Sixth Edition

PHARMACOTHERAPY

A Pathophysiologic Approach

Sixth Edition

PHARMACOTHERAPY

A Pathophysiologic Approach

Editors

Joseph T. DiPiro, PharmD, FCCP
Professor and Executive Dean, South Carolina College of Pharmacy,
University of South Carolina, Columbia, and Medical University of South Carolina, Charleston

Robert L. Talbert, PharmD, FCCP, BCPS
Professor, College of Pharmacy, University of Texas at Austin;
Professor, Departments of Medicine and Pharmacology, University of Texas Health Science Center at San Antonio, Texas

Gary C. Yee, PharmD, FCCP
Professor and Chair, Department of Pharmacy Practice, College of Pharmacy,
University of Nebraska Medical Center, Omaha, Nebraska

Gary R. Matzke, PharmD, FCP, FCCP
Professor, Department of Pharmacy and Therapeutics, School of Pharmacy,
Renal-Electrolyte Division, School of Medicine,
University of Pittsburgh, Pittsburgh, Pennsylvania

Barbara G. Wells, PharmD, FASHP, FCCP, BCPP
Dean and Professor, School of Pharmacy, The University of Mississippi, University, Mississippi

L. Michael Posey, BS Pharm
President, PENS Pharmacy Editorial and News Services, Athens, Georgia

McGRAW-HILL
Medical Publishing Division

New York   Chicago   San Francisco   Lisbon
London   Madrid   Mexico City   Milan   New Delhi
San Juan   Seoul   Singapore   Sydney   Toronto

Pharmacotherapy: A Pathophysiologic Approach, Sixth Edition

2 3 4 5 6 7 8 9 0 DOWDOW 0 9 8 7 6 5

Set ISBN 0-07-141613-7
Book p/n 0-07-146392-5
E-book download access card p/n 0-07-146393-3 and sticker p/n 0-07-146394-1
E-book ISBN 0-07-146390-9

This book is sold with codes for access to an Online Learning Center and an e-book version of the text. This book is not returnable unless the shrink-wrap and the scratch-off coating on the codes are intact.

Please tell the authors and publisher what you think of this book by sending your comments to *pharmacotherapy@mcgraw-hill.com.* Please put the author and title of the book in subject line.

This book was set in Times Roman by TechBooks, Inc.
The editors were Michael Brown, Andrew Hall, Karen G. Edmonson, and Peter J. Boyle.
The production supervisor was Richard Ruzycka.
The text designer was Joan O'Connor.
The cover designer was Elizabeth Pisacreta.
Barbara Littlewood prepared the index.
RR Donnelley was printer and binder.

This book is printed on acid-free paper.

Cover images copyright © 1999 by Obi-Tabot Tabe. The images used on the cover and spine are taken from a $9' \times 4\text{-}1/2'$ oil painting by Obi-Tabot Tabe, PharmD, a painter, graphic designer, scientific illustrator, and pharmacist. Dr. Tabe, originally from Cameroon, is a graduate of the University of Pittsburgh, School of Pharmacy. The painting incorporates the artist's impressions of concepts introduced in the pharmacy curriculum. The painting can be seen in the student lounge of Salk Hall at the university.

Cataloging-in-publication data is on file for this title at the Library of Congress.

Dedication

To those pharmacists who had the courage and perseverance to pioneer the development of the clinical practice of pharmacy.

To the contemporary pharmaceutical care practitioners who continue to expand their impact on patient outcomes and thereby serve as role models for their colleagues and students while clinging tenaciously to the highest standards of practice.

To our mentors, whose vision provided educational and training programs that encouraged our professional growth and challenged us to be innovators in our patient care, research, and educational endeavors.

To our faculty colleagues for their efforts and support for our mission to provide a comprehensive and challenging educational foundation for the clinical pharmacists of the future.

And finally to our families for the time that they have sacrificed so that this sixth edition would become a reality.

CONTENTS

Color plates appear between pages 1740 and 1741.

FOREWORD

Drug therapy often represents the best treatment for human diseases and illnesses, and the spectrum of effective medications continues to improve at a remarkable pace. This is likely to continue over the coming years, as our understanding of disease pathogenesis and molecular pharmacology rapidly expands, fueling the discovery of new classes of medication. This, coupled with impressive advances in technology and our understanding of the human genome, promises to usher in a new wave of targeted therapies and individualized medicine that may further improve the efficacy and reduce the toxicity of medications. However, most of the highly effective medications currently available for clinical use emerged from classical pharmacology and chemistry, on a foundation of incomplete knowledge of disease mechanisms. This may contribute in part to the propensity of many medications to produce adverse drug effects or to exhibit limited efficacy in a subset of patients with a given diagnosis. These imperfect medications will remain the mainstay of therapeutics for years to come.

The limited efficacy and potential toxicity of many of today's medications, coupled with the rapidly expanding portfolio of medications for disease treatment and prevention, creates enormous complexity in selecting optimal medications for individual patients. Thus, the expertise of clinically educated and trained pharmacists is increasingly important if we are to ensure patients receive the most effective medications in the doses and combinations that are optimal for them and their illnesses.

The sixth edition of *Pharmacotherapy: A Pathophysiologic Approach* contains a wealth of information that will be an invaluable resource to students and practitioners who work to expand their knowledge of pharmacotherapy and translate it into better drug therapy for individual patients. In a perfect world, every patient would benefit from the collective talents of a health care team that is fully able to integrate knowledge of disease pathogenesis and pharmacotherapy, thereby optimizing drug therapy for each individual. Such a team is incomplete without a clinical pharmacist.

How many clinical pharmacists does it take in this day and age? Can one justify 25 pharmacists for a 58-bed hospital? That's the reality at St. Jude Children's Research Hospital, where I have worked for the last 25 years. And this wasn't even seriously challenged when the "health care consultants" rolled into town 10 years ago. Why not? The reasons are multiple, yet simple in the end: Pharmacists are integrally involved in the pharmacotherapy of every patient. The medical staff would not have it any other way, and the patients deserve no less. That's as it should be everywhere, in hospitals and clinics and community pharmacies. Moreover, pharmacists have become integral to the process of defining the future state of pharmacotherapy, by bringing unique expertise to the research enterprise. That must continue as well. The pharmacists of the present and future must integrate pharmacology, pathophysiology, therapeutics, and, increasingly, genetics into complex treatment decisions.

Pharmacotherapy: A Pathophysiologic Approach is an important tool to this end. By providing pharmacy students and practicing pharmacists (plus physicians and nurses) with a comprehensive and definitive source of information about diseases and their drug treatment, it is a conduit to the clinical use of pharmacotherapeutic principles by pharmacists, which is the *sine qua non* of pharmacy practice in the twenty-first century.

Health care in the United States and other developed countries has made great progress in recent decades, yet there are many opportunities to improve the way these advances are deployed, especially drug therapy. Studies have shown that even when there are clear guidelines for appropriate use of medications for specific diseases, too many patients receive suboptimal drug therapy for too long. This is caused in part by far more drug therapy choices than most clinicians can master and also by aggressive marketing—to physicians, pharmacists, and directly to consumers—which can inappropriately shape prescribing habits. Who is to intervene in the name of rational therapeutics? The well-armed pharmacist, for one!

Reality is even more alarming when one also considers adverse drug effects. A 2000 Institute of Medicine (IOM) report documented that adverse drug effects are common in the United States, representing the sixth leading cause of death according to published meta-analyses. This is staggering news. Yet even if overstated by 100% it is an enormous concern for patients. Pharmacists must intervene and make definitive strides to reduce the adverse effects of medications, and they must be armed with pharmacotherapeutic knowledge and given time in their clinical practice to do so. This textbook serves as a source of such knowledge for those who are devoted to this end, whether they are matriculating toward their pharmacy degree or striving to advance their contributions in a busy clinical practice.

A 2001 IOM report documented a substantial gap in health care between those who receive the best and those who receive the average in health care in the United States. Recent studies have also documented that when patients exceed their cap in prescription drug coverage, they often discontinue medications or take fewer doses of prescribed therapy, even when adverse consequences can result if chronic diseases are left untreated. The cost-consequences of inadequate prescription drug coverage may well exceed the cost-savings of capping or limiting prescription drug benefits.

How might pharmacists change this equation for the better? Perhaps one approach would be to avoid the use of unnecessarily expensive medications when less expensive medications are equally effective. Another would be to help minimize the adverse economic and health care impact of adverse drug effects. The pages of this text are filled with information that could simultaneously translate into greater efficacy, lower toxicity, and more cost-effective use of medications. Pharmacists who translate this knowledge to everyday treatment decisions can play a vital role in showing not only that the best drug therapy can be safe and cost-effective, but that it does not always require the newest medication on the market. This will require a wealth of knowledge and determination by pharmacists, if they are to offset the power of marketing prescription drugs to prescribers and directly to the public. *Pharmacotherapy: A Pathophysiologic Approach* is a comprehensive scholarly effort by leading practitioners and educators who have created a definitive and unbiased resource that is based on a wealth of clinical experience and academic expertise. It offers a solid foundation for the education of future clinicians and for the practice of pharmacotherapy today, loaded with ammunition to fight the forces of irrational prescribing.

William E. Evans, PharmD
Professor of Pharmacy and Pediatrics
University of Tennessee Colleges of Pharmacy and Medicine
Director and CEO
St. Jude Children's Research Hospital
Memphis, Tennessee

FOREWORD TO THE FIRST EDITION

Evidence of the maturity of a profession is not unlike that characterizing the maturity of an individual; a child's utterances and behavior typically reveal an unrealized potential for attainment, eventually, of those attributes characteristic of an appropriately confident, independently competent, socially responsible, sensitive, and productive member of society.

Within a period of perhaps 15 or 20 years, we have witnessed a profound maturation within the profession of pharmacy. The utterances of the profession, as projected in its literature, have evolved from mostly self-centered and self-serving issues of trade protection to a composite of expressed professional interests that prominently include responsible explorations of scientific/technological questions and ethical issues that promote the best interests of the clientele served by the profession. With the publication of *Pharmacotherapy: A Pathophysiologic Approach,* pharmacy's utterances bespeak a matured practitioner who is able to call upon unique knowledge and skills so as to function as an appropriately confident, independently competent pharmacotherapeutics expert.

In 1987, the Board of Pharmaceutical Specialties (BPS), in denying the petition filed by the American College of Clinical Pharmacy (ACCP) to recognize "clinical pharmacy" as a specialty, conceded nonetheless that the petitioning party had documented in its petition a specialist who does in fact exist within the practice of pharmacy and whose expertise clearly can be extricated from the performance characteristics of those in general practice. A refiled petition from ACCP requests recognition of "pharmacotherapy" as a Specialty Area of Pharmacy Practice. While the BPS had issued no decision when this book went to press, it is difficult to comprehend the basis for a rejection of the second petition.

Within this book one will find the scientific foundation for the essential knowledge required of one who may aspire to specialty practice as a pharmacotherapist. As is the case with any such publication, its usefulness to the practitioner or the future practitioner is limited to providing such a foundation. To be socially and professionally responsible in practice, the pharmacotherapist's foundation must be continually supplemented and complemented by the flow of information appearing in the primary literature. Of course this is not unique to the general or specialty practice of pharmacy; it is essential to the fulfillment of obligations to clients in any occupation operating under the code of professional ethics.

Because of the growing complexity of pharmacotherapeutic agents, their dosing regimens, and techniques for delivery, pharmacy is obligated to produce, recognize, and remunerate specialty practitioners who can fulfill the profession's responsibilities to society for service expertise where the competence required in a particular case exceeds that of the general practitioner. It simply is a component of our covenant with society and is as important as any other facet of that relationship existing between a profession and those it serves.

The recognition by BPS of pharmacotherapy as an area of specialty practice in pharmacy will serve as an important statement by the profession that we have matured sufficiently to be competent and willing to take unprecedented responsibilities in the collaborative, pharmacotherapeutic management of patient-specific problems. It commits pharmacy to an intention that will not be uniformly or rapidly accepted within the established health care community. Nonetheless, this formal action places us on the road to an avowed goal, and acceptance will be gained as the pharmacotherapists proliferate and establish their importance in the provision of optimal, cost-effective drug therapy.

Suspecting that other professions in other times must have faced similar quests for recognition of their unique knowledge and skills I once searched the literature for an example that might parallel pharmacy's modern-day aspirations. Writing in the *Philadelphia Medical Journal,* May 27, 1899, D. H. Galloway, MD, reflected on the need for specialty training and practice in a field of medicine lacking such expertise at that time. In an article entitled "The Anesthetizer as a Speciality," Galloway commented:

> The anesthetizer will have to make his own place in medicine: the profession will not make a place for him, and not until he has demonstrated the value of his services will it concede him the position which the importance of his duties entitles him to occupy. He will be obliged to define his own rights, duties and privileges, and he must not expect that his own estimate of the importance of his position will be conceded without opposition. There are many surgeons who are unwilling to share either the credit or the emoluments of their work with anyone, and their opposition will be overcome only when they are shown that the importance of their work will not be lessened, but enhanced, by the increased safety and dispatch with which operations may be done....

It has been my experience that, given the opportunity for one-on-one, collaborative practice with physicians and other health professionals, pharmacy practitioners who have been educated and trained to perform at the level of pharmacotherapeutics specialists almost invariably have convinced the former that "the importance of their work will not be lessened, but enhanced, by the increased safety and dispatch with which" individualized problems of drug therapy could be managed in collaboration with clinical pharmacy practitioners.

It is fortuitous—the coinciding of the release of *Pharmacotherapy: A Pathophysiologic Approach* with ACCP's petitioning of BPS for recognition of the pharmacotherapy specialist. The utterances of a maturing profession as revealed in the contents of this book, and the intraprofessional recognition and acceptance of a higher level of responsibility in the safe, effective, and economical use of drugs and drug products, bode well for the future of the profession and for the improvement of patient care with drugs.

Charles A. Walton, PhD
San Antonio, Texas

PREFACE

Pharmacists and other health care professionals who evaluate, design, and recommend pharmacotherapy for the management of their patients face many new and exciting challenges in these early years of the twenty-first century. As we complete our work on the sixth edition of *Pharmacotherapy: A Pathophysiologic Approach,* we recognize just how much our tasks as editors have become equally complicated, trying to balance the need to provide accurate, thorough, and unbiased information about the treatment of diseases against the hard publishing realities of deadlines, word counts, and book length. We thus strive to keep foremost in our minds the precepts that first led us to embark on this endeavor:

- Advance the quality of patient care through optimal medication management based on sound pharmacotherapeutic principles.
- Stimulate the student to achieve higher levels of learning.
- Motivate young practitioners to enhance the breadth, depth, and quality of care they can provide to each of their patients.
- Challenge established pharmacists and other primary-care providers to learn the new concepts and refine their understanding of the basic tenets of pathophysiology and therapeutics.
- Inform the pharmacy and medical communities about the standards of medication therapy management toward which we all should strive and which all patients will one day expect and, yes, demand.

While our emphasis in past editions has been on how to incorporate diseases that were previously untreatable with pharmacologic agents, new features in this sixth edition are focused more on the realities of teaching entry-level doctor of pharmacy students and meeting their postgraduate needs. We have incorporated a number of new pedagogical devices into chapters that will enable students and practitioners to more quickly grasp the important concepts and find related passages in the text. The addition of more features to disease-oriented chapters and the inclusion of more design elements give this edition a striking new look:

- Key concepts are listed at the beginning of each chapter and are identified in the text with numbered icons so that the reader can jump to the material of interest.
- The most common signs and symptoms of diseases as manifested in typical patients are presented in highlighted Clinical Presentation tables in disease-specific chapters.
- Clinical controversies in treatment or patient management are highlighted in shaded boxes to assure that the reader is aware of these issues and how practitioners are responding to them.
- Each chapter has about 100 of the most important and current references relevant to each disease, with most published since 1997.
- For easy reference, abbreviations and acronyms and their meanings are presented at the end of each chapter.
- A glossary of the medical terms used throughout the text is tabulated and presented at the end of the book.

- Finally, the diagnostic flow diagrams, desired outcomes of treatment, dosing guidelines, monitoring approaches, and treatment algorithms that were present in the fifth edition have been refined.

This edition includes two new chapters: Documentation of Pharmacy Services, which addresses the critical need for pharmacists to record their medication therapy management interventions, and Solid-Organ Transplantation, which combines material that was previously spread throughout several organ-specific chapters.

Before writing for this edition began, each editor read chapters from other editors' sections and made suggestions for enhancement. During editing, we reviewed each passage of text—and the references cited—for continued relevance and accuracy. We made deletions, asked authors to summarize concepts more succinctly or use tables to present details more concisely, included new medications as they entered the U.S. market or emerged in other countries, and updated references. This process continued as the book entered production, and even during the review of final proofs, we continued to make changes to ensure that this book is as current and complete as is possible.

Standard formats have remained relatively unchanged since the first edition of *Pharmacotherapy.* When seeking information in the disease-oriented chapters, users will find these sections: Key Concepts, Epidemiology, Etiology, Pathophysiology, Clinical Presentation (including diagnostic considerations), Treatment (including desired outcomes, general approaches, nonpharmacologic therapy, pharmacologic therapy, and pharmacoeconomic considerations), and Evaluation of Therapeutic Outcomes.

As the world increasingly relies on electronic means of communication, we are committed to keeping *Pharmacotherapy* and its companion works, *Pharmacotherapy Casebook: A Patient-Focused Approach* and *Pharmacotherapy Handbook,* integral components of clinicians' toolboxes. With the launch of this edition the Web site with unique features designed to benefit students, practitioners, and faculty that was initiated with the fifth edition has been extensively expanded. One can now find learning objectives and self-assessment questions for each chapter on the site.

In closing, we also stop once again to acknowledge the many hours that *Pharmacotherapy*'s 200 authors contributed to this labor of love. Without their devotion to the cause of improved pharmacotherapy and dedication in maintaining the accuracy, clarity, and relevance of their chapters, this text would unquestionably not be possible. In addition, we thank Michael Brown and his colleagues at McGraw-Hill—especially Jack Farrell, Marty Wonsiewicz, and Peter Boyle—for their consistent support of the *Pharmacotherapy* family of resources, insights into trends in publishing and higher education, and the necessary and critical attention to detail so necessary in a book such as this one.

The Editors
March 2005

CONTRIBUTORS

Betty J. Abate, PharmD, BCPS
Coordinator of Drug Information Services, Hurley Medical Center, Department of Pharmacy, Farmington Hills, Michigan
Chapter 104

Val R. Adams, PharmD
Associate Professor, University of Kentucky College of Pharmacy, Oncology Clinical Specialist, Markey Cancer Center, Lexington, Kentucky
Chapter 129

Jeffrey R. Aeschlimann, PharmD
Assistant Professor, Division of Infectious Diseases, University of Connecticut School of Pharmacy, Adjunct Assistant Professor of Medicine, University of Connecticut School of Medicine, Farmington, Connecticut
Chapter 103

JV Anandan, PharmD, BCPS
Adjunct Associate Professor, Eugene Applebaum College of Pharmacy and Health Sciences, Wayne State University; Pharmacy Specialist, Department of Pharmacy Services, Detroit, Henry Ford Hospital, Detroit, Michigan
Chapter 113

Edward P. Armstrong, PharmD, BCPS, FASHP
Professor, Department of Pharmacy Practice and Science, University of Arizona, College of Pharmacy, Tucson, Arizona
Chapter 116

Jacquelyn L. Bainbridge, PharmD
Associate Professor, Department of Clinical Pharmacy, School of Pharmacy; Department of Neurology, School of Medicine, University of Colorado Health Sciences Center, Denver, Colorado
Chapter 53

Carol McManus Balmer, PharmD
Associate Professor and Director, Postgraduate Professional Education, University of Colorado School of Pharmacy, Denver, Colorado
Chapter 124

Jeffrey F. Barletta, PharmD
Critical Care Specialist, Department of Pharmacy, Spectrum Health, Grand Rapids, Michigan
Chapter 11

Jody Don Bartlett, PharmD, BCPP
Clinical Specialist in Psychiatry, Central Texas Veterans Health Care System, Waco VA Medical Center, Waco, Texas
Chapter 63

Leslie L. Barton, MD
Professor of Pediatrics, University of Arizona School of Medicine, Director, Pediatric Residency Program, University Medical Center, Tucson, Arizona
Chapter 116

Larry A. Bauer, PharmD, FCP, FCCP
Professor, Departments of Pharmacy and Laboratory Medicine, University of Washington, Seattle, Washington
Chapter 5

Jerry L. Bauman, PharmD, BCPS, FCCP, FACC
Professor, Departments of Pharmacy Practice and Medicine, University of Illinois, Chicago, Illinois
Chapter 17

Terry J. Baumann, PharmD, BCPS
Adjunct Assistant Professor, Ferris State University, Clinical Pharmacy Manager, Department of Pharmacy, Munson Medical Center, Traverse City, Michigan
Chapter 58

Rosemary R. Berardi, PharmD, FASHP, FCCP
Professor of Pharmacy, University of Michigan College of Pharmacy, Clinical Pharmacist, Gastroenterology and Liver Diseases, Department of Pharmacy, University of Michigan Health System, Ann Arbor, Michigan
Chapters 33 and 39

Richard C. Berchou, PharmD
Assistant Professor, Department of Psychiatry and Behavioral Neurosciences, Wayne State University, Detroit, Michigan
Chapter 57

Betsy Bickert, PharmD
Pediatric Oncology/Stem Cell Transplant Clinical Pharmacist, Children's Hospital of Philadelphia, Philadelphia, Pennsylvania
Chapters 100 and 131

Bradley A. Boucher, PharmD, FCCP, FCCM
Professor of Clinical Pharmacy and Associate Professor of Neurosurgery, University of Tennessee Health Sciences Center, Clinical Pharmacist, Regional Medical Center at Memphis, Memphis, Tennessee
Chapters 55 and 56

Sharya V. Bourdet, PharmD, BCPS
Clinical Assistant Professor, University of North Carolina School of Pharmacy, Clinical Specialist, Medicine Intensive Care Unit, University of North Carolina Hospitals, Chapel Hill, North Carolina
Chapter 27

Donald F. Brophy, PharmD, FCCP, BCPS
Associate Professor of Pharmacy and Medicine, Virginia Commonwealth University School of Pharmacy, Richmond, Virginia
Chapter 50

Thomas E. R. Brown, BScPhm, PharmD
Clinical Coordinator–Women's Health, and Assistant Professor, University of Toronto, Pharmacy, Sunnybrook and Women's College Health Science Centre, Toronto, Ontario, Canada
Chapter 118

Kathryn K. Bucci, PharmD, BCPS, FASHP
Clinical Education Consultant, Pfizer, Inc., Southold, New York
Chapter 77

Peter F. Buckley, MD
Professor and Chairman, Department of Psychiatry, Medical College of Georgia, Augusta, Georgia
Chapter 66

David S. Burgess, PharmD
Clinical Associate Professor, College of Pharmacy, University of Texas at Austin, Department of Pharmacology and Medicine, University of Texas Health Sciences Center at San Antonio, San Antonio, Texas
Chapter 104

Karim Anton Calis, PharmD, MPH, BCPS, BCNSP, FASHP
Clinical Professor, Department of Pharmacy Practice and Science, School of Pharmacy, University of Maryland, Baltimore Maryland, Clinical Specialist, Endocrinology and Women's Health, Coordinator, Drug Information Service, Pharmacy Department, Clinical Research Center, National Institutes of Health, Bethesda, Maryland
Chapters 75 and 80

Kimberly A. Cappuzzo, PharmD, MS
Assistant Professor of Pharmacy, Virginia Commonwealth University School of Pharmacy, Clinical Pharmacist/Geriatric Pharmacotherapy Specialist, Virginia Commonwealth University (VCU) Medical Center, Richmond, Virginia
Chapter 85

Barry L. Carter, PharmD, FCCP, BCPS
Professor and Head, Division of Clinical and Administrative Pharmacy, University of Iowa College of Pharmacy, Iowa City, Iowa
Chapter 13

Peggy L. Carver, PharmD
Associate Professor of Pharmacy, University of Michigan College of Pharmacy, Clinical Pharmacist, Infectious Diseases, University of Michigan Health System, Ann Arbor, Michigan
Chapter 119

Larisa H. Cavallari, PharmD, BCPS
Assistant Professor of Pharmacy Practice, University of Illinois at Chicago, Chicago, Illinois
Chapter 6

C. Y. Jennifer Chan, PharmD
Clinical Associate Professor in Pharmacy, University of Texas in Austin, College of Pharmacy, Clinical Associate Professor of Pediatrics, University of Texas Health Science Center in San Antonio, Clinical Manager, Pediatrics, Methodist Children's Hospital of South Texas, San Antonio, Texas
Chapter 101

Kunal Chaudhary, MD, FACP
Assistant Professor, Pennsylvania State University, Nephrologist, Lehigh Valley Hospital, Allentown, Pennsylvania
Chapter 44

Nina Han Cheigh, PharmD
Clinical Assistant Professor and Coordinator of Academic Programs, University of Illinois College of Pharmacy, Chicago, Illinois
Chapters 94 and 97

Kathy Hammond Chessman, BS, PharmD, BCNSP, BCPS
Associate Professor, Department of Pharmacy Practice and Pharmaceutical Sciences, College of Pharmacy, Medical University of South Carolina, Clinical Pharmacy Specialist, Pediatrics, Medical University of South Carolina Children's Hospital, Charleston, South Carolina
Chapters 135 and 138

Thomas W. F. Chin, BScPhm, PharmD
Clinical Pharmacy Specialist, and Assistant Professor, St. Michael's Hospital, and University of Toronto, Pharmacy and Innercity Health Programme Department, Toronto, ON, Canada
Chapter 118

Elaine Chiquette, PharmD, BCPS
Clinical Assistant Professor, University of Texas at Austin, College of Pharmacy, Medical Science Liaison, Amylin Pharmaceuticals, San Antonio, Texas
Chapter 3

Marie A. Chisholm, PharmD
Associate Professor of Pharmacy, University of Georgia College of Pharmacy, Clinical Associate Professor of Medicine, Medical College of Georgia, Augusta, Georgia
Chapter 31

Peter A. Chyka, FAACT, DABAT
Professor, Department of Pharmacy, University of Tennessee Health Science Center, Memphis, Tennessee
Chapter 10

Thomas J. Comstock, PharmD
Senior Manager, Global Medical Affairs, Nephrology Medical Communications, Amgen, Inc., Thousand Oaks, California
Chapter 41

Stephen Joel Coons, PhD
Professor, University of Arizona College of Pharmacy, Tucson, Arizona
Chapter 2

John R. Corboy, MD
Associate Professor of Neurology, University of Colorado School of Medicine, Director, University of Colorado Multiple Sclerosis Center, Denver, Colorado
Chapter 53

Elizabeth A. Coyle, PharmD
Clinical Assistant Professor, University of Houston College of Pharmacy, Clinical Specialist, Infectious Diseases, University of Texas M.D. Anderson Cancer Center, Houston, Texas
Chapter 114

M. Lynn Crismon, PharmD, FCCP, BCPP
Behrens Inc Centennial Professor of Pharmacy, Associate Dean for
Clinical Programs, Director of Psychiatric Pharmacy Program,
University of Texas at Austin College of Pharmacy, Clinical
Pharmacologist, Office of the Medical Director, Texas
Department of Mental Health and Mental Retardation,
Austin, Texas
Chapter 66

Michael A. Crouch, PharmD, BCPS
Assistant Professor, School of Pharmacy, Department of
Pharmacy Practice, Virginia Commonwealth University,
Richmond, Virginia
Chapter 109

Judy L. Curtis, PharmD, BCPP, FASHP
Assistant Director, CNS Regional Medical Services,
Janssen Medical Affairs, LLC, Owing Mills, Maryland
Chapter 71

Larry H. Danziger, PharmD
Professor, Department of Pharmacy Practice, Associate Vice
Chancellor for Research, University of Illinois at Chicago,
Chicago, Illinois
Chapter 108

Joseph F. Dasta, MSc
Professor, Division of Pharmacy Practice and Administration,
Ohio State Unviersity College of Pharmacy, Ohio State University
Medical Center, Columbus, Ohio
Chapter 23

Lisa E. Davis, PharmD, FCCP, BCPS, BCOP
Associate Professor of Clinical Pharmacy, Philadelphia College of
Pharmacy, University of the Sciences in Philadelphia,
Philadelphia, Pennsylvania
Chapter 127

Susan R. Davis, PhD, MBBS, FRACP
Director of Research, Jean Hailes Foundation, Clayton, Australia
Chapter 80

Simon de Denus, Bpharm, MSc
Invited Professor, Faculty of Pharmacy, University of Montreal,
Fellow in Cardiovascular Research, Montreal Heart Institute,
Montreal, Quebec, Canada
Chapter 16

Renee M. DeHart, PharmD, BCPS
Associate Professor, Pharmacy Practice, Samford University,
McWhorter School of Pharmacy, Clinical Pharmacy Specialist,
Medical Center East Family Practice Residency Program,
Birmingham, Alabama
Chapter 139

Jeffrey C. Delafuente, MS, FCCP, FASCP
Professor, Director of Geriatric Programs, Interim Director
Community Pharmacy Program, Virginia Commonwealth University,
Richmond, Virginia
Chapter 85

John W. Devlin, PharmD, BCPS, FCCM
Associate Professor, Northeast University School of Pharmacy,
Boston, Massachusetts, Clinical Pharmacist, Medical ICU,
Tufts-New England Medical Center, Boston, Massachusetts
Chapter 121

Lori M. Dickerson, PharmD, FCCP, BCPS
Associate Professor of Family Medicine, Assistant Residency
Program Director, Department of Family Medicine, Medical
University of South Carolina, Charleston, South Carolina
Chapter 77

Cecily V. DiPiro, PharmD
Clinical Assistant Professor, University of Georgia College of
Pharmacy, Manager, Department of Pharmacy, MCG Health System,
Augusta, Georgia
Chapter 35

Joseph T. DiPiro, PharmD, FCCP
Professor and Executive Dean, South Carolina College of Pharmacy,
University of South Carolina, Columbia, and Medical University of
South Carolina, Charleston
Chapters 34, 86, 112, and 117

Paul L. Doering, MS
Distinguished Service Professor of Pharmacy Practice, College of
Pharmacy, University of Florida, Gainesville, Florida
Chapters 64 and 65

Julie A. Dopheide, PharmD, BCPP
Associate Professor of Clinical Pharmacy, Psychiatry, and
Behavioral Sciences, Schools of Pharmacy and Medicine, University
of Southern California, Psychiatric Pharmacist Specialist,
Los Angeles and USC Medical Center, Los Angeles, California
Chapter 61

Thomas C. Dowling, PharmD, PhD
Assistant Professor, Director, Renal Clinical Pharmacology
Laboratory, University of Maryland School of Pharmacy, Baltimore,
Maryland
Chapter 41

Deepak P. Edward, MD
Associate Professor, Department of Ophthalmology,
University of Illinois at Chicago Eye and Ear Infirmary,
Chicago, Illinois
Chapter 92

Mary Elizabeth Elliott, PharmD, PhD
Associate Professor, School of Pharmacy, University of
Wisconsin–Madison, Pharmacist, Veterans Affairs Medical Center,
Madison, Wisconsin
Chapter 90

Rowland J. Elwell, PharmD
Assistant Professor of Pharmacy Practice, Albany College of
Pharmacy, Albany, New York
Chapter 45

Solveig G. Ericson, MD, PhD
Associate Professor of Medicine, West Virginia University
School of Medicine, Director, Blood and Marrow
Transplant/Hematologic Malignancy Program, WVU Hospitals,
Inc, Mary Babb Randolph Cancer Center, Morgantown,
West Virginia
Chapter 98

Brian L. Erstad, PharmD, FCCM, FCCP, FASHP
Professor, Department of Pharmacy Practice and Sciences,
College of Pharmacy, University of Arizona, Tucson, Arizona
Chapter 24

Susan C. Fagan, PharmD, BCPS, FCCP
Professor of Clinical and Administrative Pharmacy,
University of Georgia College of Pharmacy, Adjunct
Professor of Neurology, Medical College of Georgia,
Augusta, Georgia
Chapters 20 and 52

Martha P. Fankhauser, MS Pharm, FASHP, BCPP
Clinical Associate Professor, Department of Pharmacy Practice and
Science, University of Arizona, College of Pharmacy,
Tucson, Arizona
Chapters 68 and 78

Jennifer D. Faulkner, PharmD, BCPP
Clinical Practitioner Faculty, University of Texas, Clinical Pharmacy
Specialist, Psychiatry, Central Texas Veterans Health Care System,
Temple, Texas
Chapter 63

Rebecca S. Finley, PharmD, MS, FASHP
Vice President, Meniscus Educational Institute,
West Conshohocken, Pennsylvania
Chapter 126

Richard G. Fiscella, BS Pharm, MPH
Clinical Professor, Department of Pharmacy Practice, Adjunct
Assistant Professor, Department of Ophthalmology, University of
Illinois at Chicago
Chapter 92

Douglas N. Fish, PharmD, BCPS
Associate Professor and Vice Chair, Department of Clinical
Pharmacy, University of Colorado Health Sciences Center, Clinical
Specialist in Infectious Diseases/Critical Care, University of
Colorado Hospital, Denver, Colorado
Chapters 108 and 120

Courtney V. Fletcher, PharmD
Professor, Department of Pharmacy Practice, University of
Colorado Health Sciences Center, School of Pharmacy,
Denver, Colorado
Chapter 123

Edward F. Foote, PharmD, FCCP, BCPS
Chair and Associate Professor of Pharmacy, Wilkes University,
Nesbitt School of Pharmacy, Wilkes-Barre, Pennsylvania
Chapter 45

Sarah Forgie, MD, FRCP(C)
Assistant Professor, Pediatrics, Division of Infectious Diseases,
University of Alberta, Consultant, Pediatric Infectious Diseases,
Associate Director, Infection Control, Stollery Children's Hospital,
Department of Pediatrics, Faculty of Medicine and Dentistry,
Edmonton, Alberta, Canada
Chapter 107

Marlene P. Freeman, MD
Assistant Professor of Psychiatry and Obstetrics and Gynecology,
University of Arizona College of Medicine, Director, Women's
Mental Health Program, Tucson, Arizona
Chapters 68 and 78

Reginald F. Frye, PharmD, PhD
Associate Professor, Department of Pharmacy Practice, College of
Pharmacy, University of Florida, Gainesville, Florida
Chapter 48

Peter Gal, PharmD, BCPS, FCCP, FASHP
Clinical Professor, School of Pharmacy, University of North Carolina
at Chapel Hill, Director, Neonatal Pharmacotherapy Laboratory and
Fellowship Program, Department of Neonatal Medicine, Women's
Hospital of Greensboro, Greensboro, North Carolina
Chapter 28

William R. Garnett, PharmD, FCCP
Professor of Pharmacy and Neurology, Virginia Commonwealth
University, Medical College of Virginia, Richmond, Virginia
Chapter 54

Todd W. B. Gehr, MD
Professor of Internal Medicine, Chairman of Nephrology, Virginia
Commonwealth University, Medical College of Virginia,
Richmond, Virginia
Chapter 50

Barry E. Gidal, PharmD
Professor, School of Pharmacy, University of Wisconsin,
Madison, Wisconsin
Chapter 54

Mark A. Gill, PharmD
Professor of Clinical Pharmacy, University of Southern California,
Clinical Pharmacy, Los Angeles, California
Chapter 38

Mark L. Glover, PharmD
Assistant Professor, Department of Pharmacy Practice, College of
Pharmacy, Nova Southeastern University, Palm Beach Gardens,
Florida, Clinical Pharmacist/Faculty, Miami Children's Hospital,
Miami, Florida
Chapter 106

S. Diane Goodwin, PharmD, FCCP
Clinical Pharmacist, Durham Regional Hospital, Duke University
Health System, Durham, North Carolina
Chapter 120

Shelly L. Gray, PharmD, MS, BCPS
Associate Professor and Director, Geriatric Pharmacy Program,
University of Washington School of Pharmacy, Seattle, Washington
Chapter 8

David R. P. Guay, PharmD, CGP, FCP, FCCP, FASCP
Professor, Department of Experimental and Clinical Pharmacology,
University of Minnesota College of Pharmacy,
Minneapolis, Minnesota
Chapters 8 and 83

John G. Gums, PharmD
Professor of Pharmacy and Medicine, Departments of Pharmacy
Practice and Community Health and Family Medicine, Director of
Clinical Research in Family Medicine, University of Florida, Family
Practice Medical Group, Gainesville, Florida
Chapter 74

Stuart T. Haines, PharmD, BCPS, CDE, CACP, FASHP
Professor and Vice Chair, University of Maryland School of
Pharmacy, Clinical Specialist, Antithrombosis Service, University of
Maryland Medical System, Baltimore, Maryland
Chapter 19

Emily R. Hajjar, PharmD
Assistant Professor of Clinical Pharmacy, Philadelphia College of
Pharmacy, University of the Sciences in Philadelphia,
Philadelphia, Pennsylvania
Chapter 8

Philip D. Hall, PharmD, FCCP, BCPS, BCOP
Associate Professor, Department of Pharmaceutical Sciences,
Medical University of South Carolina, Clinical Specialist in
Hematology/Oncology, Hollings Cancer Center and Medical
University Hospital, Charleston, South Carolina
Chapter 84

Joseph T. Hanlon, PharmD, MS, BCPS, FASCP, FASHP
Visiting Professor, Geriatrics Division, University of Pittsburgh
School of Medicine, Pittsburgh, Pennsylvania
Chapter 8

Karen E. Hansen, MD
Assistant Professor of Medicine, University of Wisconsin, Chief of
Rheumatology at the VA Hospital, Madison, Wisconsin
Chapter 90

Michelle Sue Harkins, MD
Assistant Professor of Medicine, University of New Mexico Health
Science Center, Albuquerque, New Mexico
Chapter 29

David W. Hawkins, PharmD
Professor and Senior Associate Dean, Mercer University Southern
School of Pharmacy, Atlanta, Georgia
Chapter 91

Peggy E. Hayes, MD
President, Hayes CNS Services, LLC, San Diego, California
Chapter 67

Mary S. Hayney, PharmD, BCPS
Assistant Professor of Pharmacy, University of Wisconsin School of
Pharmacy, Madison, Wisconsin
Chapters 84 and 122

Thomas K. Hazlet, PharmD, DrPH
Associate Professor, Department of Pharmacy, University of
Washington, Pharmaceutical Outcomes Research and Policy
Program, Seattle, Washington
Chapter 9

Amy M. Heck Sheehan, PharmD
Associate Professor of Pharmacy Practice, Purdue University School
of Pharmacy, Drug Information Specialist, Clarian Health Partners,
Indianapolis, Indiana
Chapter 75

Elizabeth D. Hermsen, PharmD, MBA
Infectious Diseases Research Fellow, University of Minnesota
College of Pharmacy, Minneapolis, Minnesota
Chapter 105

Katherine C. Herndon, PharmD, BCPS
Clinical Education Consultant, Pfizer, Inc., Birmingham, Alabama
Chapter 59

David C. Hess, MD
Professor and Chairman, Department of Neurology, Medical College
of Georgia, Augusta, Georgia
Chapter 20

Paul B. Hicks, MD, PhD
Professor, Department of Psychiatry and Behavioral Science,
Texas A&M University System Health, Science Center College of
Medicine, Deputy Director, Mental Health and Behavioral
Medicine, Central Texas Veterans Health Care System,
Waco, Texas
Chapter 63

Jonathan Himmelfarb, MD
Director, Division of Nephrology and Transplantation, Maine
Medical Center, Portland, Maine
Chapter 46

Gerald A. Hladik, MD
Associate Professor of Medicine, Department of Medicine, Division
of Nephrology, University of North Carolina School of Medicine,
Chapel Hill, North Carolina
Chapter 49

Barbara J. Hoeben, PharmD
Clinical Pharmacy Flight Commander, 59th Wilford Hall Medical
Center, Lackland AFB, Texas
Chapter 22

Collin A. Hovinga, PharmD
Assistant Professor of Neurosurgery, University of Miami School of
Medicine, Neuropharmacologist, Miami Children's Hospital
Institute, Miami, Florida
Chapter 55

Thomas R. Howdieshell, MD, FACS, FCCP
Associate Professor of Surgery, Division Chief,
Trauma/Burns/Surgical Critical Care, Department of Surgery,
University of New Mexico Health Sciences Center,
Albuquerque, New Mexico
Chapter 112

Joanna Q. Hudson, PharmD, BCPS
Associate Professor of Clinical Pharmacy, Department of Pharmacy and Medicine, University of Tennessee, Memphis, Tennessee
Chapter 44

Andrea Iannucci, PharmD, BCOP
Assistant Clinical Professor, University of California, San Francisco School of Pharmacy, San Francisco, California, Oncology Clinical Specialist, University of California, Davis Medical Center, Sacramento, California
Chapter 124

Beata A. Ineck, PharmD, BCPS, CDE
Assistant Professor, University of Nebraska Medical Center, Primary Care Clinical Pharmacist, VA Nebraska Western Iowa Health Care System–Omaha Division, Omaha, Nebraska
Chapter 99

William L. Isley, MD
Associate Professor of Medicine, Mayo College of Medicine, Senior Associate Consultant, Mayo Clinic, Rochester, Minnesota
Chapter 72

Cherry W. Jackson, BS, BS Pharm, PharmD, PCPP
Professor and Assistant Dean, Admissions and Student Affairs, South University School of Pharmacy, Savannah, Georgia
Chapter 71

Mark W. Jackson, MD
Gastroenterologist, Fort Sanders Regional Hospital and Baptist Hospital of East Tennessee, Knoxville, Tennessee
Chapter 31

Thomas E. Johns, PharmD, BCPS
Clinical Assistant Professor, College of Pharmacy, University of Florida, Manager, Clinical Practice Operations, Shands Hospital at the University of Florida, Gainesville, Florida
Chapter 102

Heather J. Johnson, PharmD, BCPS
Assistant Professor, University of Pittsburgh School of Pharmacy, Department of Pharmacy and Therapeutics, Clinical Pharmacy Director, Istituto Mediterraneo Per I Trapianti, University of Pittsburgh Medical Center/Italy
Chapter 87

Julie A. Johnson, PharmD, BCPS, FCCP
Professor and Chair of Pharmacy Practice, Professor of Pharmaceutics and Medicine (Cardiology), Director, Center for Pharmacogenomics, College of Pharmacy, Gainesville, Florida
Chapter 14

Melanie S. Joy, PharmD, FCCP
Associate Professor of Medicine, Assistant Professor of Pharmacy, Division of Nephrology and Hypertension, University of North Carolina Schools of Medicine and Pharmacy, Chapel Hill, North Carolina
Chapters 43 and 49

Laura L. Jung, PharmD
Medical Writer, Syntazz Communications, Inc, Mount Holly, North Carolina
Chapter 130

Rose Jung, PharmD, BCPS
Assistant Professor, University of Colorado Health Sciences Center, School of Pharmacy, Department of Clinical Pharmacy, Clinical Specialist in Critical Care, University of Colorado Hospital, Denver, Colorado
Chapter 111

Thomas N. Kakuda, PharmD
Associate Clinical Research Scientist, and Clinical Assistant Professor, Abbott Laboratories and University of Minnesota, Minneapolis, Minnesota
Chapter 123

Sophia N. Kalantaridou, MD, PhD
Assistant Professor, Department of Obstetrics and Gynecology, University of Ioannina, School of Medicine, University Hospital, Ioannina, Greece
Chapter 80

Judith C. Kando, PharmD, BCPP
Assistant Director, CNS Regional Medical Services, Janssen Medical Affairs
Chapter 67

S. Lena Kang-Birken, PharmD
Associate Professor, Department of Pharmacy, University of the Pacific, Santa Barbara, California
Chapter 117

Salmaan Kanji, BSc Pharm, PharmD
Associate Scientist, Ottawa Health Research Institute, Clinical Specialist-Critical Care, Ottawa Hospital, General Campus, Ottawa, Ontario, Canada
Chapter 121

H. William Kelly, PharmD, BCPS
Professor Emeritus of Pharmacy and Pediatrics, University of New Mexico Health Sciences Center, Albuquerque, New Mexico
Chapter 26

Yasmin Khaliq, BSc(Pharm), PharmD
Lecturer, Department of Medicine, University of Ottawa, Drug Information Pharmacist, Ottawa Hospital, Ottawa, Ontario, Canada
Chapter 107

Mehmood A. Khan, MD, FACE
Vice President Medical and Scientific Affairs, Takeda Pharmaceuticals North America, Inc, Lincolnshire, Illinois
Chapter 140

Deborah S. King, PharmD
Associate Professor, Pharmacy Practice and Medicine, Department of Pharmacy Practice and Medicine, University of Mississippi Medical Center, Jackson, Mississippi
Chapter 59

William R. Kirchain, PharmD, CDE
Wilber and Mildred Robichaux Professor of Pharmacy, Chair,
Division of Clinical and Administrative Sciences, Xavier University
of Louisiana, College of Pharmacy, New Orleans, Louisiana
Chapter 38

Cynthia K. Kirkwood, PharmD
Associate Professor of Pharmacy, Vice Chair for Education, Virginia
Commonwealth University, Richmond, Virginia
Chapters 69 and 70

Leroy C. Knodel, PharmD
Director of Drug Information Service and Associate Professor,
Department of Pharmacology, University of Texas Health Sciences
Center at San Antonio, Clinical Associate Professor, College of
Pharmacy, University of Texas at Austin, Austin, Texas
Chapter 115

Jill M. Kolesar, PharmD, BCPS
Associate Professor, University of Wisconsin School of Pharmacy,
Faculty Supervisor-Analytical Instrumentation Laboratory,
Madison, Wisconsin
Chapter 128

Connie K. Kraus, PharmD, BCPS
Clinical Associate Professor of Pharmacy, University of Wisconsin
School of Pharmacy, Madison, Wisconsin
Chapter 76

Abhijit V. Kshirsagar, MD, MPH
Assistant Professor of Medicine, University of North Carolina at
Chapel Hill, Attending Physician UNC Hospitals, Chapel Hill,
North Carolina
Chapter 43

Vanessa J. Kumpf, PharmD, BCNSP
Clinical Specialist, Nutrishare, Inc, Elk Grove, California
Chapters 135 and 138

Janet L. Kwiatkowski, MD
Assistant Professor of Pediatrics, University of Pennsylvania School
of Medicine, Attending Hematologist, Division of Hematology,
Children's Hospital of Philadelphia, Philadelphia, Pennsylvania
Chapter 100

Thomas E. Lackner, PharmD
Professor of Pharmacy and Clinical Pharmacist Specialist in
Geriatrics, Institute for the Study of Geriatric Pharmacotherapy,
Experimental and Clinical Pharmacotherapy, University of
Minnesota, College of Pharmacy, Minneapolis, Minnesota
Chapter 83

Y. W. Francis Lam, PharmD
Associate Professor of Pharmacology and Medicine, Clinical
Associate Professor of Pharmacy, Departments of Pharmacology and
Medicine, University of Texas Health Science Center at San Antonio,
San Antonio, Texas
Chapter 6

Alan H. Lau, PharmD, FCCP
Professor, University of Illinois at Chicago College of Pharmacy,
Chicago, Illinois
Chapter 47

Helen L. Leather, B Pharm, BCPS
Clinical Assistant Professor, University of Florida, College of
Pharmacy, Clinical Pharmacy Specialist, BMT/Leukemia, Shands at
the University of Florida, Gainesville, Florida
Chapter 131

Mary W. Lee, PharmD, BCPS, FCCP
Dean and Professor of Pharmacy Practice, Midwestern University,
Chicago College of Pharmacy, Downers Grove, Illinois
Chapters 81 and 82

Timothy S. Lesar, PharmD
Director of Pharmacy, Albany Medical Center, Department of
Pharmacy, Albany, New York
Chapter 92

Stephanie M. Levine, MD
Professor of Medicine, Division of Pulmonary and Critical Care
Medicine, University of Texas Health Science Center,
San Antonio, Texas
Chapter 25

Peter A. LeWitt, MD
Professor of Neurology, Psychiatry and Behavioral Neurosciences,
Wayne State University School of Medicine, Clinical Neuroscience
Center-A Parkinson Foundation Center of Excellence,
Southfield, Michigan
Chapter 57

Catherine I. Lindblad, PharmD
Assistant Clinical Specialist and Assistant Professor, Department of
Experimental and Clinical Pharmacology, Institute for the Study of
Geriatric Pharmacotherapy, University of Minnesota College of
Pharmacy, Clinical Pharmacist Specialist in Geriatrics, Minneapolis
Veterans Affairs Medical Center, Minnneapolis, Minnesota
Chapter 8

Celeste M. Lindley, PharmD, BCPS, BCOP
Associate Professor, School of Pharmacy, University of North
Carolina, Chapel Hill, North Carolina
Chapter 125

George E. MacKinnon, III, RPh, MS, PhD, FASHP
Adjunct Professor, Thunderbird, The Garvin School of International
Management, Glendale, Arizona, Associate Medical Director, Center
for Pharmaceutical Appraisal and Outcomes Research, Abbott
Laboratories, Abbott Park, Illinois
Chapter 4

Neil J. MacKinnon, RPh, MS, PhD
Associate Professor and Merck Frosst Chair of Patient Health
Management, Dalhousie University College of Pharmacy,
Halifax, Canada
Chapter 4

Eugene H. Makela, PharmD, BCPP
Associate Professor, Department of Clinical Pharmacy, West Virginia
University School of Pharmacy, Morgantown, West Virginia
Chapter 70

Michael Malkin, MD
Assistant Clinical Director, UCLA, Director, Juvenile Court Mental
Health Services (Psychiatrist), Los Angeles County Department of
Mental Health, Los Angeles, California
Chapter 61

Patricia A. Marken, BS Pharm, PharmD, FCCP, BCPP
Chair and Professor of Pharmacy Practice, Professor of Psychiatry, School of Pharmacy and Medicine, University of Missouri–Kansas City, Kansas City, Missouri
Chapters 60 and 62

Patricia L. Marshik, PharmD
Associate Professor, University of New Mexico, Health Sciences Center, Albuquerque, New Mexico
Chapter 29

Steven J. Martin, PharmD, BCPS, FCCM
Associate Professor and Director, Infectious Diseases Research Laboratory, University of Toledo College of Pharmacy, Toledo, Ohio
Chapter 111

Barbara J. Mason, PharmD
Professor and Vice Chair, Department of Pharmacy Practice, Idaho State University College of Pharmacy, Primary Care Clinical Pharmacist, Boise Veterans Affairs Medical Center, Boise, Idaho
Chapter 99

Todd W. Mattox, PharmD, BCNSP
Clinical Assistant Professor, Department of Pharmacy Practice, University of Florida, Clinical Assistant Professor, Department of Pharmacy Practice, Nova Southeastern College of Pharmacy, Coordinator, Nutrition Support Team, H. Lee Moffitt Cancer Center and Research Institute, Tampa, Florida
Chapter 137

Gary R. Matzke, PharmD, FCP, FCCP
Professor, Department of Pharmacy and Therapeutics, School of Pharmacy, Renal-Electrolyte Division, School of Medicine, University of Pittsburgh, Pittsburgh, Pennsylvania
Chapters 46, 48, and 51

J. Russell May, PharmD, FASHP
Clinical Professor, Department of Clinical and Administrative Pharmacy, University of Georgia College of Pharmacy, Pharmacist, Medical College of Georgia Health System, Augusta, Georgia
Chapter 93

Teresa C. McCarthy, MD, MS
Assistant Professor, Department of Family Medicine and Community Health, University of Minnesota Medical School, Minneapolis, Minnesota
Chapter 8

Jeannine Sue McCune, BSPharm, PharmD
Assistant Professor, University of Washington, Seattle, Washington
Chapter 126

Timothy R. McGuire, PharmD, FCCP
Associate Professor, College of Pharmacy, University of Nebraska, Omaha, Nebraska
Chapter 132

Patrick J. Medina, PharmD, BCOP
Assistant Professor, University of Oklahoma College of Pharmacy, Oklahoma City, Oklahoma
Chapter 127

Sarah T. Melton, PharmD, BCPP
Consultant Pharmacist, Melton Healthcare Consulting, LLC, Lebanon, Virginia
Chapter 69

Renee-Claude Mercier, PharmD
Associate Professor of Pharmacy and Medicine, College of Pharmacy, University of New Mexico–Health Sciences Center, Albuquerque, New Mexico
Chapter 40

Giuseppe Micali, MD
Professor of Dermatology, Department of Dermatology, University of Catania, Catania, Italy
Chapters 95 and 96

Laura Boehnke Michaud, PharmD, BCOP
Clinical Pharmacy Specialist–Breast Oncology, Division of Pharmacy, University of Texas M.D. Anderson Cancer Center, Houston, Texas
Chapter 125

Gary Milavetz, PharmD
Associate Professor of Pharmacy and Assistant Head for Academic Affairs, Division of Clinical and Administrative Pharmacy, University of Iowa College of Pharmacy, Clinical Pharmacist, Pediatric Allergy and Pulmonary Division, University of Iowa Hospitals and Clinics, Iowa City, Iowa
Chapter 30

Patricia A. Montgomery, PharmD
Clinical Pharmacy Specialist, Mercy General Hospital, Sacramento, California
Chapter 39

Reginald H. Moore, MD
Assistant Professor, University of Texas Heath Science Center at San Antonio, Department of Pediatrics, Hematology, Oncology, & Immunization, Associate Director of Regional Sickle Cell Program Christus Santa Rosa Children's Hospital, San Antonio, Texas
Chapter 101

Bruce A. Mueller, PharmD, FCCP, BCPS
Professor and Department Chair, Clinical Sciences Department, College of Pharmacy, University of Michigan, Ann Arbor, Associate Director, Department of Pharmacy Services University of Michigan Health Systems, Ann Arbor, Michigan
Chapter 42

Stuart Munro, MD
Chair, Department of Psychiatry, University of Missouri–Kansas City, School of Medicine, Assistant Medical Director, Western Missouri Mental Health Center, Kansas City, Missouri
Chapter 60

Maria Letizia Musumeci, MD, PhD
Dermatologist, Department of Dermatology, University of Catania, Catania, Italy
Chapter 95

Milap C. Nahata, MS, PharmD
Professor of Pharmacy, Pediatrics and Internal Medicine,
Division Chairman, Pharmacy Practice and Administration,
Ohio State University College of Pharmacy, Associate Director,
Department of Pharmacy, Ohio State University Medical Center,
Columbus, Ohio
Chapter 7

Jean M. Nappi, PharmD, FCCP, BCPS
Professor of Pharmacy and Clinical Sciences, College of Pharmacy,
Medical University of South Carolina Clinical Specialist, Cardiology,
Medical University of South Carolina, Charleston, South Carolina
Chapter 18

Merlin V. Nelson, PharmD, MD
Neurologist, Department of Neurology, Affiliated Community
Medical Center, Willmar, Minnesota
Chapter 57

Fenwick T. Nichols, III, MD, FACP
Professor of Neurology, Medical College of Georgia,
Augusta, Georgia
Chapter 52

Thomas D. Nolin, PharmD, PhD
Clinical Pharmacologist, Division of Nephrology and
Transplantation, Maine Medical Center, Portland, Maine
Chapter 46

Mary Beth O'Connell, PharmD, BCPS, FCCP, FSHP
Associate Professor, Department of Pharmacy Practice, Wayne State
University, Eugene Applebaum College of Pharmacy and Health
Sciences, Detroit, Michigan
Chapter 88

Dennis R. Ownby, MD
Professor of Pediatrics and Internal Medicine, Head, Section of
Allergy and Immunology, Medical College of Georgia,
Augusta, Georgia
Chapter 86

Manjunath P. Pai, PharmD, BCPS
Assistant Professor, University of New Mexico College of Pharmacy,
Albuquerque, New Mexico
Chapter 40

Paul M. Palevsky, MD
Professor of Medicine, University of Pittsburgh School of Medicine,
Chief, Renal Section, VA Pittsburgh Healthcare System,
Pittsburgh, Pennsylvania
Chapter 51

James Paparello, MD
Clinical Assistant Professor, Feinberg School of Medicine,
Northwestern University, Evanston, Illinois
Chapter 43

Robert B. Parker, PharmD, FCCP
Associate Professor, Department of Pharmacy, University of
Tennessee, College of Pharmacy, Memphis, Tennessee
Chapter 14

Alkesh D. Patel, MD
Clinical Assistant Professor, University of Maryland, Baltimore
School of Medicine, Baltimore, Maryland, Family Physician,
University Care at Shipley's Choice, Millersville, Maryland
Chapter 79

J. Herbert Patterson, PharmD, FCCP, BCPS
Associate Professor of Pharmacy and Research Associate Professor
of Medicine, University of North Carolina at Chapel Hill, School of
Pharmacy, Chapel Hill, North Carolina
Chapter 14

Steven Z. Pavletic, MD
Principal Investigator, National Cancer Institute, Head,
Graft-versus-Host and Autoimmunity Unit, National Cancer Institute,
Bethesda, Maryland
Chapter 132

Charles A. Peloquin, PharmD
Adjoint Professor of Pharmacy and Medicine, University of Colorado,
Denver, Director, Infectious Disease Pharmacokinetics Laboratory,
National Jewish Medical and Research Center, Denver, Colorado
Chapter 110

Susan L. Pendland, MS, PharmD
Associate Professor, Section of Infectious Diseases Pharmacotherapy,
Department of Pharmacy Practice, University of Illinois at Chicago,
College of Pharmacy, Chicago, Illinois
Chapter 108

Janelle B. Perkins, PharmD, BCPS
Assistant Professor, College of Medicine, University of Florida,
Manager, BMT Clinical Research H. Lee Moffitt Cancer Center &
Research Institute, Tampa, Florida
Chapter 134

Jay I. Peters, MD
Professor of Medicine, Division of Pulmonary Diseases and Critical
Care Medicine, University of Texas Health Science Center at
San Antonio, San Antonio, Texas
Chapter 25

William P. Petros, PharmD
Mylan Chair of Pharmacology, Associate Professor of Pharmacy and
Medicine, West Virginia University Health Sciences Center,
Associate Director for Anti-Cancer Drug Development, MRB/WVU
Cancer Center, Morgantown, West Virginia
Chapter 98

Stephanie J. Phelps, PharmD, FCCP
Professor, Departments of Pharmacy and Pediatrics, Vice-Chair,
Professional Experiential Program, The University of Tennessee
Health Science Center, Director, Pharmacokinetics Service,
LeBonheur Children's Medical Center, Memphis, Tennessee
Chapters 55 and 56

Denise Walbrandt Pigarelli, PharmD
Clinical Associate Professor of Pharmacy, School of Pharmacy,
University of Wisconsin-Madison, Clinical Pharmacy Specialist,
William S. Middleton Memorial VA Hospital,
Madison, Wisconsin
Chapter 76

L. Michael Posey, BS Pharm
President, PENS Pharmacy Editorial and News Services,
Athens, Georgia
Chapter 3

Beth E. Potter, MD
Assistant Professor, Department of Family Medicine, University of
Wisconsin–Madison, Madison, Wisconsin
Chapter 76

Randall A. Prince, PharmD
Professor, College of Pharmacy, University of Houston, Adjunct
Professor of Medicine, University of Texas M. D. Anderson Cancer
Center, Houston, Texas
Chapter 114

Marsha A. Raebel, PharmD, BCPS, FCCP
Pharmacotherapy Research Manager, Clinical Research Unit, Kaiser
Permanente of Colorado, Adjoint Associate Professor, University of
Colorado Health Sciences Center School of Pharmacy,
Aurora, Colorado
Chapter 40

Daniel W. Rahn, MD
President, Medical College of Georgia, Professor of Medicine and
Rheumatology, Medical College of Georgia Hospital and Clinics,
Augusta, Georgia
Chapter 91

Hengameh H. Raissy, PharmD
Research Assistant Professor of Pediatrics, Department of Pediatrics,
University of Mexico Health Sciences Center, Albuquerque,
New Mexico
Chapter 29

J. Laurence Ransom, MD, FAAP
Clinical Associate Professor of Pediatrics, University of
North Carolina at Chapel Hill, Medical Director, Neonatal Intensive
Care Unit, Moses Cone Health System, Greensboro,
North Carolina
Chapter 28

Charles A. Reasner, II, MD, FACE, FACP
Professor of Medicine, University of Texas Health Science Center at
San Antonio, Medical Director, Texas Diabetes Institute, San
Antonio, Texas
Chapter 72

Michael D. Reed, PharmD, FCCP, FCP
Professor of Pediatrics School of Medicine, Case Western Reserve
University, Director, Pediatric Clinical Pharmacology and
Toxicology, Rainbow Babies and Children's Hospital, Pediatric
Pharmacology Division, Cleveland, Ohio
Chapter 106

Pamela D. Reiter, PharmD, BCPS
Adjoint Assistant Professor, University of Colorado, School of
Pharmacy, Clinical Pharmacy Specialist, Pediatric ICU and Trauma,
Children's Hospital, Denver, Colorado
Chapters 136 and 137

John C. Rotschafer, PharmD
Professor, Experimental and Clinical Pharmacology, University of
Minnesota, Minneapolis, Minnesota
Chapter 105

Eric S. Rovner, MD
Associate Professor of Urology, Department of Urology, Medical
University of South Carolina, Charleston, South Carolina
Chapter 83

Maria I. Rudis, PharmD, ABAT, BCPS
Assistant Professor of Clinical Pharmacy and Clinical Emergency
Medicine, School of Pharmacy and Keck School of Medicine,
University of Southern California, Los Angeles, USC School of
Pharmacy, Director, Emergency Medicine and Critical Care
Pharmacy Residency Program, Los Angeles, California
Chapter 23

Michael J. Rybak, PharmD
Associate Dean for Research, Professor of Pharmacy and Medicine,
Director, Anti-Infective Research Laboratory, Eugene Applebaum
College of Pharmacy and Health Sciences, Wayne State University,
Detroit, Michigan
Chapter 103

Gordon S. Sacks, PharmD, BCNSP, FCCP
Clinical Associate Professor, University of Wisconsin Schools of
Pharmacy and Medicine, Nutrition Support Team Coordinator,
University of Wisconsin Hospital and Clinics,
Madison, Wisconsin
Chapter 136

John V. St. Peter, PharmD, BCPS
Associate Professor, Experimental and Clinical Pharmacology,
Division of Endocrinology, University of Minnesota College of
Pharmacy, Hennepin Center for Diabetes and Endocrinology,
Hennepin County Medical Center, Minneapolis, Minnesota
Chapter 140

Lisa A. Sanchez, PharmD
President, PE Applications, Highlands Ranch, Colorado
Chapter 1

Joseph J. Saseen, PharmD, FCCP, BCPS
Associate Professor of Clinical Pharmacy and Family Medicine,
University of Colorado Health Sciences Center,
Denver, Colorado
Chapter 13

Robert R. Schade, MD
Professor, Department of Medicine, Chief, Section of
Gastroenterology and Hepatology, Medical College of Georgia,
Augusta, Georgia
Chapters 32 and 34

Mark E. Schneiderhan, PharmD, BCPP
Clinical Assistant Professor, Department of Pharmacy Practice,
University of Illinois at Chicago, Pharmacotherapist, Department of
Psychiatry, University of Illinois Medical Center, Chicago, Illinois
Chapter 60

Marieke Dekker Schoen, PharmD, BCPS
Clinical Associate Professor, Departments of Pharmacy Practice and
Medicine, Section of Cardiology, University of Illinois,
Chicago, Illinois
Chapter 17

Kristine S. Schonder, BS Pharm, PharmD
Assistant Professor, University of Pittsburgh School of Pharmacy,
Clinical Pharmacist, Thomas E. Starzl Transplantation Institute,
Pittsburgh, Pennsylvania
Chapter 87

Arthur A. Schuna, MS
Clinical Professor, University of Wisconsin School of Pharmacy,
Clinical Coordinator and Pharmacotherapist in Rheumatology,
William S. Middleton VA Medical Center, Madison, Wisconsin
Chapter 89

Rowena N. Schwartz, PharmD, BCOP
Associate Professor, School of Pharmacy, University of Pittsburgh,
Pittsburgh, Pennsylvania
Chapter 133

Laura Scuderi, MD
Resident in Dermatology, Department of Dermatology, University of
Catania, Catania, Italy
Chapter 96

Terry L. Seaton, PharmD
Professor of Pharmacy Practice, St. Louis College of Pharmacy,
Clinical Pharmacist Faculty, Mercy Family Medicine,
St. Louis, Missouri
Chapter 88

Jeffrey J. Smith, MD
Associate Professor of Pediatrics (Clinical), University of Iowa
College of Medicine, University of Iowa Hospitals and Clinics,
Iowa City, Iowa
Chapter 30

Philip H. Smith, MD
Assistant Professor of Medicine, Medical College of Georgia,
Augusta, Georgia, Children's Medical Center of Georgia, VAH
Augusta, Augusta, Georgia
Chapter 93

Roger W. Sommi, Jr., BS Pharm, PharmD, FCCP, BCPP
Professor of Pharmacy Practice and Psychiatry, University of
Missouri Kansas City, Department of Pharmacy, Kansas City, MO
Chapter 62

Christine A. Sorkness, PharmD
Professor of Pharmacy and Medicine, University of
Wisconsin–Madison, Madison, Wisconsin
Chapter 26

Sarah A. Spinler, PharmD, FCCP
Associate Professor of Clinical Pharmacy, Philadelphia College of
Pharmacy, University of the Sciences in Philadelphia,
Philadelphia, Pennsylvania
Chapter 16

William J. Spruill, PharmD
Associate Professor, Department of Clinical and Administrative
Pharmacy, College of Pharmacy, University of Georgia,
Athens, Georgia
Chapter 36

Andy Stergachis, PhD, RPh
Professor, Departments of Epidemiology and Pharmacy, Northwest
Center for Public Health Practice, University of Washington, Seattle,
Washington
Chapter 9

James J. Stragand, MD, PhD, FACG, FACP
Attending Gastroenterologist, St. Charles Medical Center,
Bend, Oregon
Chapter 37

Deborah Ann Sturpe, PharmD, BCPS
Assistant Professor, University of Maryland School of Pharmacy,
Baltimore, Maryland
Chapter 79

Carol Taketomo, PharmD
Assistant Clinical Professor of Pharmacy Practice, University of
Southern California School of Pharmacy, Pharmacy Manager,
Children's Hospital of Los Angeles, Los Angeles, California
Chapter 7

Robert L. Talbert, PharmD, FCCP, BCPS
Professor, College of Pharmacy, University of Texas at Austin;
Professor, Departments of Medicine and Pharmacology, University of
Texas Health Science Center at San Antonio, Texas
Chapters 11, 15, 21, 22, and 73

A. Thomas Taylor, PharmD
Assistant Dean and Associate Department Head, University of
Georgia College of Pharmacy, Clinical Professor of Family Medicine,
Department of Family Medicine, Medical College of Georgia School
of Medicine, Augusta, Georgia
Chapter 35

Karen A. Theesen, PharmD, BCPP
Senior Regional Medical Scientist II, Research and Development,
GlaxoSmithKline, Minneapolis, Minnesota
Chapter 61

E. Gregory Thompson, MD
Affiliate Faculty, Department of Pharmacy Practice, Idaho State
University, Meridian, Idaho, Clinical Instructor of Medicine,
University of Washington, Seattle, Washington
Chapter 99

Edward G. Timm, PharmD, MS
Senior Clinical Pharmacy Specialist, Critical Care and Adjunct
Assistant Professor, Albany Medical Center Hospital and Albany
College of Pharmacy, Albany, New York
Chapter 37

Shelly D. Timmons, MD, PhD
Neurological Surgeon, Semmes-Murphey Neurologic and Spine
Institute, Memphis, Tennessee
Chapter 56

Margaret E. Tonda, PharmD
Director of Clinical Development, Alza Corp, Mountain View,
California
Chapter 130

John Mark Tovar, PharmD
Clinical Fellow in Pharmacy and Family Medicine, Departments of
Pharmacy Practice and Community Health and Family Medicine,
University of Florida, Gainesville, Florida
Chapter 74

Curtis L. Triplitt, PharmD, CDE, BCPS
Instructor, Department of Medicine, Division of Diabetes, Clinical
Assistant Professor of Pharmacy, University of Texas Health Science
Center at San Antonio, Texas
Chapter 72

Amy Wells Valley, PharmD, BCOP
Oncology Pharmacy Specialist and Senior Consultant, Pharmacy
Healthcare Solutions, Grapevine, Texas, Clinical Assistant Professor,
University of Texas College of Pharmacy, Austin, Texas
Chapter 124

Angie Veverka, BS, PharmD
Assistant Professor of Pharmacy, Wingate University School of
Pharmacy, Wingate, North Carolina
Chapter 109

William E. Wade, PharmD, FASHP, FCCP
Professor of Pharmacy, College of Pharmacy, University of Georgia,
Athens, Georgia
Chapter 36

Sherman Jay Weaver, PharmD, MPH
Manager, Health Information and Outcomes, ACS State HealthCare
Solutions, Atlanta, Georgia
Chapter 102

Lynda S. Welage, PharmD, FCCP
Professor of Pharmacy and Associate Dean for Academic Affairs,
University of Michigan College of Pharmacy, Clinical Pharmacist,
Critical Care, Department of Pharmacy, University of Michigan
Health System, Ann Arbor, Michigan
Chapter 33

Barbara G. Wells, PharmD, FASHP, FCCP, BCPP
Dean and Professor, School of Pharmacy, University of Mississippi,
University, Mississippi
Chapters 67 and 70

Dennis P. West, PhD
Professor of Dermatology and Director, Dermatopharmacology
Program, Department of Dermatology, Northwestern University,
Chicago, Illinois
Chapters 95 and 96

Lee E. West, BS
Consultant Pharmacist, Department of Dermatology, Northwestern
University, Chicago, Illinois
Chapters 95 and 96

Dennis M. Williams, PharmD, BCPS
Associate Professor, Division of Pharmacotherapy and Experimental
Therapeutics, School of Pharmacy, University of North Carolina,
Chapel Hill, Clinical Specialist, Pulmonary Disease, UNC Hospitals,
Chapel Hill, North Carolina
Chapter 27

Dianne B. Williams, PharmD, BCPS
Clinical Assistant Professor, University of Georgia College of
Pharmacy, Durg Information Specialist MCG Health, Inc,
Augusta, Georgia
Chapter 32

Daniel M. Witt, PharmD
Adjoint Assistant Professor, University of Colorado School of
Pharmacy, Manager, Clinical Pharmacy Services, Kaiser Permanente
of Colorado Pharmacy Administration, Aurora, Colorado
Chapter 19

Jean F. Wyman, PhD, RN
Professor and Cora Medil Siehl Chair in Nursing Research,
University of Minnesota School of Nursing,
Minneapolis, Minnesota
Chapter 83

Jack A. Yanovski, MD, PhD
Head, Unit on Growth and Obesity, Developmental Endocrinology
Branch, National Institute of Child Health and Human Development,
National Institutes of Health, Bethesda, Maryland
Chapter 75

Gary C. Yee, PharmD
Professor and Chair, Department of Pharmacy Practice, College of
Pharmacy, University of Nebraska Medical Center,
Omaha, Nebraska
Chapters 129 and 134

Sunshine J. Yocom, PharmD
Assistant Professor of Pharmacy Practice, Samford University
McWhorter School of Pharmacy, Birmingham, Alabama
Chapter 139

William C. Zamboni, PharmD
Assistant Professor, Pharmaceutical Sciences and Medicine,
University of Pittsburgh Schools of Pharmacy and Medicine,
Assistant Member of Molecular Therapeutics and Drug Development
Program, University of Pittsburgh Cancer Institute,
Pittsburgh, Pennsylvania
Chapter 130

Mario Zeolla, PharmD
Assistant Professor of Pharmacy Practice, Albany College of
Pharmacy, Patient Care Pharmacist, Eckerd Patient Care Center,
Albany, New York
Chapter 19

George G. Zhanel, PharmD, PhD
Professor, Department of Medical Microbiology, University of
Manitoba, Coordinator-Antibiotic Resistance Program, Department
of Medicine, Health Sciences Centre, Microbiology Health Sciences
Centre, Winnipeg, Canada
Chapter 107

Michael R. Zile, MD, FACC
Charles Ezra Daniel Professor of Medicine, Medical University of
South Carolina, Director of MICU, Ralph H. Johnson
Department of Veterans Affairs Medical Center, Charleston,
South Carolina
Chapter 18

GUIDING PRINCIPLES OF PHARMACOTHERAPY

1. There should be a justifiable and documented indication for every medication that is used.
2. A medication should be used at the lowest dosage and for the shortest duration that is likely to achieve the desired outcome.
3. When a patient is adequately treated with a single drug, monotherapy is preferred.
4. Newly approved medications should be used only if there are clear advantages over older medications.
5. Whenever possible, the selection of a medication regimen should be based upon evidence obtained from controlled clinical trials.
6. The timing of drug administration should be considered as a possible influence on drug efficacy, adverse effects, and interactions with other drugs and food.
7. A medication regimen should be simplified as much as possible to enhance patient adherence.
8. A patient's perception of illness or the risks and benefits of therapy may affect adherence and treatment outcomes.
9. Careful observation of a patient's response to treatment is necessary to confirm efficacy, prevent, detect, or manage adverse effects, assess compliance, and determine the need for dosage adjustment or discontinuation of drug therapy.
10. A medication should not be given by injection when giving it by mouth would be just as effective and safe.
11. Before medications are used, lifestyle modifications should be made, when indicated, to obviate the need for drug therapy or to enhance pharmacotherapy outcomes.
12. Initiation of a drug regimen should be done with full recognition that a medication may cause a disease, sign, symptom, syndrome, or abnormal laboratory test.
13. When a variety of drugs are equally efficacious and equally safe, the drug that results in the lowest health care cost or is most convenient for the patient should be chosen.
14. When making a decision about drug therapy for individual patients, societal effects should be considered.
15. The possible reasons for failure of medication regimens include inappropriate drug selection, poor adherence, improper drug dose or interval, misdiagnosis, concurrent illness, interactions with foods or drugs, environmental factors, or genetic factors.

Joseph T. DiPiro, PharmD, FCCP
Barbara G. Wells, PharmD, FASHP, FCCP, BCPP
David W. Hawkins, PharmD
August 13, 2001

Sixth Edition

PHARMACOTHERAPY

A Pathophysiologic Approach

1

PHARMACOECONOMICS: PRINCIPLES, METHODS, AND APPLICATIONS

Lisa A. Sanchez

Learning Objectives and other resources can be found at *www.pharmacotherapyonline.com.*

KEY CONCEPTS

◀1 Pharmacoeconomics identifies, measures, and compares the costs and consequences of drug therapy to health care systems and society.

◀2 The perspective of a pharmacoeconomic evaluation is paramount because the study results will be highly dependent on the perspective selected.

◀3 Health care costs can be categorized as direct medical, direct nonmedical, indirect nonmedical, intangible, opportunity, and incremental costs.

◀4 Economic, humanistic, and clinical outcomes should be considered and valued using pharmacoeconomic methods, to inform local decision making whenever possible.

◀5 To compare various health care choices, economic valuation methods are used, including cost-minimization, cost-benefit, cost-effectiveness, and cost-utility analyses. These methods all provide the means to compare competing treatment options and are similar in the way they measure costs (dollar units). They differ, however, in their measurement of outcomes and expression of results.

◀6 In today's health care settings, pharmacoeconomic methods can be applied for effective formulary management, individual patient treatment, medication policy determination, and resource allocation.

◀7 When evaluating published pharmacoeconomic studies, the following factors should be considered: study objective, study perspective, pharmacoeconomic method, study design, choice of interventions, costs and consequences, discounting, study results, sensitivity analysis, study conclusions, and sponsorship.

◀8 Use of economic models and performance of pharmacoeconomic analyses on a local level both can be useful and relevant sources of pharmacoeconomic data when rigorous methods are employed, as outlined in this chapter.

Today's cost-sensitive health care environment has created a competitive and challenging workplace for clinicians. Competition for diminishing resources has necessitated that the appraisal of health care goods and services extends beyond evaluations of safety and efficacy and considers the economic impact of these goods and services on the cost of health care. A challenge for health care professionals is to provide quality patient care with minimal resources.

An interest in defining the *value* of medicine is a common thread that unites today's health care practitioners. With serious concerns about rising medication costs and consistent pressure to decrease pharmacy expenditures and budgets, clinicians/prescribers, pharmacists, and other health care professionals must answer the question, "What is the value of the pharmaceutical goods and services I provide?" *Pharmacoeconomics*, or the discipline of placing a value on drug therapy,[1] has evolved to answer this question.

Challenged to provide high-quality patient care in the least expensive way, clinicians have developed strategies aimed at containing costs. However, most of these strategies focus solely on determining the least expensive alternative rather than the alternative that represents the best value for the money. The "cheapest" alternative—with respect to drug acquisition cost—is not always the best value for patients, departments, institutions, and health care systems.

Quality patient care must not be compromised while attempting to contain costs. The products and services delivered by today's health professionals should demonstrate *pharmacoeconomic value*, that is, a balance of economic, humanistic, *and* clinical outcomes. Pharmacoeconomics can provide the systematic means for this quantification. This chapter discusses the principles and methods of pharmacoeconomics and how they can be applied to clinical pharmacy practice and thereby how they can assist in the valuation of pharmacotherapy and other modalities of treatment in clinical practice.

PRINCIPLES OF PHARMACOECONOMICS

DEFINITIONS

◀ *Pharmacoeconomics* has been defined as the description and analysis of the cost of drug therapy to health care systems and society.[2] More specifically, pharmacoeconomic research is the process of identifying, measuring, and comparing the costs, risks, and benefits of programs, services, or therapies and determining which alternative produces the best health outcome for the resource invested.[3] For most practitioners, this translates into weighing the cost of providing a pharmacy product or service against the consequences (outcomes) realized by using the product or service to determine which alternative yields the optimal outcome per dollar spent. This information can assist clinical decision makers in choosing the most cost-effective treatment options.[4]

There is a distinct relationship between pharmacoeconomics, outcomes research, and pharmaceutical care. Pharmacoeconomics is not synonymous with outcomes research. *Outcomes research* is defined more broadly as studies that attempt to identify, measure, and evaluate the results of health care services in general.[5] Outcomes research is discussed further in Chapter 2. Pharmacoeconomics is a division of outcomes research that can be used to quantify the value of pharmaceutical care products and services. *Pharmaceutical care* has been defined as the responsible provision of drug therapy for the purposes of achieving definite outcomes.[6] By accepting this as the paradigm or vision for our profession, pharmacy is accepting responsibility for managing drug therapy so that positive outcomes are produced.

Cost is defined as the value of the resources consumed by a program or drug therapy of interest. *Consequence* is defined as the effects, outputs, or outcomes of the program of drug therapy of interest. Consideration of both costs and consequences differentiates most pharmacoeconomic evaluation methods from traditional cost-containment strategies and drug-use evaluations.

PERSPECTIVES

Assessing costs and consequences—the value of a pharmaceutical product or service—depends heavily on the perspective of the evaluation. Common perspectives include those of the patient, provider, payer, and society. A pharmacoeconomic evaluation can assess the value of a product or service from single or multiple perspectives. However, clarification of the perspective is critical because the results of a pharmacoeconomic evaluation depend heavily on the perspective taken. For example, if comparing the value of alteplase (tissue plasminogen activator, or tPA) with that of streptokinase from a patient or societal perspective, tPA may be the best-value alternative because a 1% reduction in mortality rates is observed in this large population. Yet, from a small community hospital's perspective, streptokinase may represent a better value because it provides similar outcomes for less money. Once the perspective is clear, a full evaluation of the relevant costs and consequences can begin. Again, perspective is critical because the value placed on a treatment alternative will be dependent heavily on the point of view taken.

PATIENT PERSPECTIVE

Patient perspective is paramount because patients are the ultimate consumers of health care services. Costs from the perspective of patients are essentially what patients pay for a product or service, that is, the portion not covered by insurance. Consequences, from a patient's perspective, are the clinical effects, both positive and negative, of a program or treatment alternative. For example, various costs from a patient's perspective might include insurance copayments and out-of-pocket drug costs, as well as indirect costs, such as lost wages. This perspective should be considered when assessing the impact of

drug therapy on quality of life or if a patient will pay out-of-pocket expenses for a health care service.

PROVIDER PERSPECTIVE

Costs from the provider's perspective are the actual expense of providing a product or service, regardless of what the provider charges. Providers can be hospitals, managed-care organizations (MCOs), or private-practice physicians. From this perspective, direct costs such as drugs, hospitalization, laboratory tests, supplies, and salaries of health care professionals may be identified, measured, and compared. However, indirect costs may be of less importance to the provider. When making formulary management or drug-use policy decisions, the viewpoint of the health care organization should dominate.

PHARMACOECONOMIC CONTROVERSY

Surprisingly few providers are prepared to identify and measure their true economic costs. Charge data may be more readily available but usually are not reflective of the true costs of health care. Thus it can be challenging translating charges into costs. A cost-to-charge ratio may be useful in many instances. Additionally, a common proxy used for costs of medications is average wholesale price (AWP). However, realistically, there are no providers actually paying AWP for their drugs, and AWP therefore is not an accurate proxy for drug-cost data.

PAYER PERSPECTIVE

Payers include insurance companies, employers, or the government. From this perspective, costs represent the charges for health care products and services allowed, or reimbursed, by the payer. The primary cost for a payer is of a direct nature. However, indirect costs, such as lost workdays and decreased productivity, also may contribute to the total cost of health care to the payer. When insurance companies and employers are contracting with MCOs or selecting health care benefits for their employees, then the payer's perspective should be employed.

SOCIETAL PERSPECTIVE

The perspective of society is the broadest of all perspectives because it is the only one that considers the benefit to society as a whole. Theoretically, all direct and indirect costs are included in an economic evaluation performed from a societal perspective. Costs from this perspective include patient morbidity and mortality and the overall costs of giving and receiving medical care. An evaluation from this perspective also would include all the important consequences an individual could experience. In countries with nationalized medicine, society is the predominant perspective.

PHARMACOECONOMIC CONTROVERSY

Controversy surrounds the issue of study perspective. Many researchers assert that society is the only relevant and the most appropriate perspective from which to conduct a pharmacoeconomic analysis. However, in the United States, these studies can be very resource-intensive in terms of time and money. Further, organizations may need to focus solely from their own perspectives to obtain the data necessary to inform timely decision making.

TABLE 1–1. Example of Health Care Cost Categories

Cost Category	Costs
Direct medical costs	Medications
	Supplies
	Laboratory tests
	Health care professionals' time
	Hospitalization
Direct nonmedical costs	Transportation
	Food
	Family care
	Home aides
Indirect costs	Lost wages (morbidity)
	Income forgone due to premature death (mortality)
Intangible costs	Pain
	Suffering
	Inconvenience
	Grief
Opportunity costs	Lost opportunity
	Revenue forgone

COSTS

Once a perspective is chosen, the costs and consequences associated with a given product or service may be identified and measured using pharmacoeconomic methods. A comparison of two or more treatment alternatives should extend beyond a simple comparison of drug acquisition costs. Health care costs or economic outcomes can be grouped into several categories: direct medical, direct nonmedical, indirect nonmedical, and intangible costs.[7] Other costs often discussed in pharmacoeconomic evaluations include opportunity and incremental costs. Inclusion of these various cost categories, when appropriate, provides a more accurate estimate of the total economic impact of a health care program or treatment alternatives on a specific population, organization, or patient. Table 1–1 contains examples of these costs. Again, the costs that are identified, measured, and ultimately compared vary depending on the perspective.

DIRECT MEDICAL COSTS

Direct medical costs are the costs incurred for medical products and services used to prevent, detect, and/or treat a disease.[7] Direct medical costs are the fundamental transactions associated with medical care that contribute to the portion of gross national product spent on health care. Examples of these costs include drugs, medical supplies and equipment, laboratory and diagnostic tests, hospitalizations, and physician visits. Direct medical costs can be subdivided into fixed and variable costs. Fixed costs are essentially "overhead" costs (e.g., heat, rent, electricity) that are not readily influenced at the treatment level and thus remain relatively constant. For this reason, they are often not included in most pharmacoeconomic analyses. Variable costs, which change as a function of volume, include medications, fees for professional services, and supplies. As more services are used, more funding must be used to provide them.

PHARMACOECONOMIC CONTROVERSY

Should personnel costs be considered fixed or variable costs? In a hospital setting, one might consider whether switching from a drug that requires a three-times-daily versus once-daily administration truly saves time for health care personnel. Some argue that staffing is relatively constant and that such a change would not cause the hospital to reduce its overall personnel levels, whereas others maintain that such a change allows personnel to perform other activities that provide value. In times of *downsizing*, personnel often are viewed as variable costs by hospital administrators.

DIRECT NONMEDICAL COSTS

Direct nonmedical costs are any costs for nonmedical services that are results of illness or disease but do not involve purchasing medical services.[7] These costs are consumed to purchase services other than medical care and include resources spent by patients for transportation to and from health care facilities, extra trips to the emergency department, child or family care expenses, special diets, and various other out-of-pocket expenses.

INDIRECT NONMEDICAL COSTS

Indirect nonmedical costs are the costs of reduced productivity (e.g., morbidity and mortality costs).[7–9] Indirect costs are costs that result from morbidity and mortality and are an important source of resource consumption, especially from the perspective of the patient. Morbidity costs are costs incurred from missing work (i.e., lost productivity), whereas mortality costs represent the years lost as result of premature death. To estimate indirect costs, two techniques typically are used: (1) human capital (HC) and (2) willingness-to-pay (WTP) methods. The HC approach attempts to value morbidity and mortality (primarily wages and productivity) losses based on an individual's earning capacity using standard labor wage rates.[10] This approach raises an ethical dilemma because the value of a life is related directly to income. Using the WTP approach (contingent valuation), the indirect and intangible aspects of a disease can be valued. Patients are asked how much money they would be willing to spend to reduce the likelihood of illness.[11] However, the values obtained through this method may be unreliable because of the substantial differences in valuations of life that result from the subjective nature of this approach.

INTANGIBLE COSTS

Intangible costs are those of other nonfinancial outcomes of disease and medical care.[7] Examples include pain, suffering, inconvenience, and grief, and these are difficult to measure quantitatively and impossible to measure in terms of economic or financial costs. In pharmacoeconomic analyses, frequently intangible costs are identified but not quantified formally.

OPPORTUNITY COSTS

Opportunity costs represent the economic benefit forgone when using one therapy instead of the next best alternative therapy.[12] Therefore, if a resource has been used to purchase a program or treatment alternative, then the opportunity to use it for another purpose is lost. In other words, opportunity cost is the value of the alternative that was forgone.

INCREMENTAL COSTS

Incremental costs represent the additional cost that a service or treatment alternative imposes over another compared with the additional effect, benefit, or outcome it provides.[13] As medical interventions become increasingly intense, costs generally increase. However, the additional outcome gained per additional dollar spent generally decreases. At some point of increasing expenditures, there may be no additional benefits or even a reduction in outcome. Thus incremental costs are the extra costs required to purchase an additional unit of effect and provide another way to assess the pharmacoeconomic impact of a service or treatment option on a population.

CONSEQUENCES

Similar to costs, the outcomes or consequences of a disease and its treatment are an equally important component of pharmacoeconomic analyses. The manner in which consequences are quantified is a key distinction among pharmacoeconomic methods because the assessment of costs is relatively standard.

Like costs, the consequences (or outcomes) of medical care also can be categorized. One approach is to separate outcomes into three categories: economic, clinical, and humanistic. *Economic outcomes* are the direct, indirect, and intangible costs compared with the consequences of medical treatment alternatives.[14] *Clinical outcomes* are the medical events that occur as a result of disease or treatment (e.g., safety and efficacy end points).[14] *Humanistic outcomes* are the consequences of disease or treatment on patient functional status or quality of life along several dimensions (e.g., physical function, social function, general health and well-being, and life satisfaction).[14] Assessing the economic, clinical, and humanistic outcomes (ECHO) associated with a treatment alternative provides a complete model for decision making.

POSITIVE VERSUS NEGATIVE CONSEQUENCES

These consequences (outcomes) can be further categorized as positive or negative. An example of a positive outcome is a desired effect of a drug (efficacy or effectiveness measure), possibly manifested as cases cured, life-years gained, or improved health-related quality of life (HRQOL). Since all drugs have adverse effects, negative consequences also can occur with their use. A negative outcome is an undesired or adverse effect of a drug, possibly manifested as a treatment failure, an adverse drug reaction (ADR), a drug toxicity, or even death. Pharmacoeconomic evaluations should include assessments of both types of outcomes. Evaluating only positive outcomes may be misleading because of the potential detriment and expense associated with negative outcomes. Thus the balancing of positive and negative consequences is important in any pharmacoeconomic evaluation.

INTERMEDIATE AND FINAL CONSEQUENCES

Consequences also can be discussed in terms of intermediate and final outcomes. Intermediate outcomes can serve as a proxy for more relevant final outcomes. For example, achieving a decrease in low-density lipoprotein cholesterol levels with a lipid-lowering agent is an intermediate consequence that may serve as a proxy for a more final outcome such as a decrease in myocardial infarction rate.[15] Intermediate consequences are used commonly in clinical and pharmacoeconomic analyses as proxies predictive of final outcomes because their use reduces the cost and time required to conduct a trial.

METHODS OF PHARMACOECONOMICS

The pharmacoeconomic methods of evaluation are listed in Fig. 1–1. These methods or tools can be separated into two distinct categories: economic and humanistic evaluation techniques. These methods have been used in a variety of fields and are being applied increasingly to health care.[16]

ECONOMIC EVALUATION METHODS

The basic task of economic evaluation is to identify, measure, value, and compare the costs and consequences of the alternatives being considered. The two distinguishing characteristics of economic evaluation are as follows: (1) Is there a comparison of two or more alternatives? and (2) Are both costs and consequences of the alternatives examined?[17] A full economic evaluation encompasses both characteristics, whereas a partial economic evaluation addresses only one. Pharmacoeconomic evaluations conducted in today's health care settings may be either partial or full economic evaluations.

Partial economic evaluations may include simple descriptive tabulations of outcomes or resources consumed and thus require a minimum of time and effort. If only the consequences or only the costs of a program, service, or treatment are described, the evaluation illustrates an outcome or cost description. A cost-outcome or cost-consequence analysis (CCA) describes the costs and consequences of an alternative but does not provide a comparison with other treatment options.[15] Another partial evaluation is a cost analysis that compares the costs of two or more alternatives without regard to outcome.

Full economic evaluations include cost-minimization, cost-benefit, cost-effectiveness, and cost-utility analyses. Each method is used to compare competing programs or treatment alternatives. The methods are all similar in the way they measure cost (in dollars) and different in their measurement of outcomes. Although a full economic evaluation generally provides higher-quality and more useful information, the time, resources, and effort employed are also great. Thus health care practitioners and clinicians also find it necessary to employ various partial economic evaluations.

Application of economic evaluation methods to health care products and services, especially pharmaceuticals, may increase their acceptance by health care professionals and society.[18] The methods used most commonly by health care practitioners are discussed in the next sections and summarized briefly in Table 1–2.

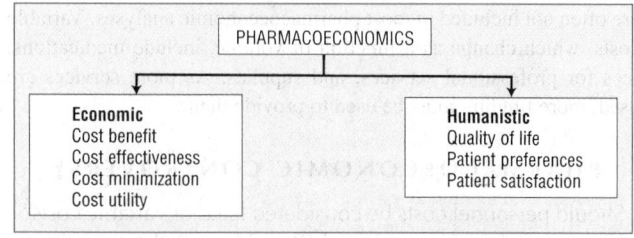

FIGURE 1–1. Components of pharmacoeconomics.

TABLE 1–2. Summary of Pharmacoeconomic Methodologies

Method	Description	Application	Cost Unit	Outcome Unit
COI	Estimates the cost of a disease on a defined population	Use to provide baseline to compare prevention/treatment options against	$$$	NA
CMA	Finds the least expensive cost alternative	Use when benefits are the same	$$$	Assume to be equivalent
CBA	Measures benefit in monetary units and computes a net gain	Can compare programs with different objectives	$$$	$$$
CEA	Compares alternatives with therapeutic effects measured in physical units; computes a C/E ratio	Can compare drugs/programs that differ in clinical outcomes and use the same unit of benefit	$$$	Natural units
CUA	Measures therapeutic consequences in utility units rather than physical units; computes a C/U ratio	Use to compare drugs/programs that are life extending with serious side effects or those producing reductions in morbidity	$$$	QALYs
QOL	Physical, social, and emotional aspects of patient's well-being that are relevant and important to the patient	Examines drug effects in areas not covered by laboratory or physiologic measurements	NA	QOL score

Key: CBA, cost-benefit analysis; CEA, cost-effectiveness analysis; CMA, cost-minimization analysis; COI, cost-of-illness evaluation; CUA, cost-utility analysis; QOL, quality of life; QALY, quality-adjusted life-year.

COST-OF-ILLNESS EVALUATION

A cost-of-illness (COI) evaluation identifies and estimates the overall cost of a particular disease for a defined population.[8] This evaluation method is often referred to as *burden of illness* and involves measuring the direct and indirect costs attributable to a specific disease. The costs of various diseases, including peptic ulcer disease, mental disorders, and cancer, in the United States have been estimated.

By successfully identifying the direct and indirect costs of an illness, one can determine the relative value of a treatment or prevention strategy. For example, by determining the cost of a particular disease to society, the cost of a prevention strategy could be subtracted from this to yield the benefit of implementing this strategy nationwide. COI evaluation is not used to compare competing treatment alternatives but to provide an estimation of the financial burden of a disease. Thus the value of prevention and treatment strategies can be measured against this illness cost. Various examples of COI studies are available in the literature, including the burden or cost of Alzheimer's disease.[19, 20]

COST-MINIMIZATION ANALYSIS

Cost-minimization analysis (CMA) involves the determination of the least costly alternative when comparing two or more treatment alternatives. With CMA, the alternatives must have an assumed or demonstrated equivalency in safety and efficacy (i.e., the two alternatives must be equivalent therapeutically). Once this equivalency in outcome is confirmed, the costs can be identified, measured, and compared in monetary units (dollars).

CMA is a relatively straightforward and simple method for comparing competing programs or treatment alternatives as long as the therapeutic equivalence of the alternatives being compared has been established. If no evidence exists to support this, then a more comprehensive method such as cost-effectiveness analysis should be employed. Remember, CMA shows only a "cost savings" of one program or treatment over another.[21]

Employing CMA is appropriate when comparing two or more therapeutically equivalent agents or alternate dosing regimens of the same agent.[21] For example, if drugs A and B are antiulcer agents and have been documented as equivalent in efficacy and incidence of adverse drug reactions (ADRs), then the costs of using these drugs could be compared using CMA. These costs should extend beyond a comparison of drug acquisition costs and include costs of drug preparation (pharmacist and technician time), administration (nursing time), and storage. When appropriate, other costs to be valued may include the cost of physician visits, number of hospital days, and pharmacokinetic consultations. The least expensive agent, considering all these costs, should be preferred. This method has been used frequently, and its application could expand given the increasing number of "me too" products and generic competition in the pharmaceutical marketplace.[22]

COST-BENEFIT ANALYSIS

Cost-benefit analysis (CBA) is a method that allows for the identification, measurement, and comparison of the benefits and costs of a program or treatment alternative. The benefits realized from a program or treatment alternative are compared with the costs of providing it. Both the costs and the benefits are measured and converted into equivalent dollars in the year in which they will occur.[8, 16] Future costs and benefits are discounted or reduced to their current value.

These costs and benefits are expressed as a ratio (a benefit-to-cost ratio), a net benefit, or a net cost. A clinical decision maker would choose the program or treatment alternative with the highest net benefit or the greatest benefit-to-cost (B/C) ratio.[9] Guidelines for the interpretation of this ratio are indicated[16, 21, 23]:

- If the B/C ratio is greater than 1, the program or treatment is of value. The benefits realized by the program or treatment alternative outweigh the cost of providing it.

- If the B/C ratio equals 1, the benefits equal the cost. The benefits realized by the program or treatment alternative are equivalent to the cost of providing it.
- If the B/C ratio is less than 1, the program or treatment is not economically beneficial. The cost of providing the program or treatment alternative outweighs the benefits realized by it.

CBA should be employed when comparing treatment alternatives in which the costs and benefits do not occur simultaneously. CBA also may be used when comparing programs with different objectives because all benefits are converted into dollars. CBA also can be used to evaluate a single program or compare multiple programs. However, valuing health benefits in monetary terms can be difficult and controversial. The expression of some health benefits as monetary units is neither appropriate nor widely accepted. Therefore, unless the benefits of a program or treatment alternative are expressed appropriately in dollars, CBA should not be employed.[21]

CBA may be an appropriate method to use in justifying and documenting the value of an existing health care service or the potential worth of a new one. For example, when a clinical pharmacy service is competing for institutional resources, CBA can provide data to document that the service yields a high return on investment compared with other institutional services competing for the same resources. However, the relative magnitude of the costs and benefits for the service must be considered when making this resource-allocation decision. If a service costs $100 to implement and results in a benefit to the hospital of $1000 and a service that costs $100,000 to implement results in a benefit of $1 million, both have a B/C ratio of 10.[21] Thus caution should be exercised when using B/C ratios and CBA as a comparison tool.

Numerous examples of CBAs have been published in the literature recently.[24–27] However, of all pharmacoeconomic evaluation methods, CBA is probably used the least. Although this method has the advantage of valuing indirect costs monetarily (using the HC and WTP approaches) and intangible benefits (using the WTP approach), the valuation of outcomes such as productivity and quality of life is difficult to perform reliably and meaningfully.[10,28]

Because of difficulties in measuring indirect and intangible benefits, many CBAs measure and quantify direct costs and direct benefits only. Some researchers assert that these should not be considered "true" CBAs because they do not take into account the indirect costs and benefits.[28]

COST-EFFECTIVENESS ANALYSIS

Cost-effectiveness analysis (CEA) is a way of summarizing the health benefits and resources used by competing health care programs so that policymakers can choose among them.[17] CEA involves comparing programs or treatment alternatives with different safety and efficacy profiles. Cost is measured in dollars, and outcomes are measured in terms of obtaining a specific therapeutic outcome. These outcomes are often expressed in physical units, natural units, or non-dollar units (lives saved, cases cured, life expectancy, or drop in blood pressure).[8,13,29]

The results of CEA are also expressed as a ratio—either as an average cost-effectiveness ratio (ACER) or as an incremental cost-effectiveness ratio (ICER). An ACER represents the total cost of a program or treatment alternative divided by its clinical outcome to yield a ratio representing the dollar cost per specific clinical outcome gained, independent of comparators. The ACER can be summarized as follows[7,13,21]:

$$\text{ACER} = \frac{\text{health care costs (\$)}}{\text{clinical outcome (not in \$)}}$$

This allows the costs and outcomes to be reduced to a single value to allow for comparison. Using this ratio, the clinician would choose the alternative with the least cost per outcome gained.[9] The most cost-effective alternative is not always the least costly alternative for obtaining a specific therapeutic objective. In this regard, cost-effectiveness need not be cost reduction but rather cost optimization.[30]

Often clinical effectiveness is gained at an increased cost. Is the increased benefit worth the increased cost? Incremental CEA may be used to determine the additional cost and effectiveness gained when one treatment alternative is compared with the next best treatment alternative.[7] Thus, instead of comparing the ACERs of each treatment alternative, the additional cost that a treatment alternative imposes over another treatment is compared with the additional effect, benefit, or outcome it provides. The ICER can be summarized as follows:

$$\text{ICER} = \frac{\text{cost}_A(\$) - \text{cost}_B(\$)}{\text{effect}_A(\%) - \text{effect}_B(\%)}$$

This formula yields the additional cost required to obtain the additional effect gained by switching from drug A to drug B.

CEA is particularly useful in balancing cost with patient outcome, determining which treatment alternatives represent the best health outcome per dollar spent, and deciding when it is appropriate to measure outcome in terms of obtaining a specific therapeutic objective. In addition, CEA may provide valuable data to support drug policy, formulary management, and individual patient treatment decisions. Globally, CEA is being used to set public policies regarding the use of pharmaceutical products (national formularies) in countries such as Australia,[31] New Zealand, and Canada.[32] These countries, along with others, including Spain, the United Kingdom, Italy, and the United States, even have their own guidelines for conducting research.

PHARMACOECONOMIC CONTROVERSY

Which ratio is the right ratio to use in pharmacoeconomic analyses? Experts differ over which ratio, ACER or ICER, is the most appropriate and useful. ACER reflects the cost per benefit of a new strategy independent of other alternatives, whereas ICER reveals the cost per unit of benefit of switching from one treatment strategy (that already may be in place) to another.[13]

COST-UTILITY ANALYSIS

Pharmacoeconomists sometimes want to include a measure of patient preference or quality of life when comparing competing treatment alternatives. Cost-utility analysis (CUA) is a method for comparing treatment alternatives that integrates patient preferences and HRQOL. CUA can compare cost, quality, and the quantity of patient-years. Cost is measured in dollars, and therapeutic outcome is measured in patient-weighted utilities rather than in physical units. Often the utility measurement used is a quality-adjusted life year (QALY) gained. QALY is a common measure of health status used in CUA, combining morbidity and mortality data.[33]

Results of CUA are also expressed in a ratio, a cost-utility ratio (C/U ratio). Most often this ratio is translated as the cost per QALY gained or some other health-state utility measurement.[8,16] The preferred treatment alternative is that with the lowest cost per QALY (or other health-status utility). QALYs represent the number of full years at full health that are valued equivalently to the number of years as experienced. For example, a full year of health in a disease-free patient would equal 1.0 QALY, whereas a year spent with a specific disease might be valued significantly lower, perhaps as 0.5 QALY, depending on the disease.

CUA is the most appropriate method to use when comparing programs and treatment alternatives that are life extending with serious side effects (e.g., cancer chemotherapy),[34] those which produce reductions in morbidity rather than mortality (e.g., medical treatment of arthritis),[30,35] and when HRQOL is the most important health outcome being examined. CUA is employed less frequently than other economic evaluation methods because of a lack of agreement on measuring utilities, difficulty comparing QALYs across patients and populations, and difficulty quantifying patient preferences. CUA is complex, and thus CUA may be limited in scope of application from a hospital or MCO perspective. Nevertheless, when comparing treatment alternatives where HRQOL is the most important health outcome being examined, CUA should be considered.

PHARMACOECONOMIC CONTROVERSY

Because QALYs and other utility measures are highly subjective, there is some disagreement among researchers regarding which scales should be preferred for measuring utility.

HUMANISTIC EVALUATION METHODS

Pharmacoeconomic evaluations also may focus on humanistic concerns. Methods for evaluating the impact of disease and treatment of disease on a patient's HRQOL, patient preferences, and patient satisfaction are all growing in popularity and application to pharmacotherapy decisions. These methods also can assist clinicians in quantifying the value of pharmaceuticals.

HRQOL has been defined as the assessment of the functional effects of illness and its consequent therapy as perceived by the patient.[36] These effects often are displayed as physical, emotional, and social effects on the patient.[17] Measurement of HRQOL usually is achieved through the use of patient-completed questionnaires. Many questionnaires are available, and most are either disease-specific or generic measures of health status.[37,38] Various overviews on HRQOL and its application to pharmacy have been published.[15,38–41] For further discussion on health outcomes and HRQOL, refer to Chapter 2.

APPLICATIONS OF PHARMACOECONOMICS

Health care practitioners, regardless of practice setting, can benefit from applying the principles and methods of pharmacoeconomics to their daily practice settings. *Applied pharmacoeconomics* is defined as putting pharmacoeconomic principles, methods, and theories into practice to quantify the *value* of pharmacy products and pharmaceutical care services used in real-world environments. Today's practitioners increasingly are required to justify the value of the products and services they provide. Applied pharmacoeconomics can provide the means or tools for this valuation.

One of the primary applications of pharmacoeconomics in clinical practice today is to aid clinical and policy decision making. Through the appropriate application of pharmacoeconomics, practitioners and administrators can make better, more-informed decisions regarding the products and services they provide. Complete pharmacotherapy decisions should contain assessments of three basic outcome areas whenever appropriate: clinical, economic, and humanistic outcomes. Traditionally, most drug therapy decisions were based solely on the clinical outcomes (e.g., safety and efficacy) associated with a treatment alternative. Over the past 10 to 15 years, it has become quite popular also to include an assessment of the economic outcomes associated with a treatment alternative. The current trend is also to

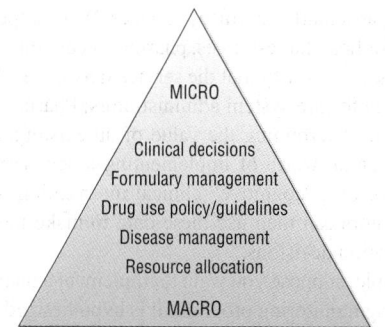

FIGURE 1–2. Decisions for pharmacoeconomic applications.

incorporate the humanistic outcomes associated with a treatment alternative, that is, to bring the patient back into this decision-making equation. This ECHO model for medical decision making has become prevalent in current health care settings.[14] In today's health care environment, it is no longer appropriate to make drug-selection decisions based solely on acquisition costs. Thus, through the appropriate application of pharmacoeconomic principles and methods, incorporating these three critical components into clinical decisions can be accomplished.

Pharmacoeconomic data can be a powerful tool to support various clinical decisions, ranging from the level of the patient to the level of an entire health care system. Figure 1–2 shows various decisions that may be supported using pharmacoeconomics, including effective formulary management, individual patient treatment, medication policy, and resource allocation.[13,21] For discussion purposes, the application of pharmacoeconomics to decision making is divided into two basic areas: drug therapy evaluation and clinical pharmacy service evaluation.

DRUG THERAPY EVALUATION

Historically, pharmacoeconomic principles and methods have been applied commonly to assist clinicians and practitioners in making more informed and complete decisions regarding drug therapy. For example, pharmacoeconomics can provide critical cost-effectiveness data to support the addition or deletion of a drug to or from a hospital formulary with or without restriction. In fact, the pharmacoeconomic assessment of formulary actions is becoming a standardized part of many pharmacy and therapeutic (P&T) committees.

Selecting the most cost-effective drugs for an organizational formulary is important. However, it is equally important to determine the most appropriate way to use and prescribe these agents. Hence, developing and implementing appropriate use guidelines or policies based on sound pharmacoeconomic data can have a great impact on influencing prescribing patterns. Further, implementing sound drug-use guidelines/policies will ensure the most appropriate and cost-effective use of pharmaceutical agents throughout the health care system.

The application of pharmacoeconomics also can be useful for making a decision about an individual patient's therapy. Evaluating the impact a drug has on a patient's HRQOL can be useful when deciding between two agents for customizing a patient's pharmacotherapy. Although this can be one of the most difficult applications of pharmacoeconomics, it is also one of the most important.

CLINICAL PHARMACY SERVICE EVALUATION

The most recent application of pharmacoeconomic principles and methods has been for justifying the value of various health care services, particularly pharmacy services. When a specific service is competing for hospital resources, pharmacoeconomics can provide the data necessary to justify that the service maximizes the resources allocated by health care system administrators. Pharmacoeconomics can be useful in determining the value of an existing service, estimating the potential worth of implementing a new service, or capturing the value of a "cognitive" clinical intervention. Practitioners and administrators can then use these data to make more informed resource-allocation decisions.

For example, suppose you want to implement a pharmacy-based therapeutic drug monitoring program. It is hypothesized that this service will improve quality of patient care and save money for the health care system. After negotiating with hospital administrators, the funding for this service is approved for a 1-year trial basis, after which you must document and justify the value of this practice. Theoretically, all the relevant costs and benefits of the program should be measured and, if appropriate, converted into dollars using CBA. Potential benefits may include decreased total drug costs and decreased incidence of ADRs. Potential program costs are primarily the salary and benefits for a pharmacist and additional laboratory tests to monitor patients. Data documenting that the benefit of this pharmacy service yields a high return on investment (ROI) should increase the probability of the program continuing to be funded by the health care system.

Unfortunately, previous reviews of the literature have revealed a disappointing number of rigorous economic evaluations of clinical pharmacy services published to date.[42-44] However, a recently published review shows that the quality of published studies finally may be increasing.[45] For example, McGhan and colleagues[42] evaluated 35 potential CBAs or CEAs of pharmacy services published before 1978 and concluded that only 5 of these studies were legitimate CBAs or CEAs. MacKeigan and Bootman[43] reviewed 22 CBAs or CEAs published between 1978 and 1987 and concluded that CBAs and CEAs have not been adopted extensively for the evaluation of clinical pharmacy services. In 1996, Schumock and associates[44] reviewed economic evaluations of pharmacy services published between 1988 and 1995. Of the studies reviewed, only 19 were considered "full" or legitimate economic analyses, and the authors concluded that although the number of articles published has increased over the years, there is still a need for improvement in the quality or rigor of study design. Despite the relatively low number of methodologically sound studies, this review also revealed some results that demonstrate the potential

value of clinical pharmacy services. Of the 109 studies evaluated, the various clinical services reviewed in this study yielded an average C/B ratio of 16:1. In 2003, these authors updated their review and included articles published from 1996 to 2000.[45] After reviewing 59 articles, these authors noted an improvement in the overall quality of the research (more studies included comparison groups and measured both costs and outcomes). Studies were conducted in hospital settings (52%), community pharmacies and clinics (41%), and community/clinic settings (18%). For the studies reporting the statistic, B/C ratios ranged from 1.74:1 to 17.01.[45]

STRATEGIES TO INCORPORATE PHARMACOECONOMICS INTO PHARMACOTHERAPY

Various strategies are available to incorporate pharmacoeconomics into pharmacotherapy. Popular strategies for applying pharmacoeconomics to assess the value of pharmaceutical products and services include using the results of published pharmacoeconomic studies, building economic models, and conducting pharmacoeconomic research.[46] Advantages and disadvantages of these strategies are summarized in Table 1–3.

USE THE PHARMACOECONOMIC LITERATURE

Quantifying the value of pharmaceuticals through pharmacoeconomics has increased in popularity. Many pharmacoeconomic analyses are published in primary medical and pharmacy literature sources. Over the past 30 or more years, the actual number of pharmacoeconomic studies published exceeded 35,000 in 1993. However, the eagerness to conduct pharmacoeconomic evaluations of drugs often exceeds the quality of these evaluations. Variations in quality and indiscriminate use of pharmacoeconomic terminology are documented in medical and pharmacy literature sources.[4,42-45,47-49] To use this literature as an aid in clinical decision making, it must be (1) critically evaluated for quality and rigor and (2) interpreted correctly. Therefore, prior to using pharmacoeconomic data to make clinical and policy decisions, decision makers should recognize the potential limitations of those data.

TABLE 1–3. Advantages and Disadvantages of Pharmacoeconomic Application Strategies

Strategy	Advantage	Disadvantage
Use published literature	Quick Inexpensive Subject to peer review Results may be from RCT Variety of results can be examined	Results from RCT Difficult to generalize results May not be comparative Misuse of pharmacoeconomic terms Variations in rigor/quality
Build an economic model	Quick Relatively inexpensive Yields organization-specific results Bridges efficacy and effectiveness Data collection is unobtrusive	Results dependent on assumptions Potential for researcher bias Controversial Reluctance of decision makers to accept results
Conduct a pharmacoeconomic study	Flexible Usually comparative Yields organization-specific data Reflects "usual care" or effectiveness Data from multiple sources can be used	Expensive Time-consuming Difficult to control and randomize Potential for patient selection bias Potential for small sample size

RCT, randomized controlled trial.

A primary consideration when evaluating and interpreting a study is the ability to generalize or transfer the results to other health care settings and countries. It can be difficult to generalize and transfer the results of a published study primarily because of wide variations in practice patterns, patient populations, and costs among health care systems and countries. Further, differences in study perspectives, data sources, and analytic styles may present a challenge for practitioners attempting to extrapolate or relate exact cost savings or cost ratios to their own practice settings. To enhance the ability to use pharmacoeconomic results published in the literature, consider the following points:

1. What is the technical merit of the study?
2. Are the results applicable to local decision making?
3. Do the results apply generally in different jurisdictions with different perspectives?[50]

Various guidelines, criteria, reviews, and consensus-based recommendations for evaluating, conducting, and reporting pharmacoeconomic literature have been published.[7,17,31,32,51–60] These guidelines and criteria have been combined and summarized into 11 categories most pertinent to pharmacotherapy.[54] A summary of these 11 criteria and pertinent questions for each category are given in Table 1–4. Each evaluation criterion is briefly discussed next.

STUDY OBJECTIVE

A clear statement of the purpose of the study should be given. This objective should be clear, concise, well defined, and measurable.

STUDY PERSPECTIVE

The researcher must select one or more perspectives (e.g., patient, provider, payer, or society) from which the analysis will be conducted.[9] This perspective should be appropriate given the scope of the pharmacoeconomic problem identified. An evaluation may be conducted from single or multiple perspectives as long as the costs and consequences identified are relevant to the perspective(s) chosen.

PHARMACOECONOMIC METHOD

It should be clear which pharmacoeconomic method was employed (CEA, CMA, CBA, or CUA), and this method should be appropriate given the problem (e.g., CMA is appropriate if comparing two alternatives equivalent in therapeutic outcome but not if the alternatives differ in therapeutic outcome). Also, a researcher may claim that a specific method was employed (e.g., CEA) but actually employ another method (e.g., CMA).

STUDY DESIGN

Pharmacoeconomic evaluations can be prospective or retrospective. Although prospective designs usually are preferred, retrospective evaluations can be rich with information and reflective of usual care. Many pharmacoeconomic evaluations today are conducted as a part of randomized, controlled clinical trials. Two cautions for interpreting pharmacoeconomic data collected in this manner include (1) costs can be protocol-driven, not necessarily reflective of using a drug in common practice,[61] and (2) control of subjects and decreased complications may yield greater costs and benefits than those observed in common practice.[51]

CHOICE OF INTERVENTIONS

All relevant treatment options that are available should be described completely or mentioned. The treatment alternatives and dosages being compared should be those used in common practice, and evidence of their effectiveness should be established. Because pharmacoeconomic methods are tools to aid in choosing among treatment

---

TABLE 1–4. Basic Criteria for Evaluation of Pharmacoeconomic Literature

Objective
What is the question(s) being considered?
Is the question clear, defined, and measurable?

Perspective
What is/are the perspective(s) of the analysis?
Is the perspective appropriate given the scope of the problem?

Pharmacoeconomic Method
What pharmacoeconomic tool was used?
Is it appropriate given the problem?
Is it actually what was conducted?

Study Design
What was the study design?
What were the data sources?
Is the evaluation suitable if carried out in a clinical trial?

Choice of Interventions
Were all appropriate alternatives considered and described?
Were any appropriate alternatives omitted?
Are the alternatives relevant to the perspective and clinical nature of the study?
Is there evidence that the alternatives' effectiveness has been established?

Costs and Consequences
What are the costs and consequences (outcomes) included?
Are the costs and outcomes relevant to the perspective chosen?

Sensitivity Analysis
Are cost ranges for significant variables tested for sensitivity?
Are the appropriate and relevant variables varied?
Do the findings follow the anticipated trend?

Conclusions
Are the conclusions of the study justified?
Is it possible to extrapolate the conclusions to daily clinical practice?

Sponsorship
Was there any bias due to the sponsorship of the study?
Do they include negative outcomes (failures, ADRs)?
How were they valued?
Were costs and consequences measured in the appropriate physical units?

Discounting
Was the study performed over time?
Were costs and consequences that occur in the future discounted to their present value?
Was any justification given for the discount rate used?

Results
Are the results accurate and practical for medical decision makers?
Were the appropriate statistical analyses performed?
Was an incremental analysis performed?
Are all the assumptions and limitations of the study discussed?

alternatives, assessing the cost of a single alternative is considered a partial economic evaluation.

COSTS AND CONSEQUENCES

All the important and relevant costs and consequences for each program or treatment alternative should be identified. The costs and consequences identified must be relevant to the study perspective(s) and measured in suitable terms using the appropriate physical units. Costs should include direct, indirect, and intangible costs. Consequences should include the positive and negative clinical and humanistic outcomes associated with the program or treatment alternative. All these costs and consequences must be valued credibly, with the data sources clearly identified.

DISCOUNTING

The comparison of programs or treatment alternatives should be made at one point in time; thus any costs and consequences not occurring in the present must be addressed. *Discounting*, or adjusting for differential timing, is the process of reducing any costs and consequences that may occur in the future back to their present value. If a study is performed over time (more than 1 year), or if future cost savings are projected, discounting should be done using an appropriate discount rate. The rate recommended by most investigators is typically 3% to 8% per annum, representing annual inflation or bank interest rates. However, the modal rates used in pharmacoeconomic evaluations appear to be 5%.

Researchers disagree about which discount rate to use, as well as about whether to discount costs and health benefits (simultaneously) using the same discount rate(s).

STUDY RESULTS

A full discussion of the study assumptions and limitations and how to interpret the results in the context of different practice settings[17] should be provided. This discussion should include all relevant issues of concern to potential users of the study. The results should show that the appropriate statistical analyses were performed. Also, it may be appropriate to express the study results in terms of increases, that is, to use incremental cost analysis (additional cost of gaining an additional benefit by using one drug over another).

SENSITIVITY ANALYSIS

It is imperative that researchers test the sensitivity of study results using sensitivity analysis. Using this method, practitioners and researchers can deal with data uncertainties and assumptions and their effect on study conclusions. *Sensitivity analysis* (SA) is the process of testing the robustness of an economic evaluation by examining changes in results. Specific variables such as percent effectiveness, incidence of ADRs, and dominant resources can be varied over a range of plausible values and the results recalculated. The four general approaches to SA are simple SA, threshold analysis, analysis of extremes, and Monte Carlo simulation analysis.[62] SA is of paramount importance because of the very common need for investigators to use assumptions and estimates for unknown variables.[49]

STUDY CONCLUSIONS

Researchers should assist the reader in extrapolating study conclusions to clinical practice. The conclusions drawn from the study results should be justified (internal validity) and able to be generalized (external validity).[54] Also, conclusions drawn from results that were *statistically* significant may or may not be *clinically* relevant, and vice versa.

SPONSORSHIP

Similar to evaluating the quality of a clinical trial, sponsorship of a pharmacoeconomic study should be considered when evaluating the quality and usefulness of that study.[52] The quality of studies conducted or funded by different companies or organizations will vary by sponsor, company, product, or evaluation, and the potential for bias should be neither ignored nor assumed. For example, many of the studies sponsored or conducted by the pharmaceutical industry to date have been academically rigorous as well as informative. A clear understanding of how to evaluate, critique, and use the pharmacoeconomic literature appropriately will minimize any potential effects of this criterion on clinical decision making.

CONTROVERSIES WITH PHARMACOECONOMIC LITERATURE

Over the years, the literature has highlighted the misuse of pharmacoeconomic terms, inconsistent reporting, and disagreement on the methods used for pharmacoeconomic analyses. Since pharmacoeconomics is a fairly new discipline that lacks strong consensus with respect to its methods and technically appropriate applications, the disagreement between leading researchers in this field has been widespread and evident.[60] Unfortunately, this has led to some external skepticism, as well as the inability of clinicians to use the findings of these analyses as extensively as they could to inform their local decision making.[60] Creating and implementing a standardized system for conducting and reporting results of pharmacoeconomic analyses are critical to minimize or eliminate some of these controversies. A review of national guidelines for various countries was published and revealed some areas of emerging standardization.[63] Such a standardized system would enhance clinicians' and decision makers' comprehension of the available data, as well as provide increased assurance that the results reported are methodologically sound.

BUILD AN ECONOMIC MODEL

Studies that *model* the economic impact of a pharmaceutical product or service on a defined population are increasing in popularity. Modeling studies use existing clinical and/or epidemiologic data to project future outcomes.[64] Use of economic models can provide support for various clinical decisions, especially those which are time-contingent.[46] Identifying assumptions regarding the treatment alternatives being compared, the patient outcomes under study, and the probability of those outcomes occurring can provide the basis for an economic simulation to assist in the medication decision-making process.

These studies can use data from various sources available within (internal) and from outside (external) a specific health care organization. Common approaches to modeling are to modify and adapt existing models or to develop a distinct model to answer a specific question.[65] Typically, economic modeling in today's practice settings employs *clinical decision analysis*, which has been defined as an explicit, quantitative, and prescriptive approach to choosing among alternative outcomes.[66,67] The tool used in decision analysis is a decision tree. A decision tree provides a framework to display graphically primary variables, including treatment options, outcomes associated with those treatment options, and probabilities of the outcomes. The researcher can then algebraically reduce all these factors into a single value, allowing for comparison.

Many examples of decision-analytic models are available in the literature, spanning many therapeutic areas, including the treatment of depression,[68] migraine,[69] type 2 diabetes,[70] and community-acquired pneumonia (CAP).[71] In fact, by 1996, more than 80 published articles had been identified that applied decision analysis to questions regarding pharmaceutical products.[72] This simple decision-analysis approach is well suited for comparisons of treatment alternatives with relatively immediate consequences, for example, treating a patient with CAP. However, chronic conditions or diseases such as chronic hepatitis C are difficult to model using simple decision trees for various reasons, including time-dependent clinical outcomes, and thus may require alternate modeling techniques.

Markov models are another method of decision analysis that provides an alternative way to arrange the decision process so that clinical outcomes and time-dependent risk changes are managed efficiently. The Markov model is designed to simulate the most important aspects of a disease and can be used to estimate the long-term clinical, humanistic, and economic dimensions of the disease.[73] There are examples of Markov models available in the literature, including estimates of the cost-effectiveness of interferon-α therapy for the treatment of chronic hepatitis C infection.[74-76] Although Markov models can be stand-alone models, they often are combined with simple decision trees to predict the long-term effects of therapies.[73] These models can be complex; thus clinicians who attempt to use these data or perform their own Markov modeling should become familiar with these techniques.[73,77]

Using an economic model can help the clinician to forecast the impact of medication-use decisions on a patient, institution, or health care system. Also, as new drugs are marketed that can displace older agents, an economic model can expedite the reappraisal process for formulary management and drug-use policy decisions.[78] For building an economic model to assist in clinical decision making, various published studies and a review can be considered.[72,79-83] Further, guidelines for economic modeling are available, and health care practitioners considering using modeling techniques should refer to them.[84-86]

CONDUCT A PHARMACOECONOMIC EVALUATION

Clinicians may need to conduct a pharmacoeconomic evaluation if there is insufficient literature, if published results cannot be extrapolated to clinical practice, or if building a model is not appropriate. Before conducting a pharmacoeconomic evaluation, clinicians should be familiar with the similarities, differences, and appropriate application of pharmacoeconomic methods (discussed earlier in this chapter).

The decision to conduct a local pharmacoeconomic study is not without its own costs. Because both time and monetary resources are consumed by these evaluations, specific pharmacy products and services for pharmacoeconomic evaluation should be targeted. Thus this strategy should be reserved for pharmacy decisions that may have a significant impact on cost or quality of care.

Conducting pharmacoeconomic research in a hospital or managed-care environment can be challenging. Lack of institutional resources, small sample sizes, difficulty randomizing, inability to compare with placebo, and difficulty generalizing results all may be limitations. For example, when asked to determine and recommend the most cost-effective antihypertensive agent for a formulary management decision, clinicians may lack monetary and time resources to conduct a scientifically rigorous study.

Conducting a pharmacoeconomic evaluation should be guided by the criteria for quality economic evaluations.[8,17,32,51-59] A 10-step process identified by Jolicoeur and associates[87] and four additional steps that I have added can provide readers with guidance for conducting a local pharmacoeconomic study.[88] This process contains 14 fundamental steps for conducting a pharmacoeconomic evaluation in a health care system and can be applied to virtually any therapeutic area or health care service. Although some of these steps are similar to the evaluation criteria detailed earlier in this chapter, they will now be discussed briefly in the context of conducting an evaluation.

STEP 1: DEFINE THE PHARMACOECONOMIC PROBLEM

A broad problem might be, "Which antiemetic regimen represents the best value for the prevention of chemotherapy-induced emesis (CIE)?" However, a more succinct and measurable problem would be, "Which regimen is the best value for preventing acute CIE in patients receiving highly emetogenic chemotherapy?"

STEP 2: ASSEMBLE A CROSS-FUNCTIONAL STUDY TEAM

The study team can provide early buy-in and additional resources for a pharmacoeconomic evaluation. Team members vary depending on the analysis but may include representatives from medicine, nursing, pharmacy, hospital administration, and information systems.

STEP 3: DEFINE THE APPROPRIATE STUDY PERSPECTIVE

Choose a study perspective(s) most relevant to the problem. For example, if the problem is as listed in step 1, then the perspective of the institution or health care system may be most appropriate.

STEP 4: IDENTIFY TREATMENT ALTERNATIVES AND OUTCOMES

Treatment alternatives can include pharmacologic and nonpharmacologic options but should include all clinically relevant alternatives. The outcomes identified should include both positive and negative clinical outcomes.

STEP 5: IDENTIFY THE APPROPRIATE PHARMACOECONOMIC METHOD TO EMPLOY

Pharmacoeconomic methods to choose from include CMA, CBA, CEA, and CUA. Employing the incorrect method can adversely affect medication decisions influencing both cost and quality of care.

STEP 6: PLACE A MONETARY VALUE ON TREATMENT ALTERNATIVES AND OUTCOMES

Placing a monetary value on treatment alternatives and outcomes includes not only drug administration and acquisition costs but also the cost of positive and negative clinical outcomes (e.g., determining the cost of ADRs and treatment failures). This can be measured prospectively or retrospectively or estimated using comprehensive databases or expert panels.

STEP 7: IDENTIFY RESOURCES TO CONDUCT STUDY IN AN EFFICIENT MANNER

Resources necessary will vary by study but may include access to medical or computerized records, average medical personnel wages, and specialty medical staff.

STEP 8: IDENTIFY PROBABILITIES THAT OUTCOMES MAY OCCUR IN THE STUDY POPULATION

What are the probabilities of the outcomes identified in step 4 actually occurring in clinical practice? Using primary literature and expert opinion, these probabilities can be obtained and may be manifested as efficacy rates and incidence of ADRs.

STEP 9: EMPLOY DECISION ANALYSIS

The use of decision analysis can assist in conducting various economic evaluations, including CEA. Although not necessary for all pharmacoeconomic evaluations, decision analysis and decision trees may provide a solid backbone or platform for the decision at hand. Using a decision tree, treatment alternatives, outcomes, and probabilities may be presented graphically and may be reduced algebraically to a single value for comparison (i.e., cost-effectiveness ratio).

When comparing antiemetic agents for the development of a policy for CIE prevention, CEA can be employed. Many of these agents differ with respect to effectiveness, safety, and cost. By performing a thorough CEA, these variables can be reduced to a single number (cost-effectiveness ratio), which will allow for a meaningful comparison. The treatment alternative with a better cost-effectiveness ratio than the others (i.e., lower cost per unit of outcome) would be selected and promoted for use.

Figure 1–3 contains an example of a decision tree illustrating how the probabilities of various outcomes can be organized. To calculate the ACER for drug A using "averaging out and folding back," these steps are followed:

1. Multiply the cost of path 1 by the probability of no ADE ($250 × 0.89). Repeat for path 2 ($400 × 0.11).
2. Add these two numbers and multiply by the probability of success ($266.50 × 0.93 = $247.80).
3. Repeat the two preceding steps for paths 3 and 4, and then add the resultant values ($247.80 + $50.50 = $298.30).
4. Add the cost of the drug to this value ($298.30 + $60), and divide by the probability of a success (93%, or 0.93); thus $358.30/0.93 = $385.
5. Repeat this process for drug B using paths 5 through 8.

Using the values in Table 1–5, another way to calculate the ACER for these treatment options is to multiply the cumulative probabilities (P) by the cumulative costs for each path, then sum the costs for each path 1 through 4 (for drug A) and 5 through 8 (for drug B), and then divide by each drug's respective effectiveness for acute CIE. On completion, the ACERs for drugs A and B are $385 and $369, respectively. Therefore, despite the 33% increase in the cost of drug B

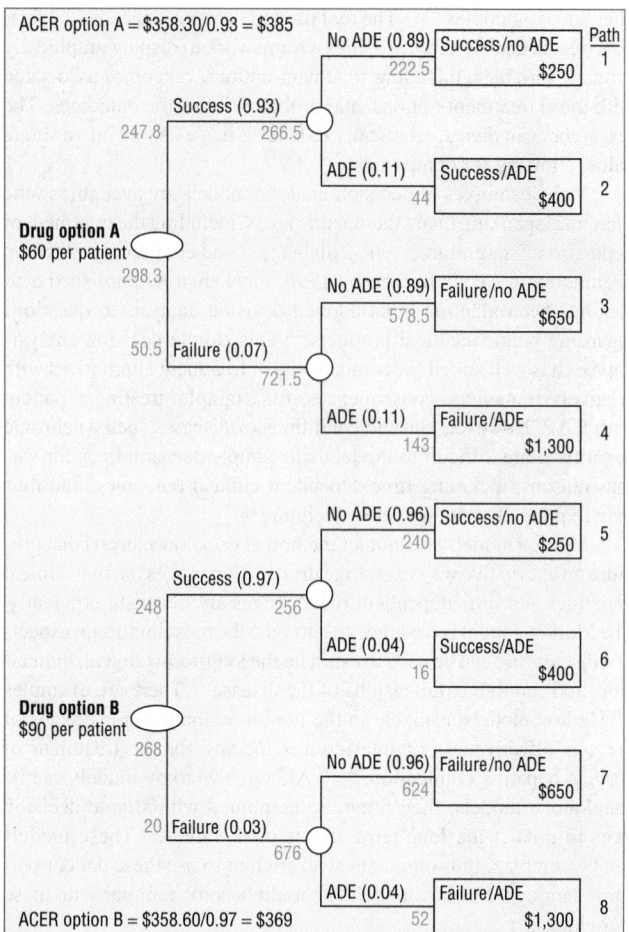

FIGURE 1–3. Example of a pharmacoeconomic decision tree comparing two drugs. *Option B* is a drug that is more specific for the target receptor in the body, is more effective, and produces fewer adverse effects than does *option A*. However, because drug *B* is more expensive than drug *A*, the cost of the added benefits must be analyzed using pharmacoeconomic techniques. This figure was completed using the safety and efficacy values for drugs *A* and *B* from Table 1–5. Values in color are calculated numbers, only included to illustrate the process of "averaging out and folding back." ACER = average cost-effectiveness ratio; ADE = adverse drug event; P = probability (a decimal fraction between 0 and 1 indicating the likelihood of a particular event occurring in a given period). *(Data from Sanchez LA, Lee JT. Applied pharmacoeconomics: Modeling data from internal and external sources. Am J Health Syst Pharm 2000;57:146–158.)*

over drug A, its increased efficacy for acute CIE and its decreased incidence of ADRs actually make it a more cost-effective option.

STEP 10: DISCOUNT COSTS OR PERFORM A SENSITIVITY OR INCREMENTAL COST ANALYSIS

Costs and consequences that occur in the future must be discounted back to their present value. Sensitive variables must be tested over a clinically relevant range and results recalculated. If appropriate, an incremental analysis of the costs and consequences should be performed.

STEP 11: PRESENT STUDY RESULTS

Results should be presented to the cross-functional team and the appropriate committees. Presentation style and content may vary depending on the audience.

TABLE 1–5. Comparison of Costs of Two Drug Options for Preventing Acute Chemotherapy-Induced Emesis

Path	Drug Cost ($)	Chemotherapy Cost ($)	Lab Cost ($)	Extra Therapy Cost ($)	Delay in Clinic Cost ($)	Hospital Cost ($)	Cumulative Cost ($)	Cumulative Probabilities	Cost of path ($)
Drug A									
1	60	200	50				310	0.827	256.37
2	60	200	100	100			460	0.102	46.92
3	60	200	100	200	150		710	0.062	44.02
4	60	200	150	300	150	500	1360	0.007	9.52
Cost of option									$356.83
Drug B									
5	90	200	50				340	0.931	316.54
6	90	200	100	100			490	0.038	18.62
7	90	200	100	200	150		740	0.028	20.72
8	90	200	150	300	150	500	1390	0.001	1.39
Cost of option									$357.27

STEP 12: DEVELOP A POLICY OR AN INTERVENTION

Take the study results and develop a policy or an intervention that can improve or maintain quality of care, possibly at a cost savings.

STEP 13: IMPLEMENT POLICY AND EDUCATE PROFESSIONALS

Spend adequate time and resources strategically implementing the policy or intervention. Educate the health care professionals most likely to be affected by this policy using various strategies, including verbal, written, and online communication.

STEP 14: FOLLOW-UP DOCUMENTATION

Once the intervention or policy has been implemented for a reasonable period of time, collect follow-up data. These data will provide feedback on the success and quality of the policy or intervention.

For additional information and hands-on practice conducting a pharmacoeconomic evaluation in the real world, practitioners should consider a recently published case study. In 2003, Okamoto[89] published a case study on conducting a pharmacoeconomic evaluation using 16 steps that readers also may find useful. In this case, clinicians are challenged to conduct a faux economic analysis from an MCO (provider) perspective to support a review of inhaled corticosteroids for formulary management purposes.

CONCLUSIONS

The principles and methods of pharmacoeconomics provide the means to quantify the value of pharmacotherapy through balancing costs and outcomes. Providing quality care with minimal resources is the future, and the future is here. By understanding the principles, methods, and application of pharmacoeconomics, health care professionals will be prepared to make better, more-informed decisions regarding the use of pharmaceutical products and services, that is, decisions that ultimately represent the best interests of the patient, the health care system, and society.

ABBREVIATIONS

ACER: average cost-effectiveness ratio
ADR: adverse drug reaction
AWP: average wholesale price
B/C ratio: benefit-to-cost ratio
CAP: community-acquired pneumonia
CBA: cost-benefit analysis
CCA: cost-consequence analysis
CEA: cost-effectiveness analysis
COI: cost of illness
CMA: cost-minimization analysis
CUA: cost-utility analysis
ECHO: economic, clinical, and humanistic outcomes
HRQOL: health-related quality of life
ICER: incremental cost-effectiveness ratio
MCO: managed-care organization
QALY: quality-adjusted life year
SA: sensitivity analysis
WTP: willingness-to-pay

Review Questions and other resources can be found at *www.pharmacotherapyonline.com.*

REFERENCES

1. Sanchez LA. Expanding the pharmacist's role in pharmacoeconomics: How and why? Pharmacoeconomics 1994;5:367–375.
2. Townsend RJ. Post-marketing drug research and development. Ann Pharmacother 1987;21:134–136.
3. Drummond M, Smith GT, Wells N. Economic Evaluation in the Development of Medicines. London, Office of Health Economics, 1988:33.
4. Lee JT, Sanchez LA. Interpretation of "cost-effective" and soundness of economic evaluations in the pharmacy literature. Am J Hosp Pharm 1991;48:2622–2627.
5. Bootman JL. Pharmacoeconomics and outcomes research. Am J Health System Pharm 1995;52(suppl 3):S16–S19.
6. Hepler CD, Strand LM. Opportunities and responsibilities in pharmaceutical care. Am J Hosp Pharm 1990;47:533–543.
7. Eisenberg JM. Clinical economics: A guide to economic analysis of clinical practices. JAMA 1989;262:2879–2886.
8. Bootman JL, Townsend RJ, McGhan WF. Principles of Pharmacoeconomics. 3rd ed. Cincinnati, Harvey Whitney Books, 2005.
9. Freund DA, Dittus RS. Principles of pharmacoeconomic analysis of drug therapy. Pharmacoeconomics 1992;1:20–32.
10. Barner J, Rascati K. Cost-benefit analysis. In Grauer D, Lee J, Odom T, et al., eds. Pharmacoeconomics and Outcomes, 2d ed. Kansas City, MO, American College of Clinical Pharmacy, 2003:115–132.

11. Blumenschein K, Johannesson M. Use of contingent valuation to place a monetary value on pharmacy services: An overview and review of the literature. Clin Ther 1999;21:1402–1417.

12. Glossary of terms used in pharmacoeconomic and quality of life analysis. Pharmacoeconomics 1992;1:151.

13. Detsky AS, Nagiie IG. A clinician's guide to cost-effectiveness analysis. Ann Intern Med 1990;113:147–154.

14. Kozma CM, Reeder CE, Schulz RM. Economic, clinical, and humanistic outcomes: A planning model for pharmacoeconomic research. Clin Ther 1993;15:1121–1132.

15. Bungay KM, Sanchez LA. Types of economic and humanistic outcomes assessments. In Grauer D, Lee J, Odom T, et al., eds. Pharmacoeconomics and Outcomes, 2d ed. Kansas City, MO, American College of Clinical Pharmacy, 2003:18–60.

16. Draugalis JR, Bootman LJ, Larson LN, McGhan WF. Current Concepts: Pharmacoeconomics. Kalamazoo, MI, Upjohn, 1989.

17. Drummond MF, Stoddart GL, Torrance GW. Methods for the Economic Evaluation of Health Care Programmes, 2d ed. Oxford, England, Oxford University Press, 1997.

18. McGhan WF. Pharmacoeconomics and the evaluation of drugs and services. Hosp Formul 1993;28:365–378.

19. Rice DP, Fox PJ, Max W, et al. The economic burden of Alzheimer's disease care. Health Affairs 1993;12(2):164–176.

20. Ernst RL, Hay JW. The U.S. economic and social costs of Alzheimer's disease revisited. Am J Public Health 1994;84:1261–1264.

21. Sanchez LA, Lee JT. Use and misuse of pharmacoeconomic terms. Top Hosp Pharm Manage 1994;13:11–22.

22. Cox E. Cost-minimization analysis. In Grauer D, Lee J, Odom T, et al. (eds.): Pharmacoeconomics and Outcomes, 2d ed. Kansas City, MO, American College of Clinical Pharmacy, 2003:103–114.

23. Sanchez LA. Pharmacoeconomic principles and methods: An introduction for hospital pharmacists. Hosp Pharm 1994;29:1035–1040.

24. Lai LL, Sorkin AL. Cost-benefit analysis of pharmaceutical care in a Medicaid population: From a budgetary perspective. J Manage Care Pharm 1998;4:303–308.

25. Schrand LM, Elliott JM, Ross MB, et al. Cost benefit analysis of RSV prophylaxis in high-risk infants. Ann Pharmacother 2001;35:1186–1193.

26. Nesbit TW, Shermock KM, Bobek MB, et al. Implementation and pharmacoeconomic analysis of a clinical staff pharmacist practice model. Am J Health Syst Pharm 2001;58:784–790.

27. Sias JJ, Cook S, Wolfe T, et al. An employee influenza immunization initiative in a large university managed care setting. J Manage Care Pharm 2001;7:219–223.

28. Zarnke KB, Levine MAH, O'Brien BJ. Cost-benefit analyses in the health-care literature: Don't judge a study by its label. Clin Epidemiol 1997;50:813–822.

29. Bootman JL, Larson LN, McGhan WF, Townsend RJ. Pharmacoeconomic research and clinical trials: Concepts and issues. Ann Pharmacother 1989;23:693–697.

30. Bootman JL. The basics of pharmacoeconomic analysis. Pharm Rep 1993;23:14–15.

31. Langley PC. The role of pharmacoeconomic guidelines for formulary approval: The Australian experience. Clin Ther 1993;15:1154–1176.

32. Detsky AS. Guidelines for economic analysis of pharmaceutical products: A draft document for Ontario and Canada. Pharmacoeconomics 1993;3:354–361.

33. Pathak DS. QALYs in health outcomes research: Representation of real preferences or another numerical abstraction? J Res Pharm Econ 1995;6:3–27.

34. Kaplan RM. Quality-of-life assessment for cost/utility studies in cancer. Cancer Treat Rep 1993;19(suppl A):85–96.

35. Gabriel SE, Campion ME, O'Fallon WM. A cost-utility analysis of misoprostol prophylaxis for rheumatoid arthritis patients receiving nonsteroidal anti-inflammatory drugs. Arthritis Rheum 1994;37:333–341.

36. Schipper H, Clinch J, Powell V. Definitions and conceptual issues. In Spilker B (ed.): Quality of Life Assessments in Clinical Trials. New York, Raven Press, 1990.

37. Spilker B. Quality of Life Assessments in Clinical Trials. New York, Raven Press, 1990.

38. Spilker B, White WSA, Simpson RJ, Tilson HN. Quality of life bibliography and indexes—1990 update. Clin Pharmacoepidemiol 1992;6:157–158.

39. Coons SJ. Quality of life assessment: Understanding its use as an outcome measure. Hosp Formul 1993;28:486–498.

40. Jaeschke R, Guyatt GH, Cook D. Quality of life instruments in the evaluation of new drugs. Pharmacoeconomics 1992;1:84–94.

41. Mackeigan LD, Pathak DS. Overview of health-related quality-of-life measures. Am J Hosp Pharm 1992;49:2236–2245.

42. McGhan WF, Rowland CR, Bootman JL. Cost-benefit and cost-effectiveness: Methodologies for evaluating innovative pharmaceutical services. Am J Hosp Pharm 1978;35:133–140.

43. MacKeigan LD, Bootman JL. A review of cost-benefit and cost-effectiveness analyses of clinical pharmacy services. J Pharm Market Manage 1988;2:63–84.

44. Schumock GT, Meek PD, Ploetz PA, Vermeulen LC. Economic evaluations of clinical pharmacy services—1988–1995. Pharmacotherapy 1996;16:1188–1208.

45. Schumock GT, Butler MG, Meek PD, et al. Evidence of economic benefit of clinical pharmacy services: 1996–2000. Pharmacotherapy 2003;23:113–132.

46. Sanchez LA. Pharmacoeconomic principles and methods: Including pharmacoeconomics into hospital pharmacy practice. Hosp Pharm 1994;29:1035–1040.

47. Doubilet P, Weinstein MC, McNeil BJ. The use and misuse of the term "cost-effective" in medicine. N Engl J Med 1986;314:253–256.

48. Bradley CA, Iskedjian M, Lanctot KL, et al. Quality assessment of economic evaluation in selected pharmacy, medical, and health economic journals. Ann Pharmacother 1995;29:681–689.

49. Udvarhelyi S, Colditz GA, Rai A, et al. Cost-effectiveness and cost-benefit analyses in the medical literature. Ann Intern Med 1992;116:238–244.

50. Mason J. The generalizability of pharmacoeconomic studies. Pharmacoeconomics 1997;11:503–514.

51. Sacristan JA, Soto J, Galende I. Evaluation of pharmacoeconomic studies: Utilization of a checklist. Ann Pharmacother 1993;27:1126–1133.

52. Hillman AL, Eisenberg JM, Pauly MV, et al. Avoiding bias in the conduct and reporting of cost-effectiveness research sponsored by pharmaceutical companies. N Engl J Med 1991;324:1362–1365.

53. McGhan WF, Lewis JV. Guidelines for pharmacoeconomic studies. Clin Ther 1992;14:486–494.

54. Sanchez LA. Pharmacoeconomic principles and methods: Evaluating the quality of published pharmacoeconomic evaluations. Hosp Pharm 1995;30:146–152.

55. Clemans K, Townsend R, Luscombe F, et al. Methodological and conduct principles for pharmacoeconomic research. Pharmacoeconomics 1995;8:169–174.

56. Task Force on Principles for Economic Analysis of Health Care Technology. Economic analysis of healthcare technology: A report on principles. Ann Intern Med 1995;122:61–70.

57. Russell LB, Gold MR, Siegel JE, et al. The role of cost-effectiveness analysis in health and medicine. JAMA 1996;276:1172–1177.

58. Weinstein MC, Siegel JE, Gold MR, et al. Recommendations of the Panel on Cost-effectiveness in Health and Medicine. JAMA 1996;276:1253–1258.

59. Siegel JE, Weinstein MC, Russell LB, et al. Recommendations for repeating cost-effectiveness analyses. JAMA 1996; 276:1339–1341.

60. Mullins CD, Flowers LR. Evaluating economic outcomes literature. In Grauer D, Lee J, Odom T, et al. (eds.): Pharmacoeconomics and Outcomes, 2d ed. Kansas City, MO, American College of Clinical Pharmacy, 2003:246–273.

61. Eisenberg JM, Glick H, Koffer H. Pharmacoeconomics: Economic evaluation of pharmaceuticals. In Strom BL (ed.): Pharmacoepidemiology. New York, Churchill-Livingstone, 1989:325–350.

62. Armstrong EP. Sensitivity analysis. In Grauer D, Lee J, Odom T, et al. (eds.): Pharmacoeconomics and Outcomes, 2d ed. Kansas City, MO, American College of Clinical Pharmacy, 2003:231–245.

63. Mullins CD, Ogilvie S. Emerging standardization in pharmacoeconomics. Clin Ther 1998;20(60):1194–1202.

64. Milne RJ. Evaluation of the pharmacoeconomic literature. Pharmacoeconomics 1994;6:337–345.

65. Sanchez LA, Lee JT. Applied pharmacoeconomics: Modeling data from internal and external sources. Am J Health Syst Pharm 2000;57:146–158.

66. Sackett DL, Haynes RB, Tugwell P. Clinical Epidemiology: A Basic Science for Clinical Medicine. Boston, Little Brown, 1985:126.

67. Barr JT, Schumacher GE. Decision analysis and pharmacoeconomic evaluations. In Bootman JL, Townsend RJ, McGhan WF (eds.): Principles of Pharmacoeconomics, 2d ed. Cincinnati, Harvey Whitney Books, 1996.

68. Jones MT, Cockrum PC. A critical review of published economic modeling studies in depression. Pharmacoeconomics 2000;17:555–583.

69. Biddle AK, Shih YC, Kwong WJ. Cost-benefit analysis of sumatriptan tablets versus usual therapy for treatment of migraine. Pharmacotherapy 2000;20:1356–1364.

70. Coyle D, Lee KM, O'Brian BJ. The role of models with economic analysis: Focus on type 2 diabetes mellitus. Pharmacoeconomics 2002;20(suppl 1):11–19.

71. Najib MM, Stein GE, Goss TF. Cost-effectiveness of sparfloxacin compared with other oral antimicrobials in outpatient treatment of community-acquired pneumonia. Pharmacotherapy 2000;20:461–469.

72. Barr JT, Schumacher GE. Using decision analysis to conduct pharmacoeconomic studies. In Spilker B, ed. Quality of Life and Pharmacoeconomics in Clinical Trials, 2d ed. Philadelphia, Lippincott-Raven, 1996.

73. Touchette D, Hartung D. Markov modeling. In Grauer D, Lee J, Odom T, et al. (eds.): Pharmacoeconomics and Outcomes, 2d ed. Kansas City, MO, American College of Clinical Pharmacy, 2003:206–230.

74. Bennett WG, Inoue Y, Beck JR, et al. Estimates of the cost-effectiveness of a single course of interferon-α2b in patients with histologically mild chronic hepatitis C. Ann Intern Med 1997;127:855–865.

75. Kim WR, Poterucha JJ, Hermans JE, et al. Cost-effectiveness of 6 and 12 months of interferon-α therapy for chronic hepatitis C. Ann Intern Med 1997;127:866–874.

76. Younossi ZM, Singer ME, McHutchison JG, Shermock KM. Cost effectiveness of interferon-α2b combined with ribavirin for the treatment of chronic hepatitis C. Hepatology 1999;30:1318–1324.

77. Briggs A, Sculpher M. An introduction to Markov modeling for economic evaluation. Pharmacoeconomics 1998;13:397–409.

78. Schecter CB. Decision analysis in formulary decision making. Pharmacoeconomics 1993;3:454–461.

79. Bjornson DC, Hiner WO, Potyk RP, et al. Effect of pharmacists on health care outcomes in hospitalized patients. Am J Hosp Pharm 1993;50:1875–1884.

80. Zabinski RA, Burke TA, Johnson J, et al. An economic model for determining the costs and consequences of using various treatment alternatives for the management of arthritis in Canada. Pharmacoeconomics 2001;19(suppl 1):49–58.

81. Harrison DL, Bootman JL, Cox ER. Cost-effectiveness of consultant pharmacists in managing drug-related morbidity and mortality at nursing facilities. Am J Health Syst Pharm 1998;55:1588–1594.

82. Kessler JM. Decision analysis in the formulary process. Am J Health Syst Pharm 1997;54(suppl 1):S5–S8.

83. Paladino JA. Cost-effectiveness comparison of cefepime and ceftazidime using decision analysis. Pharmacoeconomics 1994;5:505–512.

84. Akehurst R, Anderson P, Brazier J, et al. Consensus Conference on Guidelines on Economic Modeling in Health Technology Assessment. Decision analytic modeling in economic evaluation of health technologies: A consensus statement. Pharmacoeconomics 2000;17:443–444.

85. Brennan A, Akehurst R. Modeling in health economic evaluation. What is its place? What is its value? Pharmacoeconomics 2000;17:445–459.

86. Schulpher M, Fenwick E, Claxton K. Assessing quality in decision analytic cost-effectiveness models: A suggested framework and example of application. Pharmacoeconomics 2000;17:461–477.

87. Jolicoeur LM, Jones-Grizzle AJ, Boyer JG. Guidelines for performing a pharmacoeconomic analysis. Am J Hosp Pharm 1992;49:1741–1747.

88. Sanchez LA. Pharmacoeconomic principles and methods: Conducting pharmacoeconomic evaluations in a hospital setting. Hosp Pharm 1995;30:412–428.

89. Okamoto JL. Case study: Conducting a pharmacoeconomic evaluation. In Grauer D, Lee J, Odom T, et al. (eds.): Pharmacoeconomics and Outcomes, 2d ed. Kansas City, MO, American College of Clinical Pharmacy, 2003:394–403.

2

HEALTH OUTCOMES AND QUALITY OF LIFE

Stephen Joel Coons

Learning Objectives and other resources can be found at *www.pharmacotherapyonline.com.*

KEY CONCEPTS

◀1 The evaluation of health care is focused increasingly on assessment of the *outcomes* of medical interventions.

◀2 An essential patient-reported outcome is self-assessed function and well-being or health-related quality of life (HRQOL).

◀3 In certain chronic conditions, HRQOL may be the most important health outcome to consider in assessing treatment.

◀4 Information about the impact of pharmacotherapy on HRQOL can provide additional data for making medication-use decisions.

◀5 HRQOL instruments can be categorized as generic/general or targeted/specific.

◀6 In HRQOL research, the quality of the data-collection tool is the major determinant of the overall quality of the results.

Over the past two decades, the medical care marketplace in the United States has undergone unprecedented change.[1] This change is evidenced by a variety of developments, including an increase in investor-owned organizations, heightened competition, numerous mergers and acquisitions, increasingly sophisticated clinical and administrative information systems, and new financing and organizational structures. In this dynamic and increasingly competitive environment, there is a concern that health care quality is being compromised in the push to ◀1 contain costs. As a consequence, there has been a growing movement to focus the evaluation of health care on the assessment of the end results, or *outcomes,* associated with medical care delivery systems, as well as specific medical interventions. The primary objective of this effort is to maximize the net health benefit derived from the use of finite health care resources.[2] However, there is a serious lack of critical information as to what value is received for the tremendous amount of resources expended on medical care.[3] This lack of critical information as to the outcomes produced is an obstacle to optimal health care decision making at all levels.

HEALTH OUTCOMES

Although the implicit objective of medical care is to improve health outcomes, until relatively recently, little attention was paid to the explicit measurement of outcomes. An outcome is one of the three components of the conceptual framework articulated by Donabedian[4] for assessing and ensuring the quality of health care: *structure, process,* and *outcome.* Traditionally, the approach to evaluating health care has emphasized the structure and processes involved in medical care delivery rather than the outcomes. However, health care regulators, payers, providers, manufacturers, and patients are placing increasing emphasis on the outcomes that medical care products and services produce.[5] As stated by Ellwood,[6] outcomes research is "designed to help patients, payers, and providers make rational medical care choices based on better insight into the effect of these choices on the patient's life."

TYPES OF OUTCOMES

The types of outcomes that result from medical care interventions can be described in a number of ways. One classic list, called the *five D's,* although quite negatively worded, captures a wide range of outcomes used in assessing the quality of medical care.[7] The five D's are death, disease, disability, discomfort, and dissatisfaction.

A more comprehensive conceptual framework, the ECHO model, places outcomes into three categories: *e*conomic, *c*linical, and *h*umanistic *o*utcomes.[8] The model covers the five D's within the clinical and humanistic outcomes and provides an added economic outcomes dimension. As described by Kozma and associates,[8] *clinical outcomes* are the medical events that occur as a result of the condition or its treatment. *Economic outcomes* are the direct, indirect, and intangible costs compared with the consequences of a medical ◀2 intervention. Along with patient satisfaction, an essential humanistic or patient-reported outcome is self-assessed function and well-being, or *health-related quality of life* (HRQOL). This chapter focuses on HRQOL as an outcome of pharmacotherapeutic interventions.

QUALITY OF LIFE

DEFINITION

As mentioned earlier, one of the essential elements of outcomes research is the assessment of patient *health-related quality of life.* However, there is no consensus on the definition of quality of life (QOL) or its overall conceptual framework.[9] In the literature, the term *quality of life* has been used in a variety of ways. It has been proposed that studies of health outcomes use the term *health-related quality of life* (HRQOL) to distinguish health effects from the effects of standard of living, family life, friendships, job satisfaction, and other factors on overall quality of life.[10] Only health outcomes are discussed in this chapter, so *quality of life* and *health-related quality of life* are used interchangeably, along with *health status.*

HRQOL CONTROVERSY

Some observers question whether, when completing HRQOL instruments, respondents are able to distinguish between the impact of health versus the impact of other important life domains on their functioning and well-being.

QOL, like other aspects of the human experience, is hard to define. In much of the empirical literature, explicit definitions of QOL are rare; readers must deduce the implicit definition of QOL from the manner in which it is measured. However, some authors have provided definitions. For example, Schron and Shumaker[11] define HRQOL as "a multidimensional concept referring to a person's total well-being, including his or her psychological, social, and physical health status." Patrick and Erickson[12] propose that HRQOL is "the value assigned to duration of life as modified by the impairments, functional states, perceptions, and social opportunities that are influenced by disease, injury, treatment, or policy." Although the two definitions differ in certain respects, a conceptual characteristic they share is the multidimensionality of QOL. Although the terminology may vary with the author, commonly measured domains of HRQOL include

- Physical health and functioning
- Mental health and functioning
- Social and role functioning
- Perceptions of general well-being

HRQOL CONTROVERSY

Should symptoms of a disease or the adverse effects of treatment interventions be assessed explicitly by HRQOL instruments? Although some instruments include items addressing specific symptoms or side effects (particularly in the mental health domain), most HRQOL instruments are developed based on the premise that if a symptom or adverse effect is sufficiently problematic, it will be manifested in one or more of the measured HRQOL domains.

RELEVANCE OF QOL AS AN OUTCOME

For medical care providers, HRQOL increasingly is viewed as a therapeutic end point. An overriding factor leading to this has been the gradual shift in the focus of primary medical care from limiting mortality to limiting morbidity and the patient-reported impact of that morbidity. The pattern of illness in the United States has shifted from mostly acute disease to one in which chronic conditions predominate. In the early part of the twentieth century, many individuals died from infectious diseases for which cures (e.g., antibiotics) or effective preventive measures (e.g., vaccines, increased sanitation) were unavailable or underused. Today, although there are many diseases that may shorten life expectancy, it is more likely that a disease will have adverse health consequences leading to dysfunction and decreased well-being. For conditions that shorten life expectancy and for which there are no cures, managing symptoms and maintaining function and well-being should be the primary objectives of medical care.

Because therapeutic interventions such as medications have the potential to increase or decrease HRQOL, medical care providers must strive to achieve enhanced HRQOL as an outcome of therapy. Although it must be assumed that HRQOL always has played an implicit role in the provision of health care, it has not always been viewed as equal in importance to the more clinical or physiologic outcome parameters (e.g., blood pressure). The subjective nature of HRQOL assessment has made many people uneasy with it as a measure of the patient outcomes produced by medical treatment.[13]

However, there is growing awareness that in certain diseases, HRQOL may be the most important health outcome to consider in assessing treatment.[14] Physiologic measures may change without improving functioning and well-being. Likewise, patients may feel and function better without measurable change in physiologic values.

QOL AND PHARMACOTHERAPY

As described by Smith,[15] there are four possible QOL outcomes associated with pharmacotherapy: (1) QOL is improved, (2) QOL is actively maintained, (3) QOL is decreased, or (4) QOL remains unaffected. To assess these possible outcomes effectively, moving beyond consideration of only the biologic or physical manifestations of a disease or its treatment is essential. The use of standardized measurement tools (e.g., self-reported HRQOL instruments) to collect information regarding the impact of pharmacotherapy on the quality of patients' lives is increasing.[16,17] However, the vast majority of HRQOL claims in prescription drug advertisements continue to be based on physiologic parameters and/or clinician-assessed physical function rather than patient-reported functioning and well-being.[18]

A study by Croog and colleagues[19] was one of the first in a growing body of literature reporting the QOL impact of pharmacotherapy, specifically the use of antihypertensive agents. Along with hypertension, examples of other therapeutic areas that are receiving increasing attention are arthritis, asthma, cancer, diabetes, and HIV/AIDS.[20–25] The type of condition and type of treatment dictate the importance of HRQOL data in determining the value of pharmacotherapy. As discussed by Badia and Herdman,[26] in chronic conditions and palliative treatments (i.e., ameliorating symptoms but not curing the underlying disease), HRQOL may be the primary measure of efficacy. However, with acute conditions and curative treatments, HRQOL is likely to be secondary (although excluding it may underestimate the positive and negative impacts of the treatment).

Information about the impact of pharmacotherapy on QOL can provide additional data for making medication-use policy decisions. In fact, the Academy of Managed Care Pharmacy, in its *Format for Formulary Submissions*, states that manufacturers of pharmaceutical, biologic, and vaccine products should include outcomes data (e.g., QOL data) in their formulary submission dossiers.[27] When available, pharmacy and therapeutics committees should incorporate QOL data into the formulary and practice guideline decision-making process. HRQOL as an input to clinical decision making at the patient level is also very important. For example, alternative treatments may have equal efficacy based on traditional clinical parameters (e.g., blood pressure reduction) but produce very different effects on the patient's HRQOL. Thus a provider's selection among competing alternatives may hinge on documented differential impact on HRQOL. A perceived decrease in QOL attributed by the patient to an adverse effect of a drug may lead to a decrease in adherence to the medication regimen.[15]

MEASURING QOL

TYPES OF INSTRUMENTS

Hundreds of HRQOL instruments are available.[28–30] Table 2–1 gives a taxonomy of the different types of instruments.[31] A primary distinction among HRQOL instruments is whether they are generic or specific.

TABLE 2–1. Taxonomy of Quality-of-Life Instruments

Generic Instruments
    Health profiles
    Preference-based measures
Specific Instruments
    Disease specific (e.g., diabetes)
    Population specific (e.g., frail older adults)
    Function specific (e.g., sexual functioning)
    Condition or problem specific (e.g., pain)

Adapted from Ref. 32.

GENERIC INSTRUMENTS

Generic, or general, HRQOL instruments are designed to be applicable across all diseases or conditions, across different medical interventions, and across a wide variety of populations.[32] Table 2–2 lists the dimensions or domains of five generic instruments. In choosing or evaluating the use of an instrument, the specific dimensions of functioning and well-being covered must be considered. The instruments in Table 2–2 share common dimensions, but they also reflect the diversity and range of dimensions covered. The two main types of generic instruments are health profiles and preference-based measures.

HEALTH PROFILES

Health profiles provide an array of scores representing individual dimensions or domains of HRQOL or health status. An advantage of a health profile is that it provides multiple outcome scores that may be useful to clinicians and/or researchers attempting to measure differential effects of a condition or its treatment on various QOL domains.

TABLE 2–2. Domains Included in Selected Generic Instruments

EuroQol Group's EQ-SD[33]

Mobility	Self-care
Usual activity	Pain/discomfort
Anxiety/depression	

Nottingham Health Profile (NHP)[34]
Part I: Distress within the following domains

Emotions	Energy
Sleep	Pain
Social isolation	Mobility

Part II: Health-related problems within the following domains

Occupation	Sex life
Housework	Hobbies
Social life	Holidays
Home life	

Quality of Well-Being Scale (QWB)[35]

Symptoms/problems	Physical activity
Mobility	Social activity

Sickness Impact Profile (SIP)[36]

Sleep and rest	Home management
Eating	Recreation and pastimes
Work	Body care and movement
Ambulation	Alertness behavior
Mobility	Emotional behavior
Communication	Social interaction

Health Utilities Index (HUI)—Mark III[37]

Vision	Dexterity
Hearing	Cognition
Speech	Pain and discomfort
Ambulation	Emotion

TABLE 2–3. SF-36 Scales and Number of Items per Scale (SF-36/SF-12)

Physical functioning (10/2)
Role limitations attributed to physical problems (4/2)
Bodily pain (2/1)
General health (5/1)
Vitality (4/1)
Social functioning (2/1)
Role limitations attributed to emotional problems (3/2)
Mental health (5/2)
Health transition (1/0)

Compiled from Refs. 38 and 42.

A commonly used profile instrument is the Medical Outcomes Study 36-Item Short-Form Health Survey (SF-36).[38] This instrument includes nine health concepts or scales (Table 2–3). The SF-36 can be self-administered or administered by a trained interviewer (face to face or via telephone). This instrument has several advantages. For example, it is brief (it takes about 5–10 minutes to complete), and its reliability and validity have been documented in many clinical situations and disease states.[39,40] A means of aggregating the items into physical (PCS) and mental (MCS) component summary scores is available.[41] In addition, an abbreviated version of the SF-36 containing only 12 items (SF-12) has been introduced.[42] However, the scale scores and mental and physical component summary scores derived from the SF-12 are based on fewer items and fewer defined levels of health and, as a result, are estimated with less precision and less reliability. The loss of precision and reliability in measurement can be a problem in small samples and/or with small expected effect sizes for an intervention.

PREFERENCE-BASED MEASURES

HRQOL as assessed by preference-based measures is a single overall index score on a scale anchored by 1.0 (full health) and 0.0 (dead). Health states considered worse than dead can be reflected by negative numbers on the scale. This approach combines the measurement of an individual's health status with an adjustment for the relative desirability of or preference for that health state. The preferences are measured or assigned empirically through a variety of procedures. Although often called health state *utilities,* the term *preferences* will be used in this chapter as the broader term because it subsumes both *utilities* and *values.*[43]

Preference-based measures are useful in pharmacoeconomic research, specifically cost-utility analysis (CUA).[44] CUA, an economic technique discussed in Chapter 1, involves comparing the costs of an intervention (e.g., a medication) with its outcomes expressed in units such as quality-adjusted life years (QALYs) gained. QALYs gained is an outcome measure that incorporates both quantity and quality of life. This can be a key outcome measure, especially in diseases such as cancer, where the treatment itself can have a major impact on patient functioning and well-being. Numerous published studies have used CUA to evaluate the economic efficiency of health care interventions. A review of CUAs published from 1976 to 1997 by Neumann and colleagues[45] found that the number increased markedly during that time. Of the 228 articles reviewed, about one-third focused on pharmaceutical interventions. CUA data compiled during this extensive review can be accessed on the Web (*http://www.hsph.harvard.edu/cearegistry*).

QALYs can be produced by increases in QOL and/or length of life. Figure 2–1 represents a case in which QALYs were gained

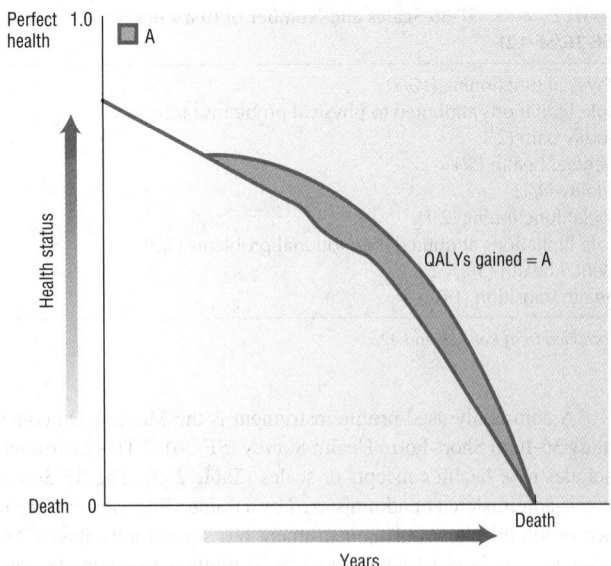

FIGURE 2–1. QALYs gained (i.e., area between the curves) as the outcome of a hypothetical health care intervention, such as a drug.

through an increase in QOL alone. The top curve represents the hypothetical life course of a cohort of individuals receiving a specific health care intervention compared with the life course of a cohort (i.e., lower curve) that did not receive the intervention. Average age at death did not differ between the two cohorts, but the intervention led to improvements in QOL in the treatment cohort. The area between the curves represents the QALYs gained through the intervention. This hypothetical case reflects a chronic disease, such as osteoarthritis, in which functioning and well-being are increased, but survival remains unchanged. Other hypothetical combinations of quality and quantity of life can be graphed in this manner. For example, an alternative scenario could reflect a temporary decrease in QOL but an increase in survival that may result from a chemotherapeutic regimen for cancer.

HRQOL CONTROVERSY

Although the QALY is the most commonly used health outcome summary measure, it is not the only one. Other conceptually equivalent outcomes include *years of healthy life* (YHL), *well years* (WYs), *health-adjusted person-years* (HAPYs), and *health-adjusted life expectancy* (HALE). An alternative concept called *healthy year equivalents* (HYEs) has been proposed as theoretically superior to QALYs, but its practical significance has been limited.

Direct Measures of Health-State Preferences
The most commonly used direct measurement techniques include visual analog scales, standard gamble, and time tradeoff.[46]

Visual Analog Scales. The *visual analog scale* is a line, typically 10 to 20 cm in length, with the end points well defined (e.g., 0 = worst imaginable health state and 100 = best imaginable health state). The respondent is asked to mark the line where he or she would place a real or hypothetical health state in relation to the two end points. In addition, since death may not always be considered the worst possible health state, the subject's placement of death on the scale in relation to the other health states must be explicitly elicited. If a subject has placed death at 0 and rates a health state at the midpoint between

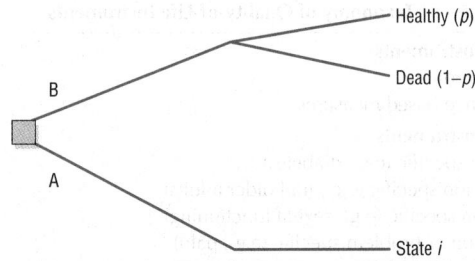

FIGURE 2–2. Standard gamble for a chronic health status. The subject is offered the choice between *A* and *B*. *A* involves the certainty of living in health state *i* (a suboptimal health state) for a specified period of time. *B* involves an intervention that could lead to full health for the same period of time or immediate death. The probabilities associated with the outcomes of healthy and dead are *p* and $1 - p$, respectively. As *p* is varied, the indifference point between choices *A* and *B* represents the utility of state *i*.

0 and 100 on the scale, that subject's preference for that health state is 0.5.

Standard Gamble. The *standard gamble* offers a choice between two alternatives: choice *A*, living in health state *i* with certainty, or choice *B*, taking a gamble on a new treatment for which the outcome is uncertain. Figure 2–2 shows this gamble.[43] The subject is told that a hypothetical treatment will lead to perfect health, for a defined remaining lifetime, with a probability of *p* or immediate death with a probability of $1 - p$. The subject can choose between remaining, for the same defined lifetime, in state *i*, which is intermediate between healthy and dead, or taking the gamble and trying the new treatment. The probability *p* is varied until the subject is indifferent between choices *A* and *B*. For example, if a subject is indifferent between the choices *A* and *B* when $p = 0.75$, the preference (i.e., utility) of state *i* is 0.75.

Time Tradeoff. Figure 2–3 represents the time-tradeoff technique for a chronic disease state.[47] Here, the subject is offered a choice of living for a variable amount of time *x* in perfect health or a defined amount of time *t* in a health state *i* that is less desirable. By reducing the time *x* of being healthy (at 1.0) and leaving the time *t* in the suboptimal health state fixed, an indifference point can be determined $(h_i = x/t)$. For example, a subject may indicate that undergoing chronic

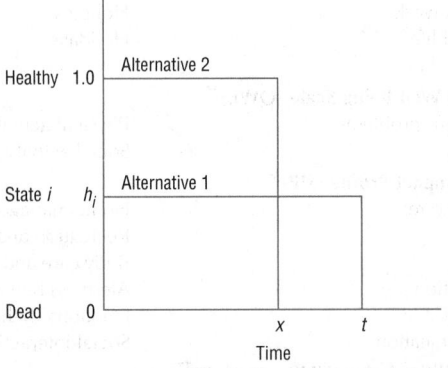

FIGURE 2–3. Time tradeoff for a chronic health state. The subject chooses between living a varying amount of time in full health (*x*) and living a specified amount of time (*t*) in state *i*. The length of time in full health is shortened until the subject is indifferent between the two choices. The value of health state *i*(*h_i*) is then calculated by dividing *x*/*t*.

hemodialysis for 2 years is equivalent to perfect health for 1 year. Therefore, the value of that health state would be 0.5 ($h_i = {}^1/_2$).

HRQOL CONTROVERSY

There is considerable debate regarding the best approach to the direct measurement, or elicitation, of health-state preferences. The empirical literature consistently shows that there are differences in the preferences derived through the different elicitation methods. Although there have been calls for the development of standardized preference-elicitation protocols, it is likely that the lack of consensus will continue into the foreseeable future.

Multiattribute Health-Status Classification Systems

In addition to direct measures, instruments are available for which the health-state preferences have been derived empirically through population studies. The instruments are administered to measure respondents' health status, which is then mapped onto a multiattribute health status classification system. Examples of such instruments include the Quality of Well-Being Scale (QWB),[35] the Health Utilities Index (HUI),[37] and the EuroQOL Group's EQ-5D.[33] Although each will be described briefly below, more thorough descriptions of these three instruments are provided elsewhere.[43,48]

The QWB is a generic HRQOL instrument that includes symptoms or problems plus three dimensions of functional health status (see Table 2–2). Standardized preference values for the health states represented by the QWB have been measured (via the category rating scale method, a technique related to visual analog scales) and validated on a general population sample.[35] The QWB was available originally only as an interviewer-administered version, but a self-administered version is now available.[49]

The HUI is another generic instrument that describes the health status of a person at a point in time in terms of his or her ability to function on a set of attributes or dimensions of health status. The HUI Mark II/III is available as a 15-item self-administered form. The measurements for the development of the health-state preference system were made with visual analog scales (VASs) and the standard gamble technique. The dimensions covered in the most recent version of the HUI (Mark III) are listed in Table 2–2.[37]

The EQ-5D was developed concurrently in five languages (Dutch, English, Finnish, Norwegian, and Swedish) by a multidisciplinary team of European researchers.[33] It was designed to be self-administered and short enough to be used in conjunction with other measures. The first of two parts classifies subjects into one of 243 health states within five dimensions. The most commonly used set of health-state preferences was estimated using the time-tradeoff technique in a random sample of adults in the United Kingdom. A set of preference weights derived from the general U.S. adult population is forthcoming. The second part of the EQ-5D is a 20-cm VAS that has end points labeled "best imaginable health state" and "worst imaginable health state" anchored at 100 and 0, respectively. Respondents are asked to indicate how they rate their own health state by drawing a line from an anchor box to that point on the VAS that best represents their own health on that day.

HRQOL CONTROVERSY

Whose preferences should be used in the calculation of QALYs for CUA? Some authors have argued that health-state preferences elicited from the general population should not

TABLE 2–4. Selected Disease-Specific Quality-of-Life Instruments

Arthritis Impact Measurement Scales (AIMS)[50]
Asthma Quality of Life Questionnaire (AQLQ)[51]
Diabetes Quality of Life (DQOL)[52]
Kidney Disease Quality of Life (KDQOL) Instrument[53]
Quality of Life in Epilepsy (QOLIE)[54]
Medical Outcomes Study HIV Health Survey (MOS-HIV)[55]

be applied to specific patient groups. However, when public resource-allocation decisions are being made, general population preferences may be the most appropriate.

SPECIFIC INSTRUMENTS

Specific or targeted instruments are intended to provide greater detail concerning particular outcomes, in terms of functioning and well-being, uniquely associated with a condition and/or its treatment. Several selected examples of disease-specific instruments are listed in Table 2–4. One of the instruments listed is the Asthma Quality of Life Questionnaire (AQLQ), a 32-item instrument developed to assess the impact of asthma on patients' everyday functioning and well-being.[51] Results from research in which the AQLQ was used have appeared in promotional materials for the salmeterol inhaler (GlaxoSmithKline). As opposed to prior prescription drug advertisements that involved predominantly physiologic-based QOL claims,[18] this was one of the first times a pharmaceutical firm has promoted a product based on data from trials involving QOL as a primary outcome measure. This is likely to occur with increasing frequency as pharmaceutical firms look for ways to demonstrate value and differentiate their products from those of the competition.[56,57] Leidy and colleagues[58] have provided useful recommendations for evaluating the validity of QOL claims for labeling and promotion of pharmaceuticals.

Although not always, disease- or condition-specific instruments can be more sensitive than a generic measure to particular changes in HRQOL secondary to the disease or its treatment. In addition, specific measures may appear to be more clinically relevant to patients and health care providers.[31]

However, a concern regarding the use of only specific instruments is that by focusing on the specific impact, the general or overall impact on functioning and well-being may be overlooked. In studies involving pharmacotherapy, the use of both a generic and a specific instrument may be the best approach. The generic instrument provides a more general outcome assessment and allows comparability across other disease states or conditions in which it has been used. An appropriately selected specific instrument should provide more detailed outcome information regarding expected changes in the particular patient population.

MEASUREMENT ISSUES

A number of issues must be considered when evaluating existing HRQOL research and/or choosing the appropriate instrument to use when designing a study involving QOL assessment. A thorough review of these issues is not within the scope of this chapter; more in-depth reviews of methodologic considerations are available in the literature.[12,59,60] Of particular concern are the psychometric properties of a chosen instrument. *Psychometrics* refers to the measurement of psychological constructs, such as QOL. Instruments should be developed and tested such that one can place confidence in the measurement made. Psychometric properties of measures (e.g., reliability and validity) are considered in the review criteria developed by the Scientific Advisory Committee of the Medical Outcomes Trust (MOT).[61] The MOT is a depository and distributor of standardized health outcomes measurement instruments. Every instrument that is proposed for addition to the MOT list of approved instruments is reviewed against a rigorous set of eight attributes. These attributes provide a useful evaluative framework. The eight attributes of an instrument addressed by the review criteria are as follows: (1) conceptual and measurement model, (2) reliability, (3) validity, (4) responsiveness, (5) interpretability, (6) respondent and administrative burden, (7) alternate forms, and (8) cultural and language adaptations.

CONCEPTUAL AND MEASUREMENT MODELS

A *conceptual model* is the rationale for and description of the concepts that a measurement instrument is intended to assess and the interrelationships of those concepts. A *measurement model* is an instrument's scale and subscale structure and the procedures followed to create scale and subscale scores. An example is the well-defined conceptual and measurement models for the scales and scale structure of the SF-36.[62] The SF-36 contains 36 items that cover nine theory-based health concepts. Eight of these health concepts are measured by multi-item scales. There is a clearly defined means of creating the individual scale scores and the physical and mental component summary scales.[41]

RELIABILITY

Reliability refers to the extent to which measures give consistent or accurate results. The purpose of evaluating the reliability of a QOL instrument is to estimate how much of the variation in a score is real as opposed to random. The two reliability assessment methods discussed most often in the HRQOL literature are internal consistency and test-retest reliability. *Internal consistency* is an assessment of the performance of items within a scale. It is a function of the number of items and their covariation.[63] Internal consistency is commonly measured using Cronbach's alpha coefficient. Alpha coefficients above 0.90 are recommended for making comparisons between individuals and above 0.70 for comparisons between groups.[64]

Test-retest reliability refers to the relationship between scores obtained from the same instrument on two or more separate occasions when all pertinent conditions remain relatively unchanged. It is usually evaluated using the intraclass correlation coefficient (ICC).[60] However, QOL is not assumed to be constant over the course of time. In fact, most clinical studies attempt to assess how QOL changes. Test-retest reliability estimates may have limited value in evaluating measures that are designed to assess a dynamic process.

Interrater reliability and *equivalent-forms reliability* are two other approaches to reliability assessment that are not used as commonly in QOL research. More in-depth discussions of these and the other reliability assessment methods are found elsewhere.[60,65]

VALIDITY

Reliability is necessary but not sufficient for valid measurement.[63] *Validity* is an estimation of the extent to which the instrument is measuring what it is supposed to be measuring. Validity is not an absolute property of an instrument. Hence a measurement instrument is not "valid," but empirical data can provide evidence to support its validity. Three types of validity commonly considered are criterion, content, and construct.

Criterion validity is demonstrated when a new measure corresponds to an established measure or observation that accurately reflects the phenomenon of interest. By definition, the criterion must be a superior measure of the phenomenon if it is to serve as a comparative norm. However, in QOL assessment, "gold standards," or criterion measures, rarely exist against which a new measure can be compared.

Content validity, which is tested infrequently statistically, refers to how adequately the questions/items capture the relevant aspects of the domain or concept being measured.

Construct validity refers to the relationship between measures purporting to measure the same underlying theoretical construct (convergent evidence) or purporting to measure different constructs (discriminant evidence). For example, convergent evidence for the validity of a new measure of emotional well-being could be established by showing a strong association between the new scale and the Beck Depression Inventory.[66] Evidence for the construct validity of other aspects of the measure might be established through comparisons with physiologic measures, organ pathology, or clinical signs.

RESPONSIVENESS

Responsiveness, or sensitivity to change, is the ability or power of the measure to detect clinically important change when it occurs.[67] Although some authors have suggested that responsiveness is a psychometric property of a measure distinct from validity,[68] others argue that responsiveness is an aspect of validity rather than a separate property.[63,69]

HRQOL CONTROVERSY

What constitutes a minimally important difference on an HRQOL measure? Although the statistical significance of a change, or difference score, is used often to denote important change, it may over- or underestimate the true impact of the disease and/or its treatment in terms of change that is perceptible and important to patients. Discussions regarding the concept of minimally important difference are appearing increasingly in the literature.

INTERPRETABILITY

Interpretability is the degree to which one can assign qualitative meaning to an instrument's quantitative scores. Interpretability is facilitated by comparison of a score or change in scores to a qualitative category that has clinical or commonly understood meaning. For example, it would be helpful to know how scale scores obtained in a specific patient sample compare with the scale scores of the general population. Ware and colleagues[62] have provided very useful U.S. population-based normative data for the SF-36.

RESPONDENT AND ADMINISTRATIVE BURDEN

Respondent burden refers to the time, energy, and other demands placed on those to whom the instrument is administered. *Administrative burden* refers to the demands placed on those who administer the instrument. A practical aspect of the measurement of HRQOL is length of the instrument or the administration time involved. Instruments should be as brief as possible without severely compromising the validity and reliability of the measurement. The longer an instrument, the greater is the respondent burden. This can lead to an individual's unwillingness or refusal to complete the instrument or to incomplete responses.

ALTERNATE FORMS

Alternate forms of an instrument include all modes of administration other than the original source instrument. Evidence should be provided that supports the comparability of the alternate mode of administration with that of the original instrument.[70] Many QOL measures can be administered in different ways. The primary modes of administration are (1) interviewer-administered, either in person or over the telephone, or (2) self-administered questionnaires.[31] Other self-completed modes include computer-based (using the keyboard or touch screen to respond) and telephone touchtone administration. Used but not recommended are proxy responders (i.e., using a health care provider, family member, or friend to respond for the subject when the subject is unable to complete the instrument). Because QOL is such a subjective concept, patients must have the opportunity to provide their perspective on the impact of illness and/or medical care on their functioning and well-being. The patient's perspective has been shown to be quite different from that of outside observers, including physicians, family members, or others close to the patient.[71]

CULTURAL AND LANGUAGE ADAPTATIONS

Methods used to achieve conceptual and linguistic equivalence of cross-culturally adapted instruments should be stated explicitly.[72] Evidence should be provided that the measurement properties of the adaptation are comparable with those of the original instrument. It is obvious that this is an extremely important issue when planning cross-national QOL assessment projects. However, it is also very important within countries that are multicultural, such as the United States.[73] Many of the English-language instruments have been developed for the dominant U.S. culture and may not be appropriate for all patients.

OTHER MEASUREMENT ISSUES

SELECTION OF AN APPROPRIATE INSTRUMENT

It is essential that the purpose of the measurement be well defined before selection of an HRQOL instrument. Is the purpose of the measurement to describe the health status or HRQOL of a patient population at a particular time or over time?[74] Is it to document change in health outcomes associated with a particular intervention? These and other questions should be answered before HRQOL instruments are selected. Too many practitioner-researchers attempting to demonstrate improvements in outcomes resulting from a pharmaceutical product or service select a commonly used generic instrument, such as the SF-36, with the expectation that it will be sufficiently responsive to changes that may occur. The best approach may be to use the SF-36 or other generic instrument in conjunction with a more targeted, disease-specific instrument.

AVAILABILITY OF INSTRUMENTS

Many HRQOL instruments are in the public domain. However, although they can be used for no or little cost, there may be a fee associated with the purchase of a user's guide or scoring manual. The MOT (*www.outcomes-trust.org*) is a source for a number of instruments, including the Duke Health Profile, QWB, MOS-HIV Health Survey, Migraine Specific Quality of Life (MSQOL), and Sickness

Impact Profile (SIP). For information on availability of the SF-36 and SF-12, go to *http://www.sf36.org*. The Functional Assessment of Chronic Illness Therapy (FACIT) Web site (*http://www.facit.org*) provides an extensive array of cancer- and chronic-disease–targeted instruments. Developers of particular instruments often can be contacted through addresses provided in other books referenced at the end of this chapter.[28–30,60]

CONCLUSIONS

The concept of HRQOL has gained increasing attention in the evaluation of the outcomes associated with medical care, including pharmacotherapy. In fact, in certain diseases, HRQOL may be the most important outcome to consider in assessing the effectiveness of health care interventions. Health care practitioners and policymakers must remember that efforts to increase length of life must not outstrip the ability to maintain or improve QOL.

HRQOL assessment is a relatively new field of endeavor, and a number of theoretical and methodologic issues remain unresolved. However, some general concepts in the measurement of HRQOL outcomes should be considered carefully when designing a study, evaluating existing research, or evaluating new programs or services. This chapter has provided only a brief overview of the concepts in an effort to sensitize students and health care practitioners to the importance of the area, as well as to provide insight as to how these concepts can and should be incorporated into their practices.

ABBREVIATIONS

AIMS: Arthritis Impact Measurement Scales
AQLQ: Asthma Quality of Life Questionnaire
CUA: cost-utility analysis
DQOL: Diabetes Quality of Life
ECHO: economic, clinical, and humanistic outcomes
FACIT: Functional Assessment of Chronic Illness Therapy
HALE: health-adjusted life expectancy
HAPYs: health-adjusted person years
HRQOL: health-related quality of life
HIV/AIDS: human immunodeficiency virus/acquired immunodeficiency syndrome
HUI: Health Utilities Index
HYEs: healthy-year equivalents
ICC: intraclass correlation coefficient
KDQOL: Kidney Disease Quality of Life instrument
MCS: mental component summary scale of the SF-36
MOS-HIV: Medical Outcomes Study HIV Health Survey
MOT: Medical Outcomes Trust
MSQOL: Migraine Specific Quality of Life
NHP: Nottingham Health Profile
PCS: physical component summary scale of the SF-36
QALY: quality-adjusted life year
QOL: quality of life
QOLIE: Quality of Life in Epilepsy
QWB: Quality of Well-Being scale
SF-36: MOS 36-Item Short-Form Health Survey
SIP: Sickness Impact Profile
VAS: visual analog scale
WY: well year
YHL: years of healthy life

Review Questions and other resources can be found at *www.pharmacotherapyonline.com.*

REFERENCES

1. Peterson MA, ed. Healthy Markets? The New Competition in Medical Care. Durham, NC, Duke University Press, 1999.
2. Gold MR, Siegel JE, Russell LB, Weinstein MC, eds. Cost-Effectiveness in Health and Medicine. New York, Oxford University Press, 1996.
3. Sloan FA, ed. Valuing Health Care: Costs, Benefits, and Effectiveness of Pharmaceuticals and Other Medical Technologies. New York, Cambridge University Press, 1996.
4. Donabedian A. Explorations in Quality Assessment and Monitoring, Vol. I: The Definition of Quality and Approaches to Its Assessment. Ann Arbor. MI, Health Administration Press, 1980.
5. Zitter M. Outcomes assessment: True customer focus comes to health care. Med Interface 1992;5:32–37.
6. Ellwood PM. Outcomes management: A technology of patient experience. N Engl J Med 1998;318:1551.
7. Lohr KN. Outcome measurement: Concepts and questions. Inquiry 1988;25:37–50.
8. Kozma CM, Reeder CE, Schulz RM. Economic, clinical, and humanistic outcomes: A planning model for pharmacoeconomic research. Clin Ther 1993;15:1121–1132.
9. Stewart AL. Conceptual and methodologic issues in defining quality of life: State of the art. Prog Cardiovasc Nurs 1992;7(2):3–11.
10. Kaplan RM, Bush JW. Health-related quality of life measurement for evaluation research and policy analysis. Health Psychol 1982;1:61–80.
11. Schron EB, Shumaker SA. The integration of health quality of life in clinical research: Experience from cardiovascular clinical trials. Prog Cardiovasc Nurs 1992;7(2):21.
12. Patrick DL, Erickson P. Health Status and Health Policy: Allocating Resources to Health Care. New York, Oxford University Press, 1993:22.
13. Schipper H, Clinch JJ, Olweny CLM. Quality of life studies: Definitions and conceptual issues. In: Spilker B, ed. Quality of Life and Pharmacoeconomics in Clinical Trials, 2d ed. Philadelphia, Lippincott-Raven, 1996:11–23.
14. Staquet M, Aaronson NK, Ahmedzai S, et al. Health-related quality of life research (editorial). Qual Life Res 1992;1:3.
15. Smith M. Medication, quality of life and compliance: The role of the pharmacist. Pharmacoeconomics 1992;1:225–230.
16. Bungay KM, Boyer JG, Steinwald AB, Ware JE Jr. Health-related quality of life: An overview. In: Bootman JL, Townsend RJ, McGhan WF, eds. Principles of Pharmacoeconomics, 2d ed. Cincinnati, Harvey Whitney Books, 1996:126–148.
17. Revicki DA, Rothman M, Luce B. Health-related quality of life assessment and the pharmaceutical industry. Pharmacoeconomics 1992;1:394–408.
18. Rothermich EA, Pathak DS, Smeenk DA. Health-related quality of life claims in prescription drug advertisements. Am J Health Syst Pharm 1996;53:1565–1569.
19. Croog SH, Levine S, Testa MA, et al. The effects of antihypertensive therapy on quality of life. N Engl J Med 1986;319:1220–1221.
20. Côté I, Grégoire J-P, Moisan J. Health-related quality-of-life measurement in hypertension: A review of randomised controlled drug trials. Pharmacoeconomics 2000;18:435–450.
21. Juniper EF. Quality of life considerations in the treatment of asthma. Pharmacoeconomics 1995;8:123–138.
22. Fairclough DL, Fetting JH, Cella D, et al. Quality of life and quality adjusted survival for breast cancer patients receiving adjuvant therapy. Qual Life Res 1999;8:723–731.
23. Testa MA, Simonson DC. Health economic benefits and quality of life during improved glycemic control in patients with type 2 diabetes mellitus: A randomized, controlled, double-blind trial. JAMA 1998;280:1490–1496.
24. Briggs A, Scott E, Steele K. Impact of osteoarthritis and analgesic treatment on quality of life of an elderly population. Ann Pharmacother 1999;33:1154–1159.
25. Delate T, Coons SJ. The use of two health-related quality-of-life measures in a sample of persons infected with human immunodeficiency virus. Clin Infect Dis 2001;32(3):e47–e52.
26. Badia X, Herdman M. The importance of health-related quality-of-life data in determining the value of drug therapy. Clin Ther 2001;23:168–175.
27. Academy of Managed Care Pharmacy. Format for Formulary Submissions, Version 2.0. Alexandria, VA, The Foundation for Managed Care Pharmacy, October 2002; available at *http://www.fmcpnet.org/fmcp.cfm? c = resources#a3.*
28. Bowling A. Measuring Health: A Review of Quality of Life Measurement Scales, 2d ed. Buckingham, England, Open University Press, 1997.
29. Bowling A. Measuring Disease: A Review of Disease-Specific Quality of Life Measurement Scales, 2d ed. Buckingham, England, Open University Press, 2001.
30. McDowell I, Newell C. Measuring Health: A Guide to Rating Scales and Questionnaires, 2d ed. New York, Oxford University Press, 1996.
31. Guyatt GH, Feeny DH, Patrick DL. Measuring health-related quality of life. Ann Intern Med 1993;118:622–629.
32. Patrick DL, Deyo RA. Generic and disease-specific measures in assessing health status and quality of life. Med Care 1989;27:S217–S232.
33. Kind P. The EuroQOL instrument: An index of health-related quality of life. In Spilker B, ed. Quality of Life and Pharmacoeconomics in Clinical Trials, 2d ed. Philadelphia, Lippincott-Raven, 1996:191–201.
34. Hunt SM, McEwen J, McKenna SP. Measuring health status: A new tool for clinicians and epidemiologists. J R Coll Gen Pract 1985;35:185–188.
35. Kaplan RM, Anderson JP. The general health policy model: An integrated approach. In Spilker B, ed. Quality of Life and Pharmacoeconomics in Clinical Trials, 2d ed. Philadelphia, Lippincott-Raven, 1996:309–322.
36. Bergner M, Bobbitt RA, Carter WB, Gilson BS. The Sickness Impact Profile: Development and final revisions of a health status measure. Med Care 1976;14:57–67.
37. Furlong WJ, Feeny DH, Torrance GW, Barr RD. The Health Utilities Index (HUI) system for assessing health-related quality of life in clinical studies. Ann Med 2001;33:375–384.
38. Ware JE Jr, Sherbourne CD. The MOS 36-Item Short-Form Health Survey (SF-36): I. Conceptual framework and item selection. Med Care 1992;30:473–483.
39. McHorney CA, Ware JE Jr, Raczek AE. The MOS 36-Item Short-Form Health Survey (SF-36): II. Psychometric and clinical tests of validity in measuring physical and mental health constructs. Med Care 1993;31:247–263.
40. McHorney CA, Ware JE Jr, Raczek AE. The MOS 36-Item Short-Form Health Survey (SF-36): III. Tests of data quality, scaling assumptions, and reliability across diverse patient groups. Med Care 1994;32:40–66.
41. Ware JE Jr, Kosinski M, Keller SD. SF-36 Physical and Mental Health Summary Scales: A User's Manual. Boston, The Health Institute, 1994.
42. Ware JE Jr, Kosinski M, Keller SD. A 12-item short-form health survey: Construction of scales and preliminary test of reliability and validity. Med Care 1996;34:220.
43. Drummond MF, O'Brien B, Stoddart GL, Torrance GW. Methods for the Economic Evaluation of Health Care Programmes, 2d ed. Oxford, England, Oxford University Press, 1997.
44. Coons SJ, Kaplan RM. Cost-utility analysis. In Bootman JL, Townsend RJ, McGhan WF, eds. Principles of Pharmacoeconomics, 2d ed. Cincinnati, Harvey Whitney, 1996:102–126.
45. Neumann PJ, Stone PW, Chapman RH, et al. The quality of reporting in published cost-utility analyses, 1976–1997. Ann Intern Med 2000;132:964–972.
46. Feeny DH, Torrance GW, Labelle R. Integrating economic evaluations and quality of life assessments. In Spilker B, ed. Quality of Life and Pharmacoeconomics in Clinical Trials, 2d ed. Philadelphia, Lippincott-Raven, 1996:85–95.
47. Torrance GW, Thomas WH, Sackett DL. Utility maximization model for evaluation of health care programmes. Health Serv Res 1972;7:118–133.
48. Coons SJ, Rao S, Keininger DL, Hays RD. A comparative review of generic quality of life instruments. Pharmacoeconomics 2000;17:13–35.

49. Kaplan RM, Sieber WJ, Ganiats TG. The quality of well-being scale: Comparison of an interviewer-administered version with a self-administered questionnaire. Psychol Health 1997;12:783–791.

50. Meenan RF, Gertman PM, Mason JH. Measuring health status in arthritis: The arthritis impact measurement scales. Arthritis Rheum 1980;23:146–152.

51. Juniper EF, Guyatt GH, Epstein RS, et al. Evaluation of impairment of health-related quality of life in asthma: Development of a questionnaire for use in clinical trials. Thorax 1992;47:76–83.

52. Parkerson GR, Connis RT, Broadhead WE, et al. Disease-specific versus generic measurement of health-related quality of life in insulin-dependent diabetic patients. Med Care 1993;7:629–639.

53. Hays RD, Kallich JD, Mapes DL, et al. Development of the kidney disease quality of life (KDQOL) instrument. Qual Life Res 1994;3:329–338.

54. Perrine KR. A new quality of life inventory for epilepsy patients: Interim results. Epilepsia 1993;34(suppl 4):S28–S33.

55. Wu AW, Revicki DA, Jacobson D, Malitz FE. Evidence for reliability, validity and usefulness of the medical outcomes study HIV health survey (MOS-HIV). Qual Life Res 1997;6:481–493.

56. Santanello NC, Baker D, Cappelleri JC, et al. Regulatory issues for health-related quality of life--PhRMA Health Outcomes Committee Workshop, 1999. Value Health 2002;5:14–25.

57. Revicki DA, Osoba D, Fairclough D, et al. Recommendations on health-related quality of life research to support labeling and promotional claims in the United States. Qual Life Res 2000;9:887–900.

58. Leidy NK, Revicki DA, Geneste B. Recommendations for evaluating the validity of quality of life claims for labeling and promotion. Value Health 1999;2:113–127.

59. Staquet MJ, Hays RD, Fayers PM. Quality of Life Assessment in Clinical Trials: Methods and Practice. Oxford, England, Oxford University Press, 1998.

60. Fayers PM, Machin D. Quality of Life: Assessment, Analysis and Interpretation. Chichester, England, Wiley, 2000.

61. Scientific Advisory Committee of the Medical Outcomes Trust. Assessing health status and quality-of-life instruments: Attributes and review criteria. Qual Life Res 2002;11:193–205.

62. Ware JE Jr, Snow KK, Kosinski M, Gandek B. SF-36 Health Survey: Manual and Interpretation Guide. Boston, The Health Institute, 1993.

63. Hays RD, Anderson R, Revicki D. Psychometric considerations in evaluating health-related quality of life measures. Qual Life Res 1993;2:441–449.

64. Nunnally J. Psychometric Theory, 2d ed. New York, McGraw-Hill, 1978.

65. Streiner DL, Norman GR. Health Measurement Scales: A Practical Guide to Their Development and Use, 2d ed. Oxford, England, Oxford University Press, 1995.

66. Beck AT, Steer RA, Brown GK. Beck Depression Inventory Manual, 2d ed (BDI-II). San Antonio, The Psychological Corporation, 1996.

67. Juniper EF, Guyatt GH, Jaeschke R. How to develop and validate a new health-related quality of life instrument. In Spilker B, ed. Quality of Life and Pharmacoeconomics in Clinical Trials, 2d ed. Philadelphia, Lippincott-Raven, 1996:49–56.

68. Guyatt G, Walter S, Norman G. Measuring change over time: Assessing the usefulness of evaluative instruments. J Chron Dis 1987;40:171–178.

69. Hays RD, Hadorn D. Responsiveness to change: An aspect of validity, not a separate dimension. Qual Life Res 1992;1:73–75.

70. Cook DJ, Guyatt GH, Juniper E, et al. Interviewer versus self-administered questionnaires in developing a disease-specific, health-related quality of life instrument for asthma. J Clin Epidemiol 1993;46:529–534.

71. Jachuck SJ, Brierly H, Jachuck S, Wilcox PM. The effect of hypotensive drugs on the quality of life. J R Coll Gen Pract 1982;32:103–105.

72. Bullinger M, Power MJ, Aaronson NK, et al. Creating and evaluating cross-cultural instruments. In Spilker B, ed. Quality of Life and Pharmacoeconomics in Clinical Trials, 2d ed. Philadelphia, Lippincott-Raven, 1996:659–668.

73. Yu J, Coons SJ, Draugalis JR, et al. Equivalence of the Chinese and U.S.-English versions of the SF-36 health survey. Qual Life Res 2003;12:449–457.

74. Fairclough DL. Design and Analysis of Quality of Life Studies in Clinical Trials. Boca Raton, FL, Chapman & Hall/CRC, 2002.

3
EVIDENCE-BASED MEDICINE

Elaine Chiquette and L. Michael Posey

Learning Objectives and other resources can be found at *www.pharmacotherapyonline.com.*

KEY CONCEPTS

◀**1** The best current evidence integrated into clinical expertise ensures optimal care for patients.

◀**2** The four steps in the process of applying evidence-based medicine (EBM) in practice are (a) formulate a clear question from a patient's problem, (b) identify relevant information, (c) critically appraise available evidence, and (d) implement the findings in clinical practice.

◀**3** The decision as to whether to implement the results of a specific study, conclusions of a review article, or another piece of evidence in clinical practice depends on the quality (i.e., internal validity) of the evidence, its clinical importance, whether benefits outweigh risks and costs, and its relevance in the clinical setting and patient's circumstances.

◀**4** EBM strategies can be applied to help in keeping current.

◀**5** EBM is realistic.

In the information age, clinicians are presented with a daunting number of diseases and possible treatments to consider as they care for patients each day. As knowledge increases and as the technology for accessing information becomes widely available, health care professionals are expected to stay current in their fields of expertise and to remain competent throughout their careers. In addition, the number of information sources for the typical practitioner has ballooned, and clinicians must sort out information from many sources: college courses and continuing education (including seminars and journals), pharmaceutical representatives, and colleagues, as well as guidelines from committees of health care facilities, governmental agencies, and expert committees and organizations.

◀**1** How does the health care professional find valid information from such a cacophony? Increasingly, clinicians are turning to the principles of evidence-based medicine (EBM) to identify the best course of action for each patient. EBM strategies help health care professionals to ferret out these gold nuggets, enabling them to integrate the best current evidence into their pharmacotherapeutic decision making. These strategies can help physicians, pharmacists, and other health care professionals to distinguish reliably beneficial pharmacotherapies from those which are ineffective or harmful. Also, EBM approaches can be applied to keep up to date and to make an overwhelming task seem more manageable.

This chapter describes for the reader the principles of EBM, offers guidance for finding EBM sources on the World Wide Web, provides a model for applying EBM in patient care, and explains how EBM strategies can help a practitioner stay current.

WHAT IS EVIDENCE-BASED MEDICINE?

EBM is an approach to medical practice that uses the results of patient care research and other available objective evidence as a component of clinical decision making. Similarly, evidence-based pharmacotherapy, defined by Etminan and colleagues,[1] is an approach to decision making whereby clinicians appraise the scientific evidence and its strength in support of their therapeutic decisions.

While few would argue against the necessity for basing clinical decisions on the best possible evidence available, considerable controversy actually surrounds the practice of EBM. Critics note that not all questions relevant to the care of a patient are of a scientific nature and that EBM favors a "cookbook" approach. In fact, EBM integrates knowledge from research with other factors affecting clinical decision making. EBM does not replace clinical judgment. Rather, it informs clinical judgment with the current best evidence. The expertise and experience of the clinician who understands the disease are crucial in determining whether the external evidence applies to the patient and whether it should be integrated in the therapeutic plan. Also, nonmedical factors affect decision making, such as the patient's preferences and readiness and the health care delivery system's characteristics.

Other critics state that EBM considers randomized, controlled trials (RCTs) as the only evidence to be used in clinical decision making. Actually, EBM seeks the best existing evidence from basic science to clinical research with which to inform clinical decision. For example, a decision about the accuracy of a diagnostic test is best informed by evidence from a cross-sectional study, not an RCT. A cohort study, not an RCT, best answers a question about prognosis. However, in selecting a treatment, the randomized trial is the best study design to provide the most accurate estimate of treatment efficacy and safety.

EBM opponents note that RCTs usually are conducted in idealized environments or situations that are not sufficiently similar to the conditions of the "real world." In addition, errors can be made when results of an RCT of one drug are extrapolated to all members of that class of drugs.[2,3]

Regardless of one's view, RCTs have confirmed the value of many therapeutic options today and have disproved or clarified the usefulness of others. For example, in 1970, observational studies had indicated a possible association between the occurrence of premature ventricular contractions (PVCs) in patients after myocardial infarction

(MI) and sudden death. As a result, the eighth edition of *Harrison's Principles of Internal Medicine* recommended the use of antiarrhythmic agents to eradicate post-MI PVCs and thereby minimize the risk of sudden death. However, an RCT tested the antiarrhythmic therapy in patients with frequent PVCs, and it showed that class 1 antiarrhythmic agents increased rather than decreased the risk of sudden death.[4,5] Today, guidelines discourage the use of antiarrhythmic agents to suppress PVCs in post-MI patients.[6]

More recently, the 1996 guidelines for the management of patients with acute MI concluded that observational studies "indicate that estrogen therapy does reduce mortality in women with moderate and severe coronary disease."[7] Subsequently, an RCT found no reduction in overall risk for nonfatal MI or coronary death with estrogen therapy. Rather, significantly more coronary events occurred during the first year of the trial among women receiving estrogen therapy compared with women taking placebo.[8] These results prompted revision of the guidelines to conclude: "On the basis of the finding of no overall cardiovascular benefit and a pattern of early increase in risk of coronary events, starting estrogen plus progestin is not recommended for the purpose of secondary prevention of coronary disease."[6]

In both these examples, conventional wisdom was wrong. Results from observational studies proved incorrect. Only through careful assessment using RCT methodology was the true estimate of the efficacy and safety of the therapeutic options discovered.

CLINICAL CONTROVERSY

In many ways, EBM is controversial, with some people feeling that it prevents the application of common sense and experience-based reasoning to clinical care. Some joke that a clinician called an EBM center and asked whether parachutes are effective when jumping from a plane. We do not know came the response—there are no randomized, controlled trials comparing jumping from a plane with and without one!

EBM ON THE WORLD WIDE WEB

For additional information and resources relevant to EBM, several comprehensive EBM sites exist on the World Wide Web. These sites include information on the history and development of EBM, glossaries of EBM terms, tutorials, training programs, software, links to EBM organizations and practice centers, guides to searching the medical literature, and results of evidence-based studies. For an excellent list of EBM links, access "Netting the Evidence: A ScHARR Introduction to Evidence Based Practice" (*http://www.shef.ac.uk/~scharr/ir/netting/*). A specialized EBM site dedicated to pharmacotherapy deserves special mention. It is provided by the Centre for Evidence-Based Pharmacotherapy (*http://www.aston.ac.uk/pharmacy/cebp/*). The mission of the center, created in 1995 by pharmacy professor Alain Li Wan Po, is to undertake research into the methodology of medicines assessment, pharmacoepidemiology, and pharmacoeconomics. In addition, the center offers postgraduate and distance learning in evidence-based pharmacotherapy.

INCORPORATING EBM INTO PHARMACOTHERAPEUTIC DECISION MAKING

The practice of EBM is to recognize an information need while caring for a patient, identify the best existing evidence to help resolve the problem, consider the evidence in light of the actual circumstances, and integrate the evidence into a medical plan. In this section, the four steps involved in applying the EBM process to a pharmacotherapeutic decision are described[9]:

1. Recognize information needs and convert them into answerable questions.
2. Conduct efficient searches for the best evidence with which to answer these questions.
3. Critically appraise the evidence for its validity and usefulness.
4. Apply the results to patient situations to best assist clinical decision making.

BUILDING A FOCUSED QUESTION

Clinicians constantly balance the benefits and risks of various therapeutic choices. The questions they face are patient-specific:

- Should clopidogrel be prescribed to this 65-year-old man with unstable angina?
- Should hormone-replacement therapy be prescribed for this postmenopausal woman?
- Is sildenafil safe in this patient with type 2 diabetes?

When searching for the best evidence to answer such questions, the questions must be rephrased with more precision and specificity. A well-formulated question includes the following elements: the patient or problem being addressed, the intervention being considered, the comparison intervention, and the outcome(s) of interest.[10] Using these four elements, the preceding questions can be reframed as follows:

- Would clopidogrel in addition to aspirin (*intervention*) prevent death or coronary events (*clinically relevant outcome*) in this patient with unstable angina (*patient with a problem*) who is currently on aspirin alone (*comparison intervention*)?
- Should we begin hormone-replacement therapy (*intervention compared with no intervention*) to prevent cardiovascular events (*outcome*) in this asymptomatic postmenopausal woman with a family history of coronary artery disease (*patient*)?
- If sildenafil is begun (*intervention*), what is the risk of myocardial ischemia (*outcome*) in this asymptomatic patient with known coronary artery disease (CAD) and newly diagnosed with type 2 diabetes (*patient*)?

The acronym *PICO* can be helpful to remember the elements of a well-balanced question[11]:

P = patient
I = intervention
C = comparison
O = outcome

Focusing the question clarifies the target of the literature search and permits use of the appropriate guides for assessing external validity, that is, the applicability of the evidence found in the study to appropriate parts of the "real world."

CONDUCTING AN EFFICIENT SEARCH

Health care professionals have four options as they try to identify the best evidence available to answer a well-framed question:

1. Ask a colleague for his or her expert opinion.
2. Review practice guidelines (evidence-based or expert-opinion–based) or a textbook for appropriate disease management.

TABLE 3–1. North American Sources of Evidence-Based Clinical Practice Guidelines

Resource/Web Address	Special Features
National Guideline Clearinghouse (NGC) (*www.guideline.gov*) NGC is a collaboration of U.S. Department of Health and Human Services and the Agency for Healthcare Research and Quality (AHRQ), in partnership with the American Medical Association (AMA) and the American Association of Health Plans (AAHP). NGC provides access to full text guidelines (when available) produced by a number of different professional medical associations and health care organizations. Each guideline is critically appraised using a standard instrument. The site permits side-by-side comparison of several guidelines.	• 966 guideline summaries • Weekly e-mail alerts • Advanced search queries based on guideline attributes • Annotated bibliography of resources relevant to guideline methodology
National Library of Medicine's Health Services/Technology Assessment Text (*http://hstat.nlm.nih.gov/hq/Hquest/screen/HquestHome/s/55240*) This World Wide Web resource is a collection of AHRQ Supported Guidelines, AHRQ Technology Assessments and Reviews, ATIS (HIV/AIDS Technical Information), NIH Warren G. Magnuson Clinical Research Studies, NIH Consensus Development Program, Public Health Service (PHS) Guide to Clinical Preventive Services and the Substance Abuse, and Mental Health Services Administration's Center for Substance Abuse Treatment (SAMHSA/CSAT) Prevention Enhancement and Treatment Improvement Protocols.	• 199 full-text guidelines • Metasearch capabilities to PubMed, Centers for Disease Control and Prevention (CDC) Prevention Guidelines Database, and National Guideline Clearinghouse • Access to quick-reference guides for clinicians and consumer brochures.
Primary Care Clinical Practice Guidelines (*http://medicine.ucsf.edu/resources/guidelines*) This Web resource offers a listing of online guidelines.	• Searchable by clinical content and organization
CDC Prevention Guidelines Database Home Page (*http://www.phppo.cdc.gov/cdcrecommends*) The site is a comprehensive collection of all the official guidelines and recommendations published by the CDC about prevention of diseases, injuries, and disabilities.	• More than 500 prevention guidelines/documents • Searchable • Sort by date, by topic, or alphabetically
Cancer Care Ontario Practice Guidelines Initiative (CCOPGI) (*http://www.cancercare.on.ca*) This Web page includes published and unpublished guidelines related to cancer care. These guidelines are created by the CCOPGI and are available full text.	• 75 guidelines • When information is scarce, evidence summaries are created to review the best evidence available
Agency for Healthcare Research and Quality's Evidence-Based Practice Centers (AHRQ EPCs) (*http://www.ahcpr.gov/clinic/epcix.htm*) AHRQ has established 12 Evidence-Based Practice Centers to analyze and synthesize the scientific literature and develop evidence reports and technology assessments on clinical topics.	• 84 evidence reports • Full text available

3. Consult electronic databases of systematic reviews and/or meta-analyses.
4. Conduct a literature search using an electronic database such as MEDLINE.

Each of these options has advantages and disadvantages, as described below.

OPTION 1

Asking an expert or colleague may provide a quick and easy answer to a clinical question. Exercise caution, however. These sources have become less reliable as the volume and complexity of medical information have grown exponentially. Colleagues may be out of date or biased by their own experiences.

OPTION 2

Online practice guidelines or current textbooks with evidence links are useful if the question relates to a common or well-established issue (e.g., *UpToDate, Harrison's Online,* and *Scientific American*

Medicine Online electronic textbooks). As their names suggest, evidence-based clinical guidelines are guided by objective data and should be preferred over expert-opinion–based guidelines that refer loosely to evidence to support their opinions. Expert-opinion guidelines vary in their scientific validity and reproducibility.[12]

One Web site—the National Guideline Clearinghouse on the Web (*http://www.guideline.gov*)—provides links to many evidence-based clinical practice guidelines. For each guideline, this comprehensive database offers a short summary of the key attributes, including the bibliographic sources, guideline developers and endorsers, status of the guidelines, and major recommendations. In addition, the site provides the ability to generate side-by-side comparisons for any combination of two or more guidelines. Table 3–1 presents an annotated list of additional resources to find and access evidence-based clinical practice guidelines.

OPTION 3

Consulting electronic databases of systematic reviews and meta-analyses is attractive because of the limited amount of time health care professionals have to research and review the literature before they answer clinical questions or reach patient care decisions. Busy health care professionals prefer summaries of information. Traditional narrative reviews are useful for broad overviews of particular therapies or diseases or for reports on the latest advances in a particular area where research may be limited.[13] However, information from narrative reviews is often gathered ad hoc, and the author's biases may enter into the process of gathering, analyzing, and reporting information.

In contrast, systematic reviews employ a comprehensive, reproducible data search and selection process to summarize all the best evidence. They follow a rigorous process to appraise and analyze the information, quantitatively (through the meta-analysis technique) or qualitatively, to best answer a defined clinical question. Systematic reviews are a useful means of assessing whether findings from multiple individual studies are consistent and can be generalized.[14]

The Cochrane Library represents one of the most comprehensive sources of systematic reviews summarizing the evidence about health care. About 2000 Cochrane reviews are currently available, and another 1441 reviews were in progress when this chapter was finalized in spring 2004. Since new reviews are added quarterly, eventually all areas of health care will be covered. The Cochrane Library includes the Database of Abstracts of Reviews of Effectiveness, which contains more than 2500 structured abstracts of good-quality published reviews about the effectiveness of health interventions. Table 3–2 lists accessible sources of systematic reviews and provides a search strategy developed by librarians at McMaster University to locate systematic reviews and meta-analyses on MEDLINE efficiently.[15]

OPTION 4

Consider conducting a literature search on an electronic database such as MEDLINE if the question relates to new developments in therapeutic options. In this case, health care professionals must consult primary literature. Dozens of electronic databases exist as primary sources of original research reports.

MEDLINE and PubMed, both produced by the National Library of Medicine (NLM), are the largest and best known bibliographic databases of biomedical journal literature. PubMed's in-process records provide basic citation information and abstracts *before* the citations are indexed with NLM's Medical Subject Headings (MeSH) Terms and added to MEDLINE. To optimize the efficiency of a clinical search, PubMed offers specialized searches using methodologic filters. These filters, based on work by Haynes and colleagues,[15] are validated search strategies to identify clinically relevant studies

TABLE 3–2. Selected Resources for Systematic Reviews

Resources	Advantages	Disadvantages
Best Evidence Electronic version of both American College of Physicians (ACP) Journal Club and Evidence-Based Medicine (http://hiru.mcmaster.ca/acpjc/acpod.htm). Available on CD-ROM.	• All review articles are systematic reviews. • Updated every 6 months • Short title includes meta-analysis or review to facilitate identification	• Includes systematic reviews from only the journal scanned by ACP Journal Club and Evidence-Based Medicine
MEDLINE Systematic review search strategy: (meta-analy$ or metanal$ or metaanal$). tw. or Meta-Analysis/or meta-analysis (pt) or (quantitativ$ review$ or quantitativ$ overview$).tw. or (systematic$ review$ or systematic$ overview$).tw. or (methodologic$ review$ or methodologic$ overview$).tw. or medline.tw. or pooled.tw.) and eng.lg. and human/ not (letter or editorial or comment).pt	• Covers more than 4000 journals • Contains 11 million citations	• One-tenth of the citations are indexed as review articles. Even fewer are indexed as systematic reviews. • Requires search strategy to identify meta-analysis or systematic reviews
Cochrane Library Electronic library of high-quality reviews (*http://www.cochrane.org*). Available on CD-ROM.	• Most comprehensive collection of systematic reviews • Updated every 3 months • Abstracts of Cochrane Reviews are available free on the Internet at *http://www.cochrane.org.*	• Limited access; not all libraries subscribe to the Cochrane Library
United Kingdom National Health Services Centre for Reviews and Dissemination (*http://agatha.york.ac.uk/welcome.htm*) Includes the Database of Abstracts of Reviews of Effectiveness (DARE), NHS Economic evaluation database, and the Health Technology Assessment (HTA) database	• The DARE Web version, which is updated monthly, is more current than the Cochrane Library version.	• NHS economic evaluation, last update 1999
Effective Health Care Bulletins *http://www.york.ac.uk/inst/crd/ehcb.htm*	• Reports of systematic reviews produced by NHS Centre for Reviews and Dissemination	• Limited number of reviews
National Institute for Clinical Excellence Part of the UK National Health Service (NHS). Provides guidelines and technology assessments to health care practitioners (*http://nice.org.uk*).	• Follows Cochrane methodology to develop technology assessments. Twenty-eight have been completed, and 38 are in progress.	• Limited number of guidelines and assessments available

TABLE 3–3. Metasearch Engines for Web-Based Health Information

Turning Research Into Practice (TRIP)
Web address: *www.update-software.com/trip/about.htm*
Sources: Fifty-eight sites categorized as evidence-based, peer-reviewed journals, guidelines, or other. Sites include top 20 medical journals, EMB sites such as Bandolier, Critically Appraised Bank, Cochrane Database of Systematic Reviews, Journal Club on the Web, Evidence-Based Medicine series, guideline and systematic review sites such as SIGN, DARE, NICE, and National Guideline Clearinghouse.
Special features: Updated monthly. Searches use keywords in the title only. Results are displayed by categories: evidence-based, peer-reviewed journals, guidelines, or other.

SUMSearch
Web address: *http://SUMSearch.uthscsa.edu*
Sources: Three Internet sites: The National Library of Medicine, the Database of Abstracts of Reviews of Effectiveness, and the National Guideline Clearinghouse.
Special features: If the first search resulted in too many or not enough hits, SUMSearch uses metasearching and contingency search techniques to query the sites again.

Search.com
Web address: *http://www.search.com*
Sources: Twenty-two Internet sites containing health and medical information. Some of these sites are American College of Physicians Online, Centers for Disease Control and Prevention, *New England Journal of Medicine*, Agency for Healthcare Research and Quality, *Journal of the American Medical Association*, PubMed, Merck, Mayo Clinic, Food and Drug Administration, World Health Organization, WebMD, and Medical Subject Headings (MeSH).
Special features: The site allows customization in choosing search engines and how to display results.

Query Server
Web address: *http://queryserver.com*
Sources: Twelve sites containing health and medical information. These sites are American Health Consultants, American Heart Association, Centers for Disease Control and Prevention, Department of Health and Human Services, Food and Drug Administration, Johns Hopkins Infectious Diseases, Leukemia and Lymphoma Society, MEDLINE, Medscape Clinical Content, Medscape News, National Institutes of Health, National Library of Medicine.
Special features: Results are sorted according to content and/or source.

that answer questions about etiology, prognosis, diagnosis, or therapy of a disease.

To facilitate the searches of multiple Internet sources, metasearching is useful. Metasearch tools launch a single query across a set of Web-based health sites. One query returns a merged and often ranked list of hits, allowing the user to search several databases at once. Table 3–3 describes the specifics of new metasearch engines available to search for Internet-based health information.

Once the evidence is gathered, the clinician needs to determine whether the identified guideline, review article, or study report will help to answer the clinical problem. This is accomplished by considering the validity and by judging the clinical relevance (usefulness) of the information.[16]

ASSESSING VALIDITY

The *external validity* refers to applicability and generalization and is outlined in the section, "Applying the Results." The remainder of this section focuses on critically appraising the quality—that is, the *internal validity*—of individual trials. The internal validity is determined by how well the trial ensures that the known and unknown risk factors are equally distributed between the treatment and control groups. To ensure validity, the conduct of the trial should minimize systematic bias and random error as much as possible to provide results that are as accurate and close to the truth as possible. Four sources of bias are possible in trials of health care interventions: selection bias, performance bias, attrition bias, and detection bias. Bias can result in an overestimation or underestimation of the effectiveness of a drug therapy and mislead the reader. While it is beyond

the scope of this chapter to present extensive details about critical appraisal, here are some questions that must be answered in assessing the internal validity of an RCT:

- *Was the subject's treatment allocation randomized?* To minimize selection bias, all participants should have an equal chance to be allocated to the treatment or control group. Randomization is the best method to create groups of similar known and unknown confounders. If important risk factors known to affect prognosis (such as disease severity or presence of comorbidities) are unevenly distributed between groups, then selection bias could falsely estimate the benefit of the intervention. Furthermore, recruiters should not know which assignment (treatment or control group) is next in line. Recruiters who assess eligibility criteria and are aware of the next random allocation may consciously or unconsciously select the healthiest patient to be enrolled in the control group or vice versa. Approaches to randomization that may allow the recruiters to manipulate the assignment include improper use of record numbers (e.g., if all odd numbers were assigned to control group), dates of birth, day of the week, or open lists of random numbers. Examples of bias-free random allocations include centralized randomization (e.g., a central office unaware of subject characteristics allocates group assignments), pharmacy-controlled randomization (assuming that the pharmacist is not recruiting the subjects), and opaque envelopes that are numbered sequentially and sealed.[17]
- *Was the study double-blinded?* To minimize performance bias (systematic differences in the care provided, apart from the intervention being evaluated), the subjects and the clinicians should be unaware of the therapy received. The double-blind

method prevents subjects or clinicians from adding any additional treatments (or cointerventions) to one of the groups. For example, clinicians who know that certain patients are receiving the therapy they perceive to be less effective (control group) may opt to check on those patients more often than is required in the study protocol. A third blind can be applied to the outcome assessor (e.g., a statistician or clinician whose role is to measure the outcome) to minimize detection bias (systematic differences in outcome assessment). The necessity for blinding outcome assessors is controversial at this time.

- *Was intention-to-treat analysis performed?* Intention-to-treat analysis means that the results from all subjects randomized in the study were accounted for and attributed to the group to which they were assigned. This strategy minimizes attrition bias and ensures that the known and unknown prognostic factors are kept equally distributed. For example, exclusion of subjects who withdrew early in treatment may bias the

comparison because the reasons people withdraw early are often related to prognosis.[18] Excluding early withdrawals from the final analysis may select the subjects most likely to get the best outcome and thereby overestimate the benefit of the intervention.

For a more detailed description of the concepts in critical appraisal, a series of articles published in the *Journal of the American Medical Association (JAMA)* provides a useful tool for practitioners who are evaluating clinical trials.[19–50] These users' guides to the medical literature—developed by The Evidence-Based Medicine Working Group, a group of clinicians at Canada's McMaster University and colleagues across North America—can help to assess the validity of primary studies as well as review articles.

Online materials to support teaching of evidence-based health care, including the Users' Guides to Evidence-Based Practice, are now supported through the Centres for Health Evidence at *http://www.cche.net.* Table 3–4 summarizes the key elements to be

---

TABLE 3–4. Checklist for Critical Appraisal of Articles Addressing Pharmacotherapeutic Decisions

Therapy
Internal validity
- Was subject's treatment allocation randomized?
- Was the study double-blinded?
- Was intention-to-treat analysis performed?
- Was the randomization successful?

Magnitude of the effect
- What was the impact of the treatment?
- How narrow is the 95% confidence interval range?
- Were clinically relevant outcomes considered?

Applicability
- Does this patient fulfill inclusion criteria for the trial?
- Do the treatment benefits outweigh the risks?

Harm
Internal validity
- Were the control subjects similar to the cases?
- Was bias minimized while measuring exposure and outcomes?
- Was length of follow-up appropriate?
- Does exposure precede the adverse outcome?
- Is there a dose-response relationship?

Magnitude of the effect
- How strong is the association between exposure and outcome?
- How precise is the estimate?
- How many patients must be exposed to the agent to cause an adverse event?

Applicability
- What is the likelihood of harm in my patient?
- What are the consequences of eliminating the agent from my patient's therapy?

Overview, Systematic Reviews, Meta-analysis
Internal validity
- Did the overview clearly state a well-formulated question?
- Were the criteria used to select articles for inclusion appropriate?
- Were all relevant studies included?
- Were included articles critically appraised for quality?
- Was bias minimized in the selection, data extraction, and analysis processes?
- Were all clinically important outcomes considered?
- Were the studies appropriately combined?

Magnitude of the effect
- What is the average effect?
- How precise are the results?

Applicability
- Are this patient's characteristics similar to the subjects included in the studies?
- Do the treatment benefits outweigh the risks?

Practice Guidelines
Internal validity
- Were the management options and outcomes clearly specified?
- Was all evidence relevant to each arm of the evidence model sought?
- Were systematic and explicit methods used to identify, select, and combine evidence?
- Were all clinically relevant outcomes evaluated?
- Is the guideline up-to-date?
- Does the guideline clearly present the evidence to support the benefit of following the recommendations?
- Has the guideline been peer-reviewed?

Magnitude of the effect
- How strong are the recommendations?
- What is the impact of uncertainty in the evidence on outcomes?

Applicability
- Are the guideline recommendations targeting my practice (e.g., family practice setting versus endocrinology setting)?
- Is my patient the intended target for this guideline?

Economic Analyses
Internal validity
- Were both costs and outcomes evaluated for all strategies considered?
- Were costs and outcomes measured and valued accurately?
- Was the potential impact of uncertainties in the analysis evaluated?
- Was the potential impact of different baseline risk in the treatment population estimated on costs and outcomes?

Magnitude of the effect
- What were the incremental costs and outcomes of each strategy considered?
- Do incremental costs and outcomes vary between selected groups of patients?
- What is the impact of sensitivity analyses on incremental cost?

Applicability
- Do the treatment benefits outweigh the treatment risk and cost?
- Are the results transferable to my practice setting (e.g., similar patient types, similar costs of resources)?

Adapted from Users' Guide Series (Refs. 19 to 50).

addressed for each type of evidence to appraise internal validity and usefulness.[19–50]

CONSIDERING CLINICAL RELEVANCE

Once the clinician has gathered all relevant studies, eliminated those which addressed other questions, and identified those with the best methods, one question remains: So what? Also known as the "who cares" test,[51] applying this admittedly crude criterion begins the process of asking oneself, "Will these findings change the way I will treat or prevent this disease in my practice—and specifically for the patient sitting in front of me right now?"

The first step in making this decision is to consider the clinical value of the beneficial outcomes reported. Are the outcomes demonstrating improvements important to the patients? For example, a drug therapy that improves left ventricular ejection fraction (a surrogate end point) does not have the same clinical value as a drug that is shown to decrease mortality or improve functional status (primary end points) in an individual with heart failure.

The usefulness of an intervention depends not only on its efficacy but also on whether the magnitude of the benefit outweighs the risks, costs, and benefits of existing alternative interventions. In this context, the number needed to treat (NNT) and the number needed to harm (NNH) are clinically useful measures. NNT and NNH describe the number of patients who need to be treated and for how long to achieve one favorable or harmful outcome, respectively (Table 3–5 illustrates the values of NNT and NNH). The NNT strategy provides a way to estimate an intervention's impact and tradeoffs and to decide whether this therapy should be implemented.

The relative risk reduction (RRR), as a measure of the magnitude of an intervention's effect, can be misleading. It does not discriminate between large and trivial absolute differences between the control and experimental groups. For example, an intervention may result in a 50% risk reduction for the adverse outcome, and this amount of decrease would sound impressive to most clinicians and patients. However, it might represent only a small difference in the risk of a rare event (e.g., 0.2% of patients in a placebo group died compared with 0.1% of patients on active drug). In contrast, a 50% risk reduction might reflect a much more meaningful difference, for instance, when 50% of placebo group died versus 25% of patients in the intervention group (an absolute difference of 25%). The RRR is the same for both examples, but the magnitude of the impact of the intervention is drastically different. The information provided by the RRR is incomplete

---

TABLE 3–5. Number Needed to Treat and Number Needed to Harm

In this example, the clinical question is whether the addition of clopidogrel to the regimen of a 65-year-old man with unstable angina who is already taking aspirin would prevent death or coronary event? A search of published trials and presented papers at scientific meetings uncovered only one relevant study. It was presented in abstract form at the American College of Cardiology meeting on March 19, 2001.

In the trial:
- 12,562 subjects with coronary syndrome were randomized to aspirin alone or aspirin plus clopidogrel.
- On average, patients were followed for 9 months.
- The primary endpoint was to prevent cardiovascular (CV) death, myocardial infarction (MI), or stroke.

To calculate the number needed to treat (NNT), first calculate the absolute risk reduction (ARR). This is the absolute difference between the event rate in the control group (CER) minus the event rate in the experimental group (EER). The NNT is the inverse of the ARR.

The trial reports that 11.47% of the aspirin alone group (control group) had MI, stroke, or CV death. In contrast, 9.28% of the aspirin plus clopidogrel (experimental group) had these events.

Control Event Rate (Aspirin-Alone Group)	Experimental Event Rate (Aspirin Plus Clopidogrel)	RRR= (CER — EER)/CER	ARR = (CER — EER)	NNT = 1/ARR
11.47%	9.28%	19%	2.19%	46

Thus the NNT is 46. That is, treating 46 patients with unstable angina for 9 months with aspirin with clopidogrel should prevent MI, stroke, or CV death in 1 patient. To balance risks versus benefits of an intervention, we can generate a similar number needed to harm to express the risks associated to the intervention.

The trial reports that 2.7% of the aspirin-alone group had major nonfatal bleeding events compared with 3.6% in the intervention group (aspirin plus clopidogrel).

To calculate the number needed to harm (NNH), first calculate the absolute risk increase (ARI). This is the absolute difference between the event rate in the experimental group (EER) minus the event rate in the control group (CER). The NNH is the inverse of the ARI.

Control Event Rate	Experimental Event Rate	ARI (Absolute Risk Increase)	NNH
2.7%	3.6%	0.9%	111

The NNH is thus 111, meaning that treating 111 patients with both drugs for 9 months would result in 1 major nonfatal bleed. Combining the NNT and NNH and projecting the results to 1000 patients would lead to this conclusion: This randomized, controlled trial suggests that treating 1000 individuals with unstable angina with the combination of aspirin plus clopidogrel would prevent 21 patients from having a stroke, MI, or CV death at the cost of 9 major nonfatal bleeding events.

because it does not take into account the baseline risk of subjects in the trial.

CLINICAL CONTROVERSY

NNT and NNH can be a bit nebulous when it comes to applying these values in clinical situations. *P* values are considered significant routinely when they fall below 0.05, but what is a good NNT in one study may not be so good in another trial. NNT and NNH provide visualizations for how much risk and benefit are present when a group of similar patients—such as those seen by a physician or cared for in a pharmaceutical care clinic—are all treated with a medication or other intervention.

APPLYING THE RESULTS

For every health care professional, the ultimate test of which studies are important and which are not comes down to the decision of how to treat each patient. Thus clinical judgment is crucial in assessing the importance of drug-therapy evidence.

Several patient-specific factors must be considered in the final analysis:

1. *Compare the patient with those in the study (similar disease state and stage, similar baseline characteristics).* This assessment should ensure that the population studied has a similar disease state and prognostic factors as the patient now being treated. For instance, the results of a trial assessing the mortality benefit of simvastatin in dyslipidemic men with known coronary artery disease would not likely apply to dyslipidemic women with no other coronary risk factors.

2. *Consider the patient's baseline risk for the outcome of interest and other potential risks associated with the therapy.* If this patient has a higher baseline risk for the outcome than the population studied, then treatment may yield an even higher benefit. In contrast, if the patient has a lower baseline risk than the population studied, then treatment-associated risks may outweigh the potential benefit. For example, premenopausal women, in general, have a lower cardiovascular mortality risk than do men. Therefore, an intervention shown to prevent cardiovascular mortality in men may result in a smaller benefit in women.

3. *Consider the patient's values, beliefs, concerns, and readiness for the intervention.* In addition, health care delivery characteristics (cost and accessibility) must be factored in. While not very long ago health care professionals were considered patriarchal figures who directed the patient's treatment, today patients are fully engaged partners in decisions about therapy. The evidence must be discussed and integrated with the specific patient's circumstances to result in successful outcomes.

KEEPING UP TO DATE BY USING EBM

◀ The same combination of clinical experience and EBM skills that enables health care professionals to resolve patient-specific pharmacotherapeutic questions also aids health care professionals' continued efforts to keep up to date. The process is the same: (1) Recognize information needs (the areas of one's practice), (2) identify literature relevant to clinical practice, (3) critically appraise the evidence for validity and utility, and (4) devise a mechanism to implement new evidence in daily practice.

As with human knowledge in general, medical information is growing exponentially. Clinicians have difficulty staying current; a few statistics explain why. The National Library of Medicine contains more than 11 million citations covering nearly 4500 biomedical journals.[52] The number of citations *doubled* in just 6 years, from 1995 to 2001. Each year, 10,000 RCTs addressing the impact of health care interventions are published. Some influence how clinicians practice, others provide preliminary evidence that is too early to act on or is irrelevant to clinical practice, and others are seriously flawed and should not be implemented. Who has time to read it all and separate the good from the bad? A literature-sorting strategy, using the EBM approach, is one solution.

First, the clinician must recognize the areas important in his or her practice (e.g., internal medicine, cardiology, nuclear medicine, nutrition, psychiatry, or pharmacokinetics). Second, scan the literature for clinically relevant studies in that area of interest or practice. These are studies addressing clinical outcomes likely to be relevant to clinical practice and possibly change prescribing behaviors, such as those which report the effect of a pharmacotherapy on quality of life, cost-effectiveness, mortality, or morbidity. In contrast, trials addressing the impact of drug therapy on surrogate end points (e.g., biochemical markers) most often are irrelevant to current clinical practice and rarely would result in a change in practice. When in a "keeping up-to-date mode," choose the studies reporting clinically relevant outcomes over those with surrogate end points. Third, critically appraise the evidence for validity and usefulness. When addressing therapeutic efficacy, RCTs are considered the "gold standard" and should be preferred over observational studies for most clinical questions. Scan the abstracts of RCTs for obvious design flaws and size of the effect before appraising further. Shaughnessy and colleagues[53] have created a formula to help determine the usefulness of medical information (Fig. 3–1). Finally, integrate the new findings into one's daily practice.

If this process seems too labor-intensive for keeping pace with the medical literature, consider an evidence-based abstraction service. These services, which have grown tremendously in the past 10 years, claim to reduce by 98% the amount of clinical literature a clinician needs to read, enabling the busy health care professional to concentrate on the 2% that is most methodologically rigorous and useful to his or her practice.[54] In general, abstraction services consist of an editorial team that scans dozens of journals, usually organized by specialty. They identify articles of potential clinical relevance, critically appraise the studies, and provide commentary on the quality/validity and clinical significance of the results reported. Table 3–6 presents a selected list of translation journals offering evidence-based abstracts of original research.

$$\text{Usefulness of Medicine Information} = \frac{\text{Relevance} \times \text{Validity}}{\text{Work Factor}}$$

FIGURE 3–1. In this usefulness formula, *relevance* represents patient-oriented evidence that matters and affects health care, *validity* refers to a true estimate of the effect, and *work factor* describes the effort required to review the information.

TABLE 3–6. Evidence-Based Abstraction Services

ACP Journal Club (*http://www.acponline.org/journals/acpjc/jcmenu.htm*)
Audience: Internal medicine, primary care
Selection criteria: Original articles, systematic reviews, English, adult, clinically relevant with important outcomes, randomized controlled trials for treatment questions
Journals scanned: 26 journals

Bandolier (*http://www.jr2.ox.ac.uk/bandolier/*)
Audience: Internal medicine
Selection criteria: Those which look remotely interesting are read, and where they are both interesting and make sense, they are summarized
Journal scanned: Each month PubMed and the Cochrane Library are searched for systematic reviews and meta-analyses published in the recent past

Evidence-Based Cardiovascular Medicine (*http://www.harcourt-international.com/journals/ebcm/*)
Audience: Cardiology (adult and pediatric)
Selection criteria: Original articles, English, clinically relevant, adult or pediatric humans randomized controlled trials, double blinded
Journals scanned: 25 journals mostly cardiology specialty journals

Evidence-Based Health Care (*http://www.harcourt-international.com/journals/ebhc/*)
Audience: Managers
Selection criteria: Articles providing evidence for decision making; articles that are likely to be widely applicable
Journals scanned: More than 50 journals mostly with economics and public health focus

Evidence-Based Medicine (*http://www.evidence-basedmedicine.com*)
Audience: Internal medicine, general and family practice, surgery, psychiatry, pediatrics, and obstetrics and gynecologists
Selection criteria: Original articles, Cochrane Reviews, randomized controlled trial or therapeutic efficacy trial, clinically relevant outcomes, 80% follow-up
Journals scanned: More than 30 journals

Evidence-Based Mental Health (*http://www.ebmentalhealth.com/*)
Audience: Mental health clinicians
Selection criteria: Original articles, Cochrane Reviews, randomized controlled trial or therapeutic efficacy trial, clinically relevant outcomes, 80% follow-up
Journals scanned: Not available

Journal Watch series (*http://www.jwatch.org/*)
Audience: General medicine, dermatology, cardiology, psychiatry, women's health, emergency medicine, infectious disease, neurology, gastroenterology (specialty Journal Watch for each audience)
Selection criteria: Not given
Journals scanned: More than 50 journals

Journal of Family Practice (*http://www.jfp.msu.edu*)
Audience: Family practice, pharmacists
Selection criteria: High-quality articles with patient-oriented outcomes that have the greatest potential to change the way that primary care clinicians practice
Journals scanned: 80 journals

Journal Club on the Web (*http://www.journalclub.org*)
Audience: Internal medicine
Selection criteria: Not given
Journals scanned: *New England Journal of Medicine, Annals of Internal Medicine, Journal of the American Medical Association, The Lancet*

CONCLUSIONS

Is EBM realistic? The needed skills for practicing EBM may appear daunting, but once acquired, they can help health care professionals to better use available resources and time by knowing how to focus a search and be more critical in what reading and information to integrate into their knowledge base. Several sites have demonstrated that EBM can be incorporated into practice successfully.[55–58]

Why practice EBM? Implementing EBM in a practice provides a framework and the skills to strengthen confidence in pharmacotherapeutic decisions and results in better communication with colleagues involved in the decision-making process. Furthermore, an evidence-based pharmaceutical care plan facilitates dialogue with patients about the rationale for the management decisions. Finally, using EBM principles enables practicing health care professionals to update their knowledge continuously.

This chapter provides tools for health care professionals to

1. Identify rapidly evidence-based clinical practice guidelines
2. Identify rapidly systematic reviews
3. Conduct validated searches to identify studies answering pharmacotherapy questions
4. Critically appraise the literature found
5. Assess relevance and applicability of the evidence

6. Develop strategies to triage the most useful literature and help to keep pace with the evidence that makes a difference in one's practice

ABBREVIATIONS

CAD: coronary artery disease
EBM: evidence-based medicine
MeSH: medical subject headings
MI: myocardial infarction
NLM: National Library of Medicine
NNH: number needed to harm
NNT: number needed to treat
PICO: patient, intervention, comparison, outcome
PVC: premature ventricular contraction
PCT: randomized, controlled trial
RRR: relative risk reduction

Review Questions and other resources can be found at *www.pharmacotherapyonline.com.*

REFERENCES

1. Etminan M, Wright JM, Carleton BC. Evidence-based pharmacotherapy: Review of basic concepts and applications in clinical practice. Ann Pharmacother 1998;32:1193–1200.
2. Swales JD. Evidence-based medicine and hypertension. J Hypertens 1999;17:1511–1516.
3. Mancia G, Zanchetti A. Evidence-based medicine: An educational instrument or a standard for implementation (editorial)? J Hypertens 1999;17:1509–1510.
4. Echt DS, Liebson PR, Mitchell B, et al. Mortality and morbidity in patients receiving encainide, flecainide or placebo: The Cardiac Arrhythmia Suppression Trial. N Engl J Med 1991;324:781–788.
5. Greene HL, Roden DM, Katz RJ, et al. The Cardiac Arrhythmia Suppression Trial: First CAST, then CAST-II. J Am Coll Cardiol 1992;19:894–898.
6. Ryan TJ, Antman EM, Brooks NH, et al. 1999 Update: ACC/AHA guidelines for the management of patients with acute myocardial infarction. A report of the American College of Cardiology/American Heart Association Task Force on Practice Guidelines (Committee on Management of Acute Myocardial Infarction). J Am Coll Cardiol 1999;34:890–911.
7. Ryan TJ, Anderson JL, Antman EM, et al. ACC/AHA guidelines for the management of patients with acute myocardial infarction: A report of the American College of Cardiology/American Heart Association Task Force on Practice Guidelines (Committee on Management of Acute Myocardial Infarction). J Am Coll Cardiol 1996;28:1328–1428.
8. Hulley S, Grady D, Bush T, et al. Randomized trial of estrogen plus progestin for secondary prevention of coronary heart disease in postmenopausal women. Heart and Estrogen/progestin Replacement Study (HERS) Research Group. JAMA 1998;280:605–613.
9. Sackett DL, Richardson SW, Rosenberg W, Haynes BR. Evidence-Based Medicine: How to Practice and Teach EBM. New York, Churchill-Livingstone, 1997.
10. Richardson WS, Wilson MC, Nishikawa J, Hayward RSA. The well-built clinical question: A key to evidence-based decisions (editorial). ACP J Club 1995;123:A12–A13.
11. Ghosh AK, Ghosh K. Enhance your practice with evidence-based medicine. Patient Care 2000;Feb:32–56.
12. Oxman A, Guyatt GH. The science of reviewing research. Ann NY Acad Sci 1993;703:125–134.
13. Mulrow CD. The medical review article: State of the science. Ann Intern Med 1987;106:485–488.
14. Mulrow CD. Rationale for systematic reviews. Br Med J 1994;309:597–599.
15. Haynes RB, Wilczynski NL, McKibbon KA, et al. Developing optimal search strategies for detecting clinically sound studies in MEDLINE. J Am Med Inform Assoc 1994;1:447–458.
16. Huth EJ. How to Write and Publish Papers in the Medical Sciences, 2d ed. Philadelphia, ISI Press, 1990:56–57.
17. Chalmers TC, Smith H Jr, Blackburn B, et al. A method for assessing the quality of a randomized control trial. Control Clin Trials 1981;2:31–49.
18. Horwitz RI, Viscoli CM, Berkman L, et al. Treatment adherence and risk of death after a myocardial infarction. Lancet 1990;336:542–545.
19. Oxman AD, Sackett DL, Guyatt GH. Users' guides to the medical literature: I. How to get started. The Evidence-Based Medicine Working Group. JAMA 1993;270:2093–2095.
20. Guyatt GH, Sackett DL, Cook DJ. Users' guides to the medical literature: II. How to use an article about therapy or prevention. A. Are the results of the study valid? Evidence-Based Medicine Working Group. JAMA 1993;270:2598–2601.
21. Guyatt GH, Sackett DL, Cook DJ. Users' guides to the medical literature: II. How to use an article about therapy or prevention. B. What were the results and will they help me in caring for my patients? Evidence-Based Medicine Working Group. JAMA 1994;271:59–63.
22. Jaeschke R, Guyatt G, Sackett DL. Users' guides to the medical literature: III. How to use an article about a diagnostic test. A. Are the results of the study valid? Evidence-Based Medicine Working Group. JAMA 1994;271:389–391.
23. Jaeschke R, Guyatt GH, Sackett DL. Users' guides to the medical literature: III. How to use an article about a diagnostic test. B. What are the results and will they help me in caring for my patients? The Evidence-Based Medicine Working Group. JAMA 1994;271:703–707.
24. Levine M, Walter S, Lee H, et al. Users' guides to the medical literature: IV. How to use an article about harm. Evidence-Based Medicine Working Group. JAMA 1994;271:1615–1619.
25. Laupacis A, Wells G, Richardson WS, Tugwell P. Users' guides to the medical literature: V. How to use an article about prognosis. Evidence-Based Medicine Working Group. JAMA 1994;272:234–237.
26. Oxman AD, Cook DJ, Guyatt GH. Users' guides to the medical literature: VI. How to use an overview. Evidence-Based Medicine Working Group. JAMA 1994;272:1367–1371.
27. Richardson WS, Detsky AS. Users' guides to the medical literature: VII. How to use a clinical decision analysis. A. Are the results of the study valid? Evidence-Based Medicine Working Group. JAMA 1995;273:1292–1295.
28. Richardson WS, Detsky AS. Users' guides to the medical literature: VII. How to use a clinical decision analysis. B. What are the results and will they help me in caring for my patients? Evidence Based Medicine Working Group. JAMA 1995;273:1610–1613.
29. Hayward RS, Wilson MC, Tunis SR, et al. Users' guides to the medical literature: VIII. How to use clinical practice guidelines. A. Are the recommendations valid? The Evidence-Based Medicine Working Group. JAMA 1995;274:570–574.
30. Wilson MC, Hayward RS, Tunis SR, et al. Users' guides to the medical literature: VIII. How to use clinical practice guidelines. B. What are the recommendations and will they help you in caring for your patients? The Evidence-Based Medicine Working Group. JAMA 1995;274:1630–1632.
31. Guyatt GH, Sackett DL, Sinclair JC, et al. Users' guides to the medical literature: IX. A method for grading health care recommendations. Evidence-Based Medicine Working Group. JAMA 1995;274:1800–1804.
32. Naylor CD, Guyatt GH. Users' guides to the medical literature: X. How to use an article reporting variations in the outcomes of health services. The Evidence-Based Medicine Working Group. JAMA 1996;275:554–558.
33. Naylor CD, Guyatt GH. Users' guides to the medical literature: XI. How to use an article about a clinical utilization review. Evidence-Based Medicine Working Group. JAMA 1996;275:1435–1439.
34. Guyatt GH, Naylor CD, Juniper E, et al. Users' guides to the medical literature: XII. How to use articles about health-related quality of life. Evidence-Based Medicine Working Group. JAMA 1997;277:1232–1237.

35. Drummond MF, Richardson WS, O'Brien BJ, et al. Users' guides to the medical literature: XIII. How to use an article on economic analysis of clinical practice. A. Are the results of the study valid? Evidence-Based Medicine Working Group. JAMA 1997;277:1552–1557.

36. O'Brien BJ, Heyland D, Richardson WS, et al. Users' guides to the medical literature: XIII. How to use an article on economic analysis of clinical practice. B. What are the results and will they help me in caring for my patients? Evidence-Based Medicine Working Group. JAMA 1997;277:1802–1806.

37. Dans AL, Dans LF, Guyatt GH, Richardson S. Users' guides to the medical literature: XIV. How to decide on the applicability of clinical trial results to your patient. Evidence-Based Medicine Working Group. JAMA 1998;279:545–549.

38. Richardson WS, Wilson MC, Guyatt GH, et al. Users' guides to the medical literature: XV. How to use an article about disease probability for differential diagnosis. Evidence-Based Medicine Working Group. JAMA 1999;281:1214–1219.

39. Guyatt GH, Sinclair J, Cook DJ, Glasziou P. Users' guides to the medical literature: XVI. How to use a treatment recommendation. Evidence-Based Medicine Working Group and the Cochrane Applicability Methods Working Group. JAMA 1999;281:1836–1843.

40. Barratt A, Irwig L, Glasziou P, et al. Users' guides to the medical literature: XVII. How to use guidelines and recommendations about screening. Evidence-Based Medicine Working Group. JAMA 1999;281:2029–2034.

41. Randolph AG, Haynes RB, Wyatt JC, et al. Users' guides to the medical literature: XVIII. How to use an article evaluating the clinical impact of a computer-based clinical decision support system. JAMA 1999;282:67–74.

42. Bucher HC, Guyatt GH, Cook DJ, et al. Users' guides to the medical literature: XIX. Applying clinical trial results. A. How to use an article measuring the effect of an intervention on surrogate end points. Evidence-Based Medicine Working Group. JAMA 1999;282:771–778.

43. McAlister FA, Laupacis A, Wells GA, Sackett DL. Users' guides to the medical literature: XIX. Applying clinical trial results. B. Guidelines for determining whether a drug is exerting (more than) a class effect. JAMA 1999;282:1371–1377.

44. Hunt DL, Jaeschke R, McKibbon KA. Users' guides to the medical literature: XXI. Using electronic health information resources in evidence-based practice. Evidence-Based Medicine Working Group. JAMA 2000;283:1875–1879.

45. McAlister FA, Straus SE, Guyatt GH, Haynes RB. Users' guides to the medical literature: XX. Integrating research evidence with the care of the individual patient. Evidence-Based Medicine Working Group. JAMA 2000;283:2829–2836.

46. McGinn TG, Guyatt GH, Wyer PC, et al. Users' guides to the medical literature: XXII. How to use articles about clinical decision rules. Evidence-Based Medicine Working Group. JAMA 2000;284:79–84.

47. Giacomini MK, Cook DJ. Users' guides to the medical literature: XXIII. Qualitative research in health care. A. Are the results of the study valid? Evidence-Based Medicine Working Group. JAMA 2000;284:357–362.

48. Giacomini MK, Cook DJ. Users' guides to the medical literature: XXIII. Qualitative research in health care. B. What are the results and how do they help me care for my patients? Evidence-Based Medicine Working Group. JAMA 2000;284:478–482.

49. Richardson WS, Wilson MC, Williams JW Jr, et al. Users' guides to the medical literature: XXIV. How to use an article on the clinical manifestations of disease. Evidence-Based Medicine Working Group. JAMA 2000;284:869–875.

50. Guyatt GH, Haynes RB, Jaeschke RZ, et al. Users' guides to the medical literature: XXV. Evidence-based medicine: Principles for applying the users' guides to patient care. Evidence-Based Medicine Working Group. JAMA 2000;284:1290–1296.

51. Huth EJ. Writing and Publishing in Medicine, 3d ed. Baltimore, Williams & Wilkins, 1999:10–12.

52. National Library of Medicine, Bethesda, MD; accessed at http://www.nlm.nih.gov/pubs/factsheets/pubmed.html, April 12, 2004.

53. Shaughnessy AF, Slawson DC, Bennet JH. Becoming an information master: A guidebook to the medical information jungle. J Fam Pract 1994;39:484–499.

54. Sackett DL, Haynes RB. 13 steps, 100 people, 1,000,000 thanks. Evidence Based Med 1997;2:101–102.

55. Ellis J, Mulligan I, Rower J, Sackett DL. Inpatient general medicine is evidence-based. Lancet 1995;346:407–410.

56. Geddes JR, Game D, Jenkins NE, et al. What proportion of primary psychiatric interventions are based on randomised evidence? Qual Health Care 1996;5:215–217.

57. Gill P, Dowell AC, Neal RP, et al. Evidence-based general practice: A retrospective study of interventions in our training practice. Br Med J 1996;312:819–821.

58. Kenny SE, Shankar KR, Rentala R, et al. Evidence-based surgery: Interventions in a regional pediatric surgical unit. Arch Dis Child 1997;76:50–53.

4

DOCUMENTATION OF PHARMACY SERVICES

George E. MacKinnon III and Neil J. MacKinnon

Learning Objectives and other resources can be found at *www.pharmacotherapyonline.com*.

KEY CONCEPTS

◀ Documentation of pharmacists' interventions and intent and their actions and impact on patient outcomes is central to the process of pharmaceutical care.

◀ Unless pharmacists in all practice settings document their activities and communicate with other health professionals, they may not be considered an essential and integral part of the health care team.

◀ Manual systems of documentation for pharmacists have been described in detail, but increasingly electronic systems are used to facilitate integration with payer records and health care systems.

◀ Integrated electronic information systems can facilitate provision of seamless care as patients move among ambulatory, acute, and long-term care settings.

◀ Federal systems of documentation are becoming increasingly important models in the United States as the Medicare Part D (oral prescription drug) benefit is implemented.

◀ Electronic medical records have several advantages over manual systems that will facilitate access by community pharmacists and their participation as fully participating members of the health care team.

As the opportunities to become more patient-focused increase and market pressures exert increased accountability for pharmacists' actions, the importance of documenting pharmacists' professional activities related to patient care will become paramount in the years to come. Processes to document the clinical activities and therapeutic interventions of pharmacists have been described extensively in the pharmacy literature, yet universal adoption of documentation throughout pharmacy practice remains inconsistent, incomplete, and misunderstood.

◀ Documentation is central to the provision of pharmaceutical care.[1] Pharmaceutical care is provided through a "system" in which feedback loops are established for monitoring purposes. This has advantages compared with the traditional medication-use process because the system enhances communication among members of the health care team and the patient. Pharmaceutical care requires responsibility by the provider to identify drug-related problems (DRPs), provide a therapeutic monitoring plan, and ensure that patients receive the most appropriate medicines and ultimately achieve their desired level of health-related quality of life (HRQOL).

To provide pharmaceutical care, the pharmacist, patient, and other providers enter a covenantal relationship that is considered to be mutually beneficial to all parties. The patient grants the pharmacist the opportunity to provide care, and the pharmacist, in turn, must accept this and the responsibility it entails. Documentation enables the pharmaceutical care model of pharmacy practice to be maximized and communicated to vested parties. Communication among sites of patient care must be accurate and timely to facilitate pharmaceutical care. As discussed by Hepler,[1] documentation supports care that is coordinated, efficient, and cooperative.

Conversely, failure to document activities and patient outcomes can directly affect patients' quality of care. There are several reasons for failure to document in the medication-use system, and these are related to the process of documentation, the specific data collected on a consistent basis, how documentation is shared (e.g., other pharmacists, health care providers, patients, insurers), and methods by which the data are shared.

In describing the medication-use system, Grainger-Rousseau and colleagues[2,3] have proposed eight essential structures, or elements, that must be in place for drug therapy to be both safe and effective (Table 4–1). When interventions are being planned to improve the medication-use system, all eight elements must be considered. When one or more of these eight essential elements are missing in the care of a patient, that patient is at a high risk of experiencing a DRP. One of these elements (number 7) is documentation and communication.

The lack of a universal reimbursement model for cognitive services provided by pharmacists can serve as a roadblock for initiating documentation; however, the opportunity to demonstrate contributions to patient outcomes and safety should serve as a catalyst for pharmacists to document their services provided in all practice settings. While a reimbursement model associated with professional services for the profession may emerge as Medicare Part D is implemented, its description is beyond the scope of this chapter. The reasons why pharmacists should document their patient care activities, along with the specific information that should be recorded, as well as examples of documentation systems and forms that have been used successfully, are illustrated in this chapter.

NEED FOR PHARMACIST DOCUMENTATION

The 1999 Institute of Medicine (IOM) Report (*To Err Is Human: Building a Safer Health System*) detailed the finding that as many as 98,000 Americans die unnecessarily every year as a result of medical

TABLE 4–1. Eight Elements of a Safe and Effective Drug Therapy System[2,3]

Element	Examples
Timely recognition of drug indications and other signs and symptoms relevant to drug use with accurate identification of underlying disease	"Correct" therapy for a late or incorrect diagnosis cannot improve a patient's quality of life
Safe, accessible, and cost-effective medicines	Safe and cost-effective (efficient) drug products must be legally and financially available
Appropriate prescribing for explicit (clear, measurable, and communicable) objectives	Explicit therapeutic objectives simplify the assessment of prescribing appropriateness and are necessary for assessing (monitoring) therapeutic outcomes
Drug product distribution, dispensing, and administration with appropriate patient advice	Including (1) ensuring that a patient actually obtained the medicine, (2) negotiating a regimen that the patient can tolerate and afford, (3) ensuring that a patient (or caregiver) can correctly use the medicine and administration devices, (4) advising to empower the patient or caregiver to cooperate in his or her own care as much as possible
Patient participation in care (intelligent adherence)	The ambulatory patient or caregiver should consent to therapeutic objectives and know the signs of therapeutic success, adverse effects, and toxicities; when to expect them; and what to do if they appear
Monitoring (problem detection and resolution)	Many failures can be detected while they are still problems and before they become adverse outcomes or treatment failures
Documentation and communication of information and decisions	Communication and documentation are necessary for cooperation in a system
Product and system performance evaluation and improvement	Practice guidelines, performance indicators, and databases are a useful approach to achieving and maintaining improved system performance (outcomes)

mistakes and errors, of which 7000 deaths were attributable to medication errors, costing upwards of $9 billion.[4] Handwritten prescriptions, orders, notes, and other methods of communication, unless transcribed electronically, are fraught with potential for misinterpretation and are error-prone. Through professional obligations, pharmacists in all settings (e.g., community, hospital, long-term care) play a pivotal role in ensuring the appropriate use of medications through prescription procurement or compounding, verification of the appropriateness of prescribed products (e.g., dose, duration, dosage form, and intended use) with prescribers, processing of prescription insurance-related claims, counseling of patients, and ultimately, follow-up and monitoring. The ability to continue to support uncompensated professional services and act as a critical safety net with respect to medication use in the health care system is now at a critical juncture and requires the profession's immediate attention and subsequent action.

Documentation is the primary method to demonstrate value within an organized health care system. More importantly, it is the accepted method by which health care providers communicate with one another with respect to patient care decision making and clinical outcomes. Thus, if pharmacists in all practice settings are not communicating data/information routinely with other providers, they may not be considered an essential and integral part of the health care team.

FORCES AFFECTING CLINICAL DOCUMENTATION

- The need for enhanced communication among health care providers
- A focus on reducing redundancy and the potential for fatal and nonfatal medical errors and preventable drug-related morbidity in all practice settings

- The emergence of electronic medical records (EMRs) in health care, thereby facilitating the sharing of data and aiding in clinical decision making
- The need to maintain secure patient and provider data while also making this information available to other key individuals
- The desire of patients to communicate more regularly with health care providers and to obtain health care information in a more convenient manner

In the community setting, pharmacists may be one of the most accessible health care providers seen by patients on a regular basis (e.g., when medications are dispensed or over-the-counter products and diagnostics are purchased). By actively participating in the management of prescribed and nonprescribed drug products, as well as monitoring associated clinical outcomes, pharmacists can make a valuable contribution to patient care and demonstrate their impact on clinical and economic outcomes. While such activities presently are occurring in community practice, the provision of timely documentation to other providers and patients alike often is lacking.

STRUCTURE AND ORGANIZATION OF DOCUMENTATION

A great deal has been written about manual documentation systems in the pharmacy literature, both in clinical practice and in education, but these systems tend to be individualized applications in which the transfer of data to other providers is nonexistent or quite limited.[5–8] Many documentation systems in pharmacy focus on the generation of reports for workload analysis or accreditation purposes. Unfortunately, the information gathered and analyzed in such applications does little, if anything, to improve patient care if it is not in a real-time format.

The principal purpose of clinical documentation is to provide a record of what a practitioner does, why it is done, and when possible, what outcomes are achieved. It is essential to document succinctly the patient-specific recommendations and actions taken by pharmacists and why these decisions were made. Functions performed by pharmacists, such as obtaining medication histories, counseling patients, performing limited patient assessment and monitoring, conducting drug regimen reviews, and providing drug information are direct services that benefit patients, pharmacists, and other health care providers in various practice settings. The provision of these services by pharmacists and their associated outcomes need to be documented and communicated on a consistent basis. Documentation that occurs in a vacuum and devoid of real-time dissemination ultimately may not benefit patient care.

KEY CHARACTERISTICS OF CLINICAL DOCUMENTATION

- The primary purpose of clinical documentation is to provide a record of what a practitioner does, why it is done, and where possible, what outcomes are achieved.
- Clinical documentation should provide a real-time trail of care provided to patients.
- Documentation systems and applications must be easy to use, portable, produce useful reports, be replicated by others consistently, and allow for knowledge sharing with other providers.

While convenient and easy to use, paper documentation forms can be time-consuming to complete accurately, are inefficient in terms of producing useful information, and often result in inconsistent reporting because there is great variance in their format and use among practitioners. Efficient and effective documentation systems capable of capturing data supporting the involvement of the profession in direct patient care activities must be developed, tested in clinical settings, and used uniformly in practice.

TYPES OF PATIENT INFORMATION TO DOCUMENT

A well-designed documentation system serves a multitude of purposes. It encompasses a complete and comprehensive archive of the patient's drug-related information, a record of pharmaceutical care interventions, and all care plans and outcomes, and it also may serve as a legal record of the care that has been provided.[9]

PROBLEM-ORIENTED MEDICAL RECORD

Information within a patient's file must be organized in a fashion that facilitates quick retrieval. One commonly used and efficient method of organization is the problem-oriented medical record (POMR) format, whereby documents within a patient's file are organized according to a list of problems.[10] This process, pioneered by Dr. Lawrence Weed, consists of four major components: a defined database, a problem list, an initial plan, and progress notes. Each document is to be filed according to the source from which it comes, typically physician orders, nursing notes, and laboratory and diagnostic results. The clinical notes for each medical problem commonly are organized according to the SOAP approach: *s*ubjective and *o*bjective data, *a*ssessment, and therapeutic *p*lan.

Subjective data are related to the identified problem and associated symptoms as described by the patient himself or herself (or in some cases by the caregivers of the patient). *Objective data* include observations made and information acquired by the health care practitioner that is determined to be relevant to the identified patient problems. The *assessment* refers to the practitioner's clinical opinion or judgment about the problem based on subjective and objective data, as well as the practitioner's previous experiences related to similar clinical problems and patients. The *plan* is the course of action deemed appropriate for each identified problem given the data available to the clinician.

DRUG-RELATED PROBLEMS

While the SOAP approach is very practical and systematic, it may not be appropriate for many pharmacists because there are limitations with respect to consistent access to certain data elements available in many practice settings. Additional concerns relate to the redundancy created in a patient record if the pharmacy documentation is to become part of an existing record. Such patient medical records are already voluminous, and only succinct, essential information needs to be added. Thus the contributions of pharmacist-generated documentation should be supportive of a patient's care plan to assist in achieving defined therapeutic objectives and/or avoiding drug-related problems (DRPs) where appropriate.[11]

DRUG-RELATED PROBLEMS

- Untreated indication
- Improper drug selection
- Subtherapeutic dosage
- Overdosage/toxicity
- Failure to receive drug
- Adverse drug reactions/events
- Interactions
- Drug use without indication

When a pharmacist identifies a DRP, it may be listed and counted among the documents for an existing problem (e.g., subtherapeutic dose of a proton pump inhibitor for treatment of an ulcer), or if the cause is not readily identifiable, it may be listed as a new problem. All patient files established by a pharmacist should contain similar basic elements. For example, to provide pharmaceutical care, such as identification of DRPs, pharmacists need specific knowledge about the patient, such as demographic characteristics, social and medical history, general appearance, health status, and third-party insurance or billing information.[9]

Currie and colleagues[12] devised a tool to assess the quality of pharmacists' documentation. These researchers created a list of data elements after a comprehensive literature search and input from practitioners and expert panels. The elements are divided into two groups: those essential to each individual patient encounter and those essential to a patient record (Table 4–2). The acquisition of each of these elements is critical to the provision of pharmaceutical care.

COMMUNICATION OF DOCUMENTATION AND FINDINGS

Once patient information has been documented appropriately, it should be made available to other health care providers for review when necessary. Without a universal electronic documentation

TABLE 4–2. Elements to Be Documented by the Pharmacist[12]

Status of Element	For Patient Encounters*	For Patient Records
Essential	Patient identifier	Patient identifier
	Date of encounter	Date of birth
	Reason for encounter	Sex
	Pharmacist identifier	Contact information
	History of present illness	Allergies and adverse drug reactions
	Relevant prescription, over-the-counter, and alternative mediations (history and compliance)	Medical problem(s), current and past
	Assessment (conclusions reached by the pharmacists after assessment of the drug therapy)	Prescription, nonprescription, and alternative medications (history and adherence)
	Plan(s)/action(s) to correct problem(s) (A listing of planned steps to achieve the goals established with the patient for the patient's drug therapy; the goal of the therapy should be implicitly or explicitly stated)	Payment method and economic situation
	Monitoring plan and follow-up (steps to monitor the outcomes of actions taken)	
To be included if relevant	Past medical history	Family history
	Family history	Social history
	Social history (diet, alcohol, tobacco use, caregiver status, etc.)	Ethnic background
	Objective information (e.g., vital signs, laboratory results, diagnostic signs or physical examination results)	Objective information (a compilation of testing results from the pharmacy practice or other testing site)
		Special needs of patient (e.g., need for assistive devices, special educational needs)
		Nonmedication therapy

*The essential elements may be present in the chart and referred to in the note and not repeated in the encounter note itself. If there is a follow-up encounter, the note could be abbreviated.

system in place for pharmacists, various means of communication (e.g., mail, fax, phone, or e-mail) can be used to communicate with other health care providers and patients where appropriate. One patient may have several patient files at different sites of care (e.g., in the hospital, in various physicians' offices, and in community pharmacies), thus complicating the manner of communication. However, it is critical to determine what information must be passed on to fellow health care workers.

An integral part of providing pharmaceutical care is monitoring patient outcomes. To follow patients effectively throughout the course of their therapy, monitoring parameters and desired outcomes must be determined and documented. Examples of monitoring parameters include reducing the blood pressure in a hypertensive post–myocardial infarction patient to less than 120/80 mm Hg and reducing the low-density lipoprotein cholesterol to less than 100 mg/dL. Properly documenting this information assists other pharmacists and health care professionals during follow-up appointments because the preestablished monitoring parameters and recommended changes (based on collected data from all providers) can be reviewed readily.

DOCUMENTATION AND SEAMLESS CARE

Although the exact terminology may vary, *seamless care* is a concept that has been viewed widely as a fundamental component of the optimal delivery of health care services. Several different health professions, including nursing, occupational therapy, and others, have published studies in which seamless care was provided within the context of their own practice environments.[13] Where seamless care is provided, effort is placed on developing multidisciplinary teams that work together across any transitions of care that may arise.[14]

In recent years, the average length of hospital stays has shortened, and consequently, patients are being discharged into the ambulatory setting and long-term care facilities at a higher level of acuity. Regrettably, in most health systems, an effective means of communication regarding patients' drug therapy has not been established across the continuum of care. Such communication is vital since drugs may be added to or discontinued from a patient's drug regimen during hospitalization, or dosing may be altered. One study that tracked changes in medications over a hospitalization period in the elderly (age 65 and over) reported that 71% of patients had at least one of their admission medications discontinued by the time they were discharged from hospital, accounting for 40% of all admission medications.[15]

Patients, caregivers, and community pharmacists may be unclear as to what medication changes have been made in the inpatient setting and the reasons for these changes. Subsequently, there may be DRPs in the patient's medication regimen that will not be identified or resolved in a timely fashion. The community pharmacist, who may fill discharge prescriptions, generally is not privy to information regarding the patient's diagnosis and laboratory test results. In essence, the community pharmacist is uninformed and at a disadvantage to monitor for future DRPs that may result from previous medication regimen alterations. A study in the United Kingdom indicated that 95.7% of community pharmacists surveyed would not even know if one of their patients had been admitted recently to a hospital.[16]

Problems stemming from care that is not seamless are not limited to patients who are moving from a hospital to the community. Equally important is the provision of seamless care from the hospital to long-term care setting and the community pharmacy to the hospital pharmacy setting.

TABLE 4–3. Seven Principles of the Australian National Seamless Care Guidelines[20]

Principle 1	It is the responsibility of the admitting institution to ensure the development and coordination of a medication discharge plan for each patient. The person responsible for coordinating the development, implementation, and monitoring of the medication discharge plan, including medication supply and medication information, should be identified as soon as practicable after admission.
Principle 2	Hospital staff should obtain an accurate medication history, including prescription and nonprescription medicines and other therapies such as herbal products, at the time of admission.
Principle 3	Hospital staff should evaluate the current medication at the time of admission, in consultation with the patient's general practitioner, with a view to (1) identifying the appropriateness and effectiveness of current medication and rationalizing current medications if appropriate, (2) paying particular attention to any problems associated with current drug therapy, including any possible relationship with the current medical conditions, and (3) documenting allergies and any previous adverse drug reactions.
Principle 4	During the hospital stay, treatment plans relating to the probable medication management during the stay and, where applicable, at discharge should be developed in consultation with the patient and/or caregiver. Hospital staff should negotiate with the patient issues relating to treatment and the development of a discharge plan, and these discussions should be documented in the patient's notes. This plan should form part of the overall care plan or critical pathway.
Principle 5	Prior to discharge, predischarge medication review and dispensing of adequate medication should take place in a planned and timely fashion. Adequate medication means sufficient medication to carry the patient through to the next arranged review or to complete course of treatment.
Principle 6	At the time of discharge, each patient should be provided with a discharge folio containing relevant information such as consumer medicine information, a medication record, patient/care plan, and information on the availability and future supply of medication.
Principle 7	No patient should be discharged from hospital until the details of the admission, medication changes, and arrangements for follow-up have been communicated to the health care provider(s) identified by the patient as being responsible for his or her ongoing care.

STUDIES INVOLVING THE EVALUATION OF DOCUMENTATION BY PHARMACISTS ACROSS THE CONTINUUM OF CARE

Several studies evaluating the impact of the provision of proper documentation by pharmacists across the continuum of care have been conducted in Australia, Canada, the United Kingdom, the United States, and beyond. Examples of such studies are presented. The examples are not meant to be a comprehensive list of all such activities but rather are reviewed to give an indication of the state of pharmacist documentation in each country.

PHARMACIST-DIRECTED DOCUMENTATION INITIATIVES IN AUSTRALIA

Pharmacist-directed documentation activities in Australia have been the center of considerable attention in recent years. The need for these services has been articulated in the *Australian Journal of Hospital Pharmacy*: "... hospital-based services developed with little thought to what happens to patients before they come to the hospital and after they leave. This has placed hospital pharmacy in a dangerously isolated position," and "presently Australia has no system that effectively manages information relating to medications. This lack of timely and accurate medication information remains a significant barrier to ensuring the quality use of medications by the community at large."[17] The Department of Pharmacy at the Royal North Shore Hospital in Sydney reported on a practice guide for the provision of pharmaceutical care that, among other things, helped to educate the patient at the time of discharge to promote seamless care as the patient returned back into the community.[18]

The Pharmacy Continuity of Care Project, a study by the Faculty of Pharmacy at the University of Sydney, promoted the use of patient discharge forms that were sent by the hospital pharmacist to (1) the community pharmacist and (2) case conferences between these two individuals and the patient's general practitioner.[19]

One of the more significant developments in Australia has been the publication of the Australian Pharmaceutical Advisory Council's *National Guidelines to Achieve the Continuum of Quality Use of Medicines Between Hospital and Community*. This 1998 publication contained seven principles that are recommended to be followed to help to attain a high level of seamless pharmaceutical care[20] (Table 4–3).

PHARMACIST-DIRECTED DOCUMENTATION INITIATIVES IN CANADA

The profession of pharmacy in Canada also has been active in documentation activities across the continuum of care. In 1994, Cameron[21] reported on the findings of a pilot project in Halifax, Nova Scotia, in which forms completed by the hospital pharmacist that contained either the rationale for inpatient medication changes or recommendations for future changes were sent to family physicians and community pharmacists. Austin[22] provided an overview of seamless care issues in Canada in 1995, including the description of a seamless care program called Palliative At-Home Care Team at the Scarborough General Hospital in Ontario. More recently, other researchers have evaluated the use of hospital discharge prescription summary forms in Halifax, Nova Scotia,[23] and Montreal, Quebec.[24] Seamless care pilot projects also have been undertaken in Calgary; Alberta; Montreal, Quebec; and Pictou County, Nova Scotia, as described in the cases at the end of this chapter.

A randomized controlled study was carried out at the Moncton Hospital in Moncton, New Brunswick, to determine the impact of a pharmacist-directed seamless care program on economic, clinical, and humanistic outcomes and processes of care.[25] A total of 253 patients (119 in the control group and 134 in the intervention group) completed the study. A mean of 3.59 drug therapy problems for seamless monitoring per intervention patient was identified, and 72.1% of these problems were scored as having a *significant* or *very significant* clinical impact level. Participating community pharmacists who were surveyed believed that seamless care service helped them to provide better pharmaceutical care and improved efficiency in their pharmacies. In conclusion, the study researchers argued that a pharmacist-directed seamless care service can effectively resolve many drug therapy problems and improve drug-related processes of care in hospital and community pharmacies. On a national level, the Canadian Society of Hospital Pharmacists and the Canadian Pharmacists Association have had a joint task force on seamless care in operation for several years.

PHARMACIST-DIRECTED DOCUMENTATION INITIATIVES IN THE UNITED KINGDOM

In the United Kingdom, some health researchers have concluded that the medication-use system requires seamless care services to improve communication and safety. A study conducted in a large general hospital in England showed that breakdowns in the present discharge system can create problems for patients.[26] Thus 13% of participants had at least one discrepancy in their take-home prescriptions transcribed from the discharge notes. When the discharge letter was compared with the discharge notes, 27% of the patients' letters had a drug discrepancy. The researchers found that the mean time for the discharge letter to arrive from the hospital to the general practitioner's office was 26.9 days, and one-half took longer than 32 days. At follow-up, 57% of patients were experiencing a DRP that by clinical pharmacists' standards required intervention.

The results of the completed surveys from 163 U.K. Trust Hospitals showed that a wide variation still exists among various institutions in their ability to meet patients' needs.[27] Pharmacists were involved in the preparation of discharge prescriptions in only one-third of the hospitals, and their impact there was close to negligible. Alarmingly, 95% of institutions did not have their clinical pharmacists communicating with their community counterparts. The authors made the following recommendations: implementation of medication compliance charts, telephone medicine help lines, additional copies of discharge prescriptions for the general practitioner and the community pharmacist, regular involvement of the pharmacist in preparation of discharge medications (checking against the ward chart), and directly faxing copies of the prescriptions (complete with reasons for changes) to the general practitioner's office.

Studies that have evaluated pharmacist-directed seamless care services in the United Kingdom have had mixed results. In a randomized controlled trial of 362 patients that evaluated the effectiveness of a pharmacy discharge plan in hospitalized older adults, no impact on patient outcomes was found.[28] A smaller study of 32 patients found a positive impact on unintentional medication discrepancies in the intervention group,[29] whereas a seamless care feasibility study was received positively by participating community pharmacists.[30] Pharmacists in the United Kingdom also have begun to take an expanded role in primary care groups, working closely with physicians and nurses.

In 1993, the Royal Pharmaceutical Society of Great Britain created checklists for pharmacists that served as a guide to the types of communication that should occur between hospital and community pharmacists regarding patients' medication and pharmaceutical needs.[31] These checklists contained information that should be completed by the community pharmacist to the hospital pharmacist on hospital admission of a patient, such as the medication history and domiciliary circumstances and known adverse drug reactions (ADRs),

and information to be provided by the hospital pharmacist to the community pharmacist, such as the medication plan.

PHARMACIST-DIRECTED DOCUMENTATION INITIATIVES IN THE UNITED STATES

Many of the activities in the United States in this area relate to initiatives regarding the expanded scope of practice of pharmacists in the hospital, community, and managed-care settings. Most states now allow pharmacists to enter into collaborative prescribing agreements with physicians. The American Society of Health-System Pharmacists' Statement on the Pharmacist's Role in Primary Care advocates a larger role for pharmacists, including participation in multidisciplinary reviews of patients' progress, initiating or modifying medication therapy on the basis of patient responses, and performing limited physical assessments.[32] The American College of Physicians–American Society of Internal Medicine also has put forward a pharmacist's scope of practice, including the pharmacist's role in collaborative practice with physicians; pharmacist involvement in patient education and hospital medical rounds; pharmacist prescribing, immunizing, and therapeutic substitution; and reimbursement for pharmacists' cognitive services.[33] This expanded scope of practice also has legal implications; as Brushwood and Belgado explain, "The expanding availability of knowledge will expand professional responsibilities—and legal duties will not be far behind."[34]

Some pharmacist-directed seamless care evaluation studies have been conducted in the United States. Community and ambulatory care pharmacists who received a referral form from the hospital pharmacist when patients were discharged believed that the form helped them to better tailor patient counseling to the needs of the patients and positively affected the pharmacist–patient relationship.[35] Two studies that evaluated the impact of a hospital pharmacist providing pharmaceutical care at the time of discharge revealed the service to be well received by physicians and nurses[36] and patients.[37] Kuehl, Chrischilles, and Sorofman reported on a novel pharmacist-directed seamless care program among ambulatory care, hospital care, and long-term care pharmacists in five pharmacies in the midwestern United States.[38] In this study of 156 patients, patient-specific information significantly increased the number of interventions by the hospital and ambulatory care pharmacists.

HOSPITAL PHARMACY TO COMMUNITY PHARMACY

Most research projects to date have focused on the transfer of information from hospital pharmacies to community-based facilities primarily involving the general practitioner and the community pharmacist. These projects have clearly addressed a real need. In a survey of community pharmacists in the United Kingdom, 95.7% indicated that they would not know if one of their patients had been admitted to a hospital, and almost one-third had never seen a copy of the discharge information provided to patients and their general practitioners.[16]

COMMUNITY PHARMACY TO HOSPITAL PHARMACY

Far fewer initiatives have focused on the transfer of information from the community pharmacist to other members of the health care team. This is unfortunate because the community pharmacist often possesses valuable patient information by virtue of seeing the patient regularly for prescription refills and other self-care needs. Developing stronger ties between the community pharmacy and other sites of care can only serve to increase communication to improve the quality of patient care delivered.

COMMUNICATION WITH PHYSICIANS

Communication between the pharmacists and a patient's physician or physicians is crucial to the delivery of high-quality care, but such relationships can be threatened by perceived turf battles and misunderstandings. As discussed by Buerger,[39] improving the pharmacist–physician relationship requires effort and understanding on the part of both parties. Various stresses inherent in health care delivery make effective communication rather challenging in certain situations. To strengthen ties between physicians and pharmacists, all parties should focus on improving their communication skills and exercising their conflict-resolution skills.[39]

COMMUNICATION WITH PATIENTS

In this era of an ever-increasing desire on the part of patients to be involved in their own health care, an increasing number of self-care products (e.g., diagnostic, pharmaceutical, and nutraceutical) in the marketplace, and advanced communication technologies available to consumers (e.g., cell phones, personal digital assistants, electronic mail, and the Internet), community pharmacists have a unique opportunity to assume a pivotal role among other health care providers and patients in communicating, interpreting, and monitoring for the desired health outcomes. While not commonplace today, pharmacists should begin to communicate more regularly with their patients with respect to their health care needs and, where possible, should refer those patients back to health care providers when necessary. For example, how often has a patient presented himself or herself to a community pharmacy describing a condition or possible DRP in which the recommendation of the pharmacist following a brief triage is to refer the patient to his or her physician or other caregivers (e.g., dentist or optometrist) for follow-up? Unfortunately, this interaction seldom involves documentation by the pharmacist to the patient or other provider involved, and more than likely, follow-up with either party is by serendipity. This situation in the medical community would result in what is commonly known as a *referral* from one health care provider to another. Clearly, anecdotal reports of patients who have presented to a pharmacist, and describe significantly negative health outcomes and possibly death were averted because of this interaction with the pharmacist. However, such actions commonly went undocumented and therefore were not reported or traceable and possibly underappreciated or undervalued. Many patients have not experienced such formal and consistent documentation from the pharmacy profession, and it would prove valuable. Once these activities are consistent and valued by patients and providers alike, this may begin to set the parameters for patient payments directly to pharmacists while ultimately contributing to beneficial health outcomes of the patients served.

BILLING CONSIDERATIONS AND DOCUMENTATION SYSTEMS

MEDICAL BILLING SYSTEMS IN THE UNITED STATES

5 The Centers for Medicare and Medicaid Services (CMS) universal claim form is used by health care providers for third-party billing related to the provision of services. This form is required by Medicare and other third-party payers in the United States and uses the *International Classification for Disease,* 9th Revision, *Clinical Modification* (ICD-9-CM) coding system by providers for reimbursement, and this system is becoming increasingly important as Medicare Part D (oral prescription drug) coverage is implemented. Categories 1 to 15 (codes 001–779) identify diseases and related common medical conditions. Category 16 (codes 780–799) designates symptoms, signs, and ill-defined conditions. Category 19 (codes 800–999) relates to injury and poisoning. Each category contains additional codes that provide greater specificity and precision in terms of the condition or illness. There are two additional subsets of codes: V codes, which are used to classify routine screening examinations, and E codes, which are related to environmental injury or illness.

Use of Current Procedural Terminology (CPT) codes or the Common Procedure Coding System is required for completion of the universal claims form. CPT codes were created to be a listing of descriptive terms and identifying codes for medical services and procedures performed. Codes 99201 to 99205 are used for an office visit with a new patient, and codes 99211 to 99215 are used for an office visit with an existing patient. The differentiation among codes used is based on the intensity of service provided by the health care provider and the time involved. While not used commonly in pharmacy, these codes have been used by pharmacists to document the provision of patient-centered services in ambulatory and community settings when completing the universal claims form for billing purposes to third-party payers.

PHARMACY BILLING SYSTEMS

Recognizing issues related to nomenclature, compatibility, and transmission of data, some organizations have created guidelines to assist in the standardization of documentation systems for pharmacy. Historically, these efforts have been centered on the outpatient arena, focusing primarily on prescription claims related to the procurement and dispensing of prescription pharmaceutical products to patients from community pharmacies and by mail order. Founded in 1976, the National Council for Prescription Drug Programs (NCPDP) developed standards that allow for electronic data interchange (EDI) among providers of pharmaceuticals (e.g., pharmacies) and third-party administrators [e.g., pharmacy benefit management (PBM) organizations] primarily for the adjudication (i.e., financial approval) of prescriptions. This adjudication historically has centered on the assessment of the formulary status of a prescribed medication, resulting in verification or denial of the prescription and resulting payment to the dispensing pharmacy.

The payment formula for pharmaceuticals (and not professional services) typically has included a discounted cost of ingredients [e.g., the average wholesale price (AWP) discounted by a given percentage] plus a dispensing fee. The dispensing fee, often in the range of $1 to $2 per prescription, is paid irrespective of the pharmacist time involved in processing the prescription (procuring/compounding the product, verifying with the prescriber patient- and product-specific concerns identified, addressing insurance-related claims issues, and conducting patient counseling/follow-up monitoring). Arguably, no uniform standard has been adopted by pharmacists and third-party administrators to allow for billing and financial compensation associated with the provision of professional services by pharmacists both in scope and in intensity of services provided.

Having a reimbursement system tied only to product dispensing is fraught with problems. For example, in community pharmacy practice, if a pharmacist provides a recommendation to discontinue therapy and this recommendation is followed, no reimbursement to the pharmacy will take place because no product would be dispensed (although the third-party administrator and the patient would save money). However, if the recommendation is ignored and the product is dispensed, the third-party payer would incur a cost related to dispensing the prescription. Clearly, the issue related to the appropriateness of the prescription is somewhat lost.

Recent efforts by the NCPDP and other professional organizations such as the National Community Pharmacists Association have recognized the need for allowing the transmission and adjudication not only of electronic prescriptions but also of requests for refills and other transactions among prescribers (e.g., physicians) and pharmacists. As a result, various initiatives have been undertaken to allow for such levels of transmission among pharmacists, physicians and other health care providers, payers, and ultimately, patients.

ROLE OF TECHNOLOGY IN CLINICAL DOCUMENTATION

Emerging technologies will have a profound effect on health care, thus offering opportunities for the pharmacy profession in maintaining constant vigilance related to the procurement, preparation, and distribution of pharmaceuticals and allowing for more consistent provision of pharmaceutical care. Digital documentation, such as computer-stored medical records or electronic medical records (EMRs), is one vehicle that, if adapted universally, would assist in enhancing the communication among providers in all settings. EMRs must be implemented by 2009 under the new Medicare Part D regulations, and this is expected to drive adoption of the new technologies by prescribers. Significant benefits to EMRs have been described as the following: (1) improved logistics and organization of the medical record to speed care and improve efficiency, (2) automatic computer review of the medical record to limit errors and control costs, and (3) systematic analysis of past clinical experience to guide future practices and policies.[40] The use of EMRs that include pharmacy-specific data (e.g., history of medication usage, both prescription and over the counter; history of refills; assessment of adherence and persistence; and other information deemed appropriate for inclusion by pharmacists) allows for improved communication, enhanced decision making, and the ability to follow up on outcomes associated with care plans.

Advances in technology can facilitate the generation and transfer of patient documentation. As more pharmacies use the Internet as a means of communication, information can be transferred quickly and accurately over greater distances. Handheld computers and specialty software allow health care practitioners to document information in an electronic format that can be transformed immediately for rapid transfer to others. Reports in the literature have described methods to assess pharmacist interventions related to medication errors,[5] the use of computer-based systems,[6] and recently, the use of personal digital assistants (PDAs) in specific patient care areas.[7] Many of these documentation systems tend to be individualized applications in which the transfer of data to other providers is not possible or quite limited. Often these systems focus on the generation of reports for workload analysis or accreditation purposes.

The internal pharmacy environment may dictate the method for data collection and documentation as well. While pharmacists in some practice settings routinely use personal computers (PCs), others tend to be more mobile, and therefore, access to portable technology is more crucial (e.g., laptops and PDAs). For example, a community pharmacist may be more likely to document his or her activities on

a PC as opposed to a PDA because the internal workflow would necessitate this. In contrast, a consultant pharmacist who travels among various long-term care facilities may prefer a portable device for documentation.

CONSIDERATIONS WHEN SELECTING ELECTRONIC DOCUMENTATION SYSTEMS FOR PHARMACISTS

- Cost to implement and support the system
- Ability to interface with pharmacy billing, dispensing, and drug information systems
- Compatibility with other operating systems in the organization
- Ability to ensure private and secure data
- Support for enhancements and updates to the software and hardware
- Compatibility with the workflow of pharmacists

Internal operating systems and their incompatibility with other operating systems present challenges as well. The inability to interface with other systems can create redundancies that potentially can lead to serious misinterpretations and mistakes in the translation of data that can compromise patient care. In choosing an electronic documentation program for pharmacists, consideration must be given to the ability to interface not only with the pharmacy system (billing and automated dispensing) but also with other electronic records throughout an organization. When a pharmacy system does not interface with the laboratory system of the EMRs of a hospital, the ability of providers to communicate effectively is reduced.

Pharmacists in community settings must communicate more regularly with hospital pharmacists, and vice versa, yet this is often not the case.[14,27] Interventions often need to be shared with other pharmacists at shift changes, transfer of patients from one care area to another, or even transfer of patients to new health systems altogether. One study assessed the use of computerized reminders to physicians to increase preventive care in inpatient settings for pneumococcal and influenza vaccinations and prophylactic heparin and prophylactic aspirin at discharge with the use of a computerized order-entry system. The investigators concluded that computerized reminders significantly increased the rate of delivery of the intended therapies.[41] Future digital technologies not only will prompt and remind practitioners of situations that require their attention but also will prevent such occurrences.

Likewise, electronic mail and the Internet can be used as vehicles to communicate not only among health care providers but also with patients. Electronic reminders aiding medication adherence, answering medication- and disease-related questions, and providing product comparisons can be sent via e-mail from pharmacy providers. Access to the Internet in the work setting, however, may be a limiting factor for many community pharmacists, in particular, those in chain pharmacies,[42] and must be overcome to allow for universal adoption in community pharmacy practice. The benefits to allowing Internet access in community pharmacies far outweigh potential concerns for inappropriate use in the work setting when patients' lives may depend on the information contained within resources available through the Internet.

PDAs are efficient tools that can be used to collect, process, and transmit data that ultimately have an impact on the care delivered to patients, although they do have limitations, such as their memory capabilities, screen size, and overall functionality.[43] In some software applications, a synchronization interface can be written to allow for an automatic link to a Web site to deposit and collate aggregate data from PDA users or directly from a computer linked to the Internet.[44] An example of an electronic documentation system is provided in the case study.

TRAINING CONSIDERATIONS FOR PHARMACISTS AND SUPPORT STAFF IN DOCUMENTATION

Pharmacists often are not comfortable in documenting their activities related to patient care within the pharmacy setting and are even more uncomfortable in communicating this information to other health care providers. All too often communications from pharmacists to physicians relate to pharmaceutical product usage and restrictions (i.e., nonformulary issues) and do not focus on patient care issues. Thus attention must be directed toward practicing pharmacists and providing them with education and training related to why documentation is necessary, how to document, and use of technology to assist in the documentation process. The training of support staff, such as pharmacy technicians, must not be overlooked because these individuals can assist in the routine collection of both pharmaceutical data and retrievable patient information (e.g., from medical charts and laboratory reports) that can be presented to pharmacists for assessment and needed follow-up.

Although the concepts of documentation are consistent irrespective of practice settings, the process by which data are collected and the tools for documentation can be quite different. Thus the training associated with documentation must be specific to the respective practice environments of pharmacists. For example, access to health care providers, medical records, laboratory data, and patients is more common in hospital pharmacy practice than in community pharmacy practice, where direct access to patients is often the only source of information. As a result, data collection, documentation, and communication with other health care providers and patients will vary based on the practice setting. However, as the use of EMRs and digital documentation becomes more common, the ability of pharmacists to interface with these systems will become less of a logistical barrier.

CONCLUSIONS

While the common maxim, "If it wasn't documented, it wasn't done," applies to all providers of health care, for the pharmacy profession, this is the mantra the profession needs to embrace if it is to remain an active and valued participant in the health care systems of industrialized countries. The profession must not wait for the creation and implementation of a universal billing system related to the provision of cognitive services by pharmacists; rather, the focus should remain centrally on the patient; one in which pharmacists universally assume a pivotal role between other health care providers and patients in communicating, interpreting, and monitoring the desired health outcomes associated with prescription and nonprescription therapies and all actions are documented and communicated effectively to all stakeholders in a convenient, consistent, and interpretable manner.

CASE STUDY

This case could be seen in either a community or hospital setting (if the prescription was a handwritten order in the medical chart of the patient).

A 59-year-old African-American man who has atrial fibrillation presents a handwritten prescription that appears to read, "warfarin sodium 25 mg PO qd." The pharmacist identifies this as too high of a dose (most likely missing the decimal point for the dose of 2.5 mg) and contacts the prescriber immediately. The pharmacist would proceed to log this intervention as shown in Fig. 4–1.

Continuing, in the box on the first "Reasons" page under the subheading of "Order Clarification," "Illegible writing" would be checked. and under "Drug Regimen Selection," "Dose" would be checked (Fig. 4–2), given that the prescription was written poorly (e.g., illegibly) and the dose appeared incorrect.

As with most interventions by pharmacists, typically, recommendations are made to health care providers, patients, or caregivers. Using the preceding example with the warfarin prescription, the box under the recommendation subheading "Medication Related" would be checked, and "Change dose" would be indicated (Fig. 4–3). In this case, additional "Patient Care Related" recommendations could have been made, such as the ordering of "laboratory tests" and "therapeutic drug monitoring."

The next step would be to check the box under the subheading "Contact" entitled, "Contact health care provider," to ensure that the illegible prescription and the incorrect dose were interpreted correctly and that the appropriate medication and strength were verified by the pharmacist and dispensed to the patient (Fig. 4–4).

With respect to outcomes, the following items would be indicated for the prescription if the prescriber agreed with (accepted) the interpretation that the prescription was in fact for "Warfarin sodium

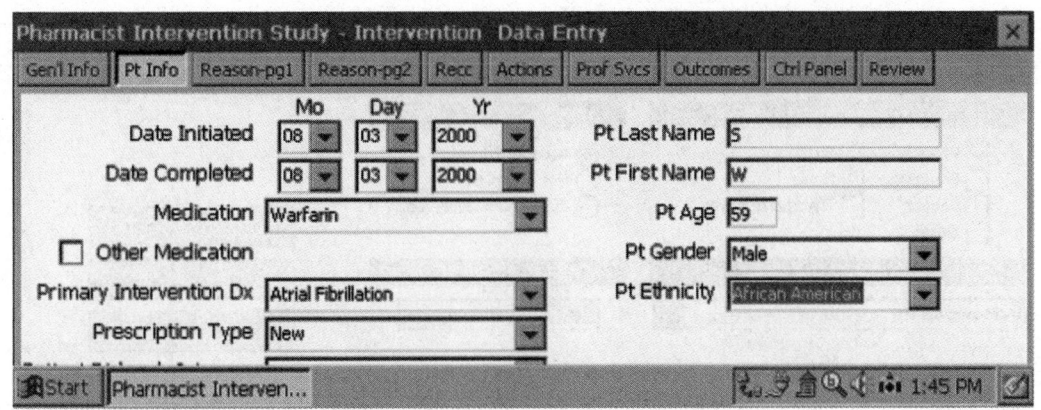

FIGURE 4–1. PSDS initial patient screen.

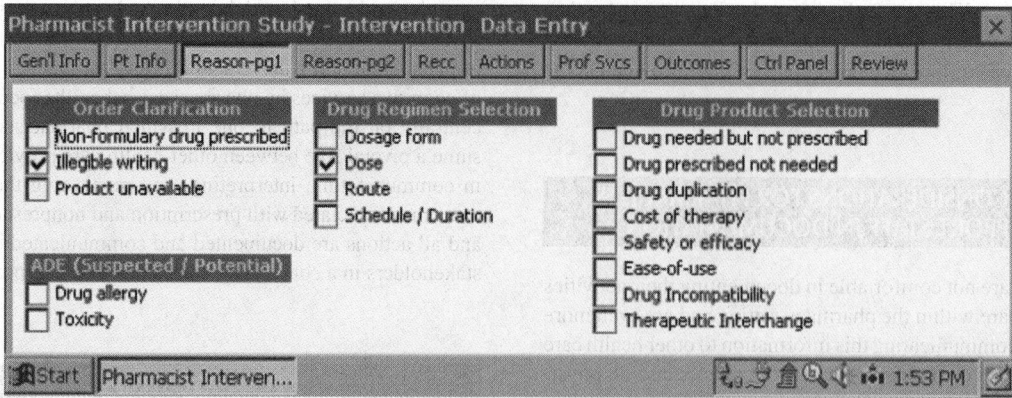

FIGURE 4-2. PSDS reason for intervention screen.

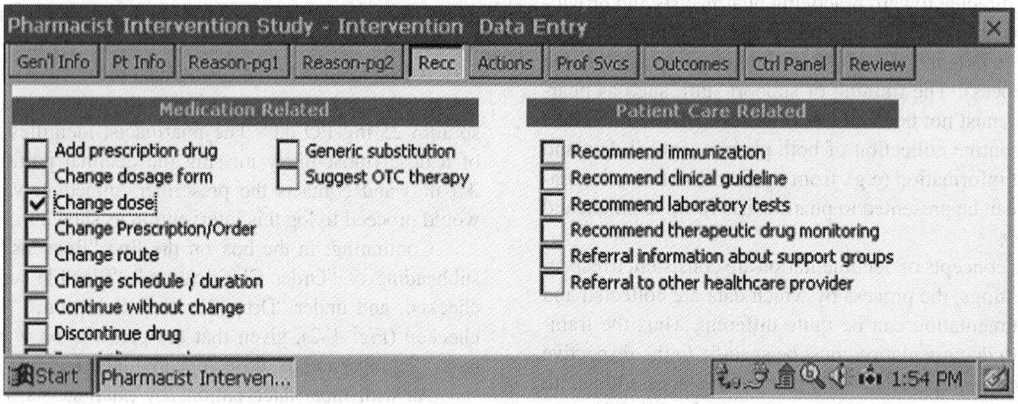

FIGURE 4-3. PSDS intervention recommendation screen.

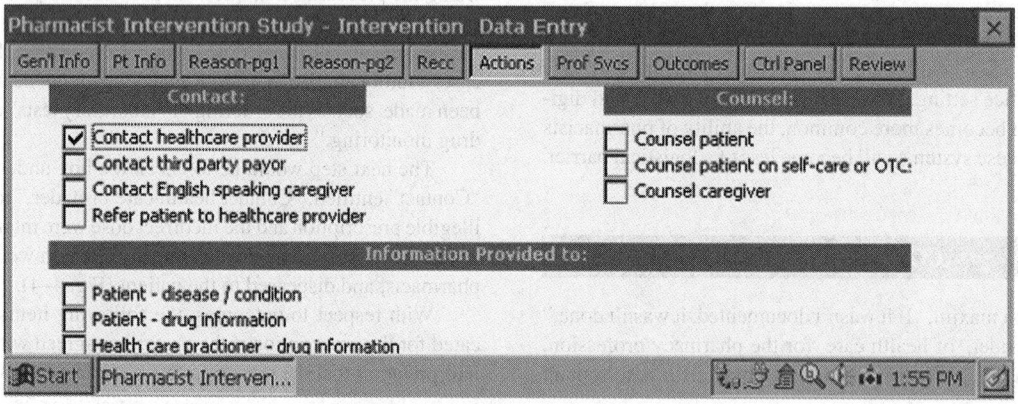

FIGURE 4-4. PSDS intervention action screen.

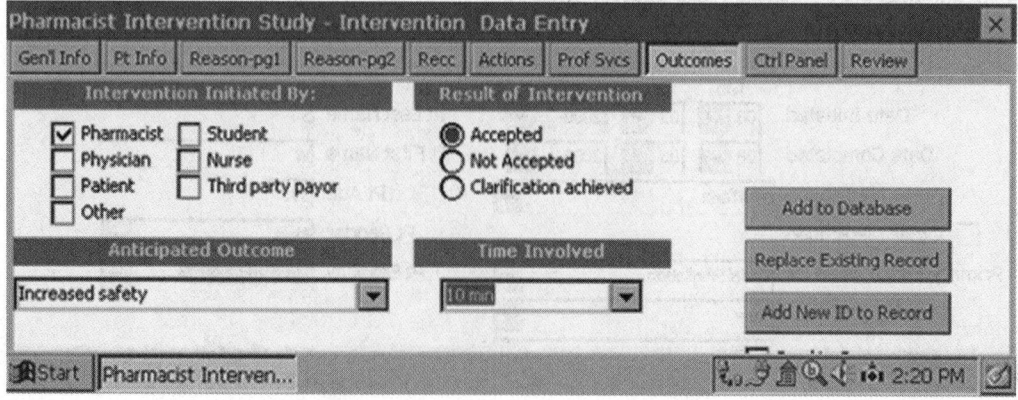

FIGURE 4-5. PSDS intervention outcomes screen.

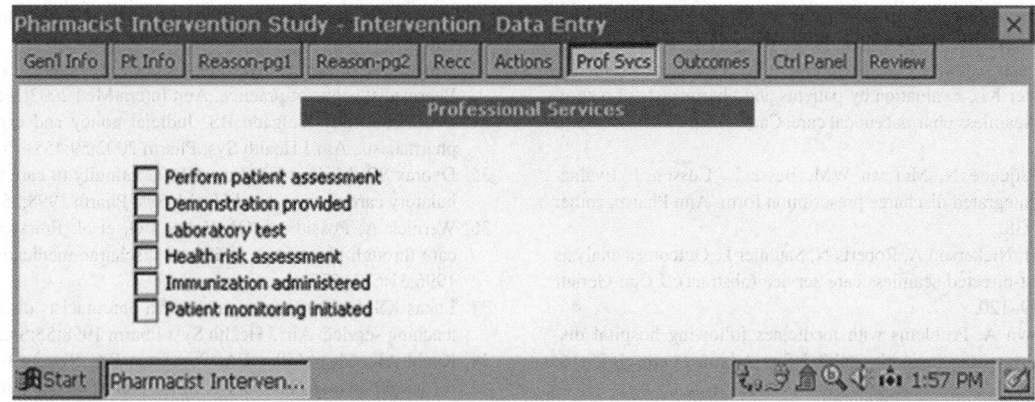

FIGURE 4–6. PSDS professional services screen.

2.5 mg PO qd" and not "Warfarin sodium 25 mg PO qd" as written in the "Result of Intervention" section. The intervention required 10 minutes of the pharmacist's time, captured in "Time Involved." It was assumed that this action by the pharmacist would have an "Anticipated Outcome" of "Increased safety" for the patient (Fig. 4–5).

In a situation where point-of-care diagnostic monitoring for anticoagulation is available to the pharmacist, under the "Professional Services" subheading, "Laboratory tests" could have been checked (Fig. 4–6).

In many instances, this interaction and others quite similar take place on a daily basis, but the valuable contributions pharmacists make in averting potentially lethal medication-related errors are never captured. More importantly, without this systematic approach to documentation of specific classes of agents, most common reasons for interventions and outcomes of recommendations would not be known or available for follow-up.

ABBREVIATIONS

DRPs: drug-related problems
HRQOL: health-related quality of life
IOM: Institute of Medicine
POMR: problem-oriented medical record
SOAP: *subjective–objective–assessment–plan*
CMS: Centers for Medicare & Medicaid Services
ICD-9-CM: *International Classification for Disease,* 9th edition, *Clinical Modification*
CPT: Current Procedural Terminology
NCPDP: National Council for Prescription Drug Programs
EDI: electronic drug interchange
AWP: average wholesale price
EMRs: electronic medical records
PDAs: personal digital assistants
PCs: personal computers

REFERENCES

1. Hepler CD, Stand LM. Opportunities and responsibilities in pharmaceutical care. Am J Hosp Pharm 1990;47:533–543.
2. Grainger-Rousseau TJ, Miralles MA, Hepler CD, et al. Therapeutic outcomes monitoring: Application of pharmaceutical care guidelines to community pharmacy. J Am Pharm Assoc 1997;NS37:647–661.
3. MacKinnon NJ. Risk assessment of preventable drug-related morbidity in older persons. Ph.D. dissertation, University of Florida, Gainesville, 1999.
4. Kohn LT, Corrigan JM, Donaldson MS, eds. To Err Is Human: Building a Safer Health System. Committee on Quality of Health Care in America, Institute of Medicine. Washington, National Academy Press, 1999.
5. Overhage JM, Lukes A. Practical, reliable, comprehensive method for characterizing pharmacists' clinical activities. Am J Health Syst Pharm 1999;56:2444–2449.
6. Sauer BL, Heeren DL, Walker RG, et al. Computerized documentation of activities of Pharm.D. clerkship students. Am J Health Syst Pharm 1997;54:1727–1732.
7. Lau A, Balen RM, Lam, R, Malyuk, DL. Using a personal digital assistant to document clinical pharmacy services in an intensive care unit. Am J Health Syst Pharm 2001;58:1229–1232.
8. MacKinnon GE III. Documenting pharmacy student interventions via scannable patient care activity records (PCAR). Pharm Educ 2002;2:191–197.
9. Rovers JP, Currie JD, Hagel HP, et al. Documentation. In Meade V, ed. A Practical Guide to Pharmaceutical Care. Washington, American Pharmaceutical Association, 1998:103–115.
10. Weed LL. Medical Records, Medical Education, and Patient Care. Cleveland, Case Western University Press, 1971.
11. Strand LM, Morley PC, Cipolle RJ, et al. Drug-related problems: Their structure and function. DICP 1990;24:1093–1097.
12. Currie J, Kuhle J, Doucette WR, et al. Quality Assessment for Documentation of Pharmaceutical Care Final Report. Iowa City, Iowa, American Pharmaceutical Foundation Quality Center, 1999.
13. Naylor MD, Brooten D, Campbell R, et al. Comprehensive discharge planning and home follow-up of hospitalized elders: A randomized controlled trial. JAMA 1999;281:613–620.
14. MacKinnon NJ, Zwicker LA. Review of seamless care: Backgrounder. In MacKinnon NJ, ed. Seamless Care: A Pharmacist's Guide to Continuous Care Programs. Ottawa, Canada, Canadian Pharmacists Association, 2003:1–12.
15. Beers MH, Dang J, Hasegawa J, et al. Influence of hospitalization on drug therapy in the elderly. J Am Geriatr Soc 1989;37:679–683.
16. Al-Rashid SA, Wright DJ, Reeves JA, Chrystyn H. Opinions about hospital discharge information: 2. Community pharmacists. J Soc Admin Pharm 2001;18:129–135.
17. Low J. Seamless care anyone. Aust J Hosp Pharm 1997;27:356–357.
18. Wilcox C, Duguid MJ. The medication chart as an integral tool in the pharmaceutical care plan. Aust J Hosp Pharm 2001;31:268–274.
19. Editorial Staff. Continuity of care between hospital and the community. Aust J Pharm 2002;83:136–138.
20. Australian Pharmaceutical Advisory Council. National Guidelines to Achieve the Continuum of Quality Use of Medicines Between Hospital and Community. Canberra: Publications Production Unit, Commonwealth Department of Health and Family Services, 1998.

21. Cameron B. The impact of pharmacy discharge planning on continuity of care. Can J Hosp Pharm 1994;47:101–119.
22. Austin Z. Towards seamless care. Hosp Pharm Pract 1995;3:17–21.
23. Cole DL, Slayter KL. Evaluation by patients and pharmacists of a summary form for seamless pharmaceutical care. Can J Hosp Pharm 1999;52:162–166.
24. Lamontagne-Paquette N, McLean WM, Besse L, Cusson J. Evaluation of a new integrated discharge prescription form. Ann Pharmacother 2001;35:935–938.
25. MacKinnon NJ, Nickerson A, Roberts N, Saulnier L. Outcomes analysis of a pharmacist-directed seamless care service (abstract). J Can Geriatr Soc 2002;5:119–120.
26. Sexton J, Brown A. Problems with medicines following hospital discharge: Not always the patient's fault? J Soc Admin Pharm 1999;16:199–207.
27. Sexton J, Ho YJ, Green CF, et al. Ensuring seamless care at hospital discharge: A national survey. J Clin Pharmcol Ther 2000;25:385–393.
28. Nazareth I, Burton A, Shulman S, et al. A pharmacy discharge plan for hospitalized elderly patients: A randomized, controlled trial. Age Ageing 2001;30:33–40.
29. Pickrell L, Duggan C, Dhillon S. From hospital admission to discharge: An exploratory study to evaluate seamless care. Pharm J 2001;267:650–653.
30. Cook H. Transfer of information between hospital and community pharmacy: A feasibility study. Pharm J 1995;254:736–737.
31. Communication Between Hospital and Community Pharmacists Concerning Patients' Medication and Pharmaceutical Needs. London, Royal Pharmaceutical Society of Great Britain, 1993.
32. American Society of Health-System Pharmacists. ASHP statement on the pharmacist's role in primary care. Am J Health Syst Pharm 1999;56:1665–1667.
33. American College of Physicians–American Society of Internal Medicine. Pharmacist scope of practice. Ann Intern Med 2002;136:79–85.
34. Brushwood DB, Belgado BS. Judicial policy and expanded duties for pharmacists. Am J Health Syst Pharm 2002;59:455–457.
35. Dvorak SR, McCoy RA, Voss GD. Continuity of care from acute to ambulatory care setting. Am J Health Syst Pharm 1998;55:2500–2504.
36. Wernick A, Possidente CJ, Keller EG, et al. Enhancing continuity of care through pharmacist review of discharge medications. Hosp Pharm 1996;31:672–676.
37. Lucas KS. Outcomes evaluation of a pharmacists discharge medication teaching service. Am J Health Syst Pharm 1998;55:S32–S35.
38. Kuehl AK, Chrischilles EA, Sorofman BA. System for exchanging information among pharmacists in different practice environments. J Am Pharm Assoc 1998;38:317–324.
39. Buerger D. Basic steps to better pharmacist–physician communication. Consult Pharm 1994;14:95–96.
40. McDonald CJ, Tierney WM. Computer-based medical records: Their future role in medical practice. JAMA 1988;259:3433–3440.
41. Dexter PR, Perkins S, Overhage JM, et al. A computerized reminder system to increase the use of preventive care for hospitalized patients. N Engl J Med 2001;345:965–970.
42. MacKinnon GE III, Mologousis NM. Preliminary survey of pharmacists' use of the Internet. Am J Health Syst Pharm 1999;56:1675–1676.
43. MacKinnon GE III. Development of a personal digital assistant application for pharmacy documentation. Pharm Educ 2003;3:11–16.
44. MacKinnon GE III. Evaluation of an Internet-based system to document pharmacy student interventions. Am J Pharm Educ 2003;67:90.

5

CLINICAL PHARMACOKINETICS AND PHARMACODYNAMICS

Larry A. Bauer

Learning Objectives and other resources can be found at *www.pharmacotherapyonline.com.*

KEY CONCEPTS

⬤1 Clinical pharmacokinetics is the discipline that describes the absorption, distribution, metabolism, and elimination of drugs in patients requiring drug therapy.

⬤2 Clearance is the most important pharmacokinetic parameter because it determines the steady-state concentration for a given dosage rate. Physiologically, clearance is determined by blood flow to the organ that metabolizes or eliminates the drug and the efficiency of the organ in extracting the drug from the bloodstream.

⬤3 The volume of distribution is a proportionality constant that relates the amount of drug in the body to the serum concentration. The volume of distribution is used to calculate the loading dose of a drug that will immediately achieve a desired steady-state concentration. The value of the volume of distribution is determined by the physiologic volume of blood and tissues and how the drug binds in blood and tissues.

⬤4 Half-life is the time required for serum concentrations to decrease by one-half after absorption and distribution are complete. Half-life is important because it determines the time required to reach steady state and the dosage interval. Half-life is a dependent kinetic variable because its value depends on the values of clearance and volume of distribution.

⬤5 The fraction of drug absorbed into the systemic circulation after extravascular administration is defined as its bioavailability.

⬤6 Most drugs follow linear pharmacokinetics, whereby steady-state serum drug concentrations change proportionally with long-term daily dosing.

⬤7 Some drugs do not follow the rules of linear pharmacokinetics. Instead of steady-state drug concentration changing proportionally with dose, serum concentration changes more or less than expected. These drugs follow nonlinear pharmacokinetics.

⬤8 Pharmacokinetic models are useful to describe data sets, to predict serum concentrations after several doses or different routes of administration, and to calculate pharmacokinetic constants such as clearance, volume of distribution, and half-life. The simplest case uses a single compartment to represent the entire body.

⬤9 Factors to be taken into consideration when deciding on the best drug dose for a patient include age, gender, weight, ethnic background, other concurrent disease states, and other drug therapy.

⬤10 Cytochrome P450 is a generic name for the group of enzymes that are responsible for most drug metabolism oxidation reactions. Several P450 isozymes have been identified, including CYP1A2, CYP2C9, CYP2C19, CYP2D6, CYP2E1, and CYP3A4.

⬤11 The importance of transport proteins in drug bioavailability and elimination is now better understood. The principal transport protein involved in the movement of drugs across biologic membranes is P-glycoprotein. P-glycoprotein is present in many organs, including the gastrointestinal tract, liver, and kidney.

⬤12 When deciding on initial doses for drugs that are renally eliminated, the patient's renal function should be assessed. A common, useful way to do this is to measure the patient's serum creatinine concentration and convert this value into an estimated creatinine clearance ($CrCl_{est}$). For drugs that are eliminated primarily by the kidney ($\geq 60\%$ of the administered dose), some agents will need minor dosage adjustments for $CrCl_{est}$ between 30 and 60 mL/min, moderate dosage adjustments for $CrCl_{est}$ between 15 and 30 mL/min, and major dosage adjustments for $CrCl_{est}$ less than 15 mL/min. Postdialysis supplemental doses of some medications also may be needed for patients receiving hemodialysis if the drug is removed by the artificial kidney.

⬤13 When deciding on initial doses for drugs that are hepatically eliminated, the patient's liver function should be assessed. The Child-Pugh score can be used as an indicator of a patient's ability to metabolize drugs that are eliminated by the liver. In the absence of specific pharmacokinetic dosing guidelines for a medication, a Child-Pugh score equal to 8 or 9 is grounds for a moderate decrease (~25%)

in initial daily drug dose for agents that are metabolized primarily hepatically ($\geq$60%), and a score of 10 or greater indicates that a significant decrease in initial daily dose ($\sim$50%) is required for drugs that are metabolized mostly hepatically.

14 For drugs that exhibit linear pharmacokinetics, steady-state drug concentration (C_{ss}) changes proportionally with dose (D). To adjust a patient's drug therapy, a reasonable starting dose is administered for an estimated three to five half-lives. A serum concentration is obtained, assuming that it will reflect C_{ss}. Independent of the route of administration, the new dose (D_{new}) needed to attain the desired C_{ss} ($C_{ss,new}$) is calculated: $D_{new} = D_{old}(C_{ss,new}/C_{ss,old})$,

where D_{old} and $C_{ss,old}$ are the old dose and old C_{ss}, respectively.

15 If it is necessary to determine the pharmacokinetic constants for a patient to individualize his or her dose, a small pharmacokinetic evaluation is conducted in the individual. Additionally, Bayesian computer programs that aid in the individualization of therapy are available for many different drugs.

16 Pharmacodynamics is the study of the relationship between the concentration of a drug and the response obtained in a patient. If pharmacologic effect is plotted versus concentration for most drugs, a hyperbola results with an asymptote equal to maximum attainable effect.

Pharmacokinetic concepts have been used successfully by pharmacists to individualize patient drug therapy for about a quarter of a century. Pharmacokinetic consultant services and individual clinicians routinely provide patient-specific drug dosing recommendations that increase the efficacy and decrease the toxicity of many medications. Laboratories routinely measure patient serum or plasma samples for many drugs, including antibiotics (e.g., aminoglycosides and vancomycin), theophylline, antiepileptics (e.g., phenytoin, carbamazepine, valproic acid, phenobarbital, and ethosuximide), methotrexate, lithium, antiarrhythmics (e.g., lidocaine, procainamide, quinidine, and digoxin), and immunosuppressants (e.g., cyclosporine and tacrolimus). Combined with a knowledge of the disease states and conditions that influence the disposition of a particular drug, kinetic concepts can be used to modify doses to produce serum drug concentrations that result in desirable pharmacologic effects without unwanted side effects. This narrow range of concentrations within which the pharmacologic response is produced and adverse effects prevented in most patients is defined as the *therapeutic range* of the drug. Table 5–1 lists the therapeutic ranges for commonly used medications.

Although most individuals experience favorable effects with serum drug concentrations in the therapeutic range, the effects of a given serum concentration can vary widely among individuals. Clinicians should never assume that a serum concentration within the therapeutic range will be safe and effective for every patient. The response to the drug, such as number of seizures a patient experiences while taking an antiepileptic agent, always should be assessed when serum concentrations are measured.

Throughout this chapter, abbreviations for various pharmacokinetic parameters are used frequently. Commonly used abbreviations are listed in Table 5–2.

TABLE 5–1. Selected Therapeutic Ranges

Drug	Therapeutic Range
Digoxin	0.5–2 ng/mL
Lidocaine	1.5–5 mcg/mL
Procainamide/*N*-acetylprocainamide	10–30 mcg/mL (total)
Quinidine	2–5 mcg/mL
Amikacin*a*	20–30 mcg/mL (peak)
	<5 mcg/mL (trough)
Gentamicin, tobramycin, netilmicin*	5–10 mcg/mL (peak)
	<2 mcg/mL (trough)
Vancomycin	20–40 mcg/mL (peak)
	5–10 mcg/mL (trough)
Chloramphenicol	10–20 mcg/mL
Lithium	0.6–1.4 mEq/L
Carbamazepine	4–12 mcg/mL
Ethosuximide	40–100 mcg/mL
Phenobarbital	15–40 mcg/mL
Phenytoin	10–20 mcg/mL
Primidone	5–12 mcg/mL
Valproic acid	50–100 mcg/mL
Theophylline	10–20 mcg/mL
Cyclosporine	150–400 ng/mL (blood)

*Using a multiple dose per day dosage schedule, single daily dose therapeutic concentrations not yet established.

TABLE 5–2. Pharmacokinetic Abbreviations

Abbreviation	Definition
Cl	Clearance
k_0	Intravenous infusion rate
C_{ss}	Steady-state concentration
D	Dose
τ	Dosage interval
F	Fraction of drug absorbed into the systemic circulation
Q	Blood flow
E	Extraction ratio
f_b	Fraction of drug in the blood that is unbound
Cl_{int}	Intrinsic clearance
$C_{ss,u}$	Steady-state concentration of unbound drug
V_D	Volume of distribution
LD	Loading dose
MD	Maintenance dose
$t_{1/2}$	Half-life
k	Elimination rate constant
k_a	Absorption rate constant
α	Distribution rate constant
β	Terminal rate constant
t'	Postinfusion time
T	Duration of infusion
AUC	Area under serum or blood concentration-versus-time curve
V_{max}	Maximum rate of drug metabolism
K_m	Serum concentration at which the rate of metabolism equals $V_{max}/2$
C_{max}	Maximum serum or blood concentration
C_{min}	Minimum serum or blood concentration
DR	Dosage rate
PGP	P-glycoprotein

CLINICAL PHARMACOKINETIC CONCEPTS

1 Clinical pharmacokinetics is the discipline that describes the absorption, distribution, metabolism, and elimination of drugs in patients requiring drug therapy. When a drug is administered extravascularly to patients, it must be absorbed across biologic membranes to reach the systemic circulation. If the drug is given orally, the drug molecules must pass through the gastrointestinal tract wall into capillaries. For transdermal patches, the drug must penetrate the skin to enter the vascular system. In general, the pharmacologic effect of the drug is delayed when it is given extravascularly because time is required for the drug to be absorbed into the vascular system.

The vascular system generally provides the "transportation" for the drug molecule to its site of activity. After the drug reaches the systemic circulation, it can leave the vasculature and penetrate the various tissues or remain in the blood. If the drug remains in the blood, it may bind to endogenous proteins such as albumin or α_1-acid glycoprotein. This binding usually is reversible, and an equilibrium is created between protein-bound drug and unbound drug. Unbound drug in the blood provides the driving force for distribution of the agent to body tissues. If unbound drug leaves the bloodstream and distributes to tissue, it may become tissue-bound, it may remain unbound in the tissue, or if the tissue can metabolize or eliminate the drug, it may be rendered inactive and/or eliminated from the body. If the drug becomes tissue-bound, it may bind to the receptor that causes its pharmacologic or toxic effect or to a nonspecific binding site that causes no effect. Again, tissue binding is usually reversible so that the tissue-bound drug is in equilibrium with unbound drug in the tissue.

Certain organs—such as the liver, gastrointestinal tract wall, and lung—possess enzymes that metabolize drugs. The resulting metabolite may be inactive or have a pharmacologic effect of its own. The blood also contains esterases, which cleave ester bonds in drug molecules and generally render them inactive.

Drug metabolism usually occurs in the liver through one or both of two types of reactions. Phase I reactions generally make the drug molecule more polar and water soluble so that it is prone to elimination by the kidney. Phase I modifications include oxidation, hydrolysis, and reduction. Phase II reactions involve conjugation to form glucuronides, acetates, or sulfates. These reactions generally inactivate the pharmacologic activity of the drug and may make it more prone to elimination by the kidney.

Other organs have the ability to eliminate drugs or metabolites from the body. The kidney can excrete drugs by glomerular filtration or by such active processes as proximal tubular secretion. Drugs also can be eliminated via bile produced by the liver or air expired by the lungs.

LINEAR PHARMACOKINETICS

6 Most drugs follow linear pharmacokinetics: Serum drug concentrations change proportionally with long-term daily dosing. For example, if a drug dose were doubled from 300 to 600 mg/day, the patient's serum drug concentration would double.

When a drug is given by continuous intravenous infusion, serum concentrations increase until an equilibrium is established between the drug dosage rate and the rate of drug elimination. At that point, the rate of drug administration equals the rate of drug elimination, and the serum concentrations therefore remain constant (Fig. 5–1). For example, if a patient were receiving a continuous intravenous infusion of theophylline at 40 mg/h, the theophylline serum concentration

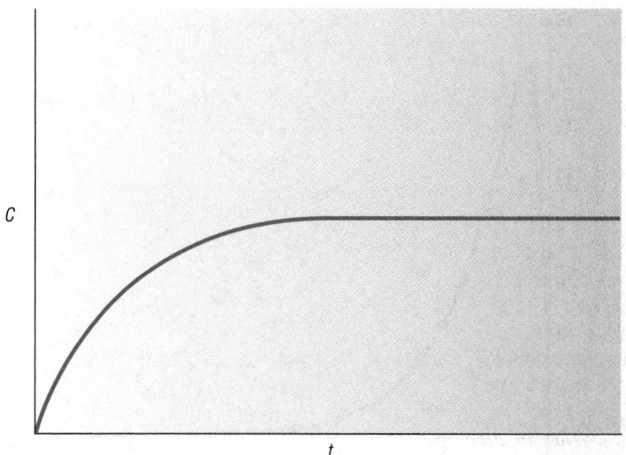

FIGURE 5–1. Normal serum concentration-time curve following a continuous intravenous infusion.

would increase until the patient's body was eliminating theophylline at 40 mg/h. When serum drug concentrations reach a constant value, steady state is achieved.

If the drug is given at intermittent dosage intervals, such as 250 mg every 6 hours, steady state is achieved when the serum-concentration-versus-time curves for each dosage interval are superimposable. The amount of drug eliminated during the dosage interval equals the dose.

BIOAVAILABILITY AND BIOEQUIVALENCE

When drugs are administered extravascularly, drug molecules must be released from the dosage form (dissolution) and pass through several biologic barriers before reaching the vascular system **5** (absorption). The fraction of drug absorbed into the systemic circulation (F) after extravascular administration is defined as its *bioavailability* and can be calculated after single intravenous and extravascular doses as[1]

$$F = \frac{D_{iv}(\text{AUC}_{0-\infty})}{D(\text{AUC}_{iv,0-\infty})}$$

where D and D_{iv} are the extravascular and intravenous doses, respectively, and $\text{AUC}_{iv,0-\infty}$ and $\text{AUC}_{0-\infty}$ are the intravenous and extravascular areas under the serum- or blood-concentration-versus-time curves, respectively, from time zero to infinity. The AUC represents the body's total exposure to the drug and is a function of the fraction of the drug dose that enters the systemic circulation via the administered route and clearance (Fig. 5–2). When F is less than 1 for a drug administered extravascularly, either the dosage form did not release all the drug contained in it, or some of the drug was eliminated or destroyed (by stomach acid or other means) before it reached the systemic circulation.

When the extravascular dose is administered orally, part of the dose may be metabolized by enzymes or removed by transport proteins contained in the gastrointestinal tract wall or liver before it reaches the systemic circulation.[2,3] This occurs commonly when drugs have a high liver extraction ratio or are subject to gastrointestinal tract wall metabolism because, after oral administration, the drug must pass through the gastrointestinal tract wall and into the portal circulation of the liver. Transport proteins are also present in the gastrointestinal tract wall that can actively pump drug molecules that already have been absorbed back into the lumen of the gastrointestinal tract. P-Glycoprotein (PGP) is the primary transport protein that

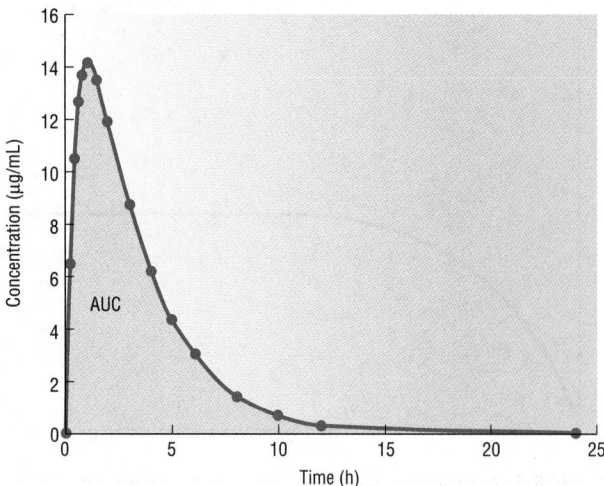

FIGURE 5–2. Area under the concentration-time curve (AUC) after the administration of an extravascular dose. The AUC is a function of the fraction of drug dose that enters the systemic circulation and clearance. AUCs measured after intravenous and extravascular doses can be used to determine bioavailability for the extravascular dose.

interferes with drug absorption by this mechanism. For example, if an orally administered drug is 100% absorbed from the gastrointestinal tract but has a hepatic extraction ratio of 0.75, only 25% of the original dose enters the systemic circulation. This first-pass effect through the liver and/or gastrointestinal tract wall is avoided when the drug is given by other routes of administration. The computation of F does not separate loss of oral drug metabolized by the first-pass effect and drug not absorbed by the gastrointestinal tract. Special techniques are needed to determine the fraction of drug absorbed orally for drugs with high liver extraction ratios or substantial gut wall metabolism.

Two different dosage forms of the same drug are considered to be bioequivalent when the $AUC_{0-\infty}$, maximum serum or blood concentrations (C_{max}), and the times that C_{max} occurs (t_{max}) are neither clinically nor statistically different. When this occurs, the serum-concentration-versus-time curves for the two dosage forms should be superimposable and therefore identical. Bioequivalence studies have become very important because many expensive drugs have become available recently in generic form. Most bioequivalence studies involve 18 to 25 healthy adults who are given the brand-name product and the generic product in a randomized, crossover study design.

CLEARANCE

Clearance (Cl) is the most important pharmacokinetic parameter because it determines the steady-state concentration for a given dosage rate. When a drug is given at a continuous intravenous infusion rate equal to k_0, the steady-state concentration (C_{ss}) is determined by the quotient of k_0 and Cl($C_{ss} = k_0$/Cl). If the drug is administered as individual doses (D) at a given dosage interval (τ), the average steady-state concentration (C_{ss}) over the dosage interval is given by the equation[4]

$$C_{ss} = \frac{F(D/\tau)}{Cl}$$

where F is the fraction of dose absorbed into the systemic vascular system. The average steady-state concentration over the dosage interval is the steady-state concentration that would have occurred had the same dose been given as a continuous intravenous infusion (e.g., 300 mg every 6 hours would produce an average C_{ss} equivalent to the

actual C_{ss} produced by a continuous infusion administered at a rate of 50 mg/h).

Physiologically, clearance is determined by (1) blood flow (Q) to the organ that metabolizes (liver) or eliminates (kidney) the drug and (2) the efficiency of the organ in extracting the drug from the bloodstream.[5] Efficiency is measured using an extraction ratio (E), calculated by subtracting the concentration in the blood leaving the extracting organ (C_{out}) from the concentration in the blood entering the organ (C_{in}) and then dividing the result by C_{in}:

$$E = \frac{C_{in} - C_{out}}{C_{out}}$$

Clearance for that organ is calculated by taking the product of Q and E (Cl = QE). For example, if liver blood flow equals 1.5 L/min and the drug's extraction ratio is 0.33, hepatic clearance equals 0.5 L/min. Total clearance is computed by summing all the individual organ clearance values. Clearance changes occur in patients when the blood flow to extracting organs changes or when the extraction ratio changes. Vasodilators such as hydralazine or nifedipine increase liver blood flow, whereas congestive heart failure and hypotension can decrease hepatic blood flow. Extraction ratios can increase when enzyme inducers increase the amount of drug-metabolizing enzyme. Extraction ratios may decrease if enzyme inhibitors inhibit drug-metabolizing enzymes or necrosis causes loss of parenchyma.

INTRINSIC CLEARANCE

The extraction ratio also can be thought of in terms of the unbound fraction of drug in the blood (f_b), the intrinsic ability of the extracting organ to clear unbound drug from the blood (Cl_{int}), and blood flow to the organ (Q)[6,7]:

$$E = \frac{f_b(Cl_{int})}{Q + f_b(Cl_{int})}$$

By substituting this equation for E, the clearance equation becomes

$$Cl = \frac{Q[f_b(Cl_{int})]}{Q + f_b(Cl_{int})}$$

Clearance changes will occur when blood flow to the clearing organ changes [in conditions where blood flow is reduced (e.g., shock, congestive heart failure) or when medications such as vasodilators increase blood flow], binding in the blood changes (e.g., if the concentration of binding proteins is low or highly protein-bound drugs are displaced), or intrinsic clearance of unbound drug changes (e.g., when metabolizing enzymes are induced or inhibited by other drug therapy or functional organ tissue is destroyed by disease processes).

If Cl_{int} is large (enzymes have a high capacity to metabolize the drug), the product of f_b and Cl_{int} is much larger than Q. When $f_b(Cl_{int})$ is much greater than Q, the sum of Q and $f_b(Cl_{int})$ in the denominator of the clearance equation almost equals $f_b(Cl_{int})$:

$$f_b(Cl_{int}) \approx Q + f_b(Cl_{int})$$

Substituting this expression in the denominator of the clearance equation and canceling common terms leads to the following expression for drugs with a large Cl_{int}: Cl $\approx Q$. In this case, clearance of the drug is equal to blood flow to the organ; such drugs are called *high-clearance drugs* and have large extraction ratios. Propranolol, verapamil, morphine, and lidocaine are examples of high-clearance drugs. High-clearance drugs such as these typically exhibit high first-pass effects when administered orally.

If Cl_{int} is small (enzymes have a limited capacity to metabolize the drug), Q is much larger than the product of f_b and Cl_{int}. When Q

is much greater than $f_b(\text{Cl}_{int})$, the sum of Q and $f_b(\text{Cl}_{int})$ in the denominator of the clearance equation becomes almost equal to Q: $Q \approx Q + f_b(\text{Cl}_{int})$. Substituting this expression in the denominator of the clearance equation and canceling common terms leads to the following expression for drugs with a small Cl_{int}: $\text{Cl} \approx f_b(\text{Cl}_{int})$. In this case, clearance of the drug is equal to the product of the fraction unbound in the blood and the intrinsic ability of the organ to clear unbound drug from the blood; such drugs are known as *low-clearance drugs* and have small extraction ratios. Warfarin, theophylline, diazepam, and phenobarbital are examples of low-clearance drugs.

As mentioned previously, the concentration of unbound drug in the blood is probably more important pharmacologically than the total (bound plus unbound) concentration. The unbound drug in the blood is in equilibrium with the unbound drug in the tissues and reflects the concentration of drug at its site of action. Therefore, the pharmacologic effect of a drug is thought to be a function of the concentration of unbound drug in the blood. The unbound steady-state concentration ($C_{ss,u}$) can be calculated by multiplying C_{ss} and f_b: $C_{ss,u} = C_{ss}f_b$. The effect that changes in Q, f_b, and Cl_{int} have on $C_{ss,u}$ and therefore on the pharmacologic response of a drug depends on whether a high- or low-clearance drug is involved. Because $\text{Cl} = Q$ for high-clearance drugs, a change in f_b or Cl_{int} does not change Cl or C_{ss} ($C_{ss} = k_0/\text{Cl}$). However, a change in unbound drug fraction does alter $C_{ss,u}$ ($C_{ss,u} = f_bC_{ss}$), thereby affecting the pharmacologic response. Plasma-protein-binding displacement drug interactions are thus very important clinically, but they are also dangerous because the changes in $C_{ss,u}$ are not reflected in changes in C_{ss}. Since laboratories usually measure only total concentrations (concentrations of unbound drug are difficult to determine), the interaction is hard to detect. If Cl_{int} changes for high-clearance drugs, Cl, C_{ss}, $C_{ss,u}$, and pharmacologic response do not change. Changes in Q cause a change in Cl; changes in C_{ss}, $C_{ss,u}$, and drug response are indirectly proportional to changes in Cl.

For low-clearance drugs, total clearance is determined by unbound drug fraction and intrinsic clearance: $\text{Cl} = f_b(\text{Cl}_{int})$. A change in Q does not change Cl, C_{ss}, $C_{ss,u}$, or pharmacologic response. However, a change in f_b or Cl_{int} does alter Cl and C_{ss} ($C_{ss} = k_0/\text{Cl}$). Changes in Cl_{int} will cause a proportional change in Cl. Changes in C_{ss}, $C_{ss,u}$, and drug response are indirectly proportional to changes in Cl. Altering f_b for low-clearance drugs produces interesting results. A change in f_b alters Cl and C_{ss} ($C_{ss} = k_0/\text{Cl}$). Since Cl and C_{ss} change in opposite directions with changes in f_b, $C_{ss,u}$ ($C_{ss,u} = f_bC_{ss}$) and pharmacologic response do not change with alterations in the fraction of unbound drug in the blood. For example, a low-clearance drug is administered to a patient until steady-state is achieved:

$$\text{Cl} = f_b(\text{Cl}_{int})$$

$$C_{ss} = \frac{k_0}{\text{Cl}}$$

Suppose that another drug is administered to the patient that displaces the first drug from plasma-protein-binding sites and doubles f_b (f_b now equals $2f_b$). Cl doubles because of the protein-binding displacement $[2\text{Cl} = 2f_b(\text{Cl}_{int})]$, and C_{ss} decreases by one-half because of the change in clearance $[1/2(C_{ss}) = k_0/(2\text{Cl})]$. $C_{ss,u}$ does not change because even though f_b is doubled, C_{ss} decreased by one-half ($C_{ss,u} = f_bC_{ss}$). The potential for error in this situation is that clinicians may increase the dose of a low-clearance drug after a protein-binding displacement interaction because C_{ss} decreased. Since $C_{ss,u}$ and the pharmacologic effect do not change, the dose should remain unaltered. Plasma-protein-binding decreases occur commonly in patients taking phenytoin. Low albumin concentrations (as in trauma or pregnant patients), high concentrations of endogenous plasma-protein-binding displacers

(as with high concentrations of bilirubin), or plasma-protein-binding drug interactions (as with concomitant therapy with valproic acid) can result in subtherapeutic total phenytoin concentrations. Despite this fact, unbound phenytoin concentrations usually are within the therapeutic range, and often the patient is responding appropriately to treatment. Thus, in these situations, unbound rather than total phenytoin serum concentrations should be monitored and used to guide future therapeutic decisions.

CLEARANCES FOR DIFFERENT ROUTES OF ELIMINATION AND METABOLIC PATHWAYS

Clearances for individual organs can be computed if the excretion the organ produces can be obtained. For example, renal clearance can be calculated if urine is collected during a pharmacokinetic experiment. The patient empties his or her bladder immediately before the dose is given. Subsequent urine production is collected until the last serum concentration (C_{last}) is obtained. Renal clearance (Cl_R) is computed by dividing the amount of drug excreted in the urine by $\text{AUC}_{0-t,\text{last}}$. Biliary and other clearance values are computed in a similar fashion.

Clearances also can be calculated for each metabolite that is formed from the parent drug. This computation is particularly useful in drug-interaction studies to determine which metabolic pathway is stimulated or inhibited. In the following metabolic scheme, the parent drug (D) is metabolized into two different metabolites (M_1, M_2) that subsequently are eliminated by the kidney (M_{1R}, M_{2R}):

$$D \xrightarrow{\text{Cl}_{FM1}} M_1 \xrightarrow{\text{kidney}} M_{1R}$$
$$\downarrow \text{Cl}_{FM2}$$
$$M_2 \xrightarrow{\text{kidney}} M_{2R}$$

To compute the formation clearance of M_1 and M_2 (Cl_{FM1}, Cl_{FM2}), urine would be collected for five or more half-lives after a single dose or during a dosage interval at steady state. The amount of metabolite eliminated in the urine is then determined. The fraction of the dose (in moles, because the molecular weights of the parent drug and metabolites are not equal) eliminated by each metabolic pathway ($f_{M1} = M_{1R}/D$ and $f_{M2} = M_{2R}/D$) can then be computed. Formation clearance for each pathway can be calculated using the following equations: $\text{Cl}_{FM1} = f_{M1}\text{Cl}_M$ and $\text{Cl}_{FM2} = f_{M2}\text{Cl}_M$, where Cl_M is the metabolic clearance for the parent drug.

VOLUME OF DISTRIBUTION

The volume of distribution (V_D) is a proportionality constant that relates the amount of drug in the body to the serum concentration (amount in body $= CV_D$). V_D is used to calculate the loading dose (LD) of a drug that will immediately achieve a desired C_{ss} (LD $= C_{ss}V_D$). However, in practice, the patient's own V_D is not known at the time the loading dose is administered. In this case, an average V_D is assumed and used to calculate a loading dose. Because the patient's V_D is almost always different from the average V_D for the drug, a loading dose does not attain the calculated C_{ss}, but it hopefully achieves a therapeutic concentration. As usual, steady-state conditions are achieved in three to five half-lives for the drug.

The numeric value for the volume of distribution is determined by the physiologic volume of blood and tissues and how the drug binds in blood and tissues[8]:

$$V_D = V_b + (f_b/f_t)V_t$$

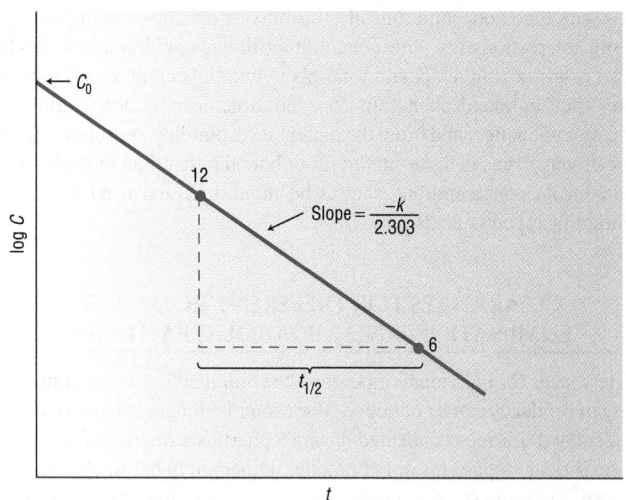

FIGURE 5–3. Calculation of the half-life of a drug following intravenous bolus dosing.

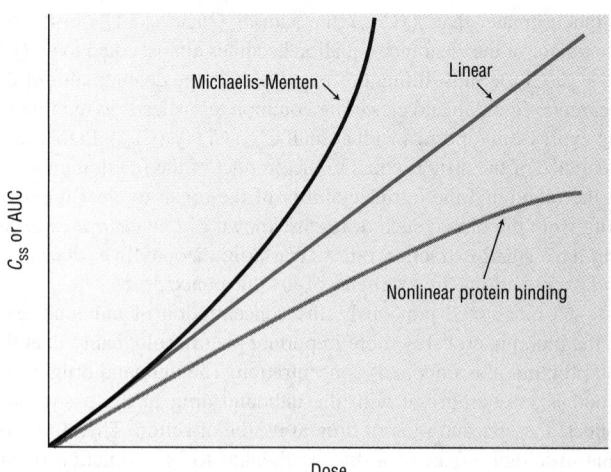

FIGURE 5–4. Relationship of dose and C_{ss} or AUC under linear and nonlinear conditions.

where V_b and V_t are the volumes of blood and tissues, respectively, and f_b and f_t are the fractions of unbound drug in blood and tissues, respectively.

HALF-LIFE

Half-life ($t_{1/2}$) is the time required for serum concentrations to decrease by one-half after absorption and distribution are complete. It takes the same amount of time for serum concentrations to drop from 200 to 100 mg/L as it does for concentrations to decline from 2 to 1 mg/L (Fig. 5–3).

Half-life is important because it determines the time required to reach steady state and the dosage interval. It takes approximately three to five half-lives to reach steady-state concentrations during continuous dosing. In three half-lives, serum concentrations are at about 90% of their ultimate steady-state values. Because most serum drug assays have about a 10% error, it is difficult to differentiate concentrations that are within 10% of each other. For this reason, many clinicians consider concentrations obtained after three half-lives to be C_{ss}.

Half-life is also used to determine the dosage interval for a drug. For instance, it may be desirable to maintain maximum steady-state concentrations at 20 mg/L and minimum steady-state concentrations at 10 mg/L. In this case, it would be necessary to administer the drug every half-life because the minimum desirable concentration is one-half the maximum desirable concentration.

Half-life is a dependent kinetic variable because its value depends on the values of Cl and V_D.[8] The equation that describes the relationship among the three variables is $t_{1/2} = 0.693 V_D/Cl$. Changes in $t_{1/2}$ can result from a change in either V_D or Cl; a change in $t_{1/2}$ does not necessarily indicate that Cl has changed. Half-life can change solely because of changes in V_D. The elimination rate constant (k) is related to the half-life by the following equation: $k = 0.693/t_{1/2}$. Both the half-life and elimination rate constant describe how quickly serum concentrations decrease in the serum or blood.

NONLINEAR PHARMACOKINETICS

MICHAELIS-MENTEN KINETICS

Some drugs do not follow the rules of linear pharmacokinetics. Instead of C_{ss} and AUC increasing proportionally with dose,

serum concentrations change more or less than expected (Fig. 5–4). One explanation for the greater than expected increase in C_{ss} and AUC after an increase in dose is that the enzymes responsible for the metabolism or elimination of the drug may start to become saturated. When this occurs, the maximum rate of metabolism (V_{max}) for the drug is approached. This is called *Michaelis-Menten kinetics*. The serum concentration at which the rate of metabolism equals $V_{max}/2$ is K_m. Practically speaking, K_m is the serum concentration at which nonproportional changes in C_{ss} and AUC start to occur when dose is increased. The Michaelis-Menten constants (V_{max} and K_m) determine the dosage rate (DR) needed to maintain a given C_{ss}: DR $= V_{max}C_{ss}/(K_m + C_{ss})$. Most drugs eliminated by the liver are metabolized by enzymes but still appear to follow linear kinetics. The reason for this disparity is that the therapeutic range for most drugs is well below the K_m of the enzyme system that metabolizes the agent. The therapeutic range is higher than K_m for some commonly used drugs. The average K_m for phenytoin is about 4 mg/L. The therapeutic range for phenytoin is usually 10 to 20 mg/L. Most patients experience Michaelis-Menten kinetics while taking phenytoin.

NONLINEAR PROTEIN BINDING

Another type of nonlinear kinetics can occur if C_{ss} and AUC increase less than expected after an increase in dose of a low-clearance drug. This usually indicates that plasma-protein-binding sites are starting to become saturated so that f_b increases with increases in dose (see Fig. 5–4). For a low-clearance drug, Cl depends on the values of f_b and Cl_{int} (Cl $= f_bCl_{int}$). When a dosage increase takes place, f_b increases because nearly all plasma-protein-binding sites are occupied and no binding sites are available. If f_b increases, Cl increases and C_{ss} increases less than expected with the dosage change ($C_{ss} = k_0/Cl$). However, $C_{ss,u}$ increases proportionally with dose because $C_{ss,u}$ depends on Cl_{int} for low-clearance drugs ($C_{ss,u} = k_0/Cl_{int}$). Valproic acid[9] and disopyramide[10] both follow saturable-protein-binding pharmacokinetics.

PHARMACOKINETIC MODELS AND EQUATIONS

Pharmacokinetic models are useful to describe data sets, to predict serum concentrations after several doses or different routes of administration, and to calculate pharmacokinetic constants such as Cl, V_D, and $t_{1/2}$.[11] Compartmental models depict the body as one

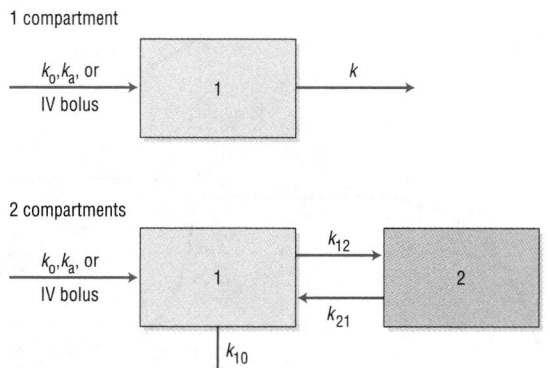

FIGURE 5–5. Visual representations of one- and two-compartment drug-distribution models.

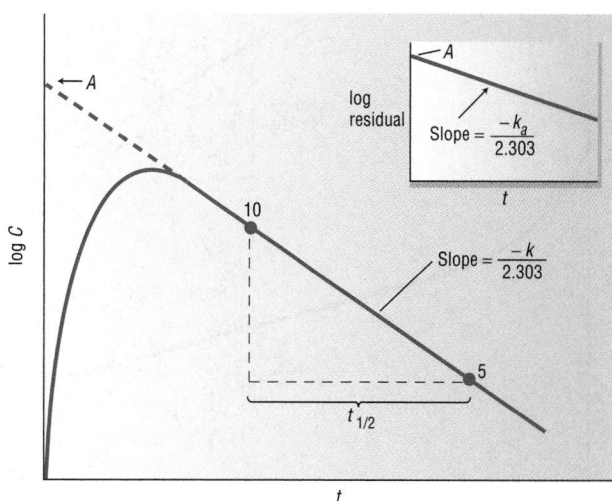

FIGURE 5–6. Calculation of the half-life of a drug following oral, intramuscular, or other extravascular dosing route.

or more discrete compartments to which drug is distributed and/or from which drug is eliminated. The shape of the serum-concentration-versus-time curve determines the number of compartments in the pharmacokinetic model and the equation used in computations (Fig. 5–5). First-order rate constants, known as *microconstants,* describe the rate of transfer from one compartment to another. Each compartment also has its own V_D. For clinical dosage adjustment purposes using drug concentrations, a one-compartment model is the most commonly used pharmacokinetic model.

ONE-COMPARTMENT MODEL

The simplest case uses a single compartment to represent the entire body (see Fig. 5–5). Drug enters the compartment by continuous intravenous infusion (k_0), absorption from an extravascular site with an absorption rate constant of k_a, or intravenous bolus (D). After an intravenous bolus, serum concentrations decline in a straight line when plotted on semilogarithmic coordinates (see Fig. 5–3). The slope of the line is $-k/2.303$; $t_{1/2}$ can be computed by determining the time required for concentrations to decrease by one-half ($t_{1/2} = 0.693/k$). The equation that describes the data is $C = (D/V_D)e^{-kt}$. V_D is calculated by dividing the intravenous dose by the y intercept (the concentration at time zero, C_0) of the graph. Cl is computed by taking the product of k and V_D. Once V_D and k are known, concentrations at any time after the dose can be computed [$C = (D/V_D)e^{-kt}$].

When an extravascular dose is given, one-compartment-model serum concentrations rise during absorption, reach C_{max}, and then decrease in a straight line with a slope equal to $-k/2.303$. The equation that describes the data is $C = \{(FDk_a)/[V_D(k_a - k)]\}(e^{-kt} - e^{-k_a t})$, where F is the fraction of the dose absorbed into the systemic circulation. The absorption rate constant (k_a) is obtained using the method of residuals.

The method of residuals is used to obtain the individual rate constants (Fig. 5–6). A is determined by extrapolating the terminal slope to the y axis; k_a can be obtained by calculating the slope or $t_{1/2}$ and using the formulas given for the intravenous bolus case. At each time point in the absorption portion of the curve, the concentration value from the extrapolated line is noted and called the *extrapolated concentration.* For each point, the actual concentration is subtracted from the extrapolated concentration to compute the *residual concentration.* When the residual concentrations are plotted on semilogarithmic coordinates, a line with y intercept equal to A and slope equal to $-k_a/2.303$ is obtained. When these values are calculated, they can be placed into the equation ($C = Ae^{-kt} - Ae^{-k_a t}$, where $A = FDk_a/[V_D(k_a - k)]$) and used to compute the serum concentration at any time after the

extravascular dose. The intercepts and rate constants also can be used to compute Cl and V_D: Cl $= FD/(A/k - A/k_a)$ and $V_D =$ Cl/k, where F is the fraction of the dose absorbed into the systemic circulation.

During a continuous intravenous infusion, the serum concentrations in a one-compartment model change according to the following function: $C = (k_0/\text{Cl})(1 - e^{-kt})$. If the infusion has been running for more than three to five half-lives, the patient will be at steady state, and Cl can be calculated (Cl $= k_0/C_{ss}$). When the infusion is discontinued, serum concentrations appear to decline in a straight line when plotted on semilogarithmic paper with a slope of $-k/2.303$. V_D is computed by dividing Cl by k (Fig. 5–7).

MULTICOMPARTMENT MODEL

After an intravenous bolus dose, serum concentrations often decline in two or more phases. During the early phases, drug leaves the bloodstream by two mechanisms: (1) distribution into tissues and (2) metabolism and/or elimination. Because the drug is leaving the bloodstream through these two mechanisms, serum concentrations decline rapidly. After tissues and blood are in equilibrium, only metabolism and/or elimination remove drug from the blood. During this terminal

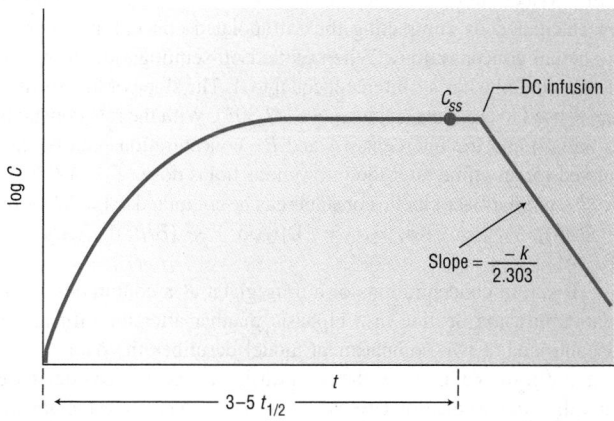

FIGURE 5–7. Achievement of steady-state serum concentrations after three to five half-lives of a drug. Note the elimination phase after discontinuance of the infusion.

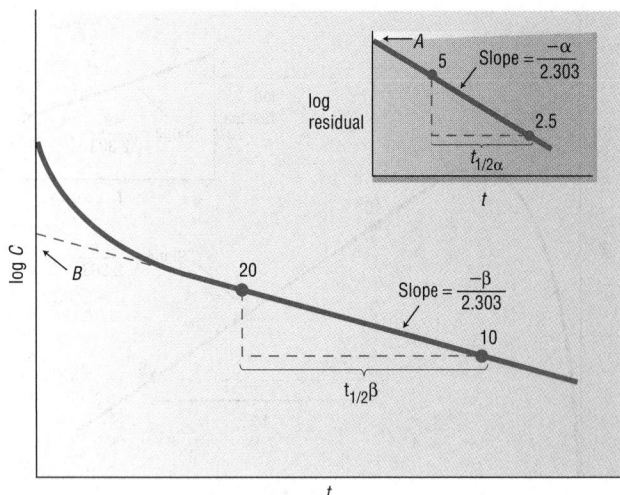

FIGURE 5–8. Calculation of α and β half-lives following intravenous dosing.

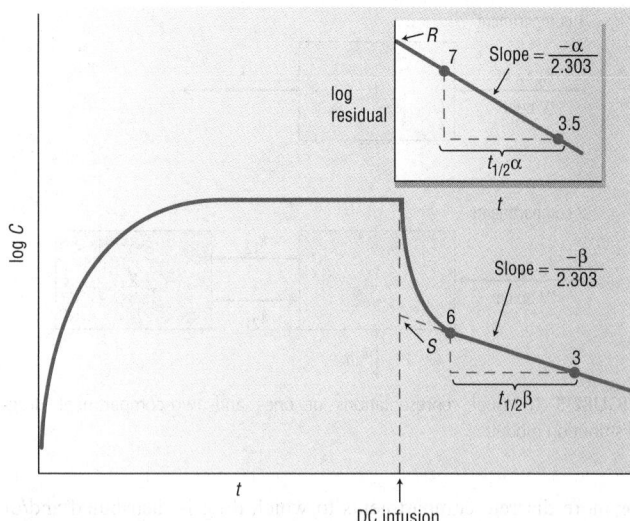

FIGURE 5–9. Calculation of α and β half-lives following a steady-state infusion.

phase, serum concentrations decline more slowly. The half-life is measured during the terminal phase by determining the time required for concentrations to decline by one-half.

After an intravenous bolus dose, serum concentrations decrease as if the drug were being injected into a central compartment that not only metabolizes and eliminates drug but also distributes drug to one or more other compartments. Of these multicompartment models, the two-compartment model is encountered most commonly (see Fig. 5–5). After an intravenous bolus injection, serum concentrations decrease in two distinct phases described by the equation:

$$C = \frac{D(\alpha - k_{21})}{V_{D_1}(\alpha - \beta)}e^{-\alpha t} + \frac{D(k_{21} - \beta)}{V_{D_1}(\alpha - \beta)}e^{-\beta t}$$

or $C = Ae^{-\alpha t} + Be^{-\beta t}$, where k_{21} is the first-order rate constant that reflects the transfer of drug from compartment 2 to compartment 1, V_{D1} is the V_D of compartment 1, $A = D(\alpha - k_{21})/[V_{D1}(\alpha - \beta)]$ and $B = D(k_{21} - \beta)/[V_{D1}(\alpha - \beta)]$. The rate constants α and β found in the exponents of the equations describe the distribution and elimination of the drug, respectively (Fig. 5–8). A and B are the y intercepts of the lines that describe drug distribution and elimination, respectively, on the log concentration-versus-time plot.

The residual line is calculated as before using the method of residuals. The terminal line is extrapolated to the y axis, and extrapolated concentrations are determined for each time point. Because actual concentrations are greater in this case, residual concentrations are calculated by subtracting the extrapolated concentrations from the actual concentrations. When plotted on semilogarithmic paper, the residual line has a y intercept equal to A. The slope of the residual line is used to compute α (slope $= -\alpha/2.303$). With the rate constants (α and β) and the intercepts (A and B), concentrations can be calculated for any time after the intravenous bolus dose ($C = Ae^{-\alpha t} + Be^{-\beta t}$), or pharmacokinetic constants can be computed: $Cl = D/[(A/\alpha) + (B/\beta)]$, $V_{D,\beta} = Cl/\beta$, $V_{D,ss} = \{D[(A/\alpha^2) + (B/\beta^2)]\}/[(A/\alpha) + (B/\beta)]^2$.

If serum concentrations of a drug given as a continuous intravenous infusion decline in a biphasic manner after the infusion is discontinued, a two-compartment model describes the data set[12,13] (Fig. 5–9). In this instance, the postinfusion concentrations decrease according to the equation $C = Re^{-\alpha t'} + Se^{-\beta t'}$, where t' is the postinfusion time ($t' = 0$ when infusion is discontinued) and $R, S, \alpha,$ and β are determined from the postinfusion concentrations using the method of residuals with the y axis set at $t' = 0$. R and S are used to compute

A and B. A and B are the y intercepts that would have occurred had the total dose given during the infusion ($D = k_0T$) been administered as an intravenous bolus dose:

$$A = \frac{RD\alpha}{k_0(1 - e^{-\alpha T})}$$

$$B = \frac{SD\beta}{k_0(1 - e^{-\beta T})}$$

where T is the duration of infusion. Once $A, B, \alpha,$ and β are known, the equations for an intravenous bolus are used to compute the pharmacokinetic constants. Often, when a drug is given as an intravenous bolus or continuous intravenous infusion, a two-compartment model is used to describe the data, but when the same agent is given extravascularly, a one-compartment model applies.[14] In this case, distribution occurs during the absorption phase, so a distribution phase is not observed.

VOLUMES OF DISTRIBUTION IN MULTICOMPARTMENT MODELS

Two different V_D values are needed as proportionality constants for drugs that require multicompartment models to describe the serum-concentration-versus-time curve. The V_D that is used to compute the amount of drug in the body during the terminal (β) portion of the curve is called $V_{D,\beta}$ (amount of drug in body $= V_{D,\beta}C$). During a continuous intravenous infusion at steady state, $V_{D,ss}$ is used to compute the amount of drug in the body (amount of drug in body $= V_{D,ss}C$). $V_{D,ss}$ is also the V_D that can be computed using the physiologic volumes of blood and tissues and the ratio of unbound drug in blood to that in tissues [$V_{D,ss} = V_b + (f_b/f_t)V_t$]. Because the value of $V_{D,\beta}$ changes when Cl changes, $V_{D,ss}$ should be used to indicate if drug distribution changes during pharmacokinetic or drug-interaction experiments.

MULTIPLE DOSING AND STEADY-STATE EQUATIONS

Any of these compartmental equations can be used to determine serum concentrations after multiple doses. The multiple-dosing factor ($1 - e^{-nK\tau})/(1 - e^{-K\tau}$), where n is the number of doses, K is the appropriate rate constant, and τ is the dosage interval, is simply multiplied by each exponential term in the equation, substituting the rate constant of each exponent for K. Time (t) is set at 0 at the beginning of each dosage interval. For example, a single-dose two-compartment intravenous bolus is calculated as follows: $C = Ae^{-\alpha t} + Be^{-\beta t}$. The equation for a multiple-dose two-compartment intravenous bolus is therefore

$$C = Ae^{-\alpha t}\frac{1 - e^{-n\alpha\tau}}{1 - e^{-\alpha\tau}} + Be^{-\beta t}\frac{1 - e^{-n\beta\tau}}{1 - e^{-\beta\tau}}$$

A single-dose one-compartment intravenous bolus is calculated as $C = (D/V_D)e^{-kt}$. For a multiple-dose one-compartment intravenous bolus, the concentration is $C = (D/V_D)e^{-kt}[(1 - e^{-nkt})/(1 - e^{-k\tau})]$.

At steady state, the number of doses becomes large, $e^{-nK\tau}$ approaches zero, and the multiple-dosing factor equals $1/(1 - e^{-K\tau})$. Therefore, the steady-state versions of the equations are simpler than their multiple-dose counterparts:

$$C = \frac{Ae^{-\alpha t}}{1 - e^{-\alpha\tau}} + \frac{Be^{-\beta t}}{1 - e^{-\beta\tau}}$$

and

$$C = \frac{(D/V_D)e^{-kt}}{1 - e^{-k\tau}}$$

for a steady-state two-compartment intravenous bolus and a steady-state one-compartment intravenous bolus, respectively.

USE OF PHARMACOKINETIC CONCEPTS FOR INDIVIDUALIZATION OF DRUG THERAPY

9 Many factors must be taken into consideration when deciding on the best drug dose for a patient. For example, the age of the patient is important because the dose (in milligrams per kilogram) for pediatric patients may be higher and for geriatric patients may be lower than the typically prescribed dose for young adults. Gender also can be a factor because males and females metabolize and eliminate some drugs differently. Patients who are significantly obese or cachectic also may require different drug doses because of clearance and volume of distribution changes. Other drug therapy that could cause drug interactions needs to be considered. Disease states and conditions may alter the drug-dosage regimen for a patient. Three disease states that deserve special mention are congestive heart failure, renal disease, and hepatic disease. Renal and hepatic diseases cause loss of organ function and decreased drug elimination and metabolism. Congestive heart failure causes decreased blood flow to organs that clear the drug from the body.

Many drug compounds are racemic mixtures of stereoisomers. In most cases, one of the isomers is more pharmacologically active than the other isomer, and each isomer may exhibit different pharmacokinetic properties. Warfarin, propranolol, verapamil, and ibuprofen are all racemic mixtures of stereoisomers. Some drug interactions inhibit or increase the elimination of only one stereoisomer. The importance of the drug interaction depends on which isomer is affected. Other drugs, such as dextromethorphan, levofloxacin, and diltiazem, are composed of just one stereoisomer.

10 Genetics also plays a role in drug metabolism. *Cytochrome P450* is a generic term for the group of enzymes that are responsible for most drug metabolism oxidation reactions. Several cytochrome P450 isozymes have been identified that are responsible for the metabolism of many important drugs (Table 5–3). CYP2C19 (P450IIC19, P450$_{mp}$, formerly included in CYP2C9) is responsible for aromatic hydroxylation of mephenytoin, and CYP2D6 (P450IID6, P450$_{db}$) oxidizes debrisoquine.[15] These subsets of the cytochrome P450 enzyme family are also responsible for the metabolism of several other drugs (CYP2D6: many tricyclic antidepressants, codeine,

TABLE 5–3. Cytochrome P450 Enzyme Family and Selected Substrates

CYP1A2	**CYP2E1**
Acetaminophen	Ethanol
Antipyrine	Isoniazid
Caffeine	
Tacrine	**CYP3A4**
Theophylline	Alfentanil
R-Warfarin	Alprazolam
	Astemizole
CYP2C9	Carbamazepine
Diclofenac	Cisapride
Hexobarbital	Cyclosporine
Ibuprofen	Diltiazem
Naproxen	Erythromycin
Phenytoin	Felodipine
Tolbutamide	Fluconazole
S-Warfarin	Itraconazole
	Ketoconazole
CYP2C19	Lidocaine
Diazepam	Lovastatin
Mephenytoin	Midazolam
Omeprazole	Nifedipine
	Quinidine
CYP2D6	Simvastatin
Codeine	Tacrolimus
Debrisoquine	Terfenadine
Dextromethorphan	Verapamil
Encainide	
Fluoxetine	
Haloperidol	
Metoprolol	
Paroxetine	
Propafenone	
Risperidone	
Thioridazine	
Venlafaxine	

metoprolol; CYP2C19: most proton pump inhibitors, sertraline, voriconazole). Both these isozymes appear to be under genetic control. As a consequence, there are "poor metabolizers" who have a defective mutant gene for the isozyme, cannot manufacture a fully functional isozyme, and therefore cannot metabolize the drug substrate very well. "Extensive metabolizers" have the standard gene for the isozyme and metabolize the drugs normally. Poor metabolizers usually are a minority of the general population. They may achieve toxic concentrations of drug when usual doses are prescribed for them or, if the active drug moiety is a metabolite, may fail to have any pharmacologic effect from the drug. The ethnic background of the patient can affect the likelihood that he or she will be a poor metabolizer.[15] For example, the incidence of poor metabolizers for CYP2D6 is about 5% to 10% for Caucasians and about 0% to 1% for Asians, whereas for CYP2C19, poor metabolizers make up about 3% to 6% of the Caucasian population and about 20% of the Asian population.

Other cytochrome P450 isozymes have been isolated.[15] CYP1A2 (P450IA2) is the enzyme that is responsible for the demethylation of caffeine and theophylline; CYP2C9 (P450IIC9) metabolizes phenytoin, tolbutamide, losartan, and ibuprofen; most antiretroviral protease inhibitors, cyclosporine, nifedipine, and atorvastatin are metabolized by CYP3A4 (P450IIIA4); and ethanol is a substrate for CYP2E1 (P450IIE1). It is important to recognize that a drug may be metabolized by more than one cytochrome P450 isozyme. While most tricyclic antidepressants are hydroxylated by CYP2D6, *N*-demethylation probably is mediated by a combination of

CYP2C19, CYP1A2, and CYP3A4. Acetaminophen appears to be metabolized by both CYP1A2 and CYP2E1. The 4-hydroxy metabolite of propranolol is produced by CYP2D6, but side-chain oxidation of propranolol is probably a product of CYP2C19. The CYP3A enzyme family comprises approximately 90% of the drug-metabolizing enzyme present in the intestinal wall but only approximately 30% of the drug-metabolizing enzyme found in the liver. The remainder of hepatic drug-metabolizing enzyme is approximately 20% for the CYP2C family, approximately 13% for CYP1A2, approximately 7% for CYP2E1, and approximately 2% for CYP2D6.

Understanding which cytochrome P450 isozyme is responsible for the metabolism of a drug is extraordinarily useful in predicting and understanding drug interactions. Some drug-metabolism inhibitors and inducers are highly selective for certain cytochrome P450 isozymes.[15] Quinidine is an extremely potent inhibitor of the CYP2D6 enzyme system[15]; a single 50-mg dose of quinidine can change a rapid metabolizer of debrisoquine into a poor metabolizer. Ciprofloxacin and zileuton inhibit whereas tobacco or marijuana smoke induce CYP1A2. Some drugs that are enzyme inhibitors are also substrates for that same enzyme system and appear to cause drug interactions by being a competitive inhibitor. For example, erythromycin is both a substrate for and an inhibitor of CYP3A4. Obviously, if one knows that a new drug is metabolized by a given cytochrome P450 enzyme system, it is logical to assume that the new drug will exhibit drug interactions with the known inducers and inhibitors of that cytochrome P450 isozyme.

11 The importance of transport proteins in drug bioavailability and elimination is now better understood. The principal transport protein involved in the movement of drugs across biologic membranes is PGP. PGP is present in many organs, including the gastrointestinal tract, liver, and kidney. If a drug is a substrate for PGP, its oral absorption may be decreased when PGP transports drug molecules that have been absorbed back into the gastrointestinal tract lumen. In the liver, some drugs are transported by PGP from the blood into the bile, where the drug is eliminated by biliary secretion. Similarly, some drugs eliminated by the kidney are transported from the blood into the urine by PGP. Digoxin is a substrate of PGP. Other possible mechanisms for drug interactions are when two drugs that are substrates for PGP compete for transport by the protein and when a drug is an inhibitor or inducer of PGP. Drug interactions involving inhibition of PGP decrease drug transportation in these organs and potentially can increase gastrointestinal absorption of orally administered drug, decrease biliary secretion of the drug, or decrease renal elimination of drug molecules. The drug interaction between amiodarone and digoxin probably involves all three of these mechanisms, and this explains why digoxin concentrations increase so dramatically in patients receiving amiodarone. Many drugs that are metabolized by CYP3A4 are also substrates for PGP, and some of the drug interactions attributed to inhibition of CYP3A4 may be due to decreased drug transportation by PGP. Drug interactions involving induction of PGP have the opposite effect in these organs and may decrease gastrointestinal absorption of orally administered drug, increase biliary secretion of the drug, or increase renal elimination of drug molecules.

SELECTION OF INITIAL DRUG DOSES

12 When deciding on initial doses for drugs that are eliminated renally, the patient's renal function should be assessed. A common, useful way to do this is to measure the patient's serum creatinine concentration and convert this value into an estimated creatinine clearance (CrCl$_{est}$). Serum creatinine values alone should not be used to assess renal function because they do not include the effects of age, body weight, or gender. The Cockcroft-Gault equation[16] is probably the most widely used method to estimate creatinine clearance (in milliliters per minute) in adults (18 years or older) who are within about 30% of their ideal body weight and have stable renal function:

$$\text{Male: } CrCl_{est} = \frac{(140 - \text{age})BW}{S_{Cr} \times 72}$$

$$\text{Female: } CrCl_{est} = \frac{0.85(140 - \text{age})BW}{S_{Cr} \times 72}$$

where BW is body weight (in kilograms), age is the patient's age (in years), 0.85 is a correction factor to account for lower muscle mass in females, and S_{Cr} is serum creatinine (in milligrams per deciliter). For children, the following estimation equations are available according to the age of the child[17]: age 0 to 1 years: CrCl$_{est}$ (in mL/min/1.73 m^2) = $(0.45 \times \text{Lt})/S_{Cr}$; age 1 to 20 years: CrCl$_{est}$ (in mL/min/1.73 m^2) = $(0.55 \times \text{Lt})/S_{Cr}$, where Lt is patient length in centimeters. Other methods to determine CrCl$_{est}$ for obese adults[18] and patients with rapidly changing renal function[19] are available. Creatinine is a by-product of muscle breakdown in the body, so none of these estimation methods work well in patients with muscle disease, such as multiple sclerosis, or diseases that alter muscle mass, such as cachexia, malnutrition, cancer, or spinal cord injury. Nomograms that adjust initial doses according to a patient's renal function are available for several drugs, including digoxin,[20] vancomycin,[21] and the aminoglycoside antibiotics.[22] For many other drugs, William M. Bennett[23,24] occasionally updates his monograph on drug dosing in renal disease, which includes suggested dosage adjustments. For drugs that are eliminated primarily by the kidney (≥60% of the administered dose), some agents will need minor dosage adjustments for CrCl$_{est}$ between 30 and 60 mL/min, moderate dosage adjustments for CrCl$_{est}$ between 15 and 30 mL/min, and major dosage adjustments for CrCl$_{est}$ less than 15 mL/min. Postdialysis supplemental doses of some medications also may be needed for patients receiving hemodialysis if the drug is removed by the artificial kidney.

13 A similar assessment of liver function should be made for drugs that are metabolized hepatically. Unfortunately, there is no single test that can estimate liver drug-metabolism capacity accurately, and those which are used do not always prove accurate. High aminotransferase (AST or SGOT and ALT or SGPT) and alkaline phosphatase concentrations usually indicate acute hepatic cellular damage and do not establish poor liver drug metabolism reliably. Abnormal values for three tests that usually indicate that drugs will be metabolized poorly by the liver are high serum bilirubin concentration, low serum albumin concentration, and a prolonged prothrombin time. Bilirubin is metabolized by the liver, and albumin and clotting factors are manufactured by the liver, so aberrant values for all three of these tests are a more reliable indicator of abnormal liver drug metabolism. The Child-Pugh score,[25] a widely used clinical classification for liver disease that incorporates clinical signs and symptoms (ascites and hepatic encephalopathy) in addition to these three laboratory tests, can be used as an indicator of a patient's ability to metabolize drugs that are eliminated by the liver. A score in excess of 10 suggests very poor liver function. As a general rule, patients with cirrhosis have the most severe decreases in liver drug metabolism. Patients with acute or chronic hepatitis often retain relatively normal or slightly decreased hepatic drug-metabolism capacity. In the absence of specific pharmacokinetic dosing guidelines for a medication, a Child-Pugh score equal to 8 to 9 is grounds for a moderate decrease (approximately 25%) in initial daily drug dose for agents that are metabolized primarily (≥60%) hepatically, and a score of 10 or greater indicates that a significant decrease in initial daily dose (approximately 50%)

TABLE 5–4. Theophylline Pharmacokinetic Parameters for Selected Disease States/Conditions

Disease State/Condition	Mean Clearance (mL/min/kg)	Mean Dose (mg/kg/h)
Children 1–9 yr	1.4	0.8
Children 9–12 yr or adult smokers	1.25	0.7
Adolescents 12–16 yr or elderly smokers (>65 yr)	0.9	0.5
Adult nonsmokers	0.7	0.4
Elderly nonsmokers (>65 yr)	0.5	0.3
Decompensated CHF, cor pulmonale, cirrhosis	0.35	0.2

Mean volume of distribution = 0.5 L/kg.
Adapted from Ref. 49.

is required for drugs that are metabolized mostly by the liver. As in any patient with or without liver dysfunction, initial doses are meant as starting points for dosage titration based on patient response and avoidance of adverse effects.

Since there are no good markers of liver function, clinicians have come to rely on pharmacokinetic parameters derived in various patient populations to compute initial doses of drugs that are eliminated hepatically. Table 5–4 contains average pharmacokinetic parameters for theophylline in several disease states. Initial doses of many liver-metabolized drugs are computed by determining which disease states and/or conditions the patient has that are known to alter the kinetics of the drug and by using these average pharmacokinetic constants to calculate doses. The patient is then monitored for therapeutic and adverse effects, and drug serum concentrations are obtained to ensure that concentrations are appropriate and to adjust doses, if necessary. The following computations illustrate the estimated intravenous loading dose and the intravenous continuous infusion necessary to achieve a theophylline concentration of 10 mg/L for a 55-year-old, 70-kg male with liver cirrhosis (mean kinetic parameters obtained from Table 5–4):

$V_D = (0.5 \text{ L/kg})(70 \text{ kg}) = 35 \text{ L}$
$LD = C_{ss}V_D = (10 \text{ mg/L})(35 \text{ L})$
$\quad = 350 \text{ mg theophylline infused over 20 to 30 min}$

$$Cl(\text{in L/h}) = \frac{(0.35 \text{ mL/min/kg})(70 \text{ kg})(60 \text{ min/h})}{1000 \text{ mL}/L}$$

$\quad = 1.5 \text{ L/h}$
$k_0 = C_{ss}Cl = (10 \text{ mg/L})(1.5 \text{ L/h})$
$\quad = 15 \text{ mg/h of theophylline to begin after loading dose is given}$

If theophylline is to be given as the aminophylline salt form, each dose would need to be changed to reflect the fact that aminophylline contains only 85% theophylline (LD = 350 mg of theophylline/0.85 = 410 mg of aminophylline infused over 20 to 30 minutes, k_0 = 15 mg/h of theophylline/0.85 = 18 mg/h of aminophylline to begin after loading dose is given).

Heart failure is often overlooked as a disease state that can alter drug disposition. Severe heart failure decreases cardiac output and therefore reduces liver blood flow. Theophylline,[26] lidocaine,[27] and drugs with high extraction ratios are compounds whose clearance declines with decreased liver blood flow. Initial dosages of these drugs should be reduced in patients with moderate to severe heart failure (New York Heart Association class III or IV) by 25% to 50% until steady-state concentrations and response can be determined.

USE OF STEADY-STATE DRUG CONCENTRATIONS

Serum drug concentrations are readily available to clinicians to use as guides for the individualization of drug therapy. The therapeutic ranges for several drugs have been identified, and it is likely that new drugs also will be monitored using serum concentrations. Although several individualization methods have been advocated for specific drugs, one simple, reliable method is used commonly. For drugs that exhibit linear pharmacokinetics, C_{ss} changes proportionally with dose. To adjust a patient's drug therapy, a reasonable starting dose is administered for an estimated three to five half-lives. A serum concentration is obtained, assuming that it will reflect C_{ss}. Independent of the route of administration, the new dose (D_{new}) needed to attain the desired C_{ss} ($C_{ss,new}$) is calculated: $D_{new} = D_{old}(C_{ss,new}/C_{ss,old})$, where D_{old} and $C_{ss,old}$ are the old dose and old C_{ss}, respectively. To use this method, $C_{ss,old}$ must reflect steady-state conditions. Often patients are noncompliant with regard to their drug dosage and therefore are not at steady state. This occurs not only in outpatients but also in hospital inpatients. Inpatients can spit out oral doses or alter the infusion rates on intravenous pump rates after the nurse leaves the hospital room. Doses also can be missed if the patient is absent from his or her room at the time medications are to be administered. If $C_{ss,old}$ is much larger or smaller than expected for the D_{old} the patient is taking, one should suspect noncompliance and repeat the serum concentration determination after another three to five half-lives or change the patient's dose cautiously and monitor for signs of toxicity or lack of effect.

MEASUREMENT OF PHARMACOKINETIC PARAMETERS IN PATIENTS

If it is necessary to determine the kinetic constants for a patient to individualize his or her dose, a small kinetic evaluation is conducted in the individual. In these cases, the number of serum concentrations obtained from the patient is held to the minimum needed to calculate accurate pharmacokinetic parameters and doses. The reason for using fewer serum drug concentration determinations is to be as cost-effective as possible because these laboratory tests generally cost $20 to $50 each.

Although many drugs follow two-compartment-model pharmacokinetics (especially after intravenous administration), a one-compartment model is used to compute kinetic parameters in patients because too many serum concentration determinations would be needed to determine accurately both the distribution and elimination phases found in the two-compartment model. Because of this, serum concentrations usually are not measured in patients during the distribution phase. Another important reason serum concentrations are not measured during the distribution phase for therapeutic drug-monitoring purposes in patients is that drug in the blood and drug in the tissues are not in equilibrium during this time so that serum concentrations do not reflect tissue concentrations. When drug serum concentrations are obtained in patients for the purpose of assessing efficacy or toxicity, it is important that they be measured in the post-distribution phase when drug in the blood is in equilibrium with drug at the site of action.

In the case where the patient has received enough doses to be at steady state, pharmacokinetic parameters can be computed using a predose minimum concentration and a postdose maximum concentration. Under steady-state conditions, serum concentrations after each dose are identical, so the predose minimum concentration is the same before each dose (Fig. 5–10). This situation allows the predose concentration to be used to compute both the patient's $t_{1/2}$ and V. If the drug was given extravascularly or has a significant distribution

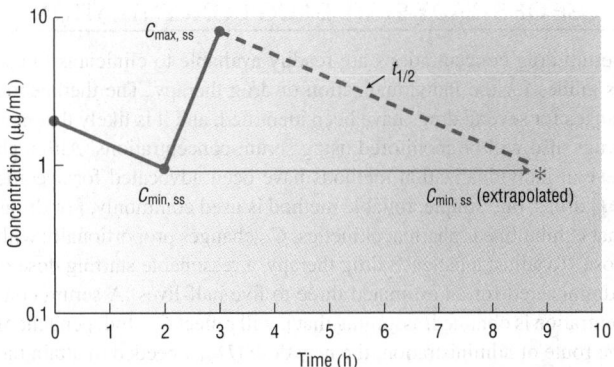

FIGURE 5–10. When a patient has received enough doses to be at steady state, steady-state maximum ($C_{max,ss}$) and minimum ($C_{min,ss}$) concentrations can be used to compute clearance, volume of distribution, and half-life. At steady state, consecutive $C_{min,ss}$ values are equal, so the predose value can be extrapolated to the time before the next dose and be used to calculate half-life (*dashed line*).

phase, the postdose concentration should be determined after absorption or distribution is finished. To ensure that steady-state conditions have been achieved, the patient needs to receive the drug on schedule for at least three to five estimated half-lives. To make sure that this is the case, inpatients should have their medication administration records checked, and the patient's nurse should be consulted regarding missed or late doses. Outpatients should be interviewed about compliance with the prescribed dosage regimen. When compliance with the dosage regimen has been verified, steady-state conditions reasonably can be assumed.

If the patient is not at steady state, an additional postdose serum concentration determination should be done to compute the patient's pharmacokinetic parameters. Ideally, the third concentration (C_3) should be acquired approximately one estimated half-life after the postdose maximum concentration. Determining serum concentrations too close together will hamper the drug assay's ability to measure differences between them, and getting the third sample too late could result in a concentration too low for the assay to detect. In this situation, the predose minimum and postdose maximum concentrations are used to compute V, and both postdose concentrations are used to calculate $t_{1/2}$ (Fig. 5–11).

After Cl, V, and $t_{1/2}$ have been computed for a patient, the dose and dosage interval necessary to achieve desired steady-state serum

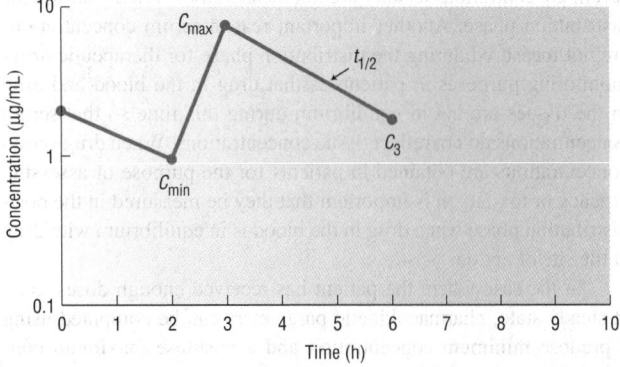

FIGURE 5–11. If a patient has not received enough doses to be at steady state, or doses have been given on an irregular schedule, the minimum concentration (C_{min}), maximum concentration (C_{max}), and an additional postdose concentration (C_3) can be used to compute clearance, volume of distribution, and half-life.

concentrations can be calculated using one-compartment-model equations. Specific examples of these methods to calculate initial doses and individualized doses using serum concentrations are discussed later in this chapter for the aminoglycoside antibiotics, vancomycin, digoxin, theophylline, phenytoin, and cyclosporine.

COMPUTER PROGRAMS

Computer programs that aid in the individualization of therapy are available for many different drugs. The most sophisticated programs use nonlinear regression to fit Cl and V_D to actual serum concentrations obtained in a patient.[28] After drug doses and serum concentrations are entered into the computer, nonlinear least-squares regression programs adjust Cl and V_D until the sum of the squared error between actual (C_{act}) and computer-estimated concentrations (C_{est}) is at a minimum [$\Sigma(C_{est} - C_{act})^2$]. Once estimates of Cl and V_D are available, doses are calculated easily.

Many programs also take into account what the Cl and V_D should be on the basis of disease states and conditions present in the patient.[29] Incorporation of expected population-based parameters allows the computer to use a limited number of serum concentrations (one or two) to provide estimates of Cl and V_D. This type of computer program is called *Bayesian* because it incorporates portions of Bayes' theorem during the fitting routine.[30] Bayesian pharmacokinetic dosing programs are used widely to adjust the dose of a variety of drugs. In the case of renally eliminated drugs (e.g., aminoglycosides, vancomycin, and digoxin), population estimates for kinetic parameters are generated by entering the patient's age, weight, height, gender, and serum creatinine concentration into the computer program. For hepatically eliminated drugs (e.g., theophylline and phenytoin), population estimates for kinetic parameters are computed using the patient's age, weight, and gender, as well as other factors that might change hepatic clearance, such as the presence or absence of disease states (e.g., cirrhosis or congestive heart failure) or other drug therapy that might cause a drug interaction. The Bayesian estimates of the pharmacokinetic parameters are then modified using nonlinear least-squares regression fits of serum concentrations to result in individualized parameters for the patient. The individualized parameters are used to compute doses for the patient that will result in desired steady-state concentrations of the drug.

AMINOGLYCOSIDES

Although aminoglycoside pharmacokinetics follow multicompartment models,[31] a one-compartment model appears sufficient to individualize doses in patients.[32] Aminoglycosides usually are given as short-term intermittent intravenous infusions and administered as a single daily dose or multiple doses per day. Initial doses for aminoglycosides can be computed using estimated kinetic parameters derived from population pharmacokinetic data. The elimination rate constant is estimated using the patient's creatinine clearance in the following formula: k (in h^{-1}) $= 0.00293(CrCl) + 0.014$, where CrCl is the measured or estimated creatinine clearance in milliliters per minute. The volume of distribution is estimated using the average population value for normal-weight (within 30% of ideal weight) individuals equal to 0.26 L/kg [$V = 0.26(Wt)$, where Wt is the patient's weight] or for obese individuals (over 30% ideal weight)[33] by taking into account the patient's excess adipose tissue: $V = 0.26[IBW + 0.4(TBW - IBW)]$, where IBW is ideal body weight [IBW_{males} (in kilograms) $= 50 + 2.3(Ht - 60)$ or $IBW_{females}$ (in kilograms) $= 45 + 2.3(Ht - 60)$, where Ht is the patient's height in inches]. Additional volume-of-distribution population estimates are available for other disease states and conditions such as cystic fibrosis,[34] ascites,[35] and neonates.[36]

Appropriate $C_{max,ss}$ and $C_{min,ss}$ values are selected for the patient based on the site and severity of the infection and the sensitivity of the known or suspected pathogen, as well as avoidance of adverse effects. For example, $C_{max,ss}$ values of 8 to 10 mg/L generally are selected for gram-negative pneumonia patients, whereas $C_{min,ss}$ values of less than 2 mg/L usually are chosen to avoid aminoglycoside-induced nephrotoxicity when tobramycin and gentamicin are prescribed using conventional multiple-daily-dosing regimens. Once appropriate steady-state serum concentrations are selected, the dosage interval required to achieve those concentrations is calculated, and τ is rounded to a clinically acceptable value (e.g., 8, 12, 18, 24, 36, or 48 hours): $\tau = [(\ln C_{max,ss} - \ln C_{min,ss})/k] + T$. Finally, a dose is computed for the patient using the one-compartment-model intermittent intravenous infusion equation at steady state, and the dose is rounded off to the nearest 5 to 10 mg:

$$D = TkV_DC_{max,ss}\frac{1 - e^{-k\tau}}{1 - e^{-kT}}$$

The Hull and Sarrubi aminoglycoside dosage nomogram (Table 5–5) is based on this dosage-calculation method and includes precalculated doses and dosage intervals for a variety of creatinine clearance values.[22] The nomogram assumes that $V_D = 0.26$ L/kg and should not be used to compute doses for disease states with altered V_D.

For extended-interval therapy, $C_{max,ss}$ values of 20–30 mg/L and $C_{min,ss}$ values less than 1 mg/L generally are accepted as appropriate for gram-negative pneumonia patients. A minimum 24-hour dosage interval is chosen for this dosing technique, and the dosing interval is increased in 12- to 24-hour increments for patients with renal dysfunction.

An example of this initial dosage scheme for a typical case is provided to illustrate the use of the various equations. Mr. JJ is a 65-year-old, 80-kg, 6-ft-tall man with the diagnosis of gram-negative pneumonia. His serum creatinine concentration is 2.1 mg/dL and is stable. Compute a conventional gentamicin dosage regimen (infused over 1 hour) that would provide approximate peak and trough concentrations of $C_{max,ss} = 8$ mg/L and $C_{min,ss} = 1.5$ mg/L, respectively. The patient is within 30% of his ideal body weight [$IBW_{male} = 50 + 2.3(72$ in $- 60) = 78$ kg] and has stable renal function, so the Cockcroft-Gault creatinine clearance estimation equation can be used: $CrCl_{est} = [(140 - 65$ yrs$)80$ kg$]/[72(2.1$ mg/dL$)] = 40$ mL/min. The patient's weight and estimated creatinine clearance are used to compute his V and k, respectively: $V = 0.26$ L/kg$(80$ kg$) = 20.8$ L; $k = 0.00293(40$ mL/min$) + 0.014 = 0.131$ h^{-1} or $t_{1/2} = 0.693/0.131$ h$^{-1}) = 5.3$ h. The dosage interval and dose for the desired serum concentrations would then be calculated: $\tau = [(\ln 8$ mg/L $- \ln 1.5$ mg/L$)/0.131$ h$^{-1}] + 1$ h $= 13.7$ h rounded to 12 h; $D = (1$ h$)(0.131$ h$^{-1})(20.8$ L$)(8$ mg/L$)[(1 - e^{-(0.131h^{-1})(12h)})/(1 - e^{-(0.131h^{-1})(1h)})] = 140$ mg. Thus the prescribed dose would be gentamicin 140 mg every 12 hours administered as a 1-hour infusion. If a loading dose were deemed necessary, it would be given as the first dose [LD = $(20.8$ L$)(8$ mg/L$) = 166$ mg rounded to 170 mg infused over 1 hour], and the first maintenance dose would be administered 12 hours (e.g., one dosage interval) later. Using the Hull and Sarrubi nomogram for the same patient, the loading dose is 160 mg (gentamicin loading dose for serious gram-negative infection is 2 mg/kg: 2 mg/kg $\times 80$ kg $= 160$ mg), and the maintenance dose is 115 mg every 12 hours (for a 12-hour dosage interval and $CrCl_{est} = 40$ mL/min, maintenance dose is 72% of the loading dose: 0.72×160 mg $= 115$ mg).

TABLE 5–5. Aminoglycoside Dosage Chart

1. Compute patient's creatinine clearance (CrCl) using Cockcroft–Gault method: CrCl = [(140 = age)BW]/(Scr × 72). Multiply by 0.85 for females.
2. Use patient's weight if within 30% of IBW; otherwise use adjusted dosing weight = IBW + [0.40(TBW = IBW)].
3. Select loading dose in mg/kg to provide peak serum concentrations in range listed below for the desired aminoglycoside antibiotic:

Aminoglycoside	Usual Loading Doses	Expected Peak Serum Concentrations
Tobramycin Gentamicin Netilmicin	1.5 to 2.0 mg/kg	4 to 10 mcg/mL
Amikacin Kanamycin	5.0 to 7.5 mg/kg	15 to 30 mcg/mL

4. Select maintenance dose (as percentage of loading dose) to continue peak serum concentrations indicated above according to desired dosage interval and the patient's creatinine clearance. To maintain usual peak/trough ratio, use dosage intervals in clear areas.

Percentage of Loading Dose Required for Dosage Interval Selected

CrCl (mL/min)	Est. Half-Life (h)	8 h (%)	12 h (%)	24 h (%)
>90	2=3	90	–	–
90	3.1	84	–	–
80	3.4	80	91	–
70	3.9	76	88	–
60	4.5	71	84	–
50	5.3	65	79	–
40	6.5	57	72	92
30	8.4	48	63	86
25	9.9	43	57	81
20	11.9	37	50	75
17	13.6	33	46	70
15	15.1	31	42	67
12	17.9	27	37	61
10[a]	20.4	24	34	56
7[a]	25.9	19	28	47
5[a]	31.5	16	23	41
2[a]	46.8	11	16	30
0[a]	69.3	8	11	21

[a]Note: Dosing for patients with CrCl ≤ 10 mL/min should be assisted by measuring serum concentrations.
Adapted from Ref. 22.

CLINICAL CONTROVERSY

Some clinicians use conventional dosing or extended-interval dosing exclusively for patients requiring aminoglycosides, whereas others use a mix of both approaches according to the perceived benefit to the patient. Definitive, authoritative recommendations to guide the choice of one method of aminoglycoside dosing over the other are not available.

If appropriate aminoglycoside serum concentrations are available, kinetic parameters can be calculated at any point in therapy. When the patient is not at steady state, serum aminoglycoside concentrations are obtained before a dose (C_{min}), after a dose administered as an intravenous infusion of about 1 hour or as a $^1/_2$-hour infusion followed by a $^1/_2$-hour waiting period to allow for drug distribution (C_{max}), and at one additional postdose time (C_3) approximately one estimated half-life after C_{max}. The $t_{1/2}$ and k values are computed using C_{max} and C_3: $k = (\ln C_{max} - \ln C_3)/\Delta t$ and $t_{1/2} = 0.693/k$, where Δt is the time that expired between the times C_{max} and C_3 were obtained. If the patient is at steady state, serum aminoglycoside concentrations are obtained before a dose ($C_{min,ss}$) and after a dose administered as an intravenous infusion of about 1 hour or as a $^1/_2$-hour infusion followed by a $^1/_2$-hour waiting period to allow for drug distribution ($C_{max,ss}$). The $t_{1/2}$ and k values are computed using $C_{max,ss}$ and $C_{min,ss}$: $k = (\ln C_{max,ss} - \ln C_{min,ss})/(\tau - T)$ and $t_{1/2} = 0.693/k$, where τ is the dosage interval and T is the dose infusion time or dose infusion time plus waiting time.

Assuming a one-compartment model, the following equation is used to compute V_D[32]:

$$V_D = \frac{(D/T)(1 - e^{-kT})}{k(C_{max} - C_{min}e^{-kT})}$$

where D is dose and T is duration of infusion. Once these are known, the dose and dosage interval (τ) can be calculated for any desired maximum C_{ss} ($C_{max,ss}$) and minimum C_{ss} ($C_{min,ss}$):

$$\tau = \frac{\ln C_{max,ss} - \ln C_{min,ss}}{k} + T$$

$$D = TkV_DC_{max,ss}\frac{1 - e^{-k\tau}}{1 - e^{-kT}}$$

The dose and dosage interval should be rounded to provide clinically accepted values (every 8, 12, 18, 24, 36, and 48 hours for dosage interval, nearest 5 to 10 mg for conventional dosing or every 24, 36, and 48 hours for dosage interval, nearest 10 to 25 mg for extended interval dosing). This method also has been used to individualize intravenous theophylline dosage regimens.[37]

To provide an example of this technique, the problem given previously will be extended to include steady-state concentrations. Mr. JJ was prescribed gentamicin 140 mg every 12 hours (infused over 1 hour) for the treatment of gram-negative pneumonia. Steady-state trough ($C_{min,ss}$) and peak ($C_{max,ss}$) values were obtained before and after the fourth dose was given (more than three to five estimated half-lives), respectively, and equaled $C_{min,ss} = 2.8$ mg/L and $C_{max,ss} = 8.5$ mg/L. Clinically, the patient was improving with decreased white blood cell counts and body temperatures and a resolving chest x-ray. However, the serum creatinine value had increased to 2.5 mg/dL. Because of this, a new dosage regimen with a similar peak (to maintain high intrapulmonary levels) but lower trough (to decrease the risk of drug-induced nephrotoxicity) concentrations was suggested. The patient's elimination rate constant and half-life can be computed using the following formulas: $k = (\ln 8.5$ mg/L $- \ln 2.8$ mg/L)/(12 h $- 1$ h$) = 0.101$ h^{-1} and $t_{1/2} = 0.693/0.101$ h$^{-1} = 6.9$ h. The patient's volume of distribution can be calculated using the following equation:

$$V = \frac{(140 \text{ mg/1 h})[1 - e^{-(0.101 \text{ h}^{-1})(1 \text{ h})}]}{(0.101 \text{ h}^{-1})\{8.5 \text{ mg/L} - [(2.8 \text{ mg/L})e^{-(0.101 \text{ h}^{-1})(1 \text{ h})}]\}} = 22.3 \text{ L}$$

Thus the patient's volume of distribution was larger and half-life was longer than originally estimated, and this led to higher serum concentrations than anticipated. To achieve the desired serum concentrations ($C_{min,ss} = 1.5$ mg/L and $C_{max,ss} = 8$ mg/L), the patient's actual kinetic parameters are used to compute a new dose and dosage interval: $\tau = [(\ln 8$ mg/L $- \ln 1.5$ mg/L)/0.101 h$^{-1}] + 1$ h $= 17.6$ h, rounded

to 18 h and

$$D = (1 \text{ h})(0.101 \text{ h}^{-1})(22.3 \text{ L})(8 \text{ mg/L})\frac{(1 - e^{-(0.101 \text{ h}^{-1})(18 \text{ h})})}{(1 - e^{-(0.101 \text{ h}^{-1})(1 \text{ h})})}$$

$$= 157 \text{ mg, rounded to 160 mg}$$

Thus the new dose would be gentamicin 160 mg every 18 hours and infused over 1 hour; the first dose of the new dosage regimen would be given 18 hours (e.g., the new dosage interval) after the last dose of the old dosage regimen.

Because aminoglycoside antibiotics exhibit concentration-dependent bacterial killing and the postantibiotic effect is longer with higher concentrations, investigators studied the possibility of giving a higher dose of aminoglycoside using an extended-dosage interval (24 hours or longer, depending on renal function). Generally, these studies have shown comparable microbiologic and clinical cure rates for many infections and about the same rate of nephrotoxicity (approximately 5% to 10%) as with conventional dosing. Ototoxicity has not been monitored using audiometry in most of these investigations, but loss of hearing in the conversational range, as well as signs and symptoms of vestibular toxicity, usually has been assessed and found to be similar to that with aminoglycoside therapy dosed conventionally. Based on these data, clinicians have begun using extended-interval dosing in selected patients. For *Pseudomonas aeruginosa* infections where the organism has an expected MIC ≈ 2 mg/L, peak concentrations between 20 and 30 mg/L and trough concentrations of less than 1 mg/L for gentamicin or tobramycin have been suggested.[38]

At the present time, there is not a consensus on how to approach concentration monitoring using this mode of administration. Some clinicians obtain steady-state peak and trough concentrations and use the kinetic equations given earlier to adjust the dose and dosage interval in order to attain appropriate target levels. Other clinicians measure only trough concentrations, trusting that the large doses administered to patients achieve adequate peak concentrations.

Also, a nomogram that adjusts extended-interval doses based on a single postdose concentration to achieve these steady-state concentration goals has been proposed (Fig. 5–12). The dose is 7 mg/kg of gentamicin or tobramycin. The initial dosage interval is set according to the patient's creatinine clearance (see Fig. 5–12). The Hartford nomogram includes a method to adjust doses based on serum concentrations. This portion of the nomogram contains average serum concentration time lines for gentamicin or tobramycin in patients with creatinine clearances of 60, 40, and 20 mL/min. A serum concentration is measured 6 to 14 hours after the first dose is given, and this concentration/time point is plotted on the graph (see Fig. 5–12). The modified dosage interval is indicated by which zone the serum concentration/time point falls in. Because cystic fibrosis patients have a different volume of distribution (0.35 L/kg) than assumed by this dosing technique and extended-interval dosing has not been tested adequately in patients with endocarditis, the Hartford nomogram should not be used in these situations.

To illustrate how the nomogram is used, the same patient example used previously will be repeated for this dosage approach. Mr. JJ is an 80-kg man with a CrCl$_{est}$ of 40 mL/min. Using the Hartford nomogram, the patient would receive gentamicin 560 mg every 36 hours (7 mg/kg $\times$ 80 kg $= 560$ mg, initial dosage interval for CrCl$_{est} = 40$ mL/min is 36 hours). Ten hours after the first dose was given, the serum gentamicin concentration is 8.2 mg/L. According to the graph contained in the nomogram, the dosage interval should be changed to 48 hours. The new dose is 560 mg every 48 hours.

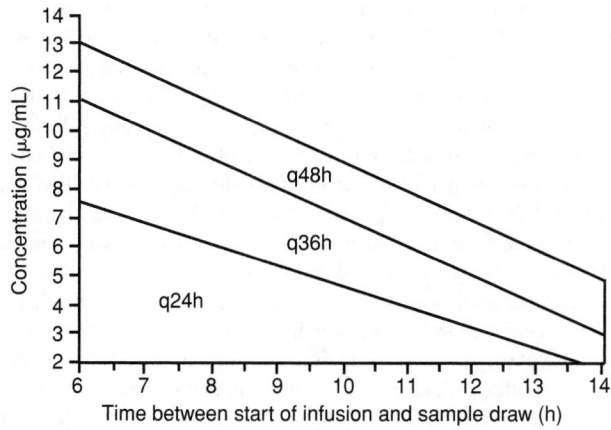

1. Administer 7 mg/kg gentamicin with initial dosage interval:

Estimated CrCl (mL/min)	Initial dosage interval
≥60 mL/min	q24h
40–59 mL/min	q36h
20–39 mL/min	q48h
<20 mL/min	Monitor serial concentrations and administer next dose when <1 μg/mL.

2. Obtain timed serum concentration 6 to 14 hours after dose (ideally first dose).

3. Alter dosage interval to that indicated by the nomogram zone (above q48h zone, monitor serial concentrations and administer next dose when <1 μg/mL)

FIGURE 5–12. Hartford nomogram for extended-interval aminoglycosides. *(Adapted with permission from ref. 38.)*

CLINICAL CONTROVERSY

"Trough only" measurement of steady-state vancomycin concentrations is becoming a mainstream method to monitor therapy. The exact range for this value is uncertain. Some clinicians recommend 5 to 10 mcg/mL, whereas others suggest 5 to 15 mcg/mL. Many clinicians continue to measure both steady-state peak and trough vancomycin concentrations.

VANCOMYCIN

Vancomycin requires multicompartment models to completely describe its serum-concentration-versus-time curves. However, if peak serum concentrations are obtained after the distribution phase is completed (usually $1/2$ to 1 hour after a 1-hour intravenous infusion), a one-compartment model can be used for patient dosage calculations. Also, since vancomycin has a relatively long half-life compared with the infusion time, only a small amount of drug is eliminated during infusion, and it is usually not necessary to use more complex intravenous infusion equations. Thus simple intravenous bolus equations can be used to calculate vancomycin doses for most patients. Although a recent review paper[39] questioned the clinical usefulness of measuring vancomycin concentrations on a routine basis, research articles[40,41] have shown potential benefits in obtaining vancomycin concentrations

TABLE 5–5. Vancomycin Dosage Chart

1. Compute patient's creatinine clearance (CrCl) using Cockcroft-Gault method: CrCl = [(140 – age)BW]/(S$_{Cr}$ × 72). Multiply by 0.85 for females.
2. Use patient's total body weight to compute doses.
3. Dosage chart designed to achieve peak serum concentrations of 30 μg/mL and trough concentrations of 7.5 μg/mL.
4. Compute loading dose of 25 mg/kg.
5. Compute maintenance dose of 19 mg/kg given at the dosage interval listed in the following chart for the patient's CrCl:

CrCl (mL/min)	Dosage Interval (Days)
≥120	0.5
100	0.6
80	0.75
60	1.0
40	1.5
30	2.0
20	2.5
10	4.0
5	6.0
0	12.0

Adapted from Ref. 45.

in selected patient populations. Some clinicians advocate monitoring only steady-state trough concentrations of vancomycin.[42] The decision to conduct vancomycin concentration monitoring should be made on a patient-by-patient basis.

Initial doses of vancomycin can be computed for adult patients using estimated kinetic parameters derived from population pharmacokinetic data. Clearance is estimated using the patient's creatinine clearance in the following equation[41]: Cl (in mL/min/kg) = 0.695(CrCl in mL/min/kg) + 0.05. The volume of distribution is computed assuming the standard value of 0.7 L/kg: $V_D = 0.7(Wt)$, where Wt is the patient's weight. In the case of obese patients, actual or total body weight is used in the calculations of clearance, but ideal body weight is used to compute volume of distribution.[44] The elimination rate constant is calculated using clearance and volume-of-distribution estimates, correcting for possible differences in units for these parameters: $k = Cl/V_D$. A nomogram that uses this type of approach for vancomycin therapy is available to determine initial doses rapidly for patients[45] (Table 5–6).

Steady-state peak and trough concentrations are chosen for the patient based on the site and severity of the infection, as well as the known or suspected pathogen and avoidance of potential side effects. $C_{max,ss}$ values of between 20 and 40 mg/L and $C_{min,ss}$ values of between 5 and 10 mg/L typically are used for patients with moderate to severe methicillin-resistant *Staphylococcus aureus, Staphylococcus epidermidis,* or penicillin-resistant enterococcal infections. After appropriate steady-state concentrations are chosen, the dosage interval required to attain those concentrations is computed, and τ is rounded to a clinically acceptable value (12, 18, 24, 36, 48, or 72 hours): $\tau = (\ln C_{max,ss} - \ln C_{min,ss})/k$. Finally, the maintenance dose is computed for the patient using a one-compartment-model intravenous bolus equation at steady state, and the dose is rounded off to the nearest 100 to 250 mg:

$$D = C_{max,ss} V_D (1 - e^{-k\tau})$$

If desired, a loading dose can be computed using the following equation:

$$LD = V_D C_{max,ss}$$

The following case will illustrate the use of this dosage methodology. Ms HJ is a 65-year-old, 68-kg, 5-ft, 4-in-tall coronary artery bypass graft surgery patient who has developed a surgical wound infection with *S. aureus* the suspected pathogen. Her serum creatinine concentration is 1.8 mg/dL and stable. Compute a vancomycin dosage regimen that would provide approximate peak (obtained 1 hour after a 1-hour infusion) and trough concentrations of 30 and 7 mg/L, respectively. The patient is within 30% of her ideal body weight [IBW$_\text{female}$ = 45 + 2.3(64 in − 60) = 54 kg] and has stable renal function, so the Cockcroft-Gault creatinine clearance estimation formula can be used: CrCl$_\text{est}$ = 0.85[(140 − 65 yrs)68 kg]/[72(1.8 mg/dL)] = 33 mL/min. The patient's weight and estimated creatinine clearance are used to calculate her estimated Cl, V_D, and k, respectively: Cl = 0.695 (33 mL/min/68 kg) + 0.05 = 0.387 mL/min/kg; V_D = 0.7 L/kg(68 kg) = 48 L; and k = [(0.387 mL/min/kg)(68 kg)(60 min/h)]/[(48 L)(1000 mL/L)] = 0.033 h^{-1} or $t_{1/2}$ = 0.693/0.033 h^{-1} = 21 h. The dosage interval, maintenance dose, and loading dose for the desired serum concentrations then can be computed: τ = (ln 30 mg/L − ln 7 mg/L)/0.033 h^{-1} = 44 h, rounded to 48 h; D = (30 mg/L) (48 L)(1 − $e^{-(0.033h^{-1})(48h)}$) = 1145 mg, rounded to 1200 mg; LD = (48 L)(30 mg/L) = 1440 mg, rounded to 1450 mg. Therefore, the prescribed doses would be vancomycin 1200 mg every 48 hours administered as a 1-hour infusion. If a loading dose was used, it would be given as the first dose, and the first maintenance dose would be administered 48 hours (one dosage interval) later. Using the Matzke nomogram for the same patient, the loading dose would be 1700 mg (vancomycin loading dose is 25 mg/kg: 25 mg/kg × 68 kg = 1700 mg), followed by a maintenance dose of 1300 mg every 48 hours (for CrCl$_\text{est}$ = 30 mL/min, maintenance dose is 19 mg/kg every 2 days: 19 mg/kg × 68 kg = 1292 mg, rounded to 1300 mg).

If appropriate vancomycin serum concentrations are available, kinetic parameters can be computed at any point in therapy. When the patient is not at steady state, serum vancomycin concentrations are obtained before a dose (C_min), after a dose administered as an intravenous infusion of 1 hour followed by a $^1/_2$- to 1-hour waiting period to allow for drug distribution (C_max), and at one additional postdose time (C_3) approximately one estimated half-life after C_max. The $t_{1/2}$ and k values are computed using C_max and C_3: k = (ln C_max − ln C_3)/Δt and $t_{1/2}$ = 0.693/k, where Δt is the time that expired between the times C_max and C_3 were obtained. If the patient is at steady state, serum vancomycin concentrations are obtained before a dose ($C_\text{min,ss}$) and after a dose administered as an intravenous infusion of about 1 hour followed by a $^1/_2$- to 1-hour waiting period to allow for drug distribution ($C_\text{max,ss}$). The $t_{1/2}$ and k values are computed using $C_\text{max,ss}$ and $C_\text{min,ss}$: k = (ln $C_\text{max,ss}$ − ln $C_\text{min,ss}$)/(τ − T_max) and $t_{1/2}$ = 0.693/k, where τ is the dosage interval and T_max is the dose infusion time plus waiting time.

Assuming a one-compartment model, the following equation is used to compute V_D:

$$V_D = \frac{D}{C_\text{max} - C_\text{min}}$$

where D is dose. Once these are known, the dose and dosage interval (τ) can be calculated for any desired maximum C_ss ($C_\text{max,ss}$) and minimum C_ss ($C_\text{min,ss}$):

$$\tau = \frac{\ln C_\text{max,ss} - \ln C_\text{min,ss}}{k}$$
$$D = C_\text{max,ss} V_D(1 - e^{-k\tau})$$

The dose and dosage interval should be rounded to provide clinically accepted values (every 12, 18, 24, 36, 48, or 72 hours for dosage interval, nearest 100 to 250 mg for dose).

To provide an example for this dosage-calculation method, the preceding problem will be extended to include steady-state concentrations. Ms HJ was prescribed vancomycin 1200 mg every 48 hours (infused over 1 hour) for the treatment of a surgical wound infection. Steady-state trough ($C_\text{min,ss}$) and peak ($C_\text{max,ss}$) values ($C_\text{max,ss}$ obtained 1 hour after the end of the infusion) were obtained before and after the the third dose was given (more than three to five estimated half-lives), respectively, and equaled $C_\text{min,ss}$ = 2.5 mg/L and $C_\text{max,ss}$ = 22.4 mg/L. Clinically, the patient had improved somewhat, but her white blood cell count was still elevated, and the patient was still febrile. Because of this, a modified dosage regimen with a $C_\text{max,ss}$ = 30 mg/L and $C_\text{min,ss}$ = 7 mg/L was suggested to maintain trough concentrations three to five times above the minimal inhibitory concentration (MIC) for the suspected pathogen. The patient's actual elimination rate constant and half-life can be calculated using the following formulas: k = (ln 22.4 mg/L − ln 2.5 mg/L)/(48 h − 2 h) = 0.048 h^{-1} and $t_{1/2}$ = 0.693/0.048 h^{-1} = 14.4 h. The patient's volume of distribution can be calculated using the following equation:

$$V_D = \frac{1200\,\text{mg}}{22.4\,\text{mg/L} - 2.5\,\text{mg/L}} = 60\,\text{L}$$

Thus the patient's volume of distribution was larger and half-life shorter than originally estimated, and this led to lower serum concentrations than anticipated. To achieve the desired serum concentrations ($C_\text{max,ss}$ = 30 mg/L and $C_\text{min,ss}$ = 7 mg/L), the patient's actual kinetic parameters are used to calculate a new dose and dosage interval:

$$\tau = \frac{\ln 30\,\text{mg/L} - \ln 7\,\text{mg/L}}{0.048\,\text{h}^{-1}}$$
$$= 30\,\text{h}, \text{ rounded to 36 h}$$
$$D = (30\,\text{mg/L})(60\,\text{L})(1 - e^{-(0.048\,\text{h}^{-1})(36\,\text{h})})$$
$$= 1480\,\text{mg, rounded to 1500 mg}$$

The new dose would be vancomycin 1500 mg every 36 hours (infused over 1 hour); the first dose of the new dosage regimen would be given 36 hours (the new dosage interval) after the last dose of the old dosage regimen.

Some clinicians measure only steady-state vancomycin trough concentrations in patients. The justification for this approach is that since vancomycin exhibits time-dependent bacterial killing, the minimum concentration is the most important with regard to therapeutic outcome. Vancomycin pharmacokinetics also support this approach because the volume of distribution is relatively stable and is not changed by many disease states or conditions. Because of this important point, it is difficult to attain peak steady-state concentrations in the toxic range when the steady-state vancomycin trough is in the therapeutic range if typical doses are used (15 mg/kg or ∼1000 mg for average-weight individuals). Also, toxic peak concentrations (generally greater than 80 to 100 mg/L) are quite a bit higher than therapeutic peak concentrations, which adds a safety margin between effective concentrations and those yielding adverse drug effects.

Coupled with trough-only vancomycin concentration monitoring is a widening of the therapeutic steady-state trough concentration range from 5 to 15 mg/L. The justification for increasing the top of the range from 10 to 15 mg/L comes from limited retrospective[41] and prospective[42] studies and until more clinical evidence is available should be reserved for severely ill patients, infections caused by bacteria with higher MICs, and patients not responding to trough concentrations within the usual 5- to 10-mg/L range.

When trough-only monitoring of vancomycin concentrations is chosen by a clinician, a simple variant of linear pharmacokinetics can be used to adjust the dose (D) and dosage interval (τ): (D_{new}/τ_{new}) = (D_{old}/τ_{old})($C_{ss,new}/C_{ss,old}$), where *new* and *old* indicate the new target trough concentration and the old measured trough concentration, respectively. This equation is an approximation of the actual new steady-state trough concentration that will be attained in the patient because, mathematically, $C_{ss,new}$ is an exponential function of τ.

An example of this approach is given in the following case. Mr. MK (72 years old, 72 kg weight, 5 ft, 9 in tall) was prescribed vancomycin 1000 mg every 12 hours (infused over 1 hour) for the treatment of an *S. epidermidis* central venous catheter infection. A steady-state trough ($C_{min,ss}$) value was obtained before the fifth dose was given (more than three to five estimated half-lives), and $C_{min,ss}$ equaled 19 mg/L. Clinically, the patient was improving, but the trough concentration was judged to be too high. Because of this, a modified dosage regimen with a $C_{min,ss}$ = 10 mg/L was suggested to maintain trough concentrations three to five times above the minimal inhibitory concentration (MIC) for the suspected pathogen: (D_{new}/τ_{new}) = (1000 mg/12 h)(10 mg/L/19 mg/L) = 44 mg/h. Because the patient is near his ideal weight, a new dose of 1000 mg can be used (D_{new}), and the new dosage interval (τ_{new}) can be computed: τ = 1000 mg/44 mg/h = 23 h, rounded to 24 h. The new prescribed dose for the patient would be 1000 mg every 24 hours.

DIGOXIN

Digoxin pharmacokinetics are best described by a two-compartment model. However, because digoxin has a long half-life compared with its dosage interval and a very long distribution phase, simple pharmacokinetic equations can be used to individualize dosing when postdistribution serum concentrations are used. Digoxin can be given as an intravenous injection and orally as elixir ($F = 0.8$), tablets ($F = 0.7$), or capsules ($F = 0.9$). When given orally, the appropriate bioavailability fraction must be used to compute the correct dose. Initial doses of digoxin can be computed using population pharmacokinetic data obtained from published studies. Digoxin clearance is estimated using the patient's creatinine clearance in the following formula[20]: Cl (in milliliters per minute) = 1.303(CrCl in milliliters per minute) + Cl_m, where Cl_m is metabolic clearance and equals 40 mL/min for patients with no or mild heart failure or 20 mL/min for patients with moderate to severe heart failure. The volume of distribution decreases with declining renal function and is estimated using the following equation[20]: V_D (in liters) = 226 + [298(CrCl in milliliters per minute)]/(29.1 + CrCl in milliliters per minute). The elimination rate constant can be computed by taking the product of Cl and V_D: $k = Cl/V_D$. For obese individuals, digoxin dosing should be based on ideal body weight.[46]

Appropriate C_{ss} values are chosen for the patient based on the disease state being treated, the goal of therapy, and avoidance of adverse effects. The inotropic effects of digoxin occur at lower concentrations than do the chronotropic effects. Therefore, initial serum concentrations of digoxin for the treatment of heart failure generally are 1 ng/mL or less and for the treatment of atrial fibrillation are 1–1.5 ng/mL. Once the appropriate C_{ss} is selected, a dose is computed for the patient: $D/\tau = (C_{ss}Cl)/F$.

An example of this initial dosage scheme is provided in the following case. Mr. PO is a 72-year-old, 83-kg, 5-ft, 11-in man admitted to the hospital for the treatment of community-acquired pneumonia. While in the hospital, Mr. PO develops atrial fibrillation, and the decision is made to treat him with digoxin to provide ventricular rate control. His serum creatinine concentration is 2.5 mg/dL and stable. Calculate an intravenous loading dose and oral maintenance dose that will achieve a C_{ss} of 1.5 ng/mL. The Cockcroft-Gault equation can be

used to estimate the patient's creatinine clearance because his serum creatinine concentration is stable and he is within 30% of his ideal weight [IBW_{male} = 50 + 2.3(71 in − 60) = 75 kg]: CrCl = [(140 − 72 yrs)83 kg]/[72(2.5 mg/dL)] = 31 mL/min. Using the estimated CrCl, both Cl and V_D can be computed:

$$Cl = 1.303(31\ \text{mL/min}) + 40 = 80\ \text{mL/min}$$

$$V_D = 226 + \frac{298(31\ \text{mL/min})}{29.1 + 31\ \text{mL/min}} = 380\ \text{L}$$

The maintenance dose will be given as digoxin tablets, so $F = 0.7$ in the dosing equation: D/τ = [(1.5 mcg/L)(80 mL/min)(60 min/h) (24 h/day)]/[0.7(1000 mL/L)] = 247 mcg/day, rounded to 250 mcg/ day. The loading dose will be given intravenously as a digoxin injection: LD = (1.5 mcg/L)(380 L) = 570 mcg, rounded to 500 mcg. The loading dose would be given 50% now (250 mcg), 25% (125 mcg) in 4 to 6 hours after monitoring the patient's heart rate and blood pressure and assessing the patient for digoxin adverse effects, and the final 25% (125 mcg) 4 to 6 hours later after monitoring the same clinical parameters. The first maintenance dose would be given one dosage interval (in this case 24 hours) after the first part of the loading dose was given.

Adjustment of digoxin doses using steady-state concentrations is accomplished using linear pharmacokinetics and dosage ratios: D_{new} = $D_{old}(C_{ss,new}/C_{ss,old})$. For example, Mr. PO's atrial fibrillation responded to digoxin therapy, and he was discharged after resolution of his pneumonia. A month later he was followed up in the clinic with moderate nausea, possibly due to digoxin toxicity. His heart rate was 55 beats per minute. A steady-state digoxin concentration was determined and reported by the clinical laboratory as 2.2 mcg/L. Compute a new dose for the patient to achieve a C_{ss} of 1.5 mcg/L. The digoxin C_{ss} and old dose would be used to calculate a new dose using the linear pharmacokinetic equation: D_{new} = 250 mcg/day[(1.5 mcg/L)/ (2.2 mcg/L)] = 170 mcg/day. This approximate average daily dose could be achieved by having the patient alternate take two 125-mcg tablets (250 mcg) and one 125-mcg tablet daily, giving an average dose equal to 187.5 mcg/day [(250 mcg + 125 mcg)/2 = 187.5 mcg/day].

THEOPHYLLINE

Theophylline disposition is described most accurately by nonlinear kinetics.[47,48] However, at the usual doses, theophylline acts as if it obeys linear kinetics in most patients. Initial theophylline doses are computed by taking a detailed medical history of the patient and noting disease states and conditions that are known to change theophylline disposition. Age, smoking of tobacco-containing products, heart failure, and liver disease are among the important factors that alter theophylline kinetic parameters and dosage requirements. Once the patient has been assessed, average theophylline kinetic parameters obtained from the literature for patients similar to the one being currently treated are used to compute either oral or intravenous doses. Dosage guidelines that take into account most common disease states and conditions that change theophylline kinetic parameters are available[49] (see Table 5–4). Once theophylline is administered, the patient is monitored for the therapeutic effect and potential adverse effects. Theophylline concentrations then are used to individualize the theophylline dose that the patient receives. An example of this approach was given previously for a patient in the section on drug dosing in patients with liver disease.

Continuous intravenous infusions of theophylline (or its salt, aminophylline) can be individualized rapidly by determining the patient's Cl before steady state occurs.[50] Assuming that the patient receives theophylline only by continuous intravenous infusion (previous doses of sustained-release oral theophylline are completely absorbed), two serum theophylline concentration determinations are done 4 hours or more apart. The infusion rate (k_0) cannot be changed between the times the samples are drawn. With one-compartment model equations, the first (C_1) and second (C_2) theophylline concentrations are used to calculate theophylline Cl:

$$Cl = \frac{2k_0}{C_1 + C_2} + \frac{2V_D(C_1 - C_2)}{(C_1 + C_2)(t_2 - t_1)}$$

V_D is assumed to be 0.5 L/kg, and t_1 and t_2 are the times at which C_1 and C_2, respectively, are obtained. Once Cl is known, k_0 can be computed easily for any desired C_{ss} ($C_{ss} = k_0/Cl$). This method probably can be applied to other drugs that are administered as continuous intravenous infusions, such as intravenous antiarrhythmics, when rapid individualization of drug dosage is desirable.

An example of this approach can be obtained by continuing the theophylline patient case from the section on drug dosing in liver disease. In this example, a 55-year-old, 70-kg man with liver cirrhosis was prescribed a loading dose of theophylline 350 mg intravenously over 20 to 30 minutes, followed by a maintenance dose of 15 mg/h of theophylline as a continuous infusion. The infusion began at 9 A.M., blood samples were obtained at 10 A.M. and 4 P.M., and the clinical laboratory reported the theophylline serum concentrations as 10.9 and 12.3 mg/L, respectively. The patient's theophylline clearance and revised continuous infusion to maintain a C_{ss} of 15 mg/L can be computed as follows (patient's V_D estimated at 0.5 L/kg):

$$Cl = \frac{2(15 \text{ mg/h})}{10.9 \text{ mg/L} + 12.3 \text{ mg/L}}$$

$$+ \frac{2(0.5 \text{ L/kg} \times 70 \text{ kg})(10.9 \text{ mg/L} - 12.3 \text{ mg/L})}{(10.9 \text{ mg/L} + 12.3 \text{ mg/L})(16 - 10 \text{ h})} = 0.59 \text{ L/h}$$

$$k_0 = C_{ss}Cl = (15 \text{ mg/L})(0.59 \text{ L/h}) = 9 \text{ mg/h theophylline}$$

If theophylline is to be given as the aminophylline salt form, the doses would need to be changed to reflect the fact that aminophylline contains only 85% theophylline ($k_0 = 9$ mg/h theophylline/0.85 = 11 mg/h aminophylline).

If continuous intravenous infusions or oral dosage regimens are given long enough for steady state to occur (three to five estimated half-lives based on previous studies conducted in similar patients), linear pharmacokinetics can be used to adjust doses for either route of administration: $D_{new} = D_{old} (C_{ss,new}/C_{ss,old})$. For example, a patient receiving 200 mg of sustained-release oral theophylline every 12 hours with a theophylline steady-state serum concentration of 9.5 mcg/mL can have the dose required to achieve a new steady-state concentration equal to 15 mcg/mL computed by applying linear pharmacokinetics: $D_{new} = 200$ mg[(15 mcg/mL)/(9.5 mcg/mL)] = 316 mg, rounded to 300 mg. Thus the new theophylline dose would be 300 mg every 12 hours.

PHENYTOIN

Phenytoin doses are very difficult to individualize because the drug follows Michaelis-Menten kinetics, and there is a large amount of interpatient variability in V_{max} and K_m. Initial maintenance doses of phenytoin in adults usually range between 4 and 7 mg/kg per day, yielding starting doses of 300 to 400 mg/day in most individuals. If needed, loading doses of phenytoin or fosphenytoin (a prodrug of phenytoin used intravenously) can be administered in adults at a dose of 15 mg/kg, which is approximately 1000 mg in many individuals. Loading doses of phenytoin can be given orally but need to be administered in divided doses separated by several hours in order to avoid decreased bioavailability and gastrointestinal intolerance (400 mg, 300 mg, and then 300 mg with each dose separated by 4 to 6 hours). Since phenytoin is metabolized hepatically, decreased doses may be needed in patients with liver disease. Because phenytoin follows dose-dependent pharmacokinetics, the half-life of phenytoin increases for a patient as the maintenance dose increases. Therefore, the time to steady-state phenytoin concentrations increases with dose. On average, at a phenytoin dose of 300 mg/day, it takes approximately 5 to 7 days to achieve steady state; at a dose of 400 mg/day, it takes approximately 10 to 14 days to achieve steady state; and at a dose of 500 mg/day, it takes approximately 21 to 28 days to achieve steady state. It should be noted that the injectable and capsule dosage forms of phenytoin are phenytoin sodium, and the labeled dosage amounts contain 92% of active phenytoin [300-mg phenytoin sodium capsules contain 276 mg (300 mg × 0.92 = 276 mg) of active phenytoin]. Unbound phenytoin concentrations are useful in patients with hypoalbuminemia (e.g., liver disease, nephrotic syndrome, pregnancy, cystic fibrosis, burns, trauma, and malnourishment, as well as the elderly), in patients in whom displacement with endogenous compounds is possible (e.g., hyperbilirubinemia, liver disease, or end-stage renal disease), or in patients receiving other drugs that may displace phenytoin from plasma-protein-binding sights (e.g., valproic acid, aspirin therapy of more than 2 g/day, warfarin, and nonsteroidal anti-inflammatory drugs with high albumin binding).

After steady state has occurred, phenytoin serum concentrations can be obtained as an aid to dosage adjustment. A simple, easy way to approximate new serum concentrations after a dosage adjustment with phenytoin is to temporarily assume linear pharmacokinetics and then add 15% to 33% for a dosage increase or subtract 15% to 33% for a dosage decrease to account for Michaelis-Menten kinetics. To avoid large disproportionate changes in phenytoin concentrations when using this empirical method, dosage adjustments should be limited to 50 to 100 mg/day. For example, Ms PP is a 35-year-old, 65-kg patient with grand mal seizures who is receiving phenytoin capsules 300 mg orally at bedtime. A steady-state concentration of 9.2 mcg/mL is measured. It is observed that her seizure frequency decreased by only about 15% and that she has had no adverse effects due to phenytoin treatment. Because of this, her phenytoin dose is increased to 400 mg orally at bedtime. The expected phenytoin steady-state concentration would be estimated using linear pharmacokinetics [$C_{new} = (D_{new}/D_{old})C_{old} = (400$ mg/300 mg)/(9.2 mcg/mL) = 12.3 mcg/mL] and then increased by 15% to 33% to account for nonlinear kinetics [$C_{new} = 1.15(12.3$ mcg/mL) = 14.1 mcg/mL or $C_{new} = 1.33$ (12.3 mcg/mL) = 16.4 mcg/mL]. Thus the patient would be expected to have a steady-state phenytoin concentration of approximately 14 to 16 mcg/mL due to the dosage increase. An alternative approach would be to use a graphic Bayesian method that allows an estimate of V_{max} and K_m from one steady-state phenytoin concentration and the prediction of new steady-state concentrations when doses are changed.[51]

Other methods used to individualize phenytoin doses involve rearrangements of the Michaelis-Menten equation [$DR = V_{max}C_{ss}/(K_m + C_{ss})$, in which DR is the dosage rate at steady state] so that two or more doses and C_{ss} values can be used to obtain graphic solutions for V_{max} and K_m. One rearrangement[52] is $DR = -K_m(DR/C_{ss}) + V_{max}$. When DR is plotted on the y axis and DR/C_{ss} is plotted on the x axis of Cartesian graph paper, a straight line with a y intercept of V_{max}

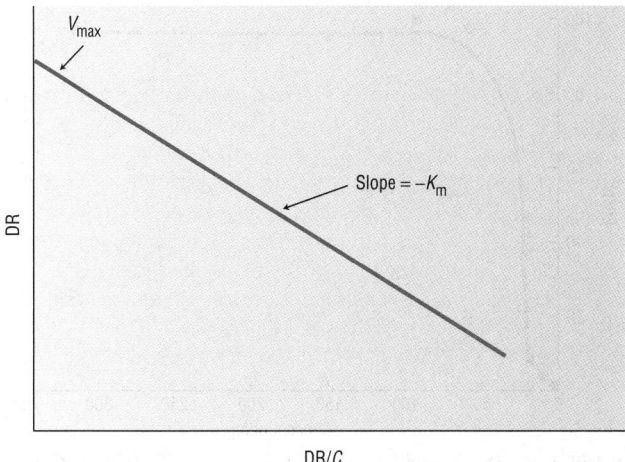

FIGURE 5–13. Relationship between dosage rate (DR) and steady-state serum concentrations (C_{ss}).

and slope equal to $-K_m$ is found (Fig. 5–13). To use this method, patients are prescribed an initial phenytoin dose, and C_{ss} is obtained. The phenytoin dose is then changed, and a second C_{ss} from the new dose is obtained. Each dose is divided by its respective C_{ss} to derive DR/C_{ss} values. The DR/C_{ss} and C_{ss} values are plotted on the graph to calculate V_{max} (y intercept) and K_m (minus slope). The steady-state Michaelis-Menten equation can be used to compute C_{ss} for a given DR or a DR for any C_{ss}.

CYCLOSPORINE

Because of the large amount of variability in cyclosporine pharmacokinetics, even when concurrent disease states and conditions are identified, many clinicians believe that the use of standard cyclosporine doses for various situations is warranted. Indeed, most transplant centers use doses that are determined employing a locally derived cyclosporine dosage protocol. The original computations of these doses were based on the pharmacokinetic dosing methods described in preceding sections and subsequently modified based on clinical experience. In general, the expected cyclosporine steady-state concentration used to compute these doses depends on the type of transplanted tissue and the posttransplantation time line. Generally speaking, initial oral doses of 8 to 18 mg/kg per day or intravenous doses of 3 to 6 mg/kg per day (one-third the oral dose to account for approximately 30% oral bioavailability) are used and vary greatly from institution to institution. For obese individuals (more than 30% over ideal body weight), ideal body weight should be used to compute initial doses.

It is likely that doses computed using patient population characteristics will not always produce cyclosporine concentrations that are expected or desirable. Additionally, there is a very high amount of interday variation in cyclosporine concentrations. Because of pharmacokinetic variability, the narrow therapeutic index of cyclosporine, and the severity of cyclosporine adverse side effects, measurement of cyclosporine concentrations is mandatory for patients to ensure that therapeutic, nontoxic levels are present. When cyclosporine concentrations are measured in patients and a dosage change is necessary, clinicians should seek to use the simplest, most straightforward method available to determine a dose that will provide safe and effective treatment. In most cases, a simple dosage ratio can be used

to change cyclosporine doses using steady-state concentrations and assuming that the drug follows linear pharmacokinetics:

$$D_{new} = D_{old} \frac{C_{ss,new}}{C_{ss,old}}$$

For example, LK is a 50-year-old, 75-kg, 5-ft, 11-in male renal transplant recipient who is receiving oral cyclosporine 400 mg every 12 hours. The current steady-state blood cyclosporine concentration is 375 ng/mL. To compute a cyclosporine dose that will provide a steady-state concentration of 200 ng/mL, linear pharmacokinetic equations can be used. The new dose to attain the desired concentration should be proportional to the old dose that produced the measured concentration (total daily dose = 400 mg/dose × 2 doses/day = 800 mg/day):

$$D_{new} = D_{old} \frac{C_{ss,new}}{C_{ss,new}} = 800 \text{ mg/day} \frac{200 \text{ ng/mL}}{375 \text{ ng/mL}} = 427 \text{ mg/day},$$

rounded to 400 mg/day

The new suggested dose would be 400 mg/day or 200 mg every 12 hours of cyclosporine capsules to be started at the next scheduled dosing time.

CLINICAL PHARMACODYNAMICS

Pharmacodynamics is the study of the relationship between the concentration of a drug and the response obtained in a patient. Originally, investigators examined the dose-response relationship of drugs in humans but found that the same dose of a drug usually resulted in different concentrations in individuals because of pharmacokinetic differences in clearance and volume of distribution. Examples of quantifiable pharmacodynamic measurements include changes in blood pressure during antihypertensive drug therapy, decreases in heart rate during β-blocker treatment, and alterations in prothrombin time or international normalized ratio during warfarin therapy.

For drugs that exhibit a direct and reversible effect, the following diagram describes what occurs at the level of the drug receptor:

Drug + receptor ↔ drug − receptor complex ↔ response

According to this scheme, there is a drug receptor located within the target organ or tissue. When a drug molecule "finds" the receptor, it forms a complex that causes the pharmacologic response to occur. The drug and receptor are in dynamic equilibrium with the drug-receptor complex.

THE E_{max} AND SIGMOID E_{max} MODELS

The mathematical model that comes from the classic drug receptor theory shown previously is known as the E_{max} model:

$$E = \frac{E_{max} \times C}{EC_{50} + C}$$

where E is the pharmacologic effect elicited by the drug, E_{max} is the maximum effect the drug can cause, EC_{50} is the concentration causing one-half the maximum drug effect ($E_{max}/2$), and C is the concentration of drug at the receptor site. EC_{50} can be used as a measure of drug potency (a lower EC_{50} indicating a more potent drug), whereas E_{max} reflects the intrinsic efficacy of the drug (a higher E_{max} indicating greater efficacy). If pharmacologic effect is plotted versus concentration in the E_{max} equation, a hyperbola results with an asymptote equal to E_{max} (Fig. 5–14). At a concentration of zero, no measurable effect is present.

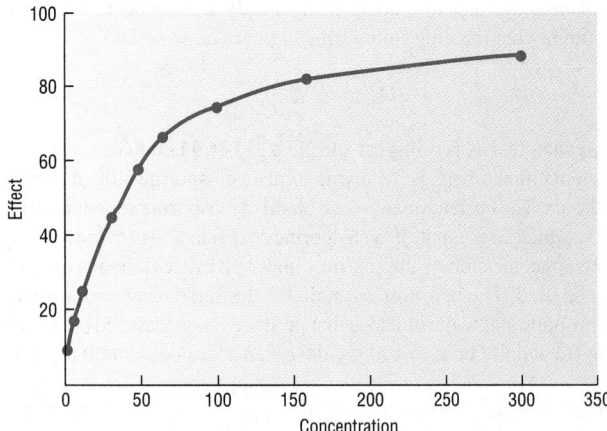

FIGURE 5–14. The E_{max} model $[E = (E_{max} \times C)/(EC_{50} + C)]$ has the shape of a hyperbola with an asymptote equal to E_{max}. EC_{50} is the concentration where effect $= E_{max}/2$.

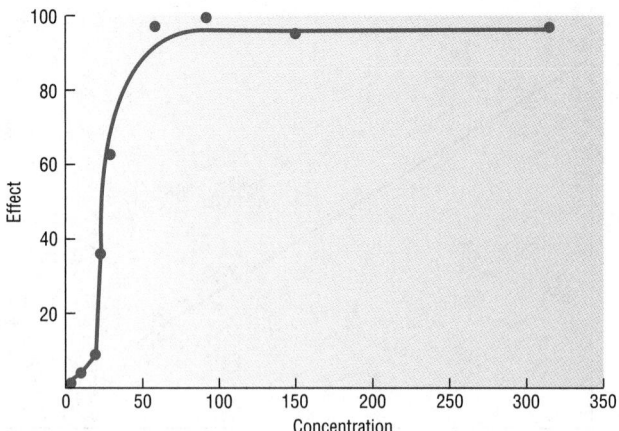

FIGURE 5–15. The sigmoid E_{max} model $[E = (E_{max} \times C^n)/(EC_{50}^n + C^n)]$ has an S-shaped curve at lower concentrations. In this example, E_{max} and EC_{50} have the same values as in Fig. 5–14.

When dealing with human studies in which a drug is administered to a patient and pharmacologic effect is measured, it is very difficult to determine the concentration of drug at the receptor site. Because of this, serum concentrations (total or unbound) usually are used as the concentration parameter in the E_{max} equation. Therefore, the values of E_{max} and EC_{50} are much different than if the drug were added to an isolated tissue contained in a laboratory beaker.

The result is that a much more empirical approach is used to describe the relationship between concentration and effect in clinical pharmacology studies. After a pharmacodynamic experiment has been conducted, concentration-effect plots are generated. The shape of the concentration-effect curve is used to determine which pharmacodynamic model will be used to describe the data. Because of this, the pharmacodynamic models used in a clinical pharmacology study are deterministic in the same way that the shape of the serum-concentration-versus-time curve determines which pharmacokinetic model is used in clinical pharmacokinetic studies.

Sometimes a hyperbolic function does not describe the concentration-effect relationship at lower concentrations adequately. When this is the case, the sigmoid E_{max} equation may be superior to the E_{max} model:

$$E = \frac{E_{max} \times C^n}{EC_{50}^n + C^n}$$

where n is an exponent that changes the shape of the concentration-effect curve. When $n > 1$, the concentration-effect curve is S- or sigmoid-shaped at lower serum concentrations. When $n < 1$, the concentration-effect curve has a steeper slope at lower concentrations (Fig. 5–15).

With both the E_{max} and sigmoid E_{max} models, the largest changes in drug effect occur at the lower end of the concentration scale. Small changes in low serum concentrations cause large changes in effect. As serum concentrations become larger, further increases in serum concentration result in smaller changes in effect. Using the E_{max} model as an example and setting $E_{max} = 100$ units and $EC_{50} = 20$ mg/L, doubling the serum concentration from 5 to 10 mg/L increases the effect from 20 to 33 units (a 67% increase), whereas doubling the serum concentration from 40 to 80 mg/L only increases the effect from 67 to 80 units (a 19% increase). This is an important concept for clinicians to remember when doses are being titrated in patients.

LINEAR MODELS

When serum concentrations obtained during a pharmacodynamic experiment are between 20% and 80% of E_{max}, the concentration-effect curve may appear to be linear (Fig. 5–16). This occurs often because lower drug concentrations may not be detectable with the analytic technique used to assay serum samples, and higher drug concentrations may be avoided to prevent toxic side effects. The equation used is that of a simple line: $E = S \times C + I$, where E is the drug effect, C is the drug concentration, S is the slope of the line, and I is the y intercept. In this situation, the value of S can be used as a measure of drug potency (the larger the value of S, the more potent the drug). The linear model can be derived from the E_{max} model. When EC_{50} is much greater than C, $E = (E_{max}/EC_{50})C = S \times C$, where $S = E_{max}/EC_{50}$.

The linear model allows a nonzero value for effect when the concentration equals zero. This may be a baseline value for the effect that is present without the drug, the result of measurement error when determining effect, or model misspecification. Also, this model does not allow the prediction of a maximum response.

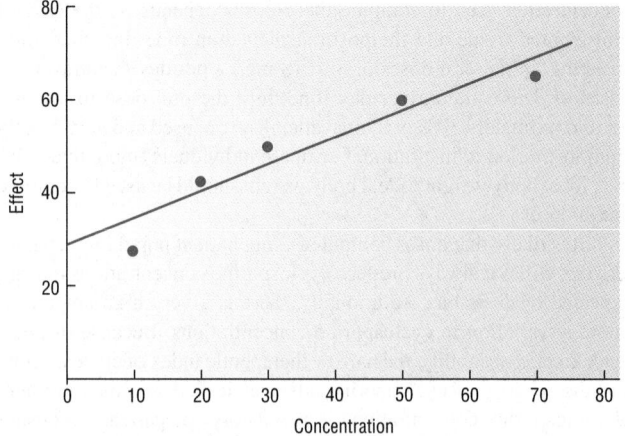

FIGURE 5–16. The linear model ($E = S \times C + I$) is often used as a pharmacodynamic model when the measured pharmacologic effect is 20% to 80% of E_{max}. In this situation, the determination of E_{max} and EC_{50} is not possible. To illustrate this, effect measurements from Fig. 5–14 between 20% and 80% of E_{max} are graphed using the linear pharmacodynamic model.

Some investigators have used a log-linear model in pharmacodynamic experiments: $E = S \times (\log C) + I$, where the symbols have the same meaning as in the linear model. The advantages of this model are that the concentration scale is compressed on concentration-effect plots for experiments where wide concentration ranges were used, and the concentration values are transformed so that linear regression can be used to compute model parameters. The disadvantages are that the model cannot predict a maximum effect or an effect when the concentration equals zero. With the increased availability of nonlinear regression programs that can compute the parameters of nonlinear functions such as the E_{max} model easily, use of the log-linear model has been discouraged.[53]

BASELINE EFFECTS

At times, the effect measured during a pharmacodynamic study has a value before the drug is administered to the patient. In these cases, the drug changes the patient's baseline value. Examples of these types of measurements are heart rate and blood pressure. In addition, a given drug may increase or decrease the baseline value. Two basic techniques are used to incorporate baseline values into pharmacodynamic data. One way incorporates the baseline value into the pharmacodynamic model; the other way transforms the effect data to take baseline values into account.

Incorporation of the baseline value into the pharmacodynamic model involves the addition of a new term to the previous equations. E_0 is the symbol used to denote the baseline value of the effect that will be measured. The form that these equations takes depends on whether the drug increases or decreases the pharmacodynamic effect. When the drug increases the baseline value, E_0 is added to the equations:

$$E = E_0 + \frac{E_{max} \times C}{EC_{50} + C}$$

$$E = E_0 + \frac{E_{max} \times C^n}{EC_{50}^n + C^n}$$

$$E = S \times C + E_0$$

When E_0 is not known with any better certainty than any other effect measurement, it should be estimated as a model parameter similar to the way that one would estimate the values of E_{max}, EC_{50}, S, or n.[54,55] If the baseline effect is well known and has only a small amount of measurement error, it can be subtracted from the effect determined in the patient during the experiment and not estimated as a model parameter. This approach can lead to better estimates of the remaining model parameters.[55] Using the linear model as an example, the equation used would be $E - E_0 = S \times C$.

If the drug decreases the baseline value, the drug effect is subtracted from E_0 in the pharmacodynamic models:

$$E = E_0 - \frac{E_{max} \times C}{IC_{50} + C}$$

$$E = E_0 - \frac{E_{max} \times C^n}{IC_{50}^n + C^n}$$

$$E = E_0 - S \times C$$

where E_{max} represents the maximum reduction in effect caused by the drug, and IC_{50} is the concentration that produces a 50% inhibition of E_{max}. These forms of the equations have been called the *inhibitory* E_{max} and *inhibitory sigmoidal* E_{max} *equations,* respectively. In this arrangement of the pharmacodynamic model, E_0 is a model parameter and can be estimated. If the baseline effect is well known and has little measurement error, the effect in the presence of the drug can be subtracted from the baseline effect and not estimated as a model

parameter. Using the inhibitory E_{max} model as an example, the formula would be $E_0 - E = (E_{max} \times C)/(IC_{50} + C)$.

When using the inhibitory E_{max} model, a special situation occurs if the baseline effect can be obliterated completely by the drug (e.g., decreased premature ventricular contractions during antiarrhythmic therapy). In this situation, $E_{max} = E_0$, and the equation simplifies to a rearrangement known as the *fractional E_{max} equation:*

$$E = E_0 \left(1 - \frac{C}{IC_{50} + C}\right)$$

This form of the model relates drug concentration to the fraction of the maximum effect.

An alternative approach to the pharmacodynamic modeling of drugs that alter baseline effects is to transform the effect data so that they represent a percentage increase or decrease from the baseline value.[55] For drugs that increase the effect, the following transformation equation would be used: percent effect$_t$ = [(treatment$_t$ − baseline)/baseline] × 100. For drugs that decrease the effect, the following formula would be applied to the data: percent inhibition$_t$ = [(baseline − treatment$_t$)/baseline] × 100. The subscript indicates the treatment, effect, or inhibition that occurred at time t during the experiment. If the study included a placebo control phase, baseline measurements made at the same time as treatment measurements (i.e., heart rate determined 2 hours after placebo and 2 hours after drug treatment) could be used in the appropriate transformation equation.[55] The appropriate model (excluding E_0) then would be used.

HYSTERESIS

Concentration-effect curves do not always follow the same pattern when serum concentrations increase as they do when serum concentrations decrease. In this situation, the concentration-effect curves form a loop that is known as *hysteresis*. With some drugs the effect is greater when serum concentrations are increasing, whereas with other drugs the effect is greater while serum concentrations are decreasing (Fig. 5–17). When individual concentration-effect pairs are joined in

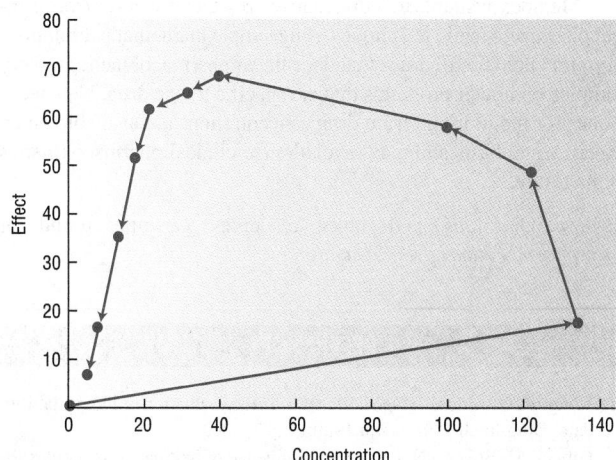

FIGURE 5–17. Hysteresis occurs when effect measurements are different at the same concentration. This is commonly seen after short-term intravenous infusions or extravascular doses where concentrations increase and subsequently decrease. Counterclockwise hysteresis loops are found when concentration-effect points are joined as time increases (*shown by arrows*) and effect is larger at the same concentration but at a later time. Clockwise hysteresis loops are similar, but the concentration-effect points are joined in clockwise order and the effect is smaller at a later time.

time sequence, this results in clockwise and counterclockwise hysteresis loops.

Clockwise hysteresis loops usually are caused by the development of tolerance to the drug. In this situation, the longer the patient is exposed to the drug, the smaller is the pharmacologic effect for a given concentration. Therefore, after an extravascular or short-term infusion dose of the drug, the effect is smaller when serum concentrations are decreasing compared with the time when serum concentrations are increasing during the infusion or absorption phase. Accumulation of a drug metabolite that acts as an antagonist also can cause clockwise hysteresis.

Counterclockwise hysteresis loops can be caused by the accumulation of an active metabolite, sensitization to the drug, or delay in time in equilibration between serum concentration and concentration of drug at the site of action. Combined pharmacokinetic-pharmacodynamic models have been devised that allow equilibration lag times to be taken into account.

CONCLUSIONS

The availability of inexpensive, rapidly achievable serum drug concentrations has changed the way clinicians monitor drug therapy in patients. The therapeutic range for many drugs is known, and it is likely that more drugs will be monitored using serum concentrations in the future. Clinicians need to remember that the therapeutic range is merely an average guideline and to take into account interindividual pharmacodynamic variability when treating patients. Individual patients may respond to smaller concentrations or require concentrations that are much greater to obtain a therapeutic effect. Conversely, patients may show toxic effects at concentrations within or below the therapeutic range. Serum concentrations should never replace clinical judgment.

Three kinetic constants determine the dosage requirements of patients. Clearance determines the maintenance dose (MD = ClC_{ss}), volume of distribution determines the loading dose (LD = V_DC_{ss}), and half-life determines the time to steady state and the dosage interval. Several methods are available to compute these parameters.

Methods available to individualize drug therapy range from clinical pharmacokinetic techniques using simple mathematical relationships that hold for all drugs that obey linear pharmacokinetics to very complex computer programs that are specific to one drug. New techniques for monitoring serum drug concentrations are available on an experimental basis and may revolutionize clinical pharmacokinetics in the future.

Review Questions and other resources can be found at *www.pharmacotherapyonline.com*.

REFERENCES

1. Koup JR, Gibaldi M. Some comments on the evaluation of bioavailability data. Drug Intell Clin Pharm 1980;14:327–330.
2. Gibaldi M, Boyes RN, Feldman S. Influence of first pass effect on availability of drugs on oral administration. J Pharm Sci 1971;60:1338–1340.
3. Wu C-Y, Benet LZ, Hebert MF, el al. Differentiation of absorption and first-pass gut and hepatic metabolism in humans: Studies with cyclosporine. Clin Pharmacol Ther 1995;58:492–497.
4. Wagner JG, Northam JI, Alway CD, el al. Blood levels of drug at the equilibrium state after multiple dosing. Nature 1965;207:1301–1302.
5. Rowland M, Benet LZ, Graham GG. Clearance concepts in pharmacokinetics. J Pharmacokinet Biopharm 1973;1:123–136.
6. Wilkinson GR, Shand DG. A physiological approach to hepatic drug clearance. Clin Pharmacol Ther 1975;18:377–390.
7. Nies AS, Shand DG, Wilkinson GR. Altered hepatic blood flow and drug disposition. Clin Pharmacokinet 1976;1:135–155.
8. Gibaldi M, Koup JR. Pharmacokinetic concepts: Drug binding, apparent volume of distribution and clearance. Eur J Clin Pharmacol 1981;20:299–305.
9. Bowdle TA, Patel IH, Levy RH, el al. Valproic acid dosage and plasma protein binding and clearance. Clin Pharmacol Ther 1980;28:486–492.
10. Lima JJ, Boudonlas H, Blanford M. Concentration-dependence of disopyramide binding to plasma protein and its influence on kinetics and dynamics. J Pharmacol Exp Ther 1981;219:741–747.
11. Gibaldi M, Perrier D. Pharmacokinetics, 2d ed. New York, Marcel Dekker, 1980.
12. Gibaldi M. Estimation of the pharmacokinetic parameters of the two-compartment open model from post-infusion plasma concentration data. J Pharm Sci 1969;58:1133–1135.
13. Loo JCK, Riegelman S. Assessment of pharmacokinetic constants from postinfusion blood curves obtained after IV infusion. J Pharm Sci 1970;59:53–55.
14. Wagner JG. Model-independent linear pharmacokinetics. Drug Intell Clin Pharm 1976;10:179–180.
15. Hansten PD, Horn JR. The Top 100 Drug Interactions: A Guide to Patient Management, 2003 ed. Edmonds, WA, H&H Publications, 2003.
16. Cockcroft DW, Gault MH. Prediction of creatinine clearance from serum creatinine. Nephron 1976;16:31–41.
17. Traub SL, Johnson CE. Comparison of methods of estimating creatinine clearance in children. Am J Hosp Pharm 1980;37:195–201.
18. Salazar DE, Corcoran GB. Predicting creatinine clearance and renal drug clearance in obese patients from estimated fat-free body mass. Am J Med 1988;84:1053–1060.
19. Jelliffe RW, Jelliffe SM. A computer program for estimation of creatinine clearance from unstable serum creatinine levels, age, sex, and weight. Math Biosci 1972;14:17–24.
20. Koup JR, Jusko WJ, Elwood CM, Kohli RK. Digoxin pharmacokinetics: Role of renal failure in dosage regimen design. Clin Pharmacol Ther 1975;18:9–21.
21. Matzke GR, McGory RW, Halstenson CE, Keane WF. Pharmacokinetics of vancomycin in patients with various degrees of renal function. Antimicrob Agents Chemother 1984;25:433–437.
22. Sarubbi FA, Hull JH. Amikacin serum concentrations: Predictions of levels and dosage guidelines. Ann Intern Med 1978;89:612–618.
23. Sivan SK, Bennett WM. Drug dosing guidelines in patients with renal failure. West J Med 1992;156:633–638.
24. Aronoff GR, Berns JS, Brier ME, el al. Drug Prescribing in Renal Failure: Dosing Guidelines for Adults, 4th ed. Philadelphia, American College of Physicians, 1999.
25. Pugh RNH, Murray-Lyon IM, Dawson JL, el al. Transection of the oesophagus for bleeding oesophageal varices. Br J Surg 1973;60:646–649.
26. Jusko WJ, Gardner MJ, Mangione A, el al. Factors affecting theophylline clearances: Age, tobacco, marijuana, cirrhosis, congestive heart failure, obesity, oral contraceptives, benzodiazepines, barbiturates, and ethanol. J Pharm Sci 1979;68:1358–1366.
27. Thomson PD, Melmon KL, Richardson JA, el al. Lidocaine pharmacokinetics in advanced heart failure, liver disease, and renal failure in humans. Ann Intern Med 1973;78:499–508.
28. Koup JR, Killen T, Bauer LA. Multiple-dose nonlinear regression analysis program: Aminoglycoside dose prediction. Clin Pharmacokinet 1983;8:456–462.
29. Sheiner LB, Beal S, Rosenberg B, el al. Forecasting individual pharmacokinetics. Clin Pharmacol Ther 1979;26:294–305.
30. Sheiner LB, Beal SL. Bayesian individualization of pharmacokinetics: Simple implementation and comparison with non-Bayesian methods. J Pharm Sci 1982;71:1344–1348.
31. Schentag JJ, Jusko WJ. Renal clearance and tissue accumulation of gentamicin. Clin Pharmacol Ther 1977;22:364–370.
32. Sawchuk RJ, Zaske DE, Cipolle RJ, el al. Kinetic model for gentamicin

dosing with the use of individual patient parameters. Clin Pharmacol Ther 1977;21:362–369.

33. Bauer LA, Edwards WAD, Dellinger EP, Simonowitz DA. Influence of weight on aminoglycoside pharmacokinetics in normal weight and morbidly obese patients. Eur J Clin Pharmacol 1983;24:643–647.

34. Bauer LA, Piecoro JJ, Wilson HD, Blouin RA. Gentamicin and tobramycin pharmacokinetics in patients with cystic fibrosis. Clin Pharm 1983; 2:262–264.

35. Sampliner R, Perrier D, Powell R, Finley P. Influence of ascites on tobramycin pharmacokinetics. J Clin Pharmacol 1984;24:43–46.

36. Zank KE, Miwa L, Cohen JL, et al. Effect of body weight on gentamicin pharmacokinetics in neonates. Clin Pharm 1984;3:170–173.

37. Pancorbo S, Sawchuk RJ, Dashe C, el al. Use of a pharmacokinetic model for individual intravenous doses of aminophylline. Eur J Clin Pharmacol 1979;16:251–254.

38. Nicolau DP, Freeman CD, Belliveau PP, el al. Experience with a once-daily aminoglycoside program administered to 2184 adult patients. Antimicrob Agents Chemother 1995;39:650–655.

39. Cantu TG, Yamanaka-Yuen NA, Lietman PS. Serum vancomycin concentrations: Reappraisal of their clinical value. Clin Infect Dis 1994;18: 533–543.

40. Welty TE, Copa AK. Impact of vancomycin therapeutic drug monitoring on patient care. Ann Pharmacother 1994;28:1335–1339.

41. Zimmermann AE, Katona BG, Plaisance KI. Association of vancomycin serum concentrations with outcomes in patients with gram-positive bacteremia. Pharmacotherapy 1995;15:85–91.

42. Karam CM, McKinnon PS, Neuhauser MM, Rybak MJ. Outcome assessment of minimizing vancomycin monitoring and dosage adjustments. Pharmacotherapy 1999;19:257–266.

43. Moellering RC Jr, Krogstad DJ, Greenblatt DJ. Vancomycin therapy in patients with impaired renal function: A nomogram for dosage. Ann Intern Med 1981;94:343–346.

44. Blouin RA, Bauer LA, Miller DD, el al. Vancomycin pharmacokinetics in normal and morbidly obese subjects. Antimicrob Agents Chemother 1982;21:575–580.

45. Matzke GR, McGory RW, Halstenson CE, Keane WF. Pharmacokinetics of vancomycin in patients with various degrees of renal function. Antimicrob Agents Chemother 1984;25:433–437.

46. Abernethy DR, Greenblatt DJ, Smith TW. Digoxin disposition in obesity: Clinical pharmacokinetic investigations. Am Heart J 1981;102: 740–744.

47. Sarrazin E, Hendeles L, Weinberger M, et al. Dose-dependent kinetics for theophylline: Observations among ambulatory asthmatic children. J Pediatr 1980;97:825–828.

48. Tang-Liu DDS, Williams RL, Riegelman S. Nonlinear theophylline elimination. Clin Pharmacol Ther 1982;31:358–369.

49. Edwards DJ, Zarowitz BJ, Slaughter RL. Theophylline In: Evans E, Schentag JJ, Jusko WJ, eds. Applied Pharmacokinetics: Principles of Therapeutic Drug Monitoring. Vancouver, WA, Applied Therapeutics, 1992.

50. Vozeh S, Kewitz G, Wenk M, et al. Rapid prediction of steady-state serum theophylline concentrations in patients treated with intravenous aminophylline. Eur J Clin Pharmacol 1980;18:473–477.

51. Vozeh S, Muir KT, Sheiner LB, Follath F. Predicting individual phenytoin dosage. J Pharmacokinet Biopharm 1991;9:131–146.

52. Ludden TM, Allen JP, Valutsky WA, el al. Individualization of phenytoin dosage regimens. Clin Pharmacol Ther 1977;21:287–293.

53. Holford NHG, Sheiner LB. Understanding the dose-effect relationship: Clinical application of pharmacokinetic-pharmacodynamic models. Clin Pharmacokinet 1981;6:429–453.

54. Schwinghammer TL, Kroboth PD. Basic concepts in pharmacodynamic modeling. J Clin Pharmacol 1988;28:388–394.

55. Sheiner LB, Stanski DR, Vozeh S, el al. Simultaneous modeling of pharmacokinetics and pharmacodynamics: Application to d-tubocurarine. Clin Pharmacol Ther 1979;25:358.

6
PHARMACOGENETICS
Larisa H. Cavallari and Y. W. Francis Lam

Learning Objectives and other resources can be found at *www.pharmacotherapyonline.com.*

KEY CONCEPTS

1 Genetic variations contribute to interpatient differences in drug response.

2 Genetic variations occur for drug metabolism, drug transporter, and drug target proteins, as well as disease-associated genes.

3 Genetic polymorphisms may be linked to drug efficacy and toxicity.

4 Pharmacogenetics is the study of the impact of genetic polymorphisms on drug response.

5 The goals of pharmacogenetics are to optimize drug efficacy and limit drug toxicity based on an individual's DNA.

6 Single-nucleotide polymorphisms are the most common variations in the human genome.

7 Gene therapy aims to cure disease caused by genetic defects by changing gene expression.

8 Inadequate gene delivery and expression and serious adverse effects are obstacles to successful gene therapy.

Great variability exists among individuals in response to drug therapy, and it is often difficult to predict how effective or safe a medication will be for a particular patient. For example, when treating a patient with hypertension, it may be necessary to try several agents or a combination of agents before achieving adequate blood pressure control with acceptable tolerability. A number of factors may influence drug response, including pharmacokinetics, age, ethnicity, and concomitant drug use. However, these alone do not predict the likelihood of drug efficacy or safety sufficiently for a given patient. For instance, identical antihypertensive therapy in two patients with similar demographic characteristics, medical histories, and concomitant drug therapy may produce inadequate blood pressure reduction in one patient and symptomatic hypotension in the other.

1 2 The observed interpatient variability in drug response may result largely from genetically determined differences in drug metabolism, drug distribution, and drug target proteins. The influence of hereditary factors on drug response was demonstrated as early as 1956 with the discovery that an inherited deficiency of glucose-6-phosphate dehydrogenase was responsible for hemolytic reactions to the antimalarial drug primaquine.[1] Variations in the genetic makeup of cytochrome P450 (CYP) and other drug-metabolizing enzymes are now well recognized as causes of interindividual differences in plasma concentrations of certain drugs. These variations may have serious implications for narrow-therapeutic-index drugs such as warfarin, phenytoin, and mercaptopurine.[2–4] More recently, interest has been generated in the associations between drug response and genetic polymorphisms for drug transporters such as P-glycoprotein and drug targets such as receptors, enzymes, and proteins involved in intracellular signal transduction. Genetic variations for drug-metabolizing enzymes and drug transporter proteins may influence drug disposition, thus altering pharmacokinetic drug properties. Drug target genes may alter pharmacodynamic mechanisms by affecting sensitivity to a drug at its target site. Finally, genes associated

with disease severity have been correlated with drug efficacy despite having no direct effect on pharmacokinetic or pharmacodynamic mechanisms.

PHARMACOGENETICS: A DEFINITION

3 4 Pharmacogenetics involves the search for genetic variations that lead to interindividual differences in drug response. The term *pharmacogenetics* often is used interchangeably with the term *pharmacogenomics.* However, pharmacogenetics generally refers to monogenetic variants that affect drug response, whereas pharmacogenomics refers to the entire spectrum of genes that interact to determine drug efficacy and safety. For example, a pharmacogenetic study would be one that examines the influence of the β_1-adrenergic receptor gene on blood pressure response to carvedilol. A pharmacogenomic study might examine the interaction between the CYP2D6, β_1-, β_2-, and α_1-adrenergic receptor genes on carvedilol effects. To date, most studies of gene-drug responses are pharmacogenetic in nature. However, given that multiple proteins are involved in determining the ultimate response to most drugs, many investigators are now taking a more pharmacogenomic approach to elucidating genetic contributions to drug response. For simplicity, this chapter treats pharmacogenetics and pharmacogenomics as synonymous.

5 The goals of pharmacogenetics are to optimize drug therapy and limit drug toxicity based on an individual's genetic profile. Thus pharmacogenetics aims to use genetic information to choose a drug, drug dose, and treatment duration that will have the greatest likelihood for achieving therapeutic outcomes with the least potential for harm in a given patient. The results of pharmacogenetic research ultimately will provide opportunities for clinicians to use genetic tests to predict individual responses to drug treatments, specifically to select medications for patients based on DNA profiles, and to develop

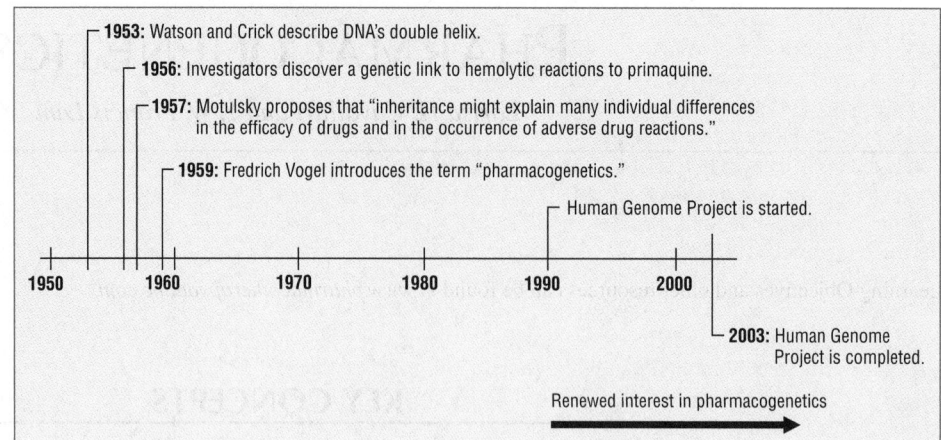

FIGURE 6–1. Timeline of genomic discoveries.

novel strategies for disease treatment and prevention based on an understanding of genetic control of cellular functions.

Although there has been considerable interest in genetic influences of drug response in recent years, pharmacogenetics is not a new area. As shown in Fig. 6–1, in 1957, shortly after the discovery of a genetic predisposition toward primaquine-induced toxicity, Arno Motulsky proposed that inheritance might underlie much of the disparity among individuals in drug response.[5] Fredrich Vogel first introduced the term *pharmacogenetics* 2 years later.[6] With the advent of the Human Genome Project in 1990 came a resurgence of interest in determining genetic contributions to drug response.

HUMAN GENOME PROJECT

In 1988, Congress commissioned the Department of Energy and the National Institutes of Health to plan and implement the Human Genome Project. The goal of the Human Genome Project was to determine the entire sequence of the human genome by 2005. The mapping of the human genome, which officially began in 1990, has led to a better understanding of genetic contributions to disease susceptibility. To encourage research and ultimately maximize the societal benefits of the Human Genome Project, sequence data from the Human Genome Project have been deposited into a freely accessible database run by the National Center for Biotechnology Information (*www.ncbi.nlm.nih.gov*). As a consequence of these shared data, research efforts in the 1990s accelerated the discovery of genetic variations affecting treatment response and development of new treatments and preventive strategies for human disease.

Largely because of advances in biotechnology, the initial working draft of the human genome sequence was completed in 2000, well ahead of schedule.[7] In April of 2003, 50 years after James Watson and Francis Crick described the double-helix structure of DNA and over 2 years ahead of schedule, researchers announced the completion of the Human Genome Project.[8] The final version contains 99% of the gene-containing sequence, with 99.9% accuracy.

Following completion of the Human Genome Project, the National Human Genome Research Institute announced its vision for the future of genomic research with the goal of improving human health and well-being.[9] One of the challenges set forth to meet this goal is to develop genome-based approaches to predict drug response. This challenge will involve the accurate, unbiased determination of genetic variants linked to drug response, advanced technology to

reduce genotyping costs, and appropriate integration of genetic testing into the therapeutic decision process. The National Human Genome Research Institute also challenges investigators to develop new, gene-based approaches to disease management, which will require a thorough understanding of genetic determinants of disease susceptibility and progression.

GENETIC CONCEPTS

The human genome contains approximately 3 billion nucleotide bases, which code for approximately 30,000 genes. Two purine nucleotide bases, adenine (A) and guanine (G), and two pyrimidine nucleotide bases, cytosine (C) and thymidine (T), are present in DNA, with purines and pyrimidines always pairing together as A-T and C-G in the two strands that make up the DNA structure. Most nucleotide base pairs are identical from person to person, with only 0.1% contributing to individual differences.

According to the central dogma, when one strand of DNA is transcribed into RNA and translated to make proteins, three consecutive nucleotides form a codon. Each codon specifies an amino acid or amino acid chain termination. For example, the nucleotide sequence, or codon, GGA specifies the amino acid glycine. The genetic code has substantial redundancy, in that two or more codons code for the same amino acid. For example, both GGA and GGC code for glycine. Amino acids are the basic constituents of proteins, which mediate all cellular functions. Only 20 different amino acids, in various arrangements, form the basic units of all the proteins in the human body.

A gene is a series of codons that specifies a particular protein. Genes contain several regions: *exons* that encode for the final protein, *introns* that consist of intervening noncoding regions, and *promoter regions* that regulate gene transcription. At each gene locus, an individual carries two alleles, one from each parent. An *allele* is defined as the sequence of nucleic acid bases at a given gene chromosomal locus. Two identical alleles make up a *homozygous* genotype, and two different alleles make up a *heterozygous* genotype. A *phenotype* refers to the outward expression of the genotype.

TYPES OF GENETIC VARIATIONS

Genetic variations occur as either rare defects or polymorphisms. *Polymorphisms* are defined as variations occurring at a frequency of at least 1% in the human population. For example, the genes encoding the CYP enzymes 2A6, 2C9, 2C19, 2D6, and 3A4 are polymorphic, with functional mutations of greater than 1% occurring in different ethnic groups. In contrast, rare mutations occur in less than 1% of the population and cause inherited diseases such as cystic fibrosis, hemophilia, and Huntington's disease. Common diseases, such as essential hypertension and diabetes mellitus, are polygenic in that multiple genetic polymorphisms likely interact to contribute to the disease susceptibility.

Single-nucleotide polymorphisms, abbreviated as SNPs and pronounced "snips," are the most common genetic variations in human DNA, occurring approximately once in every 1000 base pairs. Approximately 3.7 million SNPs have been mapped thus far in the human genome. SNPs occur when one nucleotide base pair replaces another, as illustrated in Fig. 6–2. Thus SNPs are single-base differences that exist between individuals. Nucleotide substitution results in two possible alleles. One allele, typically either the most commonly occurring allele or the allele originally sequenced, is considered the *wild type,* and the alternative allele is considered the *variant allele.*

A SNP may change the codon resulting in amino acid substitution, which may or may not alter gene expression. For example, in Fig. 6–2, guanine (G) is substituted for adenine (A) at nucleotide 46. This results in the substitution of glycine for arginine at amino acid position 16. SNPs such as this that result in amino acid substitution are referred to as *nonsynonymous.* SNPs that do not result in amino acid substitution are called *synonymous.* Referring to a previous example of redundancy in the genetic code, replacement of adenine (A) with cytosine (C) in the codon GGA is an example of a synonymous SNP because the resulting amino acid is still glycine. Synonymous SNPs usually are abbreviated based on the nucleotides involved and the nucleotide base position. For example, A1166C or A1166→C indicates that cytosine is substituted for adenine at nucleotide position 1166 of a given gene region. Nonsynonymous SNPs usually are designated by the amino acids and codon involved. For example, Arg16Gly or Arg16→Gly indicates that glycine is substituted for arginine at codon 16. If a SNP changes the expression of a protein that contributes to drug response, it may alter a patient's sensitivity to a drug or predispose a patient to adverse reactions to drug therapy.

Other examples of genetic variants include

* *Insertion-deletion polymorphisms,* in which a nucleotide or nucleotide sequence is either added to or deleted from a DNA sequence
* *Tandem repeats,* in which a nucleotide sequence repeats in tandem (i.e., if "AG" is the nucleotide repeat unit, "AGAGAGAGAG" is a five-tandem repeat)
* *Frameshift mutation,* in which there is an insertion/deletion polymorphism, and the number of nucleotides added or lost is not a multiple of 3, resulting in disruption of the gene's reading frame
* *Defective splicing,* in which an internal polypeptide segment is abnormally removed, and the ends of the remaining polypeptide chain are joined
* *Aberrant splice site,* in which processing of the protein occurs at an alternate site
* *Premature stop codon polymorphisms,* in which there is premature termination of the polypeptide chain by a stop codon (specific sequence of three nucleotides that do not code for an amino acid but rather specify polypeptide chain termination)

For more detailed information about genetic concepts, refer to the recommended genetics textbook.[10]

As mentioned earlier, most common diseases are polygenic in nature. For example, independent studies have demonstrated associations between gene variants for proteins involved in the renin-angiotensin system, sympathetic nervous system, and renal sodium transport and the risk for essential hypertension.[11] Environmental factors are also well-known risk factors for diseases such as hypertension and often interact with genetic factors to influence disease susceptibility and progression. Given the complex pathophysiology of most common diseases, genes linked to disease susceptibility will not be discussed in this chapter. Rather, this chapter will focus on genetic variations linked to responses to pharmacologic agents.

POLYMORPHISMS IN GENES FOR DRUG-METABOLIZING ENZYMES

Polymorphisms in the drug-metabolizing enzymes represent the first recognized and, so far, the most documented examples of genetic variants with consequences in drug response and toxicity. The major phase I enzymes are the CYP superfamily of isoenzymes. *N*-acetyltransferase, thiopurine *S*-methyltransferase, and glutathione *S*-transferase are examples of phase II metabolizing enzymes that exhibit genetic polymorphisms. Table 6–1 lists selected examples of polymorphic metabolizing enzymes, corresponding drug substrates, and the consequences of altered enzyme function as a result of gene mutation.

CYTOCHROME P450 ENZYMES

Currently, 57 different CYP isoenzymes have been documented to be present in humans, with 42 involved in the metabolism of xenobiotics, including drugs, and endogenous substances such as steroids and prostaglandins.[12] Fifteen of these isoenzymes are known to be involved in the metabolism of xenobiotics, and functional

---

A. "Wild type" allele

Codon	13	14	15	16	17	18	19
Nucleotide	...GCA	CCC	AAT	AGA	AGC	CAT	GCG...
Amino acid	Ala	Pro	Asn	**Arg**	Ser	His	Ala

B. "Variant" allele

Codon	13	14	15	16	17	18	19
Nucleotide	...GCA	CCC	AAT	GGA	AGC	CAT	GCG...
Amino acid	Ala	Pro	Asn	**Gly**	Ser	His	Ala

FIGURE 6–2. Nucleotide sequence of the β_2-adrenergic receptor gene from codons 13 through 19. *A.* Nucleotide sequence of the wild-type allele with adenine (A) at nucleotide position 46 (*underlined*) located in codon 16 of the β_2-adrenergic receptor gene. The AGA codon designates the amino acid arginine (Arg), with an average frequency of 39% in the human population. *B.* Nucleotide sequence of the variant allele with guanine (G) at nucleotide position 46 (*underlined*), located in codon 16. The GGA codon designates the amino acid glycine (Gly), which occurs at an average frequency of 61%. Although the Arg16 polymorphism occurs less commonly than the Gly16 polymorphism, it is referred to as the wild type because it was identified first.

TABLE 6–1. Selected Examples of Genetic Polymorphisms in Drug-Metabolizing Enzymes and Response to Drug Therapy

Genetic Variants/Genes	Drug	Drug Effect Associated with Polymorphism
CYP2D6*4, CYP2D6*5	Perhexiline	Neuropathy[18]
	Codeine	Significant reduction in analgesic effect[22,23]
	Tramadol	
CYP2D6*2 (n > l)	Tricyclic antidepressants (e.g., desipramine, nortriptyline)	Inadequate antidepressant response[29,30]
CYP2D6*10	Antipsychotics (e.g., haloperidol)	Elevated plasma concentrations and exaggerated responses[33]
CYP2C9*3	Warfarin	Hemorrhage[2]
CYP2C9, CYP2C19	Phenytoin	Phenytoin toxicity[3]
CYP2C19	Omeprazole	Improved cure rates for Helicobacter pylori[41]
Glutathione-S-transferase	Primaquine	Hemolytic reactions[1]
Thiopurine methyltransferase	Mercaptopurine	Bone marrow depression[4]
N-Acetyltransferase slow acetylator	Isoniazid	More prone to peripheral neuropathy[119]
	Procainamide	More prone to development of SLE-like syndrome[120,121]
	Hydralazine	
	Sulfonamides	Increased hematologic and gastrointestinal adverse reactions[122]
UDP-glucuronosyltransferase	Irinotecan	Increased severity of diarrhea and neutropenia in carrier of (TA)₇ TAA allele[59]

genetic polymorphism has been discovered for CYP2A6, CYP2C9, CYP2C19, CYP2D6,[13] and more recently, CYP3A4/5.[14,15] A polymorphism in the regulatory region of the gene encoding for CYP1A2[16] has been identified, but its functional importance remains to be determined.

CYP2D6

Polymorphisms in the *CYP2D6* gene are the best characterized of the CYP variants. Over the years, at least 48 gene variants and 53 alleles have been identified in the *CYP2D6* gene.[17] Nevertheless, the CYP2D6 extensive-metabolizer (EM) and poor-metabolizer (PM) phenotypes (outward expression of genotypes) can be predicted with up to 99% confidence with six genotypic variants. *CYP2D6*1* is considered the wild-type variant and exhibits normal enzyme activity. *CYP2D6*2* has the same activity as *CYP2D6*1* but is capable of duplication or amplification. Both these variants are present in EMs. The *CYP2D6*4* (defective splicing) and *CYP2D6*5* (gene deletion) variants are present in PMs and result in an inactive enzyme and absence of enzyme, respectively. The predominant variants in people of Asian and African heritage are *CYP2D6*10* (Pro34Ser) and *CYP2D6*17* (Arg296Cys), respectively, both resulting in single-amino-acid substitution and consequent reduction in enzyme activity.

Poor CYP2D6 metabolizers carry two defective alleles, such as *CYP2D6*3*, *CYP2D6*4* (more common), *CYP2D6*5*, and *CYP2D6*6*, resulting in a total absence of active enzyme and an impaired ability to metabolize CYP2D6-dependent substrates. Examples of CYP2D6 substrates include neuroleptic medications, antidepressants such as tricyclic antidepressants and mianserin, antiarrhythmic drugs such as propafenone, and β-adrenergic antagonists such as metoprolol (see Table 6–1). Depending on the importance of the affected CYP2D6 pathway to overall drug metabolism and the drug's therapeutic index, clinically significant side effects may occur in PMs as a result of elevated parent drug concentrations. For example, compared with EMs, PMs have been shown to develop

neuropathy after treatment with the antianginal agent perhexiline[18] and have experienced more adverse effects with propafenone[19] and neuroleptic agents such as perphenazine.[20,21]

The therapeutic implication of CYP2D6 polymorphism is different if the substrate in question is a prodrug. In this case, PMs would not be able to convert the drug into the therapeutically active metabolite. Two examples of prodrugs dependent on CYP2D6-mediated conversion to active forms are codeine and tramadol. Codeine and tramadol are converted by CYP2D6 to morphine and O-desmethyltramadol, respectively, and thus poor CYP2D6 metabolizers would experience little or no analgesic relief after taking these drugs.[22,23]

Although PMs are at a disadvantage from the standpoint of drug toxicity and lack of efficacy for most CYP2D6 substrates and prodrugs, data suggest that they may be "protected" from abusing opiates such as codeine, oxycodone, and hydrocodone. This is primarily based on an observation that no PMs were found among opiate-dependent subjects, which likely reflects their inability to convert these drugs of abuse into their respective "pharmacologically active" moieties.[24] Given the reduced potential for opiate abuse among CYP2D6 PMs, investigators have used daily doses of fluoxetine 20 mg, a CYP2D6 inhibitor, as adjunctive therapy in the management of opiate abuse to "metabolically convert" drug abusers who are EMs to PMs.[25]

Furthermore, the potential and magnitude of drug interactions involving competitive inhibition of CYP2D6 are much greater in EMs versus PMs, who have either deficient or absent enzyme activity.[26,27] For example, Hamelin and colleagues[28] showed that in EMs, but not PMs, hemodynamic responses to metoprolol (a CYP2D6 substrate) were pronounced and prolonged during concomitant diphenhydramine administration. Thus potent CYP2D6 inhibitors may reduce the metabolic capacity of EMs significantly so that EMs appear phenotypically as PMs.

Patients who are EMs have a wide range of CYP2D6 activity, with ultrarapid metabolizers (UMs) on one end of the spectrum and subjects with diminished activity on the other end. Both have clinical implications in terms of dosage adjustment for CYP2D6 substrates.

UMs carry a duplicated or amplified mutant allele, resulting in two or multiple copies of the functional CYP2D6*2 allele, and therefore show very high CYP2D6 activity. Nontherapeutic plasma concentrations of nortriptyline, a CYP2D6 substrate, were observed in a UM given normal doses of the drug.[29] The CYP2D6 enzyme converts nortriptyline to 10-hydroxynortriptyline, and one study demonstrated a directly proportional relationship between the number of functional CYP2D6 genes and the concentration of 10-hydroxynortriptyline after nortriptyline ingestion.[30] A patient with three copies of CYP2D6*2 was shown to require nortriptyline doses three- to fivefold higher than normally recommended to achieve therapeutic plasma concentrations (50–150 mcg/mL).[29,31] In the same report, another patient with duplicated CYP2D6*2 required twice the usual recommended daily dose (300 mg versus 25–150 mg) to achieve adequate therapeutic response.[31] The UM genotype also has been reported to affect the potential for drug interaction with paroxetine, a CYP2D6 substrate as well as a potent CYP2D6 inhibitor.[32]

The high prevalence of CYP2D6*10 (associated with lower enzyme activity) in the Asian population provides a biologic and molecular explanation for the higher drug concentrations and/or lower dosage requirements of neuroleptic medications and mianserin in people of Asian heritage.[33,34] The widespread presence of the CYP2D6*17 variant among people of African heritage suggests that native African populations would metabolize CYP2D6 substrates at a slower rate than do other ethnic or racial groups.[35,36] However, there are no current genotype- and phenotype-based data to document the need for prescribing lower doses of psychotropics and other CYP2D6 substrates in native African populations.

In addition to the therapeutic implications of genetic polymorphisms, a recent study showed that the CYP2D6 polymorphism also has an economic impact.[37] The annual cost of treating UMs and PMs (carriers of two nonfunctional CYP2D6 alleles) was $4,000–$6,000 higher than the cost of treating EMs or intermediate metabolizers (carriers of one nonfunctional allele and one allele associated with diminished activity). The cost of genotyping can be considerably less than that incurred in a patient with a serious adverse drug reaction. Brockmoller and colleagues[38] recently suggested how CYP2D6 genotyping can be used to achieve higher therapeutic success with the CYP2D6 substrate haloperidol.

CYP2C19

The principal defective alleles for the CYP2C19 genetic polymorphism are CYP2C19*2 (aberrant splice site) and CYP2C19*3 (premature stop codon), resulting in inactive CYP2C19 enzymes and the PM phenotype. The clinical implication of the CYP2C19 polymorphism has not been examined as extensively as that of the CYP2D6 polymorphism. However, PMs for the CYP2C19 polymorphism showed more than a 12-fold increase in the area under the curve (AUC) of the CYP2C19 substrate omeprazole compared with EMs.[39] In a separate study, the steady-state AUC of omeprazole and other CYP2C19 substrate proton-pump inhibitors was 5-fold higher in PMs versus EMs.[40]

The presence of a defective CYP2C19 allele has been associated with improved Helicobacter pylori cure rates after dual (omeprazole and amoxicillin)[41] or triple therapy (omeprazole, amoxicillin, and clarithromycin) with omeprazole,[42] as well as with lansoprazole.[43] This difference likely reflects the higher achievable intragastric pH in the PM group.[44] The cure rate achieved with dual therapy was 100% in PMs compared with 60% and 29% in heterozygous and homozygous EMs, respectively.[41] In two studies, EMs had H. pylori

eradication rates of 41% with dual therapy and 74% to 83% with triple therapy.[42,43] In contrast, both dual- and triple-therapy regimens produced 100% cure rates in all 15 PMs included in the same studies. Interestingly, EMs who failed initial triple therapy (lansoprazole, clarithromycin, and amoxicillin) and were retreated with high-dose lansoprazole (30 mg four times daily) and amoxicillin achieved a 97% H. pylori eradication.[45]

Similar to the CYP2D6 polymorphism, people of Asian heritage also metabolize most CYP2C19 substrates at a slower rate than do Caucasians.[46] This is a reflection of a higher prevalence of both PMs (13% to 20% versus 2% to 6% in Caucasians) and heterozygotes for the defective CYP2C19 allele in Asians.[47] This genotypic difference may explain the practice of prescribing lower diazepam dosages for patients of Chinese heritage.[48]

CYP2C9

Warfarin, phenytoin, and tolbutamide are examples of narrow-therapeutic-index drugs that are metabolized by CYP2C9. Warfarin is a racemic mixture, and the S-isomer, which possesses about three times the anticoagulant effects of the R-isomer, is metabolized by CYP2C9. CYP2C9*2 and CYP2C9*3 are the two most common CYP2C9 variants, and both exhibit single-amino-acid substitutions at positions critical for enzyme activity.[49] This could have clinically important consequences in warfarin-treated patients. For example, a 90% reduction in S-warfarin clearance was reported in CYP2C9*3 homozygotes compared with subjects homozygous for the wild-type variant.[50] In another study, an overrepresentation of CYP2C9 mutant alleles was observed in 81% of patients requiring low-dose warfarin therapy ($\leq$1.5 mg/day).[2] The low-dose group was reported to have more difficulty with warfarin induction, requiring longer hospital stays to stabilize the warfarin regimen and experiencing a higher incidence of bleeding complications. In addition, a profound therapeutic response to usual doses of warfarin was observed in a patient homozygous for the CYP2C9*3 allele, necessitating dose reduction to 0.5 mg/day.[51]

CYP2A6

A recent polymorphism was characterized for CYP2A6, with several variants identified: CYP2A6*1 (wild type), CYP2A6*2 (single-amino-acid substitution), CYP2A6*3 (gene conversion), and three gene-deletion alleles: CYP2A6*4A, CYP2A6*4B, and CYP2A6*4D.[52] Deletion of the CYP2A6 gene is very common in Asian patients,[52,53] which likely accounts for the dramatic difference in the frequency of PMs in Asian (20%) versus European and Caucasian populations ($\leq$1%). Nicotine is metabolized by CYP2A6, and the clinical relevance of the CYP2A6 polymorphism lies in management of tobacco abuse.[54] Investigators reported that nonsmokers were more likely to carry the defective CYP2A6 allele than were smokers. Smokers who had the defective CYP2A6 allele smoked fewer cigarettes and were more likely to quit.[54] The inability to metabolize nicotine, secondary to the presence of a defective CYP2A6 allele, likely leads to enhanced nicotine tolerance and increased adverse effects from nicotine. Based on these observations, CYP2A6 inhibition may have a role in the management of tobacco dependency.[55]

CYP3A4/5

Within the CYP3A subfamily, at least three isoenzymes, namely, CYP3A4, CYP3A5, and CYP3A7, have been characterized. Despite as much as 40-fold interindividual variability in its expression, functional CYP3A4 is expressed in most adults. CYP3A4 variants with amino acid substitutions in exons 7 and 12 have been associated with altered catalytic activity for a CYP3A4 substrate, nifedipine.[14] The clinical importance of this finding needs to be further elucidated and confirmed.

CYP3A5 is reported to be polymorphic in 60% of African-Americans and 33% of Caucasians. In contrast to individuals with the *CYP3A5*1* allele, subjects with variant alleles such as *CYP3A5*3* (aberrant splice site) in intron 3 have no functional CYP3A5 enzyme.[15] It remains unknown whether there are clinically used drugs that are substrates for CYP3A5 but not CYP3A4 and vice versa.

PHASE II METABOLIZING ENZYMES

The clinical relevance of genetic polymorphisms in thiopurine-*S*-methyltransferase (TPMT), dihydropyrimidine dehydrogenase (DPD), and UDP-glucuronosyl transferase (UGT) enzymes has been demonstrated in the treatment of cancer.[4,56,57] The *TPMT* gene has three mutant alleles: *TPMT*3A* (the most common), *TPMT*2*, and *TPMT*3C*. Patients who are homozygous or heterozygous for the *TPMT* mutant alleles are at higher risk for developing serious anemias during mercaptopurine treatment.[4] DPD mediates the metabolism of 5-fluorouracil, and patients with a defective allele of the *DPD* gene cannot metabolize 5-fluorouracil and thus may experience enhanced drug-related neurotoxicity.[56] The camptothecin derivative irinotecan (CPT-11) is activated by carboxylesterase to SN-38, which is a potent topoisomerase I inhibitor. SN-38 is inactivated by glucuronidation via the polymorphic UDP-glucouronosyl transferase (UGT1A1) enzyme, which may play a role in CPT-11–related toxicity. A polymorphism in the promoter region of the *UGT1A1* gene results in the *(TA)$_7$TAA* allele, which possesses lower enzyme activity than the wild-type *(TA)$_6$TAA* allele. A patient homozygous for the *(TA)$_7$TAA* allele had impaired SN-38 glucuronidation.[57] Since abnormally high SN-38 concentrations have been associated with diarrhea,[58] likely resulting from increased SN-38 excretion into the gut lumen, patients with the *(TA)$_7$TAA* allele may be predisposed to developing diarrhea with usual CPT-11 doses. This observation has been confirmed in a prospective clinical trial that demonstrated more severe diarrhea and neutropenia in patients who are homozygous or heterozygous carriers of the *(TA)$_7$TAA* allele.[59]

POLYMORPHISMS IN DRUG TRANSPORTER GENES

Certain membrane-spanning proteins facilitate drug transport across the gastrointestinal tract, drug excretion into the bile and urine, and drug distribution across the blood-brain barrier. Genetic variations for drug transport proteins may affect the distribution of drugs that serve as substrates for these proteins and alter drug concentrations at their therapeutic sites of action. P-glycoprotein is one of the most recognized of the drug transport proteins that exhibit genetic polymorphism. P-glycoprotein is an energy-dependent transmembrane efflux pump encoded by the multidrug-resistance 1 (*MDR-1*) gene. P-glycoprotein was first recognized for its ability to actively export anticancer agents from cancer cells and promote multidrug resistance to cancer chemotherapy. Later, it was discovered that P-glycoprotein is also widely distributed on normal cell types, including intestinal enterocytes, hepatocytes, renal proximal tubule cells, and endothelial cells lining the blood-brain barrier. At these locations, P-glycoprotein serves a protective role by transporting toxic substances or metabolites out of cells. P-glycoprotein also affects the distribution of some

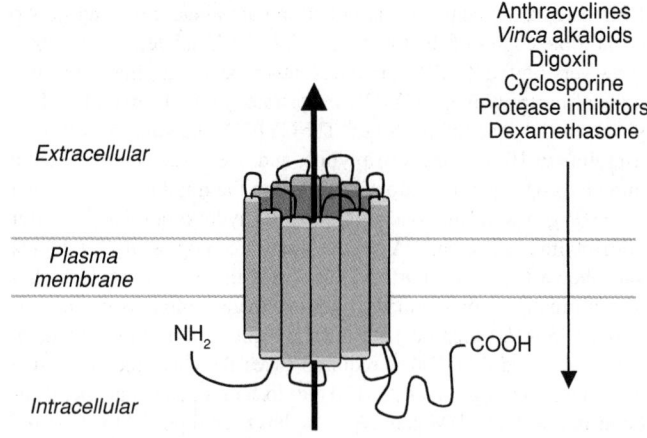

FIGURE 6–3. Active transport of drugs out of the cell by P-glycoprotein.

nonchemotherapeutic agents, including digoxin, the immunosuppressants cyclosporine and tacrolimus, and antiretroviral protease inhibitors (Fig. 6–3). Increased intestinal expression of P-glycoprotein can limit the absorption of P-glycoprotein substrates, thus reducing their bioavailability and preventing attainment of therapeutic plasma concentrations. Conversely, decreased P-glycoprotein expression may result in supratherapeutic plasma concentrations of relevant drugs and drug toxicity.

CLINICAL CONTROVERSY

Much of the data on individual variations in the multidrug resistance gene and response to P-glycoprotein substrates are inconsistent and even conflicting. The combination of multiple variations in the multidrug resistance gene eventually may prove to be a stronger predictor of drug response than any individual variation.

A number of polymorphisms have been identified in the promoter and exon regions of the *MDR-1* gene. Common SNPs occur in exons 12 (C1236T), 21 (G2677T), and 26 (C3435T). The exon 21 and 26 SNPs have been associated with intestinal MDR-1 expression, P-glycoprotein activity, and digoxin plasma concentrations in healthy volunteers.[60] These data imply that the MDR-1 genotype may be useful in predicting digoxin concentrations in patients with atrial arrhythmias or heart failure and in choosing initial digoxin doses accordingly.

The *MDR-1* exon 26 polymorphism also has been associated with plasma concentrations and clinical effects of protease inhibitors in patients infected with the human immunodeficiency virus (HIV).[61] Specifically, following therapy with efavirenz or nelfinavir for 6 months, a greater rise in CD4 cell counts was observed in individuals with the exon 26 TT genotype compared with CC homozygotes. This findings suggest a role for *MDR-1* genotyping in predicting hematologic responses to protease inhibitors and individualizing antiretroviral drug therapy for HIV-infected patients.

Other examples of polymorphic drug transporter proteins include the dipeptide transporter, organic anion and cation transporters, and L-amino acid transporter. Their effects on drug distribution are the focus of ongoing research.

POLYMORPHISMS IN DRUG TARGET GENES

Genetic polymorphisms occur commonly for drug target proteins, including receptors, enzymes, and intracellular signaling proteins. Drug target genes may work in concert with genes that affect pharmacokinetic properties to contribute to overall drug response. Table 6–2 provides examples of drug target genes linked to drug response in clinical studies. The following section highlights some of the receptor, enzyme, and cell-signaling protein genes shown to influence the efficacy and safety of various pharmacologic agents.

RECEPTOR GENOTYPES AND DRUG RESPONSE

The β_1- and β_2-adrenergic receptor genes have been the focus of much research into genetic determinants of responses to β-agonists and β-antagonists. β_1-Receptors are located in the heart and kidney, where they participate in blood pressure regulation. Two nonsynonymous SNPs commonly occur in the β_1-receptor gene at codons 49 (Ser→Gly) and 389 (Arg→Gly), and there is evidence of their involvement in blood pressure control.[62] Recently, investigators examined the influence of the β_1-receptor gene on blood pressure response to β_1-receptor blockade with metoprolol. Hypertensive patients who were homozygous for both the Ser49 and Arg389 alleles were found to have greater reductions in diastolic blood pressure with metoprolol monotherapy compared with carriers of the Gly49 and/or Gly389 alleles.[63] These data suggest that β_1-receptor genotype may be an important determinant of blood pressure response to β-blockers in the management of hypertension. Given that a significant percentage of hypertensive patients fail to derive adequate blood pressure reduction with β-blocker monotherapy,[64] the ability to predict the likelihood of response based on genotype would have important clinical implications. Specifically, β-blockers could be started in patients expected to respond well to this drug class based on their β_1-receptor genotype, whereas other classes of antihypertensive agents could be used in those expected to respond poorly to β-blockers.

β_2-Receptors are located on vascular and bronchial smooth muscle cells, where they mediate vasodilation and bronchodilation, respectively, on exposure to the β_2-receptor agonists. Inhaled β_2-agonists are the most effective agents for the acute reversal of bronchospasm; however, the magnitude of their effects varies substantially among asthmatic patients.[65] More than 11 SNPs have been identified in the β_2-receptor gene, 3 of which occur frequently and result in amino acid changes. Two common nonsynonymous SNPs are found in the gene's coding block region, at codons 16 and 27, and a third occurs upstream from the coding block in the gene's promoter region.

Three groups of investigators have examined the influence of the β_2-receptor codon 16 (Arg→Gly) polymorphism on vasodilatory response to β_2-agonist therapy. Two of these groups reported greater vasodilation with the homozygous Arg genotype, whereas the third reported greater response with the Gly/Gly form.[66–68] A fourth group of investigators found that the combination of SNPs in the gene's coding block and promoter region was a better determinant of β_2-agonist response than any individual SNP.[69] These data suggest that an individual SNP in the β_2-receptor gene is an insufficient predictor of β_2-agonist effects and that multiple receptor gene variations more accurately correlate with β_2-agonist response.

Clozapine is an example of a drug for which there is evidence that multiple receptor genes interact to influence its effects. Clozapine is an atypical antipsychotic used in the treatment of schizophrenia. Because of its potential to produce agranulocytosis in 0.5% to 2% of treated patients, clozapine is reserved for schizophrenic patients who are unresponsive to other drug therapies. However, only 30% to 60% of patients with refractory schizophrenia respond to clozapine.[70] Clozapine's effects are believed to be mediated through dopaminergic, serotoninergic, adrenergic, and histaminergic receptors in the central nervous system.[71] Although several studies have demonstrated relationships between single genetic variants for these receptor subtypes and clozapine response, the data are inconsistent.[72] In a more recent study, a combination of six polymorphisms in the histamine and serotonin 2A and 2C receptor genes and the serotonin transporter gene

TABLE 6–2. Genetic Polymorphisms in Drug Targets and Response to Drug Therapy

Gene	Drug/Drug Class	Drug Effect Associated with Polymorphism
α-Adducin	Hydrochlorothiazide	Blood pressure reduction[91] and clinical outcomes[92]
ACE	ACE inhibitors	Blood pressure reduction,[74] regression of left ventricular hypertrophy,[77] renoprotective effects,[123] drug-induced cough[81]
Angiotensinogen	ACE inhibitors	Blood pressure reduction[80]
β_1-Adrenergic receptor	β-Blockers	Blood pressure lowering[63]
β_2-Adrenergic receptor	β_2-Agonists	Bronchodilation[69,124–126]
Bradykinin B_2 receptor	ACE inhibitors	Cough[127]
Dopamine D_2 receptor	Levodopa	Peak-dose dyskinesias[128]
Dopamine D_3 receptor	Levodopa, neuroleptics	Akathisia[129]
Estrogen receptor	Estrogen	Bone mineral density[130]
Inhibitory GTP-binding protein β_3 subunit	Antidepressants	Antidepressant response[88,89]
5-Lipoxygenase	Leukotriene modifier	Change in FEV_1[131]
Combination of H_2, 5-HT_{2A}, 5-HT_{2C}, 5-HT transporter	Clozapine	Response in schizophrenia[70]
Stimulatory G-protein α subunit	β-Blockers	Blood pressure lowering[85]

Key: ACE, angiotensin-converting enzyme; H, histamine; FEV_1, forced expiratory volume in 1 second; 5-HT, serotonin.

were 77% predictive of antipsychotic response to clozapine.[70] These findings imply that, similar to other drug target gene–drug response relationships, a combination of polymorphisms, rather than any single polymorphism, provides a more accurate prediction of clozapine response.

ENZYME GENES AND DRUG RESPONSE

The angiotensin-converting enzyme (ACE) is an example of an enzyme with genetic contributions to drug response. An insertion/deletion (I/D) polymorphism in intron 16 of the ACE gene results in the presence or absence of a 287-base-pair fragment. This polymorphism has been linked consistently to plasma concentrations of ACE, the enzyme responsible for the conversion of angiotensin I to the potent vasoconstrictor angiotensin II.[73]

ACE inhibitors are among the most commonly prescribed antihypertensive agents. However, ACE inhibitors fail to sufficiently lower blood pressure in over 50% of patients.[64] Given its association with ACE concentrations, a number of investigators have examined whether the ACE I/D polymorphism contributes to the interpatient variability in ACE inhibitor response. To date, much of the data with the ACE gene and response to ACE inhibitors are inconsistent and even conflicting. While some studies have demonstrated greater blood pressure reductions with ACE inhibitor therapy among individuals with the ACE DD genotype, others have shown greater blood pressure reductions with the II genotype.[74–76] Still other investigators have reported no association between the ACE I/D genotype and the antihypertensive effects of ACE inhibition.[77,78]

Numerous proteins are involved in the complex signaling pathway of the renin-angiotensin system, and multiple genetic polymorphisms have been identified for many of these proteins (Fig. 6–4). Thus one explanation for the inconsistent and conflicting ACE gene–drug response data is that a single polymorphism contributes little to the overall response to ACE inhibition. Rather, response to ACE inhibition is best determined by a combination of multiple polymorphisms occurring in multiple genes involved in the renin-angiotensin

pathway. Indeed, other renin-angiotensin system genes, including the angiotensinogen and aldosterone synthase genes, have been correlated with antihypertensive responses to ACE inhibitors and angiotensin receptor blockers,[79,80] suggesting that ACE, angiotensinogen, aldosterone synthase, and probably other genes encoding for renin-angiotensin system proteins interact to influence ACE inhibitor response. Thus, before genotype may be used as a predictor of response to renin-angiotensin antagonists, the combination of genetic variants in the renin-angiotensin system that best determines drug response first must be elucidated.

The ACE gene also may predict the likelihood of adverse reactions of ACE inhibitors. Approximately 10% of patients receiving ACE inhibitors develop a cough that persists for the duration of treatment.[81] The ACE I/D polymorphism was correlated with the ACE inhibitor–induced cough in one small study.[81] However, a larger study found no such association.[82] Given the proven benefits of ACE inhibitors in diseases such as hypertension, diabetes, and heart failure, it is unlikely that genes associated with the ACE inhibitor–induced cough, even if validated, would influence drug prescribing. This is so because the development of a cough during ACE inhibitor treatment may be bothersome and a potential threat to drug adherence, but it is unlikely that the cough will result in any serious outcomes. Thus one should not deprive a patient of the potential benefits from ACE inhibitor therapy on the basis of a genetic predisposition for drug-induced cough.

On the other hand, in cases where an adverse drug effect may have serious consequences, knowledge of a genetic propensity for such an effect would be of great clinical significance. Angioedema is an example of a serious and potentially life-threatening adverse drug effect that may have genetic influences. Angioedema is estimated to occur in approximately 0.1% to 0.2% of ACE inhibitor–treated patients.[83] Given its infrequent occurrence, genetic data from a relatively large number of affected patients would be necessary to establish a definite genetic cause for ACE inhibitor–induced angioedema. Investigators for many multicenter clinical drug trials are now asking study participants to provide consent for the collection of genetic material so that

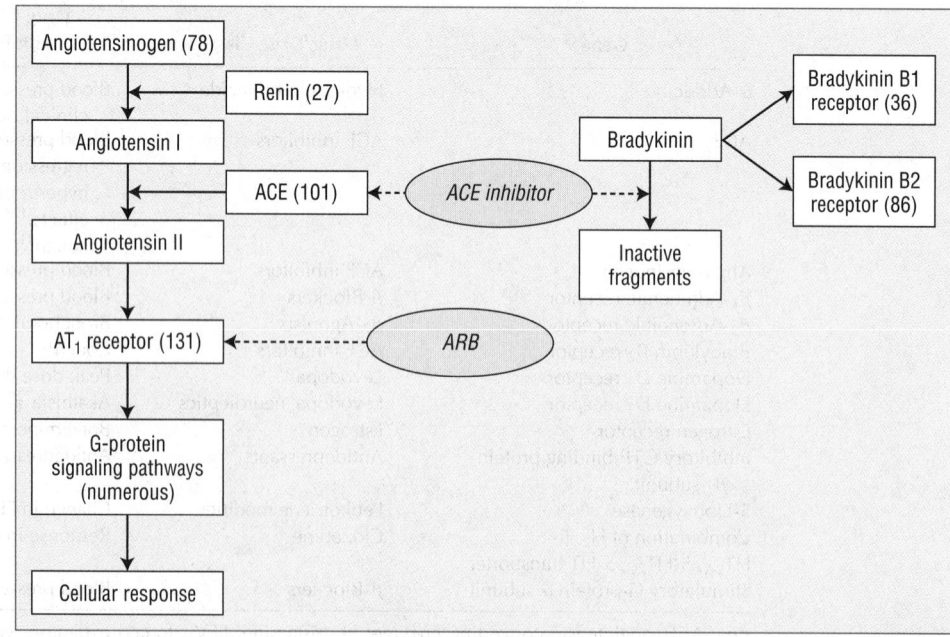

FIGURE 6–4. Single-nucleotide polymorphisms (SNPs) identified for renin-angiotensin system genes. The number of polymorphisms identified for each protein is shown in parenthesis after the protein name (*http://snp.cshl.org*). ACE, angiotensin-converting enzyme; ARB, angiotensin receptor blocker.

in the future, genetic contributions to rare but serious adverse drug effects may be elucidated.

There is evidence of racial differences in antihypertensive response to ACE inhibitors. Specifically, African-Americans in general are believed to have diminished antihypertensive responses to ACE inhibitors compared with Caucasians.[64] The frequencies of many SNPs in the renin-angiotensin system vary between African-American and white populations and may contribute to the observed racial differences in ACE inhibitor response.[84] Indeed, most racial differences in drug response probably can be attributed to racial differences in genotype frequencies, although this is yet to be determined.

GENES FOR INTRACELLULAR SIGNALING PROTEINS, ION TRANSPORTERS, AND DRUG RESPONSE

Cellular responses to many drugs are mediated through GTP-binding proteins also called *G-proteins*. The β_1-adrenergic receptor is an example of a G-protein–coupled receptor in which a stimulatory G-protein (G_s-protein) couples the receptor to intracellular signaling mechanisms to elicit a cellular response (Fig. 6–5). Receptor-coupled G_s-proteins contain α, β, and γ subunits that mediate the activation of adenylyl cyclase and the generation of cyclic AMP following receptor stimulation. A SNP in the α subunit of G_s-protein has been linked to the blood pressure response to β-blockers.[85] Whether the G_s-protein α-subunit gene interacts with the β_1-adrenergic receptor gene or other intracellular signaling-protein genes to determine β-blocker response remains to be determined.

Disturbances in G-protein–mediated signal transduction have been implicated in the pathophysiology of depressive disorders.[86] In addition, data suggest that abnormalities in signal-transduction proteins contribute to antidepressant drug response.[87] A common SNP (C825→T) occurs in the gene for the inhibitory G-protein (G_i-protein) β_3 subunit and has been associated with enhanced intracellular signal transduction. In a study of patients treated with either tricyclic antidepressants or serotonin reuptake inhibitors, the TT genotype was correlated with greater improvement in depression symptoms,[88,89] implying that the G_i-protein β_3 subunit gene may have a future role in therapeutic decisions for depression management.

There is evidence that the gene for α-adducin, a cytoskeletal protein involved in renal tubular ion transport, contributes to thiazide diuretic response. Substitution of tryptophan for glycine at codon 460 of the α-adducin gene has been associated with enhanced renal tubular sodium reabsorption.[90] Two separate studies demonstrated that hydrochlorothiazide produced greater blood pressure reductions in hypertensive individuals with at least one 460Trp allele (Trp/Trp homozygotes or Gly/Trp heterozygotes) compared with Gly/Gly homozygotes.[91] In a subsequent population-based case-control study, hypertensive patients with at least one 460Trp allele appeared to derive superior protection against stroke and myocardial infarction from diuretic therapy compared with treatment with alternative agents.[92] These findings suggest that the α-adducin genotype may be an important determinant not only of antihypertensive response to diuretic therapy but also, more important, of the effects of diuretic therapy on hypertension-related target-organ damage.

DISEASE-ASSOCIATED GENES

Numerous genes have been correlated with disease outcomes, and many of these have been found subsequently to influence response to pharmacologic disease management. These gene–drug response associations often occur despite the lack of a direct effect on pharmacokinetic or pharmacodynamic drug properties. Examples of such disease-associated genes are given below.

FACTOR V AND PROTHROMBIN GENES AND ORAL CONTRACEPTION

The use of oral contraceptives is associated with an increased risk for developing thromboembolic disorders, including deep venous thrombosis, pulmonary embolism, and thrombotic stroke. Variations in the genes for the coagulation factors prothrombin and factor V Leiden also have been identified as risk factors for thromboembolic disorders.[93,94] In case-control studies, the presence of a factor V Leiden or prothrombin gene variation significantly increased the risk for deep vein thrombosis and cerebral vein thrombosis among oral contraceptive users.[93,94] Thus it appears as though carrier status for either the prothrombin or factor V Leiden mutation markedly increases the risk of thrombosis with oral contraceptive use. These data suggest that alternative birth control measures should be employed in women with the prothrombin or factor V Leiden mutations.

CONGENITAL LONG-QT SYNDROME AND DRUG-INDUCED TORSADES DE POINTES

Drug-induced QT-interval prolongation and torsades de pointes are serious, potentially life-threatening adverse effects of many drugs. It is well recognized that many antiarrhythmic drugs can cause torsades de pointes. In addition, numerous noncardiovascular agents can induce torsades de pointes, and many have been withdrawn from the market as a result. Such drugs include the antihistamines terfenadine and astemizole, the fluoroquinolone antibiotic grepafloxacin, and the motility agent cisapride. Given the serious and unpredictable nature of torsades de pointes, there has been great interest in identifying genetic markers that predispose individuals to its occurrence.

Abnormalities in ion flux across the cardiac cell membrane resulting in an excess of intracellular positive ions and delayed ventricular repolarization are characteristic of long-QT syndromes. Mutations in genes for the pore-forming channel proteins that affect potassium and sodium transport across the cardiac cell membrane underlie congenital long-QT syndromes.[95] There is evidence that these mutations also may increase the risk for drug-induced torsades de pointes.[96,97] The ability to screen for mutations associated with drug-induced torsades de pointes would be of clinical significance in that

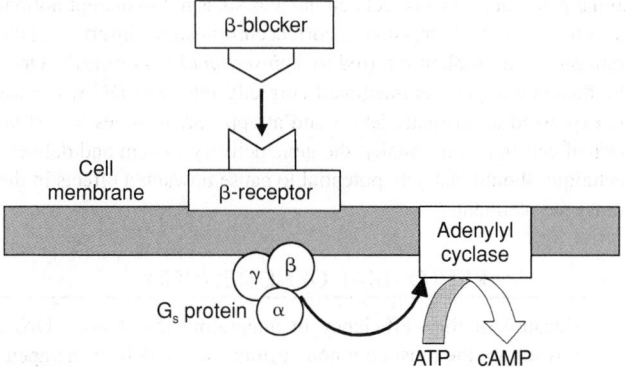

FIGURE 6–5. β_1-receptor coupled to intracellular signaling mechanisms by a stimulatory G-protein.

individuals with a genetic predisposition for this life-threatening arrhythmia could be spared exposure to potentially causative agents and treated with alternative therapies.

CORONARY DISEASE PROGRESSION GENE AND RESPONSE TO STATIN THERAPY

Several large clinical trials in patients with coronary heart disease, including the Scandinavian Simvastatin Survival Study (4S), have demonstrated significant reductions in coronary events and mortality with HMG-CoA reductase inhibitors, or statins. The gene for apolipoprotein E has been correlated with hepatic cholesterol uptake and the risk for coronary heart disease.[98] Its contribution to coronary heart disease progression and statin response was examined in the 4S population.[99] Investigators found that the variant $\varepsilon 4$ allele was associated with increased risk for all-cause mortality among placebo-treated study participants. However, no such association was observed in the simvastatin group, suggesting that simvastatin abolished the excess mortality risk associated with the $\varepsilon 4$ allele.

Several other genes have been associated with responses to statins in coronary heart disease. These include the genes for the cholesteryl ester transfer protein, which is involved in the metabolism of high-density lipoprotein cholesterol; β-fibrinogen, which influences plasma fibrinogen concentrations; and stromelysin-1, which is involved in remodeling of the extracellular matrix of atherosclerotic plaques.[100–102] In each case, the gene linked to worse disease progression or clinical outcomes also was associated with the greatest response to statin therapy. These data imply that genotype may be useful in identifying which coronary heart disease patients are at an increased risk for coronary events and death, in whom treatment with a statin would be of particular benefit.

NOVEL SITES FOR DRUG DEVELOPMENT

The discovery of genes that confer disease has led to an improved understanding of the molecular mechanisms involved in disease pathophysiology. Once associations between genes and diseases are discovered, scientists can elucidate the functions of the encoded proteins and more clearly define the consequences of genetic mutations. Insight into the genetic control of cellular functions may reveal new strategies for disease treatment and prevention.

For example, researchers have discovered that the gene for the cysteine protease calpain-10 confers susceptibility to type 2 diabetes and may serve as a new target for treatment intervention.[103] While the exact function of calpain-10 remains to be determined, it is expressed in tissues involved in the pathophysiology of type 2 diabetes mellitus, including the pancreatic islet cells, skeletal myocytes, and hepatocytes. These sites are important for controlling insulin secretion, peripheral insulin uptake, and hepatic glucose production, suggesting that the product of calpain-10 protein may influence glucose homeostasis.[104] Multiple SNPs have been identified in the calpain-10 gene, one of which has been correlated with reduced calpain-10 levels in skeletal muscle and insulin resistance.[103] The discovery of calpain-10 as a candidate gene for type 2 diabetes identifies a potential new drug target for glucose control and an opportunity to improve glucose homeostasis permanently in patients with diabetes through pharmacogenetics.

Similarly, the discovery that the apolipoprotein E gene is strongly linked to late-onset Alzheimer's disease[105] and that the α-synuclein gene is associated with Parkinson's disease[106] raises the possibility of examining these gene as targets for future drug therapy in psychiatric and neurologic diseases.

GENE THERAPY

Gene therapy has emerged as a possible approach to treating and curing disease by altering gene expression. The goal of gene therapy is to correct genetic defects permanently and thereby restore normal cellular function.

Most gene therapy techniques attempt to replace defective genes with normally functioning ones. Exogenous genes, called *transgenes*, can be transferred into either somatic (body) or germ line (egg or sperm) cells of the recipient. In somatic cell gene transfer, genetic changes do not affect future generations. In contrast, germ line cell transfer, which is currently prohibited by the Food and Drug Administration (FDA),[107] results in the passage of genetic alterations to offspring.

Initially, the focus of gene therapy was for the treatment of inherited disorders such as cystic fibrosis, sickle cell anemia, hemophilia, and adenosine deaminase deficiency.[108] Gene therapy trials were later expanded to include patients with acquired diseases such as cancer and heart disease.

The first clinical gene therapy trial began in 1990 for the treatment of adenosine deaminase deficiency.[107] B and T lymphocytes fail to develop in this autosomal recessive disease, resulting in a severe combined immunodeficiency syndrome (SCID) made famous by the "bubble boys" whose lives were confined to tents in an effort to keep them in a germ-free environment. Only two patients were included in this trial, and although both continued to demonstrate clinical improvement 10 years later, gene therapy did not cure the disease, as investigators had hoped.

Since then, the FDA has approved more than 350 clinical gene therapy trials.[108] Most of these trials involve cancer patients; however, a number of studies also target inherited disorders. The results of gene therapy trials to date have been largely disappointing, with reports of serious toxicities and few therapeutic successes.

OBSTACLES TO SUCCESS

Reasons for limited success with gene therapy include inefficient gene delivery to target cells, inadequate gene expression, and unacceptable adverse effects.[107]

Sufficient amounts of the transgene must be inserted into a sufficient number of recipient cells to produce a therapeutic response. In addition, the transgene must be inserted into the correct chromosomal position of the correct cell nucleus so as not to disrupt normal gene function and expression. Incorrect chromosomal insertion of the transgene is a problem referred to as *insertional mutagenesis*. Once the therapeutic gene is integrated correctly into host DNA, it must be expressed at adequate levels and at appropriate times to restore normal cell function. Finally, the gene delivery system and delivery technique should lack any potential to cause unwanted effects in the transgene recipient.

RETROVIRAL GENE DELIVERY

Because of their efficiency in integrating into human DNA, viruses are the most common vectors used to deliver therapeutic genes to recipient cell targets. Disease-causing genes are replaced with the desired therapeutic genes; the viral genes that control delivery mechanisms are retained.

The first viral vectors introduced were retroviruses, which are RNA viruses that integrate into the host cell genome and replicate during cell division. Thus retroviral gene transfer is capable of permanently altering gene expression. Retroviruses may be used to deliver genes through either direct infusion into target organs or ex vivo manipulation of harvested cells followed by reinfusion into the recipient. The disadvantages of retroviral vectors are the limited size of the gene they can carry, relatively low efficiency, and the risk of insertional mutagenesis. In fact, the FDA temporarily halted retroviral gene delivery into hematopoietic tissue in early 2003 after leukemia developed as a result of insertional mutagenesis in two SCID-affected children treated with retroviral gene therapy.[109]

ADENOVIRAL GENE DELIVERY

Unlike retroviruses, adenoviruses do not integrate into the host genome and thus do not replicate. As a result, genes delivered by adenoviruses are only active temporarily. Adenoviral-mediated gene therapy is employed commonly in cancer patients because permanent gene expression is unnecessary in this patient population.

Tumor cells have been infused with adenoviral vectors carrying the herpes simplex virus-1 thymidine kinase gene and then exposed to ganciclovir as a mode of cancer chemotherapy.[110] Thymidine kinase converts ganciclovir to its active, cytotoxic form, which is incorporated in the DNA of tumor cells, leading to their death. Adenoviruses can be grown in high titers and do not carry the risk of insertional mutagenesis. The major disadvantage of adenoviruses is their immunogenic potential, which has resulted in one death and prompted federal oversight of gene therapy trials.[111]

OTHER MEANS OF GENE DELIVERY

Adeno-associated viruses are human DNA-containing viruses that appear neither to cause disease in humans nor to trigger immune responses on injection. Similar to retroviruses, adeno-associated viruses are incapable of carrying a large amount of genetic material, and their use entails the risk of insertional mutagenesis. Investigators have had some success in treating hemophilia B using intramuscular injections of an adeno-associated virus vector that expresses the human coagulation factor IX gene.[112]

Scientists are also experimenting with nonviral delivery methods such as the use of direct DNA injection, liposomes, and electroporation. There has been some success with intramyocardial transfection of plasmid DNA encoding for vascular endothelial growth factor into patients with severe, intractable angina.[113] Initially, the procedure improved myocardial perfusion and angina in this patient population with few major adverse events. One year later, patients continued to report some improvement in their angina symptoms.[114]

Scientists have enjoyed few successes with gene therapy in recent years, and it is unlikely that gene therapy will progress to have a lasting impact on medicine during the next decade. Improvements in gene delivery techniques and a better understanding of molecular processes controlling gene expression are necessary before gene therapy can correct genetic defects successfully and thus cure associated diseases without inducing adverse effects. Because of limited success with traditional approaches to gene therapy, scientists are exploring other strategies, such as repairing defective genes rather than replacing them.[115] It is important that gene therapy eventually succeeds so that diseases such as Huntington's disease, sickle cell anemia, and inherited immunodeficiency disorders may be cured and their associated morbidity and mortality alleviated.

PHARMACOGENETICS

Traditionally, *genetic testing* refers to screening human genetic material to identify genotypes associated with disease susceptibility or carrier status for inherited diseases, such Huntington's disease, Alzheimer's disease, or breast cancer. This kind of testing can have profound legal, ethical, and social implications. For example, knowledge that a patient is at risk for developing a genetic disorder could result in discrimination by employers or insurance companies. In addition, this information likely would cause emotional distress for the individual at risk and his or her family members.

Within the context of pharmacogenetics, however, testing involves searching for genetic variations linked to drug efficacy or toxicity rather than to disease susceptibility. This form of testing carries little risk for ethical, legal, and social concerns. To prevent public wariness and confusion, genetic testing in reference to pharmacogenetics needs to be defined or renamed so that it can be distinguished from genetic testing for susceptibility to inherited disorders.

CLINICAL CONTROVERSY

Many individuals are wary of the term *genetic testing* because this term is usually associated with determining genetic risk for serious diseases. Therefore, clinicians may cause unnecessary anxiety among patients if they refer to the screening for genetic variants associated with drug response as genetic testing.

GENE THERAPY

Many of the ethical concerns with gene therapy center on transgenic manipulation of somatic versus germ line cells. Somatic gene therapy only affects the recipient. That is, genetic alterations introduced by gene therapy are not passed on to future generations. In contrast, with manipulation of germ line cells, alterations are passed on to future children of the treated patient. Some argue that this is unethical because it violates the rights of future generations. Thus it appears that most gene therapy in the foreseeable future will focus on somatic gene transfer.

Although pharmacogenetics provides opportunities to improve drug therapy outcomes, it likely will increase the complexity of drug prescribing. In addition to considering factors such as age, concomitant drug therapy, and renal and hepatic function, prescribers also will have to interpret the results of genetic analyses when making drug therapy decisions. Further complicating the drug-prescribing process are many medications whose effects are not determined by single polymorphisms in single genes. Rather, pharmacologic effects for most medications likely are determined by the interaction of polymorphisms in multiple genes that encode proteins involved in the various pathways of drug metabolism, distribution, and effects. For example, the immunosuppressants cyclosporine and tacrolimus are believed to be substrates for both P-glycoprotein and the CYP450 3A4 and possibly 3A5 enzymes.[116] Thus it is possible that genes for both MDR-1 and CYP450 enzymes interact to influence cyclosporine and tacrolimus distribution and plasma concentrations.

Pharmacists are broadly trained in a number of medication-related areas, including pharmacology, pharmacokinetics, and pharmacodynamics. This places pharmacists in an extremely valuable position in dealing with the complexities of the drug-decision process in the age of pharmacogenetics. Pharmacists will be in key positions to interpret the results of genetic tests, determine the ultimate effects of multiple genetic variations on drug response, and choose the most appropriate drug for a given patient based on the individual's DNA. Thus it will be essential for pharmacists to stay abreast of significant discoveries in genotype–drug response relationships and understand how best to incorporate this genomic information into pharmacotherapeutic decisions.

Recognizing the challenges in health care delivery with advancing genetic discoveries, the National Coalition for Health Professional Education in Genetics established core competencies related to genetics for health care professionals that are available through the coalition's Web site (*www.nchpeg.org*). The objective of these competencies is to encourage clinicians to incorporate genetics knowledge, skills, and attitudes into their clinical practices. Subsequently, the American Association of Colleges of Pharmacy developed recommendations to guide academic institutions in instilling these competencies in future pharmacists so that pharmacists will be prepared to provide appropriate pharmacotherapy in the age of genomics.[117]

APPLICATION OF PHARMACOGENETIC DATA TO DISEASE MANAGEMENT

Pharmacogenetics has the potential to greatly improve the pharmacologic management of disease. Clinicians may be able to predict the likelihood that an individual will respond to a particular medication based on the patient's genotype. Medications may be avoided or prescribed in lower doses with careful monitoring in patients genetically predisposed to their adverse effects. This would be of particular benefit for narrow-therapeutic-index drugs. For example, in warfarin candidates with a *CYP2C9*2* or *CYP2C9*3* allele, warfarin may be initiated at lower doses with closer monitoring. If the anticipated benefit from warfarin is low in a patient homozygous for the *CYP2C9*2* or *CYP2C9*3* alleles, it may be safer to withhold warfarin and institute alternative anticoagulant therapy.

With pharmacogenetics, it also may be possible to eliminate the trial-and-error approach to drug prescribing for many diseases. Instead, clinicians may be able to use genetic information to match the right drug to the right patient at the right dose while minimizing adverse effects. For example, the current approach to hypertension management involves the trial of various antihypertensives until blood pressure goals are achieved with acceptable drug tolerability. Commonly, the initial agent(s) fails to lower blood pressure to goal or produces intolerable adverse effects (Fig. 6–6). Trials of additional or alternative antihypertensive medications must be undertaken until treatment is deemed successful. In the interim, the patient remains hypertensive and at risk for hypertension-related target-organ damage. With pharmacogenetics, clinicians may choose the antihypertensive drug expected to provide the greatest response with the best tolerability for a particular patient based on his or her DNA. For example, if a hypertensive patient is found to have the 460Trp allele of the α-adducin gene, a thiazide diuretic may be the most appropriate initial antihypertensive agent because evidence suggests that diuretic

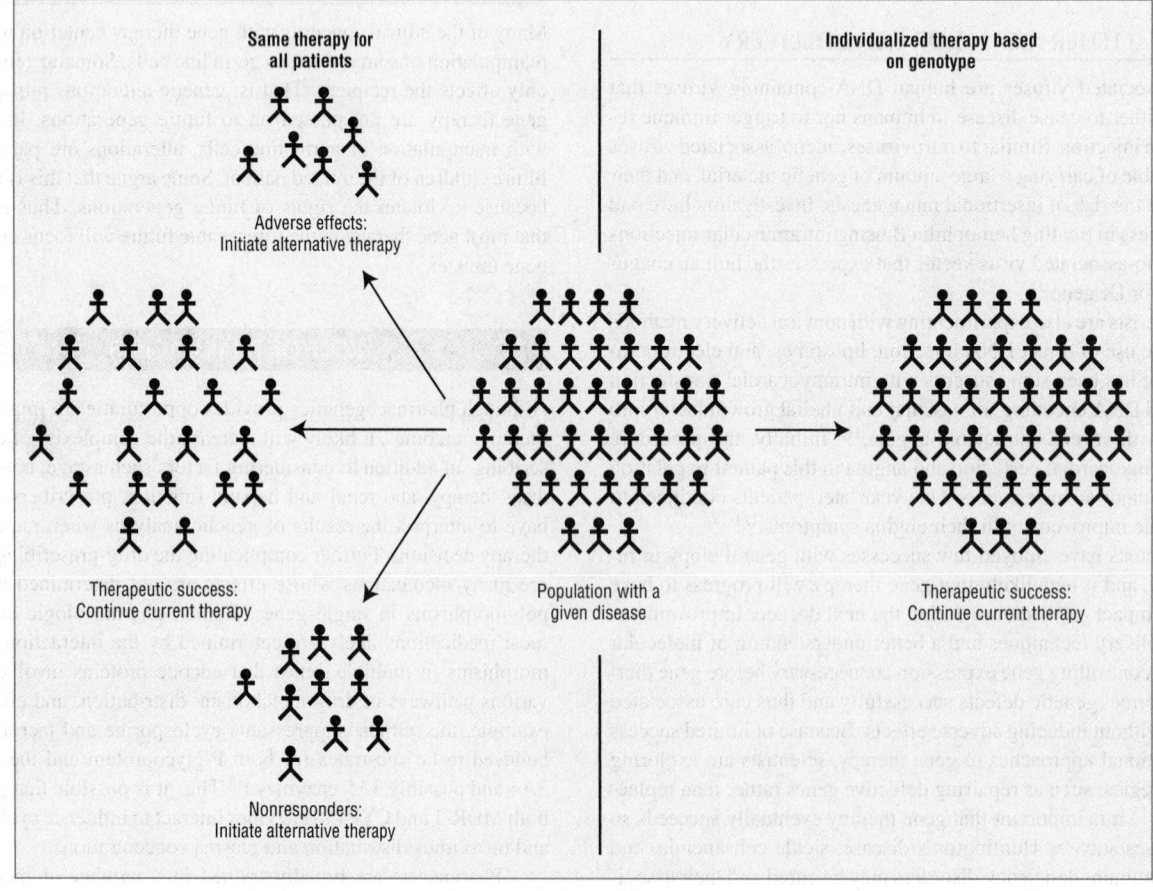

FIGURE 6–6. Current and future approaches to pharmacologic management of disease.

therapy in 460Trp allele carriers will lower blood pressure effectively and potentially improve clinical outcomes.

New drugs may be developed based on knowledge about genetic control of cellular functions. For example, the discovery that chronic myeloid leukemia (CML) was caused by chromosome translocation and consequent production of an enzyme capable of producing life-threatening lymphocyte levels led to accelerated FDA approval of Gleevec (also known as STI-571), an inhibitor of the translocation-created enzyme, for treatment of CML.[118] In addition, future drug development may focus on treating specific genetic subgroups instead of broadly treating all individuals with a particular disease. Ultimately, pharmacogenetics may improve the quality and reduce the overall costs of health care by decreasing the number of treatment failures and the number of adverse drug reactions and leading to the discovery of new genetic targets and therapeutic interventions for disease management.

CLINICAL CONTROVERSY

For some drugs, variations in genes affecting both pharmacokinetic and pharmacodynamic drug properties may interact to determine the ultimate effects from drug therapy. Thus the challenge for researchers will be to identify the combination of gene variations that best predicts response for these drugs.

ABBREVIATIONS

CYP: cytochrome P450
SNPs: single-nucleotide polymorphisms
A: adenine
C: cytosine
G: guanine
T: thymidine
EM: extensive metabolizer
PM: poor metabolizer
UM: ultrarapid metabolizer
AUC: area under the curve
TPMT: thiopurine-*S*-methyltransferase
DPD: dihydropyrimidine dehydrogenase
UGT: UDP-glucuronosyl transferase
MDR-1: multidrug resistance 1
HIV: human immunodeficiency virus
ACE: angiotensin-converting enzyme
I/D: insertion/deletion
FDA: Food and Drug Administration
SCID: severe combined immunodeficiency syndrome
CML: chronic myeloid leukemia

Review Questions and other resources can be found at *www.pharmacotherapyonline.com.*

REFERENCES

1. Alving AS, Carson PE, Flanagan CL, Ickes CE. Enzymatic deficiency in primaquine-sensitive erythrocytes. Science 1956;124:484–485.
2. Aithal GP, Day CP, Kesteven PJ, Daly AK. Association of polymorphisms in the cytochrome P450 CYP2C9 with warfarin dose requirement and risk of bleeding complications. Lancet 1999;353:717–719.
3. Mamiya K, Ieiri I, Shimamoto J, et al. The effects of genetic polymorphisms of CYP2C9 and CYP2C19 on phenytoin metabolism in Japanese adult patients with epilepsy: Studies in stereoselective hydroxylation and population pharmacokinetics. Epilepsia 1998;39:1317–1323.
4. Relling MV, Hancock ML, Rivera GK, et al. Mercaptopurine therapy intolerance and heterozygosity at the thiopurine S-methyltransferase gene locus. J Natl Cancer Inst 1999;91:2001–2008.
5. Motulsky AG. Drug reactions, enzymes and biochemical genetics. JAMA 1957;165:835–837.
6. Vogel F. Moderne Probleme der Humangenetick. Ergebn Inn Med Kinderheilk 1959;12:52–125.
7. Lander ES, Linton LM, Birren B, et al. Initial sequencing and analysis of the human genome. Nature 2001;409:860–921.
8. Human Genome Program. Genomics and Its Impact on Medicine and Society: A 2003 Primer. Washington, US Department of Energy, 2003.
9. Collins FS, Green ED, Guttmacher AE, Guyer MS. A vision for the future of genomics research. Nature 2003;422:835–847.
10. Strachan T, Read AP. Human molecular genetics, 3d ed. New York, Garland Science, 2004.
11. Ferrari P, Bianchi G. Genetic mapping and tailored antihypertensive therapy. Cardiovasc Drugs Ther 2000;14:387–395.
12. Nelson DR. Comparison of P450s from human and fugu: 420 million years of vertebrate P450 evolution. Arch Biochem Biophys 2003;409:18–24.
13. Evans WE, Relling MV. Pharmacogenomics: Translating functional genomics into rational therapeutics. Science 1999;286:487–491.
14. Sata F, Sapone A, Elizondo G, et al. CYP3A4 allelic variants with amino acid substitutions in exons 7 and 12: Evidence for an allelic variant with altered catalytic activity. Clin Pharmacol Ther 2000;67:48–56.
15. Kuehl P, Zhang J, Lin Y, et al. Sequence diversity in CYP3A promoters and characterization of the genetic basis of polymorphic CYP3A5 expression. Nature Genet 2001;27:383–391.
16. Sachse C, Brockmoller J, Bauer S, Roots I. Functional significance of a C→A polymorphism in intron 1 of the cytochrome P450 CYP1A2 gene tested with caffeine. Br J Clin Pharmacol 1999;47:445–449.
17. Marez D, Legrand M, Sabbagh N, et al. Polymorphism of the cytochrome P450 CYP2D6 gene in a European population: Characterization of 48 mutations and 53 alleles, their frequencies and evolution. Pharmacogenetics 1997;7:193–202.
18. Shah RR, Oates NS, Idle JR, et al. Impaired oxidation of debrisoquine in patients with perhexiline neuropathy. Br Med J (Clin Res Ed) 1982;284:295–299.
19. Lee JT, Kroemer HK, Silberstein DJ, et al. The role of genetically determined polymorphic drug metabolism in the beta–blockade produced by propafenone. N Engl J Med 1990;322:1764–1768.
20. Dahl-Puustinen ML, Liden A, Alm C, et al. Disposition of perphenazine is related to polymorphic debrisoquin hydroxylation in human beings. Clin Pharmacol Ther 1989;46:78–81.
21. Spina E, Ancione M, Di Rosa AE, et al. Polymorphic debrisoquine oxidation and acute neuroleptic-induced adverse effects. Eur J Clin Pharmacol 1992;42:347–348.
22. Poulsen L, Arendt-Nielsen L, Brosen K, Sindrup SH. The hypoalgesic effect of tramadol in relation to CYP2D6. Clin Pharmacol Ther 1996;60:636–644.
23. Sindrup SH, Brosen K, Bjerring P, et al. Codeine increases pain thresholds to copper vapor laser stimuli in extensive but not poor metabolizers of sparteine. Clin Pharmacol Ther 1990;48:686–693.
24. Tyndale RF, Droll KP, Sellers EM. Genetically deficient CYP2D6 metabolism provides protection against oral opiate dependence. Pharmacogenetics 1997;7:375–379.
25. Romach MK, Otton SV, Somer G, et al. Cytochrome P450 2D6 and treatment of codeine dependence. J Clin Psychopharmacol 2000;20:43–45.
26. Alfaro CL, Lam YW, Simpson J, Ereshefsky L. CYP2D6 status of extensive metabolizers after multiple-dose fluoxetine, fluvoxamine, paroxetine, or sertraline. J Clin Psychopharmacol 1999;19:155–163.
27. Alfaro CL, Lam YW, Simpson J, Ereshefsky L. CYP2D6 inhibition by fluoxetine, paroxetine, sertraline, and venlafaxine in a crossover study: Intraindividual variability and plasma concentration correlations. J Clin Pharmacol 2000;40:58–66.

28. Hamelin BA, Bouayad A, Methot J, et al. Significant interaction between the nonprescription antihistamine diphenhydramine and the CYP2D6 substrate metoprolol in healthy men with high or low CYP2D6 activity. Clin Pharmacol Ther 2000;67:466–477.

29. Bertilsson L, Aberg-Wistedt A, Gustafsson LL, Nordin C. Extremely rapid hydroxylation of debrisoquine: A case report with implication for treatment with nortriptyline and other tricyclic antidepressants. Ther Drug Monit 1985;7:478–480.

30. Dalen P, Dahl ML, Ruiz ML, et al. 10-Hydroxylation of nortriptyline in white persons with 0, 1, 2, 3, and 13 functional CYP2D6 genes. Clin Pharmacol Ther 1998;63:444–452.

31. Bertilsson L, Dahl ML, Sjoqvist F, et al. Molecular basis for rational megaprescribing in ultrarapid hydroxylators of debrisoquine. Lancet 1993;341:63.

32. Lam YW, Gaedigk A, Ereshefsky L, et al. CYP2D6 inhibition by selective serotonin reuptake inhibitors: Analysis of achievable steady-state plasma concentrations and the effect of ultrarapid metabolism at CYP2D6. Pharmacotherapy 2002;22:1001–1006.

33. Lin KM, Finder E. Neuroleptic dosage for Asians. Am J Psychiatry 1983;140:490–491.

34. Mihara K, Otani K, Tybring G, et al. The CYP2D6 genotype and plasma concentrations of mianserin enantiomers in relation to therapeutic response to mianserin in depressed Japanese patients. J Clin Psychopharmacol 1997;17:467–471.

35. Masimirembwa C, Persson I, Bertilsson L, et al. A novel mutant variant of the CYP2D6 gene (*CYP2D6*17*) common in a black African population: Association with diminished debrisoquine hydroxylase activity. Br J Clin Pharmacol 1996;42:713–719.

36. Droll K, Bruce-Mensah K, Otton SV, et al. Comparison of three CYP2D6 probe substrates and genotype in Ghanaians, Chinese and Caucasians. Pharmacogenetics 1998;8:325–333.

37. Chou WH, Yan FX, de Leon J, et al. Extension of a pilot study: Impact from the cytochrome P450 2D6 polymorphism on outcome and costs associated with severe mental illness. J Clin Psychopharmacol 2000;20:246–251.

38. Brockmoller J, Kirchheiner J, Schmider J, et al. The impact of the CYP2D6 polymorphism on haloperidol pharmacokinetics and on the outcome of haloperidol treatment. Clin Pharmacol Ther 2002;72:438–452.

39. Andersson T, Regardh CG, Lou YC, et al. Polymorphic hydroxylation of S-mephenytoin and omeprazole metabolism in Caucasian and Chinese subjects. Pharmacogenetics 1992;2:25–31.

40. Andersson T, Holmberg J, Rohss K, Walan A. Pharmacokinetics and effect on caffeine metabolism of the proton pump inhibitors, omeprazole, lansoprazole, and pantoprazole. Br J Clin Pharmacol 1998;45:369–375.

41. Furuta T, Ohashi K, Kamata T, et al. Effect of genetic differences in omeprazole metabolism on cure rates for *Helicobacter pylori* infection and peptic ulcer. Ann Intern Med 1998;129:1027–1030.

42. Tanigawara Y, Aoyama N, Kita T, et al. CYP2C19 genotype-related efficacy of omeprazole for the treatment of infection caused by *Helicobacter pylori*. Clin Pharmacol Ther 1999;66:528–534.

43. Kawabata H, Habu Y, Tomioka H, et al. Effect of different proton pump inhibitors, differences in CYP2C19 genotype and antibiotic resistance on the eradication rate of *Helicobacter pylori* infection by a 1-week regimen of proton pump inhibitor, amoxicillin and clarithromycin. Aliment Pharmacol Ther 2003;17:259–264.

44. Furuta T, Ohashi K, Kosuge K, et al. CYP2C19 genotype status and effect of omeprazole on intragastric pH in humans. Clin Pharmacol Ther 1999;65:552–561.

45. Furuta T, Shirai N, Takashima M, et al. Effect of genotypic differences in CYP2C19 on cure rates for *Helicobacter pylori* infection by triple therapy with a proton pump inhibitor, amoxicillin, and clarithromycin. Clin Pharmacol Ther 2001;69:158–168.

46. Ghoneim MM, Korttila K, Chiang CK, et al. Diazepam effects and kinetics in Caucasians and Orientals. Clin Pharmacol Ther 1981;29:749–756.

47. Kalow W. Interethnic variation of drug metabolism. Trends Pharmacol Sci 1991;12:102–107.

48. Kumana CR, Lauder IJ, Chan M, et al. Differences in diazepam pharmacokinetics in Chinese and white Caucasians: Relation to body lipid stores. Eur J Clin Pharmacol 1987;32:211–215.

49. Stubbins MJ, Harries LW, Smith G, et al. Genetic analysis of the human cytochrome P450 CYP2C9 locus. Pharmacogenetics 1996;6:429–439.

50. Takahashi H, Kashima T, Nomoto S, et al. Comparisons between in-vitro and in-vivo metabolism of (S)-warfarin: Catalytic activities of cDNA-expressed CYP2C9, its Leu359 variant and their mixture versus unbound clearance in patients with the corresponding CYP2C9 genotypes. Pharmacogenetics 1998;8:365–373.

51. Steward DJ, Haining RL, Henne KR, et al. Genetic association between sensitivity to warfarin and expression of CYP2C9*3. Pharmacogenetics 1997;7:361–367.

52. Nunoya K, Yokoi T, Kimura K, et al. A new deleted allele in the human cytochrome P450 2A6 (CYP2A6) gene found in individuals showing poor metabolic capacity to coumarin and (+)-cis-3,5-dimethyl-2-(3-pyridyl)thiazolidin-4-one hydrochloride (SM-12502). Pharmacogenetics 1998;8:239–249.

53. Nunoya KI, Yokoi T, Kimura K, et al. A new CYP2A6 gene deletion responsible for the in vivo polymorphic metabolism of (+)-cis-3,5-dimethyl-2-(3-pyridyl)thiazolidin-4-one hydrochloride in humans. J Pharmacol Exp Ther 1999;289:437–442.

54. Pianezza ML, Sellers EM, Tyndale RF. Nicotine metabolism defect reduces smoking. Nature 1998;393:750.

55. Sellers EM, Tyndale RF. Mimicking gene defects to treat drug dependence. Ann NY Acad Sci 2000;909:233–246.

56. Lu Z, Zhang R, Carpenter JT, Diasio RB. Decreased dihydropyrimidine dehydrogenase activity in a population of patients with breast cancer: Implication for 5-fluorouracil-based chemotherapy. Clin Cancer Res 1998;4:325–329.

57. Ando Y, Saka H, Asai G, et al. UGT1A1 genotypes and glucuronidation of SN-38, the active metabolite of irinotecan. Ann Oncol 1998;9:845–847.

58. Wasserman E, Myara A, Lokiec F, et al. Severe CPT-11 toxicity in patients with Gilbert's syndrome: Two case reports. Ann Oncol 1997;8:1049–1051.

59. Iyer L, Das S, Janisch L, et al. UGT1A1*28 polymorphism as a determinant of irinotecan disposition and toxicity. Pharmacogenom J 2002;2:43–47.

60. Johne A, Kopke K, Gerloff T, et al. Modulation of steady-state kinetics of digoxin by haplotypes of the P-glycoprotein *MDR1* gene. Clin Pharmacol Ther 2002;72:584–594.

61. Fellay J, Marzolini C, Meaden ER, et al. Response to antiretroviral treatment in HIV-1-infected individuals with allelic variants of the multidrug resistance transporter 1: A pharmacogenetics study. Lancet 2002;359:30–36.

62. Johnson JA, Terra SG. Beta-adrenergic receptor polymorphisms: Cardiovascular disease associations and pharmacogenetics. Pharm Res 2002;19:1779–1787.

63. Johnson JA, Zineh I, Puckett BJ, et al. Beta 1-adrenergic receptor polymorphisms and antihypertensive response to metoprolol. Clin Pharmacol Ther 2003;74:44–52.

64. Materson BJ, Reda DJ, Cushman WC. Department of Veterans Affairs single-drug therapy of hypertension study: Revised figures and new data. Department of Veterans Affairs Cooperative Study Group on Antihypertensive Agents. Am J Hypertens 1995;8:189–192.

65. Drazen JM, Israel E, Boushey HA, et al. Comparison of regularly scheduled with as-needed use of albuterol in mild asthma. Asthma Clinical Research Network. N Engl J Med 1996;335:841–847.

66. Hoit BD, Suresh DP, Craft L, et al. β_2-Adrenergic receptor polymorphisms at amino acid 16 differentially influence agonist-stimulated blood pressure and peripheral blood flow in normal individuals. Am Heart J 2000;139:537–542.

67. Cockcroft JR, Gazis AG, Cross DJ, et al. Beta(2)-adrenoceptor polymorphism determines vascular reactivity in humans. Hypertension 2000;36:371–375.

68. Gratze G, Fortin J, Labugger R, et al. Beta-2 adrenergic receptor variants affect resting blood pressure and agonist-induced vasodilation in young adult Caucasians. Hypertension 1999;33:1425–1430.

69. Drysdale CM, McGraw DW, Stack CB, et al. Complex promoter and coding region beta 2-adrenergic receptor haplotypes alter receptor expression and predict in vivo responsiveness. Proc Natl Acad Sci USA 2000; 97:10483–10488.

70. Arranz MJ, Munro J, Birkett J, et al. Pharmacogenetic prediction of clozapine response. Lancet 2000;355:1615–1616.

71. Ashby CR Jr, Wang RY. Pharmacological actions of the atypical antipsychotic drug clozapine: A review. Synapse 1996;24:349–394.

72. Masellis M, Basile VS, Ozdemir V, et al. Pharmacogenetics of antipsychotic treatment: Lessons learned from clozapine. Biol Psychiatry 2000; 47:252–266.

73. Turner ST, Schwartz GL, Chapman AB, et al. Antihypertensive pharmacogenetics: Getting the right drug into the right patient. J Hypertens 2001;19:1–11.

74. Stavroulakis GA, Makris TK, Krespi PG, et al. Predicting response to chronic antihypertensive treatment with fosinopril: The role of angiotensin-converting enzyme gene polymorphism. Cardiovasc Drugs Ther 2000;14:427–432.

75. Ohmichi N, Iwai N, Uchida Y, et al. Relationship between the response to the angiotensin-converting enzyme inhibitor imidapril and the angiotensin-converting enzyme genotype. Am J Hypertens 1997;10: 951–955.

76. Ueda S, Meredith PA, Morton JJ, et al. ACE (I/D) genotype as a predictor of the magnitude and duration of the response to an ACE inhibitor drug (enalaprilat) in humans. Circulation 1998;98:2148–2153.

77. Sasaki M, Oki T, Iuchi A, et al. Relationship between the angiotensin-converting enzyme gene polymorphism and the effects of enalapril on left ventricular hypertrophy and impaired diastolic filling in essential hypertension: M-mode and pulsed Doppler echocardiographic studies. J Hypertens 1996;14:1403–1408.

78. Kohno M, Yokokawa K, Minami M, et al. Association between angiotensin-converting enzyme gene polymorphisms and regression of left ventricular hypertrophy in patients treated with angiotensin-converting enzyme inhibitors. Am J Med 1999;106:544–549.

79. Kurland L, Melhus H, Karlsson J, et al. Aldosterone synthase (CYP11B2) −344 C/T polymorphism is related to antihypertensive response: Result from the Swedish Irbesartan Left Ventricular Hypertrophy Investigation versus Atenolol (SILVHIA) trial. Am J Hypertens 2002;15:389–393.

80. Hingorani AD, Jia H, Stevens PA, et al. Renin-angiotensin system gene polymorphisms influence blood pressure and the response to angiotensin-converting enzyme inhibition. J Hypertens 1995;13:1602–1609.

81. Takahashi T, Yamaguchi E, Furuya K, Kawakami Y. The ACE gene polymorphism and cough threshold for capsaicin after cilazapril usage. Respir Med 2001;95:130–135.

82. Zee RY, Rao VS, Paster RZ, et al. Three candidate genes and angiotensin-converting enzyme-related cough: A pharmacogenetic analysis. Hypertension 1998;31:925–928.

83. Vleeming W, van Amsterdam JG, Stricker BH, de Wildt DJ. ACE inhibitor–induced angioedema: Incidence, prevention and management. Drug Saf 1998;18:171–188.

84. Wang JG, Staessen JA. Genetic polymorphisms in the renin-angiotensin system: Relevance for susceptibility to cardiovascular disease. Eur J Pharmacol 2000;410:289–302.

85. Jia HHA, Sharma P, Hopper R, et al. Association of the G(s)alpha gene with essential hypertension and response to beta-blockade. Hypertension 1999;34:8–14.

86. Hudson CJ, Young LT, Li PP, Warsh JJ. CNS signal transduction in the pathophysiology and pharmacotherapy of affective disorders and schizophrenia. Synapse 1993;13:278–293.

87. Rasenick MM, Chaney KA, Chen J. G-protein-mediated signal transduction as a target of antidepressant and antibipolar drug action: Evidence from model systems. J Clin Psychiatry 1996;57(suppl 13):49–55; discussion 56–58.

88. Serretti A, Lorenzi C, Cusin C, et al. SSRIs antidepressant activity is influenced by G beta 3 variants. Eur Neuropsychopharmacol 2003;13:117–122.

89. Zill P, Baghai TC, Zwanzger P, et al. Evidence for an association between a G-protein beta3-gene variant with depression and response to antidepressant treatment. Neuroreport 2000;11:1893–1897.

90. Manunta P, Cusi D, Barlassina C, et al. Alpha-adducin polymorphisms and renal sodium handling in essential hypertensive patients. Kidney Int 1998;53:1471–1478.

91. Glorioso N, Manunta P, Filigheddu F, et al. The role of alpha-adducin polymorphism in blood pressure and sodium handling regulation may not be excluded by a negative association study. Hypertension 1999;34:649–654.

92. Psaty BM, Smith NL, Heckbert SR, et al. Diuretic therapy, the alpha-adducin gene variant, and the risk of myocardial infarction or stroke in persons with treated hypertension. JAMA 2002;287:1680–1689.

93. Aznar J, Vaya A, Estelles A, et al. Risk of venous thrombosis in carriers of the prothrombin G20210A variant and factor V Leiden and their interaction with oral contraceptives. Haematologica 2000;85:1271–1276.

94. Martinelli I, Sacchi E, Landi G, et al. High risk of cerebral-vein thrombosis in carriers of a prothrombin-gene mutation and in users of oral contraceptives. N Engl J Med 1998;338:1793–1797.

95. Priori SG, Barhanin J, Hauer RN, et al. Genetic and molecular basis of cardiac arrhythmias: Impact on clinical management parts I and II. Circulation 1999;99:518–528.

96. Yang P, Kanki H, Drolet B, et al. Allelic variants in long-QT disease genes in patients with drug-associated torsades de pointes. Circulation 2002;105:1943–1948.

97. Abbott GW, Sesti F, Splawski I, et al. MiRP1 forms IKr potassium channels with HERG and is associated with cardiac arrhythmia. Cell 1999;97:175–187.

98. Wilson PW, Schaefer EJ, Larson MG, Ordovas JM. Apolipoprotein E alleles and risk of coronary disease: A meta-analysis. Arterioscler Thromb Vasc Biol 1996;16:1250–1255.

99. Gerdes LU, Gerdes C, Kervinen K, et al. The apolipoprotein ε4 allele determines prognosis and the effect on prognosis of simvastatin in survivors of myocardial infarction: A substudy of the Scandinavian simvastatin survival study. Circulation 2000;101:1366–1371.

100. Kuivenhoven JA, Jukema JW, Zwinderman AH, et al. The role of a common variant of the cholesteryl ester transfer protein gene in the progression of coronary atherosclerosis. The Regression Growth Evaluation Statin Study Group. N Engl J Med 1998;338:86–93.

101. de Maat MP, Kastelein JJ, Jukema JW, et al. −455G/A polymorphism of the beta-fibrinogen gene is associated with the progression of coronary atherosclerosis in symptomatic men: Proposed role for an acute-phase reaction pattern of fibrinogen. REGRESS group. Arterioscler Thromb Vasc Biol 1998;18:265–271.

102. de Maat MP, Jukema JW, Ye S, et al. Effect of the stromelysin-1 promoter on efficacy of pravastatin in coronary atherosclerosis and restenosis. Am J Cardiol 1999;83:852–856.

103. Baier LJ, Permana PA, Yang X, et al. A calpain-10 gene polymorphism is associated with reduced muscle mRNA levels and insulin resistance. J Clin Invest 2000;106:R69–73.

104. Horikawa Y, Oda N, Cox NJ, et al. Genetic variation in the gene encoding calpain-10 is associated with type 2 diabetes mellitus. Nature Genet 2000; 26:163–175.

105. Strittmatter WJ, Saunders AM, Schmechel D, et al. Apolipoprotein E: High-avidity binding to beta-amyloid and increased frequency of type 4 allele in late-onset familial Alzheimer disease. Proc Natl Acad Sci USA 1993;90:1977–1981.

106. Polymeropoulos MH, Lavedan C, Leroy E, et al. Mutation in the alpha-synuclein gene identified in families with Parkinson's disease. Science 1997;276:2045–2047.

107. Fibison WJ. Gene therapy. Nurs Clin North Am 2000;35:757–772.

108. Williams DA, Smith FO. Progress in the use of gene transfer methods to treat genetic blood diseases. Hum Gene Ther 2000;11:2059–2066.

109. Marshall E. Gene therapy: Second child in French trial is found to have leukemia. Science 2003;299:320.

110. Morris JC, Ramsey WJ, Wildner O, et al. A phase I study of intralesional administration of an adenovirus vector expressing the HSV-1 thymidine kinase gene (AdV.RSV-TK) in combination with escalating doses of

ganciclovir in patients with cutaneous metastatic malignant melanoma. Hum Gene Ther 2000;11:487–503.

111. Marshall E. Gene therapy death prompts review of adenovirus vector. Science 1999;286:2244–2245.

112. Manno CS, Chew AJ, Hutchison S, et al. AAV-mediated factor IX gene transfer to skeletal muscle in patients with severe hemophilia B. Blood 2003;101:2963–2972.

113. Symes JF, Losordo DW, Vale PR, et al. Gene therapy with vascular endothelial growth factor for inoperable coronary artery disease. Ann Thorac Surg 1999;68:830–836; discussion 836–837.

114. Fortuin FD, Vale P, Losordo DW, et al. One-year follow-up of direct myocardial gene transfer of vascular endothelial growth factor-2 using naked plasmid deoxyribonucleic acid by way of thoracotomy in no-option patients. Am J Cardiol 2003;92:436–439.

115. Sullenger BA. Targeted genetic repair: An emerging approach to genetic therapy. J Clin Invest 2003;112:310–311.

116. Hesselink DA, van Schaik RH, van der Heiden IP, et al. Genetic polymorphisms of the CYP3A4, CYP3A5, and MDR-1 genes and pharmacokinetics of the calcineurin inhibitors cyclosporine and tacrolimus. Clin Pharmacol Ther 2003;74:245–254.

117. Johnson JA, Bootman JL, Evans WE, et al. Pharmacogenomics: A scientific revolution in pharmaceutical sciences and pharmacy practice. Report of the 2001–2002 Academic Affairs Committee. Am J Pharm Educ 2002;66:12S–15S.

118. Johnson JR, Bross P, Cohen M, et al. Approval summary: Imatinib mesylate capsules for treatment of adult patients with newly diagnosed Philadelphia chromosome–positive chronic myelogenous leukemia in chronic phase. Clin Cancer Res 2003;9:1972–1979.

119. Devadatta S, Gangadharam PRJ, Andrews RH. Peripheral neuritis due to isoniazid. Bull WHO 1960;23:587–598.

120. Henningsen NC, Cederberg A, Hanson A, Johansson BW. Effects of long-term treatment with procaine amide: A prospective study with special regard to ANF and SLE in fast and slow acetylators. Acta Med Scand 1975;198:475–482.

121. Strandberg I, Boman G, Hassler L, Sjoqvist F. Acetylator phenotype in patients with hydralazine-induced lupoid syndrome. Acta Med Scand 1976;200:367–371.

122. Pullar T, Hunter JA, Capell HA. Effect of acetylator phenotype on efficacy and toxicity of sulphasalazine in rheumatoid arthritis. Ann Rheum Dis 1985;44:831–837.

123. Jacobsen P, Rossing K, Rossing P, et al. Angiotensin-converting enzyme gene polymorphism and ACE inhibition in diabetic nephropathy. Kidney Int 1998;53:1002–1006.

124. Kotani Y, Nishimura Y, Maeda H, Yokoyama M. Beta2-adrenergic receptor polymorphisms affect airway responsiveness to salbutamol in asthmatics. J Asthma 1999;36:583–590.

125. Lima JJ, Thomason DB, Mohamed MH, et al. Impact of genetic polymorphisms of the beta2-adrenergic receptor on albuterol bronchodilator pharmacodynamics. Clin Pharmacol Ther 1999;65:519–525.

126. Martinez FD, Graves PE, Baldini M, et al. Association between genetic polymorphisms of the beta2-adrenoceptor and response to albuterol in children with and without a history of wheezing. J Clin Invest 1997;100:3184–3188.

127. Mukae S, Aoki S, Itoh S, et al. Bradykinin B(2) receptor gene polymorphism is associated with angiotensin-converting enzyme inhibitor-related cough. Hypertension 2000;36:127–131.

128. Oliveri RL, Annesi G, Zappia M, et al. Dopamine D2 receptor gene polymorphism and the risk of levodopa-induced dyskinesias in PD. Neurology 1999;53:1425–1430.

129. Eichhammer P, Albus M, Borrmann-Hassenbach M, et al. Association of dopamine D3-receptor gene variants with neuroleptic induced akathisia in schizophrenic patients: A generalization of Steen's study on DRD3 and tardive dyskinesia. Am J Med Genet 2000;96:187–191.

130. Ongphiphadhanakul B, Chanprasertyothin S, Payatikul P, et al. Oestrogen-receptor-alpha gene polymorphism affects response in bone mineral density to oestrogen in post-menopausal women. Clin Endocrinol (Oxf) 2000;52:581–585.

131. Drazen JM, Yandava CN, Dube L, et al. Pharmacogenetic association between ALOX5 promoter genotype and the response to anti-asthma treatment. Nature Genet 1999;22:168–170.

7

PEDIATRICS

Milap C. Nahata and Carol Taketomo

Learning Objectives and other resources can be found at *www.pharmacotherapyonline.com.*

KEY CONCEPTS

◀1 Children are not just "little adults," and lack of data on important pharmacokinetic and pharmacodynamic differences has led to several disastrous situations in pediatric care.

◀2 Variations in absorption of medications from the gastrointestinal tract, intramuscular injection sites, and skin are important in pediatric patients, especially in premature and other newborn infants.

◀3 The rate and extent of organ function development and the distribution, metabolism, and elimination of drugs differ not only between pediatric versus adult patients but also among pediatric age groups.

◀4 The effectiveness and safety of drugs may vary among various age groups and from one drug to another in pediatric versus adult patients.

◀5 Concomitant diseases may influence dosage requirements to achieve a targeted effect for a specific disease in children.

◀6 The myth that neonates and young children do not experience pain has led to inadequate pain management in this population.

◀7 Special methods of drug administration are needed for infants and young children.

◀8 Many medicines needed for pediatric patients are not available in appropriate dosage forms, and thus the dosage forms of drugs marketed for adults may have to be modified for infants and children, requiring assurance of potency and safety of drug use.

◀9 The pediatric medication-use process is complex and error-prone owing to multiple steps required in calculating, verifying, preparing, and administering doses.

Remarkable progress has been made in the clinical management of disease in pediatric patients. This chapter highlights important principles of pediatric pharmacotherapy that must be considered when the diseases discussed in other chapters of this book occur in pediatric patients, defined as those younger than 18 years of age. Newborn infants born before 37 weeks of gestational age are termed *premature;* those between 1 day and 1 month of age are *neonates;* 1 month to 1-year-old, *infants;* 1 year to 11 years of age, *children;* and 12 to 16 years, *adolescents.* Covered are notable examples of problems in pediatrics, pharmacokinetic differences in pediatric patients, drug efficacy and toxicity in this patient group, and various factors affecting pediatric pharmacotherapy. Specific examples of problems and special considerations in pediatric patients are cited to enhance understanding.

◀1 Infant mortality has declined from 200 per 1000 births in the nineteenth century to 75 per 1000 births in 1925 to 6.8 per 1000 births in 2001.[1] This success has resulted largely from improvements in identification, prevention, and treatment of diseases once common during delivery and the period of infancy. Although most marketed drugs are used in pediatric patients, only one-fourth of the drugs approved by the Food and Drug Administration (FDA) have indications specific for use in the pediatric population. Data on the pharmacokinetics, pharmacodynamics, efficacy, and safety of drugs in infants and children are scarce. Lack of this type of information led to such disasters as gray baby syndrome from chloramphenicol, phocomelia from thalidomide, and kernicterus from sulfonamide therapy. Gray baby syndrome was first reported in two neonates who died after excessive chloramphenicol doses (100–300 mg/kg per day); the serum

concentrations of chloramphenicol immediately before death were 75 and 100 mcg/mL. Patients with gray baby syndrome usually have abdominal distention, vomiting, diarrhea, a characteristic gray color, respiratory distress, hypotension, and progressive shock.

Thalidomide is well known for its teratogenic effects. Clearly implicated as the cause of multiple congenital fetal abnormalities (particularly limb deformities), it also can cause polyneuritis, nerve damage, and mental retardation. Isotretinoin (Accutane) is another teratogen. Because it is used to treat acne vulgaris, common in teenage patients who may be sexually active but not willing to acknowledge that activity to health care professionals, isotretinoin has presented a difficult problem in patient education since its marketing in the 1980s.

Kernicterus was reported in neonates receiving sulfonamides, which displaced bilirubin from protein-binding sites in the blood to cause a hyperbilirubinemia. This results in deposition of bilirubin in the brain and induces encephalopathy in infants.

Another area of concern in pediatrics is identifying an optimal dosage. Dosage regimens cannot be based simply on body weight or surface area of a pediatric patient extrapolated from adult data. Bioavailability, pharmacokinetics, pharmacodynamics, efficacy, and adverse-effect information can differ markedly between pediatric and adult patients, as well as among pediatric patients, because of differences in age, organ function, and disease state. Significant progress has been made in the area of pediatric pharmacokinetics during the last two decades, but few such studies have correlated pharmacokinetics with the outcomes of efficacy, adverse effects, or quality of life.

Several additional factors should be considered in optimizing pediatric drug therapy. Many drugs prescribed widely for infants and children are not available in suitable dosage forms. For example, extemporaneous liquid dosage forms of amiodarone, captopril, omeprazole, and spironolactone are prepared for infants and children who cannot swallow tablets or capsules, and injectable dosage forms of aminophylline, methylprednisolone, morphine, and phenobarbital are diluted to accurately measure small doses for infants. Alteration (dilution or reformulation) of dosage forms intended for adult patients raises questions about the bioavailability, stability, and compatibility of these drugs. Because of low fluid volume requirements and limited access to intravenous sites, special methods must be used for the delivery of intravenous drugs to infants and children. As simple as it may seem, administration of oral drugs to young patients continues to be a difficult task for nurses and parents. Similarly, ensuring adherence to pharmacotherapy in pediatric patients poses a special challenge.

Finally, the need for additional pharmacologic or therapeutic research brings up the issue of ethical justification for conducting research. The investigators proposing studies and institutional review committees approving human studies must assess the risk-benefit ratio of each study to be fair to children who are not in a position to accept or reject the opportunity to participate in the research project.

Enormous progress has been made in pharmacokinetics in pediatric patients. Two factors have contributed to this progress: (1) the availability of sensitive and specific analytic methods to measure drugs and their metabolites in small volumes of biologic fluids and (2) awareness of the importance of clinical pharmacokinetics in optimization of drug therapy. Absorption, distribution, metabolism, and elimination of many drugs are different in premature infants, full-term infants, and older children, and this topic is discussed in detail in the next few sections.

ABSORPTION

GASTROINTESTINAL TRACT

Two factors affecting the absorption of drugs from the gastrointestinal tract are pH-dependent passive diffusion and gastric emptying time. Both processes are strikingly different in premature infants compared with older children and adults. In a full-term infant, gastric pH ranges from 6 to 8 at birth but declines to 1 to 3 within 24 hours.[2] In contrast, the gastric pH is elevated in premature infants because of immature acid secretion.[3]

In premature infants, higher serum concentrations of acid-labile drugs—such as penicillin,[4] ampicillin,[5] and nafcillin[6]—and lower serum concentrations of a weak acid such as phenobarbital[7] can be explained by higher gastric pH. Because of a lack of extensive data comparing serum concentration-time profiles after oral versus intravenous drug administration, differences in the bioavailability of drugs in premature infants are poorly understood. Although little is known about the influence of developmental changes with age on drug absorption in pediatric patients, a few studies with drugs (e.g., digoxin and phenobarbital) and nutrients (e.g., arabinose and xylose) have suggested that the processes of both passive and active transport may be fully developed by about 4 months of age.[8] No data are available about the development and expression of the efflux transporter P-glycoprotein in the intestine.

Studies have shown that gastric emptying is slow in a premature infant.[9] Thus drugs with limited absorption in adults may be absorbed efficiently in a premature infant because of prolonged contact time with gastrointestinal mucosa.

INTRAMUSCULAR SITES

Drug absorption from an intramuscular site also may be altered in premature infants. Differences in relative muscle mass, poor perfusion to various muscles, peripheral vasomotor instability, and insufficient muscular contractions in premature infants compared with older children and adults can influence drug absorption from the intramuscular site. The net effect of these factors on drug absorption is impossible to predict; phenobarbital has been reported to be absorbed rapidly,[10] whereas diazepam absorption may be delayed.[11] Thus intramuscular dosing is used rarely in neonates except in emergencies or when an intravenous site is inaccessible.

SKIN

Percutaneous absorption may be increased substantially in newborns because of an underdeveloped epidermal barrier (stratum corneum) and increased skin hydration. The increased permeability can produce toxic effects after the topical use of hexachlorophene soaps and powders,[12] salicylic acid ointment, and rubbing alcohol.[13] Interestingly, a study has shown that a therapeutic serum concentration of theophylline can be achieved to control apnea in premature infants of less than 30 weeks' gestation after a topical application of gel containing a standard dose of theophylline.[14] The use of this route of administration may minimize the unpredictability of oral and intramuscular absorption and complications of intravenous drug administration for certain drugs.

DISTRIBUTION

Drug distribution is determined by the physicochemical properties of the drug itself (pK_a, molecular weight, partition coefficient) and the physiologic factors specific to the patient. Although the physicochemical properties of the drug are constant, the physiologic functions often vary in different patient populations. Some important patient-specific factors include extracellular and total body water, protein binding by the drug in plasma, and the presence of pathologic conditions modifying physiologic function. Total body water, as a percentage of total body weight, has been estimated to be 94% in the fetus, 85% in premature infants, 78% in full-term infants, and 60% in adults.[14] Extracellular fluid volume is also markedly different in premature infants compared with older children and adults; the extracellular fluid volume may account for 50% of body weight in premature infants, 35% in 4- to 6-month-old infants, 25% in children 1 year of age, and 19% in adults.[15] This conforms to the observed gentamicin distribution volumes of 0.48 L/kg in neonates and 0.20 L/kg in adults.[16] Studies have shown that the distribution volume of tobramycin is largest in the most premature infants and decreases with increases in the gestational age and birth weight of the infant.[17]

Binding of drugs to plasma proteins is also decreased in newborn infants because of the decreased plasma protein concentration, lower binding capacity of protein, decreased affinity of proteins for drug binding, and competition for certain binding sites by endogenous compounds such as bilirubin. The plasma protein binding of many drugs—including phenobarbital, salicylates, and phenytoin—is significantly less in the neonate than in the adult.[18] The decrease in plasma protein binding of drugs can increase their apparent volumes of distribution. Therefore, premature infants require a larger loading dose than older children and adults to achieve a therapeutic serum concentration of such drugs as phenobarbital[19] and phenytoin.[20]

The consequences of increased concentrations of free or unbound drug in the serum and tissues must be considered. Pharmacologic and toxic effects are related directly to the concentration of free drug in the body. Increases in free drug concentrations may result directly from decreases in plasma protein binding or indirectly from, for example, drug displacement from binding sites. The increased mortality from the development of kernicterus secondary to displacement of bilirubin by sulfisoxazole in neonates has been well documented.[21] However, because drug bound to plasma proteins cannot be eliminated by the kidney, an increase in free drug concentration also may increase its clearance.[22]

The amount of body fat is substantially lower in neonates compared with adults, which may affect drug therapy. Certain highly lipid-soluble drugs are distributed less widely in infants than in adults. The apparent volume of distribution of diazepam has ranged from 1.4 to 1.8 L/kg in neonates and from 2.2 to 2.6 L/kg in adults.[23] In recent years, the numbers of mothers breast-feeding their infants has climbed. Thus certain drugs distributed in breast milk may pose problems for the infants. The American Academy of Pediatrics recommends that bromocriptine, cyclophosphamide, cyclosporine, doxorubicin, ergotamine, lithium, methotrexate, phenindione, and all drugs of abuse (e.g., amphetamine, cocaine, heroin, marijuana, and phencyclidine, or PCP) be contraindicated during breast-feeding. Further, the use of nuclear medicines should be stopped temporarily during breast-feeding.[24] Note that these recommendations are based on limited data; other drugs taken over a prolonged period by the mother also may be toxic to the infant. For example, acebutolol, aspirin, atenolol, clemastine, phenobarbital, primidone, sulfasalazine, and 5-aminosalicylic acid have been associated with adverse effects in some nursing infants.[24,25] Unless benefits outweigh the risks, the use of any drug should be avoided by the mother during pregnancy and while breast-feeding.

METABOLISM

Drug metabolism is substantially slower in infants compared with older children and adults. There are important differences in the maturation of various pathways of metabolism within a premature infant. For example, the sulfation pathway is well developed but the glucuronidation pathway is undeveloped in infants.[26] Although acetaminophen metabolism by glucuronidation is impaired in infants compared with adults, it is partly compensated for by the sulfation pathway. The cause of the tragic chloramphenicol-induced gray baby syndrome in newborn infants is a decreased metabolism of chloramphenicol by glucuronyl transferases to the inactive glucuronide metabolite.[27] This metabolic pathway appears to be age-related[28] and may take several months to a year to develop fully. Evidence for this is the increase in clearance with age up to 1 year.[29]

Interestingly, higher serum concentrations of morphine are required to achieve efficacy in premature infants than in adults in part because infants are not able to metabolize morphine adequately to its 6-glucuronide metabolite (20 times more active than morphine).[30] This is balanced to some degree by the fact that the clearance of morphine quadruples between 27 and 40 weeks of postconceptional age.

Metabolism of drugs such as theophylline, phenobarbital, and phenytoin by oxidation is also impaired in newborn infants. The rate of metabolism, however, is more rapid with phenobarbital and phenytoin than with theophylline, perhaps owing to the involvement of different cytochrome P450 isozymes. Total clearance of phenytoin by CYP2C9 and to a lesser extent by CYP2C19 surpasses adult values by 2 weeks

of age, whereas theophylline clearance is not fully developed for several months.[18] Two additional observations should be noted about theophylline metabolism by CYP1A2 in pediatric patients. First, in premature infants receiving theophylline for the treatment of apnea, a significant amount of its active metabolite caffeine may be present, unlike in older children and adults.[18] Second, theophylline clearance in children 1 to 9 years of age exceeds the values in infants as well as adults. Thus a child with asthma often requires markedly higher doses on a weight basis of theophylline compared with an adult.[31] Because of decreased metabolism, doses of such drugs as theophylline, phenobarbital, phenytoin, and diazepam should be decreased in premature infants.

The clearance of unbound S-warfarin, a substrate of CYP2C9, was substantially greater in prepubertal children than among pubertal children and adults even after adjustment for total body weight.[32] Finally, the clearance of caffeine, metabolized by demethylation, declines to adult values when girls reach Tanner stage 2 (early puberty) and boys reach Tanner stage 4 and 5 (late puberty).[33]

ELIMINATION

Drugs and their metabolites are often eliminated by the kidney. The glomerular filtration rate may be as low as 0.6–0.8 mL/min per 1.73 m^2 in preterm infants and about 2–4 mL/min per 1.73 m^2 in term infants. The processes of glomerular filtration, tubular secretion, and tubular reabsorption determine the efficiency of renal excretion. These processes may take several weeks to 1 year after birth to develop fully.

Studies in infants have shown that tobramycin clearance during the first postnatal week may increase with an increase in gestational age.[17] In infants up to 1 month after birth, postnatal age also was correlated directly with aminoglycoside clearance.[29] Thus premature infants require a lower daily dose of drugs eliminated by the kidney during the first week of life; the dosage requirement then increases with age.

Because of immature renal elimination, chloramphenicol succinate can accumulate in premature infants. Although chloramphenicol succinate is inactive, this accumulation may be the reason for an increased bioavailability of chloramphenicol in premature infants compared with older children.[28] These data indicate that dose-related toxicity may result from an underdeveloped glucuronidation pathway, as well as increased bioavailability of chloramphenicol in premature infants.

DRUG EFFICACY AND TOXICITY

Besides the pharmacokinetic differences previously identified between pediatric and older patients, factors related to drug efficacy and toxicity also should be considered in planning pediatric pharmacotherapy. Unique pathophysiologic changes occur in pediatric patients with some disease states.

Examples of these pathophysiologic and pharmacodynamic differences are numerous. Clinical presentation of chronic asthma differs in children and adults.[34] Children present almost exclusively with a reversible extrinsic type of asthma, whereas adults have nonspecific, nonatopic bronchial irritability.[34] This explains the value of adjunctive hyposensitization therapy in the management of pediatric patients with extrinsic asthma.[35,36]

The maintenance dose of digoxin is substantially higher in infants than in adults. This is explained by a lower binding affinity of receptors in the myocardium for digoxin and increased digoxin-binding sites on neonatal erythrocytes compared with adult erythrocytes.[37] Insulin requirement is highest during adolescence because of the individual's rapid growth. Growth hormone therapy has allowed children with growth hormone deficiency to attain greater adult height. However, a recent study has shown that in "normal" short children (without growth hormone deficiency), early and rapid pubertal progression by growth hormone therapy may lead to a shorter final adult height than may have been attained naturally.[38] This emphasizes the need for identifying specific indications for the effective and safe use of drugs in pediatric patients.

Certain adverse effects of drugs are most common in the newborn period, whereas other toxic effects may continue to be important for many years of childhood. Chloramphenicol toxicity is increased in newborns because of immature metabolism and enhanced bioavailability. Similarly, propylene glycol—added to many injectable drugs, including phenytoin, phenobarbital, digoxin, diazepam, vitamin D, and hydralazine, to increase their stability—can cause hyperosmolality in infants.[39] Benzyl alcohol was a popular preservative in intravascular flush solutions until a syndrome of metabolic acidosis, seizures, neurologic deterioration, gasping respirations, hepatic and renal abnormalities, cardiovascular collapse, and death was described in premature infants. A decline in both mortality and the incidence of major intraventricular hemorrhage has been documented after the use of solutions containing benzyl alcohol was stopped in low-birth-weight infants.[40]

Tetracyclines are also contraindicated in pregnant women, nursing mothers, and children younger than 8 years of age because they can cause dental staining and defects in enamelization of deciduous and permanent teeth, as well as a decrease in bone growth.[41]

CLINICAL CONTROVERSY

Are fluoroquinolones safe in pediatric patients younger than 1 year of age? The antibiotics of the fluoroquinolone class (e.g., ciprofloxacin) are not recommended for pediatric patients or pregnant women because of an association between these drugs and development of permanent lesions of the cartilage of weight-bearing joints and other signs of arthropathy in immature animals of various species.[42] Reversible arthralgia, sometimes accompanied by synovial effusion, was associated with ciprofloxacin therapy in 1.8% of pediatric patients with cystic fibrosis.[43] Although these drugs are used to treat certain infections in pediatric populations, further safety data are needed before they can be prescribed routinely, especially in infants.

CLINICAL CONTROVERSY

Are antidepressants safe and effective in children and adolescents? Because of observations of an increased suicidality among adolescents (and adults, for that matter), experts are questioning whether these medications merely bring out an increased suicide risk that the patient has suppressed or has been too depressed to act on or actually increase the risk per se through some pharmacologic effect. Fluoxetine is the only selective serotonin reuptake inhibitor (SSRI) currently approved for use in pediatric patients in the United States. The British regulatory agency banned the use of another SSRI, paroxetine, in 2003 after analysis of the data indicated the occurrence of suicidal thoughts or episodes of self-harm at a rate of 1.5 to 3.2 times higher than that with placebo. Subsequently, the

FDA has cautioned about the use of and need for monitoring SSRI therapy in pediatric patients, and this area remained controversial when this chapter was finalized in the spring of 2004.

Some drugs may be less toxic in pediatric patients than in adults. Aminoglycosides appear to be less toxic in infants than in adults. In adults, aminoglycoside toxicity is related to both peripheral compartment accumulation and the individual patient's inherent sensitivity to these tissue concentrations.[44] Although neonatal peripheral tissue compartments for gentamicin have been reported to closely resemble those of adults with similar renal function,[16] gentamicin is rarely nephrotoxic in infants. This dissimilarity in the incidence of nephrotoxicity implies that newborn infants may have less inherent tissue sensitivity for toxicity than adults.

The differences in efficacy, toxicity, and protein binding of drugs in pediatric versus adult patients raise an important question about the acceptable therapeutic range in children. Therapeutic ranges for drugs are first established in adults and often are applied directly to pediatric patients, but specific studies should be conducted in pediatric patients to define optimal therapeutic ranges of drugs.

FACTORS AFFECTING PEDIATRIC THERAPY

DISEASES

5 Because most drugs are either metabolized by the liver or eliminated by the kidney, hepatic and renal diseases are expected to decrease the dosage requirements in patients. Nevertheless, not all diseases require lower doses of drugs; for instance, patients with cystic fibrosis require larger doses of certain drugs to achieve therapeutic concentrations.[45]

LIVER DISEASE

Because the liver is the main organ for drug metabolism, drug clearance usually is decreased in patients with hepatic disease; however, most studies on the influence of liver disease on dosage requirements have been carried out in adults, and these data may not be extrapolated uniformly to pediatric patients.

Drug metabolism by the liver depends on complex interactions among hepatic blood flow, ability of the liver to extract the drug from the blood, drug binding in the blood, and both type and severity of liver disease. Routine liver function tests—such as determinations of serum aspartate aminotransferase, serum alanine aminotransferase, alkaline phosphatase, and bilirubin levels—have not correlated consistently with drug pharmacokinetics. Further, because of different pathologic changes in various types of liver diseases, patients with acute viral hepatitis may have different abilities to metabolize drugs compared with patients with alcoholic cirrhosis.[46]

On the basis of hepatic extraction characteristics, drugs can be divided into two categories. The first category consists of drugs with a high hepatic extraction ratio (>0.7; such drugs include morphine, meperidine, lidocaine, and propranolol). Clearance of these drugs is affected by hepatic blood flow. A decreased hepatic blood flow in the presence of such disease states as cirrhosis and congestive heart failure is expected to decrease the clearance of drugs with high extraction ratios. The second category consists of drugs with a low extraction ratio (<0.2) and a low affinity for plasma proteins. Metabolism of these drugs (e.g., theophylline, chloramphenicol, and acetaminophen) is influenced mainly by hepatocellular function and not as much by changes in hepatic blood flow or plasma protein binding. One report suggested that theophylline clearance may decrease by 45% in a child with acute viral hepatitis.[47] Because of a lack of specific data on dosage adjustment in liver disease, drug therapy should be monitored closely in pediatric patients to avoid potential toxicity from excessive doses, particularly for drugs with narrow therapeutic indices.

RENAL DISEASE

Renal failure decreases the dosage requirement of drugs eliminated by the kidney. Once again, because of limited studies, dosage adjustments in pediatric patients are based largely on data obtained in adults. For many important drugs—such as aminoglycoside antibiotics—renal clearance or rate of elimination is directly proportional to the glomerular filtration rate, as measured by endogenous renal creatinine clearance.

In clinical practice, glomerular filtration rate (GFR) can be estimated from prediction equations such as the Schwartz formula, which takes into account serum creatinine concentration and the patient's height, gender, and age. The advantage of estimating GFR using the Schwartz equation is rapid determination and the avoidance of a cumbersome 24-hour urine collection.[48,49] The following formula is used to estimate GFR:

$$GFR = K \times L/S_{Cr}$$

where GFR is expressed in milliliters per minute per 1.73 m^2, K is an age-specific constant of proportionality (see below), L is the child's length in centimeters; and S_{Cr} is the serum creatinine in milligrams per deciliter.

Age	K
<1 year of age, low-birth-weight infant	0.33
<1 year of age, full-term infant	0.45
2- to 12-year-old child	0.55
13- to 21-year-old female	0.55
13- to 21-year-old male	0.70

Studies comparing the Schwartz-predicted GFR versus measured GFR noted that the Schwartz formula overestimated GFR in patients with decreasing GFR. The formula may not provide an accurate estimation of GFR in patients with rapidly changing serum creatinine concentrations, as seen in the critical care setting, in infants younger than 1 week of age, and in patients with obesity, malnutrition, or muscle wasting. Factors that interfere with serum creatinine measurement also may cause errors in estimation of GFR.

Serum drug concentrations should be monitored for drugs with narrow therapeutic indices and eliminated largely by the kidney (e.g., aminoglycosides and vancomycin) to optimize therapy in pediatric patients with renal dysfunction. For drugs with wide therapeutic ranges (e.g., penicillins and cephalosporins), dosage adjustment may be necessary only in moderate to severe renal failure.

CYSTIC FIBROSIS

Drug therapy in pediatric patients with cystic fibrosis has been reviewed.[50] For unknown reasons, these patients require increased doses of certain drugs. Studies have reported a higher clearance of such drugs as gentamicin, tobramycin, netilmicin, amikacin, dicloxacillin, cloxacillin, azlocillin, piperacillin, and theophylline in patients with cystic fibrosis compared with those without this disease; the apparent volume of distribution of certain drugs also may be altered in cystic fibrosis.[50] Severity of the illness may influence the change in dosage requirements, but this is not certain. Chapter 30 reviews these changes in detail.

OTHER DISEASES

Although specific dosage guidelines are not available, pediatric patients with gastrointestinal disease (e.g., celiac disease, gastroenteritis, and severe malabsorption) may require dosage adjustments.[45] Hypoxemia also has been shown to decrease the elimination of amikacin in low-birth-weight infants.[51] Critically ill adult and pediatric patients with severe head trauma require higher than normal doses of phenytoin in part because of increased intrinsic clearance.[52]

ISSUES IN PEDIATRIC DRUG THERAPY

PAIN MANAGEMENT

For many years, the term *pain* could not be found in the index of any major pediatric medicine or pediatric surgical textbooks.[53] The prevailing wisdom was that neonates did not experience pain owing to inadequately developed neuroendocrine systems and nerve pathways. During the last years of the twentieth century, however, many research and clinical studies were performed in the areas of pain management and assessment in neonates, infants, children, and adolescents. Today, results of these discoveries have been incorporated into clinical practice, making effective pain therapy a standard of care and pain assessment the fifth vital sign in modern pediatric practice.[54]

The basic mechanisms of pain perception in infants and children are similar to those of adults except that pain impulse transmission in neonates occurs primarily along slow-conducting, nonmyelinated C fibers rather than along myelinated Aδ fibers. In addition, less precision in pain signal transmission exists in the spinal cord, and descending inhibitory neurotransmitters are lacking. The result is that neonates and young infants may perceive pain more intensely and are more sensitive to pain than older children or adults.[55,56] It is now known that previous pain experience leads to long-term consequences such as alterations in response to a subsequent painful event.[57] Taddio and colleagues[58,59] reported that boys circumcised with the topical anesthetic EMLA had a lower pain response to subsequent immunizations than those who were circumcised without topical anesthesia. An inadequately treated initial painful procedure may decrease the effect of adequate analgesia in subsequent procedures owing to altered pain response patterns.

Children consistently report that needles and shots are what they fear most. However, with the current immunization schedule that recommends 14 to 33 injections before adolescence, interventions to decrease injection pain need to be performed (Table 7–1).

Pharmacologic pain management for medical conditions and surgical and postoperative events has progressed considerably over the past decade with the use of continuous opioid infusions, epidural anesthesia, peripheral nerve blockade, local anesthetics, nonsteroidal anti-inflammatory drugs, different routes for traditional agents (i.e., transmucosal and transdermal), and nonopioid adjuvant drugs (Table 7–2). New pain management techniques, education, research, and increasing awareness of pain management options have helped to improve the quality of life in children.

TABLE 7–1. Techniques for Minimizing Pain Caused by Injection

Pharmacologic Methods

EMLA[60] (eutectic mixture of lidocaine and prilocaine)	*Advantages:* Penetrates the skin to provide anesthesia to a depth of 5 mm; effective in decreasing the pain of IM and subcutaneous injections, venipuncture, IV cannulation, lumbar puncture, circumcision, skin-graft harvesting, and laser dermal therapy; safe and effective in newborns >37 weeks' gestation. *Disadvantages:* Requires 1 h before onset of adequate anesthesia, has a vasoconstrictive effect that may make starting IV catheters difficult, may induce methemoglobinemia.
Numby Stuff (lidocaine iontophoresis)[61]	*Advantages:* Provides dermal anesthesia to a depth of 10 mm within 10–20 min; effective in decreasing the pain of IM injection, IV cannulation, venipuncture, lumbar puncture, skin biopsy, and bone marrow aspiration. *Disadvantage:* Tingling, itching, or burning sensation from the electric current used to transport drug to the tissues.
Vapocoolant sprays (ethyl chloride or dichlorodifluoromethane)[62]	*Advantages:* Vapocoolant is sprayed directly onto the skin or applied to a cotton ball that is held on the area to be anesthetized; provides local anesthesia within 15 seconds; effective in reducing injection pain in children 4–6 years of age. *Disadvantages:* Brief duration of action so that procedure should be completed in 1 or 2 min; may not be effective in reducing injection pain in infants aged 2–6 months.
Local anesthetic (lidocaine)[63]	*Advantage:* Reduces the pain of subsequent needle insertion. *Disadvantage:* Local anesthetic injection itself is associated with pain and burning sensation
Pacifier with sucrose[64,65]	*For preterm neonates:* 0.1–0.4 mL of a 12%–24% sucrose solution (place on pacifier or the tongue 2 min before procedure). *For term neonates:* 1–2 mL of a 12%–24% sucrose solution (place on pacifier or the tongue 2 min before procedure). *Advantage:* Noninvasive method to reduce pain associated with needle insertion in infants. *Disadvantage:* Sucrose solution's effect in reducing pain gradually decreases over time.

Other Techniques

Site selection[66]	*For children older than 18 months of age:* Use of the deltoid muscle for IM injections is associated with less pain than injections administered in the thigh. *For children older than 3 years of age:* Use of the ventrogluteal area for injection is associated with less pain than the anterior thigh or dorsogluteal area.
Z-tract technique	Z-tract intramuscular injection technique is less painful (pull skin taut at the injection site, give injection, and then release the skin); use a higher-gauge needle when the injectable solution is not viscous.
Behavioral	Use of distraction methods such as blowing bubbles, providing music by headphones, relaxation, imagery, self-hypnosis, or having parents present for the procedure can be helpful.

DRUG ADMINISTRATION

Drugs often are given by the intravenous route to seriously ill patients. Flow rates and injection sites vary widely with pediatric intravenous drug delivery sets. Effective serum concentrations are expected to be achieved rapidly after drug infusion. Several studies demonstrated that the method of drug infusion has a profound influence on peak serum concentration and time to attain peak concentrations of chloramphenicol and tobramycin.[67,68] This has practical implications for routine therapeutic drug monitoring in that anticipated serum concentrations may be inaccurate, leading to unjustified, costly, and potentially harmful alterations in doses. Proper recommendations for obtaining patient specimens can be made only with the knowledge of drug characteristics and infusion method.

Intravenous drugs commonly are infused in an antegrade fashion. By this method, the doses injected at various sites of the intravenous set (e.g., a Y-site and a volumetric chamber such as Metriset Buretrol) are expected to move directly toward the patient (Fig. 7–1).

In vitro studies with gentamicin and aminophylline have shown that the delivery of these drugs may be delayed substantially depending on the flow rate and injection site.[69] These observations were confirmed with infusion of chloramphenicol succinate[67] and tobramycin.[68] These studies clearly have demonstrated that the variables of intravenous drug infusion systems (e.g., flow rate, injection site, volume of drug, and fluid volume of the tubing) can affect the serum concentrations of drugs markedly after infusions into pediatric patients. For example, mean peak serum concentrations of chloramphenicol can be 5 mcg/mL higher and occur 1 hour earlier after flashball injection compared with Buretrol injection in infants and children.[67] Similarly, the mean serum concentrations of tobramycin can be 2.3–2.5 mcg/mL higher and occur 1 to 1.5 hours earlier after an infusion from a syringe pump compared with infusions from the Y-site of a system similar to that of Fig. 7–1.[69] These differences can be important because of the narrow therapeutic indices of chloramphenicol and tobramycin. Furthermore, a lack of knowledge of these variables may result in inappropriate timing and interpretation of blood level data, leading to unnecessary dosage adjustments.

Specific gravity also can influence drug delivery at slow infusion rates.[70] For example, in vitro studies have indicated that drugs with a specific gravity lower than that of the maintenance fluid may layer at the top of the tubing, where delivery would be prolonged by laminar-flow characteristics.[70] Similarly, injections into a filter chamber, Y-site, or T-site with dead space also can prolong drug delivery.

No single infusion system is ideal for delivery of all drugs in all institutions for all patients. For example, a syringe pump with microbore tubing may be preferred for the infusion of vancomycin to neonates. Each facility must be cognizant of problems of drug delivery and develop specific guidelines for intravenous infusions.

TABLE 7–2. Opioid Administration for Acute and Severe Pain

Intermittent IV or PO bolus administration (not as needed)	Weak opioids (e.g., codeine, hydrocodone, oxycodone) often are combined with acetaminophen or a nonsteroidal anti-inflammatory agent (NSAID) for moderate pain. With dose escalation of combination oral products, be aware that the dose does not exceed recommended daily amounts for acetaminophen or ibuprofen. IV administration of codeine has been associated with allergic reactions related to histamine release. Parenteral administration of codeine is not recommended. Intermittent opioid administration is associated with wide fluctuation between peak and trough levels so that the patient may alternate between peak blood levels associated with untoward effects and trough levels associated with inadequate pain relief when treating severe pain. Oxycodone and morphine are available in a sustained-release formulation for use with chronic pain (not acute pain). Tablet must be swallowed whole and cannot be administered to patients through gastric tubes.
Intravenous continuous infusion[67,68]	Loading dose is administered to achieve rapidly a therapeutic blood level and pain relief (i.e., morphine loading dose of 0.05–0.15 mg/kg in children; 0.1 mg/kg infused over 90 min in neonates). Loading dose is followed by a maintenance continuous infusion. Doses that are considered safe in children can cause respiratory depression and seizures in neonates because of decreased clearance, immature blood-brain barrier at birth that is more permeable to morphine, and neonates have an increased unbound fraction of morphine that increases CNS effects of the drug.
PCA (patient-controlled analgesia)[69]	Gives patient some control over their pain therapy. PCA allows the patient to self-administer small opioid doses. The PCA-Plus pump allows the patient to receive a continuous infusion together with a set number of self-administered doses per hour. PCA helps to eliminate wide peak and trough fluctuations so that levels remain in a therapeutic range. Children as young as 6 or 7 years of age can master the use of PCA.
Epidural and intrathecal analgesia[70]	Effective in the management of severe postoperative, chronic, or cancer pain. Spinal opioids can be administered by a single bolus injection into the epidural or subarachnoid space or by continuous infusion via an indwelling catheter. Dosage requirement by these routes is significantly less than with IV administration (epidural opioid doses: 10-fold lower than IV doses; intrathecal opioid doses: 100-fold lower than IV doses). Morphine, hydromorphone, fentanyl, and sufentanil are effective when administered intrathecally. The most commonly used local anesthetic in continuous epidural infusions is bupivacaine. Fentanyl, morphine, or hydromorphone is usually combined with bupivacaine for epidural infusions.
Transmucosal administration	Fentanyl lozenge is absorbed transmucosally. It is useful for providing analgesia during painful procedures. Advantages of this product include rapid onset of action (within 15 min), short duration of action (60–90 min), and painless administration because no injection is needed. A common side effect is vomiting and mild to moderate oxygen desaturation. Doses of 10–15 mcg/kg provide blood levels equivalent to 3–5 mcg/kg IV.

At our institution, specific guidelines are provided for administration of each drug. These guidelines take into account various infusion rates and provide consistency of delivery with each dose. As long as the time for actual delivery can be anticipated, times to obtain blood samples can be adjusted accordingly to generate meaningful data.

ALTERATION OF DOSAGE FORMS

Many drugs used in pediatric patients are not available in suitable dosage forms. This necessitates dilution of high concentrations of drugs intended for adult patients. Examples of these drugs include atropine, carbamazepine, diazepam, digoxin, epinephrine, hydralazine, insulin, morphine, phenobarbital, and phenytoin. Volumes ranging from 0.01 to 0.1 mL must be measured to dispense these drugs for use in infants. This obviously can be associated with large errors in measurements, and such errors have caused intoxication with digoxin[71] and morphine[72] in infants. One solution to this problem is to dilute these concentrated products, but such alterations can influence the stability or compatibility of these drugs. Because of limited data, pharmacists justifiably may be reluctant to alter dosage forms of certain drugs.

Selection of the appropriate vehicle to dilute the adult dosage forms for use in pediatric patients also can be difficult. Phenobarbital sodium contains propylene glycol in the original product to improve drug stability. Because propylene glycol can cause hyperosmolality in infants,[39] further addition of this vehicle may not be wise. Because of limited access to intravenous sites in pediatric patients, drugs must be administered through the same site; however, data on their compatibility often are missing. Newborn infants often require aminoglycosides for presumed or proven sepsis and calcium gluconate to correct hypocalcemia. Tobramycin and calcium gluconate have been found to be compatible at least during a 1-hour period of administration at the same site.[72]

Administration of oral drugs continues to challenge parents and nurses. Alteration of these drugs by crushing or mixing, refusal of patients to accept the medication, and loss of drug during administration are some factors that can affect pediatric therapy. A common practice is to mix medications in applesauce, syrup, ice cream, or other vehicles just before administration to make the drugs palatable.

A number of extemporaneous formulations for oral, intravenous, and rectal administration are included in a compilation of products for use in pediatric patients.[73] A specific reference on the stability

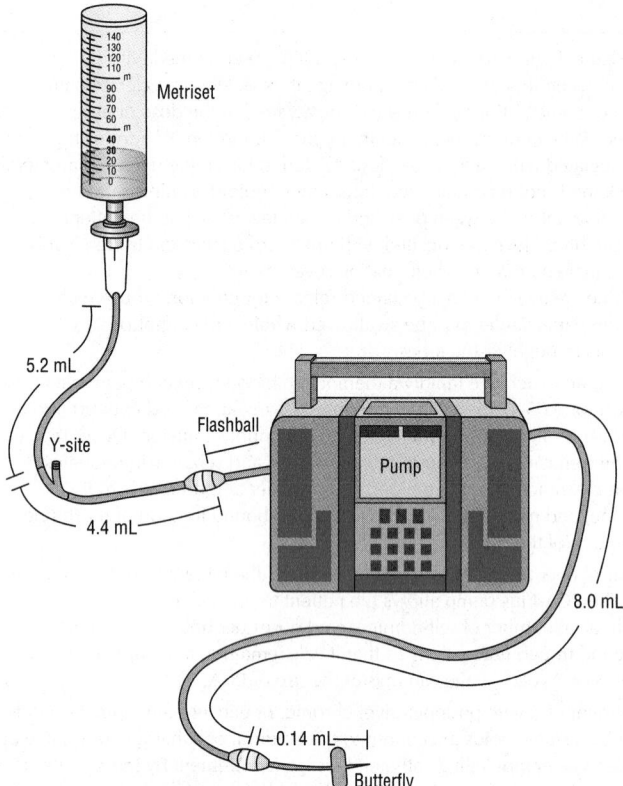

FIGURE 7–1. Schematic diagram of an intravenous set with a volumetric chamber (Metriset or Buretrol), Y-site, flashball, and butterfly. Values shown for the various components of the system are volume capacities. *(From ref. 59, with permission.)*

of many drugs of these formulations, however, is still lacking. This emphasizes the need for continued research in this area.

Drug administration into the middle ear, nose, or eye of a child requires special attention. Certain drugs (e.g., sodium valproate and morphine) can be administered rectally to infants who have limited access for intravenous drug administration or if oral drug administration cannot be accomplished.

Transdermal drug delivery can be used in pediatric patients (1) to avoid problems of drug absorption from the oral route and complications from the intravenous route and (2) to maximize duration of effect and minimize adverse effects of drugs. Unfortunately, the commercially available transdermal dosage forms (e.g., clonidine and scopolamine) are not intended for pediatric patients; these would deliver doses much higher than those needed for infants and children.

MEDICATION ADHERENCE

The issue of medication adherence is more complex in pediatric patients than in adults. The caregivers of young patients must appreciate the importance of understanding and following the prescribing information.

In one study, medication adherence was considered to be a problem in nearly 60% of adolescents (age 12–15 years with asthma). About 40% of patients had severe denial regarding their asthma and its severity. Nearly 80% of patients had preventable asthma exacerbations.[74]

Among the factors that can negatively affect adherence are poor communication between the physician and patient or parent; insufficient prescribing information; lack of understanding about the

severity of illness by the patient or parent; lack of interest, e.g., among adolescents; fear of side effects; failure of the patient or parent to remember to administer the drugs; inconvenient dosage forms or dosing schedules involving administration of three or more doses daily; and unpalatibility of drug products.[75] Studies in pediatric volunteers have been done to compare the palatability of antibiotics.[76] These data may have important implications for adherence in children.

DOSE REQUIREMENTS

Medication doses often are based on the body weight of neonates, infants, and children e.g., milligrams per kilogram of body weight per day to be given in one or more portions daily. However, certain drugs, including antineoplastic agents, may be given based on body surface area, e.g., milligrams per square meter in one or more doses daily. In either case, the total amount of weight- or surface area–based individual or daily dose in a pediatric patient, especially an adolescent, should not exceed the amount of drug indicated in an adult patient.

DRUG INTERACTIONS

Drug interaction studies generally are lacking in pediatric age groups. The data often are extrapolated from those in adult populations. Special attention should be given to adolescents, who may concurrently use alcohol, recreational/illicit drugs, or other prescription or nonprescription medications without the knowledge of the primary health care provider to avoid drug interactions.

COMPLEMENTARY AND ALTERNATIVE THERAPY

In a study of patients between 3 weeks and 18 years (mean 5.3 years) of age, 45% of caregivers were giving a product to the children; 27% had given three or more products in the past year. The most commonly used products were aloe plant/juice (44% of those reporting use of herbal therapies), echinacea (33%), and sweet oil (25%). The most dangerous combination was ephedra (which has since been withdrawn from the U.S. market) with albuterol in adolescents with asthma. Most caregivers did not recognize potential adverse effects or drug interactions associated with herbs. Friends or relatives were the main source of information for 80% of caregivers.[77]

Little is known about the efficacy of herbal products in infants, children, and adolescents. Health care professionals must ask caregivers specifically about the use of complementary and alternative treatments to minimize the adverse effects and costs associated with ineffective therapies.

MEDICATION SAFETY

The Institute of Medicine (IOM) reported that between 44,000 and 98,000 Americans die each year in hospitals from medical errors.[78] According to this report, the vast majority of medical errors that cause harm to patients are preventable. Health care professionals have a responsibility for creating a safe medication environment and reducing risk to a vulnerable pediatric population.

Pediatric medication errors commonly occur at the medication-ordering step owing to multiple calculations required with weight-based dosing and adjustments needed in providing therapy to the developing pediatric patient.[79–81] The United States Pharmacopeia (USP) Center for the Advancement of Patient Safety states that risk to patients when performing repeated calculations involving multiple steps can be minimized using computer-based algorithms.[82] Since the medication-preparation step is also a high-hazard point owing to the need for dilution or manipulation of commercially available products only available in adult doses, the USP recommends that compounded pediatric medications be prepared and labeled in the pharmacy and verified by a pharmacist. Among drug administration–related errors, wrong dose, wrong technique, and wrong drug are the three most common errors and may be related to an inability to access pediatric drug information. Risk-reduction strategies include placement of a clinical pharmacist on pediatric wards in hospitals, simplifying the process, ordering standardized concentrations and doses, implementing computerized physician order-entry systems with dose range checking, dispensing pharmacy-prepared/ready-to-administer doses, standardizing infusion equipment, and using bar-coded medications and barcoding systems that check the medication at the point of care.[81,83] Identifying and understanding the high-hazard areas or points of failure in the medication-use process will help us to design strategies to prevent problems before they arise.

CONCLUSIONS

Although tremendous progress has been made in the area of pediatric pharmacotherapy, many questions remain unanswered. The pharmacokinetics of many important drugs have been elucidated, but their pharmacodynamics have not been explored fully. Similarly, effect of disease states and patient characteristics such as genetic status have not been studied for most drugs. The effect of these factors on the development of cytochrome P450 isozymes (e.g., 3A4, 2D6, 1A2, 2C9, and 2C19) and other enzymes needs to be studied (see Chaps. 5 and 6). Similarly, comparative efficacy and safety data for many therapies are unavailable. Influence of drug therapy on clinical and economic outcomes and on quality of life needs to be studied in pediatric patients.

The development of new drugs has contributed to improved patient care. The new FDA regulations (Best Pharmaceuticals for Children Act of 2002) can require the industry to conduct studies and seek labeling of important drugs for pediatric patients. As an incentive, a 6-month patent extension and waiver of supplemental new drug application fee are offered to the industry. This should encourage the industry to develop and market more drugs for the pediatric population. However, greater emphasis also should be placed on disease prevention. Millions of children die because of preventable diseases, particularly in developing countries of the world. Administration of vaccines and control of diarrhea alone could save millions of these lives annually. However, the developed countries face different problems. The infant mortality rate in the United States is nearly twice as high among blacks as whites. Improved prenatal care, educational programs, and avoidance of alcohol, smoking, and drugs of abuse during pregnancy may decrease mortality as well as morbidity from illnesses, including acquired immunodeficiency syndrome.

Finally, efforts should be made to offer evidence-based pharmacotherapy. This is often difficult in pediatric populations when the drugs must be used outside the guidelines and indications approved by the FDA. The institutions should develop guidelines for the use of drugs in specific diseases and for the use of high-cost drugs such as colony-stimulating factors, palivizumab, dornase-α, epoetin-α, immunoglobulins, surfactants, and growth hormones.

Although much needs to be learned about the optimization of therapy, it is encouraging to witness the continued growth of knowledge in this area to improve the quality of life and survival from pharmacotherapy in pediatric patients.

ABBREVIATIONS

FDA, Food and Drug Administration
GFR, glomerular filtration rate
IOM, Institute of Medicine
SSRI, selective serotonin reuptake inhibitor
USP, United States Pharmacopeia

Review Questions and other resources can be found at *www.pharmacotherapyonline.com.*

REFERENCES

1. Infant Mortality Statistics from the 2002 Period Linked Birth/Infant Death Data Set. National Vital Statistics Report, Vol 52. Washington, U.S. Department of Health and Human Services, Centers for Disease Control and Prevention, National Center for Health Statistics, 2003:1–28.
2. Avery GB, Randolph JG, Weaver T. Gastric acidity in the first day of life. Pediatrics 1966;37:1005–1007.
3. Agunod M, Yamaguchi N, Lopex R, et al. Correlative study of hydrochloric acid, pepsin, and intrinsic factor secretion in newborns and infants. Am J Dig Dis 1969;14:400–414.
4. Huang NN, High RN. Comparison of serum levels following the administration of oral and parenteral preparations of penicillin to infants and children of various age groups. J Pediatr 1953;42:657–668.
5. Silverio J, Poole JW. Serum concentrations of ampicillin in newborn infants after oral administration. Pediatrics 1973;51:578–580.
6. O'Connor WJ, Warren GH, Edrada LS, et al. Serum concentrations of sodium nafcillin in infants during the perinatal period. Antimicrob Agents Chemother 1965;220–222.
7. Jalling B. Plasma concentrations of phenobarbital in the treatment of seizures in newborns. Acta Paediatr Scand 1975;64:514–524.
8. Kearns GL, Abdel-Rahman SM, Alander SW, et al. Drug therapy: Developmental pharmacology—Drug disposition, action, and therapy in infants and children. N Engl J Med 2003;349:1157–1167.
9. Signer E, Fridrich R. Gastric emptying in newborns and young infants. Acta Paediatr Scand 1975;64:525–530.
10. Boreus IO. Plasma concentrations of phenobarbital in mother and child after combined prenatal and postnatal administration for prophylaxis of hyperbilirubinemia. J Pediatr 1978;93:695.
11. Morselli PL. Serum levels and pharmacokinetics of anticonvulsants in the management of seizure disorders. In: Merkin B, ed. Clinical Pharmacology. Chicago, Year Book, 1978:89.
12. Tyrala FF, Hillman LS, Hillman RE, et al. Clinical pharmacology of hexachlorophene in newborn infants. J Pediatr 1977;91:481–486.
13. McFadden S, Haddow JE. Coma produced by topical application of isopropanol. Pediatrics 1969;43:622–623.
14. Evans NJ, Rutter N, Hadgraft J, et al. Percutaneous administration of theophylline in preterm infant. J Pediatr 1985;107:307–311.
15. Friis-Hansen B. Body water compartments in children: Changes during growth and related changes in body composition. Pediatrics 1961;28:169–181.
16. Haughey DB, Hilligoss DM, Grassi A, et al. Two-compartment gentamicin pharmacokinetics in premature neonates: A comparison to adults with decreased glomerular filtration rates. J Pediatr 1980;96:325–330.
17. Nahata MC, Powell DA, Durrell DE, et al. Effect of gestational age and birth weight on tobramycin kinetics in newborn infants. J Antimicrob Chemother 1984;14:59–65.
18. Roberts RJ. Pharmacologic principles in therapeutics in infants. In: Drug Therapy in Infants. Philadelphia, Saunders, 1984:3–12.
19. Pitlick W, Painter M, Pippenger C. Phenobarbital pharmacokinetics in neonates. Clin Pharmacol Ther 1978;23:346–350.
20. Painter MJ, Pippenger C, MacDonald H, et al. Phenobarbital and diphenylhydantoin levels in neonates with seizures. J Pediatr 1978;92:315–319.

21. Silverman WA, Anderson DH, Blanc WA, et al. A difference in mortality rate and incidence of kernicterus among premature infants allotted to two prophylactic antibacterial regimens. Pediatrics 1956;18:614–624.

22. Odell GB. The dissociation of bilirubin from albumin and its clinical implications. J Pediatr 1959;55:268–279.

23. Morselli PL. Clinical pharmacokinetics in neonates. Clin Pharmacokinet 1976;1:81–98.

24. Committee on Drugs, American Academy of Pediatrics. The transfer of drugs and other chemicals into human milk. Pediatrics 1994;93:137–150.

25. Anderson PO. Drugs and breast milk. J Pediatr 1995;95:957.

26. Rane A. Basic principles of drug disposition and action in infants and children. In: Yaffe JF, ed. Pediatric Pharmacology: Therapeutic Principles in Practice. New York, Grune & Stratton, 1980:7–28.

27. Weiss CF, Glazko AJ, Weston JK. Chloramphenicol in the newborn infant: A physiologic explanation of its toxicity when given in excessive doses. N Engl J Med 1960;262:787–794.

28. Nahata MC, Powell DA. Comparative bioavailability and pharmacokinetics of chloramphenicol after intravenous chloramphenicol succinate in premature infants and older patients. Dev Pharmacol Ther 1983;6:23–32.

29. Kuhn R, Nahata MC, Powell DA, et al. Netilmicin pharmacokinetics in newborn infants. Eur J Clin Pharmacol 1986;29:635–637.

30. Cha PCW, Duffy BJ, Walker JS. Pharmacokinetic-pharmacodynamic relationships of morphine in neonates. Clin Pharmacol Ther 1992;51:334–342.

31. Edwards DJ, Zarowitz BJ, Slaughter RL. Theophylline. In: Evans WE, Schentag JJ, Jusko WJ, eds. Applied Pharmacokinetics, 3d ed. Vancouver, WA, Applied Therapeutics, 1992:1–47.

32. Takahashi H, Ishikawa S, Nomoto S. et al. Developmental changes in pharmacokinetics and pharmacodynamics of warfarin enantiomers in Japanese children. Clin Pharmacol Ther 2000;68:541–555.

33. Lambert GH, Schoeller DA, Kotake AN, et al. The effect of age, gender, and sexual maturation on the caffeine breath test. Dev Pharmacol Ther 1986;9:375–388.

34. Leffert FL. The management of chronic asthma. J Pediatr 1980;97:875–885.

35. Johnston DE. Immunotherapy in children: Past, present, and future, part I. Ann Allergy 1981;46:1–7.

36. Johnston DE. Immunotherapy in children: Past, present, and future, part II. Ann Allergy 1981;46:59–66.

37. Kearin M, Kelly JG, O'Malley K. Digoxin "receptors" in neonates: An explanation of less sensitivity to digoxin than in adults. Clin Pharmacol Ther 1980;28:346–349.

38. Kawai M, Momoi T, Yorifuji, T, et al. Unfavorable effects of growth hormone therapy on the final height of boys with short stature not caused by growth hormone deficiency. J Pediatr 1997;130:205–209.

39. Glasgow AM, Boeckx RL, Miller MK, et al. Hyperosmolality in small infants due to propylene glycol. Pediatrics 1983;72:353–355.

40. Hiller JL, Benda GI, Rahatzad M, et al. Benzyl alcohol toxicity: Impact of mortality and intraventricular hemorrhage among very low birth weight infants. Pediatrics 1986;77:500–506.

41. Grossman ER, Walchek A, Freedman H. Tetracyclines and permanent teeth: The relation between dose and tooth color. Pediatrics 1971;47:567–570.

42. Walker RC, Wright AJ. The quinolones. Mayo Clin Proc 1987;62:1007–1012.

43. Chysky V, Kapla M, Hullman R, et al. Safety of ciprofloxacin in children: Worldwide clinical experience based on compassionate usage. Infection 1991;19:289–296.

44. Schentag JJ, Plaut ME, Cerra FB, et al. Aminoglycoside nephrotoxicity in critically ill surgical patients. J Surg Res 1979;26:270–279.

45. Kauffman RE, Habersange R. Modification of dosage regimens in disease states of childhood. In: Mirking BL, ed. Clinical Pharmacology and Therapeutics: A Pediatric Perspective. Chicago, Year Book, 1978:73–88.

46. Roberts RJ. Special considerations in drug therapy in infants. In: Drug Therapy in Infants. Philadelphia, Saunders, 1984:25–35.

47. Feinstein RA, Miles MV. The effect of acute viral hepatitis on theophylline clearance. Clin Pediatr 1985;24:357–358.

48. Hogg RJ, Furth S, Lemley KV, et al. National Kidney Foundation's kidney disease outcomes quality initiative clinical practice guidelines for chronic kidney disease in children and adolescents: Evaluation, classification, and stratification. Pediatrics 2003;111:1416–1421.

49. Schwartz Gj, Brion LP, Spitzer A. The use of plasma creatinine concentration for estimating glomerular filtration rate in infants, children and adolescents. Pediatr Clin North Am 1987;34:571–590.

50. Wallace CS, Hall M, Kuhn RJ. Pharmacologic management of cystic fibrosis. Clin Pharm 1993;12:657–674.

51. Myers MG, Roberts JF, Mirhig NJ. Effect of gestational age, birth weight, and hypoxemia on the pharmacokinetics of amikacin in serum of infants. Antimicrob Agents Chemother 1977;11:1027.

52. Bahal-O'Mara N, Jones R, Nahata MC, et al. Pharmacokinetics of phenytoin in children with acute neurotrauma. Crit Care Med 1995;23:1418–1424.

53. Rana SR. Pain: A subject ignored (letter). Pediatrics 1987;79:309.

54. Franch LS, Greenberg CS, Stevens B. Pain assessment in infants and children. Pediatr Clin North Am 2000;47(3):487–512.

55. Anand KJS. Consensus statement for the prevention and management of pain in the newborn. Arch Pediatr Adolesc Med 2001;155:173–180.

56. American Academy of Pediatrics at Canadian Paediatric Society. Prevention and management of pain and stress in the neonate. Pediatrics 2000;105:454–461.

57. Fitzgerald M, Anand KJS. Development neuroanatomy and neurophysiology of pain. In: Schechter NL, Berde CB, Yaster M, eds. Pain in Infants, Children and Adolescents. Baltimore, Williams & Wilkins, 1993:11–31.

58. Taddio A, Katz J, Ilersich Al, et al. Effect of neonatal circumcision on pain response during subsequent routine vaccination. Lancet 1997;349:559–603.

59. Taddio A, Ohlsson A, Einarson T, et al. A systematic review of lidocaine-prilocaine cream for neonatal circumcision pain. N Engl J Med 1997;336:1197–1201.

60. Uhari M. Eutectic mixture of lidocaine and prilocaine for alleviating vaccination pain in infants. Pediatrics 1993;92:719–721.

61. Zempsky, WT, Anand KS, Sullivan KM, et al. Lidocaine iontophoresis for topical anesthesia before intravenous line placement in children. J Pediatr 1998;132:1061–1063.

62. Reis EC, Holobukov R. Vapocoolant spray is equally effective as EMLA cream in reducing immunization pain in school aged children. Pediatrics 1997;100:5.

63. Bartfield JM, Connis P, Barbera J, et al. Buffered versus plain lidocaine as a local anesthetic for simple laceration repair. Ann Emerg Med 1990;19:1387–1390.

64. Annand KHS and International Evidenced Based Group for Neonatal Pain. Consensus statement for the prevention and management of pain in the newborn. Arch Pediatr Adolesc Med 2001;155:173–180.

65. Schechter Nl, Berde CB, Yaster M, et al. Pain in Infants, Children, and Adolescents. Baltimore, Lippincott Williams & Wilkins, 2003.

66. Keen MF. Comparison of intramuscular injection techniques to reduce site discomfort and lesions. Nurs Res 1986;35:207–210.

67. Nahata MC, Powell DA, Glazer JP, et al. Effect of intravenous flow rate and infection site on in vitro delivery of chloramphenicol succinate and in vivo kinetics. J Pediatr 1981;99:463–466.

68. Nahata MC, Powell DA, Durrell DE, et al. Effect of infusion methods on tobramycin serum concentrations in newborn infants. J Pediatr 1984;104:136–138.

69. Gould T, Robert RJ. Therapeutic problems arising from the use of intravenous route for drug administration. J Pediatr 1997;95:465–471.

70. Rajchgot P, Radde IC, MacLeod SM. Influence of specific gravity on intravenous drug delivery. J Pediatr 1981;99:658–661.

71. Berman W. Whitman V, Marks KH, et al. Inadvertent overadministration of digoxin to low birth weight infants. J Pediatr 1978;92:1024.

72. Zenk KE, Anderson S. Improving the accuracy of minivolume injections. Infusion 1982;Jan–Feb:7–11.

73. Nahata MC, Pai V, Hipple TF. Pediatric Drug Formulations, 5th ed. Cincinnati, Harvey Whitney Books, 2003:1–307.

74. Martin AJ, Campbell DA, Gluyas PA, et al. Characteristics of near-fatal asthma in childhood. Pediatr Pulmonol 1995;20:1–8.

75. Boreus LO. Drug compliance. In: Yaffe SJ, ed. Principles of Pediatric Pharmacology. New York, Churchill-Livingstone, 1982:176–192.

76. Matsui D, Barron A, Rieder MJ. Assessment of the palatability of antistaphylococcal antibiotics in pediatric volunteers. Ann Pharmacother 1996;30:586–588.

77. Lanski SL, Greenwald M, Perkins A. et al. Herbal therapy use in a pediatric emergency department population: Expect the unexpected. Pediatrics 2003;111:981–985.

78. Institute of Medicine, Committee on Quality of Health Care in American. To Err Is Human: Building a Safer Health System. Washington, National Academy Press, 2000.

79. Raju TN, Kecskes S, Thornton JP, et al. Medication errors in neonatal and paediatric intensive-care units. Lancet 1989;2:374–376.

80. Folli HL, Poole RL, Benitz WE, et al. Medication error prevention by clinical pharmacists in two children's hospitals. Pediatrics 1987;79:718–722.

81. Kaushal R, Bates DW, Landrigan C, et al. Medication errors and adverse drug events in pediatric inpatients. JAMA 2001;285:2114–2120.

82. USP Center for the Advancement of Patient Safety. USP issues recommendations for preventing medication errors in children. January 21, 2003.

83. American Academy of Pediatrics Committee on Drugs and Committee on Hospital Care. Prevention of medication errors in pediatric inpatient setting. Pediatrics 2003;112:431–436.

8

GERIATRICS

Catherine I. Lindblad, Shelly L. Gray, David R. P. Guay, Emily R. Hajjar, Teresa C. McCarthy, and Joseph T. Hanlon

Learning Objectives and other resources can be found at *www.pharmacotherapyonline.com.*

KEY CONCEPTS:

1. The population of persons 65 and older is increasing.

2. Age-related changes in physiology can affect the pharmacokinetics and pharmacodynamics of numerous drugs.

3. Improving and maintaining functional status is a cornerstone of care for elders.

4. Drug-related problems in the elderly are common and cause considerable morbidity.

5. Pharmacists can play a major role in optimizing drug therapy and preventing drug-related problems in the elderly.

Pharmacotherapy for the elderly can cure or palliate disease as well as enhance health-related quality of life (HRQOL). HRQOL considerations for the elderly include focusing on improvement in physical functioning (e.g., activities of daily living), psychological functioning (e.g., cognition, depression), social functioning (e.g., social activities, support systems), and overall health (e.g., general health perception).[1] Despite the benefits of pharmacotherapy, HRQOL can be compromised by drug-related problems. The avoidance of drug-related adverse consequences in the elderly requires health care practitioners to become knowledgeable about a number of age-specific issues. To address these knowledge needs, this chapter will discuss the epidemiology of aging; physiologic changes associated with aging, with emphasis on those which can affect the pharmacokinetics and pharmacodynamics of drugs; common clinical conditions seen in geriatric patients; epidemiology of drug-related problems in the elderly; and an approach to reduce drug-related problems through the provision of comprehensive geriatric assessment.

EPIDEMIOLOGY OF AGING

1. The older American population is very diverse and heterogeneous with respect to health status. The demographics and health characteristics of persons aged 65 to 74 years are different from those of persons 85 years of age and older, as are those of persons who are institutionalized compared with those living in the community. It is teasing apart the various threads of wellness and illness, independence and dependence, and function and dysfunction that makes the available demographic and health status data relevant for clinical practice. Understanding this diversity and growth of the older population will allow society to plan for the training, research, and resource needs necessary for future clinical practice and adequate health care.

In 2000, persons aged 65 or older accounted for 12.4% (35 million) of the total U.S. population.[2] Of those over 65 years of age, women outnumbered men and accounted for 58% of this segment of the population. The gender gap widens with increasing age in that women accounted for 70% of the cohort aged 85 years and older.[3] By 2030, it is projected that one in five (20%) Americans will

be over the age of 65 years, with 2.5% of the U.S. population aged 85 years and older. This 20% projection for persons aged 65 years and older will persist until 2050. However, the number of persons aged 85 years and older will further increase by 2050 to 5% (19 million) of the total U.S. population.[4] The increase in the number of older persons is not just due to the post-World War II birth rate but also to a declining mortality rate and overall better health among elders.[5] The decline in early death and better health of older adults arise for a variety of reasons: (1) public health measures affecting all age groups (e.g., immunizations, prenatal care), (2) advances in medical procedures and drugs, (3) promotion of a healthy lifestyle, and (4) improvements in social living conditions.[6–8] More relevant to providers of care for older Americans is life expectancy at age 65. In 2000, white women 65 years of age can expect an average additional 19.2 years of life; black women, 17.4 years; white men, 16.3 years; and black men, 14.5 years.[9] Today, if a person survives to age 85, he can expect to live another 5.6 years and she another 6.7 years.[9] Given this increase in life expectancy, it is not surprising that the number of centenarians increased from 37,306 in 1990 to 50,454 in 2000.[9] The Census Bureau has projected that this special population segment could number 834,000 by the middle of the next century.[10]

Along with changes in the life expectancy of future elders, there also will be changes in their racial/ethnic composition. In 2000, an estimated 84% of persons age 65 years and older were non-Hispanic white, 8% were non-Hispanic black, and 6% were Hispanic. By 2050, the percent of white elders will decline to 64%, and Hispanics and non-Hispanic blacks will account for 16% and 12% of the older population, respectively.[11]

Contrary to popular thinking, most older persons are self-sufficient and live in the community. However, as they age in the community, the likelihood of living alone increases, more so for women than men. Only 4.5% of older persons reside in a long-term care facility, which has decreased since 1990 (5.1%). As expected, most of the older adults residing in nursing homes are 85 years of age and older (50%), followed by persons 75 to 84 years of age (16.9%) and those 65 to 74 years of age (13.5%).[3]

An important goal in the care of older adults is to maintain independence and avoid the need for institutionalization for as long as possible. Functional loss or disability is often a final common pathway of most clinical problems in older persons, especially in those over age 75. In 2000, 28.6% of elders reported a physical disability (e.g., walking, climbing stairs, reaching, lifting, or carrying), and 9.5% reported disability with self-care or basic activities of daily living (ADLs) (e.g., dressing, bathing, getting around inside the home, feeding, toileting, and grooming).[12] Disability increases with increasing age and is higher in institutionalized older persons, where approximately 80% have some problems with mobility and 65% have difficulty controlling their bowels.[13] Segments of the population that are especially vulnerable to disability include women, minorities, and those in lower socioeconomic classes. Recent data suggest that disability rates declined significantly during the 1990s. The decline in late-life disability was greatest for limitations in instrumental activities of daily living (IADLs) (e.g., housekeeping chores, shopping, going outside, medication management) and physical disability. Conflicting evidence exists for basic ADL disability, the most severe type of disability that often leads to institutionalization.[14] Nonetheless, whether disability rates will continue to decline is debatable and depends on changes in the environment, changes in social roles, changes in the use of assistive devices, advancements in medicine and pharmacy, and changes in elders' education levels.[8]

A chronic condition, defined as an illness or impairment that cannot be cured, is often the cause of disability in the elderly. The older population compared with younger persons is more affected by chronic conditions for several reasons: (1) the types of chronic conditions common among older persons tend to be more disabling (e.g., arthritis, heart disease), (2) the conditions become more severe with aging, and (3) several conditions are likely to be present.[15]

The most common chronic conditions of older Americans depend on their residence status. For noninstitutionalized older Americans, the list has changed little in the past decade.[16] These conditions, in rank order of prevalence, include arthritis (45%), high blood pressure (34%), hearing impairments (28%), heart disease (25%), cataracts (16%), orthopedic impairments (15%), sinusitis (11%), diabetes (9%), tinnitus (8%), and visual impairments (8%).[16,17] For elderly patients admitted to a nursing home, the common primary diagnoses are cardiovascular or cerebrovascular disease, mental disorders, nervous system or sensory impairment, and complications secondary to injuries.[17] A national report released in 2000 noted that one-third of all elderly hospital admissions were due to cardiovascular disease, 14% were due to respiratory problems, 6.5% were due to fractures, and 6.3% were due to cancer.[18]

Figure 8–1 illustrates the top 10 causes of death in elders. The ranking of these causes has changed little over the last 20 years. Some important trends have emerged over the past two decades, however. First, there has been a decrease in the death rate for heart disease and stroke. This trend is secondary to the gains made in the prevention and treatment of these diseases. Second, death secondary to Alzheimer's disease has increased rapidly in recent years (9% from 1999 to 2000). This increase in rate may be because of the improvements in diagnosis and awareness in the medical community.[9]

Elders are avid consumers of medical and prescription drug resources. With older persons accounting for 36% of all hospital stays and 49% of all days of care in hospitals, elders consume almost one-third of total U.S. health care expenditures.[19] By 2030, health care spending by the U.S. population is projected to increase by 25% simply because of aging demographics.[19] Although older persons comprise 12.4% of the U.S. population, they account for 34% of all prescription drug expenditures.[20] Overall in 2002, prescription drug spending was estimated to be between $91 and $117 billion.[21] For those over the age of 65, national estimates in 2000 indicated that elders fill nearly 20 prescriptions per year and that their average expenditure for prescription drugs was $1102.[22] Nearly one-half of adults have prescription drug coverage that is limited or intermittent, and one-third of elders have no prescription benefit.[20] Hopefully, this problem with prescription coverage for elders will be addressed in the near future with an additional Medicare benefit.

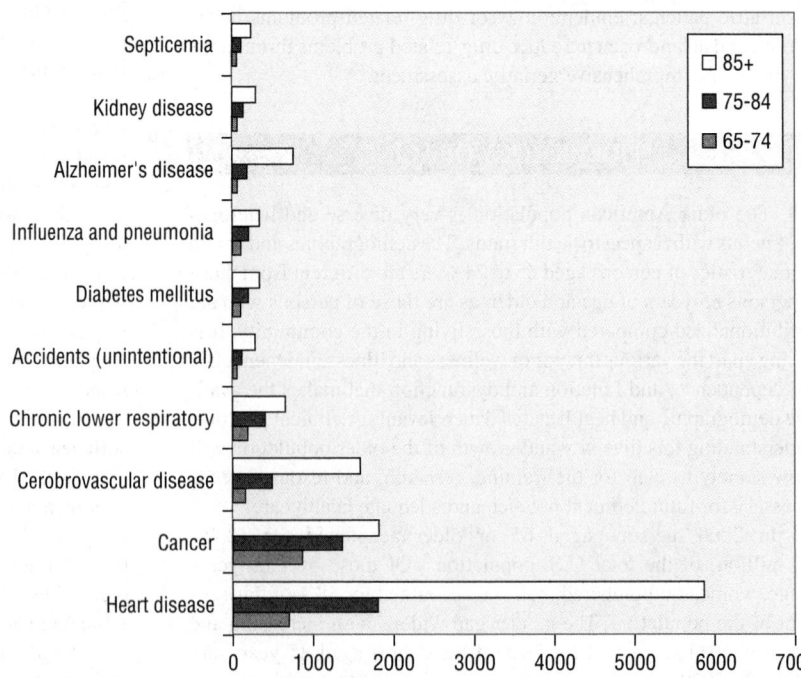

FIGURE 8–1. Leading causes of death in 2000: age-adjusted death rates. Rates per 100,000 population in specified age group. *(Data from Miniño AM, Arias E, Kochanek KD, et al. Deaths: Final Data for 2000. Natl Vital Stat Rep 2002;50:1–120.)*

HUMAN AGING AND CHANGES IN DRUG PHARMACOKINETICS AND PHARMACODYNAMICS

2 There is a progressive functional decline in many organ systems with advancing age. Table 8–1 reviews some common physiologic changes with an emphasis on those which can affect pharmacotherapy. For more detailed information, readers are referred to excellent reviews.[23,24]

Age-associated physiologic changes may cause reductions in functional reserve capacity (i.e., the ability to respond to physiologic challenges or stresses) and the ability to preserve homeostasis, thus making an elder susceptible to decompensation in a stressful situation.[25,26] To deal with physiologic challenges or stresses, an older individual may require up to 95% of his or her remaining reserve capacity.[23,24] The cardiovascular, musculoskeletal, and central nervous systems appear to be most affected.[24] Examples of impaired homeostatic mechanisms include postural or gait stability, orthostatic blood pressure responses, thermoregulation, cognitive reserve, and bowel and bladder function. An event resulting in functional impairment may involve an insult for which the body cannot compensate, and relatively small stresses may result in major morbidity and mortality.[25]

A number of age-related physiologic changes occur that potentially could affect drug pharmacokinetics and pharmacodynamics

TABLE 8–1. Physiologic Changes with Aging[23,24]

Organ System	Manifestation
Body composition	↓ Total body water
	↓ Lean body mass
	↑ Body fat
	↔ or ↓ Serum albumin
	↔ or ↑ α_1-Acid glycoprotein (↑ by several disease states)
Cardiovascular	↓ Myocardial sensitivity to beta-adrenergic stimulation
	↓ Baroreceptor activity
	↓ Cardiac output
	↑ Total peripheral resistance
Central nervous system	↓ Weight and volume of the brain
	Alterations in several aspects of cognition
Endocrine	Thyroid gland atrophies with age
	Increase in incidence of diabetes mellitus, thyroid disease
	Menopause
Gastrointestinal	↑ Gastric pH
	↓ Gastrointestinal blood flow
	Delayed gastric emptying
	Slowed intestinal transit
Genitourinary	Atrophy of the vagina due to decreased estrogen
	Prostatic hypertrophy due to androgenic hormonal changes
	Age-related changes may predispose to incontinence
Immune	↓ Cell-mediated immunity
Liver	↓ Liver size
	↓ Liver blood flow
Oral	Altered dentition
	↓ Ability to taste sweetness, sourness, and bitterness
Pulmonary	↓ Respiratory muscle strength
	↓ Chest wall compliance
	↓ Total alveolar surface
	↓ Vital capacity
	↓ Maximal breathing capacity
Renal	↓ Glomerular filtration rate
	↓ Renal blood flow
	↑ Filtration fraction
	↓ Tubular secretory function
	↓ Renal mass
Sensory	↓ Accommodation of the lens of the eye, causing farsightedness
	Presbycusis (loss of auditory acuity)
	↓ Conduction velocity
Skeletal	Loss of skeletal bone mass (osteopenia)
Skin/hair	Skin dryness, wrinkling, and changes in pigmentation, epithelial thinning, loss of dermal thickness
	↓ Number of hair follicles
	↓ Number of melanocytes in the hair bulbs

(see Table 8–1). Unfortunately, limited data are available regarding the pharmacokinetics and pharmacodynamics of individual drugs commonly used in the elderly. This information gap may improve with the implementation of Food and Drug Administration (FDA) guidelines calling for pharmacokinetic studies by pharmaceutical companies for new molecular entities likely to have significant use in the elderly.[27]

ALTERED PHARMACOKINETICS

Table 8–2 and the following discussion summarize what is known about the effect of aging on each of the four major facets of pharmacokinetics.[26,28,29]

ABSORPTION

Most drugs are given orally, and thus a number of the age-related changes in gastrointestinal physiology potentially could affect the absorption of medications. Fortunately, most drugs are absorbed via passive diffusion, and age-related physiologic changes appear to have little influence on drug bioavailability.[30] A few drugs require active transport for their absorption, and thus their bioavailability may be reduced (e.g., calcium in the setting of hypochlorhydria). However, there is evidence for a decreased first-pass effect on hepatic and/or gut wall metabolism that results in increased bioavailability and higher plasma concentrations of drugs such as propranolol and morphine.[30] Increased drug bioavailability also may be seen with the concurrent ingestion of grapefruit juice. Constituents of this product inhibit cytochrome P450 (CYP450) isoenzyme 3A4, thus decreasing first-pass metabolism and resulting in exaggerated pharmacologic effects.[31]

DISTRIBUTION

The distribution of medications in the body depends on factors such as blood flow, plasma protein binding, and body composition, each of which may be altered with age. For example, the volume of distribution of water-soluble drugs is decreased, whereas lipophilic drugs will exhibit an increased volume of distribution.[26,28,29] Changes in the volume of distribution can have a direct impact on the amount of medication that needs to be given as a loading dose.

The two major plasma proteins to which medications can bind are albumin and α_1-acid glycoprotein (AAG), and concentrations of these proteins may change with concurrent pathologies seen with increasing age.[32] For acidic drugs such as naproxen, phenytoin, tolbutamide,

and warfarin, decreased serum albumin may lead to an increase in free fraction. An increase in AAG induced by burns, cancer, inflammatory disease, or trauma may lead to a decreased free fraction of basic drugs such as lidocaine, propranolol, quinidine, and imipramine. In the absence of compromise in excretory pathways, these potential changes are unlikely to have any deleterious clinical effect. However, they may be important to consider when interpreting serum concentrations of these drugs because usually only total drug concentrations (sum of free and protein-bound drug) are reported.

METABOLISM

The liver is the major organ responsible for drug metabolism, including phase I (oxidative) and phase II (conjugative) reactions.[33] The most remarkable characteristic of liver function in the elderly is the increase in interindividual variability compared with other age groups, a feature that may obscure true age-related changes.[33] Recent data suggest that age-related declines in phase I metabolism are more likely the result of reduced liver volume rather than reduced hepatic enzymatic activity.[34] Decreased phase I metabolism (e.g., hydroxylation, dealkylation) producing decreased drug clearance and increased terminal disposition half-life ($t_{1/2}$) has been reported in elders for medications such as diazepam, piroxicam, theophylline, and quinidine. Phase II metabolism (e.g., glucuronidation, acetylation) of medications such as lorazepam and oxazepam appears to be relatively unaffected by advancing age. Hepatic enzyme induction (e.g., by rifampin, phenytoin) or inhibition (e.g., by fluoroquinolone and macrolide antimicrobials, cimetidine) does not appear to be affected by the aging process.[33,35]

Age-related decreases in liver blood flow also can decrease significantly the metabolism of high-hepatic-extraction-ratio drugs such as imipramine, lidocaine, morphine, and propranolol.[33] The effect of aging on polymorphic drug metabolism has not been well studied. Advancing age has been reported both to have no significant effect and to reduce significantly the activity of CYP450 3A4.[36,37] Other available data suggest that advancing age has no significant effect on drug acetylation or CYP450 2D6 or 2C9 isoenzyme-mediated metabolism.[38–41] Finally, a number of potential confounding factors, including race, sex, frailty, smoking, diet, and drug-drug interactions, may affect hepatic metabolism significantly in the elderly.[33]

ELIMINATION

Renal excretion is the primary route of elimination for many drugs. Although age-related reductions in glomerular filtration are well

TABLE 8–2. Age-Related Changes in Drug Pharmacokinetics[26,28,29]

Pharmacokinetic Phase	Pharmacokinetic Parameters
Gastrointestinal absorption	Unchanged passive diffusion and no change in bioavailability for most drugs ↓ Active transport and ↓ bioavailability for some drugs ↓ First-pass extraction and ↑ bioavailability for some drugs
Distribution	↓ Volume of distribution and ↑ plasma concentration of water-soluble drugs ↑ Volume of distribution and ↑ terminal disposition half-life ($t_{1/2}$) for fat-soluble drugs ↑ or ↓ Free fraction of highly plasma protein bound drugs
Hepatic metabolism	↓ Clearance and ↑ $t_{1/2}$ for some oxidatively metabolized drugs ↓ Clearance and ↑ $t_{1/2}$ of drugs with high hepatic extraction ratios
Renal excretion	↓ Clearance and ↑ $t_{1/2}$ of renally eliminated drugs and active metabolites

documented, as many as one-third of "normal" elderly subjects may have no reduction, as measured by creatinine clearance.[26,28,29] Moreover, emerging information suggests that renal tubular secretion may not decline in proportion to other renal processes.[42] The estimation of creatinine clearance, although not entirely accurate in individual patients, can serve as a useful screening approximation. One of the most commonly used equations for adults with stable renal function and whose actual weight is within 30% of their ideal body weight was created by Cockcroft and Gault[43]:

$$\text{Creatinine clearance (males)} = \frac{(140 - \text{age in years})(\text{actual body weight in kg})}{72(\text{serum creatinine in mg/dL})}$$

For females, multiply this result by 0.85.

Medications whose excretion is primarily renal and for which there is evidence of age-related reduction in renal and total body clearance include (but are not limited to) amantadine, aminoglycosides, atenolol, captopril, cimetidine, digoxin, lithium, and vancomycin. Some hepatically metabolized medications can yield active, primarily renally excreted metabolites such as N-acetylprocainamide, normeperidine, and morphine-6-glucuronide, which can accumulate with advancing age owing to reduced renal function.

CLINICAL CONTROVERSY

When estimating creatinine clearance in the elderly using the Cockcroft and Gault equation, some clinicians choose to round the value up to 1 if the patient's serum creatinine concentration is less than 1. Rounding the serum creatinine concentration may provide an underestimation of creatinine clearance and result in improper dose adjustment of renally eliminated medications. It is important to realize that the equation is merely an estimate, and attempts should be made to determine creatinine clearance accurately with certain medications (e.g., metformin).

ALTERED PHARMACODYNAMICS

There is some evidence in the elderly of altered drug response or "sensitivity." Four possible mechanisms have been suggested: (1) changes in receptor numbers, (2) changes in receptor affinity, (3) postreceptor alterations, and 4) age-related impairment of homeostatic mechanisms.[26,44,45] For example, muscarinic, parathyroid hormone, β-adrenergic, α_1-adrenergic, and μ-opioid receptors exhibit reduced density with increasing age.[26,44,45] Evidence from epidemiologic and experimental studies suggest that, independent of pharmacokinetic alterations, the elderly are more sensitive to the central nervous system effects of benzodiazepines.[26,44,45] The elderly also exhibit a greater analgesic responsiveness to opioids when compared with their younger counterparts, even when pharmacokinetic parameters are similar in the two groups.[26,44,45] In addition, the elderly demonstrate an enhanced responsiveness to anticoagulants such as warfarin and heparin, as well as thrombolytic therapy.[26,44,45] In contrast, the elderly exhibit decreased responsiveness to certain drugs (e.g., β-agonists/antagonists).[26,44,45] Also, reflex tachycardia, seen commonly with vasodilator therapy, is often blunted in the elderly, perhaps owing to dampened baroreceptor function. For some drugs (e.g., calcium channel blockers), both enhanced responsiveness (as demonstrated by greater reduction in blood pressure) and

decreased responsiveness (as demonstrated by reduced atrioventricular nodal blockade) can occur simultaneously in elders.[26,44,45]

CLINICAL GERIATRICS

Maintenance of independence and prevention of disability are primary goals in the clinical care of persons 65 years of age or older. To achieve these goals, it is necessary that all health care professionals understand the concept of functional status. Functional status is a proxy measure of a patient's ability to live independently and can be determined in part by inquiring about an elderly person's ability to perform specific tasks. As mentioned previously, there are two types of functional measurements: ADLs and the more complex IADLs.[46,47] However, to assess functional status fully, the patient's psychological state, financial resources, physical function, and social circumstances must be considered as well.[1]

One of the challenges of maintaining and improving functional status in geriatric individuals is recognizing and managing conditions frequently seen in older adults. Problems found more commonly in older persons sometimes are referred to as the "I's of geriatrics"[23] (Table 8-3). These problems are often due to underlying disease processes that may or may not be diagnosed. Examples of diseases and syndromes that can present as common problems in the elderly include Parkinson's disease, falls, hip fractures, benign prostatic hypertrophy, dementia, glaucoma, postherpetic neuralgia, and tuberculosis.

Another factor contributing to the challenge of clinical geriatrics is that approximately 50% of older patients present with atypical symptoms or complaints, making it difficult to use the classic medical model for diagnosis. For example, cardiac ischemia may present as syncope or weakness in an older person rather than the typical presentation of chest pain. Confusion may be the presenting symptom of an acute abdominal process rather than the expected severe pain, rigidity of the abdominal muscles, and leukocytosis. Serious adverse consequences may result if a diagnosis is delayed or missed because of these atypical presentations. Such unusual presentations may be due to age-related physiologic changes, the presence of multiple comorbid illnesses or compromised function, and the presence of psychological stressors.[48] Table 8-4 presents additional examples of medical illnesses that often present atypically in the elderly.[48-50] For very frail older adults, delirium, falls, and nonspecific functional decline frequently are presenting problems.[48-50]

Multiple coexisting chronic illnesses are another common threat to independence that distinguishes the elderly from younger patients. It is not unusual for elderly patients to have multiple comorbidities such as osteoarthritis, heart disease, and diabetes. Although multiple comorbidities can have a substantial impact on a patient's functional status, the mere existence of multiple diseases alone does not determine functional impairment.

TABLE 8-3. The I's of Geriatrics: Common Problems in the Elderly[23]

Immobility	Instability
Isolation	Intellectual impairment
Incontinence	Impotence
Infection	Immunodeficiency
Inanition (malnutrition)	Insomnia
Impaction	Iatrogenesis
Impaired senses	

TABLE 8–4. Atypical Disease Presentation in the Elderly[48–50]

Disease	Presentation
Acute myocardial infarction	Only about 50% present with chest pain. In general, the elderly present with weakness, confusion, syncope, and abdominal pain; however, electrocardiographic findings are similar to younger patients.
Congestive heart failure	Instead of dyspnea, the older patient may present with hypoxic symptoms, lethargy, restlessness, and confusion.
Gastrointestinal bleed	Although the mortality rate is about 10%, presenting symptoms are nonspecific, ranging from mental status change to syncope with hemodynamic collapse. Abdominal pain is often absent.
Upper respiratory infection	Older patients typically present with lethargy, confusion, anorexia, and decompensation of a preexisting medical condition. Fever, chills, and a productive cough may or may not be present.
Urinary tract infection	Dysuria, fever, and flank pain may be absent. More commonly, the elderly present with incontinence, confusion, abdominal pain, nausea/vomiting, and azotemia.

DRUG-RELATED PROBLEMS IN THE ELDERLY

Although medications used by the elderly can lead to improvement in HRQOL, negative outcomes owing to drug-related problems are considerable.[51,52] Three important and potentially preventable negative outcomes owing to drug-related problems that can occur in the elderly are adverse drug withdrawal events (ADWEs), which are clinically significant sets of symptoms or signs caused by the removal of a drug; therapeutic failure (inadequate or inappropriate drug therapy and not related to the natural progression of disease); and adverse drug reactions (ADRs), defined as a reaction that is noxious and unintended and which occurs at dosages normally used in humans for prophylaxis, diagnosis, or therapy.[53–55]

Limited data are available about the prevalence of ADWEs and therapeutic failures in the elderly. Graves and colleagues[53] reported ADWEs in 38 of 124 male outpatients who had 238 medications discontinued. Grymonpre and coworkers[54] reported that 19% of drug-associated hospital admissions in a group of older Canadians were related to therapeutic failure. ADRs occur commonly in elders, with reported rates ranging from 2.5% to 50.6% depending on the study population and methodology employed.[52] In a recent large study of more than 30,000 Medicare outpatients, Gurwitz and colleagues[56] reported that 5% experienced an ADR in a period of 1 year, with more serious reactions more likely to be preventable. ADRs and other drug-related problems (e.g., ADWEs, therapeutic failure) are major threats to the HRQOL of outpatient elders and account for billions of health care dollars per year.[52,57,58] In the nursing home setting alone, a cost-of-illness study estimated that drug-related problems (including ADRs and therapeutic failure) cost $4 billion per year.[59]

RISK FACTORS

A number of factors are believed to increase the risk of drug-related problems in the elderly, including suboptimal prescribing (e.g., overuse of medications or polypharmacy, inappropriate use, and underuse), medication errors (both dispensing and administration problems), and patient medication nonadherence (both intentional and unintentional). The following subsections address suboptimal prescribing and medication nonadherence, the most common problems.

OVERUSE

Polypharmacy can be defined as either the concomitant use of multiple drugs or the administration of more medications than are indicated clinically.[60,61] Polypharmacy is common and increasing among the elderly. Community-based surveys reveal that elders take an average of 2.7 to 4.2 prescription and nonprescription medications each day.[61,62] A recent study of community-dwelling elders in Finland reported an increase in polypharmacy, growing most in the oldest old.[63] Increased use of dietary supplements, such as herbal products, vitamins, and minerals, may add to the increase in polypharmacy. Kaufman and colleagues[64] found in a nationwide survey that 59% of women and 46% of men older than age 65 used a vitamin or mineral supplement and that 14% of these women and 11% of these men used an herbal product. The use of drugs increases to an average of 5 medications in elders who are hospitalized.[62] A recent nursing facility survey found that institutionalized elderly persons take an average of 6.69 routine medications and that 27.1% took 9 or more medications on a regular basis.[65] Drug-use studies that defined polypharmacy as use of one or more unnecessary medications showed that this occurs in 55% to 59% of elderly outpatients.[66,67] Multiple medication use has been strongly associated with ADRs.[52] Polypharmacy is also problematic for elderly patients because it may increase the risk of geriatric syndromes (e.g., falls, cognitive impairment), diminished functional status, and health care costs.[60,61,68]

INAPPROPRIATE PRESCRIBING

Inappropriate prescribing can be defined as prescribing of medications outside the bounds of accepted medical standards.[68] This phenomenon occurs commonly in elderly outpatients, as exemplified by one study in which 74% of drugs had at least one inappropriate rating based on clinical review applying explicit criteria.[66] Studies using explicit drug-use review criteria have found that between 7% and 53% of community-dwelling elders take one or more medications that have a dose, duration, duplication, or drug-interaction problem.[68,69]

Alternatively, *inappropriate prescribing* can be defined as prescribing of drugs whose use should be avoided because their risk outweighs their potential benefit.[70] Applying explicit criteria developed by Beers and colleagues, different investigators have found that between 14% and 27% of persons 65 years of age and older living in the community take one or more drugs whose use should be avoided.[70,71]

The Beers criteria were updated recently.[72] At present, it is not clear what is the best way to measure inappropriate prescribing. Global measures for detecting polypharmacy or unnecessary drug use and underuse of essential medications are needed, as well as additional studies examining drug-disease interactions and other health outcomes. Moreover, we recommend further studies of the predictive validity of evidence-based standards for measuring inappropriate medications in the elderly.

Inappropriate prescribing may pose important health risks. Limited retrospective data suggest that inappropriate prescribing is associated with drug-related hospital admissions and readmissions.[68] Hanlon and colleagues[73,74] reported on community-dwelling elderly taking any inappropriate drug as defined by drug utilization review explicit criteria from the Centers for Medicare and Medicaid Services. They found that elders with inappropriate drug use, especially those with potential drug-drug or drug-disease interactions, were more likely to report problems in basic self-care (e.g., toileting, dressing, eating, transferring, and grooming) and had more outpatient physician visits.

UNDERUSE

An important and increasingly recognized problem in elders is *underuse*, defined as the omission of drug therapy that is indicated for the treatment or prevention of a disease or condition.[75] One study found that 55% of 236 ambulatory elderly patients had one or more necessary drugs omitted because of lack of physician prescribing.[75] Another study of community-dwelling elders examined whether unrelated disorders are less likely to be treated in patients with chronic diseases.[76] They found that patients with diabetes mellitus were less likely to receive estrogen-replacement therapy, that patients with pulmonary emphysema were less likely to receive lipid-lowering medications, and that patients with psychotic syndromes were less likely to receive medications for arthritis.[76] Other investigators have focused on the omission of treatment of certain conditions such as asthma, cardiovascular disease, dyslipidemia, osteoporosis, pain, hypertension, cancer chemotherapy, and depression and underuse of angiotensin-converting enzyme (ACE) inhibitor medications in patients with congestive heart failure (CHF), anticoagulation in elderly patients with atrial fibrillation, and preventive therapy after myocardial infarction.[68,75,77]

Underuse may have an important relationship with negative health outcomes in the elderly, including functional disability, death, and health services use.[68] The risk from underuse of medication in general owing to limiting Medicaid patients' access to medications resulted in a more than doubling of the risk of admission to a nursing home.[78] Tamblyn and colleagues[79] studied the effects of a deductible and 25% coinsurance fee from medications taken by elders from Canada. This reform led to a decrease in the number of essential medications (e.g., furosemide, anticoagulants, ACE inhibitors) used by elderly patients and increasing costs owing to adverse events and emergency department visits.[79]

MEDICATION NONADHERENCE

Medication nonadherence is a common problem in the elderly.[80–82] The prevalence rate ranges from 40% to 80% of patients (mean of approximately 50%).[80–82] Overall, the elderly are adherent with about 75% of their medications.[80–82] The elderly have similar adherence to younger patients when the number of drugs taken by both groups is similar.[83] In fact, there is some evidence that adherence may be better in elders for some conditions.[84,85] What does seem to be different is that intentional nonadherence may be more common in the elderly.[86] This may be related to the occurrence of ADRs and may represent intelligent nonadherence. A study by Fincke and coworkers[87] found that elders who perceived that they were overmedicated were more likely to have decreased adherence.

Limited retrospective data suggest that nonadherence is associated with increased health services use and adverse drug reactions. A meta-analysis of studies published by Sullivan and associates[88] that included patients of all ages determined that the rate of hospital admissions owing to nonadherence was 5.5%. A study by Col and coworkers[89] evaluated 315 consecutive elderly patients admitted to a hospital and determined that 11.4% of admissions resulted from nonadherence. Gurwitz and colleagues[56] found that 21% of preventable ADRs in elderly outpatients were due to errors in patient adherence.

Given that drug-related problems are common, costly, and clinically important, how can they be prevented/managed? A solution may lie in comprehensive geriatric assessment. The term *comprehensive geriatric assessment* has been applied to geriatric evaluation and management (GEM), in which GEM clinicians manage the patient, and to consultative geriatric assessment, in which the geriatric multidisciplinary team makes recommendations to other clinicians for management of the patient. Comprehensive geriatric assessment has become a cornerstone in the care of the elderly; its effectiveness was summarized recently in a meta-analysis of 28 controlled trials and a randomized, multicenter, controlled trial of frail elderly veterans.[90,91]

Pharmacists can play a major role in optimizing pharmacotherapy for the elderly. A recent article summarized the results from 13 randomized, controlled studies that clinical pharmacy interventions can reduce drug-related problems and improve health outcomes in the elderly.[92] The following subsections provide an approach to how pharmacists in any practice setting can optimize medication use through the provision of comprehensive geriatric assessment.

HISTORY TAKING

Several potential difficulties may occur while taking medication histories from the elderly. They include (1) communication problems (impaired hearing and vision), (2) underreporting (health beliefs, cognitive impairment), (3) vague or nonspecific symptoms (altered presentation), (4) multiple diseases and medications, (5) reliance on a caregiver for the history, and (6) lack of medical records to confirm findings. Despite these potential difficulties, health care professionals should find value in pursuing the collection of this vital medication history information. The importance of inquiry regarding nonprescription medication use in the elderly cannot be stressed enough because one-third of all medications used by the ambulatory elderly are sold without a prescription, especially analgesics and laxatives.[93] Moreover, with the passage of the Dietary Supplement Health and Education Act of 1994, it is important to probe about use of dietary supplements, including vitamins and minerals, herbal agents, and products such as glucosamine and chondroitin.

TABLE 8–5. Medication Appropriateness Index[98,99]

Questions to ask about each individual medication:
1. Is there an indication for the medication?
2. Is the medication effective for the condition?
3. Is the dosage correct?
4. Are the directions correct?
5. Are the directions practical?
6. Are there clinically significant drug-drug interactions?
7. Are there clinically significant drug-disease/condition interactions?
8. Is there unnecessary duplication with other medication(s)?
9. Is the duration of therapy acceptable?
10. Is this medication the least expensive alternative compared with others of equal utility?

Asking elders and their caregivers about methods they use to keep track of medicines is also important. This will allow one to design solutions to the problems detected and prevent repeating ineffective and previously used methods.

Patients and caregivers also should be asked about risk factors for prescribing problems (e.g., multiple physicians and pharmacies) and for adherence problems (e.g., impaired hearing, vision, and cognition and ability to open safety caps, pay for medicines, and swallow medications).[94]

ASSESSING AND MONITORING DRUG THERAPY

The appropriateness of each prescribed medication should be assessed using a variety of methods.[95–97] One standardized measure that has demonstrated reliability and validity is the Medication Appropriateness Index (MAI).[98,99] The MAI consists of 10 questions that should be asked about each medication (Table 8–5).

Several other factors that are not included in the MAI also should be assessed[95]: (1) suboptimal medication choice (based on effectiveness, safety, cost, and effects on HRQOL), (2) allergy (especially for new prescriptions), (3) undertreatment, and (4) drug interactions with food or laboratory tests. Some additional factors to consider during drug regimen review include adherence, medication storage problems, laboratory monitoring, therapeutic end points, and ADRs.

CLINICAL CONTROVERSY

An increasing number of clinical trials are enrolling elderly patients. For example, we now have evidence to support the cardiac benefits of pravastatin in the elderly.[100] Clinicians must weigh the risks and benefits of adding drug therapy to a patient's drug regimen because increasing the number of drugs may decrease adherence and can lead to an increased risk of ADRs. Furthermore, a clinician must decide if it is ethical to add drug therapy in patients who may not live long enough to benefit from the medication.

DOCUMENTING PROBLEMS AND FORMULATING A THERAPEUTIC PLAN

The clinician must document the problems that have been detected, develop a therapeutic plan to resolve them, and establish reasonable therapeutic end points if these have not been set already. An important point to remember is that what may be a reasonable end point for a 40-year-old patient may not be as reasonable for an 80-year-old person when comorbidities, functional status, and life expectancy are taken into consideration.

CONSULTING THE PHYSICIAN REGARDING PROBLEMS AND CONCERNS

In some cases, the pharmacist or other health care professional must contact a patient's physician regarding problems and concerns that have been detected and documented. In discussing the patient in this context, the importance of optimizing the prescribing for elderly patients before implementing strategies to enhance their adherence cannot be overstressed. Otherwise, the adherence intervention, if effective, may result in patient harm. Similarly, in institutional settings, strategies to reduce medication administration errors may not improve patient outcomes if prescribing is not improved beforehand.

COUNSELING AND ADHERENCE AIDS

Some general factors to consider, before medication dispensing, to enhance adherence in the elderly include modifying medication schedules to fit patients' lifestyles, considering generic agents to reduce costs, using easy-to-open bottles and easy-to-swallow dosage forms, and using larger-type direction labels and auxiliary labels.[80] When dispensing medications (in particular, new medications or old ones that have changed in appearance or directions for use), both written and oral drug information should be provided to the patient and caregiver.

To improve the likelihood of adherence, the health care professional also should recruit active patient and caregiver involvement, stress the importance of adherence, and consider the use of adherence-enhancing aids (e.g., special packaging, a medication record, a drug calendar, medication boxes, magnification for insulin syringes, dose-measuring devices, and spacers for metered-dose inhalers).[101,102] In institutional settings, discussion of special considerations (e.g., medications that can be crushed and given via feeding tube) with health care professionals responsible for medication administration is also prudent.

DOCUMENTING INTERVENTIONS AND MONITORING PATIENT PROGRESS

All interventions must be documented, and the steps just outlined must be repeated over time with elderly patients. During follow-up contacts, minimum inquiry should include questions as to whether the patient has any questions or concerns regarding medicines and determining whether the therapeutic end points previously established have been achieved. Moreover, ask patients whether they are or have recently experienced any side effects, unwanted reactions, or other problems with their medications to assess potential ADRs.[52]

TARGETING HIGH-RISK ELDERLY

In busy practices, the approach outlined here may not be feasible for every patient. Therefore, practitioners may consider targeting these activities to patients at high risk for developing drug-related problems. Geriatric experts have identified 18 risk factors for drug-related problems in elderly nursing home patients.[103] These include the following medication-related factors: (1) polypharmacy (e.g., 9 or more medications or 12 or more doses per day), (2) taking specific high-risk drugs (e.g., intermediate- and long-half-life benzodiazepines, sedative-hypnotic agents, antipsychotic drugs, anticholinergic medications, opioid analgesics, and chlorpropamide), (3) certain patient characteristics (e.g., low body weight, age 85 years or older, and decreased renal function), (4) use of narrow-therapeutic-range drugs (e.g., lithium, digoxin, warfarin, and anticonvulsants), (5) a history of a prior ADR, and (6) presence of six or more illnesses. The applicability of these criteria to elderly persons in other care settings and the relationship between identification of elderly patients with these potential risk factors and actual health outcomes remain to be determined.[56]

CONCLUSION

The number of people older than age 65 years is growing in the United States and around the world, and the fastest growing segment of the American population is those over age 85. A number of physiologic changes with age affect pharmacokinetics and pharmacodynamics of drugs, especially hepatic metabolism and renal excretion. Improving and maintaining functional status and managing comorbidities are hallmarks of clinical geriatrics. Certain medical conditions are restricted to the elderly, and drug-related problems represent a major concern for this group. Innovative approaches, such as the provision of comprehensive geriatric assessment by pharmacists and other health care professionals, are needed to decrease the occurrence of these drug-related problems.

ABBREVIATIONS

HRQOL: health-related quality of life
ADLs: activities of daily living (e.g., dressing, bathing, getting around inside the home, feeding, toileting, grooming)
IADLs: instrumental activities of daily living (e.g., housekeeping chores, shopping, going outside, medication management)
FDA: Food and Drug Administration
CYP450: cytochrome P450
AAG: α_1-acid glycoprotein
ADRs: adverse drug reactions
ADWEs: adverse drug withdrawal events
ACE: angiotensin-converting enzyme
CHF: congestive heart failure
GEM: geriatric evaluation and management
MAI: Medication Appropriateness Index

Review Questions and other resources can be found at *www.pharmacotherapyonline.com.*

REFERENCES

1. Rubenstein LZ, Rubenstein LV. Multidimensional geriatric assessment. In: Tallis R, Fillit H, eds. Brocklehurst's Textbook of Geriatric Medicine, 6th ed. London, Churchill-Livingstone, 2003:291–299.
2. Hobbs F, Stoops N. Demographic Trends in the 20th Century: Census 2000 Special Reports. November Report Number CENSR-4. Washington, US Department of Commerce, Economics and Statistics Administration, US Census Bureau, 2002.
3. Hetzel L, Smith A. The 65 Years and Over Population: 2000. Census 2000 Brief. October Report Number C2KBR/01-10. Washington, US Department of Commerce, Economics and Statistics Administration, U.S. Census Bureau; 2001.
4. US Bureau of the Census. Current Population Reports: Special Studies. Washington, US Department of Commerce, Economics and Statistics Administration.1997:23–193.
5. Horiuchi S. Demography: Greater lifetime expectations. Nature 2000;405:744–745.
6. Fries JF, Green LW, Levine S. Health promotion and the compression of morbidity. Lancet 1989;1:481–483.
7. Kane RL, Ouslander JG, Abrass IB. The geriatric patient: Demography, epidemiology and health services utilization. In: Essentials of Clinical Geriatrics. 5th ed. New York, McGraw-Hill, 2004:17–33.
8. National Center for Health Statistics. Annual Report on Nation's Health Spotlights Elderly Americans. Hyattsville, MD, US Department of Health and Human Services, 1999.
9. Miniño AM, Arias E, Kochanek KD, et al. Deaths: Final data for 2000. Vital Health Stat 2002;50:1–120.
10. Velkoff VA. New Census Report Shows Exponential Growth in Number of Centenarians. Washington, National Institutes of Health, National Institute of Aging, 1999.
11. Federal Interagency Forum on Aging-Related Statistics. Older Americans 2000: Key Indicators of Well-Being; available at *www.agingstats. gov,* August 2000.
12. Waldrop J, Stern SM. Disability Status: 2000. Census 2000 Brief. March Report Number C2KBR-17. Washington, US Department of Commerce, Economics and Statistics Administration, US Census Bureau; 2003.
13. National Center for Health Statistics. Health, United States, 2000. Hyattsville, MD, US Department of Health and Human Services, 2000.
14. Freedman VA, Martin LG, Schoeni RF. Recent trends in disability and functioning among older adults in the United States: A systematic review. JAMA 2002;288:3137–3146.
15. National Academy on an Aging Society. Challenges for the 21st Century: Chronic and Disabling Conditions. Washington, Gerontological Society of America, 1999.
16. National Center for Health Statistics. Current estimates from the National Health Interview Survey, 1994. Vital Health Stat 1995;10:81–82.
17. National Center for Health Statistics. Current estimates from the National Health Interview Survey, 1996. Vital Health Stat 1999;10:81–82.
18. National Center for Health Statistics. 1998 Summary: National Hospital Discharge Survey. Washington, US Department of Health and Human Services, Centers for Disease Control and Prevention, Advance Data, 2000:316:1–8.
19. National Center for Chronic Disease Prevention and Health Promotion. Healthy Aging: Preventing Disease and Improving Quality of Life Among Older Americans: At-a-Glance 2000. Atlanta, Centers for Disease Control and Prevention, 2000.
20. Stuart B, Shea D, Briesacher B: Dynamics in drug coverage of Medicare beneficiaries: Finders, losers, switchers. Health Affairs 2001;20:86–99.
21. Henry J. Kaiser Foundation: Medicare and prescription drugs, fact sheet; available at *http://www.kff.org/content/2003/1583-06/1583-06.pdf;* accessed on August 26, 2003.
22. Stagnitti MN: MEPS Medical Expenditure Panel Survey. Statistical Brief 21: Trends in Outpatient Prescription Drug Utilization and Expenditures: 1997–2000; available at *http://www.meps.ahrq.gov/papers/ st21/stat21.htm#Introduction;* accessed on August 20, 2003.
23. Kane RL, Ouslander JG, Abrass IB. Clinical implications of the aging process. In: Essentials of Clinical Geriatrics, 5th ed. New York, McGraw-Hill, 2004:3–15.
24. Masoro EJ. Physiology of aging. In: Tallis R, Fillit H, eds. Brocklehurst's Textbook of Geriatric Medicine, 6th ed. London, Churchill-Livingstone, 2003:291–299.
25. Becker PM, Cohen HJ. The functional approach to the care of the elderly: A conceptual framework. J Am Geriatr Soc 1984;32:923–929.
26. Hammerlein A, Derendorf H, Lowenthal DT. Pharmacokinetic and pharmacodynamic changes in the elderly: Clinical implications. Clin Pharmacokinet 1998;35:49–64.
27. US Food and Drug Administration. Guideline for industry: Studies in support of special populations: Geriatrics, ICH-E7 August 1994; available at *http://www.fda.gov/cder/guidance/iche7.pdf.*
28. Chapron DJ. Drug disposition and response. In: Delafuente JC, Stewart RB, eds. Therapeutics in the Elderly, 3d ed. Cincinnati, Harvey Whitney, 2000:257–288.

29. Kinross MT, Crone P. Clinical pharmacokinetic considerations in the elderly: An update. Clin Pharmacokinet 1997;33:302–312.

30. Iber FL, Murphy PA, Connor ES. Age-related changes in the gastrointestinal system: Effects on drug therapy. Drugs Aging 1994;5:34–48.

31. Dresser GK, Bailey DG, Carruthers SG. Grapefruit juice–felodipine interaction in the elderly. Clin Pharmacol Ther 2000;68:28–34.

32. Grandison MK, Boudinot FD. Age-related changes in protein binding of drugs: Implications for therapy. Clin Pharmacokinet 2000;38:271–90.

33. Herrlinger C, Klotz U. Drug metabolism and drug interactions in the elderly. Best Prac Res Clin Gastroenterol 2001;15:897–918.

34. Sotaniemi EA, Arranto AJ, Pelkonen O, Pasanen M. Age and cytochrome P450–linked drug metabolism in humans. Clin Pharmacol Ther 1997;61:331–339.

35. Dilger K, Hofmann U, Klotz U. Enzyme induction in the elderly: Effect of rifampin on the pharmacokinetics and pharmacodynamics of propafenone. Clin Pharmacol Ther 2000;67:512–520.

36. Schwartz JB. Race not age affects erythromycin breath test results in older hypertensive men. J Clin Pharmacol 2001;41:324–329.

37. Krecic-Shepard ME, Barnas CR, Slimko J, Schwartz JB. Faster clearance of sustained release verapamil in men versus women: Continuing observations on sex-specific differences after oral administration of verapamil. Clin Pharmacol Ther 2000;68:286–292.

38. Korrapati MR, Sorkin JD, Andres R, et al. Acetylator phenotype in relation to age and gender in the Baltimore Longitudinal Study of Aging. J Clin Pharmacol 1997;37:83–91.

39. Agundez JA, Rodriguez I, Olivera M, et al. C4P2D6, NAT2 and C4P2E1 genetic polymorphisms in nonagenarians. Age Ageing 1997;26:147–151.

40. Taioli E, Mari D, Franceschi C et al. Polymorphisms of drug-metabolizing enzymes in healthy nonagenarians and centenarians: Difference at *GSTT1* locus. Biochem Biophys Res Commun 2001;280:1389–1392.

41. Brenner SS, Herrlinger C, Dilger K, et al. Influence of age and cytochrome P450 2C9 genotype on the steady-state disposition of diclofenac and celecoxib. Clin Pharmacokinet 2003;42:283–292.

42. Ujhelyi MR, Bottorff MB, Schur M, et al. Aging effects on the organic base transporter and stereoselective renal clearance. Clin Pharmacol Ther 1997;62:117–128.

43. Cockcroft DW, Gault MH. Prediction of creatinine clearance from serum creatinine. Nephron 1976;16:31–41.

44. Klotz U. Effect of age on pharmacokinetics and pharmacodynamics in man. Int J Clin Pharmacol Ther 1998;36:581–585.

45. Guay D, Artz MB, Hanlon JT, Schmader KE. The pharmacology of aging. In: Tallis R, Fillit H, eds. Brocklehurst's Textbook of Geriatric Medicine, 6th ed. London, Churchill-Livingstone, 2003:155–161.

46. Katz S, Akpom CA. A measure of primary sociobiologic functions. Int J Health Serv 1976;6:493–507.

47. Fillenbaum GG. Screening the elderly: A brief instrumental ADL measure. J Am Geriatr Soc 1985;33:698–706.

48. Fried LP, Storer DJ, King DE, et al. Diagnosis of illness presentation in the elderly. J Am Geriatr Soc 1991;39:117–123.

49. Jarrett PG, Rockwood K, Carver D, et al. Illness presentation in elderly patients. Arch Intern Med 1995;155:1060–1064.

50. Beers MH, Berkow R, eds. History and physical examination. In: Merck Manual of Geriatrics, 3d ed. Whitehouse Station, NJ, Merck, 2000:24–40.

51. Atkin PA, Veitch PC, Veitch EM, Ogle SJ. The epidemiology of serious adverse drug reactions among the elderly. Drugs Aging 1999;14:141–152.

52. Hanlon JT, Schmader K, Gray SL. Adverse drug reactions. In: Delafuente JC, Stewart RB, eds. Therapeutics in the Elderly, 3d ed. Cincinnati, Harvey Whitney, 2000:289–314.

53. Graves T, Hanlon JT, Schmader KE, et al. Adverse events after discontinuing medications in elderly outpatients. Arch Intern Med 1997;157:2205–2210.

54. Grymonpre RE, Mitenko PA, Sitar DS, et al. Drug-associated hospital admissions in older medical patients. J Am Geriatr Soc 1988;36:1092–1098.

55. Venulet J, Ham MT. Methods for monitoring and documenting adverse drug reactions. J Clin Pharmacol 1996;34:112–129.

56. Gurwitz JH, Field TS, Harrold LR, et al. Incidence and preventability of adverse drug events among older persons in the ambulatory setting. JAMA 2003;289:1107–1116.

57. Kohn L, Corrigan J, Donaldson M. Committee on Quality of Health Care in America, Institute of Medicine. To Err Is Human: Building a Safer Health System. Washington, National Academy of Sciences, 1999.

58. Ernst FR, Grizzle AJ. Drug-related morbidity and mortality: Updating the cost-of-illness model. J Am Pharm Assoc 2001;41:192–199.

59. Bootman JL, Harrison DL, Cox E. The health care cost of drug-related morbidity and mortality in nursing facilities. Arch Intern Med 1997;157:2089–2096.

60. Montamat SC, Cusack B. Overcoming problems with polypharmacy and drug misuse in the elderly. Clin Geriatr Med 1992;8:143–158.

61. Stewart RB, Cooper JW. Polypharmacy in the aged: Practical solutions. Drugs Aging 1994;4:449–461.

62. Nolan L, O'Malley K. Prescribing for the elderly, part II. J Am Geriatr Soc 1988;36:245–254.

63. Linjakumpu T, Hartikainen S, Klaukka T, Veijola J. Use of medications and polypharmacy are increasing among the elderly. J Clin Epidemiol 2002;55:809–817.

64. Kaufman DW, Kely JP, Rosenberg L, et al. Recent patterns of medication use in the ambulatory adult population of the United States: The Slone survey. JAMA 2002;287:337–344.

65. Tobias DE, Sey M. General and psychotherapeutic medication use in 328 nursing facilities: A year 2000 national survey. Consult Pharm 2001;16:54–64.

66. Schmader K, Hanlon JT, Weinberger M, et al. Appropriateness of medication prescribing in ambulatory elderly patients. J Am Geriatr Soc 1994;42:1241–1247.

67. Lipton HL, Bero LA, Bird JA, McPhee SJ. The impact of clinical pharmacists' consultations on physicians geriatric drug prescribing: A randomized, controlled trial. Med Care 1992;30:646–658.

68. Hanlon JT, Schmader KE, Ruby CM, Weinberger M. Suboptimal prescribing in older inpatients and outpatients. J Am Geriatr Soc 2001;49:200–209.

69. Hanlon JT, Schmader KE, Boult C, et al. Use of inappropriate prescription drugs by older people. J Am Geriatr Soc 2002;50:26–34.

70. Beers MH. Explicit criteria for determining potentially inappropriate medication use by the elderly: An update. Arch Intern Med 1997;157:1531–1536.

71. Liu GG, Christensen DB. The continuing challenge of inappropriate prescribing in the elderly: An update of the evidence. J Am Pharm Assoc 2002;42:847–857.

72. Fick DM, Cooper JW, Wade WE, et al. Updating the Beers criteria for potentially inappropriate medication use in older adults: Results of a US consensus panel of experts. Arch Intern Med. 2003;163:2716–2724.

73. Hanlon JT, Fillenbaum GG, Kuchibhatla M, et al. Impact of inappropriate drug use on mortality and decline in functional status in representative community dwelling elders. Med Care 2002;40:166–176.

74. Fillenbaum GG, Hanlon JT, Dowd B, et al. Impact of inappropriate drug use defined by Beers criteria on health service use (abstract). Gerontologist 2001;41(suppl 1):52.

75. Lipton HL, Bero LA, Bird JA, McPhee SJ. Undermedication among geriatric outpatients: Results of a randomized, controlled trial. Ann Rev Gerontol Geriatr 1992;12:95–108.

76. Redelmeier DA, Tan SH, Booth GL. The treatment of unrelated disorders in patients with chronic medical diseases. N Engl J Med 1998;338:1516–1520.

77. Simon SR, Gurwitz JH. Drug therapy in the elderly: Improving quality and access. Clin Pharmacol Ther 2003;73:387–393.

78. Soumerai SB, Ross-Degnan D, Avorn J, et al. Effects of Medicaid drug-payment limits on admission to hospitals and nursing homes. N Engl J Med 1991;325:1072–1077.

79. Tamblyn R, Laprise R, Hanley JA, et al. Adverse events associated with prescription drug cost-sharing among poor and elderly persons. JAMA 2001;285:421–429.

80. Ryan AA. Medication compliance and older people: A review of the literature. Int J Nurs Stud 1999;36:153–162.

81. Lipton HL, Bird JA. The impact of clinical pharmacists' consultations on geriatric patients' compliance and medical care use: A randomized, controlled trial. Gerontologist 1994;34:307–315.

82. Benner JS, Glynn RJ, Mogun H, et al. Long-term persistence in use of statin therapy in elderly patients. JAMA 2002;288:455–461.

83. German PS, Klein LE, McPhee SJ, et al. Knowledge of and compliance with drug regimens in the elderly. J Am Geriatr Soc 1982;30:568–571.

84. Park DC, Hertzog C, Leventhal H, et al. Medication adherence in rheumatoid arthritis patients: Older is wiser. J Am Geriatr Soc 1999;47:172–183.

85. Buist DSM, LaCroix AZ, Black DM, et al. Inclusion of older women in randomized clinical trials: Factors associated with taking study medication in the Fracture Intervention Trial. J Am Geriatr Soc 2000;48:1126–1131.

86. Cooper JK, Love DW, Raffoul PR. International prescription nonadherence (noncompliance) by the elderly. J Am Geriatr Soc 1982;30:329–333.

87. Fincke BG, Miller DR, Spiro A 3rd. The interaction of patient perception of overmedication with drug compliance and side effects. J Gen Intern Med 1998;13:182–185.

88. Sullivan SD, Kreling DH, Hazlet TK. Noncompliance with medication regimens and subsequent hospitalizations: Literature analysis and cost of hospitalization estimate. J Res Pharm Econ 1990;2:19–33.

89. Col N, Fanale JE, Kronholm P. The role of medication noncompliance and adverse drug reactions in hospitalizations in the elderly. Arch Intern Med 1990;150:841–845.

90. Stuck AE, Siu AL, Wieland GD, et al. Comprehensive geriatric assessment: A meta-analysis of controlled trials. Lancet 1993;342:1032–1036.

91. Cohen HJ, Feussner JR, Weinberger M, et al. A controlled trial of inpatient and outpatient geriatric evaluation and management. N Engl J Med 2002;346:905–912.

92. Hanlon JT, Lindblad CI, Gray SL. Evidence that clinical pharmacy services can have a positive impact on drug-related problems and health outcomes in community based older adults. Am J Geriatr Pharmacother 2003;1:38–43.

93. Hanlon JT, Fillenbaum GG, Ruby CM, et al. Epidemiology of over-the-counter drug use in community-dwelling elders. Drugs Aging 2001;18:123–131.

94. Ruscin JM, Semla TP. Assessment of medication management skills in older outpatients. Ann Pharmacother 1996;30:1083–1087.

95. Shelton PS, Fritsch MA, Scott MA. Assessing medication appropriateness in the elderly: A review of available measures. Drugs Aging 2000;16:437–50.

96. Morris CJ, Cantrill JA, Hepler CD, Noyce PR. Preventing drug-related morbidity: Determining valid indicators. Int J Quality Health Care 2002;14:183–198.

97. Knight EL, Avorn J. Quality indicators for appropriate medication use in vulnerable elders. Ann Intern Med 2001;135:703–710.

98. Hanlon JT, Schmader KE, Samsa GP, et al. A method for assessing drug therapy appropriateness. J Clin Epidemiol 1992;45:1045–1051.

99. Kassam R, Martin LG, Farris KB. Reliability of a modified MAI in community pharmacies. Ann Pharmacother 2003;37:40–46.

100. Shepherd J, Blauw GJ, Murphy MB, et al. PROspective Study of Pravastatin in the Elderly at Risk. Pravastatin in elderly individuals at risk of vascular disease (PROSPER): A randomized, controlled trial. Lancet 2002;360:1623–1630.

101. van Eijken M, Tsang S, Wensing M, et al. Interventions to improve medication compliance in older patients living in the community: A systematic review of the literature. Drugs Aging 2003;20:229–240.

102. Cramer JA. Enhancing patient compliance in the elderly: Role of packaging aids and monitoring. Drugs Aging 1998;12:7–15.

103. Fouts MM, Hanlon JT, Pieper CF, et al. Identification of elderly nursing facility residents at high risk for drug-related problems. Consult Pharm 1997;12:1103–1111.

9
PHARMACOEPIDEMIOLOGY

Andy Stergachis and Thomas K. Hazlet

Learning Objectives and other resources can be found at *www.pharmacotherapyonline.com.*

KEY CONCEPTS

◀ Risks and benefits are commonly identified only after a drug is used widely by the general population.

◀ Observational study designs are essential for the study of risks associated with marketed drugs.

◀ Not all associations represent cause-effect relationships.

◀ The practice of pharmacotherapy presents numerous challenges to clinicians as they apply knowledge of the benefits and risks of pharmaceuticals to individual and population-based patient care. A great deal of our understanding about the efficacy and short-term safety of drugs arises from well-controlled studies conducted during the drug development and approval process. However, many additional risks and, increasingly, additional benefits are only identified after the drug is used widely by the general population. Benefits and risks learned following a drug's approval may range from relatively minor to clinically important effects that seriously alter an individual drug's risk-benefit ratio. The association between certain appetite-suppressant drugs and primary pulmonary hypertension and valvular heart disease is an example where serious adverse effects were discovered only after these drugs had come into widespread use.[1,2] This example highlights both the inherent limitations of the drug development process and the need to study populations receiving medications obtained through usual clinical practice. The liver toxicity seen with troglitazone is another example of the valuable contribution of close monitoring to drug safety. Introduced for treatment of type 2 diabetes mellitus in 1997, troglitazone was withdrawn from the market based on reports of serious hepatocellular injury. Medical products (drugs, biologicals, and medical devices) must be monitored closely following their introduction into the marketplace, and this information has value when applied to clinical practice. The purpose of this chapter is to describe the role of pharmacoepidemiology in drug development and therapeutics and to characterize the primary methods and contemporary issues in this field.

As illustrated in Fig. 9–1, pharmaceuticals and other medical products today are developed and used within a complex system involving contributions from numerous stakeholders, including manufacturers who develop and test products, the Food and Drug Administration (FDA) through its premarketing review and approval process and postmarketing surveillance programs, health care providers, and patients.

Pharmacoepidemiology is a discipline that provides valuable information about the health and cost outcomes of drugs, devices, and biologicals, particularly after their approval for clinical use. *Pharmacoepidemiology* is defined as the study of the use of and effects of drugs in large numbers of people.[3] The field as applied to the period after a drug enters the market is referred to as *postmarketing drug*

surveillance (PMS). *Pharmacovigilance* is the science and activities relating to the detection, assessment, understanding, and prevention of adverse effects or any other drug-related problems and generally refers to the continual monitoring for unwanted effects and other safety-related aspects of marketed drugs. One of the noteworthy developments in the field of pharmacoepidemiology has been the use of automated, linked databases that permit efficient and rapid studies of drug effects, although Health Insurance Portability and Accountability Act of 1996 concerns about confidentiality of medical information may curtail future access to these data.

Epidemiologic study designs are also essential for evaluating drug safety and effectiveness in situations where it is either infeasible or unethical to assign patients randomly to active treatment or placebo. While the randomized, controlled, blinded trial (RCT) is the standard against which other designs are measured, it is often not suitable for safety questions within the domain of pharmacoepidemiology. Clinical trials conducted prior to drug approval cannot uncover every important health effect of a pharmaceutical agent. For example, the adverse health effects of drugs on the human fetus can be estimated only through observational but not experimental methods. The teratogenic effects of thalidomide and, more recently, isotretinoin were identified through observational methods. Epidemiologic studies of the patterns of drug prescribing and use are also essential to assess a drug's usefulness.[4] As a discipline, pharmacoepidemiology traditionally has concerned itself with the study of adverse drug effects. Epidemiologic study designs such as case-control and cohort studies are also used to identify beneficial effects of drugs in populations. For example, to determine the relationship between patterns of use of inhaled corticosteroids and the risk of fatal or near-fatal asthma, Suissa and colleagues[5] conducted an epidemiologic study of 30,569 residents of Saskatchewan who were dispensed three or more asthma drugs in any 1 year from September 1975 through December 1991. The authors found the death rate to be 21% lower among inhaled corticosteroid users for each additional canister used in the preceding year and an increased death rate in patients who had discontinued inhaled corticosteroid use. These findings support practice guidelines and quality performance measurements that recommend the use of inhaled anti-inflammatory agents in patients with moderate to severe asthma.

Whether or not a drug in fact achieves its desired effect in the real world, in contrast to RCTs, is referred to as its *effectiveness,*

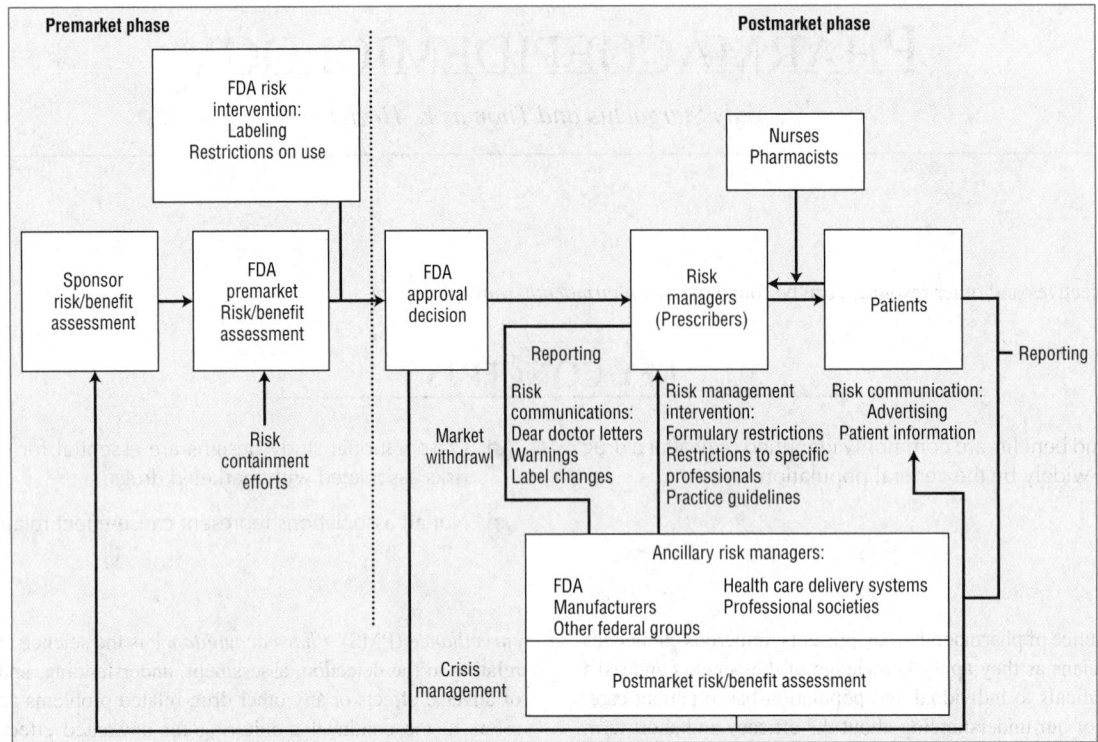

FIGURE 9-1. System for managing the risks of prescription drugs. (*From U.S. Food and Drug Admin-istration. Managing the risks from medical product use: creating a risk management framework; http://www.fda.gov/oc/tfrm/executivesummary.html; accessed May 10, 2004.*)

not efficacy. Studies of drug effectiveness generally are conducted using observational study designs, although RCTs also play a role in determining a drug's effectiveness.[6] It is recognized widely that results from an RCT offer the best evidence that a drug will perform under ideal conditions, and it is likely that the "well controlled" design of RCTs will continue to be required for new drug applications (NDAs) to the FDA. As described in regulations governing NDAs, reports of adequate and well-controlled investigations provide the primary basis for determining whether there is "substantial evidence" to support the claims of effectiveness for new drugs.[7]

However, the rigorous circumstances surrounding the design and implementation of an RCT do not necessarily extrapolate to the in-dividual patient. Fletcher and associates[8] drew a distinction between *efficacy*—Does the treatment work?—and *effectiveness*—Does the treatment's benefits outweigh its liabilities for those to whom it is offered in clinical practice?

The tension between the conflicting goals of validity in effi-cacy trials and generalizability in effectiveness trials is illustrated in Fig. 9–2. For example, in an efficacy trial, subjects are selected us-ing narrowly defined eligibility criteria and are monitored closely to ensure that they use or are exposed to the intervention in the man-ner defined in the trial's protocol and are cooperative with medical advice. In clinical practice, patients are not selected, and the manner in which the patient uses the intervention may vary widely from the intended use for which it was approved. Clinical outcomes among RCT subjects often are better than in nontrial patients.[9] Trials to evaluate therapeutic effectiveness in clinical practice are difficult or expensive for researchers. If results from an effectiveness study are inconclusive, such results could be due to a lack of the interven-tion's efficacy, patient behavior (such as lack of patient adherence), or both.

LIMITS OF KNOWLEDGE AT THE TIME OF NEW DRUG APPROVAL

The NDA process and the role of pharmacoepidemiology in the United States have evolved since the Food, Drug, and Cosmetic (FD&C) Act of 1938 was enacted into law. The FD&C Act was adopted fol-lowing the deaths of more than 100 patients of renal failure from sulfanilamide prepared in a diethylene glycol vehicle.[10] For the first time in U.S. history, the act required a drug to be proven safe under

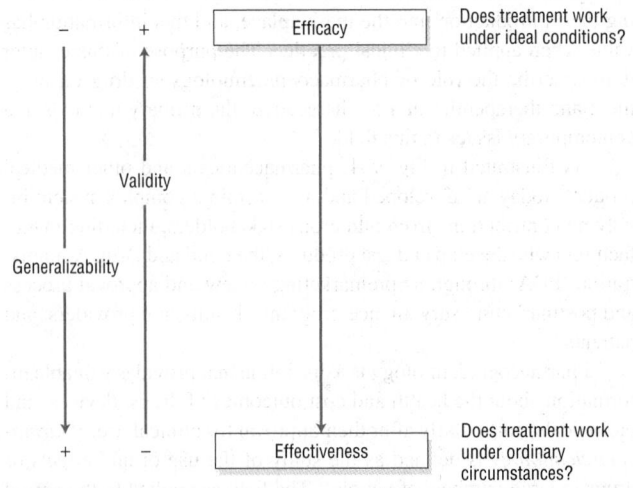

FIGURE 9–2. Schematic drawing showing the tension between conflicting goals of validity in efficacy trials and generalizability in effectiveness trials.

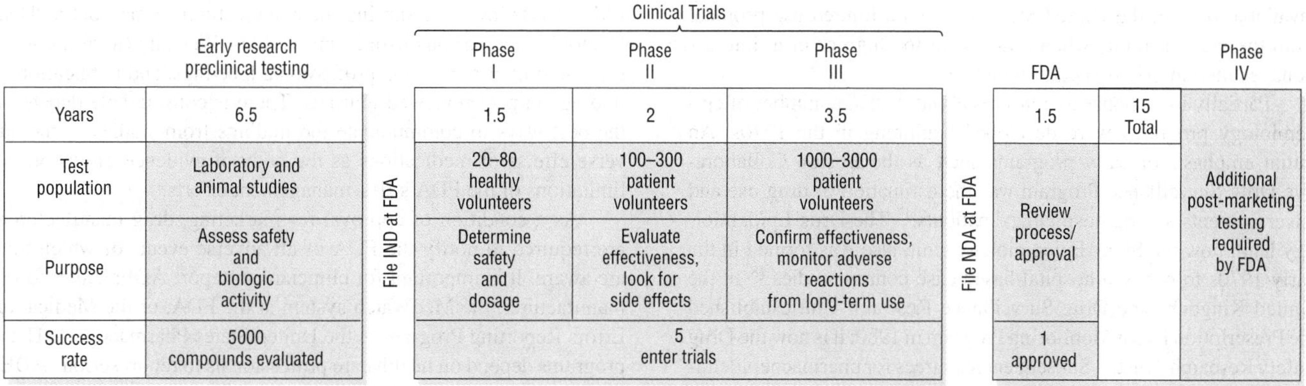

	Early research preclinical testing		Phase I	Phase II	Phase III		FDA		Phase IV
Years	6.5		1.5	2	3.5		1.5	15 Total	
Test population	Laboratory and animal studies	File IND at FDA	20–80 healthy volunteers	100–300 patient volunteers	1000–3000 patient volunteers	File NDA at FDA	Review process/ approval		Additional post-marketing testing required by FDA
Purpose	Assess safety and biologic activity		Determine safety and dosage	Evaluate effectiveness, look for side effects	Confirm effectiveness, monitor adverse reactions from long-term use				
Success rate	5000 compounds evaluated			5 enter trials			1 approved		

FIGURE 9–3. The drug development and approval process in the United States.

conditions of use intended by the manufacturer before marketing. The act also required manufacturers to conduct preclinical toxicity testing and gather and submit clinical data about drug safety to the FDA prior to drug marketing under an NDA. It also required new drugs to be labeled with adequate instructions and appropriate warnings for safe use. However, the FD&C Act required no proof of drug efficacy.

The FD&C Act was amended in 1962 following the epidemic of thalidomide-associated birth defects in Europe.[11] The Kefauver-Harris Amendments of 1962 strengthened the requirements for proof of drug safety and added a new requirement for demonstration of drug efficacy before marketing. Requiring "substantial evidence that the drug will have the effect it purports or is represented to have" resulted in the establishment of the RCT as the "gold standard" for proof of efficacy. The 1962 amendments also required manufacturers to report adverse drug events detected in the postmarketing setting to the FDA: Investigational new drug (IND) applications were required to be submitted to the FDA before clinical testing could begin. In 1985, requirements for manufacturers' adverse drug event (ADE) reporting were clarified, and specific regulations and guidelines were published to define the manufacturers' obligations in reviewing and reporting ADEs.

The Kefauver-Harris Amendments also identified explicit phases of preclinical animal testing followed by three phases of clinical testing (Fig. 9–3). In addition, a postapproval surveillance, phase IV of drug development, is now common. Today we are witnessing even more regulatory changes to the drug approval process as it pertains to pharmacoepidemiology. The Food and Drug Administration Modernization Act (FDAMA) of 1997 resulted in new provisions stating that substantial evidence of drug effectiveness may consist of data from one adequate and well-controlled clinical investigation plus confirmatory evidence. This indicates that two or more well-controlled trials (the previous standard) are not always necessary and that the FDA

should relate the number and type of trials to the specific product under development.

Phase III controlled clinical trials required by the FDA as part of the process of drug approval and labeling are the primary source of information about new drugs. Although these studies help to ensure that a drug is efficacious and does not cause unacceptable harm, premarketing studies fail to provide much of the information needed to make therapeutic decisions.[12] Table 9–1 describes the major limitations of premarketing controlled clinical trials, which lend support to the need for further evaluation of drugs after their approval for marketing by the FDA. Briefly, clinical trials performed during drug development cannot be depended on to detect rare adverse drug events and delayed adverse events. In addition, they cannot be used directly to address the performance of drugs in the populations that will use the drug in ways not studied in clinical trials because clinical trials restrict the complexity of the patients tested. Thus often not included in drug testing are many persons who are likely to receive new medicines eventually— the chronically ill, women of childbearing age, and pregnant women. Moreover, clinical trials are performed for patients with prespecified conditions. To improve the representativeness of populations included in clinical trials, the FDA has issued guidelines in support of inclusion of geriatric patients in phase II and phase III studies. Also, the FDA has issued guidelines and incentives to encourage manufacturers to provide efficacy, safety, pharmacokinetic, and pharmacodynamic information in support of the use of drugs and biologic products in pediatric and geriatric populations.

Despite the rigorous process for drug approval and regulation, several important medications have been removed from the market because of serious ADEs over the past 30 years. Examples of serious but uncommon effects include acute flank syndrome associated with suprofen,[13] the gastrointestinal effects associated with nonsteroidal anti-inflammatory drugs (NSAIDs) in the elderly,[14] troglitazone and the risk of hepatotoxicity,[15] and the adverse effects of cisapride

TABLE 9–1. Limitations of Premarketing Clinical Trials

Short duration	Premarketing studies are limited in time
	Effects that develop following chronic use or those that have a long latency period cannot be detected
Small sample size	Few drugs are studied in more than 4000 subjects before FDA approval
	Effects that occur with a frequency of less than 1/1000 are difficult to detect
Narrowly defined population	Premarketing studies generally do not include special populations, such as children, women of childbearing age, or the elderly
Narrow set of indications	Manufacturers pursue specific indications for use during premarketing studies
Limited comparison groups	The comparison group is often limited to placebo

(available only in the United States through a limited-use protocol from the manufacturer) when doses were too high or drug interactions resulted in QT-segment prolongation.[16]

Partially in response to concerns about ADEs, a number of epidemiology programs were developed beginning in the 1970s. An initial emphasis of early programs such as the Boston Collaborative Drug Surveillance Program was the estimation of drug use and adverse events among hospitalized patients.[17] The Drug Epidemiology Unit, now the Slone Epidemiology Unit, also was formed in the early 1970s to perform hospital-based case-control studies.[18] In the United Kingdom, the Drug Surveillance Research Unit established the Prescription Event Monitoring Program in 1980; it is now the Drug Safety Research Trust.[19] Subsequent resources for pharmacoepidemiology evolved from the use of Medicaid data, followed by the use of databases from health maintenance organizations (HMOs) and other population-based data sources. Since the time of the 1980 report of the Joint Commission on Prescription Drug Use, there has been considerable interest in the use of HMO records for postmarketing drug surveillance.[20] Advantages to conducting PMS in an HMO setting include the availability of an identifiable population base for the estimation of rates, the presence of a relatively stable population base, and access to medical records and computerized databases.[21] One evolution of the use of data from HMOs is the formation of the HMO Research Network, a group of 14 HMOs that facilitates health services and epidemiologic research in managed-care organizations.[22]

CLINICAL CONTROVERSY

The FDA's proposed risk-assessment guidelines identify a sponsor's responsibilities to anticipate adverse events with medical products using survey methods and other techniques during product development: Generally, a sponsor determines its product's intended use and intended population(s) during product development. Decisions as to which interactions to either explore or specifically test in clinical trials could be based on these determinations and/or surveys and epidemiologic analyses. Missing from the guidelines is an acknowledgment that many medical products are used "off label" (e.g., recent experience with gabapentin and thalidomide, whose dominant use has been off-label). What is the sponsor's obligation to assess the risk of anticipated off-label usage during drug development?

Source: Guidance for Industry Premarketing Risk Assessment, May 2004, U.S. Food and Drug Administration, http://www.fda.gov/cber/guidelines.htm; accessed May 20, 2004.

ROLE OF THE FDA AND PHARMACOEPIDEMIOLOGY

Drug development should be viewed as a process that continues even after a drug is approved for marketing. As noted in the preceding section, it is not possible to detect all potential risks and benefits during premarketing studies. The FDA's PMS program provides important information on the clinical experience of medical products. The FDA's involvement in PMS includes monitoring approved drug use, monitoring the serious ADEs associated with the use of approved drugs, and the initiation of selected epidemiologic studies to estimate the risk or test specific hypotheses.[23] One of the primary uses of findings from PMS of drugs is modification of a drug's product labeling or package insert. Other methods used to communicate the results of

PMS efforts involve requiring the manufacturer to mail out a "Dear Doctor" letter, various listings on the FDA Web site (*www.fda.gov*), presentation of findings at professional meetings, and publication of findings in peer-reviewed journals. There is considerable debate on the best ways to communicate the findings from studies of the adverse effects of medications as the body of evidence grows on the limitations of the FDA's risk-management efforts.

As a condition of approval for marketing, drug manufacturers are required to notify the FDA of all adverse events of which they are aware. It is important for clinicians to report ADEs either to the manufacturer, the MedWatch system at the FDA, or the Medication Errors Reporting Program of the United States Pharmacopeia. These programs depend on health care professionals to report serious ADEs observed in the course of their practices as part of their professional responsibility and on the lay public to volunteer information about possible ADEs. The MedWatch form can be used to report ADEs or problems related to any medical product, with the exception of those occurring with vaccines. Reports concerning vaccines should be sent to the Vaccine Adverse Event Reporting System (VAERS), a joint program of the FDA and the Centers for Disease Control and Prevention. Table 9–2 describes the FDA's MedWatch program.

The FDA provides limited funding for investigators to use large, automated databases to study the adverse effects of drugs marketed in the United States and its territories. Through its cooperative-agreements program, the FDA has encouraged the use of large databases in pharmacoepidemiology. These agreements provide the FDA with access to data on the safety of pharmaceutical agents. The objectives of these programs include the rapid and efficient

TABLE 9–2. Characteristics of the FDA's MEDWATCH Program

Report experiences with:
- Medications (durgs or biologics)
- Medical devices (including in vitro diagnostics)
- Special nutritional products (dietary supplements, medical foods, infant formulas)
- Other products regulated by the FDA

Report SERIOUS adverse events. An event is serious when the patient outcome is:
- Death
- Life threatening (real risk of dying)
- Hospitalization (initial or prolonged)
- Disability (significant, persistent, or permanent)
- Congenital anomaly
- Required intervention to prevent permanent impairment or damage

Report even if:
- You're not certain that the product caused the event
- You don't have all the details

Report product problems—quality, performance, or safety concerns—such as:
- Suspected contamination
- Questionable stability
- Defective components
- Poor packaging or labeling
- Therapeutic failures

Important numbers:
- 1-899-FDA-0178 to fax report
- 1-800-FDA-7737 to report by modem
- 1-800-FDA-1088 to report by phone, for more information, or to obtain software for reporting by modem
- 1-800-822-7967 for a VAERS form for vaccines
- FDA MedWatch Web site: http://www.fda.gov/medwatch/Download reporting forms (PDF format) MedWatch information

conduct of pharmacoepidemiologic research designed to test hypotheses, particularly those arising from the MedWatch program. Current programs receiving funding for PMS from the FDA include Vanderbilt, Harvard-Pilgrim Health, and United HealthCare. The FDA also maintains agreements for pharmacoepidemiology with Kaiser Permanente, the Veterans Administration, and the Agency for Healthcare Research and Quality's Centers for Education and Research on Therapeutics (CERTs). Even though the FDA supports cooperative agreements for PMS, historically it has lacked regulatory authority to require phase IV studies for previously approved drugs. The Prescription Drug User Fee Act Amendments of 2002 will permit fee revenues to be used for some postapproval risk-management activities for the first time (*http://www.fda.gov/oc/pdufa3/2003plan/default.htm#update;* accessed April 5, 2004).

The Food and Drug Administration Modernization Act (FDAMA) does, however, require any sponsor of a drug that agreed to conduct a postmarketing study to report annually to the FDA on the progress of its postmarketing study commitments. The FDA uses postmarketing study commitments to gather additional information about a product's safety, efficacy, or optimal use. The FDA analyzed its data as of February 2002 on postmarketing commitments, and of the 2400 drug commitments, 882 had been categorized as completed. The FDA placed on its Web site a report on all postmarketing status reports received (*http://www.accessdata.fda.gov/scripts/cder/pmc/index.cfm;* accessed April 5, 2004).

The FDA has identified efficient risk management as the primary way to make the most effective use of agency resources and address these challenges. Efficient risk management requires using the best scientific data, developing quality standards, and using efficient systems and practices that provide clear and consistent decisions and communications for the American public and regulated industry. The FDA has long led the way in the science of risk management, and this ability is more important than ever given the expanding complexity of the agency's challenges and the need to reduce the health risks facing the public at the lowest possible cost to society (*http://www.fda.gov/oc/mcclellan/strategic_risk.html;* accessed April 5, 2004).

To assist in translating information about the risks and benefits of drugs into action, the federal Agency for Healthcare Research and Quality funds studies focused on patient outcomes associated with pharmaceutical therapy. The CERTs program is a national initiative to conduct research and provide education that advances the optimal use of medical products (i.e., drugs, medical devices and biological products) (*http://www.ahrq.gov/clinic/certsovr.htm;* accessed April 5, 2004). The program, which consists of seven centers and a coordinating center, is administered as a cooperative agreement by the Agency for Healthcare Research and Quality in consultation with the FDA.

CURRENT CONTROVERSY

Hormone-replacement therapy (HRT) is an example of a widely prescribed treatment among middle-aged women that was later found to have overall health risks that exceeded its benefits. The Women's Health Initiative showed that HRT did not reduce the risk of coronary artery disease, contrary to the results of most observational studies.

ADVERSE DRUG EVENTS

The field of pharmacoepidemiology concerns itself primarily with the study of adverse drug reactions (ADRs). According to the World Health Organization, an *adverse drug reaction* is any noxious, unintended, and undesired effect of a drug that occurs at doses used in humans for prophylaxis, diagnosis, or therapy, and it implies a causal relationship between use of the drug and the noxious event.[24] ADEs, in contrast, describe an injury resulting from administration of a drug, but use of this term implies that the relationship may be coincidental or that the event is not caused solely by the drug itself but rather may relate to the circumstances surrounding use of the drug.

Virtually any drug can have adverse effects. Between 3% and 11% of hospital admissions have been attributed to adverse effects.[25] The likelihood that a patient will experience an ADE during hospitalization ranges from 1% to 44% depending on the type of hospital, the definition of an ADE, and the study methodology.[26] The economic impact of ADEs is substantial and potentially avoidable.[27,28] The incidence of serious and fatal ADRs in hospital patients was reported to be as high as 6.7% and 0.32%, respectively.[29] More recently, ADEs among older persons in the ambulatory clinical setting were studied among all Medicare enrollees cared for by a multispecialty group practice during a 1-year study period. The researchers reported an overall rate of ADEs of 50.1 per 1000 person-years, with a rate of 13.8 preventable ADEs per 1000 person-years.[30]

Although most ADEs can be anticipated, others are unpredictable, especially rare idiosyncratic reactions. ADRs have been separated into type A and B reactions. Type A reactions are expected exaggerations of a drug's known pharmacologic effects. Therefore, they usually are dose-dependent, predictable, and preventable. Type A reactions are responsible for most of the ADEs encountered. Examples include hypotension with antihypertensive agents and anticholinergic effects with tricyclic antidepressants. Type A reactions tend to occur in individuals who have one of three characteristics.[31] First, the individual may have received more of a drug than is customarily required. Second, the individual may have received a conventional dose of the drug, but he or she may metabolize or excrete the drug unusually slowly, leading to drug levels that are too high, possibly owing to concomitant disease or drug interactions. Third, the individual may have normal drug levels but for some reason is overly sensitive to them. Most type A reactions are identified prior to drug marketing and are listed in a product's labeling.

Type B reactions are idiosyncratic and tend to be unrelated to the known pharmacologic action of a drug. They usually are not related to dose, are unpredictable and uncommon, and potentially are more serious than type A reactions. They may be due to what are known as *hypersensitivity reactions* or *immunologic reactions.* Type B reactions may be the consequence of some other idiosyncratic reaction to the drug, such as an inherited susceptibility. These reactions may concentrate in certain body systems, including the liver, blood, skin, kidney, and nervous system.[32] Type B reactions represent a major focus of pharmacoepidemiologic studies of ADRs. Carcinogenic and teratogenic ADEs are considered type B reactions.

Because ADRs represent an important public health concern, institutions complying with the Joint Commission on Accreditation of Healthcare Organizations (JCAHO) are required to perform numerous steps pertaining to the surveillance and management of ADRs. They must define significant ADRs, initiate intensive assessments for ADRs meeting the institution's definition, and be able to provide evidence during accreditation surveys of sufficiently detailed follow-up on the causes of ADRs.[33] The JCAHO recently has instituted an additional requirement for reporting of sentinel events, which are those involving the occurrence of risk of death or serious physical or psychological injury. In situations where the sentinel event indicates an ongoing possibility of threat to life or safety, the JCAHO may conduct an unscheduled survey and require that the institution undertake

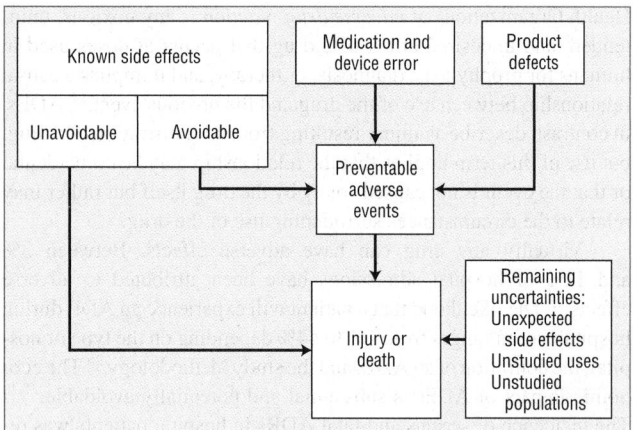

FIGURE 9–4. Sources of risk from medical products. (*From U.S. Food and Drug Administration. Managing the risks from medical product use: creating a risk management framework; http://www.fda.gov/oc/tfrm/executivesummary.html; accessed May 10, 2004.*)

extensive systems and process reviews and implement improvements to prevent recurrence of the sentinel event.

Risks from drugs and other medical products generally fall into four categories (Fig. 9–4). Most injuries and deaths associated with the use of medical products result from their known adverse effects. Some adverse effects are unavoidable, but others can be prevented or minimized by careful product choice and use. It is estimated that more than half the adverse effects from pharmaceuticals are avoidable.[34] Other sources of preventable adverse events are medication or device errors.

METHODOLOGIES FOR PHARMACOEPIDEMIOLOGIC STUDIES

A large number of study designs and methods are used to generate data on the uses and risks of new and older drugs. The types of study designs used in pharmacoepidemiology can be classified as experimental and observational. Experimental studies employ control in the assignment of individuals to exposure groups, usually through random assignment of individuals to the exposure under investigation, and then follow-up of individuals to detect the effects of exposure. For example, a recent clinical trial demonstrated that HRT does not prevent coronary heart disease in women. This randomized, controlled primary prevention trial, the Women's Health Initiative, studied 16,608 postmenopausal women aged 50 to 79 years with an intact uterus at baseline recruited by 40 U.S. clinical centers in 1993–1998. Overall health risks exceeded benefits from use of combined estrogen plus progestin for an average 5.2-year follow-up among healthy postmenopausal U.S. women.[35]

Observational epidemiologic study designs, such as case-control, cohort, and cross-sectional studies, are used extensively. Large automated databases, meta-analyses, RCTs, and hybrid designs, such as nested case-control studies, also play an important role in pharmacoepidemiology. Epidemiologic studies typically do not use randomization to determine who will receive a particular drug exposure. Rather, associations between exposure(s) and disease(s) under study are determined through the use of observational study designs and statistical analyses. Observational methods are used in most situations because ethics and cost limit the use of experimentation. For example, one would not experimentally subject individuals to certain

drugs to determine if they develop cancer. A number of methods are used to study health events associated with drug exposures. The usual approach to studying ADEs begins with the collection of spontaneous reports of drug-related morbidity or mortality.

There has been a growing interest in using computerized databases containing medical care information for pharmacoepidemiologic studies.[36] These databases usually consist of patient-level data from two or more separate files (e.g., billing files for pharmacy and medical services reimbursement) that were developed originally for clinical or administrative applications.[37] Through record linkage, person-based longitudinal files can be created on an ad hoc basis. Multipurpose databases used for pharmacoepidemiologic studies include data from managed-care organizations, the Medicaid program, the Medicare program, and geographically defined populations. In general, these databases include information on patient demographics, outpatient drugs, hospital discharge diagnoses, and ambulatory care encounters. The advantages and disadvantages of linked databases for pharmacoepidemiologic studies have been the subject of numerous publications.[38,39]

CASE REPORTS AND CASE SERIES

Case reports describe a single patient who was exposed to a drug and experienced a particular, usually adverse outcome. For example, within the first 3 months of marketing, hemolytic anemia and acute renal failure following use of the antibiotic temafloxacin were reported to the Spontaneous Report System, the predecessor of the MedWatch system. Case reports are useful for raising hypotheses about drug effects to be tested with more rigorous study designs. It is uncommon for a case report or a series of case reports to be used to make a statement about causation. Case series are collections of patients, all of whom have a single exposure, whose clinical outcomes are then evaluated and described. They are useful for quantifying the incidence of an adverse reaction, particularly for a newly approved drug. Further, case series can be useful for being certain that the incidence rate of any particular adverse effects of concern does not occur in a population that is larger than that studied prior to drug's marketing.

If the event is rare and the exposure combination is very specific, the cause of the adverse health event may be inferred from a case-series study. In most situations, however, it is necessary to compare cases with a group of controls to identify risk factors. Thus the major disadvantage of a case-series study is the lack of a comparison group. However, recent methodologic advances in the analysis of case-series data allow the estimation of relative incidence without the use of controls.[40]

CASE-CONTROL STUDIES

A case-control study assembles a group of cases (people who have the disease of interest) and controls (people who do not). The exposure histories of the cases and the controls are determined to establish the extent of association between exposure(s) of interest and disease. Case-control studies compare patients with a specific disease with a control group composed of similar people but without the disease. Case-control studies attempt to identify risk factors for a disease by examining differences in antecedent exposure variables between cases and controls. For example, one can select cases of women of childbearing age with ovarian cysts and compare them with controls, looking for differences in prior use of oral contraceptives. Such a study was performed to determine if the then newly introduced triphasic oral contraceptives were associated with functional ovarian cysts.[41]

Case-control studies have been used extensively to assess the safety of pharmaceuticals. There are many examples of case-control studies that have identified important associations between drugs and adverse health events: vaginal cancer and diethylstilbestrol, Reye's syndrome and aspirin, peptic ulcer disease and nonsteroidal anti-inflammatory drugs, and venous thromboembolism and oral contraceptives. Data from case-control studies are used to calculate an odds ratio, which is the ratio of the odds of developing the disease for exposed patients to the odds of developing the disease for unexposed patients.

A classic example is a study of diethylstilbestrol given during pregnancy and the risk of vaginal adenocarcinoma among female offspring nearly a generation later.[42] Recently, the association between use of antibiotics and the risk of breast cancer was studied in a case-control study among women enrolled in a large, nonprofit health plan. Controls were selected from health plan records and frequency matched to cases on age and length of enrollment. Cases were identified from the Surveillance, Epidemiology, and End Results Cancer Registry, whereas antibiotic use was ascertained from computerized pharmacy records.[43]

A study of hip fracture risk in relation to the prescription of benzodiazepines exemplifies a nested case-control design.[44] Hip fracture cases and controls were chosen from a large existing database on health care use among Saskatchewan residents. The use of a nested case-control design to assess the role of potential confounding factors efficiently is further illustrated in the previously cited study of inhaled corticosteroids and the risk of fatal and near-fatal asthma.[45] A nested case-control study is an efficient variation of a case-control and a cohort study. In a nested case-control study, all cases (or a sample of all cases) and only a random sample of all controls are chosen for study from the same defined population.

An advantage of the case-control design for the study of drug-outcome relationships is its efficiency for the study of rare or delayed outcomes. Compared with other strategies, the case-control study is relatively inexpensive. One potential problem with case-control studies is their susceptibility to certain types of bias, including selection bias and information bias. *Selection bias* refers to systematic differences between those selected for study and those who are not, whereas *information bias* is systematic differences in the quality of information gathered for study and comparison groups.

COHORT STUDIES

A cohort study assembles a group of persons without the disease(s) of interest at the onset of the study, ascertains the exposure status of each person, and then follows the cohort over time to determine the development of disease in exposed and nonexposed persons. Cohort studies involve a comparison of the incidence of one or more outcome events among those who received a drug or some other exposure of interest compared with the incidence of the event(s) for a comparison group. For example, much information about the risk of fatal cardiovascular diseases among oral contraceptive users has come from the Royal College of General Practitioners Oral Contraception Study, in which 23,000 oral contraceptive users were compared with 23,000 nonusers chosen from the same British general practices.[42] Death certificate records were used to ascertain instances of fatal events during the follow-up period.

Cohort studies can be prospective, as the Royal College of General Practitioners study illustrates, or retrospective. Some prospective cohort studies follow a large population over decades. For example, the Nurses Health Study was begun in 1976 to investigate the potential long-term consequences of the use of oral contraceptives and was later expanded to include diet and nutrition and their relationship with the development of chronic diseases (*http://www.channing.harvard.edu/nhs/*). Prospective cohort studies are one of the most valid types of observational study designs because exposure is measured and recorded prior to the development of the health outcome(s) of interest. Using a prospective cohort study design, Hooton and colleagues[46] determined the association between contraceptive methods and symptomatic urinary tract infections in young women. The investigators recruited sexually active young women who were starting a new method of contraception and followed them for 6 months to determine the incidence of symptomatic urinary tract infections by contraceptive method.

An alternative to the prospective cohort design is the retrospective cohort study. Retrospective cohort studies are useful when comparison cohorts of persons exposed and not exposed to drugs of interest can be identified at some time in the past from large preexisting databases and followed from that time to the present with regard to the incidence of a given outcome. Recently, Soumerai and associates[47] used a retrospective cohort design to study the determinants and adverse health outcomes of β-blocker underuse in elderly patients with myocardial infarction. Controlling for other predictors of survival, the mortality rate among β-blocker recipients was 43% less than that for the comparison group, suggesting that use of β-blockers reduces the risk of death among elderly patients with myocardial infarction.

Prospective cohort studies can provide strong evidence of associations between drugs and diseases because the exposure is assessed before the outcome occurs. However, because many cohort studies require large numbers of people followed for long periods of time, they can be expensive and, in some instances, infeasible. Retrospective or historical cohort studies can overcome these limitations if high-quality data have been collected already.

QUASI-EXPERIMENTAL STUDY DESIGNS

One of the opportunities that has emerged with increased computerization in health care is the use of large, linked databases for exploring pharmaceutical outcomes. The ability to use transaction or claims data from an insurance company or state Medicaid agency and link these data to files containing diagnostic and other patient-specific information has allowed researchers to explore outcomes questions at relatively low expense. Because these studies do not rely on random assignment of subjects, they have been described as *quasi-experimental*.[48] The typical design includes a treatment (exposed) group, a control (unexposed) group, and some type of posttest assessment for both. Although efforts may be made to match treatment and control groups for important patient characteristics, the groups are not equivalent in the sense of an RCT. A refinement to this design is one where an analysis of underlying trends—factors that could influence study outcomes and progress independent of the study—is made using time-series methods. These studies often are used to evaluate the consequences of a change of policy, such as a prescription limit, or addition or removal of a drug from the marketplace. For instance, Soumerai and associates[49] studied the effect of a prescription cap on the use of psychotropic drugs and emergency mental health services using claims data. They used pharmacy claims data collected over a 42-month period, including the 11 months that the prescription cap was in effect, and found that drug use decreased while costs to the state Medicaid program increased during the period of the cap.

Recently, a quasi-experimental design was used to study British Columbia's reference pricing policy for five therapeutic classes of drugs to determine if a worsening of health outcomes could be detected after implementation of the reference pricing policy. The

TABLE 9–3. Criteria for the Causal Nature of an Association

1. **The association makes biologic sense.** In other words, the proposed association is consistent with our knowledge of the mechanism of disease. You can use data from other human or animal studies, or data from in vitro studies.
2. **The suspected cause precedes the disease.** Even though this is self-evident, it can be overlooked when interpreting findings from certain observational studies.
3. **The association is strong.** Associations with a relative risk of less than 2.0 are considered to be weak. Risks of 2.0 to 4.0 are considered moderate, while those greater than 4.0 are strong. You also need to consider the 95% confidence interval.
4. **The association is found consistently when studied using different methods or populations.** An important characteristic of science is that a finding is reproducible.
5. **There is a dose–response relationship.** For example, there is a higher risk among persons with greater exposure to a risk factor.

authors reported that there has been no worsening of health outcomes associated with implementing the reference pricing policy.[50]

INTERPRETATION OF PHARMACOEPIDEMIOLOGIC STUDIES

Not all associations represent a cause-effect relationship. Because most epidemiologic studies of drug effects do not employ random allocation, it is important to determine if a legitimate cause-effect relationship exists. A central methodologic concern in observational studies is *confounding*—i.e., the possibility that the apparent effect of an exposure or intervention is due wholly or partly to other factors associated with it that have their own impact on the outcome of interest. Criteria have been proposed to help determine if an association is causal. The fewer criteria that are met, the less likely it is that an association is causal. Table 9–3 is adapted from the work of Hill and Stolly.[51,52] Practitioners should ask the series of questions listed in the table to interpret findings from studies to determine if an association is likely to be causal.

CONCLUSION

Pharmacoepidemiologic studies conducted during the postapproval period provide important information to assist in optimizing therapeutic responses to drugs. The aging U.S. population, the introduction of new drugs, and reimbursement policies make pharmacoepidemiology an essential part of clinical practice. Studies can provide valuable information about the relationship between therapeutic agents and adverse and beneficial health outcomes. Information from pharmacoepidemiologic studies also contributes to population-based care and drug regulatory and reimbursement decisions. At the level of individual patient care, a combination of medical and epidemiologic knowledge leads to the choice to use a particular medication. Moreover, patient monitoring to optimize the therapeutic response to drugs also involves epidemiologic data and logic to balance likely benefits against potential risks. Epidemiologic information can provide vital information regarding safety, patterns of drug use, and effectiveness to assist in the provision of evidence-based health care. New data resources and methodologies are likely to expand the field of pharmacoepidemiology. There is an inherent tradeoff between the need for more information about a drug's risks and the need to make a drug available for use. Because of limitations in the drug development process, more information emerges about a drug after its approval through PMS. The challenge—articulated in the FDA's recent "Innovation or Stagnation: Challenge and Opportunity on the Critical Path to New Medical Products"—will be to improve on this tradeoff through enhanced assessment methods for safety and utility and to better integration of these measures with manufacturing technology (*http://www.fda.gov/oc/initiatives/criticalpath/whitepaper.html;* accessed April 8, 2004).

ABBREVIATIONS

RCT: randomized, controlled trial
NDAs: new drug applications
FDA: Food and Drug Administration
FD&C Act: Food, Drug, and Cosmetic Act
IND: investigational new drug
ADE: adverse drug event
FDAMA: Food and Drug Administration Modernization Act
HMOs, health maintenance organizations
VAERS, Vaccine Adverse Event Reporting System
CERTs, Centers for Education and Research on Therapeutics
ADR, adverse drug reaction
JCAHO, Joint Commission on Accreditation of Healthcare Organizations
HRT, hormone-replacement therapy
WHI, Women's Health Initiative
PMS, postmarketing drug surveillance

Review Questions and other resources can be found at *www.pharmacotherapyonline.com.*

REFERENCES

1. Abenhaim L, Moride Y, Brenot F, et al. Appetite-suppressant drugs and the risk of primary pulmonary hypertension. N Engl J Med 1996;335:609–616.
2. Connolly HM, Crary JL, McGoon MD, et al. Valvular heart disease associated with fenfluramine-phentermine. N Engl J Med 1997;337:581–588.
3. Strom BL, ed. Pharmacoepidemiology. New York, Wiley, 1994.
4. Collett JP, Boissel JP. Pharmacoepidemiology: Epidemiologic approach to the study of drugs. Post Market Surveillance 1991;5:3–14.
5. Suissa S, Ernst P, Benayoun S, et al. Low-dose inhaled corticosteroids and the prevention of death from asthma. N Engl J Med 2000;343:332–336.
6. Strom BL, Melmon KL. The use of pharmacoepidemiology to study beneficial drug effects. In: Strom BL, ed. Pharmacoepidemiology. New York, Wiley, 1994.
7. 21 CFR Part 314.126, Adequate and well-controlled studies.
8. Fletcher RH, Fletcher SW, Wagner EH. Clinical Epidemiology, The Essentials, 3d ed. Baltimore, Williams & Wilkins, 1996.
9. Fayers PM. Generalisation from phase III clinical trials: Survival, quality of life, and health economics. Lancet 1997;350:1025–1027.
10. Geiling EMK, Cannon PR. Pathogenic effects of elixir of sulfanilamide (diethylene glycol) poisoning. JAMA 1938;111:919–926.
11. Lenz W. Malformations caused by drugs in pregnancy. Am J Dis Child 1966;112:99–106.
12. Ray WA, Griffin MR, Avorn J. Evaluating drugs after their approval for clinical use. N Engl J Med 1993;329:2029–2032.
13. Rossi AC, Bosco L, Faich GA, et al. The importance of adverse reaction reporting by physicians: Suprofen and the flank pain syndrome. JAMA 1988;259:1203–1204.
14. Griffin MR, Piper JM, Daugherty JR, et al. Nonsteroidal anti-inflammatory drug use and increased risk for peptic ulcer disease in elderly persons. Ann Intern Med 1991;114:257–263.

15. Ault A. Troglitazone may cause irreversible liver damage. Lancet 1997;350:1451.

16. Smalley W, Shatin D, Wysowski DK, et al. Contraindicated use of cisapride: Impact of Food and Drug Administration regulatory action. JAMA 2000;284:3036–3039.

17. Jick H, Miettinen OS, Shapiro S, et al. Comprehensive drug surveillance. JAMA 1970;213:1455–1460.

18. Shapiro S. Case-control surveillance. In: Strom BL, ed. Pharmacoepidemiology. New York, Wiley, 1994.

19. Inman WHW. Prescription event monitoring. Acta Med Scand Suppl 1984;683:119–126.

20. Joint Commission on Prescription Drug Use, 96th Congress. Washington, US Government Printing Office, 1980.

21. Saunders KW, Stergachis A, Von Korff M. Group Health Cooperative. In: Strom BL, ed. Pharmacoepidemiology, 2d ed. New York, Wiley, 1994:171–185.

22. Platt R, Davis R, Finkelstein J, Go AS, et al. Multicenter epidemiologic and health services research on therapeutics in the HMO Research Network Center for Education and Research on Therapeutics. Pharmacoepidemiol Drug Saf 2001;10:373–377.

23. Arrowsmith-Lowe JB, Anello C. A view from a regulatory agency. In: Strom BL, ed. Pharmacoepidemiology, 2d ed. New York, Wiley, 1994: 87–97.

24. World Health Organization. International Drug Monitoring: The Role of the Hospital. Technical Report Series No 425. Geneva, World Health Organization, 1966.

25. Beard K. Adverse reactions as a cause of hospital admission in the aged. Drugs Aging 1992;2:356–367.

26. Koch KE. Adverse drug reactions. In: Brown T, ed. Handbook of Institutional Pharmacy Practice, 3d ed. Bethesda, MD, American Society of Hospital Pharmacists, 1992:279–291.

27. Johnson JA, Bootman JL. Drug-related morbidity and mortality: A cost-of-illness model. Arch Intern Med 1995;155:1949–1956.

28. Ernst FR, Grizzle AJ. Drug-related morbidity and mortality: Updating the cost-of-illness model. J Am Pharm Assoc. 2001;41:192–198.

29. Lazarou J, Pomeranz BH, Corey PN. Incidence of adverse drug reactions in hospitalized patients: A meta-analysis of prospective studies. JAMA 1998;279:1200–1205.

30. Gurwitz JH, Field TS, Harrold LR, et al. Incidence and preventability of adverse drug events among older persons in the ambulatory setting. JAMA 2003;289:1107–1116.

31. Strom BL. In: Strom BL, ed. Pharmacoepidemiology, 2d ed. New York: Wiley, 1994:3–14.

32. Park BK, Pirmohamed M, Kitteringham NNR. Idiosyncratic drug reactions: A mechanistic evaluation of risk factors. Br J Clin Pharmacol 1992;34:377–395.

33. Joint Commission on Accreditation of Healthcare Organizations. Comprehensive Accreditation Manual for Hospitals: The Official Handbook. Oakbrook Terrace, IL, JCAHO, 1996.

34. Bates DW, Leape LL, Petrycki S. Incidence and preventability of adverse drug events in hospitalized adults. J Gen Intern Med 1993;8:289–294.

35. Rossouw JE, Anderson GL, Prentice RL, et al. Risks and benefits of estrogen plus progestin in healthy postmenopausal women: Principal results from the Women's Health Initiative randomized, controlled trial. JAMA 2002;288:321–333.

36. Strom BL, Carson JL. Use of automated databases for pharmacoepidemiology research. Epidemiol Rev 1990;12:87–107.

37. Stergachis A. Evaluating the quality of linked automated data sets for use in pharmacoepidemiology. In: Hartzema AG, Porta MS, Tilson HH, eds. Pharmacoepidemiology: An Introduction, 2d ed, Cincinnati, Harvey Whitney Books, 1991.

38. Shapiro S. The role of automated records linkage in the postmarketing surveillance of drug safety: A critique. Clin Pharmacol Ther 1989;46:371–386.

39. Faich GA, Stadel BV. The future of automated record linkage for postmarketing surveillance: A response to Shapiro. Clin Pharmacol Ther 1989;46:387–389.

40. Farrington CP, Nash J, Miller E. Case-series analysis of adverse reactions to vaccines: A comparative evaluation. Am J Epidemiol 1996;143:1165–1173.

41. Holt VL, Daling JR, Weiss NS, et al. Functional ovarian cyst risk associated with use of monophasic and triphasic oral contraceptives. Obstet Gynecol 1992;79:529–533.

42. Herbst AL, Ulfelder H, Poskanzer DC. Adenocarcinoma of the vagina: Association of maternal stilbestrol therapy with tumor appearance in young women. N Engl J Med 1971;284:878–881.

43. Velicer CM, Heckbert SR, Lampe JW, et al. Antibiotic use in relation to the risk of breast cancer. JAMA 2004;291:827–835.

44. Ray WA, Griffin MR, Downey W. Benzodiazepines of long and short elimination half-life and the risk of hip fracture. JAMA 1989;262:3303–3307.

45. Royal College of General Practitioners. Oral Contraceptives and Health. London, Pitman, 1974.

46. Hooten TM, Scholes D, Hughs JP, et al. A prospective study of risk factors for symptomatic urinary tract infection in young women. N Engl J Med 1996;335:468–474.

47. Soumerai SB, McLaughlin TJ, Spiegelman D, et al. Adverse outcomes of underuse of beta-blockers in elderly survivors of acute myocardial infarction. JAMA 1997;277:115–121.

48. Cook TD, Campbell DT. Quasi-Experimentation: Design and Analysis Issues for Field Settings. Boston, Houghton-Mifflin, 1979.

49. Soumerai SB, McLaughlin TJ, Ross-Degnan D, et al. Effects of limiting Medicaid drug-reimbursement benefits on the use of psychotropic agents and acute mental health services by patients with schizophrenia. N Engl J Med 1994;441:650–655.

50. Hazlet TK, Blough DK. Health services utilization with reference drug pricing of histamine(2) receptor antagonists in British Columbia elderly. Med Care 2002;40:640–649.

51. Hill AB. The environment and disease: Association or causation? Proc R Soc Med 1965;58:295–300.

52. Stolly PD. How to interpret studies of adverse drug reactions. Clin Pharmacol Ther 1990;48:337–339.

10

CLINICAL TOXICOLOGY

Peter A. Chyka

Learning Objectives and other resources can be found at *www.pharmacotherapyonline.com.*

KEY CONCEPTS

❶ Poisoning can result from exposure to excessive doses of any chemical, with medicines being responsible for most childhood and adult poisonings.

❷ The total number and rate of poisonings have been increasing, but preventive measures, such as child-resistant containers, have reduced mortality in young children.

❸ Immediate first aid may reduce the development of serious poisoning, and consultation with a poison control center may indicate the need for further therapy.

❹ The use of ipecac syrup, gastric lavage, and cathartics has fallen out of favor as routine therapies, whereas activated charcoal and whole-bowel irrigation are still useful for the gastric decontamination of appropriate patients.

❺ Antidotes can prevent or reduce the toxicity of certain poisons, but symptomatic and supportive care is essential for all patients.

❻ Acute acetaminophen poisoning produces severe liver injury and occasionally kidney failure. A determination of

serum acetaminophen concentration may indicate whether there is risk of hepatotoxicity and the need for acetylcysteine therapy.

❼ Anticholinesterase insecticides may produce life-threatening respiratory distress and paralysis by all routes of exposure and may be treated with symptomatic care, atropine, and pralidoxime.

❽ Calcium channel antagonists will produce severe hypotension and bradycardia on overdose and can be treated with supportive care, calcium, glucagon, and insulin.

❾ Poisoning with iron-containing drugs produces vomiting, gross gastrointestinal bleeding, shock, metabolic acidosis, and coma and can be treated with supportive care and deferoxamine.

❿ Overdoses of tricyclic antidepressants can cause arrhythmias, such as prolonged QRS intervals and ventricular dysrhythmias, coma, respiratory depression, and seizures and are treated with symptomatic care and intravenous sodium bicarbonate.

Poisoning is an adverse effect from a chemical that has been taken in excessive amounts. The body is able to tolerate and, in some cases, detoxify a certain dose of a chemical, but once a critical threshold is exceeded, toxicity results. Poisoning can produce minor local effects that are treated readily in the outpatient setting or systemic life-threatening effects that require intensive medical intervention. This spectrum of toxicity is typical for many chemicals with which humans come in contact. Virtually any chemical can become a poison when taken in sufficient quantity, but the potency of some compounds leads to serious toxicity with small quantities[1] (Table 10–1). Poisoning by chemicals includes exposures to drugs, industrial chemicals, household products, plants, venomous animals, and agrochemicals. This chapter will describe some examples of this spectrum of toxicity, outline means to recognize poisoning risk, and present principles of treatment.

EPIDEMIOLOGY

Each year poisonings account for approximately 22,000 deaths and at least 875,000 emergency department visits in the United States.[2,3] Young adults aged 25 to 44 years are at greatest risk of a poisoning death, and males have a twofold higher risk of death than females.

Nearly one-half of all poisoning deaths of adults are due to suicide. Poisoning deaths in adults most commonly involve motor vehicle exhaust (carbon monoxide), other gases or vapors, antidepressants, tranquilizers, barbiturates, alcohol, opioids, and local anesthetics, including cocaine.[3–5] Approximately 0.3% of poisoning deaths involve children under the age of 5 years. The elderly, those 75 years old and older, children under 5 years of age, and adolescents and young adults 15 to 24 years of age have the highest risk for nonfatal poisonings requiring hospitalization. The number and rates of poisoning deaths (Fig. 10–1) have been increasing steadily, with a twofold increase from 1981 to 2001.[3]

❶ There are several databases in the United States that provide different levels of insight into and documentation of the poisoning problem (Table 10–2). Poisonings documented by U.S. poison centers are compiled in the annual report of the American Association of Poison Control Centers-Toxic Exposure Surveillance System (AAPCC-TESS).[6] Although it represents the largest database on poisoning, it is not complete because it relies on individuals voluntarily contacting a poison control center. The AAPCC-TESS data set captures approximately 5% of the annual number of deaths from poisoning tabulated in death certificates.[4] Despite this shortcoming, AAPCC-TESS provides valuable insight into the characteristics and frequency of poisonings. In the 2003 AAPCC-TESS summary, 2,395,582 poisoning exposures

TABLE 10–1. Serious Toxicity in a Child Associated with Ingestion of One Mouthful or One Dosage Unit

Acids[a]	Cocaine
Anticholinesterase insecticides[a]	Colchicine
Caustics or alkalis[a]	Cyanide[a]
Cationic detergents[a]	Hydrocarbons[a]
Chloroquine	Methanol[a]
Clonidine	Phencyclidine or LSD

[a]Concentrated or undiluted form.

were reported by 64 participating poison centers that served a population of 295 million people.[6] Children younger than 6 years of age accounted for 52% of the cases. The site of exposure was the home in 93% of the cases, and a single substance was involved in 92% of the cases. An acute exposure accounted for 92% of the cases, 85% of which were unintentional or accidental exposures. Only 12% were intentional. Fatalities accounted for 1106 (0.05%) cases, of which 3% were children younger than 6 years of age. The distribution of substances most frequently involved in pediatric and adult exposures differed; however, medicines were the most frequently involved (49%) substances (Table 10–3). Seventy-four percent of the poison exposures were treated at the scene, typically a home. In summary, children account for most of the reported poisonings with morbidity, but adults account for a greater proportion of mortality from poisoning.

ECONOMIC IMPACT OF POISONING

Poisoning, which ranks as the second leading cause of injury-related death, accounted for a total lifetime cost of $8.5 billion in 1989 and, when adjusted for 2003, represented $12.6 billion annually.[7] Estimates of the lifetime cost of injury include related health care costs and lost lifetime earnings of the victim; however, they do not include the costs of suffering, reduced productivity of caregivers, or legal costs. The definition of poisoning for this economic estimate excluded poisoning from alcohol and other illicit drugs.

POISON PREVENTION STRATEGIES

The number of poisoning deaths in children has declined dramatically over the past three decades due, in part, to the implementation of several poison prevention approaches.[7,8] These include the Poison Prevention Packaging Act (PPPA) of 1970, the evolution of regional poison control centers, the application of prompt first-aid measures, improvements in overall critical care, development of less toxic product formulations, better clarity in the packaging and labeling of products, and public education on the risks and prevention of poisoning.[9] Although all these factors play a role in minimizing poisoning dangers, particularly in children, the PPPA has perhaps had the most significant influence.[8] The intent of the PPPA was to develop packaging that is difficult for children under 5 years of age to open or to obtain harmful amounts within a reasonable period of time. However, the packaging was not to be difficult for normal adults to use properly. There are a number of products and product categories for which safety packaging is required (Table 10–4). Child-resistant containers are not totally childproof and may be opened by children, which can result in poisoning. Despite the success of child-resistant containers, many adults disable the hardware or simply use no safety cap and thus place children at risk.[10] Fatigue of the packaging materials also can occur, which underscores the need for new prescription ware for refills, as required in the PPPA.[11]

Poison prevention requires constant vigilance because there are new generations of families where parents and grandparents need to be educated on poisoning risks and prevention strategies. New products and changes in product formulations also present different poisoning dangers and must be studied to provide optimal management. Strategies to prevent poisonings should consider the various psychosocial circumstances of poisoning (Table 10–5), prioritize risk groups and behaviors, and customize an intervention for specific situations.[12,13]

RECOGNITION AND ASSESSMENT

The clinician's initial responsibility is to determine whether a poisoning has occurred or if there is a potential for one to develop. Some patients provide a clear account of an exposure that has occurred with a known quantity of a specific agent. In other cases, the patient may appear with only an unexplained illness characterized by nonspecific signs and symptoms and no immediate history of ingestion. Exposure to folk remedies, dietary supplements, and environmental toxins also should be considered. Patients with suicide gestures can deliberately give an unclear history, and poisoning should be suspected routinely. Poisoning and drug overdoses should be suspected in any patient with a sudden, unexplained illness or with a puzzling combination of signs and symptoms, particularly in high-risk age groups. Nearly any

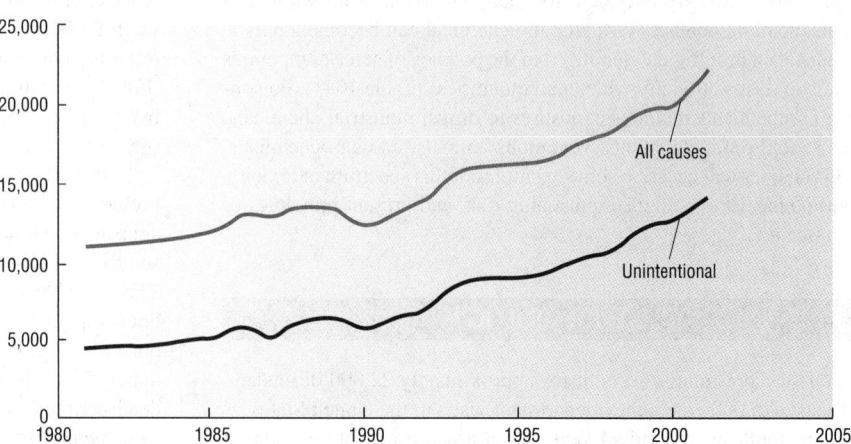

FIGURE 10–1. Deaths from all causes of poisoning and unintentional poisoning in the United States from 1981 to 2001. (*Adapted from reference 2.*)

TABLE 10–2. Strengths of Various Poisoning Databases

Database (abbreviation)	Strength
Death certificates from state health departments compiled by the National Center for Health Statistics (NCHS)	Compiles all death certificates where the cause of death was by disease or external forces. Data typically verified by laboratory and clinical observations.
National Electronic Injury Surveillance System of U.S. Consumer Product Safety Commission (NEISS)	Surveys electronically all injuries, including poisonings, treated daily at a sample of approximately 100 emergency departments. Used to identify product-related injuries.
Drug Abuse Warning Network (DAWN) of the Federal Substance Abuse and Mental Health Services Administration	Identifies substance abuse–related episodes and deaths as reported to 400 hospitals and 150 medical examiners.
The American Association of Poison Control Centers-Toxic Exposure Surveillance System (AAPCC-TESS)	Represents largest database of poisonings with high representation of children based on voluntary reporting to poison control centers.

symptom can be seen with poisoning, but some signs and symptoms are suggestive of a particular toxin exposure.[14] Compounds that produce characteristic clinical pictures (toxidromes), such as organophosphate poisoning with pinpoint pupils, rales, bradycardia, central nervous system depression, sweating, excessive salivation, and diarrhea, are most readily recognizable.[15] The recognition of chemicals responsible for acute, mass emergencies due to industrial disasters, hazardous materials accidents, or acts of terrorism may be aided by evaluating characteristic signs and symptoms.[16] Assessment of the patient may be aided by consultation with a poison control center. These centers can provide information on product composition, typical symptoms, range of toxicity, laboratory analysis, treatment options, and bibliographic references. Furthermore, the center will have specially trained physicians, pharmacists, nurses, and toxicologists on staff or on file to assist with difficult cases. Consultation with a poison control center also may identify changes in recommended therapy. A nationwide toll-free poison center access number (1-800-222-1222) routes callers to the local poison control center.

When the circumstances of a poison exposure indicate that it is minimally toxic, many poisonings can be managed successfully at the scene of the poisoning.[6] Poison control centers typically monitor the victim by telephone during the first 2 to 6 hours of the exposure to assess the patient's status and outcome of first aid.

Once a poisoning is suspected and there is a need to confirm the diagnosis for medical or legal purposes, appropriate biologic material should be sent to the laboratory for analysis. Gastric contents may contain the greatest concentration of drug, but they are difficult

to analyze. Blood or urine may be tested by qualitative screening in order to detect a drug's presence.[17,18] The results of a qualitative drug screen can be misleading owing to interfering or low-level substances (Table 10–6); it rarely guides therapy and thus has questionable value for nonspecific, general screening purposes.[17,18] Consultation with the laboratory technician and review of the assay package insert will help to determine the sensitivity and specificity of the assay. Quantitative determination of serum concentrations may be important for the assessment of some poisonings, such as those with acetaminophen, ethanol, methanol, iron, theophylline, and digoxin.[19]

PHARMACOKINETICS OF OVERDOSE

The pharmacokinetic characteristics of drugs taken in overdose may differ from those observed following therapeutic doses[20,21] (Table 10–7). These differences are due to dose-dependent changes in absorption, distribution, metabolism, or elimination; pharmacologic effects of the drug; or pathophysiologic consequences of the overdose. Dose-dependent changes may decrease the rate and extent of absorption, whereas the bioavailability of the agent may be increased due to saturation of first-pass metabolism. The distribution of a compound may be altered due to saturation of protein-binding sites. Metabolism and elimination of a compound may be retarded due to saturated biotransformation pathways leading to nonlinear elimination kinetics. Delayed gastric emptying by anticholinergic drugs or as the result of general central nervous system depression caused by many drugs may alter the rate and extent of absorption. The formation of concretions or bezoars of solid dosage forms may delay the onset, prolong the duration, or complicate the therapy of an acute overdose.[22] A combination of pharmacokinetic and pharmacodynamic factors may lead to the delayed onset of toxicity of several toxins, such as thyroid hormones, oral

TABLE 10–3. Poison Exposure by Age Group and Fatal Outcome, Ranked in Decreasing Order

Pediatric	Adult	Fatal Outcome
Medicines	Medicines	Medicines
Cosmetics and personal care items	Cleaning substances	Alcohols
Cleaning substances	Bites or envenomations	Gases and fumes
Foreign bodies	Food products or food poisoning	Chemicals
Plants	Cosmetics and personal care items	Pesticides
Pesticides	Pesticides	Cleaning substances
Arts and crafts or office supplies	Chemicals	Automotive products

From Watson.[6]

TABLE 10–4. Examples of Products Requiring Child-Resistant Closures

Acetaminophen	Kerosene
Aspirin	Methanol
Diphenhydramine	Oral prescription drugs[a]
Ethylene glycol	Permanent hair wave neutralizers containing sodium bromate
Glue removers containing acetonitrile	Sodium hydroxide
Ibuprofen	Sulfuric acid
Iron pharmaceuticals	Turpentine

[a]With certain exceptions such as nitroglycerin and oral contraceptives.

TABLE 10–5. Psychosocial Characteristics of Poisoning Patients

Children	Young Adults	Elderly
Act purposefully or are poisoned by caretaker or sibling	Intentional abuse or suicidal intent is possible	Suicidal intent or unintentional misuse
Act with developmentally appropriate curiosity	Disregard or cannot read directions	Confuse product identity and directions for use
Attracted by product appearance	Do not recognize poisoning risk	Do not recognize poisoning risk
Ingest substances that adults find unpleasant	Reluctant to seek assistance until ill	Comorbid conditions complicate toxicity
React to stressful and disrupted household	Exaggerate or misrepresent situation	Unable or unwilling to describe situation
Imitate adult behaviors (e.g., taking medicine)	Peer pressure to experiment with drugs	Multiple drugs may lead to adverse reactions

TABLE 10–7. Examples of the Influence of Drug Overdosage on Pharmacokinetic and Pharmacodynamic Characteristics

Effect of Overdosage[a]	Examples
Slowed absorption due to formation of poorly soluble concretions in the gastrointestinal tract	Aspirin, lithium, phenytoin, sustained-release theophylline
Slowed absorption due to slowed gastrointestinal motility	Benztropine, nortriptyline
Slowed absorption due to toxin-induced hypoperfusion	Procainamide
Decreased serum protein binding	Lidocaine, salicylates, valproic acid
Increased volume of distribution associated with toxin-induced acidemia	Salicylates
Slowed elimination due to saturation of biotransformation pathways	Ethanol, phenytoin, salicylates, theophylline
Slowed elimination due to toxin-induced hypothermia (<35°C)	Ethanol, propranolol
Prolonged toxicity due to formation of longer-acting metabolites	Carbamazepine, dapsone, glutethimide, meperidine

[a]Compared to characteristics following therapeutic doses or resolution of toxicity.
From Rosenberg[20] and Young-Jin.[21]

TABLE 10–6. Considerations in Evaluating the Results of Some Common Immunoassays Used for Urine Drug Screening

Drug	Detection After Stopping Use	Comments
Amphetamines	2–5 days Up to 2 weeks with prolonged or heavy use	Many sympathomimetic amines such as pseudoephedrine, ephedra, phenylephrine, fenfluramine, and phentermine may cause positive results. Other drugs such as selegiline, chlorpromazine, trazodone, bupropion, and amantadine may cause false-positive results depending on the assay.
Benzodiazepines	Up to 2 weeks Up to 6 weeks with chronic use of some drugs	The ability to detect benzodiazepines varies by drug.
Cannabinoid metabolite (marijuana)	7–10 days Up to 1–2 months with prolonged or heavy use	The extent and duration of use will affect detection time. Drugs such as ibuprofen and naproxen may cause false-positive results depending on the assay.
Cocaine metabolite (benzoylecgonine)	12–72 hours Up to 1–3 weeks with prolonged or heavy use	Cocaine is metabolized rapidly, and specific metabolites are typically the substance detected. False-positive results from "-caine" anesthetics and other drugs are unlikely.
Opioids	2–3 days typically Up to 6 days with sustained-release formulations Up to 1 week with prolonged or heavy use	Since the assay was made to detect morphine, detection of other opioids, such as codeine, oxycodone, hydrocodone, and other semisynthetic opioids, may be limited. Some synthetic opioids, e.g., fentanyl and meperidine, may not be detected. Drugs such as rifampin and some fluoroquinolones may cause false-positive results depending on the assay.
Phencyclidine	2–10 days 1 month or more with prolonged or heavy use	Drugs such as ketamine, dextromethorphan, diphenhydramine, and sertraline may cause false positive results depending upon the assay.

anticoagulants, acetaminophen, and drugs in sustained-release dosage forms.[23] Drug-induced hypoperfusion may affect drug distribution and result in reduced hepatic or renal clearance. Changes in blood pH may alter the distribution of weak acids and bases. Drug-induced renal or hepatic injury also can decrease clearance significantly. Implications of these changes for poisoning management include the delayed achievement of peak concentrations with a corresponding longer period of opportunity to remove the drug from the gastrointestinal tract. The expected duration of effects may be much greater than that observed with therapeutic doses due to continued absorption and impaired clearance. The application of pharmacokinetic variables, such as percentage protein binding and volume of distribution, from therapeutic doses may not be appropriate in poisoning cases.[20] Data on toxicokinetics often are difficult to interpret and compare because the doses and times of ingestion are uncertain, the duration of sampling is inadequate, active metabolites may not be measured, protein binding typically is not assessed, and the severity of toxicity may vary dramatically.

▶ TREATMENT: Clinical Toxicology

GENERAL APPROACHES TO TREATMENT OF THE POISONED PATIENT

▦ PREHOSPITAL CARE

▦ FIRST AID

◀3 The presence of adequate airway, breathing, and circulation should be assessed, and cardiopulmonary resuscitation should be started if needed. The most important step in preventing a minor exposure from progressing to a serious intoxication is early decontamination of the poison. Basic poisoning first-aid and decontamination measures (Table 10–8) should be instituted immediately at the scene of the poisoning. If there is any question about the potential severity of the poison exposure, a poison control center should be consulted immediately (1-800-222-1222). While awaiting transport, placing the patient on the left side may afford easier clearance of the airway if emesis occurs and may slow absorption of drug from the gastrointestinal tract.[24]

▦ IPECAC SYRUP

◀4 Ipecac syrup, a nonprescription drug, has been used in the United States for the past 50 years as a means to induce vomiting for the treatment of ingested poisons. Despite its widespread use, concerns about its effectiveness and safety have been raised recently. An expert panel of North American and European toxicologists concluded that its routine use in the emergency department should be abandoned.[25] The American Academy of Pediatrics issued a policy statement in 2003 that indicated that ipecac syrup was no longer to be used routinely to treat poisonings at home and that parents should discard any ipecac.[26] The key reason for the policy change was that research failed to show benefits in those children who were treated with ipecac syrup. It likely will take several years for these recommendations to be adopted fully by parents and health care professionals, and rare exceptions may arise.

There are several contraindications to the use of ipecac syrup.[25] If the patient is without a gag reflex; is lethargic, comatose, or convulsing; or is expected to become unresponsive within the next 30 minutes, emesis should not be induced. If a fruitful emesis has occurred spontaneously shortly after ingestion, ipecac syrup may not be necessary. Ingestions of caustics, corrosives, ammonia, and bleach are definite contraindications to ipecac-induced emesis. The ingestion of aliphatic hydrocarbons (e.g., gasoline, kerosene, and charcoal lighter fluid) typically does not require emesis. When the agent is definitely known to be nontoxic, induction of emesis is purposeless and potentially dangerous. The rapid onset of coma or seizures or the potential to exaggerate the toxic effects of the poison may preclude the use of ipecac syrup. Some examples include poisonings with diphenoxylate, propoxyphene, clonidine, tricyclic antidepressants, hypoglycemic agents, nicotine, strychnine, β-blocking agents, and calcium channel blockers. Debilitated, pregnant, and elderly patients may be further compromised by the induction of emesis.

▦ HOSPITAL TREATMENT

▦ GENERAL CARE

Supportive and symptomatic care is the mainstay of treatment of a poisoned patient. In the search for specific antidotes and methods to increase excretion of the drug, attention to vital signs and organ functions should not be neglected. Establishment of adequate oxygenation and maintenance of adequate circulation are the highest priority. Other components of the acute supportive care plan include the management of seizures, arrhythmias, hypotension, acid-base balance, fluid status, electrolyte balance, and hypoglycemia. Placement of intravenous and urinary catheters is typical to ensure delivery of fluids and drugs when necessary and to monitor urine production, respectively.

▦ GASTRIC LAVAGE

Gastric lavage involves the placement of an orogastric tube and washing out of the gastric contents through repetitive instillation and withdrawal of fluid. Gastric lavage may be considered only if a potentially toxic agent has been ingested within the past hour for most patients. If the patient is comatose or lacks a gag reflex, gastric lavage should be performed only after intubation with a cuffed or well-fitting endotracheal tube. The largest orogastric tube that can be passed (at least an

TABLE 10–8. First Aid for Poison Exposures

Inhaled Poison
Immediately get the person to fresh air. Avoid breathing fumes. Open doors and windows. If victim is not breathing, start artificial respiration.

Poison on the Skin
Remove contaminated clothing and flood skin with water for 10 minutes. Wash gently with soap and water and rinse. Avoid further contamination of victim or first aid providers.

Poison in the Eye
Flood the eye with lukewarm or cool water poured from a glass 2 or 3 inches from the eye. Repeat for 10 to 15 continuous minutes. Keep eye open, but do not force the eyelid open.

Swallowed Poison
Unless the patient is unconscious, having convulsions, or cannot swallow, give 2 to 4 ounces of water immediately and then seek further help.

external diameter of 12 mm in adults and 8 mm in children) should be used to ensure adequate evacuation, especially of undissolved tablets. Lavage should be performed with warm (37–38°C) normal saline or tap water until the gastric return is clear; this usually requires 2 to 4 L or more of fluid. Relative contraindications for gastric lavage include ingestion of a corrosive or hydrocarbon agent. Complications of gastric lavage include aspiration pneumonitis, laryngospasm, mechanical injury to the esophagus and stomach, hypothermia, and fluid and electrolyte imbalance.[27]

SINGLE-DOSE ACTIVATED CHARCOAL

Reduction of toxin absorption can be achieved by the administration of activated charcoal. It is a highly purified, adsorbent form of carbon that prevents the gastrointestinal absorption of a drug by chemically binding (adsorbing) the drug to the charcoal surface. There are no toxin-related contraindications to its use, but it is generally ineffective for iron, lead, lithium, simple alcohols, and corrosives. It is not indicated for aliphatic hydrocarbons because of the increased risk of emesis and pulmonary aspiration. Activated charcoal is most effective when given within the first few hours after ingestion, ideally within the first hour.[28] The recommended dose of activated charcoal for a child (1–12 years old) is 25 to 50 g; for an adolescent or adult it is 25 to 100 g. Children under 1 year of age may receive 1 g/kg.[9] Activated charcoal is mixed with water to make a slurry, shaken vigorously, and administered orally or by means of a nasogastric tube. Activated charcoal is contraindicated when the gastrointestinal tract is not intact. Activated charcoal is relatively nontoxic, but there are two identified risks: (1) emesis following administration and (2) pulmonary aspiration of charcoal and gastric contents leading to pneumonitis in patients with an unprotected airway or absent gag reflex.[28] Some activated charcoal products contain sorbitol, a cathartic that may be associated with an increased incidence of emesis following use.[29]

CATHARTICS

Cathartics, such as magnesium citrate and sorbitol, were thought to decrease the rate of absorption by increasing gastrointestinal elimination of the poison and the poison-activated charcoal complex, but their value is unproven. Poisoned patients do not routinely require the administration of a cathartic, and it is rarely, if ever, given without concurrent activated charcoal administration.[30] If used, a cathartic should be administered only once and only if bowel sounds are present. Infants, the elderly, and patients with renal failure should be given saline cathartics cautiously, if at all.[9,30]

CLINICAL CONTROVERSY

Activated charcoal has been promoted for use at home as a replacement for ipecac syrup, but some have contended that there is little evidence which indicates that it can be used safely and properly in this setting.

WHOLE-BOWEL IRRIGATION

Polyethylene glycol electrolyte solutions, such as GoLytely and Colyte, are used routinely as whole-bowel irrigants prior to colonoscopy and bowel surgery.[31] These solutions also can be used as a means to decontaminate the gastrointestinal tract of ingested toxins.[9,14,32] Large volumes of these osmotically balanced solutions

are administered continuously through a nasogastric or duodenal tube for 4 to 12 hours or more. They quickly cause gastrointestinal evacuation and are continued until the rectal discharge is relatively clear. This procedure may be indicated for certain patients in whom the ingestion occurred several hours prior to hospitalization and the drug still is suspected to be in the gastrointestinal tract, such as drug smugglers who swallow condoms filled with cocaine.[33] In addition, patients who have ingested delayed-release or enteric-coated drug formulations or have ingested substances such as iron that are not well adsorbed by activated charcoal may benefit from whole-bowel irrigation.[32] It should not be used in patients with a bowel perforation or obstruction, gastrointestinal hemorrhage, ileus, or intractable emesis. Emesis, abdominal cramps, and intestinal bloating have been reported with whole-bowel irrigation.[32]

CLINICAL CONTROVERSY

Some clinicians believe that whole-bowel irrigation should be used more routinely as a rapid means to evacuate the gastrointestinal tract. Others recognize that it does have a quick onset but point out that there is little proof that it makes a difference in patient outcome.

PERSPECTIVES ON GASTRIC DECONTAMINATION

Although there are a variety of options for gastric decontamination, two clinical toxicology groups (the American Academy of Clinical Toxicology and the European Association of Poison Centers and Clinical Toxicologists) have concluded that no means of gastric decontamination should be used routinely for a poisoned patient without careful consideration.[25,27,28,30,32] They indicate that therapy is most effective within the first hour and that effectiveness beyond this time cannot be supported or refuted with the available data. A clinical policy statement by the American College of Emergency Physicians concludes that although no definitive recommendation can be made on the use of ipecac syrup, gastric lavage, cathartics, or whole-bowel irrigation, activated charcoal is advocated for most patients when appropriate.[34] The clinical policy also states that ipecac syrup is rarely of value in the emergency department and that the use of whole-bowel irrigation following ingestion of substances not well adsorbed by activated charcoal is not supported by evidence. Although gastric lavage can reduce drug absorption if performed within 1 hour of ingestion, its use is not recommended routinely.[27,34,35] In recent years, the use of ipecac syrup has declined markedly in part because of its apparent lower efficacy compared with activated charcoal in minimizing drug absorption.[6,25,28] The American Academy of Pediatrics has recommended that ipecac syrup no longer be used for the treatment of poisonings at home and has called for its removal from the home.[26] Recently, activated charcoal has been promoted for the treatment of poisonings at home, but issues of safety, patient compliance, and effectiveness have not been proven in the home setting.[26,36] Poison control centers may be a source of guidance on the contemporary application of gastric decontamination techniques for a specific patient.

Enhanced Elimination

Numerous methods have been used to increase the rate of excretion of poisons from the body. Of these, only diuresis, multiple-dose activated charcoal, and hemodialysis are useful occasionally. These approaches should be considered only if the risks of the procedure are significantly outweighed by the expected benefits or if the recovery of the patient is seriously in doubt and the method has been shown to be helpful.

Diuresis

Diuresis may be used for poisons excreted predominantly by the renal route; however, most drugs and poisons are metabolized, and only a good urine flow, such as 2–3 mL/kg per hour, needs to be maintained for most patients. Fluid and electrolyte balance should be monitored closely. Ionized diuresis by altering urinary pH may increase excretion of certain chemicals that are weak acids or bases by trapping ionized drug in the renal tubule and minimizing reabsorption.[14] Alkalinization of the urine to achieve a urine pH of 7.5 or greater for poisoning by weak acids such as salicylates or phenobarbital can be achieved by the intravenous administration of sodium bicarbonate 1–2 mEq/kg over a 1- to 2-hour period. Complications of urinary alkalinization include alkalosis, fluid and electrolyte disturbances, and inability to achieve target urinary pH values.[37] Acid diuresis may enhance the excretion of weak bases, such as amphetamines, but it is rarely, if ever, used because it risks worsening rhabdomyolysis commonly associated with amphetamine overdose.[14] Generally, ionized diuresis is rarely indicated for poisoned patients because it is inefficient relative to other methods of enhancing elimination, there is a risk of unacceptable adverse effects, and the renal elimination of most drugs is not enhanced dramatically.

Multiple-Dose Activated Charcoal

Multiple doses of activated charcoal can augment the body's clearance of certain drugs by enhanced passage from the bloodstream into the gastrointestinal tract and subsequent adsorption. This process, termed charcoal intestinal dialysis or charcoal-enhanced intestinal exsorption, describes the attraction of drug molecules across the capillary bed of the intestine by activated charcoal in the intestinal lumen and subsequent adsorption of the drug to the charcoal.[38] Furthermore, it may interrupt the enterohepatic recirculation of certain drugs.[14,38] Once the drug is adsorbed to the charcoal, it is eliminated with the charcoal in the stool. The systemic clearance of several drugs has been shown to be enhanced up to severalfold.[38,39] An international toxicology group's position statement on multiple-dose activated charcoal concluded that it should be considered only if a patient has ingested a life-threatening amount of carbamazepine, dapsone, phenobarbital, quinine, or theophylline.[39] Although a prospective, randomized study of the effects of multiple-dose activated charcoal on phenobarbital-overdosed patients demonstrated increased drug elimination, no demonstrable effect on patient outcome was observed.[40]

This approach provides a rapid onset of action that is limited by blood flow and a maximal "ceiling effect" related to the dose of charcoal present in the intestine. The response to multiple-dose activated charcoal is greatest for drugs with the following characteristics: good affinity for adsorption by activated charcoal, low intrinsic clearance, sufficient residence time in the body (long serum half-life), long distributive phase, and nonrestrictive protein binding. A small volume of distribution is also desirable, but it has a marginal influence as an isolated characteristic,[41] particularly if multiple-dose activated charcoal is instituted during the toxin's distributive phase. A typical dosage schedule is 15–25 g activated charcoal every 2 to 6 hours until serious symptoms abate or the serum concentration of the toxin is below the toxic range. This procedure has been used in premature and full-term infants in doses of 1 g/kg every 1 to 4 hours. Serious complications, such as pulmonary aspiration, occur in less than 1% of patients.[42] The

risks of aspiration pneumonitis in obtunded or uncooperative patients and of intestinal obstruction in patients prone to ileus following a period of bowel ischemia, for example, after cardiopulmonary arrest in the elderly may be higher.[43] Contraindications are the same as those for single-dose charcoal.

Hemodialysis

Hemodialysis may be necessary for certain severe cases of poisoning. Dialysis should be considered when the duration of symptoms is expected to be prolonged, other pathways of excretion are unavailable, clinical deterioration is present, the drug is dialyzable, and appropriate personnel and equipment are available. Drugs that are hemodialyzable usually have a low molecular weight, are not highly or tightly protein bound, and are not highly distributed to tissues. The principles of hemodialysis for acutely ill individuals are described in Chap. 45. Hemodialysis and charcoal hemoperfusion are the most efficient methods of dialysis, but both pose serious risks related to anticoagulation, blood transfusions, loss of blood elements, fluid and electrolyte disturbances, and infection.[44] Hemodialysis may be lifesaving for methanol and ethylene glycol poisoning and effective for other poisons, such as lithium, salicylates, ethanol, and theophylline.[14,34] Charcoal hemoperfusion was popular in the 1970s and 1980s as a means to remove toxins quickly from the circulation, but this approach has fallen out of favor owing to poor results, inappropriate use for drugs with large volumes of distribution, and limited commercial availability of charcoal hemoperfusion columns. Continuous hemofiltration transports drugs across a semipermeable membrane by convection in response to hydrostatic pressure gradients.[14,44] Limited experience is reported with the use of hemofiltration for poisonings, but it may be attractive for the hemodynamically unstable patient who cannot tolerate hemodialysis.

ANTIDOTES

The search for and use of an antidote should never replace good supportive care.[34] Specific systemic antidotes are available for many common poisonings[45,46] (Table 10–9). Inadequate availability of antidotes at acute care hospitals has been noted throughout the United States and can complicate the care of a poisoned patient. An evidenced-based consensus of experts has recommended minimum stocking requirements for 16 antidotes for acute care hospitals.[47] These recommendations may provide guidance to pharmacy and therapeutics committees in establishing a hospital's antidote needs. Drugs used conventionally for nonpoisoning situations may act as antidotes to reverse acute toxicity, such as glucagon for β-adrenergic blocker or calcium channel antagonist overdose and octreotide for sulfonylurea-induced hypoglycemia.[48] As our understanding of drug toxicity increases, antidotes may have applications beyond contemporary indications, such as acetylcysteine, which has shown promise for treating approximately 25 different poisonings and adverse drug reactions.[49] The use of toxin-specific antibodies (e.g., Fab antibody fragments for digoxin[50] or crotalid snake venom[51]) has offered a new approach to the treatment of poisoning victims.

ASSESSING THE EFFECTIVENESS OF THERAPIES

Our knowledge of poisoning treatment is derived from case reports, clinical studies, human volunteer studies, animal investigations, and

TABLE 10–9. Systemic Antidotes Available in the United States

Antidote	Toxic Agent
Acetylcysteine	Acetaminophen
Atropine	Anticholinesterase insecticides
Botulism antitoxin	Botulism
Calcium EDTA	Lead
Crotalidae polyvalent antivenin	Rattlesnakes, cottonmouth snakes, copperhead snakes
Crotalidae polyvalent immune Fab	Rattlesnakes, cottonmouth snakes, copperhead snakes
Cyanide antidote kit (Amyl nitrite, sodium nitrate, and sodium thiosulfate)	Cyanide
Deferoxamine	Iron
Digoxin immune Fab	Digoxin, digitoxin
Dimercaprol	Various heavy metals
Ethanol	Ethylene glycol, methanol
Flumazenil	Benzodiazepines
Fomepizole	Ethylene glycol, methanol
Lactrodectus mactans antivenin	Black widow spider
Methylene blue	Methemoglobinemia
Micrurus fulvius antivenin	Coral snake
Nalmefene	Opioids
Naloxone	Opioids
Oxygen	Carbon monoxide
Penicillamine	Various heavy metals
Phytonadione	Anticoagulants
Pralidoxime	Organophosphate insecticides
Succimer	Lead

in vitro tests. Each of these approaches has limited applicability to the care of humans who have been poisoned. Case reports often are difficult to assess because they are uncontrolled, the histories are uncertain, and multiple therapies frequently are used. They can, however, be useful to describe unique or new toxicities or characterize adverse effects associated with a therapy. Although clinical studies may describe tens to hundreds of patients, they can exhibit serious shortcomings, such as weak randomization procedures, no laboratory confirmation or correlation with history, insufficient number of severe cases, no control group, and no quantitative measure of outcome. Extrapolation of data from human volunteer studies to patients who overdose is difficult because of potential or unknown variations in pharmacokinetics (e.g., differing dissolution, gastric emptying, and absorption rates) seen with toxic as opposed to therapeutic doses,[20,21] differences in time to institute therapy in the emergency setting, and differences in absorption in fasted human volunteers compared with the full stomach of some patients who overdose. These studies, however, provide the most controlled and objective measures of the efficacy of a treatment. Experiences from animal studies cannot be applied directly to humans because of interspecies differences in toxicity and metabolism. In vitro tests serve to screen the efficacy of some approaches, such as activated charcoal adsorption, but they do not mimic physiologic conditions sufficiently to allow direct clinical application of the findings. Despite their limitations, these data comprise the basis for the therapy of poisoned patients and are tempered with the consideration of non-poisoning-related factors such as a particular patient's underlying medical condition, age, and need for concurrent supportive measures.

CLINICAL SPECTRUM OF POISONING

Poisoning and drug overdose with acetaminophen, anticholinesterase insecticides, calcium channel blockers, iron, and tricyclic antidepressants are the focus of the remainder of this chapter because they represent commonly encountered poisonings for which pharmacotherapy is indicated. These agents also were chosen because they represent common examples with different mechanisms of toxicity, and they illustrate the application of general treatment approaches as well as some agent-specific interventions.

ACETAMINOPHEN

CLINICAL PRESENTATION

Acute acetaminophen poisoning characteristically results in hepatotoxicity[52,53] and is the leading cause of acute liver failure in the United States.[54] Clinical presentation (see below) is determined by the time required for hepatic necrosis to occur, presence of risk factors, and the ingestion of other drugs. During the first 12 to 24 hours after ingestion, nausea, vomiting, anorexia, and diaphoresis may be observed; however, many patients are asymptomatic. During the next 1 to 3 days, a latent phase of lessened symptoms, patients often have an asymptomatic rise in liver enzymes and bilirubin. Signs and symptoms of hepatic injury become manifest 3 to 5 days after ingestion and include right upper quadrant abdominal tenderness, jaundice, hypoglycemia, and encephalopathy. Prolongation of the prothrombin time worsens as hepatic necrosis progresses and may lead to disseminated intravascular coagulopathy. Patients with hepatic damage may develop hepatic coma, hepatorenal syndrome and death can occur.[52,53,55] Even in patients with severe hepatotoxicity, there are usually no resid-

ual functional or histologic abnormalities of the liver noted within 1 to 6 months of the incident.[53]

CLINICAL PRESENTATION OF ACUTE ACETAMINOPHEN POISONING

GENERAL

- No or mild nonspecific symptoms within 6 hours of ingestion

SYMPTOMS

- Nausea, vomiting, and abdominal discomfort within hours after ingestion
- Right upper abdominal quadrant tenderness typically within 1 to 2 days
- Jaundice, scleral icterus, bleeding within 3 to 10 days
- With severe poisoning, hepatic encephalopathy (delirium, coma) within 5 to 10 days

SIGNS

- Typically no signs present within first day
- Oliguria occasionally within 2 to 7 days
- Depressed reflexes and hypotension within 5 to 10 days with encephalopathy

LABORATORY TESTS

- Toxic serum acetaminophen concentration no earlier than 4 hours after ingestion by comparison with nomogram
- Elevated aspartate aminotransferase (AST), alanine aminotransferase (ALT), serum bilirubin, and international

normalization ratio (INR); hypoglycemia within 1 to 3 days
• Elevated serum creatinine and blood urea nitrogen (BUN) within 2 to 7 days

OTHER DIAGNOSTIC TESTS

• Ultrasound for hepatomegaly, if warranted

MECHANISM OF TOXICITY

Acetaminophen is metabolized in the liver primarily to glucuronide or sulfate conjugates, which are excreted into the urine with small amounts (<5%) of unchanged drug. Approximately 5% of a therapeutic dose is metabolized by the cytochrome P450 mixed-function oxygenase system, primarily CYP2E1, to a reactive metabolite, N-acetyl-p-benzoquinone-imine (NAPQI). This metabolite normally is conjugated with glutathione, a sulfhydryl-containing compound, in the hepatocyte and excreted in the urine as a mercapturate conjugate[55] (Fig. 10–2).

In an acute overdose situation, sulfate stores are depleted, shifting more drug through the cytochrome system, thereby depleting the available glutathione used to detoxify the reactive metabolite. The reactive metabolite, NAPQI, then reacts with other hepatocellular sulfhydryl compounds such as those in the cytosol, cell wall, and endoplasmic reticulum. This results in centrilobular hepatic necrosis.[55] Several other mechanisms, such as cytokine release or oxidative stress, also may be initiated by the initial cellular injury.[55]

In many cases of severe hepatotoxicity, renal injury is also present and may range from oliguria to acute renal failure. The etiology of the renal injury may be a direct effect of a toxic metabolite of acetaminophen, N-acetyl-p-benzoquinone-imine (discussed in the next section), generated by renal cytochrome oxidase or a consequence of hepatic injury resulting in hepatorenal syndrome.[56] Isolated cases of myocardial injury have been reported rarely.[57]

CAUSATIVE AGENTS

Acetaminophen, also known as paracetamol in other countries, is available widely without prescription as an analgesic and antipyretic. It is available in various oral dosage forms, including an extended-release preparation. Acetaminophen may be combined with other drugs, such as antihistamines or opioid analgesics, and marketed in cough and cold preparations, menstrual remedies, and allergy products.

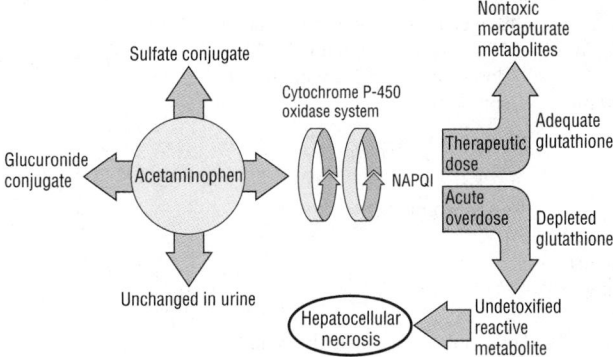

FIGURE 10–2. Pathway of acetaminophen metabolism and basis for hepatotoxicity. (NAPQI, N-acetyl-p-benzoquinone-imine, a reactive acetaminophen metabolite.)

INCIDENCE

Acetaminophen is one of the most commonly ingested drugs by small children and is used commonly in suicide attempts by adolescents and adults. The 2003 AAPCC-TESS report documented 61,755 nonfatal exposures and 147 deaths from acetaminophen, with 48% of the exposures in children younger than 6 years of age.[6]

Age-based differences in the metabolism of acetaminophen appear to be responsible for major differences in the incidence of serious toxicity. Despite the common ingestion of acetaminophen by young children, few develop hepatotoxicity from acute overdosage.[6] In children younger than 9 to 12 years of age, acetaminophen undergoes more sulfation and less glucuronidation. The reduced fraction available for metabolism by the cytochrome system may explain the rare development of serious toxicity in young children who take large overdoses. Earlier treatment intervention and spontaneous emesis also may reduce the risk of toxicity in children.

RISK ASSESSMENT

There is a risk of developing hepatotoxicity when adolescents or adults acutely ingest more than 7.5 g acetaminophen or when children acutely ingest more than 150 mg/kg.[52] The least amount reported to produce death is 10 g in an adult, but others have survived much larger doses, particularly with early treatment. Initial symptoms, if present, do not predict how serious the toxicity eventually may become.

Chronic exposure to drugs that induce the cytochrome oxidase system—specifically isoenzyme CYP2E1, which is responsible for most of the formation of NAPQI—may increase the risk of acetaminophen hepatotoxicity. Poorer outcomes have been noted in patients who chronically ingest alcohol and those receiving anticonvulsants, both known to induce CYP2E1.[53,58] Patients with chronic alcoholism have a 3.5 greater odds of mortality with acute acetaminophen poisoning.[59] Concurrent acute ingestion of alcohol and acetaminophen may decrease the risk of acetaminophen-induced hepatotoxicity by ethanol acting as a competitive substrate for CYP2E1, thus reducing NAPQI formation.[60] Ethanol co-ingestion is not advocated as a preventive measure, and it is difficult to account for its specific impact on care.

Chronic, excessive acetaminophen consumption, defined as doses exceeding the recommended daily doses of 4 g for an adult and 90 mg/kg for a child for several days, has been associated with hepatotoxicity.[53] The incidence is unknown, and the basis of this association is not well understood. Patients who are fasting or have ingested alcohol in the preceding 5 days appear to be at greater risk.[61] Young children who receive acetaminophen in excess of the recommended total daily dose of 50–75 mg/kg have a risk of developing hepatotoxicity, particularly when they have been acutely fasting as the result of a febrile illness or gastroenteritis.[62,63]

The risk of developing hepatotoxicity may be predicted from a nomogram (Fig. 10–3) based on the acetaminophen serum concentration and time after ingestion.[52] The treatment line of the nomogram (150 mcg/mL at 4 hours), which allows a margin of error in laboratory analysis and time of ingestion, should be used to make treatment decisions. The other lines on the nomogram indicate differing levels of risk for hepatotoxicity based on a multicenter study of 11,195 patients.[52]

If the plasma concentration plotted on the nomogram falls above the nomogram treatment line, indicating that hepatic damage is possible, a full course of treatment with acetylcysteine is indicated. When the results of the acetaminophen determination will be available later than 8 hours after the ingestion, acetylcysteine therapy should be

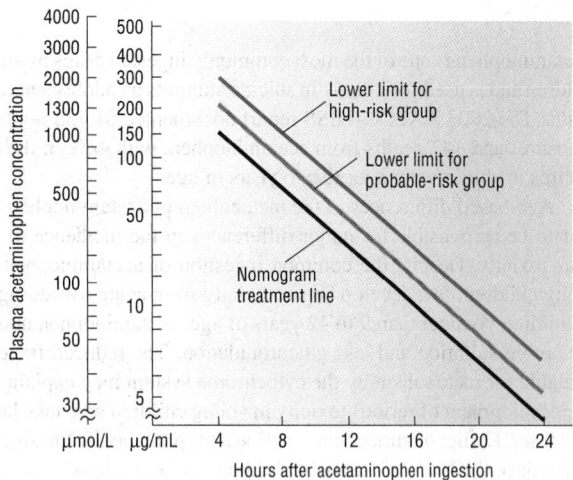

FIGURE 10–3. Nomogram for assessing hepatotoxic risk following acute ingestion of acetaminophen. *(Adapted from reference 52.)*

initiated based on the history and later discontinued if the results indicate nontoxic concentrations. The nomogram has not been evaluated and thus is not useful for assessing chronic exposure to acetaminophen. Some have advocated that patients with chronic alcoholism should be treated with acetylcysteine regardless of the risk estimation.[59]

MANAGEMENT OF TOXICITY

Therapy of an acute acetaminophen overdose depends on the amount ingested, time after ingestion, and the serum concentration of acetaminophen. When adolescents or adults ingest excessive amounts, when the history is unclear, or when an intentional ingestion is suspected, the patient must be evaluated at an emergency department and acetaminophen serum concentrations obtained. No prehospital care generally is indicated, and ipecac syrup typically is avoided. If the patient presents to the emergency department within 4 hours of the ingestion or other drugs are suspected, one dose of activated charcoal may be administered.

Acetylcysteine (also known as *N*-acetylcysteine), a sulfhydryl-containing compound, replenishes the hepatic stores of glutathione by serving as a glutathione surrogate that combines directly with reactive metabolites or by serving as a source of sulfate, thus preventing hepatic damage.[64] It should be started within 10 hours of the ingestion to be most effective.[52] Initiation of therapy 24 to 36 hours after the ingestion may be of value in some patients, particularly those with measurable serum acetaminophen concentrations.[64,65] Patients with fulminant hepatic failure may benefit through other mechanisms by the administration or initiation of acetylcysteine several days after ingestion.[64]

CLINICAL CONTROVERSY

The routine administration of acetylcysteine more than 24 hours after acetaminophen overdose has been proposed. Case reports and animal studies indicate that it is relatively safe and that its use may minimize hepatotoxicity. Although accepted criteria for its use are lacking, it may be considered for patients with fulminant hepatoxicity, when acetaminophen is still measurable in the serum, or when the ingestion was not recognized within 24 hours and liver toxicity is apparent.

Therapy should be initiated with the oral or intravenous form of acetylcysteine within 10 hours of ingestion when indicated. The oral liquid was the only approved form of acetylcysteine in the United States until the Food and Drug Administration (FDA) approved an intravenous form in 2004. Besides the means of administration, there are several notable differences[49,52,66,67] (Table 10–10). The 20-hour dosage regimen for the intravenous form is based on one used in Europe for two decades and has similar outcome to the 72-hour oral regimen.[49,68] The preference for the oral or intravenous form of acetylcysteine will evolve during the next few years of experience.

When plasma concentrations are below the nomogram treatment line, there is little risk of toxicity, protective therapy with acetylcysteine is not necessary, and further medical therapy is unnecessary for the acetaminophen overdose.[52] The acetaminophen blood sample should be drawn no sooner than 4 hours after the ingestion to ensure that peak acetaminophen concentrations have been reached.

TABLE 10–10. Comparison of Intravenous and Oral Regimens for Acetylcysteine in the Treatment of Acute Acetaminophen Poisoning

Characteristic	Intravenous	Oral
Regimen (D₅W = 5% dextrose in water for injection)	150 mg/kg in 200 mL D₅W infused over 15 minutes, then 50 mg/kg in 500 mL D₅W over 4 hours, followed by 100 mg/kg in 1000 mL D₅W over 16 hours	140 mg/kg, followed 4 hours later by 70 mg/kg every 4 hours for 17 doses diluted to 5% with juice or soft drinks
Total dose (mg/kg)	200	1330
Duration (h)	20	72
Adverse effects	Anaphylactoid reactions (rash, hypotension, wheezing, dyspnea); acute flushing and erythema in first hour of the infusion that typically resolves spontaneously	Nausea, vomiting
Ancillary therapy, if needed	Antihistamines and epinephrine for severe anaphylactic reactions	Antiemetics, e.g., metoclopramide, ondansetron, or droperidol
Tradename	Acetadote	Mucomyst
Available strength	20%	10%, 20%

If a concentration is obtained less than 4 hours after ingestion, it is uninterpretable, and a second determination should be done at least 4 hours after ingestion. Serial determinations of a serum concentration, 4 to 6 hours apart, typically are unnecessary unless there is some evidence of slowed gastrointestinal motility from other ingested drugs (e.g., opioids, antihistamines, or anticholinergic drugs) or unless an extended-release product is involved. Therapy with acetylcysteine is continued if any concentration is above the treatment line of the nomogram, and therapy is discontinued when both concentrations are below the treatment line.

Although young children have an inherently lower risk of acetaminophen-induced hepatotoxicity, these patients should be managed in the same manner as adults. When acetaminophen plasma concentrations predict that toxicity is probable, young children should receive acetylcysteine in the dosing regimen described previously.[58]

If fulminant hepatic failure develops, the approaches described in Chap. 37 should be considered. In unresponsive patients, liver transplantation is a lifesaving option.[53]

MONITORING AND PREVENTION

Baseline liver function tests (AST, ALT, bilirubin, prothrombin time), serum creatinine determination, and urinalysis should be obtained on admission and repeated at 24-hour intervals until at least 96 hours have elapsed for those at risk. Most patients with liver injury develop elevated transaminase concentrations within 24 hours of ingestion. Transaminase concentrations greater than 1000 IU/L commonly are associated with other signs of liver dysfunction and have been used as the threshold concentration in outcome studies to define severe liver toxicity.[52] The extent of transaminase elevation is not correlated directly with severity of the hepatic injury, with nonfatal cases demonstrating peak concentrations as high as 30,000 IU/L between 48 and 72 hours after ingestion.[53]

Prevention of acetaminophen poisoning is based on recognition of the maximum daily therapeutic doses, observance of general poison prevention practices, and early intervention in cases of suspected overdose.

ANTICHOLINESTERASE INSECTICIDES

CLINICAL PRESENTATION

The clinical manifestations of anticholinesterase insecticide poisoning include any or all of the following: pinpoint pupils, excessive lacrimation, excessive salivation, bronchorrhea, bronchospasm and expiratory wheezes, hyperperistalsis producing abdominal cramps and diarrhea, bradycardia, excessive sweating, fasciculations and weakness of skeletal muscles, paralysis of skeletal muscles (particularly those involved with respiration), convulsions, and coma.[69] Symptoms of anticholinesterase poisoning and their response to antidotal therapy depend on the action of excessive acetylcholinesterase at different receptor types (Table 10–11).

TABLE 10–11. Effects of Acetylcholinesterase Inhibition at Muscarinic, Nicotinic, and CNS Receptors

Muscarinic Receptors	Nicotinic–Sympathetic Neurons
Diarrhea	Increased blood pressure
Urination	Sweating and piloerection
Miosis[a]	Mydriasis[a]
Bronchorrhea	Hyperglycemia
Bradycardia[a]	Tachycardia[a]
Emesis	Priapism
Lacrimation	**Nicotinic–Neuromuscular Neurons**
Salivation	Muscular weakness
CNS Receptors (Mixed Type)	Cramps
Coma	Fasciculations
Seizures	Muscular paralysis

[a]Generally muscarinic effects predominate, but nicotinic effects can be observed.

The time of onset and severity of symptoms depend on the route of exposure, potency of the agent, and total dose received (see below). Toxic signs and symptoms develop most rapidly after inhalation or intravenous injection and slowest after skin contact. Anticholinesterase insecticides are absorbed through the skin, lungs, conjunctivae, and gastrointestinal tract. Severe symptoms can occur from absorption by any route. Within 6 hours, most patients are symptomatic, and without treatment, death may occur within 24 hours. Death typically is caused by respiratory failure owing to the combination of pulmonary and cardiovascular effects[69] (Fig. 10–4). Poisoning may be complicated by aspiration pneumonia, urinary tract infections, and sepsis.[70]

CLINICAL PRESENTATION OF ANTICHOLINESTERASE INSECTICIDE POISONING

GENERAL

- Mild symptoms may resolve spontaneously; life-threatening toxicity may develop with 1 to 6 hours of exposure

SYMPTOMS

- Diarrhea, diaphoresis, urination, miosis, blurred vision, pulmonary congestion, dyspnea, emesis, lacrimation, salivation, and shortness of breath within 1 hour
- Muscle weakness, fasciculations, and respiratory paralysis within 1 to 6 hours
- Headache, confusion, coma, and seizures possible within 1 to 6 hours

SIGNS

- Increased bronchial secretions, tachypnea, rales, and cyanosis within 1 to 6 hours

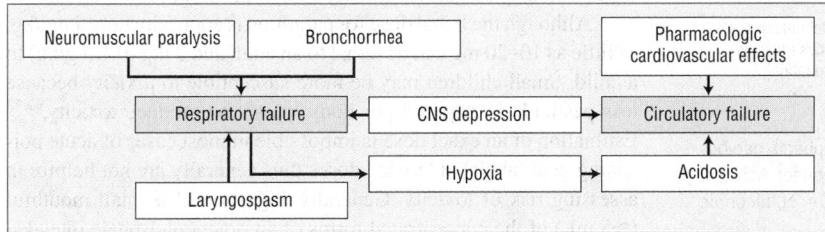

FIGURE 10–4. Pathogenesis of life-threatening effects of organophosphate poisoning.

• Bradycardia, atrial fibrillation, atrioventricular block, and hypotension within 1 to 6 hours

LABORATORY TESTS

• Depressed erythrocyte cholinesterase activity (not readily available)
• Markedly depressed serum pseudocholinesterase activity below normal range
• Altered arterial blood gases, serum electrolytes, BUN, and serum creatinine in response to respiratory distress and shock within 1 to 6 hours

OTHER DIAGNOSTIC TESTS

• Chest radiographs for progression of pulmonary edema or hydrocarbon pneumonitis in symptomatic patients
• Electrocardiogram (ECG) with continuous monitoring and pulse oximetry for complications from toxicity and hypoxia

MECHANISM OF TOXICITY

Anticholinesterase insecticides phosphorylate the active site of cholinesterase in all parts of the body.[69,71] Inhibition of this enzyme leads to accumulation of acetylcholine at affected receptors and results in widespread toxicity. Acetylcholine is the neurohormone responsible for physiologic transmission of nerve impulses from preganglionic and postganglionic neurons of the cholinergic (parasympathetic) nervous system, preganglionic adrenergic (sympathetic) neurons, the neuromuscular junction in skeletal muscles, and multiple nerve endings in the central nervous system (Fig. 10–5).

CAUSATIVE AGENTS

Anticholinesterase insecticides include organophosphate and carbamate insecticides. These insecticides are currently in widespread

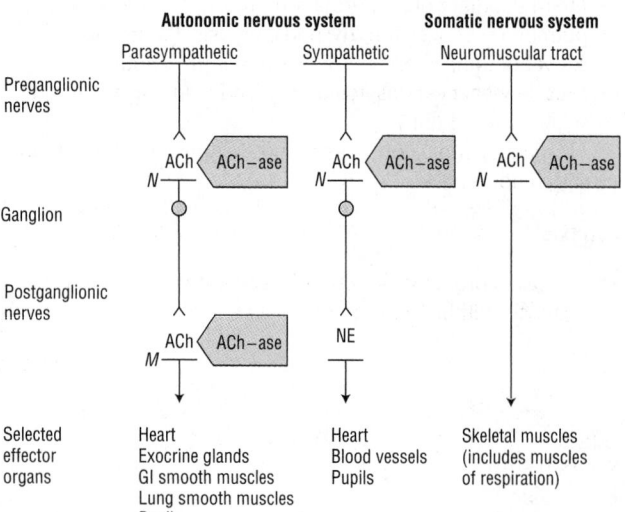

FIGURE 10–5. Organization of neurotransmitters of the peripheral nervous system and site of acetylcholinesterase action. (Ach, acetylcholine; Ach-ase, acetylcholinesterase; NE, norepinephrine; M, muscarinic receptor; N, nicotinic receptor.)

TABLE 10–12. Commonly Used Organophosphate Insecticides

Chemical Name	Product Name Examples
Agricultural Use: High Potency	
Disulfoton	Di-syston
Mevinphos	Phosdrin
Parathion	Niagara Phos Kil Dust
Animal Use: Intermediate Potency	
Coumaphos	Co-Ral, Baymix
Dichlorphos	Agridip, Muscatox
Famphur	Brevinyl, DDVP, Vapona
Phosmet	Dovip, Warbex
Trichlorfon	Prolate, Smidan
Household Use: Low Potency	
Diazinon	Security Fire Ant Killer
Malathion	Ortho Malathion Insect Spray

use throughout the world for the eradication of insects in dwellings and crops. Carbamates typically are less potent and inactivate cholinesterase in a more reversible fashion through carbamylation compared with organophosphates.[69] The prototype anticholinesterase agent is the organophosphate, which will be the focus of this discussion. A large number of organophosphates are used as pesticides (Table 10–12), and several also have been used as potent chemical warfare or terrorist agents (e.g., sarin, tabun, and VX, which are known as nerve agents).[72,74] The chemical warfare agents act like organophosphate insecticides, but as a group they are highly potent, absorbed quickly, and deadly to humans.[73,74] An anticholinesterase insecticide typically is stored in a garage, chemical storage area, or living area. Anticholinesterase agents also can be found in occupational (e.g., pest exterminators) or agricultural (e.g., crop dusters or farm workers) settings. These agents also have been used as a means for suicide or homicide.

INCIDENCE

Anticholinesterase insecticides are among the most poisonous substances commonly used for pest control and are a frequent source of serious poisoning in children and adults in rural and urban settings. The 2003 AAPCC-TESS report documented 11,332 nonfatal exposures and 19 deaths from anticholinesterase insecticides alone or in combination with other pesticides, with 31% of the exposures in children younger than 6 years of age.[6]

RISK ASSESSMENT

The triad of miosis, bronchial secretions, and muscle fasciculations should suggest the possibility of anticholinesterase insecticide poisoning and warrants a therapeutic trial of the antidote atropine. In cases of low-level exposure, failure to develop signs within 6 hours indicates a low likelihood of subsequent toxicity.[69] Ruling out other chemical exposures may be guided initially by symptoms at presentations.[16]

Although the lethal dose for parathion is approximately 4 mg/kg, as little as 10–20 mg can be lethal to an adult and 2 mg (0.1 mg/kg) to a child. Small children may be more susceptible to toxicity because less pesticide is required per body weight to produce toxicity.[69,73] Estimation of an exact dose is impossible in most cases of acute poisoning, and tabulated "toxic" doses thus generally are not helpful in assessing risk of toxicity. Generally, ingestion of a small mouthful (≈5 mL) of the concentrated forms of an organophosphate intended to be diluted for commercial or agricultural use will produce serious toxicity, whereas a mouthful of an already diluted household product such as an insecticide typically does not produce serious toxic effects.[73]

Measurement of acetylcholinesterase activity at the neuronal synapse is not feasible clinically. Cholinesterase activity can be measured in the blood as the pseudocholinesterase (butylcholinesterase) activity of the plasma and acetylcholinesterase activity in the erythrocyte. Both cholinesterases will be depressed with anticholinesterase insecticide poisoning.[69,75] Severity can be estimated roughly by the extent of depressed activity in relation to the low end of normal values. Because there are several methods to measure and report cholinesterase activity, each particular laboratory's normal range must be considered. Clinical toxicity usually is seen only after a 50% reduction in enzyme activity, and severe toxicity typically is observed with levels at 20% or less of the normal range.[71,73,75] The intrinsic activity of acetylcholinesterase may be depressed in some individuals, but the absence of any manifestations in most people does not permit the recognition of the relative deficiency in the general population. Therapy should not be delayed pending laboratory confirmation when the clinical suspicion of poisoning is present.

MANAGEMENT OF TOXICITY

People handling the patient should wear gloves and aprons to protect themselves against contaminated clothing, skin, or gastric fluid of the patient.[69,73] Because many insecticides are dissolved in a hydrocarbon vehicle, there is an additional risk of pulmonary aspiration of the hydrocarbon leading to pneumonitis. The risks and benefits of prehospital ipecac-induced emesis should be considered carefully and should involve consultation with a poison control center or clinical toxicologist. Symptomatic cases of anticholinesterase insecticide exposure typically are referred to an emergency department for evaluation and treatment.

If the poison has been ingested within the hour, gastric lavage should be considered and followed by the administration of activated charcoal. The patient with skin contamination should be washed with copious amounts of soap and water. An alcohol wash may be useful to remove residual insecticide due to its lipophilic nature. A surgical scrub kit for the hands, feet, and nails may be useful for exposure to those areas. Supportive therapy should include maintenance of an airway (including bronchotracheal suctioning), provision of adequate ventilation, and establishment of an intravenous line. Based on a history of an exposure and presence of typical symptoms, the anticholinesterase syndrome should be recognized without difficulty.

The pharmacologic management of organophosphate intoxication relies on the administration of atropine and pralidoxime.[69,71,73] Atropine has no effect on inhibited cholinesterase, but it competitively blocks the actions of acetylcholine on cholinergic and some central nervous system receptors. It thereby alleviates bronchospasm and reduces bronchial secretions. Although atropine has little effect on the flaccid muscle paralysis or the central respiratory failure of severe poisoning, it is indicated in all symptomatic patients and can be used as a diagnostic aid. It should be given intravenously and in larger than conventional doses of 0.05–0.1 mg/kg in children younger than 12 years of age and 2–5 mg in adolescents and young adults.[73] It should be repeated at 5- to 10-minute intervals until bronchial secretions and pulmonary rales resolve. Therapy may require large doses over a period of several days until all absorbed organophosphate is metabolized, and acetylcholinesterase activity is restored.

Restoration of enzyme activity is necessary for severe poisoning, characterized by reduction of cholinesterase activity to less than 20% of normal, profound weakness, and respiratory distress. Pralidoxime (Protopam), also called 2-PAM or pyridine aldoxamine methiodide, breaks the covalent bond between the cholinesterase and organophosphate and regenerates enzyme activity. Organophosphate-cholinesterase binding is reversible initially, but it gradually becomes irreversible. Therefore, therapy with pralidoxime should be initiated as soon as possible, preferably within 36 to 72 hours of exposure.[73] The drug should be given at a dose of 25–50 mg/kg up to 1 g intravenously over 5 to 20 minutes. If muscle weakness persists or recurs, the dose may be repeated after an hour and again if needed. A continuous infusion of pralidoxime has been shown to be effective in adults when administered at 3.2 mg/kg per hour preceded by a loading dose of 4 mg/kg[76] and in children at 10–20 mg/kg per hour with a loading dose of 15 to 50 mg/kg.[77] Both atropine and pralidoxime should be given together since they have complementary actions (Table 10–13). Carbamate insecticide poisonings typically do not require the administration of pralidoxime.

CLINICAL CONTROVERSY

Some references indicate that pralidoxime should be avoided in the treatment of carbamate (another type of anticholinesterase insecticide) poisoning because of reports of worsened toxicity in animals. Pralidoxime may be considered when exposure to carbamates is not known but an anticholinesterase is suspected based on symptoms or when respiratory paralysis due to nicotinic effects is not managed sufficiently by mechanical ventilation.

One of the pitfalls of therapy is the delay in administering sufficient doses of atropine or pralidoxime.[69,73] The adverse effects of atropine and pralidoxime, predictable extensions of their anticholinergic actions, are minimally important compared with the life-threatening effects of severe anticholinesterase poisoning and can be minimized easily by decreasing the dose.

TABLE 10–13. Comparative Characteristics of Atropine and Pralidoxime for Anticholinesterase Poisoning

Characteristic	Atropine	Pralidoxime
Interaction	Synergy with pralidoxime	Reduces atropine dose requirement
Indication	Any anticholinesterase agent	Typically needed for organophosphates
Primary sites of action	Muscarinic, CNS	Nicotinic > muscarinic > CNS
Adverse effects	Coma, hallucinations, tachycardia	Dizziness, diplopia, tachycardia, headache
Daily dose[a]	2–1600 mg	1–12 g
Total dose[a]	2–11, 422 mg	1–92 g

[a]Range of reported cases; higher doses may be required in rare cases.

MONITORING AND PREVENTION

Poisoned patients may require monitoring of vital signs, measurement of ventilatory adequacy such as blood gases and pulse oximetry, leukocyte count with differential to assess development of pneumonia, and chest radiographs to assess the degree of pulmonary edema or development of hydrocarbon pneumonitis. Workers involved in the formulation and application of pesticides should be monitored by periodic measurement of cholinesterase activity in their bloodstream. Untreated, anticholinesterase-depressed acetylcholinesterase activity returns to normal values in approximately 120 days.

Many anticholinesterase insecticide poisonings are unintentional as a result of misuse, improper storage, and failure to follow instructions for mixing or application, or inability to read directions for use. Training and vigilant adherence to directions may minimize some poisonings. Storing pesticides in original or labeled containers can minimize the risk of unintentional ingestion. Keeping pesticides out of children's reach may decrease the risk of childhood poisoning.[78]

CALCIUM CHANNEL BLOCKERS

CLINICAL PRESENTATION

8   Overdosage with calcium channel blockers typically results in bradycardia and hypotension (Fig. 10–6). Many patients become lethargic and may develop agitation and coma. If the degree of hypotension becomes severe or is prolonged, the secondary effects of seizures, coma, and metabolic acidosis usually develop. Pulmonary edema, nausea and vomiting, and hyperglycemia are frequent complications of calcium channel blocker overdoses. Paralytic ileus, mesenteric ischemia, and colonic infarction have been observed in patients with severe hypotension. Many symptoms become manifest within 1 to 2 hours of ingestion (see below). If a sustained-release formulation is involved, the onset of overt toxicity may be delayed by 6 to 18 hours from the time of ingestion. Severe poisoning can result in refractory shock and cardiac arrest. Death can occur within 3 to 4 hours of ingestion.[79–82]

CLINICAL PRESENTATION OF CALCIUM CHANNEL BLOCKER POISONING

GENERAL

- Life-threatening cardiac toxicity within 1 to 3 hours of ingestion, delayed by 12 to 18 hours if a sustained-release product is involved
- Increased cardiovascular toxicity with concurrent ingestion of β-adrenergic blockers or digoxin

SYMPTOMS

- Nausea and vomiting within 1 hour
- Dizziness, lethargy, coma, and seizures within 1 to 3 hours

SIGNS

- Hypotension and bradycardia within 1 to 6 hours
- Unresponsiveness and depressed reflexes within 1 to 6 hours
- Atrioventricular block, intraventricular conduction defects, and ventricular dysrhythmias on electrocardiogram

LABORATORY TESTS

- Hyperglycemia typically resolves spontaneously
- Altered arterial blood gases (metabolic acidosis), serum electrolytes, BUN, and serum creatinine in response to shock within 1 to 6 hours

OTHER DIAGNOSTIC TESTS

- Electrocardiogram with continuous monitoring and pulse oximetry to monitor for toxicity and shock
- Monitor for complications of pulmonary aspiration such as hypoxia and pneumonia by physical findings and chest radiographs

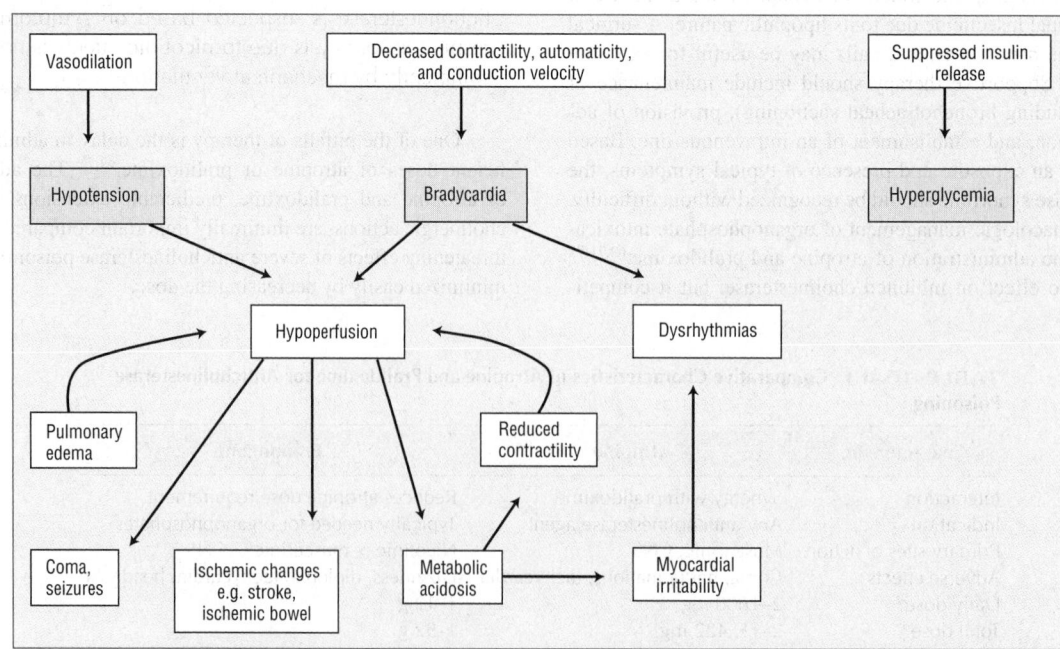

FIGURE 10–6. Pathophysiologic changes associated with calcium channel blocker poisoning.

MECHANISM OF TOXICITY

Most toxic effects of calcium channel blockers are produced by three basic actions on the cardiovascular system: vasodilation through relaxation of smooth muscles, decreased contractility by action on cardiac tissue, and decreased automaticity and conduction velocity through slow recovery of calcium channels. Calcium channel blockers interfere with calcium entry by inhibiting one or more of the several types of calcium channels and binding at one or more cellular binding sites.[83] Selectivity of these actions varies with the calcium channel blocker and provides some therapeutic distinctions (see Chap. 13), but these differences are less clear with overdosage.[82] Current experiences suggest that the signs and symptoms of calcium channel blocker toxicity are similar among the drugs in this class.

CAUSATIVE AGENTS

There are approximately a dozen calcium channel antagonists marketed in the United States for the treatment of hypertension, certain dysrhythmias, and some forms of angina (see Chaps. 13, 15, and 17). The calcium channel blockers are classified by their chemical structure as phenylalkylamines (e.g., verapamil), benzothiapines (e.g., diltiazem), and dihydropyridines (e.g., amlodipine, felodipine, nicardipine, and nifedipine). Several of these agents, namely, diltiazem, nicardipine, nifedipine, and verapamil, are formulated as sustained-release oral dosage forms or have a slow onset of action and longer half-life (e.g., amlodipine[84]), allowing once-daily administration.

INCIDENCE

In 2003, the AAPCC-TESS report documented 9650 people with a toxic exposure to a calcium channel blocker, with 339 patients exhibiting and surviving major toxic effects.[6] Fifty-seven people died. Poison control center reports have shown a steady increase in the number of cases of morbidity and mortality following calcium channel blocker overdosage.

RISK ASSESSMENT

Ingestion of doses near or in excess of 1 g of diltiazem, nifedipine, or verapamil may result in life-threatening symptoms or death in an adult.[79,85] Asymptomatic children who ingest less than 12 mg/kg of verapamil sustained release or 2.7 mg/kg of nifedipine sustained release may be monitored at home.[86] Doses associated with serious toxicity with the other agents have not been established. Patients on chronic therapy with these agents who acutely ingest an overdose may have a greater risk of serious toxicity. Elderly patients and those with underlying cardiac disease may not tolerate mild hypotension or bradycardia. Concurrent ingestion of β-adrenergic blocking drugs, digitalis, class I antiarrhythmics, and other vasodilators may worsen the cardiovascular effects of calcium channel blockers.[80,82]

MANAGEMENT OF TOXICITY

There is no accepted specific prehospital care for calcium channel blocker poisoning except to summon an ambulance for symptomatic patients. Ipecac syrup should be avoided due to the risks of seizures and coma.[82,85] The therapeutic options for the management of calcium channel blocker poisoning include supportive care, gastric decontamination, and adjunctive therapy for the cardiovascular and metabolic effects. Supportive care consists of airway protection, ventilatory support, intravenous hydration to maintain adequate urine flow, and maintenance of electrolyte and acid-base balance. Maintaining vital organ perfusion is critical for successful therapy in order to allow time for calcium channel blocker toxicity to resolve.[81,82]

Gastric lavage and a single dose of activated charcoal should be administered if instituted within 1 to 2 hours of ingestion. Besides exhibiting a slower onset of symptoms, sustained-release formulations also can form concretions in the intestine.[82,85] Whole-bowel irrigation with polyethylene glycol electrolyte solution may accelerate rectal elimination of the sustained-release tablets and should be considered routinely for ingestion of sustained-release calcium channel antagonist formulations.[32,87]

Adjunctive therapy is focused on treating hypotension, bradycardia, and resulting shock. Hypotension is treated primarily by correction of coexisting dysrhythmias (e.g., bradycardia, heart block) and implementation of conventional measures to treat decreased blood pressure. Infusion of normal saline and placement of the patient in the Trendelenburg position are initial therapy. Further fluid therapy should be guided by central venous pressure monitoring. Dopamine in conventional doses for cardiogenic shock should be considered next. If hypotension persists, dysrhythmias are present, or other signs of serious toxicity are present, calcium should be administered intravenously.[79,82]

A calcium chloride bolus test dose (10–20 mg/kg up to 1 to 3 g) is the preferred therapy for patients with serious toxicity. In adults, calcium chloride 10% can be diluted in 100 mL normal saline and infused over 5 minutes through a central venous line. If a positive cardiovascular response is achieved with this test dose, a continuous infusion of calcium chloride (20–50 mg/kg per hour) should be started. Calcium gluconate is less desirable to use because it contains less elemental calcium per milligram of final dosage form. Intravenous calcium salts can produce vomiting and tissue necrosis on extravasation.[48,82] Atropine also may be considered for treatment of bradycardia, but it is seldom sufficient as a sole therapy.[81]

If the bradycardia and hypotension are refractory to the foregoing therapy, a bolus infusion of glucagon (0.05–0.20 mg/kg) should be considered. Benefit typically is observed within 5 minutes of administration and can be sustained with a continuous intravenous infusion (0.05–0.1 mg/kg per hour) titrated to clinical response.[88] Glucagon possesses chronotropic and inotropic effects in part by stimulating adenyl cyclase and increasing cyclic AMP, which may promote intracellular entry of calcium through calcium channels. It thereby may improve hypotension and bradycardia.[48] Vomiting is not uncommon with these large doses of glucagon, and the airway should be protected to avoid pulmonary aspiration. Hyperglycemia may occur or be exacerbated in those patients receiving glucagon therapy. Hyperglycemia from calcium channel blocker toxicity or glucagon therapy typically does not require treatment with insulin. Intravenous sodium bicarbonate, however, may be necessary to establish acid-base balance and correct the metabolic acidosis that is common with serious calcium channel blocker overdoses.

An insulin infusion should be considered for severe cases of calcium channel blocker toxicity.[48,79,91] Case reports suggest that an intravenous bolus of regular insulin (0.5–1 units/kg) with 50 mL dextrose 50% (0.25 mg/kg for children) followed with a continuous infusion of regular insulin (0.5–1 units/kg per hour) may improve myocardial contractility. The effect of insulin is presently unclear, but it may improve myocardial metabolism that is adversely affected by calcium channel blocker overdoses, such as decreased cellular uptake of glucose and free fatty acids and a shift from fatty acid oxidation to carbohydrate metabolism.[79] This insulin regimen is titrated to improvement in systolic blood pressure over 100 mm Hg and heart rate over 50 beats per minute. It is used for patients with serum glucose concentrations under 200 mg/dL. Serum glucose and potassium concentrations should be monitored closely. Patients with serum potassium concentrations below 2.5 mEq/L may need supplemental potassium (20 mEq intravenous infusion). The insulin infusion is reduced gradually as signs of toxicity resolve.

Therapies with glucagon and insulin are based on animal studies and case reports; clinical trials have not been performed to date to demonstrate effectiveness.[48,79]

CLINICAL CONTROVERSY

Some clinicians believe that insulin or glucagon therapy for calcium channel antagonist poisoning should be used early in the course of therapy. Others reserve it for life-threatening symptoms not responsive to other therapy. More safety and effectiveness data are needed to define the place of these two agents in therapy.

Several lifesaving options may be warranted for patients with cardiogenic shock that is refractory to conventional therapy. Electrical cardiac pacing may restore an acceptable heart rate in patients with severe bradycardia.[82] Intraaortic balloon counterpulsation or cardiopulmonary bypass may improve shock in patients unresponsive to other therapies.[48,82,89,90]

Measures to enhance elimination from the bloodstream by hemodialysis or multiple-dose activated charcoal have not been shown to be effective and are not indicated for calcium channel blocker poisoning.[39,80,82,92]

MONITORING AND PREVENTION

Regular monitoring of vital signs and electrocardiogram is essential in suspected calcium channel blocker poisoning. Determinations of serum electrolytes, serum glucose, arterial blood gases, urine output, and renal function are indicated to assess and monitor symptomatic patients. If serious toxicity is likely to develop, overt symptoms will manifest within 6 hours of ingestion.[81,82] For ingestions of sustained-release products in toxic doses, observation for 24 hours in a critical care unit may be prudent because the onset of symptoms may be slow and delayed up to 12 to 18 hours after ingestion.[79,87,92,93] Serum concentrations of these agents in overdose patients do not correlate well with the ingested dose, degree of toxicity, or outcome.[82]

Poisonings owing to these agents are likely to increase as their therapeutic indications and use increase. These poisonings may be the result of an intentional suicide or unintentional ingestion by young children. Prevention of calcium channel blocker poisonings in children rests with the education of patients receiving these agents, particularly of grandparents and those who have children visit their homes infrequently, of their dangers on overdosage. Safe storage and use of child-resistant closures may reduce the opportunities for unintentional poisonings by children.[80]

IRON

CLINICAL PRESENTATION

In the first few hours after the ingestion of toxic amounts of iron, symptoms of gastrointestinal irritation (e.g., nausea, vomiting, and diarrhea) are common (see below). In certain severe cases, acidosis and shock can become manifest within 6 hours of ingestion. Some have observed a quiescent phase between 6 and 48 hours after ingestion where symptoms improve or abate, but this phenomenon is poorly characterized.[94] Continued gastrointestinal symptoms, poor perfusion, and oliguria should suggest the development of severe toxicity, with other effects still to become manifest. Generally, within 24 to 36 hours of the ingestion, central nervous system involvement with coma and seizures; hepatic injury characterized by jaundice, increased prothrombin time, increased bilirubin, and hypoglycemia; cardiovascular shock; and acidosis also develop.[94] Adult respiratory distress syndrome (ARDS) may develop in patients with severe cardiovascular shock and further compromise recovery.[95] Coagulopathy with decreased thrombin formation is one of the early direct effects of excessive iron concentrations, and later disturbances of coagulation (after 24 to 48 hours of ingestion) are a consequence of hepatotoxicity.[96] Mucosal injury, an iron-rich circulation, or deferoxamine therapy may promote septicemia with *Yersinia enterocolitica* during iron overdose; other bacteria or viruses also may cause septicemia.[94] Two to four weeks after the exposure, some patients experience persistent vomiting from gastric outlet obstruction as the result of pyloric and duodenal stenosis from the earlier gastric mucosal necrosis. Autopsy findings in children indicate prominent iron deposition in intestinal mucosa and periportal necrosis of the liver that correlate with the primary symptoms of serious iron poisoning.[97]

CLINICAL PRESENTATION OF IRON POISONING

GENERAL

- Gastrointestinal symptoms shortly after ingestion with possible rapid progression to shock and coma

SYMPTOMS

- Vomiting, abdominal pain, and diarrhea within 1 to 6 hours
- Lethargy, coma, seizures, bloody vomiting, bloody diarrhea, and shock within 6 to 24 hours

SIGNS

- Hypotension and tachycardia within 6 to 24 hours
- Liver dysfunction and failure possible in 2 to 5 days

LABORATORY TESTS

- Toxic serum iron concentrations beyond 500 mcg/dL
- Altered arterial blood gases and serum electrolytes associated with a high anion gap metabolic acidosis within 3 to 24 hours
- Elevated BUN, serum creatinine, AST, ALT, and INR associated with systemic toxicity within 1 to 2 days

OTHER DIAGNOSTIC TESTS

- Guaiac test of stools for the presence of blood
- Abdominal radiograph to detect solid iron tablets in gastrointestinal tract

MECHANISM OF TOXICITY

The toxicity of acute iron poisoning includes local effects on the gastrointestinal mucosa and systemic effects induced by excessive iron in the body.[94,95] Iron is irritating to the gastric and duodenal mucosa, which may result in hemorrhage and occasional perforations. Once

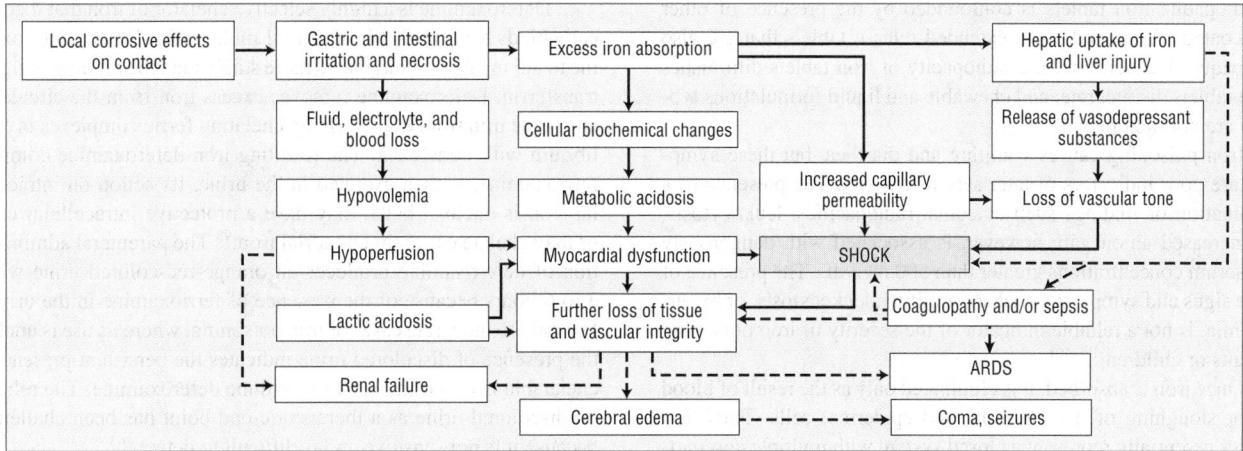

FIGURE 10–7. Pathophysiology of acute iron poisoning. Events indicated by dashed lies are not observed consistently in all serious poisonings. (ARDS, adult respiratory distress syndrome.)

absorbed, iron is taken up by tissues, particularly the liver, and acts as a mitochondrial poison. It occasionally causes hepatic injury. Iron may inhibit aerobic glycolysis and perturb the electron transport system. Further, iron may shunt electrons away from the electron transport system, thereby reducing the efficiency of oxidative phosphorylation. These biochemical factors, along with the cardiovascular effects of iron, lead to metabolic acidosis. The pathogenesis of shock is not well understood but may include the development of hypovolemia and lactic acidosis, release of endogenous vasodilators, and the direct vasodepressant effects of iron and ferritin on the circulation (see Fig. 10–7).

CAUSATIVE AGENTS

Iron poisoning results from the ingestion and absorption of excessive amounts of iron from iron tablets, multiple vitamins with iron, and prenatal vitamins. Different iron salts and formulations contain varying amounts of elemental iron (see Chap. 99). Generally, children's chewable vitamins are less likely to produce systemic iron poisoning due in part to lower iron content.

INCIDENCE

Acute iron poisoning can produce death in children and adults.[97,98] An analysis by the Consumer Products Safety Commission concluded that iron poisoning remains a significant public health threat to young children based on injury and mortality data from 1980 through 1996.[98] The 2003 AAPCC-TESS report documented 32,991 nonfatal and 4 fatal cases, respectively, of iron poisoning, with 81% of the exposures in children younger than 6 years of age. In most cases (90%), multiple vitamins with iron were the source of iron.[6]

RISK ASSESSMENT

The minimum lethal and toxic doses for acute iron poisoning are not well established. The ingestion of 10–20 mg/kg elemental iron usually elicits mild gastrointestinal symptoms. The ingestion of 20–60 mg/kg is not likely to produce systemic toxicity, and typically these patients can be managed at home with observation and administration of a glassful of fluids. Ingestions of greater than 60 mg/kg usually are associated with serious systemic toxicity and require medical attention.

Immediate psychiatric and medical intervention is indicated for adults and adolescents who acutely ingest greater than 20 mg/kg elemental iron because this suggests that the overdose was intentional.[94,95]

An abdominal radiograph (Fig. 10–8) may help to confirm the ingestion of iron tablets and indicate the need for aggressive gastrointestinal evacuation with whole-bowel irrigation. An abdominal radiograph is most useful within 2 hours of ingestion. The visualization

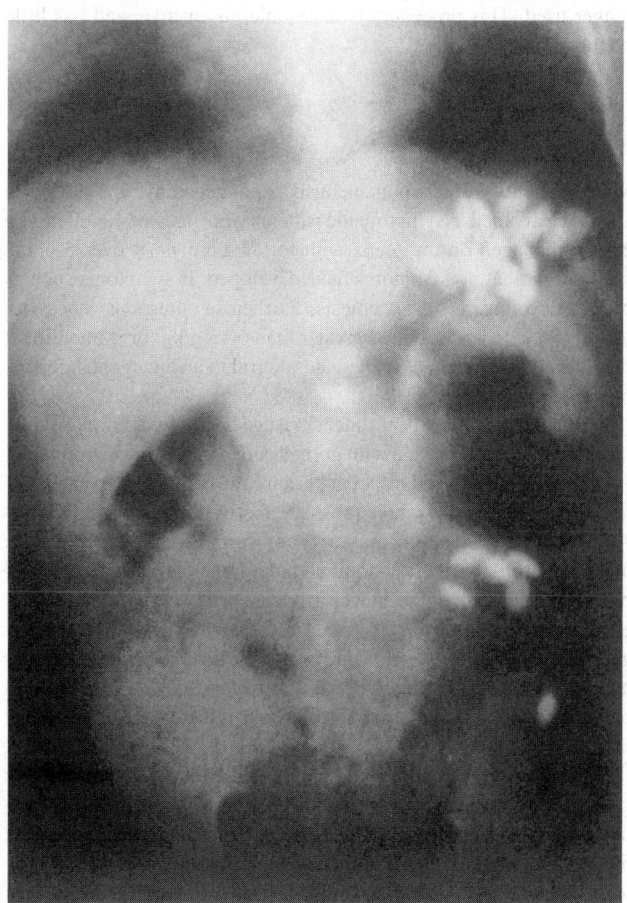

FIGURE 10–8. Abdominal radiograph of a 3-year-old boy who had ingested ferrous sulfate tablets.

of radiopaque iron tablets is confounded by the presence of other hard-coated tablets and some extended-release tablets that are also radiopaque. Furthermore, the radiopacity of iron tablets diminishes as the tablets disintegrate, and chewable and liquid formulations typically are not radiopaque.[99]

Iron poisoning causes vomiting and diarrhea, but these symptoms are poor indicators of later serious toxicity. The presence of a combination of findings such as coma, radiopacities, leukocytosis, and increased anion gap, however, is associated with dangerously high serum concentrations greater than 500 mcg/dL. The presence of single signs and symptoms, such as vomiting, leukocytosis, or hyperglycemia, is not a reliable indicator of the severity of iron poisoning in adults or children.[100,101]

Once iron is absorbed, it is eliminated only as the result of blood loss or sloughing of the intestinal and epidermal cells. Thus iron kinetics essentially represent a closed system with multiple compartments. The serum iron concentration represents a small fraction of the total-body content of iron and is at its greatest concentration in the postabsorptive and distributive phases, typically 2 to 10 hours after ingestion.[102] Serum iron concentrations in excess of 500 mcg/dL have been associated with severe toxicity, whereas concentrations below 350 mcg/dL typically are not associated with severe toxicity; however, exceptions have been reported for both thresholds.[102] Serious toxicity is best determined by assessing the development of gross gastrointestinal bleeding, metabolic acidosis, shock, and coma regardless of the serum iron concentration.[95] The serum iron concentration serves as a guide for further assessment and treatment options. The ratio of the serum iron concentration to the total iron-binding capacity previously has been advocated to assess acute iron poisoning, but it is no longer used. This procedure is unreliable, insensitive, and has little relationship to toxicity.[101]

MANAGEMENT OF TOXICITY

Many patients vomit spontaneously, and generally, ipecac syrup should be avoided. Asymptomatic patients who ingested 10–60 mg/kg can be managed on the scene with follow-up contact over 6 hours to ascertain that no symptoms have developed. If symptoms such as persistent vomiting, bloody emesis, diarrhea, or unresponsiveness develop; if the patient ingested greater than 60 mg/kg; or if intentional overdosage is suspected, immediate referral to an emergency department is indicated.[94,95]

At the emergency department, gastric lavage with normal saline can be considered. Lavage with normal saline may remove iron tablet fragments and dissolved iron, but because the lumen of the tube is often smaller than some whole tablets, effective removal is unlikely.[94] Activated charcoal administration is not warranted routinely because it adsorbs iron poorly. If abdominal radiographs reveal a large number of iron tablets, whole-bowel irrigation with polyethylene glycol electrolyte solution typically is necessary.[32] Although removal by gastrostomy has been used in a few cases,[95] early and aggressive decontamination and evacuation of the gastrointestinal tract usually will be adequate to minimize iron absorption and thereby reduce the risk of systemic toxicity.

Patients with systemic symptoms (e.g., shock, coma, or gross gastrointestinal bleeding or metabolic acidosis) should receive deferoxamine as soon as possible. If the serum iron concentration exceeds 500 mcg/dL, deferoxamine is also indicated because serious systemic toxicity is likely.[94,95] Its use is less clear in patients with serum iron concentrations in the range of 350–500 mcg/dL because many of these patients do not develop systemic symptoms.[102]

Deferoxamine is a highly selective chelator of iron that theoretically binds ferric (Fe^{3+}) iron in a 1:1 molar ratio (100 mg deferoxamine to 8.5 mg ferric iron) that is more stable than the binding of iron to transferrin. Deferoxamine removes excess iron from the circulation and some iron from transferrin by chelating ferric complexes in equilibrium with transferrin. The resulting iron-deferoxamine complex, ferrioxamine, is then excreted in the urine. Its action on intracellular iron is unclear, but it may have a protective intracellular effect or may chelate extramitochondrial iron.[95] The parenteral administration of deferoxamine produces an orange-red-colored urine within 3 to 6 hours because of the presence of ferrioxamine in the urine.[94] For mild to moderate cases of iron poisoning, where its use is unclear, the presence of discolored urine indicates the persistent presence of chelatable iron and the need to continue deferoxamine. The reliance on discolored urine as a therapeutic end point has been challenged because it is not sensitive and is difficult to detect.[103]

An initial intravenous infusion of 15 mg/kg per hour generally is indicated, although some have used up to 30 mg/kg per hour for life-threatening cases. In these situations, the dose must be titrated carefully to minimize deferoxamine-induced hypotension.[94,95,104] The rapid intravenous infusion of deferoxamine (>15 mg/kg per hour) has been associated with tachycardia, hypotension, shock, generalized erythema, and urticaria.[94,105] Anaphylaxis has been reported rarely. The use of deferoxamine for greater than 24 hours at doses used for the treatment of acute poisoning has been associated with the exacerbation or development of ARDS.[105–107] Although the manufacturer states that the total dose in 24 hours should not exceed 6 g, the basis for this recommendation is unclear, and daily doses as high as 37.1 g have been administered without incident.[104,106] Good hydration and urine output may moderate some of the secondary physiologic effects of iron toxicity and ensure urinary elimination of ferrioxamine. In the patient who develops renal failure, hemodialysis or hemofiltration does not remove excess iron, but it will remove ferrioxamine.[94]

CLINICAL CONTROVERSY

There is little evidence on how much deferoxamine should be given for iron poisoning or for how long to administer it. The dosage regimen should balance the benefits of increased iron removal in patients with exceedingly high serum iron concentrations versus the risk of developing ARDS when therapy lasts for more than 1 to 3 days.

The desired end point for deferoxamine therapy is not clear. Some have suggested that deferoxamine therapy should cease when the serum iron concentration falls below 150 mcg/dL.[95] The decline of serum iron concentrations, however, may not account for the potential cellular action of deferoxamine irrespective of its effect on iron elimination. The cessation of orange-red urine production that is indicative of ferrioxamine excretion is also not reliable because many individuals cannot distinguish its presence in the urine.[103] Considering these shortcomings, deferoxamine therapy should be continued for 12 hours after the patient is asymptomatic and the urine returns to normal color or until the serum iron concentration falls below 350 mcg/dL and approaches 150 mcg/dL.

OTHER THERAPIES

Lavage solutions of phosphate or deferoxamine have been proposed previously as a means to render iron insoluble, but they were found ineffective and dangerous.[95] Administering deferoxamine orally with activated charcoal has been shown in volunteers to decrease iron absorption, but its application to the poisoned patient requires further evaluation.[108] Deferiprone, an oral iron chelating agent, is available for the management of chronic iron overload states, but its role in the treatment of acute iron poisoning remains to be determined.[109]

MONITORING AND PREVENTION

Once a poisoning has occurred, acid-base balance (anion gap and arterial blood gases), fluid and electrolyte balance, and perfusion should be monitored. Other indicators of organ toxicity such as ALT, AST, bilirubin, prothrombin time, serum glucose and creatinine concentrations, as well as markers of physiologic stress or infection such as leukocytosis, also should be monitored.

Iron poisoning often is not recognized as a potentially serious problem by parents or victims until symptoms develop, and thus valuable time to institute treatment is lost. Parents should be made aware of the potential risks and asked to observe basic poison prevention measures. Many chewable vitamins with iron are shaped like animal or cartoon characters that can be attractive to children and can lead to poisoning. Some hard-coated iron tablets resemble candy-coated chocolates and are confused easily by children. Based on these considerations and the frequency of this poisoning, iron tablets are packaged in child-resistant containers.

TRICYCLIC ANTIDEPRESSANTS

CLINICAL PRESENTATION

10 Patients may deteriorate rapidly and progress from no symptoms to life-threatening cardiotoxicity or seizures within 1 hour.[110,111] Major symptoms of tricyclic antidepressant overdose typically are manifest within 6 hours of ingestion.[110] The principal effects of tricyclic antidepressant poisoning involve the cardiovascular system and the central nervous system and can result in arrhythmias, hypotension, coma, and seizures (see below).

CLINICAL PRESENTATION OF TRICYCLIC ANTIDEPRESSANT POISONING

GENERAL

- Sedating and cardiovascular effects observed within 1 hour of ingestion, quickly leading to life-threatening symptoms; death is possible within 1 to 2 hours

SYMPTOMS

- Lethargy, coma, and seizures occur within 1 to 6 hours
- Anticholinergic symptoms, such as dry mouth, mydriasis, urinary retention, and hypoactive bowel sounds, develop within 1 to 6 hours

SIGNS

- Tachycardia within 1 to 3 hours
- Mild hypertension early will change to severe hypotension and shock within 1 to 6 hours
- Unresponsiveness and depressed reflexes within 1 to 3 hours
- Depressed respiratory rate and depth depending on the degree of coma
- Common arrhythmias, such as prolonged QRS and QT intervals to ventricular dysrhythmias, within 1 to 6 hours

LABORATORY TESTS

- Altered arterial blood gases associated with metabolic acidosis from hypoxia and seizures
- Altered serum electrolytes, BUN, and serum creatinine in response to seizures and shock within 3 to 12 hours

OTHER DIAGNOSTIC TESTS

- Electrocardiogram with continuous monitoring and pulse oximetry to monitor for toxicity and shock
- Monitor for complications of pulmonary aspiration, such as hypoxia and pneumonia, by physical findings and chest radiograph

---

Prolongation of the QRS complex on electrocardiogram indicating nonspecific intraventricular conduction delay or bundle-branch block is the most distinctive feature of tricyclic antidepressant overdose.[111] Sinus tachycardia with rates typically under 160 beats per minute is common and does not cause serious hemodynamic changes in most patients. Ventricular tachycardia is a common ventricular arrhythmia, but it may be difficult to distinguish from sinus tachycardia in the presence of QRS complex prolongation and the apparent absence of P waves. It often occurs in patients with marked QRS complex prolongation or hypotension and may be precipitated by seizures.[111,112] High rates of mortality are associated with ventricular tachycardia; ventricular fibrillation is the terminal rhythm. Torsades de pointes is observed infrequently with tricyclic antidepressant poisoning. With massive tricyclic antidepressant overdose, slow ventricular rhythms may be observed. Hypotension is a significant factor in most cases of tricyclic antidepressant poisoning. Refractory hypotension leading to death is due to vasodilation and impaired cardiac contractility.[111] Other factors, such as extreme heart rates, intravascular volume depletion, hypoxia, hyperthermia, seizures, and acidosis, may contribute to refractory hypotension.

Coma usually is present in patients with tricyclic antidepressant poisoning and may or may not be associated with QRS complex prolongation. In severe cases, coma is sufficient to depress respirations. Delirium, manifest as agitation or disorientation, may occur early in the course of severe poisoning or with poisoning of moderate severity. Seizures often occur within 2 hours of ingestion and usually are generalized, single, and brief. Seizures may result in acidosis, hyperthermia, or rhabdomyolysis, and 10% to 20% of patients may abruptly develop cardiovascular deterioration.[111] Myoclonus also may be observed with tricyclic antidepressant overdose.

Hyperthermia often results from seizure and myoclonic activity in the presence of decreased sweating and is associated with a high incidence of neurologic sequelae and mortality. Anticholinergic symptoms, such as urinary retention, ileus, and dry mucous membranes, often are observed with tricyclic antidepressant overdose.[110,111] Pupil size is variable. Tricyclic antidepressant overdose can be staged based on the patient's symptoms and recovery time. In stage 1, patients are responsive to pain, have sinus tachycardia, and recover within 24 hours. In stage 2, seizures, coma, and cardiac conduction problems are evident; respiratory support typically is needed. Patients recover within 24 to 48 hours of ingestion. Stage 3 is characterized by the features of stage 2 with the addition of respiratory arrest, hypotension, ventricular dysrhythmias, and asystole, which may occur within 1 to 24 hours of ingestion.

Amoxapine, bupropion, and maprotiline are atypical antidepressants associated with a higher incidence of seizures on overdose; amoxapine produces minimal cardiotoxicity,[111,113] but venlafaxine has been associated with greater mortality.[114] The selective serotonin reuptake inhibitors (SSRIs) generally produce a common toxicity profile on overdose despite their structural and pharmacologic distinctions.[115] The SSRIs inhibit the presynaptic neuronal uptake of serotonin, resulting in increased synaptic serotonin levels. When ingested in excess, SSRIs rarely cause death and typically produce nausea, vomiting, diarrhea, tremor, and decreased level of consciousness.[115] Tachycardia and seizures are infrequent.[111,113,116] Serotonin syndrome is associated with the coingestion of drugs increasing serotonin levels and develops within minutes to hours of the inciting action. It is characterized by a collection of neurobehavioral (e.g., confusion, agitation, coma, seizures), autonomic (e.g., hyperthermia, diaphoresis, tachycardia, hypertension), and neuromuscular (e.g., myoclonus, rigidity, tremor, ataxia, shivering, nystagmus) signs and symptoms.[117,118] Most cases are mild and resolve spontaneously within 24 to 72 hours. Cardiac arrest, coma, and multiple-organ-system failure have been reported as consequences of serotonin syndrome.[117] Recognition of the syndrome is based on a high index of suspicion and identification of risk factors.

MECHANISM OF TOXICITY

Many of the toxic effects of tricyclic antidepressants are associated with an exaggeration of their pharmacologic action. The tricyclic antidepressants, such as type Ia antiarrhythmic drugs, inhibit the fast sodium channel so that phase zero depolarization of the myocardium is slowed.[111] This action leads to QRS complex prolongation, atrioventricular block, ventricular tachycardia, and decreased myocardial contractility. Tricyclic antidepressants also block vascular α-adrenergic receptors, resulting in vasodilation, which contributes to hypotension. Sinus tachycardia is related to the inhibition of norepinephrine reuptake and anticholinergic effects. Other anticholinergic effects include urinary retention, ileus, dry mucous membranes, and impaired sweating. Inhibition of norepinephrine reuptake also may account for the early, transient, and self-limiting elevation of blood pressure observed in some patients. The central nervous system toxicity of tricyclic antidepressants is not well understood.

CAUSATIVE AGENTS

Tricyclic antidepressants and SSRIs are used to treat a variety of behavioral conditions (see Chaps. 68 and 69). The tricyclic antidepressants include drugs such as amitriptyline, desipramine, doxepin, imipramine, and nortriptyline. Atypical agents include amoxapine, bupropion, maprotiline, nefazodone, trazodone, and venlafaxine. The SSRIs include fluoxetine, paroxetine, and sertraline. The tricyclic antidepressants are generally highly protein bound, exhibit a large volume of distribution, and possess elimination half-lives of 8 to 24 hours or more. Virtually none of the drug is eliminated unchanged in the urine. Metabolism of the parent drug produces active metabolites in most cases (e.g., amitriptyline to nortriptyline) that may contribute to toxicity after the first 12 to 24 hours.[111] Genetic polymorphism at CYP2D6 may lead to slower recovery in patients who are slow hydroxylators.[119]

INCIDENCE

Tricyclic antidepressant poisoning is a common cause of death from drug overdose.[111,112] The 2003 AAPCC-TESS report documented 12,710 patients with exposures to tricyclic antidepressants, of whom 62% were intentional overdoses. A total of 1373 people experienced a major effect, and 93 people died.[6] The SSRIs accounted for 55,871 nonfatal exposures and 106 deaths.

RISK ASSESSMENT

Ingestion of greater that 1 g of a tricyclic antidepressant (>10 mg/kg in children) typically results in life-threatening toxicity.[111] Because serious toxicity may occur within 1 to 2 hours of ingestion, prompt transport to an emergency department is crucial for overdoses. A QRS complex greater than 160 ms or progressive prolongation of the QRS complex is an indicator of toxicity such as seizures or ventricular arrhythmias and often precedes more serious symptoms.[110,112,120] The QRS complex duration should not be used as the sole indicator of risk for tricyclic antidepressant poisoning.[120] Although urine drug analyses routinely screen for tricyclic antidepressant, the qualitative result can only suggest or confirm a potential risk for the development of toxicity.

Patients with coexisting cardiovascular and pulmonary conditions (e.g., ARDS, pulmonary infection, pulmonary aspiration) may be more susceptible to the toxic effects or complications of tricyclic antidepressant poisoning. The influence of chronic exposure to tricyclic antidepressants on the risks of an acute overdose is unclear. Tricyclic antidepressants interact with other central nervous system depressant drugs, which together may lead to increased central nervous system and respiratory depression.

The risk of serotonin syndrome may be increased shortly after dosage increases of SSRIs or when drug interactions increase serotonin activity.[121] Concomitant or proximal use of SSRIs, tricyclic antidepressants, or monoamine oxidase inhibitors may cause serotonin syndrome. Further, the addition of certain drugs, such as tryptophan, dextromethorphan, cocaine, or sympathomimetics, to SSRI therapy may increase the risk of developing serotonin syndrome.[117,121]

MANAGEMENT OF TOXICITY

Once the ingestion of an overdose of tricyclic antidepressant is suspected or for any intentional ingestions, medical evaluation and treatment should be sought promptly. If the patient is symptomatic, it may be prudent to call for an ambulance owing to the rapid progression of some cases. At the emergency department, the patient should be monitored carefully, have vital signs assessed regularly, and have an intravenous line started. Supportive and symptomatic care includes oxygen, intravenous fluids, and other treatments as indicated. Prompt administration of activated charcoal may decrease the absorption of any remaining tricyclic antidepressant. It also may be useful beyond the first hour of ingestion owing to decreased gastrointestinal motility from the anticholinergic action of tricyclic antidepressants. Gastric lavage may be considered if the time of the ingestion is unknown or if it occurred within the past 1 to 2 hours. Some practitioners avoid gastric lavage altogether.[111] Ipecac syrup should be avoided in patients who ingest tricyclic antidepressants because the rapid onset of toxicity limits its usefulness. Multiple-dose activated charcoal has been shown to increase the elimination of some tricyclic antidepressants in human volunteers[39] and has been used in poisoned patients.[110,111] It may be most useful during the first 12 hours of ingestion while the drug is distributing to tissue compartments. Because the tricyclic antidepressants possess such a large volume of distribution and so little of the drug is present in the bloodstream, hemodialysis is not useful for the extracorporeal removal of tricyclic antidepressants.

Intravenous sodium bicarbonate is part of the first-line treatment of QRS complex prolongation, ventricular arrhythmias, and hypotension caused by tricyclic antidepressant overdose.[48,111,122] Typically 1–2 mEq/kg sodium bicarbonate (1 mEq/mL) is administered as a bolus infusion (usually a 50-mEq ampule in an adult) and repeated as necessary to achieve an arterial blood pH of 7.50 to 7.55 or abatement of toxicity.[110,111] A therapeutic effect usually is observed within minutes. Excessive use of sodium bicarbonate may produce dangerous alkalemia, which is by itself associated with ventricular arrhythmias.[111] The mechanism of action of sodium bicarbonate is unclear. Although some practitioners have proposed that sodium bicarbonate increases protein binding of tricyclic antidepressants, this has been discounted. Sodium may play an important role by stabilizing tricyclic antidepressant–induced changes to the sodium gradient of the myocardium.[111,123] Regardless of its action, it is effective and generally safe. Hyperventilation to produce a mild state of respiratory alkalosis has been used to treat some dysrhythmias, but it is used less widely than sodium bicarbonate.[110,111]

CLINICAL CONTROVERSY

Since intravenous sodium bicarbonate is used as therapy for certain arrhythmias and hypotension caused by tricyclic antidepressant poisoning, some practitioners have advocated its prophylactic use. There is little evidence to indicate which patients would benefit from prophylactic use. The risks of potentially producing alkalosis in a patient who is not seriously toxic should be considered.

Treatment of the complications of tricyclic antidepressant poisoning is outlined in Table 10–14 and includes pharmacologic and nonpharmacologic approaches.[110,111] Several agents generally should be avoided in the treatment of tricyclic antidepressant poisoning. Other drugs that inhibit the fast sodium channel, such as procainamide and quinidine, are contraindicated. Phenytoin has limited usefulness in treating tricyclic antidepressant seizures and has questionable efficacy in managing cardiotoxicity.[110] Physostigmine was used in the past as a treatment of tricyclic antidepressant cardiotoxicity and seizures because it antagonizes anticholinergic actions. However, physostigmine has been associated with bradycardia and asystole[111,124] and has been avoided in the contemporary treatment of tricyclic antidepressant cardiovascular or central nervous system toxicity. Flumazenil is used to antagonize the effects of benzodiazepines, but its use in the presence of a tricyclic antidepressant has been associated with the development of seizures and should be avoided.[125]

Treatment of an overdose of the atypical antidepressants and SSRIs is directed primarily toward decontamination of the gastrointestinal tract with activated charcoal, symptomatic treatment, and general supportive care. Management of the serotonin syndrome involves discontinuation of the serotinergic agent and supportive therapy. Benzodiazepines, propranolol, and cyproheptadine, a serotonin antagonist, have been used successfully.[117]

MONITORING AND PREVENTION

Measurement of vital signs, electrolytes, and blood urea nitrogen and a urinalysis are indicated for initial assessment. Patients should be monitored continuously by electrocardiogram, and a 12-lead electrocardiogram should be obtained if QRS complex prolongation is noted. If patients start to show signs of cardiotoxicity, arterial blood gases should be determined. Patients who show no signs of toxicity during 6 hours of observation and have received activated charcoal promptly require no further medical monitoring. Psychiatric evaluation is indicated for adolescents and adults. When signs of tricyclic antidepressant are present in a patient, cardiac monitoring generally is recommended for at least 24 hours after the patient is without findings.[111]

Prevention of tricyclic antidepressant poisoning poses unique challenges. Many of the dosage forms are small in size, and adults and children can consume large numbers easily. In the course of treating depression, several antidepressant agents may be tried to achieve results. By not discarding unused medicines, a storehouse of potentially deadly drugs may be available for children to discover or for the

TABLE 10–14. Treatment Options for Acute Tricyclic Antidepressant Toxicity

Toxicity	Treatment
Cardiovascular	
QRS prolongation, if progressive or greater than 0.16 s	Intravenous sodium bicarbonate to a blood pH of 7.5 even in the absence of acidosis; generally avoid other antiarrhythmic drugs
Hypotension	Intravascular fluids; intravenous sodium bicarbonate; consider norepinephrine or dopamine; treat hyperthermia, acidosis, seizures, hypokalemia; if present
Ventricular tachycardia	Intravenous sodium bicarbonate; lidocaine, overdrive pacing; treat hyperthermia, acidosis, seizures, hypokalemia; if present
Ventricular bradycardia	Epinephrine drip; cardiac pacemaker
Atrioventricular block type II, second or third degree	Cardiac pacemaker
Cardiac arrest	Advanced cardiac life support, prolonged resuscitation may be needed
Neurologic	
Seizures, agitation	Benzodiazepines (physical restraints for agitation); neuromuscular blockade may be needed if hyperthermia or acidosis are present
Coma	Endotracheal intubation; mechanical ventilation if needed
Homeostatic	
Hyperthermia	Treat seizures and agitation; consider cooling blanket, ice water lavage, and cool water mist of body
Acidosis	Intravenous sodium bicarbonate; treat hypotension, hypoventilation, seizures

despondent patient to use to attempt suicide. Although patients take tricyclic antidepressants for therapeutic relief of depression, they are also a group likely to contemplate suicide with tricyclic antidepressants. Strategies that would limit the amount of tricyclic antidepressant prescribed at one time also potentially would impair adherence to a dosage regimen and thereby compromise the therapeutic potential of these agents.[111,122] Patients with a history of suicidal gestures may be candidates for the atypical antidepressants or SSRIs, which possess less cardiotoxicity. General poison prevention measures may limit childhood poisonings, and monitoring depressed patients for suicidal ideation may identify patients at risk.[126]

ABBREVIATIONS

AAPCC-TESS: American Association of Poison Control Centers-Toxic Exposure Surveillance System
ALT: Alanine aminotransferase
ARDS: Adult respiratory distress syndrome
AST: Aspartate aminotransferase
BUN: Blood urea nitrogen
ECG: Electrocardiogram
INR: International normalization ratio
NAPQI: N-acetyl-p-benzoquinone-imine
PPPA: Poison Prevention Packaging Act (of 1970)

Review Questions and other resources can be found at *www.pharmacotherapyonline.com*.

REFERENCES

1. Bar-Oz B, Levichek A, Koren G. Medications that can be fatal for a toddler with one tablet or teaspoonful: A 2004 update. Pediatr Drugs 2004; 6:123–126.
2. Substance Abuse and Mental Health Services Administration, Office of Applied Studies. Emergency Department Trends From the Drug Abuse Warning Network, Final Estimates 1995–2002. DAWN Series D-24. DHHS Publication No. (SMA) 03-3780. Rockville, MD, Department of Health and Human Services, 2003; available at http://dawninfo.samhsa.gov/pubs_94_02/edpubs/2002final/files/EDTrendFinal02AllText.pdf; accessed on January 13, 2004.
3. Centers for Disease Control and Prevention. Web-based Injury Statistics Query and Reporting System (WISQARS) (online). Washington, National Center for Injury Prevention and Control, Centers for Disease Control and Prevention; available at *www.cdc.gov/ncipc/wisqars;* accessed on: January 13, 2004.
4. Hoppe-Roberts JH, Lloyd LM, Chyka PA. Poisoning mortality in the United States: Comparison of national mortality statistics and poison control center reports. Ann Emerg Med 2000;35:440–448.
5. Fingerhut LA, Cox CS. Poisoning mortality. Public Health Rep 1998;113:218–233.
6. Watson WA, Litovitz TL, Klein-Schwartz W, et al. 2003 Annual Report of the American Association of Poison Control Centers Toxic Surveillance System. Am J Emerg Med 2004;22:335–404.
7. Institute of Medicine. Forging a Poison Prevention and Control System. Committee on Poison Prevention and Control. Board on Health Promotion and Disease Prevention. Washington, National Academy Press, 2004.
8. Rodgers GB. The safety effects of child-resistant packaging for oral prescription drugs: Two decades of experience. JAMA 1996;275:1661–1665.
9. Shannon M. Ingestion of toxic substances by children. N Engl J Med 2000;342:186–191.

10. King WD, Palmisano PA. Ingestion of prescription drugs by children: An epidemiologic study. South Med J 1989;82:1468–1478.
11. Poison Prevention Packaging: A Textbook for Pharmacists and Physicians. Publication number 384. Washington, US Consumer Product Safety Commission, 1999; available at http://www.cpsc.gov/cpscpub/pubs/384.pdf; accessed January 9, 2004.
12. Buckley NA, Whyte IM, Dawson AH, et al. Correlations between prescriptions and drugs taken in self-poisoning. Med J Aust 1995;162:194–197.
13. Haselberger MB, Kroner BA. Drug poisoning in older patients: Preventative and management strategies. Drugs Aging 1995;7:292–297.
14. Mokhlesi B, Leiken JB, Mirray P, Corbridge TC. Adult toxicology in critical care: I. General approach to the intoxicated patient. Chest 2003;123:577–592.
15. Liang HK. Clinical evaluation of the poisoned patient and toxic syndromes. Clin Chem 1996;42:1350–1355.
16. Kales SN, Christiani DC. Acute chemical emergencies. N Engl J Med 2004;350:800–808.
17. Chyka PA. Substance abuse and toxicological tests. In: Lee M (ed). Basic Skills in Interpreting Laboratory Data, 3d ed. Bethesda, MD, American Society of Health System Pharmacists, 2004:61–86.
18. Tests for drugs of abuse. Med Lett Drug Ther 2002;44:71–73.
19. Wu AB, McKay C, Broussard LA, et al. National Academy of Clinical Biochemistry Laboratory Medicine Practice Guidelines: Recommendations for the use of laboratory tests to support poisoned patients who present to the emergency department. Clin Chem 2003;49:357–379.
20. Rosenberg J, Benowitz NL, Pond S. Pharmacokinetics of drug overdose. Clin Pharmacokinet 1981;6:161–192.
21. Young-Jin S, Shannon M. Pharmacokinetics of drugs in overdose. Clin Pharmacokinet 1992;23:93–105.
22. Taylor JR, Streetman DS, Castle SS. Medication bezoars: A literature review and report of a case. Ann Pharmacother 1998;32:940–946.
23. Bosse GM, Matyunas NJ. Delayed toxidromes. J Emerg Med 1999;17:679–690.
24. Vance MV, Selden BS, Clark RF. Optimal patient position for transport and initial management of toxic ingestions. Ann Emerg Med 1992;21:243–246.
25. Krenzelok EP, McGuigan M, Lheur P. American Academy of Clinical Toxicology, European Association of Poison Centres and Clinical Toxicologists. Position statement: Ipecac syrup. J Toxicol Clin Toxicol 1997;35:699–709.
26. Committee on Injury, Violence, and Poison Prevention. American Academy of Pediatrics policy statement: Poison treatment in the home. Pediatrics 2003:112:1180–1181.
27. Vale JA. American Academy of Clinical Toxicology, European Association of Poison Centres and Clinical Toxicologists. Position statement: Gastric lavage. J Toxicol Clin Toxicol 1997;35:711–719.
28. Chyka PA, Seger D. American Academy of Clinical Toxicology, European Association of Poison Centres and Clinical Toxicologists. Position statement: Single-dose activated charcoal. J Toxicol Clin Toxicol 1997;35:721–741.
29. McFarland AK III, Chyka PA. Selection of activated charcoal products for the treatment of poisonings. Ann Pharmacother 1993;27:358–361.
30. Barceloux D, McGuigan M, Hartigan-Go K. American Academy of Clinical Toxicology, European Association of Poisons Centres and Clinical Toxicologists. Position statement: Cathartics. J Toxicol Clin Toxicol 1997;35:743–752.
31. Oral electrolyte solutions for colonic lavage before colonoscopy or barium enema. Med Lett Drugs Ther 1985;27:39–40.
32. Tenenbein M. American Academy of Clinical Toxicology, European Association of Poison Centres and Clinical Toxicologists. Position statement: Whole bowel irrigation. J Toxicol Clin Toxicol 1997;35:753–762.
33. Traub SJ, Hoffman RS, Nelson LS. Body packing: The internal concealment of illicit drugs. N Engl J Med 2003;349:2519–2526.
34. American College of Emergency Physicians. Clinical policy for the initial approach to patients presenting with acute toxic ingestion or dermal or inhalation exposure. Ann Emerg Med 1999;33:735–761.

35. Bond GR. The role of activated charcoal and gastric emptying in gastrointestinal decontamination: A state-of-the-art review. Ann Emerg Med 2002;39:273–286.

36. McGuigan MA. Activated charcoal in the home. Clin Pediatr Emerg Med 2000;1:191–194.

37. Elenbaas RM. Critical review of forced alkaline diuresis in acute salicylism. Crit Care Q 1982;4:89–95.

38. Chyka PA. Multiple-dose activated charcoal and enhancement of systemic drug clearance: Summary of studies in animals and humans. J Toxicol Clin Toxicol 1995;33:399–405.

39. American Academy of Clinical Toxicology, European Association of Poison Centres and Clinical Toxicologists. Position statement and practice guidelines on the use of multidose activated charcoal in the treatment of acute poisoning. J Toxicol Clin Toxicol 1999;37:731–751.

40. Pond SM, Olson KR, Osterloh JD, et al. Randomized study of the treatment of phenobarbital overdose with repeated doses of activated charcoal. JAMA 1984;251:3104–3108.

41. Chyka PA, Holley JE, Mandrell TM, Sugathan P. Correlation of drug pharmacokinetics and effectiveness of multiple-dose activated charcoal therapy. Ann Emerg Med 1995;25:356–362.

42. Dorrington CL, Johnson DW, Brant R, et al. The frequency of complications associated with the use of multiple-dose activated charcoal. Ann Emerg Med 2003;42:370–377.

43. Tomaszewski C. Activated charcoal: Treatment or toxin? (editorial). Clin Toxicol 1999;37:17–18.

44. Zimmerman JL. Poisonings and overdoses in the intensive care unit: general and specific management issues. Crit Care Med 2003;31:2794–2801.

45. Bowden CA, Krenzelok EP. Clinical applications of commonly used contemporary antidotes. Drug Saf 1997;16:9–47.

46. Trujillo MH, Guerrero J, Fragachan C, Fernandez MA. Pharmacologic antidotes in critical care medicine: A practical guide for drug administration. Crit Care Med 1998;26:377–391.

47. Dart RC, Goldfrank L, Chyka PA, et al. Combined evidence-based literature analysis and consensus guidelines for stocking of emergency antidotes in the United States. Ann Emerg Med 2000;36:126–132.

48. Albertson TE, Dawson A, de Latorre F, et al. Tox-ACLS: Toxicologic-oriented advanced cardiac life support. Ann Emerg Med 2001;37:S78–S90.

49. Chyka PA, Butler AY, Holliman BJ, Herman MI. Utility of N-acetylcysteine in treating poisonings and adverse drug reactions. Drug Saf 2000;22:123–148.

50. Antman EM, Wenger TL, Butler VP, et al. Treatment of 150 cases of life-threatening digitalis intoxication with digoxin-specific Fab antibody fragments. Circulation 1990;81:1744–1752.

51. Dart RC, Seifert SA, Boyer LV, et al. A randomized multicenter trial of Crotalidae polyvalent immune Fab (ovine) antivenom for the treatment for crotaline snakebite in the United States. Arch Intern Med 2001;161:2030–2036.

52. Smilkstein MJ, Knapp GL, Kulig KW, Rumack BH. Efficacy of oral N-acetylcysteine in the treatment of acetaminophen overdose: Analysis of the national multicenter study (1976–1985). N Engl J Med 1988;319:1557–1562.

53. Makin AJ, Wendon J, Williams R. A 7-year experience of severe acetaminophen-induced hepatotoxicity (1987–1993). Gastroenterology 1995;109:1907–1916.

54. Lee WM. Acute liver failure in the United States. Semin Liver Dis 2003;23:217–226.

55. James LP, Mayeux PR, Hinson JA. Acetaminophen-induced hepatotoxicity. Drug Metab Dispos 2003;31:1499–1506.

56. Blantz RC. Acetaminophen: Acute and chronic effects on renal function. Am J Kidney Dis 1996;28(suppl 1):S3–S6.

57. Smilkstein MJ. APAP-induced heart injury? Maybe yes, maybe no. Next question. J Toxicol Clin Toxicol 1996;34:155–156.

58. Bray GP, Harrison PM, O'Grady JG, et al. Long-term anticonvulsant therapy worsens outcome in paracetamol-induced fulminant hepatic failure. Hum Exp Toxicol 1992;11:265–270.

59. Schmidt LE, Dalhoff K, Poulsen HE. Acute versus chronic alcohol consumption in acetaminophen-induced hepatoxicity. Hepatology 2002;35:876–882.

60. Lee WM. Drug-induced hepatotoxicity. N Engl J Med 2003;349:474–485.

61. Draganov P, Durrence H, Cox C, Reuben A. Alcohol-acetaminophen syndrome: Even moderate social drinkers are at risk. Postgrad Med 2000;107:189–195.

62. Heubi JE, Barbacci MB, Zimmerman HJ. Therapeutic misadventures with acetaminophen: Hepatotoxicity after multiple doses in children. J Pediatr 1998;132:22–27.

63. Kearns GL, Leeder JS, Wasserman GS. Acetaminophen intoxication during treatment: What you don't know can hurt you. Clin Pediatr 2000;39:133–144.

64. Jones AL. Mechanism of action and value of N-acetylcysteine in the treatment of early and late acetaminophen poisoning: A critical review. J Toxicol Clin Toxicol 1998;36:277–285.

65. Tucker JR. Late-presenting acute acetaminophen toxicity and the role of N-acetylcysteine. Pediatr Emerg Care 1998;14:424–426.

66. Acetadote (acetylcysteine) Injection, manufacturer's package insert. Nashville, TN, Cumberland Pharmaceuticals, February 2004.

67. Bailey B, McGuigan MA. Management of anaphylactoid reactions to intravenous N-acetylcysteine. Ann Emerg Med 1998;31:710–715.

68. Yip L, Dart RC. A 20-hour treatment for acute acetaminophen overdose (letter). N Engl J Med 2003;348: 2471–2472.

69. Reigart JR, Roberts JR. Recognition and Management of Pesticide Poisonings, 5th ed. Washington, US Environmental Protection Agency, 1999. Available at http://www.epa.gov/pesticides/safety/healthcare/handbook/handbook.pdf; accessed on January 15, 2004.

70. Sungar M, Guven M. Intensive care management of organophosphate insecticide poisoning. Crit Care 2001;5:211–215.

71. Kwong TC. Organophosphate pesticides: Biochemistry and clinical toxicology. Ther Drug Monit 2002;24:144–149.

72. Okumura T, Takasu N, Ishimatsu S, et al. Report on 640 victims of the Tokyo subway sarin attack. Ann Emerg Med 1996;28:129–135.

73. Organophosphates management. In: Toll LL, Hurlbut KM, eds. Poisindex System, Vol 119. Greenwood Village, CO, Micromedex; edition expires March 31, 2004.

74. Evison D, Hinsley D, Rice P. Chemical weapons. Br Med J 2002;324: 332–335.

75. Aygun D, Doganay Z, Altintop L, et al. Serum acetylcholinesterase and prognosis of acute organophosphate poisoning. J Toxicol Clin Toxicol 2002;40:903–910.

76. Medicis JJ, Stork CM, Howland MA, et al. Pharmacokinetics following a loading dose plus a continuous infusion of pralidoxime compared with the traditional short infusion regimen in human volunteers. J Toxicol Clin Toxicol 1996;34:289–295.

77. Farrar HC, Wells TG, Kearns GL. Use of continuous infusion of pralidoxime for treatment of organophosphate poisoning in children. J Pediatr 1990;116:658–661.

78. Pesticides: Health and Safety. Washington, US Environmental Protection Agency; available at: http://www.epa.gov/pesticides/health; accessed January 15, 2004.

79. Salhanick SD, Shannon MW. Management of calcium channel antagonist overdose. Drug Saf 2003;26:65–79.

80. Pearigen PD, Benowitz NL. Poisoning due to calcium antagonists: Experience with verapamil, diltiazem, and nifedipine. Drug Saf 1991;6:408–430.

81. Ramoska EA, Spiller HA, Winter M, Borys D. A one-year evaluation of calcium channel blocker overdoses: Toxicity and treatment. Ann Emerg Med 1993;22:196–200.

82. Kline JA. Calcium channel antagonists. In: Ford M, Delaney K, Ling L, Erickson T, eds. Clinical Toxicology. Philadelphia, Saunders, 2001:370–378.

83. Michel T, Weinfled MS. Coronary artery disease. In: Carruthers SG, Hoffman BB, Melmon KI, Nierenberg DW, eds. Clinical Pharmacology: Basic Principles in Therapeutics, 4th ed. New York, McGraw-Hill, 1999:114–131.

84. Adams BD, Browne WT. Amlodipine overdose causes prolonged calcium channel blocker toxicity. Am J Emerg Med 1998;16:527–528.

85. Calcium antagonists management. In Toll LL, Hurlburt KM, eds. Poisondex System, Vol 119. Greenwood Village, CO, Micromedex; edition expires March 31, 2004.

86. Belson MG, Gorman SE, Sullivan K, Geller RJ. Calcium channel blocker ingestions in children. Am J Emerg Med 2000;18:581–586.

87. Buckley N, Dawson AH, Howarth D, Whyte IM. Slow-release verapamil poisoning: Use of polyethylene glycol whole-bowel lavage and high-dose calcium. Med J Aust 1993;158:202–204.

88. Papadopoulos J, O'Neil MG. Utilization of a glucagon infusion in the management of a massive nifedipine overdose. J Emerg Med 2000;18:453–455.

89. Holzer M, Sterz F, Schoerkhuber W, et al. Successful resuscitation of a verapamil-intoxicated patient with percutaneous cardiopulmonary bypass. Crit Care Med 1999;27:2818–2823.

90. Durward A, Guerguerian AM, Lefebvre M, Shemie SD. Massive diltiazem overdose treated with extracorporeal membrane oxygenation. Pediatr Crit Care Med 2003;4:372–376.

91. Yuan TH, Kerns WP 2d, Tomaszewski CA, et al. Insulin-glucose as adjunctive therapy for severe calcium channel antagonist poisoning. J Toxicol Clin Toxicol 1999;37:463–474.

92. Luomanmaki K, Tiula E, Kivisto KT, Neuvonen PJ. Pharmacokinetics of diltiazem in massive overdose. Ther Drug Monit 1997;19:240–242.

93. Morimoto S, Sasaki S, Kiyama M, et al. Sustained-release diltiazem overdose. J Hum Hypertens 1999;13:643–644.

94. Fine JS. Iron poisoning. Curr Probl Pediatr 2000;30:71–90.

95. Chyka PA, Banner W Jr. Hematopoietic agents. In: Dart RC (ed). Medical Toxicology, 3d ed. Philadelphia, Lippincott Williams & Wilkins, 2004:605–614.

96. Tenenbein M, Israels SJ. Early coagulopathy in severe iron poisoning. J Pediatr 1988;113:695–697.

97. Pestaner JP, Ishak KG, Mullick FG, Centeno JA. Ferrous sulfate toxicity: A review of autopsy findings. Biol Trace Element Res 1999;69:191–198.

98. Morris CC. Pediatric iron poisonings in the United States. South Med J 2000;93:352–358.

99. Everson GW, Oukjhane K, Young LW, et al. Effectiveness of abdominal radiographs in visualizing chewable iron supplements following overdose. Am J Emerg Med 1989;7:459–463.

100. Palatnick W, Tenenbein M. Leukocytosis, hyperglycemia, vomiting, and positive x-rays are not indicators of severity of iron overdose in adults. Am J Emerg Med 1996;14:454–455.

101. Chyka PA, Butler AY. Assessment of acute iron poisoning by laboratory and clinical observations. Am J Emerg Med 1993;11:99–103.

102. Chyka PA, Butler AY, Holley JE. Serum iron concentrations and symptoms of acute iron poisoning in children. Pharmacother 1996;16:1053–1058.

103. Eisen TF, Lacouture PG, Woolf A. Visual detection of ferrioxamine color changes in urine. Vet Hum Toxicol 1988;30:369–370.

104. Peck M, Rogers J, Riverbach J. Use of high doses of deferoxamine (Desferal) in an adult patient with acute iron overdosage. J Toxicol Clin Toxicol 1982;19:865–869.

105. Howland MA. Risks of parenteral deferoxamine for acute iron poisoning. J Toxicol Clin Toxicol 1996;34:491–497.

106. Shannon M. Desferrioxamine in acute iron poisoning (letter). Lancet 1992;339:1601.

107. Tenenbein M, Kowalski S, Sienko A, et al. Pulmonary toxic effects of continuous desferrioxamine administration in acute iron poisoning. Lancet 1992;339:699–701.

108. Gomez HF, McClafferty HH, Flory D, et al. Prevention of gastrointestinal iron absorption by chelation from an orally administered premixed deferoxamine/charcoal slurry. Ann Emerg Med 1997;30:587–592.

109. Berkovitch M, Livne A, Lushkov G, et al. The efficacy of oral deferiprone in acute iron poisoning. Am J Emerg Med 2000;18:36–40.

110. Kerr GW, McGuffie AC, Wilkie S. Tricyclic antidepressant overdose: a review. Emerg Med J 2001:18:236–241.

111. Pentel PR, Keyler DE, Haddad LM. Tricyclic antidepressants and selective serotonin reuptake inhibitors. In: Haddad LM, Shannon MW, Winchester JI, eds. Clinical Management of Poisoning and Drug Overdose, 3d ed. Philadelphia, Saunders, 1998.

112. James LP, Kearns GL. Cyclic antidepressant toxicity in children and adolescents. J Clin Pharmacol 1995;35:343–350.

113. Henry JA. Epidemiology and relative toxicity of antidepressant drugs in overdose. Drug Saf 1997;16:374–390.

114. Buckley NA, McManus PR. Fatal toxicity of serotoninergic and other antidepressant drugs: analysis of United Kingdom mortality data. Br Med J 2002;325:1332–1333.

115. Barbey JT, Roose SP. SSRI safety and overdose. J Clin Psychiatry 1998;59(suppl 15):42–48.

116. Borys DJ, Setzer SC, Ling LJ, et al. Acute fluoxetine overdose: A report of 234 cases. Am J Emerg Med 1992;10:115–120.

117. Mills KC. Serotonin syndrome. Crit Care Clin 1997;13:763–783.

118. Corkeron MA. Serotonin syndrome: A potentially fatal complication of antidepressant therapy. Med J Aust 1995;163:481–482.

119. Spina E, Henthorn TK, Eleborg L, et al. Desmethylimipramine overdose: Nonlinear kinetics in a slow hydroxylator. Ther Drug Monit 1985;7:239–241.

120. Buckley NA, Chevalier S, Leditschke A, et al. The limited utility of electrocardiography variables used to predict arrhythmia in psychotropic drug overdose. Crit Care 2003;7:R102–R107; available at http://ccforum.com/content/7/5/R101; accessed on September 9, 2003.

121. Mitchell PB. Drug interactions of clinical significance with selective serotonin reuptake inhibitors. Drug Saf 1997;17:390–406.

122. Smilkstein MJ. Reviewing cyclic antidepressant cardiotoxicity: Wheat and chaff. J Emerg Med 1990;8:645–648.

123. McCabe JL, Cobaugh DJ, Mengazzi JJ, Fata J. Experimental tricyclic antidepressant toxicity: A randomized, controlled comparison of hypertonic saline solution, sodium bicarbonate, and hyperventilation. Ann Emerg Med 1998;32:329–333.

124. Suchard JR. Assessing physostigmine's contraindication in cyclic antidepressant ingestions. J Emerg Med 2003;25:185–191.

125. Weinbroum AA, Flaishon R, Sorkine P. A risk-benefit assessment of flumazenil in the management of benzodiazepine overdose. Drug Saf 1997;17:181–196.

126. US Food and Drug Administration, Center for Drug Evaluation and Research. FDA Public Health Advisory: Worsening depression and suicidality in patients being treated with antidepressant medications. Available at http://www.fda.gov/cder/drug/antidepressants/AntidepressanstPHA.htm; accessed on March 23, 2004.

11

CARDIOVASCULAR TESTING

Robert L. Talbert

Learning Objectives and other resources can be found at *www.pharmacotherapyonline.com.*

KEY CONCEPTS

◀1 A careful patient history and physical examination are extremely important in diagnosing cardiovascular disease and should be done prior to any test.

◀2 Heart sounds and heart murmurs are important in identifying heart valve abnormalities and other structural cardiac defects.

◀3 Elevated jugular venous pressure is an important sign of heart failure and may be used to assess severity and response to therapy.

◀4 Electrocardiography is useful for determining rhythm disturbances (tachy- or bradyarrhythmias) and changes in ventricular and atrial size.

◀5 Exercise stress testing provides important information concerning the likelihood and severity of coronary artery disease; changes in the electrocardiogram, blood pressure, and heart rate are used to assess the response to exercise.

◀6 Cardiac catheterization and angiography are used to assess coronary anatomy and ventricular performance.

◀7 Echocardiography is used to assess valve structure and function as well as ventricular wall motion; transesophogeal echocardiography is more sensitive for detecting thrombus and vegetations than transthoracic echocardiography.

◀8 Radionuclides such as technetium-99m and thallium-201 are used to assess wall motion and myocardial viability in patients with coronary artery disease and heart failure.

◀9 Pharmacologic stress testing is used when patients cannot perform physical exercise to assess the likelihood of coronary artery disease.

Cardiovascular disease (CVD) is present in more than 64 million Americans, and CVD has been the number one killer of men and women in the United States every year since 1900 except for 1918.[1] CVD kills nearly 2600 Americans each day and accounts for more deaths than the next five leading causes of death. Following the initial myocardial infarction (MI), 25% of men and 38% of women will die within 1 year. Also, 50% of men and 64% of women who died suddenly of CVD had no previous symptoms of this disease.[1] Although it may seem prudent to screen the population for CVD with the goal of reducing disease development, progression, and associated morbidities and mortality, currently, there are no tests with adequate sensitivity or specificity or that have been shown to have an impact on disease outcomes. An awareness of symptoms of CVD and aggressive prevention and management of risk factors are more cost-effective than expensive diagnostic tests.

A plethora of tests exist to evaluate CVD. Four properties of the CVD system can be evaluated to provide diagnostic, prognostic, and therapeutic management information. These include (1) electrical conduction, (2) pump function, (3) myocardial perfusion and vasculature competence, and (4) anatomy.[2] Multiple test modalities are available to evaluate each of these functions. Selection of the most appropriate test is complex owing to overlap in available information from different tests, paucity of comparative data between tests, and "gold standards" that may not have been challenged by new technologies and drug therapies, making extrapolation of data difficult.[2,3] For example, myocardial perfusion can be evaluated using the "gold standard" angiography but also can be measured using echocardiography (ECHO), positron-emission tomography (PET), computed tomographic (CT) scans, magnetic resonance imaging (MRI), and nuclear imaging, and it can be inferred from the exercise stress test (ET) and electrocardiogram (ECG). There is considerable debate as to how best to evaluate new tests, but for cost-effective use of tests, comparative head-to-head trials are essential. This chapter will outline each of the main groups of CVD testing modalities, highlight their advantages and disadvantages, give basic interpretation of results, and where possible, provide some comparative information. Tables 11–1 and 11–2 outline the use of different tests in CVD.

PATIENT INTERVIEW AND PHYSICAL EXAMINATION

◀1 In CVD, patient interview, history taking, and physical examination are the most important elements of patient assessment.[4–6] Technologically advanced tests can be used effectively only in conjunction with a complete physical examination and history.

The history and patient interview provide valuable insight into the patient's condition and help in the planning and interpretation of

TABLE 11–1. Types of Tests Used to Evaluate the Cardiovascular System

| | Cardiac Function[a] | | | |
	Myocardial Perfusion	Pump	Electrical Rhythm	Anatomy
Type of test	Stress tests Nuclear imaging Angiography Echocardiography	Angiography MUGA Echocardiography	ECG Electrophysiologic studies Holter monitoring	Echocardiography Angiography Intravascular ultrasound Angioscopy
Parameters evaluated	Coronary anatomy and blood flow Myocardial perfusion	Cardiac output Ejection fraction Valvular function Shunts	Rhythm Rate Conduction pathways	Chamber size Wall motion Valve function Valve structure Pericardium Coronary anatomy

[a]Not all tests for any one cardiac function are used to evaluate all parameters listed.
MUGA = multigated acquisition; ECG = electrocardiogram.

tests performed at a later date. History taking enables the examiner to establish a relationship with the patient and develop an awareness of the patient's perception of problems and quality of life and an assessment of problem acuity and severity. History taking covers elements such as chief complaint, present problems, past medical history, review of systems, and social and family history.

Primary signs and symptoms of CVD disease include chest pain, dyspnea with or without orthopnea, paroxysmal nocturnal dyspnea, cyanosis, fatigue, palpitations, cough, edema, and syncope.[4–6] During the interview and physical examination, identification and elucidation of the characteristics of and modulating factors for cardiac-related signs and symptoms are obtained.

PHYSICAL EXAMINATION

The cardiovascular physical examination is divided into four categories:

1. Global examination of the patient for signs of CVD and a review of all body systems
2. Observation and assessment of physical findings (e.g., jugular venous pressure)
3. Measurement of parameters of CVD function (pulse, blood pressure)
4. Auscultation, percussion, and palpation of the chest and related cardiac structures[4–6]

The initial part of the physical examination consists of inspection of the precordium for normal patterns of rise and fall and any abnormal markings or shape. The chest is then palpated for normal pulses, thrills (humming vibrations like the throat of a purring cat), and heaves (lifting of the chest wall). Thrills may indicate murmurs, and heaves may indicate enlargement of one of the heart chambers or an abnormal vessel such as an aneurysm. The apical pulse (also known as the *point of maximum impulse* [PMI]) is helpful to estimate heart size and rotation. This is usually located in the fifth intercostal space in the midsternal line and radiates in an arc of 1 to 2 cm. Heightened intensity and/or displacement laterally suggests left or right ventricle enlargement, and reduced intensity may be a sign of fluid overload or pericardial effusion. Factors such as obesity, large breasts, muscularity, and pulmonary disease can interfere with determination of the apical pulse. The carotid pulse is examined for its intensity and, concurrently with the apical pulse, for concordance within the cardiac cycle. Decreased carotid pulsations may be due to reduced stroke volume or atherosclerotic narrowing of the carotid artery.

TABLE 11–2. Types of Tests for Various Cardiac Disorders or Features

Feature/Disorder	CXR	Echo	Angiography	Nuclear Scan	CT	MRI	ET	ECG	PET
Ischemic	—	+++	++++	+++	++/+++[a]	++	++	++	+++
Valvular	+	++++	+++	+	+++	+++	++	+	+
Congenital	++	++++	+++	+	+++	++++	+	+	+
Anatomy	+	+++	++	+	+++	++++	—	+	+
Cardiomyopathy	+	++++	+++	++	+++	+++	—	—	++
Pericardial	+	++++	++	—	++++	++++	—	±	—
Endocarditis	—	++++[b]	+	—	++	+++	—	±	—
Masses	—	++++	+	—	+++	+++	—	—	+
Metabolism	—	—	—	+	—	—	—	—	++++
Graft patency	—	±	+++	++	+	++	++	+	+++
CA anatomy	—	—	++++	++	+	++	++	+	+
Ventricular function	—	++++	+++	++	+++	+++	+	—	++

CXR = chest x-ray; echo = echocardiography; CT = computed tomography; MRI = magnetic resonance imaging; ET = exercise testing; ECG = electrocardiogram; PET = positron emission tomography; CA = coronary artery.
[a]Ultrafast or cine-CT may be very useful in detecting ischemia based on calcium deposition.
[b]Transesophageal echocardiography is superior to transthoracic echocardiography.

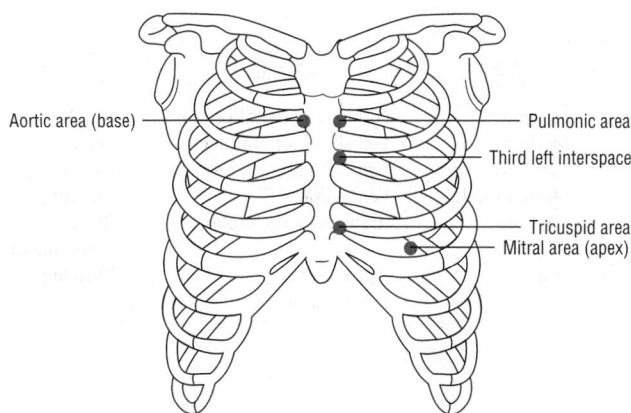

FIGURE 11–1. Schematic illustrations of topographic areas on the precordium for cardiac auscultation. Auscultatory areas do not correspond to anatomic locations of the valves but to the sites at which particular valves are heard best. *(Redrawn from Kinney MR, Packa DR (eds). Andreoli's Comprehensive Cardiac Care, 8th ed. St. Louis, Mosby, 1996, with permission.)*

HEART SOUNDS

Auscultation with a stethoscope is used to characterize heart sounds. Auscultation is conducted in a systematic manner to ensure that all sites where normal and abnormal sounds are heard are reviewed (Fig. 11–1). Respiratory pattern, various maneuvers such as handgrip and the Valsalva maneuver, sitting versus standing, and pharmacologic agents (e.g., amyl nitrate) also may be used in the evaluation of heart sounds to accentuate or diminish the intensity of these sounds. Auscultation is an acquired art and requires considerable practice to become competent.

The normal heart sounds include S_1 (first heart sound) and S_2 (second heart sound) and occur with closure of the mitral and tricuspid valves and the pulmonic and aortic valves, respectively. The sound of S_1 is thought to be generated by closure of the valvular leaflet. Other sounds, such as S_3 (third heart sound) and S_4 (fourth heart sound) and murmurs, are not considered normal but provide important diagnostic information.[4–6] Initially, the patient is examined lying partially on the left side to accentuate left-sided S_3 and S_4 and mitral murmurs, with the bell on the PMI. To identify S_1 and S_2, the patient can be examined lying or sitting. The other areas that are auscultated are the apex or base of the heart (mitral sounds), the lower left sternal border (tricuspid sounds), the second left interspace (pulmonic sounds), and the second right interspace (aortic sounds). At each of these locations, S_1 and S_2 should be heard.

Heart sounds are characterized by location, pitch, intensity, duration, and timing within the cardiac cycle. High-pitched sounds such as S_1 and S_2, murmurs of aortic and mitral regurgitation, and pericardial friction rubs are best heard with the diaphragm. The bell is preferred for low-pitched sounds such as S_3 and S_4. S_1 is heard as a click at the end of diastole and usually is synchronous with the apical pulse. The intensity of S_1 can be increased if systole begins prior to the mitral valve closing, which may occur in high-output states (e.g., exercise, tachycardia, anemia, or hyperthyroidism) and mitral valve stenosis. S_1 intensity is decreased in first-degree heart block, mitral regurgitation, states of reduced myocardial contractility (such as heart failure or coronary artery disease), obesity (difficult to hear), and systemic or pulmonary hypertension. S_2 is heard at the end of systole and is best heard at the tricuspid and mitral areas. Most of the sound arises from aortic valve closure. Heart sounds may be "spilt" if the two valves do not close synchronously. Physiologic splitting of S_1 or S_2 is

accentuated by inspiration and may disappear with expiration. Splitting of S_2 creates a pulmonic (P_2) and aortic (A_2) sound. S_2 frequently is heard as a split sound and is most predominant at the height of inspiration. Although S_1 also may be split, this is often difficult to hear.

Pathologic splitting of S_2 during expiration is described as *wide splitting, fixed splitting,* and *paradoxical splitting* and may be indicative of both stenosis and regurgitation. With right-sided heart failure, right bundle-branch block, pulmonic stenosis, or atrial septal defects, S_2 may be split owing to delayed closure of the pulmonic valve. Fixed splitting of S_2 is associated with large atrial septal defects and right ventricular failure. Increased intensity of P_2 is seen in pulmonary hypertension and dilated pulmonary arteries and with atrial septal defects. Decreased or absent P_2 occurs with aging and in pulmonic stenosis. Extra heart sounds in systole include early systolic ejection sounds and clicks and midsystolic clicks. Early ejection sounds such as aortic or pulmonic ejection sounds often are associated with valvular disease. Midsystolic to late systolic clicks usually are due to mitral valve prolapse (MVP). MVP is best heard at or medial to the apex but also may be heard at the left lower sternal border.

The S_3 heart sound, or ventricular gallop, is an abnormal low-pitched sound usually heard at the apex of the heart. It is thought to be due to rapid filling and stretching of the left ventricle when the left ventricle is somewhat noncompliant. This heart sound is characteristic of volume overloading such as in congestive heart failure (especially left-sided heart failure), tricuspid or mitral valve insufficiency, and atrial and/or ventricular septal defects. A physiologic S_3 is heard commonly in children and may persist into young adulthood. Localization of S_3 is helpful for determining heart rotation within the chest cavity.

The S_4 diastolic sound is a dull, low-pitched postsystolic atrial gallop (rapid blood flow) usually due to reduced ventricular compliance. It is best heard at the apex in the left lateral position. Like S_3, it occurs with reduced ventricular compliance and is present in conditions such as aortic stenosis, hypertension, hypertrophic cardiomyopathies, and coronary artery disease. It is less specific for congestive heart failure than S_3.

HEART MURMURS

Murmurs are auditory vibrations heard on auscultation, and they occur because of turbulent blood flow within the heart chambers or through the valves.[5,6] They are classified by timing and duration within the cardiac cycle (systolic, diastolic, and continuous), location, intensity, shape (configuration or pattern), pitch (frequency), quality, and radiation (Table 11–3).

Some murmurs are considered innocent or physiologic and result from rapid, turbulent flow of blood into the left ventricle during atrial systole and through the aorta during ventricular systole. Fever, anxiety, anemia, hyperthyroidism, and pregnancy exacerbate physiologic murmurs, and these murmurs need to be distinguished from those suggestive of valvular abnormalities.

As with heart sounds, accurate determination of murmurs requires practice. The intensity or loudness of a murmur is graded using a scale of I to VI. Grade I is so faint that it is heard only with special effort. Grade VI may be heard with the stethoscope just off the chest wall. Determinants of the grade include the amount of blood ejected across a valve, severity of the lesion, and chest anatomy.

Systolic murmurs begin with or after S_1 and end at or before S_2 depending on the origin of the murmur. They are classified based on time of onset and termination within systole: midsystolic, holosystolic (pansystolic), early, or late. Pathologic midsystolic murmurs are associated with pulmonic stenosis, aortic stenosis, and hypertrophic

TABLE 11–3. Characteristics of Heart Sounds

Type of Murmur	Examples	Location	Pitch	Radiation	Quality
Midsystolic	Aortic stenosis	2nd RICS	Medium	Neck, left sternal border	Harsh
	Pulmonic stenosis	2nd and 3rd LICS	Medium	Left shoulder and neck	Harsh
	Hypertrophic cardiomyopathy	3rd and 4th LICS	Medium	Left sternal border to apex	Harsh
Pansystolic	Mitral regurgitation	Apex	Medium to high	Left axilla	Blowing
	Tricuspid regurgitation	Lower left sternal border	Medium	Right sternum, xiphoid	Blowing
	Ventricular septal defect	3rd, 4th, and 5th LICS	High		Often harsh
Diastolic	Aortic regurgitation	2nd to 4th LICS	High	Apex	Blowing
	Mitral stenosis	Apex	Low	Little or none	

RICS = right intercostal space; LICS = left intercostal space.

cardiomyopathy. Midsystolic murmurs include obstruction to ventricular outflow, dilatation of the aortic root or pulmonary trunk, an increased flow in the great arteries, anatomic changes in the semilunar valves, and some forms of regurgitation. Holosystolic murmurs occur when blood flows from a chamber of higher pressure to one of lower pressure, such as with mitral or tricuspid regurgitation and ventricular septal defects. Early systolic murmurs are decrescendo and may be associated with ventricular septal defects, mitral regurgitation, or tricuspid regurgitation. A late systolic murmur preceded by one or more midsystolic to late systolic clicks is the hallmark of MVP. Atherosclerotic obstruction of the carotid, subclavicular, or iliofemoral artery can give rise to a crescendo-decrescendo extracardiac systolic arterial murmur.

Early diastolic murmurs are heard commonly with aortic regurgitation. This murmur begins with A_2 and generally is decrescendo, reflecting the progressive decline in volume and rate of regurgitant flow during diastole. Aortic regurgitation is best heard by having the patient lean forward while holding his or her breath and listening with the diaphragm at the midleft sternal border. Pulmonary hypertension (Graham Steell's murmur) also may cause an early diastolic murmur. Middiastolic murmurs occur across the atrioventricular valves during rapid filling and are consistent with pure mitral stenosis or mitral stenosis along with a ventricular septal defect or tricuspid regurgitation with an atrial septal defect. The Austin Flint murmur may be middiastolic or presystolic and results from antegrade flow across the mitral valve that is closing rapidly because of simultaneous left ventricular filling from aortic regurgitation. Continuous murmurs begin in systole and continue without interruption into all or part of diastole. Such murmurs are due mainly to aortopulmonary connections (e.g., patent ductus arteriosus), arteriovenous connections (e.g., arteriovenous fistula, coronary artery fistula), and disturbances of flow patterns in arteries or veins.

Anatomic correlation of murmurs may require cardiac catheterization or ECHO, where direct visualization of the blood flow abnormality and calculation of flow and chamber pressures can be obtained. PET and MRI are also possible options to evaluate flow patterns and gradients of murmurs across heart valves.

JUGULAR VENOUS PRESSURE

The jugular venous pressure (JVP) is used as a measure of right atrial pressure.[5,6] The JVP is measured in centimeters from the sternal angle and is best visualized with the patient's head rotated to the left. The JVP is described for its quality and character, effects of respiration, and patient position–induced changes. When reporting a JVP, both the measure and the patient position must be reported. The JVP can be reported as actual centimeters above the manubrium, or

this value plus 5 to 7 cm to indicate the rise of the JVP above the right ventricle. For persons in whom the central venous pressure (CVP) is normal, JVP is observed in the right internal jugular vein with the patient supine at 30 degrees or less. In the presence of an elevated CVP, the JVP is measured at 60 to 90 degrees. In patients with poor myocardial function, the accuracy of the JVP as a measure of CVP is reduced, and CVP is best measured directly by means of a Swan-Ganz catheter.

The normal JVP is a *v* wave 1 to 2 cm above the sternal ridge. If it is greater than halfway to the jaw angle, there is elevated CVP. Both the degree of elevation of the JVP and its wave flow in conjunction with the heartbeat are noted. The first wave, or *a* wave, represents atrial contraction and occurs just prior to S_1, giving rise to increased pressure. It is seen as an undulating pulsation in the internal jugular vein. The second and much larger wave, the *v* wave, represents the increased venous pressure that occurs during venous filling. To interpret the JVP accurately, the carotid pulse is palpated concurrently. The *a* wave occurs just before the pulse and the *v* wave just after. Jugular venous pressure is often elevated in heart failure, and the degree of elevation can be used to assess the severity of heart failure, and diminution of JVP can be used to assess therapy.

PERIPHERAL CIRCULATION AND ARTERIAL PULSES

Arterial pulses are evaluated and characterized bilaterally by observation, palpation, and auscultation for presence, character, pattern, and rhythm.[4–6] Various arterial pulse patterns are described: pulsus alterans (variation in amplitude beat to beat), bisferans pulse (increased arterial pulse with a double systolic peak), bigeminal pulse (reduced amplitude associated with premature ventricular beats), and paradoxical pulse (decrease in amplitude with inspiration). Although each may be associated with certain disorders (e.g., bigeminal pulse in premature ventricular contractions), none is sensitive or specific enough to be diagnostic. The status of the patient's overall peripheral circulation is recorded, especially the presence and degree of edema or skin changes suggestive of venous or arterial insufficiency. Color, condition, and integrity of the skin are also recorded, including signs of thrombophlebitis, tenderness, or swelling. Capillary refill (normal less than 2 seconds) is assessed by depressing the nail bed until it blanches and then releasing pressure and watching for the return of color, indicating blood flow.

HEART RATE

Heart rate is described by both rate and rhythm.[5,6] The arterial pulse usually is taken at the radius, but carotid or other arterial pulses may be used. In healthy individuals, the heart rate is usually assessed by counting the pulse for 15 seconds and multiplying by 4. In patients with irregular rhythms, the pulse should be taken over an extended period, approximately 1 to 2 minutes, to try to determine the patient's average pulse and rhythm.

Arterial pulses are an accurate measure of the ventricular rate in healthy persons with good ventricular function. In patients with a rapid ventricular rate—because of supraventricular tachyarrhythmias such as atrial flutter or fibrillation or rapid ventricular rates (e.g., ventricular tachycardia or premature ventricular beats)—extremity pulses (e.g., radial pulse) may be considerably slower than the true ventricular rate. A more accurate ventricular rate is determined by listening to the ventricles with the stethoscope (usually at the apex) or counting from an ECG. In patients with atrial fibrillation and a fast ventricular rate, a pulse deficit (measure of the difference in true ventricular rate and peripheral pulse rate) may exist. This may be as much as 10 to 20 beats per minute. Thus the location of the pulse (radial or apical) should be recorded. The pulse deficit will be reduced as the ventricular rate is controlled with drug therapy or normal sinus rhythm is restored.

PRACTICE GUIDELINES FOR DIAGNOSTIC AND PROGNOSTIC TESTING IN CVD TESTING

The American Heart Association (AHA) and American College of Cardiology (ACC) task force on practice guidelines publishes guidelines as to the recommended uses for many diagnostic testing methods. Such guidelines were first developed in the 1980 and are updated as more information is available. These are evidence-based recommendations that rank the indications and uses of tests into three primary classes. Class I indications are those where there is evidence or agreement that the specific procedure is useful and effective. Class II indications are those situations where there is divergence of opinion as to the usefulness of the method. Class III indications are those where there is evidence or agreement that a diagnostic test is not useful. Each class (usually class II) may be broken down into two to three subcategories. Class IIa indications are those where there is evidence or opinion in favor of the test, whereas class IIb indications are those where there is less evidence. With each class of recommendation for a specific clinical scenario, the guidelines will indicate the level of evidence for the recommendation. Level A evidence is given if the recommendation is based on the availability of multiple randomized clinical trials. Level B evidence is given if only a single randomized trial or multiple nonrandomized trials exist. Level C evidence is given if the recommendation is afforded based on expert opinion only.

Each guideline provides a preamble to indicate how it was constructed and the peer review process. These documents provide the clinician with an extensive database on the testing methodologies and are endorsed by both organizations as acceptable standards of practice.

TESTING MODALITIES

CHEST X-RAY

The chest x-ray (CXR) provides supplemental information to the physical examination and is usually the first diagnostic test in a cardiac work-up.[4–6] It does not provide details of internal cardiac structures but gives global information about position and size of the heart and chambers and surrounding anatomy. The standard CXRs for evaluation of lungs and heart are standing posteroanterior (PA) and lateral

views taken at maximal inspiration. Portable CXRs usually are less satisfactory because of penetration difficulties, patient rotation, and poor inspiratory effort.

Initial assessment of the CXR evaluates the quality of the film for patient rotation, inspiratory effort, and penetration. Rotation is assessed by evaluating symmetry of the clavicles and central placement of the carina. Inspiratory effect is considered adequate if the diaphragms are pulled below the ninth rib. Lack of inspiratory effort and obesity lead to a poor-quality CXR, which makes it more difficult to assess the presence of pleural effusions and fluid in the costophrenic angles. Where possible, comparison with previous or baseline films is done to determine the quality of film and comparison of structures.

The PA view CXR outlines the superior vena cava, right atrium on the right and left sides, aortic knob, main pulmonary artery, left atrial appendage (especially if enlarged), and left ventricle. In the lateral view, the CXR visualizes the right ventricle, inferior vena cava, and left ventricle. These structures are visualized as shadows of differing density rather than discrete structures (Fig. 11–2).

The CXR is approached from two perspectives: (1) observation and (2) clinical correlation. Observation notes gross anatomic features such as size and placement of the cardiac silhouette, definition of the cardiac border, chamber enlargement, pulmonary vasculature, air-fluid levels, and diaphragm. Cardiac enlargement is determined by the cardiothoracic (CT) ratio, which is the maximal transverse diameter of the heart divided by the maximal transverse diameter of the thorax of a PA view. Normal averages 0.45, but it may be up to 0.55 in subjects with large stroke volumes (e.g., highly trained athletes). Heart conditions such as congestive heart failure and hypertension may enlarge the heart and so the CT ratio. Individual chamber enlargement can be seen on the CXR. Right ventricle enlargement is best seen on the lateral film, where the heart appears to occupy the retrosternal space. Left atrial enlargement is suspected if there is elevation of the left bronchus or an increase in the atrial appendage bulge. Left ventricular enlargement is the most common feature identified on CXR and is seen as an elongation and downward displacement of the apex of the heart. Sometimes a characteristic "boot" or "water bottle"

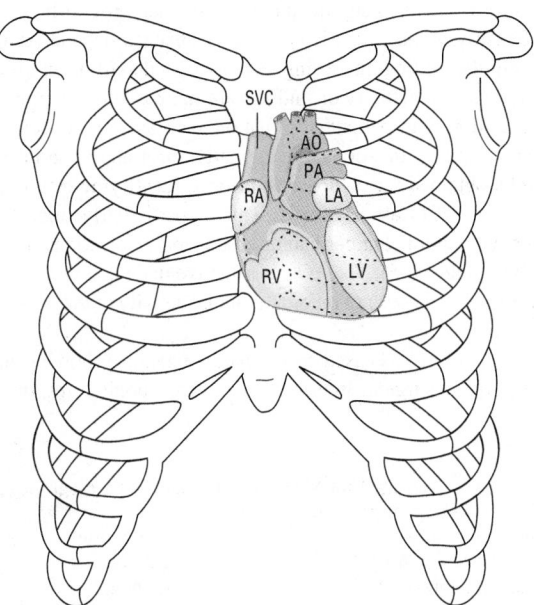

FIGURE 11–2. Schematic illustration of the parts of the heart. (AO = aorta; SVC = superior vena cava; RA = right atrium; PA = pulmonary artery; LA = left atrium; RV = right ventricle; LV = left ventricle.)

outline is seen with left ventricular enlargement, as in congestive heart failure (CHF).

The pulmonary vessels are examined for plumpness and definition of vessel walls. Decreased pulmonary flow (e.g., tetralogy of Fallot) causes central and peripheral vessels to be decreased in size. Increased pulmonary flow is associated with high-output states such as hyperthyroidism and atrial septal defects. This may lead to enlargement and tortuosity of the central and peripheral vessels. Pulmonary arterial hypertension (increased pulmonary resistance) is identified by enlargement of the central vessels and diminished peripheral vessels. Pulmonary venous hypertension usually is due to mitral stenosis or left ventricular failure. This is characterized by larger than normal vessels in the upper lung zones owing to recruitment of upper vessels from blood diverted from the lower constricted vessels (cephalization of flow).

Heart failure causes Kerley's B lines (edema of interlobular septa), which appear as thin, horizontal reticular lines in the costophrenic angles. At higher pressures, alveolar edema and pleural effusions appear in the pleural space or as blunting of the costophrenic angles. Pericardial effusions also may appear as a large heart, but because it usually occurs rapidly, there is no evidence of pulmonary venous congestion.

ELECTROCARDIOGRAM (ECG)

4 Measurement of electrical activity in the heart, now known as the *electrocardiogram* (ECG), was introduced about 75 years ago by Willem Einthoven. The ECG is simple to perform and is the most frequently used, least invasive, and cheapest cardiovascular test.[7-10] It remains the procedure of first choice for evaluation of chest pain, dizziness, or syncope. In its simplest interpretation, the ECG characterizes rhythms and conduction abnormalities. However, the ECG also provides, by inference, information about the anatomy and structures of the heart, pathophysiologic changes, and hemodynamics of the CVD system.[3,8] ECG abnormalities are often the earliest sign of adverse drug effects, ischemia, and electolyte abnormalities.

Although few ECG recordings are highly specific or sensitive to a disease state, correlation of findings with clinical and pathologic states affords the ECG significant diagnostic and prognostic capabilities. Sensitivity and specificity of ECG changes depend primarily on the clinical setting, recording technique, and skill of interpreters. Sensitivity and specificity of findings are increased by interpretation in conjunction with patient information such as age, gender, medical history, and medications. Additionally, prior and/or serial ECGs should be obtained for comparison prior to identifying new findings on a current ECG as diagnostic. This is particularly important in patients with significant cardiac disease or on medications that alter the ECG (Table 11–4). The ECG is sensitive in detecting rhythm abnormalities, but it does not record the actual activity of the conduction tissue.[7-9]

The ECG can be used to evaluate ischemia following angioplasty or other surgical interventions and to monitor responses to

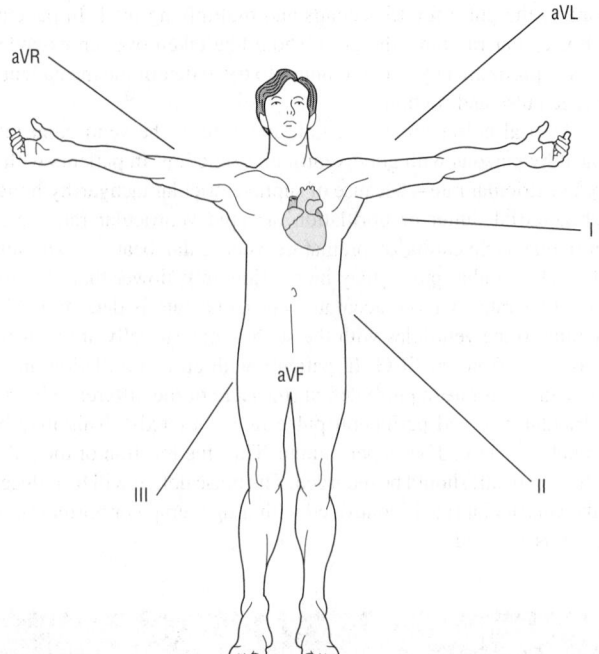

FIGURE 11–3. The torso with the six limb leads in a single frontal plane.

antiarrhythmic agents or in patients receiving drugs with potential cardiac effects. Refer to Table 11–5 for examples of conditions for which the ECG is a recommended evaluation tool.

Electrocardiography is based on the measurement of change in summated three-dimensional electrical vectors or forces that result from depolarization and repolarization of cells in the conduction system and heart muscle. The standard external 12-lead ECG uses two sets of leads: limb and chest (Fig. 11–3) The six limb leads look at the heart in a single frontal plane. Limb lead nomenclature is as follows: lead I, right arm/left arm; lead II, right arm/left leg; lead III, left arm/left leg. Altering resistances create the augmented limb leads, which are called aVR, aVL, and aVF. Unipolar chest leads are positioned across the chest and labeled V_1 to V_6. V_1 is positioned slightly to the right of the midline, and V_6 is positioned in the left midaxillary line (Fig. 11–4). Leads aVR and V_1 are considered right-sided leads, so they appear inverted, and leads aVL, I, II, V_5 and V_6 are left-sided leads, so they appear upright on the ECG. Leads II, III, and aVF are inferior leads. Leads V_1 to V_4 are anterior wall leads. Single-lead ECGs or ECG monitors frequently use lead II.

Recording of the ECG has several standard features. The paper is divided into squares of 1 mm; each 10 mm (10 small boxes) is equivalent to 1 mV. Paper speed is 25 mm/s. Each small box on the tracing paper equals 0.04 second (40 ms), and each big box is 0.2 second. If there is one QRS complex per six big boxes (6 × 0.20 second), the patient has a heart rate of 50 beats per minute, whereas one QRS per big box indicates a heart rate of 300 beats per minute.

The ECG pattern is named alphabetically and is read from left to right, beginning with the P wave. Electrical activation (depolarization) of the right and then the left atrium owing to discharge from the sinoatrial (SA) nodes causes an upward or positive deflection in lead II called the *P wave*. The normal duration of the P wave is up to 0.12 second, and it has an amplitude of 0.25 mV (i.e., 2.5 small boxes). The *PR segment* is created by passage of the impulse through the atrioventricular (AV) node and the bundle of His and its branches, and it has a duration of 0.12 to 0.21 second. The *QRS complex* primarily traces the electrical depolarization of the ventricles. Initially, there is

TABLE 11–4. Drugs That May Affect the Electrocardiogram

Digoxin	Pentamidine
Antiarrhythmics—classes I–IV	Lithium
Tricyclic antidepressants	Catecholamines (e.g.,
H_1 antagonists	dopamine, albuterol)
Methylxanthines	Diuretics (electrolyte
Doxorubicin	abnormalities)

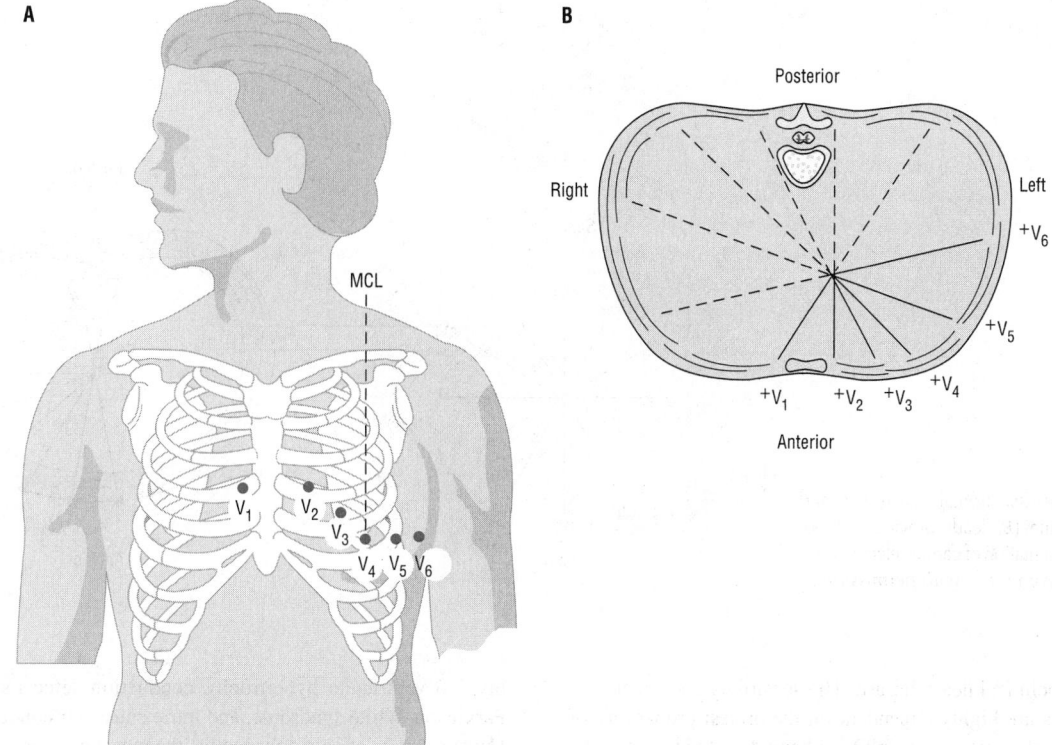

FIGURE 11–4. *A.* Electrode positions of the precordial leads (V_1 = fourth intercostal space at the right sternal border; V_2 = fourth intercostal space at the left sternal border; V_3 = halfway between V_2 and V_4; V_4 = fifth intercostal space at the midclavicular line; V_5 = anterior axillary line directly lateral to V_4; V_6 = anterior axillary space directly lateral V_5. *B.* The precordial reference figure. Leads V_1 and V_2 are called right-sided precordial leads; leads V_3 and V_4, midprecordial leads; and leads V_5 and V_6, left-sided precordial leads. *(Redrawn from Kinney MR, Packa DR (eds). Andreoli's Comprehensive Cardiac Care, 8th ed. St. Louis, Mosby, 1996, with permission.)*

a negative deflection, the *Q wave,* followed by a positive deflection, the *R wave,* and finally a negative deflection, the *S wave.* Q-wave duration is normally 0.4 second or less, and the amplitude is 25% or less of the overall height of the QRS complex. Normal duration of the QRS complex is 0.12 second. The QRS complex is positive in left-sided leads and negative in right-sided leads because the left ventricle is much thicker than the right, and the forces going left during depolarization dominate.

Following the QRS complex is a plateau phase called the *ST segment,* which extends from the end of the QRS complex (called the *J point*) to the beginning of the T wave. The ST segment is evaluated from its position relevant to the baseline, configuration, and leads where changes occur. The ST segment is normally on or slightly above the baseline. Configuration changes, convexity upward or downward, identify the presence of myocardial ischemia. Lead localization of ST-segment changes indicates the area of ischemia. The *QT interval* is measured from the start of the QRS complex to the end of the T wave. This varies with heart rate and is corrected (QTc) for heart rates greater than 60 beats per minute. The normal QTc is less than 0.42 second in men and 0.43 second in women.

Repolarization of the ventricle leads to the *T wave.* The T wave usually goes in the same direction as the QRS complex. The normal axis of the ECG is 30 degrees (above the horizontal) to +110 degrees (away from the horizontal) (Fig. 11–5). The six frontal plane (A) and the six horizontal plane (B) leads provide a three-dimensional representation of cardiac electrical activity.

The ECG is evaluated in a systematic manner to avoid omission of important characteristics. All ECGs are interpreted for the following elements: rate, general rhythm, intervals, voltage, axis, waveforms, abnormal features (e.g., Q waves), and technical aspects such as adequacy of lead placement and calibration.[8] The number of P waves and QRS complexes (*RR interval*) is also used to determine rate. QRS complexes may be more useful if heart block exists. The rhythm from the ECG is identified by the following features:

1. The rate of the QRS (>100/min is tachycardia and <60/min is bradycardia)
2. The regularity of the QRS [The presence or absence of the QRS complex with each P wave helps to identify if the rhythm is atrial or ventricular in origin and if each atrial beat (P wave) is being conducted to the ventricles. The regularity of the QRS identifies conditions such as atrial fibrillation and extra beats.]
3. Configuration of the QRS—wide or narrow—indicating if it is generated from electrical activity that arose in the atria or ventricles

Always reported are the RR, PR, QRS, and QT intervals and the duration, magnitude, and configuration of the P waves, QRS complexes, ST segments, T waves, and U waves. Computer interpretation of the ECG provides a standardized reading and records and calculates basic rhythm patterns, heart rate, and intervals but does not interpret arrhythmias. Independent review of the ECG is necessary for accurate translation of findings.[8]

In epidemiologic studies, the ECG is used to assess physical fitness, document the prevalence of ischemic heart disease (IHD),

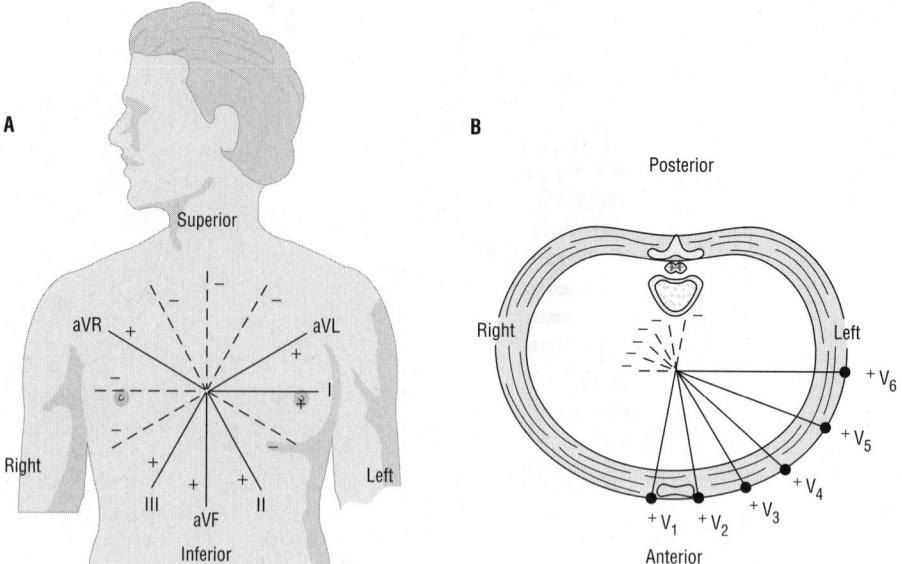

FIGURE 11–5. The six frontal plane (*A*) and six horizontal plane (*B*) leads provide a three-dimensional representation of cardiac electrical activity. *(Redrawn from ref. 7 with permission.)*

and identify subclinical heart disease. The sensitivity and specificity of ECG changes are highly dependent on the pretest probability of heart disease. As the pretest probability of heart disease increases, the sensitivity and specificity of ECG findings increase. The use and value of the ECG as a screening tool are controversial. It is only used where the diagnosis of heart disease would preclude active employment, such as in airline pilots. The ECG frequently is used in conjunction with other diagnostic tests to provide additional data, to monitor the patient, and to identify if abnormalities detected during tests correlate with ECG changes.[7,8,10]

Gating, or linkage of and simultaneous recording of an ECG and other diagnostic tests, such as ECHO and CT scans, allows for correlation of images with the cardiac cycle. Gating is either prospective, where a certain portion of the cardiac cycle is predetermined as the time during which the images are obtained, or retrospective, where the ECG and image are recorded simultaneously but independently and later matched for concurrent events. This allows multiple cardiac cycles to be overlaid, thus increasing the sensitivity to detect abnormalities.

Anomalies on the ECG include abnormal intervals, altered waveform configurations, and rate variability. Other findings give evidence for various forms of heart block, ischemia, infarction, atrial and ventricular enlargement and hypertrophy, atrial and ventricular rhythm disorders, pericarditis, metabolic abnormalities, drug-induced changes, and pacemaker-related changes. ECG patterns found on consecutive leads can help to identify where a particular conduction defect or impulse generation is occurring or anatomic problem is located. For example, ST-segment elevation in V_2 to V_6 is indicative of anterior wall myocardial infarction from occlusion of the left anterior descending coronary artery. Single-lead abnormalities most frequently are attributed to poor lead placement, position of the patient, or recording artifacts.

Examples of some common findings will be discussed briefly.[7,8] Short PR intervals are associated with the Wolff-Parkinson-White and Lown-Ganong-Levine syndromes and reflect the presence of accessory pathways. Long PR intervals are measures of heart block. The presence of a Q wave is a marker for loss of electrically functioning myocardium and suggests a prior myocardial infarction. It also may be present in congenital heart disorders, hypertrophic cardiomyopa-

thy, left ventricular hypertrophy, conduction defects such as Wolff-Parkinson-White syndrome, and intraventricular conduction defects. U waves are relatively nonspecific, the most common cause being hypertension. Bundle-branch blocks are frequent findings and indicate conduction defects in one of the bundles of His. Their presence confounds the interpretation of important ECG findings such as ischemia. Right bundle-branch block is associated with an R wave and the following abnormalities: QRS complex greater than or equal to 12 ms, delayed right ventricular forces resulting in terminal R waves in the right-sided leads and S wave in the left-sided lead, and right-sided ST-segment depression and T-wave inversion. Left bundle-branch block is characterized by the following: QRS complex greater than or equal to 12 ms, delayed left ventricular activation, loss of the normal "septal Q wave" in the left-sided leads, and left-sided ST-segment depression and T-wave inversion. Intraventricular conduction delay usually causes a wide QRS complex, and generally there are ST-segment–T-wave abnormalities.

Myocardial ischemia, ranging from injury to necrosis, results in T-wave changes, ST-segment abnormalities, and changes in the QRS complex.[7,10] Myocardial infarction results in a typical pattern of ECG changes that begins with tall peaked T waves persisting up to several hours, followed by ST-segment elevation with a coved (convexity upward) configuration, and inverted T waves. Development of a new Q wave has a high specificity but low sensitivity for acute myocardial ischemia. Q waves that are 4 ms or longer in duration and 25% or greater of the overall QRS height are considered diagnostic and occur within minutes to hours of occlusion. Although Q waves usually evolve within hours of infarction, they may not become evident for several days. The finding of new and significant Q waves on an ECG is indicative of a previous infarction. Q waves persist indefinitely in 80% to 90% of myocardial infarctions. The location of Q waves identifies the region of myocardium affected and the coronary artery blocked (e.g., inferior infarction will result in Q waves in II, III, and aVF associated with blockage in the right coronary artery). Non–Q-wave (subendocardial) myocardial infarction implies that the Q wave does not meet the diagnostic criteria for Q-wave infarction. ST-segment depression may be present.

ST-segment changes are very common and always should be compared with a previous ECG. ST-segment elevation may be seen in persons with no known coronary disease but is usually indicative of hyperacute ischemia. ST-segment depression is never considered a normal finding. ST-segment scooping (convexity downward) may be normal, but coving (convexity upward) is abnormal. Depression of the ST segment that does not return quickly to normal and changes in multiple leads suggests clinically significant heart disease. Diffuse ST-segment elevation in all leads except V_1 and aVR suggests the diagnosis of pericarditis. Exertion in normal individuals may cause J-point depression with a rapid rise of the ST segment, and this may be confused with ST-segment depression owing to the configuration. Poor R-wave progression (usually increase in size moving from V_1 to V_6) suggests anterior myocardial infarction, but smaller R waves also can occur in diseases such as chronic obstructive pulmonary disease (COPD). T-wave changes are the most frequent and most sensitive abnormality on the ECG but are also the least specific and frequently are found in persons with no heart disease.

Left atrial enlargement is characterized by a P wave that is 12 mV in lead II, or the negative component of the biphasic P wave is 4 mV in duration and 0.1 mV in depth in lead V_1. In right atrial enlargement, the P wave in lead II can exceed 0.25 mV and usually has a vertical axis. Ventricular hypertrophy results in increased deflection of the QRS complex because of the increased muscle mass. Left ventricular hypertrophy (LVH) is diagnosed from the ECG using several different sets of criteria; none are considered highly sensitive or specific. LVH often is indicative of hypertension and resulting ventricular enlargement and strain. Commonly used voltage criteria indicating LVH are summation of the S wave in V_1 and the R wave in V_5 or the S wave in V_2 and the R wave in V_6 that exceeds 3.5 mV (35 small boxes) or the R wave in lead aVL that exceeds 1.1 mV (11 small boxes). Right ventricular hypertrophy (RVH) is characterized by an R wave in V_1 that is equal to or greater than the S wave in that lead. In persons who are obese, increased voltage may not be apparent, making voltage criteria a less useful tool to identify hypertrophy. LVH also may be assessed using ECHO.

Electrolyte abnormalities have characteristic signs on the ECG and can be used as monitoring parameters. Hypokalemia may increase ventricular ectopy and causes ST-segment depression, T-wave flattening, and the appearance of a U wave (usually when the serum potassium concentration is less than 3.0 mEq/L). Hyperkalemia results in very characteristic changes in the ECG. Potassium concentrations above 6.0 mEq/L produce tall, peaked T waves. As the concentration rises further, intraventricular conduction becomes blocked, with widening of the QRS complex, and ultimately, a sine wave develops. Hypercalcemia causes a short QT interval and, occasionally, ST-segment depression, sinus arrest, and AV conduction blocks. Hypocalcemia causes a long QT interval and some broadening of the T wave. A number of drugs cause characteristic changes in the ECG that may mask interpretation of other findings. A list of commonly used drugs that may alter the ECG is given in Table 11–4. Pericardial effusion, obesity, and large breasts limit the amount of voltage that is measured on the skin surface and reduce the QRS voltage. In the presence of large pericardial effusions, rapid changes in the positive to negative deflection of the QRS complex or electrical alternans may occur because the heart is swinging on a beat-to-beat basis.

Signal-averaged ECG (SAECG) may be used to help elucidate the presence of low-amplitude bioelectrical potentials.[11] Derangements of ventricular activation and late potentials can be detected on the ECG after the QRS and ST segments and are thought to be associated with increased risk of ventricular arrhythmias. Traditional ECGs are unable to detect these potentials because they are "lost" in the noise of the ECG recording. SAECG improves the signal-to-noise ra-

tio, enabling the low-amplitude potentials to be interpreted. SAECG can be used to identify patients at risk for developing sustained ventricular tachycardia after myocardial infarction. Patients with IHD and unexplained syncope who are at risk for sustained ventricular tachycardia also may be candidates for SAECG. Other potential uses of SAECG include patients with nonischemic cardiomyopathy with sustained ventricular tachycardia, detection of acute rejection of heart transplant, and assessment of the proarrhythmia potential of antiarrhythmic drug therapy.

AMBULATORY ECG MONITORING

Ambulatory ECG monitoring (AEM), or Holter monitoring, named for its inventor, is an aid to detect, document, characterize, and evaluate arrhythmias and other ECG abnormalities over extended periods of time.[12–17] AEM provides information regarding random abnormal cardiac electrical activity during daily activity and helps relate altered electrical activity to precipitating factors and patient symptomatology. Additionally, some findings on AEM have been used to determine prognostic implications.

Although controversial, AEM is used as a diagnostic and screening tool for asymptomatic ischemia. It is difficult to interpret changes in the ST segment recorded during AEM owing to amplitude, and definitions of significant changes recorded with AEM are still in evolution. As a prognostic tool, it is used primarily to evaluate patients with known CVD who have symptoms that may be associated with an arrhythmia. It is also used in clinical trials to evaluate the efficacy of drug therapy.

Guidelines as to the recommended uses of AEM are available from AHA/ACC. The major class I indications for AEM include diagnosis in patients with symptoms suggestive of arrhythmias, prognostic delineation in patients with cardiac disease considered at risk for arrhythmia-related events, and measurement of efficacy of interventions in patients with known and characterized arrhythmias. Examples of clinical rhythm disturbances are listed in Table 11–5.

A major limitation of AEM is the amount of data collected with ECG abnormalities that are of unknown clinical significance. High day-to-day variability of frequency and type of arrhythmias means that repeat AEM may demonstrate as much as a 90% difference in

TABLE 11–5. Indications for AECG to Assess Symptoms Possibly Related to Rhythm Disturbances

Class I
Patients with unexplained syncope, near syncope, or episodic dizziness in whom the cause is not obvious
Patients with unexplained recurrent palpitation

Class IIb
Patients with episodic shortness of breath, chest pain, or fatigue that is not otherwise explained
Patients with neurological events when transient atrial fibrillation or flutter is suspected
Patients with symptoms such as syncope, near syncope, episodic dizziness, or palpitation in whom a probable cause other than an arrhythmia has been identified but in whom symptoms persist despite treatment of this other cause

Class III
Patients with symptoms such as syncope, near syncope, episodic dizziness, or palpitation in whom other causes have been identified by history, physical examination, or laboratory tests
Patients with cerebrovascular accidents, without other evidence of arrhythmia

the number of premature ventricular contractions. Little correlation of arrhythmia suppression and clinical outcomes is available. No AEM study has shown a mortality advantage when used in conjunction with antiarrhythmic drugs or devices. Following an intervention (drugs or device), at least a 63% to 95% reduction in arrhythmia frequency is required for AEM to be considered a valuable arrhythmia detection and evaluation tool. Compared with electrophysiology testing (EPS) in the Electrophysiologic Study Versus Electrocardiographic Monitoring (ESVEM) study, AEM was equivalent but not superior to EPS in the ability to select initial drug therapy.[16] The Asymptomatic Cardiac Ischemia Pilot (ACIP) study found that 75% of patients with asymptomatic evidence of ischemia on AEM had multivessel coronary artery disease on angiography.[17]

During AEM, the patient wears a portable ECG recorder that weighs about 8 to 16 oz. The recorder uses two to four chest leads (V_5 and V_3 most commonly). Additional leads do not improve the sensitivity of AEM significantly. If ST-segment changes are known to occur in certain leads, these can be used during AEM. Most AEM recordings are for 24 to 48 hours, but they can extend to weeks or months where the frequency of events related to ECG abnormalities is low. Implantable devices are used when long periods of monitoring are necessary. Currently used equipment is able to detect and analyze arrhythmias, ST-segment deviations, QRS complexes, RR intervals, and late potentials.

Three types of monitors are available: (1) continuous monitors, which record an ECG strip over the duration of the test, (2) event or intermittent recorders, which continuously monitor the ECG but only record preprogrammed abnormal ECG events or are patient-activated based on occurrence of symptoms, and (3) real-time analytical recorders, which record throughout the monitoring period and analyze each beat as it occurs. Monitors digitize, encode, and store the information in a solid-state memory or on magnetic tape. Event monitors are preprogrammed to record parameters such as the number of premature ventricular contractions and heart rate. During monitoring, the patient maintains a diary in which the occurrence, duration, and severity of symptoms (e.g., light-headedness, chest pain) are recorded, plus any specific activities undertaken, development of symptoms with the activity, and any interventions such as the taking of medication. A clocking device in the recorder allows later correlation of the patient's diary with the recorded ECG.

Evaluation and analysis of the ECG record are complex. Computer-assisted interpretation is used to scan the ECG and identify irregular rhythms, rates, and specific preprogrammed changes. The main advantage of computer analysis is to reduce interpretation of artifact recordings. Each beat recorded during AEM is evaluated for its arrhythmia potential and classified as normal or abnormal. The morphology of each QRS-T section is examined for ischemia potential, although, as indicated previously, baseline ST-segment abnormalities and adjustments in amplitude of the recording may preclude interpretation of these segments. The new ACC/AHA guidelines provide detail as to the suitability of using ST segments for analysis of ischemia.[12] Various drugs such as digoxin and the tricyclic antidepressants that cause baseline ECG abnormalities may preclude patients from being evaluated with AEM.

Sections identified by the computer as abnormal or those correlating with patient symptoms are then evaluated and characterized further (e.g., potentially pathologic rhythms) by technical personnel and physicians. Confounding factors when using AEM can arise from the patient and the device (Table 11–6). AEM is evolving rapidly, primarily related to improved technology with respect to data interpretation, signal quality, and improved understanding of the implications of ECG changes.

TABLE 11–6. Confounding Factors in Ambulatory ECG Monitoring

Patient Factors	Equipment Factors
Electrolyte abnormalities	Battery failure
Hyperventilation	Loose lead
Lead interference by patient	Mechanical failure of
Medications	recorder
Physiologic variations in	Motor failure
waveforms	Overrecording
Medications	Computer inability to detect
Patient activities (e.g., sudden exercise)	arrhythmia
Presence of atrial fibrillation	

EXERCISE STRESS TESTING (ET)

ET is a noninvasive test used to evaluate clinical and cardiovascular responses to exercise.[19–23] ET is used frequently as an initial test, in conjunction with physical examination and patient symptoms, to aid in the selection of additional testing modalities. It is a simple test that can be conducted in a physician's office and is about 20 times less expensive than an angiogram and almost three times less expensive than stress ECHO. Almost two-thirds of ETs billed to Medicare in 1996 were conducted in physicians' offices, and one-third were conducted by noncardiologists.

The ET provides diagnostic information in patients with known or suspected IHD and prognostic information in patients after myocardial infarction or revascularization. However, there are no data that support its use as a screening tool for coronary artery disease (CAD) or for detection of early CAD in asymptomatic subjects.

The principle behind ET is to increase myocardial oxygen demand above myocardial oxygen supply and coronary reserve, thereby provoking ischemia (inadequate myocardial perfusion), using exercise as a stressor. Ischemia is detected by patient symptoms, ECG changes, and/or hemodynamic changes. The type of ECG changes, leads affected, and patient performance are used as an index of severity and location of disease. ET is a very practical test in that it can assess patients' functional capacity.

Some examples of class I, II, and III indications from the ACC/AHA guidelines on ET are presented here.[20] The major class I indications are evaluation of males older than 40 years who have symptoms suggestive of CAD and risk factors for CAD or atypical symptoms suggestive of CAD. Another class I indication is to help assess prognosis and functional capacity in patients with confirmed CAD.[21] Frequently, the ET is performed following an acute myocardial infarction (AMI) for this purpose. Class II indications are patients with variant angina or women with a history of typical or atypical chest pain. Examples of class III indications are patients with simple premature ventricular contractions on a resting ECG with no other signs or symptoms of CAD. Additionally, ET is used to assess symptoms such as chest pain or breathlessness. The ET should be used only if the results are able to alter patient management or to assess patient function.

Guidelines for conducting and interpreting the tests and details of testing equipment and environment are outlined in the ACC/AHA guidelines on ET standards. ET is conducted on a treadmill or bicycle ergometer or by means of a handgrip. These dynamic methods are used to assess exercise tolerance because they induce both a volume and pressure load on the heart. Both modalities also allow the degree of stress to be delivered in a graded and calibrated manner. Treadmill walking is preferred over the ergometer because it involves more muscle mass and the $Vo_{2,max}$ achieved with cycle ergometer is 10% to 15% lower than with the treadmill.

Many protocols have been designed and validated for use with ET, but the two used most commonly are the Bruce and Naughton protocols. Protocols help to decrease inter- and intrapatient variability and allow for standardization in the interpretation of the tests. Protocols may be customized for individual patients to ensure an exercise time of 6 to 12 minutes and a heart rate of 85% to 90% of maximum predicted (adjusted for age and gender). Protocols detail gradient, speed, and rates of change of these parameters during the test.

In preparation for ET, patients fast prior to the test for a minimum of 3 hours, may not exercise 12 hours prior to the test, and must dress suitably for exercise. Baseline evaluation consists of history and physical examination, blood pressure, heart rate, and ECG. The test begins with a 1-minute warmup period to orient the patient to the equipment. Each stage of the test is maintained for at least 3 minutes. Continuous blood pressure, heart rate, and ECG recordings are obtained, with definitive readings 2 minutes into each stage. Patients are questioned 2 to 3 minutes into each stage of the test about symptoms such as headache, dizziness, and chest pain. Clinical symptoms assessed include color of skin, level of perspiration, and evidence of peripheral cyanosis and light-headedness. Patients are encouraged to exercise as vigorously as they can to ensure an optimal test result. Onset, nature, and duration of all changes in symptoms, hemodynamics, and ECG are noted. Following the test there is a cool-down period during which the patient is seated or lying and is observed for changes as described earlier.

The ET requires considerable effort, with many patients requiring encouragement to perform to the best of their ability. Some patients use the test as a personal challenge and perform better on repeated attempts. This is referred to as a *training effect* and may be a confounding factor in using ET to assess the effect of drug therapy or after interventions for IHD in clinical trials.

Interpretation of the ET requires correlation of clinical, ECG, and other parameters measured during the test with the patient's history (e.g., age, gender, concurrent risk factors, and medical history) and concomitant therapy. Results of the ET can be used as a guide to future patient management, including suitability for interventional cardiology and selection of pharmacotherapy. A positive ET is defined as 1 mm of horizontal or downsloping depression or elevation of the ST segment for 60 to 80 ms after the QRS complex. For patients with baseline ST-segment depression, combinations of abnormal responses (e.g., 2 mm of ST-segment depression with hemodynamic abnormalities) would be necessary to call a test positive. ST-segment depression of 2 mm or more, especially in conjunction with heart rates of less than 120 beats per minute, low levels of stress, or depression persisting for up to 6 minutes after the cessation of the ET, is associated with a poor prognosis. Depression of the ST segment in multiple leads is also significant. Other ECG changes include development of U waves and increased complexity and/or frequency of premature ventricular contractions or beats, especially if associated with bigeminy or periods of ventricular tachycardia.

Although ECG changes and heart rate responses are used as objective end points of an ET, patient and clinical end points are actually preferred. The use of the 85% to 90% maximally predicted heart rate is highly variable among patients and often is not achieved because of concomitant drug therapy and different levels of fitness. Symptom-limited or patient-directed tests are continued to the predetermined end point(s) unless the patient tires or certain characteristics are noted. Clinical symptoms, exhaustion, chest pain, and changes in blood pressure, heart rate, and the ECG (rhythm, configuration, and

rate) are used as end points for such *open-ended tests*. Also, patient performance, measured as exercise duration, time until symptoms, stress at which symptoms occur, and hemodynamic parameters, is a better indicator of an adequate test than heart rate response. *Close-ended testing* is the use of fixed end points such as time on the treadmill or maximal heart rate.

The product of blood pressure and heart rate (*double product*) is a measure of myocardial oxygen demand. In patients with stable angina, the double product is reproducible on repeat ETs; thus it is used as an objective parameter to follow an individual patient's disease. Inappropriate or inadequate responses in blood pressure and/or heart rate to exercise suggest heart disease. A reduction in heart rate or a flat response (failure to increase heart rate above 120 beats per minute) with increasing levels of stress has a poor prognosis. Likewise, failure to increase the systolic blood pressure or the finding of a sustained decrease of more than 10 mm Hg is also associated with a worse prognosis. Such responses indicate that the heart has an inadequate reserve to respond to stress. Patients who are unable to progress beyond stage II of the Bruce protocol have a poor prognosis and more severe IHD. Other rating scales (e.g., Borg, which measures perceived exertion) may be used in conjunction with the objective results from the ET to classify patients into high- and low-risk groups. Silent ischemia may confound the interpretation of ET because blood pressure and ECG changes may occur in the absence of symptoms.

To provide standardized comparability between tests and patients, metabolic equivalents (METs) are used as a measure of $Vo_{2,max}$. A MET is a measure of resting oxygen uptake. Activity energy demands then can be calculated in terms of METs. For example, 4 METs is equivalent to walking at 4 mi/h. The number of METs a patient can undertake without symptoms of ischemia correlates with prognosis and helps to guide appropriate management strategies. Refer to Table 11–7 for examples of METs and activity correlations. Exercise capacities of less than 5 METs are associated with a poor prognosis; those greater than 13 METs have a good prognosis despite the presence of disease.

Meta-analysis of more than 24,000 patients in 147 studies showed a mean sensitivity of 68% and specificity of 77% for ET as a diagnostic test. The specificity of ET to detect the presence of CAD, compared with angiography, is 84%. Sensitivity ranges from 40% to 90% depending on the number of vessels affected, with a mean of 66%.

As a prognostic test, ET is very popular after myocardial infarction and can be conducted within 3 days of an acute event. It can be used to determine functional capacity, assess the degree of rehabilitation, and identify patients at risk for further cardiovascular events. Immediately after myocardial infarction, a modified protocol is used; the test is terminated when a heart rate of 70% to 75% of age- and gender-predicted maximum is reached (e.g., 140 beats per minute for those under age 40 and 130 for those older than age 40) or a MET level of 5 for patients older than 40 or 7 for those younger than 40. Tests usually are done prior to discharge or within 6 weeks of infarction.

TABLE 11–7. MET Relationship to Activity and Function

METs	Level of Activity	ET Result
1	Resting	< 6 METs
2	Level walking at 2 mi/h	Symptom-limited lifestyle
4	Level walking at 4 mi/h	Sedentary lifestyle tolerated
13	Cycling 9–10 mi/h	Little or no activity-limited lifestyle
20	Shoveling heavy snow	No limitations on lifestyle

TABLE 11–8. Contraindications for Exercise Testing

Absolute	Relative
Unstable angina	Left main coronary artery disease
Syncope	Tachy- or bradyarrhythmias
<72 hours after AMI	Electrolyte abnormalities
Uncontrolled CHF	Hypertension (SBP >220 mm Hg)
Uncontrolled arrhythmias	High-degree AV block
Acute systemic illness	
Acute pulmonary embolism	
Acute myocarditis	
Thrombosis of lower extremity	

In the peri-infarction period, mortality and reinfarction rates are 0.02% and 0.09%, respectively. Patients may be stratified into low-, intermediate-, and high-risk categories depending on the evidence for ischemia and the level of exercise tolerance.

ET is relatively safe, with an estimated risk of AMI or death of 10 per 10,000 tests overall. Most adverse effects are cardiac in nature, including arrhythmias (primarily bradyarrhythmias), sudden death, hypotension, and myocardial infarction. Patients in whom ET is contraindicated are those who are unable or who should not exercise because of physiologic or psychological limitations (Table 11–8). Unstable angina is usually a contraindication to ET because of the instability of the patient's disease state and because patients cannot exercise to a satisfactory level for the test to be considered adequate. However, once such a patient is stable, ET is excellent for prognostic evaluation. In patients with untreated life-threatening arrhythmias or CHF, ET is also contraindicated. Patients with comorbid diseases such as COPD or peripheral vascular disease (PVD) may be limited in their exercise capacity, whereas lower limb amputees are unable to perform the standard treadmill test. For patients with disabilities or other medical conditions that limit their exercise capacity independent of heart disease, pharmacologic stress testing with dipyridamole, adenosine, or dobutamine is an alternative (see "Pharmacologic Stress Testing" below).

Drug therapy rarely is discontinued for the test primarily because few data exist to support better test results off drug therapy. Patients on β-blockers or calcium channel blockers may not achieve maximal heart rates, but ET helps to demonstrate patients' exercise capacity on drug therapy. Nitrates do not alter exercise capacity directly and theoretically may improve patient response because they relieve or prevent symptoms of ischemia. Digoxin interferes with interpretation of ST-segment changes, and patients rarely achieve ST-segment changes greater than 1 mm even in the face of significant ischemia. Owing to its long half-life, digoxin need not be discontinued prior to the test.

CARDIAC CATHETERIZATION AND ANGIOGRAPHY

Development of the cardiac catheterization technique was a major milestone in the diagnosis and management of CVD because it provided a physiologic and anatomic approach to assess patency of coronary vessels and hemodynamic parameters of cardiac function.[24–34] Cardiac catheterization is the technique used to gain vascular access to the coronary arteries by intravascular catheters and heart chambers. Once cardiac catheterization is complete, other diagnostic and therapeutic procedures, such as angiography, ventriculography, and percutaneous transluminal angioplasty (PTCA), and drug administration (e.g., thrombolytics) may be undertaken.

Following interventional procedures such as PTCA, catheterization with angiography can be used to evaluate efficacy of the intervention. In recurrent clinical syndromes, following a procedure, catheterization is used to help delineate a new management strategy. Catheterization is also now used commonly with PTCA and/or drug therapy in the management of acute coronary syndromes.

Additionally, catheterization allows assessment of valvular function and computation of various cardiac performance parameters such as cardiac output, stroke volume, systemic vascular resistance, cardiac chamber pressures, and blood flow. It also allows for placement of cardiac pacemakers. Drug administration during cardiac catheterization is used primarily for assessment of end points in clinical trials (e.g., thrombolytics to assess coronary artery patency), for management of events (e.g., chest pain) during catheterization, or for diagnostic purposes (e.g., ergonovine to evaluate coronary spasm). Further applications of cardiac catheterization include aortic root angiography, pulmonary angiography, retrieval of foreign bodies, and atherectomy.

More than 1 million cardiac catheterizations are performed in the United States each year, making it the second most frequent inhospital procedure. Images obtained during catheterization are stored on 35-mm cineradiographic film or are digitized, allowing comparison of studies at a later date. The ACC/AHA guidelines on angiography and PTCA describe the class I, II, and III indications for each of these procedures; examples are given in Table 11–9.[27,28] The guidelines for angiography, PTCA, and catheterization also include recommendations regarding technique, procedures, facilities, personnel, and training.

The cardiac catheterization procedure requires vascular access, usually obtained percutaneously at brachial or femoral arteries or veins. Left-sided catheterization provides access to the aorta, left ventricle, and left atrium. Right-sided catheterization enables the right side of the heart, coronary sinus, pulmonary arteries, and pulmonary wedge position to be reached. Left-sided catheterization is used for coronary angiography and ventriculography, whereas right-sided catheterization is used for determination of cardiac performance parameters.

Prior to an elective procedure, the patient is given nothing by mouth (after midnight) except for oral medications. It is not necessary to stop any medications except warfarin prior to catheterization. Patients receiving warfarin may be transitioned to low-molecular-weight

TABLE 11–9. Indications for Coronary Angiography

Class I
Patients with class III–IV angina or high risk for adverse outcomes not responding to medical therapy
Patients who have high-risk findings on noninvasive testing
Suspected abrupt closure or stent thrombosis following PTCA
Recurrent angina within 9 months of PTCA
Alternative to thrombolytic therapy in patients less than 12 hours from AMI
Class II
Patients with class III–IV angina who improve on medical therapy
Patients with CAD who fail to respond to medical therapy
Patients with CAD who cannot be risk stratified by other methodologies
Recurrent angina within 12 months of PTCA
Recurrent angina not controlled by medical therapy post PTCA
Class III
Patients after interventional procedure with no evidence of ischemia
Patients who are not candidates for or do not wish interventional procedures for revascularization
Assessment of atypical chest pain

or unfractionated heparin or anticoagulation may be discontinued depending on the clinical scenario about 3 days prior to the procedure. Heparin products are stopped about 6 hours before the procedure to allow normalization of coagulation. There are no data to support low-molecular-weight heparin during catheterization procedures because its longer half-life may increase the risk of intra- and postprocedural bleeding. Patients who require anticoagulation prior to angiography (e.g., those with acute coronary syndromes) usually are treated with unfractionated heparin or low-molecular-weight heparin.

Patients frequently develop chest pain and/or vasospasm during introduction and manipulation of catheters and injection of angiographic dyes. Nitroglycerin and/or morphine may be given for chest pain. Nitroglycerin also is used to prevent vasospasm and is given sublingually or by intravenous infusion. Sedatives, such as midazolam or other short-acting benzodiazepines, frequently are given to ensure patient comfort and safety, but the patient is awake and aware of the procedure. Patient cooperation is necessary to obtain the angiographic views and assess symptoms. The patient will be required to remain still for about 6 to 8 hours to reduce the risk of bleeding from the catheter entry site(s). Depending on the procedure, patients may be discharged the same day or within 24 hours, if stable.

Heparin products are used during procedures such as angiography, left-sided heart catheterization, and PTCA to prevent thrombotic complications. Depending on the procedure undertaken, heparin is either discontinued almost immediately following the procedure or continued for 12 to 24 hours. Heparin administration during the procedure is measured with the activated clotting time (ACT), not the partial thromboplastin time (PTT). For patients undergoing PTCA, aspirin, clopidogrel, or ticlopidine and calcium channel blockers are used prior to and following the procedure. Despite the invasive nature of the procedure, there is no consensus as to the need for prophylactic antibiotics in patients at risk for bacterial endocarditis because of valvular prostheses or a prior history of rheumatic fever. With the advent of class IIb/IIIa receptor antagonists such as tirofiban, eptifibatide, and abciximab, which have been shown to improve short- and long-term coronary artery patency rates with PTCA, patients who receive a stent also will receive one of these agents prior to, during, and/or after the procedure.

During the procedure, hemodynamic parameters, blood pressure, and heart rate are monitored continuously. ECG monitoring and intermittent 12-lead ECGs are also maintained. Measurements taken during catheterization are obtained only after hemodynamic stabilization: at baseline, following catheter movement, or during pharmacologic intervention. Information obtained during catheterization is in real time and is assumed to reflect the ongoing status of the coronary circulation. Procedurally related vasospasm may be misleading because the catheter itself is a powerful stimulus for spasm.

Complications associated with cardiac catheterization procedures and attending angiographic or interventional activities are related to the expertise and experience of the operator, with case load being a good indicator of the latter. The incidence of significant complications related to catheterization with angiography is reported to be less than 2%, with mortality about 0.11%. Patient factors such as hemodynamic stability and renal function increase risk. There are no absolute contraindications to coronary angiography, and the relative contraindications are not well substantiated (Table 11–10). In essence, clinical stability of the patient and potential benefit of the procedure in terms of future patient management predicate the importance of relative contraindications. Complication rates, especially those of a thrombotic nature, increase with the dwell time of the catheters, duration of catheterization, catheter type, and operator technique. Bleeding complications can be reduced by ensuring that patients have normal

TABLE 11–10. Contraindications of Cardiac Catheterization and Other Procedures[a]

Recent stroke	Patient noncompliance[b]
Advanced physiologic age	Digoxin intoxication
Severe anemia	Anaphylaxis to radiographic dyes
Severe hypertension	Active infection
Active gastrointestinal bleed	Severe electrolyte imbalances
Fever	Unstable condition
Other comorbid illnesses, e.g., COPD[c,d]	

[a]Primarily contraindications to procedures such as arteriography and PTCA.
[b]Patient not willing to undergo further treatment (e.g., surgery based on results of catheterization).
[c]COPD = chronic obstructive pulmonary disease.
[d]Disease states that may prohibit or increase risk of other interventions (e.g., surgery).
[e]Patients in whom emergency cardiac surgery would pose a high risk (e.g., during acute asthma or acute exacerbation of COPD).

coagulation studies prior to the procedure and remain at bed rest for several hours after the procedure and that the nursing staff undertakes good care of the catheter entry and exit sites. In the event of bleeding complications, direct pressure is required with sandbags, followed by emergency surgery if there is no resolution, to prevent further complications. Heart perforation is an uncommon but potentially lethal complication requiring emergency surgical intervention. Other complications such as a vagal reflex with hypotension, bradycardia, and nausea can occur. These occur most frequently in conjunction with patient anxiety and can be prevented or treated with atropine. An increased predisposition to myocardial infarction during and after the procedure is seen in patients with unstable angina, recent subendocardial infarction, and type 1 diabetes mellitus. After catheterization, patients may have elevated creatine phosphokinase and troponins owing to tissue damage during the procedure. There is some controversy as to how to interpret these values with respect to what they indicate regarding myocardial damage. Acute closure of a coronary vessel or myocardial ischemia is managed by return to the catheterization laboratory or cardiac surgery. All facilities should be in close liaison with a cardiothoracic surgery unit.

Angiography, which accompanies most cardiac catheterization procedures, is defined as the "radiographic visualization of coronary vessels after injection of radiopaque contrast medium." Despite the expanding role of cardiac catheterization, angiography is used most frequently to describe the presence and extent of CAD and to allow planning for medical or surgical intervention. Cardiac catheterization with angiography is the "gold standard" in the diagnosis and assessment of CAD, against which all new invasive and noninvasive tests are measured. Unlike most other procedures, angiography determines the morphology of a stenotic lesion and the degree of luminal obstruction. However, this does not relate well to physiologic or functional significance of the lesion.[34] For example, a 50% luminal occlusion not considered significant by radiologic standards may still be the lesion producing symptomatic chest pain, and a diabetic patient with significant microvascular CAD may appear to have unaffected larger arteries at angiography and yet still be at risk of a cardiac event. Angiography also assesses the presence of collateral circulation and dynamic abnormalities such as vasospasm.

The extent of disease by angiography is defined as the number of vessels, and the vessels affected are named. Angiography is able to detect lesions that occlude the vessel by as little as 20%. Occlusions of 75% or more are almost always seen on angiography. Significant narrowing is usually assumed to be 50% or more, although some studies use 70% narrowing as the cutoff point. The lesion can be measured in several ways. Considerable controversy exists as to the best methodology. During angiography, the lesion is compared visually with surrounding vessels. Inherent difficulties include individual evaluator variability and also the assumption that surrounding vessels are normal. Calipers can be used to document physical size, but generally, the degree of stenosis is reported as a percentage of narrowing. Various grading scales, such as the coronary artery score and myocardial jeopardy scores, are used, and these scores have been shown to predict long-term outcomes. Coronary artery lesions most prone to rupture and thrombosis are those with 40% to 60% narrowing, so lesions with less than 50% narrowing are not benign.

Multiple views are required to obtain a good image of the vessel; the right anterior oblique planes are used most commonly (two views at 90 degrees to each other). Lesions may be described as concentric and smooth (simple lesions) or eccentric and broad with a rough surface (complicated lesions). The number of lesions is also considered of importance to the severity and prognosis of IHD, although there is considerable variation in the accuracy of such predictions because angiographic and pathologic correlation of lesions is imperfect. The occurrence of spasm, variants in anatomy, and collateral filling also complicate interpretation of the angiogram.

Angiographic films are used to plan interventions, in particular coronary artery bypass grafting (CABG) and PTCA. They are also used during both surgery and PTCA to guide the procedure.[35,36] Ventriculographic studies may be performed during cardiac catheterization to obtain information about the contours of the heart and to assess global and segmental function. Regional wall motion, filling defects, and the presence of mural thrombi also may be visualized. During this procedure, radiopaque dye is injected into the heart chambers, and serial films are taken to follow the dye passage. Left ventricular ventriculography is a routine part of left-sided catheterization unless ventricular function information is already available from other noninvasive studies or there are specific contraindications to the procedure.

Cardiac performance is also best assessed during catheterization procedures as direct visualization of performance along with calculated parameters that can be obtained simultaneously and represent real-time values. Measured and observed parameters obtained during catheterization are used to determine cardiac performance. Contractility, as judged by wall motion and ejection fraction, can be used to assess global cardiac performance and to plan and evaluate or assess therapy.

Invasive cardiology is growing rapidly not only in terms of the numbers of patients undergoing such procedures but also in terms of the diversity of procedures. The development of electrophysiologic studies for the assessment and treatment of arrhythmias was made possible because of catheterization. The diversity of techniques is "limited only by the imagination of the physician and inventiveness of the microtechnologist."

COMPUTED TOMOGRAPHY

CT scanning is used rarely as a primary diagnostic procedure in the evaluation of CVD and function because it provides similar information as other diagnostic procedures (e.g., ECHO) and is significantly more expensive. Enhanced definition and spatial resolution of structures are possible with CT scanning, which is useful in some specific indications such as to evaluate aortic and pericardial disease and assess paracardiac and cardiac masses. More accurate determination of chamber volume and size and mass calculations of myocardial wall thickness can be obtained from CT scanning than with other methods

such as ECHO or angiography. Additionally, CT scanning acquires three-dimensional images.[37]

New techniques such as ultrafast CT (cine-CT) scanning have resolved the problems of cardiac motion that distorted conventional CT images.[38] With cine-CT scanning, complete tomograms are assembled within one cardiac cycle (50 ms), thus providing real-time images. For ultrafast CT scanners, a set event within the cardiac cycle (determined by ECG) usually is used as initiator for imaging to ensure standardization. Conventional CT scanning requires that images be correlated with the cardiac cycle by gating the CT to the ECG. Cine-CT scans examine the heart at 10 to 14 tomographic levels in 10-mm slices.

Although still in its infancy, cine-CT scanning has been proposed as a screening tool for evaluating the risk of developing obstructive CAD and as a diagnostic tool for CAD. Recent AHA/ACC guidelines address the current state of practice with this methodology. The CT scan will show localized areas of infarction and abnormal perfusion and allows quantification of the extent and density of coronary artery calcification.[40] Cine-CT scanning is more sensitive and specific than fluoroscopy in identifying the extent and density of coronary artery calcification. The calcium score (calcium density and volume of calcium) in patients older than 30 to 70 years with known CAD is significantly higher than in subjects with no CAD and appears to correlate well with the degree of coronary artery occlusion.[41]

CT scanning is more definitive and accurate in the diagnosis of aortic dissection and evaluation of the pericardium than ECHO. Diagnostic accuracy of aortic dissections with CT scanning is at least 90%. CT scanning affords definition of the edges of the intimal flap of the dissection, and true and false channels can be seen. It also demarcates the components of the myocardial wall from the inner endocardial wall through to the epicardial surface and pericardium, allowing visualization of abnormalities, such as aneurysms and thrombin. Detection of the presence of a thrombus on a CT scan is comparable in accuracy with two-dimensional ECHO. The pericardium appears as a distinct entity and can be evaluated for thickening and calcification. CT scanning is the most sensitive technique to differentiate types of pericarditis and estimate pericardial fluid volume. Compared with ECHO, CT scanning is equivocal to define loculated and hemorrhagic effusions.

In the evaluation of cardiac masses, CT scanning shows the mass as a distinct space-occupying entity. Tissue density differentiation as seen on a CT scan allows characterization of density, aiding in determination of the nature of masses. Masses as small as 0.5 to 1 cm can be identified on CT scans.

Like radionuclide assessment, contrast angiography, and ECHO, CT scanning can be used to calculate ejection fraction, left ventricular volume, and stroke volume. The blood pool is defined with intravenous iodinated contrast material. Ventricular volumes, ejection fraction, and stroke volume are determined directly from the blood pool on each image. Values obtained with CT scanning are more accurate and reproducible than those obtained on angiography and ECHO. The three-dimensional image of a CT scan also allows determination of the extent and distribution of LVH in patients with hypertrophic or congestive cardiomyopathy.

CT scanning has proven to be an effective noninvasive method to visualize congenital heart disease, but its role is challenged by the higher-resolution capacity of MRI.[42] For measuring parameters in some congenital disorders, such as evaluation of ventricular function and estimation of the volume of cardiac shunts, CT scanning still remains the evaluation method of choice.

In summary, CT scanning, especially cine-CT scanning, is a rapidly evolving technique for evaluation of CVD.[43–46] It remains an expensive alternative to other methodologies in many instances, but the high resolution and spatial capabilities mean that CT scanning offers unique properties.

POSITRON-EMISSION TOMOGRAPHY (PET)

PET is a relatively new modality for diagnostic imaging in CVD medicine.[47–54] PET has found a niche to characterize myocardial physiologic and metabolic activity, perfusion, and viability. PET can measure regional myocardial uptake of exogenous glucose and fatty acids, quantitate free fatty acid metabolism, define perfused myocardium energy source(s), and evaluate myocardial chemoreceptor sites.[50] Although many other techniques can be used similarly to evaluate myocardial function, PET images are superior in definition. The primary advantages of PET are its noninvasive nature, the ability to do repeat scans within a short period of time, such as before and after PTCA, and the reproducibility of images over time. PET is very expensive owing to the need for on-site cyclotrons for many of the radiotracers, and there is limited availability of sites that offer the technique. Cheaper forms of PET-like scanning are in development, but image resolution is less.

PET uses positron-emitting isotopes such as oxgen-15, nitrogen-13, carbon-11, and fluoride-18. These are incorporated into substances such as water, glucose analogs, or fatty acids, the metabolic substrates for myocardial tissue. For myocardial perfusion studies, rubidium-82 (^{82}Rh), nitrogen-13 ammonia ([^{13}N]H$_3$), and ^{15}O$_2$-labeled water are used. For myocardial substrate metabolism studies, [^{11}C]palmitate, [^{11}C]acetate, and [^{18}F]2-deoxyglucose (FDG) are used. All these substances have very short half-lives (<10 minutes). In the fasted state, perfused myocardium primarily uses fatty acids as energy source. Postprandially, glucose is the preferred substrate. Ischemic myocardium primarily metabolizes glucose because mitochondial fatty acid oxidation is impaired. Hence, with PET using either a fatty acid or glucose substrate, ischemic versus nonischemic areas can be defined. Frequently, PET is used in conjunction with pharmacologic stress testing to provoke ischemia, with images obtained before and after stress application.

Uptake of ^{82}Rb occurs via the Na$^+$,K$^+$-ATPase pump and occurs preferentially in viable tissue. Net uptake into tissue resolving from an ischemic insult and infarcted tissue is reduced. With a half-life of 1.26 minutes, serial images of myocardial perfusion can be taken as frequently as every 5 minutes, and a dobutamine stress test is completed within 45 minutes. Comparative studies with ET, single-photon-emission computed tomography (SPECT), and stress ECHO show PET to be more accurate in the detection of IHD. The substrate [^{13}N]H$_3$ rapidly crosses capillary membranes and is trapped in the myocardium by glutamate-glutamine reactions. This product produces high-contrast images with a sensitivity of 88% to 97% and a specificity of 90% to 100% to detect IHD. Oxygen-15–labeled water has a high extraction ratio into myocardial tissue, which appears to be independent of blood flow or the metabolic state of the myocardium. Oxygen-15–labeled water studies are done in conjunction with [^{15}O]carbon monoxide (labels red blood cells in the vascular space) studies to help eliminate some of the background activity that occurs as a result of the high extraction ratio.[54]

Tracers used for assessment of myocardial metabolism are selected based on the type of metabolism of interest: FDG traces glucose metabolism, [^{11}C]palmitate traces mitochondrial fatty acid metabolism, and [^{11}C]acetate is an indirect marker for myocardial oxygen consumption, allowing assessment of ventricular performance. [^{11}C]Palmitate is a useful marker for normal myocardial oxygen consumption because baseline energy needs of the myocardium

are met through fatty acid oxidation. Clearance of [^{11}C]palmitate is biexponential, and studies in animals and in healthy men have shown clearance to be proportional to cardiac workload and myocardial oxygen consumption. In acute ischemia, the first component of clearance is reduced and the second is increased. The use of [^{11}C]palmitate to assess myocardial metabolism in ischemic tissue is limited because there is altered transport and storage of the compound and significant backdiffusion of the agent into the vascular space.

FDG accumulates in the heart proportional to glucose use by the myocardial cell and so is a marker of cell viability. FDG studies help to identify the affected vascular bed and allow evaluation as to whether angioplasty or surgery might be used.[50] Detection of hibernating myocardium is possible because it predominantly uses glucose and can be seen readily on PET scans. Patients with a significant degree of jeopardized or hibernating myocardium identified on PET scanning then could be candidates for revascularization procedures. In contrast, a perfusion study would not show as good differentiation of infarcted versus hibernating tissue, and revascularization may not be considered. In studies of recovery of left ventricular function following revascularization, PET has a positive predictive value of 72% and a negative predictive value of 83%. PET with FDG has been used in the assessment of cardiomyopathies. In ischemic cardiomyopathy, discrete regional ischemia is seen as a patchy, nonhomogeneous uptake of the tracers; dilated cardiomyopathies show global decreased uptake of tracers.

In CAD, PET is used to assess and follow the physiologic significance of stenotic lesions. After infarction, PET myocardial substrate metabolism studies are used to evaluate the amount and activity of viable tissue around the infarcted area and the site and extent of infarction. Myocardial perfusion studies with PET identify more accurately the viable and nonviable myocardium compared with technetium and thallium. PET also quantifies regional myocardial perfusion more accurately than other modalities. When linked with physiologic or pharmacologic stress tests, PET enables evaluation of the myocardium under stress conditions. Studies in patients with more than 50% stenosis on angiography suggest that dipyridamole stress SPECT and [^{13}N]ammonia PET are comparable tests to assess coronary artery perfusion, with respective sensitivities of 98% and 96% and specificities of 88% and 81%.[51] SPECT analysis using FDG compared with PET with FDG shows comparable accuracy for the detection of CAD. Comparative studies with SPECT thallium in conjunction with bicycle ergometer or dipyridamole versus PET perfusion scanning showed comparative sensitivities (76% to 79%) but improved specificity (90% versus 82%, $p < .005$).[53,54]

The future of PET appears promising. Improved tomographic scanners, development of new radiopharmaceuticals, and improved understanding of substrate metabolism and its relationship to myocardial tissue viability will provide new dimensions to assess and evaluate myocardial function. Research enterprises are developing agents to label receptors as a tool to determine cardiovascular physiology and how altered receptor function, biochemical abnormalities, substrate metabolism, or other as yet unrecognized abnormalities impair cardiac function.

ECHOCARDIOGRAM

ECHO is the use of ultrasound to visualize anatomic structures such as the valves within the heart and to describe wall motion.[55–60] Clinically, ECHO is the most frequently used noninvasive cardiovascular test, aside from the ECG. It competes well with invasive techniques such as cardiac catheterization with angiography for the evaluation of ischemia and valvular abnormalities. ECHO is relatively cheap to perform and can be done at the bedside, in the operating room, or in the physician's office. The major disadvantages of ECHO relate to technical limitations of operator-dependent images and competition from other noninvasive technologies such as MRI and CT scanning that provide similar information with superior tissue-type resolution. ECHO is used often as an initial evaluative tool following auscultation detection of an abnormality, thus providing a baseline visual characterization. Serial determinations in a given patient, especially following a change in clinical condition or a procedure, allow evaluation of progression of disease over time.

ECHO remains the procedure of choice in the diagnosis and evaluation of a number of conditions such as valvular dysfunction (aortic and mitral stenosis and regurgitation and endocarditis), wall motion abnormalities associated with ischemia, and congenital abnormalities, such as ventricular or atrial septal defects. Images obtained from ECHO are used to estimate chamber wall thickness and left ventricle ejection fraction, assess ventricular function, and detect abnormalities of the pericardium such as effusions or thickening.

ECHO is based on the principle of differential acoustic impedance (or tissue density) and the laws of reflection and refraction. Sound waves directed across tissues from a transducer will reflect back sound waves of different frequencies. The ability of the ultrasonic beam to penetrate chest wall structures is inversely proportional to the frequency of the signal. With transthoracic ECHO, frequencies of 2.0 to 5.0 MHz are used commonly in adults, and frequencies of 3.5 to 10.0 MHz are used in children. Serial determinations in a given patient using the same conditions and ECHO images (windows) provide the best form of internal control to allow comparisons of test results. In clinical trials, echocardiograms are read and interpreted independently by two or three clinicians to provide a means of control.

Two primary approaches to ECHO are used in clinical practice. Transthoracic echocardiography (TTE) is conducted with the transducer on the chest wall, whereas transesophageal echocardiography (TEE) is conducted with the transducer in the esophagus. In TTE, several modes of operation are possible, the most common being M-mode (motion) and two-dimensional (2D) imaging. Both M-mode and 2D ECHO provide visualization of heart structures and can indicate numerous structural abnormalities such as aneurysms, wall thickness abnormalities, chamber collapse (e.g., tamponade), and valvular stenosis. TEE is used primarily for assessment of valvular anatomy and function or to image intracardiac masses such as tumors or thrombi and valvular vegetations.[59,60]

In M-mode ECHO, the transducer is placed at a single site on the chest (usually along the sternal border), and the ultrasound is directed posteriorly. M-mode ECHO records only static objects in one plane, producing a single picture of a small region of the heart, or an "icepick view." Results depend on the exact placement of the transducer with respect to the underlying structures. Conventional M-mode ECHO provides visualization of the right ventricle, left ventricle, and posterior left ventricular wall and pericardium. If the transducer is swept in an arc from the apex to the base of the heart, virtually the whole heart can be visualized, including the valves and left atrium. Images are displayed as "windows."

Two-dimensional ECHO employs multiple windows of the heart, and each view provides a wedge-shaped image. Windows most commonly used include parasternal long- and short-axis and apical two- and four-chamber views (Fig. 11–6). These views are processed onto a videotape to produce a motion picture of the heart. 2D ECHO renders increased accuracy in calculating ventricular volumes, wall thickness, and degree of valvular stenosis compared with M-mode ECHO. Patient-specific calculated parameters such as ejection fraction and wall thickness are compared with standardized values (population-

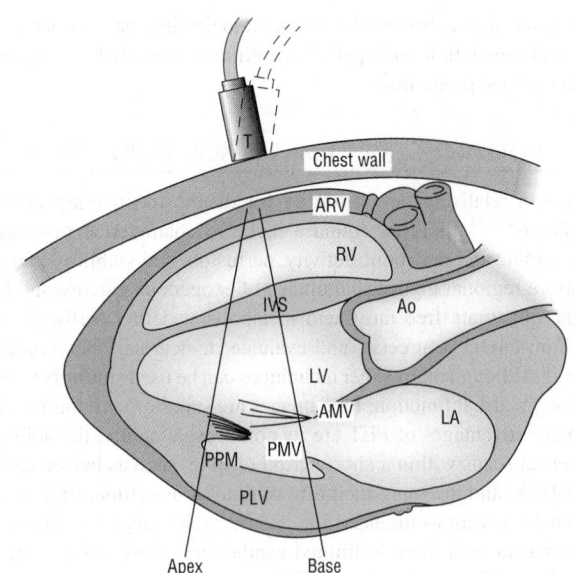

FIGURE 11–6. Schematic drawing of two-dimensional echocardiography to illustrate location of cardiac structures as "seen" by the transducer. The transducer is swept in an arc so that several pictures of the heart are obtained to generate the final electrocardiogram. *(Redrawn from Coryu BC, et al. Application of electrocardiography in acute myocardial infarction. Cardiovasc Clin 1995;2:113, with permission.)*

based) or with previously obtained values from the patient. Although ejection fraction is still commonly obtained with ECHO, it is a derived number, so it is considered subjective. Other tests to determine ejection fraction provide different numbers and highlight the difficulty of comparing results between tests. Ejection fraction from ECHO is also limited by the dimished views of total ventricular volume able to be visualized, especially in persons with distorted ventricles. Despite these limitations, ECHO remains the most common modality for ejection fraction determination.

ECHO can be used for diagnosis and prognosis and as a serial evaluation tool to assess acute and chronic ischemic heart disease and regional left ventricular function.[57] Areas of ischemic myocardium are seen on ECHO as aberrations in wall motion. Wall motion abnormalities are seen as altered thicknesses of various segments of the heart. Wall motion abnormalities are graded using descriptive terms such as *akinetic, hypokinetic, dyskinetic,* and *hyperkinetic.* It is possible to visualize the complete ventricle (in segments), allowing both global and regional left ventricular function to be assessed. Studies have shown that the locations of segmental ventricular wall motion abnormalities correspond with areas of CAD. ECHO can be linked with the various stress tests (ET, dipyridamole) to assess stress-induced structural or functional abnormalities (e.g., changes in wall motion). As a serial monitoring test, ECHO is comparable with angiography as a prognostic tool and can be used as a treatment planning tool. After myocardial infarction, ECHO is a useful noninvasive diagnostic tool for detection of ventricular aneurysms, thrombi, and pericardial effusions and can be used serially for diagnostic and prognostic information.

In TEE, the transducer is advanced into the esophagus and rests just behind the heart. The transducer also can be passed into the fundus of the stomach to obtain better images of the ventricles. Images are obtained in either the horizontal or vertical plane.[58] This is a low-risk invasive procedure and does not require routine antibiotic prophylaxis for patients at risk of developing endocarditis. Complications such as esophageal tears or perforation, esophageal burns, transient ventricular tachycardia, minor throat irritation, and transient vocal cord paralysis have been reported rarely.[59] In one series of 10,218 studies, only 1 death (0.0098%) was reported, comparable with that with esophageal gastroduodenoscopy (0.004%).[58] TEE is contraindicated in patients with esophageal abnormalities, in whom passage of the transducer might be limited (e.g., esophageal strictures or varices).

TEE yields higher resolution and improved visualization of structures, especially pulmonary veins and valves, compared with TTE. Interference of ribs, lungs, and subcutaneous tissues is reduced, enabling TEE to be more useful in patients in whom TTE is limited because of pulmonary disease, mechanical ventilation, or obesity. A high-frequency transducer (5 MHz for adults) is used, thus producing better image resolution. TEE is used for the same indications as TTE. Visualization of the heart valves—in particular, the mitral valve—is superior, allowing more accurate evaluation of both native and prosthetic valves. Clinical studies have shown that it is possible to visualize valvular vegetations as small as 5 mm with TEE. The ACC/AHA guidelines recommend TEE if the TTE is equivocal and the patient has staphylococcal bacteremia.[57] In a study comparing vegetation visualization, TEE detected vegetations in 90% of patients compared with 58% with TTE. It also can help to define complications of endocarditis such as thrombosis or valve leakage. In aortic dissection, TEE is able to identify the initial flap and origin of dissection and has an overall sensitivity and specificity of 97% and 100%, respectively. CT remains the diagnostic method of choice for aortic dissection, but TEE offers a sensitive and fast test that can be conducted in the emergency room.

Other uses of TEE include identification of cardiac thrombus, especially thrombi in the left atrium, and assessment of atrial dilation. After transient ischemic attacks or cerebrovascular accidents, TEE may enable identification of the site of cardiac emboli by providing excellent images of likely sources of such, namely, ventricular or atrial thrombus, valvular vegetation, cardiac shunts, cardiac tumors, or atrial and ventricular septal defects. In a study of almost 1500 patients with cerebral ischemia or nonvalvular atrial fibrillation, atrial thrombi were seen in 183 patients when evaluated by TEE versus only 2 patients using TTE. TEE can be used for intraoperative cardiac imaging to ascertain development of ischemia.

Another advance with ECHO has been the addition of Doppler and color-flow Doppler technology. The Doppler principle involves reflecting sound off a moving object—in the case of ECHO, the red blood cell. As the red cell moves in relation to the transducer, a frequency shift occurs in the reflected wave. Assessment with Doppler ECHO combines structural images and hemodynamic monitoring. Thus it is possible to evaluate the impact of structural disease on cardiac function and quantify the associated hemodynamics. Color enhancement allows flow direction to be visualized; different colors are used for antegrade and retrograde flow. These improve resolution of structures, identify patterns of blood flow, and allow calculation of flow gradients.

Doppler ECHO is used primarily in conjunction with traditional ECHO for analysis of valvular function or blood flow patterns. It allows measurement of transvalvular pressure gradients, valve area, and pressure changes on either side of the valve. Doppler ECHO is either continuous or pulsed; the former is used to assess pressure changes, whereas the latter is used to localize points of origin and creation of turbulent and high blood flow. Color Doppler is used to visualize blood flow (e.g., regurgitation). Turbulence associated with valvular and wall motion abnormalities can be visualized and quantified clearly. In aortic regurgitation, Doppler ECHO is the best noninvasive technique to assess the pressure and severity of regurgitation. Color-flow mapping allows tracing of the jet direction and an indication

of its volume, point of wall contact, and width. Because Doppler ECHO distinguishes different types of turbulence, it can simultaneously identify more than one type of valvular abnormality (e.g., aortic regurgitation and mitral stenosis) and the source of concomitant heart murmur.

NUCLEAR CARDIOLOGY

Nuclear cardiology continues to be a major advance as a noninvasive testing method.[61–70] Radionuclides with short half-lives, which can be used either alone or combined with other substances to form agents with particular properties, such as technetium-99m pyrophosphate, have expanded the role for nuclear imaging in cardiology. Nuclear imaging techniques have demonstrated equal sensitivity and specificity to many of the invasive "gold standard" testing modalities. The major limitations of nuclear cardiology are the availability of suitable radionuclides and correlation of nuclear images with cardiovascular function.

Despite the availability of new radionuclides, technetium-99m (^{99m}Tc) and thallium-201 (^{201}Tl) remain the two most commonly used radionuclides. [99m]Tc is ideal for clinical imaging, with a half-life of about 6 hours, a single 140-keV photon peak suitable for available imaging systems, primarily γ-ray emission, and the ability to be combined with multiple pharmaceuticals. It is generated in-house by a benchtop generator that reduces transportation costs and provides immediate availability. The short half-life means high doses and repeat injections can be given to evaluate efficacy of interventional therapy over a relatively short period of time. [201]Th has a much longer half-life of 73 hours, which prevents the use of multiple doses close together but does mean that delayed imaging is possible following administration of the agent. Uptake into cells depends on blood flow. The energy from [201]Th is x-ray, with an energy level of 69 to 83 keV. Production of thallium requires a cyclotron. Images are obtained with a conventional gamma camera.

TECHNETIUM SCANNING

Technetium scanning is used for the evaluation of blood pool and myocardial perfusion and as an infarct-avid agent to identify damaged myocardium. Analysis of the blood pool, as in a multigated angiography (MUGA), uses technetium either alone or as a red blood cell complex. The former obtains images following a bolus of technetium and traces its passage from the venous system through the heart to the aorta and is known as *first-pass angiography*. Equilibrium tests where technetium is bound to red blood cells provide an imaging time of several hours, which allows serial images to be obtained. These tests are used to determine right and left ventricular ejection fractions, detect cardiac shunts, estimate ventricular volumes, and view wall motion.[64]

Infarct-avid radionuclides such as technetium-pyrophosphate (^{99m}Tc-PYP) are used to describe the presence and extent of damaged myocardium after myocardial infarction, in suspected myocardial contusion, and following chest wall injuries. Imaging with ^{99m}Tc-PYP is applicable when myocardial infarction is suspected clinically, but patient history, ECG changes, and laboratory evidence are not definitive. Uptake of ^{99m}Tc-PYP into infarcted tissue depends on regional blood flow, myocardial calcium concentration, the degree of irreversible myocardial injury, and time after infarction. ^{99m}Tc-PYP attaches to calcium deposited in the infarcted area, so the approach is known as *hot spot scanning*. False hot spots may occur where there is necrotic myocardial tissue, as in myocarditis, myocardial abscesses, old infarctions, and myocardial trauma. Additionally, uptake has been seen during unstable angina and ventricular dyskinesia and at sites of ventricular aneurysms, suggesting that these are associated with transient low blood flow. In infarcted tissue, ^{99m}Tc-PYP levels can be as high as 18 to 20 times that of normal myocardium, which gives rise to very distinct borders between the infarcted and normal myocardium. Uptake of ^{99m}Tc-PYP into necrotic myocardium is delayed and not measurable until after about 4 hours of coronary occlusion. Scans prior to this time are usually negative and become positive about 12 hours after occlusion. Peak intensity of ^{99m}Tc-PYP is reached at 48 hours. Washout occurs over 5 to 7 days, so ^{99m}Tc-PYP is a useful late marker of infarction, especially in patients who present late or with a silent infarction. Images are viewed by comparing sternum and rib uptake with that seen in the myocardium. This type of imaging also can be used to assess graft patency after coronary artery bypass. Certain characteristics of the images obtained have been linked with various prognostic values but await confirmation in comparative and long-term prognostic trials.

Other technetium-labeled agents used include technetium-t-butyl isonitrile (^{99m}Tc-TIBI); technetium-carboxy isopropyl isonitrile (^{99m}Tc-CPI); technetium-sestamibi, also known as methoxy-isobutyl isonitrile (Tc-MIBI); and technetium-teboroxime. Technetium-sestamibi has a similar myocardial uptake pattern to thallium and produces similar results but with improved image quality because it generates a much higher photon yield. This is now popular as an alternative perfusion imaging agent to thallium. Technetium-teboroxime is still primarily an investigational agent. The main advantage of the newer technetium compounds is the lack of redistribution perfusion, allowing for delayed imaging. This is particularly useful in acute clinical settings; the radiopharmaceutical can be injected during the acute event and imaging undertaken when the patient is more stable.

THALLIUM SCANNING

Thallium is a potassium analog taken up into normal myocardium by passive diffusion and possibly by active transport via the Na$^+$,K$^+$-ATPase pump. Uptake depends on regional blood flow and in a linear fashion up to very high blood flow rates. It is used primarily for the analysis of coronary and myocardial perfusion. High thallium uptake occurs in perfused myocardium; in ischemic myocardium, uptake is reduced significantly. Scans taken during acute ischemia or following infarction show areas of poor or nil distribution of thallium corresponding to the site of ischemia. A scan repeated 4 to 6 hours after the initial scan may show a redistribution of the thallium into areas that previously had little to no thallium uptake. These defects are referred to as *partial defects,* demonstrating areas hypoperfused during "stress" but viable myocardium at rest. Redistribution occurs because there is delayed washout of thallium from poorly perfused myocardium, resulting in less contrast between the density of thallium in different areas of the heart. This gives the appearance of "redistribution" of the radionuclide into the previously ischemic area. To enhance evaluation of potential partial defects, a second injection of thallium can be used. Areas of nil distribution are called *cold spots* or *fixed defects* and reflect infarcted myocardium.

Thallium scanning with the aid of computer analysis segregates the images into anatomic regions and specifically localizes areas of dead or necrotic myocardial tissue. In conjunction with ECHO or SPECT,[66] thallium scans can correlate areas of abnormal wall motion with areas of poor perfusion. Sensitivity and specificity of thallium scanning to detect IHD disease are comparable with those of ET (75% and 80%, respectively). When used in conjunction with exercise ECG, sensitivity increases to about 80%. Thallium scanning also can be used in conjunction with ET to allow detection of lower levels of ischemia than may be determined from ECG abnormalities or patient

symptoms. Thallium is injected at the peak of the ET, and exercise continues for another 30 to 60 seconds, when the initial images are taken. Repeat images are taken at 3 to 4 hours.

Thallium scanning is useful in patients with atypical chest pain and ambiguous or false-positive ET to determine if IHD is the cause of symptoms and the ET abnormalities. Thallium scanning is also used for postoperative evaluation of revascularization or angioplasty procedures and for preoperative evaluation for prognostic stratification for persons with IHD. A normal thallium scan heralds a benign outcome, even in patients who have angiographically evident CAD. The finding of redistribution is a marker of jeopardized but viable myocardium and has been shown to have important prognostic value. Major cardiac events such as MI in patients with normal ^{201}Tl studies average less than 1% per year. The best predictor of coronary events, which correlates thallium scans with clinical significance, is the number of myocardial segments with transient (redistribution) defects.

A number of other radiopharmaceuticals have found some use in cardiovascular testing, such as labeled antimyosin antibodies.[67] Theoretically, these antibodies should be more specific markers of myocyte necrosis. The currently used antibodies are a murine Fab fragment. Phase I, II, and III trials suggest that these are highly specific for irreversibly injured myocytes, but they have limitations in terms of pharmacokinetic properties. Uptake into myocardial tissues is very slow, with a prolonged blood pool activity seen for at least 24 hours. In clinical use, the antibody is given within 24 hours of the infarction, and planar or SPECT imaging is undertaken 24 to 48 hours later. Despite the supposed specificity of the antibody to myosin, localization is more dependent on blood flow than on myosin concentration, so measurement of infarction size is not as accurate as expected. Another investigational agent, [^{123}I]phenylpentadecanoic acid, is able to assess both myocardial perfusion and metabolism by virtue of its affinity for fatty acid metabolism.[67]

PHARMACOLOGIC STRESS TESTING

Pharmacologic stress testing is an alternative to ET and ET with thallium in patients who are unable or unwilling to undergo ET.[70–77] Additionally, pharmacologic stress testing is now used more than 50% of the time to assess coronary perfusion. The pharmacologic agent produces stress by a hyperemic (vasodilator) response or by increasing myocardial oxygen demand (heart rate and myocardial contractility). Agents currently used include dipyridamole and adenosine (hyperemic stress) and dobutamine (myocardial stress). Pharmacologic stress tests can be linked to various imaging techniques such as thallium planar scanning, SPECT, MRI, and ECHO. Dobutamine is linked most frequently to ECHO, allowing quantification of wall motion abnormalities, which have been shown to correlate well with areas of ischemia.

The principle of dipyridamole and adenosine thallium imaging is related to their coronary arteriolar vasodilator properties. Dipyridamole inhibits adenosine cellular reuptake, resulting in increased concentrations of adenosine in the blood and tissues. Adenosine is a potent coronary artery vasodilator and can increase perfusion four to five times over baseline. Areas distal to a coronary artery obstruction will show a relative hypoperfusion compared with normal coronary arteries because there is reduced perfusion pressure owing to preferential perfusion of normal segments over stenotic segments. Acutely, these areas will appear as cold spots, but on the redistribution scans, the defects will fill, indicating viable but jeopardized myocardium.

Dipyridamole is given intravenously in a dose of 0.142 mg/kg per minute over 4 minutes. This dose has been shown to increase baseline coronary blood flow in the normal tissues up to four to five times over control. Some studies have used doses up to 0.84 mg/kg to enhance the vasodilator response. At the higher dose, acute adverse effects such as chest pain are more common. Adenosine for stress testing is an unlabeled use of this drug. Adenosine is given over 6 minutes at a dose of 0.140 mcg/kg per minute. At the end of infusion (dipyridamole) or after 3 minutes (adenosine), a 2.5- to 4-mCi dose of thallium is given. The maximum effect of dipyridamole occurs at 5 to 7 minutes and adenosine at about 30 seconds after the end of infusion. Imaging follows immediately and can be repeated at 24 hours (thallium scanning) to heighten the redistribution defects from fixed or partial defects.

Like exercise thallium scanning, dipyridamole and adenosine scanning or ECHO is used to detect IHD, evaluate the prognosis of patients with known disease, assess patients after MI, and as a risk-stratification method prior to vascular, cardiac, and noncardiac surgery. Pharmacologic stress testing evaluates wall motion abnormalities and perfusion defects under stress and has been shown in numerous studies to have comparable sensitivity and specificity with the traditional ET. Using planar scanning and dipyridamole, sensitivity to detect IHD ranges from 67% to 95% with a 67% to 100% specificity. A summary of 13 studies in almost 900 patients gave a pooled sensitivity of 85% and specificity of 87%. SPECT scanning has at least comparable sensitivity and slightly lower specificity to planar imaging but produces higher-quality imaging, which may enhance quantitative interpretation.

Dipyridamole testing has been shown to be safe and effective in the elderly and in those with unstable angina immediately after MI (within days). It also may be used to assess the status of revascularization procedures.[70] As a prognostic test, dipyridamole testing is very useful. In several studies, abnormal scans have shown about a 10-fold increase in event rates over 1 to 2 years of follow-up. Abnormal scans also have been shown to be an independent risk factor for myocardial infarction and death with a relative risk of 3.1. Reversible defects correlate best with events, with one study demonstrating a 4.41 relative risk for cardiac events.

Adverse effects with dipyridamole thallium testing are minimal, the main adverse effects being chest pain (with or without ischemic changes on the ECG), headache, dizziness, and nausea. Adverse effects are related to the increased adenosine activity and can be ameliorated by xanthine compounds because they are direct competitive antagonists of adenosine. Caffeine products must be avoided for about 24 hours prior to the test. Adenosine is associated with a higher incidence of adverse effects (80% versus 50%), but these are very transient, and some studies have shown that patients prefer it over dipyridamole. Both agents are relatively contraindicated in patients with a history of bronchospasm.

Dobutamine, a synthetic catecholamine, increases heart rate and cardiac output, resulting in an increase in myocardial oxygen demand. Ischemia develops in areas where stenosis prevents the increase in oxygen demand from being met with increased blood flow. Ischemia is detected by ECHO as regional wall motion abnormalities or with thallium scanning.

Dobutamine, when used as a stress test, is given in doses of 20–40 mcg/kg per minute. The dose is titrated at 3-minute intervals in increments of 10 mcg/kg per minute. If thallium is used, it is given 2 to 3 minutes before the end of infusion. Atropine 0.5–1 mg may be given to augment the heart rate response to 85% of the patient's calculated maximum. ECG and blood pressure are recorded continuously throughout the test, and ECHO recordings are made during the last minute of each dose level and during recovery.

β-Blocker and calcium channel blocker therapy may interfere with the heart rate response to dobutamine stress tests and is recommended to be discontinued prior to the test. Dobutamine stress testing is relatively well tolerated. Reasons to discontinue the test include development of severe chest pain, extensive new wall motion abnormalities, ST-segment elevation and depression suggestive of significant ischemia, tachyarrhythmias, and symptomatic reductions in blood pressure.[64,74] β-Blockers can be used to reverse most adverse effects if they persist. Dobutamine stress tests are contraindicated in patients with aortic stenosis, uncontrolled hypertension, and severe ventricular arrhythmias. Ventricular fibrillation and myocardial infarction occur at a rate of about 0.05%.

Dobutamine stress testing has been studied as a diagnostic, prognostic, and therapy assessment tool after MI and for unstable and chronic angina. One study compared dobutamine, dipyridamole, and ET with coronary angiography for diagnostic accuracy in patients with IHD and showed an overall accuracy of 87% for ET, 82% for dobutamine, and 77% for dipyridamole. A recent review of 14 studies of 942 patients for the detection of IHD with dobutamine stress testing calculated the sensitivity to be about 80% (70% to 100%) with a 75% (64% to 100%) specificity. Sensitivity is highest for detection of three-vessel disease (92%). Dobutamine-sestamibi stress testing seems to be less sensitive than thallium even for multivessel disease. Comparative studies with ET and dipyridamole ECHO show dobutamine to be more sensitive. After MI, dobutamine stress testing identifies patients at high risk of subsequent cardiac events. For patients with suspected or known IHD, a positive dobutamine stress test is an independent predictor of cardiac events, and a negative test affords protection from cardiac death.

INTRAVASCULAR ULTRASOUND

Intravascular ultrasound (IVUS) combines braided polyethylene catheter technology with miniaturized ultrasound transducers that can be inserted into a variety of vascular beds within the body, including the coronary artery vasculature.[78–81] Catheter configuration varies and may include over-the-wire, monorail, and fixed-guidewire tip configurations, resulting in different torqueability, steerability, and pushability characteristics for each type of catheter. There are two basic types of transducers, the solid-state phased array and a rotating mechanical transducer. In general, the phased-array transducers are smaller and may be mounted on more flexible catheters so that smaller vessels (such as coronary arteries) can be visualized, but they require a more complex system for image reconstruction and show more artifacts in imaging.

In contrast to angiography, IVUS provides quantitative information from within the vessel on diameter, circumference, luminal diameter, plaque volume, and percent stenosis. Qualitative information regarding the amount of plaque elevation, plaque composition (e.g., calcific, fibrous, or fatty plaque), and the presence of plaque versus thrombus, thrombus versus tumor, and aneurysm and hematoma can be provided with IVUS. IVUS is also used as a therapeutic adjunct with PTCA, atherectomy, stent or graft placement, and fibrinolysis, although routine use may not be justified.[80] These combination procedures may be monitored in real time as the procedure (e.g., atherectomy) is being performed.

CORONARY ANGIOSCOPY

Percutaneous coronary angioscopy permits direct visualization of the luminal surface of the coronary blood vessels.[82] The coronary angioscope is composed of a flexible catheter with a fiberoptic imaging bundle coupled with a video monitor and video recorder for live and archival viewing. Because a blood-free field is necessary for viewing, an occlusion catheter on the end of the catheter can be inflated for 45 to 90 seconds in a disease-free portion of the artery of interest and flushed with saline or lactated Ringer's solution to view diseased segments.

Although the role of angioscopy is still being developed, the recognized uses include guiding saphenous vein bypass graft interventions, postinterventional evaluation of lesions, identification of culprit and borderline lesions, stent deployment, and directing of procedures to achieve better outcomes with fewer complications. The limitations of angioscopy include lack of cross-sectional information, large fluid boluses to clear the field, large introducer size, and length of the procedure. Currently, this technology is not widely available, but it holds promise for future applications.

ABBREVIATIONS

A$_2$ aortic heart sound
ACC: American College of Cardiology
ACIP: Asymptomatic Cardiac Ischemia Pilot Study
AEM: ambulatory ECG monitoring; Holter monitoring
AHA: American Heart Association
CABG: coronary artery bypass grafting
CAD: coronary artery disease
CHF: congestive heart failure
COPD: chronic obstructive pulmonary disease
CT: computed tomography, cardiothoracic ratio
CVD: cardiovascular disease
CXR: chest x-ray
ECG: electrocardiogram
ECHO: echocardiography
ESVEM: electrophysiologic study versus electrocardiographic monitoring
ET: exercise stress testing
FDG: fluorine deoxyglucose
IHD: ischemic heart disease
IVUS: intravascular ultrasound
JVP: jugular venous pressure
LICS: left intercostal space
MET: metabolic equivalent
MRI: magnetic resonance imaging
MVP: mitral valve prolapse
P$_2$: pulmonic heart sound
PA: posteroanterior; pulmonary artery
PCI: percutaneous coronary intervention
PET: positron-emission tomography
PMI: point of maximum impulse
PTCA: percutaneous transluminal angioplasty
PVD: peripheral vascular disease
RICS: right intercostal space
S$_1$: first heart sound
S$_2$: second heart sound
S$_3$: third heart sound
S$_4$: fourth heart sound
SAECG: signal averaged electrocardiogram
SPECT: single-photon-emission computed tomography
Tc-MIBI: methoxy-isobutyl isonitrile; sestamibi
^{99m}Tc-PYP: technetium-99m pyrophosphate
^{99m}Tc-TIBI: technetium-t-butyl isonitrile
TEE: transesophageal echocardiography
TTE: transthoracic echocardiography
V$_{O_2}$: oxygen extraction by tissue

Review Questions and other resources can be found at *www.pharmacotherapyonline.com.*

REFERENCES

1. American Heart Association. Heart Disease and Stroke Statistics—2004 Update. Dallas, American Heart Association, 2003.
2. American Heart Association. AHA medical/scientific statement: Classification of functional capacity and objective assessment of patients with diseases of the heart. Circulation 1994;90:644–645.
3. Bernstein SJ, Hilborne LH, Leape LL, et al. The appropriateness of use of cardiovascular procedures in women and men. Arch Intern Med 1994;1554:2759–2765.
4. Braunwald E. Physical examination. In: Braunwald E, ed. Heart Disease: A Textbook of Cardiovascular Medicine, 4th ed. Philadelphia, Saunders, 1992:13–42.
5. O'Rourke RA, Braunwald E. Physical examination of the cardiovascular system. In: Fauci AS, Braunwald E, Isselbacher KJ, et al, eds. Harrison's Principles of Internal Medicine, 14th ed. New York, McGraw-Hill, 1998:1231–1237.
6. Come PC, Lee RT, Braunwald E. Noninvasive methods of cardiac examination. In: Isselbacher KJ, Braunwald E, Wilson JD, et al, eds. Harrison's Principles of Internal Medicine, 13th ed. New York, McGraw-Hill, 1994:966–972.
7. Zimetbaum PJ, Josephson ME. Use of the electrocardiogram in acute myocardial infarction. N Engl J Med 2003;348:933–940.
8. Davis D. How to Quickly and Accurately Master ECG Interpretation, 2nd ed. Philadelphia, Lippincott, 1992:89–95, 235–273.
9. Fisch C. Evolution of the clinical electrocardiogram. J Am Coll Cardiol 1989;14:1127–1138.
10. Garland JL, Wolfson AB. Routine admission electrocardiography in emergency department patients. Ann Emerg Med 1994;23:275–280.
11. ACC Expert Consensus Document. Signal-averaged electrocardiography. J Am Coll Cardiol 1996;27:238–249.
12. Kadish AH, Buxton AE, Kennedy HL, et al. ACC/AHA clinical competence statement on electrocardiography and ambulatory electrocardiography: A report of the American College of Cardiology/American Heart Association/American College of Physicians-American Society of Internal Medicine Task Force on Clinical Competence (ACC/AHA Committee to Develop a Clinical Competence Statement on Electrocardiography and Ambulatory Electrocardiography). *Circulation.* 2001;104:3169–3178.
13. Fisch C, DeSanctis RW, Dodge HT, et al. Guidelines for ambulatory electrocardiography. J Am Coll Cardiol 1989;13:249–258.
14. DiMarco JP, Philbrick JT. Ambulatory electrocardiographic (Holter) monitoring. Ann Intern Med 1990;113:77–79.
15. Resch DD. Diagnostic and prognostic value of ambulatory electrocardiographic monitoring in older patients. J Am Geriatr Soc 1996;43:66–70.
16. Reiter MJ, Karagounis LA, Mann De, et al. Reproducibility of drug efficacy predictions by Holter monitoring in the electrophysiologic study versus electrocardiographic monitoring (ESVEM) trial. Am J Cardiol 1997;79:315–322.
17. Linzer M, Yang EH, Estes M, et al. Diagnosing syncope: 1. Value of history, physical examination and electrocardiography. Ann Intern Med 1997;126:989–996.
18. Sharaf BL, Williams DO, Miele RP, et al. A detailed angiographic analysis of patients with ambulatory electrocardiographic ischemia: Results from the Asymptomatic Cardiac Ischemia Pilot (ACIP) study of angiographic core laboratory. J Am Coll Cardiol 1997;29:78–84.
19. Chaitman B. Exercise stress testing. In: Braunwald E, ed. Heart Disease: A Textbook of Cardiovascular Medicine, 4th ed. Philadelphia, Saunders, 1992:161–179.
20. Gibbons RJ, Balady GJ, Bricker JT, et al. ACC/AHA 2002 guideline update for exercise testing: A report of the American College of Cardiology/American Heart Association Task Force on Practice Guidelines (Committee on Exercise Testing), 2002. American College of Cardiology Web site (www.acc.org); accessed June 23, 2004.

21. Mark D. Prognostic value of a treadmill exercise score in outpatients with suspected coronary artery disease. N Engl J Med 1991;325:849–853.

22. Seceri S, Michelassi C. Prognostic impact of stress testing in coronary artery disease. Circulation 1991;83(suppl 3):82–89.

23. Pina IL, Balady GJ, Hanson P, et al. Guidelines for clinical exercise testing laboratories: A statement for healthcare professionals from the committee on exercise and cardiac rehabilitation, American Heart Association. Circulation 1995;91:912–921.

24. Fletcher GF, Balady G, Froelicher VF, et al. Exercise standards: A statement for healthcare professionals from the American Heart Association. Circulation 1995;91:580–615.

25. Grossman W, Barry WH. Cardiac catheterization. In: Braunwald E, ed. Heart Disease: A Textbook of Cardiovascular Medicine, 4th ed. Philadelphia, Saunders, 1992:180–205.

26. Baim DS, Grossman W. Diagnostic cardiac catheterization and angiography. In: Fauci AS, Braunwald E, Isselbacher KJ, et al, eds. Harrison's Principles of Internal Medicine, 14th ed. New York, McGraw-Hill, 1998:1247–1253.

27. Levin DC, Gardiner GA. Cardiac arteriography. In: Braunwald E, ed. Heart Disease: A Textbook of Cardiovascular Medicine, 4th ed. Philadelphia, Saunders, 1992:235–275.

28. Report of the American College of Cardiology/American Heart Association Task Force on Assessment of Diagnostic and Therapeutic Cardiovascular Procedures (Subcommittee on Cardiac Catheterization). Guidelines for cardiac catheterization and cardiac catheterization laboratories. J Am Coll Cardiol 1991;18:1149–1182.

29. Report of the American College of Cardiology/American Heart Association Task Force on Assessment of Diagnostic and Therapeutic Cardiovascular Procedures (Subcommittee on Coronary Angiography). Guidelines for coronary angiography. J Am Coll Cardiol 1987;10:935–950.

30. Walder LA, Schaller FA. Diagnostic cardiac catheterization. When is it appropriate? Postgrad Med 1995;97:37–42.

31. Ryan TJ, Bauman WB, Kennedy JW, et al. Guidelines for percutaneous transluminal coronary angioplasty: A report of the ACC/AHA Task Force on Assessment of Diagnostic and Therapeutic Cardiovascular Procedures (Committee on Percutaneous Transluminal Coronary Angioplasty). J Am Coll Cardiol 1993;22:2033–2054.

32. Foley DP, Escaned J, Strauss BH, et al. Quantitative coronary angiography (QCA) in interventional cardiology: Clinical application of QCA measurements. Prog Cardiovasc Dis 1994;36:363–384.

33. Reagan K, Boxt LM, Katz J. Introduction to coronary arteriography. Radiol Clin North Am 1994;32:419–433.

34. Gorlin R. Perspectives on invasive cardiology: The 24th Louis F. Bishop lecture. J Am Coll Cardiol 1994;23:525–532.

35. Topol EJ, Nissen SE. Our preoccupation with coronary luminology: The dissociation between clinical and angiographic findings on ischemic heart disease. Circulation 1995;92:2333–2342.

36. Landau C, Lange RA, Hillis LD. Percutaneous transluminal coronary angioplasty. N Engl J Med 1994;330:981–993.

37. Strauss BH, Escaned J, Foley DP, et al. Technological considerations and practical limitations in the use of quantitative angiography during percutaneous coronary recanalization. Prog Cardiovasc Dis 1994;36:343–362.

38. Higgins CB. Newer cardiac imaging techniques: CT, MRI. In: Braunwald E, ed. Heart Disease: A Textbook of Cardiovascular Medicine, 4th ed. Philadelphia, Saunders, 1992:312–341.

39. Higgins CB. New cardiac imaging techniques. In: Isselbacher KJ, Braunwald E, Wilson JD, et al, eds. Harrison's Principles of Internal Medicine, 13th ed. New York, McGraw-Hill, 1994:972–979.

40. Thompson BH, Stanford W. Evaluation of cardiac function with ultrafast computed tomography. Radiol Clin North Am 1995;32:537–554.

41. Lazem F, Barbir M, Banner N, et al. Coronary calcification detected by ultrafast computed tomography is a predictor of cardiac events in heart transplant recipients. Transplant Proc 1997;29:572–575.

42. Ganz W, Serafini A, Lerner D, et al. Cardiovascular magnetic resonance imaging goes beyond anatomy. Crit Rev Diagn Imaging 1995;36:479–503.

43. Hartiala J, Knuuti J. Imaging of the heart by MRI and PET. Ann Med 1995;27:35–45.

44. Hartiala J, Sakuma H, Higgins CB. Magnetic resonance imaging and spectroscopy of the human heart. Scand J Clin Lab Invest 1993;53:425–437.

45. McMillan RM. Cardiac magnetic resonance imaging. Cardiovasc Clin 2003;23:125–135.

46. De Roos A, van der Wall EE. Evaluation of ischemic heart disease by magnetic resonance imaging and spectroscopy. Radiol Clin North Am 1994;32:581–592.

47. Globits S, Higgins CB. Assessment of valvular heart disease by magnetic resonance imaging. Am Heart J 1995;129:369–381.

48. McGhie AI. Positron emission tomography. In: Raizner AE, ed. Topics in Cardiology: Indications for Diagnostic Procedures. New York, Igaku-Shoin, 1997:81–98.

49. Go RT, MacIntyre WJ, Chen EQ, et al. Current status of the clinical applications of cardiac positron emission tomography. Radiol Clin North Am 1995;32:501–520.

50. Schelbert HR. Metabolic imaging to assess myocardial viability. J Nucl Med 1994;35(suppl):8S–14S.

51. Schwaiger M, Beanlands R, vom Dahl J. Metabolic tissue characterization in the failing heart by positron emission tomography. Eur Hear J 1994;15(suppl D):14.

52. Canmici PG, Gropler RJ, Jones T, et al. The impact of myocardial blood flow quantification with PET on the understanding of heart diseases. Eur Heart J 1996;17:25–34.

53. Schwaiger M, Hutchins G. Quantification of regional myocardial perfusion by PET: Rationale and first clinical results. Eur Heart J 1995;16(suppl J):84–91.

54. Schwaiger M, Muzik O. Assessment of myocardial perfusion by perfusion emission tomography. Am J Cardiol 1991;67:35D–43D.

55. Feigenbaum H. Echocardiography. In: Braunwald E, ed. Heart Disease: A Textbook of Cardiovascular Medicine, 4th ed. Philadelphia, Saunders, 1992:64–115.

56. Popp RL. Echocardiography. In: Bennett JC, Plum F, Gill GN, et al, eds. Cecil's Textbook of Medicine, 20th ed. Philadelphia, Saunders, 1996:194–199.

57. Cheitlin MD, Armstrong WF, Aurigemma GP, et al. ACC/AHA/ASE 2003 guideline update for the clinical application of echocardiography—summary article: A report of the American College of Cardiology/American Heart Association Task Force on Practice Guidelines (ACC/AHA/ASE Committee to Update the 1997 Guidelines on the Clinical Application of Echocardiography). Circulation 2003;108:1146–1162.

58. Seward JB, Khandheria BK, Oh JK, et al. Critical appraisal of transesophageal echocardiography: Limitations, pitfalls, and complications. J Am Soc Echocardiogr 1992;5:288–305.

59. Shively BK, Gurule FT, Roldan CA, et al. Diagnostic value of transesophageal compared with transthoracic echocardiography in infective endocarditis. J Am Coll Cardiol 1991;18:391–397.

60. Birmingham GD, Rahko PS, Ballantyne F III. Improved detection of infective endocarditis with transesophageal echocardiography. Am Heart J 1992;123:774–781.

61. Klocke FJ, Baird MG, Bateman TM, et al. ACC/AHA/ASNC guidelines for the clinical use of cardiac radionuclide imaging: A report of the American College of Cardiology/American Heart Association Task Force on Practice Guidelines (ACC/AHA/ASNC Committee to revise the 1995 guidelines for the clinical use of radionuclide imaging), 2003. American College of Cardiology Web site (www.acc.org); accessed June 20, 2004.

62. Taillefer R, Amyot R, Turpin S, Lambert R. Comparison between dipyridamole and adenosine as pharmacologic coronary vasodilators in detection of coronary artery disease with thallium 201 imaging. J Nucl Cardiol 1996;3:204–211.

63. Lewin HC, Sciammarella MG, Watters TA, Alexander HG. An overview of contemporary nuclear cardiology. Curr Cardiol Rep 2004;6:13–19.

64. Sabharwal NK, Lahiri A. Role of myocardial perfusion imaging for risk stratification in suspected or known coronary artery disease. Heart 2003;89:1291–1297.

65. Mieres JH, Shaw LJ, Hendel RC, et al. A report of the American Society of Nuclear Cardiology Task Force on Women and Heart Disease (Writing Group on Perfusion Imaging in Women). J Nucl Cardiol 2003;10:95–101.

66. Picano E. Stress echocardiography: A historical perspective. Am J Med 2003;114:126–130.

67. Cerqueira MD, Lawrence A. Nuclear cardiology update. Radiol Clin North Am 2001;39:931–946.

68. Acampa W, Di Benedetto C, Cuocolo A. An overview of radiotracers in nuclear cardiology. J Nuc Cardiol 2000;7:701–707.

69. Beller GA, Zaret BL. Contributions of nuclear cardiology to diagnosis and prognosis of patients with coronary artery disease. Circulation 2000;101:1465–1478.

70. Travain MI, Wexler JP. Pharmacological stress testing. Semin Nucl Med 1999;29:298–318.

71. Verani MS. Adenosine thallium-201 myocardial perfusion scintigraphy. Am Heart J 1991;122:269–277.

72. Geleijnse ML, Fioretti PM, Roelandt JRTC. Methodology, feasibility, safety and diagnostic accuracy of dobutamine stress echocardiography. J Am Coll Cardiol 1997;30:595–606.

73. Sicari R, Picano E, Landi P, et al. Prognostic value of dobutamine-atropine stress echocardiography early after acute myocardial infarction. J Am Coll Cardiol 1997;29:254–260.

74. Greco CA, Salustri A, Seccareccia F, et al. Prognostic value of dobutamine echocardiography early after uncomplicated acute myocardial infarction: A comparison with exercise electrocardiography. J Am Coll Cardiol 1997;29:261–267.

75. Rallidis L, Cokkinos P, Tousoulis D, Nihoyannopoulos P. Comparison of dobutamine and treadmill exercise echocardiography in inducing ischemia in patients with coronary artery disease. J Am Coll Cardiol 1997;30:1660–1668.

76. Steinberg EH, Madmon L, Patel CP, et al. Long-term prognostic significance of dobutamine echocardiography in patients with suspected coronary artery disease: Results of a 5-year follow-up study. J Am Coll Cardiol 1997;29:969–973.

77. Beleslin BD, Ostojic M, Stepanovic J, et al. Stress echocardiography in the detection of myocardial ischemia: Head to toe comparison of exercise, dobutamine, and dipyridamole test. Circulation 1994;90:1168–1176.

78. Metz JA, Yock PG, Fitzgerald PJ. Intravascular ultrasound: Basic interpretation. Cardiol Clin 1997;15:1–16.

79. Benenati JF. Intravascular ultrasound: The role in diagnostic and therapeutic procedures. Cardiol Clin 1997;15:141–159.

80. Orford JL, Lerman A, Holmes DR. Routine intravascular ultrasound guidance of percutaneous coronary intervention: A critical reappraisal. J Am Coll Cardiol 2004;43:1335–1342.

81. Schwartz L, Bui S. The role of intravascular ultrasound in the diagnosis and treatment of patients with coronary artery disease. Comp Ther 2003;29:54–65.

82. Annex BH. Coronary angioscopy: Clinical applications. Cardiol Clin 1997;15:131–140.

12
CARDIOPULMONARY RESUSCITATION

Jeffrey F. Barletta

Learning Objectives and other resources can be found at *www.pharmacotherapyonline.com.*

KEY CONCEPTS

◀1 For patients in ventricular fibrillation/pulseless ventricular tachycardia (VF/PVT), rapid defibrillation is the single most important intervention that affects survival.

◀2 The purpose of using vasopressors following cardiac arrest is to increase both coronary and cerebral perfusion pressure.

◀3 Either epinephrine or vasopressin is an appropriate drug of first choice in patients with VF/PVT; if vasopressin is used, only one dose is administered.

◀4 The primary reason for the use of antiarrhythmic agents following cardiac arrest is to raise the fibrillation threshold.

◀5 Amiodarone is the only antiarrhythmic drug that has shown benefit over placebo in patients with out-of-hospital cardiac arrest.

◀6 Electrolyte abnormalities always should be assessed as a cause of refractory arrhythmias.

◀7 For pulseless electrical activity (PEA) and asystole, the primary focus should be diagnosis and identification of a reversible cause.

Cardiopulmonary arrest is the abrupt cessation of spontaneous and effective ventilation and circulation following a cardiac or respiratory event.[1] Cardiopulmonary resuscitation (CPR) provides artificial ventilation and circulation until it is possible to provide advanced cardiac life support (ACLS) and reestablish spontaneous circulation. In the United States, there are more than 450,000 victims of sudden cardiac arrest each year, with 60% to 70% occurring outside the hospital.[2]

Early attempts at resuscitation date back to the biblical era.[3] Modern-day resuscitation began in the late 1950s when it was discovered that expired air delivered via a mouth-to-mouth technique can maintain adequate oxygenation of blood.[4] Later, in 1960, Kouwenhoven and colleagues described "closed chest cardiac massage," and together with mouth-to-mouth ventilation, modern-day CPR was born.[5]

EPIDEMIOLOGY

In an adult patient, cardiopulmonary arrest usually results from the development of an arrhythmia.[2,6] Most cardiac arrests take place outside the hospital shortly after the onset of symptoms, and most patients have coronary artery disease (CAD)[7]. The most common arrhythmia is either ventricular fibrillation (VF) or pulseless ventricular tachycardia (PVT).[8,9] The number of patients with out-of-hospital cardiac arrests presenting with VF as the initial rhythm, however, has changed dramatically.[10–12] In one study, the number of patients with VF was 61% in 1980 compared with only 41% in 2000, a reduction of greater than 30%.[10] This change may be due to the aggressive treatment strategies aimed at CAD, the growing awareness of the symptoms of cardiac ischemia (shifting the occurrence of VF to in-hospital rather than out of hospital), or the overall decline in CAD-related mortality. Hospital survival for VF or PVT is approximately 3% to 40%, with higher mortality rates being observed in communities that do not have a rapid response system.[6,10,13,14]

CLINICAL PRESENTATION OF CARDIOPULMONARY ARREST

SYMPTOMS

- Anxiety, change in mental status, or unconscious
- Cold, clammy extremities
- Dyspnea, shortness of breath, or no respiration
- Chest pain
- Diaphoresis
- Nausea and vomiting

SIGNS

- Hypotension
- Tachycardia, bradycardia, irregular or no pulse
- Cyanosis
- Hypothermia
- Distant or absent heart and lung sounds

ETIOLOGY

Cardiopulmonary arrest is much less common in pediatric patients than in adults.[8] In pediatric patients, cardiopulmonary arrest is often the terminal event of progressive shock or respiratory failure.[8] The cause of cardiac arrest varies with age, the underlying health of the child, and the location of the event. Out-of-hospital arrests frequently are associated with events such as trauma, sudden infant death syndrome, drowning, poisoning, choking, severe asthma, and pneumonia. In-hospital arrests, on the other hand, are associated with sepsis, respiratory failure, drug toxicity, metabolic disorders, and arrhythmias. Pediatric out-of-hospital arrest generally presents with hypoxia and hypercarbia progressing to respiratory arrest and bradycardia and finally to asystolic cardiac arrest. In contrast to adult patients, only 10% of pediatric patients present with VF or PVT as the initial rhythm.[8] Unfortunately, survival following pediatric out-of-hospital cardiopulmonary arrest ranges only from 3% to 17%, with most survivors having a poor neurologic status.[8]

PATHOPHYSIOLOGY

There are two proposed theories describing the mechanism of blood flow during CPR.[1,15,16] The first theory, known as the *cardiac pump theory,* states that the active compression of the heart between the sternum and vertebrae creates an "artificial systole" in which intraventricular pressure increases, the atrioventricular valves close, the aortic valve opens, and blood is forced out of the ventricles. When ventricular compression ends, the decline in intraventricular pressure causes the mitral and tricuspid valves to open, and ventricular filling begins. The second, more recent theory is the *thoracic pump theory.*

The basis for this theory is the belief that blood flow results from intrathoracic pressure alterations induced by chest compressions. During compression or systole, a pressure gradient develops between the intrathoracic arteries and the extrathoracic veins, causing forward blood flow from the lungs into the systemic circulation. The heart merely acts as a passive conduit for flow. After compression ends, or diastole, intrathoracic pressure declines, and blood flow returns to the lungs.

The concept of cough CPR supports the importance of changes in intrathoracic pressure as a means of generating forward blood flow.[15,16] During vigorous coughing, intrathoracic pressures increase secondary to contractions of the diaphragm, abdominal muscles, and intracostal muscles. These pressure changes occur without direct chest compression and are sufficient to maintain consciousness. The observation that cough alone can maintain consciousness led many investigators to question the cardiac pump theory and accept the thoracic pump theory. In reality, it is likely that both models apply to the mechanism of blood flow during CPR.[16]

▶ TREATMENT: Cardiopulmonary Resuscitation

■ DESIRED OUTCOME

The goal of CPR is to return effective ventilation and circulation as quickly as possible to minimize hypoxic damage to vital organs. It is not sufficient to restore spontaneous circulation if the patient is left neurologically devastated or incurs severe morbidity in the process. Factors proved to enhance prehospital survival include the occurrence of a witnessed arrest, rapid implementation of bystander CPR, presence of VF as the initial rhythm, and early defibrillation therapy for VF.[17] In one report, the rate of survival to hospital discharge was 74% when defibrillation was performed within 3 minutes of a witnessed cardiac arrest compared with 49% when defibrillation was performed after 3 minutes ($p = .02$).[18]

Considerable controversy surrounds the identification of patient-specific factors that affect resuscitation survival. Proposed risk factors are age, concomitant diseases, initial pH, duration of resuscitation, and end-tidal carbon dioxide. The accuracy of these predictors has not been consistent in clinical studies, however.[6]

■ GENERAL APPROACH TO TREATMENT

National conferences and organized committees have played a major role in encouraging widespread competency in CPR technique. The first national conference took place in 1966 and recommended the training of health care professionals in the techniques of CPR.[3] Since then, the American Heart Association (AHA) has organized six additional national conferences to update philosophies for providing CPR and emergency cardiovascular care (ECC) to the general population. The most recent conference was the Guidelines 2000 Conference, which provided the latest set of recommendations for CPR and ECC.[8] The resuscitation guidelines are now internationally developed, as well as evidence-based, and a new intervention category has been added to the three categories originally established at the 1992 conference.[7] Class I interventions are considered to be appropriate and efficacious. Class II interventions are subdivided into those in class IIa, meaning that they are probably beneficial and efficacious, and those in class IIb, meaning that they are possibly beneficial

without causing harm. Class III interventions are considered inappropriate and potentially harmful. The Guidelines 2000 Conference added class indeterminate, meaning there is insufficient evidence to support a final class decision.

In an effort to highlight the crucial components for successful CPR, the National Council on CPR and ECC has orchestrated a "chain of survival."[7] Based on the concept that "a chain is only as strong as its weakest link," each element in the chain is essential for a successful resuscitation outcome. If one of these critical actions is neglected or delayed, survival is unlikely. The four links of the chain of survival are

1. Early access, which encompasses the events initiated after the patient's collapse to promote the arrival of paramedic personnel. Rapid emergency medical dispatch is a critical component of this link.
2. Early bystander basic life support and CPR. Basic life support is based on the assessment and application of the ABCs: airway, breathing, and circulation.
3. Early defibrillation. Because this is the most likely to improve survival, automatic external defibrillators (AED) have become more common in community settings. Public-access defibrillation (PAD), which places AEDs in the hands of trained laypersons, has the potential to become the greatest advance in the treatment of cardiac arrest since the discovery of CPR.[8] Evidence supports the value of PAD programs in locations either where the frequency of cardiac arrests is greater than 1 arrest per 1000 patient-years or where conventional paramedic services cannot ensure a call-to-shock time of less than 5 minutes.[8]
4. Early ACLS, the final link in the "chain of survival."

The idea of a team approach to cardiac resuscitation has existed since the early 1960s,[19] but it was not until the late 1960s that pharmacists began participating as cardiac resuscitation team members.[20] Defining roles for specific health care professionals, it is hoped, will make resuscitation attempts more efficient and consequently more effective. Team composition may vary among institutions, but a code team generally consists of a physician-in-charge, a surgeon, an anesthesiologist, a respiratory therapist, a nurse, and a pharmacist.[21] Table 12–1 lists the typical roles for each team member.[21]

TABLE 12–1. Responsibilities of Cardiac Resuscitation Team Members

Team Member	Responsibilities
Physician-in-charge	Team leader; determines appropriate therapy; directs and oversees order implementation including provision of CPR, electrical therapy, endotracheal intubation, intravenous access, ECG monitoring, and drug administration; arranges postresuscitation care
Surgeon	Identifies surgically correctable causes for arrest
Anesthesiologist	Performs endotracheal intubation; provides adequate oxygenation; may assist with obtaining vascular access
Respiratory therapist	Maintains adequate oxygenation and ventilation
Nurse	Records timing and outcome of therapeutic interventions; may assist with chest compressions, obtaining peripheral venous access, administering fluids and medications, acquiring blood samples for laboratory determination
Pharmacist	Prepares medications for administration; provides drug information; documents medication administration and outcomes of interventions

Adapted from: Bardas SL. Demystifying the cardiopulmonary code team response. Pharm Technol 1992;8:151–154.

VENTRICULAR FIBRILLATION AND PULSELESS VENTRICULAR TACHYCARDIA

NONPHARMACOLOGIC THERAPY

Because electrical defibrillation is the only effective method of restoring a perfusing cardiac rhythm,[22] electrical defibrillation is the most crucial link in the "chain of survival." The probability of successful defibrillation is directly related to the time interval between the onset of VF and the delivery of the first shock.[8] Generally, with each passing minute, the rate of survival decreases by 8% to 10%.[23] In one study, a 23% relative improvement in survival was observed with each 1-minute reduction in the time to defibrillation (odds ratio [OR] 0.77, 95% confidence interval [CI] 0.73–0.81).[24]

Although early defibrillation is crucial for survival following cardiac arrest, several animal studies have suggested that CPR prior to defibrillation may lead to more successful outcomes.[23] Two clinical trials have evaluated the impact of delaying defibrillation to allow for CPR in patients with out-of-hospital VF.[25,26] In the first, the provision of roughly 90 seconds of CPR prior to defibrillation was associated with an increased rate of hospital survival (compared with a historical control group) when response intervals were 4 minutes or longer (27% versus 17%; $p < .007$).[25] In the second, hospital survival rates were higher in patients with response intervals greater than 5 minutes when 3 minutes of CPR was administered prior to defibrillation (22% versus 4%; $p = .006$).[26] These trials support the theory of a three-phase time-sensitive model for resuscitation after cardiac arrest.[23] This model suggests that the optimal treatment of cardiac arrest is time-specific based on three distinct phases. These phases are the electrical phase (cardiac arrest until about 4 minutes), the circulatory phase (approximately 4 minutes to approximately 10 minutes), and the metabolic phase (after approximately 10 minutes). Successful defibrillation most likely will occur when cardiac arrest victims are in the electrical phase. On the other hand, when cardiac arrest victims are in the circulatory phase (4 to 10 minutes following cardiac arrest), global ischemia has already occurred, and immediate defibrillation may be detrimental. It may be more important to first provide some blood flow and cardiac perfusion via CPR to flush out the deleterious metabolic factors that have accumulated during ischemia.[23] Further trials are needed to evaluate this resuscitation technique.

Persons in VF or PVT should receive electrical defibrillation with at least three shocks.[8] The initial defibrillation attempt should begin with 200 J. The second and third shocks can be either the same or as high as 360 J. Repeated shocks, even at the same energy level, increase the probability of successful defibrillation. Following three unsuccessful attempts of defibrillation, the patient should receive roughly 1 minute of CPR. Endotracheal intubation and intravenous (IV) access should be obtained at this time. Once an airway is achieved, patients should be ventilated with 100% oxygen. Pharmacologic agents, such as sympathomimetics and antiarrhythmics, play a secondary role and are not recommended until an airway has been established and IV access attempted (Fig. 12–1).

PHARMACOLOGIC THERAPY

SYMPATHOMIMETICS

The use of sympathomimetics is a major part of drug therapy in CPR. The goal of using these agents is to augment both coronary and cerebral perfusion pressures during the low-flow state seen with CPR. Coronary perfusion pressures of at least 15 mm Hg are associated with a higher rate of return of spontaneous circulation (ROSC).[27] Animal studies have shown that coronary perfusion pressure averages between 10 and 15 mm Hg with CPR alone following 10 minutes of ventricular fibrillation.[28] Sympathomimetics work primarily by increasing systemic arteriolar vasoconstriction, thus improving coronary and cerebral perfusion pressure. In addition, they also maintain vascular tone, decreasing arteriolar collapse, and shunt blood to the heart and brain.

Epinephrine continues to be a drug of first choice for the treatment of VF, PVT, asystole, and pulseless electrical activity (PEA). Epinephrine is both an α- and β-receptor agonist, although its effectiveness is thought to be due to its α effects. One study evaluated the importance of α-adrenergic, β-adrenergic, and any nonadrenergic activity mediated by epinephrine in dogs.[29] The first group received epinephrine along with phenoxybenzamine (an α-blocker), whereas a second group received epinephrine along with propranolol (a β-blocker). When α-receptors were blocked, epinephrine was not successful in restoring circulation. When β-receptors were blocked, epinephrine was successful in restoring circulation in six of eight animals ($p \leq .01$). It was concluded that the efficacy of epinephrine is due to the α-adrenergic receptor stimulation and that β-stimulation is not important. It is unclear, however, whether β effects are useful or harmful during CPR. It has been shown that β-stimulation lowers the defibrillation threshold, whereas β-blockade increases it.[30] This would make epinephrine, a drug with both α and β properties, an ideal agent. Conversely, β-stimulation increases myocardial oxygen demand and can increase the severity of postresuscitation myocardial dysfunction.[31,32]

Several studies have compared the effects of pure α_1-agonists, such as phenylephrine and methoxamine, with epinephrine to

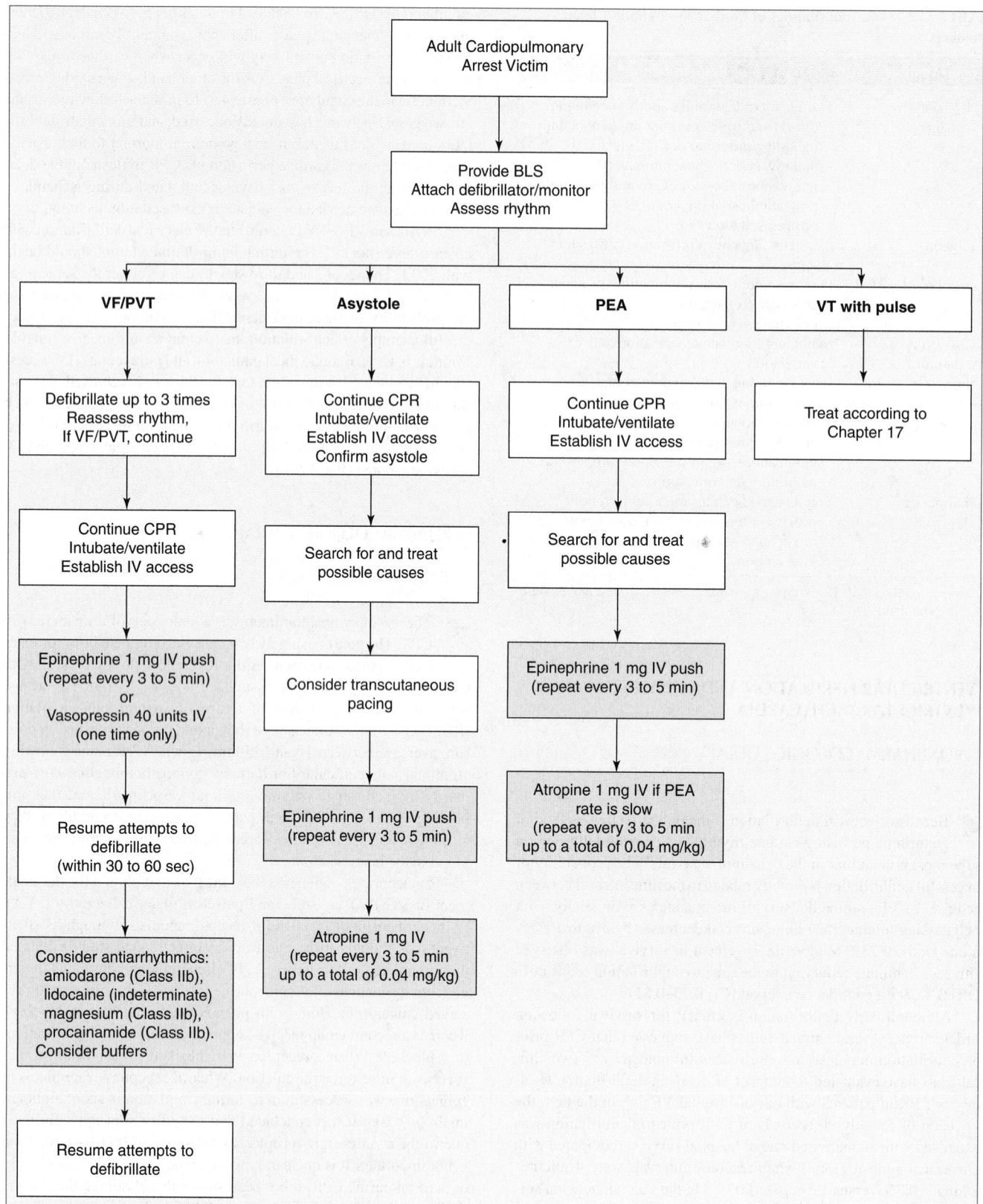

FIGURE 12–1. Treatment algorithm for adult cardiopulmonary arrest.

determine whether the β effects have a negative impact on cardiac arrest outcome. These studies have shown the use of α_1-agonists to have no long-term survival advantage over epinephrine.[33] One study found that both epinephrine (50 mcg/kg) and phenylephrine (50 mcg/kg) increased arterial blood pressure in dogs, but only epinephrine increased coronary and cerebral blood flows.[34] This study has been criticized, however, because doses were not equipotent. The primary reason that selective α_1-agonists are not superior to epinephrine is related to the α_2 effects. Agents that have potent α_2 effects (e.g., epinephrine and norepinephrine) may be more effective because the α_2-adrenergic receptors lie extrajunctionally in the intima of the blood vessels, making them more accessible to circulating catecholamines—even in low-flow states that occur during CPR.[33] Furthermore, during ischemia, the number of postsynaptic α_1-receptors decreases, which suggests a greater role for α_2-agonist activity during CPR.[35]

Another agent possessing α_2-agonist activity is norepinephrine (an α_1, α_2, β_1-agonist). Since it has been hypothesized that β_2-agonist–induced vasodilation may counteract the efficacy of α-agonist–induced vasoconstriction, investigators have compared the effects of the exogenous administration of epinephrine with those of norepinephrine in order to determine the impact of β_2-agonist activity during CPR. Callaham and associates conducted the only large-scale randomized, double-blind, prospective trial comparing the efficacy of norepinephrine with that of epinephrine in the prehospital cardiac arrest setting.[36] In this trial, 816 adults were randomized to receive standard-dose epinephrine (1 mg), high-dose epinephrine (15 mg), or high-dose norepinephrine (11 mg) after initial defibrillation attempts failed. Study end points were ROSC (i.e., measurable blood pressure or pulse for at least 5 minutes), hospital discharge rate, and neurologic status. Thirteen percent (35 of 260) of patients who received norepinephrine achieved ROSC prior to reaching the hospital. Thirteen percent (37 of 286) of patients received 15 mg epinephrine achieved ROSC compared with 8% (22 of 270) of patients randomized to receive 1 mg epinephrine ($p = .01$). Return of spontaneous circulation was not statistically different between norepinephrine and epinephrine ($p = .19$). Overall, only 1.8% (15 of 816) of all patients enrolled survived to hospital discharge. The percentages of patients discharged from the standard-dose epinephrine, high-dose epinephrine, and high-dose norepinephrine groups were not statistically different; they were 1.2%, 1.7%, and 2.6%, respectively. Neurologic survival was most favorable in the standard-dose epinephrine group; however, these differences were not statistically significant. The low number of surviving patients made it impossible to detect a meaningful difference in these two areas. Lindner and colleagues compared the efficacy of norepinephrine (1 mg) with repeated doses of epinephrine (1 mg) on the ROSC and hospital discharge rate in 50 patients.[37] In this study, there was an increase in ROSC with norepinephrine, but there was no difference in the hospital discharge rate.

A study using a swine model compared the effects of epinephrine (200 mcg/kg) and norepinephrine (80, 120, and 160 mcg/kg) on VF.[28] Compared with epinephrine, there was a trend toward improved myocardial blood flow and successful defibrillation with the two highest doses of norepinephrine. A second study, in a swine model, examined the effects of epinephrine (45 mcg/kg) and norepinephrine (45 mcg/kg) on myocardial oxygen delivery and consumption.[38] In this trial, norepinephrine reduced myocardial oxygen consumption, thereby creating a more favorable profile between myocardial oxygen supply and demand than did epinephrine. Similarly, Brown and colleagues compared the effect of epinephrine (200 mcg/kg) and three doses of norepinephrine (80, 120, and 160 mcg/kg) on cerebral blood flow in a swine model.[39] Statistically significant increases in aortic diastolic pressure and coronary perfusion pressure occurred with

epinephrine and the two highest doses of norepinephrine (120 and 160 mcg/kg). Increased blood flow to the left cerebral cortex, midbrain, pons, medulla, and cervical spinal cord also was evident with the two highest doses of norepinephrine. Epinephrine, however, improved only flow to the medulla and cervical cord compared with 80 mcg/kg norepinephrine. Although norepinephrine has demonstrated beneficial effects over epinephrine on myocardial oxygen balance and ROSC, there is no difference in survival to hospital discharge. Consequently, epinephrine remains the first-line sympathomimetic for CPR until more definitive data become available.

Considerable controversy surrounds the optimal dose of epinephrine for CPR. The standard epinephrine dose is 1 mg administered by IV push every 3 to 5 minutes.[8] This epinephrine dose was derived from animal studies (0.1 mg/kg in a 10-kg dog) and equates to approximately 0.015 mg/kg for a 70-kg human.[40] Both animal and human studies have demonstrated a positive dose-response relationship with epinephrine.[41–44] Animal studies have suggested that higher doses were necessary to improve hemodynamics and achieve successful resuscitation. These results, however, have not been replicated in human studies.[36,45–52] Collectively, these studies (Table 12–2) have shown that high-dose epinephrine may increase the initial resuscitation success rate but that overall survival is not significantly different. One study demonstrated an unfavorable neurologic outcome in patients treated with high-dose epinephrine.[53] Many of these patients would not have survived if given only standard-dose epinephrine, however, so this result may wrongfully discredit high-dose epinephrine.

The discrepancy between animal and human studies may be due to the fact that most victims of cardiac arrest have CAD, a condition not present in an animal model. In a human model, however, atherosclerotic plaques can aggravate the balance between myocardial oxygen supply and demand. Moreover, the interval from arrest to treatment in animal studies is shorter than the interval frequently reported in human studies. Since time to CPR and defibrillation are crucial variables for success, prolonging this time period can lower resuscitation rates. Because of the lack of evidence supporting high-dose epinephrine, the current guidelines recommend 1 mg IV push every 3 to 5 minutes or vasopressin as initial drug therapy for VF or PVT.[8] Tolerance to adrenergic stimulation can occur, especially when catecholamine levels are high. Therefore, if the standard dose of epinephrine is not successful, higher doses (up to 0.2 mg/kg) can be considered.

VASOPRESSIN

The algorithm for the treatment of VF/PVT now includes vasopressin. Also known as *antidiuretic hormone,* vasopressin is a potent vasoconstrictor that increases blood pressure and systemic vascular resistance. Although it acts on various receptors throughout the body, its vasoconstrictive properties are due primarily to its effects on the V_1 receptor.[54] Measurement of vasopressin levels in patients undergoing CPR has shown a high correlation between the levels of endogenous vasopressin released and the potential for ROSC.[55] In fact, in one study, plasma vasopressin concentrations were approximately three times as high in survivors compared with nonsurvivors, suggesting that vasopressin is released as an adjunct vasopressor to epinephrine in life-threatening events such as cardiac arrest.[55] Vasopressin may have several advantages over epinephrine. First, the metabolic acidosis that frequently accompanies cardiopulmonary arrest can blunt the vasoconstrictive effect of adrenergic agents such as epinephrine. This effect does not occur with vasopressin. Second, the

TABLE 12–2. Summary of Adult High-Dose Epinephrine Studies

Author	Design	Epinephrine Dosing SDE vs HDE	N	Initial Resuscitation SDE vs HDE		Hospital Discharge SDE vs HDE		Discharge Neurologic Status SDE vs HDE	
Gueugniaud et al.,[45] 1998	P, MC, R, DB	1 mg vs 5 mg, up to 15 doses	3327	601/1650 (36.4%)	678/1677[a] (40.4%)	46/1650 (2.8%)	38/1677 (2.3%)	26/46 (56.5%) Discharged without neurologic impairment	26/38 (68.4%)
Sherman et al.,[46] 1997	P, MC, R, DB	0.01 mg/kg vs 0.1 mg/kg, up to 4 doses	140	7/62 (11%)	15/78 (19%)	Not addressed		Not addressed	
Choux et al.,[47] 1995	P, R, DB	1 mg vs 5 mg, up to 15 doses	536	85/265 (32%)	96/271 (35.5%)	20/54 (37%)	23/63[b] (35.4%)	GCS≥9 (at day 3): 4/20 EEG Normal (at day 3): 1/20	3/23 3/23
Lipman et al.,[48] 1993	P, R, DB	1 mg vs 10 mg, up to 3 doses	35	11/16 (69%)	15/19 (79%)	1/16 (6.3%)	0/19 (0%)	Not addressed	
Stiell et al.,[49] 1992	P, R, DB	1 mg vs 7 mg, up to 5 doses	650	76/333 (23%)	56/317 (18%)	16/333 (5%)	10/317 (3%)	94% Remained in their best CPC on discharge	90%
Brown et al.,[50] 1992	P, MC, R, DB	0.02 mg/kg vs 0.2 mg/kg for the first dose	1280	190/632 (30%)	217/648 (33%)	26/632 (4%)	31/648 (5%)	92% Conscious at discharge (CPC = 1–3)	94%
Callaham et al.,[36] 1992	P, R, DB	1 mg vs 15 mg, up to 3 doses	556	22/270 (8%)	37/286[a] (13%)	3/270 (1.2%)	5/286 (1.7%)	2.3 Mean CPC score	3.2
Lindner et al.,[51] 1991	P, R, DB	1 mg vs 5 mg for the first dose	68	6/40 (15%)	16/28[a] (57%)	2/40 (5%)	4/28 (14%)	Not addressed	
Callaham et al.,[52] 1991	Ret	HDE: ≥ 50 mcg/kg or total dose > 2.8 mcg/kg/min	68	Not addressed		11/35 (31%)	6/33 (18.2%)	Intact:8/11 vs 4/6 Impaired: 2/11 vs 2/6 Vegetative: 1/11 vs 0/6	

[a] $p < .05$.
[b] Number of patients admitted to the hospital alive on day 3.
Abbreviations: SDE = standard dose epinephrine; HDE = high-dose epinephrine; P = prospective; MC = multicenter; R = randomized; DB = double-blind; Ret = retrospective; GCS = Glasgow Coma Scale; EEG = electroencephalogram; CPC = cerebral performance category.

stimulation of β-receptors caused by epinephrine can increase myocardial oxygen demand and complicate the postresuscitative phase of CPR. Because vasopressin does not act on β-receptors, this effect does not occur with its use.

Several animal studies have demonstrated the beneficial effect of vasopressin on coronary and cerebral blood flow.[56–58] Although vasopressin improves vital organ perfusion during VF, myocardial oxygen consumption is lower with vasopressin than with epinephrine.[59] Vasopressin also may have a beneficial effect on renal blood flow by stimulating V_2 receptors in the kidney, causing vasodilation and increased water reabsorption. With regard to splanchnic blood flow, however, most studies have shown that vasopressin has a detrimental effect compared with epinephrine.[59,60]

Unfortunately, there are limited data on vasopressin in humans. Lindner and associates evaluated the use of vasopressin in eight patients following in-hospital cardiac arrest.[61] After standard ACLS had failed, 40 units of vasopressin was administered intravenously. Spontaneous circulation returned in all eight patients, but only three survived until hospital discharge. Following these results, Lindner and colleagues conducted a prospective, randomized, controlled trial comparing vasopressin with epinephrine.[62] Forty patients who experienced out-of-hospital VF resistant to electrical defibrillation were randomized to receive either 40 units of vasopressin or 1 mg of epinephrine as the initial drug for the treatment of cardiac arrest. In the vasopressin group, 16 patients (80%) achieved ROSC, compared with 11 patients (55%) in the epinephrine group ($p = .18$). Fourteen

patients (70%) in the vasopressin group survived to hospital admission, and 12 patients (60%) survived more than 24 hours. Seven patients in the epinephrine group (35%) survived to hospital admission ($p = .06$), and 4 (20%) survived more than 24 hours ($p = .02$). There was no difference in hospital discharge rates between the groups— 8 patients (40%) in the vasopressin group and 3 patients (15%) in the epinephrine group ($p = .16$). Following administration of the study drug alone (i.e., no further ACLS), ROSC was achieved in 7 (35%) vasopressin patients compared with 2 (10%) epinephrine patients ($p < .001$). No adverse drug events secondary to vasopressin were observed. This trial showed a trend toward survival with vasopressin; however, statistical significance was evident only with survival longer than 24 hours and ROSC following use of the study drug alone.

Stiell and colleagues evaluated vasopressin and epinephrine in 200 patients with in-hospital cardiac arrest.[63] In contrast to Lindner and colleagues, no advantage was noted with vasopressin in either ROSC (60% versus 59%; $p = .97$), short-term (1-hour) survival (39% versus 35%; $p = .66$), or survival to hospital discharge (12% versus 14%; $p = .67$) compared with epinephrine. When only patients with VF were evaluated, short-term survival rates were 54% and 61% for vasopressin and epinephrine, respectively, whereas survival rates to hospital discharge were 25% and 33%. Major differences between the two trials (Stiell and colleagues[63] and Lindner and colleagues[62]) include the setting in which cardiac arrest was evaluated (in-hospital versus out of hospital), the average time from collapse to study drug administration (6.1 versus 14.5 minutes), and the

TABLE 12–3. **Initial Doses of Drugs Used in Cardiac Arrest**

Drug	Initial Dose	Comments
Epinephrine	1 mg IV every 3 to 5 minutes.	If a 1-mg dose is not successful, then high-dose epinephrine (up to 0.2 mg/kg) is acceptable.
Vasopressin	40 units IV	A single dose of vasopressin may be used in place of epinephrine following the initial three unsuccessful defibrillation attempts. If there is no response to vasopressin after 5 to 10 minutes, epinephrine therapy may resume.
Amiodarone	VF or PVT: 300 mg diluted in a volume of 20 to 30 mL of saline or D_5W by rapid infusion	Supplementary doses of 150 mg by rapid infusion may be administered for recurrent or refractory VF/VT, followed by an infusion of 1 mg/min for 6 hours and then 0.5 mg/min, to a maximum daily dose of 2 grams
Lidocaine	VF or PVT: 1.5 mg/kg IV	A continuous infusion at 2–4 mg/min is reasonable if the drug was associated with the restoration of a stable rhythm. Reappearance of an arrhythmia during a constant infusion should be treated with a small bolus dose (0.5 mg/kg) of lidocaine with an increase in the infusion rate.
Magnesium	VF or PVT: 1 to 2 grams diluted in 100 mL D_5W administered over 1 to 2 min	For treatment of torsades de pointes, a loading dose of 1 to 2 grams mixed in 50–100 mL of D_5W given over 5–60 min, followed by an infusion of 0.5–1 gram per hour.
Sodium bicarbonate	1 mEq/kg IV	Therapy should be guided by the bicarbonate concentration or calculated base deficit obtained from blood gas analysis or laboratory measurement. Complete correction of the base deficit should be avoided to minimize the risk of iatrogenically induced alkalosis.
Atropine	1 mg IV repeated as needed every 3 to 5 minutes	Maximum dose is 0.04 mg/kg. Doses less than 0.5 mg should be avoided.

Abbreviations: IV = intravenous; VF = ventricular fibrillation; PVT = pulseless ventricular tachycardia; D_5W = dextrose in water.

number of patients presenting with VF as the initial rhythm (21% versus 100%). The superior effects of vasopressin may be evident only when response times are prolonged and the effect of catecholamines is blunted.

In the largest comparative trial conducted to date, 1186 patients with out-of-hospital cardiac arrest were randomized to receive two doses of either vasopressin 40 units or epinephrine 1 mg.[64] Most patients presented with asystole (45%) or VF (40%) as their initial cardiac rhythm, and the average time to the administration of study drug was about 18 minutes. Overall, there were no significant differences between vasopressin and epinephrine in ROSC (25% versus 28%; $p = .19$), hospital admission rate (36% versus 31%; $p = .06$), or discharge rate (10% versus 10%; $p = .99$). When patients were stratified according to their initial presenting rhythm, no significant differences were noted for patients with VF or PEA. Patients with asystole, on the other hand, had a significantly higher rate of hospital admission (29% versus 20%; $p = .02$) and discharge (4.7% versus 1.5%; $p = .04$) when vasopressin was administered compared with epinephrine. In addition, a subgroup analysis of 732 patients who required additional epinephrine therapy despite the two doses of study drug revealed significant benefits in ROSC (37% versus 26%; $p = .002$), hospital admission rate (26% versus 16%; $p = .002$), and discharge rate (6.2% versus 1.7%; $p = .002$) with vasopressin. There was a trend, however, toward a poorer neurologic state or coma among the patients who survived to discharge and received vasopressin. It appears that combined therapy using both vasopressin and epinephrine was effective in restoring cardiac function but not brain function in some patients. Further research is needed in this area.

Overall, these studies suggest that vasopressin has a beneficial effect in out-of-hospital cardiac arrests or arrests secondary to asystole, situations when the effect of catecholamines may be diminished because of profound acidosis. Its usefulness for in-hospital cardiac arrest secondary to VF or PVT remains questionable. The doses for vasopressin and other agents used for cardiac arrest are listed in Table 12–3.

ANTIARRHYTHMICS

The primary reason for the use of antiarrhythmic agents following unsuccessful defibrillation and vasopressor administration is to prevent the development or recurrence of VF and PVT by raising the fibrillation threshold. There is, however, conflicting evidence and a divergence of opinion regarding the efficacy of these drugs and their place in CPR. These agents, therefore, receive either a class indeterminate or class IIb intervention classification according to the 2000 guidelines for CPR and ECC.[8]

With drugs used as a secondary intervention, there is no recommendation for a specific antiarrhythmic. Many experts feel that amiodarone, the newest antiarrhythmic added to the VF/PVT algorithm (class IIb), should be the agent of choice. Lidocaine remains on the algorithm, although its classification has been changed from a class IIb to an indeterminate intervention. Bretylium, previously the second antiarrhythmic on the VF/PVT algorithm, has been dropped from the guidelines because of the difficulty in obtaining the raw materials necessary for production. Magnesium is a class IIb intervention for polymorphic VT (torsades de pointes) and suspected hypomagnesemia. Procainamide is considered acceptable for refractory or recurrent VF/PVT (class IIb); however, its usefulness is limited by the need for a prolonged administration time, which makes it unsuitable for cardiac arrest.

Amiodarone

Although officially classified as a class III antiarrhythmic, amiodarone possesses electrophysiologic characteristics of all four Vaughn Williams classifications. Acutely, intravenous amiodarone displays mainly antiadrenergic (class II) and calcium channel blocking (class IV) properties. Consequently, hypotension, which occurs in roughly 20% of clinical trials, is a concern. This hypotension is more dependent on the rate of administration than on the amount of drug administered. A decrease in the infusion rate generally reverses hypotension induced by amiodarone.[65] The diluent used for the amiodarone solution, polysorbate 80, also may contribute to the hypotensive effect because it is known to have vasodilatory actions.[66] Amiodarone has mild negative inotropic actions as well, but its vasodilatory action usually offsets this effect, resulting in a minimal change in cardiac output.[67] Other adverse effects noted acutely include fever, elevated values on liver function tests, confusion, nausea, and thrombocytopenia.

Kudenchuk and colleagues conducted a large randomized, double-blind, placebo-controlled study evaluating amiodarone for out-of-hospital cardiac arrest (also known as the ARREST trial).[68] After receiving epinephrine 1 mg, 504 patients with cardiac arrest secondary to VF or PVT were randomized to receive either amiodarone 300 mg or placebo. Conventional ACLS was then followed. The primary end point was admission to the hospital with a spontaneously perfusing rhythm. Secondary end points included the number of precordial shocks required after administration of amiodarone or placebo, the total duration of resuscitative efforts, and the need for additional antiarrhythmics. Survival to discharge and neurologic status at discharge also were evaluated, although the trial did not have sufficient statistical power to demonstrate differences in these outcomes. Recipients of amiodarone were more likely to be resuscitated and survive to hospital admission than were recipients of placebo (44% and 34%, respectively; $p = .03$) for a relative improvement of 29%. A subgroup analysis revealed that patients whose cardiac arrest was due to VF were more likely to survive to hospital admission than those with asystole or PEA (44% and 14%, respectively; $p < .001$). There were no significant differences in number of precordial shocks, total duration of resuscitative efforts, or need for additional antiarrhythmics. ◀**5** This is the first trial to demonstrate the benefit of an antiarrhythmic agent over placebo in patients with out-of-hospital cardiac arrest.

The ALIVE trial compared amiodarone with lidocaine in patients with out-of-hospital VF.[69] Following three unsuccessful defibrillation attempts, IV epinephrine, and an additional defibrillation attempt, 347 patients were randomized to receive either amiodarone 5 mg/kg or lidocaine 1.5 mg/kg. A second dose of amiodarone 2.5 mg/kg or lidocaine 1.5 mg/kg was administered if needed. As in the ARREST trial, the primary end point was survival to hospital admission; survival to hospital discharge was a secondary outcome. Amiodarone was associated with a relative improvement of 90% in survival to hospital admission compared with lidocaine (22.8% versus 12%; OR 2.17; 95% CI 1.21–3.83; $p = .009$). Among patients who presented with either VF or PVT as their initial rhythm, survival to hospital admission was higher with amiodarone (24.8% versus 14.2%; $p = .03$). This benefit was less evident in patients who presented with a rhythm other than VF or PVT; 15.8% and 3.2% ($p = .08$) for amiodarone- and lidocaine-treated patients, respectively. Survival to hospital discharge was only 5% for patients receiving amiodarone and 3% for those receiving lidocaine ($p = .34$). The initial rhythm for all long-term survivors was VF. Amiodarone therefore has become the antiarrhythmic of first choice among many experts.[8]

Lidocaine

For many years lidocaine has been used for the treatment of ventricular arrhythmias in the setting of acute myocardial infarction (AMI). The efficacy seen in cardiac arrest, however, has not mirrored that seen in AMI. In the only published case-control trial where patients were classified according to whether they received lidocaine, no significant difference was noted in ROSC, admission to the hospital, or survival to hospital discharge between groups.[70] Similarly, a prospective study comparing the effectiveness of lidocaine with that of standard-dose epinephrine showed not only a lack of benefit with lidocaine but also a higher tendency to promote asystole.[71] In contrast, a retrospective analysis in patients with VF indicated that lidocaine was associated with a higher rate of ROSC and hospitalization ($p < .01$) but not an increase in the hospital discharge rate.[72]

Lidocaine has been shown to increase VF threshold in both the CPR and non-CPR settings.[73] Furthermore, it benefits the defibrillation threshold or the amount of energy required to convert VF to a more stable rhythm.[74] Although controversial, some studies show that lidocaine has a detrimental effect on defibrillation threshold.[75] These conflicting results may be related to drug interactions with lidocaine and the agents used for anesthesia.[75]

Lidocaine pharmacokinetics have not been studied extensively during cardiac arrest. Animal studies suggest that plasma lidocaine concentrations of at least 6 mcg/mL are necessary to achieve antifibrillatory effects, but concentrations greater than 12 mcg/mL may result in toxicity.[76] Because lidocaine metabolism depends on hepatic blood flow, lidocaine clearance may decrease following the reduction in cardiac output seen in cardiac arrest, thereby yielding toxic lidocaine concentrations.[77] Clinical trials in humans indicate that lidocaine levels are highly variable and unpredictable during cardiac arrest,[78] but they are nontoxic following ROSC and return of cardiac output.[79] In fact, a physiologically based pharmacokinetic model suggested that a 2 mg/kg dose of lidocaine may be more appropriate than the current AHA recommended dose because this dosing regimen will achieve a therapeutic concentration more rapidly.[76] Clinical trials in humans are necessary to validate this particular dosing regimen.

■ THERAPEUTIC ALTERNATIVES FOR REFRACTORY VF OR PVT

◀**6** Patients with persistent or recurrent VF or PVT following antiarrhythmic administration should be assessed for underlying electrolyte abnormalities as a cause for their refractory arrhythmia. The primary electrolyte abnormalities associated with refractory ventricular arrhythmias include hyperkalemia, hypokalemia, and hypomagnesemia.

In one study of prehospital cardiac arrests, 49% of resuscitated patients were found to be hypokalemic ($[K^+] < 3.6$ mEq/L) on hospital admission.[80] Although frequently debated, it is not yet known whether the hypokalemia most often precedes cardiac arrest or is a consequence of cardiac resuscitation.[80–82] Hypokalemia identified during cardiac arrest also may result from conditions that arise during resuscitation. For example, intracellular potassium shifts may occur secondary to metabolic derangements or to elevated circulating catecholamine concentrations.[80–82] Similarly, hypomagnesemia has been associated with ventricular arrhythmias.[83] Investigators have found that in hospitalized patients, approximately 40% of hypokalemic patients have coexisting hypomagnesemia.[84] This is important because uncorrected hypomagnesemia may prevent successful potassium repletion.[83] The value of magnesium in cardiac arrest has not been demonstrated in randomized, controlled trials, but anecdotal evidence is supportive. Therefore, the administration of magnesium is recommended only when a low level of magnesium is the suspected cause of an arrhythmia or when the patient experiences torsades de pointes.[8] Large doses of magnesium may produce hypotension but do not compromise coronary perfusion pressure because of coronary artery dilatation.[7]

THERAPEUTIC HYPOTHERMIA

Restoration of blood flow following cardiac arrest can lead to several chemical cascades and destructive enzymatic reactions that can result in cerebral injury. These reactions include free-radical production, excitatory amino acid release, and calcium shifts, leading to mitochondrial damage and apoptosis (programmed cell death).[85] Hypothermia can protect from cerebral injury by suppressing these chemical reactions, thereby reducing the production of free radicals. Various animal models have demonstrated improved functional recovery and reduced cerebral deficits with the induction of mild therapeutic hypothermia.[85] Recently, there have been two clinical trials in humans evaluating this technique.[86,87]

The first trial was conducted in nine centers in five European countries.[86] In this study, patients who had been resuscitated after cardiac arrest due to VF but remained comatose were assigned randomly to undergo therapeutic hypothermia, targeting a temperature of 32 to 34°C, for 24 hours. The primary end point was neurologic outcome within 6 months of cardiac arrest. Secondary end points were mortality (within 6 months) and complication rate within 7 days. A favorable neurologic outcome (defined as a cerebral performance category score of 1 or 2; see Table 12–4) was achieved in 55% of patients in the hypothermia group as opposed to 39% in the normothermia group ($p = .009$). Additionally, mortality rates were improved significantly in the hypothermia group (41% versus 55%; $p = .02$). Based on this difference, seven patients would need to be treated with hypothermia to prevent one death. The rate of complications (e.g., bleeding, pneumonia, sepsis, and renal failure) did not differ between the two groups (73% for the hypothermia group and 70% for the normothermia group; $p = .70$).

The second trial was conducted in four hospitals in Melbourne, Australia.[87] Entry criteria were similar to the previous trial, but the target temperature for hypothermia was 33°C, which was maintained for 12 hours. The primary outcome measure was survival to hospital discharge with good neurologic function. Forty-nine percent of

patients in the hypothermia group had good neurologic function on discharge (to either home or a rehabilitation facility) compared with 26% of patients in the normothermia group ($p = .046$). Mortality rates were similar between the two groups (51% for the hypothermia group and 68% for the normothermia group; $p = .145$). Hypothermia was associated with a lower cardiac index, higher systemic vascular resistance, and hyperglycemia.

In light of these trials, the Advanced Life Support Task Force of the International Liaison Committee on Resuscitation has recommended that unconscious adult patients with spontaneous circulation after out-of-hospital cardiac arrest be cooled to 32 to 34°C for 12 to 24 hours when the initial rhythm was VF.[85] Such cooling also may be of benefit for other rhythms or in-hospital cardiac arrest. There is insufficient evidence to make a recommendation on the use of therapeutic hypothermia in children.

NON-VF/PVT RHYTHMS: PEA AND ASYSTOLE

NONPHARMACOLOGIC THERAPY

Pulseless electrical activity (PEA) is defined as the absence of a detectable pulse and the presence of some type of electrical activity other than VF or PVT. *Asystole* is defined as the presence of a flat line on the ECG monitor. Although PEA is still classified as a "rhythm of survival," the success rate of treatment is much lower than the rates seen with VF/PVT.[10,13] The rate of survival among patients with asystole is a dismal 1% to 2%.[8,10] Successful treatment of both PEA and asystole depends almost entirely on diagnosis of the underlying cause (Table 12–5). The treatment of PEA is relatively similar to the treatment of asystole. Both conditions require CPR, intubation, and IV access. Emphasis, once again, should be placed on identifying a correctable cause. Asystole should be reconfirmed by checking a second lead on the cardiac monitor. Defibrillation should be avoided in patients with asystole because the parasympathetic discharge that occurs with defibrillation may reduce the chance of ROSC and worsen the chance of survival. If available, transcutaneous pacing can be attempted. Asystole often represents confirmation of death rather than a rhythm to be treated; therefore, withdrawal of efforts must be strongly considered.

PHARMACOLOGIC THERAPY

The primary pharmacologic agents used in the treatment of asystole are epinephrine and atropine. The recommended epinephrine dose is identical to that used for the treatment of VF/PVT.

Atropine is an antimuscarinic agent that blocks the depressant effect of acetylcholine on both the sinus and atrioventricular nodes, thus decreasing parasympathetic tone. During asystole, parasympathetic tone may increase because of the vagal stimulation that occurs secondary to intubation, the effects of hypoxia and acidosis, or alterations in the balance of parasympathetic and sympathetic control.[88] Unfortunately, there are no large randomized trials showing benefit from atropine for the treatment of asystole. Evidence is limited to small case series or retrospective reviews.[89-91]

Earlier small observational reports found some response to atropine in asystole or pulseless idioventricular rhythm but little evidence to suggest that long-term outcomes were altered.[89] In a retrospective case-control study, Stueven and colleagues found a 14% (6 of 43) success rate with atropine compared with a 0% (0 of 41) rate

---

TABLE 12–4. Assessment of Neurologic Function

A. Cerebral Performance Category[99]		
Conscious and alert with normal function or only slight disability		1
Conscious and alert with moderate disability		2
Conscious with severe disability		3
Comatose or in a persistent vegetative state		4
Brain dead		5
B. Glasgow Coma Scale[100]		
Eyes opening	Spontaneous	4
	To command	3
	To pain	2
	No response	1
Best motor response	Obeys verbal commands	6
	Localizes pain	5
	Withdraws to pain	4
	Abnormal flexion (decorticate)	3
	Extensor response (decerebrate)	2
	Flaccid	1
Verbal	Oriented	5
	Confused conversation	4
	Inappropriate words	3
	Incomprehensible sounds	2
	No response	1

TABLE 12–5. Potentially Reversible Causes of PEA and Asystole

Condition	Clues	Treatment
Hypovolemia	History, flat neck veins	Intravenous fluids
Hypoxia	Cyanosis, blood gases, airway problems	Ventilation, oxygen
Preexisting acidosis	History of bicarbonate-responsive preexisting acidosis	Sodium bicarbonate, hyperventilation
Hyperkalemia	History of renal failure, diabetes, recent dialysis, dialysis fistulas, medications	Calcium chloride, insulin, glucose, sodium bicarbonate, sodium polystyrene sulfonate, dialysis
Hypothermia	History of exposure to cold, central body temperature	Rewarming, oxygen, intravenous fluids
Drug overdose	Bradycardia, history of ingestion, empty bottles at the scene, pupils, neurologic exam	Drug screens, intubation, lavage, activated charcoal
Cardiac tamponade	History (trauma, renal failure, thoracic malignancy), no pulse with CPR, vein distention, impending tamponade-tachycardia, hypotension, low pulse pressure changing to sudden bradycardia as terminal event	Pericardiocentesis
Tension pneumothorax	History (asthma, ventilator, chronic obstructive pulmonary disease, trauma), no pulse with CPR, neck vein distention, tracheal deviation	Needle decompression
Coronary thrombosis	History, ECG, enzymes	Thrombolytics, oxygen, nitroglycerin, heparin, aspirin, morphine
Pulmonary thrombosis	History, no pulse with CPR, distended neck veins	Pulmonary arteriogram, surgical embolectomy, thrombolytics

Adapted from 1997–1999 Emergency Cardiovascular Care Programs, Advanced Cardiac Life Support. Dallas, American Heart Association, 1997.

with a control; as in previous trials, no patients survived to hospital discharge.[89] Ornato and associates published a retrospective study of 24 patients with asystole as the presenting rhythm; of the 22 patients who received atropine, asystole was abolished in 4.[90] Once again, none survived to hospital discharge. Finally, Tortolani and associates retrospectively reviewed the case histories of 123 patients with asystole.[91] Of the 101 patients who had received atropine, 24 were alive 24 hours after resuscitation. It is unclear how many survived to hospital discharge. These results show that although atropine may achieve ROSC in some instances, asystolic arrest is almost always fatal. Thus the use of atropine for this indication is not harmful, but the beneficial effect is limited.

ACID-BASE MANAGEMENT DURING CPR

Acidosis seen during cardiac arrest results from decreased blood flow and inadequate ventilation. Chest compressions generate approximately 20% to 30% of normal cardiac output, leading to inadequate organ perfusion, tissue hypoxia, and metabolic acidosis. In addition, the lack of ventilation causes retention of carbon dioxide, leading to respiratory acidosis. This combined acidosis produces not only reduced myocardial contractility and negative inotropic effect but also the appearance of arrhythmias because of a lower fibrillation threshold. In early cardiac arrest, adequate alveolar ventilation is the mainstay of control to limit the accumulation of carbon dioxide and control the acid-base imbalance.[8] With arrests of long duration, buffer therapy often is necessary.

Although sodium bicarbonate was once given routinely to reduce the detrimental effects associated with acidosis (e.g., reduced myocardial contractility), enhance the effect of epinephrine, and improve the rate of defibrillation, its use for cardiac arrest has been extremely controversial over the past several years. Unfortunately, there are few clinical data supporting sodium bicarbonate use.[92] Furthermore, sodium bicarbonate may have some detrimental effects.[92–94] The effect of sodium bicarbonate can be described by the following reaction:

$$[HCO_3^-] + [H^+] \longleftrightarrow [H_2CO_3] \longleftrightarrow [H_2O] + [CO_2]$$

When sodium bicarbonate is added to an acidic environment, this reaction will shift to the right, thereby increasing tissue and venous hypercarbia. The carbon dioxide generated by this reaction will diffuse into the cell and decrease intracellular pH. The accumulation of intracellular carbon dioxide, specifically within the myocardium, is inversely correlated with coronary perfusion pressure produced by CPR. Intracellular acidosis also will decrease myocardial contractility, further complicating the low-flow state associated with CPR.[92] Furthermore, treatment with sodium bicarbonate often overcorrects extracellular pH because sodium bicarbonate has a greater effect when the pH is closer to normal.[93] Alkalosis, created by overcorrection, causes an increase in the affinity of oxygen to hemoglobin, thus interfering with oxygen release into the tissues.

Recommendations for sodium bicarbonate vary (from class I to class III) depending on the clinical situation.[8] Sodium bicarbonate use is acceptable for patients with known, preexisting hyperkalemia (class I), preexisting bicarbonate-responsive acidosis (class IIa), overdoses of tricyclic antidepressants (class IIa), and to alkalinize the urine in aspirin and other drug overdoses (class IIa). In addition, sodium bicarbonate may be of benefit in intubated and ventilated patients with a long arrest interval (class IIb). Sodium bicarbonate may be harmful in hypercarbic acidosis, and patients with this condition should not receive it (class III).

GUIDELINES FOR DRUG ADMINISTRATION DURING EMERGENCY SITUATIONS

Several routes of administration are available for drug delivery during CPR. The routes chosen represent a compromise between the practicality of access and their apparent efficacy in introducing the necessary drug into the central circulation. The most efficacious method, obviously, is administration through a central venous catheter. Compared with peripheral administration, drug delivery via a central venous catheter results in a faster and higher peak concentration.[95] Central lines located above the diaphragm are preferable to those located below the diaphragm because of poor blood flow during CPR.[95,96] It is not practical, however, to interrupt CPR for an invasive procedure such as central line placement. Thus, if a central line is not already present, it is necessary to use a peripheral venous line. The antecubital vein is the first target for IV access.[7] Peripheral drug administration yields a peak concentration in the major systemic arteries in 1.5 to 3 minutes.[95] Circulation time is shortened by up to 40% if the drug is followed by a 20-mL fluid bolus with elevation of the extremity.[95]

In the event that neither central nor venous IV access is available, then a few drugs can be administered endotracheally. These drugs are atropine, lidocaine, and epinephrine remembered by the AHA pneumonic *ALE*.[7] Animal studies have shown that endotracheal administration mimics the effects of IV administration.[96] Human studies, on the other hand, show that drugs administered endotracheally have a lower plasma concentration with a delayed peak but a longer duration of action.[95] The endotracheal dose, therefore, should be 2 to 2.5 times larger than the IV dose.[9] Clinical trials evaluating outcomes, however, such as ROSC or survival, have failed to show any benefit using this dosing regimen.[97,98] Further trials are needed evaluating larger doses.

The technique of endotracheal drug administration markedly influences the pattern of absorption.[96] The dose first should be diluted with 10 mL sterile water or normal saline to permit distribution over the largest possible surface area. CPR should be interrupted and the dose administered beyond the tip of the endotracheal tube. Immediately, three to five forceful insufflations should follow using a bag-valve device to aerosolize the drug and enhance bioavailability.

In pediatric patients, the intraosseous route can be used temporarily if no other route is available. Lastly, the intracardiac route is no longer recommended for patients of any age because of potential complications such as myocardial laceration, coronary artery laceration, hemopericardium, and pneumopericardium.

ETHICAL AND ECONOMIC CONSIDERATIONS IN CPR

The primary objective of CPR is to obtain *neurologic survival*. Since this is often unobtainable, many health care professionals are attempting to identify patients unlikely to benefit from cardiac resuscitation. One difficulty in accomplishing this task is defining *medical futility*. The two major determinants of medical futility are length of life and quality of life.[8] An intervention that cannot increase length or quality of life is considered futile. Key factors in CPR are the disease underlying the cardiac arrest and the expected state of health after resuscitation. One important question that is debated often is how low should the chance of survival be before medical therapy is considered futile? Should it be 0.1%, 1%, or 2%? Is the chance of 1 or 2 months of life for a patient an acceptable goal? These are important questions that must be addressed when determining resuscitation status.

Unfortunately, there is no scientific evidence or scoring system that can predict the outcome following CPR. Therefore, all patients in cardiac arrest should receive resuscitation unless the patient has a "do not resuscitate" order, signs of irreversible death, or vital organ function deterioration that makes it impossible to expect any benefit from CPR—despite maximum therapy.[8] Withholding CPR attempts in these futile cases not only would decrease the number of patients left in a vegetative state with poor neurologic status but also would improve the cost-effectiveness of CPR programs. CPR is of minimal economic benefit if the only outcome following ROSC is a prolonged, expensive hospital stay.

CLINICAL CONTROVERSIES

Animal studies have suggested that higher doses of epinephrine are beneficial in improving resuscitation outcomes. Human studies, on the other hand, have not shown an advantage with higher dosing regimens.

A recommendation for a specific antiarrhythmic agent of first choice does not exist. Amiodarone, lidocaine, and procainamide are the available options.

EVALUATION OF THERAPEUTIC OUTCOMES

To gauge the success of resuscitation outcomes, therapeutic outcome monitoring should occur both during the resuscitation attempt and in the postresuscitation phase. The optimal outcome following CPR is an awake, responsive, spontaneously breathing patient. Patients must remain neurologically intact with minimal morbidity following the resuscitation if it is to be truly classified as a success. Heart rate, cardiac rhythm, and blood pressure should be assessed and documented throughout the resuscitation attempt and subsequent to each intervention. Determination of the presence or absence of a pulse is paramount to deciding which interventions may be appropriate. In addition, nonresponse to an array of suitable interventions may indicate that resuscitation is impossible.

The primary goal of resuscitation is the complete reestablishment of regional organ and tissue perfusion. Simple restoration of blood pressure and improvement in tissue gas exchange do not necessarily improve the patient's chance of survival.[8] Clinicians should consider the precipitating cause of the cardiac arrest, such as an AMI, electrolyte imbalance, or primary arrhythmia. They should review prearrest status carefully, particularly if the patient was receiving drug therapy. Laboratory investigations, including a 12-lead ECG, portable chest x-ray, measurement of arterial blood gases, and blood chemistry determinations, are necessary. Altered cardiac, hepatic, and renal function resulting from ischemic damage during the cardiopulmonary arrest warrant special attention. Neurologic function should be assessed by means of the Cerebral Performance Category and the Glasgow Coma Scale (see Table 12–4).

ABBREVIATIONS

ACLS: advanced cardiac life support
AED: automatic external defibrillator
AMI: acute myocardial infarction
CPC: cerebral performance category
CPR: cardiopulmonary resuscitation
D_5W: dextrose 5% in water
ECC: emergency cardiovascular care
ECG: electrocardiogram
GCS: Glasgow Coma Scale
IV: intravenous
PAD: public-access defibrillation
PEA: pulseless electrical activity
PVT: pulseless ventricular tachycardia
ROSC: return of spontaneous circulation
VF: ventricular fibrillation

Review Questions and other resources can be found at *www.pharmacotherapyonline.com*.

REFERENCES

1. Niemann JT. Cardiopulmonary resuscitation. N Engl J Med 1992;327: 1075–1080.
2. Zheng ZJ, Croft JB, Giles WH, Mensah GA. Sudden cardiac death in the United States, 1989 to 1998. Circulation 2001;104:2158–2163.

3. Paraskos JA. History of CPR and the role of the national conference. Ann Emerg Med 1993;22:275–280.

4. Safar P, Escarraga L, Elam JO. A comparison of the mouth-to-mouth and mouth-to-airway methods of artificial respiration with chest pressure arm-life method. N Engl J Med 1958;258:671–677.

5. Kouwenhoven WB, Jude JR, Knickerbocker GG. Closed-chest cardiac massage. JAMA 1960;173:1064–1067.

6. Thel MC, O'Connor CM. Cardiopulmonary resuscitation: Historical perspective to recent investigations. Am Heart J 1999;137:39–48.

7. 1997–1999 Emergency Cardiovascular Care Programs, Advanced Cardiac Life Support. Chicago, American Heart Association, 1997.

8. American Heart Association in collaboration with the International Liaison Committee on Resuscitation. Guidelines 2000 for cardiopulmonary resuscitation and emergency cardiovascular care: An international consensus on science. Circulation 2000;102(suppl 1):1–370.

9. Priori SG, Aliot E, Blomstrom-Lundquist C, et al. Task force on sudden cardiac death of the European Society of Cardiology. Eur Heart J 2001;22:1374–1450.

10. Cobb LA, Fahrenbruch CE, Olsufka M, Copass MK. Changing incidence of out-of-hospital ventricular fibrillation, 1980–2000. JAMA 2002;288:3008–3013.

11. Kuisma M, Repo J, Alaspaa A. The incidence of out-of-hospital ventricular fibrillation in Helsinki, Finland, from 1994 to 1999. Lancet 2001;358:473–474.

12. Herlitz J, Andersson E, Bang A, et al. Experiences from treatment of out-of-hospital cardiac arrest during 17 years in Goteborg. Eur Heart J 2000;21:1251–1258.

13. Stiell IG, Wells GA, Field BJ, et al. Improved out-of-hospital cardiac arrest survival through the inexpensive optimization of an existing defibrillation program. OPALS study phase II. JAMA 1999;281:1175–1181.

14. Bunch TJ, White RD, Gersh BJ, et al. Long-term outcomes of out-of-hospital cardiac arrest after successful early defibrillation. N Engl J Med 2003;348:2626–2633.

15. Chandra NS. Mechanisms of blood flow during CPR. Ann Emerg Med 1993;22:281–288.

16. Tucker KJ, Savitt MA, Idris A, Redberg RF. Cardiopulmonary resuscitation: Historical perspectives, physiology, and future directions. Arch Intern Med 1994;154:2141–2150.

17. Becker LB, Berg RA, Pepe PE, et al. A reappraisal of mouth-to-mouth ventilation during bystander initiated cardiopulmonary resuscitation: A statement for healthcare professionals from the ventilation working group of the basic life support and pediatric life support subcommittees, American Heart Association. Ann Emerg Med 1997;30:654–666.

18. Valenzuela TD, Roe DJ, Nichol G, et al. Outcomes of rapid defibrillation by security officers after cardiac arrest in casinos. N Engl J Med 2000;343:1206–1209.

19. Ayers SM. Preventing cardiac arrest. Crit Care Med 1994;22:189–191.

20. Edwards GA, Samuels TM. The role of the hospital pharmacist in emergency situations. Am J Hosp Pharm 1968;25:128–133.

21. Bardas SL. Demystifying the cardiopulmonary code team response. Pharm Technol 1992;8:151–154.

22. Bossaert LL. Fibrillation and defibrillation of the heart. Br J Anaesth 1997;79:203–213.

23. Weisfeldt ML, Becker LB. Resuscitation after cardiac arrest: A 3-phase time-sensitive model. JAMA 2002;288:3035–3038.

24. DeMaio VJ, Stiell IG, Wells GA, Spaite DW. Optimal defibrillation response intervals for maximum out-of-hospital cardiac arrest survival rates. Ann Emerg Med 2003;42:242–250.

25. Cobb LA, Fahrenbruch CE, Walsh TR, et al. Influence of cardiopulmonary resuscitation prior to defibrillation in patients with out-of-hospital ventricular fibrillation. JAMA 1999;281:1182–1188.

26. Wik L, Hansen TB, Fylling F, et al. Delaying defibrillation to give basic cardiopulmonary resuscitation to patients with out-of-hosptial ventricular fibrillation: A randomized trial. JAMA 2003;289:1389–1395.

27. Paradis NA, Martin GB, Rivers EP, et al. Coronary perfusion pressure and the return of spontaneous circulation in human cardiopulmonary resuscitation. JAMA 1990;263:1106–1113.

28. Robinson LA, Brown CG, Jenkins J, et al. The effect of norepinephrine versus epinephrine on myocardial hemodynamics during CPR. Ann Emerg Med 1989;18:336–340.

29. Otto CW, Yakaitis RW, Blitt CD. Mechanism of action of epinephrine in resuscitation from asphyxial arrest. Crit Care Med 1981;9:321–324.

30. Paradis NA, Koscrove EM. Epinephrine in cardiac arrest: A critical review. Ann Emerg Med 1990;19:1288–1301.

31. Ditchey RV, Lindenfeld J. Failure of epinephrine to improve the balance between myocardial oxygen supply and demand during closed-chest resuscitation in dogs. Circulation 1988;78:382–389.

32. Tang W, Weil MH, Sun S, et al. Epinephrine increases the severity of postresuscitation myocardial dysfunction. Circulation 1995;92:3089–3093.

33. Ornato JP. Use of adrenergic agonists during CPR in adults. Ann Emerg Med 1993;22:411–416.

34. Holmes HR, Babbs CF, Voorhees WD, et al. Influence of adrenergic drugs upon vital organ perfusion during CPR. Crit Care Med 1980;8:137–140.

35. Brown C, Wiklund L, Bar-Joseph G, et al. Future directions for resuscitation research: IV. Innovative advanced life support pharmacology. Resuscitation 1996;33:163–177.

36. Callaham M, Madsen CD, Barton CW, et al. A randomized clinical trial of high-dose epinephrine and norepinephrine vs standard-dose epinephrine in prehospital cardiac arrest. JAMA 1992;268:2667–2672.

37. Lindner KH, Ahnefeld FW, Grunert A. Epinephrine versus norepinephrine in prehospital ventricular fibrillation. Am J Cardiol 1991;67:427–428.

38. Lindner KH, Anhefeld FW, Schuermann W, et al. Epinephrine and norepinephrine in cardiopulmonary resuscitation: Effects on myocardial oxygen delivery and consumption. Chest 1990;97:1458–1462.

39. Brown CG, Robinson LA, Jenkins J, et al. The effect of norepinephrine versus epinephrine on regional cerebral blood flow during cardiopulmonary resuscitation. Am J Emerg Med 1989;7:278–282.

40. Redding JS, Pearson JW. Evaluation of drugs for cardiac resuscitation. Anaesthesia 1963;24:203–207.

41. Kosnik J, Jackson R, Keats S, et al. Dose-related response of aortic diastolic pressure during closed-chest massage in dogs. Ann Emerg Med 1985;14:204–208.

42. Brown CG, Werman HA, Davis EA, et al. Comparative effect of graded doses of epinephrine on regional brain blood flow during CPR in a swine model. Ann Emerg Med 1986;15:1138–1144.

43. Brunette DD, Jameson SJ. Comparison of standard versus high-dose epinephrine in the resuscitation of cardiac arrest in dogs. Ann Emerg Med 1990;19:8–11.

44. Gonzalez ER, Ornato JP, Garnett AR, et al. Dose-dependent vasopressor response to epinephrine during CPR in human beings. Ann Emerg Med 1989;18:920–926.

45. Gueugniaud P, Mols P, Goldstein P, et al. A comparison of repeated high doses and repeated standard doses of epinephrine for cardiac arrest outside the hospital. N Engl J Med 1998;339:1595–1601.

46. Sherman BW, Munger MA, Foulke GE, et al. High-dose versus standard-dose epinephrine treatment of cardiac arrest after failure of standard therapy. Pharmacotherapy 1997;17:242–247.

47. Choux C, Gueugniaud P, Barbieux A, et al. Standard doses versus repeated high doses of epinephrine in cardiac arrest outside the hospital. Resuscitation 1995;29:3–9.

48. Lipman J, Wilson W, Kobilski S, et al. High-dose adrenaline in adult in-hospital asystolic cardiopulmonary resuscitation: A double-blind randomized trial. Anaesth Intens Care 1993;21:192–196.

49. Stiell IG, Hebert PC, Weitzman BN, et al. High-dose epinephrine in adult cardiac arrest. N Engl J Med 1992;327:1045–1050.

50. Brown CG, Martin DR, Pepe PE, et al. A comparison of standard-dose and high-dose epinephrine in cardiac arrest outside the hospital. N Engl J Med 1992;327:1051–1055.

51. Lindner KH, Ahnefeld FW, Prengel AW. Comparison of standard and high-dose adrenaline in the resuscitation of asystole and electromechanical dissociation. Acta Anaesthesiol Scand 1991;35:253–256.

52. Callaham M, Barton CW, Kayser S. Potential complications of high-dose epinephrine therapy in patients resuscitated from cardiac arrest. JAMA 1991;265:1117–1122.

53. Behringer W, Kittler H, Sterz F, et al. Cumulative epinephrine dose during cardiopulmonary resuscitation and neurologic outcome. Ann Intern Med 1998;129:450–456.

54. Kelly CM, Ponzillo JJ. Vasopressin use in cardiopulmonary resuscitation. Ann Pharmacother 1997;31:1523–1525.

55. Lindner KH, Strohmenger HU, Ensinger H, et al. Stress hormone response during and after cardiopulmonary resuscitation. Anesthesiology 1992;77:662–668.

56. Wenzel V, Lindner KH, Prengel AW, et al. Vasopressin improves vital organ blood flow after prolonged cardiac arrest with postcountershock pulseless electrical activity in pigs. Crit Care Med 1999;27:486–492.

57. Wenzel V, Lindner KH, Krismer AC, et al. Repeated administration of vasopressin but not epinephrine maintains coronary perfusion pressure after early and late administration during prolonged cardiopulmonary resuscitation in pigs. Circulation 1999;99:1379–1384.

58. Wenzel V, Lindner KH, Krismer AC, et al. Survival with full neurologic recovery and no cerebral pathology after prolonged cardiopulmonary resuscitation with vasopressin in pigs. J Am Coll Cardiol 2000;35:527–533.

59. Lindner KH, Brinkmann A, Pfenninger EG, et al. Effect of vasopressin on hemodynamic variables, organ blood flow, and acid base status in a pig model of cardiopulmonary resuscitation. Anesth Analg 1993;77:427–435.

60. Voelckel WG, Lindner KH, Wenzel V, et al. Effects of vasopressin and epinephrine on splanchnic blood flow and renal function during and after cardiopulmonary resuscitation in pigs. Crit Care Med 2000;28:1083–1088.

61. Lindner KH, Prengel AW, Brinkmann A, et al. Vasopressin administration in refractory cardiac arrest. Ann Intern Med 1996;124:1061–1064.

62. Lindner KH, Dirks B, Strohmenger HU, et al. Randomized comparison of epinephrine and vasopressin in patients with out-of-hospital ventricular fibrillation. Lancet 1997;349:535–537.

63. Stiell IG, Hebert PC, Wells GA, et al. Vasopressin versus epinephrine for in-hospital cardiac arrest: A randomised, controlled trial. Lancet 2001;358:105–109.

64. Wenzel V, Krismer AC, Arntz HR, et al. A comparison of vasopressin and epinephrine for out-of-hospital cardiopulmonary resuscitation. N Engl J Med 2004;350:105–113.

65. Gonzalez ER, Kannewurf BS, Ornato JP. Intravenous amiodarone for ventricular arrhythmias: Overview and clinical use. Resuscitation 1998;39:33–42.

66. Kowey PR, Levine JH, Herre JM, et al. Randomized, double-blind comparison of intravenous amiodarone and bretylium in the treatment of patients with recurrent, hemodynamically destabilizing ventricular tachycardia or fibrillation. The Intravenous Amiodarone Multicenter Investigators Group. Circulation 1995;92:3255–3263.

67. Podrid PJ. Amiodarone: Reevaluation of an old drug. Ann Intern Med 1995;122:689–700.

68. Kudenchuk PJ, Cobb LA, Copass MK, et al. Amiodarone for resuscitation after out-of-hospital cardiac arrest due to ventricular fibrillation. N Engl J Med 1999;341:871–878.

69. Dorian P, Cass D, Schwartz B, et al. Amiodarone as compared with lidocaine for shock-resistant ventricular fibrillation. N Engl J Med 2002;346:884–890.

70. Harrison EE. Lidocaine in prehospital countershock refractory ventricular fibrillation. Ann Emerg Med 1981;10:420–423.

71. Weaver WD, Fahrenbruch CE, Johnson DD, et al. Effect of epinephrine and lidocaine therapy on outcome after cardiac arrest to ventricular fibrillation. Circulation 1990;82:2027–2034.

72. Herlitz J, Ekstrom L, Wennerblom B, et al. Lidocaine in out-of-hospital ventricular fibrillation: Does it improve survival? Resuscitation 1997;33:199–205.

73. Chow MS. Advanced cardiac life support controversy: Where do antiarrhythmic agents fit in? Pharmacotherapy 1997;17:84S–88S.

74. Kerber RE, Pandian NG, Jensen SR, et al. Effect of lidocaine and bretylium on energy requirements for transthoracic defibrillation: Experimental studies. J Am Coll Cardiol 1986;7:397–405.

75. Jaffe AS. The use of antiarrhythmics in advanced cardiac life support. Ann Intern Med 1993;22:307–316.

76. Grillo JA, Venitz J, Ornato JP. Prediction of lidocaine tissue concentration following different dose regimes during cardiac arrest using a physiologically based pharmacokinetic model. Resuscitation 2001;50:331–340.

77. Pentel P, Benowitz N. Pharmacokinetic and pharmacodynamic considerations in drug therapy of cardiac emergencies. Clin Pharmacokinet 1984;9:273–308.

78. Chow MS, Ronfeld RA, Ruggett D, Fieldman A. Lidocaine pharmacokinetics during cardiac arrest and external cardiopulmonary resuscitation. Am Heart J 1981;102:799–801.

79. Hendrie J, O'Callaghan CJ. Lidocaine pharmacokinetics after cardiac arrest and external cardiopulmonary resuscitation. Am J Cardiol 1996;78:1322–1323.

80. Thompson RG, Cobb LA. Hypokalemia after resuscitation from out-of-hospital ventricular fibrillation. JAMA 1982;248:2860–2863.

81. Ornato JP, Gonzalez ER, Starke H, et al. Incidence and causes of hypokalemia associated with cardiac resuscitation. Am J Emerg Med 1985;3:503–506.

82. Higham PD, Adams PC, Murray A, Campbell RW. Plasma potassium, serum magnesium and ventricular fibrillation: A prospective study. Q J Med 1993;86:609–617.

83. Noronha JL, Matuschak GM. Magnesium in critical illness: Metabolism, assessment, and treatment. Intens Care Med 2002;28:667–679.

84. Whang R, Flink EB, Dyckner T, et al. Magnesium depletion as a cause of refractory potassium repletion. Arch Intern Med 1985;145:1686–1689.

85. Nolan JP, Morley PT, Vanden Hoek TL, Hickey RW. Therapeutic hypothermia after cardiac arrest: An advisory statement by the Advanced Life Support Task Force of the International Liaison Committee on resuscitation. Circulation 2003;108:118–121.

86. The Hypothermia After Cardiac Arrest Study Group. Mild therapeutic hypothermia to improve the neurologic outcome after cardiac arrest. N Engl J Med 2002;346:549–556.

87. Bernard SA, Gray TW, Buist MD, et al. Treatment of comatose survivors of out-of-hospital cardiac arrest with induced hypothermia. N Engl J Med 2002;346:557–563.

88. Gonzalez ER. Pharmacologic controversies in CPR. Ann Emerg Med 1993;22:317–323.

89. Stueven HA, Tonsfeldt DJ, Thompson BM, et al. Atropine in asystole: Human studies. Ann Emerg Med 1984;13:815–817.

90. Ornato JP, Gonzalez ER, Morkunas AR, et al. Treatment of presumed asystole during prehospital cardiac arrest: Superiority of electrical countershock. Am J Emerg Med 1985;3:395–399.

91. Tortolani AJ, Risucci DA, Powell SR, et al. In-hospital cardiopulmonary resuscitation during asystole: Therapeutic factors associated with 24-hour survival. Chest 1989;96:622–626.

92. Levy MM. An evidence-based evaluation of the use of sodium bicarbonate during cardiac resuscitation. Crit Care Clin 1998;14:457–483.

93. Bjerneroth G. Tribonat: A comprehensive summary of its properties. Crit Care Med 1999;27:1009–1013.

94. Adgey AAJ. Adrenaline dosage and buffers in cardiac arrest. Heart 1998;80:412–414.

95. Vincent R. Drugs in modern resuscitation. Br J Anaesth 1997;79:188–197.

96. Gonzalez ER. Pharmacologic controversies in CPR. Ann Intern Med 1993;22:317–323.

97. Niemann JT, Stratton SJ. Endotracheal versus intravenous epinephrine and atropine in out-of-hospital "primary" and postcountershock asystole. Crit Care Med 2000;28:1815–1819.

98. Niemann JT, Stratton SJ, Cruz B, Lewis RJ. Endotracheal drug administration during out-of-hospital resuscitation: Where are the survivors? Resuscitation 2002;53:153–157.

99. Jennett B, Bond M. Assessment of outcome after severe brain damage. Lancet 1975;1:480–484.

100. Jannett B, Teasdale G. Aspects of coma after severe head injury. Lancet 1977;1:878.

13

HYPERTENSION

Joseph J. Saseen and Barry L. Carter

Learning Objectives and other resources can be found at *www.pharmacotherapyonline.com*.

KEY CONCEPTS

❶ The risk of cardiovascular morbidity and mortality is directly correlated with blood pressure (BP). Starting at a BP of 115/75 mm Hg, risk of cardiovascular disease doubles with every 20/10-mm Hg increase. Even patients with prehypertension have an increased risk of cardiovascular disease. Outcome trials have shown that antihypertensive drug therapy substantially reduces the risks of cardiovascular events and death.

❷ Essential hypertension is usually an asymptomatic condition. A diagnosis cannot be made based on one elevated BP measurement. An elevated value from the average of two or more measurements on two or more clinical encounters is needed to diagnose hypertension.

❸ The overall goal of treating hypertension is to reduce hypertension-associated morbidity and mortality. The selection of specific drug therapy is based on evidence that demonstrates risk reduction.

❹ A goal BP of less than 140/90 mm Hg is appropriate for most patients. Achieving lower BP values has not been proven to provide additional risk reduction, except in patients with diabetes or chronic kidney disease. These patients have a goal BP of less than 130/80 mm Hg.

❺ Lifestyle modifications should be prescribed in all patients with hypertension and prehypertension. However, they should never be used as a replacement for antihypertensive drug therapy in patients with hypertension.

❻ Thiazide diuretics are first-line agents for the management of hypertension in most patients. This recommendation is

supported by clinical trials showing reduced morbidity and mortality with these agents. Comparative data from the landmark clinical trial, the ALLHAT, confirm the first-line role of thiazide diuretics.

❼ Compelling indications are comorbid conditions where specific drug therapies have been shown in outcome trials to provide unique long-term benefits. Drug therapy recommendations for compelling indications are either in combination with or in place of a thiazide diuretic.

❽ Patients with diabetes are at very high risk for cardiovascular disease. All patients with diabetes and hypertension should be managed with either an angiotensin-converting enzyme (ACE) inhibitor or an angiotensin II receptor blocker (ARB), typically in combination with one or more other antihypertensive agents. Multiple agents frequently are needed to control BP.

❾ Older patients with isolated systolic hypertension are often at risk for orthostatic hypotension when drug therapy is started. This is particularly prevalent with diuretics, ACE inhibitors, and ARBs. Although overall treatment should be the same, initial doses should be very low and dose titrations gradual to minimize risk of orthostatic hypotension.

❿ Most patients require combination therapy to achieve goal BP values. Combination regimens should include a diuretic, preferably a thiazide. If a diuretic was not the first drug, it should be the second drug add-on therapy.

Hypertension is a common disease that is defined simply as persistently elevated arterial blood pressure (BP). Although elevated BP was perceived to be necessary for adequate perfusion of essential organs during the early and middle 1900s, it is now identified as one of the most significant risk factors for cardiovascular disease in the United States. Increasing awareness and diagnosis of hypertension and improving control of BP with appropriate treatment are considered critical public health initiatives to reduce cardiovascular morbidity and mortality.

The Seventh Report of the Joint National Committee on the Detection, Evaluation, and Treatment of High Blood Pressure (JNC7) is the national clinical guideline that was developed to aid clinicians in the management of hypertension.[1] This chapter reviews relevant components of this evidence-based guideline with a focus on the pharmacotherapy of hypertension. Data from the National

Health and Nutrition Examination Survey from 1999 to 2000 indicate that of the population of Americans with hypertension, 68.9% are aware that they have hypertension, and only 58.4% are on some form of antihypertensive treatment.[2] Moreover, only 34% of all patients have controlled BP, which increases to only 53.1% when only those on treatment are evaluated.[2] Therefore, there are ample opportunities for clinicians to improve the care of hypertensive patients.

EPIDEMIOLOGY

It is estimated that approximately 30% of the population (50 million Americans) has high BP ($\geq$140/90 mm Hg).[2,3] Estimates from the National Health and Nutrition Examination Survey from 1999–2000 indicate that the prevalence is 30.1% and 27.1% among men and women, respectively.[2] This represents a significant increase of 5.6% in women from 1988 to 2000, whereas the prevalence in men has remained unchanged. Prevalence rates are highest in non-Hispanic blacks (33.5%), followed by non-Hispanic whites (28.9%) and Mexican-Americans (20.7%).

BP values increase with age, and hypertension is very common in the elderly. The lifetime risk of developing hypertension among those 55 years of age and older who are normotensive is 90%.[1] Most patients have prehypertension BP values before they are diagnosed with hypertension, and most hypertension diagnoses occur between the third and fifth decades of life. Up to the age of 55 years, more men than women have hypertension. From the ages of 55 to 74 years, slightly more women have hypertension than men, with this sex difference becoming greater in the very elderly (≥75 years). In the older population (age ≥ 60 years), the prevalence of hypertension is 65.4% (estimated in 2000), which is significantly higher than the 57.9% prevalence estimated in 1988.[2]

ETIOLOGY

Hypertension is a heterogeneous medical condition. In most patients it results from unknown pathophysiologic etiology (essential or primary hypertension). While this form of hypertension cannot be cured, it can be controlled. A small percentage of patients have a specific cause of their hypertension (secondary hypertension). There are many potential secondary causes that are either concurrent medical conditions or are endogenously induced. If the cause of secondary hypertension can be identified, hypertension in these patients potentially can be cured.

ESSENTIAL HYPERTENSION

Over 90% of individuals with hypertension have essential hypertension (primary hypertension).[1] Numerous mechanisms have been identified that may contribute to the pathogenesis of this form of hypertension, so identifying the exact underlying abnormality is not possible. Hypertension often runs in families, indicating that genetic factors may play an important role in the development of essential hypertension. Data suggest that there are monogenic and polygenic forms of BP dysregulation that may be responsible for essential hypertension.[4,5] Many of these genetic traits feature genes that affect sodium balance,[5] but genetic mutations altering urinary kallikrein excretion, nitric oxide release, aldosterone excretion, other adrenal steroids, and angiotensinogen are also documented.[4] In the future, identifying individuals with these genetic traits could lead to alternative approaches to preventing or treating hypertension; however, this is not currently recommended.

SECONDARY HYPERTENSION

Fewer than 10% of patients have secondary hypertension, where either a comorbid disease or a drug is responsible for elevating BP[1] (see Table 13–1). In most of these cases, renal dysfunction resulting from chronic kidney disease or renovascular disease is the most common secondary cause.[6] Certain drugs, either directly or indirectly, can cause hypertension or exacerbate hypertension by increasing BP. The most common agents are listed in Table 13–1. Some of these agents are herbal products. Although these are not technically drugs, they have been identified as causes of elevated BP and secondary hypertension. When a secondary cause is identified, removing the offending agent or treating/correcting the underlying comorbid condition should be the first step in management.

TABLE 13–1. Secondary Causes of Hypertension

Disease	Drugs Associated with Hypertension in Humans

Chronic kidney disease
Cushing's syndrome
Coarctation of the aorta
Obstructive sleep apnea
Parathyroid disease
Pheochromocytoma
Primary aldosteronism
Renovascular disease
Thyroid disease
	Prescription drugs
	Corticosteroids,[a] ACTH
	Estrogens[a] (usually oral contraceptives with high estrogenic activity)
	Nonsteroidal anti-inflammatory drugs,[a] COX-2 inhibitors[a]
	Phenylpropanolamine[a] and analogues[a]
	Cyclosporine[a] and tacrolimus[a]
	Erythropoetin[a]
	Sibutramine[a]
	Antidepressants (especially venlafaxine), bromocriptine, buspirone,
	    carbamazepine, clozapine, desfulrane, ketamine, metoclopramide
	Clonidine/β-blocker combination
	Pheochromocytoma: β-blocker without α-blocker first
	Street Drugs and Other Natural Products
	Cocaine[a] and cocaine withdrawal[a]
	Ma huang,[a] "herbal ecstasy,"[a] other phenylpropanolamine analogues[a]
	Nicotine and withdrawal, anabolic steroids, narcotic withdrawal,
	    methylphenidate, phencyclidine, ketamine, ergotamine and other
	    ergot-containing herbal products, St. John's wort
	Food Substances
	Sodium[a]
	Ethanol[a]
	Licorice
	Tyramine-containing foods if taking a monoamine oxidase inhibitor
	Chemical Elements and Other Industrial Chemicals
	Lead, mercury, thallium and other heavy metals, lithium

[a]Agents of most clinical importance.

PATHOPHYSIOLOGY[4,7]

A clear understanding of arterial BP and regulation is needed to manage hypertension appropriately and to understand antihypertensive drug therapy mechanistically. Multiple factors that control BP are potential contributing components in the development of hypertension. These include malfunctions in either humoral (i.e., the renin-angiotensin-aldosterone system [RAAS]) or vasodepressor mechanisms, abnormal neuronal mechanisms, defects in peripheral autoregulation, and disturbances in sodium, calcium, and natriuretic hormone. Many of these factors are cumulatively affected by the multifaceted RAAS, which ultimately regulates arterial BP. It is probable that none of these factors is solely responsible for hypertension; however, most antihypertensives specifically target these mechanisms and components of the RAAS.

ARTERIAL BLOOD PRESSURE

Arterial BP is the measured pressure in the arterial wall in millimeters of mercury. Two arterial BP values are typically measured, systolic BP (SBP) and diastolic BP (DBP). SBP is achieved during cardiac contraction and represents the peak value. DBP is achieved after contraction when the cardiac chambers are filling and represents the nadir value. The difference between SBP and DBP is called the *pulse pressure* and indicates arterial wall tension. Mean arterial pressure (MAP) is the average pressure throughout the cardiac cycle of contraction. It is sometimes used clinically to represent overall arterial BP. During a cardiac cycle, two-thirds of the time is spent in diastole and one-third in systole. Therefore, the MAP can be estimated by using the following equation:

$$MAP = \frac{1}{3}(SBP) + \frac{2}{3}(DBP)$$

Arterial BP is generated hemodynamically by the interplay between blood flow and the resistance to blood flow. It is defined mathematically as the product of cardiac output (CO) and total peripheral resistance (TPR) according to the following equation:

$$BP = CO \times TPR$$

CO is the major determinant of SBP, whereas TPR largely determines DBP. In turn, CO is a function of stroke volume, heart rate, and venous capacitance. Table 13–2 lists physiologic causes of increased CO and TPR and correlates them with potential mechanisms of pathogenesis.

Under normal physiologic conditions, arterial BP fluctuates throughout the day. It typically follows a circadian rhythm, where it decreases to its lowest daily values during sleep.[8] This is followed by a sharp rise starting a few hours prior to awakening, with the high-

TABLE 13–2. Potential Mechanisms of Pathogenesis

Blood pressure is the mathematical product of cardiac output and peripheral resistance. Increased blood pressure can result from increased cardiac output and/or increased total peripheral resistance.

Increased cardiac output	Increased cardiac preload: • Increased fluid volume from excess sodium intake or renal sodium retention (from reduced number of nephrons or decreased glomerular filtration) Venous constriction: • Excess stimulation of the RAAS • Sympathetic nervous system overactivity
Increased peripheral resistance	Functional vascular constriction: • Excess stimulation of the RAAS • Sympathetic nervous system overactivity • Genetic alterations of cell membranes • Endothelial-derived factors Structural vascular hypertrophy: • Excess stimulation of the RAAS • Sympathetic nervous system overactivity • Genetic alterations of cell membranes • Endothelial-derived factors • Hyperinsulinemia resulting from obesity or the metabolic syndrome

est values occurring midmorning. BP is also increased acutely during physical activity or emotional stress.

CLASSIFICATION

The JNC7 classification of BP in adults (age $\geq$ 18 years) is based on the average of two or more properly measured BP readings from two or more clinical encounters[1] (Table 13–3). It includes four categories, with normal values considered to be an SBP of less than 120 mm Hg and a DBP of less than 80 mm Hg. Prehypertension is not considered a disease category but identifies patients whose BP is likely to increase into the classification of hypertension in the future. There are two stages of hypertension, and all patients in these categories warrant drug therapy.

Hypertensive crises are clinical situations where BP values are greater than 180/120 mm Hg.[7,9] They are categorized as either a hypertensive emergency or hypertensive urgency. *Hypertensive emergencies* are extreme elevations in BP that are accompanied by acute or progressing target-organ damage. Examples of acute target-organ injury include encephalopathy, intracranial hemorrhage, acute left ventricular failure with pulmonary edema, dissecting aortic aneurysm, unstable angina, and eclampsia or severe hypertension during pregnancy. Hypertensive emergencies require an immediate but gradual

TABLE 13–3. Classification of Blood Pressure in Adults (Age $\geq$ 18 Years)[a]

Classification	Systolic Blood Pressure (mm Hg)		Diastolic Blood Pressure (mm Hg)
Normal	Less than 120	and	Less than 80
Prehypertension[b]	120–139	or	80–89
Stage 1 hypertension	140–159	or	90–99
Stage 2 hypertension	Greater than or equal to 160	or	Greater than or equal to 100

[a] Classification determined based on the average of two or more properly measured seated BP measurements from two or more clinical encounters. If systolic and diastolic blood pressure values yield different classifications, the highest category is used for the purpose of determining a classification.

[b] For patients with diabetes mellitus or chronic kidney disease, values $\geq$130/80 mm Hg are considered above goal.

reduction in BP over a period of several minutes to several hours using intravenous antihypertensive agents. A reasonable goal is to gradually lower DBP to <110 mm Hg.[7] Abrupt BP reductions should be avoided. *Hypertensive urgencies* are high elevations in BP without acute or progressing target-organ injury. These situations require BP reductions with oral antihypertensive agents to stage 1 values over a period of several hours to several days.

CARDIOVASCULAR RISK AND BLOOD PRESSURE

Epidemiologic data clearly indicate a strong correlation between BP and cardiovascular morbidity and mortality.[10] Risk of stroke, myocardial infarction, angina, heart failure, kidney failure, or early death from a cardiovascular cause are directly correlated with BP. Starting at a BP of 115/75 mm Hg, risk of cardiovascular disease doubles with every 20/10 mm Hg increase.[1] Even within the prehypertension BP category, an increased risk of cardiovascular disease is associated with higher BP values.[11] Moreover, large-scale placebo-controlled outcome trials have shown that the increased risks of cardiovascular events and death associated with elevated BP are reduced substantially by antihypertensive therapy.[12–15]

SBP is a stronger predictor of cardiovascular disease than DBP in adults 50 years of age and older and is the most important clinical BP parameter for most patients.[1,16] Patients with DBP values less than or equal to 90 mm Hg and SBP values greater than or equal to 140 mm have *isolated systolic hypertension*. Isolated systolic hypertension is believed to result from pathophysiologic changes in the arterial vasculature consistent with aging. These changes decrease the compliance of the arterial wall and portend an increased risk of cardiovascular morbidity and mortality.

Cardiovascular risk, especially in those with isolated systolic hypertension, may be projected by calculating the pulse pressure.[17] Pulse pressure is the difference between SBP and DBP. It is believed to reflect extent of atherosclerotic disease in the elderly and is a measure of increased arterial stiffness. Higher pulse pressure values are correlated with an increased risk of cardiovascular mortality.[17]

HUMORAL MECHANISMS

Several humoral abnormalities may be involved in the development of essential hypertension. These abnormalities may involve the RAAS, natriuretic hormone, and hyperinsulinemia.

THE RENIN-ANGIOTENSIN-ALDOSTERONE SYSTEM (RAAS)

The RAAS is a complex endogenous system that is involved with most regulatory components of arterial BP. Activation and regulation are governed primarily by the kidney (Fig. 13–1). The RAAS regulates sodium, potassium, and fluid balance. Therefore, this system significantly influences vascular tone and sympathetic nervous system activity and is the most influential contributor to the homeostatic regulation of BP.

Renin is an enzyme that is stored in the juxtaglomerular cells, which are located in the afferent arterioles of the kidney. The release of renin is modulated by several factors: intrarenal factors (e.g., renal perfusion pressure, catecholamines, and angiotensin II) and extrarenal factors (e.g., sodium, chloride, and potassium).

Juxtaglomerular cells function as a baroreceptor-sensing device. Decreased renal artery pressure and kidney blood flow are sensed by these cells and stimulate secretion of renin. The juxtaglomerular apparatus also includes a group of specialized distal tubule cells

referred to collectively as the *macula densa*. A decrease in sodium and chloride delivered to the distal tubule stimulates renin release. Catecholamines increase renin release probably by directly stimulating sympathetic nerves on the afferent arterioles that, in turn, activate the juxtaglomerular cells. Decreased serum potassium and/or intracellular calcium is detected by the juxtaglomerular cells, resulting in renin secretion.

Renin catalyzes the conversion of angiotensinogen to angiotensin I in the blood. Angiotensin I is then converted to angiotensin II by angiotensin-converting enzyme (ACE). After binding to specific receptors (classified as either AT_1 or AT_2 subtypes), angiotensin II exerts biologic effects in several tissues. The AT_1 receptor is located in brain, kidney, myocardium, peripheral vasculature, and the adrenal glands. These receptors mediate most responses that are critical to cardiovascular and kidney function. The AT_2 receptor is located in adrenal medullary tissue, uterus, and brain. Stimulation of the AT_2 receptor does not influence BP regulation.

Circulating angiotensin II can elevate BP through pressor and volume effects. The pressor effects include direct vasoconstriction, stimulation of catecholamine release from the adrenal medulla, and centrally mediated increases in sympathetic nervous system activity. Angiotensin II also stimulates aldosterone synthesis from the adrenal cortex. This leads to sodium and water reabsorption that increases plasma volume, total peripheral resistance, and ultimately, BP. Clearly, any disturbance in the body that leads to activation of the RAAS could explain chronic hypertension.

The heart and brain contain a local RAAS. In the heart, angiotensin II is also generated by a second enzyme, angiotensin I convertase (human chymase). This enzyme is not blocked by ACE inhibition. Activation of the myocardial RAAS increases cardiac contractility and stimulates cardiac hypertrophy. In the brain, angiotensin II modulates the production and release of hypothalamic and pituitary hormones and enhances sympathetic outflow from the medulla oblongata.

Peripheral tissues can locally generate biologically active angiotensin peptides, which may explain the increased vascular resistance seen in hypertension. Some evidence suggests that angiotensin produced by local tissue may interact with other humoral regulators and endothelium-derived growth factors to stimulate vascular smooth muscle growth and metabolism. These angiotensin peptides may, in fact, instigate increased vascular resistance in low plasma renin forms of hypertension. Components of the tissue RAAS also may be responsible for the long-term hypertrophic abnormalities seen with hypertension (left ventricular hypertrophy, vascular smooth muscle hypertrophy, and glomerular hypertrophy).

NATRIURETIC HORMONE

Natriuretic hormone inhibits sodium and potassium ATPase and thus interferes with sodium transport across cell membranes. Inherited defects in the kidney's ability to eliminate sodium can cause an increased blood volume. A compensatory increase in the concentration of circulating natriuretic hormone theoretically could increase urinary excretion of sodium and water. However, this same hormone is also thought to block the active transport of sodium out of arteriolar smooth muscle cells. The increased intracellular concentration of sodium ultimately would increase vascular tone and BP.

INSULIN RESISTANCE AND HYPERINSULINEMIA

Evidence has linked insulin resistance and hyperinsulinemia with the development of hypertension, sometimes referred to as the *metabolic*

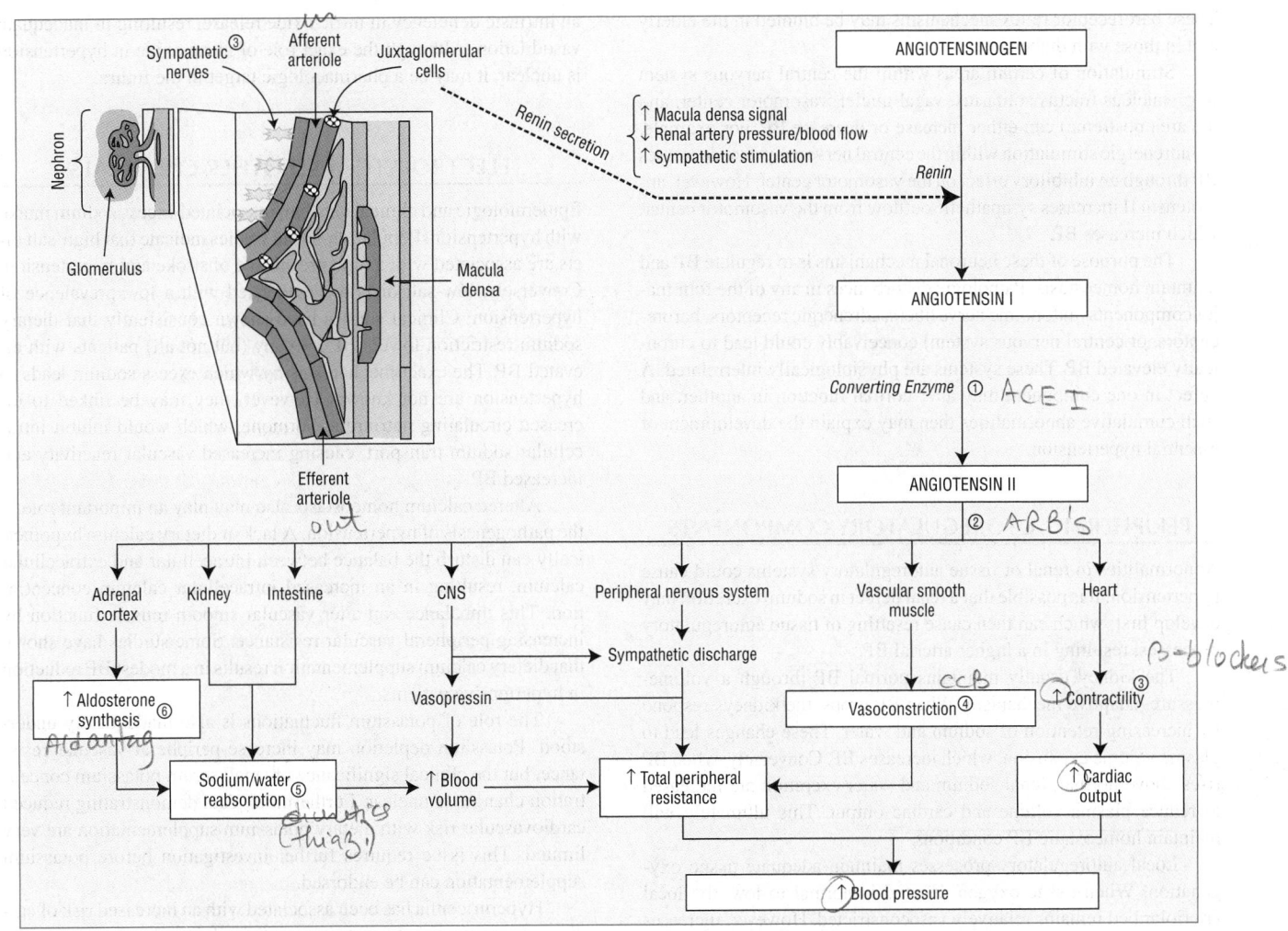

FIGURE 13–1. Diagram representing the renin-angiotensin-aldosterone system. The interrelationship between the kidney, angiotensin II, and regulation of blood pressure is depicted. Renin secretion from the juxtaglomerular cells in the afferent arteriole is one of the major regulators of this system. Sites of action for major antihypertensive agents are included (①, ACE inhibitors; ②, angiotensin II receptor blockers; ③, β-blockers; ④, calcium channel blockers; ⑤, diuretics; ⑥, aldosterone antagonists).

syndrome.[18] Hypothetically, increased insulin concentrations may lead to hypertension because of increased renal sodium retention and enhanced sympathetic nervous system activity. Moreover, insulin has growth hormone–like actions that can induce hypertrophy of vascular smooth muscle cells. Insulin also may elevate BP by increasing intracellular calcium, which leads to increased vascular resistance. The exact mechanism by which insulin resistance and hyperinsulinemia occur in hypertension is unknown. However, this association is strong because many of the criteria used to define this population (elevated blood pressure, obesity, dyslipidemia, and elevated blood glucose) are often present in hypertensive patients.[18]

NEURONAL REGULATION

The central and autonomic nervous systems are intricately involved in the regulation of arterial BP. A number of receptors that either enhance or inhibit norepinephrine release are located on the presynaptic surface of sympathetic terminals. The α and β presynaptic receptors play a role in negative and positive feedback to the norepinephrine-containing vesicles located near the neuronal ending. Stimulation

of presynaptic α-receptors (α_2) exerts a negative inhibition on norepinephrine release. Stimulation of presynaptic β-receptors facilitates further release of norepinephrine.

Sympathetic neuronal fibers located on the surface of effector cells innervate the α- and β-receptors. Stimulation of postsynaptic α-receptors (α_1) on arterioles and venules results in vasoconstriction. There are two types of postsynaptic β-receptors, β_1 and β_2. Both are present in all tissue innervated by the sympathetic nervous system. However, in some tissues, β_1-receptors predominate, and in other tissues, β_2-receptors predominate. Stimulation of β_1-receptors in the heart results in an increase in heart rate and contractility, whereas stimulation of β_2-receptors in the arterioles and venules causes vasodilation.

The baroreceptor reflex system is the major negative-feedback mechanism that controls sympathetic activity. Baroreceptors are nerve endings lying in the walls of large arteries, especially in the carotid arteries and aortic arch. Changes in arterial pressure rapidly activate baroreceptors, which then transmit impulses to the brain stem through the ninth cranial nerve and vagus nerves. In this reflex system, a decrease in arterial BP stimulates baroreceptors, causing reflex vasoconstriction and increased heart rate and force of cardiac contraction.

These baroreceptor reflex mechanisms may be blunted in the elderly and in those with diabetes.

Stimulation of certain areas within the central nervous system (e.g., nucleus tractus solitarius, vagal nuclei, vasomotor center, and the area postrema) can either increase or decrease BP. For example, α_2-adrenergic stimulation within the central nervous system decreases BP through an inhibitory effect on the vasomotor center. However, angiotensin II increases sympathetic outflow from the vasomotor center, which increases BP.

The purpose of these neuronal mechanisms is to regulate BP and maintain homeostasis. Pathologic disturbances in any of the four major components (autonomic nerve fibers, adrenergic receptors, baroreceptors, or central nervous system) conceivably could lead to chronically elevated BP. These systems are physiologically interrelated. A defect in one component may alter normal function in another, and such cumulative abnormalities then may explain the development of essential hypertension.

PERIPHERAL AUTOREGULATORY COMPONENTS

Abnormalities in renal or tissue autoregulatory systems could cause hypertension. It is possible that a renal defect in sodium excretion may develop first, which can then cause resetting of tissue autoregulatory processes, resulting in a higher arterial BP.

The kidney usually maintains normal BP through a volume-pressure–adaptive mechanism. When BP drops, the kidneys respond by increasing retention of sodium and water. These changes lead to plasma volume expansion, which increases BP. Conversely, when BP rises above normal, renal sodium and water excretion are increased to reduce plasma volume and cardiac output. This ultimately will maintain homeostatic BP conditions.

Local autoregulatory processes maintain adequate tissue oxygenation. When tissue oxygen demand is normal to low, the local arteriolar bed remains relatively vasoconstricted. However, increases in metabolic demand trigger arteriolar vasodilation that lowers peripheral vascular resistance and increases blood flow and oxygen delivery through autoregulation.

Intrinsic defects in these renal adaptive mechanisms could lead to plasma volume expansion and increased blood flow to peripheral tissues, even when BP is normal. Local tissue autoregulatory processes that vasoconstrict then would be activated to offset the increased blood flow. This effect would result in increased peripheral vascular resistance and, if sustained, also would result in thickening of the arteriolar walls. This pathophysiologic component is plausible because increased total peripheral vascular resistance is a common underlying finding in patients with essential hypertension.

VASCULAR ENDOTHELIAL MECHANISMS

Vascular endothelium and smooth muscle play important roles in regulating blood vessel tone and BP. These regulating functions are mediated through vasoactive substances that are synthesized by endothelial cells. It has been postulated that a deficiency in the local synthesis of vasodilating substances (e.g., prostacyclin and bradykinin) or excess vasoconstricting substances (e.g., angiotensin II and endothelin I) contribute to essential hypertension, atherosclerosis, and other diseases.

Nitric oxide is produced in the endothelium, relaxes the vascular epithelium, and is a very potent vasodilator. The nitric oxide system is an important regulator of arterial BP. Hypertensive patients may have an intrinsic deficiency in nitric oxide release, resulting in inadequate vasodilation. Although the exact role of nitric oxide in hypertension is unclear, it may be a pharmacologic target in the future.

ELECTROLYTES AND OTHER CHEMICALS

Epidemiologic and clinical data have associated excess sodium intake with hypertension. Population-based studies indicate that high-salt diets are associated with a high prevalence of stroke and hypertension. Conversely, low-salt diets are associated with a low prevalence of hypertension. Clinical studies have shown consistently that dietary sodium restriction lowers BP in many (but not all) patients with elevated BP. The exact mechanisms by which excess sodium leads to hypertension are not known. However, they may be linked to increased circulating natriuretic hormone, which would inhibit intracellular sodium transport, causing increased vascular reactivity and increased BP.

Altered calcium homeostasis also may play an important role in the pathogenesis of hypertension. A lack of dietary calcium hypothetically can disturb the balance between intracellular and extracellular calcium, resulting in an increased intracellular calcium concentration. This imbalance can alter vascular smooth muscle function by increasing peripheral vascular resistance. Some studies have shown that dietary calcium supplementation results in a modest BP reduction in hypertensive patients.

The role of potassium fluctuations is also inadequately understood. Potassium depletion may increase peripheral vascular resistance, but the clinical significance of small serum potassium concentration changes is unclear. Furthermore, data demonstrating reduced cardiovascular risk with dietary potassium supplementation are very limited. This issue requires further investigation before potassium supplementation can be endorsed.

Hyperuricemia has been associated with an increased risk of cardiovascular events in hypertensive patients but remains controversial because of inconsistent data. Uric acid has no physiologic function and is considered a biologic waste product. Therefore, there is no rational explanation describing why uric acid would cause cardiovascular harm. However, elevated uric acid may be viewed as a supplemental risk marker in hypertensive patients.

CLINICAL PRESENTATION

CLINICAL PRESENTATION OF HYPERTENSION

GENERAL

The patient may appear very healthy or may have the presence of additional cardiovascular risk factors:

- Age (≥55 years for men to 65 years for women)
- Diabetes mellitus
- Dyslipidemia (elevated low-density lipoprotein [LDL] cholesterol, total cholesterol or triglycerides; low high-density lipoprotein [HDL] cholesterol)
- Microalbuminuria
- Family history of premature cardiovascular disease
- Obesity (body mass index ≥ 30 kg/m^2)
- Physical inactivity
- Tobacco use

SYMPTOMS

- Most patients are asymptomatic

SIGNS

- Previous blood pressure values measured in the prehypertension or hypertension category

LABORATORY TESTS

The patient may have normal values and still have hypertension. However, some may have abnormal values consistent with either additional cardiovascular risk factors or hypertension-related damage.

- Blood urea nitrogen (BUN) and serum creatinine
- Fasting lipid panel
- Fasting blood glucose
- Serum potassium
- Urinalysis

OTHER DIAGNOSTIC TESTS

- 12-lead electrocardiogram (to detect LVH)
- Highly sensitive C-reactive protein (high concentrations are associated with increased cardiovascular risk)

TARGET-ORGAN DAMAGE

The patient may have a previous medical history or diagnostic findings that indicate the presence of hypertension-related target-organ damage:

- Brain (stroke, transient ischemic attack, dementia)
- Eyes (retinopathy)
- Heart (left ventricular hypertrophy, angina or prior myocardial infarction, prior coronary revascularization, heart failure)
- Kidney (chronic kidney disease)
- Peripheral vasculature (peripheral arterial disease)

DIAGNOSTIC CONSIDERATIONS

Hypertension is termed the "silent killer" because patients with essential hypertension are usually asymptomatic. The primary physical finding is elevated BP. The diagnosis of hypertension cannot be made based on one elevated BP measurement. The average of two or more measurements taken during two or more clinical encounters should be used to diagnose hypertension.[1] Thereafter, this BP average can be used to establish a diagnosis and then to classify the stage of hypertension present using Table 13–3.

MEASURING BLOOD PRESSURE

Sphygmomanometry

Indirect measurement of BP using a sphygmomanometer is a common routine medical screening tool that should be conducted at every health care encounter.[1] The appropriate procedure to measure BP has been described by the American Heart Association (AHA).[19] It is imperative that the measurement equipment (inflation cuff, stethoscope, manometer) meet certain national standards.[20] These standards use criteria to ensure maximum quality and precision with measurement.

The following stepwise technique is recommended[1,19]:

- Patients should refrain from smoking or caffeine ingestion for 30 minutes and be seated with the lower back supported in a chair and with their bare arm resting near heart level. Legs should be flat on the floor (not crossed). Measuring BP in the supine or standing position may be required under special circumstances (e.g., suspected orthostatic hypotension, volume depletion, or dehydration). The measurement environment should be relatively quiet and should provide privacy.
- Measurement should begin only after a 5-minute period of rest.
- A properly sized cuff (pediatric, small, regular, large, or extra large) should be used. Overestimating the actual BP can occur if the cuff is too small. The inflatable rubber bladder inside the cuff should encircle at least 80% of the arm, and the width of the cuff should be at least two-thirds the length of the upper arm.
- The palpatory method should be used to estimate the SBP:
  - Place the cuff on the upper arm, and attached it to the manometer (either a mercury or aneroid).
  - Close the inflation valve with the thumb and index finger, and inflate the cuff to 70 mm Hg, and then inflate in increments of 10 mm Hg by pumping the inflation bulb (as it is resting in the palm of your hand) with the last three fingers.
  - Simultaneously palpate the radial pulse with the first and second fingers of the opposite hand.
  - Note the pressure at which the radial pulse disappears; this is the estimated SBP.
  - Release pressure from the cuff by turning the valve counterclockwise.
- The bell (not the diaphragm) of the stethoscope should be placed on the skin of the antecubital fossa, directly over where the brachial artery is palpated. The stethoscope earpieces should be inserted appropriately. The valve should be closed with the cuff then inflated rapidly to about 30 mm Hg above the estimated SBP from the palpatory method. The value should be opened only slightly to release pressure at a rate of 2 to 3 mm Hg/s.
- The clinician should listen for Korotkoff sounds with the stethoscope. The first phase of Korotkoff sounds is the initial presence of clear tapping sounds. Note the pressure at the first recognition of these sounds. This is the SBP. As pressure continues to deflate, note the pressure when all sounds disappear (also known as the fifth Korotkoff phase). This is the DBP.
- A second measurement should be obtained after 2 minutes, and the average should be documented. If these values differ by more than 5 mm Hg, additional measurements should be collected and averaged.

In all instances, using the stethoscope bell rather than the diaphragm is recommended. Low-frequency Korotkoff sounds may not be heard clearly and accurately with the diaphragm. This is especially problematic in patients with faint or "distant" sounds.

Inaccuracies with indirect measurements result from inherent biologic variability of blood pressure, inaccuracies related to suboptimal technique, and the white coat effect.[21] BP varies with environmental temperature, the time of day and year, meals, physical activity, posture, smoking, and emotions.[8,19,22] Some patients have *white coat hypertension,* where BP values rise in a clinical setting but return to normal in nonclinical environments using home or ambulatory blood pressure measurements.[23] Interestingly, the rise in BP dissipates gradually over several hours after leaving the clinical setting. It may or may not be precipitated by other stresses in the patient's daily life. Aggressive treatment of white coat hypertension is controversial. However, patients with white coat hypertension may have increased cardiovascular risk compared with those without such BP changes.[24]

Several additional factors can result in erroneous BP measurements. *Pseudohypertension* is a falsely elevated BP measurement that is seen in elderly patients with a rigid, calcified brachial artery.[25] In these patients, the true arterial BP when measured directly intraarterially (the most accurate measurement of BP) is much lower than that measured using the indirect cuff method. The Osler's maneuver can be used to test for pseudohypertension. In this maneuver, the BP cuff is inflated above peak SBP. If the radial artery remains palpable, the patient has a positive Osler's maneuver (rigid artery), which indicates pseudohypertension.

Patients with an *auscultatory gap* may have either underestimated SBP or overestimated DBP measurements. In this situation, as the cuff pressure falls from the true SBP value, the Korotkoff sound may disappear (indicating a false DBP measurement), reappear (a false SBP measurement), and then disappear again at the true DBP value. This is often identified by using the palaptory method to estimate SBP and then inflating the cuff an additional 30 mm Hg above this estimate because the "gap" is usually less than 30 mm Hg. When an auscultatory gap is present, Korotkoff sounds usually are heard when pressure in the cuff first starts to decrease after inflation.

Patients with irregular ventricular rates (e.g., atrial fibrillation or atrial flutter) may have misleading BP values when measured indirectly. In this situation, SBP and DBP values may vary from one heartbeat to the next.

Ambulatory and Self Blood Pressure Monitoring

Twenty-four-hour ambulatory BP monitoring can document BP at frequent time intervals throughout the day.[23] Ambulatory BP values usually are lower than clinic-measured values because hypertensive patients have average values greater than 135/85 mm Hg during the day and greater than 120/80 mm Hg during sleep. Home BP measurements are collected by patients, preferably in the morning, using home monitoring devices. Either of these may be warranted in patients with suspected white coat hypertension (without hypertension-related target-organ damage) to differentiate white coat from essential hypertension.[1] Moreover, ambulatory BP monitoring may be helpful in patients with apparent drug resistance, hypotensive symptoms while on antihypertensive therapy, episodic hypertension, and autonomic dysfunction.[1]

Some data suggest that 24-hour and home BP measurements correlate better with cardiovascular risk than do conventional office-based measurements.[26,27] However, one controlled study found that ambulatory and self BP monitoring are complementary to conventional clinic-based measurements.[28] Limitations of these measurements that prohibit routine use of such technology include complexity of use, availability of devices, costs, and lack of prospective outcomes data describing normal ranges for these measurements. Although self-monitoring of BP at home is less complicated than ambulatory monitoring, patients may fail to record some high values and then actually may add lower "ghost" values that were never measured.[23]

CLINICAL EVALUATION

Frequently, the only sign of essential hypertension is elevated BP. The rest of the physical examination may be completely normal. However, a complete medical evaluation (a comprehensive medical history, physical examination, and laboratory and/or diagnostic tests) is recommended after diagnosis to (1) identify secondary causes, (2) identify other cardiovascular risk factors or comorbid conditions that may define prognosis and/or guide therapy, and (3) assess for the presence or absence of hypertension-associated target-organ damage.[1] All hypertensive patients should have the following measured prior to initiating therapy: 12-lead electrocardiogram; urinalysis; blood glucose and hematocrit; serum potassium, creatinine (with estimated glomerular filtration rate [GFR]), and calcium; and a fasting lipid panel.[1] A urinary albumin excretion or albumin/creatinine ratio is considered an optional test.

SECONDARY CAUSES

The most common secondary causes of hypertension are listed in Table 13–1. A complete medical evaluation may provide clues for diagnosing secondary hypertension. For example, patients with coarctation of the aorta may have diminished or even absent femoral pulses, and patients with renal artery stenosis may have an abdominal systolic-diastolic bruit.

Patients with secondary hypertension may complain of symptoms suggestive of the underlying disorder, but some are asymptomatic. Patients with pheochromocytoma may have a history of paroxysmal headaches, sweating, tachycardia, and palpitations. Over half these patients suffer from episodes of orthostatic hypotension. In primary aldosteronism, symptoms related to the hypokalemia usually include muscle cramps and muscle weakness. Patients with Cushing's syndrome may complain of weight gain, polyuria, edema, menstrual irregularities, recurrent acne, or muscular weakness and have several classic physical features (e.g., moon face, buffalo hump, hirsutism, and abdominal striae).

Routine laboratory tests may help to identify secondary hypertension. Baseline hypokalemia may suggest mineralocorticoid-induced hypertension. Protein, blood cells, and casts in the urine may indicate renovascular disease. Some laboratory tests are used specifically to diagnose secondary hypertension. These include: plasma norepinephrine and urinary metanephrine concentrations for pheochromocytoma, plasma and urinary aldosterone concentrations for primary aldosteronism, and plasma renin activity, captopril stimulation test, renal vein renins, and renal artery angiography for renovascular disease.

Certain medications and herbal products can result in drug-induced hypertension. The most common of these are listed in Table 13–1. For some patients, the addition of these agents can be the cause of hypertension or can exacerbate underlying hypertension. Identifying a temporal relationship between starting the suspected agent and developing elevated BP is most suggestive of drug-induced BP elevation.

NATURAL COURSE OF THE DISEASE

Essential hypertension usually is preceded by elevated BP values that are in the prehypertension category. BP values may fluctuate between elevated and normal values for an extended period of time. These changes may begin as early as the second decade of life. During this stage, many patients have a hyperdynamic circulation with increased cardiac output and normal or even low peripheral vascular resistance. As the disease progresses, peripheral vascular resistance increases, and BP elevation is sustained to the point where essential hypertension is diagnosed.

TARGET-ORGAN DAMAGE

As hypertension progresses, target-organ damage may appear. The primary organs involved are the eye, brain, heart, kidneys, and peripheral blood vessels. Cardiovascular events, cerebrovascular accidents, and kidney failure are the primary causes of morbidity and mortality in patients with hypertension. These clinical events are often preceded by the development of hypertension-association target-organ damage (see Clinical Presentation above). The probability of morbidity and mortality in hypertension is directly correlated with the severity of BP elevation.

Hypertension accelerates atherosclerosis and stimulates left ventricular and vascular hypertrophy. These pathologic changes are thought to be secondary to both a chronic pressure overload and a variety of nonhemodynamic stimuli. Some of the nonhemodynamic disturbances that have been implicated in these effects include the adrenergic system, RAAS, increased synthesis and secretion of endothelin I, and a decreased production of prostacyclin and nitric oxide. Accelerated atherogenesis in hypertension is accompanied by proliferation of smooth muscle cells, lipid infiltration into the vascular endothelium, and an enhancement of vascular calcium accumulation.

Cerebrovascular disease is a consequence of hypertension. A neurologic assessment can detect either gross neurologic deficits or a slight hemiparesis with some incoordination and hyperreflexia that are indicative of cerebrovascular disease. Stroke can result from lacunar infarcts caused by thrombotic occlusion of small vessels or intracerebral hemorrhage resulting from ruptured microaneurysms. Transient ischemic attacks secondary to atherosclerotic disease in the carotid arteries are common in hypertensive individuals.

Retinopathies can occur in hypertension and may manifest as a variety of different findings. A funduscopic examination can detect hypertensive retinopathy, which manifests as arteriolar narrowing, focal arteriolar constrictions, arteriovenous crossing changes (nicking), retinal hemorrhages and exudates, and disc edema. Accelerated arteriosclerosis, a long-term consequence of essential hypertension, can cause nonspecific changes such as increased light reflex, increased tortuosity of vessels, and arteriovenous nicking. Focal arteriolar narrowing, retinal infarcts, and flame-shaped hemorrhages usually are suggestive of an accelerated or malignant phase of hypertension. Papilledema is a swelling of the optic disc and is caused by a breakdown in autoregulation of capillary blood flow in the presence of high pressure. It is usually only present in very severe hypertension or in hypertensive emergencies.

Heart disease is the most well-identified form of target-organ damage. A thorough cardiac and pulmonary examination can identify cardiopulmonary abnormalities. Clinical manifestations include left ventricular hypertrophy, coronary heart disease (e.g., angina, prior myocardial infarction, and prior coronary revascularization), and heart failure. These complications may lead to cardiac arrhythmias, angina, myocardial infarction, and sudden death. Coronary heart disease and associated cardiac events are the most common causes of death in hypertensive patients.

The kidney damage caused by hypertension is characterized pathologically by hyaline arteriosclerosis, hyperplastic arteriosclerosis, arteriolar hypertrophy, fibrinoid necrosis, and atheroma of the major renal arteries. Glomerular hyperfiltration and intraglomerular hypertension are early stages of hypertensive nephropathy. Microalbuminuria is followed by a gradual decline in renal function. The primary renal complication in hypertension is nephrosclerosis, which is secondary to arteriosclerosis. Atheromatous disease of a major renal artery may give rise to renal artery stenosis. Although overt kidney failure is an uncommon complication of essential hypertension, it is an important cause of end-stage kidney disease, especially in African-Americans, Hispanics, and Native Americans. It is not completely understood why these ethnic groups are more at risk for kidney decline than other races.

The peripheral vasculature is considered a target organ. Physical examination of the systemic vasculature can detect evidence of atherosclerosis, which may present as bruits (in the aortic, abdominal, and peripheral arteries), distended veins, diminished or absent peripheral arterial pulses, or lower extremity edema. Peripheral arterial disease is a clinical condition that can result from atherosclerosis, which is accelerated in hypertension. Other cardiovascular risk factors (e.g., smoking) can increase the likelihood of peripheral arterial disease as well as all other forms of target-organ damage.

▶ TREATMENT: Hypertension

▦ DESIRED OUTCOMES

▦ OVERALL GOAL OF THERAPY

3 The overall goal of treating hypertension is to reduce hypertension-associated morbidity and mortality.[1] This morbidity and mortality are related to target-organ damage (e.g., cardiovascular events, cerebrovascular events, heart failure, and kidney disease). Reducing risk remains the primary purpose of hypertension therapy, and the choice of drug therapy is influenced significantly by evidence demonstrating such risk reduction.

▦ SURROGATE GOAL OF THERAPY

4 Treating hypertensive patients to achieve a desired target BP value is simply a surrogate goal of therapy. Reducing BP to target does not guarantee that target-organ damage will not occur. However, attaining target BP values is associated with a lower risk of cardiovascular disease and target-organ damage.[1,16,29,30] Targeting a goal BP value is a tool that clinicians can use easily to evaluate response to therapy and is the primary method used to determine the need for titration and regimen modification.

Most patients have a goal BP of less than 140/90 mm Hg. However, this goal is lowered to less than 130/80 mm Hg for patients with diabetes or chronic kidney disease.

> ### GOAL BP VALUES RECOMMENDED BY THE JNC7
>
> - Most patients < 140/90 mm Hg
> - Patients with diabetes < 130/80 mm Hg
> - Patients with chronic kidney disease < 130/80 mm Hg (estimated GFR < 60 mL/min, serum creatinine > 1.3 mg/dL in women or > 1.5 mg/dL in men, or albuminuria > 300 mg/day or ≥ 200 mg/g creatinine)

Some clinicians advocate attaining BP goal values that are lower than what is recommended as a modality to further reduce cardiovascular risk following the myth that "lower is better." Contrary to this, a J-curve hypothesis where lowering BP too much might increase the risk of cardiovascular events has been described.[31,32] However, these

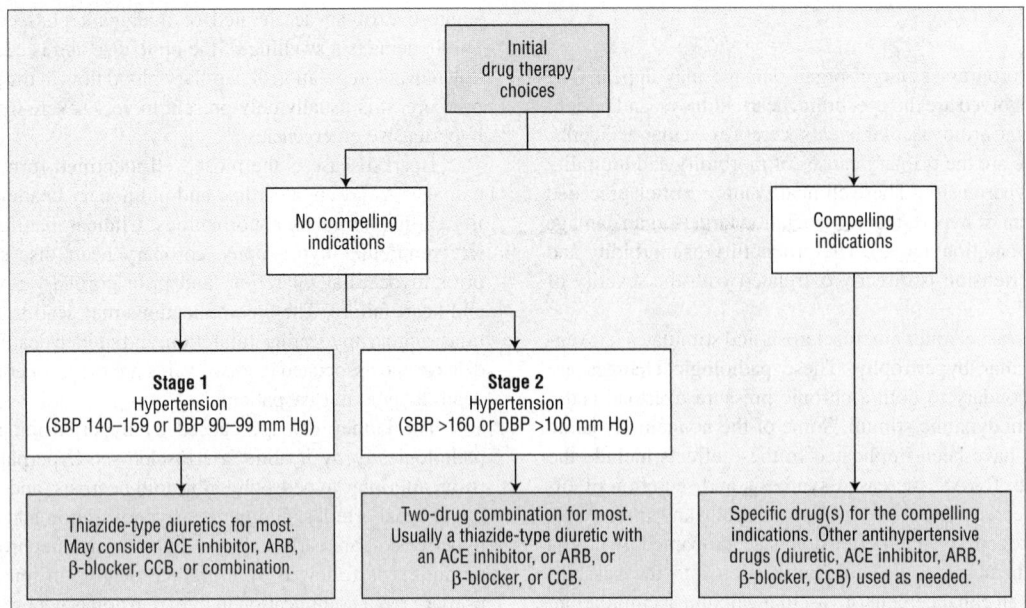

FIGURE 13–2. Algorithm for treatment of hypertension when patients are not at their goal blood pressure. *(Adapted from the JNC7.[1])*

data are based on observational studies and cannot establish a cause-and-effect relationship owing to confounding variables.

Lower-goal BP values have been evaluated prospectively in the Hypertension Optimal Treatment (HOT) trial.[29] In this study, over 18,700 patients were randomized to target DBP values of 90, 85, or 80 mm Hg or less. Although the actual DBP values achieved were 85.2, 83.2, and 81.1 mm Hg, respectively, the risk of major cardiovascular events was the lowest with a BP of 139/83 mm Hg, and lowest risk of stroke was with a BP of 142/80 mm Hg. Risk of events in subjects with either diabetes or ischemic heart disease was lowest at DBP values of less than 80 mm Hg. No J-curve relationship was seen. The HOT trial results provide evidence that support the JNC recommended goal value of less than 140/90 mm Hg for most patients and the more aggressive goal of less than 130/80 mm Hg in patients with diabetes.

GENERAL APPROACH TO TREATMENT

Although hypertension is one of the most common medical conditions, BP control rates are poor. Many hypertensive patients are at goal DBP values but continue to have elevated SBP values. It has been estimated that of the hypertensive population that is treated yet not controlled, 76.9% have an SBP greater than or equal to 140 mm Hg with DBP values less than 90 mm Hg.[33] For most hypertensive patients, attaining the SBP goal almost always ensures achievement of the DBP goal. When coupled with the fact that SBP is a better predictor of cardiovascular risk than DBP, SBP must be used as the primary clinical marker of disease control in hypertension.

After a definitive diagnosis of hypertension is made, patients should be placed on both lifestyle modifications and drug therapy concurrently. Lifestyle modification alone is considered appropriate therapy for patients with prehypertension. However, lifestyle modifications alone are not considered adequate for patients with hypertension or patients with BP goals of less than 130/80 mm Hg (those with diabetes and chronic kidney disease) who have BP values above their goal.

The choice of initial drug therapy depends on the degree of BP elevation and the presence of compelling indications (discussed later). Most patients with stage 1 hypertension should be treated initially with a thiazide-type diuretic. For most patients with more severe BP elevation (stage 2 hypertension), combination drug therapy, with one of the agents preferably being a thiazide type-diuretic, is recommended. This general approach is outlined in Fig. 13–2. There are six compelling indications where specific antihypertensive drug classes have shown evidence of unique benefits (Fig. 13–3).

NONPHARMACOLOGIC THERAPY

All patients with prehypertension and hypertension should be prescribed lifestyle modifications. Modifications that have been shown to lower BP are listed in Table 13–4. These approaches are recommended by the JNC7[1] and provide small to moderate reductions in SBP. Aside from lowering BP in patients with known hypertension, lifestyle modification can decrease the progression to hypertension in patients with prehypertension BP values.[34] In a number of hypertensive patients with relatively good BP control while on single antihypertensive drug therapy, sodium reduction and weight loss may allow withdrawal of drug therapy.[35,36]

A sensible dietary program is one that is designed to reduce weight gradually for overweight and obese patients and one that restricts sodium intake with only moderate alcohol consumption. Successful implementation of dietary lifestyle modifications by clinicians requires aggressive promotion through reasonable patient education, encouragement, and continued reinforcement. Patients may better understand the rationale for dietary intervention in hypertension if they are provided the following observations and facts:

1. Hypertension is two to three times more prevalent in overweight as compared with lean persons.
2. Over 60% of hypertensive persons are overweight.

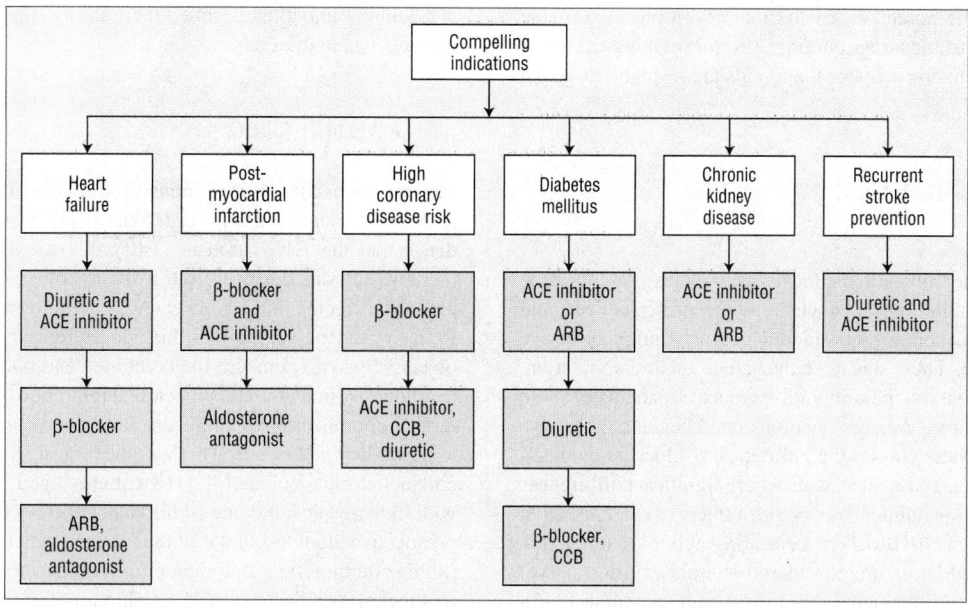

FIGURE 13–3. Compelling indications for individual drug classes. Compelling indications for specific drugs are evidenced-based recommendations from outcome studies or existing clinical guidelines. The order of drug therapies serves only as a general guidance that should be balanced with clinical judgment and patient response. Blood pressure control should be managed concurrently with the compelling indication. *(Adapted from the JNC7.[1])*

3. Weight loss, even as little as 10 pounds, can decrease BP significantly in hypertensive overweight individuals.[37]
4. Abdominal obesity is associated with the metabolic syndrome, which is a precursor to hypertension and insulin-resistance syndrome that may progress to type 2 diabetes, dyslipidemia, and ultimately, cardiovascular disease.[18]
5. Diets rich in fruits and vegetables and low in saturated fat have been shown to lower BP in hypertensive individuals.[38,39]
6. Although some hypertensive patients are not salt-sensitive, most people experience some degree of SBP reduction with sodium restriction.[40,41]

The DASH eating plan is a diet that is rich in fruits, vegetables, and low-fat dairy products with a reduced content of saturated and total fat. It is advocated by the JNC7 as a reasonable and feasible diet that is known to lower BP. The recommended restriction is less than 2.4 g (100 mEq) sodium per day. Patients should be aware of the multiple sources of dietary sodium (e.g., processed meats, soups, and table salt) so that they may follow this restriction. Excessive alcohol use can either cause or worsen hypertension. Hypertensive patients who drink alcoholic beverages should restrict their daily intake (see Table 13–4). Patients should be counseled about how much 80-proof whiskey, wine, and beer servings correlate with a drink equivalent.

Carefully designed programs of physical activity can lower BP. Regular aerobic exercise for at least 30 minutes a day most days of the week is ideal for most patients. Studies have shown that aerobic exercise, such as jogging, swimming, walking, and bicycling, can reduce BP. These benefits can occur even in the absence of weight loss. Patients should consult their physicians before starting an exercise program, especially those with target-organ disease.

Cigarette smoking is a major independent, modifiable risk factor for cardiovascular disease. Hypertensive patients who smoke should be thoroughly counseled regarding the additional risks that smoking

TABLE 13–4. Lifestyle Modifications to Prevent and Manage Hypertension

Modification	Recommendation	Approximate Systolic Blood Pressure Reduction (mm Hg)[a]
Weight reduction	Maintain normal body weight (body mass index, 18.5–24.9 kg/m^2)	5–20 per 10-kg weight loss
Adopt DASH eating plan	Consume a diet rich in fruits, vegetables, and low-fat dairy products with a reduced content of saturated and total fat	8–14
Dietary sodium restriction	Reduce daily dietary sodium intake to less than or equal to 100 mEq (2.4 g sodium or 6 g sodium chloride)	2–8
Physical activity	Regular aerobic physical activity (at least 30 minutes/day, most days of the week)	4–9
Moderate alcohol consumption	Limit consumption to less than or equal to 2 drinks/day (1 oz or 30 mL ethanol [e.g., 24 oz beer, 10 oz wine, 3 oz 80-proof whiskey] in most men and less than or equal to 1 drink/day in women and lighter-weight persons)	2–4

[a] Effects of implementing these modifications are time- and dose-dependent and could be greater for some patients.

incurs. Moreover, the potential benefits that cessation can provide should be explained to encourage quitting. Several smoking-cessation programs, pharmacotherapy options, and aids are available to assist patients.

PHARMACOLOGIC THERAPY

There are nine different antihypertensive drug classes. Diuretics, β-blockers, ACE inhibitors, angiotensin II receptor blockers, and calcium channel blockers are considered primary antihypertensive agents (Table 13–5). These agents, either alone or in combination, should be used to treat the majority of hypertensive patients because evidence from outcomes data have demonstrated benefits with these classes. Several of these classes (i.e., diuretics, β-blockers, and calcium channel blockers) have subclasses where significant differences in mechanism of action, clinical use, or side effects or evidence from outcomes studies exist. α-Blockers, central α_2-agonists, adrenergic inhibitors, and vasodilators are considered alternative drug classes that may be used in select patients after primary agents (Table 13–6).

Evidence-based medicine is a conscientious, explicit, and judicious use of current best evidence to make decisions about the care of individual patients.[42] Evidence-based practice in hypertension involves selecting specific agents based on outcomes data demonstrating a reduction in hypertension-associated target-organ damage or cardiovascular morbidity and mortality. Scientific evidence demonstrating simply BP lowering, tolerability, or costs never should be the sole justification for selecting drug therapy. When considering these factors, the most useful agents are diuretics, ACE inhibitors, angiotensin II receptor blockers, β-blockers, and calcium channel blockers. The JNC7 drug therapy recommendations are discussed throughout this section and are founded based on evidence-based medicine principles.

FIRST-LINE TREATMENT FOR MOST PATIENTS

JNC7 guidelines recommend thiazide-type diuretics whenever possible as first-line therapy for most patients.[1] Figure 13–2 displays the algorithm for the treatment of hypertension. This recommendation is specifically for those without compelling indications and is based on the best available evidence demonstrating reductions in morbidity and mortality. However, diuretics are also useful agents in hypertensive patients with compelling indications, but they are not always the first agent recommended based on the compelling indication present.

Three landmark placebo-controlled clinical trials have established the benefits of both hypertension treatment and diuretic therapy. The Systolic Hypertension in the Elderly Program (SHEP),[12] the Swedish Trial in Old Patients with Hypertension (STOP-Hypertension),[13] and the Medical Research Council (MRC) trial[14] showed significant reductions in stroke, myocardial infarction, and all-cause cardiovascular disease and mortality with thiazide diuretic–based therapy versus placebo. These trials allowed for β-blockers as add-on therapy for BP control. Newer agents (i.e., ACE inhibitors, angiotensin II receptor blockers [ARBs], and calcium channel blockers [CCBs]) were not available at the time of these studies. However, subsequent clinical trials have compared these newer antihypertensive agents (ACE inhibitors, ARBs, and CCBs) to diuretics.[43–48] These data show similar effects, but most trials used a prospective, open-label, blinded end point (PROBE) study methodology that is not double-blinded and limited their ability to prove equivalence of newer drugs to diuretics.

The ALLHAT Study[46]

The results of the Antihypertensive and Lipid-Lowering Treatment to Prevent Heart Attack Trial (ALLHAT) was the deciding evidence that the JNC7 used to justify thiazide diuretics as first-line therapy.[46] It was designed to test the hypothesis that newer antihypertensive agents (an α-blocker, ACE inhibitor, and dihydropyridine CCB) would be superior to thiazide diuretic therapy. The primary objective was to compare the combined end point of fatal coronary heart disease and nonfatal myocardial infarction. Other hypertension-related complications (e.g., heart failure and stroke) were evaluated as secondary end points. This was the largest hypertension trial ever conducted and included 42,418 patients aged 55 years and older with hypertension and one additional cardiovascular risk factor. This prospective, double-blind trial randomized patients to chlorthalidone (a thiazide diuretic), amlodipine (dihydropyridine CCB), doxazosin (α-blocker), or lisinopril (ACE inhibitor) for a mean follow-up of 4.9 years.

The doxazosin arm was terminated early when a significantly higher risk of heart failure compared with chlorthalidone was observed.[49] The other arms were continued as scheduled, and no significant differences in the primary end point were seen between chlorthalidone and either lisinopril or amlodipine. However, chlorthalidone had statistically fewer secondary end points than amlodipine (heart failure) and lisinopril (combined cardiovascular disease, heart failure, and stroke). The study conclusions were that chlorthalidone was superior in preventing one or more major forms of cardiovascular disease and was less expensive than amlodipine and lisinopril.

The ALLHAT was double-blinded and provided the most scientific rigor when compared with other comparative trials that were open label. While the JNC7 recommendations follow the ALLHAT results, the 2003 European Society of Hypertension/European Society of Cardiology guidelines for the management of arterial hypertension do not support thiazide diuretics over other primary antihypertensive classes.[50] These guidelines are founded on the principle that target-organ disease and cardiovascular risk reduction are functions of BP control that are largely independent of specific drug(s).[50] These guidelines criticize the ALLHAT, stating limitations such as lower BP values (1 to 4 mm Hg) with chlorthalidone versus other agents, especially in African-Americans; β-blockers, clonidine, and reserpine as unrealistic add-on therapies; and an overreliance on the end point of heart failure that was not systematically evaluated throughout the study.

ALLHAT was designed as a superiority study with the hypothesis that amlodipine, doxazosin, and lisinopril would be better than chlorthalidone.[51] It did not prove this hypothesis because the primary end point was not different among chlorthalidone, amlodipine, and lisinopril. Therefore, thiazides remain unsurpassed in their ability to reduce hypertension-related morbidity and mortality. A meta-analysis in 2003 supports this statement. In this analysis of 42 clinical trials representing 192,478 patients, low-dose diuretics were found to be the most effective first-line agent for preventing cardiovascular mortality.[52] The preponderance of evidence supports the JNC7 recommendation of using a thiazide-type diuretic in most patients unless there are contraindications or a compelling indication for another agent is present. Since most patients require two or more agents to control BP, a thiazide diuretic should be one of these agents unless contraindicated.

TABLE 13–5. Primary Antihypertensive Agents

Class	Subclass	Drug (Brand Name)	Usual Dose Range, mg/day	Daily Frequency	Comments
Diuretics	Thiazides	Chlorthalidone (Hygroton)	6.25–25	1	Dose in the morning to avoid nocturnal diuresis; thiazides are more effective antihypertensives than loop diuretics except in patients with severely decreased glomerular filtration rate (Estimated creatinine clearance < 30 mL/min); use usual doses to avoid adverse metabolic effects; hydrochlorothiazide and chlorthalidone are generally preferred, with 25 mg/day generally considered the maximum effective dose; chlorthalidone is nearly twice as potent as hydrochlorothiazide; have additional benefits in osteoporosis; may require additional monitoring in patients with a history of gout or hyponatremia
		Hydrochlorothiazide (Esidrix, HydroDiuril, Microzide, Oretic)	12.5–50	1	
		Indapamide (Lozol)	1.25–2.5	1	
		Metolazone (Mykrox)	0.5	1	
		Metolazone (Zaroxolyn)	2.5	1	
	Loops	Bumetanide (Bumex)	0.5–4	2	Dose in the morning and afternoon to avoid nocturnal diuresis; higher doses may be needed for patients with severely decreased glomerular filtration rate or heart failure
		Furosemide (Lasix)	20–80	2	
		Torsemide (Demadex)	5	1	
	Potassium sparing	Amiloride (Midamor)	5–10	1 or 2	Dose in the morning or afternoon to avoid nocturnal diuresis; weak diuretics that are generally used in combination with thiazide diuretics to minimize hypokalemia; since hypokalemia from low-dose thiazide diuretics is uncommon, these agents should generally be reserved for patients experiencing diuretic-induced hypokalemia; avoid in patients with chronic kidney disease (estimated creatinine clearance < 30 mL/min); may cause hyperkalemia, especially in combination with an ACE inhibitor, angiotensin-receptor blocker, or potassium supplements
		Amiloride/ hydrochlorothiazide (Moduretic)	5–10/50–100	1	
		Triamterene (Dyrenium)	50–100	1 or 2	
		Triamterene/ hydrochlorothiazide (Dyazide)	37.5–75/25–50	1	
	Aldosterone Antagonists	Eplerenone (Inspra)	50–100	1 or 2	Dose in the morning or afternoon to avoid nocturnal diuresis; eplerenone contraindicated in patients with an estimated creatinine clearance < 50 mL/min, elevated serum creatinine (> 1.8 mg/dL in women, > 2 mg/dL in men), and type 2 diabetes with microalbuminuria; avoid spironolactone in patients with chronic kidney disease (estimated creatinine clearance < 30 mL/min); may cause hyperkalemia, especially in combination with an ACE inhibitor, angiotensin-receptor blocker or potassium supplements
		Spironolactone (Aldactone)	25–50	1 or 2	
		Spironolactone/ hydrochlorothiazide (Aldactazide)	25–50/25–50	1	
Angiotensin-converting enzyme inhibitors		Benazepril (Lotensin)	10–40	1 or 2	Starting dose should be reduced 50% in patients who are on a diuretic, are volume depleted, or are very elderly due to risks of hypotension; may cause hyperkalemia in patients with chronic kidney disease or in those receiving potassium-sparing diuretics, aldosterone antagonists, or angiotensin receptor blockers; can cause acute kidney failure in patients with severe bilateral renal artery stenosis or severe stenosis in artery to solitary kidney; do not use in pregnancy or in patients with a history of angioedema
		Captopril (Capoten)	12.5–150	2 or 3	
		Enalapril (Vasotec)	5–40	1 or 2	
		Fosinopril (Monopril)	10–40	1	
		Lisinopril (Prinivil, Zestril)	10–40	1	
		Moexipril (Univasc)	7.5–30	1 or 2	
		Perindopril (Aceon)	4–16	1	
		Quinapril (Accupril)	10–80	1 or 2	
		Ramipril (Altace)	2.5–10	1 or 2	
		Trandolapril (Mavik)	1–4	1	
Angiotensin II receptor blockers		Candesartan (Atacand)	8–32	1 or 2	Starting dose should be reduced 50% in patients who are on a diuretic, are volume depleted, or are very elderly due to risks of hypotension; may cause hyperkalemia in patients with chronic kidney disease or in those receiving potassium-sparing diuretics, aldosterone antagonists, or ACE inhibitors; can cause acute kidney failure in patients with severe bilateral renal artery stenosis or severe stenosis in artery to solitary kidney; do not cause a drug cough like ACE inhibitors may; do not use in pregnancy
		Eprosartan (Teveten)	600–800	1 or 2	
		Irbesartan (Avapro)	150–300	1	
		Losartan (Cozaar)	50–100	1 or 2	
		Olmesartan (Benicar)	20–40	1	
		Telmisartan (Micardis)	20–80	1	
		Valsartan (Diovan)	80–320	1	
β-Blockers	Cardioselective	Atenolol (Tenormin)	25–100	1	Abrupt discontinuation may cause rebound hypertension; inhibit β_1 receptors at low to moderate dose, higher doses also block β_2 receptors; may exacerbate asthma when selectivity is lost; have additional benefits in patients with atrial tachyarrhythmia or preoperative hypertension
		Betaxolol (Kerlone)	5–20	1	
		Bisoprolol (Zebeta)	2.5–10	1	
		Metoprolol (Lopressor)	50–200	2	
		Metoprolol extended release (Toprol XL)	50–200	1	

TABLE 13–5. (Continued)

Class	Subclass	Drug (Brand Name)	Usual Dose Range, mg/day	Daily Frequency	Comments
	Nonselective	Nadolol (Corgard)	40–120	1	Abrupt discontinuation may cause rebound hypertension; inhibit β_1 and β_2 receptors at all doses; can exacerbate asthma; have additional benefits in patients with essential tremor, migraine headache, thyrotoxicosis
		Propranolol (Inderal)	160–480	2	
		Propranolol long-acting (Inderal LA, InnoPran XL)	80–320	1	
		Timolol (Blocadren)	10–40	1	
	Intrinsic sympathomimetic activity	Acebutolol (Sectral)	200–800	2	Abrupt discontinuation may cause rebound hypertension; partially stimulate β-receptors while blocking against additional stimulation; no clear advantage for these agents except in patients with bradycardia, who must receive a β-blocker; contraindicated in patients post-myocardial infarction; produce fewer or no metabolic side effects, but they may not be as cardioprotective as other β-blockers
		Carteolol (Cartrol)	2.5–10	1	
		Penbutolol (Levatol)	10–40	1	
		Pindolol (Visken)	10–60	2	
	Mixed α- and β-blockers	Carvedilol (Coreg)	12.5–50	2	Abrupt discontinuation may cause rebound hypertension; additional α blockade produces more orthostatic hypotension
		Labetolol (Normodyne, Trandate)	200–800	2	
Calcium channel blockers	Dihydropyridines	Amlodipine (Norvasc)	2.5–10	1	Short-acting dihydropyridines should be avoided, especially immediate-release nifedipine and nicardipine; dihydropyridines are more potent peripheral vasodilators than nondihydropyridines and may cause more reflex sympathetic discharge (tachycardia), dizziness, headache, flushing, and peripheral edema; have additional benefits in Raynaud's syndrome
		Felodipine (Plendil)	5–20	1	
		Isradipine (DynaCirc)	5–10	2	
		Isradipine SR (DynaCirc SR)	5–20	1	
		Nicardipine sustained release (Cardene SR)	60–120	2	
		Nifedipine long-acting (Adalat CC, Procardia XL)	30–90	1	
		Nisoldipine (Sular)	10–40	1	
	Non-Dihydropyridines	Diltiazem sustained-release (Cardizem SR)	180–360	2	Extended-release products are preferred for hypertension; these agents block slow channels in the heart and reduce heart rate; may produce heart block; these products are not AB rated as interchangeable on a equipotent mg-per-mg basis due to different release mechanisms and different bioavailability parameters; Cardizem LA, Covera HS, and Verelan PM have delayed drug release for several hours after dosing, when dosed in the evening can provide chronotherapeutic drug delivery starting shortly before patients awake from sleep; have additional benefits in patients with atrial tachyarrhythmia
		Diltiazem sustained-release (Cardizem CD, Cartia XT, Dilacor XR, Diltia XT, Tiazac, Taztia XT)	120–480	1	
		Diltiazem extended-release (Cardizem LA)	120–540	1 (morning or evening)	
		Verapamil sustained-release (Calan SR, Isoptin SR, Verelan)	180–480	1 or 2	
		Verapamil controlled-onset extended-release (Covera HS)	180–420	1 (in the evening)	
		Verapamil chronotherapeutic oral drug absorption system (Verelan PM)	100–400	1 (in the evening)	

COMPELLING INDICATIONS

The JNC7 report identifies six compelling indications. *Compelling indications* represent specific comorbid conditions where evidence from clinical trials supports using specific antihypertensive classes to treat both the compelling indication and hypertension. Drug therapy recommendations for compelling indications are either in combination with or in place of a thiazide diuretic (see Fig. 13–3). Data from these clinical trials have demonstrated reduction in morbidity and/or mortality that justify use in hypertensive

TABLE 13–6. Alternative Antihypertensive Agents

Class	Drug (Brand Name)	Usual Dose Range, mg/day	Daily Frequency	Comments
α₁-Blockers	Doxazosin (Cardura)	1–8	1	First dose should be given at bedtime; counsel patients to rise from sitting or laying down slowly to minimize risk of orthostatic hypotension; have additional benefits in men with benign prostatic hyperplasia
	Prazosin (Minipress)	2–20	2 or 3	
	Terazosin (Hytrin)	1–20	1 or 2	
Central α₂-agonists	Clonidine (Catapres)	0.1–0.8	2	Abrupt discontinuation may cause rebound hypertension; most effective if used with a diuretic to diminish fluid retention; clonidine patch is replaced once per week
	Clonidine patch (Catapres-TTS)	0.1–0.3	1 weekly	
	Methyldopa (Aldomet)	250–1000	2	
Peripheral adrenergic antagonist	Reserpine (generic only)	0.05–0.25	1	A very useful agent that has been used in many of the major clinical trials; should be used with a diuretic to diminish fluid retention
Direct arterial vasodilators	Minoxidil (Loniten)	10–40	1 or 2	Should be used with diuretic and β-blocker to diminish fluid retention and reflex tachycardia
	Hydralazine (Apresoline)	20–100	2 to 4	

patients with such a compelling indication. Some compelling indications have recommendations provided by other national treatment guidelines that are complimentary to the JNC7 guidelines.

Heart Failure[53]

Five drug classes are listed as compelling indications for heart failure. These recommendations specifically refer to systolic heart failure, where the primary physiologic abnormality is decreased cardiac contractility. ACE inhibitors are recommended as the first drugs of choice based on numerous outcome studies showing reduced morbidity and mortality.[53] Diuretics are also a part of first-line therapy because they provide symptomatic relief of edema by inducing diuresis. Loop diuretics often are needed, especially in patients with more advanced systolic heart failure. Evidence from clinical trials has shown that ACE inhibitors significantly modify disease progression by reducing morbidity and mortality. Although systolic heart failure was the primary disease in these studies, ACE inhibitor therapy also will control BP in patients with heart failure and hypertension. ACE inhibitors should be started with low doses in patients with heart failure, especially those in acute exacerbation. Heart failure induces a compensatory high-renin condition, and starting ACE inhibitors under this circumstance can cause a pronounced first-dose effect and possible orthostatic hypotension.

β-Blocker therapy is appropriate to further modify disease in systolic heart failure. In patients on a standard regimen of a diuretic and ACE inhibitor, β-blockers have been shown to reduce morbidity and mortality.[54,55] It is of paramount importance that β-blockers be dosed appropriately because of the risk of inducing an acute exacerbation of heart failure. They must be started in very low doses, doses much lower than those used to treat hypertension, and titrated slowly to high doses based on tolerability.

After diuretics, ACE inhibitors and β-blockers (collectively considered standard therapy), other agents may be added to further reduce cardiovascular morbidity and mortality and reduce BP if needed. Early data suggested that ARBs may be better than ACE inhibitors in systolic heart failure.[56] However, when directly compared in a well-designed prospective trial, ACE inhibitors were found to be better.[57] ARBs are acceptable as an alternative therapy for patients who cannot tolerate ACE inhibitors and possibly as add-on therapy to those already on a standard three-drug regimen.[58,59]

The addition of aldosterone antagonists can reduce morbidity and mortality in systolic heart failure.[60,61] Spironolactone has been studied in severe heart failure and has shown benefit in addition to diuretic and ACE inhibitor therapy.[60] Eplerenone, the newest aldosterone antagonist, has been studied in patients with symptomatic systolic heart failure within 3 to 14 days after an acute myocardial infarction in addition to a standard three-drug regimen.[61] Collectively, both these agents should be considered in the specific heart failure population studied but only in addition to diuretics, ACE/ARBs, and β-blockers.

Post Myocardial Infarction[62]

Hypertension is a strong risk factor for myocardial infarction. Once a patient experiences a myocardial infarction, controlling BP is essential for secondary prevention to reduce the risk of recurrent cardiovascular events. β-Blocker therapy (agents without intrinsic sympathomimetic activity [ISA]) and ACE inhibitor therapy are recommended in the American College of Cardiology/American Heart Association post–myocardial infarction guidelines.[62] β-Blockers decrease cardiac adrenergic stimulation and have been shown in clinical trials to reduce the risk of a subsequent myocardial infarction or sudden cardiac death.[63,64] ACE inhibitors have been shown to improve cardiac remodeling and cardiac function and to reduce cardiovascular events after myocardial infarction.[65,66] These two drug classes, with β-blockers first, are considered the first drugs of choice for patients who have experienced a myocardial infarction.

Eplerenone has been shown recently to reduce morbidity and mortality in patients soon after experiencing an acute myocardial infarction (within 3 to 14 days).[61] However, this supporting evidence was in patients with symptoms of acute left ventricular dysfunction (systolic heart failure). Considering that this drug has a propensity to cause significant hyperkalemia, and given the patient population studied, eplerenone should be used only in selected patients following a myocardial infarction.

High Coronary Disease Risk[62,67]

Chronic stable angina, unstable angina, and myocardial infarction are all forms of coronary disease (also known as coronary artery disease or ischemic heart disease). These are the most common forms of hypertension-associated target-organ disease. β-Blocker therapy has the most evidence demonstrating benefits in these patients. β-Blockers are first-line therapy in chronic stable angina and have the ability to reduce BP, improve myocardial oxygen consumption, and decrease demand.[1]

Long-acting CCBs traditionally have been viewed as alternatives to β-blockers in chronic stable angina. The INVEST study has compared β-blocker with diuretic therapy with nondihydropyridine CCB with ACE inhibitor therapy in this population and has shown no difference in cardiovascular risk reduction.[68] Nonetheless, the preponderance of data are with β-blockers, and they remain therapy of choice.[1,62]

For acute coronary syndromes (non–ST-segment elevation myocardial infarction and unstable angina), first-line therapy should consist of a β-blocker and an ACE inhibitor.[62] This regimen will lower BP, control acute ischemia, and reduce cardiovascular risk. Diuretics can be added thereafter if the goal BP is not achieved with first-line therapy.

CCBs (especially the nondihydropyridines diltiazem and verapamil) and β-blockers lower BP and reduce myocardial oxygen demand in patients with hypertension and high coronary disease risk. However, cardiac stimulation may occur with dihydropyridine CCBs or β-blockers with intrinsic sympathomimetic activity, making these agents less desirable. Therefore, β-blockers with intrinsic sympathomimetic activity should be avoided, and CCBs (especially dihydropyridines) should be reserved as second- or third-line therapy.

There has been concern that overtreating high BP in patients with coronary artery disease may bring about more harm than good (termed the *J-curve phenomenon*). Since coronary blood flow occurs during diastole, the rate of flow is directly influenced by the DBP. Therefore, excessively reducing DBP may compromise coronary perfusion, especially in patients with fixed coronary artery stenosis, and lead to myocardial infarction. This concern has been theoretical based on retrospective analyses, and prospective studies have not found a J-curve until DBPs were very low (<60 mm Hg). However, this controversy has resurfaced because a post-hoc subgroup analysis of the INVEST study has shown a J-curve in patients with DBP less than 84 mm Hg.

Diabetes Mellitus[1,29,30,69–72]

The primary cause of mortality in diabetes is cardiovascular disease, and hypertension management is a very important risk-reduction strategy. The BP goal in diabetes is less than 130/80 mm Hg, and five antihypertensive agents have evidence supporting their compelling indications in diabetes (see Fig. 13–3). All these agents have been shown to reduce cardiovascular events in patients with diabetes. However, risk reduction may not be equal when comparing these agents.

All patients with diabetes and hypertension should be treated with an antihypertensive regimen that includes either an ACE inhibitor or an ARB.[70] Pharmacologically, both these agents should provide nephroprotection owing to vasodilation in the efferent arteriole of the kidney. Moreover, ACE inhibitors have overwhelming data demonstrating cardiovascular risk reduction in patients with established forms of heart disease. Evidence from outcome studies has demonstrated reductions in both cardiovascular risk (mostly with ACE inhibitors) and the risk of progressive kidney dysfunction (mostly with ARBs) in patients with diabetes. There is controversy surrounding which agent is better because data support both drug classes. Nonetheless, either drug class should be used to control BP as one of the drugs in the antihypertensive regimen for patients with diabetes because multiple agents often are needed to attain goal BP values, and a thiazide diuretic is recommended as the second agent.

Some evidence indicates that ACE inhibitors and ARBs may increase insulin sensitivity. A few case reports have associated hypoglycemia with ACE inhibitor use in patients with diabetes taking oral hypoglycemic agents. While such effects could be problematic in some patients, the fact that ACE inhibitors improve insulin sensitivity is of limited clinical significance in diabetes.

β-Blockers have been shown to reduce cardiovascular risk in patients with diabetes, and these agents should be used when needed. β-Blockers have been shown in at least one study to be as effective as ACE inhibitors in protection against morbidity and mortality in patients with diabetes.[71] They are especially indicated in patients with diabetes who have suffered a myocardial infarction or have high coronary disease risk. However, β-blockers (especially nonselective agents) may mask the signs and symptoms of hypoglycemia in patients with tightly controlled diabetes because most of the symptoms of hypoglycemia (i.e., tremor, tachycardia, and palpitations) are mediated through the sympathetic nervous system. Sweating, a cholinergically mediated symptom of hypoglycemia, still should occur during a hypoglycemic episode despite β-blocker therapy. Patients also may have a delay in hypoglycemia recovery time because compensatory recovery mechanisms need the catecholamine input that is antagonized by β-blocker therapy. Finally, unopposed α-receptor stimulation during the acute hypoglycemic recovery phase (owing to endogenous epinephrine release intended to reverse hypoglycemia) may result in acutely elevated BP from vasoconstriction. Despite these potential problems, β-blockers are highly beneficial in diabetes after ACE inhibitors/ARBs and diuretics.

CCBs are useful add-on agents for BP control in hypertensive patients with diabetes. Several studies have compared an ACE inhibitor with either a dihydropyridine CCB or a β-blocker. In the studies comparing a dihydropyridine with an ACE inhibitor, the ACE inhibitor group had significantly lower rates of cardiovascular end points, including myocardial infarctions and all cardiovascular events.[73] These data do not suggest that CCBs are harmful in diabetic patients but indicate that they are not as protective as ACE inhibitors. While data are limited, nondihydropyridine CCBs (diltiazem and verapamil) appear to provide more kidney protection than the dihydropyridines.[30]

Based on the weight of all evidence, ACE inhibitors/ARBs are preferred first-line agents for controlling hypertension in diabetes. The need for combination therapy should be anticipated, and thiazide diuretics should be the second agent added in most patients to lower BP. Based on scientific evidence, β-blockers and CCBs are useful evidenced-based agents in this population but are considered add-on therapies to the aforementioned agents.

Chronic Kidney Disease[30,74]

Patients with hypertension may develop damage to either the renal tissue (parenchyma) or the renal arteries. Chronic kidney disease presents initially as microalbuminuria (30–299 mg albumin in a 24-hour urine collection) that can progress to macroalbuminuria and overt kidney failure.[75] The rate of kidney function deterioration is accelerated when both hypertension and diabetes are present.[30,75] Once patients have an estimated glomerular filtration rate (GFR) of less than 60 mL/m^2 per minute or macroalbuminuria, they have chronic kidney disease, and the risk of cardiovascular disease and progression to severe chronic kidney disease increases.[1] Strict BP control to a goal of less than 130/80 mm Hg can slow the decline in kidney function. This strict control often requires two or more antihypertensive agents.

In addition to lowering BP, ACE inhibitors and ARBs reduce intraglomerular pressure, which can provide additional benefits in further reducing the decline in renal function. ACE inhibitors and ARBs have been shown to reduce progression of chronic kidney disease in patients with diabetes[76–80] and in those without diabetes.[30,81] One of these two agents should be used as first-line therapy to control blood pressure and preserve kidney function in patients with chronic kidney disease. Some data indicate that the combination of an ACE inhibitor and an ARB may be more effective than either agent alone.[82] However, routine use of this combination in all patients with chronic kidney disease is controversial. Since these patients typically require multiple antihypertensive agents, diuretics and a third antihypertensive drug class (β-blocker or CCB) often are needed. Thiazide diuretics can be used but may not be as effective as loop diuretics when creatinine clearances are below 30 mL/min.

Patients may experience a rapid and profound drop in BP or acute kidney failure when given an ACE inhibitor or ARB. The potential to produce acute kidney failure is particularly probematic in patients with bilateral renal artery stenosis or a solitary functioning kidney with stenosis. Patients with renal artery stenosis are usually older, and the condition is more common in patients with diabetes or those who smoke. Patients with renal artery stenosis do not necessarily have evidence of renal disease unless sophisticated tests are performed. Starting with low dosages and evaluating renal function shortly after starting the drug (in 2 to 4 weeks) can minimize this risk.

Recurrent Stroke Prevention

Attaining goal BP values in patients who have experienced a stroke is considered a primary modality to reduce the risk of a second stroke. However, BP lowering should be attempted only after patients have stabilized following an acute cerebrovascular event. One clinical trial, the PROGRESS trial, showed that an ACE inhibitor in combination with a thiazide diuretic reduces the incidence of recurrent stroke in patients with a history of stroke or transient ischemic attacks.[47] Reduction in recurrent stroke was seen with this combination therapy, even in those with BP values less than 140/90 mm Hg. These data are consistent with other evidence demonstrating reduced cardiovascular risk with ACE inhibitor therapy in high-risk patients at goal BP values.[66,83]

ALTERNATIVE DRUG TREATMENTS

It is necessary to use other agents such as α-blockers, central α_2-agonists, adrenergic inhibitors, and vasodilators in some patients. Although these agents are potent, they have a much greater incidence of adverse effects. Moreover, they do not have compelling outcomes data showing reduced morbidity and mortality in hypertension. They generally are reserved for patients with resistant hypertension and ideally should be used only in combination with other primary antihypertensive agents, especially diuretics.

SPECIAL POPULATIONS[1]

Selection of drug therapy should follow the guidelines provided by the JNC7, which are summarized in Figs. 13–2 and 13–3. These should be maintained as the guiding principles of drug therapy. However, there are some patient populations where the approach to drug therapy may be slightly different or use recommended agents with tailored dosing strategies. In some cases this is so because other agents have unique properties that benefit a coexisting condition but may not be based on evidence from outcomes studies in hypertension.

Hypertension in Older People

Hypertension often presents as isolated systolic hypertension in the elderly. Epidemiologic data indicate that cardiovascular morbidity and mortality are more closely related to SBP than to DBP in patients aged 50 years and older, so this population is at high risk for hypertension-related target-organ damage.[1,16] Although several placebo-controlled trials have specifically demonstrated risk reduction in this form of hypertension, many older people with hypertension are either not treated or treated yet not controlled.[33]

The SHEP was a landmark double-blind, placebo-controlled trial that evaluated active treatment (chlorthalidone-based, with atenolol or reserpine as add-on therapy) for isolated systolic hypertension.[12] A 36% reduction in total stroke, a 27% reduction in coronary artery disease, and 55% reduction in heart failure were demonstrated versus placebo. The Systolic Hypertension–Europe (Syst-Eur) was another placebo-controlled trial that evaluated treatment with a long-acting dihydropyridine CCB.[15] Treatment resulted in a 42% reduction in stroke, 26% reduction in coronary artery disease, and 29% reduction in heart failure. Similar findings were observed in a Chinese population with isolated systolic hypertension.[84] These data clearly demonstrate reductions in cardiovascular morbidity and mortality in older patients with isolated systolic hypertension, especially with thiazide diuretics and long-acting dihydropyridine CCBs.

The very elderly population, those 80 years of age and older, has been underrepresented in clinical trials, including the SHEP and Syst-Eur studies. This population often is not treated to goal either because of a fear of lowering BP too much or because of limited data demonstrating benefit. The best available data in the very elderly come from meta-analyses.[85,86] Although these data do not show reductions in mortality, they consistently show fewer strokes with active antihypertensive treatment.

Thiazide diuretics or β-blockers have been compared with either ACE inhibitors or CCBs in elderly patients with either systolic or diastolic hypertension or both.[87] In a Swedish trial, no significant differences were seen between conventional drugs and either ACE inhibitors or CCBs. However, there were significantly fewer myocardial infarctions and cases of heart failure in the ACE inhibitor group compared with the CCB group. These data suggest that overall treatment may be more important than specific antihypertensive agents in this population.

Elderly patients are more sensitive to volume depletion and sympathetic inhibition than younger individuals. This may lead to orthostatic hypotension (see next section). In the elderly, this can increase the risk of falls because of the associated dizziness and risk of fainting. Antihypertensives such as the centrally acting agents and α-blockers should be used with caution in the elderly because they are frequently associated with dizziness and postural hypotension. Diuretics and ACE inhibitors provide significant benefits and can be used safely in the elderly, but smaller-than-usual initial doses must be used. Most authorities agree that a thiazide should be the initial antihypertensive agent in most elderly patients, especially in those with isolated systolic hypertension, and that the starting dose should be low (e.g., 12.5 mg hydrochlorothiazide).

The JNC7 goal BP recommendations are independent of age; in the elderly, they are less than 140/90 mm Hg or less than 130/80 mm Hg (for diabetes or chronic kidney disease).[1] Age-adjusted goals are not appropriate.[16] Moreover, the JNC7 recommends that treatment follow the same principles that are outlined for general care of hypertension (e.g., diuretics for most and specific drug therapies to treat compelling indications). However, initial drug doses may be lower and dosage titrations should occur over a longer period of time to minimize the risk of hypotension. An interim goal of an SBP of below 160 mm Hg may be necessary for those with a very high initial SBP, but the ultimate goal should still be an SBP of less than 140 mm Hg.

Patients at Risk for Orthostatic Hypotension

Orthostatic hypotension is a significant drop in BP when standing and can be associated with dizziness and/or fainting. It is defined as an SBP decrease of greater than 20 mm Hg or a DBP decrease of greater than 10 mm Hg when changing from supine to standing.[1] Older patients (especially those with isolated systolic hypotension) and patients with diabetes, severe volume depletion, baroreflex dysfunction, autonomic insufficiency, and those using venodilators (α-blockers, mixed α/β-blockers, nitrates, and phosphodiesterase inhibitors for erectile dysfunction) all are at increase risk of orthostatic hypotension. In patients with these risks, antihypertensive agents should be started in low doses, especially diuretics and ACE inhibitors.

Hypertension in Children and Adolescents[88]

Detecting hypertension in children requires special attention to BP measurement, and detection is based on age-determined percentiles for excessive BP.[88] Hypertensive children often have a family history of high BP, and many are overweight. Unlike hypertension in adults, secondary hypertension is much more common in children and adolescents. An appropriate work-up for secondary causes is essential if elevated BP is identified. Kidney disease (e.g., pyelonephritis, glomerulonephritis, renal artery stenosis, and renal cysts) is the most common cause of secondary hypertension in children. Pheochromocytoma and coarctation of the aorta also can produce secondary hypertension. Medical or surgical management of the underlying disorder usually normalizes BP.

Treatment recommendations are provided in the 1996 National High Blood Pressure Education Program Working Group on Hypertension Control in Children and Adolescents.[88] Nonpharmacologic treatment is the cornerstone of therapy for essential hypertension. The goal is to reduce the BP to below the 95th percentile for age. Diuretics, β-blockers, and ACE inhibitors are very effective. ACE inhibitors and ARBs are contraindicated in sexually active girls owing to potential teratogenic effect and in those who might have bilateral renal artery stenosis or unilateral stenosis in a solitary kidney. Long-acting dihydropyridine CCBs have been successfully used in children, but long-term safety is unknown.

Women

Younger women generally have a lower prevalence of hypertension than younger men. However, after the fifth decade of life, prevalence rises sharply to the point that it actually exceeds men in the sixth decade.[1] Many women on oral contraceptives have a very small but detectable increase in BP. Women with a family history of hypertension, pregnancy-induced hypertension, obesity, age greater than 35 years, kidney disease, and extended duration of use have increased susceptibility to hypertension. It appears as though BP increases are related to the progestin, not the estrogen, component of oral contraceptives. BP increases in postmenopausal women treated with hormone-replacement therapy are modest and do not preclude use in hypertensive women. Regardless, all women on oral contraceptives or hormone-replacement therapy should have their BP monitored at least every 6 months.[1]

Women receive the same benefits from antihypertensive therapy as men. However, ACE inhibitors and ARBs are contraindicated in women who intend to become pregnant because they are teratogenic. Thiazide diuretics may be especially beneficial in postmenopausal women with osteoporosis because they cause retention of calcium and have been shown to positively affect bone mineral density. Women tend to have higher rates of drug-related adverse effects than men.

Pregnancy[89]

The National High Blood Pressure Education Program Working Group Report on High Blood Pressure in Pregnancy was updated in 2000.[89] It is important to differentiate preeclampsia from chronic, transient, and gestational hypertension. Preeclampsia can lead rapidly to life-threatening complications for both mother and fetus and usually presents after 20 weeks' gestation in primigravid women. The diagnosis of preeclampsia is based on the appearance of hypertension (> 140/90 mm Hg) after 20 weeks' gestation with proteinuria. Chronic hypertension presents before 20 weeks' gestation. It is controversial whether treating elevated BP in patients with chronic hypertension in pregnancy is beneficial. Women with chronic hypertension prior to pregnancy can develop preeclampsia.

Definitive treatment of preeclampsia is delivery. Delivery is clearly indicated if pending or frank eclampsia (preeclampsia plus convulsions) is present. Otherwise, management consists of restricting activity, bed rest, and close monitoring. Salt restriction or any other measures that contract blood volume should not be employed. Antihypertensive agents are used prior to induction of labor if the DBP is greater than 105 or 110 mm Hg, with a target DBP of 95 to 105 mm Hg. Intravenous hydralazine is used most commonly, and intravenous labetalol is also effective. Immediate-release oral nifedipine has been used, but it is not approved by the Food and Drug Administration (FDA) for hypertension, and untoward fetal and maternal effects (hypotension with fetal distress) have been reported.

Many agents can be used to treat chronic hypertension in pregnancy (Table 13–7). Methyldopa is considered the drug of choice.[1] Data indicate that uteroplacental blood flow and fetal hemodynamics are stable with methyldopa. Moreover, it is viewed as very safe based on long-term follow-up data (7.5 years) that have not demonstrated adverse effects on childhood development. β-Blockers, labetalol, and

TABLE 13–7. Treatment of Chronic Hypertension in Pregnancy

Drug/Class	Comments
Methyldopa	Preferred agent based on long-term follow-up data supporting safety
β-Blockers	Generally safe, but intrauterine growth retardation reported
Labetolol	Increasingly preferred over methyldopa because of fewer side effects
Clonidine	Limited data available
Calcium channel blockers	Limited data available; no increase in major teratogenicity with exposure
Diuretics	Not first-line agents but probably safe in low doses
ACE inhibitors, angiotensin II receptor blockers	Contraindicated; major teratogenicity reported with exposure (fetal toxicity and death)

CCBs are also reasonable alternatives. ACE inhibitors and ARBs are absolutely contraindicated. Although they are pregnancy category C in the first trimester, they are category D in the second and third trimesters owing to potential teratogenicity.

African-Americans[1,3,90]

Hypertension affects African-American patients at a disproportionately higher rate, and hypertension-related target-organ damage is more prevalent than in other populations. The reasons for these differences are not fully understood. Differences in electrolyte homeostasis, GFR, sodium excretion and transport mechanisms, plasma renin activity, and BP response to plasma volume expansion may explain the higher prevalence but do not account for the increased severity. The African-American population has comparatively low plasma renin activity and increased BP response to sodium and fluid loading.

African-Americans have an increased need for combination therapy to attain and maintain BP goals.[90] The Hypertension in African American Working Group of the International Society on Hypertension in Blacks has published treatment guidelines that are similar to the JNC7.[90] Lifestyle modifications are recommended to augment drug therapy. The guidelines also support thiazide diuretics as first-line therapy for most patients and selecting specific drug therapy to treat compelling indications, if present. These guidelines aggressively promote combination therapy and recommend starting with two drugs in patients with SBP values greater than or equal to 15 mm Hg from goal. These recommendations are more stringent than the JNC7 cutoff of greater than or equal to 20 mm Hg. This more aggressive approach is reasonable considering that overall goal BP attainment rates are low in African-Americans.

BP-lowering effects of antihypertensive classes vary in African-Americans. Monotherapy with β-blockers, ACE inhibitors, or ARBs results in less BP lowering compared with Caucasian patients. This may be due to the low-renin pattern of hypertension. Even within these three drug classes, data suggest that β-blockers may have better effects on target-organ disease than ARBs.[91] Conversely, thiazide diuretics and CCBs seem to be particularly effective at lowering BP in African-Americans. When either of these two classes (especially thiazides) is used in combination with a β-blocker, ACE inhibitor, or ARB, antihypertensive response is increased significantly. Interestingly, African-Americans have a higher risk of angioedema and cough from ACE inhibitors compared with Caucasians.[90]

Despite differences in antihypertensive effects, drug therapy selection should be based on evidence, as outlined in the JNC7 guidelines. Thiazide diuretics are first-line therapy based on the preponderance of evidence. These agents just so happen to also be very effective at controlling BP in this population. Other drug therapies should be used if a compelling indication is present, even if antihypertensive effect may not be as great as with another drug class (i.e., a β-blocker is first-line therapy for BP control in an African-American patient who has suffered a myocardial infarction). Combination therapy is needed frequently in this population, and a thiazide diuretic ideally should be one of the agents used.

OTHER CONCOMITANT CONDITIONS

Most patients with hypertension have some other coexisting conditions that may influence selection or use of drug therapy. Under most circumstances, these are helpful in deciding on a particular antihypertensive agent when more than one agent is recommended to treat a compelling indication(s). In some cases, an agent should be avoided because it may aggravate a concomitant disorder. In other cases, an antihypertensive agent can be used to treat hypertension, a compelling indication, and another concomitant condition. The influence of concomitant conditions only should be complementary to and never in replacement of drug therapy choices indicated by compelling indications.

Pulmonary Disease and Peripheral Arterial Disease

Nonselective β-blockers should be avoided in hypertensive patients with asthma, chronic obstructive pulmonary disease (COPD), and peripheral vascular disease. α/β-Blockers (carvedilol and labetalol) will not result in unopposed α constriction like pure β-blockers can and may be used in peripheral arterial disease. However, similar to nonselective β-blockers, they should be avoided in patients with asthma and COPD. If a hypertensive patient with mild to moderate asthma or COPD requires a β-blocker to treat a compelling indication, a β_1-selective agent should be selected, and the lowest effective dose should be used.[92]

Dyslipidemia

Dyslipidemia (high low-density lipoprotein [LDL] cholesterol, high triglycerides, and/or low high-density lipoprotein [HDL] cholesterol) is considered a major cardiovascular risk factor. Therefore, controlling dyslipidemia is important to the overall care of hypertensive patients. Thiazide diuretics and β-blockers without intrinsic sympathomimetic activity may adversely affect serum cholesterol values, but these effects generally are transient and of no clinical consequence.[93]

α-Blockers, on the other hand, have been shown to have favorable effects (decreased LDL cholesterol and increased HDL cholesterol). However, because data from the ALLHAT show that α-blockers do not reduce cardiovascular risk as much as thiazide diuretics, this benefit is not clinically applicable.[49] ACE inhibitors and CCBs have no effect on serum cholesterol.

Left Ventricular Hypertrophy

Left ventricular hypertrophy (LVH) is an independent risk factor for cardiovascular disease and is considered a form of target-organ damage. LVH is present in about 50% of hypertensive patients. Most classes of antihypertensive agents, except vasodilators, prevent or regress LVH. Attaining goal BP values also should improve LVH. ACE inhibitors and ARBs are considered the most effective agents for regressing LVH, but data suggest that long-term diuretic use leads to the most regression. While prevention or regression of LVH is an important objective in the overall management of hypertension, it is merely a surrogate marker of reducing cardiovascular risk. Drug selections should not be made based on the potential to improve LVH at this time.

The Losartan Intevention For Endpoint (LIFE) trial was a prospective study that compared losartan versus atenolol in patients with LVH and hypertension.[45] Losartan was more effective than atenolol in reducing the combined end point of stroke, myocardial infarction, and death. When patients with diabetes from the LIFE trial were evaluated is a subanalysis, there was a significant reduction in both cardiovascular morbidity and mortality with losartan versus atenolol.[94] Despite this evidence, LVH is not considered a compelling indication for ARBs in the JNC7.

Erectile Dysfunction[95]

Most antihypertensive agents have been associated with erectile dysfunction in men. Diuretics and β-blockers traditionally have been labeled as more problematic than ACE inhibitors, ARBs, and CCBs. However, prospective long-term data from the Treatment of Mild Hypertension Study (TOMHS) and the VA Cooperative trial show no difference in the incidence of erectile dysfunction between diuretics and β-blockers versus ACE inhibitors and CCBs.[96,97] Nonetheless, if a β-blocker is necessary to treat a compelling indication, a cardioselective agent should be used. Centrally acting agents (e.g., clonidine, methyldopa, and guanethidine) are associated with higher rates of sexual dysfunction and should be avoided in men with erectile dysfunction.

Hypertensive men frequently have arterial dysfunction, which can result in erectile dysfunction. Therefore, erectile dysfunction may be associated mostly with chronic arterial changes resulting from elevated BP, and lack of control may increase the risk of erectile dysfunction. These changes are even more pronounced in hypertensive men with diabetes.

INDIVIDUAL ANTIHYPERTENSIVE AGENTS[1,7]

Diuretics[12–14,46,52,98]

Diuretics, preferably a thiazide, are fist-line agents for most patients with hypertension.[1] The best available evidence justifying this recommendation is from ALLHAT.[46] Moreover, when combination therapy is needed in hypertension to control BP, a diuretic is recommended as one of the agents used.[1] Four subclasses of diuretics are used in the treatment of hypertension: thiazides, loops, potassium-sparing agents, and aldosterone antagonists (see Table 13–5). Potassium-sparing diuretics are weak antihypertensive agents when used alone but provide an additive effect when used in combination with a thiazide or loop diuretic. Moreover, they counteract the potassium- and magnesium-losing properties of the other diuretic agents. Aldosterone antagonists (spironolactone) technically may be considered potassium-sparing agents but are more potent antihypertensives with a slow onset of activity (up to 6 weeks with spironolactone). However, they are viewed by the JNC7 as an independent class because of evidence supporting compelling indications.

The exact hypotensive mechanism of action of diuretics is not known but has been well hypothesized. The drop in BP seen when diuretics are first started is caused by an initial diuresis. Diuresis causes reductions in plasma and stroke volume, which decreases cardiac output and BP. This initial drop in cardiac output causes a compensatory increase in peripheral vascular resistance. With chronic diuretic therapy, extracellular fluid and plasma volume return to near pretreatment values. However, peripheral vascular resistance decreases to values that are lower than the pretreatment baseline. This reduction in peripheral vascular resistance is responsible for chronic antihypertensive effects.

Thiazide diuretics have additional actions that may further explain their antihypertensive effects. Thiazides mobilize sodium and water from arteriolar walls. This effect would lessen the amount of physical encroachment on the lumen of the vessel created by excessive accumulation of intracellular fluid. As the diameter of the lumen relaxes and increases, there is less resistance to the flow of blood, and peripheral vascular resistance drops further. High dietary sodium intake can blunt this effect, and a low salt intake can enhance this effect. Thiazides also are postulated to cause direct relaxation of vascular smooth muscle. This theory is based on the known mechanism of action of diazoxide, which is a direct vasodilator that is structurally related to thiazide diuretics.

Thiazides are the preferred type of diuretic for treating hypertension. In patients with adequate kidney function (estimated GFR > 30 mL/min), thiazides are the most effective diuretics for lowering BP. As kidney function declines, a more potent diuretic is needed to counteract the associated increase in sodium and water retention. In this case, a loop diuretic (e.g., furosemide dosed twice daily) should be considered. Diuretics ideally should be dosed in the morning if given once daily and in the morning and afternoon if dosed twice daily to minimize the risk of nocturnal diuresis. However, with chronic use, thiazides, potassium-sparing diuretics, and aldosterone antagonists rarely cause a pronounced diuresis.

The major pharmacokinetic differences between the various thiazides are serum half-life and duration of diuretic effect. The clinical relevance of these differences is unknown because the serum half-life of most antihypertensive agents does not correlate with the hypotensive duration of action. Moreover, diuretics may lower BP primarily through extrarenal mechanisms. Hydrochlorothiazide and chlorthalidone are the two most frequently used thiazide diuretics in landmark clinical trials that have demonstrated reduced morbidity and mortality. It was once thought that these agents were equipotent on a milligram-per-milligram basis. However, chlorthalidone appears to be 1.5 to 2.0 times more potent than hydrochlorothiazide.[99] This has been attributed to a longer half-life (45–60 hours versus 8–15 hours) and longer duration of effect (48–72 hours versus 16–24 hours) with chlorthalidone. When looking at both agents, a dose of 25 mg daily results in a mean decrease in SBP of 18 and 12 mm Hg for chlorthalidone and hydrochlorothiazide, respectively. Again, since a difference in outcomes has not been demonstrated in outcomes trials, the significance of these differences is unknown, and it is well accepted that either of these agents is reasonable to use.

Diuretics are very effective in lowering BP when used in combination with most other antihypertensive agents. This additive response is explained by two independent pharmacodynamic effects. First, when two drugs cause the same overall pharmacologic effect (BP lowering) through different mechanisms of action, their combination usually results in an additive or synergistic effect. This is especially relevant when a β-blocker or ACE inhibitor is indicated in an African-American but does not elicit sufficient antihypertensive effect. Adding a diuretic in this situation often can lower BP significantly. Second, a compensatory increase in sodium and water retention may be seen with antihypertensive agents. This problem is counteracted with the concurrent use of a diuretic.

The side effects of thiazide diuretics include hypokalemia, hypomagnesemia, hypercalcemia, hyperuricemia, hyperglycemia, hyperlipidemia, and sexual dysfunction. Loop diuretics may cause the same side effects, although the effect on serum lipids and glucose is not as significant, and hypocalcemia may occur. Short-term studies indicate that indapamide does not adversely affect lipids or glucose tolerance or cause sexual dysfunction. These side effects are all dose-related. Many of these side effects were identified when high doses of thiazides were used in the past (e.g., hydrochlorothiazide 100 mg/day). Current guidelines suggest limiting the dose of hydrochlorothiazide or chlorthalidone to 12.5–25 mg/day, which markedly reduces the risk for most metabolic side effects.

Hypokalemia and hypomagnesemia may cause muscle fatigue or cramps. However, serious cardiac arrhythmias can occur in patients with significant degrees of hypokalemia and hypomagnesemia. Patients at greatest risk are those with LVH, high coronary disease risk, previous myocardial infarction, a history of arrhythmia, or concurrently receiving digoxin. Low-dose thiazide diuretic therapy (i.e., 25 mg hydrochlorothiazide or 12.5 mg chlorthalidone daily) rarely causes significant electrolyte disturbances. Every effort should be made to keep potassium in the therapeutic range by careful monitoring because severe hypokalemia also may negate the beneficial effects of the diuretic (reducing cardiovascular events).

Diuretic-induced hyperuricemia can precipitate gout, either acute gouty arthritis or uric acid nephrolithiasis. This side effect may be especially problematic in patients with a previous history of gout. However, attacks are unlikely in patients with no previous history of gout. If gout does occur in a patient who requires diuretic therapy, allopurinol can be given to prevent gout and will not compromise the antihypertensive effects of the diuretic. High doses of thiazide and loop diuretics may increase fasting glucose and serum cholesterol values. These effects, however, usually are transient and often inconsequential.[100] Low-dose diuretic therapy is much less likely to produce these metabolic abnormalities.

Potassium-sparing diuretics can cause hyperkalemia, especially in patients with chronic kidney disease or diabetes and in patients receiving concurrent treatment with an ACE inhibitor, ARB, nonsteroidal anti-inflammatory drugs, or potassium supplements. Hyperkalemia is especially problematic for the newest aldosterone antagonist eplerenone. Since this agent is a very selective aldosterone antagonist, its propensity to cause hyperkalemia is believed to be greater than the other potassium-sparing agents and even spironolactone (the other aldosterone antagonist). Because of an increased risk of hyperkalemia, eplerenone is contraindicated in patients with impaired renal function or type 2 diabetes with proteinuria (see Table 13–5). While spironolactone may cause gynecomastia in up to 10% of patients, this occurs rarely with eplerenone.

Diuretics can be used safely with most other agents. However, concurrent administration with lithium may result in increased lithium serum concentrations. This interaction can predispose patients to lithium toxicity.

▪ Angiotensin-Converting Enzyme Inhibitors[43,48,69,87,101]

ACE inhibitors are considered second-line therapy to diuretics in most patients with hypertension.[1] The ALLHAT demonstrated less heart failure and stroke with chlorthalidone versus lisinopril.[46] This difference in stroke is consistent with another outcomes trial, the Captopril Prevention Project (CAPPP).[101] However, other outcome studies have demonstrated similar, if not better, outcomes with ACE inhibitors versus thiazide diuretics.[43,48] In the elderly, one study found that they were at least as effective when compared with diuretics and β-blockers,[87] and another study found that they were more effective.[48] In addition, ACE inhibitors have many roles for patients with hypertension and coexisting conditions. Nonetheless, most clinicians will agree that if ACE inhibitors are not first-line therapy in most patients with hypertension, they are a very close second to diuretics.

ACE facilitates the production of angiotensin II, which has a major role in the regulation of arterial BP, as depicted in Fig. 13–1. ACE is distributed in many tissues and is present in several different cell types, but its principal location is in endothelial cells. Therefore, the major site for angiotensin II production is in the blood vessels, not the kidney. ACE inhibitors block the conversion of angiotensin I to angiotensin II. This latter substance is a potent vasoconstrictor that also stimulates aldosterone secretion. ACE inhibitors also block the degradation of bradykinin and stimulate the synthesis of other vasodilating substances, including prostaglandin E_2 and prostacyclin. The observation that ACE inhibitors lower BP in patients with normal plasma renin

activity suggests that bradykinin and perhaps tissue production of ACE are important in hypertension. Increased bradykinin enhances the BP-lowering effects of ACE inhibitors but also is responsible for the side effect of dry cough. ACE inhibitors effectively prevent or regress LVH by reducing the direct stimulation by angiotensin II on myocardial cells.

The JNC7 lists six compelling indications for ACE inhibitors, indicating many evidence-based uses for this drug class (see Fig. 13–3). Several studies have shown that ACE inhibitors may be more effective at reducing cardiovascular risk than other antihypertensives. In type 2 diabetes, two studies showed that ACE inhibitors were superior to CCBs.[69,70] However, one of the U.K. Prospective Diabetes Study Group (UKPDS) trials found captopril equivalent to atenolol in preventing cardiovascular events in patients with type 2 diabetes.[71] ACE inhibitors reduce cardiovascular morbidity and mortality in patients with heart failure[53] and decrease progression of chronic kidney disease.[30] They should be first-line disease–modifying therapy in all these patients unless absolutely contraindicated.[53] In addition to β-blocker therapy, evidence shows that ACE inhibitors further reduce cardiovascular risk in chronic stable angina (the EUROPA trial)[83] and in patients after myocardial infarction (the HOPE trial).[62,66] Finally, data from the PROGRESS trial have shown reduced risk of secondary stroke with the combination of an ACE inhibitor and thiazide diuretic.[47]

There are 10 ACE inhibitors on the U.S. market (see Table 13–5). All can be dosed once daily for hypertension except captopril, which has a shorter half-life than the others. It is usually dosed two or three times daily. In addition to captopril, enalapril and lisinopril are the most frequently used ACE inhibitors. Enalapril is a prodrug that is converted to the active metabolite enalaprilat, which has a longer half-life than the parent drug, extends the duration of action, and usually allows for once-daily dosing. In some patients, especially when higher doses are used, twice-daily dosing is needed to maintain 24-hour effects. Lisinopril has an even longer duration of action and does not require metabolic conversion to exert its effect. All three are excreted in the urine, and therefore, an adjustment in dosage may be necessary in patients with severe chronic kidney disease. The absorption of captopril, but not enalapril or lisinopril, is reduced by 30% to 40% when given with food. Benazepril, captopril, fosinopril, moexipril, quinapril, ramipril, and trandolapril can provide 24-hour BP reduction with once daily dosing. Similar to enalapril, benazepril, moexipril, quinapril, and ramipril may need twice daily dosing in some patients.

ACE inhibitors are well tolerated in most patients but are not absent of side effects. ACE inhibitors decrease aldosterone and can increase potassium serum concentrations. Usually the increase in potassium is small, but hyperkalemia is possible. It is seen primarily in patients with chronic kidney disease or diabetes mellitus and in those on concomitant ARBs, nonsteroidal anti-inflammatory drugs, potassium supplements, or potassium-sparing diuretics. Judicious monitoring of potassium and serum creatinine values within 4 weeks of starting or increasing the dose of an ACE inhibitor often can identify these abnormalities before they evolve into more serious complications.

The most worrisome adverse effects of ACE inhibitors are neutropenia and agranulocytosis, proteinuria, glomerulonephritis, and acute kidney failure. Fortunately, these serious adverse effects are rare, occurring in less than 1% of patients. Preexisting kidney or connective tissue diseases increase the risk of these side effects. Bilateral renal artery stenosis or unilateral stenosis of a solitary functioning kidney renders patients dependent on the vasoconstrictive effect of angiotensin II on the efferent arteriole of the kidney, thus explaining why these patients are particularly susceptible to acute kidney failure from ACE inhibitors. Slowly titrating the dose of ACE inhibitor and judicious kidney function monitoring can minimize risk and allow for early detection of those with renal artery stenosis.

It is important to note that GFR does decrease in patients placed on ACE inhibitors or ARBs.[30] This is attributed to the inhibition of angiotensin II vasoconstriction on the efferent arteriole. This decrease in GFR often increases serum creatinine concentration, and small increases should be anticipated when monitoring patients on ACE inhibitors. Modest elevations of either up to a 35% (for baseline creatinine values of less than or equal to 3 mg/dL) or absolute increases of less than 1 mg/dL do not warrant changes.[30] If larger increases occur, ACE inhibitor therapy should be stopped or the dose reduced.

Angioedema is a serious potential complication of ACE inhibitor therapy. Although it occurs in less than 2% of the population, it is more likely in African-Americans and smokers. Symptoms include lip and tongue swelling and possibly difficulty breathing. Drug withdrawal is appropriate for all patients with angioedema, but laryngeal edema and pulmonary symptoms occur occasionally and also require epinephrine, corticosteroids, antihistamines, and/or emergent intubation to support respiration. A history of angioedema, even if not from an ACE inhibitor, precludes use of another ACE inhibitor. Cross-reactivity between ACE inhibitors and ARBs has been reported, but the exact incidence of cross-reactivity is unknown. Therefore, it is controversial whether patients with ACE inhibitor–induced angioedema should be given an ARB.

A persistent dry cough develops in up to 20% of patients and is explained pharmacologically by the inhibition of bradykinin breakdown. This cough does not cause clinical illness but is annoying to patients. It should be clearly differentiated from a wet cough associated with pulmonary edema, which may be a sign of uncontrolled heart failure. Cromolyn and sulindac have been used to treat the cough, but these options are not recommended. If an ACE inhibitor is indicated for the compelling indications of heart failure, diabetes, or chronic kidney disease, then patients with a dry cough should be switched to an ARB. Otherwise, other antihypertensive alternatives, including ARBs, should be considered.

ACE inhibitors are absolutely contraindicated in pregnancy (see "Pregnancy" section under "Special Populations") and in patients with a history of angioedema. Similar to diuretics, ACE inhibitors can increase lithium serum concentrations in patients on lithium therapy. Concurrent use of an ACE inhibitor with a potassium-sparing diuretic (including aldosterone antagonists), potassium supplements, or an ARB may result in excessive increases in potassium.

Starting doses of ACE inhibitors should be low, with even lower doses started in patients at risk for orthostatic hypotension. Acute hypotension may occur at the onset on ACE inhibitor therapy. Patients who are sodium- or volume-depleted, in heart failure exacerbation, very elderly, or on concurrent vasodilators or diuretics are at high risk for this effect (see the "Hypertension in Older People" and "Patients at Risk for Orthostatic Hypotension" sections under "Special Populations"). It is important to start with half the normal dose of an ACE inhibitor for all patients with these risk factors and to use slow dose titration. The risk of serious adverse reactions overall can be decreased approximately 50% by using a 6-week time interval between dose increases versus a 2-week interval.[102]

■ Angiotensin II Receptor Blockers[45,56–59,78–80,103–106]

Angiotensin II is generated by two enzymatic pathways: the RAAS, which involves ACE, and an alternative pathway that uses other enzymes such as chymases. ACE inhibitors inhibit only the effects of angiotensin II produced through the RAAS, whereas ARBs inhibit angiotensin II from all pathways. It is unclear how these differences affect tissue concentrations of ACE. Because of these differences, ACE inhibitors only partially block the effects of angiotensin II. ARBs directly block the angiotensin II type 1 (AT_1) receptor that mediates the known effects of angiotensin II in humans: vasoconstriction, aldosterone release, sympathetic activation, antidiuretic hormone release, and constriction of the efferent arterioles of the glomerulus. They do not block the angiotensin II type 2 (AT_2) receptor. Therefore, beneficial effects of AT_2 receptor stimulation (i.e., vasodilation, tissue repair, and inhibition of cell growth) remain intact when ARBs are used. Unlike ACE inhibitors, ARBs do not block the breakdown of bradykinin. Therefore, some of the beneficial effects of bradykinin such as vasodilation (which can enhance BP lowering), regression of myocyte hypertrophy and fibrosis, and increased levels of tissue plasminogen activator are not present with ARB therapy.

ARBs have outcomes data showing long-term reductions in progression of target-organ damage in patients with hypertension and certain compelling indications. In patients with type 2 diabetes and nephropathy, progression of nephropathy has been shown to be reduced significantly with ARB therapy.[78–80] Some benefits appear to be independent of BP lowering, suggesting that the unique benefits of ARBs are explained pharmacologically by effects on the efferent arteriole. For patients with systolic heart failure, the CHARM studies showed that ARB therapy reduces the risk of cardiovascular events when added to a stable regimen of a diuretic, ACE inhibitor, and β-blocker or as alternative therapy in ACE inhibitor–intolerant patients.[58,59] However, the ELITE studies also have shown that losartan is not superior to captopril in systolic heart failure when compared head to head.[56,57] This finding is consistent with other data in post–myocardial infarction patients (the OPTIMAAL study).[105]

Seven ARBs are marketed for the treatment of hypertension. Data from pooled analyses and direct comparisons have demonstrated that all these drugs are effective in lowering BP. They have a fairly flat dose-response curve, suggesting that increasing the dose above low or moderate levels is unlikely to result in a large degree of BP lowering. The addition of low doses of a thiazide diuretic to an ARB significantly increases antihypertensive efficacy. Similar to ACE inhibitors, most ARBs have long enough half-lives to allow for once daily dosing. However, candesartan, eprosartan, and losartan have the shortest half-lives and may require twice daily dosing for sustained BP lowering.

ARBs seem to have the lowest incidence of side effects compared with other antihypertensive agents. Since they do not affect bradykinin, they do not have an associated dry cough like ACE inhibitors. While these drugs often have been considered to be "ACE inhibitors without the cough," pharmacologic differences highlight that they could have very different effects on vascular smooth muscle and myocardial tissue that can correlate with different effects on target-organ damage and cardiovascular risk reduction when compared with ACE inhibitors. It is possible that their effects may be superior to ACE inhibitors in patients with type 2 diabetic nephropathy but may be inferior to ACE inhibitors in patients with more advanced heart disease (e.g., heart failure and after myocardial infarction). Unfortunately, there are no direct comparisons that look at long-term effects in patients with just hypertension. Regardless, their role in patients with type 2 diabetic nephropathy is well established, and they also are very reasonable alternatives in patients requiring an ACE inhibitor but who experience an intolerable cough. Using the combination of an ACE inhibitor with an ARB has not been well studied in hypertension despite demonstrated benefits of this combination in patients with heart failure and nephrotic syndrome.

Like ACE inhibitors, ARBs may cause kidney insufficiency, hyperkalemia, and orthostatic hypotention. The same precautions that apply to ACE inhibitors for patients with suspected bilateral renal artery stenosis, those on drugs that can raise the potassium level, and those on drugs that increase the risk of hypotension apply to ARBs. Cough is very uncommon. Angioedema is also less likely to occur than with ACE inhibitors, but cross-reactivity has been reported. ARBs should be used cautiously in patients with a history of angioedema but, unlike ACE inhibitors, are not contraindicated. ARBs should not be used in pregnancy.

◼ β-Blockers[43,44,46,53,62,67,71]

β-Blockers have been used in several large outcome trials in hypertension. They were recommended previously as first-line agents along with diuretics in most patients. However, in most of these trials, diuretics were the primary agents, and β-blockers were added on for additional BP lowering. Therefore, they are now considered appropriate first-line agents when there are compelling indications (after myocardial infarction or high coronary disease risk) and are evidenced-based as additional therapy for other compelling indications (heart failure and diabetes). Numerous trials have shown reduced cardiovascular risk when β-blockers are used following a myocardial infarction, during acute coronary syndrome, or in chronic stable angina. Although once considered contraindicated in heart failure, multiple studies have shown that carvedilol and metoprolol succinate reduce mortality in patients with systolic heart failure who are treated with a diuretic and an ACE inhibitor. Atenolol was even used in type 2 diabetes in the UKPDS studies and showed comparable, if not better, cardiovascular risk reduction when compared with captopril.

Several mechanisms of action have been proposed for β-adrenoceptor blockers (β-blockers), but none of them alone has been shown to be associated consistently with a reduction in arterial BP. β-Blockers have negative chronotropic and inotropic cardiac effects that reduce cardiac output, which explains some of the antihypertensive effect. However, cardiac output falls equally in patients treated with β-blockers regardless of BP lowering. Additionally, β-blockers with intrinsic sympathomimetic activity (ISA) do not reduce cardiac output, yet they lower BP and decrease peripheral resistance.

β-Adrenoceptors are also located on the surface membranes of juxtaglomerular cells, and β-blockers inhibit the release of renin. However, there is a weak association between plasma renin concentrations and antihypertensive efficacy of β-blocker therapy. Some patients with low plasma renin concentrations do respond to β-blockers. Therefore, additional mechanisms also must account for the antihypertensive effect of β-blockers. However, the ability of β-blockers to reduce plasma renin and thus angiotensin II concentrations may play a major role in their ability to reduce cardiovascular risk.

There are important pharmacodynamic and pharmacokinetic differences among the various β-blockers, but all agents provide a similar degree of BP lowering. There are three pharmacodynamic properties of the β-blockers that differentiate this class: cardioselectivity, ISA, and membrane-stabilizing effects. β-Blockers that possess a greater affinity for β_1-receptors than β_2-receptors are *cardioselective.*

Both β_1- and β_2-adrenoceptors are distributed throughout the body, but they concentrate differently in certain organs and tissues. There is a preponderance of β_1-receptors in the heart and kidney and a preponderance of β_2-receptors in the lungs, liver, pancreas, and arteriolar smooth muscle. β_1-Receptor stimuation increases heart rate, contractility, and renin release. β_2-Receptor stimulation results in bronchodilation and vasodilation. Cardioselective β-blockers are less likely to provoke bronchospasm and vasoconstriction. Also, both insulin secretion and glycogenolysis are adrenergically mediated by β_2-receptors. Blocking β_2-receptors may reduce these processes and cause hyperglycemia or blunt recovery from hypoglycemia.

Atenolol, betaxolol, bisoprolol, and metoprolol are cardioselective β-blockers. Therefore, they are safer than nonselective β-blockers in patients with asthma, COPD, peripheral arterial disease, and diabetes who have a compelling indication for a β-blocker. However, cardioselectivity is a dose-dependent phenomenon. At higher doses, cardioselective agents lose their relative selectivity for β_1-receptors and block β_2-receptors as effectively as they block β_1-receptors. The dose at which cardioselectivity is lost varies from patient to patient. In general, cardioselective β-blockers are preferred when using a β-blocker to treat hypertension.

Some β-blockers have *intrinsic sympathomimetic activity* (ISA). Acebutolol, carteolol, penbutolol, and pindolol are ISA β-blockers that act as partial β-receptor agonists. When they bind to the β-receptor, they stimulate it, but far less than a pure β-agonist. If sympathetic tone is low, as it is during resting states, β-receptors are partially stimulated by ISA β-blockers. Therefore, resting heart rate, cardiac output, and peripheral blood flow are not reduced when these types of β-blockers are used. Theoretically, ISA agents would appear to have advantages over β-blockers in patients with heart failure, sinus bradycardia, or perhaps even peripheral arterial disease. Unfortunately, they do not appear to reduce cardiovascular events as well as other β-blockers. In fact, they may increase risk after myocardial infarction or in those with high coronary disease risk. Thus agents with ISA are rarely needed.

Finally, all β-blockers exert a *membrane-stabilizing action* on cardiac cells when large enough doses are given. This activity is important when antiarrhythmic properties of the β-blockers are needed.

Pharmacokinetic differences among β-blockers relate to first-pass metabolism, serum half-lives, degree of lipophilicity, and route of elimination. Propranolol and metoprolol undergo extensive first-pass metabolism, so the dose needed to attain β-blockade with either drug varies from patient to patient. Atenolol and nadolol have relatively long half-lives and are excreted renally. The dose of these agents may need to be reduced in patients with moderate to severe chronic kidney disease. Even though the half-lives of the other β-blockers are much shorter, once daily administration may be effective because serum half-life does not correlate well with the hypotensive duration of action.

β-Blockers also vary in terms of their lipophilic properties and thus central nervous system penetration. All β-blockers cross the blood-brain barrier, but lipophilic agents penetrate to a greater extent than hydrophilic agents. Propranolol is the most lipophilic drug, and atenolol is the least lipophilic. Therefore, much higher brain concentrations of propranolol compared with atenolol are seen after equivalent doses are given. This can result in more central nervous system side effects (e.g., dizziness and drowsiness) with lipophilic agents such as propranolol. However, the lipohilic properties can provide better effects for noncardiovascular conditions such as migraine headache prevention, essential tremor, and thyrotoxicosis. BP lowering is equal among β-blockers regardless of lipophilicity.

Most side effects of β-blockers are an extension of their ability to antagonize β-adrenoceptors. β-Blockade in the myocardium can be associated with bradycardia, atrioventricular conduction abnormalities (e.g., second- or third-degree heart block), and the development of acute heart failure. The decreases in heart rate actually may benefit certain patients with atrial arrhythmias (e.g., atrial fibrillation and atrial flutter) and hypertension by both providing rate control and lowering BP. β-Blockers usually only produce heart failure if they are used in high initial doses in patients with preexisting left ventricular dysfunction (systolic heart failure) or if started in these patients during an acute heart failure exacerbation. Blockade of β_2-receptors in the lung may cause acute exacerbations of bronchospasm in patients with asthma or COPD. Blocking β_2-receptors in arteriolar smooth muscle may cause cold extremities and may aggravate intermittent claudication or Raynaud's phenomenon as a result of decreased peripheral blood flow. In addition, there is an increase of sympathetic tone during periods of hypoglycemia that may result in a significant increase in BP because of unopposed α-receptor–mediated vasoconstriction.

Abrupt cessation of β-blocker therapy can produce unstable angina, myocardial infarction, and even death in patients with high coronary disease risk. Abrupt cessation also may lead to rebound hypertension (a sudden increase in BP to the pretreatment values) or overshoot hypertension (increase in BP above pretreatment values). To avoid this, β-blockers always should be tapered gradually over 1 to 2 weeks before eventually discontinuing the drug. This acute withdrawal syndrome is believed to be secondary to progression of underlying coronary artery disease, hypersensitivity of β-adrenergic receptors because of upregulation, and increased physical activity after withdrawal of a drug that decreases myocardial oxygen requirements. In patients without coronary artery disease, abrupt discontinuation may present as sinus tachycardia, increased sweating, and generalized malaise, in addition to increased BP.

Like diuretics, β-blockers have been shown to increase serum cholesterol and glucose values, but these effects are transient and of little clinical significance. In patients with diabetes or dyslipidemia, the reduction in cardiovascular events was as great with β-blockers as with an ACE inhibitor in the UKPDS trial[71] and far superior to placebo in the SHEP trial.[12] β-Blockers can increase serum triglycerides and decrease HDL cholesterol slightly. β-Blockers with α-blocking properties (carvedilol and labetalol) produce no changes in these lipid values. Moreover, ISA β-blockers do not adversely affect these values and may even increase HDL cholesterol. However, since these are of questionable clinical significance, cardioselective agents remain the β-blockers of choice for most patients.

Calcium Channel Blockers[15,43,107,108]

CCBs are not first-line agents but are very effective antihypertensive agents, especially in African-American patients. They have compelling indications in high coronary disease risk and in diabetes. However, with these compelling indications, they are in addition to or in replacement of other antihypertensive drug classes. Some data indicated that dihydropyridines may not provide as much protection against cardiac events when compared with "conventional" therapy (diuretics and β-blockers) or ACE inhibitors in uncomplicated hypertension.[43] Since only heart failure was higher with amlodipine versus chlorthalidone in ALLHAT, differences between agents are small.[46] In patients with hypertension and diabetes, ACE inhibitors appear to be more cardioprotective than dihydropyridines.[69] Studies with the nondihydropyridine CCBs diltiazem and verapamil are limited, but the NORDIL study found diltiazem to be equivalent to diuretics and β-blockers in reducing cardiovascular events.[43] It is possible that these differences (beneficial with diltiazem and neutral with dihydropyridines) may relate to the sympathetic stimulation that can occur with dihydropyridines.

Dihydropyridine CCBs are very effective in older patients with isolated systolic hypertension. The Syst-Eur was a placebo-controlled trial that demonstrated that a long-acting dihydropyridine CCB reduced the risk of cardiovascular events markedly in isolated systolic hypertension.[15] In previous guidelines, isolated systolic hypertension was a compelling indication for a long-acting dihydropyridine CCB. The JNC7 does not list isolated systolic hypertension differently from any other form of hypertension, and diuretics remain first-line therapy. However, a long-acting dihydropyridine CCB may be considered as add-on therapy if a thiazide diuretic is not controlling BP in a patient with isolated systolic hypertension and no other compelling indications. This is especially relevant if the patient is older with SBP elevation.

Contraction of cardiac and smooth muscle cells requires an increase in free intracellular calcium concentrations from the extracellular fluid. When cardiac or vascular smooth muscle is stimulated, voltage-sensitive channels in the cell membrane are opened, allowing calcium to enter the cells. The influx of extracellular calcium into the cell releases stored calcium from the sarcoplasmic reticulum. As intracellular free calcium concentration increases, it binds to a protein, calmodulin, which then activates myosin kinase, enabling myosin to interact with actin to induce contraction. CCBs work by inhibiting influx of calcium across the cell membrane. There are two types of voltage-gated calcium channels: a high-voltage channel (L-type) and a low-voltage channel (T-type). Currently available CCBs only block the L-type channel, which leads to coronary and peripheral vasodilation.

There are two subclasses of calcium channel blockers, dihydropyridines and nondihydropyridines (see Table 13–5). They are pharmacologically very different from each other. They are all similar in their antihypertensive effectiveness, but they differ somewhat in other pharmacodynamic effects. Nondihydropyridines (verapamil and diltiazem) decrease heart rate and slow atrioventricular nodal conduction. Similar to β-blockers, these drugs also may treat supraventricular tachyarrhythmias. Verapamil produces a negative inotropic and chronotropic effect that is responsible for its propensity to precipitate or cause heart failure in high-risk patients. Diltiazem also has these effects but to a lesser extent than verapamil. All CCBs (except amlodipine) have negative inotropic effects. Dihydropyridines cause a baroreceptor-mediated reflex tachycardia because of their potent peripheral vasodilating effects, although this varies among agents within this subclass. Dihydropyridines do not alter conduction through the atrioventricular node and thus are not effective agents in supraventricular tachyarrhythmias.

Within the dihydropyridines, nifedipine rarely may cause an increase in the frequency, intensity, and duration of angina in association with acute hypotension. This effect is most likely due to a reflex sympathetic stimulation and likely is obviated by using sustained-release formulations of nifedipine. For this reason, all other dihydropyridines have an intrinsically long half-life or are provided in sustained-release formulations. Immediate-release nifedipine has been associated with an increased incidence of adverse cardiovascular effects, and it is not approved for treatment of hypertension. It should not be used to treat hypertension. Other side effects with dihydropyridines include dizziness, flushing, headache, gingival hyperplasia, peripheral edema, mood changes, and various gastrointestinal complaints. The side effects due to vasodilation such as dizziness, flushing, headache, and peripheral edema occur more frequently with all dihydropyridines than with the nondihydropyridines verapamil and diltiazem because they are less potent vasodilators.

Diltiazem and verapamil can cause cardiac conduction abnormalities such as bradycardia or atrioventricular block, but this occurs mostly with high doses. Heart failure has been reported in otherwise healthy patients secondary to negative inotropic effects. These problems occur at increased frequency in those with preexisting abnormalities in the cardiac conduction system. Both drugs can cause anorexia, nausea, peripheral edema, and hypotension. Verapamil causes constipation in about 7% of patients. This side effect also occurs with diltiazem, but to a lesser extent.

Verapamil and, to a lesser extent, diltiazem can cause drug interactions because of their ability to inhibit the cytochrome P450 3A4 isoenzyme system. This inhibition can increase the serum concentrations of other drugs that are metabolized by this isoenzyme system. Agents such as cyclosporine, digoxin, lovastatin, simvastatin, tacrolimus, and theophylline are examples of these drugs. Verapamil and dilitazem should be given very cautiously with a β-blocker for treating hypertension because there is an increased risk of heart block with these combinations. If a CCB is needed in combination with a β-blocker, a dihydropyridine should be selected because it will not increase the risk of heart block. The hepatic metabolism of CCBs, especially nifedipine, may be inhibited by ingesting large quantities of grapefruit juice and can increase pharmacologic effects.

Many different formulations of verapamil and diltiazem are currently available (see Table 13–5). Although certain sustained-release verapamil and diltiazem products may contain the same active drug (i.e., Calan SR and Verelan; both contain verapamil), they are usually not AB rated by the FDA as interchangeable on a milligram-per-milligram basis because of different biopharmaceutical release mechanisms.

Two sustained-release verapamil products (Covera HS and Verelan PM) and one diltiazem product (Cardizem LA) are chronotherapeutically designed to target the circadian changes in BP rhythm. These agents are dosed primarily in the evening so that drug is released during the morning when BP first starts to increase. The rationale behind chronotherapy in hypertension is that blunting the early-morning BP surge may result in more reduction in cardiovascular events than conventional dosing of regular antihypertensive products in the morning. However, evidence from the CONVINCE trial showed that chronotherapeutic verapamil was similar to but not better than a thiazide diuretic/β-blocker–based regimen with respect to cardiovascular events.[44]

α_1-Blockers[49]

Prazosin, terazosin, and doxazosin are selective α_1-receptor blockers. They work in the peripheral vasculature and inhibit the uptake of catecholamines in smooth muscle cells, resulting in vasodilation and BP lowering.

Doxazosin was one of the original treatment arms of the ALLHAT. However, it was stopped prematurely when statistically more secondary end points of stoke, heart failure, and cardiovascular events were seen with doxazosin compared with chlorthalidone.[49] There were no differences in the primary end point of fatal coronary heart disease and nonfatal myocardial infarction. These data suggest that thiazide diuretics are superior to doxazosin (and probably other α_1-blockers) in preventing cardiovascular events in patients with hypertension. Therefore, α_1-blockers are alternative agents that should be used in combination with one or more primary antihypertensive agent(s). α_1-Blockers can provide symptomatic benefits in men with benign prostatic hypertrophy. These agents block postsynaptic α_1-adrenergic receptors located on the prostate capsule, causing relaxation and decreased resistance to urinary outflow. However, they

should be used only in addition to other standard antihypertensive agents.

A potentially severe side effect of α_1-blockers is a first-dose phenomenon that is characterized by transient dizziness or faintness, palpitations, and even syncope within 1 to 3 hours of the first dose. This adverse reaction also can occur after dose increases. These episodes are accompanied by orthostatic hypotension and can be obviated by taking the first dose and subsequent first increased doses at bedtime. Orthostatic hypotension and dizziness may persist with chronic administration. For these reasons, these agents should be used very cautiously in elderly patients. Even though antihypertensive effects are achieved through a peripheral α_1-receptor antagonism, these agents cross the blood-brain barrier and may cause central nervous system side effects such as lassitude, vivid dreams, and depression. α_1-Blockers also may cause priapism. Sodium and water retention can occur with higher doses and sometimes even with chronic administration of low doses. Therefore, these agents are most effective when given in combination with a diuretic to maintain the hypotensive efficacy and minimize potential edema.

Central α_2-Agonists

Clonidine, guanabenz, guanfacine, and methyldopa lower BP primarily by stimulating α_2-adrenergic receptors in the brain. This stimulation reduces sympathetic outflow from the vasomotor center in the brain and increases vagal tone. It is also believed that peripheral stimulation of presynaptic α_2-receptors may further reduce sympathetic tone. Reduced sympathetic activity, together with enhanced parasympathetic activity, can decrease heart rate, cardiac output, total peripheral resistance, plasma renin activity, and baroreceptor reflexes. Although guanabenz and guanfacine are used rarely in clinical practice, clonidine is often used in resistant hypertension, and methyldopa is a first-line agent for hypertension in pregnancy.

Chronic use of centrally acting α-agonists results in sodium and water retention, which is most prominent with methyldopa. Low doses of clonidine (and guanfacine or guanabenz) can be used to treat hypertension without the addition of a diuretic. However, methyldopa should be given with a diuretic to avoid the blunting of antihypertensive effect that happens with prolonged use, except in pregnancy. Sedation and dry mouth are common side effects that typically improve with chronic use of low doses. As with other centrally acting antihypertensives, depression can occur. The incidence of orthostatic hypotension and dizziness is higher than with other antihypertensive agents, so they should be used very cautiously in the elderly. Lastly, clonidine has a relatively high incidence of anticholinergic side effects such as sedation, dry mouth, constipation, urinary retention, and blurred vision.

Abrupt cessation of central α_2-agonists may lead to rebound hypertension or overshoot hypertension. This effect is thought to be secondary to a compensatory increase in norepinephrine release after abrupt discontinuation. Methyldopa can cause hepatitis or hemolytic anemia, although this is rare. Transient elevations in serum hepatic transaminases are seen occasionally with methyldopa therapy but are clinically irrelevant unless they are greater than three times the upper limit of normal. Methyldopa should be discontinued quickly if persistent increases in serum hepatic transaminases or alkaline phosphatase are detected because this may indicate the onset of a fulminant hepatitis, which is life-threatening. A Coombs'-positive hemolytic anemia occurs in less than 1% of patients receiving methyldopa, although 20% exhibit a positive direct Coombs' test without anemia. For these reasons, methyldopa has limited use in the routine management of hypertension.

Transdermal clonidine may be associated with fewer side effects and thus better adherence than oral clonidine. This patch is applied to the skin and replaced once a week. It possesses the same BP-lowering effects as oral clonidine but avoids the high peak serum drug concentrations seen with oral dosing, which contribute to the high incidence of adverse effects. Hypertensive patients on clonidine should be taking other primary oral antihypertensive medications because clonidine is an alternative antihypertensive. Therefore, the potential advantage of improved adherence with a transdermal product is mostly hypothetical. Disadvantages of this system are cost, a 20% incidence of local skin rash or irritation, and delayed onset 2 to 3 days that requires an overlapping period of using the oral formulation if the transdermal product is replacing oral clonidine. A similar delay in offset of action is also seen when the patch is removed, so BP returns to pretreatment values over a 2- to 3-day period.

Reserpine

Reserpine lowers BP by depleting norepinephrine from sympathetic nerve endings and blocking transport of norepinephrine into its storage granules. Norepinephrine release into the synapse following nerve stimulation is reduced and results in reduced sympathetic tone, peripheral vascular resistance, and BP. Reserpine also depletes catecholamines from the brain and the myocardium, which may lead to sedation, depression, and decreased cardiac output.

Reserpine has a slow onset of action and long half-life that allows for once daily dosing. However, it may take 2 to 6 weeks before the maximal antihypertensive effect is seen. Reserpine can cause significant sodium and water retention. It should be given in combination with a diuretic (preferably a thiazide). Reserpine's strong inhibition of sympathetic activity results in increased parasympathetic activity. This effect explains why side effects such as nasal stuffiness, increased gastric acid secretion, diarrhea, and bradycardia can occur. Depression has been reported, which is a consequence of central nervous system depletion of catecholamines and serotonin. Depression may manifest as sadness, loss of appetite or self-confidence, gradual loss of energy, erectile dysfunction, or early-morning awakening. The initial reports of depression with reserpine were in the 1950s and are not consistent with current definitions of depression. Regardless, reserpine-induced depression is likely dose-related, and very high doses (above 1 mg daily) were used frequently in the 1950s. Depression is minimal when doses between 0.05 and 0.25 mg daily are used. With these low doses, the rate of depression is equal to that seen with β-blockers, diuretics, or placebo.[12]

Reserpine was used as a third-line agent in many of the landmark clinical trials that have documented its benefit in treating hypertension, including the VA Cooperative trials and, most important, the SHEP trial.[12] An analysis of the SHEP data found that reserpine was very well tolerated. The combination of a diuretic and reserpine is very effective at lowering BP, and this is a very inexpensive antihypertensive regimen.

Direct Arterial Vasodilators

The antihypertensive effects of hydralazine and minoxidil are caused by direct arteriolar smooth muscle relaxation. They exert little to no venous vasodilation. By decreasing arterial BP, they also reduce impedance to myocardial contractility. Both agents cause potent reductions in perfusion pressure that activates the baroreceptor reflexes. Activation of baroreceptors results in a compensatory increase in sympathetic outflow, which leads to an increase in heart rate, cardiac output, and renin release. Consequently, tachyphylaxis can develop, resulting in a loss of hypotensive effect, with continued use. This compensatory baroreceptor response can be counteracted by concurrent use of a β-blocker.

All patients receiving these drugs long term for hypertension generally should receive both a diuretic and a β-blocker first. Direct arterial vasodilators can precipitate angina in patients with underlying coronary artery disease unless the baroreceptor reflex mechanism is completely blocked with a β-blocker. Clonidine can be used in patients who have contraindications to β-blockers. The side effect of sodium and water retention is significant with these drugs and can be minimized with diuretic therapy (preferably thiazides).

One side effect unique to hydralazine is a dose-dependent drug-induced lupus-like syndrome. Hydralazine is eliminated by hepatic N-acetyltransferase. This enzyme displays genetic polymorphism, and slow acetylators are especially prone to develop drug-induced lupus with hydralazine. This syndrome is more common in women and is reversible on discontinuation. Drug-induced lupus may be avoided by using less than 200 mg hydralazine daily. Other side effects of hydralazine include dermatitis, drug fever, peripheral neuropathy, hepatitis, and vascular headaches. For these reasons, hydralazine has limited usefulness in the treatment of hypertension. However, it is still used with isosorbide dinitrate in patients with heart failure (especially African-Americans) and is useful in patients with severe chronic kidney disease and kidney failure.

Minoxidil is a more potent vasodilator than hydralazine. Therefore, the compensatory increases in heart rate, cardiac output, renin release, and sodium retention are even more dramatic. Sodium and water retention can be so severe with minoxidil that heart failure can be precipitated. It is even more important to coadminister a β-blocker and a diuretic with minoxidil. A loop diuretic is often more effective than a thiazide diuretic in patients treated with minoxidil. A troublesome side effect of minoxidil is hypertrichosis. Increased hair growth occurs on the face, arms, back, and chest. This drug-induced hirsutism ceases with discontinuation of the drug. Other minoxidil side effects include pericardial effusion and a nonspecific T-wave change on the electrocardiogram. Minoxidil generally is reserved for very difficult to control hypertension and patients requiring hydralazine that experience drug-induced lupus.

Other Agents

Guanethidine and guanadrel are postganglionic sympathetic inhibitors. They deplete norepinephrine from postganglionic sympathetic nerve terminals and inhibit the release of norepinephrine in response to sympathetic nerve stimulation, thus resulting in reduced cardiac output and peripheral vascular resistance. Orthostatic hypotension is common because reflex-mediated vasoconstriction is blocked. Other common side effects include erectile dysfunction, diarrhea, and weight gain. Long-term norepinephrine depletion leads to postsynaptic receptor supersensitivity. Therefore, concomitant use of tricyclic antidepressants and sympathomimetics may provoke acute severe hypertensive episodes. Because of these complications, these drugs have little to no role in the current management of hypertension.

PHARMACOECONOMIC CONSIDERATIONS

The cost of effectively treating hypertension is substantial. However, these costs can be offset by savings that would be realized by reducing cardiovascular morbidity and mortality. Cost related to treating other forms of target-organ damage (e.g., myocardial infarction and end-stage kidney failure) can drive health care costs up substantially. The cost per life-year saved from treating hypertension has been estimated to be $40,000 for younger adults and even less for older adults.[109] Treatments that cost less than $50,000 per life-year saved generally are considered favorable by health economists.

Drug costs can account for over 70% of the total cost of hypertensive care. One model for calculating the cost-effectiveness of various initial monotherapies for mild to moderate hypertension found that the cost of life-year saved ranged from $10,900 with a generic β-blocker to $72,100 with a brand-name ACE inbhitor.[109]

In a cost-minimization study that included the cost of drug acquisition, supplemental drugs, laboratory tests, clinic visits, and complications, the total costs of treating hypertension were $895 for β-blockers, $1043 for diuretics, $1165 for α-agonists, $1243 for ACE inhibitors, $1288 for α-blockers, and $1425 for CCBs.[110] Another cost-minimization analysis found that 86 middle-aged or 29 elderly hypertensive patients would need to be treated to prevent one myocardial infarction, stroke, or death.[111] The excess cost of preventing one event with a CCB or ACE inhibitor instead of a diuretic or β-blocker was $89,000 to $341,000 for a middle-aged patient and $30,000 to $115,000 for an elderly patient. Depending on the agent chosen, the added cost would be $200 to $800 per year.

A comparative analysis in 133,624 hypertensive patients aged 65 and older from a state prescription drug assistance program demonstrated that 40% of patients were prescribed pharmacotherapy that was not necessarily recommended by the JNC7 guidelines.[112] If these 40% had drug therapy modifications made to follow evidence-based treatment, a reduction in costs of $11.6 million would have been realized in the 2001 calendar year based on discounted prices. This was projected to increase to $20.5 million using usual Medicaid pricing limits.

It therefore is crucial to identify ways to reduce the cost of care without increasing the morbidity and mortality associated with uncontrolled hypertension. Using evidence-based pharmacotherapy will save costs not only by using the most effective agents. Thiazide diuretics are recommended as first-line therapy in most patients and are very inexpensive. Just using thiazides, either as monotherapy or in combination, is appropriate under almost all circumstances and aspects of hypertension management. When needed, using other generic primary antihypertensive agents (e.g., atenolol or metoprolol for β-blockers and lisinopril or enalapril for ACE inhibitors) that can be administered once daily should be considered.

CLINICAL CONTROVERSIES

Hydrochlorothiazide is used more frequently to treat hypertension than chlorthalidone despite the fact that chlorthalidone was the thiazide used in the majority of outcome trials. Chlorthalidone also is twice as potent in BP lowering on a milligram-per-milligram basis.[99] However, the clinical impact of these differences on cardiovascular morbidity and mortality is unknown.

Patients with angioedema from an ACE inhibitor also can experience this with an ARB, but the exact incidence of cross-reactivity is not known. The ACC/AHA guidelines for the management of systolic heart failure recommend ARBs as alternative therapy in patients with angioedema from an ACE inhibitor. The best available data are from the CHARM-Alternative study, where only 1 of 39 patients with ACE inhibitor–associated angioedema experienced the same reaction when treated with candesartan.[58]

Over 90% of ACE is localized in tissues and organs, and benazepril, lisinopril, quinapril, and ramipril are ACE inhibitors that have a high degree of tissue penetration. In vitro studies show that high-penetration ACE inhibitors have greater improvements in endothelial function compared with low-penetration ACE inhibitors.[113,114] However, multiple outcome trials using low- or medium-penetration ACE inhibitors have shown reduced cardiovascular morbidity and mortality, thus questioning the clinical significance of tissue penetration.

HYPERTENSIVE URGENCIES AND EMERGENCIES[1,7,9,107]

Hypertensive urgencies and emergencies both are characterized by the presence of very elevated BP, greater than 180/120 mm Hg (see "Classification" in the "Arterial Blood Pressure" section). However, the need for urgent or emergent antihypertensive therapy should be determined based on the presence of acute or immediately progressing target-organ injury but not elevated BP alone. Urgencies are not associated with acute or immediately progressing target-organ injury, whereas emergencies are.

A common error with hypertensive urgency is overly aggressively antihypertensive therapy. This treatment likely has been perpetrated by the classification terminology urgency. Hypertensive urgencies ideally are managed by adjusting maintenance therapy by adding a new antihypertensive and/or increasing the dose of a present medication. This is the preferred approach to these patients because it provides a more gradual reduction in BP. Very rapid reductions in BP to goal values should be discouraged because of potential risks. Since autoregulation of blood flow in chronically hypertensive patients occurs at a much higher range of pressures than in normotensive persons, the inherent risks of reducing BP too precipitously include cerebrovascular accidents, myocardial infarction, and acute kidney failure. All patients with hypertensive urgency should be reevaluated within no more than 7 days (preferably after 1 to 3 days).

Acute administration of a short-acting oral antihypertensive agent (captopril, clonidine, or labetolol), followed by careful observation for several hours to ensure a gradual reduction in BP, is an option for hypertensive urgency. However, there are no data supporting this approach as being absolutely needed. Oral captopril is one of the agents of choice and can be used in doses of 25–50 mg at 1- to 2-hour intervals. The onset of action of oral captopril is 15 to 30 minutes, and a marked fall in BP is unlikely to occur if no hypotensive response is observed within 30 to 60 minutes. For patients with hypertensive rebound following withdrawal of clonidine, 0.2 mg clonidine can be given initially, followed by 0.2 mg hourly until the DBP falls below 110 mm Hg or a total of 0.7 mg clonidine has been administered. A single dose may be all that is necessary. Labetolol can be given in a dose of 200–400 mg, followed by additional doses every 2 to 3 hours.

Oral or sublingual immediate-release nifedipine has been used in the office setting, nursing homes, and hospitals for acute BP lowering but is potentially dangerous. This approach produces a rapid reduction in BP. Immediate-release nifedipine should never be used for hypertensive urgencies because of reports of severe adverse events such as myocardial infarctions and strokes.[107]

TABLE 13–8. Parenteral Antihypertensive Agents for Hypertensive Emergency

Drug	Dose	Onset (minutes)	Duration (minutes)	Adverse Effects	Special Indications
Sodium nitroprusside	0.25–10 mcg/kg/min intravenous infusion (requires special delivery system)	Immediate	1–2	Nausea, vomiting, muscle twitching, sweating, thiocynate and cyanide intoxication	Most hypertensive emergencies; caution with high intracranial pressure, azotemia, or in chronic kidney disease
Nicardipine hydrochloride	5–15 mg/h intravenous	5–10	15–30; may exceed 240	Tachycardia, headache, flushing, local phlebitis	Most hypertensive emergencies except acute heart failure; caution with coronary ischemia
Fenoldopam mesylate	0.1–0.3 mcg/kg/min intravenous infusion	<5	30	Tachycardia, headache, nausea, flushing	Most hypertensive emergencies; caution with glaucoma
Nitroglycerin	5–100 mcg/min intravenous infusion	2–5	5–10	Headache, vomiting, methemoglobinemia, tolerance with prolonged use	Coronary ischemia
Enalaprilat	1.25–5 mg intravenous every 6 h	15–30	360–720	Precipitous fall in pressure in high-renin states; variable response	Acute left ventricular failure; avoid in acute myocardial infarction
Hydralazine hydrochloride	12–20 mg intravenous 10–50 mg intramuscular	10–20 20–30	60–240 240–360	Tachycardia, flushing, headache vomiting, aggravation of angina	Eclampsia
Labetalol hydrochloride	20–80 mg intravenous bolus every 10 min; 0.5–2.0 mg/min intravenous infusion	5–10	180–360	Vomiting, scalp tingling, bronchoconstriction, dizziness, nausea, heart block, orthostatic hypotension	Most hypertensive emergencies except acute heart failure
Esmolol hydrochloride	250–500 mcg/kg/min intravenous bolus, then 50–100 mcg/kg/min intravenous infusion; may repeat bolus after 5 minutes or increase infusion to 300 mcg/min	1–2	10–20	Hypotension, nausea, asthma, first-degree heart block, heart failure	Aortic dissection; perioperative

Hypertensive emergencies are those rare situations that require immediate BP reduction to limit new or progressing target-organ damage (see "Classification" in the "Arterial Blood Pressure" section). Hypertensive emergencies generally require parenteral therapy, at least initially, with one of the agents listed in Table 13–8. The goal in hypertensive emergencies is not to lower BP to less than 140/90 mm Hg; rather, a reduction in mean atrial pressure (MAP) of up to 25% within minutes to hours is the initial target. If the BP is then stable, BP can be reduced toward 160/100–110 mm Hg within the next 2 to 6 hours. Precipitous drops in BP may lead to end-organ ischemia or infarction. If patients tolerate this reduction well, additional gradual reductions toward goal BP values can be attempted after 24 to 48 hours. The exception to this guideline is for patients with an acute ischemic stroke, in whom maintaining an elevated BP is needed for a much longer period of time.

The clinical situation should dictate which intravenous medication is used to treat hypertensive emergencies. Regardless, therapy should be provided in a hospital or emergency room setting with intraarticular BP monitoring. Table 13–8 lists special indications for agents that can be used. Some of these agents are discussed in further detail below.

Nitroprusside is widely considered the agent of choice for most cases but can be problematic in patients with chronic kidney disease. It is a direct-acting vasodilator that decreases peripheral vascular resistance but does not increase cardiac output unless left ventricular failure is present. Nitroprusside can be given to treat most hypertensive emergencies, but in aortic dissection, propranolol should be given first to prevent reflex sympathetic activation. Since nitroprusside is metabolized to cyanide and then to thiocyanate, which is eliminated by the kidneys, serum thiocyanate levels should be monitored when infusions are continued longer than 72 hours. Nitroprusside should be discontinued if the concentration exceeds 12 mg/dL. The risk of thiocyanate accumulation and toxicity is increased in patients with impaired kidney function.

Fenoldopam is a dopamine-1 agonist that is a popular alternative to nitroprusside. It is used often for perioperative hypertension. Similar to nitroprusside, it has a very quick onset of action and can be titrated easily by adjusting the continuous infusion rate. Conversely, it can improve renal blood flow and is especially useful in patients with kidney insufficiency.

Intravenous nitroglycerin dilates both arterioles and venous capacitance vessels, thereby reducing both cardiac afterload and preload, which can decrease myocardial oxygen demand. It also dilates collateral coronary blood vessels and improves perfusion to ischemic myocardium. These properties make intravenous nitroglycerin ideal for the management of hypertensive emergency in the presence of myocardial ischemia. Intravenous nitroglycerin is associated with tolerance when used over 24 to 48 hours and can cause severe headache.

The hypotensive response of hydralazine is less predictable than with other parenteral agents. Therefore, its major role is in the treatment of eclampsia or hypertensive encephalopathy associated with renal insufficiency.

EVALUATION OF THERAPEUTIC OUTCOMES

ACHIEVING GOALS

The most important strategy to prevent cardiovascular morbidity and mortality in hypertension is BP control to goal values (<140/90 mm Hg for most). Modifying other cardiovascular risk factors, such as

TABLE 13–9. Fixed-Dose Combination Products

Combination	Drugs (Brand Name)	Strengths (mg/mg)	Daily Frequency
ACE inhibitor with a thiazide diuretic	Benazepril/hydrochlorothiazide (Lotensin HCT)	5/6.25, 10/12.5, 20/12.5, 20/25	1
	Captopril/hydrochlorothiazide (Capozide)	25/15, 25/25, 50/15, 50/25	1 to 3
	Enalapril/hydrochlorothiazide (Vaseretic)	5/12.5, 10/25	1
	Lisinopril/hydrochlorothiazide (Prinizide, Zestoretic)	10/12.5, 20/12.5, 20/25	1
	Moexipril/hydrochlorothiazide (Uniretic)	7.5/12.5, 15/25	1 or 2
	Quinapril/hydrochlorothiazide (Accuretic)	10/12.5, 20/12.5, 20/25	1
Angiotensin-receptor blocker with a thiazide diuretic	Candesartan/hydrochlorothiazide (Atacand HCT)	16/12.5, 32/12.5	1
	Eprosartan/hydrochlorothiazide (Teveten HCT)	600/12.5, 600/25	1
	Irbesartan/hydrochlorothiazide (Avalide)	75/12.5, 150/12.5, 300/12.5	1
	Losartan/hydrochlorothiazide (Hyzaar)	50/12.5, 100/25	1
	Olmesartan/hydrochlorothiazide (Benicar HCT)	20/12.5, 40/12.5, 40/25	1
	Telmisartan/hydrochlorothiazide (Micardis HCT)	40/12.5, 80/12.5	1
	Valsartan/hydrochlorothiazide (Diovan HCT)	80/12.5, 160/12.5	1
β-Blocker with a thiazide diuretic	Atenolol/chlorthalidone (Tenoretic)	50/25, 100/25	1
	Bisoprolol/hydrochlorothiazide (Ziac)	2.5/6.25, 5/6.25, 10/6.25	1
	Propranolol/hydrochlorothiazide (Inderide)	40/25, 80/25	2
	Propranolol LA/hydrochlorothiazide (Inderide LA)	80/50, 120/50, 160/50	1
	Metoprolol/hydrochlorothiazide (Lopressor HCT)	50/25, 100/25	1 or 2
	Nadolol/bendroflumethazide (Corzide)	40/5, 80/5	1
	Timolol/hydrochlorothiazide (Timolide)	10/25	1 or 2
ACE inhibitor with calcium channel blocker	Amlodipine/benazepril (Lotrel)	2.5/10, 5/10, 10/20	1
	Enalapril/pelodipine (Lexxel)	5/5	1
	Trandolapril/verapamil (Tarka)	2/180, 1/240, 2/240, 4/240	1 or 2

smoking, dyslipidemia, and diabetes mellitus, is also important. Lowering BP to less than 130/80 mm Hg should be targeted in patients with diabetes or chronic kidney disease. For these patients, BP lowering should be done cautiously if high-risk coronary disease risk is present to avoid precipitation of ischemic myocardial events. Moreover, routine goal BP values should be attained in elderly patients with isolated systolic hypertension, but actual BP lowering can occur at a very gradual pace over a period of several months to avoid orthostatic hypotension.

COMBINATION ANTIHYPERTENSIVE THERAPY

Starting therapy with a combination of two drugs is now recommended in patients far from their BP goal, for patients in whom goal achievement may be difficult (i.e., those with diabetes or chronic kidney disease and African-Americans), or in patients with multiple compelling indications for different antihypertensive agents. However, combination therapy is often needed to control BP in patients already on therapy, and most patients require two or more agents.[1,30,33,50]

Combination regimens for hypertension should include a diuretic, preferably a thiazide. If a diuretic was not the first drug added, it should be the second agent as add-on therapy. This method will provide additional BP lowering because most patients respond well to a two-drug regimen that includes a diuretic. Clinicians should anticipate the need for three drugs to control BP in patients with aggressive BP goals (diabetes and chronic renal disease).[30]

Diuretics, when combined with several agents (especially an ACE inhibitor, ARB, or β-blocker), can result in additive antihypertensive effects that are independent of reversing fluid retention. BP lowering from certain antihypertensive agents can activate the RAAS as a compensatory mechanism to counteract BP changes and regulate fluid loss. Most alternative antihypertensive agents (e.g., reserpine, arterial vasodilators, and centrally acting agents) need to be given with a diuretic to avoid sodium and water retention.

Many fixed-dose combination products are available commercially, and some are generic (Table 13–9). Most of these products contain a thiazide diuretic and have multiple dose strengths available. Individual dose titration is more complicated with fixed-dose combination products, but this strategy can reduce the number of daily tablets/capsules and can simplify regimens to improve adherence. This alone may increase the likelihood of achieving or maintaining goal BP values. Depending on the product, some may be less expensive to patients and to health systems.

RESISTANT HYPERTENSION

Resistant hypertension is the failure to achieve goal BP in patients who are adhering to full doses of an appropriate three-drug regimen that includes a diuretic.[1] Several causes of resistant hypertension are listed in Table 13–10. These highlight the importance of diuretic therapy in the management of hypertension. Patients should be evaluated closely to see if any of these causes can be reversed. If nothing is identified, the principle of drug therapy selection from the JNC7 still should apply.

TABLE 13–10. Causes of Resistant Hypertension

Improper BP measurement
Volume overload
• Excess sodium intake
• Volume retention from kidney disease
• Inadequate diuretic therapy
Drug-induced or other causes
• Nonadherence
• Inadequate doses
• Agents listed in Table 13–1
Associated conditions
• Obesity, excess alcohol intake
Disease causing secondary hypertension

Compelling indications, if present, should guide selection, assuming that these patients are on a diuretic. If additional therapy is needed, spironolactone and reserpine are agents with unique mechanisms of action that can be particularly effective in augmenting BP lowering.

CLINICAL MONITORING

Patients should be monitored for signs and symptoms of progressive target-organ disease (see p. 191). A careful history for chest pain (or tightness), palpitations, dizziness, dyspnea, orthopnea, headache, sudden change in vision, one-sided weakness, slurred speech, and loss of balance should be taken to assess the likelihood of cardiovascular and cerebrovascular hypertensive complications. Other clinical monitoring parameters that may be used to assess target-organ disease includes changes in funduscopic findings, LVH regression on electrocardiogram or echocardiogram, proteinuria, and changes in kidney function. These parameters should be monitored periodically because any sign of deterioration requires immediate assessment and follow-up.

Clinic-based BP monitoring remains the standard for managing hypertension. BP response should be evaluated 2 to 4 weeks after initiating or making changes in therapy. With some agents, monitoring BP 4 to 6 weeks later may better represent steady-state BP values (reserpine) or in the case of ACE inhibitors may minimize the risk of adverse effects. Once goal BP values are attained, assuming no symptoms of acute target-organ disease, BP monitoring can be done every 3 to 6 months. More frequent evaluations are required in patients with a history of poor control, nonadherence, progressive target-organ damage, or symptoms of adverse drug effects. Self-measurements of BP or automatic ambulatory BP monitoring can be useful clinically to establish effective 24-hour control. This type of monitoring may become the standard of care in the future, but the JNC7 recommends that ambulatory BP monitoring only be used in select situations such as suspected white coat hypertension. If patients are measuring their BP at home, it is important that they measure during the early morning hours for most days and then at different times of the day on alternative days of the week.

Patients should be monitored routinely for adverse drug effects. The most common side effects that attend each class of antihypertensive agents are discussed in the treatment section of this chapter, and laboratory parameters for primary agents are listed in Table 13–11. These side effects typically should occur 2 to 4 weeks after starting a new agent or increasing the dose, and laboratory tests should be repeated every 6 to 12 months in stable patients. Additional monitoring may be needed for other concomitant diseases, if present (e.g., diabetes, dyslipidemia, and gout). The occurrence of an adverse drug event may require dosage reduction or substitution with an alternative antihypertensive agent.

ADHERENCE

Hypertension is a relatively asymptomatic disease, and antihypertensive agents are not without adverse side effects. Therefore, it is imperative to assess patient adherence on a regular basis. Identification of nonadherence should be followed up with appropriate patient education and counseling. Once daily regimens are preferred in most patients to improve adherence. Although some practitioners may believe that aggressive treatment will have a negative impact on quality of life, several studies have found that most patients actually feel better once their BP is controlled. Patients on antihypertensive therapy should be questioned periodically about changes in their general health perception, energy level, physical functioning, and overall satisfaction with their treatment. At the present time, there is inadequate information to recommend any herbal therapy as a treatment strategy for hypertension. Lifestyle modifications always should be recommended and encouraged continually in patients engaging in such endeavors.

ABBREVIATIONS

ACE: angiotensin-converting enzyme
ARB: angiotensin II receptor blocker
BP: blood pressure
BUN: blood urea nitrogen
CCB: calcium channel blocker
COPD: chronic obstructive pulmonary disease
DBP: diastolic blood pressure
GFR: glomerular filtration rate
JNC7: Seventh Report of the Joint National Committee on Prevention, Detection, Evaluation, and Treatment of High Blood Pressure
ISA: intrinsic sympathomimetic activity
LVH: left ventricular hypertrophy
RAAS: renin-angiotensin-aldosterone system
SBP: systolic blood pressure

Review Questions and other resources can be found at *www.pharmacotherapyonline.com.*

REFERENCES

1. Chobanian AV, Bakris GL, Black HR, et al. Seventh Report of the Joint National Committee on Prevention, Detection, Evaluation, and Treatment of High Blood Pressure. Hypertension 2003;42:1206–1252.
2. Hajjar I, Kotchen TA. Trends in prevalence, awareness, treatment, and control of hypertension in the United States, 1988–2000. JAMA 2003;290:199–206.
3. American Heart Association. Heart Disease and Stroke Statistics—2004 Update. Dallas, American Heart Association, 2003.
4. Staessen JA, Wang J, Bianchi G, Birkenhager WH. Essential hypertension. Lancet 2003;361:1629–1641.
5. Warnock DG. Genetic forms of human hypertension. Curr Opin Nephrol Hypertens 2001;10:493–499.
6. Dosh SA. The diagnosis of essential and secondary hypertension in adults. J Fam Pract 2001;50:707–712.

TABLE 13–11. **Select Monitoring for Antihypertensive Drug Therapy**

Class	Parameters
Diuretics	Blood pressure, BUN/serum creatinine, serum electrolytes (potassium, magnesium, sodium), uric acid (for thiazides)
Aldosterone antagonists	Blood pressure, BUN/serum creatinine, serum potassium
β-Blockers	Blood pressure, heart rate
ACE inhibitors	Blood pressure, BUN/serum creatinine, serum potassium
Angiotensin II receptor blockers	Blood pressure, BUN/serum creatinine, serum potassium
Calcium channel blockers	Blood pressure; heart rate

7. Kaplan NM. Kaplan's Clinical Hypertension, 8th ed. Philadelphia, Lippincott Williams & Wilkins, 2002:1–550.

8. Smolensky MH. Chronobiology and chronotherapeutics: Applications to cardiovascular medicine. Am J Hypertens 1996;9:11S–21S.

9. Bales A. Hypertensive crisis: How to tell if it's an emergency or an urgency. Postgrad Med 1999;105:119–126, 130.

10. MacMahon S, Peto R, Cutler J, et al. Blood pressure, stroke, and coronary heart disease: 1. Prolonged differences in blood pressure: Prospective observational studies corrected for the regression dilution bias. Lancet 1990;335:765–774.

11. Vasan RS, Larson MG, Leip EP, et al. Impact of high-normal blood pressure on the risk of cardiovascular disease. N Engl J Med 2001; 345:1291–1297.

12. SHEP Cooperative Research Group. Prevention of stroke by antihypertensive drug treatment in older persons with isolated systolic hypertension: Final results of the Systolic Hypertension in the Elderly Program (SHEP). JAMA 1991;265:3255–3264.

13. Dahlof B, Lindholm LH, Hansson L, et al. Morbidity and mortality in the Swedish Trial in Old Patients with Hypertension (STOP-Hypertension). Lancet 1991;338:1281–1285.

14. MRC Working Party. Medical Research Council trial of treatment of hypertension in older adults: Principal results. Br Med J 1992;304:405–412.

15. Staessen JA, Fagard R, Thijs L, et al. Randomised double-blind comparison of placebo and active treatment for older patients with isolated systolic hypertension. The Systolic Hypertension in Europe (Syst-Eur) Trial Investigators. Lancet 1997;350:757–764.

16. Izzo JL Jr, Levy D, Black HR. Clinical advisory statement: Importance of systolic blood pressure in older Americans. Hypertension 2000;35:1021–1024.

17. Domanski M, Norman J, Wolz M, et al. Cardiovascular risk assessment using pulse pressure in the first national health and nutrition examination survey (NHANES I). Hypertension 2001;38:793–797.

18. Executive Summary of the Third Report of the National Cholesterol Education Program (NCEP) Expert Panel on Detection, Evaluation, and Treatment of High Blood Cholesterol in Adults (Adult Treatment Panel III). JAMA 2001;285:2486–2497.

19. American Heart Association. Human Blood Pressure Determination by Sphygmomanometry. Dallas, American Heart Association, 1994.

20. Prisant LM, Alpert BS, Robbins CB, et al. American national standard for nonautomated sphygmomanometers: Summary report. Am J Hypertens 1995;8:210–213.

21. Jones DW, Appel LJ, Sheps SG, et al. Measuring blood pressure accurately: New and persistent challenges. JAMA 2003;289:1027–1030.

22. Kristal-Boneh E, Harari G, Green MS. Seasonal change in 24-hour blood pressure and heart rate is greater among smokers than nonsmokers. Hypertension 1997;30:436–441.

23. Pickering T. Recommendations for the use of home (self) and ambulatory blood pressure monitoring. American Society of Hypertension Ad Hoc Panel. Am J Hypertens 1996;9:1–11.

24. Glen SK, Elliott HL, Curzio JL, et al. White-coat hypertension as a cause of cardiovascular dysfunction. Lancet 1996;348:654–657.

25. Domanski MJ, Davis BR, Pfeffer MA, et al. Isolated systolic hypertension: Prognostic information provided by pulse pressure. Hypertension 1999;34:375–380.

26. Staessen JA, Thijs L, Fagard R, et al. Predicting cardiovascular risk using conventional vs ambulatory blood pressure in older patients with systolic hypertension. Systolic Hypertension in Europe Trial Investigators. JAMA 1999;282:539–546.

27. Bobrie G, Chatellier G, Genes N, et al. Cardiovascular prognosis of "masked hypertension" detected by blood pressure self-measurement in elderly treated hypertensive patients. JAMA 2004;291:1342–1349.

28. Staessen JA, Den Hond E, Celis H, et al. Antihypertensive treatment based on blood pressure measurement at home or in the physician's office: A randomized, controlled trial. JAMA 2004;291:955–964.

29. Hansson L, Zanchetti A, Carruthers SG, et al. Effects of intensive blood-pressure lowering and low-dose aspirin in patients with hypertension: Principal results of the Hypertension Optimal Treatment (HOT) randomised trial. HOT Study Group. Lancet 1998;351:1755–1762.

30. Bakris GL, Williams M, Dworkin L, et al. Preserving renal function in adults with hypertension and diabetes: A consensus approach. National Kidney Foundation Hypertension and Diabetes Executive Committees Working Group. Am J Kidney Dis 2000;36:646–661.

31. Farnett L, Mulrow CD, Linn WD, et al. The J-curve phenomenon and the treatment of hypertension: Is there a point beyond which pressure reduction is dangerous? JAMA 1991;265:489–495.

32. Voko Z, Bots ML, Hofman A, et al. J-shaped relation between blood pressure and stroke in treated hypertensives. Hypertension 1999;34:1181–1185.

33. Hyman DJ, Pavlik VN. Characteristics of patients with uncontrolled hypertension in the United States. N Engl J Med 2001;345:479–486.

34. Appel LJ, Champagne CM, Harsha DW, et al. Effects of comprehensive lifestyle modification on blood pressure control: Main results of the PREMIER clinical trial. JAMA 2003;289:2083–2093.

35. Whelton PK, Appel LJ, Espeland MA, et al. Sodium reduction and weight loss in the treatment of hypertension in older persons: A randomized, controlled trial of nonpharmacologic interventions in the elderly (TONE). TONE Collaborative Research Group. JAMA 1998;279:839–846.

36. Kostis JB, Wilson AC, Shindler DM, et al. Persistence of normotension after discontinuation of lifestyle intervention in the trial of TONE. Trial of Nonpharmacologic Interventions in the Elderly. Am J Hypertens 2002;15:732–734.

37. National Institutes of Health. Clinical guidelines on the identification, evaluation, and treatment of overweight and obesity in adults: The evidence report. Obes Res 1998;(suppl 2):51–209S.

38. Sacks FM, Svetkey LP, Vollmer WM, et al. Effects on blood pressure of reduced dietary sodium and the Dietary Approaches to Stop Hypertension (DASH) diet. DASH-Sodium Collaborative Research Group. N Engl J Med 2001;344:3–10.

39. Appel LJ, Moore TJ, Obarzanek E, et al. A clinical trial of the effects of dietary patterns on blood pressure. DASH Collaborative Research Group. N Engl J Med 1997;336:1117–1124.

40. Chobanian AV, Hill M. National Heart, Lung, and Blood Institute Workshop on Sodium and Blood Pressure: A critical review of current scientific evidence. Hypertension 2000;35:858–863.

41. Vollmer WM, Sacks FM, Ard J, et al. Effects of diet and sodium intake on blood pressure: Subgroup analysis of the DASH-sodium trial. Ann Intern Med 2001;135:1019–1028.

42. Sackett DL, Rosenberg WM, Gray JA, et al. Evidence-based medicine: What it is and what it isn't. Br Med J 1996;312:71–72.

43. Saseen JJ, MacLaughlin EJ, Westfall JM. Treatment of uncomplicated hypertension: Are ACE inhibitors and calcium channel blockers as effective as diuretics and beta-blockers? J Am Board Fam Pract 2003;16:156–164.

44. Black HR, Elliott WJ, Grandits G, et al. Principal results of the Controlled Onset Verapamil Investigation of Cardiovascular End Points (CONVINCE) trial. JAMA 2003;289:2073–2082.

45. Dahlof B, Devereux RB, Kjeldsen SE, et al. Cardiovascular morbidity and mortality in the Losartan Intervention For Endpoint (LIFE) reduction in hypertension study: A randomised trial against atenolol. Lancet 2002;359:995–1003.

46. ALLHAT Officers and Coordinators for the ALLHAT Collaborative Research Group. Major outcomes in high-risk hypertensive patients randomized to angiotensin-converting enzyme inhibitor or calcium channel blocker vs diuretic. The Antihypertensive and Lipid-Lowering Treatment to Prevent Heart Attack Trial (ALLHAT). JAMA 2002;288:2981–2997.

47. PROGRESS Collaborative Group. Randomised trial of a perindopril-based blood-pressure-lowering regimen among 6,105 individuals with previous stroke or transient ischaemic attack. Lancet 2001;358:1033–1041.

48. Wing LM, Reid CM, Ryan P, et al. A comparison of outcomes with angiotensin-converting enzyme inhibitors and diuretics for hypertension in the elderly. N Engl J Med 2003;348:583–592.

49. Diuretic versus alpha-blocker as first-step antihypertensive therapy: Final results from the Antihypertensive and Lipid-Lowering Treatment

to Prevent Heart Attack Trial (ALLHAT). Hypertension 2003;42:239–246.

50. 2003 European Society of Hypertension-European Society of Cardiology guidelines for the management of arterial hypertension. J Hypertens 2003;21:1011–1053.

51. Davis BR, Cutler JA, Gordon DJ, et al. Rationale and design for the Antihypertensive and Lipid Lowering Treatment to Prevent Heart Attack Trial (ALLHAT). ALLHAT Research Group. Am J Hypertens 1996;9:342–360.

52. Psaty BM, Lumley T, Furberg CD, et al. Health outcomes associated with various antihypertensive therapies used as first-line agents: A network meta-analysis. JAMA 2003;289:2534–2544.

53. Hunt SA, Baker DW, Chin MH, et al. ACC/AHA guidelines for the evaluation and management of chronic heart failure in the adult: Executive summary. A report of the American College of Cardiology/American Heart Association Task Force on Practice Guidelines (Committee to revise the 1995 Guidelines for the Evaluation and Management of Heart Failure). J Am Coll Cardiol 2001;38:2101–2113.

54. Effect of metoprolol CR/XL in chronic heart failure: Metoprolol CR/XL Randomised Intervention Trial in Congestive Heart Failure (MERIT-HF). Lancet 1999;353:2001–2007.

55. Packer M, Coats AJ, Fowler MB, et al. Effect of carvedilol on survival in severe chronic heart failure. N Engl J Med 2001;344:1651–1658.

56. Pitt B, Segal R, Martinez FA, et al. Randomised trial of losartan versus captopril in patients over 65 with heart failure (Evaluation of Losartan in the Elderly Study, ELITE). Lancet 1997;349:747–752.

57. Pitt B, Poole-Wilson PA, Segal R, et al. Effect of losartan compared with captopril on mortality in patients with symptomatic heart failure: Randomised trial. The Losartan Heart Failure Survival Study ELITE II. Lancet 2000;355:1582–1587.

58. Granger CB, McMurray JJ, Yusuf S, et al. Effects of candesartan in patients with chronic heart failure and reduced left-ventricular systolic function intolerant to angiotensin-converting-enzyme inhibitors: The CHARM-Alternative trial. Lancet 2003;362:772–776.

59. McMurray JJ, Ostergren J, Swedberg K, et al. Effects of candesartan in patients with chronic heart failure and reduced left-ventricular systolic function taking angiotensin-converting-enzyme inhibitors: The CHARM-Added trial. Lancet 2003;362:767–771.

60. Pitt B, Zannad F, Remme WJ, et al. The effect of spironolactone on morbidity and mortality in patients with severe heart failure. Randomized Aldactone Evaluation Study Investigators. N Engl J Med 1999;341:709–717.

61. Pitt B, Remme W, Zannad F, et al. Eplerenone, a selective aldosterone blocker, in patients with left ventricular dysfunction after myocardial infarction. N Engl J Med 2003;348:1309–1321.

62. Braunwald E, Antman EM, Beasley JW, et al. ACC/AHA 2002 guideline update for the management of patients with unstable angina and non-ST-segment elevation myocardial infarction: Summary article. A report of the American College of Cardiology/American Heart Association task force on practice guidelines (Committee on the Management of Patients With Unstable Angina). J Am Coll Cardiol 2002;40:1366–1374.

63. A randomized trial of propranolol in patients with acute myocardial infarction: I. Mortality results. JAMA 1982;247:1707–1714.

64. Dargie HJ. Effect of carvedilol on outcome after myocardial infarction in patients with left-ventricular dysfunction: The CAPRICORN randomised trial. Lancet 2001;357:1385–1390.

65. Pfeffer MA, Braunwald E, Moye LA, et al. Effect of captopril on mortality and morbidity in patients with left ventricular dysfunction after myocardial infarction: Results of the survival and ventricular enlargement trial. The SAVE Investigators. N Engl J Med 1992;327:669–677.

66. Yusuf S, Sleight P, Pogue J, et al. Effects of an angiotensin-converting-enzyme inhibitor, ramipril, on cardiovascular events in high-risk patients. The Heart Outcomes Prevention Evaluation Study Investigators. N Engl J Med 2000;342:145–153.

67. Gibbons RJ, Abrams J, Chatterjee K, et al. ACC/AHA 2002 guideline update for the management of patients with chronic stable angina: Summary article. A report of the American College of Cardiology/American Heart Association Task Force on Practice Guidelines (Committee on

the Management of Patients With Chronic Stable Angina). Circulation 2003;107:149–158.

68. Pepine CJ, Handberg EM, Cooper-DeHoff RM, et al. A calcium antagonist vs a non-calcium antagonist hypertension treatment strategy for patients with coronary artery disease. The International Verapamil-Trandolapril Study (INVEST): A randomized, controlled trial. JAMA 2003;290:2805–2816.

69. Arauz-Pacheco C, Parrott MA, Raskin P. The treatment of hypertension in adult patients with diabetes. Diabetes Care 2002;25:134–147.

70. Arauz-Pacheco C, Parrott MA, Raskin P. Hypertension management in adults with diabetes. Diabetes Care 2004;27(suppl 1):S65–67.

71. UK Prospective Diabetes Study Group. Efficacy of atenolol and captopril in reducing risk of macrovascular and microvascular complications in type 2 diabetes: UKPDS 39. Br Med J 1998;317:713–720.

72. UK Prospective Diabetes Study Group. Tight blood pressure control and risk of macrovascular and microvascular complications in type 2 diabetes: UKPDS 38. Group. Br Med J 1998;317:703–713.

73. Pahor M, Psaty BM, Alderman MH, et al. Therapeutic benefits of ACE inhibitors and other antihypertensive drugs in patients with type 2 diabetes. Diabetes Care 2000;23:888–892.

74. 1995 update of the working group reports on chronic renal failure and renovascular hypertension. National High Blood Pressure Education Program Working Group. Arch Intern Med 1996;156:1938–1947.

75. K/DOQI clinical practice guidelines for chronic kidney disease: Evaluation, classification, and stratification. Kidney Disease Outcome Quality Initiative. Am J Kidney Dis 2002;39:S1–246.

76. Lewis EJ, Hunsicker LG, Bain RP, Rohde RD. The effect of angiotensin-converting-enzyme inhibition on diabetic nephropathy. The Collaborative Study Group. N Engl J Med 1993;329:1456–1462.

77. Heart Outcomes Prevention Evaluation Study Investigators. Effects of ramipril on cardiovascular and microvascular outcomes in people with diabetes mellitus: Results of the HOPE study and MICRO-HOPE substudy. Lancet 2000;355:253–259.

78. Brenner BM, Cooper ME, de Zeeuw D, et al. Effects of losartan on renal and cardiovascular outcomes in patients with type 2 diabetes and nephropathy. N Engl J Med 2001;345:861–869.

79. Parving HH, Lehnert H, Brochner-Mortensen J, et al. The effect of irbesartan on the development of diabetic nephropathy in patients with type 2 diabetes. N Engl J Med 2001;345:870–878.

80. Viberti G, Wheeldon NM. Microalbuminuria reduction with valsartan in patients with type 2 diabetes mellitus: A blood pressure–independent effect. Circulation 2002;106:672–678.

81. Wright JT Jr, Bakris G, Greene T, et al. Effect of blood pressure lowering and antihypertensive drug class on progression of hypertensive kidney disease: Results from the AASK trial. JAMA 2002;288:2421–2431.

82. Nakao N, Yoshimura A, Morita H, et al. Combination treatment of angiotensin-II receptor blocker and angiotensin-converting-enzyme inhibitor in non-diabetic renal disease (COOPERATE): A randomised, controlled trial. Lancet 2003;361:117–124.

83. Fox KM. Efficacy of perindopril in reduction of cardiovascular events among patients with stable coronary artery disease: Randomised, double-blind, placebo-controlled, multicentre trial (the EUROPA study). Lancet 2003;362:782–788.

84. Wang JG, Staessen JA, Gong L, Liu L. Chinese trial on isolated systolic hypertension in the elderly. Systolic Hypertension in China (Syst-China) Collaborative Group. Arch Intern Med 2000;160:211–220.

85. Gueyffier F, Bulpitt C, Boissel JP, et al. Antihypertensive drugs in very old people: A subgroup meta-analysis of randomised controlled trials. INDANA Group. Lancet 1999;353:793–796.

86. Staessen JA, Gasowski J, Wang JG, et al. Risks of untreated and treated isolated systolic hypertension in the elderly: Meta-analysis of outcome trials. Lancet 2000;355:865–872.

87. Hansson L, Lindholm LH, Ekbom T, et al. Randomised trial of old and new antihypertensive drugs in elderly patients: Cardiovascular mortality and morbidity the Swedish Trial in Old Patients with Hypertension-2 study. Lancet 1999;354:1751–1756.

88. Update on the 1987 Task Force Report on High Blood Pressure in Children and Adolescents: A working group report from the National High

Blood Pressure Education Program. National High Blood Pressure Education Program Working Group on Hypertension Control in Children and Adolescents. Pediatrics 1996;98:649–658.

89. Report of the National High Blood Pressure Education Program Working Group on High Blood Pressure in Pregnancy. Am J Obstet Gynecol 2000;183:S1–22.

90. Douglas JG, Bakris GL, Epstein M, et al. Management of high blood pressure in African-Americans: Consensus statement of the Hypertension in African-Americans Working Group of the International Society on Hypertension in Blacks. Arch Intern Med 2003;163:525–541.

91. Julius S, Alderman MH, Beevers G, et al. Cardiovascular risk reduction in hypertensive black patients with left ventricular hypertrophy: The LIFE study. J Am Coll Cardiol 2004;43:1047–1055.

92. Salpeter SR, Ormiston TM, Salpeter EE. Cardioselective beta-blockers in patients with reactive airway disease: A meta-analysis. Ann Intern Med 2002;137:715–725.

93. Lakshman MR, Reda DJ, Materson BJ, et al. Diuretics and beta-blockers do not have adverse effects at 1 year on plasma lipid and lipoprotein profiles in men with hypertension. Department of Veterans Affairs Cooperative Study Group on Antihypertensive Agents. Arch Intern Med 1999; 159:551–558.

94. Lindholm LH, Ibsen H, Dahlof B, et al. Cardiovascular morbidity and mortality in patients with diabetes in the Losartan Intervention For Endpoint (LIFE) reduction in hypertension study: A randomised trial against atenolol. Lancet 2002;359:1004–1010.

95. Barksdale JD, Gardner SF. The impact of first-line antihypertensive drugs on erectile dysfunction. Pharmacotherapy 1999;19:573–581.

96. Materson BJ, Reda DJ, Cushman WC, et al. Single-drug therapy for hypertension in men: A comparison of six antihypertensive agents with placebo. The Department of Veterans Affairs Cooperative Study Group on Antihypertensive Agents. N Engl J Med 1993;328:914–921.

97. Grimm RH Jr, Grandits GA, Prineas RJ, et al. Long-term effects on sexual function of five antihypertensive drugs and nutritional hygienic treatment in hypertensive men and women. Treatment of Mild Hypertension Study (TOMHS). Hypertension 1997;29:8–14.

98. Brater DC. Diuretic therapy. N Engl J Med 1998;339:387–395.

99. Carter BL, Ernst ME, Cohen JD. Hydrochlorothiazide versus chlorthalidone: Evidence supporting their interchangeability. Hypertension 2004;43:4–9.

100. Grimm RH Jr, Flack JM, Grandits GA, et al. Long-term effects on plasma lipids of diet and drugs to treat hypertension. Treatment of Mild Hypertension Study (TOMHS) Research Group. JAMA 1996;275:1549–1556.

101. Hansson L, Lindholm LH, Niskanen L, et al. Effect of angiotensin-converting-enzyme inhibition compared with conventional therapy on cardiovascular morbidity and mortality in hypertension: The Captopril Prevention Project (CAPPP) randomised trial. Lancet 1999;353:611–616.

102. Flack JM, Yunis C, Preisser J, et al. The rapidity of drug dose escalation influences blood pressure response and adverse effects burden in patients with hypertension: The Quinapril Titration Interval Management Evaluation (ATIME) Study. ATIME Research Group. Arch Intern Med 2000;160:1842–1847.

103. Willenheimer R, Dahlof B, Rydberg E, Erhardt L. AT$_1$-receptor blockers in hypertension and heart failure: Clinical experience and future directions. Eur Heart J 1999;20:997–1008.

104. Cohn JN, Tognoni G. A randomized trial of the angiotensin-receptor blocker valsartan in chronic heart failure. N Engl J Med 2001;345:1667–1675.

105. Dickstein K, Kjekshus J. Effects of losartan and captopril on mortality and morbidity in high-risk patients after acute myocardial infarction: The OPTIMAAL randomised trial. Optimal Trial in Myocardial Infarction with Angiotensin II Antagonist Losartan. Lancet 2002;360:752–760.

106. Lewis EJ, Hunsicker LG, Clarke WR, et al. Renoprotective effect of the angiotensin-receptor antagonist irbesartan in patients with nephropathy due to type 2 diabetes. N Engl J Med 2001;345:851–860.

107. Grossman E, Messerli FH, Grodzicki T, Kowey P. Should a moratorium be placed on sublingual nifedipine capsules given for hypertensive emergencies and pseudoemergencies? JAMA 1996;276:1328–1331.

108. Packer M, O'Connor CM, Ghali JK, et al. Effect of amlodipine on morbidity and mortality in severe chronic heart failure. Prospective Randomized Amlodipine Survival Evaluation Study Group. N Engl J Med 1996;335:1107–1114.

109. Edelson JT, Weinstein MC, Tosteson AN, et al. Long-term cost-effectiveness of various initial monotherapies for mild to moderate hypertension. JAMA 1990;263:407–413.

110. Hilleman DE, Mohiuddin SM, Lucas BD Jr, et al. Cost-minimization analysis of initial antihypertensive therapy in patients with mild-to-moderate essential diastolic hypertension. Clin Ther 1994;16:88–102; discussion 187.

111. Pearce KA, Furberg CD, Psaty BM, Kirk J. Cost-minimization and the number needed to treat in uncomplicated hypertension. Am J Hypertens 1998;11:618–629.

112. Fischer MA, Avorn J. Economic implications of evidence-based prescribing on hypertension: Can better care cost less? JAMA 2004;291:1850–1856.

113. O'Keefe JH, Wetzel M, Moe RR. Should an angiotensin-converting enzyme inhibitor be standard therapy for patients with atherosclerotic disease? J Am Coll Cardiol 2001;37:1–8.

114. Dzau VJ, Bernstein K, Celermajer D, et al. The relevance of tissue angiotensin-converting enzyme: Manifestations in mechanistic and endpoint data. Am J Cardiol 2001;88:1L–20L.

14
HEART FAILURE

Robert B. Parker, J. Herbert Patterson, and Julie A. Johnson

Learning Objectives and other resources can be found at *www.pharmacotherapyonline.com.*

KEY CONCEPTS

1 Heart failure is a clinical syndrome caused by the inability of the heart to pump sufficient blood to meet the metabolic needs of the body. Heart failure can result from any disorder that reduces ventricular filling (diastolic dysfunction) and/or myocardial contractility (systolic dysfunction). The leading causes of heart failure are coronary artery disease and hypertension. The primary manifestations of the syndrome are dyspnea, fatigue, and fluid retention.

2 Heart failure is a progressive disorder that begins with myocardial injury. In response to the injury, a number of compensatory responses are activated in an attempt to maintain adequate cardiac output, including the sympathetic nervous system, increased preload, vasoconstriction, and ventricular hypertrophy/remodeling. These compensatory mechanisms are responsible for the symptoms of heart failure and contribute to disease progression.

3 Our current understanding of heart failure pathophysiology is best described by the neurohormonal model. Activation of endogenous neurohormones, including norepinephrine, angiotensin II, aldosterone, vasopressin, and numerous proinflammatory cytokines, play an important role in ventricular remodeling and the subsequent progression of heart failure. Importantly, pharmacotherapy targeted at antagonizing this neurohormonal activation has slowed the progression of heart failure and improved survival.

4 Most patients with symptomatic heart failure should be treated routinely with four medications: an angiotensin-converting enzyme (ACE) inhibitor, a β-blocker, a diuretic, and digoxin. The benefits of these medications on slowing heart failure progression, reducing morbidity and mortality, and improving symptoms are clearly established.

5 In patients with heart failure, ACE inhibitors improve survival, slow disease progression, reduce hospitalizations, and improve quality of life. The doses for these agents should be targeted at those shown in clinical trials to improve survival. When ACE inhibitors are contraindicated or not tolerated, an angiotensin II receptor blocker or the combination of hydralazine and isosorbide dinitrate are reasonable alternatives. Patients with asymptomatic left ventricular dysfunction and/or a previous myocardial infarction (stage B of the American College of Cardiology/American Heart Association (ACC/AHA) classification scheme) also should receive ACE inhibitors, with the goal of preventing symptomatic heart failure and reducing mortality.

6 The β-blockers carvedilol, metoprolol CR/XL, and bisoprolol have been shown to prolong survival, decrease hospitalizations and the need for transplantation, and cause "reverse remodeling" of the left ventricle. These agents are recommended for all patients with symptomatic heart failure. Therapy must be instituted at low doses, with slow upward titration to the target dose.

7 Although chronic diuretic therapy frequently is used in heart failure patients, it is not mandatory and is required only in patients with peripheral edema and/or pulmonary congestion.

8 Digoxin does not improve survival in patients with heart failure but does provide symptomatic benefits, particularly in patients with moderate and severe heart failure and those with supraventricular tachyarrhythmias (e.g., atrial fibrillation). Digoxin doses should be adjusted to achieve plasma concentrations of 0.5 to 1 ng/mL; higher plasma concentrations are not associated with additional benefits but may be associated with increased risk of toxicity.

9 Aldosterone antagonism with low-dose spironolactone has been shown to reduce mortality in patients with New York Heart Association (NYHA) class III and IV heart failure and thus should be strongly considered in these patients. Given its low cost and safety profile at the doses studied, it may be reasonable to consider in other patients with symptomatic heart failure, especially those taking potassium supplementation, in whom the aldosterone antagonist might allow dose reduction or discontinuation of the potassium supplement, and should be considered strongly in patients with severe heart failure.

10 No therapy for advanced/decompensated heart failure studied to date has been shown conclusively to influence mortality. Treatment goals are directed toward restoration of systemic oxygen transport and tissue perfusion, relief of pulmonary edema, and limitation of further cardiac damage. Maximizing oral therapy and using combinations of short-acting intravenous medications with different cardiovascular actions often are needed to optimize cardiac output, relieve pulmonary edema, and limit myocardial ischemia. Invasive hemodynamic monitoring usually is required to provide immediate feedback on treatment efficacy and adverse effects.

11 Pharmacists should play an important role as part of a multidisciplinary team to optimize therapy in heart failure. The pharmacist should be responsible for such activities as optimizing regimens for heart failure drug therapy (namely, ensuring that appropriate drugs at appropriate doses are used), educating patients about the importance of adherence to their heart failure regimen (including pharmacologic and dietary interventions), screening for drugs that may exacerbate or worsen heart failure, and monitoring for adverse drug effects and drug interactions.

◄1 ◄2 Heart failure is a clinical syndrome that can result from any disorder that impairs the ability of the ventricle to fill with or eject blood, thus rendering the heart unable to pump blood at a rate sufficient to meet the metabolic demands of the body.[1] Heart failure is the final common pathway for numerous cardiac disorders, including those affecting the pericardium, heart valves, and myocardium. Diseases that adversely affect ventricular diastole (filling), ventricular systole (contraction), or both can lead to heart failure. For many years it was believed that reduced myocardial contractility, or systolic dysfunction, was the sole disturbance in cardiac function responsible for heart failure. However, it is now recognized that disturbances in relaxation (lusitropic) properties of the heart, or diastolic dysfunction, cause heart failure in 20% to 50% of patients.[2] However, regardless of the etiology of heart failure, the underlying pathophysiologic process and principal clinical manifestations (i.e., fatigue, dyspnea, and volume overload) are similar and appear to be independent of the initial cause. Historically, this disorder was commonly referred to as *congestive heart failure*; the preferred nomenclature now is *heart failure* because a patient can have the clinical syndrome of heart failure without having symptoms of congestion. This chapter will focus on treatment of patients with systolic dysfunction (with or without concurrent diastolic dysfunction), whereas Chap. 18 will focus on the treatment of heart failure with normal ejection fraction (isolated diastolic dysfunction).

EPIDEMIOLOGY

Heart failure is an epidemic public health problem in the United States. Approximately 5 million Americans have heart failure, with an additional 550,000 cases diagnosed each year.[3] Unlike most other cardiovascular diseases, the prevalence of heart failure is increasing and is expected to continue to increase over the next few decades as the population ages.[3] A large majority of patients with heart failure are elderly, with multiple comorbid conditions that influence morbidity and mortality.[2] The incidence of heart failure doubles with each decade of life and affects nearly 10% of individuals over age 75.[3] Heart failure is more common in men than in women until age 65, reflecting the greater incidence of coronary artery disease.[3] Recent results from the Framingham Heart Study showed that the incidence of heart failure in men has not changed over the last 40 years but has decreased by approximately one-third in women.[4] These differences in heart failure incidence may be due to sex-based differences in the cause of heart failure because myocardial infarction is the leading cause in men, whereas hypertension is the leading etiology in women.

Heart failure is the most common hospital discharge diagnosis in individuals over age 65.[3] Annual hospital discharges for heart failure now total nearly 1 million, a 165% increase over the last two decades.[3] Heart failure also exacts a tremendous economic impact, with this expected to increase markedly as the baby-boom generation ages. Estimates of annual expenditures for heart failure range from $24 to $50 billion, with most of these costs spent on hospitalized patients.[3,5] Thus heart failure is a major medical problem with substantial economic impact that is expected to become even more significant as the population ages.

Despite prodigious advances in our understanding of the etiology, pathophysiology, and pharmacotherapy of heart failure, the prognosis for patients with this disorder remains grim. Although the mortality rates have declined over the last 50 years, the overall 5-year survival remains approximately 50% for all patients with a diagnosis of heart failure, with mortality increasing with symptom severity.[4] For heart failure patients under age 65, 80% of men and 70% of women will die within 8 years.[3] Death is classified as sudden in about 40% of patients,[1–3] implicating serious ventricular arrhythmias as the underlying cause of death in many patients with heart failure.

ETIOLOGY

◄1 Heart failure can result from any disorder that affects the ability of the heart to contract (systolic function) and/or relax (diastolic dysfunction); common causes of heart failure are shown in Table 14–1.[6] Systolic heart failure is the classic, more familiar form of the disorder, but current estimates suggest that 20% to 50% of patients with heart failure have preserved left ventricular systolic function and suffer from diastolic dysfunction.[2] In contrast to systolic heart failure that is usually caused by previous myocardial infarction (MI), patients with diastolic heart failure typically are elderly, female, and have hypertension and diabetes.[2] However, systolic and diastolic dysfunction frequently coexist. The common cardiovascular diseases such as MI and hypertension can cause both systolic and diastolic dysfunction; thus many patients have heart failure as a result of reduced myocardial contractility and abnormal ventricular filling.

◄1 Coronary artery disease is the most common cause of systolic heart failure, accounting for nearly 70% of cases.[7] MI leads to

TABLE 14–1. Causes of Heart Failure

Systolic Dysfunction (Decreased Contractility)
- Reduction in muscle mass (e.g., myocardial infarction)
- Dilated cardiomyopathies
- Ventricular hypertrophy
  - Pressure overload (e.g., systemic or pulmonary hypertension, aortic or pulmonic valve stenosis)
  - Volume overload (e.g., valvular regurgitation, shunts, high-output states)

Diastolic Dysfunction (Restriction in Ventricular Filling)
- Increased ventricular stiffness
- Ventricular hypertrophy (e.g., hypertrophic cardiomyopathy, other examples above)
- Infiltrative myocardial diseases (e.g., amyloidosis, sarcoidosis, endomyocardial fibrosis)
- Myocardial ischemia and infarction
- Mitral or tricuspid valve stenosis
- Pericardial disease (e.g., pericarditis, pericardial tamponade)

Data from Colucci W, Braunwald E. Pathophysiology of heart failure. In: Braunwald E, Zipes DP, Libby P, eds. Heart Disease: A Textbook of Cardiovascular Medicine, 6th ed. Philadelphia, Saunders, 2001:503–533; and Wynne J, Braunwald E. The cardiomyopathies and myocarditides. In: Braunwald E, Zipes DP, Libby P, eds. Heart Disease: A Textbook of Cardiovascular Medicine, 6th ed. Philadelphia, Saunders, 2001:1751–1806.

a reduction in muscle mass owing to death of affected myocardial cells. The degree to which contractility is impaired will depend on the size of the infarction. In an attempt to maintain cardiac output, the surviving myocardium undergoes a compensatory remodeling, thus beginning the maladaptive process that initiates the heart failure syndrome. This is discussed in greater detail in the "Pathophysiology" section. Myocardial ischemia and infarction also affect the diastolic properties of the heart by slowing ventricular relaxation and increasing ventricular stiffness. Thus MI frequently results in systolic and diastolic dysfunction.

Systolic contractile dysfunction is a cardinal feature of dilated cardiomyopathies. Although the cause of reduced contractility frequently is unknown, abnormalities such as interstitial fibrosis, cellular infiltrates, cellular hypertrophy, and myocardial cell degeneration are seen commonly on histologic examination.[8]

Pressure or volume overload causes ventricular hypertrophy, which attempts to return contractility to a near-normal state. However, if the pressure or volume overload persists, the remodeling process results in alterations in the geometry of the hypertrophied myocardial cells and is accompanied by increased collagen deposition in the extracellular matrix. Thus both systolic and diastolic function may be impaired.[6] Examples of pressure overload include systemic or pulmonary hypertension and aortic or pulmonic valve stenosis. Hypertension remains an important cause and/or contributor to heart failure in many patients, particularly women, the elderly, and African-Americans.[4] The role of hypertension should not be underestimated because hypertension is an important risk factor for ischemic heart disease and thus is also present in a high percentage of the patients with this disorder. Volume overload may occur in the presence of valvular regurgitation, shunts, or high-output states such as anemia or pregnancy. Less common causes of diastolic dysfunction are listed in Table 14–1 and include infiltrative myocardial diseases, mitral or tricuspid valve stenosis, and pericardial disease.

Since ischemic heart disease and/or hypertension contribute so significantly to the development of heart failure in the majority of patients, it is important to emphasize that heart failure is a largely preventable disorder. Thus recent evidence that obesity and salt intake are important risk factors for heart failure is not surprising.[9,10] Moreover, control of blood pressure and appropriate management of other risk factors for cardiovascular disease (e.g., smoking cessation, treatment of lipid disorders, diabetes management, dietary modification, etc.) are important strategies for clinicians to implement to reduce their patients' risk of heart failure.

PATHOPHYSIOLOGY

NORMAL CARDIAC FUNCTION

To understand the pathophysiologic processes in heart failure, a basic understanding of normal cardiac function is necessary. *Cardiac output* (CO) is defined as the volume of blood ejected per unit time (L/min) and is the product of heart rate (HR) and stroke volume (SV):

$$CO = HR \times SV$$

The relationship between CO and mean arterial pressure (MAP) is

$$MAP = CO \times \text{systemic vascular resistance (SVR)}$$

Heart rate is controlled by the autonomic nervous system. Stroke volume, or the volume of blood ejected during systole, depends on preload, afterload, and contractility.[6] As defined by the Frank-Starling mechanism, the ability of the heart to alter the force of contraction

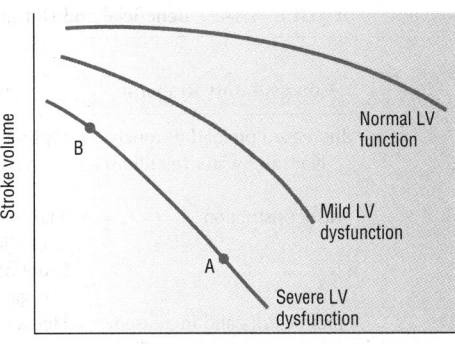

FIGURE 14–1. Relationship between stroke volume and systemic vascular resistance. In an individual with normal left ventricular (LV) function, increasing systemic vascular resistance has little effect on stroke volume. As the extent of LV dysfunction increases, the negative inverse relationship between stroke volume and systemic vascular resistance becomes more important (*B* to *A*).

depends on changes in preload. As myocardial sarcomere length is stretched, the number of cross-bridges between thick and thin myofilaments increases, resulting in an increase in the force of contraction. The length of the sarcomere is determined primarily by the volume of blood in the ventricle; therefore, left ventricular end-diastolic volume (LVEDV) is the primary determinant of preload. In normal hearts, the preload response is the primary compensatory mechanism such that a small increase in end-diastolic volume results in a large increase in cardiac output. Because of the relationship between pressure and volume in the heart, left ventricular end-diastolic pressure (LVEDP) is often used in the clinical setting to estimate preload. The hemodynamic measurement used to estimate LVEDP is the pulmonary artery occlusion pressure (PAOP). Afterload is a more complex physiologic concept that can be viewed pragmatically as the sum of forces preventing active forward ejection of blood by the ventricle. Major components of global ventricular afterload are ejection impedance, wall tension, and regional wall geometry. In patients with left ventricular systolic dysfunction, an inverse relationship exists between afterload (or SVR) and stroke volume such that increasing afterload causes a decrease in stroke volume (Fig. 14–1). Contractility is the intrinsic property of cardiac muscle describing fiber shortening and tension development.

COMPENSATORY MECHANISMS IN HEART FAILURE

Heart failure is a progressive disorder initiated by an event that impairs the ability of the heart to contract and/or relax. The index event may have an acute onset, as with MI, or the onset may be slow, as with long-standing hypertension. Regardless of the index event, the decrease in the heart's pumping capacity results in the heart having to rely on compensatory responses to maintain an adequate cardiac output.[11] These compensatory responses are (1) tachycardia and increased contractility through sympathetic nervous system (SNS) activation, (2) the Frank-Starling mechanism, whereby an increase in preload results in an increase in stroke volume, (3) vasoconstriction, and (4) ventricular hypertrophy and remodeling. Teleologically, these compensatory responses are intended to be short-term responses to maintain circulatory homeostasis after acute reductions in blood pressure or renal perfusion. However, the persistent decline in cardiac output in heart failure results in long-term activation of these compensatory responses, resulting in the complex functional, structural, biochemical, and molecular changes important for the initiation

TABLE 14–2. Beneficial and Detrimental Effects of the Compensatory Responses in Heart Failure

Compensatory Response	Beneficial Effects of Compensation	Detrimental Effects of Compensation
Increased preload (through Na^+ and water retention)	Optimize stroke volume via Frank-Starling mechanism	Pulmonary and systemic congestion and edema formation Increased MVO_2
Vasoconstriction	Maintain BP in face of reduced cardiac output Shunt blood from nonessential organs to brain and heart	Increased MVO_2 Increased afterload decreases stroke volume and further activates the compensatory responses
Tachycardia and increased contractility (due to SNS activation)	Helps maintain cardiac output	Increased MVO_2 Shortened diastolic filling time β_1-Receptor downregulation, decreased receptor sensitivity Precipitation of ventricular arrhythmias Increased risk of myocardial cell death
Ventricular hypertrophy and remodeling	Helps maintain cardiac output Reduces myocardial wall stress Decreases MVO_2	Diastolic dysfunction Systolic dysfunction Increased risk of myocardial cell death Increased risk of myocardial ischemia Increased arrhythmia risk Fibrosis

Abbreviations: SNS = sympathetic nervous system; BP = blood pressure; MVO_2 = myocardial oxygen demand.

and progression of the heart failure syndrome. The benefits and detrimental consequences of these compensatory responses are described below and are summarized in Table 14–2.

TACHYCARDIA AND INCREASED CONTRACTILITY THROUGH SNS ACTIVATION

The change in heart rate and contractility that occurs in response to a drop in cardiac output is due primarily to release of norepinephrine (NE) from adrenergic nerve terminals, although parasympathetic nervous system activity is diminished. Because cardiac output equals the product of heart rate and stroke volume, one might expect cardiac output to change linearly with heart rate, but the relationship is much more complex. Since systolic time intervals change comparatively little with changing heart rate, almost all cardiac cycle shortening occurs during diastole. Cardiac output continues to increase with heart rate until diastolic filling becomes compromised, which in the normal heart is at 170 to 200 beats per minute. When preexisting or acute diastolic dysfunction is present, however, the ventricle's need for more complete (longer) diastolic filling results in reduction of effective preload at significantly lower heart rates. Loss of atrial contribution to ventricular filling also can occur (e.g., atrial fibrillation or ventricular tachycardia), reducing ventricular performance even more. Because ionized calcium is sequestered into the sarcoplasmic reticulum and pumped out of the cell during diastole, shortened diastolic time also results in a higher average intracellular calcium concentration during diastole, increasing actin-myosin interaction, augmenting the active resistance to fibril stretch, and reducing lusitropy. Conversely, the higher average calcium concentration translates into greater filament interaction during systole, generating more tension.[6]

Increasing heart rate greatly increases myocardial oxygen demand. If ischemia is induced or worsened, both diastolic and systolic function may become impaired, and stroke volume can drop precipitously.

INCREASED PRELOAD

Augmentation of preload is another compensatory response that is activated rapidly in response to decreased cardiac output. Renal perfusion in heart failure is reduced owing to both depressed cardiac output and redistribution of blood away from nonvital organs. The kidney interprets the reduced perfusion as an ineffective blood volume, resulting in activation of the renin-angiotensin-aldosterone (RAA) system. Reduced renal perfusion and increased sympathetic tone also stimulate renin release from juxtaglomerular cells in the kidney. As shown in Fig. 14–2, renin is responsible for conversion of angiotensinogen to angiotensin I. Angiotensin I is converted to angiotensin II by angiotensin-converting enzyme (ACE). Angiotensin II also may be generated via non-ACE-dependent pathways. Angiotensin II feeds back on the adrenal gland to stimulate aldosterone release, thereby providing an additional mechanism for sodium and water retention in the kidney. As intravascular volume increases secondary to sodium and water retention, left ventricular volume and pressure (preload) increase, sarcomeres are stretched, and the force of contraction is enhanced.[6] While the preload response is the primary compensatory mechanism in normal hearts, the chronically failing heart usually has exhausted its preload reserve.[6] As shown in Fig. 14–3, increases in preload will increase stroke volume only to a certain point. Once the flat portion of the curve is reached, further increases in preload will only lead to pulmonary or systemic congestion, a detrimental result.[6] Figure 14–3 also shows that the curve is flatter in patients with left ventricular dysfunction. Consequently, a given increase in preload in a patient with heart failure will produce a smaller increment in stroke volume than in an individual with normal ventricular function.

In addition to causing symptoms of congestion, augmentation of preload in the heart failure patient will increase afterload because increasing the radius of the ventricle elevates wall tension. Because the failing ventricle is highly afterload-dependent, increases in performance augmented by preload at times may be offset by the attendant increase in afterload. Additionally, the effects of increased preload on force of contraction and afterload will increase myocardial

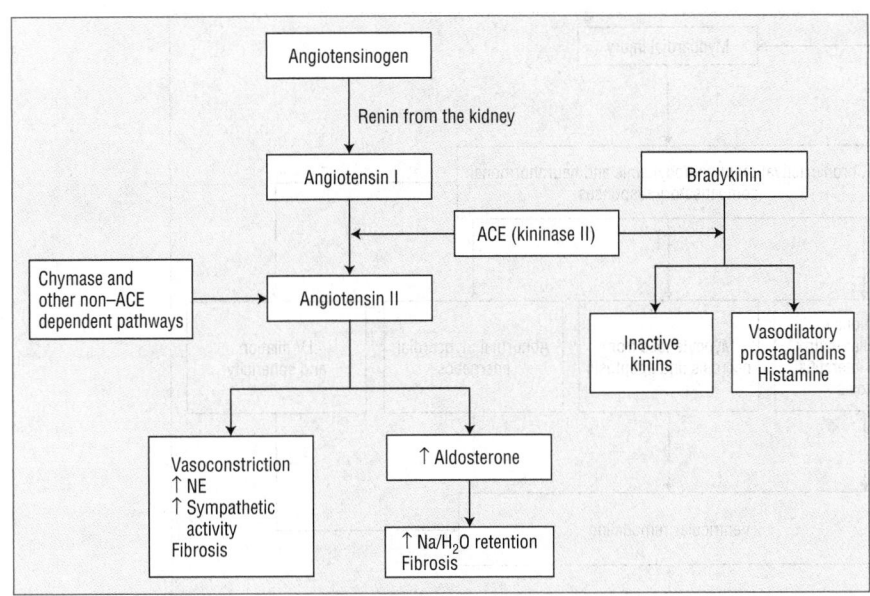

FIGURE 14–2. Physiology of the renin-angiotensin-aldosterone system. Renin produces angiotensin I from angiotensinogen. Angiotensin I is cleaved to angiotensin II by angiotensin-converting enzyme (ACE). Angiotensin II has a number of physiologic actions that are detrimental in heart failure. Note that angiotensin II can be produced in a number of tissues, including the heart, independent of ACE activity. ACE is also responsible for the breakdown of bradykinin. Inhibition of ACE results in accumulation of bradykinin, which, in turn, enhances the production of vasodilatory prostaglandins.

oxygen consumption. Thus an increase in preload can induce ischemia in the coronary patient, with subsequent lusitropic and inotropic compromise.

VASOCONSTRICTION

Vasoconstriction occurs in patients with heart failure to help redistribute blood flow away from nonessential organs to coronary and cerebral circulations to support blood pressure, which may be reduced secondary to a decrease in cardiac output (MAP = CO × SVR).[6] A number of neurohormones likely contribute to the vasoconstriction, including NE, angiotensin II, endothelin-1, and arginine vasopressin (AVP).[6] Vasoconstriction impedes forward ejection of blood from the ventricle, further depressing cardiac output and heightening the compensatory responses. Because the failing ventricle usually has exhausted its preload reserve (unless the patient is depleted intravascularly), its performance is exquisitely sensitive to changes in afterload (see Fig 14–1). Thus, increases in afterload often potentiate a vicious

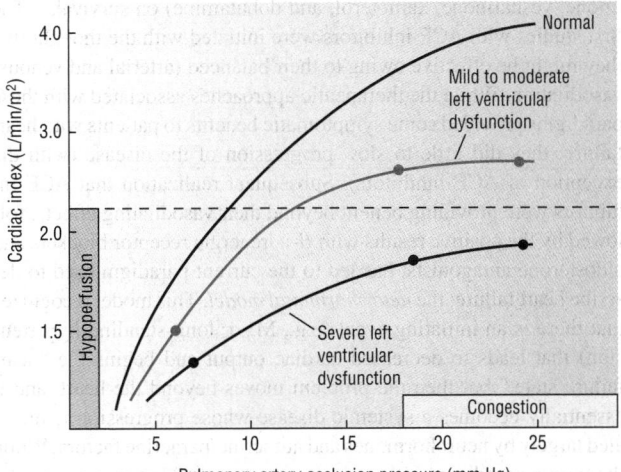

FIGURE 14–3. Relationship between cardiac output (shown as cardiac index, which is CO/BSA) and preload (shown as pulmonary artery occlusion pressure).

cycle of continued worsening and downward spiraling of the heart failure state.

VENTRICULAR HYPERTROPHY AND REMODELING[6,11]

While the signs and symptoms of heart failure are associated closely with the items just described, the progression of heart failure appears to be independent of the patient's hemodynamic status. It is now recognized that ventricular hypertrophy and remodeling are key components in the pathogenesis of progressive myocardial failure. *Ventricular hypertrophy* is a term used to describe an increase in ventricular muscle mass. *Cardiac* or *ventricular remodeling* is a broader term describing changes in both myocardial cells and extracellular matrix that result in changes in the size, shape, structure, and function of the heart. Ventricular hypertrophy and remodeling can occur in association with any condition that causes myocardial injury, including MI, cardiomyopathy, hypertension, and valvular heart disease.

Cardiac remodeling is a complex process that affects the heart at the molecular and cellular levels. Key elements in the process are shown in Fig. 14–4. Collectively, these events result in progressive changes in myocardial structure and function, such as cardiac hypertrophy, myocyte loss, and alterations in the extracellular matrix. The progression of the remodeling process leads to reductions in myocardial systolic and/or diastolic function that, in turn, lead to further myocardial injury, perpetuating the remodeling process and the decline in ventricular function. Angiotensin II, NE, endothelin, aldosterone, vasopressin, and numerous inflammatory cytokines, as well as substances under investigation, that are activated both systemically and in the heart play an important role in initiating the signal-transduction cascade responsible for ventricular remodeling.

Pressure overload (and probably hormonal activation) associated with hypertension produces a concentric hypertrophy (an increase in ventricular wall thickness without chamber enlargement). Eccentric left ventricular hypertrophy (myocyte lengthening with increased chamber size and a minimal increase in wall thickness) characterizes the hypertrophy seen in patients with systolic dysfunction or previous MI. As the myocytes undergo change, so do various

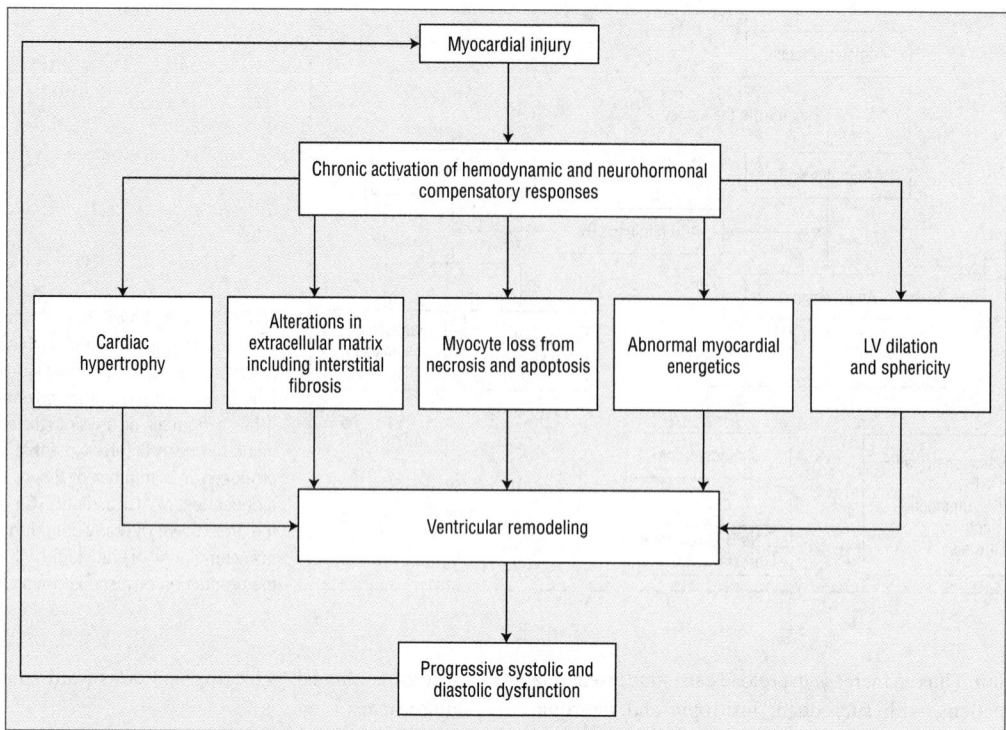

FIGURE 14–4. Key components of the pathophysiology of cardiac remodeling. Myocardial injury (e.g., myocardial infarction) results in the activation of a number of hemodynamic and neurohormonal compensatory responses in an attempt to maintain circulatory homeostasis. Chronic activation of the neurohormonal systems results in a cascade of events that affect the myocardium at the molecular and cellular levels. These events lead to the changes in ventricular size, shape, structure, and function known as *ventricular remodeling*. The alterations in ventricular function result in further deterioration in cardiac systolic and diastolic function, which further promotes the remodeling process.

components of the extracellular matrix. For example, there is evidence for collagen degradation, which may lead to slippage of myocytes, fibroblast proliferation, and increased fibrillar collagen synthesis, resulting in fibrosis and stiffening of the entire myocardium. Thus a number of important ventricular changes that occur with remodeling include changes in the geometry of the heart from elliptical to spherical, increases in ventricular mass (from myocyte hypertrophy), and changes in ventricular composition (especially the extracellar matrix) and volume, all of which likely contribute to the impairment of cardiac function. If the event that produces cardiac injury is acute (e.g., MI), the ventricular remodeling process begins immediately. However, it is the progressive nature of this process that results in continual worsening of the heart failure state and thus is now the major focus for identification of therapeutic targets. In fact, it is believed that all the heart failure therapies that have been associated with decreased mortality and/or slowing of the progression of the disease produce this effect largely through their ability to slow or reverse the ventricular remodeling process. Thus, while ventricular hypertrophy and remodeling may have some beneficial effects by helping to maintain cardiac output, they also are believed to play an essential role in the progressive nature of heart failure.

THE NEUROHORMONAL MODEL OF HEART FAILURE AND THE THERAPEUTIC INSIGHTS IT PROVIDES[6,11]

Over the years, several different paradigms have guided the therapy of heart failure. The early paradigm is often called the *cardiorenal model,* in which the problem was viewed as excess sodium and water retention, and diuretic therapy was the main therapeutic approach to combating the problem. The next paradigm was the *cardiocirculatory model,* which focused on impaired cardiac output (viewed as being due to both inadequate contractility and systemic vasoconstriction). This paradigm focused on positive inotropes and, later, vasodilators as the primary therapies to overcome the problems associated with heart failure. The inadequacy of this model to explain the progressive nature of heart failure is pointed out by the detrimental effects of positive inotropic drugs (e.g., amrinone, milrinone, enoximone, vesnarinone, xamoterol, and dobutamine) on survival.[12] The first studies with ACE inhibitors were initiated with the thought that they might be effective owing to their balanced (arterial and venous) vasodilation. While the therapeutic approaches associated with these paradigms provided some symptomatic benefits to patients with heart failure, they did little to slow progression of the disease (with the exception of ACE inhibitors). Subsequent realization that ACE inhibitors were providing benefit beyond their vasodilating effects, followed by the positive results with β-adrenergic receptor blockers and aldosterone antagonists, has led to the current paradigm used to describe heart failure: the *neurohormonal model.* This model recognizes that there is an initiating event (e.g., MI or long-standing hypertension) that leads to decreased cardiac output and begins the "heart failure state," but then the problem moves beyond the heart, and it essentially becomes a systemic disease whose progression is mediated largely by neurohormones and autocrine/paracrine factors. While the former paradigms still guide us to some extent in the symptomatic management of the disease (e.g., diuretics and digoxin), it is the latter paradigm that helps us understand disease progression and, more important, the ways to slow disease progression. In the sections that follow, important neurohormones and autocrine/paracrine factors are described with respect to their role in heart failure and its progression. The benefits of current and investigational drug therapies can be better understood through a solid understanding of the neurohormones they regulate/affect.

ANGIOTENSIN II[6,11]

Of the neurohormones and autocrine/paracrine factors that play an important role in the pathophysiology of heart failure, angiotensin II is probably the best understood. Angiotensin II has multiple actions that contribute to its detrimental effects in heart failure. Angiotensin II increases systemic vascular resistance in heart failure through direct, potent vasoconstriction. Its ability to cause release of AVP and endothelin-1 also may contribute to vasoconstriction. Angiotensin II also facilitates release of NE from adrenergic nerve terminals, heightening SNS activation. It promotes sodium retention through direct effects on the renal tubules and by stimulating aldosterone release. Its vasoconstriction of the efferent glomerular arteriole helps to maintain perfusion pressure in patients with severe heart failure or impaired renal function. Thus, in patients dependent on angiotensin II for maintenance of perfusion pressure, initiation of an ACE inhibitor or angiotensin II receptor type I blocker (ARB) causes efferent arteriole vasodilation, decreased perfusion pressure, and decreased glomerular filtration. This explains the risk of transient impairment in renal function associated with initiation of ACE inhibitor or ARB therapy. Finally, angiotensin II, as well as many of the neurohormones whose release/production is stimulated by angiotensin II, plays a central role in stimulating ventricular hypertrophy, remodeling, myocyte apoptosis (programmed cell death), and alterations in the extracellular matrix. Clinical data suggest that blocking these effects contributes substantially to the prolonged survival of ACE inhibitor– and ARB-treated heart failure patients.[13,14] The favorable effects of ACE inhibitors (and presumably ARBs) on hemodynamics, symptoms, quality of life, and survival in heart failure highlight the importance of angiotensin II in the pathophysiology of heart failure.

NOREPINEPHRINE[6,15,16]

Many of the detrimental effects of NE in heart failure were described earlier. NE plays a central role in the tachycardia, vasoconstriction, and increased contractility observed in heart failure. Plasma NE concentrations are elevated in correlation with the degree of heart failure, and patients with the highest plasma NE concentrations have the poorest prognosis. In addition to the detrimental effects described, excessive SNS activation causes downregulation of β_1-receptors, with a subsequent loss of sensitivity to receptor stimulation. Recent evidence suggests that genetic variations in the β_1- and α_{2c}-receptors, which are targets for NE's actions, may increase the risk of heart failure.[17] Excess catecholamines increase the risk of arrhythmias and can cause myocardial cell loss by stimulating both necrosis and apoptosis. Finally, NE contributes to ventricular hypertrophy and remodeling. The detrimental effects of SNS activation are further highlighted by the clinical trials of chronic therapy with β-agonists, phosphodiesterase inhibitors, or other drugs that cause SNS activation because they have been shown uniformly to increase mortality in heart failure.[12] Additionally, β-blockers, ACE inhibitors, and digoxin all help to decrease SNS activation through various mechanisms and are beneficial in heart failure. Thus it is clear that NE plays a critical role in the pathophysiology of the heart failure state.

ALDOSTERONE[18,19]

Aldosterone-mediated sodium retention and its key role in volume overload and edema have long been recognized as important components of the heart failure syndrome. Circulating aldosterone is increased in heart failure due to stimulation of its synthesis and release from the adrenal cortex by angiotensin II and to decreased hepatic clearance secondary to reduced hepatic perfusion. Although its enhancement of sodium retention is an important component of heart failure symptoms, recent studies indicate that direct effects of aldosterone on the heart may be even more important in heart failure pathophysiology. Chief among these is the ability of aldosterone to produce interstitial cardiac fibrosis through increased collagen deposition in the extracellular matrix of the heart. This cardiac fibrosis may decrease systolic function and also impair diastolic function by increasing the stiffness of the myocardium. Current research shows that extraadrenal production of aldosterone in the heart, kidneys, and vascular smooth muscle also contributes to the progressive nature of heart failure through target-organ fibrosis and vascular remodeling. Aldosterone also may increase the risk of ventricular arrhythmias through a number of mechanisms, including creation of reentrant circuits as a result of fibrosis, inhibition of cardiac NE reuptake, depletion of intracellular potassium and magnesium, and impairment of parasympathetic traffic. Recent studies with the aldosterone antagonists spironolactone[20] and eplerenone[21] produced significant reductions in mortality in patients with heart failure without appreciable effects on diuresis or hemodynamics, providing substantial evidence that the direct cardiac effects of aldosterone play an important role in heart failure pathophysiology.

NATRIURETIC PEPTIDES[22,23]

The natriuretic peptide family has three members, atrial natriuretic peptide (ANP), B-type natriuretic peptide (BNP), and C-type natriuretic peptide (CNP). ANP is stored mainly in the right atrium, whereas BNP is found mainly in the ventricles. Both are released in response to pressure or volume overload. CNP is found mainly in the brain and has very low plasma concentrations. ANP and BNP plasma concentrations are elevated in patients with heart failure and are thought to balance the effects of the RAA system by causing natriuresis, diuresis, vasodilation, decreased aldosterone release, decreased hypertrophy, and inhibition of the SNS and the RAA system.

The role of BNP as a biomarker for prognostic, diagnostic, and therapeutic use has received much recent attention. In patients with chronic heart failure, the degree of elevation in BNP levels is closely associated with increased mortality, risk of sudden death, symptoms, and hospital readmission. Current data indicate that BNP is more sensitive than NE in predicting morbidity and mortality in heart failure patients. Accurate diagnosis of decompensated heart failure in acute care settings is often difficult because many of the symptoms (e.g., dyspnea) mimic those of other disorders such as pulmonary disease or obesity. The development of a rapid bedside BNP assay has proven helpful for discriminating decompensated heart failure from these other disorders. Although larger prospective trials are needed, initial evidence indicates that BNP may be a useful marker to guide titration of heart failure therapy. Patients whose heart failure therapy was titrated to achieve lower BNP concentrations had improved outcomes (defined as a composite of death, hospital admission, or heart failure decompensation) compared with traditionally treated patients.[24] Finally, administration of recombinant human BNP (nesiritide) for short-term management of acute heart failure resulted in hemodynamic and symptomatic improvement, further supporting the role of BNP in heart failure pathophysiology.

ARGININE VASOPRESSIN[25]

AVP is a pituitary peptide hormone that plays an important role in regulation of renal water and solute excretion. AVP secretion is linked directly to changes in plasma osmolality, thus attempting to maintain body fluid homeostasis. The physiologic effects of AVP are mediated through the V_{1a} and V_2 receptors. V_{1a} receptors are located in vascular smooth muscle and in myocytes, where their stimulation by AVP results in vasoconstriction and increased cardiac contractility, respectively. V_2 receptors are located in the collecting duct of the kidney, where AVP stimulation causes reabsorption of free water.

Plasma concentrations of AVP are elevated in patients with heart failure, with the magnitude of elevation correlating with symptom severity. Importantly, current research suggests that AVP also may play a role in the pathophysiology of heart failure. Important effects associated with increased circulating AVP concentrations include (1) increased renal free water reabsorption in the face of plasma hypoosmolality, resulting in volume overload and hyponatremia, (2) increased arterial vasoconstriction, which contributes to reduced cardiac output, and, (3) stimulation of remodeling by cardiac hypertrophy and extracellular matrix collagen deposition.

Given the importance of AVP in heart failure, recent efforts have focused on the development of AVP antagonist drugs for treatment of acute and chronic heart failure. Although still investigational, the oral V_2-receptor antagonist tolvaptan reduced edema and body weight and increased urine output and serum sodium concentration without affecting heart rate, blood pressure, or renal function in volume-overloaded heart failure patients.[26] Similar effects have been reported with agents that are V_{1a}/V_2 antagonists. These results suggest that AVP antagonists may be useful in the treatment of heart failure patients with volume overload. Unlike diuretics, they appear to reduce excess fluid volume without affecting heart rate, blood pressure, renal function, or electrolytes. Thus these agents may offer a new therapeutic approach to currently available drug therapies, although additional clinical trials are needed to establish long-term efficacy and safety.

OTHER CIRCULATING MEDIATORS[27,28]

In addition to neurohormones, several proinflammatory cytokines are under extensive investigation for their role in heart failure pathophysiology. Tumor necrosis factor α (TNF-α), interleukin-6 (IL-6), and IL-1β all have been shown to be elevated in heart failure, with a direct relationship between the degree of elevation and the severity of heart failure. Of these cytokines, TNF-α is best studied for its pathophysiologic role in heart failure. TNF-α produces multiple deleterious actions, including negative inotropic effects, uncoupling β-adrenergic receptors from adenylyl cyclase (thus reducing β-receptor-mediated responses), increasing myocardial cell apoptosis, and stimulating remodeling via several mechanisms. Although these findings clearly imply a role for TNF-α in the pathophysiology of heart failure, clinical trials evaluating anti-TNF-α therapies (e.g., etanercept) have been disappointing, with no improvement in outcomes demonstrated.

The endothelin peptides are potent vasoconstrictors that may be involved in heart failure pathophysiology through a number of mechanisms. Endothelin-1 (ET-1), the best characterized of these peptides, is synthesized by endothelial and vascular smooth muscle cells, with the release of ET-1 enhanced by NE, angiotensin II, and inflammatory cytokines. Like other peptides and hormones described earlier, ET-1 plasma concentrations are elevated in heart failure and have been correlated directly with the severity of hemodynamic abnormality, symptoms, and mortality. Its arterial and venous constrictive effects increase preload and afterload, and its vasoconstriction of both efferent and afferent renal arterioles may decrease renal plasma flow and induce sodium retention. ET-1 has direct cardiotoxic effects, is a potent stimulator of cardiac myocyte hypertrophy, and has arrhythmogenic effects. It is also a positive inotrope and, like the β-agonists, over the long-term may be harmful owing to the increased myocardial energy utilization. Finally, ET-1 also appears to modulate production of many other neurohormones involved in heart failure pathophysiology, including angiotensin II, aldosterone, and NE. These findings suggest that endothelin-receptor antagonists may be beneficial in patients with heart failure. Clinical trials with several agents have shown improvements in hemodynamics and symptoms, although the more important long-term effects of endothelin-receptor blockade on heart failure progression and mortality remain unknown.

PRECIPITATING FACTORS IN HEART FAILURE DECOMPENSATION

Although significant advancements have been made in treatment, exacerbations of symptoms to the point that hospitalization is required is a common and growing problem in patients with heart failure. Hospitalization for heart failure exacerbation consumes large amounts of health care dollars and significantly impairs the patient's quality of life. Thus there is great interest in identifying and then remedying factors that increase the risk of decompensation. In patients with heart failure, appropriate therapy often can maintain them in a "compensated" state, indicating that they are relatively symptom-free. However, there are many aggravating or precipitating factors that may cause a previously compensated patient to decompensate, resulting in worsened symptoms and necessitating hospitalization. Precipitants of heart failure decompensation typically increase preload or afterload and/or decrease cardiac contractility. The resulting symptoms are typically those associated with volume overload, but in more severe cases, hypoperfusion also may be present.

Factors involved in precipitating decompensation have been evaluated prospectively in patients admitted to the hospital with heart failure.[29,30] These studies consistently show that noncompliance with drugs or diet is a common cause of heart failure exacerbation. For example, 43% of patients admitted with an acute decompensation of chronic heart failure were assessed as having dietary sodium excess, 34% had excess fluid intake (defined as >2.5 L/day), and about 24% had drug noncompliance that may have contributed to their decompensation (although not necessarily defined as the primary cause of decompensation).[30] Use of inappropriate medications such as antiarrhythmic agents or calcium channel blockers also was an important precipitant of exacerbations.

Cardiac events also may precipitate heart failure exacerbations. Myocardial ischemia and infarction are potentially reversible causes that must be considered carefully because nearly 70% of heart failure patients have coronary artery disease. It should be noted that myocardial ischemia can be either a cause or a consequence of heart failure decompensation. Revascularization should be considered in appropriate patients. Atrial fibrillation occurs in up to 10% to 30% of patients with heart failure and is associated with increased morbidity and mortality.[31] Atrial fibrillation can exacerbate heart failure through rapid ventricular response and loss of atrial contribution to ventricular filling. Conversely, decompensated heart failure can precipitate atrial fibrillation by atrial distension resulting from ventricular volume overload. Control of ventricular response, maintenance of sinus rhythm in appropriate patients, and prevention of thromboembolism are important elements in the treatment of heart failure patients with atrial fibrillation.

A number of noncardiac events may also be associated with heart failure decompensation. Pulmonary infections frequently cause worsening of heart failure. At least some of these events would be preventable with more widespread use of the pneumococcal and influenza vaccines in these patients. Recent studies suggest that anemia occurs frequently in patients with heart failure and that it is associated with reduced survival and functional status and increased risk of hospitalization.[32] Although correction of anemia with agents such as epoetin-α may improve symptoms, the effect on prognosis awaits the results of ongoing clinical trials.

What should be evident is that many of the precipitating factors are preventable, particularly through appropriate pharmacist intervention. Specifically, patient education and counseling by a pharmacist should help to decrease the most common reason for heart failure exacerbation—noncompliance with dietary sodium and water restrictions, drug therapy, or both. Pharmacists also should be able to identify and address inadequate heart failure therapy, poorly controlled hypertension, and administration of drugs that may worsen heart failure owing to their negative inotropic, cardiotoxic, or sodium-retaining properties. Specific examples of drugs that can worsen heart failure are given in Table 14–3. It should be noted that while the cyclooxygenase-2 (COX-2) inhibitors may differ from the traditional nonsteroidal anti-inflammatory drugs (NSAIDs) in their gastric ulceration effects, their effects on renal function are similar to those of NSAIDs.[33] Thus both NSAIDs and COX-2 inhibitors should be used judiciously in heart failure patients. The thiazolidinedione hypoglycemic drugs rosiglitazone and pioglitazone are associated with weight gain and the development of edema that may exacerbate heart failure. Current guidelines indicate these agents should not be used in patients with NYHA class III or IV heart failure.[1] It can be argued that heart failure exacerbations owing to noncompliance, inadequate/inappropriate drug therapy, and poorly controlled hypertension are all preventable and amenable to pharmacist intervention. Thus the value of the pharmacist's role in careful and repeated education of patients and monitoring of the drug regimen should not be underestimated. Attention to these factors may make an important contribution to reducing the risk of hospitalization and improving the quality of life of patients.

CLINICAL PRESENTATION[34]

SIGNS AND SYMPTOMS

The primary manifestations of heart failure are dyspnea and fatigue, which lead to exercise intolerance, and fluid overload, which can result in pulmonary congestion and peripheral edema. The presence of these signs and symptoms may vary considerably from patient to patient such that some patients have dyspnea but no signs of fluid retention, and others may have marked volume overload with few complaints of dyspnea or fatigue. However, many patients may have both dyspnea and volume overload. It is also important to note that these symptoms can vary considerably over time in a given patient. Historically, these signs and symptoms have been classified as being due to left ventricular failure, LVF (pulmonary congestion) or right ventricular failure, RVF (systemic congestion). Although most patients initially have LVF, the ventricles share a septal wall, and because LVF increases the workload of the right ventricle, both ventricles eventually fail and contribute to the heart failure syndrome. Because of the complex nature of this syndrome, it has become exceedingly more difficult to attribute a specific sign or symptom as caused by either RVF or LVF. Therefore, the numerous signs and symptoms associated with this disorder are collectively attributed to heart failure rather than to dysfunction of a specific ventricle.

CLINICAL PRESENTATION OF HEART FAILURE

GENERAL

Patient presentation may range from asymptomatic to cardiogenic shock.

SYMPTOMS

- Dyspnea, particularly on exertion
- Orthopnea
- Paroxysmal nocturnal dyspnea
- Exercise intolerance
- Tachypnea
- Cough
- Fatigue
- Nocturia
- Hemoptysis
- Abdominal pain
- Anorexia
- Nausea
- Bloating
- Ascites
- Mental status changes

SIGNS

- Pulmonary rales
- Pulmonary edema
- S_3 gallop
- Pleural effusion
- Cheyne-Stokes respiration
- Tachycardia

TABLE 14–3. Drugs that May Precipitate or Exacerbate Heart Failure

Negative Inotropic Effect
Antiarrhythmics (e.g., disopyramide, flecainide, and others)
β-Blockers (e.g., propranolol, metoprolol, atenolol, and others)
Calcium channel blockers (e.g., verapamil and others)
Itraconazole
Terbinafine

Cardiotoxic
Doxorubicin
Daunomycin
Cyclophosphamide

Sodium and Water Retention
NSAIDs
COX-2 inhibitors
Rosiglitazone and pioglitazone
Glucocorticoids
Androgens
Estrogens
Salicylates (high dose)
Sodium-containing drugs (e.g., carbenicillin disodium, ticarcillin disodium)

- Cardiomegaly
- Peripheral edema
- Jugular venous distension
- Hepatojugular reflux
- Hepatomegaly

LABORATORY TESTS

- BNP >100 pg/mL.
- Electrocardiogram: May be normal or could show numerous abnormalities including acute ST-T-wave changes from myocardial ischemia, atrial fibrillation, bradycardia, and left ventricular hypertrophy.
- Serum creatinine: May be increased owing to hypoperfusion. Preexisting renal dysfunction can contribute to volume overload.
- Complete blood count: Useful to determine if heart failure due to reduced oxygen-carrying capacity.
- Chest x-ray: Useful for detection of cardiac enlargement, pulmonary edema, and pleural effusions.
- Echocardiogram: Used to assess LV size, valve function, pericardial effusion, wall motion abnormalities, and ejection fraction.

Pulmonary congestion arises as the left ventricle fails and is unable to accept and eject the increased blood volume that is delivered to it. Consequently, pulmonary venous and capillary pressures rise, leading to interstitial and bronchial edema, increased airways resistance, and dyspnea. The associated signs and symptoms may include: (1) dyspnea (with or without exertion), (2) orthopnea, (3) paroxysmal nocturnal dyspnea (PND), and (4) pulmonary edema. Exertional dyspnea occurs when there is a reduction in the level of exertion that causes breathlessness. This is typically described as more breathlessness than was associated previously with a specific activity (e.g., vacuuming or stair climbing). As heart failure progresses, many patients eventually have dyspnea at rest.

Orthopnea is dyspnea that occurs with assumption of the supine position. It occurs within minutes of recumbency and is due to reduced pooling of blood in the lower extremities and abdomen. Orthopnea is relieved almost immediately by sitting upright and typically is prevented by elevating the head with pillows. A change in the number of pillows required to prevent orthopnea (e.g., a change from "two-pillow" to "three-pillow" orthopnea) suggests worsening heart failure. Attacks of PND typically occur after 2 to 4 hours of sleep; the patient awakens from sleep with a sense of suffocation. The attacks are due to severe pulmonary and bronchial congestion, leading to shortness of breath and wheezing. The reasons these attacks occur at night are unclear but may include: (1) reduced pooling of blood in the lower extremities and abdomen (as in orthopnea), (2) slow resorption of interstitial fluid from sites of dependent edema, (3) normal reduction in sympathetic activity that occurs with sleep (e.g., less support for the failing ventricle), and (4) the normal depression in respiratory drive that occurs with sleep.

Pulmonary edema is the most severe form of pulmonary congestion and is caused by accumulation of fluid in the interstitial spaces and alveoli. In heart failure patients, it is the result of increased pulmonary venous pressure. The patient experiences extreme breathlessness and anxiety and may cough pink, frothy sputum. Pulmonary edema can be terrifying for the patient, causing a feeling of suffocation or drowning.

Rales (crackling sounds heard on auscultation) are present in the lung bases owing to transudation of fluid into alveoli. The rales typically are bibasilar, but if they are heard unilaterally, they are usually right-sided. A third heart sound, or S_3 gallop, is heard frequently in patients with LVF and may be due to elevated atrial pressure and altered distensibility of the ventricle.

Systemic congestion is associated with a number of signs and symptoms. Jugular venous distension (JVD) is the simplest and most reliable sign of fluid overload. Examination of the right internal jugular vein with the patient at a 45-degree angle is the preferred method for assessing JVD. The presence of JVD more than 4 cm above the sternal angle suggests systemic venous congestion. In patients with mild systemic congestion, JVD may be absent at rest, but application of pressure to the abdomen will cause an elevation of JVD (hepatojugular reflux).

Peripheral edema is a cardinal finding in heart failure. Edema usually occurs in dependent parts of the body and thus is seen as ankle or pedal edema in ambulatory patients, although it may be manifested as sacral edema in bedridden patients. Adults typically have a 10-lb fluid weight gain before trace peripheral edema is evident; therefore, patients with acute heart failure may have no clinical evidence of systemic congestion except weight gain.

DIAGNOSIS[1]

No single test is available to confirm the diagnosis of heart failure. Because the syndrome of heart failure can be caused or worsened by multiple cardiac and noncardiac disorders, accurate diagnosis is essential for development of therapeutic strategies. Heart failure often is suspected initially in a patient based on the symptoms. These frequently will include dyspnea, exercise intolerance, fatigue, and/or fluid retention. However, it must be emphasized that signs and symptoms lack sensitivity for diagnosing heart failure because these symptoms are found frequently with other disorders such as pulmonary disease. Even in patients with known heart failure, there is poor correlation between the presence or severity of symptoms and hemodynamic abnormality.

A complete history and physical examination are essential in the initial evaluation of a patient suspected of having heart failure. Particular attention should be paid to cardiovascular risk factors and to other disorders that can cause or exacerbate heart failure. Since coronary artery disease is the cause of heart failure in nearly 70% of patients, careful attention to and evaluation of the possibility of coronary disease is essential, especially in men. The patient's volume status should be documented by assessing the body weight, JVP, and presence or absence of pulmonary congestion and peripheral edema. Laboratory testing may assist in identification of disorders that cause or worsen heart failure. The initial evaluation should include a complete blood count, serum electrolytes (including magnesium), tests of renal and hepatic function, urinalysis, lipid profile, chest x-ray, and a 12-lead electrocardiogram (ECG). There are no specific ECG findings associated with heart failure. Measurement of BNP also may assist in differentiating dyspnea caused by heart failure from other causes.[23]

Although the history, physical examination, and laboratory tests can provide important clues to the underlying cause of heart failure, imaging is required to identify any structural abnormality of the heart. In most patients, an echocardiogram is used to detect any valvular, pericardial, or myocardial abnormalities. The echocardiogram also can determine the presence of systolic and/or diastolic dysfunction and the left ventricular ejection fraction (LVEF).

▶ TREATMENT: Chronic Heart Failure

▧ DESIRED OUTCOMES

For many years, the goals of therapy in the management of chronic heart failure were to improve the patient's quality of life, reduce symptoms, reduce hospitalizations, slow progression of the disease process, and prolong survival. Although these goals are still important, identification of risk factors for heart failure development and recognition of its progressive nature have led to increased emphasis on preventing the development of this disorder. With this in mind, the most recent ACC/AHA guidelines for the evaluation and management of chronic heart failure developed a new staging system that not only recognizes the evolution and progression of the disorder but also emphasizes risk-factor modification and preventive treatment strategies.[1] This system consists of four stages (Fig. 14–5). This staging system differs from the NYHA functional classification (Table 14–4) that most clinicians are familiar with. The NYHA system is intended primarily to classify *symptomatic* heart failure according to the clinician's subjective evaluation and does not recognize preventive measures or the progression of heart failure. A patient's symptoms can change frequently over a short period of time owing to changes in medications, diet, intercurrent illnesses, etc. For example, a patient with NYHA class IV symptoms with marked volume overload could improve rapidly to class II–III with aggressive diuretic therapy. Despite these limitations, this system can be useful for monitoring patients and is used widely in heart failure studies. However, the ACC/AHA staging system provides a more comprehensive framework for evaluation, prevention, and treatment of heart failure.

▧ GENERAL MEASURES

The complexity of the heart failure syndrome necessitates a comprehensive approach to management that includes accurate diagnosis, identification and treatment of risk factors (e.g., diabetes, hypertension, and coronary artery disease), elimination or minimization of precipitating factors such as NSAIDs, and appropriate pharmacologic and nonpharmacologic therapy.

The first step in the management of chronic heart failure is to determine the etiology (see Table 14–1) and/or any precipitating factors. Treatment of underlying disorders such as anemia or hyperthyroidism may obviate the need for treatment of heart failure. Patients with valvular diseases may derive significant benefit from valve replacement or repair. Revascularization or anti-ischemic therapy in patients with coronary disease may reduce heart failure symptoms. Drugs that aggravate heart failure (see Table 14–3) should be discontinued, if possible.

Restriction of physical activity reduces cardiac workload and is recommended for virtually all patients with acute congestive symptoms. However, once the patient's symptoms have stabilized and excess fluid is removed, restrictions on physical activity are discouraged. In fact, current guidelines indicate that exercise training programs in stable heart failure patients improve exercise tolerance and functional capacity and may slow heart failure progression.[1]

Because a major compensatory response in heart failure is sodium and water retention, restriction of fluid intake and dietary sodium is an important nonpharmacologic intervention. Fluid intake

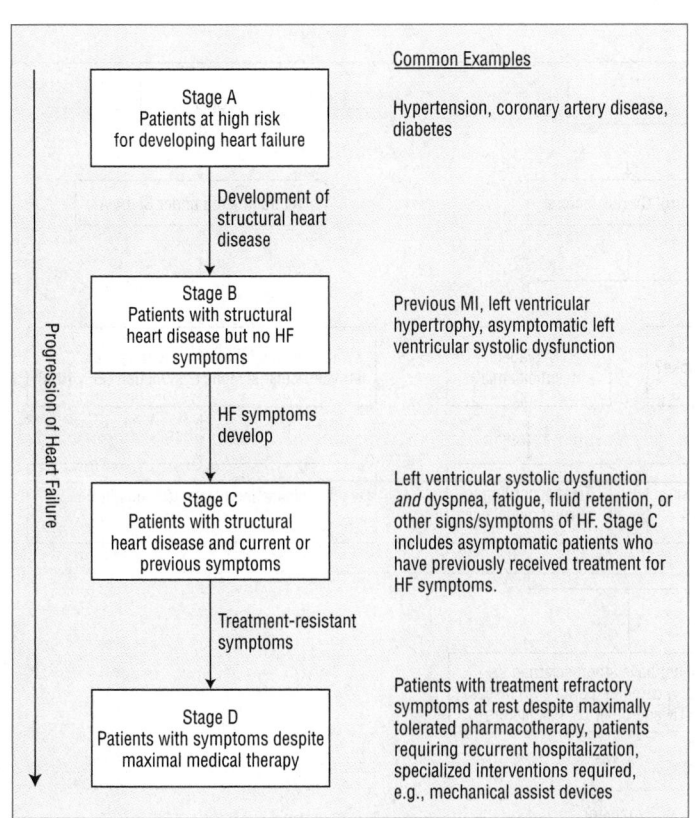

FIGURE 14–5. ACC/AHA heart failure staging system. *(Adapted with permission from Circulation 2001;104:2996–3007.)*

TABLE 14–4. New York Heart Association Functional Classification

Functional Class	Description
I	Patients with cardiac disease but without limitations of physical activities. Ordinary physical activity does not cause undue fatigue, dyspnea, or palpitations.
II	Patients with cardiac disease that results in slight limitations of physical activity. Ordinary physical activity results in fatigue, palpitations, dyspnea, or angina.
III	Patients with cardiac disease that results in marked limitation of physical activity. Although patients are comfortable at rest, less than ordinary activity will lead to symptoms.
IV	Patients with cardiac disease that results in an inability to carry on physical activity without discomfort. Symptoms of congestive heart failure are present even at rest. With any physical activity, increased discomfort is experienced.

typically is limited to a maximum of about 2 L/day from all sources. The typical American diet contains 3 to 6 g sodium per day, and this should be reduced by about half (1.5 to 2 g sodium per day). This can be accomplished by not adding salt to prepared foods and eliminating foods high in sodium (e.g., salt-cured meats, salted snack foods, pickles, soups, delicatessen meats, and processed foods). Further reductions in dietary sodium can be achieved by eliminating salt from cooking. However, this is not recommended for most heart failure patients because excessive sodium restriction produces an unpalatable diet, which leads to poor dietary compliance or compromised nutritional status. Additionally, the availability of potent diuretics makes excessive sodium restriction unnecessary in most cases. Although dietary sodium and water restriction should be instituted in all heart failure patients, pharmacologic therapy is required for slowing disease progression and prolonging survival and usually is necessary for control of symptoms. Thus all patients with systolic heart failure should be on pharmacologic therapy in addition to the nonpharmacologic therapies discussed earlier.

GENERAL APPROACH TO TREATMENT

Current ACC/AHA treatment guidelines are organized around the four identified stages of heart failure[1] (Figs 14–6 and 14–7). This staging system emphasizes the progressive nature of the disorder and targets treatment to prevent and/or slow the progression of heart failure.

TREATMENT OF STAGE A HEART FAILURE (SEE FIG. 14–6)

Patients in stage A do not have structural heart disease or symptoms but are at high risk for developing heart failure because of the presence of risk factors. The emphasis here is on identification and modification of these risk factors to prevent the development of structural heart disease and subsequent heart failure. Commonly encountered risk factors include hypertension, diabetes, and coronary artery disease. Although each of these disorders individually increases risk, they frequently coexist in many patients and act synergistically to foster the development of heart failure. Effective control of blood pressure reduces the risk

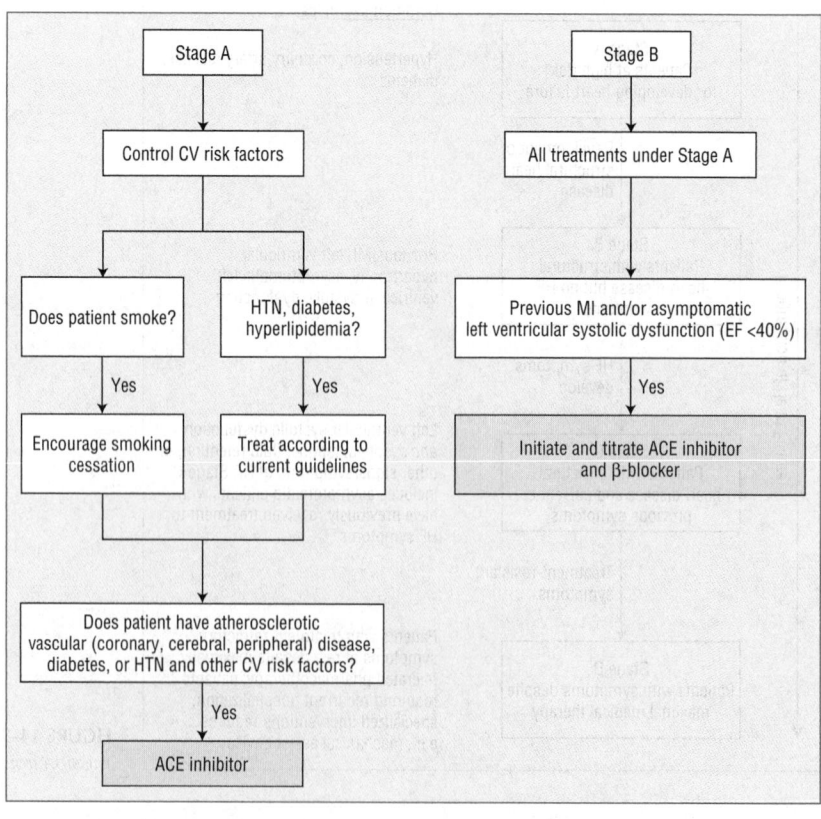

FIGURE 14–6. Treatment algorithm for patients with ACC/AHA stages A and B heart failure. *(Adapted with permission from Circulation 2001;104:2996–3007.)*

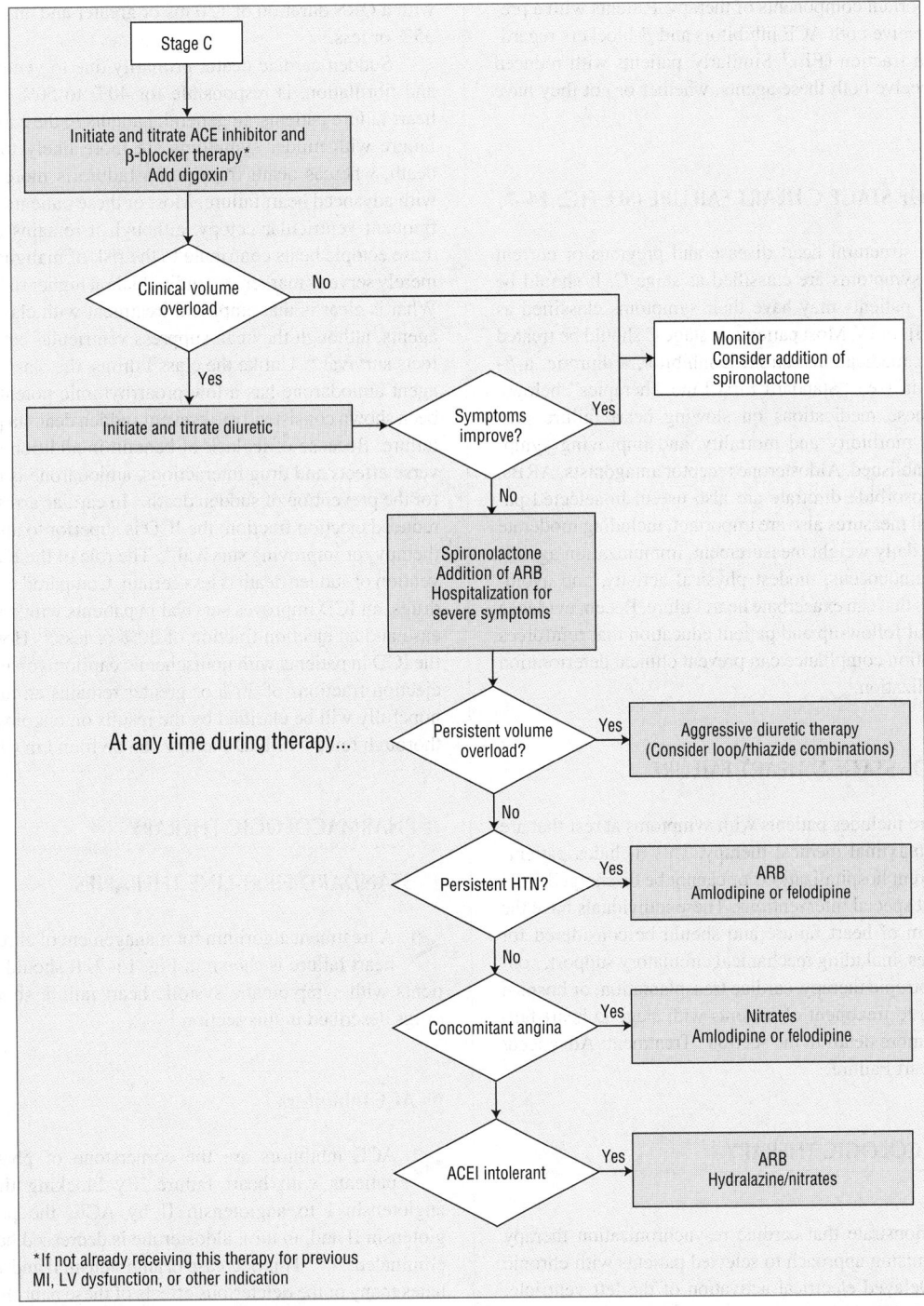

FIGURE 14–7. Treatment algorithm for patients with ACC/AHA stage C heart failure. *(Adapted with permission from Circulation 2001;104:2996–3007.)*

of developing heart failure by approximately 50%.[35] Control of hyperglycemia reduces the risk of end-organ damage and may decrease the risk of heart failure. Appropriate management of coronary artery disease and its associated risk factors is also important, including treatment of hyperlipidemia according to published guidelines and smoking cessation. Although treatment must be individualized, ACE inhibitors should be strongly considered for antihypertensive therapy in patients with multiple vascular risk factors.[1,36,37] Diuretics and β-blockers also are useful in this setting.

TREATMENT OF STAGE B HEART FAILURE (SEE FIG. 14–6)

Patients in stage B have structural heart disease but do not have heart failure symptoms. This group includes patients with left ventricular hypertrophy or fibrosis, previous MI, valvular disease, or left ventricular systolic dysfunction. These individuals are at risk for developing heart failure, and treatment is targeted at minimizing additional injury and preventing or slowing the remodeling process. In addition to the treatment measures outlined in stage A, ACE inhibitors and β-blockers are important components of therapy. Patients with a previous MI should receive both ACE inhibitors and β-blockers regardless of the ejection fraction (EF).[1] Similarly, patients with reduced EFs also should receive both these agents, whether or not they have had a MI.[1]

TREATMENT OF STAGE C HEART FAILURE (SEE FIG. 14–7)

Patients with structural heart disease and previous or current heart failure symptoms are classified as stage C. It should be noted that stage C patients may have their symptoms classified as NYHA class I, II, III, or IV. Most patients in stage C should be treated routinely with four medications: an ACE inhibitor, a diuretic, a β-blocker, and digoxin (see "Standard First-Line Therapies" below). The benefits of these medications on slowing heart failure progression, reducing morbidity and mortality, and improving symptoms are clearly established. Aldosterone receptor antagonists, ARBs, and hydralazine-isosorbide dinitrate are also useful in selected patients. Other general measures also are important, including moderate sodium restriction, daily weight measurement, immunization against influenza and pneumococcus, modest physical activity, and avoidance of medications that can exacerbate heart failure. Recent evidence suggests that careful follow-up and patient education that reinforces dietary and medication compliance can prevent clinical deterioration and reduce hospitalization.[1]

TREATMENT OF STAGE D HEART FAILURE

Stage D heart failure includes patients with symptoms at rest that are refractory despite maximal medical therapy. This includes patients who undergo recurrent hospitalizations or cannot be discharged from the hospital without special interventions. These individuals have the most advanced form of heart failure and should be considered for specialized therapies, including mechanical circulatory support, continuous positive inotropic therapy, cardiac transplantation, or hospice care. The approach to treatment of patients with stage D heart failure is discussed in more detail in the section "Treatment: Advanced/ Decompensated Heart Failure."

NONPHARMACOLOGIC THERAPY

Recent studies demonstrate that cardiac resynchronization therapy (CRT) offers a promising approach to selected patients with chronic heart failure.[38,39] Delayed electrical activation of the left ventricle, characterized on the ECG by a QRS duration that exceeds 120 ms, occurs in approximately one-third of patients with moderate to severe systolic heart failure. Since the left and right ventricles normally activate simultaneously, this delay results in asynchronous contraction of the left and right ventricles, which contributes to the hemodynamic abnormalities of this disorder. Implantation of a specialized biventricular pacemaker to restore synchronous activation of the ventricles can improve ventricular contraction and hemodynamics. Recent trials show improvements in exercise capacity, NYHA classification, quality of life, hemodynamic function, and hospitalizations.[38,39] A device that combined CRT with an implantable cardioverter-defibrillator (ICD) improved survival in addition to functional status.[39] CRT is currently indicated only in NYHA class III–IV patients receiving optimal medical therapy (ACE inhibitors, diuretics, β-blockers, and digoxin) and

with a QRS duration of 120 ms or greater and an ejection fraction of 35% or less.

Sudden cardiac death, primarily due to ventricular tachycardia and fibrillation, is responsible for 40% to 50% of the mortality in heart failure patients. In general, patients in the earlier stages of heart failure with milder symptoms are more likely to die from sudden death, whereas death from pump failure is more frequent in those with advanced heart failure. Most of these patients have complex and frequent ventricular ectopy, although it remains unknown whether these ectopic beats contribute to the risk of malignant arrhythmias or merely serve as markers for individuals at higher risk for sudden death. What is clear is that empirical treatment with class I antiarrhythmic agents, although they can suppress ventricular ectopy, adversely affects survival.[40] Unlike the class I drugs, the class III antiarrhythmic agent amiodarone has a low proarrhythmic potential, but it has not been shown consistently to prevent sudden death in patients with heart failure. Because of its lack of benefit, in addition to its multiple adverse effects and drug interactions, amiodarone is not recommended for the prevention of sudden death.[1] In cardiac arrest survivors with a reduced ejection fraction, the ICD is superior to antiarrhythmic drug therapy for improving survival.[41] The role of the ICD in primary prevention of sudden death is less certain. Compared with antiarrhythmic drugs, an ICD improves survival in patients with coronary artery disease and an ejection fraction of 30% or less.[41] However, the role of the ICD in patients with nonischemic cardiomyopathy and those with ejection fractions of 30% or greater remains an unsettled issue and hopefully will be clarified by the results on ongoing clinical trials. A thorough review of ICD therapy can be found in Chap. 17.

PHARMACOLOGIC THERAPY

STANDARD FIRST-LINE THERAPIES

A treatment algorithm for management of chronic (i.e., stage C) heart failure is shown in Fig. 14–7. It should be noted that patients with symptomatic systolic heart failure should be on all the drugs described in this section.[1]

ACE Inhibitors

ACE inhibitors are the cornerstone of pharmacotherapy of patients with heart failure. By blocking the conversion of angiotensin I to angiotensin II by ACE, the production of angiotensin II and, in turn, aldosterone is decreased but not completely eliminated.[42–44] This decrease in angiotensin II and aldosterone attenuates many of the deleterious effects of these neurohormones, including reducing ventricular remodeling, myocardial fibrosis, myocyte apoptosis, cardiac hypertrophy, NE release, vasoconstriction, and sodium and water retention.[42,45] Thus ACE inhibitor therapy appears to play an important role in preventing angiotensin II–mediated progressive worsening of myocardial function. The endogenous vasodilator bradykinin, which is inactivated by ACE, is also increased by ACE inhibitors, along with the release of vasodilatory prostaglandins and histamine.[42,45] The precise contribution of the effects of ACE inhibitors on bradykinin and vasodilatory prostaglandins is unclear. However, the persistence of clinical benefits with ACE inhibitors despite the fact that angiotensin II and aldosterone levels return to pretreatment levels suggests that this is a potentially important effect.[43,44]

Numerous placebo-controlled trials have documented the favorable effects of ACE inhibitor therapy on hemodynamic variables, clinical status, and symptoms in heart failure.[5,45,46] Hemodynamic effects observed with long-term therapy include significant increases in cardiac index, stroke work index, and stroke volume index, as well as significant reductions in left ventricular filling pressure, SVR, MAP, and heart rate. Significant improvements in clinical status, functional class, exercise tolerance, and left ventricular size also are well documented. When compared with placebo, patients treated with ACE inhibitors have fewer treatment failures, fewer hospitalizations, and fewer increases in diuretic dosages.[1,5,46] The acute response to ACE inhibitor therapy is greater in patients with high levels of plasma renin activity. However, long-term hemodynamic and clinical responses to ACE inhibition cannot be predicted from the plasma renin activity or from response to the initial dose of ACE inhibitor.

The beneficial effect of ACE inhibitors on mortality has been documented conclusively, with numerous trials showing a 20% to 30% relative reduction in mortality with ACE inhibitor therapy compared with placebo.[46] A long-term (12-year) follow-up of the Studies of Left Ventricular Dysfunction (SOLVD) prevention and treatment trials demonstrated sustained survival benefits in patients treated with enalapril.[47] In addition to improving survival, ACE inhibitors also reduce the combined risk of death or hospitalization, slow the progression of heart failure, and reduce the rates of reinfarction.[46] The benefits of ACE inhibitor therapy are independent of the etiology of heart failure (ischemic versus nonischemic) and are observed in patients with mild, moderate, or severe symptoms. ACE inhibitors clearly are superior to vasodilator therapy with hydralazine-isosorbide dinitrate.[48]

The most common cause of heart failure is ischemic heart disease, where MI results in loss of myocytes, followed by ventricular dilatation and remodeling. Captopril, ramipril, and trandolapril all have been shown to benefit post-MI patients whether they are initiated early (within 36 hours) and continued for 4 to 6 weeks[49] or started later and administered for several years.[46] Collectively, these studies indicate that ACE inhibitors after MI improve overall survival, decrease the development of severe heart failure, and reduce reinfarction and heart failure hospitalization rates.[46,49] The benefit occurs within the first few days of therapy and persists during long-term treatment. The effects are most pronounced in higher-risk patients, such as those with symptomatic heart failure or reduced EFs, with 20% to 30% reductions in mortality reported in these patients.[46,49] Post-MI patients without heart failure symptoms or decreases in EF also benefit from ACE inhibitors, but the magnitude of this effect is less pronounced, with all-cause mortality reduced by 7% to 11%.[49]

In addition to their benefits in patients with established heart failure, ACE inhibitors also are effective for prevention of heart failure. The SOLVD prevention trial showed that enalapril decreased the risk of hospitalization for worsening heart failure and reduced the composite end point of death and heart failure hospitalization in patients with asymptomatic left ventricular dysfunction.[50,51] The development of diabetes mellitus, an important risk factor for cardiovascular disease that also increases morbidity and mortality in heart failure patients, is reduced by enalapril in patients with chronic heart failure.[52] In a post-hoc analysis of the Heart Outcomes Prevention Evaluation (HOPE) trial, ramipril reduced the development of new-onset heart failure by nearly 25% in patients with normal EFs and no symptoms of heart failure.[36]

Despite the overwhelming benefit demonstrated with ACE inhibitors, there is substantial evidence that these agents are underused and underdosed in patients with heart failure.[53–55] These data indicate that significant numbers of heart failure patients do not receive ACE inhibitors, and of those who are receiving these agents, many may be taking lower than recommended doses.[53–55] The most common reasons cited for underuse or underdosing are concerns about safety and adverse reactions to ACE inhibitors, especially in patients with underlying renal dysfunction or hypotension. The use of ACE inhibitors in patients with renal insufficiency is particularly relevant because it occurs in 25% to 50% of heart failure patients and is associated with an increased risk of mortality.[56,57] Recent evidence indicates that ACE inhibitors in post-MI patients with decreased left ventricular function may be more effective in patients with renal insufficiency.[58] In this retrospective cohort study, nearly 21,000 Medicare patients with confirmed MIs and EFs of less than 40% on hospital discharge were studied. In patients receiving an ACE inhibitor at hospital discharge, those with a serum creatinine level of greater than 3 mg/dL had a 37% increase in 1-year survival compared with only a 16% increase in patients with a serum creatinine level of less than 3 mg/dL. Since many heart failure patients have concomitant disorders (e.g., diabetes, hypertension, or previous MI) that also may be affected favorably by ACE inhibitors, renal dysfunction should not be a contraindication to ACE inhibitor use in patients with left ventricular dysfunction. However, these patients should be monitored carefully for the development of acute renal failure and/or hyperkalemia, with special attention to risk factors associated with this complication of ACE inhibitor therapy.[56,57]

No dose-dependent differences in mortality have been reported for ACE inhibitors. In the ATLAS trial, over 3000 patients with NYHA class II–IV heart failure and an EF of 30% or less were randomized to receive either low-dose (2.5–5 mg/day) or high-dose (32.5–35 mg/day) lisinopril for a median of 45 months.[59] No differences in mortality were found between the high- and low-dose groups. However, the composite end point of death or hospitalization for any cause was reduced significantly by 12% and heart failure hospitalizations decreased by 24% in the high-dose group. In many positive trials of other heart failure therapies (e.g., β-blockers, aldosterone antagonists), intermediate ACE inhibitor doses generally were used as background therapy. These results emphasize that clinicians should attempt to use ACE inhibitor doses proven to be beneficial in clinical trials, but if these doses are not tolerated, lower doses can be used with the knowledge that there are likely only small differences in efficacy between the high and low doses.

In summary, the evidence that ACE inhibitors improve symptoms, slow disease progression, and decrease mortality in heart failure is unequivocal. As such, all patients with documented left ventricular dysfunction, irrespective of symptomatology, should receive ACE inhibitors unless there are contraindications or intolerance is present.[1]

β-Blockers

It may seem paradoxical that within this chapter β-blockers are listed as drugs that may exacerbate or worsen heart failure (see Table 14–3) and as standard therapy for the management of chronic heart failure, but both are true. Initiation of β-blocker therapy at normal doses in patients with heart failure has the potential to lead to symptomatic worsening or decompensation owing to the drug's negative inotropic effect. However, there is also overwhelming evidence that if stable patients are initiated on low doses of a β-blocker, with slow upward dose titration over several weeks, they can expect to derive significant benefits. As such, the ACC/AHA guidelines on the management of heart failure recommend that β-blockers should be used in all patients with stable systolic heart failure unless they have a contraindication or have been shown clearly to be unable to tolerate β-blockers.[1] Patients should receive a β-blocker even if their symptoms are well controlled with diuretic and ACE inhibitor therapy because they remain at risk for progression of disease. Additionally, it is not essential that ACE inhibitor doses are optimized prior to initiation of β-blocker therapy because patients are more likely to accrue benefit from addition of a β-blocker than from an increase in their ACE inhibitor dose.[1]

β-Blockers have been studied extensively, with data on more than 10,000 participants of placebo-controlled trials. Carvedilol, metoprolol controlled release/extended release (CR/XL), and bisoprolol are the best studied of the β-blockers in heart failure. Each has been studied in large populations, with a primary study end point of mortality, and each has been shown to reduce mortality significantly compared with placebo. The CIBIS-II trial studied bisoprolol in over 2600 patients, most of whom had class III heart failure. The study was stopped prematurely because of the 34% reduction in mortality associated with bisoprolol.[60] Post-hoc analyses showed a 44% reduction in sudden death and a 26% reduction in death due to worsening heart failure. The data from the largest β-blocker mortality trial to date, Metoprolol CR/XL Randomised Intervention Trial in Congestive Heart Failure (MERIT-HF), were very similar to those with bisoprolol. In this study, nearly 4000 patients were randomized to metoprolol CR/XL (Toprol XL) or placebo.[61] Most of the patients had class II or III heart failure. Again, the study was halted prematurely because of a 34% reduction in total mortality, with a 41% reduction in sudden death and a 49% reduction in death from worsening heart failure. Multiple post-hoc subgroup analyses suggested that all analyzed subgroups benefited from the therapy.

Following publication of these trials, the value of β-blockers in class II and III heart failure patients was clear, and they became standard therapy in these patients. However, there remained questions about their value or safety in patients with class IV heart failure. The Carvedilol, Prospective, Randomized, Cumulative Survival (COPERNICUS) trial was designed to test carvedilol in the severe heart failure population and, like the other studies, was stopped prematurely because of the drug's significant survival benefit.[62] Specifically, carvedilol produced a 35% relative reduction in mortality and an impressive 7.1% absolute reduction in mortality (from 18.5% to 11.4%). Thus there is now clear evidence of benefit with β-blockers in all patients with symptomatic systolic heart failure.

In addition to data on the effects of β-blockers on survival, there are data showing improvements in numerous other end points. All the large clinical trials have shown β-blockers to produce 15% to 20% reductions in all-cause hospitalization and 25% to 35% reductions in hospitalizations for worsening heart failure.[60,63,64] The positive effects of β-blockers on the left ventricle systolic function also have been very consistent across studies. Following several weeks to months of therapy, β-blockers have been documented consistently to increase EFs by 5 to 10 units (e.g., from an EF of 20% to 25% or 30%), to decrease ventricular mass, to improve the sphericity of the ventricle, and to reduce systolic and diastolic volumes (LVESV and LVEDV).[65,66] These effects are often collectively called *reverse remodeling,* referring to the fact that they return the heart toward more normal size, shape, and function.

While the effects of β-blockers on survival prolongation and left ventricular reverse remodeling could be argued to be greater than those of any other drugs used in heart failure, this is not the case for their symptomatic benefits. Many, but not all studies, have shown improvements in the NYHA functional class, patient symptom scores or quality-of-life assessments (such as the Minnesota Living with Heart Failure Questionnaire), and exercise performance, as assessed by the 6-minute walk test.[63–66] Thus it is important to educate patients that they will not necessarily notice dramatic symptomatic improvements with β-blocker therapy. However, even in the absence of symptomatic improvement, positive effects on disease progression and survival are still anticipated.

A number of potential mechanisms have been suggested to explain the beneficial effects of β-blockers in heart failure patients. Although not clearly elucidated, it seems likely that the mechanisms of benefit include antiarrhythmic effects, slowing or reversing the detrimental ventricular remodeling caused by sympathetic stimulation, decreased myocyte death from catecholamine-induced necrosis or apoptosis, and prevention of fetal gene expression and the other detrimental effects of SNS activation described earlier.[1,67]

■ *Use of β-Blockers in Heart Failure.* An important aspect to the safe use of β-blockers in heart failure is initiation of therapy at a low dose, with slow upward dose titration. Current guidelines recommend initiation of therapy once patients have been relatively stable for several weeks. However, a recent study indicated that initiation of carvedilol therapy before discharge in patients hospitalized for decompensated heart failure increased the number of patients treated with β-blockers compared with usual care and did not increase the risk of serious adverse effects.[68] Typically, starting doses have been 1/10 to 1/20 the final dose, with doses doubling no more frequently than every 2 weeks until the target dose is reached. The starting and target doses are described in Table 14–5. As shown in the table, the starting dose for bisoprolol is 1.25 mg/day. However, the smallest commercially available tablet of bisoprolol is a scored 5-mg tablet. Since the starting dosage of bisoprolol is not readily available, this drug is the least commonly used of the three agents, and it is not approved by the Food and Drug Administration (FDA) for use in heart failure.

Clinical questions about how high the dose should be are also common. There is strong evidence with carvedilol and metoprolol CR/XL that decreases in hospitalization depend on β-blocker dose, with greater benefit seen at higher doses.[69,70] The data suggest that lower doses may prolong survival but that the benefits may be greater with higher doses.[69] It appears that an important guide to therapy is the patient's heart rate, and lower doses might be judged reasonable if the heart rate provides evidence of β-blockade.[69] Thus it seems important to make every effort to titrate patients to target doses when possible, although there are benefits over placebo at lower doses; thus any dose of β-blocker is likely to provide some benefit.

Education of patients about β-blocker therapy is also particularly important to ensure the greatest likelihood for success. It is essential that patients understand that there will be a long, slow upward titration of dose to attempt to get them to a specific target. They also need to be aware of the benefits of β-blocker therapy and that the β-blocker may make them feel worse during the initiation phase. If they understand the benefits, they are less likely to discontinue

TABLE 14–5. Initial and Target Doses for β-Blockers Used in Treatment of Heart Failure

Drug	Initial Dose[a]	Target Dose
Bisoprolol[b]	1.25 mg qd	10 mg qd
Carvedilol[b]	3.125 mg bid	25 mg bid[d]
Metoprolol succinate CR/XL[b]	12.5–25 mg qd[c]	200 mg qd

[a] Doses should be doubled approximately every 2 weeks or as tolerated by the patient until the highest tolerated or target dose is reached.
[b] Regimens proven in large trials to reduce mortality.
[c] In MERIT-HF, the majority of class II patients were given 25 mg/day, whereas the majority of class III patients were given 12.5 mg/day as their starting dose.
[d] Target dose for patients >85 kg is 50 mg bid.

therapy if they do have some worsening of heart failure symptoms during the dose-titration phase. Nearly all patients can tolerate some dose of a β-blocker, and with good communication between the patient and health care provider(s), initiation of β-blocker therapy is likely to be successful.

Details regarding selection of a specific β-blocker are contained in the "Drug Class" section of this chapter. Based on the clinical trial data to date, there is some clarity on this issue. First, it seems clear that any assumptions about class effect should not be made and that therapy should be limited to carvedilol, metoprolol CR/XL, or bisoprolol. Additionally, the data provide reasonable evidence that it is inappropriate to assume that the cheaper immediate-release formulation of metoprolol tartrate will provide benefits equivalent to those of metoprolol CR/XL. And given that bisoprolol is not available in the necessary starting doses, the choice typically is limited to either carvedilol or metoprolol CR/XL. Many clinicians consider carvedilol to be the agent of choice, but there is no compelling evidence that it is superior to metoprolol CR/XL or bisoprolol. Please see the "Drug Class" section of this chapter for a more detailed discussion on the Carvedilol Or Metoprolol European Trial (COMET) comparing carvedilol with immediate-release metoprolol.

In summary, the data provide clear evidence that β-blockers slow the progression of heart failure, evidenced by reductions in mortality and hospitalizations. Many patients also will have improvements in quality of life associated with β-blocker therapy, although this is not a universal finding. Based on these data, β-blockers are recommended as standard therapy for all patients with systolic dysfunction, irrespective of the severity of their symptoms.

Diuretics[71–73]

The compensatory mechanisms in heart failure stimulate excessive sodium and water retention, often leading to signs and symptoms of systemic and pulmonary congestion. Consequently, diuretic therapy is recommended for all patients with clinical evidence of fluid retention. Among the drugs used for management of heart failure, the diuretics are most rapid in producing symptomatic benefits. The majority of patients with heart failure will require chronic diuretic therapy to control their fluid status, and as such, diuretics represent a cornerstone of heart failure therapy. However, because they do not alter disease progression (or prolong survival), they are not considered mandatory therapy. Thus patients who do not have fluid retention would not require diuretic therapy.

The primary goal of diuretic therapy is to reduce symptoms associated with fluid retention and pulmonary congestion, improve quality of life, and reduce hospitalizations from heart failure. They accomplish this by decreasing edema and pulmonary congestion through reduction of preload. Although preload is a determinant of cardiac output, the Frank-Starling curve (see Fig. 14–3) shows that patients with congestive symptoms have reached the flat portion of the curve. A reduction in preload improves symptoms but has little effect on the patient's stroke volume or cardiac output until the steep portion of the curve is reached. However, diuretic therapy must be used judiciously because overdiuresis can lead to a reduction in cardiac output and symptoms of dehydration.

Once diuretic therapy is initiated, dosage adjustments are based on symptomatic improvement and daily body weight. Change in body weight is a sensitive marker of fluid retention or loss, and it is recommended that patients monitor their status by taking daily morning body weights. Patients who gain a pound per day for several consecutive days or 3 to 5 lb in a week should contact their health care provider for instructions (which often will be to increase the diuretic dose temporarily). Such action often will allow patients to prevent a decompensation that requires hospitalization.

Thiazide Diuretics. Thiazide diuretics such as hydrochlorothiazide block sodium and chloride reabsorption in the distal convoluted tubule (approximately 5% to 8% of filtered sodium). The thiazides therefore are relatively weak diuretics and infrequently are used alone in heart failure. However, as is reviewed in detail in the section "Treatment: Advanced/Decompensated Heart Failure" under "Diuretic Resistance," thiazides or the thiazide-like diuretic metolazone can be used in combination with loop diuretics to promote a very effective diuresis.

Loop Diuretics. Loop diuretics are the most widely used diuretics in heart failure. They act in the thick ascending limb of the loop of Henle, where 20% to 25% of filtered sodium normally is reabsorbed. Because loop diuretics are highly bound to plasma proteins, they are not highly filtered at the glomerulus. They reach the tubular lumen by active transport via the organic acid transport pathway. Competitors for this pathway (probenecid or organic by-products of uremia) can inhibit delivery of loop diuretics to their site of action and decrease effectiveness. Loop diuretics also induce a prostaglandin-mediated increase in renal blood flow, which contributes to their natriuretic effect. Coadministration of NSAIDs and COX-2 inhibitors blocks this prostaglandin-mediated effect and can diminish diuretic efficacy. Unlike thiazides, loop diuretics maintain their effectiveness in the presence of impaired renal function, although higher doses are necessary to obtain adequate delivery of the drug to the site of action.

Heart failure is one of the disease states in which the maximal response to loop diuretics is reduced. This is believed to be the result of increased proximal or distal tubule reabsorption of sodium, which might occur owing to increased expression and activity of the Na-K-2Cl transporter.[71] As a consequence, doses above the recommended ceiling doses produce no additional diuresis. Thus, once these doses are reached, it is recommended to give the diuretic more frequently for additional effect rather than to give progressively higher doses. The appropriate chronic dose is that which maintains the patient at a stable dry weight without symptoms of dyspnea. Ranges of doses of loop diuretics and recommended ceiling doses are shown in Table 14–6.

Digoxin

In 1785, William Withering was the first to report extensively on the use of foxglove, or *Digitalis purpurea,* for the treatment of dropsy (i.e., edema). Although digitalis glycosides have been in clinical use for more than 200 years, not until the 1920s were they clearly demonstrated to have a positive inotropic effect on the heart. Furthermore, it was not until the late 1980s that clinical trials were conducted to critically evaluate the role of digoxin in the therapy of chronic heart failure. The results of the Digitalis Investigation Group (DIG) trial helped to clarify the role of digoxin in this setting.[74] The view of digoxin also has shifted over the past decade. While historically it was considered to be useful in heart failure because of its positive inotropic effects, it now seems clear that its real benefits in heart failure are related to its neurohormonal modulating effects.

Clinical Efficacy and Role in Therapy. The efficacy of digoxin in patients with heart failure and supraventricular tachyarrhythmias such as atrial fibrillation is well established and widely accepted.[75,76]

TABLE 14–6. Loop Diuretics: Use in Heart Failure

	Furosemide	Bumetanide	Torsemide
Usual daily dose (PO)	20–160 mg/day	0.5–4 mg/day	10–80 mg/day
Ceiling dose[a]			
Normal renal function	80–160 mg	1–2 mg	20–40 mg
CL_{CR}: 20–50 mL/min	160 mg	2 mg	40 mg
CL_{CR}: <20 mL/min	400 mg	8–10 mg	100 mg
Bioavailability	10–100% Average, 50%	80–90%	80–100%
Affected by food	Yes	Yes	No
Half-life	0.3–3.4 h	0.3–1.5 h	3–4 h

[a]Ceiling dose: single dose above which additional response is unlikely to be observed.
Adapted from Am J Med Sci. 2000; 319:38–50.

Its role in heart failure patients with normal sinus rhythm has been considerably more controversial. Until the 1980s, most data supporting efficacy of digoxin in these patients came from anecdotal evidence and seriously flawed or uncontrolled studies. Since then, a number of clinical trials have shown that digoxin improves LVEF, quality of life, exercise tolerance, and heart failure symptoms.[75,76] However, these studies involved small numbers of patients followed for short time periods, with many of the patients being withdrawn from preexisting digoxin treatment on entering the trial. Although these trials demonstrated hemodynamic and symptomatic improvement in heart failure patients receiving digoxin, an unresolved issue was the unknown effect of digoxin on mortality. This was of particular concern given the increased mortality seen with other positive inotropic drugs and finally led to organization and performance of the DIG trial to determine the effects of digoxin on survival in patients with heart failure in sinus rhythm.[74]

The DIG trial was a double-blind, randomized, placebo-controlled trial with the primary end point of all-cause mortality.[74] Patients ($n = 6800$) with heart failure symptoms and an EF of 45% or less were eligible and followed for a mean of 37 months. Most patients received background therapy with diuretics and ACE inhibitors. The mean serum digoxin concentration achieved was 0.8 ng/mL after 12 months of therapy. No significant difference in all-cause mortality was found between patients receiving digoxin and placebo (34.8% and 35.1%, respectively). A trend toward lower mortality due to worsening heart failure was observed in the digoxin group, although this was offset by a trend toward an increased mortality from other cardiovascular causes (presumably arrhythmias) in patients receiving digoxin. Hospitalizations for worsening heart failure were reduced 28% by digoxin compared with placebo ($p < .001$), whereas hospitalizations for other cardiovascular causes were increased in the digoxin group. In all, 64.3% of digoxin-treated patients were hospitalized compared with 67.1% of patients receiving placebo ($p = .006$). Therefore, DIG is the first trial to show that a positive inotropic agent does not increase mortality in patients with heart failure.

Although digoxin does not improve survival in heart failure patients, multiple post-hoc analyses of data from studies evaluating the effect of digoxin withdrawal have helped to clarify the role of digoxin use for patients in sinus rhythm.[75,76] Collectively, these studies suggested that the drug produces important symptomatic benefits and that digoxin withdrawal increased the risk of treatment failure and deterioration of exercise capacity and EF. Furthermore, the risk of symptomatic exacerbation of heart failure after digoxin discontinuation was highest in patients with the most severe symptoms.[75,76] Based on this evidence, digoxin is now recommended for use in patients with stage C heart failure, along with ACE inhibitors, β-blockers, and diuretics, to improve symptoms and clinical status.[1]

The appropriate dose or target plasma concentration for digoxin also has been clarified by recent trials. One reported that an increase in the digoxin plasma concentration from a mean of 0.67 to 1.22 ng/mL resulted in only a minor increase in EF (23.7% to 27.1%) but no improvement in symptoms, exercise tolerance, or neurohormone levels.[77] Another study found that an increase in digoxin plasma concentration from 0.8 to 1.5 ng/mL produced no additional effect on EF and likewise did not improve other hemodynamic variables or indices of neurohormonal function.[78] Two recent retrospective analyses of the combined PROVED/RADIANCE database[79] and the DIG trial database[80] offer additional insights as to the clinical benefit of low serum digoxin concentrations in heart failure patients. While all patients in the PROVED and RADIANCE trials who continued to take digoxin did significantly better than those who were withdrawn, those who had plasma digoxin concentrations between 0.5 and 0.9 ng/mL were just as likely to be free of worsening heart failure as those with higher plasma concentrations. Retrospective analysis of the DIG trial database suggests that a serum digoxin concentration of 0.5 to 0.8 ng/mL may be associated with a reduction in mortality, whereas higher concentrations may increase mortality.[80] In another post-hoc analysis of the DIG trial, digoxin therapy was associated with an increased risk of death in women but not men.[81]

These results suggest that most of the benefit from digoxin is achieved at low plasma concentrations and that little additional effect is achieved with higher doses. Thus, for most patients, the target digoxin plasma concentration should be 0.5 to 1 ng/mL. This more conservative target also would be expected to decrease the risk of adverse effects from digoxin toxicity. In most patients with normal renal function, this plasma concentration range can be achieved with a daily dose of 0.125 mg. Patients with decreased renal function, the elderly, or those receiving interacting drugs (e.g., amiodarone) should receive 0.125 mg every other day. In patients with atrial fibrillation and a rapid ventricular response, the historic practice of increasing digoxin doses (and plasma concentrations) until rate control is achieved is no longer recommended. Digoxin alone is often ineffective to control ventricular response in patients with atrial fibrillation, and increasing the dose only increases the risk of toxicity. A recent study showed that digoxin combined with carvedilol is superior to either agent alone for controlling ventricular response in patients with atrial fibrillation and heart failure.[82] Therefore, it should be dosed similarly irrespective of whether the patient is in sinus rhythm or atrial fibrillation. Adequate rate control can be achieved by adding a β-blocker or amiodarone. Several equations and nomograms have been proposed to estimate digoxin maintenance doses based on estimated renal function for a particular patient and population pharmacokinetic parameters. These methods are reviewed extensively elsewhere.[83] In the absence of supraventricular tachyarrhythmias, a loading dose is not indicated because digoxin is a mild inotropic agent that will produce gradual effects over several hours, even after loading.

Digoxin's place in the pharmacotherapy of chronic heart failure therefore can be summarized for two patient groups. In patients with heart failure and supraventricular tachyarrhythmias such as atrial fibrillation, it should be considered early in therapy to help control ventricular response rate. For patients in normal sinus rhythm, although digoxin does not improve survival, its effects on symptom reduction and quality-of-life improvement are evident in patients with mild to severe heart failure. Therefore, it should be used together with other standard heart failure therapies, including diuretics, ACE inhibitors, and β-blockers, in patients with symptomatic heart failure. Clinicians may want to consider adding digoxin after instituting β-blocker therapy so that the potential bradycardic effect of digoxin does not preclude the use of a β-blocker.

OTHER HEART FAILURE THERAPIES

Aldosterone Antagonists

Spironolactone has long been recognized as an inhibitor of aldosterone that produces a weak, potassium-sparing diuretic effect. However, only recently have the cardiovascular effects of aldosterone been understood. As discussed in detail under "Pathophysiology" above, aldosterone is now recognized as a neurohormone that plays an important role in ventricular remodeling, particularly by causing increased collagen deposition in the extracellular matrix and thus causing cardiac fibrosis. Based on this knowledge, the effects of aldosterone antagonism by spironolactone were studied in 1600 patients with class III (with recent hospitalization) or class IV heart failure. This study (called RALES) tested addition of spironolactone 25 mg daily versus placebo to standard heart failure therapy, which included ACE inhibitor, a diuretic, and digoxin.[20] Owing to the timing of this trial, the benefits of β-blockers were not appreciated fully, and only 10% of patients were taking β-blockers. Patients with a serum creatinine concentration above 2.5 mg/dL or a serum potassium concentration above 5 mEq/L were excluded. The study was stopped prematurely after an average of 24 months of follow-up because of the significant reduction in mortality associated with spironolactone. Specifically, spironolactone was associated with a 30% reduction in total mortality, a 36% reduction in death due to progressive heart failure, and a 29% reduction in sudden deaths. Spironolactone also produced significant reductions in hospitalizations for cardiac causes and hospitalizations for heart failure. Active therapy also was associated with significant improvements in symptoms, as assessed by changes in NYHA functional class.

The low dose of spironolactone in the RALES study was well tolerated. The most common adverse effect was gynecomastia, which occurred in 10% of men on spironolactone and 1% of men on placebo, although only 10 patients (1.7% of men) in the spironolactone group discontinued therapy because of gynecomastia. It also produced statistically significant, although probably clinically unimportant, increases in serum creatinine and serum potassium levels of 0.05 to 0.10 mg/dL and 0.30 mEq/L, respectively. Serious hyperkalemia was not different between groups, occurring in 1% on placebo and 2% on spironolactone.

More recently, the EPHESUS trial evaluated the effect of an aldosterone-selective receptor antagonist eplerenone in patients with left ventricular dysfunction after MI.[21] Eplerenone or placebo was added to usual therapy (ACE inhibitor, β-blocker, aspirin, and diuretics in the majority) in 6642 patients, and similar to the RALES trial, patients were excluded who had serum creatinine concentrations of greater than 2.5 mg/dL or serum potassium concentrations of greater than 5 mEq/L. In this study, eplerenone was associated with a 13% reduction in death from any cause, with the greatest survival benefit appearing to be a reduction in sudden death from cardiac causes. And while there was no evidence for a reduction in hospitalizations from all causes, there was a 23% reduction in the risk of hospitalization from heart failure. Owing to the receptor-selective nature of eplerenone, it was not associated with gynecomastia. However, there was a significant difference in the incidence of serious hyperkalemia, occurring in 5.5% of eplerenone- and 3.9% of placebo-treated patients.

While the clinical trial evidence suggests minimal risk associated with aldosterone antagonists in the setting of heart failure, the data from clinical practice suggest a different picture. Several studies have highlighted that the risk of serious hyperkalemia and worsening renal function are much higher than observed in the clinical trials.[84,85] These data suggest that 25% to 40% of patients develop hyperkalemia (>5 mEq/L) and that 10% to 12% develop serious hyperkalemia (>6 mEq/L). This may be due, in part, to failure of clinicians to consider the patient's renal function, to reduce or stop the patient's potassium supplementation, or to monitor renal function and potassium concentration closely once the aldosterone antagonist is initiated. However, even in closely monitored patients, the risk of hyperkalemia may remain high, particularly in the elderly and those with very low EFs.[84] Thus, if a clinician is to use an aldosterone antagonist, it must be done cautiously, with careful monitoring of renal function and potassium concentration and with avoidance of use in patients with significant renal impairment or high-normal potassium levels.

The benefits of aldosterone antagonists in heart failure appear to be due largely to their neurohormonal inhibition, namely, inhibition of aldosterone's actions in the heart. Specifically, the benefits are believed to be due to the ability of these agents to inhibit aldosterone-mediated cardiac fibrosis and thus ventricular remodeling.[86] And while spironolactone historically has been viewed as a diuretic, this is believed to contribute little to its benefits in heart failure in part because the doses used have minimal diuretic effect.[20] Thus, as with ACE inhibitors and β-blockers, the data on aldosterone antagonists also support the neurohormonal model of heart failure.

Taken together, the RALES and EPHESUS trials provide evidence of benefit from aldosterone antagonists at the two extremes of the heart failure spectrum, namely, after MI (NYHA class I) and NYHA class IV. While the benefits of aldosterone antagonists in patients with class II or stable class III heart failure have not been studied, it would be reasonable to speculate that benefit might exist. The place of aldosterone antagonists in therapy remains to be fully elucidated; however, it seems reasonable to consider their addition to standard therapy in patients who are similar to those enrolled in the RALES and EPHESUS trials. For patients who fall outside the populations studied in these clinical trials, there are no clear guidelines on aldosterone antagonist use. For such patients, it might be reasonable to consider use of an aldosterone antagonist if the patient requires potassium supplementation. The premise for use in this setting would be that reduction or elimination of the potassium supplement might be possible and that there also would be potential for additional benefit with respect to altering the disease course. Addition of spironolactone to class II or III heart failure patients who remain symptomatic despite optimal therapy is also a reasonable consideration.

TABLE 14–7. Clinical Trials of Candesartan in Heart Failure

Trial	Drug	Patient Population	Primary End Point	Results (%) Drug	Results (%) Placebo	Adjusted Hazard Ratio	p Value
CHARM-Added	Candesartan vs. placebo	Symptomatic HF and EF ≤ 40% on ACE inhibitors	CV death or hospital admission for HF	37.9	42.3	0.85	0.01
CHARM-Alternative	Candesartan vs. placebo	Symptomatic HF and EF ≤ 40%, ACE inhibitor intolerant	CV death or hospital admission for HF	33.0	40.0	0.70	<0.0001
CHARM-Preserved	Candesartan vs. placebo	Symptomatic HF and EF ≥ 40%	CV death or hospital admission for HF	22.0	24.3	0.86	0.051
CHARM-Overall	Candesartan vs. placebo	Combined from preceding three trials	All-cause mortality	23.0	25	0.90	0.032

Angiotensin II Receptor Blockers

5 The use of angiotensin II receptor blockers (ARBs) in heart failure has generated great interest and controversy. The crucial role of the RAA system in heart failure development and progression is well established, as are the benefits of RAA system inhibition with ACE inhibitors. However, chronic administration of ACE inhibitors can result in *ACE escape,* with increased circulating angiotensin II, NE, and aldosterone.[20,43,44] In addition, angiotensin II can be formed in a number of tissues, including the heart, through non-ACE-dependent pathways (e.g., chymase, cathepsin, and kallikrein).[14,87] Therefore, blockade of the detrimental effects of angiotensin II by ACE inhibition is incomplete. In addition, troublesome adverse effects of ACE inhibitors such as cough are linked to accumulation of bradykinin associated with these agents.[13] The ARBs block the angiotensin II receptor subtype AT_1, preventing the deleterious effects of angiotensin II, regardless of its origin. They do not appear to affect bradykinin.[14,87] By inhibiting both the formation of angiotensin II and its effects on the AT_1 receptor, combination therapy with an ACE inhibitor and an ARB offers a theoretical advantage over either agent used alone by more complete blockade of the deleterious effects of angiotensin II. Also, by directly blocking AT_1 receptors, ARBs would allow unopposed stimulation of AT_2 receptors, causing vasodilation and inhibition of ventricular remodeling.[14,87] Because the bradykinin-related adverse effects of ACE inhibitors such as angioedema and cough lead to drug discontinuation in some patients, the potential for an ARB to produce similar clinical benefits with fewer side effects is of great interest. Whether ARBs add incremental benefit to current established therapies or are superior (or equivalent) to ACE inhibitors is the focus of several clinical trials.

Initial studies indicate that ARBs and ACE inhibitors produce similar hemodynamic effects and that combination therapy improves exercise capacity, ventricular function, quality of life, and neurohormones in heart failure patients.[14,87] The ELITE II trial was the first to compare the effects of an ARB (losartan) with those of an ACE inhibitor (captopril) on all-cause mortality in patients with NYHA class II–IV heart failure.[88] No significant difference in mortality between the two groups was observed, although losartan was better tolerated than captopril. The Val-HeFT trial evaluated whether the addition of valsartan to standard background heart failure therapy (which included an ACE inhibitor in 93% and a β-blocker in 35% of patients) improved survival.[89] The addition of valsartan had no effect on all-cause mortality but produced a 13% reduction in morbidity and mortality (principally due to reductions in heart failure hospitalizations). Subgroup analysis showed that the benefits were greatest in patients not receiving background ACE inhibitor therapy, and detrimental effects were found in those who had valsartan added to ACE inhibitor and β-blocker. Based on these results, valsartan is now approved for use in patients intolerant to ACE inhibitors. Although this study suggests a benefit of combined ARB-ACE inhibitor therapy, it does not provide clear support for use of the combination, especially in patients receiving β-blocker therapy.

The Candesartan in Heart Failure: Assessment of Reduction in Mortality and Morbidity (CHARM) trials were designed as three studies to compare candesartan with placebo in patients with symptomatic heart failure[90] (Table 14–7). Both the CHARM-Added[91] and the CHARM-Alternative[92] trials found significant reductions in the primary end point of cardiovascular death or hospitalization for heart failure in patients receiving candesartan, although the benefit was modest in CHARM-Added. By the end of the CHARM-Added trial, over 60% of patients were receiving β-blocker therapy, but unlike the Val-HeFT trial, no adverse interaction with β-blockers was detected. No significant benefit of candesartan was observed in the CHARM-Preserved trial.[93] Overall, candesartan was well tolerated, but its use was associated with an increased risk of hypotension, hyperkalemia, and renal dysfunction.

The Valsartan in Acute Myocardial Infarction Trial (VALIANT) compared the effects of valsartan, captopril, and the combination of the two agents in post-MI patients with symptomatic heart failure, left ventricular dysfunction, or both.[94] The primary end point of total mortality occurred in 19.3% of patients receiving valsartan and captopril, 19.5% of captopril-treated patients, and 19.9% of the valsartan-treated group. Thus, in this high-risk post-MI population, valsartan was as effective as captopril in reducing the risk of death, but combination therapy only increased the risk of adverse effects and did not improve survival compared with monotherapy with either agent.

The ACC/AHA guidelines, developed before the Val-HeFT, CHARM, and VALIANT trials were completed, indicate that ARBs should not be considered equivalent or superior to ACE inhibitors and that they should be considered in patients who are intolerant of ACE inhibitors.[1] Collectively, the results of these trials clearly support this recommendation. For patients unable to tolerate an ACE inhibitor, usually due to intractable cough or angioedema, an ARB is a safe and effective alternative, although caution still should be exercised when it is used in patients with angioedema from ACE inhibitors. ARBs are not an alternative in patients with hypotension, hyperkalemia, or renal insufficiency secondary to ACE inhibitors because they are as likely to cause these adverse effects. The specific drugs and doses proven to be effective in clinical trials should be used. The role of ARBs as an adjunct to ACE inhibitors remains controversial.

The CHARM-Added trial found that the addition of candesartan to ACE inhibitor and β-blocker therapy produced incremental reductions in cardiovascular death and hospitalizations for heart failure but did not improve overall survival.[91] In contrast, VALIANT found no benefit from the addition of valsartan to ACE inhibitor treatment in post-MI patients, and post-hoc analysis of Val-HeFT suggested potential harm in patients receiving both ACE inhibitors and β-blockers.[89,94] These results suggest that the addition of an ARB to optimal heart failure therapy (ACE inhibitors, β-blockers, diuretics, etc.) offers, at best, marginal benefits with increased risk of adverse effects. Thus, until additional data are available, ACE inhibitor and β-blocker therapy should be optimized first before considering the addition of an ARB.

Nitrates and Hydralazine

Nitrates and hydralazine were combined originally in the treatment of heart failure because of their complementary hemodynamic actions. Nitrates, by activating guanylate cyclase to increase cyclic guanosine monophosphate (cGMP) in vascular smooth muscle, are primarily venodilators, thus producing reductions in preload.[42] Hydralazine is a direct-acting vasodilator that acts predominantly on arterial smooth muscle to reduce SVR and increase stroke volume and cardiac output (see Fig 14–1); its effects on preload are minimal.[42] Recent evidence suggests that these agents also may have beneficial effects in heart failure beyond their hemodynamic actions by inhibiting the ventricular remodeling process, preventing nitrate tolerance, and attenuating cellular mechanisms associated with heart failure progression.[1,5]

Compared with placebo, the combination of hydralazine and isosorbide dinitrate (ISDN) reduced mortality in patients receiving diuretics and digoxin (but not ACE inhibitors or β-blockers).[95] However, another trial comparing the combination with an ACE inhibitor found that mortality was lower in the ACE inhibitor group.[48] Adverse effects (primarily headache and gastrointestinal complaints) with combined hydralazine-ISDN were common, limiting their use in many patients. Patient compliance also was an important issue because hydralazine-ISDN therapy was given four times daily in these trials. Whether less frequent administration provides equivalent benefit is unknown.

Current guidelines recommend that hydralazine-ISDN should not be used instead of ACE inhibitors as standard therapy in heart failure or substituted for ACE inhibitors in patients who are tolerating an ACE inhibitor.[1] The combined use of hydralazine-ISDN may be considered a therapeutic option in patients unable to take an ACE inhibitor or an ARB because of renal insufficiency, hyperkalemia, or possibly hypotension. However, it should be anticipated that compliance with this regimen will be poor and the risk of adverse effects high. Therefore, given the proven benefits and low risk of adverse effects, many clinicians now prefer ARBs in patients who cannot tolerate an ACE inhibitor. There are no controlled trials evaluating the benefits of adding hydralazine-ISDN therapy to patients who remain symptomatic despite ACE inhibitor and/or β-blocker treatment.

TREATMENT OF CONCOMITANT DISORDERS

Heart failure is often accompanied by other disorders whose natural history or therapy may affect morbidity and mortality. In selected patients, optimal management of these concomitant disorders may have a profound impact on heart failure symptoms and outcomes.

Hypertension

Although ischemic heart disease has replaced hypertension as the most common cause of heart failure, still nearly two-thirds of heart failure patients currently have hypertension or a previous history of hypertension.[1] Hypertension can contribute directly to the development of heart failure and also contributes indirectly by increasing the risk of coronary artery disease. Pharmacotherapy of hypertension in patients with heart failure initially should involve agents that can treat both disorders, such as ACE inhibitors, β-blockers, and diuretics. If control of hypertension is not achieved after optimizing treatment with these agents, the addition of an ARB or a second-generation calcium channel blocker such as amlodipine (or possibly felodipine) should be considered. Medications that should be avoided include the calcium channel blockers with negative inotropic effects (e.g., verapamil, diltiazem, and most dihydropyridines) and direct-acting vasodilators (e.g., minoxidil) that cause sodium retention.

Angina

Coronary artery disease is the most common heart failure etiology. Appropriate management of coronary artery disease and its risk factors is thus an important strategy for the prevention and treatment of heart failure. Coronary revascularization should be strongly considered in patients with both heart failure and angina.[1] Pharmacotherapy of angina in patients with heart failure should use drugs that can treat both disorders successfully. Nitrates and β-blockers are effective antianginal agents and are the preferred agents for patients with both disorders because they may improve hemodynamics and clinical outcomes.[1] It should be noted that the antianginal effectiveness of these agents may be significantly limited if fluid retention is not controlled with diuretics. Similar to their use in hypertension, both amlodipine and felodipine appear to be safe to use in this setting.

Atrial Fibrillation

Atrial fibrillation is the most frequently encountered arrhythmia, and it is found commonly in patients with heart failure, affecting 10% to 50% of patients.[96] The high incidence of atrial fibrillation in the heart failure population is not surprising because each of these two disorders predisposes to the other, and they share many risk factors, including coronary artery disease and hypertension. The presence of atrial fibrillation in patients with heart failure is associated with a worse long-term prognosis. The combination of atrial fibrillation and heart failure may exert a number of detrimental effects that include increased risk of thromboembolism secondary to stasis of blood in the atria, a reduction in cardiac output owing to loss of the atrial contribution to ventricular filling, and hemodynamic compromise from the rapid ventricular response. Moreover, heart failure exacerbations and atrial fibrillation are linked closely, and it is often difficult to determine which disorder caused the other. For example, worsening heart failure results in volume overload, which, in turn, causes atrial distension and increases the risk of atrial fibrillation. Similarly, atrial fibrillation with a rapid ventricular response can reduce cardiac output and lead to heart failure exacerbation. Thus optimal management of both conditions is required, with careful attention paid to control of ventricular response and anticoagulation for stroke prevention (see Chap. 17).

Because of the close association between atrial fibrillation, heart failure exacerbations, and hospitalizations, many clinicians prefer maintenance of sinus rhythm with antiarrhythmic drugs to the rate-control approach in the treatment of patients with both disorders. However, it must be noted that the benefits of restoring and maintaining sinus rhythm remain unclear in this population and is not without risk. Although the recently completed AFFIRM study showed no difference in outcomes between the rhythm-control and rate-control approaches, less than 10% of the patients in this study had significant left ventricular dysfunction.[97] An ongoing clinical trial should help to clarify the best approach to these difficult to manage patients.[96] In general, amiodarone is the preferred agent if the rhythm-control approach is taken. Although it has many noncardiac toxicities, amiodarone does not have cardiodepressant or significant proarrhythmic effects. Dofetilide also appears to be safe and effective in this population. Class I antiarrhythmics should be avoided.

Diabetes Mellitus

Diabetes is highly prevalent in the heart failure population, with current estimates indicating that it is present in approximately one-third of heart failure patients.[1,98] Diabetes may contribute directly to systolic or diastolic dysfunction, as well as indirectly by contributing to the development of coronary artery disease. Diabetes is an independent risk factor for developing heart failure, and its presence is associated with a hastened progression of heart failure and worse prognosis.

Pharmacotherapy of diabetes in heart failure patients is complicated by concerns about adverse effects with metformin and the thiazolidinedione (TZD) drugs (rosiglitazone and pioglitazone). The beneficial effects of these agents on glucose control and cardiovascular risk factors lead to their widespread use in patients with heart failure despite the warnings in the product labeling against their use in heart failure.[99] Metformin is contraindicated for use in patients with heart failure requiring pharmacologic treatment because of the risk of lactic acidosis. Although the mechanisms are presently unclear, the TZDs are associated with weight gain, peripheral edema, and heart failure. The TZD package insert indicates that these agents should not be used in patients with class III or IV heart failure because they may cause intravascular volume expansion and heart failure exacerbation. Most clinical trials with these drugs excluded patients with moderate to severe heart failure; thus the evidence supporting this precaution comes mainly from retrospective analyses and case reports. Because of the potential risk, a recent consensus statement indicates that TZDs should not be used in patients with NYHA class III or class IV heart failure.[98] TZDs should be used cautiously in patients with class I or II symptoms, and close observation is needed to detect weight gain, edema formation, or heart failure exacerbation.[98]

DRUG CLASS INFORMATION

ACE Inhibitors

A number of ACE inhibitors are available currently in the United States; those approved for use in heart failure are summarized in Table 14–8. The major differences in the ACE inhibitors are not in their pharmacologic properties but in their pharmacokinetic properties. Although it appears that mortality reduction with ACE inhibitors is probably a drug class effect, not all ACE inhibitors FDA approved for treatment of heart failure have been tested for their effects on mortality in heart failure. Thus it seems most prudent to use those agents which have been documented to prolong survival because the dose required for this effect has been documented. Table 14–8 also contains a summary of the target doses for survival benefit.

To minimize the risk of hypotension and renal insufficiency, ACE inhibitor therapy should be started with low doses, followed by gradual titration to the target doses as tolerated.[1] Asymptomatic hypotension should not be considered a contraindication to initiation of an ACE inhibitor. Renal function and serum potassium concentration should be evaluated within 1 to 2 weeks after therapy is started with periodic assessments, especially after dose increases. Careful attention to appropriate doses of diuretics is important because fluid overload may blunt the beneficial effects of ACE inhibitors, and overdiuresis increases the risk of hypotension and renal insufficiency. After titration of the drug to the target dose, most patients tolerate chronic therapy with few complications. Although symptoms may improve within a few days of initiating therapy, it may take weeks to months before the full benefits are apparent. Even if symptoms do not improve, long-term ACE inhibitor therapy should be continued to reduce the risk of mortality and hospitalization.

Because of the high prevalence of coronary artery disease in patients with heart failure, aspirin frequently is coadministered with ACE inhibitors. Several retrospective cohort analyses suggest that aspirin may attenuate the hemodynamic and mortality benefits of ACE inhibitors.[100] The postulated mechanism of this interaction involves opposing effects on synthesis of vasodilatory prostaglandins. The ACE inhibitor–mediated increase in bradykinin increases the synthesis of vasodilatory prostaglandins that have favorable hemodynamic benefits in heart failure. Because of aspirin's effect

TABLE 14–8. ACE Inhibitors Approved for Use in Heart Failure

Generic Name	Brand Name	Initial Dose	Target Dosing Survival Benefit[a]	Prodrug	Elimination[b]
Captopril	Capoten	6.25 mg tid	50 mg tid	No	Renal
Enalapril	Vasotec	2.5–5 mg bid	10 mg bid	Yes	Renal
Lisinopril	Zestril, Prinivil	2.5–5 mg qd	20–40 mg qd[c]	No	Renal
Quinapril	Accupril	10 mg bid	20–40 mg bid[d]	Yes	Renal
Ramipril	Altace	1.25–2.5 mg bid	5 mg bid	Yes	Renal
Fosinopril	Monopril	5–10 mg qd	40 mg qd[d]	Yes	Renal/hepatic
Trandolapril	Mavik	0.5–1 mg qd	4 mg qd	Yes	Renal/hepatic

[a] Target doses associated with survival benefits in clinical trials.
[b] Primary route of elimination.
[c] Note that in the ATLAS trial,[57] no significant difference in mortality was found between low dose (~5 mg/day) and high dose (~35 mg/day) lisinopril therapy.
[d] Effects on mortality have not been evaluated.
Abbreviations: tid = three times daily; bid = twice daily; qd = once daily.

on prostaglandin synthesis, this potentially beneficial action of ACE inhibitors may be negated. However, in contrast with studies that showed an ACE inhibitor–aspirin interaction, other investigators have found no interaction[101,102] or that the effect of aspirin is dose-related.[103] Since there is no prospective evidence confirming an interaction between these agents, it is currently recommended that the decision to use each of these medications be made based on whether an individual patient has indications for each drug. Use of aspirin doses of 160 mg/day or less may be considered.

Adverse Effects of ACE Inhibitors. The primary adverse effects of ACE inhibitor therapy are secondary to their major pharmacologic effects of angiotensin II suppression and increased bradykinin. The reductions in angiotensin II are associated with hypotension and functional renal insufficiency, which are the most common adverse effects observed with ACE inhibitors. Hypotension may be asymptomatic or manifested as dizziness, light-headedness, presyncope, or syncope. It occurs most commonly early in therapy or after an increase in dose, although it may occur at any time during treatment. Risk factors for hypotension include hyponatremia (serum sodium concentration <130 mEq/L), hypovolemia, and overdiuresis.[1] The occurrence of hypotension may be minimized by initiating therapy with lower ACE inhibitor doses and/or temporarily withholding or reducing the dose of diuretic and liberalizing salt intake.[1] An often-overlooked solution to hypotension is to space the administration times of vasoactive medications (e.g., diuretics and β-blockers) throughout the day so that these medications are not all administered at or near the same time. Many patients who experience symptomatic hypotension early in therapy are still good candidates for long-term treatment if risk factors for low blood pressure are addressed.

Functional renal insufficiency is manifested as increases in serum creatinine and blood urea nitrogen. As cardiac output and renal blood flow decline, renal perfusion is maintained by the vasoconstrictor effect of angiotensin II on the efferent arteriole. Patients most dependent on this system for maintenance of renal perfusion (and therefore most likely to develop functional renal insufficiency with ACE inhibitors) are those with severe heart failure, hypotension, hyponatremia, volume depletion, and concomitant use of NSAIDs.[56,57] Sodium depletion (usually secondary to diuretic therapy) is the most important factor in the development of functional renal insufficiency with ACE inhibitor therapy. Renal insufficiency therefore can be minimized in many cases by reduction in diuretic dosage or liberalization of sodium intake. In some patients, the serum creatinine concentration will return to baseline levels without a reduction in ACE inhibitor dose.[56] Since renal dysfunction with ACE inhibitors is secondary to alterations in renal hemodynamics, it is almost always reversible on discontinuation of the drug.[56,57]

Careful dose titration can minimize the risks of hypotension and transient worsening of renal function. Thus usual initial doses should be about one-fourth the final target dose, with slow upward dose titration over several days based on blood pressure and serum creatinine concentration. In certain patients, especially hospitalized patients who seem at high risk for hypotension or worsening of renal function, it also may be advisable to initiate therapy with a short-acting agent such as captopril. This will help to minimize the duration of adverse effects should they occur. Once the patient is stabilized on ACE inhibitor therapy with captopril, he or she then can be switched to a longer-half-life drug.

Retention of potassium with ACE inhibitor therapy can occur and is due to the reduced feedback of angiotensin II to stimulate aldosterone release. Hyperkalemia is most likely to occur in patients with renal insufficiency and in those taking concomitant

potassium supplements, potassium-containing salt substitutes, or potassium-sparing diuretic therapy, especially if they have diabetes.[57] The more widespread use of aldosterone antagonists (e.g., spironolactone) in patients with heart failure may increase the risk of hyperkalemia.[104]

A dry, hacking cough occurs with a similar frequency (5% to 15% of patients) with all the agents and is related to bradykinin accumulation. The cough is usually nonproductive, occurs within the first few months of therapy, resolves within 1 to 2 weeks of drug discontinuation, and reappears with rechallenge. Cough occurs in up to 40% of patients with heart failure independent of ACE inhibitor use, although ACE inhibitors increase its incidence significantly. However, in large clinical trials, only about 1% of participants discontinued ACE inhibitor therapy because of cough. Because cough is a bradykinin-mediated effect, replacement of ACE inhibitor therapy with an ARB would be reasonable in patients who cannot tolerate the cough. Angioedema is a rare but potentially life-threatening complication that is also believed to be related to bradykinin accumulation. Use of ACE inhibitors is contraindicated in patients with a history of angioedema. Rash and dysgeusia are troublesome side effects of ACE inhibitor therapy that appear to be more common with high doses; the rash may resolve with continued therapy.

β-Blockers

Metoprolol CR/XL, carvedilol, and bisoprolol all have been shown to reduce mortality in heart failure and are the β-blockers discussed here. The initial and target doses are shown in Table 14–5. Metoprolol is a lipophilic β_1-selective blocker, bisoprolol is a hydrophilic β_1-selective blocker, and carvedilol is a nonselective β-blocker with α_1-blocker and antioxidant effects. Despite some studies aimed at addressing the issue, there is no clear evidence that these pharmacologic differences have any important effects on the outcomes associated with β-blockers in heart failure. However, their pharmacologic differences may aid in selection of a specific agent. For example, the α_1-blockade of carvedilol causes more hypotension and dizziness than metoprolol or bisoprolol.[105] Thus metoprolol or bisoprolol may be preferred in patients with low blood pressure or in whom dizziness would be especially problematic. Conversely, carvedilol may be preferred in patients whose blood pressure is poorly controlled because it would be expected to have a greater antihypertensive effect than the others.

Bisoprolol is eliminated about 50% by renal elimination, whereas metoprolol and carvedilol are essentially completely metabolized and undergo extensive hepatic first-pass metabolism. Both metoprolol and carvedilol are also substrates for the cytochrome P450 2D6, which is known to be polymorphic. Thus the 7% of the white population and 1% to 2% of the Asian-American and African-American populations who are CYP2D6 poor metabolizers would be expected to have more pronounced effects than anticipated at the usual doses of carvedilol and metoprolol.

An important issue regarding use of β-blockers in heart failure is whether the benefits seen represent a class effect, and if not, which drug(s) should be used. The evidence that benefits of β-blockers in heart failure should not be viewed as a class effect is fairly strong. Specifically, a study powered for mortality reduction showed that bucindolol was no different from placebo.[106] There has been much debate since publication of this trial about why this particular β-blocker failed to show benefit, but most practitioners now believe it relates to ancillary properties of the drug that were counterproductive in heart failure, namely, intrinsic sympathomimetic activity or central sympatholytic effects.[107,108] Unlike many other drug classes, the various β-blockers have differing receptor selectivities and other ancillary properties. As such, it is even more critical for β-blockers than other drug classes to confine use to agents that have proven efficacy in clinical trials.

There also has been much debate about whether carvedilol is superior to metoprolol or bisoprolol and whether immediate-release metoprolol has equivalent efficacy to metoprolol CR/XL, the formulation studied in the MERIT-HF trial. Despite the differing properties of carvedilol versus metoprolol or bisoprolol, the clinical trials data provided little evidence for superiority of one drug over another. Specifically, mortality reduction versus placebo for each of these drugs was identical (34% to 35%). Yet questions persist about potential superiority of carvedilol, in part because it appears to be superior in its effects on certain parameters, such as change in EF, and certain hemodynamic responses at peak exercise.[65,66]

To address the issue of superiority of carvedilol, a head-to-head clinical trial (COMET) of carvedilol versus immediate-release metoprolol tartrate was undertaken.[109] Consistent with the hypothesis that carvedilol tartrate has superior effects, this trial showed that mortality was 17% lower in patients treated with carvedilol 25 mg twice daily than in those treated with immediate-release metoprolol 50 mg twice daily. While this trial may have been expected to settle the debate, there were several concerns with the design of the study. First, the study did not use metoprolol CR/XL, the formulation that had been shown previously to be superior to placebo. It had long been thought that the pharmacokinetic profile of metoprolol CR/XL, which provides more sustained β-blockade, might make this formulation superior to immediate-release metoprolol. More significant were the concerns that the doses used in COMET did not provide equivalent β-blockade.[110] Specifically, it was felt that the dosing of carvedilol was much more aggressive than that of metoprolol. This is supported in part by the fact the target metoprolol dose in COMET was 100 mg/day (50 mg twice daily), whereas the target metoprolol dose in the MERIT-HF trial was 200 mg/day. While there are differences in the first-pass effects of the CR/XL and immediate-release formulations, it still seems likely that the degree of β-blockade achieved in COMET with immediate-release metoprolol 50 mg twice daily is less than that achieved in the MERIT-HF trial with metoprolol CR/XL 200 mg/day or that achieved by carvedilol 25 mg twice daily. Thus the question about whether carvedilol is superior to metoprolol CR/XL at similar β-blocking doses remains and is one that is not likely to be answered by a subsequent clinical trial.

Thus the clinical trial data suggest that we should only use drugs that have been shown superior to placebo in large mortality trials. And while some clinicians would argue superiority of carvedilol, it seems clear that what is most important is that one of the three proven β-blockers is used in all heart failure patients.

Diuretics[73]

Loop diuretics, as described earlier, represent the typical diuretic therapy for patients with heart failure due to their potency and, as such, are the only diuretics discussed here. There are currently three loop diuretics available that are used routinely: furosemide, bumetanide, and torsemide. They share many similarities in their pharmacodynamics, with their differences being largely pharmacokinetic in nature. Relevant information on the loop diuretics is shown in Table 14–6. Following oral administration, the peak effect with all the agents occurs in 30 to 90 minutes, with duration of 2 to 3 hours (slightly longer for torsemide). Following intravenous administration, the diuretic effect begins within minutes. All three drugs are

highly (>95%) bound to serum albumin and enter the nephron by active secretion in the proximal tubule. The magnitude of effect is determined by the peak concentration achieved in the nephron, and there is a threshold concentration that must be achieved before any diuresis is seen.

The biggest difference between the agents is bioavailability. Bioavailability of bumetanide and torsemide is essentially complete (80% to 100%), whereas furosemide bioavailability exhibits marked intra- and interpatient variability. Furosemide bioavailability ranges from 10% to 100%, with an average of 50%. Thus, if bioequivalent intravenous and oral doses are desired, oral furosemide doses should be approximately double that of the intravenous dose, whereas intravenous and oral doses are the same for torsemide and bumetanide. Coadministration of furosemide and bumetanide with food can decrease bioavailability significantly, whereas food has no effect on bioavailability of torsemide. The intraabdominal congestion that can occur in heart failure also may slow the rate (and thus decrease the peak concentration) of furosemide, which can reduce the diuretic's efficacy. Thus furosemide is most problematic with respect to rate and extent of absorption and the factors that influence it, whereas torsemide has the least variable bioavailability.

Recent data suggest that these differences in bioavailability and variability may have clinical implications. For example, several studies have suggested that torsemide is absorbed reliably and is associated with better outcomes than the more variably absorbed furosemide.[111,112] And while the costs of torsemide exceed those of furosemide, pharmacoeconomic analyses suggest that the costs of care are similar or less with torsemide.[112] These data require confirmation in controlled, double-blinded clinical trials but provide preliminary evidence that the more reliably absorbed loop diuretics may be superior to furosemide.

As noted in the previous section on diuretics, the loop diuretics exhibit a ceiling effect in heart failure, meaning that once the ceiling dose is reached, no additional response is achieved by increasing the dose. Thus, when this dose is reached, additional diuresis is achieved by giving the drug more often or by giving combination diuretic therapy. The ceiling doses are listed in Table 14–6. While some heart failure patients take their diuretic once per day, many will take it twice per day and a small percentage three times per day. Multiple daily dosing is somewhat common in heart failure because of the ceiling-dose effects and to achieve a more sustained diuresis throughout the day. When dosed two or three times daily, the first dose is usually given first thing in the morning and the final dose in late afternoon/early evening.

Diuretics cause a variety of metabolic abnormalities, with severity related to the potency of the diuretic. The reader is referred to Chap. 13 for a detailed discussion on the adverse effects of diuretic therapy. The most common metabolic disturbance associated with both thiazide and loop diuretics is hypokalemia, which in heart failure patients may be exacerbated by hyperaldosteronism. Hypokalemia in these patients also is accompanied frequently by hypomagnesemia, and since adequate magnesium is necessary for entry of potassium into the cell, magnesium supplementation also is necessary sometimes in order to correct the hypokalemia. Hypokalemia is especially worrisome in the setting of heart failure because it can precipitate ventricular arrhythmias, a common mode of death for these patients. Digoxin-associated arrhythmias are also more common with concurrent hypokalemia. Concomitant ACE inhibitor and/or aldosterone antagonist therapy may help to minimize diuretic-induced hypokalemia because these drugs tend to increase serum potassium concentration through their effects on aldosterone. Nonetheless, the serum potassium concentration should be monitored closely in heart failure patients and supplemented appropriately when needed.

TABLE 14–9. Clinical Pharmacokinetics of Digoxin

Oral bioavailability	
Tablets	0.5–0.9 (0.65)[a]
Elixir	0.75–0.85 (0.80)
Capsules	0.9–1.0 (0.95)
Onset of action	
Oral	1.5–6 h
Intravenous	15–30 min
Peak effect	
Oral	4–6 h
Intravenous	1.5–4 h
Terminal half-life	
Normal renal function	36 h
Anuric patients	5 d
Volume of distribution at steady state	7.3 L/kg
Fraction unbound in plasma	0.75–0.80
Fraction excreted unchanged in urine	0.65–0.70

[a] Range and mean value in parentheses.
Data from Reuning RH, Geraets DR, Rocci ML, Vlasses PH. Digoxin. In: Evans WE, Schentag JJ, Jusko WJ, eds. Applied Pharmacokinetics: Principles of Therapeutic Drug Monitoring, 3d ed. Spokane, WA, Applied Therapeutics, 1992: 20-1–20-48.

Digoxin

Pharmacology. Digoxin exerts its positive inotropic effect by binding to sodium- and potassium-activated adenosine triphosphatase (Na^+,K^+-ATPase or sodium pump).[75,76] Inhibition of Na^+,K^+-ATPase decreases outward transport of sodium and leads to increased intracellular sodium concentrations. Higher intracellular sodium concentrations favor calcium entry and reduce calcium extrusion from the cell through effects on the sodium-calcium exchanger.[75] The result is increased storage of intracellular calcium in the sarcoplasmic reticulum and, with each action potential, a greater release of calcium to activate contractile elements. Digoxin also has beneficial neurohormonal actions. These effects occur at low plasma concentrations, where little inotropic effect is seen, and are independent of inotropic activity.[75,76] Unlike other positive inotropes that increase intracellular cAMP, digoxin attenuates the excessive SNS activation present in heart failure patients.[75,76] Although the precise mechanism is unknown, a digoxin-mediated reduction in central sympathetic outflow and improvement in impaired baroreceptor function appear to play an important role.[75,76] Because mortality and progression of heart failure are linked to the extent of SNS activation, these sympathoinhibitory effects may be an important component of the clinical response to the drug. Chronic heart failure is also marked by autonomic dysfunction, most notably suppression of the parasympathetic (vagal) system.[75] Digoxin increases parasympathetic activity in heart failure patients and leads to a decrease in heart rate, thus enhancing diastolic filling.[75,76] The vagal effects also result in slowed conduction and prolongation of atrioventricular node refractoriness, thus slowing the ventricular response in patients with atrial fibrillation. Because atrial fibrillation is a common complication of heart failure, the combined positive inotropic, neurohormonal, and negative dromotropic effects of digoxin can be particularly beneficial for such patients. The overall

TABLE 14–10. Digoxin Drug Interactions

Drug	Mechanism/Effect	Suggested Clinical Management
Amiodarone	Inhibits P-glycoprotein resulting in decrease in renal and nonrenal clearance; can increase SDC by 70–100%	Monitor SDC and adverse effects; anticipate the need to reduce the dose by 50%
Antacids	Concurrent administration may decrease digoxin bioavailability by 20–35%	Space doses at least 2 h apart or avoid concurrent use if possible
Cholestyramine, colestipol	Bind digoxin in gut and decrease bioavailability 20–35%; also may decrease enterohepatic recycling	Space doses at least 2 h apart or avoid concurrent use if possible
Diuretics	Thiazides or loop diuretics may cause hypokalemia and hypomagnesemia, thereby increasing the risk of digitalis toxicity	Monitor and replace electrolytes if necessary
Erythromycin, clarithromycin, tetracycline	Alter gut bacterial flora; bioavailability and SDC increase 40–100% in about 10% of patients who extensively metabolize digoxin in the gut, also may be due to inhibition of P-glycoprotein by macrolides	Monitor SDC and anticipate the need to reduce the dose; avoid concurrent use if possible
Ketoconazole, itraconazole	Decrease in renal and nonrenal clearance by inhibition of P-glycoprotein; SDC may increase by 50–100%	Monitor SDC and anticipate the need to reduce the dose by 50%
Kaolin-pectin	Large dose (30–60 mL) may decrease digoxin bioavailability by about 60%	Space doses at least 2 h apart or avoid concurrent use if possible
Metoclopramide	Increase in gut mobility may decrease bioavailability of slowly dissolving tablets; unknown significance	Effect is minimized by administration of digoxin capsules
Neomycin, sulfasalazine	Decrease in bioavailability by 20–25%	Space doses at least 2 h apart or avoid concurrent use if possible
Propafenone	Decrease in renal clearance; SDC may increase 30–40%	Monitor SDC and anticipate the need to reduce the dose
Quinidine	Inhibits P-glycoprotein resulting in decrease in renal and nonrenal clearance; also displacement of digoxin from tissue binding sites with decrease in the volume of distribution; SDC generally increases about twofold.	Monitor SDC and adverse effect the need to reduce dose by 50%
Spironolactone	Decrease in renal and nonrenal clearance; also interference with some digoxin assays thus increasing apparent SDC	Monitor SDC and anticipate the need to reduce dose; check assay for interference
Verapamil	Inhibits P-glycoprotein resulting in decrease in renal and nonrenal clearance, SDC may increase 70–100%	Monitor SDC and anticipate the need to reduce the dose by 50%; consider using another calcium channel blocker

SDC = serum digoxin concentration.

response to digoxin is usually an increase in cardiac index, a decrease in SVR, PAOP, and plasma NE, but relatively little change in arterial blood pressure.[75,76]

Pharmacokinetics.

Numerous studies of digoxin pharmacokinetics have been published and are summarized in Table 14–9.[83] Digoxin has a large volume of distribution and is extensively bound to various tissues, most notably to Na^+,K^+-ATPase in skeletal and cardiac muscles. Because it does not distribute appreciably to body fat, loading doses of digoxin (when necessary) should be calculated based on estimates of lean body weight. There is a long "distribution phase" after administration of oral or intravenous digoxin, resulting in a lag time before maximum pharmacologic response is observed (see Table 14–9). Transiently elevated serum digoxin concentrations (SDCs) during the distribution phase are not associated with increased therapeutic or adverse effects, although they can mislead the clinician who is unaware of the timing of blood sampling relative to the previous digoxin dose. Consequently, blood samples for measurement of SDCs should be collected at least 6 hours and preferably 12 hours or more after the last dose.

In patients with normal renal function, 60% to 80% of a dose of digoxin is eliminated unchanged in urine via glomerular filtration and tubular secretion. The terminal half-life of digoxin is approximately 1.5 days in subjects with normal renal function but approximately 5 days in anuric patients (see Table 14–9). Recent evidence indicates that the drug efflux transporter P-glycoprotein (P-gp) plays an important role in the bioavailability, renal and nonrenal clearance, and drug interactions with digoxin.[113] Clinically important pharmacokinetic/pharmacodynamic drug interactions are summarized in Table 14–10. An extensive review of the pharmacokinetics and pharmacodynamics of digoxin is available.[83]

Adverse Effects.

Digoxin can produce a variety of cardiac and noncardiac adverse effects, but it is usually well tolerated by most patients[75,76] (Table 14–11). Noncardiac adverse effects frequently involve the central nervous system or gastrointestinal system but also may be nonspecific (e.g., fatigue or weakness). Cardiac manifestations include numerous different arrhythmias that are believed to be caused by multiple electrophysiologic effects (see Table 14–11). Cardiac arrhythmias may be the first evidence of toxicity in a patient (before any noncardiac symptoms occur). Rhythm disturbances are of particular concern because patients with chronic heart failure are already at increased risk for sudden cardiac death presumably owing

TABLE 14–11. Signs and Symptoms of Digoxin Toxicity

Noncardiac (Mostly CNS) Adverse Effects
Anorexia, nausea, vomiting, abdominal pain
Visual disturbances, such as halos, photophobia, problems with color perception (i.e., red-green or yellow-green vision), scotomata
Fatigue, weakness, dizziness, headache, neuralgia, confusion, delirium, psychosis

Cardiac Adverse Effects[a,b]
Ventricular arrhythmias
Premature ventricular depolarizations, bigeminy, trigeminy, ventricular tachycardia, ventricular fibrillation
Atrioventricular (AV) block
First degree, second degree (Mobitz type I), third degree
AV junctional escape rhythms, junctional tachycardia
Atrial arrhythmias with slowed AV conduction or AV block
Particularly paroxysmal atrial tachycardia with AV block
Sinus bradycardia

[a]Some adverse effects may be difficult to distinguish from the signs/symptoms of heart failure.
[b]Digoxin toxicity has been associated with almost every known rhythm abnormality (only the more common manifestations are listed).
Compiled from Circulation 1999;99:1265–1270; Prog Cardiovasc Dis. 2002;44:251–266; and from Reuning RH, et al: Digoxin. In: Evans WE, Schentag JJ, Jusko WJ, eds. Applied Pharmacokinetics: Principles of Therapeutic Drug Monitoring, 3rd ed. Spokane, WA, Applied Therapeutics, 1992:20-1–20-48.

to ventricular arrhythmias. Patients at increased risk of toxicity include those with impaired renal function, decreased lean body mass, the elderly, and those taking interacting drugs. Hypokalemia, hypercalcemia, and hypomagnesemia will predispose patients to cardiac manifestations of digoxin toxicity. Thus concomitant therapy with diuretics may lead to electrolyte abnormalities and increase the likelihood of cardiac arrhythmias. Similarly, hypothyroidism, myocardial ischemia, and acidosis also will increase the risk of cardiac adverse effects. Although digoxin toxicity is associated commonly with plasma concentrations greater than 2 ng/mL, clinicians should remember that digoxin toxicity is based on the presence of symptoms rather than a specific plasma concentration. Usual treatment of digoxin toxicity includes drug withdrawal or dose reduction and treatment of cardiac arrhythmias and electrolyte abnormalities. In patients with life-threatening digoxin toxicity, purified digoxin-specific Fab antibody fragments provide reversal of adverse effects within 1 hour in over 90% of patients.

▶ TREATMENT: Advanced/Decompensated Heart Failure[114,115]

As discussed previously, the number of patients with heart failure is substantial and continues to increase. Although mortality from heart failure has improved, the growing number of patients with the disorder and the progressive nature of the syndrome have led to substantial increases in hospitalizations for heart failure.[3] Recent data indicate that nearly 1 million patients are hospitalized annually for heart failure, resulting in significant morbidity, reduced quality of life, and consumption of large quantities of health care resources.[3] In fact, the majority of costs for the treatment of heart failure are attributed to patients admitted to the hospital. Inpatient admission for heart failure exacerbations is associated with an increased risk of subsequent hospitalization and decreased long-term survival.[114]

A number of descriptive terms have been used to identify this group of patients. Patients with *advanced, end-stage,* or *refractory heart failure* are those with persistent symptoms despite optimal therapy with ACE inhibitors, β-blockers, diuretics, and digoxin (i.e., stage

D in the ACC/AHA classification scheme).[114,115] The terms *decompensated heart failure* and *exacerbation of heart failure* refer to patients with acute worsening of their baseline symptoms that is usually caused by volume overload and/or hypoperfusion. Irrespective of the term used, these forms of severe heart failure may be caused by progression of the underlying disorder or by other intercurrent events that result in worsening of the patient's symptoms. Early identification and aggressive management of patients with advanced heart failure hopefully will reduce morbidity, mortality, and cost of care.

PATHOPHYSIOLOGY AND CLINICAL PRESENTATION

Patients requiring intensive therapy for advanced heart failure may present via several pathways. Patients with chronic progressive heart failure can become refractory to available oral therapy and decompensate following a relatively mild insult (e.g., dietary indiscretion), from medical noncompliance, from a noncardiac concurrent illness (e.g., infection), or simply from a progressive reduction in cardiac output (*low-output syndrome*). A new cardiac event, such as recurrent MI, atrial fibrillation, myocarditis, or acute valvular insufficiency, also can cause a stable patient to decompensate. A third group of patients consists of those with acute massive MI whose initial presentation is severe heart failure. Regardless of their presentation, these patients represent the most advanced stage of heart failure.

The general pathophysiologic determinants of myocardial systolic (preload, afterload, or inotropy) and diastolic function (ventricular compliance or lusitropic function) in these patients are essentially the same as described earlier in this chapter. However, the severity of their symptoms, lack of cardiopulmonary reserve, and potential for adverse responses to intervention make successful treatment of these patients a challenge.

GENERAL APPROACH TO TREATMENT

The overall goals of therapy in the patient with advanced/decompensated heart failure are to relieve symptoms of congestion and edema and improve the hemodynamic profile so that the patient can be discharged in a compensated (euvolemic) state on oral drug therapy. Although diuretic, vasodilator, and positive inotrope therapy can be very effective at achieving these goals, their efficacy must be balanced against the potential for serious toxicity. Thus another important goal is to minimize the risks of pharmacologic therapy. Maintenance of vital organ perfusion to preserve renal function and prevent additional myocardial injury is as important a goal as is prevention of diuretic-induced electrolyte depletion, hypotension from vasodilators, and myocardial ischemia and arrhythmias from positive inotropes.

A careful history and physical examination are key components in the diagnosis of decompensated heart failure. The history should focus on the potential etiologies of heart failure; the presence of any precipitating factors; onset, duration, and severity of symptoms; and a careful medication history. Important elements of the physical examination include vital signs, cardiac auscultation for heart sounds and murmurs, pulmonary examination for the presence of rales, the presence of peripheral edema, and weight. The JVP is a reliable indicator of the patient's volume status and should be evaluated carefully on admission and followed closely as an indicator of the efficacy of diuretic therapy.

The development of a bedside assay for plasma BNP has focused considerable attention on the use of BNP as an aid in the diagnosis of suspected heart failure. Plasma BNP concentration is positively correlated with the degree of left ventricular dysfunction and heart failure, and this assay is now used frequently in acute care settings to assist in the differential diagnosis of dyspnea [heart failure versus asthma, chronic obstructive pulmonary disease (COPD), or infection]. Recent studies found that an elevated BNP concentration is an independent predictor of heart failure as the cause of dyspnea and that in patients with decompensated heart failure, an elevated pre-hospital discharge BNP concentration is associated with an increased risk of death or readmission.[116,117] Additional research is ongoing to better characterize the role of BNP measurement in the diagnosis and treatment of heart failure.

Patients should be admitted to an intensive care unit (ICU) for decompensated heart failure when they show signs of significant systemic hypoperfusion (e.g., severe fatigue, shortness of breath at rest, hypotension, altered mental status, or decreased renal function), develop pulmonary vascular congestion requiring mechanical ventilation, manifest symptomatic sustained tachyarrhythmias, or require potent intravenous vasoactive or inotropic drugs or mechanical ventricular assistance. However, most patients do not require ICU admission and are admitted to a monitored unit or general medical floor. Reversible or treatable causes of the patient's decompensation, such as a thyroid disorder or anemia, should be addressed and corrected. The need for drugs that may aggravate heart failure (e.g., calcium channel blocking drugs, antiarrhythmics, and NSAIDs) should be evaluated carefully and discontinued when possible.

The first step in the management of advanced heart failure is to ascertain that optimal treatment with oral medications has been achieved. If fluid retention is evident on physical examination, aggressive diuresis should be accomplished. Although increasing the dose of oral diuretic may be effective in some cases, the use of intravenous diuretics frequently is necessary. Most patients should be receiving digoxin at a low dose prescribed to achieve a trough serum concentration of 0.5 to 1 ng/mL.[1] Additionally, every effort should be made to optimally treat the patient with an ACE inhibitor. Although β-blockers generally should not be started during this period of instability, it is desirable to continue their administration, if possible, in patients who are receiving them on a chronic basis. However, discontinuation occasionally may be necessary because some patients with advanced heart failure may not be able to tolerate target doses of both ACE inhibitors and β-blockers.

There are two general approaches to maximize therapy in the advanced/decompensated heart failure patient. One is to use simple clinical parameters (i.e., signs and symptoms, blood pressure, and renal function), and the other is to use invasive hemodynamic monitoring. However, it is frequently necessary to combine the two approaches.

PRINCIPLES OF THERAPY BASED ON CLINICAL PRESENTATION[114,115,118]

Appropriate medical management of the patient presenting with advanced heart failure is aided by determination of whether the patient has signs and symptoms of fluid overload ("wet" heart failure) or low cardiac output ("dry" heart failure).[115,118] Most patients present with congestion (or the wet profile). Symptoms of an elevated filling pressure include orthopnea and dyspnea with minimal exertion and can lead to systemic symptoms such as gastrointestinal discomfort, ascites, and peripheral edema. Patients with no or minimal fluid overload (or the dry category of advanced heart failure) may have symptoms that are more difficult to distinguish. This is a syndrome of low cardiac output and is characterized principally by fatigue and other symptoms not commonly attributed to cardiac causes, such as poor appetite, nausea, and early satiety. Moreover, these patients frequently exhibit worsening renal function and a decline in serum sodium level. Many patients will present with signs and symptoms of both types of advanced heart failure. In these patients, low-output symptoms may not be obvious until congestion is treated. Based on the assessment of wet versus dry heart failure, the algorithm in Fig. 14–8 may be considered.

PRINCIPLES OF THERAPY BASED ON HEMODYNAMIC SUBSETS

Patients with severe heart failure may have critically reduced cardiac output, usually with low arterial blood pressure and systemic hypoperfusion resulting in organ system dysfunction (i.e., cardiogenic

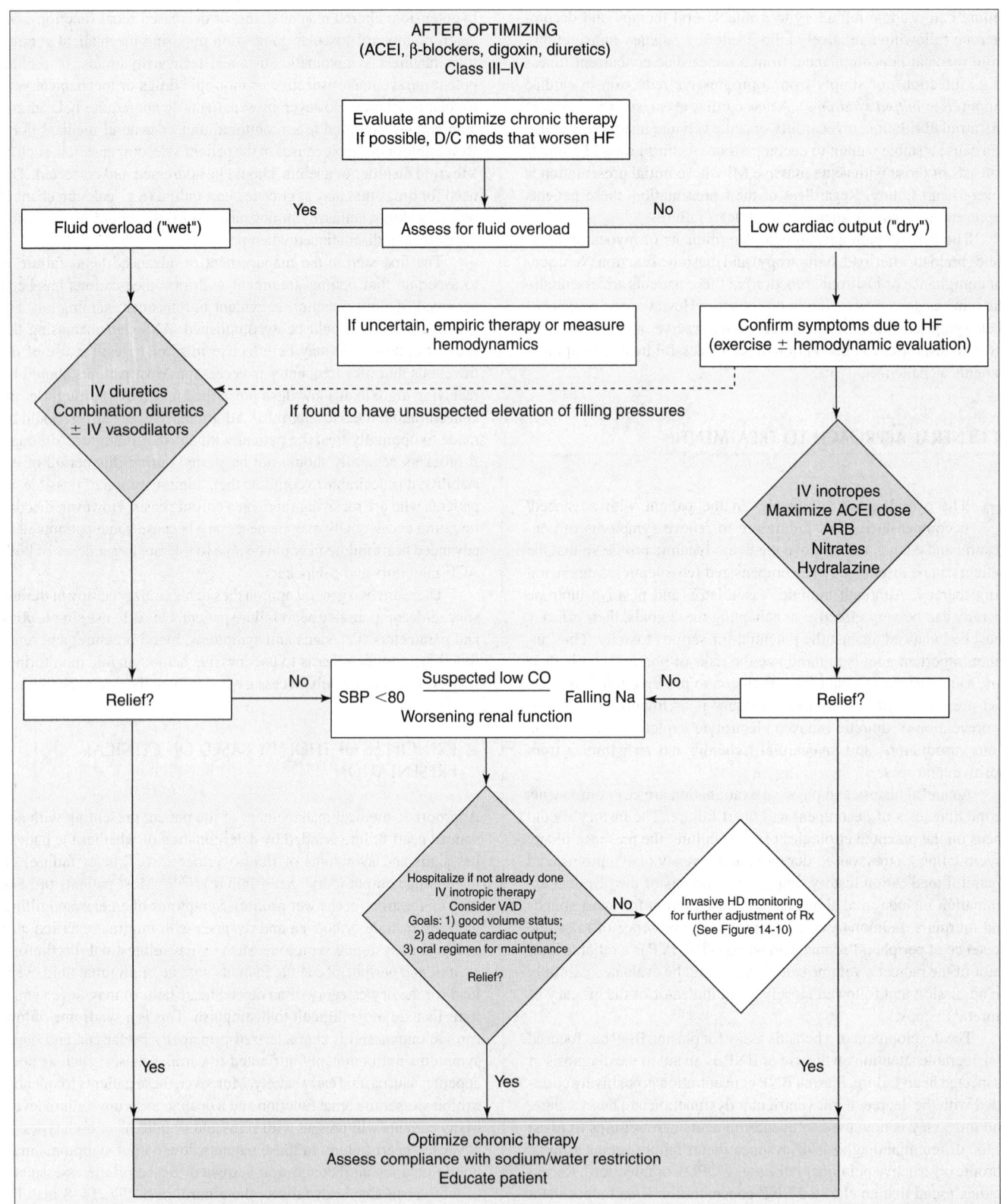

FIGURE 14–8. General treatment algorithm for advanced/decompensated heart failure based on clinical presentation. Intravenous vasodilators that may be used include nitroglycerin, nesiritide, and nitroprusside. *(Adapted with permission from Am Heart J 1998;135:S293–309.)*

shock). They also may demonstrate pulmonary edema with hypoxemia, respiratory acidosis, and markedly increased work of breathing. Since cardiopulmonary support must be instituted and adjusted rapidly, immediate assessment of the results of an intervention limits risks and makes adjustments in therapy more prompt. ECG monitoring, continuous pulse oximetry, urine flow monitoring, and automated sphygmomanometric blood pressure recording are now the minimal noninvasive standard of care for critically ill patients with cardiopulmonary decompensation. Peripheral or femoral arterial catheters provide continuous and accurate assessment of arterial pressure.

Hemodynamic Monitoring

The role of invasive hemodynamic monitoring for improving outcomes in patients with severe heart failure remains controversial. No guidelines or consensus statements are available to identify optimal hemodynamic end points or which patients may benefit from invasive monitoring. Although the routine use of invasive monitoring has come under scrutiny, its efficacy and safety in individual patients with advanced heart failure seem well established. Hemodynamic monitoring often provides essential information necessary to achieve optimal drug therapy in patients with a confusing or complicated clinical picture and during dose titration of rapidly acting medications. Invasive monitoring should be considered in patients with cardiogenic shock, refractory hypotension or heart failure symptoms, uncertain volume status, or declining renal function.

Invasive hemodynamic monitoring usually is performed with a flow-directed pulmonary artery (PA) or Swan-Ganz catheter placed percutaneously through a central vein and advanced through the right side of the heart and into the PA. Inflation of a balloon proximal to the end port allows the catheter to "wedge," yielding the PAOP, which estimates the pulmonary venous (left atrial) pressure and, in the absence of intracardiac shunt or mitral valve or pulmonary disease, left ventricular diastolic pressure. Additionally, cardiac output may be measured and systemic vascular resistance (SVR) calculated. Normal values for hemodynamic parameters are listed in Table 14–12.

In addition to the clinical presentation, invasive hemodynamic monitoring helps in the selection of appropriate medical therapy, as well as in the classification of patients into specific subsets. These *hemodynamic subsets* were first proposed for patients with left ventricular dysfunction following an acute MI but also are applicable

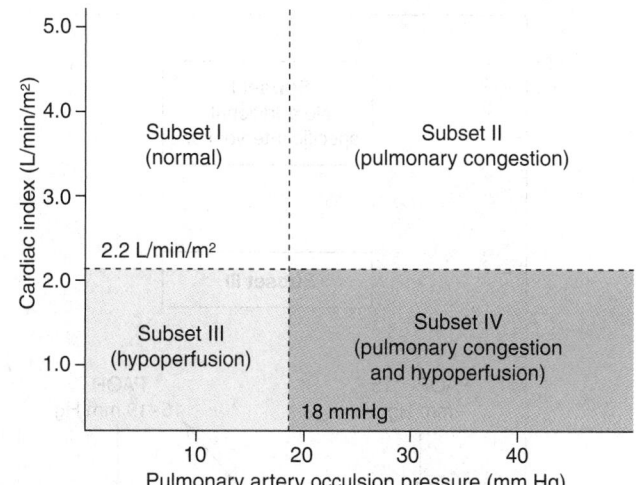

FIGURE 14–9. Hemodynamic subsets of heart failure based on cardiac index and pulmonary artery occlusion pressure. *(Adapted with permission from N Engl J Med 1976;295:1356–1362.)*

to patients with acute or severe heart failure from other causes[119] (Fig. 14–9). This hemodynamic classification has four subsets and is based on a cardiac index above or below 2.2 L/m² per minute and a PAOP above or below 18 mm Hg. A treatment algorithm, based on hemodynamic subsets, is shown in Fig. 14–10.

Subset I

Patients in hemodynamic subset I have a cardiac index and PAOP within generally acceptable ranges and have the lowest mortality of any subset. These patients do not need immediate specific interventions other than maximizing oral therapy and monitoring. It should be emphasized that patients with significant left ventricular dysfunction still may present in subset I because normal compensatory mechanisms and/or appropriate drug therapy at least partially may correct an otherwise abnormal hemodynamic profile.

Subset II

As shown in Fig. 14–9, patients in subset II have an adequate cardiac index but a PAOP greater than 18 mm Hg. These patients are likely to have pulmonary congestion (i.e., wet heart failure) secondary to increased hydrostatic pressure in the pulmonary capillaries but no evidence of peripheral hypoperfusion. The primary goal of therapy in these patients is to reduce pulmonary congestion by lowering PAOP. However, it is critically important that PAOP not be decreased excessively so as to cause a significant decrease in cardiac index. Although the normal range of PAOP is 5 to 12 mm Hg for individuals without cardiac dysfunction, higher pressures of 15 to 18 mm Hg frequently are necessary for heart failure patients to optimize cardiac index while avoiding pulmonary congestion. Generally, the PAOP can be lowered to the range of 15 to 18 mm Hg with relatively little decrease in cardiac index because the Frank-Starling curve is flatter at higher PAOP values, particularly in patients with heart failure. Intravenous administration of agents that reduce preload (i.e., loop diuretics, nitroglycerin, or nesiritide) is the most appropriate acute therapy to achieve the therapeutic goal for patients in subset II. These agents will produce a very

TABLE 14–12. Hemodynamic Monitoring: Normal Values

Central venous (right atrial) pressure, mean	<5 mm Hg
Right ventricular pressure	25/0 mm Hg
Pulmonary artery pressure	25/10 mm Hg
PAP, mean	<18 mm Hg
Pulmonary artery occlusion pressure, mean	<12 mm Hg
Systemic arterial pressure	120/80 mm Hg
Mean arterial pressure	90–110 mm Hg
Cardiac index	2.8–4.2 L/min/m²
Stroke volume index	30–65 mL/beat/m²
Systemic vascular resistance	900–1400 dyn·s·cm⁻⁵
Pulmonary vascular resistance	150–250 dyn·s·cm⁻⁵
Arterial oxygen content	20 mL/dL
Mixed venous oxygen content	15 mL/dL
Arteriovenous oxygen content difference	3–5 mL/dL

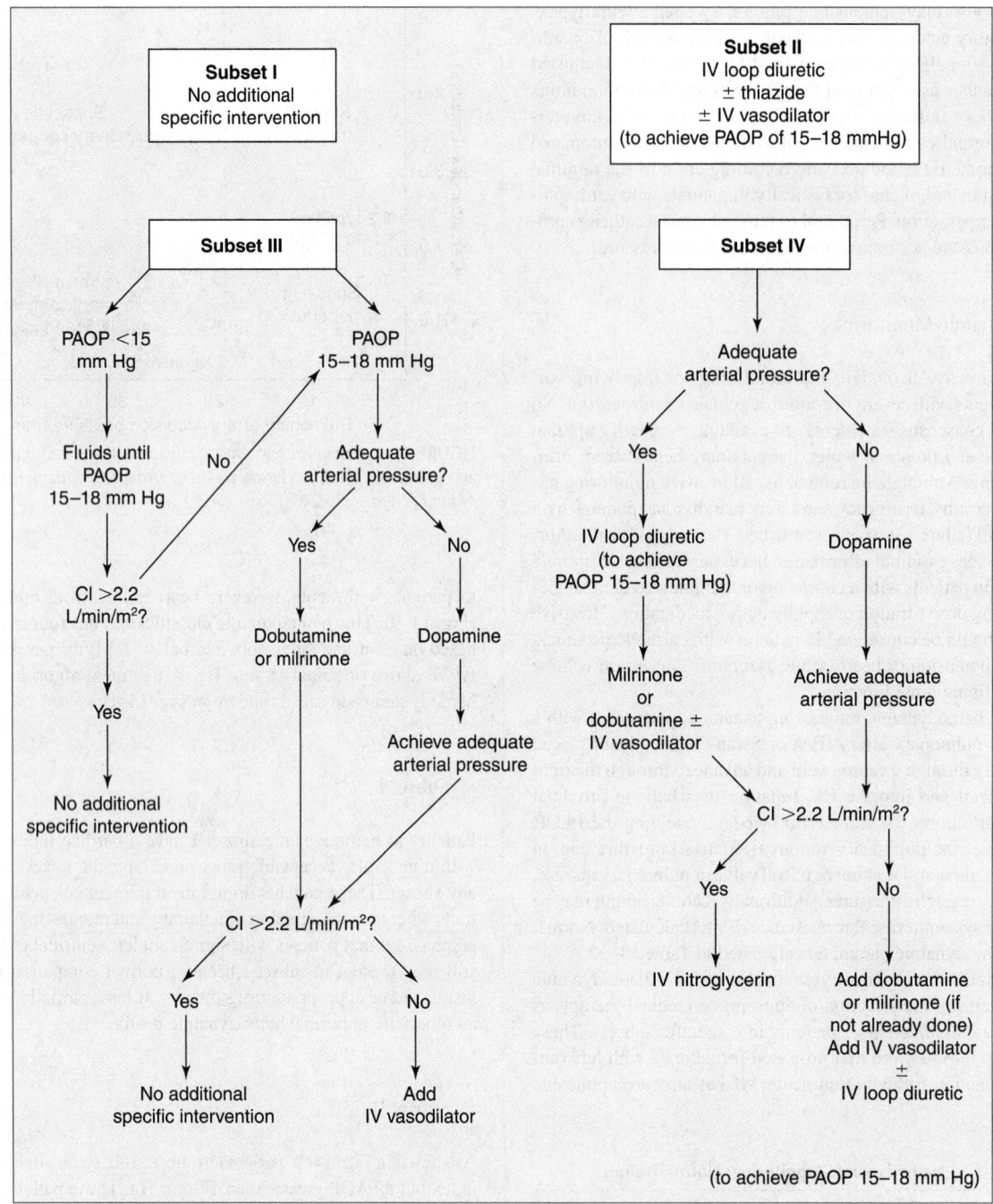

FIGURE 14–10. General treatment algorithm for patients with advanced/decompensated heart failure based on hemo-dynamic monitoring and hemodynamic subsets. Intravenous vasodilators that may be used include nitroglycerin, nesiritide, and nitroprusside.

rapid decrease in preload, although signs and symptoms of pulmonary congestion may take longer to resolve.

Subset III

Patients in hemodynamic subset III have a cardiac index of less than 2.2 L/m² per minute but without an abnormally elevated PAOP (see Fig 14–9). These patients usually will present without evidence of

pulmonary congestion, but the low cardiac index will result in signs and symptoms of peripheral hypoperfusion (i.e., decreased urine output, weakness, peripheral vasoconstriction, and weak pulses). The mortality rate of subset III patients is reported to be four times higher than that of patients without hypoperfusion.[119] Although the treatment goal is to alleviate the signs and symptoms of hypoperfusion by increasing cardiac index and perfusion to essential organs, therapy will differ among patients. If the PAOP is significantly below 15 mm Hg, initial therapy will be to administer intravenous fluids to provide a more optimal left ventricular filling pressure of 15 to 18 mm Hg and consequently improve cardiac index. When there is only mild left ventricular dysfunction, intravenous fluid administration may be all that is necessary to achieve a cardiac index above 2.2 L/m² per minute. However, many patients will have significant left ventricular dysfunction and a depressed Frank-Starling relationship despite adequate preload (i.e., PAOP of 15 to 18 mm Hg). In these patients, intravenously administered positive inotropic agents (e.g., dobutamine or milrinone) and/or arterial vasodilators (e.g., nitroprusside or nitroglycerin) often are necessary to achieve an adequate cardiac index. It is noteworthy that many positive inotropic drugs also will have arterial vasodilating activity (see specific drug classes that follow).

Subset IV

Patients with a cardiac index of less than 2.2 L/m² per minute and a PAOP higher than 18 mm Hg are in hemodynamic subset IV. These patients have the worst prognosis of any subset and illustrate the typical hemodynamic profile for the patient hospitalized for severe heart failure.

Because of severe pump failure, these patients cannot maintain an adequate cardiac index despite the elevated left ventricular filling pressure and increased myocardial fiber stretch. These patients will present with signs and symptoms of both wet and low-output heart failure. The treatment goals are to alleviate these signs and symptoms by increasing cardiac index above 2.2 L/m² per minute and reducing PAOP to 15–18 mm Hg while maintaining an adequate mean arterial pressure. Thus therapy will involve a combination of agents used for subset II and subset III patients to achieve these goals (i.e., combination of diuretic plus positive inotrope). These targets may be difficult to achieve and will necessitate careful monitoring and individualization of drug therapy. Nitroprusside is a particularly useful agent in this setting because of its mixed arterial-venous vasodilating effects. In the presence of significant hypotension, inotropic agents with vasopressor activity may be required initially to achieve an adequate perfusion pressure to essential organs and then can be combined, if necessary, with diuretics and/or vasodilators to obtain the desired hemodynamic effects and clinical response.

PHARMACOLOGIC THERAPY OF ADVANCED OR DECOMPENSATED HEART FAILURE

Unfortunately, the treatment of advanced heart failure has not improved substantially in the past decade owing in large part to the lack of clinical trial data in this population. The pharmacotherapeutic agents used to treat patients with decompensated heart failure rarely, if ever, produce a single cardiovascular action. Even when intended for a single purpose (e.g., a positive inotrope), other drug effects (e.g., tachycardia, vasodilation, or vasoconstriction) may either add to the therapeutic effect or cause adverse events that negate or even outweigh the intended therapeutic benefit. It often can be difficult to anticipate how an individual patient will respond to a given intervention. For this reason, hemodynamic monitoring can be useful, and many drugs are considered first-line therapy owing in part to their short half-lives and ease of titration. The description of expected drug actions outlined below should be viewed as a general guide to the clinician, who must reassess the patient continuously for desired outcomes. Table 14-13 contains a summary of the expected hemodynamic effects of the various drugs discussed below.

DIURETICS

Intravenous loop diuretics, including furosemide, bumetanide, and torsemide, are used in the management of advanced heart failure, with furosemide the most widely studied and used agent in this setting. Bolus administration of diuretics decreases preload by functional venodilation within 5 to 15 minutes and later (>20 minutes) via sodium and water excretion, thereby improving pulmonary congestion.[73,120] However, the acute reduction in venous return may severely compromise effective preload in patients with significant diastolic dysfunction or intravascular depletion. This results in a reflex increase in sympathetic activation, renin release, NE, and AVP elevations and the expected consequences of arteriolar and coronary constriction, tachycardia, and increased PAOP and myocardial oxygen consumption.[73] Unlike arterial dilators and positive inotropic agents, diuretics do not cause an upward shift in the Frank-Starling curve or increase

TABLE 14-13. Usual Hemodynamic Effects of Intravenous Agents Commonly Used for Treatment of Acute/Severe Heart Failure[a]

Drug	Dose	HR	MAP	PAOP	CO	SVR
Dopamine	0.5–3 mcg/kg/min	0	0	0	0/+	−
Dopamine	3–10 mcg/kg/min	+	+	0	+	0
Dopamine	>10 mcg/kg/min	+	+	+	+	+
Dobutamine	2.5–20 mcg/kg/min	0/+	0	−	+	−
Amrinone	5–10 mcg/kg/min	0/+	0/−	−	+	−
Milrinone	0.375–0.75 mcg/kg/min	0/+	0/−	−	+	−
Nitroprusside	0.25–3 mcg/kg/min	0/+	0/−	−	+	−
Nitroglycerin	5–200 mcg/min	0/+	0/−	−	0/+	0/−
Furosemide	20–80 mg; repeated as needed up to 4–6 times/d	0	0	−	0	0
Enalaprilat	0.25–2.5 mg q6–8h	0	0/−	−	+	+
Nesiritide	Bolus: 2 mcg/kg; Infusion: 0.01 mcg/kg/min	0	0/−	−	+	−

[a] See text for a more detailed description of the interpatient variability in response.
+ = increase; − = decrease; 0 = no change; HR = heart rate; MAP = mean arterial pressure; PAOP = pulmonary artery occlusion pressure; CO = cardiac output; SVR = systemic vascular resistance.

cardiac index significantly in most patients (see Table 14–13). Excessive preload reduction with diuretics can lead to a decline in cardiac output (see Fig 14–3). Thus diuretics must be used judiciously to obtain the desired improvement in symptoms of congestion while avoiding a reduction in cardiac output.

Diuretic Resistance

Occasionally, patients respond poorly to large doses of loop diuretics, and heart failure is the most common clinical setting in which diuretic resistance is observed.[120] The mechanisms responsible for diuretic resistance in heart failure patients appear to be both pharmacokinetic and pharmacodynamic. The bioavailability of furosemide is relatively normal in heart failure patients, but the rate of absorption is prolonged approximately twofold, and peak concentrations are about half of normal. Because loop diuretics have a sigmoid-shaped urine concentration-response curve, prolonged absorption may result in concentrations that fail to reach the steep portion of this curve, resulting in diminished responsiveness. Thus diuretic resistance with oral therapy may be overcome by giving larger oral doses, converting to intravenous administration, or combining a thiazide diuretic with the loop diuretic.[120]

Despite normal pharmacokinetics following intravenous administration, diuretic resistance is also observed with this route, suggesting an important pharmacodynamic component to diuretic resistance. The decreased responsiveness in heart failure patients is explained in part by the high concentrations of sodium reaching the distal tubule as a result of the blockade of sodium reabsorption in the loop of Henle. As a consequence, the distal tubule hypertrophies, increasing its ability to reabsorb sodium.[120] In addition, low cardiac output, reduced renal perfusion, and subsequent decreased delivery of drug to the kidney also may contribute to resistance.

Several maneuvers can be attempted to overcome diuretic resistance. Treatment of heart failure by other agents (e.g., positive inotropes or afterload reducers) may improve diuresis by increasing cardiac output and renal perfusion. Administration of low doses of dopamine with the hope of enhancing diuresis is also a common practice. However, recent data suggest that the addition of dopamine to furosemide provides no additional diuresis.[121] Larger intravenous bolus doses may achieve concentrations closer to the top of the concentration-response curve, or a continuous intravenous infusion may be used to maintain more constant concentrations in the steep portion of the concentration-response curve. Recent studies of continuous-infusion furosemide suggest a greater natriuretic effect and no difference in metabolic adverse effects when compared with the same total daily dose given by intravenous bolus.[122] Infusions also may limit adverse hemodynamic events.

Another approach to improving diuresis is addition of a second diuretic with a different mechanism of action. Combining a loop diuretic with a distal tubule blocker such as metolazone or hydrochlorothiazide can produce a synergistic diuretic effect.[120] The synergism is not a pharmacokinetic interaction but is related to the increased delivery of sodium to the distal convoluted tubule. Enhanced sodium delivery to (and reabsorption in) the distal tubule then can be blocked by the thiazide-type diuretic. Thus, when thiazide-type diuretics are added to a loop diuretic, they block more than their normal 5% to 8% of filtered sodium, and the combination results in synergistic natriuresis.[120]

The loop diuretic–thiazide combination generally should be reserved for the inpatient setting, where the patient can be monitored closely, because it can induce a profound diuresis with severe sodium, potassium, and volume depletion. When used in the outpatient setting, very low doses or only occasional doses of the thiazide-type diuretic should be used along with close follow-up (weight, vital signs, dizziness) to avoid serious adverse events.

POSITIVE INOTROPIC AGENTS[114,123]

Drugs that increase intracellular cAMP are the only positive inotropic agents currently approved for the treatment of acute heart failure. β-Agonists activate adenylate cyclase through stimulation of β-adrenergic receptors, with the enzyme then catalyzing the conversion of ATP to cAMP. Phosphodiesterase inhibitors raise cAMP concentrations by reducing its degradation. Thus both drug classes increase intracellular cAMP, which enhances phospholipase (and subsequently phosphorylase) activity, increasing the rate and extent of calcium influx during systole and enhancing contractility. Additionally, cAMP enhances reuptake of calcium by the sarcoplasmic reticulum during diastole, improving active relaxation. The receptor activities of the β-agonists are summarized in Table 14–14. Although rarely used in management of heart failure, the receptor effects of epinephrine, NE, and isoproterenol are provided for reference.

Digoxin has little, if any, place in the acute treatment of patients with advanced heart failure who are hemodynamically unstable. The delay in peak inotropic effect, limited inotropic effect, long duration of action, and potential toxicity (arrhythmic, vasoconstrictive, neurologic) are disadvantages in the acute setting. However, in patients with acute decompensation who are taking digoxin as part of their chronic therapy, it is generally unnecessary to adjust the dose or discontinue its use unless changes in renal function increase the risk of toxicity.

Although a number of parenteral agents have been used for the treatment of patients with advanced heart failure, dobutamine and milrinone have emerged as the two drugs administered most commonly. These drugs differ in their mechanisms of action and resulting pharmacologic effects and provide advantages and disadvantages in any given patient.

TABLE 14–14. Relative Effects of Adrenergic Drugs on Receptors

Drug	α_1	β_1	β_2	Dopamine$_1$
Norepinephrine	++++	++++	0	0
Epinephrine	++++	++++	++	0
Dopamine^a	++++	++++	++	++
Isoproterenol	0	++++	++++	0
Dobutamine^b	+	++++	++	0

^{a} See text for a more detailed description of the dose-dependent hemodynamic effects.
^{b} Combined effects of the commercially available racemic mixture (see text).

■ Dobutamine[123]

Dobutamine, a synthetic catecholamine, is a β_1- and β_2-receptor agonist with some α_1-agonist effects (see Table 14–14). Unlike dopamine, dobutamine does not cause release of NE from nerve terminals. The overall hemodynamic effects of dobutamine are the result of its effects on adrenergic receptors and reflex-mediated actions. Its β_2-receptor-mediated effects are greater than those of dopamine, and β_2-receptor-mediated vasodilation will tend to offset some of the α_1-receptor-mediated vasoconstriction. Thus the net vascular effect is usually vasodilation. The positive inotropy is primarily a β_1-receptor-mediated effect. Cardiac β_1-receptor stimulation by dobutamine causes an increase in contractility but generally no significant change in heart rate and may provide an explanation for the apparently more modest chronotropic actions of dobutamine compared with dopamine.

The overall hemodynamic effects of dobutamine are those of a potent inotropic agent with vasodilating action. Initial doses of 2.5–5 mcg/kg per minute can be increased progressively to 20 mcg/kg per minute or higher based on clinical and hemodynamic responses. Cardiac index is increased because of inotropic stimulation, arterial vasodilation, and a variable increase in heart rate. Because of the offsetting changes in arteriolar resistance and cardiac index, dobutamine usually will cause relatively little change in mean arterial pressure compared with the more consistent increase observed with dopamine. This smaller effect on blood pressure is beneficial in patients with heart failure and ischemic heart disease because it will minimize the increase in myocardial oxygen demand. More important, dobutamine appears to improve coronary blood flow by augmenting coronary perfusion pressure, increasing diastolic filling time, vasodilating coronary vessels, and unloading the left ventricle. However, the absence of a consistent hypertensive effect with dobutamine is a disadvantage in patients with heart failure and significant hypotension. Dobutamine's vasodilating action usually will decrease PAOP, making it particularly useful in the presence of low cardiac index and an elevated left ventricular filling pressure.

Attenuation of dobutamine's hemodynamic effects has been reported after 72 hours of continuous infusion and may be a consequence of downregulation of β_1-adrenergic receptors or uncoupling of β_2-adrenergic receptors from adenylate cyclase. However, it is unlikely that total loss of effect occurs with chronic administration. The evidence for this, although anecdotal, is the large number of patients (especially those awaiting transplant) who are "dobutamine-dependent" and experience hemodynamic deterioration when discontinuation is attempted. Thus, when dobutamine therapy is discontinued, it should be tapered off rather than stopped abruptly to prevent decompensation. Receptor downregulation should occur during long-term therapy with any β-agonist, and cross-tolerance with dopamine would be predicted. Full sensitivity to β-agonists should be restored 7 to 10 days after drug withdrawal. The maximum inotropic effects of dobutamine are diminished in patients with severe heart failure compared with those without heart failure. The mechanism of this tolerance is decreased myocardial β-receptor density and uncoupling from G-protein, which is caused by chronically elevated circulating catecholamine concentrations in heart failure patients.

In some patients, dobutamine (or milrinone) dose reduction or discontinuation results in acute decompensation, and these patients then may require placement of an indwelling intravenous catheter for continuous therapy. This approach may be used to "bridge" patients awaiting cardiac transplantation and also may be used to facilitate the discharge of patients who are not transplant candidates but who cannot be weaned from inotrope therapy. The use of continuous outpatient dobutamine therapy should be considered only after multiple unsuccessful attempts to maximize oral therapy. Although effective for symptom palliation, it should be realized that the risk of mortality is likely increased. In contrast, the use of regularly scheduled intermittent dobutamine infusions at home or in an outpatient clinic is not recommended in the current guidelines.[1]

■ Milrinone and Amrinone[123]

Both milrinone and amrinone are bipyridine derivatives that inhibit phosphodiesterase III, an enzyme responsible for the breakdown of cAMP to AMP. The subsequent increase in intracellular cAMP levels leads to an increase in intracellular calcium concentration and increased myocardial contractility. These agents produce similar pharmacologic and hemodynamic effects during intravenous administration. Amrinone was the prototype drug in this group, but its use has been supplanted largely by milrinone owing to the more frequent occurrence of thrombocytopenia with amrinone. Both positive inotropic and arterial and venous vasodilating effects contribute to the therapeutic response in heart failure patients; hence these drugs have been referred to as *inodilators*. The relative balance of these pharmacologic effects may vary in a particular patient with dose and underlying cardiovascular pathology.

During intravenous administration, there is an increase in stroke volume (and therefore cardiac output) with little change in heart rate (see Table 14–13). Despite the increase in cardiac index, mean arterial pressure generally remains constant because of the concomitant decrease in arteriolar resistance. However, the vasodilating effects may predominate in certain patients and lead to a decrease in blood pressure and a reflex tachycardia. The drugs lower PAOP by venodilation and thus are particularly useful in patients with a low cardiac index and an elevated left ventricular filling pressure. Such a reduction in preload, however, can be hazardous for patients without excessive filling pressure (especially those with symptoms of dry heart failure), leading to a decrease in cardiac index. Such an effect would blunt the improvement in cardiac output that otherwise would be produced by the positive inotropic and arterial dilating actions. These drugs should be used cautiously as single agents in severely hypotensive heart failure patients because they will not increase and may even decrease arterial blood pressure. The results of controlled studies comparing dobutamine with amrinone or milrinone indicate that these agents produce generally similar hemodynamic effects to dobutamine. A clinically insignificant but greater increase in heart rate with dobutamine is the most consistent difference in these studies.

Milrinone and amrinone have longer terminal elimination half-lives than adrenergic agonists. The average milrinone half-life in healthy subjects is about 1 hour and for amrinone is 2 to 4 hours. This roughly doubles in patients with heart failure.[124] These long elimination half-lives may be a disadvantage in this patient population because a loading dose may be necessary to obtain a prompt initial response, minute-to-minute titrations in dose cannot be made based on response, and adverse effects (arrhythmias or hypotension) will persist longer after drug discontinuation. The usual loading dose for milrinone is 50 mcg/kg administered over 10 minutes and for amrinone is 0.75 mg/kg administered over 2 to 3 minutes. However, if rapid hemodynamic changes are not necessary, the loading dose should be eliminated owing to the risk of hypotension and patients simply started on the maintenance infusion. The maintenance infusion for milrinone is 0.5 mcg/kg per minute (range 0.375 to 0.75 mcg/kg per minute) and for amrinone it is 5 to 10 mcg/kg per minute. Over 80% of a dose of milrinone is excreted unchanged in urine, and unlike amrinone, its infusion rate should be decreased by 50% to 70% in patients with significant renal impairment.

In addition to undesirable hemodynamic effects, the most notable adverse events associated with inodilators are arrhythmias, hypotension, and thrombocytopenia. Thrombocytopenia is reported to occur in 2.4% of patients who have received intravenous amrinone, with decreased platelet survival from nonimmunologic platelet damage as the postulated mechanism. This adverse effect is dose-dependent and generally completely reversible within 5 to 7 days of drug discontinuation. The incidence of thrombocytopenia associated with milrinone therapy is very low (<0.5%). Milrinone therefore is preferable to amrinone because of its better side-effect profile. Patients who receive either drug should be monitored for signs of bleeding and have platelet counts determined before and during therapy.

Well-designed studies comparing clinical outcomes of milrinone treatment with those of other inotropes are limited. A recent retrospective analysis in patients with decompensated heart failure found no differences in clinical end points between dobutamine and milrinone, although the cost of dobutamine therapy was significantly less than milrinone.[125] In a prospective, randomized trial comparing milrinone and dobutamine as a pharmacologic "bridge" to cardiac transplantation, these agents produced similar hemodynamic and clinical outcomes, but again, drug costs favored dobutamine.[126] The combination of dobutamine and a bipyridine produces additive effects on cardiac index and PAOP reduction, suggesting this regimen as an option in patients who have dose-limiting adverse effects with either class of drugs. It is unclear, however, if this combination provides a therapeutic advantage over the combination of a positive inotrope and a traditional pure vasodilator such as nitroprusside.

A recent study with milrinone points out the risk of routine administration of inotropic therapy to patients admitted to the hospital with an acute exacerbation of heart failure. Although this approach is not supported by clinical trial data, many patients without signs or symptoms of hypoperfusion receive milrinone or other inotropic therapy with the belief that the hemodynamic effects may shorten hospitalization and improve clinical outcomes. Designed to evaluate this strategy, the OPTIME CHF trial was a randomized, double-blind trial that compared the effects of milrinone and placebo in patients hospitalized with an acute exacerbation of chronic heart failure who, in the investigator's opinion, did not require inotropic therapy.[127] The 949 patients received a 48-hour infusion of milrinone 0.5 mcg/kg per minute with no loading dose or placebo. No difference between milrinone and placebo was found in the primary end point of the number of days patients were hospitalized for cardiovascular causes within 60 days of randomization. However, adverse events were more common in the milrinone group. Sustained hypotension requiring intervention (10.7% versus 3.2%; $p < .001$) and new onset of atrial fibrillation or flutter (4.6% versus 1.5%; $p = .004$) occurred more frequently in patients receiving milrinone. These results add to the growing concern about the use of inotropic drugs in patients with decompensated heart failure and strongly suggest that milrinone, and probably other inotropes, should not be used routinely for the treatment of acute heart failure exacerbations. Although the routine use of milrinone should be discouraged, clinicians should be aware that inotropic therapy may be needed in selected patients, such as those with low cardiac output states with organ hypoperfusion or with cardiogenic shock. Generally, milrinone should be considered for patients who are receiving chronic β-blocker therapy because its positive inotropic effect does not involve stimulation of β-receptors. Although it appears that β-agonists such as dobutamine still exert some beneficial effects in patients on β-blocker therapy, it is expected that higher than normal doses of these drugs would be needed to achieve the desired pharmacologic effect. Therefore, milrinone may provide a theoretical advantage in β-blocker-treated patients.

Dopamine[123]

Although dopamine generally should be avoided in the treatment of advanced heart failure, there are two clinical scenarios where its pharmacologic actions may be preferable to dobutamine or milrinone. The first is a patient with marked systemic hypotension or cardiogenic shock in the face of elevated ventricular filling pressures, where dopamine in doses greater than 5 mcg/kg per minute may be necessary to raise central aortic pressure. The second use, although somewhat controversial, is to directly attempt to improve renal function in a patient with inadequate urine output despite volume overload and high ventricular filling pressures. Low doses (1 to 3 mcg/kg per minute) traditionally have been administered for this indication. As discussed earlier, however, there are no data to support this commonly employed practice.

Dopamine, the endogenous precursor of NE, exerts its effects by directly stimulating adrenergic receptors as well as causing release of NE from adrenergic nerve terminals. Dopamine produces dose-dependent hemodynamic effects because of its relative affinity for α_1-, β_1-, β_2-, and D_1-receptors (vascular dopaminergic) (see Table 14–14). The following dose-dependent actions are intended as a general guide to the clinician.

Positive inotropic effects mediated primarily by β_1-receptors become more prominent with dopamine doses of 3 to 10 mcg/kg per minute. Cardiac index is increased because of an increase in stroke volume and a variable increase in heart rate, which is partially dose-dependent. There is usually little change in SVR, presumably because neither vasodilation (D_1- and β_2-receptor–mediated) nor vasoconstriction (α_1-receptor-mediated) predominates. Renal effects of dopamine still may be evident at these higher doses and are caused by a combination of D_1-mediated renovascular effects, increased cardiac index, and altered sodium tubular reabsorption. At doses above 10 mcg/kg per minute, chronotropic and α_1-receptor-mediated vasoconstricting effects become more prominent. Mean arterial pressure usually increases because of an increase in both cardiac index and SVR (see Table 14–13). The vasoconstricting effects of higher doses could indirectly limit the increase in cardiac index by increasing afterload and PAOP, thus complicating the management of patients with preexisting high afterload. In such patients, alternative agents (e.g., dobutamine or milrinone) or the addition of diuretics and/or vasodilators may be necessary.

Dopamine, particularly at higher doses, may alter several parameters that increase myocardial oxygen demand (increased heart rate, contractility, and systolic pressure) and potentially decrease myocardial blood flow (coronary vasoconstriction and increased wall tension), worsening ischemia in some patients with coronary artery disease. Arrhythmogenesis is also more common at higher doses.

VASODILATORS

Activation of the SNS, the RAA system, AVP, and other mediators all cause vasoconstriction and increased SVR. In patients with heart failure, stroke volume varies inversely with SVR such that an increase in peripheral resistance leads to a severe decline in stroke volume and cardiac output (see Fig. 14–1).

Vasodilators typically are described by their prominent site of action (arterial or venous). Arterial vasodilators act as impedance-reducing agents and usually cause an increase in cardiac output. Venodilators act as preload reducers by increasing venous capacitance, reducing symptoms of pulmonary congestion in patients with high cardiac filling pressures. Mixed vasodilators act on both resistance and capacitance vessels, reducing congestive symptoms while increasing cardiac output. Nitroprusside, nitroglycerin, and now nesiritide are the most widely studied and commonly used intravenous vasodilating agents in acute/severe heart failure. Other vasodilators have shown either tachyphylaxis, excessive reflex tachycardia, or refractory hypotension compromising coronary blood flow; they are rarely, if ever, used in this setting.

Nitroprusside[124]

Sodium nitroprusside, a mixed arterial-venous vasodilator, acts on vascular smooth muscle, increasing synthesis of nitric oxide to produce its balanced vasodilating action. As such, it both increases cardiac index and decreases venous pressure. Nitroprusside's effects on these parameters are qualitatively similar to those produced by dobutamine and phosphodiesterase inhibitors despite the fact that it has no direct inotropic activity (see Table 14–13). However, nitroprusside generally causes a greater decrease in PAOP, SVR, and blood pressure than these agents. Mean arterial pressure may remain fairly constant but often decreases depending on the relative increase in cardiac output and reduction in arteriolar tone. Hypotension is an important dose-limiting adverse effect of nitroprusside and other vasodilators. Therefore, this drug is used primarily in patients who have a significantly elevated SVR.

Patients with normal left ventricular function will not have an increase in stroke volume when SVR falls because the normal ventricle is fairly insensitive to small changes in afterload. Consequently, these patients experience a significant decrease in blood pressure after administration of arterial vasodilators. This explains why nitroprusside is a potent antihypertensive agent in patients without heart failure but causes less hypotension and reflex tachycardia in patients with left ventricular dysfunction. Nonetheless, even a modest increase in heart rate could have adverse consequences in patients with underlying ischemic heart disease and/or resting tachycardia, and close monitoring is necessary during therapy.

Nitroprusside has been studied extensively and shown to be effective in the short-term management of patients with severe heart failure in a variety of settings (i.e., acute MI, valvular regurgitation, after coronary bypass surgery, decompensated chronic heart failure). Generally, nitroprusside will not worsen and may improve the balance between myocardial oxygen demand and supply. This is mainly due to a decrease in oxygen demand caused by the lowering of left ventricular wall tension and a possible increase in subendocardial blood flow resulting from decreased LVEDP. However, an excessive decrease in systemic arterial pressure can reduce coronary perfusion and worsen ischemia, leading to increased risk of coronary steal.

Nitroprusside has a rapid onset of action and a duration of action of less than 10 minutes, necessitating its administration by continuous intravenous infusion. This allows for precise dose titration based on measured clinical and hemodynamic parameters. It, like other vasodilators used in heart failure, should be initiated at a low dose (0.1 to 0.2 mcg/kg per minute) to avoid excessive hypotension and then increased by small increments (0.1 to 0.2 mcg/kg per minute) every 5 to 10 minutes as needed and tolerated. Usually effective doses range from 0.5 to 3 mcg/kg per minute. A rebound phenomenon has been reported after abrupt withdrawal of nitroprusside in patients with heart failure and is apparently due to reflex neurohormonal activation during therapy. If renal perfusion pressure is compromised by the drug, salt and water retention can contribute to volume expansion and tachyphylaxis; this is seen typically only in patients with chronic hypertension, baseline azotemia, or when therapeutic augmentation of cardiac output during therapy is minimal. When stopping nitroprusside and switching to oral drugs, it is usually advisable to taper doses slowly. Nitroprusside can cause cyanide and thiocyanate toxicity, but these are very unlikely when doses of less than 3 mcg/kg per minute are administered for less than 3 days, except in patients with a serum creatinine level greater than 3 mg/dL.

Nitroglycerin

Intravenous nitroglycerin is often considered the preferred agent for preload reduction in patients with severe heart failure. Because of its short half-life, intravenous nitroglycerin is administered by continuous infusion. Its major hemodynamic actions are reductions in preload and PAOP via functional venodilation and mild arterial vasodilation that is particularly evident in patients with heart failure and elevated SVR or when given in doses approaching 200 mcg/min (see Table 14–13). Intravenous nitroglycerin is used primarily as a preload reducer for patients with pulmonary congestion and low-normal cardiac output or in combination with inotropic agents for patients with severely depressed systolic function and pulmonary edema. Combination therapy with nitroglycerin and dobutamine or dopamine produces complementary effects to increase cardiac index and decrease PAOP. In higher doses, nitroglycerin displays potent coronary vasodilating properties and beneficial effects on myocardial oxygen demand and supply, making it the vasodilator of choice for patients with severe heart failure and ischemic heart disease.

Nitroglycerin should be initiated at a dose of 5 to 10 mcg/min (0.1 mcg/kg per minute) and increased every 5 to 10 minutes as necessary and tolerated. Hypotension and an excessive decrease in PAOP are important dose-limiting side effects. Maintenance doses usually vary from 35 to 200 mcg/min (0.5 to 3 mcg/kg per minute), although doses over 1000 mcg/min (15 mcg/kg per minute) have been used in rare cases. Tolerance to the hemodynamic effects of nitroglycerin may develop over 12 to 72 hours of continuous administration, but some patients have a sustained response. Neither nitroglycerin nor nitroprusside should be used in the presence of elevated intracranial pressure because either may worsen cerebral edema in this setting.

Nesiritide[22,128]

Nesiritide is the first new drug approved for the treatment of decompensated heart failure since milrinone. Manufactured by recombinant techniques, it is identical to the endogenous human BNP secreted by the ventricular myocardium in response to volume overload. Exogenous administration of nesiritide mimics the vasodilatory and natriuretic actions of the endogenous peptide by stimulating natriuretic peptide receptor A, which leads to increased levels of cGMP in target tissues. In small clinical trials, nesiritide produces venous and arterial vasodilation, increases natriuresis and diuresis, and decreases cardiac filling pressures, blood pressure, and SNS and RAA system activity. Unlike nitroglycerin or dobutamine, tolerance does not develop to nesiritide's pharmacologic actions. It does not affect cAMP or stimulate β-receptors, mechanisms that are thought to contribute to the myocardial toxicity associated with the positive inotropic drugs. Thus, as shown in a recent comparative trial, nesiritide does not have the proarrhythmic effects associated with dobutamine.[129] Nesiritide is eliminated by several pathways, including the natriuretic peptide receptor C on target tissues, proteolytic cleavage by neutral endopeptidase, and renal filtration. Its elimination half-life of 18 minutes is considerably longer than that of other vasodilators or β-agonists.

The VMAC trial was a randomized, double blind trial that compared the effects of nesiritide, intravenous nitroglycerin, or placebo in patients with decompensated heart failure and dyspnea receiving standard background therapy.[130] Patients received pulmonary artery catheterization at the discretion of the investigators. The primary end points were the patient's self-assessment of dyspnea (all patients) and the change in PAOP at 3 hours after the start of the study drug infusion (only in patients with a pulmonary artery catheter). Although nesiritide reduced dyspnea at 3 hours compared with placebo, no difference between nesiritide and nitroglycerin was found. In patients with a pulmonary artery catheter, nesiritide reduced PAOP by a mean of 5.8 mm Hg, which was significantly greater than the reduction with nitroglycerin (3.8 mm Hg) or placebo (2 mm Hg). This small but statistically significant difference between nesiritide and nitroglycerin was maintained for 24 hours, although this did not result in differences in dyspnea. The most frequently reported adverse effect was headache, which occurred more often with nitroglycerin (20%) than with nesiritide (8%). A similar frequency of asymptomatic and symptomatic hypotension was reported with nesiritide and nitroglycerin. However, because the elimination half-life of nesiritide is longer than that of nitroglycerin (18 versus 2–3 minutes), the duration of hypotensive episodes with nesiritide was significantly longer than those with nitroglycerin (2.2 versus 0.7 hours). Although not the primary end point of the trial, 30-day follow-up of the patients found no differences between the nesiritide and nitroglycerin groups in hospital readmissions, death, or other serious adverse events.

The precise role of nesiritide in the pharmacotherapy of decompensated heart failure remains controversial. Much of this controversy centers on the marginal hemodynamic benefits and the lack of improvement in mortality or other clinical outcomes with nesiritide compared with nitroglycerin (or nitroprusside) balanced against nesiritide's significantly greater costs (~$450 for a 24-h nesiritide infusion compared with $10 to $15 for nitroglycerin). Nesiritide does offer several potential therapeutic advantages, including beneficial neurohormonal effects, use without invasive hemodynamic monitoring, administration in outpatient settings (e.g., emergency departments) with the goal of preventing hospital admission, and low proarrhythmic potential compared with inotropes. Disadvantages of nesiritide include the risk of sustained hypotension, the cost, and the lack of improvement in important clinical outcomes. Given these questions on the role of nesiritide, the use of this medication varies considerably among institutions, with many developing specific criteria for its use. Nesiritide may be most useful in the treatment of patients with volume overload (i.e., warm and wet) and systolic blood pressure greater than 90 mm Hg who fail to respond adequately to intravenous diuretics and/or vasodilators such as nitroglycerin.

MECHANICAL CIRCULATORY SUPPORT[131]

INTRAAORTIC BALLOON PUMP

The intraaortic balloon pump (IABP) is a frequently used form of mechanical circulatory assistance and typically is employed in patients with advanced heart failure who do not respond adequately to drug therapy, those with intractable myocardial ischemia, or patients in cardiogenic shock. The IABP consists of a polyethylene balloon mounted on a catheter that is usually inserted percutaneously into the femoral artery, and the balloon is then advanced into the descending thoracic aorta. During counterpulsation, the balloon is synchronized with the ECG so that it inflates during diastole and displaces aortic blood, thus increasing aortic diastolic pressure and coronary perfusion. The balloon deflates just prior to opening of the aortic valve during systole and causes a sudden decrease in aortic pressure, allowing the left ventricle to pump against reduced arterial impedance. IABP support results in increased cardiac index, coronary artery perfusion, and myocardial oxygen supply, accompanied by decreased myocardial oxygen demand. Thus it is particularly useful for short-term use in patients with decompensated heart failure in the setting of myocardial ischemia (evolving infarction, patients awaiting emergency coronary bypass surgery). It is also used in hemodynamically unstable patients to stabilize them prior to insertion of a left ventricular assist device that will serve as a bridge to cardiac transplantation when inotropic drugs are no longer effective. Intravenous vasodilators and inotropic agents generally are used in conjunction with the IABP to maximize hemodynamic and clinical benefits.

VENTRICULAR ASSIST DEVICES

A number of different ventricular assist devices (VADs) are available or under investigation. These pumps are surgically implanted and assist, or in some cases replace, the pumping functions of the right and/or left ventricles. VADs are currently used to provide short-term hemodynamic support in patients experiencing an acute event (e.g., acute MI accompanied by cardiogenic shock or patients who cannot be weaned from cardiopulmonary bypass after cardiac surgery) in which ventricular recovery is anticipated. There is also strong interest in longer-term use of these devices in patients whose ventricular function is unlikely to recover. Here, VADs are being used as a bridge to cardiac transplantation and for palliative therapy (so-called destination therapy) in lieu of continuous inotropic therapy in patients who are not transplant candidates. Also, several models of total artificial hearts are currently under investigation for use as a bridge to transplant or for destination therapy.

SURGICAL THERAPY

Orthotopic cardiac transplantation remains the best therapeutic option for patients with chronic, irreversible NYHA class IV heart failure, with a 5-year survival of approximately 60% to 70% in well-selected patients. Unfortunately, the shortage of acceptable donor hearts has resulted in an average waiting time for transplant of more than 6 months, with only about one in five approved potential recipients receiving a heart before succumbing to their disease. Another large percentage of patients is rejected from consideration for transplant because of age, concurrent illnesses, psychosocial factors, and other reasons. See Chap. 87 for additional details on cardiac transplantation. The shortage of donor hearts has prompted development of new surgical techniques, including ventricular aneurysm resection, mitral valve repair, and myocardial cell transplantation, which have resulted in variable degrees of symptomatic improvement. Further development of these and other techniques may offer additional options in patients who are not transplant candidates.

PHARMACOECONOMIC CONSIDERATIONS

Heart failure imposes a tremendous economic burden on the health care system. In patients over age 65, it is the most common reason for hospitalization, with hospital admission rates for this disorder continuing to increase. Heart failure is also associated with 30% to 50% readmission rates during the 3 to 6 months after initial discharge. Current estimates of costs of heart failure treatment in the United States exceed $40 billion, with most of the costs associated with hospitalization.[1,3] The prevalence of heart failure and the costs associated with patient care are expected to increase as the population ages and as survival from ischemic heart disease is improved. Thus approaches to improve the quality and cost-effectiveness of care for these patients may have a significant impact on health care costs.

Studies to assess the cost-effectiveness of drug therapy for heart failure have been reviewed recently.[132] Carvedilol reduced the number of heart failure–related hospital admissions compared with placebo, resulting in a significant savings in hospital costs. The cost per life-year saved with carvedilol was $12,799, which is similar to that of other medical therapies.[132] β-Blockers reduced Medicare costs by approximately $6000 per patient, primarily owing to a reduction in the rates of hospitalization, and resulted in reduced hospital and physician revenue.[133] In the DIG trial, patients treated with digoxin had fewer hospitalizations for heart failure, but digoxin produced an absolute decrease of only 2.8% in hospitalizations for any cause.[74] Although no prospective economic analyses have been performed, studies using decision-analysis techniques indicate that ACE inhibitors are cost-effective.[132] While not providing direct cost estimates, number needed to treat (NNT) is often a useful index that provides a sense of the cost-effectiveness of a given therapy. In the case of the ACE inhibitors and β-blockers, the NNT to prevent one death has ranged from 7 to 20 patients for the ACE inhibitor studies (including most of the post-MI studies) and from 14 to 26 patients for the β-blocker studies. These numbers compare favorably with and in fact are superior to most other cardiovascular therapies. In the case of both drug classes, the benefits are greater (NNT lower) for the patients with more severe heart failure.

As the management of heart failure has become increasingly complex, the development of disease-management program approaches that use multidisciplinary teams has attracted significant interest.[132,134] These programs use several broad approaches, including heart failure specialty clinics and/or home-based interventions. Most are multidisciplinary and may include physicians, advanced practice nurses, dieticians, and pharmacists. In general, the programs focus on optimization of drug and nondrug therapy, patient and family education and counseling, exercise and dietary advice, intense follow-up by telephone or home visits, and monitoring and management of signs and symptoms of decompensation. Collectively, studies evaluating this disease-management approach have reported fewer hospitalizations, improved functional capacity and symptoms, reduced health care costs, and improved patient satisfaction and quality of life compared with usual care.[132,134] The improvement in outcome in these studies may be related to better adherence to heart failure treatment guidelines by cardiologists compared with other physicians.[135]

Pharmacists can play an important role in the multidisciplinary team management of heart failure.[136,137] Compared with conventional treatment, pharmacist intervention that included medication evaluation and therapeutic recommendations, patient education, and follow-up telephone monitoring reduced hospitalizations for heart failure. Adherence to guideline-recommended therapy was improved by pharmacist intervention. Thus the role and cost benefits of pharmacist involvement in the multidisciplinary care of heart failure

patients are now apparent and should include optimizing doses of heart failure drug therapy, screening for drugs that exacerbate heart failure, monitoring for adverse drug effects and drug interactions, educating patients, and patient follow-up.

CLINICAL CONTROVERSIES

There is now reasonable evidence that immediate-release metoprolol tartrate is inferior to carvedilol, but controversy remains about the equivalency of metoprolol succinate CR/XL (Toprol-XL) and carvedilol. Some practitioners believe that the evidence suggests that carvedilol is superior, whereas others believe that any of the drugs (bisoprolol, carvedilol, or metoprolol CR/XL) are appropriate for management of chronic heart failure.

Some clinicians advocate the use of aldosterone antagonists in essentially all patients with symptomatic heart failure or post-MI left ventricular dysfunction. Others believe that they should be reserved for those who remain symptomatic with NYHA class IIIb or IV heart failure.

The role of nesiritide in patients with acute decompensated heart failure remains controversial. The debate focuses primarily on the efficacy and increased cost of nesiritide compared with other vasodilators (i.e., nitroglycerin). Although a more rapid improvement in hemodynamics was observed with nesiritide therapy compared with nitroglycerin, this advantage was not apparent after 24 hours of treatment. Because of the marginal efficacy advantage over nitroglycerin, coupled with the substantially higher cost of nesiritide, many institutions restrict the use of nesiritide to patients failing to respond to nitroglycerin or other vasodilators. Others advocate nesiritide as the treatment of choice in this patient population.

EVALUATION OF THERAPEUTIC OUTCOMES

CHRONIC HEART FAILURE

Although mortality is an important end point, it does not give a complete measure of the overall effects of the disease on patient outcomes because many patients are hospitalized repeatedly for heart failure exacerbations and continue to survive. Thus some of the more important therapeutic outcomes in heart failure management, such as prolonged survival or prevention or slowing of the progression of heart failure, cannot be quantified in an individual patient. However, after appropriate diagnostic evaluation to determine the etiology of heart failure, ongoing clinical assessment of patients typically focuses on three general areas: (1) evaluation of functional capacity, (2) evaluation of volume status, and (3) laboratory evaluation.

The evaluation of functional capacity should focus on the presence and severity of symptoms the patient experiences during activities of daily living and how those symptoms affect these activities. Questions directed toward the patient's ability to perform specific activities may be more informative than general questions about what symptoms the patient may be experiencing. For example, ask patients if they can participate in exercise, climb stairs, get dressed without stopping, check the mail, or clean the house. Another important component of assessment of functional capacity is to ask patients what activities they would like to do but are now unable to perform.

Assessment of volume status is a vital component of the ongoing care of patients with heart failure. This evaluation provides the clinician with important information about the adequacy of diuretic therapy. Since the cardinal signs and symptoms of heart failure are caused by excess fluid retention, the efficacy of diuretic treatment is readily evaluated by the disappearance of these signs and symptoms. The physical examination is the primary method for the evaluation of fluid retention, and specific attention should be focused on the patient's body weight, extent of jugular venous distension, presence of hepatojugular reflux, presence and severity of pulmonary congestion, and peripheral edema. Specifically, in a patient with pulmonary congestion, monitoring is indicated for resolution of rales and pulmonary edema and improvement or resolution of dyspnea on exertion (DOE), orthopnea, and PND. For patients with systemic congestion, a decrease or disappearance of peripheral edema, JVD, and hepatojugular reflux is sought. Other therapeutic outcomes include an improvement in exercise tolerance and fatigue, decreased nocturia, and a decrease in heart rate. Clinicians also will want to monitor blood pressure and ensure that the patient does not develop symptomatic hypotension as a result of drug therapy. Body weight is a sensitive marker of fluid loss or retention, and patients should be counseled to weigh themselves daily, reporting changes to their health care provider so that adjustments can be made in diuretic doses. It should be noted that, particularly with β-blocker therapy, symptoms may worsen initially and that it may take weeks to months of treatment before patients notice improvement in symptoms. Also, patients and health care providers should be aware that heart failure progression may be slowed even though symptoms have not resolved.

Routine monitoring of serum electrolytes and renal function is required in patients with heart failure. Assessment of serum potassium is especially important because hypokalemia is a common adverse effect of diuretic therapy and is associated with an increased risk of arrhythmias and digoxin toxicity. Serum potassium monitoring is also required because of the risk of hyperkalemia associated with ACE inhibitors, ARBs, and aldosterone antagonists. A serum potassium concentration of 4 mEq/L or greater should be maintained, with some evidence suggesting that it should be 4.5 mEq/L or greater.[138] Assessment of renal function (BUN and serum creatinine) is also an important end point for monitoring diuretic and ACE inhibitor therapy. Common causes of worsening renal function in patients with heart failure include overdiuresis, adverse effects of ACE inhibitor or ARB therapy, and hypoperfusion.

ADVANCED/DECOMPENSATED HEART FAILURE

Assessment of adequacy of therapy in the advanced heart failure patient can be separated into two general categories: initial improvement of physiologic parameters and safe discharge from the ICU following conversion to a chronic oral therapeutic regimen. Both goals must be achieved because hemodynamic improvement has not correlated with prolonged symptom improvement or enhanced survival.

Initial stabilization requires achievement of adequate arterial oxygen saturation and content. Cardiac index and blood pressure must be sufficient to ensure adequate organ perfusion, as assessed by alert mental status, creatinine clearance sufficient to prevent metabolic azotemic complications, hepatic function adequate to maintain synthetic and excretory functions, a stable heart rate (generally between 50 and 110 beats per minute) and rhythm (predominately sinus rhythm, rate-stabilized atrial fibrillation or flutter, or paced rhythm), absence of ongoing myocardial ischemia or infarction, skeletal muscle and skin blood flow sufficient to prevent ischemic injury, and normal arterial pH (7.34 to 7.47) with a normal serum lactate concentration. Although these goals are achieved most often with a cardiac index greater than 2.2 L/m^2 per minute, a mean arterial blood pressure greater than 60 mm Hg, and a PAOP of 25 mm Hg or greater, the absolute values are highly variable and depend on chronicity of ill-

ness, efficacy of chronic compensatory mechanisms, previous chronic therapy, and concurrent illness.

Discharge from the ICU requires maintenance of the preceding parameters in the absence of ongoing intravenous infusion therapy, mechanical circulatory support, or positive-pressure ventilation. Some patients may achieve this goal with markedly lower blood pressure or higher filling pressure than suggested earlier; hence numerical goals cannot always be substituted for clinical status. Nonpharmacologic treatments aimed at the precipitants of a patient's heart failure exacerbation include permanent pacing, CRT with or without ICD, coronary angioplasty or valvuloplasty, pericardial drainage, cardiac surgery (coronary bypass, valve replacement or reconstruction, closure of intracardiac shunts), or even cardiac transplantation to achieve initial stabilization, definitive therapy, or both.

Note Added in Proof. The European Society of Cardiology released new treatment guidelines in February 2005 for the diagnosis and treatment of acute heart failure. (Nieminen MS, Bohm M, Cowie MR, et al. Executive summary of the guidelines on the diagnosis and treatment of acute heart failure. The Task Force on Acute Heart Failure of the European Society of Cardiology. Eur Heart J 2005;26: 384–416.)

ADDENDUM

Since the final preparation of this chapter, the results from two recently published clinical trials provide important information for clinicians involved in the pharmacotherapy of heart failure. The first trial examined prescribing rates for spironolactone and hospital admission rates for hyperkalemia in approximately 1.3 million elderly patients in the Ontario Drug Benefit Program before and after publication of the RALES trial.[139] Immediately after publication of RALES, the spironolactone prescription rate increased nearly fivefold. Similarly, the rates of hospitalization for hyperkalemia and hyperkalemia-associated deaths increased by threefold. These results indicate that the use of spironolactone was widely embraced and that important clinical trial results can be rapidly translated into clinical practice. However, these findings also confirm earlier case reports that spironolactone-induced hyperkalemia occurs more frequently in clinical practice than in clinical trials. Risk factors for hyperkalemia with aldosterone antagonists include the elderly, renal insufficiency, diabetes, concomitant use of ACE inhibitors, potassium supplements, NSAIDs, or β-blockers, high doses of aldosterone antagonists, and inadequate laboratory monitoring. Appropriate patient selection and monitoring are keys to minimizing the risk of hyperkalemia with the aldosterone antagonists.

Post-hoc analyses of several clinical trials collectively suggested African-Americans with heart failure responded better to the combination of isosorbide dinitrate plus hydralazine than to ACE inhibitors. These findings served as the basis for the African-American Heart Failure Trial (A-HeFT) that compared the effects of isosorbide dinitrate combined with hydralazine, when added to standard background heart failure pharmacotherapy (ACE inhibitors or ARBs, β-blockers, diuretics, and digoxin), to placebo in patients self-identified as African-Americans.[140] The investigational study medication was a fixed-dose combination of isosorbide and hydralazine (BiDil) containing 20 mg of isosorbide and 37.5 mg of hydralazine in one tablet that was administered three times daily. The dose could be increased to two tablets three times daily if no drug-related adverse effects were present. The trial was terminated early due to a 40% reduction in all-cause mortality in patients receiving isosorbide and hydralazine compared to placebo. Hospitalizations for heart failure were reduced and quality of life was improved by the combination product. However, patients receiving isosorbide plus hydralazine were more likely to experience headaches or dizziness compared to those receiving placebo. The mechanism(s) for these beneficial effects remains uncertain but are likely linked to nitric oxide donation from isosorbide and a hydralazine-mediated reduction in oxidative stress leading to an overall increase in nitric oxide availability. These results suggest, but do not confirm, that nitric oxide may play a protective role in attenuating myocardial hypertrophy and remodeling. Whether the benefits of isosorbide and hydralazine are specific for African-Americans or if other racial or ethnic groups may also benefit remains to be determined. Although not incorporated into current heart failure treatment guidelines, these results suggest that the addition of isosorbide dinitrate and hydralazine to standard therapy should be strongly considered in African-Americans with heart failure.

ABBREVIATIONS

ACC: American College of Cardiology
ACE: angiotensin-converting enzyme
AHA: American Heart Association
ANP: atrial natriuretic peptide
ARB: angiotensin receptor blocker
AVP: arginine vasopressin
BNP: B-type natriuretic peptide
cAMP: cyclic adenosine monophosphate
CNP: C-type natriuretic peptide
CO: cardiac output
COPD: chronic obstructive pulmonary disease
COX-2: cyclooxygenase-2
EF: ejection fraction
ET: endothelin
HTN: hypertension
IABP: intraaortic balloon pump
ICD: implantable cardioverter-defibrillator
ICU: intensive care unit
JVD: jugular venous distension
LVEDV: left ventricular end-diastolic volume
LVEDP: left ventricular end-diastolic pressure
LVEF: left ventricular ejection fraction
LVF: left ventricular failure
MI: myocardial infarction
NE: norepinephrine
NSAID: nonsteroidal anti-inflammatory drug
NYHA: New York Heart Association
PA: pulmonary artery
PAOP: pulmonary artery occlusion pressure
P-gp: P-glycoprotein
RAA: renin-angiotensin-aldosterone
RVF: right ventricular failure
SDC: serum digoxin concentration
SVR: systemic vascular resistance
TNF-α: tumor necrosis factor-α
TZD: thiazolidinedione
VAD: ventricular assist device

Review Questions and other resources can be found at *www.pharmacotherapyonline.com.*

REFERENCES

1. Hunt SA, Baker DW, Chin MH, et al. ACC/AHA Guidelines for the evaluation and management of chronic heart failure in the adult: Executive summary. A report of the American College of Cardiology/American Heart Association Task Force on Practice Guidelines (Committee to Revise the 1995 Guidelines for the Evaluation and Management of Heart Failure): Developed in collaboration with the International Society for Heart and Lung Transplantation; endorsed by the Heart Failure Society of America. Circulation 2001;104:2996–3007.
2. Jessup M, Brozena S. Heart failure. N Engl J Med 2003;348:2007–2018.
3. American Heart Association. 2004 Heart and Stroke Statistical Update. Dallas, AHA, 2003.
4. Levy D, Kenchaiah S, Larson MG, et al. Long-term trends in the incidence of and survival with heart failure. N Engl J Med 2002;347:1397–1402.
5. Klein L, O'Connor CM, Gattis WA, et al. Pharmacologic therapy for patients with chronic heart failure and reduced systolic function: Review of trials and practical considerations. Am J Cardiol 2003;91:18F–40F.
6. Colucci W, Braunwald E. Pathophysiology of heart failure. In: Braunwald E, Zipes DP, Libby P, eds. Heart Disease: A Textbook of Cardiovascular Medicine, 6th ed. Philadelphia, Saunders, 2001:503–533.
7. Gheorghiade M, Bonow RO. Chronic heart failure in the United States: A manifestation of coronary artery disease. Circulation 1998;97:282–289.
8. Wynne J, Braunwald E. The cardiomyopathies and myocarditides. In: Braunwald E, Zipes DP, Libby P, eds. Heart Disease: A Textbook of Cardiovascular Medicine, 6th ed. Philadelphia, Saunders, 2001:1751–1806.
9. He J, Ogden LG, Bazzano LA, et al. Dietary sodium intake and incidence of congestive heart failure in overweight US men and women: First National Health and Nutrition Examination Survey Epidemiologic Follow-up Study. Arch Intern Med 2002;162:1619–1624.
10. Kenchaiah S, Evans JC, Levy D, et al. Obesity and the risk of heart failure. N Engl J Med 2002;347:305–313.
11. Mann DL. Mechanisms and models in heart failure: A combinatorial approach. Circulation 1999;100:999–1008.
12. Felker GM, O'Connor CM. Inotropic therapy for heart failure: An evidence-based approach. Am Heart J 2001;142:393–401.
13. Brown NJ, Vaughan DE. Angiotensin-converting enzyme inhibitors. Circulation 1998;97:1411–1420.
14. Patterson JH. Angiotensin II receptor blockers in heart failure. Pharmacotherapy 2003;23:173–182.
15. Colucci WS. The effects of norepinephrine on myocardial biology: Implications for the therapy of heart failure. Clin Cardiol 1998;21:I20–24.
16. Colucci WS, Sawyer DB, Singh K, Communal C. Adrenergic overload and apoptosis in heart failure: Implications for therapy. J Card Fail 2000;6:1–7.
17. Small KM, Wagoner LE, Levin AM, et al. Synergistic polymorphisms of β_1- and α_{2C}-adrenergic receptors and the risk of congestive heart failure. N Engl J Med 2002;347:1135–1142.
18. Weber KT. Aldosterone in congestive heart failure. N Engl J Med 2001;345:1689–1697.
19. Lijnen P, Petrov V. Induction of cardiac fibrosis by aldosterone. J Mol Cell Cardiol 2000;32:865–879.
20. Pitt B, Zannad F, Remme WJ, et al. The effect of spironolactone on morbidity and mortality in patients with severe heart failure: Randomized Aldactone Evaluation Study Investigators. N Engl J Med 1999;341:709–717.
21. Pitt B, Remme W, Zannad F, et al. Eplerenone, a selective aldosterone blocker, in patients with left ventricular dysfunction after myocardial infarction. N Engl J Med 2003;348:1309–1321.
22. Adams KF Jr, Mathur VS, Gheorghiade M. B-type natriuretic peptide: from bench to bedside. Am Heart J 2003;145:S34–46.
23. de Lemos JA, McGuire DK, Drazner MH. B-type natriuretic peptide in cardiovascular disease. Lancet 2003;362:316–322.
24. Troughton RW, Frampton CM, Yandle TG, et al. Treatment of heart failure guided by plasma aminoterminal brain natriuretic peptide (N-BNP) concentrations. Lancet 2000;355:1126–1130.
25. Lee CR, Watkins ML, Patterson JH, et al. Vasopressin: A new target for the treatment of heart failure. Am Heart J 2003;146:9–18.

26. Gheorghiade M, Niazi I, Ouyang J, et al. Vasopressin V_2-receptor block-ade with tolvaptan in patients with chronic heart failure: Results from a double-blind, randomized trial. Circulation 2003;107:2690–2696.

27. Mann DL. Inflammatory mediators and the failing heart: Past, present, and the foreseeable future. Circ Res 2002;91:988–998.

28. Spieker LE, Luscher TF. Will endothelin receptor antagonists have a role in heart failure? Med Clin North Am 2003;87:459–474.

29. Tsuyuki RT, McKelvie RS, Arnold JM, et al. Acute precipitants of congestive heart failure exacerbations. Arch Intern Med 2001;161:2337–2342.

30. Michalsen A, Konig G, Thimme W. Preventable causative factors leading to hospital admission with decompensated heart failure. Heart 1998;80:437–441.

31. Wang TJ, Larson MG, Levy D, et al. Temporal relations of atrial fibrillation and congestive heart failure and their joint influence on mortality: The Framingham Heart Study. Circulation 2003;107:2920–2925.

32. Horwich TB, Fonarow GC, Hamilton MA, et al. Anemia is associated with worse symptoms, greater impairment in functional capacity and a significant increase in mortality in patients with advanced heart failure. J Am Coll Cardiol 2002;39:1780–1786.

33. Bleumink GS, Feenstra J, Sturkenboom MC, Stricker BH. Nonsteroidal anti-inflammatory drugs and heart failure. Drugs 2003;63:525–534.

34. Givertz M, Colucci W, Braunwald E. Clinical aspects of heart failure: High-output failure; pulmonary edema. In: Braunwald E, Zipes DP, Libby P, eds. Heart Disease: A Textbook of Cardiovascular Medicine, 6th ed. Philadelphia, Saunders, 2001:534–561.

35. Chobanian AV, Bakris GL, Black HR, et al. The Seventh Report of the Joint National Committee on Prevention, Detection, Evaluation, and Treatment of High Blood Pressure: The JNC 7 report. JAMA 2003;289:2560–2572.

36. Arnold JM, Yusuf S, Young J, et al. Prevention of Heart Failure in Patients in the Heart Outcomes Prevention Evaluation (HOPE) study. Circulation 2003;107:1284–1290.

37. Yusuf S, Sleight P, Pogue J, et al. Effects of an angiotensin-converting-enzyme inhibitor, ramipril, on cardiovascular events in high-risk patients. The Heart Outcomes Prevention Evaluation Study Investigators. N Engl J Med 2000;342:145–153.

38. Abraham WT, Hayes DL. Cardiac resynchronization therapy for heart failure. Circulation 2003;108:2596–2603.

39. Bristow MR, Saxon LA, Boehmer J, et al. Cardiac-resynchronization therapy with or without an implantable defibrillator in advanced chronic heart failure. N Engl J Med. 2004;350:2140–2150.

40. Echt DS, Liebson PR, Mitchell LB, et al. Mortality and morbidity in patients receiving encainide, flecainide, or placebo. The Cardiac Arrhythmia Suppression Trial. N Engl J Med 1991;324:781–788.

41. DiMarco JP. Implantable cardioverter-defibrillators. N Engl J Med 2003;349:1836–1847.

42. Ooi H, Colucci W. Pharmacological treatment of heart failure. In: Hardman JG, Limbird LE, eds. Goodman and Gilman's The Pharmacological Basis of Therapeutics. New York, McGraw Hill, 2001:901–932.

43. Jorde UP, Ennezat PV, Lisker J, et al. Maximally recommended doses of angiotensin-converting enzyme (ACE) inhibitors do not completely prevent ACE-mediated formation of angiotensin II in chronic heart failure. Circulation 2000;101:844–846.

44. Jorde UP, Vittorio T, Katz SD, et al. Elevated plasma aldosterone levels despite complete inhibition of the vascular angiotensin-converting enzyme in chronic heart failure. Circulation 2002;106:1055–1057.

45. Bristow M, Port J, Kelly R. Treatment of heart failure: Pharmacological methods. In: Braunwald E, Zipes DP, Libby P, eds. Heart Disease: A Textbook of Cardiovascular Medicine, 6th ed. Philadelphia, Saunders, 2001:562–599.

46. Flather MD, Yusuf S, Kober L, et al. Long-term ACE-inhibitor therapy in patients with heart failure or left-ventricular dysfunction: A systematic overview of data from individual patients. ACE-Inhibitor Myocardial Infarction Collaborative Group. Lancet 2000;355:1575–1581.

47. Jong P, Yusuf S, Rousseau MF, et al. Effect of enalapril on 12-year survival and life expectancy in patients with left ventricular systolic dysfunction: A follow-up study. Lancet 2003;361:1843–1848.

48. Cohn JN, Johnson G, Ziesche S, et al. A comparison of enalapril with hydralazine-isosorbide dinitrate in the treatment of chronic congestive heart failure. N Engl J Med. 1991;325:303–310.

49. ACE Inhibitor Myocardial Infarction Collaborative Group. Indications for ACE inhibitors in the early treatment of acute myocardial infarction: Systematic overview of individual data from 100,000 patients in randomized trials. Circulation 1998;97:2202–2212.

50. The SOLVD Investigators. Effect of enalapril on mortality and the development of heart failure in asymptomatic patients with reduced left ventricular ejection fractions. N Engl J Med 1992;327:685–691.

51. Dries DL, Strong MH, Cooper RS, Drazner MH. Efficacy of angiotensin-converting enzyme inhibition in reducing progression from asymptomatic left ventricular dysfunction to symptomatic heart failure in black and white patients. J Am Coll Cardiol 2002;40:311–317.

52. Vermes E, Ducharme A, Bourassa MG, et al. Enalapril reduces the incidence of diabetes in patients with chronic heart failure: Insight from the Studies Of Left Ventricular Dysfunction (SOLVD). Circulation 2003;107:1291–1296.

53. Echemann M, Zannad F, Briancon S, et al. Determinants of angiotensin-converting enzyme inhibitor prescription in severe heart failure with left ventricular systolic dysfunction: The EPICAL study. Am Heart J 2000;139:624–631.

54. Roe CM, Motheral BR, Teitelbaum F, Rich MW. Angiotensin-converting enzyme inhibitor compliance and dosing among patients with heart failure. Am Heart J 1999;138:818–825.

55. Stafford RS, Radley DC. The underutilization of cardiac medications of proven benefit, 1990 to 2002. J Am Coll Cardiol 2003;41:56–61.

56. Shlipak MG. Pharmacotherapy for heart failure in patients with renal insufficiency. Ann Intern Med 2003;138:917–924.

57. Schoolwerth AC, Sica DA, Ballermann BJ, Wilcox CS. Renal considerations in angiotensin converting enzyme inhibitor therapy: A statement for healthcare professionals from the Council on the Kidney in Cardiovascular Disease and the Council for High Blood Pressure Research of the American Heart Association. Circulation 2001;104:1985–1991.

58. Frances CD, Noguchi H, Massie BM, et al. Are we inhibited? Renal insufficiency should not preclude the use of ACE inhibitors for patients with myocardial infarction and depressed left ventricular function. Arch Intern Med 2000;160:2645–2650.

59. Packer M, Poole-Wilson PA, Armstrong PW, et al. Comparative effects of low and high doses of the angiotensin-converting enzyme inhibitor, lisinopril, on morbidity and mortality in chronic heart failure. ATLAS Study Group. Circulation 1999;100:2312–2318.

60. The Cardiac Insufficiency Bisoprolol Study II (CIBIS-II): A randomised trial. Lancet 1999;353:9–13.

61. Effect of metoprolol CR/XL in chronic heart failure: Metoprolol CR/XL Randomised Intervention Trial in Congestive Heart Failure (MERIT-HF) (see comments). Lancet 1999;353:2001–2007.

62. Packer M, Coats AJ, Fowler MB, et al. Effect of carvedilol on survival in severe chronic heart failure. N Engl J Med 2001;344:1651–1658.

63. Packer M, Fowler MB, Roecker EB, et al. Effect of carvedilol on the morbidity of patients with severe chronic heart failure: Results of the carvedilol prospective, randomized, cumulative survival (COPERNICUS) study. Circulation 2002;106:2194–2199.

64. Hjalmarson A, Goldstein S, Fagerberg B, et al. Effects of controlled-release metoprolol on total mortality, hospitalizations, and well-being in patients with heart failure: The Metoprolol CR/XL Randomized Intervention Trial in congestive heart failure (MERIT-HF). MERIT-HF Study Group. JAMA 2000;283:1295–1302.

65. Kukin ML, Kalman J, Charney RH, et al. Prospective, randomized comparison of effect of long-term treatment with metoprolol or carvedilol on symptoms, exercise, ejection fraction, and oxidative stress in heart failure. Circulation 1999;99:2645–2651.

66. Metra M, Nodari S, Parrinello G, et al. Marked improvement in left ventricular ejection fraction during long-term β-blockade in patients with

chronic heart failure: Clinical correlates and prognostic significance. Am Heart J 2003;145:292–299.

67. Bristow MR. Mechanistic and clinical rationales for using beta-blockers in heart failure. J Card Fail 2000;6:8–14.

68. Gattis WA, O'Connor CM, Gallup DS, et al. Predischarge initiation of carvedilol in patients hospitalized for decompensated heart failure: Results of the Initiation Management Predischarge: Process for Assessment of Carvedilol Therapy in Heart Failure (IMPACT-HF) trial. J Am Coll Cardiol 2004;43:1534–1541.

69. Wikstrand J, Hjalmarson A, Waagstein F, et al. Dose of metoprolol CR/XL and clinical outcomes in patients with heart failure: Analysis of the experience in metoprolol CR/XL randomized intervention trial in chronic heart failure (MERIT-HF). J Am Coll Cardiol 2002;40:491–498.

70. Bristow MR, Gilbert EM, Abraham WT, et al. Carvedilol produces dose-related improvements in left ventricular function and survival in subjects with chronic heart failure. MOCHA Investigators. Circulation 1996;94:2807–2816.

71. Shankar SS, Brater DC. Loop diuretics: From the Na-K-2Cl transporter to clinical use. Am J Physiol Renal Physiol 2003;284:F11–21.

72. Kramer BK, Schweda F, Riegger GA. Diuretic treatment and diuretic resistance in heart failure. Am J Med 1999;106:90–96.

73. Brater DC. Pharmacology of diuretics. Am J Med Sci 2000;319:38–50.

74. The Digitalis Investigation Group. The effect of digoxin on mortality and morbidity in patients with heart failure. N Engl J Med 1997;336:525–533.

75. Hauptman P, Kelly R. Digitalis. Circulation 1999;99:1265–1270.

76. Eichhorn EJ, Gheorghiade M. Digoxin. Prog Cardiovasc Dis 2002;44:251–266.

77. Gheorghiade M, Hall VB, Jacobsen G, et al. Effects of increasing maintenance doses of digoxin on left ventricular function and neurohormones in patients with chronic heart failure treated with diuretics and angiotensin-converting enzyme inhibitors. Circulation 1995;92:1801–1807.

78. Slatton ML, Irani WN, Hall SA, et al. Does digoxin provide additional hemodynamic and autonomic benefits in patients with mild to moderate heart failure and normal sinus rhythm? J Am Coll Cardiol 1997;29:1206–1213.

79. Adams KF, Gheorghiade M, Uretsky BF, et al. Clinical benefits of low serum digoxin concentrations in heart failure. J Am Coll Cardiol 2002;39:946–953.

80. Rathore SS, Curtis JP, Wang Y, et al. Association of serum digoxin concentration and outcomes in patients with heart failure. JAMA 2003;289:871–878.

81. Rathore SS, Wang Y, Krumholz HM. Sex-based differences in the effect of digoxin for the treatment of heart failure. N Engl J Med 2002;347:1403–1411.

82. Khand AU, Rankin AC, Martin W, et al. Carvedilol alone or in combination with digoxin for the management of atrial fibrillation in patients with heart failure? J Am Coll Cardiol. 2003;42:1944–1951.

83. Reuning RH, Geraets DR, Rocci ML, et al. Digoxin. In: Evans WE, Schentag JJ, Jusko WJ, eds. Applied Pharmacokinetics: Principles of Therapeutic Drug Monitoring, 3rd ed. Spokane, WA, Applied Therapeutics, 1992:20-1-20-48.

84. Bozkurt B, Agoston I, Knowlton AA. Complications of inappropriate use of spironolactone in heart failure: When an old medicine spirals out of new guidelines. J Am Coll Cardiol 2003;41:211–214.

85. Svensson M, Gustafsson F, Galatius S, et al. Hyperkalaemia and impaired renal function in patients taking spironolactone for congestive heart failure: Retrospective study. Br Med J 2003;327:1141–1142.

86. Zannad F, Dousset B, Alla F. Treatment of congestive heart failure: Interfering the aldosterone–cardiac extracellular matrix relationship. Hypertension 2001;38:1227–1232.

87. Burnier M, Brunner HR. Angiotensin II receptor antagonists. Lancet 2000;355:637–645.

88. Pitt B, Poole-Wilson PA, Segal R, et al. Effect of losartan compared with captopril on mortality in patients with symptomatic heart failure: Randomised trial. The Losartan Heart Failure Survival Study ELITE II. Lancet 2000;355:1582–1587.

89. Cohn JN, Tognoni G. A randomized trial of the angiotensin-receptor blocker valsartan in chronic heart failure. N Engl J Med 2001;345:1667–1675.

90. Pfeffer MA, Swedberg K, Granger CB, et al. Effects of candesartan on mortality and morbidity in patients with chronic heart failure: The CHARM-Overall programme. Lancet 2003;362:759–766.

91. McMurray JJ, Ostergren J, Swedberg K, et al. Effects of candesartan in patients with chronic heart failure and reduced left-ventricular systolic function taking angiotensin-converting-enzyme inhibitors: The CHARM-Added trial. Lancet 2003;362:767–771.

92. Granger CB, McMurray JJ, Yusuf S, et al. Effects of candesartan in patients with chronic heart failure and reduced left-ventricular systolic function intolerant to angiotensin-converting-enzyme inhibitors: The CHARM-Alternative trial. Lancet 2003;362:772–776.

93. Yusuf S, Pfeffer MA, Swedberg K, et al. Effects of candesartan in patients with chronic heart failure and preserved left-ventricular ejection fraction: The CHARM-Preserved Trial. Lancet 2003;362:777–781.

94. Pfeffer MA, McMurray JJ, Velazquez EJ, et al. Valsartan, captopril, or both in myocardial infarction complicated by heart failure, left ventricular dysfunction, or both. N Engl J Med 2003;349:1893–1906.

95. Cohn JN, Archibald DG, Ziesche S, et al. Effect of vasodilator therapy on mortality in chronic congestive heart failure: Results of the Veterans Administration Cooperative Study. N Engl J Med 1986;316:1547–1552.

96. The AF-CHF Trial Investigators. Rationale and design of a study assessing treatment strategies of atrial fibrillation in patients with heart failure: The Atrial Fibrillation and Congestive Heart Failure (AF-CHF) trial. Am Heart J 2002;144:597–607.

97. Wyse DG, Waldo AL, DiMarco JP, et al. A comparison of rate control and rhythm control in patients with atrial fibrillation. N Engl J Med 2002;347:1825–1833.

98. Nesto RW, Bell D, Bonow RO, et al. Thiazolidinedione use, fluid retention, and congestive heart failure: A consensus statement from the American Heart Association and American Diabetes Association. Circulation 2003;108:2941–2948.

99. Masoudi FA, Wang Y, Inzucchi SE, et al. Metformin and thiazolidinedione use in Medicare patients with heart failure. JAMA 2003;290:81–85.

100. Nawarskas JJ, Spinler SA. Does aspirin interfere with therapeutic efficacy of angiotensin-converting enzyme inhibitors in hypertension or congestive heart failure? Pharmacotherapy 1998;18:1041–1052.

101. Teo KK, Yusuf S, Pfeffer M, et al. Effects of long-term treatment with angiotensin-converting-enzyme inhibitors in the presence or absence of aspirin: A systematic review. Lancet 2002;360:1037–1043.

102. Aumegeat V, Lamblin N, de Groote P, et al. Aspirin does not adversely affect survival in patients with stable congestive heart failure treated with angiotensin-converting enzyme inhibitors. Chest 2003;124:1250–1258.

103. Guazzi M, Brambilla R, Reina G, et al. Aspirin-angiotensin-converting enzyme inhibitor coadministration and mortality in patients with heart failure: A dose-related adverse effect of aspirin. Arch Intern Med 2003;163:1574–1579.

104. Wrenger E, Muller R, Moesenthin M, et al. Interaction of spironolactone with ACE inhibitors or angiotensin receptor blockers: Analysis of 44 cases. Br Med J 2003;327:147–149.

105. Metra M, Giubbini R, Nodari S, et al. Differential effects of beta-blockers in patients with heart failure: A prospective, randomized, double-blind comparison of the long-term effects of metoprolol versus carvedilol. Circulation 2000;102:546–551.

106. The Beta-Blocker Evaluation of Survival Trial Investigators. A trial of the beta-blocker bucindolol in patients with advanced chronic heart failure. N Engl J Med 2001;344:1659–1667.

107. Bristow M. Antiadrenergic therapy of chronic heart failure: Surprises and new opportunities. Circulation 2003;107:1100–1102.

108. Andreka P, Aiyar N, Olson LC, et al. Bucindolol displays intrinsic sympathomimetic activity in human myocardium. Circulation 2002;105:2429–2434.

109. Poole-Wilson PA, Swedberg K, Cleland JGF, et al. Comparison of carvedilol and metoprolol on clinical outcomes in patients with chronic heart failure in the Carvedilol Or Metoprolol European Trial (COMET): Randomised, controlled trial. Lancet 2003;362:7–13.

110. Wikstrand J, Fagerberg B, Goldstein S, et al. COMET: A proposed mechanism of action to explain the results and concerns about dose. Lancet 2003;362:1076–1077.

111. Murray MD, Deer MM, Ferguson JA, et al. Open-label randomized trial of torsemide compared with furosemide therapy for patients with heart failure. Am J Med 2001;111:513–520.

112. Young M, Plosker GL. Torasemide: A pharmacoeconomic review of its use in chronic heart failure. Pharmacoeconomics 2001;19:679–703.

113. Matheny CJ, Lamb MW, Brouwer KR, Pollack GM. Pharmacokinetic and pharmacodynamic implications of P-glycoprotein modulation. Pharmacotherapy 2001;21:778–796.

114. Jain P, Massie BM, Gattis WA, et al. Current medical treatment for the exacerbation of chronic heart failure resulting in hospitalization. Am Heart J 2003;145:S3–17.

115. Nohria A, Lewis E, Stevenson LW. Medical management of advanced heart failure. JAMA 2002;287:628–640.

116. Maisel AS, Krishnaswamy P, Nowak RM, et al. Rapid measurement of B-type natriuretic peptide in the emergency diagnosis of heart failure. N Engl J Med 2002;347:161–167.

117. Logeart D, Thabut G, Jourdain P, et al. Predischarge B-type natriuretic peptide assay for identifying patients at high risk of readmission after decompensated heart failure. J Am Coll Cardiol 2004;43:635–641.

118. Stevenson LW, Massie BM, Francis GS. Optimizing therapy for complex or refractory heart failure: A management algorithm. Am Heart J 1998;135:S293–309.

119. Forrester JS, Diamond G, Chatterjee K, Swan HJC. Medical therapy of acute myocardial infarction by application of hemodynamic subsets. N Engl J Med 1976;295:1356–1362.

120. Brater DC. Diuretic therapy in congestive heart failure. CHF 2000;6:197–210.

121. Vargo DL, Brater DC, Rudy DW, Swan SK. Dopamine does not enhance furosemide-induced natriuresis in patients with congestive heart failure. J Am Soc Nephrol 1996;7:1032–1037.

122. Dorman TPJ, van Meyel JJM, Gerlag PGG, et al. Diuretic efficacy of high dose furosemide in severe heart failure: Bolus injection versus continuous infusion. J Am Coll Cardiol 1996;28:376–382.

123. Leier CV, Binkley PF. Parenteral inotropic support for advanced congestive heart failure. Prog Cardiovasc Dis 1998;41:207–224.

124. Kirsten R, Nelson K, Kirsten D, Heintz B. Clinical pharmacokinetics of vasodilators, part II. Clin Pharmacokinet 1998;35:9–36.

125. Yamani MH, Haji SA, Starling RC, et al. Comparison of dobutamine-based and milrinone-based therapy for advanced decompensated congestive heart failure: Hemodynamic efficacy, clinical outcome, and economic impact. Am Heart J 2001;142:998–1002.

126. Aranda JM, Schofield RS, Pauly DF, et al. Comparison of dobutamine versus milrinone therapy in hospitalized patients awaiting cardiac transplantation: A prospective, randomized trial. Am Heart J 2003;145:324–329.

127. Cuffe MS, Califf RM, Adams KF, et al. Short-term intravenous milrinone for acute exacerbation of chronic heart failure: A randomized, controlled trial. JAMA 2002;287:1541–1547.

128. Zineh I, Schofield RS, Johnson JA. The evolving role of nesiritide in advanced or decompensated heart failure. Pharmacotherapy 2003;23:1266–1280.

129. Burger AJ, Horton DP, LeJemtel T, et al. Effect of nesiritide (B-type natriuretic peptide) and dobutamine on ventricular arrhythmias in the treatment of patients with acutely decompensated congestive heart failure: The PRECEDENT study. Am Heart J 2002;144:1102–1108.

130. The VMAC Investigators. Intravenous nesiritide vs nitroglycerin for treatment of decompensated congestive heart failure: A randomized, controlled trial. JAMA 2002;287:1531–1540.

131. Radovancevic B, Vrtovec B, Frazier OH. Left ventricular assist devices: An alternative to medical therapy for end-stage heart failure. Curr Opin Cardiol 2003;18:210–214.

132. Weintraub WS, Cole J, Tooley JF. Cost and cost-effectiveness studies in heart failure research. Am Heart J 2002;143:565–576.

133. Cowper PA, DeLong ER, Whellan DJ, et al. Economic effects of beta-blocker therapy in patients with heart failure. Am J Med 2004;116:104–111.

134. Moser DK, Mann DL. Improving outcomes in heart failure: It's not unusual beyond usual care. Circulation 2002;105:2810–2812.

135. Philbin EF, Jenkins PL. Differences between patients with heart failure treated by cardiologists, internists, family physicians, and other physicians: Analysis of a large, statewide database. Am Heart J 2000;139:491–496.

136. Gattis WA, Hasselblad V, Whellan DJ, O'Connor CM. Reduction in heart failure events by the addition of a clinical pharmacist to the heart failure management team. Arch Intern Med 1999;159:1939–1945.

137. Whellan DJ, Gaulden L, Gattis WA, et al. The benefit of implementing a heart failure disease management program. Arch Intern Med 2001;161:2223–2228.

138. Macdonald JE, Struthers AD. What is the optimal serum potassium level in cardiovascular patients? J Am Coll Cardiol 2004;43:155–161.

139. Juurlink DN, Mamdani MM, Lee DS, et al. Rates of hyperkalemia after publication of the Randomized Aldactone Evaluation Study. N Engl J Med 2004;351:543–551.

140. Taylor AL, Ziesche S, Yancy C, et al. Combination of isosorbide dinitrate and hydralazine in blacks with heart failure. N Engl J Med 2004;351:2049–2057.

15

ISCHEMIC HEART DISEASE

Robert L. Talbert

Learning Objectives and other resources can be found at *www.pharmacotherapyonline.com*.

KEY CONCEPTS

◀1 Ischemic heart disease (IHD) is caused primarily by coronary atherosclerosis, a very common disease in the U.S. population, and results in an imbalance between oxygen supply and demand with resulting ischemia.

◀2 Chest pain is the cardinal symptom of ischemia due to coronary artery disease (CAD).

◀3 Risk-factor identification and modification are important for individual patients with known or suspected IHD and as a population-based policy to reduce the impact of this disease.

◀4 Major risk factors that can be altered include dyslipidemia (high total and low-density lipoprotein [LDL] cholesterol, low high-density lipoprotein [HDL] cholesterol, and high triglycerides), smoking, glycemic control in diabetes mellitus, hypertension, and adoption of therapeutic lifestyle changes (exercise, weight reduction, and reduced cholesterol and saturated fat in the diet).

◀5 Chronic stable angina should be managed initially with β-blockers because they provide better symptomatic control at least as well as nitrates or calcium channel blockers and decrease the risk of recurrent myocardial infarction (MI) and CAD mortality.

◀6 Nitroglycerin and other nitrate products are useful for prophylaxis of angina when patients are undertaking activities known to provoke angina; however, when angina is occurring on a regular, routine basis, chronic prophylactic therapy should be instituted.

◀7 Although calcium channel blockers are effective as monotherapy, they generally are used in combination with β-blockers or as monotherapy if patients are intolerant of β-blockers; most patients with moderate to severe angina will require two drugs to control their symptoms.

◀8 Pharmacologic management is as effective as revascularization (PTCA, CABG, etc.) if one or two vessels are involved, and there are no differences in survival, recurrent MI, or other measures of effectiveness.

◀9 Multivessel involvement, especially if the patient has left main coronary artery disease or left main equivalent disease, or two- to three-vessel involvement with significant left ventricular dysfunction is best managed with revascularization.

◀10 Percutaneous transluminal angioplasty (PTCA) and coronary artery bypass grafting (CABG) produce similar results overall, but certain patient subsets (e.g., diabetics) should have CABG done.

The pathogenesis of ischemic heart disease (IHD), which is also known as *coronary artery disease* (CAD), is now known to be atherosclerosis of the epicardial vessels. This process begins early in life, often not being clinically manifest until the middle-aged years and beyond. IHD may present as an acute coronary syndrome (ACS), which includes unstable angina, non–ST-segment-elevation myocardial infarction (NSTEMI), and ST-segment-elevation myocardial infarction (STEMI), and MI diagnosed by biomarkers only, chronic stable exertional angina pectoris, and ischemia without clinical symptoms or owing to coronary artery vasospasm (variant or Prinzmetal's angina). Other manifestations of atherosclerosis include heart failure, arrhythmias, cerebrovascular disease (stroke), and peripheral vascular disease. The American Heart Association (AHA) recently published management guidelines for stable and unstable angina.[1–3]

EPIDEMIOLOGY

The syndrome of angina pectoris is reported to occur with an average annual incidence rate (number of new cases per time period per total number of persons in the population for the same time period) of about 1.5% (range 0.1 to 5 per 1000) depending on the patient's age, gender, and risk-factor profile.[4] The presenting manifestation in women is more commonly angina, whereas men more frequently have MI as the initial event. Estimates of the incidence and prevalence of angina are not entirely accurate owing to waxing and waning of symptoms; angina may disappear in up to 30% of patients with angina that is less severe and of recent onset.

Cardiovascular diseases (CVD) claimed 949,619 lives, or 1 of every 2.5 deaths, in the United States in 1998.[5] More than 2600 Americans die of CVD each day, or on average of 1 death every 33 seconds. In 1998, the death rates from CVD were 532.0 (per 100,000) for black males, 419.3 for white males, 400.7 for black females, and 294.9 for white females.[5] CAD was responsible for 459,841 deaths (or 48%) from CVD. Men die earlier from IHD and acute myocardial infarction (AMI) than women, and aging of both sexes is associated with a higher incidence of these afflictions. The disparity in mortality from IHD between men and women decreases with aging, being about four to five times more common in men in their mid-30s to a preponderance of female deaths in the very elderly.

TABLE 15–1. Criteria for Determination of the Specific Activity Scale Functional Class[a]

	Any Yes	No
1. Can you walk down a flight of steps without stopping (4.5–5.2 MET)?	Go to 2	Go to 4
2. Can you carry anything up a flight of 8 steps without stopping (5–5.5 MET)? Or can you:	Go to 3	Class III
a. Have sexual intercourse without stopping (5–5.2 MET)		
b. Garden, rake, weed (5.6 MET)		
c. Roller skate, dance fox trot (5–6 MET)		
d. Walk at a 4 mi/h rate on level ground (5–6 MET)		
3. Can you carry at least 24 lb up 8 steps (10 MET)? Or can you:	Class I	Class II
a. Carry objects that weigh at least 80 lb (18 MET)		
b. Do outdoor work, shovel snow, spade soil (7 MET)		
c. Do recreational activites such as skiing, basketball, touch football, squash, handball (7–10 MET)		
d. Jog/walk 5 mi/h (9 MET)		
4. Can you shower without stopping (3.6–4.2 MET)? Or can you:	Class III	Go to 5
a. Strip and make bed (3.9–5 MET)		
b. Mop floors (4.2 MET)		
c. Hang washed clothes (4.4 MET)		
d. Clean windows (3.7 MET)		
e. Walk 2.5 mi/h (3–3.5 MET)		
f. Bowl (3–4.4 MET)		
g. Play golf, walk and carry clubs (4.5 MET)		
h. Push power lawn mower (4 MET)		
5. Can you dress without stopping because of symptoms (2–2.3 MET)?	Class III	Class IV

[a]MET, metabolic equivalents of activity.

From Goldman L, Hashimoto B, Cook F, et al. Comparative reproducibility and validity of systems for assessing cardiovascular functional class: Advantages of a new specific activity scale. Circulation 1981;64:1228, with permission.

Data from the Framingham Study showed that the prevalence was 5.9% for the 16-year period studied from earlier reports.[6] More recent data from the Framingham Study showed that the prevalence in a 1970 cohort followed for 10 years was about 1.5% for women and 4.3% for men aged 50 to 59 years at inception.[4] The AHA estimates that the prevalence of angina was 6.4 million in 1998.[5] Other interesting trends noted include a 21% decline in the incidence of cardiovascular disease in women but only a 6% decline in men over two cohorts from 1950 and 1970. Cardiovascular mortality was reduced by 59% in women and 53% in men from the same cohorts. The risk of developing IHD is not the same worldwide. Countries such as Japan and France are on the low end of the spectrum, whereas Finland, Northern Ireland, Scotland, and South Africa have very high rates.[7,8]

Angina may be classified according to symptom severity, disability induced, or a specific activity scale (Tables 15–1 and 15–2). The specific activity scale developed by Goldman and coworkers[9] may be preferable because it has been shown to be equal to or better than the New York Heart Association (NYHA) or Canadian Cardiovascular Society (CCS) functional classifications for reproducibility and provides better agreement with treadmill testing.

An important determinate of outcome for the angina patient is the number of vessels obstructed. Twelve-year survivals from the Coronary Artery Surgery Study (CASS) for patients with zero-, one-, two-, and three-vessel disease were 88%, 74%, 59%, and 40%, respectively.[10] Other factors that increase the risk of death in medically managed patients include the presence of heart failure (or markers such as poor ventricular wall motion and low ejection fraction), smoking, left main or left main equivalent CAD, diabetes, and prior MI. Twelve-year survivals for patients with at least one diseased vessel and ejection fractions in the ranges of 50% to 100%, 35% to 49%, and 0% to 34% are 73%, 54%, and 21%, respectively. Of particular note, patients with left main CAD (or left main equivalent) are at extremely high risk and constitute a unique group for therapeutic consideration.[11] In the CASS, at 15 years of follow-up, 37% of the surgery group and 27% of the medical group are surviving; median survival is 13.3 years and 6.7 years, respectively ($p < .0001$). If systolic function was normal, then median survival and percent surviving were not different between the surgery and medical groups (median survival of about 15 years). Patients screened but not randomized to CASS had similar survival rates, suggesting that results from randomized patients may be applicable to more generalized populations as

TABLE 15–2. Grading of Angina Pectoris by the Canadian Cardiovascular Society Classification System

Class	Description of Stage
Class I	Ordinary physical activity does not cause angina, such as walking, climbing stairs. Angina occurs with strenuous, rapid, or prolonged exertion at work or recreation.
Class II	Slight limitation or ordinary activity. Angina occurs on walking or climbing stairs rapidly, walking uphill, walking or stair climbing after meals, or in cold, or in wind, or under emotional stress, or only during the few hours after wakening. Walking more than two blocks on the level and climbing more than one flight of ordinary stairs at a normal pace and in normal condition.
Class III	Marked limitations of ordinary physical activity. Angina occurs on walking one to two blocks on the level and climbing one flight of stairs in normal conditions and at a normal pace.
Class IV	Inability to carry on any physical activity without discomfort—anginal symptoms may be present at rest.

From Campeau L. Grading of angina (letter). Circulation 1976;54:522–523, with permission.

a measure of external reliability. Other factors that predict outcome in ACS include age, heart rate, systolic blood pressure, ST-segment depression, signs of heart failure, and cardiac enzymes (also called *biomarkers*).[12]

ETIOLOGY AND PATHOPHYSIOLOGY

The pathophysiology that underlies this disease process is dynamic, evolutionary, and complex. An understanding of the determinants of myocardial oxygen demand (MVO$_2$), regulation of coronary blood flow, the effects of ischemia on the mechanical and metabolic function of the myocardium, and how ischemia is recognized is important in understanding the rationale for the selection and use of pharmacotherapy for IHD.

Ischemia may be defined as lack of oxygen and decreased or no blood flow in the myocardium. In contrast, *anoxia*, defined as the absence of oxygen to the myocardium, results in continued perfusion with washout of acid by-products of glycolysis, thereby preserving the mechanical and metabolic status of the heart to a greater extent than does ischemia for short periods of time.

DETERMINANTS OF OXYGEN DEMAND

The major determinants of MVO$_2$ are (1) heart rate, (2) contractility, and (3) intramyocardial wall tension during systole. Overall, intramyocardial wall tension is thought to be the most important among these three factors. Since the consequences of IHD are a result of increased demand in the face of a fixed supply of oxygen in most situations, alterations in MVO$_2$ are critically important in producing ischemia and for interventions intended to alleviate ischemia. MVO$_2$ cannot be measured directly in patients; however, an indirect assessment that correlates reasonably well with MVO$_2$ as determined in experimental animal models is the *tension-time index* (TTI). This is a measure of the area under the curve of the left ventricular (LV) pressure curve. Tension in the ventricle wall is a function of the radius of the left ventricle and intraventricular pressure. These factors are related through Laplace's law, which states that wall stress is related directly to the product of intraventricular pressure and internal radius and inversely to wall thickness multiplied by a factor of 2. Increasing systemic blood pressure or ventricular dilatation would increase wall tension and oxygen demand, whereas ventricular hypertrophy would tend to minimize increasing MVO$_2$. Clinical application of these principles has led to the use of the double product (DP), which is heart rate (HR) multiplied by systolic blood pressure (SBP) (DP = HR × SBP). Although this is a clinically useful indirect estimate of MVO$_2$, it does not consider changes in contractility (an independent variable), and because only changes in pressure are considered with the DP, volume loading of the left ventricle and increased MVO$_2$ related to ventricular dilation are underestimated.

REGULATION OF CORONARY BLOOD FLOW

Coronary blood flow is influenced by multiple factors; however, the caliber of the resistance vessels delivering blood to the myocardium and MVO$_2$ are the prime determinants in the occurrence of ischemia. The anatomy of the vascular bed will affect oxygen supply and, subsequently, myocardial metabolism and mechanical function.

ANATOMIC FACTORS

The normal coronary system (see Fig. 15–1 for normal anatomy) consists of large epicardial or surface vessels (R$_1$) that normally

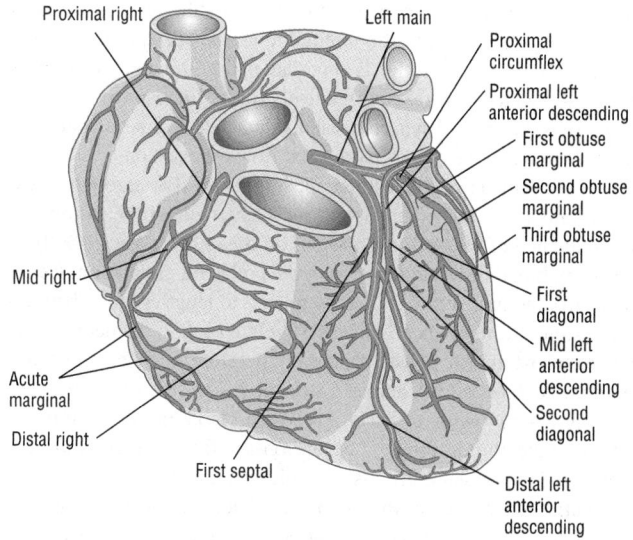

Sternocostal aspect

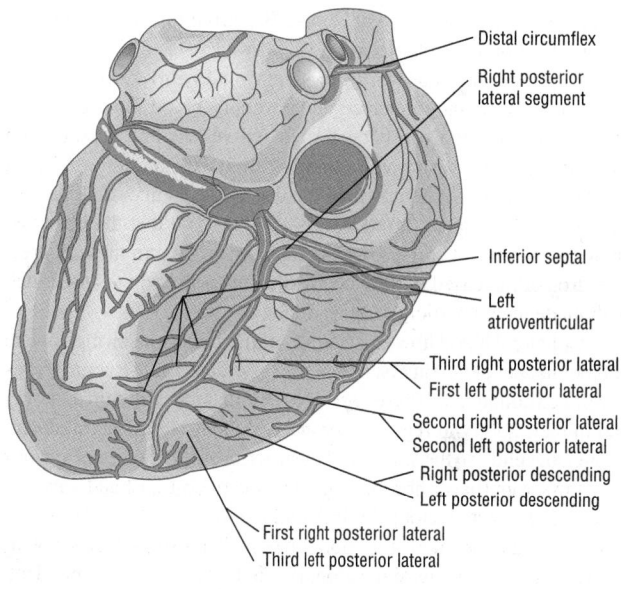

Diaphragmatic aspect

FIGURE 15–1. Coronary artery anatomy with sternocostal and diaphragmatic views.

offer little intrinsic resistance to myocardial flow and intramyocardial arteries and arterioles (R$_2$), which branch into a dense capillary network (about 4000 capillaries/mm^2) to supply basal blood flow of 60 to 90 mL/min per 100 g of myocardium. R$_1$ and R$_2$ are in series, and total resistance is the algebraic sum; however, under normal circumstances, the resistance in R$_2$ is much greater. Myocardial blood flow is inversely related to arteriolar resistance and directly related to the coronary driving pressure. The arterioles dynamically alter their intrinsic tone in response to demands for oxygen and other factors, and as a result, myocardial oxygen delivery and myocardial oxygen demand are tightly coupled in a rapidly responsive system.

Atherosclerotic lesions encroaching on the luminal cross-sectional area of the larger epicardial vessels (R$_1$) transform the relationships among R$_1$, R$_2$, and blood flow. As resistance increases in R$_1$ owing to occlusion, R$_2$ can vasodilate to maintain coronary blood flow. This response is inadequate with greater degrees of obstruction, and the coronary flow reserve afforded by R_2 vasodilation is insufficient to meet oxygen demand (also referred to as *autoregulation*). The extent of functional obstruction is important in the limitation of coronary blood flow, and the presence of relatively severe stenosis (>70%) may provoke ischemia and symptoms at rest, whereas less severe stenosis may allow a reserve of coronary blood flow for exertion.[13]

The diameter of the lesion impeding blood flow through a vessel is important, but other factors such as length of the lesion and the influence of pressure drop across an area of stenosis also affect coronary blood flow and function of the collateral circulation. Resistance to flow in a vessel is directly related to length of the obstructing lesion, but resistance is inversely related to the diameter of the vessel to the fourth power. Diameter therefore is much more important. As blood flows across a stenotic lesion, the pressure drops (energy losses) owing to friction between blood and the lesion and owing to the abrupt turbulent expansion as blood emerges from the stenosis. This pressure drop is dynamic and directly related to flow, giving rise to a resistance that is not fixed but rather fluctuates as flow is changed. This relationship can affect collateral blood flow and its response to exercise dramatically, resulting in what has been called *coronary steal*. A similar situation also may occur when the epicardial or subepicardial vessels "steal" blood flow from the endocardium in the presence of a stenotic lesion.

Large and small coronary arteries may undergo dynamic changes in coronary vascular resistance and coronary blood flow. Dynamic coronary obstruction can occur in normal vessels and vessels with stenosis, in which vasomotion or spasm may be superimposed on a fixed stenosis. Although it is possible that these changes may be "active" in small coronary arteries, it is also possible that the observed changes may reflect collapse owing to poststenotic intraluminal pressure drop or increased intramyocardial compressive forces associated with inadequate ventricular relaxation.

Collateral blood flow exists to a certain extent from birth as native collaterals, but persisting ischemia may promote collateral growth as developed collaterals. These two types of collaterals differ in anatomy and in their ability to regulate coronary blood flow. Collateral development depends on the severity of obstruction, the presence of various growth factors (basic fibroblast growth factor [b-FGF] and vascular endothelial growth factor [VEGF]), endogenous vasodilators (e.g., nitrous oxide and prostacyclin), hormones such as estrogen, and potentially, exercise. Collateral development is highly species-dependent, and this should be considered when reading experimental literature.

METABOLIC REGULATION

Coronary blood flow is closely tied to oxygen needs of the heart. Changes in oxygen balance lead to very rapid changes in coronary blood flow. Although a number of mediators may contribute to these changes, the most important ones are likely to be adenosine, other nucleotides, nitric oxide, prostaglandins, CO_2, and H^+. Adenosine, which is formed from adenosine triphosphate (ATP) and adenosine monophosphate (AMP) under conditions of ischemia and stress, is a potent vasodilator that links decreased perfusion to metabolically induced vasodilation, or *reactive hyperemia*. The synthesis and release of adenosine into coronary sinus venous effluent occur within seconds of coronary artery occlusion, and about 30% of the hyperemic response can be blocked by metabolic blockers of adenosine.[14]

ENDOTHELIAL CONTROL OF CORONARY VASCULAR TONE

The vascular endothelium, a single-cell tissue with an enormous surface area separating the blood from vascular smooth muscle of the artery wall, is capable of a broad range of metabolic functions. The endothelium functions as a protective surface for the artery wall, and as long as it remains intact and functional, it promotes vascular smooth muscle relaxation and inhibits thrombogenesis and atherosclerotic plaque formation; damaged endothelium reacts to numerous stimuli with vasoconstriction, thrombosis, and plaque formation. The vascular endothelium of the coronary arteries synthesizes large molecules such as fibronectin, interleukin-1, tissue plasminogen activator, and various growth factors. Small molecules that are also produced include prostacyclin, platelet-activating factor, endothelin-1, and endothelium-derived relaxing factor (EDRF) that is now characterized as nitric oxide. EDRF is synthesized from L-arginine via nitric oxide synthase and released by shear force on the endothelium, as well as through interaction with many biochemical stimuli such as acetylcholine, histamine, arginine, catecholamines, arachidonic acid, adenosine diphosphate (ADP), endothelin-1, bradykinin, serotonin, and thrombin.[14] EDRF or nitric oxide then causes relaxation of the underlying smooth muscle and may be thought of as a paracrine homeopathic defense mechanism against noxious stimuli. Denudation or loss of the vascular endothelium results in loss of EDRF and this protective mechanism. Loss of the endothelial cell layer and function may occur secondary to physical disruption (e.g., percutaneous transluminal angioplasty [PTCA]), factors impinging from the vascular side (cyanide from smoke), or disruption of the intimal-medial layers (oxidized low-density lipoprotein). Impaired endothelial function may be related to the development of premature atherosclerosis based on recent family studies. Endothelial function may be improved with angiotensin-converting enzyme (ACE) inhibitors, statins, and exercise.

FACTORS EXTRINSIC TO THE VASCULAR BED

Blood flow to the coronary arteries arises from orifices located immediately distal to the aorta valve. Perfusion pressure is equal to the difference between the aortic pressure at an instantaneous point in time minus the intramyocardial pressure. Coronary vascular resistance is influenced by phasic systolic compression of the vascular bed. The driving force for perfusion therefore is not constant throughout the cardiac cycle. Opening of the aortic valve also may lead to a Venturi effect, which can slightly decrease perfusion pressure. If perfusion pressure is elevated for a period of time, coronary vascular resistance declines, and blood flow increases; however, continued perfusion pressure increases lead, within limits, to a return of coronary blood flow back toward baseline levels through autoregulation.

Alterations in intramyocardial wall tension throughout the cardiac cycle also will impose significant changes in coronary blood flow. Diastole is the period during which coronary artery filling can occur owing to these pressure differences, and little or no coronary blood flow occurs to the left ventricle during systole. The extent of pressure development in the ventricle and heart rate have a major effect on the development of wall tension, time for diastolic coronary artery filling, and myocardial oxygen demand.

Under normal conditions, the average global distribution of blood flow between the epicardial and endocardial layer is about 1:1 at rest and remains approximately even during exercise secondary to autoregulatory changes. Regional disparity of blood flow distribution does exist normally, and these disparities are magnified in the presence of diseased coronary arteries and with increased cardiac work as the vasodilator reserve in the resistance vessels of the subendocardium layers is exhausted. Factors that favor a reduction in subendocardial blood flow include decreased perfusion pressure owing to decreased diastolic blood pressure or coronary artery obstruction by atherosclerotic plaques with or without vasomotion, abbreviation of diastole (increased heart rate), and increased intraventricular diastolic pressure (e.g., valvular obstruction to flow).

Extravascular resistance may decrease coronary blood flow, primarily during systole. This effect is much more pronounced in the left ventricle compared with the right ventricle. When the effect of increased contractility is separated from the effect of ventricular pressure, about 75% of extravascular resistance is accounted for by passive stretch in equilibrium with ventricular pressure, whereas only 25% results from active myocardial contraction.

FACTORS INTRINSIC TO THE VASCULAR BED

Metabolic factors, myogenic responses, neural reflexes, and humoral substances within the vascular bed of the coronary circulation function in an orchestrated fashion to maintain relative consistency in blood flow to the myocardium in the face of imposed changes in perfusion pressures. Autoregulation, mediated primarily through the effects of myogenic responses and metabolic factors, is thought to be responsible for maintaining regional blood flow in a narrow range while systemic pressure varies over a range of approximately 50 to 150 mm Hg.

Myogenic control (also known as the *Bayliss effect*) of coronary artery tone occurs when the vessel is stretched secondary to an increase in pressure and contracts to return blood flow to normal. It is thought that the myogenic response to stretching in coronary arteries is a modest one and that metabolic factors such as nitric oxide play a much larger role in autoregulation.

There are three well-studied metabolic factors that have the ability to modify coronary artery resistance and blood flow at the local level. Basal coronary blood flow meets oxygen demands of 8 to 10 mL/min per 100 g of myocardium with essentially complete extraction of oxygen from the blood. As cardiac output or mean arterial blood pressure increases, the increased demand for oxygen is met by increasing blood flow because little additional oxygen is available from hemoglobin. Decreased oxygen availability causes vasodilation of vascular smooth muscle and relaxation of precapillary sphincters, which increase tissue oxygen and help to maintain blood flow on a regional basis.

At perfusion pressures below 60 mm Hg, since the coronary arteries are maximally dilated and the buffering effect of autoregulation has reached its capacity, further reduction in coronary blood flow will decrease perfusion pressure and tissue oxygenation. It is thought that autoregulation works more efficiently in the epicardial layers than in the subendocardial layers, and this may contribute to coronary steal.

Neural components that participate in the regulation of coronary blood flow include the sympathetic nervous system, the parasympathetic nervous system, coronary reflexes, and possibly, central control of coronary blood flow. Within the sympathetic system, stimulation of the stellate ganglion elicits coronary vasodilation, which is associated with tachycardia and enhanced contractility. This indirect coronary vasodilation is secondary to increased MVO_2 related to increased heart rate, contractility, and aortic pressure and occurs following stellate stimulation. The direct effect of the sympathetic system is α_1-mediated vasoconstriction at rest and during exercise. Other receptor types, α_2 and β_1, have little influence on tone, whereas β_2-stimulation produces a modest vasodilatory effect. Although coronary atherosclerosis may decrease blood flow secondary to obstruction, severe coronary atherosclerosis and obstruction also may increase the sensitivity of coronary arteries to the effects of α_1-stimulation and vasoconstriction.

Vagal stimulation within the parasympathetic system produces a small to moderate increase in coronary blood flow, which involves the coronary efferent and afferent parasympathetic components (Bezold-Jarish reflex). Indirectly, vasoconstriction may result, with vagal stimulation as the result of bradycardia and decreased contractility reducing myocardial oxygen demand.

Coronary reflexes have an undetermined role in the regulation of coronary blood flow. Based on experimental data, coronary reflexes that may be important include the baroreceptor, the chemoreceptor, the Bezold-Jarish reflex, and the pulmonary inhalation reflex.

FACTORS LIMITING CORONARY PERFUSION

During exercise and pacing, as MVO_2 increases, coronary vascular resistance can be reduced to about 25% of basal values, which results in a four- to fivefold increase in coronary blood flow. The cross-sectional area can be reduced by about 80% prior to any mechanical or biochemical changes in the myocardium, reflecting a margin of safety for coronary blood flow. The extent of cross-sectional obstruction, the length of the lesion, lesion composition, and the geometry of the obstructing lesion each can affect flow across coronary arteries with atherosclerosis. Bernoulli's theorem states that the pressure drop across a lesion is directly related to the length of the lesion and inversely related to the radius of the lesion to the fourth power; critical stenosis occurs when the obstructing lesion encroaches on the luminal diameter and exceeds 70%. Lesions creating obstructions of 50% to 70% may reduce blood flow; however, these obstructions are not consistent, and vasospasm and thrombosis superimposed on a "noncritical" lesion may lead to clinical events such as MI.[15] If the lesion enlarges from 80% to 90%, resistance in that vessel is tripled. Coronary reserve is diminished at about 85% obstruction owing to vasoconstriction. Exaggerated responsiveness can be seen when the coronary stenosis reaches this critical level, and vasoactive substances such as prostaglandins, thromboxanes, and serotonin may play more of a role in the regulation of coronary vascular tone and thrombosis.

Little reserve exists for coronary blood flow, and a relatively small reduction of 10% to 20% results in decreased myocardial fiber shortening as the first evidence for abnormal function. The subendocardial layers are affected to a greater extent than the epicardium by ischemia, considering changes in fiber shortening, arteriovenous (AV) difference in oxygen saturation, and lactate production. A reduction of 80% gives rise to akinesis, and a 95% reduction of coronary blood flow produces dyskinesis during contraction of the ventricles. Although these abnormalities of contraction are associated with transient impaired function, depletion of high-energy phosphate compounds and ultrastructural changes may last for days even after transient ischemia; this has been referred to as *stunned myocardium.* Chronic hypoperfusion may lead to *hibernation,* in which ventricular function is impaired over longer time intervals. Hibernating myocardium can be differentiated from necrosis with various techniques (see Chap. 10), and revascularization of hibernating myocardium is useful in improving ventricular function. Regional loss of contractility may impose a burden on the remaining myocardial tissue, resulting in heart failure, increased MVO_2, and rapid depletion of blood flow reserve. Consequently, zones of tissue with marginal blood flow may develop in a lateral or transmural fashion; such development puts this tissue at risk for more severe damage if the ischemic episode persists or becomes more severe. Nonischemic areas of myocardium may compensate for the severely ischemic and border zones of ischemia by developing more tension than usual in an attempt to maintain cardiac output. At the cellular level, ischemia and the attendant acidosis are thought to alter calcium release from storage sites such as the sarcolemma and the sarcoplasmic reticulum, as well as inhibiting the binding of calcium to

CLINICAL PRESENTATION OF ANGINA

GENERAL

- Many episodes of ischemia do not cause symptoms of angina (silent ischemia).
- Patients often have a reproducible pattern of pain or other symptoms that appear after a specific amount of exertion.
- Increased frequency, severity, duration, and symptoms at rest suggest an unstable angina pattern, and the patient should seek help immediately.

SYMPTOMS

- Sensation of pressure or burning over the sternum or near it, often but not always radiating to the left jaw, shoulder, and arm; also, chest tightness and shortness of breath.
- Pain usually lasting from 0.5 to 30 minutes, often with a visceral quality (deep location).
- Precipitating factors include exercise, cold environment, walking after a meal, emotional upset, fright, anger, and coitus.
- Relief occurs with rest and nitroglycerin.

SIGNS

- Abnormal precordial (over the heart) systolic bulge
- Abnormal heart sounds

LABORATORY TESTS

- Typically, no laboratory tests are abnormal; however, if the patient has intermediate- to high-risk features for unstable angina, electrocardiographic changes are seen, and serum troponin or creatine kinase concentrations may become abnormal (Table 15–3).
- Patients are likely to have laboratory test abnormalities for the risk factors for IHD, such as elevated total and low-density lipoprotein (LDL) cholesterol, low high-density lipoprotein (HDL) cholesterol, impaired fasting glucose or elevated glucose concentration, high blood pressure, and elevated C-reactive protein. Hemoglobin should be checked to make sure that the patient is not anemic.

OTHER DIAGNOSTIC TESTS

- A resting electrocardiogram (ECG) followed by an exercise tolerance test usually are the first tests done in stable patients.
- A chest x-ray should be done if the patient has heart failure symptoms.
- Cardiac imaging using radioisotopes to detect ischemic myocardium and measure ventricular function are done commonly when revascularization is being considered.
- Echocardiography also may be used to assess ventricular wall motion at rest or during stress.
- Cardiac catheterization and coronary arteriography are used to determine coronary artery anatomy and if the patient would benefit from angioplasty, coronary artery bypass grafting (CABG), or other revascularization procedures.

troponin, thereby impairing the association of actin and myosin. The clinical correlates of these cellular biochemical events leading to the development of LV or right ventricular (RV) dysfunction include an S_3 gallop, dyspnea, orthopnea, tachycardia, fluctuating blood pressure, transient murmurs, and mitral or tricuspid regurgitation.

Calcium accumulation and overload secondary to ischemia impair ventricular relaxation as well as contraction. This is apparently a result of impaired calcium uptake after systole from the myofilaments, leading to a less negative decline in the pressure in the ventricle over time. Impaired relaxation is associated with enhanced diastolic stiffness, decreased rate of wall thinning, and slowed pressure decay, producing an upward shift in the ventricular pressure-volume relationship; put more simply, MVO_2 is likely to be increased secondary to increased wall tension. Impairment of both diastolic and systolic function leads to elevation of the filling pressure of the left ventricle.

CLINICAL PRESENTATION AND DIAGNOSIS

Important aspects of the clinical history for chest pain for patients with angina include the nature or quality of the pain, precipitating factors, duration, pain radiation, and the response to nitroglycerin or rest. Because there can be considerable variation in the manifestations of angina, it is more accurate to refer to these symptoms as an *anginal syndrome*. For some patients with significant CAD, the presenting symptoms may differ from the classic symptoms, yet the symptoms are due to ischemic pain, and these are often referred to as *anginal equivalents*. Obtaining an accurate and detailed family history is useful in placing symptoms in perspective. Significant positive information includes premature coronary heart disease (<55 years in men and <65 years in women), as manifested as fatal and nonfatal MI, stroke, and peripheral vascular disease, and other risk factors such as hypertension, smoking, familial lipid disorders, and diabetes mellitus. Typical pain radiation patterns include anterior chest pain (96%), left upper arm pain (83.7%), left lower arm pain (29.3%), and neck pain at some time (22%). Pain from other areas is less common. Ischemia detected by ECG monitoring is more likely to be detected in the morning hours (6 AM to 12 noon) than other periods throughout the day. Patients suffering from variant or Prinzmetal's angina secondary to coronary spasm are more likely to experience pain at rest and in the early morning hours. Prinzmetal's anginal pain usually is not brought on by exertion or emotional stress nor relieved by rest; and the ECG pattern is that of current injury with ST-segment elevation rather than depression.

It is also important to differentiate the pattern of pain for stable angina from that of unstable angina. Unstable angina may be stratified into categories of risk ranging from high to low[16] (see Table 15–3). Ischemia also may be painless or "silent" in 60% to 100% of patients depending on the series cited and the patient population.[17] In patients with myocardial ischemia, approximately 70% of the episodes of documented ischemia are painless, as determined by ambulatory ECG monitoring, and the ST-segment changes associated with these episodes can be ST elevation or depression. The mechanism of silent ischemia is unclear, but studies have shown that patients not experiencing pain have altered pain perception, with the threshold and tolerance for pain being higher than those of patients who have pain more frequently. Although diabetics tend to have more extensive CAD than nondiabetics do and may suffer from autonomic neuropathy, asymptomatic ischemia is not more prevalent based on the Asymptomatic Cardiac Ischemia Pilot (ACIP) study.[18] Altered endorphin release is a plausible explanation, but investigations with naloxone to block endorphins do not consistently show altered pain thresholds to various stimuli compared with patients with symptomatic ischemia, and

TABLE 15–3. Short-Term Risk of Death or Nonfatal MI in Patients with Unstable Angina

Feature	High Risk (At least 1 of the following features must be present)	Intermediate Risk (No high-risk feature but must have 1 of the following)	Low Risk (No high- or intermediate-risk feature but may have any of the following)
History	Accelerating tempo of ischemic symptoms in preceding 48 h	Prior MI, peripheral or cerebrovascular disease, or CABG, prior aspirin use	
Character of pain	Prolonged ongoing (>20 min), rest pain	Prolonged (>20 min), rest angina, now resolved, with moderate or high likelihood of CAD	New-onset CCS class III or IV angina in the past 2 weeks without prolonged (>20 min) rest pain but with moderate or high likelihood of CAD
Clinical findings	Pulmonary edema, most likely due to ischemia New or worsening MR murmur S_3 or new/worsening rales Hypotension, bradycardia, tachycardia Age >75 yrs		
ECG	Angina at rest with transient ST-segment changes > 0.05 mV Bundle-branch block, new or presumed new	T-wave inversions > 0.2 mV Pathologic Q waves	Normal or unchanged ECG during an episode of chest discomfort
Cardiac markers	Markedly elevated (e.g., TnT or TnI > 0.1 ng/mL)	Slightly elevated (e.g., TnT > 0.01 but <0.1 ng/mL)	Normal

Abbreviations: MI = myocardial infarction; CABG = coronary artery bypass grafting; CAD = coronary artery disease; CCS = Canadian Cardiovascular Society; MR = mitral regurgitation; ECG = electrocardiogram; TnT = troponin T; TnI = troponin I

patients with asymptomatic ischemia do not necessarily have impaired somatic pain sensitivity.[19] Alternatively, adenosine and substance P release during ischemia and mechanical stretch on coronary arteries may play a role in the perception of pain.

Last, it should be recognized that the threshold for pain owing to exertion is fixed in some patients and variable in others and that the amount of exercise or stress necessary to provoke symptoms can change over time. A fixed threshold for the induction of pain or ECG evidence of ischemia means that these indicators of ischemia occur at the same or nearly so, doubling the rate-pressure product. This is apparently owing to at least two factors. Over long periods of time, atherosclerosis may progress, leading to more severe stenosis, reduced oxygen supply, and less of an increase in demand to precipitate ischemic symptoms. Once stenotic lesions reach a critical level of about 80% or greater, vasomotion, vasospasm, and thrombotic occlusion become significant factors impairing blood flow to the myocardium. Consequently, anatomic considerations and vasoactive substances may interact to provide an environment amenable to changing thresholds for the production of angina.

There appears to be little relationship between the historical features of angina and the severity or extent of coronary artery vessel involvement. Therefore, one may speculate that severe symptoms might be associated with multivessel disease, but no predictive markers exist on a routine basis.

Chest pain may resemble pain arising from a variety of noncardiac sources, and the differential diagnosis of anginal pain from other etiologies may be quite difficult based on history alone. Table 15–4 outlines other common problems that may present with episodic chest pain. Although much less common, nonatherosclerotic etiologies of CAD do exist and should be excluded with appropriate tests. The clinical classification of chest pain encompasses typical angina, including (1) substernal chest pain with a characteristic quality and duration that is (2) provoked by exertion or emotional stress and (3) relieved by rest or nitroglycerin; atypical angina meets two of the characteristics for typical angina, and noncardiac chest pain meets one or fewer of the typical angina characteristics.[1]

There are few signs apparent on physical examination to indicate the presence of CAD, and usually only the cardiovascular system reveals any useful information. Elevated heart rate or blood pressure can yield an increased DP and may be associated with angina, and it would be important to correct extreme tachycardia or hypertension if present. Other noncardiac physical findings that suggest that significant cardiovascular disease may be associated with angina include abdominal aortic aneurysms or peripheral vascular disease. Cardiac examination findings in CAD are noted in Table 15–5. During an angina attack, these findings may appear or become more prominent, making them more valuable if present.

In addition to screening for CVD risk factors (see Table 21–7), other recommended tests include hemoglobin, fasting glucose, fasting lipoprotein panel, resting ECG, and chest x-ray in patients with signs or symptoms of heart failure, valvular heart disease, pericardial disease, or aortic dissection/aneurysm.[1] Hemoglobin is assessed to ensure adequate oxygen-carrying capacity. Fasting glucose determinations to exclude diabetes and glucose monitoring for concurrent diabetes should be performed routinely. Lipids are assessed as total, LDL, and HDL cholesterol and triglycerides[20] (see Chap. 21). Other risk factors that may be important for some patients include C-reactive protein, homocysteine level, evidence of *Chylamdia* infection, and elevations in lipoprotein (a), fibrinogen, and plasminogen activator inhibitor.[21,22] Cardiac enzymes all should be normal in stable angina. Troponin T or I, myoglobin, or creatinine phosphokinase-MB isoform may be elevated in patients with unstable angina, and interventions such as anticoagulation and antiplatelet therapy have been shown to reduce cardiac end points when these markers for injury are elevated[23] (see Table 15–3).

Patients presenting with chest pain are stratified into chronic stable angina or having features of intermediate- or high-risk unstable angina (Fig. 15–2; see also Table 15–3). These features include rest pain lasting more than 20 minutes, age greater than 65 years, ST-segment and T-wave changes, and pulmonary edema. Patients with ACS (unstable angina, NSTEMI, and STEMI) are managed differently from those with chronic stable angina.

TABLE 15–4. Differential Diagnosis of Episodic Chest Pain Resembling Angina Pectoris

	Duration	Quality	Provocation	Relief	Location	Commet
Effort angina	5–15 min	Visceral (pressure)	During effort or emotion	Rest, NTG	Substernal, radiates	First episode vivid
Rest angina	5–15 min	Visceral (pressure)	Spontaneous (?with exercise)	NTG	Substernal, radiates	Often nocturnal
Mitral prolapse	Min–hours	Superficial (rarely visceral)	Spontaneous (no pattern)	Time	Left anterior	No pattern, variable
Esophageal reflux	10 min–1 h	Visceral	Spontaneous, cold liquids, exercise, lying down	Foods, antacids, H$_2$ blockers, proton pump inhibitors, NTG	Substernal, radiates	Mimics angina
Peptic ulcer	Hours	Visceral, burning	Lack of food, "acid" foods	Foods, antacids, H$_2$ blockers, proton pump inhibitors	Epigastric, substernal	
Biliary disease	Hours	Visceral (wax and wane)	Spontaneous, food	Time, analgesia	Epigastric, radiates	Colic
Cervical disk	Variable (gradually subsides)	Superficial	Head and neck, movement and palpation	Time, analgesia	Arm, neck	Not relieved by rest
Hyperventilation	2–3 min	Visceral	Emotion, tachypnea	Stimulus removed	Substernal	Facial paraesthe
Musculoskeletal	Variable	Superficial	Movement, palpation	Time, analgesia	Multiple	Tenderness
Pulmonary	30 min	Visceral (pressure)	Often spontaneous	Rest, time bronchodilator	Subsernal	Dyspneic

NTG = nitroglycerin.

TABLE 15–5. Cardiac Findings in Patients with Coronary Artery Disease

Sign	Clinical Significance	Frequency
Abnormal precordial systolic bulge	Left ventricular wall motion abnormality	Not usually present unless patient has sustained a prior MI (especially anterior wall) or is experiencing angina at time of examination
Decreased intensity of S$_1$	Decrease in left ventricular contractility	Difficult to evaluate in resting state, but can be commonly demonstrated during angina
Paradoxical splitting of S$_2$	Left ventricular wall motion abnormality	Very uncommon but occasionally noted during angina
S$_3$ (ventricular gallop)	Increased left ventricular diastolic pressure, with or without clinical CHF	Not usually present unless patient sustained extensive MI; may occasionally be present during angina
S$_4$ (atrial gallop)	Reduced ventricular compliance ("stiff heart")	Common; very common in patients who have sustained a prior MI as well as during angina
Apical systolic murmur (in absence of rheumatic mitral regurgitation or Barlow's syndrome)	Papillary muscle dysfunction	Not usually present unless patient has sustained prior MI
Diastolic murmur (in absence of aortic regurgitation)	Coronary artery stenosis	Rare

Abbreviations: S$_1$ = first heart sound; S$_2$ = second heart sound; S$_3$ = third heart sound; S$_4$ = fourth heart sound; MI = myocardial infarction; CHF = congestive heart failure.
From Cohn PF, ed. Diagnosis and Therapy of Coronary Artery Disease, 2d ed. Boston, Martinus Nijhoff, 1985:101, with permission.

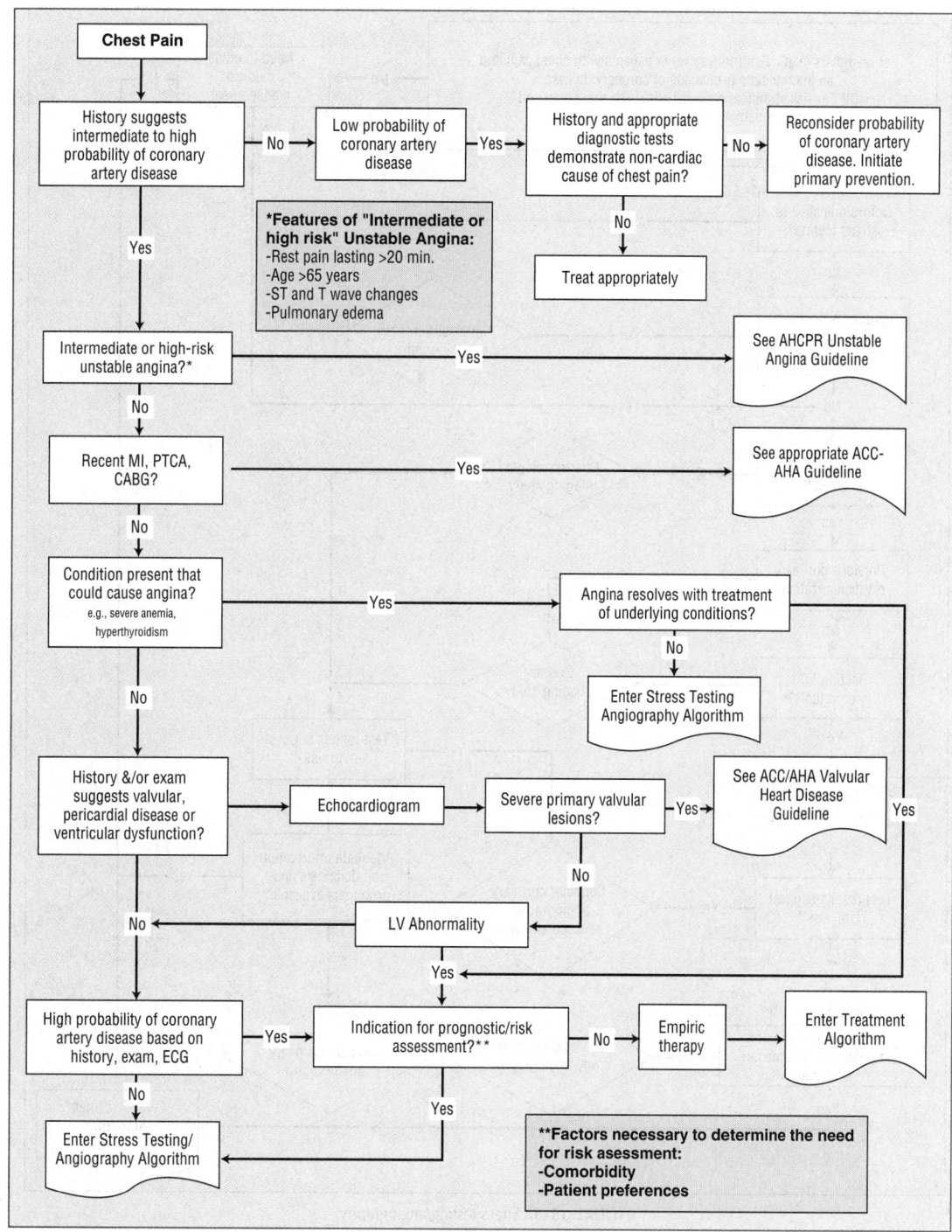

FIGURE 15–2. Clinical assessment (AHCPR = Agency for Health Care Policy and Research).

DIAGNOSTIC TESTS (See Chap. 11)

ELECTROCARDIOGRAM

The ECG is normal in about one-half of patients with angina who are not experiencing an acute attack. Typical ST-T–wave changes include depression, T-wave inversion, and ST-segment elevation. Forms of ischemia other than exertional angina may have ECG manifestations that are different; variant angina is associated with ST-segment elevation, whereas silent ischemia may produce elevation or depression. Significant ischemia is associated with ST-segment depression

of greater than 2 mm, exertional hypotension, and reduced exercise tolerance.

EXERCISE TOLERANCE TESTING[24]

Exercise tolerance (stress) testing (ETT) is recommended for patients with intermediate pretest probability of CAD based on age, gender, and symptoms, including those with complete right bundle branch block or less than 1 mm of rest ST-segment depression (Fig. 15–3). Although ETT is insensitive for predicting coronary artery anatomy, it does correlate well with outcome, such as the likelihood of

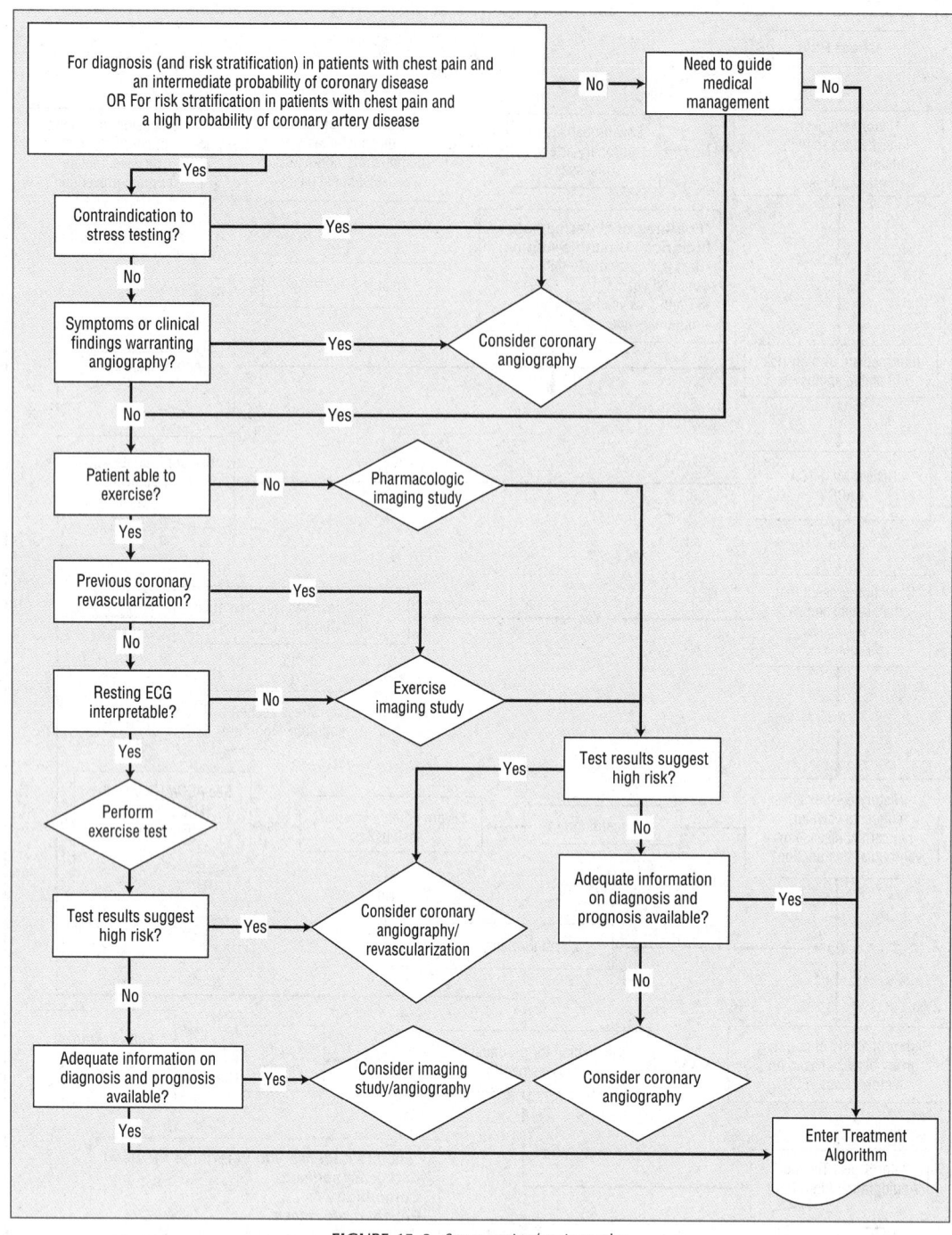

FIGURE 15–3. Stress testing/angiography.

progressing to angina, the occurrence of acute MI, and cardiovascular death. Ischemic ST-segment depression that occurs during ETT is an independent risk factor for cardiac events and cardiovascular mortality. Thallium (^{201}Tl) myocardial perfusion scintigraphy may be used in conjunction with ETT to detect reversible and irreversible defects in blood flow to the myocardium because it is more sensitive than ETT.

CARDIAC IMAGING

Radionuclide angiocardiography (performed with technetium-99m, a radioisotope) is used to measure ejection fraction, regional ventricular performance, cardiac output, ventricular volumes, valvular regurgitation, asynchrony or wall motion abnormalities, and intracar-

diac shunts.[25] Technetium pyrophosphate scans are used routinely for the detection and quantification of acute MI (see Chap. 11). Positron-emission tomography (PET) is useful for quantifying ischemia with metabolically important substrates such as oxygen, carbon, and nitrogen. Other metabolic probes use radiolabeled fatty acids and glucose to study metabolic processes that may be deranged during ischemia in animals and for investigative purposes in humans.

A new method using ultrarapid computed tomography (spiral CT, ultrafast CT, electron-beam CT) minimizes artifact owing to motion of the heart during contraction and relaxation and provides a semiquantitative assessment of calcium content in coronary arteries.[26] Calcium scores greater than 150 provide a sensitivity of 74% and specificity of 89%, and this method may be cost-effective compared with ETT.

ECHOCARDIOGRAPHY

Echocardiography is useful if patients have history or physical examination suggestive of valvular pericardial disease or ventricular dysfunction. For patients unable to exercise, pharmacologic stress echocardiography (dobutamine, dipyridamole, or adenosine) or pacing may be done to identify abnormalities during stress.

CARDIAC CATHETERIZATION AND CORONARY ARTERIOGRAPHY

Cardiac catheterization and angiography in patients with suspected CAD are used diagnostically to document the presence and severity of disease, as well as for prognostic purposes. High-risk features during ETT suggesting the need for coronary angiography include early and significant (≥ 2 mm) changes on the ECG during ETT, as well

as multiple lead involvement, prolonged recovery from ischemia, low workload performance, abnormal blood pressure response (reduction in blood pressure), or ventricular arrhythmias. Multiple defects with thallium scans, as well as lung uptake during exercise or postexercise ventricular cavity dilation, are also high-risk indications for catheterization. Interventional catheterization is used for thrombolytic therapy in patients with acute MI and for the management of patients with significant CAD to relieve obstruction through PTCA, atherectomy, laser treatment, or stent placement. Catheterization and angiography may be done after coronary artery bypass grafting (CABG) to determine if the graft has closed or if CAD has progressed. Coronary artery intravascular ultrasound (IVUS) is useful for directly imaging anatomy, calcified and fatty plaques, and thrombosis superimposed on plaque, as well as for determining patency following revascularization procedures. IVUS guidance of stent implantation may result in more effective stent expansion compared with angiographic guidance alone.[27]

▶ TREATMENT: Ischemic Heart Disease

▥ DESIRED OUTCOME

The short-term goals of therapy for IHD are to reduce or prevent the symptoms of angina that limit exercise capability and impair quality of life. Long-term goals of therapy are to prevent CHD events such as MI, arrhythmias, and heart failure and to extend the patient's life. Since there is little evidence that revascularization procedures such as angioplasty and CABG extend life, the primary focus should be on altering the underlying and ongoing process of atherosclerosis through risk-factor modification while providing symptomatic relief through the use of nitrates, β-blockers, and calcium channel blockers for anginal symptoms.

▥ RISK-FACTOR MODIFICATION

❸ Primary prevention of ischemic heart disease through the identification and modification of risk factors prior to the initial morbid event would be the optimal management approach and should result in a significant impact on the prevalence of IHD. However, early recognition of some risk factors may not be possible in all cases, and in others, the patient may not be willing to undertake intervention until overt evidence of CAD is apparent. Secondary intervention continues to be pursued more commonly by both health care professionals and patients, and it is important to recognize this type of intervention as effective in reducing subsequent morbidity and mortality. The presence of risk factors in individual patients plays a major role in determining the occurrence and severity of IHD.[20] Risk factors are additive in nature and can be classified as alterable or unalterable (see Table 21–7). Unalterable risk factors include gender; age; family history or genetic composition; environmental influences such as climate, air pollution, and trace metal composition of drinking water; and to some extent, diabetes mellitus. Improved glycemic control reduces the microvascular complications of diabetes mellitus (see Chap. 72) and reduces coronary end points; however, based on the Diabetes Control and Complications study, the reduction was impressive (40 versus 23 major events) but not significant because the trial was underpowered **❹** to detect these changes.[28] Risk factors that can be altered include smoking, hypertension, hyperlipidemia, obesity, sedentary lifestyle, hyperuricemia, psychosocial factors such as stress and type A behavior patterns, and the use of certain drugs that may be detrimental, including progestins, corticosteroids, and cyclosporine.

Cigarette smoking is common; nearly 50 million people are regular smokers in this country, and the risk for IHD is increased by about 1.8 in active smokers and by about 1.3 in those exposed to passive or environmental smoke.[29] Approximately 430,700 Americans die each year from smoking-related illnesses, and one in five deaths owing to CVD are attributable to smoking.[5] Risk owing to smoking is related to the number of cigarettes smoked per day and the duration of smoking. Passive smoking in angina pectoris patients has been shown to decrease exercise time.[7] Pipe and cigar smokers are at increased risk compared with nonsmokers, but their risk is somewhat less than that of cigarette smokers.[30] The direct effects of cigarette smoke that are detrimental to patients with angina include (1) elevated heart rate and blood pressure from nicotine, which increases MVO_2, and impaired myocardial oxygen delivery owing to carboxyhemoglobin generation from carbon monoxide inhalation in smoke, (2) the negative inotropic effect of carboxyhemoglobin, (3) increased platelet adhesiveness and promotion of aggregation, resulting in thrombotic tendencies owing to nicotine and carboxyhemoglobin, (4) lowered threshold for ventricular fibrillation during ischemia owing to carboxyhemoglobin, and (5) impaired endothelial function owing to smoking.[31] Similar changes have been noted for marijuana smoking as well. Smoking also accelerates the risk for myocardial infarction, sudden death, cerebrovascular disease, peripheral vascular disease, and hypertension, and it reduces HDL concentrations. Clearly, primary prevention is needed for this risk factor, and much of the education effort to discourage initiation of smoking should be targeted to teenagers. Techniques for cessation of smoking that may be useful include aversive conditioning, group programs, self-help programs, hypnosis, "cold turkey," and the use of nicotine substitutes (lobeline) or other sources of nicotine (Nicorette chewing gum and transdermal nicotine systems) for short-term substitution during withdrawal syndrome. Cessation of smoking reduces the incidence of coronary events to about 15% to 25% of that associated with continued smoking, and these benefits are noted within 2 years of cessation.[32]

Hypertension, whether labile or fixed, borderline or definite, casual or basal, systolic or diastolic, at any age regardless of gender is the most common and a powerful contributor to atherosclerotic coronary vascular disease.[33] Morbidity and mortality increase progressively with the degree of elevation of either systolic or diastolic pressure and pulse pressure, and no discernible critical value exists (see Chap. 13). Numerous trials have documented the reduction in risk associated with blood pressure lowering; however, most of these studies show that mortality and morbidity reduction is a result of fewer strokes and less renal failure and heart failure. The reduction in coronary heart disease end points is significant but not as dramatic. The reasons for this are unclear but perhaps relate to the multifactorial etiology of IHD.

Hypercholesterolemia is a significant cardiovascular risk factor, and risk is related directly to the degree of cholesterol elevation.[20] As with hypertension, there is no critical value that defines risk, but rather, risk is related incrementally to the degree of elevation and the presence of other risk factors (see Chap. 21 for a detailed discussion). A fasting lipoprotein panel should be obtained in all patients with known CAD. The goals for total, LDL, and HDL cholesterol and triglycerides are discussed in Chap. 21. All patients should undertake therapeutic lifestyle changes. Reductions in LDL cholesterol for primary prevention and secondary intervention have been shown to reduce total and CAD mortality and stroke, as well as the need for interventions such as PTCA and CABG. Supplemental vitamin E or other antioxidants reduce the susceptibility of LDL cholesterol to oxidation, but clinical trial data have failed to show any benefit with supplementation.[34]

The prevalence of obesity, defined as greater than 20% over ideal body weight, ranges from 7.4% to 17% in men and from 9.6% to 34.7% in women in this country. Body mass index, weight (in kilogams) divided by height (in meters) squared, greater than about 32 is associated with an increased mortality ratio compared with individuals of normal body weight, and the objective for patients with IHD is to maintain or reduce to a normal body weight. This may be accomplished through dietary modification, exercise, pharmacologic therapy, or surgical therapy. Frequently associated with obesity is a sedentary lifestyle, and inactivity may contribute to higher blood pressure, elevated blood lipid levels, and insulin resistance associated with glucose intolerance in diabetics (insulin resistance syndrome). Exercise to the level of about 300 kcal three times a week is useful in improving maximal oxygen uptake, improving cardiorespiratory efficiency, promoting collateral artery formation, and promoting potential alterations in the risk of ventricular fibrillation, coronary thrombosis, and improved tolerance to stress. Epidemiologic studies have found that mortality is related directly to resting heart rate and a low heart rate difference between resting and maximal exercise heart rates and inversely related to exercise heart rate.[35] Although a regular exercise program may not reduce CVD mortality, participants feel better, and their overall cardiovascular risk may be reduced.[36]

Competitiveness, intense striving for achievement, easily provoked hostility, a sense of urgency about doing things quickly and being punctual, impatience, abrupt and rapid speech and gestures, and concentration on self-selected goals to the point of not perceiving and attending to other aspects of the environment are traits that characterize the behavioral pattern known as the *type A* or *coronary-prone personality*. Although the issue is somewhat controversial, type A individuals may have increased cardiovascular risk, with risk ratios ranging from insignificant to three times that of a matched population. The mechanism by which personality affects the cardiovascular system is not understood but may reflect the activity of the sympathetic system and enhanced responsiveness of other stress hormones when compared with non–type A personalities.

Alcohol ingestion in small to moderate amounts (<40 g/day of pure ethanol) reduces the risk of CAD; however, consumption of large amounts (>50 g/day) or binge drinking of alcohol is associated with increased mortality from stroke, cancer, vehicular accidents, and cirrhosis. The mechanisms for the presumed protective effects of alcohol are not known, but the effects may be related to increased HDL levels, impaired platelet function, or associations between the amount of alcohol ingested and personality type. Whatever the relationship, it is well to remember that alcohol drinking is implicated in over 40% of all fatal automobile accidents and that consumption of alcohol predisposes to hepatic cirrhosis, the sixth to seventh most common cause of death in middle age in the United States. With this in mind, it seems illogical to suggest alcohol ingestion as a prophylactic measure for CAD but rather advise moderation in alcohol consumption, if it is the preference of the individual.

Thiazide diuretics have been shown to elevate serum cholesterol and triglyceride levels, whereas β-blockers tend to lower HDL and raise LDL slightly; however, a direct association between these drugs and cardiovascular risk is tenuous and based on aggregating results rather than randomized clinical trials. Conjugated equine estrogen alone or in combination with progestin lowers LDL and raises HDL based on the Postmenopausal Estrogen/Progestin Interventions (PEPI) study.[37] Unfortunately, the HERS trial showed no benefit of hormone-replacement therapy (HRT) for secondary intervention and increased risk for thromboembolism.[38] In secondary intervention, HRT or estrogen alone in women after hysterectomy found that hormonal therapy health risks exceeded benefits as well.[39] Unopposed estrogen is the optimal regimen for elevation of HDL, but the high rate of endometrial hyperplasia restricts use to women without a uterus. In women with a uterus, estrogen with cyclic medroxyprogesterone has the most favorable effect on HDL and no excess risk of endometrial hyperplasia. Use of oral contraceptives in women who smoke and are over the age of 35 years increases the risk of MI, stroke, and venous thromboembolism by threefold or higher. Alternative forms of contraception and cessation of smoking should be promoted in these patients. The risk for nonsmoking oral contraceptive users under the age of 35 is very small. The relative risk of breast cancer is increased but in the absence of risk factors for breast cancer, the relative risk is approximately 1.3 (30% increase). Coffee consumption also has been linked to CAD, and caffeine does transiently elevate blood pressure; however, the overall risk, if any, appears to be low. Although thiazide diuretics and β-blockers (nonselective without intrinsic sympathomimetic activity) may elevate both cholesterol and triglycerides by some 10% to 20%, and these effects may be detrimental, no objective evidence exists from prospective, well-controlled studies to support avoiding these drugs at this time. This controversy is most pertinent in the treatment of mild hypertension, and it is discussed in greater detail in Chap. 13.

► TREATMENT: Stable Exertional Angina Pectoris

The current national guidelines recommend that all patients be given the following unless contraindications exist: (1) aspirin, (2) β-blockers with prior MI, (3) angiotensin-converting enzyme (ACE) inhibitor to patients with CAD and diabetes or LV systolic dysfunction, (4) LDL-lowering therapy with CAD and an LDL concentration greater than130 mg/dL (*Note:* this is likely to be lowered to less than 100 mg/dL after recent statin trials have shown benefit; see Chap. 21), (5) sublingual nitroglycerin for immediate relief of angina, (6) calcium antagonists or long-acting nitrates for reduction of symptoms when β-blockers are contraindicated, (7) calcium antagonists or long-acting nitrates in combination with β-blockers when initial treatment with β-blockers is not successful, and (8) calcium antagonists or long-acting nitrates as a substitute for β-blockers if initial treatment with β-blockers leads to unacceptable side effects.[1]

After assessing and manipulating the alterable risk factors, as discussed previously, the next intervention that could be undertaken is the institution of a regular exercise program. Training is possible in many patients with angina, and the observed benefits include decreased heart rate and systolic blood pressure and increased ejection fraction and duration of exercise. Although the mechanism of these effects has been debated, improved overall cardiovascular and muscular conditions are probably most important. Improved production of nitric oxide and coronary vasomotion may account partially for the beneficial effects of exercise. The intensity of exercise influences training, and more vigorous programs provide better overall results.[14,40] Obviously, an exercise program should be undertaken with caution and in a graded fashion with adequate supervision.

5 Chronic prophylactic therapy for patients with more than one angina episode per day also may be instituted with β-adrenergic blocking agents, and in many instances, β-blockers may be preferable because of less frequent dosing and other properties inherent in β-blockade (e.g., potential cardioprotective effects, antiarrhythmic effects, lack of tolerance, and antihypertensive effects), as well as their antianginal effects and documented protective effects in post-MI patients.[1] Patients who continue to smoke have reduced antianginal efficacy of β-blockers. This may be due to enhanced hepatic metabolism of drugs that are eliminated through this route or related to the effects of smoking on MVO_2 and oxygenation.

The one characteristic that is relevant is the duration of effect on the DP. β-Blockers with longer half-lives (e.g., nadolol) are more likely to affect the DP for a longer period of time and require fewer doses per day. The choice of β-blocker for angina rests on selecting the appropriate dose to achieve the goals outlined for heart rate and DP and choosing an agent that is well tolerated by individual patients and of acceptable cost. Selective use may incorporate ancillary properties, but these are secondary considerations in overall drug product selection. Patients most likely to respond well to β-blockade are those who have a high resting heart rate and those having a relatively fixed anginal threshold. In other words, their symptoms appear at the same level of exercise or workload on a consistent basis. Symptoms appearing with variable workloads suggest fluctuations in myocardial oxygen supply, perhaps due to coronary artery vasomotion, and these patients are more likely to respond to calcium channel antagonists.

6 Nitrate therapy should be the first step in managing acute attacks for patients with chronic stable angina if the attacks are infrequent (i.e., a few times per month) or for prophylaxis of symptoms when undertaking activities known to precipitate attacks. In general, if angina occurs no more often than once every few days, then sublingual nitroglycerin tablets or spray or buccal products may be sufficient to allow the patient to maintain an adequate lifestyle. For episodes of "first effort" angina occurring in a predictable fashion, nitroglycerin may be used in a prophylactic manner with the patient taking 0.3 to 0.4 mg sublingually about 5 minutes prior to the anticipated time of activity. Nitroglycerin spray may be useful when inadequate saliva is produced to rapidly dissolve sublingual nitroglycerin or if a patient has difficulty opening the container. Most patients have a response that lasts about 30 minutes or so, but this is subject to interindividual variability.

When angina occurs more frequently than once a day, a chronic prophylactic regimen using β-blockers as the first line of therapy should be considered (see Fig. 15–4 for a stable angina algorithm). Chronic prophylactic therapy with long-acting forms of nitroglycerin (oral or transdermal), isosorbide dinitrate, 5-mononitrate, and pentaerythritol trinitrate may be effective; however, the development of tolerance is a major limiting step in their continued effectiveness. Since long-acting nitrates are not as effective as β-blockers and do not have beneficial effects, monotherapy with nitrates should not be first-line therapy unless β-blockers and calcium channel blockers are contraindicated or not tolerated.

As described previously, providing a nitrate-free interval of 8 hours per day or longer appears to be the most promising approach to maintaining the efficacy of chronic nitrate therapy. Oral administration of nitrates is susceptible to a saturable first-pass effect; therefore, larger doses can produce a measurable hemodynamic effect, and dose titration should be based on these changes in the DP. There are few well-controlled studies comparing oral or sublingual nitrate efficacy, and the choice among these products should be based on familiarity with the preparation, cost, and patient acceptance.

7 Calcium channel antagonists have the potential advantage of improving coronary blood flow through coronary artery vasodilation, as well as decreasing MVO_2, and they may be used instead of β-blockers for chronic prophylactic therapy. However, in chronic stable angina, comparative trials of long-acting calcium channel blockers with β-blockers do not show significant differences in response.[41,42] They are as effective as β-blockers and are most useful in patients who have a variable threshold for exertional angina. Calcium antagonists may provide better skeletal muscle oxygenation, resulting in decreased fatigue and better exercise tolerance. Additionally, if contraindications exist to β-blocker therapy, calcium antagonists can be used safely in many patients. The available calcium channel blockers appear to have similar efficacy in the management of chronic stable angina.

Differences in their electrophysiology, peripheral and central hemodynamic effects, and adverse-effect profiles are useful in selecting the appropriate agent. Patients with conduction abnormalities and moderate to severe LV dysfunction (ejection fraction <35%) should not be treated with verapamil, whereas amlodipine may be used safely in many of these patients. Diltiazem has significant effects on the atrioventricular node and can produce heart block in patients with preexisting conduction disease or when other drugs, such as digoxin or β-blockers, with effects on conduction are used concurrently. Nifedipine may cause excessive heart rate elevation, especially if the patient is not receiving a β-blocker, and this may offset the beneficial effect it has on MVO_2. Gingival hyperplasia also has been reported with nifedipine, and some dental authorities say that this may be seen in as many as 20% of patients on nifedipine. Bepridil prolongs the QT interval in patients with certain conditions (e.g., hypokalemia, advanced age, and preexisting QT-interval prolongation), and because of this potential proarrhythmic effect, it is indicated only in patients who have been inadequately controlled with other antianginal therapy.

Case-control studies with calcium blockers suggest an increased risk for MI and cancer.[43,44] The relationship to cancer appears to be weak to nonexistent, whereas the risk for MI is probably real and related to the type of drug used and the relationship to recent MI. Shorter-acting calcium blockers can activate the sympathetic nervous system and in patients with recent MI or significant CAD may induce ischemia. This effect has not been shown for longer-acting products. The hemodynamic effect of calcium antagonists is complementary to β-blockade, and consequently, combination therapy is rational, but clinical trial data do not support the notion that combination therapy is always more effective.[41,45]

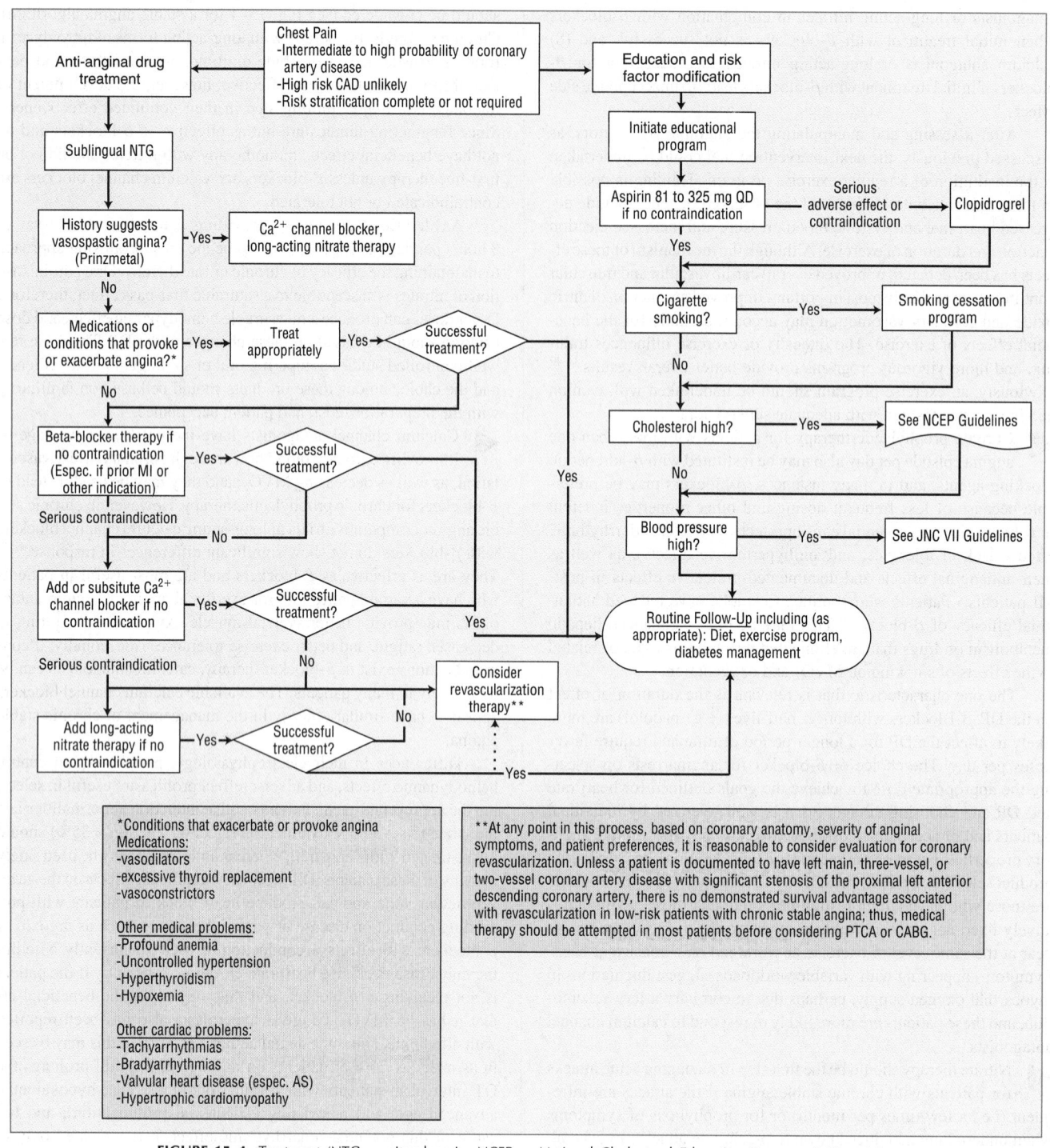

FIGURE 15–4. Treatment (NTG = nitroglycerin; NCEP = National Cholesterol Education Program; JNC = Joint National Committee; AS = aortic stenosis).

NONPHARMACOLOGIC THERAPY

REVASCULARIZATION

The decision to choose percutaneous coronary intervention (PCI) or CABG for revascularization is based on the extent of CAD (number of vessels and location/amount of stenosis) and ventricular function. The recommended mode of coronary revascularization is outlined in Table 15–6.[16]

The largest randomized trial of PCI versus CABG is the Bypass Angioplasty Revascularization (BARI) trial conducted in 1829 patients with two- or three-vessel disease; 64% of these patients had an admitting diagnosis of unstable angina (UA), and 19% were diabetic.[46] Seven-year survival for the total population was 84.4% for CABG and 80.9% for PTCA ($p = .043$). Patients with diabetes mellitus undergoing CABG had improved survival compared with nondiabetics (76.4% CABG and 55.7% PTCA; $p = .0011$). Among the remaining 1,476 patients without treated diabetes, survival was

TABLE 15–6. Recommended Mode of Coronary Revascularization

Extent of Disease	Treatment	Class/Level of Evidence
Left main disease,[a] candidate for CABG	CABG	I/A
	PCI	III/C
Left main disease, not a candidate for CABG	PCI	IIb/C
Three-vessel disease with EF < 0.50	CABG	I/A
Multivessel disease including proximal LAD with EF < 0.50 or treated diabetes	CABG	I/A
	PCI	IIb/B
Multivessel disease with EF > 0.50 and without diabetes	PCI	I/A
One- or two-vessel disease without proximal LAD but with large areas of myocardial ischemia or high-risk criteria on noninvasive testing (see text)	CABG or PCI	I/B
One-vessel disease with proximal LAD	CBAG or PCI	IIa/B
One- or two-vessel disease without proximal LAD with small area of ischemia or no ischemia on noninvasive testing	CABG or PCI	III/C
Insignificant coronary stenosis	CABG or PCI	III/C

[a]≥50% diameter stenosis.

Abbreviations: CABG = coronary artery bypass grafting: PCI = percutaneous coronary intervention; EF = ejection fraction; LAD = left anterior descending coronary artery. Class I evidence means conditions for which there is evidence and/or general agreement that a given procedure or treatment is useful and effective. Class IIa evidence means conditions for which there is conflicting evidence and/or divergence of opinion about usefulness/efficacy of a procedure or treatment. Class IIa indicates that the weight of evidence/opinion is in favor of usefulness/efficacy. Class IIb indicates that the usefulness/efficacy is less well established. Class III indicates that the evidence and/or general agreement that the procedure/treatment is not useful or effective and may be harmful. Level A evidence is derived from multiple randomized clinical trials with large numbers of patients. Level B evidence is derived from limited number of trials with small numbers of patients or from nonrandomized trials or observational studies. Level C evidence is based on expert opinion. *From Braunwald E, Antman EM, Beasley JW, et al. ACC/AHA guidelines for the management of patients with unstable angina and non-ST-segment elevation myocardial infarction: A report of the American College of Cardiology/American Heart Association Task Force on Practice Guidelines (Committee on the Management of Patients with Unstable Angina). J Am Coll Cardiol 2000;36:970–1062, with permission.*

virtually identical by assigned treatment (86.4% CABG, 86.8% PTCA; $p = .72$). The PTCA group had substantially higher subsequent revascularization rates than the CABG group (59.7% versus 13.1%; $p < .001$); however, the changes between the 5- and 7-year rates were similar for the two groups. Insulin-requiring diabetics seem to be at the highest risk, and CABG is the revascularization procedure of choice for this population.[47] In a large observational study by Hannan and colleagues, patients with proximal left anterior descending coronary artery (LAD) lesions and multivessel disease had higher survival rates with CABG than with PTCA.[48] High-risk patients who should be considered for CABG over PCI are those with LV systolic dysfunction, patients with diabetes, and those with two-vessel disease with severe proximal LAD involvement or severe three-vessel or left main artery disease[16] (Table 15–7). AWESOME (Angina With Extremely Serious Operative Mortality) is a large, randomized trial comparing PTCA with CABG, and the results should further define which method of revascularization is best for patients with refractory ischemia and high risk of adverse outcomes.[49]

PCI has been used successfully in the management of UA.[50–52] PTCA involves the insertion of a guidewire and inflatable balloon into the affected coronary artery and enlarging the lumen of the artery by stretching the vessel wall. This frequently causes atheroma plaque fracture by stretching inelastic components and denuding the endothelium, resulting in loss of nitric oxide and other vasodilators and exposure of plaque contents to the vascular compartment. Consequently, immediate vascular recoil, platelet adhesion and aggregation, mural thrombus formation, and smooth muscle proliferation and synthesis of extracellular matrix may give rise to acute occlusion and early or late restenosis.[53,54] The presence of coronary artery spasm and intraluminal thrombus, common occurrences in UA, increases the hazard

of these complications. The advent of combination therapy with aspirin, unfractionated heparin (UFH) or low-molecular-weight heparin (LMWH), and glycoprotein (GP) IIb/IIIa receptor antagonists and coronary artery stents has reduced the occurrence of early reocclusion and late restenosis dramatically.[16,50] Patients best suited for PTCA are those with recent onset of worsening of angina without a long history of symptoms. Angiographic characteristics associated with these clinical findings that allow the greatest probability of success for PTCA are severe, discrete, proximal lesions found in a large epicardial vessel subtending a moderate or large area of viable myocardium and have high risk. Patients with focal saphenous vein graft lesions who are poor candidates for reoperation have a class IIa recommendation for PCI. Class IIb indications include patients with one or more lesions to be dilated in vessels subtending a less than moderate area of viable myocardium and patients with multivessel disease and proximal LAD lesions, diabetes, or abnormal LV function.[50]

Candidates for PTCA also must be suited for CABG because a small percentage of procedures results in emergency CABG. Success of PCI may be defined as angiographic success (TIMI 3 flow and less than 20% residual stenosis), procedural success (lack of in-hospital clinical complications), and clinical success (anatomic and procedural success with relief of ischemic pain for at least 6 months). In trials of invasive versus conservative strategies (medical management) using PCI, death, or MI is less frequent in some trials but not all.[51,55–57] Numerous studies support the use of IIb/IIIa receptor antagonists in addition to aspirin and UFH or LMWH, and as described previously, abciximab was superior to tirofiban in the only comparative study available.[16,50] The initial success rate for PTCA in UA is approximately 80% to 90%, but these patients are at risk for

TABLE 15–7. Recommendations for Primary Coronary Intervention Based on Angina Classification

Class I	Class IIa	Class IIb	Class III
Class I Angina			
Patients who do not have treated diabetes with asymptomatic ischemia or mild angina with one or more significant lesions in one or two coronary arteries suitable for PCI with a high likelihood of success and a low risk of morbidity and mortality	The same clinical and anatomic requirements for class I, except the myocardial area at risk is of moderate size or the patient has treated diabetes	Patients with asymptomatic ischemia or mild angina with three or more coronary arteries suitable for PCI with a high likelihood of success and a low risk of morbidity	Patients with asymptomatic ischemia or mild angina who do not meet the criteria listed under class I or II and who have a. Only a small area of viable myocardium at risk b. No objective evidence of ischemia c. Lesions that have a low likelihood of successful dilation d. Mild symptoms that are unlikely to be due to myocardial ischemia e. Factors associated with increased risk of morbidity or mortality f. Left main disease g. Insignificant disease
The vessels to be dilated must subtend a large area of viable myocardium		The vessels to be dilated must subtend at least a moderate area of viable myocardium In the physician's judgment, there should be evidence of myocardial ischemia such as ECG exercise testing, stress nuclear imaging, stress echocardiography, ambulatory ECG monitoring, or intracoronary physiologic measurements	
Class II-IV Angina, UA/NSTEMI			
Patients with one or more significant lesions in one or more coronary arteries suitable for PCI with a high likelihood of success and a low risk of morbidity and mortality	Patients with focal saphenous vein graft lesions or multiple stenoses who are poor candidates for reoperative surgery	Patient has one or more lesions to be dilated with reduced likelihood of success or the vessel(s) subtend less than moderate area of viable myocardium	Patient has no evidence or myocardial injury or ischemia on objective testing and has not had a trial of medical therapy or has a. Only a small area of myocardium at risk b. All lesions or the culprit lesion to be dilated with morphology with a low likelihood of success c. A high risk of procedure-related morbidity or mortality
The vessel(s) to be dilated should subtend a moderate or large area of viable myocardium and have high risk		Patients with two- or three-vessel disease, with significant proximal LAD CAD and treated diabetes or abnormal LV function	Patients with insignificant coronary stenosis (e.g., <50% diameter)
			Patients with left main CAD who are candidates for CABG

Note: See Table 15–6 for definitions for class I to III recommendations.
Abbreviations: PCI = primary coronary intervention; ECG = electrocardiogram; LAD = left anterior descending coronary artery; CAD = coronary artery disease; LV = left ventricular; CABG = coronary artery bypass grafting.
From ACC/AHA guidelines of percutaneous coronary interventions (revision of the 1993 PTCA guidelines): Executive summary. A report of the American College of Cardiology/American Heart Association Task Force on Practice Guidelines. J Am Coll Cardiol 2001;37:22391–lxvi, with permission.

more complications than are those with stable angina because of the underlying pathophysiology.

In the event of prolonged chest pain and ischemic ECG changes unrelieved by nitrate therapy or calcium channel antagonists, one may assume total occlusion of a coronary vessel, and steps should be taken to restore blood flow with either PCI or CABG.

CORONARY ARTERY BYPASS GRAFTING

Following the introduction of saphenous vein graft replacement for the severely occluded coronary arteries by Favorolo and Garrett in 1967, coronary artery bypass grafting (CABG) became an accepted and commonly used approach for the management of IHD. The objectives in performing CABG are twofold: (1) to reduce the number of symptomatic anginal attacks not controlled with medical management or PCI and improve the lifestyle of the patient and (2) to reduce the mortality associated with CAD. Surgery is effective in providing pain relief in large numbers of patients, with about 70% to 95% being pain-free at 1 year and 46% to 55% being pain-free at 5 years. This compares favorably with medical management, with which only about 30% are free of symptoms at 5 years. Mortality at 10 years from the largest published studies is 26.4% with CABG and 30.5% with medical management ($p = .03$), but there are significant differences based on subgroup analysis (e.g., left main coronary artery disease versus one-vessel without a proximal LAD lesion).[58] The second objective is met in certain patients, and this has been addressed in three large, well-controlled trials of bypass surgery. These three studies, the Veterans Administration (VA) study, the European Cooperative Surgery Study (ECSS), and the Coronary Artery Surgery Study (CASS), are not directly comparable because the inclusion and exclusion criteria for entry into each study were different and patients were followed for different periods of time. They also have been criticized for not being representative of the population that may be candidates for surgery, lacking women or late-middle-aged and elderly patients, and for crossover of medically managed patients to the surgical group. A major change in medical practice that influences the interpretation of these older studies is the common procedure of stent placement at the time of angioplasty.[59] There are about 20 different types of stents available, and their use is associated with greater luminal diameter after angioplasty, fewer acute reocclusions, and less restenosis after stent placement. Consequently, the validity of generalizing the results from these studies to routine practice has been questioned, but these studies are useful for providing a basis for decisions concerning surgery.

Current class I recommendations for CABG in asymptomatic or mild angina patient include significant (>50%) left main coronary artery stenosis, left main equivalent (≥70% stenosis of the proximal LAD and proximal left circumflex artery), and three-vessel disease, especially in patients with an LV ejection fraction of less than 0.50.[58] Class IIa recommendations for CABG are proximal LAD stenosis with one- or two-vessel disease and class IIb one- or two-vessel disease not involving the proximal LAD. In stable angina, class I recommendations are the same as for mild angina with the following additions: one- or two-vessel disease without significant proximal LAD stenosis but with a large area of viable myocardium and high-risk criteria in noninvasive testing and disabling angina despite maximal medical therapy when surgery can be performed with acceptable risk. Class IIb recommendations in stable angina include proximal LAD stenosis with one-vessel disease and one- or two-vessel disease without significant proximal LAD stenosis but with a moderate area of viable myocardium and ischemia on noninvasive testing. The indications for CABG in UA/NSTEMI were described previously. In STEMI, CABG is indicated for ongoing ischemia/infarction not responsive to maximal medical therapy (class IIb).

In patients with poor LV function, CABG is employed for the same indications as in mild angina for class I. Class IIa recommendations include poor LV function with significant viable, noncontracting, revascularizable myocardium without any of the aforementioned anatomic patterns (e.g., left main coronary artery disease). CABG is useful in patients with life-threatening ventricular arrhythmia in the presence of left main coronary artery disease and three-vessel disease (class I), in bypassable one- or two-vessel disease causing life-threatening ventricular arrhythmias, and in proximal LAD disease with one- or two-vessel disease (class IIa).

CABG also may be used for patients who have failed PTCA if there is ongoing ischemia or threatened occlusion with significant myocardium at risk and in patients with hemodynamic compromise (class I). Class IIa recommendations for failed PTCA include a foreign body in a crucial anatomic position and hemodynamic compromise in patients with impairment of the coagulation system and without a previous sternotomy. CABG may be repeated in patients with a previous CABG if disabling angina exists despite maximal noninvasive therapy (class I) and if a large area of myocardium is threatened and is subtended by bypassable distal vessels (class IIa).

The need for nitrates and β-blockers clearly is reduced by surgery, with only 30% of CABG patients requiring chronic medication, in contrast to 70% of their medical counterparts who receive anginal drugs. Employment status after surgery has been shown in CASS to be more dependent on the pretreatment status than on an effect induced by the treatment arm, and about 70% of patients are employed before and after surgery. Recent follow-up analyses of these studies suggest that patients who have diabetes or peripheral vascular disease, who are African-Americans, or who continued to smoke are at high risk for CAD events, and diabetics in particular are more likely to have a better outcome with CABG than with PTCA.[46,60,61] The overall benefit noted after CABG is similar in men and women, and elderly patients appear to have outcomes similar to younger patients.

Operative mortality is reported to range from 1% to 3% and is related to the number of vessels involved and preoperative ventricular function. Patients in CASS with one-, two-, or three-vessel disease had operative mortalities of 1.4%, 2.1%, and 2.8%, respectively. The relationship to LV ejection fraction follows a similar trend, with patients with ejection fractions of greater than 50%, 20% to 40%, and less than 20% having operative mortality rates of 1.9%, 4.4%, and 6.7%, respectively. Perioperative infarction averages 5% depending on the sensitivity of the method for assessment, and the occurrence of an infarct reduces long-term survival. Neurologic dysfunction is relatively common postoperatively in CABG patients (~6%), but many of the deficits are insignificant clinically and resolve with time. Fatal brain damage occurs in 0.3% to 0.7%, stroke in about 5%, and ophthalmologic defects in 25%, but only 3% have clinically apparent field defects. Peripheral nerve lesions (12%) and brachial plexopathy (7%) are also reported to occur. Other complications include constrictive pericarditis (0.2%), cellulitis at the site of the vein graft, and mediastinal infections (1% to 4%).

Graft patency influences the success for symptom control and survival, and the mechanism for early graft occlusion is probably different from that associated with late closure. Early occlusion is related to platelet adhesion and aggregation, whereas late occlusion may be related to endothelial proliferation and progression of atherosclerosis. Patency of grafts early on after the CABG is reported to range from 88% to 97% in at least one graft and 58% to 81% in all grafts at 1 year. Long-term patency based on the CASS Montreal Heart Institute experience suggests that 60% to 67% of all grafts remain patent at 5 to 11 years. Antiplatelet therapy has been demonstrated to improve early and late patency rates and probably should be used in all patients who do not have any contraindications. Aspirin with or without other antiplatelet agents (dipyridamole) reduces the late development of vein graft occlusions. Late graft closure is related to elevated lipid levels and the progression of atherosclerosis in the grafted vessels as well as the native circulation. Elevation of very low-density lipoprotein (VLDL), LDL, and LDL apolipoprotein B is correlated with disease progression and graft closure. Aggressive lipid lowering can stabilize the progression of CAD and may induce regression in selected coronary artery segments within a patient following CABG. Cessation of smoking is an important preoperative and postoperative objective, as well as in the management of other coronary risk factors (e.g., hypertension), and institution of a supervised daily exercise program is recommended. Internal mammary artery grafts should be used for revascularizing the LAD system when possible owing to better graft survival and clinical outcomes.

Valvular heart disease can coexist with CAD, although this is relatively uncommon with rheumatic valve disease, usually the mitral valve, and more common with aortic stenosis and regurgitation. Angina may occur in 35% to 65% of patients with aortic stenosis or regurgitation and, if severe, may be the cause of angina in the absence of CAD. Patients being evaluated for possible CABG also should be evaluated for valvular disease to determine if valve replacement needs to be performed along with bypass grafting.

■ PERCUTANEOUS TRANSLUMINAL CORONARY ANGIOPLASTY[62]

Since the introduction into clinical cardiology of PTCA[63,64] by Gruentzig in 1977, this procedure has gained rapid acceptance as a safe and effective means of managing CAD. It is estimated that more than 750,000 PCI procedures are done each year in this country, and 525,000 of them are PTCAs. The proposed mechanisms of reduced stenosis with PTCA include (1) compression and redistribution of the atherosclerotic plaque, (2) embolization of plaque contents, (3) aneurysm formation, and (4) disruption of the plaque and arterial wall with distortion and tearing of the intima and media, which leads to denudation of the endothelium, platelet adhesion and aggregation, thrombus formation, and smooth muscle proliferation. Of these mechanisms, the last one is felt to be the most important, but the others may contribute to opening of the lesions in some situations.

The indications for PTCA have been provided by the ACC/AHA and now span single- or multivessel disease as well as asymptomatic and symptomatic patients[50] (see Table 15–7). PTCA generally is not useful if only a small area of viable myocardium is at risk, when ischemia cannot be demonstrated, with borderline (<50%) stenosis or with lesions that are difficult to dilate, or in patients who are at high risk for morbidity or mortality or both (e.g., left main or equivalent disease or three-vessel disease). PTCA alone or in conjunction or sequentially with thrombolysis for acute MI is discussed in Chap. 16. Stent placement accompanies balloon angioplasty in about 80% of cases in the United States. The current recommendations for PCI are provided in Table 15–7 based on class of angina.

Assessment of outcome with PCI can be based on several angiographic, procedural, and clinical outcomes, as discussed previously. The success of PCI depends on the experience of the operator (i.e., high volume, better outcome), on complicating factors for the patient (including the number of vessels to be dilated), and on technical advances in the equipment used (e.g., steerable and low-profile catheters). The acute success rate for opening of uncomplicated stenotic lesions ranges from 96% to 99% with the combined balloon-device–pharmacologic approach in experienced hands, and angina is decreased or eliminated in about 80% of cases. The success rate in totally occluded lesions is somewhat less (~65%). Mortality at 1 year is 1% and 2.5% for single-vessel disease and multiple-vessel involvement, respectively, reflecting the good prognosis associated with this degree of CAD. At 10 years, survival is 95% and 81% for single- and multiple-vessel disease, respectively.[50] Most patients remain event-free (no death, MI, or CABG) for an extended period.

Symptomatic status, as measured by the NYHA classification, is improved in many patients. Restenosis is noted in 32% to 40% of patients after balloon angioplasty at 6 months, and half these patients will have symptoms associated with restenosis.[50] A few late restenotic events occur, but most restenosis occurs within the first 6 months. Anatomic factors that predict restenosis include lesions greater than 20 mm in length, excessive tortuosity of the proximal segment, extremely angulated segments (>90 degrees), total occlusions more than 3 months old and/or bridging collaterals, inability to protect the major side branches, and degenerated vein grafts with friable lesions. Clinical factors that predict worse outcome include diabetes, advanced age, female gender, UA, heart failure, and multivessel disease. A four-variable scoring system that predicts cardiovascular collapse for failed PTCA includes percentage of myocardium at risk (e.g., >50% viable myocardium at risk and LV ejection fraction <25%), preangioplasty percent diameter stenosis, multivessel CAD, and diffuse disease in the dilated segment or a high myocardial jeopardy score.[50] Strut thickness of the stent influences restenosis as well, and thicker struts are associated with angiographic and clinical restenosis.[65]

The overall complication rate ranges from 2% to 21% depending on the lesion type.[52] Coronary occlusion, dissection, or spasm occurs in 4% to 8% of patients, whereas Q-wave MI occurs in 1.6% to 4.8%.[50] Prolonged angina and ventricular tachycardia or fibrillation occurs in 6.9% and 2.3%, respectively. In-hospital mortality ranges from 0.7% to 2.5% overall, and high-risk events for mortality include ventricular arrhythmias and myocardial infarction. The frequency of urgent CABG because of complications ranges from 0.4% to 5.8%.[50]

Antiplatelet therapy with aspirin 81 to 325 mg/day given at least 2 hours prior to angioplasty is currently recommended. If patients are sensitive to aspirin, clopidogrel and ticlopidine are acceptable alternatives. Most centers now use clopidogrel owing to adverse effects. In elective settings, clopidogrel should be started at least 72 hours in advance of the procedure to allow for maximal antiplatelet effects. Alternatively, a loading dose of clopidogrel (300 to 600 mg) may be given to achieve a more rapid antiplatelet effect.[66] The combination of aspirin and clopidogrel currently is recommended for patients undergoing angioplasty and stenting, and this combination is safer and superior to antiplatelet therapy plus anticoagulation with warfarin-like drugs.[67] Follow-up for up to 4 years from the Intracoronary Stenting and Antithrombotic Regimen (ISAR) trial shows that the benefit of combined antiplatelet therapy evident after 30 days is maintained after 4 years.[68] Aspirin is an incomplete inhibitor of platelet aggregation, and combination therapy with aspirin and a GP IIb/IIIa receptor antagonist for PCI has shown a relative risk reduction of 37.5% for death and nonfatal MI at 30 days, favoring GP IIb/IIIa receptor antagonists over placebo (absolute rates of 5.5% versus 8.9% based on PCI trials of EPIC, IMPACT-II, EPILOG, CAPTURE, RESTORE, and EPISTENT).[50] High-risk patients and those having a stent placed are most likely to benefit from GP IIb/IIIa receptor antagonist use. Patients presenting with elevated cardiac biomarkers are also more likely to receive benefit from GP IIb/IIIa receptor antagonists than patients with normal levels of biomarkers.[69] In the only comparative trial (TARGET), abciximab was superior to tirofiban.[70]

During PTCA, patients usually are heparinized to prevent immediate thrombus formation at the site of arterial injury and on coronary guidewires and catheters; anticoagulation is continued for up to 24 hours. The intensity of anticoagulation is monitored using the activated clotting time (ACT), and the targeted range for ACT is 250 to 300 seconds (HemoTec device) in the absence of GP IIb/IIIa receptor antagonist use.[50] When GP IIb/IIIa receptor antagonists are not used, UFH is given as an intravenous bolus of 70 to 100 IU/kg to achieve a target ACT of 200 seconds. The loading dose is lowered to 50 to 70 IU/kg when GP IIb/IIIa receptor antagonists are given. Target ACT for eptifibatide and tirofiban is less than 300 seconds during angioplasty; postprocedural UFH infusions are not recommended during GP IIb/IIIa receptor antagonist therapy. Some authors have advocated heparin alternatives such as hirudin or hirulog, but there is no apparent long-term advantage with these agents.[71-73]

Mechanisms that result in restenosis include acute lumen loss owing to "recoil," mural thrombosis formation and smooth muscle cell proliferation with synthesis of extracellular matrix.[64] Approaches to preventing restenosis may be aimed at altering the underlying mechanisms. Recoil and loss of luminal diameter may be reduced by the use of stent placement; however, this beneficial effect is offset by an increased number of vascular complications. Cracking of the plaque leads to severe damage to the arterial wall, exposure of collagen, and endothelial dysfunction. These factors promote mural thrombi, and the propensity for thrombus formation is related in part to the composition of the plaque, as well as to the depth of injury. Combination therapy with aspirin, heparin, and GP IIb/IIIa receptor antagonists is recommended to minimize acute occlusion, and numerous clinical trials document the efficacy of this combined approach.[50] Unfortunately, antithrombotic therapy (i.e., warfarin, aspirin, dipyridamole, prostacyclin, UFH, hirudin, or antiplatelet combinations) has little effect on long-term restenosis rates.[74] Other pharmacologic interventions that have failed to alter restenosis include β-blockers, ACE inhibitors, calcium channel blockers, and omega-3 fatty acids. Pharmacologic therapy for which some evidence exists that restenosis may be prevented include investigational antiproliferative agents (e.g., trapidil, angiopeptin, and tranilast),[75-77] cilostanzol,[78] valsartan (angiotensin-receptor blocker)[79] enoxaparin,[80] and possibly ticlopidine.[81] One of the most promising approaches is the use of brachytherapy (local gamma or beta irradiation of the stent and surrounding tissue).[53,82] Intracoronary irradiation with iridium-192 resulted in lower rates of clinical and angiographic restenosis and the need for revascularization (43.8% versus 28.2% assigned to iridium-192; $p = .02$), although it also was associated with a higher rate of late thrombosis, resulting in an increased risk of MI. If the problem of late thrombosis within the stent can be overcome, intracoronary irradiation with iridium-192 may become a useful approach to the treatment of in-stent restenosis.[83]

Alternatives to PTCA include directional coronary atherectomy (DCA), excimer laser, rotational atherectomy (Rotablator), and intracoronary stents or some combination of these interventions.[84] Based on randomized trials, DCA produces greater initial luminal diameter but results in a higher rate of postprocedural complications such as non–Q-wave MI and death and is more expensive. Consequently, PTCA is considered to be superior to DCA for most patients. Tissue debulking with DCA is useful for in-stent restenosis,

particularly for diabetic patients.[85] The use of abciximab may improve these results.[86] Excimer laser angioplasty followed by balloon angioplasty or rotational atherectomy provides no benefit over balloon angioplasty alone.[87]

When medical therapy, PTCA, and CABG have been compared, low-risk patients with single-vessel CAD and normal LV function had greater alleviation of symptoms with PTCA than with medical treatment; mortality rates and rates of MI were unchanged. In high-risk patients (risk was defined by severity of ischemia, number of diseased vessels, and presence of LV dysfunction), improvement in survival was greater with CABG than with medical therapy. In moderate-risk patients with multivessel CAD (most had two-vessel disease and normal LV function), PTCA and CABG produced equivalent mortality rates and rates of MI.

PHARMACOLOGIC THERAPY (TABLE 15–8)

Historically, about 30% of anginal syndrome symptoms have responded regardless of which therapy was instituted. These observations stem from two problems inherent in clinical trials undertaken to assess the efficacy of any therapy for angina: (1) adequate trial design incorporating appropriate controls and washout periods and (2) assessment of treatment effects using objective measures of efficacy, including improvement in exercise performance, resting and ambulatory ECG improvement in ischemic changes, and other objective tests to address other aspects of myocardial function or metabolism. The use of pain episode frequency and nitroglycerin consumption is subjective, and their use as sole measures of efficacy should be avoided. Objective assessment using ETT has shown that placebo does not provide improvement in patients with exertional angina, substantiating this as a valid means to assess efficacy.

β-ADRENERGIC BLOCKING AGENTS[88]

Decreased heart rate, decreased contractility, and a slight to moderate decrease in blood pressure with β-adrenergic receptor antagonism reduce MVO$_2$. The predominant receptor type in the heart is the β_1-receptor, and competitive blockade minimizes the influence of endogenous catecholamines on the chronotropic and inotropic state of

TABLE 15–8. Recommendations for Pharmacologic Management of Patients Undergoing PCI

Drugs	Class I Angina	Class II–IV Angina, UA/NSTEMI	Transmural MI Acute-Phase MI	Hospital After Thrombolysis	Management Phase
Aspirin	I[a]	I	I	I	I
Clopidogrel[b]	I[e]	I	I	I	I[d]
Warfarin[c]	III	III	III	II	I[f]
GP blockers[g]	II	I	II	I	III
UFH/LMWH	I	I	I	II	III

[a]Roman numerals refer to ACC/AHA class recommendations for use. See Table 15–6 for definitions.
[b]In conjunction with stenting.
[c]To be given 24–48 hours before planned stenting, if possible.
[d]To be given 2–4 weeks after stent placement.
[e]In patients without atrial fibrillation or other preexisting clinical indications.
[f]Patients with anterior myocardial wall motion abnormalities or LV thrombus.
[g]Every indication may not apply to all available agents.

Abbreviations: PCI = primary coronary intervention; UA = unstable angina; NSTEMI = non–ST-segment myocardial infarction; MI = myocardial infarction; GP = glycoprotein receptor; UFH = unfractionated heparin; LMWH = low-molecular-weight heparin.
From ACC/AHA guidelines of percutaneous coronary Interventions (revision of the 1993 PTCA guidelines): Executive summary. A report of the American College of Cardiology/American Heart Association Task Force on Practice Guidelines. J Am Coll Cardiol 2001;37:2239i–lxvi, with permission.

TABLE 15–9. Effect of Drug Therapy on Myocardial Oxygen Demand[a]

	Heart Rate	Myocardial Contractility	LV Wall Tension — Systolic Pressure	LV Wall Tension — LV Volume
Nitrates	⇑	0	⇓	⇓⇓
β-Blockers	⇓⇓	⇓	⇓	⇑
Nifedipine	⇑	0 or ⇓	⇓⇓	0 or ⇓
Verapamil	⇓	⇓	⇓	0 or ⇓
Diltiazem	⇓⇓	0 or ⇓	⇓	0 or ⇓

[a]Calcium channel antagonists and nitrates also may increase myocardial oxygen supply through coronary vasodilation. Diastolic function also may be improved with verapamil, nifedipine, and perhaps, diltiazem. These effects may vary from those indicated in the table depending on individual patient baseline hemodynamics.
Abbreviation: LV = left ventricular.

the myocardium. These beneficial effects may be countered to some degree by the increased ventricular volume and ejection time seen with β-blockade; however, the overall effect of β-blockers in patients with effort-induced angina is a reduction in oxygen demand (Table 15–9). The β-blockers do not improve oxygen supply, and in certain instances, unopposed α-adrenergic stimulation following the use of β-blockers may lead to coronary vasoconstriction. For patients with chronic exertional stable angina, β-blockers improve symptoms about 80% of the time, and objective measures of efficacy demonstrate improved exercise duration and delay in the time at which ST-segment changes and initial or limiting symptoms occur. β-Blockers do not alter the rate-pressure product (DP) for maximal exercise, therefore substantiating reduced demand rather than improved supply as the major consequence of their actions. Reflex tachycardia from nitrate therapy can be blunted with β-blocker therapy, making this a common and useful combination. Although β-blockade may decrease exercise capacity in healthy individuals or in patients with hypertension, it may allow angina patients previously limited by symptoms to perform more exercise and ultimately to improve overall cardiovascular performance through a training effect. Ideal candidates for β-blockers include patients in whom physical activity figures prominently in their anginal attacks, those who have coexisting hypertension, those with a history of supraventricular arrhythmias or post-MI angina, and those who have a component of anxiety associated with angina.[89] β-Blockers also may be used safely in angina and heart failure, as described in Chap. 14.

Pertinent pharmacokinetics for the β-blockers includes half-life and route elimination, which are reviewed in Chap. 13. Drugs with longer half-lives need to be dosed less frequently than drugs with shorter half-lives; however, disparity exists between half-life and duration of action for several β-blockers (e.g., metoprolol), and this may reflect attenuation of the central nervous system–mediated effects on the sympathetic nervous system, as well as the direct effects of this category on heart rate and contractility. Renal and hepatic dysfunction can affect the disposition of β-blockers, but these agents are dosed to effect, either hemodynamic or symptomatic, and route of elimination is not a major consideration in drug selection. Guidelines for the use of β-blockers in treating angina include the objective of lowering resting heart rate to 50 to 60 beats per minute and limiting maximal exercise heart rate to about 100 beats per minute or less. It also has been suggested that exercise heart rate should be no more than about 20 beats per minute or a 10% increment over resting heart rate with modest exercise. Because β-blockade is competitive, circulating catecholamine

concentrations vary depending on the intensity of exercise and other factors, and cholinergic tone may be important in controlling resting heart rate in some patients, these guidelines are general in nature. These effects generally are dose- and plasma concentration–related, and for propranolol, plasma concentrations of 30 ng/mL are needed for a 25% reduction in anginal frequency. Initial doses of β-blockers should be at the lower end of the usual dosing range and titrated to response, as indicated earlier.

There is little evidence to suggest superiority of any β-blocker; however, the duration of β-blockade depends in part on the half-life of the agent used, and those with longer half-lives may be dosed less frequently. Of note, propranolol may be dosed twice a day in most patients with angina, and the efficacy is similar to that seen with more frequent dosing. The ancillary property of membrane-stabilizing activity is irrelevant in the treatment of angina, and intrinsic sympathomimetic activity appears to be detrimental in rest or severe angina because the reduction in heart rate would be minimized, therefore limiting a reduction in MVO_2. Cardioselective β-blockers may be used in some patients to minimize adverse effects such as bronchospasm in asthmatic or chronic obstructive pulmonary disease patients, intermittent claudication, and sexual dysfunction. It should be remembered that cardioselectivity is a relative property, and the use of larger doses (e.g., metoprolol 200 mg/day) is associated with loss of selectivity and with adverse effects. Patients with angina after acute MI are particularly good candidates for β-blockade both because anginal symptoms may be treated as well as reducing the risk of post-MI reinfarction and because mortality has been demonstrated with timolol, propranolol, and metoprolol (see Chap. 16). Combined β-nonselective and α-selective blockade with labetalol may be useful in some patients with marginal LV reserve, and fewer deleterious effects on coronary blood flow are seen when compared with other β-blockers. Extension of pharmacologic effect is the underlying reason for many of the adverse effects seen with β-blockade. Hypotension, heart failure, bradycardia and heart block, bronchospasm, peripheral vasoconstriction and intermittent claudication, and altered glucose metabolism are directly related to β-adrenoreceptor antagonism. Patients with preexisting LV dysfunction who use other negative inotropic agents are most prone to developing overt heart failure, and in the absence of these agents, heart failure is uncommon (<5%). Other drugs that depress conduction are additive to β-blockade, and intrinsic conduction system disease predisposes the patient to conduction abnormalities. Altered glucose metabolism is most likely to be seen in insulin-dependent diabetics, and β-blockade obscures the symptoms of hypoglycemia, except for sweating. β-Blockers also may aggravate the lipid abnormalities seen in patients with diabetes; however, these changes are dose-related, are more common with normal baseline lipids than with dyslipidemia, and may be of short-term significance only.

One of the more common reasons for discontinuation of β-blocker therapy is related to central nervous system adverse effects of fatigue, malaise, and depression. Cognition changes seen with β-blockers are usually minimal and comparable with those of other categories of drugs based on studies done in hypertension.[90,91] Abrupt withdrawal of β-blocker therapy in patients with angina has been associated with increased severity and number of pain episodes and MI. The mechanism of this effect is unknown but may be related to increased receptor sensitivity or disease progression during therapy that becomes apparent following discontinuation of β-blockade. In any event, tapering of β-blocker therapy over about 2 days should minimize the risk of withdrawal reactions for patients in whom therapy is being discontinued. β-Adrenoreceptor blockade is effective in chronic exertional angina as monotherapy and in combination with nitrates and/or calcium channel antagonists. β-Blockers should be the first-line drug in chronic angina requiring daily maintenance therapy because β-blockers are more effective in reducing episodes of silent ischemia, reducing early-morning peak of ischemic activity, and improving mortality after Q-wave MI than nitrates or calcium channel blockers[41] (see Fig. 15–4). If β-blockers are ineffective or not tolerated, then monotherapy with a calcium channel blocker or combination therapy if monotherapy is ineffective for either alone may be instituted. Patients with severe angina, rest angina, or variant angina (i.e., a component of coronary artery spasm) may be better treated with calcium channel blockers or long-acting nitrates.

▧ NITRATES[92,93]

Nitroglycerin has a well-documented role in the alleviation of anginal attacks when used as rapidly absorbed and readily available preparations by the oral and intravenous routes (Table 15–10; see also Fig. 15–4). Sublingual, buccal, or spray products are the products of choice for this indication. Prevention of symptoms may be accomplished by the prophylactic use of oral or transdermal products; however, concern has been expressed over the long-term efficacy of many of these preparations and the development of tolerance. Nitrates have multiple potential mechanisms of action, and for a given patient, it is not always clear which of these is most important. In general, the major action appears to be mediated indirectly through a reduction in myocardial oxygen demand secondary to venodilation and arterial-arteriolar dilation, leading to a reduction in wall stress from reduced ventricular volume and pressure (see Table 15–8).

Systemic venodilation also promotes increased flow to deep myocardial muscle by reducing the gradient between intraventricular pressure and coronary arteriolar (R_2) pressure. Direct actions on the coronary circulation include dilation of large and small intramural coronary arteries, collateral dilation, coronary artery stenosis dilation, abolition of normal tone in narrowed vessels, and relief of spasm; these actions occur even if the endothelium is denuded or dysfunctional. It is likely that depending on the underlying pathophysiology, different mechanisms become operative. For example, in the presence of a 60% to 70% stenosis, venodilation with MVO_2 reduction is most important; however, with higher-grade lesions, direct effects on the coronary circulation and vessel tone are the predominant effects. Although the cellular mechanism of vasodilation by nitrates is not entirely understood, organic nitrates are converted intracellularly to nitric oxide (EDRF) and 5-nitrosothiol via interaction with sulfhydryl groups.

Nitric oxide, and perhaps 5-nitrosothiol, activates soluble guanylate cyclase to increase intracellular concentrations of cyclic GMP. Increased cyclic GMP induces a sequence of protein phosphorylation associated with reduced intracellular calcium release from the sarcoplasmic reticulum or reduced permeability to extracellular calcium and, consequently, smooth muscle relaxation.

Pharmacokinetic characteristics common to the organic nitrates used for angina include a large first-pass effect of hepatic metabolism, short to very short half-lives (except for isosorbide mononitrate), large volumes of distribution, high clearance rates, and large interindividual variations in plasma or blood concentrations. Pharmacodynamic-pharmacokinetic relationships for the entire class remain poorly defined, presumably owing to methodologic difficulty in characterizing the parent drug and metabolite concentrations at or within vascular smooth muscle and secondary to counterregulatory or adaptive mechanisms from the drug's effects, as well as the occurrence of tolerance. Nitroglycerin is extracted by a variety of tissues and metabolized locally; differential extraction and metabolite generation occur depending on the tissue site. There are also numerous technical problems limiting the generation of reliable pharmacokinetic parameter estimates, including the following: assay sensitivity; arterial-venous extraction gradients and therefore extrahepatic metabolism; in vitro degradation, drug adsorption to polyvinyl chloride tubing and syringes; potentially saturable metabolism; accumulation of metabolites (some of which are active) with multiple doses; postural and exercise-induced changes in pharmacokinetics; and a number of variables associated with transdermal delivery, including the delivery system (matrix, membrane-limited, ointment), vehicle used, surface area and thickness of application, site application, and other skin variables (e.g., temperature and moisture content). Nitroglycerin concentrations are affected by the route of administration, with the highest concentrations usually obtained with intravenous administration and the lowest seen with lower oral doses. Peak concentrations with sublingual nitroglycerin appear within 2 to 4 minutes, with the oral route producing peaks at about 15 to 30 minutes and the transdermal route producing peaks at 1 to 2 hours. The half-life of nitroglycerin is 1 to 5 minutes regardless of route, hence the potential advantage of sustained-release and transdermal products. Transdermal nitroglycerin does produce sufficient concentrations for acute hemodynamic effects to occur, and these concentrations are maintained for long intervals; however, the hemodynamic and antianginal effects are minimal after 1 week or less with chronic, continuous (24 h/day) therapy. Isosorbide dinitrate (ISDN) is metabolized to isosorbide 2-mono- and 5-mononitrate (isosorbide mononitrate [ISMN]). ISMN is well absorbed, has a half-life of about 5 hours, and may be given once or twice daily depending on the product chosen. Multiple, larger doses of ISDN lead to disproportionate increases in the area under the plasma time profile curve, suggesting that metabolic pathways are being saturated or that metabolite accumulation may influence the disposition of ISDN. Little pharmacokinetic information is available for other nitrate compounds.

Nitrate therapy may be used to terminate an acute anginal attack, to prevent effort- or stress-induced attacks, or for long-term prophylaxis, usually in combination with β-blockers or calcium channel blockers. Sublingual nitroglycerin 0.3 to 0.4 mg will relieve pain in about 75% of patients within 3 minutes, with another 15% becoming pain-free in 5 to 15 minutes. Pain persisting beyond about 20 to 30 minutes following the use of two or three nitroglycerin tablets is suggestive of ACS, and the patient should be instructed to seek emergency aid. Patients should be instructed to keep nitroglycerin in the original, tightly closed glass container and to avoid mixing it with other medications because mixing may reduce nitroglycerin adsorption and vaporization. Additional counseling should include the

TABLE 15–10. Nitrate Products

Product	Onset (min)	Duration	Initial Dose
Nitroglycerin			
IV	1–2	3–5 min	5 μg/min
Sublingual/lingual	1–3	30–60 min	0.3 mg
PO	40	3–6 h	2.5–9 mg tid
Ointment	20–60	2–8 h	1/2–1 in
Patch	40–60	>8 h	1 patch
Erythritol tetranitrate	5–30	4–6 h	5–10 mg tid
Penterythritol tetranitrate	30	4–8 h	10–20 mg tid
Isosorbide dinitrate			
Sublingual/chewable	2–5	1–2 h	2.5–5 mg tid
PO	20–40	4–6 h	5–20 mg tid
Isosorbide mononitrate	30–60	6–8 h	20 mg qd, bid[a]

[a]Product-dependent.

facts that nitroglycerin is not an analgesic but rather that it partially corrects the underlying problem and that repeated use is not harmful or addicting. Patients also should be aware that enhanced venous pooling in the sitting or standing position may improve the effect as well as the symptoms of postural hypotension and that inadequate saliva may slow or prevent tablet disintegration and dissolution. An acceptable, albeit expensive, alternative is lingual spray, which may be more convenient and has a shelf life of 3 years compared with the 6 months or so for some forms of nitroglycerin tablets. Chewable, oral, and transdermal products are acceptable for the long-term prophylaxis of angina; however, considerable controversy surrounds their use, and it appears that the development of tolerance or adaptive mechanisms limits the efficacy of all chronic nitrate therapies regardless of route. Dosing of the longer-acting preparations should be adjusted to provide a hemodynamic response, and as an example, this may require doses of oral ISDN ranging from 10 to 60 mg as often as every 3 to 4 hours owing to tolerance or first-pass metabolism, and similar large doses are required for other products. Nitroglycerin ointment has a duration of up to 6 hours, but it is difficult to apply in a cosmetically acceptable fashion over a consistent surface area, and response varies depending on the epidermal thickness, vascularity, and amount of hair. Percutaneous adsorption of nitroglycerin ointment may occur unintentionally if someone other than the patient applies the ointment, and limiting exposure through the use of gloves or some other means is advisable. Peripheral edema also may impair the response to nitroglycerin because venodilation cannot increase capacitance to a maximum, and pooling may be reduced. Transdermal patch delivery systems were approved on the basis of sustained and equivalent plasma concentrations to other forms of therapy. Trials required by the Food and Drug Administration using transdermal patches as a continuous 24-hour delivery system revealed a lack of efficacy for improved exercise tolerance. Subsequently, large, randomized, double-blind, placebo-controlled trials of intermittent (10 to 12 hours on, 12 to 14 hours off) transdermal nitroglycerin therapy in chronic stable angina demonstrated modest but significant improvement in exercise time after 4 weeks for the highest doses at 8 to 12 hours after patch placement.[94] Subjective assessment methods for nitrate effects include reduction in the number of painful episodes and the amount of nitroglycerin consumed. Objective assessment includes the resolution of ECG changes at rest, during exercise, or with ambulatory ECG monitoring. Because nitrates work primarily through a reduction in MVO_2, the DP can be used to optimize the dose of sublingual and oral nitrate products. It is important to realize that reflex tachycardia may offset the beneficial reduction in systolic blood pressure, and calculation of the observed changes is necessary. The DP is best assessed in the sitting position and at intervals of 5 to 10 minutes and 30 to 60 minutes following sublingual and oral therapy, respectively. Owing to the placebo effect, the unpredictable and variable course of angina, the numerous pharmacologic effects of nitroglycerin, diurnal variation in pain patterns, stringent investigative protocols, and interindividual sensitivity to nitroglycerin, assessment with transdermal and sustained-release products is difficult. ETT provides valuable information concerning efficacy and mechanism of action for nitrates, but its use usually is reserved for clinical investigation rather than for routine patient care. Most ETT studies have shown nitrates to delay the onset of ischemia (ST-segment changes or initial chest discomfort) at submaximal exercise, but the threshold for maximal exercise is unaltered, suggesting a reduction in oxygen demand rather than an improved oxygen supply. More sophisticated studies of myocardial function such as wall motion abnormalities and myocardial metabolism could be used to document efficacy, but these studies are generally only for investigative purposes.

Adverse effects of nitrates are related most commonly to an extension of their pharmacologic effects and include postural hypotension with associated central nervous system symptoms, headaches, and flushing secondary to vasodilation and occasional nausea from smooth muscle relaxation. If hypotension is excessive, coronary and cerebral filling may be compromised, leading to MI and stroke. While reflex tachycardia is most common, bradycardia with nitroglycerin has been reported. Other noncardiovascular adverse effects include rash with all products but particularly with transdermal nitroglycerin, the production of methemoglobinemia with high doses given for extended periods, and measurable concentrations of ethanol (intoxication has been reported) and propylene glycol (found in the diluent) with intravenous nitroglycerin.

Tolerance with nitrate therapy was first described in 1867 with the initial experience using amyl nitrate for angina and later was widely recognized in munitions workers who underwent withdrawal reactions during periods of absence from exposure. Tolerance to nitrates is associated with a reduction in tissue cyclic GMP, which results from decreased production (guanylate cyclase) and increased breakdown via cyclic GMP-phosphodiesterase and increased superoxide levels. One proposed mechanism for the lack of cyclic GMP is lack of conversion of organic nitrates to nitric oxide owing to depletion of intracellular sulfhydryl cofactors (cysteine) in cells following chronic exposure to nitrates. This effect is more pronounced on the venous system than on the arterial system. Activation of neurohormonal systems following vasodilation with nitrates may result in vasoconstriction and sodium retention. The major systems thought to be involved in this second mechanism are the sympathoadrenal axis and the renin-angiotensin system. Concomitant use of captopril (25 mg three times daily) may attenuate the increased sensitivity to phenylephrine and angiotensin II noted in patients with stable CAD.[95,96] Nitroglycerin administration is accompanied by a fall in hematocrit (caused by hemodilution rather than renal water conservation) and intravascular volume expansion, minimizing the ability of nitrates to decrease ventricular filling pressures as a third mechanism of tolerance. Logically, a diuretic would minimize this mechanism; however, Parker and colleagues[97] found no effect on the development of tolerance to continuous transdermal nitroglycerin. Diuretic therapy itself has important antianginal effects and improves exercise capacity in patients with stable angina.[97] Supplemental vitamin E also has been studied to restore cyclic GMP production and the vasodilatory response to nitroglycerin.[98] Most of the published information from controlled trials examining nitrate tolerance have been done with either ISDN or transdermal nitroglycerin, and these studies demonstrate the development of tolerance within as few as 24 hours of therapy.

While the onset of tolerance is rapid, the offset may be just as rapid, and one alternative dosing strategy to circumvent or minimize tolerance is to provide a daily nitrate-free interval of 6 to 8 hours. Studies with a variety of nitrate preparations and dosing schedules demonstrate that this approach is useful and that the nitrate-free interval should be a minimum of 8 hours and perhaps 12 hours for even better effects.[94] Another concern for intermittent transdermal nitrate therapy is the occurrence of rebound ischemia during the nitrate-free interval. Freedman and colleagues[99] found more silent ischemia during the patch-free interval during a randomized, double-blind, placebo-controlled trial than during the placebo patch phase, although others have not noted this effect. ISDN, for example, should not be used more often than three times per day if tolerance is to be avoided. Interestingly, hemodynamic tolerance does not always coincide with antianginal efficacy, but this is not well studied.

Nitrates may be combined with other drugs for anginal therapy, including β-adrenergic blocking agents and calcium channel antagonists. These combinations usually are instituted for chronic prophylactic therapy based on complementary or offsetting mechanisms of action (see Table 15–9). Combination therapy generally is used in patients with more frequent symptoms or symptoms not responding to β-blockers alone (nitrates plus β-blockers or calcium channel blockers), in patients intolerant of β-blockers or calcium channel blockers, and in patients having an element of vasospasm leading to decreased supply (nitrates plus calcium blockers).[100]

CALCIUM CHANNEL ANTAGONISTS[101]

Modulation of calcium entry into vascular smooth muscle and myocardium, as well as a variety of other tissues, is the principal action of the calcium antagonists. The cellular mechanism of these drugs is not completely understood, and it differs among the available classes of the phenylalkylamines (verapamil-like), dihydropyridines (nifedipine-like), benzothiazepines (diltiazem-like), bepridil, and a recent class referred to as *T-channel blockers*. Receptor-operated channels stimulated by norepinephrine and other neurotransmitters and potential-dependent channels activated by membrane depolarization control the entry of calcium and, consequently, the cytosolic concentration of calcium responsible for activation of the actin-myosin complex, leading to contraction of vascular smooth muscle and myocardium. In the myocardium, calcium entry triggers the release of intracellular stores of calcium to increase cytosolic calcium, whereas in smooth muscle, calcium derived from the extracellular fluid may do this directly. Binding proteins within the cell, calmodulin and troponin, after binding with calcium, participate in phosphorylation reactions, leading to contraction. Decreased calcium availability, through the actions of calcium antagonists, inhibits these reactions.

Direct actions of the calcium antagonists include vasodilation of systemic arterioles and coronary arteries, leading to a reduction in arterial pressure and coronary vascular resistance, as well as depression of the myocardial contractility and conduction velocity of the sinoatrial (SA) and atrioventricular (AV) nodes (see Chap. 17). Reflex β-adrenergic stimulation overcomes much of the negative inotropic effect, and depression of contractility becomes apparent clinically only in the presence of LV dysfunction and when other negative inotropic drugs are used concurrently. Verapamil and diltiazem cause less peripheral vasodilation than nifedipine, and consequently, the risk of myocardial depression is greater with these two agents. Conduction through the AV node is predictably depressed with verapamil and diltiazem, and they must be used with caution in patients with preexisting conduction abnormalities or in the presence of other drugs with negative chronotropic properties. Bepridil, in addition to having calcium channel–blocking properties, also has class I and III antiarrhythmic activity. MVO_2 is reduced with all the calcium channel antagonists because of reduced wall tension secondary to reduced arterial pressure and, to a minor extent, depressed contractility (see Table 15–9). Heart rate changes depend on the drug used and the state of the conduction system. Nifedipine generally increases heart rate or causes no change, whereas either no change or decreased heart rate is seen with verapamil and diltiazem because of the interaction of these direct and indirect effects. In contrast to the β-blockers, calcium channel antagonists have the potential to improve coronary blood flow through areas of fixed coronary obstruction by inhibiting coronary artery vasomotion and vasospasm. Beneficial redistribution of blood flow from well-perfused myocardium to ischemic areas and from epicardium to endocardium also may contribute to improvement in ischemic symptoms. Overall, the benefit provided by calcium channel antagonists is related to reduced MVO_2 rather than improved oxygen supply based

on lack of alteration in the rate-pressure product at maximal exercise in most studies performed to date. However, as CAD progresses and vasospasm becomes superimposed on critical stenotic lesions, improved oxygen supply through coronary vasodilation may become more important.

Absorption of the calcium channel antagonists is excellent, and large, variable first-pass metabolism results in oral bioavailability ranging from about 20% to 50% or greater for diltiazem, nicardipine, nifedipine, verapamil, felodipine, and isradipine. Amlodipine and bepridil have a range of bioavailability of approximately 60% to 80%. Saturation of this effect may occur with verapamil and diltiazem, resulting in greater amounts of drug being absorbed with chronic dosing. Nifedipine may have slow or fast absorption patterns, and the ingestion of food delays and impairs its absorption, as well as potential enhanced absorption in elderly patients. This variability in absorption produces fluctuations in the hemodynamic response with nifedipine. Sublingual nifedipine is used frequently to provide a more rapid response; however, the rationale for this application is suspect because little nifedipine is absorbed from the buccal mucosa, and the swallowed drug is responsible for the observed plasma concentrations. Absorption of verapamil in sustained-release products may be influenced by food, and when it is used in the fasted state, dose dumping may occur, resulting in high peak concentrations with some products. The sustained-release products for nifedipine, verapamil, and diltiazem are approved primarily for the treatment of hypertension (see Chap. 13). The presence of severe liver disease (e.g., alcoholic liver disease with cirrhosis) has been shown to reduce the first-pass metabolism of verapamil, and this shunting of drug around the liver gives rise to higher plasma concentrations and lower dose requirements in these patients. Interestingly, this effect appears to be stereoselective for the more active isomer of verapamil. Verapamil also may reduce liver blood flow; however, evidence for this reduction is based primarily on animal experiments. Few data are available regarding the influence of liver disease on the kinetics of calcium blockers; however, these drugs undergo extensive hepatic metabolism, with little unchanged drug being excreted renally, and liver disease can be expected to alter the pharmacokinetics. Nifedipine has no active metabolites, whereas norverapamil possesses 20% or less activity of the parent compound. Desacetyldiltiazem has not been studied in humans, but canine studies suggest that its potency ranges from 100% to 40% of the parent compound for various cardiovascular effects; the clinical importance of these observations remains to be determined. With chronic dosing of verapamil and diltiazem, apparent saturation of metabolism occurs, producing higher plasma concentrations of each drug than those seen with single-dose administration. Consequently, the elimination half-life for verapamil is prolonged, and less frequent dosing intervals may be used in some patients. The elimination half-life for diltiazem is also somewhat prolonged, and the half-life of desacetyldiltiazem is longer than that of the parent drug. However, it is not clear if less frequent dosing may be used. Bepridil also undergoes hepatic elimination, and an active metabolite, 4-hydroxyphenyl bepridil, is produced; the parent compound has a long half-life of 30 to 40 hours. Nifedipine does not accumulate with chronic dosing; however, it is eliminated via oxidative pathways that may be polymorphic, and slow and fast metabolizers have been described for nifedipine. Most of the calcium channel blockers are eliminated via cytochrome P (CYP) 3A4 and other CYP isoenzymes, and many inhibit CYP 3A4 activity as well.[102] Renal insufficiency has little or no effect on the pharmacokinetics of these three drugs. Although disease alterations in kinetics have been described, the most important quantitative alteration is the influence of liver disease on bioavailability, and elimination has been shown to reduce the clearance of verapamil and diltiazem. Thus dosing in this population should be done with caution. Altered protein binding owing to renal disease, decreased protein concentration, or increased α_1-acid glycoprotein has been noted, but the clinical import of these changes is unknown.

Good candidates for calcium channel blockers in angina include patients with contraindications to or intolerance of β-blockers, those with coexisting conduction system disease (except for verapamil and diltiazem), those with Prinzmetal's angina (vasospastic or variable-threshold angina), those with peripheral vascular disease, those with severe ventricular dysfunction (amlopidine is probably the calcium channel blocker of choice, and others need to be used with caution if the ejection fraction is less than 40%), and those with concurrent hypertension.

In the diabetic substudy of the Heart Outcomes Prevention Evaluation (HOPE), 9297 high-risk men and women 55 years of age and older with previous cardiovascular disease or diabetes plus one risk factor were randomly assigned to ramipril (up to 10 mg/day), vitamin E (400 IU/day), their combination, or matching placebos.[103] During the mean follow-up of 4.5 years, there were 482 (10.4%) patients with MI and unexpected cardiovascular death in the ramipril group compared with 604 (12.9%) in the placebo group.[103] Ramipril was associated with a trend toward fewer fatal MIs and unexpected deaths[103] and with a significant reduction in nonfatal MIs [5.6% versus 7.2%; relative risk ratio (RRR) 23% (CI 9%–34%)]. This study and others suggest that ACE inhibitors provide significant protection against the long-term consequences of IHD.

■ INVESTIGATIONAL AGENTS

Ranolazine is a novel antianginal agent currently under investigation as monotherapy and adjunct therapy for the treatment of chronic stable angina. Although the mechanism of action of ranolazine is not understood completely, it is believed to involve a reduction in fatty acid oxidation, ultimately leading to a shift in myocardial energy production from fatty acid oxidation to glucose oxidation. Because the oxidation of glucose requires less oxygen than the oxidation of fatty acids, ranolazine can help to maintain myocardial function in times of ischemia. In addition, ranolazine does not affect blood pressure, heart rate, or cardiac conduction significantly. Ranolazine has been shown to improve exercise time as monotherapy or in combination with traditional antianginal agents.[104,105]

Therapeutic angiogenesis aims to deliver an angiogenic growth factor or cytokine to the myocardium to stimulate collateral blood vessel growth throughout the ischemic tissue. The angiogenic factor may be administered as a recombinant protein or as a transgene within a plasmid or gene-transfer vector. An example of this approach is the intracoronary administration of the adenoviral gene for fibroblast growth factor (Ad5FGF-4) to determine if therapeutic angiogenesis could improve myocardial perfusion compared with placebo.[106] In a study of 52 patients with stable angina and reversible ischemia, Ad5FGF-4 decreased the ischemic defect by 21% ($p < .001$), as determined by single-photon-emission computed tomography (SPECT) imaging.[106] More trials are needed before angiogenesis becomes a standard therapy.

Selective 5-HT subtype 3 receptor (5-HT$_3$) antagonists may have potential in the treatment of the pain associated with MI. MCI-9042 (sarpogrelate) or other 5-HT$_{2A}$ antagonists may have clinical potential for the treatment of vasospastic angina, IHD, reperfusion injury, and hindlimb ischemia. Several modulators of 5-HT (5-HT transporter inhibitors and 5-HT$_{1B}$ and 5-HT$_{2B}$ antagonists) may have potential alone or in combination in the treatment of pulmonary hypertension.[107]

Tedisamil is a bradycardic agent because of its ability to inhibit transient outward current (I_{to}) in atria. Tedisamil inhibits I_{to}, potassium current (I_K), $I_{K(ATP)}$, and the protein kinase A–activated chloride channel in ventricles, as well as vascular I_K and Ca^{2+}-activated I_K ($I_{K(Ca)}$). As compared with atenolol, tedisamil produced a prolongation of the QTc interval (+31 versus 8 ms) at initial values of 0.408 ± 0.018 seconds with the PQ and QRS intervals remaining unaltered. In patients with stable angina, tedisamil (100 mg twice daily) as compared with atenolol (50 mg twice daily) generated similar hemodynamic, neurohumoral, and anti-ischemic effects.[108]

Markers of systemic inflammation (e.g., C-reactive protein [CRP] and interleukin-6 [IL-6]) have been proposed to be "nontraditional" risk factors for cardiovascular disease in patients with type 2 diabetes mellitus. Matrix metalloproteinase-9 (MMP-9) has been implicated in the pathogenesis of atherosclerotic plaque rupture, which raises the possibility of the use of MMP-9 levels as a marker for future MI or UA. In vitro and animal studies suggest that thiazolidinediones can reduce the expression of these markers. Rosiglitazone reduces serum levels of MMP-9 and the proinflammatory marker CRP in patients with type 2 diabetes, which indicates potentially beneficial effects on overall cardiovascular risk.[109] The management of UA and NSTEMI is covered in detail in Chap. 16.

▶ TREATMENT: Coronary Artery Spasm and Variant Angina Pectoris (Prinzmetal's Angina)

Prinzmetal, in his original description of variant angina pectoris, noted the waxing and waning course of this syndrome associated with ST-segment elevation and that it resolves most commonly without progression to MI. Patients who develop variant angina are usually younger and have fewer coronary risk factors but more commonly smoke than patients with chronic stable angina. Hyperventilation, exercise, and exposure to cold may precipitate variant angina attacks, or there may be no apparent precipitating cause. The onset of chest discomfort is usually in the early morning hours. The exact cause of variant angina is not well understood but may be an imbalance between endothelium-produced vasodilator factors (e.g., prostacyclin and nitric oxide) and vasoconstrictor factors (e.g., endothelin and angiotensin II), as well as an imbalance of autonomic control characterized by parasympathetic dominance.[110]

The diagnosis of variant angina is based on ST-segment elevation during transient chest discomfort (usually at rest) that resolves when

the chest discomfort diminishes in patients who have normal or nonobstructed coronary lesions. In the absence of ST-segment elevation, a provocative test using ergonovine, acetylcholine, or methacholine may be used to precipitate coronary artery spasm, ST-segment elevation, and typical symptoms. Nitrates and calcium antagonists should be withdrawn prior to provocative testing. Provocative testing should not be used in patients with high-grade lesions. Hyperventilation also may be used to provoke spasm, and patients with positive a hyperventilation test are more likely to have a higher frequency of attacks, multivessel disease, and a high degree of AV block or ventricular tachycardia.

Optimization of therapy includes dose titration using sufficiently high doses to obtain clinical efficacy without unacceptable adverse effects in individual patients. All patients should be treated for acute attacks and maintained on prophylactic treatment for 6 to 12 months following the initial episode. The occurrence of serious arrhythmias during attacks is associated with a greater risk of sudden death, and these patients should be treated more aggressively and for prolonged periods. For patients without arrhythmias who become asymptomatic and remain so for several months after treatment has been instituted, withdrawal of therapy may be safe after first ascertaining that disease activity is quiescent. Aggravating factors such as alcohol or cocaine use and cigarette smoking should be eliminated when instituting treatment.

Nitrates have been the mainstay of therapy for the acute attacks of variant angina and coronary artery spasm for many years. Most patients respond rapidly to sublingual nitroglycerin or isosorbide dinitrate; however, intravenous and intracoronary nitroglycerin may be very useful for patients not responding to sublingual preparations. In particular, vasospasm provoked by ergonovine may require intracoronary nitroglycerin. Although studies with nitrates generally show them to be efficacious, high does often are required, and it is unclear if they reduce mortality. Because calcium antagonists may be more effective, have few serious adverse effects in effective doses, and can be given less frequently than nitrates, some clinicians consider them the agents of choice for variant angina.

Nifedipine, verapamil, and diltiazem are all equally effective as single agents for the initial management of variant angina and coronary artery spasm. Dose titration is important to maximize the response with calcium antagonists. Comparative trials are few in number and do not reveal significant differences among these three drugs for variant angina. Patients unresponsive to calcium antagonists alone may have nitrates added. Combination therapy with nifedipine-diltiazem or nifedipine-verapamil has been reported to be useful in patients unresponsive to single-drug regimens. This is probably rational because, at the cellular level, the drugs have different receptors, but the combination of verapamil-diltiazem should be used cautiously owing to their potential additive effects on contractility and conduction.

β-Adrenergic blockade has little or no role in the management of variant angina according to most authorities.[111] Although not all studies report increased painful episodes of variant angina with the addition of β-blockers, they may induce coronary vasoconstriction and prolong ischemia, as documented by continuous ECG monitoring. Other approaches to therapy attempting to modify sympathetic/parasympathetic tone include α-antagonists, anticholinergics, plexectomy, surgical interruption of the sympathetic innervation of the heart, thromboxane receptor antagonism, prostacyclin, lipoxygenase inhibition, and ticlopidine, but these drugs or procedures do not occupy a major place in therapy at the present time.

▶ TREATMENT: Silent Ischemia[17]

The objective in the treatment of silent myocardial ischemia is to reduce the total number of ischemic episodes, both symptomatic and asymptomatic, regardless of the direction of ST-segment shift. The incidence of silent ischemia in the general, asymptomatic population is not known. Significant day-to-day variability in the number of episodes, the duration of ischemia, and the amount of ST-segment deviation complicates both the understanding of this process and the utility of various therapeutic interventions. Silent ischemia in patients with known CAD is common ($\sim$80% of all ischemic episodes) and associated with the extent of disease, as well as a high risk for MI and sudden death when compared with symptomatic episodes of ischemia. Although the underlying mechanisms for silent ischemia continue to be defined, increased physical activity, activation of the sympathetic nervous system, increased cortisol secretion, increased coronary artery tone, and enhanced platelet aggregation owing to endothelia dysfunction leading to intermittent coronary obstruction may be additive in lowering the threshold for ischemia. Platelet aggregability is increased in the morning hours (7 to 11 AM), corresponding to circadian rhythms noted for the peak frequency of ischemia, acute MI, and sudden death. Silent ischemia is associated with ST-segment elevation or depression and frequently occurs without antecedent changes in heart rate or blood pressure, suggesting that this form of ischemia is a result of primary reduction in oxygen supply. Silent ischemia is classified into class I, patients who do not experience angina at any time, and class II, patients who have both asymptomatic and symptomatic ischemia. Patients with silent ischemia have a defective warning system for angina pain that may encourage excessive myocardial demand. Regardless of the exact mechanism, there is increasing concern that painless ischemia carries considerable risk for myocardial perfusion defects, detrimental hemodynamic changes, arrhythmogenesis, and sudden death. Silent ischemia is associated with reduced survival and increased need for PTCA and CABG, as well as increased risk of acute MI.[112] Because it is apparently very common in some settings, major emphasis should be placed on its management. A consensus has not been reached for the most appropriate method of detecting and quantifying the magnitude of silent ischemia; however, ambulatory ECG monitoring is felt by many to be the most useful tool at the present time.

The initial step in management is to modify the major risk factors for IHD—hypertension, hypercholesterolemia, and smoking—and data from the Multiple Risk Factor Intervention Trial (MRFIT) show these interventions to be useful in patients with silent ischemia. In a subset of the study population that had abnormal baseline exercise ECG responses, the special intervention group had a 57% reduction in coronary heart disease death (22.2 of 1000 versus 51.8 of 1000) and a reduction in sudden death resulting from cessation of smoking and lowering of blood pressure and cholesterol when compared with the usual-care group.

The Asymptomatic Cardiac Ischemia Pilot study (ACIP), a randomized trial of medical therapy versus revascularization (PTCA or CABG), at the 2-year follow-up demonstrated that total mortality was 6.6% in the angina-guided strategy (i.e., therapy based on symptoms), 4.4% in the ischemia-guided strategy (based on ECG changes), and 1.1% in the revascularization strategy ($p < .02$). The rate of death or MI was 12.1% in the angina-guided strategy, 8.8% in the ischemia-guided strategy, and 4.7% in the revascularization strategy ($p < .04$).[113] The rate of death, MI, or recurrent cardiac hospitalization was 41.8% in the angina-guided strategy, 38.5% in the ischemia-guided strategy, and 23.1% in the revascularization strategy ($p < .001$). Post-MI patients and those with a high level of sympathetic nervous system activity are perhaps the best candidates for β-blocker therapy.

Calcium channel antagonists alone and in combination have been shown to be effective in reducing symptomatic and asymptomatic ischemia; however, they do not interrupt the diurnal surge in ischemia observed on ambulatory monitoring, and in general, they are somewhat less effective than β-blockers for silent ischemia.[114,115] Nifedipine in particular seems to provide less protection and provides wide fluctuations in response, with approximate reductions in the number of episodes ranging from 0% to 93% and in duration from 23% to 65% unless combined with β-blockers. Fewer studies are available with other calcium blockers, and comparative trials are uncommon.

Earlier studies have shown that combination therapy with calcium channel blockers and β-blockers provides a better response than calcium channel blockers and nitrates or monotherapy.[116,117]

Surgical intervention using CABG does not appear warranted in asymptomatic patients without significant CAD. Based on the CASS 12-year follow-up results, survival following CABG was enhanced in men with three-vessel disease compared with medical therapy (61% versus 46%) but not for women (45% versus 50%) with silent ischemia.[118] The role for PTCA is promising in silent ischemia, and improvement in exercise tolerance and freedom from MI, CABG, and PTCA for new lesions or death may be seen in patients becoming asymptomatic after PTCA. However, exercise-induced silent myocardial ischemia is seen frequently early after successful PTCA and is more prevalent in patients undergoing multivessel angioplasty and incomplete revascularization. Both silent and symptomatic ischemia early after PTCA are predictors of an unfavorable prognosis.

▶ TREATMENT: Syndrome X[119]

Syndrome X refers to the occurrence of effort angina and exercise-induced ECG changes with a normal coronary arteriogram and no evidence of structural (stenosis) or functional (spasm) abnormalities. Although the basis for this syndrome is not yet established, it is thought that syndrome X may be a result of inducible myocardial ischemia caused by impaired functional coronary reserve at the microvascular level of intramural prearteriolar vessels.[120] It has been proposed that this defect is caused by defective prearteriolar regulation of blood flow into the arteriolar bed with subsequent focal, sustained, compensatory release of adenosine; excessive local concentrations of adenosine are then responsible for the pain seen in this syndrome. Cardiomyopathy and left bundle block may result from ischemia in some patients. Follow-up studies have shown that the occurrence of left bundle branch block in response to stress is associated with a greater likelihood of deterioration of LV performance, whereas stress-induced ST-segment depression does not predict a detrimental outcome in ventricular function. Esophageal abnormalities may be seen in these patients, and acid refluxing into the esophagus may reduce coronary blood flow.

α-Adrenergic blockers are much less effective in many studies in syndrome X than in exertional angina, and one characteristic, if present, that may predict a good response to β-blockers is increased sympathetic nervous system activity.[121] ACE inhibitors have been shown to improve coronary reserve, exercise capacity, and exercise time in patients with microvascular angina.[122,123] Estrogen-replacement therapy in postmenopausal women has been shown to restore endothelial responsiveness to acetylcholine, and this has potential in the management of syndrome X patients.[124]

PHARMACOECONOMIC CONSIDERATIONS

Pharmacoeconomic studies have been performed primarily in patients with acute coronary syndromes and only with LMWHs, GP IIb/IIIa receptor antagonists, and statins.[125] Most of the studies on LMWHs have been cost-minimization analyses and have focused on enoxaparin sodium because this is the only LMWH proven to be superior to UFH. Several analyses show that, compared with UFH plus aspirin, enoxaparin sodium provides cost savings both during hospitalization (30 days) and at 1-year follow-up. These cost savings are mainly attributable to fewer cardiac interventions, shorter hospital stays, and lower administrative costs. Indeed, the clinical and economic advantages of enoxaparin sodium have led to its recommendation in recent guidelines as the antithrombotic agent of choice for CAD. Most of the economic analyses of GP IIb/IIIa inhibitors have been cost-effectiveness analyses.[126] Such analyses indicate that the high acquisition costs of these drugs may be at least partially offset by reductions in other costs if a noninvasive approach to risk stratification is used. Furthermore, use of GP IIb/IIIa inhibitors appears to give favorable cost-effectiveness ratios compared with other accepted therapies, such as fibrin-specific thrombolytic therapy, in the cardiovascular field, particularly in high-risk patients and those undergoing PCI. However, more comprehensive economic data on the GP IIb/IIIa inhibitors are needed.

Atorvastatin when used in ACS has been shown to reduce events, and this offsets the upfront acquistion costs.[126] The total expected cost was (British) £784.05 per patient in the placebo cohort and £851.59 per patient in the atorvastatin cohort, resulting in an incremental cost of £67.54 per patient in the atorvastatin group. The cost per event avoided was £1762.04. A third of the cost of atorvastatin treatment was offset within 16 weeks by the cost savings resulting from the reduction in the number of events in the atorvastatin cohort compared with the placebo cohort.

Aspirin and clopidogrel have been evaluated for secondary prevention of CHD, and clopidogrel is only cost-effective for patients who cannot take aspirin.

CLINICAL CONTROVERSIES

Once patients with angina develop symptoms sufficient for pharmacologic therapy on a daily basis, the initial prophylactic therapy recommended is a β-blocker. There is a paucity of comparative, long-term clinical trials of β-blockade versus calcium channel blockers to determine which is superior for survival benefit. β-Blockers are recommended first-line therapy because of their efficacy in post-MI patients and favorable adverse-effect profile.

There is continuing controversy whether the vasculoprotective effects of the ACE inhibitors are seen with only tissue-selective ACE inhibitors or if this effect extends across the entire class. Quantitative differences in lipophilicity and enzyme-binding capabilities do exist among the ACE inhibitors, and optimal doses for therapeutic benefit must be established in large-scale clinical trials.

The use of high-sensitivity CRP in diagnosis and risk stratification in IHD has gained support in recent years, but not all studies consistently demonstrate improved sensitivity and specificity in the diagnosis of CAD.

EVALUATION OF THERAPEUTIC OUTCOMES

Improved symptoms of angina, improved cardiac performance, and improvement in risk factors all may be used to assess the outcome of treatment of IHD and angina. Symptomatic improvement in exercise capacity (longer duration) or fewer symptoms at the same level of exercise is subjective evidence that therapy is working. Once patients have been optimized on medical therapy, symptoms should improve over 2 to 4 weeks and remain stable until the disease progresses. There are several instruments [e.g., the Seattle Angina Questionnaire, the Specific Activity Scale (see Table 15–1), and the Canadian Classification System (see Table 15–2)] that could be used to improve the reproducibility of symptom assessment.[1] If the patient is doing well, then no other assessment may be necessary. Objective assessment is obtained through increased exercise duration on ETT and the absence of ischemic changes on ECG or deleterious hemodynamic changes. Echocardiography and cardiac imaging also may be used; however, owing to their expense, they are used only if a patient is not doing well to determine if revascularization or other measures should be undertaken. Coronary angiography may be used to assess the extent of stenosis or restenosis after angioplasty or CABG.

Review Questions and other resources can be found at *www.pharmacotherapyonline.com.*

REFERENCES

1. Gibbons RJ, Abrams J, Chatterjee K, et al. ACC/AHA 2002 guideline update for the management of patients with chronic stable angina: Summary article. A report of the American College of Cardiology/American Heart Association Task Force on Practice Guidelines (Committee on the Management of Patients With Chronic Stable Angina). Circulation 2003;107:149–158.
2. Gibbons RJ, Balady GJ, Bricker TJ, et al. ACC/AHA 2002 guideline update for exercise testing: Summary article. A report of the American College of Cardiology/American Heart Association Task Force on Practice Guidelines (Committee to Update the 1997 Exercise Testing Guidelines). J Am Coll Cardiol 2002;40:1531–1540.
3. Braunwald E, Antman EM, Beasley JW, et al. ACC/AHA 2002 guideline update for the management of patients with unstable angina and non-ST-segment elevation myocardial infarction: Summary article. A report of the American College of Cardiology/American Heart Association Task Force on Practice Guidelines (Committee on the Management of Patients with Unstable Angina). J Am Coll Cardiol 2002;40:1366–1374.
4. Sytkowski PA, D' Agostino RB, Belanger A, Kannel WB. Sex and time trends in cardiovascular disease incidence and mortality: The Framingham Heart Study, 1950–1989. Am J Epidemiol 1996;143:338–350.
5. American Heart Association. 2001 Heart and Stroke Statistical Update. Dallas, AHA, 2000:1–33.
6. Kannel WB. Natural history of angina pectoris in the Framingham Study: Prognosis and survival. Am J Cardiol 1972;29:154–163.
7. Menotti A, Keys A, Blackburn H, et al. Comparison of multivariate predictive power of major risk factors for coronary heart diseases in different countries: Results from eight nations of the Seven Countries Study, 25-year follow-up. J Cardiovasc Risk 1996;3:69–75.
8. Keys A. Mediterranean diet and public health: Personal reflections. Am J Clin Nutr 1995;61:1321S–1323S.
9. Goldman L, Hashimoto B, Cook F, et al. Comparative reproducibility and validity of systems for assessing cardiovascular functional class: Advantages of a new specific activity scale. Circulation 1981;64:1227–1234.
10. Emond M, Mock MB, Davis KB, et al. Long-term survival of medically treated patients in the Coronary Artery Surgery Study (CASS) Registry. Circulation 1994;90:2645–2657.
11. Caracciolo EA, Davis KB, Sopko G, et al. Comparison of surgical and medical group survival in patients with left main coronary artery disease: Long-term CASS experience. Circulation 1995;91:2325–2334.
12. Boersma E, Pieper KS, Steyerberg EW, et al. Predictors of outcome in patients with acute coronary syndromes without persistent ST-segment elevation: Results from an international trial of 9461 patients. The PURSUIT Investigators. Circulation 2000;101:2557–2567.
13. Epstein SE CRI, Talbot TL. Hemodynamic principles in the control of coronary blood flow. Am J Cardiol 1985;56:4E–10E.
14. Gielen S, Schuler G, Hambrecht R. Exercise training in coronary artery disease and coronary vasomotion. Circulation 2001;103:E1–6.
15. Libby P. Coronary artery injury and the biology of atherosclerosis: Inflammation, thrombosis, and stabilization. Am J Cardiol 2000;86:3J–8J.
16. Braunwald E, Antman EM, Beasley JW, et al. ACC/AHA guidelines for the management of patients with unstable angina and non-ST-segment elevation myocardial infarction: Executive summary and recommendations. A report of the American College of Cardiology/American Heart Association Task Force on Practice Guidelines (Committee on the Management of Patients with Unstable Angina). Circulation 2000;102:1193–1209.
17. Cohn PF. Silent myocardial ischemia and infarction. In: Goldhaber SZ, Gounameaux H, eds. Fundamental and Clinical Cardiology. New York, Marcel Dekker, 2000:1–327.
18. Caracciolo EA, Chaitman BR, Forman SA, et al. Diabetics with coronary disease have a prevalence of asymptomatic ischemia during exercise treadmill testing and ambulatory ischemia monitoring similar to that of nondiabetic patients: An ACIP database study. ACIP Investigators. Asymptomatic Cardiac Ischemia Pilot Investigators. Circulation 1996;93:2097–2105.
19. Glusman M, Coromilas J, Clark WC, et al. Pain sensitivity in silent myocardial ischemia. Pain 1996;64:477–483.
20. Expert Panel on Detection EaToHBCiA. Executive summary of the Third Report of the National Cholesterol Education Program (NCEP) Expert Panel on Detection, Evaluation, and Treatment of High Blood Cholesterol in Adults (ATP III). JAMA 2001;285:2486–2497.
21. Hoeg JM. Evaluating coronary heart disease risk: Tiles in the mosaic. JAMA 1997;277:1387–1390.
22. Ridker PM, Morrow DA. C-reactive protein, inflammation, and coronary risk. Cardiol Clin 2003;21:315–325.
23. O' Rourke RA, Hochman JS, Cohen MC, et al. New approaches to diagnosis and management of unstable angina and non-ST-segment elevation myocardial infarction. Arch Intern Med 2001;161:674–682.
24. Gibbons RJ, Balady GJ, Bricker JT, et al. ACC/AHA 2002 guideline update for exercise testing: Summary article. A report of the American College of Cardiology/American Heart Association Task Force on Practice Guidelines (Committee to Update the 1997 Exercise Testing Guidelines). Circulation 2002;106:1883–1892.
25. Klocke FJ, Baird MG, Lorell BH, et al. ACC/AHA/ASNC guidelines for the clinical use of cardiac radionuclide imaging: Executive summary. A report of the American College of Cardiology/American Heart Association Task Force on Practice Guidelines (ACC/AHA/ASNC Committee to Revise the 1995 Guidelines for the Clinical Use of Cardiac Radionuclide Imaging). J Am Coll Cardiol 2003;42:1318–1333.
26. Raggi P, Callister TQ, Cooil B, et al. Evaluation of chest pain in patients with low to intermediate pretest probability of coronary artery disease by electron beam computed tomography. Am J Cardiol 2000;85:283–288.
27. Fitzgerald PJ, Oshima A, Hayase M, et al. Final results of the Can Routine Ultrasound Influence Stent Expansion (CRUISE) study. Circulation 2000;102:523–530.
28. Anonymous. Effect of intensive diabetes management on macrovascular events and risk factors in the Diabetes Control and Complications Trial. Am J Cardiol 1995;75:894–903.
29. Smith CJ, Fischer TH, Sears SB. Environmental tobacco smoke, cardiovascular disease, and the nonlinear dose-response hypothesis. Toxicol Sci 2000;54:462–472.
30. Wald NJ, Watt HC. Prospective study of effect of switching from cigarettes to pipes or cigars on mortality from three smoking related diseases (see comments). BMJ 1997;314:1860–1863.
31. Vogel RA. Coronary risk factors, endothelial function, and atherosclerosis: A review. Clin Cardiol 1997;20:426–432.
32. Russell LB, Carson JL, Taylor WC, et al. Modeling all-cause mortality: Projections of the impact of smoking cessation based on the

NHEFS. NHANES I Epidemiologic Follow-up Study. Am J Public Health 1998;88:630–636.

33. Kannel WB. Blood pressure as a cardiovascular risk factor: Prevention and treatment. JAMA 1996;275:1571–1576.

34. Yusuf S, Dagenais G, Pogue J, et al. Vitamin E supplementation and cardiovascular events in high-risk patients. The Heart Outcomes Prevention Evaluation Study Investigators. N Engl J Med 2000;342:154–160.

35. Sandvik L, Erikssen J, Ellestad M, et al. Heart rate increase and maximal heart rate during exercise as predictors of cardiovascular mortality: A 16-year follow-up study of 1960 healthy men. Coronary Artery Dis 1995;6:667–679.

36. Dorn J, Naughton J, Imamura D, Trevisan M. Results of a multicenter randomized clinical trial of exercise and long-term survival in myocardial infarction patients: The National Exercise and Heart Disease Project (NEHDP). Circulation 1999;100:1764–1769.

37. Subbiah MT. Mechanisms of cardioprotection by estrogens. Proc Soc Exp Biol Med 1998;217:23–29.

38. Hulley S, Grady D, Bush T, et al. Randomized trial of estrogen plus progestin for secondary prevention of coronary heart disease in postmenopausal women. Heart and Estrogen/progestin Replacement Study (HERS) Research Group. JAMA 1998;280:605–613.

39. Rossouw JE, Anderson GL, Prentice RL, et al. Risks and benefits of estrogen plus progestin in healthy postmenopausal women: Principal results from the Women's Health Initiative randomized, controlled trial. JAMA 2002;288:321–333.

40. Ades PA, Coello CE. Effects of exercise and cardiac rehabilitation on cardiovascular outcomes. Med Clin North Am 2000;84:251–265, x–xi.

41. Pehrsson SK, Ringqvist I, Ekdahl S, et al. Monotherapy with amlodipine or atenolol versus their combination in stable angina pectoris. Clin Cardiol 2000;23:763–770.

42. Fox KM, Mulcahy D, Findlay I, et al. The Total Ischaemic Burden European Trial (TIBET): Effects of atenolol, nifedipine SR and their combination on the exercise test and the total ischaemic burden in 608 patients with stable angina. The TIBET Study Group. Eur Heart J 1996;17:96–103.

43. Howes LG, Edwards CT. Calcium antagonists and cancer: Is there really a link? Drug Saf 1998;18:1–7.

44. Opie LH, Yusuf S, Kubler W. Current status of safety and efficacy of calcium channel blockers in cardiovascular diseases: A critical analysis based on 100 studies. Prog Cardiovasc Dis 2000;43:171–196.

45. Knight CJ, Fox KM. Amlodipine versus diltiazem as additional antianginal treatment to atenolol. Centralised European Studies in Angina Research (CESAR) Investigators. Am J Cardiol 1998;81:133–136.

46. Anonymous. Seven-year outcome in the Bypass Angioplasty Revascularization Investigation (BARI) by treatment and diabetic status. J Am Coll Cardiol 2000;35:1122–1129.

47. Weintraub WS, Stein B, Kosinski A, et al. Outcome of coronary bypass surgery versus coronary angioplasty in diabetic patients with multivessel coronary artery disease. J Am Coll Cardiol 1998;31:10–19.

48. Hannan EL, Racz MJ, McCallister BD, et al. A comparison of three-year survival after coronary artery bypass graft surgery and percutaneous transluminal coronary angioplasty. J Am Coll Cardiol 1999;33:63–72.

49. Morrison DA, Sethi G, Sacks J, et al. A multicenter, randomized trial of percutaneous coronary intervention versus bypass surgery in high-risk unstable angina patients. The AWESOME (Veterans Affairs Cooperative Study 385, Angina With Extremely Serious Operative Mortality Evaluation) investigators from the Cooperative Studies Program of the Department of Veterans Affairs. Controlled Clin Trials 1999;20:601–619.

50. Smith SC Jr, Dove JT, Jacobs AK, et al. ACC/AHA guidelines for percutaneous coronary intervention (revision of the 1993 PTCA guidelines): Executive summary. A report of the American College of Cardiology/American Heart Association Task Force on Practice Guidelines (Committee to Revise the 1993 Guidelines for Percutaneous Transluminal Coronary Angioplasty). Endorsed by the Society for Cardiac Angiography and Interventions. Circulation 2001;103:3019–3041.

51. Williams DO, Braunwald E, Thompson B, et al. Results of percutaneous transluminal coronary angioplasty in unstable angina and non-Q-wave myocardial infarction: Observations from the TIMI IIIB Trial. Circulation 1996;94:2749–2755.

52. Keelan ET, Nunez BD, Grill DE, et al. Comparison of immediate and long-term outcome of coronary angioplasty performed for unstable angina and rest pain in men and women. Mayo Clin Proc 1997;72:5–12.

53. Kaluza GL, Mazur W, Raizner AE. Basic science review: Radiotherapy for prevention of restenosis. Cathet Cardiovasc Intervent 2001;52:518–529.

54. Cutlip DE. Stent thrombosis: Historical perspectives and current trends. J Thromb Thrombol 2000;10:89–101.

55. Pepine CJ. An ischemia-guided approach for risk stratification in patients with acute coronary syndromes. Am J Cardiol 2000;86:27M–35M.

56. Boden WE, O'Rourke RA, Crawford MH, et al. Outcomes in patients with acute non-Q-wave myocardial infarction randomly assigned to an invasive as compared with a conservative management strategy. Veterans Affairs Non-Q-Wave Infarction Strategies in Hospital (VANQWISH) Trial Investigators. N Engl J Med 1998;338:1785–1792.

57. Anonymous. Invasive compared with non-invasive treatment in unstable coronary-artery disease: FRISC II prospective, randomised multicentre study. FRagmin and Fast Revascularisation during InStability in Coronary artery disease Investigators. Lancet 1999;354:708–715.

58. Eagle KA, Guyton RA, Davidoff R, et al. ACC/AHA guidelines for coronary artery bypass graft surgery: Executive summary and recommendations. A report of the American College of Cardiology/American Heart Association Task Force on Practice Guidelines (Committee to Revise the 1991 Guidelines for Coronary Artery Bypass Graft Surgery). Circulation 1999;100:1464–1480.

59. Colombo A, Tobis J. Techniques in Coronary Artery Stenting. London, Martin Dunitz, 2000:1–422.

60. Jacobs AK, Kelsey SF, Brooks MM, et al. Better outcome for women compared with men undergoing coronary revascularization: A report from the Bypass Angioplasty Revascularization Investigation (BARI). Circulation 1998;98:1279–1285.

61. Taylor HA Jr, Mickel MC, Chaitman BR, et al. Long-term survival of African Americans in the Coronary Artery Surgery Study (CASS). J Am Coll Cardiol 1997;29:358–364.

62. Smith SC Jr, Dove JT, Jacobs AK, et al. ACC/AHA guidelines of percutaneous coronary interventions (revision of the 1993 PTCA guidelines): Executive summary. A report of the American College of Cardiology/American Heart Association Task Force on Practice Guidelines (Committee to Revise the 1993 Guidelines for Percutaneous Transluminal Coronary Angioplasty). J Am Coll Cardiol 2001;37:2215–2239.

63. Solomon AJ, Gersh BJ. Management of chronic stable angina: Medical therapy, percutaneous transluminal coronary angioplasty, and coronary artery bypass graft surgery. Lessons from the randomized trials. Ann Intern Med 1998;128:216–223.

64. Landzberg BR, Frishman WH, Lerrick K. Pathophysiology and pharmacological approaches for prevention of coronary artery restenosis following coronary artery balloon angioplasty and related procedures. Prog Cardiovasc Dis 1997;39:361–398.

65. Kastrati A, Mehilli J, Dirschinger J, et al. Intracoronary Stenting and Angiographic Results: Strut Thickness Effect On Restenosis Outcome (ISAR-STEREO) trial. Circulation 2001;103:2816–2821.

66. Bertrand ME, Rupprecht HJ, Urban P, et al. Double-blind study of the safety of clopidogrel with and without a loading dose in combination with aspirin compared with ticlopidine in combination with aspirin after coronary stenting: The Clopidogrel Aspirin Stent International Cooperative Study (CLASSICS). Circulation 2000;102:624–629.

67. Schomig A, Neumann FJ, Walter H, et al. Coronary stent placement in patients with acute myocardial infarction: Comparison of clinical and angiographic outcome after randomization to antiplatelet or anticoagulant therapy. J Am Coll Cardiol 1997;29:28–34.

68. Schuhlen H, Kastrati A, Pache J, et al. Sustained benefit over four years from an initial combined antiplatelet regimen after coronary stent placement in the ISAR trial. Intracoronary Stenting and Antithrombotic Regimen. Am J Cardiol 2001;87:397–400.

69. Heeschen C, van Den Brand MJ, Hamm CW, Simoons ML. Angiographic findings in patients with refractory unstable angina according to troponin T status. Circulation 1999;100:1509–1514.

70. Topol EJ, Moliterno D, Herrmann HC, et al. Comparison of two platelet glycoprotein IIb/IIIa inhibitors, tirofiban and abciximab, for the prevention of ischemic events with percutaneous coronary revascularization. N Engl J Med 2001;344:1888–1894.

71. Shah PB, Ahmed WH, Ganz P, Bittl JA. Bivalirudin compared with heparin during coronary angioplasty for thrombus-containing lesions. J Am Coll Cardiol 1997;30:1264–1269.

72. Anonymous. A clinical trial comparing primary coronary angioplasty with tissue plasminogen activator for acute myocardial infarction. The Global Use of Strategies to Open Occluded Coronary Arteries in Acute Coronary Syndromes (GUSTO IIb) Angioplasty Substudy Investigators. N Engl J Med 1997;336:1621–1628.

73. Bittl JA, Strony J, Brinker JA, et al. Treatment with bivalirudin (Hirulog) as compared with heparin during coronary angioplasty for unstable or postinfarction angina. Hirulog Angioplasty Study Investigators. N Engl J Med 1995;333:764–769.

74. Lefkovits J, Topol EJ. Pharmacological approaches for the prevention of restenosis after percutaneous coronary intervention. Prog Cardiovasc Dis 1997;40:141–158.

75. Kosuga K, Tamai H, Ueda K, et al. Effectiveness of tranilast on restenosis after directional coronary atherectomy. Am Heart J 1997;134:712–718.

76. Emanuelsson H, Beatt KJ, Bagger JP, et al. Long-term effects of angiopeptin treatment in coronary angioplasty: Reduction of clinical events but not angiographic restenosis. European Angiopeptin Study Group. Circulation 1995;91:1689–1696.

77. Holmes D, Fitzgerald P, Goldberg S, et al. The PRESTO (Prevention of Restenosis with Tranilast and Its Outcomes) protocol: A double-blind, placebo-controlled trial. Am Heart J 2000;139:23–31.

78. Kozuma K, Hara K, Yamasaki M, et al. Effects of cilostazol on late lumen loss and repeat revascularization after Palmaz-Schatz coronary stent implantation. Am Heart J 2001;141:124–130.

79. Peters S, Gotting B, Trummel M, et al. Valsartan for prevention of restenosis after stenting of type B2/C lesions: The VAL-PREST trial. J Invas Cardiol 2001;13:93–97.

80. Kiesz RS, Buszman P, Martin JL, et al. Local delivery of enoxaparin to decrease restenosis after stenting: Results of initial multicenter trial. Polish-American Local Lovenox NIR Assessment study (The POLONIA study). Circulation 2001;103:26–31.

81. Steinhubl SR, Ellis SG, Wolski K, et al. Ticlopidine pretreatment before coronary stenting is associated with sustained decrease in adverse cardiac events: Data from the Evaluation of Platelet IIb/IIIa Inhibitor for Stenting Trial (EPISTENT). Circulation 2001;103:1403–1409.

82. Verin V, Popowski Y, de Bruyne B, et al. Endoluminal beta-radiation therapy for the prevention of coronary restenosis after balloon angioplasty. The Dose-Finding Study Group. N Engl J Med 2001;344:243–249.

83. Leon MB, Teirstein PS, Moses JW, et al. Localized intracoronary gamma-radiation therapy to inhibit the recurrence of restenosis after stenting. N Engl J Med 2001;344:250–256.

84. Ellis SG, Holmes DR Jr (eds.). Strategic Approaches in Coronary Interventional. Philadelphia, Lippincott Williams & Wilkins, 1999:1–622.

85. Moustapha A, Assali AR, Sdringola S, et al. Percutaneous and surgical interventions for in-stent restenosis: Long-term outcomes and effect of diabetes mellitus. J Am Coll Cardiol 2001;37:1877–1882.

86. Ghaffari S, Kereiakes DJ, Lincoff AM, et al. Platelet glycoprotein IIb/IIIa receptor blockade with abciximab reduces ischemic complications in patients undergoing directional coronary atherectomy. EPILOG Investigators. Evaluation of PTCA to Improve Long-term Outcome by c7E3 GP IIb/IIIa Receptor Blockade. Am J Cardiol 1998;82:7–12.

87. Appelman YE, Piek JJ, van der Wall EE, et al. Evaluation of the long-term functional outcome assessed by myocardial perfusion scintigraphy following excimer laser angioplasty compared to balloon angioplasty in longer coronary lesions. Int J Cardiac Imag 2000;16:267–277.

88. Goldstein S. Beta-blocking drugs and coronary heart disease. Cardiovasc Drugs Ther 1997;11:219–225.

89. Carbajal EV, Deedwania PC. Contemporary approaches in medical management of patients with stable coronary artery disease. Med Clin North Am 1995;79:1063–1084.

90. Prince MJ, Bird AS, Blizard RA, Mann AH. Is the cognitive function of older patients affected by antihypertensive treatment? Results from 54 months of the Medical Research Council's trial of hypertension in older adults. BMJ 1996;312:801–805.

91. Rosenthal J, Bahrmann H, Benkert K, et al. Analysis of adverse effects among patients with essential hypertension receiving an ACE inhibitor or a beta-blocker. Cardiology 1996;87:409–414.

92. Darius H. Role of nitrates for the therapy of coronary artery disease patients in the years beyond 2000. J Cardiovasc Pharmacol 1999;34:S15–20; discussion S29–31.

93. Thadani U. Oral nitrates: More than symptomatic therapy in coronary artery disease? Cardiovasc Drugs Ther 1997;11:213–218.

94. Parker JO, Amies MH, Hawkinson RW, et al. Intermittent transdermal nitroglycerin therapy in angina pectoris: Clinically effective without tolerance or rebound. Minitran Efficacy Study Group. Circulation 1995;91:1368–1374.

95. Pizzulli L, Hagendorff A, Zirbes M, et al. Influence of captopril on nitroglycerin-mediated vasodilation and development of nitrate tolerance in arterial and venous circulation. Am Heart J 1996;131:342–349.

96. Heitzer T, Just H, Brockhoff C, et al. Long-term nitroglycerin treatment is associated with supersensitivity to vasoconstrictors in men with stable coronary artery disease: Prevention by concomitant treatment with captopril. J Am Coll Cardiol 1998;31:83–88.

97. Parker JD, Parker AB, Farrell B, Parker JO. Effects of diuretic therapy on the development of tolerance to nitroglycerin and exercise capacity in patients with chronic stable angina. Circulation 1996;93:691–696.

98. Watanabe H, Kakihana M, Ohtsuka S, Sugishita Y. Randomized, double-blind, placebo-controlled study of supplemental vitamin E on attenuation of the development of nitrate tolerance. Circulation 1997;96:2545–2550.

99. Freedman SB, Daxini BV, Noyce D, Kelly DT. Intermittent transdermal nitrates do not improve ischemia in patients taking beta-blockers or calcium antagonists: Potential role of rebound ischemia during the nitrate-free period. J Am Coll Cardiol 1995;25:349–355.

100. Parmley WW. Optimal treatment of stable angina. Cardiology 1997;88:27–31.

101. Opie LH. First-line drugs in chronic stable effort angina: The case for newer, longer-acting calcium channel blocking agents. J Am Coll Cardiol 2000;36:1967–1971.

102. Katoh M, Nakajima M, Shimada N, et al. Inhibition of human cytochrome P450 enzymes by 1,4-dihydropyridine calcium antagonists: Prediction of in vivo drug-drug interactions. Eur J Clin Pharmacol 2000;55:843–852.

103. Dagenais GR, Yusuf S, Bourassa MG, et al. Effects of ramipril on coronary events in high-risk persons: Results of the Heart Outcomes Prevention Evaluation Study. Circulation 2001;104:522–526.

104. Chaitman BR, Skettino SL, Parker JO, et al. Anti-ischemic effects and long-term survival during ranolazine monotherapy in patients with chronic severe angina. J Am Coll Cardiol 2004;43:1375–1382.

105. Chaitman BR, Pepine CJ, Parker JO, et al. Effects of ranolazine with atenolol, amlodipine, or diltiazem on exercise tolerance and angina frequency in patients with severe chronic angina: A randomized, controlled trial (see comment). JAMA 2004;291:309–316.

106. Grines CL, Watkins MW, Mahmarian JJ, et al. A randomized, double-blind, placebo-controlled trial of Ad5FGF-4 gene therapy and its effect on myocardial perfusion in patients with stable angina. J Am Coll Cardiol 2003;42:1339–1347.

107. Doggrell SA. The role of 5-HT on the cardiovascular and renal systems and the clinical potential of 5-HT modulation. Exp Opin Invest Drugs 2003;12:805–823.

108. Mitrovic V, Miskovic A, Strau M, et al. Hemodynamic, antiischemic, and neurohumoral effects of tedisamil and atenolol in patients with coronary artery disease. Cardiovasc Drugs Ther 2000;14:511–521.

109. Haffner SM, Greenberg AS, Weston WM, et al. Effect of rosiglitazone treatment on nontraditional markers of cardiovascular disease in patients with type 2 diabetes mellitus. Circulation 2002;106:679–684.

110. Sakata K, Miura F, Sugino H, et al. Assessment of regional sympathetic nerve activity in vasospastic angina: Analysis of iodine-123-labeled metaiodobenzylguanidine scintigraphy. Am Heart J 1997;133: 484–489.

111. Lanza GA, Pedrotti P, Pasceri V, et al. Autonomic changes associated with spontaneous coronary spasm in patients with variant angina. J Am Coll Cardiol 1996;28:1249–1256.

112. Conti CR, Geller NL, Knatterud GL, et al. Anginal status and prediction of cardiac events in patients enrolled in the Asymptomatic Cardiac Ischemia Pilot (ACIP) study. ACIP investigators. Am J Cardiol 1997;79:889–892.

113. Davies RF, Goldberg AD, Forman S, et al. Asymptomatic Cardiac Ischemia Pilot (ACIP) study two-year follow-up: Outcomes of patients randomized to initial strategies of medical therapy versus revascularization (see comments). Circulation 1997;95:2037–2043.

114. Singh N, Mironov D, Goodman S, et al. Treatment of silent ischemia in unstable angina: A randomized comparison of sustained-release verapamil versus metoprolol. Clin Cardiol 1995;18:653–658.

115. Dwivedi SK, Saran RK, Mittal S, et al. Silent ischemic interval on exercise test is a predictor to drug therapy: A randomized crossover trial of metoprolol versus diltiazem in stable angina. Clin Cardiol 2001;24:45–49.

116. Pratt CM, McMahon RP, Goldstein S, et al. Comparison of subgroups assigned to medical regimens used to suppress cardiac ischemia (the Asymptomatic Cardiac Ischemia Pilot [ACIP] study). Am J Cardiol 1996;77:1302–1309.

117. Davies RF, Habibi H, Klinke WP, et al. Effect of amlodipine, atenolol and their combination on myocardial ischemia during treadmill exercise and ambulatory monitoring. Canadian Amlodipine/Atenolol in Silent Ischemia Study (CASIS) investigators. J Am Coll Cardiol 1995;25:619–625.

118. Weiner DA, Ryan TJ, Parsons L, et al. Significance of silent myocardial ischemia during exercise testing in women: Report from the Coronary Artery Surgery Study. Am Heart J 1995;129:465–470.

119. Ali O, Smart FW, Nguyen T, Ventura H. Recent developments in microvascular angina. Curr Atheroscler Rep 2001;3:149–155.

120. Bellamy MF, Goodfellow J, Tweddel AC, et al. Syndrome X and endothelial dysfunction. Cardiovasc Res 1998;40:410–417.

121. Lanza GA, Colonna G, Pasceri V, Maseri A. Atenolol versus amlodipine versus isosorbide-5-mononitrate on anginal symptoms in syndrome X. Am J Cardiol 1999;84:854–856, A8.

122. Motz W, Strauer BE. Improvement of coronary flow reserve after long-term therapy with enalapril. Hypertension 1996;27:1031–1038.

123. Nalbantgil I, Onder R, Altintig A, et al. Therapeutic benefits of cilazapril in patients with syndrome X. Cardiology 1998;89:130–133.

124. Roque M, Heras M, Roig E, et al. Short-term effects of transdermal estrogen replacement therapy on coronary vascular reactivity in postmenopausal women with angina pectoris and normal results on coronary angiograms. J Am Coll Cardiol 1998;31:139–143.

125. Bosanquet N, Jonsson B, Fox KA. Costs and cost effectiveness of low molecular weight heparins and platelet glycoprotein IIb/IIIa inhibitors in the management of acute coronary syndromes. Pharmacoeconomics 2003;21:1135–1152.

126. Plosker GL, Ibbotson T. Eptifibatide: A pharmacoeconomic review of its use in percutaneous coronary intervention and acute coronary syndromes. Pharmacoeconomics 2003;21:885–912.

16

ACUTE CORONARY SYNDROMES

Sarah A. Spinler and Simon de Denus

Learning Objectives and other resources can be found at *www.pharmacotherapyonline.com*.

KEY CONCEPTS

❶ The cause of an acute coronary syndrome (ACS) is the rupture of an atherosclerotic plaque with subsequent platelet adherence, activation, aggregation, and activation of the clotting cascade. Ultimately, a clot forms and is composed of fibrin and platelets.

❷ The American Heart Association (AHA) and the American College of Cardiology (ACC) recommend strategies or guidelines for ACS patient care for ST-segment- and non-ST-segment-elevation ACS.

❸ Patients with ischemic chest discomfort and suspected ACS are risk-stratified based on a 12-lead electrocardiogram (ECG), past medical history, and results of creatine kinase (CK) MB and troponin biochemical marker tests.

❹ The diagnosis of myocardial infarction (MI) is confirmed based on the results of the CK MB and troponin tests.

❺ Three key features identifying high-risk patients with non-ST-segment-elevation ACS are a Thrombolysis in Myocardial Infarction (TIMI) risk score of 5 to 7, the presence of ST-segment depression on ECG, and positive CK MB or troponin.

❻ Early reperfusion therapy with either primary percutaneous coronary intervention (PCI) or administration of a fibrinolytic agent is the recommended therapy for patients presenting with ST-segment-elevation ACS.

❼ In addition to reperfusion therapy, additional pharmacotherapy that all patients with ST-segment-elevation ACS and without contraindications should receive within the first day of hospitalization and preferably in the emergency department are intranasal oxygen (if oxygen saturation is low),

aspirin, sublingual nitroglycerin, intravenous nitroglycerin, intravenous followed by oral β-blockers, and unfractionated heparin (UFH).

❽ High-risk patients with non-ST-segment-elevation ACS should undergo early coronary angiography and revascularization with either PCI or coronary artery bypass graft (CABG) surgery.

❾ In the absence of contraindications, all patients with non-ST-segment-elevation ACS should be treated in the emergency department with intranasal oxygen (if oxygen saturation is low), aspirin, sublingual nitroglycerin, intravenous nitroglycerin, intravenous followed by oral β-blockers, and either unfractionated heparin (UFH) or a low-molecular-weight heparin (enoxaparin preferred). Most patients should receive additional therapy with clopidogrel. High-risk patients also should receive a glycoprotein IIb/IIIa receptor blocker.

❿ Following MI, all patients, in the absence of contraindications, should receive indefinite therapy with aspirin, a β-blocker and an angiotensin-converting enzyme (ACE) inhibitor for secondary prevention of death, stroke, and recurrent infarction. Most patients will receive a statin to reduce low-density lipoprotein cholesterol to less than 70 to 100 mg/dL. Anticoagulation with warfarin should be considered for patients at high risk of death, reinfarction, or stroke.

⓫ Secondary prevention of death, reinfarction, and stroke is more cost-effective than primary prevention of coronary heart disease (CHD) events.

Since the early 1900s cardiovascular disease (CVD) has been the leading cause of death. Acute coronary syndromes (ACSs), including unstable angina (UA) and myocardial infarction (MI), are forms of coronary heart disease (CHD) that constitute the most common ❶ cause of CVD death.[1] The cause of an ACS is the rupture of an atherosclerotic plaque with subsequent platelet adherence, activation, aggregation, and activation of the clotting cascade. Ultimately, a clot forms and is composed of fibrin and platelets. Correspondingly, pharmacotherapy of ACS has advanced to include combinations of fibrinolytics, antiplatelets, and anticoagulants with more traditional therapies such as nitrates and β-adrenergic blockers. Pharmacother-

apy is integrated with reperfusion therapy and revascularization of the culprit coronary artery through interventional means such as percutaneous coronary intervention (PCI) and coronary artery bypass graft ❷ (CABG) surgery. The American Heart Association (AHA) and the American College of Cardiology (ACC) recommend strategies or guidelines for ACS patient care for ST-segment- and non-ST-segment-elevation ACS. These joint practice guidelines are based on a review of available clinical evidence, have graded recommendations based on the weight and quality of evidence, and are updated periodically. The guidelines form the cornerstone for quality patient care of the ACS patient.[2,3]

EPIDEMIOLOGY

Each year more than 1 million Americans will experience an ACS, and 239,000 will die of an MI.[1] In the United States, more than 7.6 million living persons have survived an MI.[1] Chest discomfort is the most frequent reason for patient presentation to emergency departments, with up to 7 million emergency department visits, or approximately 3% of all emergency department visits, linked to chest discomfort and possible ACS. CHD is the leading cause of premature, chronic disability in the United States. The cost of CHD is high, with more than $10 billion being paid to Medicare beneficiaries in 1999, or more than $10,000 per MI hospital stay. The average length of hospital stay for MI in 1999 was 5.6 days.[1]

Much of the epidemiologic data regarding ACS treatment and survival come from the National Registry of Myocardial Infarction (NRMI), the Global Registry of Acute Coronary Events (GRACE), and statistical summaries of U.S. hospital discharges prepared by the AHA. In patients with ST-segment-elevation ACS, in-hospital death rates are approximately 7% for patients who are treated with fibrinolytics and 16% for patients who do not receive reperfusion therapy. In patients with non-ST-segment-elevation MI, in-hospital mortality is less than 5%. In-hospital mortality and 1-year mortality are higher for women and elderly patients. In the first year following MI, 38% of women and 25% of men will die, most from recurrent infarction.[1] At 1 year, rates of mortality and reinfarction are similar between ST-segment-elevation and non-ST-segment-elevation MI.

Approximately 30% of patients develop heart failure at some time during their hospitalization for MI. In-hospital death rates for patients who present with or develop heart failure are more than three-fold higher than for those who do not.[4]

Because reinfarction and death are major outcomes following ACS, therapeutic strategies to reduce morbidity and mortality, particularly use of coronary angiography, revascularization, and pharmacotherapy, will have a significant impact on the social and economic burden of CHD is the United States.

ETIOLOGY

In this section we will discuss the formation of atherosclerotic plaques, the underlying cause of coronary artery disease (CAD) and ACS in most patients. The process of atherosclerosis starts early in life. Its earliest stage, endothelial dysfunction, progresses over the ensuring decades into plaque formation and atherosclerosis.[5] A number of factors are directly responsible for the development and progression of endothelial dysfunction and atherosclerosis, including hypertension, age, male gender, tobacco use, diabetes, obesity, elevated plasma homocysteine concentrations, and dyslipidemias.[5,6]

Endothelial dysfunction is characterized by an imbalance between vasodilating (including nitric oxide and prostacyclin) and vasoconstricting (including endothelin-1, angiotensin II, and norepinephrine) substances resulting in an increase in vascular reactivity. This also leads to an imbalance between procoagulant (plasminogen activator inhibitor-1 and tissue factor) and anticoagulant (tissue plasminogen activator and protein C) substances, thereby promoting platelet aggregation and thrombus formation. Furthermore, endothelial dysfunction is characterized by an increase in the expression of leukocyte adhesion molecules, which promotes the migration of inflammatory cells in the subintimal vessel wall.[6] Finally, endothelial dysfunction increases the permeability of the endothelium to low-density lipoprotein (LDL) cholesterol and inflammatory cells that promote their migration and infiltration in the subintimal vessel wall.[6,7]

Taken together, all these factors contribute to the evolution of endothelial dysfunction to the formation of fatty streaks in the coronary arteries and eventually to atherosclerotic plaques.

PATHOPHYSIOLOGY

SPECTRUM OF ACS

Acute coronary syndromes (ACSs) is a term that includes all clinical syndromes compatible with acute myocardial ischemia resulting from an imbalance between myocardial oxygen demand and supply.[3] In contrast to stable angina, an ACS results primarily from diminished myocardial blood flow secondary to an occlusive or partially occlusive coronary artery thrombus. ACSs are classified according to electrocardiographic changes into ST-segment-elevation ACS (ST-elevation MI [STEMI]) or non-ST-segment-elevation ACS (non-ST-elevation MI [NSTEMI] and unstable angina [UA]) (Fig. 16–1). NSTEMI differs from UA in that ischemia is severe enough to produce myocardial necrosis, resulting in the release of a detectable amount of biochemical markers, mainly troponins T or I and creatine kinase (CK) myocardial band (MB) from the necrotic myocytes, in the bloodstream.[3] The clinical significance of serum markers will be discussed in more details in later sections of this chapter. Following an STEMI, pathologic Q waves are seen frequently on the electrocardiogram (ECG), whereas such an ECG manifestation is seen less commonly in patients with NSTEMI.[7] The presence of Q waves usually indicates transmural MI.

PLAQUE RUPTURE AND CLOT FORMATION

The predominant cause of ACS, in more than 90% of patients, is atheromatous plaque rupture, fissuring, or erosion of an unstable atherosclerotic plaque that encompasses less than 50% of the coronary lumen prior to the event rather than a more stable 70% to 90% stenosis of the coronary artery.[3] Stable stenoses are characteristic of stable angina. Plaques that are more susceptible to rupture are characterized by an eccentric shape, a thin fibrous cap (particularly in the shoulder region of the plaque), large fatty core, a high content in inflammatory cells such as macrophages and lymphocytes, and limited amounts of smooth muscle. Inflammatory cells promote the thinning of the fibrous cap through the release of proteolytic enzymes, particularly matrix metalloproteinases.[7]

Following plaque rupture, a partially occlusive or completely occlusive thrombus, a clot, forms on top of the ruptured plaque. The thrombogenic contents of the plaque are exposed to blood elements. Exposure of collagen and tissue factor induce platelet adhesion and activation, which promote the release of platelet-derived vasoactive substances, including adenosine diphosphate (ADP) and thromboxane A_2 (TXA_2).[8] These produce vasoconstriction and potentiate platelet activation. Furthermore, during platelet activation, a change in the conformation in the glycoprotein (GP) IIb/IIIa surface receptors of platelets occurs that cross-links platelets to each other through fibrinogen bridges. This is considered the final common pathway of platelet aggregation. Other substances known to promote platelet aggregation include serotonin, thrombin, and epinephrine.[8] Inclusion of platelets gives the clot a white appearance. Simultaneously, the extrinsic coagulation cascade pathway is activated as a result of exposure of blood components to the thrombogenic lipid core and endothelium, which are rich in tissue factor. This leads to the production of thrombin (factor IIa), which converts fibrinogen to fibrin through enzymatic activity.[8] Fibrin stabilizes the clot and traps red blood cells, which give the clot a red appearance. Therefore, the clot is composed of cross-linked platelets and fibrin strands.[8]

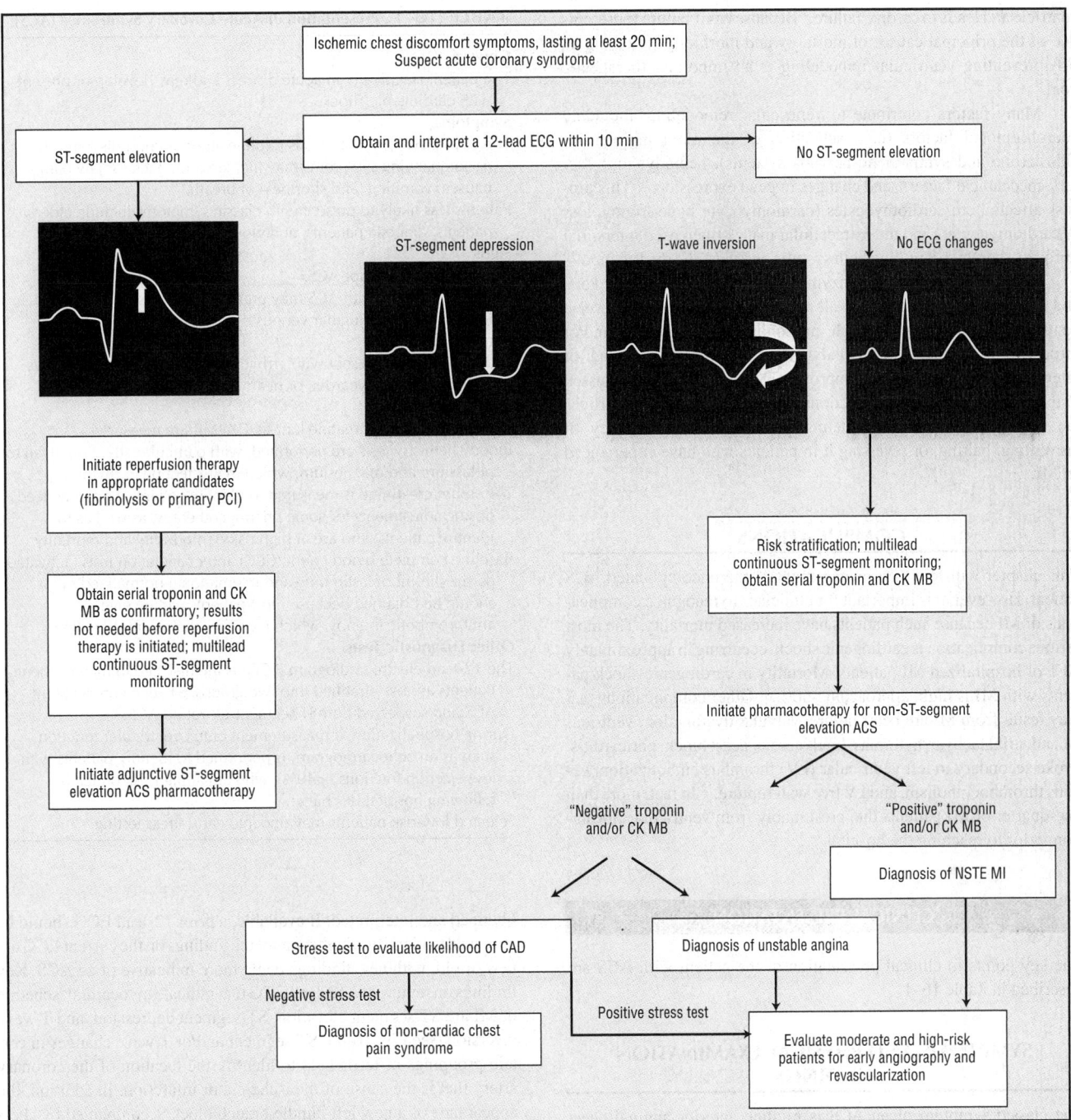

FIGURE 16–1. Evaluation of the acute coronary syndrome patient. ACS = acute coronary syndrome; CAD = coronary artery disease; CK = creatine kinase; ECG = electrocardiogram; PCI = percutaneous coronary intervention; Positive = above the MI decision limit; Negative = below the MI decision limit.

A thrombus containing more platelets than fibrin, or a "white" clot, generally produces an incomplete occlusion of the coronary lumen and is more common in non-ST-segment-elevation ACS. In patients presenting with an ST-segment-elevation ACS, the vessel generally is completely occluded by a "red" clot that contains larger amounts of fibrin and red blood cells but a smaller amount of platelets compared with a "white" clot.[2] As will be discussed later on in this chapter, the composition of the clot influences the selection of the combinations of antithrombotic agents used in ST-segment- and non-ST-segment-elevation ACS. Finally, myocardial ischemia can re-sult from the downstream embolization of microthrombi and produce ischemia with eventual necrosis.[2]

VENTRICULAR REMODELING FOLLOWING AN ACUTE MI

Ventricular remodeling is a process that occurs in several cardiovascular conditions, including heart failure and following an MI. It is characterized by changes in the size, shape, and function of the left ventricle and leads to cardiac failure.[9] Because heart failure represents one of the principal causes of mortality and morbidity following an MI, preventing ventricular remodeling is an important therapeutic goal.[9]

Many factors contribute to ventricular remodeling, including neurohormonal factors (e.g., activation of the renin-angiotensin-aldosterone and sympathetic nervous systems), hemodynamic factors, mechanical factors, and changes in gene expression.[10] This process affects both cardiomyocytes (cardiomyocyte hypertrophy, loss of cardiomyocytes) and the extracellular matrix (increased interstitial fibrosis), thereby promoting both systolic and diastolic dysfunction.[10]

Angiotensin-converting enzyme (ACE) inhibitors, β-blockers, and aldosterone antagonists are all agents that slow down or reverse ventricular remodeling through neurohormonal blockage and/or through improvement in hemodynamics (decreasing preload or afterload).[9] These agents also improve survival and will be discussed in more detail in subsequent sections of this chapter. This underlines the importance of the remodeling process and the urgency of preventing, halting, or reversing it in patients who have experienced an MI.

COMPLICATIONS

This chapter will focus on management of the uncomplicated ACS patient. However, it is important for clinicians to recognize complications of MI because such patients have increased mortality. The most serious complication is cardiogenic shock, occurring in approximately 10% of hospitalized MI patients. Mortality in cardiogenic shock patients with MI is high, approaching 60%.[11] Other complications that may result from MI are heart failure, valvular dysfunction, ventricular and atrial tachyarrhythmias, bradycardia, heart block, pericarditis, stroke secondary to left ventricular (LV) thrombus embolization, venous thromboembolism, and LV free wall rupture.[12] In fact, more than one-quarter of MI patients die, presumably from ventricular fibrillation, prior to reaching the hospital.[1]

CLINICAL PRESENTATION

The key points in clinical presentation of the patient with ACS are described in Table 16–1.

SYMPTOMS AND PHYSICAL EXAMINATION FINDINGS

The classic symptom of an ACS is midline anterior anginal chest discomfort, most often either at rest, severe new-onset, or increasing angina that is at least 20 minutes in duration. The chest discomfort may radiate to the shoulder, down the left arm, to the back, or to the jaw. Associated symptoms that may accompany the chest discomfort include nausea, vomiting, diaphoresis, or shortness of breath. All health care professionals should review these warning symptoms with patients at high risk for CHD. On physical examination, no specific features are indicative of ACS.

TWELVE-LEAD ELECTROCARDIOGRAM (ECG)

There are key features of a 12-lead ECG that identify and risk-stratify a patient with an ACS. Within 10 minutes of presentation to an emergency department with symptoms of ischemic chest discomfort (or preferably pre-hospital) a 12-lead ECG should be

TABLE 16–1. Presentation of Acute Coronary Syndromes (ACS)

General

The patient is typically in acute distress and may develop or present with cardiogenic shock.

Symptoms

The classic symptom of ACS is midline anterior chest discomfort. Accompanying symptoms may include arm, back, or jaw pain; nausea; vomiting; and shortness of breath.

Patients less likely to present with classic symptoms include elderly patients, diabetic patients, and women.

Signs

No signs are classic for ACS.

However, patients with ACS may present with signs of acute heart failure, including jugular venous distension and an S_3 sound on auscultation.

Patients also may present with arrhythmias and therefore may have tachycardia, bradycardia, or heart block.

Laboratory Tests

Troponin I or T and creatine kinase (CK) MB are measured.

Blood chemistry tests are performed, with particular attention given to potassium and magnesium, which may affect heart rhythm.

The serum creatinine is measured to identify patients who may need dosing adjustments for some pharmacotherapy, as well as to identify patients who are at high risk of morbidity and mortality.

Baseline complete blood count (CBC) and coagulation tests (activated partial thromboplastin time and international normalized ratio) should be obtained because most patients will receive antithrombotic therapy, which increases the risk for bleeding.

Other Diagnostic Tests

The 12-lead electrocardiogram (ECG) is the first step in management. Patients are risk-stratified into two groups, ST-segment-elevation ACS and suspected non-ST-segment-elevation ACS.

During hospitalization, a measurement of left ventricular function, such as an echocardiogram, is performed to identify patients with low ejection fractions (<40%), who are at high risk of death following hospital discharge.

Selected low-risk patients may undergo early stress testing.

obtained and interpreted. If available, a prior 12-lead ECG should be reviewed to identify whether or not the findings on the current ECG are new or old, with new findings being more indicative of an ACS. Key findings on review of a 12-lead ECG that indicate myocardial ischemia or MI are ST-segment elevation, ST-segment depression, and T-wave inversion (see Fig. 16–1). ST-segment and/or T-wave changes in certain groupings of leads help to identify the location of the coronary artery that is the cause of the ischemia or infarction. In addition, the appearance of a new left bundle branch block accompanied by chest discomfort is highly specific for acute MI. About one-half of patients diagnosed with MI present with ST-segment elevation on their ECG, with the remainder having ST-segment depression, T-wave inversion, or in some instances, no ECG changes. Some parts of the heart are more "electrically silent" than others, and myocardial ischemia may not be detected on a surface ECG. Therefore, it is important to review findings from the ECG in conjunction with biochemical markers of myocardial necrosis, such as troponin I or T, and other risk factors for CHD to determine the patient's risk for experiencing a new MI or having other complications.

BIOCHEMICAL MARKERS

 Biochemical markers of myocardial cell death are important for confirming the diagnosis of MI. *Evolving MI* is defined by the

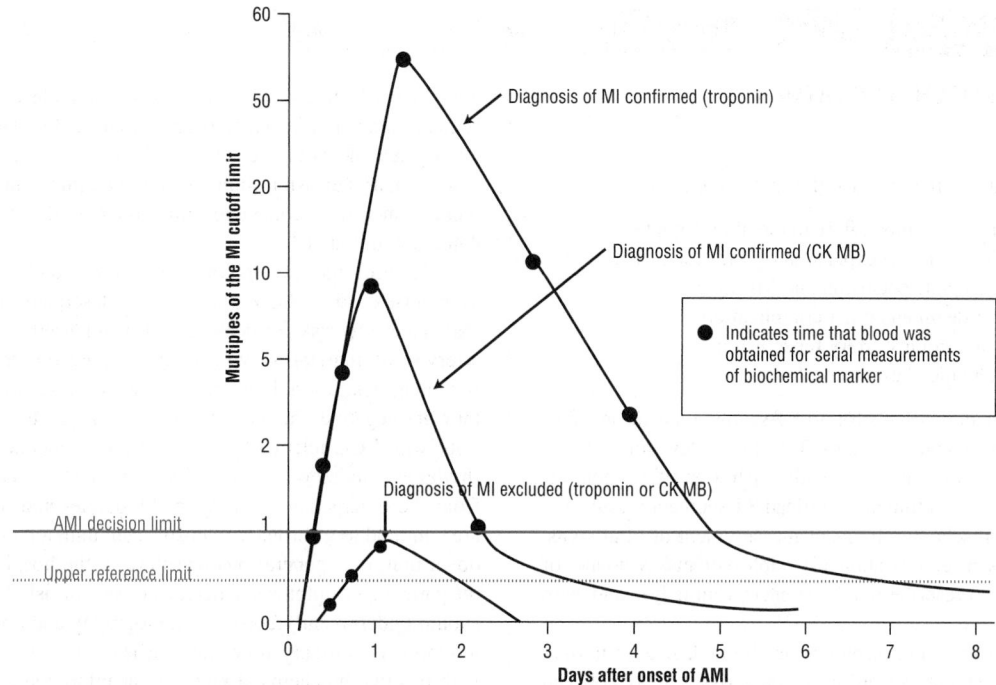

FIGURE 16–2. Biochemical markers in suspected acute coronary syndrome.

ACC as "typical rise and gradual fall (troponin) or more rapid rise and fall (CK MB) of biochemical markers of myocardial necrosis."[13] Troponin and CK MB rise in the blood following the onset of complete coronary artery occlusion subsequent myocardial cell death. Their time course is depicted in Fig. 16–2. Typically, blood is obtained from the patient at least three times, once in the emergency department and two additional times over the next 12 to 24 hours, in order to measure troponin and CK MB. A single measurement of a biochemical marker is not adequate to exclude a diagnosis of MI because up to 15% values that were below the level of detection initially (a negative test) are above the level of detection (a positive test) in the subsequent hours. An MI is identified if at least one troponin value is greater than the MI decision limit (set by the hospital laboratory) or two CK MB results are greater than the MI decision limit (set by the hospital laboratory). While troponins and CK MB appear in the blood within 6 hours of infarction, troponins stay elevated in the blood for up to 10 days, whereas CK MB returns to normal values within 48 hours. Therefore, if a patient is admitted with elevated troponin and CK MB concentrations and several days later experiences recurrent chest discomfort, the troponin will be less sensitive to detect new myocardial damage because it would still be elevated. If early reinfarction is suspected, CK MB concentration determination is the preferred diagnostic test.[13]

RISK STRATIFICATION

5 Patient symptoms, past medical history, ECG, and troponin or CK MB determinations are used to stratify patients into low, medium, or high risk of death or MI or likelihood of failing pharmacotherapy and needing urgent coronary angiography and percutaneous coronary intervention (PCI). Initial treatment according to risk stratification is depicted in Fig. 16–1. Patients with ST-segment elevation are at the highest risk of death. Initial treatment of ST-segment-elevation ACS should proceed without evaluation of the troponin or CK MB levels because these patients have a greater than 97% chance of having an MI subsequently diagnosed with biochemical markers. The ACC/AHA defines a target time to initiate reperfusion treatment of within 30 minutes of hospital presentation for fibrinolytics and within 90 minutes or less from presentation for primary PCI.[3] The sooner the infarct-related coronary artery is opened for these patients, the lower is their mortality, and the greater is the amount of myocardium that is preserved.[14,15] While all patients should be evaluated for reperfusion therapy, not all patients may be eligible. Indications and contraindications for fibrinolytic therapy are described in the treatment section of this chapter. Fewer than 15% of hospitals in the United States are equipped to perform primary PCI. If patients are not eligible for reperfusion therapy, additional pharmacotherapy for ST-segment-elevation patients should be initiated in the emergency department, and the patient should be transferred to a coronary intensive care unit. The typical length of stay for a patient with uncomplicated STEMI is 3 to 5 days.

Risk stratification of the patient with non-ST-segment-elevation ACS is more complex because in-hospital outcomes for this group of patients vary, with reported rates of death of 0% to 12%, reinfarction of 0% to 3%, and recurrent severe ischemia of 5% to 20%.[16] Not all patients presenting with suspected non-ST-segment-elevation ACS will even have CAD. Some will be diagnosed eventually with nonischemic chest discomfort.

Newer markers that identify patients at high risk of mortality or reinfarction that are under development but have not been incorporated currently into routine patient care include C-reactive protein,[5] a maker of vascular inflammation; elevated serum creatinine or reduced creatinine clearance, identifying patients with chronic kidney disease[17]; and brain (B-type) natriuretic peptide (BNP),[18] which is released predominately from ventricular myocytes in response to cell stretch as the infarct remodels. Dialysis patients have a 1-year mortality rate of more than 40% following a first MI.[17]

▶ TREATMENT: Acute Coronary Syndromes

▦ GENERAL APPROACH TO TREATMENT

The short-term goals of treatment for the ACS patient are

1. Early restoration of blood flow to the infarct-related artery to prevent infarct expansion (in the case of MI) or prevent complete occlusion and MI (in UA)
2. Prevention of death and other complications
3. Prevention of coronary artery reocclusion
4. Relief of ischemic chest discomfort

General treatment measures for all ST-segment-elevation ACSs and high- and intermediate-risk non-ST-segment-elevation patients include admission to hospital, oxygen administration (if oxygen saturation is low, <90%), continuous multilead ST-segment monitoring for arrhythmias and ischemia, frequent measurement of vital signs, bed rest for 12 hours in hemodynamically stable patients, avoidance of Valsalva maneuver (prescribe stool softeners routinely), and pain relief.

Because risk varies and resources are limited, it is important to triage and treat patients according to their risk category. Initial approaches to treatment of the ST-segment-elevation and non-ST-segment-elevation ACS patient are outlined in Fig. 16–1. Patients with ST-segment elevation are at high risk of death, and efforts to reestablish coronary perfusion should be initiated immediately. Reperfusion therapy should be considered immediately and adjunctive pharmacotherapy initiated.[3]

Features identifying low-, moderate-, and high-risk non-ST-segment-elevation ACS patients are described in Table 16–2.[19] Patients at low risk for death or MI or for needing urgent coronary artery revascularization typically are evaluated in the emergency department, where serial biochemical marker tests are obtained, and if they are negative, the patient may be admitted to a general medical floor with ECG telemetry monitoring for ischemic changes and arrhythmias, undergo a noninvasive stress test, or may be discharged from the emergency department. Moderate- and high-risk patients are admitted to a coronary intensive care unit, an intensive care step-down unit, or a general medical floor in the hospital depending on the patient's symptoms and perceived level of risk. High-risk patients should undergo early coronary angiography and revascularization if a significant coronary artery stenosis is found. Moderate-risk patients with positive biochemical markers for infarction typically also will

TABLE 16–2. TIMI Risk Score for Non-ST-Segment-Elevation Acute Coronary Syndromes

Past Medical History	Clinical Presentation
Age ≥65 years	ST-segment depression (≥0.5 mm)
≥3 Risk factors for CAD	≥2 Episodes of chest discomfort
Hypercholesterolemia	within the past 24 hours
HTN	Positive biochemical marker for
DM	infarction[b]
Smoking	
Family history of premature CHD[a]	
Known CAD (≥50% stenosis of coronary	
artery)	
Use of aspirin within the past 7 days	

Using the TIMI Risk Score

One point is assigned for each of the seven medical history and clinical presentation findings.
The score (point) total is calculated, and the patient is assigned a risk for experiencing the composite end point of death, myocardial infarction, or urgent need for revascularization as follows:

High Risk	Medium Risk	Low Risk
TIMI risk score 5–7 points	TIMI risk score	TIMI risk score
Other Ways to Identify High-Risk Patients	3–4 points	0–2 points
Other findings that alone or in combination may identify a high-risk patient:		
• ST-segment depression		
• Positive biochemical marker for infarction		
• Deep symmetric T-wave inversions (≥2 mm)		
• Acute heart failure		
• DM		
• Chronic kidney disease		
• Refractory chest discomfort despite maximal pharmacotherapy for ACS		
• Recent MI within the past 2 weeks		

ACS = acute coronary syndrome; CAD = coronary artery disease; CHD = coronary heart disease; DM = diabetes mellitus; HTN = hypertension; MI = myocardial infarction; TIMI = Thrombolysis in Myocardial Infarction.
[a]As defined in Chapter 21.
[b]A positive biochemical marker for infarction is a value of troponin I, troponin T, or creatine kinase MB of greater than the MI detection limit.

undergo angiography and revascularization during hospital admission. Moderate-risk patients with negative biochemical markers for infarction also may undergo angiography and revascularization or first undergo a noninvasive stress test, with only patients with a positive stress test proceeding to angiography.

Following risk stratification, pharmacotherapy for non-ST-segment-elevation ACS is initiated. Urgent (within 24 hours) coronary angiography and revascularization of the infarct-related coronary artery with PCI or CABG surgery is considered for moderate- and high-risk patients[2] (see Fig. 16–1 and Table 16–2).

NONPHARMACOLOGIC THERAPY

PRIMARY PERCUTANEOUS CORONARY INTERVENTION (PCI) FOR ST-SEGMENT-ELEVATION ACS

6 Either fibrinolysis or immediate primary PCI is the treatment of choice for reestablishing coronary artery blood flow for patients with ST-segment-elevation ACS when the patient presents within 3 hours of symptom onset and both options are available at the institution. For primary PCI, the patient is taken from the emergency department to the cardiac catheterization laboratory and undergoes coronary angiography with either balloon angioplasty or placement of a bare metal or drug-eluting intracoronary stent. Additional details regarding angioplasty and intracoronary stenting are provided in Chap. 15. Results from a recent meta-analysis of trials comparing fibrinolysis with primary PCI indicate a lower mortality rate with primary PCI.[20] One reason for the superiority of primary PCI compared with fibrinolysis is that more than 90% of occluded infarct-related coronary arteries are opened with primary PCI compared with less than 60% of coronary arteries with currently available fibrinolytics.[21] In addition, the intracranial hemorrhage and major bleeding risks from primary PCI are lower than following fibrinolysis. An invasive strategy of primary PCI is generally preferred in patients presenting to institutions with skilled interventional cardiologists and a catheterization laboratory immediately available, in patients with cardiogenic shock, in patients with contraindications to fibrinolytics and in patients presenting with symptom onset greater than 3 hours.[3] A quality indicator in the care of MI patients with ST-segment elevation is the time from hospital presentation to the time that the occluded artery is opened with PCI. This "door-to-primary PCI time" should be ≤90 minutes[3,22] (Table 16–3). Unfortunately, most hospitals do not have interventional cardiology services capable of performing primary PCI 24 hours a day. Therefore, only 7% of MI patients are currently treated with primary PCI.

PCI during hospitalization for STEMI also may be appropriate in other patients following STEMI, such as those in whom fibrinolysis is not successful, those presenting later in cardiogenic shock patients with life-threatening ventricular arrhythmias, and those with persistent rest ischemia or signs of ischemia on stress testing following MI.[3,21] The strategy of routine angiography and revascularization in all ST-segment-elevation patients later (after hospital day 1) during hospitalization is controversial.

PERCUTANEOUS CORONARY INTERVENTION IN NON-ST-SEGMENT-ELEVATION ACS

8 The most recent non-ST-segment-elevation ACC/AHA clinical practice guidelines recommend early coronary angiography with either PCI or CABG revascularization as an early treatment for

TABLE 16–3. Quality Patient Care Indicators for Acute Myocardial Infarction

ST-Segment-Elevation Myocardial Infarction
Eligible patients receiving any type of reperfusion therapy
Primary percutaneous coronary intervention within 90 minutes of hospital presentation
Initiation of fibrinolysis within 30 minutes of hospital presentation
ST-Segment-Elevation or Non-ST-Segment-Elevation Myocardial Infarction
Within the first 24 hours
   Administration of aspirin
   Administration of β-blocker
At or before hospital discharge
   Smoking-cessation counseling
   Lipid panel measurement
   Aspirin prescription
   β-Blocker prescription
   Angiotensin-converting enzyme inhibitor prescription (if ejection fraction <40%)

Note: Increasing compliance (approaching 100% of patients) with each factor indicates excellence in patient care. Achievement of indicators is reported to U.S. governmental agencies (e.g., Centers for Medicare and Medicaid Services, Veterans Affairs Health System), managed-care organizations (e.g., National Committee for Quality Assurance), and hospital accrediting bodies (e.g., Joint Commission on the Accreditations of Healthcare Organizations). *From refs. 2 and 37.*

high- and moderate-risk non-ST-segment-elevation ACS patients.[2] Several recent clinical trials support an "early invasive strategy" with PCI or CABG versus a "medical stabilization management strategy" whereby coronary angiography with revascularization is reserved for patients with symptoms refractory to pharmacotherapy and patients with signs of ischemia on stress testing.[23] An early invasive approach results in fewer MIs, and less need for additional revascularization procedures over the next year following hospitalization, and is less costly than the conservative medical stabilization approach.[23]

ADDITIONAL TESTING AND RISK STRATIFICATION

At some point during hospitalization but prior to discharge, patients with MI should have their LV function evaluated for risk stratification.[2,3] The most common way LV function is measured is using an echocardiogram to calculate the patient's LV ejection fraction (EF). LV function is the single best predictor of mortality following MI. Patients with LVEFs of less than 40% are at highest risk of death. Patients with ventricular fibrillation or sustained ventricular tachycardia more than 2 days following MI and those with LVEFs <30% measured at least 1 month following STEMI and 3 months after coronary artery revascularization with either PCI or CABG benefit from placement of an implantable cardioverter-defibrillator (ICD).[3] The Multicenter Automatic Defibrillator Implantation II trial (MADIT) demonstrated a 29% reduction in mortality in patients with a history of MI, low LVEFs, and no history of symptomatic ventricular arrhythmias who received prophylactic implantation of an ICD.[24] Additional discussion of the role of ICDs in the management of high-risk patients and those with ventricular arrhythmias may be found in Chap. 17.

Predischarge stress testing (see Fig. 16–1) may be indicated in moderate- or low-risk patients in order to determine which patients would benefit from coronary angiography to establish the diagnosis of CAD and also in patients following MI to predict intermediate and long-term risk of recurrent MI and death.[25] In most cases, patients with a positive stress test indicating coronary ischemia will then undergo coronary angiography and subsequent revascularization of significantly occluded coronary arteries. Exercise stress testing, most often with the addition of a radionuclide imaging agent, is preferred over nonpharmacologic stress testing because it evaluates the workload achieved with exercise, as well as the occurrence of ischemia. If a patient has a negative exercise stress test for ischemia, the patient is at low risk for subsequent CHD events. Therefore, exercise stress testing has high negative predictive value. Additional discussion of the types of stress testing may be found in Chap. 11.

Patients admitted for ACS should have a fasting lipid panel drawn within the first 24 hours of hospitalization because following that period, values for cholesterol, an acute-phase reactant may be falsely low. Initiation of pharmacotherapy with a statin is common for all ACS patients and does not depend on the results of this lipid panel, however.

■ EARLY PHARMACOLOGIC THERAPY FOR ST-SEGMENT-ELEVATION ACS

Pharmacotherapy for early treatment of ACS is outlined in Fig. 16–3. According to the ACC/AHA ST-segment-elevation ACS practice guidelines, early pharmacotherapy of ST-segment elevation should include intranasal oxygen (if oxygen saturation is <90%), sublingual (SL) followed by intravenous (IV) nitroglycerin (NTG), aspirin, an IV β-blocker, unfractionated heparin (UFH), and fibrinolysis in eligible candidates. Morphine is administered to patients with refractory angina as an analgesic and a venodilator that lowers preload. These agents should be administered early, while the patient is still in the emergency department. Dosing and contraindications for SL and IV NTG, aspirin, IV β-blockers, UFH, and fibrinolytics are listed in Table 16–4.[2,3,26]

■ FIBRINOLYTIC THERAPY

Administration of a fibrinolytic agent is indicated in patients with ST-segment-elevation ACS presenting to hospital within 24 hours of the onset of chest discomfort who have at least 1 mm of ST-segment elevation in two or more contiguous ECG leads.[3] The mortality benefit of fibrinolysis is highest with early administration and diminishes after 12 hours. Fibrinolytic therapy is preferred over primary PCI in patients presenting within 3 hours of symptom onset where there is a delay to primary PCI because of a delay in access to a cardiac catheterization laboratory or a delay in obtaining patient vascular access which would result in a "door-to-primary PCI" delay that would be greater

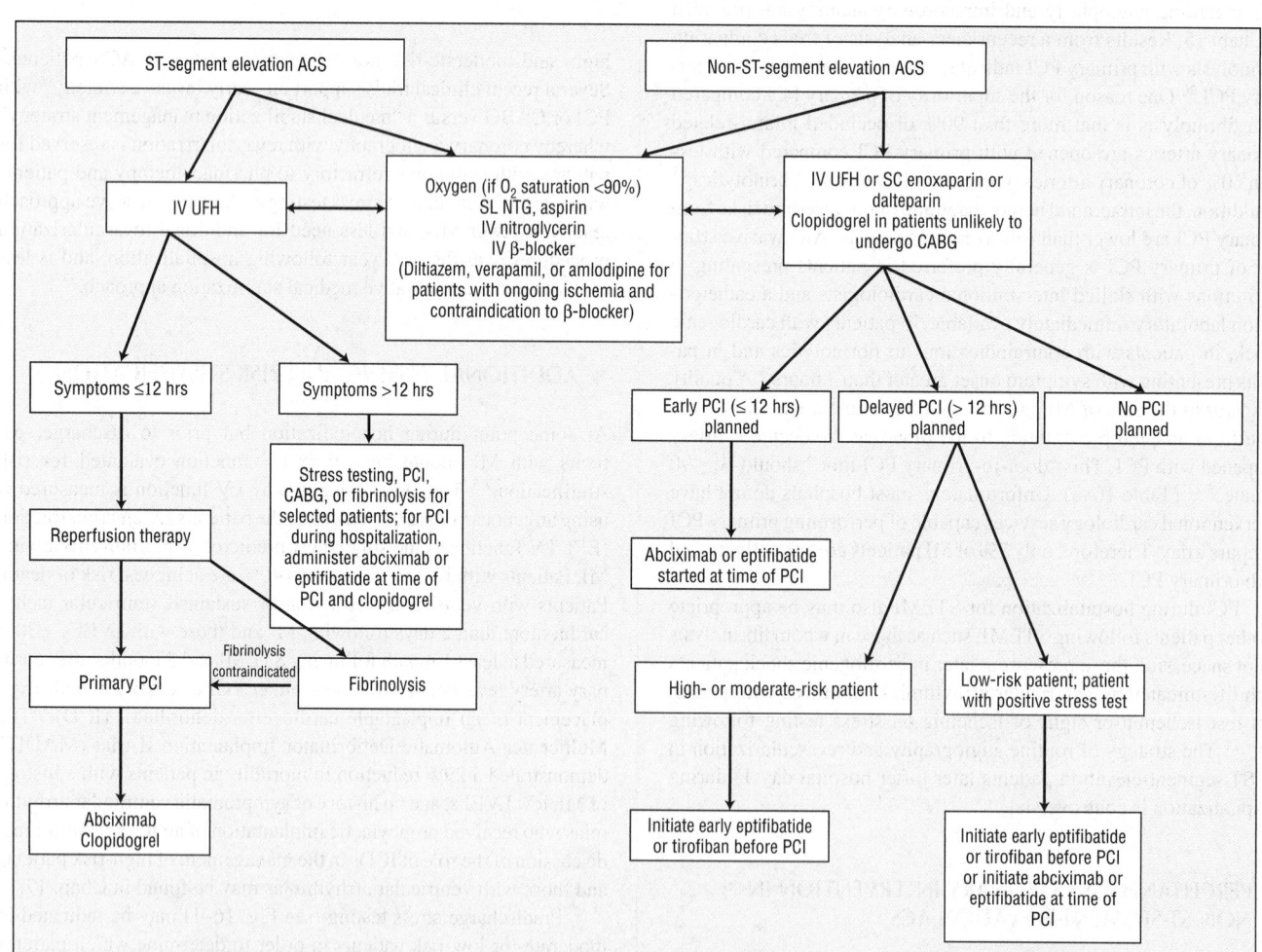

FIGURE 16–3. Initial pharmacotherapy for acute coronary syndromes (ACS). CABG = coronary artery bypass graft; IV = intravenous; PCI = percutaneous coronary intervention; SC = subcutaneous; SL = sublingual; UFH = unfractionated heparin.

TABLE 16–4. Pharmacotherapy for Acute Coronary Syndrome (ST-Segment-Elevation and Non-ST-Segment-Elevation)

Drug	Clinical Condition and ACC/AHA Guideline Recommendation	Contraindications[a]	Dose
Aspirin	STE ACS, class I recommendation[b] for all patients NSTE ACS, class I recommendation for all patients	Hypersensitivity Active bleeding Severe bleeding risk	160–162 mg on hospital day 1 75–162 mg daily starting hospital day 2 and continued indefinitely
Clopidogrel	STE ACS, class I recommendation in patients allergic to aspirin NSTE ACS, class I recommendation for all hospitalized patients in whom a noninterventional approach is planned In PCI in STE and NSTE ACS, class I recommendation	Hypersensitivity Active bleeding Severe bleeding risk	300–600 mg loading dose on hospital day 1 followed by a maintenance dose of 75 mg PO qd starting on hospital day 2 Administer indefinitely in patients with an aspirin allergy (class I recommendation) Administer for at least 9 months in medically managed patients with NSTE ACS (class I recommendation) Administer for at least 30 days to 1 year in patients with STE or NSTE ACS (class I recommendation) undergoing PCI If possible, withhold for at least 5 days in patients whom CABG is planned to decrease bleeding risk (class I recommendation)
Unfractionated heparin (UFH)	STE ACS, class I recommendation in patients undergoing PCI and for patients treated with alteplase, reteplase, or tenecteplase, class IIa recommendation for patients not treated with fibrinolytic therapy NSTE ACS, class I recommendation in combination with aspirin PCI, class I recommendation	Active bleeding History of heparin-induced thrombocytopenia Severe bleeding risk Recent stroke	For STE ACS administer 60 units/kg IV bolus (maximum 4000 μ) followed by a constant IV infusion at 12 units/kg/h (maximum 1000 units/h) For NSTE ACS administer 60–70 units/kg IV (maximum 5000 μ) bolus followed by a constant IV infusion of 12–15 units/kg/h (maximum 1000 μ/hr) Titrated to maintain aPTT between 1.5 to 2.5 times control for NSTE ACS and 50 to 70 s in STE ACS The first aPTT should be measured at 4 to 6 h for NSTE ACS and STE ACS in patients not treated with thrombolytics The first aPTT should be measured at 3 h in patients with STE ACS who are treated with thrombolytics
Low-molecular-weight heparin	STE ACS, class IIb recommendation for patients <75 yrs old treated with fibrinolytics, class IIa for patients not undergoing reperfusion therapy NSTE ACS, class I recommendation in combination with aspirin, class IIa recommendation over UFH in patients without renal failure who are not anticipated to undergo coronary artery bypass graft surgery within 24 h	Active bleeding History of heparin-induced thrombocytopenia Severe bleeding risk Recent stroke Cr_{CL} <10 mL/min (enoxaparin) Cr_{CL} <30 mL/min (dalteparin)	Enoxaparin 1 mg/kg SC q12h ($Cr_{CL} \geq 30$ mL/min) Enoxaparin 1 mg/kg SC q24h (Cr_{CL} 10–29 mL/min) Dalteparin 120 IU/kg SC q12h (maximum single bolus dose of 10,000 units)
Fibrinolytics	STE ACS, class I recommendation in patients age <75 yrs presenting within 12 h following the onset of symptoms, class IIa recommendation in patients age 75 yrs and older, class IIa in patients presenting between 12 and 24 h following the onset of symptoms with continuing signs of ischemia. NSTE ACS: class III recommendation	Absolute and relative contraindications as per Table 16-5	Streptokinase: 1.5 million units IV over 60 min Alteplase: 15 mg IV bolus followed by 0.75 mg/kg IV over 30 min (max 50 mg) followed by 0.5 mg/kg (max 35 mg) over 60 min (max dose = 100 mg) Reteplase: 10 units IV × 2, 30 min apart Tenecteplase <60 kg = 30 mg IV bolus 60–69.9 kg = 35 mg IV bolus 70–79.9 kg = 40 mg IV bolus 80–89.9 kg = 45 mg IV bolus ≥90 kg = 50 mg IV bolus

(continued)

TABLE 16–4. (Continued)

Drug	Clinical Condition and ACC/AHA Guideline Recommendation	Contraindications[a]	Dose			
			Drug with/ without PCI	**Dose for PCI**	**Dose for NSTE ACS**	**Adjustment for Renal Insufficiency or Obesity**
Glycoprotein IIb/IIIa receptor blockers	NSTE ACS, class IIa recommendation for either tirofiban or eptifibatide for patients with either continuing ischemia, elevated troponin or other high-risk features, class I recommendation for patients undergoing PCI, class IIb recommendation for patients without high-risk features who are not undergoing PCI	Active bleeding Prior stroke Thrombocytopenia Renal dialysis (eptifibatide)	Abciximab	0.25 mg/kg IV bolus followed by 0.125 mcg/kg/min (maximum 10 mcg/min) for 12 h	Not recommended	None
	STE ACS, class IIa for abciximab for primary PCI and class IIb for either tirofiban or eptifibatide for primary PCI		Eptifibatide	180 mcg/kg IV bolus × 2, 10 min apart with an infusion of 2 mcg/kg/min started after the first bolus for 18–24 h	180 mcg/kg IV bolus followed by an infusion of 2 mcg/kg/min for 18–24 h	Reduce maintenance infusion to 1 mcg/kg/min for patients with serum creatinine 2 or estimated Cr_{CL} <50 mL/min; patients weighing 121 kg should receive a maximum infusion rate of 22.6 mg per bolus and a maximum infusion rate of 15 mg/h
			Tirofiban	Not recommended	0.4 mcg/kg IV infusion for 30 min followed by an infusion of 0.1 mcg/kg/min for 18–24 h	Reduce bolus dose to 0.2 mcg/kg/min and the maintenance infusion to 0.05 mcg/kg/min for patients with creatinine clearance <30 mL/min

TABLE 16–4. (Continued)

Drug	Clinical Condition and ACC/AHA Guideline Recommendation	Contraindications[a]	Dose
Nitroglycerin	STE and NSTE ACS, class I indication in patients whose symptoms are not fully relieved with three sublingual nitroglycerin tablets and initiation of β-blocker therapy, in patients with large infarctions, those presenting with heart failure or those who are hypertensive on presentation	Hypotension Sildenafil or vardenafil within 24 h or tadalifil within 48 h	0.4 mg SL, repeated every 5 min × 3 doses 5 to 10 mcg/min by continuous infusion Titrated up to 75 to 100 mcg/min until relief of symptoms or limiting side effects (headache or hypotension with a systolic blood pressure <90 mm Hg or more than 30 percent below starting mean arterial pressure levels if significant hypertension is present) Topical patches or oral nitrates and acceptable alternatives for patients without ongoing or refractory symptoms
Beta-blockers[c]	STE and NSTE ACS, class I recommendation in all patients without contraindications, class II b recommendation for patients with moderate left ventricular failure with signs of heart failure provided they can be closely monitored.	PR ECG segment >0.24 seconds Second- or third-degree atrioventricular (AV) block Heart rate <60 beats per min Systolic blood pressure <90 mm Hg Shock Left ventricular failure with congestive heart failure Severe reactive airway disease	*Target resting heart rate 50–60 beats per min* *Metoprolol* 5 mg increments by slow (over 1 to 2 min) IV administration Repeated every 5 min for a total initial dose of 15 mg Followed in 1 to 2 h by 25–50 mg by mouth every 6 h If a very conservative regimen is desired, initial doses can be reduced to 1–2 mg Alternatively, initial intravenous therapy may be omitted *Propranolol* 0.5–1 mg IV dose Followed in 1 to 2 h by 40–80 mg PO every 6 to 8 h Alternatively, initial intravenous therapy may be omitted *Atenolol* 5 mg IV dose Followed 5 min later by a second 5 mg IV dose and then 50–100 mg PO every day initiated 1 to 2 h after the intravenous dose Alternatively, initial intravenous therapy may be omitted *Esmolol* Starting maintenance dose of 0.1 mg/kg/min IV Tritration in increments of 0.05 mg/kg/min every 10 to 15 min as tolerated by blood pressure until the desired therapeutic response has been obtained, limiting symptoms develop, or a dose of 0.20 mg/kg/min is reached Optional loading dose of 0.5 mg/kg may be given by slow IV administration (2 to 5 min) for more rapid onset of action Alternatively, initial intravenous therapy may be omitted
Calcium channel blockers	STE ACS class IIa recommendation and NSTE ACS class I recommendation for patients with ongoing ischemia who are already taking adequate doses of nitrates and β-blockers or in patients with contraindications to or intolerance to β-blockers (diltiazem or verapamil for STE ACS and diltiazem, verapamil or amlodipine for NSTE ACS) NSTE ACS, class IIb recommendation for diltiazem for patients with AMI	Pulmonary edema Evidence of left ventricular dysfunction Systolic blood pressure <100 mm Hg PR ECG segment >0.24 seconds for diltiazem or verapamil Second- or third-degree AV block for diltiazem or verapamil Heart rate <60 beats per minute for diltiazem or verapamil	Diltiazem 120–240 mg sustained-release once daily Verapamil 80–240 mg sustained-release once daily Nifedipine 30–120 mg sustained-release once daily Amlodipine 5–10 mg once daily

(continued)

TABLE 16–4. (Continued)

Drug	Clinical Condition and ACC/AHA Guideline Recommendation	Contraindications[a]	Dose		
ACE inhibitors	STE ACS, class I recommendation within the first 24 hrs after hospital presentation for patients with anterior wall infarction, clinical signs of heart failure and those with EF <40% in the absence of contraindications, class IIa recommendation for all other patients in the absence of contraindications NSTE ACS, class I recommendation for patients with heart failure, left ventricular dysfunction and EF <40%, hypertension or type 2 diabetes mellitus Consider in all patients with CAD Indicated indefinitely for all post-AMI patients	Systolic blood pressure <100 mm Hg History of intolerance to an ACE inhibitor Bilateral renal artery stenosis Serum potassium >5.5 mEq/L	**Drug** Captopril Enalapril Lisinopril Ramipril Trandolapril	**Initial Dose (mg)** 6.25–12.5 2.5–5 2.5–5 1.25–2.5 1	**Target Dose (mg)** 50 twice daily to 50 three times daily 10 twice daily 10–20 once daily 5 twice daily or 10 once daily 4 once daily
Angiotensin receptor blockers	STE ACS, class I recommendation in patients with clinical signs of heart failure or EF <40% and intolerant of an ACE inhibitor, class IIa in patients with clinical signs of heart failure or EF <40% and no documentation of ACE inhibitor intolerance	Systolic blood pressure <100 mmg Hg Bilateral renal artery stenosis Serum potassium >5.5 mEq/L	**Drug** Candesartan Valsartan	**Initial Dose (mg)** 4–8 40	**Target Dose (mg)** 32 once daily 160 twice daily
Aldosterone antagonist	STE ACS, class I recommendation for patients with AMI and ejection fraction ≤40% and either heart failure symptoms or a diagnosis of diabetes mellitus.	Hypotension Serum potassium >5 mEq/L	**Drug** Eplerenone Spironolactone	**Initial Dose (mg)** 25 12.5	**Maximum Dose (mg)** 50 once daily 25–50 once daily
Morphine sulfate	STE and NSTE ACS, class I recommendation for patients whose symptoms are not relieved after three serial sublingual nitroglycerin tablets or whose symptoms recur with adequate anti-ischemic therapy	Hypotension Respiratory depression Confusion Obtundation	2–5 mg IV dose May be repeated every 5 to 30 min as needed to relieve symptoms and maintain patient comfort		

[a]Allergy or prior intolerance contraindication for all categories of drugs listed in this chart.

[b]Class I recommendations are conditions for which there is evidence and/or general agreement that a given procedure or treatment is useful and effective.

Class II recommendations are those conditions for which there is conflicting evidence and/or a divergence of opinion about the usefulness/efficacy of a procedure or treatment. For Class IIa recommendations, the weight of the evidence/opinion is in favor of usefulness/efficacy. Class IIb recommendations are those for which usefulness/efficacy is less well established by evidence/opinion.

[c]Choice of the specific agent is not as important as ensuring that appropriate candidates receive this therapy. If there are concerns about patient intolerance due to existing pulmonary disease, especially asthma, selection should favor a short-acting agent, such as propranolol or metoprolol or the ultra short-acting agent, esmolol. Mild wheezing or a history of chronic obstructive pulmonary disease should prompt a trial of a short-acting agent at a reduced dose (e.g., 2.5 mg intravenous metoprolol, 12.5 mg oral metoprolol, or 25 mcg/kg/min esmolol as initial doses) rather than complete avoidance of beta-blocker therapy.

ACC = American College of Cardiology; ACE = angiotensin-converting enzyme inhibitor; AHA = American Heart Association; AMI = acute myocardial infarction; CAD = coronary artery disease; EF = ejection fraction; IV = intravenous; Cr_{CL} = creatinine clearance; SC = subcutaneous.

Adapted from ref. 26; updated with information from ref. 3.

TABLE 16–5. Indications and Contraindications to Fibrinolytic Therapy: ACC/AHA Guidelines for Management of Patients with ST-Segment-Elevation Myocardial Infarction

Indications

Ischemic chest discomfort at least 20 minutes in duration but 12 hours or less since symptom onset

ST-segment elevation of at least 1 mm in height in two or more contiguous leads

New or presumed new left bundle branch block

Absolute Contraindications

Active internal bleeding (not including menses)

Previous intracranial hemorrhage at any time; ischemic stroke within 3 months

Known intracranial neoplasm

Known structural vascular lesion (example arteriovenous malformation)

Suspected aortic dissection

Significant closed head or facial trauma within 3 months

Relative Contraindications

Severe, uncontrolled hypertension on presentation (blood pressure >180/110 mm Hg)

History of prior ischemic stroke >3 months, dementia, or known intracranial pathology not covered above under absolute contraindications

Current use of anticoagulants

Known bleeding diathesis

Traumatic or prolonged (>10 min) CPR or major surgery (<3 weeks)

Noncompressible vascular puncture (such as a recent liver biopsy or carotid artery puncture)

Recent (within 2–4 weeks) internal bleeding

For prior streptokinase administration, prior administration (5 days–2 years), or prior allergic reactions

Pregnancy

Active peptic ulcer

History of severe, chronic poorly controlled hypertension

INR = international normalized ratio; CPR = cardiopulmonary resuscitation. *From ref.*[3]

than 90 minutes.[3] Other indications and contraindications for fibrinolysis are listed in Table 16–5.[3] It is not necessary to obtain the results of biochemical markers before initiating fibrinolytic therapy. Because administration of fibrinolytics results in clot lysis, patients at high risk for major bleeding, including intracranial hemorrhage, have either relative or absolute contraindications. Patients presenting with an absolute contraindication likely will not receive fibrinolytic therapy, and primary PCI is preferred. Patients with a relative contraindication may receive fibrinolytic therapy if the perceived risk of death from the MI is higher than the risk of major hemorrhage. For every 1000 patients with anterior wall MI, treatment with fibrinolysis saves 37 lives compared with placebo. For patients with inferior wall MI, who generally have smaller MIs and are at lower risk of death, treatment with fibrinolysis saves 8 lives per 1000 patients treated.[14]

Fibrinolytic therapy is controversial in patients older than 75 years of age. More than 60% of all MI deaths occur in this group. Benefit, in terms of absolute mortality reduction compared with placebo, varies from approximately 1% to 9%, with some observational studies suggesting higher mortality in the very elderly treated with fibrinolysis compared with no fibrinolysis. Stroke rates also grow in number with increasing patient age. While the intracranial hemorrhage rate is approximately 1% in younger patients, it is 2% in older patients. There is no excess risk of stroke in patients younger than 55 years of age, of whereas patients older than 75 years of age experience an excess of 8 strokes per 1000 patients treated.[14] However, the ACC/AHA practice guidelines recommend the use of fibrinolytics for this age group, provided that the patient has no contraindications.[3] A 1% absolute mortality benefit is felt to be clinically significant, and the benefit in terms of lives saved per 1000 patients treated has been reported to range from 10 to 80 in patients older than age of 75 years.[14] Because older patients may have cognitive impairment, careful history taking and assessment weighing the bleeding risk versus the benefit must be performed prior to administration of fibrinolysis.

The comparative pharmacology of commonly prescribed fibrinolytics is described in Table 16–6.[26] According to the ACC/AHA

TABLE 16–6. Comparison of Fibrinolytic Agents

Agent	Fibrin Specificity	TIMI-3 Blood Flow, Complete Perfusion at 90 min	Systemic Bleeding Risk/ICH Risk	Administration	Approximate Cost per Patient (MI Dosing)	Other Approved Uses
Streptokinase	+	35%	+++/+	Infusion over 60 min	$400	Pulmonary embolism, deep vein thrombosis, arterial thromboembolism, clearance of an occluded arteriovenous catheter
Alteplase (rt-PA)	+++	50%–60%	++/++	Bolus followed by infusions over 90 min, weight-based dosing	$2400	Pulmonary embolism, stroke, clearance of an occluded arteriovenous catheter
Reteplase (rPA)	++	50%–60%	++/++	2 bolus doses, 30 min apart	$2400	
Tenecteplase (TNK-tPA)	++++	50%–60%	+/++	Single bolus dose, weight-based dosing	$2400	

ICH = intracranial hemorrhage; MI = myocardial infarction; TIMI = Thrombolysis in Myocardial Blood Flow (TIMI-3 blood flow indicates complete perfusion of the infarct artery)
Adapted from ref. 26 with permission.

ST-segment-elevation ACS practice guideline, a more fibrin-specific agent, such as alteplase, reteplase, or tenecteplase, is preferred over a non-fibrin-specific agent, such as streptokinase.[3] Fibrin-specific fibrinolytics open a greater percentage of infarct arteries when measured in patients undergoing emergent angiography. Because an early open artery results in smaller infarcts, administration of fibrin-specific agents should result in lower mortality. This concept has been termed the *open-artery hypothesis*. In a large clinical trial, administration of alteplase reduced mortality by 1% (absolute reduction) and costs about $30,000 per year of life saved compared with streptokinase.[27] Two other trials compared alteplase with reteplase and alteplase with tenecteplase and found similar mortality between agents.[28,29] Therefore, either alteplase, reteplase, or tenecteplase is acceptable as a first-line agent. Most hospitals have at least two agents on their formulary. Most often, formulary decisions are based on frequency of use of fibrinolytics for other approved indications, with alteplase having the most indications of the fibrin-specific agents. Administration considerations also guide formulary decision making and choice for patient treatment with tenecteplase given as a single, weight-based dose and reteplase given as two fixed doses without weight adjustment. Therefore, both tenecteplase and reteplase are easier to administer than alteplase.

Intracranial hemorrhage and major bleeding are the most serious side effects of fibrinolytic agents (see Table 16–6). The risk of intracranial hemorrhage is higher with fibrin-specific agents than with streptokinase. Models are available for use in clinical practice to predict an individual patient's risk of intracranial hemorrhage following administration of a fibrinolytic.[3] The risk of systemic bleeding other than intracranial hemorrhage is higher with streptokinase than with other, more fibrin-specific agents.[27]

Only 20% to 40% of patients presenting with ST-segment-elevation ACS receive fibrinolysis compared with 7% receiving primary PCI.[30,31] Therefore, many patients do not receive early reperfusion therapy. The primary reason for lack of reperfusion therapy is that most patients present more than 12 hours after the time of symptom onset.[31] Of those presenting within the first 12 hours, the main reason that patients fail to receive fibrinolysis is the contraindication of prior stroke.[30] The percentage of eligible patients who receive reperfusion therapy is a quality indicator of care in patients with MI[27] (see Table 16–3). The "door-to-needle time," the time from presentation to start of fibrinolytic therapy, is another quality indicator[27] (see Table 16–3). While the ACC/AHA guidelines recommend a door-to-needle time of less than 30 minutes, the average in the United States currently is approximately 37 minutes.[31] Therefore, health care professionals can work to shorten administration times.

ASPIRIN

Based on several randomized trials, aspirin has become the preferred antiplatelet agent in the treatment of all ACSs.[2,3] Early aspirin administration to all patients without contraindications within the first 24 hours of hospital admission is a quality care indicator[27] (see Table 16–3). The antiplatelet effects of aspirin are mediated by inhibiting the synthesis of thromboxane A_2 through an irreversible inhibition of platelet cyclooxygenase-1.[32] Following the administration of a non-enteric-coated formulation, aspirin rapidly (<10 minutes) inhibits thromboxane A_2 production in the platelets. Aspirin also has anti-inflammatory actions, which decrease C-reactive protein and also may contribute to its effectiveness in ACS.[32] In patients undergoing PCI, aspirin prevents acute thrombotic occlusion during the procedure.

The Second International Study of Infarct Survival (ISIS-2), which studied the impact of streptokinase and aspirin (162.5 mg/day) either alone or in combination, is a landmark clinical trial that convincingly demonstrated the value of aspirin in patients with ST-segment-elevation ACS.[33] In this trial ($n = 17,187$), patients receiving aspirin demonstrated a lower risk of 35-day vascular mortality compared with placebo (9.4% versus 11.8%; $p < .0001$). The use of aspirin was not associated with any increase in major bleeding, although the incidence of minor bleeding was increased. Furthermore, the combination of aspirin plus streptokinase reduced mortality compared with placebo, as well as compared with either agent alone, thereby highlighting the additive effects of combination antithrombotic therapy. Because of its important role in the treatment of the MI patient, aspirin administration within the first 24 hours of hospital admission in patients without contraindications is a quality indicator of care[27] (see Table 16–3).

In patients experiencing an ACS, an initial dose equal to greater than 160 mg nonenteric aspirin is necessary to achieve a rapid platelet inhibition[32,33] (see Table 16–4). This first dose can be chewed in order to achieve high blood concentrations and platelet inhibition rapidly.[2,3] The notion of chewing aspirin came from the use of an enteric-coated formulation of aspirin in the ISIS-2 trial in order to break the enteric coating to ensure more rapid effect.[33] Current data suggest that although an initial dose 160 to 325 mg is required, long-term therapy with doses of 75 to 150 mg daily are as effective as higher doses and that doses of less than 325 mg daily are associated with a lower rate of bleeding.[34,35] The major bleeding rate associated with chronic aspirin administration in doses of less than 100 mg/day is 1.1%, whereas the frequency with doses of more than 100 mg/day is 1.7%.[35] Therefore, a daily maintenance dose of 75 to 160 mg is recommended in order to inhibit the 10% of the total platelet pool that is regenerated daily.[2]

Although the risk of major bleeding, particularly gastrointestinal bleeding, appears to be reduced by using low-dose aspirin,[32] low-dose aspirin, taken chronically, is not free of adverse effects. Patients should be counseled on the potential risk of bleeding.[34,36] In order to minimize the risk of bleeding, the use of aspirin with other agents that can induce bleeding, including clopidogrel and warfarin, should be avoided, unless the combination is clinically indicated and the increased risk of bleeding has been considered in evaluating the potential benefit of using such a combination. Other gastrointestinal disturbances, including dyspepsia and nausea, are infrequent when low-dose aspirin is used.[32] The ACC/AHA STE ACS guidelines specifically recommend that ibuprofen not be administered on a regular basis for pain relief concurrently with aspirin due to a reported drug interaction with aspirin whereby ibuprofen blocks aspirin's antiplatelet effects.[3] Finally, although some concern has been voiced regarding the possible increased risk of hemorrhagic stroke in patients taking aspirin,[37] this risk appears to be very small and is outweighed by the benefit in reducing the risk of ischemic stroke and other vascular events.[38] The risk of hemorrhagic stroke appears to be minimal in patients with adequate blood pressure control.[14] Aspirin therapy should be continued indefinitely.

THIENOPYRIDINES

Clopidogrel is recommended to be administered to patients with ST-segment-elevation ACS if they have an aspirin allergy[3] (see Table 16–4). Although aspirin is effective in the setting of ACS, it is a relatively weak platelet inhibitor that blocks platelet aggregation through only one pathway. The thienopyridines clopidogrel and ticlopidine are antiplatelet agents that mediate their antiplatelet effects through a blockade of ADP receptors on platelets.[39] Because ticlopidine is associated with the occurrence of neutropenia that requires frequent monitoring of the complete blood count (CBC) during the first 3 months of use,[40] clopidogrel is the preferred thienopyridine for ACS and PCI patients.

Although clopidogrel and ticlopidine have not been studied as monotherapy for ST-segment-elevation ACS, their use as an alternative, second-line agent for patients who are allergic to aspirin seems reasonable. Their efficacy as single antiplatelet agents used without aspirin has been demonstrated in various settings, including UA,[41] and in secondary prevention of vascular events in patients with a recent MI, stroke, or symptomatic peripheral vascular disease.[42] Studies evaluating the combination of clopidogrel with aspirin in patients with ST-segment-elevation ACS are ongoing.

At this point, the combination of clopidogrel and aspirin should be reserved for non-ST-segment-elevation patients and those patients undergoing PCI.[2,21] A more detailed discussion of clopidogrel administration in patients undergoing PCI may be found in Chap. 15. For PCI, clopidogrel is administered as a 300- to 600-mg loading dose followed by a 75 mg/day maintenance dose, in combination with aspirin, to prevent subacute stent thrombosis and long-term events such as the composite end point of death, MI, or need to undergo repeat PCI.[2,21] The most frequent side effects of clopidogrel are nausea, vomiting, and diarrhea, which occur in approximately 5% of patients. Rarely, thrombotic thrombocytopenic purpura has been reported with clopidogrel.[40] The most serious side effect of clopidogrel is bleeding, which will be discussed in more detail in the section "Pharmacotherapy for Non-ST-Segment-Elevation ACS."

GLYCOPROTEIN IIB/IIIA RECEPTOR INHIBITORS

Abciximab is a first-line GP IIb/IIIa receptor inhibitor for patients undergoing primary PCI[3,21,43] who have not received fibrinolytics. It should not be administered for medical management of the ST-segment-elevation ACS patient who will not be undergoing PCI. Abciximab is preferred over eptifibatide and tirofiban in this setting because abciximab is the most common GP IIb/IIIa receptor inhibitor studied in primary PCI trials.[3,21,43] Abciximab, in combination with aspirin, a thienopyridine, and UFH (administered as an infusion for the duration of the procedure), has been shown to reduce the risk of reinfarction[44,45] and need for repeat PCI [43] in ST-segment-elevation ACS clinical trials.

Dosing and contraindications for abciximab are described in Table 16–4. GP IIb/IIIa receptor inhibitors block the final common pathway of platelet aggregation, namely, cross-linking of platelets by fibrinogen bridges between the GP IIb and IIIa receptors on the platelet surface. Abciximab typically is initiated at the time of PCI, and the infusion is continued for 12 hours. Administration of a GP IIb/IIIa receptor inhibitor increases the risk of bleeding, especially if it is given in the setting of recent (<4 hours) administration of fibrinolytic therapy.[43–45] An immune-mediated thrombocytopenia occurs in approximately 5% of patients.[46]

Some trials suggest that early administration of abciximab results in early opening of the coronary artery, making primary PCI easier for the interventional cardiologist. Clinical trials performed to date suggest that the combination of early administration of a reduced dose of a fibrinolytic agent in combination with abciximab does not reduce mortality and increases the risk of bleeding, including intracranial hemorrhage, in elderly patients with ST-segment-elevation ACS.[44,45] Additional clinical trials of combined antithrombotic therapy for ST-segment-elevation PCI patients are ongoing.

ANTICOAGULANTS

UFH, administered as a continuous infusion, is a first-line anticoagulant for the treatment of patients with ST-segment-elevation ACS, both for medical therapy and for patients undergoing PCI.[3,21] UFH binds to antithrombin and then to clotting factors Xa and IIa (thrombin). Anticoagulant therapy should be initiated in the emergency department and continued for 24 hours or longer in patients who will be bridged over to receive chronic warfarin anticoagulation following acute MI.[3] In the United States, UFH typically is continued until the patient has undergone PCI during the hospitalization for ST-segment-elevation ACS. UFH dosing is described in Table 16–4. The dose of the UFH infusion is adjusted frequently to a target activated partial thromboplastin time (aPTT) (see Table 16–4). When coadministered with a fibrinolytic, aPTTs above the target range are associated with an increased rate of bleeding, whereas aPTTs below the target range are associated with increased mortality and reinfarction.[47] UFH is discontinued immediately after the PCI procedure.

A meta-analysis of small randomized studies from the 1970s and 1980s suggests that UFH reduces mortality by approximately 17%.[3] Other beneficial effects of anticoagulation are prevention of cardioembolic stroke, as well as venous thromboembolism, in MI patients.[3] If a fibrinolytic agent is administered, UFH is given concomitantly with alteplase, reteplase, and tenecteplase, but UFH is not administered to patients receiving the non-fibrin-selective agent streptokinase because no benefit of combined therapy can be demonstrated.[48] Rates of reinfarction are higher if UFH is not given in combination with the fibrin-selective agents.[48]

Besides bleeding, the most frequent adverse effect of UFH is an immune-mediated clotting disorder, heparin-induced thrombocytopenia, which occurs in up to 5% of patients treated with UFH. Heparin-induced thrombocytopenia is less common in patients receiving low-molecular-weight heparins (LMWHs).[49]

LMWHs have not been studied in the setting of primary PCI. LMWHs, like UFH, bind to antithrombin and inhibit both factor Xa and IIa. However, because their composition is mostly short saccharide chain lengths, they preferentially inhibit factor Xa over factor IIa, which requires larger chain lengths for binding and inhibition. Limited data, primarily with enoxaparin, suggest that LMWHs may be an alternative to UFH. Pooled data from smaller ST-segment-elevation ACS trials suggest that enoxaparin is associated with similar safety and reduced reinfarction when coadministered with fibrinolytics (and aspirin).[50] A larger trial evaluating enoxaparin versus UFH in combination with fibrinolytics for ST-segment-elevation ACS is ongoing.

NITRATES

One SL nitroglycerin (NTG) tablet should be administered every 5 minutes for up to three doses to relieve myocardial ischemia. If patients have previously been prescribed sublingual NTG and ischemic chest discomfort persists for more than 5 minutes after the first dose, the patient should be instructed to contact emergency medical services before self-administering subsequent doses in order to activate emergency care sooner. IV NTG then should be initiated in all patients with an ACS who do not have a contraindication and who have persistent ischemic symptoms, heart failure, or uncontrolled blood pressure, and should be continued for approximately 24 hours after ischemia is relieved[3] (see Table 16–4). Importantly, other life-saving therapy, such as ACE inhibitors or β-blockers, should not be witheld because the mortality benefit of nitrates is unproven. Nitrates promote the release of nitric oxide from the endothelium, which results in venous and arterial vasodilation. Venodilation lowers preload and myocardial oxygen demand. Arterial vasodilation may lower blood pressure, thus reducing myocardial oxygen demand. Arterial vasodilation also relieves coronary artery vasospasm, dilating coronary arteries to improve myocardial blood flow and oxygenation. Nitrates play a limited role in the treatment of ACS patients because two large, randomized clinical trials failed to show a mortality benefit for IV followed by oral nitrate therapy in acute MI.[51,52] The most significant adverse effects of nitrates are tachycardia, flushing, headache, and hypotension. Nitrate administration is contraindicated in patients who have received oral phosphodiesterase-5 inhibitors, such as sildenafil and vardenafil within the past 24 hours and tadalafil within the past 48 hours.

β-BLOCKERS

IV bolus doses or oral doses of a β-blocker should be administered early in the care of patients with ST-segment-elevation ACS and then an oral β-blocker continued indefinitely. Early administration of a β-blocker within the first 24 hours of hospitalization in patients lacking a contraindication is a quality care indicator[27] (see Table 16–3). In ACS, the benefit of β-blockers results mainly from the competitive blockade of β_1-adrenergic receptors located on the myocardium. β_1-Blockade produces a reduction in heart rate, myocardial contractility, and blood pressure, decreasing myocardial oxygen demand. In addition, the reduction in heart rate increases diastolic time, thus improving ventricular filling and coronary artery perfusion.[53] As a result of these effects, β-blockers reduce the risk for recurrent ischemic, infarct size, risk of reinfarction, and occurrence of ventricular arrhythmias in the hours and days following MI.[53]

Landmark clinical trials have established the role of early β-blocker therapy in reducing MI mortality. Most of these trials were performed in the 1970s and 1980s before routine use of early reperfusion therapy. In the First International Study of Infarct Survival (ISIS-1), 16,027 patients with a suspected MI were randomized to IV atenolol 5 to 10 mg followed by atenolol 100 mg daily for 7 days or to no treatment.[54] After 7 days, vascular death was reduced by 15% ($p < .04$). The benefit was apparent after 1 day of treatment ($p < .003$), reflecting the ability of β-blockers to prevent early reinfarction and sudden death. In the Metoprolol In Acute Myocardial Infarction (MI-AMI) trial, 5778 patients with a suspected MI were randomized to IV metoprolol followed by oral metoprolol or placebo, and mortality was reduced from 4.9% to 4.3%[55] ($p = NS$), and the occurrence of early progression to Q-wave MI also was reduced ($p = .024$).[56]

Data regarding the acute benefit of β-blockers in MI in the reperfusion era is derived mainly from the Thrombolysis in Myocardial Infarction (TIMI) II trial.[57] In this trial, patients with ST-segment-elevation ACS were randomized to either IV metoprolol to be given as soon as possible following fibrinolytic administration followed by oral metoprolol or oral metoprolol deferred until day 6. Early administration of metoprolol was associated with a significant decrease in recurrent ischemia and early reinfarction. Patients receiving fibrinolytic therapy within 2 hours of symptom onset demonstrated the greatest benefit from early metoprolol administration. Based on the results of these trials, early administration of β-blockers (to patients without contraindications) within the first 24 hours of hospital admission is a standard of quality patient care[27] (see Table 16–3).

The most serious side effects of β-blocker administration early in ACS are hypotension, bradycardia, and heart block. While initial acute administration of β-blockers is not appropriate for patients who present with decompensated heart failure, initiation of β-blockers may be attempted before hospital discharge is most patients following

treatment of acute heart failure. It cannot be underemphasized that diabetes mellitus does not constitute a contraindication to β-blockers. Although the use of β-blockers may mask symptoms of hypoglycemia, except sweating, diabetics greatly benefit from β-blocker administration because they are at high risk of recurrent events.[53] In patients in whom a major concern exists regarding a possible intolerance to β-blockers, such as patients with chronic obstructive pulmonary disease, a short acting β-blocker, such as metoprolol or esmolol, should be administered intravenously initially.[53] β-Blockers are continued indefinitely.

CALCIUM CHANNEL BLOCKERS

Administration of calcium channel blockers in the setting of ST-segment-elevation ACS is reserved for patients who have contraindications to β-blockers and is used for relief of ischemic symptoms.[3] Patients prescribed calcium channel blockers for treatment of hypertension who are not receiving β-blockers and who do not have a contraindication to β-blockers should have the calcium channel blocker discontinued and a β-blocker initiated. Calcium channel blockers inhibit calcium influx into myocardial and vascular smooth muscle cells, causing vasodilatation. Although all calcium channel blockers produce coronary vasodilatation and decrease blood pressure, other effects are more heterogeneous between agents. Dihydropyridine calcium channel blockers (e.g., amlodipine, felodipine, and nifedipine) primarily produce their anti-ischemic effects through peripheral vasodilatation with no clinical effects on atrioventricular (AV) node conduction and heart rate. Diltiazem and verapamil, on the other hand, have additional anti-ischemic effects by reducing contractility and AV nodal conduction and slowing heart rate.[58]

Current data suggest little benefit on clinical outcomes beyond symptom relief for dihydropyridine calcium channel blockers in the setting of ACS.[58] Moreover, the use of first-generation short-acting dihydropyridines, such as nifedipine, should be avoided because they appear to worsen outcomes through their negative inotropic effects, induction of reflex sympathetic activation, tachycardia, and increased myocardial ischemia.[58]

Although earlier trials suggested that verapamil and diltiazem may provide improved benefit in selected patients, the large Incomplete Infarction Trial of European Research Collaborators Evaluating Prognosis post-Thrombolysis (INTERCEPT) has dampened the interest for the use of diltiazem in patients receiving fibrinolytics.[59] In this trial, the use of extended-release diltiazem had no effect on the 6-month risk of cardiac death, MI, or recurrent ischemia. Therefore, the role of verapamil or diltiazem appears to be limited to relief of ischemia-related symptoms or control of heart rate in patients with supraventricular arrhythmias for whom β-blockers are contraindicated or ineffective.[2,3]

Adverse effects and contraindications of calcium channel blockers are described in Table 16–4. Verapamil, diltiazem, and first-generation dihydropyridines also should be avoided in patients with acute decompensated heart failure or LV dysfunction because they can worsen heart failure and potentially increase mortality secondary to their negative inotropic effects. In patients with heart failure requiring treatment with a calcium channel blocker, amlodipine is the preferred agent.[60,61]

Two groups of patients may benefit from calcium channel blockers as opposed to β-blockers as initial therapy. Cocaine-induced ACS and variant (or Prinzmetal's) angina are two conditions in which coronary vasospasm plays an important role.[2,3,58] Calcium channel blockers and/or NTG generally are considered the agents of choice in these patients because they can reverse the coronary spasm by inducing smooth muscle relaxation in the coronary arteries. In contrast, β-blockers generally should be avoided in these patients unless there is uncontrolled sinus tachycardia (>100 beats per minute) or severe uncontrolled hypertension (systolic blood pressure greater than 150 mm Hg) following cocaine use because β-blockers actually may worsen vasospasm through an unopposed β_2-blocking effect on the smooth muscle cells.[2]

EARLY PHARMACOTHERAPY FOR NON-ST-SEGMENT-ELEVATION ACS

In general, early pharmacotherapy for non-ST-segment-elevation ACS (see Fig. 16–3) is similar to that for ST-segment-elevation ACS with four exceptions:

1. Fibrinolytic therapy is not administered.
2. Clopidogrel should be administered, in addition to aspirin, to most patients.
3. GP IIb/IIIa receptor blockers are administered to high-risk patients for medical therapy as well as for PCI patients.
4. There are no standard quality indicators for patients with non-ST-segment-elevation ACS who are not diagnosed with MI.

⑨ According to the ACC/AHA non-ST-segment-elevation ACS practice guidelines, early pharmacotherapy for non–ST-segment elevation should include intranasal oxygen (if oxygen saturation is <90%), SL followed by IV NTG, aspirin, an IV β-blocker, and UFH or, preferably, LMWH. Morphine is also administered to patients with refractory angina, as described previously. These agents should be administered early, while the patient is still in the emergency department. Dosing and contraindications for SL and IV NTG, aspirin, IV β-blockers, UFH, and LMWHs are listed in Table 16–4.[2,26]

FIBRINOLYTIC THERAPY

Fibrinolytic therapy is not indicated in any patient with non-ST-segment-elevation ACS, even those who have positive biochemical markers (e.g., troponin) that indicate infarction. Because the risk of death from MI is lower in patients with non-ST-segment-elevation ACS, whereas the risk for life-threatening adverse effects, such as intracranial hemorrhage, with fibrinolytics is similar between patients with ST-segment-elevation and non-ST-segment-elevation ACS, the risks of fibrinolytic therapy outweigh the benefit for non-ST-segment-elevation ACS patients. In fact, increased mortality has been reported with fibrinolytics compared with controls in clinical trials where fibrinolytics have been administered to patients with non-ST-segment-elevation ACS (patients with normal or ST-segment-depression ECGs).[14]

ASPIRIN

Aspirin reduces the risk of death or developing MI by about 50% (compared with no antiplatelet therapy) in patients with non-ST-segment-elevation ACS.[34] Therefore, aspirin remains the cornerstone of early treatment for all ACSs. Dosing of aspirin for non-ST-segment-elevation ACS is the same as that for ST-segment-elevation ACS (see Table 16–4). Aspirin is continued indefinitely.

THIENOPYRIDINES

For patients with non-ST-segment-elevation ACS, the addition of clopidogrel started on the first day of hospitalization as a 300- to 600-mg loading dose followed the next day by 75 mg/day orally is recommended for most patients.[2] Although the use of aspirin in ACS is the mainstay of antiplatelet therapy, morbidity and mortality following an ACS remains high. Researchers explored whether or not combining two oral antiplatelet agents with different mechanisms of action, aspirin and clopidogrel, would result in additional clinical benefit over using aspirin alone. Efficacy and safety of this dual antiplatelet therapy were demonstrated in the Clopidogrel in Unstable Angina to Prevent Recurrent Events (CURE) trial.[62] In CURE, 12,562 patients with unstable angina or an NSTEMI randomized to a loading dose of 300 mg clopidogrel followed by a daily dose of 75 mg or placebo in addition to aspirin for a mean duration of 9 months. Clopidogrel reduced the combined risk of death from cardiovascular causes, nonfatal MI, or stroke from 11.4% to 9.4% compared with placebo, mainly through a reduction in the risk of MI. Cardiovascular mortality was similar between groups. Because this study was conducted primarily in Canada and in Europe, patients routinely did not undergo angiographic evaluation, and fewer than 50% of patients eventually underwent PCI. Although a subsequent analysis of non-ST-segment-elevation patients undergoing PCI[63] suggested benefit for the prolonged use of clopidogrel in these patients, the applicability of these results was limited by its observational nature and the low use of a GP IIb/IIIa receptor antagonist, considered a standard of PCI care in the United States. In addition, there was no statistical benefit demonstrated for event reductions between 30 days and 1 year. Administration of clopidogrel for at least 30 days in patients undergoing intracoronary stenting is a standard of care.[21]

Results from a second trial in PCI patients, the Clopidogrel for the Reduction of Events During Observation (CREDO) trial,[64] in which patients treated with long-term clopidogrel (1 year), demonstrated a lower risk of death, MI, or stroke compared with patients receiving only 28 days of clopidogrel (8.5% versus 11.5%; $p = .02$). However, the interpretation of this study is limited in that the control group did not receive a loading dose of clopidogrel on the first day. Whether or not treatment with clopidogrel should be extended to more than 1 year is currently being investigated in a large, randomized trial. Therefore, based on the results of these three clinical trials, clopidogrel is indicated for at least 9 months in non-ST-segment-elevation ACS patients who do not undergo PCI or CABG (medical management) and for at least 30 days in patients receiving bare metal intracoronary stents.

The major concern when combining two antiplatelet agents is the increased risk of bleeding. In CURE, the risk of major bleeding was increased in patients receiving clopidogrel plus aspirin compared with aspirin alone (3.7% versus 2.7%; $p = .001$).[62] A post-hoc analysis of CURE revealed that the rate of major bleeding depends on the dose of aspirin and showed that doses equal to or less than 100 mg daily reduced the risk of bleeding with similar efficacy when compared with higher doses.[65] Therefore, using a low dose of aspirin (75–100 mg/day) for maintenance therapy is recommended when aspirin is used in combination with clopidogrel.

In patients undergoing CABG, major bleeding was increased in patients having the procedure within 5 days of clopidogrel discontinuation (9.6% versus 6.3%; $p = .06$) but not in patients for which clopidogrel was discontinued more than 5 days before the procedure.[62] Aspirin was continued up to and after CABG. Therefore, in patients scheduled for CABG, clopidogrel should be withheld at least 5 days and preferably 7 days before the procedure.[2]

The timing of initiation of clopidogrel for a patient presenting with non-ST-segment-elevation ACS is controversial. Although it is clear that clopidogrel should be initiated as soon as possible in patients being treated with a noninterventional strategy or in patients who have a contraindication to aspirin, the need to delay CABG for 5 to 7 days following clopidogrel has led many to suggest that clopidogrel administration should be delayed until coronary angiography is performed and the need for CABG is excluded. This is particularly relevant in centers in which the waiting time for CABG is less than 5 days. However, existing data also suggest that early treatment with clopidogrel before angiography is performed reduces the number of cardiovascular events following the procedure.[64] Therefore, others have advocated the expanded use of early clopidogrel in all patients experiencing a non-ST-segment-elevation ACS.

A pragmatic yet non-evidence-based approach suggests that in centers in which patients can undergo coronary angiography within 24 hours of admission, it is reasonable to wait until after angiography is performed and it has been determined that a CABG will not be performed before clopidogrel is initiated.[2]

GLYCOPROTEIN IIB/IIIA RECEPTOR INHIBITORS

Administration of tirofiban or eptifibatide is recommended for high-risk non-ST-segment-elevation ACS patients as medical therapy without planned revascularization, and administration of either abciximab or eptifibatide is recommended for non-ST-segment-elevation ACS patients undergoing PCI. Administration of tirofiban or eptifibatide is also indicated in patients with continued or recurrent ischemia despite treatment with aspirin and an anticoagulant.[2] The pharmacologic similarities and differences between GP IIb/IIIa receptor inhibitors are reviewed in Chap. 15. As discussed in Chap. 15, the benefits of GP IIb/IIIa receptor inhibitors in PCI is well established, and they are considered first-line agents to reduce the risk of reinfarction and the need for repeat PCI.[21]

Two large clinical trials highlight their role in the setting of ACS and PCI. In the Platelet Glycoprotein IIb/IIIa in Unstable Angina: Receptor Suppression Using Integrilin Therapy (PURSUIT) trial ($n = 10,948$), eptifibatide added to aspirin and UFH and continued for up to 72 hours reduced the combined end point of death or MI at 30 days (14.2% versus 15.7%) compared with aspirin and UFH alone.[66] In the Platelet Receptor Inhibition in Ischemic Syndrome Management in Patients Limited by Unstable Signs and Symptoms (PRISM-PLUS) study ($n = 1915$), tirofiban added to aspirin and UFH and continued for up to 72 hours reduced the rate of death, MI, or refractory ischemia at 7 days compared with aspirin and UFH alone.[67] However, in these and other trials of GP IIb/IIIa inhibitors for non-ST-segment-elevation ACS, the benefit was limited to patients undergoing PCI and not those treated without interventional therapy.[68] This concept was proven in the Global Use of Strategies to Open Occluded Arteries (GUSTO) IV trial ($n = 7800$), in which medical therapy with abciximab continued for up to 48 hours failed to demonstrate benefit and trended toward worsened outcomes.[69] Therefore, medical therapy with GP IIb/IIIa receptor inhibitors is reserved for higher-risk patients, such as those with positive troponin or ST-segment depression, and patients who have continued or recurrent ischemia despite other antithrombotic therapy.[2] Patients undergoing PCI in these trials received several hours to days of pretreatment with the GP IIb/IIIa receptor blocker before proceeding to PCI.

The role of GP IIb/IIIa receptor antagonists in patients with non-ST-segment-elevation ACS undergoing PCI also was evaluated in two large clinical trials that used GP IIb/IIIa receptor blockers initiated at the time of PCI. In the Enhanced Suppression of the Platelet IIb/IIIa Receptor with Integrilin Therapy Trial (ESPRIT) ($n = 1024$), eptifibatide in combination with aspirin and UFH reduced the rate of death or MI up to 1 year in patients undergoing PCI.[70] The benefits of treatment in ACS subgroup were more pronounced compared with the stable angina subgroup, thereby establishing a role for eptifibatide in the ACS PCI patient.

Only one trial has compared two GP IIb/IIIa receptor blockers with each other. In the Do Tirofiban and ReoPro Give Similar Efficacy Outcomes Trial (TARGET), tirofiban, at a different dose from that used in the PRISM-PLUS study, was compared with abciximab in patients undergoing PCI.[71,72] In the subgroup of patients with ACS, there was a statistically significant reduction in the composite end point of death, nonfatal MI, or need for repeat PCI at 30 days in patients randomized to receive abciximab compared with tirofiban (6.3% versus 9.3%).[71] While the numerical benefit of a 3% absolute risk reduction was maintained at 6 months, it approached but was no longer statistically significant (hazard ratio 1.19, abciximab better than tirofiban, 95% confidence internal 0.99–1.42).[72] Therefore, while there is an early benefit to administering abciximab, perhaps it is not sustained. Following TARGET, the dose of tirofiban that was used in that trial has been shown to be ineffective at inhibiting platelet aggregation during the PCI procedure.[73] Therefore, tirofiban cannot be recommended for PCI unless the patient has been treated with tirofiban for several hours to days prior to PCI and adequate inhibition of platelet aggregation can be ensured. If a GP IIb/IIIa receptor blocker is initiated while the patient is undergoing the procedure, abciximab or eptifibatide should be used because the most appropriate tirofiban dose is not known at this time.

As emphasized in the ACC/AHA guidelines, the benefits of GP IIb/IIIa receptor blockers are greater in patients undergoing PCI. A recent meta-analysis estimates that 30 adverse outcomes (either death or MI) are prevented for every 1000 patients treated with a GP IIb/IIIa receptor blocker before PCI, whereas only 4 events are prevented for medical management of non-ST-segment-elevation ACS patients using GP IIb/IIIa receptor blockers without PCI.[74] This translates into a number needed to treat 32 patients to prevent 1 event if a GP IIb/IIIa receptor blocker is administered before PCI and 250 patients to prevent 1 event if it is administered as medical therapy without PCI.[74]

Doses and contraindications to GP IIb/IIIa receptor blockers are described in Table 16–4, and common adverse effects are described in the preceding section. Administration of intravenous GP IIb/IIIa receptor blockers in combination with aspirin and an anticoagulant results in major bleeding rates of 3.6%[35] but no increased risk of intracranial hemorrhage in the absence of concomitant fibrinolytic treatment. The risk of thrombocytopenia with tirofiban and eptifibatide appears to be lower than that with abciximab. Bleeding risks appear similar among agents. However, major bleeding with the combination of aspirin, heparin, and a GP IIb/IIIa inhibitor is higher (approximately 3% to 4%) than using a heparin plus aspirin (<2%).

ANTICOAGULANTS

Either UFH or LMWHs should be administered to patients with non-ST-segment-elevation ACS. Therapy should be continued for up to 48 hours or until the end of the angiography or PCI procedure. In patients initiating warfarin therapy, UFH or LMWHs should be continued until the international normalization ratio (INR) with warfarin is in the therapeutic range. Data supporting the addition of UFH to aspirin stems from a meta-analysis of six randomized trials demonstrating a 33% reduction in the risk of death or MI at 6 weeks with UFH plus aspirin compared with aspirin alone.[75] One trial compared the LMWH dalteparin plus aspirin with aspirin alone and found a 60% reduction in death or MI at 6 days.[76] Three clinical trials have compared UFH with LMWHs for medical management of NSTE ACS.[77–79] Two trials in a total of approximately 7000 patients demonstrated a 15% reduction in the composite end point of death, MI, or recurrent ischemia with enoxaparin compared with UFH.[77,78] One trial with dalteparin in approximately 1400 patients demonstrated similar outcomes between dalteparin and UFH.[79] The results from these trials also showed no increased risk of major bleeding with LMWHs compared with UFH.[77–79] Minor bleeding, mostly injection-site hematomas, was increased because the LMWHs are given by subcutaneous injection, whereas UFH is administered by continuous infusion.[77–79] Because of a reduction in event rates compared with UFH, enoxaparin was mentioned as "preferred" over UFH in the ACC/AHA clinical practice guidelines.[2]

Previously, lack of data with LMWHs in non-ST-segment-elevation ACS patients undergoing PCI has limited their use in this setting. Traditionally, interventional cardiologists monitor the degree of anticoagulation of UFH using the activated clotting time (ACT) in the cardiac catheterization laboratory. Because LMWHs have only a small effect on increasing the ACT owing to their preferential effect on activated factor X inhibition, the ACT cannot be used to monitor LMWH efficacy or toxicity. One large clinical trial of enoxaparin compared with UFH in this setting found similar efficacy with a slightly higher risk of major bleeding with enoxaparin. This trial was confounded by a large number of patients who received both UFH and enoxaparin. The authors concluded that the use of enoxaparin has similar reduction in death or MI compared to UFH. Enoxaparin is an option that may be initiated and then continued through PCI, but switching between UFH and enoxaparin should be avoided.[80]

The risk of major bleeding with UFH or LMWHs is higher in patients undergoing angiography because there is an associated risk of hematoma at the femoral access site. Major bleeding rates in these patients are less than or equal to 2%. The risk of heparin-induced thrombocytopenia is lower in some, but not all, clinical trials with LMWHs compared with UFH.

Because LMWHs are eliminated renally and patients with renal insufficiency generally have been excluded from clinical trials, some practice protocols recommend UFH for patients with creatinine clearance rates of less than 30 mL/min. (Creatinine clearance is calculated based on total patient body weight.) However, recent recommendations for dosing adjustment of enoxaparin in patients with creatinine clearances between 10 and 30 mL/min are now listed in the product manufacturer's label (see Table 16–4). Administration of LMWHs should be avoided in dialysis patients. UFH is monitored and the dose adjusted to a target aPTT, whereas LMWHs are administered by a fixed, weight-based dose. Other dosing information and contraindications are described in Table 16–4.

NITRATES

SL followed by IV NTG should be administered to all patients with non-ST-segment-elevation ACS in the absence of contraindications (see Table 16–4). The mechanism of action, dosing, contraindications, and adverse effects are the same as described in the section "Early Pharmacotherapy for ST-Segment-Elevation ACS" above. IV NTG typically is continued for approximately 24 hours following ischemia relief. The mechanism of action, dosing, contraindications, and adverse effects are the same as described in the section "Early Pharmacotherapy for ST-Segment-Elevation ACS" above.

β-BLOCKERS

IV followed by oral β-blockers should be administered to all patients with non-ST-segment-elevation ACS in the absence of contraindications. The mechanism of action, dosing, contraindications, and adverse effects are the same as described in the section "Early Pharmacotherapy for ST-Segment-Elevation ACS" above. β-Blockers are continued indefinitely.

CALCIUM CHANNEL BLOCKERS

As described above, calcium channel blockers should not be administered to most patients with ACS. Their role is a second-line treatment for patients with certain contraindications to β-blockers and those with continued ischemia despite β-blocker and nitrate therapy. They are a first-line therapy in patients with Prinzmetal's vasospastic angina and those with cocaine-associated ACS. Administration of either amlodipine, diltiazem, or verapamil is preferred.[2] Agent selection based on heart rate and LV dysfunction (diltiazem and verapamil contraindicated in patients with bradycardia, heart block, or systolic heart failure) is described in more detail in the section "Early Pharmacotherapy for ST-Segment-Elevation ACS" above. Dosing and contraindications are described in Table 16–4.

SECONDARY PREVENTION FOLLOWING MI

The long-term goals following MI are to

1. Control modifiable CHD risk factors
2. Prevent the development of systolic heart failure
3. Prevent recurrent MI and stroke
4. Prevent death, including sudden cardiac death

Pharmacotherapy that has been proven to decrease mortality, heart failure, reinfarction, or stroke should be initiated prior to hospital discharge for secondary prevention. Guidelines from the ACC/AHA suggest that following MI from either ST-segment-elevation ACS or non-ST-segment-elevation ACS, patients should receive indefinite treatment with aspirin, a β-blocker, and an ACE inhibitor.[2,3] For patients with non-ST-segment-elevation ACS, most should receive clopidogrel, in addition to aspirin, for up to 9 months.[2] Selected patients also will be treated with long-term warfarin anticoagulation. Newer therapies include eplerenone, an aldosterone antagonist. For all ACS patients, treatment and control of modifiable risk factors such as hypertension, dyslipidemia, and diabetes mellitus are essential. Most patients with CHD will require drug therapy for hyperlipidemia, usually with a statin (hydroxymethylglutaryl coenzyme A reductase inhibitor). Benefits and adverse effects of long-term treatment with these medications are discussed in more detail below.

ASPIRIN

Aspirin decreases the risk of death, recurrent MI, and stroke following MI. An aspirin prescription at hospital discharge is a quality care indicator in MI patients[27] (see Table 16–3). The clinical value of aspirin in secondary prevention of ACS and other vascular diseases was demonstrated in a large number of clinical trials. Following an

MI, aspirin is expected to prevent 36 vascular events per 1000 patients treated for 2 years.[32] Because the benefit of antiplatelet agents appears to be sustained for at least 2 years following an MI,[34] all patients should receive aspirin indefinitely, or clopidogrel in patients with a contraindication to aspirin.[2,3]

The risk of major bleeding from chronic aspirin therapy is approximately 2% and is dose-related. Aspirin doses of 75 to 150 mg are not less effective than doses of 160 to 325 mg and may have lower rates of bleeding. Therefore, chronic doses of 75 to 162 mg are now recommended.[3]

CLOPIDOGREL

For patients with non-ST-segment-elevation ACS, clopidogrel decreases the risk of developing either death, MI, or stroke. The benefit is primarily in reducing the rate of MI.[62] The ACC/AHA guidelines suggest a duration of therapy of 9 months[2] because this was the average duration of treatment in the CURE trial.[62] Patients who have undergone a PCI with stent implantation may receive clopidogrel for up to 12 months.[64] The benefits of clopidogrel therapy in PCI are discussed in more detail in Chap. 15.

Because of the risk of bleeding with clopidogrel and aspirin doses higher than 100 mg, low-dose aspirin should be administered concomitantly.[65] Although not specifically studied, longer duration of therapy with clopidogrel plus aspirin may be considered for patients with many recurrent vascular events such as stroke, MI, or recurrent ACS. In addition, patients with concomitant peripheral arterial disease or CABG surgery may benefit from combined therapy with aspirin and clopidogrel to prevent CHD events.[42]

ANTICOAGULATION

Warfarin should be considered in selected patients following an ACS, including patients with a left ventricular thrombus, patients demonstrating extensive ventricular wall motion abnormalities on cardiac echocardiogram, and patients with a history of thromboembolic disease or chronic atrial fibrillation.[3] A more detailed discussion regarding the use of warfarin is available in Chap. 19.

Because of the importance of thrombus formation in the pathophysiology of ACS and the findings from several studies suggesting residual thrombus at the site of plaque rupture even months following an MI, anticoagulants, primarily warfarin, have been the subject of many clinical trials in patients following an ACS. These trials have produced varying and inconsistent results. Because the intensity of anticoagulation varied among these trials, it is important to take into consideration the intensity of the anticoagulation when interpreting these trials.

Data from two large, randomized trials demonstrate that the use of low, fixed-dose warfarin (mean INR 1.4) combined with aspirin[81] or of low-intensity anticoagulation (mean INR 1.8) monotherapy[82] provides no significant clinical benefit compared with aspirin monotherapy but significantly increases the risk of major bleeding. Therefore, warfarin therapy targeted to an INR of less than 2 cannot be recommended for secondary prevention of CHD events following MI.

Subsequently, in two large, randomized trials, a strategy of combining intermediate-intensity anticoagulation (target INR 2–2.5) with low-dose aspirin reduced the combined end point of death, MI, or stroke in patients following MI compared with aspirin alone. The

Antithrombotics in Secondary Prevention of Events in Coronary Thrombosis 2 (ASPECT-2)[83] and the Wafarin Re-Infarction Study 2 (WARIS-2)[84] reported that warfarin alone targeted to a high-intensity INR and medium-intensity warfarin plus low-dose aspirin were superior to aspirin alone in preventing the combined end point of death, MI, or stroke. The target INRs in the high-intensity warfarin monotherapy group were 3 to 4[83] and 2.8 to 4.2,[84] respectively. The target INR in the more effective medium-intensity warfarin and low-dose aspirin group was 2 to 2.5 in both trials. No significant differences in efficacy were observed between the combination of medium-intensity anticoagulation and low-dose aspirin and monotherapy with high-intensity anticoagulation.

The use of warfarin in combination with aspirin was associated with an increased risk of minor and major bleeding. Furthermore, patients in the warfarin groups were two to three times more likely to discontinue their treatment. Since the trials were analyzed as intention to treat, the treatment effect of warfarin probably is greater, but the long-term bleeding risks may be greater as well. A meta-analysis of seven clinical trials of secondary prevention with aspirin, warfarin, and the combination suggested that the risk of cardiovascular death, MI, or stroke was reduced by 3.3% (absolute risk reduction 15.9% versus 12.6%) and reported the risk of major bleeding to be increased by 1.3% (absolute risk 3% versus 1.7%) for a net benefit of 2%.[85] Many consider this net benefit for a composite end point to be small in comparison with the large management issues related to warfarin therapy, such as INR monitoring and drug interactions. WARIS-2 and ASPECT-2 were conducted in the Netherlands and in Norway, two countries renowned for the quality of their anticoagulation programs and clinics, thereby limiting generalization of the findings. Furthermore, because a large proportion of ACS patients in North America undergo coronary revascularization with subsequent stent implementation, patients require a combination of aspirin and clopidogrel to prevent stent thrombosis, a platelet-dependent phenomenon that warfarin does not effectively prevent.[86] Therefore, because of the complexity of managing current anticoagulants, the use of warfarin is unlikely to gain wide acceptance. Despite the superiority of warfarin plus aspirin over aspirin alone, it is not currently recommended as a preferred regimen by any professional association practice guidelines in the absence of the conditions for selected patients outlined previously.

β-BLOCKERS, NITRATES, AND CALCIUM CHANNEL BLOCKERS

Current treatment guidelines recommend that following an ACS, patients should receive a β-blocker indefinitely[2,3] whether they have residual symptoms of angina or not.[87] β-Blocker prescription at hospital discharge in the absence of contraindications is a quality care indicator[27] (see Table 16–3). Overwhelming data support the use of β-blockers in patients with a previous MI. Data from a systematic review of long-term trials of patients with recent MI demonstrate that the number needed to treat for 1 year with a β-blocker to prevent one death is only 84 patients.[88] Because the benefit from β-blockers appears to be maintained for at least 6 years following an MI,[89] it is recommended that all patients receive β-blockers indefinitely in the absence of contraindications or intolerance.[2,3] Currently, there are no data to support the superiority of one β-blocker over another, although the only β-blocker with intrinsic sympathomimetic activity that has been shown to be beneficial following MI is acebutolol.[90]

Although β-blockers should be avoided in patients with decompensated heart failure from LV systolic dysfunction complicating an MI, clinical trial data suggest that it is safe to initiate β-blockers prior to hospital discharge in these patients once heart failure symptoms have resolved.[91] These patients actually may benefit more than those without LV dysfunction.[92]

Despite the overwhelming benefit demonstrated in clinical trials, β-blockers are still widely underused, perhaps because clinicians fear that patients will experience adverse reactions, including depression, fatigue, and sexual dysfunction. A recent systematic review of 15 trials that included more than 35,000 patients demonstrated that withholding β-blocker therapy in such a group was not founded because β-blockers do not significantly increase the risk of depression and only modestly increase the risk of fatigue and sexual dysfunction.[93]

In patients who cannot tolerate or have a contraindication to a β-blocker, a calcium channel blocker can be used to prevent anginal symptoms but should not be used routinely in the absence of such symptoms.[2,3,87] Finally, all patients should be prescribed short-acting SL NTG or lingual NTG spray to relieve any anginal symptoms when necessary and should be instructed on its use.[2,3] Chronic long-acting nitrate therapy has not been shown to reduce CHD events following MI. Therefore, IV NTG is not followed routinely by chronic, long-acting oral nitrate therapy in ACS patients who have undergone revascularization unless the patient has chronic stable angina or significant coronary stenoses that were not revascularized.[87]

ACE INHIBITORS AND ANGIOTENSIN RECEPTOR BLOCKERS

ACE inhibitors should be initiated in all patients following MI to reduce mortality, decrease reinfarction, and prevent the development of heart failure.[2,3] Dosing and contraindications are described in Table 16–4. The benefit of ACE inhibitors in patients with MI most likely comes from their ability to prevent cardiac remodeling. Other proposed mechanisms include improvement in endothelial function, a reduction in atrial and ventricular arrhythmias, and promotion of angiogenesis, leading to a reduction in ischemic events. The largest reduction in mortality is observed for patients with LV dysfunction [low LV ejection fraction (EF)] or heart failure symptoms. The use of ACE inhibitors in relatively unselected patients without a contraindication to ACE inhibitors may be expected to save 5 lives per 1000 patients treated for 30 days.[94] Long-term studies in patients with LV systolic dysfunction with or without heart failure symptoms demonstrate greater benefit because mortality reductions are larger (23.4% versus 29.1%; $p < .0001$) such that only 17 patients need treatment to prevent 1 death, with 57 lives saved for every 1000 patients treated.[95] ACE inhibitor prescription at hospital discharge following MI, in the absence of contraindications, to patients with depressed LV function (ejection fraction $< 40\%$) is currently a quality care indicator, and there are plans to make administration of an ACE inhibitor in all patients without contraindications a quality care indicator.[27] (see Table 16–3).

Early initiation (within 24 hours) of an *oral* ACE inhibitor appears to be crucial during an acute MI because 40% of the 30-day survival benefit is observed during the first day, 45% from days 2 to 7, and approximately and only 15% from days 8 to 30.[94] However, current data do not support the early administration of *intravenous* ACE inhibitors in patients experiencing an MI because mortality may be increased.[96] Hypotension should be avoided because coronary artery filling may be compromised. Because the benefits of ACE inhibitor

administration have been documented out to 3 years following MI,[27] administration should continue indefinitely.

More recent data suggest that all patients with CAD, not just ACS or heart failure patients, benefit from an ACE inhibitor. In the Heart Outcome Prevention Evaluation (HOPE) trial, ramipril significantly reduced the risk of death, MI, or stroke in high-risk patients aged 55 years or older with chronic CAD or with diabetes and one cardiovascular risk factor.[97] The more recent EUropean trial On Reduction Of Cardiac Events With Perindopril In Stable Coronary Artery Disease (EUROPA) extended the benefit of chronic therapy with ACE inhibitors to patients with stable CAD at lower risk of cardiovascular events compared with patients from the HOPE trial.[98] In the EUROPA trial, patients randomized to perindopril experienced a lower risk of the combined end point of cardiovascular death, MI, or cardiac arrest compared with patients randomized to placebo. Therefore, based on the extensive benefit of ACE inhibitors in patients with CAD, their routine use should be considered in all patients following an ACS in the absence of a contraindication.

Besides hypotension, the most frequent adverse reaction to an ACE inhibitor is cough, which may occur in up to 30% of patients. Patients with ACE inhibitor cough and either clinical signs of heart failure or LVEF less than 40% may be prescribed an angiotensin-receptor blocker (ARB).[3] Both candesartan and valsartan have improved outcomes in clinical trials in patients with heart failure.[99,100] Other less common but more serious adverse effects of ACE inhibitors include acute renal failure, hyperkalemia, and angioedema. Although some data have suggested that aspirin use may decrease the benefits from ACE inhibitor treatment, a systematic review of more than 20,000 patients demonstrated that ACE inhibitors improve outcome irrespective of treatment with aspirin.[101]

LIPID-LOWERING AGENTS

There are now overwhelming data supporting the benefits of statins in patients with CAD in the prevention of total mortality, cardiovascular mortality, and stroke. According to the National Cholesterol Education Program (NCEP) Adult Treatment Panel recommendations, all patients with CAD should receive dietary counseling and pharmacologic therapy in order to reach a low-density lipoprotein (LDL) cholesterol concentration of less than 100 mg/dL, with statins being the preferred agents to lower LDL cholesterol.[102] Results from landmark clinical trials have demonstrated unequivocally the value of statins in secondary prevention following MI in patients with moderate to high cholesterol levels. These trials, which included only patients with stable CAD, showed that the benefit of statins appears approximately after 1 year of treatment.[102] Although the primary effect of statins is to decrease LDL cholesterol, statins are believed to produce many non-lipid-lowering or "pleiotropic" effects. These effects, which include improvement in endothelial dysfunction, anti-inflammatory and antithrombotic properties, and a decrease in matrix metalloproteinase activity, may be relevant in patients experiencing an ACS and result in short-term (<1 year) benefit.[6] Newer recommendations from the NCEP give an optional goal of an LDL cholesterol of less than 70 mg/dL.[103] This recommendation is based upon a large clinical trial evaluating recurrence of major cardiovascular events in patients with a history of an ACS occurring within the past 10 days. This trial documented the benefit of lowering LDL cholesterol to, on average, 62 mg/dL, with 80 mg of atorvastatin compared to 95 mg/dL in patients treated with pravastatin 40 mg daily.[104] Whether or not a statin should be used routinely in all patients irrespective of their baseline LDL cholesterol level is currently being investigated, but preliminary data from the Heart Protection Study suggests that patients benefit from statin therapy irrespective of their baseline LDL cholesterol level.[105]

In addition, early initiation in patients with ACS appears to increase long-term adherence with statin therapy, which should result in clinical benefit.[107] Recent data suggest that long-term adherence to statins in patients with an ACS and in patients with chronic CAD is poor, with less than 50% of patients being compliant with their statin regimen 2 years following drug initiation.[105] Therefore, in patients with an ACS, statin therapy initiation should not be delayed, and statins should be prescribed at or prior to discharge in most patients.

A fibrate derivative or niacin should be considered in selective patients with a low high-density lipoprotein (HDL) cholesterol concentration (<40 mg/dL) and/or a high triglyceride level (>200 mg/dL). In a large, randomized trial in men with established CAD and low levels of HDL cholesterol, the use of gemfibrozil (600 mg twice daily) significantly decreased the risk of nonfatal MI or death from coronary causes.[108]

Additional discussion, dosing, monitoring, and adverse effects of using lipid-lowering drugs for secondary prevention may be found in Chap. 21.

FISH OILS (MARINE-DERIVED OMEGA-3 FATTY ACIDS)

Eicosapentaenoic acid (EPA) and docosahexaenoic acid (DHA) are omega-3 polyunsaturated fatty acids that are most abundant in fatty fish such as sardines, salmon, and mackerel. Epidemiologic and randomized trials have demonstrated that a diet high in EPA plus DHA or supplementation with these fish oils reduces the risk of cardiovascular mortality, reinfarction, and stroke in patients who have experienced an MI.[109] Although the exact mechanism responsible for the beneficial effects of omega-3 fatty acids has not been clearly elucidated, potential mechanisms include triglyceride-lowering effects, antithrombotic effects, retardation in the progression of atherosclerosis, endothelial relaxation, mild antihypertensive effects, and reduction in ventricular arrhythmias.[109]

The GISSI-Prevenzione trial, the largest randomized trial of fish oils published to date, evaluated the effects of open-label EPA plus DHA in 11,324 patients with recent MI who were randomized to receive 850 to 882 mg/day of n-3 polyunsaturated fatty acid (EPA plus DHA), 300 mg vitamin E, both, or neither.[110] The use of EPA plus DHA reduced the risk of death, nonfatal acute MI, or nonfatal stroke, whereas the use of vitamin E had no significant impact on this combined clinical end point. Therefore, based on current data, the AHA recommends that CHD patients consume approximately 1 g EPA plus DHA per day, preferably from oily fish.[109] Because oil content in fish varies, the number of 6-oz servings of fish that would need to be consumed to provide 7 g EPA plus DHA per week varies from approximately 4 to more than 14 for secondary prevention. The average diet only contains one-tenth to one-fifth the recommended amount.[109] Supplements should be considered in selected patients who do not eat fish, have limited access to fish, or who cannot afford to purchase fish. Approximately three 1-g fish oil capsules per day should be consumed to provide 1 g omega-3 fatty acids depending on the brand of supplement.[109] Finally, current guidelines suggest that higher doses of EPA plus DHA (2 to 4 g/day) also can be considered for the management of hypertriglyceridemia.[109]

Adverse effects from fish oils include fishy aftertaste, nausea, and diarrhea.[109]

OTHER MODIFIABLE RISK FACTORS

Smoking cessation, control of hypertension, weight loss, and tight glucose control for patients with diabetes mellitus, in addition to treatment of dyslipidemia, are important treatments for secondary prevention of CHD events.[3] Smokers should be instructed to stop smoking. A recent systematic review has highlighted that smoking cessation is accompanied by a significant reduction in all-cause mortality in patients with CAD.[111] Smoking cessation counseling at the time of discharge following MI is a quality care indicator[27] (see Table 16–3). The use of nicotine patches or gum or of bupropion alone or in combination with nicotine patches should be considered in appropriate patients.[3] Hypertension should be strictly controlled according to published guidelines.[112] Patients who are overweight should be educated on the importance of regular exercise, healthy eating habits, and of reaching and maintaining an ideal weight.[113] Finally, because diabetics have up to a fourfold increased risk of mortality compared with nondiabetics, the importance of tight glucose control, as well as other CHD risk factor modification, cannot be understated.[114]

NEW THERAPIES FOR SECONDARY PREVENTION: ALDOSTERONE ANTAGONISTS

Administration of an aldosterone antagonist, either eplerenone or spironolactone, should be considered within the first 2 weeks following MI in all patients already receiving an ACE inhibitor who have an EF of 40% or less and either heart failure symptoms or a diagnosis of diabetes mellitus to reduce mortality.[3] Aldosterone plays an important role in heart failure and MI because it promotes vascular and myocardial fibrosis, endothelial dysfunction, hypertension, LV hypertrophy, sodium retention, potassium and magnesium loss, and arrhythmias. Aldosterone blockers have been shown in experimental and human studies to attenuate these adverse effects.[115] As discussed in Chap. 14, the benefit of aldosterone blockade in patients with stable, severe heart failure was highlighted in the Randomized Aldactone Evaluation Study (RALES), where spironolactone decreased the risk of all-cause mortality.[116]

Eplerenone, like spironolactone, is an aldosterone blocker that blocks the mineralocorticoid receptor. In contrast to spironolactone, eplerenone has no effect on the progesterone or androgen receptor, thereby minimizing the risk of gynecomastia, sexual dysfunction, and menstrual irregularities.[115] The Eplerenone Post-Acute Myocardial Infarction Heart Failure Efficacy and Survival Study (EPHESUS) evaluated the effect of aldosterone antagonism in patients with an MI complicated by heart failure or LV dysfunction. Patients ($n = 6642$) were randomized 3 to 14 days following the MI to eplerenone or placebo.[117] Eplerenone significantly reduced the risk of mortality (14.4% versus 16.7%; $p = .008$). Data from EPHESUS suggest that eplerenone reduced mortality from sudden death, heart failure, and MI. Eplerenone also reduced the risk of hospitalizations for heart failure. Most patients in EPHESUS also were being treated with aspirin, a β-blocker, and an ACE inhibitor. Approximately half the patients also were receiving a statin. Therefore, the mortality reduction observed was in addition to that of standard therapy for secondary CHD prevention. These benefits were obtained at the expense of an increased risk of severe hyperkalemia (5.5% versus 3.9%; $p = .002$), defined as a potassium concentration equal or greater than 6 mmol/L. Patients with a serum creatinine concentration of greater than 2.5 mg/dL or a serum potassium concentration of greater than 5 mmol/L at baseline were excluded. The risk of hyperkalemia was particularly alarming in patients with a creatinine clearance of less than 50 mL/min. This highlights the importance of close monitoring of potassium level and renal function in patients being treated with eplerenone. There was no increase in gynecomastia, breast pain, or impotence.

The results from EPHESUS have raised the question of which aldosterone blocker, spironolactone or eplerenone, should be used preferentially. Currently, there are no data to support that the more selective but more expensive eplerenone is superior to or should be preferred to the less expensive generic spironolactone unless a patient has experienced gynecomastia, breast pain, or impotence while receiving spironolactone. Finally, it should be noted that hyperkalemia is just as likely to appear with both these agents.

THERAPIES NOT USEFUL AND POTENTIALLY HARMFUL FOLLOWING MI

Administration of hormone-replacement therapy (HRT) to all women following MI does not prevent recurrent CHD events and may be harmful.[118,119] Postmenopausal women already taking estrogen plus progestin should not continue, especially while at bedrest in hospital, owing to an increased risk of venous thromboembolism.[3] Administration of vitamin E for secondary prevention is ineffective following MI.[120,121] Similarly, because of the uniformly disappointing results from trials evaluating the protective effects of vitamins, the U.S. Preventive Services Task Force has published a statement concluding that there was insufficient evidence to recommend the use of supplements of vitamins A, C, or E, multivitamins with folic acid, or a combination of antioxidants to prevent CVDs. Furthermore, they conclude against the use of β-carotene supplementation, particularly in heavy smokers, because of an apparent increased risk of lung cancer.[122]

PHARMACOECONOMIC CONSIDERATIONS

The risks of CHD events, such as death, recurrent MI, and stroke, are higher for patients with established CHD and a history of MI than for patients with no known CHD. Because the costs for chronic preventative pharmacotherapy are the same for primary and secondary prevention, whereas the risk of events is higher with secondary prevention, secondary prevention is more cost-effective than primary prevention of CHD. Pharmacotherapy that has demonstrated cost-effectiveness to prevent death in ACS and post-MI patients includes fibrinolytics, aspirin, GP IIb/IIIa receptor blockers, β-blockers, ACE inhibitors, statins, and gemfibrozil.[123] Studies documenting cost-effectiveness of ACS and secondary prevention are based on the landmark clinical trials discussed throughout this chapter. The cost-effectiveness ratio of administering streptokinase compared with no reperfusion therapy is $2000 to $4000 per year of life saved, whereas administering alteplase compared with streptokinase has a cost-effectiveness ratio of about $33,000 per year of life saved.[123,124] While no formal cost-effectiveness analyses on aspirin therapy have been performed, the profound benefit in ACS, accompanied by its low cost, makes aspirin intuitively cost-effective.[125] The cost-effectiveness of β-blockers is less than $5000 per year of life saved for patients at highest risk of death and less than $15,000 for patients at lower risk of death, with β-blockers being cost-savings in some scenarios.[126,127] ACE inhibitor cost-effectiveness ratios range from $3000 to $5000 per year of life gained following MI.[128] Other studies have suggested that even in relatively unselected low-risk MI patients, the highest cost-effectiveness ratio is approximately $40,000 per year of life saved.[129] Lipid-lowering therapy with statins has a secondary prevention cost-effectiveness ratio of between $4500 and $9500 per year of life saved,[130] whereas gemfibrozil has a cost-effectiveness ratio of less than $17,000 per year of life saved.[131] In patients with non-ST-segment-elevation ACS, the cost per life year added for eptifibatide treatment in U.S. patients ranges from $13,700 to $16,500.[132] Newer therapies such as fish oils also have demonstrated cost-effectiveness, with a cost-effectiveness ratio of approximately $28,000 per year of life gained.[133] Because cost-effectiveness ratios of less than $50,000 per added life-year are considered economically attractive from a societal perspective,[123] pharmacotherapy as outlined earlier for ACS and secondary prevention are standards of care because of their efficacy and cost attractiveness to payers.

CLINICAL CONTROVERSIES

1. Administration of fibrinolytic agents to patients older than 75 years of age:
   a. Clinical trials have not been conducted specifically in this age group.
   b. Number of relative contraindications is likely larger than in younger patients.
   c. Risk of intracranial hemorrhage and bleeding is higher.
   d. Benefit may be larger but not well documented.
2. Spironolactone administration rather than eplerenone following MI in patients with an EF of 40% or less, either diabetes mellitus, or signs of heart failure:
   a. Spironolactone is the standard of care for patients with LV dysfunction and New York Heart Association class III or IV heart failure symptoms regardless of cause (ischemic or nonischemic cardiomyopathy).
   b. Spironolactone has not been studied specifically in acute MI.
   c. Eplerenone is more expensive than spironolactone.
   d. Eplerenone causes less gynecomastia, breast pain, and sexual dysfunction.
   e. The frequency of hyperkalemia is similar between eplerenone and spironolactone.

EVALUATION OF THERAPEUTIC OUTCOMES

The monitoring parameters for *efficacy* of nonpharmacologic and pharmacotherapy for both ST-segment-elevation and non-ST-segment-elevation ACS are similar:

- Relief of ischemic discomfort
- Return of ECG changes to baseline
- Absence or resolution of heart failure signs

Monitoring parameters for recognition and prevention of *adverse effects* from ACS pharmacotherapy are described in Table 16–7. In general, the most common adverse reactions from ACS therapies are hypotension and bleeding. Treatment for bleeding and hypotension involves discontinuation of the offending agent(s) until symptoms

TABLE 16–7. Therapeutic Drug Monitoring for Adverse Effects of Pharmacotherapy for Acute Coronary Syndromes

Drug	Adverse Effects	Monitoring
Aspirin	Dyspepsia, bleeding, gastritis	Clinical signs of bleeding[a]; gastrointestinal upset; baseline CBC and platelet count; CBC platelet count every 6 months
Clopidogrel	Bleeding, thrombocytopenia (rare)	Clinical signs of bleeding[a]; baseline CBC and platelet count; CBC and platelet count every 6 months following hospital discharge
Unfractionated heparin	Bleeding, heparin-induced thrombocytopenia	Clinical signs of bleeding[a]; baseline CBC and platelet count; aPTT every 6 hour until target then every 24 hours; CBC and platelet count daily
Low-molecular-weight heparins	Bleeding, heparin-induced thrombocytopenia	Clinical signs of bleeding[a]; baseline CBC and platelet count; daily CBC, platelet count every 3 days (minimum, preferably every day); S_{Cr} daily
Fibrinolytics	Bleeding, especially intracranial hemorrhage	Clinical signs of bleeding[a]; baseline CBC and platelet count; mental status every 2 hours for signs of intracranial hemorrhage; daily CBC
Glycoprotein IIb/IIIa receptor blockers	Bleeding, acute, profound thrombocytopenia	Clinical signs of bleeding[a]; baseline CBC and platelet count; daily CBC; platelet count at 4 hours after initiation then daily
Intravenous nitrates	Hypotension, flushing, headache, tachycardia	BP and HR every 2 hours
β-Blockers	Hypotension, bradycardia, heart block, bronchospasm, heart failure, fatigue, depression, sexual dysfunction, nightmares, and masking hypoglycemia symptoms in diabetics	BP, RR, HR, 12-lead ECG, and clinical signs of heart failure every 5 min during bolus intravenous dosing; BP, RR, HR, and clinical signs of heart failure every shift during oral administration during hospitalization; then BP and HR every 6 months following hospital discharge
Diltiazem/verapamil	Hypotension, bradycardia, heart block, heart failure, gingival hyperplasia	BP and HR every 8 hours during oral administration during hospitalization; then every 6 months following hospital discharge; dental exam and teeth cleaning every 6 months
Amlodipine	Hypotension, dependent peripheral edema, gingival hyperplasia	BP and HR every 8 hours during oral administration during hospitalization; then every 6 months following hospital discharge; dental exam and teeth cleaning every 6 months
Angiotensin-converting enzyme inhibitors (ACEIs) and angiotensin receptor blockers	Hypotension, cough (with ACEIs), hyperkalemia, prerenal azotemia, angioedema	BP every 2 hours × 3 for first dose; then every 8 hours during oral administration during hospitalization; then once every 6 months following hospital discharge; baseline S_{Cr}; daily S_{Cr} while hospitalized then every 6 months; baseline serum potassium concentration; then daily if taking concomitant potassium supplements, spironolactone, or eplerenone or if renal insufficiency; potassium concentration every 6 months following discharge unless taking concomitant eplerenone (see below) or spironolactone; counsel patient on throat, tongue, and facial swelling
Eplerenone	Hypotension, hyperkalemia	BP and HR every 8 hours during oral administration during hospitalization; then once every 6 months; baseline S_{Cr} and serum potassium concentration; S_{Cr} and potassium at 48 h; then at one month then 6 months following hospital discharge
Warfarin	Bleeding, skin necrosis	Clinical signs of bleeding[a]; baseline CBC and platelet count; CBC and platelet count every 6 months following hospital discharge; baseline aPTT and INR; daily INR until two consecutive INRs are within the target range; then once weekly × 2 weeks; then every month
Morphine	Hypotension, respiratory depression	BP and RR 5 min after each bolus dose

ACEIs = angiotensin-converting enzyme inhibitors; aPTT = activated partial thromboplastin time; BP = blood pressure; CBC = complete blood count; HR = heart rate; INR = international normalized ratio; RR = respiratory rate; S_{Cr} = serum creatinine.

[a]Note: Clinical signs of bleeding include bloody stools, melena, hematuria, hemetemesis, bruising, and oozing from arterial or venous puncture sites.

resolve. Severe bleeding resulting in hypotension secondary to hypovolemia may require blood transfusion.

ABBREVIATIONS

ACC: American College of Cardiology
ACE: angiotensin-converting enzyme
ACS: acute coronary syndrome
ACT: activated clotting time
ADP: adenosine diphosphate
AHA: American Heart Association
aPTT: activated partial thromboplastin time
ARB: angiotensin-receptor blocker
ASPECT: Antithrombotics in Secondary Prevention of Events in Coronary Thrombosis BNP brain (B-type) natriuretic peptide
CABG: coronary artery bypass graft
CBC: complete blood count
CK: creatine kinase
CREDO: Clopidogrel for the Reduction of Events During Observation
CURE: Clopidogrel in Unstable Angina to Prevent Recurrent Events
CVD: cardiovascular disease
DHA: docosahexaenoic acid
ECG: electrocardiogram
EF: ejection fraction
EPA: eicosapentaenoic acid
EPHESUS: Eplerenone Post-Acute Myocardial Infarction Heart Failure Efficacy and Survival Study
ESPRIT: Enhanced Suppression of the Platelet IIb/IIIa Receptor with Integrilin Therapy Trial
EUROPA: EUropean trial On Reduction Of Cardiac Events With Perindopril In Stable Coronary Artery Disease
GRACE: Global Registry of Acute Coronary Events
GUSTO: Global Use of Strategies to Open Occluded Arteries
HOPE: Heart Outcomes Prevention Evaluation
INR: international normalized ratio
INTERCEPT: Incomplete Infarction Trial of European Research Collaborators Evaluating Prognosis post-Thrombolysis
ISIS-1: First International Study of Infarct Survival
ISIS-2: Second International Study of Infarct Survival
IV: intravenous
LDL: low-density lipoprotein
LMWH: low-molecular-weight heparin
LVEF: left ventricular ejection fraction
MB: myocardial band
MI: myocardial infarction
MIAMI: Metoprolol In Acute Myocardial Infarction
NRMI: National Registry of Myocardial Infarction
NTG: nitroglycerin
PCI: percutaneous coronary intervention
PRISM-PLUS: Platelet Receptor Inhibition in Ischemic Syndrome Management in Patients Limited by Unstable Signs and Symptoms
PURSUIT: Platelet Glycoprotein IIb/IIIa in Unstable Angina: Receptor Suppression Using Integrilin Therapy
RALES: Randomized Aldactone Evaluation Study
SL: sublingual
TARGET: Do Tirofiban and ReoPro Give Similar Efficacy Outcomes Trial
TIMI: Thrombolysis in Myocardial Infarction
TXA$_2$: thromboxane A$_2$
UA: unstable angina
UFH: unfractionated heparin
WARIS: Warfarin Re-Infarction Study

Review Questions and other resources can be found at *www.pharmacotherapyonline.com.*

REFERENCES

1. American Heart Association. Heart Disease and Stroke Statistics—2003 Update. Dallas, TX, American Heart Association, 2002.
2. Braunwald E, Antman EM, Beasley JW, et al. ACC/AHA 2002 guideline update for the management of patients with unstable angina and non-ST-segment-elevation myocardial infarction: Summary article. A report of the American College of Cardiology/American Heart Association Task Force on Practice Guidelines (Committee on the Management of Patients With Unstable Angina). J Am Coll Cardiol 2002;40:1366–1374.
3. Antman EM, Anbe DT, Armstrong PW, Bates ER, et al. ACC/AHA guidelines for the management of patients with ST-elevation myocardial infarction: Executive summary. A report of the American College of Cardiology/American Heart Association Task Force on Practice Guidelines (Committee to revise the 1999 Guidelines for the Management of Patients with Acute Myocardial Infarction). Circulation 2004;110: 588–636 .
4. Spencer FA, Meyer TE, Gore JM, Goldenberg RJ. Heterogeneity in the management and outcomes of patients with acute myocardial infarction complicated by heart failure: The National Registry of Myocardial Infarction. Circulation 2002;105:2605–2610.
5. Ross R. Atherosclerosis: An inflammatory disease. N Engl J Med 1999;340:115–126.
6. de Denus S, Spinler SA. Early statin therapy for acute coronary syndromes. Ann Pharmacother 2002;36:1749–1758.
7. Libby P. Current concepts of the pathogenesis of the acute coronary syndromes. Circulation 2001;104:365–372.
8. Ruberg FL, Leopold JA, Loscalzo J. Atherothrombosis: Plaque instability and thrombogenesis. Prog Cardiovasc Dis 2003;44:381–394.
9. St John Sutton M, Ferrari VA. Prevention of left ventricular remodeling after myocardial infarction. Curr Treat Options Cardiovasc Med 2002;4:97–108.
10. Mann DL. Mechanisms and models in heart failure: A combinatorial approach. Circulation 1999;100:999–1008.
11. Goldberg RJ, Gore JM, Thompson CA, Gurwitz JH. Recent magnitude of and temporal trends (1994–1997) in the incidence and hospital death rates of cardiogenic shock complicating acute myocardial infarction: The second National Registry of Myocardial Infarction. Am Heart J 2001; 141:65–72.
12. Lavie CJ, Gersh BJ. Mechanical and electrical complications of acute myocardial infarction. Mayo Clin Proc 1990;65:709–730. Erratum in Mayo Clin Proc 1990;65:1032.
13. The Joint European Society of Cardiology/American College of Cardiology Committee. Myocardial infarction redefined: A consensus document of the joint European Society of Cardiology/American College of Cardiology Committee for the Redefinition of Myocardial Infarction. J Am Coll Cardiol 2000;36:959–969.
14. Fibrinolytic Therapy Trialists' (FTT) Collaborative Group. Indications for fibrinolytic therapy in suspected myocardial infarction: Collaborative overview of early mortality and major morbidity results from all randomized trials of more than 1000 patients. Lancet 1994;343:311–322.
15. Berger P, Ellis SG, Holmes DR Jr, et al. Relationship between delay in performing direct coronary angioplasty and early clinical outcome in patients with acute myocardial infarction: Results from the Global Use of Strategies to Open Occluded Arteries in Acute Coronary Syndromes (GUSTO-IIb) trial. Circulation 1999;100:14–20.
16. Steg PG, Goldberg RJ, Gore JM, et al. Baseline characteristics, management practices, and in-hospital outcomes of patients hospitalized with acute coronary syndromes in the Global Registry of Acute Coronary Events (GRACE). Am J Cardiol 2002;90:358–363.

17. Townsend R. Cardiac mortality in chronic kidney disease: A clearer perspective. Ann Intern Med 2002;137:615–616.

18. de Lemos JA, Morrow DA. Brain natriuretic peptide measurement in acute coronary syndromes: Ready for clinical application? Circulation 2002;106:2868–2870.

19. Antman EM, Cohen M, Bernink PJ, et al. The TIMI risk score for unstable angina/non-ST-segment-elevation MI: A method for prognostication and therapeutic decision-making. JAMA 2000;284:835–842.

20. Weaver WD, Simes RJ, Betriu A, et al. Comparison of primary coronary angioplasty and intravenous thrombolytic therapy for acute myocardial infarction: A quantitative review. JAMA 1997;278:2093–2098.

21. Smith SC Jr, Dove JT, Jacobs AK, et al. ACC/AHA guidelines for percutaneous coronary intervention (revision of the 1993 PTCA guidelines). J Am Coll Cardiol 2001;37:2215–2239.

22. Spertus JA, Radford MJ, Every NJ, et al. Challenges and opportunities in quantifying the quality of care for acute myocardial infarction: Summary from the Acute Myocardial Infarction Working Group of the American Heart Association/American College of Cardiology First Scientific Forum on Quality of Care and Outcomes Research in Cardiovascular Disease and Stroke. Circulation 2003;107:1681–1691.

23. Fox KAA, Poole-Wilson PA, Henderson RA, et al. Interventional versus conservative treatment for patients with unstable angina or non-ST-elevation myocardial infarction: The British Heart Foundation RITA 3 randomised trial. Lancet 2002; 360:743–751.

24. Moss AJ, Zareba W, Hall WJ. Prophylactic implantation of a defibrillator in patients with myocardial infarction and reduced ejection fraction. N Engl J Med 2002;346:877–883.

25. Bertrand ME, Simoons ML, Fox KAA. Management of acute coronary syndromes in patients presenting without persistent ST-segment elevation. The Task Force on the Management of Acute Coronary Syndromes of the European Society of Cardiology. Eur Heart J 2002;23:1809–1840.

26. Spinler SA. Acute coronary syndromes. In: Shumock GT, Brundage DM, Chapman MM, et al, eds. Pharmacotherapy Self-Assessment Program, Book 1: Cardiovascular I, Cardiovascular II, 5th ed. Kansas City, American College of Clinical Pharmacy, 2004.

27. The Global Use of Strategies to Open Occluded Coronary Arteries (GUSTO) Investigators. An international randomized trial comparing four thrombolytic strategies for acute myocardial infarction. N Engl J Med 1993;329:673–682.

28. The Global Use of Strategies to Open Occluded Coronary Arteries (GUSTO III) Investigators. A comparison of reteplase with alteplase for acute myocardial infarction. N Engl J Med 1997;337:1118–1123.

29. Assessment of the Safety and Efficacy of a New Thrombolytic (ASSENT-2) Investigators. Single-bolus tenecteplase compared with front-loaded alteplase in acute myocardial infarction: The ASSENT-2 double-blind, randomized trial. Lancet 1000;354:716–722.

30. Gryzbowski M, Clements EA, Parsons L, et al. Mortality benefit of immediate revascularization of acute ST-segment-elevation myocardial infarction in patients with contraindications to thrombolytic therapy: A propensity analysis. JAMA 2003;290:1891–1898.

31. Rogers WJ, Canto JG, Lambrew CT, et al. Temporal trends in the treatment of over 1.5 million patients with myocardial infarction in the U.S. from 1990 through 1999. J Am Coll Cardiol 2000;36:2056–2063.

32. Awtry EH, Loscalzo J. Aspirin. Circulation 2000;101:1206–1218.

33. ISIS-2 (Second International Study of Infarct Survival) Collaborative Group. Randomised trial of intravenous streptokinase, oral aspirin, both, or neither among 17,187 cases of suspected acute myocardial infarction: ISIS-2. Lancet 1988;2:349–360.

34. Antiplatelet Trialists' Collaboration. Collaborative meta-analysis of randomised trials of antiplatelet therapy for prevention of death, myocardial infarction, and stroke in high risk patients. Br Med J 2002;324:71–86.

35. Serebruany VL, Malinin AI, Sane DC, et al. The risk of bleeding complications with antiplatelet agents: A meta-analysis of 338,191 patients enrolled in 50 randomized controlled trials (abstract). Eur Heart J 2003;24:671.

36. Aspirin for the primary prevention of cardiovascular events: Recommendation and rationale. Ann Intern Med 2002;136:157–160.

37. He J, Whelton PK, Vu B, Klag MJ. Aspirin and risk of hemorrhagic stroke: A meta-analysis of randomized, controlled trials. JAMA 1998; 280:1930–1935.

38. Collaborative overview of randomised trials of antiplatelet therapy: I. Prevention of death, myocardial infarction, and stroke by prolonged antiplatelet therapy in various categories of patients. Antiplatelet Trialists' Collaboration. Br Med J 1994;308:81–106.

39. Mehta SR, Yusuf S. Short- and long-term oral antiplatelet therapy in acute coronary syndromes and percutaneous coronary intervention. J Am Coll Cardiol 2003;41:79S–88S.

40. Bertrand ME, Rupprecht HJ, Urban P, et al. Double-blind study of the safety of clopidogrel with and without a loading dose in combination with aspirin compared with ticlopidine in combination with aspirin after coronary stenting: the clopidogrel aspirin stent international cooperative study (CLASSICS). Circulation 2000;102:624–629.

41. Balsano F, Rizzon P, Violi F, et al. Antiplatelet treatment with ticlopidine in unstable angina: A controlled multicenter clinical trial. The Studio della Ticlopidina nell'Angina Instabile Group. Circulation 1990;82:17–26.

42. CAPRIE Steering Committee. A randomised, blinded trial of clopidogrel versus aspirin in patients at risk of ischaemic events (CAPRIE). Lancet 1996;348:1329–1339.

43. Eisenberg MJ, Jamal S. Glycoprotein IIb/IIIa inhibition in the setting of acute ST-segment-elevation myocardial infarction. J Am Coll Cardiol 2003;42:1–6.

44. The GUSTO V Investigators. Reperfusion therapy for acute myocardial infarction with fibrinolytic therapy or combination reduced fibrinolytic therapy and platelet glycoprotein IIb/IIIa inhibition: The GUSTO V randomised trial. Lancet 2001;357:1905–1914.

45. The Assessment of the Safety and Efficacy of a New Thrombolytic Regimen (ASSENT) 3 Investigators. Efficacy and safety of tenecteplase in combination with enoxaparin, abciximab, or unfractionated heparin: The ASSENT-3 randomised trial in acute myocardial infarction. Lancet 2001;358:605–613.

46. Dasgupta H, Blankenship JC, Wood C, et al. Thrombocytopenia complicating treatment with intravenous glycoprotein IIb/IIIa receptor inhibitors: A pooled analysis. Am Heart J 2000;140:206–211.

47. Granger CB, Hirsh J, Califf RM, et al. Activated partial thromboplastin time and outcome after thrombolytic therapy for acute myocardial infarction. Circulation 1996;93:870–878.

48. Gruppo Italioano per Lo Studio della Sopravvivenza Nell'infarcto Myocardio. GISSI-2: A factorial randomised trial of alteplase versus streptokinase and heparin versus no heparin among 12,490 patients with acute myocardial infarction. Lancet 1990;336:65–71.

49. Young SK. New treatment options for heparin-induced thrombocytopenia. J Pharm Pract 2002;15:305–317.

50. Theroux P, Welsh RC. Meta-analysis of randomized trials comparing enoxaparin versus unfractionated heparin as adjunctive therapy to fibrinolysis in ST-elevation acute myocardial infarction. Am J Cardiol 2003;91:860–864.

51. Gruppo Italioano per Lo Studio della Sopravvivenza Nell'infarcto Myocardio. GISSI-3: Effects of lisinopril and transdermal glyceryl trinitrate singly and together on 6-week mortality and ventricular function after acute myocardial infarction. Lancet 1994;343:1115–1122.

52. ISIS-4 (Fourth International Study of Infarct Survival Collaborative Group). ISIS-4: A randomised factorial trial assessing early oral captopril, oral mononitrate, and intravenous magnesium sulphate in 58,050 patients with suspected acute myocardial infarction. Lancet 1995;345:669–685.

53. Gheorghiade M, Goldstein S. β-Blockers in the post-myocardial infarction patient. Circulation 2002;106:394–398.

54. First International Study of Infarct Survival Collaborative Group. Randomised trial of intravenous atenolol among 16,027 cases of suspected acute myocardial infarction: ISIS-1. Lancet 1986;2:57–661.

55. Metoprolol in acute myocardial infarction (MIAMI). A randomised, placebo-controlled international trial. Eur Heart J 1985;6:199–226.

56. The MIAMI Trial Research Group. Metoprolol in acute myocardial infarction: Development of myocardial infarction. Am J Cardiol 1985;56:23G–26G.

57. Roberts R, Rogers WJ, Mueller HS, et al. Immediate versus deferred beta-blockade following thrombolytic therapy in patients with acute myocardial infarction: Results of the Thrombolysis in Myocardial Infarction (TIMI) IIB study. Circulation 1991;83:422–437.

58. Abernethy DR, Schwartz JB. Calcium-antagonist drugs. N Engl J Med 1999;341:1447–1457.

59. Boden WE, van Gilst WH, Scheldewaert RG, et al. Diltiazem in acute myocardial infarction treated with thrombolytic agents: A randomised, placebo-controlled trial. Incomplete Infarction Trial of European Research Collaborators Evaluating Prognosis post-Thrombolysis (INTERCEPT). Lancet 2000;355:1751–1756.

60. Pitt B, Byington RP, Furberg CD, et al. Effect of amlodipine on the progression of atherosclerosis and the occurrence of clinical events. PREVENT Investigators. Circulation 2000;102:1503–1510.

61. Packer M, O'Connor CM, Ghali JK, et al. Effect of amlodipine on morbidity and mortality in severe chronic heart failure: Prospective Randomized Amlodipine Survival Evaluation Study Group. N Engl J Med 1996;335:1107–1114.

62. Yusuf S, Zhao F, Meta SR, et al. Effects of clopidogrel in addition to aspirin in patients with acute coronary syndromes without ST-segment elevation. N Engl J Med 2001;345:494–502.

63. Mehta SR, Yusuf S, Peters RJ, et al. Effects of pretreatment with clopidogrel and aspirin followed by long-term therapy in patients undergoing percutaneous coronary intervention: The PCI-CURE study. Lancet 2001;358:527–533.

64. Steinhubl SR, Berger PB, Mann JT 3d, et al: Early and sustained dual oral antiplatelet therapy following percutaneous coronary intervention: A randomized, controlled trial. JAMA 2002;288:2411–2420.

65. Peters RJ, Mehta SR, Fox KA, et al. Effects of aspirin dose when used alone or in combination with clopidogrel in patients with acute coronary syndromes: Observations from the clopidogrel in unstable angina to prevent recurrent events (CURE) study. Circulation 2003;108:1682–1687.

66. The PURSUIT Trial Investigators. Inhibition of platelet glycoprotein IIb/IIIa with eptifibatide in patients with acute coronary syndromes. N Engl J Med 1998;339:436–443.

67. Platelet Receptor Inhibition in Ischemic Syndrome Management in Patients Limited by Unstable Signs and Symptoms (PRISM-PLUS) Study Investigators. Inhibition of the platelet glycoprotein IIb/IIIa receptor with tirofiban in unstable angina and non-Q-wave myocardial infarction. N Engl J Med 1998;338:1488–1497.

68. Watson RD, Chin BS, Lip GY. Antithrombotic therapy in acute coronary syndromes. Br Med J 2002;325:1348–1351.

69. The GUSTO-IV ACS Investigators. Effect of glycoprotein IIb/IIIa receptor blocker abciximab on outcome in patients with acute coronary syndromes without early coronary revascularization: The GUSTO-IV ACS randomised trial. Lancet 2001;357:1915–1924.

70. O'Shea JC, Buller CE, Cantor WJ, et al. Long-term efficacy of platelet glycoprotein IIb/IIIa integrin blockade with eptifibatide in coronary stent intervention. JAMA 2002;287:618–621.

71. Topol EJ, Moliterno DJ, Herrmann HC, et al. Comparison of two platelet glycoprotein IIb/IIIa inhibitors tirofiban and abciximab for the prevention of ischemic events with percutaneous coronary revascularization. N Engl J Med 2001;344:1888–1894.

72. Moliterno DJ, Yakubov SJ, DiBattiste PM, et al. Outcomes at 6 months for the direct comparison of tirofiban and abciximab during percutaneous coronary revascularization with stent placement: the TARGET follow-up study. Lancet 2002;360:355–360.

73. Soffer D, Moussa I, Karatepe M, et al. Suboptimal inhibition of platelet aggregation following tirofiban bolus in patients undergoing percutaneous coronary intervention for unstable angina pectoris. Am J Cardiol 2003;91:872–875.

74. Roffi M, Chew DP, Mukherjee D, et al. Platelet glycoprotein IIb/IIIa inhibitors in acute coronary syndromes: A meta-analysis of all major randomised clinical trials. Eur Heart J 2002;23:1408–1411.

75. Oler A, Whooley MA, Oler J. Grady D. Adding heparin to aspirin reduces the incidence of myocardial infarction and death in patients with unstable angina: A meta-analysis. JAMA 1996;276:811–815.

76. Fragmin During Instability in Coronary Artery Disease Study Group. Low-molecular-weight heparin during instability in coronary artery disease. Lancet 1996;347:561–568.

77. Klein W, Buchwald A, Hillis SE, et al. Comparison of low-molecular-weight heparin with unfractionated heparin acutely and with placebo for 6 weeks in the management of unstable coronary artery disease: Fragmin in Unstable Coronary Artery Disease Study (FRIC). Circulation 1997;96:61–68.

78. Antman EM, McCabe CH, Gurfinkle EP, et al. Enoxaparin prevents deaths and cardiac ischemic events in unstable angina/non-Q-wave myocardial infarction: Results of the Thrombolysis in Myocardial Infarction (TIMI 11B) trial. Circulation 1999;100:1593–1601.

79. Cohen M, Demers C, Gurfinkle EP, et al. A comparison of low-molecular-weight heparin with unfractionated heparin for unstable coronary artery disease. N Engl J Med 1997;337:447–452.

80. The Synergy Trial Investigators. Enoxaparin versus unfractionated heparin in high-risk patients with non-ST-segment elevation acute coronary syndromes managed with an intended early invasive strategy. JAMA 2004;292:45–54.

81. Coumadin Aspirin Reinfarction Study (CARS) Investigators. Randomised, double-blind trial of fixed low-dose warfarin with aspirin after myocardial infarction. Lancet 1997;350:389–396.

82. Fiore LD, Ezekowitz MD, Brophy MT, et al. Department of Veterans Affairs Cooperative Studies Program Clinical Trial comparing combined warfarin and aspirin with aspirin alone in survivors of acute myocardial infarction: Primary results of the CHAMP study. Circulation 2002;105:557–563.

83. van Es RF, Jonker JJ, Verheugt FW, et al. Aspirin and coumadin after acute coronary syndromes (the ASPECT-2 study): A randomised, controlled trial. Lancet 2002;360:109–113.

84. Hurlen M, Abdelnoor M, Smith P, et al. Warfarin, aspirin, or both after myocardial infarction. N Engl J Med 2002;347:969–974.

85. Anand SS, Yusuf S. Oral anticoagulants in patients with coronary artery disease. J Am Coll Cardiol 2003;41:62S–69S.

86. Leon MB, Baim DS, Popma JJ, et al. Clinical trial comparing three antithrombotic-drug regimens after coronary-artery stenting. Stent Anticoagulation Restenosis Study Investigators. N Engl J Med 1998;339:1665–1671.

87. Gibbons RJ, Abrams J, Chatterjee K, et al. ACC/AHA 2002 guideline update for the management of patients with chronic stable angina: Summary article. A report of the American College of Cardiology/American Heart Association Task Force on Practice Guidelines (Committee on the Management of Patients With Chronic Stable Angina). J Am Coll Cardiol 2003;41:159–168.

88. Freemantle N, Cleland J, Young P, et al. β-Blockade after myocardial infarction: Systematic review and meta regression analysis. Br Med J 1999;318:1730–1737

89. Pedersen TR. Six-year follow-up of the Norwegian Multicenter Study on Timolol after Acute Myocardial Infarction. N Engl J Med 1985;313:1055–1058.

90. Cucherat M, Boissel JP, Leizorovicz A. Persistent reduction of mortality for five years after one year of acebutolol treatment initiated during acute myocardial infarction. The APSI Investigators. Acebutolol et Prevention Secondaire de l'Infarctus. Am J Cardiol 1997;79:587–589.

91. Dargie HJ. Effect of carvedilol on outcome after myocardial infarction in patients with left-ventricular dysfunction: The CAPRICORN randomised trial. Lancet 2001;357:1385–1390.

92. Houghton T, Freemantle N, Cleland JG, et al. Are beta-blockers effective in patients who develop heart failure soon after myocardial infarction? A meta-regression analysis of randomised trials. Eur J Heart Fail 2000;2:333–340.

93. Ko DT, Hebert PR, Coffey CS, et al. Beta-blocker therapy and symptoms of depression, fatigue, and sexual dysfunction. JAMA 2002;288:351–357.

94. ACE Inhibitor Myocardial Infarction Collaborative Group. Indications for ACE inhibitors in the early treatment of acute myocardial infarction: Systematic overview of individual data from 100,000 patients in randomized trials. Circulation 1998; 97:2202–2212.

95. Flather MD, Yusuf S, Kober L, et al. Long-term ACE inhibitor therapy in patients with heart failure or left ventricular dysfunction: A systematic overview of data from individual patients. ACE Inhibitor Myocardial Infarction Collaborative Group. Lancet 2000;355:1575–1581.

96. Swedberg K, Held P, Kjekshus J, et al. Effects of the early administration of enalapril on mortality in patients with acute myocardial infarction: Results of the Cooperative New Scandinavian Enalapril Survival Study II (CONSENSUS II). N Engl J Med 1992;327:678–684.

97. Yusuf S, Sleight P, Pogue J, et al. Effects of an angiotensin-converting enzyme inhibitor, ramipril, on cardiovascular events in high-risk patients. The Heart Outcomes Prevention Evaluation Study Investigators. N Engl J Med 2000;342:145–153.

98. Fox KM. Efficacy of perindopril in reduction of cardiovascular events among patients with stable coronary artery disease: Randomised, double-blind, placebo-controlled, multicentre trial (the EUROPA study). Lancet 2003;362:782–788.

99. Pfeffer MA, McMurray JJV, Velazquez EJ, et al. Valsartan, captopril, or both in myocardial infarction complicated by heart failure, left ventricular dysfunction, or both. N Engl J Med 2003;349:1893–1906.

100. Granger CB, McMurray JV, Yusuf S, et al., eds. CHARM Investigators and Committees. Effects of candesartan in patients with chronic heart failure and reduced left-ventricular systolic function intolerant to angiotensin-converting-enzyme inhibitors: CHARM Alternative trial. Lancet 2004;362:772–776.

101. Teo KK, Yusuf S, Pfeffer M, et al. Effects of long-term treatment with angiotensin-converting enzyme inhibitors in the presence or absence of aspirin: A systematic review. Lancet 2002;360:1037–1043.

102. Executive Summary of the Third Report of the National Cholesterol Education Program (NCEP) Expert Panel on Detection, Evaluation, and Treatment of High Blood Cholesterol in Adults (Adult Treatment Panel III). JAMA 2001;285:2486–2497.

103. Grundy SM, Cleeman JI, Bairey Merz, CN, et al., eds. Coordinating Committee of the National Cholesterol Education Program, Endorsed by the National Heart, Lung, and Blood Institute, American College of Cardiology Foundation, and American Heart Association. Implications of Recent Clinical Trials for the National Cholesterol Education Program Adult Treatment Panel III Guidelines. Circulation 2004;110:227–239.

104. Cannon CP, Braunwald E, McCabe CH, et al. Pravastatin or Atorvastatin Evaluation and Infection Therapy: Thrombolysis in Myocardial Infarction 22 Investigators. Intensive versus moderate lipid lowering with statins after acute coronary syndromes. N Engl J Med 2004;350:1495–1504.

105. Anonymous. MRC/BHF Heart Protection Study of cholesterol lowering with simvastatin in 20,536 high-risk individuals: A randomised placebo-controlled trial. Lancet 2002;360:7–22.

106. Muhlestein JB, Horne BD, Bair TL, et al. Usefulness of in-hospital prescription of statin agents after angiographic diagnosis of coronary artery disease in improving continued compliance and reduced mortality. Am J Cardiol 2001;87:257–261.

107. Jackevicius CA, Mamdani M, Tu JV. Adherence with statin therapy in elderly patients with and without acute coronary syndromes. JAMA 2002;288:462–467.

108. Rubins HB, Robins SJ, Collins D, et al. Gemfibrozil for the secondary prevention of coronary heart disease in men with low levels of high-density lipoprotein cholesterol. Veterans Affairs High-Density Lipoprotein Cholesterol Intervention Trial Study Group. N Engl J Med 1999;341:410–418.

109. Kris-Etherton PM, Harris WS, Appel LJ. Fish consumption, fish oil, omega-3 fatty acids, and cardiovascular disease. Circulation 2002;106:2747–2757.

110. Gruppo Italiano per lo Studio della Sopravvivenza nell'infarcto miocardio. Dietary supplementation with n-2 fatty acids and vitamin E after myocardial infarction: Results of GISSI-Prevenzione trial. Lancet 1999;354:447–455.

111. Critchley JA, Capewell S. Mortality risk reduction associated with smoking cessation in patients with coronary heart disease: A systematic review. JAMA 2003;290:86–97.

112. Chobanian AV, Bakris GL, Black HR, et al. The seventh report of the Joint National Committee on Prevention, Detection, Evaluation, and Treatment of High Blood Pressure: The JNC7 Report. JAMA 2003;289:2560–2572.

113. Thompson PD, Bucner D, Pina IL, et al. Exercise and physical activity in the prevention and treatment of atherosclerotic cardiovascular disease: A statement from the Council on Clinical Cardiology (Subcommittee on Exercise, Rehabilitation and Prevention) and the Council on Nutrition, Physical Activity, and Metabolism (Subcommittee on Physical Activity). Circulation 2003;107:3109–3116.

114. American Diabetes Association. Standards of medical care for patients with diabetes mellitus. Diabetes Care 2003;26(suppl 1):S33–50.

115. Zillich AJ, Carter BL. Eplerenone: A novel selective aldosterone blocker. Ann Pharmacother 2002;36:1567–1576.

116. Pitt B, Zannad F, Remme WJ, et al. The effect of spironolactone on morbidity and mortality in patients with severe heart failure. Randomized Aldactone Evaluation Study Investigators. N Engl J Med 1999;341:709–717.

117. Pitt B, Remme W, Zannad F, et al. Eplerenone, a selective aldosterone blocker in patients with left ventricular dysfunction after myocardial infarction. N Engl J Med 2003;348:1309–1321.

118. Hulley S, Grady D, Bush T, et al. Randomized trial of estrogen plus progestin for secondary prevention of coronary heart disease in postmenopausal women. JAMA 1998;280:605–613.

119. Writing Group for the Women's Health Initiative Investigators. Risks and benefits of estrogen plus progestin in health postmenopausal women: Principal results from the Women's Health Initiative Randomized Controlled Trial. JAMA 2002;288:321–333.

120. GISSI-Prevenzione Investigators. Dietary supplementation with n-3 polyunsaturated fatty acids and vitamin E after myocardial infarction: Results of the GISSI-Prevenzione Trial. Lancet 1999;354:447–455.

121. The Heart Outcomes Prevention Evaluation Study Investigators. Vitamin E supplementation and cardiovascular risk in high-risk patients. N Engl J Med 2000;342:154–160.

122. U.S. Preventive Services Task Force. Routine vitamin supplementation to prevent cancer and cardiovascular disease: Recommendations and rationale. Ann Intern Med 2003;139:51–55.

123. Mark DB. Medical economics in cardiovascular medicine. In: Topol EJ, Califf RM, Isner J, et al, eds. Textbook of Cardiovascular Medicine. Philadelphia, Lippincott Williams & Wilkins, 2003:957–979.

124. Hlatky MA, Califf RM, Naylor CD, et al. Cost effectiveness of thrombolytic therapy with tissue plasminogen activator as compared with streptokinase for acute myocardial infarction. N Engl J Med 1996;332:1418–1424.

125. Eccles M, Freemantle N, Mason J, et al. North of England evidence based guideline development project: Guideline on the use of aspirin as secondary prophylaxis for vascular disease in primary care. Br Med J 1998;316:1303–1309.

126. Phillips KA, Shlipak MG, Coxson P, et al. Health and economic benefits of increased beta-blocker use following myocardial infarction. JAMA 2001;284:2748–2754.

127. Phillips KA, Shiplak MG, Coxson P, et al. Health and economic benefits of increased beta-blocker use following myocardial infarction. JAMA 2000;284:2748–2754.

128. McMurray JJ, McGuire A, Davie AP, Hughs D. Cost-effectiveness of different ACE inhibitor treatment scenarios post-myocardial infarction. Eur Heart J 1997;18:1411–1415.

129. Franzosi MG, Maggioni AP, Santoro E. Cost-effective analysis of early lisinopril use with acute myocardial infarction: Results from GISSI-3 trial. Pharmacoeconomics 1998;13:337–346.

130. Grover SA, Coupal L, Paquet S, Zowall H. Cost-effectiveness of 3-hydroxy-3-methylglutaryl-coenzyme A reductase inhibitors in the secondary prevention of cardiovascular disease: Forecasting the incremental benefits of preventing coronary and cerebrovascular events. Arch Intern Med 1999;159:593–600.

131. Nyman JA, Martinson MS, Nelson D, et al. Cost-effectiveness of gemfibrozil for coronary heart disease patients with low levels of high-density lipoprotein cholesterol: The Department of Veterans Affairs High-Density Lipoprotein Cholesterol Intervention Trial. Arch Intern Med 2002;162:177–182.

132. Mark DB, Harrington RA, Lincoff AM, et al. Cost effectiveness of platelet glycoprotein IIb/IIIa inhibition with eptifibatide in patients with non-ST-segment-elevation acute coronary syndromes. Circulation 2000;101:366–371.

133. Franzosi MG, Brunetti M, Marchioli R, et al. Cost-effectiveness analysis of n-3 polyunsaturated fatty acids (PUFA) after myocardial infarction: Results from Gruppo Italiano per lo Studio della Sopravvivenza nell'Infarcto (GISSI)-Prevenzione Trial. Pharmacoeconomics 2001: 19:411–420.

17

ARRHYTHMIAS

Jerry L. Bauman and Marieke Dekker Schoen

Learning Objectives and other resources can be found at *www.pharmacotherapyonline.com.*

KEY CONCEPTS

◀1 The use of antiarrhythmic drugs in the United States is declining because of major trials that show increased mortality with their use in several clinical situations, the realization of proarrhythmia as a significant side effect, and the advancing technology of nondrug therapies such as ablation and the internal cardioverter-defibrillator.

◀2 Antiarrhythmic drugs frequently cause side effects and are complex in their pharmacokinetic characteristics. The therapeutic range of these agents provides only a rough guide to modifying treatment; it is preferable to attempt to define an individual's effective (or target) concentration and match that during long-term therapy.

◀3 The most commonly prescribed antiarrhythmic drug is now amiodarone. This agent is effective in terminating and preventing a wide variety of symptomatic tachycardias but is plagued by frequent side effects and therefore requires close monitoring. The most concerning toxicity is pulmonary fibrosis; side-effect profiles of the intravenous (acute, short-term) and oral (chronic, long-term) forms differ.

◀4 In patients with atrial fibrillation, therapy traditionally has been aimed at controlling ventricular response (e.g., digoxin, calcium antagonists, and β-blockers), preventing thromboembolic complications (e.g., warfarin and aspirin), and restoring and maintaining sinus rhythm (e.g., antiarrhythmic drugs and direct-current cardioversion). Recent studies show that there is no need to pursue strategies aggressively to maintain sinus rhythm (e.g., long-term antiarrhythmic drugs); rate control alone is often sufficient in patients who can tolerate it.

◀5 Paroxysmal supraventricular tachycardia is usually due to reentry in or proximal to the atrioventricular (AV) node or AV reentry incorporating an extra nodal pathway; common tachycardias can be terminated acutely with AV nodal

blocking agents such as adenosine, and recurrences can be prevented by ablation with radiofrequency current.

◀6 Patients with Wolff-Parkinson-White (WPW) syndrome may have several different tachycardias that are treated acutely by different strategies: orthodromic reentry (adenosine), antidromic reentry (adenosine or procainamide), and atrial fibrillation (procainamide or amiodarone). AV nodal blocking drugs are contraindicated with WPW syndrome and atrial fibrillation.

◀7 Because of the results of the Cardiac Arrhythmia Suppression Trials and other trials, antiarrhythmic drugs (except β-blockers) should not be used routinely in patients with prior myocardial infarction (MI) or left ventricular (LV) dysfunction and minor ventricular rhythm disturbances (e.g., premature ventricular complexes).

◀8 Patients with hemodynamically significant ventricular tachycardia or ventricular fibrillation not associated with an acute MI who are resuscitated successfully (electrical cardioversion, pressors, amiodarone) are at high risk for death and should receive implantation of an internal cardioverter-defibrillator.

◀9 The clinical approach to patients with left ventricular dysfunction and nonsustained ventricular tachycardia is a major remaining controversy, with three divergent strategies: invasive electrophysiologic studies with possible internal cardioverter-defibrillator implantation, empirical amiodarone therapy, and conservative (no treatment beyond β-blockers) management. Invasive electrophysiologic studies can aid in deciding among these strategies, particularly in patients with coronary artery disease.

◀10 Life-threatening proarrhythmia generally takes two forms: sinusoidal or incessant monomorphic ventricular tachycardia (type Ic agents) and torsade de pointes (type Ia or III agents and others such as select antihistamines).

The heart has two basic properties, namely, an electrical property and a mechanical property. The synchronous interaction between these two properties is complex, precise, and relatively enduring. The study of the electrical properties of the heart has grown at a steady rate, interrupted by periodic salvos of scientific breakthroughs. Einthoven's pioneering work allowed graphic electrical tracings of cardiac rhythm and probably represents the first of these breakthroughs. This discov-

ery (of the surface electrocardiogram [ECG]) has remained the cornerstone of diagnostic tools for cardiac rhythm disturbances. Since then, intracardiac recordings and programmed cardiac stimulation have advanced our understanding of arrhythmias, whereas microelectrode, voltage clamp, and patch clamping techniques have allowed considerable insight into the electrophysiologic actions and mechanisms of antiarrhythmic drugs. Certainly, the new era of molecular biology and mapping of the human genome promises even greater insights into mechanisms (and potential therapies) of arrhythmias. Noteworthy in this regard is the discovery of genetic abnormalities in the ion channels that control electrical repolarization (heritable long-QT syndromes) or depolarization (Brugada syndrome).

The clinical use of drug therapy started with the use of digitalis and then quinidine, followed somewhat later by a surge of new agents in the 1980s. A theme of drug discovery during this decade initially was to find orally absorbed lidocaine congeners (such as mexilitene and tocainide), and later the emphasis was on drugs with extremely potent effects on conduction, i.e., flecainide-like agents. The most recent focus of investigational antiarrhythmic drugs is the potassium channel blockers, with dofetilide being the most recently approved in the United States. Previously, there was some expectation that advances in antiarrhythmic drug discovery would lead to a highly effective and nontoxic agent that would be effective for a majority of patients (the so-called magic bullet). Instead, significant problems with drug toxicity and proarrhythmia have resulted in a decline in the overall volume of antiarrhythmic drug usage in the United States since 1989. The other phenomenon that has contributed significantly to the decline in drug usage is the development of extremely effective nondrug therapies. Technical advances have made it possible to permanently interrupt reentry circuits with radiofrequency ablation, which renders long-term antiarrhythmic drug use obsolete in certain arrhythmias. Further, refinement of the internal cardioverter-defibrillators continues to advance at an impressive rate, and this, combined with the now known hazards of drugs, has led most clinicians to choose this form of therapy as the first-line treatment of serious, recurrent ventricular arrhythmias. What does the future hold for the use of antiarrhythmic drugs? Certainly, new knowledge and technological advances have forced investigators and clinicians to rethink the concept of traditional membrane-active drugs. Although some degree of enthusiasm exists for some of the newer or investigational agents, the overall impact of these drugs has yet to be determined.

The purpose of this chapter is to review the principles involved in both normal and abnormal cardiac conduction and to address the pathophysiology and treatment of the more commonly encountered arrhythmias. Certainly, many volumes of complete text could be (and have been) devoted to basic and clinical electrophysiology. Therefore, this chapter briefly addresses those principles necessary for clinicians.

ARRHYTHMOGENESIS

NORMAL CONDUCTION

Electrical activity is initiated by the sinoatrial (SA) node and moves through cardiac tissue via a treelike conduction network. The SA node initiates cardiac rhythm under normal circumstances because this tissue possesses the highest degree of automaticity or rate of spontaneous impulse generation. The degree of automaticity of the SA node is largely influenced by the autonomic nervous system in that both cholinergic and sympathetic innervations control sinus rate. Most tissues within the conduction system also possess varying degrees of inherent automatic properties. However, the rates of spontaneous impulse generation of these tissues are less than that of the SA node. Thus these latent automatic pacemakers are continuously overdriven by impulses arising from the SA node (primary pacemaker) and therefore do not become clinically apparent.

From the SA node, electrical activity moves in a wavefront through an atrial specialized conducting system and eventually gains entrance to the ventricle via an atrioventricular (AV) node and a large

bundle of conducting tissue referred to as the *bundle of His*. Aside from this AV nodal–Hisian pathway, a fibrous AV ring that will not permit electrical stimulation separates the atria and ventricles. The conducting tissues bridging the atria and ventricles are referred to as the *junctional areas*. Again, this area of tissue (junction) is largely influenced by autonomic input and possesses a relatively high degree of inherent automaticity (about 40 beats per minute, less than that of the SA node). From the bundle of His, the cardiac conduction system bifurcates into several (usually three) bundle branches: one right bundle and two left bundles. These bundle branches further arborize into a conduction network referred to as the *Purkinje system*. The conduction system as a whole innervates the mechanical myocardium and serves to initiate excitation-contraction coupling and the contractile process. After a cell or group of cells within the heart is stimulated electrically, a brief period of time follows in which those cells cannot be excited again. This time period is referred to as the *refractory period*. As the electrical wavefront moves down the conduction system, the impulse eventually encounters tissue refractory to stimulation (recently excited) and subsequently dies out. Then the SA node recovers, fires spontaneously, and begins the process again.

Prior to cellular excitation, an electrical gradient exists between the inside and the outside of the cell membrane. At this time, the cell is polarized. In atrial and ventricular conducting tissue, the intracellular space is about 80 to 90 mV negative with respect to the extracellular environment. The electrical gradient just prior to excitation is referred to as *resting membrane potential* (RMP) and is the result of differences in ion concentrations between the inside and the outside of the cell. At RMP, the cell is polarized primarily by the action of active membrane ion pumps, the most notable of these being the sodium-potassium pump. For example, this specific pump (in addition to other systems) attempts to maintain the intracellular sodium concentration at 5–15 mEq/L and the extracellular sodium concentration at 135–142 mEq/L and the intracellular potassium concentration at 135–140 mEq/L and the extracellular potassium concentration at 3–5 mEq/L. RMP can be calculated by using the Nernst equation:

$$RMP = -61.5 \log \frac{[\text{ion outside}]}{[\text{ion inside}]}$$

Electrical stimulation (or depolarization) of the cell will result in changes in membrane potential over time or a characteristic action potential curve (Fig. 17–1). The action potential curve results from the transmembrane movement of specific ions and is divided into

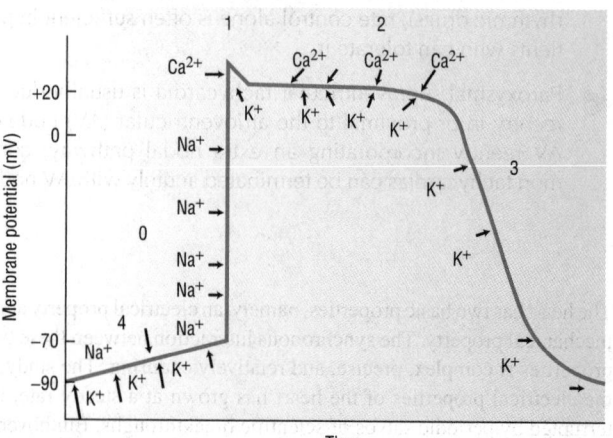

FIGURE 17–1. Purkinje fiber action potential showing specific ion flux responsible for the change in membrane potential.

different phases. Phase 0, or initial, rapid depolarization of atrial and ventricular tissues, is due to an abrupt increase in the permeability of the membrane to sodium influx. This rapid depolarization more than equilibrates (overshoots) the electrical potential, resulting in a brief initial repolarization, or phase 1. Phase 1 (initial depolarization) is due to a transient and active potassium efflux. Calcium begins to move into the intracellular space at about –60 mV (during phase 0), causing a slower depolarization. Calcium influx continues throughout phase 2 of the action potential (plateau phase) and is balanced to some degree by potassium efflux. Calcium entrance (only through L-channels in myocardial tissue) distinguishes cardiac conducting cells from nerve tissue and provides the critical ionic link to excitation-contraction coupling and the mechanical properties of the heart as a pump (see Chap. 14). The membrane remains permeable to potassium efflux during phase 3, resulting in cellular repolarization. Phase 4 of the action potential is the gradual depolarization of the cell and is related to a constant sodium leak into the intracellular space balanced by a decreasing (over time) efflux of potassium. The slope of phase 4 depolarization determines, in large part, the automatic properties of the cell. As the cell is slowly depolarized during phase 4, an abrupt increase in sodium permeability occurs, allowing the rapid cellular depolarization of phase 0. The juncture of phase 4 and phase 0, where rapid sodium influx is initiated, is referred to the *threshold potential* of the cell. The level of threshold potential also regulates the degree of cellular automaticity.

Not all cells in the cardiac conduction system rely on sodium influx for initial depolarization. Some tissues depolarize in response to a slower inward ionic current caused by calcium influx. These calcium-dependent tissues are found primarily in the SA and AV nodes (both L- and T-channels) and possess distinct conduction properties in comparison with the sodium-dependent fibers. Calcium-dependent cells generally have a less negative RMP (–40 to –60 mV) and a slower conduction velocity. Furthermore, in calcium-dependent tissues, recovery of excitability outlasts full repolarization, whereas in sodium-dependent tissues, recovery is prompt after repolarization. These two types of electrical fibers also differ dramatically in how drugs modify their conduction properties (see below).

Ion conductance across the lipid bilayer of the cell membrane occurs via the formation of membrane pores or channels (Fig. 17–2).

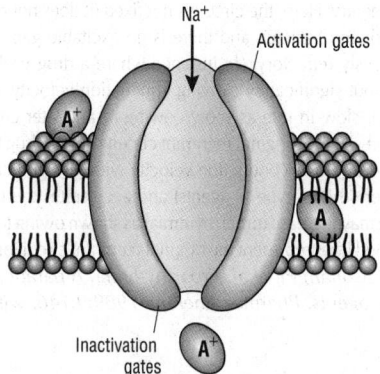

FIGURE 17–2. Lipid bilayer, sodium channel, and possible sites of action of the type I agents (*A*). Type I antiarrhythmic drugs theoretically may inhibit sodium influx at an extracellular, intramembrane, or intracellular receptor sites. However, all approved agents appear to block sodium conductance at a single receptor site by gaining entrance to the interior of the channel from an intracellular route. Active ionized drugs block the channel predominantly during the activated or inactivated state and bind and unbind with specific time constants (described as fast on/off, slow on/off, and intermediate).

Selective ion channels probably form in response to specific electrical potential differences between the inside and the outside of the cell (voltage dependence). The membrane itself consists of both organized and disorganized lipids and phospholipids in a dynamic sol-gel matrix. During ion flux and electrical excitation, changes in this sol-gel equilibrium occur and permit the formation of activated ion channels. Besides channel formation and membrane composition, intrachannel proteins or phospholipids, referred to as *gates*, also regulate the transmembrane movement of ions. These gates are thought to be positioned strategically within the channel to modulate ion flow (see Fig. 17–2). Each ion channel conceptually has two types of gates: an activation gate and an inactivation gate. The activation gate opens during depolarization to allow the ion current to enter or exit from the cell, and the inactivation gate closes to stop ion movement. When the cell is in a rested state, the activation gates are closed, and the inactivation gates are open. The activation gates then open to allow ion movement through the channel, and the inactivation gates later close to stop ion conductance. Therefore, the cell cycles between three states: resting, activated or open, and inactivated or closed. Activation of SA and AV nodal tissue depends on a slow depolarizing current through calcium channels and gates, whereas activation of atrial and ventricular tissue depends on a rapid depolarizing current through sodium channels and gates.

ABNORMAL CONDUCTION

The mechanisms of tachyarrhythmias classically have been divided into two general categories: those resulting from an abnormality in impulse generation, or "automatic" tachycardias, and those resulting from an abnormality in impulse conduction, or "reentrant" tachycardias. Automatic tachycardias depend on spontaneous impulse generation in latent pacemakers and may be due to several different mechanisms. Experimentally, chemicals such as digitalis glycosides and catecholamines and conditions such as hypoxemia, electrolyte abnormalities (e.g., hypokalemia), and fiber stretch (e.g., cardiac dilatation) may lead to an increased slope of phase 4 depolarization in cardiac tissues other than the SA node. These factors, which lead experimentally to abnormal automaticity, are also known to be arrhythmogenic in clinical situations. The increased slope of phase 4 causes heightened automaticity of these tissues and competition with the SA node for dominance of cardiac rhythm. If the rate of spontaneous impulse generation of the abnormally automatic tissue exceeds that of the SA node, then an automatic tachycardia may result. Automatic tachycardias have the following characteristics: (1) The onset of the tachycardia is not related to an initiating event such as a premature beat, (2) the initiating beat is usually identical to subsequent beats of the tachycardia, (3) the tachycardia cannot be initiated by programmed cardiac stimulation, and (4) onset of the tachycardia usually is preceded by a gradual acceleration in rate and termination by a deceleration in rate. Clinical tachycardias owing to the classic forms of enhanced automaticity, as just described, are not as common as once thought. Examples are sinus tachycardia and junctional tachycardia.

Triggered automaticity is also a possible mechanism for abnormal impulse generation. Briefly, *triggered automaticity* refers to transient membrane depolarizations that occur during repolarization (early after-depolarizations [EADs]) or after repolarization (delayed afterdepolarizations [DADs]) but prior to phase 4 of the action potential. After-depolarizations may be related to abnormal calcium and sodium influx during or just after full cellular repolarization. Experimentally, early after-depolarizations may be precipitated by hypokalemia, type Ia antiarrhythmic drugs, or slow stimulation rates—any factor that blocks the ion channels (e.g., potassium) responsible

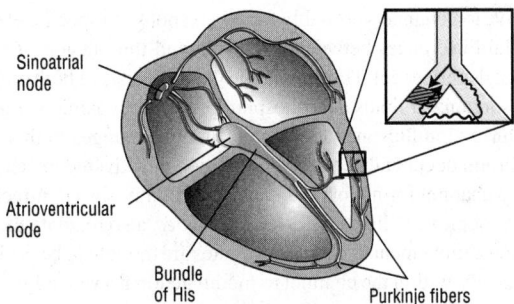

FIGURE 17–3. Conduction system of the heart. The magnified portion shows a bifurcation of a Purkinje fiber traditionally explained as the etiology of reentrant ventricular tachycardia. A premature impulse travels to the fiber, damaged by heart disease or ischemia. It encounters a zone of prolonged refractoriness (area of unidirectional block) (*cross-hatched area*) but fails to propagate because it remains refractory to stimulation from the previous impulse. However, the impulse may slowly travel (*squiggly line*) through the other portion of the Purkinje twig and will "reenter" the cross-hatched area if the refractory period is concluded and it is now excitable. Thus the premature impulse never meets refractory tissue; circus movement ensues. If this site stimulates the surrounding ventricle repetitively, clinical reentrant ventricular tachycardia results.

for cellular repolarization. EADs provoked by drugs that block potassium conductance and delay repolarization are the underlying cause of torsade de pointes. Late after-depolarizations may be precipitated by digitalis or catecholamines and suppressed by calcium channel inhibitors and have been suggested as the mechanism for multifocal atrial tachycardia, digitalis-induced tachycardias, and exercise-provoked ventricular tachycardia. Triggered automatic rhythms possess some of the characteristics of automatic tachycardias and some of the characteristics of reentrant tachycardias (described below).

As mentioned previously, the impulse originating from the SA node in an individual with sinus rhythm eventually meets previously excited and thus refractory tissue. Reentry is a concept that involves indefinite propagation of the impulse and continued activation of previously refractory tissue. There are three conduction requirements for the formation of a viable reentrant focus: two pathways for impulse conduction, an area of unidirectional block (prolonged refractoriness) in one of these pathways, and slow conduction in the other pathway (Fig. 17–3). Usually a critically timed premature beat initiates reentry. This premature impulse enters both conduction pathways but encounters refractory tissue in one of the pathways at the area of unidirectional block. The impulse dies out because it is still refractory from the previous (sinus) impulse. Although it fails to propagate in one pathway, the impulse may still proceed in a forward direction (antegrade) through the other pathway because of this pathway's relatively shorter refractory period. The impulse may then proceed through a loop of tissue and "reenter" the area of unidirectional block in a backward direction (retrograde). Because the antegrade pathway has slow conduction characteristics, the area of unidirectional block has time to recover its excitability. The impulse can proceed retrograde through this (previously refractory) tissue and continue around the loop of tissue in a circular fashion. Thus the key to the formation of a reentrant focus is crucial conduction discrepancies in the electrophysiologic characteristics of the two pathways. The reentrant focus may excite surrounding tissue at a rate greater than that of the SA node, and a clinical tachycardia results. This model is anatomically determined in that there is only one pathway for impulse conduction with a fixed circuit length. Another model of reentry, referred to as a *functional reentrant loop* or *leading circle model* also may occur[1] (Fig. 17–4).

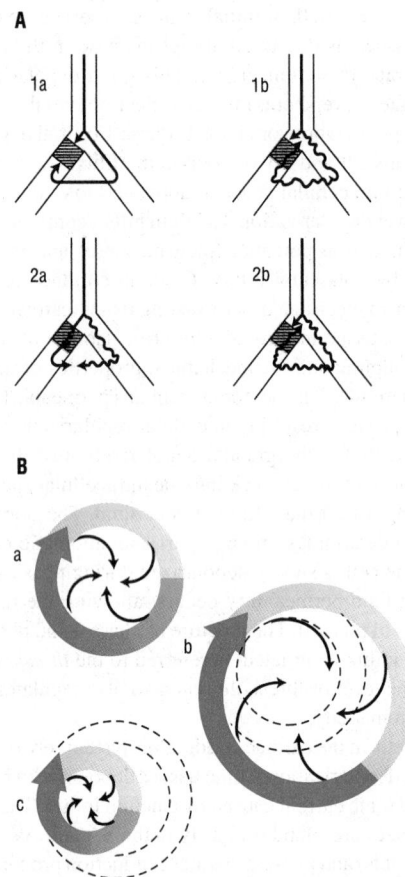

FIGURE 17–4. *A.* Possible mechanism of proarrhythmia in the anatomic model of reentry. (*1a*) Nonviable reentrant loop owing to bidirectional block (*shaded area*). (*1b*) Instance where a drug slows conduction velocity without significantly prolonging the refractory period. The impulse is now able to reenter the area of unidirectional block (*shaded area*) because slowed conduction through the contralateral limb allows recovery of the block. A new reentrant tachycardia may result. (*2a*) Nonviable reentrant loop owing to a lack of a unidirectional block. (*2b*) Instance where a drug prolongs the refractory period without significantly slowing conduction velocity. The impulse moving antegrade meets refractory tissue (*shaded area*), allowing for unidirectional block. A new reentrant tachycardia may result. *B.* Mechanism of reentry and proarrhythmia. (*a*) Functionally determined (*leading circle*) reentrant circuit. This model should be contrasted with anatomic reentry. Here, the circuit is not fixed (it does not necessarily move around an anatomic obstacle), and there is no excitable gap. All tissue inside is held continuously refractory. (*b*) Instance where a drug prolongs the refractory period without significantly slowing conduction velocity. The tachycardia may terminate or slow in rate as shown owing to a greater circuit length. The dashed lines represent the original reentrant circuit prior to drug treatment. (*c*) Instance where a drug slows conduction velocity without significantly prolonging the refractory period (i.e., type Ic agents) and accelerates the tachycardia. The tachycardia rate may increase (proarrhythmia) as shown owing to a shorter circuit length. The dashed lines represent the original reentrant circuit prior to drug treatment. *(From McCollam PL et al. Proarrhythmia: A paradoxic response to antiarrhythmic agents. Pharmacotherapy 1989;9:146, with permission.)*

In a functional reentrant focus, the length of the circuit may vary depending on the conduction velocity and recovery characteristics of the impulse. The area in the middle of the loop is continually kept refractory by the inwardly moving impulse. The length of the circuit is not fixed but is the smallest circle possible such that the leading edge of the wavefront is continuously exciting tissue just as it recovers; i.e., the head of the impulse nearly catches its tail. It differs from the anatomic model in that the leading edge of the impulse is not preceded by an excitable gap of tissue, and it does not have an obstacle in the middle nor a fixed anatomic circuit. Clinically, many reentrant foci probably have both anatomic and functional characteristics. In the figure-eight model, a zone of unidirectional block is present; allowing for two impulse loops that join and reenter the area of block in a retrograde fashion to form a pretzel-shaped reentrant circuit. This model combines functional characteristics with an excitable gap. All these theoretical models require a critical balance of refractoriness and conduction velocity within the circuit and, as such, have helped to explain the effects of drugs on terminating, modifying, and causing cardiac rhythm disturbances.

What causes reentry to become clinically manifest? Reentrant foci may occur at any level of the conduction system: within the branches of the specialized atrial conduction system, within the Purkinje network, and even within portions of the SA and AV nodes. The anatomy of the Purkinje system is felt to provide a suitable substrate for the formation of microreentrant loops and often is used as a model to facilitate understanding of reentry concepts (see Fig. 17–4). Of course, reentry usually does not occur in normal, healthy conduction tissue, and therefore, various forms of heart disease or conduction abnormalities usually must be present before reentry becomes manifest. In other words, the various forms of heart disease can result in changes in conduction in the pathways of a suitable reentrant substrate. An often-used example is reentry occurring as a consequence of ischemic or hypoxic damage: With inadequate cellular oxygen, cardiac tissue resorts to anaerobic glycolysis for adenosine triphosphate (ATP) production. As high-energy phosphate concentration diminishes, the activity of the transmembrane ion pumps declines, and the RMP rises. This rise in RMP causes inactivation in the voltage-dependent sodium channel, and the tissue begins to assume slow conduction characteristics. If changes in conduction parameters occur in a discordant manner owing to varying degrees of ischemia or hypoxia, then a reentry circuit may become manifest. Furthermore, an ischemic, dying cell liberates intracellular potassium, which also causes a rise in the RMP. In other cases, reentry may occur as a result of anatomic or functional variants in the normal conduction system. For instance, patients may possess two (instead of one) conduction pathways near or within the AV node or have an anomalous extranodal AV pathway that possesses different electrophysiologic characteristics from the normal AV nodal pathway. Reentry in these cases may occur within the AV node or encompass both atrial and ventricular tissue (see below). Reentrant tachycardias have the following characteristics: (1) The onset of the tachycardia is usually related to an initiating event (i.e., premature beat), (2) the initiating beat is usually different in morphology from subsequent beats of the tachycardia, (3) initiation of the tachycardia is usually possible with programmed cardiac stimulation, and (4) the initiation and termination of the tachycardia are usually abrupt without an acceleration or deceleration phase. There are many examples of reentrant tachycardias including atrial flutter and AV nodal or AV reentry and recurrent ventricular tachycardia.

ANTIARRHYTHMIC DRUGS

In a theoretical sense, drugs may have antiarrhythmic activity by directly altering conduction in several ways. First, a drug may depress the automatic properties of abnormal pacemaker cells. An agent may do this by decreasing the slope of phase 4 depolarization and/or by elevating threshold potential. If the rate of spontaneous impulse generation of the abnormally automatic foci becomes less than that of

the SA node, normal cardiac rhythm can be restored. Second, drugs may alter the conduction characteristics of the pathways of a reentrant loop.[1,2] An agent may facilitate conduction (shorten refractoriness) in the area of unidirectional block, allowing antegrade conduction to proceed. On the other hand, an antiarrhythmic agent may further depress conduction (prolong refractoriness) in either the area of unidirectional block or in the pathway with slowed conduction and a relatively shorter refractory period. If refractoriness is prolonged in the area of unidirectional block, retrograde propagation of the impulse is not permitted, causing a "bidirectional" block. In the anatomic model, if refractoriness is prolonged in the pathway with slow conduction, antegrade conduction of the impulse is not permitted through this route. In either case, drugs that reduce the discordance and cause uniformity in conduction properties of the two pathways may suppress the reentrant substrate. In the functionally determined model, if refractoriness is prolonged without significantly slowing conduction velocity, the tachycardia may terminate or slow in rate owing to a greater circuit length (see Fig. 17–4). There are other possible ways to stop reentry. For example, a drug may eliminate the critically timed premature impulse that triggers reentry, or a drug may slow conduction velocity to such an extent that conduction is extinguished.

Antiarrhythmic drugs have specific electrophysiologic actions that alter cardiac conduction in patients with or without heart disease. These actions form the basis of grouping antiarrhythmic agents into specific categories based on their electrophysiologic actions in vitro. Vaughan Williams proposed the most frequently used classification system[2] (Table 17–1). This classification has been criticized because (1) it is incomplete and does not allow for the classification of agents such as digoxin or adenosine, (2) it is not pure, and many agents have properties of more than one class of drugs, (3) it does not incorporate drug characteristics such as mechanisms of tachycardia termination/prevention, clinical indications, or side effects, and (4) agents become "labeled" within a class, although they may be distinct in many regards.[3] These criticisms formed the basis for an attempt to reclassify antiarrhythmic agents based on a variety of basic and clinical characteristics (called the *Sicilian gambit*[3]). Nonetheless, the Vaughan Williams classification remains the most frequently used system despite many proposed modifications and alternative systems. The type Ia drugs such as quinidine, procainamide, and disopyramide slow conduction velocity, prolong refractoriness, and decrease the automatic properties of sodium-dependent (normal and diseased) conduction tissue. Therefore, the type Ia agents can be effective in automatic tachycardias by decreasing the rate of spontaneous impulse generation of atrial or ventricular foci. In reentrant tachycardias, these drugs generally depress conduction and prolong refractoriness, theoretically transforming the area of unidirectional block into a bidirectional block. Clinically, type Ia drugs are broad-spectrum antiarrhythmics, being effective for both supraventricular and ventricular arrhythmias.

Historically, lidocaine and phenytoin were categorized separately from quinidine-like drugs. This was due to early work demonstrating that lidocaine had distinctly different electrophysiologic actions. In normal tissue models, lidocaine generally facilitates actions on cardiac conduction by shortening refractoriness and having little effect on conduction velocity. Thus it was postulated that these agents could improve antegrade conduction, eliminating the area of unidirectional block. Of course, arrhythmias usually do not arise from normal tissue, leading investigators to study the actions of lidocaine and phenytoin in ischemic and hypoxic tissue models. Interestingly, studies have shown these drugs to possess quinidine-like properties in diseased tissues. Therefore, it is probable that lidocaine acts in clinical

TABLE 17–1. Classification of Antiarrhythmic Drugs

Type	Drug	Conduction Velocity[a]	Refractory Period	Automaticity	Ion Block
Ia	Quinidine	↓	↑	↓	Sodium (intermediate)
	Procainamide				Potassium
	Disopyramide				
Ib	Lidocaine	0/↓	↓	↓	Sodium (fast on/off)
	Mexiletine				
	Tocainide				
Ic	Flecainide	↓↓	0	↓	Sodium (slow on/off)
	Propafenone[c]				Potassium[e]
	Moricizine[d]				
II[b]	β-Blockers	↓	↑	↓	Calcium (indirect)
III	Amiodarone[f]	0	↑↑	0	Potassium
	Bretylium[c]				
	Dofetilide				
	Sotalol[c]				
	Ibutilide				
IV[b]	Verapamil	↓	↑	↓	Calcium
	Diltiazem				

[a]Variables for normal tissue models in ventricular tissue.
[b]Variables for SA and AV nodal tissue only.
[c]Also has type II β-blocking actions.
[d]Classification controversial.
[e]Not clinically manifest.
[f]Also has sodium, calcium, and β-blocking actions; see Table 17–2.

tachycardias in a similar fashion to the type Ia drugs, i.e., accentuated effects in diseased ischemic tissues leading to bidirectional block in a reentrant circuit by prolonging refractoriness. Lidocaine and similar agents have accentuated effects in ischemic tissue owing to the local acidosis and potassium shifts that occur during cellular hypoxia. Changes in pH alter the time that local anesthetics occupy the sodium channel receptor and therefore affect the agent's electrophysiologic actions. In addition, the intracellular acidosis that ensues owing to ischemia could cause lidocaine to become "trapped" within the cell, allowing increased access to the receptor. The type Ib agents such as lidocaine (and structural analogues such as tocainide and mexiletine) are considerably more effective in ventricular arrhythmias than in supraventricular arrhythmias.

The third group of type I drugs, type Ic drugs, includes propafenone, flecainide, and moricizine. These agents profoundly slow conduction velocity while leaving refractoriness relatively unaltered. Type Ic drugs theoretically eliminate reentry by slowing conduction to a point where the impulse is extinguished and cannot propagate further. Although the type Ic drugs are effective for both ventricular and supraventricular arrhythmias, their use for ventricular arrhythmias has been limited by the risk of proarrhythmia (see below).

Type I drugs exert their effects on a subcellular basis by inhibiting the transmembrane influx of sodium. In essence, type I agents can be referred to as *sodium channel blockers*. The receptor site for the antiarrhythmics is probably inside the sodium channel so that, in effect, the drug plugs the pore. The agent may gain access to the receptor either via the intracellular space through the membrane lipid bilayer or directly through the channel. There are several principles inherent in antiarrhythmic-sodium channel receptor theories, and these are listed below.[4]

1. Type I antiarrhythmics have predominant affinity for a particular state of the channel, e.g., during activation or inactivation. For example, lidocaine and flecainide block sodium current primarily when the cell is in the inactivated state, whereas quinidine is predominantly an open (or activated) channel blocker.

2. Type I antiarrhythmics have specific binding and unbinding characteristics to the receptor. For example, lidocaine binds to and dissociates from the channel receptor quickly (termed *fast on/off*), but flecainide has very slow on/off properties. This explains why flecainide has such potent effects on slowing ventricular conduction, but lidocaine has little effect on normal tissue (at normal heart rates). In general, the type Ic drugs are slow on/off, the type Ib drugs are fast on/off, and type Ia drugs are intermediate in their binding kinetics.

3. Type I antiarrhythmics possess rate dependence; i.e., sodium channel blockade and slowed conduction are greatest at fast heart rates and least during bradycardia. For slow on/off drugs, sodium channel blockade is evident at normal rates (60 to 100 beats per minute), but for fast on/off agents, slowed conduction is apparent only at rapid rates of stimulation.

4. Type I antiarrhythmics (except phenytoin) are weak bases with a $pK_a > 7$ and block the sodium channel in their ionized form. Therefore, pH will alter these actions: Acidosis will accentuate and alkalosis diminishes sodium channel blockade.

5. Type I antiarrhythmics appear to share a single receptor site in the sodium channel. It should be noted, however, that a number of type I drugs have other electrophysiologic properties. For instance, quinidine has potent potassium channel blocking activity (manifest predominantly at low concentrations), as does N-acetylprocainamide (manifest predominantly at high concentrations), the primary metabolite of procainamide. Additionally, propafenone has β-blocking actions.

These principles are important in understanding additive drug combinations (e.g., quinidine and mexiletine), antagonistic combinations (e.g., flecainide and lidocaine), and potential antidotes to excess sodium channel blockade (e.g., sodium bicarbonate or propranolol). They also explain a number of clinical observations, such as why lidocaine-like drugs are relatively ineffective for supraventricular tachycardia. The type Ib drugs are fast on/off, inactivated sodium blockers; atrial cells, however, have a very brief inactivated phase relative to ventricular tissue.

The β-adrenergic antagonists are classified as type II antiarrhythmic drugs. For the most part, the clinically relevant acute antiarrhythmic mechanisms of the β-blockers result from their antiadrenergic actions. Because the SA and AV nodes are heavily influenced by adrenergic innervation, β-blockers would be most useful in tachycardias in which these nodal tissues are abnormally automatic or are a portion of a reentrant loop. These agents are also helpful in slowing ventricular response in atrial tachycardias (e.g., atrial fibrillation) by their effects on the AV node. Furthermore, some tachycardias are exercise-related or are precipitated by states of high sympathetic tone (perhaps through triggered activity), and β-blockers may be useful in these instances. β-Adrenergic stimulation results in increased conduction velocity, shortened refractoriness, and increased automaticity of the nodal tissues; β-adrenergic blockers will antagonize these effects. Propranolol is often noted to have "local anesthetic" or quinidine-like activity; however, suprapharmacologic concentrations usually are required to elicit this action. In the nodal tissues, β-blockers interfere with calcium entry into the cell by altering catecholamine-dependent channel integrity and gating kinetics. In sodium-dependent atrial and ventricular tissue, β-blockers shorten repolarization somewhat but otherwise have little direct effect. The antiarrhythmic properties of β-blockers observed with long-term, chronic therapy in patients with heart disease are less well understood. While it is clear that β-blockers decrease the likelihood of sudden death (presumably arrhythmic death) after myocardial infarction (MI), why this is so remains unclear but may relate to the complex interplay of changes in sympathetic tone, damaged myocardium, and ventricular conduction. In patients with heart failure, drugs such as β-blockers and angiotensin-converting enzyme (ACE) inhibitors may prevent arrhythmias such as atrial fibrillation that are linked to poor cardiac function by improving ventricular performance over time.[5,6]

Type III antiarrhythmics include agents that specifically prolong refractoriness in atrial and ventricular tissue. This class includes very different drugs: bretylium, amiodarone, sotalol, ibutilide, and recently, dofetilide; they share the common effect of delaying repolarization by blocking potassium channels. The electrophysiologic actions of bretylium are related to its multifaceted pharmacology.

Bretylium is structurally similar to guanethidine and can, likewise, cause an initial increase in catecholamine release from the adrenergic neuron. This action potentially may affect arrhythmogenesis by an indirect mechanism—an increase in coronary blood flow and myocardial perfusion—that reverses ischemia-related arrhythmias (similar to epinephrine's action in a patient with ventricular fibrillation). After causing catecholamine release, bretylium then causes an uncoupling of autonomic nerve stimulation from the release step, resulting in antiadrenergic effects. Theoretically, bretylium also may be antiarrhythmic by these sympatholytic actions. Nonetheless, bretylium prolongs repolarization owing to blockade of potassium conductance independent of the sympathetic nervous system, and many researchers feel that these direct actions account for its clinical effectiveness. Bretylium increases the ventricular fibrillation threshold and seems to have selective antifibrillatory but not antitachycardic effects. In other words, bretylium can be effective in ventricular fibrillation, but it is often ineffective in ventricular tachycardia.

In contrast, amiodarone and sotalol are effective in most tachycardias. Amiodarone displays electrophysiologic characteristics consistent with each class within the Vaughan Williams scheme; it is a sodium channel blocker with relatively fast on/off kinetics, has noncompetitive, nonselective β-blocking actions, blocks potassium channels, and also has a small degree of calcium antagonist activity (Table 17–2). At normal heart rates and with chronic use, its predominant effect is to prolong repolarization. On intravenous administration, its onset is relatively quick (unlike the oral form), and β-blockade predominates initially. Theoretically, amiodarone, like type I agents, may interrupt the reentrant substrate by transforming an area of unidirectional block into an area of bidirectional block. However, electrophysiologic studies using programmed cardiac stimulation imply that amiodarone may leave the reentrant loop intact. Rather, it is possible that amiodarone abolishes the premature impulse that usually triggers the reentry process. In addition, the potent β-blocking properties of amiodarone may contribute significantly to its acute and chronic efficacy. The impressive effectiveness of amiodarone, coupled with its low proarrhythmic potential, has challenged the notion that selective ion channel blockade by antiarrhythmic agents is preferable. Sotalol is a potent inhibitor of outward potassium movement during repolarization and also possesses β-blocking actions. Indeed, it was first synthesized as a nonselective β-antagonist but now has evolved into the prototypical type III agent on which most investigational agents are based. Ibutilide and, more recently, dofetilide have been approved for the conversion and prevention of atrial fibrillation, respectively; these agents are structurally similar to sotalol. Both possess type III activity by blocking the rapid component of the delayed potassium rectifier current (I_{Kr}).

TABLE 17–2. Time Course and Electrophysiologic Effects of Amiodarone

Class	Mechanism	EP	ECG	IV			PO
Type I	Na$^+$ block	↑ HV	↑ QRS	0	+	+	++
Type II	β-Block	↑ AH	↑ PR ↓ HR	++	++	++	++
Type III	K$^+$	↑ VERP ↑ AERP	↑ QT	0	+	++	++++
Type IV	Ca^{2+} block[a]	↑ AH	↑ PR	+	+	+	+
				Min–hrs	Hrs–days	Days–wks	Wks–mos

[a]Rate-dependent.
HV = His-ventricle interval; AH = atria-His interval; VERP = ventricular effective refractory period; AERP = atrial effective refractory period; HR = heart rate; EP = electrophysiologic actions; ECG = electrocardiographic effects.

There are a number of different potassium channels that function during normal conduction, but the most relevant in terms of approved and investigational antiarrhythmic drugs is the delayed rectifier current (I_K) responsible for phase 2 and 3 repolarization. Subcurrents make up I_K; an ultrarapid component I_{Kur}, a rapid component I_{Kr}, and a slow component I_{Ks}. N-acetylprocainamide (NAPA) and dofetilide selectively block I_{Kr}, whereas amiodarone and azimilide (investigational) block both I_{Kr} and I_{Ks}. The clinical relevance of selectively blocking components of the delayed rectifier current remains to be determined. Potassium current blockers (particularly those with selective I_{Kr}-blocking properties) display "reverse use-dependence"; i.e., their effects on repolarization are greatest at low heart rates. Sotalol and drugs like it also appear to be much more effective in preventing ventricular fibrillation (in dog models) than the traditional sodium blockers. They also decrease defibrillation threshold in contrast to type I agents, which tend to increase this parameter. This could be important in patients with automatic internal defibrillators because concurrent therapy with type I drugs may require more energy for successful cardioversion or, worse, render it ineffective in terminating the tachycardia. The Achilles' heel of all type III agents is an extension of their underlying ionic mechanism, i.e., by blocking potassium and delaying repolarization they also may cause proarrhythmia in the form of torsade de pointes.

The calcium channel antagonists comprise the type IV antiarrhythmic category. At least two types of calcium channels are operative in SA and AV nodal tissues: an L-type channel and a T-type channel. Therefore, both L-channel blockers (verapamil and diltiazem) and selective T-channel blockers (mibefradil—previously approved but withdrawn from the market) will slow conduction, prolong refractoriness, and decrease automaticity (e.g., owing to early or late afterdepolarizations) of the calcium-dependent tissue in the SA and AV nodes. Therefore, these agents are effective in automatic and reentrant tachycardias, which arise from or use the SA or AV nodes. In atrial tachycardias, these drugs can slow ventricular response (e.g., atrial fibrillation) by slowing AV nodal conduction. Furthermore, because calcium entry seems to be integral to exercise-related tachycardias and/or tachycardias owing to some forms of triggered automaticity, preliminary evidence shows effectiveness in these types of arrhythmias. In all likelihood, verapamil and diltiazem work at different receptor sites because of their dissimilar chemical structures and pharmacologic actions. Nifedipine (or any of the dihydropyridine calcium antagonists) does not have significant antiarrhythmic activity because a reflex increase in sympathetic tone owing to vasodilation counteracts this agent's direct negative dromotropic action. Calcium antagonists can shorten repolarization slightly in normal sodium-dependent tissue but otherwise have little effect.

All antiarrhythmic agents currently available have an impressive side-effect profile (Table 17–3). A considerable percentage of patients cannot tolerate long-term therapy with these drugs, and chances are good that an agent will have to be discontinued because of side effects. In one trial,[7] over 50% of patients had to discontinue long-term procainamide (mostly due to a lupus-like syndrome) after MI. In another study,[8] disopyramide caused anticholinergic side effects in about 70% of patients. Flecainide and disopyramide may precipitate congestive heart failure in a significant number of patients with underlying left ventricular (LV) dysfunction; they should not be used in patients with systolic heart failure.[9] The type Ib agents such as tocainide and mexiletine cause neurologic and/or gastrointestinal

TABLE 17–3. Side Effects of Antiarrhythmic Drugs

Amiodarone	CNS, corneal microdeposits/blurred vision, optic neuropathy/neuritis, GI, aggravation of underlying ventricular arrhythmias, torsade de pointes, bradycardia or AV block, bruising without thrombocytopenia, pulmonary fibrosis, hepatitis, hypothyroidism, hyperthyroidism, photosensitivity, blue-gray skin discoloration, myopathy, hypotension and phlebitis (IV use)
Bretylium	Hypotension, GI
Disopyramide	Anticholinergic symptoms, GI, torsade de pointes, heart failure, aggravation of underlying conduction disturbances and/or ventricular arrhythmias, hypoglycemia, hepatic cholestasis
Dofetilide	Torsades de pointes
Flecainide	Blurred vision, dizziness, headache, GI, bronchospasm,[a] aggravation of underlying
Propafenone	heart failure, conduction disturbances or ventricular arrhythmias
Ibutilide	Torsades de pointes, hypotension
Lidocaine	CNS, seizures, psychosis, sinus arrest, aggravation of underlying conduction disturbances
Mexiletine	CNS, psychosis, GI, aggravation of underlying conduction disturbances or ventricular arrhythmias
Moricizine	Dizziness, headache, GI, aggravation of underlying conduction disturbances or ventricular arrhythmias
Procainamide	Systemic lupus erythematosus, GI, torsade de pointes, aggravation of underlying heart failure, conduction disturbances or ventricular arrhythmias, agranulocytosis
Quinidine	Cinchonism, diarrhea, GI, hypotension, torsade de pointes, aggravation of underlying heart failure, conduction disturbances or ventricular arrhythmias, hepatitis, thrombocytopenia, hemolytic anemia
Sotalol	Fatigue, GI, depression, torsades de pointes, bronchospasm, aggravation of underlying heart failure, conduction disturbances or ventricular arrhythmias
Tocainide	CNS, psychosis, GI, aggravation of underlying conduction disturbances or ventricular arrhythmias, rash/arthralgias, pulmonary infiltrates, agranulocytosis, thrombocytopenia

[a]Propafenone only.
GI = nausea, anorexia; CNS = confusion, paresthesias, tremor, ataxia, etc.

TABLE 17–4. Pharmacokinetics of Antiarrhythmic Drugs

Drug	Bioavailability (%)	Primary Route of Elimination[a]	Substrate[c]	Inhibitor[c]	$V_{D,ss}$ (L/kg)	Protein Binding (%)	$t_{1/2}^{d}$	Therapeutic Range (mg/L)
Quinidine	70–80	H	CYP3A4	CYP2D6 P-GP	2–3.5	80–90	5–9 h	2–6
Procainamide	75–95	H/R	NAT CYP2D6		1.5–3	10–20	5–6 h (SAs) 2–3 h (FAs)	4–15
Disopyramide	70–95	H/R	CYP3A4		0.8–2	50–80	4–8 h	2–6
Lidocaine	20–40	H	CYP3A4 CYP2D6		1–2	65–75	1–3 h	1.5–5
Mexiletine	80–95	H	CYP2D6 CYP1A2	CYP1A2	5–12	60–75	12–20 h (PMs) 7–11 h (EMs)	0.8–2
Tocainide	90–95	H	PH II, gluc		1.5–3	10–30	12–15 h	4–10
Moricizine	34–38	H	CYP1A2?		6–11	92–95	2–4 h	—
Flecainide	90–95	H/R	CYP2D6		8–10	35–45	14–20 h (PMs) 10–14 h (EMs)	0.3–2.5
Propafenone[b]			CYP2D6 CYP3A4					
	11–39	H	CYP1A2		2.5–4	85–95	10–25 h (PMs) 3–7 h (EMs)	1.0–2.5
Amiodarone	22–88	H	CYP3A4 CYP2C8	CYP1A2 CYP2C9 CYP2D6 CYP3A4 P-GP	70–150	95–99	15–100 d	1.0–2.5
Sotalol	90–95	R			1.2–2.4	30–40	10–20 h	—
Dofetilide	85–95	R/H	CYP3A4		2.5–3.5	60–70	6–10 h	—
Ibutilide	—	H			6–12	40–50	3–6 h	—
Bretylium	15–20	R			4–8	Negligible	5–10 h	0.5–2
Verapamil	20–40	H	CYP3A4 CYP1A2	CYP3A4 P-GP	1.5–5	95–99	4–12 h	>0.05
Diltiazem	35–50	H	CYP3A4	CYP3A4 P-GP	3–5	70–85	4–10 h	>0.05

[a]H, hepatic; R, renal.
[b]Variables for parent compound (not 5-OH-propafenone).
[c]CYP = cytochrome P450 isoenzyme; NAT = N-acetyltransferase; P-GP = P-glycoprotein; PII, gluc = phase II glucuronidation.
[d]PMs = poor metabolizers; EMs = extensive metabolizers; SAs = slow acetylators; FAs = fast acetylators.

toxicity in a high percentage of patients. Tocainide, specifically, has been reported to cause both pulmonary fibrosis and leukopenia, the significance of which came to light after Food and Drug Administration (FDA) approval. Clearly, the most frightening adverse effects related to antiarrhythmic drugs are the aggravation of underlying ventricular arrhythmias or the precipitation of new (and life-threatening) ventricular arrhythmias[10] (see below).

Amiodarone has taken a prominent place in the treatment of both chronic and acute arrhythmias and is now the most commonly prescribed antiarrhythmic drug. Once considered a drug of last resort, it is now the first drug considered in many symptomatic tachycardias. Yet amiodarone is a peculiar and complex drug, displaying unusual pharmacologic effects, pharmacokinetics, dosing schemes, and multisystem side effects. Amiodarone has an extremely long elimination phase and large volume of distribution; therefore, onset of action with the oral form is delayed (days to weeks) despite a loading regimen, and effects persist long (months) after discontinuation. Amiodarone inhibits most cytochrome P450 enzymes (and P-glycoprotein), resulting in many common drug interactions (e.g., it will cause digoxin levels to approximately double, and one must reduce the maintenance dose of warfarin by one-third to one-half). Acute administration usually is tolerated well by patients, but severe toxicities may result with chronic use. Severe bradycardia (sometimes requiring pacing to allow the patient to remain on amiodarone), hyper-

and hypothyroidism, photosensitivity, and a blue-gray skin discoloration on exposed areas are common. Hepatitis (uncommon) and pulmonary fibrosis (5% to 10% of patients) have caused death.[11,12] These side effects mandate close and continued monitoring (e.g., liver enzymes, thyroid function tests, eye examinations, chest x-rays, and pulmonary function tests) and have led to a proliferation of "amiodarone clinics" designed just for patients receiving this agent on a chronic basis.[13]

The pharmacokinetics of the antiarrhythmic agents are summarized in Table 17–4, and a nomogram for estimating effective dosages of the oral forms (except amiodarone) is shown in Fig. 17–5. Dosing recommendations for the intravenous forms are shown in Table 17–5.

SUPRAVENTRICULAR ARRHYTHMIAS

The common supraventricular tachycardias that often require drug treatment are (1) atrial fibrillation or atrial flutter, (2) paroxysmal supraventricular tachycardia, and (3) automatic atrial tachycardias. Other common supraventricular arrhythmias that usually do not require drug therapy include premature atrial complexes (PACs), wandering atrial pacemaker, sinus arrhythmia, and sinus tachycardia. As an example, PACs rarely cause symptoms and never cause hemodynamic compromise, and therefore, drug therapy usually is not

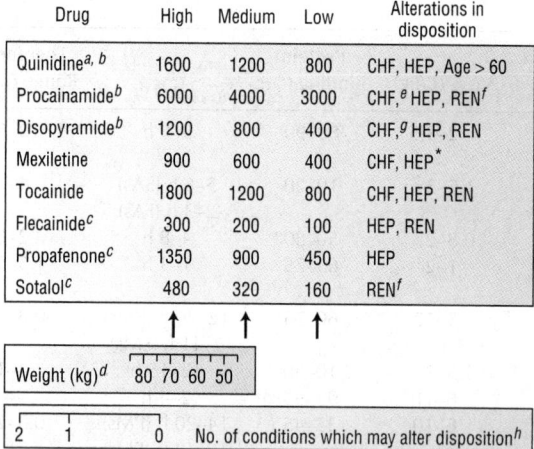

Drug	High	Medium	Low	Alterations in disposition
Quinidine[a, b]	1600	1200	800	CHF, HEP, Age > 60
Procainamide[b]	6000	4000	3000	CHF,[e] HEP, REN[f]
Disopyramide[b]	1200	800	400	CHF,[g] HEP, REN
Mexiletine	900	600	400	CHF, HEP[*]
Tocainide	1800	1200	800	CHF, HEP, REN
Flecainide[c]	300	200	100	HEP, REN
Propafenone[c]	1350	900	450	HEP
Sotalol[c]	480	320	160	REN[f]

Weight (kg)[d]   80 70 60 50

2   1   0   No. of conditions which may alter disposition[h]

FIGURE 17–5. Nomogram for estimating effective doses of commonly used oral antiarrhythmic drugs for acute efficacy testing. The dosages are grouped into high, medium, and low categories based on commonly used regimens and commercially available dosage forms. The dosages for each drug are listed as milligrams per day and are expected to result in the average steady-state concentrations shown in Table 17–2. Abbreviations: CHF = congestive heart failure; HEP = hepatic disease; REN = renal insufficiency (creatinine clearance < 50 mL/min). [a]Sulfate salt equivalents.
[b]Sustained-release forms may allow less fluctuation in concentrations.
[c]Best to initiate low-dose regimens in all patients and escalate slowly.
[d]Ideal body weight.
[e]Conflicting data regarding alteration in disposition.
[f] Significant accumulation of active metabolites or patent in renal disease limit use.
[g]Disopyramide not recommended in congestive heart failure.
[h]Use 1 for each suspected alteration but 2 where indicated (*).

Use of nomogram:
Step 1. Connect a straight line from the bar indicating the number of alterations in disposition, through the patient's weight to the base of the box.
Step 2. Approximate daily dosage is shown directly above the arrow. When the line connects between the arrows, use the crossbars between the arrows to choose high, medium, or low dosages or estimate an intermediate amount. Exercise caution when choosing dosages in the high range.
Example: A 70-kg patient with poor LV function (i.e., CHF) and frequent paroxysmal episodes of atrial fibrillation is to be treated with oral quinidine. A straight line drawn between 1 on the conditions bar and 70 kg on the weight bar will intersect near the center arrow on the box. Directly above the point of intersection are the medium dosage ranges; quinidine sulfate can be initiated at 1200 mg/day or 300 mg every 6 hours in this patient. *(From Bauman JL, Schoen MD, Hoon TJ. Practical optimisation of antiarrhythmic drug therapy using pharmacokinetic principles. Clin Pharmacokinet 1991;20:151–166, with permission.)*

indicated. Likewise, sinus tachycardia is usually the result of underlying metabolic or hemodynamic disorders (such as infection, dehydration, hypotension, etc.), and therapy should be directed at the underlying cause, not at the tachycardia per se. Of course, there are exceptions to these suggestions. For example, sinus tachycardia may be deleterious in patients after cardiac surgery or MI. In another unusual tachycardia termed *nonparoxysmal sinus tachycardia*, chronically elevated heart rates may cause alterations in LV function. In these instances, antiarrhythmic drugs such as β-blockers indeed may be indicated. Stated in another way, although many arrhythmias generally do not require therapy, clinical judgment and patient-specific variables play an important role in this decision. Nevertheless, for the purpose of this discussion, only the tachycardias usually requiring antiarrhythmic drug therapy as listed above will be addressed.

TABLE 17–5. Intravenous Antiarrhythmic Dosing

Drug	Clinical Situation	Dose
Amiodarone	Recurrent VT/VF	150 mg/10 min IV push 1 mg/min for 6 h, then 0.5 mg/min infusion
Bretylium	Cardiac arrest Acute VF	300 mg IV push 5 mg/min IV push (may repeat to total dose 30 mg/kg) 1–2 mg/min infusion if needed
Diltiazem	PSVT; rate control AF	0.25 mg/kg IV push (may repeat with 0.35 mg/kg) 5–15 mg/h infusion
Ibutilide	Termination AF	1 mg/10 min IV push (may repeat if needed)
Lidocaine	VT/VF	100 mg IV push (may repeat up to total dose 300 mg) (limit total to 200 mg if CHF present) 2–4 mg/min infusion (1–2 mg/min if liver disease or CHF)
Procainamide	AF, VT	15–18 mg/kg at 20–50 mg/min load 1–6 mg/min infusion
Verapamil	PSVT; rate control AF	5 mg IV push (may repeat up to 20 mg) 5–15 mg/h infusion

CLINICAL PRESENTATION: SUPRAVENTRICULAR TACHYCARDIA

ATRIAL FIBRILLATION/FLUTTER

GENERAL

These rhythms are usually not directly life-threatening, nor do they generally cause hemodynamic collapse or syncope, but 1:1 atrial flutter (ventricular response ~300 beats per minute) is an exception. Also, patients with underlying forms of heart disease that are heavily reliant on atrial contraction to maintain adequate cardiac output (e.g., mitral stenosis and obstructive cardiomyopathy) will display more severe symptoms of atrial fibrillation/flutter.

SYMPTOMS

Most often patients complain of rapid beat rate/palpitations and/or worsening symptoms of heart failure (shortness of breath, fatigue). Medical emergencies are severe heart failure (i.e., pulmonary edema, hypotension) or atrial fibrillation occurring in the setting of acute MI.

DIAGNOSTIC TESTS/SIGNS (ECG)

Atrial fibrillation is an irregularly irregular supraventricular rhythm with no discernible, consistent atrial activity (*p* waves). Ventricular response is usually 120–180 beats per minute, and the pulse is irregular. Atrial flutter is (usually) a regular supraventricular rhythm with characteristic flutter waves (or sawtooth pattern) reflecting more organized atrial activity. Commonly, ventricular rate is in factors of 300 beats per minute (e.g., 150, 100, or 75 beats per minute).

PSVT DUE TO REENTRY

GENERAL

These rhythms can be transient, resulting in few, if any, symptoms, or prolonged and life-threatening, causing hemodynamic collapse.

SYMPTOMS

Patients frequently complain of intermittent episodes of rapid heart rate/palpitations that start and stop abruptly, usually without provocation (but occasionally during exercise). Severe symptoms include syncope. Often (in particular, those with AV nodal reentry) patients complain of a chest pressure or a fullness in the neck sensation. This is due to simultaneous AV contraction with the right atrium contracting against a closed tricuspid valve. Life-threatening symptoms (syncope, hemodynamic collapse) are associated with extremely rapid rate (e.g., >200 beats per minute) and atrial fibrillation associated with an accessory AV pathway.

DIAGNOSTIC TESTS/SIGNS (ECG)

Most commonly, PSVT is a rapid, narrow-QRS-complex tachycardia, regular in rhythm, that starts and stops abruptly. Atrial activity, although present, is difficult to ascertain on surface ECG because P waves are "buried" within the QRS complex or T wave.

ATRIAL FIBRILLATION AND ATRIAL FLUTTER

MECHANISMS AND BACKGROUND

Atrial fibrillation and atrial flutter are common supraventricular tachycardias. These tachycardias occur more often in men, especially elderly men. In the general population, the overall prevalence of atrial fibrillation is about 0.4% (independent of gender and age), and this increases with age (e.g., more than 6% in patients older than 80 years of age).[14] About 10% to 30% of patients with heart failure have had episodes of atrial fibrillation.[14] These arrhythmias may present as a chronic, established tachycardia, an acute tachycardia, or a self-terminating paroxysmal form. The following semantics and definitions are sometimes used[14,15]: *acute atrial fibrillation* (onset within 48 hours), *paroxysmal atrial fibrillation* (terminates spontaneously in less than 7 days), *recurrent atrial fibrillation* (two or more episodes), *persistent atrial fibrillation* (duration longer than 7 days and does not terminate spontaneously), and *permanent atrial fibrillation* (does not terminate with attempts at pharmacologic or electrical cardioversion). Atrial fibrillation is characterized as an extremely rapid (400 to 600 atrial beats per minute) and disorganized atrial activation. With this disorganized atrial activity, there is a loss of the contribution of atrial contraction (atrial kick) to forward cardiac output. Supraventricular impulses penetrate the AV conduction system in variable degrees, resulting in an irregular activation of the ventricles and an *irregularly irregular* pulse. The AV junction will not conduct most of the supraventricular impulses, causing ventricular response to be considerably slower (120 to 180 beats per minute) than the atrial rate. Atrial flutter occurs less frequently than atrial fibrillation but is similar in its precipitating factors, consequences, and drug-therapy approach (exceptions noted below). This arrhythmia is characterized by rapid (270 to 330 atrial beats per minute) but regular atrial activation. The slower and regular electrical activity results in a regular ventricular response and a pulse that is in approximate factors of 300 beats per minute (i.e., 1:1 AV conduction = ventricular rate of 300 beats per minute;

2:1 AV conduction = ventricular rate of 150 beats per minute; 3:1 AV conduction = ventricular rate of 100 beats per minute). Atrial flutter may occur in two distinct forms (type I and type II). Type I flutter is the more common classic form with atrial rates of approximately 300 beats per minute and the typical "sawtooth pattern" of atrial activation, as shown by the surface ECG. Type II flutter tends to be faster, being somewhat of a hybrid between classic atrial flutter and atrial fibrillation. Although the ventricular response usually has a regular pattern, atrial flutter with varying degrees of AV block or that occurs with episodes of atrial fibrillation ("fib-flutter") can cause an irregular ventricular rate and pulse.

It is generally accepted that the predominant mechanism of atrial fibrillation and atrial flutter is reentry. Atrial fibrillation appears to result from multiple atrial reentrant loops (or wavelets), and atrial flutter is due to a single, dominant reentrant substrate (counterclockwise circus movement around the tricuspid annulus). Atrial fibrillation or flutter usually occurs in association with forms of organic heart disease that causes atrial distension. Forms of heart disease that commonly lead to atrial stretch and precipitate atrial fibrillation or flutter include

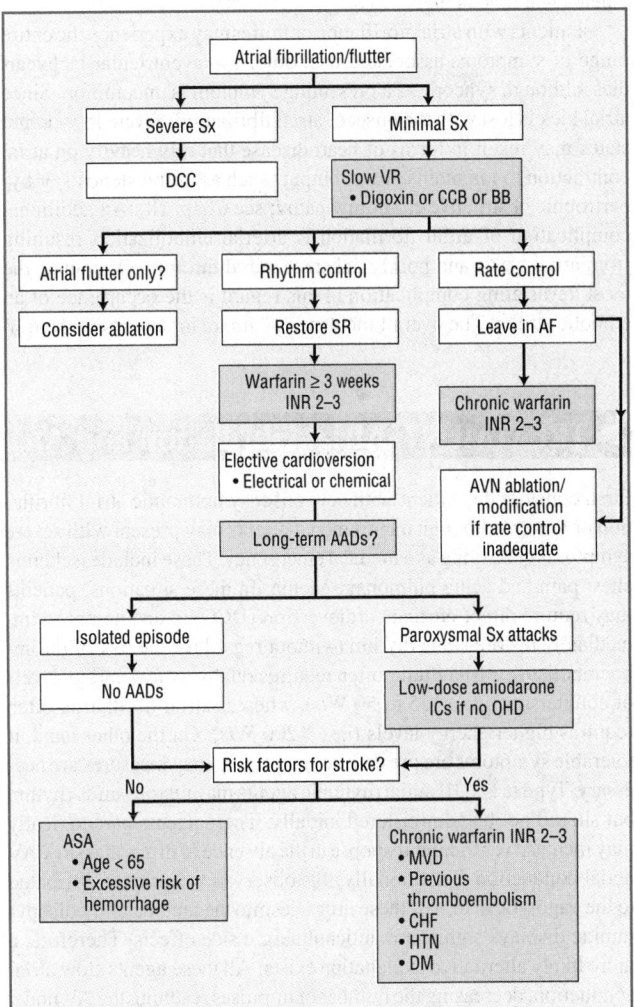

FIGURE 17–6. Algorithm for the treatment of atrial fibrillation and atrial flutter. Sx = symptoms; AVN = AV node; DCC = direct-current cardioversion; CCB = calcium channel antagonist (verapamil or diltiazem); BB = β-blocker; ASA = aspirin; OHD = organic heart disease; AADs = antiarrhythmic drugs; INR = international normalized ratio; MVD = mitral valve disease; CHF = congestive heart failure; HTN = hypertension; DM = diabetes mellitus.

ischemia or infarction, hypertensive heart disease, valvular disorders such as mitral stenosis, mitral insufficiency, congenital abnormalities such as septal defects, and primary myocardial disease such as dilated or hypertrophic cardiomyopathy. Disorders that cause right atrial stretch and are associated with atrial fibrillation or flutter include acute pulmonary embolus and chronic lung disease resulting in pulmonary hypertension and cor pulmonale. It is sometimes said that "atrial fibrillation begets atrial fibrillation." That is, the arrhythmia tends to perpetuate itself; long episodes are more difficult to terminate, perhaps due to tachycardia-induced changes in atrial function (mechanical and/or electrical "remodeling"). Atrial fibrillation also may occur in association with states of high adrenergic tone such as thyrotoxicosis, alcohol withdrawal, sepsis, or excessive physical exertion. Established or paroxysmal atrial fibrillation occurring without identifiable heart disease or known precipitating factors is termed *lone atrial fibrillation*. Other states in which patients are predisposed to episodes of atrial fibrillation are the presence of an anomalous AV pathway (i.e., Kent bundle) and sinus node dysfunction (i.e., tachy-brady or sick sinus syndrome). Finally, although unusual, some patients have atrial fibrillation that appears to be perpetuated by states of high cholinergic tone; episodes occur after meals or during sleep when vagal tone is high.

Patients with atrial fibrillation or flutter may experience the entire range of symptoms associated with other supraventricular tachycardias, although syncope as a presenting symptom is uncommon. Since atrial kick is lost with the onset of atrial fibrillation, severe low-output states may result in forms of heart disease that rely heavily on atrial contraction to maintain cardiac output (such as mitral stenosis or hypertrophic obstructive cardiomyopathy; see Chap. 18). An additional complication of atrial fibrillation is arterial embolization resulting from atrial stasis and poorly adherent mural thrombi. Of course, the most devastating complication in this regard is the occurrence of an embolic stroke. The overall incidence of stroke in patients with atrial fibrillation not receiving antithrombotic therapy is about 3% to 6% per year.[16,17] Patients with concurrent mitral stenosis or severe systolic heart failure and atrial fibrillation are at particularly high risk for cerebral embolism. Other risk factors for stroke identified from recent trials are increasing age, history of hypertension, previous transient ischemic event or stroke, and diabetes.[17] Stroke can precede the onset of documented atrial fibrillation, probably due to undetected paroxysms prior to the onset of established atrial fibrillation. In contrast, young patients (age younger than 60 years) with atrial fibrillation in whom precipitating factors cannot be identified (i.e., lone atrial fibrillation) have a low risk of embolic stroke.[17] The risk of stroke in patients with only atrial flutter traditionally has been felt to be low, prompting some to recommend only aspirin for prevention of thromboembolism. However, since isolated atrial flutter is relatively uncommon and the risk of stroke is not as well established (as it is for the more common atrial fibrillation), more recent recommendations suggest using the identical guidelines for both atrial fibrillation and atrial flutter.[15,18]

MANAGEMENT

The traditional approach to the treatment of atrial fibrillation can be organized into several sequential goals: (1) Evaluate the need for acute treatment (usually administration of drugs that slow ventricular rate), (2) contemplate methods to restore sinus rhythm, taking into consideration the risks (e.g., thromboembolism), and (3) consider ways to prevent the long-term complications of atrial fibrillation such as arrhythmia recurrences and thromboembolism. A time-honored presumption, recently challenged, lies within this strategy; i.e., long-term maintenance of sinus rhythm is a desirable goal. Nevertheless, a discussion of the management and drug therapy of atrial fibrillation/flutter follows, organized according to these goals. An algorithm for the management of atrial fibrillation is shown in Fig. 17–6.

▶ TREATMENT: Atrial Fibrillation and Atrial Flutter

First, consider the patient with new-onset symptomatic atrial fibrillation or flutter. Although uncommon, patients may present with severe symptoms qualifying as a medical emergency. These include ischemic chest pain and acute pulmonary edema. In these situations, patients may require direct-current cardioversion (DCC) in an attempt to immediately restore sinus rhythm (without regard for the risk of thromboembolism). Atrial flutter often requires relatively low energy levels of countershock (i.e., 25 to 50 W/s), whereas atrial fibrillation often requires higher energy levels (i.e., >200 W/s). On the other hand, if tolerable symptoms are present, no such emergency measures are necessary. Type Ia and III antiarrhythmic agents may restore sinus rhythm but should not be administered initially. These agents paradoxically may increase ventricular response in the absence of drugs that slow AV nodal conduction. Traditionally, this observation has been attributed to the vagolytic action of these drugs despite the fact that only disopyramide displays significant anticholinergic side effects. Therefore, a more likely alternative explanation exists: All these agents slow atrial conduction, decreasing the number of impulses reaching the AV node, and as a result, the AV node paradoxically allows more impulses to gain entrance to the ventricular conduction system (increasing ventricular rate).

Because of this phenomenon and the lack of need for immediate restoration of sinus rhythm, drugs that slow conduction and increase refractoriness in the AV node should be used as initial therapy. Loading dosages of digoxin historically have been recommended as first-line treatment to slow ventricular rate, particularly in patients with heart failure. However, the place of digoxin in therapy has been questioned in both the acute and chronic settings.[19,20] Digoxin is sometimes ineffective and often slow in onset; although an initial decrease in ventricular response sometimes can be observed within 1 hour of intravenous administration, full control (resting heart rate of less than 80 beats per minute and less than 110 beats per minute during moderate exercise) usually is not achieved for 24 to 48 hours. Digoxin will not restore sinus rhythm, although spontaneous termination of atrial fibrillation may occur in some patients during the loading procedure. As mentioned previously, patients can present at two ends of the spectrum (i.e., either severely symptomatic or with no or mild symptoms), and often they present somewhere in between. Consequently, clinical judgment is necessary in choosing the proper treatment strategy. For example, intravenous calcium antagonists (e.g., diltiazem or verapamil) provide an alternative approach, allowing for a rapid decrease in ventricular rate and symptomatic relief without the need for DCC.[21,22] Because control of ventricular response can be transient, verapamil or diltiazem can be given as an initial intravenous bolus, followed by a continuous infusion titrated to heart rate. Although digoxin in the past has been considered the drug of first choice to slow ventricular rate, many practitioners now choose calcium antagonists in most patients with atrial fibrillation or flutter. Further, atrial fibrillation or flutter precipitated by states of high adrenergic tone, such as thyrotoxicosis, is often resistant to digoxin therapy (digoxin slows AV nodal conduction primarily through vagotonic mechanisms). In these cases, intravenous β-blockers (e.g., propranolol or esmolol) can be highly effective and should be considered first.

Although β-blockers and calcium channel blockers have taken a more prominent role in acutely controlling rate in patients with rapid atrial fibrillation or flutter, a cautionary note must be made. That is, most patients with these tachycardias also have concomitant symptoms of heart failure, and these two forms of drug therapy may worsen the situation initially. Usually, a prompt decline in rate and increase in stroke volume balances the decrease in contractility seen with β-blockers or calcium channel blockers such that heart failure symptoms remain unchanged. However, occasionally, severe reactions and hypotension may occur; one study implies that diltiazem may be safer than verapamil.[22]

Patients may present with a slow ventricular response (in the absence of AV nodal–blocking drugs) and thus do not require therapy with digoxin, verapamil, or esmolol. This type of presentation should alert the clinician to the possibility of preexisting SA or AV nodal conduction disease such as sick sinus syndrome. DCC should not be attempted in these patients without a temporary pacemaker in place (see below).

■ RESTORATION OF SINUS RHYTHM?

After treatment with AV nodal–blocking agents and a subsequent decrease in ventricular response, the patient should be evaluated for the possibility of restoring sinus rhythm if atrial fibrillation persists. Within the context of this evaluation, several factors should be considered. First, many patients convert spontaneously to sinus rhythm without intervention, obviating therapy needed to achieve this goal. For instance, atrial fibrillation occurs frequently as a complication of cardiac surgery and often reverts spontaneously to sinus rhythm without therapy. Second, restoring sinus rhythm is not a necessary or realistic goal in some patients. Important in this regard is the recent publication of a number of trials,[23,24] including the National Institutes of Health (NIH)–sponsored Atrial Fibrillation Follow-up Investigation of Rhythm Management (AFFIRM)[23] that compared strategies to maintain sinus rhythm with those just to control ventricular rate, allowing atrial fibrillation to remain. In AFFIRM, patients were randomized to receive rate-control therapy only or to drug therapy designed to achieve and maintain sinus rhythm. Rate-control treatment involved AV nodal–blocking drugs (e.g., digoxin, β-blockers, and/or calcium channel blockers) first and then nondrug treatment (AV nodal ablation with pacemaker implantation) if necessary to control rates. Treatment with type I or type III antiarrhythmic drugs (e.g., amiodarone, sotalol, and then propafenone were used most frequently) was used to maintain sinus rhythm. Cumulative mortality was not statistically different between the two strategies but tended ($p = .08$) to be higher in the group given antiarrhythmic drugs to maintain sinus rhythm. The results of other similar large multicenter trials are consistent with those of AFFIRM.[24] Clearly, these important findings temper the old approach of aggressively attempting to maintain sinus rhythm. Many, if not most, patients now can be allowed to remain in atrial fibrillation, chronically treated with AV nodal–blocking

agents to control ventricular response (e.g., resting rate of approximately 80 beats per minute or less). Often, long-term therapy with digoxin alone for this purpose will not control exercise-related increases in ventricular response and tachycardia symptoms. In these patients, small doses of calcium antagonists or β-blockers can be added; the need for these ancillary agents can be evaluated readily by treadmill exercise testing or by simple ambulation. Alternatively, β-blockers alone can be used to control rate on a chronic basis. Since most patients with atrial fibrillation also have heart failure, β-blockers can control rate and improve systolic function. Occasionally, patients may be encountered who are highly refractory to AV nodal–blocking agents (including combination drug therapy), and ventricular response remains rapid. Aggressive attempts to lower rate are necessary; chronic tachycardias can result in a progressive decline in LV function causing so called tachycardia cardiomyopathy. Hence, in drug-refractory patients, ablation or modification of the AV node by a transvenous catheter delivering radiofrequency current is indicated.[25] This procedure often completely blocks conduction from the atrium to the ventricle, requiring the concurrent implantation of a permanent pacemaker with a ventricular lead. If it is decided in a given patient not to restore sinus rhythm but rather to allow atrial fibrillation to remain, one additional treatment consideration should be considered. That is, these individuals must remain on anticoagulant or antiplatelet therapy for at least as long as the atrial fibrillation remains; they are at continued risk for thromboembolic complications.

In which patients should restoration of sinus rhythm be considered? Post-AFFIRM, this decision is left to clinical judgment, but one could imagine that several groups of patients should undergo electrical or pharmacologic cardioversion. These include patients who are judged to have a relatively low chance of recurrence (e.g., first episodes of lone atrial fibrillation in young individuals or transient states of high sympathetic tone) or those with troublesome symptoms despite adequate rate control.

In patients in whom it is decided to restore sinus rhythm, one must consider that this very act (independent of the method chosen) places the patient at risk for thromboembolism. The reason for this is that the return of sinus rhythm restores an effective contraction, which may dislodge poorly adherent thrombi. Anticoagulation prior to cardioversion prevents clot growth and the formation of new thrombi and allows existing thrombi to become organized and well adherent to the atrial wall. This form of preventative therapy has been shown to prevent stroke associated with cardioversion, but several weeks of anticoagulation is necessary. Therefore, current recommendations are to institute warfarin treatment (international normalization ratio [INR] 2 to 3) for at least 3 weeks prior to cardioversion. The common clinical scenario is to discharge the patient from the hospital, monitor the patient on an ambulatory basis, and readmit for elective cardioversion after this time period.[17] After restoration of sinus rhythm, full atrial contraction does not occur immediately. Rather, it returns gradually to a maximum contractile force over a 3- to 4-week period. Therefore, warfarin should be continued for at least 1 month after effective cardioversion and return of sinus rhythm (see below).

There are several exceptions to this recommended process of anticoagulation. In patients with atrial fibrillation of less than 48 hours' duration, anticoagulation prior to cardioversion probably is not necessary because there has not been sufficient time to form atrial thrombi. However, in most presentations of atrial fibrillation, the exact time of onset is unclear. In the past, patients with atrial flutter were felt to be at low risk for stroke, but current consensus recommendations give strong consideration to treating atrial flutter in the same way as atrial fibrillation, i.e., generally at least 3 weeks of anticoagulation prior to elective cardioversion.[14,17] Transesophageal echocardiography (TEE) is also being used as a tool to stratify which patients may require anticoagulation prior to DCC from those who may not. If an atrial thrombus or severe stasis ("smoke") is not noted on TEE, then perhaps these patients can be cardioverted without the mandatory 3 weeks of warfarin pretreatment. Initial data are promising and seemingly cost-effective, obviating the need for more than 3 weeks of prior warfarin treatment and subsequent readmission to the hospital. The use of TEE in this manner has been compared with the conventional 3 weeks of anticoagulation before cardioversion in patients with atrial fibrillation.[26] In this large multicenter, randomized trial, the incidence of thromboembolic events was not different between the two strategies, but bleeding episodes were higher in the 3 weeks of warfarin group. Patients in the TEE strategy group had a higher success rate of achieving sinus rhythm probably because it is more difficult to terminate atrial fibrillation the longer a patient remains in it (i.e., "atrial fibrillation begets atrial fibrillation"). These impressive data will more than likely place the use of TEE in patients with atrial fibrillation in a much more prominent role.

After prior anticoagulation or TEE, the methods available to restore sinus rhythm can be considered (in those patients in whom maintenance of sinus rhythm is the goal). There are two methods of restoring sinus rhythm in patients with atrial fibrillation or flutter: pharmacologic cardioversion and DCC. Which of these is the method of choice generally is a matter of clinical preference, but it should be noted that international consensus guidelines recommend that DCC be considered first.[14] Indeed, in one economic analysis, DCC as first-line therapy was less costly than the strategy of trying a drug first (such as ibutilide) and then proceeding to DCC in the event of drug failure.[27] Nonetheless, some clinicians elect to use antiarrhythmic drugs first and then resort to DCC in the event that these agents fail. Nearly all type Ia, Ic, and III agents have been demonstrated to possess some effectiveness in terminating atrial fibrillation, but because of the risk of proarrhythmia, they should be initiated in a monitored inpatient setting. A meta-analysis supported by the Agency for Healthcare Research and Quality (AHRQ) and published treatment guidelines from international cardiology groups both summarize the effectiveness and level of evidence of antiarrhythmic drugs to restore sinus rhythm. In sum, there is relatively strong evidence for efficacy the type III pure I_K blockers (e.g., ibutilide and dofetilide) and the type Ics (e.g., flecainide and propafenone).[14,28] Oral loading doses of the type Ic antiarrhythmic (e.g., propafenone 600 mg as a single dose) have been demonstrated to be effective compared with placebo and provide a simple regimen.[29] Intravenous or oral amiodarone may both control ventricular rate (because of calcium and β-blocking actions) and restore sinus rhythm. Although often chosen, intravenous amiodarone is expensive, appears only modestly effective in restoring sinus rhythm, and has a delayed onset of action (days to weeks).[30] The disadvantages of pharmacologic cardioversion are the risk of significant side effects such as drug-induced torsade de pointes,[31] the inconvenience of drug-drug interactions (e.g., digoxin-quinidine or digoxin-amiodarone), and the fact that drugs generally are less effective when compared with DCC. The advantages of DCC are that it is quick and more often successful. The disadvantages of DCC are the need for prior sedation/anesthesia and a risk (albeit small) of serious complications such as sinus arrest or ventricular arrhythmias. Contrary to past beliefs, DCC carries very little risk in patients receiving digoxin without evidence of digitalis toxicity.

LONG-TERM COMPLICATIONS

There are two forms of therapy that the clinician must consider in each patient: long-term antithrombotic therapy to prevent stroke and long-term antiarrhythmic drugs to prevent recurrences of atrial fibrillation. Consider the issue of antithrombotic therapy first. In the past, patients with atrial fibrillation were not anticoagulated routinely (unless there was a history of stroke or concurrent mitral valve disease) because it was felt that the risk of warfarin exceeded its potential (though unknown) benefit. More recently, a large number of randomized, placebo-controlled trials designed to evaluate this issue have been published. All possess relatively similar findings, and many were terminated prematurely because of a significant effect in the treatment group (warfarin). In all, these studies culminated in the American College of Chest Physicians Consensus Conference[17] on antithrombotic therapy recommending the following: Warfarin (INR 2.0–3.0, target = 2.5) should be prescribed to all patients with atrial fibrillation who are at high risk for stroke (i.e., rheumatic valvular disease, previous history of thromboembolism, age greater than 75 years, LV dysfunction, or hypertension); those at low risk (age less than 65 years without discernible cardiovascular disease or lone atrial fibrillation) should receive aspirin 325 mg/day. In analyzing these recommendations, it becomes apparent that there is an intermediate-risk group, i.e., those with atrial fibrillation aged 65 to 75 years with minor risk factors for stroke (e.g., diabetes, coronary artery disease, or thyrotoxicosis). In these patients a careful risk-benefit assessment should be made between aspirin and warfarin, balancing the risk of stroke and hemorrhage on an individual basis. The current recommendation is that warfarin or aspirin should be continued until sinus rhythm has been maintained for at least 4 weeks, but this may be altered in the future. It has been shown that many patients have undetected recurrences of atrial fibrillation, placing the patient at risk for stroke. In other words, the clinician may think that sinus rhythm has been maintained, but in fact, brief, self-terminating episodes may have occurred.[32] Adding fuel to this cautionary note were the results of AFFIRM[23]: Thromboembolism rates were similar in patients with permanent atrial fibrillation (rate-control arm) and in *those in sinus rhythm*. Therefore, many practitioners now will continue warfarin treatment indefinitely even in patients who have appeared to remain successfully in sinus rhythm.

Clearly, in patients with permanent atrial fibrillation or documented, recurrent paroxysms, antithrombotic therapy should be continued indefinitely. Pharmacoeconomic analyses tend to support the use of aspirin only in patients with atrial fibrillation without risk factors for stroke.[33] Warfarin is more cost-effective in patients at risk for the complications of recurrent atrial fibrillation. New strategies to prevent stroke and thromboembolism more effectively are being evaluated continuously, including the use of new direct thrombin inhibitors which do not require intensive INR monitoring and dosage adjustment. One such agent, ximelagatran, though effective[34] was recently rejected by the FDA for use in the United States (it is available in Europe) mainly because of concerns about liver toxicity.

The second form of chronic therapy to be considered (at least in those patients in whom maintenance of sinus rhythm is a goal) is antiarrhythmic drugs to prevent recurrences of atrial fibrillation. With some exceptions (postoperative situations), atrial fibrillation often recurs after initial cardioversion because most patients have irreversible underlying heart or lung disease. Large atrial size, poor LV function, and the presence of long-standing atrial fibrillation are factors that make the restoration and maintenance of sinus rhythm difficult, if not impossible. Nevertheless, historically, many clinicians have attempted aggressively to maintain sinus rhythm by prescribing oral antiarrhythmic drugs (usually quinidine) to prevent these recurrences despite the fact that only small studies with conflicting results have evaluated this approach. To evaluate the efficacy of quinidine in preventing atrial fibrillation, a well-known meta-analysis of the existing literature was completed.[35] This meta-analysis demonstrated that indeed more patients remain in sinus rhythm with quinidine therapy (compared with placebo), although about 50% have recurrences of atrial fibrillation within a year despite quinidine. However, this reported effectiveness was at the cost of an associated increase in mortality (presumably due to proarrhythmia) in the quinidine-treated patients. These disturbing results (published soon after the CAST[36]) became widely quoted and highly visible, making clinicians question the wisdom of long-term prevention of recurrences of atrial fibrillation with antiarrhythmic drugs. Although the results were questioned because some of the reported causes of death in the treated patients could not be directly attributed to quinidine, subsequent studies[37] tended to support the findings of the meta-analysis.

These results, coupled with the recent findings of AFFIRM,[23] question the need to use antiarrhythmic drugs to prevent recurrences of atrial fibrillation. Perhaps this practice should now be totally abandoned, allowing patients to remain in atrial fibrillation once recurrences happen with strategies only to control rate and prevent thromboembolism. While it is true that these data certainly have led to a less aggressive approach, patients with paroxysmal atrial fibrillation and intolerable symptoms during recurrences do require antiarrhythmic drugs to prevent attacks.

Although nearly every type I or III antiarrhythmic drug has some published evidence of effectiveness in preventing recurrences of atrial fibrillation, amiodarone is clearly the most effective agent and now the most frequently chosen despite its impressive toxicity. Initially, uncontrolled studies[38] indicated that low doses (100 to 200 mg/day) of amiodarone are effective. Later, in a comparative trial,[39] amiodarone was shown to be superior to either sotalol or propafenone in maintaining sinus rhythm. Further, in a substudy of AFFIRM,[23] amiodarone was demonstrated to be the most effective antiarrhythmic agent of those used in the study.

Alternatives to amiodarone include the type Ic drugs (e.g., flecainide and propafenone) and the type III I_{Kr} blockers (e.g., sotalol and dofetilide). Because of the risk of proarrhythmia, the type Ic drugs should be reserved for those without heart disease (i.e., lone atrial fibrillation). Sotalol has been shown to be at least as effective as quinidine in preventing recurrences of atrial fibrillation.[40] However, treatment with either quinidine or sotalol is associated with a similar incidence of torsade de pointes. Since this form of proarrhythmia occurs primarily with higher doses of sotalol (quinidine usually causes torsade de pointes at low or therapeutic concentrations), it may be predicted more easily and therefore avoided. Nonetheless, it is possible that sotalol increases mortality in patients with atrial fibrillation similar to quinidine, and this requires further study.[41]

The newest type III agent, dofetilide, is effective in preventing recurrences of atrial fibrillation[42] but has not been compared directly with amiodarone. In a large multicenter trial,[43] dofetilide (dose adjusted for renal function and QT interval) was more effective than placebo in maintaining sinus rhythm (about 40% to 60% at 1 year). Like sotalol and quinidine, dofetilide has significant potential to cause torsade de pointes (in a dose-related fashion), and because of this, we believe that dofetilide should not be considered first-line therapy for recurrent atrial fibrillation at this time.

In view of important studies implying increased mortality due to antiarrhythmic drugs such as quinidine and the results of AFFIRM, we suggest the following approach: Reserve chronic antiarrhythmic drugs only for patients with documented paroxysmal atrial fibrillation associated with intolerable symptoms. Those with an isolated episode should not receive chronic preventative therapy. In terms of drug choice, we feel that low-dose amiodarone should be given preference as the agent of first choice for most patients. After appropriate oral loading doses, patients should receive 200 mg/day on a chronic basis. If this dose has prevented recurrences, one may attempt to reduce it to 100 mg/day, but more data are required on this practice. Although the methods of oral amiodarone loading vary considerable, we recommend 800 mg/day for 1 week, followed by 400 mg/day for 1 month before initiation of the 200 mg/day maintenance dose for patients with recurrent atrial fibrillation. As second-line treatment in those who cannot tolerate amiodarone, sotalol or dofetilide can be considered. For patients with symptomatic recurrences of atrial fibrillation but no evidence of organic heart disease (e.g., recurrent lone atrial fibrillation), type Ic drugs such as flecainide and propafenone are highly effective and could be used safely as first-line drugs.

Nondrug forms of therapy designed to maintain sinus rhythm are either currently in use or actively being investigated. For patients who have "pure" (i.e., not associated with concurrent atrial fibrillation) type I atrial flutter, ablation of the reentrant substrate with radiofrequency current (see below) is highly effective (approximately 80%).[44] Recent guidelines place ablation as first-line treatment to prevent recurrences.[14,45] For patients with atrial fibrillation, an innovative surgical procedure referred to as the *maze operation* has been used for over a decade.[46] Because of its highly complex nature, the maze was reserved for highly drug-refractory patients. Some have attempted to replicate the ideas of the maze procedure by using catheter ablation technologies. Success has been varied, and complications include recurrences of atrial fibrillation, new atrial flutter, and thromboembolism. Interestingly, a subset (often those with lone atrial fibrillation) of patients with paroxysmal atrial fibrillation appears to have their episodes initiated from premature beats that arise in the pulmonary veins. In these cases, ablation (see later) of the pulmonary venous foci or pulmonary vein isolation can result in prevention of recurrences in a high percentage of patients.[47,48] Some believe these initial promising findings could lead to ablation being a first-line approach in the future.

PAROXYSMAL SUPRAVENTRICULAR TACHYCARDIA DUE TO REENTRY

Paroxysmal supraventricular tachycardia (PSVT) arising by reentrant mechanisms includes arrhythmias caused by AV nodal reentry, AV reentry incorporating an anomalous AV pathway, SA nodal reentry, and intraatrial reentry. AV nodal reentry and AV reentry are by far the most common of these tachycardias.

MECHANISMS

The underlying substrate of AV nodal reentry is the functional division of the AV node into two (or more) longitudinal conduction pathways, or dual AV nodal pathways.[49] Most practitioners now believe that there are not two distinct anatomic pathways inside the AV node itself. Rather, it is likely that a fanlike network of perinodal fibers inserts into the AV node and represents the second pathway. The two

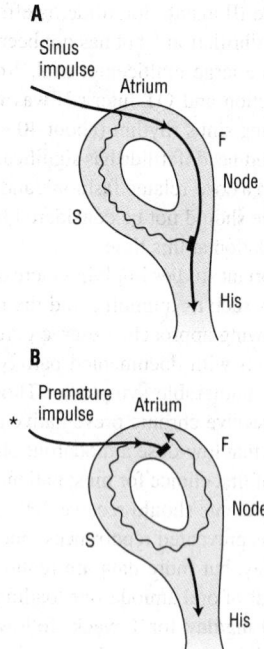

FIGURE 17–7. Reentry mechanism of dual-AV-nodal- pathway PSVT. *A.* Sinus rhythm. The impulse travels from the atrium through the fast pathway (F) and then to the His-Purkinje system. The impulse also travels through the slow pathway (S) but is stopped when refractory tissue is encountered. *B.* Dual-AV-nodal reentry. A critically timed premature impulse (*) is stopped in the fast pathway (because of prolonged refractoriness) but is able to travel antegrade down the slow pathway and retrograde through the fast pathway.

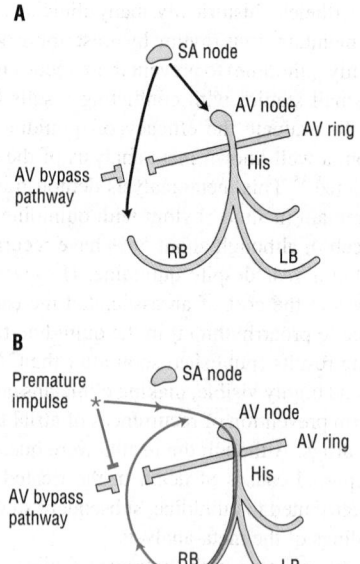

FIGURE 17–8. Reentry mechanism for AV-accessory-pathway PSVT in Wolff-Parkinson-White syndrome. *A.* Sinus rhythm. The impulse travels from the atrium to the ventricle by two pathways—the AV node and an accessory bypass pathway. *B.* AV reentry. A critically timed premature impulse (*) is stopped in the Kent bundle (because of prolonged refractoriness) but travels antegrade through the AV node and retrograde through the Kent bundle.

pathways possess key differences in conduction characteristics: One is a fast conducting pathway with a relatively long refractory period (fast pathway), and the other is a slower conducting pathway with a shorter refractory period (slow pathway). The presence of dual pathways does not necessarily imply that the patient will have clinical PSVT. In fact, it is estimated that between 10% and nearly 50% of patients have discernible dual pathways, but the incidence of PSVT is considerably lower.[49] Sustenance of the tachycardia depends on the critical electrophysiologic discrepancies and the ability of one pathway (usually the slow) to allow repetitive antegrade conduction and the ability of the other pathway (usually the fast) to allow repetitive retrograde conduction. During sinus rhythm, a patient with dual pathways conducts supraventricular impulses antegrade through both pathways. Electrical activity reaches the distal common pathway at the level of or above the bundle of His and continues to depolarize the ventricles in an antegrade direction. Conduction proceeds via the two pathways but reaches the distal common pathway first through the fast AV nodal route (Fig. 17–7). For this reason, a short PR interval is sometimes observed during sinus rhythm.

PSVT due to AV nodal reentry may occur by the following sequence of events: The occurrence of an appropriately timed premature impulse penetrates the AV node but is blocked in the fast pathway that is still refractory from the previous beat. However, the slow pathway, which has a shorter refractory period, permits antegrade conduction of the premature impulse. By the time the impulse has reached the distal common pathway, the fast pathway has recovered its excitability and now will permit retrograde conduction. The impulse reaches the common proximal pathway, preceded by an excitable gap of tis-

sue, and reenters the slow pathway. A reentrant circuit that does not require atrial or ventricular tissue is completed within (or nearly so) the AV node, and a tachycardia is thereby initiated (see Fig. 17–7). The common form of this tachycardia uses the slow pathway for antegrade conduction and the fast pathway for retrograde conduction; an uncommon form exists in which the reentrant impulse travels in the opposite direction.

AV reentrant tachycardia depends on the presence of an anomalous, or accessory, extranodal pathway that bypasses the normal AV conduction pathway. Several different types of accessory pathways have been described, depending on the specific anatomic areas they connect (e.g., atrioventricular bundles or nodoventricular tracts); some are also referred to as *eponyms,* such as the Kent bundle. A Kent bundle is an extranodal AV connection that is associated with the Wolff-Parkinson-White (WPW) syndrome. During sinus rhythm (Fig. 17–8), patients with WPW syndrome depolarize the ventricles simultaneously through both AV pathways (AV nodal pathway and the Kent bundle), creating a fusion pattern on the early portion of the QRS complex (delta wave). The degree of ventricular "preexcitation" depends on the contribution of antegrade ventricular activation through the accessory pathway. Patients may have an accessory pathway that is not evident on surface ECG or a "concealed" Kent bundle. These concealed accessory pathways often are incapable of antegrade conduction and can only accept electrical stimulation in a retrograde fashion. The ECG expression of preexcitation (delta wave) depends on the location of the accessory pathway, the distance from the wavefront of sinus activation, and the conduction characteristics of the various structures involved. It should be noted that (similar to patients with dual AV nodal pathways) not all patients with preexcitation with an accessory AV pathway are capable of having clinical PSVT.

Patients with an accessory AV pathway may have three forms of supraventricular tachycardia: orthodromic reentry, antidromic reentry, and/or atrial fibrillation or flutter. AV reentrant PSVT usually occurs by the following sequence of events: Analogous to AV nodal reentry, two pathways (the normal AV nodal pathway and the accessory AV pathway) exist that have different electrophysiologic characteristics. The AV nodal pathway usually has a relatively slower conduction velocity and shorter refractory period, and the accessory pathway has a faster conduction velocity and a longer refractory period. A critically timed premature impulse may block in the accessory pathway because it is still refractory from the previous sinus beat. However, the AV nodal pathway with its relatively shorter refractory period may accept antegrade conduction of the premature impulse. Meanwhile, the accessory pathway may recover its excitability and now allow retrograde conduction. A macroreentrant tachycardia is thereby initiated in which the antegrade pathway is the AV nodal pathway, the distal common pathway is the ventricle, the retrograde pathway is the accessory pathway, and the proximal common pathway is the atrium (Fig. 17–8). This sequence of events (down node, up Kent), termed *orthodromic PSVT,* is the common variety of reentry in patients with an accessory AV pathway, resulting in a narrow QRS tachycardia. In the uncommon variety (down Kent, up node), conduction proceeds in the opposite direction, resulting in a wide QRS tachycardia termed *antidromic PSVT.* Patients with WPW syndrome can have a third type of tachycardia, namely, atrial fibrillation. The mechanism for its occurrence is unknown, but the occurrence of this arrhythmia can be very serious, and sudden death is well described. Since atrial fibrillation is an extremely rapid atrial tachycardia, conduction can proceed down the accessory AV pathway, resulting in a very fast ventricular response or even ventricular fibrillation. Unlike the AV nodal pathway, the refractory period of the accessory bundle shortens in response to rapid stimulation rates.

Sinus node reentry or intraatrial reentry occur less commonly, and neither is as well described as AV nodal or AV reentry. Aside from a characteristic abrupt onset and termination, coupled with subtle changes in P-wave morphology, these tachycardias can be difficult to diagnose. Electrophysiologic studies may be necessary to determine the ultimate mechanism of the PSVT.

► TREATMENT: Paroxysmal Supraventricular Tachycardia

Both pharmacologic and nonpharmacologic methods have been used to treat patients with PSVT. Drugs used in the treatment of PSVT can be divided into three broad categories: (1) those which directly or indirectly increase vagal tone to the AV node such as digoxin, (2) those which depress conduction through slow calcium-dependent tissue such adenosine, β-blockers, and calcium channel blockers, and (3) those which depress conduction through fast sodium-dependent tissue such quinidine, procainamide, disopyramide, and flecainide. Drugs within these categories alter the electrophysiologic characteristics of the reentrant substrate so that PSVT cannot be sustained.[50,51] In PSVT due to AV nodal reentry, type I antiarrhythmic drugs such as procainamide act primarily on the retrograde fast pathway. Digoxin and propranolol may work on either the retrograde fast or the antegrade slow limb. Verapamil, diltiazem, and adenosine prolong conduction time and increase refractoriness primarily in the slow antegrade pathway of the reentrant loop. In PSVT due to AV reentry incorporating an extranodal pathway, type I drugs increase refractoriness in the fast accessory pathway or within the His-Purkinje system. Propranolol, digoxin, adenosine, and verapamil all act by their effects on the AV nodal (antegrade, slow) portion of the reentrant circuit. Regardless of the mechanism, treatment measures are directed at first terminating an acute episode of PSVT and then preventing symptomatic recurrences of PSVT.

As in any rapid reentrant tachycardia resulting in severe symptoms (e.g., syncope, near syncope, anginal chest pain, and severe heart failure), synchronized DCC is the treatment of choice. Even at low energy levels (e.g., 25 W/s), DCC for PSVT is almost always effective in quickly restoring sinus rhythm and correcting symptomatic hypotension. Patients with only mild to moderate symptoms usually do not require DCC, and nondrug measures that increase vagal tone to the AV node can be used first. Unilateral carotid sinus massage, Valsalva maneuver, ice water facial immersion, induced retching, and other more elaborate vagomimetic measures often are successful in terminating PSVT, although carotid massage and Valsalva maneuver are the simplest, least obtrusive, and most frequently used of these techniques.

In the event that these methods fail, drug therapy is the next option. A therapeutic approach to the acute therapy of the different forms of reentrant PSVT is presented in Fig. 17–9. This approach is based on analysis of the electrocardiographic characteristics of the rhythm because PSVT is not always discernible from other arrhythmias, and some forms of PSVT require different treatment. In patients with a narrow-QRS-complex, regular arrhythmia (AV nodal reentry or orthodromic AV reentry), intravenous verapamil (5 to 10 mg), intravenous diltiazem (15 to 25 mg), and adenosine (6 to 12 mg) all are equally efficacious; any may be chosen as the agent of first choice. About 80% to 90% of PSVT episodes will revert to sinus rhythm within 5 minutes of intravenous verapamil, diltiazem, or adenosine therapy.[52] Verapamil has the advantage in terms of cost, being available in generic formulations, whereas adenosine (although it has a higher frequency of side effects) may be safer because of its ultrashort duration of action. Adenosine should not be used in patients with severe asthma; rapid reinitiation of PSVT also may occur.

The most recent guidelines for emergency care from the American Heart Association[53] and practice guidelines from the American College of Cardiology/American Heart Association/European Society of Cardiology[45] both promote adenosine as the drug of first choice in patients with PSVT. This recommendation is particularly important when treating a patient who presents with a wide-QRS-complex, regular tachycardia that may be ventricular tachycardia or PSVT (antidromic AV reentry or because of aberrancy). Because of its short duration of action (seconds), adenosine will not cause the severe and prolonged hemodynamic compromise seen in patients with ventricular tachycardia who were mistakenly treated with verapamil and suffer from its negative inotropic effects and vasodilator properties.[54] If in fact the arrhythmia is PSVT, adenosine likely will terminate it. An alternative treatment for this type of patient is intravenous procainamide, which works on the fast sodium-dependent extranodal pathway as well as for ventricular tachycardia. Likewise, intravenous procainamide or perhaps amiodarone (particularly in patients with LV dysfunction) should be used for the patient who presents with a wide-QRS-complex, irregular arrhythmia who is hemodynamically

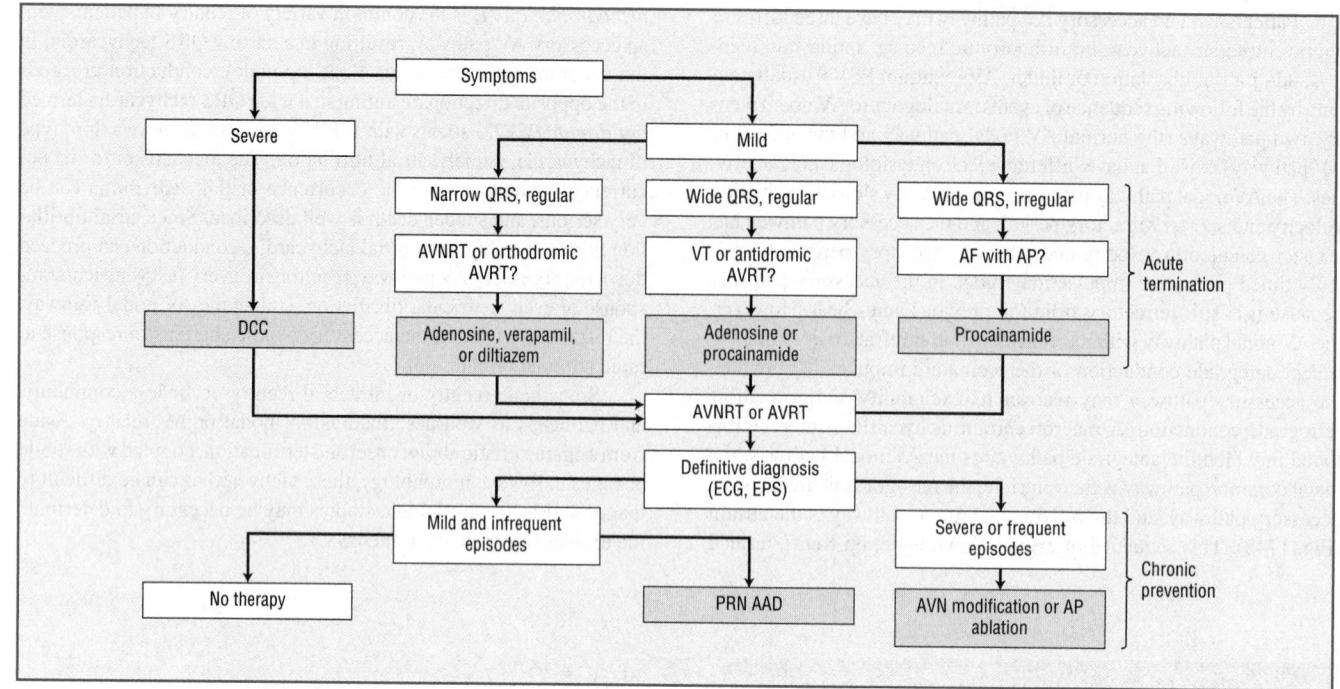

FIGURE 17–9. Algorithm for the treatment of acute (*above*) PSVT and chronic prevention of recurrences (*below*). DCC = direct current cardioversion, AVNRT = AV nodal reentrant tachycardia, AVRT = AV reentrant tachycardia, VT = ventricular tachycardia, AF = atrial fibrillation, AP = accessory pathway, ECG = electrocardiographic monitoring, EPS = electrophysiologic studies, PRN = as needed, AAD = antiarrhythmic drugs. Note: For empirical bridge therapy prior to radiofrequency ablation procedures, calcium antagonists (or other AV nodal blockers) should not be used if the patient has AV reentry with an accessory pathway.

stable.[45] This rhythm could represent atrial fibrillation with ventricular activation through an extranodal pathway. Administration of intravenous verapamil or adenosine to these patients could result in a paradoxical increase in ventricular response, causing severe symptoms that require cardioversion. These agents (particularly long-acting AV nodal–blockers such as verapamil, diltiazem, and digoxin) are to be considered contraindicated in this specific setting.

Once the acute episode of PSVT is terminated, a decision on long-term preventive therapy must follow. Most patients require long-term therapy; preventive treatment is indicated if (1) frequent episodes occur that necessitate therapeutic intervention (i.e., emergency room visits or interference with the patient's lifestyle) or (2) infrequent but severely symptomatic symptoms occur. For patients in whom a preventive treatment is deemed necessary, two methods of management have been used: preventative drug therapy and ablation.

There are a number of ways to develop an effective drug regimen for patients with recurrent PSVT. A trial-and-error approach on an ambulatory basis may be considered for patients with frequently recurrent, mildly symptomatic PSVT. Ambulatory ECG recordings (Holter) or telephonic transmissions of cardiac rhythm (event monitors) can be used to objectively document the efficacy or failure of drug therapy. Drugs known to be effective in preventing recurrences of PSVT are the AV nodal–blocking agents (e.g., digoxin, β-blockers, calcium channel blockers, or combinations of these agents) and the type Ic drugs (e.g., flecainide and propafenone). There are patterns of drug response in patients with PSVT; the tachycardia behaves as if it has a "weak link." That is, patients who respond to agents that act on one limb of the reentrant loop are less likely to respond to drugs that block conduction on the other limb. For instance, in a patient with AV nodal reentry, one first may choose a calcium channel blocker or β-blocker (to affect the antegrade slow pathway). If symptomatic recurrences are documented subsequently, then it may be prudent to switch to a type Ic drug such as flecainide (to affect the retrograde fast pathway) in an attempt to find the weak link, or susceptible pathway. There are other considerations. Patients with evidence of preexcitation (delta waves during sinus rhythm) should not be treated only with AV nodal–blocking agents. If atrial fibrillation were to occur, these agents would facilitate rapid conduction over the accessory pathway. Also, the trial-and-error method for determining drug effectiveness has inherent shortcomings. If the PSVT episodes are infrequent, a considerable time period may be consumed before an effective regimen is realized, or if the patient has moderate to severe symptoms associated with PSVT, he or she may experience several troublesome episodes before the correct agent is identified. Therefore, serial testing of antiarrhythmic agents by invasive electrophysiologic techniques has been used to determine effective long-term therapy in patients with sporadic and/or symptomatic PSVT, and this method represents the third treatment strategy. Basically, the patient's clinical tachycardia is replicated in the laboratory by inserting appropriately timed premature extra stimuli via a transvenous right-sided heart catheter. The patient is first studied off of antiarrhythmic therapy; induction of the tachycardia by premature stimuli by programmed stimulation serves as a control study. Then, over a period of several days, specific drugs are administered in a serial fashion and tested for efficacy in preventing the induction of PSVT.[50,51]

Regardless of the method for choosing long-term therapy, chronic antiarrhythmic drug treatment in these often young, otherwise healthy patients is problematic. Besides the necessity of taking daily medication possibly for life, antiarrhythmic drugs are not well tolerated, sometimes precipitate severe side effects, and commonly ◀5 are ineffective. For these reasons, nondrug therapies have been pioneered. One such procedure, namely, transcutaneous catheter ablation using radiofrequency current on the PSVT substrate has altered the traditional treatment of these patients dramatically (Fig. 17–10). Radiofrequency energy delivered through a transvenous or arterial catheter causes small, discrete lesions through thermal energy. During invasive electrophysiologic studies, portions of the reentrant circuit can be located (or "mapped") by the use of a number of catheters. Once this is completed, radiofrequency energy is applied, creating thermal injury in the tissue necessary for reentry. In this way, the substrate for reentry is destroyed, "curing" the patient of recurrent episodes of PSVT and obviating the need for chronic drug therapy. Historically, ablation procedures were reserved for drug-refractory patients because they necessitated open-heart surgery. However, breakthroughs in technology have allowed, first, transvenous catheter approaches and then, later, the use of radiofrequency (rather than direct-current) energy. Complications, although unusual, include tamponade, pericarditis, valvular insufficiency, and AV block. Radiofrequency ablation is highly effective, preventing the recurrences of PSVT in 85% to 98% of patients.[55,56] The procedure was used originally in patients with WPW syndrome.[55] In this syndrome, the extranodal pathway often is located at the left lateral free wall of the left ventricle (see Fig. 17–10). After the pathway is located, the catheter is put as close to the site as possible, and radiofrequency current is applied to make small burns in the tissue. Ablation of the extranodal connection occurs promptly, and evidence of preexcitation (delta waves) disappears. Thereafter, a similar approach was developed for patients with AV nodal reentry, placing the catheter in the coronary sinus, proximal to the AV node.[56] The preferred method in these individuals is to apply small amounts of radiofrequency current to the slow pathway of the reentrant circuit in order to modify its properties enough so that PSVT cannot recur.

It has been suggested that *all* patients with symptomatic PSVT undergo radiofrequency catheter ablation.[57] This is so because it is highly effective and curative, rarely resulting in complications, and obviates the need for chronic antiarrhythmic drug therapy. In other words, it should be considered in *any* patient who previously would have been considered for chronic antiarrhythmic drug treatment. Radiofrequency ablation is also a cost-effective approach (in the long term) because, if effective, the costs of drugs and repeated hospital visits are avoided. In one cost-effectiveness analysis, radiofrequency ablation improved quality of life and reduced lifetime medical expenditures by nearly $30,000 compared with chronic drug treatment.[58]

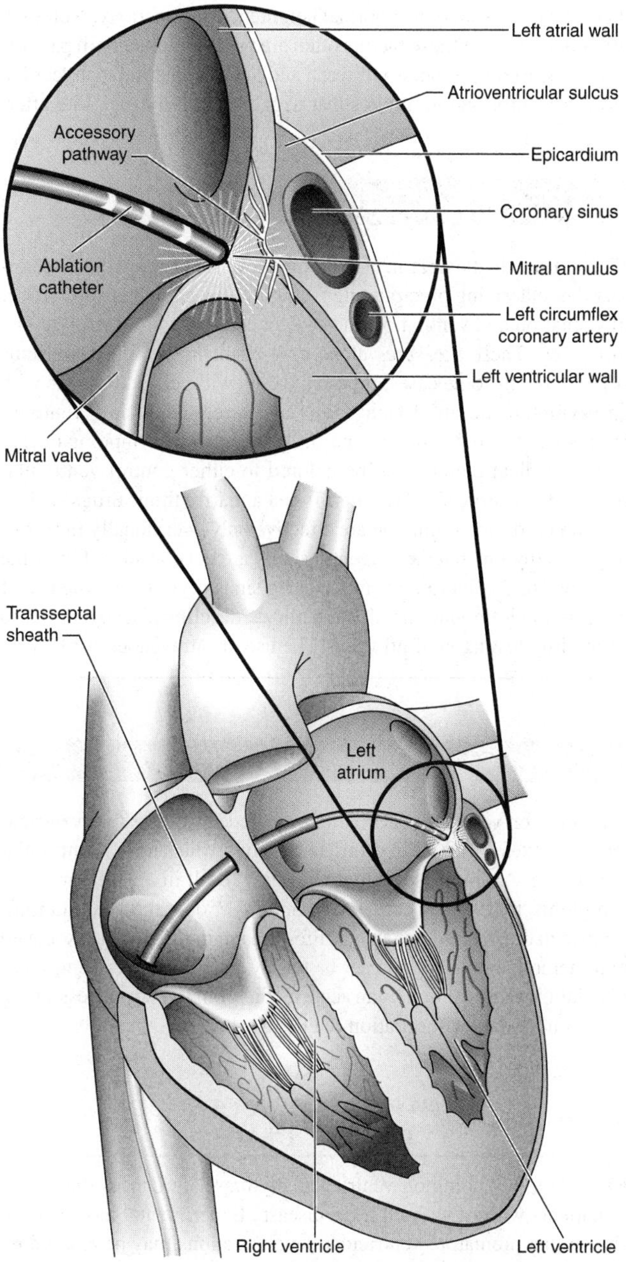

FIGURE 17–10. Drawing showing catheter placement for radiofrequency ablation of left free wall accessory pathway. Here, the retrograde arterial approach is taken, although a venous (atrial) transseptal puncture also has been used. *(From Lerman BB, Basson CT. High-risk patients with ventricular preexcitation: A pendulum in motion. N Engl J Med 2003;349:1787–1789, with permission)*

AUTOMATIC ATRIAL TACHYCARDIAS

Automatic atrial tachycardias such as multifocal atrial tachycardia appear to arise from supraventricular foci that have enhanced automatic properties.[59] It is presumed that multifocal atrial tachycardia is the result of multiple ectopic atrial pacemakers, which account for the variable and differing P-wave morphology. In unifocal atrial tachycardia (sometimes referred to as *ectopic atrial tachycardia*), a single P-wave morphology different from that of sinus rhythm is recorded. In either case, the underlying, precipitating disorder present in the majority (60% to 80%) of these patients is severe pulmonary disease. Other disease states associated with these arrhythmias include acute infection (pneumonia and sepsis) and dilated congestive cardiomyopathy. It should be noted that young patients without associated precipitating factors rarely may present with rapid atrial tachycardias from unknown etiologies. In these cases, long-standing tachycardias cause the cardiomyopathic state. Effective treatment of the tachycardia may result in reversal of LV dysfunction. Traditionally, many factors (e.g., electrolyte disturbances, hypoxia, catecholamines, and tissue stretch) have caused an elevated slope of phase 4 depolarization and theoretically resulted in abnormal heightened automaticity. Noteworthy is that many of these factors often are present clinically in patients with concurrent pulmonary disease and automatic atrial tachycardia. However, information implies that triggered activity (i.e., late after-depolarizations) is a more likely mechanism in the genesis of these tachycardias. Atrial tachycardias with AV block or a slow ventricular response should alert the clinician to the possibility of digitalis toxicity.

▶ TREATMENT: Automatic Atrial Tachycardia

The first step in the treatment of automatic atrial tachycardia is to correct the underlying precipitating factors.[59] One should ensure proper oxygenation and ventilation and correct acid-base or electrolyte disturbances. These measures alone may result in the return of sinus rhythm, but in some cases, the tachycardia will persist. Patients with an asymptomatic atrial tachycardia and a relatively slow ventricular response usually require no drug therapy. In symptomatic patients, medical therapy can be tailored to either control ventricular response or restore sinus rhythm. Type I antiarrhythmic drugs such as procainamide and quinidine are effective only occasionally in restoring sinus rhythm, but these agents usually are not considered first-line therapy. DCC is ineffective in restoring sinus rhythm, and the use of programmed stimulation will not replicate the clinical tachycardia, so serial drug testing is of no value. The use of intravenous β-blockers to slow ventricular response usually is contraindicated because of the frequent coexistence of bronchospastic pulmonary disease or uncompensated heart failure. Digoxin has been used but is controversial because of its ability to increase the automatic properties of atrial tissue, and the high sympathetic state of these patients frequently overrides the vagotonic effects of digoxin, rendering it ineffective. Calcium antagonists such as verapamil are most effective and now may be considered first-line drug therapy.[60] Interestingly, verapamil seems to decrease ventricular response by altering atrial automaticity, not by slowing AV nodal conduction.[60] Intravenous magnesium (independent of serum magnesium concentration) also can be effective, but high doses are required, and the effects are transient, rendering it impractical.[59] Both verapamil and parenteral magnesium probably act by suppressing calcium-mediated late after-depolarizations (LADs).

VENTRICULAR ARRHYTHMIAS

The common ventricular arrhythmias include (1) premature ventricular complexes (PVCs), (2) ventricular tachycardia, and (3) ventricular fibrillation. Again, these arrhythmias may result in a wide variety of symptoms. PVCs often cause no symptoms or only mild palpitations. Ventricular tachycardia may be a life-threatening situation associated with hemodynamic collapse or be totally asymptomatic. Ventricular fibrillation, by definition, is an acute medical emergency necessitating cardiopulmonary resuscitation (CPR).

PVCs AND PREVENTION OF SUDDEN CARDIAC DEATH

PVCs are very common ventricular rhythm disturbances that occur in patients with or without heart disease. Experimental models have shown that premature ventricular depolarizations may be elicited by abnormal automaticity, triggered activity, or reentrant mechanisms. It has become well known that PVCs can be observed commonly in apparently healthy individuals. However, PVCs occurring in overtly normal subjects without discernible heart disease seem to have little, if any, prognostic significance. PVCs occur more frequently and in more complex forms (see below) in patients with detectable heart disease than in healthy individuals. The prognostic meaning of PVCs has been well studied in patients with MI (acute or remote) with several consistent themes. Patients with some forms of PVCs (see below) are at higher risk for sudden death than if they did not have these minor rhythm disturbances. *Sudden cardiac death* can be defined as unexpected death occurring in a patient within 1 hour of experiencing symptoms. Studies of patients who experienced sudden cardiac death (and happened to be wearing an ECG monitor at the time) often demonstrate the cause to be ventricular fibrillation preceded by a short run of ventricular tachycardia and frequent PVCs.[61] Therein lies the basis of the so-called PVC hypothesis; i.e., preventing more minor arrhythmias such as PVCs may prevent the occurrence of sudden death.

CLINICAL PRESENTATION: VENTRICULAR ARRHYTHMIAS

PVCs
PVCs are non-life-threatening and usually asymptomatic. Occasionally, patients will complain of palpitations or uncomfortable beats. Since the PVC, by definition, occurs early, and the ventricle contracts when it is incompletely filled, patients do not feel the PVC. Rather, the next beat (after the PVC and a compensatory pause) usually is responsible for the patient's symptoms.

VENTRICULAR TACHYCARDIA (VT)
The symptoms of VT (monomorphic VT or torsade de pointes), if prolonged (i.e., sustained), can vary from nearly completely asymptomatic to pulseless hemodynamic collapse. Fast rates and underlying poor ventricular function will result in more severe symptoms. Symptoms of nonsustained, self-terminating VT also correlate with duration of episodes (e.g., patients with 15-second episodes will be more symptomatic than those with three-beat episodes).

VENTRICULAR FIBRILLATION (VF)
By definition, VF results in hemodynamic collapse, syncope, and cardiac arrest. Cardiac output and blood pressure are not recordable.

SIGNIFICANCE

Historically, investigators promoted the concept that patients in the acute phase of MI may have types of PVCs that are predictive of ventricular fibrillation and sudden cardiac death. These types of PVCs were referred to as *warning arrhythmias* and include frequent ectopy (>5 per minute), multiform configuration (different morphology), couplets (two in a row), and R-on-T phenomenon (PVCs occurring during the repolarization phase of the preceding sinus beat in the vulnerable period of ventricular recovery). However, using sophisticated monitoring techniques, it has become apparent that almost all patients have warning arrhythmias in the acute infarct setting. In patients who experience ventricular fibrillation, warning arrhythmias are no more common than in those without ventricular fibrillation. Therefore, warning arrhythmias observed during acute MI are neither a sensitive nor a specific predictive tool in determining which patients will have ventricular fibrillation. Hence, in patients with acute MI, there is little need to direct drug therapy specifically at PVC suppression. Studies have shown that effective prevention of ventricular fibrillation in the acute MI setting may be achieved without the abolition of PVCs. The inability of PVCs (warning arrhythmias) to predict the occurrence of ventricular fibrillation, coupled with the lack of correlation between a drug's effectiveness in preventing ventricular fibrillation and suppressing PVCs, forms the basis of suggesting antiarrhythmic drug prophylaxis (e.g., lidocaine and magnesium) for all patients with an uncomplicated acute MI (see below).

On the other hand, data strongly imply that PVCs documented in the convalescence period of MI do carry important long-term prognostic significance.[62] PVCs occurring after an MI seem to be a risk factor for patient death that is independent of the degree of LV dysfunction or the extent of coronary atherosclerosis. Lown and Wolff[63] have developed a grading scale for classifying different types of PVCs. The grading scale is as follows: grade 0, no ectopy; grade I, less than 30 PVCs/h of uniform morphology; grade II, more than 30 PVCs/h of uniform morphology; grade III, multiform PVCs; grade Iva, couplets; grade Ivb, 3 or more consecutive PVCs (nonsustained ventricular tachycardia); and grade V, R-on-T phenomenon. A common assumption is that the higher grades of PVCs within this classification system imply a higher risk of subsequent arrhythmogenic death. It should be emphasized that this assumption has never been proven. Ruberman and coworkers[62] devised a simple alternative classification based on the significance of simple or benign (infrequent and monomorphic) versus complex PVCs (all other types in the Lown classification). These investigators found that the presence of complex ventricular ectopy in the setting of ischemic heart disease was associated with a higher incidence of cardiac death (but not necessarily arrhythmogenic death). One can see that within the controversy of the significance of PVCs is a basic question: Are complex forms of PVCs simply an unimportant marker of underlying structural heart disease, or are PVCs an important electrical disorder that should be addressed independently?

▶ TREATMENT: Premature Ventricular Complexes

Because PVCs without associated heart disease, in apparently healthy individuals, carry little or no risk, drug therapy is unnecessary. However, owing to the prognostic significance of complex PVCs in patients with heart disease, the use of antiarrhythmic drug therapy to suppress them has been controversial. Traditionally, many clinicians supported aggressive drug therapy designed to suppress a high percentage of PVCs based on the Lown grading system. The underlying premise of this approach is to attempt to eliminate a risk factor for cardiac death in patients with coronary disease, namely, the presence of complex PVCs. However, others have favored a more conservative approach and have disregarded drug therapy in the absence of significant symptoms. The initial CAST results[36] clearly support the latter conservative approach.

▩ THE CARDIAC ARRHYTHMIA SUPPRESSION TRIAL (CAST)

◀ The CAST[36,64] was initiated by the NIH in 1987 to determine if suppression of ventricular ectopy with encainide, flecainide, or moricizine could decrease the incidence of death from arrhythmia in patients who had suffered an MI. Entrance criteria included documented MI between 6 days and 2 years prior to enrollment and six or more PVCs per hour without runs of ventricular tachycardia greater than 15 beats in length. Also, patients were required to have an ejection fraction of 55% or less if recruited within 90 days of MI or 40% or less if recruited 90 days or more after MI. Patients with an ejection fraction of less than 30% were randomized only to encainide or moricizine. Patients were randomized to receive drug therapy or placebo after demonstrating PVC suppression with one of the agents. The drug and dose were determined during an open-label dose-titration phase that preceded randomization.

In April 1989, a routine preliminary review of the study by the Safety and Monitoring Board revealed alarming results, and the study was interrupted. The results showed that compared with placebo, treatment with encainide or flecainide was associated with a significantly higher rate of total mortality and death due to arrhythmia, presumably due to drug-induced proarrhythmia (Fig. 17–11). Analysis of the moricizine arm indicated neither harm nor benefit from this therapy; therefore, only this portion of the study was allowed to continue as CAST II.[64] However, later (July 1991), CAST II also was stopped prematurely; there was a trend toward an increase in mortality in moricizine-treated patients. This was particularly true during the initiation of moricizine therapy (dose-titration phase) but was not observed during the chronic treatment phase. The overall results of the two CASTs prove conclusively that patients with PVCs after MI do not benefit from chronic antiarrhythmic drug therapy (beyond the

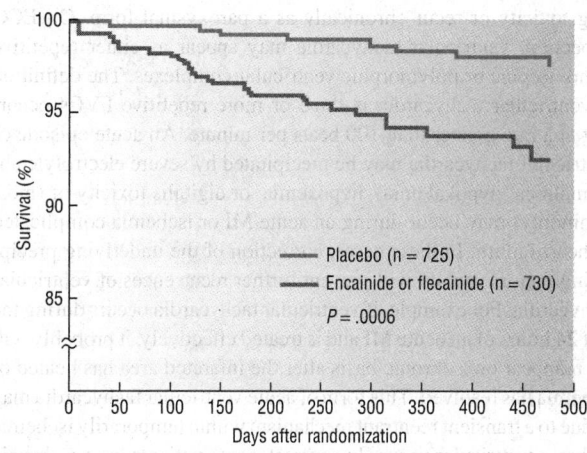

FIGURE 17–11. Life table curves from the CAST, specifically for patients receiving encainide or flecainide (*lighter line*) and matching placebo (*darker line*). Note the divergent slopes of each line implying sustained risk of death (presumed proarrhythmia). (*From the CAST Investigators. Preliminary report: Effect of encainide and flecainide on mortality in a randomized trial of arrhythmia suppression after myocardial infarction. N Engl J Med 1989;321:406–412, with permission.*)

general use of β-blocking agents) and that, in fact, such therapy is detrimental. The study also puts into perspective the risk associated with the use of antiarrhythmic therapy and the need to carefully select only patients with a defined therapeutic benefit.

Although now more than 15 years old, the CAST is considered one of the most important trials ever undertaken by the NIH, and it has had a tremendous influence on the overall approach to the treatment of tachycardias, in addition to a far-reaching impact on new drug development. The results have colored the long-term use of all antiarrhythmics, causing a broad skepticism in the risk-benefit ratio of this class of drugs. Pharmaceutical companies, as a result, have shifted their drug discovery and investigative efforts away from potent sodium channel blockers. As immediate fallout, encainide was withdrawn from the market, and another pharmaceutical manufacturer decided not to market the type Ic agent indecainide despite FDA approval. These findings also provided additional fuel for the pursuit of nondrug therapies for tachycardias, such as ablation and implantable devices.

Despite the discouraging results of the CAST, post-MI patients with complex ventricular ectopy remain at risk for death. Other drugs besides type Ic drugs have been studied, including sotalol. Sotalol is marketed as a racemic mixture of a D- and L-isomer; both are type III potassium blockers, but the L-isomer has β-blocking actions. Chronic therapy with D-sotalol was studied in patients with remote MI complicated by complex ectopy in the Survival With Oral D-Sotalol (SWORD) trial.[65] Unlike in the CAST, D-sotalol treatment was not designed to cause PVC suppression, yet (as in the CAST) the trial was halted prematurely because of excessive mortality in the treatment arm. Again, the presumed reason for this observation was D-sotalol-related proarrhythmia. Currently, only two antiarrhythmic

drugs have been shown *not* to increase mortality with long-term use: amiodarone and dofetilide. A number of trials[66,67] have shown amiodarone to decrease the incidence of sudden (or arrhythmic) death but not total mortality in post-MI patients with complex ventricular ectopy. A meta-analysis of all trials (6553 combined patients) demonstrated a reduction in total mortality (by 13%) with long-term amiodarone therapy.[68] It is unclear if these findings can be attributed to one property (e.g., β-blocking) or a combination of amiodarone's complex pharmacologic effects on conduction. Noteworthy is that in two major studies patients treated with amiodarone *and* a β-blocker generally did better than when no β-blocker was used.[66,67] Clearly, because of its impressive adverse-effect profile and its inability to improve survival, amiodarone cannot be recommended routinely in patients with heart disease such as remote MI and complex PVC's. Two randomized, controlled trials[69,70] have shown chronic therapy with dofetilide to have no effect on overall mortality in patients who have suffered MI with LV dysfunction. Dofetilide (not approved for prevention of sudden death) caused torsade de pointes in about 5% of patients, necessitating a protocol amendment with dosage adjustments during both trials (particularly in those with renal disease because the primary route of elimination is through the kidney).

How should the clinician approach the patient with documented asymptomatic PVCs? Clearly, attempts to suppress asymptomatic PVCs should not be made with any antiarrhythmic drug. Indeed, those at risk for arrhythmic death (recent MI, LV dysfunction, complex PVCs) should not be given *any* type I or III antiarrhythmic agent routinely.[71] Of the antiarrhythmic drugs in the Vaughn Williams classification, only β-blockers have been proven conclusively to prevent overall mortality in these patients, and therefore, chronic drug therapy should be restricted to these agents.

VENTRICULAR TACHYCARDIA

MECHANISMS AND TYPES OF VENTRICULAR TACHYCARDIA

Ventricular tachycardia is a wide-QRS-complex tachycardia that may occur acutely as a result of metabolic abnormalities, ischemia, or drug toxicity or recur chronically as a paroxysmal form. On ECG inspection, ventricular tachycardia may appear as either repetitive monomorphic or polymorphic ventricular complexes. The definition of ventricular tachycardia is three or more repetitive PVCs occurring at a rate greater than 100 beats per minute. An acute episode of ventricular tachycardia may be precipitated by severe electrolyte abnormalities (hypokalemia), hypoxemia, or digitalis toxicity or (most commonly) may occur during an acute MI or ischemia complicated by heart failure. In these cases, correction of the underlying precipitating factors usually will prevent further recurrences of ventricular tachycardia. For example, if ventricular tachycardia occurs during the first 24 hours of an acute MI and is treated effectively, it probably will not reappear on a chronic basis after the infarcted area has healed or ischemia has resolved. This form of acute ventricular tachycardia may be due to a transient reentrant mechanism within temporarily ischemic or dying ventricular tissue. In contrast, some patients have a chronic recurrent form of ventricular tachycardia that is almost always associated with some type of underlying organic heart disease. Common examples are paroxysmal ventricular tachycardia associated with idiopathic dilated cardiomyopathy or remote MI with a LV aneurysm. Indeed, LV dysfunction and aneurysm formation are risk factors for the development of ventricular tachycardia on a recurrent basis after

MI. In chronic, recurrent ventricular tachycardia, microreentry within the distal Purkinje network is presumed to be responsible for the underlying substrate in a large majority of patients (see Fig. 17–3). Theoretically, electrophysiologic discrepancies occur as a result of structural damage and heart disease within the ventricular conducting system. The reentrant circuit may possess both anatomically determined and functional properties coursing through normal tissue, damaged tissue, and around islands of necrosed tissue. In a minority of patients, macro reentrant circuits may be responsible for recurrent ventricular tachycardia, including reentry incorporating the bundle branches.

Patients with acute ventricular tachycardia associated with a precipitating factor often suffer severe symptoms requiring immediate treatment measures. *Chronic recurrent ventricular tachycardia* also may cause severe hemodynamic compromise, but sometimes only mild symptoms that are generally well tolerated result. *Sustained ventricular tachycardia* is that which requires therapeutic intervention to restore a stable rhythm or lasts a relatively long time (usually greater than 30 seconds). *Nonsustained ventricular tachycardia* (NSVT) is that which self-terminates after a brief duration (usually less than 30 seconds). If the patient has ventricular tachycardia more frequently than sinus rhythm (i.e., ventricular tachycardia is the dominant rhythm), this is referred to as *incessant ventricular tachycardia*. *Exercise-induced ventricular tachycardia* is that which occurs during times of high sympathetic tone such as physical exertion. *Monomorphic ventricular tachycardia* has a consistent QRS configuration, whereas *polymorphic ventricular tachycardia* has varying QRS complexes. A characteristic type of polymorphic ventricular tachycardia, in which the QRS complexes appear to undulate around a central axis

TABLE 17–6. Heritable Polymorphic Ventricular Tachycardia

Syndrome	Channel Defect	Mutant Gene	Characteristics	Treatment
LQTS$_1$	$\downarrow I_{Ks}$	KVLQT1	SD/TdP with exercise	BB/ICD
LQTS$_2$	$\downarrow I_{Kr}$	HERG	SD/TdP with arousal	BB/ICD
LQTS$_3$	$\uparrow I_{Na}+$ during plateau/ repolarization	SCN5A	SD/TdP at rest/sleep	Mexilitine/ICD
Brugada	$\downarrow I_{Na}+$	SCN5A	SD/PMVT or VF at rest/ sleep in Asian males	ICD

LQTS = long-QT syndrome; SD = sudden death; TdP = torsade de pointes; PMVT = polymorphic ventricular tachycardia; VF = ventricular fibrillation; BB = β-blocker; ICD = internal cardioverter-defibrillator.
Note: LQTS can be provoked by potassium channel blockers (e.g., quinidine, sotalol), and Brugada syndrome can be provoked by potent sodium channel blockers (e.g., cocaine, flecainide). LQTS$_3$ and Brugada may coexist.

and is associated with evidence of delayed ventricular repolarization (long QT interval or prominent U waves), is referred to as *torsade de pointes.*

Most but not all forms of recurrent ventricular tachycardia occur in patients with extensive heart disease. Ventricular tachycardia occurring in a patient without heart disease is sometimes referred to as *idiopathic ventricular tachycardia* and may take several forms.[72–74] Fascicular tachycardia arises from a fascicle of the left bundle branch (usually posterior) and usually is not associated with severe underlying heart disease. Calcium channel blockers (but not adenosine) are effective in terminating an acute episode of fascicular ventricular tachycardia. Ventricular outflow tract tachycardia (usually originating from the right ventricular outflow tract and thus abbreviated RVOT) originates from near the pulmonic valve (or uncommonly the aortic) and also occurs in patients with normal LV without discernible cardiac disease.[74] Unlike other forms of ventricular tachycardia, RVOT often terminates with adenosine and may be prevented with β-blockers and/or calcium channel blockers.

Some unusual forms of ventricular tachycardia are congenital or heritable (Table 17–6). Torsade de pointes can be associated with heritable defects in the flux of ions that govern ventricular repolarizaton. Although seven syndromes have been described, the more common examples are long-QT-interval syndromes (LQTS) 1 (depressed I_{Ks}), 2 (depressed I_{Kr}), and 3 (enhanced inward Na$^+$ flux during repolarization).[75,76] Polymorphic ventricular tachycardia (without a long QT interval) or ventricular fibrillation also may occur owing to a heritable defect in the sodium channel. This is the case in Brugada syndrome, described as a typical ECG pattern (ST-segment elevation in leads V$_1$–V$_3$) during sinus rhythm and associated with sudden death, commonly in males of Asian descent.[77] It has been estimated that Brugada syndrome accounts for about 40% of all cases of ventricular fibrillation in patients without heart disease.

▶ TREATMENT: Ventricular Tachycardia

Consider the patient with the more common form of sustained monomorphic ventricular tachycardia, i.e., a patient with structural heart disease, usually ischemic in nature. As with other rapid tachycardias, the initial management of an acute episode of ventricular tachycardia requires a quick assessment of the patient's status and symptoms. If severe symptoms are present, then DCC should be instituted to restore sinus rhythm immediately. An investigation should be made into possible precipitating factors, and these should be corrected, if possible. The diagnosis of acute MI should be entertained. If the episode of ventricular tachycardia is felt to be an isolated electrical event associated with a transient initiating factor (such as acute MI or digitalis toxicity), there is no need for long-term antiarrhythmic therapy once the precipitating factors are corrected (e.g., an infarct has healed and the patient is stable). Nevertheless, the patient should be monitored closely for possible recurrences of ventricular tachycardia.

Patients presenting with an acute episode of ventricular tachycardia associated with only mild symptoms can be treated initially with antiarrhythmic drugs (DCC should be readily available). The reader is referred to the most recent Guidelines for Cardiopulmonary Resuscitation and Emergency Cardiac Care put forth by the American Heart Association.[53] Intravenous amiodarone now usually is chosen first in this situation. Intravenous procainamide or lidocaine are suitable alternatives, although in one small study procainamide was shown to be superior to lidocaine in terminating ventricular tachycardia.[78] DCC should be instituted if the patient's status deteriorates, ventricular tachycardia degenerates to ventricular fibrillation, or drug therapy fails. As an alternate to DCC, a transvenous pacing wire can be inserted and ventricular tachycardia terminated by overdrive pacing methods.

Once an acute episode of sustained ventricular tachycardia has been terminated successfully by electrical or pharmacologic means and an acute MI has been ruled out, the possibility of paroxysmal ventricular tachycardia reappearing on a recurrent basis should be considered. This possibility often can be confirmed by the use of invasive electrophysiologic studies using programmed ventricular stimulation. Management of a patient with chronic recurrent sustained ventricular tachycardia deserves considerable attention. Because such a patient is at extremely high risk for death, trial-and-error attempts to find effective therapy is unwarranted. Two methods using surrogate end points have been used: (1) inability to induce sustained ventricular tachycardia with programmed extrastimuli by invasive electrophysiologic studies and (2) suppression of ventricular ectopy by serial 24-hour continuous ECG (Holter) monitoring.

Electrophysiologic studies using programmed stimulation incorporate the concepts of reentry in order to replicate the patient's clinical tachycardia in a controlled laboratory setting. The patient is admitted to the hospital (often to an intensive care unit) and strips of the clinical tachycardia are analyzed carefully. All antiarrhythmic drugs are discontinued, and (after the systemic elimination of these drugs) the patient is brought to the electrophysiology laboratory in the nonsedated state. Here, transvenous multipolar catheters, which can both pace the heart and record electrical activity, are inserted into the right

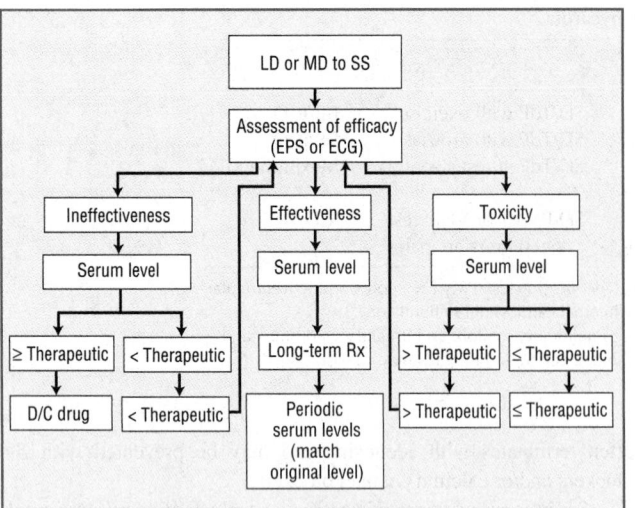

FIGURE 17–12. Algorithm for the clinical approach to therapeutic drug monitoring of antiarrhythmic drugs. EPS = electrophysiologic study; ECG = continuous electrocardiographic monitoring; D/C = discontinue drug.

side of the heart. Next, attempts to replicate the clinical tachycardia are made by the insertion of early beats and/or pacing methods via programmed stimulation. If replication of the clinical tachycardia is achieved, this initial study (without drug therapy) serves as a control that can be compared with subsequent studies on drug therapy. Once ventricular tachycardia is induced by programmed stimulation, it can be terminated by programmed stimulation, overdrive pacing, or DCC depending on the patient's status. Antiarrhythmic drugs then can be administered serially, and the electrophysiologic study is repeated (at presumed drug steady state). If a patient has sustained ventricular tachycardia induced during the control study, then the inability to reproduce ventricular tachycardia or the induction of only brief, self-terminating episodes of ventricular tachycardia (usually less than 15 beats) generally predicts that the drug will be effective in preventing recurrent episodes on a long-term basis. When ventricular tachycardia is rendered noninducible with drug therapy, a serum drug level determination should be done immediately. This serum level then serves as the patient's target level for chronic oral therapy (Fig. 17–12). Efforts should be directed at keeping the serum level at or above this target to prevent recurrence of the arrhythmia.[79]

Although this method can be efficacious in determining effective antiarrhythmic drug therapy in patients with recurrent ventricular tachycardia, it has several drawbacks besides its invasive nature. Foremost in this regard is that the yield for finding an effective drug is low. Sustained monomorphic ventricular tachycardia can be rendered noninducible or nonsustained in only 20% to 25% of patients. Therefore, the clinician frequently must search for other therapeutic options or settle for other treatment end points such as slower and more tolerable inducible ventricular tachycardia. Amiodarone is clearly the most effective (about 50% effective after 2 years) agent in patients with recurrent ventricular tachycardia; however, electrophysiologic drug testing does not necessarily predict the clinical efficacy of amiodarone. Patients may have continued inducibility of ventricular tachycardia on amiodarone despite long-term success. Indeed, empirical amiodarone has been compared with therapy with other agents guided by electrophysiologic testing in patients as high risk for recurrent ventricular tachycardia.[80] In this trial, amiodarone therapy without invasive testing was superior in preventing cardiac

death and recurrences of severe ventricular arrhythmias at all time points.

Older trials that seemingly demonstrated that serial drug testing identifies effective chronic agents always lacked a control group (i.e., patients rendered noninducible after treatment with an antiarrhythmic drug who are not treated chronically with that agent). This obviously was done because of ethical concerns but raises the possibility that noninducibility simply identifies low-risk patients, independent of drug treatment.

The second method used to determine therapy for patients with chronic recurrent sustained ventricular tachycardia is the use of serial Holter monitors with drug testing. The surrogate end point in this case is the suppression of ventricular ectopy and total abolition of NSVT compared with control (drug-free) recordings. This method was not used routinely in the United States; initial small studies[81] demonstrated a superiority of invasive electrophysiologic testing over serial Holter recordings. Nonetheless, enough controversy was generated to initiate a large study to compare the two methods of drug testing. The Electrophysiologic Study Versus Electrocardiographic Monitoring (ESVEM) trial[82,83] enrolled patients with documented clinical ventricular tachycardia/ventricular fibrillation, inducible ventricular tachycardia, and frequent ventricular ectopy. These patients were randomized to electrophysiologic studies or serial Holter recordings to test up to seven antiarrhythmic drugs (i.e., imipramine, mexiletine, pirmenol, procainamide, quinidine, propafenone, and sotalol). Holter testing had a greater yield of identifying effective agents, and there was no statistical difference between this method and electrophysiologic testing in terms of ventricular tachycardia recurrence or sudden death. Although patients with poor LV systolic function could not receive it in the ESVEM trial, sotalol proved to be the most effective drug in the trial. The relatively impressive results in the ESVEM trial with racemic sotalol contrasted with the poor results of its D-isomer in the SWORD trial (albeit in a different population) speaks strongly for the importance of chronic treatment with β-blockers in patients with serious ventricular arrhythmias. Regardless of the methods of drug testing, recurrence rate of ventricular tachycardia in the ESVEM was high (20% to 50% per year depending on the drug chosen). These findings and the impressive side-effect profiles of antiarrhythmic agents have led investigators to study nondrug approaches to the treatment of recurrent ventricular tachycardia/ventricular fibrillation.[84]

❽ Some centers have had excellent results with the surgical excision of the ventricular tachycardia focus in appropriate candidates for this extensive procedure. With the aid of endocardial mapping techniques, procedures such as ventricular aneurysectomy, encircling ventriculotomy, and cryo- or laser ablation can abolish the arrhythmogenic substrate successfully. Less invasive techniques such as catheter-guided ablation with radiofrequency current also have been used. This approach is highly effective (~90%) in idiopathic ventricular tachycardia (RVOT or fascicular ventricular tachycardia) but less so in recurrent ventricular tachycardia associated with a cardiomyopathic processes or remote MI with LV aneurysm. In the latter patients, ablation usually is regarded as second-line therapy after other methods have failed. The introduction of and advances in the implantable automatic cardioverter-defibrillator (ICD), coupled with its demonstrated effectiveness, have obviated the need for serial drug testing (by invasive or noninvasive methods) and many risky surgical procedures[85] (Fig. 17–13). Early ICDs required a thoracotomy for placement and were programmed to tachycardia rate. Once the patient's rate rose to a certain level, a series of internal defibrillations was delivered. Although effective in terminating ventricular tachycardia/ventricular fibrillation, inappropriate shocks sometimes were

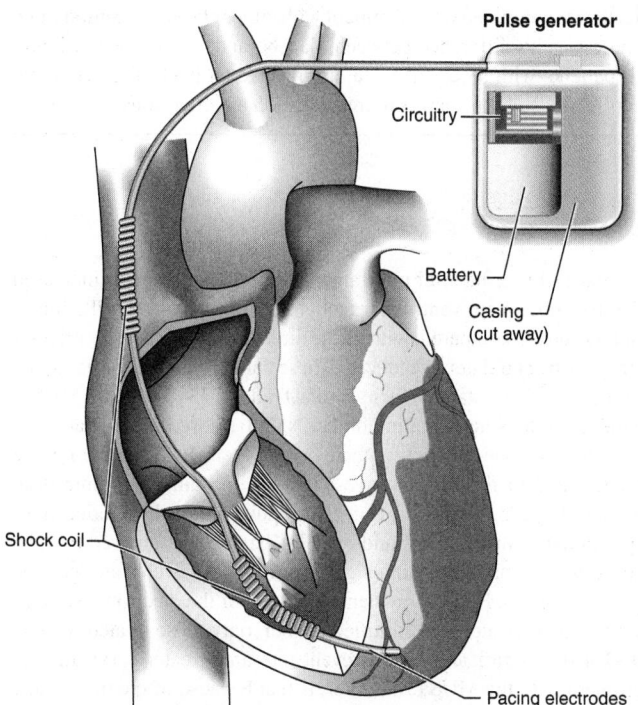

Pulse generator

Circuitry

Battery

Casing
(cut away)

Shock coil

Pacing electrodes

FIGURE 17–13. Drawing showing automatic implantable cardioverter-defibrillators with newer methods of device placement. It shows an endocardial lead system where the leads are placed transvenously without the need for a thoracotomy. The generator is now small enough to be placed in the pectoral region of the chest. *(From DiMarco,[85] with permission.)*

delivered for supraventricular tachycardias or NSVT. Further, a pulse generator was placed in the abdomen with a relatively short battery life in these early models. ICD technology has expanded rapidly[85] so that now the newer devices employ a "tiered-therapy approach"; i.e., new ICDs provide in a sequential fashion: programmed stimulation, overdrive pacing, and then low-energy (<5 J) synchronized shocks before unsynchronized internal defibrillation (10–30 J) is employed as a last step. In addition, backup bradycardia pacing and extended battery lives have made these devices much more attractive. All models store recordings during delivery of pacing shocks; this is extremely important in discerning appropriate from inappropriate shocks and in documenting recurrences of the patient's tachycardia. Importantly, transvenous insertion techniques not requiring a thoracotomy are now being used routinely and the pulse generator is now small enough to implant in the pectoral region of the chest (see Fig. 17–13).

Most would agree that the ICD is a highly effective method in preventing sudden death due to recurrent ventricular tachycardia or ventricular fibrillation,[86] although several problems remain. First, the device and implantation are expensive. The actual device, implantation procedure, electrophysiologic studies, hospitalization, and physician fees are costly and, considering the expanding indications, place a great burden on the health care system. Second, many patients (as high as 50%) end up receiving antiarrhythmic drugs (usually amiodarone or sotalol[87]) in addition to the ICD. Here, the end point of drug therapy is different from that without the ICD; i.e., the drugs do not necessarily need to prevent all sustained recurrences because the ICD is there as a backup. Antiarrhythmic drugs are prescribed in this instance to decrease the frequency of ventricular tachycardia/ventricular fibrillation episodes and NSVT, minimize patient discomfort, and save battery life. Each patient should be individualized, and antiarrhyth-

mic drugs should be administered in those with frequent ventricular tachycardia and shocks. If antiarrhythmic drugs are added to ICD therapy, one should note that many agents alter defibrillation thresholds, and therefore, the device should be reprogrammed to account for this.[88]

Which is better, antiarrhythmic drugs or the ICD? The use of the ICD in patients with remote MI, LV dysfunction, and at least one episode of ventricular fibrillation or sustained ventricular tachycardia was compared with chronic antiarrhythmic drug (>90% empirical amiodarone) therapy in the Antiarrhythmic-drug versus Internal Defibrillator (AVID) trial.[89] The trial was stopped early because of a demonstrated superiority of the ICD; patients in the ICD group had a better overall survival (75% versus 64% at 3 years). In other words, in this important study, the ICD was superior to the most effective drug known, namely, amiodarone. Other large multicenter trials comparing the ICD with amiodarone in patients with a history of ventricular fibrillation and/or sustained ventricular tachycardia have shown similar results, with the ICD reducing overall mortality by 20% to 25%.[90,91] Despite the high costs, these results provide strong support for the aggressive use of the ICD in patients at high risk for recurrent life-threatening ventricular arrhythmias. ICD implantation can be cost-effective, particularly in patients with poor LV function (depending on the indication, about $30,000 per life-year saved).[92] Although nearly all clinicians now consider the ICD as first-line treatment in patients with a history of recurrent sustained ventricular tachycardia/ventricular fibrillation (i.e., used as "secondary" prevention), there is at least one possible patient group that may do as well with drug therapy alone. In the AVID trial, patients with only mild LV dysfunction (EF > 35%) treated with amiodarone (especially with a β-blocker) did just as well as if they were treated with an ICD. It is possible that this specific subgroup of patients could be treated without an ICD.

The indications for implantation of an ICD have expanded considerably[92] (Table 17–7). Initially, its efficacy was evaluated in patients who had already suffered a documented episode of ventricular tachycardia or ventricular fibrillation (secondary prevention), but now primary prevention trials have been published[93] or are being planned. These results will help clinicians in choosing the proper therapy for patients with life-threatening arrhythmias. For instance, the Sudden Cardiac Death in Heart Failure Trial (SCD-Heft) is a primary prevention trial that evaluated survival in patients with LV dysfunction

---

TABLE 17–7. Current Indications for ICD Implantation[a]

1. Documented recurrent VT or VF
2. Patients successfully resuscitated from cardiac arrest (due to VT or VF) not due to an identifiable, reversible cause (e.g., AMI, severe electrolyte disturbances)
3. Syncope with sustained VT or VF induced at electrophysiologic study by programmed stimulation
4. NSVT, CAD (remote MI), LV dysfunction, and sustained VT or VF induced at electrophysiologic study by programmed stimulation
5. Heritable polymorphic VT (congenital long-QT syndromes or Brugada syndrome)
6. Severe LV dysfunction (EF < 30%) and remote MI

[a]Summarized from national guidelines[71] to include indications where there is clear evidence (class I) or conflicting evidence but the weight of it is in favor of implantation (class Ia) or evidence from large randomized trials may never be completed but there is clinical consensus (heritable polymorphic VT).
[b]Primary prevention; all others are secondary prevention.
VT = ventricular tachycardia; VF = ventricular fibrillation; AMI = acute myocardial infarction; MI = myocardial infarction; LV = left ventricular; NSVT = nonsustained ventricular tachycardia; CAD = coronary artery disease; EF = ejection fraction.

(ejection fraction ≤ 35%) at risk for sudden death treated with amiodarone or an ICD.[94] This important study, although completed, has not been published in full form at the time of this writing. Preliminary results show that ICD implantation resulted in a significantly lower death rate compared with treatment with either placebo or amiodarone (there was no difference between placebo and amiodarone). Should all patients with severe heart failure receive an ICD? The economic implications of the answer to this question are enormous.

▶ TREATMENT: Nonsustained Ventricular Tachycardia (NSVT)

At this time, it is clear that patients with complex ventricular ectopy should not be treated with type I or III antiarrhythmic drugs and that those with recurrent sustained ventricular tachycardia definitely require some form of preventative treatment, generally an ICD with or without amiodarone, but the approach to NSVT remains an area of controversy. Obviously, patients with long symptomatic episodes require drug therapy, but most have asymptomatic NSVT. Asymptomatic NSVT can be documented frequently in patients with poor LV function of ischemic or nonischemic origin, and epidemiologic data indicate that patients with NSVT and coronary disease are at increased risk for sudden death.[95] However, owing in part to the results of the CAST and other similar trials with antiarrhythmic drugs, clinicians have sought clearer risk stratification before initiating drug therapy.

Traditionally, there are three strategies to approach the treatment of NSVT: (1) conservative (no antiarrhythmic drug treatment beyond β-blockers), (2) empirical amiodarone, and (3) aggressive, i.e., electrophysiologic studies with possible insertion of an ICD. A number of early studies[96,97] have suggested that tests such as electrophysiologic studies could be used to determine long-term risk in patients with NSVT. For instance, Wilbur and colleagues[96] demonstrated that post-MI patients with NSVT and inducible sustained ventricular tachycardia after programmed stimulation were at increased risk for subsequent ventricular tachycardia/ventricular fibrillation or sudden death compared with those in whom sustained ventricular tachycardia could not be induced. These data provide the basis for the Multicenter Unsustained Tachycardia Trial (MUST).[97] In the MUST, patients with asymptomatic clinical NSVT (more than 3 beats), inducible sustained ventricular tachycardia, and LV dysfunction were randomized to the conservative approach (no antiarrhythmic drug therapy beyond β-blockers) or electrophysiologically guided therapy (antiarrhythmic drugs and/or ICD). The results showed that the conservative approach had a significantly higher event rate (cardiac arrest or death). However, when the results of the electrophysiologically guided group were stratified further, only those treated with an ICD had a significantly lower event rate and greater survival. One problem with the MUST, however, is that because of the time frame that the trial was initiated (1989), nearly 50% of patients received type I antiarrhythmic drugs or drugs that are now known not to improve survival in patients with coronary disease and ventricular arrhythmias; only 10% received the most effective agent in this setting, amiodarone.

In summary, most patients with coronary disease, LV dysfunction and NSVT should undergo electrophysiologic studies. If

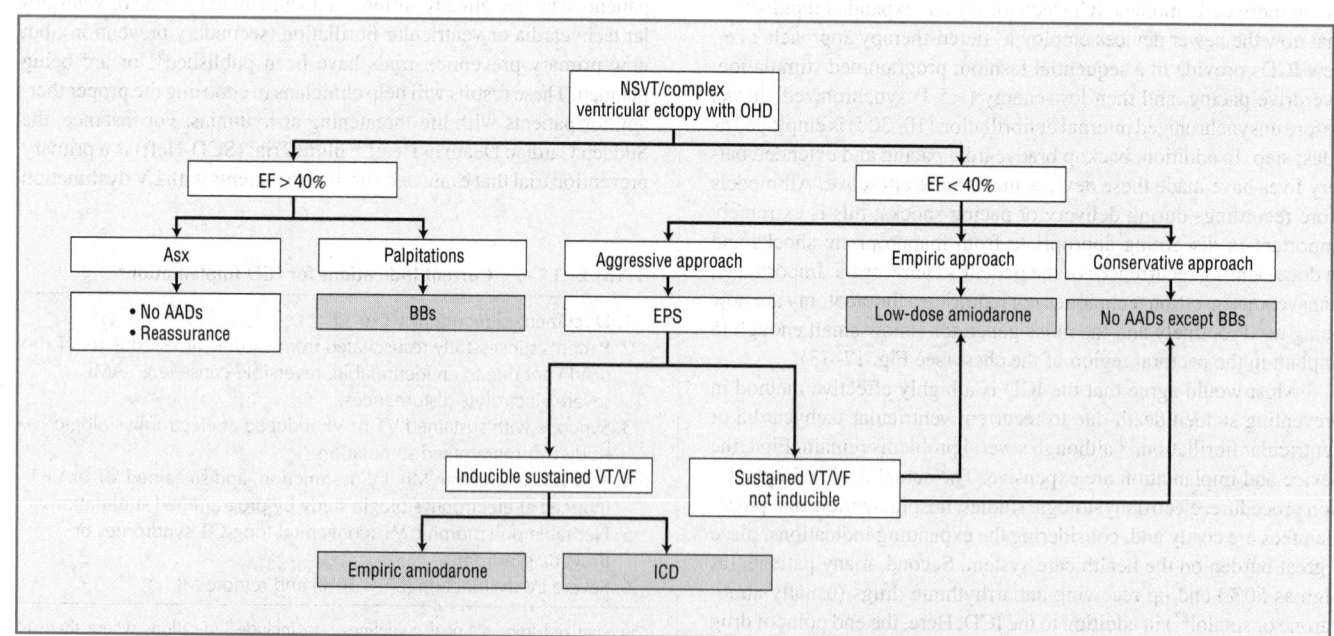

FIGURE 17–14. An algorithm for management of patients with ventricular ectopy or nonsustained ventricular tachycardia (NSVT) in patients with organic heart disease (OHD). In patients with significant LV dysfunction (EF < 40%), the type of OHD will influence the therapeutic pathway. Patients with ischemic heart disease will be treated more aggressively and those with idiopathic cardiomyopathy will be treated more conservatively (i.e., less commonly ICD and more commonly amiodarone). EF = ejection fraction; EPS = electrophysiologic studies; VT/VF = ventricular tachycardia/ventricular fibrillation; ICD = implantable cardioverter-defibrillator; F/U = follow-up; BB = β-blockers; AADs = antiarrhythmic drugs.

these patients do not have inducible sustained ventricular tachycardia/ventricular fibrillation, no antiarrhythmic drug therapy targeted specifically to the arrhythmia should be given on a chronic basis. On the other hand, if sustained ventricular tachycardia/ventricular fibrillation is inducible, chronic preventative therapy is warranted (Fig. 17–14). Because of the results of trials such as MUST and others,[98] many such patients will receive an ICD. For patients with NSVT but with idiopathic cardiomyopathy of nonischemic origin, the use of an ICD cannot be recommended routinely. In a recent trial,[99] there was no difference in mortality or quality of life between treatment with empirical amiodarone and ICD implantation in these patients. Treatment with amiodarone was associated with lower cost, although 50% of patients randomized to amiodarone had to have it discontinued owing to side effects. There was no placebo in this trial, and mortality was surprisingly low, so it is conceivable that no therapy (drug or device) could have been as successful. Nonetheless, these results show the importance of the form of underlying heart disease in patients with ventricular tachycardia or NSVT.

VENTRICULAR PROARRHYTHMIA

All antiarrhythmic agents have the potential to aggravate existing arrhythmias or to cause new arrhythmias. It is believed that antiarrhythmic drugs may cause proarrhythmia in 5% to 20% of patients.[10] Although drug-induced arrhythmias have been recognized for several years, it has only been recently that this adverse effect has gained widespread attention. Many definitions for proarrhythmia have been proposed; however, in simplest terms, it indicates the development of a significant new arrhythmia (such as ventricular tachycardia, ventricular fibrillation, or torsade de pointes) or worsening of an existing arrhythmia (episodes are longer, faster, or more frequent). As with all arrhythmias, the consequences of proarrhythmia are varied. Some patients who develop proarrhythmia may be totally asymptomatic, others may notice a worsening of symptoms, and some may die suddenly from this side effect. The development of proarrhythmia results from the same mechanisms that cause arrhythmias in general (e.g., quinidine-induced torsade de pointes due to early afterdepolarizations) or from an alteration in the underlying substrate owing to the antiarrhythmic agent (e.g., development of an accelerated tachycardia due to flecainide, which decreases conduction velocity without significantly altering the refractory period)[10] (see Fig. 17–4). The diagnosis of proarrhythmia is sometimes difficult to make because of the variable nature of the underlying arrhythmias. However, in all cases, the agent should be discontinued if proarrhythmia is detected or suspected.

INCESSANT MONOMORPHIC VENTRICULAR TACHYCARDIA

The prototypical form of proarrhythmia due to the type Ic drugs is a rapid, sustained, monomorphic ventricular tachycardia with a characteristic sinusoidal QRS pattern that is often resistant to resuscitation with cardioversion or overdrive pacing. It is sometimes referred to as *sinusoidal* or *incessant ventricular tachycardia* and is the result of excessive sodium channel blockade and slowed conduction. Sinusoidal ventricular tachycardia attributed to type Ic drugs was thought to occur within the first several days of drug initiation; however, the results of the CAST indicate that the risk may exist as long as the agent is continued. Patient factors that definitely predispose to this form of proarrhythmia are the presence of (1) underlying ventricular arrhythmias, (2) ischemic heart disease, and (3) poor LV function. Provocation of proarrhythmia caused by type Ic drugs is sometimes reported during exercise; this is more than likely due to augmented slowed conduction at rapid heart rates (i.e., rate-dependent sodium blockade). The incidence of proarrhythmia is greatest in patients with all three risk factors (approximately 10% to 20%) and extremely uncommon in those without risks, such as patients with good LV function and supraventricular tachycardias. In one study with patients with risk factors, the incidence of death caused by proarrhythmia from encainide and flecainide was approximately the same as the chance of

long-term effectiveness.[100] Other factors that have a less defined association with proarrhythmia are elevated antiarrhythmic serum concentrations and rapid dosage escalation. It has also been proposed that the presence of underlying ventricular conduction delays may pose a risk. As mentioned earlier, this arrhythmia is resistant to resuscitation; however, some practitioners have had success with intravenous lidocaine (competes for the sodium channel receptor) or the administration of sodium bicarbonate (reverses the excessive sodium channel blockade).

TORSADE DE POINTES

As defined previously, torsade de pointes (TdP) is a rapid form of polymorphic ventricular tachycardia (Fig. 17–15) that is associated with evidence of delayed ventricular repolarization (long QT interval or prominent U waves) on surface ECGs. It is important to note that most forms of polymorphic ventricular tachycardia occurring in the setting of a normal QT interval are similar to monomorphic ventricular tachycardia in terms of etiology and treatment strategies (thus a long QT interval is crucial to the diagnosis of TdP). TdP may occur in association with hereditary syndromes or may be acquired (e.g., caused by drugs or diseases). The underlying etiology in both cases is delayed ventricular repolarization due to blockade of potassium conductance. It is possible, however, that some individuals have a partially expressed form of these congenital syndromes but may never suffer TdP unless some other external factor (e.g., drugs or diseases) further delay ventricular repolarization. Acquired forms of TdP are associated with electrolyte disturbances (e.g., hypokalemia or hypomagnesemia), subarachnoid hemorrhage, myocarditis, liquid protein diets, arsenic poisoning, hypothyroidism, or most commonly, drug therapy (notably phenothiazines, antihistamines, antidepressants, and antiarrhythmics) (Table 17–8). The type Ia (especially quinidine) and type III I_{Kr} blockers are most notorious for precipitating TdP; type Ib and Ic drugs rarely, if ever, cause it. Quinidine-induced TdP occurs in 4% to 8% of patients treated with this agent. Associated features of quinidine-induced TdP have been identified and can be summarized as follows[31]: (1) low to "therapeutic" quinidine serum concentrations without other evidence of quinidine-related toxicity such as prolonged QRS duration, (2) concurrent organic heart disease, commonly ischemic, (3) evidence of mild delayed repolarization (prolonged QT interval) prior to quinidine therapy, (4) documentation usually within 1 week of initiating therapy, (5) high incidence of cross-sensitivity (recurrence of TdP) with other type Ia antiarrhythmic agents but not type Ib or Ic drugs or amiodarone, (6) frequent coexisting electrolyte disturbances such as hypokalemia or hypomagnesemia, (7) a characteristic long-short initiating sequence (so-called pause dependence) of the episode of TdP (see Fig. 17–15), and (8) female gender. However, none of these associations is an absolute prerequisite to the occurrence of quinidine syncope and TdP. For instance, although usually documented early in the course of therapy,

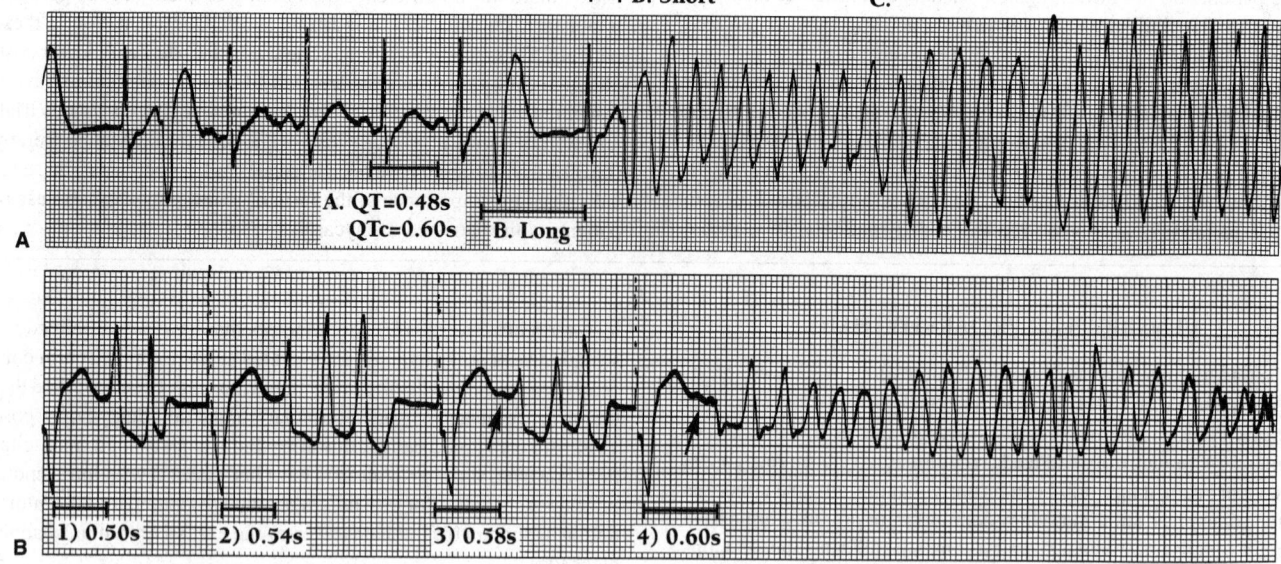

FIGURE 17–15. A. Torsade de pointes in a patient receiving procainamide. Note several characteristic features: (a) prolonged QT interval prior to torsade de pointes; (b) long–short initiating sequence—extra ventricular beat with a pause followed by a supraventricular beat followed by another premature ventricular beat on the preceding T wave, which initiates torsade de pointes; (c) polymorphic, undulating QRS morphology rate of 250 beats per minute. **B.** Torsade de pointes caused by quinidine. The reader should note a couplet and two triplets, which follow each extra systolic pause. The pause gets progressively longer until it is long enough to result in an episode of sustained torsade de pointes. Also, as the pause lengthens, discernible U waves (labeled ↑) (EADs?) begin to appear. The amplitude of the U wave is somewhat greater with the longest pause. *(From Bauman JL: Drug safety: Cardiac arrhythmias. Antihistamine update symposium. Hospital Medicine 1995; 31:24, with permission.)*

TABLE 17–8. Some Reported Causes of QT Prolongation and Torsades de Pointes

Conditions	Pimozide
Congenital long QT syndromes	Thioridazine
Myocarditis	Toxins
Myocardial ischemia/infarction	Organophosphate insecticides
Severe bradycardia due to AV block,	Arsenic
<50 beats per minute	Antihistamines
Hypokalemia	Terfenadine[a]
Severe hypothermia	Astemizole[a]
Hypomagnesemia	Antibiotics
Hypothyroidism	Pentamidine
Cardiomyopathy	Clarithromycin
Subarachnoid hemorrhage	Erythromycin
Drugs	Trimethoprim-sulfamethoxazole
Antiarrhythmic/vasodilating drugs	Grepafloxacin[a]/sparfloxacin
Quinidine	Miscellaneous
Procainamide	Liquid protein diets[b]
N-Acetylprocainamide	Corticosteroids[b]
Disopyramide	Diuretics[b]
Amiodarone	Vasopressin
Dofetilide	Quinine
Sotalol	Chloroquine
Ibutilide	Chloral hydrate
Bepridil[a]	Cisipride[a]
Psychotropics	Sumitriptan
Phenothiazines	Tacrolimus
Tricyclic and tetracyclic antidepressants	Tamoxifen
Haloperidol/droperidol	

[a]Withdrawn from market due to torsade de pointes.
[b]Due, more than likely, to severe electrolyte imbalance.

patients may suffer TdP during chronic quinidine treatment.[101] Most of these associations also occur with TdP caused by drugs besides quinidine. One important exception is that other drug-related causes of TdP usually occur in association with high concentrations and doses, e.g., sotalol, dofetilide, and N-acetylprocainamide. Quinidine's ability to block I_{Kr} is manifest clinically at low concentrations; at higher concentrations, its sodium-blocking properties predominate. Other agents that block I_{Kr} usually do so in a concentration-dependent fashion. Of the type Ia or III antiarrhythmic drugs, amiodarone is the least frequent cause of TdP; the incidence is estimated at 1% or less.

Drug-induced TdP has become an extremely visible hazard plaguing new drugs, sometimes resulting in public health disasters. For instance, cisapride, astemizole, and terfenadine are potent potassium channel blockers that were withdrawn from the market because of TdP. All these agents are metabolized rapidly to active moieties by cytochrome P450 (CYP) 3A4. However, in the presence of drugs that block the CYP3A4 isozyme (e.g., ketoconazole, erythromycin, and diltiazem), accumulation of the parent compounds (which are potent I_{Kr} blockers) results in TdP, and death may result.[102] Because of these experiences, all new drug entities under investigation should be screened for their ability to block I_{Kr}, delay repolarization and provoke TdP prior to approval.

Much has been learned about the underlying etiology of TdP. Basic defects (e.g., genetic, drugs, or diseases) that delay repolarization by influencing ion movement (usually by blocking potassium efflux) provoke early after-depolarizations (EADs) preferentially in cells deep in the heart muscle (termed M cells). EADs in these M cells, in turn, trigger reentry and TdP. Drugs that cause TdP usually delay ventricular repolarization in an inhomogeneous way (termed *dispersion of refractoriness*), and this facilitates the formation of multiple reentrant loops in the ventricle.[103]

▶ TREATMENT: Torsade de Pointes

Acute treatment of TdP is different from treatment for the more common acute monomorphic ventricular tachycardia (or polymorphic VT with a normal QT interval). For an acute episode of TdP, most patients will require and respond to DCC. However, TdP tends to the paroxysmal in nature and often will recur rapidly after countershock. Therefore, after the initial restoration of a stable rhythm, therapy designed to prevent recurrences of TdP should be instituted. Drugs that further prolong repolarization such as intravenous procainamide are absolutely contraindicated. Lidocaine usually is ineffective. Intravenous magnesium sulfate, by suppressing early after-depolarizations, is now considered the drug of choice in preventing recurrences of TdP.[104] If ineffective, treatment strategies designed to increase heart rate, shorten ventricular repolarization, and prevent the pause dependency should be initiated—either temporary transvenous pacing (105–120 beats per minute) or pharmacologic pacing (isoproterenol or epinephrine infusion). All agents that prolong the QT interval should be discontinued, and exacerbating factors (such as hypokalemia or hypomagnesemia) should be corrected.

VENTRICULAR FIBRILLATION

BACKGROUND AND PREVENTION WITH ACUTE MI

Ventricular fibrillation is electrical anarchy of the ventricle resulting in no cardiac output and cardiovascular collapse. Death will ensue rapidly if effective treatment measures are not taken. Patients who die abruptly (within 1 hour of initial symptoms) and unexpectedly (i.e., sudden death) usually have ventricular fibrillation recorded at the time of death.[61] Sudden cardiac death accounts for about 400,000 deaths per year or 1000 deaths per day in the United States. Sudden cardiac death occurs most commonly in patients with ischemic heart disease and primary myocardial disease associated with LV dysfunction, less commonly in those with WPW syndrome and mitral valve prolapse, and occasionally, in those without associated heart disease (e.g., Brugada syndrome). Patients who have sudden cardiac death (not associated with acute MI) but survive because of appropriate CPR often have inducible sustained ventricular tachycardia and/or ventricular fibrillation during electrophysiologic studies.[105] These individuals are at high risk for the recurrence of ventricular tachycardia and/or ventricular fibrillation.

In contrast, patients who have ventricular fibrillation associated with acute MI (i.e., during the first 24 hours after symptom appearance) usually have little risk of recurrence. Of all patients who die from an acute MI, approximately 50% die suddenly prior to hospitalization. Ventricular fibrillation associated with acute MI can be subdivided into two types: primary ventricular fibrillation and complicated or secondary ventricular fibrillation. Primary ventricular fibrillation occurs in an uncomplicated MI not associated with heart failure; secondary ventricular fibrillation occurs in an MI complicated by heart failure. The time course, incidence, mechanisms, treatment, and complications of these two forms of ventricular fibrillation are different. For example, about 2% to 6% patients with acute MI suffer primary ventricular fibrillation within 24 hours of chest pain, but the risk of ventricular fibrillation declines rapidly over time and is nearly zero after the initial 24-hour period. Complicated ventricular fibrillation does not follow such a predictable time course and may occur in the late infarction period. The premise of prophylactic antiarrhythmic drugs administered to all patients with uncomplicated MI is based on (1) the inability to predict which patients are at risk for primary ventricular fibrillation and (2) the predictable time course of primary ventricular fibrillation (in contrast with complicated ventricular fibrillation). Of the prophylactic therapies used, lidocaine has been the debated and studied most widely. Lie and coworkers[106] performed the classic study showing the effectiveness of lidocaine in preventing primary ventricular fibrillation. Although lidocaine reduced the incidence of ventricular fibrillation significantly compared with placebo, there was not a decrease in total mortality between the groups. This fact and the effectiveness of rapidly instituted DCC in modern coronary care units with sophisticated monitoring techniques have caused most practitioners to reject the notion of prophylactic lidocaine administration for all patients with uncomplicated MI. In support of this, two meta-analyses[107,108] concluded against the routine use of prophylactic lidocaine because of a trend toward increased mortality in lidocaine-treated patients[107] and the declining incidence of primary ventricular fibrillation documented in recent years (in the acute coronary intervention era with rapid treatment with β-blockade, thrombolytics, and acute coronary intervention).[108]

The use of intravenous magnesium sulfate also has been entertained for the prevention of ventricular fibrillation during the acute infarct period. Small trials implying effectiveness subsequently were incorporated into a meta-analysis.[109] This meta-analysis found a decrease in the incidence of ventricular tachycardia/ventricular fibrillation and a reduction in total mortality with magnesium therapy. A subsequent large multicenter trial[110] found similar results, although most of the decrease in mortality was (surprisingly) attributed to heart failure deaths rather than deaths due to ventricular arrhythmias. These results would lead one to conclude that magnesium sulfate should be administered routinely to patients with suspected MI because of its ease of administration and safety. However, data from another large trial (ISIS-4) apparently have verified no such effectiveness of magnesium therapy in this setting.[111] Hence prophylactic magnesium also cannot be recommended. Indeed, no therapies (i.e., lidocaine, magnesium, or other antiarrhythmic drugs) have shown a conclusive benefit in preventing ventricular fibrillation in the acute infarct period, and this form of therapy cannot be recommended at this time.

▶ TREATMENT: Ventricular Fibrillation

A patient with ventricular fibrillation (with or without associated myocardial ischemia) should be managed according to the American Heart Association's recommendations for advanced cardiac life support (ACLS).[52] Summarizing, DCC should be instituted immediately and repeated twice (if unsuccessful) prior to drug therapy. If DCC does not restore a stable rhythm, vasopressin or epinephrine should be administered prior to the next DCC. It has been debated whether the standard dose of epinephrine (1 mg) is sufficient (see Chap. 11). A large multicenter trial[112] found "high dose" epinephrine (0.2 mg/kg) to not affect success or survival (compared with 0.02 mg/kg) of patients with cardiac arrest (including ventricular fibrillation). A recent comparative trial[113] found vasopressin (40 units twice) and epinephrine to be of equal efficacy in patients with ventricular fibrillation (in patients with asystole, however, vasopressin was superior). Nevertheless, if vasopressin or epinephrine (coupled with DCC) is unsuccessful, an antiarrhythmic drug should be selected and administered, and then DCC should be repeated as necessary. It appears clear from the most recent ACLS guidelines that intravenous amiodarone is now the antiarrhythmic drug of first choice in most situations of patients with ventricular fibrillation. Unlike its oral counterpart, intravenous amiodarone has a quick onset of action and may be effective in 40% to 60% of patients with ventricular tachycardia or ventricular fibrillation refractory to lidocaine. The promotion of intravenous amiodarone to the first antiarrhythmic drug used during ventricular fibrillation (and the corresponding demotion of lidocaine) is the result of (1) a lack of data demonstrating the effectiveness of other agents, (2) the Amiodarone in out-of-hospital Resuscitation of REfractory Sustained ventricular Tachycardia (ARREST) study,[114] and (3) the Amiodarone versus Lidocaine In prehospital Ventricular Fibrillation Evaluation (ALIVE) study.[115] In the ARREST,[114] significantly more patients receiving 300 mg amiodarone intravenously survived to hospital admission than did a corresponding placebo group. Noteworthy was that the survival to hospital *discharge* was no different (although the study was not powered to determine this end point). In the ALIVE,[115] amiodarone was more effective than lidocaine in increasing survival to hospital admission in patients with out-of-hospital ventricular fibrillation. Again, there were no differences in survival to hospital discharge between the groups. Nonetheless, these results stimulated a change (away from lidocaine and toward amiodarone) in the treatment of acute ventricular fibrillation. Indeed, amiodarone may be the only drug used during cardiac arrest caused by ventricular fibrillation because the new guidelines also suggest that only *one* antiarrhythmic agent be given to patients with ventricular fibrillation. This is in contrast to the tradition of adding drugs if the first fails (e.g., lidocaine, then bretylium, then procainamide, etc.).

Once the patient is resuscitated successfully, antiarrhythmics should be continued until the patient's rhythm and overall status is stable. If the episode of ventricular fibrillation was associated with acute ischemia, long-term antiarrhythmic drugs probably are unnecessary, but the patient should be monitored closely for recurrence of ventricular tachycardia and/or ventricular fibrillation. If, on the other hand, ventricular fibrillation was not associated with acute MI (or a known precipitating factor), the patient should undergo invasive electrophysiologic studies and (depending on the results) probably ICD implantation (Fig. 17–16).

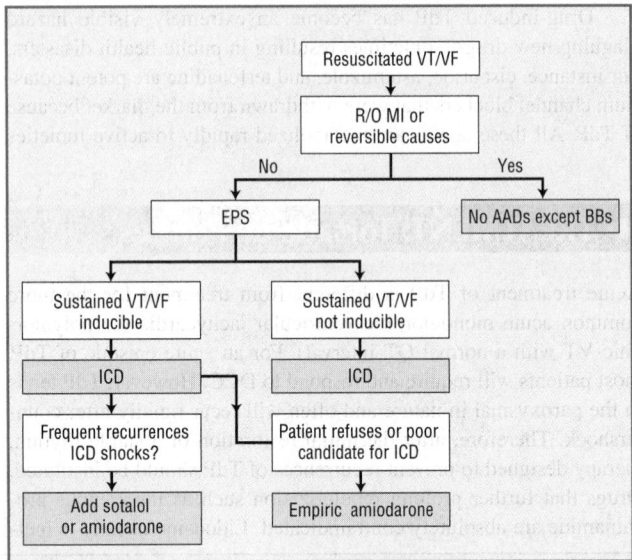

FIGURE 17–16. Example of an approach to the management of survivors of cardiac arrest (resuscitated VT/VF). Reversible causes of cardiac arrest (e.g., electrolyte abnormalities, acute phase of MI) should be treated with specific therapy. AADs = antiarrhythmic drugs; BBs = β-blockers; EPS = invasive electrophysiologic studies; ICD = implantable cardioverter - defibrillator; VT/VF = ventricular tachycardia/ventricular fibrillation; MI = myocardial infarction.

BRADYARRHYTHMIAS

SINUS NODE DYSFUNCTION

The preceding sections reviewed the pathophysiology and treatment of tachyarrhythmias, and this section serves to briefly consider the bradyarrhythmias. For the most part, the symptoms of bradyarrhythmias result from a decline in cardiac output. Because cardiac output decreases as heart rate decreases (to a point), patients experience symptoms in association with hypotension, such as dizziness, syncope, fatigue, and confusion. If LV dysfunction exists, patients may have an exacerbation of congestive heart failure symptoms. Except in the case of recurrent syncope, these symptoms are often subtle and nonspecific.

SINUS BRADYCARDIA

Sinus bradyarrhythmias (heart rate <60 beats per minute) is a common finding, especially in young, athletically active individuals, and usually is neither symptomatic nor requires therapeutic intervention. On the other hand, some patients, particularly the elderly, have sinus node dysfunction. This may be the result of underlying organic heart disease and the normal aging process, which, over time, attenuate SA nodal function. *Sick sinus syndrome* refers to this process resulting in symptomatic sinus bradycardia and/or periods of sinus arrest.[116,117] Sinus node dysfunction usually is reflective of diffuse conduction disease, and accompanying AV block is not uncommon. Furthermore, symptomatic bradyarrhythmias may be accompanied by alternating periods of paroxysmal tachycardias such as atrial fibrillation. In this instance, atrial fibrillation sometimes presents with a rather slow ventricular response (in the absence of AV nodal–blocking drugs) because of diffuse conduction disease. The occurrence of alternating bradyarrhythmias and tachyarrhythmias is referred to as the *tachy-brady syndrome*. The occurrence of paroxysmal atrial fibrillation in a patient with sinus node dysfunction may be due to underlying heart disease with atrial dysfunction or to atrial escape in response to reduced sinus node automaticity. In fact, because the rate of impulse generation by the sinus node generally is depressed or may fail altogether, other automatic pacemakers within the conduction system may "rescue" the sinus node. These rescue rhythms often present as paroxysmal atrial rhythms (e.g., atrial fibrillation) or as a junctional escape rhythm.

The treatment of sinus node dysfunction involves the elimination of symptomatic bradycardia and the possibility of managing alternating tachycardias such as atrial fibrillation. In general, the long-term therapy of choice is a permanent dual-chamber or ventricular pacemaker. Pacemaker therapy,[92] however, should be reserved for patients with significant symptoms. In other words, the aim of pacing is not to correct ECG findings but to improve the patient's symptoms and quality of life.

Drugs that are employed commonly to treat supraventricular tachycardias should be used with caution, if at all, in the absence of a functioning pacemaker.[116] Type I agents such quinidine can suppress the escape or rescue rhythms that appear in severe sinus bradycardia or sinus arrest. In this way, they may transform an asymptomatic patient with bradycardia into a symptomatic one. It is also important to remember that the addition of type I antiarrhythmic agents can affect pacemaker threshold and result in loss of capture if the pacemaker is not interrogated and adjusted appropriately.[88] Other drugs that depress SA or AV nodal function such as β-blockers or calcium channel antagonists also may exacerbate bradycardia significantly. Even agents with indirect sympatholytic actions such as α-methyldopa or clonidine may worsen sinus node dysfunction. Digitalis use in these patients is controversial, but in most cases, it can be used safely.

OTHER CAUSES

Another reason for paroxysmal bradycardia and sinus arrest that is not due directly to sinus node dysfunction is carotid sinus hypersensitivity.[118,119] Again, this syndrome occurs commonly in the aged with underlying heart disease. Symptoms occur when the carotid sinus is stimulated, resulting in an accentuated baroreceptor reflex. Thus the patient may experience paroxysmal episodes of dizziness or syncope because of sinus arrest caused by either 1) increased vagal tone and sympathetic withdrawal (cardioinhibitory type), 2) drop in systemic blood pressure owing to sympathetic withdrawal (vasodepressor type), or 3) both (mixed cardioinhibitory and vasodepressor

types). The diagnosis can be confirmed by performing carotid sinus massage with ECG and blood pressure monitoring in controlled conditions. Symptomatic carotid sinus hypersensitivity also should be treated with permanent pacemaker therapy.[118] However, some patients, particularly those with a significant vasodepressor component, still experience syncope or dizziness. In these cases, α-adrenergic stimulants such as midodrine, sometimes in combination (and caution) with β-blockers to achieve maximal α-sympathetic stimulation, can be tried in addition to the pacemaker.[119]

Vasovagal syndrome, by causing bradycardia, sinus arrest, and/or hypotension, is the cause of syncope in many patients who present with recurrent fainting of unknown origin.[120,121] By history, many individuals can recount rare instances of fainting spells at times of duress or fear. These are most often due to vasovagal syncope. However, some of these patients have extremely frequent, unexpected syncopal episodes that interfere with their quality of life and cause physical danger (sometimes referred to as *neurocardiogenic syncope syndrome* or *malignant vasovagal syndrome*). Vasovagal syncope is presumed to be a neurally mediated paradoxical reaction involving stimulation of cardiac mechanoreceptors (i.e., Bezold-Jarisch reflex). Forceful contraction of the ventricle (e.g., as with adrenergic stimulation), coupled with low ventricular volumes (e.g., with upright posture or dehydration), provides a powerful stimulus for cardiac mechanoreceptors. Syncope results from the spontaneous development of transient hypotension (sympathetic withdrawal) and bradycardia (vagotonia). However, the true mechanism of vasovagal syncope remains to be determined definitively. For instance, patients with denervated hearts (e.g., heart transplant recipients) still can experience this form of syncope. This observation has led some to question the ultimate role of the Bezold-Jarisch reflex in these patients.[122] Regardless, patients believed to have frequent episodes of vasovagal syncope have been evaluated and diagnosed using the upright body-tilt test, a potent stimulus for the development of vasovagal symptoms. Although used commonly, the sensitivity and reproducibility of this test have been questioned.

Vasovagal syncope usually can be treated successfully with oral β-blockers. Although these agents may seem inappropriate to treat a syndrome resulting from vasodilation and bradycardia, the therapeutic approach is designed to block an inappropriate vasovagal reaction. β-Blockers act by inhibiting the sympathetic surge that causes forceful ventricular contraction and precedes the onset of hypotension and bradycardia. Drug testing with intravenous esmolol or metoprolol during repeat head-up tilt tests has been used to predict the long-term response of oral β-blockers.[123] Other drugs that have been used successfully (with or without β-blockers) include anticholinergic agents (e.g., scopolamine patches and disopyramide), α-adrenergic agonists (e.g., midodrine), adenosine analogs (e.g., theophylline and dipyridamole), and selective serotonin receptor antagonists (e.g., sertroline and fluoxetine).[124] Permanent pacing has been used for patients with malignant vasovagal syncope, but its routine use is controversial. More information is required, particularly comparative trials with effective agents, in order to make definitive conclusions regarding the place of these alternatives to β-blockers in this disorder. Chronic pacing has been used with some success but should be reserved for drug-refractory patients.[92,124]

ATRIOVENTRICULAR BLOCK

Conduction delay or block may occur in any area of the AV conduction system: the AV node, the His bundle, or the bundle branches. AV block usually is categorized into three different types based on surface ECG

TABLE 17–9. Forms of Atrioventricular Block

Type	Criteria
First-degree block	Prolonged PR interval (>0.2 s), 1:1 AV conduction
Second-degree block	
Mobitz I	Progressive PR prolongation until QRS is dropped, <1:1 AV conduction
Mobitz II	Random nonconducted beats (absence of QRS), <1:1 AV conduction
Third-degree block	AV dissociation, absence of AV conduction

findings (see Table 17–9). First-degree AV block is 1:1 AV conduction with a prolonged PR interval. Second-degree AV block is divided into two forms: Mobitz I AV block (Wenkebach periodicity) is less than 1:1 AV conduction with progressively lengthening PR intervals until a ventricular complex is dropped; Mobitz II AV block is intermittently dropped ventricular beats in a random fashion without progressive PR-interval lengthening. Third-degree AV block is complete heart block where AV conduction is totally absent (AV dissociation). By using intracardiac His bundle ECGs, the actual site of conduction delay/block can be correlated to the preceding diagnoses. First-degree AV block usually represents prolonged conduction in the AV node. Mobitz I, second-degree AV block is also usually due to prolonged conduction in the AV node. Indeed, Wenkebach periodicity is a normal AV nodal response to rapid supraventricular stimulation or high vagal tone. In contrast, Mobitz II AV block is usually due to conduction disease below the AV node (i.e., His bundle). Third-degree AV block may be due to disease at any level of the AV conduction system: complete AV nodal block, His bundle block, or trifasicular block. The ventricle will beat independently of the atria (AV dissociation), and the rate of ventricular activation and QRS-complex configuration are determined by the site of AV block. The usual degree of automaticity of ventricular pacemakers declines progressively as impulses move down the conduction system. Therefore, the ventricular escape rate in cases of trifasicular block will be significantly less than in complete AV nodal block.

AV block may be found in patients without underlying heart disease, such as trained athletes or during sleep when vagal tone is high. Also, AV block may be transient where the underlying etiology is reversible, such as in myocarditis, myocardial ischemia, after cardiovascular surgery, or during drug therapy. β-Blockers, digitalis, or calcium antagonists may cause AV block primarily in the AV nodal area. Type I antiarrhythmic agents may exacerbate conduction delays below the level of the AV node (sodium-dependent tissue). In other cases, AV block may be irreversible, such as that owing to acute MI, rare degenerative diseases, primary myocardial disease, or congenital forms.

The cornerstone to the acute treatment of acute symptomatic bradycardia or AV block is temporary pacing, either through a transvenous wire or, in the event of an emergency, by transcutaneous leads.[53,92] Intravenous atropine (0.5–1 mg) should be given as the leads for pacing are being placed. Drugs such as atropine will facilitate the effectiveness of transcutaneous pacing. In the past, isoproterenol infusion frequently was chosen for this purpose but now is not recommended because of its vasodilating properties and its ability to increase myocardial oxygen consumption (particularly during acute MI). Sympathomimetic infusions such as epinephrine and dopamine can be used in the event of atropine failure and are particularly effective in sinus bradycardia/arrest and AV nodal block. These agents usually will not help when the site of AV block is below the AV node (e.g., Mobitz II or trifasicular AV block).

Patients with chronic symptomatic AV block should be treated with the insertion of a permanent pacemaker. Patients without symptoms sometimes can be followed closely without the need for a pacemaker. The reader is referred to national consensus guidelines for pacemaker implantation, last updated in 2002.[92] Because symptoms often correlate with the ventricular rate and the ventricular rate corresponds to the site of block, pacemaker therapy usually is necessary in distal AV blocks such as that occurring in the His bundle or the bundle branches. Patients with acute MI and evidence of new AV block or conduction disturbances often will require the insertion of a temporary transvenous pacemaker. AV block occurs more commonly as a complication of inferior wall infarcts because of high degree of vagal innervation at this site, and the coronary blood flow to the nodal areas usually supplies the inferior wall. However, the AV block may be only transient, obviating the need for permanent pacing. In patients with chronic AV conduction disturbances, intracardiac recordings (His bundle ECGs) sometimes are used to document the actual site of block and define the potential need for and specific type of pacemaker therapy.

EVALUATION OF THERAPEUTIC AND ECONOMIC OUTCOMES

Generally, patients who suffer from tachyarrhythmias can be monitored for one or several possible therapeutic outcomes. Obviously, the presence or recurrence of any arrhythmia can be documented by electrocardiographic means, e.g., surface ECG, Holter monitor, or event monitor. Further, patients may experience a decrease in blood pressure that may result in symptoms that range from light-headedness to abrupt syncope depending on the rate of the arrhythmia and the status of the underlying heart disease. For some patients, the potential alteration in hemodynamics may result in death if the arrhythmia is not detected and treated immediately. Besides these clinical outcomes, many patients with tachyarrhythmias experience alterations in quality of life caused by troublesome recurrent symptoms of the arrhythmia or to side effects of therapy. And finally, there are the economic considerations of medical or surgical intervention, continued medical care, and chronic drug or nondrug treatment.[125,126] Most of the studies are limited to the use of nondrug therapies such as the ICD or radiofrequency ablation.[45,92] Since that technology is evolving rapidly, what is not very cost-effective now indeed may be in the next several years. For example, original cost-effectiveness analysis of the ICD showed it to be highly sensitive to the life of the generator, yet newer-generation devices have made significant advances not only in the size but also with regard to battery life. More recent data on the effect of the ICD on mortality, coupled with the declining costs of an ICD, imply that the device is indeed cost-effective in certain subsets of patients, not unlike well-proven drug therapies used for other disorders.[92] Other nondrug treatments such as radiofrequency for PSVT not only improve quality of life but also save money on medical expenditures compared with chronic drug therapy.[45]

There are some therapeutic outcomes that are unique to certain arrhythmias. For instance, patients with atrial fibrillation or flutter need to be monitored for thromboembolism and for complications of anticoagulation therapy (bleeding, drug interactions) prescribed to prevent it. However, the most important monitoring parameters for most patients fall into the following categories: (1) mortality (total and arrhythmic), (2) arrhythmia recurrence (duration, frequency, symptoms), (3) hemodynamic consequences (rate, blood pressure, symptoms), and (4) treatment complications (need for alternative or additional drugs, devices, or surgery) (see Table 17–10). When evaluating

TABLE 17–10. Outcomes: Arrhythmias

Mortality
  Total, all-cause
  Arrhythmic death (i.e., sudden)
Recurrences documented by ECG
  Time to recurrence
  Frequency of recurrences
Tolerance
  Symptoms
  Blood pressure
  Rate of tachycardia
Surrogate markers of efficacy, such as
  Number of PVCs/day
  Inducibility of tachycardia with programmed stimulation
Necessity of nondrug interventions (e.g., ICD)
ICD shocks
Side effects of drugs/treatment complications
Quality of life
Economics
Outcomes specific to tachycardia (e.g., ventricular rate, systemic
  embolism in atrial fibrillation)

the arrhythmia literature, care should be taken to consider real outcomes. For example, total mortality is more meaningful than only sudden death rates; it is possible that an intervention prevents arrhythmic death, but patients die from other causes, leaving all-cause mortality unaltered. Likewise, surrogate markers of drug efficacy (e.g., noninducible tachycardia, suppression of minor arrhythmias, etc.) should be judged with a degree of skepticism. One should ask oneself, did the treatment make patients live longer (reduce mortality)? Did it make them feel better (improve humanistic outcomes or quality of life)? And/or was it economically worth it (cost-effective)?

ABBREVIATIONS

ACLS: advanced cardiac life support
AF: atrial fibrillation
AFFIRM: Atrial Fibrillation Follow-up Investigation of Rhythm
  Management
ALIVE: Amiodarone versus Lidocaine In pre-hospital Ventricular
  fibrillation Evaluation
ARREST: Amiodarone in out-of hospital Resuscitation of
  Refractory Ventricular Tachycardia Trial
AV: atrioventricular
AVID: Antiarrhythmic drug Versus Internal Defibrillator trial
CAST: Cardiac Arrhythmia Suppression Trial
DCC: direct-current cardioversion
EADs: early after-depolarizations
ESVEM: Electrophysiologic Study Versus Electrocardiographic
  Monitoring trial
ICD: implantable cardioverter-defibrillator
LADs: late after-depolarizations
LQTS: long-QT syndrome
MI: myocardial infarction
MUST: Multicenter Unsustained Tachycardia Trial
NAPA: N-acetylprocainamide
NSVT: nonsustained ventricular tachycardia
PACs: premature atrial complexes
PSVT: paroxysmal supraventricular tachycardia
PVCs: premature ventricular complexes

RMP: resting membrane potential
RVOT: right ventricular outflow tachycardia
SA: sinoatrial
SCD-HeFT: Sudden Cardiac Death in Heart Failure Trial
SWORD: Survival With ORal D-sotalol
TdP: torsade de pointes
TEE: transesophageal echocardiography
VF: ventricular fibrillation
VT: ventricular tachycardia
WPW syndrome: Wolff-Parkinson-White syndrome

Review Questions and other resources can be found at *www.pharmacotherapyonline.com.*

REFERENCES

1. Alice MA, Bonke FIM, Schopman FJG. Circus movement in rabbit atrial muscle as a mechanism of tachycardia: III. The "leading circle" concept: A new model of circus movement in cardiac tissue without the involvement of an anatomic obstacle. Circ Res 1977;41:9–18,
2. Vaughan Williams EM. A classification of antiarrhythmic actions reassessed after a decade of new drugs. J Clin Pharmacol 1984;24:129–147.
3. Working Group on Arrhythmias of the European Society of Cardiology. The Sicilian gambit: A new approach to the classification of antiarrhythmic drugs based upon their actions on arrhythmogenic mechanisms. Circulation 1991;84:1831–1851.
4. Hondeghem LM, Katzung BG. Antiarrhythmic agents: The modulated receptor mechanism of action of sodium and calcium channel-blocking drugs. Ann Rev Pharmacol Toxicol 1984;24:387–423.
5. MERIT-HF Study Group. Effect of metoprolol CR/XL in chronic heart failure: Metoprolol CR/XL Randomized Intervention Trial in Congestive Heart Failure (MERIT-HF). Lancet 1999;353:2001–2007.
6. Kumagi K, Nakashima H, Urata H, et al. Effects of angiotensin II type I receptor antagonists on electrical and structural remodeling in atrial fibrillation. J Am Coll Cardiol 2002;41:2197–2204.
7. Kosowsky BD, Taylor J, Lown B, et al. Long-term procaine amide following acute myocardial infarction. Circulation 1973;47:1204–1210.
8. Bauman JL, Gallastegui J, Strasberg B, et al. Long-term therapy with disopyramide phosphate: Side effects and effectiveness. Am Heart J 1986;111:654–660.
9. Podrid PJ, Schoeneburger A, Lown B. Congestive heart failure caused by oral disopyramide. New Engl J Med 1980;302:614–617.
10. McCollam PL, Parker RB, Beckman KJ, et al. Proarrhythmia: A paradoxic response to antiarrhythmic agents. Pharmacotherapy 1989;9:144–153.
11. Dusman RE, Stanton MS, Miles WM, et al. Clinical features of amiodarone-induced pulmonary toxicity. Circulation 1990;82:51–59.
12. Podrid PJ. Amiodarone: Reevaluation of an old drug. Ann Intern Med 1995;122:689–700.
13. Sanoski C, Schoen MD, Gonzalez RD, et al. Rational, development and outcomes of a multidisciplinary clinic for patients receiving chronic oral amiodarone. Pharmacotherapy 1998;18:1465–1515.
14. Fuster V, Ryden LE, Asinger RW, et al. ACC/AHA/ESC Guidelines for the management of patients with atrial fibrillation. A report of the American College of Cardiology/American Heart Association Task Force on Practice Guidelines and the European Society of Cardiology Committee for Practice Guidelines and Policy Conferences (Committee to Develop Guidelines for the Management of Patients with Atrial Fibrillation). J Am Coll Cardiol 2001;38:1231–1265.
15. Levy S, Camm AJ, Saksena S, et al. International consensus on nomenclature and classification of atrial fibrillation: A collaborative project of the Working Group on Arrhythmias and the Working Group on Cardiac Pacing of the European Society of Cardiology and the North American Society of Pacing and Electrophysiology. Europace 2003;5:119–122.

16. Atrial Fibrillation Investigators. Risk factors for stroke and efficacy of antithrombotic therapy in atrial fibrillation: Analysis of pooled data from five randomized controlled trials. Arch Intern Med 1994;154:1449–1457.

17. Albers GW, Dalen J, Laupacis A, et al. Antithrombotic therapy in atrial fibrillation. Chest 2001;119:194S–206S.

18. Wyndham CRC. Atrial fibrillation: The most common arrhythmia. Tex Heart Inst J 2000;27:257–267.

19. Falk RH, Leavitt JI. Digoxin for atrial fibrillation: A drug whose time has gone? Ann Intern Med 1991;114:573–575.

20. Roberts SA, Diaz C, Nolan PE, et al. Effectiveness and costs of digoxin treatment for atrial fibrillation and flutter. Am J Cardiol 1993;72:567–573.

21. Ellenbogen KA, Dias VC, Plumb VJ, et al. A placebo-controlled trial of continuous intravenous diltiazem infusion for 24-hour heart rate control during atrial fibrillation and atrial flutter: A multicenter study. J Am Coll Cardiol 1991;18:891–897.

22. Phillips BG, Gandhi AJ, Sanoski CA, et al. Comparison of intravenous diltiazem and verapamil for the acute treatment of atrial fibrillation and flutter. Pharmacotherapy 1997;17:1238–1245.

23. The Atrial Fibrillation Follow-up Investigation of Rhythm Management (AFFIRM) Investigators. A comparison of rate control and rhythm control in patients with atrial fibrillation. N Engl J Med 2003;347:1825–1833.

24. Van Gelder IC, Hagens VE, Bosker HA, et al. The Rate Control Versus Electrical Cardioversion for Persistent Atrial Fibrillation Study Group: A comparison of rate control and rhythm control in patients with recurrent persistent atrial fibrillation. New Engl J Med 2002;347:1834–1840.

25. Feld GK, Fleck P, Fujimura O, et al. Control of rapid ventricular response by radiofrequency catheter modification of the atrioventricular node in patients with medically refractory atrial fibrillation. Circulation 1994;90:2299–2307.

26. Klein AL, Grimm RA, Murray D, et al. Use of transesophageal echocardiography to guide cardioversion in patients with atrial fibrillation. N Engl J Med 2001;344:1411–1420.

27. Murdock DK, Schumock GT, Kaliebe J, et al. Clinical and case comparison of ibutilide and direct-current cardioversion for atrial fibrillation and flutter. Am J Cardiol 2000;85:503–506.

28. Management of New Onset Atrial Fibrillation: Summary, Evidence Report/Technology Assessment, Number 12. AHQR Publication No 00-E006. Rockville, MD, Agency for Healthcare Research and Quality, May 2000.

29. Boriani G, Biffi M, Alessandro C, et al. Oral propafenone to convert recent-onset atrial fibrillation in patients with and without underlying heart disease: A randomized, controlled trial. Ann Intern Med 1997;126:621–625.

30. Hilleman DE, Spinler SA. Conversion of recent-onset atrial fibrillation with intravenous amiodarone: A meta-analysis of randomized controlled trials. Pharmacotherapy 2002;22:66–74.

31. Bauman JL, Bauernfeind RA, Hoff JV, et al. Torsade de pointes due to quinidine: Observations in 31 patients. Am Heart J 1984;107:425–430.

32. Israel CW, Gronefeld G, Ehrlich JR, et al. Long-term risk of recurrent atrial fibrillation as documented by an implantable monitoring device: Implications for optimal patient care. J Am Coll Cardiol 2004;43:47–52.

33. Gage BF, Cardinally AB, Abers GW, Owens DR. Cost-effectiveness of warfarin and aspirin for prophylaxis of stroke in patients with nonvalvular atrial fibrillation. JAMA 1995;274:1839–1845.

34. SPORTIF III Investigators. Stroke prevention with the oral direct thrombin inhibitor ximelagatran compared with warfarin in patients with nonvalvular atrial fibrillation (SPORTIF III): Randomized, controlled trial. Lancet 2003;362:1691–1698.

35. Coplen SE, Antman EM, Berlin JA, et al. Efficacy and safety of quinidine therapy for maintenance of sinus rhythm after cardioversion: A meta-analysis of randomized control trials. Circulation 1990;82:1106–1116.

36. Echt DS, Liebson PR, Mitchell B, et al. Mortality and morbidity in patients receiving encainide, flecainide, or placebo: The cardiac arrhythmia suppression trial. N Engl J Med 1991;324:781–788.

37. Flaker GC, Blackshear JL, McBride R, et al. Antiarrhythmic drug therapy and cardiac mortality in atrial fibrillation. J Am Coll Cardiol 1992;20:527–532.

38. Gosselink ATM, Crijns HJM, VanGelder IC, et al. Low-dose amiodarone for maintenance of sinus rhythm after cardioversion of atrial fibrillation or flutter. JAMA 1992;267:3289–3292.

39. Roy D, Talajic M, Dorian P, et al. Amiodarone to prevent recurrence of atrial fibrillation. Canadian Trial of Atrial Fibrillation Investigators. N Engl J Med 2000;324:913–920.

40. Juul-Moller S, Edvardsson N, Rehnqvist-Ahlberg N. Sotalol versus quinidine for the maintenance of sinus rhythm after direct current conversion of atrial fibrillation. Circulation 1990;82:1932–1939.

41. Southworth MR, Zarembski D, Viana M, Bauman JL. Comparison of sotalol versus quinidine for maintenance of normal sinus rhythm in patients with chronic atrial fibrillation. Am J Cardiol 1999;83:1629–1632.

42. Pedersen OD, Bagger H, Keller N, et al. Efficacy of dofetilide in the treatment of atrial fibrillation-flutter in patients with reduced left ventricular function. The Danish Investigation of Arrhythmia and Mortality ON Dofetilide (DIAMOND) substudy. Circulation 2001;104:292–296.

43. Singh S, Zoble RG, Yellen L, et al. Efficacy and safety of oral dofetilide in converting and maintaining sinus rhythm in patients with chronic atrial fibrillation or atrial flutter. The Symptomatic Atrial Fibrillation Investigative Research on Dofetilide (SAFIRE-D) study. Circulation 2000;102:2385–2390.

44. Fischer B, Haissaguerre M, Garrigues S, et al. Radiofrequency catheter ablation of common atrial flutter in 80 patients. J Am Coll Cardiol 1995;25:1365–1372.

45. Blomstrom-Lundgrist C, Scheimanman MM, Aliot EM, et al. ACC/AHA/ESC guidelines for the management of patients with supraventricular arrhythmias. A report of the American College of Cardiology/American Heart Association Task Force and the European Society of Cardiology Committee for Practice Guidelines. J Am Coll Cardiol 2003;42:1493–1531.

46. Cox JL, Schuessler RB, Loppas DG, Boineau JP. An $8\frac{1}{2}$-year clinical experience with surgery for atrial fibrillation. Ann Surg 1996;224:267–275.

47. Chen SA, Hsieh MH, Tai CT, et al. Initiation of atrial fibrillation by ectopic beats originating from the pulmonary veins: Electrophysiologic characteristics, pharmacologic responses and the effects of radiofrequency ablation. Circulation 1999;80:1527–1535.

48. Pappone C, Rasario S, Augello G, et al. Mortality, morbidity and quality of life after circumferential pulmonary vein ablation for atrial fibrillation: Outcomes from a controlled, nonrandomized long-term study. J Am Coll Cardiol 2003;42:185–197.

49. Sung RJ, Lauer MR, Chun H. Atrioventricular node reentry: Current concepts and new perspectives. PACE 1994;17:1413–1430.

50. Bauernfeind RA, Wyndham CR, Dhingra RC, et al. Serial electrophysiologic testing of multiple drugs in patients with atrioventricular nodal reentrant paroxysmal tachycardia. Circulation 1980;62:1341–1349.

51. Wu D, Amat-Y-Leon F, Simpson R, et al. Electrophysiological studies with multiple drugs in patients with atrioventricular reentrant tachycardias utilizing an extra nodal pathway. Circulation 1977;56:727–736.

52. DiMarco JP, Miles W, Akhtar M, et al. Adenosine for paroxysmal supraventricular tachycardia: Dose ranging and comparison with verapamil. Assessment in placebo-controlled, multicenter trials. Ann Intern Med 1990;1113:104–110.

53. The American Heart Association in collaboration with the International Liaison Committee on Resuscitation. Guidelines 2000 for cardiopulmonary resuscitation and emergency cardiovascular care. Circulation 2000;102(8):I1–I384.

54. Rankin AC, McGovern BA. Adenosine or verapamil for the acute treatment of supraventricular tachycardia? Ann Intern Med 1991;114:513–515.

55. Jackman WM, Wang Z, Friday KJ, et al. Catheter ablation of accessory atrioventricular pathways (Wolff-Parkinson-White syndrome) by radiofrequency current. N Engl J Med 1991;324:1605–1611.

56. Jackman WM, Beckman KJ, McClelland JH, et al. Treatment of supraventricular tachycardia due to atrioventricular nodal reentry by

radiofrequency catheter ablation of slow pathway conduction. N Engl J Med 1992;327:313–318.

57. Scheinman MM. Radiofrequency catheter ablation for patients with supraventricular tachycardia. PACE 1993;16:671–679.

58. Cheng CH, Sanders GD, Hlatky MA, et al. Cost effectiveness of radiofrequency ablation for supraventricular tachycardia. Ann Intern Med 2000;133:864–876.

59. McCord J, Borzak S. Multifocal atrial tachycardia. Chest 1998;113:203–209.

60. Levine JH, Michael JR, Guarnier T. Treatment of multifocal atrial tachycardia with verapamil. N Engl J Med 1985;312:21–25.

61. Bayes deLuna A, Coumel P, LeClercq IF. Ambulatory sudden cardiac death: Mechanisms of production of fatal arrhythmia on the basis of data from 157 cases. Am Heart J 1989;117:151–159.

62. Ruberman W, Weinblatt E, Goldberg JD, et al. Ventricular premature beats and mortality after myocardial infarction. N Engl J Med 1977;297:750–757.

63. Lown B, Wolf M. Approaches to sudden death from coronary heart disease. Circulation 1971;44:130–142.

64. The Cardiac Arrhythmia Suppression Trial II Investigators. Effect of the antiarrhythmic agent moricizine on survival after myocardial infarction. N Engl J Med 1992;327:227–233.

65. Waldo AL, Camm AJ, deRuyter H, et al. Effect of D-sotalol on mortality in patients with left ventricular dysfunction and remote myocardial infarction. Lancet 1996;348:7–12.

66. Julian DG, Camm AJ, Frangin G, et al. Randomized trial of effect of amiodarone on mortality in patients with left ventricular dysfunction after recent myocardial infarction: EMIAT. Lancet 1997;349:667–674.

67. Cairns JA, Connolly SJ, Roberts R, et al. Randomized trial of outcome after myocardial infarction in patients with frequent or repetitive ventricular premature depolarizations: CAMIAT. Lancet 1997;349:675–682.

68. Amiodarone Trials Meta-Analysis Investigators. Effect of prophylactic amiodarone on mortality after acute myocardial infarction and in congestive heart failure: Meta-analysis of individual data from 6,500 patients in randomized trials. Lancet 1997;350:1417–1424.

69. Torp-Pederson C, Moller M, Bloch-Thomsen PE, et al. Dofetilide in patients with congestive heart failure and left ventricular dysfunction. N Engl J Med 1999;341:857–865.

70. Kober L, Block-Thomsen PE, Moller M, et al. Effect of dofetilide in patients with recent myocardial infarction and left ventricular dysfunction: A randomized trial. Lancet 2000;356:2052–2058.

71. Hilleman DE, Bauman JL. Role of antiarrhythmic therapy in patients at risk for sudden cardiac death: An evidence-based review. Pharmacotherapy 2001;21:556–575.

72. Edhouse J, Morris F. Broad complex tachycardia, part 1. Br Med J 2002;312:719–722.

73. Edhouse J, Morris F. Broad complex tachycardia, part II. Br Med J 2002;324:776–779.

74. Cole CR, Marrouche NF, Natale A. Evaluation and management of ventricular outflow tract tachycardias. Card Electrophysiol Rev 2002;6:442–447.

75. Moss AJ. Long-QT syndrome. JAMA 2003;289:2041–2044.

76. Kass RS, Moss AJ. Long-QT syndrome: Novel insights into the mechanisms of cardiac arrhythmias. J Clin Invest 2003;112:810–815.

77. Antzelevitch C, Brugada P, Brugada J, et al. Brugada syndrome, 1992–2002: A historical perspective. J Am Coll Cardiol 2003;41:1665–1671.

78. Gorgels A, van den Dool A, Hofs A, et al. Comparison of procainamide and lidocaine in terminating sustained monomorphic ventricular tachycardia. Am J Cardiol 1996;78:43–46.

79. Bauman JL, Schoen MD, Hoon TJ. Practical optimization of antiarrhythmic drug therapy using pharmacokinetic principles. Clin Pharmacokinet 1991;20:151–166.

80. The Cascade Investigators. Randomized antiarrhythmic drug therapy in survivors of cardiac arrest (the CASCADE Study). Am J Cardiol 1993;72:280–287.

81. Mitchell LB, Duff HJ, Manyari DE, et al. A randomized clinical trial of the noninvasive and invasive approaches to drug therapy of ventricular tachycardia. N Engl J Med 1987;317:1681–1687.

82. Mason JW and the Electrophysiologic Study versus Electrocardiographic Monitoring Investigators. A comparison of electrophysiologic testing with Holter monitoring to predict antiarrhythmic drug efficacy for ventricular tachyarrhythmias. N Engl J Med 1993;329:445–451.

83. Mason JW and the Electrophysiologic Study versus Electrocardiographic Monitoring Investigators. A comparison of seven antiarrhythmic drugs in patients with ventricular tachyarrhythmias. N Engl J Med 1993;329:452–458.

84. Zipes DP. Cardiac electrophysiology: Promises and contributions. J Am Coll Cardiol 1989;13:1329–1352.

85. DiMarco JP. Implantable cardioverter-defibrillators. N Engl J Med 2003;349:1836–1847.

86. Powell AC, Fuchs T, Finklestein DM, et al. Influence of implantable cardioverter-defibrillators on long-term prognosis of survivors of out-of-hospital cardiac arrest. Circulation 1993;88:1083–1092.

87. Pacifico A, Hohnloser SH, Williams JH, et al. Prevention of implantable-defibrillator shocks by treatment with sotalol. N Engl J Med 1999;340:1855–1862.

88. Tworek DA, Nazari J, Ezri M, Bauman JL. Interference by antiarrhythmic agents with the function of electrical cardiac devices. Clin Pharm 1992;11:48–56.

89. Moss AJ, Hall WJ, Cannom DS, et al. Improved survival with an implanted defibrillator in patients with coronary disease at high risk for ventricular arrhythmia. N Engl J Med 1996;335:1933–1940.

90. Connolly SJ, Gene M, Roberts TS, et al. Cardiac Implantable Defibrillator Study (CIDS): A randomized trial of the implantable cardioverter-defibrillator against amiodarone. Circulation 2000;101:1297–1302.

91. Kuck KH, Cappato R, Siebels J, et al. Randomized comparison of antiarrhythmic drug therapy with implantable defibrillators in patients resuscitated from cardiac arrest: The Cardiac Arrest Study Hamburg (CASH). Circulation 2000;102:748–754.

92. Gregoratos G, Abrams J, Epstein AE. ADD/AHA/NASPE 2002 guidelines update for implantation of cardiac pacemakers and antiarrhythmic devices. A report of the American College of Cardiology/American Heart Association Task Force on Practice Guidelines (ACC/AHA/NASPE Committee on Pacemaker Implantation). Circulation 2002;106:2145–2161.

93. Moss AJ, Zareba W, Hall WJ, et al. Prophylactic implantation of a defibrillator in patients with myocardial infarction and reduced ejection fraction. N Engl J Med 2002;346:877–883.

94. Tanne JH. Benefits of implantable cardiac defibrillators in heart failure are confirmed. Br Med J 2004;328:664.

95. Mitra RL, Buxton AE. The clinical significance of nonsustained ventricular tachycardia. J Cardiovasc Electrophys 1993;4:490–496.

96. Wilber DJ, Olshansky B, Moran JF, et al. Electrophysiological testing and nonsustained ventricular tachycardia: Use and limitations in patients with coronary artery disease and impaired ventricular function. Circulation 1990;82:350–358.

97. Buxton AE, Leek KL, DiCarlo L, et al. Electrophysiologic testing to identify patients with coronary artery disease who are at risk for sudden death. Multicenter Unsustained Tachycardia trial. N Engl J Med 2000;342:1937–1945.

98. Moss AJ, Hall WJ, Cannom DS, et al. Improved survival with an implantable defibrillator in patients with coronary disease at high risk for ventricular arrhythmia. N Engl J Med 1996;335:1933–1940.

99. Strickberger SA, Hummel JD, Bartlett TG, et al. Amiodarone versus implantable cardioverter-defibrillator: randomized trial in patients with nonischemic dilated cardiomyopathy and asymptomatic nonsustained ventricular tachycardia. AMIOVIRT. J Am Coll Cardiol 2003;41:1707–1712.

100. Herre JM, Titus C, Oeff M, et al. Inefficacy and proarrhythmic effects of flecainide and encainide for sustained ventricular tachycardia and ventricular fibrillation. Ann Intern Med 1990;113:671–676.

101. Oberg KC, O'Toole MF, Gallastegui JL, Bauman JL. "Late" proarrhythmia due to quinidine. Am J Cardiol 1994;74:192–194.

102. Bauman JL. The role of pharmacokinetics, drug interactions and pharmacogenetics in the acquired long QT syndrome. Eur Heart J 2001;3:K93–100.

103. Antzelevitch C. Heterogeneity of cellular repolarization in LQTS: The role of M cells. Eur Heart J 2001;3:K2–K16.

104. Tzivoni D, Banai S, Schuger C, et al. Treatment of torsade de pointes with magnesium sulfate. Circulation 1987;77:392–397.

105. Ruskin JN, DiMarco JP, Garan H. Out-of-hospital cardiac arrest: Electrophysiologic observation and selection of long-term antiarrhythmic therapy. N Engl J Med 1980; 03:607–613.

106. Lie KI, Wellens HJJ, Van Capelle FJ. Lidocaine in the prevention of primary ventricular fibrillation. N Engl J Med 1974;291:1324–1326.

107. MacMahon S, Collin R, Peto R, et al. Effects of prophylactic lidocaine in suspected acute myocardial infarction: An overview of results from the randomized, controlled trials. JAMA 1988;260:1910–1916.91.

108. Antman EM, Berlin JA. Declining incidence of ventricular fibrillation in myocardial infarction: Implications for the prophylactic use of lidocaine. Circulation 1992; 86:764–773.

109. Horner SM. Efficacy of intravenous magnesium in acute myocardial infarction in reducing arrhythmias and mortality: Meta-analysis of magnesium in acute myocardial infarction. Circulation 1992;86:774–779.

110. Woods KL, Fletcher S, Roffe C, Haider Y. A randomized trial of intravenous magnesium sulfate in suspected acute myocardial infarction: Results of the second Leicester Intravenous Magnesium Intervention Trial (LIMIT-2). Lancet 1992;339:1553–1558.

111. Sleight P. Vasodilators after myocardial infarction: ISIS IV. Am J Hypertens 1994;7:1025–1055.

112. Brown CG, Martin DR, Pepe PE, et al. A comparison of standard-dose and high dose epinephrine in cardiac arrest outside the hospital. N Engl J Med 1992;327:1051–1055.

113. Wenzel V, Krismer AC, Arnz R, et al. A comparison of vasopressin and epinephrine for out-of-hospital cardiopulmonary resuscitation. N Engl J Med 2004;350:105–113.

114. Kudenchuk PJ, Cobb LA, Copass MK, et al. Amiodarone for resuscitation after out-of-hospital cardiac arrest due to ventricular fibrillation. N Engl J Med 1999;341:871–878.

115. Dorian P, Schwartz B, Cooper R, et al. Amiodarone as compared with lidocaine for shock-resistant ventricular fibrillation. N Engl J Med 2002; 346:884–890.

116. Talano JV, Euler D, Randall WC, et al. Sinus node dysfunction: An overview with emphasis on autonomic and pharmacologic consideration. Am J Med 1978;64:773–781.

117. Sneddon JF, Camm AJ. Sinus node disease: Current concepts in diagnosis and therapy. Drugs 1992;44:728–737.

118. Sugrue DD, Gersh BJ, Holmes DR, et al. Symptomatic "isolated" carotid sinus hypersensitivity: Natural history and results of treatment with anticholinergic drugs or pacemaker. J Am Coll Cardiol 1986;7: 158–162.

119. Strasberg B, Sagie A, Erdman S, et al. Carotid sinus hypersensitivity and the carotid sinus syndrome. Prog Cardiovasc Dis 1989;31:379–391.

120. Milstein S, Reyes WJ, Benditt DG. Upright body tilt for evaluation of patients with recurrent, unexplained syncope. PACE 1989;12: 117–124.

121. Almquist A, Goldenberg I, Milstein S. Provocation of bradycardia and hypotension by isoproterenol and upright posture in patients with unexplained syncope. N Engl J Med 1990;320:346–351.

122. Somers VK, Abboud FM. Neurocardiogenic syncope. Adv Intern Med 1996;41:399–435.

123. Sra JS, Vishnubhakta S, Murthy S, et al. Use of intravenous esmolol to predict efficacy of oral beta-adrenergic blocker therapy in patients with neurocardiogenic syncope. J Am Coll Cardiol 1992;19:402–408.

124. Zagga M, Massumi A. Neurally mediated syncope. Tex Heart Inst J 2000; 27:268–272.

125. Kupersmith J, Holmes-Novner M, Hogan A, et al. Cost-effectiveness analysis in heart disease: I. General principles. Prog Cardiovasc Dis 1994; 37:161–184.

126. Kupersmith J, Holmes-Novner M, Hogan A, et al. Cost-effectiveness analysis in heart disease: III: Ischemia, congestive heart failure, and arrhythmias. Prog Cardiovasc Dis 1995;37:307–346.

18

DIASTOLIC HEART FAILURE AND THE CARDIOMYOPATHIES

Jean M. Nappi and Michael R. Zile

Learning Objectives and other resources can be found at *www.pharmacotherapyonline.com.*

KEY CONCEPTS

1 Diastolic heart failure is a frequent cause of congestive heart failure (prevalence 35% to 50%) and has a significant effect on mortality (25% to 35% 5-year mortality rate) and morbidity (50% 1-year readmission rate).

2 Hypertension is a common cause of diastolic heart failure.

3 The diagnosis of diastolic heart failure can be made when a patient has (1) both symptoms and signs on physical examination of congestive heart failure and (2) preserved left ventricular (LV) function.

4 Treatment should be targeted at symptom reduction, causal clinical disease, and underlying basic mechanisms. Patients with diastolic heart failure may be treated differently than those with systolic dysfunction.

5 Symptom-targeted therapy includes decreasing pulmonary venous pressure, maintaining atrial contraction and atrioventricular (AV) synchrony, and reducing heart rate. Exercise tolerance is increased by reducing exercise-induced increases in blood pressure and heart rate.

6 Disease-targeted therapy includes preventing or treating myocardial ischemia and preventing or regressing LV hypertrophy.

7 Future directions may include modifying neurohumoral activation, inhibiting endothelin, and altering intracellular mechanisms and extracellular matrix structures.

8 Treatment strategies for patients with hypertrophic cardiomyopathy (HCM) are aimed at improving symptoms and preventing sudden cardiac death.

9 Patients with hypertrophic cardiomyopathy (HCM) who are at high risk for sudden cardiac death should receive an implantable cardioverter-defibrillator (ICD).

10 Patients with HCM who are symptomatic may benefit from β-blockade or verapamil.

11 Antibiotic prophylaxis for endocarditis is appropriate for HCM patients with evidence of outflow obstruction.

DIASTOLIC HEART FAILURE

Heart failure (HF) may be caused by a primary abnormality in systolic function, diastolic function, or both. Making the distinction is important because the prevalence, prognosis, and treatment of HF may be quite different depending on whether the predominant mechanism causing the symptoms is systolic or diastolic dysfunction. Some clinical studies have reported that as many as 30% to 50% of patients with congestive heart failure have preserved left ventricular (LV) function, making diastolic heart failure (DHF) very common.[1] In addition, abnormalities in diastolic function also can play an important role in the development of symptoms in patients with cardiomyopathy and systolic heart failure (SHF).

DHF can be defined as a condition in which myocardial relaxation and filling are impaired and incomplete. The ventricle is unable to accept an adequate volume of blood from the venous system, does not fill at low pressure, and/or is unable to maintain normal stroke volume. In its most severe form, DHF results in overt symptoms of congestive heart failure (CHF). In modest DHF, symptoms of dyspnea

and fatigue occur only during stress or activity, when heart rate and/or end-diastolic volume increase. In its mildest form, DHF can be manifested as a slow or delayed pattern of relaxation and filling with little or no elevation in diastolic pressure and few or no cardiac symptoms. The congestive symptoms that occur with DHF are a manifestation of increased pulmonary venous pressures. DHF is caused by impaired myocardial relaxation and/or increased diastolic stiffness. When CHF is caused by a predominant abnormality in diastolic function, the ventricular chamber is not enlarged, and the ejection fraction (EF) is normal.[2] Figure 18–1 demonstrates the pressure-volume relationship in a patient with normal versus abnormal diastolic function. Changes in the myocardium are associated with a shift upward and to the left of the pressure-volume curve so that for any increase in LV volume, diastolic pressure rises to a much greater level than normally would occur. Clinically, patients present with reduced exercise tolerance and dyspnea when they have elevated LV diastolic pressures. Patients with DHF have a predominant abnormality in diastolic function, whereas patients with SHF have a predominant abnormality in systolic function of the left ventricle.[3]

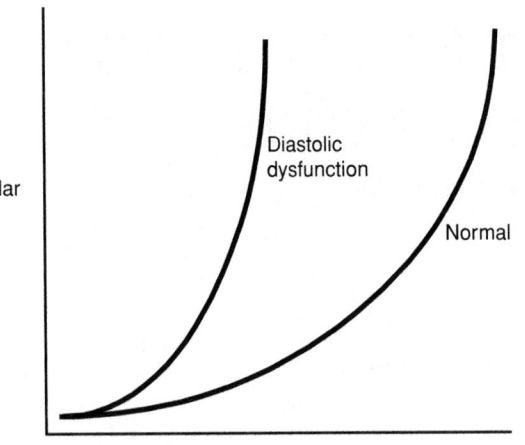

FIGURE 18–1. The diastolic pressure-volume relationship in a normal patient (*right*) and a patient with diastolic dysfunction (*left*).

EPIDEMIOLOGY

Recent studies suggest that as many as one-third to one-half of patients presenting with overt CHF have a preserved EF.[4,5] The prevalence of DHF depends on a number of determinants: patient age, patient gender, study design, the particular population under consideration, and EF. It is important to recognize that these determinants are not independent but interdependent. The most important determinant appears to be patient age. DHF is relatively uncommon in young and middle-aged patients. The prevalence of DHF increases with age, approximating 15% in patients younger than 60 years of age, 35% in patients between 60 and 70 years of age, and 50% in patients over 70 years of age. Prospective community-based studies showed that in patients over 70 years of age, the prevalence of DHF approaches 50%.[6,7]

ETIOLOGY

Several disorders can impair ventricular function and play a role in the development of DHF. DHF is seen often in patients with hypertension, coronary artery disease (CAD), valvular heart disease, and hypertrophic cardiomyopathies. Hypertension is the most common underlying cardiovascular disorder in patients with DHF.[1] There are several proposed mechanisms by which hypertension may impair diastolic function. Hypertension can alter diastolic function through its effects on (1) wall tension, (2) myocardial hypertrophy and fibrosis, and (3) small vessel structure and function, and (4) by predisposing to epicardial CAD. An association between impaired LV filling and subnormal high-energy phosphate metabolism has been shown in hypertensive patients, even in the absence of left ventricular hypertrophy (LVH).[8]

LVH plays a central role in the adaptation of the myocardium to pressure overload. Severe and long-standing pressure overload has been associated with phenotypic alterations at the myocyte level, which differs from the physiologic hypertrophy seen in athletes.[9] Long-term chronic pressure overload stimulates cardiac growth and collagen production, which lead to an increase in myocardial mass and structural remodeling. The results of these changes are an increase in myocardial stiffness and a decrease in diastolic filling.

Diastolic dysfunction has been reported to be present in 90% of patients with CAD.[9] Patients with CAD, such as (1) patients with

exercise-induced ischemia but normal function at rest, (2) patients with myocardial stunning, and (3) patients with previous myocardial infarction (MI), all may exhibit signs of diastolic dysfunction.

PATHOPHYSIOLOGY

The pathologic disease processes that cause DHF include myocardial ischemia with or without epicardial CAD, pressure overload hypertrophy, and genetic hypertrophy. Hypertrophy consequent to the physiologic adaptation to pregnancy, hypertrophy that occurs in athletes, and volume-overload hypertrophy do not cause abnormalities in diastolic function and do not result in the development of DHF.

Hypertrophic cardiomyopathy (HCM) is a prototype for DHF. The grossly thickened myocardium, structural changes, and interstitial fibrosis severely alter the passive elastic properties of the myocardium. Patients with HCM and LV outflow obstruction are sensitive to small changes in volume such that a small decrease in filling pressure can lead to a decrease in LV end-diastolic volume and a dramatic fall in stroke volume and cardiac output.

The basic mechanisms by which pressure-overload hypertrophy and genetic hypertrophy cause DHF include extramyocardial factors and factors intrinsic to the myocardium, which include changes in the cardiac muscle cell and in the extracellular matrix that surrounds the cardiomyocyte[2,10,11] (Table 18–1). Intracellular processes such as changes in calcium homeostasis, contractile and noncontractile proteins, energetics, and the cytoskeleton contribute to abnormalities in myocardial relaxation and stiffness. Changes in the extracellular matrix, particularly changes in fibrillar collagen, alter relaxation and stiffness. In addition to the cardiomyocyte and the extracellular matrix, local myocardial neuroendocrine activation can impair relaxation and increase stiffness. Activation of neurohormones such as the renin-angiotensin-aldosterone system may act directly to alter diastolic properties or act indirectly by altering calcium homeostasis. Finally, extramyocardial changes in loading conditions and changes in heterogeneity occur in hypertrophied ventricles and contribute to changes in relaxation and stiffness so that even when the myocardium itself is normal, changes in these extramyocardial factors can cause abnormalities in diastolic function.[12]

Myocardial ischemia, particularly in the subendocardial region, is common when ventricular hypertrophy is present. Slow or delayed myocardial relaxation and perivascular fibrosis can affect coronary blood flow and coronary blood flow reserve adversely. This may contribute to the development of myocardial ischemia and sudden death.[5,13] Therefore, myocardial ischemia may be part of clinical syndrome of DHF even if there is no epicardial CAD.

Endothelial dysfunction is associated with the progression of myocardial diastolic dysfunction in patients with CAD.[14] Both in the acute manifestation of myocardial ischemia and within the chronic consequences of myocardial fibrosis, epicardial CAD is frequently the underlying pathologic cause of DHF.[9,15,16] Myocardial ischemia caused either by an acute decrease in supply or an increase in demand (exercise and tachycardia) results in impaired relaxation and an acute increase in myocardial stiffness.[16] Chronic coronary occlusions may result in myocardial fibrosis, remodeling, and DHF. It is clear that the same basic mechanisms causing diastolic dysfunction in the presence of pressure-overload hypertrophy also underlie changes produced by CAD.

DIAGNOSIS

 The criteria used to make the diagnosis of DHF remain controversial. However, making the diagnosis accurately is extremely

TABLE 18–1. Potential Pathologic Mechanisms of Diastolic Heart Failure

Mechanisms Directly Affecting Myocardial Tissue

Cardiomyocyte	Increase in intracellular calcium, producing calcium overload
	Myofilaments
	Increased troponin-C calcium binding and increased myofilament calcium sensitivity
	Cytoskeleton
	Changes in cytoskeletal proteins
	Energetics
	Decrease in ATP availability, leading to a decreased rate or extent of actomyosin dissociation
Extracellular matrix	Increased content of fibrillar collagen
	Thickening of existing fibrillar collagen
	Decreased MMP and/or increased TIMP
Neurohormones	Increased renin-angiotensin-aldosterone
	Increased endothelin
Extramyocardial Mechanisms	
Increased hemodynamic load: preload or afterload	
Increased heterogeneity	
Systemic neurohormones	Increased levels of angiotensin II
Pericardium	The pericardium may have a constraining effect as LV filling pressure and end-diastolic volume increase.

MMP = matrix metalloproteinase; TIMP = tissue inhibitor of MMP; LV = left ventricular.

important. Guidelines from the European Society of Cardiology propose that three requirements must be present to make the diagnosis of DHF: (1) symptoms or signs of CHF, (2) normal systolic function, and (3) abnormal diastolic function (e.g., abnormal relaxation, filling, distensibility, or stiffness).[17] The first two requirements appear to be well justified; the third requirement may not be.[3]

CLINICAL PRESENTATION: DIASTOLIC HEART FAILURE

SYMPTOMS

- Exertional dyspnea
- Orthopnea
- Exercise intolerance

SIGNS

- Pulmonary congestion (rales)
- Exaggerated rise in blood pressure and heart rate in response to exercise

ECHOCARDIOGRAPHY OR CATHETERIZATION

- Normal (or increased) ejection fraction
- Normal (or decreased) cardiac output
- Increased LV pressure
- Pulmonary venous hypertension
- LV hypertrophy and/or concentric remodeling
- Abnormal LV relaxation and increased LV chamber stiffness

LABORATORY TESTS

- Increased BNP levels

Vasan and Levy proposed criteria for DHF according to the degree of diagnostic certainty.[18] Three conditions would be met for a definite diagnosis of DHF: (1) definitive evidence of CHF, (2) objective evidence of normal LV systolic function within 72 hours of a CHF event, and (3) objective evidence of LV diastolic dysfunction. If the third criterion is lacking, then the patient would have *probable* DHF. If the objective evidence for normal systolic function is not apparent at the time of the CHF event and there is no conclusive information on LV dysfunction, then the patient would be classified as having *possible* DHF.

With few exceptions, DHF cannot be distinguished from SHF on the basis of the history, physical examination, chest x-ray, and electrocardiogram (ECG) alone. The frequency with which patients have symptoms of HF and signs of HF on physical examination or chest x-ray is not dependent on whether they have SHF or DHF.[5] Patients with DHF are often elderly, hypertensive females.[19] In one study, patients with DHF had a higher prevalence of hypertension with higher systolic, diastolic, and pulse pressures when compared with control patients and patients with SHF.[20]

The data from a number of studies demonstrate that signs and symptoms of CHF do not predict EF. In contrast, they do predict the presence of increased LV diastolic pressure. The question then becomes whether the increase in LV diastolic pressure occurs in association with normal LV volume and EF, as would occur in DHF, or whether the increase in LV diastolic pressure occurs in association with an increased LV volume and decreased EF, as would occur with SHF. Therefore, determining whether CHF is caused by systolic or diastolic dysfunction requires some estimate of LV size and EF. These measurements can be made using echocardiography, radionuclide ventriculography, or contrast ventriculography. When a patient presents with dyspnea, pulmonary rales, and radiographic evidence of pulmonary venous hypertension, the detection of normal LV end-diastolic volume and normal EF supports the diagnosis of DHF. Conditions such as mitral stenosis, pulmonary disease, sleep apnea, anemia, cirrhosis, hypothyroidism, and drug-induced fluid retention must be ruled out because they can cause similar symptoms.[21]

B-type natriuretic peptide (BNP) is a cardiac neurohormone secreted from the myocardium in response to increases in ventricular volume and pressure. It is used frequently as an aid in the differential diagnosis of dyspnea. The Breathing Not Properly study evaluated 452 patients with echocardiography within 30 days of an emergency department visit. Of those 452 patients, 165 (36.5%) had an EF greater than 45% (mean EF 59%).[22] In these patients with preserved EF who had been admitted to the hospital for dyspnea, BNP levels were significantly lower than those found in patients with SHF (413 versus 821 pg/mL). However, there was considerable overlap in the BNP levels in patients with DHF compared with those without HF, making BNP levels less useful. Furthermore, the sensitivity, specificity, and predictive accuracy of BNP levels in DHF are limited in part because BNP is altered by age, gender, and other factors.

PROGNOSIS

The prognosis in patients with DHF, although less ominous than in patients with SHF, is worse than that of age-matched control patients.

The 5-year mortality of patients with DHF approximates 25%, although mortality rates as high as 13% over a 6-month period have been reported.[4,23,24] In comparison, the annual mortality of patients with SHF approximates 10% to 15%, whereas age-matched control mortality approaches 1%. In patients with DHF, the prognosis is also affected by the clinical pathologic etiology causing the disease. When patients with CAD are excluded, the annual mortality for DHF approximates 2% to 3%.[6] In addition to the clinical pathologic etiology causing CHF, another important determinant of mortality is age. In patients older than 70 years of age, the mortality rates for DHF and SHF are similar.[6] Of note, non-Caucasian patients with DHF may have a higher mortality rate than Caucasian patients.[23]

The mode of death appears similar in patients with systolic versus diastolic HF. Sudden death and death from progressive pump failure occurred with equal frequency in systolic versus diastolic HF patients. Morbidity from DHF is quite high, requiring frequent outpatient visits, hospital admissions, and the expenditure of significant health care resources. The 1-year readmission rate approaches 50% in patients with DHF. This morbidity rate is nearly identical to that of patients with SHF.[4,25]

▶ TREATMENT: Diastolic Heart Failure

The general principles used to guide the treatment of SHF are based on numerous large, randomized, double-blind, multicenter trials. Until recently, no such randomized trials had been performed in patients with DHF. Consequently, the guidelines for the management of DHF are based primarily on clinical investigations in relatively small groups of patients, clinical experience, and concepts based on the knowledge and understanding of the pathophysiology of the disease process. The treatment regimen outlined below (Table 18–2) applies to patients with DHF who have clear manifestations of congestion either at rest or with exertion. Whether treatment of asymptomatic diastolic dysfunction confers any benefit has not been examined.

■ DESIRED OUTCOME

Treatment should be targeted at reducing symptoms, principally those of increased pulmonary venous pressure. Treatment should include decreasing diastolic pressure by decreasing LV volume, maintaining atrial contraction, and reducing heart rate. If symptoms are controlled, the need for hospitalization is reduced. Second, treatment should be targeted at the pathologic diseases that cause DHF. For example, CAD, hypertensive heart disease, and aortic stenosis provide relatively specific therapeutic targets, such as lowering blood

TABLE 18–2. General Approach to Treatment of Diastolic Heart Failure

Symptom-Targeted Treatment		
Decrease pulmonary venous pressure	Reduce left ventricular volume	Diuretics, salt restriction
	Maintain atrial contraction	Cardioversion of atrial fibrillation
	Reduce heart rate	β-Blockers, diltiazem, verapamil
Improve exercise tolerance	As above	
Use positive inotropic agents with caution		
Disease-Targeted Treatment		
Prevent/treat myocardial ischemia		β-Blockers, diltiazem, verapamil, nitrates
Prevent/regress ventricular hypertrophy		Antihypertensive therapy
Mechanism-Targeted Treatment		
Modify myocardial and extramyocardial mechanisms		Possibly ACE inhibitors or ARBs, diuretics, spironolactone
Modify intracellular and extracellular mechanisms		Possibly ACE inhibitors or ARBs, spironolactone

ACE = angiotensin-converting enzyme; ARBs = angiotensin-receptor blockers.

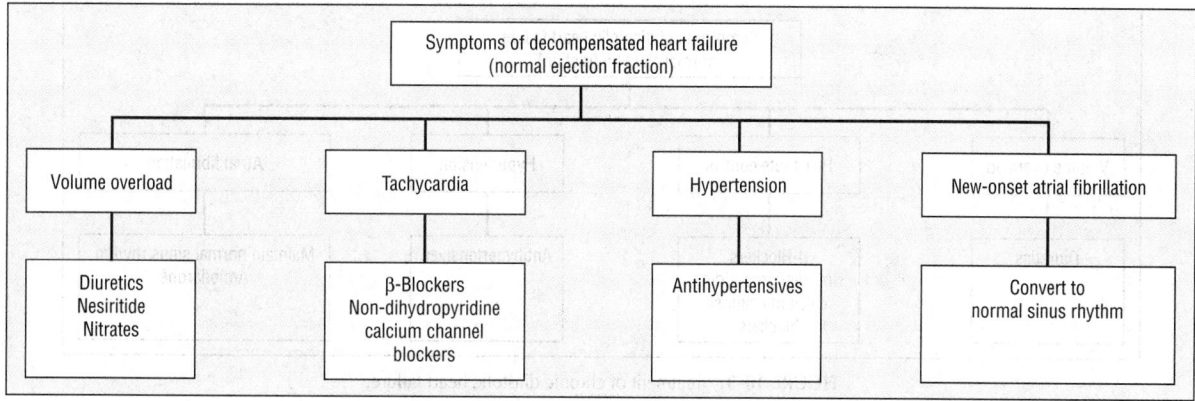

FIGURE 18–2. Treatment of acute decompensated diastolic heart failure.

pressure, inducing LVH regression, performing aortic valve replacement, and treating ischemia by increasing myocardial blood flow and reducing myocardial oxygen demand. Third, treatment should be targeted at the underlying mechanisms that are altered by the disease processes just mentioned.[26]

NONPHARMACOLOGIC THERAPY

DIET AND LIFESTYLE

The initial effort in the treatment of DHF is aimed at decreasing symptoms. The first step in this effort is to decrease pulmonary congestion by decreasing LV volume using sodium and fluid restriction. A low-sodium diet (<2 g/day) and moderate fluid restriction will help to prevent volume overload. Both sodium and fluid restriction must be done with care. Excessive restriction can lead to hypotension, low-output state, and/or renal insufficiency. Daily weights may help to assess volume status. Dietary and lifestyle factors that decrease the risk of development of epicardial CAD and high blood pressure should be encouraged.

EXERCISE

Moderate aerobic exercise to improve cardiovascular conditioning is beneficial to maintain a slower heart rate, improve cardiac reserve, and maintain skeletal muscle function. Isometric exercise should be avoided.[27]

INTERVENTIONAL/SURGICAL PROCEDURES

An important step in symptom-targeted therapy that acts to decrease pulmonary venous pressures is to maintain atrial contraction and atrioventricular (AV) synchrony. Maintaining atrial contraction and AV synchrony is important both in preserving normal cardiac output and in keeping LV diastolic pressure low. Chemical or electrical cardioversion of persistent atrial tachyarrhythmias will decrease diastolic pressure, increase cardiac output, and resolve pulmonary edema. An AV sequential pacemaker should be used to treat bradyarrhythmias in patients requiring pacing.

Therapy also should be aimed at preventing or treating the underlying pathologic cause of DHF. Aortic valve replacement should be performed in symptomatic patients with pressure-overload

hypertrophy caused by aortic stenosis. Revascularization should be performed in selected patients with DHF caused by CAD-induced myocardial ischemia. In addition, myocardial oxygen consumption and myocardial blood flow should be increased using medical treatment, including nitrates, β-blockers, and calcium channel blockers.

INDICATIONS FOR HOSPITALIZATION

Patients with DHF may present with an acute onset of pulmonary edema. There are a number of potential causes for the acute decompensation of these patients, including: volume overload, uncontrolled hypertension, acute myocardial ischemia, progressive valvular disease (aortic stenosis), and new-onset or uncontrolled tachyarrhythmias. Treatment strategies for these patients eventually may include the need for surgery, as in the case of valvular disease.

The initial management focuses on relieving pulmonary congestion and maintaining oxygenation (Fig. 18–2). Intravenous diuretic agents and nesiritide for patients are effective for volume overload. Caution must be exercised to avoid overdiuresis or an excessive lowering of LV end-diastolic volume, which can lead to a decrease in stroke volume. Morphine and nitroglycerin also are effective in reducing LV end-diastolic pressure.[28]

A study involving patients who required emergency treatment for pulmonary edema assessed the association of clinical findings with prognosis or outcome.[29] In this study of 186 patients, 40% had no recognized precipitating factor identified for their hospitalization. Patients who responded to diuretic therapy with a good urine output had a better outcome than patients who did not respond as well. This study did not examine whether prognosis was related to the presence of systolic or diastolic heart failure. Based on this information, diuretics are appropriate first-line therapeutic agents for acute decompensation and pulmonary edema.

PHARMACOLOGIC TREATMENT

DRUG TREATMENTS OF FIRST CHOICE

With a few notable exceptions, many of the drugs used to treat systolic heart failure are in fact the same as those used to treat DHF (Fig. 18–3). However, the rationale for their use, the pathophysiologic process that is being altered by the drug, and the dosing regimen may be entirely different depending on whether the patient has systolic or diastolic

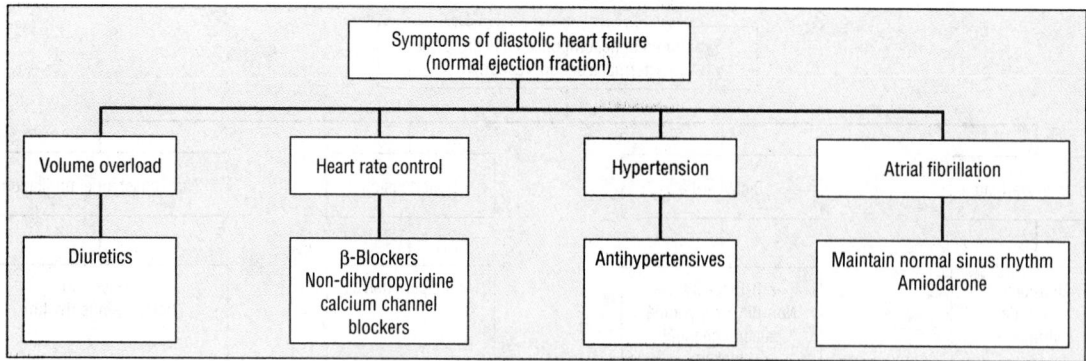

FIGURE 18–3. Treatment of chronic diastolic heart failure.

HF. For example, β-blockers are recommended for the treatment of both SHF and DHF. In DHF however, β-blockers are used to decrease heart rate, increase diastolic duration, and modify the hemodynamic response to exercise. In SHF, β-blockers are used in the long run to increase inotropic state and modify LV remodeling. Diuretics also are used in the treatment of both SHF and DHF. However, the doses of diuretics used to treat DHF are in general much smaller than the dose used in SHF. Antagonists of the renin-angiotensin-aldosterone system are useful in lowering blood pressure and reducing LVH. Some drugs, however, are used only to treat either SHF or DHF but not both. Calcium channel blockers such as diltiazem, nifedipine, and verapamil have little utility in the treatment of SHF. In contrast, each of these has been proposed as being useful in the treatment of DHF.

PUBLISHED GUIDELINES

In 2001, the American College of Cardiology and the American Heart Association released a revision to the 1995 guidelines for the evaluation and management of heart failure.[30] In general, the guidelines recommend treating comorbid conditions by controlling heart rate and blood pressure, alleviating causes of myocardial ischemia, and reducing volume.

GENERAL INFORMATION

Although dozens of trials evaluating pharmacologic therapy have been conducted in patients with SHF, there are few trials focusing on patients with isolated DHF. In fact, most published HF trials have specifically excluded patients with a preserved EF. There are a few published studies and several trials underway that are examining various agents in the treatment of DHF. With these studies and others that are currently under development, an effective treatment for DHF will be defined more completely.

There were almost 1000 patients with EF greater than 45% in the Digitalis Investigation Group (DIG) trial who were randomized to either digoxin or placebo.[25] After 37 months of follow-up, the mortality rate was identical in each group (23.4%). There was no statistically significant difference in the combined end point of death or hospitalization owing to worsening HF in the DHF patients who were receving digoxin (risk ratio 0.82; 95% confidence interval 0.63–1.07). In contrast, in patients with SHF, digoxin reduced hospitalization owing to worsening heart failure by 28% ($p < .001$).

The CHARM-Preserved trial was one of three studies evaluating the use of candesartan in heart failure. The CHARM-Preserved

trial investigated the effects of candesartan, an angiotensin-receptor blocker (ARB), versus placebo in over 3000 patients with New York Heart Association (NYHA) functional class II–IV symptoms of HF and an EF of greater than 40%.[31] The two groups were well matched for medical treatment at the times of randomization. Candesartan had no effect on mortality in the patients with DHF. On the composite end point of cardiovascular death or hospitalization for worsening HF, there was a 14% relative risk reduction ($p = .051$) using an adjusted hazards ratio. Hospital readmissions for CHF were reduced by 16% ($p = .047$) using an adjusted hazards ratio. The data were analyzed by intention to treat, and it should be noted that by the end of the study, 22% of the candesartan-treated patients had discontinued the medication. As expected, there were more adverse events (e.g., hypotension, hyperkalemia, and increase in serum creatinine concentration) in the candesartan group. Interestingly, there was a significant reduction in the number developing diabetes in the patients receiving candesartan. It appears that for a cardiovascular patient with DHF, the addition of candesartan to a typical medical regimen including angiotensin-converting enzyme (ACE) inhibitors, β-blockers, diuretics, digoxin, and calcium channel blockers provides a modest reduction in the need for hospitalization owing to worsening HF.

ALTERNATIVE DRUG TREATMENT

As a result of the controversy regarding the diagnosis of DHF, the development and design of large clinical trials have been hindered. At this point in time, most antihypertensive agents would be acceptable forms of therapy for hypertensive heart disease, with the exception of α-blockers (e.g., doxasosin). In the Antihypertensive and Lipid-Lowering Treatment to Prevent Heart Attack Trial (ALLHAT), the doxazosin treatment arm was dropped because patients randomized to doxazosin had an increased risk of developing HF and stroke when compared with the chlorthalidone arm.[32]

SPECIAL POPULATIONS

DHF is associated with hypertension and aging, making it a common diagnosis in elderly Caucasian women. Since these women are often frail, with low muscle mass, their creatinine clearance and renal function may be compromised. Special care must be taken in selecting and titrating doses of drugs, as well as in monitoring serum creatinine and electrolytes, when using diuretics, ACE inhibitors, and ARBs.

Diabetes is often a comorbid condition in patients with HF. Since the thiazolidinediones (pioglitazone and rosiglitazone) are associated with fluid retention, caution is warranted when initiating these drugs in patients with a history of DHF. Thiazolidinediones should be discontinued in patients with symptoms related to volume overload.

DRUG CLASS INFORMATION

DIURETICS

Diuretics can provide symptom-targeted therapy by acting to decrease systemic and LV volume. By decreasing LV diastolic volumes, LV pressures slide down the curvilinear diastolic pressure-volume relationship toward a lower, less steep portion of the curve. As pressure throughout diastole falls, mean diastolic pressure, pulmonary capillary wedge pressure, and pulmonary venous pressure fall. These agents effectively reduce the central blood volume, lower diastolic pressures, and thus alleviate the symptoms of the congestive state. Diuretics can provide disease-targeted therapy by decreasing blood pressure and favorably affecting the myocardial oxygen supply-versus-demand ratio. Lower LV diastolic pressures may increase subendocardial blood flow, preventing or alleviating the imbalance between myocardial oxygen supply and demand (see Fig. 18–1). Diuretics alone and especially in combination with other antihypertensive drugs are an effective approach to therapy.

Treatment with diuretics should be initiated at low doses in order to avoid hypotension and fatigue. Hypotension can be a significant problem in the treatment of DHF because these patients have a very steep LV diastolic pressure-volume curve such that a small change in volume causes a large change in filling pressure and cardiac output. After the acute treatment of DHF has been completed, long-term treatment should include small to moderate doses of diuretics (furosemide 20 to 40 mg/day orally or hydrochlorothiazide 25 mg/day orally). If prompt and sustained diuresis is not achieved, the dosage of a single diuretic should be increased, or a loop and thiazide or thiazide-like diuretic should be used in combination. Aldosterone antagonists such as spironolactone and eplerenone may be especially effective in long-term use because of their potassium-sparing effects and because their antagonism of renin-angiotensin-aldosterone system activation may alter intra- and extramyocardial mechanisms causing abnormalities in diastolic function.[33] Thiazide diuretics generally are ineffective in patients with a creatinine clearance of less than 30 mL/min.

Excessive diuresis may result in hypotension, low-output syndrome, and worsening renal insufficiency. In some cases, loop diuretics may be withdrawn safely from elderly patients without any worsening of HF symptoms and with improvement in symptoms of orthostatic hypotension.[34] Electrolyte imbalances, including hypokalemia and hypomagnesemia, are common with diuretics. Carbohydrate intolerance and hyperuricemia are dose-related adverse drug reactions seen with thiazide diuretics. Spironolactone can cause hyperkalemia and gynecomastia. Eplerenone may be used as an alternative to spironolactone in patients who complain of gynescomastia. In general, diuretic agents are very cost-effective agents in the management of DHF.

NITRATES

Similar to diuretics, nitrates can provide symptom-targeted therapy by acting to decrease LV volume by increasing venous capacitance. In addition, nitrates can provide disease-targeted therapy by providing anti-ischemic effects in patients with DHF owing to CAD.

Like diuretics, therapy should be initiated at low doses in order to avoid hypotension. Isosorbide dinitrate 10 mg three or four times daily, isosorbide mononitrate (Imdur) 30 mg/day, nitroglycerin paste 1/2 to 1 inch every 4 to 6 hours, and nitroglycerin patch 0.1 to 0.2 mg/h applied each day are common initial doses. Doses can be increased during long-term therapy and titrated against symptoms. Nitrate tolerance has not been studied in this patient population but probably occurs. Similar to diuretics, nitrates can cause hypotension and a low-output syndrome. Headaches are common but may be less frequent with continued use.

Sublingual nitroglycerin tablets or nitroglycerin spray may be used for patients who develop shortness of breath with mild exercise, and they may be used much in the same way as in patients with ischemic symptoms. Nitroglycerin will decrease LV end-diastolic volume resulting in relief of breathlessness.

β-ADRENERGIC BLOCKERS

β-Blockers can provide symptom-targeted therapy by decreasing heart rate and can provide disease-targeted therapy by treating high blood pressure and CAD. By decreasing heart rate and increasing the duration of diastole, β-blockers can help to lower and maintain low pulmonary venous pressures. Tachycardia is poorly tolerated in patients with DHF for several reasons. First, rapid heart rates cause an increase in myocardial oxygen demand and a decrease in coronary perfusion time. This rapid rate can promote ischemic diastolic dysfunction even in the absence of epicardial CAD, especially in patients with LVH. Second, there may be incomplete relaxation between cardiac cycles, resulting in an increase in diastolic pressure relative to volume. Thus LV distensibility is reduced. Third, a rapid rate reduces diastolic filling time and ventricular filling. Fourth, hearts with diastolic dysfunction exhibit a flat or even negative relaxation rate versus frequency relationship. Thus, as heart rate increases in these hearts, relaxation does not become augmented and may become slower and incomplete, causing diastolic pressures, especially early in diastole, to increase.[26] For these and other reasons, most clinicians use β-blockers (and calcium channel blockers) to prevent excessive tachycardia and produce a relative bradycardia in patients with diastolic dysfunction. However, excessive bradycardia can result in a fall of cardiac output despite an increase in LV filling. Such considerations underscore the need for individualizing therapeutic interventions that affect heart rate. While the optimal heart rate must be individualized, an initial goal might be a resting heart rate of approximately 60 beats per minute with a blunted exercise-induced increase in heart rate not to exceed 110 beats per minute.[26]

There is no evidence to suggest that there is a specific therapeutic advantage to one β-blocker over another. Selective and nonselective β-blockers appear equally effective in DHF. β-Blockers with intrinsic sympathomimetic activity (ISA) may be less effective because they slow the heart rate less. In general, it is not necessary to start the drug at an extremely low dose and titrate the β-blocker in a slow, progressive fashion in DHF, as it is in SHF. Since the population is older, it is prudent to start with a moderate dose of β-blockers, such as metoprolol 25 mg twice daily or atenolol 25 mg/day and titrate to a higher dose with a treatment target of a heart rate of approximately 60 beats per minute.

Prinzmetal's vasospastic angina, bronchospastic chronic obstructive pulmonary disease (COPD), asthma, occlusive peripheral vascular disease, type I diabetes mellitus that is prone to hypoglycemia, heart block, and excessive bradycardia are contraindications to β-blockers. The main side effects of β-blockers are depression, fatigue, bradycardia, bronchospasm, and impotence. Many of the β-blockers are eliminated via hepatic metabolism and may be affected by other drugs that either inhibit (e.g., cimetidine and verapamil) or enhance (e.g., barbiturates) hepatic enzymes. Since the doses are titrated to patient response, these interactions are managed easily. Several β-blockers (e.g., propranolol, metoprolol, atenolol, nadolol, and timolol) are available as generic formulations, making them very cost-effective.

CALCIUM CHANNEL BLOCKERS (CCBs)

CCBs can provide symptom-targeted treatment by decreasing heart rate and increasing exercise tolerance. They can provide disease-targeted treatment by treating high blood pressure and CAD. However, the beneficial effect of these agents on exercise tolerance is not always paralleled by improved LV diastolic function or increased relaxation rate.[26] Nonetheless, a number of small clinical trials have shown that the use of these agents results in both short- and long-term improvement in exercise capacity in patients with DHF.[35]

Of the CCBs, the nondihydropyradines (verapamil and diltiazem) are the most effective because they lower heart rate in addition to lowering blood pressure.[36] Nifedipine, because of its strong vasodilator properties, tends to cause hypotension and reflex tachycardia. In addition, nifedipine causes peripheral edema. These characteristics make it less useful in DHF. Amlodipine is also effective because it reduces blood pressure. Initial doses are verapamil 120 to 240 mg/day, diltiazem 90 to 120 mg/day, and amlodipine 2.5 mg/day.

Heart block is a contraindication for the nondihydropyridines. The most common side effects are bradycardia and heart block (for the nondihydropyridines). Peripheral edema and headache are also common. Nondihydropyridines exacerbate bradycardic effects of β-blockers, and verapamil raises digoxin serum concentrations by 70%. Diltiazem raises cyclosporine serum concentrations. Intravenous calcium salts inhibit the pharmacologic effect of CCBs. Generic formulations or similar products, but not necessarily generic equivalents to the original brand names, are available for verapamil, nifedipine, and diltiazem.

NEUROHUMORAL ANTAGONISTS

Both basic and clinical studies suggest that DHF is associated with activation of systemic and local cardiac neuroendocrine systems such as the renin-angiotensin-aldosterone system. One mechanism causing fluid retention and the increases in central and systemic volume in patients with DHF is activation of these neuroendocrine systems. Therefore, treatment for DHF should include agents such as ACE inhibitors, ARBs, and aldosterone antagonists that attenuate the fluid retention caused by neuroendocrine activation. In addition to promoting fluid retention, neuroendocrine activation can have direct effects on cellular and extracellular mechanisms that contribute to the development of DHF. Modulation of neuroendocrine activation may provide mechanism-targeted treatment by decreasing fibroblast activity and interstitial fibrosis, improving intracellular calcium handling, and decreasing myocardial stiffness. Finally, renin-angiotensin-aldosterone system antagonists provide disease-targeted treatment by treating hypertension.[26,37]

The mechanisms that evoke activation of the neuroendocrine system remain incompletely understood in patients with DHF. A number of factors have been suggested. Myocardial ischemia, uncontrolled hypertension, and excessive dietary sodium or sodium-retaining medications may contribute to neuroendocrine activation. Limited distensibility of the atria may attenuate the secretion of atrial natriuretic factor and thereby reduce its diuretic effect. In others, low systemic vascular resistance and/or low arterial pressure may contribute to an increase in renin-angiotensin-aldosterone system activation and salt and water retention. Elevated venous pressure may cause renal sodium retention directly. The reduction in blood volume that follows the use of diuretics triggers an increase in sympathetic tone and further activation of the renin-angiotensin-aldosterone system. Such neurohormonal activation can lead to vasoconstriction and a worsening of the congestive state. Some vasodilators, particularly nitrates and pure arteriolar vasodilators, evoke a similar response. By contrast, ACE inhibitors (and β-blockers) blunt neurohormonal activation and decrease the salt and water retention that complicates the treatment of CHF.

ANGIOTENSIN-CONVERTING ENZYME (ACE) INHIBITORS

ACE inhibitors can provide symptom-targeted treatment by decreasing LV volume and directly improving relaxation. They can provide disease-targeted treatment by treating high blood pressure, preventing LVH, promoting regression, and preventing fibrosis. Treatment of high blood pressure with ACE inhibitors has been shown to normalize load, prevent and/or regress LV hypertrophy, correct the abnormality in intracellular processes, and modify the extracellular matrix response.[38] ACE inhibitors may reduce the incidence of HF by 23% among patients with CAD and preserved EF.[39]

A small, prospective, double-blind, randomized trial compared lisinopril with hydrochlorothiazide in 35 patients with primary hypertension, LVH, and LV diastolic dysfunction.[40] After 6 months of therapy, lisinopril caused regression of myocardial fibrosis and improved LV diastolic function, although LVH was unchanged.

At this time, there is no evidence to suggest advantage of one ACE inhibitor over another. Their effects appear to be a class effect. Initial doses should be small to moderate in order to avoid hypotension, especially if the patient examination does not indicate volume overload. Examples of initial starting doses are captopril 6.25 mg three times daily, enalapril 2.5 mg/day, or lisinopril 2.5 mg/day.

Severe renal failure, history of angioedema, and pregnancy are contraindications to ACE inhibitors. Hyperkalemia, persistent cough, hypotension, taste disturbances, and worsening renal function are common side effects but are managed by decreasing the dose or discontinuing the drug.

ANGIOTENSIN-RECEPTOR BLOCKERS (ARBs)

ARBs can provide symptom-targeted treatment by decreasing LV pressure, decreasing LV volume, and increasing exercise tolerance. They can provide disease-targeted treatment by lowering blood pressure. As mentioned previously, the CHARM-Preserved trial showed a reduction in hospitalizations for worsening HF in patients receiving candesartan in addition to usual treatment.[31]

Losartan was evaluated in a randomized, double-blind, placebo-controlled trial in 20 patients with diastolic dysfunction.[41] In this trial, losartan or placebo was added to the current medical regimen for a 2-week period. Patients enrolled in the study had a marked hypertensive response to exercise, an EF of greater than 50%, and no evidence of ischemia on stress echocardiogram. The blood pressure at rest was well controlled (143/79 mm Hg), but the mean peak systolic blood pressure after 11 minutes of exercise was 226 mm Hg. The resting systolic and diastolic blood pressures were not changed with placebo or losartan. However, the peak systolic blood pressure with losartan was reduced to 193 mm Hg compared with placebo (217 mm Hg) and baseline (226 mm Hg). Losartan increased exercise time, NYHA class, and quality of life as assessed by the modified Minnesota Living with Heart Failure Survey.

The specific mechanism of the losartan-induced improvement is not known. However, angiotensin II slows the rate of LV relaxation and increases LV diastolic pressures. In a 2-week period of time, there was no evidence of improved diastolic function. Losartan did slow the increase in systolic blood pressure during exercise and decreased the peak systolic blood pressure by a mean of 33 mm Hg. Although the patients had no evidence of myocardial ischemia, losartan may have improved endothelial function and coronary perfusion.

No ARB has yet been shown to have any major advantage over another. Initial doses of candesartan start at 4 mg/day, irbesartan 150 mg/day, losartan 25 mg/day, telmisartan 40 mg/day, and valsartan 80 mg/day. As with the ACE inhibitors, ARBs are contraindicated in pregnancy. The side effects of ARBs are similar to those of ACE inhibitors, but they are not associated with persistent cough.

ALDOSTERONE ANTAGONISTS

Aldosterone antagonists can provide symptom-targeted treatment by decreasing LV volume. They can provide disease-targeted treatment by decreasing the fibrosis that accompanies LVH. An analysis of the RALES study found that spironolactone significantly decreased the levels of serum markers for cardiac collagen turnover. The benefit from spironolactone was seen in patients with the higher level collagen synthesis markers. This was the first study to show that serum levels of markers of cardiac collagen synthesis were associated with a poor clinical outcome and could be decreased with spironolactone. This property distinguishes spironolactone from other diuretics that have no effect on myocardial necrosis or collagen turnover.

Like other diuretics, spironolactone should be initiated at a low dose and increased to treat symptoms. Spironolactone may be initiated at doses of 12.5 to 25 mg/day. Spironolactone should be avoided in severe renal failure. Hyperkalemia and gynecomastia are the most common side effects. Eplerenone is a viable alternative to spironolactone in patients complaining of sex hormone–related side effects.[33]

POSITIVE INOTROPIC AGENTS

Positive inotropic agents, like β-agonists and phosphodiesterase inhibitors, generally are not used in the treatment of patients with isolated DHF because the LV ejection fraction is preserved and there appears to be little potential for a beneficial effect. Positive inotropic agents have the potential to worsen DHF by adversely affecting energetics, inducing ischemia, raising heart rate, and inducing arrhythmias.[26] In contrast to long-term use, positive inotropic drugs may be beneficial in the short-term treatment of pulmonary edema associated with DHF. These agents can enhance sarcoplasmic reticular function, promote more rapid and complete relaxation, increase splanchnic blood flow, increase venous capacitance, and facilitate diuresis.[26] However, these agents should be used with caution, if they are used at all, because the risk-benefit ratio is not clearly established.

DIGITALIS DERIVATIVES

Digoxin, by inhibiting the Na^+,K^+-potassium-ATPase pump, augments intracellular calcium and thereby augments contractile state. In this manner, digoxin produces an increase in systolic energy demands while adding to a relative calcium overload in diastole. These effects may not be apparent clinically under many circumstances, but during hemodynamic stress or ischemia, digoxin may promote or contribute to diastolic dysfunction.[26] Therefore, until recently, and with the exception of patients with chronic atrial fibrillation (to slow ventricular rate), digoxin was not used in the treatment of DHF. However, results of the DIG trial suggested that even patients with a normal EF may have fewer symptoms and fewer hospitalizations if they are treated with digoxin.[25] This salutary effect was not likely a result of digoxin's effect on inotropy but rather of its blunting of neuroendocrine activation. Others have found that patients treated chronically with digoxin have higher levels of serum markers associated with excessive extracellular matrix turnover.[42] Whether this is due to digoxin or to the condition for which digoxin is being used remains unclear.

PHARMACOECONOMIC CONSIDERATIONS

Frequent admission to the hospital is common in patients with DHF. Unfortunately, there are no pharmacoeconomic data associated with the only large clinical outcome trial (CHARM-Preserved) published to date. Since DHF is primarily a disease of the elderly, comorbid conditions will create challenges in any trial designed. At the present time, cost to the patient should be considered because adherence to an antihypertensive regimen is paramount to a beneficial outcome.

CLINICAL CONTROVERSIES

- Digoxin may not be beneficial in patients with isolated DHF who are in normal sinus rhythm.
- Drugs that antagonize the renin-angiotensin-aldosterone system may be the preferred antihypertensive drugs for patients with DHF.

EVALUATION OF THERAPEUTIC OUTCOMES

The end points used in assessing effective therapies for DHF include mortality, hospitalization for worsening HF, functional status or quality-of-life indicators, and cost. Other end points may target underlying mechanisms of disease, such as calcium homeostasis or regression of fibrosis. A number of clinical trials are underway that will address this important clinical problem.

CARDIOMYOPATHIES

Diastolic dysfunction plays a role in the presentation of some types of cardiomyopathy. The cardiomyopathies represent a variety of diseases affecting the myocardium in either a diffuse or multifocal manner that frequently results in HF. The terminology and classification used for the cardiomyopathies are confusing owing to overlap among the diseases and/or classification schemes. Cardiomyopathies sometimes are defined according to etiology or as primary or secondary

TABLE 18–3. Characteristics of the Cardiomyopathies

	Dilated	Hypertrophic	Restrictive
Myocardial mass	$\uparrow \rightarrow \uparrow\uparrow$	$\uparrow\uparrow\uparrow$	nl$\rightarrow\uparrow$
Ventricular cavity size	$\uparrow\uparrow \rightarrow \uparrow\uparrow\uparrow\uparrow$	$\downarrow\downarrow \rightarrow$ nl	nl$\rightarrow\downarrow$
Contractile function	$\downarrow\downarrow\downarrow$	$\uparrow\uparrow \rightarrow \downarrow$	nl$\rightarrow\downarrow$
LV filling pressure	$\uparrow\uparrow$	nl$\rightarrow\uparrow$	$\uparrow$
Chest x-ray	Moderate to marked cardiac enlargement	Mild to moderate cardiac enlargement	Mild cardiac enlargement
Electrocardiogram	ST-segment and T-wave abnormalities	ST-segment and T-wave abnormalities Left ventricular hypertrophy	Low voltage, conduction defects
Echocardiogram	LV dilatation and dysfunction	Asymmetric septal hypertrophy Systolic anterior motion of the mitral valve	Increased LV wall thickness possible
Radionuclide studies	LV dilatation and dysfunction	Vigorous systolic function	Normal systolic function

$\uparrow$ = increased; $\downarrow$ = decreased; nl = normal; LV = left ventricular.

forms. *Primary* cardiomyopathies are disorders in which either the structure or function of the myocardium is affected in the *absence* of other known causes of heart disease or systemic diseases known to affect the heart. *Secondary* forms of cardiomyopathy are conditions in which the myocardial abnormality is due to a recognized factor. Infectious agents, inflammation, metabolic disorders, infiltrative diseases, and toxins are a few of the causative factors of secondary cardiomyopathy.[43]

Frequently, a specific etiology is not evident. Therefore, another commonly used categorization of the cardiomyopathies is based on the structural and/or functional abnormalities present. The three groups of cardiomyopathies usually are described as dilated (congestive), hypertrophic, and restrictive. An understanding of the pathophysiologic basis for each type of cardiomyopathy leads to a rational selection of drug therapy or other treatment modality. The characteristics for each of the types of cardiomyopathy are presented in Table 18–3. The distinction among the cardiomyopathies is not absolute, and there is some overlap in the functional abnormalities.

In dilated cardiomyopathy, the cardinal feature is dilatation of the ventricles. Systolic function is abnormal, leading to a decreased cardiac output. In patients with hypertrophic cardiomyopathy (HCM), the ventricular cavity is not dilated, and the ventricular muscle mass is increased. Ventricular cavity size is normal or decreased, and systolic function often is preserved. Patients with HCM may have an obstructive or nonobstructive form. Patients with restrictive cardiomyopathy have inadequate ventricular compliance causing diastolic dysfunction owing to endocardial and/or myocardial disease. The clinical presentation is similar to that of constrictive pericarditis.

Other terms are encountered frequently in discussions of patients with cardiomyopathy. *Familial cardiomyopathy* is used to denote a condition found in more than one family member. Genetic predisposition may occur in all three functional types. *Ischemic cardiomyopathy* is another frequently used term. Patients with occlusive atherosclerotic CAD and LV dysfunction are said to have ischemic cardiomyopathy. Ischemic cardiomyopathy is not a true cardiomyopathy because there is an identifiable cause of the ventricular muscle dysfunction.

HYPERTROPHIC CARDIOMYOPATHY

Hypertrophic cardiomyopathy is a primary myocardial disorder characterized by a hypertrophied and nondilated left ventricle existing in the absence of known causes of LVH.[44] HCM is inherited as an autosomal dominant trait caused by mutations in any of 10 genes.[44,45] The distribution of the hypertrophy is usually asymmetric, meaning

that segments of the left ventricle are thickened to varying degrees. There also may be enlargement of the atria, thickening of the mitral valve leaflets, and fibrotic areas within the ventricular wall. In the past, the terms of *idiopathic hypertrophic subaortic stenosis* (IHSS) and *hypertrophic obstructive cardiomyopathy* (HOCM) were used to describe patients with HCM with an outflow obstruction. These terms are used less frequently now because they overemphasize the obstructive component of the disease, which is present in a minority of patients.[45]

EPIDEMIOLOGY

Recent epidemiologic investigations estimate the prevalence of phenotypically expressed HCM in the general adult population to be approximately 0.2% (1 in 500).[45] Therefore, HCM is the most common genetic cardiovascular disease. However, many individuals have a mutant gene but go undetected.

ETIOLOGY

The genetic predisposition to HCM is thought to be an autosomal dominant trait with variable penetrance. Owing to the wide variability of presentation, not all cases in a family may be detected. HCM usually is caused by mutations in the genes for β-myosin heavy chain, myosin-binding protein C, and cardiac troponin T.[45,46]

PATHOPHYSIOLOGY

HCM appears to have several different pathophysiologic mechanisms leading to similar clinical manifestations, although the prognoses for patients will vary. The pathophysiology of HCM is a complex relationship among several factors, including: (1) asymmetric LVH, (2) diastolic dysfunction, (3) dynamic obstruction of the outflow tract, and (4) myocardial ischemia. Each of these components contributes to the overall presentation of the patient to a varying degree.

Left Ventricular Hypertrophy

The hypertrophy seen in HCM usually is diffuse and involves the septum and LV anterolateral free wall to a greater degree than the posterior segment. Asymmetric septal hypertrophy is a sensitive marker for HCM but is not specific for this disorder. In patients with outflow obstruction, the basal septum usually is markedly thickened at the level of the mitral valve. In patients with nonobstructive HCM, the outflow tract is larger, and the septal hypertrophy that occurs has a more distal or apical distribution.

Cellular disorganization is a common histologic finding in HCM. Morphologic abnormalities are found at the gross, microscopic, and ultrastructural levels. The disarray of myocytes may contribute to diastolic and systolic dysfunction, as well as serving as a nidus for ventricular arrhythmias.[45] The degree of LVH is associated with a worse clinical course. The presence of hypertrophy correlates directly with MI, HF, stroke, and ventricular arrhythmias.[47] Spirito and colleagues found that the magnitude of LVH was directly related to the risk of sudden cardiac death.[48]

Diastolic Dysfunction

Diastolic dysfunction is the most common abnormality found in patients with HCM. Approximately 80% of patients will exhibit symptoms associated with diastolic dysfunction. Studies of the left ventricle led to the realization that diastolic dysfunction is the result of abnormalities in relaxation, distensibility (compliance), and filling. The abnormalities of diastolic function can be both regional and global and lead to an incoordination of contraction and relaxation. β-Adrenergic stimulation can aggravate these abnormalities, whereas β-blockade may diminish them.[43,49]

Abnormalities in filling are also associated with changes in chamber stiffness that occur in HCM. This stiffness may be the result of myocardial fibrosis, cellular disorganization, or increased myocardial mass. The decreased distensibility leads to an abnormally steep slope of the diastolic pressure-volume curve such that an increase in LV volume results in a disproportionate increase in diastolic pressure.

Myocardial relaxation is an energy-dependent process that is sensitive to episodes of ischemia. Diastolic resequestration of calcium ions by the sarcoplasmic reticulum is an energy-dependent process. In the event of ischemia, the sequestration of calcium is inhibited, allowing the calcium to continue its interaction with the myofibrillar contractile proteins. CCBs have been used with some success in patients with diastolic dysfunction.[43]

Systolic Function and Outflow Tract Obstruction

Abnormalities of systolic function also occur in patients with HCM. The hypertrophied left ventricle may cause a powerful but sometimes uncoordinated contraction presumably owing to the abnormal architecture of the myocardium. The increase seen in the LV wall thickness results in decreased wall stress during systole. Therefore, the left ventricle contracts against a decreased afterload so that the left ventricle is described as being *hyperdynamic*. EF often is increased.

Considerable controversy has surrounded the issue of the importance of outflow tract obstruction in conjunction with HCM. The presence of a gradient (the systolic pressure difference between the body and the outflow tract of the left ventricle) is indicative of a dynamic obstruction of the LV outflow tract. Outflow tract gradients occur in about 25% of patients with HCM.[50] The obstruction that occurs usually shows spontaneous variability and may be reduced by interventions that decrease myocardial contractility. The gradient can be augmented by factors that increase contractility[43] (Table 18-4). LV outflow tract obstruction at rest has been found to be a predictor of progression to severe HF symptoms, stroke, and death.[50]

Myocardial Ischemia

Chest pain in the absence of CAD is a common symptom of patients with HCM. However, it is appropriate to consider typical CAD in any patient with HCM if they have the usual risk factors for atherosclerosis.[43,45,51] There are several mechanisms proposed for the myocardial ischemia seen in this patient population. There may be inadequate capillary density in relation to the increased LV muscle mass. The small intramural coronary arteries may be abnormally narrowed

TABLE 18–4. Factors Known to Affect Outflow Gradients in HCM

Factors That Diminish Gradients
Decreasing myocardial contractility
  β-Blocking drugs
  Verapamil
Increasing ventricular volume
Increasing arterial pressure
Factors That Enhance Gradients
Increasing myocardial contractility
  Exercise
  Inotropic agents
Decreasing ventricular volume
Decreasing arterial pressure

or excessively compressed during systole. Impaired relaxation during diastole may inhibit blood flow to the subendocardium. Once myocardial ischemia develops, further increases in LV filling pressure may occur, which, in turn, leads to more ischemia. Repeated episodes of ischemia may be responsible for progressive myocyte loss and fibrosis. The subendocardium is at greatest risk for ischemic damage owing to the lower capillary density and higher oxygen demand secondary to wall tension.[43]

DIAGNOSIS

It may be difficult to make the diagnosis of HCM because the disorder may be confused with CAD, aortic stenosis, or mitral regurgitation. Patients with HCM can be young and physically active. The physical signs of the cardiac examination depend on the presence of a systolic pressure gradient within the left ventricle. If a gradient is present, a late-onset systolic murmur is heard often. The murmur is intensified by standing and the Valsalva maneuver and lessened with squatting or handgrip. Very rarely, some patients develop an end-stage LV dilatation and a declining LV ejection fraction, which is often confused with idiopathic dilated cardiomyopathy.

Echocardiography is used to confirm the diagnosis. The diagnosis of HCM is made with two-dimensional echocardiography, with the usual criteria being LV wall thickness greater than or equal to 15 mm.[51] Magnetic resonance imaging (MRI) of the entire left ventricle may add valuable information, especially if the echocardiogram is of suboptimal quality.

The development of or increase in a murmur suggests progression of disease, but disappearance of a murmur does not imply improvement. In fact, disappearance of a murmur may herald further impairment of systolic function. Some patients will progress to CHF owing to atrial fibrillation, mitral regurgitation, or MI. If SHF develops, the patient has a poor prognosis.

CLINICAL PRESENTATION: HYPERTROPHIC CARDIOMYOPATHY

GENERAL
The clinical presentation varies widely, ranging from no symptoms to severe symptoms of angina, HF, and/or sudden cardiac death. The severity of symptoms corresponds to the degree of LVH, but this relationship is not absolute.

SYMPTOMS

- Dyspnea
- Chest pain
- Fatigue

- Palpitations
- Presyncope
- Syncope

SIGNS

- Systolic murmur

ELECTROCARDIOGRAM

- LV hypertrophy
- ST-segment and T-wave abnormalities

ECHOCARDIOGRAM

- Increased myocardial mass

PROGNOSIS

The clinical course for a patient with HCM should be viewed in terms of the specific subtypes of the disease spectrum. Patients fall into one of several relatively discrete pathways: (1) high risk for sudden death, (2) symptoms of DHF, including syncope, (3) progression toward advanced end-stage HF, and (4) atrial fibrillation and its sequelae.[51] Of major concern is the incidence of sudden cardiac death among patients with HCM. Approximately 10% to 20% of HCM patients are at increased risk for sudden death. The mechanism responsible for sudden cardiac death is thought to be related to an electrically unstable myocardium leading to complex ventricular arrhythmias. Less often, sudden death may be the result of hemodynamic changes. The onset of atrial fibrillation in the face of severe LV diastolic dysfunction may result in a significant decrease in stroke volume. This decrease in cardiac output could lead acute LV failure, MI, or sudden death. Sudden death can be a complication, especially in young athletes with

TABLE 18–5. Risk Factors Associated with Sudden Cardiac Death in HCM

Prior cardiac arrest
Spontaneous sustained ventricular tachycardia
Positive family history of premature death related to HCM
Multiple syncopal or near-syncopal episodes, especially if associated with exertion
Multiple and repetitive or prolonged episodes of nonsustained ventricular tachycardia
Marked left ventricular hypertrophy
Hypotensive blood pressure response to exercise

HCM. It is recommended that young patients with HCM refrain from competitive athletics.[51]

Quantification of the risk of sudden death remains elusive for patients with HCM. The clinical markers associated with an increased risk for sudden death (Table 18–5) have a high negative predictive value. The absence of all these markers can be used to develop a profile for a patient at low risk of sudden death. The magnitude of hypertrophy appears to be a strong predictor, with the cumulative risk nearly zero for patients with a wall thickness of 19 mm or less.[48] Young patients with severe hypertrophy (wall thickness > 30 mm) are at a high risk for sudden death even if they are asymptomatic. A high LV outflow tract pressure gradient (>30 mm Hg) is a strong predictor for older patients.[52] Presentation of HCM in the latter decades of life is common. Patients who present with HCM at an advanced age (>65 years) usually have a prognosis that is no different from that of age- and gender-matched controls. Elderly patients with HCM tend to have mild degrees of LVH, and their symptoms are not severe.[53] Since systolic hypertension and diastolic HF are common in the elderly, the diagnosis of HCM may be challenging. However, marked LVH out of proportion to blood pressure, unusual patterns of LVH, or an outflow obstruction at rest strongly suggests HCM.[51]

▶ TREATMENT: Hypertrophic Cardiomyopathy

▦ DESIRED OUTCOMES

Because there are no known means available to prevent HCM, the focus must be on methods to minimize the consequences of the disorder.

▦ GENERAL APPROACH TO TREATMENT

The treatment of HCM is designed to reduce symptoms, improve exercise tolerance, retard disease progression, and improve prognosis. Agents that decrease contractility, improve diastolic dysfunction, reduce ischemia, and suppress arrhythmias have been used with some success (Fig. 18–4). In 2003, the American College of Cardiology in conjunction with the European Society of Cardiology published a consensus document on HCM.[51]

▦ NONPHARMACOLOGIC THERAPY

Surgical treatment generally is reserved for patients who are refractory to medical management, have an outflow gradient of 50 mm Hg or more, a very thick ventricular septum, and high LV pressures. Surgical

intervention is designed to relieve the outflow obstruction and the elevated LV pressures. The surgeon accomplishes this by performing a myectomy, or removal of excess tissue. The procedure results in a reduction in LV filling pressures and a long-term improvement in symptoms. However, early mortality rates of up to 5% have been reported.[49,51] Other complications may include septal perforation and late occurrence of CHF.

The results of uncontrolled studies suggested that dual-chamber pacing decreased LV outflow gradients and improved symptoms. Subsequent controlled trials were not able to replicate the initial findings but demonstrated more modest improvement. Consequently, the American College of Cardiology, the American Heart Association, and the North American Society of Pacing and Electrophysiology (ACC/AHA/NASPE) have issued guidelines suggesting pacing for severely symptomatic patients who have failed medical management (class IIb recommendation, or one in which the efficacy is less well established by evidence).[54]

Ablation of the myocardium using alcohol is another alternative to surgery. Septal ablation with alcohol results in the same type of outcomes as seen with myectomy. Long-term follow-up is limited because this procedure has been used for less than a decade. Since it is a percutaneous procedure (similar to cardiac catheterizations), it is being done more frequently than myectomy.[51] There is some concern that the risk for arrhythmia-related cardiac events may increase following alcohol ablation. Long-term follow-up is needed to assess this risk. Complete heart block is a common complication of septal

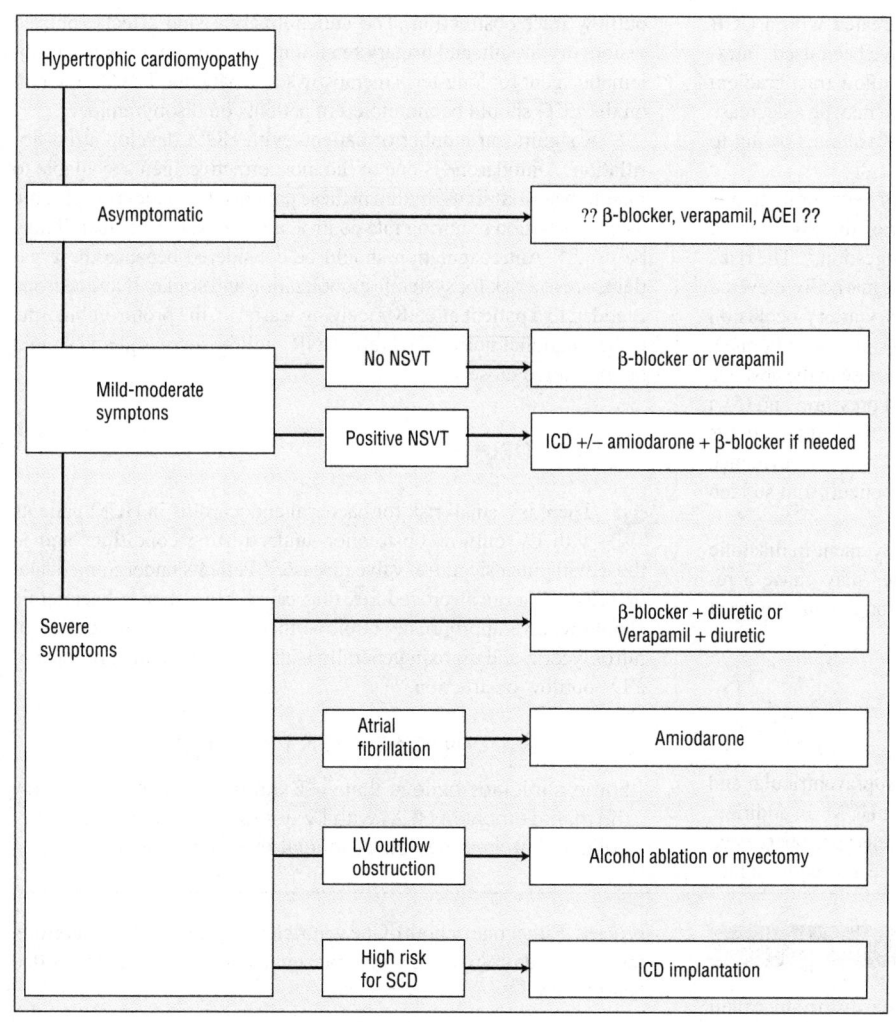

FIGURE 18–4. Treatment algorithm for hypertrophic cardiomyopathy. ACEI = angiotensin-converting enzyme inhibitor; NSVT = nonsustained ventricular tachycardia; ICD = implantable cardioverter-defibrillator; LV = left ventricular; SCD = sudden cardiac death.

ablation (14% in one case series) and requires a permanent pacemaker if it occurs.[55]

IMPLANTABLE CARDIOVERTER-DEFIBRILLATOR (ICD)

Sudden death is the most worrisome outcome of HCM, and the ICD is the most effective treatment for the prevention of sudden death.[56] It is difficult to know when to implant an ICD, especially in a young patient diagnosed with HCM. Patients who are candidates for an ICD for primary prevention will be young and relatively asymptomatic. The ACC/AHA/NASPE 2002 guidelines have designated the ICD for primary prevention of sudden death (class IIb recommendation) and for secondary prevention following cardiac arrest (class I recommendation, where there is evidence or general agreement that the procedure is beneficial).[54] Conducting a clinical trial to provide evidence for a higher-level recommendation for primary prevention is unlikely to occur.[56]

PHARMACOLOGIC THERAPY

β-BLOCKING AGENTS

β-Blocking agents have been used in obstructive and nonobstructive forms of HCM since the 1960s. Approximately one-third to one-half of patients with angina, dyspnea, light-headedness, or syncope will have a favorable response to these agents.[43] Doses of up to 480 mg/day of propranolol or its equivalent are used. Resting heart rate should be 60 beats per minute, and the maximum exercise heart rate should be less than 120 beats per minute. The mechanism by which β-blockade is beneficial is by inhibiting sympathetic stimulation of the heart. Myocardial oxygen demand is reduced by decreasing heart rate, LV contractility, and myocardial wall stress during systole. Outflow tract obstruction may be minimized with β-blockade, especially under conditions of stress or exercise, when sympathetic stimulation is high.

CALCIUM CHANNEL BLOCKING AGENTS

Patients who have an inadequate response to β-blockade may respond to verapamil.[46] Doses of verapamil up to 480 mg/day have beneficial effects on symptoms.[51] There are several reasons why CCBs may be of benefit to patients with HCM. Increased calcium concentrations have been shown to play a role in prolonging the ventricular action potential, as well as the duration of isometric contraction and relaxation. Patients with HCM have a hyperdynamic ventricle in systole and delayed relaxation and decreased compliance during diastole. CCBs decrease the myocardial oxygen demand, resulting in an improved balance between oxygen supply and demand; therefore, diastolic function may be improved.

Most patients with HCM who have been treated with a CCB have received verapamil, although others also have been used. Intravenous verapamil has been noted to reduce the outflow tract gradient in patients with obstructive HCM. The mechanism may be a decrease in systolic function, as well as an increase in LV volumes owing to an enhanced LV diastolic filling.

The adverse effects associated with the use of verapamil include constipation, sinus node blockade, prolongation of the PR interval, AV dissociation, hypotension, and pulmonary congestion.[43] The risks may outweigh the benefits in patients with (1) a markedly elevated pulmonary capillary wedge pressure or pulmonary artery occlusion pressure, (2) a history of paroxysmal nocturnal dyspnea or orthopnea, (3) sick sinus syndrome or significant AV nodal disease in the absence of a permanent pacemaker, (4) low systolic blood pressure, and (5) a substantial outflow gradient. Verapamil should be avoided in patients with heart failure owing to systolic dysfunction.[51] There is no evidence that either β-blockade or verapamil protects the patient from sudden cardiac death.

Studies using other CCBs are limited. Improvement in diastolic dysfunction may occur, but the dihydropyridines may cause a reflex increase in heart rate or hypotension or worsen the outflow tract gradient.

ANTIARRHYTHMIC AGENTS

Disopyramide has been used in treating both the supraventricular and ventricular arrhythmias occurring in patients with HCM. In addition, the negative inotropic effect and the ability to increase peripheral vascular resistance attributed to disopyramide have been used to reduce

outflow tract obstruction. The anticholinergic side effects (blurred vision, dry mouth, and urinary retention) make disopyramide a problematic agent for long-term therapy in some patients. The QT interval on the ECG should be monitored in patients on disopyramide.[51]

A significant number of patients with HCM develop atrial fibrillation. Amiodarone is one of the most effective agents available to maintain normal sinus rhythm in these patients. For patients in chronic atrial fibrillation requiring rate control, a β-blocker or verapamil may be used.[45] Anticoagulation should be considered because these patients are at a risk for systemic embolization and stroke. If amiodarone is added to a patient already receiving warfarin, the prothrombin time or international normalized ratio (INR) will be increased and should be monitored closely.

OTHER DRUGS

There is a small risk for bacterial endocarditis in HCM patients with LV outflow obstruction under resting conditions and in those with intrinsic mitral valve disease.[51] Patients undergoing dental or selected surgical procedures that cause blood-borne bacteremia should receive appropriate antibiotic therapy. The administration of nitroglycerin and digoxin generally is discouraged in the presence of a LV outflow obstruction.[51]

CLINICAL CONTROVERSY

Some clinicians believe that ACE inhibitors have no role in the management of HCM with LV outflow obstruction. Others believe that they may be beneficial by limiting hypertrophy.

EVALUATION OF THERAPEUTIC OUTCOMES

The goal of treatment of patients with HCM is primarily to reduce their symptoms of dyspnea and exercise intolerance. Either β-blockers or CCBs may be used. If a β-blocker is chosen, it is best to use an agent that does not have intrinsic sympathomimetic activity. The dose should be maximized. If the patient does not tolerate a β-blocker or has a contraindication to the use of a β-blocker, then verapamil may be tried. Patients should be monitored for resolution of symptoms and an increase in exercise tolerance. Resolution of symptoms may take months to occur. In addition, both β-blockers and CCBs may cause hypotension and conduction abnormalities. β-Blockers may worsen pulmonary function. If dyspnea continues with maximal doses of a β-blocker or CCB, a diuretic agent or a nitrate may be added with caution. Patients who are at high risk for sudden cardiac death should be considered candidates for an ICD.

For patients with a significant obstruction to LV outflow who do not respond to medical management, a surgical approach may be necessary. Septal myectomy and alcohol ablation have been employed. These approaches generally are reserved for patients who have an outflow gradient of more than 50 mm Hg and/or severe symptoms and who have failed an adequate trial of medical therapy.

RESTRICTIVE CARDIOMYOPATHY

Restrictive cardiomyopathy is primarily an abnormality of diastolic function that results in impaired filling and increases in ventricular end-diastolic pressures with normal or decreased diastolic volume. It is associated with normal systolic function early in the course of the disease but a decrease in systolic function later in the disease

process. Either one or both of the ventricles may be affected; therefore, restrictive cardiomyopathy may present as either left- or right-sided heart failure.[57]

CLINICAL PRESENTATION: RESTRICTIVE CARDIOMYOPATHY

SYMPTOMS

- Dyspnea
- Orthopnea
- Fatigue
- Edema
- Ascites
- Chest pain

SIGNS

- Significant jugular venous distention
- Mitral and/or tricuspid regurgitant murmurs
- Thromboembolic complications
- Kussmaul's sign may be present

ELECTROCARDIOGRAM

- Atrial arrhythmias
- Tachy-brady syndrome
- Conduction abnormalities

EPIDEMIOLOGY AND ETIOLOGY

Restrictive cardiomyopathy is the type of cardiomyopathy encountered least frequently in Western countries. Since the occurrence of restrictive cardiomyopathy is rare, the natural course of the disease is not well characterized, and reports on prognosis have been highly variable. Restrictive cardiomyopathies may be classified as either myocardial or endomyocardial. The myocardial types may be noninfiltrative, infiltrative, or storage diseases. The endomyocardial types are due to endomyocardial fibrosis, hypereosinophilic syndrome, carcinoid heart disease, metastatic cancers, radiation, and anthracycline toxicity or secondary to drugs known to cause fibrosis.[57]

Restrictive myocardial disease may result from several local or systemic disorders. Amyloidosis, hemochromatosis, scleroderma, carcinoid, sarcoidosis, diabetes, pseudoxanthoma elasticum, and endomyocardial fibrosis have been known to cause restrictive cardiomyopathy. The most common cause of restrictive cardiomyopathy in the industrialized world is amyloidosis, whereas endomyocardial fibrosis is a common cause in tropical areas of the world. There may be a genetic predisposition to idiopathic restrictive cardiomyopathy.[57]

The cause of the disease, the severity of HF symptoms, and the presence of cardiac thrombi and arrhythmias are factors that affect long-term survival. Children diagnosed with restrictive cardiomyopathy have a worse prognosis than adults and should be considered for early cardiac transplantation.[58]

PATHOPHYSIOLOGY

The major hemodynamic abnormality in restrictive cardiomyopathy is a limitation in ventricular filling leading to increased filling pressures. The cavity size and wall thickness of the ventricles are usually normal. Atrial dimensions often are increased. Thrombi are found frequently in the cardiac chambers. Patients have signs and symptoms consistent with CHF. The abnormality is similar to what is seen in pericardial disease causing constriction or tamponade.

DIAGNOSIS

The diagnosis of restrictive cardiomyopathy should be considered in any patient who presents with signs and symptoms of CHF but has only mild cardiomegaly. Differentiation from constrictive pericarditis is important because pericardectomy is an effective form of treatment for constrictive pericarditis.

▶ TREATMENT: Restrictive Cardiomyopathy

The treatment of restrictive cardiomyopathy is complex because of the heterogeneity of the pathophysiologic abnormalities. Diuretics are used for the symptoms of venous congestion in the presence of restrictive cardiomyopathy, but caution is advised because these patients require high filling pressures to maintain an adequate stroke volume and cardiac output. Hypotension and hypoperfusion may occur as a result of the excessive use of diuretics. Because systolic function is often normal, digoxin is of little benefit and may be proarrhythmic. Amiodarone may be used to maintain normal sinus rhythm in patients who have episodes of atrial fibrillation. Anticoagulation is needed to decrease the risk of systemic embolization, particularly in patients with atrial fibrillation, valvular regurgitation, and low cardiac output. In the case of hemachromatosis, chelation therapy and/or repeated phlebotomy may be of benefit. Treatment with corticosteroids and cytotoxic drugs has been used with some success in the early phase of endomyocardial fibrosis and eosinophilic cardiomyopathy.[57]

EVALUATION OF THERAPEUTIC OUTCOMES

The first step in assessing and treating a patient with restrictive cardiomyopathy is to rule out constrictive pericarditis because the two conditions have a similar presentation. Constrictive pericarditis is treated easily with surgery, whereas patients with restrictive cardiomyopathy have a varied approach to therapy depending on the etiology of their disorder. The treatment is aimed at relieving the symptoms associated with high filling pressures. This is achieved generally through the use of diuretics. Diuretic therapy should be initiated with low doses. Normalization of filling pressures is not possible or desirable. Patients' symptoms should be monitored for improvement. Excessive diuresis will result in an inadequate cardiac output. Chelation therapy has been advocated for patients with hemochromatosis. Prednisone has been suggested for patients with sarcoidosis. There is no curative treatment for restrictive cardiomyopathy.

Review Questions and other resources can be found at *www.pharmacotherapyonline.com.*

REFERENCES

1. Yamamoto K, Wilson DJ, Canzanello VJ, Redfield MM. Left ventricular diastolic dysfunction in patients with hypertension and preserved systolic dysfunction. Mayo Clin Proc 2000;75:148–155.
2. Zile MR. Diastolic dysfunction and heart failure in hypertrophied hearts. Congest Heart Fail 1998;4:32–42.
3. Zile MR. Heart failure with preserved ejection fraction: Is this diastolic heart failure? J Am Coll Cardiol 2003;41:1519–1522.
4. Smith GL, Masoudi FA, Vaccarino V, et al. Outcomes in heart failure patients with preserved ejecion fraction. J Am Coll Cardiol 2003;41:1510–1518.
5. Torosoff M, Philbin EF. Improving outcomes in diastolic heart failure. Postgrad Med 2003;113:51–58.
6. Zile MR, Brutsaert DL. New concepts in diastolic dysfunction and diastolic heart failure, part I. Circulation 2002;105:1387–1393.
7. Redfield MM, Jacobsen SJ, Burnett JC, et al. Burden of systolic and diastolic ventricular dysfunction in the community: Appreciating the scope of the heart failure epidemic. JAMA 2003;289:194–202.
8. Lamb HJ, Beyerbacht HP, van der Laarse A, et al. Diastolic dysfunction in hypertensive heart disease. Circulation 1999;99:2261–2267.
9. Mandinov L, Eberli FR, Seiler C, Hess OM. Diastolic heart failure. Cardiovasc Res 2000;45;813–825.
10. Zile MR, Richardson K, Cowles MK, et al. Constitutive properties of adult mammalian cardiac muscle cells. Circulation 1998;98:567–579.
11. Tian R, Nascimben L, Ingwall JS, Lorell BH. Failure to maintain a low ADP concentration impairs diastolic function in hypertrophied rat hearts. Circulation 1997;96:1313–1319.
12. Zile MR, Brutsaert DL. New concepts in diastolic dysfunction and diastolic heart failure, part II. Circulation 2002;105:1503–1508.
13. Cecchi F, Olivotto I, Gistri R, et al. Coronary microvascular dysfunction and prognosis in hypertrophic cardiomyopathy. N Engl J Med 2003;349:1027–1035.
14. Ma LN, Zhao SP, Gao M, et al. Endothelial dysfunction associated with left ventricular diastolic dysfunction in patients with coronary heart disease. Int J Cardiol 2000;72:275–279.

15. Cannon RO. Assessing risk in hypertrophic cardiomyopathy. N Engl J Med 2003;349:1016–1018.
16. Paulus WJ, Bronzwaer JGF, de Bruyne B, Grossman W. Different effects of "supply" and "demand" ischemia on left ventricular diastolic function in humans. In: Gaasch WH, LeWinter MM, eds. Left Ventricular Diastolic Dysfunction and Heart Failure. Philadelphia, Lea & Febiger, 1994:286.
17. European Study Group on Diastolic Heart Failure. How to diagnose diastolic heart failure. Eur Heart J 1998;19:990–1003.
18. Vasan RS, Levy D. Defining diastolic heart failure: A call for standardized diagnostic criteria. Circulation 2000;101:2118–2121.
19. Jessup M, Brozena S. Heart failure. N Engl J Med 2003;348;2007–2018.
20. Kitzman DW, Little WC, Brubaker PH, et al. Pathophysiological characterization of isolated diastolic heart failure in comparison to systolic heart failure. JAMA 2002;288:2144–2150.
21. Massie BM. Natriuretic peptide measurements for the diagnosis of "nonsystolic" heart failure. J Am Coll Cardiol 2003;41:2018–2021.
22. Maisel AS, McCord J, Nowak RM, et al. Bedside B-type natriuretic peptide in emergency diagnosis of heart failure with reduced or preserved ejection fraction. J Am Coll Cardiol 2003;41:2010–2017.
23. O'Connor AM, Gattis WA, Shaw L, et al. Clinical characteristics and long-term outcomes of patients with heart failure and preserved systolic function. Am J Cardiol 2000;86:863–867.
24. MacCarthy PA, Kearney MT, Nolan J, et al. Prognosis in heart failure with preserved left ventricular systolic function: Prospective cohort study. BMJ 2003;327:78–79.
25. The Digitalis Investigation Group. The effect of digoxin on mortality and morbidity in patients with heart failure. N Engl J Med 1997;336:525–533.
26. Zile MR: Diastolic heart failure: Diagnosis, prognosis, treatment. Minerva Cardiol 2003;51:131–142.
27. Pina IL, Apstein CS, Balady GJ, et al. Exercise and heart failure. Circulation 2003;107:1210–1225.
28. Gaasch WH, Zile MR. Left ventricular diastolic dysfunction and diastolic heart failure. Ann Rev Med 2004;55: 373–394.
29. LeConte P, Countant V, N'Guyen JM, et al. Prognostic factors in acute cardiogenic pulmonary edema. Am J Emerg Med 1999;17:329–332.
30. Hunt SA, Baker DW, Chin MH, et al. ACC/AHA guidelines for the evaluation and management of chronic heart failure in the adult: A report of the American College of Cardiology/American Heart Association Task Force on Practice Guidelines. American College of Cardiology Web site: http://www.acc.org/clinical/guidelines/failure/hf_index.htm; accessed September 15, 2003.
31. Yusuf S, Pfeffer M, Swedberg K, et al. Effects of candesartan in patients with chronic heart failure and preserved left-ventricular ejection fraction: The CHARM-Preserved Trial. Lancet 2003;362:777–781.
32. The ALLHAT Officers and Coordinators for the ALLHAT Collaborative Research Group. Major cardiovascular events in the hypertensive patients randomized to doxazosin vs chlorthalidone: The Antihypertensive and Lipid-Lowering Treatment to Prevent Heart Attack Trial (ALLHAT). JAMA 2000;283:1967–1975.
33. Davis KL, Nappi JM. The cardiovascular effects of eplerenone, a new selective aldosterone receptor antagonist. Clin Ther 2003;25:2647–2668.
34. van Kraaij DJW, Jansen RWMM, Bouwels LHR, et al. Furosemide withdrawal in elderly heart failure patients with preserved left ventricular systolic function. Am J Cardiol 2000;85:1461–1466.
35. Udelson JE, Bonow RO. Left ventricular diastolic function and calcium channel blockers in hypertrophic cardiomyopathy. In: Gaasch WH, Le Winter MM, eds. Left Ventricular Diastolic Dysfunction and Heart Failure. Philadelphia, Lea & Febiger, 1994:465.
36. Lefrandt JD, Heitmann J, Sevre K, et al. Contrasting effects of verapamil and amlodipine on cardiovascular stress response in hypertension. Br J Clin Pharmacol 2001;52:687–692.
37. Weber KT. Aldosterone in congestive heart failure. N Engl J Med 2001;345:1689–1697.
38. Hoit BD, Walsh RA. Diastolic function in hypertensive heart disease. In: Gaasch WH, LeWinter MM, eds. Left Ventricular Diastolic Dysfunction and Heart Failure. Philadelphia, Lea & Febiger, 1994:354.
39. Baker DW. Prevention of heart failure. J Cardiac Failure 2002;8:333–346.
40. Brilla CG, Funck RC, Rupp H. Lisinopril-mediated regression of myocardial fibrosis in patients with hypertensive heart disease. Circulation 2000;102:1388–1393.
41. Warner JG, Metzger C, Kitzman DW, et al. Losartan improves exercise tolerance in patients with diastolic dysfunction and a hypertensive response to exercise. J Am Coll Cardiol 1999;33:1567–1572.
42. Zannad F, Alla F, Dousset B, et al. Limitation of excessive extracellular matrix turnover may contribute to survival benefit of spironolactone therapy in patients with congestive heart failure: Insights from the randomized aldactone evaluation study. Circulation 2000;102:2700–2706 (erratum appears in Circulation 2001;103:476).
43. Wynne J, Braunwald E. The cardiomyopathies and myocarditides. In: Braunwald E, Zipes DP, Libby P, eds. Heart Disease: A Textbook of Cardiovascular Medicine, 6th ed. Philadelphia, Saunders, 2001:1751–1806.
44. Roberts R, Sigwart U. New concepts in hypertrophic cardiomyopathies, part I. Circulation 2001;104:2113–2116.
45. Maron BJ. Hypertrophic cardiomyopathy: A systematic review. JAMA 2002;287:1308–1320.
46. Spirito P, Seidman CE, McKenna WJ, Maron BJ. The management of hypertrophic cardiomyopathy. N Engl J Med 1997;336:775–785.
47. St. John Sutton M, Epstein JA. Hypertrophic cardiomyopathy: Beyond the sarcomere. N Engl J Med 1998;338:1303–1304.
48. Spirito P, Bellone P, Harris KM, et al. Magnitude of left ventricular hypertrophy and risk of sudden death in hypertrophic cardiomyopathy. N Engl J Med 2000;342:1778–1785.
49. Robets R, Sigwart U. New concepts in hypertrophic cardiomyopathies, part II. Circulation 2001;104:2249–2252.
50. Maron MS, Olivotto I, Betocchi S, et al. Effects of left ventricular outflow tract obstruction on clinical outcome in hypertrophic cardiomyopathy. N Engl J Med 2003;348:295–303.
51. Maron BJ, McKenna WJ, Danielson GK, et al. ACC/ESC clinical expert consensus document on hypertrophic cardiomyopathy: A report of the American College of Cardiology Task Force on Clinical Expert Consensus Documents and the European Society of Cardiology Committee for Practice Guidelines (Committee to Develop an Expert Consensus Document on Hypertrophic Cardiomyopathy). J Am Coll Cardiol 2003;42: 1687–1713.
52. Maki S, Ikeda H, Muro A, et al. Predictors of sudden cardiac death in hypertrophic cardiomyopathy. Am J Cardiol 1998;82:774–778.
53. Maron BJ, Casey SA, Hauser RG, Aeppli DM. Clinical course of hypertrophic cardiomyopathy with survival to advanced age. J Am Coll Cardiol 2003;42:882–888.
54. Gregoratos G, Abrams J, Epstein AE, et al. ACC/AHA/NASPE 2002 guideline update for implantation of cardiac pacemakers and antiarrhythmia devices: A report of the American College of Cardiology/American Heart Association Task Force on Practice Guidelines (ACC/AHA/NASPE Committee on Pacemaker Implantation). Circulation 2002;106:2145–2161.
55. Chang SM, Nagueh SF, Spencer WH, Lakkis NM. Complete heart block: Determinants and clinical impact in patients with hypertrophic obstructive cardiomyopathy undergoing nonsurgical septal reduction therapy. J Am Coll Cardiol 2003;42:296–300.
56. Maron BJ, Estes M, Maron MS, et al. Primary prevention of sudden death as a novel treatment strategy in hypertrophic cardiomyopathy. Circulation 2003;107:2872–2875.
57. Kushwaha S, Fallon JT, Fuster V. Restrictive cardiomyopathy. N Engl J Med 1997;336:267–276.
58. Weller RJ, Weintraub R, Addonizio LJ, et al. Outcome of idiopathic restrictive cardiomyopathy in children. Am J Cardiol 2002;90:501–506.

19
VENOUS THROMBOEMBOLISM

Stuart T. Haines, Mario Zeolla, and Daniel M. Witt

Learning Objectives and other resources can be found at *www.pharmacotherapyonline.com.*

KEY CONCEPTS

1. The risk of venous thromboembolism (VTE) is related to several easily identifiable factors, including age, major surgery (particularly orthopedic procedures of the lower extremities), previous VTE, trauma, malignancy, and hypercoagulable states. These risks are additive.

2. The diagnosis of VTE must be confirmed by an objective test.

3. Antithrombotic therapies require meticulous and systematic monitoring as well as ongoing patient education. Well-organized anticoagulation management services improve the quality of patient care and reduce overall cost.

4. Bleeding is the most common adverse effect associated with anticoagulant drugs. A patient's risk of major hemorrhage is related to the intensity and stability of therapy, concurrent drug use, history of gastrointestinal bleeding, risk of fall/trauma, recent surgery, and age.

5. Warfarin is prone to numerous clinically important drug-drug and drug-food interactions.

6. At the time of hospital admission, all patients should receive prophylaxis against VTE that corresponds to their level of risk. Prophylaxis should be continued throughout the period of risk.

7. In the absence of contraindications, the treatment of VTE initially should include a rapid-acting anticoagulant (e.g., unfractionated heparin [UFH], a low-molecular-weight heparin [LMWH], or fondaparinux) overlapped with warfarin for at least 5 days and until the patient's international normalized ratio (INR) is greater than 2.0. Anticoagulation therapy should be continued for a minimum of 3 months. The duration of anticoagulation therapy should be based on the patient's risk of VTE recurrence and major bleeding.

8. Most patients with an uncomplicated deep vein thrombosis (DVT) can be managed safely on an outpatient basis.

9. Heparin-induced thrombocytopenia (HIT) frequently goes unrecognized and is associated with a high risk of thrombosis and mortality. HIT is diagnosed based on clinical and laboratory data. It requires aggressive treatment with a direct thrombin inhibitor.

Venous thromboembolism (VTE) is a potentially fatal disorder and a significant national health problem in our aging society.[1,2] Although it can strike young, otherwise healthy adults, it occurs most frequently in patients who sustain multiple traumas, undergo major surgery, are immobile for a lengthy period of time, or have a hypercoagulable disorder. Resulting from clot formation within the venous circulation (Fig. 19–1), VTE is manifested as deep vein thrombosis (DVT) and pulmonary embolism (PE). Death from pulmonary embolism can occur within minutes of the onset of symptoms, before effective treatment can be given.

Unfortunately, the disease is often clinically silent and the first manifestation may be sudden death. In some case series, 80% of patients who died suddenly had some evidence of pulmonary embolism at the time of autopsy.[3] Beyond the symptoms produced by the acute event, the long-term sequelae of VTE, such as the postthrombotic syndrome and recurrent thromboembolic events, also cause substantial pain and suffering.[1]

The treatment of VTE is fraught with substantial risks.[4] Antithrombotic drugs require precise dosing and meticulous monitoring.[5–8] Systematic approaches to drug-therapy management substantially reduce the risks, but bleeding remains an all too common

and serious complication of administering antithrombotic drugs.[8,9] Therefore, the prevention of VTE in at-risk patients is paramount to improving outcomes.[3] When there is a suspicion of VTE, the rapid and accurate diagnosis of the disorder is critical to making appropriate treatment decisions.[10] The optimal use of antithrombotic drugs requires not only an in-depth knowledge of their pharmacology and pharmacokinetic properties but also a comprehensive approach to patient management.[6,11]

EPIDEMIOLOGY

The true incidence of VTE in the general population is unknown because a substantial portion of patients, perhaps greater than 50%, have clinically silent disease. An estimated 2 million people in the United States develop VTE each year; 600,000 are hospitalized, and 60,000 die.[12] The estimated annual direct medical costs of managing the disease are well over $1 billion and growing. The best available data indicate the age-adjusted annual incidence of symptomatic VTE in Caucasians to be 117 per 100,000.[13] The incidence of VTE nearly doubles in each decade of life over the age of 50 and is slightly higher

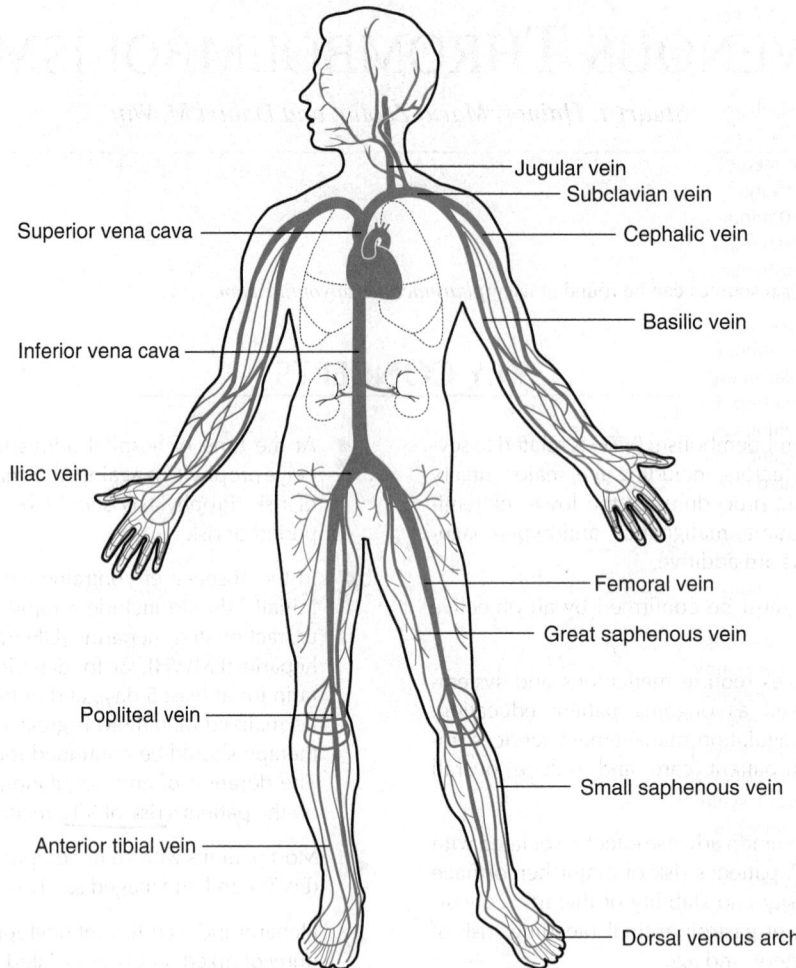

FIGURE 19–1. Venous circulation.

in men. The age-adjusted incidence of PE has declined slightly in recent years, presumably because of heightened awareness of VTE, effective prevention strategies, early diagnosis, and prompt treatment. However, as the population ages, the total number of cases of DVT and PE continues to climb.

Relatively little is known about the risk of VTE in ethnic populations. African-Americans appear to be at somewhat higher risk of VTE than are Americans of predominantly European ancestry, whereas Hispanic-Americans may be somewhat protected.[14] Asian-Americans and Pacific Islanders appear to have a strikingly lower incidence of VTE.

The incidence of VTE in specific high-risk patient populations has been studied extensively.[3] Patients who sustain multiple trauma or undergo an orthopedic procedure involving a lower extremity are at particularly high risk, with the incidence of VTE often exceeding 50% in the absence of effective prophylaxis. Among those undergoing major surgeries other than procedures involving the lower extremities, the incidence of VTE is 20% to 40% when one or more other risk factors are present, such as age over 60 years. The long-term incidence of VTE among patients who have a prior history of VTE or who have metastatic cancer is extremely high.[15,16] Likewise, the incidence of VTE after myocardial infarction, stroke, and spinal cord injury is high.[3] Several disorders of hypercoagulability also have been linked to a high lifetime incidence of VTE.[17,18]

ETIOLOGY

A number of factors increase the risk of developing VTE (Table 19–1). These risk factors are additive and can be identified easily in clinical practice. A prior history of venous thrombosis is perhaps the strongest risk factors for recurrent VTE, presumably because of the destruction of venous valves and obstruction of blood flow caused by the initial event.[19] Rapid blood flow has an inhibitory effect on thrombus formation, but a slow rate of flow reduces the clearance and dilution of activated clotting factors in the zone of injury and slows the influx of regulatory substances. Stasis tips the delicate balance of procoagulation and anticoagulation in favor of thrombogenesis. The rate of blood flow in the venous circulation, particularly in the deep veins of the lower extremities, is relatively slow. Valves in the deep veins of the legs, as well as contraction of the calf and thigh muscles, facilitate the flow of blood back to the heart and lungs. Damage to the venous valves and prolonged periods of immobility result in venous stasis. Vessel obstruction, either from external compression or a thrombus, also promotes clot propagation. Reduced venous blood flow explains, at least in part, why numerous medical conditions and surgical procedures are associated with an increased risk of VTE (see Table 19–1). Greater than normal blood viscosity, as seen in myeloproliferative disorders such as polycythemia vera, for example, also may contribute to slowed blood flow and thrombus formation.

TABLE 19–1. Risk Factors for Venous Thromboembolism

Risk Factor	Example
Age	Risk doubles with each decade after age 50
✱ History of VTE	Strongest known risk factor for DVT and PE
Venous stasis	Major medical illness (e.g., CHF, MI)
	Major surgery (e.g., general anesthesia >30 minutes)
	Paralysis (e.g., stroke, spinal cord injury)
	Polycythemia vera
	Obesity
	Varicose veins
Vascular injury	Major orthopedic surgery (e.g., knee and hip replacement)
	Trauma (esp. fractures of the pelvis, hip, or leg)
	Indwelling venous catheters
Hypercoagulable states	Malignancy, diagnosed or occult
	Activated protein C resistance/factor V Leiden
	Prothrombin (20210A) gene mutation
	Protein C deficiency
	Protein S deficiency
	Antithrombin (AT) deficiency
	Factor VIII excess (>90th percentile)
	Factor XI excess (>90th percentile)
	Antiphospholipid antibodies
	Dysfibrinogenemia
	Hyperhomocysteinemia
	Plasminogen activator inhibitor (PAI-1) excess
	Inflammatory bowel disease
	Nephrotic syndrome
	Pregnancy/postpartum
Drug therapy	Estrogen-containing oral contraceptive pills
	Estrogen-replacement therapy
	Selective estrogen-receptor modulators (SERMs)
	Heparin-induced thrombocytopenia (HIT)

From refs. 3, 17, and 18.

A growing list of hereditary deficiencies, gene mutations, and acquired diseases has been linked to hypercoagulability[17,18] (see Table 19–1). Activated protein C resistance is the most common genetic disorder of hypercoagulability, with a prevalence rate approaching 5% among community-dwelling Caucasians and a rate as high as 40% among those who suffer an idiopathic DVT or who have a strong family history of VTE. Although these patients have normal plasma concentrations of protein C, they often have a mutation on factor V that renders it resistant to degradation by activated protein C. This mutation is known as *factor V Leiden,* named after the city of Leiden, Holland, where the defect was initially reported. The prothrombin 20210A mutation also appears to be a relatively common defect, occurring in as many as 3% of healthy individuals of southern European ancestry and 16% of those with an idiopathic DVT. Although less common, inherited deficiencies of the natural anticoagulants protein C, protein S, and antithrombin place patients at a high lifetime risk for VTE. Conversely, excessively high concentrations of factors VIII, IX, and XI also increase the risk of VTE. Given the prevalence of these inherited abnormalities in the general population, some patients have multiple genetic defects that have additive effects in terms of increasing the lifetime thrombotic risk.

Acquired disorders of hypercoagulability may result from malignancy, the presence of antiphospholipid antibodies, and estrogen use. The strong link between cancer and thrombosis has been recognized since the late 1800s.[20] Tumor cells secrete a number of procoagulant substances that activate the coagulation cascade. Further, patients with cancer often have suppressed levels of protein C, protein S, and antithrombin. It has been postulated that cancer cells use thrombotic mechanisms to recruit a blood supply (angiogenesis), metastasize, and create a barrier against host defense mechanisms. Antiphospholipid antibodies, most commonly found in patients with autoimmune disorders such as systemic lupus erythematosus (SLE) and inflammatory bowel disease, can cause venous and arterial thrombosis.[17] These antibodies are also associated with repeated pregnancy loss due to placental thrombosis. The precise mechanism by which the antiphospholipid antibodies provoke thrombosis is unclear, but they appear to activate the coagulation cascade and platelets, as well as to inhibit the anticoagulant activity of proteins C and S. Estrogen-containing contraceptives, estrogen-replacement therapy, and the selective estrogen-receptor modulators (SERMs) all have been linked to venous thrombosis.[21] Women with an underlying disorder of hypercoagulability are at particularly high risk of developing venous thrombosis while taking estrogens. While the mechanisms are not clearly understood, estrogens increase serum clotting factor concentrations and induce activated protein C resistance. Increased serum estrogen concentrations may explain, in part, the increased risk of VTE observed during pregnancy and the immediate postpartum period.[22]

PATHOPHYSIOLOGY

The arrest of bleeding following vascular injury, or hemostasis, is essential to life.[23,24] Within the vascular system, blood remains in a fluid state, transporting oxygen, nutrients, plasma proteins, and waste. With vascular injury, a dynamic series of reactions involving a complex interplay of thrombogenic and antithrombotic stimuli results in the local formation of a hemostatic plug that seals the vessel wall and prevents further blood loss (Table 19–2 and Figs. 19–2, 19–3, and 19–4). A disruption of this delicate system of checks and balances may lead to inappropriate clot formation within the blood vessel that

TABLE 19–2. Factors Regulating Hemostasis and Thrombosis

	Thrombogenic	Antithrombotic
Vessel wall	Exposed subendothelium	Heparan sulfate
	Tissue factor	Dermatan sulfate
	Plasminogen activator inhibitor–1 (PAI–1)	Thrombomodulin
		Tissue plasminogen activator (t-PA)
		Urokinase plasminogen activator (u-PA)
Circulating elements	Platelets	Antithrombin (AT)
	Platelet activating factor (PAF)	Heparin cofactor II
	Clotting factors	Protein C
	Prothrombin (Factor II)	Protein S
	Fibrinogen (Factor I)	Plasminogen
	von Willebrand factor (vWF)	Tissue factor pathway inhibitor
	α_2-Antiplasmin	Proteolytic enzymes
Blood flow	Slow rate of flow	Fast rate of flow
	Turbulent flow	Laminar flow

From ref. 23.

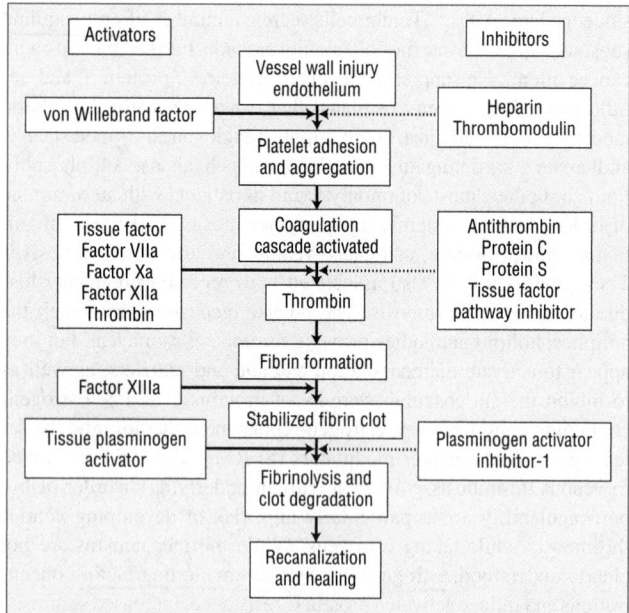

FIGURE 19–2. Hemostasis and thrombosis.

subsequently obstructs blood flow or embolizes to a distant vascular bed. In the late 1800s, Dr. Rudolf Virchow, a German pathologist, recognized the role played by blood vessels, circulating elements in the blood, and the speed of blood flow in the regulation of clot formation[23] (see Table 19–2). Alterations in any one of these elements, known today as *Virchow's triad,* may lead to pathologic clot formation.

Under normal circumstances, the endothelial cells that form the intima of vessels maintain blood flow by producing a number of substances that inhibit platelet adherence, prevent the activation of the coagulation cascade, and facilitate fibrinolysis.[23,24] Vascular injury can expose the subendothelium (see Fig. 19–3). Platelets readily adhere to the subendothelium, using glycoprotein Ib receptors found on their surfaces and facilitated by von Willebrand factor. This causes platelets to become activated, releasing a number of procoagulant substances into the local circulation that stimulate platelets to expose glycoprotein IIb-IIIa receptors. These receptors allow the platelets to adhere to one another, resulting in platelet aggregation. In addition, the damaged vascular tissue releases tissue factor, also known as *tissue thromboplastin,* which activates the extrinsic pathway of the coagulation cascade (see Fig. 19–4).

The coagulation cascade is a stepwise series of enzymatic reactions that results in the formation of a fibrin mesh.[23,24] Clotting factors

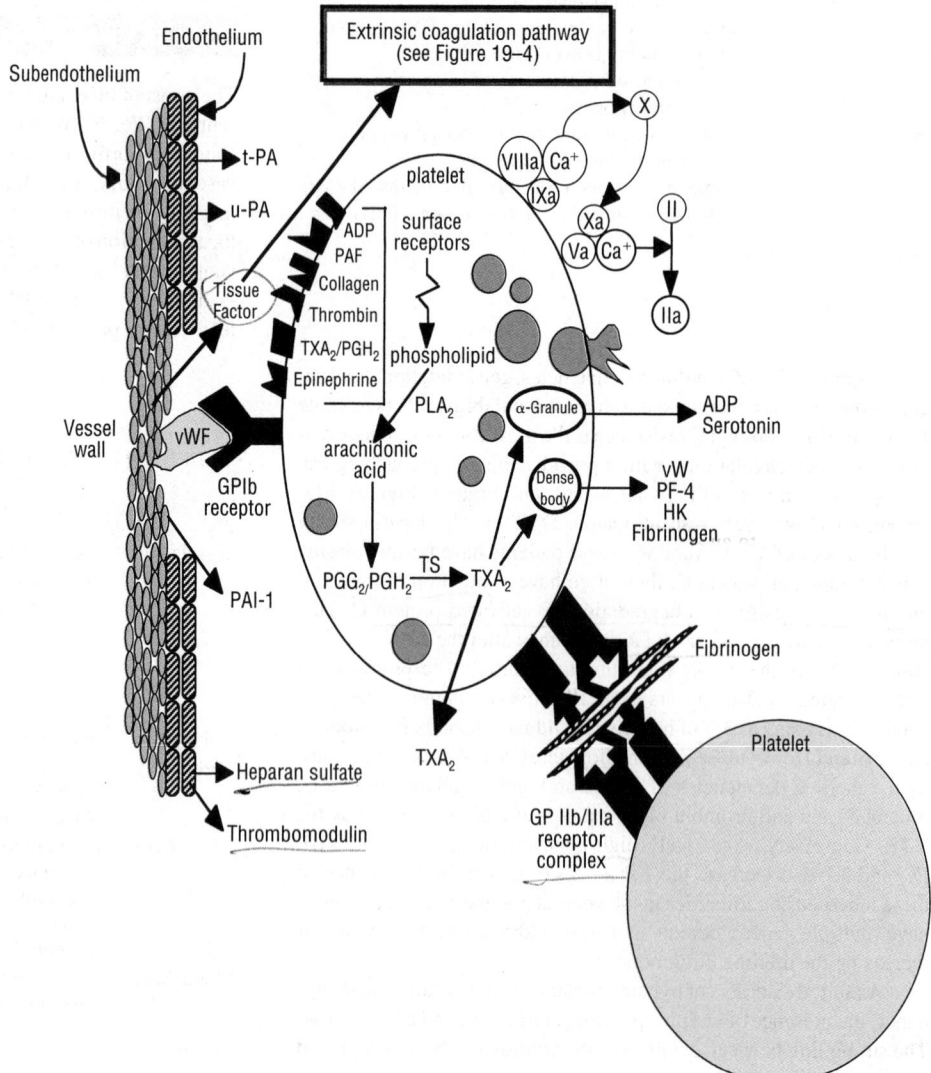

FIGURE 19–3. Vascular injury and thrombosis. ADP = adenosine diphosphate; CO = cyclooxygenase; GP Ib = glycoprotein Ib; GP IIb/IIa = glycoprotein IIb/IIa; HK = high-molecular-weight kininogen; PAF = platelet-activating factor; PAI-1 = plasminogen activator inhibitor; PF-4 = platelet factor-4; PGG/PGH = prostaglandins; PGI = prostacyclin; PLA = phospholipase A; TS = thromboxane synthetase; TXA₂ = thromboxane A₂; t-PA = tissue plasmogen activator; u-PA = urokinase plasmogen activator; vWF = von Willebrand factor.

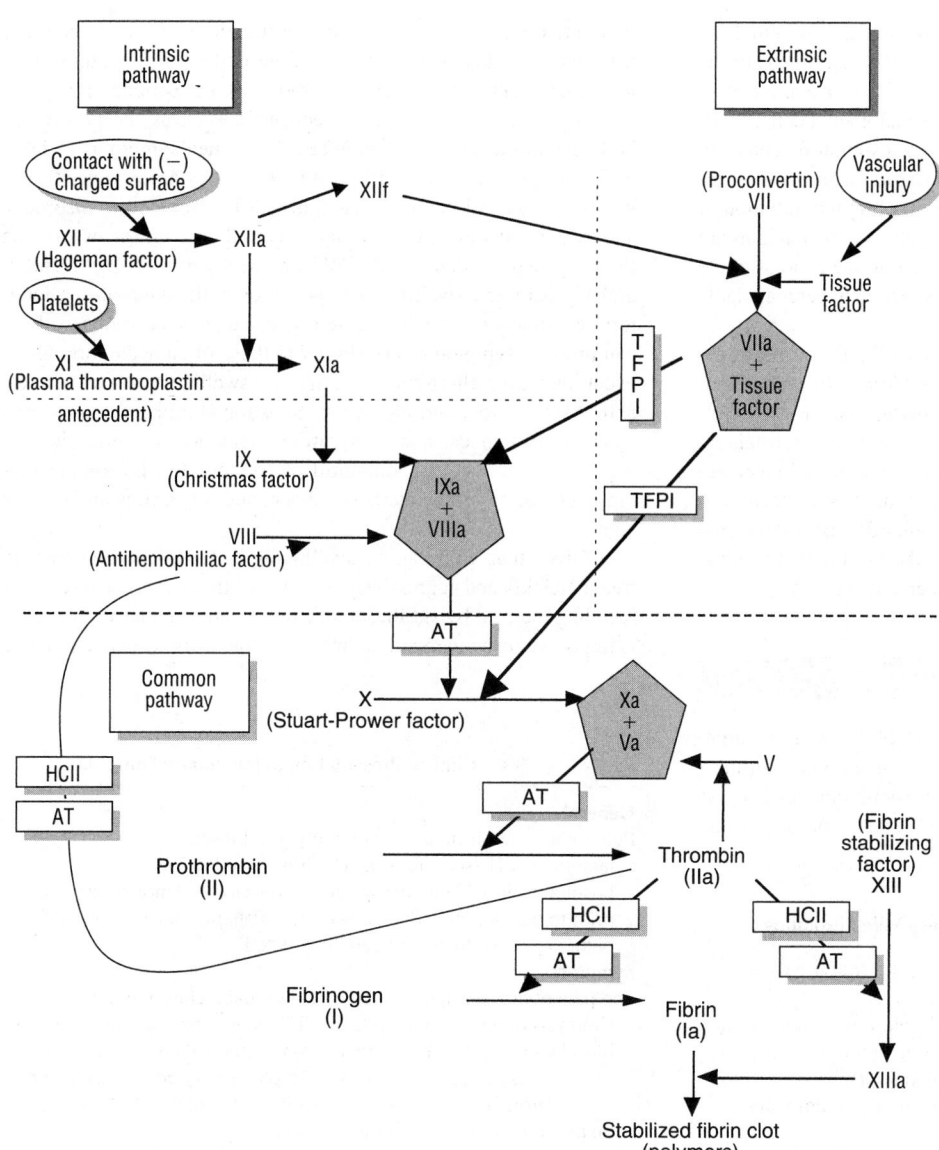

FIGURE 19–4. Coagulation cascade. AT = antithrombin; HCII = heparin cofactor II; TFPI = tissue factor pathway inhibitor.

circulate in the blood in inactive forms. Specific stimuli convert an inactive precursor into an active form that, in turn, converts the next precursor in the sequence. It was once believed that all clotting factors were proteolytic enzymes, known as *zymogens*. It is now known that factors V and VIII have no enzymatic activity themselves but rather serve as cofactors that greatly accelerate the enzymatic activity of their respective partners. The final steps in the cascade are the conversion of prothrombin to thrombin and fibrinogen to fibrin. Thrombin plays a key role in the coagulation cascade; it is responsible not only for the production of fibrin but also for the conversion of factors V and VIII, creating a positive-feedback loop that greatly accelerates the production of more thrombin. Additionally, thrombin enhances platelet aggregation through its interactions with the glycoprotein IIb-IIIa receptor.

Traditionally, the coagulation cascade has been divided into three distinct parts: the intrinsic, extrinsic, and common pathways[23,24] (see Fig. 19–4). This artificial division is somewhat misleading because there are numerous interactions among the three pathways. The extrinsic pathway, sometimes referred to as the *tissue factor pathway,* appears to be the principal mechanism that triggers the coagulation

cascade. Tissue factor, released from the subendothelium, forms a complex with factor VIIa. The factor VIIa–tissue factor complex activates factor X in the common pathway and factor IX in the intrinsic pathway. The intrinsic pathway may begin in several ways. Negatively charged surfaces in contact with the blood will activate factor XII, and activated platelets can convert factor XI. Both the intrinsic and extrinsic pathways meet at a common point with the activation of factor X. With its partner, factor Va, factor Xa converts prothrombin (II) to thrombin (IIa), which then cleaves fibrinogen to form fibrin monomers. Finally, as the fibrin monomers reach a critical concentration, they begin to precipitate and polymerize to form fibrin strands. Factor XIIIa covalently bonds these strands to one another.

Normally, a number of tempering mechanisms control coagulation[23,24] (see Table 19–2 and Fig. 19–2). Without effective self-regulation, the coagulation cascade would proceed unabated until all the clotting factors and platelets were consumed. Thus the intact endothelium adjacent to the damaged tissue actively secretes several antithrombotic substances. As its name implies, thrombomodulin modulates thrombin activity by converting protein C to its active form. When joined with its cofactor, protein S, protein C enzymatically inactivates factors Va and VIIIa. Activated protein C also stimulates the release of tissue plasminogen activator (t-PA). Antithrombin is a circulating protein that inhibits thrombin and factor Xa. Heparan sulfate, a heparin-like compound secreted by endothelial cells, exponentially accelerates antithrombin activity. By a similar mechanism, heparin cofactor II also inhibits thrombin. Tissue factor pathway inhibitor (TFPI) plays an important role by regulating the initiation of the coagulation cascade. When these self-regulatory mechanisms are intact, the formation of the fibrin clot is limited to the zone of tissue injury. However, disruptions in the system, so-called hypercoagulable states, often result in thrombosis.[23,24]

The fibrinolytic protein plasmin degrades the fibrin mesh into soluble end products collectively known as *fibrin split products* or *fibrin degradation products.*[23,24] The fibrinolytic system is also under the control of a series of stimulatory and inhibitory substances. Tissue plasminogen activator (t-PA) and urokinase plasminogen activator (u-PA) convert plasminogen to plasmin. Plasminogen activator inhibitor-1 (PAI-1) inhibits the plasminogen activators, and α_2-antiplasmin inhibits plasmin activity. Aberrations in the fibrinolytic system also have been linked to hypercoagulability.

CLINICAL PRESENTATION AND DIAGNOSIS

Although a thrombus can form in any part of the venous circulation, the majority begin in the lower extremities. Once formed, a venous thrombus may either (1) remain asymptomatic, (2) lyse spontaneously, (3) obstruct the venous circulation, (4) propagate into more proximal veins, (5) embolize, or (6) act in any combination of these ways.[10] Most patients with VTE never develop symptoms from the acute event.[25] However, even those who experience no symptoms may suffer long-term consequences, such as the postthrombotic syndrome and recurrent VTE. Even when symptoms of DVT or PE are present (Tables 19–3 and 19–4), they are nonspecific.[1,26] It is extremely difficult to distinguish VTE from other disorders, and additional objective tests are required to confirm or exclude the diagnosis. Patients with DVT frequently present with unilateral leg pain and swelling. The postthrombotic syndrome, a long-term complication of DVT caused by damage to the venous valves, can produce symptoms very similar to those of an acute thrombotic event, including chronic lower extremity swelling, pain, tenderness, skin discoloration, and ulceration. Symptomatic PE often produces dyspnea, tachypnea, and tachycardia. Hemoptysis, while distressing, occurs in less than one-third of patients. Cardiovascular collapse, characterized by cyanosis, shock, and oliguria, is an ominous sign.

Given that VTE can be debilitating or fatal, it is important to treat it quickly and aggressively.[2,10] On the other hand, because major bleeding induced by antithrombotic drugs can be equally harmful, it is important to avoid treatment when the diagnosis is not a reasonable

TABLE 19–3. Clinical Presentation of Deep Vein Thrombosis (DVT)

General

Venous thromboembolism most commonly develops in patients with identifiable risk factors (see Table 19–1) during or following a hospitalization. Many patients, perhaps the majority, have asymptomatic disease. Patients may die suddenly of pulmonary embolism.

Symptoms

The patient may complain of leg swelling, pain, or warmth. Symptoms are nonspecific, and objective testing must be performed to establish the diagnosis.

Signs

- The patient's superficial veins may be dilated, and a "palpable cord" may be felt in the affected leg.
- The patient may experience pain in back of the knee when the examiner dorsiflexes the foot of the affected leg.

Laboratory Tests

- Serum concentrations of D-dimer, a by-product of thrombin generation, usually are elevated.
- The patient may have an elevated erythrocyte sedimentation rate (ESR) and white blood cell (WBC) count.

Diagnostic Tests

- Duplex ultrasonography is the most commonly used test to diagnosis DVT. It is a noninvasive test that can measure the rate and direction of blood flow and visualize clot formation in proximal veins of the legs. It cannot reliably detect small blood clots in distal veins. Coupled with a careful clinical assessment, it can rule in or out the diagnosis in the majority of cases.
- Venography (also known as phlebography) is the "gold standard" for the diagnosis of DVT. However, it is an invasive test that involves injection of radiopaque contrast dye into a foot vein. It is expensive and can cause anaphylaxis and nephrotoxicity.

TABLE 19–4. Clinical Presentation of Pulmonary Embolism

General

Pulmonary embolism most commonly develops in patients with risk factors for VTE (see Table 19–1) during or following a hospitalization. While many patients develop a symptomatic DVT prior to developing a PE, many do not. Patients may die suddenly before effective treatment can be initiated.

Symptoms

The patient may complain of cough, chest pain, chest tightness, shortness of breath, or palpitation. The patient may spit or cough up blood (hemoptysis). When PE is massive, the patient may complain of dizziness or light-headedness. Symptoms may be confused with a myocardial infarction or pneumonia, and objective testing must be performed to establish the diagnosis.

Signs

The patient may have tachypnea (increased respiratory rate) and tachycardia (increased heart rate). The patient may appear diaphoretic (sweaty). The patient's neck veins may be distended. In massive PE, the patient may appear cyanotic and may become hypotensive. In such cases, oxygen saturation by pulse oximetry or arterial blood gas likely will indicate that the patient is hypoxic. In the worse case, the patient may go into circulatory shock and die within minutes.

Laboratory Tests

- Serum concentrations of D-dimer, a by-product of thrombin generation, usually are elevated.
- The patient may have an elevated erythrocyte sedimentation rate (ESR) and white blood cell (WBC) count.

Diagnostic Tests

- Ventilation-perfusion ($\dot{V}/\dot{Q}$) and computed tomographic (CT) scans are the most commonly used tests to diagnosis PE. A $\dot{V}/\dot{Q}$ scan measures the distribution of blood and airflow in the lungs. When there is a large mismatch between blood and airflow in one area of the lung, there is a high probability that the patient has a PE. Spiral CT scans can detect emboli in the pulmonary arteries.
- Pulmonary angiography is the "gold standard" for the diagnosis of PE. However, it is an invasive test that involves injection of radiopaque contrast dye into the pulmonary artery. The test is expensive and associated with a significant risk of mortality.

certainty. Assessment of the patient's status should focus on a search for risk factors in the patient's medical history[27] (see Table 19–1). Venous thrombosis is uncommon in the absence of risk factors, and the effects of these risks are additive. Conversely, even when the symptoms are mild or vague, VTE should be strongly suspected in those with multiple risk factors.

❷ Because radiographic contrast studies are the most accurate and reliable methods for the diagnosis of VTE, they are considered the "gold standards" in clinical trials.[10] Contrast venography allows visualization of the entire venous system in the lower extremity and abdomen. Pulmonary angiography allows visualization of the pulmonary arteries. The diagnosis of VTE can be made if there is a persistent intraluminal filling defect observed on multiple x-ray films. Contrast studies are expensive, invasive procedures that are technically difficult to perform and evaluate. Severely ill patients are often unable to tolerate the procedure, and many develop hypotension and cardiac arrhythmias. Furthermore, the contrast medium is irritating to vessel walls and toxic to the kidneys. For these reasons, noninvasive tests, such as ultrasonography, computed tomographic (CT) scans, and the ventilation-perfusion ($\dot{V}/\dot{Q}$) scan, are used frequently in clinical practice for the initial evaluation of patients with suspected VTE.[1,10]

Despite its pitfalls, clinical assessment improves the diagnostic accuracy of a noninvasive test.[1,10] Simple assessment checklists can be used to stratify patients into high, moderate, and low probability of a DVT or PE (Table 19–5). Patients with a high pretest probability of VTE have a greater than 60% chance of having VTE compared with only 5% in the low pretest probability group. Clinical assessment can rule in or rule out the diagnosis of VTE with reasonable certainty when its results are concordant with those of a noninvasive test.[1,10,26] In patients with a moderate pretest probability of VTE and an abnormal lower extremity ultrasonogram, the diagnosis of VTE can be reasonably concluded. If the results of the clinical assessment and the ultrasonogram are discordant, venography or angiography should be performed to make the definitive diagnosis.

TABLE 19–5. Clinical Assessment Models for DVT and PE

Clinical Feature	Score
Pretest Probability of DVT	
Tenderness along entire deep vein system	1.0
Swelling of the entire leg	1.0
Greater than 3-cm difference in calf circumference	1.0
Pitting edema	1.0
Collateral superficial veins	1.0
Risk factors present:	
Active cancer	1.0
Prolonged immobility or paralysis	1.0
Recent surgery or major medical illness	1.0
Alternative diagnosis likely (ruptured Baker's cyst, rheumatoid arthritis, superficial thrombophlebitis, or infective cellulitis)	−2.0
Score ≥3 = high probability; 1–2 = moderate probability; ≤0 = low probability	
Pretest Probability of PE	
Clinical features of deep vein thrombosis	3.0
Recent prolonged immobility or surgery	1.5
Active cancer	1.0
History of deep vein thrombosis or pulmonary embolism	1.5
Hemoptysis	1.0
Resting heart rate > 100 beats per minute	1.5
No alternative explanation for acute shortness of breath or chest pain	3.0
Score ≥6 = high probability; 2–6 = moderate probability; ≤1.5 = low probability	

From refs. 1 and 10.

▶ TREATMENT: Venous Thromboembolism

PHARMACOLOGIC AGENTS USED IN THE MANAGEMENT OF VTE

UNFRACTIONATED HEPARIN (UFH)

Since the 1930s, clinicians have used unfractionated heparin (UFH) for the prevention and treatment of thrombosis.[7] McLean discovered UFH in 1916 when he found that an extract of dog liver was an inhibitor of coagulation.[28] While it has been known since 1939 that UFH requires a "heparin cofactor" to produce an anticoagulant effect, it was not until 1968 that antithrombin (previously known as antithrombin III) was identified and isolated. Soon thereafter it was recognized that UFH greatly accelerated the activity of antithrombin. Commercially available UFH preparations are derived from bovine lung or porcine intestinal mucosa. Although some differences exist between those two preparations, no differences in antithrombotic activity have been demonstrated. Today, UFH and the low-molecular-weight heparins (LMWHs) are the mainstays for the acute treatment of arterial and venous thrombosis.[7]

Pharmacology

UFH is a heterogeneous mixture of sulfated glycosaminoglycans of variable lengths and pharmacologic properties[28] (Table 19–6). Each heparin molecule is composed of repetitive units of D-glycosamine and uronic acid. The molecular weights of these molecules range from 5000 to 30,000 Da, with a mean of 15,000 Da.[7] The anticoagulant profile and clearance of each UFH molecule varies based on its length. The smaller chains are cleared less rapidly than their longer counterparts.

The anticoagulant effect of UFH is mediated through a specific pentasaccharide sequence on the heparin molecule that binds to antithrombin, provoking a conformational change[7] (Fig. 19–5). Only one-third of the UFH molecules possess the unique pentasaccharide sequence with affinity for antithrombin.[7] The UFH-antithrombin complex is 100 to 1000 times more potent as an anticoagulant compared with antithrombin alone. Antithrombin inhibits the activity of several clotting factors, including factors IXa, Xa, and XIIa and thrombin[7] (see Fig. 19–4). Through its action on thrombin, the UFH-antithrombin complex also inhibits the thrombin-induced activation of factors V and VIII.[7] UFH prevents the growth and propagation of a formed thrombus and allows the patient's own thrombolytic system to degrade the clot.

Factors IIa and Xa are the most sensitive to inhibition by the UFH-antithrombin complex. In order to inactivate thrombin, the heparin molecule must form a ternary complex bridging between antithrombin and thrombin[7] (see Fig. 19–5). Only molecules that contain more than 18 saccharides are able to bind to both antithrombin and thrombin simultaneously. Smaller heparin molecules cannot facilitate

TABLE 19–6. Comparison of the Chemical and Pharmacokinetic Properties of Antithrombotic Drugs Used for VTE

Agent (Trade Name)	FDA-Approved (2004)	Method of Preparation	Mean Molecular Weight (Da)	Plasma Half-Life	Anti-Xa–Anti-IIa activity	Bioavailability
Unfractionated Heparin	Yes	Extracted from porcine gut mucosa or beef lung	≈15,000	30–90 min (dose dependent)	1:1	SC: 30–70% (dose dependent)
Low-Molecular-Weight Heparins (LMWHs)						
Ardeparin (Normiflo)	Yes (no longer marketed in U.S.)	Peroxidative depolymerization	≈6,000	200 min	1.9:1	SC: 90%
Dalteparin (Fragmin)	Yes	Nitrous acid depolymerization	≈6,000	119–139 min	2.7:1	SC: 87%
Enoxaparin (Lovenox)	Yes	Benzylation and alkaline depolymerization	≈4,200	129–180 min	3.8:1	SC: 92%
Nadroparin (Fraxiparine)	No (available in Canada and Mexico)	Nitrous acid depolymerization	≈4,500	132–162 min	3.6:1	SC: 99%
Tinzaparin (Innohep)	Yes	Heparinase digestion	≈4,500	111–234 min	2.8:1	SC: 90%
Heparinoid						
Danaparoid (Orgaran)	Yes (no longer marketed in U.S.)	Extracted from porcine gut mucosa	≈6,500	22–24 h	20:1	SC: 95%
Anti-Factor Xa Inhibitors						
Fondaparinux (Arixtra)	Yes	Synthetic	1,728	15–18 h	100% anti-Xa	SC: 100%
Indraparinux (SanOrg 34006)	No	Synthetic	≈1700	≈80 h	100% anti-Xa	SC: 100%
Direct Thrombin Inhibitors (DTIs)						
Argatroban (Argatroban)	Yes	Synthetic	509	30–50 min	100% anti-IIa	
Bivalrudin (Angiomax)	Yes	Semi-synthetic	2180	25 min	100% anti-IIa	
Desirudin (Iprivask)	Yes	Recombinant DNA technology	6964	120 min	100% anti-IIa	SC: >90%
Lepirudin (Refludan)	Yes	Recombinant DNA technology	6980	80 min	100% anti-IIa	SC: 70%
Ximelagatran (Exanta)	No	Synthetic	474	3–5 h	100% anti-IIa	Oral: 40–45%
Vitamin K antagonists						
Warfarin (Coumadin)	Yes	Synthetic	330	40 h	1:1	Oral: 90–100%

From refs. 23, 41, 119, and 120.

the interaction between antithrombin and thrombin.[7] In contrast, the inactivation of factor Xa does not require UFH to form a bridge with antithrombin. It only requires that UFH bind to antithrombin using the specific pentasaccharide sequence. Heparin molecules with as few as five saccharide units are able to catalyze the inhibition of factor Xa.[7] Heparin uncouples from antithrombin after it has produced its effect and quickly recouples with another antithrombin molecule. Because of its relatively large size, the UFH-antithrombin complex is incapable of inactivating thrombin or factor Xa within a formed clot or bound to surfaces. At high doses, UFH also binds to heparin cofactor II, further inhibiting the activity of thrombin.[7] UFH increases the release of TFPI from vascular endothelium, augmenting its inhibitory effect on factor Xa.[7] UFH, especially high-molecular-weight heparin fractions, also binds to platelets and inhibits platelet aggregation.

Pharmacokinetics

UFH is not absorbed reliably when taken orally because of its large molecular size and anionic structure. The bioavailability and biologic activity of UFH are limited by its propensity to bind to plasma proteins, platelet factor-4 (PF-4), macrophages, fibrinogen, lipoproteins, and endothelial cells.[7,28] This may explain the substantial inter- and intrapatient variability observed in the anticoagulation response to UFH. Patients who are acutely ill or have active thrombosis have rapid changes in the circulating levels of these heparin-binding proteins.

These patients often appear to have "heparin resistance," requiring relatively high doses of UFH to achieve a therapeutic response.[7]

The subcutaneous bioavailability of UFH is dose-dependent and ranges from 30% at low doses to as much as 70% at high doses. Higher doses presumably saturate protein-binding sites, thereby permitting a larger proportion to reach the systemic circulation. The onset of anticoagulant effect is usually evident 1 to 2 hours after subcutaneous injection.[7] Because of its unpredictable absorption and delayed onset when administered subcutaneously, heparin should be administered intravenously when the patient requires rapid anticoagulation. A continuous intravenous infusion is preferable. Intermittent intravenous boluses produce relatively high peaks in anticoagulation activity and have been associated with a greater risk of major bleeding.[7] Intramuscular administration is discouraged because the absorption is erratic, and it may result in large hematomas.

The volume of distribution of UFH is similar to blood volume ($V_D = 60$ mL/kg).[7] The dose required to achieve a therapeutic anticoagulation response is correlated to weight. Obese patients do not have a proportional increase in blood volume relative to body weight. However, it is unclear if the patient's actual or adjusted body weight should be used when calculating initial heparin doses for obese patients.

UFH has a dose-dependent half-life of approximately 30 to 90 minutes but may be prolonged to as much as 150 minutes when given in high doses to some patients.[7] There are two primary mechanisms for the elimination of UFH.[7,28] The relative contribution of each mechanism to the total clearance of heparin is related to the

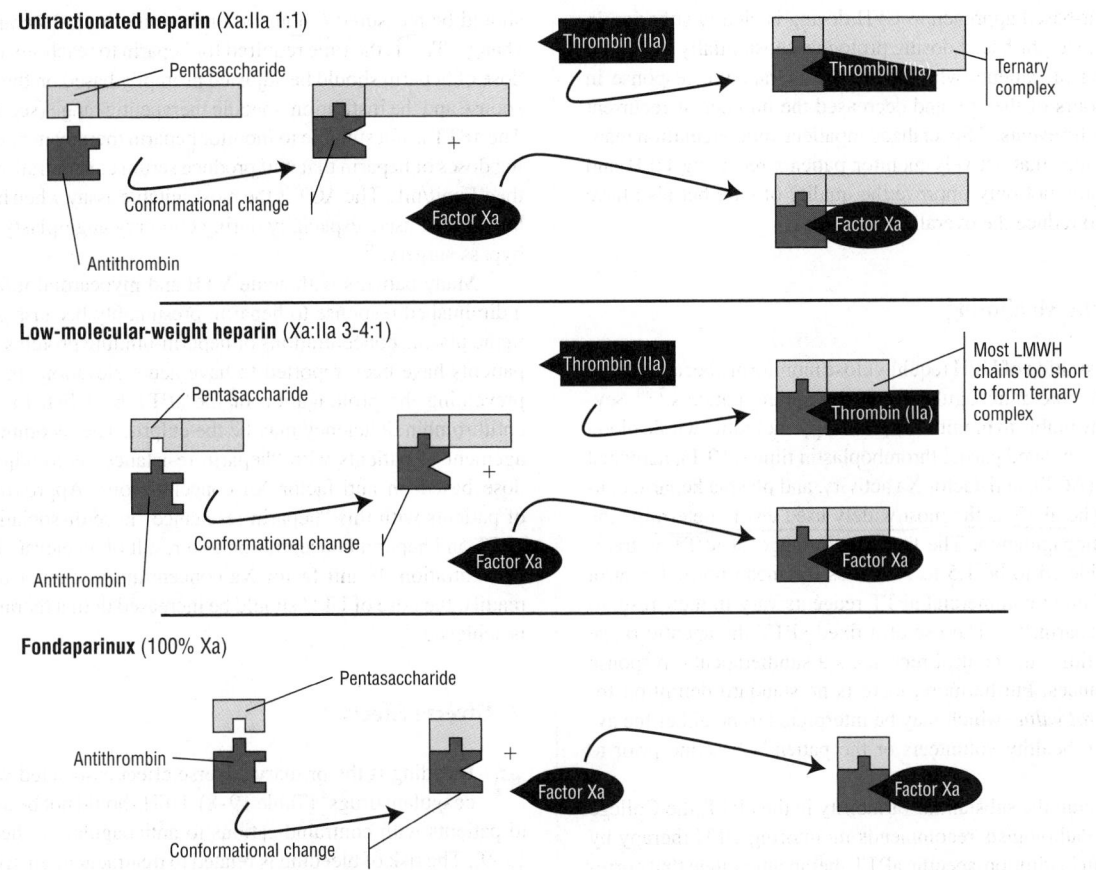

FIGURE 19–5. Pharmacologic activity of unfractionated heparin, low-molecular-weight heparins, and fondaparinux. AT = antithrombin.

dose and size of the UFH molecules. One mechanism is a rapid but saturable zero-order process. Heparinases and desulfatases enzymatically inactivate heparin molecules bound to endothelial cells and macrophages, reducing them to smaller and less sulfated molecules. Heparin is also eliminated renally. This first-order process is slower and nonsaturable. Low doses of UFH are cleared principally by the saturable, rapid zero-order mechanism, whereas the renal route predominates at very high doses. With typical regimens, a combination of the two mechanisms is used to eliminate UFH. Renal and hepatic dysfunction reduces the rate of clearance of UFH. Patients with active thrombosis may eliminate UFH more rapidly, possibly because of increased binding to acute-phase reactants.

Dose and Administration

The dose and route of administration for UFH heparin are based on the indication, the therapeutic goals, and the patient's individual response to therapy.[7] The dose of UFH is expressed in units of activity. The number of units per milligram is variable and depends on the manufacturing process.[28] For the prevention of VTE, UFH is given by subcutaneous injection in the abdominal fat layer. The typical dose for prophylaxis is 5000 units every 8 to 12 hours. When immediate and full anticoagulation is required, a weight-based intravenous bolus dose followed by a continuous infusion is preferred[7,29] (Table 19–7). While some clinicians continue to use the time-honored "standard" dosing regimen consisting of a 5000-unit bolus followed by an infusion rate of 1000 to 1200 units per

TABLE 19–7. Weight-Based[a] Dosing for UFH Administered by Continuous Intravenous Infusion

Indication	Initial Loading Dose	Initial Infusion Rate
DVT/PE	80–100 units/kg Maximum = 10,000 units	17–20 units/kg/h Maximum = 2300 units/h

aPTT (s)	Maintenance Infusion Rate Dose Adjustment
<37 (or >12 s below institution-specific therapeutic range)	80 units/kg bolus; then increase infusion by 4 units/kg/h
37–47 (or 1–12 s below institution-specific therapeutic range)	40 units/kg bolus; then increase infusion by 2 units/kg/h
48–71 (within institution-specific therapeutic range)	No change
72–93 (or 1–22 s above institution-specific therapeutic range)	Decrease infusion by 2 units/kg/h
>93 (or >22 s above institution-specific therapeutic range)	Hold infusion for 1 h; then decrease by 3 units/kg/h

[a]Use actual body weight for all calculations. Adjusted body weight may be used for obese patients (>130% of IBW).
From refs. 7 and 29.

hour, a weight-based approach to UFH dosing is clearly superior. In clinical trials, weight-based dosing protocols substantially increased the proportion of patients who achieved a therapeutic response in the first 24 hours of therapy and decreased the number of recurrent thromboembolic events.[29] Specialized inpatient anticoagulation management services that actively monitor patients receiving UFH and warfarin therapy not only improve the quality of care but also have been shown to reduce the overall cost of care.[9]

Therapeutic Monitoring

Administration of UFH requires close monitoring because of the unpredictable anticoagulant response among patients.[7,30] Several tests are available to monitor UFH therapy, including whole blood clotting time, activated partial thromboplastin time (aPTT), activated clotting time (ACT), anti-factor Xa activity, and plasma heparin concentrations. The aPTT is the most widely used test to determine the degree of anticoagulation. The therapeutic range of aPTT is traditionally considered to be 1.5 to 2.5 times the mean normal control value.[7,30] Different commercial aPTT reagents vary in their responsiveness to heparin.[31,32] The use of a fixed aPTT therapeutic range of 1.5 to 2.5 times the control represents a subtherapeutic response in many instances. Furthermore, there is no standard definition for the term *control value,* which may be interpreted to be either the average aPTT in healthy volunteers or the patient's baseline prior to treatment.

Recognizing the substantial variability in the aPTT, the College of American Pathologists recommends monitoring UFH therapy by establishing an institution-specific aPTT therapeutic range that correlates with a plasma heparin concentration of 0.2 to 0.4 units/mL by a protamine titration assay or 0.3 to 0.7 units/mL by an amidolytic anti-factor Xa assay.[30] Ideally, this should be done by comparing aPTT measurements with heparin levels or antifactor Xa activity in plasma samples obtained from patients treated with heparin. Alternatively, but considered a less reliable method, the aPTT reagent can be calibrated by adding heparin at several clinically relevant concentrations in vitro to several plasma samples.

The use of aPTT has several limitations.[7,31] First, the aPTT does not reliably correlate with heparin concentrations because factors such as reagent sensitivity, temperature, collection methods, and hemodilution produce variability. Second, the turnaround time in most institutions is relatively slow because of the time required to collect and process the sample in a central laboratory. Third, while the aPTT can measure the intensity of anticoagulation when the heparin concentration is 0.1–1 units/mL, it is prolonged beyond measurable limits when the concentration exceeds 1 unit/mL. Fourth, the lower-molecular-weight heparin fragments accumulate but have little effect on the aPTT in vivo.[7,31] Lastly, the data supporting the currently recommended heparin concentration therapeutic range are not robust. Despite these problems, most experts advocate using the aPTT to monitor UFH provided that institution-specific therapeutic ranges are defined.[31,32]

When used in full therapeutic doses, UFH must be monitored to determine the appropriate dose to administer.[7,30] The choice of assay is based on clinician preference and institutional availability. The aPTT remains the most commonly used test to monitor UFH therapy in North America. In some European countries, anti-factor Xa heparin activity is used commonly. The aPTT should be measured prior to the initiation of therapy to determine the patient's baseline. When administered by intravenous infusion, the response to therapy should be measured 6 hours after the initiation of therapy or a dose change. This is the time required for heparin to reach steady state. The dose of heparin should be adjusted promptly based on the patient's response and the institution-specific therapeutic range (see Table 19–7). The aPTT is not suitable to monitor heparin therapy in patients requiring doses of heparin that will produce serum concentrations of greater than 1 unit/mL. The ACT is the most suitable assay when high doses of heparin are used, especially during coronary angioplasty or coronary bypass surgery.[30]

Many patients with acute VTE and myocardial infarction have a diminished response to heparin, presumably because of variations in the plasma concentrations of heparin-binding proteins.[7,28,33] Some patients have been reported to have acute elevations in factor VIII, preventing the prolongation of the aPTT by UFH. In some cases, antithrombin deficiency may be the culprit. The recommended management of patients with "heparin resistance" is to adjust the UFH dose based on anti-factor Xa concentrations. Approximately 50% of patients with this "heparin resistance" have dissociation between aPTT and heparin concentration as a result of an elevated factor VIII concentration. If anti-factor Xa concentrations cannot be measured readily, the dose of UFH should be increased until a therapeutic aPTT is achieved.

Adverse Effects

Bleeding is the primary adverse effect associated with all anticoagulant drugs[4] (Table 19–8). UFH should not be administered to patients with contraindications to anticoagulation therapy (Table 19–9). The risk of bleeding is related to treatment intensity. Low-dose subcutaneous UFH is associated with a minimal risk of major bleeding. The rates of major bleeding for patients with VTE receiving full therapeutic doses of UFH via intravenous infusion for 5 to 10 days range from 2% to 4%, and the rate of fatal bleeding ranges from approximately 0% to 2%.[4] The presence of concomitant bleeding risks such as thrombocytopenia, the use other antithrombotic therapy, and a preexisting source of bleeding increase the risk of UFH-induced hemorrhage. The risk of bleeding also increases with age. Recent surgery, hemostatic defects, heavy alcohol consumption, renal failure, peptic ulcers, and neoplasms also increase the risk of major bleeding while receiving UFH.

The most common sites for bleeding are the gastrointestinal and urinary tracts, as well as soft tissues. Bruising at the site of injection is common. Local irritation, mild pain, erythema, histamine-like

TABLE 19–8. Risk Factors for Major Bleeding While Taking Anticoagulation Therapy

Anticoagulation intensity (e.g., INR > 4.0)
Initiation of therapy (first few days and weeks)
Unstable anticoagulation response
Age > 65 years
Concurrent antiplatelet drug or NSAID use
History of gastrointestinal bleeding
Recent surgery or trauma
Fall
Heavy alcohol use
Renal failure
Cerebrovascular disease
Malignancy

From ref. 4.

TABLE 19–9. Contraindications to Anticoagulation Therapy

General
Active bleeding
Hemophilia or other hemorrhagic tendencies
Severe liver disease with elevated baseline PT
Severe thrombocytopenia (platelet count < 20,000/mm^3)
Malignant hypertension
Inability to meticulously supervise and monitor treatment
Product-Specific Contraindications
UFH
  Hypersensitivity to UFH
  History of heparin-induced thrombocytopenia (HIT)
LMWHs
  Hypersensitivity to LMWH, UFH, pork products, methylparaben,
    or propylparaben
  History of HIT or suspected HIT
Fondaparinux
  Hypersensitivity to fondaparinux
  Severe renal insufficiency (creatinine clearance < 30 mL/min)
Lepirudin
  Hypersensitivity to hirudins
Argatroban
  Hypersensitivity to argatroban
Warfarin
  Hypersensitivity to warfarin
  Pregnancy
  History of warfarin-induced skin necrosis
  Inability to obtain follow up PT/INR measurements
  Inappropriate medication use or lifestyle behaviors

From ref. 6.

reactions, and hematoma can occur. The calcium UFH preparation has been reported to cause hematoma less frequently than the sodium preparation.

Thrombocytopenia, defined as a platelet count less than 150,000/mm^3, is common with UFH therapy.[34] Up to 30% of patients have some appreciable decline in their platelet count. Thrombocytopenia occurs more frequently with UFH preparations derived from bovine lung tissue than those from porcine gut. Two distinct clinical presentations for thrombocytopenia can occur during heparin therapy. Heparin-associated thrombocytopenia (HAT) is a benign, transient, and mild phenomenon generally occurring within the first few days of treatment in the heparin-naïve patient. Platelet counts rarely drop below 100,000/mm^3 in patients with HAT and recover with continued therapy. On the other hand, heparin-induced thrombocytopenia (HIT) is a serious drug-induced problem requiring immediate intervention (see "Heparin-Induced Thrombocytopenia" section). Platelet counts must be monitored every 1 to 2 days, and the patient should be evaluated rigorously for HIT if the platelet count drops by more than 50% or to below 100,000/mm^3.

Hypersensitivity reactions involving chills, fever, urticaria, and rarely, bronchospasm, nausea, vomiting, and shock have been reported in patients with HIT. Cutaneous necrosis is a rare but serious complication of UFH therapy that can occur in the setting of HIT.

Long-term UFH has been reported to cause alopecia, priapism, and suppressed aldosterone synthesis with subsequent hyperkalemia. The use of UFH for longer than 1 month has been associated with significant bone loss and may lead to osteoporosis.[7]

Few drug interactions have been reported with UFH. Concurrent use with other antithrombotic drugs, thrombolytics, and antiplatelet agents will increase the risk of bleeding, however.

Management of Bleeding and Excessive Anticoagulation

Hemorrhage can occur at any site in patients receiving UFH, and close monitoring for signs and symptoms of bleeding is crucial.[4,7] In addition to an appropriate coagulation study to measure the response to UFH, it is necessary to monitor hemoglobin, hematocrit, and blood pressure regularly. Bleeding can produce a wide variety of symptoms, depending on the site of hemorrhage. Symptoms may include severe headache, joint pain, chest pain, abdominal pain, swelling, tarry stools, frank hematuria, or the passage of bright red blood through the rectum. Life-threatening bleeding owing either to a significant volume loss or to the location (e.g., bleeding into a critical space) must be recognized swiftly and treated immediately. Critical areas include intracranial, pericardial, and intraocular sites, as well as the adrenal gland.

When major bleeding occurs, UFH should be discontinued immediately, and the underlying source of bleeding should be identified and treated.[28] Intravenous protamine sulfate, 1 mg/100 units of UFH up to a maximum of 50 mg can be administered to reverse the anticoagulant effects of UFH. Protamine sulfate has intrinsic anticoagulation activity, but when administered with UFH, it forms a stable salt that results in the loss of anticoagulation activity of both drugs. Protamine sulfate neutralizes UFH in 5 minutes, and its activity persists for 2 hours. It should be given by slow intravenous infusion over 10 minutes. In cases of large heparin overdoses or in patients with renal failure, a "rebound" effect may occur, with a return of some anticoagulant activity several hours after the administration of protamine sulfate. Therefore, the patient's coagulation status should be monitored closely. Multiple doses of protamine sulfate may be necessary if hemorrhage continues.

Use in Special Populations

UFH is the anticoagulant of choice during pregnancy.[7,22] Although UFH appears to be safer for pregnant women than warfarin, it is not without risks. UFH use has been associated with stillbirths and prematurity. UFH should be used cautiously during the last trimester of pregnancy and the peripartum period owing to the risk of maternal hemorrhage. UFH is not excreted in breast milk and thus is considered safe to use by women who are breast-feeding.

For the treatment of acute thrombosis in children, the dosage of UFH is 50 units/kg bolus followed by a continuous infusion at 20,000 units/m^2 per day.[35] Alternatively, an initial loading dose of 75 units/kg over 10 minutes followed by a maintenance dose of 28 units/kg per hour for infants up to 12 months of age and 20 units/kg per hour for children 1 year of age or older may be used.

LOW-MOLECULAR-WEIGHT HEPARINS

Produced by either chemical or enzymatic depolymerization (see Table 19–6), LMWHs are fragments of UFH.[7,28] They are heterogeneous mixtures of sulfated glycosaminoglycans with approximately one-third the molecular weight of UFH. Although all the LMWHs share similarities in their mechanisms of action with UFH, their molecular weight distributions vary, resulting in differences in their activity against factor Xa and thrombin, affinity for plasma proteins, propensity to release TFPI, and duration of activity.[7] The mean molecular weight of the LMWHs is product-specific. These agents have

TABLE 19-10. Indications and Doses for the Low-Molecular Weight Heparins (LMWHs)

Indication	Enoxaparin	Dalteparin	Tinzaparin
Hip replacement surgery (prophylaxis)	30 mg SC q 12 h initiated 12–24 h after surgery[a] OR 40 mg SC q 24 h initiated 12 h prior to surgery[a] Extended prophylaxis may be given for up to 3 weeks[a]	2,500 units SC given 2 h prior to surgery, followed by 2,500 units the evening after surgery and at least 6 h after first dose, then 5,000 units SC q 24 h[a] OR 5,000 units SC q 24 h initiated the evening prior to surgery[a]	750 units/kg SC q 24 h initiated the evening prior to surgery or 12 h after surgery OR 4,500 units SC q 24 h initiated 12 h prior to surgery
Knee replacement surgery (prophylaxis)	30 mg SC q 12 h initiated 12–24 h prior to surgery[a]		75 units/kg SC q 24 h initiated the evening prior to surgery or 12 h after surgery
Abdominal surgery (prophylaxis)	40 mg SC q 24 h initiated 2 h prior to surgery[a]	2,500 units SC q 24 h initiated 1–2 h prior to surgery[a] Patients with malignancy: 5,000 units SC the evening prior to surgery, then 5,000 units SC q 24 h[a] OR 2,500 units SC 1–2 h prior to surgery, then 2,500 units 12 h after surgery followed by 5,000 units SC q 24 h[a]	3500 units SC q 24 hrs initiated 1–2 hrs prior to surgery
Acute medical illness (prophylaxis)	40 mg SC q 24 h[a]	2,500 units SC q 24 h	
Trauma (prophylaxis)	30 mg SC q 12 h starting 12–36 hours after injury		
DVT treatment (with or without PE)	1 mg/kg SC q 12 h[a] OR 1.5 mg/kg SC q 24 h[a]	100 units/kg SC q 12 h OR 200 units/kg SC q 24 h	175 units/kg SC q 24 h[a]
Unstable angina or non-Q-wave MI	1 mg/kg SC q 12 h[a]	100 units/kg SC q 12 h (maximum dose 10,000 units)[a]	

[a]Dose approved by the Food and Drug Administration for indication.
SC = subcutaneous; DVT = deep vein thrombosis; PE = pulmonary embolism; MI = myocardial infarction.
From ref. 3.

several advantages over UFH, including (1) predictable anticoagulation dose response, (2) improved subcutaneous bioavailability, (3) dose-independent clearance, (4) longer biologic half-life, (5) lower incidence of thrombocytopenia, and (6) a reduced need for routine laboratory monitoring.

Currently, there are three LMWH products available in the United States. The usefulness of LMWHs has been evaluated extensively for a wide array of indications, including the treatment of acute coronary syndromes, DVT, and PE, as well as the prevention of VTE in several high-risk populations. The Food and Drug Administration (FDA)–approved indications and doses for the LMWHs are product-specific (Table 19–10). The LMWHs largely have replaced UFH for the prevention and treatment of VTE in some hospitals. However, institutional resources and individual patient needs should determine their precise role in the management of VTE.

Pharmacology

The LMWHs prevent the growth and propagation of formed thrombi. Like UFH, the LMWHs enhance and accelerate the activity of antithrombin which binds to a specific pentasaccharide sequence.[36] Approximately 20% of the LMWH molecules contain the specific sequence necessary to interact with antithrombin compared with nearly 30% for UFH. The principal difference in the pharmacologic activity of the LMWHs and UFH is their relative inhibition of factor Xa and thrombin (IIa). Owing to their smaller chain length, the LMWHs have limited activity against thrombin (see Fig. 19–5). Fewer than 50% of the LMWH molecules have the requisite chain length to bind antithrombin and thrombin simultaneously. For this reason, the LMWHs have proportionally greater anti-factor Xa activity. The ratio of anti-factor Xa–IIa activity varies between 4:1 and 2:1. By comparison, UFH has an anti-factor Xa–IIa activity ratio of 1:1. Like UFH, the LMWHs cause the endothelium to release TFPI, which is believed to enhance the inhibition of factor Xa and to inactivate factor VIIa.

Pharmacokinetics

Compared with UFH, the LMWHs have a more predictable anticoagulation response. The improved pharmacokinetic profile of LMWHs is the result of reduced binding to proteins and cells.[7] The bioavailability of LMWHs varies between 85% and 99% when it is administered subcutaneously, whereas the absorption of UFH is relatively poor and erratic. The subcutaneous bioavailability of the LMWH products differs only slightly. The peak anticoagulation effect is seen in 3 to 5 hours.

The renal route is the predominant mode of elimination for the LMWHs.[7,28] Consequently, their biologic half-life may be prolonged in patients with renal impairment. Longer heparin chains bind to macrophages and are degraded rapidly. Therefore, anti-factor Xa activity, which is mediated by smaller heparin molecules, persists longer than antithrombin activity. The plasma half-life of the LMWH preparations is two to four times longer than that of UFH. The clearance of LMWHs is independent of dose.

Dosing and Administration

The LMWHs are given in fixed or weight-based doses based on the product and indication[7,28] (see Table 19–10). The dose for enoxaparin is expressed in milligrams, whereas dalteparin and tinzaparin doses are expressed in units of anti-factor Xa activity. Although they can be given by continuous intravenous infusion, the LMWHs generally are given by subcutaneous injection in the abdominal area while the patient is in a supine position. The clinician or patient pinches a layer of skin between the thumb and forefinger and then introduces the entire length of the needle into a skin fold at a 90-degree angle. Injection sites should be alternated between right and left sides. Following subcutaneous administration, the drug is absorbed slowly, resulting in sustained antithrombotic activity over several hours.

The dosing interval for the LMWHs is every 12 or 24 hours depending on the indication and product. Larger doses are given once daily and produce significantly higher peak plasma concentrations. Given that the elimination half-life of the LMWHs is prolonged in patients with severe renal impairment, high doses may lead to a significant accumulation in these patients. Enoxaparin should be dosed once daily in patients with creatinine clearances of less than 30 mL/min.[37] Given that few published data are available regarding the use of LMWHs in the setting of renal insufficiency, some experts recommend measuring anti-factor Xa activity if therapy is continued for more than a few days.

For the prevention of VTE, the LMWHs have been studied in a variety of high-risk circumstances, including orthopedic surgery, abdominal surgery, acute spinal cord injury, neurosurgery, multiple trauma, and critical illness.[3] The effectiveness of the LMWHs has been evaluated extensively for the treatment of VTE in hospitalized patients and used in the outpatient management of DVT.[12] They are also a reasonable alternative to warfarin therapy in cancer patients with recurrent VTE and circumstances where a prothrombin time/international normalized ratio (PT/INR) cannot be obtained routinely.

Therapeutic Monitoring

The LMWHs achieve a predictable anticoagulant response when given subcutaneously. Therefore, routine laboratory monitoring is unnecessary to guide the dosing of these agents. The PT, the ACT, and the aPTT are minimally affected by LMWHs.[7] Prior to initiation of LMWH, a baseline PT/INR, aPTT, complete blood count (CBC) with platelet count, and serum creatinine concentration determination should be obtained. Most experts recommend monitoring the CBC every 5 to 10 days during the first 2 weeks of LMWH therapy and every 2 to 4 weeks thereafter.

While several methods to monitor LMWHs have been explored, measurement of anti-factor Xa activity has been the most widely used method in clinical practice. Routine anti-factor Xa activity measurement is not necessary in a patient whose condition is stable and uncomplicated.[7] Although very limited data support the use of laboratory monitoring to guide LMWH therapy, measuring anti-factor Xa activity may be helpful in patients who have significant renal impairment (e.g., creatinine clearance of less than 30 mL/min), weigh less than 50 kg, have morbid obesity (e.g., BMI ≥ 40 kg/m^2 or weigh ≥ 120 kg), or require prolonged therapy (e.g., >14 days). Periodic anti-factor Xa activity monitoring also may be useful in women treated with a LMWH during pregnancy because of changing pharmacokinetic variables (e.g., volume of distribution and renal function).[22] Patients who are at very high risk of bleeding or thrombotic recurrence also may benefit from anti-factor Xa monitoring to avoid periods of over- or underanticoagulation. Newborns have unpredictable pharmacokinetic profiles and therefore may require monitoring to ensure adequate therapy.

When anti-factor Xa activity is used to monitor LMWH therapy, the sample should be drawn approximately 4 hours after the subcutaneous injection, during the peak period of anti-factor Xa activity.[7] A calibrated LMWH heparin should be used to establish the standard curve for the assay. The therapeutic range for anti-factor Xa activity is not well defined and to date has not been correlated clearly with efficacy or the risk of bleeding.[38] For the treatment of VTE, an acceptable target range is 0.5 to 1.0 unit/mL. Specific algorithms for dosing adjustments based on anti-factor Xa activity are not available at the present time.

Adverse Effects

As with UFH, bleeding is the most common adverse effect of the LMWHs.[4,7] Although not demonstrated consistently in clinical trials, the frequency of major bleeding is purported to be less with the LMWHs than with UFH.[7,39] This difference may be due in part to their reduced effects on platelet function, endothelial cells, and microvascular permeability. The incidence of major bleeding reported in clinical trials is less than 3% and varies among the LMWH preparations, their indication for use, patient population, and dose administered. Minor bleeding, particularly at the site of injection, occurs frequently with LMWH use. Several cases of epidural and spinal hematoma resulting in long-term or permanent paralysis have been reported with the use of enoxaparin during spinal and epidural anesthesia or spinal puncture.[37] The risk of these events is higher with the use of in-dwelling epidural catheters and concomitant use of drugs that affect hemostasis. Epidural catheters should be removed only after a minimum of 12 hours has elapsed after the last dose of the LMWH, and any subsequent dose should be given at least 2 hours later.

If major bleeding occurs in a patient receiving an LMWH, it is recommended that protamine sulfate be administered intravenously.[7] However, because of its limited binding to the shorter LMWH chains, protamine sulfate cannot neutralize their anticoagulant effects completely. When given in equimolar concentrations, protamine sulfate neutralizes an estimated 60% to 75% of the antithrombotic activity. The recommended dose of protamine sulfate is 1 mg/1 mg of enoxaparin or 1 mg/100 anti-factor Xa units of dalteparin or tinzaparin administered in the previous 8 hours. If the LMWH dose was given in the previous 8 to 12 hours, a 0.5-mg dose of protamine should be given for every 100 anti-factor Xa units. The use of protamine sulfate is not recommended if the LMWH was administered more than 12 hours earlier.

While thrombocytopenia can occur with the use of a LMWH, the incidence of HIT is substantially lower than that observed with the use of UFH.[7,34] The explanation may lie in the reduced propensity of the LMWHs to bind to platelets and platelet factor-4 (PF-4). The

LMWHs exhibit nearly 100% cross-reactivity with heparin antibodies in vitro.[34] Therefore, the LMWHs should be avoided in patients with an established diagnosis or history of HIT. Platelet counts must be monitored periodically in all patients receiving a LMWH, and thrombocytopenia of any degree should be evaluated promptly.

The risk of osteoporosis appears to be substantially lower with the LMWHs compared with UFH. The LMWHs have not caused appreciable changes in bone mineral density after several months of use.[22] They have been used in a limited number of patients with established heparin-induced osteoporosis. Although these reports are promising, it cannot be concluded that the LMWHs have no effect on bone formation until well-designed clinical trials are available.

Use in Special Populations

There is growing experience with the use of LMWHs during pregnancy.[22] The LMWHs do not cross the placenta. According to the results of a few large case series, the LMWH appear to be relatively safe to use during pregnancy and are an attractive alternative to UFH when long-term anticoagulation therapy is required. Furthermore, the LMWHs do not appear to affect bone formation. Dalteparin, enoxaparin, and tinzaparin are classified as FDA pregnancy category B. The safety and effectiveness of the LMWHs to treat VTE in children and infants has not been studied extensively.[35] Limited data exist on enoxaparin. The recommended treatment dose for enoxaparin in patients younger than 1 year of age is 1.5 mg/kg every 12 hours and 1 mg/kg every 12 hours in children 1 year of age or older. Until more data are available, it is prudent to monitor anti-factor Xa activity periodically in these special populations during long-term use.

DANAPAROID

Danaparoid is a glycosaminoglycan that is structurally distinct from but mechanistically related to heparin.[7] It is a mixture of three sulfated glycosaminoglycans: heparan (84%), dermatan (12%), and chondroitin (4%). Like heparin, danaparoid's anticoagulant activity is mediated, in part, through its interaction with antithrombin. Compared with the LMWHs, danaparoid is fivefold more selective for factor Xa. It is approved by the FDA for the prevention of VTE in patients undergoing elective hip replacement surgery. Historically, danaparoid was used primarily for the treatment of thrombosis in patients who developed HIT. In 2002, the manufacturer discontinued the distribution of danaparoid, citing shortages in the United States.[38]

FONDAPARINUX

Pharmacology

Fondaparinux, also known as pentasaccharide, is a synthetic molecule consisting of the five critical saccharide units that bind specifically but reversibly to antithrombin[40,41] (see Fig. 19–5). Fondaparinux is the first in a class of anticoagulants that selectively inhibits factor Xa activity.[42] Similar to UFH and the LMWHs, fondaparinux prevents thrombus generation and clot formation by indirectly inhibiting factor Xa activity through its interaction with antithrombin. When fondaparinux binds to antithrombin, it causes a conformational change in antithrombin's active site and catalyzes anti-factor Xa activity by about 300-fold. Fondaparinux is not destroyed during this process and is released to bind many other antithrombin molecules. Unlike UFH and the LMWHs, fondaparinux has no direct effect on thrombin activity at therapeutic plasma concentrations. Selective inhibition of factor Xa may provide more efficient control over fibrin generation while preserving thrombin's regulatory functions in the control of hemostasis. Fondaparinux has no known effect on platelet function.

Pharmacokinetics

Fondaparinux is absorbed rapidly and completely following subcutaneous administration (absolute bioavailability 100%).[40,42] Peak plasma concentrations are achieved in approximately 2 hours after a single dose and 3 hours with repeated once-daily dosing. It is distributed primarily in blood. At therapeutic concentrations, fondaparinux is highly and specifically bound to antithrombin. It does not bind to red blood cells or other plasma proteins, including albumin, glycoprotein, platelets, or PF-4. Fondaparinux is eliminated primarily unchanged in the urine. It is contraindicated in patients with severe renal function impairment (creatinine clearance < 30 mL/min) due to an increased risk for bleeding. The terminal elimination half-life is 17 to 21 hours and is independent of the patient's age or sex.[40] The anticoagulant effect of fondaparinux persists for 2 to 4 days following discontinuation of the drug in patients with normal renal function. Fondaparinux has no known pharmacokinetic drug interactions. However, concurrent use with other antithrombotic agents increases the risk of hemorrhage.

Dose and Administration

Fondaparinux is approved by the FDA for the prevention of VTE following orthopedic surgery (e.g., hip fracture, hip replacement, and knee replacement) and for the treatment of DVT and PE.[40] In the setting of VTE prevention, the dose of fondaparinux is 2.5 mg injected subcutaneously once daily starting 6 to 8 hours following surgery. It is important to avoid initiating fondaparinux too soon because there is a significant relationship between the timing of the first dose and the frequency of major bleeding complications. Patients who weigh less than 50 kg should not be given fondaparinux for VTE prophylaxis. The usual duration of therapy is 5 to 9 days, but fondaparinux may be given as extended prophylaxis following hospital discharge for up to 21 days.[43] Fondaparinux has been evaluated for the treatment of DVT and PE in two phase III clinical trials.[44,45] For the treatment of DVT or PE, the dose of fondaparinux is 7.5 mg given subcutaneously once daily. Patients who weigh more than 100 kg should be given 10 mg once daily, and those who weigh less than 50 kg should receive only 5 mg daily.

Similar to the LMWHs, fondaparinux is administered into the fatty tissue of the abdominal wall. Patients should be instructed to pinch a fold of skin at the injection site and hold it throughout the injection. The needle should be inserted at a 90-degree angle. Injection sites should be alternated from side to side.[40]

Therapeutic Monitoring

A CBC should be measured at baseline and monitored periodically to detect the possibility of occult bleeding.[40] Baseline kidney function should be determined and monitored closely in patients at risk of developing renal failure. Fondaparinux should be discontinued if the creatinine clearance drops below 30 mL/min. Signs and symptoms of bleeding should be monitored daily, particularly in patients with a baseline creatinine clearance of between 30 and 50 mL/min. If neuraxial anesthesia has been used, patients should be monitored closely for signs and symptoms of neurologic impairment.

Fondaparinux does not alter coagulation tests such as the aPTT and PT. The role of anti-factor Xa monitoring during fondaparinux is not well defined. Patients receiving fondaparinux therapy do not require routine coagulation testing.

Adverse Effects

The primary adverse effect associated with fondaparinux therapy is bleeding.[40,46] The rate of major bleeding in the VTE prophylaxis trials was approximately 2% to 3%. The risk of major bleeding appears to be related to weight; therefore, in patients who weigh less than 50 kg, fondaparinux is contraindicated for VTE prophylaxis, and the treatment dose is only 5 mg every 24 hours. Similar to UFH and the LMWHs, fondaparinux should be used with extreme caution in patients with neuraxial anesthesia or following a spinal puncture owing to the risk for spinal or epidural hematoma formation. Unlike UFH and the LMWHs, fondaparinux does not cause heparin-induced thrombocytopenia and does not produce cross-sensitivity in vitro.[47] A specific antidote to reverse the antithrombotic activity of fondaparinux is not currently available, but several potential products have been evaluated.[42]

Use in Special Populations

Fondaparinux has been used safely in elderly patients, but the risk of major bleeding increases with age (1.8% in patients younger than 65 years of age, 2.2% in patients 65 to 74 years of age, and 2.7% in patients 75 years of age or older).[40] This is an important consideration because many patients who undergo orthopedic surgery are elderly. Elderly patients are also more likely to have decreased renal function, and careful assessment of renal status should be conducted prior to initiating therapy. Fondaparinux is contraindicated in patients with a creatinine clearance of less than 30 mL/min.

Fondaparinux is a pregnancy category B drug.[40] There is very limited information regarding fondaparinux use during pregnancy. The drug is excreted in the milk of lactating rats, but excretion in human milk is unknown. Until more data become available, UFH and the LMWHs should remain the agents of choice in pregnant patients. Fondaparinux use in pediatric populations has not been studied.

IDRAPARINUX

Idraparinux is an analog of fondaparinux that has a very long duration of effect (see Table 19–6) and has been developed to be administered once weekly by subcutaneous injection.[48] Idraparinux is currently undergoing phase III clinical trials evaluating its utility for both the acute and long-term management of VTE.[49]

DIRECT THROMBIN INHIBITORS

A relatively new class of very potent anticoagulant agents, the direct thrombin inhibitors (DTIs), includes lepirudin, desirudin, bivalirudin, argatroban, and ximelagatran (see Table 19–6). These agents have been studied for a number of indications, including the prophylaxis and treatment of VTE, acute coronary syndromes, and HIT.[49] Given

their immediate onset of action, good oral bioavailability, wide therapeutic window, fixed dosing, and promising results from early clinical trials, oral DTIs could revolutionize the treatment of VTE in the next 5 years.[11,49]

Pharmacology and Pharmacokinetics

The direct thrombin inhibitors, as their name implies, interact directly with the thrombin molecule[49] (Fig. 19–6). The agents in this class differ in terms of their molecular weight, chemical structure, and binding to the thrombin molecule. Unlike the UFH, the LMWHs, and fondaparinux, DTIs do not require antithrombin to have antithrombotic activity. They are capable of inhibiting both circulating and clot-bound thrombin, a potential advantage over UFH and the LMWHs. Further, DTIs have not been shown to induce immune-mediated thrombocytopenia and have been used widely for the treatment of HIT.

Hirudin, the prototype of this class, was isolated from the salivary secretions of the medicinal leech (*Hirudo medicinalis*).[41] Mass production of several synthetic hirudin analogs with the potential for wide clinical application only became possible with the advent of recombinant DNA technology. Lepirudin, a recombinant analog of hirudin, is a 65-amino-acid polypeptide that irreversibly binds with high specificity to thrombin. The hirudins (i.e., lepirudin, desirudin, and bivalirudin) form a noncovalent bond in a 1:1 ratio with the catalytic and fibrinogen binding sites on the thrombin molecule (see Fig. 19–6). These agents must be administered parenterally, either by continuous intravenous infusion or by subcutaneous injection.[41,50] The primary route of elimination for lepirudin is through renal excretion, and systemic clearance is directly proportional to the glomerular filtration rate. Dose adjustment is required in the setting of impaired renal function, a potential disadvantage of this agent. Many patients develop antibodies to lepirudin. Up to 40% of patients treated with lepirudin for 10 days or more will develop antibodies. However, antibody formation has not been associated with adverse clinical outcomes.[51]

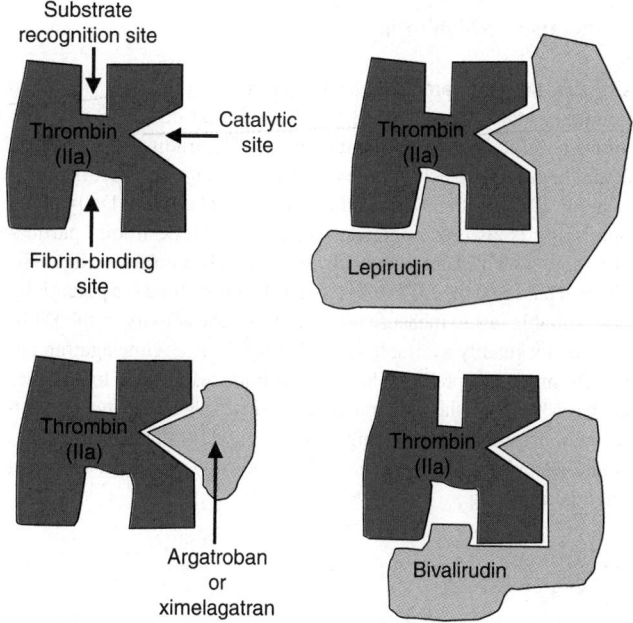

FIGURE 19–6. Pharmacologic activity of lepirudin, bivalirudin, argatroban, and ximelagatran.

Bivalirudin, formerly known as hirulog, is a semisynthetic 20-amino-acid polypeptide analog of recombinant hirudin approved by the FDA for use in patients with unstable angina undergoing percutaneous transluminal angioplasty (PCTA).[52] Unlike lepirudin, bivalirudin is a reversible inhibitor of thrombin and provides transient antithrombotic activity with an estimated 20- to 30-minute half-life.[49,53] This difference may reduce the risk of bleeding and antibody production. Approximately 20% of an intravenous dose of bivalirudin is eliminated in the urine. The manufacturer recommends reducing the dose by 20% to 60% in patients with renal impairment and monitoring the ACT closely.[52]

Desirudin is a recombinant hirudin analog administered by subcutaneous injection approved by the FDA in 2003 for the prevention of venous thrombosis in patients undergoing elective hip surgery. For acute myocardial infarction and unstable angina, desirudin has been given via continuous intravenous infusion.[50] Similar to lepirudin, desirudin is eliminated renally, and patients with moderate to severe renal impairment require dosage reductions. Antihirudin antibodies have been documented with desirudin, but the incidence appears to be lower than with lepirudin.

Argatroban differs from the hirudins in that it is a small synthetic molecule derived from arginine that reversibly binds only to the active catalytic site of thrombin. Its small size relative to other DTIs enables it to inhibit both clot-bound and soluble thrombin, offering a potential therapeutic advantage over other agents in its class. Argatroban is eliminated primarily by hydroxylation and aromatization in the liver to inactive metabolites. A small percentage is excreted unchanged in the bile. Dosage adjustment is required in patients with hepatic impairment.

Ximelagatran is a prodrug converted by hydrolysis and reduction in the liver to melagatran, the active moiety.[53] Unlike other DTIs, ximelagatran has good oral bioavailability that does not appear to be affected by food. Peak ximelagatran plasma concentrations are seen within 120 minutes following an oral dose, providing relatively rapid antithrombotic activity.[54] The elimination half-life is approximately 3 to 5 hours, therefore requiring twice-daily administration. Ximelagatran is eliminated primarily in the urine.

Therapeutic Monitoring

Although the DTIs produce changes in the PT, the aPTT is used to monitor a patient's response to lepirudin and argatroban.[51,55] After obtaining baseline coagulation studies, doses of lepirudin and argatraban should be titrated to achieve the institution-specific therapeutic range or an aPTT of 1.5 to 3.0 times the mean normal control. Daily aPTT monitoring is also recommended for patients on desirudin, particularly those with impaired renal function.[50] Bivalirudin doses should be adjusted based on the ACT.[52] The eccarin clotting time is a potentially more suitable test to measure the antithrombotic activity of the DTIs, but it is not readily available in the United States. Ximelagatran appears to produce a predictable antithrombotic response in fixed doses and has a relatively large therapeutic window.[49,54] Consequently, routine anticoagulation monitoring is not required for this agent. A CBC should be obtained at baseline and periodically thereafter to detect potential bleeding.

Adverse Effects

Contraindications for use of the DTIs and risk factors for bleeding are similar to those of other antithrombotic drugs (see Table 19–9).

Hemorrhage is the most serious and common adverse effect related to the DTIs.[34] In studies evaluating the use of lepirudin for the treatment of patients with HIT, the incidence of major bleeding was relatively high (13% to 17%).[51] However, no fatal or intracranial bleeding events occurred. A slightly lower rate of major hemorrhage was reported in HIT trials using argatroban (approximately 5%), and similarly, there were no reports of fatal or intracranial bleeding. Bleeding complications with desirudin were similar to those with enoxaparin in a trial of patients undergoing elective hip surgery. Serious bleeding occurred in less than 1% of all patients in the trial.[50] Minor bleeding and small reductions in red blood cell counts occurred relatively frequently but typically did not require drug discontinuation. There are no known agents that reverse the activity of the DTIs. Nonhemorrhagic effects such as fever, nausea, vomiting, and allergic reactions occur infrequently.

Ximelagatran was associated with a relative high incidence (6% to 9%) of elevated liver function tests (LFTs) in phase III clinical trials. In most cases, this effect was reversible with continued use. However, a very small percentage (<1%) of patients may have had severe, irreversible liver injury. In 2004, the FDA denied approval of ximelagatran until more safety data are available and an effective risk management strategy is developed.

Drug-Drug and Drug-Food Interactions

The concurrent use of DTIs and thrombolytic agents substantially increases the bleeding risk, particularly intracranial hemorrhage, and should be undertaken with great caution. Warfarin and antiplatelet agents can be initiated concurrently with these agents. Because the DTIs prolong the PT and INR, close monitoring for bleeding complications is required. Few pharmacokinetic drug interactions with this class of agents are known. Drugs that alter renal function could prolong lepirudin and desirudin activity. Drugs that inhibit liver enzymes have the potential to interact with argatroban. However, erythromycin did not alter argatroban pharmacokinetics appreciably in healthy volunteers in one small study.[56]

Use in Special Populations

Lepirudin and argatroban are classified by the FDA as pregnancy category B drugs, but they should be used cautiously in women of childbearing age because experience is very limited.[51,55] Desirudin is classified as pregnancy category C with no controlled trials in pregnant women.[50] Lepirudin has been evaluated in a small number of children. Further study is required to develop dosing guidelines in patients with renal and hepatic insufficiency.

WARFARIN

The most widely prescribed anticoagulant in North American is warfarin sodium (Coumadin). It was discovered serendipitously in the early 1940s at the University of Wisconsin after hemorrhagic deaths occurred in cattle eating spoiled sweet clover.[6] Warfarin is approved by the FDA for the prevention and treatment of VTE as well as for the prevention of thromboembolic complications associated with atrial fibrillation, heart valve replacement, and myocardial infarction. Because of its narrow therapeutic index, predisposition to drug and food interactions, and propensity to cause hemorrhage, warfarin requires

LMWH
UFH- growth & propagation
w- initial formation & propag.

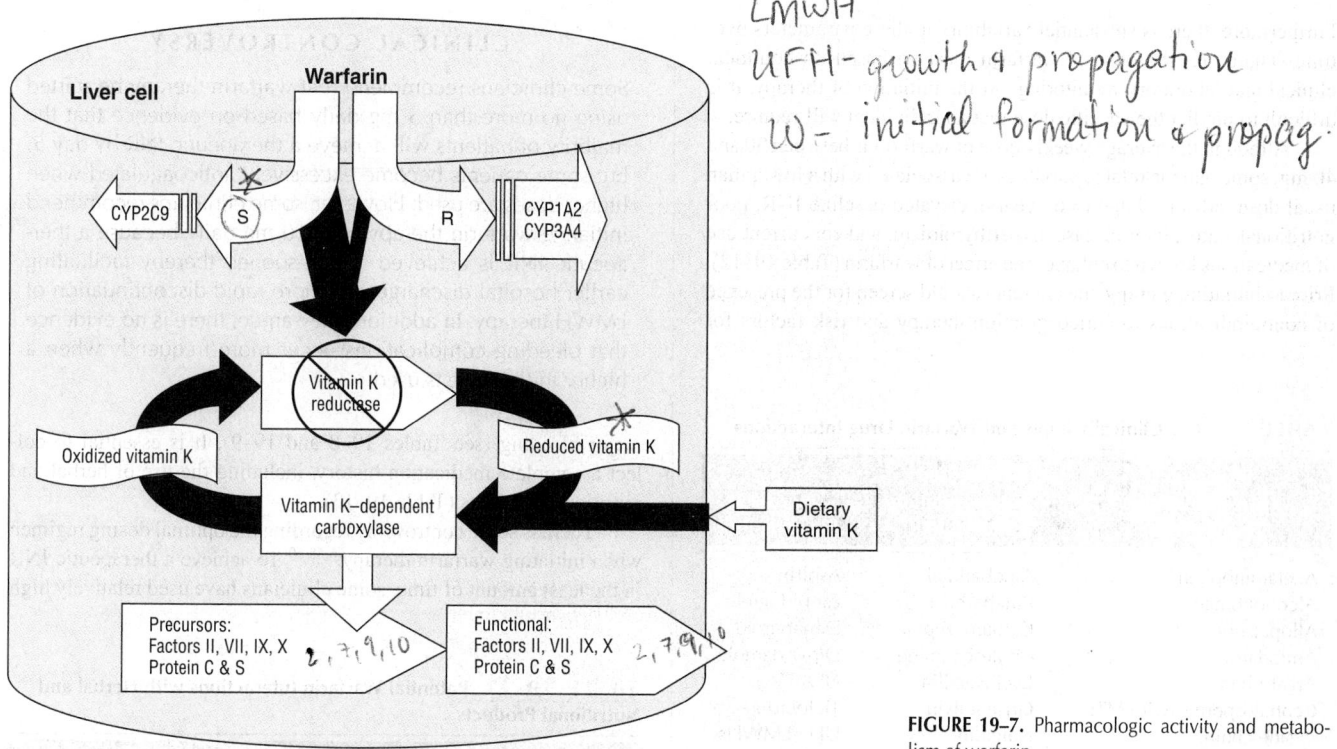

FIGURE 19–7. Pharmacologic activity and metabolism of warfarin.

continuous patient monitoring and education in order to achieve optimal outcomes.

Pharmacology

Warfarin exerts its anticoagulation effect by inhibiting the enzymes responsible for the cyclic interconversion of vitamin K in the liver[23] (Fig. 19–7). Reduced vitamin K is a cofactor required for the carboxylation of the vitamin K–dependent coagulation proteins, namely, factors II (prothrombin), VII, IX, and X, as well as the endogenous anticoagulant proteins C and S. Carboxylation of the N-terminal region of these proteins in the liver is required for biologic activity. By inhibiting the supply of vitamin K to serve as a cofactor in the production of these proteins, warfarin indirectly slows their rate of synthesis. Warfarin has no direct affect on previously circulating clotting factors or previously formed thrombus. The time required for warfarin to achieve its pharmacologic effect depends on the elimination half-lives of the coagulation proteins[5] (see Table 19–11). Given that prothrombin has a 2- to 3-day half-life, warfarin's full antithrombotic effect is not achieved for 8 to 15 days after initiation of therapy. By suppressing the production of clotting factors, warfarin prevents the initial formation and propagation of thrombus.

Pharmacokinetics

Commercially available warfarin is a racemic mixture of *R*- and *S*-isomers.[5,6] The *S*-isomer is two to five times more potent that the *R*-isomer. Rapidly and extensively absorbed from the gastrointestinal track, warfarin reaches peak plasma concentration in approximately 90 minutes, with a bioavailability of greater than 90% following oral administration. In plasma, both the *R*- and *S*-isomers are bound extensively (97% to 99%) to albumin. Warfarin undergoes stereoselective metabolism via CYP1A2, -2C9, -2C19, -2C18, and -3A4 isoenzymes in the liver (see Fig. 19–7). The pharmacokinetic parameters of warfarin, particularly hepatic metabolism, vary substantially between individuals. Genetic variations in the 2C9 isoenzyme are relatively common (up to 35% in some studies), and patients with the CYP2C9*2 and CYP2C9*3 polymorphisms require significantly lower doses of warfarin.[57] Given the relatively greater potency of *S*-warfarin, drugs that induce or inhibit the CPY2C isoenzymes are more likely to cause a clinically significant effect.[5] These and other pharmacokinetic variations in warfarin metabolism likely explain the large interpatient dose-response seen with warfarin in clinical practice.

Dosing and Administration

The dose of warfarin is patient-specific, based on the desired intensity of anticoagulation and the patient's individual response.[5,6] There is tremendous interpatient variability with regard to the pharmacodynamic response and pharmacokinetic disposition of warfarin.

TABLE 19–11. Biologic Half-Life of Vitamin K–Dependent Coagulation Proteins

Protein	Half-life (Hours)
Prothrombin (factor II)	60–100
Factor VII	4–6
Factor IX	20–30
Factor X	24–40
Protein C	8–10
Protein S	40–60

From ref. 23.

Furthermore, there is substantial variability in these parameters over time. Therefore, the dose of warfarin must be based on continual clinical and laboratory monitoring. At the initiation of therapy, it is difficult to predict the specific dose that an individual will require.

Although the average weekly dose of warfarin is between 30 and 40 mg, some patient-related variables are associated with a lower than usual dose: advanced age (>65 years), elevated baseline INR, poor nutritional status, liver disease, hyperthyroidism, and concurrent use of medications known to enhance the effect of warfarin (Table 19–12). Prior to initiating therapy, the clinician should screen for the presence of contraindications to anticoagulation therapy and risk factors for

TABLE 19–12. Clinically Important Warfarin Drug Interactions

Increased Anticoagulation Effect (⇑ INR)	Decreased Anticoagulation Effect (⇓ INR)	Increased Bleeding Risk
Acetaminophen	Amobarbital	Aspirin
Alcohol binge	Butabarbital	Clopidogrel
Allopurinol	Carbamazepine	Danaparoid
Amiodarone	Cholestyramine	Dipyridamole
Argatroban	Dicloxacillin	NSAIDs
Cephalosporins (with MTP side chain)	Griseofulvin	Ticlopidine
	Nafcillin	UFH/LMWHs
Chloral hydrate	Phenobarbital	
Chloramphenicol	Phenytoin	
Cimetidine	Primidone	
Ciprofloxacin	Rifabutin	
Clofibrate	Rifampin	
Danazol	Secobarbital	
Disulfiram	Sucralfate	
Doxycycline	Vitamin K	
Erythromycin		
Fenofibrate		
Fluconazole		
Fluorouracil		
Fluoxetine		
Fluvoxamine		
Gemfibrozil		
Influenza vaccine		
Isoniazid		
Itraconazole		
Lovastatin		
Metronidazole		
Miconazole		
Moxalactam		
Neomycin		
Norfloxacin		
Ofloxacin		
Omeprazole		
Phenylbutazone		
Piroxicam		
Propafenone		
Propoxyphene		
Quinidine		
Sertraline		
Sulfamethoxazole		
Sulfinpyrazone		
Tamoxifen		
Testosterone		
Vitamin E		
Zafirlukast		

NSAIDs = nonsteroidal anti-inflammatory drugs.
Compiled from ref. 5.

major bleeding (see Tables 19–8 and 19–9). It is essential to collect a complete medication history, including the use of herbal and nutritional products (Table 19–13).

There is some controversy regarding the optimal dosing regimen when initiating warfarin therapy.[6,58,59] To achieve a therapeutic INR in the least amount of time, some clinicians have used relatively high

TABLE 19–13. Potential Warfarin Interactions with Herbal and Nutritional Products

Increased Anticoagulation Effect (Increase Bleeding Risk or ⇑ INR)	Decreased Anticoagulation Effect (⇓ INR)
Angelica root	Coenzyme Q$_{10}$
Arnica flower	Ginseng
Anise	Green tea
Asafoetida	St. John's wort
Bogbean	
Borage seed oil	
Bromelain	
Capsicum	
Celery	
Chamomile	
Clove	
Danshen	
Devil's claw	
Dong quai	
Fenugreek	
Feverfew	
Garlic	
Ginger	
Ginkgo	
Horse chestnut	
Licorice root	
Lovage root	
Meadowsweet	
Onion	
Parsely	
Papain	
Passionflower herb	
Poplar	
Quassia	
Red clover	
Rue	
Sweet clover	
Tumeric	
Willow bark	
Vitamin E	

From ref. 70.

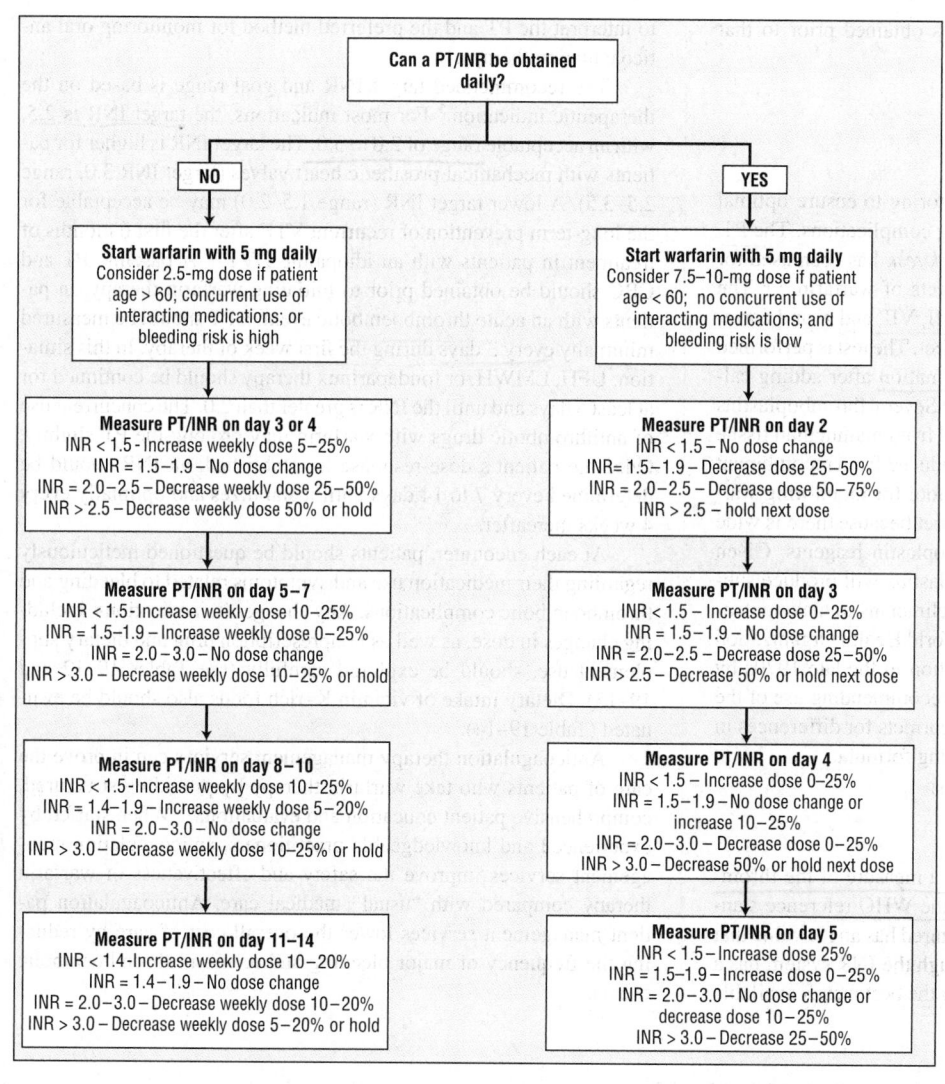

FIGURE 19–8. Initiation of warfarin therapy. PT = prothrombin time; INR = international normalized ratio.

doses of warfarin (10 or 15 mg) and then adjusted the dose based on the patient's response. Recent studies in patients with atrial fibrillation comparing a 5-mg initial dose with a 10-mg dose called into the question this practice.[60] Although a 10-mg dose produced a more rapid response in the INR, many patients became excessively anticoagulated. However, a more recent study in patients with acute venous thrombosis refutes these findings.[58]

While data on the optimal induction regimen are conflicting, there is a pharmacodynamic rationale for avoiding doses larger than 10 mg.[5] Large doses result in a more rapid depression in factor VII concentrations.[60] This early response to therapy may give the clinician a false impression that a therapeutic INR has been achieved after only 2 or 3 days. It is important to remember that patients are not truly anticoagulated at this point because a significant reduction in prothrombin concentrations requires at least 5 days to occur. Large doses also may increase the theoretical risk for early thrombotic complications, such as warfarin-induced skin necrosis. After the initiation of warfarin therapy, protein C becomes depleted rapidly, but prothrombin concentrations will remain near normal for several days. If protein C concentrations are severely suppressed relative to prothrombin, there is a potential for inducing a hypercoagulable state.

For most patients, initiating therapy with 5 mg daily and adjusting the dose based on response will produce therapeutic INRs in 4 to 5 days (Fig. 19–8). Lower or higher starting doses may be acceptable based on patient-related factors and how quickly follow-up laboratory monitoring can be performed. Several dosing nomograms have been developed and have been evaluated prospectively.[6,58–61] For patients with acute venous thrombosis, UFH, UFH, LMWH, or fondaparinux should be overlapped with warfarin therapy for at least 4 to 5 days regardless of whether the target INR has been achieved earlier.[12]

Warfarin therapy can be initiated safely on an outpatient basis, provided that there is no urgent need for anticoagulation (i.e., prevention of venous thrombosis). Given that laboratory monitoring is performed less frequently in the outpatient setting, warfarin therapy should be undertaken a bit more cautiously. In most circumstances, the initial dose should not exceed the anticipated maintenance dose. The response to therapy should be measured every 3 to 5 days until stabilized. The full antithrombotic effect may require up to 15 days to be achieved.[5]

When adjusting the dose of warfarin, the clinician should allow sufficient time for changes in the INR to occur.[6] In general, dose changes should not be made more frequently than every 3 days. Doses should be adjusted by calculating the weekly dose and reducing or increasing the weekly dose by 5% to 25%. The effect of a small dose change may not become evident for 5 to 7 days; therefore, patients should not have follow-up PT tests obtained prior to that time.

Therapeutic Monitoring

Warfarin requires frequent laboratory monitoring to ensure optimal therapeutic outcomes and minimize bleeding complications. The PT, also known as the *protime* and *one-step quick test,* has been used for decades to monitor the anticoagulation effects of warfarin.[5,62] The PT measures the biologic activity of factors II, VII, and X and correlates well with warfarin's anticoagulation effect. The test is performed by measuring the time required for clot formation after adding calcium and a thromboplastin to citrated plasma. Several thromboplastins are available commercially and are extracted from mammalian tissue rich in tissue factor (e.g., rabbit brain) or produced from recombinant human tissue factor. Although an effective tool for monitoring warfarin therapy, the PT is problematic to interpret because there is wide variability in the sensitivity of the thromboplastin reagents. Given the same blood sample, different thromboplastins will produce substantially different results that may prompt clinicians to make potentially inappropriate dosing decisions. The World Health Organization (WHO) addressed the need for standardization in the late 1970s by developing a reference thromboplastin and recommending use of the INR to monitor warfarin therapy. The INR corrects for differences in thromboplastin reagents through the following formula:

$$INR = \left(\frac{PT^{Patient}}{PT^{Control}} \right)^{ISI}$$

The International Sensitivity Index (ISI) is a measure of the thromboplastin's responsiveness compared with the WHO reference standard. Each thromboplastin reagent manufactured has an ISI value that should be used to calculate the INR. Although the INR system has a number of potential problems, it is currently the best means available to interpret the PT and the preferred method for monitoring oral anticoagulation therapy.

The recommended target INR and goal range is based on the therapeutic indication.[5] For most indications, the target INR is 2.5, with an acceptable range of 2.0 to 3.0. The target INR is higher for patients with mechanical prosthetic heart valves (target INR 3.0, range 2.5–3.5). A lower target INR (range 1.5–2.0) may be acceptable for the long-term prevention of recurrent VTE after the first 6 months of treatment in patients with an idiopathic DVT.[63] A baseline PT and CBC should be obtained prior to initiating warfarin therapy. In patients with an acute thromboembolic event, a PT should be measured minimally every 3 days during the first week of therapy. In this situation, UFH, LMWH, or fondaparinux therapy should be continued for at least 5 days and until the INR is greater than 2.0. The concurrent use of antithrombotic drugs with warfarin may prolong the PT slightly. Once the patient's dose-response is established, an INR should be determined every 7 to 14 days until it stabilizes and optimally every 4 weeks thereafter.

At each encounter, patients should be questioned meticulously regarding their medication use and symptoms related to bleeding and thromboembolic complications. Any changes in medications, including changes in dose, as well as nonprescription drug and dietary supplement use, should be explored carefully (see Tables 19–12 and 19–13). Dietary intake of vitamin K–rich foods also should be evaluated (Table 19–14).

Anticoagulation therapy management services can improve the care of patients who take warfarin therapy by providing structured, comprehensive patient education and evaluation.[6,8] When staffed by experienced and knowledgeable practitioners, anticoagulation management services improve the safety and effectiveness of warfarin therapy compared with "usual" medical care. Anticoagulation patient management services lower the overall cost of care by reducing the frequency of major bleeding and recurrent thromboembolic events.

TABLE 19–14. Vitamin K Content of Select Foods[a]

Very High (>200 mcg)	High (100–200 mcg)	Medium (50–100 mcg)	Low (<50 mcg)
Brussels sprouts	Basil	Apple, green	Apple, red
Chick pea	Broccoli	Asparagus	Avocado
Collard greens	Canola oil	Cabbage	Beans
Coriander	Chive	Cauliflower	Breads, grains
Endive	Coleslaw	Mayonnaise	Carrot
Kale	Cucumber (w/peel)	Nuts, pistachio	Celery
Lettuce, red leaf	Green onion/scallion	Squash, summer	Cereal
Parsley	Lettuce, butterhead		Coffee
Spinach	Mustard greens		Corn
Swiss chard	Soybean oil		Cucumber (w/o peel)
Tea, black			Dairy products
Tea, green			Eggs
Turnip greens			Fruit (varies)
Watercress			Lettuce, iceberg
			Meats, fish, poultry
			Pasta
			Peanuts
			Peas
			Potato
			Rice
			Tomato

[a]Approximate amount of vitamin K per 100 g (3.5-oz.) serving.
From ref. 69.

Portable PT monitoring devices have enhanced patient management. Not only do these devices permit clinicians to do "real time" therapeutic drug monitoring, but they also enable patients to engage in self-testing at home.[64] Self-monitoring, in its simplest form, requires the patient to report the test results to a health care professional. In such arrangements, the clinician continues to make warfarin-dosing decisions. Highly motivated and sophisticated patients can be trained to manage themselves, independently altering the dose of warfarin therapy based on their INR results. Patients who engage in INR self-monitoring and warfarin self-management report high levels of satisfaction with care and maintain the INR within the therapeutic range more frequently than those managed by "usual care." Home INR testing and self-management are clearly not for everyone, however. It requires careful patient selection and considerable education. Unfortunately, PT monitoring systems remain relatively expensive and rarely are covered by medical insurance.

Adverse Effects

Warfarin's primary adverse effect is bleeding. Hemorrhagic complications, ranging from mild to life-threatening, can occur at any site in the body. Although warfarin is not believed to cause bleeding per se, it can "unmask" an existing lesion or enable a massive hemorrhage from an ordinarily minor bleeding source. The gastrointestinal tract is the most frequent site of bleeding. Bruising on the arms and legs is commonplace, but a painful hematoma may necessitate the temporary discontinuation of therapy. Intracranial hemorrhage is the most serious and feared complication related to warfarin therapy, often resulting in permanent disability or death.

The annual incidence of major bleeding ranges from 1% in highly selected patients who are managed carefully to greater than 10% in patients managed in less structured environments, according to some studies.[4,6,8] There are no universally accepted criteria for defining a bleeding event as major or minor. Most studies have defined major bleeding as any bleeding event that required hospitalization, transfusion of 2 units of blood or plasma, or leads to a greater than 2 gm/dL drop in hematocrit. Bleeding that does not meet the criteria for a major hemorrhage generally is considered to be minor. Minor bleeding is very common. Few studies have prospectively evaluated the incidence of minor bleeding, but it is likely to be greater than 15% annually even in the most expertly managed patients.

Several risk factors for bleeding while taking anticoagulation therapy have been identified[4] (see Table 19–8). Intensity of anticoagulation therapy appears to be the most powerful risk factor. Patients whose target INR is greater than 3.0 have twice the incidence of major bleeding compared with those with a goal range of 2.0 to 3.0. The risk of intracranial hemorrhage increases significantly when the INR remains greater than 4.0 for prolonged periods of time. Patients given low-intensity warfarin therapy (goal INR 1.3–1.9) have a level of anticoagulation that is insufficient protection against thrombosis for most indications. Wide variability in the anticoagulation response, as seen in patients with very unstable INR values, also appears to be associated with an increased risk of bleeding. The risk of hemorrhage is greatest during the first few weeks of therapy; however, bleeding can occur at any time, and the cumulative incidence increases steadily over time.

Nonhemorrhagic adverse effects associated with warfarin are uncommon but can be serious when they do occur.[65] The purple toe syndrome, manifested as a purplish discoloration of the toes, is an extremely rare event reported in a small percentage of patients receiving warfarin. The etiology of this unusual phenomenon is unknown, but it is thought to be the result of cholesterol microembolization into the arterial circulation of the toes.

Warfarin-induced skin necrosis is an uncommon but very serious dermatologic reaction that is manifested by a painful maculopapular rash and ecchymosis or purpura that subsequently progresses to necrotic gangrene. It appears most frequently in areas of the body rich in subcutaneous fat, such as the breasts, thighs, buttocks, and abdomen. The incidence of warfarin-induced skin necrosis is less than 0.1%. It occurs most commonly in middle-aged women who are being treated for acute venous thrombosis. Although symptoms generally appear during the first week of therapy, it has been reported in a small number of patients who had taken warfarin for months and even years. The pathogenesis of warfarin-induced skin necrosis is not clearly understood. Many believe that it is the result of imbalances between procoagulant and anticoagulant proteins occur early in the course of warfarin therapy, resulting in capillary thrombosis and secondary hemorrhages. The observation that patients with deficiency of protein C or protein S appear to be at greater risk for warfarin-induced skin necrosis supports this theory. Warfarin-induced skin necrosis also has been reported in patients with other disorders of hypercoagulability, such as antithrombin deficiency and antiphospholipid antibodies. Patients who receive large "loading" doses of warfarin also may be at greater risk. It is recommended that heparin therapy be overlapped for a minimum of 7 days when initiating therapy in any patient suspected of having a hypercoagulable state or who has a strong family history of venous thrombosis. If the diagnosis of skin necrosis is suspected, warfarin therapy should be discontinued immediately, vitamin K administered, and full-dose UFH or LMWH therapy initiated. Warfarin therapy should be restarted with extreme caution in patients with a history of skin necrosis, if at all.

Gastrointestinal side effects of warfarin therapy are uncommon and usually self-limited. Because warfarin interferes with vitamin K metabolism, there has been some theoretical concern that it may adversely affect bone formation and cause osteoporosis with long-term use.[66] To date, the association between warfarin and osteoporosis is inconclusive, and the risk of fracture appears to be negligible.

Management of Bleeding and Excessive Anticoagulation

Specific recommendations for the management of patients with an elevated INR are published by the American College of Chest Physicians (ACCP) Consensus Conference on Antithrombotic Therapy[6] (Fig. 19–9). Patients with a mildly elevated INR (3.5 to 5.0) should be examined for signs and symptoms of bleeding, as well as for factors that increase bleeding risk. In this circumstance, either reducing the dose of warfarin or withholding one or two doses will manage most patients safely. When a swift reduction in an elevated INR is required, oral or intravenous vitamin K_1 (phytonadione) can be given.[6,67,68] In the absence of major bleeding, the oral route of administration is preferred. While the intravenous route produces a more rapid reversal, it is associated with rare but serious anaphylactoid reactions. If the INR is between 5 and 9, doses of warfarin should be withheld or may be combined with a low dose of oral vitamin K (1 to 5 mg). Low doses of oral vitamin K will reduce the INR consistently within 24 hours without making the patient refractory to warfarin therapy. Overcorrection of the INR in a patient who is not bleeding is unnecessary but common. Simply withholding warfarin will result in correction of INRs between 5 and 9 within 36 to 48 hours for most patients. The decision to administer vitamin K should be individualized based on the patient's bleeding risk and the underlying indication for anticoagulation therapy. Vitamin K should be used with caution in patients

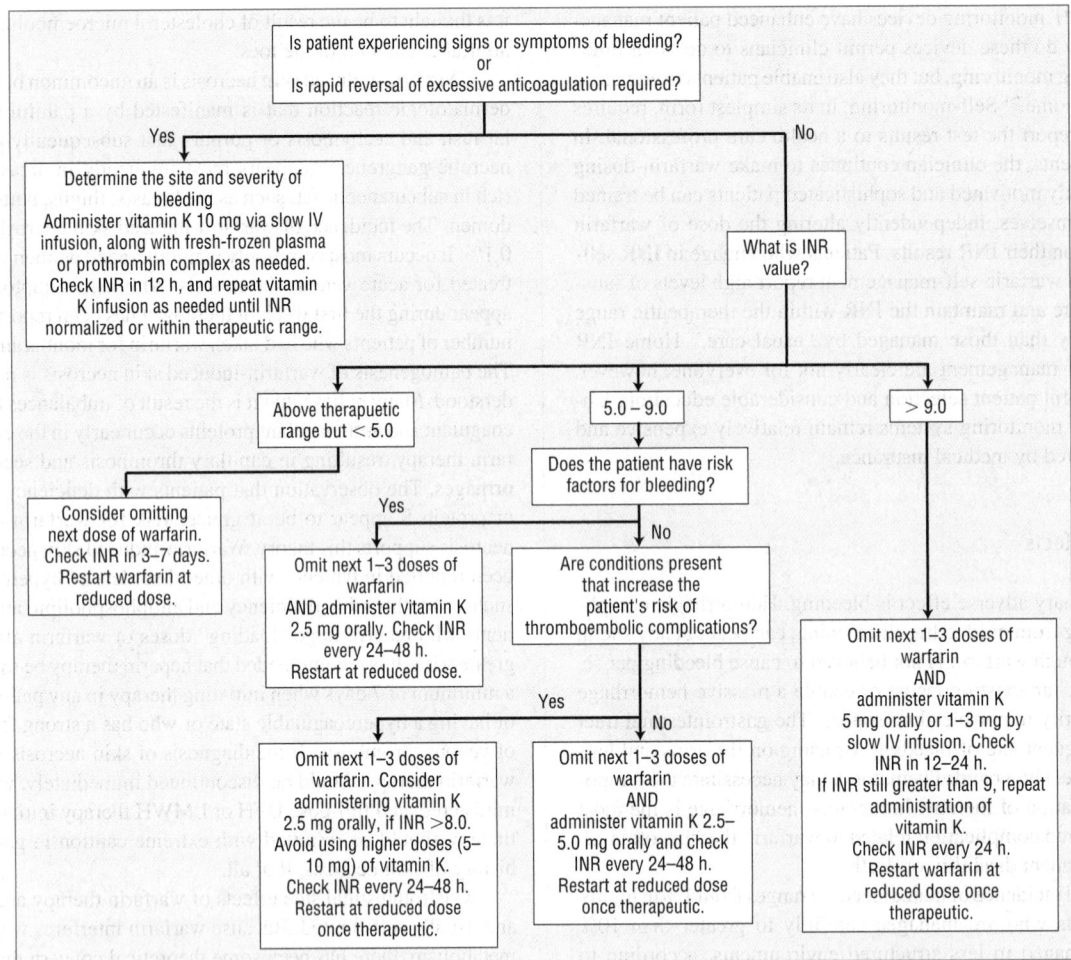

FIGURE 19–9. Management of an elevated international normalized ratio (INR) in patients taking warfarin. Dose reductions should be made by determining the weekly warfarin dose and reducing the weekly dose by 10% to 25% based on degree of INR elevation. Conditions that increase the risk of thromboembolic complications include history of hypercoagulability disorders (e.g., protein C or S deficiency, presence of antiphospholipid antibodies, antithrombin deficiency, activated Protein C resistance), arterial or venous thrombosis within the previous month, thromboembolism associated with malignancy, and mechanical mitral valve in conjunction with atrial fibrillation, previous stroke, poor ventricular function, or coexisting mechanical aortic valve.

at high risk of recurrent thromboembolism because of the possibility of INR overcorrection. Conversely, simply withholding warfarin therapy may not lower a high INR quickly enough in patients at high risk for developing bleeding complications. If the INR is greater than 9, a 5 mg oral dose of vitamin K is recommended. High doses of vitamin K (e.g., 10 mg) have been associated with prolonged resistance to warfarin and the occurrence of thromboembolic complications. In the event of a serious or life-threatening bleed, intravenous vitamin K should be administered, as well as fresh frozen plasma or clotting factor concentrates.

Drug-Drug and Drug-Food Interactions

The pharmacokinetic and pharmacodynamic properties of warfarin, coupled with its narrow therapeutic index, predispose this agent to numerous clinically important food and drug interactions[5,69] (see Tables 19–12, 19–13, and 19–14). Vitamin K can reverse warfarin's pharmacologic activity, and many foods contain sufficient vitamin K to reduce the anticoagulation effect of warfarin if a patient consumes them in large portions or repetitively in a short period of time.[69] Patients should be given a list of vitamin K–rich foods and instructed to maintain a relatively consistent intake. It is important to stress consistency and moderation rather than absolute abstinence. Abrupt changes in vitamin K intake should be considered when unexplained changes in the INR occur. Alternative sources of vitamin K, such as multivitamins and nutritional supplements (e.g., Sustical or Ensure), should also be considered. Patients who require parenteral nutrition should not receive a weekly bolus dose of vitamin K if they are taking warfarin therapy.

Pharmacokinetic drug interactions with warfarin are due primarily to alterations in hepatic metabolism or binding to plasma proteins. Drugs that inhibit or induce the CYP2C9, -1A2, and -3A4 isoenzymes have the greatest potential to significantly alter the response to warfarin therapy. Protein-binding displacement interactions can also occur. However, in the absence of hepatic disease or a diminished capacity to metabolize warfarin, changes in protein binding result in only transient changes in the INR. Drugs that alter hemostasis, platelet function, or the clearance of clotting factors (e.g., thyroid hormone replacement) can alter the response to warfarin therapy or increase the risk of bleeding by pharmacodynamic mechanisms.

The explosive increase in the use of herbal and alternative therapies in North America has raised concern regarding their potential to interact with warfarin therapy.[70] Although there are a growing number of case reports and some in vivo data, the clinical importance of specific warfarin-herbal interactions remains unclear. All patients on warfarin therapy should be questioned regarding the use of herbal drugs and dietary supplements. Clinicians should advise patients on warfarin therapy to seek information about potential interactions with warfarin whenever they start to take a new drug product, whether it is prescribed or purchased over the counter. If there is a known drug interaction or doubt about its potential to alter the response to warfarin, more frequent PT testing following the initiation of the new agent is prudent.

Use in Special Populations

In the absence of a clear and compelling indication, warfarin should not be used during pregnancy because of the potential for fetal hemorrhage and teratogenic complications.[22] Warfarin crosses the placenta and has been associated with several embryopathies, particularly central nervous system abnormalities, which have occurred throughout gestation. The FDA has designated warfarin a pregnancy category X agent. Because UFH and the LMWHs are large molecules that do not cross the placental barrier, they are considered the drugs of choice for anticoagulation during pregnancy. Warfarin is excreted in the breast milk in very low concentrations and generally is considered safe to use by women who are breast-feeding.

Patients scheduled to undergo major surgery or other invasive procedures often require temporary discontinuation of warfarin therapy.[6] The decision to withhold warfarin therapy should be based on the type of surgical procedure being performed and the patient's risk of bleeding and thromboembolism. Warfarin therapy generally should not be discontinued in patients undergoing minimally invasive procedures such as dental work.[71] If the bleeding risk from the procedure is considerable, warfarin should be stopped 4 to 5 days prior to the procedure to allow the INR to return to near-normal values. Alternatively, warfarin can be stopped and a low dose (2.5 mg) of oral vitamin K may be given 2 days prior to the procedure.[6] Patients at moderate or high risk of thromboembolism (i.e., DVT or PE in the previous month) should be given so-called "bridge therapy" with UFH or a LMWH before and/or after the procedure.

Warfarin use among elderly patients is increasingly common. While the drug has been studied extensively in this population, some debate still remains regarding the relative risks of warfarin therapy in the elderly.[4] Data supporting the notion that age increases hemorrhagic risk are somewhat conflicting. Age greater than 75 years has been associated with an increased risk of intracranial hemorrhage, but the overall incidence of major bleeding is similar to that in younger users. Elderly patients may be more prone to excessive anticoagulation due to nutritional deficiencies, comorbidities, and multiple drug interactions. Furthermore, they are often at greater risk for falls. Although they often derive the greatest benefit from anticoagulation therapy, elderly patients should be monitored with greater vigilance, and warfarin dose changes should be made more cautiously.

GENERAL APPROACH TO THE PREVENTION OF VTE

Given that VTE is often clinically silent and potentially fatal, strategies to prevent DVT in at-risk populations will have the greatest impact on patient outcomes.[3] To rely on the early diagnosis and treatment of VTE is unacceptable because many patients will die before treatment can be initiated. Furthermore, even clinically silent disease is associated with long-term morbidity from the postphlebitic syndrome and predisposes the patient to future thromboembolic events. Despite an immense body of literature that overwhelmingly supports the widespread use of pharmacologic and nonpharmacologic strategies to prevent VTE, prophylaxis is underutilized in most hospitals.[3,72] Even when prophylaxis is given, many patients receive prophylaxis that is less than optimal. Educational programs and clinical decision-support systems have been shown to improve the appropriate use of VTE prevention methods.[3]

❻ The goal of an effective VTE prophylaxis program is to identify all patients at risk, determine each patient's level of risk, select and implement regimens that provide sufficient protection for the level of risk, and avoid or limit complications from the selected regimens. Since hospitalized patients are frequently at high risk for VTE, screening all patients prior to or at the time of admission to determine their level of risk is the first step in an effective prophylaxis program. The risk-classification criteria and recommended prophylaxis strategies promulgated by the ACCP Conference on Antithrombotic Therapy are used widely in North America[3] (Table 19–15). Several pharmacologic and nonpharmacologic methods are effective for preventing VTE, and these can be used alone or in combination. Nonpharmacologic methods improve venous blood flow by mechanical means, whereas drug therapy counteracts the propensity for thrombus formation by dampening the coagulation cascade.

NONPHARMACOLOGIC STRATEGIES

Resumption of ambulation as soon as possible following surgery has been shown to reduce the incidence of VTE in low-risk patients.[3] Walking increases venous blood flow and promotes the flow of natural antithrombotic factors into the lower extremities. During prolonged surgeries, electrical calf muscle stimulation devices that mimic the pumping action produced during ambulation can be beneficial. Although these devices can reduce the risk of DVT by more than 50%, their use is painful, and they can be used only when the patient is under general anesthesia. Continuous passive motion devices and plantar compression systems are also available, but their effectiveness is not certain.

Graduated compression stockings reduce the incidence of VTE by approximately 60% following general surgery, neurosurgery, and stroke.[3,73] Compression stockings work by increasing the velocity of venous blood flow. They apply a graded amount of pressure, with the greatest amount of pressure applied at the ankle. Inexpensive and safe, they are an excellent choice when pharmacologic interventions are either contraindicated or difficult to monitor adequately. When combined with pharmacologic interventions, graduated compression stockings have an additive effect. Some patients are unable to wear compression stockings because of the size or shape of their legs, however.

Similar to graduated compression stockings, intermittent pneumatic compression (IPC) devices increase the velocity of blood flow

TABLE 19–15. Risk Classification and Consensus Guidelines for VTE Prevention

Level of Risk	Calf Vein Thrombosis,%	Symptomatic PE,%	Fatal PE,%	Prevention Strategies
Low				
Minor surgery, age < 40 years, and no clinical risk factors	2	0.2	0.002	Ambulation
Moderate				
Major or minor surgery, age 40–60 years, and no clinical risk factors	10–20	1–2	0.1–0.4	UFH 5000 units SC q12h
Major surgery, age < 40 years, and no clinical risk factors				Dalteparin 2500 units SC q24h
				Enoxaparin 40 mg SC q24h
Minor surgery, with clinical risk factor(s)				Tinzaparin 3500 units SC q24h
Acutely ill (e.g., MI, ischemic stroke, CHF exacerbation), and no clinical risk factors				IPC
				Graduated compression stockings
High				
Major surgery, age > 60 years, and no clinical risk factors	20–40	2–4	0.4–1.0	UFH 5000 units SC q8h
Major surgery, age 40–60 years, with clinical risk factor(s)				Dalteparin 5000 units SC q24h
				Enoxaparin 40 mg SC q24h
Acutely ill (e.g., MI, ischemic stroke, CHF exacerbation), with risk factor(s)				Tinzaparin 75 units/kg SC q24h
				IPC
Highest				
Major lower extremity orthopedic surgery	40–80	4–10	0.2–5	Adjusted dose UFH SC q8h (aPTT > 36 s)
Hip fracture				
Multiple trauma				Dalteparin 5000 units SC q24h
Major surgery, age > 40 years, and prior history of VTE				Desirudin 15 mg SC q12h
				Enoxaparin 30 mg SC q12h
Major surgery, age > 40 years, and malignancy				Fondaparinux 2.5 mg SC q24h
				Tinzaparin 75 units/kg SC q24h
Major surgery, age > 40 years, and hypercoagulable state				Warfarin (INR = 2.0–3.0)
Spinal cord injury or stroke with limb paralysis				IPC with UFH 5000 units SC q8h

IPC = intermittent pneumatic compression.
From ref. 3.

in the lower extremities.[3,74] The technique involves the sequential inflation of a series of cuffs wrapped around the patient's legs. Using graded pressure, the cuffs inflate in 1- to 2-minute cycles continually throughout the day from the ankles to the thighs. IPC has been shown to reduce the risk of VTE by more than 60% following general surgery, neurosurgery, and orthopedic surgery.[3] There is some theoretical concern that external compression may dislodge a previously formed clot.[75] Although IPC is well tolerated and safe to use in patients who have contraindications to pharmacologic therapies, it does have a few drawbacks. It is more expensive than the use of graduated compression stockings, it is a relatively cumbersome technique, and some patients may have difficulty sleeping while using it.[3] Like graduated compression hose, IPC can increase the effectiveness of pharmacologic prophylaxis.

Inferior vena cava (IVC) filters, also known as Greenfield filters, provide short-term protection against pulmonary embolism in very high-risk patients by preventing the embolization of a thrombus formed in the lower extremities into the pulmonary circulation.[3,76,77] Percutaneous insertion of a filter into the IVC is a minimally invasive procedure performed via fluoroscopy. Despite the widespread use of IVC filters, there are very limited data regarding their effectiveness and long-term safety. The evidence suggests that IVC filters, particularly in the absence of effective antithrombotic therapy, increase the long-term risk of recurrent DVT. In the only randomized clinical trial examining the short- and long-term effectiveness of the filters in patients with a documented proximal DVT, treatment with IVC filters in combination with anticoagulation therapy reduced the risk of PE by more than 75% during the first 12 days following insertion.[77] However, this benefit was not sustained during 2 years of follow-up, and the long-term risk of recurrent DVT was nearly twofold higher in those who received a filter. Although IVC filters can reduce the short-term risk of PE in patients at highest risk, they should be reserved for patients in whom other prophylactic strategies cannot be used. Further, to reduce the long-term risk of VTE in association with IVC filters, pharmacologic prophylaxis is necessary, and warfarin therapy should begin as soon as the patient is able to tolerate it.

PHARMACOLOGIC STRATEGIES

Several pharmacologic interventions have been evaluated extensively in numerous randomized clinical trials.[3] Appropriately selected drug therapies can reduce the incidence of VTE dramatically following hip replacement, knee replacement, general surgery, myocardial infarction, and ischemic stroke (see Table 19–15). The choice of agent and dose to use for VTE prevention must be based on the patient's level of risk for thrombosis and bleeding complications, as well as cost and the availability of an adequate drug therapy monitoring system.

CLINICAL CONTROVERSY

A recent and widely publicized study found that "low dose" warfarin (INR goal range 1.5 to 2.0) was substantially more effective than placebo for the long-term treatment of patients with an idiopathic DVT following an initial 6 months of "full intensity" therapy (INR goal range 2.0 to 3.0). However, another study found that long-term "full intensity" warfarin was more effective than the "low dose" regimen. Whereas the full-intensity warfarin appears to be slightly more effective in terms of recurrent VTE, the lower-intensity regimen is easier to manage and requires less frequent monitoring (every 8 weeks rather than every 3 to 4 weeks). It remains unclear whether the tradeoff in terms of reduced quality of life justifies long-term "full intensity" treatment.

Although a meta-analysis by the Antiplatelet Trialists' Collaboration challenges this view, most randomized, controlled trials fail to show a significant benefit from aspirin therapy in the prevention of VTE.[3,78] The ACCP Consensus Conference continues to recommend against the use of aspirin as the primary method of VTE prophylaxis. Antiplatelet drugs clearly reduce the risk of coronary artery and cerebrovascular events in patients with arterial disease, but aspirin produces a very modest reduction in VTE following orthopedic surgeries of the lower extremities. The relative contribution of platelets in the pathogenesis of venous thrombosis compared with that of arterial thrombosis can explain the reason for this difference. Venous thrombosis results primarily from venous stasis, whereas arterial thrombosis is most often the result of vascular wall injury.

The most extensively studied agents for the prevention of VTE are UFH, the LMWHs, and fondaparinux.[3,46] The LMWHs and fondaparinux provide superior protection against VTE compared with low-dose UFH.[3,46] Their more predictable absorption when given by subcutaneous injection may be the explanation. Even so, UFH remains a highly effective, cost-conscious choice for many patient populations, provided that it is given in the appropriate dose (see Table 19–15). Low-dose UFH (5000 units every 12 hours or every 8 hours) given subcutaneously has been shown to reduce the risk of VTE by 55% to 70% in patients undergoing a wide range of general surgical procedures and following a myocardial infarction or stroke. For the prevention of VTE following hip and knee replacement surgery, the effectiveness of low-dose UFH is considerably lower.[3] Adjusted-dose UFH therapy provided subcutaneously, which requires dose adjustments to maintain the aPTT at the high end of the normal range, appears to be substantially more effective than low-dose UFH in the highest-risk patient populations. However, adjusted-dose UFH has been studied in only a few relatively small clinical trials and requires frequent laboratory monitoring. The LMWHs and fondaparinux appear to provide a high degree of protection against VTE in most high-risk populations. The appropriate prophylactic dose for each LMWH product is indication-specific (see Table 19–10). There is no evidence that one LMWH is superior to another for the prevention of VTE. Fondaparinux was significantly more effective than enoxaparin in several clinical trials that enrolled patients undergoing high-risk orthopedic procedures but has not been shown to reduce the incidence of symptomatic pulmonary embolism or mortality.[46] To provide optimal protection, some experts believe that the LMWHs should be initiated prior to surgery.[3,79]

Warfarin is a commonly used option for the prevention of VTE following orthopedic surgeries of the lower extremities.[3] The evidence is equivocal regarding the relative effectiveness of warfarin compared with the LMWHs for the prevention of clinically important VTE events in the highest-risk populations. When used to prevent VTE, the dose of warfarin must be adjusted to maintain an INR between 2.0 and 3.0. Oral administration and low drug cost give warfarin some advantages over the LMWHs and fondaparinux. However, warfarin does not achieve its full antithrombotic effect for several days, requires frequent monitoring and periodic dosage adjustments, and carries a substantial risk of major bleeding. For these reasons, warfarin is reserved for the highest-risk patients. Furthermore, warfarin should be recommended only when a well-developed monitoring system is available.[6]

The optimal duration for VTE prophylaxis following surgery is not well established.[3,80] Prophylaxis should be given throughout the period of risk. For general surgical procedures and medical conditions, once the patient is able to ambulate regularly and other risk factors are no longer present, prophylaxis can be discontinued. Because of the relatively high incidence of VTE in the first month following hospital discharge among patients who have undergone a lower extremity orthopedic procedure, extended prophylaxis following hospital discharge with either an LMWH, fondaparinux, or warfarin appears to be beneficial. Most clinical trials support the use of antithrombotic therapy for 21 to 35 days following total hip replacement, hip fracture repair, and knee replacement surgeries.[43,81,82]

▪ PHARMACOECONOMIC CONSIDERATIONS

Only a handful of studies have formally evaluated the cost-effectiveness of VTE prevention strategies. The acquisition costs of graduated compression stockings, heparin, and warfarin are considerably less than those of the LMWHs, DTIs, and fondaparinux. However, the acquisition cost for drug therapy is relatively small when compared with the overall cost of care. Economic analyses must take into account the efficacy of the strategy, treatment complications, and monitoring costs.

Determination of the cost-effectiveness of VTE prophylaxis is based on the premise that a reduction in future VTE events will reduce future costs.[83] Furthermore, the incremental cost per patient will decrease proportionally with an increase in the frequency of VTE in the population. Stated another way, the cost of providing prophylaxis to 1000 patients will decline as the incidence of VTE in the given population increases. More expensive and effective strategies, therefore, become more cost-effective in higher-risk populations. In populations at low risk for VTE, early ambulation appears to be the most cost-effective strategy. In populations at moderate risk, the use of graduated compression stockings, the least expensive intervention, results in a lower overall cost of care, whereas low-dose UFH is estimated to increase the cost by $50 (1990 U.S. dollars) per patient when compared with no prophylaxis.[84] This compares favorably with the incremental costs associated with other routinely employed preventative measures. While the LMWHs provide slightly greater reductions in the risk of VTE in patients at moderate risk of VTE, the additional cost is estimated to be $107 (1999 U.S. dollars) per patient when compared with low-dose UFH.[85] Whether universal use of LMWHs in moderate-risk patients is a cost-effective strategy remains controversial.

In high-risk patients, the cost-effectiveness of prevention is far greater because the incidence of VTE is higher. Following hip replacement surgery, regardless of the strategy selected, prophylaxis saves money when compared with no prophylaxis.[83] The LMWHs and fondaparinux slightly increase the total mean cost of care after total hip and knee replacement when compared with low-dose

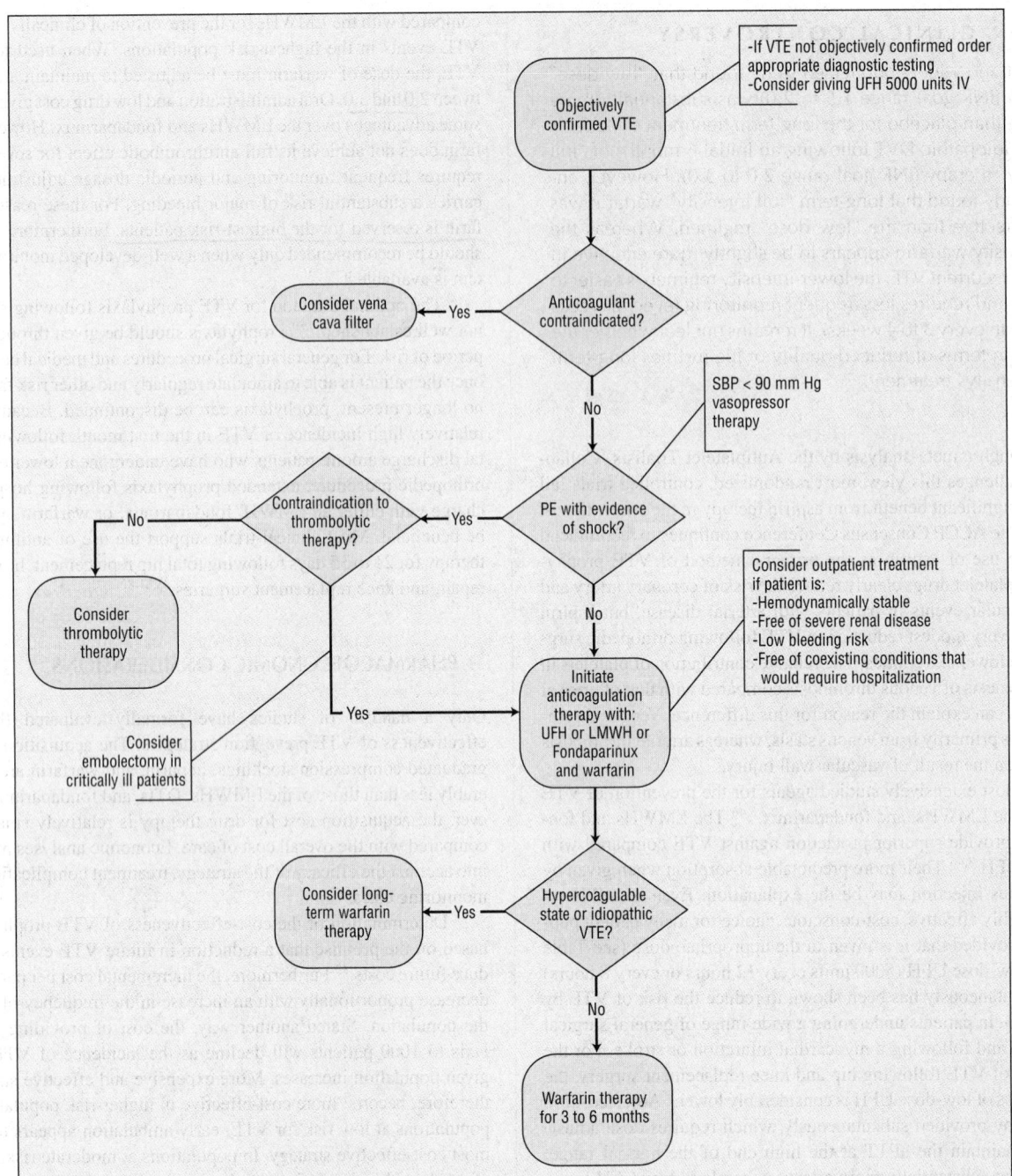

FIGURE 19–10. Treatment of venous thromboembolism.

UFH and warfarin.[86,87] However, because of their superior effectiveness, the LMWHs have a significantly lower cost per DVT and PE avoided.[83] Based on typical drug acquisition costs, the LMWHs and fondaparinux appear to be a cost-effective choice in the highest-risk patient populations.[88]

GENERAL APPROACH TO THE TREATMENT OF VTE

Anticoagulation therapy remains the mainstay of treatment for VTE. DVT and PE are manifestations of the same disease process and are treated similarly.[12] Full "therapeutic" doses of antithrombotic drugs not only prevent thrombus extension and embolization but also reduce the risk of long-term sequelae such as the postthrombotic syndrome, pulmonary hypertension, and recurrent thromboembolism.[12,89] The standard approach is to initiate therapy with UFH by continuous intravenous infusion or a LMWH by subcutaneous injection and to make the transition to warfarin for maintenance therapy (Fig. 19–10 and Table 19–16). Newer approaches using ximelagatran alone or fondaparinux plus warfarin have been investigated recently in phase III clinical trials[11,44,45,90] (Table 19–17). In rare circumstances, elimination of the obstructing thrombus is warranted, and the use of venous thrombectomy or thrombolysis can be considered.[12] IVC interruption with a filter is also an option in those

TABLE 19–16. Consensus Guidelines for VTE Treatment

	Recommendation	Grade[a]
Acute anticoagulation	Acute treatment of DVT or PE should be with LMWH, fondaparinux, intravenous UFH, or adjusted-dose subcutaneous UFH.	1A
	The dose of UFH should be sufficient to prolong the aPTT to a range that correlates to an anti-Xa activity of 0.3 to 0.6 units mL.	1C+
	LMWH or fondaparinux are preferred over UFH.	1A
	A LMWH is preferred in patients with cancer.	1A
Duration of acute treatment	Treatment with UFH, LMWH, or fondaparinux should be overlapped with warfarin for at least 5 days and can be stopped when the INR is >2.0. Most patients should have warfarin started at the same time as UFH, LMWH, or fondaparinux.	1C
	Patients with cancer should be treated with a LMWH for at least 6 months.	1A
	A longer period of heparin therapy (approximately 10 days) is recommended for massive PE or severe iliofemoral thrombosis.	1C
Long-term anticoagulation	Oral anticoagulation therapy (target INR 2.5; range 2.0–3.0) should be continued for at least 3 months. If oral anticoagulation therapy is contraindicated (e.g., pregnancy), a treatment dose of LMWH or adjusted-dose UFH should be used.	1A
	Patients with an idiopathic VTE, an inherited disorder of hypercoagulability, or antiphospholipid antibodies should be treated for at least 6 to 12 months and considered for indefinite therapy.	1A
	Patients with two or more episodes of documented DVT should be treated indefinitely.	1A

[a]Refers to grade of recommendation (1A = strong recommendation applying to most patients without reservation; 1C = intermediate-strength recommendation that may change when stronger evidence becomes available; 1C+ = strong recommendation that applies to most patients in most circumstances. *From ref. 12.*

with contraindications to anticoagulation therapy or in whom anticoagulant therapy has failed.

Once the diagnosis of VTE has been confirmed objectively (see "Clinical Presentation and Diagnosis" section), anticoagulant therapy with either UFH, LMWH, or fondaparinux should be instituted as soon as possible. Although LMWHs and fondaparinux are highly effective and can be administered in the outpatient setting, most patients in the United States continue to receive intravenous UFH for the initial treatment of VTE.[11] The decision to initiate therapy with an LMWH or fondaparinux on an outpatient basis should

be based on institutional resources and patient-specific variables (Table 19–18).

UNFRACTIONATED HEPARIN (UFH)

The parenteral administration of UFH followed by warfarin has been the conventional treatment of patients with VTE for more than 40 years.[11,89,91] Although UFH can be given by either subcutaneous or intravenous injection, continuous intravenous infusion is preferable

TABLE 19–17. Emerging Treatment Options for VTE: Major Findings from Recent Phase III Clinical Trials

Trial	Treatments	Duration of Trial	Recurrent VTE	Major Bleeding
Matisse-DVT[44]	Fondaparinux 7.5 mg SC q24h versus enoxaparin 1 mg/kg SC q12h All patients received warfarin (INR = 2.0–3.0) for 3 months	3 months	3.9% versus 4.1% (p = NS)	1.1% versus 1.2% (p = NS)
Matisse-PE[45]	Fondaparinux 7.5 mg SC q24h versus adjusted-dose UFH IV infusion All patients received warfarin (INR = 2.0–3.0) for 3 months	3 months	2.4% versus 3.6% (p = NS)	1.3% versus 1.1% (p = NS)
Thrive treatment[90]	Ximelagatran 36 mg PO q12h for 6 months versus enoxaparin 1 mg/kg SC q12h followed by warfarin (INR = 2.0–3.0) for 6 months	6 months	2.0% versus 2.1% (p = NS)	1.3% versus 2.2% (p = NS)

TABLE 19–18. Outpatient Treatment Protocol for Venous Thrombosis (Kaiser Permanente of Colorado)

Target Population	Inclusion/exclusion criteria for outpatient VTE treatment
Inclusion	Patients with objectively diagnosed VTE
Relative exclusion	Patients with clinical evidence of pulmonary embolus or suspected embolism who are hemodynamically stable
Exclusion	Arterial thromboembolism or patients who are currently receiving dialysis, actively bleeding, have had recent (within 2 weeks) major surgery/trauma, or have other severe uncompensated co-morbid conditions
Recommended Procedure	May vary depending on the patient's clinical condition

A. Confirm diagnosis of VTE by objective testing
   1. Venous ultrasound
   2. V̇/Q̇ scan
   3. CT scan
B. Day 1
   1. Baseline laboratory evaluation
      a. Prothrombin time (PT) and calculated international normalized ratio (INR)
      b. Activated partial thromboplastin time (aPTT)
      c. Serum creatinine (Cr_S)
      d. Complete blood count (CBC) with platelets
   2. Medication
      a. LMWH or fondaparinux injections
         i. Enoxaparin 1 mg/kg SC q12h or
         ii. Enoxaparin 1.5 mg/kg SC q24h (not recommended for patients with cancer and obese patients)
         iii. Dalteparin 100 units/kg SC q12h or
         iv. Dalteparin 200 units/kg SC q24h or
         v. Tinzaparin 175 units/kg SC q24h or
         vi. Fondaparinux 7.5 mg SC q24h (5 mg if < 50 kg and 10 mg if > 100 kg)
      b. Warfarin sodium 5–10 mg orally every evening
      c. Pain medication if necessary (avoid NSAIDs)
   3. Patient education
      a. Clinical pharmacy/nursing
         i. Educate patient regarding the importance of proper monitoring of anticoagulation therapy and indications for additional medical evaluation. Document activities in the medical record.
         ii. Teach patient how to self-administer LMWH or fondaparinux (if patient or family member unwilling or unable to self-administer LMWH injection, visiting nurse services should be arranged). Initial LMWH or fondaparinux injection should be administered in the medical office or hospital.
         iii. Instruct patient regarding local therapy: elevation of affected extremity, localized heat, antiembolic exercises (flexion/extension of ankle for lower extremity VTE, or hand squeezing/relaxation for upper extremity VTE).
      b. Pharmacy operations
         i. Provide back up for clinical pharmacy/nursing. Reinforce patient education regarding indication, use, monitoring, side effects, and drug interactions with antithrombotic therapy
         ii. Repackage LMWH or fondaparinux syringes (if indicated) in patient-specific doses and dispense 5 to 7 days of therapy.
         iii. Screen patient's pharmacy profile for potential drug-drug interactions with anticoagulation therapy.
      c. Clinical pharmacy anticoagulation service (CPAS) enrollment
         i. The physician should forward outpatient VTE treatment orders to the anticoagulation service.
C. Day 2
   1. Laboratory evaluation: Not required on day 2 of therapy.
   2. Medications: Continue LMWH or fondaparinux and warfarin as directed.
   3. Anticoagulation service
      a. Contact patient and evaluate for symptoms of PE, clot extension, and/or bleeding.
      b. Arrange for visiting nursing services if family or family member is having difficulty with outpatient therapy.
      c. Continue reduced activity as long as pain persists (when possible, elevate extremity); increase activity as tolerated.
      d. Document activities in medical record.
D. Day 3
   1. Laboratory evaluation: Check INR.
   2. Medications: Continue LMWH or fondaparinux and warfarin as directed.
   3. Anticoagulation service
      a. Contact patient and evaluate for symptoms of PE, clot extension, and/or bleeding.
      b. Interpret results of INR and adjust dose of warfarin to achieve a target INR of 2.5.
      c. Patient activity: Continue reduced activity as long as pain persists (when possible, elevate extremity); increase activity as tolerated.
      d. Document activities in medical record.
E. Day 4
   1. Laboratory evaluation: Check INR.
   2. Medications: Continue LMWH or fondaparinux and warfarin as directed.
   3. Anticoagulation service
      a. Contact patient and evaluate for symptoms of PE, clot extension, and/or bleeding.
      b. Interpret results of INR and adjust dose of warfarin to achieve a target INR of 2.5.
      c. Patient activity: No restrictions; if pain increases, contact anticoagulation service or provider.
      d. Document activities in medical record.

TABLE 19–18. (Continued)

F. Day 5
 1. Laboratory evaluation: Check INR and CBC with platelets.
 2. Medications: Continue LMWH or fondaparinux if indicated and warfarin as directed.
 3. Anticoagulation service
  a. Contact patient and evaluate for symptoms of PE, clot extension, and/or bleeding.
  b. Interpret results of INR and adjust dose of warfarin to achieve a target INR of 2.5.
  c. Patient activity: No restrictions; if pain increases, contact CPAS or provider.
  d. Document activities in medical record.
G. Day 6
 1. Laboratory evaluation: Check INR.
 2. Medications: Continue LMWH or fondaparinux if indicated and warfarin as directed.
 3. Anticoagulation service
  a. Contact patient and evaluate for symptoms of PE, clot extension, and/or bleeding.
  b. Interpret results of INR and adjust dose of warfarin to achieve a target INR of 2.5.
  c. If LMWH or fondaparinux has not been discontinued, continue until INR > 2.0.
  d. Patient activity: No restrictions; if pain increases, contact CPAS or provider.
  e. Document activities in medical record.

because of improved dosing precision and a lower risk of major bleeding[12] (see Table 19–7). The aPTT or a suitable coagulation study should be used to monitor the effect of UFH. The infusion rate should be adjusted to maintain an appropriate therapy range corresponding to a heparin concentration of 0.2 to 0.4 units/mL or an anti-factor Xa level of 0.3 to 0.7 units/mL. Weight-based dosing of UFH achieves a therapeutic aPTT in the vast majority of patients in the first 24 hours[11,29] (see Table 19–7). Failure to give a sufficient dose of heparin increases the risk of VTE recurrence. Intravenous UFH requires hospitalization with frequent monitoring and dose adjustment.[12] Well-organized inpatient anticoagulation management services have been shown to improve patient care by increasing the proportion of aPTT values in the therapeutic range, reducing the length of hospital stay, and lowering total hospital costs when compared with usual care.[9] However, despite the widespread use of weight-based dosing protocols, as many as 25% of patients still fail to achieve an adequate response to UFH therapy.[11] There is also evidence that UFH does not prevent thrombus progression in some patients with DVT. These limitations of UFH in the acute treatment of VTE have led to the use of alternative agents.

■ LOW-MOLECULAR-WEIGHT HEPARIN

Because of their improved pharmacokinetic and pharmacodynamic profile, as well as ease of use, the LMWHs have replaced UFH for the treatment of VTE in many institutions. The LMWHs given subcutaneously in fixed, weight-based doses (see Table 19–10) are at least as effective as UFH given intravenously for the treatment of VTE.[12] A number of meta-analyses comparing LMWHs with UFH in the treatment of VTE have been conducted.[12,39] These analyses demonstrate no differences in clinically important end points, including recurrent VTE, PE, major or minor bleeding, and thrombocytopenia. Surprisingly, patients who received LMWH have a significantly lower mortality rate. The reduction in mortality was seen primarily in patients with cancer. The explanation for this survival advantage is unknown, but studies are underway to further examine this observation.[92] There appears to be no difference in the risk of recurrent VTE among patients who are treated on an inpatient or outpatient basis with an LMWH for DVT.[39] However, outpatient treatment was associated with a slightly greater risk of major bleed, indicating the need for close monitoring

when LMWH is given in this setting. There appears to be no difference in the efficacy or safety of once-daily versus twice-daily dosing regimens.[39,93] However, a subgroup analysis in one study suggested that patients with cancer and obese patients have higher recurrence rates with once-daily enoxaparin.[93]

CLINICAL CONTROVERSY

Some clinicians advocate strict criteria for the outpatient management of VTE in order to minimize the potential for treatment failure and bleeding complications. These criteria often exclude patients with cancer and the morbidly obese. Proponents of a less restrictive approach argue that strict exclusion criteria unnecessarily withhold outpatient treatment with LMWHs or fondaparinux from those patients who may benefit the most; namely, those with cancer. Each health care system must develop outpatient DVT criteria that fit its resources, philosophy, and patient population best.

Given the predictable response and the reduced need for laboratory monitoring with the LMWHs, stable patients with DVT who have normal vital signs, low bleeding risk, and no other comorbid conditions requiring hospitalization can be discharged early or treated entirely on an outpatient basis[12,94] (see Table 19–18). The efficacy and safety of LMWHs in the home-based treatment of proximal DVT was established initially in large clinical studies.[91] The results of randomized, controlled clinical trials, as well as the experience of several successful outpatient DVT treatment programs in a variety of health care settings, have led to an increased acceptance of outpatient management.[11,91,94] Indeed, surveys of patients who received outpatient DVT treatment indicate a high degree of satisfaction and comfort, with 96% preferring at-home treatment.

Patients presenting with PE and no evidence of hemodynamic instability are at low risk of subsequent morbidity and mortality. Recent evidence suggests that patients with submassive PE who are hemodynamically stable can be managed safely as outpatients with LMWHs or fondaparinux. However, hemodynamically unstable patients with PE should be admitted and treated with intravenous UFH.[92] Patients with PE who present with shock have the highest risk of mortality and require aggressive interventions such as volume expansion,

TABLE 19–19. Patient Education for Outpatient VTE Therapy

General Information Regarding VTE and the Goals of Treatment

Anticoagulant medications injections and tablets have been prescribed to prevent the blood clot from growing larger so that the body can begin to dissolve the clot.

Your body may be able to completely dissolve the clot, but in some cases the clot never goes completely away; even with adequate anticoagulation therapy, some people will have chronic pain and swelling in the affected extremity; people who have had one clot are at increased risk of having future clots.

Warfarin tablets take several days to begin to work; LMWH or fondaparinux injections work right away, so at first, LMWH or fondaparinux injections and warfarin tablets are used together.

When the warfarin has become effective, you will be able to stop the LMWH or fondaparinux injections; you will continue to take warfarin tablets for 3 to 6 months or more to prevent blood clots from returning.

It is important for you to administer your LMWH or fondaparinux and warfarin exactly as directed.

Subcutaneous Injection Technique

You must learn to give yourself a subcutaneous injection of LMWH or fondaparinux. Alternatively, you may have a family member or visiting nurse give it to you.

If your LMWH or fondaparinux syringes were filled by the manufacturer, they can be stored at room temperature; if your syringes were filled by the pharmacy, they should be stored in the refrigerator; if you were instructed to fill your own syringes, you should prepare the syringe immediately prior to injecting its contents.

If you see a bubble in the syringe, do not try to get it out; you may accidentally squirt out part of your dose.

Choose an injection site on your abdomen; clean the area with alcohol; then position an uncapped syringe at a 90-degree angle; pinch the skin, stick the needle in as far as it will go, and gently but firmly push the plunger down; this will inject the medicine into the skin; when all the medication has been injected, remove the needle and dispose of it in an appropriate container.

You likely will experience a burning sensation when the medication is injected; this will go away after a few minutes.

Rotate injection sites from side to side; do not inject into the same site more than once; avoid the area around your navel; do not inject into any bruises.

Blood Test Monitoring

Regular blood tests will be required to make sure that your medication is working properly.

The prothrombin time tells how quickly your blood forms a clot; it is used to tell how well warfarin is working.

The INR is a way to standardize the prothrombin time between laboratories; your goal INR range is between 2.0 and 3.0; if your INR is less than 2.0, you are at higher risk for clotting, if your INR is greater than 3.0, you are at higher risk for bleeding; your dose of warfarin will be adjusted based on the results of this test.

You will need to have a complete blood count test before you begin therapy and after you have been on LMWH or fondaparinux for about 5 days; this will help detect internal bleeding and the occurrence of a rare side effect of heparin therapy that can decrease a component of your blood called platelets.

Warfarin Information

Each strength of warfarin has a unique color; each time your refill your prescription, make sure that your new tablets are the same color as the ones you have been taking; if they are not the same color, ask your pharmacist why.

Warfarin should be taken at approximately the same time each day.

The most common and serious side effect of warfarin is bleeding; you should be careful to avoid situations or activities that increase your risk of injury; apply direct pressure to control bleeding from superficial cuts.

Warfarin has many drug interactions; always check with your provider before taking any new medications (including over-the-counter medication and dietary supplements).

Foods rich in vitamin K (green leafy vegetables, etc.) may interfere with warfarin; you do not need to avoid foods rich in vitamin K, but you should try to maintain consistent dietary habits.

Alcohol can increase your risk for bleeding and interfere with warfarin therapy; drink alcohol in moderation (one to two drinks per day); avoid binge drinking.

Contact Your Provider If You Experience:

Persistent bleeding from a cut or scrape

Blood in your urine

Blood in your stool

Persistent nose bleeding

Increased swelling or pain in your affected extremity

Go to the Emergency Department If You Experience:

Shortness of breath

Chest pain

Coughing up blood

Black, tarry-appearing stool

Severe headache of sudden onset

Slurred speech

LMWH = low-molecular-weight heparin.

vasopressor therapy, intubation, and mechanical ventilation, in addition to antithrombotic therapy.[95]

Not all patients are appropriate candidates for outpatient VTE treatment. At a minimum, patients must be reliable or have adequate caregiver support.[12] Patients and their caregivers must be willing and active participants in the outpatient management of VTE (Table 19–18 and Table 19–19). Patients who are unable or decline at-home treatment should be admitted to the hospital. These patients may opt subsequently for early discharge on LMWH or fondaparinux. Daily patient contact either in person or via telephone is essential to identify potential complications and to address questions and concerns promptly. During daily contacts, patients must be asked about symptoms that may indicate bleeding, thrombus extension, and PE.[94] Once acute treatment with a LMWH or fondaparinux has been transitioned to long-term warfarin therapy (approximately 5 to 10 days), patient contact can occur less frequently.

FONDAPARINUX

Fondaparinux has been shown in two recent clinical trials to be a safe and effective alternative to enoxaparin and intravenous UFH for the treatment of VTE (see Table 19–17). In the MATISSE DVT trial, a fixed-dose regimen of fondaparinux (7.5 mg/day) given by subcutaneous injection was compared with the standard weight-adjusted dosing of enoxaparin (1 mg/kg every 12 hours) for the acute treatment of DVT followed by 3 months of warfarin therapy. In the MATISSE PE trial, fondaparinux (7.5 mg subcutaneously every 24 hours) was compared with UFH administered by intravenous infusion. In both trials, the dose of fondaparinux was increased to 10 mg subcutaneously every 24 hours for patients who weighed more than 100 kg and reduced to 5 mg every 24 hours for those who weighed less than 50 kg. Fondaparinux received FDA approval for the acute treatment of DVT and PE in 2004.

CLINICAL CONTROVERSY

In a series of large, well-designed phase III clinical trials, fondaparinux was superior to enoxaparin for the prevention of VTE in patients undergoing lower extremity orthopedic surgery. However, the rate of symptomatic PE and death was not different between the two treatments in any of these studies. Furthermore, fondaparinux has not been compared with warfarin for the prevention of VTE in high-risk patients. Based on these findings, some experts contend that fondaparinux offers no clinical advantages over enoxaparin or warfarin. In addition, although there was no difference in the risk of major hemorrhage seen in the clinical trials compared with enoxaparin, some clinicians worry about the potential for bleeding with fondaparinux because it has a long half-life and cannot be reversed with protamine sulfate. Despite these concerns, some experts believe that fondaparinux should be used preferentially because asymptomatic DVTs and PEs may increase the future risk of recurrent thrombotic events and the postthrombotic syndrome.

WARFARIN

Warfarin monotherapy is an unacceptable choice for the acute treatment of VTE because it does not produce a rapid anticoagulation effect and is associated with a high incidence of recurrent thromboembolism.[91] However, warfarin is very effective in the long-term management of VTE and should be started concurrently with UFH, LMWH, or fondaparinux therapy.[12] The acute treatment regimen should overlap with warfarin therapy for at least 5 days and until a therapeutic INR has been achieved. The initial dose of warfarin should be 5 to 10 mg (see Fig. 19–8), and it should be adjusted periodically to achieve and maintain an INR between 2.0 and 3.0.

The appropriate duration of warfarin maintenance therapy requires careful consideration of the circumstances surrounding the initial thromboembolic event, the presence of ongoing thromboembolic risk factors, and the risk of bleeding.[12] A major consideration in determining the risk of recurrent VTE once anticoagulation therapy is stopped is whether the initial thrombotic event was associated with a transient or reversible risk factor (e.g., trauma, prolonged immobility, surgery, pregnancy, estrogen use, or major medical illness). For patients in this situation, the risk of recurrence is relatively small, approximately 3% per year, and only short-term anticoagulation treatment is warranted.[12] Six to 12 weeks of warfarin therapy is sufficient for patients with symptomatic isolated calf vein DVT.[12] For patients with a proximal vein DVT, warfarin should be continued for at least 3 months. If the patient has a large iliofemoral DVT or PE, most experts recommend at least 6 months of therapy.[96] If the patient has ongoing risk factors for recurrent VTE, such as malignancy, antiphospholipid antibodies, or an inherited disorder of hypercoagulability, the risk of recurrence during the first year after stopping treatment exceeds 10%.[97] In this situation, long-term anticoagulation therapy should be considered. Several recent clinical trials provide clear evidence that long-term treatment with warfarin reduces the risk of recurrent VTE by 70% to 90% in patients with inherited deficiencies of coagulation factors (e.g., protein C or S and antithrombin) or an idiopathic VTE.[63,97,98] Similar results have been observed with the long-term use of ximelagatran.[99] The optimal duration for long-term anticoagulation therapy for patients with ongoing risk factors for VTE or an idiopathic VTE remains unknown.[63,98] The benefit of continuing warfarin therapy longer than 2.5 years has not been studied. Further, the data supporting long-term warfarin therapy in patients with factor V Leiden, prothrombin *20210A* gene mutation, increased factor VIII activity, and hyperhomocysteinemia is less compelling. For patients with stable INRs who are able to obtain follow-up blood tests at recommended intervals and who are at low risk for developing bleeding complications, long-term anticoagulation therapy can be continued indefinitely but should be reassessed annually. A decision with the patient to continue anticoagulation therapy should consider the patient's long-term prognosis, financial resources, lifestyle, and quality of life. For patients who are unable to keep follow-up appointments every 3 to 4 weeks, low-intensity warfarin therapy (goal INR 1.5 to 2.0) can be considered following the first 6 months of therapy.[63]

THROMBOLYSIS AND THROMBECTOMY

Most cases of VTE require only anticoagulation therapy. In some cases, however, removal of the occluding thrombus by either pharmacologic or surgical means may be warranted.[12] There is a relative paucity of data supporting either thrombolysis or thrombectomy in the management of VTE, and more study clearly is needed to clarify their precise role.[100] Thrombolytic agents are proteolytic enzymes that enhance the conversion of plasminogen to plasmin, which subsequently degrades the fibrin matrix.

Thrombolytic therapy for DVT was once believed to improve long-term outcomes by preventing the postthrombotic syndrome.[12] While thrombolytic therapy has been shown to improve venous patency, clinical trials have failed to demonstrate any sustained benefit from the routine use of thrombolytic therapy. There is no evidence that thrombolytic therapy is superior to anticoagulation therapy alone in preventing the postthrombotic syndrome. Patients who present with massive DVT and limb gangrene despite anticoagulation therapy are candidates for thrombolysis (Table 19–20). Some authorities recommend thrombolytic treatment for patients with massive iliofemoral venous thromboembolism who are at low risk for bleeding. Catheter-directed instillation of a thrombolytic agent directly into the clot has been used in recent years.[101] The risk of bleeding associated with catheter-directed drug administration appears to be less than systemic

TABLE 19–20. Thrombolysis for the Treatment of VTE

Thrombolytic therapy should be reserved for patients who present with shock, hypotension, right ventricular strain, or massive DVT with limb gangrene.

Diagnosis must be confirmed objectively before initiating thrombolytic therapy.

Thrombolytic therapy is most effective when administered as soon as possible after PE diagnosis, but benefit may extend up to 14 days after symptom onset.

Approved PE Thrombolytic Regimens

Streptokinase 250,000 units intravenously over 30 minutes followed by 100,000 units/h for 24 h[a]

Urokinase 4400 units/kg intravenously over 10 min followed by 4400 units/kg/h for 12 to 24 h[a]

Alteplase 100 mg intravenously over 2 h

Factors that increase the risk of bleeding must be evaluated before thrombolytic therapy is initiated (i.e., recent surgery, trauma or internal bleeding, uncontrolled hypertension, recent stroke or intracranial hemorrhage).

Baseline laboratory tests should include CBC and blood typing in case transfusion is needed.

UFH should not be used during thrombolytic therapy. The aPTT or any other anticoagulation parameter should not be monitored during the thrombolytic infusion.

aPTT should be measured following the completion of thrombolytic therapy.

If aPTT is less than 2.5 times control value, UFH infusion should be started and adjusted to maintain aPTT in therapeutic range.

If aPTT is greater than 2.5 times control value, remeasure every 2 to 4 hours and start UFH infusion when aPTT is less than 2.5.

Avoid phlebotomy, arterial puncture, and other invasive procedures during thrombolytic therapy to minimize the risk of bleeding.

[a]Two-hour infusions of streptokinase and urokinase are as effective and safe as alteplase.
From ref. 102.

administration. Prospective clinical trials are necessary to clarify the clinical utility of catheter-directed thrombolysis in the treatment of DVT.

In the management of acute PE, alteplase, streptokinase, and urokinase all have been shown to restore pulmonary artery patency more rapidly than UFH alone.[102] However, this early benefit does not improve long-term patient outcomes. One week following acute treatment, clot lysis and vessel patency are similar with or without thrombolytic therapy. Thrombolytic therapy has never been shown to improve morbidity or mortality but has been associated with a substantial risk of hemorrhage. Admittedly, clinical trials to date have been underpowered to detect a benefit from thrombolytic therapy. The association of thrombolytic therapy with hemorrhage is particularly problematic because PE frequently occurs following a surgical procedure and the risk of bleeding is high.[101] Given the relative lack of data to support their routine use, thrombolytic agents should be reserved for patients with PE who are most likely to benefit (see Table 19–20). Patients who have hemodynamic compromise, as evidenced by significant hypotension (systolic blood pressure 90 mm Hg or less) or severe right ventricular strain due to a large clot burden, may benefit from thrombolytic therapy.[12,102] Between 5% and 10% of patients diagnosed with PE present with shock. Mortality among these patients is as high as 50%, thus justifying the risks associated with thrombolytic therapy. Although thrombolytic therapy for patients with massive PE manifested by shock and cardiovascular collapse is considered the standard of care, only one trial has demonstrated a mortality benefit.[95] A significant number of hemodynamically stable patients with PE have evidence of right ventricular dysfunction and appear to be at higher risk for recurrent PE and death when treated with heparin alone.[102] Some experts believe that thrombolytic therapy is beneficial in patients with evidence of right ventricular dysfunction because it restores pulmonary blood flow and reduces pulmonary artery pressure. However, convincing data are lacking.[95,102]

Although it is an uncommon choice, venous thrombectomy is a reasonable approach to remove a massive obstructive thrombus in a patient with significant iliofemoral venous thrombosis, particularly if the patient is either not a candidate for, or has not responded to, thrombolysis.[12] In cases of chronic PE—where persistent emboli produce progressive pulmonary hypertension, hypoxemia, and right-sided heart failure—surgical embolectomy offers greater benefit than

anticoagulants and may be the treatment of choice. The surgical technique has been refined over the past 20 years. The procedure uses a balloon catheter to extract the thrombus while the patient is under general anesthesia. Fluoroscopy and venography guide the procedure. Balloon angioplasty, with or without stent placement, can be used if a focal iliac vein stenosis is discovered. Full-dose anticoagulation therapy is essential during the entire operative and postoperative periods. These patients still need chronic anticoagulation therapy for the usual recommended duration.

VENA CAVA INTERRUPTION

Anticoagulation therapy is the accepted standard for treating DVT and PE. However, an IVC filter may be indicated in special situations when anticoagulants are ineffective or unsafe, including (1) in patients with an absolute contraindication to anticoagulation therapy due to active bleeding or anticipated bleeding from a predisposing lesion, (2) in patients with a massive PE who survive but in whom recurrent embolism may be fatal, or (3) in patients who have recurrent VTE despite adequate anticoagulation therapy.[103] Interruption of the IVC can be accomplished with an occlusive filter, often called a Greenfield filter, inserted percutaneously through the femoral or jugular vein. There is little evidence to support the widespread use of IVC filters. IVC filters have not been shown to reduce the risk of rehospitalization for PE. Indeed, the permanent IVC interruption appears to increase the long-term risk for recurrent DVT presumably owing to the accumulation of thrombus on the filter resulting in venous stasis.[103] Whether patients with permanent IVC filters should receive anticoagulant therapy remains unresolved, but many clinicians opt to continue warfarin therapy indefinitely whenever possible. Given these concerns, retrievable filters that can be removed after the period of greatest risk for PE have been developed.

ANCILLARY THERAPY

In addition to anticoagulant therapy for patients with proximal DVT, wearing graduated compression stockings can reduce the risk of developing the postthrombotic syndrome by as much as 50%.[89] To be

TABLE 19–21. UFH and LWMH Use During Pregnancy

Acute treatment	**LMWH** Enoxaparin 1 mg/kg SC q12h or 1.5 mg/kg q24h or Dalteparin 100 units/kg SC q12h or 200 units/kg q24h or Tinzaparin 175 units/kg SC q24h or **UFH** Initiate using weight-based intravenous therapy, and adjust dose to achieve therapeutic aPTT for at least 5 days. Transition to SC adjusted-dose UFH administered q8–12h with midinterval aPTT in the therapeutic range.[a]
Long-term treatment[b]	**LMWH** Maintain initial LMWH dose regimen throughout pregnancy or Alter LMWH dose in proportion to any weight change (usually gain) or Obtain monthly anti-Xa level measurements 4 to 6 hours after morning dose and adjust LMWH dose to achieve an anti-Xa level of 0.5 to 1.2 units/mL if twice-daily dosing or 1.0 to 2.0 units/mL if once-daily dosing or **UFH** Obtain monthly aPTT at the midpoint of the dosing interval and adjust UFH dose as indicated.
Issues at time of delivery	**Elective induction of labor** Discontinue UFH or LMWH 24 hours prior to induction. Initiate therapeutic doses of UFH by IV infusion and discontinue 4 to 6 hours prior to expected time of delivery if risk of recurrent VTE is deemed high. **Spontaneous labor** For LMWH, if there is a reasonable expectation that significant anticoagulant effect will be present at time of delivery, (1) epidural should be avoided, and (2) reversal with protamine sulfate may be considered. For UFH, monitor the aPTT and reverse with protamine sulfate if aPTT is prolonged near the time of delivery. **Postpartum** Commence UFH or LMWH as soon as safely possible (usually 12 hours following delivery). Concurrently initiate warfarin therapy and discontinue UFH or LMWH when the INR is 2.0 or greater. Continue anticoagulants for at least 4 weeks following delivery. Warfarin can be used safely by women who are breast-feeding.

[a]Anti-Xa monitoring is preferred because the relationship between aPTT and heparin levels differs in pregnant compared with nonpregnant patients.
[b]As pregnancy progresses, the volume of distribution of LMWH changes; golmerular filtration rate increases, and most women gain weight.
From ref. 121.

effective, graduated compression stockings must fit properly. Antiembolic leg exercise also may be useful. To perform the exercise, patients should elevate the legs above the hips (7 to 10 degrees) with feet supported. The patient then flexes one foot at a time back and forth for 3 to 5 minutes or until the calf muscle group is fatigued. This exercise should be repeated four to six times daily.[104] Patients also should be instructed not to remain in a sitting position for more than 20 minutes without ambulating briefly or stretching the leg for a few minutes.

Strict bed rest traditionally was recommended following acute DVT based on the assumption that leg movement would dislodge the clot, resulting in PE. However, the evidence contradicts this assumption. Ambulation in conjunction with graduated compression stockings results in faster reduction in pain and swelling with no apparent increase in the rate of clot embolization.[12] Patients should be encouraged to ambulate as much as their symptoms permit. If pain and swelling increase with ambulation, the patient should be instructed to lie down and elevate the affected leg until symptoms subside.

TREATMENT OF VTE IN SPECIAL POPULATIONS

Pregnancy

The use of anticoagulation therapy for the treatment of DVT or PE in pregnant women is common.[22] UFH and LMWHs are the preferred

anticoagulants for use during pregnancy (Table 19–21). They do not cross the placenta, and evidence suggests that they are safe for the fetus.[22,105] Warfarin should be avoided because it crosses the placenta and can produce fetal bleeding, central nervous system abnormalities, and embryopathy. The DTIs also cross the placenta. To date, fondaparinux has not been formally evaluated in pregnant patients.

Long-term UFH therapy has been linked to significant bone loss and osteoporosis, requires multiple daily injections, and must be monitored frequently (every 1 to 2 weeks) throughout pregnancy. Because of these limitations, many experts recommend the use of LMWHs over UFH throughout pregnancy.[22]

Pediatric Patients

VTE in children has become increasingly common secondary to prematurity, cancer, trauma, surgery, congenital heart disease, and SLE.[35] Children often develop DVTs associated with an indwelling central venous catheter. In contrast to adults, children rarely develop idiopathic VTE.

Anticoagulation with UFH and warfarin remains the most frequently used approach for the treatment of VTE in pediatric patients.[35] The recommended target aPTT and INR ranges, as well as the duration of therapy, are extrapolated from clinical trials in adults. The recommended initial bolus dose of UFH is 75 to 100 units/kg given intravenously over 10 minutes, followed by a maintenance infusion of 28 units/kg per hour for infants 2 to 12 months of age and 20 units/kg per hour for children 1 year of age or older. Subsequent adjustments should be made every 4 to 6 hours to maintain the aPTT within the institution-specific therapeutic range. The usual warfarin starting dose is 0.2 mg/kg, with a maximum of 10 mg.[35,106] Infants require higher doses of warfarin per kilogram to maintain a therapeutic INR compared with teenagers and adults (mean doses 0.33 mg/kg, 0.09 mg/kg, and 0.04 to 0.08 mg/kg, respectively). The INR target range is 2.0 to 3.0. Frequent INR monitoring and warfarin dose adjustments typically are required. When compared with adults, only 10% to 20% of pediatric patients can be monitored safely once monthly. Obtaining coagulation monitoring tests in pediatric patients is problematic because many have poor or nonexistent venous access. To address this problem, many clinicians recommend using finger-stick blood samples with a portable PT monitor. Since LMWHs have low drug-interaction potential, are less likely to cause HIT or osteoporosis, and require less frequent laboratory testing, they are an attractive alternative in pediatric patients.[35] Enoxaparin, dalteparin, tinzaparin, and reviparin have been evaluated in pediatric patients. Most experts recommend that anti-factor Xa activity be monitored and the dose adjusted to maintain anti-factor Xa levels between 0.5 and 1.0 unit/mL. Compared with adults, children younger than 2 to 3 years of age or weighing less than 5 kg have higher per-kilogram dose requirements to achieve a "therapeutic" response. The doses of LMWH for older children generally are similar to the weight-adjusted doses used in adults.[35] Warfarin can be initiated concurrently with UFH or LMWH therapy. Therapy should be overlapped for a minimum of 5 days and until the INR is therapeutic. Warfarin should be continued for at least 3 months. Thrombolysis and thrombectomy have been employed successfully in pediatric patients, but published data are very limited.

Patients with Cancer

VTE is a frequent complication of malignancy.[92] Further, compared with patients without cancer, the rate of recurrent VTE in patients with cancer is threefold higher, and the risk of bleeding is two- to sixfold higher.[107] Several meta-analyses and one randomized clinical trial comparing LMWH with UFH for the treatment of VTE have shown a survival advantage for patients with cancer who received LMWHs. While the reduction in mortality may be attributable to a decline in fatal PE, several other mechanisms have been postulated, including altering tumor angiogenesis and metatasis.[20] In vitro data suggest that small to midsized heparin molecules have antiangiogenic properties. Warfarin therapy in cancer patients is often complicated by drug interactions (e.g., chemotherapy and antibiotics) and the need to frequently interrupt therapy for invasive procedures (e.g., thoracentesis, percutaneous biopsy, and abdominal paracentesis).[107] Maintaining stable INR control is more difficult in this patient population due to nausea, anorexia, and vomiting.

Two recent randomized trials provide evidence that long-term LMWH therapy for VTE in cancer patients significantly decreases the rate of recurrent VTE without increasing bleeding risks compared with traditional therapy with oral anticoagulants.[108,109] In one relatively small study in cancer patients with VTE, fixed-dose subcutaneous enoxaparin for 3 months appeared to be more effective than conventional warfarin therapy, with only 10.5% of enoxaparin-treated patients compared with 21% warfarin-treated patients reaching the composite outcome of major bleeding and recurrent VTE ($p = .09$).[108] In the Comparison of LMWH versus Oral Anticoagulation Therapy for the Prevention of Recurrent Venous Thrombosis (CLOT) trial, continuous treatment with dalteparin for 6 months was compared with conventional therapy with dalterparin followed by warfarin in cancer patients following an acute VTE.[109] The probability of recurrent VTE was reduced by nearly 50% in the long-term dalteparin treatment group, from 17.4% to 8.8% ($p = .0017$). There was no difference in the rate of major bleeding. While this provides compelling data that cancer patients should be given LMWH instead of warfarin for the long-term treatment of VTE, the economic implications of this strategy have not yet been evaluated. In the absence of insurance coverage to offset the relatively high cost of long-term LMWH therapy, most patients are unable to afford it.

PHARMACOECONOMIC CONSIDERATIONS

Hospitalization is the main cost driver in the management of VTE.[94] Although the drug acquisition cost for the LMWHs is substantially higher than UFH, avoiding hospitalization dramatically decreases the overall costs of VTE treatment. A number of cost-effectiveness analyses using decision modeling suggest that the treatment of DVT with LMWHs is more cost effective than the treatment with UFH in both inpatient and outpatient settings.[110] Based on this decision model, the LMWHs will reduce overall health care cost if as few as 8% of patients are treated entirely on an outpatients basis or 13% of patients are discharged from the hospital early.

HEPARIN-INDUCED THROMBOCYTOPENIA

Heparin-induced thrombocytopenia (HIT) is an uncommon but extremely serious adverse effect associated with heparin use.[34,111] The immune-mediated platelet activation and thrombin generation seen during HIT can lead to severe and unusual thrombotic complications. Morbidity and mortality associated with HIT are disturbingly high—up to 50% of patients who develop the disorder will suffer a thrombotic complication or die within 30 days in the absence of treatment. The diagnosis of HIT is based on clinical and laboratory findings that confirm heparin antibody formation and platelet activation. To prevent the thrombotic complications associated with HIT, prompt discontinuation of heparin and initiation of an alternative anticoagulant therapy is imperative.

ETIOLOGY AND PATHOPHYSIOLOGY OF HIT

Two types of thrombocytopenia associated with heparin use have been described.[7,34,111] As many as of 25% of patients receiving heparin therapy develop a benign, mild reduction in platelet counts referred to as *non-immune-mediated heparin-associated thrombocytopenia* (HAT) or previously called *HIT type 1*. HAT produces a transient fall in platelet count that occurs early, typically between days 2 and 4, during the course of therapy. The degree of thrombocytopenia is usually mild, with platelet counts rarely going below 100,000/mm^3. It is not necessary to discontinue heparin therapy in these patients because platelet counts generally rebound to baseline values despite continued use. The exact mechanism of HAT is unknown, but it may be the result of platelet aggregation, a dilutional effect, or diminished platelet

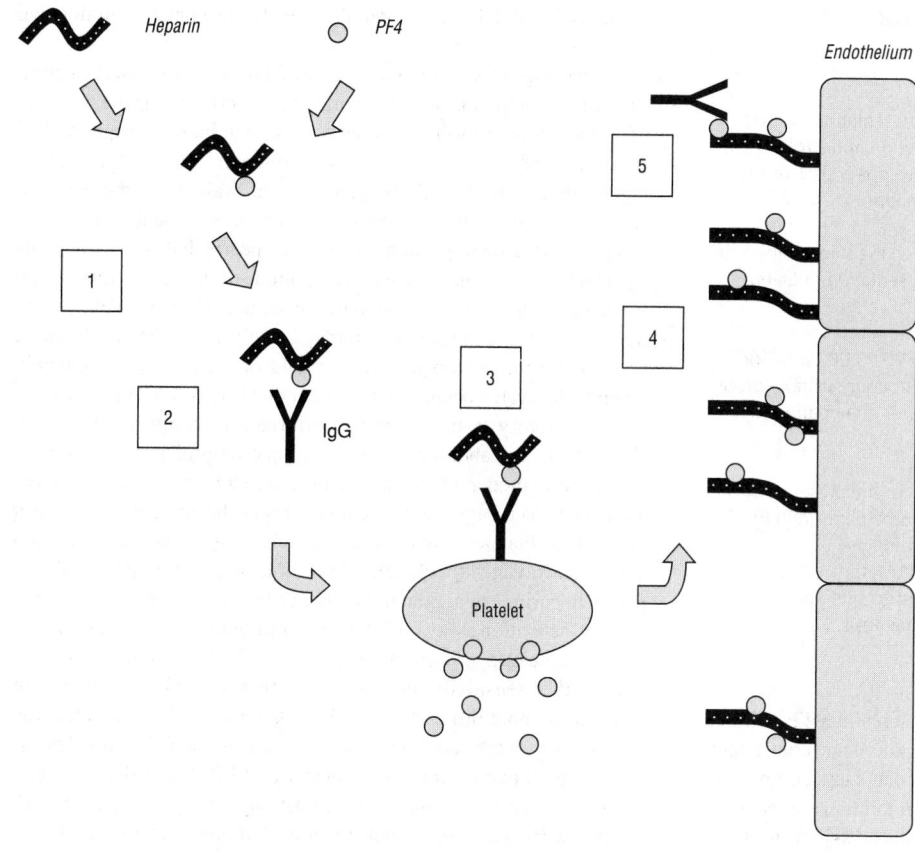

FIGURE 19–11. Pathogenesis of heparin-induced thrombocytopenia.

production often seen in acutely ill patients. No clinical sequelae are associated with this benign phenomenon.

The second type of thrombocytopenia associated with heparin use is known as *immune-mediated HIT* (formally known as *HIT type 2*).[7,34,111] HIT is a severe pathologic adverse effect of heparin with a significant potential to cause thrombotic complications. The time course and magnitude of thrombocytopenia associated with HIT differ from those of HAT. Platelets counts typically begin to fall after 5 or more days of continuous heparin use, most often between days 7 and 14 of therapy. The development of thrombocytopenia can be delayed up to 20 days in patients naive to heparin therapy. Conversely, so-called rapid-onset HIT can occur in 24 to 48 hours in patients with recent exposure to heparin (i.e., in the previous 3 to 6 months).[112] Platelet counts commonly fall below 100,000/mm^3 but rarely nadir lower than 20,000/mm^3. In some cases, overt thrombocytopenia may not occur, but a drop in platelet count greater than 50% from baseline is considered indicative of HIT.

The frequency of immune-mediated HIT is related most powerfully to the duration and type of heparin used and, to a lesser extent, to the dose and route of administration.[111] The incidence of HIT associated with intravenous full-dose UFH given for prolonged periods is significantly higher than that of low-dose subcutaneous UFH or LMWHs. The estimated overall incidence of HIT after 5 days of UFH use is 1% to 3%, but the cumulative incidence may be as high as 6% after 14 days of continuous intravenous use. LMWHs are associated with a significantly lower risk of HIT (<1%).[7,113]

The pathogenesis of HIT involves an immunoglobulin-mediated response to the heparin molecule leading to platelet activation and thrombin generation[111] (Fig. 19–11). With platelet activation, there is release of PF-4 from platelet granules. Heparin binds to PF-4 (1), forming a negatively charged polysaccharide molecule that is highly

antigenic and stimulates the production of IgG antibodies (2). Although heparin-induced antibody formation occurs in 10% to 20% of patients treated with heparin, most of these patients never develop HIT. In patients who develop HIT, the heparin–PF-4–IgG complexes bind to the Fc receptor on platelets (3), leading to further platelet activation and the release of PF-4 and procoagulant microparticles from platelet granules. In addition, PF-4 and heparin-like molecules bind to the surface of endothelial cells, resulting in antibody-induced endothelial cell damage and the release of tissue factor (4,5). The net result of this cascade of events is an increased risk of thrombotic events secondary to platelet activation, endothelial damage, and thrombin generation despite moderate to severe thrombocytopenia. Antibodies to the heparin–PF-4 complex are transient, but the exact duration of continued immunogenicity is unknown.

CLINICAL PRESENTATION AND DIAGNOSIS OF HIT

Thrombotic complications are the most common clinical sequelae of HIT[34] (Table 19–22). The incidence of thrombosis is as high as 50% in patients with laboratory-confirmed immune-mediated thrombocytopenia. Thrombosis may occur in patients with seemingly mild thrombocytopenia, but platelet counts invariably have dropped more than 50% from baseline. This syndrome is poorly recognized, and many, perhaps most, patients diagnosed with HIT initially presented with thrombosis. Even among those who are diagnosed prior to the development of thrombosis, the prognosis is poor. In one case series of patients who were diagnosed with HIT without thrombosis, the cumulative incidence of thrombosis over the next 30 days was greater than 50% despite the discontinuation of heparin therapy.[114]

Venous thrombosis is the most common thrombotic complication associated with HIT, and most patients develop proximal DVT.[114]

TABLE 19–22. Presentation of Heparin-Induced Thrombocytopenia (HIT)

General
Venous thromboembolism is the most common presentation of HIT, although arterial events (e.g., myocardial infarction and stroke) can occur. HIT should be suspected if a patient develops a DVT or PE while or soon after receiving unfractionated heparin.

Symptoms and Signs
Thromboembolic events secondary to HIT produce the same signs and symptoms as those of other etiologies (see "Presentation of Deep Venous Thrombosis and Pulmonary Embolism").

Laboratory Tests
The patient's platelet count typically will be below 100,000/mm^3 or drop more than 50% from baseline. The platelet count usually drops after 5 days of UFH therapy but may drop sooner if the patient has been given heparin in the past 6 months.

Other Diagnostic Tests
An enzyme-linked immunosorbent assay (ELISA) for the presence of antibodies to the heparin–PF-4 complex should be performed to confirm the diagnosis. Functional assays including the heparin-induced platelet-activation assay (HIPAA), the serotonin-release assay (SRA), and the platelet-aggregation assay (PAA) also may be performed to confirm the diagnosis.

A large percentage of patients develop asymptomatic VTE. PE occurs in 25% of patients with thrombotic complications and contributes significantly to mortality. Arterial thrombosis occurs less commonly. Limb artery occlusion, stroke, and myocardial infarction are the most commonly reported arterial events. Heparin-induced skin lesions occur in 10% to 20% of patients with HIT. Lesions range from painful, localized erythematous plaques to widespread dermal necrosis. Amputation in such cases frequently is required. Mortality from HIT may be as high as 36% in patients with acute thrombosis. The relatively high frequency of thrombotic complications and poor outcomes associated with HIT emphasize the need for prompt recognition and diagnosis.

The diagnosis of immune-mediated HIT is made based on clinical findings supplemented by laboratory tests confirming the presence of antibodies to heparin or platelet activation induced by heparin.[34,111] While thrombocytopenia is the most common initial event suggesting the diagnosis of HIT, clinicians should evaluate all the potential causes. New thrombosis shortly after the development of thrombocytopenia is a distinguishing feature in nearly half of all patients with HIT.[114] The time course and magnitude of thrombocytopenia are the features distinguishing immune-mediated HIT from HAT. Acute thrombosis and skin lesions also may occur prior to the development of overt thrombocytopenia. HIT should be suspected immediately when these events occur in any patient on UFH or LMWH therapy.

Laboratory testing must be performed to confirm the diagnosis of HIT.[115] Laboratory testing is very helpful in patients with only mild to moderate thrombocytopenia in whom HIT is suspected. Two types of assays are available to detect the presence of heparin antibodies. Platelet activation assays, also known as *functional assays,* confirm in vitro platelet activation in the presence of therapeutic heparin levels. Functional assays include the heparin-induced platelet-activation assay (HIPAA), the serotonin-release assay (SRA), and the platelet-aggregation assay (PAA). The HIPAA and SRA tests have higher sensitivity and specificity than the PAA assay but are technically more difficult to perform. Antigen assays that detect the presence of specific antibodies against the heparin–PF-4 complex using enzyme-linked immunosorbent assays (ELISA) are also available. These tests have reasonably high sensitivity and specificity. The optimal test for laboratory confirmation of immune-mediated HIT is unclear. The most readily available test with the greatest sensitivity and specificity should be used. The combined use of functional and ELISA assays may reduce false-negative results. When results of one test are negative or indeterminate in patients suspected of HIT, another test should be considered.

▶ TREATMENT: Heparin-Induced Thrombocytopenia

▨ GENERAL APPROACHES TO THE TREATMENT OF HIT

The ACCP has established recommendations for the treatment of HIT.[7] Once the diagnosis of HIT is established or strongly suspected, *all* sources of heparin, including heparin flushes, should be discontinued, and an alternative anticoagulant agent should be initiated[7,34,111] (Fig. 19–12). Even in the absence of thrombosis, patients with HIT are at extremely high risk for developing serious thrombotic complications over the next 30 days without treatment. The time required for laboratory results to be reported can be prolonged. It is crucial that patients be anticoagulated by some other means to prevent new thrombosis. Anticoagulant agents that rapidly inhibit thrombin activity and are devoid of significant cross-reactivity with heparin–PF-4 antibodies are the drugs of choice for the management of HIT.[34] In cases of severe or life-threatening thrombosis, surgical extraction of thrombi may be required. Limited data exist regarding the use of thrombolytic therapy in severe HIT with thrombosis. The use of warfarin for long-term anticoagulation in HIT with thrombosis patients is recommended. However, care must be taken when initiating warfarin in these patients because the risk of inducing further thrombosis secondary to inhibition of proteins C and S is possible.

▨ PHARMACOLOGIC TREATMENT OPTIONS

DTIs are the drugs of choice for the treatment of HIT with or without thrombosis (Table 19–23). For the treatment of HIT, lepirudin and argatroban are administered by intravenous infusion.[7,34] Lepirudin and argatroban should be titrated based on aPTT testing with a target of 1.5 to 3.0 times the normal control or the institution-specific therapeutic range. The comparative efficacy of these agents has not been evaluated formally, and they are considered equally suitable for the initial treatment of HIT. Some clinicians prefer argatroban because it has a shorter half-life, modest bleeding risk, and lower cost compared with lepirudin. Fondaparinux is an attractive option for the management of HIT, but it has not yet been studied systematically for this indication. If the oral DTIs receive FDA approval, they may prove to be the ideal agents for the acute and long-term management of patients with HIT. Patient-related factors, such as the presence of renal or hepatic dysfunction, as well as institutional preference, availability, and cost, should be used to determine the most appropriate agent. The LMWHs are not recommended for use in HIT because they have nearly 100% cross-reactivity with heparin-antibodies by in vitro testing.[34]

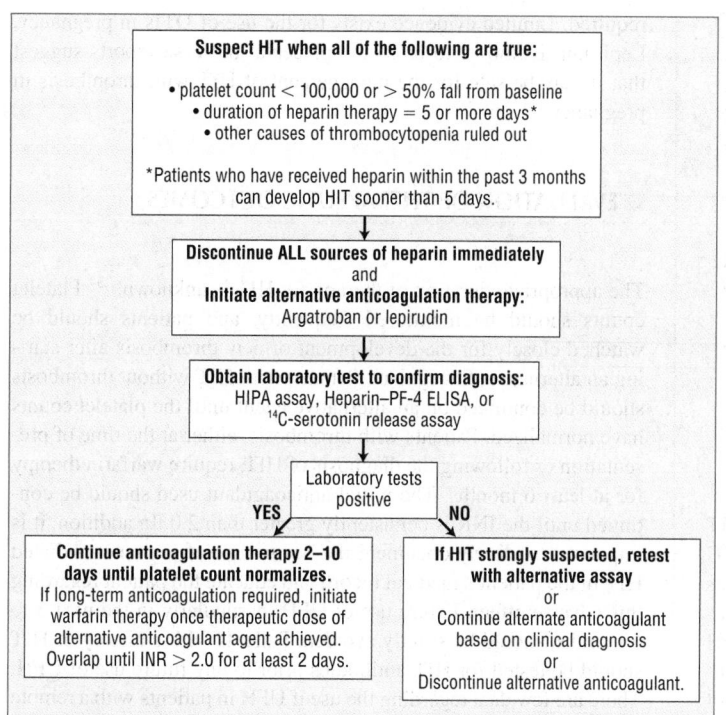

FIGURE 19–12. Treatment of heparin-induced thrombocytopenia (HIT). HIPA assay = heparin-induced platelet activation assay; ELISA = enzyme-linked immunosorbent assay; INR = international normalized ratio.

The use of warfarin during the initial treatment of HIT is potentially dangerous.[34,116] The rapid reduction in protein C concentrations induced early in the course of warfarin therapy further increases the risk of thrombosis in patients with HIT. This concern is supported by the observation that several patients with HIT have developed venous limb gangrene when treated with warfarin alone. Patients with venous limb gangrene had relatively high INRs after the initiation of warfarin therapy and presumably had rapid depletion of protein C. However, one case series found a low incidence of venous limb gangrene among HIT patients treated with low to moderate dose of warfarin.[117] Despite conflicting data, warfarin is not recommended for the initial treatment of patients diagnosed with HIT.[7,34] However, patients requiring long-term anticoagulation for the management of HIT can use warfarin safely. The appropriate timing for initiating warfarin in these patients remains unclear. A conservative approach is to withhold warfarin until the patient is stabilized and platelet counts have rebounded above 100,000/mm³. This may prevent the development of further thrombotic adverse events due to protein C depletion. Therapy should be overlapped with a DTI until the thrombocytopenia has resolved and the full anticoagulant effect of warfarin has been achieved. Initial doses of warfarin greater than 5 mg should be strictly avoided in these patients.

TABLE 19–23. Recommended Dose and Monitoring Parameters for Direct Thrombin Inhibitors to Treat Heparin-Induced Thrombocytopenia

Agent	Dose	Monitoring Parameters	Clinical Considerations
Lepirudin	0.4 mg/kg slow IV bolus, followed by 0.15 mg/kg/h IV infusion	Obtain baseline PT, aPTT, CBC, and serum Cr; check aPTT 4 hours after initiation and adjust dose to achieve aPTT of 1.5–3.0 times control; once stable, monitor aPTT q12h.	Initial dose must be reduced in patients with renal impairment. Antihirudin antibodies can occur in up to 40% of patients and can lead to reduced clearance. Concomitant warfarin requires dose adjustment.
Argatroban	2 mcg/kg/min continuous IV infusion	Obtain baseline PT and aPTT; monitor aPTT 2 hours after initiation, and adjust dose to achieve therapeutic aPTT	Reduce initial dose to 0.5 mcg/kg/min for those with hepatic impairment. Will cause significant elevation in PT/INR; concurrent warfarin therapy requires special management.

The management of pregnant patients with a history of HIT who require anticoagulation therapy presents a challenge. Both UFH and LMWH are the anticoagulants of choice for pregnant patients requiring anticoagulation therapy.[22] Women who develop HIT during pregnancy or have a recent history of HIT cannot use UFH safely. LMWHs, while known to be cross-reactive with HIT antibodies, may be considered an option, but continuous monitoring of platelet count, clinical parameters, and laboratory evidence of HIT is required. Limited evidence exists for the use of DTIs in pregnancy. Lepirudin is known to cross the placenta, but case reports suggest that it may be safe for the management of HIT with thrombosis in pregnancy.[118]

■ EVALUATION OF THERAPEUTIC OUTCOMES

The appropriate duration of therapy for HIT is unknown.[7,34] Platelet counts should be monitored frequently, and patients should be watched closely for the development of new thrombosis after starting an alternate anticoagulant. Patients with HIT without thrombosis should be continued on an alternative agent until the platelet counts have normalized. Patients with thrombosis, either at the time of presentation or following the diagnosis of HIT, require warfarin therapy for at least 6 months. The initial anticoagulant used should be continued until the INR is persistently greater than 2.0. In addition, it is important to clearly document the occurrence of immune-mediated HIT in the patient's medical record and educate the patient regarding this adverse effect. Future use of UFH, particularly in the next 3 to 6 months, should be strictly avoided. Patients with a history of HIT should be tested for HIT antibodies prior to any future use of UFH. There are few data regarding the use if UFH in patients with a remote history of HIT.[118]

ABBREVIATIONS

ACCP: American College of Chest Physicians
AT: antithrombin
DTI: direct thrombin inhibitor
DVT: deep vein thrombosis
ESR: erythrocyte sedimentation rate
FDA: Food and Drug Administration
HIT: heparin-induced thrombocytopenia
INR: international normalized ratio
IPC: intermittent pneumatic compression
LMWH: Low-molecular-weight heparin
t-PA: tissue plasminogen activator
PAF: platelet activating factor
PAI-1: plasminogen activator inhibitor-1
aPTT: activated partial thromboplastin time
PE: pulmonary embolism
PF-4: platelet factor-4
PT: prothrombin time
UFH: unfractionated heparin
VTE: venous thromboembolism
WBC: white blood cell
vWF: von Willebrand factor

Review Questions and other resources can be found at *www.pharmacotherapyonline.com.*

REFERENCES

1. Turpie AGG, Chin BSP, Lip GYH. Venous thromboembolism: Pathophysiology, clinical features, and prevention. Br Med J 2002;325:887–890.
2. Goldhaber SZ. Pulmonary Embolism. N Engl J Med 1998;339:93–104.
3. Geerts WH, Pineo GF, Heit JA, et al. Prevention of venous thromboembolism: The Seventh ACCP Conference on Antithrombotic and Thrombolytic Therapy. Chest 2004;126:338S–400S.
4. Levine MN, Raskob G, Beyth RJ, Kearon C, Schulman S. Hemorrhagic complications of anticoagulant treatment: The Seventh ACCP Conference on Antithrombotic and Thrombolytic Therapy. Chest 2004; 126:287S–310S.
5. Hirsh J, Dalen JE, Anderson DR, et al. Oral anticoagulants: Mechanism of action, clinical effectiveness, and optimal therapeutic range. Chest 2001;119:8–21S.
6. Ansell J, Hirsh J, Poller L, et al. The pharmacology and management of the vitamin K antagonists: The Seventh ACCP Conference on Antithrombotic and Thrombolytic Therapy. Chest 2004;126:204S–33S.
7. Hirsh J, Raschke R. Heparin and low-molecular-weight heparin: The Seventh ACCP Conference on Antithrombotic and Thrombolytic Therapy. Chest 2004;126:188S–203S.
8. Chiquette E, Amato MG, Bussey HI. Comparison of an anticoagulation clinic with usual medical care: Anticoagulation control, patient outcomes, and health care costs. Arch Intern Med 1998;158:1641–1647.
9. Mamdani MM, Racine E, McCreadie S, et al. Clinical and economic effectiveness of an inpatient anticoagulation service. Pharmacotherapy 1999;19:1064–1074.
10. Haines ST, Bussey HI. Diagnosis of deep vein thrombosis. Am J Health Syst Pharm 1997;54:66–74.
11. Hyers TM. Management of venous thromboembolism: Past, present, and future. Arch Intern Med 2003;163:759–768.
12. Büller HR, Agnelli G, Hull RD, et al. Antithrombotic therapy for venous thromboembolic disease: The Seventh ACCP Conference on Antithrombotic and Thrombolytic Therapy. Chest 2004;126:401S–28S.
13. Silverstein MD, Heit JA, Mohr DN, et al. Trends in the incidence of deep vein thrombosis and pulmonary embolism: A 25-year population-based study. Arch Intern Med 1998;158:585–593.
14. White RH, Zhou H, Romano PS. Incidence of idiopathic deep venous thrombosis and secondary thromboembolism among ethnic groups in California. Ann Intern Med 1998;128:737–740.
15. Heit JA, Mohr DN, Silverstein MD, et al. Predictors of recurrence after deep vein thrombosis and pulmonary embolism: A population-based cohort study. Arch Intern Med 2000;160:761–768.
16. Levitan N, Dowlati A, Remick SC, et al. Rates of initial and recurrent thromboembolic disease among patients with malignancy versus those without malignancy: Risk analysis using Medicare claims data. Medicine 1999;78:285–291.

17. Thomas RHMD. Hypercoagulability syndromes. Arch Intern Med 2001;161:2433–2439.

18. Federman DG, Kirsner RS. An update on hypercoagulable disorders. Arch Intern Med 2001;161:1051–1056.

19. Hansson PO, Sorbo J, Eriksson H. Recurrent venous thromboembolism after deep vein thrombosis: Incidence and risk factors. Arch Intern Med 2000;160:769–774.

20. Prandoni P, Piccioli A, Girolami A. Cancer and venous thromboembolism: An overview. Haematologica 1999;84:437–445.

21. Rosendaal FR, Helmerhorst FM, Vandenbroucke JP. Female hormones and thrombosis. Arterioscler Thromb Vasc Biol 2002;22:201–210.

22. Bates SM, Greer IA, Hirsh J, Ginsberg JS. Use of antithrombotic agents during pregnancy: The Seventh ACCP Conference on Antithrombotic and Thrombolytic Therapy. Chest 2004;126:627S–44S.

23. Haines ST, Bussey HI. Thrombosis and the pharmacology of antithrombotic agents. Ann Pharmacother 1995;29:892–905.

24. Dahlback B. Blood coagulation. Lancet 2000;355:1627–1632.

25. Meignan M, Rosso J, Gauthier H, et al. Systematic lung scans reveal a high frequency of silent pulmonary embolism in patients with proximal deep venous thrombosis. Arch Intern Med 2000;160:159–164.

26. Kahn SR. The clinical diagnosis of deep venous thrombosis: Integrating incidence, risk factors, and symptoms and signs. Arch Intern Med 1998;158:2315–2323.

27. Wells PS, Hirsh J, Anderson DR, et al. Accuracy of clinical assessment of deep-vein thrombosis. Lancet 1995;345:1326–1330.

28. Bick RL. Heparin and low-molecular-weight heparins. In: Bick RL, ed. Disorders of Thrombosis and Hemostasis: Clinical and Laboratory Practice. Philadelphia, Lippincott Williams & Wilkins, 2002: 359–377.

29. Raschke RA, Reilly BM, Guidry JR, et al. The weight-based heparin dosing nomogram compared with a "standard care" nomogram. Ann Intern Med 1993;119:874–881.

30. Olson JD, Arkin CF, Brandt JT, et al. College of American Pathologists Conference XXXI on laboratory monitoring of anticoagulation therapy: Laboratory monitoring of unfractionated heparin therapy. Arch Pathol Lab Med 1998;122:782–788.

31. Bussey HI. Problems with monitoring heparin anticoagulation. Pharmacotherapy 1999;19:2–5.

32. Volles DF, Ancell CJ, Michael KA, et al. Establishing an institution-specific therapeutic range. Am J Health Syst Pharm 1998;55:2002–2006.

33. Brill-Edwards P. Heparin resistance. In: Ginsberg JS, Kearon CJH, eds. Clinical Decisions in Thrombosis and Hemostasis. Hamilton, Ontario, Canada, BC Decker, 1998:117–122.

34. Warkentin TE, Barkin RL. Newer strategies for the treatment of heparin-induced thrombocytopenia. Pharmacotherapy 1999;19:181–195.

35. Monagle P, Chan A, Massicotte P, Chalmers E, Michelson AD. Antithrombotic therapy in children: The Seventh ACCP Conference on Antithrombotic and Thrombolytic Therapy. Chest 2004;126:645S–687S.

36. Crowther MA, Ginsberg JS. Practical aspects of anticoagulant therapy. In: Colman R, Hirsch J, Marder V, et al, eds. Hemostasis and Thrombosis: Basic Principles and Clinical Practice. Philadelphia, Lippincott Williams & Wilkins, 2001:1497–1516.

37. Aventis. Lovenox Prescribing Information. Available at *http://www. aventispharma-us.com/PIs/lovenox_TXT.html;* accessed on July 5, 2004.

38. Rosenbloom D, Ginsberg JS. Arguments against monitoring levels of anti-factor Xa in conjunction with low-molecular-weight heparin therapy. Can J Hosp Pharm 2002;55:15–19.

39. Dolovich L, Ginsberg JS, Douketis J, et al. A meta-analysis comparing low-molecular-weight heparins with unfractionated heparin in the treatment of venous thromboembolism. Arch Intern Med 2000;160: 181–188.

40. Sanofi-Sythelabo. Arixtra Prescribing Information. Available at *http:// www.accessdata.fda.gov/scripts/cder/drugsatfda/index.cfm?fuseaction= Search.Label_ApprovalHistory#apphist;* accessed on July 2, 2004.

41. Weitz JI, Hirsh J. New anticoagulant drugs. Chest 2001;119:95–109S.

42. Keam SJ, Goa KL. Fondaparinux sodium. Drugs 2002;62:1673–1685.

43. Eriksson BI, Lassen MR. Duration of prophylaxis against venous thromboembolism with fondaparinux after hip fracture surgery: A multicenter, randomized, placebo-controlled, double-blind study. Arch Intern Med 2003;163:1337–1342.

44. Buller HR, Davidson BL, Decousus H, et al. Fondaparinux or enoxaparin for the initial treatment of symptomatic deep venous thrombosis: A randomized trial. Ann Intern Med 2004;140:867–873.

45. Buller HR, Davidson BL, Decousus H, et al. Subcutaneous fondaparinux versus intravenous unfractionated heparin in the initial treatment of pulmonary embolism. N Engl J Med 2003;349:1695–1702.

46. Turpie AG, Bauer KA, Eriksson BI, Lassen MR. Fondaparinux vs enoxaparin for the prevention of venous thromboembolism in major orthopedic surgery: A meta-analysis of 4 randomized double-blind studies. Arch Intern Med 2002;162:1833–1840.

47. Ahmad S, Jeske WP, Walenga JM, et al. Synthetic pentasaccharides do not cause platelet activation by antiheparin-platelet factor 4 antibodies. Clin Appl Thromb Hemost 1999;5:259–266.

48. Herbert JM, Herault JP, Bernat A, et al. Biochemical and pharmacological properties of SANORG 34006, a potent and long-acting synthetic pentasaccharide. Blood 1998;91:4197–4205.

49. Weitz JI, Crowther MA. New anticoagulants: Current status and future potential. Am J Cardiovasc Drugs 2003;3:201–209.

50. Matheson AJ, Goa KL. Desirudin: A review of its use in the management of thrombotic disorders. Drugs 2000;60:679–700.

51. Berlex Laboratories. Refludan Prescribing Information, October 2002. Available at *http://www.refludan.com/product/index.htm;* accessed on July 5, 2004.

52. The Medicines Company. Angiomax Prescribing Information. Available at *http://www.angiomax.com/%7Eproducts_content/PN1002–6.pdf;* accessed on July 2, 2004.

53. Nutescu EA, Wittkowsky AK. Direct thrombin inhibitors for anticoagulation. Ann Pharmacother 2004;38:99–109.

54. Gustafsson D, Elg M. The pharmacodynamics and pharmacokinetics of the oral direct thrombin inhibitor ximelagatran and its active metabolite melagatran: A mini-review. Thromb Res 2003;109(suppl 1): S9–15.

55. Smith Kline Glaxo. Argatroban Prescribing Information, November 2003. Available at *http://us.gsk.com/products/assets/us_argatroban.pdf;* accessed on July 2, 2004.

56. Swan SK, St. Peter JV, Lambrecht LJ, Hursting MJ. Comparison of anticoagulant effects and safety of argatroban and heparin in healthy subjects. Pharmacotherapy 2000;20:756–770.

57. Tabrizi AR, Zehnbauer BA, Borecki IB, et al. The frequency and effects of cytochrome P450 (CYP) 2C9 polymorphisms in patients receiving warfarin. J Am Coll Surg 2002;194:267–273.

58. Kovacs MJ, Rodger M, Anderson DR, et al. Comparison of 10 mg and 5 mg warfarin initiation nomograms together with low-molecular-weight heparin for outpatient treatment of acute venous thromboembolism: A randomized, double-blind, controlled trial. Ann Intern Med 2003; 138:714–719.

59. Roberts GW, Helboe T, Nielsen CB, et al. Assessment of an age-adjusted warfarin initiation protocol. Ann Pharmacother 2003;37:799–803.

60. Crowther MA, Ginsberg JB, Kearon C, et al. A randomized trial comparing 5 mg and 10 mg warfarin loading doses. Arch Intern Med 1999; 159:46–48.

61. Pengo V, Biasiolo A, Pegoraro C. A simple scheme to initiate oral anticoagulant treatment in outpatients with nonrheumatic atrial fibrillation. Am J Cardiol 2001;88:1214–1216.

62. Fairweather RB, Ansell J, van den Besselaar AM, et al. College of American Pathologists Conference XXXI on laboratory monitoring of anticoagulant therapy: Laboratory monitoring of oral anticoagulant therapy. Arch Pathol Lab Med 1998;122:768–781.

63. Ridker PM, Goldhaber SZ, Danielson E, et al. Long-term, low-intensity warfarin therapy for the prevention of recurrent venous thromboembolism. N Engl J Med 2003;348:1425–1434.

64. Ansell JE. Empowering patients to monitor and manage oral anticoagulation therapy. JAMA 1999;281:182–183.

65. Gallerani M, Manfredini R, Moratelli S. Non-haemorrhagic adverse reactions of oral anticoagulant therapy. Int J Cardiol 1995;49:1–7.

66. Booth SL, Mayer J. Warfarin use and fracture risk. Nutr Rev 2000;58: 20–22.

67. Patel RJ, Witt DM, Saseen JJ, et al. Randomized, placebo-controlled trial of oral phytonadione for excessive anticoagulation. Pharmacotherapy 2000;20:1159–1166.

68. Crowther MA, Douketis JD, Schnurr T, et al. Oral vitamin K lowers the international normalized ratio more rapidly than subcutaneous vitamin K in the treatment of warfarin-associated coagulopathy: A randomized, controlled trial. Ann Intern Med 2002;137:251–254.

69. Booth SL, Centurelli MA. Vitamin K: A practical guide to the dietary management of patients on warfarin. Nutr Rev 1999;57:288–296.

70. Heck AM, DeWitt BA, Lukes AL. Potential interactions between alternative therapies and warfarin. Am J Health Syst Pharm 2000;57:1221–1227.

71. Dunn AS, Turpie AG. Perioperative management of patients receiving oral anticoagulants: A systematic review. Arch Intern Med 2003;163:901–908.

72. Stratton MA, Anderson FA, Bussey HI, et al. Prevention of venous thromboembolism: adherence to the 1995 American College of Chest Physicians consensus guidelines for surgical patients. Arch Intern Med 2000;160:334–340.

73. Agu O, Hamilton G, Baker D. Graduated compression stockings in the prevention of venous thromboembolism. Br J Surg 1999;86:992–1004.

74. Hooker JA, Lachiewicz PF, Kelley SS. Efficacy of prophylaxis against thromboembolism with intermittent pneumatic compression after primary and revision total hip arthroplasty. J Bone Joint Surg 1999;81:690–696.

75. Siddiqui AU, Buchman TG, Hotchkiss RS. Pulmonary embolism as a consequence of applying sequential compression device on legs in a patient asymptomatic of deep vein thrombosis. Anesthesiology 2000;92:880–882.

76. Velmahos GC, Kern J, Chan LS, et al. Prevention of venous thromboembolism after injury: An evidence-based report: II. Analysis of risk factors and evaluation of the role of vena caval filters. J Trauma 2000;49:140–144.

77. Decousus H, Leizorovicz A, Parent F, et al. A clinical trial of vena caval filters in the prevention of pulmonary embolism in patients with proximal deep-vein thrombosis. N Engl J Med 1998;1998:409–415.

78. Antiplatelet Trialists' Collaboration. Collaborative overview of randomised trials of antiplatelet therapy: III. Reduction in venous thrombosis and pulmonary embolism by antiplatelet prophylaxis among surgical and medical patients. BMJ 1994;308:235–246.

79. Hull RD, Brant RF, Pineo GF, et al. Preoperative vs postoperative initiation of low-molecular-weight heparin prophylaxis against venous thromboembolism in patients undergoing elective hip replacement. Arch Intern Med 1999;159:137–141.

80. Eikelboom JW, Quinlan DJ, Douketis JD. Extended-duration prophylaxis against venous thromboembolism after total hip or knee replacement: A meta-analysis of the randomised trials. Lancet 2001;358:9–15.

81. Heit JA, Elliott CG, Trowbridge AA, et al. Ardeparin sodium for extended out-of-hospital prophylaxis against venous thromboembolism after total hip or knee replacement: A randomized, double-blind, placebo-controlled trial. Ann Intern Med 2000;132:853–861.

82. Prandoni P, Bruchi O, Sabbion P, et al. Prolonged thromboprophylaxis with oral anticoagulants after total hip arthroplasty: A prospective, controlled, randomized study. Arch Intern Med 2002;162:1966–1971.

83. Davidson BL, Sullivan SD, Kahn SR, et al. The economics of venous thromboembolism prophylaxis: A primer for clinicians. Chest 2003;124:393–396S.

84. Corditz GA. Cost-effectiveness of prevention. In: Scurr JH, ed. Prevention of Venous Thromboembolism. London, Med-Orion, 1994:403–420.

85. Etchells E, McLeod RS, Geerts W, et al. Economic analysis of low-dose heparin vs the low-molecular-weight heparin enoxaparin for prevention of venous thromboembolism after colorectal surgery. Arch Intern Med 1999;159:1221–1228.

86. Hawkins DW, Langley PC, Krueger KP. Pharmacoeconomic model of enoxaparin versus heparin for prevention of deep vein thrombosis after total hip replacement. Am J Health Syst Pharm 1997;54:1185–1190.

87. Posnett J, Gordois A. Cost-effectiveness of fondaparinux vs enoxaparin as prophylaxis against venous thromboembolism following orthopaedic surgery. Value Health 2002;5:444.

88. Wade WE, Spruill WJ, Leslie RB. Cost analysis: Fondaparinux versus preoperative and postoperative enoxaparin as venous thromboembolic event prophylaxis in elective hip arthroplasty. Am J Orthop 2003;32:201–205.

89. Turpie AGG, Chin BSP, Lip GYH. Venous thromboembolism: Treatment strategies. BMJ 2002;325:948–950.

90. American Society of Hematology. Use of new direct thrombin inhibitor may be as effective as current standard treatment. Available at http://www.hematology.org/news/press/press_120803_5.cfm; accessed on July 5, 2004.

91. Hirsh J, Bates SM. Clinical trials that have influenced the treatment of venous thromboembolism: A historical perspective. Ann Intern Med 2001;134:409–417.

92. Lee AY, Levine MN. Venous thrombosis and cancer: Risks and outcomes. Circulation 2003;107:I-17–I-21.

93. Merli GJ, Spiro TE, Olson C, et al. Subcutaneous enoxaparin once or twice daily compared with intravenous unfractionated heparin for treatment of venous thromboembolic disease. Ann Intern Med 2001;134:191–202.

94. Tillman DJ, Charland SL, Witt DM. Effectiveness and economic impact associated with a program for outpatient management of acute deep vein thrombosis in a group model health maintenance organization. Arch Intern Med 2000;160:2926–2932.

95. Wood KE. Major pulmonary embolism: Review of a pathophysiologic approach to the golden hour of hemodynamically significant pulmonary embolism. Chest 2002;121:877–905.

96. Agnelli G, Prandoni P, Becattini C, et al. Extended oral anticoagulant therapy after a first episode of pulmonary embolism. Ann Intern Med 2003;139:19–25.

97. Agnelli G, Prandoni P, Gabriella M, et al. Three months versus one year of oral anticoagulant therapy for idiopathic deep venous thrombosis. N Engl J Med 2001;345:165–169.

98. Kearon C, Ginsberg JS, Kovacs MJ, et al. Comparison of low-intensity warfarin therapy with conventional-intensity warfarin therapy for long-term prevention of recurrent venous thromboembolism. N Engl J Med 2003;349:631–639.

99. Schulman S, Wahlander K, Lundstrom T, et al. Secondary prevention of venous thromboembolism with the oral direct thrombin inhibitor ximelagatran. N Engl J Med 2003;349:1713–1721.

100. Dalen JE. Pulmonary embolism: What have we learned since Virchow? Treatment and prevention. Chest 2002;122:1801–1817.

101. Horne MK 3d, Chang R. Thrombolytic therapy for deep venous thrombosis? JAMA 1999;282:2164–2166.

102. Arcasoy SM, Kreit JW. Thrombolytic therapy of pulmonary embolism: A comprehensive review of current evidence. Chest 1999;115:1695–1707.

103. White RH, Zhou H, Kim J, Romano PS. A population-based study of the effectiveness of inferior vena cava filter use among patients with venous thrombosis. Arch Intern Med 2000;160:2033–2041.

104. Bick RL. Proficient and cost-effective approaches for the prevention and treatment of venous thrombosis and thromboembolism. Drugs 2000;60:575–595.

105. Sanson B, Lensing AWA, Prins MH, et al. The use of low-molecular-weight heparins in pregnancy: A systematic review. Thromb Haemost 1999;81:668–672.

106. Buck ML. Anticoagulation with warfarin in infants and children. Ann Pharmacother 1996;30:1316–1322.

107. Levine MN, Lee AY, Kakkar AK. From Trousseau to targeted therapy: New insights and innovation in thrombosis and caner. J Thromb Haemost 2003;1:1456–1463.

108. Meyer G, Marjanovic Z, Valcke J, Lorcerie B. Comparison of low-molecular-weight heparin and warfarin for the secondary prevention of venous thromboembolism in patients with cancer. Arch Intern Med 2001;162:1729–1735.

109. Lee AY, Levine MN, Baker RI, et al. Low-molecular-weight heparin versus a coumarin for the prevention of recurrent venous thromboembolism in patients with cancer. N Engl J Med 2003;349:146–153.

110. Gould MK, Dembitzer AD, Sanders GD, Garber AM. Low-molecular-weight heparins compared with unfractionated heparin for treatment of

acute deep venous thrombosis: A cost-effectiveness analysis. Ann Intern Med 1999;130:789–799.

111. Warkentin TE. Heparin-induced thrombocytopenia: A clinicopathologic syndrome. Thromb Haemost 1999;82:439–447.

112. Warkentin TE, Kelton JG. Temporal aspects of heparin-induced thrombocytopenia. N Engl J Med 2001;344:1286–1292.

113. Warkentin TE, Levine MN, Hirsh J, et al. Heparin-induced thrombocytopenia in patients treated with low-molecular-weight heparin or unfractionated heparin. N Engl J Med 1995;332:1330–1335.

114. Januzzi JL Jr, Jang IK. Heparin induced thrombocytopenia: Diagnosis and contemporary antithrombin management. J Thromb Thrombol 1999;7:259–264.

115. Warkentin TE. Platelet count monitoring and laboratory testing for heparin-induced thrombocytopenia. Arch Pathol Lab Med 2002;126:1415–1423.

116. Warkentin TE, Elavathil LJ, Hayward CP, et al. The pathogenesis of venous limb gangrene associated with heparin-induced thrombocytopenia. Ann Intern Med 1997;127:804–812.

117. Wallis DE, Quintos R, Wehrmacher W, Messmore H. Safety of warfarin anticoagulation in patients with heparin-induced thrombocytopenia. Chest 1999;116:1333–1338.

118. Messmore H, Jeske W, Wehrmacher W, Walenga J. Benefit-risk assessment of treatments for heparin-induced thrombocytopenia. Drug Saf 2003;26:625–641.

119. Pharmacia & UpJohn Company. Fragmin Prescribing Information. Available at *http://www.fragmin.com/documents/fragmin.pdf;* accessed on July 5, 2004.

120. Pharmion. Innohep Prescribing Information. Available at *http://www.innohepusa.com/corporateweb/innohepus/home.nsf/AttachmentsByTitle/FullPrescribingInformationforInnohep.pdf/$FILE/FullPrescribingInformationforInnohep.pdf;* accessed on July 5, 2004.

121. Ginsberg JS, Bates SM. Management of venous thromboembolism during pregnancy. J Thromb Haemost 2003;1:1435–1442.

20

STROKE

Susan C. Fagan and David C. Hess

Learning Objectives and other resources can be found at *www.pharmacotherapyonline.com*.

KEY CONCEPTS

◀1 Stroke is one of the leading killers of individuals worldwide.

◀2 Stroke can be either ischemic (88%) or hemorrhagic (12%).

◀3 Carotid endarterectomy should be performed in ischemic stroke patients with 70% to 99% stenosis of the ipsilateral carotid artery, provided that it is done in an experienced center.

◀4 Early reperfusion (<3 hours from onset) with tissue plasminogen activator (tPA) has been shown to reduce the ultimate disability due to ischemic stroke.

◀5 Antiplatelet therapy is the cornerstone of secondary prevention of ischemic stroke.

◀6 Warfarin is the drug of choice for secondary prevention of cardioembolic stroke.

◀7 Blood pressure lowering is effective in both the primary and secondary prevention of both ischemic and hemorrhagic stroke regardless of blood pressure.

◀8 Blood pressure lowering in the acute stroke period (first 7 days) may result in decreased cerebral blood flow and worsened symptoms.

◀9 Statin therapy is recommended for all ischemic stroke patients, regardless of baseline cholesterol, to reduce stroke recurrence.

◀1 Stroke is a leading killer worldwide and the third leading cause of death in the United States, behind cardiovascular disease and all cancers. Despite improvements in the stroke mortality rates in the second half of the twentieth century, stroke occurs in more than 700,000 individuals per year and results in 150,000 deaths.[1] Recent advances in our knowledge of the pathophysiology of stroke have led to evidence-based recommendations on the management of the stroke patient.

EPIDEMIOLOGY

There are currently 4.6 million stroke survivors in the United States, and stroke is the leading cause of adult disability.[1] Approximately 20% of patients in nursing homes have had a stroke,[2] and stroke is also a leading diagnosis in inpatient rehabilitation. Owing in part to the need for these expensive posthospitalization care environments, stroke is also one of the most expensive diseases in the United States, with annual costs greater than $50 billion.[1] Current projections are that death due to stroke will increase exponentially in the next 30 years owing to aging of the population and our inability to control risk factors.[3]

Stroke risk is increased above that of the general population in the elderly male individuals and in African-Americans.[1] In addition, geographic disparity in stroke incidence exists, such that several areas of the southeastern United States have stroke mortality rates more than twice that of the national average.[4] This phenomenon, originally describing areas of the coastal Carolinas and Georgia, has been named the "Stroke Belt."

ETIOLOGY AND CLASSIFICATION

◀2 Stroke can be either ischemic or hemorrhagic (88% and 12%, respectively, of all strokes in the 2003 American Heart Association report).[1] A classification of stroke by mechanism is given in Figure 20–1. Hemorrhagic strokes include subarachnoid hemorrhage, intracerebral hemorrhage, and subdural hematomas. Subarachnoid hemorrhage occurs when blood enters the subarachnoid space (where cerebrospinal fluid is housed) owing to either trauma, rupture of an intracranial aneurysm, or rupture of an arteriovenous malformation (AVM). By contrast, intracerebral hemorrhage occurs when a blood vessel ruptures within the brain parenchyma itself, resulting in the formation of a hematoma. These types of hemorrhages very often are associated with uncontrolled high blood pressure and sometimes antithrombotic or thrombolytic therapy. Subdural hematomas refer to collections of blood below the dura (covering of the brain), and they are caused most often by trauma. Hemorrhagic stroke, although less common, is significantly more lethal than ischemic stroke, with 30-day case-fatality rates that are two to six times higher.[5]

Ischemic strokes are due either to local thrombus formation or to embolic phenomenon, resulting in occlusion of a cerebral artery. Atherosclerosis, particularly of the cerebral vasculature, is a causative factor in most cases of ischemic stroke, although 30% are cryptogenic. Emboli can arise either from intra- or extracranial arteries (including the aortic arch) or, as is the case in 20% of all ischemic strokes, the heart. Cardiogenic embolism is presumed to have occurred if the patient has concomitant atrial fibrillation, valvular heart disease, or any other condition of the heart that may lead to clot formation.[6] Distinguishing between cardiogenic embolism and other causes of

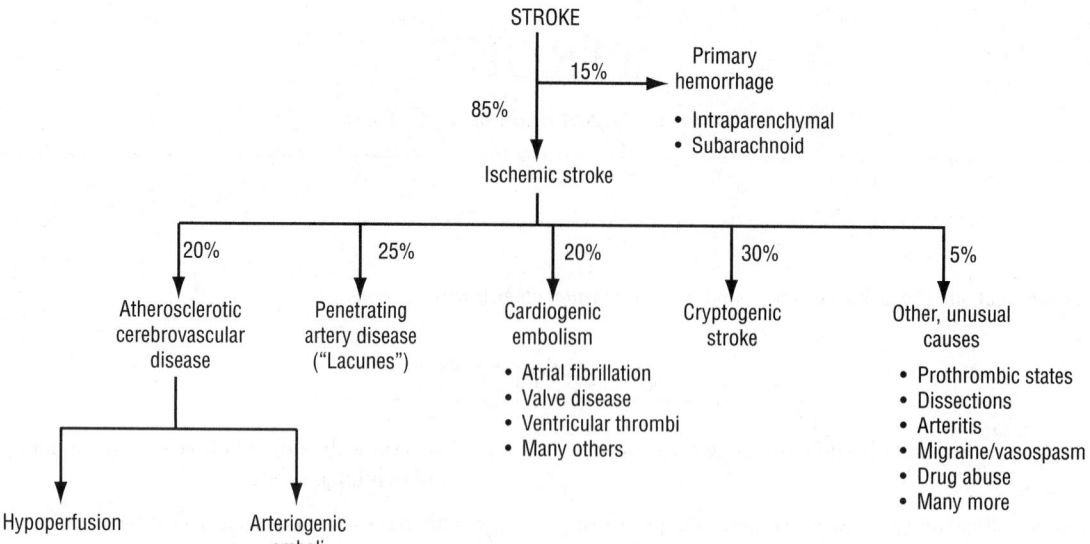

FIGURE 20–1. A classification of stroke by mechanism with estimates of the frequency of various categories of abnormalities. Approximately 30% of ischemic strokes are cryptogenic.

ischemic stroke is important in determining long-term pharmacotherapy in a given patient.

RISK FACTORS

Risk factors for stroke can be subdivided into nonmodifiable and modifiable. The main risk factors of stroke are listed in Table 20–1. An individual's risk of having a stroke increases substantially as he or she ages, with a doubling of risk for each decade after age 55. Men are at a higher risk of stroke than women when matched for age, but women who suffer from a stroke are more likely to die from

it.[1] Ethnicity is another nonmodifiable risk factor for stroke, with African-Americans, Asian-Pacific Islanders, and Hispanics experiencing higher death rates than their Caucasian counterparts.[1,4]

The most important modifiable risk factor for stroke is hypertension.[1] The treatment of hypertension, beginning in the mid-twentieth century, is thought to be primarily responsible for the drastic reduction in stroke death rates between 1950 and 1980 in the United States.[4] A second very important risk factor for stroke is cardiac disease. Patients with coronary artery disease, congestive heart failure, left ventricular hypertrophy, and especially atrial fibrillation are at increased risk of stroke.[7–9] In fact, the presence of atrial fibrillation is one of the most potent risk factors for ischemic stroke, with stroke

TABLE 20–1. Risk Factors in Ischemic Stroke

Single Risk Factors	Alcohol
Nonmodifiable risk factors or risk markers	Illicit drug use—cocaine, heroin, amphetamines, LSD, PCP and
Age	others linked with stroke
Gender	Lifestyle factors—associated with stroke risk
Race	Obesity
Ethnicity	Physical inactivity
Heredity	Diet
Potentially modifiable	Acute triggers—emotional stress
Hypertension—single most important risk factor for ischemic	Oral contraceptives—positive only with estrogen content >50 μg
stroke	Migraine—risk not clear
Cardiac disease	Hemostatic and inflammatory factors—fibrinogen linked to
Atrial fibrillation—most important and treatable cardiac	increased risk; elevated hematocrit and sickle cell disease are
cause of stroke	positive risk factors
Mitral stenosis	Homocysteine—still under study, but hyperhomocysteinemia may
Mitral annular calcification	be related to increased stroke risk
Left atrial enlargement	Asymptomatic carotid stenosis
Structural abnormalities such as atrial-septal aneurysm	Subclinical disease—aortic arch atheromas
Myocardial disease	**Multiple Risk Factors—Stroke Is Increased by the Presence of Multiple**
1% to 6% of myocardial infarction patients develop a	**Risk Factors**
stroke	Framingham profile
Transient ischemic attacks—major independent risk factor	Elevated systolic blood pressure
Diabetes—independent risk factor	Elevated serum cholesterol
Hypercholesterolemia—positive risk factor for extracranial	Glucose intolerance
atherosclerosis but link still under study for ischemic stroke	Cigarette smoking
Cigarette smoking	Left ventricular hypertrophy

rates from 5% to 20% per year depending on the patient's comorbid conditions.[10,11] Other known risk factors for atherosclerosis are also known to place patients at risk of stroke. Diabetes mellitus, hypercholesterolemia, and cigarette smoking are known atherogenic states that lead to cerebrovascular disease and ischemic stroke.[7–9,12]

PATHOPHYSIOLOGY

ISCHEMIC STROKE

In carotid atherosclerosis, progressive accumulation of lipids and inflammatory cells in the intima of the affected arteries, combined with hypertrophy of arterial smooth muscle cells, results in plaque formation. Eventually, sheer stress may result in plaque rupture, collagen exposure, platelet aggregation, and clot formation. The clot may remain in the vessel, causing local occlusion, or travel distally as an embolism, eventually lodging downstream in a cerebral vessel. In the case of cardiogenic embolism, stasis of blood in the atria or ventricles of the heart leads to the formation of local clots that can become dislodged and travel directly through the aorta to the cerebral circulation. The final result of both thrombus formation and embolism is an arterial occlusion, decreasing cerebral blood flow and causing ischemia distal to the occlusion.[13]

Normal cerebral blood flow averages 50 mL/100 g per minute, and this is maintained over a wide range of blood pressures (mean arterial pressures of 50 to 150 mm Hg) by a process called *cerebral autoregulation.* Cerebral blood vessels dilate and constrict in response to changes in blood pressure, but this process can be impaired by atherosclerosis and acute injury, such as stroke. When local cerebral blood flow decreases below 20 mL/100 g per minute, ischemia ensues, and when further reductions below 12 mL/100 g per minute persist, irreversible damage to the brain occurs, and this is called *infarction.* Tissue that is ischemic but maintains membrane integrity is referred to as the ischemic *penumbra* because it usually surrounds the infarct core. This penumbra is potentially salvageable through therapeutic intervention.

Reduction in the provision of nutrients to the ischemic cell eventually leads to depletion of the high-energy phosphates (e.g., ATP) necessary for the maintenance of membrane integrity. Subsequently, extracellular potassium accumulates at the same time that sodium and water are sequestered intracellularly, leading to cell swelling and eventual lysis. Electrolyte imbalance also leads to depolarization of the cell and influx of calcium into the cell. The increase in intracellular calcium results in the activation of lipases, proteases, and endonucleases and the release of free fatty acids from membrane phospholipids. The depolarization of the neuron leads to the release of excitatory amino acids, such as glutamate and aspartate, that perpetuate the neuronal damage when released in excess. The accumulation of free fatty acids, including arachidonic acid, results in the formation of prostaglandins, leukotrienes, and free radicals. In ischemia, the magnitude of free-radical production overwhelms normal scavenging systems, leaving these reactive molecules to attack cell membranes and contribute to the mounting intracellular acidosis. All these events occur within 2 to 3 hours of the onset of ischemia and contribute to the ultimate cell death.[13]

Later targets for intervention in the pathophysiologic process involved after cerebral ischemia include the influx of activated inflammatory cells, starting from 2 hours after the onset of ischemia and lasting for several days. Also, the initiation of apoptosis, or programmed cell death, is thought to occur many hours after the acute insult and may interfere with recovery and repair of brain tissue.[14]

HEMORRHAGIC STROKE

The pathophysiology of hemorrhagic stroke is not as well studied as that of ischemic stroke. However, it is known that the presence of blood in the brain parenchyma causes damage to the surrounding tissue through the mechanical effect it produces (mass effect) and the neurotoxicity of the blood components and their degradation products.[5] Compression of the tissue surrounding the hematoma also may lead to secondary ischemia in some cases. Approximately 30% of intracerebral hemorrhages continue to enlarge over the first 24 hours, and clot volume is the most important predictor of outcome, regardless of location.[15] Much of the early mortality of hemorrhagic stroke (up to 50% at 30 days) is due to the abrupt increase in intracranial pressure that can lead to herniation and death.[1]

CLINICAL PRESENTATION (INCLUDING DIAGNOSTIC CONSIDERATIONS)

Stroke is a term used to describe an abrupt-onset focal neurologic deficit that lasts at least 24 hours and is of presumed vascular origin. A *transient ischemic attack* (TIA) is the same but lasts less than 24 hours and usually less than 30 minutes. The abrupt onset and the duration of the symptoms are determined through the history. The use of sensitive imaging techniques (magnetic resonance imaging) has revealed that symptoms lasting more than 1 hour and less than 24 hours, although technically TIAs, are associated with infarction, making TIA and minor stroke clinically indistinguishable. The location of the central nervous system injury and its reference to a specific arterial distribution in the brain are determined through the neurologic examination and confirmed by imaging studies such as computed tomographic (CT) scanning and magnetic resonance imaging (MRI). The main arterial supply to the brain is illustrated in Figure 20–2. Further diagnostic tests are performed to identify the cause of the patient's stroke and to design appropriate therapeutic strategies to prevent further events.[16]

CLINICAL PRESENTATION OF STROKE

GENERAL

- The patient may not be able to reliably report the history owing to cognitive or language deficits. A reliable history may have to come from a family member or another witness.

SYMPTOMS

- The patient may complain of weakness on one side of the body, inability to speak, loss of vision, vertigo, or falling. Ischemic stroke is not usually painful, but patients may complain of headache, and with hemorrhagic stroke, it can be very severe.

SIGNS

- Patients usually have multiple signs of neurologic dysfunction, and the specific deficits are determined by the area of the brain involved.
- Hemi- or monoparesis occurs commonly, as does a hemisensory deficit.
- Patients with vertigo and double vision are likely to have posterior circulation involvement.

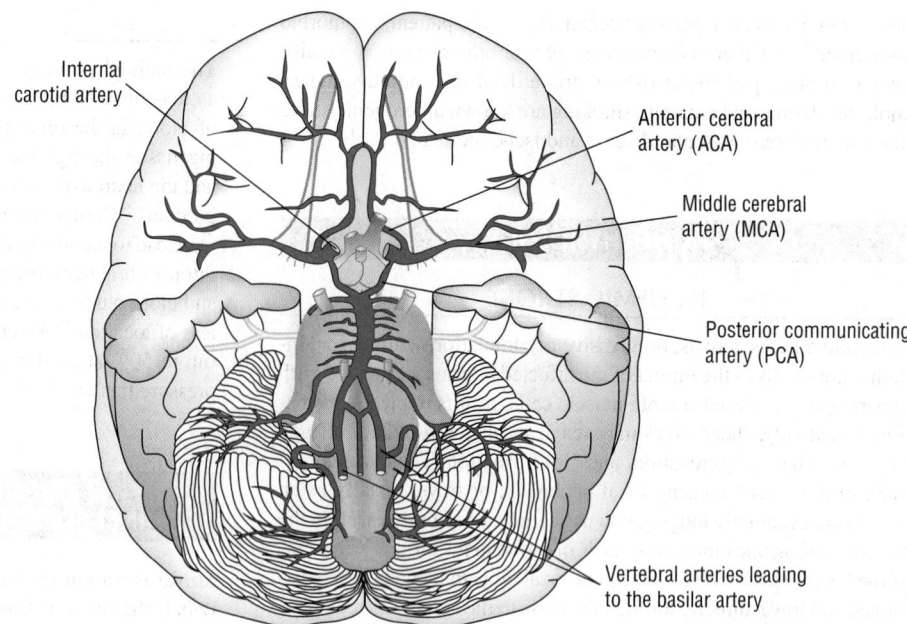

FIGURE 20–2. Main arterial blood supply to the brain.

- Aphasia is seen commonly in patients with anterior circulation strokes.
- Patients also may suffer from dysarthria, visual field defects, and altered levels of consciousness.

LABORATORY TESTS

- Tests for hypercoagulable states (protein C deficiency, antiphospholipid antibody) should be done only when the cause of the stroke cannot be determined based on the presence of well-known risk factors for stroke. Protein C, protein S, and antithrombin III are best measured in the "steady state," not in the acute stage. Antiphospholipid antibodies as measured by anticardiolipin antibodies, β_2-glycoprotein I, and lupus anticoagulant screen are of higher yield than protein C, protein S, and antithrombin III but should be reserved for patients who are young (<50 years), have had multiple venous/arterial thrombotic events, or have livedo reticularis (a skin rash).

OTHER DIAGNOSTIC TESTS

- CT scan of the head will reveal an area of hyperintensity (white) in the area of hemorrhage and will be normal or hypointense (dark) in the area of infarction. The CT scan may take 24 hours (and rarely longer) to reveal the area of infarction.
- MRI of the head will reveal areas of ischemia with higher resolution and earlier than the CT scan. Diffusion-weighted imaging (DWI) will reveal an evolving infarct within minutes.
- Carotid Doppler (CD) studies will determine whether the patient has a high degree of stenosis in the carotid arteries supplying blood to the brain (extracranial disease).
- The electrocardiogram (ECG) will determine whether the patient has atrial fibrillation, a potent etiologic factor for stroke.
- A transthoracic echocardiogram (TTE) will determine whether valve abnormalities or wall motion abnormalities are sources of emboli to the brain. A "bubble test" can be done to look for an intraatrial shunt indicating an atrial septal defect or a patent foramen ovale.
- A transesophageal echocardiogram (TEE) is a more sensitive test for thrombus in the left atrium. It is effective at examining the aortic arch for atheroma, a potential source of emboli.
- Transcranial Doppler (TCD) will determine whether the patient is likely to have intracranial arterial sclerosis (e.g., middle cerebral artery stenosis).

▶ TREATMENT: Stroke

■ DESIRED OUTCOME

The goals of treatment of acute stroke are (1) to reduce the ongoing neurologic injury and decrease mortality and long-term disability, (2) prevent complications secondary to immobility and neurologic dysfunction, and (3) prevent stroke recurrence. Primary prevention of stroke is reviewed elsewhere.[9]

■ GENERAL APPROACH TO TREATMENT

The initial approach to the patient with a presumed acute stroke is to ensure that the patient is supported from a respiratory and cardiac standpoint and to quickly determine whether the lesion is ischemic or hemorrhagic based on a CT scan. Ischemic stroke patients presenting within hours of the onset of their symptoms should be evaluated for

TABLE 20–2. Blood Pressure Treatment Guidelines in Acute Ischemic Stroke Patients[17]

Treatment	Received tPA	Did Not Receive tPA
None	<180/105	<220/120
Labetolol IV[a] or Nicordipine IV[b]	180–230/105–120	>220/121–140
Nitroprusside[c]	Diastolic >140	Diastolic >140

[a]Labetolol IV = 10–20 mg, doubled every 10–20 minutes, to a maximum of 300 mg. Also can use an infusion of 2–8 mg/min.
[b]Nicordipine IV = infusion starting at 5 mg/hr up to 15 mg/hr.
[c]Nitroprusside IV = infusion starting at 0.5 mcg/kg/min, with continuous arterial BP monitoring.

reperfusion therapy. Patients with elevated blood pressure should remain untreated unless their blood pressure exceeds 220/120 mm Hg or they have evidence of aortic dissection, acute myocardial infarction (AMI), pulmonary edema, or hypertensive encephalopathy. If blood pressure is treated, short-acting parenteral agents, such as labetalol, nicordipine, and nitroprusside, are favored. Current recommendations regarding management of arterial hypertension in stroke patients is given in Table 20–2.[17]

In patients with hemorrhagic stroke, an assessment of whether the patient is a candidate for surgical intervention via an endovascular or craniotomy approach should be made. Once the patient is out of the hyperacute phase, attention is placed on preventing worsening, minimizing complications, and instituting appropriate secondary prevention strategies. The acute phase of the stroke includes the first week after the event.[17]

NONPHARMACOLOGIC THERAPY

ISCHEMIC STROKE

Surgical interventions in the acute ischemic stroke patient are limited. In certain cases of ischemic cerebral edema owing to a large infarction, craniectomy to release some of the rising pressure has been tried. In cases of significant swelling associated with a cerebellar infarction, surgical decompression can be lifesaving. Beyond surgical intervention, however, the use of an organized, multidisciplinary approach to stroke care that includes early rehabilitation has been shown to be very effective in reducing the ultimate disability owing to ischemic stroke. In fact, the use of "stroke units" has been associated with outcomes similar to those achieved with early thrombolysis when compared with usual care.[17]

In secondary prevention, carotid endarterectomy of an ulcerated and/or stenotic carotid artery is a very effective way to reduce stroke incidence and recurrence in appropriate patients and in centers where the operative morbidity and mortality are low. In fact, in ischemic stroke patients with 70% to 99% stenosis of an ipsilateral internal carotid artery, recurrent stroke risk can be reduced by up to 48% compared with medical therapy alone when combined with aspirin 325 mg daily.[18] In patients in whom the risk of endarterectomy is thought to be excessive, carotid stenting may be effective in reducing recurrent stroke risk but is less invasive.[19] Carotid stenting is still considered investigational, however, and issues remain regarding the optimal methods and patients for this procedure.

HEMORRHAGIC STROKE

In patients with subarachnoid hemorrhage owing to a ruptured intracranial aneurysm or an AVM, surgical intervention to either clip or ablate the offending vascular abnormality substantially reduces mortality owing to rebleeding.[20] In the case of primary intracerebral hemorrhage, however, the benefits of surgery are less well documented. Although many patients undergo surgical treatment of intracerebral hematomas, the procedures have not been studied adequately in clinical trials.[5,15] Insertion of an extraventricular drain (EVD) and subsequent monitoring of intracranial pressure are done commonly and are the least invasive of the procedures done in these patients. Surgical decompression of a hematoma is more controversial, except when it is a last option in a life-threatening situation. Guidelines have been developed for the use of surgical intervention in the treatment of intracerebral hemorrhage, but they are limited in their impact by the lack of clinical trial data to support them.[15]

PHARMACOLOGIC THERAPY

ISCHEMIC STROKE

Drug Treatments of First Choice: Published Guidelines

The Stroke Council of the American Stroke Association has created and published guidelines that address the management of acute ischemic stroke.[17] In general, the only two pharmacologic agents recommended with a grade A recommendation are intravenous tissue plasminogen activator (tPA) within 3 hours of onset and aspirin within 48 hours of onset.

Early reperfusion (<3 hours from onset) with intravenous tPA has been shown to reduce the ultimate disability due to ischemic stroke.[21] Caution must be exercised when using this therapy, and adherence to a strict protocol is essential to achieving positive outcomes.[17] The essentials of the treatment protocol can be summarized as (1) stroke team activation, (2) onset of symptoms within 3 hours, (3) CT scan to rule out hemorrhage, (4) meet inclusion and exclusion criteria (Table 20–3), (5) administer tPA 0.9 mg/kg over 1 hour, with 10% given as initial bolus over 1 minute, (6) avoid antithrombotic (anticoagulant or antiplatelet) therapy for 24 hours, and (7) monitor the patient closely for response and hemorrhage.[17]

Early aspirin therapy also has been shown to reduce long-term death and disability[22,23] but should never be given within 24 hours of the administration of tPA because it can increase the risk of bleeding in such patients.[17]

The premier guidelines for the use of antithrombotic therapy in the secondary prevention of ischemic stroke are the American College of Chest Physicians (ACCP) guidelines, which are updated every 3 years.[6] It is clear that antiplatelet therapy is the cornerstone of secondary prevention of ischemic stroke and should be used in noncardioembolic strokes. All three currently used agents, aspirin, clopidogrel, and extended-release dipyridamole plus aspirin (ERDP + ASA), are considered first-line antiplatelet agents by the ACCP. In patients with atrial fibrillation and a presumed cardiac source of embolism, warfarin is the antithrombotic agent of first choice. Current recommendations regarding the acute treatment and secondary prevention of stroke are given in Table 20–4.

TABLE 20–3. Inclusion and Exclusion Criteria for Alteplase Use in Acute Ischemic Stroke

Inclusion Criteria (all YES boxes must be checked before treatment) YES

☐ Age 18 years or older

☐ Clinical diagnosis of ischemic stroke causing a measurable neurologic deficit

☐ Time of symptom onset well established to be less than 180 minutes before treatment would begin

Exclusion Criteria (all NO boxes must be checked before treatment) NO

☐ Evidence of intracranial hemorrhage on noncontrast head CT

☐ Only minor or rapidly improving stroke symptoms

☐ High clinical suspicion of subarachnoid hemorrhage even with normal CT

☐ Active internal bleeding (e.g., GI/GU bleeding within 21 days)

☐ Known bleeding diathesis, including but not limited to platelet count <100,000/mm³

☐ Patient has received heparin within 48 hours and had an elevated APTT

☐ Recent use of anticoagulant (e.g., warfarin) and elevated PT (>15 sec)/INR

☐ Intracranial surgery, serious head trauma, or previous stroke within 3 months

☐ Major surgery or serious trauma within 14 days

☐ Recent arterial puncture at noncompressible site

☐ Lumbar puncture within 7 days

☐ History of intracranial hemorrhage, arteriovenous malformation, or aneurysm

☐ Witnessed seizure at stroke onset

☐ Recent acute myocardial infarction

☐ SBP >185 mm Hg or DBP >110 mm Hg at time of treatment

GENERAL INFORMATION REGARDING SAFETY AND EFFICACY (INCLUDING PIVOTAL CLINICAL TRIALS)

tPA

The effectiveness of intravenous (IV) tPA in the treatment of ischemic stroke was demonstrated in the National Institutes of Neurologic Disorders and Stroke (NINDS) rt-PA Stroke Trial, published in 1995.[21]

In 624 patients treated in equal numbers with either tPA 0.9 mg/kg IV or placebo within 3 hours of the onset of their neurologic symptoms, 39% of the treated patients achieved an "excellent outcome" at 3 months compared with 26% of the placebo patients. An "excellent outcome" was defined as minimal or no disability by several different neurologic scales. This beneficial effect was reported despite a 10-fold increase in the risk of symptomatic intracerebral hemorrhage in the tPA-treated patients (0.6% versus 6.4%). Overall mortality was not different between the two groups (17% with tPA and 21% with placebo). Patients with very severe symptoms at baseline (NIH Stroke Scale [NIHSS] > 20) and early ischemic changes on CT scan were shown to be at highest risk for the development of symptomatic intracranial hemorrhage. Even in patients at highest risk for bleeding, however, those receiving tPA had better outcomes at 90 days than those who received placebo.[21] The publication of the NINDS trial results significantly changed the way in which acute stroke is managed in the community, promoting the development of acute stroke teams and emphasis on the early diagnosis and treatment of acute stroke. Currently, only 2% to 3% of ischemic stroke patients in the United States receive tPA, primarily owing to failure of patients to present in time to facilities equipped to administer the therapy safely.[24,25] Hemorrhage rates associated with tPA use in the community have been reported to be similar to those reported in the NINDS trial (5%),[24] but significantly higher rates (up to 15%) have been reported when a strict protocol is not followed.[25]

Aspirin

❺ The use of early aspirin to reduce long-term death and disability owing to ischemic stroke is supported by two large, randomized clinical trials. In the International Stroke Trial (IST),[23] aspirin 300 mg/day significantly reduced stroke recurrence within the first 2 weeks without effect on early mortality, resulting in a significant decrease in death and dependency at 6 months. In the Chinese Acute Stroke Trial (CAST),[22] aspirin 160 mg/day reduced the risk of recurrence and death in the first 28 days, but long-term death and disability were not different than with placebo. In both trials, a small but significant increase in hemorrhagic transformation of the infarction was demonstrated. Overall, the beneficial effects of early aspirin have been embraced and adopted into clinical guidelines.

TABLE 20–4. Recommendations for Pharmacotherapy of Ischemic Stroke

	Primary Agents	Alternatives
Acute Treatment	tPA 0.9 mg/kg IV[6,17] (maximum 90 kg) over 1 hour in selected patients within 3 hours of onset. ASA 160–325 mg daily[6,17] started within 48 hours of onset	tPA (various doses) intraarterially up to 6 hours after onset in selected patients
Secondary Prevention Noncardioembolic	Aspirin 50–325 mg daily[6] Clopidogrel 75 mg daily[6] Asprin 25 mg + extended-release dipyridamole 200 mg twice daily[6]	Ticlopidine 250 mg twice daily[6]
Cardioembolic (esp. atrial fibrillation)	Warfarin (INR = 2.5)[6]	
All	ACE inhibitor + diuretic or ARB[45] blood pressure lowering[33,34] Statin[39]	

Antiplatelet Agents

All patients who have had an acute ischemic stroke or TIA should receive long-term antithrombotic therapy for secondary prevention.[6] In patients with noncardioembolic stroke, this will be some form of antiplatelet therapy. In a recent meta-analysis, the overall benefit of antiplatelet therapy in patients with atherothrombotic disorders was estimated to be 22%.[26] Aspirin is the best-studied of the available agents and, until recently, was considered the sole first-line agent. However, published literature has supported the use of clopidogrel and the aspirin plus extended-release dipyridamole combination product (ERDP + ASA) as additional first-line agents in secondary stroke prevention.

The efficacy of clopidogrel as an antiplatelet agent in atherothrombotic disorders was demonstrated in the CAPRIE trial.[27] In this study of more than 19,000 patients with a history of either myocardial infarction (MI), stroke, or peripheral arterial disease (PAD), clopidogrel 75 mg/day was compared with aspirin 325 mg/day for its ability to decrease MI, stroke, or cardiovascular death. In the final analysis, clopidogrel was slightly (8% relative risk reduction [RRR]) more effective than aspirin ($p = .043$) and had a similar incidence of adverse effects. It is not associated with the blood dyscrasias (neutropenia) common with its congener, ticlopidine, and is used widely in patients with atherosclerosis.

In the European Stroke Prevention Study 2 (ESPS-2), aspirin 25 mg and extended-release dipyridamole (ERDP) 200 mg twice daily were compared alone and in combination with placebo for their ability to reduce recurrent stroke over a 2-year period.[28] In a total of more than 6600 patients, all three treatment groups were shown to be superior to placebo—aspirin alone, 18% RRR; ERDP alone, 16% RRR; and the combination, 37% RRR. Importantly, this study was the first to show a significant benefit of combination antiplatelet therapy in stroke prevention, with the combination demonstrating a significant advantage over the aspirin-alone group (23% RRR; $p = .006$) and the ERDP-alone group (24% RRR; $p = .002$). Headache resulting in discontinuation occurred in about 15% of the ERDP groups (four times more common than in the placebo group), and the aspirin-treated patients, even at the low dose of 50 mg/day, experienced significantly more bleeding than the other groups. The combination of aspirin 25 mg and ERDP 200 mg twice daily is a highly effective treatment to prevent recurrence in patients with stroke or TIA. No data exist on the ability of this combination to reduce MI and/or cardiovascular death in patients with other indications for antiplatelet therapy.

Warfarin

Warfarin is the most effective treatment for the prevention of stroke in patients with atrial fibrillation.[10,11,29,30] In patients with atrial fibrillation and a recent history of stroke or TIA, the risk of recurrence places these patients in one of the highest risk categories known. In the European Atrial Fibrillation Trial (EAFT), 669 patients with nonvalvular atrial fibrillation (NVAF) and a prior stroke or TIA were randomized to either warfarin (INR = 2.5–4), aspirin 300 mg/day, or placebo. Patients in the placebo group experienced stroke, MI, or vascular death at a rate of 17% per year compared with 8% per year in the warfarin group and 15% per year in the aspirin group. This represents a 53% reduction in risk with anticoagulation.[10] Subsequent studies in the primary prevention of stroke in patients with NVAF have demonstrated that targeting an international normalization ratio (INR) of 2.5 prevents stroke with the lowest bleeding risk (SPAF III); therefore,

a target INR of 2.5 is recommended in the secondary prevention of stroke.[11,29,30]

Use of warfarin in the secondary prevention of noncardioembolic stroke was addressed in the Warfarin Aspirin Recurrent Stroke Study.[31] In 2206 patients with recent stroke, warfarin (INR = 1.4–2.8) was not superior to aspirin 325 mg/day in the prevention of recurrent events. This led many clinicians to abandon the practice of using warfarin as an alternative agent in patients who suffered recurrent events while on antiplatelet therapy in favor of combination or alternate antiplatelet therapy.

Blood Pressure Lowering

Elevated blood pressure is very common in ischemic stroke patients, and treatment of hypertension in these patients is associated with a decreased risk of stroke recurrence.[32] In the PROGRESS study, a multinational stroke population (40% Asian) was randomized to receive either blood pressure lowering with the angiotensin-converting enzyme (ACE) inhibitor perindopril (with or without the thiazide diuretic indapamide) or placebo.[33] Treated patients achieved an overall 9/4 mm Hg blood pressure reduction, and this was associated with a 28% reduction in stroke recurrence. In the patients who received the combination treatment (clinician's discretion), the blood pressure lowering achieved was 12/5 mm Hg, and this was associated with an even larger reduction in stroke recurrence (43%). Similar results were achieved in patients with and without hypertension. Based on the results of this study and other evidence of the tolerability and vascular protective properties of the ACE inhibitors, the Joint National Committee (JNC7) recommends an ACE inhibitor and a diuretic for the reduction of blood pressure in patients with stroke or TIA.[34] Blood pressure lowering in the acute stroke period (first 7 days) may result in decreased cerebral blood flow and worsened symptoms; therefore, recommendations are limited to patients out of the acute stroke period.

Statins

The statins have been shown to reduce the risk of stroke by approximately 30% in patients with coronary artery disease and elevated plasma lipids.[35–37] The National Cholesterol Education Program (NCEP) considers ischemic stroke or TIA to be a coronary "equivalent" and has recommended the use of statins to achieve a low-density lipoprotein (LDL) concentration of less than 100 mg/dL.[38] More recently, the Heart Protection Study was published, and it provided evidence that simvastatin 40 mg/day reduced stroke risk in high-risk individuals (including patients with prior stroke) by 25% ($p < .0001$), even in patients with LDL concentrations of less than 116 mg/dL.[39] The investigators also showed that this practice is extremely safe, with an excess incidence of myopathy of 0.01%. The study even recommended abandoning the routine monitoring of liver function tests in these individuals because elevations are rarely significant or sustained. Other evidence in primary prevention of patients with hypertension suggests that similar stroke risk reduction can be achieved with other statins in patients with normal total cholesterol values.[40] Statin therapy is an effective way to reduce stroke risk and should be considered in all ischemic stroke patients.

Heparin for Prophylaxis of Deep Vein Thrombosis (DVT)

The use of low-molecular-weight heparins or low-dose subcutaneous unfractionated heparin (5000 units twice daily) can be recommended for the prevention of DVT in hospitalized patients with decreased mobility owing to their stroke and should be used in all but the most minor strokes.[6]

ALTERNATIVE DRUG TREATMENTS

ASPIRIN PLUS CLOPIDOGREL

In the MATCH study, clopidogrel in combination with aspirin 75 mg daily was no better than clopidogrel alone in secondary stroke prevention.[43] However, the combination has been studied in patients with acute coronary syndromes and patients undergoing percutaneous coronary interventions and shown to be significantly more effective than aspirin alone in reducing MI, stroke, and cardiovascular death.[41,42] Also, when clopidogrel was used with aspirin, the risk of life-threatening bleeding increased from 1.3% to 2.6%.[43] This combination can only be recommended in patients with ischemic stroke and a recent history of MI or other coronary events and only with ultra-low-dose aspirin to minimize bleeding risk.[44]

ANGIOTENSIN II RECEPTOR ANTAGONISTS (ARBS)

Angiotensin II receptor antagonists (ARBs) also have been shown to reduce the risk of stroke. In the LIFE study, losartan and metoprolol were compared for their ability to reduce blood pressure and prevent cardiovascular events in a group of severely hypertensive patients.[45] Despite similar reductions in blood pressure of approximately 30/16 mm Hg, the losartan group experienced a 24% reduction in the risk of stroke. The ARBs should be considered in patients unable to tolerate ACE inhibitors (LIFE) after acute ischemic stroke.

HEPARINS

The use of full-dose unfractionated heparin in the acute stroke period has never been proved to positively affect stroke outcome, and it significantly increases the risk of intracerebral hemorrhage.[6] Trials of low-molecular-weight heparins or heparinoids have been largely negative and do not support their routine use in stroke patients.[46–48] Other potential but unproven uses for treatment doses of either unfractionated or low-molecular-weight heparins include bridge therapy in patients being initiated on warfarin, carotid dissection, or continuous worsening of ischemia despite adequate antiplatelet therapy.[6]

TICLOPIDINE

Ticlopidine is a thienopyridine antiplatelet agent, similar in structure and mechanism of action to clopidogrel. It has been shown to reduce the risk of stroke by 30% compared with placebo and by 21% compared with aspirin 325 mg/day in patients at risk.[6] The use of ticlopidine has been severely restricted by its side-effect profile, however. It causes bone marrow suppression, rash, diarrhea, and elevation of the serum cholesterol concentration. Neutropenia occurs in up to 2% of patients and generally is reversible. More problematic, however, is the increased risk of aplastic anemia and thrombotic thrombocytopenic purpura.[49] Ticlopidine 250 mg twice daily is still available as an alternative in patients who fail or are intolerant of other therapies but is rarely needed.

DRUG CLASS INFORMATION

Aspirin

Aspirin exerts its antiplatelet effect by irreversibly inhibiting cyclooxygenase, which, in platelets, prevents conversion of arachidonic acid to thromboxane A_2 (TXA_2), which is a powerful vasoconstrictor and stimulator of platelet aggregation. Platelets remain impaired for their life span (5 to 7 days) after exposure to aspirin. Aspirin also inhibits prostacyclin (PGI_2) activity in the smooth muscle of vascular walls. PGI_2 inhibits platelet aggregation, and the vascular endothelium can synthesize prostacyclin such that the platelet antiaggregating effect is maintained. The suppression of PGI_2 production by aspirin has been found to be dose- and duration-related; the higher the dose, the longer the cyclooxygenase production is suppressed. Therefore, the lower the aspirin dose, the less effect on prostacyclin.[6] The optimal dose of aspirin is still under study, but it should be the dose that inhibits TXA_2 with the least amount of prostacyclin inhibition. It has been shown that an aspirin dose of 325 mg/day will inhibit TXA_2 but will not significantly inhibit PGI_2 production. There is probably a point at which lower doses of aspirin do not completely block TXA_2, and recent studies indicate that the lowest effective dose may be in the range of 50 mg/day.[50] Upper gastrointestinal (GI) discomfort and bleeding are the most common adverse effects of aspirin and have been shown to be dose-related. The highest rates of GI bleeding (5%) have been reported in patients receiving 1200 mg/day as compared with rates of 2% in patients taking the more commonly prescribed, 300 mg/day. Upper GI symptoms are much more common than frank bleeding, however, with 40% of patients affected at 1200 mg/day and 25% at 300 mg/day.[51] In the ESPS-2 study, even 50 mg/day of aspirin was associated with a twofold increase in bleeding over the placebo group.[28]

Low doses (<100 mg) of aspirin quickly inhibit cyclooxygenase in all the platelets in the circulation. Therefore, the onset of the antiplatelet effect of aspirin is less than 60 minutes.[52] It has been reported, however, that some patients either have or develop "aspirin resistance" and may require higher doses to achieve the desired antiplatelet effect.[53] Despite this, routine testing for aspirin resistance is not recommended. It was observed recently that administration of ibuprofen prior to the administration of a daily aspirin dose prohibits the aspirin from binding irreversibly to the cyclooxygenase and may decrease its antiplatelet effect.[54] Current recommendations are to administer aspirin at least 2 hours before ibuprofen or to wait at least 4 hours after an ibuprofen dose.

Extended-Release Dipyridamole plus Aspirin

Early studies of the role of dipyridamole in stroke prevention failed to show a benefit over that realized by aspirin alone. Dipyridamole, in high doses, is thought to inhibit platelet aggregation by inhibiting phophodiesterase, leading to accumulation of cyclic adenosine monophosphate (cAMP) and cyclic guanosine monophosphate (cGMP) intracellularly, which prevent platelet activation. In addition, dipyridamole also enhances the antithrombotic potential of the vascular wall.[55] The ESPS-2 demonstrated the efficacy of high-dose extended-release dipyridamole alone and in combination with aspirin in secondary stroke prevention.[28] This was the first study to demonstrate the benefits of combination antiplatelet therapy in stroke prevention (the combination was significantly more effective than either agent alone). The extended-release formulation of dipyridamole is important in that it allows twice-daily administration and higher doses to be tolerated in patients. The use of immediate-release generic dipyridamole in combination with regular aspirin, in order to reduce costs, is unproven and should be discouraged.

In the ESPS-2, 25% of the patients who received combination dipyridamole and aspirin discontinued the therapy early, and the rate of discontinuation owing to headache was more than three times as common (10%) as in the aspirin-alone group (3%). Other reasons for discontinuation were GI problems. Slow initiation of ERDP + ASA at one capsule at bedtime daily for 2 or 3 days can be tried in order to lessen headache symptoms. The headache due to ERDP + ASA is mostly self-limiting and decreases after several days.[56]

Clopidogrel

Clopidogrel has a unique platelet antiaggregatory effect in that it is an inhibitor of the adenosine diphosphate (ADP) pathway of platelet aggregation and inhibits known stimuli to platelet aggregation.[6,27] This effect causes an alteration of the platelet membrane and interference with the membrane-fibrinogenic interaction leading to a blocking of the platelet glycoprotein IIb/IIIa receptor. A time lag of 3 to 7 days before the antiplatelet effect is maximal should be expected. The tolerability of clopidogrel 75 mg/day is at least as good as medium-dose (325 mg/day) aspirin, and GI bleeding is less.[27] Clopidogrel is associated with an increased risk of diarrhea and rash, but discontinuation rates owing to adverse effects are similar to those with aspirin 325 mg/day (5.3% to 6%, respectively).[27] There is no excess neutropenia in patients taking clopidogrel, and rates of thrombotic thrombocytopenic purpura probably are no greater than background rates.[57]

Clopidogrel is a thienopyridine prodrug and needs to be biotransformed by the liver to an active metabolite. Evidence suggests that the enzyme responsible for the conversion is human cytochrome P450 3A4 (CYP3A4) and that the platelet effects of clopidogrel may be diminished in patients receiving agents that inhibit this enzyme.[58] Although high doses of the lipophilic statins atorvastatin and simvastatin may diminish the effectiveness of clopidogrel to inhibit platelet aggregation in vitro, there does not appear to be any adverse effect on atherothrombotic event rates.[59] Concomitant administration of clopidogrel with lipophilic statins is often recommended.

Ticlopidine

Ticlopidine, another thienopyridine, inhibits activation of the ADP receptor on the platelet, as does clopidogrel. However, in contrast to clopidogrel, ticlopidine possesses a significant side-effect profile and is costly. Side effects include suppression of bone marrow, rash and diarrhea, and elevation of serum cholesterol levels. Neutropenia may occur in up to 2% of patients but is reversible on discontinuation of therapy.[6] Postmarketing surveillance of the compound revealed an excess in the number of cases of serious blood dyscrasias such as thrombotic thrombocytopenic purpura (TTP).[48] Monitoring is required because of these side effects, and it is recommended that patients have complete blood counts (CBCs) with differentials every 2 weeks for 3 months. More than 50% of patients report at least one side effect, with GI complaints being the most common. Drug interactions may occur with digoxin, theophylline, and antacids, and these effects should be monitored. Ticlopidine was relegated to third-line status in stroke prevention owing to its adverse-event profile.[6] Ticlopidine (500 mg/day) in two divided doses of 250 mg is used rarely but can be recommended as an alternative antiplatelet therapy in extreme cases of intolerance to the other options available.

INVESTIGATIONAL STRATEGIES

REPERFUSION

Various investigations aimed at shortening the time required to open the occluded cerebral artery and preserve its patency are underway in acute ischemic stroke patients.[64] Strategies being tried include longer-acting fibrinolytic agents, intraarterial fibrinolysis with tPA and other agents, endovascular clot removal using mechanical and laser-guided approaches, and use of the glycoprotein IIB/IIIA receptor antagonists, both alone and in combination with fibrinolysis. In addition, investigators are trying to identify, using sensitive MRI techniques, which patients may benefit from reperfusion at time points outside the approved 3-hour time window. Undoubtedly, efforts to reperfuse the ischemic brain will continue to be explored, so more patients will be eligible for this therapy.

NEUROPROTECTION AND NEURORESTORATION

Although many different neuroprotective agents have been studied in clinical trials of acute ischemic stroke, none has been successful.[65] The only strategy that has been shown to provide neuroprotection in patients has been hypothermia.[66] Currently, clinical trials are underway to optimize the mechanism of cooling the ischemic brain (intravascular coils versus surface cooling) and rewarming the patient after hypothermia. Despite discouraging results in previous attempts, however, there is still great interest in developing pharmacologic agents that provide neuroprotection. Some of the most promising agents include free-radical scavengers, anti-inflammatory agents, and agents with multiple proposed mechanisms of protection (e.g., albumin infusions).[67] In addition, hope still exists that clinicians will be able to enhance the reparative process of the brain (neurorestoration) through targeted neurorehabilitation and the use of neural and cell transplantation.[68]

HEMORRHAGIC STROKE

There are currently no proven pharmacologic strategies for treating intracerebral hemorrhage (ICH).[15] Medical guidelines for the management of blood pressure, raised intracranial pressure, and other medical complications of ICH are those required for the management of any acutely ill patient in a neurointensive care unit.

Subarachnoid hemorrhage (SAH) owing to aneurysm rupture is associated with a high incidence of delayed cerebral ischemia (DCI) in the 2 weeks following the bleeding episode. Vasospasm of the cerebral vasculature is thought to be responsible for DCI and occurs between 4 and 21 days after the bleed, peaking at days 5 through 9.[20] The calcium channel blocker nimodipine is recommended to reduce the incidence and severity of neurologic deficits owing to DCI. Nimodipine at a dose of 60 mg every 4 hours should be initiated on diagnosis and continued for 21 days in all SAH patients. Administration of nimodipine therapy is complicated by a fairly high incidence of hypotension. This can be managed by reducing the dosing interval to 30 mg every 2 hours (same daily dose), reducing the total daily dose (30 mg every 4 hours), and maintaining intravascular volume and pressor therapy.[20]

PHARMACOECONOMIC CONSIDERATIONS

Cost-analysis data on the NINDS trial with tPA estimates that total health care costs (including acute and long-term costs) could be reduced by almost $5 million for every 1000 patients treated with tPA. Although tPA is expensive, when the total health care costs are factored in, savings can accrue to the health care system as a direct result of appropriate tPA therapy.[60]

In antithrombotic prophylaxis for atrial fibrillation, warfarin therapy was evaluated using quality-adjusted life-years saved (QALYs).[61] It was found that in patients with atrial fibrillation and one additional risk factor, warfarin therapy cost $8000 per QALY saved. In high-risk patients, those with atrial fibrillation and two or more risk factors, warfarin use was estimated to save $6200 in costs from stroke and TIA. Costs of monitoring and hemorrhages from warfarin were estimated to be $5500, thus showing a positive savings from warfarin use. Those without risk factors were much more costly to treat at an estimated $370,000 per QALY saved when compared with aspirin treatment. Warfarin is cost-effective in high-risk patients, particularly if the hemorrhagic side effects are lower relative to the stroke risk. For comparison purposes, hypertension screening is estimated to cost $10,000 to $50,000 per QALY saved. A Swedish study reported the cost-effectiveness of primary stroke prevention in atrial fibrillation patients with oral anticoagulants or aspirin based on four published clinical trials.[62] The authors found that the total cost per stroke prevented was a $16 savings if the intracerebral bleeding was 0.3% and $43 if the bleeding rate was 2%. At a bleeding complication rate of 1.3%, warfarin would prevent 1000 strokes per year and save about $29 million. The cost-effectiveness of the various first-line antiplatelet agents have been compared as well.[63] Without a doubt, aspirin, owing to its extremely low acquisition cost (pennies daily), is cost saving. In other words, it reduces costs at the same time as saving

QALYs. The use of clopidogrel or ERDP + ASA is associated with higher efficacy but significantly greater costs as well (up to $3 daily). Despite this, both options have been deemed "cost-effective" when administered to a 65-year-old patient with a history of stroke or TIA for the prevention of recurrence. In a recent analysis, ERDP + ASA was associated with $5000 to $15,000 per QALY (adjusted for the acquisition cost) and clopidogrel was $26,580 per QALY. Any cost per QALY less than $50,000 is thought to be "cost-effective."[63] These estimates are extremely dependent on the assumptions made in the model. Cost-effectiveness in an individual patient is much more difficult to discern.

Primary prevention strategies that address the risk factors for ischemic stroke can be powerful in reducing the costs of stroke. Many of the stroke risk factors can be modified and some eliminated at very low costs (lifestyle changes), therefore developing risk-factor-reduction strategies may be the most cost-effective measure of all. More research is needed in identifying the cost-effectiveness of other forms of acute stroke treatment.

CLINICAL CONTROVERSIES

The use of full-dose unfractionated heparin in the management of acute ischemic stroke remains controversial despite years of debate and a lack of evidence supporting its use. Proponents of the therapy cite strong anecdotal evidence of positive responses in selected patients who have never been studied in clinical trials.

The use of intracranial angioplasty and stenting is strongly supported in the few institutions where the technology exists. Whether these procedures should be attempted in patients outside clinical trials remains controversial.

The use of surgical evacuation of intracranial hemorrhage with and without instillation of fibrinolytic agents is

TABLE 20–5. Monitoring the Stroke Patient

	Treatment	Parameter(s)	Frequency	Comments
Ischemic stroke	tPA	BP, neurologic function, bleeding	Every 15 min × 1 h; every 0.5 h × 6 h; every 1 h × 17 h; every shift after	
	Aspirin	Bleeding	Daily	
	Clopidogrel	Bleeding	Daily	
	ERDP/ASA	Headache, bleeding	Daily	
	Ticlopidine	CBC, bleeding, diarrhea	CBC every 2 weeks × 3 months; other, daily	
	Warfarin	Bleeding, INR, Hb/Hct	INR daily × 3 days; weekly until stable; monthly	
Hemorrhagic stroke		BP, neurologic function, ICP	Every 2 h in ICU	Many patients require intervention with short-acting agents to reduce BP to <180 mm Hg systolic
	Nimodipine (for SAH)	BP, neurologic function, fluid status	Every 2 h in ICU	
All		Temperature, CBC	Temp. every 8 h; CBC daily	For infectious complications such as UTI or pneumonia
		Pain (calf or chest)	Every 8 h	For DVT, MI, acute headache
		Electrolytes and ECG	Up to daily	For fluid and electrolyte imbalances, cardiac rhythm abnormalities
	Heparins for DVT prophylaxis	Bleeding, platelets	Bleeding daily, platelets if suspected thrombocytopenia	

controversial. Although fervently pursued in select centers and countries, indications and outcomes are not known. Results of ongoing clinical trials may assist in settling this controversy.

EVALUATION OF THERAPEUTIC OUTCOMES

MONITORING OF THE PHARMACEUTICAL CARE PLAN

Patients with acute stroke should be monitored intensely for the development of neurologic worsening (recurrence or extension), complications (thromboembolism or infection), or adverse effects from pharmacologic or nonpharmacologic interventions. The most common reasons for deterioration in a stroke patient are (1) extension of the original lesion—ischemic or hemorrhagic—in the brain, (2) development of cerebral edema and raised intracranial pressure, (3) hypertensive emergency, (4) infection (urinary and respiratory most common), (5) venous thromboembolism (deep venous thrombosis and pulmonary embolism), (6) electrolyte abnormalities and cardiac rhythm disturbances (can be associated with brain injury), and (7) recurrent stroke.

The approach to monitoring the stroke patient is summarized in Table 20–5. Customization of the plan should be made for each patient based on his or her comorbidities and ongoing disease processes.

ABBREVIATIONS

ACE: angiotensin-converting enzyme
ADP: adenosine diphosphate
ARB: angiotensin II receptor blocker
ATP: adenosine triphosphate
AVM: arteriovenous malformation
cAMP: cyclic adenosine monophosphate
CAST: Chinese Acute Stroke Trial
CBC: complete blood count
CD: carotid Doppler
cGMP: cyclic guanosine monophosphate
CT scan: computed tomographic scan
CYP3A4: cytochrome P450 3A4
DCI: delayed cerebral ischemia
EAFT: European Atrial Fibrillation Trial
ECG: electrocardiogram
ERDP + ASA: extended-release dipyridamole plus aspirin
GI: gastrointestinal
ICH: intracerebral hemorrhage
INR: international normalized ratio
IST: International Stroke Trial
JNC: Joint National Committee
LDL: low-density lipoprotein
MI: myocardial infarction
MRI: magnetic resonance imaging
NCEP: National Cholesterol Education Program
NIHSS: National Institutes of Health Stroke Scale
NINDS: National Institute of Neurologic Disorders and Stroke
NVAF: nonvalvular atrial fibrillation
PAD: peripheral arterial disease
PGI$_2$: prostacyclin
QALY: quality-adjusted life-year

RRR: relative risk reduction
SAH: subarachnoid hemorrhage
TCD: transcranial Doppler
TIA: transient ischemic attack
TTP: thrombotic thrombocytopenic purpura
TXA$_2$: thromboxane A$_2$
tPA: tissue plasminogen activator

Review Questions and other resources can be found at *www.pharmacotherapyonline.com.*

REFERENCES

1. American Heart Association. Heart Disease and Stroke Statistics—2003 Update. Dallas, American Heart Association, 2002.
2. Quilliam BJ, Lapane KL. Clinical correlates and drug treatment of residents with stroke in long-term care. Stroke 2001;32:1385–1393.
3. Elkins JS, Johnston SC. Thirty-year projections for deaths from ischemic stroke in the United States. Stroke 2003;34:2109–2113.
4. Cooper R, Cutler J, Desvigne-Nickens P, et al. Trends and disparities in coronary heart disease, stroke, and other cardiovascular diseases in the United States: Findings of the National Conference on Cardiovascular Disease Prevention. Circulation 2000;102:3137–3147.
5. Fayad PB, Awad IA. Surgery for intracerebral hemorrhage. Neurology 1998;51(suppl 3):S69–73.
6. Albers GW, Amerenco P, Easton JD, et al. Antithrombotic and thrombolytic therapy for ischemic stroke: The seventh ACCP Conference on Antithrombotic and Thrombolytic Therapy. Chest 2004;126(3 suppl): 483S–512S.
7. Helgason CM, Wolf PA. American Heart Association Prevention Conference IV: Prevention and rehabilitation of stroke. Circulation 1997;96:701–707.
8. Straus SE, Majumdar SR, McAlister FA. New evidence for stroke prevention (scientific review). JAMA 2002;288:1388–1395.
9. Gorelick PB, Sacco RL, Smith DB, et al. Prevention of a first stroke: A review of guidelines and a multidisciplinary consensus statement from the National Stroke Association. JAMA 1999;281:1112–1120.
10. European Atrial Fibrillation Trial Study Group. Secondary prevention in nonrheumatic atrial fibrillation after transient ischaemic attack or minor stroke. Lancet 1993;342:1255–1262.
11. Hart RG, Halperin JL, Pearce LA, et al. Lessons from the stroke prevention in atrial fibrillation trials. Ann Intern Med 2003;138:831–838.
12. Wolf PA. Fifty years at Framingham: Contributions to stroke epidemiology. Adv Neurol 2003;92:165–172.
13. Dirnagl U, Iadecola C, Moskowitz MA. Pathobiology of ischemic stroke: An integrated view. Trends Neurosci 1999;22:391–397.
14. Feuerstein GZ, Wang X. New opportunities for stroke prevention and therapeutics: A hope from anti-inflammatory drugs? In: Feuerstein GZ, ed. Inflammation and Stroke. Basel, Birkhauser-Verlag, 2001.
15. Broderick JP, Adams HP, Barsan W, et al. Guidelines for the management of spontaneous intracerebral hemorrhage: A statement for healthcare professionals from a special writing group of the Stroke Council, American Heart Association. Stroke 1999;30:905–915.
16. Greenberg DA, Aminoff MJ, Simon RP, eds. Stroke. In: Clinical Neurology, 5th ed. New York, McGraw-Hill, 2002:282–316.
17. Adams HP, Adams RJ, Brott T, et al. Guidelines for the early management of patients with ischemic stroke: A scientific statement from the Stroke Council of the American Stroke Association. Stroke 2003;34:1056–1083.
18. Cina CA, Clase CM, Haynes RB. Carotid endarterectomy for symptomatic carotid stenosis (Cochrane Review on CD-ROM). Oxford, England, Cochrane Library Update Software, 2001; issue 1.
19. Hanel RA, Xavier AR, Kirmani JF, et al. Management of carotid artery stenosis: Comparing endarterectomy and stenting. Curr Cardiol Rep 2003; 5:153–159.

20. Miller J, Diringer M. Management of aneurysmal subarachnoid hemorrhage. Neurol Clin 1995;13:451–478.

21. The National Institute of Neurological Disorders and Stroke rt-PA Stroke Study Group. Tissue plasminogen activator for acute ischemic stroke. New Engl J Med 1995;333:1581–1587.

22. Chinese Acute Stroke Trial (CAST) Collaborative Group. CAST: A randomized, placebo-controlled trial of early aspirin use in 20,000 patients with acute ischemic stroke. Lancet 1997;349:1641–1649.

23. International Stroke Trial Collaborative Group. The International Stroke Trial (IST): A randomized trial of aspirin, subcutaneous heparin, both, or neither among 19,435 patients with acute ischemic stroke. Lancet 1997; 349:1560–1581.

24. Albers GW, Bates VE, Clark WM, et al. Intravenous tissue-type plasminogen activator for treatment of acute stroke: The Standard Treatment with Alteplase to Reverse Stroke (STARS) study. JAMA 2000;283:1145–1150.

25. Katzan IL, Furlan AJ, Lloyd LE, et al. Use of tissue-type plasminogen activator for acute ischemic stroke: The Cleveland area experience. JAMA 2000;283:1189–1191.

26. Antithrombotic Trialists' Collaboration. Collaborative meta-analysis of randomized trials of antiplatelet therapy for prevention of death, myocardial infarction, and stroke in high risk patients. BMJ 2002;324:71–86.

27. CAPRIE Steering Committee. A randomized, blinded trial of clopidogrel versus aspirin in patients at risk of ischaemic events (CAPRIE). Lancet 1995;348:1329–1339.

28. Diener HC, Cunha L, Forbes C, et al. European Stroke Prevention Study 2: Dipyridamole and acetylsalicylic acid in the secondary prevention of stroke. J Neurol Sci 1996;143:1–13.

29. American Society of Health-System Pharmacists. ASHP therapeutics position statement on antithrombotic therapy in chronic atrial fibrillation. Am J Health Syst Pharm 1998;55:376–381.

30. Hart RG, Benevente O, McBride R, Pearce LA. Antithrombotic therapy to prevent stroke in patients with atrial fibrillation: A meta-analysis. Ann Intern Med 1999;131:492–501.

31. Mohr JP, Thompson JLP, Lazar RM, et al. A comparison of warfarin and aspirin for the prevention of recurrent ischemic stroke. N Engl J Med 2001;345:1444–1451.

32. Gueyffer F, Boissel JP, Bouttie F, et al, for the INDANA Project Collaborators. Effect of antihypertensive treatment in patients having already suffered from stroke: Gathering of the evidence. Stroke 1997;28:2557–2562.

33. PROGRESS Collaborative Group. Randomized trial of perindopril-based blood-pressure-lowering regimen among 6105 individuals with previous stroke or transient ischaemic attack. Lancet 2001;358:1033–1041.

34. Chobanian AV, Bakris GL, Black HR, et al. The Seventh Report of the Joint National Committee on Prevention, Detection, Evaluation, and Treatment of High Blood Pressure. The JNC7 Report. JAMA 2003;2560–2572.

35. Hebert PR, Gaziano JM, Chan KS, Hennekens CH. Cholesterol lowering with statin drugs, risk of stroke, and total mortality: An overview of randomized trials. JAMA 1997;278:313–321.

36. Scandinavian Simvastatin Survival Study Group. Randomized trial of cholesterol lowering in 4444 patients with coronary heart disease: The Scandinavian Simvastatin Survival Study (4S). Lancet 1994;344:1383–1389.

37. Byrington RP, Davis BR, Plehn JF, et al. Reduction of stroke events with pravastatin: The Prospective Pravastatin Pooling (PPP) Project. Circulation 2001;103:387–392.

38. Executive Summary of the Third Report of the National Cholesterol Education Program (NCEP) Expert Panel on Detection, Evaluation, and Treatment of High Blood Cholesterol in Adults (Adult Treatment Panel III). JAMA 2001;285:2486–2497.

39. Heart Protection Study Collaborative Group. MRC/BHF Heart Protection Study of cholesterol lowering with simvastatin in 20,536 high-risk individuals: A randomized, placebo-control trial. Lancet 2002;360:7–22.

40. Sever PS, Dahlof B, Poulter NR, et al. Prevention of coronary and stroke events with atorvastatin in hypertensive patients who have average or lower-than-average cholesterol concentrations in the Anglo-Scandinavian Cardiac Outcomes Trial: Lipid Lowering Arm (ASCOT-LLA): A multicentre randomized controlled trial. Lancet 2003;361:1149–1158.

41. Yusuf S, Zhao F, Mehta SR, et al. Effects of clopidogrel in addition to aspirin in patients with acute coronary syndromes without ST-segment elevation. N Engl J Med 2001;54:1022–1028.

42. Steinhubl SR, Berger PB, Mann JT, et al. Early and sustained dual oral antiplatelet therapy following percutaneous coronary intervention: A randomized, controlled trial. JAMA 2002;288:2411–2420.

43. Diener HC, Bogousslavsky J, Brass LM, et al. Aspirin and clopidogrel compared with clopidogrel alone after recent ischemic stroke or transient ischaemic attack in high-risk patients (MATCH): Randomized, double-blind, placebo-controlled trial. Lancet 2004;364:331–337.

44. Peters RJG, Mehta SR, Fox KAA, et al. Effects of aspirin dose when used alone or in combination with clopidogrel in patients with acute coronary syndromes: Observations from the clopidogrel in unstable angina to prevent recurrent events (CURE) study. Circulation 2003;108:1682–1687.

45. Dahlof B, Devereux RB, Kjeldsen SE, et al. Cardiovascular morbidity and mortality in the Losartan Intervention for Endpoint Reduction in Hypertension Study (LIFE). Lancet 2002;359:995–1003.

46. The Publications Committee for the Trial of ORG 10172 in Acute Stroke Treatment (TOAST) Investigators. Low-molecular-weight heparinoid, ORG 10172 (danaparoid), and outcome after acute ischemic stroke: a randomized, controlled trial. JAMA 1998;279:1265–1272.

47. Bath PM, Lidenstrom E, Boysen G, et al. Tinzaparin in acute ischaemic stroke (TAIST): A randomized, aspirin-controlled trial. Lancet 2001;358:702–710.

48. Berge E, Abdelnoor M, Nakstad PH, et al. Low-molecular-weight heparin versus aspirin in patients with acute ischaemic stroke and atrial fibrillation: A double-blind, randomised study. HAEST Study Group. Heparin in Acute Embolic Stroke Trial. Lancet 2000;355:1205–1210.

49. Bennett CL, Davidson CJ, Raisch DW, et al. Thrombotic thrombocytopenic purpura associated with ticlopidine in the setting of coronary artery stents and stroke prevention. Arch Intern Med 1999;159:2524–2528.

50. Food and Drug Administration. FDA approves new prescribed uses for aspirin. FDA Talk Paper 1998; October 21; T98-76; www.fda.gov/bbs/topics/ANSWERS/ANS00919.html.

51. Farrell B, Godwin J, Richards S, Warlow C. The United Kingdom transient ischaemic attack (UK-TIA) aspirin trial: Final results. J Neurol Neurosurg Psychiatry 1991;54:1044–1054.

52. Serebruany VL, Malinin AI, Sane DC. Rapid platelet inhibition after a single capsule of Aggrenox: Challenging a conventional full-dose aspirin antiplatelet advantage? Am J Hematol 2003;72:280–281.

53. Eikelboom JW, Hankey GJ. Aspirin resistance: A new independent predictor of vascular events? J Am Coll Cardiol 2003;41:966–968.

54. Catella-Lawson F, Reilly MP, Kapoor SC, et al. Cyclooxygenase inhibitors and the antiplatelet effects of aspirin. N Engl J Med 2001;345:1809–1817.

55. Eisert WG. Near-field amplification of antithrombotic effects of dipyridamole through vessel wall cells. Neurology 2001;57(suppl 2):S20–23.

56. Theis JG, Deichsel G, Marshall S. Rapid development of tolerance to dipyridamole-associated headaches. Br J Clin Pharm 1999;48:750–755.

57. Bennett CL, Connors JM, Carwile JM, et al. Thrombotic thrombocytopenic purpura associated with clopidogrel. N Engl J Med 2000;342:1773–1777.

58. Lau WC, Waskell LA, Watkins PB, et al. Atorvastatin reduces the ability of clopidogrel to inhibit platelet aggregation: A new drug-drug interaction. Circulation 2003;107:32–37.

59. Saw J, Steinhubl SR, Berger PB, et al. Lack of adverse clopidogrel-atorvastatin clinical interaction from secondary analysis of a randomized, placebo-controlled clopidogrel trial. Circulation 2003;108:921–924.

60. Fagan SC, Morgenstein LB, Peitta A, et al. Cost effectiveness of tissue plasminogen activate for acute ischemic stroke. Neurology 1998;50:883–890.

61. Gage BF, Cardinalli AB, Albers GW, Owens DK. Cost-effectiveness of warfarin and aspirin for prophylaxis of stroke in patients with nonvalvular atrial fibrillation. JAMA 1995;274:1839–1845.

62. Gustafsson C, Asplund K, Britton M, et al. Cost-effectiveness of stroke prevention in atrial fibrillation. BMJ 1992;305:1457–1460.

63. Sarasin FP, Gaspoz JM, Bournameaux H. Cost-effectiveness of new antiplatelet regimens used as secondary prevention of stroke or transient ischemic attack. Arch Intern Med 2000;160:2773–2778.

64. Broderick JP, Hacke W. Treatment of acute ischemic stroke: I. Recanalization strategies. Circulation 2002;106:1563–1569.

65. Kidwell CS, Liebeskind DS, Starkman S, Saver JL. Trends in acute ischemic stroke trials through the 20th century. Stroke 2001;32:1349–1359.

66. Broderick JP, Hacke W. Treatment of acute ischemic stroke: II. Neuroprotection and medical management. Circulation 2002;106:1736–1740.

67. Gladstone DJ, Black SE, Hakim AM. Toward wisdom from failure: Lessons from neuroprotective stroke trials and new therapeutic directions. Stroke 2002;33:2123–2136.

68. Kondziolka D, Wechsler L, Goldstein S, et al. Transplantation of cultured human neuronal cells for patients with stroke. Neurology 2000;55:565–569.

21

HYPERLIPIDEMIA

Robert L. Talbert

Learning Objectives and other resources can be found at *www.pharmacotherapyonline.com.*

KEY CONCEPTS

◀1 Hypercholesterolemia, elevated low-density lipoprotein (LDL), and low high-density lipoprotein (HDL) are unequivocally linked to increased risk for coronary heart disease and cerebrovascular morbidity and mortality; LDL is the primary target.

◀2 Multiple genetic abnormalities and environmental factors are involved in clinical lipid abnormalities, and routinely used clinical laboratory measurements do not define the underlying abnormalities.

◀3 Initial therapy for any lipoprotein disorder is therapeutic lifestyle changes with restricted intake of total and saturated fat and cholesterol and a modest increase in polyunsaturated fat intake, along with a program of regular exercise and weight reduction if needed.

◀4 If pharmacologic therapy is insufficient after therapeutic lifestyle changes, lipid-lowering agents should be chosen based on the specific lipoprotein disorder presentation and the severity of the lipid abnormality.

◀5 Considering compliance, adverse effects, and effectiveness, statins are the drugs of choice for patients with hypercholesterolemia because they are the most potent form of monotherapy and are cost-effective in patients with known

coronary artery disease (CAD) or multiple risk factors and in high-risk primary prevention patients.

◀6 Patients not responding to statin monotherapy may be treated with combination therapy for hypercholesterolemia but should be monitored closely because of an increased risk for adverse effects and drug interactions.

◀7 Hypertriglyceridemia usually responds well to niacin, gemfibrozil, or high-dose/potency statins (e.g., atorvastatin or simvastatin); niacin should be used cautiously in diabetics because of worsening glycemic control.

◀8 Low HDL cholesterol is addressed with lifestyle modifications such as smoking cessation and increased exercise; niacin and gemfibrozil can increase HDL cholesterol significantly as well.

◀9 Reductions in elevated total cholesterol and LDL cholesterol reduce coronary heast disease mortality and total mortality; increasing HDL reduces coronary heart disease events as well. Aggressive treatment of hypercholesterolemia results in fewer patients progressing to myocardial infarction, angina, and stroke and reduces the need for interventions such as coronary artery bypass grafting and percutaneous transluminal coronary angioplasty.

Cholesterol, triglycerides, and phospholipids are the major lipids in the body, and they are transported as complexes of lipid and proteins known as *lipoproteins.* Plasma lipoproteins are spherical particles with surfaces that consist largely of phospholipid, free cholesterol, and protein and cores that consist mostly of triglyceride and cholesterol ester. The three major classes of lipoproteins found in serum are low-density lipoproteins (LDLs), high-density lipoproteins (HDLs), and very low-density lipoproteins (VLDLs). Intermediate-density lipoprotein resides between VLDL and LDL and is included in the LDL measurement in routine clinical measurement. Abnormalities of plasma lipoproteins can result in a predisposition to coronary, cerebrovascular, and peripheral vascular arterial disease. Accumulating evidence over the last decades had linked elevated total and LDL and reduced HDL to the development of coronary heart disease (CHD). Premature coronary atherosclerosis, leading to the manifestations of ischemic heart disease (see Chap. 15), is the most common and significant consequence of hyperlipidemia. The National Cholesterol Education Program (NCEP) Adult Treatment Panel III (ATP III) published its third report summarizing these data and giving recommendations for the management of hypercholesterolemia in adults.[1]

This report modifies earlier recommendations and provides a new way of risk-stratifying patients based on multiple risk factors and the presence of diabetes and the metabolic syndrome.[1,2] The American Heart Association (AHA) also provides guidelines for primary and secondary prevention of CHD.[3–5]

Total cholesterol and LDL cholesterol increase throughout life in men and women, representing an atherogenic pattern characteristic of Western society diets (Fig. 21–1).[6] Based on the National Health and Nutrition Examination Survey (NHANES 1999–2000) and the ATP III guidelines, slightly more than 50% or nearly 105 million American adults over 20 years of age have total cholesterol levels of 200 mg/dL or higher.[1,6,7] Only about one-third are aware that they have hypercholesterolemia, and 12% were on therapy for hypercholesterolemia.[6] Changes in the NCEP guidelines have increased the number of persons eligible for therapeutic lifestyle changes (TLCs) or lipid-lowering therapy by millions. NCEP estimates that only 26% of patients have an optimal LDL cholesterol (<100 mg/dL) and that large numbers of patients are either untreated or undertreated.[1,8] Unfortunately, the patients at highest risk are less likely to be treated to desirable levels of LDL.[9] Although these numbers seem staggering in their enormity,

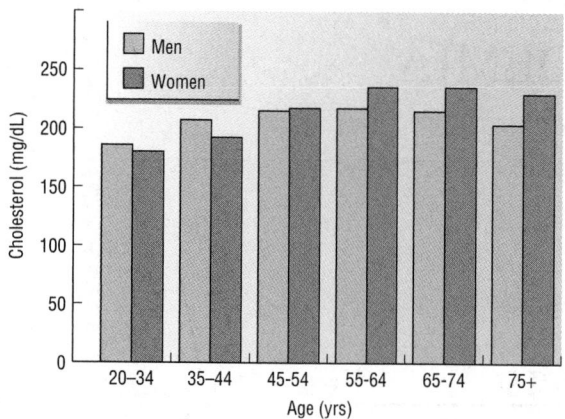

FIGURE 21–1. Serum cholesterol in men and women 20 years of age and older based on the 3rd National Health and Nutrition Survey.[6]

substantial progress has been made, and the number of Americans with a desirable blood cholesterol level (<200 mg/dL) has risen to 49% from 45% in the earlier survey (1976–1980), whereas the average total cholesterol level in this country has fallen from 220 mg/dL in 1960 to 1962 to 203 mg/dL in 1988–1994.[6] Unfortunately, there has been little change in total cholesterol between 1994 and 2000.[6] Patients who are at risk but who have not yet experienced their first cardiovascular or cerebrovascular event (e.g., myocardial infarction [MI]) are termed *primary prevention,* whereas those with manifest vascular disease are termed *secondary intervention.*

Data from the Framingham Study and from other studies demonstrate that the risk for developing cardiovascular disease is related to the degree of total cholesterol and LDL elevation in a graded, continuous fashion.[10,11] Hypercholesterolemia is additive to the other nonlipid risk factors for CHD, including cigarette smoking, hypertension, diabetes, low HDL levels, and electrocardiographic (ECG) abnormalities. The presence of established CHD or prior MI increases the risk of MI five to seven times that seen in men or women without CHD, and LDL is a significant predictor of subsequent morbidity and mortality.[10] About 50% of all MIs and at least 70% of CHD deaths occur in patients with known CHD, and these patients therefore should be a target for screening, identification, and treatment. Unfortunately, the identification of patients at high risk because of hypercholesterolemia or other lipid disorders is too frequently overlooked because blood lipid levels are not always evaluated in this population even after an event such as MI.[10]

A comparison of the United States with other countries shows similar relationships between total cholesterol and LDL and an inverse relationship with HDL and coronary artery disease (CAD) mortality.[12] On a positive note, the U.S. mortality rate is midway among the countries studied, and this country has had the greatest decline in CAD mortality (35% to 40%) in men and women over the last 10 years compared with other countries. A decline in the prevalence of hypercholesterolemia in certain segments of the U.S. population parallels these trends in mortality.[1] LDL and the ratio of LDL to HDL also have been used to assess risk, but their use adds little information to total cholesterol alone unless HDL is abnormally high or low. HDL transports cholesterol from lipid-laden foam cells to the liver. HDL has been shown to be protective for the occurrence of CHD, and an inverse relationship exists between CHD and HDL levels.[13]

LDL, is enriched with cholesterol esters and is smaller, denser, and more atherogenic than less-dense VLDL. Routine measurement of triglycerides cannot distinguish between the types of VLDL

present in plasma. Elevation of triglyceride-rich lipoproteins is associated with low HDL, and this ratio predicts increased risk. The 8-year follow-up of the Copenhagen male study found a clear gradient of risk of ischemic heart disease (IHD) with increasing triglyceride levels within each level of HDL cholesterol. When compared with the lowest tertile of triglyceride concentrations, the highest tertile had 2.2 relative risk for IHD, and the relationship extended across all concentrations of HDL.[14] The Helsinki Heart Study shows that hypertriglyceridemia and low HDL levels are associated with obesity (body mass index [BMI] > 26 kg/m^2), smoking, sedentary lifestyle, blood pressure of 140/90 mm Hg or greater, and a blood glucose concentration above 4.4 mmol/L and that the benefit of gemfibrozil (risk reduction 68%, *p* < .03) was confined largely to overweight subjects.[15] Hypertriglyceridemia in certain instances—e.g., diabetes mellitus, nephrotic syndrome, and chronic renal disease and perhaps in women—is associated with increased cardiovascular risk. This is thought to be a consequence of the presence of atherogenic lipoproteins and of hypertriglyceridemia being a marker for them, since triglycerides usually are not independently predictive for CHD.[16]

LIPOPROTEIN METABOLISM AND TRANSPORT

Cholesterol and triglycerides, as the major plasma lipids, are essential substrates for cell membrane formation and hormone synthesis and provide a source of free fatty acids.[17] *Hyperlipidemia* is defined as an elevation of one or more of cholesterol, cholesterol esters, phospholipids, or triglycerides. Lipids, being water immiscible, are not present in free form in the plasma but rather circulate as lipoproteins. *Hyperlipoproteinemia* describes an increased concentration of the lipoprotein macromolecules that transport lipids in the plasma. The density of plasma lipoproteins is determined by their relative content of protein and lipid. Density, composition, size, and electrophoretic mobility divide lipoproteins into four classes (Table 21–1).

LDL has been further divided into LDL$_1$, or intermediate-density lipoprotein (density 1.006–1.019 g/mL), and LDL$_2$ (1.019–1.063 g/mL). LDL$_2$ is the major LDL component in plasma, and it carries 60% to 70% of the total serum cholesterol. HDL has been subfractionated into HDL$_2$ (density 1.063–1.125 g/mL) and HDL$_3$ (1.125–1.21 g/mL). Fluctuations in HDL usually are caused by alterations in the levels of HDL$_2$. HDL normally carries about 20% to 30% of the total cholesterol. VLDL also has been subdivided into three classes, and it carries about 10% to 15% of serum cholesterol and most of the triglyceride in the fasting state. VLDL is the precursor for LDL, and VLDL remnants also may be atherogenic. Table 21–2 shows the characteristics of the protein constituent of lipoproteins known as *apolipoproteins.*

Chylomicrons, large triglyceride-rich particles containing apolipoprotein B-48, B-100, and E, are formed from dietary fat solubilized by bile salts in intestinal mucosal cells (Fig. 21–2). Chylomicrons normally are not present in the plasma after a fast of 12 to 14 hours and are catabolized by lipoprotein lipase (LPL), which is activated by apolipoprotein C-II, in the vascular endothelium and hepatic lipase to form chylomicron remnants. The remnants that contain apolipoprotein E (see Fig. 21–2) are taken up by the "remnant receptor," which may be an LDL-receptor–related protein, in the liver. Free cholesterol is liberated intracellularly after attachment to the remnant receptor. Chylomicrons also function to deliver dietary triglyceride to skeletal muscle and adipose tissue. During the catabolism of nascent chylomicrons to remnants, triglyceride is converted to free fatty acids and apolipoproteins A-I, A-II, A-IV (free in plasma), C-I, C-II, and

TABLE 21–1. Composition of Lipoprotein Isolated from Normal Subjects

Lipoprotein Class	Density Range (g/mL)	Diameter (nm)	Protein	Triglyceride	Free	Ester	Phospholipid
					Cholesterol		
Chylomicrons	<0.94	75–1200	1–2	80–95	1–3	2–4	3–9
VLDL	0.94–1.006	30–80	6–10	55–80	4–8	16–22	10–20
LDL	1.006–1.063	18–25	18–22	5–15	6–8	45–50	18–24
HDL	1.063–1.21	5–12	45–55	5–10	3–5	15–20	20–30

VLDL = very low-density lipoprotein; LDL = low-density lipoprotein; HDL = high-density lipoprotein.

C-III, and phospholipids are transferred to HDL. Apolipoproteins E and C-II are transferred to chylomicrons from HDL and eventually back through these metabolic events. Hepatic VLDL synthesis is regulated in part by diet and hormones and is inhibited by uptake of chylomicron remnants in the liver. VLDL is secreted from the liver and serially converted via LPL to intermediate-density lipoprotein (IDL) and finally to LDL. VLDL receptors are found in adipose tissue and muscle and bear close homology to the structure of LDL receptors.

LDL, the major cholesterol transport lipoprotein, having virtually only apolipoprotein B-100, is mostly derived from VLDL catabolism and cellular synthesis. When fasting and when normal subjects are on low-fat intake, most cholesterol is synthesized and used in the extrahepatic organs, whereas most of the cholesterol carried by LDL is taken up by the liver for catabolism.[17] In patients with homozygous familial hypercholesterolemia, enhanced synthesis of LDL may occur because LDL clearance is reduced as a consequence of the lack of LDL receptors. LDL is catabolized through interaction of cell surface receptors found on liver, adrenal, and peripheral cells (including fibroblasts and smooth muscle cells). These cells recognize apolipoprotein B-100 on LDL, and after binding to a receptor on the cell membrane, LDL is internalized and degraded. In the normal fasting state, approximately 70% of LDL is cleared through receptor-dependent mechanism, although this is highly dependent on the availability and type of saturated and mono- or polyunsaturated fat from dietary sources. Ingestion of cholesterol and saturated fatty acids such as C12:0, C14:0, and C16:0 is associated with reduction in LDL receptor activity, increased LDL production rate, and elevation in LDL plasma concentration. Receptor-independent mechanisms are also involved to a lesser extent in the catabolism of LDL, and these receptors are present in many tissues but are most active in animals in the adrenals and ovary.[17] Increased intracellular cholesterol resulting from LDL catabolism inhibits the activity of 3-hydroxy-3-methylglutaryl coenzyme A reductase (HMG-CoA reductase),

TABLE 21–2. Characteristics and Functions of Apolipoproteins

Apolipoprotein	Lipoprotein Density Class	Approximate Plasma Concentration (mg/dL)	Approximate Molecular Weight (kDa)	Reported Functions	Major Site of Synthesis
A-I	Chylomicrons, HDL	120	28	Cofactor with LCAT, structural protein on HDL, ligand for HDL receptor	Liver, intestine
A-II	Chylomicrons, HDL	35	17	Structural protein for HDL, ligand for HDL receptor	Liver
A-IV	Chylomicrons, 1.21B	15	46	Possibly facilitates transfer of other apos between HDL and chylomicrons	Intestine
ApoLp(a)	LDL, HDL	10	500±	Bound to B-100, high homology with plasminogen, may prevent LDL uptake by B, E receptor	Liver
B-100	VLDL, LDL, IDL	100	540	Necessary for assembly and secretion of VLDL from the liver, structural protein of VLDL, IDL, LDL, ligand for LDL receptor	Liver
B-48	Chylomicrons	Trace	264	Necessary for assembly and secretion of chylomicrons from the small intestine	Intestine
C-I	Chylomicrons, VLDL, HDL	7	6.6	Cofactor with LCAT, may inhibit hepatic uptake of chylomicron and VLDL remnants	Liver
C-II	Chylomicrons, VLDL, HDL	4	8.9	Activator of LPL	Liver
C-III	Chylomicrons, VLDL, HDL	13	8.8	Inhibitor with LPL, may inhibit hepatic uptake of chylomicron and VLDL remnants	Liver
D	HDL	6	32	?	?
E2–E4	Chylomicrons, VLDL, HDL	5	34	Ligand for several lipoproteins to LDL receptor, LRP, and possibly to a separate hepatic apo E receptor	Liver

LCAT = lecithin-cholesterol acyltransferase; HL = hepatic lipase; IDL = intermediate-density lipoprotein; LRP = LDL receptor-related protein. Other abbreviations are in Table 21–1.

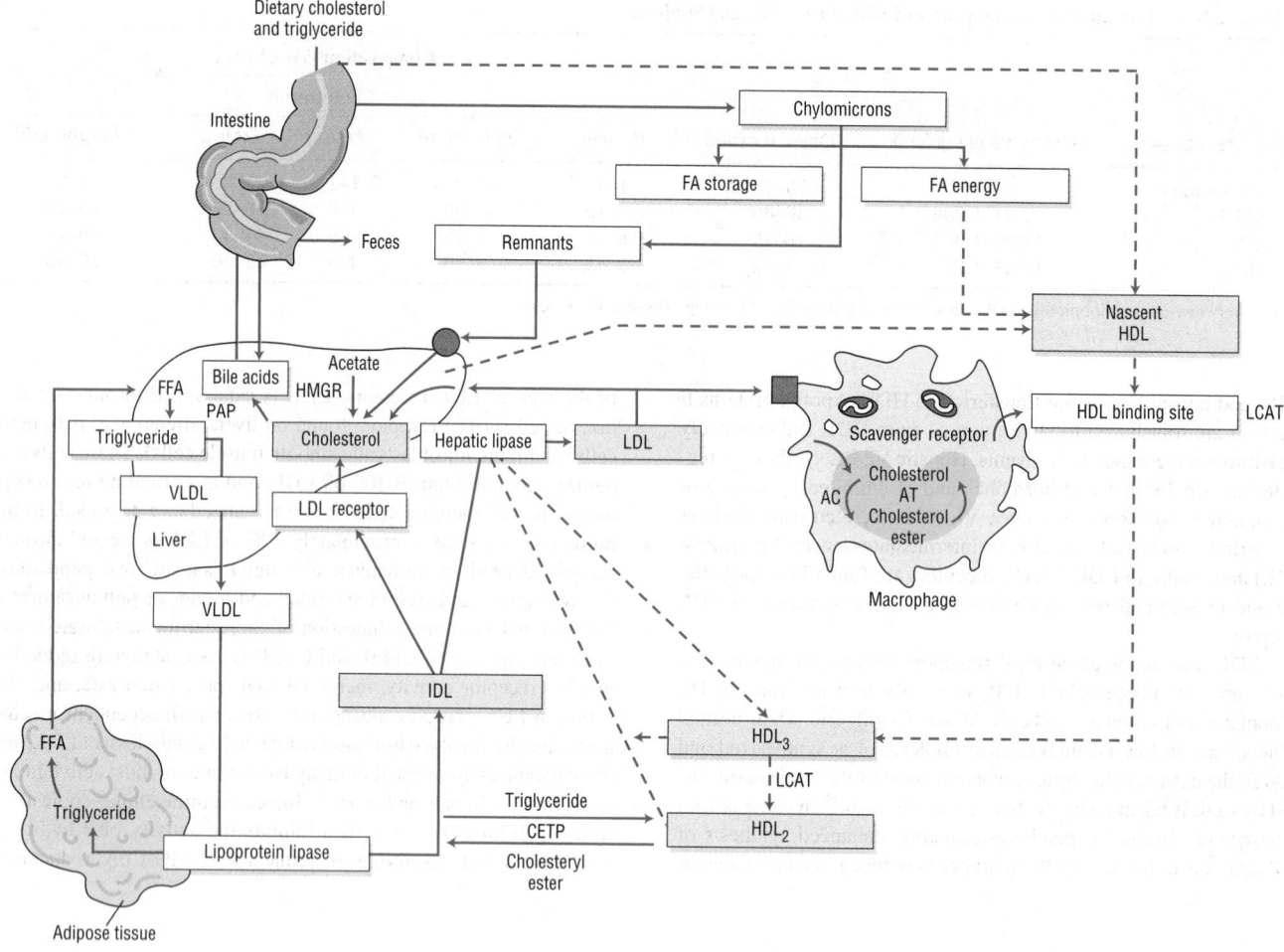

FIGURE 21–2. Overview of lipoprotein metabolism. (ACAT = acyl CoA:cholesterol acyltransferase; CETP = cholesteryl ester transfer protein; FA = fatty acid; FFA = free fatty acid; HMGR = HMG CoA reductase; LCAT = lecithin:cholesterol acyltransferase; PAP = phosphatidic acid phosphatase). *(From Ref. 17 with permission.)*

the rate-limiting enzyme for intracellular cholesterol biosynthesis (Fig. 21–3). Additional consequences of increased intracellular cholesterol include reduced synthesis of LDL receptors, which limits subsequent cholesterol uptake from the plasma, and accelerated activity of acyl coenzyme-A:cholesterol acyltransferase (ACAT) to facilitate cholesterol storage within cells. LDL cholesterol also may be excreted into bile and become part of the enterohepatic pool or may be lost in the stool. Lp(a) is a cholesterol-rich lipoprotein similar to LDL in composition and density and with close homology to fibrinogen; it is reported to be an important independent risk factor for the development of premature cardiovascular disease.

Nascent HDL is derived from liver and gut synthesis primarily in the form of apolipoprotein A-I phospholipid disks. Esterification of free cholesterol in nascent HDL and from peripheral tissues to cholesteryl esters by lecithin: cholesterol acyltransferase (LCAT) results in the production of HDL$_3$. Further addition of tissue cholesterol to HDL$_3$ results in the formation of HDL$_2$. HDL$_2$ also can be formed from remodeling of chylomicrons and VLDL catabolism. HDL$_2$ may be converted back to HDL$_3$ by the action of hepatic lipase and by the transfer of cholesteryl esters to the liver, LDL, and VLDL. Apolipoprotein A-I production is increased by estrogens, leading to higher HDL levels in women and in individuals receiving estrogen. Transfer of excess cholesterol from peripheral tissues by HDL is called

reverse cholesterol transport. Putative HDL receptors in peripheral cells facilitate the uptake of cholesterol by HDL, which transfers cholesterol to either VLDL and LDL or to the liver for secretion into bile or conversion into bile acids. These processes serve to rid peripheral tissue (e.g., coronary arteries) of excessive amounts of cholesterol and account for some of the protective effects noted with increasing HDL in women and other factors that elevate HDL levels. Variants of the cholesteryl ester transfer protein (CETP) have been demonstrated in humans, and the *B1/B1* genotype is associated with lower HDL and progression of coronary atherosclerosis. Inhibition of CETP leads to elevations in HDL, and this may prove to be an important therapeutic approach for the future if the HDL produced is fully functional in the process of reverse cholesterol transport.[18,19]

The response-to-injury hypothesis states that risk factors such as oxidized LDL, mechanical injury to the endothelium (e.g., percutaneous transluminal angioplasty), excessive homocysteine, immunologic attack, or infection-induced (e.g., *Chlamydia,* herpes simplex virus 1) changes in endothelial and intimal function lead to endothelial dysfunction and a series of cellular interactions that culminate in atherosclerosis.[20] C-reactive protein (CRP) is an acute-phase reactant and a marker for inflammation; it may be useful in identifying patients at risk for developing CAD.[21] The eventual outcomes of this atherogenic cascade are clinical events such as angina, MI, arrhythmias,

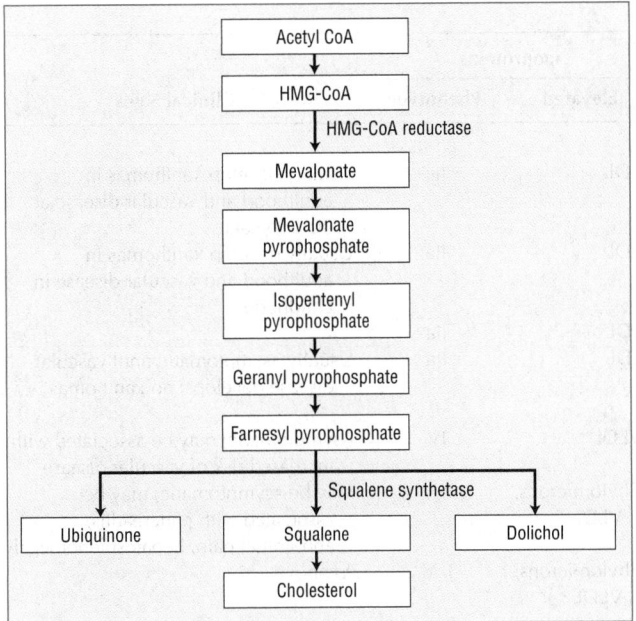

FIGURE 21–3. Biosynthetic pathway for cholesterol. The rate-limiting enzyme in this pathway is 3-hydroxy-3-methylglutaryl coenzyme A reductase (HMG-CoA reductase).

stroke, peripheral arterial disease, abdominal aortic aneurysm, and sudden death. Atherosclerotic lesions are thought to arise from transport and retention of plasma LDL cholesterol through the endothelial cell layer into the extracellular matrix of the subendothelial space. Once in the artery wall, LDL is chemically modified through oxidation and nonenzymatic glycation. Mildly oxidized LDL then recruits monocytes into the artery wall, which become transformed into macrophages. Macrophages have tremendous potential for accelerating LDL oxidation and apolipoprotein B accumulation and altering the receptor-mediated uptake of LDL into the artery wall from the usual LDL receptor to a "scavenger receptor" not regulated by cell content of cholesterol. Oxidized LDL increases plasminogen inhibitor levels (promotion of coagulation), induces the expression of endothelin (vasoconstrictive substance), inhibits the expression of nitric oxide (a vasodilator and platelet inhibitor), and is toxic to macrophages if highly oxidized. As oxidation of biologically active lipids proceeds, other lipids such as lysophosphatidylcholine, hydroperoxides, aldehydic breakdown products of fatty acids, and oxysterol are formed, which continue the reaction within the tissue. These events lead to a massive accumulation of cholesterol. The cholesterol-laden cells are called *foam cells;* foam cells are the earliest recognized cells of the arterial fatty streak.

Oxidized LDL provokes an inflammatory response, which is mediated by a number of chemoattractants and cytokines. Examples of each that appear to be involved at different stages of lesion development include monocyte chemoattractant protein 1 (MCP-1), monocyte colony-stimulating factor (M-CSF), *gro,* vascular cell adhesion molecule (VCAM-1), E-selectin (ELAM-1), intercellular adhesion molecule (ICAM-1), platelet-derived growth factor (PDGF), vascular endothelial growth factor (VEGF), transforming growth factors (TGF-α and TGF-β); interleukin-1 and interleukin-6 (IL-1, IL-6), and the ratio of interleukin-10 and interleukin-12 (IL-10, IL-12). It appears that some of these factors (e.g., MCP-1 and M-CSF) participate early in the process of monocyte-macrophage attachment and transmigration across the endothelium, whereas others (PDGF and

VCAM-1) promote later lesion growth.[22] The extent of oxidation and the inflammatory response are under genetic control of a major gene termed *Ath*-1 based on murine model studies. The process of aging may lead to lipoproteins that are more susceptible to oxidation and have longer resident time in the vascular compartment.[23] Two proteins associated with HDL—apolipoprotein J (apoJ) and paraxonase (PON)—appear to play an important role in minimizing the oxidation of LDL cholesterol.[24] Increased recognition of the role of these growth-regulatory molecules provides the possibility of future directions for antagonists to regulatory molecules such as PDGF, TGF-β, and the interleukins. Repeated injury and repair within an atherosclerotic plaque eventually leads to a fibrous cap protecting the underlying core of lipids, collagen, calcium, and inflammatory cells such as T-lymphocytes. Maintenance of the fibrous plaque is critical to preventing plaque rupture and subsequent coronary thrombosis. An imbalance between plaque synthesis and degradation may lead to a weakened or vulnerable plaque prone to rupture. The fibrous cap may become weakened through decreased synthesis of the extracellular matrix or increased degradation of the matrix. The cytokine interferon-γ, produced by T-lymphocytes, inhibits the ability of smooth-muscle cells to synthesize collagen, a structurally important component of the fibrous cap. A family of enzymes known as *matrix metalloproteinases* can degrade all major constituents of the vascular extracellular matrix: collagen, elastin, and proteoglycans.[22]

Lipoprotein disorders are classified into six categories, which are commonly used for phenotypic description of hyperlipidemia (Table 21–3). Specific genetic defects with disrupted protein, cell, and organ function give rise to several disorders within each family of lipoproteins (Table 21–4). In other words, an elevated cholesterol level does not necessarily equate with familial hypercholesterolemia, or type IIa, because cholesterol also may be elevated in other lipoprotein disorders, and the lipoprotein pattern does not describe the underlying genetic defect. The preceding discussion has focused on primary or genetic hyperlipoproteinemia; it should be remembered that secondary forms exist and that several drugs also may elevate lipid levels (Table 21–5). These secondary forms of hyperlipidemia should be managed initially by correcting the underlying abnormality, including modification of drug therapy when appropriate.

Familial hypercholesterolemia is characterized by (1) a selective elevation in the plasma level of LDL, (2) deposition of LDL-derived cholesterol in tendons (xanthomas) and arteries (atheromas), and (3) inheritance as an autosomal dominant trait, with homozygotes affected more severely than heterozygotes. Homozygotes (prevalence 1 in 1 million) have severe hypercholesterolemia (650–1000 mg/dL), with the early appearance of cutaneous xanthomas and fatal CHD generally before age 20. The primary defect in familial hypercholesterolemia is the inability to bind LDL to the LDL receptor (LDL-R)

TABLE 21–3. Frederickson-Levy-Lees Classification of Hyperlipoproteinemia

Type	Lipoprotein Elevation
I	Chylomicrons
IIa	LDL
IIb	LDL + VLDL
III	IDL (LDL$_1$)
IV	VLDL
V	VLDL + chylomicrons

LDL = low-density lipoprotein; VLDL = very low-density lipoprotein; IDL = intermediate-density lipoprotein.

TABLE 21–4. Lipoprotein Disorders

Lipid Phenotype	Plasma Lipid Levels, mmol/L (mg/dL)	Lipoproteins Elevated	Lipoproteins Phenotype	Clinical Signs
Isolated Hypercholesterolemia				
Familial hypercholesterolemia	Heterozygotes TC = 7–13 (275–500)	LDL	IIa	Usually develop xanthomas in adulthood and vascular disease at 30–50 years
	Homozygotes TC > 13 (>500)	LDL	IIa	Usually develop xanthomas in adulthood and vascular disease in childhood
Familial defective apo B100	Heterozygotes TC = 7–13 (275–500)	LDL	IIa	
Polygenic hypercholesterolemia	TC = 6.5–9 (250–350)	LDL	IIa	Usually asymptomatic until vascular disease develops; no xanthomas
Isolated Hypertriglyceridemia				
Familial hypertriglyceridemia	TG = 2.8–8.5 (250–750)	VLDL	IV	Asymptomatic; may be associated with increased risk of vascular disease
Familial LPL deficiency	TG > 8.5 (750)	Chylomicrons, VLDL	I, V	May be asymptomatic; may be associated with pancreatitis, abdominal pain, hepatosplenomegaly
Familial apo CII deficiency	TG > 8.5 (>750)	Chylomicrons, VLDL	I, V	As above
Hypertriglyceridemia and Hypercholesterolemia				
Combined hyperlipidemia	TG = 2.8–8.5 (250–750); TC = 6.5–13 (250–500)	VLDL, LDL	IIb	Usually asymptomatic until vascular disease develops; familial form also may present as isolated high TG or an isolated high LDL cholesterol
Dysbetalipoproteinemia	TG = 2.8–8.5 (250–750); TC = 6.5–13 (250–500)	VLDL, IDL; LDL normal	III	Usually asymptomatic until vascular disease develops; may have palmar or tuboeruptive xanthomas

TC = total cholesterol; TG = triglycerides; LPL = lipoprotein lipase.

or, rarely, a defect of internalizing the LDL-R complex into the cell after normal binding. Homozygotes have essentially no functional LDL receptors. This leads to a lack of LDL degradation by cells and unregulated biosynthesis of cholesterol, with total cholesterol and LDL cholesterol levels being inversely proportional to the deficit in LDL receptors. Heterozygotes have only about one-half the normal number of LDL receptors, total cholesterol levels in the range of 300–600 mg/dL, and cardiovascular events beginning in the third and fourth decades of life.

Familial LPL deficiency is a rare, autosomal recessive trait characterized by a massive accumulation of chylomicrons and a corresponding increase in plasma triglycerides, or a type I lipoprotein pattern. VLDL concentration is normal. The presenting manifestations include repeated attacks of pancreatitis and abdominal pain, eruptive cutaneous xanthomatosis, and hepatosplenomegaly beginning in childhood. Symptom severity is proportional to dietary fat intake and, consequently, to the elevation of chylomicrons. LPL normally is released from vascular endothelium or by heparin and hydrolyzes chylomicrons and VLDL (see Fig. 21–3). Diagnosis is based on low or absent enzyme activity with normal human plasma or apolipoprotein C-II, a cofactor of the enzyme. Accelerated atherosclerosis is not associated with this disease. Abdominal pain, pancreatitis, eruptive xanthomas, and peripheral polyneuropathy characterize type V (VLDL and chylomicrons). Symptoms may occur in childhood, but usually the disorder is expressed at a later age. The risk of atherosclerosis is increased with this disorder. These patients commonly are obese, hyperuricemic, and diabetic, and alcohol intake, exogenous estrogens, and renal insufficiency tend to be exacerbating factors.

Patients with familial type III hyperlipoproteinemia (also called *dysbetalipoproteinemia, broad-band,* or *β-VLDL*) develop these clinical features after 20 years of age: xanthoma striata palmaris (yellow discoloration of the palmar and digital creases), tuberous or tuboeruptive xanthomas (bulbous cutaneous xanthomas), and severe atherosclerosis involving the coronary arteries, internal carotids, and abdominal aorta. A defective structure of apolipoprotein E does not allow normal hepatic surface receptor binding of remnant particles derived from chylomicrons and VLDL (known as IDL); aggravating factors such as obesity, diabetes, or pregnancy may promote overproduction of apo-B–containing lipoproteins. Although homozygosity for the defective allele (E_2/E_2) is common (1 in 100), only 1 in 10,000 express the full-blown picture, and interaction with other genetic or environmental factors, or both, is needed to produce clinical disease.

Familial combined hyperlipidemia is characterized by elevations in total cholesterol and triglycerides, decreased HDL, increased apolipoprotein B, and small, dense LDL.[25] It is associated with premature CHD and may be difficult to diagnose because the lipid levels do not consistently display the same pattern.

Type IV hyperlipoproteinemia is common and occurs in adulthood primarily in patients who are obese, diabetic, and hyperuricemic and do not have xanthomas. It may be secondary to alcohol ingestion and can be aggravated by stress, progestins, oral contraceptives, thiazides, or β-blockers. Two genetic patterns occur in type IV hyperlipoproteinemia: familial hypertriglyceridemia, which does not carry a great risk for premature CAD, and familial combined hyperlipidemia, which is associated with increased risk of cardiovascular disease.

Rare forms of lipoprotein disorders may include hypobetalipoproteinemia, abetalipoproteinemia, Tangier disease, LCAT deficiency (fish-eye disease), cerebrotendinous xanthomatosis (CTX),

TABLE 21–5. Secondary Causes of Lipoprotein Abnormalities

Hypercholesterolemia	Hypothyroidism
	Obstructive liver disease
	Nephrotic syndrome
	Anorexia nervosa
	Acute intermittent porphyria
	Drugs: Progestins, thiazide diuretics, glucocorticoids, β-blockers, isotretinoin, protease inhibitors, cyclosporine, mirtazapine, sirolimus
Hypertriglyceridemia	Obesity
	Diabetes mellitus
	Lipodystrophy
	Glycogen storage disease
	Ileal bypass surgery
	Sepsis
	Pregnancy
	Acute hepatitis
	Systemic lupus erythematosus
	Monoclonal gammopathy: multiple myeloma, lymphoma
	Drugs: Alcohol, estrogens, isotretinoin, beta blockers, glucocorticoids, bile-acid resins, thiazides; asparaginase, interferons, azole antifungals, mirtazapine, anabolic steroids, sirolimus, bexarotene
Hypocholesterolemia	Malnutrition
	Malabsorption
	Myeloproliferative diseases
	Chronic infectious diseases: AIDS, tuberculosis
	Monoclonal gammopathy
	Chronic liver disease
Low HDL	Malnutrition
	Obesity
	Drugs: non-ISA β-blockers, anabolic steroids, probucol, isotretinoin, progestins

and sitosterolemia. Most of these rare lipoprotein disorders do not result in premature atherosclerosis, with the exceptions of familial LCAT deficiency, cerebrotendinous xanthomatosis, and sitosterolemia with xanthomatosis. Their treatment consists of dietary restriction of plant sterols (sitosterolemia with xanthomatosis) and chenodeoxycholic acid (CTX) or, potentially, blood transfusion (LCAT deficiency).

CLINICAL PRESENTATION

GENERAL

- Most patients are asymptomatic for many years prior to clinically evident disease.
- Patients with the metabolic syndrome may have three or more of the following: abdominal obesity, atherogenic dyslipidemia, raised blood pressure, insulin resistance with or without glucose intolerance, prothrombotic state, or proinflammatory state.

SYMPTOMS

- None to chest pain, palpitations, sweating, anxiety, shortness of breath, loss of consciousness or difficulty with speech or movement, abdominal pain, and sudden death.

SIGNS

- None to abdominal pain, pancreatitis, eruptive xanthomas, peripheral polyneuropathy, high blood pressure, body mass index greater than 30 kg/m^2, or waist size greater than 40 inches in men (35 inches in women).

LABORATORY TESTS

- Elevations in total cholesterol, LDL, triglycerides, apolipoprotein B, and C-reactive protein.
- Low HDL.

OTHER DIAGNOSTIC TESTS

- Lipoprotein(a), homocysteine, serum amyloid A, and small, dense LDL (pattern B).
- Various screening tests for manifestations of vascular disease (ankle-brachial index, exercise testing, magnetic resonance imaging) and diabetes (fasting glucose, oral glucose tolerance test).

PATIENT EVALUATION

A fasting lipoprotein profile (FLP) including total cholesterol, LDL cholesterol, HDL cholesterol, and triglycerides should be measured in all adults 20 years of age or older at least once every 5 years.[1] If the profile is obtained in the nonfasted state, only total cholesterol and HDL cholesterol will be usable because LDL cholesterol usually is a calculated value; if total cholesterol is 200 mg/dL or more, or if HDL cholesterol is less than 40 mg/dL, a follow-up fasting lipoprotein profile should be obtained. After a lipid abnormality is confirmed (Table 21–6), major components of the evaluation are the history (including age, gender, and if female, menstrual and estrogen-replacement status), physical examination, and laboratory investigations. A complete history and physical examination should assess (1) presence or absence of cardiovascular risk factors (Table 21–7) or definite cardiovascular disease in the individual, (2) family history of

TABLE 21–6. Classification of Total, LDL, and HDL Cholesterol and Triglycerides

Total cholesterol	
<200 mg/dL	Desirable
200–239 mg/dL	Borderline high
≥240 mg/dL	High
LDL cholesterol	
<100 mg/dL	Optimal
100–129 mg/dL	Near or above optimal
130–159 mg/dL	Borderline high
160–189 mg/dL	High
≥190 mg/dL	Very high
HDL cholesterol	
<40 mg/dL	Low
≥60 mg/dL	High
Triglycerides	
<150 mg/dL	Normal
150–199 mg/dL	Borderline high
200–499 mg/dL	High
≥500 mg/dL	Very high

HDL = high-density lipoproteins; LDL = low-density lipoproteins.

TABLE 21–7. Major Risk Factors (Exclusive of LDL Cholesterol) that Modify LDL Goals[a]

Age
  Men: ≥45 years
  Women: ≥55 years or premature menopause without
    estrogen-replacement therapy
Family history of premature CHD (definite myocardial infarction or
  sudden death before 55 years of age in father or other male
  first-degree relative or before 65 years of age in mother or other
  female first-degree relative)
Cigarette smoking
Hypertension (≥140/90 mm Hg or on antihypertensive medication)
Low HDL cholesterol (<40 mg/dL)[b]

[a]Diabetes is regarded as a coronary heart disease (CHD) risk equivalent; LDL =
low-density lipoprotein; HDL = high-density lipoprotein.
[b]HDL cholesterol (60 mg/dL) counts as a "negative" risk factor; its presence
removes one risk factor from the total count.

premature cardiovascular disease or lipid disorders, (3) presence or absence of secondary causes of lipid abnormalities, including concurrent medications (see Table 21–5), and (4) presence or absence of xanthomas or abdominal pain or history of pancreatitis, renal or liver disease, peripheral vascular disease, abdominal aortic aneurysm, or cerebral vascular disease (e.g., carotid bruits, stroke, or transient ischemic attack). An important change in the ATP III guidelines is that diabetes mellitus is regarded as a CHD risk equivalent.[1] The presence of diabetes in patients without known CHD is associated with the same level of risk as patients without diabetes but having confirmed CHD.[26] ATP III identifies three categories of risk that modify the goals and modalities of LDL-lowering therapy (Table 21–8). The highest category is known CHD or CHD risk equivalents, which is defined as the risk for major coronary events equal to or greater than established CHD; that is, more than 20% per 10 years (2% per year). The next category consists of patients with multiple (2 +) risk factors in which 10-year risk for CHD is 20% or less. The lowest risk category is persons with 0 to 1 risk factor, which is usually associated with a 10-year risk of CHD of less than 10%. Risk is estimated from Framingham risk scores.[2] Risk is estimated based on the patient's age, LDL cholesterol or total cholesterol level, blood pressure, the presence of diabetes, and smoking status (see Table 21–7). This approach for a single patient is referred to as *case finding* or *patient-based,* whereas large-scale screening and recommendations for the general populace, health care providers, and the food industry are called a *population-based approach.*

Measurement of plasma cholesterol (which is about 3% lower than serum determinations), triglyceride, and HDL cholesterol levels after a 12-hour or longer fast is important because triglycerides may be elevated in nonfasted individuals; total cholesterol is only modestly affected by fasting. Analytic and biologic variability can have a major impact on the measurement and interpretation of cholesterol (or any other laboratory test). Analytic variability can be minimized through the use of adequate quality control procedures, including internal training, routine calibration and monitoring, and external proficiency testing. Even with these measures, the coefficient of variability in the best procedures acceptably can be up to 5%, and when combined with average biologic variability, total variability may be as high as about 22%. Analytic variability with desktop equipment generally is greater in the fingerstick capillary blood methods, usually yielding measurements less than those from a clinical laboratory, and this technology should be considered for use only as a screening method. Reliance on desktop methods can result in misclassification of 7% to 14% of patients if capillary blood is used. Two determinations 1 to 8 weeks apart with the patient on a stable diet and weight and in the absence of acute illness are recommended to minimize variability and to obtain a reliable baseline.[1] If the total cholesterol level is greater than 200 mg/dL, a second determination is recommended, and if the values are more than 30 mg/dL apart, the average of three values should be used. Familiarity with the method and quality control procedures employed by local laboratories are essential for interpretation of reported values. If the physical examination and history are insufficient to diagnose a familial disorder, then agarose-gel lipoprotein electrophoresis is useful to determine which class of lipoproteins is affected. If the triglyceride levels are below 400 mg/dL and neither type III hyperlipidemia nor chylomicrons are detected by electrophoresis, then one can calculate VLDL and LDL concentrations: VLDL = triglyceride/5; LDL = total cholesterol − (VLDL + HDL).

Because total cholesterol is comprised of cholesterol derived from LDL, VLDL, and HDL, determination of HDL is useful when total plasma cholesterol is elevated. HDL may be elevated by moderate alcohol ingestion (less than two drinks per day), physical exercise, smoking cessation, weight loss, oral contraceptives, phenytoin, and terbutaline. Smoking, obesity, a sedentary lifestyle, and drugs such as β-blockers lower HDL. Only exercise and smoking cessation could be recommended as interventions for low HDL concentrations. Niacin and gemfibrozil also increase HDL concentrations.

The range of lipid concentrations represents a population mean plus or minus 2 standard deviations and does not define the risk of disease. Reference values for plasma total, LDL, and HDL cholesterol

TABLE 21–8. LDL Cholesterol Goals and Cutpoints for Therapeutic Lifestyle Changes (TLCs) and Drug Therapy in Different Risk Categories

Risk Category	LDL Goal (mg/dL)	LDL Level at Which to Initiate TLCs (mg/dL)	LDL Level at Which to Consider Drug Therapy (mg/dL)
CHD or CHD risk equivalents (10-year risk >20%)	<100	≥100	≥130 (100–129: drug optional)[a]
2+ Risk factors (10-year risk ≤20%)	<130	≥130	10-year risk 10–20%: ≥130 10-year risk <10%: ≥160
0–1 Risk factor[b]	<160	≥160	≥190 (160–189: LDL-lowering drug optional)

[a]Some authorities recommend use of LDL-lowering drugs in this category if an LDL cholesterol level of less than 100 mg/dL cannot be achieved by TLCs. Others prefer use of drugs that primarily modify triglycerides and HDL, e.g., nicotinic acid or fibrates. Clinical judgment also may call for deferring drug therapy in this subcategory.
[b]Almost all people with 0–1 risk factor have a 10-year risk of less than 10%; thus 10-year risk assessment in people with 0–1 risk factor is not necessary.
LDL = low-density lipoprotein; CHD = coronary heart disease.

TABLE 21–9. Classification of Total and Low-Density Lipoprotein Cholesterol Levels in Children and Adolescents from Families with Hypercholesterolemia or Premature Cardiovascular Disease[a]

Category	Total Cholesterol (mg/dL)	LDL Cholesterol (mg/dL)	Dietary Intervention
Acceptable	<170	<110	Recommended population eating pattern
Borderline	170–199	110–129	Step 1 diet prescribed and other risk factor interventions
High	≥200	≥130	Step 1 diet prescribed and then step 2 diet if necessary

[a]For use in children with a definite family history of premature (<50 years in females; <60 years in males) coronary heart disease, including diagnostic coronary arteriography, angioplasty, coronary artery bypass grafting, myocardial infarction, angina pectoris, peripheral vascular disease, or cerebrovascular disease before age 55 years. Screening also should be done in the offspring of a parent or sibling with blood cholesterol of 240 mg/dL or greater or, in the absence of family history, the presence of other risk factors (e.g., corticosteroid use, juvenile diabetes mellitus, hypothyroidism or other renal, endocrine, or hepatic disease known to affect cholesterol level).
From Expert Panel. National Cholesterol Education Program. Report of the Expert Panel on Blood Cholesterol Levels in Children and Adolescents. Pediatrics 1998;101:141–147.

concentrations for men and women, as well as various ethnic groups, are available from the NHANES III.[6] Cholesterol and triglycerides increase throughout life until about the fifth decade for men and the sixth decade for women. Past these ages, total cholesterol and LDL plateau and fall slightly. HDL tends to fall slightly with time and more rapidly after menopause in women. Institution of a population-based approach to cholesterol reduction should shift the entire curve to the left, and the potential reduction in cardiovascular mortality would be proportional to mean reductions at any cholesterol concentration.

Based on a careful review of the experimental pathologic, genetic, and epidemiologic evidence relating to the relationship between blood cholesterol levels and CHD, the ATP III of the NCEP recommends that a fasting lipoprotein profile and risk factor assessment be used in the initial classification of adults.[1] If total cholesterol concentration is less than 200 mg/dL, then the patient has a *desirable blood cholesterol level* (see Table 21–6). Cholesterol levels between 200 and 239 mg/dL are classified as *borderline-high blood cholesterol levels,* and assessment of risk factors (see Table 21–7) is needed to more clearly define disease risk. Blood cholesterol levels of 240 mg/dL and above are classified as *high blood cholesterol levels.* If the total cholesterol concentration is below 200 mg/dL and the HDL is above 40 mg/dL, no further follow-up is recommended for patients without known CHD and who have fewer than two risk factors. In patients with evidence of CHD or other clinical atherosclerotic disease, the LDL goal is less than 100 mg/dL, and most patients will require diet and/or drug intervention. Decisions regarding classification and management are based on the LDL cholesterol levels as outlined in Table 21–8. An increasing number of persons have the metabolic syndrome that is characterized by abdominal obesity, atherogenic dyslipidemia (elevated triglycerides, small LDL particles, low HDL cholesterol), raised blood pressure, insulin resistance (with or without glucose intolerance), and prothrombotic and proinflammatory states. ATP III recognizes the metabolic syndrome as a secondary target of

risk-reduction therapy after LDL cholesterol has been addressed, and if the metabolic syndrome is present, the patient is considered to have a CHD risk equivalent.

The Expert Panel on Children and Adolescents of the NCEP recommends screening in higher-risk children (positive family history or parental high blood cholesterol ≥ 240 mg/dL).[27] The rationale, in part, for this approach is based on the recognition that atherosclerosis begins in the childhood and adolescent years, as documented in the Pathobiologic Determinants of Atherosclerosis in Youth (PDAY) and the Bogalusa studies.[28] Similarly, if children with high blood lipids or lipoprotein levels are identified and the levels in the parents are unknown, the parents should be screened as well because they are likely to be at high risk. Racial and gender differences do exist in the determination of lipoprotein fractions, and these factors should be considered in screening. Use of the serum cholesterol level alone may be of insufficient specificity or sensitivity depending on the cut points used in screening, and other discretionary factors, such as hypertension, smoking, obesity, high-fat diet, and use of cholesterol-raising medication, may be needed to correctly identify children at risk. Table 21–9 presents these recommendations. Presently, children older than age 10 years are candidates for drug therapy if a trial of diet (6 months to 1 year) proves to be inadequate and the LDL cholesterol level remains above 190 mg/dL or above 160 mg/dL if two or more risk factors or CHD is present in the child or adolescent or if there is a history of premature CHD. The Dietary Intervention Study in Children (DISC) in pubertal children found that a fat-restricted diet modestly lowered LDL cholesterol level and maintained psychological well-being.[29] Bile acid sequestrants are the recommended drugs for this population.[30] The long-term consequences of drug therapy in this population are unknown. In special instances, familial hypercholesterolemia (particularly the homozygous form) or the existence of CHD or two or more risk factors in the child would prompt the earlier institution of drug therapy after a trial of dietary intervention.[31]

▶ TREATMENT: Hyperlipidemia

■ DESIRED OUTCOMES

The goals of therapy expressed as LDL cholesterol levels and the level of initiation of therapeutic lifestyle change (TLC) and drug therapy are provided in Tables 21–8 and Tables 21–9 for adults and

children, respectively. While these goals are surrogate end points, the primary reason to institute TLC and drug therapy is to reduce the risk first or recurrent events such as MI, angina, heart failure, ischemic stroke, or other forms of peripheral arterial disease such as carotid stenosis or abdominal aortic aneurysm.

GENERAL APPROACH

Establishing targeted changes and outcomes with consistent reinforcement of goals and measures at follow-up visits to attain goals are important to reduce barriers for optimizing TLC and pharmacologic therapy. TLC should be implemented in all patients prior to considering drug therapy. The components of TLC include reduced intakes of saturated fats and cholesterol, dietary options to reduce LDL such as plant stanols and sterols and increased soluble fiber intake, weight reduction, and increased physical activity. In general, physical activity of moderate intensity 30 minutes per day for most days of the week should be encouraged. Patients with known CAD or at high risk should be evaluated before undertaking vigorous exercise. Weight and body mass index (BMI) should be measured at each visit, and lifestyle patterns to induce a weight loss of 10% should be discussed in persons who are overweight. All patients also should be counseled to stop smoking and to meet the Joint National Committee 7 (JNC7) guidelines for control of hypertension.

NONPHARMACOLOGIC THERAPY

Individualized diet counseling that provides acceptable substitutions for unhealthy foods and ongoing reinforcement by a registered dietitian are necessary for maximal effect. The objectives of dietary therapy are to decrease the intake of total fat, saturated fatty acids (i.e., saturated fat), and cholesterol progressively and to achieve a desirable body weight. Typical American diets now include 13% to 20% of total calories from saturated fat and a cholesterol intake of 350–450 mg/day, both in excess of a "heart healthy" diet for normal Americans, let alone patients with a lipid disorder. Excessive dietary intake of cholesterol and saturated fatty acids leads to decreased hepatic clearance of LDL and deposition of LDL and oxidized LDL in peripheral tissues. The targeted saturated fatty acids have carbon chain lengths of 12 (lauric acid), 14 (myristic acid), and 16 (palmitic acid). The rationale for using a nutritionally balanced low-fat, low-cholesterol diet for the treatment of hypercholesterolemia is based on these principles: (1) It represents a reasonable extension of the diet recommended for the general public, (2) it progressively decreases the major cholesterol-raising constituent of the diet, (3) it precludes large intakes of polyunsaturated fats, and (4) it facilitates weight reduction by removing foods of high caloric density.

Dietary expertise in providing a wide range of options and suggestions in the preparation of food can make the difference between a good or an inadequate response to diet. Information concerning eating out in a healthy fashion and advice for shopping are also important factors for success in diet therapy. An example is being aware of products with misleading labels such as coffee creamers that state they contain "no cholesterol" when they may contain hydrogenated (saturated) fats or oils (e.g., palmitic acid, palm kernel oil, or coconut oil), which makes them undesirable because of their saturated fat content. Variations in polyunsaturated and saturated fat and cholesterol intake influence the LDL concentration, but the amount of cholesterol has been found to have a greater effect than the proportion of polyunsaturated or saturated fat. There also were racial differences in elevations of LDL, with high saturated fat diets being greater in whites than in other racial groups. The isomeric form of fatty acids is also important. Fatty acids with the *cis* configuration are the preferred substrate for the ACAT reaction and significantly increase hepatic LDL receptor clearance while reducing LDL cholesterol production rate.

TABLE 21–10. Macronutrient Recommendations for the TLC Diet

Component[a]	Recommended Intake
Total fat	25–35% of total calories
Saturated fat	<7% of total calories
Polyunsaturated fat	Up to 10% of total calories
Monounsaturated fat	Up to 20% of total calories
Carbohydrates[b]	50–60% of total calories
Cholesterol	<200 mg/day
Dietary fiber	20–30 g/day
Plant sterols	2 g/day
Protein	Approximately 15% of total calories
Total calories	To achieve and maintain desirable body weight

[a]Calories from alcohol not included.
[b]Carbohydrates should derive from foods rich in complex carbohydrates, such as whole grains, fruits, and vegetables.

The *trans* isomeric form cannot be used by ACAT and is biologically inactive with no effect on LDL concentration.[17]

Ideally, therapeutic TLC, including reduced intake of saturated fats and cholesterol, increased stanol/sterol and fiber intake, weight reduction, and increased physical activity, should be used to attain lower LDL cholesterol levels and to achieve reductions in CHD risk (Table 21–10). TLC may obviate the need for drug therapy, augment LDL-lowering drug therapy, and allow for lower doses. Weight control plus increased physical activity reduces risk beyond LDL cholesterol lowering, is the primary management approach for the metabolic syndrome, and raises HDL and reduces non-HDL cholesterol. Many persons should be given a 3-month trial (two visits spaced 6 weeks apart) of dietary therapy and TLC before advancing to drug therapy unless patients are at very high risk (e.g., severe hypercholesterolemia, known CHD, CHD risk equivalents, multiple risk factors, and strong family history). Although changes in blood lipid levels may occur before 3 months, adoption of a different eating pattern may require a longer period of time. It is important to involve all family members, especially if the patient is not the primary person preparing food. The NCEP and AHA both have excellent Internet-based resources to aid patients in altering their diet in a culturally sensitive manner (e.g., *http://www.americanheart.org/presenter.jhtml?identifier= 1200009* and *http://www.nhlbi.nih.gov/health/index.htm*). If all the recommended dietary changes from NCEP were instituted, the estimated reduction, on average, in LDL would range from 20% to 30%.[1] Adherence to diet and interindividual variability in macronutrient intake obviously would influence the eventual LDL level achieved. Based on the NHANES data, less than one-half of the patients who should be instructed on heart-healthy diet receive any dietary instructions.

Other dietary interventions or diet supplements may be useful in certain patients with lipid disorders. Increased intake of soluble fiber in the form of oat bran, pectins, certain gums, and psyllium products can result in useful adjunctive reductions in total and LDL cholesterol, but these dietary alterations or supplements should not be substituted for more active forms of treatment. Total daily fiber intake should be about 20 to 30 g/day, with about 25%, or 6 g/day, being soluble fiber.[1] Studies with psyllium seed in doses of 10 to 15 g/day show reductions in total and LDL cholesterol ranging from about 5% to 20%.[32] They have little or no effect on HDL cholesterol or triglyceride concentrations. These products also may be useful in managing constipation associated with the bile acid sequestrants. Psyllium binds cholesterol in the gut but also reduces hepatic production and clearance. Fish oil supplementation provides an increased amount of the omega-3 polyunsaturated fatty acids such as eicosapentaenoic acid and docosahexaenoic acid. In epidemiologic studies, ingestion of large amounts of cold water fish is associated with a reduction in CHD risk, but it is unclear whether the same advantage is conferred with commercially prepared fish oil products. Each 20 g/day ingestion of fish lowers CHD risk by 7%, and eating fish once weekly or more should reduce CHD mortality.[33] Fish oil supplementation has a fairly large effect in reducing triglycerides and VLDL cholesterol, but it either has no effect on total and LDL cholesterol or may cause elevations in these fractions. Other actions of fish oil may account for its protective effects. These effects include quantitative and qualitative alterations in the synthesis of prostanoid substances, changes in immune function and cellular proliferation, and potential antioxidative actions.[34] Responses noted with fish oil are further discussed under drug therapy.

Fat substitutes such as Olestra (Olean, sucrose polyester; Procter and Gamble), a mixture of hexa-, hepta-, and octaesters formed from the reaction of sucrose with long-chain fatty acids, are approved by the Food and Drug Administration (FDA) as a nondigestible, non-absorable, noncaloric fat substitute for snack foods. Olestra is heat-stable, an advantage over several other fat substitutes, enabling it to be used in the preparation of fried and baked foods. It is similar in composition to triglycerides, but Olestra is not hydrolyzed in the gastrointestinal tract by pancreatic lipase and, consequently, is not taken up by the intestinal mucosa. The principal adverse effects associated with Olestra use are bloating, flatulence, diarrhea, and "anal leakage." Because of the ability of Olestra to solubilize lipophilic substances, there has been concern over potential drug interactions in which lipophilic drugs (e.g., digitoxin, cyclosporin, or colchicine) or vitamins (vitamins A, D, E, and K) are solubilized in Olestra and excreted in the feces.

Recent studies have demonstrated the LDL-lowering effect of plant sterols, which are isolated from soybean and tall pine tree oils. Ingestion of 2 to 3 g/day will reduce LDL by 6% to 15%.[1] Plant sterols can be esterified to unsaturated fatty acids (creating sterol esters) to increase lipid solubility. Hydrogenating sterols produces plant stanols and, with esterification, stanol esters. The efficacy of plant sterols and plant stanols is considered to be comparable. Because lipids are needed to solubilize stanol/sterol esters, they are usually available in commercial margarines. The presence of plant stanols/sterols is listed on the food label. When margarine products are used, persons must be advised to adjust caloric intake to account for the calories contained in the products. Benecol (McNeil), as an example, is a butter-like spread that contains a plant stanol ester, an ingredient that can lower cholesterol and which is derived from plant stanols found naturally in small amounts in foods such as wheat, rye, and corn.

Drug therapy is indicated following an adequate trial of TLC changes as outlined in Tables 21–8 and Tables 21–9.

PHARMACOLOGIC THERAPY

There are now numerous randomized, double-blinded clinical trials demonstrating that reduction of LDL reduces CHD event rates in primary prevention, secondary intervention, and angiographic trials.[13,15,35–37] Generally speaking, for every 1% reduction in LDL, there is a 1% reduction in CHD event rates.[1] However, if treatment extends beyond the typical duration of a clinical trial (2–5 years), the accumulated benefit could be greater. Elevations of HDL of 1% result in approximately 2% reduction in CHD events.[15] Of interest, angiographic trials, which typically cause small changes in luminal

diameter (e.g., about a 0.04-mm difference in change between placebo and active treatment), result in fewer clinical events such as MI or the need for revascularization.[37] This unexpected finding suggests that plaque size and luminal encroachment by plaque may be less important than the effects that cholesterol lowering may have on the activity in the plaque and endothelial dysfunction. These studies provide a strong rationale for attempting to lower plasma cholesterol and LDL levels in patients with hypercholesterolemia.

4 Although many efficacious lipid-lowering drugs exist, none is effective in all lipoprotein disorders, and all such agents are associated with some adverse effects.[38] Lipid-lowering drugs can be divided broadly into agents that decrease the synthesis of VLDL and LDL, agents that enhance VLDL clearance, agents that enhance LDL catabolism, agents that decrease cholesterol absorption, agents that elevate HDL, or some combination of these characteristics (Table 21–11). Table 21–12 lists recommended drugs of choice for each lipoprotein phenotype and alternate agents. Table 21–13 lists available products and their doses.

Treatment of type I hyperlipoproteinemia is directed toward reduction of chylomicrons derived from dietary fat with the subsequent reduction in plasma triglycerides. Total daily fat intake should be no more than 10 to 25 g, or approximately 15% of total calories. Secondary causes of hypertriglyceridemia (see Table 21–5) should be excluded, or if present, the underlying disorder should be treated appropriately. Type V hyperlipoproteinemia also requires a stringent restriction of the fat component of dietary intake; in addition, drug therapy is indicated, as outlined in Table 21–12, if the response to diet alone is inadequate. Medium-chain triglycerides, which are absorbed without chylomicron formation, may be used as a dietary supplement for caloric intake if needed for types I and V. Hepatic fibrosis has been reported with medium-chain triglycerides. Omega-3 fatty acids may be useful in lipoprotein lipase deficiency in some patients. In patients with apolipoprotein C-II deficiency, infusion of plasma may normalize plasma triglyceride levels.

Primary hypercholesterolemia (i.e., familial hypercholesterolemia, familial combined hyperlipidemia, and type IIa hyperlipoproteinemia) is treated with the bile acid resins (BARs) or sequestrants (colestipol, cholestyramine, and colesevelam), HMG-CoA reductase inhibitors (statins), niacin, or eztimibe. Of these choices, statins are first choice because they are the most potent LDL-lowering agents. Statins interrupt the conversion of HMG-CoA to mevalonate, the rate-limiting step in de novo cholesterol biosynthesis, by inhibiting HMG-CoA reductase (see Fig. 21–3). Currently available products include lovastatin, pravastatin, simvastatin, fluvastatin, and atorvastatin. Rosuvastatin is the most potent statin currently on the market. Table 21–14 lists the pharmacokinetic properties of the statins.[39] The plasma half-lives for all the statins are reported to be short, except for atorvastatin and rosuvastatin, and this may account for their potency.[40] In CURVES, the largest head-to-head comparison of statins, atorvastatin was found to be the most potent drug for lowering total cholesterol and LDL cholesterol prior to the introduction of rosuvastatin, with reductions in LDL cholesterol of 38%, 46%, 51%, and 54% for the 10-, 20-, 40-, and 80-mg doses, respectively.[41] Metabolic studies with statins in normal volunteers and in patients with hypercholesterolemia suggest reduced synthesis of LDL cholesterol, as well as enhanced catabolism of LDL mediated through LDL receptors, as the principal mechanisms for lipid-lowering effects. Total and LDL cholesterol are reduced in a dose-related fashion by 30% or more on average when added to dietary therapy, with the effects being more pronounced in nonfamilial than in familial hypercholesterolemia.

6 Combination therapy with bile acid sequestrants and lovastatin is rational because LDL receptor numbers are increased, leading

TABLE 21–11. Effects of Drug Therapy on Lipids and Lipoproteins

Drug	Mechanism of Action	Effects on Lipids	Effects on Lipoproteins	Comment
Cholestyramine, colestipol, and colesevelam	↑LDL catabolism ↓Cholesterol absorption	↓Cholesterol	↓LDL ↑VLDL	Problem with compliance; binds many coadministered acidic drugs
Niacin	↓LDL and VLDL Synthesis	↓Triglyceride and cholesterol	↓VLDL, ↓LDL, ↑HDL	Problems with patient acceptance; good in combination with bile acid resins; extended-release niacin causes less flushing and is less hepatotoxic than sustained-release niacin
Probucol	↑LDL clearance	↓Cholesterol	↓LDL and HDL	Lowers HDL; modest efficacy but inhibits LDL oxidation and facilitates reverse cholesterol transport
Gemfibrozil, fenofibrate, clofibrate	↑VLDL clearance ↓VLDL synthesis	↓Triglyceride and cholesterol	↓VLDL, ↓LDL, ↑HDL	Clofibrate causes cholesterol gallstones; modest LDL lowering; raises HDL; gemfibrozil inhibits glucuronidation of simvastatin, lovastatin, and atorvastatin
Lovastatin, pravastatin, simvastatin, fluvastatin, atorvastatin, rosuvastatin	↑LDL catabolism; inhibit LDL synthesis	↓Cholesterol	↓LDL	Highly effective in heterozygous familial hypercholesterolemia and in combination with other agents
Ezetimibe	Inhibits cholesterol absorption across the intestinal border	↓Cholesterol	↓LDL	Few adverse effects; effects additive to other drugs

to greater degradation of LDL cholesterol, intracellular synthesis of cholesterol is inhibited, and enterohepatic recycling of bile acids is interrupted. Combination therapy with a statin plus eztimibe is also rational because eztimibe inhibits cholesterol absorption across the gut border and adds 12% to 20% further reduction when combined with a statin or other drugs.[42,43] In the Expanded Clinical Evaluation of Lovastatin (EXCEL) in more than 8000 patients, lovastatin reduced LDL cholesterol by 24% to 40% when given in doses ranging from

TABLE 21–12. Lipoprotein Phenotype and Recommended Drug Treatment

Lipoprotein Type	Drug of Choice	Combination Therapy
I	Not indicated	—
IIa	Statins	Niacin or BAR
	Cholestyramine or colestipol	Statins or niacin
	Niacin	Statins or BAR Ezetimibe
IIb	Statins	BAR or fibrates or niacin
	Fibrates	Statins or niacin or BAR[a]
	Niacin	Statins or fibrates Ezetimibe
III	Fibrates	Statins or niacin
	Niacin	Statins or fibrates Ezetimibe
IV	Fibrates	Niacin
	Niacin	Fibrates
V	Fibrates	Niacin
	Niacin	Fish oils

[a]BARs are not used as first-line therapy if triglycerides are elevated at baseline because hypertriglyceridemia may worsen with BARs alone.
BAR = bile acid resins; fibrates include gemfibrozil or fenofibrate.

20 mg once daily to 40 mg twice daily.[44] Constipation in placebo-treated patients occurred in 4.7% of patients, whereas lovastatin was associated with constipation in 4.2% to 7.7% of patients (20 mg twice a day). Elevation of serum transaminase levels (primarily alanine aminotransferase) to greater than three times the upper limit of normal and associated muscle symptoms (myopathy) were most common at higher doses (40 mg given twice a day)—1.5% compared with placebo at 0.1%. Creatine kinase (CK) concentrations greater than 10 times the upper limit of normal and muscle symptoms occurred in 0% of the placebo group versus 0.2% of the lovastatin group, and any elevation of CK was highest at 40 mg given twice a day, 3.5% versus 1.6% for placebo. Meta-analyses of placebo-controlled studies with statins demonstrate a low risk of abnormal alanine amino-transferase (ALT) or CK levels and a low risk of myopathy with or without rhabdomyolysis.[45] Lens opacities have been reported with lovastatin; however, in the age groups studied, these abnormalities are common and tend to wax and wane with time irrespective of drug therapy, and no statistical association is known to exist. As a category of monotherapy, the HMG-CoA reductase inhibitors are the most potent total and LDL cholesterol–lowering agents and among the best tolerated.[35,36,46–49] Recently, a potential mechanism for poor response to statin therapy was described.[50] Poor responders had a low basal rate of cholesterol synthesis that may be secondary to a genetically determined increase in cholesterol absorption, possibly mediated by apolipoprotein E4 or by polymorphisms in the HMG-CoA reductase gene.[39,40] Interestingly, statins may reduce the risk of cancer based on observational studies.[51]

The primary action of BARs is to bind bile acids in the intestinal lumen, with a concurrent interruption of enterohepatic circulation of bile acids and a markedly increased excretion of acidic steroids in the feces. This decreases the bile acid pool size and stimulates hepatic synthesis of bile acids from cholesterol. Depletion of the hepatic pool of cholesterol results in an increase in cholesterol biosynthesis and an increase in the number of LDL receptors on the hepatocyte membrane.

TABLE 21–13. Comparison of Drugs Used in the Treatment of Hyperlipidemia

Drug	Manufacturer	Dosage Forms	Usual Daily Dose	Maximum Daily Dose
Cholestyramine (Questran)	BMS	Bulk powder/4-g packets	8 g tid	32 g
Cholestyramine (Questran Light)	BMS	Bulk powder/4-g packets		
Cholestyramine (Cholybar)	Parke-Davis	4 g resin per bar		
Colestipol hydrochloride (Colestid)	Upjohn	Bulk powder/5-g packets	10 g bid	30 g
Colesevelam (Welchol)	Sankyo	625-mg tablets	1875 mg bid	4375 mg
Niacin	Various	50-, 100-, 250-, and 500-mg tablets; 125-, 250-, and 500-mg capsules	2 g tid	9 g
Extended-release niacin (Niaspan)	Kos	500-, 750-, and 1000-mg tablets	500 mg	2000 mg
Extended-release niacin + lovastatin (Advicor)[a]	Kos	Niacin/lovastatin 500-mg/20-mg tablets Niacin/lovastatin 750-mg/20-mg tablets Niacin/lovastatin 1000-mg/20-mg tablets	Niacin/lovastatin 500 mg/20 mg	Niacin/lovastatin 1000 mg/20 mg
Clofibrate (Atromid-S)	Wyeth-Ayerst	500-mg capsules	1 g bid	2 g
Fenofibrate (Tricor)	Abbott, various	43-, 67-, 87-, 134-, and 200-mg capsules (micronized); 48-, 54-, 145- and 160-mg tablets	54 mg or 67 mg	201 mg
Gemfibrozil (Lopid)	Parke-Davis	600-mg capsules	600 mg bid	1.2 g
Lovastatin (Mevacor)	MSD	20- and 40-mg tablets	20–40 mg	80 mg
Pravastatin (Pravachol)	Bristol-Myers Squibb	10- and 20-mg tablets	10–20 mg	40 mg
Simvastatin (Zocor)	MSD	5-, 10-, 20-, 40-, and 80-mg tablets	10–20 mg	80 mg
Atorvastatin (Lipitor)	Pfizer	10-mg tablets	10 mg	80 mg
Rosuvastatin (Crestor)	Astra-Zeneca	5- and 10-mg tablets	5 mg	40 mg
Ezetimibe (Zetia)	MSD	10-mg tablet	10 mg	10 mg
Atorvastatin/amlodipine (Caduet)	Pfizer	Atorvastatin/amlodipine 10 mg/5 mg Atorvastatin/amlodipine 20 mg/5 mg Atorvastatin/amlodipine 40 mg/5 mg Atorvastatin/amlodipine 80 mg/5 mg Atorvastatin/amlodipine 10 mg/10 mg Atorvastatin/amlodipine 20 mg/10 mg Atorvastatin/amlodipine 40 mg/10 mg Atorvastatin/amlodipine 80 mg/10 mg	Atovastatin/amlodipine 10 mg/5 mg	Atovastatin/amlodipine 80 mg/10 mg
Pravastatin/aspirin (Pravigard PAC)	BMS	Pravastatin/aspirin 20 mg/81 mg Pravastatin/aspirin 20 mg/325 mg Pravastatin/aspirin 40 mg/81 mg Pravastatin/aspirin 40 mg/325 mg Pravastatin/aspirin 80 mg/81 mg Pravastatin/aspirin 80 mg/325 mg		
Simvastatin/ezetimibe (Vytorin)	Merck/Schering-Plough	Simvastatin/ezetimibe 10 mg/10 mg Simvastatin/ezetimibe 20 mg/10 mg Simvastatin/ezetimibe 40 mg/ 10 mg	Simvastatin/ezetimibe 20 mg/10 mg	Simvastatin/ezetimibe 40 mg/10 mg

[a]The manufacturer does not recommend use of the fixed combination as initial therapy of primary hypercholesterolemia or mixed dyslipidemia. It is specifically indicated in patients receiving lovastatin alone plus diet who require an additional reduction in triglyceride levels or increase in HDL cholesterol levels; it is also indicated in those treated with niacin alone who require additional decreases in LDL cholesterol.

bid = twice daily; probucol is no longer on the market in the United States; gemfibrozil, fenofibrate, and lovastatin are available as generic products; BMS = Bristol-Myers Squibb; MSD = Merck Sharp & Dohme.

TABLE 21–14. Pharmacokinetics of the Statins

Parameter	Lovastatin	Simvastatin	Pravastatin	Fluvastatin	Atorvastatin	Rosuvastatin
Isoenzyme	3A4	3A4	None	2C9	3A4	2C9/2C19
Lipophilic	Yes	Yes	No	Yes	Yes	No
Protein binding (%)	>95	95–98	~50	>90	96	88
Active metabolites	Yes	Yes	No	No	Yes	Yes
Elimination half-life (hr.)	3	2	1.8	1.2	7–14	13–20

Isoenzyme refers to the specific isoenzyme in the cytochrome P450 system that is responsible for the metabolism of each drug. Pharmacokinetic parameters in this table are based on studies and reviews presented in the literature.

The increased number of receptors stimulates an enhanced rate of catabolism from plasma and lowers LDL levels. Cholesteryl ester transfer protein (CETP), which is correlated with total and LDL cholesterol concentrations, is also reduced by BARs, perhaps by interfering with hepatic microsomal cholesterol content.[53] Patients with homozygous familial hypercholesterolemia genetically lack the ability to increase synthesis of LDL receptors, and bile acid resins generally are ineffective. The increase in hepatic cholesterol biosynthesis may be paralleled by increased hepatic VLDL production, and consequently, bile acid resins may aggravate hypertriglyceridemia in patients with combined hyperlipidemia. Gastrointestinal complaints of constipation, bloating, epigastric fullness, nausea, and flatulence are reported most commonly.[1] With intensive education, patients can learn to tolerate resins on a long-term basis, as evidenced by adherence in clinical trials to active drug regimens, but in routine clinical practice, 40% or more of patients will discontinue therapy within 1 year.[54,55] These adverse effects can be managed by increasing the fluid intake, modifying the diet to increase bulk, and using stool softeners. The other major limiting complaint is the gritty texture and bulk; these problems may be minimized by mixing the powder with orange drink or juice. Tablet forms of bile acid sequestrants should help in improving compliance with this form of therapy, whereas the bar form does not improve compliance.[30] Other potential adverse effects include impaired absorption of fat-soluble vitamins A, D, E, and K, hypernatremia and hyperchloremia, gastrointestinal obstruction, and reduced bioavailability of acidic drugs such as coumarin anticoagulants, digitoxin, nicotinic acid, thyroxine, acetaminophen, hydrocortisone, hydrochlorothiazide, loperamide, and possibly iron. Hyperchloremic metabolic acidosis, hypernatremia, and gastrointestinal obstruction have been reported almost exclusively in children, and malabsorption of fat-soluble vitamins is probably most common with high doses (e.g., 30 g/day of cholestyramine) of the BARs. Drug interactions may be avoided by alternating administration times with an interval of 6 hours or greater between the BAR and other drugs. Colestipol and cholestyramine have comparable side effects, but colestipol may have better palatability because it is odorless and tasteless. Colesevelam is the newest BAR, and total and LDL cholesterol reduction is dose-related. The adverse effects are similar qualitatively to the older BARs but may occur less often. Because of adverse effects occurring commonly with BARs at higher doses, BARs are used increasingly in combination with other drugs because low doses are tolerated well, and they work in a complementary fashion with other agents.

Niacin (nicotinic acid) also may be used in primary hypercholesterolemia in combination with bile acid sequestrants or as monotherapy for this disorder and others (see Table 21–12). Niacin reduces the hepatic synthesis of VLDL, which, in turn, leads to a reduction in the synthesis of LDL. Factors responsible for decreased production of VLDL include inhibition of lipolysis with a decrease in free fatty acids in plasma, decreased hepatic esterification of triglycerides, and a possible direct effect on the hepatic production of apolipoprotein B. The complementary action of niacin and bile acid sequestrants to increase catabolism and decrease synthesis of LDL may account for the additive effects of this combination in hyperlipidemia. Niacin also increases HDL by reducing its catabolism. Niacin selectively decreases hepatic removal of HDL apoA-I but not removal of cholesterol esters, thereby increasing the capacity of retained apoA-I to augment reverse cholesterol transport in isolated hepatic cells. The principal use of niacin is for mixed hyperlipemia or as a second-line agent in combination therapy for hypercholesterolemia. It is also considered to be the first-line agent or an alternative for the treatment of hypertriglyceridemia and diabetic dyslipidemia.[56,57] There are numerous smaller trials suggesting that lower doses of niacin may be combined with statins or gemfibrozil to minimize adverse effects and maximize response. These combinations require careful monitoring because interactions do occur.

Niacin has many adverse drug reactions that occur commonly; fortunately, most of the symptoms and biochemical abnormalities seen do not require discontinuation of therapy. Cutaneous flushing and itching appear to be prostaglandin-mediated and can be reduced by aspirin 325 mg given shortly before niacin ingestion.[1] Flushing seems to be related to rising plasma concentrations of niacin; taking the dose with meals and slowly titrating the dose upward may minimize these effects. Gastrointestinal intolerance and flushing are common problems. Acanthosis nigricans, a darkening of the skin in skinfold areas and an external marker of insulin resistance, may be seen with high doses of niacin. Sustained-release products may minimize these complaints in some patients, but controlled trials with regular-release products do not demonstrate much of a difference between sustained- and regular-release products. The only legend form of niacin, Niaspan (Kos), is an extended-release form with pharmacokinetics intermediate between instant and sustained-release products that are sold as food supplements rather than legend products. In controlled trials, Niaspan is reported to have fewer dermatologic reactions and has a low risk for hepatoxicity.[58,59] Potentially important laboratory abnormalities occurring with niacin therapy include elevated liver function tests, hyperuricemia, and hyperglycemia. Recent experience with niacin in diabetes suggests that some diabetic patients do not have worsened glycemic control with dose titration and sustained-release products.[60] With less than 3 g/day, the degree of liver function test elevation generally is not marked and often is transient, and a temporary reduction in dosage frequently corrects the problem. Niacin-associated hepatitis is more common with sustained-release preparations, and their use should be restricted to patients intolerant of regular-release products.[60] Sustained-release products often are more expensive, and given the lack of data for reduced adverse effects and the increased incidence of hepatitis, regular-release products always should be used first. Preexisting gout and diabetes may be exacerbated by niacin; these patients should be monitored more closely, and their medication should be titrated appropriately. Patients with well-controlled type 2 diabetes mellitus do not have significant changes in glycemic control with niacin at doses of 2 g/day or less.[62,63] Niacin is contraindicated in patients with active liver disease. Dry eyes and other ophthalmologic complaints are also noted occasionally. Concomitant alcohol and hot drinks may magnify flushing and pruritus with niacin, and they should be avoided at the time of ingestion. Nicotinamide should not be used in the treatment of hyperlipidemia because it does not lower cholesterol or triglyceride levels effectively.

Combined hyperlipoproteinemia (type IIb) may be treated with statins, niacin, or gemfibrozil to lower LDL cholesterol without elevating VLDLs and triglycerides. Niacin is the most effective agent and may be combined with a bile acid sequestrant. BARs alone in this disorder may elevate VLDLs and triglycerides, and their use as single agents for treating combined hyperlipoproteinemia should be avoided. Fibric acid (e.g., gemfibrozil, fenofibrate, or clofibrate) monotherapy is effective in reducing VLDL, but a reciprocal rise in LDL may occur, and total cholesterol values may remain relatively unchanged. Gemfibrozil reduces the synthesis of VLDL and, to a lesser extent, apolipoprotein B, with a concurrent increase in the rate of removal of triglyceride-rich lipoproteins from plasma. Plasma HDL concentrations may rise 10% to 15% or more with fibrates. Ezetimibe also could be used in combination therapy in type IIb. Gastrointestinal complaints with fibric acid derivatives occur in 3% to 5% of patients, rash in 2% of patients, dizziness in 2.4% of patients, and transient elevations in transaminase and alkaline phosphatase levels in 4.5% and 1.3% of patients, respectively. Similar to clofibrate, gemfibrozil may enhance the formation of gallstones associated with an increase in the lithogenic index; however, the rate is low (0.6%) and similar to that seen with placebo in the Helsinki Heart Study.[15] Other studies have found the relative risk for gallstones to be 1.7.[64] Fibric acid derivatives may potentiate the effects of oral anticoagulants, and the prothrombin time and international normalized ratio should be monitored very closely with this combination.

Type III hyperlipoproteinemia may be treated with fibric acid derivatives or niacin. Although clofibrate has been suggested as the drug of choice for this disorder, given the lack of data supporting its efficacy in altering cardiovascular mortality in the major studies on hypercholesterolemia and its numerous, well-documented, and serious adverse effects, it is reasonable to consider niacin, gemfibrozil, or fenofibrate prior to the use of clofibrate. Clofibrate increases the activity of lipoprotein lipase and reduces to a lesser extent the synthesis or secretion of VLDL from the liver into the plasma. Clofibrate is less effective than gemfibrozil or niacin in reducing VLDL production. The most disturbing aspects of clofibrate's adverse effects are its potential to induce gallstones (4.7%, clofibrate; 0.54%, placebo), promote ventricular ectopy, and potentially cause gastrointestinal malignancy, resulting in a greater overall mortality than placebo alone.[1] A myositis syndrome of myalgia, weakness, stiffness, malaise, and elevations in creatinine phosphokinase and aspartate aminotransaminase is seen with the fibric acid derivatives, and it seems to be more common in patients with renal insufficiency. Enhanced hypoglycemic effects are reported to occur when fibric acid derivatives are given to patients on sulfonylurea compounds, but the mechanisms for these interactions are not well understood. Rifampin, a hepatic enzyme inducer of oxidative pathways, may induce the metabolism of clofibrate, but the long-term consequences are unknown.

Three fibric acid derivatives (clofibrate, gemfibrozil, and fenofibrate) are approved in the United States; however, several others are under development or are being used in Europe, including bezafibrate and ciprofibrate. All reduce LDL cholesterol by 20% to 25% in heterozygous familial hypercholesterolemia. The response of LDL cholesterol, HDL cholesterol, and triglycerides to this category of drug is very dependent on the specific lipoprotein type (e.g., type IIa versus IIb) and the baseline triglyceride concentration.[68]

As a potential alternative therapy for this phenotype, numerous epidemiologic and normal volunteer studies have found that diets high in omega-3 polyunsaturated fatty acids (from fish oil), mostly commonly eicosapentaenoic acid, reduce cholesterol, triglycerides, LDL cholesterol, and VLDL cholesterol and may elevate HDL cholesterol.[17,33] The effects of fish oil on lipoprotein metabolism are mediated through a reduction in VLDL production and suppression of VLDL apolipoprotein B. In patients with hypertriglyceridemia, either type IIb or type V phenotype, a diet high in omega-3 fatty acids given for 4 weeks reduced cholesterol 27% and 45% and triglyceride 64% and 79%, respectively.[33] A diet high in eicosapentaenoic acid given to hyperlipidemic hemodialysis patients resulted in significant decreases in cholesterol and triglycerides for as long as 13 weeks. Fish oil supplementation may be most useful in patients with hypertriglyceridemia; however, its role in treatment is not well defined. Potential complications of fish oil supplementation, such as thrombocytopenia and bleeding disorders, have been noted, especially with high doses (eicosapentaenoic acid 15–30 g/day), and well-controlled trials are needed to determine if fish oils are safe and effective before their use may be broadly recommended. Based a recent meta-analysis, fish consumption lowers the risk of CHD, but nutraceuticals have not been tested adequately.[33]

Combination drug therapy may be considered after adequate trials of monotherapy and for patients documented to be compliant with the prescribed regimen. Two or three lipoprotein profiles at 6-week intervals should confirm lack of response prior to initiation of combination therapy. Cholestyramine may be added in patients with fasting hypertriglyceridemia, but it should not be used as the initial drug because triglycerides are likely to increase. Contraindications to and drug interactions with combined therapy should be screened carefully, as well as consideration of the extra cost of drug product and monitoring that may be required. In general, a statin and a BAR or niacin with a BAR provides the greatest reduction in total and LDL cholesterol. Regimens intended to increase HDL levels should include either gemfibrozil or niacin, and it should be remembered that statins combined with either of these drugs may result in a greater incidence of hepatotoxicity or myositis. This is particulary important for statins that are eliminated via cytochrome P450 3A4 or through glucuronidation.[39,65] Familial combined hyperlipidemia may respond better to a fibric acid and a statin than to a fibric acid and a BAR.[66,67]

Severe forms of hypercholesterolemia—such as familial hypercholesterolemia, familial defective apolipoprotein B-100, severe polygenic hypercholesterolemia, familial combined hyperlipidemia, and familial dysbetalipoproteinemia (type III)—may require more intensive therapy. In particular, familial hypercholesterolemia patients often require combination therapy (two or three drugs) and are managed with surgical therapy (partial ileal bypass), plasmapheresis (LDL-apheresis), and liver transplantation (to replace LDL receptors).

HYPERTRIGLYCERIDEMIA

It is important to remember that lipoprotein pattern types I, III, IV, and V are associated with hypertriglyceridemia and that these primary lipoprotein disorders and underlying diseases should be excluded prior to implementing therapy (see Table 21–5). A positive family history of CHD is important in identifying patients at risk for premature atherosclerosis.[16,68] If a patient with CHD has elevated triglycerides, the associated abnormality is probably a contributing factor to CHD and should be treated.[56]

High serum triglycerides (see Tables 21–6 and Tables 21–12) should be treated by achieving desirable body weight, consumption of a low saturated fat and cholesterol diet, regular exercise, smoking cessation, and restriction of alcohol (in selected patients). ATP III identifies the sum of LDL + VLDL (termed *non-HDL* [total cholesterol–HDL]) as a secondary target of therapy in persons with high triglycerides (≥200 mg/dL). This approach is used when triglycerides exceed 200 mg/dL and accounts for atherogenic particles carried in VLDL and remnant particles. The goal for non-HDL in persons with high serum triglycerides can be set at 30 mg/dL higher than that for LDL on the premise that a VLDL level of 30 mg/dL or less is normal. In patients with borderline high triglycerides but with accompanying risk factors of established CHD disease, family history of premature CHD, concomitant LDL elevation or low HDL, and genetic forms of hypertriglyceridemia associated with CHD (familial dysbetalipoproteinemia, familial combined hyperlipidemia), drug therapy with niacin should be considered. Niacin may be used cautiously in diabetics based on the results of the ADMIT trial, which found that triglycerides were reduced by 23%, HDL cholesterol was increased by 29%, there was only a slight increase in glucose (mean 8.7 mg/dL), and there was no change in hemoglobin A$_{1c}$.[63] Alternative therapies include gemfibrozil, statins, and fish oil.[70,71] Fibrates may increase LDL, and their use in borderline high triglyceridemia requires careful monitoring to detect this deleterious change in lipid profile. Statins also may be used because they provide modest reductions in triglycerides and modest elevations in HDL. Higher doses of atorvastatin and fluvastatin may reduce HDL as well as LDL and triglycerides.[72] The goal of therapy in this situation is to lower triglycerides and VLDL particles that may be atherogenic, increase HDL, and reduce LDL.

Very high triglycerides are associated with pancreatitis and other consequences of the chylomicron syndrome. At this level of elevation of triglycerides, a genetic form of hypertriglyceridemia often coexists with other causes of elevated triglycerides such as diabetes. Dietary fat restriction (10% to 20% of calories as fat), weight loss, alcohol restriction, and treatment of the coexisting disorder are the basic elements of management. Drugs useful in hypertriglyceridemia include gemfibrozil, niacin, and higher-potency statins (e.g., atorvastatin, rosuvastatin, and simvastatin). Gemfibrozil is the preferred drug in diabetics because of the effect of niacin on glycemic control unless the newer extended-release forms are used. Fenofibrate may be preferred in combination with statin therapy because it does not impair glucuronidation and minimizes potential drug interactions. Success in treatment is defined as a reduction in triglycerides below 500 mg/dL.[1]

LOW HDL CHOLESTEROL

Low HDL is a strong independent risk predictor of CHD. The ATP III redefined low HDL cholesterol as less than 40 mg/dL but specified no goal for HDL cholesterol raising.[1] Low HDL may be a consequence of insulin resistance, physical inactivity, type 2 diabetes, cigarette smoking, very high carbohydrate intake, and certain drugs (see Table 21–5). In low HDL, the primary target remains LDL according to the ATP III, but emphasis shifts to weight reduction, increased physical activity, and smoking cessation and, if drug therapy is required, to fibric acid derivatives and niacin. Niacin has the potential for the greatest increase in HDL, and the effect is more pronounced with regular or immediate-release forms than with sustained-release forms.[61]

DIABETIC DYSLIPIDEMIA

Diabetic dyslipidemia is characterized by hypertriglyceridemia, low HDL, and LDL that is minimally elevated. Small, dense LDL (pattern B) in diabetes is more atherogenic than larger, more buoyant forms of LDL (pattern A); routine lipoprotein profiles do not differentiate between pattern A and pattern B.[72] Diabetes in the ATP III is a CHD risk equivalent, and the primary target is LDL, with a goal of treatment being to lower LDL cholesterol to less than 100 mg/dL.[1] When the LDL concentration is greater than 130 mg/dL, most patients will require simultaneous therapeutic lifestyle changes and drug therapy. When the LDL cholesterol concentration is between 100 and 129 mg/dL, intensifying glycemic control, adding drugs for the atherogenic dyslipidemia (fibric acid derivatives and niacin), and intensifying LDL cholesterol–lowering therapy are options. Because the primary target is LDL cholesterol in diabetic dyslipidemia, statins are considered by many to be the initial drugs of choice.[1,28] The relative risk reduction for CHD in diabetics versus nondiabetics was greater in the West of Scotland (37% versus 20%),[35] AFCAPS/TexCAPS (43% versus 36%),[47] CARE (25% versus 23%),[48] and 4S (55% versus 32%) trials.[36] All statins are fairly comparable in triglyceride lowering, and because statins differ in potency for LDL reduction, a ratio of LDL reduction to triglyceride reduction can be applied. Statin therapy may

protect against the development of diabetes, but the observations from the West of Scotland study with pravastatin need to be confirmed in a prospective trial.[73] The most recent trial of LDL lowering in type 2 diabetes mellitus is the Collaborative Atorvastatin Diabetes Study (CARDS).[74] This was a randomized, double-blind, placebo comparison of atorvastatin 10 mg/day versus placebo in 2838 diabetes patients to reduce first CHD events. Baseline LDL concentration was 118 mg/dL, and with atorvastatin, LDL concentration fell by 46 mg/dL. The primary end point, a composite of acute CHD death, nonfatal MI, hospitalized unstable angina, resuscitated cardiac arrest, coronary revascularization, or stroke, was reduced by 37%. This study suggests that all diabetics should have an LDL concentration that is much lower than 100 mg/dL, and these results are consistent with the Heart Protection Study analysis of diabetic patients.[75]

Fenofibrate, according to the DIAS trial, reduced the angiographic progression of CAD in type 2 diabetes.[76] Fewer CHD events were seen with fenofibrate compared with placebo, but the difference was not significant. Fibric acids principally lower VLDL and triglycerides while increasing HDL with only modest lowering of total and LDL cholesterol; on occasion, fibric acid derivatives may increase LDL levels. Fibric acid derivatives tend to improve glucose tolerance, in contrast to niacin; the greatest effect has been seen with bezafibrate. The Helsinki Heart Study found gemfibrozil to be most effective in diabetic dyslipidemia.[15] Although the effect of statins on triglycerides and HDL abnormalities commonly seen in diabetes is less than with fibric acids, the subgroup analyses cited earlier suggest that they reduce CHD risk significantly. Cholestyramine in diabetic patients may result in lower LDL levels, but VLDL and triglyceride levels, which are commonly elevated in diabetes, may be further increased in this population. Resins may aggravate constipation, which is common in diabetics. As demonstrated in the ADMIT and ADVENT trials, immediate- and extended-release niacins are very effective in raising HDL concentrations and lowering triglyceride and LDL concentrations.[62,63]

SPECIAL CONSIDERATIONS

ELDERLY

Hypercholesterolemia is an independent risk factor for CHD in the elderly (>65 years old), as it is in the younger patient. The attributable risk, which is the difference in absolute rates of CHD between segments of the population with higher or lower serum cholesterol levels, increases with age. Older patients potentially benefit to a greater extent from cholesterol lowering than younger populations. Data from studies of elderly men in a variety of settings are consistent with a relative risk of at least 1.5 in the highest compared with the lowest quartile of cholesterol levels.[75] Treatment of hypercholesterolemia in the elderly may bring about a comparable reduction in absolute risk to that obtained in younger persons.[1] Subgroup analyses of the West of Scotland (primary) and 4S (secondary) intervention studies show that elderly patients have lower CHD risk reduction (relative risk reduction of 27% and 29%, respectively) as compared with younger patients (relative risk reduction of 40% and 39%, respectively).[35,36] The Framingham Study suggests that elderly women are at higher risk because of high blood cholesterol levels, but no other large studies included women; and their risks or benefits from cholesterol reduction are not well defined. Primary prevention in younger patients requires about 2 years before reduction in CHD risk is apparent, and this lag time should be taken into consideration in patient selection for therapy. Nonlipid CHD risk factors do not decline in relative risk with aging, and aggressive management of the modifiable nonlipid risk factors is important in older patients. High-risk elderly patients are less likely to be prescribed statins, and their potent benefits are not realized.[78] Because most women with CHD are elderly and also at risk for osteoporosis, they are logical candidates for diet therapy with consideration of calcium intake consistent with osteoporosis prevention, exercise, and perhaps estrogen-replacement therapy. Recent evidence suggests that statins may reduce the risk of osteoporosis; however, there are conflicting data from various studies.[79]

Drug therapy in principle differs little from that in younger patients, and older patients respond to lipid-lowering drugs as well as younger patients.[80,81] Based on the Heart Protection Study with more elderly patients than any other trial, simvastatin 40 mg/day produced the same CHD event rate reduction in patients over 70 years of age as in younger patients.[81] The gain in life expectancy may be small depending on age at the start of treatment and magnitude of cholesterol reduction.[82] Changes in body composition, renal function, and other physiologic changes of aging may make older patients more susceptible to adverse effects of lipid-lowering drug therapy. In particular, older patients are more likely to have constipation (bile acid resins), skin and eye changes (niacin), gout (niacin), gallstones (fibric acid derivatives), and bone/joint disorders (fibric acid derivatives, statins). Therapy should be started with lower doses and titrated up slowly to minimize adverse effects.

WOMEN

Cholesterol is an important determinant of CHD in women, but the relationship is not as strong as that seen in men. HDL may be a more important predictor of disease in women.[83,84] LDL and HDL genetic regulation in women and men does not appear to be different. Based on the Nurses' Health Study, obesity is an important determinant of CHD in women, with the relative risk being 3.3 in the highest Quetelet index (weight in kilograms divided by the square of the height in meters) as compared with the lowest category (i.e., <21 versus ≥29); low HDL levels usually accompany obesity.[85] No major differences exist in the influence of exercise, alcohol ingestion, and smoking on lipid levels between men and women. Women in the highest tertile of cholesterol appear to be more responsive to dietary therapy than those in the lower tertiles and more responsive than formulas based on men predict.

Based on the HERS[86] and WHI[87,88] trials, recently published national guidelines recommended similar types of lifestyle and risk factor goals and interventions as recommended by NCEP for the entire population.[83] Hormone therapy may continue to have a role for postmenopausal symptoms; however, a notable exception is hormone-replacement therapy and heart protection. Combined estrogen plus progestin hormone therapy should not be initiated to prevent cardiovascular disease (CVD) in postmenopausal women. Combined estrogen plus progestin hormone therapy should not be continued to prevent CVD in postmenopausal women. Other forms of menopausal hormone therapy (e.g., unopposed estrogen) should not be initiated or continued to prevent CVD in postmenopausal women pending the results of ongoing trials.[83]

Cholesterol and triglyceride levels rise progressively throughout pregnancy, with an average increment in cholesterol of 30 to 40 mg/dL occurring around the thirty-sixth to thirty-ninth weeks. Triglyceride levels may go up by as much as 150 mg/dL. Drug therapy is not instituted, nor is it usually continued, during pregnancy. If the patient is very high risk, a BAR may be considered because there is no systemic drug exposure.[1] Statins are category X and are contraindicated. Ezetimibe might be an alternative because it is a category C drug (animal

studies have shown that the drug exerts teratogenic or embryocidal effects, and there are no adequate, well-controlled studies in pregnant women, or no studies are available in either animals or pregnant women) but no data are available in humans. Dietary therapy is the mainstay of treatment, with emphasis on maintaining a nutritionally balanced diet as per the needs of pregnancy.

CHILDREN

Drug therapy in children is not recommended until the age of 10 years or older, and the guidelines for institution of therapy and the goals of therapy are different from those in adults[27] (see Table 21–9). Younger children generally are managed with TLCs until after the age of 2 years.[89,90] Bile acid sequestrants are used in children because they minimize the risks of systemic toxicity.[30] Some literature does exist suggesting that resins and perhaps statins are safe and effective in children.[31,89,90] Severe forms of hypercholesterolemia (e.g., familial hypercholesterolemia) may require more aggressive treatment.

CONCURRENT DISEASE STATES

Nephrotic syndrome, end-stage renal disease and nephrotic syndrome, and hypertension compound the risk of dyslipidemia and may present difficult-to-treat lipid abnormalities. Abnormalities of lipoprotein metabolism in the nephrotic syndrome include elevated total and LDL cholesterol, Lp(a), VLDL, and triglycerides. The apolipoprotein C-III to C-II ratio is elevated, consistent with greater lipoprotein lipase inhibitor activity, and the extent of hypoalbuminemia is correlated with dyslipidemia. The basic abnormality appears to be one of overproduction of LDL-apoB from VLDL rather than reduced clearance of LDL cholesterol and related proteins. Protein restriction and a "vegan" diet correct lipid abnormalities to some extent. Statins have been shown to be effective in reducing elevated total and LDL cholesterol in the nephrotic syndrome, although the levels usually do not return to normal.[91] The pharmacokinetics of gemfibrozil are apparently not altered by renal insufficiency, and it is effective in lowering total cholesterol by about 15% for this disorder.[92] Fenofibrate reduces remnant lipoproteins. Fibric acid derivatives and statins reduce small, dense LDL cholesterol by different mechanisms, suggesting a potential role for combination therapy to optimize lowering of small, dense LDL cholesterol and remnant lipoproteins.[93]

Renal insufficiency without proteinuria leads to hypertriglyceridemia, slightly elevated total and LDL cholesterol (particularly with chronic ambulatory peritoneal dialysis), and low HDL levels (especially during hemodialysis). These abnormalities are thought to be caused by a deficiency in apolipoprotein C-II, perhaps as a result of sustained use of heparin during hemodialysis and depletion of lipoprotein lipase, carbohydrate-induced obesity and hypertriglyceridemia, loss of carnitine during hemodialysis, use of acetate buffer (acetate is a precursor to fatty acid synthesis) during hemodialysis, and decreased LCAT activity during hemodialysis. Dialysis does not correct the lipid abnormalities. Renal transplantation may correct lipid abnormalities in some patients, but in others, the use of transplantation-related medications such as corticosteroids, cyclosporine, and certain antihypertensive agents (see Chaps. 13 and 87) may aggravate the lipid abnormalities. Cyclosporine interferes with the metabolism of statins metabolized by cytochrome P450 3A4 (Table 21–14), and patients need to be observed closely for myositis and worsening renal function. Of interest, correction of lipid abnormalities may improve renal hemodynamics. Pravastatin and fluvastatin may be safer than other statins, but this needs to be validated in larger, long-term trials. Diet will modify lipoprotein levels and polyunsaturated fatty acids may have a role in impeding the progression of renal disease as well as the cardiovascular complications. Bile acid sequestrants do not correct the lipid abnormalities seen in renal insufficiency. Lovastatin or its active metabolite may accumulate in renal insufficiency, and lower doses of reductase inhibitors should be used to avoid adverse effects. Gemfibrozil may be used with caution because its pharmacokinetics are unchanged, and it lowers triglycerides and increases HDL.[65] Statins (simvastatin, lovastatin, and atorvastatin) and fibric acid derivatives may increase the risk of severe myopathy, and attention to symptoms of myositis is needed. Niacin also may be useful in nondiabetic patients with renal insufficiency.

Hypertensive patients have a greater than expected prevalence of high blood cholesterol levels, and conversely, patients with hypercholesterolemia have a higher than expected prevalence of hypertension caused by the metabolic syndrome. Recommendations for the management of hypertension in patients with hypercholesterolemia include avoiding the use of drugs that elevate cholesterol such as diuretics and β-blockers and using agents that are either lipid-neutral or that may reduce cholesterol slightly[1] (see Chap. 13). Bile acid sequestrants may bind to thiazide diuretics and some β-blockers and may interfere with their absorption; reaction may be avoided by giving the antihypertensive 1 hour before or 4 hours after the resin. Niacin may magnify the hypotensive effects of vasodilators.

OTHER THERAPIES

Partial ileal bypass has been used in severe heterozygous and homozygous familial hypercholesterolemia; however, it is ineffective in the latter case. Ileal bypass removes the site of bile acid reabsorption, depleting the bile acid pool and increasing the catabolism of cholesterol. A randomized trial of diet versus surgery, called Program On the Surgical Control of the Hyperlipidemias (POSCH), reported

that total and LDL cholesterol were decreased (23.3% and 37.7%, respectively) and HDL increased (4.3%) in patients who had undergone ileal bypass for hypercholesterolemia.[97] Overall death was delayed by nearly 3 years ($p = .032$) and CHD mortality was delayed by nearly 4 years ($p = .046$) by surgery as compared with the control group. Revascularization procedures were delayed by an average of 7 years ($p < .001$). Postoperative diarrhea was more common in the surgical group, as was the rate of kidney stones (4% versus 0.4%), gallstones (10% versus 2%), and bowel obstruction (13.5% versus 3.6%).

Portacaval shunts have been used to decrease the formation of LDL cholesterol, and reductions of 10% to 20% have been reported. Plasma exchange combined with niacin was found to reduce plasma cholesterol levels by about 50% in homozygous familial hypercholesterolemia over 5 years, and coronary atherosclerosis did not progress, as documented by angiography. LDL-apheresis, selective removal of LDL cholesterol via a filtering system, and statin therapy are effective in lowering LDL cholesterol and appear to affect the progression of vascular disease. LDL-apheresis may be combined with statin therapy for greater effect. Combined liver and heart transplantation in homozygous familial hypercholesterolemia reduces total and LDL cholesterol concentrations from about 1100 and 900 mg/dL to about 300 and 185 mg/dL prior to and after surgery, respectively. Liver transplantation replaced the missing LDL receptors, enhanced catabolism, and reduced lipoprotein synthesis in this patient.

SUMMARY OF MAJOR STUDIES

Primary and secondary prevention diet and drug trials have been performed to determine whether lowering of cholesterol will prevent CHD; Tables 21–15 and Tables 21–16 summarize these trials. A number of earlier angiographic studies demonstrated that cholesterol reduction leads to regression of atherosclerosis and plaque stabilization. Most of the primary and secondary studies were double-blinded, randomized, and placebo-controlled, lasting for 5 years or

TABLE 21–15. Primary Prevention Trials with Lipid-Lowering Drugs

Trial	F/U (years)	n	Treatment	Control Events	Treatment Events	p Value	RRR	ARR	NNT
AFCAPS/TexCAPS	5	6605	Lovastatin 20–40 mg	5.5%	3.5%	<0.001	36.4%	2.0%	50
Helsinki	5	4081	Gemfibrozil 1200 mg	4.1%	2.7%	<0.02	34.0%	1.4%	71
LRC-CPPT	7.4	3806	Cholestyramine 24 g	9.8%	8.1%	<0.05	17.3%	1.7%	59
Oslo	5	1232	Diet + smoking cessation	4.2%	2.5%	0.03	40.5%	1.7%	59
WOSCOPS	4.9	6595	Pravastatin 40 mg	7.8%	5.5%	<0.001	29.5%	2.3%	43
ALLHAT	4.8	10,355	Usual care Pravastatin 40 mg	10.4%	9.3%	0.16	9%	1.1%	91
WHI	5.2	16,608	Usual care Diet, CEE 0.625 mg + MPA 2.5 mg	1.5%	1.9%	0.05	1.29[a]	0.4%	200[b]
WHI	5.2	16,608	Usual care Diet, CEE 0.625 mg	3.7%	3.3%	NS	9%	0.4%	250
CARDS	4	2838	Atorvastatin 10 mg	9.0%	5.8%	0.001	37%	3.2%	32

[a]HR = hazard ratio. The risk of CHD was increased by 29%.
[b]Number needed to harm since CEE + MPA was worse than placebo.
AFCAPS/TexCAPS = Air Force/Texas Coronary Atherosclerosis Prevention Study (Downs et al., 1998); Helsinki = The Helsinki Heart Study (Frick et al., 1987); LRC-CPPT = The Lipid Research Clinics Coronary Primary Prevention Trial (Insull et al., 1984); Oslo = The Oslo Study (Hjermann et al., 1988); WOSCOPS = The West of Scotland Coronary Prevention Study (Shepherd et al., 1995); ALLHAT = Antihypertensive and Lipid-Lowering Treatment to Prevent Heart Attack Trial; approximately 13–15% of patients had a history of coronary heart disease (CHD); events are CHD events only; WHI = Women's Health Initiative; RRR = relative risk reduction; ARR = absolute risk reduction; NNT = number needed to treat; NA = not available; CEE = conjugated equine estrogen; MPA = medroxyprogesterone acetate; CARDS = Collaborative Atorvastatin Diabetes Study (presented at the 2004 American Diabetes Association meeting).

TABLE 21–16. Secondary Prevention Trials with Lipid-Lowering Drugs

Trial	F/U (years)	n	Treatment	Control Events	Treatment Events	p Value	RRR	ARR	NNT
VA-HIT	5.1	2531	Gemfibrozil 1200 mg	21.7%	17.3%	0.006	22%	4.4%	23
AVERT	1.5	341	Atorvastatin 80 mg	21%	13%	0.048	38%	8%	12
CARE	5	4159	Pravastatin 40 mg	13.2%	10.2%	0.003	22.7%	3.0%	33
CDP	5	8341	Niacin 3 g + clofibrate 1.8 g	20.9%	20.6%	NS	1.4%	0.3%	333
HERS	4.1	2673	Estrogen 0.625 mg + progestin 2.5 mg	12.7%	12.5%	0.91	1.6%	0.2%	500
LIPID	7.4	3806	Pravastatin 40 mg	9.8%	8.1%	<0.05	17.3%	1.7%	59
4S	5	4444	Simvastatin 20 mg	11.5%	8.2%	0.0003	28.7%	3.3%	30
WHO	5.3	15,745	Clofibrate 1.6 g	3.9%	3.1%	<0.005	20.5%	0.8%	125
BIP	6.2	3090	Placebo Bezafibrate 400 mg	15.0%	13.6%	0.26	9.3%	1.4%	72
TIMI-22	2	4162	Pravastatin 40 mg Atorvastatin 80 mg	26.3% (P)	22.4% (A)	0.005	16%	3.9%	26
HPS	5	20,536	Simvastatin 40 mg	14.7%	12.9%	0.003	13%	1.8%	56
MIRACL		3086	Atorvastatin 80 mg	17.4%	14.8%	0.048	16%	2.6%	39
PROSPER	3	5804	Pravastatin 40 mg	16.2%	14.1%	0.014	24%	2.1%	48

VA-HIT = Veterans Administration-High-Density Lipoprotein Cholesterol (HDL-C) Intervention Trial; AVERT = The Atorvastatin Versus Revascularization Treatments; CARE = Cholesterol and Recurrent Events (Melendez et al., 1996); CDP = Coronary Drug Project (Berge et al., 1975); HERS = Heart and Estrogen Replacement Study (Hulley et al., 1998); LIPID = Long-Term Intervention with Pravastatin in Ischaemic Disease Study (MacMahon et al., 1995); 4S-Scandinavian Simvastatin Survival Study (Pederson et al., 1994); WHO = World Health Organization (Committee of Principal Investigators, 1978); BIP = Bezafibrate Infarction Prevention; TIMI-22 = Thrombolysis in Myocardial Infarction Study 22; also known as the PROVE-IT trial (Cannon et al., 2004); HPS = Heart Protection Study; results expressed as all-cause mortality (HPS Collaborative Group, 2002); MIRACL = Myocardial Ischemia Reduction with Aggressive Cholesterol Lowering (Schwartz et al., 2001); PROSPER = PROspective Study of Pravastatin in the Elderly at Risk; RRR = relative risk reduction; ARR = absolute risk reduction; NNT = number needed to treat.

longer, and most had sufficient patient numbers to be meaningful. Exceptions to these qualifications were seen in the early studies, such as the Newcastle and Edinburgh trials, which were small and generally did not show much benefit; and the Coronary Drug Project (CDP) using dextrothyroxine, which was terminated early owing to adverse effects on CHD mortality. The Helsinki Heart Study, using gemfibrozil, resulted in a reduction in nonfatal MI, which was the primary contributor to reduced CHD incidence[15] (see Table 21–15).

Total and LDL cholesterol concentrations were reduced an average of 13.4% and 20.3%, respectively, by cholestyramine in the LRC-CPPT, and the reduction of lipid levels was related to the amount of drug ingested (e.g., 1 to 2 packets, 5.4% reduction in total cholesterol, versus 5 or more packets, 19.0% reduction).[98] The prescribed dose of cholestyramine was 24 g, or 6 packets, per day. The cholestyramine group experienced a 19% reduction in risk ($p < .05$) of the primary end point—definite CHD death and/or definite nonfatal MI—reflecting a 24% reduction in definite CHD death and a 19% reduction in nonfatal MI. Other end points were reduced by 25%, 20%, and 21% for new positive exercise tests, angina, and coronary bypass surgery, respectively. Death from all causes was not significantly reduced by cholestyramine secondary to more accidents and violence in this group. The mean falls in total and LDL cholesterol concentrations in the cholestyramine group were 8% and 12% relative to levels in placebo-treated men, providing evidence that for every 1% reduction in cholesterol, a 2% decline in CHD mortality can be realized.

In AFCAPS/TexCAPS, a primary prevention trial conducted in 6605 men and women aged 57 to 63 years with average total cholesterol and LDL concentrations (<221 mg/dL and <150 mg/dL, respectively) who were treated with lovastatin 20–40 mg/day for 5.2 years, a 37% reduction ($p < .001$) was shown in the risk for first acute major coronary event (fatal or nonfatal MI, unstable angina, or sudden cardiac death).[47] The need for revascularization procedures also was reduced by 33% ($p < .001$). The implications of this trial are enormous; potentially millions of "normal" people could benefit

from lipid lowering with statins based on these results. The number of patients who need to be treated (NNT; see Table 21–15) for primary prevention ranges from 43 in the West of Scotland trial to 71 in the Helsinki Heart Study. This range is within the typical boundary used for treatment decisions and described previously; cost-effectiveness is achieved routinely in patients with moderate to high risk. The Antihypertensive and Lipid-Lowering Treatment to Prevent Heart Attack Trial (ALLHAT-LLT) tested pravastatin 40 mg/day versus placebo in hypertensive patients with at least one CHD risk factor. Pravastatin did not reduce either all-cause mortality or CHD significantly when compared with usual care in older participants with well-controlled hypertension and moderately elevated LDL cholesterol. The results may be due to the modest differential in total cholesterol (9.6%) and LDL cholesterol (16.7%) between pravastatin and usual care compared with prior statin trials supporting cardiovascular disease prevention.[99] The long-awaited Women's Health Initiative trial proved to be disappointing, with no beneficial effects on CHD event reduction in the hormone-replacement arm (conjugated equine estrogens [CEE] + medroxgprogesterone), or the CEE alone arm compared with placebo.[87,88] Women did experience greater risk for thromboembolism and a slight increase in breast cancer and a reduced risk of hip fracture. Consequently, hormone-replacement therapy can no longer be recommended for cardiovascular protection.[83]

Niacin in the CDP significantly reduced definite, nonfatal MI as compared with placebo (10.1% versus 13.9%), whereas clofibrate did not reduce death from any cause or nonfatal or fatal MI at the 5-year follow-up period.[100] Clofibrate did increase the rate of definite or suspected fatal or nonfatal pulmonary embolism or thrombophlebitis compared with placebo (5.8% versus 3.6%) after adjusting for baseline characteristics for total follow-up.[100] Other findings with clofibrate that occurred more frequently than with placebo included intermittent claudication, arrhythmias, palpable spleen, cholelithiasis (including cholecystectomy), and more frequent use of anticoagulants. Skin reactions, gastrointestinal complaints, and the use of gout medication were more common with niacin than with placebo. The 5-year total mortalities were 20.0% for clofibrate and 20.9% for placebo. The 5-year total mortality for niacin was 21.2%. Long-term follow-up of the CDP has shown a reduction in total mortality with niacin that occurred 9 years after the drug had been stopped.[100] The mechanism for this effect is unclear.

One of the most important studies published in the last few years is the 4S trial, a secondary intervention trial in a large number of patients.[35] Simvastatin, 20–40 mg/day, reduced LDL cholesterol by 35% and reduced the risk of death from any cause by 30%. Coronary deaths also were reduced with simvastatin (relative risk 0.58; confidence interval, 0.46–0.73). Therapy also was shown to be effective in women (18% to 19% of patients enrolled) and in the elderly ($\geq$60 years). Indeed, the relative risk of death or major coronary event was reduced to a greater extent in the elderly than in younger patients. Death from noncardiovascular causes was similar for simvastatin and placebo (2.1% and 2.2%, respectively). The survival curves for simvastatin and placebo began to separate at 1 year and became more divergent with additional follow-up. The 4S study clearly demonstrates the benefit in cholesterol lowering and placates long-held fears of death from non-CHD causes. The Long-term Intervention with Pravastatin in Ischemic Disease (LIPID) study ($N = 7498$ men and 1516 women) has investigated the effect of pravastatin on CHD mortality in patients with prior MI or unstable angina and a mean cholesterol level of 219 mg/dL over 6 years.[101] Pravastatin reduced the risk of CHD mortality by 24% (8.3% versus 6.4%; $p = .0004$) and total mortality by 23% (14.1% versus 11.0%; $p = .00002$); stroke also was reduced by 20% (4.3% versus 3.5%; $p = .22$), as was the need for coronary artery bypass grafting (11.3% versus 8.9%; $p = .0001$) or percutaneous transluminal coronary angioplasty (5.3% versus 4.4%; $p = .04$).

The Veterans Administration High-Density Lipoprotein Intervention Trial (VA-HIT) was a double-blind trial that compared gemfibrozil (1200 mg/day) with placebo in 2531 men with CHD, an HDL cholesterol level of 40 mg/dL or less, and an LDL cholesterol level of 140 mg/dL or less.[13] The primary study outcome was nonfatal MI or death from coronary causes. The median follow-up was 5.1 years. At 1 year, the mean HDL cholesterol level was 6% higher, the mean triglyceride level was 31% lower, and the mean total cholesterol level was 4% lower in the gemfibrozil group than in the placebo group. LDL cholesterol levels did not differ significantly between the groups. A primary event occurred in 21.7% of the patients assigned to placebo and in 17.3% of the patients assigned to gemfibrozil. The overall reduction in the risk of an event was 4.4 percentage points, and the reduction in relative risk was 22% ($p = 0.006$). This trial presents the strongest evidence to date that raising HDL cholesterol level and lowering triglyceride level reduce the risk for CHD.

The Heart and Estrogen/Progestin Replacement Study (HERS) was undertaken to determine whether estrogen plus progestin therapy alters the risk for CHD events in postmenopausal women with established CAD.[86] A total of 2763 women (mean age 66.7 years)

with CAD who were younger than 80 years and postmenopausal with an intact uterus were randomized to receive either 0.625 mg CEEs plus 2.5 mg medroxyprogesterone acetate in 1 tablet daily ($n = 1380$) or a placebo of identical appearance ($n = 1383$). Follow-up averaged 4.1 years. The primary outcome was the occurrence of nonfatal MI or CHD death. There were no significant differences between groups in the primary outcome or in any of the secondary cardiovascular outcomes. More women in the hormone group than in the placebo group experienced venous thromboembolic events and gallbladder disease. Based on the finding of no overall cardiovascular benefit and a pattern of early increase in risk of CHD events, the authors did not recommend starting this treatment for the purpose of secondary prevention of CHD. In this study of secondary intervention of relatively elderly postmenopausal women, there was no evidence of benefit from hormone-replacement therapy (HRT), and only an increase in thromboembolism was seen. If women are on HRT at the time of event, then they should be given a choice to continue. HRT in the Women's Health Initiative did not prevent CHD events with or without hysterectomy, and HRT can no longer be recommended for primary or secondary intervention[87,88] (see Table 21–15).

The Atorvastatin Versus Revascularization Treatments (AVERT) study compared atorvastatin 80 mg/day with percutaneous transluminal coronary angioplasty.[102] The follow-up period was 18 months. Of the patients who received aggressive lipid-lowering treatment with atorvastatin, 13% had ischemic events compared to 21% of the patients who underwent angioplasty. The incidence of ischemic events thus was 36% lower in the atorvastatin group over an 18-month period ($p = 0.048$, which was not statistically significant after adjustment for interim analyses). This reduction in events was because of a smaller number of angioplasty procedures, coronary artery bypass operations, and hospitalizations for worsening angina (the most common end point). As compared with the patients who were treated with angioplasty and usual care, the patients who received atorvastatin had a significantly longer time to the first ischemic event ($p = 0.03$). In low-risk patients with stable CAD, aggressive lipid-lowering therapy is at least as effective as angioplasty and usual care in reducing the incidence of ischemic events.

In the PROSPER study, in men and women in the age range of 70 to 82 years it was found that pravastatin 40 mg/day reduced CHD events by 24%, with no effect on cognitive function.[103] The most recent trial, TIMI-22 (also known as PROVE-IT, Pravastatin or Atorvastatin Evaluation and Infection Therapy) enrolled 4162 patients who had been hospitalized for an acute coronary syndrome within the preceding 10 days and compared 40 mg pravastatin daily (standard therapy) with 80 mg atorvastatin daily (intensive therapy).[104] An intensive lipid-lowering statin regimen with atorvastatin 80 mg/day provided greater protection against death or major cardiovascular events than does a standard regimen. This study clearly points to "lower is better" for LDL concentration and likely will lead to a revision in guideline goals to lower LDL levels.

PHARMACOECONOMIC CONSIDERATIONS

The clinical benefits of lipid-lowering therapy for primary and secondary intervention are now well established based on the results of the AFCAPS/TexCAPS, 4S, and other studies showing a reduction in CHD morbidity and mortality. The balance of benefits and costs has been examined in a few studies.[82,95] The cost per year of life saved has been estimated to range from less than $10,000 to over $1 million dollars depending on the presence or absence of CHD, age of the patient, baseline total or LDL cholesterol level and reduction in cholesterol,

and number of risk factors present. In general, intervention in patients with known CHD, those who have CHD risk equivalents, or those with a 10-year risk of 10% to 20% are cost-effective with statin therapy, whereas other types of therapy may be cost-effective if certain assumptions concerning compliance, efficacy, and so forth are met. The range for secondary intervention based on the 4S study is $3800 for a 70-year-old man with a high cholesterol level to $27,400 per year of life gained for a middle-aged woman with an average cholesterol level.[82] In contrast, primary prevention in men based on the West of Scotland trial averages about $35,000 per year of life gained.[95] These studies demonstrate that primary and secondary interventions are well within the accepted boundary of less than $50,000 for a medical intervention to be considered cost-effective. Based on the specific lipoprotein phenotype, fibric acid derivatives, niacin, or combination therapy of statins plus BAR may be cost-effective. Cost-effectiveness is maximized by treating high-risk patients and those with established CHD.

Specialty lipid clinics have become increasingly popular, and many use pharmacists to provide direct patient care in this setting. An interesting recent analysis shows that a specialty clinic may be more expensive ($659 ± $43 versus $477 ± $42 per patient; $p < .001$) than usual care. However, the overall cost-effectiveness is improved when expressed as program costs per unit (mmol/L) reduction in the LDL cholesterol, a measure of cost-effectiveness that was significantly lower for specialized care ($758 ± $58 versus $1058 ± $70: $p = .002$) because more patients achieve their targeted goal.[95] Project ImPACT demonstrated that pharmacists working collaboratively with patients and physicians can improve persistence and compliance and that nearly two-thirds of patients achieved their NCEP lipid goal.[96]

CLINICAL CONTROVERSIES

The optimal LDL level has been hotly debated for more than 10 years. Based on a few recent trials, the optimal LDL level may need to redefined below the current goal (<100 mg/dL). An update from ATP III suggests that an LDL of <70 mg/dL is a therapeutic option in very high-risk patients (known CHD + ≥risk factors).[105]

Statins differ in their pharmacokinetic properties and in pleotropic effects (i.e., non–lipid-lowering). The contribution of lipid lowering alone (a class effect) versus other effects (anti-inflammatory, antithrombotic, etc.) continues to create controversy.

The role of nontraditional risk factors (hsCRP, homocysteine, etc.) is continuing to be clarified and may lead to recommendations for the use of these tests in patient evaluation.

EVALUATION OF THERAPEUTIC OUTCOMES

Short-term evaluation of therapy for hyperlipidemia is based on response to diet and drug treatment, as measured in the clinical laboratory by total cholesterol, LDL cholesterol, HDL cholesterol, and triglyceride levels for patients being treated for primary intervention, as well as on response to secondary intervention. The interval for follow-up depends on the severity of illness, and patients with known CAD or multiple risk factors should be monitored more closely. Less commonly used laboratory measurements include C-reactive protein, homocysteine, apolipoprotein B, and Lp(a) levels. Because many patients being treated for primary hyperlipidemia have no symptoms and may not have any clinical manifestations of a genetic lipid disorder such as xanthomas or eruptions, monitoring and outcome are solely laboratory-based. In patients treated for secondary intervention, symptoms of atherosclerotic cardiovascular disease, such as angina or intermittent claudication, may improve over months to years. If patients have xanthomas or other external manifestations of hyperlipidemia, these lesions should regress with therapy. Lipid measurements should be obtained in the fasted state to minimize interference from chylomicrons, and once the patient is stable, monitoring is needed at intervals of 6 months to 1 year. The goals for LDL and HDL cholesterol levels are provided in Tables 21–8 and Tables 21–9.

Patients with multiple risk factors and established CHD also should be monitored and evaluated for progress in managing their other risk factors such as hypertension, smoking cessation, exercise and weight control, and glycemic control if diabetic. The goals are to maintain a blood pressure of below 130/85 mm Hg or less (presence of diabetes or renal insufficiency), stop smoking, maintain an ideal body weight, exercise for at least 20 minutes three or more times per week, and keep the plasma glucose concentration below 100 mg/dL (threshold for glucose intolerance). Invasive evaluation, such as cardiac catheterization, is useful in patients with established CHD and typically is used for planning revascularization rather than monitoring of lipid-lowering therapy.

Evaluation of dietary therapy is part of the outcome evaluation for treating hyperlipidemia, and the assistance of a dietitian is recommended. Use of diet diaries and recall survey instruments enable information about diet to be collected in a systematic fashion and may improve patient adherence to dietary recommendations. Patients on resin therapy should have an FLP panel checked every 4–8 weeks until a stable dose; triglycerides should be checked at a stable dose to ensure they have not increased. Niacin requires baseline liver function tests and tests for uric acid and glucose; repeat tests are appropriate at doses of 1000 to 1500 mg/day. Symptoms of myopathy or diabetes-like symptoms should be investigated and may require CK or glucose determinations; more frequent monitoring in diabetics may be necessary. An FLP 4 to 8 weeks after the initial dose or dose changes with statins is appropriate. Liver function tests should be obtained at baseline and periodically thereafter based on package insert information; recognized experts believe that monitoring for hepatotoxicity and myopathy should be symptom-triggered.[45] Ezetimibe requires little specific monitoring.

ABBREVIATIONS

4S: Scandinavian Simvastatin Survival Study
ACAT: acyl CoA: cholesterol acyltransferase
AFCAPS/TexCAPS: Air Force/Texas Coronary Atherosclerosis Prevention Study
AHA: American Heart Association
ALLHAT-LLT: Antihypertensive and Lipid-Lowering Treatment to Prevent Heart Attack Trial
ALT: Alanine aminotransferase
apoJ: apolipoprotein J
ARR: Absolute risk reduction
ATP III: Adult Treatment Panel III
AVERT: Atrovastatin Versus Revascularization Treatments
BAR: Bile acid resin
bid: Twice daily
BIP: Bezafibrate Infarction Prevention
BMI: Body mass index
BMS: Bristol-Myers Squibb
CAD: Coronary artery disease
CARDS: Collaborative Atorvastatin Diabetes Study
CARE: Cholesterol and Recurrent Events
CDP: Coronary Drug Project
CEE: Conjugated equine estrogen
CETP: Cholesteryl ester transfer protein
CHD: Coronary heart disease
CK: Creatine kinase
CRP: C-reactive protein
CTX: Cerebrotendinous xanthomatosis
CVD: Cardiovascular disease
DISC: Dietary Intervention Study in Children
ECG: Electrocardiogram

ELAM-1: E-selectin
EXCEL: Expanded Clinical Evaluation of Lovastatin
FA: Fatty acid
FDA: Food and Drug Administration
FFA: Free fatty acid
FLP: Fasting lipoprotein profile
HDL: High-density lipoproteins
HDL-C: High-density lipoprotein cholesterol
HERS: Heart and Estrogen/Progestin Replacement Study
HL: Hepatic lipase
HMG-CoA reductase: 3-hydroxy-3-methylglutaryl coenzyme A
    reductase
HMGR: 3-hydroxy-3-methylglutaryl coenzyme A reductase
HPS: Heart Protection Study
HR: Hazard ratio
HRT: Hormone-replacement therapy
ICAM-1: Intercellular adhesion molecule
IDL: Intermediate-density lipoprotein
IHD: Ischemic heart disease
IL: Interleukin
JNC7: Joint National Committee 7
LCAT: Lecithin:cholesterol acyltransferase
LDL: Low-density lipoprotein
LDL-R: Low-density lipoprotein receptor
LIPID: Long-Term Intervention with Pravastatin in Ischemic
    Disease
LPL: Lipoprotein lipase
LRC-CPPT: Lipid Research Clinics Coronary Primary Prevention
    Trial
LRP: Low-density lipoprotein receptor-related protein
MCP-1: Monocyte chemoattractant protein 1
M-CSF: Monocyte colony-stimulating factor
MI: Myocardial infarction
MIRACL: Myocardial Ischemia Reduction with Aggressive
    Cholesterol Lowering
MPA: Medroxyprogesterone acetate
MSD: Merck Sharp & Dohme
NA: Not available
NCEP: National Cholesterol Education Program
NHANES: National Health and Nutrition Examination Survey
NNT: Number needed to treat
PAP: Phosphatidic acid phosphatase
PDAY: Pathobiologic Determinants of Atherosclerosis in Youth
PDGF: Platelet-derived growth factor
PON: paraxonase
POSCH: Program on the Surgical Control of the Hyperlipidemias
PROSPER: Prospective Study of Pravastatin in the Elderly at Risk
PROVE-IT: Pravastatin or Atorvastatin Evaluation and Infection
    Therapy
RRR: Relative risk reduction
TC: Total cholesterol
TG: Triglycerides
TGF: Transforming growth factor
TIMI-22: Thrombolysis in Myocardial Infarction Study 22
TLC: Therapeutic lifestyle change
VA-HIT: Veterans Administration High-Density Lipoprotein
    Cholesterol (HDL-C) Intervention Trial
VCAM-1: Vascular cell adhesion molecule
VEGF: Vascular endothelial growth factor
VLDL: Very low-density lipoproteins
WHI: Women's Health Initiative
WHO: World Health Organization
WOSCOPS: West of Scotland Coronary Prevention Study

Review Questions and other resources may be found at *www.pharmacotherapyonline.com.*

REFERENCES

1. National Cholesterol Education Program (NCEP) Expert Panel on Detection, Evaluation, and Treatment of High Blood Cholesterol in Adults (Adult Treatment Panel III). Third Report of the National Cholesterol Education Program (NCEP) Expert Panel on Detection, Evaluation, and Treatment of High Blood Cholesterol in Adults (Adult Treatment Panel III): Final Report. Circulation 2002;106:3143–31421.
2. Grundy SM, Pasternak R, Greenland P, et al. Assessment of cardiovascular risk by use of multiple-risk-factor assessment equations. *Circulation* 1999;100–101:1481–1492.
3. Smith SC Jr, Greenland P, Grundy SM. Prevention Conference V: Beyond secondary prevention: Identifying the high-risk patient for primary prevention: Executive summary. Circulation 2000;101:111–116.
4. Pearson TA, Blair SN, Daniels SR, et al. AHA guidelines for primary prevention of cardiovascular disease and stroke: 2002 update. Circulation 2002;106:388–391.
5. Mosca L, Appel LJ, Benjamin EJ, et al. Evidence-based guidelines for cardiovascular disease prevention in women. Circulation 2004;109: 672–693.
6. Ford ES, Mokdad AH, Giles WH, Mensah GA. Serum total cholesterol concentrations and awareness, treatment and control of hypercholesterolemia among US adults. Circulation 2003;107:2185–2189.
7. American Heart Association. Heart Disease and Stroke Statistics—2004 Update. Dallas, American Heart Association, 2003.
8. Foley KA, Massing MW, Simpson RJ Jr, et al. Population implications of changes in lipid management in patients with coronary heart disease. Am J Cardiol 2004;93:193–195.
9. Pearson TA, Laurora I, Chu H, Kafonek S. The Lipid Treatment Assessment Project (L-TAP). Arch Intern Med 2000;160:459–467.
10. Menotti A, Keys A, Blackburn H, et al. Comparison of multivariate predictive power of major risk factors for coronary heart diseases in different countries: Results from eight nations of the Seven Countries Study, 25-year follow-up. J Cardiovasc Risk 1996;3:69–75.
11. Kannel WB, Wilson PW. Comparison of risk profiles for cardiovascular events: Implications for prevention. Adv Intern Med 1997;42:39–66.
12. Sytkowski PA, D'Agostino RB, Belanger A, Kannel WB. Sex and time trends in cardiovascular disease incidence and mortality: The Framingham Heart Study, 1950–1989. Am J Epidemiol 1996;143:338–350.
13. Rubins HB, Robins SJ, Collins D, et al. Gemfibrozil for the secondary prevention of coronary heart disease in men with low levels of high-density lipoprotein cholesterol. Veterans Affairs High-Density Lipoprotein Cholesterol Intervention Trial Study Group. N Engl J Med 1999; 341:410–418.
14. Jeppesen J, Hein HO, Suadicani P, Gyntelberg F. Triglyceride concentration and ischemic heart disease: An eight-year follow-up in the Copenhagen Male Study. Circulation 1998;97:1029–1036.
15. Huttunen JK, Manninen V, Manttari M, et al. The Helsinki Heart Study: Central findings and clinical implications. Ann Med 1991;23:155–159.
16. Austin MA, McKnight B, Edwards KL, et al. Cardiovascular disease mortality in familial forms of hypertriglyceridemia: A 20-year prospective study. Circulation 2000;101:2777–2782.
17. Dietschy JM. Dietary fatty acids and the regulation of plasma low-density lipoprotein cholesterol concentrations. J Nutr 1998;128:444S–448S.
18. Brousseau ME, Schaefer EJ, Wolfe ML, et al. Effects of an inhibitor of cholesteryl ester transfer protein on HDL cholesterol. N Engl J Med 2004;350:1505–1515.
19. Clark RW, Sutfin TA, Ruggeri RB, et al. Raising high-density lipoprotein in humans through inhibition of cholesteryl ester transfer protein: An initial multidose study of torcetrapib. Arterioscler Thromb Vasc Biol 2004; 24:490–497.
20. Ross R. Cellular and molecular studies of atherogenesis. Atherosclerosis 1997;131:S3–4.

21. Pearson TA, Menash GA, Alexander RW, et al. Markers of inflammation and cardiovascular disease. Circulation 2003;107:499–511.

22. Libby P, Schoenbeck U, Mach F, et al. Current concepts in cardiovascular pathology: The role of LDL cholesterol in plaque rupture and stabilization. Am J Med 1998;104:14–18S.

23. Reaven PD, Napoli C, Merat S, Witztumc JL. Lipoprotein modification and atherosclerosis in aging. Exp Gerontol 1999;34:527–537.

24. Turban S, Fuentes F, Ferlic L, et al. A prospective study of paraxonase gene Q/R192 polymorphism and severity, progression and regression of coronary atherosclerosis, plasma lipid levels, clinical events and response to fluvastatin. Atherosclerosis 2001;154:633–640.

25. Veerkamp MJ, de Graaf J, Hendriks JCM, et al. Nomogram to diagnose familial combined hyperlipidemia on the basis of results of a 5-year follow-up study. Circulation 2004;109:2980–2985.

26. Grundy SM, Howard B, Smith S Jr, et al. Prevention conference VI: Diabetes and cardiovascular disease. Executive summary. Circulation 2002;105:2231–2239.

27. North American Academy of Pediatrics, Committee on Nutrition. Cholesterol in childhood. Pediatrics 1998;101:141–147.

28. Strong JP, Malcom GT, Oalmann MC, Wissler RW. The PDAY Study: Natural history, risk factors, and pathobiology. Pathobiological determinants of atherosclerosis in youth. Ann NY Acad Sci 1997;811:226–235; discussion 235–237.

29. Obarzanek E, Hunsberger SA, Van Horn L, et al. Safety of a fat-reduced diet: The Dietary Intervention Study in Children (DISC). Pediatrics 1997;99:687–694.

30. McCrindle BW, O'Neill MB, Cullen-Dean G, Helden E. Acceptability and compliance with two forms of cholestyramine in the treatment of hypercholesterolemia in children: A randomized, crossover trial. J Pediatr 1997;130:266–273.

31. Lambert M, Lupien PJ, Gagne C, et al. Treatment of familial hypercholesterolemia in children and adolescents: Effect of lovastatin. Canadian Lovastatin in Children Study Group. Pediatrics 1996;97:619–628.

32. Spence JD, Huff MW, Heidenheim P, et al. Combination therapy with colestipol and psyllium mucilloid in patients with hyperlipidemia. Ann Intern Med 1995;123:493–499.

33. He KH, Song Y, Daviglus ML, et al. Accumulated evidence on fish consumption and coronary heart disease mortality: A meta-analysis of cohort studies. Circulation 2004;109:2705–2711.

34. Harris WS. N-3 fatty acids and human lipoprotein metabolism: An update. Lipids 1999;34:S257–258.

35. Shepherd J, Cobbe SM, Ford I, et al. Prevention of coronary heart disease with pravastatin in men with hypercholesterolemia. West of Scotland Coronary Prevention Study Group. N Engl J Med 1995;333:1301–1307.

36. Anonymous. Randomised trial of cholesterol lowering in 4444 patients with coronary heart disease: The Scandinavian Simvastatin Survival Study (4S). Lancet 1994;344:1383–1389.

37. Brown BG, Zhao XQ, Chait A, et al. Simvastatin and niacin, antioxidant vitamins, or the combination for the prevention of coronary disease. N Engl J Med. 2001;345:1583–1592.

38. Xydakis AM, Jones PH. Toxicity of antilipidemic agents: Facts and fictions. Curr Atheroscler Rep 2003;5:403–410.

39. Bottorff M, Hansten P. Long-term safety of hepatic hydroxymethyl glutaryl coenzyme A reductase inhibitors: The role of metabolism-monograph for physicians. Arch Intern Med 2000;160:2273–2280.

40. Naoumova RP, Dunn S, Rallidis L, et al. Prolonged inhibition of cholesterol synthesis explains the efficacy of atorvastatin. J Lipid Res 1997;38:1496–1500.

41. Jones P, Kafonek S, Laurora I, Hunninghake D. Comparative dose efficacy study of atorvastatin versus simvastatin, pravastatin, lovastatin, and fluvastatin in patients with hypercholesterolemia (the CURVES study). Am J Cardiol 1998;81:582–587.

42. Melani L, Mills R, Hassman D, et al. Efficacy and safety of ezetimibe coadministered with pravastatin in patients with primary hypercholesterolemia: A prospective, randomized, double-blind trial. Eur Heart J 2003;24:717–728.

43. Davidson MH, McGarry T, Bettis R, et al. Ezetimibe coadministered with simvastatin in patients with primary hypercholesterolemia. J Am Coll Cardiol 2002;40:2125–2134.

44. Bradford RH, Shear CL, Chremos AN, et al. Expanded Clinical Evaluation of Lovastatin (EXCEL) study results: Two-year efficacy and safety follow-up. Am J Cardiol 1994;74:667–673.

45. Gotto AM Jr. Safety and statin therapy. Arch Intern Med 2003;163:657–659.

46. Pedersen TR, Berg K, Cook TJ, et al. Safety and tolerability of cholesterol lowering with simvastatin during 5 years in the Scandinavian Simvastatin Survival Study. Arch Intern Med 1996;156:2085–2092.

47. Downs JR, Clearfield M, Weis S, et al. Primary prevention of acute coronary events with lovastatin in men and women with average cholesterol levels. JAMA 1998;279:1615–1622.

48. Sacks FM, Pfeffer MA, Moye LA, et al. The effect of pravastatin on coronary events after myocardial infarction in patients with average cholesterol levels. Cholesterol and Recurrent Events Trial investigators. N Engl J Med 1996;335:1001–1009.

49. Anonymous. The effect of aggressive lowering of low-density lipoprotein cholesterol levels and low-dose anticoagulation on obstructive changes in saphenous-vein coronary-artery bypass grafts. The Post Coronary Artery Bypass Graft Trial Investigators. N Engl J Med 1997;336:153–162.

50. O'Neill FH, Patel DD, Knight BL, Clare KY. Determinants of variable response to statin treatment in patients with refractory familial hypercholesterolemia. Arterioscler Thromb Vasc Biol 2001;21:832–837.

51. Chasman DI, Posada D, Subrahmanan L, et al. Pharmacogenetic study of statin therapy and cholesterol reduction. JAMA 2004;291:2821–2827.

52. Graaf MR, Beiderbeck AB, Egberts ACG, et al. The risk of cancer in users of statins. J Clin Oncol 2004;22:2388–2394.

53. Carrilho AJ, Medina WL, Nakandakare ER, Quintao EC. Plasma cholesteryl ester transfer protein is lowered by treatment of hypercholesterolemia with cholestyramine. Clin Pharmacol Ther 1997;62:82–88.

54. Konzem SL, Gray DR, Kashyap ML. Effect of pharmaceutical care on optimum colestipol treatment in elderly hypercholesterolemic veterans. Pharmacotherapy 1997;17:576–583.

55. Tsuyuki RT, Bungard RJ. Poor adherence with hypolipidemic drugs: A lost opportunity. Pharmacotherapy 2001;21:627–635.

56. Grundy SM. Consensus statement: Role of therapy with "statins" in patients with hypertriglyceridemia. Am J Cardiol 1998;81:1B–6B.

57. American Diabetes Association. Dyslipidemia management in adults with diabetes. Diabetes Care 2004;27:S68–71.

58. Guyton JR, Blazing MA, Hagar J, et al. Extended-release niacin vs gemfibrozil for the treatment of low levels of high-density lipoprotein cholesterol. Niaspan-Gemfibrozil Study Group. Arch Intern Med 2000;160:1177–1184.

59. Goldberg A, Alagona P Jr, Capuzzi DM, et al. Multiple-dose efficacy and safety of an extended-release form of niacin in the management of hyperlipidemia. Am J Cardiol 2000;85:1100–1105.

60. McKenney J. New prespectives on the use of niacin in the treatment of lipid disorders. Arch Intern Med 2004;164:697–705.

61. McKenney JM, Proctor JD, Harris S, Chinchili VM. A comparison of the efficacy and toxic effects of sustained- vs immediate-release niacin in hypercholesterolemic patients. JAMA 1994;271:672–677.

62. Grundy SM, Vega GL, McGovern ME, et al. Efficacy, safety, and tolerability of once-daily niacin for the treatment of dyslipidemia associated with type 2 diabetes: Results of the assessment of diabetes control and evaluation of the efficacy of niaspan trial Arch Intern Med 2002;162:1568–1576.

63. Elam MB, Hunninghake DB, Davis KB, et al. Effect of niacin on lipid and lipoprotein levels and glycemic control in patients with diabetes and peripheral arterial disease: The ADMIT study. A randomized trial. Arterial Disease Multiple Intervention Trial. JAMA 2000;284:1263–1270.

64. Caroli-Bosc FX, Le Gall P, Pugliese P, et al. Role of fibrates and HMG-CoA reductase inhibitors in gallstone formation: Epidemiological study in an unselected population. Dig Dis Sci 2001;46:540–544.

65. Prueksaritanount T, Zhao JJ, Ma B, et al. Mechanistic studies on metabolic interactions between gemfibrozil and statins. J Pharmacol Exp Ther 2002;301:1042–1051.

66. Athyros VG, Papageorgiou AA, Hatzikonstandinou HA, et al. Safety and efficacy of long-term statin-fibrate combinations in patients with refractory familial combined hyperlipidemia. Am J Cardiol 1997;80:608–613.

67. Guerin M, Bruckert E, Dolphin PJ, et al. Fenofibrate reduces plasma cholesteryl ester transfer from HDL to VLDL and normalizes the atherogenic, dense LDL profile in combined hyperlipidemia. Arterioscler Thromb Vasc Biol 1996;16:763–772.

68. Sveger T, Flodmark CE, Nordborg K, et al. Hereditary dyslipidaemias and combined risk factors in children with a family history of premature coronary artery disease. Arch Dis Child 2000;82:292–296.

69. Yang CY, Gu ZW, Xie YH, et al. Effects of gemfibrozil on very-low-density lipoprotein composition and low-density lipoprotein size in patients with hypertriglyceridemia or combined hyperlipidemia. Atherosclerosis 1996;126:105–116.

70. Sheu WH, Jeng CY, Lee WJ, et al. Simvastatin treatment on postprandial hypertriglyceridemia in type 2 diabetes mellitus patients with combined hyperlipidemia. Metabolism 2001;50:355–359.

71. Bakker-Arkema RG, Davidson MH, Goldstein RJ, et al. Efficacy and safety of a new HMG-CoA reductase inhibitor, atorvastatin, in patients with hypertriglyceridemia. JAMA 1996;275:128–133.

72. Krauss RM. Atherogenic lipoprotein phenotype and diet-gene interactions. J Nutr 2001;131:340–343S.

73. Freeman DJ, Norrie J, Sattar N, et al. Pravastatin and the development of diabetes mellitus: Evidence for a protective treatment effect in the West of Scotland Coronary Prevention Study. Circulation (Online) 2001; 103:357–362.

74. Colhoun HM, Betteridge DJ, Durrington PN, et al. Primary prevention of cardiovascular disease with atorvastatin in type 2 diabetes in the Collaborative Atorvastatin Diabetes Study (CARDS): Multicentre randomised placebo-controlled trial. Lancet 2004; 364:685–696.

75. Heart Protection Study Collaborative Group. MRC/BHF Heart Protection Study of cholesterol-lowering with simvastatin in 5963 people with diabetes: A randomized, placebo-controlled trial. Lancet 2003;361: 2005–2016.

76. Anonymous. Effect of fenofibrate on progression of coronary-artery disease in type 2 diabetes: The Diabetes Atherosclerosis Intervention Study, a randomised study. Lancet 2001;357:905–910.

77. Kannel WB. Cardiovascular risk factors in the elderly. Coronary Artery Dis 1997;8:565–575.

78. Ko DT, Mandani M, Alter D. Lipid-lowering therapy with statins in high-risk elderly patients: The treatment-risk paradox. JAMA 2004;291: 1864–1870.

79. Reid IR, Hague W, Emberson J, et al. Effect of pravastatin on frequency of fracture in the LIPID study: Secondary analysis of a randomised, controlled trial. Long-term intervention with pravastatin in ischaemic disease. Lancet 2001;357:509–512.

80. Grundy SM, Cleeman JI, Rifkind BM, Kuller LH. Cholesterol lowering in the elderly population: Coordinating Committee of the National Cholesterol Education Program. Arch Intern Med 1999;159: 1670–1678.

81. Heart Protection Study Collaborative Group. MRC/BHF Heart Protection Study of cholesterol lowering with simvastatin in 20,536 high-risk individuals: A randomized, placebo-controlled trial. Lancet 2002;360: 7–22.

82. Johannesson M, Jonsson B, Kjekshus J, et al. Cost-effectiveness of simvastatin treatment to lower cholesterol levels in patients with coronary heart disease. Scandinavian Simvastatin Survival Study Group. N Engl J Med 1997;336:332–336.

83. Mosca L, Appel LJ, Benjamin E, et al. Evidence-based guidelines for cardiovascular disease prevention in women. Circulation 2004;109: 672–693.

84. Welty FK. Cardiovascular disease and dyslipidemia in women. Arch Intern Med 2001;161:514–522.

85. Abate N. Obesity and cardiovascular disease: Pathogenetic role of the metabolic syndrome and therapeutic implications. J Diabetes Comp 2000;14:154–174.

86. Hulley S, Grady D, Bush T, et al. Randomized trial of estrogen plus progestin for secondary prevention of coronary heart disease in postmenopausal women. Heart and Estrogen/progestin Replacement Study (HERS) Research Group. JAMA 1998;280:605–613.

87. Women's Health Initiative Investigators. Risks and benefits of estrogen plus progestin in healthy postmenopausal women. JAMA 2002;288: 321–333.

88. Women's Health Initiative Investigators. Effects of conjugated equine estrogen in postmenopausal women with hysterectomy. JAMA 2004; 291:1701–1712.

89. Tonstad S. A rational approach to treating hypercholesterolaemia in children: Weighing the risks and benefits. Drug Saf 1997;16:330–341.

90. Knipscheer HC, Boelen CC, Kastelein JJ, et al. Short-term efficacy and safety of pravastatin in 72 children with familial hypercholesterolemia. Pediatr Res 1996;39:867–871.

91. Toto RD, Grundy SM, Vega GL. Pravastatin treatment of very-low-density, intermediate-density and low-density lipoproteins in hypercholesterolemia and combined hyperlipidemia secondary to the nephrotic syndrome. Am J Nephrol 2000;20:12–17.

92. Samuelsson O, Attman PO, Knight-Gibson C, et al. Effect of gemfibrozil on lipoprotein abnormalities in chronic renal insufficiency: A controlled study in human chronic renal disease. Nephron 1997;75:286–294.

93. Deighan CJ, Caslake MJ, McConnell M, et al. Comparative effects of cerivastatin and fenofibrate on the atherogenic lipoprotein phenotype in proteinuric renal disease. J Am Soc Nephrol 2001;12:341–348.

94. Caro J, Klittich W, McGuire A, et al. The West of Scotland coronary prevention study: Economic benefit analysis of primary prevention with pravastatin. Br Med J 1997;315:1577–1582.

95. Schectman G, Wolff N, Byrd JC, et al. Physician extenders for cost-effective management of hypercholesterolemia. J Gen Intern Med 1996; 11:277–286.

96. Bluml BM, McKenney JM, Cziraky MJ. Pharmaceutical care services and results in project ImPACT: Hyperlipidemia. J Am Pharm Assoc 2000; 40:157–165.

97. Buchwald H, Campos CT, Boen JR, et al. Disease-free intervals after partial ileal bypass in patients with coronary heart disease and hypercholesterolemia: Report from the Program on the Surgical Control of the Hyperlipidemias (POSCH). J Am Coll Cardiol 1995;26:351–357.

98. Anonymous. The Lipid Research Clinics Coronary Primary Prevention Trial results: I. Reduction in incidence of coronary heart disease. JAMA 1984;251:351–364.

99. The ALLHAT Officers and Coordinators for the ALLHAT Collaborative Research Group. The Antihypertensive and Lipid-Lowering Treatment to Prevent Heart Attack Trial (ALLHAT-LLT). JAMA 2002;288: 2998–3007.

100. Canner PL, Berge KG, Wenger NK, et al. Fifteen-year mortality in Coronary Drug Project patients: Long-term benefit with niacin. J Am Coll Cardiol 1986;8:1245–1255.

101. Anonymous. Prevention of cardiovascular events and death with pravastatin in patients with coronary heart disease and a broad range of initial cholesterol levels. The Long-Term Intervention with Pravastatin in Ischaemic Disease (LIPID) Study Group. N Engl J Med 1998;339: 1349–1357.

102. Pitt B, Waters D, Brown WV, et al. Aggressive lipid-lowering therapy compared with angioplasty in stable coronary artery disease. Atorvastatin versus Revascularization Treatment Investigators. N Engl J Med 1999;341:70–76.

103. Shepherd J, Blauw GJ, Murphy MB, et al. Pravastatin in elderly individuals at risk of vascular disease. Lancet 2002;360:1623–1630.

104. Cannon CP, Braunwald E, McCabe CH, et al. Pravastatin or Atorvastatin Evaluation and Infection Therapy-Thrombolysis in Myocardial Infarction 22 Investigators. Comparison of intensive and moderate lipid lowering with statins after acute coronary syndromes. N Engl J Med 2004; 350:1495–1504.

105. Grundy SM, Cleeman JI, Merz CNB, et al. Implications of recent clinical trials for the National Cholesterol Education Program Adult Treatment Panel III guidelines. Circulation 2004;110:227–239.

22

PERIPHERAL ARTERIAL DISEASE

Barbara J. Hoeben and Robert L. Talbert

Learning Objectives and other resources can be found at *www.pharmacotherapyonline.com.*

KEY CONCEPTS

❶ The prevalence of peripheral arterial disease is dependent upon age and the presence of traditional risk factors for cardiovascular disease and many patients are undiagnosed; undiagnosed patients have substantial risk for coronary and cerebrovascular events.

❷ The clinical presentation of peripheral arterial disease is variable and includes a range of symptoms. The two most common characteristics of peripheral arterial disease are intermittent claudication and pain at rest in the lower extremities.

❸ The ankle-brachial index (ABI) is a simple, noninvasive, quantitative test that has been proven to be a highly sensitive and specific tool in the diagnosis of peripheral arterial disease.

❹ As with any athlerosclerotic condition, several risk factors play an important role in the morbidity and mortality of peripheral vascular disease. Many of these risk factors are

modifiable with the help of various nonpharmacologic and pharmacologic interventions.

❺ Nonpharmacologic interventions such as smoking cessation and walking exercise programs have the ability to positively impact several of the pathophysiologic abnormalities present in patients with peripheral arterial disease.

❻ Data proving that antiplatelet therapies can prevent or delay the progression of peripheral arterial disease are currently unavailable. However, aspirin therapy has repeatedly been proven to significantly reduce serious vascular events in these "high-risk" patients and, in the absence of contraindications, is highly recommended.

❼ After appropriate exercise therapy and therapeutic lifestyle changes have been implemented, patients who continue to experience severe intermittent claudication may benefit from additional pharmacologic therapy with cilostazol.

Peripheral arterial disease (PAD), the most common form of peripheral vascular disease, is a manifestation of progressive narrowing of arteries due to atherosclerosis.[1] PAD is associated with elevated risk of cardiovascular disease (CVD) morbidity and mortality, even in the absence of prior history of acute myocardial infarction (AMI), stroke, or other manifestations of CVD.[1,2] Patients with PAD have approximately the same relative risk of death from CVD as do patients with a history of coronary or cerebrovascular disease, and PAD should be considered a surrogate marker of subclinical coronary artery disease (CAD) and other vascular territories.[1,3,4] The treatment of PAD focuses on decreasing the functional impairment caused by symptoms of intermittent claudication through nonpharmacologic and pharmacologic therapy and by minimizing the impact of other cardiovascular risk factors.[5]

EPIDEMIOLOGY

❶ The National Health and Nutrition Examination Survey (NHANES) found that the prevalence of PAD among adults age 40 years and older in the United States was 4.3% using the definition of an ankle-brachial index (ABI) of less than 0.9 in either leg.[2] The prevalence of PAD is highly dependent on age, being infrequent in younger individuals and common in older individuals (Fig. 22–1). In age- and gender-adjusted logistic regression analyses, black race/ethnicity (odds ratio [OR] 2.83) current smoking (OR 4.46), diabetes (OR 2.71), hypertension (OR 1.75), hypercholesterolemia (OR 1.68)

and impaired renal function (estimated glomerular filtration rate less than 60 ml/min/1.73 m^2) (OR 2.00) were associated with more prevalent PAD.[2,6] Individuals with PAD are also more likely to have a self-reported history of any CAD or cardiovascular disease but interestingly, no association with elevated body mass index. The relative risk of death from CVD in patients with PAD is reported to range from 2 to 5.1 in patients with or without CVD and 2.9 to 5.7 in patients with known CVD.[7] Cardiovascular disease accounts for 75% of all deaths in patients with PAD.[8] It is important to recognize that the risk of death is approximately the same in men and women and is elevated even in asymptomatic patients. Patients with critical leg ischemia who have the lowest ABI values have an annual mortality of 25%.[9]

More than 5 million (estimated range 4 to 7 million) adults age 40 years or more have PAD and 95% of individuals with PAD have at least one cardiovascular risk factor; the majority of patients have multiple risk factors for CVD.[2] Based on the PAD Awareness, Risk, and Treatment: New Resources for Survival (PARTNERS) program, the prevalence of PAD in primary care practices is high, yet physician awareness of the PAD diagnosis is relatively low.[10] In this cross-sectional study, PAD was detected in 29% of 6979 patients and 83% of the patients were aware of their diagnosis but only 49% of their patients' physicians were aware. The reason for this observation is that patient self-report of symptoms and the use of questionnaires to detect PAD are not sufficiently sensitive and specific to reproducibly diagnosis PAD and the cardinal symptom of PAD, intermittent claudication, is present in the minority of patients (1 to 27%).[7] A simple ABI measurement will identify a large number of patients with previously

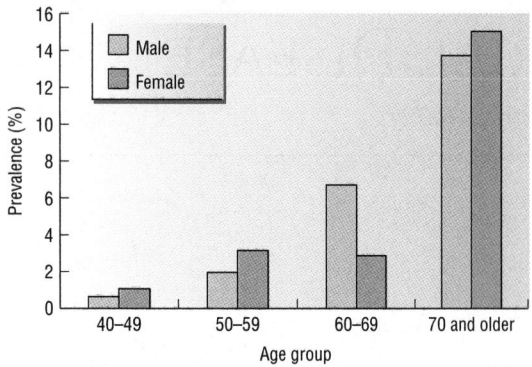

FIGURE 22–1. Prevalence of PAD by age and gender.

unrecognized PAD. Atherosclerosis risk factors were very prevalent in PAD patients, but these patients received less intensive treatment for lipid disorders and hypertension and were prescribed antiplatelet therapy less frequently than were patients with CVD. These results demonstrate that underdiagnosis of PAD in primary care practice may be a barrier to effective secondary prevention of the high ischemic cardiovascular risk associated with PAD.[10] Because of the systemic nature of atherosclerosis and the high risk of ischemic events, patients with PAD should be considered for secondary prevention strategies including aggressive risk-factor modification and antiplatelet drug therapy.[7,11,13]

ETIOLOGY AND PATHOPHYSIOLOGY

PAD is most commonly a manifestation of systemic atherosclerosis in which the arterial lumen of the lower extremities becomes progressively occluded by atherosclerotic plaque.[8] The major risk factors for the development of atherosclerosis are older age (greater than 40 years), cigarette smoking, diabetes mellitus, hypercholesterolemia, hypertension and hyperhomocysteinemia.[7,8] The arteries most commonly involved, in order of occurrence, are the femoropopliteal-tibial, aortoiliac, carotid and vertebral, splenic and renal, and brachiocephalic.[14] Familial hypercholesterolemia (FH) leading to hypercholesterolemia and elevated low-density lipoprotein (LDL) levels is associated with accelerated development of atherosclerosis earlier and with more severe symptoms (e.g., intermittent claudication) and abnormal blood flow studies compared to controls.[15] Intima-media thickness can be used as a surrogate phenotype for cardiovascular risk in FH and carotid and/or femoral artery atherosclerosis results in increased intima-media thickness and it is correlated to cardiovascular risk in FH patients compared with normolipidemic individuals.

CLINICAL PRESENTATION AND DIAGNOSIS

The clinical presentation of PAD is variable and includes a range of symptoms from no symptoms at all (typically early

in the disease) to pain and discomfort. The two most common characteristics of PAD are intermittent claudication (IC) and pain at rest in the lower extremities.[16–18] IC is generally regarded as the primary indicator of PAD and has been described as fatigue, discomfort, cramping, pain, or numbness in the affected extremities (typically the buttock, thigh or calf) during exercise and is resolved within a few minutes by resting.[16,17,19–21] Resting pain typically occurs later in the disease when the blood supply is not adequate to perfuse the extremity (critical limb ischemia). This most often can be felt at night, while the patient is lying in bed, in the feet (typically the toes or heel).[16–18]

As with any good medical encounter, a detailed patient history of symptoms and atherosclerosis risk factors (e.g., smoking, hypertension, hyperlipidemia, and diabetes) can be helpful in the diagnosis of PAD. Unfortunately, as illustrated by the PARTNERS program, providers who rely on a history alone will miss approximately 85% to 90% of patients with PAD.[19] Therefore, examination of the patient is vital to proper diagnosis. Requesting that the patient remove socks and shoes may reveal nonspecific signs of decreased blood flow to the extremities (i.e. cool skin temperature, shiny skin, thickened toenails, lack of hair on the calf, feet and/or toes) or, in severe cases, visible sores or ulcers that are slow to heal and may even be black in appearance.[16–18,22,23]

An important criterion for the accurate diagnosis of PAD is the exclusion of other conditions that possess similar signs and symptoms. A differential diagnosis should rule out other neurologic conditions (e.g., peripheral neuropathy), inflammatory conditions (e.g., arthritis) and vascular conditions (e.g., deep venous thrombosis) which may mimic PAD.[17,21,24]

The ABI is a simple, noninvasive, quantitative test that has been proven to be a highly sensitive and specific ($\geq$90%) tool in the diagnosis of PAD.[19,25–27] To measure the ABI, the patient lies in the supine position as the systolic blood pressure is measured at the brachial arteries on both arms and the dorsalis pedis and posterior tibial arteries of the legs with a standard sphygmomanometer and a continuous-wave Doppler device. The pressures obtained at the dorsalis pedis and posterior tibial arteries are averaged and divided by the mean measurement taken at the left and right brachial arteries.[7,22,28,29] An ABI of 1 is considered normal while a measurement under 0.9 is consistent with PAD. Further, the range of 0.7 to 0.9 correlates with mild PAD, 0.4 to 0.7 indicates moderate disease, and under 0.4 denotes severe PAD.[8,20,28] In addition to providing diagnostic information, the ABI measurement has been shown to be a strong predictor of future cardiovascular events associated with PAD.[30] The ABI can also be useful after a test of exercise tolerance (e.g., 5 minutes on a treadmill or 30 to 50 repetitions of heel raises). Patients with PAD will have a significant drop in the ABI after exercise while pain with a normal or unchanged ABI can rule out PAD and suggest to the provider that an alternate diagnosis exists.[8,20,22]

Alternatively, arteriography is an expensive, invasive test that may be used to diagnose PAD. However, as ABI is a sufficient means of diagnosis, arteriography is not necessary or encouraged.[16,21,26]

▶ TREATMENT: Peripheral Arterial Disease

▤ GOALS OF TREATMENT

Due to the fact the PAD is the result of atherosclerotic plaque formation in the arteries that results in decreased blood flow to the legs,

several of the treatment goals for these patients involve the reduction of confounding variables that attribute to the disease process, progress, and eventual outcome. Specific goals should include increasing maximal walking distance, duration and pain-free walking, improving control of comorbid conditions contributing to the morbidity of the condition (i.e. hypertension, hyperlipidemia, and diabetes), improvement in overall quality of life and reduction in cardiovascular complications and death.

GENERAL APPROACH TO TREATMENT

4   As with any athlerosclerotic condition, several risk factors play an important role in the morbidity and mortality of PAD. Thankfully, many of these risk factors are modifiable with the help of various nonpharmacologic and pharmacologic interventions.

NONPHARMACOLOGIC THERAPY

Smoking Cessation

5   It has been thoroughly documented that cigarette smoking not only increases the risk of developing PAD and other cardiovascular disorders, but that the duration and quantity smoked can negatively impact disease progression (i.e. increase the risk of amputation) and increase mortality.[7,24,30–35] As a result, providers must advise patients to quit and should offer nonpharmacologic and pharmacologic means to aid the patient in that goal. Individual or group behavior modification therapy with or without the addition of certain antidepressants (i.e., bupropion) or nicotine replacement therapies (i.e., gum or patches) has been proven effective in numerous studies. Reassessment of smoking status and progress encouragement at each encounter can help to reemphasize to the patient the vital importance of this lifestyle change.

Exercise

5   Walking exercise programs for patients with PAD have been proven to result in an increase in walking duration and distance, an increase in pain-free walking, and a delayed onset of claudication by 179%.[23,24,32,33,36–41] Walking, or any aerobic exercise program conducted under the supervision of a healthcare provider, has the ability to positively impact several of the pathophysiologic abnormalities present in patients with PAD. Benefits of exercise programs include improving diabetes and lipid management, reducing weight, improving blood viscosity and flow, and reducing blood pressure.[5] The type of aerobic activity recommended, as well as the duration and frequency of the activity, should be individually designed on a patient-to-patient basis.

Surgical Interventions

Various surgical procedures are available for patients with severe, debilitating claudication who have attempted, and failed, other means of nonpharmacologic and pharmacologic therapy. The TransAtlantic Inter-Society Consensus (TASC) document on peripheral arterial disease is very clear on the recommendations for invasive therapy.[23] First, there must be a lack of adequate response to exercise therapy and risk factor modification. Second, the patient must have severe disability from intermittent claudication resulting in impairment of daily activities. Third, there must be a thorough evaluation of the risks versus benefits of an invasive intervention including probability of success, the anticipated future course of the disease if an intervention is not

performed, as well as an evaluation of concomitant disease states.[23] The decision to attempt percutaneous revascularization is often made with the guidance of diagnostic angiography. Angiography can help to identify the location and size of lesions and provide valuable information as to the likelihood of success with surgical revascularization.[23]

Percutaneous transluminal angioplasty (PTA) is an example of an invasive treatment for PAD. A randomized controlled clinical trial performed by Whyman and colleagues determined that in a 2 years' postintervention, the PTA outcomes on maximum walking distance and ABI were not significantly different than in patients that had only received daily low-dose ASA ($p > 0.05$).[42] Nevertheless, patients who had received PTA had significantly fewer occluded arteries ($p = 0.003$), but the true clinical significance of this finding was not able to be realized in the time allotted for the study.

Stent placement in PAD patients has also been an area of study and controversy. A meta-analysis examining the use of stent placement versus PTA for the treatment of aortoiliac occlusive disease determined that, although stent placement and PTA yielded similar complication and mortality rates, posttreatment ABI were more improved with stents (0.87 with PTA and 0.76 with stents, $p < 0.03$) and the risk of long-term failure was 39% less with stent placement.[43] However, other studies have not demonstrated improvement in patency rates in peripheral arteries versus PTA alone.[16] The TASC document provides specific recommendations for PTA, with or without stenting, depending on how diffuse the disease process is, the number and size of the lesions, and the location of the lesions.[23]

For patients with severe IC resulting in critical leg ischemia, physicians may need to discuss alternate surgical interventions including aortofemoral bypass, femoralpopliteal bypass, or even amputation.[16,17,32]

PHARMACOLOGIC THERAPY

Hypertension

Hypertension (HTN) is a major risk factor for PAD and can lead to AMI, stroke, heart failure (HF), and death.[41] Current guidelines recommend the treatment goal for blood pressure in patients with PAD to mirror those in patients with documented cardiovascular disease (CVD), 130/85 mm Hg.[31,41] Although, the Heart Outcomes Prevention Evaluation study (HOPE trial), demonstrated that angiotensin-converting-enzyme (ACE) inhibitors reduced not only blood pressure, but other cardiovascular events (e.g., AMI, stroke, and death) in high-risk patients, including those with PAD, no specific class of antihypertensives are recommended over another for the treatment of hypertension in patients with PAD. Therefore, selection of drug therapy for hypertension should be made on the basis of comorbid disease states, drug costs and availability, drug allergies, or other possible limiting factors. For example, patients with documented CAD may receive a dual benefit by the selection of a beta-blocker while calcium-channel-blockers may be desired in a patient with concomitant Raynaud's phenomenon.[31,41,44] Dosing, monitoring guidelines and contraindications for specific agents may be found in Chapter 13, *Hypertension*.

Hyperlipidemia

Although it has been shown that a reduction in lipid levels can reduce the progression of PAD and the severity of claudication, the current recommendations for the management of hyperlipidemia in PAD are based on only a few small studies and sub-hoc analyses from larger trials.[7,31,45,46] However, PAD is considered by the Expert Panel on Detection, Evaluation, and Treatment of High Blood Cholesterol in Adults (Adult Treatment Panel III, or ATP III) to be in the category of highest risk, or a coronary heart disease (CHD) risk equivalent. Therefore, it was recommended by the Expert Panel that levels of LDL be maintained at <100 mg/dL and non-high-density lipoprotein (HDL) levels (total cholesterol—HDL cholesterol) at <130 mg/dL.[45] Clinical trials have been conducted since the time of this recommendation, specifically the Heart Protection Study (HPS)[47] and the Pravastatin or Atorvastatin Evaluation and Infection—Thrombolysis in Myocardial Infarction (PROVE IT)[48] trial, that have lead many clinical experts to now recommend an LDL goal of <70 mg/dL for additional retardation of atherosclerotic plaque formation in persons considered to be at very high risk, including patients with PAD.[16] Regardless of the goal, LDL chosen, initiation of patient therapeutic lifestyle changes (TLC) (i.e., reduction in saturated fat, weight reduction, and increased physical activity) are vital to achieving these recommendations.[13,45] Unfortunately, in many cases, TLC alone will not achieve the desired goals.

Several options are available for the initiation of drug therapy for LDL-lowering in patients with PAD. Statins, bile acid sequestrants, and nicotinic acid are all effective treatment options. However, in most cases, statins are the preferred starting agent in this patient population.[19,32,45,47] As proven in the Heart Protection Study, simvastatin demonstrated potent action in reducing not only LDL, but also provided a significant reduction in cardiovascular events overall as well (e.g., AMI, stroke, and death).[47] Additionally, if an increase in HDL levels is also necessary, niacin should be considered alone or in combination with a statin without the fear of worsening glucose metabolism, as previously believed.[7,17,24,44,49] Dosing, monitoring guidelines and contraindications for specific agents may be found in Chapter 21, *Hyperlipidemia*.

Diabetes Mellitus

A recent meta-analysis of over 95,000 diabetic patients provided additional support for the accepted premise that glycemic control serves as a risk factor for cardiovascular disease.[50] The analysis demonstrated an increasing risk of death from cardiovascular events as blood glucose concentrations increased, with the same relationship observed even at levels below the threshold of clinically defined diabetes mellitus. This relationship is just one illustration of the criticality of good glycemic control. Due to the high prevalence of PAD among diabetic patients, the American Diabetes Association recommends ABI screening of all diabetics above 50 years of age for PAD.[51] Due to the presence of peripheral neuropathy, patients with diabetes may be less likely to experience or report symptoms of PAD and the first sign may be as drastic as the appearance of a gangrenous foot ulcer. Therefore, although there is currently a lack of randomized-controlled studies illustrating that the degree of glycemic control is predictive of the extent of PAD present, it is recommended that all patients with concomitant diabetes and PAD maintain good glycemic control, as evidenced by a hemoglobin A-1c level of <7%.[7,23,24,31,33,51,52] Oral antidiabetic agents, insulin regimens, as well as other pharmacologic and nonpharmacologic strategies to reduce the risk of complications associated with diabetes mellitus are discussed at length in Chapter 72, Diabetes Mellitus.

ANTIPLATELET DRUG THERAPY (See Table 22–1)

Aspirin (ASA)

By far, the most compelling evidence for the use of any pharmacologic agent in PAD can be found with ASA. The Antithrombotic Trialists' Collaboration (ATC) conducted a meta-analysis of 195 randomized trials, composed of over 135,000 patients at high risk for occlusive arterial disease, and concluded that low-dose ASA (75 to 160 mg) and medium-dose ASA (160 to 325 mg/day) lead to a significant reduction in serious vascular events (12%) in "high-risk" patients, such as those with PAD.[53] It was also noted in this analysis that the risk of major extracranial bleed was similar between the low-dose and medium-dose regimens.

More recently, Tran and Anand conducted a systematic review of the literature in an effort to summarize the best evidence for oral antiplatelet therapy in patients with cerebrovascular disease, CAD, and PAD.[54] This review included 111 trials (42 of which included patients with PAD, n = 9214) and concluded that patients with PAD should use ASA (160 to 325 mg/day) or clopidogrel (75 mg/day) when ASA is not tolerated or contraindicated.[54,55] This is in concordance with the recommendations of the Seventh American College of Chest Physicians (ACCP) Conference on Antithrombotic and Thrombolytic Therapy which recommends lifelong ASA (75 to 325 mg/day) over clopidogrel, ticlopidine, and no antithrombotic therapy in patients with PAD.[56] Unfortunately, no data are currently available from large, clinical, randomized trials that ASA, or any other antiplatelet therapies, can actually prevent or delay the progression of PAD.[56]

ASA + Dipyridamole Extended-Release (ER) (Aggrenox)

The ATC also examined the use of dipyridamole ER in combination with ASA in "high risk" patients, such as those with PAD. Their meta-analysis of 25 trials (over 10,000 patients) concluded that the addition of dipyridamole to aspirin led to an additional reduction in serious vascular events over ASA alone (6%), however, this reduction was unable to reach statistical significance ($p = 0.32$).[53,54] It should also be taken into consideration that most of the reduction in nonfatal stroke in this analysis came from one trial, and these data are not replicated in the other studies.[53,55,57] The addition of dipyridamole to ASA may cause an increased risk of bleeding and gastrointestinal side effects when compared to placebo and should not be used with CAD.[57]

Clopidogrel (Plavix)

The ATC meta-analysis also reviewed the effectiveness of clopidogrel 75 mg/day in "high risk" patients, including those with PAD. The Collaboration concluded that although clopidogrel was able to reduce serious vascular events by 10%, this was significantly less than the reduction seen with ASA (12%, $p = 0.03$), as described previously.[53] Included in this meta-analysis was the report from the Clopidogrel versus ASA in Patients at Risk of Ischemic Events (CAPRIE) trial which had concluded that clopidogrel (75 mg daily) was more effective than ASA (325 mg daily) in preventing vascular events in "high risk" patients. In comparison to the ASA therapy, the clopidogrel regimen resulted in an overall reduction in ischemic stroke, MI or vascular death from 5.83% to 5.32% ($p = 0.043$). This difference was even more pronounced in the subgroup analysis of PAD patients (clopidogrel therapy led to a significant reduction of 4.86% versus 3.71% in the ASA group, $p = 0.0028$).[4,25,30] It must be noted that clopidogrel

TABLE 22-1. Pharmacotherapy Options for Patients with PAD[4,18,24,25,53,55,56,67-72]

Agent	Daily Dose (oral)	Mechanism of Action (MOA)	Side Effects	Contraindications	Level of Evidence[†]
Aspirin	81–325 mg	Irreversibly inhibits prostaglandin cyclooxygenase in platelets, prevents formation of thromboxane A_2	Gastrointestinal upset and/or bleeding	Active bleeding; hemophilia; thrombocytopenia	With coronary or cerebrovascular (Grade 1A), without (Grade 1C+)
Dipyridamole ER (Aggrenox)	400 mg (+ aspirin 50 mg)	May act by inhibiting platelet aggregation (complete MOA unknown)	Angina; dyspnea; hypotension; headache; dizziness	Active bleeding; CAD ("coronary steal syndrome")	Recommendation for use not specified in report
Cilostazol (Pletal)*	100 mg BID	Phosphodiesterase inhibitor, suppresses platelet aggregation; direct artery vasodilator	Fever: infection; tachycardia	All CHF patients (decreased survival)	With IC (Grade 2A)
Clopidogrel (Plavix)	75 mg	Inhibits binding of ADP analogues to its platelet receptor causing irreversible inhibition of platelets	Chest pain; purpura generalized pain; rash	Active pathological bleeding (i.e., peptic ulcer, intracranial hemorrhage)	Recommend clopidogrel over no antiplatelet therapy (Grade 1C+)
Pentoxifylline (Trental)	1.2 g	Alters RBC flexibility; decreases platelet adhesion; reduces blood viscosity; decreases fibrinogen concentration	Dyspnea; nausea; vomiting; headache; dizziness	Recent retinal or cerebral hemorrhage; active bleeding	Not recommended in patients with IC (Grade 1B)
Ticlopidine (Ticlid)	500 mg	Inhibits binding of ADP analogues to its platelet receptor causing irreversible inhibition of platelets	Leukopenia; rash; thrombocytopenia; neutropenia; agranulocytosis; aplastic anemia	Active bleeding; hemophilia; thrombocytopenia	Clopidogrel recommended over ticlopidine (Grade 1C+)

Abbreviations: ER, extended-release; mg, milligrams; g, grams; BID, twice-daily; ADP, adenosine 5′-diphosphate; RBC, red blood cell; CAD, coronary artery disease; CHF, congestive heart failure; IC, intermittent claudication.

*Cilostazol should be used in combination with antiplatelet therapy.

[†]Grades of recommendation for antithrombotic and thrombolytic therapy is part of the Seventh ACCP Conference on Antithrombotic and Thrombolytic Therapy.[73]

is significantly more expensive than ASA therapy, not only in drug costs, but clopidogrel remains a by-prescription-only medication and, thus, requires a physician visit to obtain a prescription for the medication. It is for all these reasons that the current recommendations list clopidogrel as a first-line agent, but only in cases where ASA therapy is either not tolerated or contraindicated.[53,55]

Ticlopidine (Ticlid)

Although ticlopidine has the same mechanism of action as clopidogrel and possesses a similar molecular structure, the results of clinical trials among the two agents are strikingly different.[18] The Swedish Ticlopidine Multicenter Study (STIMS) had determined that ticlopidine therapy (500 mg/day) was able to reduce total mortality in comparison to placebo in patients with intermittent claudication ($p = 0.015$).[18,58,59] Regardless, the once promising results seen with ticlopidine therapy have now been overshadowed by the severe hematologic side effects unique to this agent. Other agents, namely clopidogrel, are now used in its stead.[7,24,33]

INTERMITTENT CLAUDICATION (See Table 22-1)

Cilostazol (Pletal)

In a head-to-head, randomized, placebo-controlled study in 698 patients with moderate-to-severe claudication, Dawson and colleagues assigned patients to cilostazol (100 mg twice a day), pentoxifylline (400 mg 3 times a day), or placebo in an effort to improve maximal walking distance.[60] After 24 weeks, the cilostazol group demonstrated a 54% mean increase in distance versus pentoxifylline which demonstrated only a 30% mean increase ($p < 0.001$).[60] Similarly, a meta-analysis of 8 randomized, double-blind, placebo-controlled, parallel-design trials supported this conclusion with a reported increase in maximal walking distance and pain-free walking distance over placebo with cilostazol at doses of 50 mg and 100 mg twice-daily ($p < 0.05$ for all).[61] Regrettably, improvement in walking distance has appeared to come with a price (in addition to the high drug cost); cilostazol has a "black box" warning from the Food and Drug Administration (FDA) warning providers not to use this medication in patients with PAD and coexisting heart failure.[31] If patients with PAD are not candidates for surgical interventions to improve severe intermittent claudication, and after appropriate exercise therapy and therapeutic lifestyle changes have been implemented, the Seventh ACCP Conference on Antithrombotic and Thrombolytic Therapy then suggests the use of this agent.[56]

Pentoxifylline (Trental)

Unlike cilostazol, pentoxifylline has produced less promising results in clinical trials. An illustration of this is the randomized, placebo-controlled trial by Dawson and colleagues mentioned above.[60] Not only did cilostazol outperform pentoxifylline in improvement in walking distance, the improvement seen with pentoxifylline was no different from placebo ($p = 0.82$).[60] This nonsignificant improvement in walking distance has been observed in other studies as well.[7,62] Meanwhile, other meta-analyses of pentoxifylline in comparison to placebo for the improvement of maximal walking distance, have shown some minimal improvement over placebo, but the average effects were relatively small.[7,63–66] For these reasons, the Seventh ACCP Conference on Antithrombotic and Thrombolytic Therapy does not recommend the use of this agent.[56]

▓ EVALUATION OF THERAPEUTIC OUTCOMES

It is vital that the patient be counseled on the evaluation measures that will be used to monitor the outcomes of therapeutic interventions for PAD. Various laboratory measurements will assess patient progress in glycemic control (i.e., hemoglobin A1C) and lipid management (i.e., total cholesterol, LDL, HDL, and non-HDL cholesterol), while blood pressure checks in the clinic and patient home blood pressure monitoring can assess the effectiveness of antihypertensive therapy. Repeat exercise treadmill walking testing should be repeated at regular intervals (i.e., quarterly to biannually) to assess improvement or decline in walking duration and distance, as well as the time to pain onset while performing this activity. Repeat ABI measurements should be assessed at each patient visit to determine if there has been stabilization or progression of the disease process. Most importantly to many patients, simple concern and questioning about improvements to their daily quality of life will highlight your concern for their well-being and aid in an overall picture of the patient's general state of health.

▓ ABBREVIATIONS

ABI: ankle-brachial index
ACCP: American College of Chest Physicians
ACE: angiotensin-converting-enzyme
AMI: acute myocardial infarction
ASA: aspirin (acetylsalicylic acid)
ATC: Antithombotic Trialists' Collaboration
ATP III: Expert Panel on Detection, Evaluation, and Treatment of High Blood Cholesterol in Adults (Adult Treatment Panel III)
CAD: coronary artery disease
CHD: coronary heart disease
CVD: cardiovascular disease
FDA: Food and Drug Administration
HF: heart failure
HOPE: Heart Outcomes Prevention Evaluation study
HPS: Heart Protection Study
HTN: hypertension
IC: intermittent claudication
NHANES: National Health and Nutrition Examination Survey
OR: odds ratio
PAD: peripheral arterial disease
PARTNERS: PAD Awareness, Risk, and Treatment: New Resources for Survival
PTA: percutaneous transluminal angioplasty
STIMS: Swedish Ticlopidine Multicenter Study
TASC: TransAtlantic Inter-Society Consensus
TLC: therapeutic lifestyle changes

Review Questions and other resources can be found at *www.pharmacotherapyonline.com.*

▓ REFERENCES

1. Hiatt WR. Sounding the PAD alarm. GPs can diagnose peripheral artery disease with a simple ankle-and-arm blood pressure test. Health News 2004;10(4).
2. Selvin E, TP E. Prevalence of and risk factors for peripheral arterial disease in the United States. Results from the National Health and Nutrition Examination Survey, 1999–2000. Circulation 2004;110:738–743.
3. Newman AB, Shemanski L, Manolio TA, et al. Ankle-arm index as a predictor of cardiovascular disease and mortality in the Cardiovascular Health Study. The Cardiovascular Health Study Group. Arteriosclerosis, Thrombosis & Vascular Biology 1999;19:538–545.
4. Committee CS. A randomised, blinded, trial of clopidogrel versus aspirin in patients at risk of ischaemic events (CAPRIE). CAPRIE Steering Committee. Lancet 1996:1329–1339.
5. Stewart KJ, Hiatt WR, Regensteiner JG, Hirsch AT. Exercise training for claudication. N Engl J Med 2002;347:1941–1951.
6. O'Hare AM, Glidden DV, Fox CS, Hsu CY. High prevalence of peripheral arterial disease in persons with renal insufficiency: results from the National Health and Nutrition Examination Survey 1999–2000. Circulation 2004;109:320–323.
7. Hiatt WR. Medical treatment of peripheral arterial disease and claudication. N Engl J Med 2001;344:1608–1621.
8. Mohler ER, 3rd. Peripheral arterial disease. Identification and implications. Arch Int Med 2003;163(2306–2314).
9. Dormandy JA, Murray GD. The fate of the claudicant–a prospective study of 1969 claudicants. Euro J Vasc Surg 1991;5:131–133.
10. Hirsch AT, Hiatt WR, Committee PS. PAD awareness, risk, and treatment: new resources for survival—the USA PARTNERS program. Vasc Med 2001;6(3 Suppl):9–12.
11. Chobanian AV, Bakris GL, Black HR, et al. The Seventh Report of the Joint National Committee on Prevention, Detection, Evaluation, and Treatment of High Blood Pressure: the JNC 7 report. JAMA 2003;289:2560–2572.
12. National Cholesterol Education Program Expert Panel: Third Report of the National Cholesterol Education Program (NCEP) Expert Panel on Detection, Evaluation, and Treatment of High Blood Cholesterol in Adults (Adult Treatment Panel III) final report. Circulation 2002;106:3143–3421.
13. Grundy S, Cleeman J, Merz CB, et al: Implications of recent clinical trials for the National Cholesterol Education Program Adult Treatment Panel III Guidelines. Circulation 2004;110:227–239.
14. Jackson M, Clagett G. Antithrombotic therapy in peripheral arterial occlusive disease. Chest 2001;119(Suppl):283S–299S.
15. Hutter C, Austin M, Humphries S. Familial hypercholesterolemia, peripheral arterial disease, and stroke: A HuGE minireview. Amer J Epidemiol 2004;160:430–435.
16. Creager MA: Peripheral arterial disease. In Federman DD, Dale DC (eds): ACP Medicine. New York, WebMD, 2004.
17. Hiatt W, Nehler MR: Peripheral arterial disease. In, Cassel CK (ed): Geriatric Medicine: An Evidence Based Approach, 4 ed. New York, Spring-Verlag, 2003.
18. Hiatt WR. Preventing atherothrombotic events in peripheral arterial disease: the use of antiplatelet therapy. J Int Med 2002;251:193–206.
19. Hirsch AT, Criqui MH, Treat-Jacobson D, et al. Peripheral arterial disease detection, awareness, and treatment in primary care. JAMA 2001; 286:1317–1324.
20. Dormandy JA, Rutherford RB. Management of peripheral arterial disease (PAD). TASC Working Group. TransAtlantic Inter-Society Consensus (TASC). J Vasc Surg 2000;31(1 Pt 2):S1–S296.
21. Carman TL, Fernandez BB, Jr. A primary care approach to the patient with claudication. Am Fam Physician 2000;61(4):1027–1032, 1034.
22. Schmieder FA, Comerota AJ. Intermittent claudication: magnitude of

the problem, patient evaluation, and therapeutic strategies. Am J Cardiol 2001;87:3D–13D.

23. Group TW. Management of peripheral arterial disease (PAD). Trans-Atlantic Inter-Society Consensus (TASC). Section B: intermittent claudication. Euro J Vasc Endovasc Surg 2000; 19(Suppl A):S47–S114.

24. Gey DC, Lesho EP, Manngold J. Management of peripheral arterial disease. Am Fam Physician 2004;69:525–532.

25. Aronow W. Management of peripheral arterial disease of the lower extremities in elderly patients. J Gerontology 2004;59A:172–177.

26. Criqui MH. Systemic atherosclerosis risk and the mandate for intervention in atherosclerotic peripheral arterial disease. Am J Cardiol 2001;88:43J–47J.

27. Yao ST, Hobbs JT, Irvine WT. Ankle systolic pressure measurements in arterial disease affecting the lower extremities. Br J Surg 1969;56:676–679.

28. McDermott MM, Greenland P, Liu K, et al. The ankle brachial index is associated with leg function and physical activity: the Walking and Leg Circulation Study. Ann Int Med 2002;136:873–883.

29. McDermott MM, Criqui MH, Liu K, et al. Lower ankle/brachial index, as calculated by averaging the dorsalis pedis and posterior tibial arterial pressures, and association with leg functioning in peripheral arterial disease. J Vasc Surg 2000;32:1164–1171.

30. Belch JJ, Topol EJ, Agnelli G, et al. Critical issues in peripheral arterial disease detection and management: a call to action. Arch Intern Med 2003;163:884–892.

31. Hiatt WR. Pharmacologic therapy for peripheral arterial disease and claudication. J Vasc Surg 2002;36:1283–1291.

32. Burns P, Gough S, Bradbury AW. Management of peripheral arterial disease in primary care. Br Med J 2003;326:584–588.

33. Regensteiner JG, Hiatt WR. Current medical therapies for patients with peripheral arterial disease: a critical review. Am J Med 2002;112:49–57.

34. Kannel WB, Shurtleff D. National Heart and Lung Institute, National Institutes of Health. The Framingham Study: cigarettes and the development of intermittent claudication. Geriatrics 1973;28:61–68.

35. Tierney S, Fennessy F, Hayes DB. ABC of arterial and vascular disease: secondary prevention of peripheral vascular disease. Br Med J 2000;320:1262–1265.

36. Gardner AW, Katzel LI, Sorkin JD, Goldberg AP. Effects of long-term exercise rehabilitation on claudication distances in patients with peripheral arterial disease: a randomized controlled trial. J Cardiopulm Rehabil 2002;22:192–198.

37. Gardner AW, Katzel LI, Sorkin JD, et al. Exercise rehabilitation improves functional outcomes and peripheral circulation in patients with intermittent claudication: a randomized controlled trial. J Am Geriatr Soc 2001;49:755–762.

38. Langbein WE, Collins EG, Orebaugh C, et al. Increasing exercise tolerance of persons limited by claudication pain using polestriding. J Vasc Surg 2002;35:887–893.

39. Falcone RA, Hirsch AT, Regensteiner JG, et al. Peripheral arterial disease rehabilitation: a review. J Cardiopulm Rehabil 2003;23:170–175.

40. Tan KH, De Cossart L, Edwards PR. Exercise training and peripheral vascular disease. Br J Surg 2000;87:553–562.

41. Chobanian AV, Bakris GL, Black HR, et al. The Seventh Report of the Joint National Committee on Prevention, Detection, Evaluation, and Treatment of High Blood Pressure: The JNC 7 Report. JAMA 2003;289:2560–2571.

42. Whyman MR, Fowkes FG, Kerracher EM, et al. Is intermittent claudication improved by percutaneous transluminal angioplasty? A randomized controlled trial. J Vasc Surg 1997;26:551–557.

43. Bosch J, Hunink M. Meta-analysis of the results of percutaneous transluminal angioplasty and stent placement for aortoiliac occlusive disease (published erratum appears in Radiology 1997 Nov;205[2]:584). Radiology 1997;204:87–96.

44. McDermott MM. Peripheral arterial disease: epidemiology and drug therapy. Am J Geriatr Cardiol 2002;11:258–266.

45. Expert Panel on Detection E, and Treatment of High Blood Cholesterol in Adults. Executive Summary of the Third Report of the National Cholesterol Education Program (NCEP) Expert Panel on Detection, Evaluation, and Treatment of High Blood Cholesterol in Adults (Adult Treatment Panel III). JAMA 2001;285:2486–2497.

46. Leng GC, Price JF, Jepson RG. Lipid-lowering for lower limb atherosclerosis. Cochrane Database Syst Rev 2000;2(CD000123).

47. MRC/BHF Heart Protection Study of cholesterol lowering with simvastatin in 20536 high-risk individuals: a randomised placebo-controlled trial. Lancet 2002;360:7–22.

48. Cannon CP, Braunwald E, McCabe CH, et al. Intensive versus Moderate Lipid Lowering with Statins after Acute Coronary Syndromes. N Engl J Med 2004;350:1495–1504.

49. Elam MB, Hunninghake DB, Davis KB, et al. Effect of niacin on lipid and lipoprotein levels and glycemic control in patients with diabetes and peripheral arterial disease: The ADMIT study: a randomized trial. JAMA 2000;284:1263–1270.

50. Coutinho M, Gerstein H, Wang Y, Yusuf S. The relationship between glucose and incident cardiovascular events. A metaregression analysis of published data from 20 studies of 95,783 individuals followed for 12.4 years. Diabetes Care 1999;22:233–240.

51. Association AD. Peripheral arterial disease in people with diabetes. Diabetes Care 2003;26(12):3333–3341.

52. Creager MA, Luscher TF, Cosentino F, Beckman JA. Diabetes and vascular disease: pathophysiology, clinical consequences, and medical therapy: Part I. Circulation 2003;108:1527–1532.

53. Collaboration AT. Collaborative meta-analysis of randomised trials of antiplatelet therapy for prevention of death, myocardial infarction, and stroke in high risk patients. Br Med J 2002;324:71–86.

54. Tran H, Anand SS. Oral antiplatelet therapy in cerebrovascular disease, coronary artery disease, and peripheral arterial disease. JAMA 2004;292:1867–1874.

55. Moore TD, Linn WD, O'Rourke RA. Hot Topic: Current evidence for the use of antiplatelet therapy in cerebrovascular ideas, coronary artery disease, and peripheral arterial disease. McGraw-Hill Companies, 2004. (Accessed 29 October, 2004, at http://cardiology.accessmedicine.com.)

56. Clagett GP, Sobel M, Jackson MR, Lip GYH, Tangelder M, Verhaeghe R. Antithrombotic therapy in peripheral arterial occlusive disease: The Seventh ACCP Conference on Antithrombotic and Thrombolytic Therapy. Chest 2004;126(3 suppl):609S-26.

57. Diener HC, Cunha L, Forbes C, et al. European Stroke Prevention Study 2. Dipyridamole and acetylsalicylic acid in the secondary prevention of stroke. J Neurol Sci 1996;143:1–13.

58. Janzon L. The STIMS trial: the ticlopidine experience and its clinical applications. Swedish Ticlopidine Multicenter Study. Vasc Med 1996;1:141–143.

59. Janzon L, Bergqvist D, Boberg J, et al. Prevention of myocardial infarction and stroke in patients with intermittent claudication; effects of ticlopidine. Results from STIMS, the Swedish Ticlopidine Multicentre Study. J Int Med 1990;227:301–308.

60. Dawson DL, Cutler BS, Hiatt WR, et al. A comparison of cilostazol and pentoxifylline for treating intermittent claudication. Am J Med 2000;109:523–530.

61. Thompson PD, Zimet R, Forbes WP, Zhang P. Meta-analysis of results from eight randomized, placebo-controlled trials on the effect of cilostazol on patients with intermittent claudication. Am J Cardiol 2002;90:1314–1319.

62. Lindgarde F, Jelnes R, Bjorkman H, et al. Conservative drug treatment in patients with moderately severe chronic occlusive peripheral arterial disease. Scandinavian Study Group. Circulation 1989;80:1549–1556.

63. Girolami B, Bernardi E, Prins MH, et al. Treatment of intermittent claudication with physical training, smoking cessation, pentoxifylline, or nafronyl: a meta-analysis. Arch Int Med 1999;159:337–345.

64. Radack K, Wyderski RJ. Conservative management of intermittent claudication. Ann Int Med 1990;113:135–146.

65. Ernst E. Pentoxifylline for intermittent claudication. A critical review. Angiology 1994;45:339–345.

66. Hood SC, Moher D, Barber GG. Management of intermittent claudication with pentoxifylline: meta-analysis of randomized controlled trials. J Can Med Assoc 1996;155:1053–1059.

67. Mills DC, Puri R, Hu CJ. Clopidogrel inhibits the binding of ADP

analogues to the receptor mediating inhibition of platelet adenylate cyclase. Arterioscler Thromb 1992;12:430–436.

68. Plavix package insert. In: (Bristol-Myers Squibb/Sanofi—U.S.); Rev 11/97, Rec 2/98.

69. USP DI Editorial Group. "S" Monographs; Salicylates (systemic); Aspirin. In USP DI ® Drug Information for the Health Care Professional, 24 ed. Taunton, MA: Micromedex Inc, 2004.

70. USP DI Editorial Group. "D" Monographs; Dipyridamole (Systemic). In USP DI ® Drug Information for the Health Care Professional, 24 ed. Taunton, MA: Micromedex Inc.; 2004.

71. USP DI Editorial Group. "P" Monographs; Pentoxifylline (Systemic). In: USP DI ® Drug Information for the Health Care Professional. 24th ed. Taunton, Massachusetts: Micromedex Inc.; 2004.

72. USP DI Editorial Group. "C" Monographs; Cilostazol (Systemic). In: USP DI ® Drug Information for the Health Care Professional. 24th ed. Taunton, Massachusetts: Micromedex Inc.; 2004.

73. Guyatt G, Schunemann HJ, Cook D, Jaeschke R, Pauker S. Applying the Grades of Recommendation for Antithrombotic and Thrombolytic Therapy: The Seventh ACCP Conference on Antithrombotic and Thrombolytic Therapy. Chest 2004;126(3 suppl):179S-87.

23

USE OF VASOPRESSORS AND INOTROPES IN THE PHARMACOTHERAPY OF SHOCK

Maria I. Rudis and Joseph F. Dasta

Learning Objectives and other resources can be found at *www.pharmacotherapyonline.com.*

KEY CONCEPTS

◀1 Continuous hemodynamic monitoring either with an arterial catheter or with a pulmonary artery (or central venous) catheter with central venous oxygen saturation measurement should be used early and throughout the course of septic shock to assess intravascular fluid status and ventricular filling pressures, determine cardiac output, and monitor arterial and venous oxygenation. They also should be used for monitoring the response to drug therapy and guide dosage titration.

◀2 Early goal-directed therapy with aggressive fluid resuscitation in the emergency department within the first 6 hours of presentation improves survival in sepsis and septic shock.

◀3 Derangements in adrenergic receptor sensitivity or activity frequently result in resistance to vasopressor and inotropic therapy in critically ill patients. These changes may be a function of endogenous catecholamine concentrations, dose/duration of exposure to and type of exogenously administered vasopressors, stage of septic shock, preexisting illness, and other factors.

◀4 In refractory septic shock, the rational use of vasopressor or inotropic agents should be guided by receptor activity, pharmacologic characteristics, and regional and systemic hemodynamic effects of the drug and should be tailored to the patient's physiologic needs. Pharmacologically sound combinations of agents should be initiated early to optimize response.

◀5 Goals of therapy with vasopressors and inotropes should be predetermined and should optimize regional perfusion to tissues (e.g., cardiac, renal, mesenteric, and periphery). This can be accomplished by continuous or intermittent measurements. Central venous oxygen saturation ($SvcO_2$) should be maintained in excess of 70%. Arbitrarily targeting vasopressor and inotrope therapy to supranormal global oxygen transport variables cannot be recommended because there is no clear benefit, and morbidity may be increased.

◀6 Much higher dosages of all vasopressors and inotropes than recommended traditionally are required to improve the hemodynamic and oxygen transport variables in septic shock.

◀7 Dose titration and monitoring of vasopressor and inotropic therapy should be guided by the "best clinical response" while observing for and minimizing evidence of myocardial ischemia (e.g., tachydysrhythmias, electrocardiographic changes), renal (decreased glomerular filtration rate and/or urine output), splanchnic/gastric (low pHi, bowel ischemia), or peripheral (cold extremities) hypoperfusion, and worsening of Pao_2, pulmonary artery opening pressure (PAOP), and other hemodynamic variables.

◀8 Dopamine typically is used as an initial vasopressor agent for hemodynamic support but is limited by its ability to increase cardiac output (by only 35%). Its use is frequently complicated by tachycardia and tachydysrhythmias and occasionally by an increase in PAOP. In contrast to norepinephrine, it decreases splanchnic oxygen use. Low-dose dopamine should not be used to prevent renal failure.

◀9 Phenylephrine may be a particularly useful alternative in those who cannot tolerate tachycardia or tachydysrhythmia with dopamine or norepinephrine or in patients with known underlying myocardial dysfunction.

◀10 Epinephrine appears to be effective as a single agent and as an add-on agent. It is particularly useful in the young, in patients with otherwise healthy myocardia, and potentially when used early in the course of treatment. However, because it causes a significant increase in lactate and worsening of splanchnic oxygen utilization, it is not the agent of first choice in septic shock. It also should be used cautiously in patients with a history of coronary artery disease (CAD) or underlying cardiac disturbances.

◀11 Therapy with vasopressors and inotropes is continued until the myocardial depression and vascular hyporesponsiveness of septic shock improve, usually measured in hours to days. Discontinuation of vasopressor or inotropic therapy should be executed slowly; therapy should be "weaned" to avoid a precipitous worsening in regional and systemic hemodynamics.

TABLE 23–1. Hemodynamic and Oxygen-Transport Monitoring Parameters

Parameter	Normal Value
Blood pressure (systolic/diastolic)	100–130/70–85 mm Hg
Mean arterial pressure (MAP)	80–100 mm Hg
Pulmonary artery pressure (PAP)	25/10 mm Hg
Mean pulmonary artery pressure (MPAP)	12–15 mm Hg
Central venous pressure (CVP)	8–12 mm Hg
Pulmonary artery occlusion pressure (PAOP)	12–15 mm Hg*
Heart rate (HR)	60–80 beats/min
Cardiac output (CO)	4–7 L/min
Cardiac index (CI)	2.8–3.6 L/min/m^2
Stroke volume index (SVI)	30–50 mL/m^2
Systemic vascular resistance index (SVRI)	1300–2100 dyne · s/m^2 · cm^5
Pulmonary vascular resistance index (PVRI)	45–225 dyne · s/m^2 · cm^5
Arterial oxygen saturation (Sao$_2$)	97% (range 95–100)
Mixed venous oxygen saturation (Svo$_2$)	70–75%
Arterial oxygen content (Cao$_2$)	20.1 vol% (range 19–21)
Venous oxygen content (Cvo$_2$)	15.5 vol% (range 11.5–16.5)
Oxygen content difference (C[a-v]o$_2$)	5 vol% (range 4–6)
Oxygen consumption index (Vo$_2$)	131 mL/min/m^2 (range 100–180)
Oxygen delivery index (Do$_2$)	578 mL/min/m^2 (range 370–730)
Oxygen extraction ratio (O$_2$ER)	25% (range 22–30)
Mucosal pH (pHi)	7.40 (range 7.35–7.45)
Index (I)	Parameter indexed to body surface area

*These normal values may not necessarily be the same as optimal values needed to optimize the management of a critically ill patient.

Shock is an acute, generalized state of inadequate perfusion of critical organs that can produce serious pathophysiologic consequences, including death. Thirty years ago, mortality from septic or cardiogenic shock exceeded 70%.[1] Currently, approximately 10% of patients are admitted to hospitals with severe sepsis or experience cardiogenic shock following a myocardial infarction, with mortality rates of at least 30% to 50% despite enhanced treatment modalities and sophisticated monitoring techniques.[1,2] This chapter will review the theory and current status of hemodynamic monitoring and will present an update on the optimal use of inotropes and vasopressor drugs in shock states.[3,4]

Hemodynamic and perfusion monitoring can be categorized into two broad areas: global and regional monitoring. Global parameters, such as systemic blood pressure and pulse oximetry, assess perfusion and oxygen utilization of the entire body. Regional monitoring techniques, such as tonometry, focus on flow and subsequent changes in metabolism of individual organs and tissues. Normal values for commonly monitored parameters are listed in Table 23–1.

GLOBAL PERFUSION MONITORING

ARTERIAL BLOOD PRESSURE MEASUREMENT

Arterial blood pressure is the product of cardiac output and systemic vascular resistance. Conditions that may lower blood pressure in the critically ill include cardiac failure or hypovolemia (by lowering of cardiac output) and vasodilation (by sepsis, drugs, or neurotrauma).

Arterial blood pressure can be determined by noninvasive and invasive methods. All noninvasive blood pressure monitoring techniques depend on the use of an occluding cuff. Systolic and diastolic blood pressures are further determined by auscultation, palpation (systolic pressure only), oscillometry, or Doppler technique (systolic pressures most reliable). Auscultation is the most commonly used method outside the intensive care unit (ICU). Its use, however, is limited in patients with hypovolemia, hypothermia, or cardiogenic shock when pulses or Korotkoff sounds may be difficult to hear. Similar constraints exist for the palpation and oscillometric methods. However, oscillometry is preferred in edematous patients. Oscillometry measures blood pressure by sensing arterial blood pressure changes, or oscillations, against an inflated cuff. Rapid changes in oscillation amplitude correspond to systolic and diastolic pressure. It is the only noninvasive method to measure mean arterial pressure even in low-flow states and lends itself to automatic cycling and serial measurements (every 1 to 3 minutes) that do not require operator intervention, a key component in ICU monitoring. The use of narrow cuffs or cuffs applied too loosely can result in falsely high readings, whereas wide cuffs may produce falsely low readings.[5] Fingertip devices offer another avenue for continuous indirect blood pressure measurement, but their accuracy in ICU patients may be significantly diminished by concurrent administration of vasoactive drugs.

The use of invasive arterial catheters makes it possible to measure arterial blood pressures continuously, as well as to obtain blood samples for blood gas monitoring. The radial artery is the most commonly used vessel, but the dorsalis pedis, femoral, brachial, and axillary arteries and the umbilical artery in the newborn also can be accessed. This method of blood pressure monitoring is a standard technique against which all other methods are compared. Major complications of peripheral artery catheterization include infection and distal ischemia. Acute distal ischemia and catheter-related bacteremia occur in less than 1% of catheter insertions. This translates into 2.9% of bloodstream infections per 1000 catheter-days.[6] Ischemia is most common in patients with multiple or prolonged arterial cannulations, hypertension, or vasopressor therapy.[5] Invasive techniques are labor-intensive, require aseptic techniques, and offer potential sources of equipment errors, such as length and quality of tubing, air bubbles, stopcocks, thrombus formation, tube kinking, and placement of transducer. Hypertension, advanced age, and atherosclerosis also may affect the accuracy of invasive blood pressure readings.[7]

CENTRAL VENOUS CATHETER

The central venous catheter is used to measure the central venous pressure (CVP), to obtain venous blood gas samples, and to administer drugs or fluids directly to the central circulation. A triple-lumen catheter frequently is used, whereby drugs with known incompatibility can be administered. Blood volume, venous wall compliance, right-sided cardiac function, intraabdominal and intrathoracic pressure, and vasopressor therapy affect CVP. The CVP is not a reliable estimate of blood volume but can be used to qualitatively assess blood volume changes in patients during the early phases of fluid resuscitation. Sustained elevated pressures may indicative of fluid overloading. There are few data supporting the use of CVP monitoring in the ICU. However, initial reports in septic patients suggest that CVP monitoring of fluid therapy during shock was associated with an over 50% reduction in mortality.

PULMONARY ARTERY CATHETER

◀ Pulmonary artery catheterization, introduced in 1970, is a routinely performed bedside procedure in many ICUs. With this catheter, also known as the *Swan-Ganz catheter*, the practitioner can obtain multiple cardiovascular parameters, including central venous, pulmonary artery, and pulmonary artery occlusive pressures and cardiac output. Mixed-venous blood samples from the pulmonary artery also may be obtained. In an effort to reduce blood loss from samples, many clinicians are using special pulmonary artery catheters, called a *fiberoptic catheter*, that measure mixed-venous oxygen saturation (SvO_2). Hence trends in the venous oxygen saturation can be observed, and necessary action can be taken, if needed. Most important, inflation of the balloon at the catheter tip occludes the pulmonary artery, isolates the distal catheter tip from the right side of the heart, and allows the user to measure the pulmonary capillary "occlusive" pressure (PAOP), an approximate measure of the left ventricular (LV) end-diastolic volume and a major determinant of LV preload. Ideally, the pulmonary artery catheter should be positioned fluoroscopically; however, satisfactory placement also may be obtained by observing pulmonary artery pressure readings during catheter advancement. Proper positioning in the lower lung (zone 3) is essential to measure PAOP and to prevent distal pulmonary artery collapse. Poor wedging may be caused by catheter migration, patient movement, mechanical ventilation, or eccentric balloon inflation. Pulmonary artery catheters equipped with a distal thermistor also allow measurement of cardiac output by thermodilution. Rapid injection of saline solutions via the right atrial port allows complete mixing of blood with injectate, and the resulting change in blood temperature is measured in the pulmonary artery. From the temperature change, the patient's cardiac output can be calculated. Newer pulmonary artery catheters contain a temperature coil that intermittently warms the blood in the right ventricle for near-continuous cardiac output measurement. Significant tricuspid regurgitation, an intracardiac shunt, and significant positive end-expiratory pressure (PEEP) decrease the validity of cardiac output measurements. The most common complications of pulmonary artery catheterization include mural thrombus formation (14% to 91%), transient ventricular tachydysrrhythmias (11% to 63%), pulmonary infarction (1% to 7%), pulmonary artery rupture (0.06% to 2.0%), and sepsis (0.3% to 0.5%).[8] Most pulmonary artery catheters are heparin-bonded, and the relative risk of infection is 2.6 per 1000 patient days, similar to central venous catheters, 2.3 per 1000 patient days.[6] Despite its ubiquitous use, much controversy surrounds the utility and safety of the pulmonary artery catheter, including issues surrounding correct placement and impact of the device on patient outcome.[9] As a result, recommendations have been made to standardize and monitor physician and nurse education on proper use of the catheter (see *www.pacep.org*), to conduct clinical trials assessing the safety and efficacy of the catheter, and to evaluate new device technology on patient outcome.[8] The most recent guidelines suggest a careful evaluation of the indications and the risk of placing a pulmonary artery catheter for the resuscitation of critically ill patients.[10]

◁ The optimal PAOP needs to be individualized for each patient. Administering a fluid bolus followed by simultaneous PAOP and cardiac output (CO) measurements with the goal of increasing the PAOP until the CO does not change can be accomplished and is based on Starling's law of the heart. However, clinical experience suggests that most patients have an optimal response to PAOP values in the range of 12 to 15 mm Hg.

OXYGEN TENSION AND SATURATION MONITORING

Arterial oxygen pressure (PaO_2) and saturation (SaO_2) may be measured invasively by obtaining an arterial blood sample. Arterial blood gases measured by conventional arterial sampling are considered

standard, but their accuracy and usefulness are affected by poor sampling techniques, transportation and analysis delays, analyzer accuracy, sample cellular metabolism, and inability to trend results. Indwelling fiberoptic and electrochemical systems allow continuous monitoring and trend analyses of blood pH, PaO_2, and $PaCO_2$ while decreasing patient blood loss owing to frequent sampling. Unfortunately, studies evaluating the in vitro accuracy of these devices may not apply to the ICU environment. The indwelling sensors may exhibit lower PaO_2, higher $PaCO_2$, and lower pH than central arterial blood when peripheral flow is diminished. Furthermore, sensor contact with blood vessel wall and vigorous arterial line flushing also will diminish sensor accuracy.

◁ Mixed venous oxygen saturation (SvO_2) depends on cardiac output, oxygen demand, hemoglobin, and arterial oxygen saturation. It may be measured in patients with a pulmonary artery catheter. Initially, critically ill septic patients may present with a low SvO_2 value (<70%) indicating a high extraction of oxygen by tissues and a lack of adequate oxygen delivery to tissues. In patients with sepsis and other conditions who present with a low SvO_2 value, prompt, rapid intervention should be undertaken to increase oxygen delivery to tissues with a goal of an SvO_2 of greater than 70% to 75%.[11] As sepsis progresses, however, SvO_2 values may exceed 70% to 75%. This occurs because of a maldistribution of blood flow and a lack of extraction of oxygen in the arteriolar beds.

◁ Central venous oxygen saturation ($ScvO_2$) is a less invasive measure of venous oxygen saturation because the catheter is placed at the junction of the inferior and superior venae cavae and only requires a central line rather than a pulmonary artery catheter. It is as accurate as SvO_2. Concentrations of $ScvO_2$ of less than 70% reliably indicate inadequate oxygenation in shock states and detect subclinical ("cryptic") shock much earlier than hypotension.[12] Targeting fluid and hemodynamic resuscitation to achieve $ScvO_2$ concentrations of greater than 70% to 75% may be a more sensitive indicator of the extent of global tissue hypoxia, as well as a more sensitive measure of the adequacy of hemodynamic resuscitation than vital signs, including systolic, diastolic, and mean arterial blood pressures.[13] Targeting resuscitation to achieve $ScvO_2$ concentrations of greater than 70% to 75% is associated with improved survival in patients with sepsis and septic shock.[12]

OXYGEN DELIVERY AND CONSUMPTION

The concept of tissue oxygen debt as a determinant of organ damage in critical illness was proposed over 10 years ago. In normal individuals, oxygen consumption (VO_2 or VO_2I, indexed to body surface area) depends on oxygen delivery (DO_2 or DO_2I, indexed to body surface area) up to a certain critical level (VO_2 flow dependency). At this point, tissue oxygen requirements apparently have been satisfied, and further increases in DO_2 will not alter VO_2 (VO_2 flow independency) (Fig. 23–1). Although animal models of sepsis have substantiated this relationship, studies in critically ill humans show a continuous,

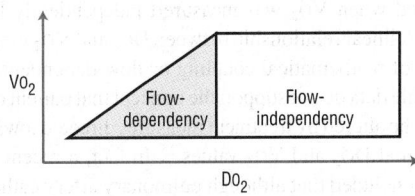

FIGURE 23–1. Relationship between oxygen consumption (VO_2) and oxygen delivery (DO_2).

pathologic dependence relationship of VO_2 on DO_2. Furthermore, ICU survivors exhibited higher DO_2 and VO_2 values than nonsurvivors. This became the basis for targeting supranormal DO_2 and VO_2 values in the treatment of ICU patients.[14] However, a recent meta-analysis of randomized clinical trials involving 1016 adult ICU patients failed to show that achievement of this goal improved patient mortality.[15] This may have been due in part to the heterogeneous nature of the ICU patients studied, lack of study blinding, crossover patients (control patients who achieve supranormal DO_2 and VO_2 values by themselves), or lack of adequate control of cointerventions.

The debate continues in more homogeneous patient populations. In high-risk surgical patients, supranormal DO_2 values decreased mortality. Two recent randomized studies further evaluated the effect of increasing DO_2I values to above 600 mL/m^2 per minute in a homogeneous population of elderly surgical patients with systemic inflammatory response syndrome (SIRS), sepsis, severe sepsis, or septic shock with conflicting results. Yu and colleagues[16] demonstrated that the intervention group had a significant increase in survival at 24 hours (21% versus 52%; $p = .01$) compared with the control group in patients between 50 and 75 years of age. This benefit was not seen in those older than 75 years of age. The authors suggested that the combination of increasing DO_2 and maintaining the oxygen extraction ratio (O_2ER) below 25% without a changing VO_2 may be helpful in maintaining or improving the reserve of the body to meet the oxygen demands. This may be true particularly in older patients who have a lower baseline VO_2. In the second study, the same intervention revealed a significant reduction in 60-day survival in high-risk elderly surgical patients randomized to have their DO_2 increased to the preceding levels.[17] Thus it remains unclear that the mechanism of benefit of supranormal DO_2 in these patients is prevention and reversal of tissue hypoxia. A recent review of alternative potential mechanisms of beneficial effect of supranormal DO_2 suggests that catecholamines exert anti-inflammatory actions by modulating cytokine response.[18] In general, catecholamines inhibit the inflammatory cytokine (e.g., tumor necrosis factor α [TNF-α]) production and may enhance anti-inflammatory cytokine (e.g., interleukin-6 and interleukin-10) production.[18] The actions of epinephrine on these cytokines are blocked by propranolol and thus are mediated by adrenergic β-receptors. These data must be interpreted with caution because most studies have used animal or cell models of sepsis, have pretreated patients with vasopressors prior to endotoxin infusion, and have used doses that may not always be clinically relevant. A further problem with goal-directed therapy to supranormal oxygen transport values is the fact that the apparent linear relationship between DO_2 and VO_2 has been questioned because both share variables and that this so-called mathematical coupling can produce artifactual relationships between variables. The DO_2 and VO_2 indexed parameters are calculated as follows:

$$DO_2 = CI \times CaO_2$$

$$VO_2 = CI \times (CaO_2 - CvO_2)$$

where CI is the cardiac index, CaO_2 is the arterial oxygen content, and CvO_2 is the mixed venous oxygen content.

However, variable relationships between DO_2 and VO_2 have been observed when VO_2 was measured independently by indirect calorimetry. A linear relationship between DO_2 and VO_2 therefore may be the result of mathematical coupling or flow-dependent VO_2. Currently available data do not support the concept that patient outcome or survival may be altered by treatment measures directed toward achieving supranormal DO_2 and VO_2 values.[15] In fact, a recent consensus conference concluded that although pulmonary artery catheterization is useful to guide therapy, routinely increasing cardiac index to predetermined supranormal values does not improve outcome.[3] Furthermore, achievement of a supranormal DO_2 does not ensure parallel improvements in regional organ blood flow and oxygenation.[19] The VO_2/DO_2 ratio (oxygen extraction ratio, or O_2ER) can be used to assess adequacy of perfusion and metabolic response. Patients who are able to increase VO_2 when DO_2 is increased show improved survival. However, low VO_2 and O_2ER values are indicative of poor oxygen utilization and lead to greater mortality.[15] Another approach that may decrease the effect of mathematical coupling and provide individualized therapy may lie in titrated therapy, with sequential measurements of DO_2 and VO_2 to achieve VO_2 flow independency along with normalization of blood lactate and hemodynamic parameters.

The most recent data regarding goal-directed therapy in the hemodynamic support of sepsis relates to the importance of achieving predetermined parameters early in the management of sepsis. In a meta-analysis of early (defined as 8 to 12 hours postoperatively or before the development of organ failure) versus late (defined as after the onset of organ failure) resuscitative efforts in patients stratified according to severity of illness [determined by the control group mortality as greater than 20% (12 studies) or less than 15% (9 studies)] and targeting to supranormal oxygen transport variables, the data suggest that timing of resuscitation matters.[20] Early goal-directed therapy reduces both mortality and the development of organ failure in studies in which patients were more severely ill and when therapeutic interventions produced differences in oxygen delivery. Moreover, outcome was not improved significantly in less severely ill patients (control mortalities group less than 15% and normal oxygen delivery values as goals) or when therapy did not improve oxygen delivery.[20]

In a recent prospective, randomized, controlled sepsis trial, Rivers and colleagues[12] demonstrated a significant improvement in survival (30.5% versus 46.5%; $p < .001$) in patients with severe sepsis and septic shock randomized to receive therapy based on goal-directed hemodynamic end points for at least 6 hours in the emergency department. They used a strategy of administering fluids rapidly to achieve a central venous pressure of 8 to 12 mm Hg, maintain a hematocrit above 30%, and use of dobutamine to achieve an $ScvO_2$ of greater than 70%. This approach demonstrates the benefits of initiating therapy early in the course of sepsis and directs therapy toward clearly defined goals in a consistent manner.

BLOOD LACTATE

Lactate is a metabolic product of pyruvate, and its production is increased under anaerobic conditions, such as may occur during shock. Blood lactate concentrations are used as a diagnostic and prognostic tool in sepsis; they are also used to measure the repayment of oxygen debt to tissues.[11] It is a useful tool to be used together with DO_2 and VO_2 because these measures change independently of one another.[14] Serial lactate concentrations may show better correlation with outcome than oxygen transport parameters and may be superior to hemodynamic markers in determining adequacy of restoration of systemic oxygenation.[11] However, there are several caveats to guide the use of lactate concentrations in septic patients. First, lactate may accumulate in patients with other conditions, such as significant liver dysfunction or acute respiratory distress syndrome, who are not in shock. Second, both well-perfused and poorly perfused tissues contribute to arterial and mixed venous lactate concentrations and therefore are not reflective of regional perfusion. Third, although increased lactate concentrations have been correlated with increased mortality, the utility of blood lactate measurements in guiding therapy has not been demonstrated clearly. Serial blood lactate measurements are more useful than single isolated measurements.

REGIONAL PERFUSION MONITORING

GASTROINTESTINAL TONOMETRY

Blood pressures, cardiac output, blood lactate, and global oxygen homeostasis parameters do not offer information as to individual organ function. The measurement of regional perfusion to detect inadequate tissue oxygenation has focused on the splanchnic circulation because it is sensitive to changes in blood flow and oxygenation for several reasons. First, the normally large majority of blood flow to the gut mucosa is redistributed toward the serosa and muscularis. Second, the gut may have a higher critical DO_2 threshold than other organs. Third, the tip of the villus has a countercurrent oxygen-exchange mechanism, rendering it very sensitive to reduction in regional blood flow and oxygenation.[11] Gastric tonometry measures gut luminal PCO_2 at equilibrium by placing a saline- or air-filled gas-permeable balloon in the gastric lumen. Assuming that CO_2 permeates freely among tissues and that the arterial bicarbonate (HCO_3^-) concentration is equal to that of the gut mucosa, the intramucosal pH (pHi) may be calculated using the Henderson-Hasselbalch equation:

$$pHi = 6.1 \log (HCO_3^-) 0.03 \times PCO_2$$

Increases in mucosal PCO_2 and calculated decreases in pHi are associated with mucosal hypoperfusion and perhaps increased mortality.[21] The calculation of pHi can be confounded by increases in luminal PCO_2, such as may occur when buffering antacids are used. Histamine-2-receptor antagonists or proton pump inhibitors may be used instead. The presence of respiratory acid-base disorders, systemic bicarbonate administration, arterial blood gas measurement errors, enteral feeding solutions, blood, or stool in the gut may confound pHi determinations.[22] Gastric tonometry may be performed using either a saline- or air-filled balloon. The time delay (30 minutes) associated with equilibration of saline inside the balloon makes this method inconvenient for routine bedside monitoring. An air-filled balloon requires a shorter equilibrium time, is simpler to use, and is equally accurate.[23]

The clinical utility of gastric tonometry, however, remains uncertain. Clinical trials of pHi-directed therapy have not been able to show consistently that it reduces mortality in critically ill patients.[21] However, patients with a normal pHi (>7.35) on ICU admission who subsequently received pHi-guided treatment to increase DO_2 experienced a 38% reduction in mortality. The incidence of multiple organ failure and mortality were not statistically different between the groups, although this may have been due to a small sample size. Many clinicians believe that gastric mucosal PCO_2 may be more accurate than pHi. Furthermore, because mucosal PCO_2 is influenced by arterial PCO_2, consensus is that the mucosal-arterial PCO_2 difference (PCO_2 gap) is likely the optimal measurement.[21]

Recent evidence suggests that the most proximal part of the gastrointestinal (GI) tract, the sublingual mucosa, may be an acceptable location to monitor regional perfusion and PCO_2. One device recently has gained Food and Drug Administration (FDA) approval and consists of a catheter placed sublingually for the determination of sublingual PCO_2 (PslCO_2). A small study of 22 critically ill patients with and without sepsis and septic shock attempted to validate the usefulness of sublingual capnography. They measured simultaneous gastric and sublingual PCO_2, along with traditional hemodynamic parameters. The sublingual PCO_2 correlated well with mucosal PCO_2; however,

the initial sublingual-to-arterial PCO_2 gap was a better predictor of mortality than mucosal-to-arterial PCO_2 gap. This pilot study needs to be expanded before this technology becomes part of routine practice, but it offers the possibility of a noninvasive measurement of regional perfusion.[24]

VASOPRESSORS AND INOTROPES

Vasopressors and inotropes in septic shock are required when volume resuscitation fails to maintain adequate blood pressure (mean arterial pressure [MAP] $\geq$ 65 mm Hg), when the PAOP is optimized to 12 to 15 mm Hg, and organs and tissues remain hypoperfused. However, vasopressors may be needed temporarily in the presence of inadequate filling pressures to treat life-threatening hypotension.[3] The clinician must decide on the choice of agent, therapeutic end points, and the safe and effective doses of vasopressors and inotropes to be used. This section reviews adrenergic receptor pharmacology, exogenous catecholamine use, and alterations in receptor function in the critically ill. It also provides guidelines for the clinical use of adrenergic agents, optimization of pharmacotherapeutic outcomes, and minimization of adverse effects in critically ill patients with septic shock.

It should be noted that agents other than catecholamines have been used as inotropes and vasopressors in shock states. These include phosphodiesterase III inhibitors, naloxone, nitric oxide synthase inhibitors, calcium sensitizers, and vasopressin. However, the focus of this chapter is on catecholamines.

RECEPTOR PHARMACOLOGY

Comparative receptor activity of endogenous and exogenously administered catecholamines is summarized in Table 23–2. Endogenous catecholamines are responsible for regulation of vascular and bronchiolar smooth muscle tone and myocardial contractility. These effects are mediated by sympathetic adrenergic receptors of the autonomic nervous system located in the vasculature, myocardium, and bronchioles. Postsynaptic adrenoceptors are located at or near the synaptic junction. These receptors can be activated by naturally circulating or exogenous catecholamines (e.g., norepinephrine, epinephrine, and phenylephrine), whereas presynaptic adrenoceptors are stimulated by locally released neurotransmitters (e.g., norepinephrine) and are controlled by a negative-feedback mechanism.

Figure 23–2 depicts adrenoceptor–G protein interaction. β- and dopamine (DA)$_1$–adrenoceptor agonists activate the stimulatory G protein, Gs, which dissociates from the receptor and activates membrane-bound adenyl cyclase (AC). α_2- and DA$_2$-agonists activate the inhibitory G protein, Gi, which dissociates from the receptor and blocks AC. AC converts adenosine triphosphate (ATP) to cyclic adenosine monophosphate (cAMP), which stimulates protein kinases, resulting in alterations in cellular functions.

The heart contains primarily postsynaptic β_1-receptors, which cause increased rate and force of contraction when stimulated. This effect appears to be mediated by activation of adenylate cyclase and subsequent generation and accumulation of cAMP. Stimulation of postsynaptic cardiac α_1-receptors causes a significant increase in contractility without an increase in rate, an effect apparently not mediated by cAMP. The increased contractility is more pronounced at lower heart rates and has a slower onset and longer duration in comparison with β_1-mediated inotropic response. Presynaptic α_2-adrenoceptors also are found in the heart and appear to be activated by norepinephrine released by the sympathetic nerve itself. Their activation inhibits further norepinephrine release from the nerve terminal.

TABLE 23–2. Adrenergic and Dopaminergic Receptor Pharmacology and Organ Distribution

Effector Organ	Receptor Subtype	Physiologic Response
Heart		
SA node	β_1, β_2	Increased heart rate
Atria	β_1, β_2	Increased contractility
		Increased conduction velocity
AV node	β_1, β_2	Increased automaticity
		Increased conduction velocity
His-Purkinje system	β_1, β_2	Increased automaticity
		Increased conduction velocity
Ventricles	$\beta_1, \beta_2, \alpha_1$	Increased contractility
		Increased conduction velocity
		Increased automaticity
		Increased rate idioventricular pacemaker cells
Arterioles		
Coronary	$\alpha_1, \alpha_2; \beta_2, DA_1$	Constriction, dilatation
Skin and mucosa	α_1, α_2	Constriction
Skeletal muscle	$\alpha_1; \beta_2$	Constriction, dilatation
Cerebral	α_1	Constriction (slight)
Pulmonary	$\alpha_1; \beta_2$	Constriction, dilatation
Abdominal viscera (mesentery)	$\alpha_1; \beta_2, DA_1$	Constriction, dilatation
Renal	$\alpha_1, \alpha_2; \beta_1, \beta_2, DA_1$	Constriction, dilatation
Veins (systemic)	$\alpha_1, \alpha_2; \beta_2$	Constriction, dilatation
Lungs		
Trachial/bronchial smooth muscle	β_2	Relaxation
Bronchial glands	$\alpha_1; \beta_2$	Decrease, increase secretion
Stomach		
Motility & tone	$\alpha_1, \alpha_2; \beta_2$	Decrease (usually)
Sphincter	α_1	Contraction (usually)
Intestine		
Motility and tone	$\alpha_1, \alpha_2; \beta_1, \beta_2$	Decrease
Sphincters	α_1	Contraction
Secretions	α_2	Inhibition (?)
Kidney		
Renin secretion	α_1	Decrease
Skeletal muscle	β_2	Increased contractility, glyconeogenesis, K^+ uptake
Liver	α_1, β_2	Glycogenolysis and gluconeogenesis

Adapted from refs. 104 and 105.

Both presynaptic and postsynaptic adrenoceptors are present in the vasculature. Postsynaptic α_1- and α_2-receptors mediate vasoconstriction, whereas postsynaptic β_2-receptors induce vasodilation. Presynaptic α_2-receptors inhibit norepinephrine release in the vasculature as well. Presynaptic β_1-adrenoceptors promote neurotransmitter release. Stimulation of peripheral DA_1-receptors produces renal, coronary, and mesenteric vasodilation and a natriuretic response. Stimulation of DA_2-receptors inhibits norepinephrine release from sympathetic nerve endings and prolactin release and may induce nausea and vomiting. DA_1- and DA_2-receptor stimulation also

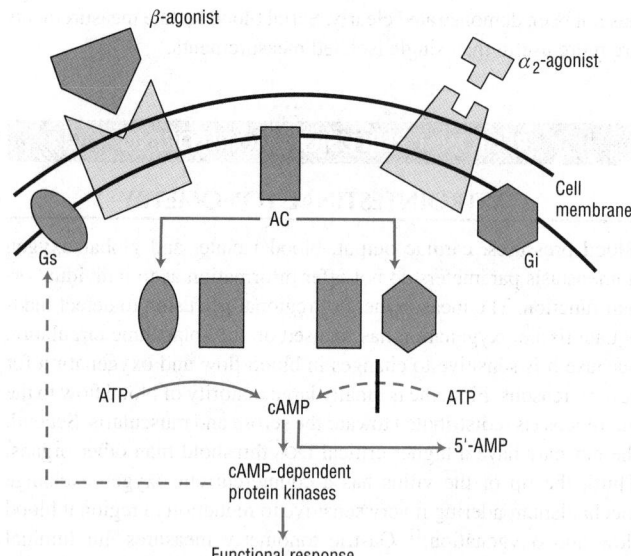

FIGURE 23–2. Adrenoceptor–G protein interaction. AC = adenylate cyclase; α-agonist = α-adrenergic receptor agonist; ATP = adenosine triphosphate; β_1-agonist = β-adrenergic receptor agonist; cAMP = cyclic adenosine monophosphate; Gs = G stimulatory protein; Gi = G inhibitory protein. (*Adapted with permission from ref. 106.*)

suppresses peristalsis and may precipitate ileus. Cloning techniques have identified novel DA_1- and DA_2-like receptors, but their function beyond positive and negative AC coupling to the α-subunit of the G proteins has yet to be determined.

ALTERED ADRENOCEPTOR FUNCTION: IMPLICATIONS FOR THE CRITICALLY ILL

Most of the work describing receptor function and associated clinical pharmacology has been done either in animal models or human volunteers. In critically ill septic patients, derangements in adrenergic receptor activity may result in resistance to exogenous catecholamine administration.[25,26] This "desensitization" frequently is characterized by myocardial and vascular hyporesponsiveness to high dosages of inotropes and vasopressor agents. Prolonged exposure of vascular endothelial tissue to vasopressor drugs (α-adrenergic agonists) or hormones (catecholamines) may produce this attenuation in response. Increased endogenous catecholamine concentrations have been reported in endotoxemic and other critically ill patients, suggesting an acquired β-adrenergic receptor defect and desensitization of β-adrenergic receptors and alteration in voltage-sensitive calcium channels.[25,26] Although the problem in critically ill patients may lie in decreased β-receptor activity or density, in patients with septic shock, the catecholamine concentrations are even higher, and thus abnormalities in β-adrenergic receptor function are greater, with associated reductions in myocardial cyclic monophosphate concentrations. The worsened receptor abnormality may be explained by defects distal to the receptor site, such as an uncoupling of the β-adrenergic receptor from AC or a dysfunction in the regulatory G protein unit of the AC system.[25,26]

Mediators other than catecholamines (e.g., circulating cytokines) may be responsible for these distal alterations. Macrophage-derived interleukin-1 (IL-1) and TNF-α produce impaired coupling of β-adrenergic receptors to adenylate cyclase.[25,26] Septic shock patients have exhibited impaired β-adrenergic receptor stimulation of cAMP associated with myocardial hyporesponsiveness to various vasopressors and inotropes.[25,26] However, increased chronotropic sensitivity to β-adrenergic stimulation with hypersensitivity of the adenylate cyclase system to isoproterenol stimulation also has been reported in animal models of bacteremia and endotoxemia. In the presence of intrinsic myocardial dysfunction and increased metabolic demands, this dysfunctional adrenergic system is incapable of mobilizing functional cardiac reserve to maintain adequate myocardial performance.[25,26] Functional adrenergic receptor changes have been reported at various stages of sepsis, and thus adrenergic receptor sensitivity may be time-dependent during progression of sepsis to septic shock. The findings are not always consistent in various animal models of sepsis and in critically ill septic patients. For example, in an in vivo rodent model of sustained endotoxemia (48 hours) and continuous parenteral nutrition simulating advanced critical illness, Dickerson and colleagues showed no difference in α_1-adrenergic maximal responsiveness (in MAP) to phenylephrine.[27] Time-dependent alterations in the production of endothelium-derived nitric oxide, a potent vasodilator, may explain the apparent differences in vascular reactivity to phenylephrine during the phases of endotoxemia.[27] These findings suggest that the clinical response to vasopressor and inotropic agents is variable during the stages of hemodynamic, myocardial, and peripheral vascular derangements of septic shock. In contrast, in critically ill septic patients in the ICU (24 to 48 hours from hospital admission), β-adrenertic receptor changes were already present, although the progression of desensitization of receptors earlier in sepsis was not quantified.[26] In summary, α- and β-adrenergic receptor derangements may vary among patients and during each bacteremic insult, and therefore, doses of catecholamines vary from patient to patient and during the insult. For these reasons, these drugs should be dosed to clinical end points and not arbitrary maximal doses.

CLINICAL PHARMACOLOGY OF CATECHOLAMINES

The receptor selectivity of clinically used vasopressors and inotropes and hemodynamic effects are listed in Table 23–3. In general, these drugs are rapidly acting with short durations of action. As such, these drugs are given as continuous infusions. Careful monitoring and calculation of infusion rates are advised because dosing adjustments are made frequently, and varying admixtures and concentrations are used in volume-restricted patients.

Dopamine often is recommended as the initial catecholamine in sepsis because it increases blood pressure by increasing myocardial contractility and vasoconstriction. Dopamine has been described to have dose-related receptor activity at DA_1-, DA_2-, β_1-, and α_1-receptors. Unfortunately, this dose-response relationship has not been confirmed in critically ill patients. In patients with septic shock, there is a great overlap of hemodynamic effects even at doses as low as 3 mcg/kg per minute.[28] Tachydysrhythmias are common owing to the release of endogenous norepinephrine by dopamine entering the sympathetic nerve terminal. Dopamine may increase the PAOP through pulmonary vasoconstriction.[29] This drug also may depress ventilation and worsen hypoxemia in patients dependent on the hypoxic ventilatory drive.

Dobutamine, a synthetic catecholamine, is primarily a selective β_1-agonist with mild β_2- and vascular α_1 activity, resulting in strong positive inotropic activity without concomitant vasoconstriction. In comparison with dopamine, dobutamine produces a larger increase in cardiac output and is less arrhythmogenic.[30] Ruffolo and colleagues[31] showed that α_1-adrenoceptors in the heart are directly stimulated by the (−) isomer of dobutamine and that the β_1- and β_2-agonist activity resides in the (+) isomer.[31] This suggests that the strong inotropic action of dobutamine is a function of its structure, the additive effect of the cardiac α_1- and β_1-agonist activity, and a relatively weak chronotropic effect limited to the (+) isomer action on the β-receptors. Clinically, the increased myocardial contractility and subsequent reflex reduction in sympathetic tone leads to a decrease in systemic vascular resistance (SVR). Even though dobutamine is used optimally for low cardiac output states with high filling pressures or in cardiogenic shock, vasopressors may be needed to counteract arterial vasodilation.

Norepinephrine is a combined α- and β-agonist but mainly produces vasoconstriction primarily via its more prominent α effects on all vascular beds, thus increasing SVR. Norepinephrine administration generally produces either no change or some increase in cardiac output.[32,33]

Phenylephrine is a pure α_1-agonist and is believed to increase blood pressure through vasoconstriction. Given the presence of cardiac α_1-receptors, phenylephrine also may increase contractility and cardiac output.[34]

Epinephrine exerts combined α- and β-agonist effects. At the high epinephrine infusion rates used in septic shock, predominantly

TABLE 23–3. Receptor Pharmacology of Selected Inotropic and Vasopressor Agents Used in Septic Shock*

Agent	α_1	α_2	β_1	β_2	DA[†]
Dobutamine (500 mg/250 mL D_5W or NS)					
2–10 mcg/kg/min	+	0	++++	++	0
>10–20 mcg/kg/min	++	0	++++	+++	0
Dopamine (800 mg/250 mL D_5W or NS)					
1–3 mcg/kg/min	0	0	+	0	++++
3–10 mcg/kg/min	0/+	0	++++	++	++++
>10–20 mcg/kg/min	+++	0	++++	+	0
Epinephrine (2 mg/250 mL D_5W or NS)					
0.01–0.05 mcg/kg/min	++	++	++++	+++	0
>0.05 mcg/kg/min	++++	++++	+++	+	
Norepinephrine (4 mg/ 250 mL D_5W or NS)					
0.02–3 mcg/kg/min (2–20 mcg/min)	+++	+++	+++	+/++	0
Phenylephrine (50 mg/250 mL D_5W or NS)					
0.5–9 mcg/kg/min	+++	+	?	0	0

* Activity ranges from no activity (0) to maximal (++++) activity or ? when activity is not known.

[†]DA = dopaminergic.

Adapted from ref. 63.

α-adrenergic effects are seen, and SVR and MAP are increased. Epinephrine traditionally has been reserved as the vasopressor of last resort owing to peripheral vasoconstriction, particularly in the splanchnic and renal beds.[35,36]

CLINICAL USE OF VASOPRESSORS AND INOTROPES

Traditionally, a few vasopressors and inotropes have been used for hemodynamic support: dopamine, dobutamine, epinephrine, norepinephrine, and phenylephrine. Optimizing MAP as the goal of vasopressor therapy does not uniformly correlate with a decrease in mortality in septic shock.[13] Historically, significant concerns about the adverse effects of the vasopressors limited their use. The recent focus on goal-directed therapy, with optimization of oxygen transport variables to supranormal values, also has yielded poor results in patients with septic shock.[15] In fact, normalization of systemic DO_2 and VO_2, whether spontaneously or by design, is associated with improved outcome and is not dependent on administration of vasopressor agents. Part of our inability to detect an improvement with vasopressor or inotrope therapy may result from our limited ability to quantify regional tissue perfusion. However, use of early aggressive goal-directed therapy to av $SvCO_2$ value of greater than 70% has been shown to reduce mortality in patients with sepsis and septic shock.[12]

Dose titration and monitoring of vasopressor and inotropic therapy should be guided by the "best clinical response." Clinically effective dosing of vasopressors and inotropes in septic shock often requires much larger doses than those recommended by the manufacturer. These large infusion rates must be tempered with the development of adverse effects. The goal is to use the minimally effective infusion rate while minimizing evidence of myocardial ischemia (e.g., tachydysrhythmias, electrocardiographic changes), renal (decreased glomerular filtration rate and/or urine output), splanchnic/gastric (low pHi, bowel ischemia), or peripheral (cold extremities) hypoperfusion, and worsening of PaO_2, PAOP, and other hemodynamic variables.

Therapy with vasopressors and inotropes is continued until the myocardial depression and vascular hyporesponsiveness (i.e., blood pressure) of septic shock improve, usually measured in hours to days. Discontinuation of vasopressor or inotropic therapy should be executed slowly; therapy should be "weaned" to avoid a precipitous worsening in regional and systemic hemodynamics. Careful monitoring of global and regional end points also should be geared toward discontinuation of vasopressors and inotropes as soon as the patient is hemodynamically stable. This requires moment-by-moment observation. Because vasopressors and inotropes often are started while the patient is not yet optimally volume-resuscitated, clinicians should reevaluate the intravascular volume status continuously in order to be able to wean the patient from the vasopressor as soon as possible. Doses should be titrated carefully downward approximately every 10 minutes to determine if the patient is able to tolerate gradual withdrawal and eventual discontinuation of the vasopressor and/or inotrope. Discontinuation of the agents may occur only minutes to hours after their initiation or may take days to weeks. Septic shock requiring vasopressor and/or inotropic support usually resolves within a week.

ADVERSE EFFECTS

Catecholamine vasopressors may result in adverse peripheral vasoconstrictive, metabolic, and dysrhythmogenic effects that limit or outweigh their positive effects on the central circulation.[37] Norepinephrine, phenylephrine, and epinephrine can produce a lactic acidosis secondary to excessive constriction in peripheral arterioles,

enhanced glycogenolysis, or as a result of mobilization of lactate from peripheral tissues as a result of improved oxygenation. Additionally, excessive peripheral vasoconstriction may cause ischemia or necrosis of already poorly perfused are as such as the skin and the mesenteric and splanchnic circulations.[35,38] Some of these profound vasoconstrictive effects have been compounded by the use of epinephrine and phenylephrine in septic shock patients, who are significantly hypovolemic. These agents are used in the context of late septic shock, where hypotension is refractory to less selective vasoconstrictors (e.g., norepinephrine or dopamine) such that very large doses of epinephrine or phenylephrine are required with little or no benefit. Myocardial ischemia and dysrhythmias may occur in patients with CAD, atherosclerosis, cardiomyopathies, LV hypertrophy, congestive heart failure, and underlying dysrhythmias owing to their inability to tolerate β_1 cardiac stimulation that mediates increases in cardiac output. The effect is usually the opposite, however, in healthy myocardium and in young patients. β_1 cardiac stimulation is well tolerated, ventricular filling pressures decrease, and cardiac output and DO_2 increase, with a resulting increase in peripheral perfusion. An extensive review of the dysrrhythmogenic potential of the catecholamine vasopressors reveals a variety of resulting atrial and ventricular arrhythmias.[30] Sympathomimetic vasopressors also have been found to occupy neutrophil β_2-receptors (e.g., epinephrine) and directly scavenge oxygen free radicals (e.g., dopamine and dobutamine).[39] These effects may be either beneficial or deleterious by dampening harmful effects of oxygen free radical–mediated tissue injury or by reducing neutrophilic defense against bacteria. At clinically relevant concentrations, dopamine inhibits in vitro endothelial adhesion molecule expression of E-selectin.[40] This and other adhesion molecules mediate leukocyte interaction with and adherence to endothelial cells, which is implicated in enhancing sepsis-induced multiple-organ failure and lung injury in many animal models.[39,40] Epinephrine, dopamine, and other β-adrenergic agonists can inhibit production of TNF-α by neutrophils or expression of cellular adhesion molecules such as E-selectin by increasing cAMP, but the mechanism is more complex than previously thought.[40,41]

Vasopressor catecholamines have the potential to cause extravasation-associated tissue damage if infusions infiltrate during peripheral administration. In the event of infiltration, an α-receptor antagonist such as phentolamine (10 mg in 10 mL saline) should be injected intradermally to reverse local vasoconstriction. As such, it is recommended to administer vasopressor drugs into a large central vein.

DOPAMINE

Dopamine is frequently the initial vasopressor used in septic shock. Doses of 5 to 10 mcg/kg per minute are initiated to improve MAP. Most studies in patients with septic shock have shown that at these doses dopamine increases CI by improving contractility and heart rate, resulting primarily from its β_1 effects. It increases arterial pressure and SVR as a result of both the increased cardiac output and, at higher doses (>10 mcg/kg per minute), as a result of the α_1 effects.

The clinical utility of dopamine as a vasopressor in the setting of septic shock is limited because large doses frequently are necessary to maintain cardiac output and blood pressure. At doses exceeding 20 mcg/kg per minute, there is limited further improvement in cardiac performance and regional hemodynamics. Its clinical use frequently is hampered by tachycardia and tachydysrhythmias, which may lead to myocardial ischemia. Although tachydysrhythmias theoretically should not be expected to occur until 5 to 10 mcg/kg per minute of dopamine, these β_1 effects are observed with doses as low as 3 mcg/kg per minute. They seem to be more prevalent in patients who are inadequately resuscitated (hypovolemic), in the elderly, in those who have preexisting or concurrent cardiac ischemia or dysrhythmias, and in patients currently receiving other dysrhythmogenic agents, including vasopressors and inotropes.

Other adverse effects limiting the use of dopamine in patients with septic shock are increases in PAOP, pulmonary shunting, and decreases in PaO_2.[29] The increase in PAOP may be due to changes in diastolic volumes from decreased cardiac compliance or increased venous return to the heart by α-adrenergic receptor–mediated venoconstriction. This may affect gas exchange and decrease PaO_2. The increase in pulmonary shunting also may result from acute enhancement of pulmonary blood flow to nonhomogeneous lung regions. Thus dopamine should be used with caution in patients with elevated preload because the drug may worsen pulmonary edema. In the instance of high filling pressures, tachycardia, or tachydysrhythmias in the presence or absence of refractory hypotension, dopamine should be replaced by another vasopressor or inotrope such as norepinephrine, dobutamine, phenylephrine, or epinephrine, depending on the desired effect. Lastly, immune suppression of T-cell proliferation and pituitary hormone secretion and blunting of growth and thyroid hormones and prolactin secretion are also potentially clinically significant unwanted neuroendocrine effects of dopamine.

The effect of dopamine on global oxygen transport variables parallels the hemodynamic effects. Although dopamine improves global DO_2 in septic patients, it appears to compromise tissue oxygen extraction in the splanchnic and mesenteric circulations by α_1-mediated vasoconstriction. Indeed, despite increasing systemic DO_2 and VO_2, large doses of dopamine worsen pHi and the PCO_2 gap. This is reflected by a decrease or lack of change in regional VO_2 and a decrease in tissue O_2ER. Dopamine at low or pressor doses impairs gastric motility in critical illness[42] and may aggravate gut ischemia in septic shock.[35,43,44] Jakob and colleagues[45] evaluated the effects of dopamine on systemic and regional blood flow and metabolism in 9 septic and 11 cardiac surgery patients. Dopamine was started at 1 mcg/kg per minute and increased until the cardiac output increased by 25%. Systemic and splanchnic hemodynamics and oxygen transport were measured at baseline and 90 minutes after increasing the cardiac output. Dopamine infusion at a mean dose of 4 mcg/kg per minute increased splanchnic blood flow in the cardiac surgery and septic patients. Splanchnic VO_2 increased in cardiac surgery patients but decreased in septic patients. The reduction in splanchnic oxygen consumption by dopamine in sepsis suggests an impairment of hepatosplanchnic metabolism despite an increase in regional perfusion.

Although splanchnic blood flow and DO_2 may increase with dopamine, there is no preferential increase in the splanchnic perfusion as a fraction of cardiac output and systemic increases in DO_2.[46,47] One study found an inverse relationship between fractional splanchnic flow at baseline and the change in fractional splanchnic blood flow such that dopamine was effective in increasing the fractional splanchnic blood flow in those in whom it was normal but worsened it in those with high baseline values, such as occurs with redistribution of regional blood flow in septic shock.[46] Clinically, it is difficult to distinguish prospectively either subset of patients.

Currently, there is insufficient evidence to promote the use of dopamine as a first-line agent because regional hemodynamics, oxygen transport variables, and functional parameters of improved organ perfusion are not improved in a sustained manner and may be negatively impaired. The negative findings of using low-dose dopamine (see below) and the deleterious effects of inotropic and vasopressor doses of dopamine on regional hemodynamics and oxygen transport are raising a controversy over whether dopamine should be considered the first-line vasopressor agent in patients with severe sepsis or septic shock.[35,48] It still may be reasonable to use dopamine empirically in a hypotensive patient in whom a pulmonary arterial catheter has not been inserted and in whom the cause of hypotension—low cardiac output or vasodilation—is yet undetermined.[3]

LOW-DOSE DOPAMINE

In the critical care setting, low doses (1 to 3 mcg/kg per minute) of dopamine sometimes are used in patients with septic shock receiving vasopressors with or without oliguria. The goal of therapy is to prevent or reverse renal vasoconstriction caused by other pressors, to prevent oliguric renal failure, or to convert it to nonoliguric renal failure. Dopamine has been shown to increase renal blood flow and increased urine output owing to either its dopaminergic effect at low doses, its natriuretic effects (inhibition of the Na^+/K^+-adenosine triphosphate of renal tubular cells), or an increase in CI.[49,50] In normal volunteers, the addition of dopamine to incremental doses of norepinephrine may blunt norepinephrine-induced renal vasoconstriction, thereby maintaining renal blood flow, natriuresis, urine output,[28,51] and in one study, glomerular filtration.[51] In oliguric patients, dopamine may increase fractional excretion of sodium and increase urine output. These effects also have been observed during the course of dopamine administration in nonseptic oliguric patients,[52] as well as in oliguric[46,53] and nonoliguric[36,47,49] patients with septic shock. For this reason, dopamine is sometimes added in low doses to other vasopressors or inotropes (e.g., norepinephrine). Despite this practice, evidence supporting low-dose dopamine in preserving kidney function in oliguria with or without septic shock or in reversing vasopressor-induced vasoconstriction in septic shock is lacking and limited to small underpowered studies.[36,49,50,53–56]

Furthermore, tolerance to the vasodilatory effects of dopamine after 24 to 48 hours is evident in nonoliguric patients with sepsis syndrome and has been reported in others.[56,57] The lack of response to dopamine in septic shock patients on vasopressors and the tolerance that develops in responders to low-dose dopamine may be explained in part by time- and disease-dependent desensitization of the dopamine receptors[56,57]; this may not occur in those with sepsis syndrome[56] or normal volunteers.[28] Furthermore, differences in the extent of preexisting vasodilation and the pathophysiology of renal dysfunction in oliguric and septic shock patients also may contribute to the inconsistent responses seen to the administration of low doses of dopamine.

Two recent studies, however, help put to rest the debate surrounding low-dose dopamine. Kellum and colleagues[58] performed a meta-analysis to determine if low-dose dopamine reduces the incidence or severity of acute renal failure, need for dialysis, or mortality in patients with critical illness. Among 17 randomized clinical trials ($n = 854$), low-dose dopamine did not prevent mortality (relative risk 0.90; 95% confidence interval 0.44–1.83; $p = .92$), onset of acute renal failure (relative risk 0.81; 95% confidence interval 0.55–1.19; $p = .34$), or need for dialysis (relative risk 0.83; 95% confidence interval 0.55–1.24; $p = .42$). There was sufficient statistical power to exclude any large ($>50\%$) effect of dopamine on the risk of acute renal failure or need for dialysis. One adequately designed prospective, controlled trial has been conducted with low-dose dopamine in oliguric renal failure in critically ill patients. This study was not cited in the aforementioned meta-analysis owing to the lag in publication. Bellomo and colleagues[53] randomized 328 critically ill patients with early renal dysfunction to either low-dose dopamine (2 mcg/kg per minute) or placebo, with the primary end point being peak SCr. At the end of the study, there were no differences in peak SCr or other renal outcomes such as increase in SCr, need for renal replacement therapies, improvement in urine output, time to recovery of normal renal function or survival, ICU stay, hospital stay, or development of arrhythmias. On the basis of available evidence, it can be concluded that low-dose dopamine for the treatment or prevention of acute renal failure cannot be justified and should be eliminated from routine clinical use.[53,58]

NOREPINEPHRINE

Norepinephrine was first used three decades ago for the treatment of hypotensive states prior to the development of the newer synthetic catecholamines dopamine and dobutamine. Traditionally, norepinephrine was viewed as causing significant peripheral tissue vasoconstriction, which could selectively impair regional flow and thus DO_2 to the renal and splanchnic beds. However, recent clinical studies of norepinephrine support the primary use of norepinephrine to restore blood pressure in septic shock.[32,59] In fact, in a retrospective study of 100 ICU patients treated with norepinephrine for severe hypotension and evidence of end-organ hypoperfusion unresponsive to both fluid resuscitation and dopamine treatment, early norepinephrine administration was associated with the lowest mortality rate.[60] However, in patients with increased sequential organ failure assessment (SOFA) scores and associated multiorgan failure, treatment with norepinephrine no longer offered an advantage. Early aggressive vasopressor support may be key to a positive outcome in septic shock.

In clinical practice, however, norepinephrine often is initiated after vasopressor doses of dopamine (4 to 20 mcg/kg per minute) alone or in combination with dobutamine (5 mcg/kg per minute) fail to achieve desired goals.[3] Doses of dopamine and dobutamine are kept constant or stopped altogether, or in some instances, dopamine is kept at low doses for purported renal protection. It may be more rational to use norepinephrine because it is more potent than dopamine and is more effective at increasing MAP. It has combined strong α_1 activity and less potent β_1-agonist effects while maintaining the vasodilatory effects of β_2-receptor stimulation.

Norepinephrine infusions may be titrated to preset goals of MAP (usually >70 mm Hg), improvement in peripheral perfusion (to restore urine output or decrease blood lactate), and/or achievement of desired oxygen transport variables while not compromising cardiac index. Norepinephrine 0.01 to 2 mcg/kg per minute reliably and predictably improves hemodynamic parameters to "normal" or "supranormal" values in most patients with septic shock. As with other vasopressors, norepinephrine doses that exceed those recommended by the manufacturer are needed in critically ill patients with septic shock to achieve predetermined goals. A significant increase in MAP generally is accompanied by an increase in SVR. In contrast to dopamine, heart rate generally does not increase significantly with norepinephrine because of diminished stimulation of cardiac β_1-receptors in septic shock.[33,61] In a study of 10 patients with septic shock in whom norepinephrine doses were increased to 23, 31, and 47 mcg/min to maintain MAPs of 65, 75, and 85 mm Hg, the mean heart rates at these doses were 95, 101, and 105 beats per minute, respectively.[33] Norepinephrine has been shown to produce no change or some increase in the cardiac index in septic shock.[32] In the same study by LeDoux and colleagues,[33] the increasing doses of norepinephrine required for the three levels of MAP resulted in a progressive increase in the cardiac index (mean values 4.7, 5.3, and 5.5 L/m^2 per minute, respectively).[33] In contrast to dopamine, with norepinephrine, there is no change in PAOP.[62]

Whereas the effects on MAP, SVR, cardiac index, and heart rate appear to be desirable and more predictable, the effect of norepinephrine on urine output may depend on concurrently administered vasoactive agents.[62] Concurrent inotropic support with dobutamine and dopamine or low doses of dopamine precludes attributing any beneficial effects to norepinephrine alone. An increase in urine output may be due to increased renal perfusion pressure secondary to the increases in MAP and the SVR index, especially given that norepinephrine has a greater vasoconstrictive effect on the efferent arteriole of the kidney than on the afferent arteriole.

The effect of norepinephrine on oxygen transport parameters is variable and depends on baseline values and concurrently administered vasoactive agents. In most of the studies, either an increase or no change in DO_2 is seen with no change in O_2ER, particularly when mean DO_2 values were "supranormal" prior to therapy.[63] In all but one study,[64] patients had received dobutamine and/or dopamine prior to initiation of goal-directed therapy with norepinephrine. Martin and colleagues[64] found norepinephrine alone to be superior to dopamine in achieving and maintaining for at least 6 hours preset hemodynamic and oxygen transport variables (93% versus 31% of patients, $p < .001$). The authors suggested that differences between the two agents resulted from norepinephrine's combined increase in VO_2 and decrease in lactate concentrations owing to correction of splanchnic ischemia and efficient hepatic clearance of lactate or owing to a preferential increase in DO_2 to areas of greatest oxygen demand, thus optimizing O_2ER.

Recently, Martin and colleagues,[59] in a prospective, observational cohort study of 97 adult patients with septic shock, determined that the use of norepinephrine to provide hemodynamic support was associated with a significant decrease in hospital mortality [day 7: 28% versus 40% ($p < .005$); day 28: 55% versus 82% ($p < .001$), and hospital discharge: 62% versus 84% ($p < .001$)].[59] Using stepwise logistic regression analysis, norepinephrine was found to be the only factor associated with significantly improved survival ($p = .03$). Despite the drawback of lack of randomization, this is the first study to demonstrate a survival benefit with any vasopressor. In a subsequent interventional study, Martin and colleagues[32] showed that the addition of norepinephrine in patients with dobutamine-resistant septic shock resulted in significant improvements (40%) in cardiac index and stroke volume index during a 4-hour study period.[32] This occurred despite an increase in LV afterload, suggesting that either a positive inotropic effect or the correction of systemic hypotension was responsible. The authors further speculated that older patients may benefit from a combined α- and β-vasopressor versus a pure β-agonist (i.e., dobutamine) given the higher incidence of coronary disease and compromised ventricles. By virtue of restored MAP and hence coronary perfusion, cardiac index is increased in older patients, whereas in younger patients with less coronary artery disease and a higher cardiac index at baseline, norepinephrine acts primarily as a vasopressor. In younger patients in this study, norepinephrine did not significantly increase cardiac index or stroke volume index.

Taken together, these recent data suggest that norepinephrine potentially should be repositioned as the vasopressor of choice in patients in septic shock because of its multiple benefits: (1) It may decrease mortality in septic shock, (2) it attenuates inappropriate vasodilation and low global oxygen extraction, (3) it attenuates myocardial depression at unchanged or increased cardiac output and increased coronary blood flow, (4) it improves renal perfusion pressure and renal filtration, (5) it improves splanchnic perfusion, and (6) it is less likely than other vasopressors to cause tachycardias and tachydysrhythmias.[59,61,65]

DOBUTAMINE

Dobutamine is an inotrope with vasodilatory properties (a so-called inodilator), and it is used in the treatment of septic and cardiogenic shock to increase cardiac index. In septic shock, LV ejection fraction (EF) and right ventricular function are depressed despite a high cardiac index, whereas ventricular volumes and compliance are increased. Stroke index is maintained by an increased heart rate and ventricular dilatation. In survivors, the myocardial depression is reversible and normalizes at 5 to 10 days after the onset of sepsis.[66] Dobutamine has been shown to increase stroke index, left ventricular stroke work index (LVSWI), and thus cardiac index and DO_2 without increasing PAOP in septic shock in animals, in human volunteers, and in controlled studies of human septic shock.[63]

Most prospective, randomized, controlled studies of goal-directed therapy with dobutamine were performed for septic shock in surgical and medically critically ill patients refractory to concurrently administered vasopressors (dopamine and/or norepinephrine).[63] The oxygen transport effects may not be significant or may be transient, particularly during prolonged infusions. It appears that achievement of supranormal oxygen transport values with dobutamine in hyperdynamic septic shock refractory to fluid resuscitation and vasopressors is of little value as compared with treatment to normal values. In addition, administration of dobutamine to achieve these high values has resulted in an unchanged or an increased mortality and a greater incidence of adverse effects,[67] with the exception of a study in older nonseptic high-risk surgical patients.[17] Results in medical and surgical patients may differ owing to differences in time of starting dobutamine infusion, the duration of the infusion, and dosages administered. Subgroups of patients with septic shock (6% to 34%) among critically ill, high-risk trauma and surgical patients have small and insignificant changes in DO_2, VO_2, O_2ER, and cardiac index.[68] The lack of response may be related to late treatment (>72 hours after surgery) resulting in irreversible changes owing to hypoperfusion and hypoxia. In a group of medical patients, the lack of sustained effect may have been attributed to the fact that very large doses were needed to achieve the desired effects over a longer treatment period (72 hours). The requirement for vasopressor support with dopamine may have decreased the oxygen extraction ratio (O_2ER) and negated the beneficial effects of increased delivery with dobutamine. Oxygen extraction ratio, mixed venous oxygen tension, and relative changes in SVR were not reported. In populations of medical and surgical patients, dobutamine did not increase the likelihood of patients achieving supranormal oxygen transport variables.[63] Continuation of dobutamine until death or resolution of acute illness resulted in an increased mortality despite an increase in the mean area under the DO_2 curve.[67] This is explained in part by the fact that no change in VO_2 was seen, and thus O_2ER decreased. Also, much higher doses of dobutamine were used in this study as compared with the previous study (5 to 200 versus 5 to 20 mcg/kg per minute). Seventeen of the 50 patients in the experimental group received 50 mcg/kg per minute or more of dobutamine at some time during the study. Despite these high doses, 35 of 50 patients (70%) were unable to achieve the predetermined goals. Infact, dose increments of dobutamine were limited by complications in half the dobutamine patients in the treatment group, with tachycardia, ischemic changes on ECG, hypertension, and tachydysrhythmias, despite the absence of preexisting cardiac abnormalities.[67]

Recent studies have focused on the effects of dobutamine on gastric mucosal flow and the splanchnic circulation. The addition of dobutamine (held constant at 5 mcg/kg per minute) to norepinephrine improves gastric mucosal perfusion without increasing cardiac index.[69] This is consistent with findings that dobutamine may improve pHi and mucosal perfusion in septic patients.[70] The addition of dobutamine to epinephrine-treated patients has been shown to improve gastric mucosal perfusion, as measured by improvements in pHi, arterial lactate concentrations, and PCO_2 gap.[71] Duranteau and colleagues'

findings likely were related to a blood flow redistribution toward gastric mucosal.[69] This effect may be due to either an increase in the fraction of the cardiac output that was distributed to the global hepatosplanchnic blood flow[71] and/or to a redistribution of blood flow within gastric wall layers toward mucosal by "stealing" blood away from the muscularis potentially owing to the greater β_2-mediated vasodilatation attributable to norepinephrine. This hypothesis is supported by two other recent investigations.[72,73]

In these studies, a constant dose of dobutamine (5 mcg/kg per minute) was added to norepinephrine and compared with either epinephrine and norepinephrine alone to determine comparative effects on systemic and regional hemodynamics and oxygen transport variables.[72,73] At the same increase in MAP, there was no significant difference in the systemic hemodynamic variables between the treatment groups. The combination of dobutamine-norepinephrine resulted in a lower increase in heart rate compared with the other groups. There was no difference among each group in DO_2I. Arterial lactate concentrations dropped significantly with norepinephrine-dobutamine as compared with dopamine and epinephrine infusions. Norepinephrine-dobutamine infusion was associated with a higher pHi compared with epinephrine infusion, but the differences were not statistically different. The difference between gastric and arterial PCO_2 with norepinephrine-dobutamine tended to be lower compared with those obtained with dopamine, epinephrine, and norepinephrine alone. The authors concluded that for the same level of MAP as the therapeutic goal in patients with septic shock, norepinephrine-dobutamine improved gastric mucosal perfusion and tissue oxygen utilization.

Dobutamine should be started with doses ranging 2.5 to 5 mcg/kg per minute. Although generally a dose response may be seen, recent evidence suggests that doses in excess of 5 mcg/kg per minute may provide limited beneficial effects on oxygen transport values and hemodynamics and may increase adverse cardiac effects.[74] If given to patients who are intravascularly depleted, dobutamine will result in hypotension and a reflexive tachycardia. Pathophysiologic factors influence dosing requirements and pharmacokinetic parameters over the time course of the illness and the duration of the infusion. Decreases in PaO_2 and increases in PVO_2, as well as myocardial adverse effects such as tachycardia, ischemic changes on electrocardiogram, tachydysrhythmias, and hypotension, are seen.[67] Thus infusion rates should be guided by clinical end points. Dobutamine, like other inotropes, usually is given until there is an improvement in myocardial function with resolution of the septic episode or when dose-limiting side effects are seen.

PHENYLEPHRINE

Despite its purported use in refractory septic shock, very little information is published regarding the clinical efficacy of phenylephrine. Nevertheless, it is an attractive agent for use in sepsis owing to its selective α-agonism and primarily vascular effects and its rapid onset and short duration of action. It is generally initiated at dosages of 0.5 mcg/kg per minute and may be titrated quickly to desired effect.

There are three clinical trials using phenylephrine in septic shock evaluating 38 patients. Phenylephrine (0.5 to 9 mcg/kg per minute), when used alone or in combination with dobutamine or low doses of dopamine, improves blood pressure and myocardial performance in fluid-resuscitated septic patients.[75] Incremental doses of phenylephrine over 3 hours result in linear dose-related increases in MAP, SVR, heart rate, and stroke index when administered as a single agent in stable, nonhypotensive but hyperdynamic, volume-resuscitated surgical ICU patients. In septic shock, phenylephrine did not impair cardiac index, PAOP, or peripheral perfusion.[34,76] Yamazaki and colleagues[75] showed that although its administration resulted in improved myocardial performance in hyperdynamic, normotensive septic patients, phenylephrine worsened it in cardiac controls.[75] At a dosage of 70 mcg/min, phenylephrine improved cardiac index and MAP by increasing venous return to the heart (increase in CVP and stroke index) and by acting as a positive inotrope because SVR did not change. There was a clinically insignificant decrease in heart rate (3 beats per minute). However, in cardiac patients, myocardial performance worsened as a result of an increase in MAP and SVR and a decrease in cardiac index with no change in heart rate. Although these results suggest caution, it is noteworthy that the cardiac indices of the two groups were not comparable at baseline.

In septic shock, phenylephrine appears to increase global tissue oxygen use, although there is conflicting information regarding the relationship of the oxygen-transport variables with increases in MAP and cardiac index.[34,76] Increases in VO_2 appear to be dissociated from DO_2, representing an increase in O_2ER because the cardiac index remains unchanged. Increases in VO_2 may result from redistribution of blood flow to previously underperfused areas, improving oxygen use as a result of changes in MAP and SVR. With phenylephrine administration, no organ dysfunction was documented, and evidence of globally improved peripheral tissue perfusion was seen as the lactic acid concentration fell or remained unchanged, and urine output increased significantly at increased or maximal VO_2. An increased O_2ER may contribute to improved tissue use.[34,76] In one small study, measured DO_2 and VO_2 values paralleled MAP in most patients.[76] As with epinephrine, phenylephrine doses (1.3 to 3.7 mcg/kg per minute) required to achieve goals of therapy were significantly higher than those traditionally recommended for use. When phenylephrine (0.5 mcg/kg per minute) was titrated to a plateau in VO_2 or the appearance of adverse cardiac effects, there was a greater than 15% increase in DO_2 and VO_2. When combined with dobutamine, phenylephrine resulted in a more consistent and statistically significant increase in both DO_2 and VO_2. However, these observations may be biased because baseline DO_2 and VO_2 values were somewhat higher in patients who did not require dobutamine (5 of 11). In a second study, Flancbaum and colleagues[34] evaluated the use of phenylephrine as a single agent without another cardiotonic agent in 10 septic, hyperdynamic surgical ICU patients.[34] Eight patients had a clinically significant increase (>15%)in VO_2 with variable doses of phenylephrine, whereas DO_2 increased in only three patients. Phenylephrine predictably increased MAP but not VO_2 in a dose-dependent fashion in the surgical patient population.

There are very few data regarding the effect of phenylephrine on regional hemodynamics and oxygen-transport variables. When phenylephrine replaced norepinephrine in patients with septic shock, it selectively reduced splanchnic blood flow and thus splanchnic DO_2 and splanchnic lactate uptake rate without changing the overall splanchnic VO_2.[77] Because all these parameters normalized when norepinephrine was reinstated, these data suggest that exogenous β-adrenergic stimulation (norepinephrine) may determine hepatosplanchnic perfusion and oxygen availability but not utilization in septic shock. This study also demonstrated that while the phenylephrine-induced reduction in splanchnic DO_2 reduced the de novo synthesis of glucose (a highly oxygen-dependent pathway in the periportal region), it did not affect the formation of MEGX, a metabolite of lidocaine (a cytochrome P450–dependent pathway in the perivenous region), suggesting that the latter metabolic activity is not so dependent on oxygen and is retained in septic shock, reflecting the heterogeneity of metabolic function in different areas of the liver.[77]

The available data on hemodynamics, oxygen-transport variables, and mortality with phenylephrine in septic shock patients may not be generalizable owing to the small numbers of patients evaluated. Adverse effects such as tachydysrhythmias are notably infrequent with phenylephrine, particularly when it is used as a single agent or with higher doses, and this is due to the fact that phenylephrine does not exert any activity on $β_1$-adrenergic receptors. It is unclear, however, how sustained the beneficial effects may be with longer administrations of phenylephrine.[34] In an experimental animal model, however, sustained endotoxemia (48 hours) does not result in desensitization of $α_1$-adrenergic responsiveness when phenylephrine is used.[27] Other mechanisms may be responsible for the ineffectiveness of vasopressors during advanced sepsis. Phenylephrine may be a particularly useful alternative in patients who cannot tolerate tachycardia or tachydysrhythmias with dopamine or norepinephrine, in patients with known underlying myocardial dysfunction, and in patients who are refractory to dopamine or norepinephrine (owing to β-adrenergic receptor desensitization). As with other vasopressors, phenylephrine is continued until resolution of the hemodynamic instability associated with the septic episode and is weaned when patients are stable clinically.

EPINEPHRINE

By convention, epinephrine has been reserved as a last-line agent in hemodynamic support of sepsis. There are very few objective data evaluating its comparative efficacy in early sepsis, with most studies examining the effects of epinephrine in refractory septic shock.[63] Despite this, epinephrine is an acceptable choice as a single agent owing to its combined vasoconstrictor and inotropic effects. Epinephrine infusion rates of 0.04 to 1 mcg/kg per minute alone increase hemodynamic and oxygen-transport variables to "supranormal" values without adverse effects in patients without CAD. In 69 patients evaluated in five studies, epinephrine alone or combined with either dobutamine or low doses of dopamine achieved the desired outcomes.[27,63] Large doses (0.5 to 1 mcg/kg per minute) often were required when epinephrine was added to other agents. Smaller doses (0.10 to 0.50 mcg/kg per minute) are effective if dobutamine and dopamine infusions are kept constant potentially owing to exposure to less β-receptor stimulation and thus less receptor desensitization. The same holds true when epinephrine is used as a first-line agent and when it is used in younger patients. A linear dose-response curve is seen, with a rapid improvement of hemodynamic variables and oxygen delivery. Although DO_2 increases mainly as a function of consistent increases in cardiac index and a more variable increase in SVR, VO_2 may not increase, and O_2ER may fall. A transient fall in pHi may be seen during the epinephrine administration, and this impairment in gastric mucosal perfusion can be counteracted in part by dobutamine. Furthermore, lactate concentrations may rise during the first few hours of epinephrine therapy; however, they normalize over the ensuing 24 hours in survivors.[63] The increase in lactate may be a result of worsened oxygen delivery to the liver (and subsequent anaerobic metabolism) or to the hepatosplanchnic circulation or, alternately, may be due to a direct increase by epinephrine in calorigenesis and breakdown of glycogen and lactate production. There is evidence, however, to suggest that epinephrine, in contrast to dopamine, may increase the proportion of total cardiac output delivered to the splanchnic circulation, although VO_2 is not increased sufficiently to increase O_2ER. In contrast, when epinephrine is compared with a short infusion (2 hours) of a combination of norepinephrine and dobutamine, it preferentially decreases splanchnic oxygen delivery, worsens pHi, and increases systemic lactate concentration without increasing

VO_2. Methodologic limitations of many of these studies included nonrandomized crossover periods, potentially leading to pharmacologic carry-over; failure of patients to achieve a steady state before crossover, and the use of time-dependent response measures. It is also unclear whether patients were comparable at baseline—whether they had received the same or other vasoactive agents before the study period and for how long.[78]

Since data on the effects of vasopressors on splanchnic circulation in humans are limited and are confounded by the use of multiple agents used concurrently, DeBacker and colleagues[38] conducted a study in which regional hemodynamic effects of three catecholamine vasopressors were evaluated individually in septic shock patients. A convenience sample of 20 patients with septic shock was divided into two groups: moderate shock, in which the MAP was >65 mm Hg with dopamine at doses between 10 and 20 mcg/kg per minute, and a severe group, in which MAP was less than 65 mm Hg. Following a stable dose of dopamine, patients were randomized either to norepinephrine or epinephrine initially and then the other agent following a period of at least 45 minutes with each agent. Systemic and regional measurements were taken for each drug. The moderate shock group revealed minimal differences between the agents. However, in the severe shock group, epinephrine resulted in a higher DO_2 and VO_2 but a lower absolute and fractional splanchnic blood flow. Although the PCO_2 gap was not different, indocyanine green (ICG) clearance was lower with epinephrine compared with norepinephrine. No detrimental effects on the splanchnic circulation were found with dopamine. This study concluded that epinephrine titrated to blood pressure in patients with severe septic shock causes deterioration in splanchnic circulation and induces changes in splanchnic metabolism. Given that these changes are likely deleterious, high-dose epinephrine should be avoided in severe septic shock patients.[38]

Three other recent studies compared epinephrine with either norepinephrine alone or norepinephrine in combination with dobutamine to determine their comparative effects on systemic and regional hemodynamics and oxygen-transport variables.[69,72,73] The first study was a prospective, randomized study of two parallel groups. Sequin and colleagues[72] compared epinephrine with the combination of norepinephrine-dobutamine on gastric perfusion, systemic and pulmonary hemodynamics, hepatic function, and blood gases in 22 patients with septic shock. Epinephrine or norepinephrine was started at a dose of 0.1 mcg/kg per minute and increased by 0.2 mcg/kg per minute every 5 minutes to reach an MAP of 70 to 80 mm Hg. Dobutamine was infused continuously at 5 mcg/kg per minute. At the same increase in MAP, there was no significant difference in the systemic or pulmonary hemodynamic and blood gas variables between the treatment groups. Epinephrine tended to induce greater increases in cardiac index and oxygen transport compared with norepinephrine-dobutamine. Epinephrine also significantly increased gastric mucosal blood flow compared with norepinephrine-dobutamine without modifying ICG clearance. The effects seen with epinephrine were mostly likely the result of an increase in the cardiac index.

The two other studies are prospective, randomized crossover studies performed in dopamine-resistant volume-replete patients with septic shock.[69,73] The design and results of the two studies are fairly similar. In the study by Duranteau and colleagues,[69] epinephrine and norepinephrine were titrated to an MAP of 70 to 80 mm Hg. Epinephrine and the combination of norepinephrine and dobutamine both produced a significant increase in heart rate compared with norepinephrine alone. Epinephrine also significantly increased the cardiac index and oxygen delivery compared with norepinephrine alone. Oxygen consumption and oxygen extraction did not change throughout the study. For the same level of MAP, epinephrine and

the combination of norepinephrine-dobutamine induced a greater increase in mucosal perfusion than did norepinephrine alone. The same ratio between gastric mucosal perfusion and DO_2 was observed with norepinephrine-dobutamine and with epinephrine or norepinephrine alone, but because the pHi and PCO_2 improved more with norepinephrine-dobutamine than with epinephrine or norepinephrine alone, the differences were not statistically different. These results can be explained by the vasodilatory effect of dobutamine on gastric mucosal microcirculation resulting in a redistribution of blood flow toward the mucosa.[69] The results of this study suggest that epinephrine does not have beneficial effects on the gastric mucosa.

In the third study, dosages of dopamine, epinephrine, norepinephrine, and norepinephrine-dobutamine also were adjusted to an MAP of >70 mm Hg.[73] Epinephrine induced a significant increase in heart rate compared with the other three groups and a higher cardiac index compared with norepinephrine alone as well as with norepinephrine-dobutamine. There was no difference among the groups in DO_2 index. However, O_2ER values were lower with epinephrine infusion compared with the other three groups. Arterial lactate concentrations dropped significantly with norepinephrine-dobutamine as compared with dopamine and epinephrine infusions. Norepinephrine-dobutamine infusion was associated with a higher pHi compared with epinephrine infusion, but the differences were not statistically significant. The difference between gastric and arterial PCO_2 with norepinephrine-dobutamine tended to be lower than that with dopamine, epinephrine, or norepinephrine alone. The authors concluded that for the same level of MAP as the therapeutic goal in patients with septic shock, the administration of dopamine, norepinephrine, epinephrine, or norepinephrine-dobutamine improved systemic hemodynamics effectively. However, epinephrine and dopamine had deleterious effect on oxygen metabolism, and similar to the study by Duranteau and colleagues, norepinephrine-dobutamine improved gastric mucosal perfusion and tissue oxygen utilization. Again, this study reinforces some undesirable effects of epinephrine on regional hemodynamics and oxygen utilization.

It is important to note that despite the large doses used in all the studies discussed, clinically important dysrhythmias or cardiac ischemia were reported rarely in patients of any age or underlying cardiac status. Nevertheless, caution must be exercised before considering epinephrine in managing hypoperfusion in hypodynamic patients with CAD, in whom ischemia, chest pain, and myocardial infarction may result. Based on the current evidence, epinephrine should be avoided in septic shock. Although it effectively increases cardiac output and oxygen delivery, is has deleterious effects on the splanchnic circulation. If it is used as a second-line agent in septic shock, factors that may influence successful therapy with epinephrine may include the time from the onset of septic shock to effective therapy and the age of the population.

EXPERIMENTAL THERAPIES

NITRIC OXIDE SYNTHASE INHIBITORS

Nitric oxide (NO) is a short-acting, potent vasodilator derived from the enzymatic oxidation of arginine. Its production is under control of nitric oxide synthase (NOS). This enzyme is present (expressed) in two forms: a constitutive form (ecNOS) and an inducible form (iNOS). Small amounts of NO normally are produced by the vascular endothelium under the control of ecNOS for the physiologic control of vascular tone and blood flow distribution. Under pathophysiologic conditions such as stimulation by lipopolysaccharide or cytokines, iNOS becomes diffusely expressed, producing large amounts of NO. The latter has been implicated in the cardiovascular failure of septic shock.[79,80]

Pharmacologic inhibition of NO production has been investigated as an adjunct to standard therapies of septic shock. L-Arginine analogs such as monomethyl-L-arginine (L-NMMA) and L-arginine-methylester (L-NAME) are competitive inhibitors of NOS and have been shown to increase blood pressure and partially restore vascular reactivity in experimental and human septic shock.[81] However, because these arginine analogs nonselectively block ecNOS and iNOS, their use has been associated with extensive vasoconstriction, decreased cardiac output, and regional hypoperfusion, thus promoting organ failure and mortality.[79,80] Some S-substituted thiourea derivatives have demonstrated both in vitro and in vivo (rodent) dose-dependent selectivity for iNOS inhibition. Recently, Rosselet and associates[79] demonstrated that low doses (0.1 mg/kg per hour) of S-methyl-isothiourea (SMT), a selective inhibitor of NO, were superior to norepinephrine in the treatment of rat endotoxic shock. These doses of SMT prevented hypotension by maintaining cardiac index without increasing the SVR index, as did norepinephrine. However, only low doses of SMT limited the development of lactic acidosis.

CORTICOSTEROIDS

The use of corticosteroids in the treatment of septic shock has been a topic of controversy for many years. A meta-analysis of early studies of steroids in sepsis demonstrated a lack of benefit and potential harm in sepsis and septic shock.[82,83] There is a renewed interest in corticosteroid use because of the increased awareness of adrenocortical insufficiency in critically ill patients with septic shock.[84] Relative adrenal insufficiency has been defined as a poor adrenal response [<250 nmol/L (9 mcg/dL) irrespective of the initial serum cortisol level] to a dose of synthetic adrenocorticotropic hormone (ACTH), indicating a low functional reserve of the adrenal cortex.[84] Although absolute insufficiency is rare, relative adrenocortical insufficiency in the presence of normal or high cortisol concentrations at baseline is present in 30% to 50% of patients with septic shock and is associated with a poor outcome.[85]

Since the two meta-analyses in 1995, five prospective, randomized, controlled trials of low-dose corticosteroids in vasopressor-dependent septic shock patients ($n = 505$) have been published.[86-90] These studies used moderate physiologic doses (200 to 300 mg/day) of hydrocortisone. A meta-analysis of these studies showed that steroid therapy was associated with an overall improvement in survival rate (odds ratio [OR] 1.52, 95% confidence interval [CI] 1.03–2.27; $p = .036$) and shock reversal (OR 4.79, 95% CI 2.07–11.11; $p = .001$). These effects were beneficial in both responders and nonresponders to corticotrophin stimulation testing ($p = .63$ and $p = .75$, respectively).[91] These studies also showed that low-dose corticosteroid administration improves hemodynamics and reduces the duration of vasopressor support.[86-90] All these studies differ from earlier studies in that steroids were administered later in septic shock (23 hours versus less than 2 hours; $p = .02$). In these studies, steroids were administered longer (6 days versus 1 day; $p = .004$), doses were tapered, lower doses were used (hydrocortisone equivalents 1209 mg versus 23,975 mg; $p = .01$), all patients received high doses of catecholamine vasopressors, and control groups had higher mortality rates (mean 57% versus 34%; $p = .03$).[91] Since only one of the five studies showed a mortality benefit of low-dose steroids in septic shock, further research is required to confirm this finding.[90]

In order to understand further the interaction between vasopressors and corticosteroids, Bellissant and colleagues[92] evaluated the hydrocortisone-phenylephrine MAP dose-response relationship in 12 septic shock patients within 3 hours of ICU admission and in normal controls.[92] The hyporesponsiveness to phenylephrine was related to alterations in vascular and not central activity (no alteration in baroreflex sensitivity). The corticosteroid effects were deemed not to be related to sympathetic or renin-angiotensin system activation nor to NO pathways because no significant relationship was found between pharmacodynamic parameters and circulating catecholamines, renin, aldosterone, or nitrite/nitrate concentrations. More indirect mechanisms or effect on adrenergic receptor activity could not be excluded by the methods used by the investigators. Current proposed mechanisms of the vasoconstrictor effect of corticosteroids may include increasing the number and stimulating the function of α_1- and β-adrenergic receptors. In addition, corticosteroids may attenuate the production of mediators responsible in part for the vasodilatation and hyperdynamic state of sepsis (perhaps indirectly through inducible NO inhibition and/or improved binding affinity of the cortisol receptor).[93]

Given the current data, corticosteroids may be administered to patients with septic shock on high doses of vasopressors for prolonged periods of time if (1) reversible causes of hypotension are eliminated, (2) relative/absolute corticosteroid deficiency is determined with corticotropin stimulation testing, and (3) corticosteroids are used for at least 5 to 7 days and then are reduced progressively.[84]

VASOPRESSIN

Vasopressin is emerging as a potentially useful therapy in the hemodynamic support of vasodilatory septic shock. Case series and small clinical trials have reported its use in patients who remain hypotensive on vasopressors.[94,95] Arginine vasopressin has little pressor activity in normal subjects but markedly increases blood pressure when sympathetic nerve function is impaired, including in septic shock. Unlike the catecholamine vasopressors, vasopressin is a direct vasoconstrictor agent and does not have inotropic or chronotropic effects. As a result, it may decrease cardiac output and hepatosplanchnic flow. In fact, studies of vasopressin in septic shock generally do not enroll patients with a cardiac index of less than 2 to 2.5 L/m^2 per minute.

The term *relative vasopressin deficiency* is used to describe the fact that vasopressin concentrations appear to be elevated early in septic shock and then fall to normal or low concentrations as shock progresses.[96] Normally, in the presence of hypotension, vasopressin concentrations would be expected to be elevated. Thus vasopressin administration in low "replacement" doses (0.01–0.04 unit/min) to patients with vasodilatory septic shock receiving high doses and long courses of norepinephrine successfully increases arterial blood pressure and SVR index. In addition, vasopressin has been shown to increase urine flow rates most likely owing to increased renal perfusion and arterial pressure. In the majority of patients in case series, vasopressor therapy (e.g., norepinephrine or dopamine) was tapered successfully and discontinued early. No clinical or laboratory signs of cardiac or mesenteric ischemia were observed, nor was PAOP or oxygenation adversely affected.[95] In a double-blinded, placebo-controlled trial in vasodilatory shock in trauma patients requiring vasopressors, a vasopressin infusion (0.04 unit/min) significantly improved arterial pressure owing to peripheral vasoconstriction and permitted the withdrawal of catecholamine vasopressors (norepinephrine, phenylephrine, and/or dopamine).[97] All patients receiving vasopressin survived the 24-hour study period and had all other catecholamine vasopressors withdrawn and blood pressure maintained solely with a low-dose vasopressin infusion.

Although vasopressin may be a useful agent in the treatment of refractory septic shock in low doses, it should not be used in doses exceeding 0.04 unit/min and/or in patients with hypovolemia, cardiogenic shock, or septic shock with myocardial depression because cardiac output may be adversely affected, including the development of myocardial ischemia and cardiac arrest.[94,97–99] There is concern that vasopressin may have deleterious effects on the hepatosplanchnic circulation in humans.[3] In addition, there are no randomized, blinded, placebo-controlled trials showing improvement in long-term outcomes such as mortality and length of hospital stay. The Canadian Critical Care Trials Group is conducting such a study, and results are expected in 2005. Until further safety data and larger efficacy trials are completed, vasopressin is not recommended as a replacement for norepinephrine or dopamine in septic shock but may be considered in patients who are refractory to catecholamine vasopressors despite adequate fluid resuscitation and should be administered in doses not exceeding 0.01–0.04 unit/min.[4]

TERLIPRESSIN

Terlipressin, a prodrug converted into lysine vasopressin, has been used recently in septic shock patients.[100] This drug has a half-life of 6 hours and acts via vascular V_{1a} receptors and renal tubular V_2 receptors.[37] In one report, terlipressin 1 mg was given intravenously to 15 patients with norepinephrine-resistant septic shock.[101] Terlipressin was shown to increase MAP at 30 minutes, which lasted for 24 hours. Despite a decrease in cardiac output, terlipressin increased gastric mucosal perfusion, urine output, and creatinine clearance. These preliminary findings suggest that a clinical trial should be conducted that evaluates mortality, in addition to hemodynamic effects.

LEVOSIMENDAN

Levosimendan is a novel inotropic calcium-sensitizing drug. In advanced congestive heart failure, it improves cardiac contractility by sensitizing troponin C to calcium. It has been used recently in a porcine model of endotoxin-induced septic shock, in which pretreatment with levosimendan improved cardiac output and systemic and gut oxygen delivery.[102] There are currently two ongoing clinical trials of levosimendan in septic shock. The role of levosimendan in the supportive management of circulatory failure in sepsis remains to be determined.

GENERAL CONCLUSIONS AND RECOMMENDATIONS

The choice of vasopressor or inotropic agent in septic shock should be made according to the needs of the patient (Fig. 23–3). The traditional algorithm suggests a stepwise approach first using dopamine and then norepinephrine; dobutamine is added for low cardiac output states, and occasionally, epinephrine and phenylephrine are used when necessary. Although this approach is empirical, it is used broadly in clinical practice and has been justified by a desire to avoid strong vasoconstriction and by the sense of safety resulting from graded doses of dopamine. This dose-response relationship, however, has never been established in the critically ill. In addition, recent observations of improved outcomes with norepinephrine and decreased regional perfusion with dopamine are calling into question the use of dopamine as a first-line agent.

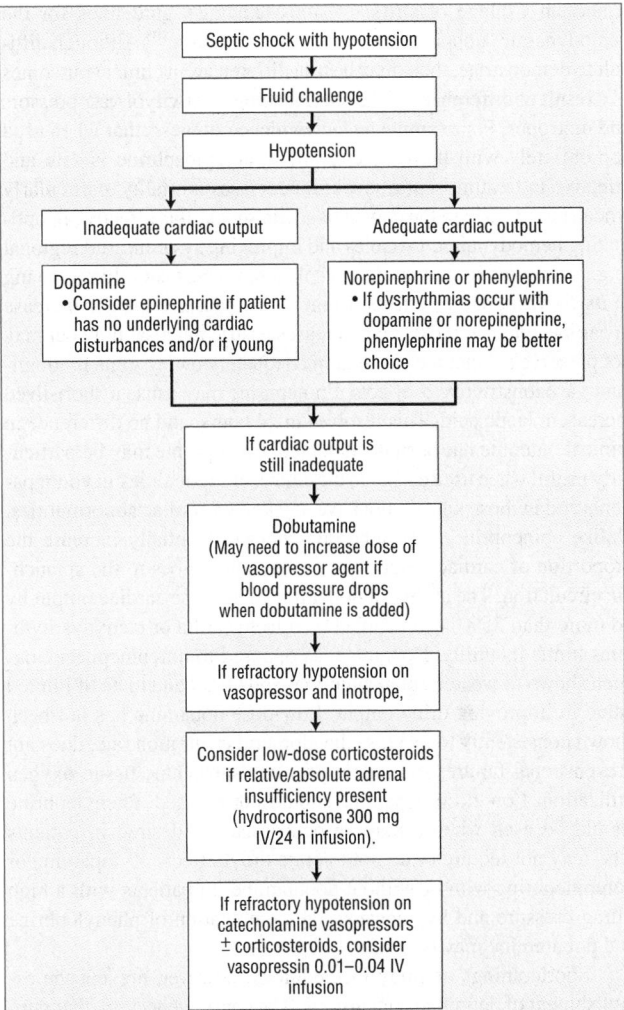

FIGURE 23–3. Algorithmic approach to the use of vasopressors and inotropes in septic shock. Algorithmic approach is intended to be used in conjunction with clinical judgment, hemodynamic monitoring parameters, and therapy end points, as discussed in the text. *(Modified from ref. 3.)*

Although goal-directed therapies to supranormal values cannot be recommended, developing a strategy to titrate therapy early in the course of illness to normal values is an acceptable approach. For all catecholamine vasopressors, larger doses than those recommended traditionally are required for goal-directed therapy to MAP and for normalization of oxygen-transport variables, DO_2, and VO_2. Attainment of supranormal DO_2 and VO_2 values is difficult in most patients, even if large doses are used. Patients who develop supranormal DO_2 and VO_2 values have a lower mortality, but whether this is achieved intrinsically or with exogenous administration of vasopressors/inotropes appears inconsequential. Goal-directed therapy to supranormal oxygen-transport variables therefore cannot be recommended because little or no benefit has been demonstrated to date. Further work is required to better elucidate the differential effects of vasopressors on regional hemodynamic and oxygen-transport values as measures of local tissue perfusion.

The algorithmic approach (see Fig. 23–3) that we recommend regarding the use of vasopressors and inotropes in the hemodynamic support of critically ill septic patients is consistent with the recommendations made in the Surviving Sepsis Campaign[4] and the

American College of Critical Care Medicine's guidelines for the hemodynamic support of adult patients with sepsis.[103] Although difficult to demonstrate, there may be true differences in clinical outcomes as a result of differences in the pharmacologic activity of vasopressors and inotropes. For example, recent evidence suggests that when used appropriately with fluid replenishment, norepinephrine is safe and effective in treating septic shock; it decreases mortality, particularly when started early in the course of septic shock. It is effective in optimizing hemodynamic variables and improving systemic and regional (e.g., renal, gastric mucosal, and splanchnic) perfusion likely owing to its β_2 vasodilatory effects. Epinephrine causes a greater increase in cardiac index and Do_2 and increases gastric mucosal flow but may not preserve splanchnic circulation adequately owing to its predominant vasoconstrictive α effects. Epinephrine may cause a short-lived increase in lactic acid. This resolves in 24 hours, and no difference in clinical outcome has been documented. Epinephrine may be particularly useful when used earlier in the course of septic shock in young patients and in those who do not have any known cardiac abnormalities. Unlike epinephrine, dopamine does not preferentially increase the proportion of cardiac output that preferentially goes to the splanchnic circulation. The ability of dopamine to increase cardiac output by no more than 35% accompanied by a tachycardia or tachydysrhythmias limits its utility. Dopamine, as opposed to norepinephrine, has been shown to worsen splanchnic Vo_2 and O_2ER and to be of limited value in improving urine output. Low-dose dopamine has not been shown consistently to increase the glomerular filtration rate, does not prevent renal failure, and indeed worsens splanchnic tissue oxygen utilization. Low-dose dopamine should not be used. Phenylephrine should be used when a pure vasoconstrictor is desired in patients who may not require or do not tolerate the β effects of dopamine or norepinephrine with or without dobutamine. In patients with a high filling pressure and hypotension, the combination of phenylephrine and dobutamine may be useful.

Shortcomings of study methodology, however, prevent the establishment of definitive conclusions. The consequences are that published guidelines for the management of severe sepsis and septic shock use many grade E (expert and consensus opinion, case series, case reports) recommendations. Short infusions (not exceeding 2 hours) during studies may show differences that are not clinically significant at 24 hours or more, as demonstrated for epinephrine and dobutamine. Clinically, vasopressors and inotropes are used for hours to days. Also, variable times at which a study is initiated with respect to the stage of sepsis or septic shock, the inherent differences in circulating catecholamine concentrations, and changes in receptor activity all may be confounding factors, as may be the prestudy duration and type of exogenous catecholamine administration.

Recent data with moderate doses of corticosteroids (200 to 300 mg/day) infused over 5 to 7 days may reverse septic shock and dependency on vasopressor agents, particularly in patients with relative adrenal insufficiency. Data are still needed regarding optimal dosing and the effect on outcomes such as mortality. Initial uncontrolled studies with vasopressin suggest a potential role in the management of vasopressor-refractory septic shock patients, although further data are needed.

Further pharmacotherapeutic and outcomes studies are still required to elucidate the place in therapy that individual vasopressors and inotropes or their combinations occupy in the supportive care of patients with bacteremia or septic shock. As supportive therapy, it is imperative that primary therapy aimed at the source of (antimicrobials) and consequences of (anticytokines) infection be initiated quickly to afford the patient the best chance of survival. Once this is accomplished, then we will need to direct our efforts to pharmacoeconomics and the cost-effectiveness of these therapies.

Review Questions and other resources can be found at *pharmacotherapyonline.com.*

REFERENCES

1. Balk RA. Severe sepsis and septic shock: Definitions, epidemiology, and clinical manifestations. Crit Care Clin 2000;16:179–192.
2. Hollenberg SM, Kavinsky CJ, Parrillo JE. Cardiogenic shock. Ann Intern Med 1999;131:47–59.
3. Practice parameters for hemodynamic support of sepsis in adult patients in sepsis. Crit Care Med 2004;32:1928–1948.
4. Dellinger RP, Carlet JM, Masur H, et al. Surviving sepsis campaign guidelines for management of severe sepsis and septic shock. Crit Care Med 2004;32:858–873.
5. Ahrens T. Hemodynamic monitoring. Crit Care Nurs Clin North Am 1999;11:19–31.
6. O'Grady N, Alexander M, Dellinger E, et al. Guidelines for the prevention of intravascular catheter-related infections. Clin Infect Dis 2002;35:1281–1307.
7. Headley JM. Invasive hemodynamic monitoring: Applying advanced technologies. Crit Care Nurs Q 1998;21:73–84.
8. Bernard GR, Sopko G, Cerra F, et al. Pulmonary artery catheterization and clinical outcomes: National Heart, Lung, and Blood Institute and Food and Drug Administration Workshop Report. Consensus Statement. JAMA 2000;283:2568–2572.
9. Prentice D, Ahrens T. Controversies in the use of the pulmonary artery catheter. J Cardiovasc Nurs 2001;15:1–5.
10. Practice guidelines for pulmonary artery catheterization: An updated report by the American Society of Anesthesiologists Task Force on Pulmonary Artery Catheterization. Anesthesiology 2003;99:988–1014.
11. Vincent JL. Hemodynamic support in septic shock. Intensive Care Med 2001;27:S80–92.
12. Rivers E, Nguyen B, Havstad S, et al. Early goal-directed therapy in the treatment of severe sepsis and septic shock. N Engl J Med 2001;345:1368–1377.
13. Rady MY, Rivers EP, Nowak RM. Resuscitation of the critically ill in the ED: responses of blood pressure, heart rate, shock index, central venous oxygen saturation, and lactate. Am J Emerg Med 1996;14:218–225.
14. Yu M. Oxygen transport optimization. New Horizons 1999;7:46–53.
15. Heyland DK, Cook DJ, King D, et al. Maximizing oxygen delivery in critically ill patients: A methodologic appraisal of the evidence. Crit Care Med 1996;24:517–524.
16. Yu M, Burchell S, Hasaniya NW, et al. Relationship of mortality to

increasing oxygen delivery in patients ≥50 years of age: A prospective, randomized trial. Crit Care Med 1998;26:1011–1019.

17. Lobo SM, Salgado PF, Castillo VG, et al. Effects of maximizing oxygen delivery on morbidity and mortality in high-risk surgical patients. Crit Care Med 2000;28:3396–3404.

18. Uusaro A, Russell JA. Could anti-inflammatory actions of catecholamines explain the possible beneficial effects of supranormal oxygen delivery in critically ill surgical patients? Intensive Care Med 2000; 26:299–304.

19. Meier-Hellmann A, Reinhart K, Bredle DL, et al. Epinephrine impairs splanchnic perfusion in septic shock. Crit Care Med 1997;25:399–404.

20. Kern JW, Shoemaker WC. Meta-analysis of hemodynamic optimization in high-risk patients. Crit Care Med 2002;30:1686–1692.

21. Chapman MV, Mythen MG, Webb AR, Vincent JL. Report from the meeting: Gastrointestinal tonometry: State of the art, 22–23 May 1998, London, UK. Intensive Care Med 2000;26:613–622.

22. Temmesfeld-Wollbruck B, Mayer K, Grimminger F. Assessment of intestinal tissue oxygenation: The canary sings—But what does the twitter tell us? Intensive Care Med 2000;26:1025–1027.

23. Barry B, Mallick A, Hartley G, et al. Comparison of air tonometry with gastric tonometry using saline and other equilibrating fluids: An in vivo and in vitro study. Intensive Care Med 1998;24:777–784.

24. Marik PE. Sublingual capnography: A clinical validation study. Chest 2001;120:923–927.

25. Bernardin G, Kisoka RL, Delporte C, et al. Impairment of beta-adrenergic signaling in healthy peripheral blood mononuclear cells exposed to serum from patients with septic shock: Involvement of the inhibitory pathway of adenylyl cyclase stimulation. Shock 2003;19:108–112.

26. Bernardin G, Strosberg AD, Bernard A, et al. Beta-adrenergic receptor–dependent and –independent stimulation of adenylate cyclase is impaired during severe sepsis in humans. Intensive Care Med 1998;24:1315–1322.

27. Dickerson RN, Lima JJ, Kuhl DA, et al. Effect of sustained endotoxemia on α_1-adrenergic responsiveness in parenterally fed rats. Pharmacotherapy 1998;18:170–174.

28. Richer M, Robert S, Lebel M. Renal hemodynamics during norepinephrine and low-dose dopamine infusions in man. Crit Care Med 1996;24:1150–1156.

29. Jindal N, Hollenberg SM, Dellinger RP. Pharmacologic issues in the management of septic shock. Crit Care Clin 2000;16:233–249.

30. Tisdale JE, Patel R, Webb CR, et al. Electrophysiologic and proarrhythmic effects of intravenous inotropic agents. Prog Cardiovasc Dis 1995;38:167–180.

31. Ruffolo R. Cardiovascular adrenoceptors: Physiology and critical care implications. In: Chernow B, Brater DC, Holaday JW, eds. The Pharmacological Approach to the Critically Ill Patient. Baltimore, Williams & Wilkins, 1994:167–181.

32. Martin C, Viviand X, Arnaud S, et al. Effects of norepinephrine plus dobutamine or norepinephrine alone on left ventricular performance of septic shock patients. Crit Care Med 1999;27:1708–1713.

33. LeDoux D, Astiz ME, Carpati CM, Rackow EC. Effects of perfusion pressure on tissue perfusion in septic shock. Crit Care Med 2000; 28:2729–2732.

34. Flancbaum L, Dick M, Dasta J, et al. A dose-response study of phenylephrine in critically ill, septic surgical patients. Eur J Clin Pharmacol 1997; 51:461–465.

35. Meier-Hellmann A, Sakka SG, Reinhart K. Catecholamines and splanchnic perfusion. Schweiz Med Wochenschr 2000;130:1942–1947.

36. Day NP, Phu NH, Mai NT, et al. Effects of dopamine and epinephrine infusions on renal hemodynamics in severe malaria and severe sepsis. Crit Care Med 2000;28:1353–1362.

37. Dunser M, Wenzel V, Mayr A, Hasibeder W. Management of vasodilatory shock. Drugs 2003;63:237–256.

38. De Backer D, Creteur J, Silva E, Vincent JL. Effects of dopamine, norepinephrine, and epinephrine on the splanchnic circulation in septic shock: Which is best? Crit Care Med 2003;31:1659–1667.

39. Weiss M, Schneider EM, Tarnow J, et al. Is inhibition of oxygen radical production of neutrophils by sympathomimetics mediated via beta-2 adrenoceptors? J Pharmacol Exp Ther 1996;278:1105–1113.

40. Fortenberry JD, Huber AR, Owens ML. Inotropes inhibit endothelial cell surface adhesion molecules induced by interleukin-1β. Crit Care Med 1997;25:303–308.

41. van der Poll T, Calvano SE, Kumar A, et al. Epinephrine attenuates downregulation of monocyte tumor necrosis factor receptors during human endotoxemia. J Leukoc Biol 1997;61:156–160.

42. Dive A, Foret F, Jamart J, et al. Effect of dopamine on gastrointestinal motility during critical illness. Intensive Care Med 2000;26:901–907.

43. Meier-Hellmann A, Sakka S, Reinhart K. [Aspects in monitoring and treatment of gastrointestinal underperfusion in sepsis: Diagnosis and therapy of gastrointestinal underperfusion in sepsis]. Anasthesiol Intensivmed Notfallmed Schmerzther 1998;33(suppl 2):S60–69.

44. Yu M. A peek at renal blood flow, renal function, and oxygen consumption with epinephrine and dopamine therapy. Crit Care Med 2000; 28:1661–1663.

45. Jakob SM, Ruokonen E, Takala J. Effects of dopamine on systemic and regional blood flow and metabolism in septic and cardiac surgery patients. Shock 2002;18:8–13.

46. Meier-Hellmann A, Bredle DL, Specht M, et al. The effects of low-dose dopamine on splanchnic blood flow and oxygen uptake in patients with septic shock. Intensive Care Med 1997;23:31–37.

47. Olson D, Pohlman A, Hall JB. Administration of low-dose dopamine to nonoliguric patients with sepsis syndrome does not raise intramucosal gastric pH nor improve creatinine clearance. Am J Respir Crit Care Med 1996;154:1664–1670.

48. Reinhart K, Sakka SG, Meier-Hellmann A. Haemodynamic management of a patient with septic shock. Eur J Anaesthesiol 2000;17:6–17.

49. Girbes AR, Patten MT, McCloskey BV, et al. The renal and neurohumoral effects of the addition of low-dose dopamine in septic critically ill patients. Intensive Care Med 2000;26:1685–1689.

50. Ichai C, Soubielle J, Carles M, et al. Comparison of the renal effects of low to high doses of dopamine and dobutamine in critically ill patients: A single-blind randomized study. Crit Care Med 2000;28:921–928.

51. Hoogenberg K, Smit AJ, and Girbes AR. Effects of low-dose dopamine on renal and systemic hemodynamics during incremental norepinephrine infusion in healthy volunteers. Crit Care Med 1998;26:260–265.

52. Rudis MI and Zarowitz BJ. Low-dose dopamine in acute oliguric renal failure. Am J Med 1997;102:320–322.

53. Bellomo R, Chapman M, Finfer S, et al. Low-dose dopamine in patients with early renal dysfunction: A placebo- controlled randomised trial. Australian and New Zealand Intensive Care Society (ANZICS) Clinical Trials Group. Lancet 2000;356:2139–2143.

54. Klahr S, Miller SB. Acute oliguria. New Engl J Med 1998;338:671–675.

55. Marik PE, Iglesias J. Low-dose dopamine does not prevent acute renal failure in patients with septic shock and oliguria. NORASEPT II Study Investigators. Am J Med 1999;107:387–390.

56. Lherm T, Troche G, Rossignol M, et al. Renal effects of low-dose dopamine in patients with sepsis syndrome or septic shock treated with catecholamines. Intensive Care Med 1996;22:213–219.

57. Ichai C, Passeron C, Carles M, et al. Prolonged low-dose dopamine infusion induces a transient improvement in renal function in hemodynamically stable, critically ill patients: A single-blind, prospective, controlled study. Crit Care Med 2000;28:1329–1335.

58. Kellum JA, Decker JM. Use of dopamine in acute renal failure: A meta-analysis. Crit Care Med 2001;29:1526–1531.

59. Martin C, Viviand X, Leone M, and Thirion X. Effect of norepinephrine on the outcome of septic shock. Crit Care Med 2000;28:2758–2765.

60. Abid O, Akca S, Haji-Michael P, Vincent JL. Strong vasopressor support may be futile in the intensive care unit patient with multiple organ failure. Crit Care Med 2000;28:947–949.

61. Groeneveld AB, Girbes AR, Thijs LG. Treating septic shock with norepinephrine. Crit Care Med 1999;27:2022–2023.

62. Redl-Wenzl EM, Armbruster C, Edelmann G, et al. The effects of norepinephrine on hemodynamics and renal function in severe septic shock states. Intensive Care Med 1993;19:151–154.

63. Rudis MI, Basha MA, Zarowitz BJ. Is it time to reposition vasopressors and inotropes in sepsis? Crit Care Med 1996;24:525–537.

64. Martin C, Papazian L, Perrin G, et al. Norepinephrine or dopamine for the treatment of hyperdynamic septic shock? Chest 1993;103:1826–1831.

65. Sharma VK, Dellinger RP. The International Sepsis Forum's controversies in sepsis: My initial vasopressor agent in septic shock is norepinephrine rather than dopamine. Crit Care 2003;7:3–5.

66. Parrillo JE. Myocardial depression during septic shock in humans. Crit Care Med 1990;18:1183–1184.

67. Hayes MA, Timmins AC, Yau EH, et al. Elevation of systemic oxygen delivery in the treatment of critically ill patients. N Engl J Med 1994; 330:1717–1722.

68. Shoemaker WC, Appel PL, Kram HB. Oxygen transport measurements to evaluate tissue perfusion and titrate therapy: dobutamine and dopamine effects. Crit Care Med 1991;19:672–688.

69. Duranteau J, Sitbon P, Teboul JL, et al. Effects of epinephrine, norepinephrine, or the combination of norepinephrine and dobutamine on gastric mucosa in septic shock. Crit Care Med 1999;27:893–900.

70. Rudis MI, Chant C. Update on vasopressors and inotropes in septic shock. J Pharm Practice 2001;15:124–134.

71. Reinelt H, Radermacher P, Fischer G, et al. Effects of a dobutamine-induced increase in splanchnic blood flow on hepatic metabolic activity in patients with septic shock. Anesthesiology 1997;86:818–824.

72. Seguin P, Bellissant E, Le Tulzo Y, et al. Effects of epinephrine compared with the combination of dobutamine and norepinephrine on gastric perfusion in septic shock. Clin Pharmacol Ther 2002;71:381–388.

73. Zhou SX, Qiu HB, Huang YZ, et al. Effects of norepinephrine, epinephrine, and norepinephrine-dobutamine on systemic and gastric mucosal oxygenation in septic shock. Acta Pharmacol Sin 2002;23: 654–658.

74. De Backer D, Moraine JJ, Berre J, et al. Effects of dobutamine on oxygen consumption in septic patients: Direct versus indirect determinations. Am J Respir Crit Care Med 1994;150:95–100.

75. Yamazaki T, Shimada Y, Taenaka N, et al. Circulatory responses to afterloading with phenylephrine in hyperdynamic sepsis. Crit Care Med 1982;10:432–435.

76. Gregory JS, Bonfiglio MF, Dasta JF, et al. Experience with phenylephrine as a component of the pharmacologic support of septic shock. Crit Care Med 1991;19:1395–1400.

77. Reinelt H, Radermacher P, Kiefer P, et al. Impact of exogenous beta-adrenergic receptor stimulation on hepatosplanchnic oxygen kinetics and metabolic activity in septic shock. Crit Care Med 1999;27:325–331.

78. Uusaro A, Takala J. Vasoactive drugs and splanchnic perfusion in septic shock. Crit Care Med 1998;26:1458–1460.

79. Rosselet A, Feihl F, Markert M, et al. Selective iNOS inhibition is superior to norepinephrine in the treatment of rat endotoxic shock. Am J Respir Crit Care Med 1998;157:162–170.

80. Griffiths MJ, Messent M, Curzen NP, Evans TW. Aminoguanidine selectively decreases cyclic GMP levels produced by inducible nitric oxide synthase. Am J Respir Crit Care Med 1995;152:1599–1604.

81. Grover R, Zaccardelli D, Colice G, et al. An open-label dose escalation study of the nitric oxide synthase inhibitor N(G)-methyl-L-arginine hydrochloride (546C88), in patients with septic shock. Crit Care Med 1999;27(5):913–922.

82. Lefering LR, Neugebauer EAM. Steroids controversy in sepsis and septic shock: A meta-analysis. Crit Care Med 1995;23:1294–1303.

83. Cronin L, Cook DJ, Carlet J, et al. Corticosteroid treatment for sepsis: A critical appraisal and meta-analysis. Crit Care Med 1995;23:1430–1409.

84. Bollaert PE. Stress doses of glucocorticoids in catecholamine dependency: A new therapy for a new syndrome? Intensive Care Med 2000; 26:3–5.

85. Spijkstra JJ, Girbes AR. The continuing story of corticosteroids in the treatment of septic shock. Intensive Care Med 2000;26:496–500.

86. Bollaert PE, Charpentier C, Levy B, et al. Reversal of late septic shock with supraphysiologic doses of hydrocortisone. Crit Care Med 1998; 26:645–650.

87. Briegel J, Forst H, Haller M, et al. Stress doses of hydrocortisone reverse hyperdynamic septic shock: A prospective, randomized, double-blind, single-center study. Crit Care Med 1999;27:723–732.

88. Keh D, Boehnke T, Weber-Cartens S, et al. Immunologic and hemodynamic effects of "low-dose" hydrocortisone in septic shock: A double-blind, randomized, placebo-controlled, crossover study. Am J Respir Crit Care Med 2003;167:512–520.

89. Yildiz O, Doganay M, Aygen B, et al. Physiological-dose steroid therapy in sepsis. Crit Care 2002;6:251–258.

90. Annane D, Sebille V, Charpentier C, et al. Effect of treatment with low doses of hydrocortisone and fludrocortisone on mortality in patients with septic shock. JAMA 2002;288:862–871.

91. Minneci PC, Deans KJ, Banks SM, et al. Dose-dependent effects of steroids on survival rates and shock during sepsis: A meta-analysis (abstract). Crit Care Med 2003;31:A20.

92. Bellissant E, Annane D. Effect of hydrocortisone on phenylephrine: Mean arterial pressure dose-response relationship in septic shock. Clin Pharmacol Ther 2000;68:293–303.

93. Burry LD, Wax RS. Role of corticosteroids in septic shock. Ann Pharmacother 2004;38:464–472.

94. Landry DW, Levin HR, Gallant EM, et al. Vasopressin pressor hypersensitivity in vasodilatory septic shock. Crit Care Med 1997;25:1279–1282.

95. Landry DW, Levin HR, Gallant EM, et al. Vasopressin deficiency contributes to the vasodilation of septic shock. Circulation 1997;95:1122–1125.

96. Sharshar T, Blanchard A, Paillard M, et al. Circulating vasopressor levels in septic shock. Crit Care Med 2003;31:1752–1758.

97. Malay MB, Ashton RC Jr, Landry DW, Townsend RN. Low-dose vasopressin in the treatment of vasodilatory septic shock. J Trauma 1999; 47:699–703.

98. Holmes CL, Patel BM, Russell JA, Walley KR. Physiology of vasopressin relevant to management of septic shock. Chest 2001;120:989–1002.

99. Holmes CL, Walley KR, Chittock DR, et al. The effects of vasopressin on hemodynamics and renal function in severe septic shock: A case series. Intensive Care Med 2001;27:1416–1421.

100. O'Brien A, Clapp L, Singer M. Terlipressin for norepinephrine-resistent septic shock. Lancet 2002;359:1209–1210.

101. Morelli A, Rocco M, Conti G, et al. Effects of terlipressin on systemic and regional haemodynamics in catecholamine-treated hyperkinetic septic shock. Intensive Care Med 2004;30:597–604.

102. Oldner A, Konrad D, Weitzberg E, et al. Effects of levosimendan, a novel inotropic calcium-sensitizing drug, in experimental septic shock. Crit Care Med 2001;29:2185–2193.

103. Practice parameters for hemodynamic support of sepsis in adult patients in sepsis. Task Force of the American College of Critical Care Medicine, Society of Critical Care Medicine. Crit Care Med 1999;27:639–660.

104. Hoffman BB, Taylor P. Neurotransmission: The autonomic and somatic motor nervous system. In: Hardman JG, Limbird LE, Gilman AG, eds. Goodman & Gilman's The Pharmacological Basis of Therapeutics, 10th ed. New York, McGraw-Hill, 2001:115–153.

105. Hoffman BB. Catecholamines, sympathomimetic drugs and adrenergic receptor antagonists. In: Hardman JG, Limbird LE, Gilman AG, eds. Goodman & Gilman's The Pharmacological Basis of Therapeutics, 10th ed. New York, McGraw-Hill, 2001:215–268.

106. Zaritsky AL. Catecholamines, inotropic medications, and vasopressor agents. In: Chernow B, Brater DC, Holaday JW, eds. The Pharmacological Approach to the Critically Ill Patient, 3d ed. Baltimore, Williams & Wilkins, 1994:387–404.

24
HYPOVOLEMIC SHOCK

Brian L. Erstad

Learning Objectives and other resources can be found at *www.pharmacotherapyonline.com.*

KEY CONCEPTS

◀1 Plasma does not have to be lost from the body for hypovolemic shock to occur.

◀2 Patients may die from hypovolemic shock despite having normal serum electrolyte concentrations.

◀3 While the Starling equation of fluid transport is useful for understanding the factors involved in fluid shifting between compartments, it is not a practical tool for use in the clinical setting.

◀4 Patients may have complications and death owing to reperfusion injury, as well as the initial insult.

◀5 The clinical presentation of patients with hypovolemic shock can vary substantially depending on concomitant disease states, medications, and cause of hypovolemia.

◀6 The initial monitoring of a patient with suspected volume depletion always should include vital signs, urine output, mental status, and physical examination.

◀7 The need for intravenous rehydration in children is often overestimated.

◀8 Crystalloid (sodium-containing) solutions should be used for most forms of circulatory insufficiency that are associated with hemodynamic instability.

◀9 Crystalloid solutions are preferred over colloid solutions for circulatory insufficiency owing to decreased plasma volume.

◀10 With adequate fluid administration, medications usually are not needed for the patient with circulatory insufficiency owing to decreased plasma volume.

This chapter discusses the assessment and management of hypovolemic shock. Depending on the classification scheme being used for shock, spinal and anaphylactic shock may be considered separately from hypovolemic shock because fluid loss from the body is not necessary for their occurrence. For example, there are distributive forms of shock, such as spinal shock resulting from loss of sympathetic activity, and anaphylactic shock, resulting from increased vascular permeability.[1] Although these forms of shock are not discussed in detail, it is important to note that the initial therapy for both is the same as for hypovolemic shock (i.e., adequate volume replacement) because circulating volume is decreased. In this regard, adequate fluid resuscitation to maintain circulating blood volume is a common principle in managing all forms of shock.

EPIDEMIOLOGY

It is estimated that approximately 1 million deaths per year occur in the United States in patients with shock.[2] The number is much higher when one considers that all causes of death ultimately result in circulatory failure (i.e., the last stage of shock). It is much more difficult to estimate the number of patients with reversible organ dysfunction or patients with end-organ damage who survived an episode of hypovolemic shock. Part of the problem is defining when progressive circulatory insufficiency results in the loss of normal compensatory responses by the body, which could reverse the processes leading to irreversible organ dysfunction. This loss of appropriate compensation varies from patient to patient and is not always readily apparent during the initial patient presentation.

ETIOLOGY

◀1 Hypovolemic shock may result from a number of problems, including plasma loss, sequestered fluid within a compartment in the body (e.g., third-spacing), thermal injury, and various forms of dehydration. Plasma loss may occur from hemorrhage or from sustained gastrointestinal or urinary losses that are insufficiently replaced. In some cases, such as in postoperative patients, a number of these problems may occur at the same time. For example, a patient may have had blood loss secondary to trauma or surgery, with additional fluid being third-spaced postoperatively. The third-spaced fluid may occur as tissue edema in the gastrointestinal tract with a concomitant ileus. As the example of third-spaced fluid indicates, fluid (i.e., plasma) does not have to be lost from the body for a person to develop hypovolemic shock.

Dehydration may result from primary water deficiency, usually because of decreased intake, but in some instances (e.g., diabetes insipidus) it may result from increased losses of water. In general, the term *dehydration* implies intracellular and interstitial fluid depletion, in contrast to *volume depletion,* which implies extracellular, and particularly intravascular, sodium and water loss. In the case of primary water deficit, cell dehydration occurs, with delayed circulatory failure from decreased circulatory volume with ongoing losses.[3] Initially, the patient may be thirsty and possibly have some mental status changes, such as confusion. If the cellular dehydration occurs slowly, intracellular substances, referred to as *idiogenic osmols,* develop that limit progressive complications (e.g., cerebral edema or coma). With combined water and salt deficiencies, such as might occur with gastrointestinal losses (e.g., diarrhea), interstitial and intravascular depletion is an early occurrence. Fortunately, dehydration is relatively easy to prevent with routine vigilance and water replacement compared with some of the other causes of shock.

PATHOPHYSIOLOGY

2 Hypovolemic shock is often described in terms of monitoring parameters such as lowered blood pressure, but patients with shock may die despite normal surrogate markers of circulatory insufficiency. Therefore, an appropriate definition should mention the underlying problem, which is inadequate tissue perfusion resulting from circulatory failure. In the case of hypovolemic shock, the cause of the altered perfusion is fluid (or volume) depletion resulting from trauma, surgery, thermal injury, or some form of dehydration. Figure 24–1 provides a simplified view of the pathophysiology of circulatory insufficiency. Cell damage and death may occur from the primary insult or from reperfusion injury. The latter problem is associated most frequently with trauma and blood loss that cause the release of a multitude of mediators of inflammation and injury that have complex interactions. Cells have varying responses to hypoxia, ranging from astrocytes that quit functioning almost immediately to hepatic cells that may function for several hours after injury.[3] Left unmitigated, cell death occurs.

The body attempts to compensate for volume depletion beginning with autoregulatory changes involving smaller blood vessels. When the cause of circulatory insufficiency continues unabated, local mechanisms eventually fail to provide adequate compensation, and macrocirculatory changes ensue. Approximately 75% of blood volume is contained in venous capacitance vessels, with gravity being the major impedance to flow back to the heart.[3] With increasing volume depletion, blood flow to the heart (preload) is decreased, with subsequent activation of baroreceptors and chemoreceptors leading to sympathetic discharge. Also, fluid shifting from the interstitial space to the intravascular space occurs through a phenomenon known as *transcapillary refill,* and hormones (e.g., adrenocorticotropic hormone, angiotensin, catecholamines, and vasopressin) that cause sodium and water retention by the kidneys are released. The phenomenon of transcapillary refill means that the body can have fluid losses exceeding normal plasma volume. These responses cause alterations in stroke volume, heart rate, and peripheral vascular resistance so that blood pressure and hence tissue perfusion can be maintained.

The microcirculatory changes associated with shock are complex and difficult to study. Although some mediators such as endothelin-1 cause vasoconstriction, other mediators, such as adenosine and nitric oxide, yield vasodilation.[4] These changes result in hypoperfusion or hyperperfusion depending on the area. As these microcirculatory changes fail to maintain adequate organ perfusion, more widespread sympathetic nervous system activation and vasoconstriction ensue.

The factors involved in fluid shifting between the intravascular and interstitial spaces are described by the modified Starling equation:

$$J_V = K_{f,c} \left[(P_c - P_t) - \sigma(\pi_c - \pi_t) \right]$$

where J_V = net transvascular flow rate (cannot be measured in the clinical setting)

$K_{f,c}$ = capillary filtration coefficient for fluids (cannot be measured in the clinical setting)

P_c = capillary hydrostatic pressure (indirectly estimated in the clinical setting, e.g., pulmonary artery occlusive pressure)

P_t = tissue hydrostatic pressure (cannot be measured in the clinical setting)

σ = reflection coefficient for proteins (cannot be measured in the clinical setting)

π_c = plasma colloid osmotic pressure (not usually measured in the clinical setting, but technology is available)

π_t = tissue colloid osmotic pressure (cannot be measured in the clinical setting)

Proteins act as oncotic agents in each of these spaces to attract fluid, whereas hydrostatic forces push fluid into or out of the vessels. The equation has distinct permeability values for water and protein because each crosses the vascular membrane at a different rate. **3** Although the Starling equation is useful to practitioners in terms of understanding the factors involved in fluid shifting between compartments, the rate and direction of transvascular flow cannot be calculated accurately in the clinical setting because most factors cannot be measured directly.

The body's compensatory mechanisms may have beneficial and harmful consequences. For example, if preload is not substantially decreased, cardiac output can be increased approximately fivefold by increases in stroke volume or heart rate.[1] Although this may be useful for providing blood flow to inadequately perfused tissues, it may cause large (e.g., fourfold) increases in oxygen consumption by the heart that could aggravate preexisting ischemia in patients with underlying coronary artery disease (CAD). Another example is the sympathetic nervous system–mediated vasoconstriction that causes blood to shift

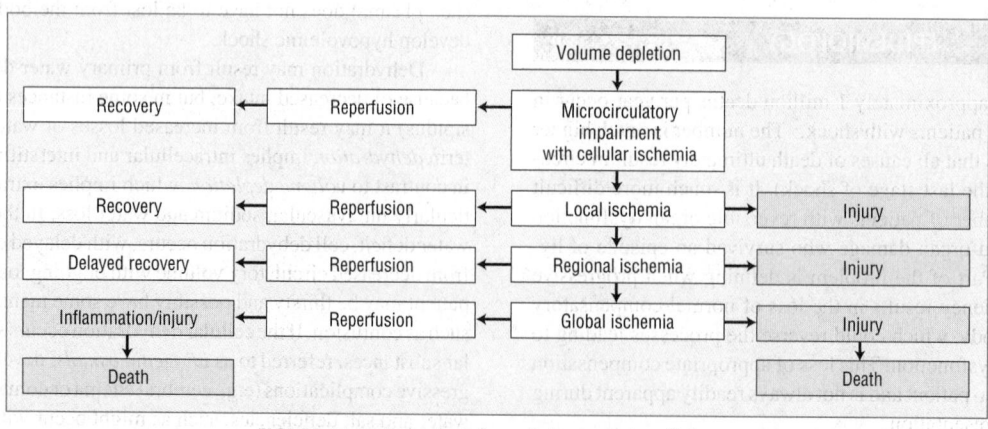

FIGURE 24–1. Pathophysiology of circulatory insufficiency.

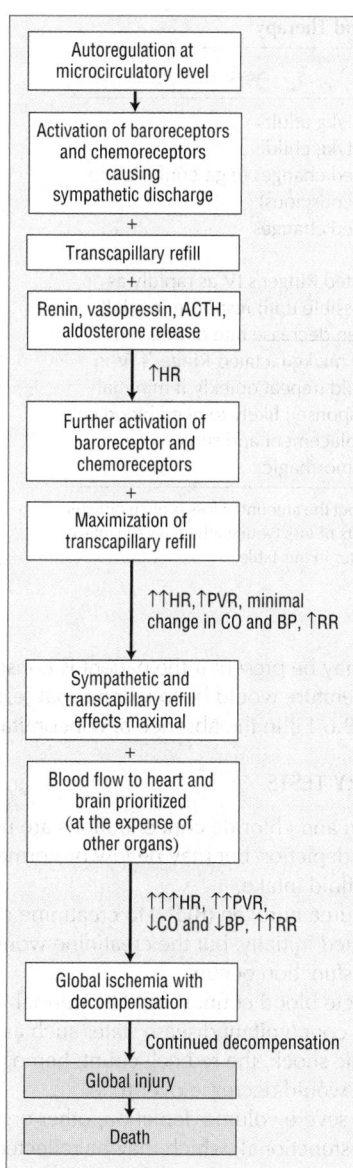

FIGURE 24–2. Activation of compensatory mechanisms with loss of circulatory volume. Certain stages may be absent depending on a number of factors, such as age, preexisting disease states, and cause of circulatory insufficiency. BP = blood pressure; CO = cardiac output; HR = heart rate; PVR = peripheral vascular resistance; RR = respiratory rate.

Although the basic pathophysiology is similar for the various causes of hypovolemic shock, there are unique considerations relative to each. For example, whereas isolated head injuries associated with trauma typically do not result in substantial blood loss or shock, pelvic fractures may sequester several liters of blood as hematoma formation.[5] Patients with traumatic or thermal injuries, as well as postoperative patients, may have substantial fluid accumulation in sites where it cannot be readily transferred back into blood vessels (i.e., third-spaced fluid) for maintaining pressure. With these types of injuries, prompt control of compressible bleeding sources with rapid patient transfer to the hospital for definitive treatment may preclude the cascade of events leading to shock. Indeed, with trauma patients, a "scoop and run" approach is used in most urban hospitals that places a priority on rapid transport to a hospital.[6]

In the case of hemorrhagic shock, prompt attention must be given to cell, as well as plasma, losses. Red blood cells lost during the bleeding episode may lead to ischemic damage in vital organs. Packed red blood cell transfusions may be needed to increase the oxygen-carrying capacity of the blood because oxygen transport is a function not only of cardiac output but also of hemoglobin concentration and saturation and of hemoglobin affinity for oxygen.

Clotting factors and platelets are also lost in hemorrhage. The resulting bleeding problems may be aggravated by the dilutional effect of fluid resuscitation on clotting factor activity. Fresh-frozen plasma that contains necessary clotting factors and platelets is often needed in massive blood loss to restore adequate coagulation. On the other hand, trauma patients are at increased risk for deep venous thrombosis and pulmonary embolism caused by multiple factors, including vessel damage, abnormal blood flow patterns, and the hypercoagulable state associated with injury. Therefore, some form of venous thromboembolism prophylaxis usually is indicated in multiple-trauma patients or patients with severe single-system injuries (e.g., spinal cord damage).

The pathophysiology becomes more complicated if the severity of shock is sufficient to require admission to the intensive care unit (ICU) after initial resuscitation or surgery. Most patients admitted to the ICU have a systemic inflammatory response syndrome (SIRS), which is the body's response to injury. This syndrome is defined by a number of hypermetabolic changes reflected in the patient's temperature, white blood cell count and differential, and respiratory and heart rates. The stress response involves complex interactions between the nervous system and immunomodulating substances and has similar (if not the same) harmful and helpful consequences described with reperfusion following shock.[7] If the underlying problems are left untreated, the patient with SIRS may develop multiple-organ dysfunction syndrome (MODS) during the final stages of illness.

CLINICAL PRESENTATION

The initial presentation of patients with suspected volume depletion can vary markedly depending on factors such as age, concomitant disease states and medications, and the etiology and rapidity of depletion (see Clinical Presentation box at the end of this chapter). Intravascular depletion as a consequence of blood loss is signified by postural vital sign changes, and such measurements should be performed unless the diagnosis is obvious, as in the case of bleeding associated with trauma.[8] Early signs and symptoms of dehydration and intravascular depletion caused by gastrointestinal or urinary losses often are relatively nonspecific. Plasma volume losses of less than 10 mL/kg of body weight usually are associated with minor signs

from the skin, skeletal muscle, and some internal organs such as the kidneys and gastrointestinal tract to organs (e.g., heart and brain) that are less tolerant of inadequate flow. If the vasoconstriction continues unabated, the hypoperfused organs eventually become damaged. Figure 24–2 provides an overview of the compensatory changes that occur with a loss of circulating blood volume.

In addition to the more acute implications of hypovolemia and attendant complications, reperfusion damage is likely to occur particularly after prolonged resuscitation attempts. In addition to oxygen free radical damage of cell membranes, a number of cellular (e.g., white blood cells and platelets) and humoral (e.g., procoagulants, anticoagulants, complement, and kinins) components are activated, causing the release of other inflammatory mediators.[4] The resulting reperfusion injury may range from readily reversible organ dysfunction to multiple-organ failure and death.

TABLE 24–1. Acute Circulatory Insufficiency: Initial Presentation and Therapy*

	Mild	Severe
Plasma/blood loss	10 mL/kg adult 20 mL/kg child	30 mL/kg adult 35 mL/kg child
Mental status/level of consciousness	None—small changes (e.g., anxious, irritable)	Marked changes (e.g., confusion to unconscious)
Vital signs/orthostatic changes	Minor changes	Marked changes
Therapy	20 mL/kg lactated Ringer's IV* over 10–15 min Unlikely to need blood cell replacement even if hemorrhagic loss	Lactated Ringer's IV as rapidly as possible until response in adult, then decrease rate of infusion 20 mL/kg lactated Ringer's IV in child (repeat quickly if minimal response); likely to need blood cell replacement and surgery if hemorrhagic

*Patients may have intermediate degrees of volume loss in addition to those listed, but the amount of loss is often difficult to quantify. The presentations may also vary greatly in patients with similar amounts of loss (young athlete vs sedentary, elderly person). Refer to text for a more in-depth discussion of some of the guidelines in this table.

and symptoms of distress. Larger losses are not likely to be well tolerated (Table 24–1), particularly in patients older than 65 years of age. An 18-year-old athlete and a 65-year-old sedentary individual are likely to have a much different response to a similar amount of fluid loss. The young patient may lose one-fourth of his or her circulating blood volume with minimal changes in arterial blood pressure and a relatively low heart rate. However, the elderly patient may have orthostatic changes in blood pressure that are not well tolerated by organs such as the kidneys.[3] Unfortunately, this same elderly patient may not have common signs and symptoms of volume depletion such as skin turgor changes or thirst but instead may have more subtle changes (e.g., mental status alterations).[9]

CLINICAL PRESENTATION OF HYPOVOLEMIC SHOCK

GENERAL

- The initial presentation of adult patients with suspected volume depletion could vary markedly depending on factors such as age, concomitant disease states and medications, and the etiology and rapidity of depletion.
- Plasma volume losses of less than 10 mL/kg of body weight usually are associated with minor signs and symptoms of distress.

SYMPTOMS

- Patients may present with thirst, nausea, anxiousness, weakness, light-headedness, and dizziness.
- Patients may report scanty urine output and dark-yellow-colored urine.

SIGNS

With more severe volume loss:

- Patients would have marked increases in heart rate (e.g., >120 beats per minute) and respiratory rate (e.g., >30 breaths per minute).
- Blood pressure would be decreased (e.g., systolic blood pressure < 90 mm Hg).
- Mental status changes or unconsciousness may occur.

- Agitation may be present if the patient is conscious.
- Body temperature would be low or normal [e.g., 36° to 37°C (96.8° to 98.6°F)] in the absence of concomitant infection.

LABORATORY TESTS

- The sodium and chloride concentrations are usually high with acute depletion but may be low or normal depending on type of fluid intake.
- The blood urea nitrogen (BUN) to creatinine ratio is likely to be elevated initially, but the creatinine would increase as renal dysfunction occurs.
- The complete blood count should be normal in the absence of concomitant disease states such as infection; in hemorrhagic shock, the red cell count, hemoglobin, and hematocrit would decrease over time.
- With more severe volume depletion, other organs may become dysfunctional, which may be reflected in laboratory testing (e.g., elevated transaminases with hepatic dysfunction).

OTHER DIAGNOSTIC TESTS

- Urine output would be decreased to less than 0.5 to 1 mL/hour.

The diagnosis of dehydration and intravascular depletion in children is complicated by difficulties in obtaining an accurate history. In younger children, parental observations are important for estimating fluid deficits and deciding whether hospitalization is necessary. Fortunately, there are prospective data that suggest that parental histories are predictive of acidosis and the need for hospitalization.[10]
    ❻ Regardless of patient age or preexisting conditions, the initial monitoring of a patient with suspected volume depletion should include the following noninvasive parameters: vital signs, urine output, mental status, and physical examination (Fig. 24–3).
    While the presenting signs and symptoms of circulatory insufficiency are variable, patients usually will have decreased blood pressure, increased heart and respiratory rates, and a normal or low-normal temperature (e.g., 36° to 37°C [96.8° to 98.6°F]) in the absence of infection, exposure to extremes of temperature, and medications that

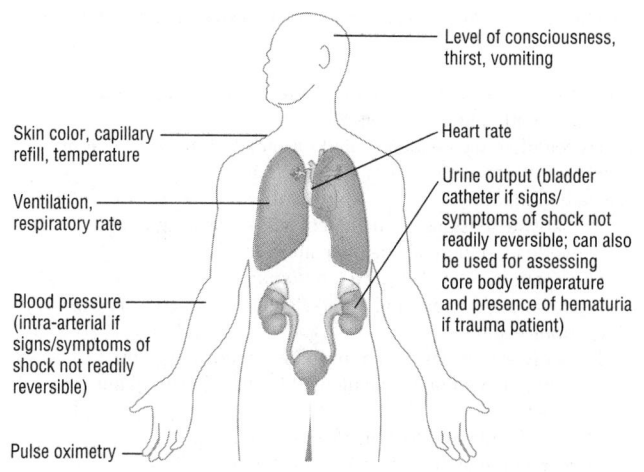

FIGURE 24–3. Noninvasive assessment of circulatory insufficiency.

impair thermoregulation. As mentioned earlier, recordings of vital signs must be interpreted in light of known or suspected baseline conditions. For example, alcohol, β-blockers, butyrophenones such as haloperidol, diuretics, and medications with anticholinergic effects may impair thermoregulation.[11] Medications such as β-blockers and calcium channel blockers may alter resting blood pressure and heart rate, as well as the subsequent response to therapeutic interventions.

Although a blood pressure reading of 110/70 mm Hg (systolic/diastolic) may be acceptable in many patients, it may be inadequate in a patient with preexisting hypertension who normally has a blood pressure of 170/105 mm Hg. At the other extreme, patients with very low blood pressure may have inaudible or inaccurate determinations with cuff (sphygmomanometric) measurements. Chapter 13 details

blood pressure measurement (e.g., cuff size, position). In this case, intraarterial monitoring is indicated. As a noninvasive tool, the respiratory rate may correlate better than the heart rate with volume loss, but respiratory rate often is not used.[3] The respiratory rate may be elevated because of anxiety or as a compensatory mechanism for the metabolic acidosis caused by lactic acidosis associated with poor tissue perfusion.

Although the kidneys continually produce urine, the bladder stores the urine for intermittent elimination. For the initial diagnosis and management of acute circulatory insufficiency, a catheter can be inserted into the bladder for measuring urine output. In contrast to thirst, which is a relatively insensitive indicator of volume depletion, urine output is generally diminished with inadequate fluid administration and increases with appropriate resuscitation. This presumes, of course, that acute renal failure or medications such as diuretics are not altering the expected response. Adults should produce at least 0.5 to 1 mL/kg per hour of urine, whereas children up to 12 years of age should produce at least 1 mL/kg per hour (2 mL/kg per hour if younger than 1 year of age).[5]

Mental status changes associated with volume depletion, if present, may range from subtle fluctuations in mood to unconsciousness. Although the latter finding typically is indicative of more severe depletion, less dramatic findings should not be interpreted as indicating mild fluid deficits. Losses of 4 L of plasma volume may be associated only with lassitude in an otherwise healthy adult patient.[3] Similar interpretation difficulties must be considered when performing the initial physical examination. An orderly progression from warm, reddish skin with appropriate capillary refill (rapid return of blood flow to the extremity after removal of compression) to cold, cyanotic discoloration with impaired refill may not occur. Also, dry mucous membranes in elderly patients may be caused by mouth breathing or anticholinergic medications and not by fluid depletion.[9]

▶ TREATMENT: Hypovolemic Shock

▨ DESIRED OUTCOME

The desired outcomes of therapy for circulatory insufficiency that has led to hypovolemic shock are to prevent further progression of the disease with subsequent organ damage and, to the extent possible, to reverse organ dysfunction that has already taken place.

▨ GENERAL APPROACH TO TREATMENT

Milder forms of volume depletion may be managed in outpatient settings. For example, supplemental fluids can be added to the usual estimated daily requirements of 30 to 35 mL/kg in patients older than 12 years of age with dehydration. Commercially available carbohydrate/electrolyte drinks generally are more palatable than water and may promote earlier recovery.[9] When the dehydration involves substantial losses of salt as well as water, additional sodium may need to be added to these drinks because they usually contain 50 mEq/L or less of sodium. This is less than the amounts of sodium (e.g., 90 to 120 mEq/L) generally recommended for rehydration.[12] The additional sodium will increase osmolarity, but this does not appear to delay gastric emptying.[13] Also, guidelines for oral rehydration of children with acute diarrhea are available, which, if used appropriately, may prevent future hospitalization.[14] Intravenous rehydration of

children in outpatient settings has been accomplished, but patients must be selected carefully.[15] Outpatient rehydration of children usually is recommended for those with uncomplicated (e.g., vomiting less than 48 hours) acute gastroenteritis and relatively mild dehydration after the exclusion of more severe illnesses such as bowel obstruction. ◀ The need for intravenous rehydration often is overestimated. In a randomized trial conducted in a pediatric emergency department, children receiving oral rehydration for acute gastroenteritis had shorter lengths of stay than those receiving intravenous rehydration (225 versus 358 minutes; $p < .01$).[16] Furthermore, there was a trend toward decreased hospital admissions in the oral compared with the intravenous rehydration group (11% versus 25%; $p = .2$).

Hospitalization is indicated in more severe forms of circulatory insufficiency. If access to the circulatory system for fluids and medication administration was not obtained prior to hospitalization, this should be a priority. Venous access generally is obtained during the preliminary examination process that includes the ABCs of life support (i.e., airway, breathing, and circulation), assessment of vital signs and mental status, and determination of urine output after catheterization. Whenever large-volume fluid resuscitation is expected, as in hemorrhagic shock, it is desirable to have at least two intravenous catheters. Because flow is a function of tubing length and catheter diameter, large-bore peripheral intravenous lines are preferred over longer central lines. Unfortunately, vascular access in some patients may be problematic, and other routes (e.g., intraosseous infusion in children) may be necessary.[5] One interesting method of fluid administration that has been investigated in elderly patients is subcutaneous infusion, or hypodermoclysis. This route of administration is not used commonly probably because of concerns of adverse effects that were found in early studies that used excessively hypotonic or hypertonic solutions. Although alternative methods of fluid administration, such as hypodermoclysis are desirable, there is a need for well-conducted trials before such methods can be recommended for routine use.

PHARMACOLOGIC THERAPY

Dextrose-in-water solutions may be appropriate for uncomplicated dehydration caused by water deprivation, but crystalloid (sodium-containing) solutions should be used for forms of circulatory insufficiency that are associated with hemodynamic instability. In the latter situation, intravenous solutions with sodium concentrations approximating normal serum sodium values usually are indicated because they cause more expansion of the intravascular and interstitial spaces compared with dextrose solutions (Table 24–2). Lactated Ringer's and normal saline solutions are examples of such crystalloid solutions, although lactated Ringer's solution is the preferred solution according to some published guidelines (see Advanced Trauma Life Support Guidelines) because it is unlikely to cause the hyperchloremic metabolic acidosis that is seen with infusion of large amounts of normal saline[5] (Table 24–3). A "large" amount of fluid does not mean the typical bolus volumes used as fluid challenges in critically ill patients. Isolated boluses (e.g., 500 mL in patients older than 18 years of age) are unlikely to cause substantial changes in blood pressure or acid-base balance.[17]

Although lactated Ringer's solution does contain lactate, it does not cause substantial elevations in circulating lactate concentrations

TABLE 24–3. Adverse Effects of Plasma Expanders: Crystalloids

Normal saline
  Primarily extensions of pharmacologic actions (e.g., fluid overload, dilutional coagulopathy)
  Hyperchloremic metabolic acidosis (has 154 mEq/L of chloride)
  Hypernatremia (has 154 mEq/L of sodium)
Lactated Ringer's
  Primarily extensions of pharmacologic actions (e.g., fluid overload, dilutional coagulopathy)
  Hyponatremia (has 130 mEq/L of sodium)
  Aggravation of preexisting hyperkalemia (has 4 mEq/L of potassium)
Hypertonic saline
  Primarily extensions of pharmacologic actions (e.g., fluid overload; dilutional coagulopathy; intracellular volume depletion)
  Hypernatremia (has 513 mEq/L of sodium)
  Hyperchloremia (has 513 mEq/L of chloride)

when used as a resuscitation solution.[18] However, blood samples for lactate determinations drawn through catheters (arterial and venous) that have not been cleared appropriately may have spurious increases or decreases in lactate concentrations because of retained lactated Ringer's and nonlactated solutions (e.g., varying concentrations of dextrose-in-water or sodium chloride), respectively.[19] Therefore, blood samples for lactate concentration determinations should be drawn from a catheter that has been cleared adequately (e.g., 5 mL) of infusate after temporarily stopping the fluid infusion.

While a number of pharmacologic therapies show promise in animal models of shock, few demonstrate success in subsequent trials involving patients with shock. In large part this is a result of the lack of acceptable animal models of shock that mimic the pathophysiology of patients.[20] In cases in which a relevant animal model is available, care

TABLE 24–2. Fluid Distribution and Major Indications[a]

Fluid	Intracellular	Interstitial	Intravascular	Major Indication
Normal saline or lactated Ringer's	None	750 mL	250 mL	Intravascular repletion in symptomatic patients
3% sodium chloride	→	750 mL+	250 mL+	Small amounts (e.g., 250 mL) have been used in conjunction with normal saline or lactated Ringer's for severe intravascular depletion in adults
5% dextrose/ 0.45% sodium chloride	333 mL	500 mL	167 mL	Maintenance fluid in euvolemic or dehydrated (sodium and water loss) patients with mild signs/symptoms of volume depletion
5% dextrose	667 mL	250 mL	83 mL	Dehydration (primarily water loss) in patients with mild signs/symptoms of volume depletion
5% albumin	None	None	1000 mL[b]	Intravascular repletion in symptomatic patients
25% albumin	→	→	1000 mL+[b]	Smaller amounts (e.g., 50–100 mL or by continuous infusion in adults) titrated to response in hypovolemic patients with excess total body water

[a]Based on the administration of 1 L of each solution (*which may not be an appropriate amount for clinical use*); numbers are approximations; arrows indicate direction of fluid shift and plus signs indicate fluid retention in that compartment.
[b]After distribution, 60% of albumin (and associated fluid) is in interstitial compartment and 40% is in intravascular compartment.

must be taken in extrapolating the information to forms of shock other than the one under study. This may be the problem with naloxone, which has been shown to raise blood pressure in some studies of shock but not in others.[21] In light of the lack of other demonstrated pharmaceutical interventions, fluids remain the mainstay of therapy, although their use is not devoid of controversy.

Larger-molecular-weight solutions (i.e., >30,000) known as *colloids* have been recommended in conjunction with or as replacements for crystalloid solutions. Examples of colloids used as plasma expanders include albumin, hetastarch, and dextran. Albumin is known as a *monodisperse colloid* because all its molecules are of the same molecular weight (~67,000), whereas hetastarch and dextran solutions are *polydisperse compounds* with molecules of varying molecular weights [*average* molecular weights of 450,000 (range 10,000 to 1 million) for hetastarch and 40,000 (range 10,000 to 90,000) or 70,000 to 75,000 (range 20,000 to 200,000) for dextran-40 or dextran-70 or -75, respectively]. This has important implications for the distribution of the products because lower-molecular-weight substances are retained in the intravascular space for a shorter period of time as a result of more rapid leakage across the vessel membrane. The theoretical usefulness of colloids is based on their increased molecular weight (average molecular weight in the case of hetastarch and dextran) that corresponds to increased intravascular retention time in the absence of increased capillary permeability compared with crystalloids. Even in patients with intact capillary permeability, the colloid molecules eventually will leak through the membrane. In the case of albumin, approximately 60% of the albumin molecules (and associated fluid) are contained in the interstitial space within 5 days of exogenous administration. In patients with altered permeability (e.g., acute respiratory distress syndrome), the leakage of albumin from the intravascular to the interstitial space may occur within hours, not days.

Albumin is available in 5% and 25% concentrations. Plasma protein fraction has oncotic actions similar to a 5% albumin solution, which is not surprising because albumin is the predominant protein in this product. When given in equipotent amounts, albumin is much more costly than crystalloid solutions. Additionally, the 5% and 25% albumin solutions typically are priced in such a way that there is no cost savings associated with dilution of the 25% product to make a 5% concentration. The 5% albumin solution is relatively *iso-oncotic*, which means that it does not pull fluid into the compartment in which it is contained. In contrast, 25% albumin is referred to as *hyperoncotic* albumin because it tends to pull fluid into the compartment containing the albumin molecules. In general, the 5% albumin solution is used for hypovolemic states. The 25% solution should not be used for acute circulatory insufficiency unless it is used in combination with other fluids or unless it is being used in patients with excess total body water but intravascular depletion as a means of pulling fluid into the intravascular space. An example of the latter condition would be cirrhosis with ascites in which total body water is substantially increased, but the patient is hypotensive as a consequence of lack of intravascular volume. This use of hyperoncotic albumin presumes that there is evidence of adverse effects associated with this excess water such as interstitial fluid accumulation in the lungs. Although appealing theoretically, improved outcomes related to the fluid shifting associated with hyperoncotic albumin have not been documented in randomized, controlled trials. Additionally, the effect is temporary because the albumin crosses the vascular membrane over time.

Hetastarch 6% has comparable plasma expansion to a 5% albumin solution but is usually less expensive, which accounts for much of its use. Most of the trials comparing albumin with hetastarch for volume expansion have found no significant differences in clinically important outcomes (e.g., mortality). Few trials have directly compared hetastarch with crystalloid solutions for intravascular expansion. Although hetastarch often is stated as being contraindicated in bleeding disorders, it has been most studied in patients with blood loss (e.g., trauma and perioperative patients). Hetastarch should be avoided in situations in which short-term impairments in hemostasis could have dire consequences, such as in patients undergoing cardiopulmonary bypass surgery and patients with intracranial bleeding. Hetastarch may aggravate bleeding through mechanisms specific to this colloid (e.g., decreased factor VIII activity). These mechanisms have not been well elucidated and often are difficult to distinguish from the dilutional effects on clotting factors caused by all plasma expanders. Hetastarch may cause elevations in serum amylase concentrations but does not cause pancreatitis.

Dextran-40, dextran-70, and dextran-75 are available for use as plasma expanders in the United States. The numbers refer to the average molecular weight of the solutions. In general, dextran solutions are not used as often as albumin or hetastarch solutions for plasma expansion possibly because of concerns related to aggravation of bleeding (i.e., anticoagulant actions related to inhibiting stasis of microcirculation) and anaphylaxis that is more likely to occur with the higher-molecular-weight solutions. However, both these concerns can be reduced if proper attention is paid to patient selection and, in the case of bleeding, published dosing guidelines with regard to the amounts of these products that should be infused. There are few comparative trials involving the dextran solutions, but the intravascular expansion within hours after infusion is approximately equal to the amount of dextran infused.

The crystalloid versus colloid debate was intensified when a meta-analysis by a well-respected group (Cochrane) found an overall increase in mortality associated with albumin using pooled results of randomized investigations.[22] The meta-analysis involved 30 randomized trials with 1419 patients (relative risk of death with albumin versus no administration or crystalloid administration 1.68, 95% confidence interval 1.26–2.23). For hypovolemia (caused by blood loss in the majority of studies), the risk of death associated with albumin administration was not quite statistically significant (relative risk 1.46, 95% confidence interval 0.97–2.22). However, the most comprehensive meta-analysis to date did not find increased mortality attributable to albumin when looking at overall mortality (relative risk of death 1.11, 95% confidence interval 0.95–1.28) or for any category of indications.[23] Furthermore, a landmark investigation involving almost 7000 critically ill patients (conducted after the previously mentioned meta-analyses) did not find statistically significant differences in 28-day mortality between patients resuscitated with either normal saline or 4% albumin.[24] This multicenter, randomized, double-blind investigation, referred to as the Saline versus Albumin Fluid Evaluation (SAFE) study, involved a heterogeneous group of ICU patients, so clinicians must be cautious when extrapolating the results to more specific patient populations. With this caution in mind, this trial provides strong evidence that crystalloid solutions should be considered first-line therapy in patients with hypovolemic shock.

SPECIAL POPULATIONS

Trauma/Perioperative Patients

The need for the immediate treatment of hemorrhagic circulatory insufficiency with plasma expanders (i.e., crystalloids or colloids) seems obvious, but no large, well-controlled trials in humans have been conducted that support this practice. To the contrary, there is evidence to suggest that fluid resuscitation beyond minimal levels (i.e., mean arterial pressure > 40–60 mm Hg) is harmful. One prospective study involving 598 adult patients with gunshot or stab wound injuries to the torso and systolic blood pressure measurements of 90 mm Hg or less found that delayed fluid resuscitation until operation was associated with increased survival and discharge from the hospital ($p =$ .04).[25] Although concerns were expressed about the comparability of the immediate and delayed resuscitation groups, particularly because true randomization did not take place, a follow-up randomized trial was conducted to verify the findings. There were no differences in survival (four deaths in each group) in the second trial regardless of whether systolic blood pressure was titrated to greater than 100 mm Hg or to 70 mm Hg.[26] Both studies were conducted in populated urban areas with approximately 2 hours from the time of injury to operation. Therefore, the results may not be applicable to rural areas with extended transport times. There is also a concern in applying the results of these investigations to patients with certain kinds of single-system injuries, particularly head trauma, where cerebral perfusion pressure is of primary importance. While the applicability of these studies to other populations and settings is debatable, the *presumption* of benefits from immediate plasma expansion in all preoperative patients with circulatory insufficiency caused by hemorrhage is no longer valid. Instead, the initial priority should be surgical control of the bleeding source.

Despite the studies suggesting that vigorous prehospital resuscitation is not helpful and possibly harmful, hypertonic solutions have several characteristics that make them attractive for acute resuscitation. The intravascular and interstitial expansion resulting from the administration of these solutions is much greater than the volume infused by emergency personnel.

CLINICAL CONTROVERSY

Some clinicians believe that hypertonic solutions should be used for the resuscitation of patients with head injuries who have concomitant circulatory insufficiency.

By causing redistribution (i.e., pulling fluid) from the intracellular space, hypertonic solutions cause rapid expansion of the intravascular compartment, which is essential for vital organ perfusion. In head-injured patients, this redistribution should decrease intracranial pressure because the vessels of the brain are more impermeable to sodium ions than vessels in other areas of the body.[27] Additionally, hypertonic saline solutions have beneficial immunomodulating actions when compared with more isotonic solutions in experiments with animals.[28,29]

Potential adverse effects associated with hypertonic fluid administration for circulatory insufficiency include cellular crenation and damage caused by the dramatic fluid shifts, as well as peripheral vein destruction from their high osmolality. Also, in the case of hypertonic sodium chloride solutions, there are the possibilities of neurologic damage from hypernatremia and hyperchloremic metabolic acidosis from hyperchloremia. In the limited number of studies conducted in humans to date, such adverse effects have been uncommon and apparently of little clinical importance.[30,31]

Unfortunately, beneficial outcome data attributable to administration of these hypertonic solutions also have been lacking.[32] Most of these studies were conducted in prehospital and emergency department settings using 250 mL 7.5% sodium chloride with or without 6% dextran-70. A meta-analysis of randomized, controlled trials found no statistical difference between the survival rates of patients receiving the hypertonic saline solutions and those receiving standard isotonic crystalloid solutions.[33] Part of the explanation for this finding may

be related to supplemental crystalloid fluids that were given routinely to patients in both the treatment and control groups, which probably would increase the number of patients needed to demonstrate a statistically significant difference in mortality. Until the concerns regarding efficacy and toxicity of these solutions have been resolved, normal saline could be considered as an alternative for head-injured patients when a hypertonic solution is desirable because it contains 154 mmol/L of both sodium and chloride. Given their relatively poor intravascular expansion and association with poor outcome in animal models of closed head injury, hypotonic solutions should be avoided in this population.[34]

In addition to crystalloid solutions, colloids have been used for plasma expansion in patients with hemorrhagic circulatory insufficiency. In the United States, albumin and starch (i.e., hetastarch) derivatives are used most commonly, although dextran solutions also are available commercially.

CLINICAL CONTROVERSY

Some clinicians believe that colloid solutions have advantages beyond crystalloid solutions that justify their use for patients with hypovolemic shock.

The theoretical advantage of these compounds is their prolonged intravascular retention time compared with crystalloid solutions. In contrast to isotonic crystalloid solutions that have substantial interstitial distribution within minutes of intravenous administration, colloids remain in the intravascular space for hours or days depending on factors such as capillary permeability.

The colloids, in particular albumin, are expensive solutions. Therefore, it is difficult to justify the additional cost of colloidal products unless the benefit-to-risk ratio is substantially greater than that associated with inexpensive crystalloid solutions. This does not appear to be the case based on randomized, controlled studies and meta-analyses comparing colloid and crystalloid solutions for acute circulatory insufficiency.[35] Because other colloids, such as hetastarch, almost always have been compared with albumin and not with crystalloid solutions in published clinical studies (with no clinically important differences being found), there is no reason to suspect that these other colloids have any unique advantages as volume expanders. Adverse effects associated with colloids appear to be uncommon and generally are extensions of their pharmacologic activity (Table 24–4), but this is also true of crystalloids. The benefit-to-risk ratio appears to be similar for colloids and crystalloids; thus, based on cost, crystalloids are preferred for initial treatment of circulatory insufficiency.

The preceding discussion has dealt primarily with acute circulatory insufficiency, but there are other considerations with regard to fluid replacement in elective surgical procedures. Preoperative fluid deficits may be associated with increased perioperative morbidity, some of which (e.g., drowsiness, dizziness) may be reduced by appropriate fluid administration prior to surgery.[36] However, care must be taken to avoid overhydration in the perioperative period because excess fluid will lead to weight gain and decreased pulmonary function.[37] There is some evidence to suggest that fluid restriction on the day of surgery may reduce postoperative morbidity. In one randomized, multicenter trial, use of a restricted intraoperative and postoperative intravenous fluid protocol led to significantly fewer cardiopulmonary (7% versus 24%; $p = .007$) and wound (16% versus 31%; $p = .04$) complications.[38]

Another consideration in the patient with injuries or surgery is the potential need for blood product administration (Table 24–5) to

TABLE 24–4. Adverse Effects of Plasma Expanders: Colloids

Albumin
  Primarily extensions of pharmacologic actions (e.g., fluid overload; dilutional coagulopathy; crystalloids are usually needed with 25% albumin in hypovolemic states to prevent intracellular volume depletion and renal failure)
  Amino acid profile and catabolism alterations (clinical significance?); potential protein overload if given with exogenous protein (e.g., parenteral nutrition)
  Anaphylactoid/anaphylaxis (life-threatening reactions rare; higher in patients with IgA deficiency)
  Infectous complications (all reported cases have been associated with improper handling by manufacturer or institution; no reported cases of HIV or hepatitis transmission)
  Interactions with medications and nutrients (clinical significance varies)
  Metal loading, particularly aluminum (long-term administration in patients with renal failure)
  Negative inotropic effect, reductions in ionized calcium concentrations?
  Pyrogenic reactions?
Hetastarch
  Primarily extensions of pharmacologic actions (e.g., fluid overload; dilutional coagulopathy)
  Bleeding (decreases factor VIII/C activity; not recommended in patients with severe bleeding conditions such as subarachnoid hemorrhage)
  Macroamylase formation may cause elevation in blood amylase that leads to inaccurate diagnosis of pancreatitis
Dextrans
  Primarily extensions of pharmacologic actions (e.g., fluid overload; dilutional coagulopathy)
  Anaphylaxis (increased incidence with increased molecular weight)
  Bleeding (sometimes used for anticoagulant activity so not recommended in patients with severe bleeding)

---

replace oxygen-carrying and clotting functions. Although a small group of trauma patients responds to the initial fluid bolus and remain stable, most patients respond initially and then deteriorate.[5] The latter patients, as well as patients undergoing blood loss associated with surgery, frequently need blood components such as packed red blood cells. In the case of the latter component, red blood cells contain hemoglobin that delivers oxygen to tissues. Neither crystalloids nor colloids perform this function.

Blood products are not risk-free. For example, there is the rare but important risk of virus transmission (e.g., HIV, hepatitis). The administration of blood products has its own risks. For example, citrate that is added to stored blood to prevent coagulation may bind to

TABLE 24–5. General Indications for Blood Products in Acute Circulatory Insufficiency Due to Hemorrhage*

Packed red blood cells
  Increase oxygen-carrying capacity of blood—usually indicated in patients with continued deterioration after volume replacement or obvious exsanguination; needs to be warmed, particularly when used in children
Fresh-frozen plasma
  Replacement of clotting factors—generally overused; indicated if ongoing hemorrhage in patients with PT/PTT > 1.5 times normal, severe hepatic disease, or other bleeding diathesis
Platelets
  Used for bleeding due to severe thrombocytopenia (i.e., platelet count < 10,000 mcL) or rapidly dropping platelet counts as would occur with massive bleeding
Other products
  Components such as cryoprecipitate and factor VIII are generally not indicated in acute hemorrhage, but rather are used after specific deficiencies are identified

* Although whole blood could be used for large-volume blood loss, most hospitals use component therapy, and use crystalloids or colloids for plasma expansion.
PT, prothrombin time; PTT, partial thromboplastin time.

calcium, resulting in hypocalcemia. In contrast, potassium and phosphate concentrations are often elevated in stored blood, particularly when hemolysis has occurred during storage. Additionally, administration of excessive blood products may be counterproductive. In the case of red blood cells, attempts to raise the hematocrit to high-normal or supranormal concentrations may decrease oxygen delivery by increasing blood viscosity.[3] Although there is no optimal hematocrit value for all patients, a minimum hematocrit concentration of 30% (equivalent to a hemoglobin concentration of 10%) traditionally has been used as the threshold for transfusion, particularly in patients at risk for ischemia, such as those with CAD. The use of a more liberal transfusion strategy has been called into question with the publication of a randomized, multicenter trial involving critically ill patients that found 30-day mortality to be similar whether patients were transfused at a hemoglobin concentration of 7 or 10 g/dL (18.7% versus 23.3%, respectively; $p = .11$).[39] The mortality during hospitalization was significantly lower in the restrictive group (22.2% versus 28.1%; $p = .05$). While the investigators were cautious about extrapolating the results of this investigation to patients with myocardial ischemia, the study does question the use of a liberal transfusion strategy for critically ill patients.

Other issues that must be considered with blood product administration include monitoring for transfusion-related reactions and attention to appropriate warming, particularly when large volumes are given to pediatric patients, because hypothermia is associated with increased fluid requirements and mortality.[40]

The periodic shortages, high costs, and adverse effect concerns related to blood products have prompted investigations of alternative "bloodless" strategies. In addition to the use of more restrictive transfusion thresholds, as mentioned previously, these strategies have included hemoglobin-based oxygen carriers and perfluorocarbon compounds to deliver oxygen to tissues.[41] Other strategies have aimed at reducing blood loss through the use of improved procedural and surgical techniques, as well as the administration of hemostatic medications.[42,43]

Patients with Thermal Injuries

There are a number of formulas for estimating fluid requirements in thermally injured patients, but there is little reason to choose one over another based on well-controlled studies. In general, the amount of loss corresponds to the size of the thermal injury.[3] Approximately 3 to 4 mL/kg of isotonic fluid (lactated Ringer's solution) for each percent burn can be used for calculating the expected fluid requirements for the first 24 hours after the burn. For example, a 60-kg person with 30% body surface area (BSA) burns is expected to require 5400 to 7200 mL of fluid over the initial 24 hours. Regardless of the calculated deficit, fluids should be administered until adequate tissue perfusion has been documented or adverse effects (e.g., pulmonary edema) occur. Crystalloids are preferred as initial therapy for burn victims because there is no substantial evidence that colloids mobilize edematous fluid, and there is a theoretical concern that extravascular fluid accumulation might be prolonged by the oncotic actions of albumin and other colloid products that have leaked through vessel walls.[44] Additionally, there is no evidence that colloids reduce mortality in patients with thermal injuries.[22] Some novel therapies for thermal resuscitation are currently under study. For example, in a prospective study involving patients with more than 30% BSA burns, antioxidant therapy with extremely high doses on intravenous vitamin C (66 mg/kg per hour for 24 hours) reduced resuscitation fluid requirements and wound edema.[45] The proposed mechanism is reduction in free radical–induced increases in capillary permeability.

CLINICAL CONTROVERSY

The appropriate use of invasive hemodynamic monitoring tools such as right-sided heart catheterization in patients with hypovolemic shock is controversial.

ONGOING MONITORING

Although the monitoring of patients in the emergency department is relatively straightforward, it becomes much more controversial in other settings such as the ICU. This is particularly true with regard to the value of right-sided heart catheterization (also known as pulmonary artery or Swan-Ganz catheterization). However, most clinicians would agree that certain forms of monitoring are important because patients in the postresuscitation phase of management are at risk for various complications secondary to ischemia. A more complete discussion of invasive and noninvasive hemodynamic monitoring is found in Chapter 23.

One form of monitoring that may take place in the emergency and operating rooms, as well as in the ICU, requires placement of a central venous pressure (CVP) line. Monitoring of CVP provides the clinician with an indirect and insensitive yet useful estimate of the relationship between increased right atrial pressure and cardiac output.[5]

A number of laboratory tests are indicated for the subacute monitoring of shock. These include a renal battery for assessing possible electrolyte alterations and kidney perfusion (e.g., blood urea nitrogen and creatinine). Among other things, a complete blood count will enable assessment of possible infection (white blood cell count), oxygen-carrying capacity of the blood (hemoglobin, hematocrit), and ongoing bleeding (hemoglobin, hematocrit, and platelet count). The prothrombin time (PT) and partial thromboplastin time (PTT) will give an indication of the ability of the blood to clot because, in the case of hemorrhagic shock, clotting factors are lost and diluted. An increasing lactate concentration (arterial, mixed venous, or central venous)[46] and base deficit are consistent with inadequate perfusion leading to anaerobic metabolism with accumulation of lactic acid. These tests often are considered the optimal end points of resuscitation in certain populations such as trauma patients.[47] Additionally, lactate clearance is a useful predictor of survival in children and adults.[48,49] Other tests may be indicated if organ dysfunction is likely. For example, when blood flow to the liver is interrupted because of sustained hypotension, a condition known as *shock liver* may occur. In this condition, the transaminases on a liver panel may be markedly elevated in the first couple of days after marked hypotension, although the concentrations should decrease over time.[3] Along with laboratory testing, a more extensive history can be obtained during the subacute monitoring period.

The value of pulmonary artery catheters has been debated hotly since their introduction. Such catheters are placed to obtain various oxygen-transport variables, some of which cannot be determined reliably from peripheral or other central vessels.[50] The debate was intensified when early studies suggested improved outcomes when cardiac output and other oxygen-transport variables were raised to supranormal levels, the monitoring of which required placement of a pulmonary artery catheter. Subsequent studies using similar monitoring parameters associated with pulmonary artery catheterization gave conflicting results.[51]

The controversy led to consensus conferences[52] and workshops,[53] the development of organizational guidelines,[54] and the publication of a meta-analysis (which found a statistically significant reduction in *morbidity* using pulmonary artery catheters to guide therapy).[55] Ultimately, a large randomized, controlled trial involving pulmonary artery catheters was conducted in high-risk surgical patients.[56] The trial involved 1994 patients. The mortality was almost identical for the catheter and control groups (7.8% versus 7.7%, 95% confidence interval 2.3 to 2.5). There were no episodes of pulmonary embolism in the catheter group and eight episodes in the control group ($p = .004$). This trial is important not only because of the implications for high-risk surgical patients but also because it allows future trials to be conducted in other patient populations without some of the ethical issues raised about such trials in the past.

Part of the concern regarding pulmonary artery catheterization relates to interpretation of its results by inexperienced practitioners. Studies in both Europe and the United States found that one of two physicians incorrectly interpreted a tracing from a pulmonary artery catheter.[57] This could explain some of the results of studies finding no benefits to pulmonary artery catheterization or, in some cases, worse outcomes in the pulmonary artery catheterization group by actions taken as a result of inaccurate measurements or misinterpretation of information obtained from the monitoring process.

Complications related to pulmonary artery catheter insertion, maintenance, and removal include damage to vessels and organs during insertion, arrhythmias, infections, and thromboembolic damage. To avoid the complications associated with pulmonary artery catheterization, other less invasive tools were developed to obtain similar information. For example, cardiac output determinations have been made by Doppler, bioimpedance, dye, and ionic dilution techniques, although such measurements would not provide other data that are obtained routinely with pulmonary artery catheters (e.g., left-sided heart-filling pressure).[58] Additionally, advances in pulmonary artery catheter technology that expand the information obtained from such monitoring (e.g., mixed venous oxyhemoglobin) are under investigation.[59] However, given the lack of well-defined outcome data associated with pulmonary artery catheterization, its use is best reserved for complicated cases of shock not responding to conventional fluid and medication therapies.

Commonly measured and calculated hemodynamic and oxygen-transport indices associated with invasive monitoring are primarily global indicators of tissue perfusion. There have been attempts to find regional and local indicators of hypoperfusion so that circulatory insufficiency could be treated before overt shock occurs. One focus of recent research has been monitoring modalities involving the gastrointestinal tract.

Although the literature is fairly consistent concerning low pHi values (gastric intramucosal pH) being predictive of death, pHi-guided therapy to decrease mortality has not been demonstrated.[60] Additionally, there are a number of technical considerations that remain to be resolved when using pHi or, more recently, capnometry (luminal Pco2 tonometry) for monitoring and therapy.[61] Despite these concerns, measures of regional tissue oxygenation continue to be investigated through a variety of novel monitoring techniques.[62]

In addition to regional monitoring of tissue perfusion, local methods of monitoring are also being studied. For example, subcutaneous measurement of tissue oxygen pressure shows promise in preliminary investigations. It is unlikely that regional and local measurements will replace more global indicators of perfusion but rather that the methods will complement each other.

ONGOING MANAGEMENT

Proper attention to plasma expansion must be continued into the intraoperative and postoperative periods. A number of neurohormonal changes take place that affect urine output, and patients may have substantial third-spacing of fluid depending on the operation and the preexisting condition of the patient. Furthermore, postoperative patients are prone to hyponatremia from renal generation of electrolyte-free water and from antidiuretic hormone release.[63] As in acute resuscitation, the administration of hypotonic solutions in the perioperative period does not prevent the decrease in extracellular volume that often occurs. Therefore, although excess fluid administration is to be avoided in the perioperative setting, isotonic crystalloid solutions should be used when fluids are indicated to prevent intravascular depletion and circulatory insufficiency.

Of the randomized studies comparing albumin with crystalloid solutions in the perioperative period, the majority found no statistically significant differences between groups.[64] The significant differences that have been found have involved isolated hemodynamic or respiratory variables with no obvious clinical correlates (e.g., duration of mechanical ventilation). Therefore, albumin (and other colloids) cannot be recommended for the prevention or initial treatment of circulatory insufficiency, although their use may be appropriate in

patients who are not responding to crystalloids and are developing problems such as interstitial fluid accumulation. Practice guidelines published by a consortium of academic medical centers reflect this recommendation, but colloids continue to be used widely.[65]

In general, medications are not indicated in the initial therapy of hypovolemic shock. With hypovolemia, the body's natural response is to increase cardiac output and to constrict blood vessels to maintain blood pressure. There is no reason why most patients should need inotropic or vasoactive agents, assuming that fluid therapy is adequate. For that matter, there is no evidence that these medications improve outcome in patients with hypovolemic shock. However, once the cause of acute circulatory insufficiency has been stopped or treated and fluids have been optimized, some patients continue to have signs and symptoms of inadequate tissue perfusion. This may be caused by reperfusion injury. Although the search for a cryptogenic source (e.g., intraabdominal bleeding in a trauma patient) should continue, the clinician may need to administer medications to improve perfusion.

Pressor agents such as norepinephrine and high-dose dopamine are to be avoided, if possible, because they may increase blood pressure at the expense of peripheral tissue ischemia. Some sources use stronger language and state that vasopressors are contraindicated in certain forms of shock (e.g., hemorrhagic).[5] This does not help the clinician who is treating a patient with unstable blood pressure despite massive fluid replacement and increasing interstitial fluid accumulation. In such situations, inotropic agents such as dobutamine are preferred if blood pressure is adequate (e.g., systolic blood pressure ≥ 90 mm Hg) because they should not aggravate the existing vasoconstriction. The inotropic agents are justified by presumed inadequate cardiac output for the specific situation, although the measured values may be in the normal range.[3]

When pressure cannot be maintained with inotropic agents, or when inotropic agents with vasodilatory properties cannot be used because of inadequate blood pressure concerns, pressors may be required as a last resort. In general, the need for pressors is predictive of the development of MODS and increased length of hospital stay.[66] Although the response to pressor agents may be variable in hypovolemic shock, there does not appear to be resistance as a consequence of altered receptor response, as is sometimes seen in patients with septic shock.[3] Potent vasoconstrictors such as norepinephrine and phenylephrine should be given through central veins because of the possibility of extravasation and necrosis with peripheral administration.

A number of interesting treatments for shock are under investigation, including autotransfusion for removing harmful cytokines from the body. Various alternatives to conventional blood components are also being studied, such as stroma-free hemoglobin and perfluorocarbon compounds, as virus-free alternatives to red blood cell transfusion. Hopefully, these will be useful adjuncts to adequate volume replacement, which is the primary therapeutic intervention in managing acute circulatory insufficiency owing to volume depletion.

PHARMACOECONOMIC CONSIDERATIONS

The primary therapy for hypovolemic shock is fluid replacement. The institutional cost of 1 L of most crystalloid solutions is less than $1. Assuming that such fluids are used, it is the associated costs of personnel and equipment that become the primary economic considerations in the resuscitation of patients with hypovolemic shock. However,

as mentioned, many clinicians recommend that colloid plasma expanders (e.g., albumin, hetastarch, or dextrans) be used to replace some or all of the standard crystalloid solutions. Although the costs of these solutions vary depending on contractual arrangements as might occur with purchasing groups, in general, albumin solutions are more expensive than hetastarch and dextran products. All these solutions are markedly more costly than crystalloid solutions; in some cases, there are 50- to 100-fold differences, even when used in equipotent amounts.

The only recent trial that investigated albumin use on a large-scale basis was an observational study involving 15 academic medical centers in the United States. Based on previously published guidelines, 62% of albumin use was defined as inappropriate at a cost of $124,939.[67] Presuming equal efficacy and toxicity (as available studies indicate) between crystalloid and colloid solutions, cost-minimization analysis clearly indicates the economic advantages of the crystalloids.

Because medications are not simply alternatives to crystalloids but rather are used when crystalloid therapy has been optimized, there is little reason to compare medication and fluid therapies from an economic perspective. Furthermore, there are no economic comparisons

of the various inotropic and vasopressor medications used in the treatment of hypovolemic shock.

EVALUATION OF THERAPEUTIC OUTCOMES

Figure 24–4 is an algorithm that summarizes many of the treatment principles discussed in this chapter. The algorithm is an example of one approach to the adult patient presenting with hypovolemic shock. It presumes that initial rehydration attempts (i.e., outpatient or prehospital) were unsuccessful in restoring circulation. Obviously, modifications may be needed for patient-specific forms of hypovolemic shock. Other limitations of the algorithm should be recognized, particularly the decisions to add or to substitute colloid or

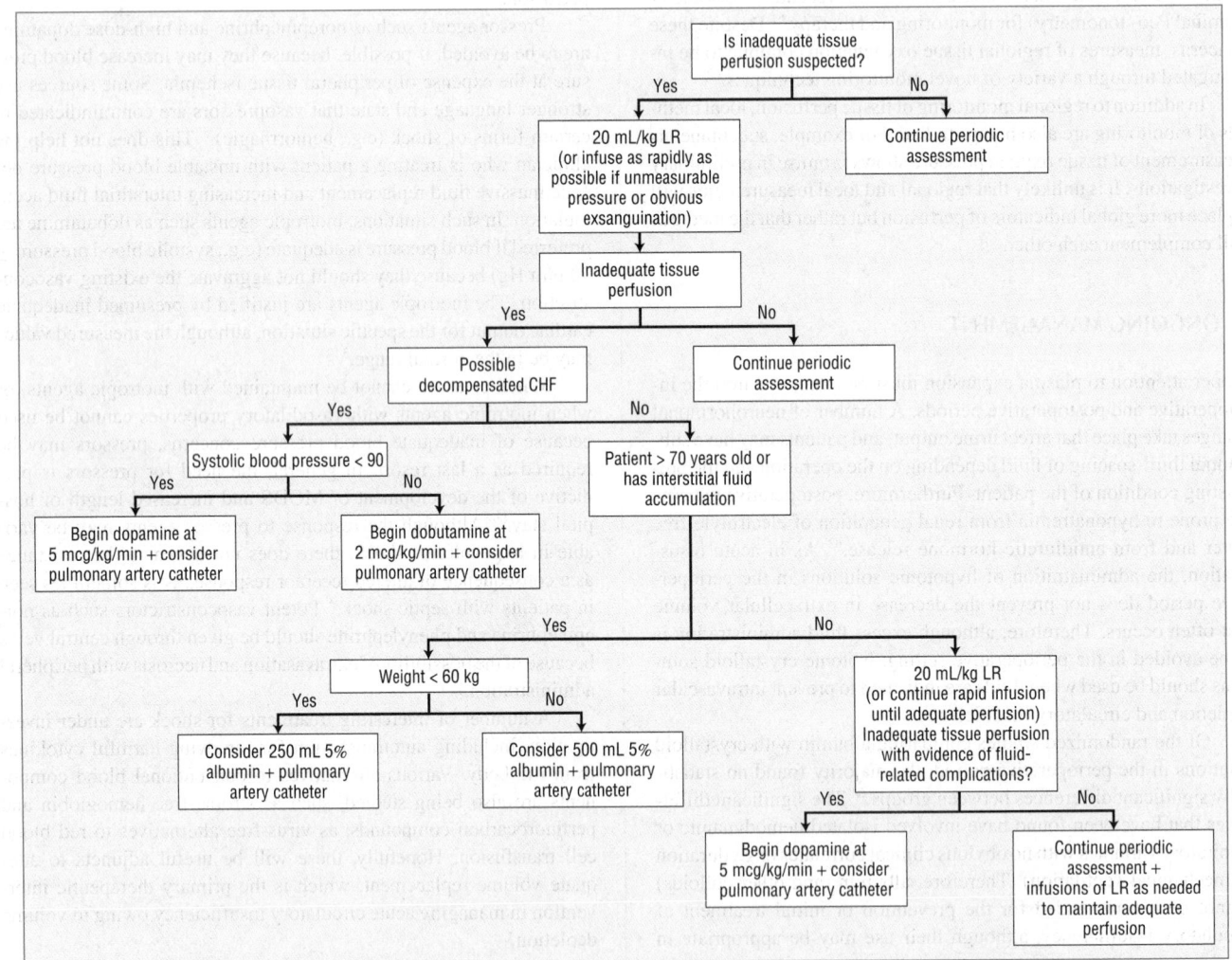

FIGURE 24–4. Hypovolemia protocol for adults. This protocol is not intended to replace or delay therapies such as surgical intervention or blood products for restoring oxygen-carrying capacity or hemostasis. If available, some measurements may be used in addition to those listed in the algorithm, such as mean arterial pressure or pulmonary artery catheter recordings. The latter may be used to assist in medication choices (e.g., agents with primary pressor effects may be desirable in patients with normal cardiac outputs, whereas dopamine or dobutamine may be indicated in patients with suboptimal cardiac outputs). Lower maximal doses of the medications in this algorithm should be considered when pulmonary artery catheterization is not available. CHF = congestive heart failure; LR = lactated Ringer's solution. Colloids that may be substituted for albumin are hetastarch 6% and dextran-40. See text for an in-depth discussion of these and other issues involved in this protocol.

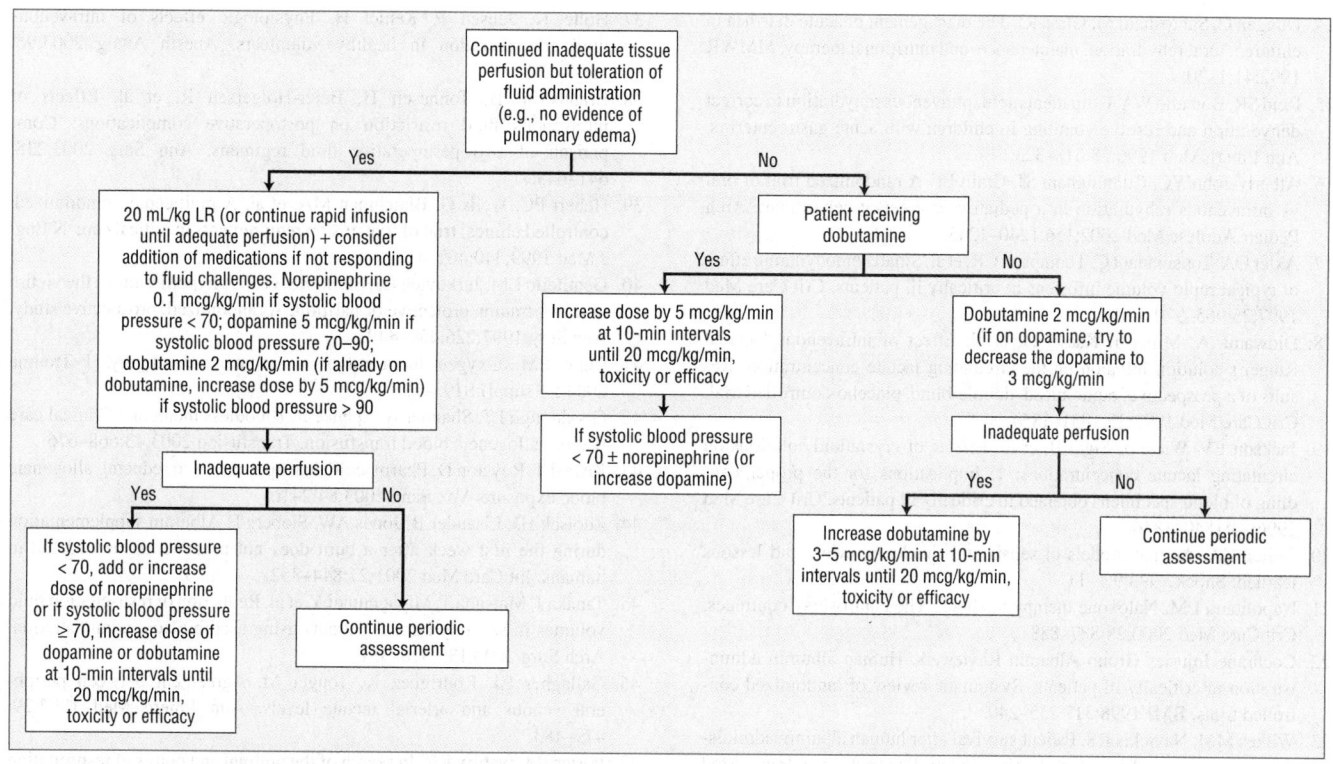

FIGURE 24–5. Ongoing management of inadequate tissue perfusion. CHF = congestive heart failure; LR = lactated Ringer's solution.

medication therapies when crystalloid solutions are not yielding desired results and when to perform pulmonary artery catheterization for more invasive monitoring. Medications become more important for the ongoing management of hypovolemic shock, particularly when the patient is unresponsive to fluids (Fig. 24–5). Additionally, it is hoped that the options for more complicated cases of hypovolemic shock do not detract from the primary effective resuscitative measure for most patients—fluid.

ABBREVIATIONS

SIRS: systemic inflammatory response syndrome
MODS: multiple-organ dysfunction syndrome
CAD: coronary artery disease
BSA: body surface area
CVP: central venous pressure
PT: prothrombin time
PTT: partial thromboplastin time
pHi: gastric intramucosal pH

Review Questions and other resources can be found at *www.pharmacotherapyonline.com.*

REFERENCES

1. Jimenez EJ. Shock. In: Civetta JM, Taylor RW, Kirby RR, eds. Critical Care, 3d ed. Philadelphia, Lippincott-Raven, 1997:359–387.
2. Shoemaker WC. Temporal physiologic patterns of shock and circulatory dysfunction based on early descriptions by invasive and noninvasive monitoring. New Horizons 1996;4:300–318.
3. Ramsay G, Boom S. Pathophysiology and management of shock. In: Cuschieri A, Giles GR, Moossa AR, eds. Essential Surgical Practice, 3d ed. Oxford, England, Butterworth-Heinemann, 1995:72–89.
4. Marzi I. Hemorrhagic shock: Update in pathophysiology and therapy. Acta Anaesthesiol Scand 1997;111(suppl):42–44.
5. American College of Surgeons Committee on Trauma. Shock. In: Advanced Trauma Life Support for Doctors: Instructor Course Manual, 6th ed. Chicago, American College of Surgeons, 1997:97–117.
6. Richardson JD. What's new in trauma and burns? J Am Coll Surg 1997;184:210–216.
7. Plank LD, Hill GL. Sequential metabolic changes following induction of systemic inflammatory response in patients with severe sepsis or major blunt trauma. World J Surg 2000;24:630–638.
8. McGee S, Abernethy WB, Simel DL. Is this patient hypovolemic? JAMA 1999;281:1022–1029.
9. Weinberg AD, Minaker KL, and the Council on Scientific Affairs, American Medical Association. Dehydration: Evaluation and management in older patients. JAMA 1995;274:1552–1556.
10. Porter SC, Fleisher GR, Kohane IS, Mandl KD. The value of parental report for diagnosis and management of dehydration in the emergency department. Ann Emerg Med 2003;41:196–205.
11. Anonymous. Prevention and treatment of heat injury. Med Lett 2003;45:58–60.
12. Tarrosa V, Stoner G, George L, Fleming CR. Alterations needed to optimize sodium content in commercially available oral rehydration solutions. Presented at the 21st Clinical Congress of Nutrition, Practice Poster, American Society of Parenteral and Enteral Nutrition, San Francisco, January 1997.
13. Brouns F, Senden J, Beckers EJ, Saris WHM. Osmolarity does not affect the gastric emptying rate of oral rehydration solutions. J Parenter Enter Nutr 1995;19:403–406.

14. Duggan C, Santosham M, Glass RI. The management of acute diarrhea in children: Oral rehydration, maintenance, and nutritional therapy. MMWR 1992;41:1–20.

15. Reid SR, Bonadio WA. Outpatient rapid intravenous rehydration to correct dehydration and resolve vomiting in children with acute gastroenteritis. Ann Emerg Med 1996;28:318–323.

16. Atherly-John YC, Cunningham SJ, Crain EF. A randomized trial of oral vs intravenous rehydration in a pediatric emergency department. Arch Pediatr Adolesc Med 2002;156:1240–1243.

17. Axler OA, Tousiganant C, Thompson CR, et al. Small hemodynamic effect of typical rapid volume infusions in critically ill patients. Crit Care Med 1997;25:965–970.

18. Didwania A, Miller J, Kassel D, et al. Effect of intravenous lactated Ringer's solution infusion on the circulating lactate concentration: Results of a prospective, randomized, double-blind, placebo-controlled trial. Crit Care Med 1997;25:1851–1854.

19. Jackson EV, Wiese J, Sigal B, et al. Effects of crystalloid solutions on circulating lactate concentrations: 1. Implications for the proper handling of blood specimens obtained in critically ill patients. Crit Care Med 1996;24:1840–1846.

20. Deitch EA. Animal models of sepsis and shock: A review and lessons learned. Shock 1998;9:1–11.

21. Napolitano LM. Naloxone therapy in shock: The controversy continues. Crit Care Med 2000;28:887–888.

22. Cochrane Injuries Group Albumin Reviewers. Human albumin administration in critically ill patients: Systematic review of randomized controlled trials. BMJ 1998;317:235–240.

23. Wilkes MM, Navickis RS. Patient survival after human albumin administration: A meta-analysis of randomized, controlled trials. Ann Intern Med 2001;135:149–164.

24. The SAFE Study Investigators. A comparison of albumin and saline for fluid resuscitation in the intensive care unit. N Engl J Med 2004;350:2247–2256.

25. Bickell WH, Wall MJ, Pepe PE, et al. Immediate versus delayed fluid resuscitation for hypotensive patients with penetrating torso injuries. N Engl J Med 1994;331:1105–1109.

26. Dutton RP, Mackenzie CF, Scalea TM. Hypotensive resuscitation during active hemorrhage: Impact on in-hospital mortality. J Trauma 2002;52:1141–1146.

27. Prough DS, Zornow MH. Solutions in search of problems. Crit Care Med 1996;24:1104–1105.

28. Kramer GC. Hypertonic resuscitation: Physiologic mechanisms and recommendations for trauma care. J Trauma 2003;54(suppl):S89–99.

29. Rhee P, Koustova E, Alam HB. Searching for the optimal resuscitation method: Recommendations for the initial fluid resuscitation of combat casualties. J Trauma 2003;54(suppl):S52–62.

30. Vassar MJ, Fischer RP, O'Brien PE, et al. A multicenter trial for resuscitation of injured patients with 7.5% sodium chloride: The effect of added dextran 70. Arch Surg 1993;128:1003–1013.

31. Suarez JI, Qureshi AI, Bhardwa A, et al. Treatment of refractory intracranial hypertension with 23.4% saline. Crit Care Med 1998;26:1118–1122.

32. Valadka AB, Robertson CS. Should we be using hypertonic saline to treat intracranial hypertension? Crit Care Med 2000;28:1245–1246.

33. Wade CE, Kramer GC, Grady JJ, et al. Efficacy of hypertonic 7.5% saline and 6% dextran-70 in treating trauma: A meta-analysis of controlled studies. Surgery 1997;122:609–616.

34. Gurevich B, Talmore D, Artru AA, et al. Brain edema, hemorrhagic necrosis volume, and neurological status with rapid infusion of 0.45% saline or 5% dextrose in 0.9% saline after closed head trauma in rats. Anesth Analg 1997;84:554–559.

35. Rizoli SB. Crystalloids and colloids in trauma resuscitation: A brief overview of the current debate. J Trauma 2003;54(suppl):S82–88.

36. Holte K, Kehlet H. Compensatory fluid administration for preoperative dehydration: Does it improve outcome? Acta Anaesthesiol Scand 2002;46:1089–1093.

37. Holte K, Jensen P, Kehlet H. Physiologic effects of intravenous fluid administration in healthy volunteers. Anesth Analg 2003;96:1504–1509.

38. Brandstrup B, Tonnesen H, Beier-Holgersen R, et al. Effects of intravenous fluid restriction on postoperative complications: Comparison of two perioperative fluid regimens. Ann Surg 2003;238:641–648.

39. Hebert PC, Wells G, Blajchman MA, et al. A multicenter, randomized, controlled clinical trial of transfusion requirements in critical care. N Engl J Med 1999;340:409–417.

40. Gentileilo LM, Jurkovich GJ, Stark MS, et al. Is hypothermia in the victim of major trauma protective or harmful? A randomized, prospective study. Ann Surg 1997;226:439–449.

41. Cohn SM. Oxygen therapeutics in trauma and surgery. J Trauma 2003;54(suppl):S193–198.

42. Goodnough LT, Shander A, Spence R. Bloodless medicine: Clinical care without allogeneic blood transfusion. Transfusion 2003;43:668–676.

43. Kovesi T, Royston D. Pharmacological approaches to reducing allogeneic blood exposure. Vox Sang 2003;84:2–10.

44. Zdolsek HJ, Lisander B, Jones AW, Sjoberg F. Albumin supplementation during the first week after a burn does not mobilise tissue oedema in humans. Int Care Med 2001;27:844–852.

45. Tanaka J, Matsuda T, Miyagantani Y, et al. Reduction of resuscitation fluid volumes in severely burned patients using ascorbic acid administration. Arch Surg 2000;135:326–331.

46. Gallagher EJ, Rodriguez K, Touger M. Agreement between peripheral venous and arterial lactate levels. Ann Emerg Med 1997;29:479–483.

47. Porter JM, Ivatury RR. In search of the optimal end points of resuscitation in trauma patients: A review. J Trauma Inj Infect Crit Care 1998;44:908–914.

48. Husain FA, Martin MJ, Mullenix PS, et al. Serum lactate and base deficit as predictors of mortality and morbidity. Am J Surg 2003;185:485–491.

49. Hatherill M, Waggie Z, Purves L, et al. Mortality and the nature of metabolic acidosis in children with shock. Int Care Med 2003;29:286–291.

50. Edwards JD, Mayall RM. Importance of the sampling site for measurement of mixed venous oxygen saturation in shock. Crit Care Med 1998;26:1356–1360.

51. Yu M. Oxygen transport optimization. New Horizons 1999;7:46–53.

52. Taylor RW, Ahrens T, Beilin Y, et al. Pulmonary artery consensus conference: Consensus statement. Crit Care Med 1997;25:190–200.

53. Bernard GR, Sopko G, Cerra F, et al. Pulmonary artery catheterization and clinical outcomes. JAMA 2000;283:2568–2572.

54. American Society of Anesthesiologists Task Force on Pulmonary Artery Catheterization. Practice guidelines for pulmonary artery catheterization. Anesthesiology 2003;99:988–1014.

55. Ivanov R, Allen J, Calvin JE. The incidence of major morbidity in critically ill patients managed with pulmonary artery catheters: A meta-analysis. Crit Care Med 2000;28:615–619.

56. Sandham JD, Hull RD, Brant RF, et al. A randomized, controlled trial of the use of pulmonary-artery catheters in high-risk surgical patients. N Engl J Med 2003;348:5–14.

57. Ginosar Y, Thijs LG, Sprung CL. Raising the standard of hemodynamic monitoring: Targeting the practice or the practitioner? Crit Care Med 1997;25:209–211.

58. Peruzzi WT. Hemodynamic monitoring: Does the end justify the means? Crit Care Med 1997;25:1767–1768.

59. Burchell SA, Yu M, Takiguchi SA, Ohta RM. Evaluation of a continuous cardiac output and mixed venous oxygen saturation catheter in critically ill surgery patients. Crit Care Med 1997;2:388–391.

60. Gomersall CD, Joynt GM, Freebairn RC, et al. Resuscitation of critically ill patients based on the results of gastric tonometry: A prospective, randomized, controlled trial. Crit Care Med 2000;28:607–614.

61. Groeneveld ABJ, Kolkman JJ. Factors affecting gastrointestinal luminal Pco_2 tonometry. Int Care Med 1999;25:249–251.

62. Siegemund M, van Bommel J, Ince C. Assessment of regional tissue oxygenation. Int Care Med 1999;25:1044–1060.

63. Steele A, Gowrishankar M, Abrahamson S, et al. Postoperative hyponatremia despite near-isotonic saline infusion: A phenomenon of desalination. Ann Intern Med 1997;126:20–25.

64. Erstad BL. Concerns with defining appropriate uses of albumin by meta-analysis. Am J Health Syst Pharm 1999;56:1451–1454.

65. Fox DL, Vermeulen LC. UHC Technology Assessment: Albumin, Nonprotein Colloid, and Crystalloid Solutions. University Health System Consortium, Oak Brook, IL, May 2000.

66. Goncalves JA, Hydo LJ, Barie PS. Factors influencing outcome of prolonged norepinephrine therapy for shock in critical surgical illness. Shock 1998;10:231–236.

67. Yim JM, Vermeulen LC, Erstad BL, et al. Albumin and nonprotein colloid solution use in US academic health centers. Arch Intern Med 1995;155:2450–2455.

25

INTRODUCTION TO PULMONARY FUNCTION TESTING

Jay I. Peters and Stephanie M. Levine

Learning Objectives and other resources can be found at *www.pharmacotherapyonline.com.*

KEY CONCEPTS

1️⃣ Normal ventilation- perfusion ratio. The function of the lung is to maintain Po_2 and Pco_2 within the normal range. This is accomplished by matching 1 mL mixed venous blood with 1 mL fresh air ($\dot{V}/\dot{Q} = 1$). Normally, there is less ventilation ($\dot{V}$) than perfusion ($\dot{Q}$), and the $\dot{V}/\dot{Q}$ ratio is 0.8.

2️⃣ The air in the lung is divided into four compartments: tidal volume—the air exhaled during quiet breathing; inspiratory reserve volume—the maximal air inhaled above tidal volume; expiratory reserve volume—the maximum air exhaled below tidal volume; and residual volume—the air remaining in the lung after maximal exhalation. The sum of all four components is called the total lung capacity.

3️⃣ Obstructive lung disease is defined as an inability to get air out of the lung and is identified on spirometry when the FEV_1/FVC (amount of air forcefully exhaled in 1 second/ total amount of air that can be exhaled during a forced exhalation) is less than 70% to 75%.

4️⃣ Reversible airway obstruction is common in asthma and chronic obstructive pulmonary disease (COPD). An increase in FEV_1 after an inhaled β-agonist of 12% and greater than 0.2 L suggests an acute bronchodilator response.

5️⃣ Restrictive lung disease is defined as an inability to get air into the lung. It is best defined as a reduction in total lung capacity (TLC) but is suspected when the forced vital capacity (FVC) is low and the FEV_1/FVC is normal.

6️⃣ Restrictive lung disease can be produced by a number of defects: increased elastic recoil (interstitial lung disease), respiratory muscle weakness (myasthenia gravis), mechanical restrictions (pleural effusion), and poor effort.

The primary function of the respiratory system is to maintain normality of arterial blood gases, that is, the PaO_2 and $PaCO_2$ (the arterial pressure of oxygen and carbon dioxide). To accomplish this task, several processes must be accomplished, including alveolar ventilation, pulmonary perfusion, ventilation-perfusion matching, and gas transfer across the alveolar-capillary membrane. Alveolar ventilation is achieved by the cyclic process of air movement in and out of the lung. During inspiration, the inspiratory muscle contracts and generates negative pressure in the pleural space. This pressure gradient between the mouth and the alveoli draws fresh air (tidal volume) into the lung. Approximately one-third of the inspired gas stays in the conducting airways (dead space), whereas two-thirds reaches the alveoli.

1️⃣ The human lung contains a series of branching, progressively tapering airways that originate at the glottis and terminate in a matrix of thin-walled alveoli. Coursing through this matrix of alveoli is a rich network of capillaries that originates from the pulmonary arterioles and terminates in the pulmonary venules. The adequacy of respiration in each gas exchange unit depends on the opposition of a thin film of mixed venous blood with just the right amount of fresh alveolar gas. During "ideal" gas exchange, there is uniform blood flow and uniform ventilation; accordingly, there is no alveolar-arterial PO_2 difference [$P(A-a) O_2$ gradient, sometimes called the A–a gradient]. Gas exchange is not perfect, however, even in the normal lung. Normally, there is less alveolar ventilation than pulmonary blood flow, and the overall ventilation-perfusion ratio is 0.8 (not 1.0).

Normal expiration is a passive process, and when the inspiratory muscles end their contraction, the elastic recoil of the lung pulls the lung back to its original size and shape. This process makes the alveolar pressure positive relative to the pressure at the mouth, and air flows out of the lung. During inspiration, the respiratory muscles must overcome the elastic properties of the lung (elastic recoil) and the resistance to airflow by the airways. During expiration, the flow of air is determined primarily by the elastic recoil and airway resistance.

Different pulmonary function tests (PFTs) are used to evaluate the physiologic process of the respiratory system. Physiologic abnormalities that can be measured by pulmonary function testing include obstruction to airflow, restriction of lung size, and decrease in the transfer of gas across the alveolar-capillary membrane. Abnormal values on PFTs are those outside the range of values obtained from a group of normal individuals matched according to age, height, sex, and race. A PFT is labeled abnormal when the results fall outside the range in which 95% of people the same age, height, and sex would be found (95% confidence interval). This definition is arbitrary and may misclassify a small percentage of normal individuals as having lung dysfunction, as well as missing some patients with mild pulmonary disease. Therefore, clinical correlation and serial pulmonary function testing may be necessary for optimal interpretation of PFTs.

Potential uses of pulmonary function testing include the evaluation of patients with known or suspected lung disease; the evaluation of symptoms such as chronic cough, dyspnea, or chest tightness; monitoring the effects of exposure to dust, chemicals, or pulmonary toxic drugs; risk stratification prior to surgery; monitoring of the effectiveness of therapeutic interventions; and objective assessment of impairment or disability.[1]

DEFINITIONS OF LUNG VOLUMES AND EXPIRATORY FLOWS

The air within the lung at the end of a forced inspiration can be divided into four compartments or lung volumes (Fig. 25–1). The volume of air exhaled during normal quiet breathing is termed *tidal volume* (V_T). The maximal volume of air inhaled above tidal volume is called the *inspiratory reserve volume* (IRV), and the maximal air exhaled below tidal volume is called the *expiratory reserve volume* (ERV). The *residual volume* (RV) is the amount of air remaining in the lungs after a maximal exhalation.

The combinations or sums of two or more lung volumes are termed *capacities* (see Fig. 25–1). *Vital capacity* (VC) is the maximal amount of air that can be exhaled after a maximal inspiration. It is equal to the sum of the IRV, V_T, and ERV. When measured on a forced expiration, it is called the *forced vital capacity* (FVC). When measured over an exhalation of at least 30 seconds, it is called the *slow vital capacity* (SVC, VC). The VC is approximately 75% of the *total lung capacity* (TLC), and when the SVC is within the normal range, a significant restrictive disorder is unlikely. Normally, the values for SVC and FVC are very similar unless airway obstruction is present.

The TLC is the volume of air in the lung after the maximal inspiration and is the sum of the four primary lung volumes (IRV, V_T, ERV, and RV). Its measurement is difficult because the amount of air remaining in the chest after maximal exhalation (RV) must be measured by indirect methods. The definition of restrictive lung disease is based on a reduction in TLC (i.e., an inability to get air into the lung or restriction to air movement on inhalation).

The *functional residual capacity* (FRC) is the volume of air remaining in the lungs at the end of a quiet expiration. FRC is the normal resting position of the lung and occurs when there is no contraction of either inspiratory or expiratory muscles and is normally 40% of TLC. *Inspiratory capacity* (IC) is the maximal volume of air that can be inhaled from the end of a quiet expiration and represents the sum of V_T and IRV.

The FVC, which represents the total amount of air than can be exhaled, can be expressed as a series of timed volumes. The *forced expiratory volume in 1 second* (FEV_1) is the volume of air exhaled during the first second of the FVC maneuver. Although the FEV_1 is a volume, it conveys information on obstruction because it is measured over a known time interval. The FEV_1 depends on the volume of air within the lung and the effort during exhalation; therefore, it can be diminished by a decrease in TLC or by a lack of effort. A more sensitive way to measure obstruction is to express the FEV_1 as a ratio of FVC. This ratio is independent of the patient's size or the TLC; therefore, the FEV_1/FVC is a specific measure of airway obstruction with or without restriction. Normally, this ratio is 75% or greater, and any value below 70% to 75% suggests obstruction.

Because *flow* is defined as the change in volume with time, forced expiratory flow may be determined graphically by dividing the volume change by the time change. The *forced expiratory flow* (FEF) *during 25% to 75% of FVC* ($FEF_{25\%-75\%}$) represents the mean flow during the middle half of the FVC. The $FEF_{25\%-75\%}$, formerly called the *maximal midexpiratory flow* (MMEF), is reported frequently to assess small airways. The 95% confidence limit is so wide that the $FEF_{25\%-75\%}$ has limited utility in the early diagnosis of small airways disease in an individual subject. The *peak expiratory flow* (PEF), also called *maximum forced expiratory flow* (FEF_{max}), is the maximum flow obtained during the FVC. This measurement is used often in the outpatient management of asthma because it can be measured with inexpensive peak flow meters.

SPIROMETRY/FLOW-VOLUME LOOP

Spirometry is the most widely available and useful PFT. It takes only 15 to 20 minutes, carries no risks, and provides information about obstructive and restrictive disease. Spirometry allows for the measurement of all lung volumes and capacities except RV, FRC, and TLC and allows assessment of FEV_1 and $FEF_{25\%-75\%}$. Spirometry measurements can be reported in two different formats—standard spirometry (Fig. 25–2) and the flow-volume loop (Fig. 25–3). In standard spirometry, the volumes are recorded on the vertical (y) axis and the time on the horizontal (x) axis. In flow-volume loops, volume is plotted on the horizontal (x) axis, and flow (derived from volume/time) is plotted on the vertical (y) axis. The shape of the flow-volume loop can be helpful in differentiating obstructive and restrictive defects and in the diagnosis of upper airway obstruction (Fig. 25–4). This curve gives a visual representation of obstruction because the expiratory descent becomes more concave with worsening obstruction.

LUNG VOLUMES

Spirometry measures three of the four basic lung volumes but cannot measure RV (residual volume). RV must be measured to determine the TLC. TLC should be measured anytime there is a reduced VC. In

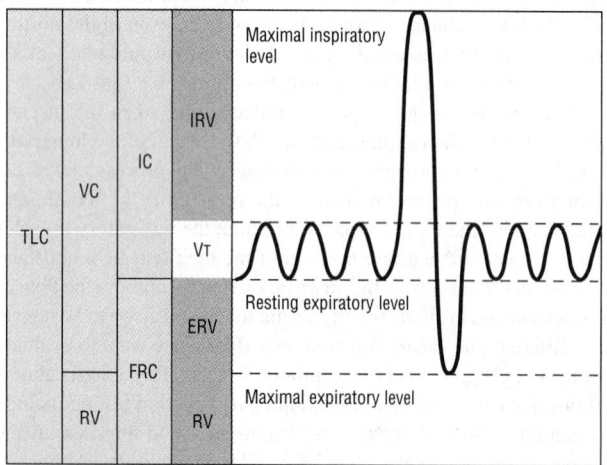

FIGURE 25–1. Lung volumes and capacities. ERV = expiratory reserve volume; FRC = functional residual capacity; IC = inspiratory capacity; IRV = inspiratory reserve volume; RV = residual volume; TLC = total lung capacity; VC = vital capacity; V_T = tidal volume.

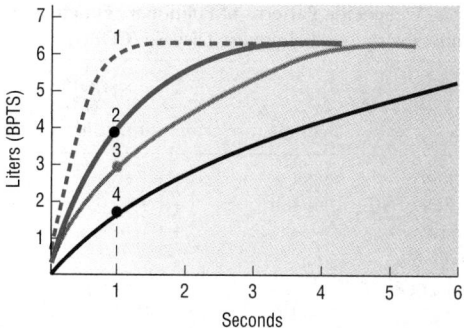

FIGURE 25–2. Standard spirometry. Curve 1 is for a normal subject with a normal FEV_1; curve 2 is the FEV_1 in a patient with mild airways obstruction; curve 3 is for a patient with moderate airways obstruction; curve 4 is a patient with severe airways obstruction; BPTS = body temperature saturated with water vapor.

the setting of chronic obstructive pulmonary disease (COPD) with a low VC, measurement of TLC can help to determine whether there is a superimposed restrictive disorder. There are four methods to measure TLC: helium dilution, nitrogen washout, body plethysmography, and chest x-ray measurement (planimetry). The first two methods are called *dilution techniques* and only measure lung volumes in communication with the upper airway. In patients with airway obstruction who have trapped air, dilution techniques will underestimate the actual volume of the lungs. Planimetry measures the circumference of the lungs on the posteroanterior view and lateral views of a chest x-ray and estimates the total lung volume.

Body plethysmography, or body box, is the most accurate technique for lung volume determinations. It measures all the air in the lungs, including trapped air. The principle of the measurement of the body box is Boyle's gas law ($P_1V_1 = P_2V_2$): A volume of gas in a closed system varies inversely with the pressure applied to it. The changes in alveolar pressure are measured at the mouth, as well as pressure changes in the body box. The volume of the body box is known. Lung volumes can be determined measuring the changes in pressures caused by panting against a closed shutter.[2] The measurement of lung volumes provides useful information about elastic recoil of the lungs. If elastic recoil is increased (as in interstitial lung disease),

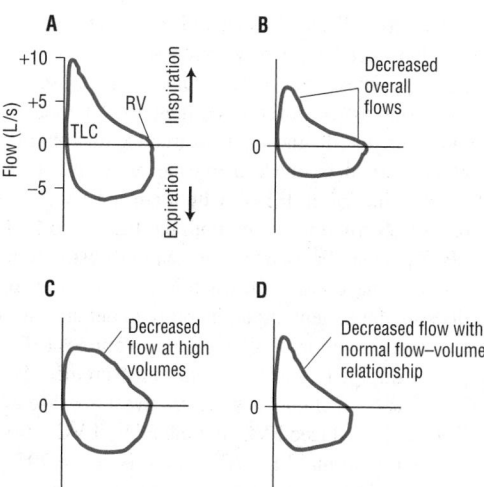

FIGURE 25–4. *A.* Flow-volume loop depicting mild obstruction characterized by decrease flow at low lung volumes. *B.* Moderate airflow obstruction characterized by a more concave curve. *C.* Variable intrathoracic obstruction in which peak flow is decreased at higher lung volumes with normalization of curve at lower lung volumes. *D.* Restrictive lung disease with a curve that is decreased in width but with a normal shape.

the lung volumes (TLC) are reduced. When the elastic recoil is reduced (as in emphysema), the lung volumes are increased.

CARBON MONOXIDE DIFFUSING CAPACITY

The diffusing capacity of the lungs (D_L) is a measurement of the ability of a gas to diffuse across the alveolar-capillary membrane. Carbon monoxide is the usual test gas because it is not normally present in the lungs and is much more soluble in blood than in lung tissue. When the diffusing capacity is determined with carbon monoxide, the test is called the *carbon monoxide diffusing capacity* (D_{LCO}). Because the D_{LCO} is directly related to the alveolar volume (V_A), it is frequently normalized to this value (D_L/V_A), which allows for its interpretation in the presence of abnormal lung volumes (e.g., after surgical lung resection).

The diffusing capacity will be reduced in all clinical situations in which there is impairment of gas transfer from the alveoli to capillary blood.[2,3] Common conditions that reduce the D_{LCO} include lung resection, emphysema (loss of functioning alveolar-capillary units), and interstitial lung disease (thickening of the alveolar-capillary membrane). Normal PFTs with a reduced D_{LCO} should suggest the possibility of pulmonary vascular disease (e.g., pulmonary embolus) but also can be seen with anemia, early interstitial lung disease, and mild *Pneumocystis carinii* (PCP) infection in AIDS patients.

OBSTRUCTIVE LUNG DISEASE

Obstructive lung disease implies a reduced capacity to get air through the conducting airways and out of the lungs. This reduction in airflow may be caused by a decrease in the diameter of the airways (bronchospasm), a loss of their integrity (bronchomalacia), or a reduction in the elastic recoil (emphysema) with a resulting decrease in the driving pressure. The most common diseases associated with obstructive pulmonary functions are asthma, emphysema, and chronic bronchitis; however, bronchiectasis, infiltration of the bronchial wall by tumor or granuloma, aspiration of a foreign body, and bronchiolitis

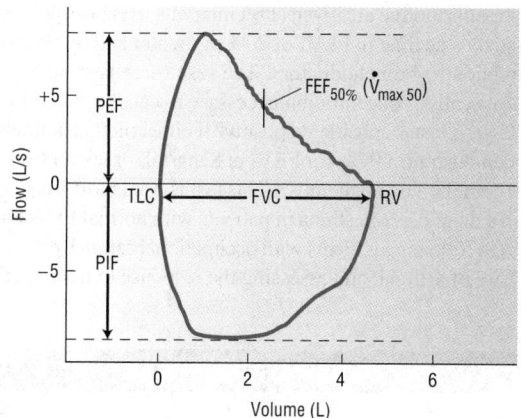

FIGURE 25–3. Normal flow-volume loop. Flows are measured on the vertical (*y*) axis, and lung volumes are measured on the horizontal (*x*) axis. FVC can be read from the tracing as the maximal horizontal deflection. Instantaneous flow (V_{max}) at any point in FVC also can be measured directly. FVC = forced vital capacity.

also cause obstructive PFTs. The standard test used to evaluate airway obstruction is the forced-expiratory spirogram.

Standard spirometry and flow-volume loop measurements include many variables; however, according to American Thoracic Society guidelines, the diagnosis of obstructive and restrictive ventilatory defects should be made using the basic measurements of spirometry.[3] A reduction in FEV_1 (with a normal FVC) establishes the diagnosis of obstruction. When both the FEV_1 and FVC are reduced, the FEV_1 cannot be used to assess airway obstruction because such patients may have either obstruction or restriction. In restrictive lung disease, the patient has an inability to get air into the lung, which results in a reduction of all expiratory volumes (FEV_1, FVC, and SVC). In obstructed patients, a better measurement is the ratio of the FEV_1 to FVC. Patients with restrictive lung disease have a reduced FEV_1 and a reduced FVC, but the FEV_1/FVC ratio remains normal. Although a normal FEV_1/FVC ratio is above 70% to 75%, the ratio is age-dependent, and slightly lower values may be normal in older patients. Caution should be used in interpreting obstruction when the ratio of FEV_1/FVC is below normal but the FEV_1 and FVC are both within the normal range because this pattern can be seen with healthy, athletic subjects. In screening spirometry, performed in office practice, the FEV_6 (the amount of air forcefully exhaled in 6 seconds) may be used in place of the FVC. The FEV_6 is a more reproducible number when obtained by less skilled personnel. The measurement of $FEF_{25\%-75\%}$ is also abnormal in patients with obstructive airways disease. In general, this test has so much variability that it adds little to the measurement of FEV_1 and FEV_1/FVC ratio. The $FEF_{25\%-75\%}$ has been of value in monitoring lung transplant patients for graft rejection,[4] and a reduced value may be an early indicator of acute rejection.

Although there is no standardization for interpretation of severity of obstruction, most pulmonary laboratories state that an FEV_1/FVC ratio of less than 70% of the predicted value is diagnostic for obstruction, and the degree of obstruction then is based on the percent predicted of the FEV_1. An FEV_1 of less than 60% of the predicted value is moderate obstruction, and less than 40% of the predicted value is severe obstruction. In patients with obstruction, a dose of a bronchodilator (e.g., albuterol or isoproterenol) by metered-dose inhaler is given during the initial examination. An increase in the FEV_1 of more than 12% and greater than 0.2 L suggest an acute bronchodilator response.[3] Because bronchodilator responsiveness is variable over time, the lack of an acute bronchodilator response should not preclude a 6- to 8-week trial of bronchodilators and/or corticosteroids.

Although all patients with obstructive lung disease of any etiology will have reduced flow rates on forced exhalation, the pattern on PFTs may be helpful in differentiating among the various etiologies (Table 25–1). Asthma is characterized by variable obstruction that often improves or resolves with appropriate therapy. Since asthma is an inflammatory disorder of the airways (predominantly large airways), the diffusing capacity of carbon monoxide (D_{LCO}) is normal. Most patients with acute asthma have a bronchodilator response of over 15% to 20%; however, this response is also seen in 20% of patients with COPD. These patients are said to have asthmatic bronchitis. Chronic bronchitis may be limited to the airways, but the vast majority of patients with chronic bronchitis and airway obstruction have a mixture of bronchitis and emphysema and have a reduction in D_{LCO}. Therefore, D_{LCO} is the best PFT in separating asthma from COPD.

After the diagnosis of obstructive airways disease is established, the course and response to therapy are best followed by serial spirometry. The multicenter Lung Health Study demonstrated an abnormally rapid decline (90–150 mL/year) in patients with COPD who continue

TABLE 25–1. Specific Patterns of Pulmonary Function in Patients with Chronic Obstructive Pulmonary Disease (COPD)

	Asthma	COPD Chronic Bronchitis	COPD Emphysema
Decreased FEV_1	++++	++++	++++
Decreased FEV_1/FVC	++++	++++	++++
Increased airway resistance	++++	++++	+
Decreased D_{LCO}	—	—/++[a]	++++
Response to bronchodilators	++++	+[b]	—[b]

[a]Most smokers with chronic bronchitis have reduced D_{LCO}.
[b]Twenty percent of patients with COPD have large (++++) bronchodilator response.

D_{LCO} = diffusing capacity of carbon monoxide; FEV_1 = forced expiratory volume after 1 second; FVC = forced vital capacity.

to smoke.[5] Smoking cessation often resulted in an increase in FEV_1 during the first year and a near-normal rate of decline (30–50 mL/year) in subsequent years.

AIRWAY HYPERREACTIVITY

Airway *hyperreactivity* or *hyperresponsiveness* is defined as an exaggerated bronchoconstrictor response to physical, chemical, or pharmacologic stimuli. Individuals with asthma, by definition, have hyperresponsive airways. Recently, the Lung Health Study Group[6] observed nonspecific hyperresponsiveness in a significant number of patients with COPD. This group of patients with airway hyperreactivity appears to have a worse prognosis and an accelerated rate of decline in FEV_1.

Some patients with asthma (especially cough-variant asthma) present with no history of wheezing and normal PFTs. The diagnosis of asthma still can be established by demonstrating hyperresponsiveness to provocative agents. The two agents used most widely in clinical practice are methacholine and histamine. Other agents used for bronchial provocation include distilled water, cold air, and exercise. During a typical bronchoprovocation test, a baseline FEV_1 is measured after the inhalation of isotonic saline, and then increasing doses of methacholine are given at set intervals. Hyperresponsiveness is defined by a decline in FEV_1 of 20% or greater and by reversibility of obstruction to bronchodilators. The result can best be expressed as the provocative concentration necessary to cause a fall in FEV_1 of 20% (PC_{20}). A test is considered positive if either methacholine or histamine demonstrate a PC_{20} for FEV_1 at 8 mg/mL or less or fewer than 60 to 80 cumulative breath units.[7] This test is used most frequently to establish a diagnosis of asthma in patients with normal PFTs but may be useful in following patients with occupational asthma, establishing the severity of asthma, and assessing the response to treatment.

UPPER AIRWAY OBSTRUCTION

Obstruction of airflow by abnormalities in the upper airway often go undiagnosed or misdiagnosed because of improper interpretation of the PFTs. The patients have obstructive physiology and often are misclassified as having asthma or COPD. The shape of the flow-volume

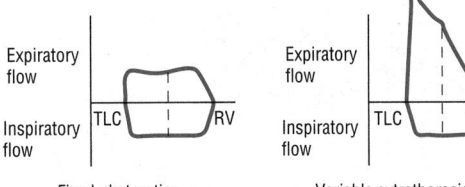
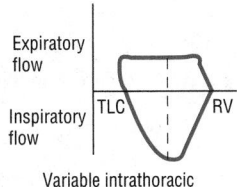

Fixed obstruction

Variable extrathoracic obstruction

Variable intrathoracic obstruction

FIGURE 25–5. Maximum expiratory flow-volume curves from patients with fixed obstruction, variable extrathoracic obstruction, and variable intrathoracic obstruction. RV = residual volume; TLC = total lung capacity.

loop, which includes inspiratory and expiratory flow-volume curves, and the ratio of the expiratory and inspiratory flow at 50% of vital capacity ($FEF_{50\%}/FIF_{50\%}$) may be useful in the diagnosis of upper airway obstruction.[8]

The shape of the flow-volume curve differs depending on whether the obstruction is fixed or variable (Fig. 25–5). Fixed lesions, as in strictures from previous intubations or tracheostomy, cause a uniform caliber of the airway during inspiration and expiration. With variable lesions, however, the airway caliber changes with changes in intrathoracic pressure. Variable lesions are subclassified into variable intrathoracic and variable extrathoracic. If the lesion is intrathoracic, as with tumors of the trachea, the negative pressure generated during inspiration opens the obstruction, whereas the positive pressure during expiration worsens the obstruction. If there is variable extrathoracic obstruction, as with vocal cord dysfunction, the negative pressure within the airways will pull the vocal cord toward the midline and potentiate the obstruction. In this case, there will be a plateau on the inspiratory limb on the flow-volume loop, and the $FEF_{50\%}/FIF_{50\%}$ will be greater than 1. Typical flow-volume curves from upper airway obstruction are shown in Figure 25–4.

Another test used to distinguish upper airway obstruction from COPD and asthma is the $FEV_1/FEV_{0.5}$ (FEV at 1 second/FEV at 0.5 second). This ratio is usually greater than 1.5 in patients with upper airway obstruction.[9] This is so because the $FEV_{0.5}$ is proportionately more reduced in upper airway obstruction because forced expiration measured at 0.5 second better reflects obstruction at high lung volumes. The abnormality seen on the flow-volume loop has been referred to as "straightening" of the curve during early expiration.

RESTRICTIVE LUNG DISEASE

5 *Restrictive lung disease* is defined as an inability to get air into the lungs and to maintain normal lung volumes. Restrictive lung disease reduces all the subdivisions of lung volumes (IRV, V_T, ERV, and RV) without reducing airflow. These patients have normal airway resistance, and their FEV_1/FVC ratio is greater than 75%.

Although *restriction* could be defined as a reduction in vital capacity (VC or FVC) with a normal FEV_1/FVC ratio, poor effort also will reduce FVC with a normal FEV_1/FVC ratio. A reduction in the TLC is the most accurate measurement of restrictive lung function. As mentioned previously, TLC can be measured by various techniques. The gas dilution methods (i.e., helium dilution and nitrogen washout) are unable to measure gas trapped in cysts or bullae and may underestimate the true lung volume. Therefore, TLC is best measured by plethysmography. Most restrictive lung disease is associated with impairment or destruction of the alveolar capillary membrane, and therefore, the D_{LCO} is reduced in most patients with restrictive lung disease. The reduction in D_{LCO} may occur prior to a reduction in lung volumes and is used as a marker of early interstitial (restrictive)

lung disease. The D_{LCO} may be abnormal even with a normal chest x-ray, and thin-cut computed tomographic (CT) scans of the chest may be required to diagnose early interstitial lung disease. Because peribronchiolar inflammation and fibrosis occur in patients with restrictive parenchymal lung disease, the $FEF_{25\%-75\%}$ may be reduced and fail to respond to bronchodilators.

The severity of restrictive disease has not been standardized; however, many laboratories classify patients with a reduced TLC into mild (TLC $\leq$ 80%), moderate (TLC $\leq$ 65%), and severe (TLC $\leq$ 50%). These definitions are completely arbitrary because a patient with obstructive lung disease may start with a TLC of 120% and subsequently develop a moderately severe restrictive lung disease while maintaining a TLC within the normal range. On flow-volume loop, patients with restrictive disease have normal-shaped curves with a reduction in the height and width of the curve because the peak expiratory flow rate (PEFR) and VC both depend on the amount of air within the lung prior to performing expiratory maneuvers (see Fig. 25–3).

6 Restrictive lung function can be produced by increased elastic recoil of the lung parenchyma (interstitial lung disease), respiratory muscle weakness, mechanical restrictions (chest wall deformities), and/or poor effort. Table 25–2 lists common causes of restrictive lung disease.

Restrictive lung function from parenchymal lung disease usually can be differentiated from processes causing mechanical

TABLE 25–2. Causes of Restrictive Lung Disease

Interstitial lung diseases
    Idiopathic pulmonary fibrosis
    Sarcoidosis
    Collagen vascular disease
    Pneumoconiosis
    Drug-induced lung disease
    Pulmonary edema
Infiltrative lung diseases
    Granulomatosis
    Tumor
Pleural diseases
    Pleural effusion
    Fibrothorax
    Pneumothorax
Chest wall diseases
    Kyphoscoliosis
    Ankylosing spondylitis
    Neuromuscular disease
Miscellaneous causes
    Obesity
    Pregnancy
    Ascites
    Paralyzed diaphragm
Lung resection

TABLE 25–3. Patterns of Pulmonary Function

| | Obstructive Lung Disease | | Restrictive Lung Disease | |
	Asthma	COPD	Parenchymal Disease	Chest Bellows Disease
FVC	Nl or I	Nl or I	D	D
FEV_1	D	D	D	D
FEV_1/FVC	<75%	<75%	≥75%	≥75%
TLC	Nl or I	Nl or I	D	D
RV/TLC	Nl or I	Nl or I	Nl	I
Airway resistance	I	I	Nl	Nl
D_{LCO}	Nl	D	D	Nl

D = decreased; I = increased; Nl = normal.

restriction as a result of chest bellows malfunction (Table 25–3). Restrictive parenchymal diseases are associated with a reduction in alveolar volume and an increase in lung elastic recoil. All lung volumes, as well as the D_{LCO}, are reduced. The RV/TLC ratio (normal ≤ 30%) and measurements of maximal inspiratory pressure (MIP; normal = −75 cm H_2O males, −50 cm H_2O females) remain normal. In addition, these patients exhibit mild resting hypoxemia that worsens with exercise. Monitoring gas exchange during exercise may be the most sensitive test for detecting progression of interstitial lung disease.[10]

Mechanical restriction caused by chest bellows malfunction may result from chest wall or skeletal deformity, loss of neuromuscular function, fibrosis of the pleural space, and abdominal overdistension causing upward displacement of the diaphragm, as well as decreased diaphragm movement. The most common pulmonary function pattern seen in these patients is a decrease in TLC and VC with only a slight decrease in RV. The RV is maintained in these diseases because lung compliance remains normal. The D_{LCO} is normal or only minimally reduced, and the D_{LCO}/V_A (corrected for alveolar volume) is normal. The RV/TLC ratio is often increased in patients with restrictive chest bellows disease. Patients with neuromuscular disease also have reduced respiratory muscle function with a reduction in their MIP.

PULMONARY GAS EXCHANGE

The essential function of the lungs is to maintain blood gas homeostasis. Arterial blood gas measurement plays an important role in the diagnosis and management of patients with pulmonary disease and should be ordered whenever hypoxemia, hypercapnia (CO_2 retention), and/or acid-base disorders are suspected clinically. Every time arterial blood gas determinations are ordered, the A–a gradient (the difference between the partial pressure of oxygen in the alveolus and the partial pressure of oxygen in arterial blood) should be calculated. This is done by computer on all automated blood gas machines, and a normal $P(A–a)O_2$ can be approximated for sea level breathing room air by multiplying the age by 0.3. The presence of hypoxemia with a normal A–a gradient usually implies alveolar hypoventilation (e.g., sedative overdose). Most patients develop hypoxemia secondary to mismatching of ventilation and perfusion, and the $P(A–a)O_2$ will be significantly elevated.

Pulse oximetry is used widely in clinical practice to monitor arterial saturation (SpO_2). A pulse oximeter is a small battery-operated device that is placed on the finger or the earlobe. This device emits and reads the reflected light from capillary blood, estimating the saturation. Although very useful clinically, SpO_2 is only an estimate of the arterial saturation, and the actual arterial oxygen saturation (SaO_2) can be ±4% of the oximetry reading. The error may be even greater with a saturation of less than 88%. Pulse oximeters do not measure carboxyhemoglobin, and the SpO_2 may be overestimated significantly in patients with smoke inhalation or recent smokers. An initial validation of pulse oximetry with direct measurement of SaO_2 is recommended in any critically ill patient.

EXERCISE TESTING

Cardiopulmonary exercise testing allows for assessment of the multiple organs involved in exercise and has benefits over the assessment of either the cardiac or pulmonary system alone. The major indications for exercise testing are dyspnea on exertion, evaluation of exercise-induced bronchospasm, and suspected arterial desaturation during exercise.[11,12] Exercise testing also can be useful in the evaluation of ventilatory or cardiovascular limitations to work, assessment of general fitness or conditioning, evaluation of disability, establishment of safe levels for exercise, evaluation of drug therapy, determining the need and liter flow for supplemental oxygen therapy during exercise, assessment of the effects of a rehabilitation program, and as a preoperative assessment before lung resection.[11–13]

Tests for general fitness include the 6-minute walking distance and the Harvard step test.[11,13] For the 6-minute walking distance, the subject simply walks a predetermined route or circuit as fast as possible for 6 minutes. The greater the distance covered, the better are the patient's general fitness and exercise tolerance. For the Harvard step test, the subject steps up and down on a 20-in step at a set rate for 5 minutes. A 1-minute rest period is followed by measurement of the subject's recovery heart rate. The lower the recovery heart rate, the better is the subject's general fitness.

Exercise testing sometimes is done to determine if exercise results in arterial oxygen desaturation (SaO_2 < 90%).[12,13] This may be useful to quantify the level of exertion the patient can perform during the activities of daily living, as well as in determining appropriate levels of supplemental oxygen therapy. Typically, this test is done using a treadmill or cycle ergometer. A baseline measurement of arterial blood gas values or pulse oximetry is followed by up to 6 minutes of exercise, during which time the patient is monitored for oxygen desaturation using pulse oximetry. If significant desaturation occurs (saturation ≤88% to 90%), the test is terminated. In the event of oxygen desaturation, the test may be repeated to determine the level of supplemental oxygen therapy needed to compensate for the desaturation that otherwise would occur.

CHAPTER 25 INTRODUCTION TO PULMONARY FUNCTION TESTING 501

TABLE 25–4. Indications and Contraindications for Exercise Testing

Indications

Dyspnea upon exertion
Exercise-induced bronchospasm
Suspected arterial desaturation with exercise
Evaluation of ventilatory limitations to exercise
Evaluation of cardiac limitations to exercise
Assessment of general fitness or conditioning
Evaluation of cardiopulmonary disability
Establishment of safe levels for exercise
Evaluation of drug therapy
Determining appropriate use of supplemental oxygen therapy
Assessment of the effect of a rehabilitation program
Evaluation of specific disease states or conditions (e.g., asthma; COPD; interstitial lung disease; pulmonary vascular disorders; coronary artery disease; other vascular disorders; neuromuscular disorders; obesity; anxiety-induced hyperventilation)
Assessment before resection

Contraindications

Pa_{O_2} less than 40 mm Hg on room air
Pa_{CO_2} greater than 70 mm Hg
FEV_1 less than 30% of predicted
Recent (within 4 weeks) myocardial infarction
Unstable angina pectoris
Second- or third-degree heart block
Rapid ventricular/atrial arrhythmias
Orthopedic impairment
Severe aortic stenosis
Congestive heart failure
Uncontrolled hypertension
Limiting neurologic disorders
Dissecting/ventricular aneurysms
Severe pulmonary hypertension
Thrombophlebitis or intracardiac thrombi
Recent systemic or pulmonary embolus
Acute pericarditis

Exercise tolerance tests or cardiopulmonary stress testing may include the measurement of oxygen consumption ($\dot{V}_{O_2}$), carbon dioxide production ($\dot{V}_{CO_2}$), minute volume ($\dot{V}_E$), oxygen saturation via pulse oximeter (Sp_{O_2}), heart rate, blood pressure, and recording or monitoring of the subject's electrocardiogram (ECG). During exercise, oxygen consumption ($\dot{V}_{O_2}$) increases with workload in a linear fashion until a maximum oxygen consumption level is reached ($\dot{V}_{O_2,max}$). Consequently, $\dot{V}_{O_2,max}$ is a measure of an individual's muscular work capacity.[11-13] Normal $\dot{V}_{O_2,max}$ is about 1700 mL/min for a sedentary person and up to 5800 mL/min in a trained athlete.[13] This compares with a resting $\dot{V}_{O_2}$ of about 250 mL/min. Ventilatory equivalents for oxygen and carbon dioxide and O_2 pulse are often calculated. Ventilatory equivalent for oxygen is a measure of the efficiency of the ventilatory pump at various workloads[11,13] and is calculated as follows:

$$\text{Ventilatory equivalent for } O_2 = \dot{V}_E/\dot{V}_{O_2}$$

A normal ventilatory equivalent for oxygen is 20 to 30.[11,13]

O_2 pulse is an estimate of oxygen consumption per cardiac cycle and may be decreased with cardiac problems. O_2 pulse can be calculated as follows:

$$O_2 \text{ pulse} = (\dot{V}_{O_2} \times 1000)/\text{heart rate}$$

A normal O_2 pulse is 2.5 to 4.0 mL per beat at rest, increasing to 10 to 15 mL per beat during strenuous exercise.[11,13]

The anaerobic threshold is the point during strenuous exercise at which anaerobic metabolism and lactic acid production begin.[11,13] Carbon dioxide production ($\dot{V}_{CO_2,max}$) increases with exercise at about the same rate as $\dot{V}_{O_2}$, until the subject's anaerobic threshold is reached. From that point on, $\dot{V}_{CO_2}$ increases faster than $\dot{V}_{O_2}$, and this change can be used to estimate the anaerobic threshold. A breath-by-breath plot of the ventilatory equivalents for O_2 and CO_2 also can be used to determine the anaerobic threshold. Anaerobic threshold is a measure of fitness in normal subjects, and aerobic training can delay the anaerobic threshold.[11,13]

For exercise-tolerance testing, the subject typically is subjected to either a constant work load (steady-state tests) or an increasing work load (progressive multistage tests) using a cycle ergometer or treadmill.[11,13] With the progressive multistage tests, the subject is exercised until exhaustion or the occurrence of an adverse reaction, at which point the test is stopped. Safety during exercise testing is of major importance, and rigorous guidelines for the termination of the test should be followed. Both types of tests can be used to determine $\dot{V}_{O_2,max}$. A limit to exercise, as indicated by a decrease in $\dot{V}_{O_2,max}$, can be as a result of (1) poor conditioning, (2) a pulmonary limitation, (3) a cardiac limitation, or (4) poor effort. In the case of poor conditioning, Sp_{O_2} and O_2 pulse will be normal. With a pulmonary limitation to exercise, Sp_{O_2} will be reduced, and O_2 pulse will be normal. With a cardiac limitation to exercise, Sp_{O_2} will be normal, and O_2 pulse reduced. Table 25–4 summarizes the indications and contraindications for exercise testing. Table 25–5 summarizes the findings during maximum exercise associated with poor conditioning, pulmonary limitations to exercise, and cardiac limitations to exercise.

Review Questions and other resources can be found at *www.pharmacotherapyonline.com.*

TABLE 25–5. Typical Findings During Maximum Exercise with Poor Conditioning, Pulmonary Limitations to Exercise, and Cardiac Limitations to Exercise

Test Parameter	Poor Conditioning	Pulmonary Limitation	Cardiac Limitation
$\dot{V}_{O_2max}$	↓	↓	↓
Sp_{O_2}	N	↓	N
O_2 pulse	N or ↓	N or ↓	↓
Anaerobic threshold	↓ or N	↓ or N	↓
Ventilatory reserve* (MVV-V_{Emax})	N	↓	N or ↑

*Ventilatory reserve = Maximum voluntary ventilation (MVV) − minute volume during maximum exercise (V_{Emax}).
N = normal.
(Adapted from Madama VE. Pulmonary function testing and cardiopulmonary stress testing. Albany, NY, Delmar, 1993.)

REFERENCES

1. Renzessi AA Jr, Bleeker, ER, Eppler, GR, et al. Evaluation of impairment/disability secondary to respiratory disorders. Am Rev Respir Dis 1986;133:1205–1209.
2. Crapo RO. Pulmonary function testing. N Engl J Med 1994;331:25–30.
3. Crapo RO, Hankinson JL, Irvin C, et al. American Thoracic Society statement: Standardization of spirometry—1994 update. Am J Respir Crit Care Med 1995;152:1107–1136.
4. Levine SM, Peters JI, Jenkinson SG. Lung transplantation and lung volume reduction surgery. In: George RB, Light RW, Matthaw MA, eds. Chest Medicine: Essentials of Pulmonary and Critical Care Medicine, 4th ed. Philadelphia, Lippincott Williams & Wilkins, 2000;208–232.
5. Anthonisen NR, Connett JE, Kiley JP, et al. Effects of smoking intervention and the use of an inhaled anticholinergic bronchodilator on the rate of decline of FEV_1: The Lung Health Study. JAMA 1994;272:1497–1505.
6. Tashkin DP, Altose MD, Bleeker ER, et al. The Lung Health Study: Airway responsiveness to inhaled methacholine in smokers with mild to moderate airflow limitation. Am Rev Respir Dis 1992;145:301–310.
7. Crapo RO, Casaburi R, Coates AL, et al. American Thoracic Society statement: Guidelines for methacholine and exercise challenge testing—1999. Am J Respir Crit Care Med 2000;161:309–329.
8. Acres JC, Kryger MH. Upper airway obstruction. Chest 1981;80:207–211.
9. Bright P, Miller MR, Franklyn JA, et al. The use of a neural network to detect upper airway obstruction caused by goiter. Am J Respir Crit Care Med 1998;157:1885–1891.
10. Leith DE, Brown R. ERS/ATS Workshop Series: Human lung volumes and the mechanisms that set them. Eur Respir J 1999;13:468–472.
11. Wasserman K, Hansen JE, Sue DY, Whipp BJ. Principles of Exercise Testing and Interpretation: Including Pathophysiology and Clinical Applications, 3d ed. Philadelphia, Lippincott Williams & Wilkins, 1999.
12. Ruppel GE. Manual of Pulmonary Function Testing. St. Louis, Mosby, 1994.
13. ATS/ACCP Statement on Cardiopulmonary Exercise Testing. Am J Respir Crit Care Med 2003;167:211–277.

26
ASTHMA
H. William Kelly and Christine A. Sorkness

Learning Objectives and other resources can be found at *www.pharmacotherapyonline.com*.

KEY CONCEPTS

◀1 Asthma is a disease of increasing prevalence that is a result of genetic predisposition and environmental interactions.

◀2 Asthma is primarily a chronic inflammatory disorder of the airways of the lung characterized by T-helper cell type 2 (Th2)–lymphocyte–mediated immune response for which there is no known cure or primary prevention.

◀3 Asthma is characterized by either the intermittent or persistent presence of highly variable degrees of airway obstruction from airway wall inflammation and bronchial smooth muscle constriction.

◀4 The inflammatory process in asthma is treated most

effectively with corticosteroids, with the inhaled corticosteroids having the greatest efficacy for persistent asthma.

◀5 Bronchial smooth muscle constriction is prevented or treated most effectively with inhaled β_2-adrenergic receptor agonists.

◀6 Variability in response to medications requires individualization of therapy within existing evidence-based guidelines for management.

◀7 Ongoing patient education, including avoidance of triggers and self-management techniques, is essential for optimal patient outcomes.

Asthma has been known since antiquity, yet it is a disease that still defies precise definition. The word *asthma* is of Greek origin and means "panting." More than 2000 years ago, Hippocrates used the word *asthma* to describe episodic shortness of breath; however, the first detailed clinical description of the asthmatic patient was made by Aretaeus in the second century.[1] An expert panel of the National Institutes of Health, the National Asthma Education and Prevention Program (NAEPP), has provided the following working definition of asthma[2]:

> Asthma is a chronic inflammatory disorder of the airways in which many cells and cellular elements play a role, in particular, mast cells, eosinophils, T-lymphocytes, macrophages, neutrophils, and epithelial cells. In susceptible individuals, this inflammation causes recurrent episodes of wheezing, breathlessness, chest tightness, and coughing, particularly at night or in the early morning. These episodes are usually associated with widespread but variable airflow obstruction that is often reversible either spontaneously or with treatment. The inflammation also causes an associated increase in the existing bronchial hyperresponsiveness to a variety of stimuli.

This definition encompasses the important heterogeneity of the clinical presentation of asthma by describing the scientific and clinically accepted characteristics of asthma.

EPIDEMIOLOGY

◀1 An estimated 14 to 15 million persons in the United States have asthma (about 5% of the population).[3] Asthma is the most common chronic disease among children in the United States, with

approximately 5 million children affected. Over the past two decades in the United States, the prevalence of asthma has increased by 75%, whereas the rate in children younger than age 5 has increased 160%.[3] In the United States, as in other Western industrialized countries, the prevalence of asthma has reached epidemic proportions. Asthma accounts for 1.6% of all ambulatory care visits (13.7 million) and results in more than 470,000 hospitalizations and 2 million emergency department visits per year.[3] Asthma is the third leading cause of preventable hospitalization in the United States, and hospitalizations for asthma among children 0 to 17 years of age have increased 4.5% per year, whereas total hospitalizations for all causes in children actually decreased.[4] Children have the highest prevalence of asthma, at 68.6 per 1000 population younger than 18 years of age. Asthma accounts for more than 10 million missed school days per year.[4] The prevalence of disabling asthma in children has increased 232% over the past 20 years compared with a 113% increase from all other chronic conditions in childhood. In young children (0 to 10 years of age), the risk of asthma is greater in boys than in girls, becomes about equal during puberty, and then is greater in women than in men.[3]

Ethnic minorities continue to share the burden of asthma disproportionately. African-Americans and Hispanics have a higher prevalence than whites, but this appears to be a result of urbanization and not race or socioeconomic status.[5] African-Americans are three times as likely to be hospitalized and approximately 2.5 times more likely to die from asthma.[3] In addition, African-Americans and Puerto Ricans living in inner cities are four times more likely to experience emergency department visits than whites.[3] These patterns are likely a result of poor access to care.

The estimated cost of asthma in the United States in 1998 was $12.6 billion.[6] The average societal burden of asthma (including both direct and indirect medical expenditures) in the United States averages $640 per patient per year, with direct medical expenditures accounting for 40% to 50% of total costs.[6] Emergency care of acute asthma exacerbations makes up the largest portion of direct medical costs. In 1997, an estimated cost of $1 billion dollars per year in lost productivity accrued from parents staying home to care for their children.[6]

The natural history of asthma is still not well defined. Although asthma can occur at any time, it is principally a pediatric disease, with most patients being diagnosed by 5 years of age and up to 50% of children having symptoms by 2 years of age.[2] Between 30% and 70% of children with asthma will improve markedly or become symptom-free by early adulthood; chronic disease persists in about 30% to 40% of patients, and generally 20% or less develop severe chronic disease.[2] Atopic status is the strongest indicator of a poor prognosis, although initial severity also predicts severity as an adult.[7] Diminished lung growth may occur in children with uncontrolled severe asthma. Low lung function and increased bronchial hyperresponsiveness are independent risk factors for low lung function in early adulthood.[8]

In adults, most longitudinal studies have suggested a more rapid rate of decline in lung function in asthmatics than in normal volunteers, primarily reflected in forced expiratory volume in 1 second (FEV_1).[7] However, the annual decline in FEV_1 is less than in smokers or in patients with a diagnosis of emphysema. In general, asthmatics with less frequent attacks and normal lung function on initial assessment have higher remission rates, whereas smokers have the lowest remission and highest relapse rates.[7] The level of bronchial hyperresponsiveness (BHR) tends to predict the rate of decline in FEV_1, with a greater decline with high levels of BHR.[8] Thus airways obstruction in asthma not only may become irreversible but also may worsen over time owing to airway remodeling (see below).[9]

Although both the prevalence and the morbidity from asthma are increasing, the death rate from asthma in the United States appears to have reached a plateau of about 5000 deaths per year and may be on the decline.[3] Despite the relatively low number of asthma deaths, 80% to 90% are preventable.[2] Most deaths from asthma occur outside the hospital, and death is rare after hospitalization. The most common cause of death from asthma is inadequate assessment of the severity of airways obstruction by the patient or physician and inadequate therapy. The most common cause of death in hospitalized patients is also inadequate or inappropriate therapy. Thus the key to prevention of death from asthma, as advocated by the NAEPP, is education.[2]

ETIOLOGY

◀ Asthma is at least a partially heritable complex syndrome that requires a gene-by-environment interaction for phenotypic expression. Epidemiologic studies strongly support the concept of a genetic predisposition to the development of asthma.[10] Genetic factors account for 35% to 70% of the susceptibility. Asthma represents a complex genetic disorder in that the asthma phenotype is likely a result of polygenic inheritance or different combinations of genes. Initial searches were focused on establishing links between atopy (genetically determined state of hypersensitivity to environmental allergens) and asthma, but more recent genome-wide searches have found linkages with genes for metalloproteinases (e.g., *ADAM33*).[10,11] Thus, although genetic predisposition to atopy is a significant risk factor for developing asthma, not all atopic individuals develop asthma, nor do all asthmatics exhibit atopy.

Environmental risk factors for the development of asthma include socioeconomic status, family size, exposure to secondhand tobacco smoke in infancy and in utero, allergen exposure, urbanization, and decreased exposure to common childhood infectious agents.[12] Currently, the so-called hygiene hypothesis that proposes that genetically susceptible individuals develop allergies and asthma by allowing the allergic immunologic system (Th2-lymphocytes) to develop instead of the immunologic system used to fight infections (Th1-lymphocytes) is being used to explain the increase of asthma in Western countries.[9,10] The first 2 years of life appear to be most important for the exposures to produce an alteration in the immune response system. Support for the hygiene hypothesis for asthma comes from studies demonstrating a lower risk for asthma in children who live on farms and are exposed to high levels of bacteria, in those with a large number of siblings, in those with early enrollment into child care, in those with exposure to cats and dogs early in life, or in those with exposure to fewer antibiotics.[10,12]

Risk factors for early (<3 years of age) recurrent wheezing associated with viral infections include low birth weight, male gender, and parental smoking. However, this early pattern is due to smaller airways, and these risk factors are not necessarily risk factors for asthma in later life.[7] Atopy is the predominant risk factor for children to have continued asthma.[7] Asthma can occur in adults later in life. Occupational asthma in previously healthy individuals emphasizes the effect of environment on the development of asthma.[13] The heterogeneity of the asthma phenotype appears most obvious when listing the diverse triggers of bronchospasm in asthmatic subjects[2,10] (Table 26–1). The various triggers have relative degrees of importance from patient to patient. This variety should serve as ample evidence that asthma is likely to be as complex genetically.

Environmental exposures are the most important precipitants of severe asthma exacerbations[2,10] (see Table 26–1). Epidemics of severe asthma in cities have followed exposures to high concentrations of aeroallergens.[2] Viral respiratory tract infections remain the single most significant precipitant of severe asthma in children and are an important trigger in adults as well.[2,10] Other possible factors include air pollution, sinusitis, food preservatives, and drugs.

TABLE 26–1. List of Agents and Events Triggering Asthma

Respiratory infection
  Respiratory syncytial virus (RSV), rhinovirus, influenza, parainfluenza, *Mycoplasma pneumonia*
Allergens
  Airbone pollens (grass, trees, weeds), house-dust mites, animal danders, cockroaches, fungal spores
Environment
  Cold air, fog, ozone, sulfur dioxide, nitrogen dioxide, tobacco smoke, wood smoke
Emotions
  Anxiety, stress, laughter
Exercise
  Particularly in cold, dry climate
Drugs/preservatives
  Aspirin, NSAIDs (cyclooxygenase inhibitors), sulfites, benzalkonium chloride, β-blockers
Occupational stimuli
  Bakers (flour dust); farmers (hay mold); spice and enzyme workers; printers (arabic gum); chemical workers (azo dyes, anthraquinone, ethylenediamine, toluene diisocyanates, polyvinyl chloride); plastics, rubber, and wood workers (formaldehyde, western cedar, dimethylethanolamine, anhydrides)

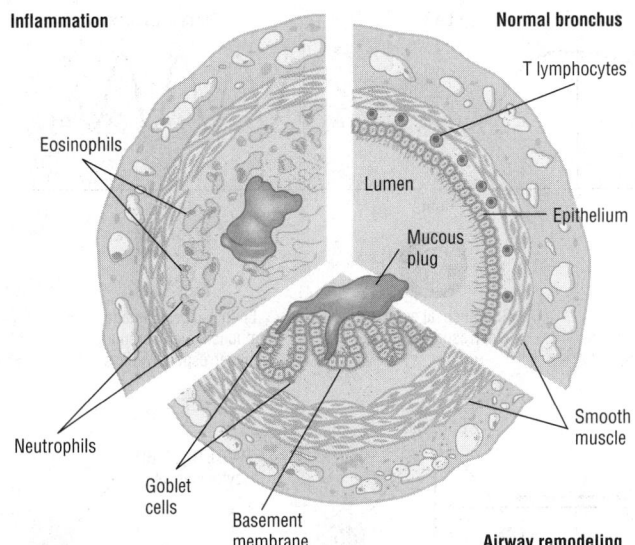

Inflammation

Eosinophils

Neutrophils

Goblet cells

Basement membrane

Normal bronchus

T lymphocytes

Lumen

Mucous plug

Epithelium

Smooth muscle

Airway remodeling

FIGURE 26–1. Representative illustration of the pathology found in the asthmatic bronchus compared with a normal bronchus (*upper right*). Each section demonstrates how the lumen is narrowed. Hypertrophy of the basement membrane, mucus plugging, smooth muscle hypertrophy, and constriction contribute (*lower section*). Inflammatory cells infiltrate, producing submucosal edema, and epithelial desquamation fills the airway lumen with cellular debris and exposes the airway smooth muscle to other mediators (*upper left*).

PATHOPHYSIOLOGY

The major characteristics of asthma include a variable degree of airflow obstruction (related to bronchospasm, edema, and hypersecretion), BHR, and airways inflammation (Fig. 26–1). Evidence of inflammation arose from the studies of nonspecific BHR, bronchoalveolar lavage (BAL), bronchial biopsies, and induced sputum, as well as from postmortem observations of patients with asthma who died from an attack of asthma or from other causes. To understand the pathogenetic mechanisms that underlie the many variants of asthma, it is critical to identify factors that initiate, intensify, and modulate the inflammatory response of the airways and to determine how these immunologic and biologic processes produce the characteristic airways abnormalities. Immune responses mediated by IgE antibodies are of foremost importance.

ACUTE INFLAMMATION

Inhaled allergen challenge models contribute most to our understanding of acute inflammation in asthma.[14] Inhaled allergen challenge in allergic patients leads to an early-phase allergic reaction that, in some cases, may be followed by a late-phase reaction. The activation of cells bearing allergen-specific IgE initiates the early-phase reaction. It is characterized primarily by the rapid activation of airway mast cells and macrophages. The activated cells rapidly release proinflammatory mediators such as histamine, eicosanoids, and reactive oxygen species that induce contraction of airway smooth muscle, mucus secretion, and vasodilatation.[14] The bronchial microcirculation has an essential role in this inflammatory process. Inflammatory mediators induce microvascular leakage with exudation of plasma in the airways.[14] Acute plasma protein leakage induces a thickened, engorged, and edematous airway wall and a consequent narrowing of the airway lumen. Plasma exudation may compromise epithe-

lial integrity, and the presence of plasma in the lumen may reduce mucus clearance.[14] Plasma proteins also may promote the formation of exudative plugs mixed with mucus and inflammatory and epithelial cells. Together these effects contribute to airflow obstruction (Fig. 26–1).

The late-phase inflammatory reaction occurs 6 to 9 hours after allergen provocation and involves the recruitment and activation of eosinophils, CD4+ T cells, basophils, neutrophils, and macrophages.[14] There is selective retention of airway T cells, the expression of adhesion molecules, and the release of selected proinflammatory mediators and cytokines involved in the recruitment and activation of inflammatory cells.[14] The activation of T cells after allergen challenge leads to the release of T-helper cell type 2 (Th2)–like cytokines that may be a key mechanism of the late-phase response.[14] The release of preformed cytokines by mast cells is the likely initial trigger for the early recruitment of cells. This cell type may recruit and induce the more persistent involvement by T cells.[14] The enhancement of nonspecific BHR usually can be demonstrated after the late-phase reaction but not after the early-phase reaction following allergen or occupational challenge.

CHRONIC INFLAMMATION

Airways inflammation has been demonstrated in all forms of asthma, and an association between the extent of inflammation and the clinical severity of asthma has been demonstrated in selected studies.[7] It is accepted that both central and peripheral airways are inflamed.

In asthma, all cells of the airways are involved and become activated (Fig. 26–2). Included are eosinophils, T cells, mast cells, macrophages, epithelial cells, fibroblasts, and bronchial smooth muscle cells. These cells also regulate airway inflammation and initiate the process of remodeling by the release of cytokines and growth factors.[15]

EPITHELIAL CELLS

Bronchial epithelial cells traditionally have been considered as a barrier, participating in mucociliary clearance and removal of noxious agents. However, epithelial cells also participate in inflammation by the release of eicosanoids, peptidases, matrix proteins, cytokines, and nitric oxide (NO). Epithelial cells can be activated by IgE-dependent mechanisms, viruses, pollutants, or histamines. In asthma, especially fatal asthma, extensive epithelial shedding occurs. The functional consequences of epithelial shedding may include heightened airways responsiveness, altered permeability of the airway mucosa, depletion of epithelial-derived relaxant factors, and loss of enzymes responsible for degrading proinflammatory neuropeptides. The integrity of airway epithelium may influence the sensitivity of the airways to various provocative stimuli. Epithelial cells also may be important in the regulation of airway remodeling and fibrosis.[15,16]

EOSINOPHILS

Eosinophils play an effector role in asthma by release of proinflammatory mediators, cytotoxic mediators, and cytokines.[15] Circulating eosinophils migrate to the airways by cell rolling, through interactions with selectins, and eventually adhere to the endothelium through the binding of integrins to adhesion proteins (vascular cell adhesion molecule 1 [VCAM–1] and intercellular adhesion molecule 1 [ICAM–1]). As eosinophils enter the matrix of the membrane, their survival is prolonged by interleukin 5 (IL-5) and

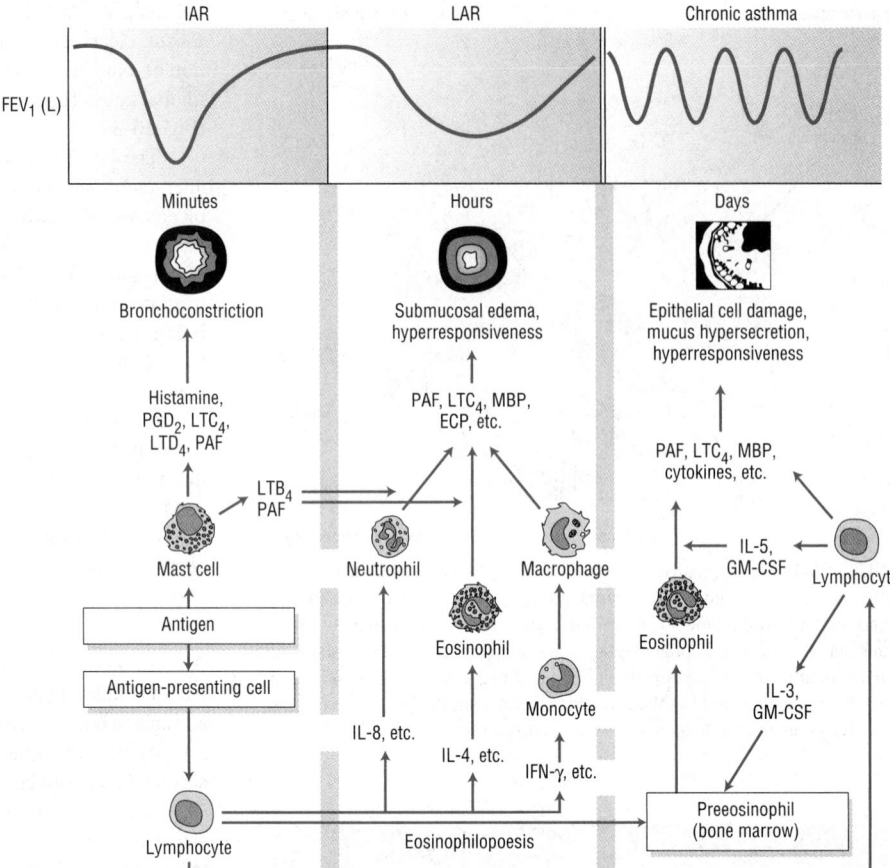

FIGURE 26–2. Diagrammatic presentation of the relationship between inflammatory cells, lipid and preformed mediators, inflammatory cytokines, and proposed pathogenesis and clinical presentation in asthma. See text for details. PG = prostaglandin; LT = leukotriene; PAF = platelet-activating factor; IL = interleukin; MBP = major basis protein; GM-CSF = granulocyte-macrophage colony-stimulating factor.

granulocyte-macrophage colony-stimulating factor (GM-CSF). On activation, eosinophils release inflammatory mediators such as leukotrienes and granule proteins to injure airway tissue.[15]

LYMPHOCYTES

Mucosal biopsy specimens from patients with asthma contain lymphocytes, many of which express surface markers of inflammation. There are two types of T-helper CD4+ cells. Type 1 T-helper (Th1) cells produce IL-2 and interferon-γ (IFN-γ), both essential for cellular defense mechanisms. Th2 cells produce cytokines (IL-4, -5, -6, -9, and -13) that mediate allergic inflammation. It is known that Th1 cytokines inhibit the production of Th2 cytokines, and vice versa. It is hypothesized that allergic asthmatic inflammation results from a Th2-mediated mechanism (an imbalance between Th1 and Th2 cells).[15]

TH1 AND TH2 CELL IMBALANCE

It has been postulated that the Th1/Th2 imbalance contributes to the cause and evolution of atopic diseases, including asthma. The T-cell population in the cord blood of newborn infants is skewed toward a Th2 phenotype.[7,15] The extent of the imbalance between Th1 and Th2 cells (as indicated by diminished IFN-γ production) during the neonatal phase may predict the subsequent development of allergic disease, asthma, or both. It has been suggested that infants at high risk of asthma and allergies should be exposed to stimuli that upregulate Th1-mediated responses in order to restore the balance during a critical time in the development of the immune system and the lung.[7]

The basic premise of the hygiene hypothesis is that the newborn's immune system is skewed toward Th2 cells and needs timely and appropriate environmental stimuli to create a balanced immune response. Factors that enhance Th1-mediated responses include infection with *Mycobacterium tuberculosis,* measles virus, and hepatitis A virus; increased exposure to infections through contact with older siblings; attendance at day care during the first 6 months of life; and a reduction in the production of IFN-γ. Restoration of the balance between Th1 and Th2 cells may be impeded by frequent administration of oral antibiotics, with concomitant alterations in gastrointestinal flora. Other factors favoring the Th2 phenotype include Western lifestyle, urban environment, diet, and sensitization to house dust mites and cockroaches. Immune "imprinting" may begin in utero by transplacental transfer of allergens and cytokines. The validity of the hygiene hypothesis has been challenged and will continue to generate intense debate.[7]

MAST CELLS

Mast cell degranulation is important in the initiation of immediate responses following exposure to allergens.[2] Mast cells are found throughout the walls of the respiratory tract, and increased numbers of these cells (three- to fivefold) have been described in the airways of asthmatics with an allergic component. Once binding of allergen to cell-bound IgE occurs, mediators such as histamine; eosinophil and neutrophil chemotactic factors; leukotrienes C$_4$, D$_4$, and E$_4$; prostaglandins; platelet-activating factor; and others are released from mast cells (see Fig. 26–2). Histologic examination has revealed decreased numbers of granulated mast cells in the airways of patients who have died from acute asthma attacks, suggesting that mast cell degranulation is a contributing factor in the progression of the disease. Mast cell degranulation is believed to be an integral cause of exercise-induced bronchospasm (EIB) following either drying or cooling of the airways.[15]

ALVEOLAR MACROPHAGES

The primary function of alveolar macrophages in the normal airway is to serve as "scavengers," engulfing and digesting bacteria and other foreign materials. They are found in large and small airways, ideally located for affecting the asthmatic response. A number of mediators produced and released by macrophages have been identified, including platelet-activating factor, leukotriene B_4, leukotriene C_4, and leukotriene D_4.[15] Additionally, alveolar macrophages are able to produce neutrophil chemotactic factor and eosinophil chemotactic factor, which, in turn, further the inflammatory process.

NEUTROPHILS

The role of neutrophils in the pathogenesis of asthma remains somewhat unclear because they normally may be present in the airways and usually do not infiltrate tissues showing chronic allergic inflammation despite the potential to participate in late-phase inflammatory reactions. However, high numbers of neutrophils have been reported to be present in the airways of patients who died from sudden-onset fatal asthma.[7] This suggests that neutrophils may play a pivotal role in the disease process, at least in the sudden-onset fatal cases and in some patients with long-standing or corticosteroid-dependent asthma. The neutrophil also can be a source for a variety of mediators, including platelet-activating factor, prostaglandins, thromboxanes, and leukotrienes, that contribute to BHR and airway inflammation.

FIBROBLASTS AND MYOFIBROBLASTS

Fibroblasts are found frequently in connective tissue. Human lung fibroblasts may behave as inflammatory cells on activation by IL-4 and IL-13. The myofibroblast may contribute to the regulation of inflammation via the release of cytokines and to tissue remodeling. In asthma, myofibroblasts are increased in numbers beneath the reticular basement membrane, and there is an association between their numbers and the thickness of the reticular basement membrane.[16]

INFLAMMATORY MEDIATORS

Associated with asthma for many years, histamine is capable of inducing smooth muscle constriction and bronchospasm and is thought to play a role in mucosal edema and mucus secretion.[2] Lung mast cells are an important source of histamine. The release of histamine can be stimulated by exposure of the airways to a variety of factors, including physical stimuli (such as exercise) and relevant allergens.[2] Histamine is involved in acute bronchospasm following allergen exposure; however, other mediators such as leukotrienes are also involved.

Besides histamine release, mast cell degranulation releases interleukins, proteases, and other enzymes that activate the production of other mediators of inflammation. Several classes of important mediators, including arachidonic acid and its metabolites (i.e., prostaglandins, leukotrienes, and platelet-activating factor), are derived from cell membrane phospholipids.

Once arachidonic acid is released, it can be broken down by the enzyme cyclooxygenase to form the prostaglandins. A further breakdown product, prostaglandin D_2, has been well characterized and is a potent bronchoconstricting agent. It is unlikely that prostaglandin D_2 can produce sustained effects on airway function or inflammation; however, its role in asthma remains to be determined. Sim-

ilarly, prostaglandin $F_{2\alpha}$ is a potent bronchoconstrictor in patients with asthma and can enhance the effects of histamine.[2] However, its pathophysiologic role in asthma is unclear. Another cyclooxygenase product, prostacyclin (prostaglandin I_2), is known to be produced in the lung. It is unclear whether prostaglandin I_2 is important as a bronchoconstricting agent in humans; however, it may contribute to inflammation and edema owing to its effects as a vasodilator.

Thromboxane A_2 is produced by alveolar macrophages, fibroblasts, epithelial cells, neutrophils, and platelets within the lung.[15] Indirect evidence from animal models suggests that thromboxane A_2 may have several effects, including bronchoconstriction, involvement in the late asthmatic response, and involvement in the development of airway inflammation and BHR. Potent and specific thromboxane synthetase inhibitors will be crucial tools for understanding the role of thromboxanes in asthma.

The 5-lipoxygenase pathway of arachidonic acid breakdown is responsible for production of the class of compounds called *cysteinyl leukotrienes* (LTs).[15] Leukotrienes C_4, D_4, and E_4 (cysteinyl LTs) constitute the slow-reacting substance of anaphylaxis (SRS-A). These leukotrienes are liberated during inflammatory processes in the lung. Leukotrienes D_4 and E_4 share a common receptor (LTD_4 receptor) that, when stimulated, produces bronchospasm, mucus secretion, microvascular permeability, and airway edema.

Thought to be produced by macrophages, eosinophils, and neutrophils within the lung, platelet-activating factor (PAF) is involved in the mediation of bronchospasm, sustained induction of BHR, edema formation, and chemotaxis of eosinophils.[15]

ADHESION MOLECULES

An important step in the inflammatory process is the adhesion of the various cells to each other and the tissue matrix to facilitate infiltration and migration of these cells to the site of inflammation. To promote this, cell membranes express a number of glycoproteins, or adhesion molecules. Adhesion molecules have additional functions involved in the inflammatory process aside from promoting cell adhesion, including activation of cells and cell-cell communication, and promoting cellular migration and infiltration.[2] The many adhesion molecules are divided into families on the basis of their chemical structure. These families are the integrins, cadherins, immunoglobulin supergene family, selectins, vascular adressins, and carbohydrate ligands.[15] Those thought to be important in inflammation include the integrins, immunoglobulin supergene family, selectins, and carbohydrate ligands, including ICAM-1 and VCAM-1.[15] Adhesion molecules are found on a variety of cells, such as neutrophils, monocytes, lymphocytes, basophils, eosinophils, granulocytes, platelets, endothelial cells, and epithelial cells, and can be expressed or activated by the many inflammatory mediators present in asthma.[15]

CLINICAL CONSEQUENCES OF CHRONIC INFLAMMATION

Chronic inflammation is associated with nonspecific BHR and induces asthma exacerbations. Exacerbations are characterized by symptoms or worsening of asthma over a period of days or even weeks. Although the inflammatory nature of chronic asthma is not completely understood, corticosteroids remain the most potent anti-inflammatory drugs for use in the treatment of asthma.

Hyperresponsiveness of the airways to physical, chemical, and pharmacologic stimuli is a hallmark of asthma.[2] BHR also occurs in some patients with chronic bronchitis and allergic rhinitis.[2] Normal healthy subjects also may develop a transient BHR after viral respiratory infections or exposure to ozone. However, the degree of BHR is quantitatively greater in asthmatic patients than in other groups. Bronchial responsiveness of the general population fits a unimodal distribution that is skewed toward increased reactivity. Patients with clinical asthma represent the extreme end of the distribution. The degree of BHR within asthmatics correlates with the clinical course of their disease and medication requirement necessary to control symptoms.[2] Patients with mild symptoms or in remission demonstrate lower levels of responsiveness, although still greater than the normal population.

Our current understanding recognizes that the increased BHR seen in asthma is at least in part owing to an inflammatory response within the airways. Early investigations found correlations with inflammatory cells in BAL fluids and degree of BHR.[2] Newer evidence suggests that airways remodeling, subepithelial fibrosis, or collagen deposition correlates with BHR.[16] Although the precise link is not known, BHR is in part related to the extent of inflammation in the airways.

REMODELING OF THE AIRWAYS

Acute inflammation is a beneficial, nonspecific response of tissues to injury and generally leads to repair and restoration of the normal structure and function. In contrast, asthma represents a chronic inflammatory process of the airways followed by healing. The end result may be an altered structure referred to as a *remodeling of the airways*.[16] Repair involves replacement of injured tissue by parenchymal cells of the same type and replacement by connective tissue and its maturation into scar tissue. In asthma, the repair process can be followed by complete or altered restitution of airways structure and function, presenting as fibrosis and an increase in smooth muscle and mucus gland mass.[16]

The precise mechanisms of remodeling of the airways are under intense study. Airways remodeling is of concern because it may represent an irreversible process that can have more serious sequelae such as the development of chronic obstructive pulmonary disease (COPD).[2] Recent observations in children with asthma (aged 5 to 12 years) suggest that prevention of the progressive loss of lung function in childhood may require recognition and treatment of the disease during the first 5 years of life.[7] Whether there is a mechanistic link between this loss of airway function and structural remodeling of the airway in early life is unknown.

MUCUS PRODUCTION

The mucociliary system is the lung's primary defense mechanism against irritants and infectious agents. Mucus, composed of 95% water and 5% glycoproteins, is produced by bronchial epithelial glands and goblet cells.[7] The lining of the airways consists of a continuous aqueous layer controlled by active ion transport across the epithelium in which water moves toward the lumen along the concentration gradient. Catecholamines and vagal stimulation enhance the ion transport and fluid movement. Mucus transport depends on the viscoelastic properties of the mucus. Mucus that is either too watery or too viscous will not be transported optimally. The exudative inflammatory process and sloughing of epithelial cells into the airway lumen impair mucociliary transport. The bronchial glands are increased in size and the goblet cells are increased in size and number in asthma. Expectorated mucus from patients with asthma tends to have a high viscosity. The mucus plugs in the airways of patients who died in status asthmaticus are tenacious and tend to be connected by mucous strands to the goblet cells. Asthmatic airways also may become plugged with

casts consisting of epithelial and inflammatory cells. Although it is tempting to speculate that death from asthma attacks is a result of the mucus plugging resulting in irreversible obstruction, there is no direct evidence for this. Autopsies of asthmatics who died from other causes have shown similar pathology. In addition, some subjects who have died of sudden severe asthma did not show the characteristic mucus plugging on necropsy.[7]

AIRWAY SMOOTH MUSCLE

The smooth muscle of the airways does not form a uniform coat around the airways but is wrapped around in a connecting network best described as a spiral arrangement.[15] The muscle contraction displays a sphincteric action that is capable of completely occluding the airway lumen. The airway smooth muscle extends from the trachea through the respiratory bronchioles. When expressed as a percentage of wall thickness, the smooth muscle represents 5% of the large central airways and up to 20% of the wall thickness in the bronchioles. Total smooth muscle mass decreases rapidly past the terminal bronchioles to the alveoli, so the contribution of smooth muscle tone to airway diameter in this region is relatively small. In the large airways of asthmatics, smooth muscle may account for 11% of the wall thickness. It is possible that the increased smooth muscle mass of the asthmatic airways is important in magnifying and maintaining BHR in chronic asthma. However, it appears that the hypertrophy and hyperplasia are secondary processes caused by chronic inflammation and are not the primary cause of BHR.[7]

NEURAL CONTROL/NEUROGENIC INFLAMMATION

The airway is innervated by parasympathetic, sympathetic, and nonadrenergic inhibitory nerves.[2] Parasympathetic innervation of the smooth muscle consists of efferent motor fibers in the vagus nerves and sensory afferent fibers in the vagus and other nerves.[15] The normal resting tone of human airway smooth muscle is maintained by vagal efferent activity. Maximum bronchoconstriction mediated by vagal stimulation occurs in the small bronchi and is absent in the small bronchioles. The nonmyelinated C fibers of the afferent system lie immediately beneath the tight junctions between epithelial cells lining the airway lumen.[15] These endings probably represent the irritant receptors of the airways. Stimulation of these irritant receptors by mechanical stimulation, chemical and particulate irritants, and pharmacologic agents such as histamine produces reflex bronchoconstriction.[15]

The nonadrenergic, noncholinergic (NANC) nervous system has been described in the trachea and bronchi. Substance P, neurokinin A, neurokinin B, and vasoactive intestinal peptide (VIP) are the best characterized neurotransmitters in the NANC nervous system.[15] VIP is an inhibitory neurotransmitter in the system. Inflammatory cells in asthma can release peptidases that can degrade VIP, producing exaggerated reflex cholinergic bronchoconstriction. NANC excitatory neuropeptides such as substance P and neurokinin A are released by stimulation of C-fiber sensory nerve endings. The NANC system may play an important role in amplifying inflammation in asthma by releasing nitric oxide (NO).

NITRIC OXIDE

NO is produced by cells within the respiratory tract. It has been thought to be a neurotransmitter of the NANC nervous system.[17] Endogenous NO is generated from the amino acid L-arginine by the enzyme NO synthase.[17] There are three isoforms of NO synthase.

One isoform is induced in response to proinflammatory cytokines, inducible NO synthase (iNOS), in airway epithelial cells and inflammatory cells of asthmatic airways.[17] NO produces smooth muscle relaxation in the vasculature and bronchials; however, it appears to amplify the inflammatory process and is unlikely to be of therapeutic benefit. Recent investigations measuring exhaled NO concentrations have suggested that it may be a useful measure of ongoing lower airways inflammation in patients with asthma and for measuring effectiveness of therapy.[17]

CLINICAL PRESENTATION

CHRONIC ASTHMA

Classic asthma is characterized by episodic dyspnea associated with wheezing; however, the clinical presentation of asthma is as diverse as the number of triggering events (see Clinical Presentation 1). Although wheezing is the characteristic symptom of asthma, the medical literature is replete with the warning that "not all that wheezes is asthma." A wheeze is a high-pitched, whistling sound created by turbulent airflow through an obstructed airway, so any condition that produces significant obstruction can result in wheezing as a symptom. In addition, "all of asthma does not wheeze" is an equally justifiable warning. Patients may present with a chronic persistent cough as their only symptom.[2]

CLINICAL PRESENTATION
CHRONIC AMBULATORY ASTHMA

GENERAL
Asthma is a disease of exacerbation and remission, so the patient may not have any signs or symptoms at the time of exam.

SYMPTOMS
The patient may complain of episodes of dyspnea, chest tightness, coughing (particularly at night), wheezing, or a whistling sound when breathing. These often occur in association with exercise, but also occur spontaneously or in association with known allergens.

SIGNS
Expiratory wheezing on auscultation, dry hacking cough, or signs of atopy (allergic rhinitis and/or eczema) may occur.

LABORATORY
Spirometry demonstrates obstruction (FEV_1/FVC less than 80%) with reversibility following inhaled β_2-agonist administration (at least a 12% improvement in FEV_1).

OTHER DIAGNOSTIC TESTS
A fall in FEV_1 of at least 20% following 6 minutes of near maximal exercise. Elevated eosinophil count and IgE concentration in blood. Elevated FeNO (greater than 12ppb). Positive methacholine challenge (PC_{20} FEV_1 less than 12.5 mg/mL).

There is no single test that can diagnose asthma. The diagnosis is based primarily on a good history[2] (Table 26–2). The patient may have a family history of allergy or asthma or have symptoms of allergic rhinitis.[2] Reversibility of airways obstruction following administration of an inhaled short-acting β_2-agonist provides confirmation but is not by itself diagnostic. Patients with normal values of spirometry can be challenged by exercise or substances that produce

TABLE 26–2. Sample Questions[a] for the Diagnosis and Initial Assessment of Asthma

A "yes" answer to any question suggests that asthma diagnosis is likely. In the past 12 months, . . .

- Have you had a sudden severe episode or recurrent episodes of coughing, wheezing (high-pitched whistling sounds when breathing out), or shortness of breath?
- Have you had colds that "go to the chest" or take more than 10 days to get over?
- Have you had coughing, wheezing, or shortness of breath during a particular season or time of the year?
- Have you had coughing, wheezing, or shortness of breath in certain places or when exposed to certain things (e.g., animals, tobacco smoke, perfumes)?
- Have you used any medications that help you breathe better? How often?
- Are the symptoms relieved when the medications are used?

In the past 4 weeks, have you had coughing, wheezing, or shortness of breath . . .

- At night that has awakened you?
- In the early morning?
- After running, moderate exercise, or other physical activity?

[a] *These questions are recommended by the NAEPP but have not been formally validated.*

---

bronchoconstriction, such as methacholine, to determine if they have hyperresponsive airways, but again, positive challenges are not diagnostic. Newer tests of inflammation in the airways such as induced sputum eosinophil counts and fraction of exhaled nitric oxide (FeNO) are consistent with but not diagnostic of asthma.

Asthma has a widely variable presentation from chronic daily symptoms to only intermittent symptoms. The intervals between symptoms can be days, weeks, months, or years. Asthma also can vary as to its severity. The NAEPP has provided a means of classifying asthma that is presented in Table 26–3.[2] The intermittent and/or chronic nature of symptoms does not necessarily determine the severity of symptoms during exacerbations. The severity is determined by lung function and symptoms prior to therapy, as well as by the amount of medication required to control the patient's symptoms. Patients can present with a range from mild intermittent symptoms that require no medications or only occasional use of short-acting inhaled β_2-agonists to severe chronic asthma symptoms despite receiving multiple medications. In addition, patients can change severity classifications based on exposures to triggering substances.

SEVERE ACUTE ASTHMA

Uncontrolled asthma, with its inherent variability, can progress to an acute state where inflammation, airways edema, excessive accumulation of mucus, and severe bronchospasm result in a profound airways narrowing that is poorly responsive to usual bronchodilator therapy[2,10] (see Clinical Presentation 2). Although this progression is the most common scenario, some patients experience rapid onset or hyperacute attacks.[2,10] Hyperacute attacks are associated with neutrophilic as opposed to eosinophilic infiltration and resolve rapidly with bronchodilator therapy, suggesting that smooth muscle spasm is the major pathogenic mechanism.[10] In most cases, emergency department visits for severe acute asthma represent the failure of an adequate therapeutic regimen for chronic asthma. Underutilization of anti-inflammatory drugs and excessive reliance on short-acting inhaled β_2-agonists are

TABLE 26–3. Classification of Asthma Severity: Clinical Features Before Treatment

	Symptoms	Lung Function[a]
Step 1 Mild Intermittent	Daytime ≤ 2 times/wk Asymptomatic between exacerbations Exacerbations brief (from a few hours to a few days); intensity may vary Nocturnal ≤ 2 times/mo	FEV_1 or PEF ≥ 80% PEF variability < 20%
Step 2 Mild Persistent	Daytime > 2 times/wk but < 1 time/day Exacerbations may affect activity Nocturnal > 2 times/mo	FEV_1 or PEF ≥ 80% PEF variability 20% to 30%
Step 3 Moderate Persistent	Daily symptoms Daily use of inhaled, short-acting β_2-agonists Exacerbations affect activity Exacerbations ≥ 2 times/wk; may last days Nocturnal > 1 time/wk	FEV_1 or PEF > 60% to < 80% PEF variability > 30%
Step 4 Severe Persistent	Continual symptoms Limited physical activity Frequent exacerbations Nocturnal frequent	FEV_1 or PEF ≤ 60% PEF variability > 30%

[a]The presence of one of the features of severity is sufficient to place a patient in that category. An individual should be assigned to the most severe grade in which any feature occurs. The characteristics noted are general and may overlap because asthma is highly variable. Furthermore, an individual's classification may change over time. Patients at any level of severity can have mild, moderate, or severe exacerbations. Some patients with intermittent asthma experience severe and life-threatening exacerbations separated by long periods of normal lung function and no symptoms.

CLINICAL PRESENTATION
SEVERE ACUTE ASTHMA

GENERAL
An episode can progress over several days or hours (usual scenario) or progresses rapidly over 1 to 2 hours.

SYMPTOMS
The patient is anxious in acute distress and complains of severe dyspnea, shortness of breath, chest tightness, or burning. The patient is only able to say a few words with each breath. Symptoms are unresponsive to usual measures (inhaled β_2-agonist administration.

SIGNS
Signs include expiratory and inspiratory wheezing on auscultation (breath sounds may be diminished with very severe obstruction), dry hacking cough, tachypnea, tachycardia, pale or cyanotic skin, hyperinflated chest with intercostal and supraclavicular retractions, hypoxic seizures if very severe, normal or slightly elevated temperature.

LABORATORY
PEF and/or FEV_1 less than 50% of normal predicted values. Decreased arterial oxygen (PaO_2), and O_2 saturations by pulse oximetry (SaO_2 less than 90% on room air is moderate to severe). Decreased arterial or capillary CO_2 if mild, but in the normal range or increased in moderate to severe obstruction.

OTHER DIAGNOSTIC TESTS
Blood gases to assess metabolic acidosis (lactic acidosis) in severe obstruction. Complete blood count if there are signs of infection (fever and purulent sputum). Serum electrolytes as therapy with β_2-agonist and corticosteroids can lower serum potassium and magnesium and increase glucose. Chest radiograph if signs of consolidation on auscultation.

the major risk factors for severe exacerbations.[2] A blunted perception of airway obstruction may predispose certain asthmatics to fatal attacks.[2] This may occur more commonly in patients who have labile asthma (fluctuation of daily peak flows of 50% or greater).

EXERCISE-INDUCED BRONCHOSPASM

During vigorous exercise, pulmonary functions (FEV_1 and peak expiratory flow [PEF]) in asthmatic patients increase during the first few minutes but then begin to decrease after 6 to 8 minutes (Fig. 26–3).[18] Exercise-induced bronchospasm (EIB) is defined as a drop in FEV_1 of greater than 15% to 20% of baseline (pre-exercise value).[2,18] Most

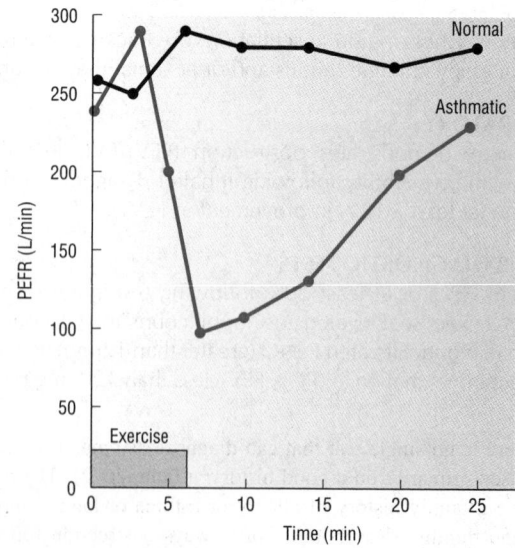

FIGURE 26–3. Typical responses to exercise in a normal subject and an asthmatic subject. Note the initial bronchodilation. PEFR = peak expiratory flow rate.

studies suggest that 70% to 90% of asthmatics experience EIB.[2] exact pathogenesis of EIB is unknown, but heat loss and/or water loss from the central airways appears to play an important role.[18] EIB is provoked more easily in cold, dry air, and warm, humid air can blunt or block it.[18] A number of studies have demonstrated increased plasma histamine and tryptase concentrations during EIB, suggesting a role for mast cell degranulation.[18]

A refractory period following EIB lasts up to 3 hours after exercise. During this period, repeat exercise of the same intensity produces either no decrease in pulmonary function or a drop of less than 50% of the initial response.[18] The refractory period is thought to be caused by an acute depletion of mast cell mediators and time required for their repletion. Patients with known refractoriness to exercise will still respond to histamine, so acute hyporesponsiveness of airway smooth muscle does not appear to be a factor.[18]

Exercise-induced bronchospasm is believed to be a reflection of the increased BHR of asthmatics. A correlation, though not perfect, exists between EIB and reactivity to histamine and methacholine.[18] Other patient groups with bronchial hyperresponsiveness (e.g., after viral infection, cystic fibrosis, or allergic rhinitis) show bronchoconstriction after exercise to a lesser degree (5% to 10%) than asthmatics (20% to 40%).[18] Patients will not always demonstrate the same sensitivity. During periods of remission, they often have a decreased sensitivity to the same degree of exercise. Finally, a number of children and adults with EIB are otherwise normal, without symptoms or abnormal pulmonary function except in association with exercise. Elite athletes have a higher prevalence of EIB than the general population.[18]

NOCTURNAL ASTHMA

Worsening of asthma during sleep is referred to as *nocturnal asthma*. Patients with nocturnal asthma exhibit significant falls in pulmonary function between bedtime and awakening.[2,10] Typically, their lung function reaches a nadir at 3 to 4 A.M. Although the pathogenesis of this phenomenon is unknown, it has been associated with diurnal patterns of endogenous cortisol secretion and circulating epinephrine.[10] Direct evidence for an inflammatory component to nocturnal asthma includes increased circulating histamine and activated eosinophils and leukotriene excretion at night associated with increased hyperresponsiveness to methacholine.[10]

Numerous other factors that may affect nocturnal worsening of asthma, including allergies and improper environmental control, gastroesophageal reflux, and sinusitis, also must be considered when evaluating these patients.[2] Most experts consider nocturnal asthma to be a sign of inadequately treated persistent asthma.[2,10]

FACTORS CONTRIBUTING TO ASTHMA SEVERITY

VIRAL INFECTIONS

Viral infections are primarily responsible for exacerbations of asthma.[2] Viral upper respiratory tract infections are a major precipitant of acute asthma in children, being involved in up to 20% to 40% of acute episodes.[2] Infants are particularly susceptible to airways obstruction and wheezing with viral infections because of their small airways. The most common cause of exacerbations in both children and adults is the common rhinovirus.[2] Other viruses isolated include respiratory syncytial virus (RSV), parainfluenza virus, coronavirus, and influenza viruses. The inflammatory response to viral infection is thought to be associated directly with the increasing BHR. Certain viruses (RSV and parainfluenza virus) are capable of inducing spe-

cific IgE antibodies, and rhinovirus can activate eosinophils directly in asthmatics. The increase in asthma symptoms and BHR that occurs may last for days or weeks following resolution of the symptoms of the viral infection. The NAEPP recommends annual influenza vaccinations for patients with asthma.[2]

ENVIRONMENTAL AND OCCUPATIONAL FACTORS

Agents and events and the mechanisms that are known to trigger asthma are listed in Table 26–1.[2,10] The general mechanisms are unknown but presumably are the result of epithelial damage and inflammation in the airway mucosa. Ozone and sulfur dioxide, common components of air pollution, have been used to induce BHR in animals. Exposure to 0.2 ppm ozone for 2 to 3 hours can induce bronchoconstriction and increase BHR in asthmatics.[2,10] Sulfur dioxide in the ambient atmosphere is highly irritating. It presumably induces bronchoconstriction through mast cell or irritant-receptor involvement.[10] Asthma produced by repeated prolonged exposure to industrial inhalants is a significant health problem. It has been estimated that occupational asthma accounts for 2% of all asthmatic persons.[13] Persons with occupational asthma have the typical symptoms of asthma with cough, dyspnea, and wheeze. Typically, the symptoms are related to work and improve on weekends and during vacations.[13] In some instances, symptoms may persist even after termination of exposure.[13]

PSYCHOLOGICAL FACTORS

Emotions and stress rarely can precipitate attacks of asthma but more commonly worsen an attack in progress.[2] Bronchoconstriction from psychological factors appears to be mediated primarily through excess parasympathetic input. Atropine has been shown to block experimental psychogenic bronchoconstriction. It is most important to emphasize to patients and to parents of asthmatic children that asthma is not an emotional disease; however, calming influences and relaxation techniques may benefit the patient who becomes severely emotionally distraught during an asthma attack.

SINUSITIS AND RHINITIS

Disorders of the upper respiratory tract, particularly sinusitis and rhinitis, have been linked with asthma for many years. As many as 40% to 50% of asthmatics have abnormal sinus radiographs.[2] However, chronic sinusitis may just represent a nonbacterial coexisting condition with allergic asthmatics because the histologic changes in the paranasal sinuses are similar to those seen in the lung and nose.[2] Some studies have shown that asthma symptoms improve with treatment of sinusitis. The mechanism by which sinusitis aggravates asthma is unknown. The treatment of allergic rhinitis with inhaled corticosteroids and cromolyn but not antihistamines will reduce BHR in asthmatic patients.[2] It has been postulated that transport of mucus chemotactic factors and inflammatory mediators from nasal passages during allergic rhinitis into the lung may accentuate BHR.

GASTROESOPHAGEAL REFLUX

Gastroesophageal reflux has been associated with asthma for many years.[2,10] Nocturnal asthma may be associated with nighttime reflux.[10] Reflux of acidic gastric contents into the esophagus is thought to initiate a vagally mediated reflex bronchoconstriction.[10] Also of concern is that most medications that decrease airways smooth muscle tone have a relaxant effect on gastroesophageal sphincter tone as well. The therapeutic approach most commonly taken for patients with gastroesophageal reflux and asthma is to initiate standard antireflux therapy and observe the asthma symptoms.[2]

MENSTRUATION-RELATED ASTHMA

Premenstrual worsening of asthma has been reported in as many as 30% to 40% of women in some studies, whereas worsening of pulmonary functions has been reported even in women not aware of worsening symptoms.[19] The pathophysiology is uncertain because estrogen replacement in postmenopausal women has been shown to worsen asthma, whereas estradiol and progesterone administration have been variably reported to improve or have no effect on asthma in women with premenstrual asthma.[19,20] Studies would indicate that, in general, bronchial responsiveness and symptoms improve in asthmatics during pregnancy.[10] The clinical significance of menstruation-related asthma is still unclear because some studies have reported that up to 50% of emergency department visits by women were premenstrual, whereas others have reported no association with menstrual phase.[19,21]

FOODS, DRUGS, AND ADDITIVES

Documentation in the literature of food allergens as triggers for asthma is not available.[10] However, additives, specifically sulfites used as preservatives, can trigger life-threatening asthma exacerbations. Beer, wine, dried fruit, and open salad bars in particular have high concentrations of metabisulfites.[2] Severe oral corticosteroid-dependent patients should be warned about ingesting foods processed with sulfites. Another additive producing bronchospasm is benzalkonium chloride, which is found as a preservative in some nebulizer solutions of antiasthmatic drugs.[22]

Aspirin and other nonsteroidal anti-inflammatory drugs can precipitate an attack in up to 20% of adults with asthma.[23] The mechanism is related to cyclooxygenase inhibition, and 5-lipoxygenase inhibition can prevent the symptoms.[23] The prevalence increases with age. The greatest frequency occurs in severe corticosteroid-dependent asthmatics in their fourth and fifth decades who also have perennial rhinitis and nasal polyposis (presence of several polyps).[23] Other drugs that do not precipitate bronchospasm but which prevent its reversal are the β-blocking agents.[2,10]

▶ TREATMENT: Asthma

▦ AEROSOL THERAPY FOR ASTHMA

◀4 ◀5 Aerosol delivery of drugs for asthma has the advantage of being site-specific and thus enhancing the therapeutic ratio.[2,24] Inhalation of short-acting β_2-agonists provides more rapid bronchodilation than either parenteral or oral administration, as well as the greatest degree of protection against EIB and other challenges.[25] Inhaled corticosteroids produce a greater reduction of BHR than corticosteroids administered systemically.[2] Specific agents (e.g., cromolyn, nedocromil, formoterol, salmeterol, and ipratropium) are only effective by inhalation.[2,24] Given the international ban on the production and use of chlorofluorocarbons (CFCs), the manufacturers of CFC-propelled metered-dose inhalers (MDIs) are developing new devices for delivering topically active medication.[2,24] Therefore, an understanding of aerosol drug delivery is essential to optimal asthma therapy. Table 26–4 lists the factors determining lung deposition of therapeutic aerosols.

▦ DEVICE DETERMINANTS OF DELIVERY

Devices used to generate therapeutic aerosols include jet nebulizers, ultrasonic nebulizers, MDIs, and dry-powder inhalers (DPIs).

TABLE 26–4. Factors Determining Lung Deposition of Aerosols

Device	Device Factors	Patient Factors
Metered-dose inhaler (MDI)	Canister held inverted	Inspiratory flow (slow, deep)
	Formulation (CFC, HFA, solution, suspension)	Breath-holding
	Actuator cleanliness	Coordinating actuation with inhalation
	Addition of a spacer device	Priming and shaking the device
Dry-powder inhaler (DPI)	Device cleanliness	Inspiratory flow (deep, forceful)
	Resistance to inhalation	Tilting head back
	Humidity	Maintaining parallel to ground once activated
Jet nebulizer (small volume)	Volume fill (3–6 mL)	Inspiratory flow (slow, deep)
	Gas flow (6–12 L/min)	Breath-holding
	Dead-space volume	Tapping nebulizer
	Open versus closed system	
	Thumb-activating valve	
	Mouthpiece versus facemask	
Ultrasonic nebulizer	Volume fill	Inspiratory flow (slow, deep)
	Not effective for suspensions	Breath-holding
	Mouthpiece versus facemask	Tapping nebulizer
Spacer device	Volume (≥650 mL)	Inspiratory flow (slow, deep)
	One-way valves	Time between actuation and inhalation (<5 s)
	Holding chamber versus opened-ended	Cleaning with detergent to reduce static
	Metal versus plastic	Multiple actuations decrease delivery
	Mouthpiece versus facemask	Coordination of actuation and inhalation for the simple open-tube spacers

The single most important device factor determining the site of aerosol deposition is particle size.[24] Devices for delivering therapeutic aerosols generate particles with aerodynamic diameters from 0.5 to 35 microns.[24] Particles larger than 10 microns deposit in the oropharynx, particles between 5 and 10 microns deposit in the trachea and large bronchi, particles 1 to 5 microns in size reach the lower airways, and particles smaller than 0.5 microns act as a gas and are exhaled. In asthma, the airways, not the alveoli, are the target for delivery. Respirable particles are deposited in the airways by three mechanisms: (1) inertial impaction, (2) gravitational sedimentation, and (3) Brownian diffusion.[24] The first two mechanisms are the most important for therapeutic aerosols and probably are the only factors that can be manipulated by patients.

Each delivery device within a classification generates specific aerosol characteristics, so extrapolation of delivery data from one device cannot be done for the other devices in the class. For instance, MDIs can deliver 5% to 50% of the actuated dose; DPIs, 10% to 30% of the labeled dose; and nebulizers, 2% to 15% of the starting dose.[24] MDIs and DPIs are portable and convenient, unlike nebulizers. MDIs consist of a pressurized canister with a metering valve; the canister contains active drug, low-vapor-pressure propellants such as chlorofluorocarbon (CFC) or hydrofluoroalkane (HFA), cosolvents, and/or surfactants.[24] With any change in these components, the Food and Drug Administration (FDA) considers it to be a new drug that requires stability, safety, and efficacy studies prior to approval. The drug is either in solution or a suspended micronized powder. In order to disperse the suspension for accurate delivery, the canister must be shaken. The metering chamber measures a liquid volume, and therefore, the device must be held with the valve stem downward so that the chamber is covered with liquid[24] (Fig. 26–4). When the canister is actuated, the device releases the propellant and drug in a forceful spray whose particles are large (mass median aerodynamic diameter [MMAD] = 45 microns)[24] (see Fig. 26–4). As evaporation occurs, the particle size is reduced to a final MMAD of 0.5 to 5.5 microns depending on the MDI. The aerosol cloud of a CFC-propelled MDI extends at least 10 in beyond the MDI at the lowest MMAD, and that of an HFA-propelled MDI extends about 6 in.[24]

The breath-actuated MDI Autohaler, is cocked with a lever to "load" the dose of medication, a baffle is opened by inspiratory pressure, and the dose is expelled from the canister metering chamber.[24] While the need for hand-lung coordination for proper actuation is reduced significantly with breath-actuated MDIs, these devices do not allow the use of a spacer device.

Spacer devices are used frequently with an MDI to decrease oropharyngeal deposition and enhance lung delivery.[2,26] However, not all spacer devices produce similar effects. The design of spacers varies from simple open-ended tubes that separate the MDI from the mouth to holding chambers with one-way valves that open during inhalation (the preferred system). The purpose of a spacer is to allow evaporation of the propellant prior to inhalation. Use of a spacer allows inhalation after actuation of the device, obviating the need for good hand-lung coordination, and permits a greater number of drug particles to achieve a respirable droplet size.[26] Additionally, the large particles that normally would deposit in the oropharynx "rain out" in the spacer.[26] All the available spacers significantly reduce oropharyngeal deposition from MDIs, with the holding-chamber devices being superior to the open-ended tubes.[26] This reduction in oropharyngeal deposition is an important factor in reducing local adverse effects (i.e., hoarseness and thrush) from inhaled corticosteroids.[24] The change in lung delivery depends on both the MDI and the drug, where one spacer device may enhance delivery with one MDI preparation and decrease delivery with others.[26] Finally, over time, holding chambers can build up static electricity that attracts small particles to the sides of the chamber, significantly reducing aerosol availability. It is recommended that spacers be washed weekly with household detergent, with a single rinse, and allowed to drip dry.[24]

Dry micronized powders can be inhaled directly into the lung. Four DPIs for asthma are available for use in the United States (i.e., Diskus, Rotahaler, Turbuhaler, and Aerolizer), with others under development.[24] Each has unique characteristics with advantages and disadvantages (Table 26–5). The primary advantage of DPIs is that they are breath-actuated and require minimal hand-lung coordination.[26] Some DPIs are more flow-dependent than others.[26] Thus, similar to MDIs and spacers, delivery data from one DPI cannot be extrapolated to another.

Nebulizers come in two basic types, the jet nebulizer and the ultrasonic nebulizer. Jet nebulizers produce an aerosol from a liquid solution or suspension placed in a cup. A tube connected to a stream of compressed air or oxygen flows up through the bottom and draws the liquid up an adjacent open-ended tube.[24] The air and liquid strike a baffle, creating a droplet cloud that is then inhaled.[24] Ultrasonic nebulizers produce an aerosol by vibrating liquid lying above a transducer at speeds of about 1 mHz.[24] Both produce similar degrees of lung deposition, with the exception that ultrasonic nebulizers are ineffective for nebulizing micronized suspensions.[26] The aerosol output and lung delivery vary significantly among the commercially available jet nebulizers even when operated in the same manner.[24] Increasing fill volume will increase the total amount of drug delivered; however, it also will take longer for the patient to nebulize the dose.[24] The MMAD of the droplets is related directly to the gas flow, with flows of 5 to 12 L/min providing an aerosol cloud with an MMAD of 4 to 8 microns for most jet nebulizers.[26]

■ PATIENT DETERMINANTS OF DELIVERY (See Table 26–4)

◀6◀ ◀7◀ The most important patient factor determining aerosol deposition is inspiratory flow.[2,24] High inspiratory flows increase the degree of deposition owing to impaction of particles of any size, thereby increasing deposition centrally (i.e., throat and large airways) and decreasing peripheral deposition. Holding chambers enhance the clinical efficacy in patients with poor hand-lung coordination but may offer no advantage in patients who can use an MDI optimally alone.[24] Optimal inspiratory flow for most MDIs is slow and deep (approximately 30 L/min).[24] In general, DPIs require

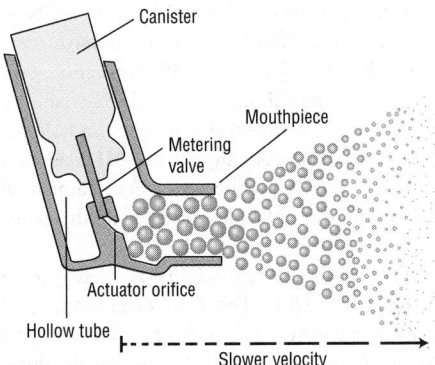

FIGURE 26–4. Illustration of a metered-dose inhaler demonstrating the particle size difference as the aerosol cloud extends outward.

TABLE 26–5. Characteristics of Various Inhalation Devices

Device	Drugs	Breath-Activated	Dose Counter	Other Excipients	Disadvantages
CFC MDI	All classes	No	No	Propellants, surfactants	Requires coordination of actuation and inhalation Large pharyngeal deposition Difficult to teach
HFA-MDI	Albuterol	No	No	Propellants, surfactants, cosolvents	Same as CFC MDI
	Beclomethasone	No	No		
Autohaler MDI	Pirbuterol	Yes	No	CFC propellant, surfactant	Requires rapid inhalation to activate
MDI plus holding chamber	All classes	No	No		More expensive than MDI alone; less portable; some payers will not pay; inconsistent effect on delivery
Jet nebulizers	All classes except long-acting β_2-agonists	No	—	Preservatives in some solutions	Significant interbrand variability; expensive and time-consuming; less efficient than MDIs; contamination possible; preparations may be light- and temperature-sensitive (short shelf-life)
Ulrasonic nebulizer	Cromolyn solution short acting β_2-agonist solutions	No	—	Preservatives in some solutions	Same as for jet nebulizers plus cannot be used for suspensions
Rotahaler	Albuterol	Yes	—	Lactose filler	Single-dose capsule; requires high inspiratory flow
Turbuhaler	Budesonide	Yes	Indicator for last 20 doses	No	Requires high inspiratory flow (60 L/min). Pharyngeal deposition. Not approved for <6 years of age
Diskus	Fluticasone Salmeterol Fluticasone/salmeterol	Yes	Yes	Lactose filler	Not approved for <4 years of age
Aerolizer	Formoterol	Yes	—	Lactose filler	Single-dose capsules. Not approved for <5 years of age Requires high inspiratory flow (≥60 L/min)
Twisthaler	Mometasone	Yes	Yes	Lactose filler	Not approved for <12 years of age

higher inspiratory flows (≥60 L/min) and a change in inhalation technique (i.e., deep, forceful inspiration) for optimal actuation, which, in turn, increases the amount of drug delivered to the larger central airways.[26] However, this difference in delivery may not produce clinically significant differences.[24] Patients should be cautioned not to exhale into DPIs because this causes loss of dose and moistens the dry powder, causing aggregation into larger particles. Patient factors that cannot be controlled include interpatient variability in airway geometry (particularly the differences between children and adults)[26] and the effects of bronchospasm, edema, and mucus hypersecretion. Mild obstruction increases aerosol deposition; however, severe obstruction probably leads to increased central deposition from impaction.[24] The absolute delivery to the lung is not as important as consistency of delivery, assuming that a sufficient dose to produce the desired therapeutic effect is achieved. No single inhalation device is the best for all patients. Table 26–5 lists the differing characteristics of inhalation devices.

Appropriate inhalation technique is essential to achieve optimal drug delivery and therapeutic effect.[2,10] The components are illustrated in Figure 26–5. Approximately 50% to 80% of a dose from MDIs and DPIs impacts on the oropharynx and is then swallowed;

the rest is either left in the device or exhaled.[26] It is important that actuation occurs during inhalation, although the time during inspiration is unimportant.[2,26] Although radiolabeled studies indicate improved delivery by holding the actuator 2 to 3 cm in front of an open mouth to allow more evaporation and less impaction, physiologic studies with bronchodilators have failed to document an advantage for this method.[24] Many patients do not use their MDIs optimally, and patient instruction with demonstration is the most effective means of improving inhaler technique.[2,24,26] Even with instruction, up to 30% of patients, particularly young children and the elderly, cannot master the use of an MDI. For these patients, attachment of a holding-chamber device to the MDI or use of a breath-actuated MDI can improve efficacy significantly.[2,24] Mouth rinsing following treatment with MDI- and DPI-inhaled corticosteroids is important to minimize local effects and oral absorption.[26]

Delivery from high-resistance DPIs is more flow-dependent than from low-resistance DPIs. The Turbuhaler device has a greater flow dependency than the Aerolizer and the Diskus.[24,26] Children 6 to 12 years of age received approximately one-half the dose of radiolabeled budesonide via Turbuhaler than those older than 12 years of age, whereas children younger than 6 years of age received

Steps for Using Your Inhaler

Please demonstrate your inhaler technique at every visit.

1. Remove the cap and hold inhaler upright.
2. Shake the inhaler.
3. Tilt your head back slightly and breathe out slowly.
4. Position the inhaler in one of the following ways (A or B is optimal, but C is acceptable for those who have difficulty with A or B. C is required for breath-activated inhalers):

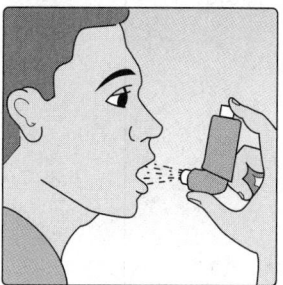
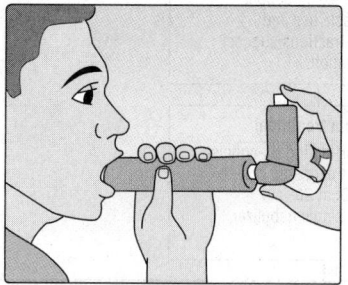
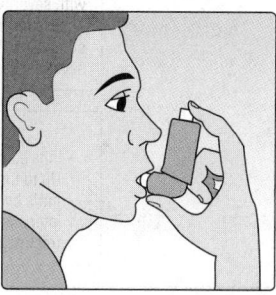
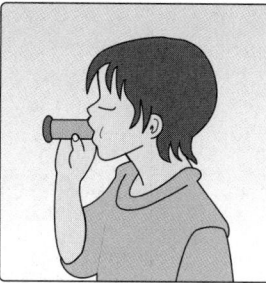

A Open mouth with inhaler 1 to 2 inches away.

B Use spacer/holding chamber (that is recommended especially for young children and for people using corticosteroids).

C In the mouth. Do not use for corticosteroids.

D NOTE: Inhaled dry powder capsules require a different inhalation technique. To use a dry powder inhaler, it is important to close the mouth tightly around the mouthpiece of the inhaler and to inhale rapidly.

5. Press down on the inhaler to release medication as you start to breathe in slowly.
6. Breathe in slowly (3 to 5 seconds).
7. Hold your breath for 10 seconds to allow the medicine to reach deeply into your lungs.
8. Repeat puff as directed. Waiting 1 minute between puffs may permit second puff to penetrate your lungs better.
9. Spacers/holding chambers are useful for all patients. They are particularly recommended for young children and older adults and for use with corticosteroids.

Avoid common inhaler mistakes. Follow these inhaler tips:

• Breathe out *before* pressing your inhaler.
• Inhale *slowly.*
• Breathe in through your mouth, not your nose.
• Press down on your inhaler at the *start* of inhalation (or within the first second of inhalation).
• Keep inhaling as you press down on inhaler.
• Press your inhaler only *once* while you are inhaling (one breath for each puff).
• Make sure you breathe in evenly and deeply.

NOTE: Other inhalers are becoming available in addition to those illustrated above. Different types of inhalers require different techniques.

FIGURE 26–5. Instructions for inhaler use from the NAEPP Expert Panel Report 2.[2]

one-quarter of the dose.[26] The Aerolizer and the Diskus deliver about 15% of the dose to the airways, and this appears to be similar at both 30 and 60 L/min inspiratory flows; both have been approved for children aged 5 and 4 years, respectively.[7,26]

► TREATMENT: Severe Acute Asthma

The primary goal is prevention of life-threatening asthma by early recognition of signs of deterioration and early intervention. As such, the principal goals of treatment include[2]

• Correction of significant hypoxemia
• Rapid reversal of airflow obstruction
• Reduction of the likelihood of recurrence of severe airflow obstruction
• Development of a written action plan in case of a further exacerbation

These goals are best achieved by early initiation of treatment and close monitoring of objective measures of oxygenation and lung function.[2] Early response to treatment as measured by the improvement in FEV_1 at 30 minutes following inhaled β_2-agonists is the best predictor of outcome.[27] Providing adequate oxygen supplementation to maintain oxygen (O_2) saturations above 90% (or above 95% in pregnant women) is essential. In children younger than 6 years of age, in whom lung function measures are difficult to obtain, a combination of objective (e.g., oxygen saturation, capillary CO_2, respiratory rate, and heart rate) and subjective measures may be used to assess severity.[2,10]

The primary therapy of acute exacerbations is pharmacologic, which includes inhaled short-acting β_2-agonists and, depending on the severity, systemic corticosteroids and O_2 (Figs. 26–6 and 26–7). It is important that therapy not be delayed, so the initial history and physical examination should be obtained while initial therapy is being provided. Patients at risk for life-threatening exacerbations require special attention. Risk factors include a history of previous severe asthma exacerbations (e.g., hospitalizations, intubations, or hypoxic seizures), complicating illnesses (e.g., cardiac disease, diabetes, illicit drug use, or psychosis), use of more than two canisters per month of short-acting inhaled β_2-agonists, and current intake of oral corticosteroids or recent withdrawal from oral corticosteroids.[10]

A complete blood count may be appropriate for patients with fever or purulent sputum, but many patients will have a leukocytosis

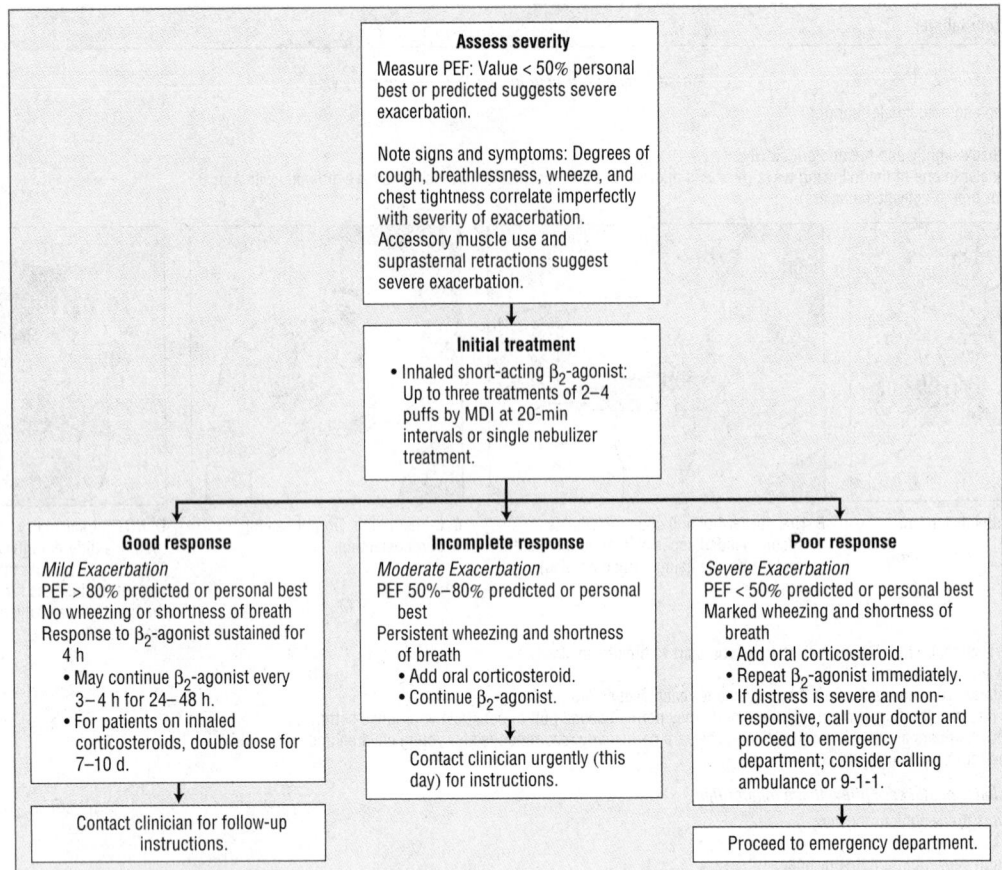

Assess severity

Measure PEF: Value < 50% personal best or predicted suggests severe exacerbation.

Note signs and symptoms: Degrees of cough, breathlessness, wheeze, and chest tightness correlate imperfectly with severity of exacerbation. Accessory muscle use and suprasternal retractions suggest severe exacerbation.

Initial treatment
- Inhaled short-acting β_2-agonist: Up to three treatments of 2–4 puffs by MDI at 20-min intervals or single nebulizer treatment.

Good response

Mild Exacerbation
PEF > 80% predicted or personal best
No wheezing or shortness of breath
Response to β_2-agonist sustained for 4 h
- May continue β_2-agonist every 3–4 h for 24–48 h.
- For patients on inhaled corticosteroids, double dose for 7–10 d.

Contact clinician for follow-up instructions.

Incomplete response

Moderate Exacerbation
PEF 50%–80% predicted or personal best
Persistent wheezing and shortness of breath
- Add oral corticosteroid.
- Continue β_2-agonist.

Contact clinician urgently (this day) for instructions.

Poor response

Severe Exacerbation
PEF < 50% predicted or personal best
Marked wheezing and shortness of breath
- Add oral corticosteroid.
- Repeat β_2-agonist immediately.
- If distress is severe and non-responsive, call your doctor and proceed to emergency department; consider calling ambulance or 9-1-1.

Proceed to emergency department.

FIGURE 26–6. Home management of acute asthma exacerbation. Patients at risk for asthma-related death should receive immediate clinical attention after initial treatment. Additional therapy may be required. *(From ref. 2.)*

from a viral infection or secondary to corticosteroid administration. Routine chest radiographs have not been shown to be of value unless physical findings suggestive of consolidations or pneumothoraces are present.[2] Serum electrolytes should be monitored if high-dose continuous inhaled or systemic β_2-agonists are to be used because they can produce transient decreases in potassium, magnesium, and phosphate.[27] The combination of high-dose β_2-agonists and systemic corticosteroids occasionally may result in excessive elevations of glucose.[27]

Initial response should be achieved within minutes, and most patients experience significant improvement within the first 30 to 60 minutes of therapy, with most patients doubling their FEV_1 or PEF.[28] In patients ultimately admitted to the hospital, only a 10% to 20% predicted improvement is seen within the first 2 hours. Hypoxemia, primarily a result of ventilation-perfusion mismatch, is immediately correctable by low-flow oxygen.[2] While reversal of lung function into the normal range may take 12 to 24 hours, complete restoration takes much longer—up to 3 to 7 days.[10,27] A strategy to prevent recurrence such as systemic corticosteroids and PEF monitoring should be used.[2,10] It is essential to provide the patient with a self-management plan that includes a written action plan for dealing with exacerbations. Patients at risk for severe exacerbations should be taught how to use a peak-flow meter and monitor morning peak flows at home.[2,10] In young children, an increased respiratory rate, increased heart rate, and inability to speak more than one or two words between breaths are signs of severe obstruction.[2] Oxygen saturations by pulse oximetry and peak flows should be measured in all patients not

completely responding to initial intensive inhaled β_2-agonist therapy. Initially, on admission, the peak flows or clinical symptoms should be monitored every 2 to 4 hours. Prior to discharge from the emergency department or hospital, the patient should be given a sufficient supply of prednisone, taught the purpose of the medications and proper inhaler technique, and given an appointment for a follow-up visit.[2]

Early recognition of deterioration and aggressive treatment are the keys to successful treatment of acute asthma exacerbations. Thus patient and/or parent education teaching self-management skills and written action plans for early institution of therapy for acute exacerbations improve outcomes.[7] For more moderate to severe patients, this therapeutic plan also may include the availability of oral prednisone to begin at home.[2] Easy access by telephone to health care providers is also needed. Because of the rapid progression to severe asthma that can occur, patients and parents should be encouraged to communicate promptly with their asthma care provider during an exacerbation. Systemic corticosteroids and aggressive use of inhaled β_2-agonists continue to be the cornerstones of therapy for acute severe asthma exacerbations.[2]

Figures 26–6 and 26–7 illustrate the recommended therapies for the treatment of acute asthma exacerbations in home and emergency department/hospital settings, respectively.[2] The dosages of the drugs for acute severe asthma are provided in Table 26–6.[2,7] Institutions should strongly consider developing critical-pathways/treatment algorithms for their emergency departments because their implementation has been shown to improve outcomes and decrease the cost of care.[27]

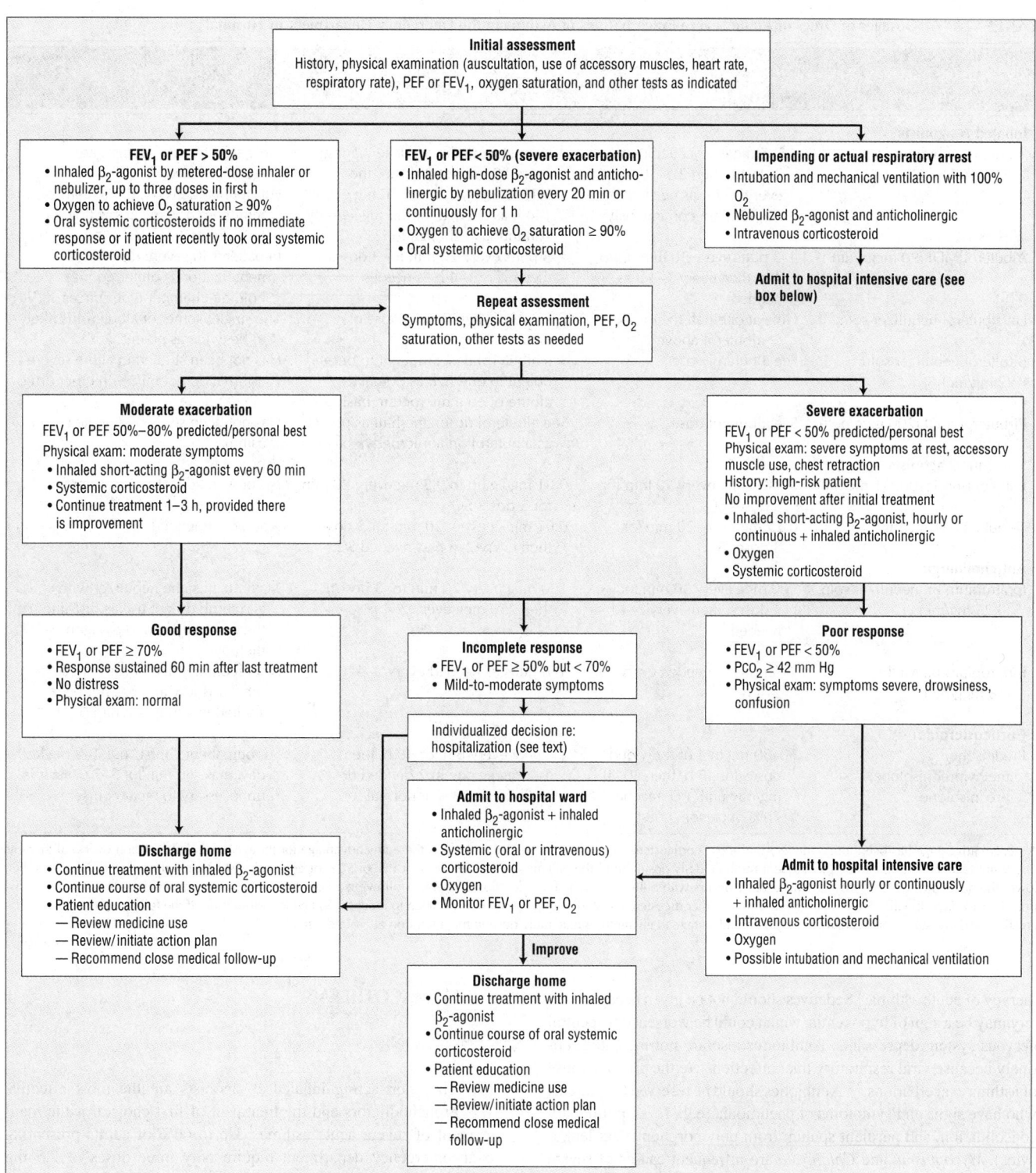

FIGURE 26–7. Emergency department and hospital care of acute asthma exacerbations. *(From ref. 2.)*

NONPHARMACOLOGIC THERAPY

Infants and young children may be mildly dehydrated owing to increased insensible loss, vomiting, and decreased intake.[2] Unless dehydration has occurred, increased fluid therapy is not indicated in acute asthma management because the capillary leak from cytokines and increased negative intrathoracic pressures may promote edema in the airways.[2] Correction of significant dehydration is always indicated, and the urine specific gravity may help to guide therapy in young children, in whom the state of hydration may be difficult to determine.[27] Chest physical therapy and mucolytics are not indicated in the

TABLE 26–6. Dosages of Drugs of Acute Severe Exacerbations of Asthma in the Emergency Department or Hospital

Medications	Dosages		Comments
	>6 Years Old	≤6 Years Old	
Inhaled β-agonists			
Albuterol nebulizer soln. (5 mg/mL)	2.5–5 mg every 20 min for 3 doses, then 2.5–10 mg every 1–4 h as needed, or 10–15 mg/h continuously	0.15 mg/kg (minimum dose 2.5 mg) every 20 min for 3 doses, then 0.15–0.3 mg/kg up to 10 mg every 1–4 h as needed, or 0.5 mg/kg/h by continuous nebulization	Only selective β2-agonists are recommended. For optimal delivery, dilute aerosols to minimum of 4 mL at gas flow of 6–8 L/min
Albuterol MDI (90 mcg/puff)	4–8 puffs every 30 min up to 4 h, then every 1–4 h as needed	4–8 puffs every 20 min for 3 doses, then every 1–4 h as needed	In patients in severe distress, nebulization is preferred; use holding-chamber-type spacer
Levalbuterol nebulizer soln.	Give at one-half the mg dose of albuterol above	Give at one-half the mg dose of albuterol above	The single isomer of albuterol is likely to be twice as potent
Bitolterol nebulizer soln. (2 mg/mL)	See albuterol dose	See albuterol dose; thought to be as potent to one-half as potent as albuterol on a microgram basis	Has not been studied in acute severe asthma; do not mix with other drugs
Pirbuterol MDI (200 mcg/puff)	See albuterol dose	See albuterol dose; one-half as potent as albuterol on a microgram basis	Has not been studied in acute severe asthma
Systemic β-agonists			
Epinephrine 1:1000 (1 mg/mL)	0.3–0.5 mg every 20 min for 3 doses SQ	0.01 mg/kg up to 0.5 mg every 20 min for 3 doses SQ	No proven advantage of systemic therapy over aerosol
Terbutaline (1 mg/mL)	0.25 mg every 20 min for 3 doses SQ	0.01 mg/kg every 20 min for 3 doses, then every 2–6 h as needed SQ	Not recommended
Anticholinergics			
Ipratropium Br. nebulizer soln. (0.25 mg/mL)	500 mcg every 30 min for 3 doses, then every 2–4 h as needed	250 mcg every 20 min for 3 doses, then 250 mcg every 2–4 h	May mix in same nebulizer with albuterol; do not use as first-line therapy; only add to β2-agonist therapy
Ipratropium Br. MDI (18 mcg/puff)	4–8 puffs as needed every 2–4 h	4–8 puffs as needed every 2–4 h	Not recommended because dose in inhaler is low and has not been studied in acute asthma
Corticosteroids			
Prednisone, methylprednisolone, prednisolone	60–80 mg in 3 or 4 divided doses for 48 h, then 30–40 mg/day until PEF reaches 70% of personal best	1 mg/kg every 6 h for 48 h, then 1–2 mg/kg/day in 2 divided doses until PEF is 70% of normal predicted	For outpatient "burst" use 1–2 mg/kg/day, max. 60 mg, for 3–7 days; it is unnecessary to taper course

Note: No advantage has been found for very-high-dose corticosteroids in acute severe asthma, nor is there any advantage for intravenous administration over oral therapy. The usual regimen is to continue the frequent multiple daily dosing until the patient achieves an FEV_1 or PEF of 50% of personal best or normal predicted value and then lower the dose to twice-daily dosing. This usually occurs within 48 hours. The final duration of therapy following a hospitalization or emergency department visit may be from 7 to 14 days. If patients are then started on inhaled corticosteroids, studies indicate there is no need to taper the systemic steroid dose. If the follow-up therapy is to be given once daily, studies indicate there may be an advantage to giving the single daily dose in the afternoon at around 3 PM.

therapy of acute asthma.[2] Sedatives should not be given because anxiety may be a sign of hypoxemia, which could be worsened by central nervous system depressants. Antibiotics also are not indicated routinely because viral respiratory tract infections are the primary cause of asthma exacerbations.[2,7] Antibiotics should be reserved for patients who have signs and symptoms of pneumonia (e.g., fever, pulmonary consolidation, and purulent sputum from polymorphonuclear leukocytes). *Mycoplasma* and *Chlamydia* are infrequent causes of severe asthma exacerbations but should be considered in patients with high oxygen requirements.[7]

Respiratory failure or impending respiratory failure as measured by rising $PaCO_2$ (>45 mm Hg) or failure to correct hypoxemia with supplemental oxygen therapy is treated with intubation and mechanical ventilation. In order to prevent barotrauma and pneumothoraces from excess positive pressure, it is recommended that controlled hypoventilation or permissive hypercapnia be used (correcting the hypoxemia, PaO_2 > 60 mm Hg, but allowing the $PaCO_2$ to rise to the high 60 mm Hg range).

PHARMACOTHERAPY

β2-AGONISTS

The short-acting inhaled β2-agonists are the most effective bronchodilators and the treatment of first choice for the management of severe acute asthma.[2] Up to 66% of adults presenting to an emergency department require only three doses of 2.5 mg nebulized albuterol to be discharged.[28] Most well-controlled clinical trials have demonstrated equal to greater efficacy and greater safety of aerosolized β2-agonists over systemic administration regardless of the severity of obstruction.[27] Systemic adverse effects, hypokalemia, hyperglycemia, tachycardia, and cardiac dysrhythmias are more pronounced in patients receiving systemic β2-agonist therapy. Children younger than 2 years of age achieve clinically significant responses from nebulized albuterol.[2,27] Effective doses of aerosolized β2-agonists can be delivered successfully through mechanical ventilator circuits to infants, children, and adults in respiratory failure secondary to severe airways obstruction.[26]

Frequent administration of inhaled β_2-agonists (every 20 minutes or continuous nebulization) has been found to be superior to the same dosage administered at 1-hour intervals.[27] In the subset of more severely obstructed patients, continuous nebulization decreases the hospital admission rate, provides greater improvement in the FEV_1 and PEF, and reduces duration of hospitalization when compared with intermittent (hourly) nebulized albuterol in the same total dose.[29] Thus continuous nebulization is recommended for patients having an unsatisfactory response (achieving less than 50% of normal FEV_1 or PEF) following the initial three doses (every 20 minutes) of aerosolized β_2-agonists and potentially for patients presenting initially with PEF or FEV_1 values of less than 30% of predicted normal.[27]

The doses of inhaled β_2-agonists for severe acute asthma (see Table 26–6) have been derived empirically. The β_2-agonists follow a log-linear dose-response curve.[25] In addition, the dose-response curve is shifted to the right by more severe bronchospasm or by increased concentrations of bronchospastic mediators, which is characteristic of functional antagonists.[30] The ability to increase the dose of the short-acting aerosolized β_2-agonists by as much as five- to ten-fold over doses producing adequate bronchodilation in chronic stable asthmatics is what contributes to their efficacy in reversing the bronchospasm of acute severe asthma.[27] The nebulizer dose of inhaled β_2-agonists for children often is listed on a weight basis (milligrams per kilogram). However, a fixed minimal dose (2.5 mg albuterol or equivalent), as opposed to a weight-adjusted dose, is more appropriate in younger children because children younger than 5 years of age receive a lower lung dose.[26] Adults dosed on a weight basis demonstrate excessive cardiac stimulation, so they have fixed maximal doses[27] (see Table 26–6). Initial doses of inhaled β_2-agonists can produce vasodilation, worsening ventilation-perfusion mismatch, slightly lowering oxygen saturation or Pao_2. High-doses of inhaled β_2-agonists can produce a decrease in serum potassium concentration, an increase in heart rate, and an increase in serum glucose concentration. However, both children and adults receiving continuously nebulized β_2-agonists have demonstrated decreased heart rates as their lung function improves.[27,29] Thus an elevated heart rate is not an indication to use lower doses or to avoid using inhaled β_2-agonists.

Some controversy exists concerning the most cost-effective delivery system (MDI plus holding chamber versus nebulization) to be used in treating severe acute asthma in the emergency department and hospital (see below).[24,31] The DPIs are currently not indicated for the treatment of severe acute asthma exacerbations. Patients with more severe obstruction may not be able to generate sufficient peak inspiratory flows for adequate delivery.[27]

CORTICOSTEROIDS

Systemic corticosteroids are indicated in all patients with acute severe asthma not responding completely to initial inhaled β_2-agonist administration (every 20 minutes for three to four doses).[2] Intravenous therapy offers no therapeutic advantage over oral administration.[2] This therapy usually is continued until hospital discharge. Tapering the dose in acute asthma following discharge from the hospital appears unnecessary, provided that patients are prescribed inhaled corticosteroids for outpatient therapy.[2] Most patients achieve 70% of predicted normal FEV_1 within 48 hours and 80% of predicted by 6 days after plateauing by day 3. Thus, maintaining systemic corticosteroid courses for 10 to 14 days may be unnecessarily long in

some patients. Indeed, many patients not admitted to the hospital respond to 3- to 5-day courses of systemic corticosteroids. Short courses of oral prednisone (3 to 10 days) have been effective in preventing hospitalizations in infants and young children.[2] It is recommended that a full dose of the corticosteroid be continued until the patient's peak flow reaches 80% of predicted normal or personal best.[2]

Multiple daily dosing of systemic corticosteroids for the initial therapy of acute asthma exacerbations appears warranted because receptor-binding affinities of lung corticosteroid receptors are decreased in the face of airway inflammation.[27] However, patients with less severe exacerbations may be treated adequately with once-daily administration. High-dose and very-high-pulse-dose corticosteroid regimens have not been shown to enhance the outcomes in severe acute asthma but are associated with a higher likelihood of side effects.[27]

A recommended practice is to increase or double the dose of inhaled corticosteroids in patients who are experiencing a deterioration of their asthma control to prevent an exacerbation that requires emergency care.[2] Studies of inhaled corticosteroids (ICSs) in acute exacerbations of asthma have provided conflicting results. Currently, there is insufficient evidence supporting efficacy in the emergency department setting.[32] However, there is some evidence that prescribing ICSs on discharge from the emergency department reduces the risk of relapse.[10] This policy seems like a reasonable recommendation because inflammation is the underlying cause of deterioration in most cases.

ANTICHOLINERGICS

Inhaled ipratropium bromide generally produces a further improvement in lung function of 10% to 15% over inhaled β_2-agonists alone. In children and adults, multiple-dose ipratropium bromide added to initial therapy also produced a reduced hospitalization rate in the subset of patients with an FEV_1 of less than 30% of predicted at baseline.[33,34] Ipratropium bromide, a quaternary amine, is poorly absorbed and produces minimal or no systemic effects. Care should be used when administering ipratropium bromide by nebulizer. If a tight mask or mouthpiece is not used, the ipratropium bromide that deposits in the eyes may produce pupillary dilatation and difficulty in accommodation. Ipratropium bromide is not a vasodilator, so unlike β_2-agonists it will not worsen ventilation-perfusion mismatch.[27]

ALTERNATIVE THERAPIES

The emergency department use of aminophylline, a moderate bronchodilator, for acute asthma has not been recommended for a number of years.[2] Clinical trials of aminophylline in adults and children hospitalized with acute asthma have not reported sufficient evidence of efficacy (improvement in lung function and reduced hospital stay) but have reported an increased risk of adverse effects.[27] However, two studies of aminophylline in children with severe disease suggested a possible small benefit in reducing intensive care unit admissions.[27] Adverse effects of theophylline include nausea and vomiting and potentiation of the cardiac effects of the inhaled β_2-agonists.

Magnesium sulfate is a moderately potent bronchodilator that is similar to aminophylline, producing relaxation of smooth muscle and central nervous system depression.[35] The use of intravenous magnesium sulfate in patients presenting to the emergency department is controversial (see below).[35] The adverse effects of magnesium sulfate include hypotension, facial flushing, sweating, nausea, loss of deep tendon reflexes, and respiratory depression.[27] Patients have required dopamine to treat the hypotension.[27]

Helium is an inert gas of low density with no pharmacologic properties that can lower resistance to gas flow and increase ventilation because the low density decreases the pressure gradient needed to achieve a given level of turbulent flow, converting turbulent flow to laminar flow.[27] Helium is given as a mixture of helium and oxygen (heliox), usually 60% to 70% helium with 30% to 40% oxygen.[27] As with a number of experimental approaches, heliox was reported to be efficacious in initial nonrandomized clinical trials. However, the small number of randomized, controlled trials completed to date have failed to document efficacy.[36] Although heliox is free of adverse effects, its use is limited to patients with a low inspired oxygen requirement because the decrease in density generally is insignificant clinically with less than 60% helium.[27]

The inhalational anesthetics halothane, isoflurane, and enflurane all have been reported to have a positive effect in children and adults with severe asthma that is unresponsive to standard medical therapy.[27] The proposed mechanisms for inhalational anesthetics include direct action on bronchial smooth muscle, inhibition of airway reflexes, attenuation of histamine-induced bronchospasm, and interaction with β_2-adrenergic receptors.[27] Well-controlled trials with these agents have not been completed. Potential adverse effects include myocardial depression, vasodilation, arrhythmias, and depression of mucociliary function. In addition, the practical problem of delivery and scavenging these agents in the intensive care environment as opposed to the operating room is a concern. The use of volatile anesthetics cannot be recommended based on insufficient evidence of efficacy.

Ketamine has been recommended for rapid induction of anesthesia in patients with asthma who require intubation and mechanical ventilation.[27] Ketamine is thought to produce bronchodilation from a combination of an increase in circulating catecholamines, direct smooth muscle relaxation, and inhibition of vagal flow.[27] Anecdotal reports have suggested that ketamine is useful as a short-term adjunct in severe acute asthma; controlled trials have not provided sufficient evidence of efficacy, however. Ketamine has several significant adverse effects, including the anesthesia emergence reaction, which can alter mood and cause delirium. These emergence phenomena occur in at least 25% of patients over 16 years of age; the incidence seems to be much lower in younger patients.[27] Other risks include an increase in heart rate, arterial blood pressure, and cerebral blood flow because of its sympathetic effects.[27]

SPECIAL POPULATIONS

Infants and children younger than 4 years of age may be at greater risk of respiratory failure than older children and adults. Although treated with the same drugs, these younger children require the use of a facemask as opposed to a mouthpiece for delivery of aerosolized medication. Use of the facemask reduces delivery of drug to the lung by one-half so that a minimal dose is recommended as opposed to a weight-adjusted dose.[26] The facemask should be sized appropriately and should fit snugly over the nose and mouth. Use of the "blow by" method, where the therapist or parent places the mask or extension tubing near the child's nose and mouth, should be discouraged because holding the mask as few as 2 cm from the patient's face reduces lung delivery of the aerosol by 80%.[26]

DRUG CLASS INFORMATION

SHORT-ACTING β_2-AGONISTS

The β_2-agonists are the most effective bronchodilators available. The β_2-adrenergic receptors are transmembrane proteins consisting of clusters of seven helices of amino acids that form the ligand-binding core.[30] The human β_2-adrenergic receptors are polymorphic in structure, with the most common polymorphisms in the amino terminus of the receptor at amino acid positions 16 (encoding either arginine [Arg] or glycine [Gly]) and 27 (encoding either glutamine [Gln] or glutamic acid [Glu]).[37] Some of the polymorphisms determine responsiveness to β_2-agonists, whereas others may act as disease modifiers (see below).[37] Stimulation of β_2-adrenergic receptor activates cytoplasmic G proteins, which, in turn, activate adenylyl cyclase to produce cyclic adenosine monophosphate (cAMP), generally thought to be responsible for the bulk of activity through activation of various proteins by cAMP-dependent protein kinase (PKA).[37] This activation, in turn, decreases unbound intracellular calcium, producing smooth muscle relaxation, mast cell membrane stabilization, and skeletal muscle stimulation.[25] Despite the fact that β_2-agonists are potent inhibitors of mast cell degranulation in vitro, they do not inhibit the late asthmatic response to allergen challenge or the subsequent bronchial hyperresponsiveness.[2,25] Long-term administration of β_2-agonists does not reduce BHR, confirming a lack of significant anti-inflammatory activity.[25] β_2-Adrenergic stimulation also activates Na^+,K^+-ATPase, produces gluconeogenesis, and enhances insulin secretion, resulting in a mild to moderate decrease in serum potassium concentration by driving potassium intracellularly.[25] The chronotropic response to β_2-agonists is mediated in part by baroreceptor reflex mechanisms as a result of the drop in blood pressure from vascular smooth muscle relaxation, as well as by direct stimulation of cardiac β_2-receptors and some β_1 stimulation at high concentrations.[25] Table 26–7 lists the pharmacologic effects of adrenergic receptor stimulation. Because β_1-receptor stimulation produces excessive cardiac stimulation, resulting in cardiac arrhythmias, and because the inotropic effect enhancing myocardial oxygen consumption leads to myocardial necrosis, there

TABLE 26–7. Pharmacologic Responses to Sympathomimetic Agonists

Tissue	Receptor Type	Response
Airways	β_2	Smooth muscle relaxation (bronchodilation), increased ciliary beat, increased serous secretion, and inhibition of mast cell degranulation
	α	Smooth muscle contraction (bronchoconstriction?)
Heart	β_1	Inotropic and chronotropic
	β_2	Chronotropic
Vasculature	β_2	Vasodilation, decrease microvascular leakage
	α	Vasoconstriction
Skeletal	β_2	Increased neuromuscular transmission (tremor and increased strength of contraction)
Uterus	β_2	Relaxation (tocolysis)
Metabolic	α, β_1	Glycogenolysis, lipolysis
	β_2	Gluconeogenesis, hypokalemia, increased lactate production

TABLE 26–8. Relative Selectivity, Potency, and Duration of Action of the β-Adrenergic Agonists

Agent	Selectivity		Potency, $\beta_2{}^a$	Duration of Action[b]		Oral activity
	β_1	β_2		Bronchodilation (h)	Protection (h)[c]	
Isoproterenol	++++	++++	1	0.5–2	0.5–1	No
Metaproterenol	+++	+++	15	3–4	1–2	Yes
Isoetharine	++	+++	6	0.5–2	0.5–1	No
Albuterol	+	++++	2	4–8	2–4	Yes
Bitolterol	+	++++	5	4–8	2–4	No
Pirbuterol	+	++++	5	4–8	2–4	Yes
Terbutaline	+	++++	4	4–8	2–4	Yes
Formoterol	+	++++	0.24	≥12	6–12	Yes
Salmeterol	+	++++	0.5	≥12	6–>12	No

[a]Relative molar potency to isoproterenol: 15 = lowest potency.
[b]Median durations with the highest value after a single dose and lowest after chronic administration.
[c]Protection refers to the prevention of bronchoconstriction induced by exercise or nonspecific bronchial challenges.

is no rationale for using non–β_2-selective agonists in the treatment of asthma.[25]

Table 26–8 compares the various β-adrenergic agonists used in asthma in terms of selectivity, potency, oral activity, and duration of action. The β_2-agonists are functional or physiologic antagonists in that they relax airway smooth muscle regardless of the mechanism for constriction.[30] When administered in equipotent doses, all the short-acting drugs produce the same intensity of response; the only differences are in duration of action and cardiac toxicity.[2,25] The catecholamine derivatives all have the disadvantage of rapid inactivation of their 3,4-hydroxyl catechol group from catechol-O-methyltransferase found in the gastrointestinal tract, rendering them orally inactive. In addition, catecholamines are taken up rapidly into tissues by secondary uptake mechanisms that limit their receptor occupancy and thus have a shorter duration of action.[25] All the β_2-agonists are more bronchoselective when administered by the aerosol route.[25] Aerosol administration of the short-acting β_2-agonists provides more rapid response and greater protection against provocations that induce bronchospasm such as exercise and allergen challenges than does systemic administration.[25] Differences in myocardial effects are discernible between selective and nonselective agents even when administered as aerosols, particularly at the higher doses used for severe acute asthma. The β_2-agonists also differ in efficacy or ability to activate the β-adrenergic receptors. Full agonists include the catecholamines, metaproterenol, and formoterol.[30] Partial agonists include albuterol, terbutaline, pirbuterol, and salmeterol.[30] The principal differences between full and partial agonists is that full agonists require a lower fraction of receptor occupancy to produce their maximum effect and more easily produce receptor desensitization.[30]

All synthetic β_2-agonists are 1:1 racemic mixtures of two mirror images (enantiomers) owing to an asymmetric or chiral carbon.[30,38] Since most physiologic functions (receptor occupancy and activation and enzymatic metabolism) are stereoselective, the (R)-enantiomers of the β_2-agonists are the most pharmacologically active isomer.[37] While it was felt initially that the (S)-enantiomers were essentially inactive owing to the 1000-fold potency difference between the enantiomers, studies in animal models and isolated in vitro tissue preparations have suggested that the (S)-enantiomers may be proinflammatory and could induce BHR.[39] However, evidence that this occurs consistently in humans or is clinically relevant is lacking (see below).[38] The pharmacokinetics are stereoselective as well, although not as predictable. (R)-Albuterol is metabolized more rapidly than (S)-albuterol, which could lead to accumulation of (S)-albuterol with continued dosing.[38] This accumulation is more exaggerated with oral

dosing, as would be expected from a drug with a high first-pass effect.[30] On the other hand, (S)-terbutaline is eliminated more rapidly than (R)-terbutaline.[30]

Both the intensity and duration of response are dose-dependent, and more important, the dose-response relationship is dynamic.[25] At increasing levels of baseline bronchoconstriction (irrespective of the stimulus), the dose-response curve is shifted to the right, and the duration of bronchodilation is decreased.[30] This shift is reflected in the need for higher, more frequent doses in acute asthma exacerbations; the duration of protection against significant provocation is much less than the duration of bronchodilation in chronic stable asthma[25] (see Table 26–8).

Chronic administration of β_2-agonists leads to downregulation (decreased number of β_2 receptors) and a decreased binding affinity for these receptors.[25,30] Systemic corticosteroid therapy can both prevent and partially reverse this phenomenon.[2,25] However, the use of inhaled corticosteroids appears to have minimal ability to prevent tolerance to β_2-agonists.[30] The homozygous Gly-16 form of the receptor downregulates to a much greater extent compared with the homozygous Arg-16 form of the receptor.[37] The heterozygous Arg-16/Gly-16 is intermediately desensitized compared with the homozygous Gly-16 form. On the other hand, glutamate substitution at codon 27 (Glu-27) protects against downregulation compared with the glutamine form (Gln-27) of the receptor.[37] However, the Gly-16 overcomes any protective effect of Glu-27.[37] Tolerance primarily reduces duration of bronchodilation as opposed to peak response. A significantly greater tolerance develops in other tissues (e.g., lymphocytes and cardiac and skeletal muscle) compared with the lung primarily as a result of the surplus β_2 receptors found in respiratory smooth muscle.[25] Tolerance to the extrapulmonary effects (cardiac stimulation and hypokalemia) may account for a lack of significant cardiac effects with retention of the bronchodilator response despite chronic inhaled β_2-agonist therapy, whereas tolerance to mast cell stabilization may be a drawback to chronic use.[25] Thus chronic β_2-agonist administration produces a tolerance of minimal clinical significance that is overcome easily by increasing the dose or by administering corticosteroids.[2,25] Most of the tolerance occurs within a week of regular administration and does not worsen with continued administration. As would be expected from a receptor phenomenon, tolerance is a cross-tolerance to all β_2-agonists.[25,30] Whether or not regular use of short-acting inhaled β_2-agonists produces worsening of asthma in a subset of patients remains controversial (see below), but it does not appear to occur in the entire population.[40] However, regular treatment (four times daily) does not improve symptom control over as-needed use.[41]

TABLE 26–9. Pharmacodynamic/Pharmacokinetic Comparison of the Corticosteroids

Systemic	Anti-inflammatory Potency	Mineralcorticoid Potency	Duration of Biologic Activity (h)	Elimination Half-Life (h)
Hydrocortisone	1	1.0	8–12	1.5–2.0
Prednisone	4	0.8	12–36	2.5–3.5
Methylprednisolone	5	0.5	12–36	3.3
Dexamethasone	25	0	36–54	3.4–4.0

ICS	Receptor Binding Affinity	Topical Skin Blanching	Oral Bioavailability (%)	Systemic Clearance (L/h)	Half-Life (h) IV/Inhaled
BDP/BMP	0.4/13.5	600/400	15–20	UK	0.5/1.5–6.5
BUD	9.4	980	11	55–84	2.8/2.0
FLU	1.8	330	20	58	1.6/1.6
FP	18	1200	≤1	66	7.8/14.4
MF	27[a]	UK	<1	53	5.8/UK
TAA	3.6	330	23	45–69	2.0/3.6

Note: Receptor binding affinities and topical skin blanching are relative to dexamethasone equal to 1. UK = unknown.
[a]MF studied in a different receptor system. Value estimated from relative values of BDP, TAA, and FP in that system.
BUD, budesonide; FLU, flunisolide; FP, fluticasone; MF, mometasone; TA, triamcinolone; BDP, beclomethasone.

In conclusion, the inhaled short-acting selective β_2-agonists are indicated for the treatment of intermittent episodes of bronchospasm. They are the first treatment of choice for acute severe asthma and exercise-induced bronchospasm.[2,25] They inhibit EIB in a dose-dependent fashion and provide complete protection for a 2-hour period following inhalation with varying levels of patient-dependent protection over 4 hours.[25] Although the regular administration of β_2-agonists slightly decreases the effect, two inhalations prior to exercise still essentially blocks exercise-induced bronchospasm completely (1% versus 5% drop in FEV_1).[42]

■ SYSTEMIC CORTICOSTEROIDS

The corticosteroids are the most effective anti-inflammatories available to treat asthma.[2,7,10] Actions useful in treating asthma include (1) increasing the number of β_2-adrenergic receptors and improving the receptor responsiveness to β_2-adrenergic stimulation, (2) reducing mucus production and hypersecretion, (3) reducing BHR, and (4) preventing and reversing airway remodeling.[9,10] The glucocorticoid receptor is found in the cytoplasm of most cells throughout the body, explaining the multiple effects of systemic corticosteroids. There is no difference between glucocorticoid receptors found throughout the body; however, genetic differences between glucocorticoid receptors from different individuals may determine some of the variations in response.[43] The corticosteroids are lipophilic, readily cross the cell membrane, and combine with the glucocorticoid receptor. The activated complex then enters the nucleus, where it acts as a transcription factor leading to gene activation or suppression.[44] This leads to specific mRNA production, resulting in increased production of anti-inflammatory mediators; suppression of several proinflammatory cytokines such as IL-1, GM-CSF, IL-3, IL-4, IL-5, IL-6, and IL-8, reducing inflammatory cell activation, recruitment, and infiltration; and decreasing vascular permeability.[44] In addition, the activated glucocorticoid receptor complex can act directly with cytoplasmic transcription factors, nuclear factor κB, and activating protein 1 to prevent the action of proinflammatory cytokines on the cell.[44]

Owing to the mechanism that modifies gene expression, the time required to see the particular effect depends on the time required for new protein synthesis, decreased formation of the particular mediator, and resolution of the inflammatory response.[44] Generally, the cellular and biochemical effects are immediate, but varying amounts of time are required to produce a clinical response. β_2-Receptor density increases within 4 hours of corticosteroid administration.[44] Improved responsiveness to β_2-agonists occurs within 2 hours.[27] In severe acute asthma, 4 to 12 hours may be required before any clinical response is noted.[27] Reversal of seasonally increased BHR requires at least 1 week of therapy.[44] The chronic use of corticosteroids does not induce a state of corticosteroid dependence. Nor is there evidence of tolerance produced by chronic administration.

The corticosteroids used in asthma are compared in Table 26–9.[45] Besides acute severe asthma, systemic corticosteroids are also recommended for the treatment of impending episodes of severe asthma unresponsive to bronchodilator therapy.[2,10] The effects of corticosteroids in asthma are dose- and duration-dependent. This pattern is true for the adverse effects as well (Table 26–10). The clinician must balance the toxicity of chronic systemic corticosteroid therapy continually with control of asthma symptoms. Because short-term (1 to 2 weeks) high-dose corticosteroids (1 to 2 mg/kg per day of prednisone) do not produce serious toxicities, the ideal use is to administer the systemic corticosteroids in a short "burst" and then to maintain the patient on appropriate long-term control therapy with inhaled corticosteroids (discussed below).[2,10] In general, therapy for more than 5 days at doses that exceed the usual physiologic endogenous cortisol

TABLE 26–10. Adverse Effects of Chronic Systemic Glucocorticoid Administration

Hypothalamic–pitutitary-adrenal suppression	Hypertension
	Skin striae
Growth retardation	Impaired wound healing
Skeletal muscle myopathy	Inhibition of leukocyte and
Osteoporosis/fractures	monocyte function
Aseptic necrosis of bone	Subcutaneous tissue atrophy
Pancreatitis	Glaucoma
Pseudotumor cerebri	Posterior subcapsular cataracts
Psychiatric disturbances	Moon facies
Sodium and water retention	Central redistribution of fat
Hypokalemia/hyperglycemia	

production will cause temporary aberration in adrenal cortisol release.[27] However, this hypothalamic-pituitary-adrenal (HPA) axis suppression is short-lived (1 to 3 days) and readily reversible following short bursts (10 days or less) of pharmacologic doses.[27] A maximum number of short bursts that a patient can receive probably exists, after which chronic corticosteroid side effects occur. Patients receiving at least eight bursts ($\geq$10 days each) were shown to have a similar decrease in trabecular bone density as patients on daily or alternate-day corticosteroids over 1 year.[27] Children who received four or more bursts of prednisone exhibited a subnormal response to hypoglycemic stress or adrenocorticotropic hormone (ACTH) administration.[27] Very short courses (3 to 5 days) have been effective in reducing hospitalization from acute exacerbations.[2,10] Use of the shorter-acting corticosteroids such as prednisone will produce less adrenal suppression than the longer-acting dexamethasone.

ANTICHOLINERGICS

The anticholinergic agents have a long history of use for asthma, but they do not have a Food and Drug Administration (FDA)–approved indication for asthma.[2,10] Anticholinergics are competitive inhibitors of muscarinic receptors.[46] Unlike β_2-agonists, they are not functional antagonists; they only reverse cholinergic-mediated bronchoconstriction.[33] Normal bronchial tone is maintained through parasympathetic innervation of the airways via the vagus nerve. A number of the triggers and mediators of asthma (i.e., histamine, prostaglandins, sulfur dioxide, exercise, and allergens) produce bronchoconstriction in part through vagal reflex mechanisms.[2] Studies of asthmatics consistently demonstrate that anticholinergics are effective bronchodilators, although not as effective as β_2-agonists. Anticholinergics attenuate but do not block allergen-induced asthma in a dose-dependent fashion and have no effect on BHR.[2]

Ipratropium bromide is a nonselective muscarinic receptor blocker, and blockade of inhibitory muscarinic receptors theoretically could result in an increased release of acetylcholine and overcome the block on the smooth muscle receptors (M_3).[46] Only the quaternary ammonium derivatives such as ipratropium bromide should be used because they have the advantage of poor absorption across mucosae and the blood-brain barrier. This results in negligible systemic effects with a prolonged local effect (i.e., bronchodilation). In addition, the quaternary compounds do not appear to produce a decrease in mucociliary clearance.[46] Ipratropium bromide has a duration of action of 4 to 8 hours. Both intensity and duration of action are dose-dependent. Time to reach maximum bronchodilation is considerably slower than from aerosolized short-acting β_2-agonists (2 hours versus 30 minutes). However, this is of little clinical consequence because some bronchodilation is seen within 30 seconds, 50% of maximum response occurs within 3 minutes, and 80% of maximum is reached within 30 minutes.[46] Ipratropium bromide is only indicated as adjunctive therapy in severe acute asthma not completely responsive to β_2-agonists alone because it does not improve outcomes in chronic asthma.[2,10]

PHARMACOECONOMICS

The number of emergency department visits for asthma exceeds the number of hospitalizations by approximately four times, yet the annual expenditures for emergency department visits ($478.6 million) is significantly less than the estimated $1.8 billion spent on inpatient hospital services for patients with acute severe asthma.[6] Thus, reducing the number of patients requiring hospitalizations is a primary goal of therapy. Inpatient services have declined as a percentage of total medical expenditures primarily as a result of decreasing duration of hospitalizations.[6] Since the primary drugs used to treat severe acute asthma are available generically, drug costs account for only a small portion of the overall costs of care. Few of the therapies used in the management of acute severe asthma have been evaluated formally for their pharmacoeconomic impact. One evaluation based on a meta-analysis of inhaled anticholinergics added to inhaled β_2-agonists in children with acute severe asthma suggested that this approach was cost-effective and would reduce overall costs by reducing hospitalizations.[47] In children with acute severe asthma admitted to an intensive care unit, the use of continuously nebulized albuterol resulted in a decreased cost of care compared with intermittent nebulization.[27]

CLINICAL CONTROVERSIES

Some clinicians believe that intravenous magnesium sulfate is effective for the treatment of severe acute asthma unresponsive to standard doses of inhaled β_2-agonists in the emergency department. This is based on subset analyses of two studies showing that patients with the most severe obstruction following initial inhaled β_2-agonists decreased hospitalizations with magnesium treatment compared with placebo.[35] However, the subset with severe obstruction is the one demonstrating an improved response to the addition of ipratropium bromide and continuous nebulization of inhaled β_2-agonists. Listed as experimental by the NAEPP,[2] the Global Initiative in Asthma (GINA) guidelines state that it can be considered for use in patients with severe episodes with a poor response to initial inhaled β_2-agonists.[10]

Numerous studies have shown that the inhaled β_2-agonists administered by MDI plus holding chamber provide a similar outcome in severe acute asthma as administration by jet nebulizers.[31] Proponents of administration by MDI plus holding chambers argue that it is more cost-effective and so should replace nebulizer therapy. However, appropriate cost analyses have yet to be performed.[24] Nor have there been comparisons in the most severe subsets, where combination therapy and continuous nebulization are recommended.[27] Current practice should be based on the comfort level of the clinical staff until sufficient data are available to warrant a wholesale recommendation of one method.

EVALUATION OF THERAPEUTIC OUTCOMES

Figures 26–6 and 26–7 provide the monitoring parameters for severe acute asthma. Lung function, either spirometry or peak flows, should be monitored 5 to 10 minutes after each treatment.[2] Oxygen saturations can be easily monitored continuously with pulse oximetry. For young children and infants, pulse oximetry, lung auscultation, and observation of the presence of supraclavicular retractions is useful.[2,27] The majority of patients will respond within the first hour of initial inhaled β_2-agonists regardless of history of home administration of drug. Patients not achieving an initial response should be monitored every 0.5 to 1 hour. Depending on whether there is a standard emergency department or a special unit for severe acute asthma, the decision to admit to the hospital should be made within 4 to 6 hours of entry to the emergency department. The mean duration of hospitalization following admission is 2 to 3 days. Frequency of monitoring depends on the severity of the exacerbation. With mild exacerbations, monitor lung function every 2 to 3 hours and severe exacerbations every 0.5 to 1 hour.

▶ TREATMENT: Chronic Asthma

The diagnosis of chronic asthma is made primarily by history and confirmatory spirometry (see Clinical Presentation above).[2,10] The NAEPP has provided a list of questions that would lead to the diagnosis of asthma[2] (see Table 26–2). In the older child and adult patient in whom spirometric evaluations can be performed, failure of pulmonary functions to improve acutely does not necessarily rule out asthma. Patients with long-standing disease or substantial inflammation may require an intensive, prolonged course of bronchodilators and glucocorticoids before reversibility is detected.[2,10] If baseline spirometry is normal, challenge testing with exercise, histamine, or methacholine can be used to elicit BHR.[2] Patients with significant symptoms and/or an FEV_1 of less than 65% of predicted normal should not be challenged. Studies for atopy such as serum IgE and sputum and blood eosinophil determinations are not necessary to make the diagnosis of asthma, but they may help differentiate asthma from chronic bronchitis in adults. Clinically, this distinction is often difficult to make. Some patients with chronic bronchitis may have a reversible component, and some patients with long-standing severe chronic asthma may have significant irreversible damage and obstruction. Very high peripheral blood eosinophil counts may point to the diagnosis of allergic bronchopulmonary aspergillosis (ABPA) or other hypereosinophilic syndromes.[10] Skin testing is of no value in diagnosing asthma but is useful in identifying triggers.[2] In small infants unable to perform spirometry, the diagnosis is more difficult. They may demonstrate hyperinflation on the chest roentgenogram.[2] Radiologic examination is helpful in ruling out other causes of wheezing (e.g., foreign-body aspiration, parenchymal lung disease, cardiac disease, and congenital anomalies).[2] In place of pulmonary functions, the parents should be given a diary card to record symptoms and precipitating events.

GOALS OF MANAGEMENT

The NAEPP has provided the following goals for chronic asthma management[2]:

1. Maintain normal activity levels (including exercise and other physical activity).
2. Maintain (near) normal pulmonary functions.
3. Prevent chronic and troublesome symptoms (e.g., coughing or breathlessness in the night, in the early morning, or after exertion).
4. Prevent recurrent exacerbations of asthma, and minimize the need for emergency department visits or hospitalizations.
5. Provide optimal pharmacotherapy with minimal or no adverse effects.
6. Meet patients' and families' expectations of satisfaction with asthma care.

Toward these goals, every effort should be made to decrease the patient's baseline BHR and prevent it from increasing.

NONPHARMACOLOGIC THERAPY

Although the mainstay of the management of asthma is pharmacologic therapy, it is likely to fail without attending to the nonpharmacologic therapy issues. Figure 26–8 depicts the stepwise approach to asthma therapy recommended in the newest update by the NAEPP.[7] It is important to note that the nonpharmacologic aspects of therapy are incorporated into the steps. The guidelines were designed to give primary health care providers a framework with which to develop the proper approach to the individualized therapy of patients. The heterogeneity of asthma demands an individualized approach to therapy with the basic goals of therapy as primary outcome measures.[2,7]

The knowledge that inflammation plays a primary role in the pathogenesis of asthma has led to the conviction that the focus of therapy is the prevention and suppression of the underlying inflammation.[2,7,10] Thus current therapeutic options in asthma consist of acute reliever medications used for acute exacerbations and long-term control medications used for the prevention of symptoms and exacerbations and the suppression of inflammation.[2] The currently accepted approach is to use drugs that suppress the inflammatory response as primary long-term control therapy, thereby reducing the degree of BHR and improving long-term control and outcomes in asthma by preventing airway remodeling.[2,7,10]

The development of a partnership in care through patient education and the teaching of patient self-management skills should be the cornerstone of any treatment program.[2,10] There are a number of published self-management programs for children and adults available through local American Lung Association chapters, as well as asthma treatment centers, and nationally through the NAEPP and the Asthma and Allergy Foundation of America.[2,10] Asthma self-management programs have been shown to improve patient adherence to medication regimens, improve self-management skills, and improve use of health care services.[2,7] The objective of these programs is to develop a partnership relationship between the patient and the health care provider. Table 26–11 lists the key educational messages recommended by the NAEPP.[2]

Self-management programs instruct patients in the pathogenesis of asthma and the appropriate use of their medications but focus principally on teaching patients to recognize triggers for their asthma and how to recognize early signs of deterioration. Use of objective measurement of airflow obstruction with a home peak-flow meter is integral to many of the programs.[2,10] However, routine peak-flow monitoring in and of itself does not improve patient outcomes.[7]

The NAEPP now advocates the use of peak-flow meters only for patients with moderate and severe persistent asthma.[2] The NAEPP also has recommended a system based on a traffic light scenario (based on percentage of normal predicted values or personal best values): The green zone is equal to 80% to 100%, the yellow zone is equal to 50% to 79%, and the red zone is less than 50%. The yellow zone is cautionary and requires increasing as-needed bronchodilator use and either increasing the anti-inflammatory dose or beginning prednisone

Classify Severity: Clinical Features Before Treatment or Adequate Control			Medications Required to Maintain Long-Term Control
	Symptoms/Day Symptoms/Night	PEF or FEV$_1$ PEF Variability	Daily Medications

STEP 4
 Severe
 Persistent
	Continual
	 Frequent
		≤60%
		 >30%
			• **Preferred treatment:**
			 – **High-dose inhaled corticosteroids**
			   AND
			 – **Long-acting inhaled β$_2$-agonists**
			   AND, ifneeded,
			 – Corticosteroid tablets or syrup long term (2 mg/kg/day,
			   generally do not exceed 60 mg per day). (Make repeat
			   attempts to reduce systemic corticosteroids and
			   maintain control with high-dose inhaled corticosteroids.)

STEP 3
 Moderate
 Persistent
	Daily
	 >1 night/week
		>60% – <80%
		 >30%
			• **Preferred treatment:**
			 – **Low-to-medium dose inhaled corticosteroids and**
			   long-acting inhaled β$_2$-agonists.
			 • Alternative treatment (listed alphabetically):
			 – Increase inhaled corticosteroids within medium-dose range
			   OR
			 – Low- to medium-dose inhaled corticosteroids and either
			   leukotriene modifier or theophylline.
			
			 If needed (particularly in patients with recurring severe exacerbations):
			 • **Preferred treatment:**
			 – **Increase inhaled corticosteroids within medium-dose**
			   range and add long-acting inhaled β$_2$-agonists.
			 • Alternative treatment:
			 – Increase inhaled corticosteroids within medium-dose range
			   and add either leukotriene modifier or theophylline.

STEP 2
 Mild
 Persistent
	>2/week but < 1x/day
	 >2 nights/month
		≥80%
		 20–30%
			• **Preferred treatment:**
			 – **Low-dose inhaled corticosteroids.**
			 • Alternative treatment (listed alphabetically): cromolyn,
			   leukotriene modifier, nedocromil, OR sustained release
			   theophylline to serum concentration of 5–15 mcg/mL.

STEP 1
 Mild
 Intermittent
	≤2days/week
	 ≤2 nights/month
		≥80%
		 <20%
			• No daily medication needed.
			 • Severe exacerbations may occur, separated by long periods
			   of normal lung function and no symptoms. A course of
			   systemic corticosteroids is recommended.

Quick Relief
 All Patients
			• Short-acting bronchodilator: 2–4 puffs short-acting inhaled β$_2$-agonists as needed for symptoms.
			 • Intensity of treatment will depend on severity of exacerbation; up to 3 treatments at 20-minute
			   intervals or a single nebulizer treatment as needed. Course of systemic corticosteroids may be needed.
			 • Use of short-acting β$_2$-agonists >2 times a week in intermittent asthma (daily, or increasing use in
			   persistent asthma) may indicate the need to initiate (increase) long-term-control therapy.

↓ STEP DOWN
Review treatment every 1 to 6 months; a gradual stepwise reduction in treatment may be possible.

↑ STEP UP
If control is not maintained, consider step up. First, review patient medication technique, adherence, and environmental control.

Goals of Therapy: Asthma Control

• Minimal or no chronic symptoms day or night
• Minimal or no exacerbations
• No limitations on activities; no school/work missed
• Maintain (near) normal pulmonary function
• Minimal use of short-acting inhaled β$_2$-agonist
• Minimal or no adverse effects from medications

Note

• The stepwise approach is meant to assist, not replace, the clinical decisionmaking required to meet individual patient needs.
• Classify severity: assign patient to most severe step in which any feature occurs (PEF is % of personal best; FEV$_1$ is % predicted).
• Gain control as quickly as possible (consider a short course of systemic corticosteroids); then step down to the least medication necessary to maintain control.
• Minimize use of short-acting inhaled β$_2$-agonists. Over reliance on short-acting inhaled β$_2$-agonists (e.g., use of short-acting inhaled β$_2$-agonist everyday, increasing use or lack of expected effect, or use of approximately one canister a month even if not using it every day) indicates inadequate control of asthma and the need to initiate or intensify long-term control therapy.
• Provide education on self-management and controlling environmental factors that make asthma worse (e.g., allergens and irritants).
• Refer to an asthma specialist if there are difficulties controlling asthma or if step 4 care is required. Referral may be considered if step 3 care is required.

FIGURE 26–8. Stepwise approach for managing asthma in adults and children older than 5 years of age. *(From ref. 2.)*

TABLE 26–11. Key Educational Messages for Patients

Basic facts about asthma
- The contrast between asthmatic and normal airways
- What happens to the airways in an asthma attack

Roles of medications
- How medications work
  Long-term control: medications that prevent symptoms, often by reducing inflammation
  Quick relief: short-acting bronchodilator relaxes muscles around airways
- Stress importance of long-term-control medications and not to expect quick relief from them

Skills
- Inhaler use (patient demonstrate)
- Spacer and holding chamber use
- Symptom monitoring, peak flow monitoring, and recognizing early signs of deterioration

Environmental control measures
- Identifying and avoiding environmental precipitants or exposures

When and how to take rescue actions
- Responding to changes in asthma severity (daily self-management plan and action plan)

if not improved, whereas the red zone warrants contacting the patient's health care provider.[2] This approach can assist the patient and health professional in determining the next level of therapy.

Patient education is essential before monitoring can be effective. Patient education has proved successful regardless of the health professional who provided the information (physician, nurse, or pharmacist). The NAEPP advocates significant involvement of the primary health care provider in the educational process. The provision of written treatment plans enhances the success of education and peak-flow monitoring and is considered an essential component of care.[2] Samples of clinically tested written action plans are available from the NAEPP Expert Panel Report 2.[2]

In patients with known allergic triggers for their asthma, allergen avoidance has resulted in an improvement in symptoms, a reduction in medication use, and a decrease in BHR.[2,10] Relatively simple environmental controls for patients with house dust mite allergy such as removing carpeting from bedrooms, washing sheets in hot water ($>130°F$), and using plastic pillow and mattress covers can reduce symptoms and need for medications.[2,10] Obvious environmental triggers (i.e., warm-blooded animals, cockroaches), if the patient is sensitive, should be avoided; however, there is very little evidence that extensive environmental controls (i.e., home air-filtering systems and chemicals for killing house dust mites) are of any value.[2] Although allergen avoidance has proved beneficial, immunotherapy (allergy shots) is not efficacious in asthma, although a proven and accepted therapy for allergic rhinitis.[2,10]

Patients who smoke should be encouraged to stop. Parents of children with asthma should stop or at least not smoke around their children.[2,10]

PHARMACOLOGIC THERAPY

The current NAEPP recommendations for therapy of chronic asthma are illustrated in Figure 26–8.[7] Regardless of the long-term control therapy, all patients need to have quick-relief medication in the form of short-acting inhaled β_2-agonists available for acute

symptoms. The inhaled corticosteroids are considered the preferred long-term control therapy for persistent asthma in all patients.[7,10] This new recommendation follows an evidence-based report by the NAEPP.[7] Low- to medium-dose inhaled corticosteroids reduce BHR, improve lung function, and reduce severe exacerbations leading to emergency department visits and hospitalizations. They are more effective than either cromolyn, nedocromil, theophylline, or the leukotriene antagonists.[7] In addition, the inhaled corticosteroids are the only therapy that reduces the risk of dying from asthma.[48]

In the low to medium doses recommended by the NAEPP guidelines (Table 26–12), inhaled corticosteroids have been proved to be safe for long-term administration.[43] The principal adverse effect at low to medium doses is delayed growth in children that appears to be about 1 to 2 cm in the first year of therapy, is not progressive, and does not appear to prevent attainment of predicted adult height.[43] The inhaled corticosteroids do not appear to increase the risk of osteoporosis in the elderly or glaucoma and cataracts except at high doses[7,43] (see Table 26–12). It is unknown whether the inhaled corticosteroids can reduce airway remodeling and loss of lung function found in some patients with persistent asthma. Studies demonstrating a reduction in some aspects of airway remodeling used high doses of inhaled corticosteroids.[9] They do not enhance lung growth in children 5 to 12 years of age when administered for 4 to 6 years, nor do they induce remission of asthma because BHR and other measures of inflammation return to pretreatment levels on discontinuation of therapy.[49]

Although short-term studies of the alternative long-term control therapies (e.g., cromolyn, leukotriene antagonists, nedocromil, and theophylline) demonstrate improvement in symptoms, lung function, and as-needed short-acting inhaled β_2-agonist use, they do not reduce BHR, suggesting minimal anti-inflammatory activity.[7] Few of these therapies have been assessed in long-term clinical trials. The evidence suggests minimal to no differences in efficacy between these alternatives. Therefore, the NAEPP lists them in alphabetical order to show no preference of one over the other.[7] Of interest, the GINA guidelines, established in cooperation with the National Institutes of Health and the World Health Organization, list the alternatives based on costs because the World Health Organization is concerned with providing therapies to third world countries.[10] As a result, theophylline is listed first as the least expensive and leukotriene antagonists last as the most expensive.[10]

The most significant change in the NAEPP guidelines update in 2002 is the recommendation that the combination of inhaled corticosteroids and long-acting inhaled β_2-agonists is the preferred treatment for step 3 moderate persistent asthma.[7] This change is based on strong evidence of superiority of the combination over doubling the dose of inhaled corticosteroids. In addition, this combination has been shown to be superior to the adding of leukotriene antagonists to inhaled corticosteroids.[7] The addition of theophylline to inhaled corticosteroids is no more effective than doubling the dose of the inhaled corticosteroids on lung function and not as effective at reducing severe asthma exacerbations.[7] The combination of inhaled corticosteroid and long-acting inhaled β_2-agonists is more effective at reducing severe asthma exacerbations than doubling the dose of inhaled corticosteroids in moderate persistent asthma; however, increasing the dose of inhaled corticosteroid fourfold into the high-dose range also will result in a significant reduction in exacerbations.[50] However, doses of inhaled corticosteroids in the high range significantly enhance the risk of toxicity. Thus high doses of inhaled corticosteroids plus long-acting inhaled β_2-agonists are reserved for patients with step 4 severe persistent asthma.[7]

TABLE 26–12. Available Inhaled Corticosteroid Products, Lung Delivery, and Comparative Doses

ICS	Product	Lung Delivery[a]
Beclomethasone dipropionate (BDP)	42 mcg/actuation CFC MDI, 200 actuations	4–10%
	40 and 80 mcg/actuation HFA MDI, 120 actuations	55–60%
Budesonide (BUD)	200 mcg/dose DPI, Turbuhaler, 200 doses	32% (16–59%)
	200 and 500-mcg ampules, 2 mL each	6%
Flunisolide (FLU)	250 mcg/actuation CFC MDI, 100 actuations	32%
Fluticasone propionate (FP)	44, 110, and 220 mcg/actuation CFC MDI, 120 actuations	26–30%
	50, 100, and 250 mcg/dose DPI, Rotadisk, 4 doses	15% (13–18%)
	50, 100, and 250 mcg/dose DPI, Diskus, 60 doses	15%
Mometasone furoate (MF)	200 and 400 mcg/dose DPI, Twisthaler, 14, 30, 60, and 120 doses	Unknown
Triamcinolone acetonide (TAA)	100 mcg/actuation CFC MDI, 240 actuations with spacer	22%

	Comparable Daily doses (mcg)		
	Low Dose, Child/Adult	*Medium Dose, Child/Adult*	*High Dose, Child/Adult*
BDP			
CFC MDI	84–336/168–504	336–672/504–840	>672/>840
HFA MDI	40–160/80–240	160–320/240–400	>320/>400
BUD			
DPI	100–200/200–400	200–400/400–800	>400/>800
Nebules	250–500/UK	500–1000/UK	>1000/UK
FLU, CFC MDI	500–750/500–1000	750–1250/1000–2000	>1250/>2000
FP			
CFC MDI	88–176/88–264	176–440/264–660	>440/>660
DPIs	100–200/100–300	200–400/300–600	>400/>600
MF, DPI	UK/200–400	UK/400–800	UK/>800
TAA, CFC MDI	400–800/400–1000	800–1200/1000–2000	>1200/>2000

[a]Lung delivery from in vivo radiolabel scintigraphy or pharmacokinetic studies.

Although the addition of a third controller medication is often used clinically in patients requiring step 4 therapy, there are few studies evaluating this practice.[7] Leukotriene antagonists added to high-dose inhaled corticosteroids and long-acting inhaled β_2-agonists do not improve outcomes.[7] None of the other long-term controllers has been evaluated in this scenario. Omalizumab or anti-IgE has received FDA approval for use in corticosteroid-dependent, severe asthma. Thus patients with severe asthma and atopy with an elevated IgE concentration would be candidates for omalizumab.[51]

■ SPECIAL POPULATIONS

Children 5 years of age and younger have not been studied adequately. Thus many of the recommendations in this age group are based on extrapolation of data from older children and adults.[7] The few studies of inhaled corticosteroids in this younger group are supportive. The nebulized formulation of budesonide gained FDA approval from three pivotal efficacy and safety trials.[7] The FDA approval for montelukast in children younger than age 6 was based on safety and pharmacokinetic studies establishing doses but not on efficacy trials.[7] Not all trials of cromolyn in this younger group have demonstrated efficacy.[7] Theophylline has not been evaluated adequately, except for pharmacokinetics.[7] Combination therapy of any kind has not been studied except for a small number of patients down to 4 years of age on inhaled corticosteroids plus long-acting inhaled β_2-agonists.[7] The FDA approval of the Advair Diskus 100/50 in patients 4 to 11 years of age was based on extrapolation of efficacy data from patients older than 12 years of age and by safety and efficacy data from a study of the Advair Diskus 100/50 in children with asthma aged 4 to 11 years.

The recommendations for children 5 years of age and younger differ slightly from the recommendations for older children and adults. For step 3 therapy, both medium-dose inhaled corticosteroids as monotherapy and the combination of inhaled corticosteroids plus long-acting inhaled β_2-agonists are considered preferred.[7] However, there is no more evidence for a significant dose-response to the inhaled corticosteroids in this age group than there is for combination therapy.

Owing to the increased risk of osteoporosis in the elderly, patients requiring high doses of inhaled corticosteroids should have their bone mineral density determinations followed and appropriate therapies for osteoporosis instituted if necessary.[43]

Asthma affects 7% of pregnant women, making it potentially the most common serious medical condition to complicate pregnancy.[52] Maternal asthma has been reported to increase the risk of perinatal mortality, preeclampsia, preterm birth, and low-birth-weight infants.[52] More severe asthma is associated with increased risks, whereas better-controlled asthma is associated with decreased risks.

A systematic review of the evidence on the safety of asthma medications has been conducted by drug class.[52] This review concluded that it is safer for pregnant women with asthma to be treated with asthma medications than for them to have asthma exacerbations.[52] Proper monitoring and control of asthma should enable a woman with asthma to maintain a normal pregnancy with little or no risk to her or her fetus.

A stepwise approach to managing asthma during pregnancy and lactation has been published, with low-dose inhaled corticosteroids recommended as preferred treatment for step 2 and the addition of long-acting β-agonists added in step 3 and step 4.[52] Budesonide is considered the preferred inhaled corticosteroid to initiate because it has the greatest safety data from the Swedish Birth Registry.[52] Albuterol is considered the preferred rescue therapy.[52]

DRUG CLASS INFORMATION

INHALED CORTICOSTEROIDS

The mechanism of action of the corticosteroids has been reviewed (see above). The principal advantage of the inhaled corticosteroids (ICSs) is their high topical potency to reduce inflammation in the lung and low systemic activity.[43–45] The ICSs have high anti-inflammatory potency, approximately 1000-fold greater than endogenous cortisol, and differ from each other by as much as four- to sixfold.[44] However, potency differences, which are simply a measure of binding affinity to the receptor, can be overcome simply by giving different microgram dosages of drug. Aerosol delivery of the preparations is remarkably variable, ranging from 10% to 60% of the nominal dose (i.e., that dose which leaves an actuator for an MDI or, in the case of a DPI, that which is released on actuation of the inhaler).[24,45] Different devices for the same chemical entity may result in twofold differences in delivery, such as with fluticasone propionate and budesonide, or as much as eightfold with beclomethasone dipropionate (BDP) preparations.[45] Thus the delivery method can make a significant difference in the relative comparable dose.[2,45]

The ICSs beclomethasone dipropionate, budesonide, flunisolide, fluticasone propionate, and triamcinolone acetonide that are currently available for use are compared and listed in Table 26–12. The ICSs have pharmacokinetic differences that result in different topical/systemic activity.[44,45] Most evidence is consistent with log-linear dose-response curves for both indirect and direct responses.[43] The log-linear nature of the dose-response curve for corticosteroid activity raises the issue of how much of a difference in dose (or lung delivery) or potency is detectable. The dose-response curves for the ICSs are relatively flat primarily because all the measures used to assess efficacy (lung function, BHR, symptoms, and as-needed short-acting inhaled β_2-agonist use) are downstream events from the anti-inflammatory activity.[44] In general, it takes a fourfold difference in potency or dose to detect clinically significant differences. The table of comparative doses (see Table 26–12) is based on extensive comparative clinical trials.[7] Clinical comparative doses take into consideration potency differences as well as lung delivery differences from the various devices.

Since the glucocorticoid receptors within the various tissues are the same, differences in the pharmacokinetic profile are required to produce differences in the topical-systemic effect ratio (therapeutic index).[43] Pharmacokinetic properties that enhance improved topical selectivity include rapid systemic clearance, poor oral bioavailability, and long residence time in the lung.[43] Owing to their high lipophilicity, systemic clearance of the available ICSs is very rapid, approaching the rate of liver blood flow.[43] However, the ICSs differ markedly in their oral bioavailability, although they all undergo rather extensive first-pass metabolism to less active substances when absorbed[45] (see Table 26–9). The ICSs produce dose-dependent systemic effects from a combination of the orally absorbed fraction and the fraction absorbed from the lung[43–45] (Table 26–13). Essentially all the drug that reaches the lung is absorbed systemically; thus a slow absorption from the lung results in an apparent long elimination half-life and enhances topical selectivity by lowering the systemic concentration.[45] The potential advantage of the drugs with low oral bioavailability is obviated by using a spacer device with the MDI for the drugs with higher oral bioavailability because appropriate spacers reduce the oral dose by 80%.[24] The use of holding chambers also can increase systemic activity by increasing lung delivery of drugs not absorbed significantly orally.[43] If this increase in lung deposition is twofold or less, it will increase systemic activity without producing a clinically important

TABLE 26–13. Effects of Inhaled Corticosteroids

Beneficial Effects	Potential Adverse Effects
Decrease eosinophil numbers	Growth retardation, skeletal muscle myopathy
Decrease mast cell numbers	Osteoporosis, fractures and aseptic necrosis of hip
Decrease T-lymphocyte cytokine production	Posterior subcapsular cataract formation and glaucoma
Inhibit transcription of inflammatory genes in airway epithelium	Adrenal axis suppression, immunosuppression
Reduce endothelial cell leak	Impaired wound healing, easy bruising, skin striae
Upregulate β_2-receptor production	Hyperglycemia/hypokalemia, hypertension
Reduce airway epithelial subbasement membrane thickening	Psychiatric disturbances

increase in efficacy, thus decreasing the therapeutic index.[43] Mouth rinsing and spitting also will reduce the oral availability and are particularly useful for DPI devices.[2,24]

The response to ICSs is somewhat delayed. Most patients' symptoms will improve in the first 1 to 2 weeks of therapy and will reach maximum improvement in 4 to 8 weeks. Improvement in baseline FEV_1 and PEFs may require 3 to 6 weeks for maximum improvement, whereas improvement in BHR requires 2 to 3 weeks and approaches maximum in 1 to 3 months but may continue to improve over 1 year.[44] Most of the improvement in these parameters occurs at low to medium doses, and there is a large variability in response, with 10% of patients not demonstrating an improvement in either parameter.[53] Whether these nonresponders also show no improvement in rates of exacerbations is unknown. Maximum decrease in exhaled nitric oxide occurs within 2 to 3 weeks.[54] Sensitivity to exercise challenge decreases after 4 weeks of therapy.[44] Although single doses do not inhibit the immediate asthmatic response to antigen challenge, continued therapy for 1 week partially suppresses the response. These two latter effects are likely due to a reduction in mucosal mast cells.[44]

Local adverse effects from ICSs include oropharyngeal candidiasis and dysphonia that are dose-dependent. The dysphonia appears to be due to a local corticosteroid-induced myopathy of the vocal cords.[2] The use of a spacer device can decrease oropharyngeal deposition and thus decrease the incidence and severity of local side effects.[24] In infants who require delivery through a facemask, the parent should clean the nasal-perioral area with a damp cloth following each treatment to prevent topical candidal infections.

Systemic adverse effects can occur with any of the ICSs given in a sufficiently high dose.[43] Long-term adverse effects of greatest concern include growth suppression in children, osteoporosis, cataracts, and adrenal insufficiency and crisis.[43] Of these, only growth retardation occurs in low to medium doses. However, the growth reduction appears to be transient in that growth velocity is reduced in the first 6 months to 1 year of therapy and then returns to normal.[43] The effect is small (1 to 2 cm total) and not cumulative, and current studies suggest that attainment of predicted adult height is not affected.[7,43] The suppression of the hypothalamic-pituitary-adrenal axis and decreased bone mineralization are dose-dependent and do not appear to be significant clinically except at high doses.[43] The risks of these adverse effects are all dose-dependent and depend on the therapeutic index of each ICS and its delivery device. The effect of delivery device is illustrated by fluticasone propionate, which has both the greatest therapeutic index when administered by DPI and the lowest therapeutic index when administered by MDI plus holding chamber.[43]

Most patients with moderate disease can be controlled with twice-daily dosing of most ICSs.[2,10] Twice-daily dosing produces less thrush than three- to four-times-daily dosing regimens. In milder asthma, once-daily dosing is often sufficient to maintain control.[44] Some of the newer products have gained once-daily dosing indications for step-down therapy once initial control is established.[44] Chronobiologic dosing studies have demonstrated that dosing at 3 to 5 P.M. improves efficacy and may decrease adverse effects; however, this is a very difficult time to achieve for working adults and school children.[7] There does not appear to be any specific pharmacologic or pharmacokinetic aspect of the ICSs that allows for once-daily dosing because all the agents studied (both the older low-potency and newer high-potency ICSs) have been effective, provided that patients had relatively mild to moderate asthma.[45] More severe patients require multiple daily dosing. The inflammatory response of asthma has been shown to inhibit steroid-receptor binding.[45] This provides strong theoretical evidence for initially beginning patients on higher and more frequent doses and then tapering down once control has been achieved. This approach is recommended by the NAEPP.[2]

LONG-ACTING INHALED β₂-AGONISTS

The two long-acting β_2-agonists, formoterol and salmeterol, provide long-lasting bronchodilation (12 or more hours) when administered as aerosols[30] (see Table 26–8). Unlike the more water-soluble short-acting β_2-agonists, the long-acting agents are lipid-soluble, readily partitioning into the outer phospholipid layer of the cell membrane.[30] Salmeterol is more β_2-selective than albuterol and more bronchoselective by virtue of its property of remaining in the lung tissue cell membrane, which produces its longer duration.[30] However, both formoterol and salmeterol will produce dose-dependent systemic β_2-agonist effects.[30]

The principal differences between formoterol and salmeterol is that formoterol has a more rapid onset of action (similar to that of albuterol), and formoterol is a full agonist, whereas salmeterol is a partial agonist. These differences are unlikely to produce clinically significant differences because both are recommended for chronic therapy only in combination with ICSs.[7,10] They are available singly and as fixed-dose combinations with ICSs (see below). Patients should be warned that salmeterol is ineffective for acute severe asthma because it can take up to 20 minutes for onset and 1 to 4 hours for maximum bronchodilation following inhalation.[2,7] Patients need to be counseled to continue to use their short-acting inhaled β_2-agonists for acute exacerbations while receiving the long-acting inhaled β_2-agonists.

Long-acting inhaled β_2-agonists are indicated as preferred therapy for step 3 as adjunctive therapy to low to medium doses of ICSs and for step 4 in combination with medium to high doses of ICSs.[7] Combination treatment with both an ICS and a long-acting β_2-agonist provides greater asthma control than increasing the dose of ICS alone while at the same time reducing the frequency and perhaps the severity of exacerbations.[55] Since they are devoid of anti-inflammatory activity, the long-acting inhaled β_2-agonists should not be used as monotherapy for asthma. Recent evidence suggests that patients treated with monotherapy are at an increased risk for severe exacerbations.[56] Additionally, a large and so far unpublished study of the effect of adding salmeterol to usual treatment for asthma in the general population has been halted prematurely owing to poor trial enrollment

and an increased risk of asthma-related deaths in African-American patients receiving salmeterol. Whether this was due to greater asthma severity or undertreatment with inhaled corticosteroids was difficult to discern.[57]

As with short-acting β_2-agonists, tolerance is produced with chronic administration. Long-term trials have shown no diminution in bronchodilator response but a partial loss of the initial bronchoprotective effect against methacholine or histamine challenge by salmeterol.[55] In particular, the duration of protection against EIB following a single dose of salmeterol is up to 9 hours but is reduced to less than 4 hours following regular treatment.[55] Following regular treatment with salmeterol and formoterol, decreased protection against nonspecific bronchoprovocation with methacholine also occurs, although it provides greater protection than placebo.[55] Responsiveness to short-acting β_2-agonists has been reported to be slightly decreased but easily overcome by increasing the dose (by approximately one puff) following chronic therapy with long-acting β_2-agonists.[55]

There is ample evidence that the use of a long-acting β_2-agonist in combination with ICS therapy does not mask inflammation.[50,55] A meta-analysis of studies comparing the addition of salmeterol to ICS therapy versus at least a doubling of ICS dose demonstrates that rather than increasing asthma exacerbations, the number of these events was reduced.[58] There are few data on the efficacy of long-acting β-agonists (LABAs) on asthma exacerbation rates in pediatric patients, but studies are ongoing.[59]

METHYLXANTHINES

Methylxanthines have been used for asthma therapy for over 50 years but their use in recent years has declined markedly owing to the high risk of severe life-threatening toxicity and numerous drug interactions, as well as decreased efficacy compared with ICSs and long-acting inhaled β_2-agonists. Theophylline, the primary methylxanthine of interest, is a moderately potent bronchodilator with mild anti-inflammatory properties.[2,10] Like the β_2-agonists, the methylxanthines are functional antagonists of bronchospasm; however, their clinical utility is limited by their low therapeutic index.[2] Theophylline as a sustained-release product is the preferred oral preparation, whereas its complex with ethylenediamine (aminophylline) is the preferred injectable product owing to increased solubility.[60]

The mechanism by which theophylline produces bronchodilation appears to be through nonselective phosphodiesterase inhibition.[60] Inhibition of phosphodiesterase results in increased cAMP and cyclic guanosine monophosphate (cGMP) concentrations. The phosphodiesterase (PDE) isoenzymes currently thought to be important for theophylline's clinical effects are isoenzymes III, predominant in airway smooth muscle, and IV, important in inflammatory cell regulation such as mast cells, neutrophils, eosinophils, and T-lymphocytes.[60] Selective PDE isoenzyme IV inhibitors, however, have no significant effects in clinical asthma. Theophylline is a competitive antagonist of adenosine and stimulates endogenous catecholamine release.[60] These latter two effects are important determinants of toxic symptoms of excess theophylline.[2,60]

Theophylline, like the β_2-agonists, has a log-linear dose-response curve.[60] Most chronic stable asthmatics will obtain significant bronchodilation when the serum theophylline concentration reaches 5 mcg/mL, and most patients will have no toxic symptoms with serum concentrations of less than 15 mcg/mL.[2,60] The percentage of patients experiencing adverse effects increases sharply as concentrations exceed 15 mcg/mL. As with the β_2-agonists, the dose-response curves for smooth muscle relaxation by theophylline are

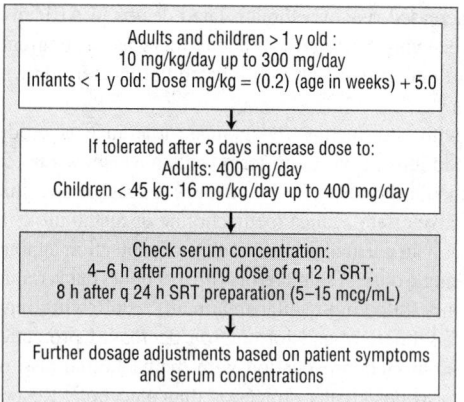

FIGURE 26–9. Algorithm for slow titration of theophylline dosage and guide for final dosage adjustment based on serum theophylline concentration measurement. For infants younger than 1 year of age, the initial daily dosage can be calculated by the following regression equation: Dose (mg/kg) = (0.2) (age in weeks) + 5.0. Whenever side effects occur, dosage should be reduced to a previously tolerated lower dose.

dynamic and shifted to the right in the face of increasing contractile stimuli.[27] This probably explains theophylline's relative lack of bronchodilatory effect in acute severe asthma.[2,27] The severity of theophylline's toxicity precludes even doubling the usual dosage. Toxicities include caffeine-like effects of nausea, vomiting, tachycardia, jitteriness, and difficulty sleeping to more severe toxicities such as cardiac tachyarrythmias and seizures. Death has occurred in children receiving their usual doses of theophylline during acute systemic viral illnesses.[60]

Routine monitoring of serum concentrations is essential for the safe and effective use of theophylline.[2,10] Theophylline is eliminated primarily by metabolism via the hepatic cytochrome P450 mixed-function oxidase microsomal enzymes (primarily the CYP1A2 and CYP3A3 isozymes), with 10% or less excreted unchanged in the kidney.[60] Theophylline clearance is age-dependent, with 1- to 9-year-olds having the highest systemic clearances and therefore requiring the largest dosages (on a weight basis). However, even within the same age groups, theophylline clearance can vary two- to threefold.[60] Figure 26–9 gives a dosing and monitoring schedule for theophylline. Factors affecting theophylline's hepatic metabolism are listed in Table 26–14.[2] Only drugs or diseases that produce a 20% or greater

inhibition or a 50% or greater induction of theophylline metabolism are likely to result in clinically significant interactions.[60]

Sustained-release theophylline is less effective than ICSs and no more effective than oral sustained-release β_2-agonists, cromolyn or leukotriene antagonists.[7] The addition of theophylline to ICSs is similar to doubling the dose of the ICS and is overall less effective than the long-acting inhaled β_2-agonists as adjunctive therapy.[7]

CROMOLYN SODIUM AND NEDOCROMIL SODIUM

Cromolyn sodium and nedocromil sodium are pharmacologically similar.[2] They are classified as mast cell stabilizers, and the principal difference appears to be potency, with 4 mg nedocromil by MDI equivalent to 10 mg cromolyn.[2,61] However, there is no apparent difference in the clinical efficacy between these two drugs.[2] They inhibit the early and late asthmatic response to allergen challenge, as well inhibit exercise-induced bronchospasm.[2,10] Treatment prevents the usual rise in bronchial hyperresponsiveness with specific pollen seasons, but long-term treatment produces minimal to no change in baseline bronchial hyperresponsiveness.[7,61] They inhibit neurally mediated bronchoconstriction, through C-fiber sensory nerve stimulation in the airways, although neither drug has a bronchodilatory effect.[10]

Cromolyn and nedocromil are only effective by inhalation and are available as MDIs, whereas cromolyn also is available as a nebulizer solution. The pharmacokinetics of both drugs are very similar. They are not bioavailable orally, but the portion of the dose that reaches the lung is absorbed completely.[61] Absorption from the airway is significantly slower than elimination (hours versus minutes). The short duration in the lung likely limits their efficacy. Both the intensity and duration of protection against various challenges are dose-dependent.[61] Higher doses produce greater and more prolonged protection.

Both drugs are remarkably nontoxic. No evidence of mutagenesis or teratogenesis has been found for cromolyn. Cough and wheeze have been reported following inhalation of each, and bad taste and headache following nedocromil are reported.[2] The taste from nedocromil is sufficiently bad in some patients (approximately 20%) to preclude them from taking the drug.[61] Tolerance to cromolyn or nedocromil has not been demonstrated. Neither are ICS-sparing agents.

Cromolyn and nedocromil are no more or less effective than theophylline or the leukotriene antagonists for persistent asthma.[7]

TABLE 26–14. Factors Affecting Theophylline Clearance

Decreased Clearance	% Decrease	Increased Clearance	% Increase
Cimetidine	−25 to −60	Rifampin	+53
Macrolides	−25 to −50	Carbamazepine	+50
Erythromycin, TAO,		Phenobarbital	+34
clarithromycin		Phenytoin	+70
Allopurinol	−20	Charcoal-broiled meat	+30
Propranolol	−30		
Quinolones	−20 to −50	High-protein diet	+25
Ciprofloxacin,		Smoking	+40
enoxacin,			
pefloxacin			
Interferon	−50	Sulfinpyrazone	+22
Thiabendazole	−65	Moricizine	+50
Ticlopidine	−25	Aminoglutethimide	+50
Zileuton	−35		
Systemic viral illness	−10 to −50		

Neither cromolyn nor nedocromil is as effective as the ICSs for controlling persistent asthma.[7,49] Neither is as effective as the inhaled β_2-agonists for preventing exercise-induced bronchospasm but can be used in conjunction for patients not responding completely to the inhaled β_2-agonists.[18]

Most patients will experience an improvement in 1 to 2 weeks, but it may take longer to achieve maximum benefit. Patients initially should receive cromolyn or nedocromil four times daily, and then only after stabilization of symptoms may the frequency be reduced to two times daily for nedocromil and three times daily for cromolyn. Only the nebulizer solution should be used for children younger than 5 years of age.[2]

LEUKOTRIENE MODIFIERS

Two clinically distinct cysteinyl leukotriene receptor antagonists (zafirlukast and montelukast) and one inhibitor of leukotriene synthesis (zileuton) have been available in the United States since 1996 for both children and adults with persistent asthma.[62] In challenge studies, they reduce allergen-, exercise-, cold-air hyperventilation-, irritant-, and aspirin-induced asthma.[63] Clinical use of zileuton is limited owing to the need for four-times-daily dosing, the potential for elevated liver enzymes (especially in the first 3 months of therapy), and the potential inhibition of drugs metabolized by the CYP3A4 isoenzymes.[62,63]

In clinical trials, the LTD_4 receptor antagonists (zafirlukast and montelukast) have demonstrated efficacy in adults and children with persistent asthma. These drugs improve pulmonary function tests (FEV_1 and PEF), decrease nocturnal awakenings and β_2-agonist use, and improve asthma symptoms.[62,63] A major advantage is that they are effective orally, administered once or twice a day, and contribute to patient adherence and satisfaction with therapy.[62] However, they are less effective in asthma than low doses of ICSs, although some patients (even those with severe disease) may have useful clinical improvement.[64] For example, in 533 patients (>15 years old) with persistent asthma, treatment with fluticasone 176 mcg by MDI twice daily improved mean morning FEV_1 at end point by 22.9% versus montelukast 10 mg daily improvements of 14.5% ($p < .001$).[64] All other asthma outcomes were improved to a greater extent by fluticasone therapy. It is not yet possible to predict which patients respond best to leukotriene modifiers, although there is some evidence that patients with aspirin-sensitive asthma do well, as predicted by studies showing increased cysteinyl leukotriene production in these patients.[63] It is possible that genetic polymorphisms in the 5-lipooxygenase (5-LO) or LTC_4 synthase pathways or in cys-LT_1 receptors might predict better responders in the future.[63] Antileukotrienes also have modest efficacy in allergic rhinitis.

In general, the LTD_4 receptor antagonists are well tolerated and do not appear to have serious class-specific effects. In the early 6-month zafirlukast trials, nonrespiratory or laboratory abnormalities did not occur with greater frequency in the treatment group than in the placebo groups. However, postmarketing surveillance reports include elevations in serum aminotransferase concentrations and clinical hepatitis (thought to be rare).[65] An idiosyncratic syndrome similar to the Churg-Strauss syndrome, with marked circulating eosinophilia, heart failure, and associated eosinophilic vasculitis, has been reported in a small number of patients treated with zafirlukast or montelukast.[65] The majority of these patients had been receiving high-dose inhaled or oral corticosteroids and were able to reduce the dose as a consequence of the LTD_4 receptor antagonists. It is unclear whether the increased reports are due to increased case findings among patients with asthma prescribed a new drug or whether the syndrome is related to glucocorticoid dose reduction or an idiosyncratic effect of leukotriene modifiers in general. Whatever the cause, it appears to be a rare syndrome, with an estimated incidence of fewer than 1 case per 15,000 to 20,000 patient-years of treatment.[65] Montelukast has been prescribed widely worldwide owing to its approval for use in young children. Churg-Strauss syndrome has not been reported in children, and the drug has been very well tolerated and palatable (4- and 5-mg chewable cherry tablets).[65]

COMBINATION CONTROLLER THERAPY: ICS/LABA VERSUS ICS/LT RECEPTOR AGONISTS

Whereas ICS therapy is considered the most effective anti-inflammatory treatment, in cases of moderate to severe persistent asthma, the addition of a second long-term control medication to ICS therapy is one recommended treatment option. A combination-product inhaler (Advair) was developed to treat both the inflammatory and bronchoconstrictive components of asthma by delivering a dose of fluticasone (100, 250, or 500 mcg) with a fixed dose of salmeterol (50 mcg). Advair, in a variety of clinical trials in persistent asthma, was superior to the individual components at the same doses, comparable with concurrent therapy at the same doses, had a rapid onset of effect (within 1 week), and demonstrated clinical benefits that improved over the duration of the studies. Importantly, salmeterol therapy allows reduction in ICS dosage by 50% in patients with persistent asthma.[7,55] Further, salmeterol plus low-dose fluticasone has been found to be more effective than higher-dose fluticasone alone in reducing asthma exacerbations in patients with persistent asthma.[55] The ability to detect deteriorating asthma and the severity of exacerbation were similar between groups.

Leukotriene receptor agonists also have been found to be successful as additive therapy in patients inadequately controlled on ICS alone and as ICS-sparing therapy.[7] However, the magnitude of these benefits is less than those reported with the addition of long-acting β_2-agonists (LABAs).[7]

ANTI-IGE (OMALIZUMAB)

Omalizumab is the first anti-IgE antibody approved for the treatment of asthma not well controlled on high doses of ICSs.[66] Omalizumab is a composite of 95% human and 5% antihuman murine IgE sequences. The mouse protein becomes part of the receptor complex and thus is shielded from exposure to the immune system and presents a low risk for an anaphylactic response.[66]

Omalizumab is administered subcutaneously and has a slow absorption rate; peak serum concentration is achieved in 3 to 14 days.[66] It is eliminated primarily through the reticuloendothelial system and has an elimination half-life of 17 to 22 days; serum free IgE levels return to baseline in about 3 weeks.[66]

The dosage of omalizumab is determined by the patient's baseline total serum IgE level (international units per milliliter) and body weigh (kilograms).[66] Doses range from 150 to 375 mg and are given at either 2- or 4-week intervals. No further adjustments for variations in total serum IgE are required, and patients receive a consistent dose for the duration of treatment.[66] Omalizumab has been studied in patients aged 12 to 74 years and appears to be safe and efficacious.[66] It is only indicated for corticosteroid-dependent atopic patients requiring oral corticosteroids or on high-dose ICSs with continued symptoms and high IgE levels.

▇ MISCELLANEOUS THERAPIES

▇ METHOTREXATE

Low-dose methotrexate (15 mg/week) used for inflammatory diseases, psoriatic and rheumatoid arthritis, and polymyositis has been used to reduce the systemic steroid dose in patients with severe steroid-dependent asthma.[67] Double-blind, placebo-controlled trials have given decidedly mixed results, with half the studies showing no effect.[68] A meta-analysis determined that a statistically significant reduction (mean 4.37 mg/day prednisone, or 23% of the original dose) can be achieved.[67] The mechanism of action is unknown but may be anti-inflammatory or immunomodulatory effects. Methotrexate inhibits chemotaxis of neutrophils, inhibits leukotriene B$_4$–induced adherence to endothelium, and inhibits the proinflammatory activity of IL-1. Low-dose weekly methotrexate is not without hazard. Both hepatotoxicity and pulmonary fibrosis have been reported in patients receiving similar therapy for psoriasis and rheumatoid arthritis.[67] No evidence for induction of asthma remission exists because patients' corticosteroid requirement returns on discontinuation of the methotrexate. Methotrexate still should be considered experimental and should be reserved for only severe steroid-dependent asthmatics under the care of specialties. Patients require careful monitoring, including periodic liver biopsies. Owing to the marginal effect of methotrexate, the risk-benefit should be evaluated carefully prior to institution.

▇ OTHER AGENTS

As a result of the inflammatory nature of asthma and the risk of toxicities from corticosteroids, a number of the drugs with anti-inflammatory or immunomodulatory activity such as hydroxychloroquine, dapsone, gold, intravenous gamma-globulin, cyclosporine, and colchicine have been studied in severe steroid-dependent asthma with mixed results.[2,67]

▇ FUTURE THERAPIES

Agents that are now in development for asthma focus on the treatment of allergic inflammation.[68,69] Examples include inhibitors of eosinophilic inflammation, drugs that may inhibit allergen presentation, and inhibitors of Th2 cells. Multiple cytokines have been implicated in allergic inflammation, and several possible inhibiting approaches are being explored. These range from drugs that inhibit cytokine synthesis (cyclosporin A and tacrolimus), humanized blocking antibodies to cytokines or their receptors, soluble receptors to mop up secreted cytokines, receptor antagonists, and drugs that block the signal-transduction pathways activated by cytokines.[68] Specifically, humanized monoclonal antibodies to IL-5 and nebulized soluble IL-4 receptors have been tested but have been disappointing to date.[68,69]

PHARMACOECONOMIC CONSIDERATIONS

Of the estimated $12.6 billion cost of asthma in the United States in 1998, direct medical expenditure accounted for 58% of the total, with emergency care (emergency department and inpatient hospital care) reaching $2.5 billion and prescription medications ($3.2 billion) as the single largest direct medical expenditure.[6] A cost-of-illness approach takes in all measurable costs; both indirect costs or costs to society and direct medical costs are considered. Using this approach, the cost per patient per year in 1994 in the United States was $756, a slight decrease in inflation-adjusted expenditures over the past 10 years.[6] Indirect costs such as lost work and death accounted for two-thirds of these expenditures.

The medication cost increase over the past 10 years resulted from a doubling of prescribed medications, as well as a 169% increase in unit cost per medication, presumably owing to a shift to more expensive anti-inflammatory drugs consistent with the recommendations of the NAEPP guidelines.[2] Asthma severity obviously has an impact on cost of care. Studies from health-maintenance organizations suggest that up to 45% of the cost of asthma is accrued by 10% of the patients, primarily as a result of emergency care.[70]

Numerous studies have demonstrated the cost-effectiveness of patient education programs for asthma, particularly those providing guided self-management.[70] Several studies have reported positive results from pharmacist interventions reducing overall cost of care.[70] Similar studies have demonstrated the cost-effectiveness of specialist care compared with generalist care. However, the results of these trials may be confounded by changes in prescribing as part of the overall program. Indeed, use of ICSs reduces both morbidity, particularly hospitalizations, and mortality in asthma patients.[48,71]

The NAEPP recommendations provide numerous alternatives for long-term controllers in mild to moderate persistent asthma, and few studies have compared their relative cost-effectiveness. This is important because outside the realm of randomized clinical trials that evaluate efficacy, other factors such as concern about adverse effects and adherence to therapy may alter the overall clinical effectiveness. Use of ICSs in children has produced a cost of $9.45 per symptom-free day gained and in adults $5.00 per symptom-free day.[70] More recently, retrospective analyses of large managed-care-linked pharmacy claims and health care utilization databases has allowed direct comparisons of the various long-term controllers in a general population to assess clinical effectiveness and cost-effectiveness. These studies have confirmed comparative randomized clinical trials showing ICSs to be significantly more cost-effective than leukotriene antagonists despite slightly better compliance with the leukotriene antagonists.[72,73] In addition, the combination of long-acting inhaled β_2-agonists and ICSs lowers health care utilization and total health care costs compared with the combination of a leukotriene antagonist and an ICS.[74]

CLINICAL CONTROVERSY

The potential for chronic use of inhaled β_2-agonists to worsen asthma has been a concern for over 30 years. Large multicenter double-blind, placebo-controlled trials with both mild and moderate persistent asthma did not show that regular administration short-acting inhaled β_2-agonists worsened asthma.[10,41] However, recent studies genotyping patients at the β-receptor suggest that homozygous Arg-16 patients (who make up about 16% of the population) are predisposed to worsening asthma with regular administration as measured by lower morning PEFs.[40,75] This phenomenon does not appear to occur with as-needed therapy with short-acting β_2-agonists. It is yet unknown if regular treatment with long-acting inhaled β_2-agonists is of similar concern. These patients still respond acutely to the β_2-agonists, so whether they should avoid all β_2-agonists is speculative. Since the use of short-acting inhaled β_2-agonists does not improve control of symptoms, they should be used only as needed for symptoms.[2]

EVALUATION OF THERAPEUTIC OUTCOMES

The desired outcomes have been described previously. Control of asthma is defined as achieving a minimal need for "rescue" short-acting β_2-agonists (ideally none), no acute episodes, no limitations on activity, no emergency care visits, no nocturnal symptoms, normal (or near-normal) pulmonary functions (FEV_1 and PEF), minimal to no medication side effects, and satisfaction of the patient and family with asthma care. Depending on the severity of the patient's asthma, compromises from the ideal control are made, and the best possible outcome balancing disease control and possible adverse effects from the drugs is attempted.

Monitoring consists of quantitating the use of inhaled short-acting β_2-agonists, days of limited activity, and number of symptoms (especially nocturnal). The NAEPP recommends yearly spirometric studies. In moderate to severe persistent asthma, once-daily (on awakening) peak-flow monitoring is recommended. Patients also should be asked about exercise tolerance. All patients on inhaled drugs should have their inhalation delivery technique evaluated periodically—monthly initially and then every 3 to 6 months.

Following initiation of anti-inflammatory therapy or an increase in dosage, most patients should begin experiencing a decrease in symptoms in 1 to 2 weeks and achieve maximum symptomatic improvement within 4 to 8 weeks. The use of higher doses or more potent ICS agents may accelerate the process. Improvement in FEV_1 and PEF should follow a similar time frame; however, a decrease in BHR, as measured by morning PEF, PEF variability, and exercise tolerance, may take longer and improve over 1 to 3 months.[2] Patients should be informed that following a viral respiratory infection, they may experience increased exercise intolerance for up to 4 weeks.

Initial visits with the patient should focus on the patient's concerns, expectations, and goals of treatment. Basic education should focus on asthma as a chronic lung disease, the types of medications, and how they are to be used. Inhaler technique is taught, as is when to seek medical advice. Written action plans should be provided. The first follow-up visit should be in 2 to 4 weeks. At that time, the educational messages of the first visit should be repeated, as well as questions about the patient's current medications and any difficulties related to the therapy.

CONCLUSION

Asthma is a complicated disease with a multitude of clinical presentations. The exact defect in asthma has not been defined, and it may be that asthma is a common presentation of a heterogeneous group of diseases. Asthma is defined and characterized by excessive reactivity of the bronchial tree to a wide variety of noxious stimuli. The reaction is characterized by bronchospasm, excessive mucus production, and inflammation. The central role of inflammation in inducing and maintaining BHR is now becoming widely appreciated and studied. The goal of asthma therapy is to normalize, as much as possible, the patient's life and prevent chronic irreversible lung changes. Drugs are the mainstay of asthma therapy. The goal of drug therapy is to use the minimum amount of medications possible to completely control the disease. In chronic asthma, therapy should be aimed at both bronchospasm and inflammation in order to produce the best results. Patients should be followed and monitored diligently for toxicities. Although death from asthma is an uncommon event, the most common cause of death is underassessment of the severity of obstruction either by the patient or by the clinician; the next common cause is undertreatment. A cornerstone of any therapy is education and the realization that most asthma deaths are avoidable.

ABBREVIATIONS

ABPA: allergic bronchopulmonary aspergillosis
ACTH: adrenocorticotropic hormone
Arg: arginine
BAL: bronchoalveolar lavage
BHR: bronchial hyperresponsiveness
CFC: chlorofluorocarbon
cAMP: cyclic adenosine monophosphate
CYP: Cytochrome P450
DPI: dry powder inhaler
EIB: exercise-induced bronchospasm
FDA: Food and Drug Administration
FeNO: fraction of exhaled nitric oxide
FEV_1: forced expiratory volume in 1 second
FVC: forced vital capacity
GINA: Global Initiative for Asthma
Gln: glutamine
Glu: glutamic acid
Gly: glycine
GM-CSF: granulocyte-macrophage colony-stimulating factor
HFA: hydrofluoroalkane
ICAM-1: intercellular adhesion molecule 1
ICSs: inhaled corticosteroids
IgE: immunoglobulin E
IL: interleukin
iNOS: inducible nitric oxide synthase
MDI: metered-dose inhaler
MMAD: mass median aerodynamic diameter
NAEPP: National Asthma Education and Prevention Program
NANC: nonadrenergic, noncholinergic
NO: nitric oxide
PAF: platelet-activating factor
PEF: peak expiratory flow
PKA: protein kinase
RSV: respiratory syncytial virus
T cells: thymically derived lymphocytes
VCAM-1: vascular cell adhesion molecule 1
VIP: vasoactive intestinal peptide

Review Questions and other resources can be found at *www.pharmacotherapyonline.com.*

REFERENCES

1. Rosenblatt MB. History of bronchial asthma. In: Weiss EB, Segal MS, Stein M, eds. Bronchial Asthma: Mechanisms and Therapeutics, 2d ed. Boston, Little, Brown, 1976:5–17.
2. NHLBI, National Asthma Education and Prevention Program, Expert Panel Report 2. Guidelines for the Diagnosis and Management of Asthma. NIH Publication No. 97-4051. Bethesda, MD, US Department of Health and Human Services, 1997.
3. CDC National Center for Health Statistics. Asthma Prevalence, Health Care Use and Mortality, 2000–2001. Bethesda, MD, US Department of Health and Human Services, January 2003; *http://www.cdc.gov/nchs/products/pubs/pubd/hestats/asthma/asthma.htm*; accessed September 2003.

4. Akinbami LJ, Schoendorf KC. Trends in childhood asthma: Prevalence, health care utilization, and mortality. Pediatrics 2002;110:315–322.

5. Aligne CA, Auinger P, Byrd RS, Weitzman M. Risk factors for pediatric asthma: Contributions of poverty, race, and urban residence. Am J Respir Crit Care Med 2000;162:873–877.

6. Weiss KB, Sullivan SD. The health economics of asthma and rhinitis: I. Assessing the economic impact. J Allergy Clin Immunol 2001;107:3–8.

7. National Institutes of Health, National Heart, Lung, and Blood Institute. National Asthma Education and Prevention Program. Expert Panel Report: Guidelines for the diagnosis and management of asthma update on selected topics 2002. J Allergy Clin Immunol 2002;110:S142–219.

8. Grol MH, Gerritsen J, Vonk JM, et al. Risk factors for growth and decline of lung function in asthmatic individuals up to age 42 years: A 30-year follow-up study. Am J Respir Crit Care Med 1999;160:1830–1837.

9. Bousquet J, Jeffery PK, Busse WW, et al. Asthma: From bronchoconstriction to airways inflammation and remodeling. Am J Respir Crit Care Med 2000;161:1720–1745.

10. National Institutes of Health, National Heart, Lung, and Blood Institute. Global Initiative for Asthma (GINA). Global Strategy for Asthma Management and Prevention Revised (2002). NHLBI/WHO Workshop Report. NIH publication No. 02-3659. Bethesda, MD, US DEpartment of Health and Human Services, 2002.

11. Van Eerdewegh P, Little RD, Dupuis J, et al. Association of the ADAM33 gene with asthma and bronchial hyperresponsiveness. Nature 2002;418:426–430.

12. von Mutius E. The environmental predictors of allergic disease. J Allergy Clin Immunol 2000;105:9–19.

13. Malo J-L, Chan-Yeung M. Occupational asthma. J Allergy Clin Immunol 2001;108:317–328.

14. Kay AB. Allergy and allergic diseases: First of two parts. N Engl J Med 2001;344:30–37.

15. Busse WW, Lemanske RF Jr. Asthma. N Engl J Med 2001;344:350–362.

16. Elias JA, Zhu Z, Chupp G, Homer RJ. Airway remodeling in asthma. J Clin Invest 1999;104:1001–1006.

17. Kharitonov SA, Barnes PJ. Exhaled markers of pulmonary disease. Am J Respir Crit Care Med 2001;163:1693–1702.

18. McFadden ER Jr. Exercise-induced airway narrowing. In: Adkinson Jr NF, Yunginger JW, Busse WW, et al, eds. Middleton's Allergy: Principles and Practice, 6th ed. St Louis, Mosby, 2003:1323–1332.

19. Alberts WM. "Circa menstrual" rhythmicity and asthma. Chest 1997;111:840–842.

20. Chandler MH, Schuldheisz HS, Phillips BA, Muse KN. Premenstrual asthma: The effect of estrogen on symptoms, pulmonary function, and β_2-receptors. Pharmacotherapy 1997;17:224–234.

21. Zimmerman JL, Woodruff PG, Clark S, Camargo CA Jr, MARC Investigators. Relation between phase of menstrual cycle and emergency department visits for acute asthma. Am J Respir Crit Care Med 2000;162:512–515.

22. Beasely R, Burgess C, Holt S. Call for a worldwide withdrawal of benzalkonium chloride from nebulizer solutions. J Allergy Clin Immunol 2001;107:222–223.

23. Szczeklik A, Stevenson D. Aspirin-induced asthma: Advances in pathogenesis and management. J Allergy Clin Immunol 1999;104:5–13.

24. Dolovich MA, MacIntyre NR, Dhand R, et al. Consensus conference on aerosols and delivery devices. Respir Care 2000;45:588–776.

25. Nelson HS. β-Adrenergic bronchodilators. N Engl J Med 1995;333:499–506.

26. Kelly HW. Aerosol delivery. In: Murphy S, Kelly HW, eds. Pediatric Asthma. Lung Biology in Health and Disease Series 126. New York, Marcel Dekker, 1999:463–487.

27. Kelly HW, Murphy SJ. The management of acute severe asthma in children. In: Busse WW, Holgate S, eds. Asthma and Rhinitis, 2d ed. Boston, Blackwell Science, 2001:1944–1960.

28. Strauss L, Hejal R, Galan G, et al. Observations on the effects of aerosolized albuterol in acute asthma. Am J Respir Crit Care Med 1997;155:454–458.

29. Camargo CA Jr, Spooner CH, Rowe BH. Continuous versus intermittent beta-agonists in the treatment of acute asthma (Cochrane Review). In: The Cochrane Library 2003;4.

30. Jenne JW, Kelly HW. β_2-Agonists. In: Murphy S, Kelly HW, eds. Pediatric Asthma. New York, Marcel Dekker, 1999:279–326.

31. Cates C, Rowe BH, Bara A. Holding chambers versus nebulisers for beta-agonist treatment of acute asthma (Cochrane Review). In: The Cochrane Library 2002;2.

32. Edmonds ML, Camargo CA Jr, Pollack CV Jr, et al. Early use of inhaled corticosteroids in the emergency department the treatment of acute asthma (Cochrane Review). In: The Cochrane Library 2003;3.

33. Plotnick LH, Ducharme FM. Should inhaled anticholinergics be added to β_2-agonists for treating acute childhood and adolescent asthma? A systematic review. Br Med J 1998;317:971–977.

34. Rodrigo GJ, Rodrigo C. The role of anticholinergics in acute asthma treatment: An evidence-based evaluation. Chest 2002;121:1977–1987.

35. Rowe BH, Bretzlaff JA, Bourdon C, et al. Intravenous magnesium sulfate treatment for acute asthma in the emergency department: A systematic review of the literature. Ann Emerg Med 2000;36:181–190.

36. Rodrigo GJ, Rodrigo C, Pollack CV, Rowe B. Use of helium-oxygen mixtures in the treatment of acute asthma: A systematic review. Chest 2003;123:891–896.

37. Liggett SB. β_2-Adrenergic receptor pharmacogenetics. Am J Respir Crit Care Med 2000;161:S197–201.

38. Waldeck B. Enantiomers of bronchodilating β_2-adrenoceptor agonists: Is there a cause for concern? J Allergy Clin Immunol 1999;103:742–748.

39. Berger WE. Levalbuterol: Pharmacologic properties and use in the treatment of pediatric and adult asthma. Ann Allergy Asthma Immunol 2003;90:583–592.

40. Israel E, Drazen JM, Liggett SB, et al. The effect of polymorphisms of the β_2-adrenergic receptor on the response to regular use of albuterol in asthma. Am J Respir Crit Care Med 2000;162:75–80.

41. Dennis SM, Sharp SJ, Vickers MR, et al. Regular inhaled salbutamol an asthma control: The TRUST randomised trial. Lancet 2000;355:1675–1679.

42. Inman MD, O'Byrne PM. The effect of regular inhaled albuterol on exercise-induced bronchoconstriction. Am J Respir Crit Care Med 1996;153:65–69.

43. Kelly HW. Potential adverse effects of the inhaled corticosteroids. J Allergy Clin Immunol 2003;112:469–478.

44. Pederson S, O'Byrne P. A comparison of the efficacy and safety of inhaled corticosteroids in asthma. Allergy 1997;52(suppl 39):1–34.

45. Kelly HW. Pharmacology of inhaled glucocorticoids: Comparative properties. Immunol Allergy Clin North Am 1999;19:725–738.

46. Campbell SC. Clinical aspects of inhaled anticholinergic therapy. Respir Care 2000;45:864–867.

47. Lord J, Ducharme FM, Stamp RJ, et al. Cost-effectiveness analysis of inhaled anticholinergics for acute childhood and adolescent asthma. Br Med J 1999;319:1470–1471.

48. Suissa S, Ernst P, Benayoun S, et al. Low-dose inhaled corticosteroids and the prevention of death from asthma. N Engl J Med 2000;343:332–336.

49. Childhood Asthma Management Program Research Group. Long-term effects of budesonide or nedocromil in children with asthma. N Engl J Med 2000;343:1054–1063.

50. Pauwels RA, Löfdahl CG, Postma DS, et al. Effect of inhaled formoterol and budesonide on exacerbations of asthma. N Engl J Med 1997;337:1405–1411.

51. Owen CE. Anti-immunoglobulin E therapy for asthma. Pulm Pharmacol Ther 2002;15:417–424.

52. National Institutes of Health, National Heart, Lung and Blood Institute. NAEPP Expert Panel Report Managing Asthma During Pregnancy: Recommendations for Pharmacologic Treatment—Update 2004. NIH Publication No. 04-5246, March 2004.

53. Szefler SJ, Martin RJ, King TS, et al. Significant variability in response to inhaled corticosteroids for persistent asthma. J Allergy Clin Immunol 2002;109:410–418.

54. Kharitonov SA, Barnes PJ. Exhaled markers of pulmonary disease. Am J Respir Crit Care Med 2001;163:1693–1722.

55. Nelson HS. Advair: Combination treatment with fluticasone propionate/salmeterol in the treatment of asthma. J Allergy Clin Immunol 2001;107:397–416.

56. Lazarus SC, Boushey HA, Fahy JV et al. Long-acting β_2-agonist montherapy vs continued therapy with inhaled corticosteroids in patients with persistent asthma: A randomized controlled trial. JAMA 2001;285:2583–2593.

57. Data on file, GlaxoSmithKline (SLGA 5011).

58. Shrewsbury S, Pyke S, Britton M. A meta-analysis of increasing inhaled steroid or adding salmeterol in symptomatic asthma (MIASMA). Br Med J 2000;320:1368–1373.

59. Bisgaard H. Effect of long-acting β_2-agonists on exacerbation rates of asthma in children. Pediatr Pulmonol 2003;36:391–398.

60. Blake K. Theophylline. In: Murphy SA, Kelly HW, eds. Pediatric Asthma. New York, Marcel Dekker, 1999:363–431.

61. Sorkness CA. Cromolyn, nedocromil, leukotriene modifiers, and alternative anti-inflammatory agents in the treatment of pediatric asthma. In: Murphy SA, Kelly HW, eds. Pediatric Asthma. New York, Marcel Dekker, 1999:433–462.

62. Sorkness CA. Leukotriene receptor antagonists in the treatment of asthma. Pharmacotherapy 2001;21:34S–37S.

63. Drazen JM, Israel E, O'Byrne PM. Treatment of asthma with drugs modifying the leukotriene pathway. N Engl J Med 1999;340:197–206.

64. Busse W, Raphael GD, Galant S, et al. Low-dose fluticasone propionate compared with montelukast for first-line treatment of persistent asthma: A randomized clinical trial. J Allergy Clin Immunol 2001;107:461–468.

65. Price D. Tolerability of montelukast. Drugs 2000;59(suppl 1):35–42.

66. DeKorte CJ. Current and emerging therapies for the management of chronic inflammation asthma. Am J Health Syst Pharm 2003;60:1949–1961.

67. Marin MG. Low-dose methotrexate spares steroid usage in steroid-dependent asthmatic patients: A meta-analysis. Chest 1997;112:29–33.

68. Barnes PJ. New directions in allergic diseases: Mechanism based anti-inflammatory therapies. J Allergy Clin Immunol 2000;106:5–16.

69. Hendeles L, Asmus M, Chesrown S. Evaluation of cytokine modulators for asthma. Paediatr Respir Rev 2003;4(suppl 1):S105–110.

70. National Asthma Education and Prevention Program. Task force report on the cost effectiveness, quality of care, and financing of asthma care. Am J Respir Crit Care Med 1996;154(Suppl):S81–130.

71. Donahue JG, Weiss ST, Livingston JM, et al. Inhaled steroids and the risk of hospitalization for asthma. JAMA 1997;277:887–891.

72. Stempel DA, Meyer JW, Stanford RH, Yancey SW. One-year claims analysis comparing inhaled fluticasone propionate with zafirlukast for the treatment of asthma. J Allergy Clin Immunol 2001;107:94–98.

73. Stempel DA, Mauskopf J, McLaughlin T, et al. Comparison of asthma costs in patients starting fluticasone propionate compared to patients starting montelukast. Respir Med 2001;95:227–234.

74. Stempel DA, O'Donnell JC, Meyer JW. Inhaled corticosteroids plus salmeterol or montelukast: Effects on resource utilization and costs. J Allergy Clin Immunol 2002;109:433–439.

75. Taylor DR, Drazen JM, Herbison GP, et al. Asthma exacerbations during long term beta agonist use: Influence of β_2-adrenoceptor polymorphism. Thorax 2000;55:762–767.

27
CHRONIC OBSTRUCTIVE PULMONARY DISEASE

Sharya V. Bourdet and Dennis M. Williams

Learning Objectives and other resources can be found at *www.pharmacotherapyonline.com*.

KEY CONCEPTS

❶ Chronic obstructive pulmonary disease (COPD) is a progressive disease characterized by airflow limitation that is not fully reversible and is associated with an abnormal inflammatory response of the lungs to noxious particles or gases.

❷ COPD includes the terms *chronic bronchitis* and *emphysema*. Chronic bronchitis is defined in clinical terms, whereas emphysema is defined in terms of anatomic pathology. Because most patient exhibit some features of each disease, the current emphasis of COPD pathophysiology is on small airway disease and parenchymal damage that contributes to chronic airflow limitation.

❸ Mortality from COPD has increased steadily over the past three decades; it currently is the fourth leading cause of death in the United States.

❹ The primary cause of COPD is cigarette smoking. Other risks include a genetic predisposition, environmental exposures (including occupational dusts and chemicals), and air pollution.

❺ Smoking cessation is the only management strategy proven to slow progression of COPD.

❻ Oxygen therapy has been shown to reduce mortality in selected patients with COPD. Oxygen therapy is indicated for patients with a resting Pao_2 of less than 55 mm Hg or a Pao_2 of less than 60 mm Hg and evidence of right-sided heart failure, polycythemia, or impaired neurologic function.

❼ Bronchodilators are the mainstay of drug therapy for COPD. Pharmacotherapy is used to relieve patient symptoms and improve quality of life. The selection of bronchodilator therapy should be based on patient-specific factors.

❽ The role of inhaled corticosteroid therapy in COPD is not well established. Patients with severe COPD and frequent exacerbations may benefit from inhaled corticosteroids.

❾ Treatment of acute exacerbations of COPD include intensification of bronchodilator therapy and a short course of systemic corticosteroids.

❿ Antimicrobial therapy should be used during acute exacerbations of COPD if the patient exhibits at least two of the following: increased dyspnea, increased sputum volume, and increased sputum purulence.

Chronic obstructive pulmonary disease (COPD) is a chronic disease of the airways characterized by the gradual progressive loss of lung function. The prevalence and mortality of COPD have increased over the past two decades. Currently, COPD is the fourth leading cause of death in the United States. Although treatment guidelines for the management of COPD have been available for many years, concerns have been expressed that the recommendations were largely opinions and were not evidenced-based.

In order to standardize the care of patients with COPD and present evidence-based recommendations, the National Heart, Lung, and Blood Institute (NHLBI) and the World Health Organization (WHO) launched the Global Initiative for Chronic Obstructive Lung Disease (GOLD) in 2001.[1] This report was updated in August 2003. The goals of the GOLD organization are to increase awareness of COPD and reduce morbidity and mortality associated with the disease. The consensus group has proposed the following working definition for COPD:

❶ *Chronic obstructive pulmonary disease* is a disease state characterized by airflow limitation that is not fully reversible. The airflow limitation is usually both

progressive and associated with an abnormal inflammatory response of the lungs to noxious particles or gases.[1]

The most common conditions comprising COPD are chronic bronchitis and emphysema. Chronic bronchitis is a condition with chronic or recurrent excessive mucus secretion into the bronchial tree with cough that is present on most days for at least 3 months of the year for at least 2 consecutive years in a patient in whom other causes of chronic cough have been excluded.[2] While chronic bronchitis is defined in clinical terms, emphysema is defined in terms of anatomic pathology. Emphysema classically was defined on histologic examination at autopsy. Because this histologic definition is of limited clinical value, emphysema also has been defined as abnormal permanent enlargement of the airspaces distal to the terminal bronchioles accompanied by destruction of their walls yet without obvious fibrosis.[2]

❷ The new consensus guidelines have moved away from chronic bronchitis and emphysema as descriptive subsets of COPD. This is based on the observation that the majority of COPD is caused by a common risk factor (cigarette smoking), and most patients exhibit features of both chronic bronchitis and emphysema. Therefore, emphasis is currently placed on the pathophysiologic features of small airways

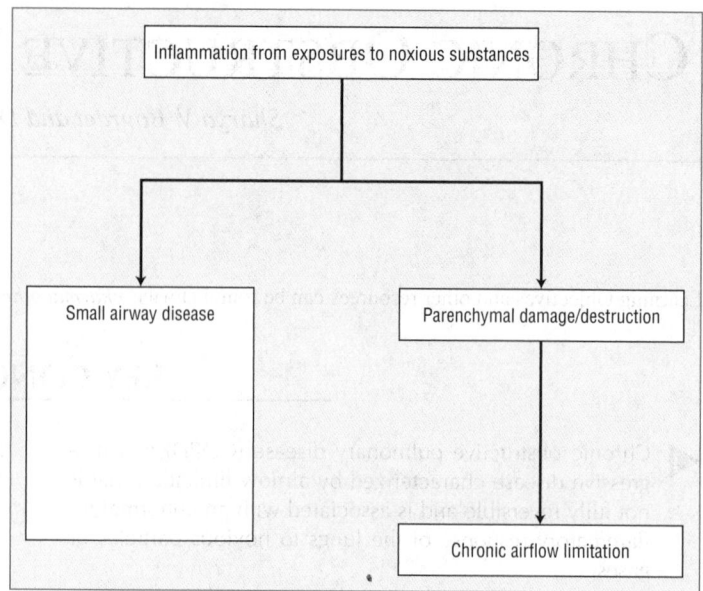

FIGURE 27–1. Mechanisms for developing chronic airflow limitation in COPD. *(From ref. 1.)*

disease and parenchymal destruction as contributors to chronic airflow limitation. Most patients with COPD demonstrate features of both problems. Chronic inflammation affects the integrity of the airways and causes damage and destruction of the parenchymal structures. This results in the chronic airflow limitation that characterizes COPD (Fig. 27–1).

EPIDEMIOLOGY

Data from the National Health Interview Survey in 2001 indicate that 12.1 million people over age 25 years in the United States have COPD.[3] Over 9 million of these individuals have chronic bronchitis; the remaining number have emphysema or a combination of both diseases. However, there is evidence that this estimate is low. According to national surveys, the true prevalence of people with symptoms of chronic airflow obstruction may exceed 24 million.[4]

COPD is the fourth leading cause of death in the United States, exceeded only by cancer, heart disease, and cerebrovascular accidents. In 2000, over 119,000 deaths in the United States and 2.74 million deaths worldwide were attributed to COPD. It is the only leading cause of death to increase over the last 30 years and is projected to be the third leading cause by 2020.[5] Overall, the mortality rate is higher in males; however, the female death rate has doubled over the last 25 years, and the number of female deaths exceeded male deaths in 2000. The mortality rate is higher in whites compared with blacks.[5]

Cigarette smoking is the primary cause of COPD, and although the prevalence of cigarette smoking has declined compared with 1965, approximately 25% of individuals in the United States currently smoke. The trend of increasing COPD mortality likely reflects the long latency period between smoking exposure and complications associated with COPD.

The mortality of COPD is significant; however, morbidity associated with the disease has significant impact on patients, their families, and the health care system. COPD represents the second leading cause of disability in the United States. Individuals with COPD have approximately double the number of hospital stays, days of restricted activity, and days of being confined to bed compared with people

without COPD.[5] In 2000, there were over 15 million physician office visits, 1.5 million emergency room visits, and 726,000 hospitalizations due to COPD. Comparison of these data with those of recent years reflects a steady continuing increase.[6]

According to the NHLBI, the economic impact of COPD was $23 billion in 2000 and $32 billion in 2002, including $18 billion in direct costs.[5] It is estimated that by 2020, COPD will be the fifth most burdensome disease, as measured by disability-adjusted life years lost due to illness.

ETIOLOGY

Cigarette smoking is the primary modifiable risk factor for the development of COPD; however, the disease can be attributed to a combination of risk factors that results in lung injury and tissue destruction. The risk factors associated with the development of COPD can be divided into host factors and environmental factors (Table 27–1), and commonly, the interaction between these risks leads to expression of the disease. Host factors, such as genetic predisposition, may not be modifiable but are important for identifying patients at high risk of developing the disease. Environmental factors, such as tobacco smoke and occupational dust and chemicals, are modifiable factors that, if avoided, may reduce the risk of disease development.

Environmental exposures associated with COPD are particles that are inhaled by the individual and result in inflammation and cell injury. Exposure to multiple environmental toxins increases the risk of COPD. In such cases, it is helpful to assess an individual's total

TABLE 27–1. Risk Factors for Development of Chronic Obstructive Pulmonary Disease (COPD)

Exposures	Host Factors
Environmental tobacco smoke	Genetic predisposition (AAT deficiency)
Occupational dusts and chemicals	Airway hyperresponsiveness
Air pollution	Impaired lung growth

burden of inhaled particles. For example, an individual who smokes and works in a textile factory has a higher total burden of inhaled particles than an individual who smokes and has no occupational exposure.

Cigarette smoking is the most common risk factor among industrialized countries and accounts for 85% to 90% of cases of COPD.[1] Components of tobacco smoke activate inflammatory cells, which produce and release the inflammatory mediators characteristic of COPD. Although the risk is lower in pipe and cigar smokers, it is still higher than in nonsmokers. Age of starting, total pack-years, and current smoking status are predictive of COPD mortality. However, only 15% to 20% of all smokers go on to develop COPD, and not all smokers who have equivalent smoking histories develop the same degree of pulmonary impairment, suggesting that other host and environmental factors contribute to the degree of lung dysfunction. Nevertheless, the rate of loss of lung function is determined primarily by smoking status and history.[2] Children and spouses of smokers are also at increased risk of developing significant pulmonary dysfunction by passive smoking, also known as *environmental tobacco smoke* or *secondhand smoke.*

Occupational exposures are also important risk factors for COPD and, in nonindustrialized countries, may be more common than cigarette smoking. These exposures include dust and chemicals such as vapors, irritants, and fumes. Reduced lung function and deaths from COPD are higher for individuals who work in gold and coal mining, in the glass or ceramic industries with exposure to silica dust, and in jobs that expose them to cotton dust or grain dust, toluene diisocyanate, or asbestos. Other occupational risk factors include chronic exposure to open cooking or heating fires.

It is unclear whether or not air pollution alone is a significant risk factor for the development of COPD in smokers and nonsmokers with normal lung function. However, in individuals with existing pulmonary dysfunction, significant air pollution worsens symptoms. As evidence for this, emergency department visits are increased during higher-intensity periods of air pollution.

Individuals exposed to the same environmental risk factors do not have the same chance of developing COPD, suggesting that host factors play an important role in pathogenesis.[1,2] While many not yet identified genes may influence the risk of developing COPD, the best documented genetic factor is a hereditary deficiency of α_1-antitrypsin (AAT). AAT-associated emphysema is an example of a pure genetic disorder inherited in an autosomal recessive pattern. The consequences of AAT deficiency are discussed in the pathophysiology section below as protease-antiprotease imbalance. True AAT deficiency accounts for less than 1% of COPD cases.[2]

AAT is a plasma protein that protects cells, especially those in the lung, from destruction by elastase released by neutrophils. In individuals with the most common allele (M), plasma levels of AAT are approximately 30 micromolar (150 mg/dL). The protective effect of AAT in the lungs is significantly diminished when plasma levels are less than 10 micromolar.[7] AAT is an acute-phase reactant, and the serum concentration can be quite variable. Typically, reference range concentrations are 80–200 mg/dL (16–40 micromolar).

Several types of AAT deficiency have been identified and are due to mutations in the AAT gene. Two main gene variants, S and Z, have been identified. In patients who are homozygous with the S variant, AAT levels are at least 60% of those of normal individuals. These patients usually do not have an increased risk of COPD compared with normal individuals. Patients with homozygous Z deficiency (ZZ) have AAT levels that are 10% of those of normal individuals, while patients with heterozygous Z variant (SZ) have levels closer to 40% of those of normal individuals. Homozygous Z patients have a higher

risk of developing COPD compared with heterozygous Z patients.[8] A history of cigarette smoking increases this risk. A small number of patients have a null, null phenotype and are at high risk for developing emphysema because they produce virtually no AAT.

Patients with AAT deficiency develop COPD at an early age (20 to 50 years) primarily owing to an accelerated decline in lung function. Compared with an average annual decline in forced expiratory volume in 1 second (FEV_1) of 25 mL/year in healthy nonsmokers, patients with homozygous Z deficiency have been reported to have declines of 54 mL/year for nonsmokers and 108 mL/year for current smokers.[8] Patients developing COPD at an early age or those with a strong family history of COPD should be screened for AAT deficiency. If the concentration is low, phenotype testing (DNA) should be performed.

Two additional host factors that may influence the risk of COPD include airway hyperresponsiveness and lung growth. Individuals with airway hyperresponsiveness to various inhaled particles may have an accelerated decline in lung function compared with those without airway hyperresponsiveness. Additionally, individuals who do not attain maximal lung growth owing to low birth weight, prematurity at birth, or childhood illnesses may be at risk for COPD in the future.[1]

PATHOPHYSIOLOGY

COPD is characterized by chronic inflammatory changes that lead to destructive changes and the development of chronic airflow limitation. The process involves not only the airways but also extends to the pulmonary vasculature and lung parenchyma. The inflammation of COPD is often referred to as neutrophilic in nature, but macrophages and CD8+ lymphocytes also play major roles.[9,10] The inflammatory cells release a variety of chemical mediators, of which tumor necrosis factor α (TNF-α), interleukin 8 (IL-8), and leukotriene B$_4$ (LTB$_4$) play major roles.[1,11] The actions of these cells and mediators are complementary and redundant, leading to the widespread destructive changes. The stimulus for activation of inflammatory cells and mediators is an exposure to noxious particles and gas through inhalation. The most common etiologic factor is exposure to environmental tobacco smoke, although other chronic inhalational exposures can lead to similar inflammatory changes.

Other processes that have been proposed to play a major role in the pathogenesis of COPD include oxidative stress and an imbalance between aggressive and protective defense systems in the lungs (proteases and antiproteases).[9] These processes may be the result of ongoing inflammation or occur as a result of environmental pressures and exposures (Fig. 27–2).

An altered interaction between oxidants and antioxidants present in the airways is responsible for the increased oxidative stress present in COPD. Increases in markers (e.g., hydrogen peroxide and nitric oxide) of oxidants are seen in the epithelial lining fluid.[1] The increased oxidants generated by cigarette smoke react with and damage various proteins and lipids, leading to cell and tissue damage. Oxidants also promote inflammation directly and exacerbate the protease-antiprotease imbalance by inhibiting antiprotease activity.

The consequences of an imbalance between proteases and antiproteases in the lungs was described over 40 years ago when the hereditary deficiency of the protective antiprotease AAT was discovered to result in an increased risk of developing emphysema prematurely. This enzyme (AAT) is responsible for inhibiting several protease enzymes, including neutrophil elastase. In the presence of

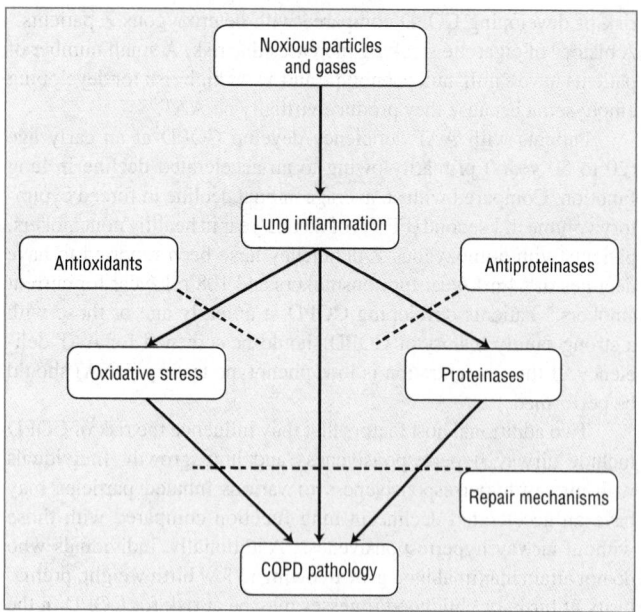

FIGURE 27–2. Pathogenesis of COPD. *(From ref. 1.)*

Pathologic changes of COPD are widespread, affecting large and small airways, lung parenchyma, and the pulmonary vasculature.[1] An inflammatory exudate is often present that leads to an increase in the number and size of goblet cells and mucus glands. Mucus secretion is increased, and ciliary motility is impaired. There is also a thickening of smooth muscle and connective tissue in the airways. Inflammation is present in central and peripheral airways. The chronic inflammation results in a repeated injury and repair process that leads to scarring and fibrosis. Diffuse airway narrowing is present and is more prominent in smaller peripheral airways.

Parenchymal changes affect the gas-exchanging units of the lungs, including the alveoli and pulmonary capillaries. The distribution of destructive changes varies depending on the etiology. Most commonly, smoking-related disease results in centrilobular emphysema that primarily affects respiratory bronchioles. Panlobular emphysema is seen in AAT deficiency and extends to the alveolar ducts and sacs.

The vascular changes of COPD include a thickening of pulmonary vessels and often are present early in the disease. These changes can be attributed to chronic inflammation and may lead to endothelial dysfunction of the pulmonary arteries. Later, structural changes lead to an increase in pulmonary pressures, especially during exercise. In severe COPD, secondary pulmonary hypertension leads to the development of right-sided heart failure.

Mucus hypersecretion is present early in the course of the disease and is associated with an increased number and size of mucus-producing cells. The presence of chronic inflammation perpetuates the process, although the resulting airflow obstruction and chronic airflow limitation may be reversible or irreversible. The various causes of airflow obstruction are summarized in Table 27–3.

Airflow limitation is assessed through spirometry, which represents the "gold standard" for diagnosing and monitoring COPD. The hallmark of COPD is a reduction in the ratio of FEV_1 to forced vital capacity (FVC) to less than 70%.[1,12] The FEV_1 generally is reduced, except in very mild disease, and the rate of FEV_1 decline is greater in COPD patients compared with normal subjects.

The impact of the numerous pathologic changes in the lung perturbs the normal gas-exchange and protective functions of the lung. Ultimately, these are exhibited through the common symptoms of COPD, including dyspnea and a chronic cough productive of sputum. As the disease progresses, abnormalities in gas exchange lead to hypoxemia and/or hypercapnia; although there often is not a strong relationship between pulmonary function and arterial blood gas results.

unopposed activity, elastase attacks elastin, a major component of alveolar walls.[1]

In the inherited form of emphysema, there is an absolute deficiency of AAT. In cigarette smoking–associated emphysema, the imbalance is likely associated with increased protease activity or reduced activity of antiproteases. Activated inflammatory cells release several proteases other than AAT, including cathepsins and metalloproteinases (MMPs). In addition, oxidative stress reduces antiprotease (or protective) activity.

It is helpful to differentiate inflammation occurring in COPD from that present in asthma because the response to anti-inflammatory therapy differs. The inflammatory cells that predominate differ between the two conditions, with neutrophils playing a major role in COPD and eosinophils and mast cells in asthma. Mediators of inflammation also differ with LTB_4, IL-8, and TNF-α predominating in COPD, compared with LTD_4, IL-4, and IL-5 among the numerous mediators modulating inflammation in asthma.[1] Characteristics of inflammation for the two diseases are summarized in Table 27–2.

TABLE 27–2. Features of Inflammation in COPD Compared with Asthma

	COPD	Asthma
Cells	Neutrophils	Eosinophils
	Large increase in macrophages	Small increase in macrophages
	Increase in CD8+ T lymphocytes	Increase in CD4+ Th2 lymphocytes
		Activation of mast cells
Mediators	LTB_4	LTD_4
	IL-8	IL-4, IL-5
	TNF-α	(Plus many others)
Consequences	Squamous metaplasia of epithelium	Fragile epithelium
	Parenchymal destruction	Thickening of basement membrane
	Mucus metaplasia	Mucus metaplasia
	Glandular enlargement	Glandular enlargement
Response to treatment	Glucocorticosteroids have variable effect	Glucocorticosteroids inhibit inflammation

From ref. 1.

TABLE 27–3. Etiology of Airflow Limitation in COPD

Reversible

Presence of mucus and inflammatory cells and mediators in bronchial
    secretions

Bronchial smooth muscle contraction in peripheral and central
    airways

Dynamic hyperinflation during exercise

Irreversible

Fibrosis and narrowing of airways

Reduced elastic recoil with loss of alveolar surface area

Destruction of alveolar support with reduced patency of small airways

Significant changes in arterial blood gases usually are not present until the FEV_1 is less than 1 L.[1] In these patients, hypoxemia and hypercapnia can become chronic problems. Initially, when hypoxemia is present, it usually is associated with exercise. However, as the disease progresses, hypoxemia at rest develops. Patients with severe COPD can have a low arterial oxygen tension (PaO_2 = 45 to 60 mm Hg) and an elevated arterial carbon dioxide tension ($PaCO_2$ = 50 to 60 mm Hg). The hypoxemia is attributed to hypoventilation ($\dot{V}$) of lung tissue relative to perfusion ($\dot{Q}$) of the area. This low $\dot{V}/\dot{Q}$ ratio will progress over a period of several years, resulting in a consistent decline in the PaO_2. Some COPD patients lose the ability to increase the rate or depth of respiration in response to persistent hypoxemia. Although this is not completely understood, the decreased ventilatory drive may be due to abnormal peripheral or central respiratory receptors responses. This relative hypoventilation subsequently leads to hypercapnia. In this case, the central respiratory response to a chronically increased $PaCO_2$ can be blunted. These changes in PaO_2 and $PaCO_2$ are subtle and progress over a period of many years; as a result, the pH usually is nearly normal because the kidneys compensate by retaining bicarbonate. If acute respiratory distress develops, such as might be seen in pneumonia or a COPD exacerbation with impending respiratory failure, the $PaCO_2$ may rise sharply, and the patient presents with an uncompensated respiratory acidosis.

The consequences of long-standing COPD and chronic hypoxemia include the development of secondary pulmonary hypertension that progresses slowly if appropriate treatment of COPD is not initiated. Pulmonary hypertension is the most common cardiovascular complication of COPD and can result in cor pulmonale, or right-sided heart failure.[13]

The elevated pulmonary artery pressures are attributed to vasoconstriction (in response to chronic hypoxemia), vascular remodeling, and loss of pulmonary capillary beds. If elevated pulmonary pressures are sustained, cor pulmonale can develop, characterized by hypertrophy of the right ventricle in response to increases in pulmonary vascular resistance.

The risks of cor pulmonale include venous stasis with the potential for thrombosis and pulmonary embolism. Another important systemic consequence of COPD is a loss of skeletal muscle mass and general decline in the overall health status.

PATHOPHYSIOLOGY OF EXACERBATION

The natural history of COPD is characterized by recurrent exacerbations associated with increased symptoms and a decline in overall health status. Because many patients experience chronic symptoms, the diagnosis of an exacerbation is based, in part, on subjective mea-sures and clinical judgment. A working definition of a COPD exacerbation is a sustained worsening of the patient's condition from the stable state and beyond normal day-to-day variations that is acute in onset and necessitates a change in regular medication.[14]

There are limited data about pathology during exacerbations owing to the nature of the disease and the condition of patients; however, inflammatory mediators including neutrophils and eosinophils are increased in the sputum. Chronic airflow limitation is a feature of COPD and may not change remarkably even during an exacerbation.[1]

The primary physiologic change is often a worsening of arterial blood gas results owing to poor gas exchange and increased muscle fatigue. In a patient experiencing a severe exacerbation, profound hypoxemia and hypercapnia can be accompanied by respiratory acidosis and respiratory failure.

CLINICAL PRESENTATION

The diagnosis of COPD is made based on the patient's symptoms, including cough, sputum production, and dyspnea, and a history of exposure to risk factors such as tobacco smoke and occupational exposures. Patients may have these symptoms for several years before dyspnea develops and often will not seek medical attention until dyspnea is significant. The common features noted at presentation are summarized in Table 27–4.

The presence of airflow limitation should be confirmed with spirometry. Spirometry represents a comprehensive assessment of lung volumes and capacities. The hallmark of COPD is an FEV_1/FVC ratio of less than 70%, which indicates airway obstruction, and a postbronchodilator FEV_1 of less than 80% of predicted confirms the presence of airflow limitation that is not fully reversible.[1] An improvement in FEV_1 of less than 12% following inhalation of a rapid-acting bronchodilator is considered to be evidence of irreversible airflow obstruction. Reversibility of airflow limitation is measured by a bronchodilator challenge, which is described in Table 27–5. The use of peak expiratory flow measurements is not adequate for the diagnosis of COPD owing to low specificity and the high degree of effort dependence; however, a low peak expiratory flow is consistent with COPD. A comprehensive discussion about spirometry can be found in Chapter 25.

TABLE 27–4. Clinical Presentation of COPD

Symptoms

Chronic cough

Sputum production

Dyspnea

Exposure to Risk Factors

Tobacco smoke

α_1-Antitrypsin deficiency

Occupational hazards

Physical Examination

Cyanosis of mucosal membranes

Barrel chest

Increased resting respiratory rate

Shallow breathing

Pursed lips during expiration

Use of accessory respiratory muscles

Diagnostic Tests

Spirometry with reversibility testing

Radiograph of chest

Arterial blood gas (not routine)

TABLE 27-5. Procedures for Reversibility Testing

Preparation

Tests should be performed when patients are clinically stable and free from respiratory infection.

Patients should not have taken inhaled short-acting bronchodilators in the previous 6 hours, long-acting β-agonists in the previous 12 hours, or sustained-release theophylline in the previous 24 hours.

Spirometry

FEV_1 should be measured before bronchodilator is given.

Bronchodilators can be given by either metered-dose inhaler or nebulization.

Usual doses are 400 mcg of β-agonist, 80 mcg of anticholinergic, or the two combined.

FEV_1 should be measured again 30–45 minutes after bronchodilator is given.

Results

An increase in FEV_1 that is both greater than 200 mL and 12% above the prebronchodilator FEV_1 is considered significant.

From ref. 1.

Spirometry is also used to determine the severity of the disease, along with an assessment of symptoms and the presence of complications. Currently, the GOLD consensus guidelines suggests a five-stage classification system, which includes patients at risk for developing COPD (Table 27–6).

Patients at risk (stage 0) have normal spirometry but experience chronic symptoms of cough or sputum production and a history of exposure to risk factors. Patients in the remaining four stages of classification all exhibit the hallmark finding of airflow obstruction, i.e., a reduction in the FEV_1/FVC ratio to less than 70%. FVC is the total amount of air exhaled after a maximal inhalation. The extent of reduction in FEV_1 further defines the patient with mild, moderate, severe, or very severe disease.[1]

Most patients who present in the milder stages of COPD will have a normal physical examination. In later stages of the disease, when airflow limitation is severe, patients may have cyanosis of mucosal

TABLE 27-6. Classification of COPD Severity

Stage 0: At Risk

May have one or more symptoms of chronic cough, sputum production, or dyspnea

Exposure to risk factors

Normal spirometry

Stage I: Mild

$FEV_1/FVC < 70\%$

$FEV_1 \geq 80\%$

With or without symptoms

Stage II: Moderate

$FEV_1/FVC < 70\%$

$50\% < FEV_1 < 80\%$

With or without symptoms

Stage III: Severe

$FEV_1/FVC < 70\%$

$30\% < FEV_1 < 50\%$

With or without symptoms

Stage IV: Very Severe

$FEV_1/FVC < 70\%$

$FEV_1 < 30\%$ or $<50\%$ with presence of chronic respiratory failure or right heart failure

From ref. 1.

membranes, development of "barrel chest" due to hyperinflation of the lungs, an increased respiratory rate and shallow breathing, and changes in breathing mechanics such as pursing of the lips to help with expiration or use of accessory respiratory muscles.

PROGNOSIS

The average rate of decline of FEV_1 is the most useful objective measure to assess the course of COPD. The average rate of decline in FEV_1 for healthy, nonsmoking patients owing to age alone is 25 to 30 mL/year. The rate of decline for smokers is steeper, especially for heavy smokers compared with light smokers. The decline in pulmonary function is a steady curvilinear path. The more severely diminished the FEV_1 at diagnosis; the steeper is the rate of decline. Greater numbers of years of smoking and number of cigarettes smoked also correlate with a steeper decline in pulmonary function.[15] Conversely, the rate of decline of blood gases has not been shown to be a useful parameter to assess progression of the disease. Patients with COPD should have spirometry performed at least annually to assess disease progression.

The survival rate of patients with COPD is highly correlated to the initial level of impairment in the FEV_1 and age. Other less important factors include degree of reversibility with bronchodilators, resting pulse, perceived physical disability, diffusing capacity (D_{LCO}), cor pulmonale, and blood gas abnormalities. A rapid decline in pulmonary function tests indicates a poor prognosis. Median survival is approximately 10 years when the FEV_1 is 1.4 L, 4 years when the FEV_1 is 1.0 L, and about 2 years when the FEV_1 is 0.5 L.

While arterial blood gas (ABGs) measurements are important, they do not carry the prognostic value of pulmonary function tests. Measurement of arterial blood gases is more useful in patients with severe disease and is recommended for all patients with an FEV_1 of less than 40% of predicted or those with signs of respiratory failure or right-sided heart failure.[1]

CLINICAL PRESENTATION OF COPD EXACERBATION

Because of the subjective nature of defining an exacerbation of COPD, the criteria used among clinicians varies widely; however, most rely on a change in one or more of the following clinical findings: worsening symptoms of dyspnea, increase in sputum volume, or increase in sputum purulence. Common presentation features are listed in Table 27–7. Patients using rapid-acting bronchodilators may report an

TABLE 27-7. Clinical Presentation of COPD Exacerbation

Symptoms

Increased sputum volume

Acutely worsening dyspnea

Chest tightness

Presence of purulent sputum

Increased need for bronchodilators

Malaise, fatigue

Decreased exercise tolerance

Physical Examination

Fever

Wheezing, decreased breath sounds

Diagnostic Tests

Sputum sample for Gram stain and culture

Chest radiograph to evaluate for new infiltrates

TABLE 27–8. Staging Acute Exacerbations of COPD[a]

Mild (type 1)	One cardinal symptom[a] plus at least one of the following: URTI[b] within 5 days, fever without other explanation, increased wheezing, increased cough, increase in respiratory or heart rate >20% above baseline
Moderate (type 2)	Two cardinal symptoms[a]
Severe (type 3)	Three cardinal symptoms[a]

[a]Cardinal symptoms include worsening of dyspnea, increase in sputum volume, and increase in sputum purulence.
[b]URTI = upper respiratory tract infection.

increase in the frequency of use. Exacerbations are commonly staged as mild, moderate, or severe according to the criteria summarized in Table 27–8.[16]

An important complication of a severe exacerbation is acute respiratory failure. In the emergency department or hospital, an ABG usually is obtained to assess the severity of an exacerbation. The diagnosis of acute respiratory failure in COPD is made on the basis of an acute change in the ABGs. Defining acute respiratory failure as a PaO_2 of less than 50 mm Hg or a $PaCO_2$ of greater than 50 mm Hg often may be incorrect and inadequate because these values may not represent a significant change from a patient's baseline values. A more precise definition is an acute drop in PaO_2 of 10 to 15 mm Hg or any acute increase in $PaCO_2$ that decreases the serum pH to 7.3 or less.[17] Additional acute clinical manifestations of respiratory failure include restlessness, confusion, tachycardia, diaphoresis, cyanosis, hypotension, irregular breathing, miosis, and unconsciousness.

PROGNOSIS

COPD exacerbations are associated with significant morbidity and mortality. While mild exacerbations may be managed at home, mortality rates are higher for patients admitted to the hospital. In one study of patients hospitalized with COPD exacerbations, in-hospital mortality ranged from 6% to 8% but increased to 23% to 35% for the first year after hospital discharge.[18] Many patients experiencing an exacerbation do not have a return to their baseline clinical status for several weeks, significantly affecting their quality of life. Additionally, as many as half the patients originally hospitalized for an exacerbation are readmitted within 6 months.[19]

▶ TREATMENT: Chronic Obstructive Pulmonary Disease

▦ DESIRED OUTCOMES

Given the nature of COPD, a major focus in health care should be on prevention. However, in patients with a diagnosis of COPD, the primary goal is to prevent or minimize progression. Specific goals of management are listed in Table 27–9.

Optimally, these goals can be accomplished with minimal risks or side effects. The therapy of the patient with COPD is multifaceted and includes pharmacologic and nonpharmacologic strategies. Appropriate measures of effectiveness of the management plan include continued smoking cessation, symptom improvement, reduction in FEV_1 decline, reduction in the number of exacerbations, improvements in physical and psychological well-being, and reduction in mortality, hospitalizations, and days lost from work.

Unfortunately, most treatments for COPD have not been shown to improve survival or to slow the progressive decline in lung function. However, many therapies do improve pulmonary function and quality of life and reduce exacerbations and duration of hospitalization. Several disease-specific quality-of-life measures are available to assess the overall efficacies of therapies for COPD, including the Chronic Respiratory Questionnaire (CRQ) and the St. George's Respiratory Questionnaire (SGRQ). These questionnaires measure the impact of various therapies on such disease variables as severity of dyspnea and level of activity; they do not measure impact of therapies on survival. While early studies of COPD therapies focused primarily on improvements in pulmonary function measurements such as FEV_1, there is a trend toward greater use of these disease-specific quality-of-life measures to evaluate the benefits of therapy on larger clinical outcomes.

▦ GENERAL APPROACH TO TREATMENT

To be effective, the clinician should address four primary components of management: Assess and monitor the condition, avoidance of or reduced exposure to risk factors, manage stable disease, and treat exacerbations. These components are addressed through a variety of nonpharmacologic and pharmacologic approaches.

▦ NONPHARMACOLOGIC THERAPY

Patients with COPD should receive education about their disease, treatment plans, and strategies to slow progression and prevent complications.[1] Advice and counseling about smoking cessation are essential, if applicable. Because the natural course of the disease leads to respiratory failure, the clinician should address end-of-life decisions and advanced directives prospectively with the patient and family.[20]

▦ SMOKING CESSATION

◀5 A primary component of COPD management is avoidance of or reduced exposure to risk factors. Exposure to environmental tobacco smoke is a major risk factor, and smoking cessation is the most effective strategy to reduce the risk of developing COPD and to slow or stop disease progression. The cost-effectiveness of smoking-cessation interventions compares favorably with interventions made for other major chronic diseases.[21] The importance of smoking

TABLE 27–9. Goals of COPD Management

Prevent disease progression
Relieve symptoms
Improve exercise tolerance
Improve overall health status
Prevent and treat exacerbations
Prevent and treat complications
Reduce morbidity and mortality

TABLE 27–10. Treating Tobacco Use and Dependence: Public Health Service Report (2000) Major Findings and Recommendations

Tobacco dependence should be recognized as a chronic condition requiring repeated treatment until permanent abstinence is achieved.

Effective treatments for tobacco dependence are available and should be offered to all tobacco users.

Clinicians and health care systems should ensure mechanisms to identify, document, and treat all tobacco users in the system.

Brief treatment interventions for tobacco dependence should be offered to all tobacco users at a minimum.

There is a strong dose-response relationship between the intensity of tobacco dependence counseling and its effectiveness.

The most effective types of counseling and behavioral therapies are (1) practical counseling employing problem solving and skills training, (2) social support as part of treatment, and (3) social support outside of treatment.

Numerous pharmacotherapies have been proven to be effective for smoking cessation and should be offered in the absence of contraindications. These include sustained-release bupropion, nicotine gum, nicotine inhaler, nicotine nasal spray, and nicotine patch.

Tobacco dependence treatments are effective and cost-effective compared with other medical and disease-prevention measures.

TABLE 27–11. Five-Step Strategy for Smoking-Cessation Program (5 A's)

Ask	Use systematic approach to identify all tobacco users.
Advise	Urge all tobacco users to quit.
Assess	Determine willingness to make a cessation attempt.
Assist	Provide support for the patient to quit smoking.
Arrange	Schedule follow-up and monitor for continued abstinence.

All clinicians should take an active role in assisting patients with tobacco dependence in order to reduce the burden on the individual, his or her family, and the health care system. It is estimated that over 75% of smokers want to quit and that one-third have made a serious effort. Yet complete and permanent tobacco cessation is difficult.[22] Counseling that is provided by clinicians is associated with greater success rates than self-initiated efforts.[23]

The PHS guidelines recommend that clinicians take a comprehensive approach to smoking-cessation counseling. Advice should be given to smokers even if they have no symptoms of smoking-related disease or if they are receiving care for reasons unrelated to smoking. Clinicians should be persistent in their efforts because relapse is common among smokers owing to the chronic nature of dependence. Brief interventions (3 minutes) of counseling are proven effective. However, it must be recognized that the patient must be ready to stop smoking because there are several stages of decision making. Based on this, a five step intervention program is proposed (Table 27–11).

There is strong evidence to support the use of pharmacotherapy to assist in smoking cessation when counseling alone is not sufficient. Agents that are considered first line are listed in Table 27–12. Precautions to consider before using bupropion include a history of seizures or an eating disorder. Nicotine-replacement therapies are contraindicated in patients with unstable coronary artery disease, active peptic ulcers, or recent myocardial infarction or stroke. Nicotine patch, bupropion, and the combination of bupropion and the nicotine patch were compared with placebo in a controlled trial.[25] The treatment groups that received bupropion had higher rates of smoking cessation than the groups that received placebo or the nicotine patch. The addition of the nicotine patch to bupropion slightly improved the smoking-cessation rate compared with bupropion monotherapy. Second-line agents are less effective or associated with greater side effects; however, they may be useful in selected clinical situations. These therapies include clonidine and nortriptyline, a tricyclic antidepressant.

Behavioral modification techniques or other forms of psychotherapy also may be helpful in assisting in smoking cessation. Programs that address the many issues associated with smoking (i.e., learned behaviors, environmental influences, and chemical dependence) using a team approach are more likely to be successful. The

cessation cannot be overemphasized. Smoking cessation leads to decreased symptomatology and slows the rate of decline of pulmonary function even after significant abnormalities in pulmonary function tests have been detected ($FEV_1/FVC < 60\%$).[15] As confirmed by the Lung Health Study, smoking cessation is the only intervention proven at this time to affect long-term decline in FEV_1 and slow the progression of COPD.[22] In this 5-year prospective trial, smokers with early COPD were randomly assigned to one of three groups: smoking-cessation intervention plus inhaled ipratropium three times a day, smoking-cessation intervention alone, or no intervention. Smokers who underwent smoking-cessation intervention had fewer respiratory symptoms and a smaller annual decline in FEV_1 compared with smokers who had no intervention. However, this study also demonstrated the difficulty in achieving and sustaining successful smoking cessation.

Every clinician has a responsibility to assist smokers in smoking-cessation efforts. A clinical practice guideline for treating tobacco dependence from the U.S. Public Health Service (PHS) was updated in 2000.[23] The major findings and recommendations of that report are summarized in Table 27–10. In 2004, a report from the Surgeon General on the health consequences of smoking broadened the scope of the detrimental effects of cigarette smoking, indicating that "Smoking harms nearly every organ of the body, causing many diseases and reducing the health of smokers in general."[24]

TABLE 27–12. First-Line Pharmacotherapies for Smoking Cessation

Agent	Usual Dose	Duration	Common Complaints
Bupropion SR	150 mg orally daily for 3 days, then twice daily	12 weeks, up to 6 months	Insomnia, dry mouth
Nicotine gum	2–4 mg gum prn, up to 24 pieces daily	12 weeks	Sore mouth, dyspepsis
Nicotine inhaler	6–16 cartridges daily	Up to 6 months	Sore mouth and throat
Nicotine nasal spray	8–40 doses daily	3 to 6 months	Nasal irritation
Nicotine patches	Various, 7–21 mg every 24 hours	Up to 8 weeks	Skin reaction, insomnia

role of alternative-medicine therapies in smoking cessation is controversial. Hypnosis may aid in improving abstinence rates when added to a smoking-cessation program but appears to give little benefit when used alone. Acupuncture has not been shown to contribute to smoking cessation and is not recommended.[2]

PULMONARY REHABILITATION

Exercise training is beneficial in the treatment of COPD to improve exercise tolerance and to reduce symptoms of dyspnea and fatigue.[1] Pulmonary rehabilitation programs are an integral component in the management of COPD and should include exercise training along with smoking cessation, breathing exercises, optimal medical treatment, psychosocial support, and health education. High-intensity training (70% maximal workload) is possible even in advanced COPD patients, and the level of intensity improves peripheral muscle and ventilatory function. Studies have demonstrated that pulmonary rehabilitation with exercise three to seven times per week can produce long-term improvement in activities of daily living, quality of life, and exercise tolerance in patients with moderate to severe COPD.[26] Programs using less intensive exercise regimens (two times per week) have not been shown to be of benefit.[27]

IMMUNIZATIONS

Vaccines can be considered as pharmacologic agents; however, their role is described here in reducing risk factors for COPD exacerbations. Because influenza is a common complication in COPD that can lead to exacerbations and respiratory failure, an annual vaccination with the inactivated intramuscular influenza vaccine is recommended. Immunization against influenza can reduce serious illness and death by 50% in COPD patients.[28] Influenza vaccine should be administered in the fall of each year (October and November) during regular medical visits or at vaccination clinics. There are few contraindications to influenza vaccine except for a patient with a serious allergy to eggs. Oral anti-influenza agents (e.g., amantadine, rimantadine, and oseltamivir) can be considered for patients with COPD during an outbreak for patients who have not been immunized; however, these therapies are less effective and cause more side effects.[29]

The polyvalent pneumococcal vaccine, administered one time, is widely recommended for people from 2 to 64 years of age who have chronic lung disease and for all people older than 65 years. Thus COPD patients at any age are candidates for vaccination. Although evidence for the benefit of the pneumococcal vaccine in COPD is not strong, the argument for continued use is that the current vaccine provides coverage for 85% of pneumococcal strains causing invasive disease and the increasing rate of resistance of pneumococcus to selected antibiotics. Currently, administering the vaccine remains the standard of practice and is recommended by the Centers for Disease Control and Prevention and the American Lung Association.[30] Repeated vaccination with the 23-valent product is not recommended for patients aged 2 to 64 years with chronic lung disease; however, revaccination is recommended for patients over 65 years of age if the first vaccination was more than 5 years earlier and the patient was younger than age 65.

LONG-TERM OXYGEN THERAPY

6 The use of supplemental oxygen therapy increases survival in COPD patients with chronic hypoxemia. Although long-term oxygen has been used for many years in patients with advanced COPD, it was not until 1980 that data became available documenting its benefits. At that time, the Nocturnal Oxygen Therapy Trial Group published its data comparing nocturnal oxygen therapy (NOT; 12 h/day) with continuous oxygen therapy (COT; average of 20 h/day).[31] Among patients who were followed for at least 12 months, the results revealed a mortality rate in the NOT group that was nearly double that of the COT group (51% versus 26%). Statistical estimates of the COT group suggest that COT may have added 3.25 years to a COPD patient's life. Additional data from the Nocturnal Oxygen Therapy Trial Group revealed that COT patients had fewer (but statistically insignificant) hospitalizations, improved quality of life and neuropsychological function, reduced hematocrit, and decreased pulmonary vascular resistance.[31]

The decline in mortality with oxygen therapy was further substantiated in 1981 in a study by the British Medical Research Council that compared 15 h/day of oxygen versus no supplemental oxygen in COPD patients.[32] Patients receiving oxygen therapy for at least part of the day had lower rates of mortality than those not receiving oxygen. Recent analyses have shown that long-term oxygen therapy provides even more benefit in terms of survival after at least 5 years of use, and it improves the quality of life of these patients by increasing walking distance and neuropsychological condition and reducing time spent in the hospital.[33]

Before patients are considered for long-term oxygen therapy, they should be stabilized in the outpatient setting, and pharmacotherapy should be optimized. Once this is accomplished, long-term oxygen therapy should be instituted if either of two conditions exists:

1. A resting PaO_2 of less than 55 mm Hg
2. Evidence of right-sided heart failure, polycythemia, or impaired neuropsychiatric function with a PaO_2 of less than 60 mm Hg

The most practical means of administering long-term oxygen is with the nasal cannula, at 1 to 2 L/min which provides 24% to 28% oxygen. The goal is to raise the PaO_2 above 60 mm Hg. Patient education about flow rates and avoidance of flames (i.e., smoking) is of the utmost importance.

There are three different ways to deliver oxygen, including (1) in liquid reservoirs, (2) compressed into a cylinder, and (3) via an oxygen concentrator. Although conventional liquid oxygen and compressed oxygen are quite bulky, smaller, portable tanks are available to permit greater patient mobility. Oxygen concentrator devices separate nitrogen from room air and concentrate oxygen. These are the most convenient and the least expensive method of oxygen delivery. Oxygen-conservation devices are available that allow oxygen to flow only during inspiration, making the supply last longer. These may be particularly useful to prolong the oxygen supply for mobile patients using portable cylinders. However, the devices are bulky and subject to failure.

ADJUNCTIVE THERAPIES

In addition to supplemental oxygen, adjunctive therapies to consider as part of a pulmonary rehabilitation program are psychoeducational care and nutritional support. Psychoeducational care (such as relaxation) has been associated with improvement in the functioning and well-being of adults with COPD.[34] The role of nutritional support in patients with COPD is controversial. Several studies have shown an association between malnutrition, low body mass index (BMI), and impaired pulmonary status among patients with COPD. However, in

	0: At risk	I: Mild	II: Moderate	III: Severe	IV: Very severe
Characteristics	• Chronic symptoms • Exposure to risk factors • Normal spirometry	• $FEV_1/FVC < 70\%$ • $FEV_1 \geq 80\%$ • With or without symptoms	• $FEV_1/FVC < 70\%$ • $50\% > FEV_1 < 80\%$ • With or without symptoms	• $FEV_1/FVC < 70\%$ • $30\% > FEV_1 < 50\%$ • With or without symptoms	• $FEV_1/FVC < 70\%$ • $FEV_1 < 30\%$ or presence of chronic respiratory failure or right heart failure
	Avoidance of risk factor(s); influenza vaccination pneumococcal vaccine				
		Add short-acting bronchodilator when needed			
			Add regular treatment with one or more long-acting bronchodilators *Add* rehabilitation		
				Add inhaled glucocorticosteroids if repeated exacerbations	
					Add long-term oxygen if chronic respiratory failure *Consider* surgical treatments

FIGURE 27–3. Recommended therapy of stable COPD. *(From ref. 1.)*

a recent meta-analysis, the effect of nutritional support on outcomes in COPD was small and was not associated with improved anthropometric measures, lung function, or functional exercise capacity.[35]

PHARMACOLOGIC THERAPY

Currently, there is no medication available for the treatment of COPD that has been shown to modify the progressive decline in lung function or prolong survival.[1] Thus a primary goal of pharmacotherapy is to control patient symptoms and reduce complications, including the frequency and severity of exacerbations and improving the overall the health status and exercise tolerance of the patient.

Pharmacotherapy focuses on the use of bronchodilators to control symptoms. There are several classes of bronchodilators to choose from, and no single class has been proven to provide superior benefit over other available agents. The initial and subsequent choice of medications should be based on the specific clinical situation and patient characteristics. Medications can be used as needed or on a scheduled basis depending on the clinical situation, and additional therapies should be added in a stepwise manner depending on the response and severity of disease. Considerations should be given to individual patient response, tolerabilility, adherence, and economic factors. A stepwise approach to the management of COPD has been proposed based on the stage of disease severity (Fig. 27–3).

BRONCHODILATORS

Bronchodilator classes available for the treatment of COPD include β_2-agonists, anticholinergics, and methylxanthines. There is no clear benefit to one agent or class over others, although inhaled therapy generally is preferred. In general, it can be more difficult for patients with COPD to use inhalation devices effectively compared with other populations owing to advanced age and the presence of other comorbidities. Clinicians should advise, counsel, and observe patient technique with the devices frequently and consistently.

Bronchodilators generally work by reducing the tone of airway smooth muscle, thus minimizing airflow limitation. In patients with COPD, the clinical benefits of bronchodilators include increased exercise capacity, decreased air trapping in the lungs, and relief of symptoms such as dyspnea. However, use of bronchodilators may not be associated with significant improvements in pulmonary function measurements such as FEV_1. In general, side effects of bronchodilator medications are related to their pharmacologic effects and are dose-dependent. Because COPD patients are older and more likely to have comorbid conditions, the risk for side effects and drug interactions is higher compared with patients with asthma.

Sympathomimetics (β_2-Agonists)

A number of sympathomimetic agents are available in the United States. They vary in selectivity, route of administration, and duration of action. In COPD management, sympathomimetic agents with β_2-selectivity, or β_2-agonists, should be used as bronchodilators. β_2-Agonists cause bronchodilation by stimulating the enzyme adenyl cyclase to increase the formation of cyclic adenosine monophosphate (cAMP). cAMP is responsible for mediating relaxation of bronchial smooth muscle, leading to bronchodilation. In addition, they may improve mucociliary clearance. Although shorter-acting and less selective β-agonists are still used widely (e.g., metaproterenol, isoetharine, isoproterenol, and epinephrine), they should not be used owing to their shorter duration of action and increased cardiostimulatory effects. Selective β_2-agonists such as albuterol, levalbuterol, bitolterol, formoterol, pirbuterol, salmeterol, and terbutaline are preferred for therapy.

Sympathomimetics are available in inhaled, oral, and parenteral dosage forms. The preferred route of administration is by inhalation. The use of oral and parenteral β-agonists in COPD is discouraged because they are no more effective than a properly used metered-dose inhaler (MDI) or dry-powder inhaler (DPI), and the incidence of systemic adverse effects such as tachycardia and hand tremor is greater. Administration of β_2-agonists in the outpatient and emergency room settings via inhalers (MDIs or DPIs) is at least as effective as nebulization therapy and usually favored for reasons of cost and convenience.[36-38] Chapter 26 includes a complete description of the devices used for delivering aerosolized medication and a comparison β_2-agonist therapies.

Albuterol is the most frequently used β_2-agonist. It is available as an oral and inhaled preparation. Albuterol is a racemic mixture of (R)-albuterol that is responsible for the bronchodilator effect and (S)-albuterol that has no therapeutic effect. (S)-Albuterol is considered by some clinicians to be inert, whereas others believe that it may be implicated in worsening airway inflammation and antagonizing the response to (R)-albuterol. Levalbuterol is a single-isomer formulation of (R)-albuterol. A retrospective evaluation of levalbuterol versus albuterol use in patients with asthma and COPD concluded that levalbuterol offered significant advantages over albuterol for hospitalized patients.[39] Other clinicians feel that there are no significant differences between the products and that the use of levalbuterol is not justified owing to its higher acquisition cost.[40] The effects of a single dose of levalbuterol have been compared with those of albuterol and ipratropium plus albuterol in patients with COPD. No significant differences in pulmonary function improvements or adverse effects were noted.[41]

In COPD patients, β_2-agonists exert a rapid onset of effect, although the response generally is less than that seen in asthma. Short-acting inhaled β_2-agonists cause only a small improvement in FEV_1 acutely but may improve respiratory symptoms and exercise tolerance despite the small improvement in spirometric measurements.[42-44] Patients with COPD can use quick-onset β_2-agonists as needed for relief of symptoms or either short- or long-acting β_2-agonists on a scheduled basis to prevent or reduce symptoms. The duration of action of short-acting β_2-agonists is 4 to 6 hours.

Long-acting, inhaled β_2-agonists offer the benefit of a long duration of action without loss of effectiveness. Salmeterol and formoterol can be dosed every 12 hours and provide bronchodilation throughout the dosing interval. Formoterol has an onset of action similar to albuterol, whereas salmeterol has a slower onset; however, both agents are indicated for sustained bronchodilation and not for acute relief of symptoms. In clinical studies, long-acting inhaled β_2-agonists provide similar or superior improvements in lung function, exacerbation rates, and symptom improvements compared with short-acting bronchodilators.[45-47] There is a growing body of literature to support the use of the long-acting agents in patient with frequent and persistent symptoms. For patients using β_2-agonists on a scheduled basis, long-acting agents such as formoterol and salmeterol are more convenient because of reduced dosing frequency but are also more expensive.[1] The long-acting therapies should be considered when patients demonstrate a frequent need for short-acting agents.

Anticholinergics

When given by inhalation, anticholinergics such as ipratropium or atropine produce bronchodilation by competitively inhibiting cholinergic receptors in bronchial smooth muscle. This activity blocks acetylcholine, with the net effect being a reduction in cyclic guanosine monophosphate (cGMP), which normally acts to constrict bronchial smooth muscle. Muscarinic receptors on airway smooth muscle include M_1, M_2, and M_3 subtypes. Activation of M_1 and M_3 receptors by acetylcholine results in bronchoconstriction; however, activation of M_2 receptors inhibits further acetylcholine release.

Until recently, ipratropium has been the only available anticholinergic agent for COPD. Atropine has a tertiary structure and is absorbed readily across the oral and respiratory mucosa, whereas ipratropium has a quaternary structure that is absorbed poorly. The lack of systemic absorption of ipratropium greatly diminishes the anticholinergic side effects such as blurred vision, urinary retention, nausea, and tachycardia associated with atropine. Ipratropium bromide is available as an MDI and a solution for inhalation. It provides a peak effect in 1.5 to 2 hours and has a duration of effect of 4 to 6 hours. Ipratropium has a slower onset of action and a more prolonged bronchodilator effect compared with standard β_2-agonists. Because of the slower onset of effect (15 to 20 minutes compared with 5 minutes for albuterol), it may be less suitable for as-needed use; however, it is often prescribed in that manner. Clinicians differ about preference in choosing the initial short-acting bronchodilator therapy for the patient with COPD. Both a short-acting β_2-agonist and ipratropium represent reasonable choices for initial therapy.

The role of inhaled anticholinergics in COPD is well established.[48-52] However, results from the Lung Health Study showed that treatment with ipratropium did not affect the progressive decline in lung function.[22] Studies comparing ipratropium with inhaled β_2-agonists have generally reported similar improvements in pulmonary function. Others report a modest benefit with ipratropium, including a lower incidence of side effects such as tachycardia.[49-51]

Although the recommended dose of ipratropium is 2 puffs four times a day, there is evidence for a dose-response, so the dose can be titrated upward often to 24 puffs a day. Ipratropium has been shown to increase maximum exercise performance in stable COPD patients with doses of 8 to 12 puffs prior to exercise but not with doses of 4 puffs or less.[52-53] During sleep, ipratropium also has been shown to improve arterial oxygen saturation and sleep quality.[54] Ipratropium is well tolerated. The most frequent patient complaints are dry mouth, nausea, and an occasional metallic taste.

Tiotropium bromide, which was released in the United States in 2004, is a long-acting quaternary anticholinergic agent. This agent blocks the effects of acetylcholine by binding to muscarinic receptors in airway smooth muscle and mucus glands, blocking the cholinergic effects of bronchoconstriction and mucus secretion. Tiotropium dissociates slowly from M_1 and M_3 receptors, allowing prolonged bronchodilation. The dissociation from M_2 receptors is much faster, allowing inhibition of acetylcholine release. Binding studies of tiotropium in the human lung show that it is approximately 10-fold more potent than ipratropium and protects against cholinergic bronchoconstriction for greater than 24 hours.[55]

When inhaled, tiotropium is minimally absorbed into the systemic circulation and results in bronchodilation within 30 minutes, with a peak effect in 3 hours. Bronchodilation persists for at least 24 hours. In the United States, it is delivered via the HandiHaler, a single-load, dry-powder, breath-actuated device. Because it acts locally, tiotropium is well tolerated, with the most common complaint being a dry mouth. Other anticholinergic side effects that are reported include constipation, urinary retention, tachycardia, blurred vision, and precipitation of narrow-angle glaucoma symptoms.

As a new therapy for COPD, tiotropium was evaluated as an addition to standard COPD medications in a 1-year, placebo-controlled, double-blind study involving over 900 subjects. Tiotropium 18 mcg/day improved the FEV_1 response an average of 12% (trough) to 22% (peak) when added to standard therapy.[56]

The efficacy and safety of tiotropium administered via a DPI were compared with ipratropium administered four times daily by MDI in a multicenter, double-blind study that followed patients for 1 year.[57] Patients who received once-daily tiotropium demonstrated significantly greater improvements in lung function and selected quality-of-life scores, decreased dyspnea, and fewer exacerbations compared with patients who received ipratropium. There were no differences in side effects between the two agents.

As a newly available agent, tiotropium is expected to compete with long-acting inhaled β_2-agonists for COPD management. Once-daily tiotropium has been compared with twice-daily salmeterol in two placebo-controlled trials of 6 months' duration. Tiotropium reduced asthma exacerbations and hospital admissions and improved quality of life, whereas both active treatments improved lung function and reduced dyspnea.[58] In another 6-month randomized, controlled trial of patients with COPD, patients were randomized to receive either tiotropium once daily by DPI, salmeterol twice daily by MDI, or placebo.[59] Patients receiving tiotropium had greater improvements in trough FEV_1 and dyspnea scores than those receiving salmeterol. Patients also were more likely to have improvements in quality-of-life indicators with tiotropium than with salmeterol. However, no differences in frequency of exacerbations were noted among the three groups.

Inhaled anticholinergic therapies have an important role in the management of COPD. Ipratropium is available as an MDI (individually and in combination with albuterol) delivering 18 mcg per puff and as a solution for nebulization at 200 mcg/mL. Tiotropium is available as a DPI at 18 mcg per dose. Tiotropium became available in mid-2004. However, based on efficacy and convenience, it likely will play a major role in COPD management.

Combination Anticholinergics and Sympathomimetics

Combination regimens of bronchodilators are used often in the treatment of COPD, especially as the disease progresses and symptoms worsen over time. Combining bronchodilators with different mechanisms of action allows the lowest possible effective doses to be used and reduces potential adverse effects from individual agents.[1] Combinations of both short- and long-acting β_2-agonists with ipratropium have been shown to provide added symptomatic relief and improvements in pulmonary function.[60-62]

A combination of albuterol and ipratropium (Combivent) is available as an MDI in the United States for chronic maintenance therapy of COPD. This product offers the obvious convenience of two classes of bronchodilators in a single inhaler. Future combination inhalation products may contain long-acting β_2-agonists with tiotropium to reduce the need for frequent dosing. In a preliminary single-dose study, the combination of tiotropium and formoterol resulted in a faster and greater improvement in FEV_1 compared with either treatment alone.[63]

Methylxanthines

Methylxanthines, including theophylline and aminophylline, have been available for the treatment of COPD for at least five decades and at one time were considered first-line therapy. However, in the past 20 years, with the advent of long-acting inhaled β_2-agonists and inhaled anticholinergics, they are no longer considered first-line therapy. Inhaled bronchodilator therapy is preferred for COPD. Because of the risk for drug interactions and the significant intrapatient and interpatient variability in dosage requirements, theophylline therapy generally is considered in patients who are intolerant or unable to use an inhaled bronchodilator.

The methylxanthines may produce bronchodilation through numerous mechanisms, including (1) inhibition of phosphodiesterase, thereby increasing cAMP levels, (2) inhibition of calcium ion influx into smooth muscle, (3) prostaglandin antagonism, (4) stimulation of endogenous catecholamines, (5) adenosine receptor antagonism, and (6) inhibition of release of mediators from mast cells and leukocytes.[64]

Chronic theophylline use in patients with COPD has been shown to exert improvements in lung function, including vital capacity (VC), FEV_1, minute ventilation, and gas exchange.[65] Subjectively, theophylline has been shown to reduce dyspnea, increase exercise tolerance, and improve respiratory drive in COPD patients.[65,66] Other nonpulmonary effects of theophylline that may contribute to improved overall functional capacity in patients with COPD include improved cardiac function and decreased pulmonary artery pressure.[65]

Although theophylline is available in a variety of oral dosage forms, sustained-release preparations are most appropriate for the long-term management of COPD. These products have the advantages of improving patient compliance and achieving more consistent serum concentrations over rapid-release theophylline and aminophylline preparations. However, caution must be used in switching from one sustained-release preparation to another because there are considerable variations in sustained-release characteristics.[66] Aside from intravenous aminophylline, there is no need to use any of the various salts forms of theophylline.

Regular use of methylxanthines has not been shown to have either a beneficial or a detrimental effect on the progression of COPD. However, methylxanthines may be added to the treatment plan of patients who have not achieved an optimal clinical response to ipratropium and an inhaled β_2-agonist. Studies suggest that adding theophylline to a combination of albuterol and ipratropium provides added benefit for stable COPD patients, supporting the hypothesis that there is a synergistic bronchodilator effect.[67-69] The efficacy of combination therapy with salmeterol and theophylline for patients with COPD was reported to improve pulmonary function and reduce dyspnea better than either treatment alone.[70] Combination treatment also was associated with a reduced number of exacerbations only when compared with the theophylline group, suggesting that the salmeterol component was responsible for this beneficial effect.

As is the case with other bronchodilator therapy, parameters other than objective measurements, such as FEV_1, should be monitored to assess efficacy of theophylline in COPD. Subjective parameters, such as perceived improvements in symptoms of dyspnea, and exercise tolerance, become increasingly important in assessing the acceptability of methylxanthines for COPD patients. Although objective improvement may be minimal, patients may experience an improvement in clinical symptoms, and thus benefit to the individual may be meaningful.

The role of theophylline in COPD is as maintenance therapy in the non-acutely ill patient. Therapy can be initiated at 200 mg twice daily and titrated upward every 3 to 5 days to the target dose. Most patients required daily doses of 400 to 900 mg. Dosage adjustments generally should be made based on serum concentration results. Traditionally, the therapeutic range of theophylline was identified as 10 to 20 mcg/mL; however, because of the frequency of dose-related side effects and the relatively minor benefit of higher concentrations, a more conservative therapeutic range of 8 to 15 mcg/mL often is targeted. This is especially preferable in the elderly. When concentrations are measured, trough measurements are most appropriate.

Once a dose is established, serum concentrations should be monitored once or twice a year unless the patient's disease worsens, medications that interfere with theophylline metabolism are added to therapy, or toxicity is suspected. The most common side effects of theophylline therapy are related to the gastrointestinal system, the cardiovascular system, and the central nervous system. Side effects are dose-related; however, there is overlap in side effects between the therapeutic and toxic ranges. Minor side effects include dyspepsia, nausea, vomiting, diarrhea, headache, dizziness, and tachy-cardia. More serious toxicities, especially at toxic concentrations, include arrhythmias and seizures.

Factors that decrease theophylline clearance and lead to reduced maintenance-dose requirements include advanced age, bacterial or viral pneumonia, left or right ventricular failure, liver dysfunction, hypoxemia from acute decompensation, and use of drugs such as cimetidine, macrolides, and fluoroquinolone antibiotics. Factors that may enhance theophylline clearance and result in the need for higher maintenance doses include tobacco and marijuana smoking, hyperthyroidism, and the use of such drugs as phenytoin, phenobarbital, and rifampin.

CORTICOSTEROIDS

Corticosteroid therapy has been studied and debated in COPD therapy for half a century; however, owing to the poor risk-benefit ratio, chronic systemic corticosteroid therapy should be avoided if possible.[1] Because of the potential role of inflammation in the pathogenesis of the disease, clinicians hoped that corticosteroids would be promising agents in COPD management. However, their use continues to be debated, especially in the management of stable COPD.

The anti-inflammatory mechanisms whereby corticosteroids exert their beneficial effect in COPD include (1) reduction in capillary permeability to decrease mucus, (2) inhibition of release of proteolytic enzymes from leukocytes, and (3) inhibition of prostaglandins. Unfortunately, the clinical benefits of systemic corticosteroid therapy in the chronic management of COPD are often not evident, and the risk of toxicity is extensive and far-reaching. Currently, the appropriate situations to consider corticosteroids in COPD include (1) short–term systemic use for acute exacerbations and (2) inhalation therapy for chronic stable COPD.

The role of oral steroid use in chronic stable COPD patients was evaluated in a meta-analysis over a decade ago.[71] Investigators concluded that only a small fraction (10%) of COPD patients treated with steroids showed clinically significant improvement in baseline FEV_1 (increase of 20%) compared with those treated with placebo. While a small number of COPD patients are considered responders to oral steroids, many of these patients actually may have an asthmatic, or reversible, component to their disease. The best predictors for response to oral steroids is the presence of eosinophils on sputum examination ($\geq$3%) and a significant response on pulmonary function tests to sympathomimetics.[72] Both the presence of eosinophils in sputum and the responsiveness to sympathomimetics suggest an asthmatic component to the disease process and thus may explain the clinical benefit seen with steroids.

Long-term adverse effects associated with systemic corticosteroid therapy include osteoporosis, muscular atrophy, thinning of the skin, development of cataracts, and adrenal suppression and insufficiency. The risks associated with long-term steroid therapy are much greater than the clinical benefits. If a decision to treat with long-term systemic corticosteroids is made, the lowest possible effective dose should be given once per day in the morning to minimize the risk of adrenal suppression. If therapy with oral agents is required, an alternate-day schedule should be used.

Previously, a common clinical practice was to administer a short course (2 weeks) of oral corticosteroids as a trial to predict which patients would benefit from chronic oral or inhaled corticosteroids. There is now sufficient evidence suggesting that this practice is not effective in predicting a long-term response to inhaled corticosteroid and should not be recommended.[73]

The use of chronic inhaled corticosteroid therapy has been of interest for the past decade. Inhaled corticosteroids have an improved risk-benefit ratio compared with systemic corticosteroid therapy. Using the model for asthma, it was hoped that the inhalation of potent corticosteroid would result in high local efficacy and limited systemic exposure and toxicity.

In the latter part of the 1990s, several large international trials were initiated to evaluate the effect on inhaled corticosteroids in COPD. Unfortunately, the results of these major clinical trials failed to demonstrate any benefit from chronic treatment with inhaled corticosteroids in modifying long-term decline in lung function that is characteristic of COPD. Therefore, the role of inhaled corticosteroids in COPD continues to be debated in the literature, unlike asthma, where their use is clearly advocated. Much of the debate centers on the appropriate outcome measures in this population of patients.

During the last decade, several studies of inhaled corticosteroids in COPD were designed to detect a benefit on slowing the progressive loss of lung function, but the results were disappointing.[74–80] None of the large national or international trials were able to demonstrate a benefit of high-dose inhaled corticosteroid therapy on this primary outcome. However, inhaled corticosteroids have been associated with other important benefits in some patients, including a decrease in exacerbation frequency and improvements in overall health status.[76,80] Clinicians continue to debate the most appropriate and relevant outcome measure to evaluate in COPD studies. Based on the results of clinical trials, consensus guidelines suggest that inhaled corticosteroid therapy should be considered for symptomatic patients with stage III or IV disease (FEV_1 <50%) who experience repeated exacerbations.[1,81] These are the patients who demonstrated benefit in clinical trials and in whom a trial of inhaled corticosteroid therapy is warranted. There are also data from epidemiologic studies that suggest that chronic treatment with inhaled corticosteroids is associated with a lower risk of rehospitalization for a broader group of patients with COPD. Thus the debate about the appropriate role for this anti-inflammatory therapy continues.

Although a dose-response relationship for inhaled corticosteroids has not been demonstrated in COPD, the major clinical trials employed moderate to high doses for treatment. Side effects of inhaled corticosteroids are relatively mild compared with the toxicity from systemic therapy. Hoarseness, sore throat, oral candidiasis, and skin bruising have been reported in the clinical trials. Severe side effects, such as adrenal suppression, osteoporosis, and cataract formation, have been reported less frequently than with systemic corticosteroids, but clinicians should monitor patients who are receiving high-dose chronic therapy.[82,83]

COMBINATION THERAPY: BRONCHODILATORS AND INHALED CORTICOSTEROIDS

Following the disappointing results of chronic inhaled corticosteroid studies and the progressive decline in lung function, investigators became interested in the combination of potent anti-inflammatory therapies and long-acting bronchodilators. Subsequently, several studies have shown an additive benefit with long-acting bronchodilators.[84–87] In various studies, combination therapy with salmeterol plus fluticasone or formoterol plus budesonide was associated with greater improvements in clinical outcomes such as FEV_1, health status, and frequency of exacerbations compared with inhaled corticosteroids or long-acting bronchodilators alone. The availability of combination inhalers (e.g., salmeterol plus fluticasone) makes administration of both inhaled corticosteroids and long-acting bronchodilators more convenient for patients and decreases the total number of inhalations needed daily. Most of these studies were performed and published after the large international corticosteroid trials. Further clinical investigations are warranted; however, the combination therapies are prescribed increasingly in clinical practice, and additional products that combine these two therapeutic classes are anticipated.

α_1-ANTITRYPSIN REPLACEMENT THERAPY

In patients with inherited AAT deficiency–associated emphysema, treatment focuses on reduction of risk factors such as smoking, symptomatic treatment with bronchodilators, and augmentation therapy with replacement AAT. Augmentation therapy consists of weekly infusions of pooled human AAT to maintain AAT plasma levels over 10 micromolar. Clinical evidence for slowing lung function decline or improving outcomes with augmentation therapy is sparse. One observational study followed patients in the National Registry of Severe AAT Deficiency over a period of several years and documented clinical outcomes. In this study, patients who received weekly augmentation therapy with purified AAT had slower declines in FEV_1 and decreased mortality compared with patients who never received augmentation therapy.[8] However, this was an observational study of patients, not a randomized, placebo-controlled trial, so direct cause-and-effect relationships cannot be concluded. One randomized, placebo-controlled study of patients with severe AAT deficiency (ZZ phenotype) did show a significant reduction in lung tissue loss and destruction as measured by computed tomographic (CT) scan in patients receiving augmentation therapy.[88] Other measures of lung function and mortality were not recorded.

The recommended dosing regimen for replacement AAT is 60 mg/kg administered intravenously once a week at a rate of 0.08 mL/kg per minute, adjusted to patient tolerance. It has been estimated that this form of augmentation therapy will have an annual cost of $20,000 to $30,000 per patient.[89] There have been repeated problems with supply of this biologic replacement therapy (derived from pooled blood donors) related to production difficulty and contamination issues. Currently, there are three products available (Prolastin, Aralast, and Zemaira), which should minimize this problem in the future.

▶ TREATMENT: COPD Exacerbation

■ DESIRED OUTCOMES

The goals of therapy for patients experiencing exacerbations of COPD are (1) prevention of hospitalization or reduction in hospital stay, (2) prevention of acute respiratory failure and death, and (3) resolution of exacerbation symptoms and a return to baseline clinical status and quality of life. Various therapeutic options are summarized in Table 27–13. Pharmacotherapy consists of intensification of bronchodilator therapy and a short course of systemic corticosteroids. Antimicrobial therapy is indicated in the presence of selected symptoms. Since the frequency and severity of exacerbations are closely related to each patient's overall health status, all patients should receive optimal chronic treatment, including smoking cessation, appropriate pharmacologic therapy, and preventative therapy such as vaccinations.

■ NONPHARMACOLOGIC THERAPY

■ CONTROLLED OXYGEN THERAPY

Oxygen therapy should be considered for any patient with hypoxemia during an exacerbation. Caution must be used, however, because many patients with COPD rely on mild hypoxemia to trigger their drive to breathe. In normal, healthy individuals, the drive to breathe is triggered by carbon dioxide accumulation. In patients with COPD who retain carbon dioxide as a result of their disease progression, hypoxemia rather than hypercapnia becomes the main trigger for their respiratory drive. Overly aggressive administration of oxygen to patients with chronic hypercapnia may result in respiratory depression and respiratory failure. Oxygen therapy should be used to achieve a PaO_2 of greater than 60 mm Hg or oxygen saturation of greater than

TABLE 27–13. Therapeutic Options for Acute Exacerbations of COPD

Therapy	Comments

Antibiotics	Recommended if two or more of the following are present:
	  Increased dyspnea
	  Increased sputum production
	  Increased sputum purulence

Corticosteroids	Oral or intravenous therapy may be used. If intravenous is used, it should be changed to oral after improvement in pulmonary status. If continued longer than 14 days, then the dose should be tapered to avoid HPA axis suppression.
Bronchodilators	MDIs and DPIs equal in efficacy to nebulization. β-Agonists also may increase mucociliary clearance. Long-acting β-agonists should not be used for quick relief of symptoms or on an as-needed basis.
Controlled oxygen therapy	Titrate oxygen to desired oxygen saturation (>90%). Monitor arterial blood gas for development of hypercapnia.
Noninvasive mechanical ventilation	Consider for patients with acute respiratory failure. Not appropriate for patients with altered mental status, severe acidosis, respiratory arrest, or cardiovascular instability.

90%. However, an ABG should be obtained after oxygen initiation to monitor carbon dioxide retention owing to hypoventilation.

▧ NONINVASIVE MECHANICAL VENTILATION

Noninvasive positive-pressure ventilation (NPPV) provides ventilatory support with oxygen and pressurized airflow using a face or nasal mask with a tight seal but without endotracheal intubation. There have been numerous trials reporting the benefits of NPPV in patients with acute respiratory failure due to COPD exacerbations. In one meta-analysis of eight studies, NPPV was associated with lower mortality, lower intubation rates, shorter hospital stays, and greater improvements in serum pH in 1 hour compared with treatment with usual care alone.[90] The benefits seen with NPPV generally can be attributed to a reduction in the complications that often arise with invasive mechanical ventilation. Not all patients with COPD exacerbations are appropriate candidates for NPPV. Patients with altered mental status may not be able to protect their airway and thus may be at increased risk for aspiration. Patients with severe acidosis (pH <7.25), respiratory arrest, or cardiovascular instability should be not be considered for NPPV. Patients failing a trial of NPPV or those considered poor candidates may be considered for intubation and mechanical ventilation.

▧ PHARMACOLOGIC THERAPY

▧ BRONCHODILATORS

During exacerbations, intensification of bronchodilator regimens is used commonly. The doses and frequency of bronchodilators are increased to provide symptomatic relief. Short-acting β_2-agonists are preferred owing to rapid onset of action. Anticholinergic agents may be added if symptoms persist despite increased doses of β_2-agonists. In fact, combinations of these agents are employed often, although data are lacking about the benefit versus higher doses of one agent. Bronchodilators may be administered via MDIs or nebulization with equal efficacy. Nebulization may be considered for patients with severe dyspnea who are unable to hold their breath after actuation of an MDI. Clinical evidence supporting the use of theophylline during exacerbations is lacking, and thus theophylline generally should be avoided. However, addition of one of these agents may be considered for patients not responding to other therapies. The risk of adverse effects such as cardiac arrhythmias should be considered and serum levels monitored closely.

▧ CORTICOSTEROIDS

Until recently, the literature supporting the use of corticosteroids in acute exacerbations of COPD was sparse. However, since 1996, five studies have been performed that document the value of systemic corticosteroids in exacerbations of COPD.[91–95] The Systemic Corticosteroids in Chronic Obstructive Pulmonary Disease Exacerbations (SCCOPE) trial evaluated three groups of patients hospitalized for exacerbations of COPD.[91] The first group received an 8-week course of corticosteroids given as methylprednisolone 125 mg intravenously every 6 hours for 72 hours, followed by once-daily oral prednisone (60 mg on days 4 through 7, 40 mg on days 8 through 11, 20 mg on days 12 through 43, 10 mg on days 44 through 50, and 5 mg on days 51 through 57). The second group received a 2-week course given as

methylprednisolone 125 mg intravenously every 6 hours for 72 hours, followed by oral prednisone (60 mg on days 5 through 7, 40 mg on days 8 through 11, and 20 mg on days 12 through 15) and placebo on days 16 through 57. The third group received placebo for all 57 days of study. Rates of treatment failure and hospital stay were significantly higher in the placebo group than in either treatment group at 30 and 90 days. Groups randomized to corticosteroid treatment also had a significantly shorter length of hospital stay compared with the placebo group. The 8-week regimen was not found to be superior to the 2-week regimen. Significant treatment benefits were no longer evident at 6 months.

Davies and colleagues[92] evaluated the oral use of corticosteroids in hospitalized patients with acute exacerbations of COPD. Patients received either 30 mg/day oral prednisolone or placebo for 14 days. Patients who were treated with corticosteroids had a significantly more rapid improvement in FEV_1 and a shorter hospital stay than did patients who received placebo. There was no significant difference between groups at 6-week follow-up.

In total, results from these trials suggest that patients with acute exacerbations of COPD should receive a short course of intravenous or oral corticosteroids. However, because of the large variability in dosage ranges, the optimal dose and duration of corticosteroid treatment are not known. It appears that short courses (9 to 14 days) are as effective as longer courses and have a lower risk of associated adverse effects owing to less time of exposure. Several trials used high initial doses of steroids before tapering to a lower maintenance dose. Adverse effects such as hyperglycemia, insomnia, and hallucinations may occur at higher doses. Depending on the clinical status of the patient, treatment may be initiated at a lower dose or tapered more quickly if these effects occur. If steroid treatment is continued for greater than 2 weeks, a tapering oral schedule should be employed to avoid hypothalamic-pituitary-adrenal (HPA) axis suppression.

▧ ANTIMICROBIAL THERAPY

Most acute exacerbations of COPD are thought to be caused by viral or bacterial infections. However, as many as 30% of exacerbations are caused by unknown factors.[1] A meta-analysis of nine studies evaluating the effectiveness of antibiotics in treating exacerbations of COPD determined that patients receiving antibiotics had a greater improvement in peak expiratory flow rate than those who did not.[96] ❿ This meta-analysis concluded that antibiotics are of most benefit and should be initiated if at least two of the following three symptoms are present: increased dyspnea, increased sputum volume, and increased sputum purulence. The utility of sputum Gram stain and culture is questionable because some patients have chronic bacterial colonization of the bronchial tree between exacerbations.

The emergence of drug-resistant organisms has mandated that antibiotic regimens be chosen judiciously. Selection of empirical antimicrobial therapy should be based on the most likely organism(s) thought to be responsible for the infection based on the individual patient profile. The most common organisms for any acute exacerbation of COPD are *Hemophilus influenzae, Moraxella catarrhalis, Streptococcus pneumoniae,* and *Hemophilus parainfluenzae.* More virulent bacteria may be present in patients with more complicated acute exacerbations of COPD, including drug-resistant pneumococci, β-lactamase-producing *H. influenzae* and *M. catarrhalis,* and enteric gram-negative organisms, including *Pseudomonas aeruginosa.* Table 27–14 summarizes recommended antimicrobial therapy for exacerbations of COPD and the most common organisms based on patient presentation.[97]

TABLE 27–14. Recommended Antimicrobial Therapy in Acute Exacerbations of COPD

Patient Characteristics	Likely Pathogens	Recommended Therapy

Uncomplicated exacerbations
    < 4 exacerbations per year
    No comorbid illness
    FEV$_1$ > 50% of predicted
	S. pneumoniae
	H. influenzae
	M. catarrhalis
	H. parainfluenzae
	Resistance uncommon
		Macrolide (azithromycin, clarithromycin)
		Second- or third-generation cephalosporin
		Doxycycline
		Therapies not recommended^a:
		TMP/SMX, amoxicillin, first-generation cephalosporins, and erythromycin

Complicated exacerbations
    Age ≥ 65 > 4 exacerbations per year
    FEV$_1$ < 50% but > 35% of predicted
	As above plus drug-resistant pneumococci, β-lactamase–producing H. influenzae and M. catarrhalis
	Some enteric gram-negatives
		Amoxicillin/clavulanate
		Fluoroquinolone with enhanced pneumococcal activity (levofloxacin, gatifloxacin, moxifloxacin)

Complicated exacerbations with risk of P. aeruginosa
    Chronic bronchial sepsis^b
    Need for chronic Corticosteroid therapy
    Resident of nursing home
    > 4 exacerbations per year
    FEV$_1$ > 35% of predicted
	As above plus P. aeruginosa	Fluoroquinolone with enhanced pneumococcal and P. aeruginosa activity (levofloxacin, gatifloxacin, moxifloxacin)
		IV therapy if required:
		β-lactamase resistant penicillin with antipseudomonal activity
		Third- or fourth-generation cephalosporin with antipseudomonal activity

^{a}TMP/SMX should not be used due to increasing pneumococcal resistance; amoxicillin and first-generation cephalosporins are not recommended due to β-lactamase susceptibility; and erythromycin is not recommended due to insufficient activity against H. influenzae.
^{b}In sepsis, double antipseudomonal coverage should be considered (e.g., addition of aminoglycoside).
Adapted from ref. 87.

Therapy with antibiotics generally should be continued for at least 7 to 10 days. Studies evaluating shorter treatment courses (usually 5 days) with the fluoroquinolones, second- and third-generation cephalosporins, and macrolide antimicrobials have demonstrated comparable efficacy with the longer treatment regimens.[98] If the patient deteriorates or does not improve as anticipated, hospitalization may be necessary, and more aggressive attempts should be made to identify potential pathogens responsible for the exacerbation.

COMPLICATIONS

COR PULMONALE

Cor pulmonale is right-sided heart failure secondary to pulmonary hypertension. Long-term oxygen therapy and diuretics have been the mainstays of therapy for cor pulmonale. Increasing the PaO$_2$ above 60 mm Hg with supplemental oxygen therapy decreases pulmonary hypertension and thus decreases the force against which the right ventricle has to work. While diuretics may help decrease fluid overload, caution should be used because patients with significant right-sided heart failure are highly dependent on preload for cardiac output. Therefore, the decision to use diuretics must be based on a risk-benefit ratio. Digitalis glycosides have no role in the treatment of cor pulmonale.

Other pharmacologic agents that have been investigated to treat cor pulmonale include hydralazine, calcium channel blockers,

angiotensin-converting enzyme inhibitors, and angiotensin II antagonists. However, there is insufficient evidence to offer guidelines for the role of these agents in COPD patients with cor pulmonale.

POLYCYTHEMIA

Polycythemia secondary to chronic hypoxemia in COPD patients can be improved by either oxygen therapy or periodic phlebotomy if oxygen therapy alone is not sufficient. COT was shown by the Nocturnal Oxygen Therapy Trial Group to reduce hematocrit values in treated patients.[31] Acute phlebotomy is indicated if the hematocrit is above 55% to 60% and the patient is experiencing central nervous system effects suggestive of sludging from high blood viscosity. Long-term oxygen then can be used to maintain a lower hematocrit.

OTHER PHARMACOLOGIC CONSIDERATIONS

A number of other treatments have been explored over the years. Among these therapies, there is either insufficient evidence to warrant recommending their use, or they have been proven to not be beneficial in the management of COPD. A brief summary is provided because the clinician likely will encounter patients who are receiving or inquire about these treatments.

SUPPRESSIVE ANTIMICROBIAL AGENTS

Because COPD patients often are colonized with bacteria and experience recurrent exacerbations of their condition, a common practice employed in the past has been the use of low-dose antimicrobial therapy as preventative or prophylaxis against these acute exacerbations. However, clinical studies over the past 40 years have failed to demonstrate any benefit from this practice.[1] The role of antimicrobial therapy is limited to acute exacerbations of COPD meeting specific criteria.

EXPECTORANTS AND MUCOLYTICS

Adequate water intake generally is acceptable to maintain hydration and assist in the removal of airway sections. Beyond this, the regular use of mucolytics or expectorants for COPD patients has no proven benefit.[99] This includes the use of saturated solutions of potassium iodide, ammonium chloride, acetylcysteine, and guaifenesin.

RESPIRATORY STIMULANTS

There is no role for respiratory stimulants in the long-term management of COPD.[1] Agents that have shown some utility in the acute setting include amiltrine and doxapram. However, amiltrine is available only in Europe, and its usefulness is limited by neurotoxicity. Doxapram is available for intravenous use only and may be no better than intermittent NPPV.

SURGICAL INTERVENTION

Recent trials have evaluated the effect of bilateral lung volume reduction surgery (LVRS) for management of severe COPD. Short-term trials comparing the effects of pulmonary rehabilitation plus LVRS with pulmonary rehabilitation alone reported that the combination of treatments resulted in greater improvements in lung function, gas exchange, and quality of life at 3 months.

Only recently have data evaluating the long-term effect of LVRS compared with pulmonary rehabilitation been published. The National Emphysema Treatment Trial (NETT), a prospective, randomized trial evaluating the long-term effects of LVRS plus pulmonary rehabilitation compared with pulmonary rehabilitation alone, followed 1218 patients for 3 years.[100] The primary end points for the study were mortality and maximal exercise capacity 2 years after randomization. Secondary end points included pulmonary function, distance walked in 6 minutes, and quality-of-life measurements. At an interim analysis, patients with an FEV_1 of less than 20% of predicted or a carbon monoxide diffusing capacity of less than 20% of predicted were noted to be at high risk of death after surgery and subsequently were excluded from the study. Results of the study showed no mortality benefit

with LVRS compared with pulmonary rehabilitation alone. Patients undergoing surgery had improved exercise capacity, lung function, and quality of life at 2 years, but these patients also had a higher risk of short-term morbidity and mortality associated with the surgery. A subgroup analysis of the study noted that patients with predominately upper-lobe emphysema and low exercise capacity undergoing surgery had lower mortality rates at 2 years compared with patients treated with medical therapy alone. Because of the costs and risks associated with LVRS, more studies are needed to better determine the ideal surgical candidates and identify subgroups of patients that would benefit most from surgery.

DIETARY SUPPLEMENTS

There has been increasing interest in the role of antioxidants, including vitamins E and C and β-carotene, in reducing the frequency of exacerbations. It is postulated that they may be beneficial in COPD as a result of an imbalance between oxidants and antioxidants that has been considered in the pathogenesis of smoking-induced lung disease. However, there is no good evidence that antioxidant therapies improve COPD symptoms or slow disease progression.

INVESTIGATIONAL THERAPIES

Based on the knowledge about the importance of neutrophilic inflammation in COPD and potential therapeutic benefit of inhibition of neutrophil activity, a number of anti-inflammatory compounds are being explored. Specifically, agents inhibiting leukotriene B$_4$, neutrophil elastase, and phosphodiesterases currently are being evaluated. To date, studies evaluating leukotriene-modifying therapies have been disappointing. Further studies are needed to evaluate the clinical benefit of such inhibitors in patients with COPD.

Phosphodiesterase 4 (PDE4) is the major phosphodiesterase found in airway smooth muscle cells and inflammatory cells and is responsible for degrading cAMP. Inhibition of PDE4 results in relaxation of airway smooth muscle cells and decreased activity of inflammatory cells and mediators such as TNF-α and IL-8. Two PDE$_4$ inhibitors have reached clinical trials, cilomilast and roflumilast. Cilomilast has been evaluated in several human trials and has been shown to improve expiratory airflow as measured by FEV_1 in patients with COPD when given at a dose of 15 mg twice daily for 6 weeks. Future studies of cilomilast should evaluate its effects on other clinical outcomes such as health status, exacerbation frequency, and progression of disease.

Neutrophil elastase is implicated in the induction of bronchial disease, causing structural changes in lungs, impairment of mucociliary clearance, and impairment of host defenses. Protease inhibitors, namely, inhibitors of neutrophil elastase, are being investigated currently for the treatment of COPD.

PHARMACOECONOMIC CONSIDERATIONS

The overall cost of therapy is an important consideration in contemporary medical practice. Meaningful cost analysis goes beyond the cost of the medication itself and incorporates the impact of a given therapeutic agent on overall health care cost. Because of the relative lack of benefit among objective outcome measures in COPD

clinical trials, pharmacoeconomic studies can be useful in decision making about pharmacotherapy options. Pharmacoeconomic analyses in COPD, although limited, are available regarding antibiotic use in acute exacerbations and some therapies for management of chronic stable COPD.

Grossman and colleagues[101] conducted a trial investigating the use of aggressive antimicrobial therapy (ciprofloxacin) compared with usual antibiotic therapy (defined as any nonquinolone) in the treatment of acute exacerbations of COPD. Overall, the results indicated no preference for either treatment arm. However, in patients who were categorized as high risk (severe underlying lung disease, more than four exacerbations per year, duration of bronchitis greater than 10 years, elderly, significant comorbid illness), the use of aggressive antibiotic therapy was associated with improved clinical outcome, higher quality of life, and fewer costs. The results of this study are consistent with Table 27–14, which suggests that higher-risk patients are likely to have more resistant strains of organisms and thus require more aggressive antimicrobial treatment.

Friedman and colleagues[102] conducted a post hoc pharmacoeconomic evaluation of two multicenter, randomized trials comparing the combination of ipratropium and albuterol with both drugs used as monotherapy. Patients who received a combination of ipratropium and albuterol had lower rates of exacerbations, lower overall treatment costs, and improved cost-effectiveness compared with either drug used alone. With the introduction of new bronchodilator therapies, and with no clearly consistent advantage of one class of agents over another, pharmacoeconomic analyses may be useful for clinicians in determining the most appropriate therapy for their patients.

CLINICAL CONTROVERSIES

Albuterol is one of the most commonly prescribed medications in the United States. Albuterol is a 50/50 racemic mixture of (R)-albuterol and (S)-albuterol, with the (R)-isomer responsible for all the therapeutic effect. A single-isomer product, levalbuterol, claims clinical superiority based on the absence of the (S)-isomer, which may have detrimental effects in the airway and antagonistic effects on the active isomer. However, the acquisition cost of levalbuterol is significantly higher than that of generic albuterol. The advantages of using the single-isomer product in clinical practice are not clear.

A combination product of a long-acting inhaled β-agonist (salmeterol) and an inhaled corticosteroid agent (fluticasone) is one of the most commonly prescribed medications for lung disease, including COPD. However, in expert guidelines, inhaled corticosteroids are indicated only for patients with more severe disease who experience frequent exacerbations. Many patients now receiving therapy with the combination inhaler may be candidates for bronchodilator therapy alone.

The role of systemic corticosteroids for acute exacerbations of COPD has been clarified in recent years. However, the appropriate dosage regimen is not well established. Regimens range from initial high doses (methylprednisolone 125 mg every 6 hours) to more conservative dosing (prednisone 40–60 mg/day).

Consensus guidelines indicate that bronchodilator therapy is the focus of pharmacotherapy for COPD. However, there is no clear choice for the initial agent. For patients with daily but not persistent symptoms, either ipratropium or albuterol offers advantages as initial therapy. Both also have limitations if chosen as the initial therapy.

EVALUATION OF THERAPEUTIC OUTCOMES

To evaluate therapeutic outcomes of COPD effectively, the practitioner must first delineate between chronic stable COPD and acute exacerbations. In chronic stable COPD, pulmonary function tests should be assessed periodically and with any therapy addition, change

in dose, or deletion of therapy. Because objective improvements often are minimal, subjective assessments are important. Other outcome parameters are commonly evaluated, including dyspnea score, quality-of-life assessments, and exacerbation rates, including visits to the emergency department or hospitalization. In acute exacerbations of COPD, white blood cell count, vital signs, chest x-ray, and changes in frequency of dyspnea, sputum volume, and sputum purulence should be assessed at the onset and throughout treatment of an exacerbation. In more severe exacerbations, ABGs and oxygen saturation also should be monitored. As with any drug therapy, patient adherence to therapeutic regimens, side effects, potential drug interactions, and subjective measures of quality of life also must be evaluated.

ABBREVIATIONS

AAT: α_1-antitrypsin
BMI: body mass index
COPD: chronic obstructive pulmonary disease
D_{LCO}: diffusion capacity for carbon monoxide
DPI: dry powder inhaler
FEV_1: forced expiratory volume in 1 second
FVC: forced vital capacity
GOLD: Global Initiative for Chronic Obstructive Lung Disease
Hg: mercury
LVRS: lung volume reduction surgery
MDI: metered-dose inhaler
NHLBI: National Heart, Lung and Blood Institute
NPPV: noninvasive positive-pressure ventilation
PaO_2: pressure exerted by oxygen gas in arterial blood
$PaCO_2$: pressure exerted by carbon dioxide gas in arterial blood
WHO: World Health Organization

Review Questions and other resources can be found at *www.pharmacotherapyonline.com*.

REFERENCES

1. National Heart, Lung, and Blood Institute, World Health Organization. Global Strategy for the Diagnosis, Management, and Prevention of Chronic Obstructive Pulmonary Disease. April 2001 (updated 2003); available at *www.goldcopd.com;* accessed June 2004.
2. American Thoracic Society. Standards for the diagnosis and care of patients with chronic obstructive pulmonary disease. Am J Respir Crit Care Med 1995;152:S77–120.
3. National Center for Health Statistics. National Health Interview Survey. Hyattsville, MD, US Department of Health and Human Services, CDC, NCHS, 2001; available at *www.cdc.gov/nchs/nhis.htm;* accessed June 2004.
4. Mannino DM, Homa DM, Akinbami LJ, et al. Chronic obstructive pulmonary disease surveillance—United States, 1971–2000. Surveillance Summaries, August 2, 2002. MMWR 2002;51:1–16.
5. Chronic Obstructive Pulmonary Disease: Data Fact Sheet. US Department of Health and Human Services, National Institutes of Health, NHLBI, NIH Publication 03-5529, March 2003.
6. Mannino DM. COPD epidemiology, prevalence, morbidity and mortality, and disease heterogeneity. Chest 2002;121:121–126S.
7. Stockley RA. Alpha-1-antitrypsin deficiency: What next? Thorax 2000;55:614–618.
8. Alpha-1-Antitrypsin Deficiency Registry Study Group. Survival and FEV_1 decline in individuals with severe deficiency of alpha-1-antitrypsin. Am J Respir Crit Care Med 1998;158:49–59.
9. Barnes PJ. Chronic obstructive pulmonary disease. New Engl J Med 2000;343:269–280.
10. Stockley RA. Neutrophils and the pathogenesis of COPD. Chest 2002;121:151–155S.

11. Hill AT, Bayley D, Stockely RA. The interrelationship of sputum inflammatory markers in patients with chronic bronchitis. Am J Respir Crit Care Med 1999;160:893–898.

12. Fabbri LM, Hurd SS, Gold Scientific Committee. Global strategy for the diagnosis, management, and prevention of COPD: 2003 update. Eur Respir J 2003;22:1–2.

13. MacNee W. Pathophysiology of cor pulmonale in chronic obstructive pulmonary disease, part 2. Am J Respir Crit Care Med 1994;150: 1158–1168.

14. Rodriguez-Roisin R. Toward a consensus definition for COPD exacerbations. Chest 2000;117(suppl 2):398–401S.

15. Celli BR. The importance of spirometry in COPD and asthma. Chest 2000;117:15–19S.

16. Anthonisen NR, Manfreda J, Warren CPW, et al. Antibiotic therapy in exacerbations of chronic obstructive pulmonary disease. Ann Intern Med 1987;106:196–204.

17. Honig EG, Ingram RH. Chronic bronchitis, emphysema, and airways obstruction. In: Fauci AS, Braunwald E, Isselbacher KJ, et al, eds. Harrison's Principles of Internal Medicine, 14th ed. New York, McGraw-Hill, 1998:1451–1460.

18. Groenewegen KH, Schols AMW, Wouters EFM. Mortality and mortality-related factors after hospitalization for acute exacerbation of COPD. Chest 2003;124:459–467.

19. Bach PB, Brown C, Gelfand SE, McCrory DC. Management of acute exacerbations of chronic obstructive pulmonary disease: A summary and appraisal of published evidence. Ann Intern Med 2001;134:600–620.

20. Heffner JE, Fahy B, Hilling L, Barbieri C. Outcomes of advanced directive education of pulmonary rehabilitation patients. Am J Respir Crit Care Med 1997;155:1055–1059.

21. Parrott S, Godfrey C, Raw M, et al. Guidance for commissioners on the cost-effectiveness of smoking cessation interventions. Health International Authority. Thorax 1998;53(suppl 5):S1–38.

22. Anthonisen NR, Connett JE, Kiley JP, et al. Effects of smoking intervention and the use of an inhaled anticholinergic bronchodilator on the rate of decline of FEV$_1$: The Lung Health Study. JAMA 1994;272:1497–1505.

23. The Tobacco Use and Dependence Clinical Practice Guideline Panel, Staff, and Consortium Representatives. A clinical practice guideline for treating tobacco use and dependence. JAMA 2000;283:244–254.

24. *http://www.cdc.gov/tobacco/sgr/sgr_2004/pdf/executivesummary.pdf.*

25. Jorenby DE, Leischow SJ, Nides MA, et al. A controlled trial of sustained-release bupropion, a nicotine patch or both for smoking cessation. New Engl J Med 1999;340:685–691.

26. Bredstrup KE, Ingemann Jensen J, Holm S, Bengtsson B. Out-patient rehabilitation improves activities of daily living, quality of life and exercise tolerance in chronic obstructive pulmonary disease. Eur Respir J 1997;10:2801–2806.

27. Ringbaek TJ, Broendum L, Hemmingsen K, et al. Rehabilitation of patients with chronic obstructive pulmonary disease: Exercise twice a week is not sufficient! Respir Med 2000;94:150–154.

28. Nichol KL, Margolis KL, Wourenma J, Von Sternberg T. The efficacy and cost effectiveness of vaccination against influenza among elderly persons living in the community. New Engl J Med 1994;331:778–784.

29. Centers for Disease Control and Prevention. Prevention and control of influenza: recommendations of the Advisor Committee on Immunization Practices (ACIP). MMWR 2004;53:1–44.

30. Nuorti, PJ, Butler JC, Breiman RF. Prevention of pneumococcal disease. MMWR 1997;46:1–24.

31. Nocturnal Oxygen Therapy Trial Group. Continuous or nocturnal oxygen therapy in hypoxemic chronic obstructive lung disease. Ann Intern Med 1980;93:391–398.

32. Medical Research Council Working Party. Long-term domiciliary oxygen therapy in chronic hypoxic cor pulmonale complicating chronic bronchitis and emphysema. Lancet 1981;1:681–685.

33. O'Donohue WJ. Home oxygen therapy. Med Clin North Am 1996;80: 611–622.

34. Devine EC, Pearcy J. Meta-analysis of the effects of psychoeducational care in adults with chronic obstructive pulmonary disease. Patient Educ Couns 1996;29:167–178.

35. Ferreira IM, Brooks D, Lacasse Y, et al. Nutritional support for individuals with COPD: A meta-analysis. Chest 2000;117:672–678.

36. Mandelberg A, Chen E, Noviski N, Priel IE. Nebulized wet aerosol treatment in emergency department: Is it essential? Comparison with large spacer device for metered-dose inhaler. Chest 1997;112:1501–1505.

37. Ikeda A, Nishimura K, Koyama H, et al. Comparison of the bronchodilator effects of salbutamol delivered via a metered-dose inhaler with spacer, a dry-powder inhaler, and a jet nebulizer in patients with chronic obstructive pulmonary disease. Respiration 1999;66:119–123.

38. Turner MO, Patel A, Ginsburg S, Fitzgerald JM. Bronchodilator delivery in acute airflow obstruction. Arch Intern Med 1997;157:1736–1744.

39. Truitt T, Witko J, Halpern M. Levalbuterol compared to racemic albuterol: efficacy and outcomes in patients hospitalized with COPD or asthma. Chest 2003;123:128–135.

40. Asmus MJ, Hendeles L. Levalbuterol nebulizer solution: Is it worth five times the cost of albuterol? Pharmacotherapy 2000;20:123–129.

41. Datta D, Vitale A, Lahiri B, ZuWallack R. An evaluation of nebulized levalbuterol in stable COPD. Chest 2003;124:844–849.

42. O'Donnel DE, Lam M, Webb KA. Measurement of symptoms, lung hyperinflation, and endurance during exercise in chronic obstructive pulmonary disease. Am J Respir Crit Care Med 1998;158:1557–1565.

43. Boyd G, Morice AH, Pounsford JC, et al. An evaluation of salmeterol in the treatment of chronic obstructive pulmonary disease (COPD). Eur Respir J 1997;10:815–821.

44. Grove A, Lipworth BJ, Reid P, et al. Effects of regular salmeterol on lung function and exercise capacity in patients with chronic obstructive airways disease. Thorax 1996;51:689–693.

45. Mahler DA, Donohue JF, Barbee RA, et al. Efficacy of salmeterol xinafoate in the treatment of COPD. Chest 1999;115:957–965.

46. Rennard SI, Anderson W, ZuWallack R, et al. Use of a long-acting β_2-agonist, salmeterol xinafoate, in patients with chronic obstructive pulmonary disease. Am J Respir Crit Care Med 2001;163:1087–1092.

47. van Noord JA, Smeets JJ, Raaijmakers JAM, et al. Salmeterol versus formoterol in patients with moderately severe asthma: Onset and duration of action. Eur Respir J 1996;9:1684–1688.

48. Schapira RM, Reinke LF. The outpatient diagnosis and management of chronic obstructive pulmonary disease: Pharmacotherapy, administration of supplemental oxygen, and smoking cessation techniques. J Gen Intern Med 1995;10:40–55.

49. Friedman M. A multicenter study of nebulized bronchodilator solutions in chronic obstructive pulmonary disease. Am J Med 1996;100(suppl 1A):30S–39S.

50. Wiggins J. The role of anticholinergics in "stable" chronic obstructive pulmonary disease: Unanswered questions. Respiration 1994;61: 303–304.

51. Colice GL. Nebulized bronchodilators for outpatient management of stable chronic obstructive pulmonary disease. Am J Med 1996;100(suppl 1A):11–18S.

52. Ikeda A, Nishimura K, Koyama H, et al. Dose-response study of ipratropium bromide aerosol on maximum exercise performance in stable patients with chronic obstructive pulmonary disease. Thorax 1996;51: 48–53.

53. Tsukino M, Nishimura K, Ikeda A, et al. Effects of theophylline and ipratropium bromide on exercise performance in patients with stable chronic obstructive pulmonary disease. Thorax 1998;53:269–273.

54. Martin RJ, Bartelson BL, Smith P, et al. Effect of ipratropium bromide treatment on oxygen saturation and sleep quality in COPD. Chest 1999;115:1338–1345.

55. Barnes PJ. The pharmacological properties of tiotropium. Chest 2000;117:63–66S.

56. Casaburi R, Mahler DA, Jones PW, et al. A long-term evaluation of once daily inhaled tiotropium in chronic obstructive pulmonary disease. Eur Resp J 2002;19:217–224.

57. Vincken W, Van Noord JA, Greefhorst APM, et al. Improved health outcomes in patients with COPD during one year treatment with tiotropium. Eur Respir J 2002;19:209–216.

58. Brusasco V, Hodder R, Miravitlles M, et al. Health outcomes following treatment for six months with once daily tiotropium compared with twice daily salmeterol in patients with COPD. Thorax 2003;58:399–404.

59. Donohue JF, van Noord JA, Bateman ED, et al. A 6-month placebo-controlled study comparing lung function and health status changes in COPD patients treated with tiotropium or salmeterol. Chest 2002;122: 47–55.

60. van Noord JA, de Munck DRAJ, Bantje TA, et al. Long-term treatment of chronic obstructive pulmonary disease with salmeterol and the additive effect of ipratropium. Eur Respir J 2000;15:880–885.

61. Combivent Inhalation Aerosol Study Group. In chronic obstructive pulmonary disease, a combination of ipratropium and albuterol is more effective than either agent alone. Chest 1994;105:1411–1419.

62. D'Urzo AD, De Salvo MC, Ramirez-Rivera A, et al. In patients with COPD, treatment with a combination of formoterol and ipratropium is more effective than a combination of salbutamol and ipratropium. Chest 2001;119:1347–1356.

63. Cazzola M, Marco FD, Santus P, et al. The pharmacodynamic effects of single inhaled doses of formoterol, tiotropium and their combination in patients with COPD. Pulm Pharmacol Ther 2004;17:35–39.

64. Barnes PJ. Theophylline: new perspectives for and old drug. Am J Respir Crit Care Med 2003;167:813–818.

65. Vaz Fragoso CA, Miller MA. Review of the clinical efficacy of theophylline in the treatment of chronic obstructive pulmonary disease. Am Rev Respir Dis 1993;147:S40–47.

66. Ramsdell J. Use of theophylline in the treatment of COPD. Chest 1995; 107:206–209S.

67. Man GC, Chapman KR, Ali SH, Darke AC. Sleep quality and nocturnal respiratory function with once-daily theophylline (Uniphyl) and inhaled salbutamol in patients with COPD. Chest 1996;110:648–653.

68. Nishimura K, Koyama H, Ikeda A, et al. The additive effect of theophylline on a high-dose combination of inhaled salbutamol and ipratropium bromide in stable COPD. Chest 1995;107:718–723.

69. Karpel JP, Kotch A, Zinny M, et al. A comparison of inhaled ipratropium, oral theophylline plus inhaled beta agonist, and the combination of all three in patients with COPD. Chest 1994;105:1089–1094.

70. ZuWallack RL, Mahler DA, Reilly D, et al. Salmeterol plus theophylline combination therapy in the treatment of COPD. Chest 2001;119: 1661–1670.

71. Callahan CM, Dittus RS, Katz BP. Oral corticosteroid therapy for patients with stable chronic obstructive pulmonary disease: A meta-analysis. Ann Intern Med 1991;114:216–223.

72. Pizzichini E, Pizzichini MM, Gibson P, et al. Sputum eosinophilia predicts benefit from prednisone in smokers with chronic obstructive bronchitis. Am J Respir Crit Care Med 1998;158:1511–1517.

73. Senderovitz T, Vestbo J, Frandsen J, et al. Steroid reversibility test followed by inhaled budesonide or placebo in outpatients with stable chronic obstructive pulmonary disease. The Danish Society of Respiratory Medicine. Respir Med 1999;93:715–718.

74. Pauwels RA, Claes-Goran L, Latinen LA, et al. Long-term treatment with inhaled budesonide in persons with mild chronic obstructive pulmonary disease who continue smoking. New Engl J Med 1999;340:1948–1953.

75. Vestbo J, Sorenson T, Lange P, et al. Long-term effect of inhaled budesonide in mild and moderate chronic obstructive pulmonary disease: A randomized, controlled trial. Lancet 1999;353:1819–1823.

76. Burge PS, Calverley PM, Jones PW, et al. Randomised, double-blind, placebo-controlled study of fluticasone propionate in patients with moderate to severe chronic obstructive pulmonary disease: The ISOLDE trial. Br Med J 2000;320:1297–1303.

77. Nishimura K, Koyama H, Ikeda A, et al. The effect of high-dose inhaled beclomethasone dipropionate in patients with stable COPD. Chest 1999;115:31–37.

78. Weir DC, Bale GA, Bright P, Sherwood Burge P. A double-blind placebo-controlled study of the effect of inhaled beclomethasone dipropionate for 2 years in patients with nonasthmatic chronic obstructive pulmonary disease. Clin Exp Allergy 1999;29(suppl 2):125–128.

79. Paggiaro PL, Dahle R, Bakran I, et al. Multicentre, randomized, placebo-controlled trial of inhaled fluticasone propionate in patients with chronic obstructive pulmonary disease. International COPD Study Group. Lancet 1998;351:773–780.

80. The Lung Health Study Research Group. Effect of inhaled triamcinolone on the decline in pulmonary function in chronic obstructive pulmonary disease. New Engl J Med 2000;343:1902–1909.

81. Jones PW, Willits LR, Burge PS, Calverley PM. Disease severity and the effect of fluticasone propionate on chronic obstructive pulmonary disease exacerbations. Eur Respir J 2003;21:68–73.

82. Lipworth BJ. Systemic adverse effects of inhaled corticosteroid therapy: A systematic review and meta-analysis. Arch Intern Med 1999;159: 941–955.

83. van Grunsven PM, van Schayck CP, Derenne JP, et al. Long-term effects of inhaled corticosteroids in chronic obstructive pulmonary disease: A meta-analysis. Thorax 1999;54:7–14.

84. Calverly P, Pauwels R, Vestbo, J, et al. Combined salmeterol and fluticasone in the treatment of chronic obstructive pulmonary disease: A randomized, controlled trial. Lancet 2003;361:449–456.

85. Szafranski W, Cukier A, Ramirez A, et al. Efficacy and safety of budesonide/formoterol in the management of chronic obstructive pulmonary disease. Eur Respir J 2003;21:74–81.

86. Mahler DA, Wire P, Horstman D, et al. Effectiveness of fluticasone propionate and salmeterol combination delivered via the Diskus device in the treatment of chronic obstructive pulmonary disease. Am J Respir Crit Care Med 2002;166:1084–1091.

87. Hanania NA, Darken P, Horstman D, et al. Efficacy and safety of fluticasone proprionate (250 mcg) and salmeterol (50 mcg) combined in the Diskus inhaler for the treatment of COPD. Chest 2003;124:834–843.

88. Dirksen A, Dijkman JH, Madsen F, et al. A randomized clinical trial of alpha-1-antitrypsin augmentation therapy. Am J Respir Crit Care Med 1999;160:1468–1472.

89. MacDonald JL, Johnson CE. Pathophysiology and treatment of α_1-antitrypsin deficiency. Am J Health Syst Pharm 1995;52:481–489.

90. Lightowler JV, Wedzicha JA, Elliott MW, et al. Noninvasive positive pressure ventilation to treat respiratory failure resulting from exacerbations of chronic obstructive pulmonary disease: Cochrane systemic review and meta-analysis. Br Med J 2003;326:185–189.

91. Niewoehner DE, Erbland ML, Deupree RH, et al. Effect of systemic glucocorticoids on exacerbations of chronic obstructive pulmonary disease. Department of Veterans Affairs Cooperative Study Group. New Engl J Med 1999;340:1941–1947.

92. Davies L, Angus RM, Calverley PMA. Oral corticosteroids in patients admitted to hospital with exacerbations of chronic obstructive pulmonary disease: A prospective, randomised, controlled trial. Lancet 1999;354:456–460.

93. Thompson WH, Nielson CP, Carvalho P, et al. Controlled trial of oral prednisone in outpatients with acute COPD exacerbation. Am J Respir Crit Care Med 1996;154:407–412.

94. Sayiner A, Aytemur ZA, Cirit M, et al. Systemic glucocorticoids in severe exacerbations of COPD. Chest 2001;119:726–730.

95. Aaron SD, Vandemheen KL, Hebert P, et al. Outpatient oral prednisone after emergency treatment of chronic obstructive pulmonary disease. New Engl J Med 2003;348:2618–2625.

96. Saint S, Bent S, Vittinghoff E, Grady D. Antibiotics in chronic obstructive pulmonary disease exacerbations: A meta-analysis. JAMA 1995;273:957–960.

97. Niederman MS. Antibiotic therapy for exacerbations of chronic bronchitis. Semin Respir Infect 2000;15:59–70.

98. Chodosh S, DeAbate C, Haverstock D, et al. Short-course moxifloxacin therapy for treatment of acute bacterial exacerbations of chronic bronchitis. Respir Med 2000;94:18–27.

99. Poole PJ, Black PN. Mucolytic agents for chronic bronchitis or chronic obstructive pulmonary disease. Cochrane Database Syst Rev 2000;2 (*www.updatusa.com*).

100. National Emphysema Treatment Trial Research Group. New Engl J Med 2003;348:2059–2073.

101. Grossman RF, Mukerjee J, Vaughan D, et al. A one-year community-based health economic study of ciprofloxacin versus usual antibiotic treatment in acute exacerbations of chronic bronchitis. Chest 1998;113:131–141.

102. Friedman M, Serby CW, Menjoge SS, et al. Pharmacoeconomic evaluation of a combination of ipratropium plus albuterol compared with ipratropium alone and albuterol alone in COPD. Chest 1999;115:635–641.

28
ACUTE RESPIRATORY DISTRESS SYNDROME

Peter Gal and J. Laurence Ransom

Learning Objectives and other resources can be found at *www.pharmacotherapyonline.com.*

KEY CONCEPTS

❶ Neonatal respiratory distress syndrome (RDS) is predominantly a disease of surfactant deficiency.

❷ Antenatal steroids markedly reduce the incidence of neonatal RDS and some other complications of prematurity.

❸ Surfactant prophylaxis and replacement therapy markedly reduce RDS-related pulmonary morbidity and mortality.

❹ Acute respiratory distress syndrome (ARDS) is a syndrome presenting with bilateral pulmonary infiltrates, high oxygen requirements (Pa_{O_2}/F_{IO_2} <200 mm Hg), and noncardiogenic pulmonary edema.

❺ Acute lung injury (ALI) is similar to ARDS but with milder gas exchange abnormalities (i.e., Pa_{O_2}/F_{IO_2} <300 mm Hg).

❻ Causes of ARDS may be pulmonary or extrapulmonary, and responses to interventions may differ with etiology.

❼ Mechanical ventilation is the foundation for treatment and prevention of ARDS.

❽ For both RDS and ARDS, ventilator maneuvers to minimize barotrauma and volutrauma are critical to management. Ventilator management remains more an art than a science.

❾ Anti-inflammatory therapies (pharmacologic and nutrition) offer theoretical therapeutic advantages for managing ARDS, but compelling evidence describing when and how to use them is not yet available.

This chapter addresses the problems of acute respiratory distress syndromes in neonates, children, and adults. Abbreviations are used throughout the text, and a glossary for physiology, diseases, and drugs is presented in Table 28–1. Descriptions of ventilator-related terms are provided in Tables 28–2 and 28–3. Because the physiology of neonatal respiratory distress syndrome (RDS) and acute respiratory distress syndrome (ARDS) has some differences, these diseases will be discussed separately.

NEONATAL RESPIRATORY DISTRESS SYNDROME (RDS)

❶ RDS, historically known as *hyaline membrane disease* (HMD), is more appropriately termed *surfactant-deficiency RDS*. RDS is associated with considerable morbidity and mortality. Before 35 weeks' gestation, the risk of RDS and the severity of disease increase with greater degree of prematurity and, in the absence of appropriate antenatal interventions, occurs in over 50% of newborns of 30 weeks' or less gestation. The Vermont Oxford Network experience for 1999 describes over 27,000 neonates below 1500 g from 325 neonatal intensive care unit (NICU) sites.[1] The annual report noted that RDS occurred in over 80% of premature infants below 1000 g and that there was a gradual decline to about 42% of neonates with birth weights between 1400 and 1500 g.

RDS is attributed primarily to insufficient formation and differentiation of type II pneumocytes with consequent impaired production and release of surfactant. Pulmonary surfactant contains phospholipids that function at the air-liquid interface in the alveolus to lower surface tension, thus preventing alveolar collapse. In the face of surfactant deficiency, atelectasis and impaired gas exchange occur. Additionally, alveolar transudation of protein-rich fluid forms a hyaline membrane, giving rise to the term *hyaline membrane disease.*[2]

Epithelial sodium channel (ENaC) maturation also appears important in RDS. In utero, fluid is actively secreted into lungs via chloride channels. At birth, the ENaC takes over, and fluid is actively reabsorbed from the lungs. In premature infants, immaturity of the ENaC results in failure to reabsorb lung fluid, with consequent pulmonary edema.[3] In term infants, this conversion occurs at birth in response to circulating catecholamines. Failure of the conversion to occur in preterm infants results in an inability to clear alveolar fluid and consequent pulmonary edema.[3]

Measurement of lung maturation in amniotic fluid using biochemical markers of surfactant deficiency is an important consideration in preventive and therapeutic interventions, as well as in predicting the likelihood of developing RDS. Measurement of surfactant components in amniotic fluid using either the ratio of lecithin to sphingomyelin (L/S ratio) or phosphatidylglycerol (PG) have been particularly useful for confirming lung maturity. PG is the better test because, unlike the L/S ratio, it is reliable in the presence of blood, meconium, or maternal diabetes. Also, turnaround time for PG is more rapid.[4] A positive PG test or L/S ratio is associated with a sensitivity of 95% to 99% and a positive predictive value of 97% to 98%. Both tests suffer from limited specificity (50% to 70%) and limited negative predictive value (54% to 56%). Thus a test result indicating immaturity does not ensure development of RDS, but a test indicating maturity makes RDS very unlikely.[4] RDS severity and risk are made worse by a variety of perinatal factors, including perinatal hypoxia or asphyxia, acidosis, cold stress, patent ductus arteriosus, and maternal diabetes mellitus. These factors may further compromise

TABLE 28–1. Glossary of Terms and Abbreviations

ENaC	Epithelial sodium channel
L/S ratio	Lecithin/sphingomyelin ratio
PG	Phosphatidylglycerol
CXR	Chest x-ray
RDS	Neonatal respiratory distress syndrome
HMD	Hyaline membrane disease
PIE	Pulmonary interstitial emphysema
BPD	Bronchopulmonary dysplasia
IVH	Intraventricular hemorrhage
PVL	Periventricular leukomalacia
PDA	Patent ductus arteriosus
NEC	Necrotizing enterocolitis
ARDS	Acute respiratory distress syndrome
ALI	Acute lung injury
PCWP	Pulmonary capillary wedge pressure
CO	Cardiac output
TRH	Thyrotropin releasing hormone
SRT	Surfactant replacement therapy
PFC	Perfluorocarbon
NO	Nitric oxide
ABG	Arterial blood gas
Pao_2	Arterial blood gas oxygen
$Paco_2$	Arterial blood gas carbon dioxide
Sao_2	Oxygen saturation
Mvo_2	Mixed venous saturation
ECMO	Extracorporeal membrane oxygenation
VILI	Ventilator-induced lung injury
MODS	Multiple organ dysfunction syndrome

pulmonary blood supply, consequently causing death of an already limited number of type II alveolar cells and limiting surfactant production.

Chronic intrauterine stress, on the contrary, lowers the risk of RDS by promoting lung maturation, perhaps by increasing endogenous glucocorticoid concentrations.[2]

CLINICAL PRESENTATION

The presentation of neonatal RDS is summarized in Table 28–4 and is illustrated in Fig. 28–1. A number of neonatal disorders may mimic and be indistinguishable from RDS, the most important being sepsis caused by group B β-hemolytic *Streptococcus*, pneumococcus, or gram-negative bacilli. Sepsis is a common concurrent problem with RDS and may alter the response to therapy.[5] All neonates with suspected RDS should be evaluated for sepsis. Antibiotics should be used until sepsis can be ruled out or a full therapeutic course is completed. Other etiologies for RDS include transient tachypnea of the newborn, spontaneous pneumothorax, congenital cyanotic heart disease, and diaphragmatic hernia.

PREVENTION

Several perinatal/antenatal interventions can be adopted to prevent or minimize the severity of RDS. These include optimizing care at labor and delivery and control of maternal diseases to avoid factors known to predispose to RDS. Additionally, drug therapy to delay premature delivery (tocolytics) or to assist with lung maturation (steroids) can be instituted (Fig. 28–2). Early initiation of antibiotics to treat bacterial vaginosis and trichomoniasis also has been associated with significant reduction in preterm births.[6,7]

Tocolysis can be expected to delay delivery for 2 to 7 days.[6] However, this may provide sufficient time to resolve a reversible etiology or promote fetal lung maturation. Up to 80% of women with presumptive preterm labor will not have a preterm delivery. Recently it was suggested that measuring fetal fibronectin to identify patients unlikely to have a preterm delivery may be better than treating all patients with symptoms of preterm labor or waiting for cervical changes that will reduce the likelihood of successful inhibition of labor.[6] Contraindications to tocolytic therapy include fetal death or lethal abnormality, eclampsia, abruptio placentae, and proven chorioamnionitis. Relative contraindications are preeclampsia, severe chronic hypertension, renal disease, heart disease, fetal distress, and fetal growth retardation. Of the tocolytics commonly used (i.e., β-sympathomimetics, calcium channel blockers, magnesium sulfate, and nonsteroidal anti-inflammatory drugs [NSAIDs]), none has clear advantages over the others, but different profiles for maternal and fetal toxicities must be considered.[6,8] Only short courses of tocolytics can be justified to allow time to control the cause of preterm labor or to administer antenatal corticosteroids. Prolonged maintenance therapy has the same results as placebo.[6,8]

TABLE 28–2. Glossary of Terms for Ventilator Settings and Management

Et	Expiratory time; in the ventilatory cycle, the amount of time devoted to exhalation.
It	Inspiratory time; in the ventilatory cycle, the amount of time devoted to inspiration.
I:E	Ratio of inspiratory time to expiratory time; in a normal, spontaneously breathing patient, this is 1:1.5.
Pao_2	Partial pressure of oxygen present in arterial blood; normal level for adults is 80–100 mm Hg; normal level for premature babies is 50–70 mm Hg.
$Paco_2$	Partial pressure of carbon dioxide present in arterial blood; normal is 35–45 mm Hg, but higher levels are acceptable to minimize ventilator support.
PEEP	Positive end-expiratory pressure; positive pressure at the end of exhalation designed to prevent alveoli from collapsing during expiration.
PIP	Peak inspiratory pressure; the maximum level of pressure achieved by the ventilator during inspiration.
IMV	Intermittent mandatory ventilation; a mode of ventilation designed to deliver a preset inspiratory rate; continuous flow of gas is available for patient's spontaneous breaths.
Fio_2	Fraction (percentage) of inspired oxygen.
TV	Tidal volume; volume of gas delivered during a single inspiration.
MAP	Mean airway pressure; a constant distending pressure.
Hz	Hertz; normally described as cycles per second, this is the number of breaths per minute.
FRC	Functional residual capacity; the volume of air remaining in the lung after normal expiration.
Amp	Amplitude; a wavelike change in pressure centered around a mean airway pressure.
Sigh	A breath that recruits and maintains alveolar patency, used in HFJV; similar to pressure provided with PIP.
CWF	Chest wiggle factor; a clinical observation ensuring appropriate chest wall movement with HFOV.
BPM	Breaths per minute.

TABLE 28–3. Mechanical Ventilator Types and Modes of Ventilation

CMV	Controlled mechanical ventilation; a ventilator mode in which RR + TV are under machine, rather than, patient control.
AC	Assist control; mode in which patient receives a full TV if the patient breathes over the ventilator.
PC	Pressure control; ventilator delivers a TV until a certain pressure is achieved.
SIMV	Synchronized intermittent mandatory ventilation; a ventilator breath "synchronized" with patient's inspiratory effort.
PS	Pressure support; pressure on inspiration designed to assist generation of tidal volume.
IRV	Inverse ratio ventilation; ventilator mode in which inspiratory time is prolonged in comparison to expiration time. Used to decrease plateau pressure and improve oxygenation.
HFOV	High-frequency oscillatory ventilation; a mechanical diphragm produces oscillations superimposed on a constant gas flow. Can provide from 180 to 900 breaths per minute. Both inspiration and expiration are actively promoted.
HFJV	High-frequency jet ventilation; small volumes of air are released in a pulsating fashion through a jet nozzle, and directed down the airway in a patient simultaneously receiving conventional ventilation. Can provide from 240 to 660 breaths per minute. Inspiration is active, but expiration is passive, predisposing to air trapping.
HFFI	High-frequency flow interruption; similar to HFJV, but air pulses are delivered at lower pressures and volumes.
HFPPV	High-frequency positive-pressure ventilation; conventional mechanical ventilation at faster-than-usual rates.
PPAV	Patient proportional assist ventilation; a collective term describing ventilators using patient-controlled rates and tidal volumes.
OH	Oxygen hood; a clear plastic enclosure placed over a nonintubated infant to allow humidification of room air (21% F_{IO_2} or increased F_{IO_2}).

Fetal lung maturation can be accelerated with antenatal corticosteroids. The National Institutes of Health (NIH) consensus conference in 1994 concluded that all fetuses between 24 and 34 weeks' gestation at risk for preterm delivery should receive corticosteroids regardless of gender, race, maternal infection, and availability of surfactant. A report by the National Institutes of Child Health and Development Neonatal Research Network noted that antenatal steroid use was associated with fewer pulmonary problems and mortality.[9] Many women who are appropriate candidates are still untreated.[9] Treatment with three or more courses of antenatal steroids is discouraged because of concerns for impaired fetal growth and long-term neurodevelopmental delays, although further studies to evaluate the validity of this conclusion are needed.[10] Use of one or two courses of antenatal steroid therapy is relatively devoid of toxicity and markedly improves neonatal morbidity and mortality. Betamethasone appears to provide superior benefits to dexamethasone.[11] The odds ratio (95% confidence interval [CI]) for developing RDS is reduced to 0.49 (95% CI 0.41–0.6) if steroids are started 24 hours to 7 days before

TABLE 28–4. Presentation of Neonatal RDS

General

The patient will appear in acute respiratory distress, which will worsen progressively to respiratory failure. Fluid retention, edema, and oliguria are common in the first 48 hours of untreated RDS.

Signs and Symptoms

Within the first few hours of life the patient will have expiratory grunting, intercostal respiratory retractions, use of accessory neck muscles, paradoxical seesaw respirations, tachycardia, pallor, cyanosis, and progressively increased oxygen requirements.

Laboratory Tests

Obstetricians may obtain amniotic fluid to measure the lecithin-sphingomyelin (L/S) ratio or phosphatidylglycerol (PG) to determine fetal lung maturity.

Since infection may cause RDS, a sepsis work-up is needed, i.e., WBC with differential, and blood culture. Arterial blood gases and oxygen saturation monitors can be used to evaluate for adequate oxygenation.

Other

Chest x-ray consistent with RDS shows a characteristic reticulogranular (ground-glass) pattern to the peripheral lung fields. The collapse of small airspaces around the large airways traps air in the large airways, making them easily visible. These are called *air bronchograms*. In severe RDS, lungs may appear as a total whiteout. Progression of RDS should be monitored with repeat chest x-rays. If echocardiography is performed to evaluate for presence of a patent ductus ateriosus, the elevated pulmonary pressure may cause shunting right to left through the ductus arteriosus.

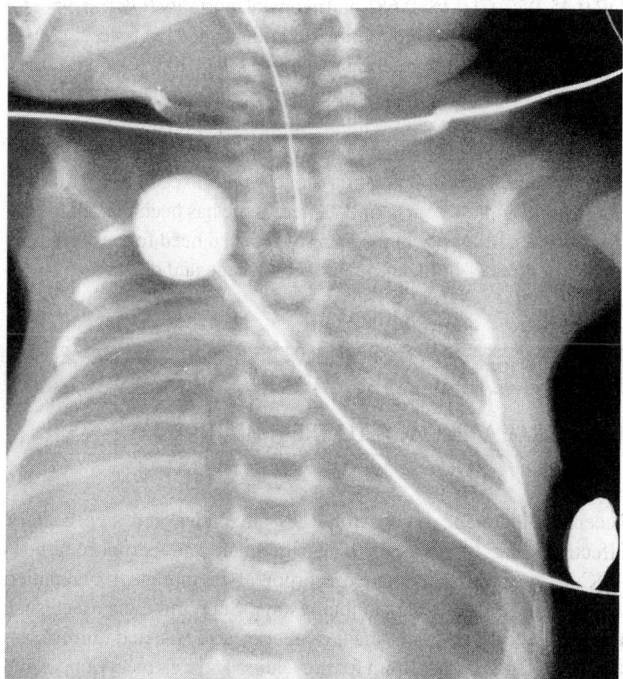

FIGURE 28–1. Chest x-ray demonstrating surfactant-deficient respiratory distress syndrome with ground glass appearance and air bronchograms.

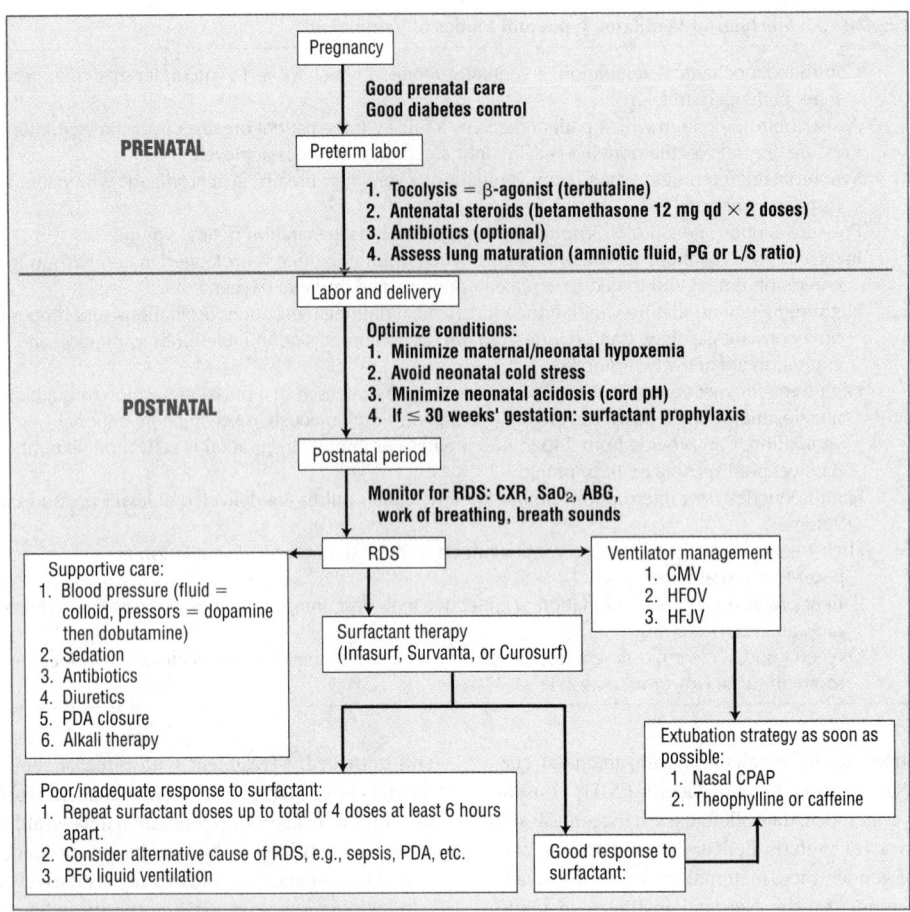

FIGURE 28–2. Algorithm for prevention and treatment of neonatal RDS.

delivery. Even if treatment is started less than 24 hours or more than 7 days from delivery, risk is still reduced (odds ratio [OR] 0.69, 95% CI 0.50–0.94).[10] Antenatal steroids also reduced the risk of intraventricular hemorrhage (OR 0.5, 95% CI 0.3–0.9), necrotizing enterocolitis (OR 0.35, 95% CI 0.18–0.68), and neonatal mortality (OR 0.6, 95% CI 0.5–0.8).[9,10] An estimated number of patients needed to treat (NNT) to prevent RDS in one preterm infant of less than 30 weeks' gestation, where RDS occurs in 50% of untreated cases, is 6 patients.[10,11] One report estimated that over $3000 was saved per treated neonate and that if treatment rates increased to 60%, annual savings in health care costs from initial hospitalization alone would exceed $157 million. Even an incomplete course of betamethasone has been proven to provide benefits, primarily in the areas of reduced need for vasopressors and lower rates of intraventricular hemorrhage and death.[11]

Use of thyrotropin-releasing hormone (TRH) as an adjunct to antenatal corticosteroids was thought to further accelerate fetal lung maturation.[12] However, the Australian Collaborative Trial of Antenatal Thyrotropin-Releasing Hormone (ACTOBAT) study failed to show additional benefits from TRH 200 mcg every 12 hours. The frequencies of RDS (relative risk [RR] 1.17, 95% CI 1.00–1.36) and need for ventilation (RR 1.15, 95% CI 1.01–1.31) were not reduced, and treatment was associated with maternal nausea, vomiting, and light-headedness. Of more concern was the 12-month follow-up report in which TRH treatment was associated with motor delays (OR 1.51, 95% CI 1.11–2.05), sensory impairment (OR 2.00, 95% CI 1.06–3.74), social delays (OR 1.41, 95% CI 1.01–1.95), and severe neurodevelopmental impairment (OR 1.75, 95% CI 1.07–2.87).[13] At this point, antenatal TRH treatment cannot be advised.

▶ TREATMENT: Neonatal Respiratory Distress Syndrome

■ GENERAL APPROACH TO TREATMENT

Recently, treatment options for RDS have advanced significantly. Effective drug therapies include surfactant and perfluorocarbons (PFCs). Nitric oxide and extracorporeal membrane oxygenation (ECMO) have been used as final resorts. Supportive therapies such as mechanical ventilation, management of acidosis, and diuresis are also important. An algorithm for prevention and treatment of neonatal RDS is presented in Fig. 28–2.

■ NONPHARMACOLOGIC THERAPY

■ VENTILATOR THERAPY

Positive-pressure ventilation (PPV) provides vital support to maintain adequate ventilation and oxygenation during the acute phase of RDS. Effective PPV is accomplished by generating a pressure that exceeds the "closing" pressure of the lung. Ventilation modes delivering this positive pressure are conventional mechanical ventilation (CV), high-frequency ventilation (HFV), patient proportional

TABLE 28–5. Ventilator Management and Considerations in RDS

Ventilator Type	Setting	Normal Initial Settings		Advantages	Disadvantages
		<1500 g	>1500 g		
CMV	PIF (cm H_2O)	18–20	20–22	High inspiratory pressures allow "popping open" of alveoli	Larger tidal volumes and inspiratory pressures causing lung injury
	Target TV (mL/kg)	4–6	6–8		
	PEEP (cm H_2O)	4	4–5		
	IMV (bpm)	40–60	40–60		
CPAP	(cm H_2O)	5–7	6–8	Little barotrauma/volutrauma	Lack of tidal volume
HFOV	MAP (cm H_2O)	7–10	8–12	Less risk of volutrauma/barotrauma	Risk for IVH/PVL?
				Increased alveolar recruitment	Unable to give aerosolized respiratory medications
					Hypotension
				Approved for air-leak syndromes	Increased mucostasis?
				Simple to operate	
	Amplitude	To appropriate CWF			
	Hz	15	15		
HFJV	PIP (cm H_2O)	18–20	20–22	Increased CO_2 removal	Risk for IVH/PVL?
					Two machines
					Increased gas trapping
					Unable to give respiratory medicines
	PEEP (cm H_2O)	4–5	4–5		
	Sigh rate (bpm)	5–10	5–10		
	Rate (bpm)	420	420		
PPAV	Rate (bpm)	20–30	10–20	Less barotrauma due to "synchronizing" with patient's own breath	Lack of clinical experience
SIMV				Patient-sensitive	
				Reduced need for sedation	
	Volume (mL/kg)	8–15	10–15		

assist ventilation (PPAV), synchronized intermittent mandatory ventilation (SIMV), and continuous positive airway pressure (CPAP).[2] As ventilator technology advances, hybrids of the different ventilation modes also have been tried. A comprehensive review describing these modes of ventilation is beyond the scope of this chapter, and we recommend the reader to an excellent text.[14]

The increased neonatal survival seen today can be credited, in part, to the extensive technological advances in respiratory care, including mechanical ventilation. CV, employed since the early 1970s, is based on delivering a volume of air (tidal volume [TV]) by using inspiratory and expiratory pressures (positive inspiratory pressure/positive end-expiratory pressure [PIP/PEEP]) at a specific rate (intermittent mandatory ventilation [IMV]).[15] Although successful, CV-induced lung morbidity has required continual assessment of ventilator modes that decrease baro- and volutrauma. A summary of these ventilation modes is given in Table 28–5, with the range of typical initial settings listed. Evidence is not yet compelling to recommend a preferred ventilator mode. The improved outcomes in premature infants also can be attributed to better understanding of neonatal physiology, most notably oxygen delivery optimization and cerebral protective effects of carbon dioxide. The oxygen-hemoglobin dissociation curves in neonates are shifted to the left as compared with adults, resulting in target PaO_2 values of 50 to 75 mm Hg and SaO_2 values greater than 90%. Whether oxygen saturation targets of 70% to 90% will become more acceptable is an area of future debate. One study of preterm infants of 28 or fewer weeks' gestation compared neonates ventilated to target oxygen saturations of 70% to 90% with those targeted to 88% to 98%.[17] Survival rates and cerebral palsy rates at 1 year were the same, but the lower saturation group had an average of 17 fewer days on mechanical ventilation and 56 fewer days on supplemental oxygen. In addition, complications of retinopathy of prematurity requiring

cryotherapy were one-fourth as frequent. This approach needs additional studies before it can be applied more broadly.

Allowing $PaCO_2$ to exceed 50 or even 60 mm Hg (called *permissive hypercapnia*) is a good strategy, provided that the blood pH remains acceptable, because it means that less aggressive ventilator pressures are needed. Too aggressive ventilation can result in hypocarbia, which is associated with periventricular leukomalacia and consequent neurodevelopmental delays. The more comprehensive understanding of neonatal physiology allows the clinician to use improved ventilator technologies and select strategies that allow for the most appropriate fit for the circumstance. For example, although CV remains a good choice for many neonates, those with pulmonary air leaks probably are managed more safely with high-frequency oscillatory ventilation (HFOV). Increasingly, HFOV using a "high volume" strategy, which avoids atelectasis, is being considered the preferred first-line ventilator therapy. This must be tempered by an inability of studies to show differences in outcomes between CV and HFOV. Since rapid and early ventilator weaning is becoming popular, and given that the optimal approach to weaning from HFOV is unknown, the pendulum may shift back to CV when prophylactic surfactant is used, and rapid advancement to extubation is anticipated.

The goals of CV are to achieve appropriate arterial blood gas parameters (PaO_2 of 50 to 75 mm Hg, $PaCO_2$ of 40 to 60 mm Hg, pH of 7.28 to 7.40), chest expansion (diaphragm position on an inspiratory film at ribs eight to nine), and avoidance of toxicities. Often a tradeoff of either higher FIO_2 or higher PIP must be made. Using permissive hypercapnea so that less aggressive ventilator pressures are needed appears the safer approach, but data proving this bias are lacking.

Such decisions thus involve clinician bias and the "art" of medicine rather than being based on a strong scientific basis.

Early conversion from ventilator modes requiring endotracheal intubation to nasal CPAP, even in infants as young as 25 weeks' gestation, is associated with reduced chronic lung disease at 28 days (NNT = 6).[15] This is aided markedly by concurrent use of methylxanthines to increase respiratory drive (NNT = 3.7 in infants < 1000 g).[16]

CLINICAL CONTROVERSY

Clinicians disagree on the best ventilator approach for managing RDS while avoiding chronic lung disease. There is consensus, however, that all modes of positive-pressure ventilation damage lungs and that patients should be extubated as soon as possible.

■ PHARMACOLOGIC THERAPY

■ SURFACTANT THERAPY

Surfactant replacement therapy (SRT) is widely accepted as the most clinically acceptable and cost-effective approach to the treatment of RDS. Clinical trials have been carried out worldwide using an array of artificial, modified natural, and natural surfactants. Natural surfactants are either processed extracts of minced lungs or extracts of lavaged surfactant, which affects the surfactant protein makeup of the preparation. The differences in preparations can be discerned from key components and dosing strategies, which are summarized in Table 28–6.

Natural human surfactant contains 85% phospholipids, 10% neutral lipids, and 5% surfactant proteins or apolipoproteins. Animal surfactants have similar protein and lipid content. Surfactant is synthesized in type II pneumocytes in the alveoli. After secretion, the major route of clearance is via reuptake by type II cells. Small quantities are removed by absorption into the lymphatics and clearance by alveolar macrophages. After reuptake into the type II cells, the phospholipids are either recycled for secretion or degraded and reused to synthesize new phospholipids.[18,19]

Most exogenous surfactants incorporate dipalmitoyl phosphatidylcholine (DPPC), which constitutes 45% to 70% of endogenous lung surfactant and is the major phospholipid causing the low surface tension of surfactant. Other phospholipids, mainly phosphatidyl ethanolamine, phosphatidyl glycerol, phosphatidylinositol, and sphingomyelin, are responsible for adsorbing to the air-liquid interface. Four surfactant proteins (SP-A, SP-B, SP-C, and SP-D) comprise 2% to 5% of the weight of natural surfactant.[18,19] SP-A appears to regulate pulmonary surfactant turnover, formation of tubular myelin, and immune regulation. Since natural surfactant products undergo an organic solvent extraction procedure, no substantial quantities of SP-A are present in these products. SP-B appears to be involved in the formation of tubular myelin. It is also the most active hydrophobic protein in improving the surface activity of surfactant, perhaps by increasing the lateral stability of the phospholipid layer. Increasing SP-B content of surfactant preparations is associated with increased activity and resistance to inactivation by various endogenous substances. Genetic deficiency of SP-B in full-term infants results in death from respiratory failure. SP-C is speculated to be involved in the spreadability and surface activity of surfactant by increasing the adsorption of DPPC and other phospholipids to the air-liquid interface. SP-D function is unknown, but it has the structure of lectins and proteins responsible for bacterial opsonization.[18,19]

When given in the delivery room as prophylaxis, natural surfactant can be given as a single bolus down the endotracheal tube, although the manufacturers still recommend divided doses using the same procedure as for treatment.[20] For neonates with established RDS

TABLE 28–6. Exogenous Surfactants Used for the Treatment of Neonate with Respiratory Distress Syndrome

Surfactant Type Dose (mg/kg)/Volume (mL/kg)	Source	Components	Concentration (g/L)	Initial Dose (mg/kg)
Artificial surfactants				
Pulmactant (ALEC) 100/1.2	Synthetic	DPPC, unsaturated phosphatidylglycerol	100	100
Colfosceril palmitate (Exosurf) 67.5/5	Synthetic	DPPC, hexadecanol, tyloxapol	13.5	67.5
Human surfactants				
Human 60/3	Aminotic fluid whole surfactant	Surfactant lipids, SP-A, SP-B (2.0–5.0%), SP-C, SP-D	20	60–70
Animal surfactants				
Calfactant (Infasurf) 100/3	Calf lung lavage	Surfactant lipids, SP-B (1.7%), SP-C	25	100
CLSE 100/3	Calf lung lavage	Surfactant lipids, SP-B (1.7%), SP-C	30	90
SFRI 1 (Alveofact) 50/1.2	Cow lung lavage	Surfactant lipids, SP-B (1.7%), SP-C	45	50
Poractant alfa (Curosurf) Dose 1: 200/2.5 Doses 2–4 100/1.25	Minced pig lung extract purified by chromatography	Lung phospholipids, SP-B (0.2%), SP-C	80	200
Surfacten (Surfactant-TA) 100/4	Minced cow lung extract + synthetic lipids	Lung lipids + DPPC, tripalmitin, palmitic acid	30	100
Beractant (Survanta) 100/4	Minced cow lung extract + synthetic lipids acid,	Lung lipids + DPPC, tripalmitin, palmitic acid, SP-B (<0.1%), SP-C	25	100

ALEC = artificial lung expanding compound; CLSE = calf lung surfactant extract; DPPC = dipalmitoyl phosphatidylcholine; SP-A = surfactant protein A; SP-B = surfactant protein B; SP-C = surfactant protein C. Doses reported per milligram of phospholipid and milliliter of surfactant product.

who are stabilized on the ventilator, surfactant is best administered via a sideport in the endotracheal adapter in two bolus fractional doses at a 45-degree upward tilt angled to the right and then left.[20] Animal studies confirm that the bolus technique delivers and distributes surfactant evenly. Use of the slow infusion technique delivered surfactant primarily to the upper lobes,[18] and nebulized surfactant concentrated in select pockets of each lobe, resulting in areas of hypo- and hyperinflation.[18]

Several issues have been addressed in the Cochrane Database Systematic Reviews and other useful publications to help direct optimal therapeutic approaches. These include synthetic versus natural surfactants, comparison of available natural surfactants, optimal timing for initiating surfactant therapy, and single versus multiple dosing strategies.[2,18,19,21-26] Outcome measures examined during surfactant trials include oxygen and ventilator requirements, severity of RDS, RDS mortality, total mortality, pneumothorax and other air-leak syndromes, pulmonary interstitial emphysema (PIE), bronchopulmonary dysplasia (BPD), and complications some investigators associate with surfactant therapy, such as intraventricular hemorrhage (IVH), pulmonary hemorrhage, and patent ductus arteriosus (PDA). In general, the primary benefits are more rapid resolution and milder course of RDS and lower risk of pneumothorax, death, or chronic lung disease (also referred to as *bronchopulmonary dysplasia*).

Several surfactant products are available currently in the United States. All represent natural surfactant preparations from different sources (Table 28–7). The only previously available synthetic surfactant in the United States was colfosceril (Exosurf). While there were clear therapeutic benefits to this product, it did not compare favorably with natural surfactant extracts.[2,18,21] A meta-analysis of 11 direct-comparison trials showed that compared with synthetic surfactant, natural surfactant reduced the risk of: pneumothorax (RR 0.63, 95% CI 0.53 to 0.75) and mortality (RR 0.87, 95% CI 0.76 to 0.98). Risks for other important clinical or toxic end points were not increased with either preparation.[21] Exosurf was withdrawn from the market because of insufficient efficacy. Comparisons of natural surfactants are more complex. Theoretically, the surfactant with the most surfactant proteins and fastest onset of action should be the best.[18] This was demonstrated for prevention of death in an animal study. However, direct comparisons of beractant with the faster-acting calfactant failed to demonstrate differences in death at discharge. It is important to recognize that the study was powered to find a 25% difference, and smaller differences may have been missed.[18] Benefits noted with calfactant in this comparison study in the prophylaxis arm were longer duration of effect, resulting in less frequent and fewer doses, and shorter duration of mechanical ventilation and supplemental oxygenation with prophylactic surfactant therapy. A larger multicenter trial repeating the earlier comparison trial is ongoing. At this point, no clear advantage can be advocated for the different surfactant products. Since onset of effect and potency are not identical, the products should not be interchanged without earlier monitoring of arterial blood gases for calfactant and poractant to avoid overventilation and the associated risk of pulmonary damage, periventricular leukomalacia, and intraventricular hemorrhage.

The optimal time to initiate surfactant is also controversial. Options are RDS prophylaxis administration in the delivery room or later administration in the NICU when the diagnosis of RDS can be made clearly and the position of the endotracheal tube for surfactant delivery can be confirmed. The advantage of prophylaxis is that the drug is more evenly distributed in the lung, and excess ventilator support is avoided.[2,18,19] Disadvantages to the use of prophylaxis are that administration errors are more likely owing to poor placement of the endotracheal tube and unnecessary exposure and costs for patients who would not have developed RDS. Alternatively, waiting for the diagnosis of RDS before treatment with surfactant results in unnecessary exposure to increased ventilator pressures and oxygen supplementation, which are associated with greater pulmonary damage and the costs associated with subsequent management.[2,18] A meta-analysis of eight studies comparing RDS prophylaxis with treatment with surfactant demonstrated a benefit to prophylaxis in infants of fewer than 30 weeks' gestation. Benefits included a decrease in the incidence of neonatal mortality (RR 0.61, 95% CI 0.48 to 0.77), mortality prior to hospital discharge (RR 0.75, 95% CI 0.59 to 0.96), bronchopulmonary dysplasia (RR 0.87, 95% CI 0.77 to 0.97), pneumothorax (RR 0.62, 95% CI 0.42 to 0.89), and pulmonary interstitial emphysema (RR 0.54, 95% CI 0.36 to 0.82).[22] If prophylactic surfactant therapy in the delivery room is used in favor of rescue therapy, the NNT to avoid one death prior to discharge is 20 patients. In reports of recent trials using surfactant rescue[22,24] in newborns weighing 501 to 1500 g in over 5000 patients, only 45% actually required treatment. Alternatively, over 80% of neonates with birth weights below 1000 g had RDS in the 1999 Vermont Oxford Network experience reporting on over 27,000 neonates with birth weights below 1500 g. Neonates below 1000 g would be expected to benefit more from a prophylactic surfactant dosing approach. Any surfactant treatment approach provides multiple outcome benefits.

The optimal dose of exogenous surfactant remains uncertain. Controlled trials comparing single and multiple doses of surfactant have shown multiple doses to reduce the incidence of pneumothorax and neonatal mortality significantly.[25] Meta-analysis of studies comparing single to multiple doses of natural surfactant identified two studies. Multiple doses reduced the risk of pneumothorax (RR 0.51, 95% CI 0.30 to 0.88) and showed a trend toward reduced mortality (RR 0.63 95% CI 0.39 to 1.02). Both reports are in relatively larger newborns (mostly more than 30 weeks' gestation), and the benefits may be different in light of the increased use of antenatal steroids, which enhance surfactant response in preterm infants, and the predominant

TABLE 28–7. Relative Risks for Potential Beneficial and Adverse Effects of Synthetic and Natural Surfactants

Outcome	\multicolumn{4}{Synthetic Surfactant}				\multicolumn{4}{Natural Surfactant}			
	No.	Prophylaxis	No.	Rescue	No.	Prophylaxis	No.	Rescue
Pneumothorax	5	0.64 (0.49–0.89)	3	0.52 (0.42–0.65)	9	0.31 (0.22–0.44)	12	0.34 (0.27–0.44)
BPD	5	1.09 (0.80–1.47)	3	0.68 (0.46–0.99)	7	0.88 (0.67–1.17)	10	1.01 (0.81–1.27)
Death	7	0.67 (0.52–0.88)	3	0.47 (0.30–0.74)	9	0.60 (0.42–0.85)	11	0.59 (0.47–0.74)
Death + BPD	3	0.82 (0.63–1.08)	2	0.65 (0.50–0.82)	7	0.64 (0.49–0.84)	10	0.66 (0.53–0.82)
All IVH	4	0.94 (0.73–1.21)	2	0.77 (0.62–0.97)	8	0.95 (0.73–1.24)	10	0.94 (0.76–1.15)
Severe IVH		1.05 (0.86–1.18)				0.91 (0.72–1.14)		
PDA	5	1.27 (1.03–1.57)	3	0.73 (0.60–0.88)	9	1.16 (0.89–1.50)	12	0.96 (0.79–1.18)
Pulmonary bleed	4	3.12 (1.54–6.32)	3	1.49 (0.57–3.79)	2	0.73 (0.31–1.69)	2	1.25 (0.74–2.13)

use of surfactant in neonates below 1000 g. The use of multiple doses makes physiologic sense because animal studies suggest that much of the initial surfactant dose is inhibited by soluble proteins and other factors in the small airways and alveoli. Multiple doses may overcome this initial inactivation. Many clinicians use up to four doses of natural surfactant based on clinical need. A typical strategy is repeating surfactant doses if after 6 hours or more from the previous dose the patient continues to require mechanical ventilation and the FIO_2 exceeds 30% or 40%, depending on the clinician's preference.

Despite the high success rates, 20% of neonates fail to respond to treatment. Factors associated with poor response include sepsis, pneumonia, PDA, congenital heart disease, pulmonary hypertension, meconium aspiration, and pulmonary hypoplasia.[2,19] Whether retreatment of RDS with surfactant after resolution of these factors is useful is currently unknown.

Although surfactant appears to be generally well tolerated, some possible toxicities and associated problems include bradycardia, airway obstruction, and oxygen desaturation during administration; pulmonary hemorrhage; intraventricular hemorrhage (IVH); and the theoretical risk of allergy to natural surfactants,[18,21,23,24] although antibodies were absent in over 1400 Survanta-treated neonates.[24]

Problems during administration appear to be related to the volume of surfactant delivered, so surfactants using lower administration volumes may be better tolerated. Surfactant treatment is also associated with higher likelihood of clinically significant PDA. Pulmonary edema is associated with PDA. The pink respiratory secretions are thought to represent hemorrhagic pulmonary edema owing to capillary leakage of blood rather than the serious pulmonary hemorrhage seen in 10% to 45% of neonates with RDS in the presurfactant era.[23] Early closure of the PDA may minimize the risk of hemorrhagic pulmonary edema, as well as optimize surfactant response. While the relationship of IVH to surfactant use is controversial, cerebral blood flow velocity has been shown to be altered in some studies.[18] The risks of surfactants causing periventricular leukomalacia (PVL), a marker of hypoxic-ischemic brain injury, is poorly understood, but two trials[25,26] comparing calfactant and colfosceril found increased risk with calfactant (OR 2.03, 95% CI 1.09 to 3.80).[25] A theoretical basis for this is the more rapid and greater pulmonary beneficial effects with calfactant, resulting in overventilation and hypocarbia, because this is associated with decreased cerebral blood flow. If this is the correct cause, a more intense respiratory monitoring approach and aggressive ventilator weaning can avoid the problem. This trend needs to be assessed for all surfactants in additional studies that better measure this important prognostic marker for neurodevelopment.

Pharmacoeconomics of SRT

The pharmacoeconomic impact of SRT is examined in several reports.[27–29] SRT has lowered RDS mortality by at least 30%. From 1989 to 1990 (when Exosurf was introduced), 80% of the decline in infant mortality nationwide was attributable directly to SRT.[27] The reduction in resource use resulted in projected savings (using 1991 dollars) of $5800 in survivors and $4400 in infants who died.[27] Survanta use was projected to save $3300 in hospital resources for infants surviving to 28 days.[28] Savings as high as $18,000 in total hospital charges per surviving infant were projected in one analysis.[29] Each RDS- or treatment-related adverse outcome confers cost to health care. Although new therapeutic approaches may improve RDS outcomes, it is unethical to perform placebo-controlled trials for RDS, so these estimates will be difficult to reconsider.

Although data are limited, the number of neonates with RDS needed to treat with SRT to avoid selected RDS-related complications is estimated in Table 28–7. Use of prophylactic surfactant in combination with new respiratory strategies to extubate neonates rapidly to nasal CPAP is not measured in these economic analyses, and it is likely that the economic savings are larger than reported in these studies if this strategy is applied to neonates born at 30 weeks or less of gestation.

CLINICAL CONTROVERSY

Most authors agree that surfactant prophylaxis is a good strategy for neonates below 30 weeks' gestational age. However, considerable disagreement exists for patients who are 30 to 32 weeks' gestation. If prophylaxis is not used, then early surfactant treatment of neonates developing RDS is necessary.

LIQUID VENTILATION WITH PERFLUOROCHEMICALS

An investigational but highly promising approach to treating refractory RDS is the use of partial liquid ventilation, also called *perfluorocarbon-associated gas exchange* (PAGE).[30,31] Studies with perflubron, a PFC, have reported a dramatic increase in partial pressure of oxygen in arterial blood (PaO_2) and dynamic lung compliance within 1 hour of starting therapy, and treatment resulted in prevention of RDS-associated deaths.[31] PFCs are inert liquids in which oxygen and carbon dioxide are highly soluble. PFCs have low surface tension and are distributed evenly throughout the lung at low inflation pressures. The surface tension with PFCs at the alveolar air-liquid interface is markedly lower than seen with air ventilation, allowing for markedly lower ventilator pressures and a reduced risk of barotrauma.[30,31] Clinically, PFCs have been dosed by instillation into the endotracheal tube through the sideport at a rate of 1 mL/kg per minute without interrupting mechanical gas ventilation until a column of fluid is welled up in the endotracheal tube. This volume of PFC is felt to represent the infant's liquid functional residual capacity (FRC). Fluid that evaporates is replaced hourly to maintain this liquid FRC.[30,32]

In animal studies, PFCs also offered a vehicle for improved drug delivery via the lungs.[30,32] Addition of exogenous surfactant to PFC ventilation appears to improve surfactant delivery and enhance response to PFCs and surfactant in animals,[30,31] although studies in humans are unavailable. Adverse events associated with PFC use are mild and manageable, although long-term studies are lacking. Problems include endotracheal tube obstruction, hypoxic episodes, pneumothorax or fluorothorax (i.e., PFC leakage into the pleural space), and pulmonary hemorrhage.[30] These are not necessarily causal relationships, and overall, PFCs have been remarkably toxicity-free. The limited experience with PFCs and PAGE requires that this therapy be viewed as a promising but investigational option in RDS unresponsive to surfactant.

NITRIC OXIDE

Nitric oxide (NO) is a natural endothelium-derived relaxing factor that is important in regulating vascular tone, especially the pulmonary vasculature. Under normal physiologic conditions, NO is synthesized in endothelial cells and released into the vascular smooth muscle, where it stimulates cyclic GMP for vascular dilatation. At birth, NO helps in the transition from the markedly elevated pulmonary pressures in utero to normal pulmonary pressures and respiratory function.

Clinical studies have demonstrated the benefits of NO in persistent pulmonary hypertension of the newborn, meconium aspiration syndrome, and RDS.[2,33,34] An exogenous NO product and delivery system was approved by the Food and Drug Administration (INOmax and INOvent; INO Therapeutics, Inc.). Dosages of 5 to 80 parts per million (ppm) usually are targeted. While inhaled NO therapy was effective in term and near-term infants with respiratory failure, it has not appeared beneficial in preterm neonates, although further studies are justified.[2,33,34] Potential toxicities are few but include methemoglobinemia, inhibited platelet aggregation, and severe acute pulmonary edema secondary to the NO_2 oxidant metabolite. Further studies are needed to examine the clinical impact of this adjunctive therapy and the cost-benefit ratio as well.

SUPPORTIVE PHARMACOTHERAPY

Supportive pharmacotherapy in RDS is aimed at alleviating pain and discomfort, minimizing ventilator complications, and correcting any metabolic and/or fluid imbalance.

Narcotics/Benzodiazepines

Appropriate pharmacologic treatment is effective in alleviating pain and discomfort in neonates. Many ventilator-induced complications are secondary to asynchrony between ventilator rates and patient-driven respirations, resulting in pneumothorax and increased cerebral pressures that may promote IVH. Avoidance of these serious adverse effects can be accomplished by nonpharmacologic methods (e.g., positive-pressure assisted ventilation [PPAV]) or through the use of sedative and paralytic agents. A comprehensive review of sedation in neonates is available[35]; therefore, the following discussion will be limited. The most commonly used analgesics and sedative agents are morphine, fentanyl, and lorazepam. Studies have shown a significantly greater percentage of ventilator time in synchrony and a decrease in catecholamine levels in neonates who receive narcotics routinely. A recent comparison of morphine and fentanyl in this patient population showed fentanyl to have a better side-effect profile at equivalent efficacy.[36] One concern is that studies examining fentanyl have shown an increase in ventilator support, tolerance, and physiologic dependence effects with long-term use.[36]

All narcotics are expected to have this problem. The most common side effects demonstrated with narcotics include decreased gastrointestinal motility and risk of hypotension. Lorazepam is the preferred sedative agent in the absence of pain owing to its fast onset of action, its lack of hemodynamic toxicities, and its low risk of metabolite accumulation in comparison with diazepam. Midazolam continuous infusion is a reasonable alternative, although more costly and requiring additional fluid, which may be detrimental in a patient predisposed to PDA. Muscle paralysis has been used to reduce ventilator fighting and the consequent complications. However, its role in RDS has diminished owing to adverse effects (e.g., edema and hypoventilation). If paralysis is induced, assessment of sedation and seizures is confounded. Consequently, concurrent phenobarbital serum concentrations of 40 mg/L are recommended. Independent of

agent use, it is imperative to establish target sedation and pain scores to guide the clinical team in optimizing drug dosage. The use of sedation scores provides a mechanism to adjust drug dosing to effect, which maximizes effectiveness while limiting complications.

Acidosis

Acidosis is associated with a number of physiologic effects that increase the severity of RDS, including increased pulmonary vascular resistance, impaired synthesis of surfactant, reduced cardiac output, and depressed ventilation. Consequently, measures that reduce the risk of acidosis, such as prevention of hypoxemia, hypotension, and excessive blood loss through venipuncture and minimizing oxygen consumption through careful temperature control, are critical. Correction of metabolic acidosis with sodium bicarbonate or 0.3 M tromethamine (THAM) is recommended when blood pH falls below 7.25 and base excess is 5 or less. Patients should not receive sodium bicarbonate in congestive heart failure or any other conditions where sodium administration worsens the clinical condition. Patients receiving THAM should be monitored for episodes of apnea and bradycardia, which may worsen following administration. THAM should be avoided in uremic or anuric patients and should not be given via umbilical artery catheter.

Diuretics

Pulmonary edema is a prominent feature of RDS. The severity of RDS is correlated with the presence of factors that cause pulmonary edema. This is not unexpected because excess fluid in the alveolar and interstitial spaces impairs pulmonary gas exchange, lowers lung compliance, and reduces FRC. Prevention of fluid overload and pulmonary edema is critical to minimize the risk of opening the ductus arteriosus and the need for high ventilatory pressures. Pulmonary edema can benefit from PEEP because of redistribution of fluid from airspaces to interstitial tissue and improvement in gas exchange. Oliguria is well recognized during the early stages of RDS. A meta-analysis of six trials concluded that routine use of a diuretic, furosemide, to correct oliguria was not shown to improve markers of ventilation, oxygenation, or mortality.[37] The potential benefits of furosemide must be weighed against its risks, especially electrolyte imbalance. Furosemide also promotes prostaglandin synthesis, which may increase the risk of developing a PDA, although the meta-analysis did not document an increased risk.[37] The intermittent use of furosemide 1 to 2 mg/kg when pulmonary edema is thought to play a clinical role is justified and often beneficial clinically.

Methylxanthines

Extubation from mechanical ventilation as soon as possible is essential to minimize the toxicity of pressure and oxygen to lungs. Methylxanthines have been shown to facilitate successful extubation. In a meta-analysis of the benefits of methylxanthines, neonates weighing less than 1000 g were able to remain extubated more often if a methylxanthine was used concurrently with CPAP.[18]

CONCLUSIONS

Advances in prevention and reversal of RDS have had considerable impact on morbidity and mortality from RDS. Systematic reviews such as those published by the Cochrane Collaboration[39] provide frequent revisions of the evidence for the therapeutic options to treat RDS. These allow implementation of best practices to minimize the incidence and severity of RDS and its sequelae. Nevertheless, chronic lung disease, although less severe, continues to occur in 10% to 45% of neonates depending on the institution studied. The challenge for the future is to manage effectively the 20% of neonates with RDS responding poorly to surfactant. Institutions need to use multidisciplinary committees to enhance proficiency with therapies that will further reduce long-term pulmonary sequelae associated with RDS. Ensuring surfactant availability at all preterm deliveries so that prophylactic surfactant treatment can be used when appropriate, rapid extubation to nasal CPAP, and use of methylxanthines to facilitate extubation are useful NICU policies. Finally, if more than one surfactant is used in an institution, the pharmacodynamic differences between surfactants must be understood to optimize timing of arterial blood gas measurements to guide ventilator weaning and thus avoid serious sequelae from under- or overventilation.

ACUTE RESPIRATORY DISTRESS SYNDROME (ARDS)

Acute respiratory distress syndrome (formerly known as *adult respiratory distress syndrome*) was first described in 1967 in 12 patients presenting with acute respiratory distress, cyanosis refractory to oxygen therapy, decreased lung compliance, and diffuse infiltrates seen on chest x-ray.[40] Although the clinical description is similar to neonatal RDS, the underlying pathophysiology and ultimate morbidity and mortality differ considerably. A proper diagnostic definition of ARDS and acute lung injury (ALI) is necessary in order for clinical trials to include appropriate patients. Efforts to arrive at a standard definition were initially made in 1971, modified in 1988, and revised again in 1994.[40] Establishing epidemiologic data is influenced by the definition used. Comparing results across clinical trials has been confounded by the lack of a standardized definition. Designing a controlled, prospective study is difficult because there are so many variables and possible measures of response, although pulmonary morbidity and death are frequent end points. Limited patient numbers in clinical trials have resulted in insufficient power to detect potentially important but modest benefits of therapies. Recently, attention has focused on the systemic inflammatory response syndrome (SIRS) and the ablation of such response in limiting lung dysfunction, with mixed results.[41–47] In this situation, biochemical markers of the disease process also may prove useful for comparisons of clinical and therapeutic interventions. Management of ARDS is still primarily supportive, with a general focus on ventilator management, prevention or limitation of pulmonary tissue damage, hemodynamic support, and prevention of multiorgan dysfunction syndrome (MODS).

EPIDEMIOLOGY AND ETIOLOGY

Accurate estimation of the incidence of ARDS has been confounded historically by variation in definition parameters. In an effort to standardize definitions, the 1994 American-European Consensus Conference (AECC) provided the clinical definition of ARDS: (1) acute onset of arterial hypoxemia with a PaO_2/FIO_2 ratio of less than 200 mm Hg, (2) bilateral infiltrates on frontal chest radiograph consistent with pulmonary edema, and (3) pulmonary wedge pressure of 18 mm Hg or less without clinical evidence of left atrial hypertension.[40,46] A broader term attempting to encompass patients with milder gas exchange abnormalities ($PaO_2/FIO_2 < 300$ mm Hg) is ALI. The 1994 consensus definitions were designed to develop homogeneity for epidemiologic and clinical research aspects; however, it is now recognized that these definitions are a temporary solution for a complex disease state.[41] While this definition has the advantages that it is easy to use and recognizes the spectrum of the clinical disorder, it fails to recognize the cause or the presence or absence of multiorgan dysfunction.[42]

The most recent estimates, using the AECC criteria and data from the NIH-sponsored ARDS network, identified an incidence of ALI/ARDS at the 20 hospitals studied of 2.2 cases per ICU bed per year (range 0.7 to 5.8) and 11.2 to 22.4 cases per 10^5 person-years.[52] These data are extrapolated from the American Hospital Association national survey of hospitals registry of the number of adult ICU beds, burn ICU beds, and cardiac ICU beds.[52] Alternatively, the incidence may be as high as 75 per 100,000.[40] In absolute terms, about 150,000 people in the United States develop ARDS or ALI annually.[49,50]

Certain groups are predisposed to developing ARDS, and the risks vary within these groups. Patients with aspiration pneumonia or sepsis are at the highest risk for developing ARDS.[53] Other causes of ARDS include pneumonia, pulmonary contusion, fat emboli, inhalational injury, near-drowning, severe trauma with shock, multiple transfusions of blood products, acute pancreatitis, cardiopulmonary bypass, and drug overdose.[42]

Mortality associated with ARDS typically has been 40% to 60% in case series but appears to be declining to 34% to 36% in more recent reports.[40,54] The explanation for this is unclear.[54] Subgroup analysis suggests that patients with trauma-induced ARDS are more likely to survive than those with an infectious etiology.[54] The constellation of underlying pathophysiologic conditions and the individual response to the inflammatory cascade appears to place the underlying subgroups at higher or lower risks for mortality.[55]

Morbidity in survivors appears to persist for several months. Pulmonary function appears to return to normal by 6 months, but muscle wasting and fatigue persist for at least 12 months, especially in the patients with more complications and requiring systemic glucocorticoids during the critical illness.[45]

PATHOPHYSIOLOGY

Damage to the alveolar epithelium and the microvascular endothelium compromises the alveolar-capillary barrier and results in influx of protein-rich edema fluid during the acute phase of ALI and ARDS. The extent of alveolar epithelial injury is predictive of outcome. Epithelial injury is thought to predispose to progression of the disease process in five ways: (1) increased fluid permeability resulting in alveolar flooding, (2) type II pneumocyte damage impairing removal of edema fluid from alveoli, (3) type II pneumocyte injury reducing surfactant production, (4) damaged epithelial barrier predisposing to systemic infection, and (5) disorganized or insufficient epithelial repair possibly leading to fibrosis.[40,42] After the acute phase of ALI or ARDS, there may be rapid resolution of the disorder, or it may progress to a fibrosing alveolitis. This fibrotic process may begin early in the disease course and be detectable histologically as early as 5 days after onset of the disease. Proinflammatory cell mediators, especially interleukin 1 (IL-1)–receptor antagonist, soluble tumor necrosis factor receptor, and autoantibodies against IL-8, IL-10, and IL-11, are thought to stimulate this cascade of events.[40] The inflammatory process is thought to reflect a balance between proinflammatory cytokines and anti-inflammatory mediators.[40] Neutrophils predominate in the pulmonary edema fluid and bronchoalveolar fluid obtained from affected patients. Neutrophils release oxidants, proteases, leukotrienes, platelet-activating factor, and other proinflammatory molecules that may play a role in causing lung injury. However, the importance of neutrophils in this cascade of lung damage was called into question recently because ALI and ARDS also occur in neutropenic patients and do not occur more frequently in patients with pneumonia who are treated with therapies to increase the number of circulating neutrophils.[40] Cytokine-mediated proinflammatory response appears to be further enhanced in association with ventilator-induced lung injury (VILI). The cascade of proinflammatory cytokine release is thought to be stimulated by alveolar overdistension and possibly by

---

TABLE 28–8. Presentation of ARDS

General

The patient will have a medical problem known to cause ARDS and exhibit refractory hypoxemia.

Signs and Symptoms

Progressive respiratory failure due to poor oxygenation.

Laboratory Tests

Arterial blood gas (ABG) and arterial blood oxygen saturation (Sao_2) monitoring are necessary.
Pao_2/Fio_2 ratio less than 200 (ARDS) or 300 (ALI).

Other

Pulmonary artery catheter to measure pulmonary wedge pressure, which should be normal ($\leq$18 mm Hg).

Chest x-ray shows bilateral pulmonary infiltrates with pulmonary edema.

CT scan to detect underlying conditions and help to evaluate pulmonary response to ventilatory and positioning maneuvers.

---

cyclic opening and closing of atelectatic alveoli.[40,57] This can result not only in local pulmonary effects but also in a systemic inflammatory response with multiple systemic organ failure.[58] No single mediator or clinical feature adequately predicts which patient will develop ARDS. One postulate is that a genetic predisposition for lung injury when combined with inflammatory mediators may contribute to this lack of predictive value.[56] Nonetheless, inflammatory mediators compromise the pulmonary endothelium, resulting in increased protein permeability across endothelial and epithelial cells. This results in arterial hypoxemia and bilateral radiographic infiltrates from a protein-rich edema that is a chemotactant for further inflammatory mediators. The "leakage" of fluid into the pulmonary interstitium results in three physiologic alterations: (1) an impairment of tissue integrity that compromises normal expansion of alveolar tissue, (2) a physical impairment of oxygen–carbon dioxide exchange on an alveolar level, and (3) inactivation of endogenous surfactant resulting in alveolar collapse and development of pulmonary ventilation-perfusion mismatch. Not all areas of the lung are equally affected. Fluid-filled alveoli, atelectasis, and consolidation occur primarily in dependent lung zones, whereas other areas may be relatively spared.[59] This creates problems with mechanical ventilation because positive pressure can overdistend normal alveoli while trying to open other atelectatic alveoli.

CLINICAL PRESENTATION

Clinical and diagnostic assessment of ARDS is summarized in Table 28–8. The clinical presentation of ARDS is associated most often with concomitant factors that can complicate the differential diagnosis. As such, ARDS presents clinically as refractory hypoxemia (blood oxygen saturation <90%) with bilateral pulmonary infiltrates on chest radiography. However, chest radiographs may be interpreted differently for the diagnosis of ARDS even among experienced intensivists.[58] To assist with the diagnosis of ARDS, computed tomography (CT) is being used with increased regularity to detect underlying conditions such as abscesses, surgical emphysema, and pneumothorax. Further, CT has been used to evaluate pulmonary response to ventilatory and positioning maneuvers.[59]

▶ TREATMENT: Acute Respiratory Distress Syndrome

▦ DESIRED OUTCOME

No effective therapy is available to treat the underlying pathophysiology of ARDS. Thus initial therapy is focused on maintaining adequate oxygenation and tissue perfusion. Identifying and appropriately managing the precipitating factors and minimizing nosocomial complications related to infection, ventilator management, and other interventions also play prominent roles. Prevention of MODS is important because studies have shown that mortality is linked to a variety of factors, including nonpulmonary organ dysfunction.[42,61] Finally, investigational pharmacologic therapies to attenuate the inflammatory response may be a part of the clinician's approach to the ARDS patient. Treatment options are outlined in Fig. 28–3.

▦ VENTILATOR MANAGEMENT

◀ The cornerstone for the treatment of ARDS is mechanical ventilation. This area of management is evolving rapidly owing to newer ventilator technologies and improved understanding of lung physiology and VILI. Traditionally, ventilator management has focused on giving patients a tidal volume sufficient to maintain normal arterial blood gas values for $Paco_2$ or pH. Often this has required supraphysiologic tidal volumes of 10 to 15 mL/kg of predicted ideal body weight (normal physiologic volume is 7 to 8 mL/kg).[50] It has become apparent that a "high volume" approach causes excessive distension of normally aerated portions of affected lungs with consequent release of inflammatory mediators. This is one mechanism thought to perpetuate ALI as well as nonpulmonary organ damage. Several investigators have tried a "low volume" strategy and administered tidal volumes of 6 mL/kg.[42,61–64] The Acute Respiratory Distress Syndrome Network compared ventilator strategies using a traditional tidal volume approach, i.e., initial tidal volume of 12 mL/kg, and adjusted to give a plateau pressure (measured after a 0.5-second pause at the end of inspiration) of 45 to 50 cm H_2O, with a "low volume" strategy, i.e., initial tidal volume 6 mL/kg, and adjusted to give a plateau pressure of 25 to 30 cm H_2O.[61] Both groups used a volume-assist-control ventilator mode until the patient was weaned from the ventilator or until day 28 of the study. The ratio for the duration of inspiration to the duration of expiration (I:E ratio) was set at 1.1 to 1.3. Ventilator settings were adjusted overall to achieve target goals for arterial blood pH of 7.3 to 7.45 and Pao_2 of 55 to 80 mm Hg or oxygen saturation of 88% to 95%. This study, which included over 400 patients in each treatment group, showed that the "low volume" strategy reduced mortality significantly (31.0% versus 39.8%), increased the percentage breathing without assistance by day 28 (65.7% versus 55.0%), reduced the

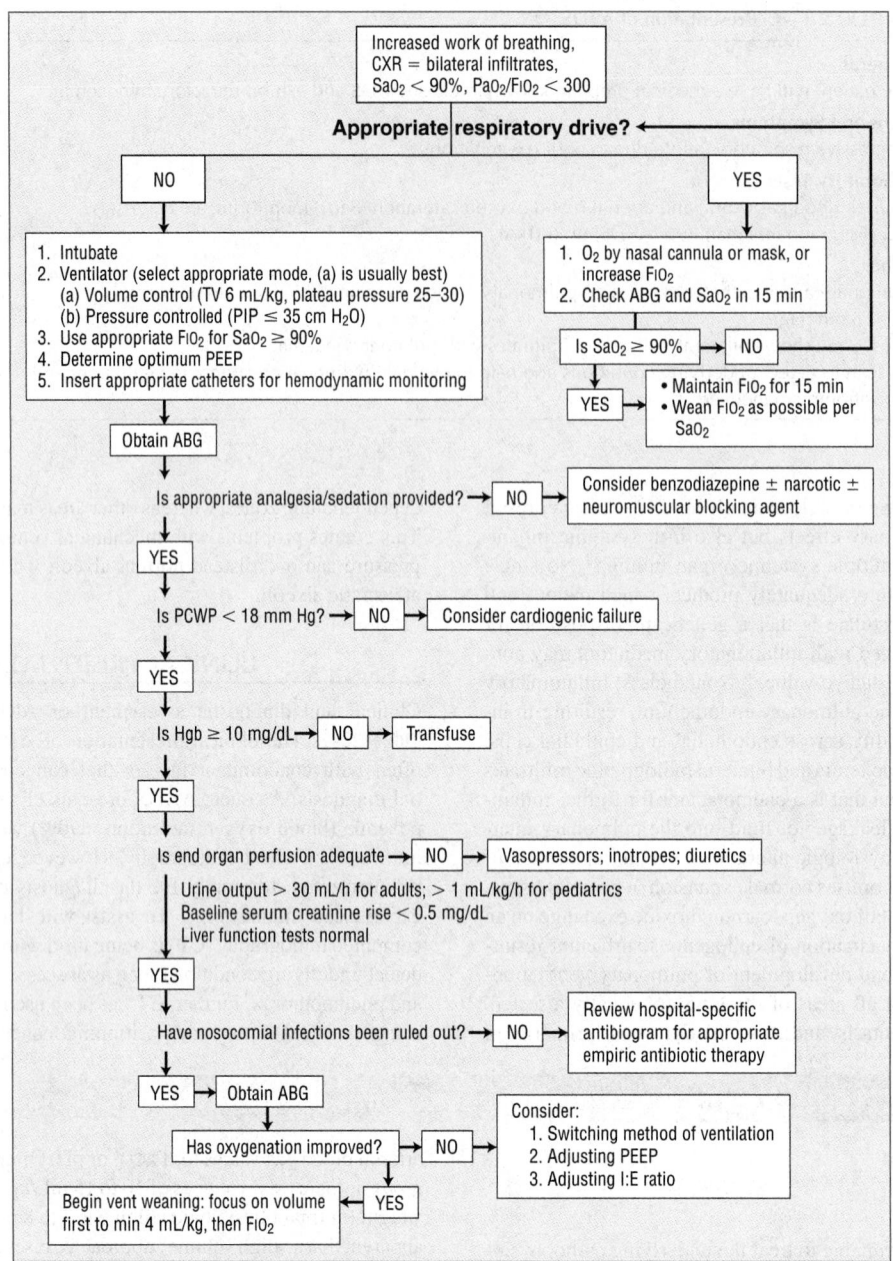

FIGURE 28–3. Algorithm for treatment of ARDS and ALI.

number of days without ventilator use during the first 28 days (12 ± 11 versus 10 ± 11), and reduced days without failure of nonpulmonary organs (15 ± 11 versus 12 ± 11). Day 3 IL-6 plasma concentrations were lower in the "low volume" strategy group, supporting the clinical findings.[61] This approach using gentler ventilation with adjunctive therapies to maintain acceptable arterial blood oxygenation and pH also was embraced in the accompanying editorial.[64] Interpretation of the data using a "low volume" strategy is confounded by inconsistent results among the five published clinical trials comparing this approach with conventional ventilator approaches.[75] A meta-analysis of these studies indicated that positive results were noted in two trials with relatively high tidal volumes in the control groups (i.e., ≥10 mL/kg), but when tidal volumes more typical of clinical practice were applied (i.e., 8–9 mL/kg), no significant differences were found. The ethics of exposing control patients to unnecessarily high tidal volumes to study the value of the "high volume" versus "low volume"

strategies resulted in a serious controversy and delayed funding of other clinical trials proposed by the prestigious ARDS Network for an indefinite period.[50] The best way to proceed with subsequent clinical trials remains controversial, but most clinicians regard a "low volume" strategy as the current best practice. The risk with using a "low volume" strategy is that it may result in lung derecruitment, atelectasis, and promotion of inflammatory response. Also, this approach of using higher PEEP and lower tidal volumes with conventional ventilation may lead to hypoventilation and respiratory acidosis. This could lead to increased need for sedation or neuromuscular blockade.[40,50] Myopathy and neuropathy are recognized increasingly as a concern with prolonged neuromuscular blocker use, especially when systemic steroids are used concurrently.

A new approach called the *alveolar recruitment maneuver* (ARM) has been used successfully in patients with extrapulmonary causes of ARDS but is less successful if the etiology is pulmonary.[60]

ARM requires that the tidal volume be delivered in a prolonged manner as an extended sigh lasting about 1 minute and that PEEP be increased in a gradual and reciprocal manner with the tidal volume to keep the newly recruited alveoli open. This maneuver can improve oxygenation but also carries many risks related to lung damage and decreased cardiac output. Patient position is important because ARM is less effective when patients are in the prone position.[60] Prone position, however, generally may be the preferred position because PaO_2 is typically higher in ventilated patients, possibly due to better recruitment of alveoli. Since ventilator management is as much of an art as a science, only individuals experienced with ventilator modes and options should oversee selection of ventilator strategy and changes in ventilator settings in such a life-threatening situation.

Clinicians caring for critically ill patients must have a rudimentary understanding of the technical aspects of mechanical ventilation to optimize therapy. Therefore, the following section simply provides an overview of ventilator technology and issues. Mechanical ventilation management is based on evaluations of respiratory and hemodynamic measurements. Arterial blood gas (ABG) determination is a key component to the respiratory management of ARDS because it describes perfusion (pH), oxygenation (PaO_2), and degree of ventilation ($PaCO_2$). In addition, the ABG determination allows assessment of the acid-base balance of a patient to differentiate whether acidosis or alkalosis is from metabolic, respiratory, or mixed etiologies so that the appropriate management can be implemented. Acid-base disorders are discussed extensively in Chapter 53. Appropriate lung distension is evaluated by clinical observation of chest wall expansion and radiography, notably the chest x-ray. Chest x-rays also provide important information, including endotracheal tube placement, severity of lung disease, markers of pulmonary toxicity, presence of air leaks, and an estimation of heart size.

The goal of mechanical ventilation is to provide adequate oxygen delivery while promoting the removal of CO_2. The target SaO_2 traditionally has been greater than 90% on the lowest possible FIO_2. In light of the recent study using low-tidal-volume ventilator strategy, slightly lower oxygen saturation and more liberal use of the FIO_2 to avoid increased ventilator pressures should be tolerated. The use of ventilatory maneuvers that achieve these end points while minimally disrupting the anatomic and physiologic aspects of respiratory and hemodynamic function is another goal. For the purpose of this discussion, there are six main types of ventilator management. A brief explanation of each follows. In reality, a number of hybrids between different ventilator modes also exist.

CONTROL-MODE VENTILATION (CMV)

CMV administers a breath independent of the patient's efforts. Ventilator settings determine the end of inspiration and the beginning of expiration (the I:E ratio, normally 1:2). PEEP is used to prevent alveolar collapse at the end of expiration. The "best PEEP" is determined clinically by monitoring the patient's oxygenation and most often is between 10 and 15 cm H_2O. PEEP rarely should exceed 20 cm H_2O. The tidal volume associated with the breath is independent of the patient and is set between 6 and 15 mL/kg of ideal weight. However, if highly compliant endotracheal tubing is used, higher volumes may be warranted. Risk associated with this form of ventilation is overdistension with possible pneumothorax. Some clinicians advocate an I:E ratio of 1:1, which purportedly allows use of more PEEP without pushing up peak inspiratory pressure or plateau pressure. This is reasonable in patients unless they have chronic obstructive pulmonary disease (COPD).

ASSIST-CONTROL VENTILATION (ACV)

ACV uses a mechanically set rate for breaths per minute but does allow patient-initiated breaths. The ventilator senses a patient's "trigger" of an inspiratory phase by noting a change in pressure within the endotracheal tubing. After such a trigger, the patient receives a full-tidal-volume inspiration. In the absence of a patient's inspiratory effort, the machine will deliver a programmed number of breaths per minute. Disadvantages of ACV include discomfort in "conforming" to predetermined tidal volumes while being alert enough to generate an inspiratory effort. Another disadvantage associated with the delivery of a complete-tidal-volume breath is the increased likelihood of developing respiratory alkalosis.

INTERMITTENT MANDATORY VENTILATION (IMV)/ SYNCHRONIZED INTERMITTENT MANDATORY VENTILATION (SIMV)

Intermittent mandatory ventilation (IMV) is a form of mechanical ventilation that not only delivers a preset number of breaths per minute but also allows the patient to breathe spontaneously between mechanical breaths. Thus, as the patient begins to initiate an increasing number of breaths, the preset mechanical IMV number can be dialed down. This form of ventilation allows the patient to increase his or her work of breathing; thus it is ideal for patients who are weaning from mechanical ventilation. An evolution of IMV is SIMV, which allows for the mechanical breaths to coincide with the inspiratory effort generated by the patient. Although functionally similar, SIMV prevents the "stacking" of breaths that may lead to higher peak airway pressures and higher intrathoracic pressures. The use of SIMV for the initial phase of ARDS is not indicated because patients generally are unable to initiate an inspiratory effort nor maintain such effort for a prolonged period of time.

PRESSURE-CONTROL VENTILATION (PCV)

PCV is a time-cycled ventilation that limits inspiratory pressures, thereby maximizing alveolar pressure. Ventilation is independent of the patient's effort but depends on pulmonary compliance. Thus there is a reduced likelihood of overdistension and pulmonary tissue damage because inspiration is limited once the predetermined peak pressure is obtained. Thus it is assumed that VILI is reduced.

PRESSURE-SUPPORT VENTILATION (PSV)

PSV is a type of mechanical ventilation that uses a patient's inspiratory effort and supplements to a select level of positive airway pressure. The patient controls the ventilatory rate and inspiratory assist time, whereas the PSV supplements inspiratory flow and tidal volume. Because PSV is heavily reliant on the patient's effort, this form of ventilation may not be optimal in patients unable to generate sufficient effort. However, it is the modality of choice in patients who are unable to synchronize with other modes of support.

HIGH-FREQUENCY VENTILATION (HFV)

HFV has been mentioned as a ventilator option for neonatal RDS (see Table 28–2). The basic concept for its use in ARDS is that the pressure-volume curve in ARDS creates a narrow window of safety for PPV. If staying between the points of low inflection (where at-electasis occurs) and high inflection (where overdistension occurs) is the goal, then theoretically HFV, which delivers small, frequent tidal volumes, should be an optimal ventilator strategy. However, initial clinical trials of HFV in patients with ARDS have failed to demonstrate superior outcomes, giving little incentive at this time for clinicians to switch from control-mode ventilation.[65] Advocates for HFV have noted several problems in the studies failing to find HFV superior to control-mode ventilation. The most serious flaw cited is that the studies lacked sufficient statistical power to recognize modest benefits. One recent editorial[65] noted that only 447 patients thus far had been included in all HFV studies combined. The authors point out that about 500 patients would be needed for each arm of the study (total 1000 patients) to detect a 10% reduction in mortality. Only the "low volume" strategy study with control-mode ventilation published by the ARDS Network[74] approaches this. Another criticism is that early studies used a "low pressure/low volume" strategy that permit-ted pressures below the lower inflection point, allowing for the shear stress associated with repeated collapse and opening of terminal air-ways. This strategy would promote inflammatory mediator release and would be unlikely to improve outcomes. Ventilation using sufficient PEEP to recruit alveoli above the lower inflection point combined with HFV to deliver small tidal volumes warrants an appropriately designed and powered clinical trial.[65] Finally, ventilator technology for HFV has been insufficient to support proper use of this ventilator mode in adults. High-frequency oscillatory ventilation (HFOV) seems most appropriate because it promotes expiration as well as inspiration and avoids air trapping. A newer high-frequency oscillatory ventilator (3100B Ventilator, SensorMedics) purportedly is able to provide the extended levels of continuous distending pressures needed to follow a "high volume" strategy necessary for HFOV to succeed in adults with ARDS.[65] HFOV is more established in infants and children with res-piratory distress, where smaller endotracheal tube sizes are used. In adults, HFOV is recommended primarily when oxygen requirements exceed 60% and mean airway pressure is 20 cm H_2O or greater or PEEP is >15 cm H_2O.[65] Theoretically, this strategy would provide the most physiologic ventilator approach because both airway col-lapse and overdistension can be avoided while gradually recruiting and opening atelectatic alveoli. Clinical trials testing this ventilator are in progress. If HFOV is used, it is important to ensure no sig-nificant obstruction of the airway with blood or mucus because this greatly impedes delivery of the oscillatory waveform.[65]

VILI AND OTHER COMPLICATIONS

Irreversible loss of disease control or serious ventilator-related tox-icities through oxygen toxicity, barotrauma, and volutrauma can occur if ventilatory management is not monitored and optimized continuously.[40,46,57] These ventilator-related toxicities may occur even with appropriate ventilator management, and minimizing these toxicities is one of the major goals of ventilator management.

Despite increasing evidence that pressure is more damaging to lungs than oxygen toxicity, oxygen supplementation remains a seri-ous concern in ARDS as well as RDS. Toxicity occurs as a result of oxygen-derived free radicals. The combination of high O_2 concentra-tions with the underlying lung damage may create a proinflammatory condition that further worsens underlying lung damage. There does not appear to be a universally accepted duration of exposure or O_2 con-centration that correlates with lung damage, thereby suggesting that disease severity and individual susceptibility are the most important factors.[40,56] However, with the increasing attention to pressure-related

lung damage, oxygen toxicity may be the lesser evil if compromises must be made to achieve adequate oxygenation.

ARDS does not affect the lung uniformly; there are consolidated and necrotic areas not available for gas exchange, areas of collapse that may be recruited, and normal alveolar components. It has been re-ported that in severe cases of ARDS the inflation capacity of the lungs may be less that one-third normal.[34,51] Although traditional ventilator management has described tidal volumes of 10 to 15 mL/kg, consoli-dated or collapsed areas of the lung volume will "shunt" to areas of least resistance, i.e., alveoli that are not collapsed. Thus areas of hyper-inflation can be located next to hypoinflation within the lung field. Fur-thermore, these areas of altered ventilation may not be evident in gross examination of mean airway pressure because this parameter is calcu-lated under passive inflation.[43] The volutrauma of ARDS is a result of regional overdistension of alveolar components and generally occurs in patients with a static pressure greater than 30 mm Hg. The risk of volutrauma occurs later in the course of ARDS presumably because of the uneven degradation of the lung structure creating areas of weak-ened tissue and increased risk for alveolar disruption.[66] As mentioned earlier, a low-tidal-volume strategy appears to be the safer course.

In addition to the damage incurred with tidal volume, barotrauma can ensue. The shearing force of a tidal volume associated with alveo-lar collapse and reinflation is an important aspect of VILI.[56] Thus the employment of PEEP can limit this barotrauma. In addition, PEEP can limit the FIO_2 needed for adequate oxygen saturation. PEEP is a pressure applied by the ventilator that prevents complete lung emp-tying at end expiration, increasing lung volume. This improved gas exchange redistributes (but does not decrease) lung water. The con-cept behind the ability of PEEP to reduce lung injury stems from the prevention of continued alveolar collapse and reopening with con-sequent inflammation and worsening ARDS.[42] However, finding the "best PEEP" can be challenging because too much volume remaining in the alveoli can cause overdistension and damage, with possible hemodynamic effects. One additional adverse consequence of a ven-tilator strategy that uses a large tidal volume is the translocation of bacteria and endotoxins with subsequent systemic sequelae.[67,68]

CLINICAL CONTROVERSY

The best ventilator approach for managing ARDS remains controversial. Most practitioners agree that lower tidal vol-umes are better, but the definition of *lower* is confusing. Fur-thermore, the proper, ethical way to study ventilator inter-ventions for ARDS has been challenged and must be resolved before additional studies of ARDS interventions can continue.

PERFUSION MANAGEMENT

Tissue perfusion is a critical component of ARDS. In order to opti-mize oxygen dissociation on a cellular level, appropriate tissue perfu-sion is required. In addition, adequate perfusion supplies glucose and electrolytes while eliminating metabolic by-products. Clinical mon-itoring of the ARDS patient requires assessment of perfusion in two capacities: hemodynamic/fluid support and end-organ function.

HEMODYNAMIC AND FLUID MANAGEMENT

Theoretically, improving oxygen supply should improve oxygen de-livery to the tissues. Although the validity of this direct relationship

TABLE 28-9. Hemodynamic and Fluid Support Decisions in ARDS

PCWP	MAP	CO	Tissue Hypoxia	Therapeutic Maneuver
Decreased	Decreased	Decreased	Yes	Fluid bolus
Decreased	Decreased	Increased	Yes	Vasopressor ± fluid bolus
Decreased	Decreased	Increased	No	Vasopressor
Decreased	Increased	Increased	No	Diuresis and negative fluid balance
Decreased	Increased	Decreased	Yes	After-load reducer
Decreased	Increased	Decreased	No	After-load reducer and negative balance

has been scrutinized, most clinicians optimize cardiac output in ARDS patients to ensure adequate perfusion by using fluids, blood transfusions, inotropic agents, and afterload-reducing agents. In addition to the ABG and hemoglobin determinations, hemodynamic parameters such as cardiac output, pulmonary artery obstruction pressure, and mean arterial pressure are monitored to determine which agent is most appropriate to improve perfusion. These parameters, combined with evaluation of tissue hypoxia, contribute extensively to the fluid-management decisions of ARDS (Table 28-9). The importance of appropriate fluid management cannot be overstated. Sufficient intravascular volume is needed for adequate perfusion. On the other hand, keeping patients relatively dry to avoid a persistent positive fluid balance is important to reduce the likelihood of pulmonary edema, which is associated with a poorer prognosis.[40] A clinical trial involving 19 treated and 18 control patients examined the value of 25 g albumin 25% given over 20 to 40 minutes plus furosemide 1 mg/mL given as a continuous infusion every 8 hours (dose titrated to weight loss) for 5 days given to hypoproteinemic patients with ALI.[49] This small double-blind trial demonstrated the albumin plus furosemide group to achieve significantly greater weight loss (10 versus 4.7 kg) and serum albumin (1.9 versus 0.7 g/dL), increases in oxygenation at 24 hours (89% versus 50%), with an apparent plateau effect by the third study day; and reversal of the diagnosis of ALI/ARDS (53% versus 11%). The study had too few patients to detect modest differences in major clinical outcomes such as ventilator dependence or mortality. An important caveat to these results was that most ALI cases were caused by an extrapulmonary etiology (mainly trauma), which the authors caution may be more associated with pulmonary edema and alveolar collapse and thus may be more amenable to diuretic therapy. Pressors also may offer theoretical benefits because catecholamines such as isoproterenol and dopamine may upregulate epithelial sodium channels and thus help to reduce pulmonary edema.[67] A randomized trial of restricted versus liberal fluid management was initiated by the National Institutes of Health ARDS Network.[50]

PERFUSION AND PREVENTION OF END-ORGAN DAMAGE

Another marker of sufficient tissue perfusion can be clinical assessment of end-organ function. As mentioned previously, prevention of MODS is an important factor in reducing ARDS-associated mortality. Clinically, assessments of urine output and serum electrolytes are important aspects of renal function monitoring, whereas liver function tests (aminotransferases AST and ALT) are important laboratory parameters for monitoring hepatic function. Central nervous system assessment can be difficult in the ARDS patient and is confounded by concurrent drug therapies (e.g., sedatives, narcotics, etc.) that alter neurologic status.

Stress-induced gastrointestinal bleeding is another complication of ARDS. Mechanical ventilation, altered gastric blood flow, and coagulopathy are indications for stress ulcer prophylaxis.[41] However, considerable controversy exists as to the role of pH-altering drugs for stress prophylaxis and the relationship with nosocomial pneumonia. Given the considerable risk of mortality with gastrointestinal bleeding in patients with ARDS, it is our opinion that prophylactic agents should be used. There does not appear to be a uniform clinical advantage of either histamine antagonists or proton pump inhibitors; therefore, selection should be based on costs.

Nosocomial Pneumonia

Nosocomial pneumonia in ARDS patients causes mortality in 67% of patients versus 23% of patients without pneumonia. Prevention and early treatment are critical to decreasing ARDS mortality. Ventilator-associated pneumonia correlates directly with length of mechanical ventilation.[69] Diagnosis of ventilator-associated pneumonia is difficult because no diagnostic method, even protected specimen brush, correlates with microbiologic results on autopsy or affects mortality.[70] Mechanically ventilated patients are always colonized with pathogenic organisms. When clinical findings suggest ventilator-associated pneumonia, the causative organism correlates with the organism colonizing the upper airway and should be the target of antimicrobial therapy.[71]

Gastric colonization does not correlate with ventilator-associated pneumonia and mortality differences. Attempts to decontaminate the gastrointestinal tract have not become established norms.[71] Antibiotic use carries the risk of acquiring multiresistant organisms, which can adversely affect hospital and community antibiograms. Based on the epidemiologic and financial costs of resistant organisms generated with such a procedure, its routine practice cannot be advocated.

Catheter-Related Infection

ARDS patients are also at risk for the development of catheter-related infections, especially bacteremia, which is life-threatening. Appropriate hospital hygiene and the standard use of sterile technique are of extreme importance in preventing infections. Catheter-related infections are dealt with elsewhere in this text (see Chap. 137). Diagnosis of catheter-related infections can be difficult, although most clinicians agree that semiquantitative cultures of removed catheters are helpful. Catheter-associated organisms usually are gram-positive bacteria, namely, *Staphylococcus* spp. Catheter removal and antimicrobial therapy are cornerstones of treatment.

Nutritional Support

Parenteral nutrition is often necessary in seriously ill ARDS patients because blood flow to the gastrointestinal tract is limited. Enteral nutrition is preferred if tolerable, even in small amounts. The advantages of enteral feedings include decreased need for central catheter access, increased gastrointestinal access, increased gastrointestinal blood flow decreasing the risk of gut contamination, and decreased risk for ulceration. It is important for the clinician to remember that using a high amount of intravenous carbohydrates as the major source of caloric intake increases the production of carbon dioxide, which can further complicate management of the ARDS patient. Interest has increased in the potential benefits of selected enteral nutritional approaches. Use of an enteral formula containing eicosapentaenoic acid (EPA, fish oil), γ-linolenic acid (GLA, borage oil), and antioxidants was compared recently with a standard ready-to-feed high-fat, low-carbohydrate (corn oil base) formula.[72] This preliminary trial reported that both formulas were well tolerated by most patients and resulted in fewer days on the ventilator and in the ICU and fewer instances of new organ failures. The authors speculated that the benefits were due to the anti-inflammatory effects of the EPA + GLA formulation. This formula contained polyunsaturated long-chain fatty acids (PUFAs) with an N-6:N-3 ratio of 1:1 (compared with 54:1 for the standard formulation). A subsequent trial with EPA + GLA (Oxepa) showed that patients fed this formula for 4 to 7 days had reduced inflammatory mediators and markers of inflammation in bronchoalveolar lavage fluid and increased oxygenation.[73] For patients who can tolerate enteral feedings, formulas with lipid content high in N-3 PUFAs are worth considering.

▓ INVESTIGATIONAL THERAPIES

Various therapies have been evaluated to reverse or limit the pulmonary damage associated with ARDS. These entities range from inhibiting the underlying etiology (e.g., antiendotoxin immunotherapy) to altering inflammatory mediators (e.g., cyclooxygenase inhibitors) to directly improving oxygenation (e.g., NO and surfactant). To date, no single therapy has uniformly demonstrated benefits in clinical trials. These trials have been summarized in a comprehensive review.[41] The failure to prove clinical benefits to the various therapies should not discourage further research on any approach. A subsequent editorial challenges the negative findings in these large trials and tries to reconcile the promising experimental evidence with the trial outcomes.[74] The author questions the definitions used for ARDS and the end point of death as perhaps issues to resolve. Most studies also suffer from problems with insufficient patient numbers to ensure the validity of negative findings, inappropriate selection of drug-delivery technique (as in the case of surfactant[76]), and uncertainty about optimal dosing. Nevertheless, some recent studies performed by the National Institutes of Health ARDS Network and other multicenter groups involved large patient numbers and placebo-controlled trials. These studies failed to show improved outcomes for mortality, pulmonary and nonpulmonary organ morbidity, and measures of interleukins or other markers of inflammation.

At this juncture, despite laboratory experiments raising expectations of benefits and in some cases experiential reports favorable to the therapy, studies to date have failed to demonstrate substantial benefits with systemic glucocorticoids, liposomal prostaglandin E_1, inhaled NO, ketoconazole, procysteine, and lisofylline.[41]

Synthetic surfactant (Exosurf) was studied in a placebo-controlled trial of patients with ARDS.[75,77] While this therapy also failed to show benefits, the drug was aerosolized over 5 days to administer 240 mL Exosurf. Since aerosolized surfactant is poorly delivered and was shown recently to be ineffective in neonates with RDS, this trial cannot be considered of value in gauging the efficacy of surfactant for ARDS. Also, natural surfactants that also have surfactant proteins may be a better choice. Phase III studies using a recombinant SP-C-based surfactant showed reduced mortality for the subgroup of patients with ARDS secondary to direct insults, although no benefit was seen for the total study population.[77] It is important to consider etiologies for ARDS when future clinical trials are designed.

Systemic glucocorticoids have been tried for the prevention of ARDS in patients with septic shock, for accelerating resolution of acute ARDS, and for prevention of fibroproliferation.[42] Short courses of high-dose systemic steroids generally have been ineffective in preventing ARDS in patients with septic shock or resolution of ARDS. In fact, a theoretical risk of a net proinflammatory state may be created in the setting of preformed and released inflammatory cytokines increasing cytokine receptors and resumption of cytokine production after steroids are withdrawn.[42]

While apparently ineffective during the acute phase of ARDS, prolonged glucocorticoid therapy may have a role in patients with ARDS who remain unimproved for 7 days. Therapy at this point is targeting the fibrosing alveolitis phase of the disease.[42,76] In a small trial, methylprednisolone was started at 2 mg/kg per day and tapered gradually over 32 days.[43] Treatment was associated with significant reduction in mortality, lung injury score, and multiorgan dysfunction. The prolonged high-dose methylprednisolone course differs from studies of glucocorticoids during the acute phase of ARDS. The study investigators challenge the negative findings for early steroid use on the basis of their findings. Ultimately, steroid use remains controversial but probably should be considered investigational and potentially harmful during the acute phase of ARDS.

Selective pulmonary vasodilation, particularly in patients with severe refractory hypoxemia, is being studied as an adjunctive therapy for ARDS.[78] Inhaled NO is the most studied. Studies using doses ranging from 1.25 to 80 ppm have demonstrated short-term benefits in oxygenation but no sustained improvement in outcomes such as days requiring mechanical ventilation or mortality.

In pediatric patients with ARDS, extracorporeal membrane oxygenation (ECMO) has been used.[46] These patients have been part of larger cohorts identified as respiratory failure. Anecdotally, practitioners observe the greatest benefit in the sickest patients. Prospective studies are needed to confirm clinical impression. The benefits of ECMO for adults with ARDS seem less optimistic.[46]

A large number of additional therapies have been or are under review. These therapies include nonsteroidal anti-inflammatory agents, proinflammatory agents (GM-CSF), antiadhesion molecules, gene therapy, antiendotoxin therapy, and antioxidants (e.g., superoxide dismutase).[43] Therapies will continue to focus on the early interventions to prevent the progressive downward spiral of lung injury, inflammation, and hypoxemia.

EVALUATION OF OUTCOMES AND MONITORING PLANS

Mortality, ICU stay, and duration of mechanical ventilation are common outcome measures used in ARDS studies. However, there is considerable debate not only on the definition of ARDS but also on the usefulness of these markers or other surrogate markers in determining efficacy of ARDS therapies.

Monitoring ventilatory parameters, ABGs, and oxygen saturation assists in determination of illness severity and provides

TABLE 28–10. Monitoring Parameters for ARDS

Hemodynamic	Ventilator Status	Infection	End-Organ Damage
PCWP	F_{IO_2}	White blood cells/differential	BUN
Cardiac output/index	Pa_{O_2}	Chest x-ray findings	Creatinine
Oxygen saturation (Sa_{O_2})	Sa_{O_2}	Temperature	Urine output
Mixed venous oxygenation (Mv_{O_2})	Mv_{O_2}	Cultures	Liver function tests
Hemoglobin/hematocrit	Plateau pressure	Changes in color/quality sputum	PT/PTT
Urine output	Respiratory effort/rate	New onset hypotension	
		Abdominal examination	
		Number of central catheter days	

rudimentary end points of perfusion. For example, most clinicians agree that maintaining an oxygen saturation of more than 90% is important. Effects of inotropic agents, blood products, and vasopressors must be measured to optimize oxygenation. Thus appropriate monitoring of invasive hemodynamic parameters (i.e., pulmonary artery obstruction pressure) through a pulmonary artery catheter is critical in appropriate management of the ARDS patient. Radiographically, ARDS cannot be distinguished from cardiogenic pulmonary edema; therefore, a pulmonary artery catheter is almost essential. In addition, because ventilatory maneuvers can reduce cardiac output (excessive PEEP), appropriate hemodynamic monitoring can be essential for establishing appropriate ventilator settings. A summary of monitoring parameters for patients with ARDS can be found in Table 28–10.

CONCLUSIONS

ARDS-related mortality remains very high. Therapy is primarily supportive but requires extensive comprehension of the underlying pathophysiology to ensure optimal pharmacotherapy. Separation of the illness into pulmonary and extrapulmonary etiologies may become necessarily to develop proper strategies for research and therapeutic interventions. Vigilance in monitoring ventilatory and hemodynamic end points to prevent MODS is the priority, with prevention of secondary complications such as pneumonia and catheter-related infections very significant. Designing research that is both ethically acceptable and clinically sound remains a difficult and controversial issue.

Review Questions and other resources can be found at *www.pharmacotherapyonline.com*.

REFERENCES

1. Vermont Oxford Network Annual Database Summary, 1999. Burlington, VT, Vermont Oxford Network, 2000.
2. Rodriguez RJ. Management of respiratory distress syndrome: An update. Respir Care 2003;48:279–287.
3. Barker PM, Gowen CW, Lawson EE, Knowles MR. Decreased sodium ion absorption across nasal epithelium of very premature infants with respiratory distress syndrome. J Pediatr 1997;130:373–377.
4. Piper JM. Lung maturation in diabetes in pregnancy: If and when to test. Semin Perinatol 2002;26:206–209.
5. Herting E, Gefeller O, Land M, et al. Surfactant treatment of neonates with respiratory failure and group B streptococcal infection. Members of the Collaborative European Multicenter Study Group. Pediatrics 2000;106:957–964.
6. Management of preterm labor. ACOG Practice Bulletin No. 43. Obstet Gynecol 2003;101:1039–1047.
7. Leitich H, Brunbauer M, Bodner-Adler B, et al. Antibiotic treatment of bacterial vaginosis in pregnancy: A meta-analysis. Am J Obstet Gynecol 2003;188:752–758.
8. Berkman ND, Thorp JM, Lohr KN, et al. Tocolytic treatment for the management of preterm labor: A review of the evidence. Am J Obstet Gynecol 2003;188:1648–1659.
9. St John EB, Carlo WA. Respiratory distress syndrome in VLBW infants: Changes in management and outcomes observed by the NICHD Neonatal Research Network. Semin Perinatol 2003;27:288–292.
10. Crowley P. Prophylactic corticosteroids for preterm birth. Cochrane Database Syst Rev 2003;1.
11. Elimian A, Figueroa R, Spitzer AR, et al. Antenatal corticosteroids: Are incomplete courses beneficial? Obstet Gynecol 2003;102:352–355.
12. Crowther CA, Alfirevic Z, Haslam RR. Prenatal thyrotropin-releasing hormone for preterm birth. Cochrane Database Syst Rev 2003;1.
13. Crowther CA, Hiller JE, Studs DS, et al. Australian Collaborative Trial of Antenatal Thyrotropin-Releasing Hormone: Adverse effects at 12-month follow-up. Pediatrics 1997;99:311–317.
14. Goldsmith JP, Karotkin EH. Assisted Ventilation of the Neonate, 3d ed. Philadelphia, Saunders, 1996.
15. Halliday HL. Towards earlier neonatal extubation. Lancet 2000;355:2091–2092.
16. Henderson-Smart DJ, Davis PG. Prophylactic methylxanthines for extubation in preterm infants. Cochrane Database Syst Rev 2003;1.
17. Tin W, Milligan DWA, Pennefather P, Hey E. Pulse oximetry, severe retinopathy, and outcome at one year in babies less than 28 weeks gestation. Arch Dis Child Fetal Neonatal Ed 2001;84:F106–110.
18. Nguyen TN, Cunsolo SM, Gal P, Ransom JL. Infasurf and curosurf: Theoretical and practical considerations with surfactants. J Pediatr Pharmacol Ther 2003;8:97–114.
19. Merrill JD, Ballard RA. Pulmonary surfactant for neonatal respiratory disorders. Curr Opin Pediatr 2003;15:149–154.
20. Zola EM, Gunkel JH, Chan RK, et al. Comparison of three dosing procedures for administration of bovine surfactant to neonates with respiratory distress syndrome. J Pediatr 1993;122:453–459.
21. Soll RF, Blanco F. Natural surfactant extract versus synthetic surfactant for neonatal respiratory distress syndrome (systematic review). Cochrane Database Syst Rev 2001;2.
22. Soll RF, Morley CJ. Prophylactic versus selective use of surfactant for preventing morbidity and mortality in preterm infants (systematic review). Cochrane Neonatal Review Group. Cochrane Database Syst Rev 2001;2.
23. Spafford PS, Kendig JW, Maniscalco WM. Use of natural surfactants to prevent and treat respiratory distress syndrome. Semin Perinatol 1993;17:285–294.
24. Verder H, Robertson B, Greisen G, et al. Surfactant therapy and nasal continuous positive airway pressure for newborns with respiratory distress syndrome. N Engl J Med 1994;331:1051–1055.
25. Soll RF. Multiple-versus single-dose natural surfactant extract for severe respiratory distress syndrome (systematic review). Cochran Neonatal Review Group. Cochrane Database Syst Rev 2000;3.
26. Hudak ML, Martin DJ, Egan EA, et al. A multicenter randomized masked comparison trial of synthetic surfactant versus calf lung surfactant

extract in the prevention of neonatal respiratory distress syndrome. J Pediatr 1996;128:396–406.

27. Schwartz RM, Luby AM, Scalon JW, et al. Effect of surfactant on morbidity, mortality, and resource use in newborn infants weighing 500 to 1500 g. N Engl J Med 1994;330:913–936.

28. Soll RF, Jacobs J, Pashko S, Thomas R. Cost-effectiveness of beractant in the prevention of respiratory distress syndrome. Pharmacoeconomics 1993;4:278–286.

29. Maniscalco WM, Kendig JW, Shapiro DL. Surfactant replacement therapy: Impact on hospital charges for premature infants with respiratory distress syndrome. Pediatrics 1989;83:1–6.

30. Greenspan JS, Wolfson MR, Shaffer TH. Liquid ventilation. Semin Perinatol 2000;24:396–405.

31. Leach CL, Greenspan JS, Rubenstein SD. Partial liquid ventilation with perflubron in premature infants with severe respiratory distress syndrome. N Engl J Med 1996;335:761–767.

32. Tarczy-Hornoch P, Hildebrandt J, Mates EA. Effects of exogenous surfactant on lung pressure-volume characteristics during liquid ventilation. J Appl Physiol 1996;80:1764–1771.

33. Kinsella JP, Walsh WF, Bose CL, et al. Inhaled nitric oxide in premature neonates with severe hypoxaemic respiratory failure: A randomised, controlled trial. Lancet 1999;354:1061–1065.

34. Kinsella JP, Abman SH. Inhaled nitric oxide: Current and future uses in neonates. Semin Perinatol 2000;24:387–395.

35. Jacqz-Aigrain E, Burtin P. Clinical pharmacokinetics of sedatives in neonates. Clin Pharmacokinet 1996;31:423–443.

36. Saarenmaa E, Huttunen P, Leppaluoto J, et al. Advantages of fentanyl over morphine in analgesia for ventilated newborn infants after birth: A randomized trial. J Pediatr 1999;134:144–150.

37. Orsini AJ, Leef KH, Costarino A, et al. Routine use of fentanyl infusions for pain and stress reduction in infants with respiratory distress syndrome. J Pediatr 1996;129:140–145.

38. Brion LP, Soll RF. Diuretics for respiratory distress syndrome in preterm infants (systematic review). Cochrane Neonatal Review Group. Cochrane Database Syst Rev 2003;1.

39. Sinclair JC, Haughton DE, Bracken MB, et al. Cochrane neonatal systematic reviews: A survey of the evidence for neonatal therapies. Clin Perinatol 2003;30:285–304.

40. Ware LB, Matthay MA. The acute respiratory distress syndrome. N Engl J Med 2000;342:1334–1349.

41. Artigas A, Bernard GR, Carlet J, et al., and the Consensus Committee. The American-European consensus on ARDS: 2. Ventilatory, pharmacologic, supportive therapy, study design strategies, and issues related to recovery and remodeling. Am J Respir Crit Care Med 1998;157:1332–1347.

42. Thompsom BT. Clucocorticoids and acute lung injury. Crit Care Med 2003;31(suppl):S253–257.

43. Meduri GU, Headley AS, Golden E, et al. Effect of prolonged methylprednisolone therapy in unresolving acute respiratory distress syndrome: A randomized, controlled trial. JAMA 1998;280:159–165.

44. NIH ARDS Network. Ketoconazole does not reduce mortality in patients with the acute respiratory distress syndrome. JAMA 2000;283:1995–2002.

45. Herridge MS, Cheung AM, Tansey CM, et al. One-year outcomes in survivors of the acute respiratory distress syndrome. N Engl J Med 2003;348:683–693.

46. Anderson MR. Update on pediatric acute respiratory distress syndrome. Respir Med 2003;48:261–278.

47. Abraham E, Matthay MA, Dinarello CA, et al. Consensus conference definitions for sepsis, septic shock, acute lung injury and acute respiratory distress syndrome: time for a reevaluation. Crit Care Med 2000;28:232–235.

48. American Lung Association. Acute respiratory distress syndrome. In: Lung Disease Data, 1998–1999. New York, American Lung Association. 1998:45–46.

49. Martin G, Mangialardi RJ, Wheeler AP, et al. Albumin and furosemide therapy in patients with acute lung injury. Crit Care Med 2002;30:2175–2182.

50. Steinbrook R. How best to ventilate? Trial design and patient safety in studies of the acute respiratory distress syndrome. N Engl J Med 2003;384:1393–1401.

51. Fein AM. Acute lung injury and acute respiratory distress syndrome in sepsis and septic shock. Crit Care Clin 2000;16:289–317.

52. Goss CH, Brower RG, Hudson LD, Rubenfeld GD. Incidence of acute lung injury in the United States. Crit Care Med 2003;31:1607–1611.

53. Pugin J, Verghese G, Widmer M, Matthay MA. The alveolar space is the site of intense inflammatory and profibrotic reactions in the early phase of acute respiratory distress syndrome. Crit Care Med 1999;27:304–312.

54. Ranieri VM, Suter PM, Tortorella C, et al. Effect of mechanical ventilation on inflammatory mediators in patients with acute respiratory distress syndrome: A randomized, controlled trial. JAMA 1999;282:54–61.

55. Slutsky AS, Tremblay LN. Multiple system organ failure: Is mechanical ventilation a contributing factor? Am J Respir Crit Care Med 1998;157:1721–1725.

56. Villar J, Flores C, Mendez-Alvarez S. Genetic susceptibility to acute lung injury. Crit Care Med 2003;31(suppl):S272–275.

57. Bohn, D. Lung salvage and protection ventilatory techniques. Pediatr Clin North Am 2001;48:553–572.

58. Meade MO, Cook RJ, Guyatt GH, et al. Interobserver variation in interpreting chest radiographs for the diagnosis of acute respiratory distress syndrome. Am J Respir Crit Care Med 2000;161:85–90.

59. Rouby J, Puybasset L, Nieszkowska A. Acute respiratory distress syndrome: Lessons from computed tomography of the whole lung. Crit Care Med 2003;31(suppl):S285–295.

60. Lim C, Jung H, Koh Y, et al. The effect of alveolar recruitment maneuver in early acute respiratory distress syndrome according to anti-derecruitment strategy, etiologic category of diffuse lung injury, and body position of the patient. Crit Care Med 2003;31:411–418.

61. The Acute Respiratory Distress Syndrome Network. Ventilation with lower tidal volumes as compared with traditional volumes for acute lung injury and the acute respiratory distress syndrome. N Engl J Med 2000;342:1301–1308.

62. Eichacker PQ, Gerstenberger EP, Banks SM, et al. Meta-analysis of acute lung injury and acute respiratory distress syndrome trials testing low tidal volumes. Am J Resp Crit Care Med 2002;166:1510–1514.

63. Tobin MJ. Culmination of an era in research on the acute respiratory distress syndrome. New Engl J Med 2000;342:1360–1361.

64. Herridge MS, Slutsky AS, Colditz GA. Has high-frequency ventilation been inappropriately discarded in adult acute respiratory distress syndome? Crit Care Med 1998;26:2073–2077.

65. Derdak S. High-frequency oscillatory ventilation for acute respiratory distress syndrome in adult patients. Crit Care Med 2003;31(suppl):S317–323.

66. Murphy DB, Cregg N, Tremblay L, et al. Adverse ventilatory strategy causes pulmonary-to-systemic translocation of endotoxin. Am J Respir Crit Care Med 2000;162:27–33.

67. Dada L, Sznajder JI. Mechanisms of pulmonary edema clearance during acute hypoxemic respiratory failure: Role of the Na,K-ATPase. Crit Care Med 2003;31(suppl):S248–252.

68. Bonten MJ, Bergmans DC, Ambergen AW, et al. Risk factors for pneumonia and colonization of respiratory tract and stomach in mechanically ventilated ICU patients. Am J Respir Crit Care Med 1996;154:1339–1346.

69. Torres A, El-Ebiary M, Padro L, et al. Validation of different techniques for the diagnosis of ventilator-associated pneumonia. Am J Crit Care Med 1994;149:324–331.

70. DeLatorre FL, Pont T, Ferrer A, et al. Patterns of tracheal colonization during mechanical ventilation. Am J Respir Crit Care Med 1995;152:1028–1033.

71. D'Amico R, Pifferi S, Leonetti C, et al. Effectiveness of antibiotic prophylaxis in critically ill adult patients: Systematic review of randomized controlled trials. Br Med J 1998;316:1275–1285.

72. Gadek JE, DeMichele SJ, Karlstad MD, et al. Effect of enteral feeding with eicosapentaenoic acid, linolenic acid, and antioxidants in patients with acute respiratory distress syndrome. Crit Care Med 1999;27:1409–1420.

73. Pacht ER, DeMichele SJ, Nelson JL, et al. Enteral nutrition with eicos-apentaenoic acid, gamma-linolenic acid, and antioxidants reduces alveolar inflammatory mediators and protein influx in patients with acute respiratory distress syndrome. Crit Care Med 2003;31:491–500.

74. Brochard L, Brun-Buisson C. Clinical trials in acute respiratory distress syndrome: What is ARDS? Crit Care Med 1999;27:1657–1658.

75. Anzueto A, Baughman RP, Guntupalli KK, et al. Aerosolized surfactant in adults with sepsis-induced acute respiratory distress syndrome. N Engl J Med 1996;334:1417–1421.

76. Brun-Buisson C, Brochard L. Corticosteroid therapy in acute respiratory distress syndrome: Better late than never? JAMA 1998;280:182–183.

77. Lewis JF, Brackenbury A. Role of exogenous surfactant in acute lung injury. Crit Care Med 2003;31(suppl):S324–328.

78. Mehta S, MacDonald R, Hallett DC, et al. Acute oxygenation response to inhaled nitric oxide when combined with high-frequency oscillatory ventilation in adults with acute respiratory distress syndrome. Crit Care Med 2003;31:383–389.

29
DRUG-INDUCED PULMONARY DISEASES

Hengameh H. Raissy, Michelle Harkins, and Patricia L. Marshik

Learning Objectives and other resources can be found at *www.pharmacotherapyonline.com.*

KEY CONCEPTS

❶ Select populations may be more susceptible to toxicities associated with specific agents.

❷ Primary treatment is discontinuation of the offending agent and supportive care.

The manifestations of drug-induced pulmonary diseases span the entire spectrum of pathophysiologic conditions of the respiratory tract. As with most drug-induced diseases, the pathologic changes are nonspecific. Therefore, the diagnosis is often difficult and, in most cases, is based on exclusion of all other possible causes. In addition, the true incidence of drug-induced pulmonary disease is difficult to assess as a result of the pathologic nonspecificity and the interaction between the underlying disease state and the drugs.

Considering the physiologic and metabolic capacity of the lung, it is surprising that drug-induced pulmonary disease is not more common. The lung is the only organ of the body that receives the entire circulation. In addition, the lung contains a heterogeneous population of cells capable of various metabolic functions, including *N*-alkylation, *N*-dialkylation, *N*-oxidation, reduction of *N*-oxides, and *C*-hydroxylation.

Evaluation of epidemiologic studies on adverse drug reactions provides a perspective of the importance of drug-induced pulmonary disease. In a 2-year prospective survey of a community-based general practice, 41% of 817 patients experienced adverse drug reactions.[1] Four patients, or 0.5% of the total respondents, experienced adverse respiratory symptoms. Respiratory symptoms occurred in 1.2% of patients experiencing adverse drug reactions. In a recent retrospective analysis of clinical case series in France, 898 patients had reported drug allergy, with a bronchospasm incidence of 6.9%. When these patients were rechallenged with the suspected drug, only 241 (17.6%) tested positive. The incidence of bronchospasm in patients with positive provocation test was 7.9%.[2]

Adverse pulmonary reactions are uncommon in the general population but are among the most serious reactions, often requiring intervention. In a study of 270 adverse reactions leading to hospitalization from two populations, 3.0% were respiratory in nature.[3] Of the reactions considered to be life-threatening, 12.3% were respiratory. An early report on death caused by drug reactions from the Boston Collaborative Drug Surveillance Program indicated that 7 of 27 drug-induced deaths were respiratory in nature.[4] This was confirmed in a follow-up study in which 6 of 24 drug-induced deaths were respiratory in nature.[5]

DRUG-INDUCED APNEA

Apnea may be induced by central nervous system (CNS) depression or respiratory neuromuscular blockade (Table 29–1). Patients with chronic obstructive airway disease, alveolar hypoventilation, and chronic carbon dioxide retention have an exaggerated respiratory depressant response to narcotic analgesics and sedatives. In addition, the injudicious administration of oxygen in patients with carbon dioxide retention can worsen ventilation-perfusion mismatching, producing apnea.[6] Although the benzodiazepines are touted as causing less respiratory depression than barbiturates, they may produce a profound additive or synergistic effect when taken in combination with other respiratory depressants. Combining intravenous diazepam with phenobarbital to stop seizures in an emergency department frequently results in admissions to an intensive care unit for a short period of assisted mechanical ventilation, regardless of the drug administration rate. Too rapid intravenous administration of any of the benzodiazepines, even without coadministration of other respiratory depressants, will result in apnea. The risk appears to be the same for the various available agents (diazepam, lorazepam, and midazolam). Respiratory depression and arrests resulting in death and hypoxic encephalopathy have occurred following rapid intravenous administration of midazolam for conscious sedation prior to medical proce-

❶ dures. This has been reported more commonly in the elderly and the chronically debilitated or in combination with opioid analgesics. Concurrent use of inhibitors of cytochrome P450 3A4 with benzodiazepines are likely to lead to greater risk of respiratory depression.

❶ Prolonged apnea may follow administration of any of the neuromuscular blocking agents used for surgery, particularly in patients with hepatic or renal dysfunction. In addition, persistent neuromuscular blockade and muscle weakness have been reported in critically ill patients receiving neuromuscular blockers continuously for more than 2 days to facilitate mechanical ventilation.[7] This has resulted in delayed weaning from mechanical ventilation and prolonged ICU stays. The prolonged neuromuscular blockade has been confined principally to pancuronium and vecuronium in patients with renal disease. Both agents have pharmacologic active metabolites that are excreted renally. The persistent muscular weakness is less well defined but appears to represent an acute myopathy.[7] High-dose corticosteroids appear to produce a synergistic effect, supported by animal studies showing that corticosteroids at dosages greater than or equal to 2 mg/kg per day of prednisone produce atrophy in denervated muscle.[8] The fluorinated corticosteroids (e.g., triamcinolone) appear to be more myopathic.[9] Dose-dependent respiratory muscle weakness has been reported in chronic obstructive pulmonary

TABLE 29–1. Drugs That Induce Apnea

Central Nervous System Depression

Narcotic analgesics	F[a]
Barbiturates	F
Benzodiazepines	F
Other sedatives and hypnotics	I
Tricyclic antidepressants	R
Phenothiazines	R
Ketamine	R
Promazine	R
Anesthetics	R
Antihistamines	R
Alcohol	I
Fenfluramine	R
L-Dopa	R
Oxygen	R

Respiratory Muscle Dysfunction

Aminoglycoside antibiotics	I
Polymyxin antibiotics	I
Neuromuscular blockers	I
Quinine	R
Digitalis	R

Myopathy

Corticosteroids	F
Diuretics	I
Aminocaproic acid	R
Clofibrate	R

[a]Relative frequency of reactions: F = frequent; I = infrequent; R = rare.

TABLE 29–2. Drugs That Induce Bronchospasm

Anaphylaxis (IgE-Mediated)		Anaphylactoid Mast-Cell Degranulation	
Penicillins	F[a]	Narcotic analgesics	I
Sulfonamides	F	Ethylenediamine	R
Serum	F	Iodinated-radiocontrast media	F
Cephalosporins	F	Platinum	R
Bromelin	R	Local anesthetics	I
Cimetidine	R	Steroidal anesthetics	I
Papain	F	Iron–dextran complex	I
Pancreatic extract	I	Pancuronium bromide	R
Psyllium	I	Benzalkonium chloride	I
Subtilase	I	**Pharmacologic Effects**	
Tetracyclines	I	β-Adrenergic receptor blockers	I–F
Allergen extracts	I		
L-Asparaginase	F	Cholinergic stimulants	I
Pyrazolone analgesics	I	Anticholinesterases	R
Direct Airway Irritation		α-Adrenergic agonists	R
Acetate	R	Ethylenediamine tetraacetic acid (EDTA)	R
Bisulfite	F		
Cromolyn	R	**Unknown Mechanisms**	
Smoke	F	ACE inhibitors	I
N-Acetylcysteine	F	Anticholinergics	R
Inhaled steroids	I	Hydrocortisone	R
Precipitating IgG Antibodies		Isoproterenol	R
		Monosodium glutamate	I
α-Methyldopa	R	Piperazine	R
Carbamazepine	R	Tartrazine	R
Spiramycin	R	Sulfinpyrazone	R
Cyclooxygenase Inhibition		Zinostatin	R
		Losartan	R
Aspirin/NSAIDs	F		
Phenylbutazone	I		
Acetaminophen	R		

[a]Relative frequency of reactions: F = frequent; I = infrequent; R = rare.

disease (COPD) and asthma patients receiving repeated short courses of oral prednisone in the previous 6 months.[10]

Respiratory failure has been known to occur following local spinal anesthesia. Apnea from respiratory paralysis and rapid respiratory muscle fatigue has followed the administration of polymyxin and aminoglycoside antibiotics.[6] The mechanism appears to be related to the complexation of calcium and its depletion at the myoneural junction. Intravenous calcium chloride has been variably effective in reversing the paralysis.[6] The aminoglycosides competitively block neuromuscular junctions. This has resulted in life-threatening apnea when neomycin, gentamicin, streptomycin, or bacitracin has been administered into the peritoneal and pleural cavities.[6] The aminoglycosides will produce an additive blockade and ventilatory paralysis with curare or succinylcholine and in patients with myasthenia gravis or myasthenic syndromes.[6] Intravenous administration of aminoglycosides has resulted in respiratory failure in babies with infantile botulism. Treatment consists of ventilatory support and administration of an anticholinesterase agent (neostigmine or edrophonium).[6]

DRUG-INDUCED BRONCHOSPASM

Bronchoconstriction is the most common drug-induced respiratory problem. Bronchospasm can be induced by a wide variety of drugs through a number of disparate pathophysiologic mechanisms (Table 29–2). Regardless of the pathophysiologic mechanism, drug-induced bronchospasm is almost exclusively a problem of patients with preexisting bronchial hyperreactivity (e.g., asthma, chronic obstructive lung disease).[11] By definition, all patients with nonspecific bronchial hyperreactivity will experience bronchospasm if given sufficiently high doses of cholinergic or anticholinesterase agents. Severe asthmatics with a high degree of bronchial reactivity may wheeze following the inhalation of a number of particulate substances, such as the

lactose in dry-powder inhalers (DPIs) and inhaled corticosteroids, presumably through direct stimulation of the central airway irritant receptors. Other pharmacologic mechanisms for inducing bronchospasm include β_2-receptor blockade and nonimmunologic histamine release from mast cells and basophils.[11] A large number of agents are capable of producing bronchospasm through immunoglobulin (IgE)–mediated reactions.[11] These drugs can become a significant occupational hazard for pharmacists, nurses, and pharmaceutical industry workers.[11]

ASPIRIN-INDUCED BRONCHOSPASM

Aspirin sensitivity or intolerance occurs in 4% to 20% of all asthmatics.[12] The frequency of aspirin-induced bronchospasm increases with age. Patients older than 40 years have a frequency approximately four times that of patients younger than 20 years.[12] The frequency increases to 14% to 23% in patients with nasal polyps.[12] Women predominate over men, and there is no evidence for a genetic or familial predisposition.[13]

The classic description of the aspirin-intolerant asthmatic includes the triad of severe asthma, nasal polyps, and aspirin intolerance. The typical patient experiences intense vasomotor rhinitis, which may or may not be associated with aspirin exposure, beginning during the third or fourth decade of life.[14] Over a period of months, nasal polyps begin to appear, followed by severe asthma exacerbated by aspirin.

Bronchospasm typically begins within minutes to hours following ingestion of aspirin and is associated with rhinorrhea, flushing of the head and neck, and conjunctivitis.[14] The reactions are severe and often life-threatening.

All aspirin-sensitive asthmatics do not fit the classic "aspirin triad" picture, and not all patients with asthma and nasal polyps develop sensitivity to aspirin.[13] In most cases, aspirin-sensitive asthmatics are clinically indistinguishable from the general population of asthmatics except for their intolerance to aspirin and other nonsteroidal anti-inflammatory drugs (NSAIDs). Aspirin-induced asthmatics are not at higher risk of having fatal asthma if aspirin and other NSAIDs are avoided.[15]

Diagnosis of aspirin-induced asthma requires a detailed medical history. The definitive diagnosis is made by aspirin provocation tests, which may be done via different routes.[13,16] An oral provocation test is used commonly where threshold doses of aspirin induce a positive reaction measured by a drop in forced expiratory volume in 1 second (FEV_1) and/or the presence of symptoms.[16,17] A nasal provocation test is done by the application of one dose of lysine-aspirin, and aspirin sensitivity is manifested with clinical symptoms of watery discharge and a significant fall in inspiratory nasal flow.[16,17] When lysine-aspirin bronchoprovocation was compared with oral aspirin provocation, both methods were equally sensitive.[18]

PATHOGENESIS

Aspirin-induced asthma is correctly classified as an idiosyncratic reaction in that the pathogenesis is still unknown. Patients with aspirin intolerance have increased plasma histamine concentrations after ingestion of aspirin and elevated peripheral eosinophil counts.[13,14] All attempts to define an immunologic mechanism have been unsuccessful. Chemically similar drugs such as salicylamide and choline salicylate do not cross-react, whereas a large number of chemically dissimilar NSAIDs do produce reactions.[13,14] Table 29–3 lists the analgesics that do and do not cross-react with aspirin.

TABLE 29–3. Tolerance of Anti-Inflammatory and Analgesic Drugs in Aspirin-Induced Asthma

Cross-Reactive Drugs	Drugs With No Cross-Reactivity
Diclofenac	Acetaminophen[a]
Diflunisal	Benzydamine
Fenoprofen	Chloroquine
Flufenamic acid	Choline salicylate
Flurbiprofen	Corticosteroids
Hydrocortisone hemisuccinate	Dextropropoxyphene
Ibuprofen	Phenacetin[a]
Indomethacin	Salicylamide
Ketoprofen	Sodium salicylate
Mefenamic acid	
Naproxen	
Noramidopyrine	
Oxyphenbutazone	
Phenylbutazone	
Piroxicam	
Sulindac	
Sulfinpyrazone	
Tartrazine	
Tolmetin	

[a]A very small percentage (5%) of aspirin-sensitive patients react to acetaminophen and phenacetin.

The currently accepted hypothesis of aspirin-induced asthma is that aspirin intolerance is integrally related to inhibition of cyclooxygenase. This is supported by the following evidence: (1) All NSAIDs that inhibit cyclooxygenase produce reactions, (2) the degree of cross-reactivity is proportional to the potency of cyclooxygenase inhibition, and (3) each patient with aspirin sensitivity has a threshold dose for precipitating bronchospasm that is specific for the degree of cyclooxygenase inhibition produced, and once established, the dose of another cyclooxygenase inhibitor needed to induce bronchospasm can be estimated.[14]

The mechanism by which cyclooxygenase inhibition produces bronchospasm in susceptible individuals is unknown. Arachidonic acid metabolism through the 5-lipoxygenase pathway may lead to the excess production of leukotrienes C_4 and D_4.[15] Leukotrienes C_4, D_4, and E_4 produce bronchospasm and promote histamine release from mast cells,[14] whereas the administration of leukotriene receptor antagonists and 5-lipoxygenase inhibitors ablate the pulmonary and nonpulmonary responses to aspirin in aspirin-sensitive asthmatics.[19] The precise mechanism by which augmented leukotriene production occurs is unknown, and available hypotheses do not explain why only a small number of asthmatic patients react to aspirin and NSAIDs.

DESENSITIZATION

Patients with aspirin sensitivity can be desensitized. The ease of desensitization correlates with the sensitivity of the patient.[14] Highly sensitive patients who react initially to less than 100 mg aspirin require multiple rechallenges to produce desensitization.[13] Desensitization usually persists for 2 to 5 days following discontinuance, with full sensitivity reestablished within 7 days.[13] Cross-desensitization has been established between aspirin and all NSAIDs tested to date. Because patients may experience life-threatening reactions, desensitization should be attempted only in a controlled environment by personnel with expertise in handling these patients. In addition, there have been reports of patients who have failed to maintain a desensitized state despite continued aspirin administration.[13] The chronic asthma symptoms have improved markedly in a number of aspirin-sensitive asthmatics who have undergone desensitization.[13]

CROSS-SENSITIVITY WITH FOOD AND DRUG ADDITIVES

Up to 80% of aspirin-sensitive asthmatics will have an adverse reaction to the yellow azo dye tartrazine (FD&C Yellow No. 5), which is used widely for coloring foods, drinks, drugs, and cosmetics.[12] However, the studies reporting high cross-reactivity were poorly controlled and often used only subjective criteria.[12,20] In double-blind, placebo-controlled trials using pulmonary function testing, sensitivity to tartrazine has proved to be a rare event.[20] Tartrazine sensitivity appears to occur only in aspirin-intolerant patients at a prevalence of 2%.[20] Although rare, owing to the severity of reaction and widespread use of tartrazine, the Food and Drug Administration (FDA) has required labeling for the products containing this dye.[21] The likely mechanism is dose-related histamine release, and the clinical presentation is the same as the reaction to aspirin in aspirin-sensitive patients.[21]

Reactions to other azo dyes, monosodium glutamate, parabens, and nonazo dyes have been reported much less frequently than reactions to tartrazine and have been equally difficult to confirm with controlled challenges.[20] Positive reactions to sodium benzoate, a food preservative, have been reported in as many as 23% of aspirin-sensitive individuals.[12] Acetaminophen is a weak inhibitor of cyclooxygenase. As such, approximately 5% of aspirin-sensitive asthmatics will experience reactions to acetaminophen.[12] Most aspirin-sensitive asthmatics can use acetaminophen as a safe alternative to aspirin. There is a growing body of evidence that selective COX-2 inhibitors may be used safely in aspirin-sensitive patients,[22–25] but long-term studies with these agents should be undertaken to confirm their safe use in aspirin-sensitive patients. At this point, the package inserts of these agents state that they are contraindicated for aspirin-sensitive asthmatics.[22–25] Sporadic cases of worsening bronchospasm and anaphylaxis have been reported in aspirin-sensitive asthmatics receiving intravenous hydrocortisone succinate, but such reactions have not been reported with use of other corticosteroids.[13] It is not known whether it is the hydrocortisone or the succinate that is the problem.

▶ TREATMENT: Aspirin-Sensitive Asthma

Therapy of aspirin-sensitive asthmatics takes one of two general approaches: desensitization or avoidance. Avoidance of triggering substances seldom alters the clinical course of patients' asthma. The therapy of asthma has been nonspecific; however, in theory, 5-lipoxygenase inhibitors such as zileuton or leukotriene antagonists should provide specific therapy. A few studies have investigated use of leukotriene modifiers to prevent aspirin-induced bronchospasm in aspirin-sensitive asthmatic patients.[26–28] Pretreatment with zileuton in eight aspirin-sensitive asthmatic patients protected them from the same threshold provoking doses of aspirin.[26] However, larger, escalating doses of aspirin above the threshold challenge doses were not examined in this study. Furthermore, when doses of aspirin were escalated above the threshold provocative doses, zileuton did not prevent formation of leukotrienes.[27] In a similar study, pretreatment with montelukast 10 mg/day did not protect patients when aspirin doses were increased above their threshold doses.[28] In a recent study, the mean provoking dose of aspirin did not differ in the asthmatics who were taking leukotriene modifiers and the control group (60.4 mg versus 70.3 mg, respectively).[29] Although initial studies suggested that leukotriene modifiers blocked aspirin-induced reactions, it is now apparent that they merely shift the dose-response curve to the right, leaving the patient at risk at higher doses. Thus even patients who might benefit from leukotriene modifiers should avoid aspirin and all NSAIDs. A case of ibuprofen 400 mg–induced asthma was reported in an asthmatic patient on zafirlukast 20 mg twice daily.[30] Furthermore, most of the challenge studies are based on incremental doses of aspirin or NSAIDs, and exposure of patients to full clinical doses of aspirin or NSAIDs can overcome the antagonistic effect of leukotriene modifiers. The respiratory symptoms can be decreased but not prevented by pretreatment with antihistamines, cromolyn, and nedocromil.[13,31] The long-term asthma control of patients with aspirin sensitivity does not differ from that for other asthmatics. There is no evidence to support that aspirin-sensitive asthmatics respond better to leukotriene modifiers. In a double-blind, randomized, placebo-controlled study, aspirin-sensitive asthmatic patients on montelukast showed a 10% improvement in FEV_1 compared with the placebo group.[32] Similar results were reported when montelukast was compared with placebo in patients with intermittent or persistent asthma.[33]

β-BLOCKERS

β-Adrenergic receptor blockers comprise the other large class of drugs that can be hazardous to a person with asthma. Even the more cardioselective agents such as acebutolol, atenolol, and metoprolol have been reported to cause asthma attacks.[11] Patients with asthma may take nonselective and β_1-selective blockers without incident for long periods; however, the occasional report of fatal asthma attacks resistant to therapy with β-agonists should provide ample warning of the dangers inherent in β-blocker therapy.[11]

If a patient with bronchial hyperreactivity requires β-blocker therapy, one of the selective β_1-blockers (e.g., acebutolol, atenolol, metoprolol, or pindolol) should be used at the lowest possible dose. Celiprolol and betaxolol appear to possess greater cardioselectivity than currently marketed drugs.[34,35] Fatal status asthmaticus has occurred with the topical administration of the nonselective timolol maleate ophthalmic solution for the treatment of open-angle glaucoma.[36] Early investigations with ophthalmic betaxolol suggest that it is well tolerated even in timolol-sensitive asthmatics.[37,38]

SULFITES

Severe, life-threatening asthmatic reactions following consumption of restaurant meals and wine have occurred secondary to ingestion of the food preservative potassium metabisulfite.[20] Sulfites have been used for centuries as preservatives in wine and food. As antioxidants, they prevent fermentation of wine and discoloration of fruits and vegetables caused by contaminating bacteria.[39] Previously, sulfites had been given "generally recognized as safe" status by the FDA. Sensitive patients react to concentrations ranging from 5 to 100 mg, amounts that are consumed routinely by anyone eating in restaurants. Consumption of sulfites in U.S. diets is estimated to be 2 to 3 mg/day in the home with 5 to 10 mg per 30 mL of beer or wine consumed.[20] Anaphylactic or anaphylactoid reactions to sulfites in nonasthmatics are extremely rare. In the general asthmatic population, reactions to sulfites are uncommon. Approximately 5% of steroid-dependent asthmatics demonstrate sensitivity to sulfiting agents, but the prevalence is only around 1% in non–steroid-dependent asthmatic patients.[39]

MECHANISM

Three different mechanisms have been proposed to explain the reaction to sulfites in asthmatic patients.[39] The first is explained by the inhalation of sulfur dioxide, which produces bronchoconstriction in all asthmatics through direct stimulation of afferent parasympathetic irritant receptors. Furthermore, inhalation of atropine or the ingestion of doxepin protects sulfite-sensitive patients from reacting to the ingestion of sulfites. The second theory, IgE-mediated reaction, is supported by reported cases of sulfite-sensitive anaphylaxis reaction in patients with positive sulfite skin test. Finally, a reduced concentration of sulfite oxidase enzyme (the enzyme that catalyzes oxidation of sulfites to sulfates) compared with normal individuals has been demonstrated in a group of sulfite-sensitive asthmatics.

A number of pharmacologic agents contain sulfites as preservatives and antioxidants. The FDA now requires warning labels on drugs containing sulfites. Most manufacturers of drugs for the treatment of asthma have discontinued the use of sulfites. In addition, labeling is required on packaged foods that contain sulfites at 10 ppm or more, and sulfiting agents are no longer allowed on fresh fruits and vegetables (excluding potatoes) intended for sale.

Pretreatment with cromolyn, anticholinergics, and cyanocobalamin have protected sulfite-sensitive patients.[39,40] Presumably, pharmacologic doses of vitamin B_{12} catalyze the nonenzymatic oxidation of sulfite to sulfate.

OTHER PRESERVATIVES

Both ethylenediamine tetraacetic acid (EDTA) and benzalkonium chloride used as stabilizing and bacteriostatic agents, respectively, can produce bronchoconstriction.[41] In addition to producing bronchoconstriction, EDTA potentiates the bronchial responsiveness to histamine.[41] These effects presumably are mediated through calcium chelation by EDTA. Benzalkonium chloride is more potent than EDTA, and its mechanism appears to be a result of mast cell degranulation and stimulation of irritant C fibers in the airways.[41]

The bronchoconstriction from benzalkonium chloride can be blocked by cromolyn but not the anticholinergic ipratropium bromide.[42] Benzalkonium chloride is found in the commercial multiple-dose nebulizer preparations of ipratropium bromide and beclomethasone dipropionate marketed in the United Kingdom and Europe and is presumed to be in part responsible for paradoxical wheezing following administration of these agents.[41–43] Benzalkonium chloride is also found in albuterol nebulizer solutions marketed in the United States and has been implicated as a possible cause of paradoxical wheezing in infants receiving this preparation.[41] The effect of these agents on FEV_1 when used in the amount administered for treatment of acute asthma was evaluated in subjects with stable asthma.[44] Patients were assigned randomly to inhale up to four 600-mcg nebulized doses of EDTA and benzalkonium chloride and normal saline. The change in FEV_1 was not different between EDTA and the placebo group; however, benzalkonium chloride was associated with a statistically significant decrease in FEV_1 compared with placebo. It is important to consider that these agents are always used in combination with bronchodilators and β_2-agonists, which are potent mast cell stabilizers, and the anecdotal reports have not yet been confirmed with controlled investigations.[41,42]

CONTRAST MEDIA

Iodinated radiocontrast materials are the most common cause of anaphylactoid reactions producing bronchospasm.[45] The reader is referred to Chap. 86 for a discussion of this topic.

NATURAL RUBBER LATEX ALLERGY

Allergy to natural rubber latex, first reported in 1989 in the United States, is a common cause of occupational allergy for health care workers.[46] Natural rubber is a processed plant product from the commercial rubber tree, *Hevea brasiliensis*.[47] Latex allergens are proteins found in both raw latex and the extracts used in finished rubber products. Latex gloves are the largest single source of exposure to the protein allergens.[47]

The reported prevalence of latex allergy depends on the sample population. In the general population, latex allergy is less than 1%; however, the prevalence increases in health care workers to 5% to 15%.[47] Risk factors for latex allergy include frequent exposure to rubber gloves, history of atopic disease, and presence or history of hand dermatitis. Patients with spina bifida are at an increased risk of latex allergy with incidence of 24% to 60% due to early and repeated exposure to rubber devices during the surgical procedures.[47]

Clinical manifestations of latex allergy range from contact dermatitis and urticaria, rhinitis and asthma, and reported cases of anaphylaxis.[46,47] The early manifestation of rubber allergy is contact urticaria, which is an IgE-mediated reaction to rubber proteins following direct contact with the medical devices: mainly rubber gloves.[47] Contact dermatitis may occur within 1 to 2 days. Contact dermatitis is a cell-mediated delayed-type hypersensitivity reaction to the additive chemical component of rubber products.[47] Rhinitis and asthma may follow inhalation of allergens by cornstarch powder used to coat the latex gloves. Asthma caused by occupational exposure is seen mostly in atopic patients with histories of seasonal and perennial allergies and asthma.[47] There are also isolated cases of wheezing secondary to latex exposure in patients without a history of asthma.[47]

The diagnosis of latex allergy is based on the presence of latex-specific IgE, as well as symptoms consistent with IgE-mediated reactions.[48] The mainstay of therapy for latex allergy is avoidance. The FDA requires appropriate labeling for all medical devices containing natural rubber latex to ensure avoidance and a latex-free environment. The role of pretreatment with antihistamines, corticosteroids, and allergen immunotherapy remains to be determined.[47,48] Two randomized, placebo-controlled clinical trials have evaluated the role of specific immunotherapy in the treatment of latex allergy.[49,50] Although both studies have shown an improvement of cutaneous and rhinitis reactions, systemic reactions were observed, and bronchoconstriction did not improve. At this time, immunotherapy remains investigational for the treatment of latex allergy.

ANGIOTENSIN-CONVERTING ENZYME INHIBITOR–INDUCED COUGH

Cough has become a well-recognized side effect of angiotensin-converting enzyme (ACE) inhibitor therapy. According to spontaneous reporting by patients, cough occurs in 1% to 10% of patients receiving ACE inhibitors, with a preponderance of females. In a retrospective analysis, 14.6% of women had cough compared with 6.0% of the men on ACE inhibitors. It is suggested that women have a lower cough threshold, resulting in their reporting this adverse effect more commonly than men.[51] Studies specifically evaluating cough caused by ACE inhibitors have reported a prevalence of 19% to 25%.[52,53] Patients receiving ACE inhibitors had a 2.3 times greater likelihood of developing cough than a similar group of patients receiving diuretics.[52] Patients with hyperreactive airways do not appear to be at greater risk.[53] African-Americans and Chinese have a higher incidence of cough.[51] When different disease states were compared, 26% of patients with heart failure had ACE inhibitor–induced cough compared with 14% of those with hypertension.[51] Cough can occur with all ACE inhibitors.[54]

The cough typically is dry and nonproductive, persistent, and not paroxysmal.[54] The severity of cough varies from a "tickle" to a debilitating cough with insomnia and vomiting. The cough can begin within 3 days or have a delayed onset of up to 12 months following initiation of ACE inhibitor therapy.[54] The cough remits within 1 to

4 days of discontinuing therapy but rarely can last up to 4 weeks and recur with rechallenge.[54] Patients should be given a 4-day withdrawal to determine if the cough is induced by ACE inhibitors. The chest x-ray is normal, as are pulmonary function tests (spirometry and diffusing capacity). Bronchial hyperreactivity, as measured by histamine and methacholine provocation, may be worsened in patients with underlying bronchial hyperreactivity such as asthma and chronic bronchitis. However, bronchial hyperreactivity is not induced in others.[54,55] The cough reflex to capsaicin is enhanced but not to nebulized distilled water or citric acid.[54]

The mechanism of ACE inhibitor–induced cough is still unknown. ACE is a nonspecific enzyme that also catalyzes the hydrolysis of bradykinin and substance P (see Chap. 24) that produce or facilitate inflammation and stimulate lung irritant receptors.[54] ACE inhibitors also may induce cyclooxygenase to cause the production of prostaglandins. NSAIDs, benzonatate, inhaled bupivacaine, theophylline, baclofen, thromboxane A_2 synthase inhibitor,[51,56] and cromolyn sodium all have been used to suppress or inhibit ACE inhibitor–induced cough.[54,57] The cough generally is not responsive to cough suppressants or bronchodilator therapy. No long-term trials evaluating different treatment options for ACE inhibitor–induced cough exist. Cromolyn sodium may be considered first because it is the most studied agent and has minimal toxicity.[51] The preferred therapy is withdrawal of the ACE inhibitor and replacement with an alternative antihypertensive agent. Owing to their decrease in ACE inhibitor–induced side effects, angiotensin II receptor antagonists often are recommended in place of an ACE inhibitor; however, there are rare reports of this agent inducing bronchospasm.[58] The clinical trials suggest that angiotensin II receptor antagonists have the same incidence of cough as placebo. Furthermore, when angiotensin II receptor antagonists were compared with ACE inhibitors, cough occurred much less frequently. Reduction in the incidence of cough with angiotensin II receptor antagonists is likely due to the lack of effect on clearance of bradykinin and substance P.[59] The use of alternative therapies to treat ACE inhibitor–induced cough generally is not recommended.[4]

PULMONARY EDEMA

Pulmonary edema may result from the failure of any of a number of homeostatic mechanisms. The most common cause of pulmonary edema is an increase in capillary hydrostatic pressure because of left ventricular failure. Excessive fluid administration in compensated and decompensated heart failure patients is the most frequent cause of iatrogenic pulmonary edema. Besides hydrostatic forces, other homeostatic mechanisms that may be disrupted include the osmotic and oncotic pressures in the vasculature, the integrity of the alveolar epithelium, interstitial pulmonary pressure, and the interstitial lymph flow.[6] The edema fluid in cardiogenic pulmonary edema contains a low amount of protein, whereas noncardiogenic pulmonary edema fluid has a high protein concentration.[6] This indicates that noncardiogenic pulmonary edema results primarily from disruption of the alveolar epithelium. The reader is referred to Chap. 28 for a detailed discussion of this topic.

The clinical presentation of pulmonary edema includes persistent cough, tachypnea, dyspnea, tachycardia, rales on auscultation, hypoxemia from ventilation-perfusion imbalance and intrapulmonary shunting, widespread fluffy infiltrates on chest roentgenogram, and decreased lung compliance (stiff lungs). Noncardiogenic pulmonary edema may progress to hemorrhage; cellular debris collects in the alveoli, followed by hyperplasia and fibrosis with a residual restrictive mechanical defect.[6]

NARCOTIC-INDUCED PULMONARY EDEMA

The most common drug-induced noncardiogenic pulmonary edema is produced by the narcotic analgesics[6] (Table 29–4). Narcotic-induced pulmonary edema is associated most commonly with intravenous heroin use but also has occurred with morphine, methadone, meperidine, and propoxyphene use.[6,60] There also have been a few reported cases associated with the use of the opiate antagonist naloxone and nalmefene, a long-acting opioid antagonist.[61,62] The mechanism is unknown but may be related to hypoxemia similar to the neurogenic pulmonary edema associated with cerebral tumors or trauma or a direct toxic effect on the alveolar capillary membrane.[60] Initially thought to occur only with overdoses, most evidence now supports the theory that narcotic-induced pulmonary edema is an idiosyncratic reaction to moderate as well as high narcotic doses.[60]

Patients with pulmonary edema may be comatose with depressed respirations or dyspnea and tachypnea. They may or may not have other signs of narcotic overdose. Symptomology varies from cough and mild crepitations on auscultation with characteristic radiologic findings to severe cyanosis and hypoxemia even with supplemental

TABLE 29–4. Drugs That Induce Pulmonary Edema

Cardiogenic Pulmonary Edema	
Excessive intravenous fluids	F[a]
Blood and plasma transfusions	F
Corticosteroids	F
Phenylbutazone	R
Sodium diatrizoate	R
Hypertonic intrathecal saline	R
β_2-Adrenergic agonists	I
Noncardiogenic Pulmonary Edema	
Heroin	F
Methadone	I
Morphine	I
Oxygen	I
Propoxyphene	R
Ethchlorvynol	R
Chlordiazepoxide	R
Salicylate	R
Hydrochlorothiazide	R
Triamterene + hydrochlorothiazide	R
Leukoagglutinin reactions	R
Iron–dextran complex	R
Methotrexate	R
Cytosine arabinoside	R
Nitrofurantoin	R
Dextran 40	R
Fluorescein	R
Amitriptyline	R
Colchicine	R
Nitrogen mustard	R
Epinephrine	R
Metaraminol	R
Bleomycin	R
Iodide	R
Cyclophosphamide	R
VM-26	R

[a]Relative frequency of reactions: F = frequent; I = infrequent; R = rare.

oxygen. Symptoms may appear within minutes of intravenous administration but may take up to 2 hours to occur, particularly following oral methadone.[60] Hemodynamic studies in the first 24 hours have demonstrated normal pulmonary capillary wedge pressures in the presence of pulmonary edema.

Clinical symptoms generally improve within 24 to 48 hours and radiologic clearing occurs in 2 to 5 days, but abnormalities in pulmonary function tests may persist for 10 to 12 weeks. Therapy consists of naloxone administration, supplemental oxygen, and ventilatory support if required. Mortality is less than 1%.[60]

OTHER DRUGS THAT CAUSE PULMONARY EDEMA

A paradoxical pulmonary edema has been reported in a few patients following hydrochlorothiazide ingestion but not any other benzthiazide diuretic.[6] Acute pulmonary edema rarely has followed the injection of high concentrations of contrast medium into the pulmonary circulation during angiocardiography.[6] Rare occurrences of pulmonary edema have followed the intravenous administration of bleomycin, cyclophosphamide, and vinblastine.[6]

The selective β_2-adrenergic agonists terbutaline and ritodrine have been reported to induce pulmonary edema when used as tocolytics.[6] This disorder commonly occurs 48 to 72 hours after tocolytic therapy.[62] This has never occurred with their use in asthma patients, even in inadvertent overdosage. This reaction may result from excess fluid administration used to prevent the hypotension from β_2-mediated vasodilation or the particular hemodynamics of pregnancy. In a review of 330 patients who received tocolytic therapy and were monitored closely for their fluid status, no episode of pulmonary edema was reported.[62]

IL-2, a cytokine used alone or in combination with cytotoxic drugs, has been reported to induce pulmonary edema. Although other cytokines have been associated with pulmonary edema, the problem is most significant with IL-2. A weight gain of 2 kg has been reported after treatment with IL-2.[62]

Pulmonary edema has occurred occasionally with salicylate overdoses. The serum salicylate concentrations are often greater than 45 mg/dL, and the patients have other signs of toxicity, although some cases have been associated with concentrations in the usual therapeutic range.[60]

PULMONARY EOSINOPHILIA

Pulmonary infiltrates with eosinophilia (Loeffler's syndrome) have been associated with nitrofurantoin, *para*-aminosalicylic acid, methotrexate, sulfonamides, tetracycline, chlorpropamide, phenytoin, NSAIDs, and imipramine[6,63] (Table 29–5). The disorder is characterized by fever, nonproductive cough, dyspnea, cyanosis, bilateral pulmonary infiltrates, and eosinophilia in the blood.[6] Lung biopsy has revealed perivasculitis with infiltration of eosinophils, macrophages, and proteinaceous edema fluid in the alveoli. The symptoms and eosinophilia generally respond rapidly to withdrawal of the offending drug.

Sulfonamides were first reported as causative agents in users of sulfanilamide vaginal cream.[6] *para*-Aminosalicylic acid frequently produced the syndrome in tuberculosis patients being treated with this agent.[6] There have been nine reported cases associated with sulfasalazine use in inflammatory bowel disease.[63] The drug as-

TABLE 29–5. Drugs That Induce Pulmonary Infiltrates with Eosinophilia (Loeffler's Syndrome)

Drug	Freq	Drug	Freq
Nitrofurantoin	F[a]2	Tetracycline	R
para-Aminosalicylic acid	F	Procarbazine	R
Sulfonamides	I	Cromolyn	R
Penicillins	I	Niridazole	R
Methotrexate	I	Gold salts	R
Imipramine	I	Chlorpromazine	R
Chlorpropamide	R	Naproxen	R
Carbamazepine	R	Sulindac	R
Phenytoin	R	Ibuprofen	R
Mephenesin	R		

[a]Relative frequency of reactions: F = frequent; I = infrequent; R = rare.

sociated most frequently with this syndrome is nitrofurantoin.[6,60] Nitrofurantoin-induced lung disorders appear to be more common in postmenopausal women.[60] Lung reactions made up 43% of 921 adverse reactions to nitrofurantoin reported to the Swedish Adverse Drug Reaction Committee between 1966 and 1976.[63] No apparent correlation exists between duration of drug exposure and severity or reversibility of the reaction.[63] Most cases occur within 1 month of therapy. Typical symptoms include fever, tachypnea, dyspnea, dry cough, and less commonly, pleuritic chest pain. Radiographic findings include bilateral interstitial infiltrates, predominant in the bases and pleural effusions 25% of the time. Although there are anecdotal reports that steroids are beneficial, the usual rapid improvement following discontinuation of the drugs brings the utility of steroids into question. Complete recovery usually occurs within 15 days of withdrawal.

A few cases of pulmonary eosinophilia have been reported in asthmatics treated with cromolyn.[6,63] The significance of this is unknown in light of the occasional spontaneous occurrence of pulmonary eosinophilia in asthmatic patients. Cases of acute pneumonitis and eosinophilia have been reported to occur with phenytoin and carbamazepine therapy.[63] Patients have had other symptoms of hypersensitivity, including fever and rashes. The symptoms of dyspnea and cough subside following discontinuation of the drug.

OXYGEN TOXICITY

Because of the similarity to pulmonary fibrosis, oxygen-induced lung toxicity is reviewed briefly. More extensive reviews on this topic have been published.[64,65]

The earliest manifestation of oxygen toxicity is substernal pleuritic pain from tracheobronchitis.[65] The onset of toxicity follows an asymptomatic period and presents as cough, chest pain, and dyspnea. Early symptoms usually are masked in ventilator-dependent patients. The first noted physiologic change is a decrease in pulmonary compliance caused by reversible atelectasis. Then decreases in vital capacity occur, followed by progressive abnormalities in carbon monoxide diffusing capacity.[65] Decreased inspiratory flow rates, reflected in the need for high inspiratory pressures in ventilator-dependent patients, occur as the fractional concentration of inspired oxygen requirement increases. The lungs become progressively stiffer as the ability to oxygenate becomes more compromised.

The fraction of inspired oxygen and duration of exposure are both important determinants of the severity of lung damage. Normal human volunteers can tolerate 100% oxygen at sea level for 24 to 48 hours with minimal to no damage.[64] Oxygen concentrations of

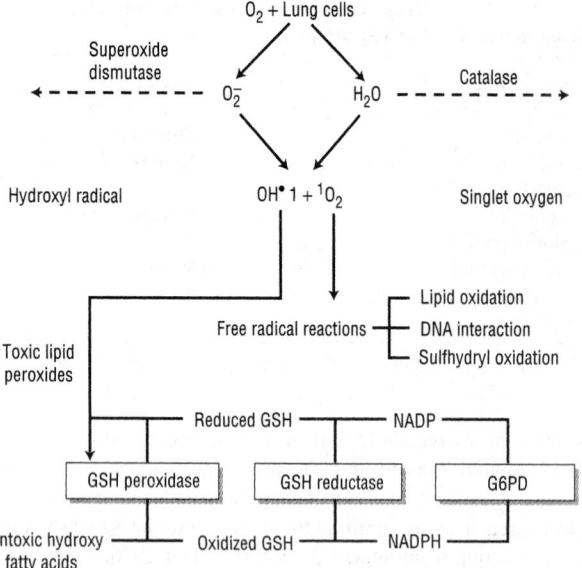

FIGURE 29–1. Schematic of the interaction of oxygen radicals and the antioxidant system. GSH = glutathione; G6PD = glucose-6-phosphate dehydrogenase; NADP = nicotinamide-adenine dinucleotide phosphate; NADPH = reduced NADP.

TABLE 29–6. Drugs That Induce Pneumonitis and/or Fibrosis

Oxygen	F[a]	Chlorambucil	R
Radiation	F	Melphalan	R
Bleomycin	F	Lomustine and semustine	R
Busulfan	F	Zinostatin	R
Carmustine	F	Procarbazine	R
Hexamethonium	F	Teniposide	R
Paraquat	F	Sulfasalazine	R
Amiodarone	F	Phenytoin	R
Mecamylamine	I	Gold salts	R
Pentolinium	I	Pindolol	R
Cyclophosphamide	I	Imipramine	R
Practolol	I	Penicillamine	R
Methotrexate	I	Phenylbutazone	R
Mitomycin	I	Chlorphentermine	R
Nitrofurantoin	I	Fenfluramine	R
Methysergide	I		
Azathioprine, 6-mercaptopurine	R		

[a]Relative frequency of reactions: F = frequent; I = infrequent; R = rare.

less than 50% are well tolerated even for extended periods. Inspired oxygen concentrations between 50% and 100% carry a substantial risk of lung damage, and the duration required is inversely proportional to the fraction of inspired oxygen.[64] Underlying disease states may alter this relationship. Lung damage may not be lasting and may improve months to years after the exposure.[66,67]

Oxygen-induced lung damage generally is separated into the acute exudative phase and the subacute or chronic proliferative phase. The acute phase consists of perivascular, peribronchiolar, interstitial, and alveolar edema with alveolar hemorrhage and necrosis of pulmonary endothelium and type I epithelial cells.[64] The proliferative phase consists of resorption of the exudates and hyperplasia of interstitial and type II alveolar lining cells. Collagen and elastin deposition in the interstitium of alveolar walls then leads to thickening of the gas-exchange area and the fibrosis.[64]

The biochemical mechanism of the tissue damage during hyperoxia is the increased production of highly reactive, partially reduced oxygen metabolites[65] (Fig. 29–1). These oxidants normally are produced in small quantities during cellular respiration and include the superoxide anion, hydrogen peroxide, the hydroxyl radical, singlet oxygen, and hypochlorous acid.[65] Oxygen free radicals normally are formed in phagocytic cells to kill invading microorganisms, but they also are toxic to normal cell components. The oxidants produce toxicity through destructive redox reactions with protein sulfhydryl groups, membrane lipids, and nucleic acids.[65]

The oxidants are products of normal cellular respiration that are normally counterbalanced by an antioxidant defense system that prevents tissue destruction. The antioxidants include superoxide dismutase, catalase, glutathione peroxidase, ceruloplasmin, and α-tocopherol (vitamin E). Antioxidants are ubiquitous in the body. Hyperoxia produces toxicity by overwhelming the antioxidant system. There is experimental evidence that a number of drugs and chemicals produce lung toxicity through increasing production of oxidants (e.g., bleomycin, cyclophosphamide, nitrofurantoin, and paraquat) and/or by inhibiting the antioxidant system (e.g., carmustine, cyclophosphamide, and nitrofurantoin).[68,69]

PULMONARY FIBROSIS

A large number of drugs have been associated with chronic pulmonary fibrosis with or without a preceding acute pneumonitis (Table 29–6). The cancer chemotherapeutic agents make up the largest group and have been the subject of numerous reviews.[68,69] Although the mechanisms by which all the drugs produce pneumonitis and/or fibrosis are not known, the clinical syndrome, pulmonary function abnormalities, and histopathology present a relatively homogeneous pattern.[68] The histopathologic picture closely resembles oxidant lung damage, and in some experimental cases, oxygen enhances the pulmonary injury.[60] Although the terms *pulmonary fibrosis* or *interstitial pneumonitis* have been used widely to describe pneumonia after bone marrow transplantation, in 1991, a National Institutes of Health workshop recommended that the term *idiopathic pneumonia syndrome* (IPS) should be used to avoid histopathologic terms and to define the inherent heterogeneity of this disorder.[70] IPS accounts for more than 40% of deaths related to bone marrow transplantation.[70] Suggested causes of IPS include radiation or chemotherapy regimens prior to transplantation, graft-versus-host disease, unrecognized infections, and other inflammation-related lung injuries.[71,72] IPS is characterized by dyspnea, hypoxemia, nonproductive cough, diffuse alveolar damage, and interstitial pneumonitis in the absence of lower respiratory infection. IPS has been reported early and late, up to 24 months after bone marrow transplantation.[72]

The lung damage following ingestion of the contact herbicide paraquat classically resembles hyperoxic lung damage. Hyperoxia accelerates the lung damage induced by paraquat. Lung toxicity from paraquat occurs following oral administration in humans and aerosol administration and inhalation in experimental animals.[69] The pulmonary specificity of paraquat results in part from its active uptake into lung tissue. Paraquat readily accepts an electron from reduced nicotinamide-adenine dinucleotide phosphate and then is reoxidized rapidly, forming superoxide and other oxygen radicals.[69] The toxicity may be a result of nicotinamide-adenine dinucleotide phosphate depletion (see Fig. 29–1) and/or excess oxygen free-radical generation with lipid peroxidation. Treatment with exogenous superoxide dismutase has had limited and conflicting results.[69]

A number of furans have been shown to produce oxidant injury to lungs.[69] Occasionally, patients with acute nitrofurantoin lung toxicity will progress to a chronic reaction leading to fibrosis, and

TABLE 29–7. Possible Causes of Pulmonary Fibrosis

Idiopathic pulmonary fibrosis (fibrosing alveolitis)
Pneumoconiosis (asbestosis, silicosis, coal dust, talc berylliosis)
Hypersensitivity pneumonitis (molds, bacteria, animal proteins,
   toluene diisocyanate, epoxy resins)
Smoking
Sarcoidosis
Tuberculosis
Lipoid pneumonia
Systemic lupus erythematosus
Rheumatoid arthritis
Systemic sclerosis
Polymyositis/dermatomyositis
Sjögren's syndrome
Polyarteritis nodosa
Wegener's granuloma
Byssinosis (cotton workers)
Siderosis (arc welders' lung)
Radiation
Oxygen
Chemicals (thioureas, trialkylphosphorothioates, furans)
Drugs (see Tables 29–5, 29–6, and 29–8)

rarely, a patient may develop chronic toxicity without an antecedent acute reaction. Like paraquat, nitrofurantoin undergoes cyclic reduction and reoxidation that may produce superoxide radicals or deplete nicotinamide-adenine dinucleotide phosphate. In addition, nitrofurantoin inhibits glutathione reductase, an enzyme involved in the glutathione antioxidant system (see Fig. 29–1). Table 29–7 provides a list of possible nondrug causes of pulmonary fibrosis.

DRUGS ASSOCIATED WITH PULMONARY FIBROSIS

ANTINEOPLASTICS

A number of cancer chemotherapeutic agents produce pulmonary fibrosis. In an excellent review,[68] six predisposing factors for the development of cytotoxic drug–induced pulmonary disease were described: (1) cumulative dose, (2) increased age, (3) concurrent or previous radiotherapy, (4) oxygen therapy, (5) other cytotoxic drug therapy, and (6) preexisting pulmonary disease. Drugs that are directly toxic to the lung would be expected to show a dose-response relationship. Dose-response relationships have been established for bleomycin, busulfan, and carmustine (BCNU).[68] Bleomycin and busulfan exhibit threshold cumulative doses below which a very small percentage of patients exhibit toxicity, but carmustine shows a more linear relationship.[69] Older patients appear to be more susceptible, possibly as a result of a decrease in the antioxidant defense system.

Excessive irradiation produces a pneumonitis and fibrosis thought to be caused by oxygen free-radical formation.[68] Evidence for synergistic toxicity with radiation exists for bleomycin, busulfan, and mitomycin.[68] Hyperoxia has shown synergistic toxicity with bleomycin, cyclophosphamide, and mitomycin.[68] Carmustine, mitomycin, cyclophosphamide, bleomycin, and methotrexate all appear to show increased lung toxicity when they are part of multiple-drug regimens.

NITROSOUREAS

BCNU is associated with the highest incidence of pulmonary toxicity (20% to 30%).[68] The lung pathology generally resembles that

produced by bleomycin and busulfan. Unique to BCNU is the finding of fibrosis in the absence of inflammatory infiltrates. BCNU preferentially inhibits glutathione reductase, the enzyme required to regenerate glutathione, thus reducing glutathione tissue stores.[68,69] The patients present with dyspnea, tachypnea, and nonproductive cough that may begin within a month of initiation of therapy but may not develop for as long as 3 years.[68] Most patients receiving BCNU develop fibrosis that may remain asymptomatic or become symptomatic any time up to 17 years after therapy.[73] The cumulative dose has ranged from 580 to 2100 mg/m^2.[69] The disease is usually slowly progressive with a mortality rate from 15% to greater than 90% depending on the study and period of follow-up. In a retrospective study, the risk factors for development of IPS and prognostic factors for outcomes were evaluated in 94 patients with relapsed Hodgkin's disease treated with BCNU containing high-dose chemotherapy and hematopoietic support. The risk factors for pulmonary fibrosis and mortality were female sex and dose of BCNU, with all deaths reported in those who received BCNU at doses of more than 475 mg/m^2.[74] Rapid progression and death within a few days occur in a small percentage of patients.[68] Corticosteroids do not appear to be effective in reducing damage.[68] Other nitrosoureas, lomustine, and semustine also have been reported to produce lung damage in patients receiving unusually high doses.[68]

BLEOMYCIN

Bleomycin is the best-studied cytotoxic pulmonary toxin. Because of its lack of bone marrow suppression, pulmonary toxicity is the dose-limiting toxicity of bleomycin therapy. The incidence of bleomycin lung toxicity is about 4%, which may be affected by the following risk factors: bleomycin cumulative dose, age, high concentration of inspired oxygen, radiation therapy, and multidrug regimens, particularly those with cyclophosphamide.[62] Age at the time of treatment with bleomycin may be a risk factor as well; patients younger than 7 years of age at the time of receiving bleomycin therapy are more likely to develop pulmonary toxicity compared with older subjects.[62] The cumulative dose above which the incidence of toxicity significantly increases is 450 to 500 units.[68] However, rapidly fatal pulmonary toxicity has occurred with doses as low as 100 units.[68]

Experimentally, bleomycin generates superoxide anions, and the lung toxicity is increased by radiation and hyperoxia.[68] Pretreatment with superoxide dismutase and catalase reduces toxicity in experimental animals.[68] Bleomycin also oxidizes arachidonic acid, which may account for the marked inflammation. Bleomycin also may affect collagen deposition by its stimulation of fibroblast growth.[68] Combination of bleomycin with other cytotoxic agents, particularly regimens containing cyclophosphamide, may predispose patients to pulmonary damage.

There are two distinct clinical patterns of bleomycin pulmonary toxicity. Chronic progressive fibrosis is the most common; acute hypersensitivity reactions occur infrequently. Patients present with cough and dyspnea. The first physiologic abnormality seen is a decreased diffusing capacity of carbon monoxide.[68] Chest radiographs show a bibasilar reticular pattern, and gallium scans show marked uptake in the involved lung.[68] Chest radiographic changes lag behind pulmonary function abnormalities. Spirometry tests before each bleomycin dose are not predictive of toxicity. The single-breath diffusing capacity of carbon monoxide is the most sensitive indicator of bleomycin-induced lung disease. Although it is not absolutely predictive, a drop of 20% or greater in the diffusing capacity of carbon monoxide is an indication for using alternative therapies.[68]

The prognosis of bleomycin lung toxicity has improved due to early detection, but the mortality rate is approximately 25%. Mild cases respond to discontinuation of bleomycin therapy.[62] Corticosteroid therapy appears to be helpful in patients with acute pneumonitis, although there have been no controlled trials. Patients with chronic fibrosis would be less likely to respond. Although corticosteroids have been used for a number of drug-induced pulmonary problems, a study in mice showing a potential for worsening of lung damage when administered early during the repair stage should sound a word of caution against their indiscriminate use.[75]

MITOMYCIN

Mitomycin is an alkylating antibiotic that produces pulmonary fibrosis at a frequency of 3% to 12%.[68] The mechanism is unknown, but oxygen and radiation therapy appear to enhance the development of toxicity.[68] The clinical presentation and symptoms are the same as for bleomycin. The mortality rate is about 50%. Early withdrawal of the drug and administration of corticosteroids appear to improve the outcome significantly.

ALKYLATING AGENTS

A number of alkylating agents have been associated with pulmonary fibrosis (see Table 29–5). The incidence of clinical toxicity is around 4%, although subclinical damage is apparent in up to 46% of patients at autopsy. The mechanism of toxicity is unknown; however, epithelial cell damage that triggers the arachidonic acid inflammatory cascade may be the initiating event.[68] The clinical presentation is insidious, with 4 years being the average duration of therapy before the onset of symptoms.[68] Patients present with low-grade fever, weight loss, weakness, dyspnea, cough, and rales.[68] Pulmonary function tests initially show abnormal diffusion capacity followed by a restrictive pattern (low vital capacity). The histopathologic findings are nonspecific. The prognosis is one of slow progression with a mean survival of 5 months following diagnosis.[68] Although there is no direct dose-dependent correlation, patients receiving less than 500 mg busulfan do not develop the syndrome without concomitant radiation or use of other pulmonary toxic chemotherapeutic agents.[68] There are anecdotal reports of beneficial responses to corticosteroids, but no controlled studies have been done.

Cyclophosphamide infrequently produces pulmonary toxicity. More than 20 well-documented cases have been reported to date. In animal models, cyclophosphamide produces reactive oxygen radicals. High oxygen concentrations produce synergistic toxicity with cyclophosphamide. The duration of therapy before the onset of symptoms is highly variable, and there may be a delay of several months between the onset of symptoms and discontinuation of the drug.[68] Cyclophosphamide may potentiate carmustine lung toxicity.[68] Clinical symptoms usually consist of dyspnea on exertion, cough, and fever. Inspiratory crackles and the bibasilar reticular pattern typical of cytotoxic drug–induced radiographic changes are present. Histopathologic changes are also nonspecific. Approximately 60% of patients recover. Corticosteroid therapy has been reported to be beneficial; however, death despite corticosteroid administration also has been reported.

Chlorambucil, melphalan, and uracil mustard also have been associated with pulmonary fibrosis. Of the alkylating agents, only nitrogen mustard and thiotepa have not been reported to cause fibrotic pulmonary toxicity.[68]

ANTIMETABOLITES

Methotrexate was first reported to induce pulmonary toxicity in 1969.[68] The pulmonary toxicity to methotrexate is unique in that discontinuation is not always necessary, and reinstitution of the drug may not produce recurrence of symptoms.[6] Methotrexate pulmonary toxicity most commonly appears to result from hypersensitivity,[63] and it can occur 3 or more years following methotrexate therapy.[76] Age, sex, underlying pulmonary disease, duration of therapy, or smoking is not associated with an increased risk of pneumonitis with methotrexate.[76] Serial pulmonary function tests did not help to identify pneumonitis in patients receiving methotrexate before the onset of clinical symptoms.[76] Reductions in diffusing capacity of carbon monoxide and lung volumes are the most common manifestations of methotrexate lung toxicity.[62] Pulmonary edema and eosinophilia are common, and fibrosis occurs in only 10% of the patients who develop acute pneumonitis.[68] Systemic symptoms of chills, fever, and malaise are common before the onset of dyspnea, cough, and acute pleuritic chest pain. Methotrexate also has been associated with granuloma formation.[68]

The prognosis of methotrexate-induced pulmonary toxicity is good, with a 1% or less mortality rate.[63] Pulmonary toxicity has followed intrathecal as well as oral administration and has occurred after single doses as well as long-term daily and intermittent administration.[68] Pneumonitis has been reported to occur up to 4 weeks following discontinuation of therapy.[68] Numerous anecdotal reports have claimed dramatic benefit from corticosteroid therapy. It is unknown whether intermittent (weekly) dosing, as is done for rheumatoid arthritis, decreases the risk of methotrexate-induced pulmonary toxicity because pneumonitis has occurred with this form of dosing.

Rarely, azathioprine and its major metabolite 6-mercaptopurine have been reported to produce an acute restrictive lung disease. Procarbazine, a methylhydrazine associated more commonly with Loeffler's syndrome, rarely has been associated with pulmonary fibrosis.[63] The vinca alkaloids vinblastine and vindesine have been reported to produce severe respiratory toxicity in association with mitomycin. The incidence with the combination is 39% and may represent a true synergistic effect between these agents.[68]

NONCYTOTOXIC DRUGS

Pulmonary fibrosis associated with the ganglionic-blocking agent hexamethonium was first reported in 1954[6] (see Table 29–6). Patients developed extreme dyspnea after several months on the drug. Pathologic findings were consistent with bronchiectasis, bronchiolectasis, and fibrosis.[6] This phenomenon has occurred occasionally with use of the other ganglionic blockers (i.e., mecamylamine and pentolinium).[6]

In 1959, radiographic changes characteristic of diffuse pulmonary fibrosis were reported in 87% of 31 patients who had taken phenytoin for 2 years or more.[60] Since then, studies have been conflicting. If phenytoin does produce chronic fibrosis, it would appear to be a relatively rare event.

Gold salts (sodium aurothiomalate) used in the treatment of rheumatoid arthritis have produced pulmonary fibrosis with cough, dyspnea, and pleuritic pain 5 to 16 weeks following institution of therapy.[60] Pulmonary function tests show a restrictive defect, and patients generally have an eosinophilia. The reactions improve on discontinuation of the gold therapy and recur promptly on reexposure. The pulmonary deficit may not resolve completely.

AMIODARONE

Amiodarone, a benzofuran derivative, produces pulmonary fibrosis when used for supraventricular and ventricular arrhythmias[77] (see Table 29–6). The duration of amiodarone therapy before the onset of symptoms has ranged from 4 weeks to 6 years.[60,77] The estimated incidence is 1 in 1000 to 2000 treated patients per year. The clinical course is variable, ranging from acute onset of dyspnea with rapid progression into severe respiratory failure and death caused by slowly developing exertional dyspnea over a few months. Patients generally improve on discontinuation of the drug.[77] The majority of patients develop reactions while taking maintenance doses greater than 400 mg daily for more than 2 months or smaller doses for more than 2 years. The risk of amiodarone pulmonary toxicity is higher during the first 12 months of therapy even at a low dosage.[78] Other risk factors include cardiopulmonary surgery combined with the administration of high concentrations of oxygen.[78] Routine spirometry does not appear to be predictive of patients at risk.[79] Carbon monoxide diffusing capacity studies are sensitive indicators of amiodarone pulmonary toxicity but have only a 21% positive predictive value.[79] Clinical findings include exertional dyspnea, nonproductive cough, weight loss, and occasionally low-grade fever.[60,79] Radiographic changes are nondiagnostic and consist of diffuse bilateral interstitial changes consistent with a pneumonitis. Pulmonary function abnormalities include hypoxia, restrictive changes, and diffusion abnormalities.

The mechanism of amiodarone-induced pulmonary toxicity is multifactorial. Amiodarone and its metabolite can damage lung tissue directly by a cytotoxic process or indirectly by immunologic reactions.[78] Amiodarone is an amphiphilic molecule that contains both a highly apolar aromatic ring system and a polar side chain with a positively charged nitrogen atom.[77] Amphiphilic drugs characteristically produce a phospholipid storage disorder in the lungs of experimental animals and humans.[69] Chlorphentermine, an anorectic, is the prototype amphiphilic compound. The mechanism is currently believed to be the inhibition of lysosomal phospholipases.[69] The inflammation and fibrosis are thought to be a late finding resulting from nonspecific inflammation following the breakdown of phospholipid-laden macrophages.[77]

In a review of 39 cases, 9 patients died, and the remaining 30 patients had resolution of abnormalities after withdrawal of the drug.[77] Some patients have had resolution with lowering of the dosage, and therapy has been reinstituted at lower doses without problems in others. Of the patients who died, one-half received corticosteroids. There have been reports of a protective effect with prophylactic corticosteroids and other reports of patients developing amiodarone lung toxicity while on corticosteroids.[77] At this time, any benefit of corticosteroids is unclear because most patients improve after stopping the drug.

PULMONARY HYPERTENSION

Pulmonary hypertension is a rare disorder, occurring with an approximate incidence of 1 to 2 cases per 1 million in the general population.[80] With progression of the disease, right ventricular afterload increases, and the ability to increase cardiac output with activity decreases. This progresses to right-sided heart failure and death.[81]

Patients with pulmonary hypertension often complain of exertional dyspnea, chest pain, and syncope. Due to the nonspecific nature of these symptoms and lack of a noninvasive diagnostic test for detecting pulmonary hypertension, there are often delays in the diagnosis of the disease, frequently up to a year after the onset of symptoms.[81]

The factors leading to the development of pulmonary hypertension are unclear, although associations with portal hypertension and pregnancy have been detected. Obesity by itself may double the risk of pulmonary hypertension.[82] Additionally, the use of cocaine or oral contraceptives, infection with the human immunodeficiency virus (HIV), the use of anorexic agents,[83] hepatic cirrhosis, genetic susceptibility, and female sex in the third to fourth decades of life also have been implicated as predisposing factors.[82] Exposure of patients to fenfluramine or dexfenfluramine has been associated with 20% of all diagnosed cases of pulmonary hypertension.[82]

The first reports of the association between pulmonary hypertension and the use of anorexic agents occurred in the late 1960s and early 1970s in western Europe when the drug aminorex was used for weight reduction.[84] The incidence of pulmonary hypertension returned to baseline after the drug was removed from the market. In the early 1990s, an association between fenfluramine use and pulmonary hypertension was established.[85] Shortly thereafter, the International Primary Pulmonary Hypertension Study Group investigated the potential role of anorexic agents in causing pulmonary hypertension.[83] Included in this multinational case-control study were 95 patients with pulmonary hypertension and 355 controls from general practices matched for gender and age. The use of anorexic agents, primarily fenfluramine and dexfenfluramine, within the last year was associated with an increased risk of pulmonary hypertension with an odds ratio of 10:1. When anorexic drugs were used for a total of more than 3 months, the odds ratio increased to 23:1.

In a 12-year observational study, 62 patients with fenfluramine-associated pulmonary hypertension were compared with 125 sex-matched patients with pulmonary hypertension unrelated to the use of fenfluramine derivatives. In most of the cases (81%), fenfluramine derivatives were used for at least 3 months. The time frame between the initiation of the therapy and the onset of dyspnea ranged from 27 days to 23 years. Both the fenfluramine-associated pulmonary hypertension group and the control group had similar levels of New York Heart Association functional class and symptoms, as well as an overall survival rate of 50% in 3 years.[86]

The mechanism by which anorexic agents cause pulmonary hypertension is unknown. Studies have shown that fenfluramine, dexfenfluramine, and aminorex inhibit potassium channels in isolated pulmonary artery smooth muscle cells in rats, which results in vasoconstriction. Potassium channel activity is altered in pulmonary artery smooth muscle cells obtained from patients with pulmonary hypertension, leading to speculation that anorexic agents may cause vasoconstriction followed by vascular growth and remodeling.[81] Another potential mechanism involves serotonin, which has been found in increased levels in patients with pulmonary hypertension.[81] Serotonin can be stored in the platelet when serotonin plasma concentration is high. Serotonin acts as a pulmonary vasoconstrictor when it is released from the platelets.[82]

Patients with pulmonary hypertension associated with anorexic use may experience a considerable improvement in their condition or possibly even remission within 1 to 3 months following discontinuation of the drug.[82,87] Pharmacologic agents used in the treatment of pulmonary hypertension include high dosage of calcium channel blockers and anticoagulants.[80] Epoprostenol, also known as *prostacyclin*, a strong vasodilator of all vascular beds was approved for the long-term therapy of pulmonary hypertension in 1995.[88] Additionally, lung and heart lung transplantations have played a role in the treatment of pulmonary hypertension. However, the 4-year survival rate is less than 60% in pulmonary hypertension patients receiving any transplant.[88] Bosentan, an endothelain receptor antagonist indicated for primary pulmonary hypertension, also may have a role, but currently, no studies exist describing its use.

In September 1997, the FDA requested the manufacturers of fenfluramine and dexfenfluramine to voluntarily withdraw their products from the market. This was done following case reports of valvular heart disease in patients taking either medication as monotherapy or in combination with another anorexic agent, phentermine. Because no association has been found between phentermine alone and valvular heart disease, it is still available. Isolated case reports of pulmonary hypertension and phentermine monotherapy have been reported,[89,90] but present data do not support an association. Although fenfluramine and phentermine were both approved by the FDA to be used as anorectic agents, the combination therapy, "fen-phen," was never approved.

MISCELLANEOUS PULMONARY TOXICITY

Drugs may produce serious pulmonary toxicity as part of a more generalized disorder. The pleural thickening, effusions, and fibrosis that occur as an extension of the retroperitoneal fibrotic reactions of methysergide and practolol or as part of a drug-induced lupus syndrome are the most common examples (Table 29–8).

Methysergide therapy for prophylaxis of poorly controlled migraine headache occasionally results in pulmonary toxicity associated with pleural effusions. The patients develop pleural pain, dyspnea, and fever. Chest radiography reveals a uniform hazy shadowing over the lower lung fields, and a loud pleural rub is heard on auscultation.[6] The mechanism is unknown, and most patients improve with discontinuation of the drug. Pleural and pulmonary fibrosis has been reported in one patient taking pindolol, a β-blocker structurally similar to practolol, an agent known to produce fibrosis.[60] Acute pleuritis with pleural effusions and fibrosis is a prominent manifestation of drug-induced lupus syndrome. Procainamide is associated with the largest number of pulmonary reactions, with 46% of patients with the lupus

syndrome developing pulmonary complications.[6] Symptoms include pleuritic pain and fever with muscle and joint pain. Chest radiographs show bilateral pleural effusions and linear atelectasis. Patients have a positive antinuclear antibody test. Symptoms usually resolve within 6 weeks of drug withdrawal.[6]

Hydralazine is the next most common cause of lupus syndrome. Most patients who develop pleuropulmonary manifestations have antecedent symptoms of generalized lupus.[6] Other drugs that produce the lupus syndrome include isoniazid and phenytoin. Phenytoin also can produce hilar lymphadenopathy as part of a generalized pseudolymphoma or lymphadenopathy syndrome.[6]

MONITORING THERAPEUTIC OUTCOMES

Monitoring for drug-induced pulmonary diseases consists primarily of having a high index of suspicion that a particular syndrome may be drug-induced. Most hypersensitivity or allergic reactions (bronchospasm) occur rapidly, within the first 2 weeks of therapy with the offending agent, and reverse rapidly with appropriate therapy (e.g., withdrawal of the offending agent and administration of corticosteroids and bronchodilators). Dyspnea associated with Loeffler's syndrome and acute pulmonary edema syndromes also improve rapidly in 1 to 2 days. However, some residual defect in diffusion capacity and the roentgenogram may persist for a few weeks. It is probably unnecessary to do follow-up spirometry or diffusion capacity determinations in these patients unless there is some concern that the syndrome will progress to pulmonary fibrosis (through the use of bleomycin or nitrofurantoin).

The routine monitoring of patients receiving known pulmonary toxins with dose-dependent toxicity such as amiodarone, bleomycin, or carmustine is still controversial. For chronic fibrosis, the diffusing capacity of carbon monoxide is the most sensitive test and may be useful in patients receiving bleomycin for detecting and preventing further deterioration of lung function with continued administration. Carmustine lung toxicity may be delayed up to 10 years following administration, and routine monitoring has not proved preventive. Monitoring patients receiving amiodarone in doses greater than 400 mg/day every 4 to 6 months may prove useful in detecting early disease that requires lowering the amiodarone or stopping the drug. Because there is no evidence of a cumulative dose effect once it has been established that the patient can tolerate the elevated dose, continued routine monitoring past the first year is unnecessary.

TABLE 29–8. Drugs That May Induce Pleural Effusions and Fibrosis

Idiopathic	
Methysergide	F[a]
Practolol	F
Pindolol	R
Methotrexate	R
Nitrofurantoin	R
Owing to Drug-Induced Lupus Syndrome	
Procainamide	F
Hydralazine	F
Isoniazid	R
Phenytoin	R
Mephenytoin	R
Griseofulvin	R
Trimethadione	R
Sulfonamides	R
Phenylbutazone	R
Streptomycin	R
Ethosuximide	R
Tetracycline	R
Pseudolymphoma Syndrome	
Cyclosporine	R
Phenytoin	R

[a]Relative frequency of reactions: F = frequent; I = infrequent; R = rare.

ABBREVIATIONS

ACE: angiotensin-converting enzyme
CNS: central nervous system
COPD: chronic obstructive pulmonary disease
DPIs: dry-powder inhalers
EDTA: ethylenediamine tetraacetic acid
FDA: Food and Drug Administration
FEV_1: forced expiratory volume in 1 second
HIV: human immunodeficiency virus
IPS: idiopathic pneumonia syndrome
NSAIDs: nonsteroidal anti-inflammatory drugs

Review Questions and other resources are available at *www.pharmocotherapyonline.com.*

REFERENCES

1. Martys CR. Adverse reactions to drugs in general practice. Br Med J 1979;2:1194–1197.

2. Messaad D, Sahla H, Benahmed S, Godard P, et al. Drug provocation tests in patietns with a history suggesting an imeediate drug hypersensitivity reaction. Ann Intern Med 2004;140:1001–1006.

3. Levy M, Kewitz H, Altwein W, et al. Hospital admissions due to adverse drug reactions: A comparative study from Jerusalem and Berlin. Eur J Clin Pharmacol 1980;17:25–31.

4. Shapiro S, Slone D, Lewis GP, et al. Fatal drug reactions among medical inpatients. JAMA 1971;216:467–472.

5. Porter J, Jick H. Drug-related deaths among medical inpatients. JAMA 1977;237:879–881.

6. Brewis RAL. Respiratory disorders. In: Davies DM, ed. Textbook of Adverse Drug Reactions, 2d ed. New York, Oxford University Press, 1981: 154–178.

7. Hansen-Flaschen J, Cowen J, Raps EC. Neuromuscular blockade in the intensive care unit: More than we bargained for. Am Rev Respir Dis 1993; 147:234–236.

8. Lieu F, Powers SK, Herb RA, et al. Exercise and glucocorticoid-induced diaphragmatic myopathy. J Appl Physiol 1993;75:763–771.

9. Dekhuijzen PNR, Gayan-Ramirez G, de Bock V, et al. Triamcinolone and prednisolone affect contractile properties and histopathology of rat diaphragm differently. J Clin Invest 1993;92:1534–1542.

10. Decramer M, Lacquet LM, Fagard R, et al. Corticosteroids contribute to muscle weakness in chronic airflow obstruction. Am J Respir Crit Care Med 1994;150:11–16.

11. Fisher HK. Drug-induced asthma syndromes. In: Weiss EB, Segal MS, Stein M, eds. Bronchial Asthma: Mechanisms and Therapeutics, 3d ed. Boston, Little, Brown, 1993:938–949.

12. Settipane GA. Aspirin and allergic diseases: A review. Am J Med 1983;74(suppl 6a):102–109.

13. Stevenson DD. Diagnosis, prevention, and treatment of adverse reactions to aspirin and nonsteroidal anti-inflammatory drugs. J Allergy Clin Immunol 1984;74:617–622.

14. Szczeklik A, Gryglewski RJ. Asthma and antiinflammatory drugs: Mechanisms and clinical patterns. Drugs 1983;25:533–543.

15. Matsuse H, Shimoda T, Matsua N, et al. Aspirin-induced asthma as a risk factor for asthma mortality. J Asthma 1997;34:314–317.

16. Szczezklik A, Nizankowaska E. Clinical features and diagnosis of aspirin induced asthma. Thorax 2000;55(Suppl 2):S42–44.

17. Dahlen B, Melillo G. Inhalation challenge in ASA-induced asthma. Respir Med 1998;92:378–384.

18. Dahlen B, Zetterstrom O. Comparison of bronchial and per oral provocation with aspirin in aspirin-sensitive asthmatics. Eur Respir J 1990;3: 527–534.

19. Lee TH. Mechanism of bronchospasm in aspirin-sensitive asthma. Am Rev Respir Dis 1993;148:1442–1443.

20. Mathison DA, Stevenson DD, Simon RA. Precipitating factors in asthma: Aspirin, sulfites, and other drugs and chemicals. Chest 1985;87(suppl): 50–54.

21. American Academy of Pediatrics, Committee on Drugs. "Inactive" ingredients in pharmaceutical products: Update. Pediatrics 1997;99:268–278.

22. Yoshida S, Ishizaki Y, Onuma K, et al. Selective cyclooxygenase 2 inhibitor in patients with aspirin-induced asthma. J Allergy Clin Immunol 2000;106:1201–1202.

23. Szczeklik A, Niankowska E, Bochenek G, et al. Safety of a specific COX-2 inhibitor in aspirin-induced asthma. Clin Exp Allergy 2001;31:219–225.

24. Dahlen B, Szczeklik A, Murray JJ. Celecoxib in patients with asthma and aspirin intolerance. N Engl J Med 2001;344:142.

25. Stevenson DD, Simon RA. Lack of cross-reactivity between rofecoxib and aspirin-sensitive patients with asthma. J Allergy Clin Immunol 2001; 108:47–51.

26. Israel E, Fischer A, Rosenberg M, et al. The pivotal role of 5-lipoxygenase products in the reaction of aspirin-sensitive asthmatics to aspirin. Am Rev Respir Dis 1993;148:1447–1451.

27. Paul JD, Simon RA, Daffern PJ, et al. Lack of effect of the 5-lipoxygenase inhibitor zileuton in blocking oral aspirin challenges in aspirin-sensitive asthmatics. Ann Allergy Asthma Immunol 2000;85:40–45.

28. Stevenson DD, Simon RA, Mathison DA, Christiansen SC. Montelukast is only partially effective in inhibiting aspirin response in aspirin-sensitive asthmatics. Ann Allergy Asthma Immunol 2000;85:477–482.

29. Berges-Gimeno MP, Simon RA, Stevenson DD. The effect of leukotriene-modifier drugs on aspirin-induced asthma and rhinitis reactions. Clin Exp Allergy 2002;32:1491–1496.

30. Menendez R, Venzor J, Ortiz G. Failure of zafirlukast to prevent ibuprofen-induced anaphylaxis. Ann Allergy Asthma Immunol 1998;80: 225–226.

31. Robuschi M, Gambaro G, Setini P, et al. Attenuation of aspirin-induced bronchoconstriction by sodium cromoglycate and nedocromil sodium. Am J Respir Crit Care Med 1997;155:1461–1464.

32. Dahlen S, Malmstrom K, Nizankowska E, et al. Improvement of aspirin-intolerant asthma by montelukast, a leukotriene antagonist: A randomized, double-blind, placebo-controlled trial. Am J Respir Crit care Med 2002;165:9–14.

33. Reiss TF, Chervinsky P, Dockhorn RJ, et al. Montelukast, a once-daily leukotriene receptor antagonist, in the treatment of chronic asthma: A multicenter, randomized, double-blind trial. Arch Intern Med 1998;158: 1213–1220.

34. Riddell JG, Shanks RG. Effects of betaxolol, propranolol, and atenolol on isoproterenol-induced β-adrenoceptor responses. Clin Pharmacol Ther 1985;38:554–559.

35. Hauck RW, Schulz CH, Emslander HP, Bohm M. Pharmacological actions of the selective and non-selective β-adrenoeceptor antagonists celiprolol, bisoprolol and propranolol on human bronchi. Br J Pharmacol 1994;113:1043–1049.

36. Fraunfeder FT, Barker AF. Respiratory effects of timolol. N Engl J Med 1984;311:1441.

37. Dunn TL, Gerber MJ, Shen AS, et al. The effect of topical ophthalmic instillation of timolol and betaxolol on lung function in asthmatic subjects. Am Rev Respir Dis 1986;133:264–268.

38. Anonymous Systemic adverse reactions with betaxolol eye drops. Med J Austral 1995;162:84.

39. Simon RA. Update on sulfite sensitivity. Allergy 1998;53:78–79.

40. Anibarro B, Caballero T, Garcia-Ara C, et al. Asthma with sulfite intolerance in children: A blocking study with cyanocobalamine. J Allergy Clin Immunol 1992;90:103–109.

41. Beasley R, Rafferty P, Holgate ST. Adverse reactions to the nondrug constituents of nebulizer solutions. Br J Clin Pharmacol 1988;25:283–287.

42. Zhang YG, Wright WJ, Tam WK, et al. Effect of inhaled preservatives on asthmatic subjects: II. Benzalkonium chloride. Am Rev Respir Dis 1990;141:1405–1408.

43. Beasley R, Fishwick, D, Miles JF, et al. Preservatives in nebulizer solutions: risks without benefit. Pharmacotherapy 1998;18:130–139.

44. Asmus MJ, Barros MD, Liang J, et al. Pulmonary function response to EDTA, an additive in nebulized bronchodilators. J Allergy Clin Immunol 2001;107:68–72.

45. Greenberger PA. Contrast media reactions. J Allergy Clin Immunol 1984; 74:600–605.

46. Tilles SA. Occupational latex allergy: Controversies in diagnosis and prognosis. Ann Allergy Asthma Immunol 1999;83:640–644.

47. Yuninger JW. Natural rubber latex allergy. In: Middleton E Jr, Reed CE, Ellis EF, et al, eds. Allergy Principles and Practice, 5th ed. St Louis, Mosby, 1998;1073–1078.

48. Poley GE, Slater JE. Latex allergy. J Allergy Clin Immunol 2000;105: 1054–1062.

49. Leynadier F, Herman D, Vervolet D, Andre C. Specific immunotherapy with a standardized latex extract versus placebo in allergic health care workers. J Allergy Clin Immunol 2000;106;585–590.

50. Sastre J, Fernandez-Nieto M, Rico P, et al. Specific immunotherapy with a standardized latex extract in allergic workers: A double-blind, placebo-controlled study. J Allergy Clin Immunol 2003;111:985–994.

51. Luque CA, Ortiz MV. Treatment of ACE inhibitor–induced cough. Pharmacotherapy 1999;19:804–810.

52. Sebastian JL, McKinney WP, Kaufman J, et al. Angiotensin-converting enzyme inhibitors and cough: Prevalence in an outpatient medical clinic population. Chest 1991;99:36–39.

53. Simon SR, Black HR, Moser M, Berland WE. Cough and ACE inhibitors. Arch Intern Med 1992;152:1698–1700.

54. Israili ZH, Hall WD. Cough and angioneurotic edema associated with angiotensin-converting enzyme inhibitor therapy: A review of the literature and pathophysiology. Ann Intern Med 1992;117:234–242.

55. Kaufman J, Casanova JE, Riendl P, et al. Bronchial hyperreactivity and cough due to angiotensin-converting enzyme inhibitors. Chest 1989;95:544–548.

56. Malini PL, Strocchi E, Zanardi M, et al. Thromboxane antagonism and cough induced by angiotensin-converting enzyme inhibitor. Lancet 1997;350:15–18.

57. Allen TL, Gora-Harper ML. Cromolyn sodium for ACE inhibitor–induced cough. Ann Pharmacother 1997;31:773–775.

58. Dicpinigaitis PV, Thomas SA, Sherman MB, et al. Losartan-induced bronchospasm. J Allergy Clin Immunol 1996;98:1128–1130.

59. Pylypchuk GB. ACE inhibitor–versus angiotensin II blocker–induced cough and angioedema. Ann Pharmacother 1998;32:1060–1066.

60. Cooper JAD, White DA, Matthay RA. Drug-induced pulmonary disease: 2. Noncytotoxic drugs. Am Rev Respir Dis 1986;133:488–505.

61. Henderson CA, Reynolds JE. Acute pulmonary edema in a young male after intravenous nalmefene. Anesth Analg 1997;84:218–219.

62. Copper JA Jr. Drug-induced lung disease. Adv Intern Med 1997;42:231–268.

63. Obermiller T, Lakshminarayan S. Drug-induced hypersensitivity reactions in the lung. Immunol Allergy Clin North Am 1991;11:575–594.

64. Frank L, Massaro D. Oxygen toxicity. Am J Med 1980;69:117–126.

65. Jackson RM. Pulmonary oxygen toxicity. Chest 1985;88:900–905.

66. Elliott CG, Rasmusson BY, Crapo RO, et al. Prediction of pulmonary function abnormalities after adult respiratory distress syndrome (ARDS). Am Rev Respir Med 1987;135:634–638.

67. Neff TA, Stocker R, Frey HR, et al. Long-term assessment of lung function in survivors of severe ARDS. Chest 2003;123:845–853.

68. Cooper JAD, White DA, Matthay RA. State of the art: Drug-induced pulmonary disease: 1. Cytotoxic drugs. Am Rev Respir Dis 1986;133:321–340.

69. Kehrer JP, Kacew S. Systematically applied chemicals that damage lung tissue. Toxicology 1985;35:251–293.

70. Clark JG, Hansen JA, Hertz MI, et al. Idiopathic pneumonia syndrome after bone marrow transplantation. Am Rev Respir Dis 1993;147:1601–1606.

71. Wiedemann HP. Toward an understanding of idiopathic pneumonia syndrome after bone marrow transplantation. Crit Care Med 1999;27:2040–2041.

72. Quabeck K. The lung as a critical organ in marrow transplantation. Bone Marrow Transplant 1994;14:S19–28.

73. O'Driscoll BR, Hasleton PS, Taylor PM, et al. Active lung fibrosis up to 17 years after chemotherapy with carmustine (BCNU) in childhood. N Engl J Med 1990;323:378–382.

74. Rubio C, Hill ME, Milan S, et al. Idiopathic pneumonia syndrome after high-dose chemotherapy for relapsed Hodgkin's disease. Br J Cancer 1997;75:1044–1048.

75. Jantz MA, Sahn SA. Corticosteroids in acute respiratory failure. Am J Respir Crit Care Med 1999;160:1079–1100.

76. Lynch JP, McCune WJ. Immunosuppressive and cytotoxic pharmacotherapy for pulmonary disorders. Am J Crit Care Med 1997;155:395–420.

77. Rakita L, Sobol SM, Mostow N, et al. Amiodarone pulmonary toxicity. Am Heart J 1983;106:906–914.

78. Jessurun GAJ, Boersma WG, Crijns HJGM. Amiodarone-induced pulmonary toxicity: Predisposing factors, clinical symptoms and treatment. Drug Safety 1998;18:339–344.

79. Gleadhill IC, Wise RA, Schonfeld SA, et al. Serial lung-function testing in patients treated with amiodarone: A prospective study. Am J Med 1989;86:4–10.

80. Rubin LJ. Primary pulmonary hypertension. N Engl J Med 1997;336:111–117.

81. McCann UD, Seiden LS, Rubin LJ, Ricaurte GA. Brain serotonin neurotoxicity and primary pulmonary hypertension from fenfluramine and dexfluramine: A systematic review of the evidence. JAMA 1997;278:666–672.

82. Vivero LE, Anderson PO, Clark RF. Pharmacology in emergency medicine: A close look at fenfluramine and dexfenfluramine. J Emerg Med 1998;16:197–295.

83. Abenhaim L, Moride Y, Brenot F, et al. Appetite-suppressant drugs and the risk of primary pulmonary hypertension. N Engl J Med 1996;335:609–616.

84. Gurtner HP. Aminorex and pulmonary hypertension: A review. Cor Vasa 1985;27:160–171.

85. Brenot F, Herve P, Petitpretz P, et al. Primary pulmonary hypertension and fenfluramine use. Br Heart J 1993;70:537–541.

86. Simonneau G, Fartoukh M, Sitbon O, et al. Primary pulmonary hypertension associated with the use of fenfluramine derivatives. Chest 1998;114:195–199S.

87. Nall KC, Rubin LJ, Lipskind S, Sennesh JD. Reversible pulmonary hypertension associated with anorexigen use. Am J Med 1991;91:97–99.

88. Bever KA, Perry PJ. Dexfenfluramine hydrochloride: an anorexigenic agent. Am J Health Syst Pharm 1997;54:2059–2072.

89. Heuer L, Benoit W, Heydrich D. Diagnostic error: Pulmonary hypertension caused by an appetite suppressant (Mirapront). Chir Praxis 1978;23:497–504.

90. Schnabel KF, Schultz V, Busch S, Just H. Drug-induced primary vascular pulmonary hypertension. Med Welt (Stuttgart) 1976;27:1300–1303.

30
CYSTIC FIBROSIS

Gary Milavetz and Jeffrey J. Smith

Learning Objectives and other resources can be found at *www.pharmacotherapyonline.com.*

KEY CONCEPTS

1. Cystic fibrosis (CF) is a disorder of chloride ion transport in epithelial cells. It especially affects the cells that line the pulmonary and gastrointestinal systems, although the functions of other exocrine glands are also altered.

2. The chloride ion transport dysfunction results in thickened secretions that typically lead to obstruction, infection, and inflammation in the airways. These, in turn, lead to most of the morbidity and mortality associated with CF.

3. Thickened secretions from the pancreas lead to deficiencies of digestive enzymes and bicarbonate, which lead to maldigestion of foodstuffs. This maldigestion leads to malabsorption and malnutrition.

4. Treatment of the gastrointestinal component includes pancreatic enzyme replacement plus vitamin, nutrient, and caloric supplementation aimed at providing adequate nutritional needs.

5. Airway obstruction and pulmonary infection occur as a result of bacterial colonization and infection, thickened secretions, and inflammation.

6. Acute antibiotic treatment is aimed at bacterial eradication, whereas chronic treatment slows the progression of the disease. *Pseudomonas aeruginosa* is the most common pathogen found in patients with CF.

7. The progression of pulmonary disease is prevented by a two-pronged approach: (1) Reducing or eradicating inflammation to decrease cellular and tissue alterations. (2) Sterilizing the pulmonary tree to reduce the bacterial infection and colonization associated with the disease.

8. Gene therapy may be the treatment of the future, but it has not demonstrated beneficial effects yet.

9. The goal of therapy of CF is to slow or stop the progression of the disease and allow young patients to grow and develop normally. Although the pathophysiologic goal is similar in adulthood, the overall goal is to have as normal a lifestyle as possible.

Cystic fibrosis (CF) is the most common lethal genetic disease in the Caucasian population. The disease mainly involves the exocrine glands and thus affects a number of organ systems (Table 30–1). The more common manifestations of this disease involve the gastrointestinal and pulmonary systems, with premature mortality associated with the latter. Most of the pathology results from a defect in electrolyte transport caused by a loss of functional chloride channels in epithelial cells. The protean nature of this disease dictates that care be multidisciplinary with a wide variety of therapeutic interventions.

EPIDEMIOLOGY

CF is inherited through an autosomal (Mendelian) recessive mode. Of a couple with each parent being a carrier (heterozygous for the trait), a child has a one-in-four chance of having the disease, a one-in-two chance of being a carrier, and a one-in-four chance of being normal (having neither the disease nor the trait). The incidence of CF is greatest in the Caucasian population; it occurs in about 1 in every 2000 live births in the United States.[1] Thus the incidence of the trait (carrier state) in this group is about 5%. The frequency of this disease is considerably less in other races, occurring in about 1 in 17,000 blacks and 1 in 90,000 Asians.[2]

After years of intensive research, the cystic fibrosis gene was identified and cloned in 1989.[3–5] The gene is located on the long arm of chromosome 7 and codes for a protein called the *cystic fibrosis transmembrane regulator* (CFTR). This membrane protein functions as a chloride channel involved in the transport of electrolytes and water. Over 1000 cystic fibrosis–associated mutations within the CF gene have been described, but the most common mutation involves a 3-base-pair deletion that results in the absence of a phenylalanine residue at position 508 of the CFTR protein.[3–5] This common mutation, referred to as the ΔF_{508} allele, is present in about 70% of patients in the United States. The mutations have been divided into four classes: class I, defective protein production; class II, defective protein processing; class III, defective channel regulation; and class IV, defective channel conductance.[6] Patients homozygous for the ΔF_{508} mutation, which falls primarily into class II, tend to be diagnosed at an earlier age owing to a greater frequency of pancreatic insufficiency (99% versus 72% in heterozygotes and 36% in patients with other genotypes).[7,8]

PATHOPHYSIOLOGY

CF is a disease of epithelia, especially the cells lining the intestinal tract, pancreatic ducts, hepatobiliary tree, vas deferens, sweat ducts,

TABLE 30–1. Organ Involvement in Cystic Fibrosis

Organ System/Organ	Abnormality	Consequence
Gastrointestinal		
Pancreas	Digestive enzyme deficiency	Maldigestion
		Malnutrition
	Insulin deficiency	Glucose intolerance
Intestines	Viscous secretions	Obstruction
Liver	Biliary cirrhosis/fatty infiltration	Portal hypertension/ esophageal varices
Pulmonary	Viscous secretions	Chronic obstruction
	Infection	Endobronchial infection
Sweat glands	Failure to reabsorb sodium	Hyponatremia
Reproductive	Obstruction of epididymis, vas deferens, and seminal vesicles	Aspermia
	Viscous cervical mucus	Decreased fertility
Hematologic	Chronic disease?	Anemia
Bone and joint	Unknown	Arthritis, osteopenia

and airway lumen. In the normal state, these epithelial cells can transport chloride through CFTR chloride channels, with sodium and water accompanying this ion flux. Chloride transport through CFTR channels is activated by protein kinases in response to an increase in the intracellular second messenger, cyclic adenosine 3′,5′-monophosphate (cAMP).[9] In cystic fibrosis, a loss of functional CFTR chloride channels leads to defective cAMP-stimulated chloride transport; in most epithelia this defect results in decreased chloride secretion and increased sodium absorption (Fig. 30–1). Defective electrolyte transport is thought to alter the volume or composition of the fluid secreted by the pancreas, hepatobiliary tree, reproductive tract, sweat gland, and airways.

GASTROINTESTINAL TRACT

The gastrointestinal tract may be involved in CF with either intestinal obstruction or deficient secretion of digestive enzymes by the pancreas. In 10% to 16% of CF patients, the first gastrointestinal manifestation of the disease is small bowel obstruction that is evident shortly after birth and known as *meconium ileus*. In these patients, the basic electrolyte transport defect is thought to cause abnormally tenacious meconium that cannot be evacuated. A similar condition, known as *distal intestinal obstruction syndrome* or *meconium ileus equivalent,* occurs in older CF patients; it is also thought to result from abnormally tenacious gastrointestinal secretions and fecal impaction. Other intestinal complications include intussusception, volvulus, gastroesophageal reflux, atresia, perforation, giant cystic meconium peritonitis, and rectal prolapse.

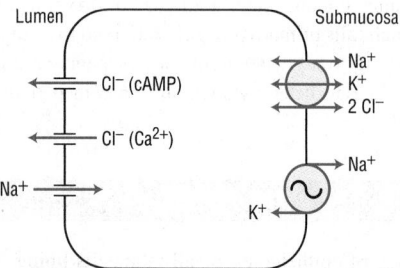

FIGURE 30–1. Electrolyte transport in the airway epithelial cell. CFTR is the cyclic-3′,5′-AMP (cAMP)–dependent chloride channel.

A relative deficiency of pancreatic digestive enzymes (pancreatic achylia) is present with most genotypes and is apparent clinically in 85% of patients. Pancreatic lesions including fibrosis, fatty replacement, and cyst formation are secondary to obstruction of small pancreatic ducts by thickened secretions and cellular debris. Inspissated eosinophilic material may accumulate in the acini and ductules. As a result, the volume of pancreatic secretions and the concentration of pancreatic enzymes and bicarbonate are reduced. Affected enzyme concentrations include trypsin, chymotrypsin, carboxypeptidase, amylase, and lipase. This leads to a maldigestion of ingested nutrients, including fats and protein. Increased fecal loses of bile acids (binding to undigested fecal fat decreases enterohepatic recycling) also may contribute to fat maldigestion.

Because of the lipase deficiency, fat-soluble vitamin (A, D, E, and K) deficiencies may occur. Whether lipase activity or bile acids (e.g., in micelle formation) are involved in fat-soluble vitamin absorption with steatorrhea is unclear. Vitamin B_{12} and zinc deficiencies also may occur as a result of pancreatic enzyme deficiency. Although pancreatic involvement is predominantly exocrine in nature, insulin deficiency with glucose intolerance also occurs in CF patients, especially as they advance in age. Carbohydrate intolerance is characterized by low insulin concentrations and enhanced peripheral sensitivity to insulin but not by the presence of islet cell or anti-insulin antibodies. Carbohydrate intolerance in CF is not usually associated with the ketosis as commonly occurs in type 1 diabetes. This complication involves an increase in the number of insulin receptors with decreased affinity for insulin. Despite a concomitant increase in tissue affinity for insulin, 8% of CF children over 12 years of age require insulin therapy.

The liver can be involved in CF. Biliary cirrhosis secondary to bile duct obstruction occurs in as many as 18% of patients, whereas fatty infiltration occurs in about 30% of patients in a pattern unrelated to nutritional status. Bile ducts may be obstructed by inspissated mucus, which may lead to focal or multilobar cirrhosis.[10] Such hepatic involvement can occur at any age but is more common with advancing age and can lead to portal hypertension, esophageal varices, and hypersplenism. The most common laboratory abnormality associated with hepatic involvement is elevated serum hepatic isoenzymes (gamma-glutamyltranspeptidase, alanine aminotransferase, aspartate aminotransferase, and alkaline phosphatase).[11,12]

PULMONARY SYSTEM

The pulmonary manifestations of CF result from an incompletely characterized defect in innate host defenses at the airway surface, including an exaggerated inflammatory response, defective bactericidal activity, and altered mucus clearance. It is unclear which step initiates the disease process, but it eventually leads to chronic airway infection, inflammation, and obstruction. The combination of persistent obstruction along with inflammation often leads to air trapping, atelectasis, and eventually bronchiectasis that progresses until respiratory insufficiency develops. The lung disease usually progresses from small airway obstruction to more generalized airway obstruction and finally toward a component of restrictive lung disease as individual segments become completely obstructed and nonfunctional. Hyperinflation or dilation of the airspaces is a common finding. Furthermore, persistent obstruction of the small airways with mucus, an excellent culture medium for microorganisms, may facilitate the growth of bacteria within an extracellular matrix or biofilm, making the infection relatively resistant to antibiotics. Although bacterial infections are thought to be a major contributor to CF airway disease, viruses and other nonbacterial pathogens also play an important pathologic role.[13–15] Environmental factors, such as exposure to tobacco smoke, also may contribute.[16]

The three most common bacterial pathogens isolated from the respiratory secretions (sputum) of CF patients are *Staphylococcus aureus, Pseudomonas aeruginosa,* and *Hemophilus influenzae,* with *P. aeruginosa* usually predominating throughout life. *Proteus, Klebsiella* spp., and *Stenotrophomonas maltophilia* are observed less frequently. Mucoid strains (alginate producers) of *P. aeruginosa* commonly observed in CF may be particularly resistant to antibiotics,[17] as are nonmotile forms. The isolation of *Burkholderia cepacia* from the sputum of CF patients has become more common at some CF centers. The significance of this contagious organism varies from one patient to the next. Three fairly distinct syndromes associated with this *B. cepacia* have been described, these being asymptomatic colonization, chronic deterioration with intermittent fever and weight loss, and rapid, usually fatal deterioration.[18] The nature of the initially cultured oropharyngeal flora in patients younger than 2 years of age has prognostic significance. The finding of *P. aeruginosa* or *P. aeruginosa* plus *S. aureus* in initial cultures appears related to increased morbidity and mortality, respectively.[19]

The presence of these bacteria contributes to the destructive changes in the airways of CF patients by direct damage from bacterial toxins and the body's immune reaction to these bacteria. For example, *P. aeruginosa* expresses number of extracellular toxins, proteases, hemolysins, and exopolysaccharides that may be responsible for direct airway damage, increased mucin production by the airway epithelium, and the production of immune complexes (IgG and IgM) that may contribute to local damage. Elevated levels of such mediators as granulocyte elastase, tumor necrosis factor α, interleukins 1 and 2, and related complexes with associated inhibitors have been well documented in CF patients. One inflammatory mediator that clearly contributes to pulmonary pathophysiology is neutrophil elastase. Present in excess, it overwhelms and neutralizes native antiproteases (α_1-antitrypsin and secretory leukocyte protease inhibitor [SLPI]), destroys structural fibers, and inhibits complement-mediated phagocytosis and antipseudomonal antibodies. Combined with other inflammatory mediators, a self-sustaining vicious cycle leading to progressive and often permanent tissue damage is established. The neutrophil influx that is part of this cycle results in release of neutrophil-derived DNA, which is thought to contribute to sputum viscosity. The occasional presence of *Aspergillus fumigatus* in the sputum of these patients also may contribute to the pulmonary pathology because it can induce a steroid-responsive allergic reaction.

The consequence of these pulmonary processes is a decrease in gas exchange by the lungs. The challenge of moving air through obstructed airways often requires the use of accessory muscles, resulting in an increased anteroposterior chest diameter (also referred to as *barrel chest*), a flattened diaphragm, and pulmonary hypertension. The increased work of breathing in these patients produces a relative exercise intolerance and increased resting energy expenditure. Hemoptysis secondary to bronchiectasis occurs but is seldom massive. Other respiratory complications include gastroesophageal reflux, pneumothorax, and right-sided heart failure (cor pulmonale) secondary to pulmonary hypertension. Although seldom overt clinically, the findings of right ventricular hypertrophy, increased heart weight, and right atrial and right ventricular chamber dilatation usually are present at autopsy. Digital clubbing, a common finding in CF as well as other chronic pulmonary conditions, may be related to chronic hypoxia.

The upper respiratory tract is also involved commonly in CF. Sinusitis and nasal polyposis occur in 90% and 50% of patients, respectively.[20] Sinusitis is chronic in character, and acute symptoms are unusual. Although its etiology is not entirely clear, sinusitis may result from obstruction of the sinus ducts, thus preventing drainage. The bacteria generally isolated in these cases include *P. aeruginosa, H. influenzae,* streptococci, and anaerobes. Usually, the same strain of *P. aeruginosa* found in the lungs is present in the upper airways (nasopharynx and sinuses), which may represent a reservoir for the pathogen.

SWEAT GLANDS

Abnormally high concentrations of sodium and chloride are found in the sweat of CF patients owing to defective chloride absorption across the water-impermeable sweat duct epithelium. This forms the basis for measuring sweat chloride concentration as a diagnostic test for CF. This defect in salt absorption rarely causes clinical symptoms except in warmer environments or during hot weather, when excessive sweating may lead to salt depletion; this clinical problem can be prevented by supplementing the diet with salt. In the sweat coil where salt and water are excreted into the gland lumen, sodium and chloride are not excreted at abnormally high concentrations in CF because chloride is secreted through chloride channels other than CFTR. However, as sweat progresses through the sweat duct toward the skin surface, chloride absorption across the water-impermeable epithelium is reduced because of a loss of CFTR chloride channels. Similar abnormalities can be seen in the excretions of the salivary glands.

REPRODUCTIVE SYSTEM

About 95% of males with CF are sterile because of obstruction of the epididymis, vas deferens, and seminal vesicles resulting in aspermia. There is late maturation of the reproductive system with delayed onset of puberty in both sexes. Females also have reduced fertility owing to the production of abnormal cervical mucus. Menstrual irregularity and oligomenorrhea are also common. Nonetheless, owing to greater life expectancy in these patients, increasing numbers are becoming mothers. In these individuals, the course and tolerance of pregnancy are related to the progravid nutritional and pulmonary status.

HEMATOLOGIC SYSTEM

Anemia is observed in some CF patients despite chronic hypoxia. The apparent deficient erythroid response occurs, at least in part, from disturbances in erythropoietin regulation and iron availability (impaired gastrointestinal absorption). Despite chronic hypoxia in some patients with CF, erythropoietin concentrations are normal or low. The condition is characterized by decreased hematocrit and serum ferritin, increased carboxyhemoglobin, and normal or low hemoglobin. Vitamin E concentrations may be normal. Many patients may have iron deficiency owing to decreased dietary intake, malabsorption, or blood loss.

BONES AND JOINTS

Arthritis may occur in CF and can take one of several forms.[21] The arthritis may be either mono- or polyarticular and usually is nondestructive. An episodic form is most common and may be due to immune complexes formed in response to the chronic pulmonary infections. Hypertrophic osteoarthropathy occurs in CF, as it does in association with other pulmonary diseases. The incidence of arthritis may be increasing as median survival age increases. Osteopenia and osteoporosis also occur more frequently in adults with CF. The causes of the resulting bone demineralization are multifactorial and include vitamin D malabsorption, decreased vitamin D conversion (via sunlight), delayed puberty and endocrine development, poor nutrition, limited physical activity, and chronic acidosis.

CLINICAL PRESENTATION

The clinical findings of CF develop as a direct consequence of the pathophysiologic processes just described. Thus the clinical findings can be conveniently subdivided by organ system.

GASTROINTESTINAL SYSTEM

Intestinal symptoms usually are secondary to either intestinal obstruction or maldigestion of nutrients. Obstruction, manifested as meconium ileus, distal intestinal obstruction syndrome, or intussusception, causes abdominal distension, pain, vomiting, or a change in stool output.

More commonly, the gastrointestinal symptoms of CF are caused by maldigestion of food, causing steatorrhea and malnutrition. The stools are foul, odorous, bulky, greasy, and more frequent in number; rectal prolapse may occur, especially in the presence of excessive weight loss. The stool's high fat content results from a relative lipase deficiency. Perhaps the most significant consequence of maldigestion is malnutrition; that is, CF children characteristically fall below their age-related norms for both weight and height.

PULMONARY SYSTEM

The respiratory symptoms of CF usually are those of obstructive airway disease such as coughing, sputum production, labored breathing, wheezing, retractions, pleurisy, and cyanosis. Digital clubbing is a common finding thought to be associated with bronchiectasis. Increased anteroposterior chest diameter, a flattened diaphragm, and hyperaeration may be noted on chest roentgenogram.

The respiratory status usually follows a cyclic pattern from a state of relative well-being to one of acute pulmonary deterioration theoretically paralleling the course of the airway infection. There may be significant declines in pulmonary function, referred to as *acute respiratory exacerbations* and generally associated with symptoms of bacterial endobronchial infection. Common pathogens found in the lungs of a CF patient include: *S. aureus, H. influenzae,* and *P. aeruginosa.* Less common pathogens include: *S. maltophilia* and *B. cepacia,* which used to be referred to as *P. cepacia.* Increased coughing, increased sputum production, changes in sputum character (e.g., thicker and darker in color), tachypnea, dyspnea, increasing oxygen requirement, and a decrease in exercise tolerance are common. Symptoms of chronic sinusitis and nasal polyposis may include nasal obstruction, pain over affected sinuses, and anosmia.

Concomitantly, laboratory testing of peripheral blood may reveal an increased white blood count with increased polymorphonuclear leukocytes and immature forms consistent with an acute infection. Tests of pulmonary function often demonstrate both intermittent and persistent decreases in forced vital capacity (FVC) and forced expiratory volume at 1 second (FEV_1) and increased residual volume (RV). Tests of small airway function are more markedly affected as the pulmonary disease progresses. Arterial blood gases may reveal hypoxia or hypercapnia as the disease progresses.

OTHER SIGNS AND SYMPTOMS

The relative insulin deficiency observed in older CF patients is often asymptomatic and only detected during annual laboratory testing. However, CF-related diabetes may present as a recent decline in weight without the typical gastrointestinal symptoms of malabsorption. It also may present as untreated cases of diabetes mellitus type 2.

Cor pulmonale usually is not evident clinically unless signs of left-sided heart failure ensue, although enlargement in cardiac size may be noted on routine chest roentgenogram prior to that time. Signs and symptoms of anemia and arthritis in CF patients do not differ from those owing to other chronic diseases.

Excess losses of sodium and chloride in the sweat of CF patients seldom results in symptoms of heat prostration, but this phenomenon may cause a "salty" taste on the skin.

DIAGNOSIS

The diagnosis of CF usually is made on the basis of elevated sweat chloride concentrations (sweat chloride testing) and may be confirmed with CFTR mutational analysis. Another test, recording the potential difference across the nasal epithelium, usually is reserved for cases in which the results of sweat testing and mutational analysis are nondiagnostic.[22] For sweat chloride determination, two samples of sweat are collected with the use of pilocarpine iontophoresis, and the concentration of chloride in each sample is measured. Duplicate sweat chloride concentrations of 60 mEq/L or more are considered diagnostic of CF. However, a number of disorders, such as adrenal insufficiency, hypothyroidism, protein-calorie malnutrition, anorexia nervosa, ectodermal dysplasia, mucopolysaccharidosis, nephrosis with edema, type 1 glycogen storage disease, familial hypoparathyroidism syndrome, fucosidosis, nephrogenic diabetes insipidus, and Mauriac syndrome, may be associated with elevated sweat chloride concentrations, but generally these conditions do not present a problem in the differential diagnosis of CF. Ninety-eight percent of CF patients will have a sweat chloride concentration 60 mEq/L or greater. The remaining 2% usually have sweat chloride concentrations between 50 and 60 mEq/L, and the test may have to be repeated one or more times to obtain definitive results. Nevertheless, the results of sweat testing alone may not be able to confirm the presence or absence of CF. The presence of chronic obstructive respiratory disease (COPD) or exocrine pancreatic insufficiency and/or a positive family history of the disease also may provide additional support for the diagnosis. Genetic (*CFTR* mutation) analysis and recording of nasal transepithelial potential difference may be helpful in making a diagnosis. Genetic (*CFTR* mutation) analysis may be used to confirm the diagnosis in utero or to detect heterozygotes (carriers), with obvious implications for genetic counseling. Newborn screening for the disease has been adopted in some states, although the benefits of making a presymptomatic diagnosis on long-term outcome are still being assessed.[23]

COURSE

CF is a heterogeneous disease in terms of initial presentation, organ involvement, and clinical course. Some children are diagnosed at birth because of meconium ileus, which occurs in about 16% of people with CF. Neonatal screening programs are increasing, but the benefits of presymptomatic diagnosis are still being assessed; prenatal diagnosis is early in its implementation. Most patients are diagnosed by 1 year of age because of a history of steatorrhea and poor weight gain. The median age at diagnosis is 7 months, and most patients are diagnosed by 12 years of age.[24]

The course of the disease after diagnosis varies from one patient to another. A patient may have a rapid downhill course from early pulmonary involvement, whereas another may suffer only from gastrointestinal complaints for many years without significant pulmonary symptoms. Although the expected life span of CF patients has increased to over 30 years of age in the last two decades, some patients still die early in life secondary to a fulminant pulmonary process. Still others, owing to minimal involvement and a mild course, may not be diagnosed until their second decade of life. The increased longevity now realized with early diagnosis and aggressive treatment may have led to an increase in formerly less common complications such as diabetes and hepatic disease. Two-year mortality rates above 50% are associated with an FEV_1 of less than 30% of predicted, a PaO_2 of <50 mm Hg, or a PCO_2 of >50 mm Hg.[25]

▶ TREATMENT: Cystic Fibrosis

DESIRED OUTCOME

The desired pharmacotherapeutic outcomes for CF are both long and short term. In the long term, one obviously tries to halt or delay progression of the disease to allow for normal growth and development. In the short term, acute problems must be dealt with. The ultimate goal of pharmacotherapy for the gastrointestinal involvement of CF is optimal nutrition. On a day-to-day basis, normal bowel habits, continued weight gain, and normal vitamin levels are desirable. The goal of therapy for the pulmonary component is to reduce the signs and symptoms of airway infection, inflammation, and obstruction. Thus antibiotic, anti-inflammatory, bronchodilator, and mucolytic therapies are geared toward treating the complications that compromise lung function. For an acute pulmonary exacerbation, a return of pulmonary function to the preexacerbation status is the central goal of therapy.

GENERAL APPROACH TO TREATMENT

The Cystic Fibrosis Foundation has published clinical guidelines for the diagnosis and care of CF patients, including applicable pharmacotherapy.[26] The following information is generally in agreement with those guidelines, although it may contain more current information. The interested reader is referred to that publication for more detail on the drug treatment of CF and its various complications.

GASTROINTESTINAL SYSTEM

The treatment of gastrointestinal involvement ultimately is aimed at correcting the nutritional deficit present in many patients.[27] In addition to pancreatic enzyme replacement and other drug therapy described below, nutritional supplementation is employed frequently. Nutritional interventions range from behavioral modification to nocturnal feedings via gastrostomies.[28]

Pancreatic Enzyme Supplementation

The backbone of gastrointestinal therapy in CF is pancreatic enzyme replacement or supplementation. The preferred products are microencapsulated pancreatic enzymes, although powders are marketed and are useful in patients unable to swallow capsules or to otherwise use the microencapsulated beads they contain. Microencapsulated products protect the contained enzymes from destruction by gastric acid and may be given in much lower doses than their predecessors, which were susceptible to acid breakdown. Most contemporary enzyme-replacement products vary mainly in enzyme content per capsule, with lipase content being the chief variable. Representative products and their contents are presented in Table 30–2. Infants are normally given 2000 to 4000 lipase units per 120 mL of formula or breast milk, which provides 450 to 900 lipase units per gram of ingested fat. In general, patients require 500 to 4000 lipase units per gram of ingested fat, with the average pediatric or adult patient requiring 1800 units per

TABLE 30–2. Pancreatic Enzyme Products

| Trade Name | Manufacturer | Enzyme Content (Units) | | | Form[a] |
		Lipase	Protease	Amylase	
Cotazym	Organon	8000	30,000	30,000	C
Cotazym-S		5000	20,000	20,000	ECM
Creon	Reid-Rowell	8000	13,000	30,000	ECM
Ilozyme	Adria	11,000	30,000	30,000	T
Ku-Zyme	Schwarz Pharma	8000	30,000	30,000	C
Pancrease	McNeil	4000	25,000	20,000	ECM
Pancrease MT4		4000	12,000	12,000	ECM
Pancrease MT10		10,000	30,000	30,000	ECM
Pancrease MT16		16,000	48,000	48,000	ECM
Pancrelipase	Geneva	4000	25,000	20,000	ECM
Protilase	Rugby	4000	25,000	20,000	ECM
Ultrase MT12	Scandipharm	12,000	39,000	39,000	ECM
Ultrase MT20		20,000	65,000	65,000	ECM
Ultrase MT24		24,000	78,000	78,000	ECM
Viokase	Robins	8000	30,000	30,000	T
Viokase		16,800	70,000	70,000	P[b]
Zymase	Organon	12,000	24,000	24,000	ECM

[a]Dosage form: C = capsule; ECM = enteric-coated microspheres or beads; T = tablet; P = powder.
[b]Viokase powder, units of enzymes per 700 mg.

gram of fat. Enzymes also may be dosed based on weight, with an initial dose of 1000 lipase units being administered per kilogram of body weight per meal. One-half that amount is administered with snacks.

Before the introduction of microencapsulated enzyme products, various maneuvers were used to circumvent or overcome the problem of acid breakdown. The most obvious of these was to administer large quantities of enzyme product. Enteric-coated (microencapsulated) pancreatic enzymes largely have solved this problem. The occasional patient may yet require large quantities of even the microencapsulated enzyme product. Whether such difficulties are caused by residual acid breakdown or perhaps low pH in the upper small intestine (secondary to deficient bicarbonate excretion by the pancreas) resulting in a failure to dissolve the coating of the microencapsulated beads is unknown. Defective enteric coating on some generic brands also has been described and led to Food and Drug Administration (FDA) reclassification of these products, which now require bioequivalence data. Histamine H_2-receptor antagonists and proton pump inhibitors have been used to reduce the enzyme dose when residual acid breakdown of enzymes or impaired neutralization of gastric acid is suspected. Another possible maneuver is to administer both microencapsulated and non-enteric-coated enzyme products (e.g., powder) concomitantly.

For patients who are unable to swallow capsules, the contents may be emptied into applesauce, jelly, or some other nonalkaline vehicle, provided that the patient does not chew the microencapsulated beads. Side effects of pancreatic enzyme products are uncommon. Perianal irritation resembling diaper rash may occur in infants fed excess quantities of enzyme powders. Hyperuricosuria also has been reported to occur secondary to pancreatic enzyme use, apparently related to their high purine content. Proximal colonic stricture (fibrosing colonopathy) is a dose-related side effect associated with lipase doses in excess of 24,000 units/kg per day.[29]

Vitamin Supplementation

Patients should receive multivitamin tablets daily to provide adequate water-soluble vitamins along with reasonable amounts of vitamins D and K. While clinically evident fat-soluble vitamin deficiencies are unusual in patients taking adequate pancreatic enzymes and receiving a balanced diet, obvious vitamin K deficiency, manifested as bleeding diathesis, can occur. Demineralization of bone also has been described, and vitamin E deficiency has been related to neurologic dysfunction. In addition, appropriate laboratory tests (serum carotene, vitamin E, and cholecalciferol concentrations) often will help to document other deficiencies, leading to recommendations for additional supplementation of these vitamins. Water-miscibilized vitamin A, 4000 international units (IU) per day, and vitamin E, 100 to 400 IU/day, also should be administered either singly or in the form of a water-miscibilized combination product (containing vitamins A, D, E, and K). Vitamin K, in a dose of 5 mg twice weekly, should be given to patients with prolonged prothrombin times. It also should be noted that appropriately adjusted doses of fat-soluble preparations may be more cost-effective than their water-miscible counterparts (e.g., 800 IU fat-soluble vitamin E versus 200 IU water-miscible vitamin E).[30]

Treating Meconium Ileus and Distal Intestinal Obstruction Syndrome

The treatment of meconium ileus or distal intestinal obstruction syndrome sometimes can be limited to the use of enemas with iso-osmolar contrast material. Unfortunately, surgery (bowel resection and primary anastomosis) is often necessary to treat meconium ileus and prevent its complications. Distal intestinal obstruction syndrome usually responds to management by oral or nasogastric administration of electrolyte lavage solutions. The adequacy of pancreatic enzyme dosage also should be reassessed in the face of distal intestinal obstruction.

Prevention and Treatment of Cirrhosis

Ursodeoxycholic acid, a bile acid with choleretic properties, has been shown to produce morphologic and functional improvement in affected patients. The effects are dose-related, and 15–20 mg/kg per day has been used, sometimes in combination with taurine supplementation.[31] Administering this agent prophylactically to patients at risk for liver disease, if feasible, has been proposed.[32]

CARDIOVASCULAR SYSTEM

Various modalities have been used in attempts to treat pulmonary hypertension and secondary cor pulmonale of CF. These treatments, which include the use of vasodilators, inotropic agents, and diuretics, all have resulted in limited and transient effects. This is most likely due to the fact that none of these modes of therapy addresses the underlying cause of the cor pulmonale—hypoxia. Likewise, supplemental (often nocturnal) oxygen treatment also has failed to affect mortality rates or disease progression, although it does appear to prevent oxygen desaturation that occurs with exercise, as well as that occurring during sleep. Thus the most beneficial approach may be to attempt to improve oxygenation with aggressive pulmonary therapy.

PULMONARY SYSTEM

Management of the pulmonary component of CF can be broken down into three general areas: anti-obstructive, anti-inflammatory, and anti-infective therapy.[33]

Anti-Obstructive Therapy

The cornerstone of pulmonary therapy is percussion and postural drainage, which aids in the clearance of pulmonary mucus and is performed once or twice daily in "healthy" patients and as often as six times daily during acute pulmonary exacerbations. New flutter devices also may be useful adjuncts in this regard. A flutter device is a hand-held unit that produces vibrations in the airways when exhaled through. These vibrations loosen and facilitate the removal of mucus and secretions from the airways. Percussion is sometimes preceded by nebulizer therapy, during which nebulized sterile water or 0.9% sodium chloride solution is inhaled to liquefy pulmonary secretions. Bronchodilators may be added to the nebulizer solution to prevent bronchospasm, and mucolytic agents (e.g., N-acetylcysteine; Mucomyst, Mead Johnson) may be added to liquefy pulmonary secretions or enhance mucus clearance. The effects of bronchodilators administered by inhalation can be demonstrated with pulmonary function testing; however, the efficacy of mucolytic agents is not readily demonstrated. Moreover, many patients prefer not to use N-acetylcysteine because of its unpleasant taste and odor and because it may induce bronchospasm. Normal saline and sodium bicarbonate solutions may be administered by aerosol as aids to sputum expectoration, but documentation of efficacy is elusive.

Recombinant human DNase has been approved for use in CF. When given by inhalation (2.5 mg once or twice daily), recombinant human (rh) DNase reduces the viscosity of CF sputum and leads to statistically significant, though modest, improvement in pulmonary function.[34] More important, the regular use of rhDNase may help to decrease the incidence of (or lengthen the time between) respiratory exacerbations and thereby improve quality of life and indirectly decrease the overall costs of care in patients with mild to moderate disease. Should these outcomes be borne out in additional long-term studies, especially before the onset of clinical symptoms, this therapy may be justified as a way to prevent or delay the progression of pulmonary disease.

Because some CF patients have a component of reactive airways disease that may contribute to their pulmonary disease, systemic bronchodilators such as theophylline and β-agonists may provide some benefit. Recurrent wheezing or dyspnea that improves with bronchodilators represents a legitimate indication for these agents. However, responsiveness to such agents (>15% improvement in FEV_1) should be documented before a protracted course is begun. Standard antiasthmatic doses of most bronchodilators should be appropriate for CF patients, but theophylline clearance may differ in CF fibrosis patients, and bioavailability of some products may be decreased, sometimes necessitating the use of higher-than-usual doses.[35] Because of the necessity of pharmacokinetic monitoring and its involvement in a number of common drug interactions, theophylline should be considered second-line bronchodilator therapy at most in these patients. Because CF patients are at high risk to develop complications from influenza, the influenza vaccine should be administered on a yearly basis, and amantadine prophylaxis or treatment may be indicated as well.

Anti-Inflammatory Therapy

In an attempt to block the consequences of the inflammatory component of this disease, corticosteroid therapy has been evaluated. Results of preliminary trials were encouraging, and a large, multicenter, placebo-controlled trial found that alternate-day prednisone treatment at 2 mg/kg had beneficial effects on pulmonary function, but it also had undesirable effects on linear growth and glucose metabolism.[36] Further analysis of the data from this same study suggested that the benefits of a 1 mg/kg dose might outweigh the risks.[37] Data concerning the efficacy of inhaled corticosteroids are scant. A long-term trial of oral ibuprofen indicates a beneficial effect in young CF patients with good lung function by slowing the rate of progression of pulmonary disease.[38] Unfortunately, therapeutic drug monitoring (periodic determination of ibuprofen serum concentrations) is required.

Antibiotic Therapy

Young children with CF have an extended period of time, perhaps months or years, when they have no evidence of airway infection. Later, they develop a mild airway infection or early bacterial colonization, often without associated symptoms. However, bronchoalveolar lavage fluid reveals evidence of infection and inflammation (high neutrophil count with a predominance of proinflammatory cytokines). Eventually, they develop a chronic airway infection that cannot be eradicated fully even with prolonged use of systemic or topical antibiotics. This scenario is best explained by the ability of bacteria such as *P. aeruginosa* to achieve high-density growth within small airways, whereby they become organized into a community that grows more slowly and secretes an extracellular matrix that protects the bacteria from local host defenses and/or most antibiotics. This complex growth pattern is referred to as a *biofilm community*. Acute exacerbations of CF are thought to involve satellite foci of bacterial proliferation that stimulate mucus production in response to bacterial exoproducts, worsen airway obstruction, and suppress the appetite owing to the host's proinflammatory response.

Because of the complexities of bacterial infections in CF, antibiotics are used with three different goals in mind. First, before an infection develops, the primary goal is to detect infections early in their course so that treatment is successful at preventing the bacteria from developing into a biofilm community (bacterial eradication). Second, once biofilm growth has become established, the primary goal is to use antibiotics to prevent rapid bacterial proliferation (bacterial suppression) to avoid excess sputum production, decreased lung function, and the concomitant loss of appetite and weight. Finally, once an acute exacerbation has developed, the primary goal is to eliminate bacterial proliferation, reduce the bacterial load and the degree of sputum production, return lung function to the preexacerbation (target) value, improve nutritional intake, and correct any weight losses (treatment of acute exacerbations).

However, the use of antibiotics in CF is somewhat controversial and certainly challenging. Controversy exists because innate host defenses in CF certainly may be sufficient to eliminate most pathogens, including *P. aeruginosa*, from the airways. Without antibiotics, some patients with CF appear to go many years before they develop typical airway infections caused by *P. aeruginosa*. In addition, some CF patients have transiently positive throat and bronchoalveolar lavage (BAL) cultures for *P. aeruginosa* that resolve without exogenous antibiotics. Thus it is unclear when antibiotics actually are needed to help eradicate these pathogens. Moreover, once bacterial eradication with antibiotics is accomplished, will some other organism soon initiate another airway infection? In other words, are the early stages of bacterial colonization merely a marker for a decrease in host defenses? Does this decrease in host defense persist, suggesting that repeated courses of antibiotics will be required regardless of whether eradication therapy was successful? The answers to these questions remain unknown, and thus the use of antibiotics in CF lung disease is controversial.

The chronic use of antibiotics to suppress bacteria in CF is controversial because antibiotic resistance may be induced or enhanced. Suppressive therapy is prescribed with the intention of prolonging the time between acute exacerbations and to slow the rate of progression of lung disease. Although attractive intuitively, this practice is not supported by well-designed clinical trials.[39] Moreover, the practice of routine, quarterly administration of intravenous courses of antibiotics used at some European centers still lacks proof of efficacy.[40] Aerosolized tobramycin (TOBI) daily for 1 to 2 months has been shown to eradicate *P. aeruginosa* from the airways of recently infected patients with CF.

Antibiotic treatment for acute pulmonary exacerbations usually results in clinical improvement without eliminating bacteria from the sputum. In this case, the antibiotics are thought to lessen the bacterial burden within the airways and thereby inhibit the quantity of exotoxins produced or the degree of host inflammation against the bacteria or their exoproducts.[41] The failure to eradicate the organism suggests that bacteria may be colonizing the airway surface rather than penetrating the tissues as a pathogen. The bacteria may remain viable within an environment protected from the antibiotics, such as enclosed within a biofilm community. It also suggests the possibility that antibiotics may not be essential for the treatment of acute exacerbations. One study comparing antibiotic therapy with placebo indicated that antibiotics are not essential for recovery from an acute exacerbation.[42] However, the study size was small and only included patients with mild to moderate disease; thus these results may not be applicable to all acute exacerbations. These results are also consistent with the notion that viral infections, air pollutants, irritants, allergens, or some other factors play a role in clinical exacerbations.

Finding known bacterial pathogens at high density in airway secretions, along with the clinical setting of increased cough, increased sputum production that is thicker and darker than baseline, and a significant decrease in lung function and loss of appetite and exercise tolerance, supports the addition of antibiotics to treat this clinical exacerbation. However, deciding to start antibiotic therapy leads to a number of other important, and sometimes perplexing, issues. These include the selection of the best antibiotic(s) for the individual patient, the optimal route of administration, the best dosage and dosage regimen to use (especially in light of altered pharmacokinetics in patients with CF and the potential emergence of antibiotic-resistant bacteria), and the identification of appropriate end points of therapy.

Selection of Antibiotic.

Suppressive therapy may be accomplished with the use of common orally administered antibiotics such as trimethoprim-sulfamethoxazole, amoxicillin–clavulanic acid, or one of the many oral cephalosporins. Specific therapy for acute exacerbations is directed at proven or likely pathogens such as *P. aeruginosa* and *S. aureus* and usually includes aminoglycoside and extended-spectrum penicillin. Since most *S. aureus* encountered are β-lactamase producers, use of an extended-spectrum penicillin–β-lactamase inhibitor combination (e.g., ticarcillin-clavulanate) will help to avoid the necessity of triple-drug therapy. Single-agent therapy with newer antibiotics, especially on an outpatient basis, is employed frequently at some centers where significant resistance to these agents has not yet emerged. Such agents would include ceftazidime, aztreonam, and ciprofloxacin. However, the evidence supporting the clinical superiority of two-drug combinations over single-agent therapy leads many clinicians to always treat with combinations.[43–46] The fact that such combinations are sometimes synergistic in vitro and the possibility that they may act to suppress or delay the emergence of resistance provides attractive rationale for their use. Further, in vitro synergism has been reported to persist even in the face of resistance to one of the single agents in a given combination.[47] Lastly, monodrug therapy has been met with rapid emergence of resistance.[48]

Unlike other cases of lower respiratory tract infection, organism-specific drug treatment may be based on results from sputum cultures in CF patients because good agreement between sputum and thoracotomy cultures has been demonstrated.[49] Typically, such results will lead one to prescribe or recommend aminoglycoside–extended-spectrum penicillin combinations, although other antibiotics such as ciprofloxacin and older agents such as colistin also may play a role. While the complete eradication of *S. aureus* and *H. influenzae* is a practical goal or end point of antibiotic therapy, the total eradication of *Pseudomonas* spp. is infrequent and transient. Thus, once a patient has been colonized/infected with *P. aeruginosa*, it is prudent to assume that it is always present regardless of culture results. Consistent with these infectious phenomena, the complete resolution of pulmonary signs and symptoms becomes less and less likely as the disease progresses. *B. cepacia* and *S. maltophilia* generally are resistant to most antibiotics. These bacteria may be susceptible to trimethoprim-sulfamethoxazole or chloramphenicol. *B. cepacia* from CF patients frequently is susceptible to ceftazidime, whereas some

TABLE 30–3. Changes in Pharmacokinetics in Cystic Fibrosis[38,50]

Agent	$\beta t_{1/2}$	V_d	Cl_B	Cl_R
Antibiotics				
Methicillin	NC	I	I	I
Cloxacillin	D	I	I	I
Dicloxacillin	I	NR	NR	I
Azlocillin	D	I	I	NR
Piperacillin	D	I	I	NR
Ticarcillin	D	NC	I	I
Aztreonam	D	I	I	I
Ceftazidime	D	I	I	I
Imipenem	NC	I	I	NR
Trimethoprim-sulfamethoxazole	D/D	NC/NC	I/I	I/NC
Gentamicin	NC	I	I	NR
Tobramycin	NC	I	I	NC
Amikacin	NC	I	I	I
Netilmicin	NC	I	I	NR
Fleroxacin	D	D	I	D
Other				
Theophylline	D	I	I	I
Furosemide	NC	NC	I	NC
Acetaminophen	NC	NR	I	NR

$\beta t_{1/2}$ = elimination half-life; V_d = apparent volume of distribution; Cl_B = total body clearance, Cl_R = renal clearance; D = decreased; I = increased; NC = no change; NR = not reported.
From refs. 38 and 50.

strains of *S. maltophilia* may be susceptible to other agents such as doxycycline and piperacillin.

Selection of Dose-Altered Pharmacokinetics.

Although altered pharmacokinetics in CF are not limited to antibiotics (Table 30–3), this drug class has been the studied most extensively.[50] As is true for theophylline, many CF patients have increased total body clearance for many antibiotics, including the aminoglycosides, some of the β-lactams, and trimethoprim-sulfamethoxazole. Thus higher doses of these agents may be necessary to produce therapeutic concentrations (Table 30–4). Unfortunately, these alterations in pharmacokinetics are neither consistent nor predictable. Why the pharmacokinetics of these antibiotics are different in CF patients is unknown. It appears that for many β-lactam antibiotics, increased total body clearance could be accounted for by increased renal clearance. However, it should be pointed out that renal function, as reflected by glomerular filtration rate and renal blood flow, is not different in CF patients as compared with non-CF controls.[51] Moreover, a concomitant increase in renal clearance does not completely explain the increase in total body clearance of aminoglycosides, leading some to speculate about extrarenal pathways for elimination. In any event, increased total body clearance dictates higher doses in many but not all patients. However, a range of dosage requirements should be expected, consistent with a range in the variation of pharmacokinetics in these patients. For example, experience with netilmicin revealed a dosage requirement range of 7–17 mg/kg per day to achieve peak concentrations (one-half hour after the end of a drug infusion) of 8 mcg/mL or greater.[52] The mean dosage requirement in this study was approximately 12 mg/kg per day. Peak concentrations of this magnitude are felt to be necessary to treat pneumonia caused by gram-negative bacteria adequately.[53,54] Variations in hepatic metabolic activity or in phenotypic distribution of metabolic polymorphisms may explain some pharmacokinetic differences in CF.[55,56]

TABLE 30–4. Antibiotic Doses in Cystic Fibrosis

Antibiotic	Dose (mg/kg/d)	Regimen	Adult Maximum Dose (g/d)
Parenteral Antibiotics			
Tobramycin,[a] gentamicin,[a] or netilmicin[a]	6–9	q8 h	NA
Amikacin[a]	20–30	q8 h	NA
Azlocillin	400	q4–6 h	24
Aztreonam	200	q6 h	8
Ceftazidime	150	q8 h	6
Colistin	2.5–6	q6–8 h	NA
Imipenem	45–100	q6 h	4
Nafcillin	100	q4–6 h	6
Ticarcillin or ticarcillin/clavulanate	400	q4–6 h	18
Piperacillin	400	q4–6 h	18
Oral Antibiotics			
Amoxicillin	20	q8 h	
Amoxicillin/clavulanate	20	q6 h	
Ciprofloxacin[b]	1500 mg/d	q12 h	1.5
Cephalexin	50–100	q6–8 h	6
Dicloxacillin	80–100	q6 h	6
Trimethoprim-sulfamethoxazole	10–15[c]	q12 h	0.64[c]
Inhaled Antibiotics			
Colistin	150 mg/d	q6–12 h	NA
Gentamicin or tobramycin	600–1800 mg/d	q12 h	NA
Polymixin B	250 mg/d	q6–12 h	NA

[a]Starting doses; adjust to desired serum concentrations based on dose/serum concentration relationship.
[b]Adult dose.
[c]Based on trimethoprim.

Although alterations in pharmacokinetics of antibiotics may correlate with the severity of pulmonary disease,[57,58] it is not possible to predict changes in antibiotic pharmacokinetics in CF patients based on markers of clinical status or disease progression. Attempts to correlate antibiotic pharmacokinetics with Shwachman score (a gross method for quantitation of disease status) have been unsuccessful.[59,60] Attempts to guide aminoglycoside dosing often are based on measured serum concentrations during a course of therapy. However, this method also may meet with mixed success owing to changing pharmacokinetics of this family of antibiotics during an acute pulmonary exacerbation.[61] This observation should not, however, deter one from attempts to adjust doses to desirable concentrations based on serum concentration determinations and subsequent pharmacokinetic calculations.

▨ *Alternate Routes of Administration.* An additional route of antibiotic administration that is intuitively attractive in patients with CF is by inhalation of aerosolized solution. Such a route of administration should, theoretically, deliver the drug to the actual site of infection and perhaps avoid systemic toxicity. Certainly many classes of antibiotics including β-lactams, aminoglycosides, and polymyxins have been administered to CF patients in this fashion, often in conjunction with systemic antibiotics. However, until recently, no clear effect or advantage had been demonstrated consistently. Early studies suffered from lack of controls, small sample size, and a failure to ensure that the respiratory equipment used would, in fact, guarantee that drug is delivered to the small airways. In a subsequent placebo-controlled, multicenter trial, 600 mg tobramycin administered by aerosol three times daily was found to produce a small but statistically significant improvement in FEV_1, forced vital capacity (FVC), forced expiratory volume from 25% to 75% of vital capacity ($FEF_{25\%-75\%}$), *P. aeruginosa* density in sputum, and peripheral white blood cell count.[62] This

being recognized, appropriate clinical circumstances for this form of therapy (type and condition of patient), length of therapy, and frequency of therapy remain to be clarified. One-half this dose is apparently also effective, and a 300-mg dose is the current norm. If such doses are to be used, preservative-free antibiotic preparations should be used. The efficacy of smaller doses of inhaled aminoglycosides remains unproven.

▨ *Bacterial Resistance.* As already noted, emergence of antimicrobial resistance seems to follow the introduction and use of a new antibiotic.[48] *P. aeruginosa* can exhibit many resistance mechanisms, revealed as resistance to quinolones (altered DNA gyrase target site), β-lactams (production of Bush group 1 β-lactamase), aminoglycosides (decreased permeability and modifying enzymes), and carbapenems (decreased permeability). *B. cepacia* is inherently resistant to most antibiotics. Methicillin-resistant staphylococci are increasingly common in institutional settings and will become a more pervasive problem in CF populations. These phenomena require close attention to susceptibility reports in selecting therapy and the avoidance of unnecessary or unnecessarily protracted courses of antibiotic therapy.

▨ *Recommendations for Antibiotic Therapy.* Despite these inherent difficulties, a number of recommendations regarding the use of systemic antibiotics in CF can be made. The selection of antibiotics should be based on specific culture and susceptibility results. When instituting empirical therapy in the absence of culture results, the clinician can be guided by the most recent laboratory data or institute therapy based on likely pathogens in the patient's age group. Aminoglycosides should be dosed initially at the upper end of the normal dosage range (e.g., 6 to 7.5 mg/kg per day for tobramycin), and serum concentrations should be determined so that dosage can be adjusted appropriately to achieve peak concentrations of at least 8 mcg/mL. It should be kept in mind that aminoglycoside serum half-lives may lengthen during the course of treatment so that a constant relationship between dose and serum concentration may not exist. Upward adjustments in dosage therefore should be made with some degree of caution and should be followed with further determination of serum concentrations. Once-daily administration of aminoglycosides is gaining popularity, as in other settings. Obviously, such a dosing practice would result in much larger peak concentrations than those mentioned earlier. Comparative efficacy and safety of such dosing regimens in CF patients have not yet been elucidated fully, but this practice is likely to be employed increasingly as CF-specific data are generated.

β-Lactam antibiotics such as extended-spectrum penicillins should be prescribed with aminoglycosides to take advantage of their frequent synergy and to prevent the emergence of resistance. These agents should be prescribed in large doses to delay stepwise resistance. Ticarcillin, azlocillin, and piperacillin should be prescribed in a dose of at least 350 mg/kg per day divided into four to six doses. For patients with *P. aeruginosa* and *S. aureus,* the combination of an aminoglycoside and ticarcillin-clavulanate or piperacillin-tazobactam is appropriate. Selection among these agents should be based on local susceptibility patterns and cost considerations. The possible increased incidence of fever and exanthema with the newer penicillins should be kept in mind.[63] Aztreonam would be a safe and effective β-lactam to use in patients experiencing these serum sickness–like reactions to the penicillins.[64] In older patients with *P. aeruginosa* isolates with broad resistance patterns, the clinician should work closely with the microbiology laboratory to identify effective agents or combinations. The potential use of older agents with unique mechanisms of action, such as colistin, should not be overlooked.

Oral antibiotics may be prescribed in symptomatic outpatients with susceptible pathogens in their sputum. Agents with activity against common pathogens such as *S. aureus* and *H. influenzae* are useful in this setting. These typically include such antibiotics as first-generation cephalosporins, trimethoprim-sulfamethoxazole, and amoxicillin–clavulanic acid. The use of such agents on a "prophylactic" basis is discouraged because the data available at present suggest that a beneficial effect does not outweigh the risk of development of resistance among the common bacterial pathogens of CF.[65] The 4-fluoroquinolone antibiotic ciprofloxacin possesses potent activity against most CF pathogens and has been evaluated in adult patients undergoing pulmonary exacerbations. Although not conclusive because of shortcomings in the studies, available data suggest that this oral agent is as effective as standard intravenous therapy.[66] The availability of a potent oral antipseudomonal agent poses a number of potential uses in the CF population. However, it should be kept in mind that repeated or long-term use likely will lead to resistance and that antibiotics play only a supportive role in the treatment of these patients. Thus oral antibiotic therapy, regardless of efficacy, does not negate the need for other forms of therapy, which are often best administered in the hospital setting. It also should be pointed out that although ciprofloxacin appears to be safe in patients less younger 18 years of age with little evidence of joint or cartilage toxicity,[67] this agent should be used with caution in the younger population.

Treatment of Other Pulmonary Complications

The drug and nondrug treatments of the most serious of pulmonary complications, including pulmonary hypertension, right-sided heart failure, respiratory failure, pneumothorax, and hemoptysis, are beyond the scope of this chapter. In general, the therapeutic approach does not vary substantively from that for other respiratory diseases.

EVALUATION OF THERAPEUTIC OUTCOMES

GASTROINTESTINAL

The patient's nutritional status should be monitored closely on both short- and long-term bases. Height, weight, and BMI should be followed with time; anthropometric measurements give more precise information. The adequacy of pancreatic enzyme replacement can be assessed grossly by following stool patterns with the goal of normal number per day and normal consistency. Any evidence of steatorrhea may indicate suboptimal enzyme therapy. A more precise method would involve assessment of fat quantities in the stool. If a patient does not respond to normal doses of enzyme supplement, other factors that can cause similar symptoms (e.g., bloating, abdominal pain, and symptomatic steatorrhea) should be considered. These would include lack of adherence with directions for taking the enzymes, outdated enzymes, dietary factors such as excessive fruit juice consumption, high-fat meals, and concomitant gastrointestinal disease (e.g., enteric bacterial or parasitic infection, celiac disease, and inflammatory bowel disease). Vitamin status can be assessed though serum monitoring of fat-soluble vitamin concentrations.

PULMONARY

Pulmonary status can be monitored with a combination of clinical observation and examination and a variety of laboratory tests. Over the long run, pulmonary function usually is followed with spirometry, lung volumes, and oxygenation. Physical examination should focus on signs and symptoms of upper and lower respiratory tract infection. In addition, exercise tolerance, recent character of sputum production, and oxygen requirements are key to long- and short-term assessment. With antibiotic and bronchodilator treatment of acute respiratory exacerbations, a return to preexacerbation clinical status, based on physical examination or pulmonary function testing, becomes a practical end point for antimicrobial treatment. Although the goal of bacterial eradication is desirable, other attainable end points may be more reasonable, as discussed earlier. Bacterial density in sputum, sputum DNA and protein content, and C-reactive protein all have proven value as monitoring parameters but may not be available at some centers. Of the objective parameters, pulmonary function tests correlate best with clinical observations and scoring systems.[68] Response to intravenous antibiotics and aggressive chest physiotherapy, as measured by FEV_1 at the end of 1 week of treatment, has been used to predict total length of therapy necessary. In patients whose FEV_1 had recovered more than 40% at the end of 1 week, a total of 2 weeks of therapy generally was sufficient.[69] Little has been done by way of pharmacodynamic studies in treating CF. Therefore, symptomatic improvement is largely relied on to assess the relative success of antibiotic therapy. Oral antibiotic therapy also should be limited in length with specific end points, such as decreased cough and/or improved pulmonary function, identified as treatment commences.

NEW DIRECTIONS IN THERAPY

Now that the gene and gene product of CF have been identified, gene therapy becomes an obvious potential for treatment.[70] Research to date has centered on introduction of the correct gene into affected tissues. Viral vectors, chiefly adenovirus, have been studied in animal models, and human trials are under way. Liposomes may represent another useful delivery mode to introduce the correct gene.

Other novel approaches to therapy are currently being investigated and, for the most part, are directed at the inflammatory component of the disease or the basic cellular defect. Protease inhibitors hold potential in this condition for reasons cited earlier. α_1-Antitrypsin administered by aerosol shows promise, as does secretory leukocyte protease inhibitor (SLPI) and other antiproteases.[71–73] Azithromycin, perhaps not functioning as an antibiotic, slow the rate of progression of lung disease in patients chronically infected with *P. aeruginosa*.[74] In an attempt to directly approach the cellular defect in CF, the diuretic amiloride had been shown to possess positive activity in improving respiratory secretion rheology and clearance,[75] presumably by blocking excessive sodium reabsorption, but was found to be no more effective than placebo in a large-scale, controlled trial. At a similar level, the secretagogues adenosine and uridine triphosphate (ATP and UTP) have been shown to increase chloride excretion in the epithelial cells of CF patients.[76] The combination of amiloride and UTP (thereby both blocking sodium absorption and stimulating chloride secretion) also may promote clearance of airway secretions.[77] Other experimental therapies interact with the defects in CFTR production or processing. Studies with phenylbutyrate (which increases the amount of functional protein that reaches the cell surface), 8-cyclopentyl-1,3-dipropylxanthine (CPX), milrinone (a phosphodiesterase inhibitor), and genistein (a tyrosine-kinase inhibitor), each of which activate mutant CFTR, and low-concentration gentamicin (which suppresses certain premature stop mutations in *CFTR*) are all active.

It is hoped that some, if not all, of these approaches will provide viable additions to our pharmacologic armamentarium for this disease. For older, more severely affected patients who may not be able to benefit from such advances, organ transplants (single-lung, double-lung, heart-lung) are more widely available and reasonably successful.[78]

CONCLUSION

Pharmacotherapeutic intervention plays an important role in the management of these patients but is complex. The clinician is as yet faced with many unresolved issues in attempting to apply sound therapeutic principles in this population. Although close attention should be paid to pharmacologic treatment, the approach to these patients should be multifaceted and multidisciplinary in character. In addition to the involvement of such pediatric subspecialties as pulmonology, gastroenterology, pharmacology, and infectious diseases, contributions from such areas as nutrition support and social work should be a regular and ongoing part of the management effort.

ABBREVIATIONS

ATP: adenosine triphosphate
BAL: bronchoalveolar lavage
BMI: body mass index

CF: cystic fibrosis
CFTR: cystic fibrosis transmembrane regulator
$FEF_{25\%-75\%}$: forced expiratory volume from 25 to 75% of vital capacity
FEV_1: forced expiratory volume at 1 second
FVC: forced vital capacity
PaO_2: partial pressure of arterial oxygen
$PaCO_2$: partial pressure of arterial carbon dioxide
SLPI: secretory leukocyte protease inhibitor
UTP: uridine triphosphate

Review Questions and other resources are available at *www.pharmocotherapyonline.com.*

REFERENCES

1. Steinberg AG, Brown DC. On the incidence of cystic fibrosis of the pancreas. Am J Hum Genet 1960;12:416–424.
2. Wright SE, Morton NE. Genetic studies on cystic fibrosis in Hawaii. Am J Hum Genet 1968;20:157–169.
3. Rommens JM, Iannuzzi MC, Kerem B, et al. Identification of the cystic fibrosis gene: Chromosome walking and jumping. Science 1989;245:1059–1065.
4. Riordan JR, Rommens JM, Kerem B, et al. Identification of the cystic fibrosis gene: Cloning and characterization of complementary DNA. Science 1989;245:1066–1073.
5. Kerem B, Rommens JM, Buchanan JA, et al. Identification of the cystic fibrosis gene: Genetic analysis. Science 1989;245:1073–1080.
6. Welsh MJ, Smith AE. Molecular mechanisms of CFTR chloride channel dysfunction in cystic fibrosis. Cell 1993;73:1251–1254.
7. Kerem E, Corey M, Kerem B, et al. The relationship between genotype and phenotype in cystic fibrosis: Analysis of the most common mutation (ΔF_{508}). N Engl J Med 1991;323:1517–1522.
8. Mohon RT, Wagener JS, Abman SH, et al. Relationship of genotype to early pulmonary function in infants with cystic fibrosis identified through neonatal screening. J Pediatr 1993;122:550–555.
9. Collins FC. Cystic fibrosis: Molecular biology and therapeutic implications. Science 1992;256:774–779.
10. Feigelson J, Anagnostopoulos C, Poquet M, et al. Liver cirrhosis: Therapeutic implications and long term follow-up. Arch Dis Child 1993;68:653–657.
11. Goldman, MJ, Anderson GM, Stolzenberg ED, et al. Human β-defensin-1 is a salt-sensitive antibiotic in lung that is inactivated in cystic fibrosis. Cell 1997;88:553–560.
12. Pier GB, Grout M, Zaida TS, et al. Role of mutant CFTR in hypersusceptibility of cystic fibrosis patients to lung infections. Science 1996;271:64–67.
13. Wang EEL, Prober CG, Manson B, et al. Association of respiratory viral infections with pulmonary deterioration in patients with cystic fibrosis. N Engl J Med 1984;311:1653–1658.
14. Abman SH, Ogle JW, Butler-Simon N, et al. Role of respiratory syncytial virus in early hospitalizations for respiratory distress of young infants with cystic fibrosis. J Pediatr 1988;113:826–830.
15. Pribble CG, Black PG, Bosso JA, et al. Clinical manifestations of exacerbations of cystic fibrosis associated with nonbacterial infections. J Pediatr 1990;117:200–204.
16. Campbell PW, Parker RA, Roberts BT, et al. Association of poor clinical status and heavy exposure to tobacco smoke in patients with cystic fibrosis who are homozygous for the F_{508} deletion. J Pediatr 1992;120:261–264.
17. May TB, Shinabarger D, Maharaj R, et al. Alginate synthesis by *Pseudomonas aeruginosa*: A key pathogenic factor in chronic pulmonary infections of cystic fibrosis patents. Clin Microbiol Rev 1991;4:191–206.
18. Isles A, Maclusky I, Corey M, et al. *Pseudomonas cepacia* infection in cystic fibrosis: An emerging problem. J Pediatr 1984;104:206–210.

19. Hudson VL, Wielinski CL, Regelmann WE. Prognostic implications of initial oropharyngeal bacterial flora in patients with cystic fibrosis diagnosed before the age of two years. J Pediatr 1993;122:854–860.

20. Triglia JM, Belus JF, Dessi P, et al. Rhinonasal manifestations of cystic fibrosis. Ann Otolaryngol Chir Cervicofac 1993;110:98–102.

21. Lawrence JM, Moore TL, Madson KL, et al. Arthropathies of cystic fibrosis: Case reports and review of the literature. J Rheumatol 1993;20(suppl 38):12–15.

22. Rosenstein BJ, Cutting GR. The diagnosis of cystic fibrosis: A consensus statement. J Pediatr 1998;132:589–595.

23. Newborn screening for cystic fibrosis: A paradigm for public health genetics policy development. Proceedings of a 1997 workshop. MMWR Morb Mortal Wkly Rep 1997;46:1–24.

24. FitzSimmons SC. The changing epidemiology of cystic fibrosis. J Pediatr 1993;122:1–9.

25. Kerem E, Reisman J, Corey M, et al. Prediction of mortality in patients with cystic fibrosis. N Engl J Med 1992;326:1187–1191.

26. Clinical Practice Guidelines for Cystic Fibrosis Committee. Clinical Practice Guidelines for Cystic Fibrosis. Bethesda, MD, Cystic Fibrosis Foundation, 1997.

27. Riedel BD. Gastrointestinal manifestations of cystic fibrosis. Pediatr Ann 1997;26:235–241.

28. Ramsey BW, Farrell PM, Pencharz P, et al. Nutritional assessment and management in cystic fibrosis. Am J Clin Nutr 1992;55:108–116.

29. FitzSimmons SC, Burkhart GA, Borowitz D, et al. High-dose pancreatic-enzyme supplements and fibrosing colonopathy in children with cystic fibrosis. N Engl J Med 1997;336:1283–1289.

30. Nasr SZ, O'Leary MH, Hillerman C. Correction of vitamin E deficiency with fat-soluble versus water-miscible preparations of vitamin E in patients with cystic fibrosis. J Pediatr 1993;122:810–812.

31. Colombo C, Battezzati PM, Podda M, et al. Ursodeoxycholic acid for liver disease associated with cystic fibrosis: A double-blind multicenter trial. Hepatology 1996;23:1484–1490.

32. Columbo C, Grazia M, Ferrari M, et al. Analysis of risk factors for the development of liver disease associated with cystic fibrosis. J Pediatr 1994;124:393–399.

33. Ramsey BW. Management of pulmonary disease in patients with cystic fibrosis. N Engl J Med 1996;335:179–188.

34. Fuchs HJ, Borwitz DS, Christainsen DH, et al. Effect of aerosolized recombinant human DNase on exacerbations of respiratory symptoms and on pulmonary function in patients with cystic fibrosis. N Engl J Med 1994;331:637–642.

35. Spino M. Pharmacokinetics of drugs in cystic fibrosis. Clin Rev Allergy 1991;9:169–210.

36. Rosenstein BJ, Eigen H. Risks of alternate-day prednisone in patients with cystic fibrosis. Pediatrics 1991;87:245–246.

37. Eigen H, Rosenstein BJ, FitzSimmons S, et al. A multicenter study of alternate-day prednisone therapy in patients with cystic fibrosis. J Pediatr 1995;126:515–523.

38. Konstan MW, Byard PJ, Hoppel CL, et al. Effect of high-dose ibuprofen in patients with cystic fibrosis. N Engl J Med 1995;332:848–854.

39. Beardsmore CS, Thompson JR, Williams A, et al. Pulmonary function in infants with cystic fibrosis: The effect of antibiotic treatment. Arch Dis Child 1994;71:133–137.

40. Jensen T, Pedersen SS, Høiby N, et al. Use of antibiotics in cystic fibrosis: The Danish approach. Antibiot Chemother 1989;42:237–246.

41. Grimwood K, Semple RA, Rabin HR, et al. Elevated exoenzyme expression by *Pseudomonas aeruginosa* is correlated with exacerbations of lung disease in cystic fibrosis. Pediatr Pulmonol 1993;15:135–139.

42. Gold R, Carpenter S, Heurter H, et al. Randomized trial of ceftazidime versus placebo in the management of acute respiratory exacerbations in patients with cystic fibrosis. J Pediatr 1987;111:907–913.

43. Parry MF, Neu HC, Merlino M, et al. Treatment of pulmonary infections in patients with cystic fibrosis: A comparative study of ticarcillin and gentamicin. J Pediatr 1977;90:144–148.

44. Møller NE, Høiby N. Antibiotic treatment of chronic *Pseudomonas aeruginosa* infection in cystic fibrosis patients. Scand J Infect Dis 1981;24(suppl):87–91.

45. Friis B. Chemotherapy of chronic infections with mucoid *Pseudomonas aeruginosa* in lower airways of patients with cystic fibrosis. Scand J Infect Dis 1979;11:211–217.

46. Krause PJ, Young LS, Cherry JD, et al. The treatment of exacerbations of pulmonary disease in cystic fibrosis: Netilmicin compared with netilmicin and carbenicillin. Curr Ther Res 1979;25:609–617.

47. Aronoff SC, Klinger JD. In vitro activities of aztreonam, piperacillin and ticarcillin combined with amikacin against amikacin-resistant *Pseudomonas aeruginosa* and *P. cepacia* isolates from children with cystic fibrosis. Antimicrob Agents Chemother 1984;25:279–280.

48. Bosso JA, Allen JE, Matsen JM. Changing susceptibility of *Pseudomonas aeruginosa* isolates from cystic fibrosis patients with the clinical use of newer antibiotics. Antimicrob Agents Chemother 1989;33:526–528.

49. Thomassen MJ, Klinger JD, Badger SJ, et al. Cultures of thoracotomy specimens confirm usefulness of sputum cultures in cystic fibrosis. J Pediatr 1984;104:352–356.

50. Lindsay CA, Bosso JA. Optimization of antibiotic therapy in cystic fibrosis patients. Clin Pharmacokinet 1993;24:496–506.

51. Spino M, Chai RP, Isles AF, et al. Assessment of glomerular filtration rate and effective renal plasma flow in cystic fibrosis. J Pediatr 1985;107:64–70.

52. Bosso JA, Townsend PL, Herbst JJ, et al. Pharmacokinetics and dosage requirements of netilmicin in cystic fibrosis patients. Antimicrob Agents Chemother 1985;28:829–831.

53. Moore RD, Smith CR, Lietman PS. Association of aminoglycoside plasma levels with therapeutic outcome in gram-negative pneumonia. Am J Med 1984;77:657–662.

54. Noone P, Parsons MC, Pattison JR, et al. Experience in monitoring gentamicin therapy during treatment of serious gram-negative sepsis. Br J Med 1974;1:477–481.

55. Kearns GL. Hepatic drug metabolism in cystic fibrosis: Recent developments and future directions. Ann Pharmacother 1993;27:74–79.

56. Bosso JA, Liu Q, Evans WE, et al. CYP2D6, *N*-acetylation, and xanthine oxidase activity in cystic fibrosis. Pharmacotherapy 1996;16:749–753.

57. MacDonald NE, Anas NG, Peterson RG, et al. Renal clearance of gentamicin in cystic fibrosis. J Pediatr 1983;103:985–990.

58. Nahata MC, Lubion AH, Visconti JA. Cephalexin pharmacokinetics in patients with cystic fibrosis. Dev Pharmacol Ther 1984;7:221–228.

59. Spino M, Chai RP, Isles AF, et al. Cloxacillin absorption and disposition in cystic fibrosis. J Pediatr 1984;105:829–835.

60. Jacobs RF, Trang JM, Kearns GL, et al. Ticarcillin/clavulanic acid pharmacokinetics in children and young adults with cystic fibrosis. J Pediatr 1985;106:1001–1007.

61. Bosso JA, Relling MV, Townsend PL, et al. Intrapatient variations in aminoglycoside disposition in cystic fibrosis. Clin Pharmacol 1987;6:54–58.

62. Ramsey BW, Dorkin HL, Eisenberg JD, et al. Efficacy of aerosolized tobramycin in patients with cystic fibrosis. N Engl J Med 1993;328:1740–1746.

63. Møller NE, Eriksen KR, Feddersen C, et al. Chemotherapy against *Pseudomonas aeruginosa* in cystic fibrosis: A study of carbenicillin, azlocillin, or piperacillin in combination with tobramycin. Eur J Respir Dis 1982;63:130–139.

64. Jensen T, Koch C, Pedersen SS, et al. Aztreonam for cystic fibrosis patients who are hypersensitive to other β-lactams. Lancet 1987;1:1319–1320.

65. Beardsmore CS, Thompson JR, Williams A, et al. Pulmonary function in infants with cystic fibrosis. Arch Dis Child 1994;71:133–137.

66. Bosso JA. Use of ciprofloxacin in cystic fibrosis patients. Am J Med 1989;87(suppl 5A):123–127S.

67. Høiby N, Pedersen SS, Jensen T, et al. Fluoroquinolones in the treatment of cystic fibrosis. Drugs 1993;45(suppl 3):98–101.

68. Bosso JA, Walker KB. Lack of correlation between objective indicators and clinical-response scores during antimicrobial therapy for acute pulmonary exacerbations of cystic fibrosis. Clin Pharm 1988;7:897–901.

69. Rosenberg SM, Schramm CM. Predictive value of pulmonary function testing during pulmonary exacerbations in cystic fibrosis. Pediatr Pulmonol 1993;16:227–235.

70. Rosenfeld MA, Collins FS. Gene therapy for cystic fibrosis. Chest 1996;109:241–252.

71. McElvaney NG, Hubbard RC, Birrer P, et al. Aerosol α_1-antitrypsin treatment for cystic fibrosis. Lancet 1991;337:392–394.

72. McElvaney NG, Nakamura H, Birrer P, et al. Modulation of airway inflammation in cystic fibrosis: In vivo suppression of interleukin 8 levels on the respiratory epithelial surface by aerosolization of recombinant secretory leukoprotease inhibitor. J Clin Invest 1992;90:296–301.

73. Meyer KC, Kewandeski JR, Zimmerman JJ, et al. Human neutrophil elastase and elastase/alpha$_1$-antiprotease complex in cystic fibrosis. Am Rev Respir Dis 1991;144:580–585.

74. Saiman L, Marshall BC, Mayer-Hamblett N, et al. Azithromycin in patients with cystic fibrosis chronically infected with *Pseudomonas aeruginosa*: A randomized controlled trial. JAMA 2003;290:1749–1756.

75. Knowles MR, Church NL, Waltner WE, et al. A pilot study of aerosolized amiloride for the treatment of lung disease in cystic fibrosis. N Engl J Med 1990;322:1189–1194.

76. Knowles MR, Clarke LL, Boucher RC. Activation by extracellular nucleotides of chloride secretion in the airway epithelia of patients with cystic fibrosis. N Engl J Med 1991;325:533–538.

77. Bennett WD, Olivier KN, Zeman KL, et al. Effect of uridine 5′-triphosphate plus amiloride on mucociliary clearance in adult cystic fibrosis. Am J Respir Crit Care Med 1996;153:1796–1801.

78. Yankaskas JR, Westerman JH, Thompson JT, et al. Improved results of lung transplantation for patients with cystic fibrosis. J Thorac Cardiovasc Surg 1995;109:224–234.

31
EVALUATION OF THE GASTROINTESTINAL TRACT

Marie A. Chisholm and Mark W. Jackson

KEY CONCEPTS

◀1 The patient history is key to evaluating GI problems and should include the problem onset, the setting in which it developed, and its presentation.

◀2 A complete physical exam should be performed with detailed attention to the overall condition of the patient and focused attention should be given to the patient's abdomen.

◀3 Contrast agents such as barium sulfate are effective in examining the GI tract for structural diseases.

◀4 The upper GI series involves radiographic visualization of the esophagus, stomach, and small intestine; whereas the lower GI series involves visualization of the colon and rectum.

◀5 Enteroclysis is used to evaluate the small bowel by introducing contrast agents by tube through the nose or mouth.

◀6 GI ultrasonography, computed tomography, and magnetic resonance imaging provide images of the gallbladder, liver, pancreas, and abdominal wall.

◀7 Radionuclide imaging is useful to visualize the liver, spleen, bile ducts, gallbladder, and gut.

◀8 The endoscope, an illuminated optical instrument, revolutionized the diagnosis and management of GI disorders with common endoscopic studies including esophagogastroduodenoscopy, colonoscopy, sigmoidoscopy, and endoscopic retrograde cholangiopancreatography.

◀9 There is an evolving role for capsule endoscopy (an encapsulated camera swallowed by the patient that takes pictures of the GI tract) in the assessment of the small bowel.

The gastrointestinal (GI) tract is composed of organs and tissues that have diverse forms and functions. It includes the esophagus, stomach, small intestine, large intestine, colon, rectum, biliary tract, gallbladder, liver, and pancreas. Despite the rapid proliferation of technology for the diagnosis of digestive diseases, the patient history and physical examination still hold central roles. When combined with a thorough patient history and physical examination, diagnostic procedures are essential in the evaluation of GI disorders. This chapter describes the most commonly used tools available in clinical practice to evaluate patients with GI diseases.

SYMPTOMS OF GASTROINTESTINAL DYSFUNCTION

A variety of symptoms can arise from GI dysfunction. Common GI symptoms include heartburn, abdominal pain, dyspepsia, nausea, vomiting, diarrhea, constipation, and gastrointestinal bleeding. Signs and symptoms of malabsorption, hepatitis, and GI infection are also commonly seen. The next sections describe methods that are commonly used to assess patients with GI complaints. For specific details concerning each GI disease state, please consult that particular chapter in this book.

PATIENT HISTORY

◀1 A comprehensive patient history is the cornerstone in the evaluation of a patient with digestive complaints. A clear, detailed, chronologic account of the patient's problems should be ascertained. This account should include the onset of the problem, the setting in which it developed, and its manifestations. The onset of the problem often provides important information that helps to confirm diagnosis. For example, biliary pain, such as that encountered with symptomatic gallstone disease, typically evolves over minutes and lasts for hours, but pain caused by pancreatitis evolves over hours and lasts for days. The setting is always relevant as it provides clues to the possible origin of the disorder. For example, is the patient an alcoholic (liver disease, esophageal varices, or pancreatitis)? Does the patient have severe atherosclerosis (mesenteric ischemia)? Is the patient immunosuppressed (opportunistic infection)? Also aiding in the differential diagnosis is identification of factors that alleviate or exacerbate the principal symptom. For instance, ingesting a meal often relieves the pain of duodenal ulcer, but worsens that of gastric ulcer. The health care professional should ask questions that address the potential etiologic possibilities, including motility disorders, structural diseases, malignancies, infections, psychosocial factors, dietary factors, and travel-associated diseases.[1,2] Questions concerning past medical and

TABLE 31–1. General Questions in a Gastrointestinal History

1. Tell me about the problem that you are experiencing. When did it start?
2. Where is your pain located? Please point to the area where you feel pain. What were you doing when the pain occurred? How rapidly did the pain come on? Is your pain constant or intermittent? What factors exacerbate or alleviate your pain? Does the pain awaken you at night?
3. What medications are you taking to help the pain? How much do you take? Do these medications work?
4. What other medications are you currently taking? Why are you taking them?
5. Have you recently had a change in dietary intake? If so, please describe. Can you draw any correlation between the foods that you eat and your GI complaint?
6. Have you recently had a change in bowel habits? Have you experienced any diarrhea or constipation lately? Do you experience painful bowel movements?
7. Have you experienced any nausea or vomiting lately? If so, please describe conditions centered around this event.
8. Have you experienced any recent change in weight? Was this intentional? How many pounds have you gained or lost and over what time period did this occur? How has your appetite been?
9. Have you passed any blood from your rectum or vomited blood? Have you noticed any dark, tarry stools?
10. Have you had any acid indigestion?
11. Do you have difficulty swallowing?
12. Has anyone in your family experienced similar GI complaints? If so, please describe. Does anyone in your family have a history of GI disorders, including cancer of the GI tract?
13. Describe your past medical history, including illnesses and surgeries.
14. Please describe any past injuries that you have experienced.
15. Have you recently traveled outside of the United States? If so, where? When? How long did you stay? What kind of living conditions did you experience? What foods and drinks did you ingest?

TABLE 31–2. Drugs That May Commonly Cause Gastrointestinal Injury

Gastrointestinal Mucosal Injury	Liver Damage (Continued)
Aspirin	Isoniazid
Bisphosphonates	Ketoconazole
Chemotherapeutic agents	Methotrexate
Corticosteroids	Methyldopa
Ethacrynic acid	Monoamine oxidase
Ethanol	inhibitors
Gentian violet	Niacin
Iron preparations	Nifedipine
Isoproterenol	Nitrofurantoin
Nonsteroidal anti-inflammatory agents	Phenytoin
Pancrease supplementation	Propylthiouracil
Potassium chloride	Pyridium
Reserpine	Rifampin
Warfarin	Salicylates
Jaundice	Sulfonamides
Acetohexamide	Tetracycline
Androgens	Verapamil
Chlorpropamide	Warfarin
Corticosteroids	Zidovudine
Erythromycin	**Pancreatitis**
Estrogens	Azathioprine
Ethanol	Corticosteroids
Gold salts	Didanosine
Nitrofurantoin	Estrogens
Phenothiazines	Ethacrynic acid
Warfarin	Ethanol
Liver Damage	Furosemide
Acetaminophen	Metronidazole
Allopurinol	Opiates
Aminosalicylic acid	Pentamidine
Dapsone	Sulindac
Erythromycin	Sulfonamides
Ethanol	Tetracycline
Glyburide	Thiazides

family history detailing illnesses, surgeries, injuries, and habits are extremely valuable (Table 31–1). Because many drugs have been reported to cause GI injury, a patient's medication history is also vital (Table 31–2).

PHYSICAL EXAMINATION

Because the organ systems of the body interact and may provide important data needed for diagnosis, it is necessary to perform a thorough physical examination.[3] A global evaluation of the patient should be performed with notable attention to appearances and vital signs because they may suggest clues to the patient's overall condition and stability. Careful examination of the abdomen is also an essential part of the work-up. Examination of the abdomen is classically approached by inspection, auscultation, percussion, and palpation. Inspection of the abdomen may reveal scars, hernias, bulges, or peristalsis. Auscultation is mainly focused on analysis of bowel sounds and identification of bruits. Percussion of the abdomen allows for detection of tympany, measurement of visceral organs, and detection of ascites. Palpation may allow the clinician to identify tenderness, rigidity, masses, and hernias. A digital rectal examination is used to detect masses, tenderness, and assess muscle tone. Stool on the examiner's glove obtained during rectal examination is often subjected to hemoccult testing for the indirect detection of occult blood.[2,3]

LABORATORY AND MICROBIOLOGIC TESTS

Laboratory and microbiologic tests may be used to (a) assess organ function, (b) screen for certain GI disorders, and (c) evaluate the effectiveness of therapy. To achieve an accurate diagnosis and provide the best care, it is important to assess the patient's fluid and electrolyte status, nutritional status, and abdominal organ function. A serum chemistry panel provides clinicians with valuable information. For example, serum creatinine (S_{Cr}) and blood urea nitrogen (BUN) are often used as a measure of hydration status, as well as serving as indicators for renal function. Elevations in S_{Cr} and BUN may be indicative of renal dysfunction or dehydration, and bleeding from the GI tract may lead to elevations in BUN. Albumin levels can be used to assess the patient's nutritional and hydration status and provide information concerning hepatic and renal function. Specifically, low albumin may be indicative of malnutrition, hepatic dysfunction, nephrotic syndromes, or protein-losing enteropathies such as Crohn's disease and ulcerative colitis. Serum measurements of sodium, chloride, and potassium are useful to determine electrolyte abnormalities associated with diarrheal illnesses. A complete blood count (CBC) helps to provide information concerning infection, malignancy, bone marrow suppression, anemia, and blood loss.[4]

Specific laboratory blood tests are used as screening tools for certain GI disorders. For example, measurements of serum aspartate transaminase (AST) and alanine transaminase (ALT) are elevated in most diseases of the liver, and serum alkaline phosphatase and bilirubin are often elevated in hepatobiliary disorders. Because prothrombin time is related to hepatocyte synthesis of vitamin K–dependent clotting factors, it serves as an indirect measure of hepatic function. When evaluating patients with suspected pancreatitis, serum and urine measurements of amylase and lipase are important, because these will be elevated in most patients with acute pancreatitis (see Chap. 39).

Microbiologic studies are useful in evaluating patients with unexplained diarrhea, abdominal pain, and suspected GI infections. Microbiologic studies of the stool may be used to detect the presence of bacteria and parasites. Pathogens most often responsible for infectious diarrhea and enteritis include bacteria such as *Shigella, Salmonella, Escherichia coli,* and *Yersinia;* viruses such as cytomegalovirus, especially in AIDS patients; and parasites such as *Entamoeba histolytica* and *Giardia lamblia.*[5] Because *Helicobacter pylori* is a significant factor associated with peptic ulcer disease and gastritis, identification of this organism is critical in evaluating patients experiencing dyspepsia (see Chap. 33).

DIAGNOSIS

The patient history, physical examination, and routine laboratory tests are extremely useful in establishing a diagnosis, but frequently a more specific study is required to confirm or disprove a clinical suspicion. The most appropriate diagnostic test depends on the anatomic region involved, the suspected abnormality, patient preference, the patient's overall condition, and clinical manifestations of the patient. The next sections outline the most frequently used diagnostic studies and procedures and their roles in evaluating the GI tract.

RADIOLOGY

Radiologic procedures rely on the differential absorption of radiation of adjacent tissues to highlight anatomy and pathology. Radiologic procedures important in evaluating the GI tract include plain radiography, upper GI series, lower GI series, and enteroclysis.[6,7]

PLAIN RADIOGRAPHY OF THE GI SYSTEM

Radiographic evaluation of the GI tract often starts with plain films of the abdomen, which are straightforward, uncontrasted radiographs.[7] Specific abdominal structures that may be identified include the kidney, ureters, and bladder (KUB); esophagus; stomach; intestine; stones; and vessels. Plain films are often used to evaluate abdominal pain. Clinicians frequently employ plain radiographic fluoroscopy to guide and position other instruments that are used to evaluate and treat GI disorders; an example is the manipulation of dilation devices to treat esophageal strictures. Bowel obstruction and perforation are especially well identified by this technique.

CONTRAST AGENTS

Many different types of contrast agents are available. Two types of contrast agents commonly used to enhance visualization of the GI tract are barium sulfate and aqueous iodinated compounds. Barium sulfate is the contrast agent of choice for studying the esophagus, stomach, and intestine, except in special clinical situations.[7] Barium sulfate is not generally absorbed, and constipation is the most frequent adverse effect reported with its use. Two widely used iodinated contrast agents for visualizing the GI tract are diatrizoate meglumine and diatrizoate sodium. Unlike barium, these agents are relatively nontoxic if inadvertently introduced into the peritoneal cavity; therefore the main indication for use of iodinated agents in GI radiography is

for suspected bowel perforation. Because iodinated contrast agents are hyperosmolar, they possess the potential to cause severe diarrhea, dehydration, and electrolyte imbalances. Nephrotoxicity associated with iodinated contrast agents may occur and is generally self-limited.[7,8] Allergies and hypersensitivity reactions such as rashes associated with contrast agents are possible and should be monitored and treated accordingly.

UPPER GI SERIES

The upper GI series refers to the radiographic visualization of the esophagus, stomach, and small intestine. Patient preparation for an upper GI usually consists of instructing patients to refrain from eating or drinking 8 to 12 hours prior to testing, thereby allowing the upper GI tract to empty. A contrast agent such as barium sulfate is administered to the patient at the beginning of the study. The observed swallowing of the contrast agent permits visualization and monitoring of esophageal structural and motor functions. This phase of the procedure is most often referred to as a barium swallow. As the contrast medium flows into the stomach and small intestine, several regional radiographic films are taken in order to inspect these areas. This tracking of contrast agents through the small intestine is referred to as the small bowel follow-through. The upper GI series with the small bowel follow-through includes the examination of the esophagus to the distal end of the small intestine, and is useful to evaluate and detect obstructions, tumors, ulcers, and abnormal intestinal loops. The upper GI series with small bowel follow-through commonly uncovers gastric cancer, peptic ulcer disease, esophagitis, gastric outlet obstruction, and Crohn's disease (Fig. 31–1).

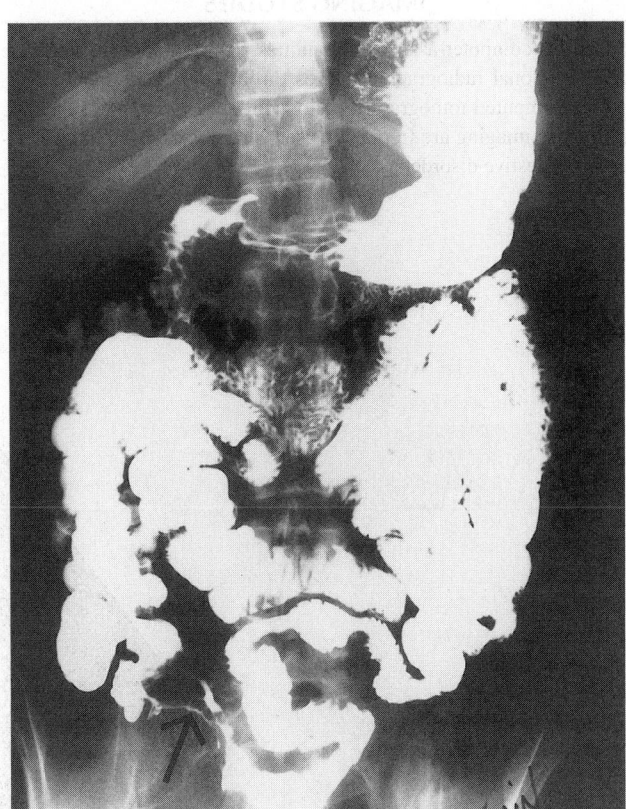

FIGURE 31–1. Upper GI series with small bowel follow-through demonstrating narrowed distal terminal ileum and separation of small bowel loops (*arrow*). These findings are consistent with Crohn's disease.

LOWER GI SERIES

The lower GI series is used to examine the colon and rectum. Patients complaining of lower abdominal pain, constipation, or diarrhea are often referred for a lower GI series. Before the procedure the colon is prepared by instructing the patient to refrain from eating or drinking 8 to 12 hours before the procedure, and by administering bowel-cleansing agents such as bisacodyl, magnesium citrate, magnesium hydroxide, or polyethylene glycol-electrolyte solution. During a lower GI series, a barium sulfate enema is given to contrast the terminal large intestine and rectum. The lower GI series is useful to detect and evaluate enterocolitis, obstructions, volvulus, and mucosal and structural lesions.[7] The lower GI series is commonly used to diagnose Crohn's disease, ulcerative colitis, colon cancers, and diverticulitis.

SMALL BOWEL ENTEROCLYSIS

Enteroclysis or small bowel enema refers to the technique of direct small bowel introduction of a contrast agent through a tube inserted through the patient's mouth or nose. Intermittent radiographic films are taken of the small bowel as the contrast agent flows distally (Fig. 31–2). Because enteroclysis provides detailed imaging, it is an accurate method for evaluating the small bowel and for detecting small mucosal lesions that may be overlooked on the traditional small bowel follow-through.[9] Methylcellulose is used to enhance the detail of the small intestine in enteroclysis, thereby improving visualization. Patient preparation for this procedure involves instructing patients to refrain from eating or drinking 8 to 12 hours before testing and administering bowel-cleansing agents. The most frequent disorder evaluated by enteroclysis is obscure GI bleeding.

IMAGING STUDIES

By using computer-assisted techniques, it is possible to generate cross-sectional radiographic images through the body. Ultrasonography, computed tomography, radionuclide scanning, and magnetic resonance imaging are frequently used imaging procedures for evaluating digestive disorders.

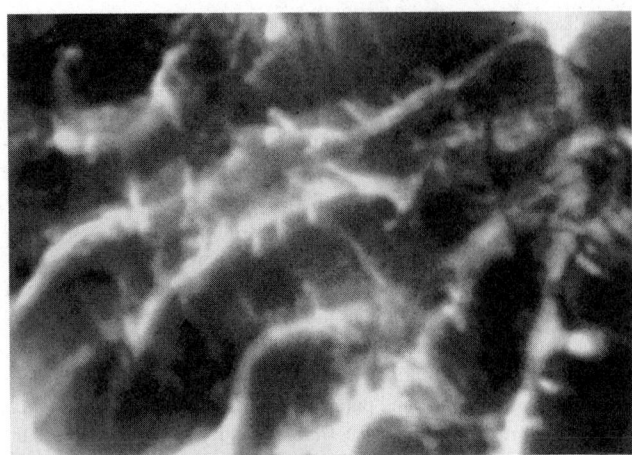

FIGURE 31–2. Normal small bowel enteroclysis. Contrast agents are instilled into the small bowel to highlight tumors, strictures, or other lesions. In this image, one can identify the normal circular folds.

ULTRASONOGRAPHY

Ultrasonography provides images of deeper structures such as the gallbladder, liver, pancreas, and abdominal wall. The clinician is able to image slices of the GI tract by directing a narrow beam of high-energy sound waves into the body and recording the reflections from the various organs and structures. Because ultrasonography is noninvasive, relatively inexpensive, requires no ionizing radiation, and can be performed with a portable unit, it is a well-accepted and useful technology. It accurately depicts gallstones and gallbladder, and hepatobiliary and pancreatic diseases (Fig. 31–3). When combined with Doppler technologies, ultrasonography may image GI vascularity. Ultrasonography is limited by the presence of bowel gas and excessive amounts of body fat.[10,11]

COMPUTED TOMOGRAPHY

Computed tomography (CT) or computed axial tomography (CAT) scans provide detailed images of the GI system in which transverse

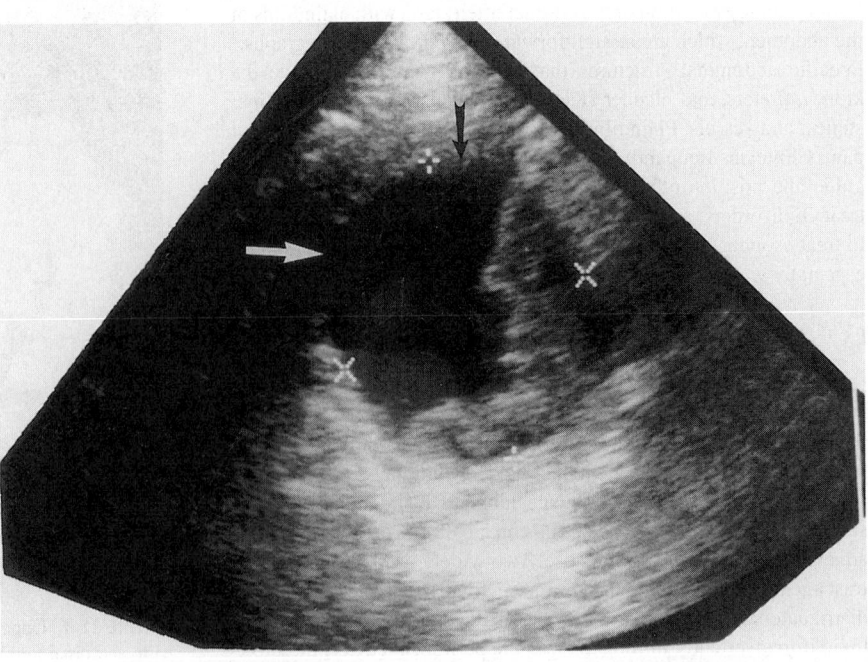

FIGURE 31–3. Abdominal ultrasound demonstrating a chronic pancreatic pseudocyst (*arrows*).

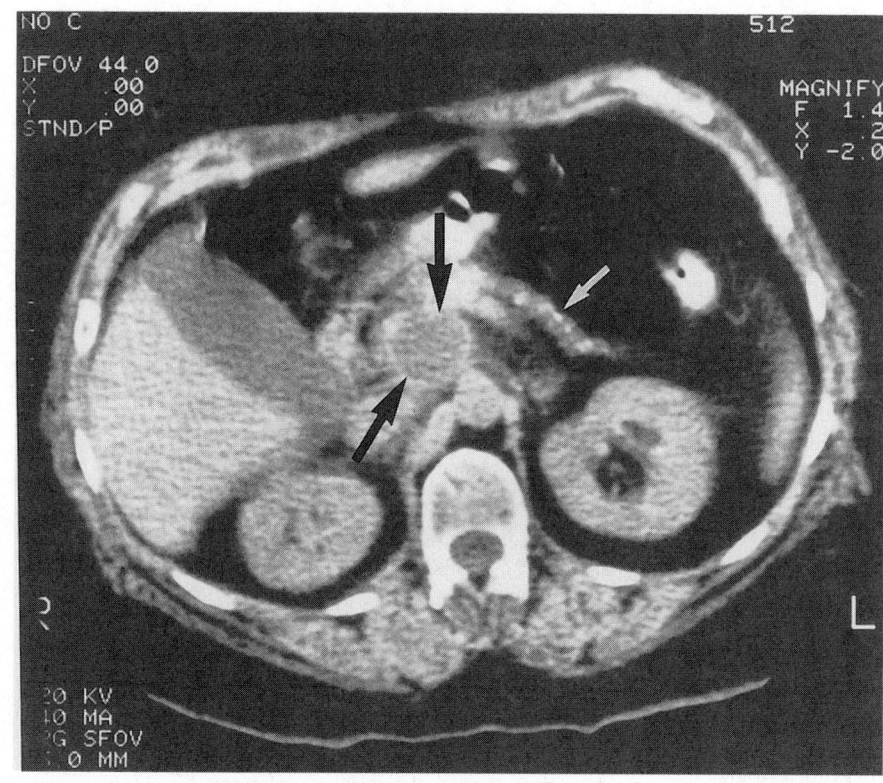

FIGURE 31–4. CT scan of the abdomen showing pancreatitis with calcification (*white arrow*) and pancreatic pseudocyst (*black arrows*).

planes of tissue are swept by a radiographic beam and a computer analysis of the variance in absorption produces a precise reconstructed image of that area.[6] Contrast agents may be added in a CT procedure to illuminate specific hollow structures and vascularity of the GI tract. The abdominal CT displays organs from the diaphragm down to the pelvic brim, and is especially valuable for detecting GI diseases of the liver, pancreas, spleen, and colon. Patient preparation for CT includes refraining from eating or drinking for a minimum of 4 hours before the test. The remarkable detail that CT offers in imaging organs and tissues adds to its popularity for evaluation of the GI system. CT is useful in the identification of liver cancer, pancreatitis, pancreatic cancer, intra-abdominal abscesses, and cysts (Fig. 31–4).[10] Unlike ultrasonography, patient body size or the presence of gas does not limit the quality of imaging with CT.

RADIONUCLIDE IMAGING

Radionuclide imaging involves intravenous injections of a radiopharmaceutical imaging agent and the use of a computerized detection camera to gather images. Although the choice of a radiopharmaceutical agent depends on the specific organ or function being studied, the most commonly used agent is technetium (Tc-99m) tagged to a carrier molecule. Radiographic imaging is useful to visualize the liver and spleen (liver-spleen scan), bile ducts, gallbladder (HIDA [hepatoiminodiacetic acid] scan), and gut (bleeding scan).[10] Cysts, abscesses, tumors, and obstructions are detected and displayed as areas of differential uptake of radioactivity (Fig. 31–5).[6] Radionuclide bleeding scans may detect hemorrhages and may assist in localization.

MAGNETIC RESONANCE IMAGING

Magnetic resonance imaging (MRI) places the patient in close proximity to a high-strength magnetic field through which pulses of

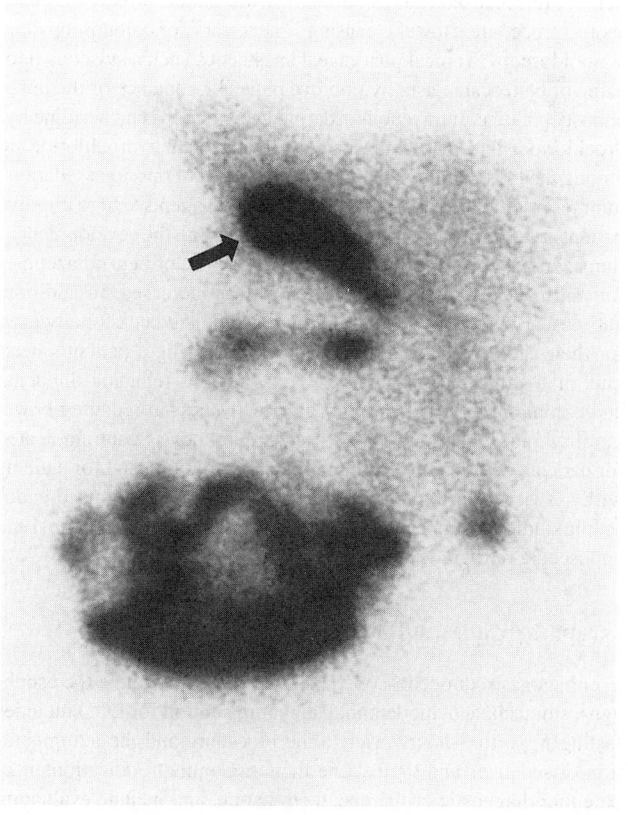

FIGURE 31–5. HIDA scan demonstrating normal gallbladder (*arrow*).

radiofrequency radiation are projected, thereby exciting the nuclei of hydrogen, phosphorus, oxygen, and other elements. The radiofrequency signals are manipulated and recorded by a computer, and a two-dimensional image representing a section of the patient is produced.[10] MRI has greater sensitivity to identify liver tumors than ultrasonography, CT, or radionuclide imaging. Although currently MRI is not as popular as other imaging techniques because of limited availability, expense, and problems associated with the use of powerful magnetic fields, its use is predicted to increase in the future.[11]

ARTERIOGRAPHY

Arteriography of the gut depicts the configuration of visceral blood vessels after intravenous administration of a contrast medium. Arteriography may be employed for detecting tumors and bleeding lesions and therapeutic applications, including embolization of bleeding vessels, fistulas, and inoperable tumors.[10]

ENDOSCOPY

Refinement in optical engineering and fiber optics has made possible the development of the endoscope, which has revolutionized the management of GI disorders. An endoscope is an illuminated optical instrument designed to inspect the interior of the GI tract. Endoscopes enable the practitioner to inspect intraluminal mucosal lesions and to obtain biopsies and washings for cytology studies. Upper GI tract endoscopy (esophagogastroduodenoscopy) is capable of inspecting the esophagus, stomach, and proximal small bowel. Lower GI tract endoscopy of the rectum and colon may be accomplished by colonoscopy or sigmoidoscopy. Endoscopy can also be used to perform many therapeutic procedures.

Preparation for endoscopic examinations includes instructing patients to refrain from eating or drinking 8 to 12 hours prior to the endoscopic procedure. Bowel cleansing is necessary for colonoscopy and sigmoidoscopy. Topical pharyngeal anesthetics such as viscous lidocaine or benzocaine usually improve patient acceptance of the upper endoscopic tube. Intravenous sedating agents such as meperidine hydrochloride, diazepam, lorazepam, and midazolam hydrochloride are among the most common agents used to induce "conscious sedation" minutes prior to the endoscopy. These sedating agents tend to improve patient acceptance and ease of the procedure. With the development of flumazenil, a benzodiazepine antagonist, the use of benzodiazepines for mild sedation during GI procedures has increased. In addition, antimuscarinic agents such as atropine sulfate are occasionally used for their cardiovascular effects, such as increasing a patient's heart rate, or for their antispasmodic effects, such as reducing duodenal and colonic motility. Because of its effectiveness at reducing bowel motility, glucagon is also often used. Endoscopy is contraindicated for patients with severe respiratory or cardiac failure, and for patients with suspected perforated viscera. The most commonly used endoscopic studies are upper endoscopy, colonoscopy, sigmoidoscopy, and endoscopic retrograde cholangiopancreatography.

ESOPHAGOGASTRODUODENOSCOPY

Esophagogastroduodenoscopy (EGD) is used to examine the esophagus, stomach, and duodenum. Patient preparation for EGD includes fasting for 6 to 8 hours prior to the procedure and the administration of sedatives and topical anesthetics. Common indications may be either diagnostic or therapeutic in nature, and include evaluating suspected upper GI bleeding, obstructions, upper abdominal pain,

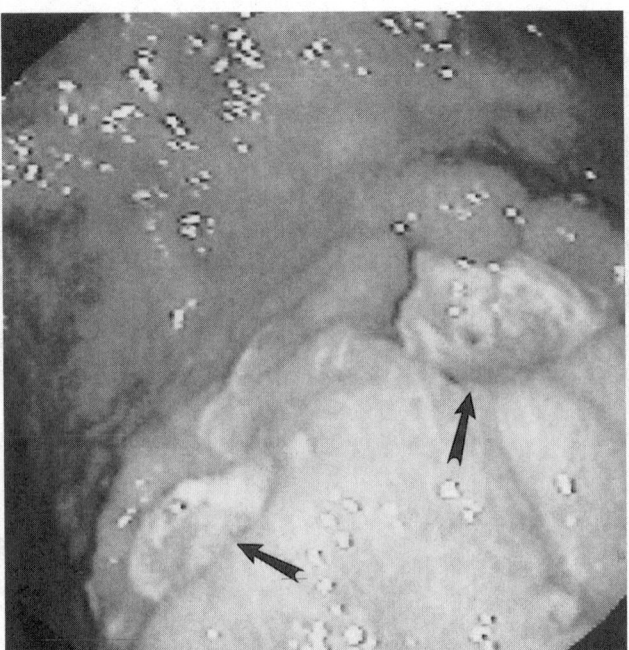

FIGURE 31–6. Deep "punched out" gastric ulcers (*arrows*) as shown by EGD.

persistent vomiting, and radiographic abnormalities.[12] EGD commonly uncovers peptic ulcers and other lesions (Fig. 31–6).

COLONOSCOPY

Colonoscopy permits direct examination of the large intestine and rectum. To prepare for colonoscopy, the patient should fast for about 8 hours prior to the examination, and bowel cleansing should be completed. Agents such as midazolam and meperidine are usually given to produce conscious sedation. Similarly to upper GI endoscopy, indications for lower GI endoscopy can be either diagnostic or therapeutic in nature, and include evaluation and detection of abnormalities visualized by radiography, as well as GI hemorrhage, colonic lesions, volvulus, ulcerative colitis, Crohn's disease, diverticulitis, and excision of colonic polyps.[13]

SIGMOIDOSCOPY

Sigmoidoscopy is used to evaluate the sigmoid colon and rectum (Fig. 31–7). Flexible sigmoidoscopy has virtually replaced rigid sigmoidoscopy because of increased patient comfort and superior performance. The major indication for this examination is to evaluate symptoms related to the colon or rectum, and to conduct screening of asymptomatic patients for colon polyps or cancer. Patient preparation involves instructing patients to abstain from eating or drinking 8 to 12 hours prior to the procedure and administering bowel-cleansing agents. Anoscopy is especially useful in evaluating the anus. The major indications for anoscopic examination include symptoms related to the anus and rectum, such as bleeding, protrusions or swelling, pain, and severe itching. Patients undergoing sigmoidoscopy or anoscopy generally do not require sedation.

ENDOSCOPIC RETROGRADE CHOLANGIOPANCREATOGRAPHY

Endoscopic retrograde cholangiopancreatography (ERCP) is an important procedure that is used to evaluate and treat diseases of the biliary tree and pancreas. By injecting contrast agents through a catheter

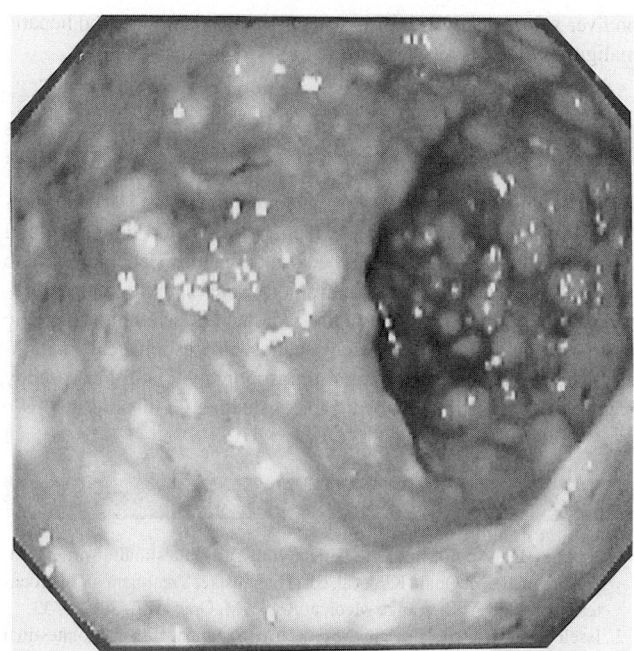

FIGURE 31–7. Sigmoidoscopic photograph revealing the light-raised lesions of antibiotic-associated pseudomembranous colitis.

placed in the pancreaticobiliary ducts during ERCP, abnormalities such as obstructions, calculi, and strictures can be examined. ERCP also allows for the use of therapeutic techniques such as the removal of ductal stones, stenting of strictures, and sphincterotomy. Preparation for ERCP consists of conscious sedation and glucagon to relax gut motility. Common reasons for ERCP include detection and evaluation of pancreatic malignancy, pancreatitis, biliary obstruction, bile duct stones, jaundice, and patients whose clinical presentation suggests biliary disease (Fig. 31–8).

CAPSULE ENDOSCOPY

Capsule endoscopy allows the visualization of the small intestine, and consists of a vitamin-pill–sized video camera that is swallowed and acts as an endoscope. While the video capsule travels naturally through the digestive tract, images are transmitted to a recording device. Patients return the recording device to the practitioner so that the images can be downloaded to a computer and evaluated. Eventually, the camera is naturally excreted and not retrieved.[14]

MISCELLANEOUS TESTS

ESOPHAGEAL MANOMETRY

Esophageal manometry is used to evaluate diseases of the esophagus by assessing esophageal motor functions. Common indications for this procedure include dysphagia and obscure chest pain. A special catheter equipped with pressure transducers is placed into the esophagus to measure esophageal pressures and peristalsis. Provocative testing with pharmacologic agents such as edrophonium chloride, a cholinergic muscle stimulant, may be used to precipitate esophageal pain during this procedure. Typical indications for esophageal manometry include evaluating esophageal dysmotility, nonobstructive dysphagia, obscure chest pain, scleroderma, intestinal pseudo-obstruction, achalasia, and aiding in positioning instruments such as pH probes.

AMBULATORY pH MONITORING

Gastric fluid pH monitoring in patients who complain of gastroesophageal reflux may be necessary. Indications for pH monitoring include evaluating atypical chest pain and severe or unusual reflux disorders. Ambulatory 24-hour pH monitoring is an elegant way to link esophageal acid exposure, as detected by a probe in the esophagus, with patient symptoms. The pH probe is placed approximately 5 cm above the distal esophagus. Because intraesophageal pH is normally higher (pH ≥6) than that of the stomach (pH approximately 1 to 3), the pH probe will record a decrease in pH if gastroesophageal reflux occurs. The ambulatory 24-hour pH study links the patient's symptom to an acid event (Fig. 31–9).

The Bernstein test, another procedure used to measure gastric fluid pH, is less expensive than ambulatory pH monitoring. This procedure requires inserting a nasogastric (NG) tube and administrating

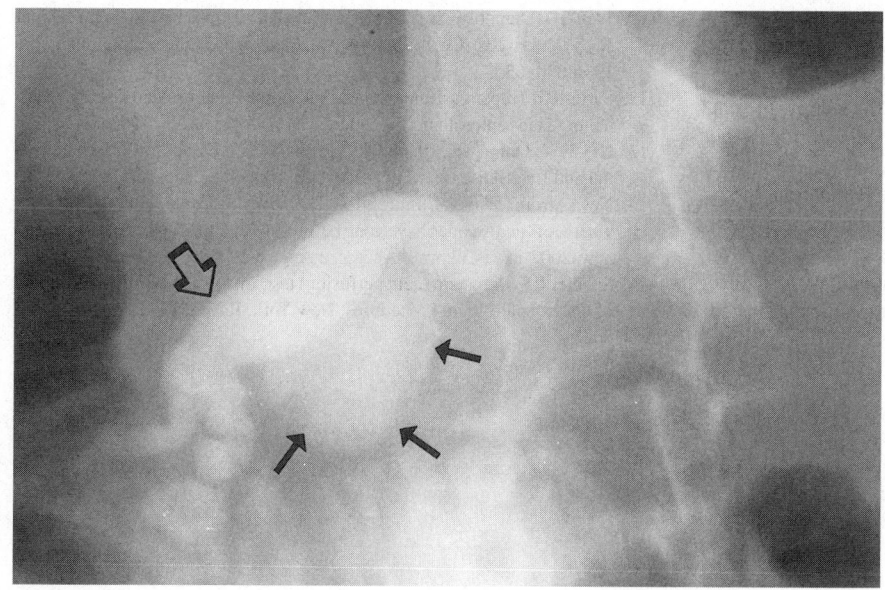

FIGURE 31–8. ERCP demonstrating a dilated, irregular pancreatic duct with areas of stricturing (*large arrow*). A pancreatic pseudocyst is visible immediately adjacent to the spine (*small arrows*).

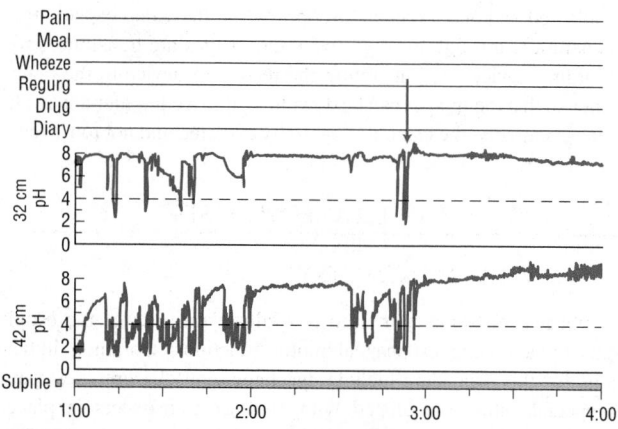

FIGURE 31–9. Ambulatory pH monitoring. The pH recordings from two esophageal probes are plotted over a 3-hour interval. Notice that the patient's symptom of regurgitation correlates with a low pH (<4) event (*arrow*).

alternating dripped solutions of normal saline and 0.1 N hydrochloric acid (HCl) into the esophagus via the NG tube. If patient symptoms are reproduced by the acid perfusion and not the saline, the study is considered abnormal and indicative of acid hypersensitivity.[15]

ENDOSCOPIC ULTRASONOGRAPHY

In recent years, endoscopic ultrasonography has emerged as a useful adjunct in the diagnosis and staging of gastroenterologic disorders. The instrument itself functions very much like a typical upper endoscope but with the added feature of an ultrasound transducer. The examiner is then able to see the regional anatomy and pathology beneath the mucosa. The major advantage of this procedure is its capability to deliver the ultrasound transducer to close proximity of deep tissues for enhanced image resolution. In clinical practice, endoscopic ultrasound is highly useful in detecting and defining gastrointestinal and pancreatic malignancies. It also plays a role in the diagnosis of submucosal lesions and small pancreatic malignancies. Endoscopic ultrasound guidance of fine-needle biopsy is increasingly performed.

LAPAROSCOPY

Laparoscopy uses a tube-like device with an elaborate optical system that permits distinct visualization of the peritoneal cavity. General anesthesia is often given and a surgical incision is made in the abdomen to allow the passage of the laparoscope. The exterior of the liver, gallbladder, spleen, peritoneum, diaphragm, and pelvic organs may be clearly examined during the laparoscopic examination. Similar to the other endoscopic techniques mentioned, biopsies and therapeutic interventions may be performed during the laparoscopy. Reasons for doing laparoscopy include evaluating patients with ascites, abdominal masses, chronic abdominal pain, abnormalities indicated

on liver-spleen scan, liver diseases, obstructive jaundice, and hepatic malignancy.

CONCLUSIONS

Evaluation of the GI tract begins with a careful history and comprehensive physical examination. It then proceeds in a deliberate and thoughtful manner to establish the correct diagnosis and appropriate management. Laboratory and microbiologic tests, radiography, ultrasonography, computed tomography, radionuclide scanning, magnetic resonance imaging, arteriography, endoscopy, esophageal manometry, pH monitoring, endoscopic ultrasonography, and laparoscopy have definite roles in diagnosing and evaluating GI disorders.

REFERENCES

1. Kearney DJ. Approach to the patient with gastrointestinal disorders. In: Friedman SL, McQuaid KR, et al, eds. Diagnosis & Treatment in Gastroenterology. New York, Lange Medical Books/McGraw-Hill, 2003:1–33.
2. Isselbacher KJ, Podolsky DK. Approach to the patient with gastrointestinal disease. In: Wilson JD, Braunwald E, et al, eds. Harrison's Principles of Internal Medicine. New York, McGraw-Hill, 1991:1213–1216.
3. Bates B. A Guide to Physical Examination. Philadelphia, Lippincott, 1994.
4. Jacobs DS, Demott WR, Finley PR, et al. Laboratory Test Handbook. Cleveland, Lexi-Comp, 1994.
5. Guerrant RL. Principles and syndromes of enteric infection. In: Mandell GL, Douglas RG, et al, eds. Principles and Practice of Infectious Diseases. New York, Churchill Livingstone, 1990:837–851.
6. Novelline RA. Squire's Fundamentals of Radiology. Cambridge, Harvard University Press, 1997.
7. Cohen AJ. Radiologic general diagnostic and imaging studies of the small and large bowel. In: Gitnick G, ed. Principles and Practice of Gastroenterology and Hepatology. Stamford, CT, Appleton & Lange, 1994:411–432.
8. Smith CR, Petty BG. Specific complications of medical management. In: Harvey AM, Johns RT, et al, eds. The Principles and Practice of Medicine. Stamford, CT, Appleton & Lange, 1988:1155–1162.
9. Miller RE, Sellink JL. Enteroclysis: The small bowel enema. How to succeed and how to fail. Gastrointest Radiol 1979;4:269–283.
10. Friedman LS, Needleman L. Hepatobiliary imaging. In: Wilson JD, Braunwald E, et al, eds. Harrison's Principles of Internal Medicine. New York, McGraw-Hill, 1991:1303–1308.
11. Wall SD. Diagnostic imaging procedures in gastro-enterology. In: Bennet JC, Plum F, eds. Cecil Textbook of Medicine. Philadelphia, Saunders, 1996:630–635.
12. Sartor RB Upper gastrointestinal endoscopy. In: Drossman DA, ed. Manual of Gastroenterologic Procedures. New York, Raven, 1993:131–139.
13. Hay DW, Onion SK. Blackwell's Primary Care Essentials: Gastrointestinal and Liver Disease. Malden, MA, Blackwell Science, 2002:363.
14. News from Mayo Clinic in Jacksonville. Capsule endoscopy goes where few endoscopes have gone before, 2002. http:www.mayoclinic.org/news2002-jax/1432.html. Accessed August 29, 2003.
15. Sandler RS. Bernstein (acid perfusion) test. In: Drossman DA, ed. Manual of Gastroenterologic Procedures. New York, Raven, 1993:56–60.

32

GASTROESOPHAGEAL REFLUX DISEASE

Dianne B. Williams and Robert R. Schade

Learning Objectives and other resources can be found at *www.pharmacotherapyonline.com*.

KEY CONCEPTS

◄1 Patients should be assessed for symptoms, such as heartburn, and for signs and symptoms of complications that require immediate medical attention, such as dysphagia or bleeding.

◄2 Endoscopy is used to evaluate mucosal damage from gastroesophageal reflux disease (GERD) and assess for the presence of Barrett's esophagus (BE); 24-hour ambulatory pH testing or a therapeutic trial of a proton pump inhibitor are useful for diagnosing GERD in patients with persistent symptoms or atypical symptoms; manometry is useful in evaluating motility and before antireflux surgery.

◄3 The goals of treatment of GERD are to alleviate symptoms, to decrease the frequency of recurrent disease, to promote healing of mucosal injury, and to prevent complications.

◄4 Treatment of GERD involves a stepwise approach determined by disease severity and includes lifestyle changes and patient-directed therapy (phase I); pharmacologic treatment with nonprescription and prescription medications (phase II); and interventional approaches such as antireflux surgery or endoluminal therapies (phase III).

◄5 Patients with typical GERD symptoms should be treated with lifestyle modifications and a trial of empiric acid-

suppression therapy. Those who do not respond to empiric therapy or who have more complicated symptoms should undergo diagnostic tests.

◄6 Interventional approaches (antireflux surgery or endoluminal therapies) offer an alternative treatment for refractory GERD or when pharmacologic management is undesirable.

◄7 Acid suppression is the mainstay of GERD treatment. H_2-receptor antagonists in divided doses are effective in less severe GERD. Proton pump inhibitors provide the greatest relief of symptoms and highest rates of healing, especially in patients with erosive disease or moderate to severe symptoms.

◄8 Many patients with GERD will relapse if medication is withdrawn, so long-term maintenance treatment is required. A proton pump inhibitor is the drug of choice for maintenance of patients with moderate to severe GERD.

◄9 Patient medication profiles should also be reviewed for drugs that may aggravate GERD. Patients should be monitored for adverse drug reactions and potential drug-drug interactions of drugs used to treat GERD. Finally, patients should be assessed for compliance to their therapeutic regimen.

Gastroesophageal reflux disease (GERD) is a common medical disorder and patients with this condition are seen by clinicians from various specialties. GERD refers to any symptomatic clinical condition or histologic alteration that results from episodes of gastroesophageal reflux. Gastroesophageal reflux is the retrograde movement of gastric contents from the stomach into the esophagus. When the esophagus is repeatedly exposed to refluxed material for prolonged periods of time, inflammation of the esophagus (reflux esophagitis) occurs, and in some cases it can progress to erosion of the squamous epithelium of the esophagus (erosive esophagitis). Complications of long-term reflux may include the development of strictures, Barrett's esophagus, or adenocarcinoma of the esophagus. Gastroesophageal reflux associated with disease processes in organs other than the esophagus, such as the lungs, is referred to as atypical (or extra-esophageal) GERD.[1] Severe reflux symptoms associated with normal endoscopic findings are referred to as symptomatic GERD, nonerosive reflux disease (NERD), or endoscopy-negative reflux disease (ENRD).

Many patients suffering from mild GERD do not go on to develop erosive esophagitis and are often managed with lifestyle changes, antacids, and nonprescription histamine (H_2)-receptor

antagonists or nonprescription proton pump inhibitors. Those with more severe symptoms (with or without endoscopic findings) predictably follow a course of relapsing disease requiring more intensive treatment with acid-suppressive therapy followed by long-term maintenance therapy.[2] Interventional therapies including antireflux surgery and endoluminal therapies offer an alternative to medical management for those patients who fail therapy or for those patients in whom medical management is undesirable.

EPIDEMIOLOGY

Gastroesophageal reflux disease occurs in both adults and children. Although mortality associated with GERD is rare (1 death per 100,000 patients), GERD symptoms have a greater impact on quality of life than do duodenal ulcers, untreated hypertension, mild congestive heart failure, angina, or menopause.[3,4]

The true prevalence and incidence of GERD is difficult to assess because (a) many patients do not seek medical treatment, (b) symptoms do not always correlate well with severity of disease, and (c) there is no standardized definition or universal gold standard method for diagnosing the disease.[3]

Approximately 44% of the American population suffer from GERD symptoms monthly, and more than 20% suffer with symptoms on a weekly basis.[5] Despite the prevalence of GERD, many patients choose not to seek medical help from a physician and self-treat with nonprescription medications or consult only with their pharmacist. This may be due to their lack of understanding of symptoms of GERD, including heartburn, or it may be due to some financial or personal reason. Heartburn is the hallmark symptom of GERD and is generally described as a substernal sensation of warmth or burning rising up from the abdomen that may radiate to the neck. It may be waxing and waning in character. Interestingly, as many as 46% of patients with mild disease will heal spontaneously with self-medication, and another 31% will show significant improvement, indicating a relatively benign process in patients with minimal symptoms.[6]

Conversely, the presence of symptoms in patients who do seek medical advice does not always correlate well with the presence of esophageal inflammation or erosion. Of the 20% to 40% of patients who experience heartburn, 30% to 79% of these patients will have evidence of esophagitis.[7] On the other hand, many patients with esophageal damage may not experience symptoms, or they may present with atypical symptoms.[8] Finally, the lack of a standardized definition and universal gold standard for diagnosing GERD presents another obstacle in assessing epidemiologic data.

The prevalence of GERD varies depending on the geographic region, but appears highest in Western countries.[3] The prevalence increases in adults older than 40 years of age. Except during pregnancy and possibly nonerosive reflux disease, there does not appear to be a major difference in incidence between men and women. Heartburn is a common complaint during pregnancy. NERD may occur more commonly in women and in patients who are approximately a decade younger than patients who develop erosive disease. Although gender does not generally play a major role in the development of GERD, it is an important factor in the development of Barrett's esophagus (BE), a complication of GERD in which the normal squamous epithelium is replaced with specialized columnar epithelium. BE is most prevalent in caucasian adult males in Western countries.

PATHOPHYSIOLOGY

The key factor in the development of GERD is the retrograde movement of acid or other noxious substances from the stomach into the esophagus.[9] In some cases, gastroesophageal reflux is associated with defective lower esophageal sphincter (LES) pressure or function. Patients may have decreased gastroesophageal sphincter pressures related to (a) spontaneous transient LES relaxations, (b) transient increases in intra-abdominal pressure, or (c) an atonic LES—all of which may lead to the development of gastroesophageal reflux. Problems with other normal mucosal defense mechanisms such as anatomic factors, esophageal clearance, mucosal resistance, gastric emptying, epidermal growth factor, and salivary buffering may also contribute to the development of GERD. Aggressive factors that may promote esophageal damage upon reflux into the esophagus include gastric acid, pepsin, bile acids, and pancreatic enzymes. Thus the composition and volume of the refluxate as well as duration of exposure are the most important aggressive factors in determining the consequences of gastroesophageal reflux. Rational therapeutic regimens in the treatment of gastroesophageal reflux are designed to maximize normal mucosal defense mechanisms and attenuate the aggressive factors.

Several complications may occur with gastroesophageal reflux, including esophagitis, esophageal strictures, Barrett's esophagus, and adenocarcinoma of the esophagus. Strictures are common in the distal esophagus and are generally 1 to 2 cm in length. The use of nonsteroidal anti-inflammatory drugs (NSAIDs) or aspirin has been implicated as an additional risk factor that may contribute to the development or worsening of esophageal strictures.[10] Although GERD may lead to esophageal bleeding, the blood loss is usually chronic and low grade in nature, but can lead to anemia. In some patients, the reparative process leads to the replacement of the squamous epithelial lining of the esophagus by specialized columnar-type epithelium. This condition, known as Barrett's esophagus, is more likely to occur in those patients with a long history (years) of symptomatic reflux that in many cases improves without intervention.[11] Barrett's esophagus can be found in 3.5% to 12% of patients undergoing first-time endoscopy for reflux symptoms, and the prevalence is probably higher in patients with more severe or complicated disease.[12] Patients with BE have a greater than 30% incidence of esophageal stricture formation. Additionally, the risk of esophageal adenocarcinoma is 30 to 60 times higher in patients with BE as compared to the general population.[13] Interestingly, the risk of esophageal adenocarcinoma could be increased in patients with long-standing frequently recurring reflux symptoms (heartburn and regurgitation) despite the presence or absence of BE.[13]

LOWER ESOPHAGEAL SPHINCTER PRESSURE

The LES is a manometrically defined zone at the distal esophagus with an elevated basal resting pressure. The sphincter is normally in a tonic, contracted state, preventing the reflux of gastric material from the stomach, but relaxes on swallowing to permit the free passage of food into the stomach.

Mechanisms by which defective LES pressure may cause gastroesophageal reflux are threefold. First, and probably most importantly, reflux may occur following spontaneous transient LES relaxations that are not associated with swallowing.[14] Although the exact mechanism is unknown, esophageal distention, vomiting, belching, and retching have all been shown to cause relaxation of the LES. While not thought to contribute significantly to erosive esophagitis, these transient relaxations, which are normal postprandially, may play an important role in intermittent nonerosive reflux.[2] Transient decreases in sphincter pressure are responsible for approximately 65% of the reflux episodes in patients with GERD. The propensity to develop gastroesophageal reflux secondary to transient decreases in LES pressure is probably dependent on numerous factors, including the degree of sphincter relaxation, efficacy of esophageal clearance, patient position (more common in recumbent position), gastric volume, and intragastric pressure. Second, reflux may occur following transient increases in intra-abdominal pressure (stress reflux).[9] An increase in intra-abdominal pressure such as that occurring during straining, bending over, coughing, eating, or a Valsalva maneuver may overcome a weak LES, and thus may lead to reflux. Third, the LES may be atonic, thus permitting free reflux as seen in patients with scleroderma, for instance. Although transient relaxations are more likely to occur when there is normal LES pressure, the latter two mechanisms are more likely to occur when the LES pressure is decreased by such factors as fatty foods, gastric distention, smoking, or certain medications.[9] Table 32–1 lists medications and foods that affect lower esophageal sphincter pressures.[15] Various foods aggravate esophageal reflux by decreasing LES pressure or by precipitating symptomatic reflux by direct mucosal irritation (e.g., spicy foods, orange juice, tomato juice, and coffee).

Pregnancy, treated achalasia, and scleroderma are conditions in which reflux is common. There are many postulated reasons for the

TABLE 32–1. Foods and Medications That May Worsen GERD Symptoms

Decreased lower esophageal sphincter pressure

Foods

Fatty meal	Garlic
Carminatives (peppermint, spearmint)	Onions
Chocolate	Chili peppers
Coffee, cola, tea	

Medications

Anticholinergics	Isoproterenol
Barbiturates	Narcotics (meperidine, morphine)
Benzodiazepines (diazepam)	
Caffeine	Nicotine (smoking)
Dihydropyridine calcium channel blockers	Nitrates
Dopamine	Phentolamine
Estrogen	Progesterone
Ethanol	Theophylline

Direct irritants to the esophageal mucosa

Foods

Spicy foods	Tomato juice
Orange juice	Coffee

Medications

Alendronate	Quinidine
Aspirin	Potassium chloride
Iron	
Nonsteroidal anti-inflammatory drugs	

Adapted from Weinberg and Kadish.[15]

increased incidence of heartburn during pregnancy, including hormonal effects on esophageal muscle, LES tone, and physical factors (increased intra-abdominal pressure) resulting from an enlarging uterus.[16]

A decrease in LES pressure resulting from any of the previously mentioned causes is not always associated with gastroesophageal reflux. Likewise, individuals who experience decreases in sphincter pressures, and subsequently reflux, do not always develop GERD. The other natural defense mechanisms (anatomic factors, esophageal clearance, mucosal resistance, and other gastric factors) must be evoked to explain this phenomenon.

ANATOMIC FACTORS

Proposed anatomic factors contributing to reflux can be categorized into valvular mechanisms, extrinsic compression, a segment of the esophagus in the chest, mucosal choke, and spiral stretch mechanisms. Disruption of the normal anatomic barriers by a hiatal hernia was once thought to be a primary etiology of gastroesophageal reflux and esophagitis. Now it appears that a more important factor related to the presence or absence of symptoms in patients with hiatal hernia is the LES pressure. The size of a hiatal hernia is proportional to the frequency of transient LES relaxations.[17] Patients with hypotensive LES pressures and large hiatal hernias are more likely to experience gastroesophageal reflux following abrupt increases in intra-abdominal pressure, compared to patients with a hypotensive LES and no hiatal hernia. Although anatomic factors are still considered significant by some, the diagnosis of hiatal hernia is currently considered a separate entity with which gastroesophageal reflux may or may not simultaneously occur.

ESOPHAGEAL CLEARANCE

In many patients with GERD, the problem is not that they produce too much acid, but that the acid produced spends too much time in contact with the esophageal mucosa. Approximately 50% of GERD patients with esophagitis have a prolonged acid clearance time from the esophagus.[9] This is not surprising, because the symptoms and/or severity of damage produced by gastroesophageal reflux are partially dependent on the duration of contact between the gastric contents and the esophageal mucosa.[18] This contact time is in turn dependent on the rate at which the esophagus clears the noxious material, as well as the frequency of reflux. The esophagus is cleared by primary peristalsis in response to swallowing, or by secondary peristalsis in response to esophageal distention and gravitational effects. Swallowing contributes to esophageal clearance by increasing salivary flow. Saliva contains bicarbonate that buffers the residual gastric material on the surface of the esophagus. The production of saliva decreases with increasing age, making it more difficult to maintain a neutral intra-esophageal pH. Therefore esophageal damage due to reflux occurs more often in the elderly, and similarly in patients with Sjögren's syndrome or xerostomia.[19] Swallowing is also decreased during sleep, making nocturnal GERD a problem in many patients.

MUCOSAL RESISTANCE

Within the esophageal mucosa and submucosa there are mucus-secreting glands. The mucus secreted by these glands may contribute to the protection of the esophagus.[20] Bicarbonate moving from the blood to the lumen can neutralize acidic refluxate in the esophagus. When the mucosa is repeatedly exposed to the refluxate in GERD, or if there is a defect in the normal mucosal defenses, hydrogen ions diffuse into the mucosa, leading to the cellular acidification and necrosis that ultimately cause esophagitis.[9] In theory, mucosal resistance may be related not only to esophageal mucus, but also to tight epithelial junctions, epithelial cell turnover, nitrogen balance, mucosal blood flow, tissue prostaglandins, and the acid-base status of the tissue.[20] Saliva is also rich in epidermal growth factor, stimulating cell renewal.

GASTRIC EMPTYING

Delayed gastric emptying can contribute to gastroesophageal reflux. An increase in gastric volume may increase both the frequency of reflux and the amount of gastric fluid available to be refluxed. Gastric volume is related to the volume of material ingested, rate of gastric secretion, rate of gastric emptying, and amount and frequency of duodenal reflux into the stomach. Factors that increase gastric volume and/or decrease gastric emptying, such as smoking and high-fat meals, are often associated with gastroesophageal reflux. This partially explains the prevalence of postprandial gastroesophageal reflux. Fatty foods may increase postprandial gastroesophageal reflux by increasing gastric volume, delaying the gastric emptying rate, and decreasing the LES pressure. Patients with gastroesophageal reflux, particularly infants, may have a defect in antral motility. The delay in emptying may promote regurgitation of feedings, which might in turn contribute to two common complications of GERD in infants (i.e., failure to thrive and pulmonary aspiration).[21]

COMPOSITION OF REFLUXATE

The composition, pH, and volume of the refluxate are the most important aggressive factors in determining the consequences of gastroesophageal reflux. In animals, acid has two primary effects when it refluxes into the esophagus. First, if the pH of the refluxate is less than 2, esophagitis may develop secondary to protein denaturation. In addition, pepsinogen is activated to pepsin at this pH and may also cause esophagitis. Duodenogastric reflux esophagitis or "alkaline" refers to esophagitis induced by the reflux of bilious and pancreatic fluid. The term *alkaline esophagitis* may be a misnomer in that the refluxate may be either weakly alkaline or acidic in nature. An increase in gastric bile concentrations may be caused by duodenogastric reflux due to a generalized motility disorder, or slower clearance of the refluxate or following surgery.[22]

Although bile acids have both a direct irritant effect on the esophageal mucosa and an indirect effect of increasing hydrogen ion permeability of the mucosa, symptoms are more often related to acid reflux than to bile reflux. Esophageal pH monitoring demonstrates that severity of disease is related to degree of esophageal acid exposure and not so much to bile exposure. Specifically, the percentage of time that the esophageal pH is below 4 is greater for patients with severe disease as compared to those with mild disease.[23,24] However, esophageal pH monitoring in conjunction with 24-hour bile monitoring has been associated with a higher incidence of BE in patients with both acid and alkaline reflux.[22] More study is needed to substantiate this finding. Nevertheless, the combination of acid, pepsin, and/or bile is a potent refluxate in producing esophageal damage.

The pathophysiology of gastroesophageal reflux is a complex cyclic process. It is difficult, if not impossible, to determine which occurs first: gastroesophageal reflux leading to defective peristalsis with delayed clearing, or an incompetent LES pressure leading to gastroesophageal reflux. Understanding the factors associated with the development of GERD provides insight into the treatment modalities currently used to manage a patient who suffers from the disease.

CLINICAL PRESENTATION

Patients with GERD may display symptoms described as (a) typical, (b) atypical, or (c) complicated. Table 32–2 summarizes each of these clinical presentations of GERD.[11] The severity of

TABLE 32–2. Clinical Presentation of GERD

Typical symptoms: May be aggravated by activities that worsen gastroesophageal reflux such as recumbent position, bending over, or eating a meal high in fat.

- Heartburn
- Water brash (hypersalivation)
- Belching
- Regurgitation

Atypical symptoms: In some cases, these extraesophageal symptoms may be the only symptoms present, making it more difficult to recognize GERD as the cause, especially when endoscopic studies are normal.

- Nonallergic asthma
- Chronic cough
- Hoarseness
- Pharyngitis
- Chest pain
- Dental erosions

Complicated symptoms: These symptoms may be indicative of complications of GERD such as Barrett's esophagus, esophageal strictures, or esophageal cancer.

- Continual pain
- Dysphagia
- Odynophagia
- Bleeding
- Unexplained weight loss
- Choking

From Schindelbeck et al.[30]

the symptoms of gastroesophageal reflux does not always correlate with the degree of esophagitis, but it does correlate with the duration of reflux. It is important to distinguish GERD symptoms from those of other diseases, especially when chest pain or pulmonary symptoms are present. Interestingly, approximately 50% of patients presenting with chest pain who have a normal electrocardiogram have GERD.[9] Similarly, 53% of patients with asthma have GERD.[25] Patients presenting with asthma (especially nocturnal asthma) that is poorly responsive to standard medical therapies should be evaluated to determine if GERD contributes to their symptoms.[11] Pulmonary symptoms result from either direct irritation of the vagus nerve when refluxed acid comes in contact with the esophageal mucosa, causing bronchospasm (the reflex theory); or less commonly from aspiration of the refluxate into the lungs, causing chemical irritation that manifests as pneumonia or pulmonary fibrosis (the reflux theory).[26]

Patients who are not adequately treated for GERD may go on to develop complications from long-term acid exposure. Long-term, recurrent reflux symptoms that are not adequately treated may lead to the development of Barrett's esophagus and may be an independent risk factor for the development of esophageal adenocarcinoma.[13] Esophageal strictures may be present in patients presenting with dysphagia. However, these symptoms may occur in other esophageal disorders such as esophageal diverticulum, achalasia, obstruction, esophageal spasm, esophageal infections, scleroderma, and malignancy. The presence of complicated symptoms should be further investigated to differentiate other diseases as the cause.

The tests that are useful in diagnosing GERD include endoscopy, 24-hour ambulatory pH monitoring, proton pump inhibitor administration as a diagnostic tool, and manometry.

The most useful tool in the diagnosis of gastroesophageal reflux is the clinical history, including both presenting symptoms and associated risk factors. Patients presenting with mild, typical symptoms of reflux (heartburn and regurgitation) do not usually require invasive esophageal evaluation. These patients generally benefit from an initial trial of lifestyle modifications and patient-directed nonprescription drug therapies. A clinical diagnosis of GERD can be assumed in patients who respond to appropriate therapy.[27]

Endoscopy is the preferred technique for assessing the mucosa for esophagitis and for the presence of complications such as Barrett's esophagus.[27] It enables visualization and biopsy of the esophageal mucosa. Although less expensive than endoscopy, barium radiography lacks the sensitivity and specificity needed to accurately determine the presence of mucosal injury or to distinguish between BE and esophagitis.[27] For these reasons barium radiography has limited use in the routine diagnosis of GERD.[27]

In patients with atypical symptoms, 24-hour ambulatory pH monitoring may be the only way to objectively prove the symptoms are reflux-related. Ambulatory pH monitoring may also be useful in patients who are on what is considered adequate therapy, but whose symptoms are not improving. However, GERD that is truly refractory to medical therapy is uncommon.[27] Continuous pH monitoring can be performed by passing a small pH probe intranasally and placing it approximately 5 cm above the LES.[19] Patients keep a diary of symptoms and these are correlated with the pH measurement corresponding to the time the symptom was reported. In addition to correlating symptoms to abnormal esophageal acid exposure, 24-hour ambulatory pH monitoring also documents the percentage of time the intraesophageal pH is low and determines the frequency and severity of reflux.[19,27] Problems with esophageal pH monitoring arise when different methods are used to perform the test or a patient's baseline differs significantly from the standard baseline. Additionally, pH monitoring is not readily available in many institutions. The empiric

TABLE 32–3. Endoscopic Classification of Esophagitis

Grade 0	Normal esophageal mucosa
Grade 1	Erythema or diffusely red mucosa and edema causing accentuated folds
Grade 2	Isolated round or linear erosions extending from the gastroesophageal junction upwards, not involving the entire circumference
Grade 3	Confluent erosions extending around the entire circumference or superficial ulceration without stenosis
Grade 4	Complicated cases; erosions as above, plus deep ulcerations, strictures, or columnar epithelium–lined esophagus

From Savary and Miller.[34]

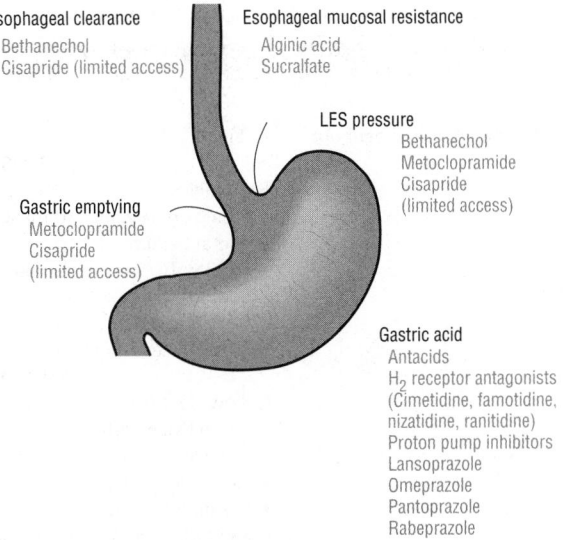

FIGURE 32–1. Therapeutic interventions in the management of gastroesophageal reflux disease. Pharmacologic interventions are targeted at improving defense mechanisms or decreasing aggressive factors. (LES, lower esophageal sphincter.)

use of standard dose, or even double-dose, omeprazole as a therapeutic trial for diagnosing the presence of GERD may be as beneficial as ambulatory 24-hour pH monitoring in diagnosing GERD. This approach is less expensive, more convenient, and more readily available than ambulatory pH monitoring, and has shown promise in patients with typical and atypical symptoms of GERD as well.[28–32] It seems to be especially useful in those patients in whom other gastrointestinal disorders such as esophageal erosions, peptic ulcers, and carcinomas, have been ruled out by endoscopy, but symptoms are still present. Preliminary results have also been promising in patients with extraesophageal symptoms.[33] Problems with using a proton pump inhibitor as a diagnostic tool include lack of a standardized dosing regimen and duration of the diagnostic trial.

Esophageal manometry to evaluate motility should be performed in any patient who is a candidate for antireflux surgery.[27] Esophageal manometry is useful in determining which surgical procedure is best for the patient. To perform manometry, a multilumen tube is passed into the stomach and the pressures are measured as the tube is pulled back across the lower esophageal sphincter, esophagus, and pharynx.

Several systems have been used to classify severity of GERD; a common grading scale is shown in Table 32–3.[34] Although endoscopy is a highly specific test, it is not extremely sensitive. In mild cases of GERD, the esophageal mucosa may appear relatively normal; however, obtaining mucosal biopsies may increase diagnostic yield. In addition, noninflammatory GERD and major motor disorders may be missed by endoscopy.

TREATMENT

DESIRED OUTCOMES

Therapeutic modalities used in the treatment of gastroesophageal reflux are targeted at reversing the various pathophysiologic abnormalities. The goals of treatment are to (a) alleviate or eliminate the patient's symptoms; (b) decrease the frequency or recurrence and duration of gastroesophageal reflux; (c) promote healing of the injured mucosa; and (d) prevent the development of complications. Therapy is directed at augmenting defense mechanisms that prevent reflux and/or decrease the aggressive factors that worsen reflux or mucosal damage (Fig. 32–1). Specifically, therapy is directed at (a) decreasing the acidity of the refluxate; (b) decreasing the gastric volume available to be refluxed; (c) improving gastric emptying; (d) increasing LES pressure; (e) enhancing esophageal acid clearance; and (f) protecting the esophageal mucosa.

▶ TREATMENT: Gastroesophageal Reflux Disease

■ GENERAL APPROACH TO TREATMENT

The treatment of GERD is categorized into one of the following modalities: (1) lifestyle changes and patient-directed therapy with antacids, nonprescription H₂-receptor antagonists, and/or nonprescription proton pump inhibitors; (2) pharmacologic intervention primarily with standard or high-dose acid-suppressing agents; (3) and interventional therapies (antireflux surgery or endoluminal therapies) (Table 32–4). The initial therapeutic modality used is in part dependent on the patient's condition (frequency of symptoms, degree of esophagitis, and presence of complications). Historically, a step-up approach has been used, starting with noninvasive lifestyle modifications and patient-directed therapy, and progressing to pharmacologic management or interventional approaches.[6,8,9] A step-down approach, starting with a proton pump inhibitor given once or twice daily instead of an H₂-receptor antagonist, and then stepping down to

the lowest degree of acid suppression needed to control symptoms, is also effective. Neither the "step-up" nor "step-down" approach has superior efficacy or cost effectiveness over the other. The clinician should determine the most appropriate approach for an individual patient.[27] Whichever method is used, every attempt should be made to aggressively control symptoms and to prevent relapses early in the course of the patient's disease in order to prevent the complications that are seen with long-standing symptomatic GERD.[35] In patients with moderate to severe GERD, starting with a proton pump inhibitor as initial therapy is advocated because of its superior efficacy over H₂-receptor antagonists.

Dietary and lifestyle modifications and education about factors that may worsen GERD symptoms should be discussed with the patient.[27] Table 32–5 lists many of the lifestyle changes that are included in phase I therapy.[8,36] Although most patients do not respond to lifestyle changes alone, the importance of maintaining these lifestyle changes throughout the course of GERD therapy should

TABLE 32–4. Therapeutic Approach to GERD

Patient Presentation	Recommended Treatment Regimen	Comments
Phase I Intermittent, mild heartburn	A. Lifestyle Changes **PLUS** B. Antacids • Maalox or Mylanta 30 mL as needed or after meals and at bedtime • Maalox TC 5–10 mL as needed or after meals and at bedtime • Gaviscon 2 tabs after meals and at bedtime • Calcium carbonate (500 mg) 2–4 tablets as needed **AND/OR** C. Low-dose OTC H_2-receptor antagonists (each taken up to twice daily) • Cimetidine 200 mg • Famotidine 10 mg • Nizatidine 75 mg • Ranitidine 75 mg **OR** OTC proton pump inhibitor (taken once daily) • Omeprazole 20 mg	Lifestyle changes should be started initially and continued throughout the course of treatment. If symptoms are unrelieved with lifestyle changes and OTC medications after 2 weeks, begin pharmacologic therapy (phase II therapy).
Phase II Symptomatic relief of GERD	A. Lifestyle modifications **PLUS** B. Standard doses of H_2-receptor antagonists for 6–12 weeks • Cimetidine 400 mg twice daily • Famotidine 20 mg twice daily • Nizatidine 150 mg twice daily • Ranitidine 150 mg twice daily **OR** B. Proton pump inhibitors for 4–8 weeks. All are given once daily. • Esomeprazole 20 mg • Lansoprazole 15 mg • Omeprazole 20 mg • Pantoprazole 40 mg • Rabeprazole 20 mg	For typical symtoms, treat empirically with phase II therapy. Mild GERD can usually be treated effectively with H_2-receptor antagonists. Patients with moderate to severe symptoms should receive a proton pump inhibitor as initial therapy. If symptoms are relieved, treat recurrences on an as-needed basis. If symptoms recur frequently, consider maintenance therapy (MT) with the lowest effective dose. Note: Most patients will require standard doses for MT.
Healing of erosive esophagitis or treatment of patients presenting with moderate to severe symptoms or complications	A. Lifestyle modifications **PLUS** B. Proton pump inhibitors for 4–16 weeks (up to twice daily) • Esomeprazole 20–40 mg daily • Lansoprazole 30 mg daily • Omeprazole 20 mg daily • Rabeprazole 20 mg daily • Pantoprazole 40 mg daily **OR** B. High-dose H_2-receptor antagonist for 8–12 weeks • Cimetidine 400 mg four times daily or 800 mg twice daily • Famotidine 40 mg twice daily • Nizatidine 150 mg four times daily • Ranitidine 150 mg four times daily	For atypical symtoms, obtain endoscopy (if possible) to evaluate mucosa. Give a trial of a proton pump inhibitor or an H_2-receptor antagonist. If symptoms are relieved, consider MT. Proton pump inhibitors are the most effective maintenance therapy in patients with atypical symptoms, complicated symptoms, and erosive disease. Patients not responding to phase II therapy, including those with persistent atypical symptoms, should be evaluated via ambulatory 24-hour pH monitoring to confirm the diagnosis of GERD (if possible). If GERD is present, consider phase III therapy.
Phase III	Interventional therapies (antireflux surgery or endoluminal therapies)	Manometry should be performed in anyone who is a candidate for surgery.

TABLE 32–5. Nonpharmacologic Treatment of GERD with Lifestyle Modifications

- Elevate the head of the bed (increases esophageal clearance). Use 6- to 8-inch blocks under the head of the bed. Sleep on a foam wedge
- Dietary changes
  Avoid foods that may decrease lower esophageal sphincter pressure (fats, chocolate, alcohol, peppermint, and spearmint)
  Avoid foods that have a direct irritant effect on the esophageal mucosa (spicy foods, orange juice, tomato juice, and coffee)
  Include protein-rich meals in diet (augments lower esophageal sphincter pressure)
  Eat small meals and avoid eating immediately prior to sleeping (within 3 h if possible) (decreases gastric volume)
  Weight reduction (reduces symtoms)
- Stop smoking (decreases spontaneous esophageal sphincter relaxation)
- Avoid alcohol (increases amplitude of the lower esophageal sphincter, peristaltic waves, and frequency of contraction)
- Avoid tight-fitting clothes
- Discontinue, if possible, drugs that may promote reflux (calcium channel blockers, β-blockers, nitrates, theophylline)
- Take drugs that have a direct irritant effect on the esophageal mucosa with plenty of liquid if they cannot be avoided (tetracyclines, quinidine, and KCl, iron salts, aspirin, nonsteroidal anti-inflammatory drugs)

Compiled From Kitchin and Castell [8] and Richter and Castell.[36]

be stressed to the patient on a routine basis, no matter what other therapeutic modality is used. Patients with mild or infrequent symptoms may see improvement with the inexpensive nonprescription H_2-receptor antagonists, antacids, or alginic acid.

After 2 weeks, if patients are not responding to lifestyle changes and to patient-directed therapy, they are generally started on a pharmacologic treatment regimen consisting of an acid-suppressing agent. Acid-suppressing therapy with proton pump inhibitors or H_2-receptor antagonists are the mainstay of GERD treatment. Patients presenting with more severe symptoms (with or without esophageal erosions) or with erosive esophagitis should be started on a proton pump inhibitor as initial therapy, because it provides the most rapid symptomatic relief and healing of esophagitis in the highest percentage of patients.[27] H_2-receptor antagonists in divided doses are effective in patients with mild GERD.[27] Patients not responding to standard doses of H_2-receptor antagonists may require higher doses and/or more frequent dosing, because improvement correlates with the extent and duration of acid suppression.[11] Standard H_2-receptor antagonist doses may be increased to two to four times the normal dose. If this is necessary, it is more cost effective to switch to a proton pump inhibitor.

Prokinetic agents offer an alternative to standard doses of H_2-receptor antagonists in mild to moderate nonerosive GERD, but may not be as effective as acid-suppressing agents and can be more expensive. Combining prokinetic agents with acid-suppressing drugs offers only modest improvements in symptoms over standard doses of H_2-receptor antagonists and should not be routinely recommended. These agents improve defects related to esophagogastric motility, such as decreased LES pressure, decreased esophageal clearance, or delayed gastric emptying. Unfortunately, the availability of a prokinetic agent that has an acceptable adverse effect profile is lacking. Cisapride has been removed from the market for general use because of reports of cardiac arrhythmias (torsades de pointes) and is currently available

only through a limited access program from the manufacturer. For this reason, it is no longer routinely used in managing patients with GERD. The use of other prokinetic agents such as metoclopramide and bethanechol is limited by their adverse effect profile. Mucosal protectants such as sucralfate have a very limited role in the treatment of GERD.

Maintenance therapy is generally necessary to control symptoms and to prevent complications. In patients with more severe symptoms (with or without esophageal erosions), or in patients with other complications, maintenance therapy with a proton pump inhibitor is most effective. Routine use of combination therapy has no role in maintenance therapy of GERD. GERD that is refractory to adequate acid suppression is rare. In these cases, the diagnosis should be confirmed through further diagnostic tests before long-term, high-dose therapy or interventional approaches (antireflux surgery or endoluminal therapies) are considered.[27] Interventional approaches may also be considered a maintenance option in certain patients with established GERD.[27]

NONPHARMACOLOGIC THERAPY

Nonpharmacologic treatment of GERD includes lifestyle modifications, which should be started initially and continued throughout the treatment course for GERD, and interventional approaches (antireflux surgery or endoluminal therapies).

LIFESTYLE MODIFICATIONS

The most common lifestyle changes that a patient should be educated about include (a) weight loss; (b) elevation of the head of the bed; (c) eating smaller meals and avoidance of eating 3 hours prior to sleeping (d) avoidance of foods or medications that exacerbate GERD; (e) smoking cessation; and (f) avoidance of alcohol (see Table 32–5). Obese patients were 2.8 times more likely to experience GERD symptoms than patients who were not obese.[37] While there are limited data indicating that reflux occurs more often with obesity, it would seem logical that the increased intra-abdominal pressure and dietary habits of obese patients would predispose them to reflux.[2] Therefore weight loss and a low-fat diet is recommended. A meal high in fat will decrease LES pressure for 2 hours or more postprandially. In contrast, a high-protein, low-fat meal will elevate LES pressure. Elevating the head of the bed about 6 to 8 inches with a foam wedge under the mattress (not just elevating the head with pillows) decreases nocturnal esophageal acid contact time and should be recommended.[9] Many foods may worsen the symptoms of GERD. Fats and chocolate can decrease LES pressure, while citrus juice, tomato juice, coffee, and pepper may irritate damaged endothelium. It is important to evaluate patient profiles and to identify potential medications that may exacerbate GERD symptoms. Medications, such as anticholinergics, barbiturates, calcium channel blockers, and theophylline decrease LES pressure. Other medications including aspirin, iron, NSAIDs, quinidine, potassium chloride, and bisphosphonates act as direct contact irritants to the esophageal mucosa.

Patients taking bisphosphonates (e.g., alendronate) should be instructed to drink 6 to 8 ounces of plain tap water and remain upright for at least 30 minutes following administration. Proper patient education can help prevent dysphagia or esophageal ulceration. Patients should be closely monitored for worsening symptoms when any of these medications are started. If symptoms worsen, alternative therapies may be warranted. The clinician must weigh the risks and benefits of continuing a drug known to worsen GERD and esophagitis. Smoking can cause aerophagia, which leads to increased belching and regurgitation.[2] However, data are lacking to show that symptoms improve in patients who quit smoking. Nevertheless, patients with GERD should be encouraged to quit smoking. Alcohol, although not thought to play a role in severe disease, decreases LES pressure and may exacerbate symptoms such as heartburn.[2]

Many patients are noncompliant with lifestyle modifications, and even those who do comply generally continue to have symptoms requiring acid-suppression therapy. Nonetheless, it is important to regularly stress the value of lifestyle modification.

INTERVENTIONAL APPROACHES

Antireflux Surgery

6 Surgical intervention is a viable alternative for selected patients with well-documented GERD.[27] The goal of antireflux surgery is to re-establish the antireflux barrier, to position the lower esophageal sphincter within the abdomen where it is under positive (intra-abdominal) pressure, and to close any associated hiatal defect.[38] It should be considered in patients (a) who fail to respond to pharmacologic treatment; (b) who opt for surgery despite successful treatment because of lifestyle considerations, including age, time, or expense of medications; (c) who have complications of GERD (BE, strictures, or grade 3 or 4 esophagitis); or (d) who have atypical symptoms and reflux documented on 24-hour ambulatory pH monitoring.[38]

Surgical procedures include Nissen, Belsey, Toupet, and Hill fundoplication operations. The procedure chosen depends on the surgeon's expertise and preference, as well as on anatomic considerations.[38] In general, 90% of patients have symptom resolution following successful open Nissen fundoplication. Because of the diminished surgical complications with the newer laparoscopic surgical procedures (Nissen fundoplication being one of the most commonly performed procedures), the role of surgery in the long-term management of GERD has become more appealing. The major complications with antireflux surgery include gas bloat syndrome (inability to belch or vomit), dysphagia, vagal denervation, splenic trauma, and very rarely, death.[1] In contrast, death has not occurred due to pharmacologic treatment with a proton pump inhibitor. Antireflux surgery has been found to be superior to medical management (with an H_2-receptor antagonist or prokinetic agent). However, similar comparisons with proton pump inhibitors are lacking. A preliminary study of 310 patients who were initially controlled on omeprazole 40 mg daily found antireflux surgery to be slightly superior to omeprazole 20 mg daily at 3 years.[39] Omeprazole doses of 40 to 60 mg were found to be equally efficacious to antireflux surgery. Long-term effectiveness of antireflux surgery ranges from 5 to 20 years.[27]

CLINICAL CONTROVERSY

Some clinicians believe that patients should be offered the newer endoscopic interventions instead of proton pump inhibitors for long-term maintenance of GERD. While the newer endoscopic therapies provide good results and less recovery time than surgery, the long-term effects are still not known. Conversely, many patients prefer not to have to take medication indefinitely, and in some cases still complain of symptoms despite drug therapy.

Endoluminal Therapies

Several new endoluminal approaches to the management of GERD have recently been developed.[40] These techniques include endoscopic suturing to produce a plication, endoluminal application of radiofrequency heat energy resulting in tissue injury or nerve ablation (the Stretta procedure), and endoscopic injection of a biopolymer known as Enteryx at the gastroesophageal junction. These techniques are relatively new, and although FDA-approved, their exact role in the management of GERD has yet to be determined.

Endoscopic gastroplastic plication of folds of the gastroesophageal junction is accomplished using a suturing device introduced by mouth with endoscopic assistance, and it enhances the barrier function of the gastroesophageal junction. Preliminary reports suggest that following the procedure there is a significant reduction in symptoms of heartburn and regurgitation, and that the quality-of-life scores improve. There has been a reported reduction in the use of other acid-suppressing medications such as proton pump inhibitors in the population treated.

The Stretta device delivers radiofrequency energy through specialized needles placed into the submucosal tissue of the esophagus while monitoring esophageal mucosal surface temperatures. This results in tissue injury leading to increased collagen deposition and scarring at the gastroesophageal junction, potentially increasing LES pressure and reducing gastroesophageal reflux. Again, the primary outcome has been reduction in symptomatic heartburn and improvement in quality of life. Although acid exposure time was reduced, proton pump inhibitor use is continued in approximately 15% of patients at 6 months, and 30% of patients at 12 months. Because of the paucity of sufficient study data, it is unclear what the role of this device will be in the management of patients with symptomatic GERD.

Therapy of gastroesophageal reflux through injection of bulking agents into the gastroesophageal junction has been tried using bovine collagen or polytetrafluoroethylene. More recently, the injection of ethylene vinyl alcohol copolymer (Enteryx) has been approved by the FDA for the treatment of GERD. In this technique, the polymer is injected through a needle placed through the endoscope into the tissue at the esophagogastric junction. The exact mechanism of action for this technique is not known, although reduction in transient LES pressure has been demonstrated. The overall safety of this procedure has been excellent with no major complications being reported. Among the 70% to 80% of treated patients who responded, most were able to discontinue proton pump inhibitor use.

PHARMACOLOGIC THERAPY

ANTACIDS AND ANTACID-ALGINIC ACID PRODUCTS

Patients should be educated that antacids are an appropriate component of treating mild GERD, even though documentation of their efficacy in placebo-controlled clinical trials is lacking.[6] Although the literature is somewhat controversial on the superiority of antacids to placebo, physicians and patients clearly consider antacids to be effective for immediate symptomatic relief, and antacids are often used concurrently with other acid-suppressing therapies. Maintaining the intragastric pH above 4 decreases the activation of pepsinogen to pepsin, a proteolytic enzyme. Also, neutralization of gastric fluid leads to increased LES pressure. Patients who require frequent use of antacids for chronic symptoms should be treated with prescription acid-suppressing therapy because their illness is considered more significant.

An antacid product combined with alginic acid is not a potent neutralizing agent and does not enhance LES pressure; however, it does form a highly viscous solution that floats on the surface of the gastric contents. This viscous solution is thought to serve as a protective barrier for the esophagus against reflux of gastric contents. It also reduces the frequency of the reflux episodes.[41] The combination product usually relieves symptoms associated with reflux.[42,43] Efficacy data indicating endoscopic healing are lacking.

Antacid or antacid combination products may cause gastrointestinal adverse effects (diarrhea or constipation, depending on the product), alterations in mineral metabolism, and acid-base disturbances. Aluminum-containing antacids may bind to phosphate in the gut and lead to bone demineralization. In addition, antacids interact with a variety of drugs by altering gastric pH, increasing urinary pH, adsorbing medications to their surfaces, providing a physical barrier to absorption, or forming insoluble complexes with other medications.[44] Antacids have clinically significant drug interactions with tetracycline, ferrous sulfate, isoniazid, quinidine, sulfonylureas, and quinolone antibiotics. Antacid-drug interactions are influenced by composition, dose, and dosage schedule of the antacid, as well as by the formulation.

Dosage recommendations for antacids in the management of GERD are somewhat difficult to derive from the literature (see Table 32–4 for general dosing guidelines). Doses range from hourly to an as-needed basis. In general, antacids have a short duration of action, which necessitates frequent administration throughout the day to provide continuous neutralization of acid. Typical doses are two tablets or one tablespoonful four times daily—after meals and at bedtime. Taking antacids after meals can increase the duration of action from about 1 hour to about 3 hours; however, nighttime acid suppression cannot be maintained with bedtime doses.

ACID SUPPRESSION WITH H_2-RECEPTOR ANTAGONISTS (CIMETIDINE, FAMOTIDINE, NIZATIDINE, AND RANITIDINE)

Acid-suppressing therapies are the mainstay of treatment of GERD. H_2-receptor antagonists in divided doses are effective in treating patients with mild to moderate GERD.[27] The majority of the trials assessing the efficacy of standard doses of H_2-receptor antagonists indicate that symptomatic improvement is achieved in an average of 60% of patients after 12 weeks of therapy.[27] However, endoscopic healing rates tend to be lower, an average of 50%.[27]

The efficacy of H_2-receptor antagonists in the management of GERD is extremely variable and is frequently lower than desired. Response to the H_2-receptor antagonists appears to be dependent on the (a) severity of disease, (b) dosage regimen used, and (c) duration of therapy. These factors are important to keep in mind when comparing various clinical trials and/or assessing a patient's response to therapy.

The severity of esophagitis at baseline has a profound impact on the patient's response to H_2-receptor antagonists. For symptomatic relief of mild GERD, low-dose, nonprescription H_2-receptor antagonists may be beneficial. For nonerosive disease, H_2-receptor antagonists are generally given at standard doses twice daily. Patients not responding to standard doses may be hypersecreters of gastric acid, requiring higher doses.[6] For these patients and those with erosive disease, higher doses and/or dosing four times daily (cimetidine 800 mg twice daily, famotidine 40 mg twice daily, nizatidine 150 mg four times daily, or ranitidine 150 mg four times daily) provide better acid control, especially after mealtime acid surges.[2] Although higher doses of H_2-receptor antagonists may provide higher symptomatic and

endoscopic healing rates, limited information exists regarding the safety of these regimens, and they can be less effective and more costly than once-daily proton pump inhibitors. Unlike duodenal ulcer disease, in which the duration of therapy is relatively short (e.g., 4 to 6 weeks), prolonged courses (8 weeks or more) of H_2-receptor antagonists are frequently required in the treatment of GERD.

Because all of the H_2-receptor antagonists have similar efficacy, selection of the specific agent to use in the management of GERD should be based on factors such as differences in pharmacokinetics, safety profile, and cost. In general, the H_2-receptor antagonists are well tolerated. The most common adverse effects are headache, somnolence, fatigue, dizziness, and either constipation or diarrhea. Patients should be monitored for the presence of adverse effects as well as potential drug interactions, especially when on cimetidine. Cimetidine may inhibit the metabolism of theophylline, warfarin, phenytoin, nifedipine, or propranolol, among others. An alternate H_2-receptor antagonist should be selected if the patient is on any of these medications.

ACID SUPPRESSION WITH PROTON PUMP INHIBITORS (ESOMEPRAZOLE, LANSOPRAZOLE, OMEPRAZOLE, PANTOPRAZOLE, AND RABEPRAZOLE)

Proton pump inhibitors are superior to H_2-receptor antagonists in treating patients with moderate to severe GERD. This includes not only those patients with erosive esophagitis or complicated symptoms (BE or strictures), but also those patients with nonerosive GERD who have moderate to severe symptoms. In these patient populations, relapse is common and long-term maintenance therapy is generally indicated. Comparable doses of proton pump inhibitors are omeprazole 20 mg = esomeprazole 20 mg = lansoprazole 30 mg = rabeprazole 20 mg = pantoprazole 40 mg per day. Symptomatic relief is seen in approximately 83% of patients treated with a proton pump inhibitor, while the endoscopic healing rate at 8 weeks is 78%.[27] All of the proton pump inhibitors are generally well tolerated, while the newer agents, esomeprazole, pantoprazole, and rabeprazole, appear less likely to cause significant drug interactions. In general, all of these agents are safe and effective and the choice of a particular agent will most likely be based on cost.

Proton pump inhibitors block gastric acid secretion by inhibiting gastric H^+/K^+-adenosine triphosphatase in gastric parietal cells.[45] This produces a profound, long-lasting antisecretory effect capable of maintaining the gastric pH above 4, even during acid surges seen postprandially.[2,9] While the proton pump inhibitors have the same mechanism of action, there are slight differences in their actual binding to the cysteine residues in the proton pump.

A correlation appears to exist between the percentage of time the gastric pH remains above 4 during the 24-hour period and healing erosive esophagitis. Lansoprazole 15 mg and 30 mg daily, omeprazole 20 mg daily, and ranitidine 150 mg four times daily were compared in suppressing gastric acid secretion in 29 healthy men.[46] After 5 days, the mean 24-hour gastric pH values for lansoprazole 30 mg, 15 mg, omeprazole, and ranitidine were 4.53, 3.97, 4.02, and 3.59, respectively. The percentage of time the pH remained above 4 for the lansoprazole 30 mg, 15 mg, omeprazole, and ranitidine groups were 63%, 48%, 51%, and 38%, respectively. This difference was statistically different for the lansoprazole 30-mg group. A similar study also showed that lansoprazole 30 mg maintained a higher 24-hour gastric pH as compared with omeprazole 20 mg.[47]

Rabeprazole appears to have a faster onset of action after the first dose and maintains the gastric pH >4 for a higher percentage of time during a 24-hour period as compared with omeprazole (45% vs

25%). The percentage of time the gastric pH values remained above 4 by day 8 was 60.3% and 50.4%, respectively. However, this was only significant on the first day of therapy.[48] Another study showed rabeprazole 20 mg and 40 mg increased mean gastric pH to 4.2 and 4.7, respectively. The percentage of time the esophageal pH was <4 was decreased and fewer reflux episodes were noted with both doses.[49]

During a 5-day study of 38 GERD patients, esomeprazole 20 mg and 40 mg maintained intragastric pH >4 for a significantly longer time as compared to omeprazole 20 mg (13 hours, 18 hours, and 11 hours, respectively).[50] The 24-hour median intragastric pH was also significantly higher in both the esomeprazole 20 mg and 40 mg groups as compared with omeprazole 20 mg (4.1, 4.9, and 3.6, respectively).

Proton pump inhibitors are superior to H_2-receptor antagonists both in their ability to control symptoms and to heal esophagitis in patients with GERD.[51] They are also more cost effective in patients with severe disease. A meta-analysis of 43 double-blind or single-blind trials with various drug classes in patients with erosive esophagitis found that healing was highest with proton pump inhibitors as compared with H_2-receptor antagonists (83.6% vs 51.9%).[51] Symptom relief was achieved in 77% of patients on a proton pump inhibitor as compared with 48% of patients on an H_2-receptor antagonist. Both healing and symptom relief occurred almost twice as fast when a proton pump inhibitor was used. Even with mild esophagitis (grade 1 or 2), omeprazole was still superior to high-dose ranitidine.[52] In a study of 446 patients with grade 1 or 2 esophagitis, omeprazole 20 mg daily was more effective at relieving symptoms than was ranitidine 150 mg four times daily. Sixty-one percent and 74% of patients were symptom-free at 4 weeks and 8 weeks, respectively, in the omeprazole group, as compared with 31% and 50% in the ranitidine group, respectively.

There are a few trials comparing proton pump inhibitors to each other. In general, healing rates at 4 weeks and 8 weeks are similar; lansoprazole and rabeprazole, however, may relieve symptoms faster after the first dose when compared to omeprazole. This is especially true when the higher dose of lansoprazole (30 mg daily) is compared to omeprazole 20 mg.[53] Both daytime and nighttime symptoms, as well as pain severity, were reported to be significantly better with lansoprazole 30 mg, as compared with omeprazole 20 mg or lansoprazole 15 mg, after the first dose. Healing rates at 4 weeks and 8 weeks were similar. Symptom relief was similar when a higher dose of omeprazole (40 mg daily) was compared with lansoprazole 30 mg.[54]

Esomeprazole, is the S-isomer of omeprazole and may offer greater acid suppression and improved healing rates as compared with the other proton pump inhibitors. Esomeprazole was compared with omeprazole in 1960 patients with endoscopy-confirmed grade 2 reflux esophagitis.[55] The number of patients healed at 8 weeks were 94% (esomeprazole 40 mg), 90% (esomeprazole 20 mg), and 87% (omeprazole 20 mg) ($p < 0.05$). Healing at 4 weeks and improvement in heartburn was also considered superior in the esomeprazole 40 mg group as compared with the omeprazole 20 mg group. More experience with using this agent in clinical practice will clarify its role in the treatment of patients with GERD.

Rabeprazole 20 mg daily was compared with omeprazole 20 mg daily and found to be equally efficacious at 4 and 8 weeks in healing erosive esophagitis. Symptom relief (both frequency and intensity) was similar in both groups.[56]

Similar results were seen when pantoprazole 40 mg was compared with omeprazole 20 mg in 286 patients with mild to moderate reflux esophagitis. Healing rates were 74% and 78%, respectively, after 4 weeks; and 90% and 94%, respectively, after 8 weeks of treatment. Symptom relief was similar for both groups.[57] More pub-

lished trials are needed with pantoprazole and rabeprazole, especially with long-term use.

Omeprazole (40 to 60 mg daily) and lansoprazole (30 to 60 mg daily) also appear to be effective in healing esophagitis and esophageal ulcers in patients with gastroesophageal reflux complications.[58,59] When patients with complications of GERD (BE, strictures, or failed antireflux surgery) who were refractory to high-dose H_2-receptor antagonist therapy received omeprazole 40 mg daily, all patients were healed during 20 weeks of therapy.[58]

Whether proton pump inhibitors can actually reverse BE remains a topic for debate. The use of high-dose omeprazole (40 mg twice daily) caused partial regression of BE, but no change was noted in patients receiving ranitidine 150 mg twice daily.[60] Others propose that these islands of normal squamous cells that appear in patients with BE after high-dose proton pump inhibitors may be covering gastric mucosa and may mask the development of cancerous changes in the mucosa.[61] It is unknown whether regression of BE reduces the risk of adenocarcinoma in someone who already has BE, but aggressive therapy aimed at adequate suppression of acid reflux early in the course of a patient's disease may help to prevent the development of BE.

The proton pump inhibitors are usually well tolerated; however, potential adverse effects include headache, dizziness, somnolence, diarrhea, constipation, and nausea. The frequency of adverse events appears to be similar to that seen with the H_2-receptor antagonists. Concern and controversy regarding the safety of therapy with a proton pump inhibitor are based on the proton pump inhibitor's ability to cause hypergastrinemia and gastric carcinoid tumors in rats. After nearly a decade of experience with the proton pump inhibitors, gastric carcinoid tumors have not been directly linked to omeprazole use in humans.[6]

Drug interactions with the proton pump inhibitors vary with each agent. All proton pump inhibitors can decrease the absorption of drugs such as ketoconazole or itraconazole, which require an acidic environment to be absorbed. All proton pump inhibitors are metabolized by the cytochrome P450 system to some extent, specifically by the CYP2C19 and CYP3A4 enzymes. However, no interactions with lansoprazole, pantoprazole, or rabeprazole have been seen with CYP2C19 substrates such as diazepam, warfarin, or phenytoin.[35] Esomeprazole does not appear to interact with warfarin or phenytoin, and an interaction with diazepam is generally not considered clinically relevant. Pantoprazole is also metabolized by a cytosolic sulfotransferase and is therefore less likely to have significant drug interactions compared with the other proton pump inhibitors.[62] While generally not causing major concern, omeprazole has the potential to inhibit the metabolism of warfarin, diazepam, and phenytoin; and lansoprazole may decrease theophylline concentrations.

Drug interactions with omeprazole are of particular concern in patients who are considered "slow metabolizers," as found in approximately 3% of the caucasian population. Unfortunately, it is unclear which patients have the polymorphic gene variation that makes them slow metabolizers.[62] Like omeprazole, the metabolism of esomeprazole may also be altered in patients with this polymorphic gene variation. Rabeprazole increases digoxin trough concentrations by approximately 20%.[62] Patients on potentially interacting drugs should be monitored closely for potential problems.

The proton pump inhibitors degrade in acidic environments and are therefore formulated in a delayed-release capsule or tablet formulation. Lansoprazole, esomeprazole, and omeprazole contain enteric-coated (pH-sensitive) granules in a capsule form. In patients unable to swallow the capsule or in pediatric patients, the contents of the capsule can be mixed in applesauce or placed in orange juice. If a patient has a nasogastric tube, the contents of an omeprazole capsule can be mixed in 8.4% sodium bicarbonate solution. Esomeprazole can be mixed with water. Lansoprazole comes in a packet for oral suspension and a delayed-release orally disintegrating tablet. While these dosage forms are beneficial for those who cannot swallow the capsule, such as elderly or pediatric patients, it should not be placed through a nasogastric tube. Patients taking pantoprazole or rabeprazole should be instructed not to crush, chew, or split the delayed-release tablets. Pantoprazole is available in an intravenous formulation, which offers an alternative route of administration for patients unable to take an oral proton pump inhibitor. It should be emphasized that the intravenous product is not more efficacious than oral proton pump inhibitors and will be significantly more expensive. Careful patient selection will be necessary to avoid the tremendous cost anticipated from the use of this product. An injectable form of lansoprazole is expected to be approved within the year. Patients should be instructed to take their proton pump inhibitor in the morning, 15 to 30 minutes before breakfast to maximize efficacy, because these agents inhibit only actively secreting proton pumps.[2,62] Food may decrease the absorption of lansoprazole. If dosed twice daily, the second dose should be administered approximately 10 to 12 hours after the morning dose and prior to a meal or snack.[35]

PROKINETIC AGENTS

The efficacy of the prokinetic agents cisapride, metoclopramide, and bethanechol has been evaluated in the treatment of GERD. The inferior efficacy and side effect profiles associated with metoclopramide and bethanechol, as compared with cisapride, limit their use in the treatment of GERD. Cisapride, on the other hand, has comparable efficacy to H_2-receptor antagonists in treating patients with mild esophagitis. Unfortunately, cisapride is no longer available for routine use because of life-threatening arrhythmias when it is combined with certain medications and other disease states. Prokinetic agents have also been used as adjunctive therapy with an H_2-receptor antagonist. The only scenario in which this combination is appropriate is in a patient with GERD who has a known or suspected motility disorder, or in a patient who has failed high-dose proton pump inhibitor therapy.

Cisapride

The efficacy of cisapride appears similar to that of the H_2-receptor antagonists in patients with mild esophagitis. However, cisapride generally costs more than the H_2-receptor antagonists and offers no real advantage, especially in patients with normal GI motility. Because this agent is no longer available for routine use in GERD, an evaluation of clinical trials is not included. Three treatment protocols are available through the manufacturer, Janssen. One protocol is a pediatric outpatient study, the second protocol is an adult outpatient study, and the third protocol is an inpatient neonatal study. Physicians must register as investigators and patients must be enrolled just as with any other study protocol. More information can be obtained from the company.

Metoclopramide

Metoclopramide, a dopamine antagonist, increases LES pressure in a dose-related manner, and accelerates gastric emptying in gastroesophageal reflux patients. Unlike cisapride, however, metoclopramide does not improve esophageal clearance. Metoclopramide

provides symptomatic improvement for some patients with gastroesophageal reflux disease; however, substantial data indicating that metoclopramide provides endoscopic healing are lacking. In addition, metoclopramide's side effect profile and the incidence of tachyphylaxis with continued use limits its usefulness in treating many patients with GERD. The risk of adverse effects is much greater in patients with renal dysfunction because the drug is primarily eliminated by the kidneys. Contraindications include Parkinson's disease, mechanical obstruction, concomitant use of other dopamine antagonists, anticholinergic agents, and pheochromocytoma.

MUCOSAL PROTECTANTS

Sucralfate, a nonabsorbable aluminum salt of sucrose octasulfate, has very limited value in the treatment of GERD. Sucralfate has similar healing rates as H_2-receptor antagonists for patients with mild esophagitis.[63] However, sucralfate is less effective than higher doses of H_2-receptor antagonists in patients with refractory esophagitis.[63] Overall, the efficacy of sucralfate varies greatly among the studies. The wide range of response rates may in part be related to patient population, baseline degree of esophagitis, duration of treatment, dose used, or sucralfate formulation used. Sucralfate cannot be routinely recommended for use in the treatment of anything but the mildest cases of GERD.

COMBINATION THERAPY

Combination therapy with an acid-suppressing agent and a prokinetic agent or a mucosal protectant agent would seem logical given the multifactorial nature of the disease, particularly in light of the disappointing results seen with many monotherapy regimens. However, sufficient data to support combination therapy are limited, and this approach should not be routinely recommended unless a patient has esophagitis plus motor dysfunction occurring concurrently or if the patient has failed high-dose proton pump inhibitor therapy. Most studies suggest that combination therapy offers only modest improvements over standard doses of H_2-receptor antagonists alone. Therefore patients not responding to standard doses of H_2-receptor antagonists should have their dose of H_2-receptor antagonists increased or be switched to a proton pump inhibitor instead of adding a prokinetic agent. Monotherapy with a proton pump inhibitor is not only more efficacious in patients not responding to an H_2-receptor antagonist or prokinetic agent alone, but it also improves compliance with once-daily dosing and is ultimately more cost effective.

MAINTENANCE THERAPY

Although healing and/or symptomatic improvement may be achieved via many different therapeutic modalities, a large percentage of patients with gastroesophageal reflux will relapse following discontinuation of therapy, especially those with more severe disease.[64] Follow-up studies indicate that 70% to 90% of patients will relapse within 1 year of discontinuation of therapy, regardless of what therapeutic regimen had been used to induce remission.[64] Patients who have symptomatic relapse following discontinuation of therapy or lowering of dose, including patients with complications such as BE, strictures, or hemorrhage, should be considered for long-term maintenance therapy to prevent complications or worsening of esophageal function.[9] The goal of maintenance therapy is to improve quality of life by controlling the patient's symptoms and preventing complications.[6] These goals cannot generally be achieved by decreasing the dose of the therapeutic modality used for initial healing or switching to a less potent acid-suppressing agent. Most patients will require standard doses to prevent relapses.[65] Patients should be counseled on the importance of complying with lifestyle changes and long-term maintenance therapy in order to prevent recurrence or worsening of disease.[6]

H$_2$-receptor antagonists may be effective maintenance therapy for patients with mild disease.[2] Although cisapride was an effective maintenance therapy, it is no longer an option unless it is obtained through the limited access program from the manufacturer. The proton pump inhibitors are the drugs of choice for maintenance treatment of moderate to severe esophagitis.[66] Lower doses of a proton pump inhibitor or alternate-day dosing may be effective in some patients with less-severe disease, thereby allowing titration in some cases.[2] Preliminary data with esomeprazole suggest that "on demand" maintenance therapy for patients with endoscopy-negative GERD may be effective.[67,68] However, patients with more severe disease and/or complications should be maintained on omeprazole 20 mg daily, lansoprazole 30 mg daily, rabeprazole 20 mg daily, or esomeprazole 20 mg daily. Long-term chronic use of higher doses of proton pump inhibitors is not indicated unless the patient has complicated symptoms, has high-grade erosive esophagitis per endoscopy, or has had further diagnostic evaluation to determine the level of acid exposure. Many institutions allow the use of normal-dose proton pump inhibitors by all physicians, but limit the use of high-dose proton pump inhibitors to gastroenterologists. Antireflux surgery and other endoluminal procedures may also be considered a viable alternative to long-term drug therapy for maintenance of healing in patients who are candidates.

Maintenance Therapy with Proton Pump Inhibitors

In a comparison of maintenance regimens, omeprazole (20 mg daily) alone or in combination with cisapride (10 mg three times daily) was significantly more effective in preventing recurrence of erosive GERD than was ranitidine (150 mg three times daily) alone or cisapride (10 mg three times daily) alone.[66] Omeprazole was also effective in patients with complicated forms (grades 3 and 4) of esophagitis.

Omeprazole and lansoprazole in doses of 20 mg and 30 mg daily, respectively, decreased relapse rates significantly.[65,66] At 1 year, relapse rates were 15% and 10%, respectively. Both omeprazole and lansoprazole were superior to H$_2$-receptor antagonists in maintaining Lansoprazole 15 mg daily was compared to lansoprazole 30 mg daily or ranitidine 300 mg twice daily in preventing recurrence of reflux esophagitis.[69] At 12 months, relapse rates were 31%, 20%, and 68% for lansoprazole 15 mg, 30 mg, and ranitidine 300 mg, respectively. Lansoprazole 15 mg and 30 mg daily were comparable in maintaining

treatment phase for grade 1 or 2 esophagitis, patients were randomized to receive maintenance therapy with omeprazole 10 mg daily or ranitidine 150 mg twice daily. At 1 year, 68% of patients on omeprazole were in remission, as compared with 39% of patients receiving ranitidine. Even at a lower dose, omeprazole was superior to ranitidine for maintenance therapy.

Preliminary placebo-controlled studies with esomeprazole indicate that maintenance of erosive esophagitis healing occurs in 54% to 94% of patients after 6 months of 10-mg to 40-mg doses of esomeprazole.[70,71] Doses of 20 mg to 40 mg were superior to the 10-mg dose. Studies are needed comparing esomeprazole to the other proton pump inhibitors in maintenance therapy for GERD.

Omeprazole 20 mg (given on the weekend) was compared to omeprazole 20 mg daily and ranitidine 150 mg twice daily. The relapse rate at 12 months was 68%, 11%, and 75%, respectively, indicating that weekend regimens are ineffective in preventing recurrence.[72] Long-term studies are needed with pantoprazole, but it should be effective as maintenance therapy for GERD.

Long-term use of the proton pump inhibitors indicates that they are safe, with no evidence of carcinoid tumors directly linked to their use. Prolonged hypergastrinemia leading to the development of colonic polyps, and potentially adenocarcinoma, was also a concern that has proven unfounded with long-term use of proton pump inhibitors.[73] However, the role of *Helicobacter pylori* status in patients with GERD is a concern. One study showed that patients treated with proton pump inhibitors had a higher incidence of atrophic gastritis that was linked to the development of gastric cancer.[1] In this study, 30% of patients treated with omeprazole over an average of 5 years developed atrophy, whereas none of a cohort group that received antireflux surgery developed atrophy within the same time frame.[74] Most of the patients who developed atrophic gastritis had concomitant *H. pylori* infection. On the other hand, the presence of *H. pylori* infection may actually have a protective effect against GERD, and clearing the infection may be associated with a worsening of GERD symptoms.[75] The FDA recently stated that there was insufficient evidence linking proton pump inhibitor use to atrophic gastritis, intestinal metaplasia, or gastric cancer.[76] As a consequence of the controversy surrounding *H. pylori* and GERD, specific guidelines on how to handle these patients are lacking. Most clinicians would probably opt to eradicate *H. pylori* infections once detected. Further studies are needed to determine the role of *H. pylori* in patients with GERD.

Maintenance Therapy with H$_2$-Receptor Antagonists

The studies evaluating the efficacy of the H$_2$-receptor antagonists in maintaining GERD patients in remission have been disappointing. Currently, ranitidine 150 mg twice daily is the only H$_2$-receptor antagonist regimen that is FDA approved for maintenance of healing of erosive esophagitis.

SPECIAL POPULATIONS CONSIDERATIONS

ATYPICAL GERD SYMPTOMS

Patients presenting with atypical symptoms may require higher doses and longer treatment courses as compared with patients with typical symptoms. These patients are best diagnosed with ambulatory pH testing or an empiric trial with a proton pump inhibitor.[77] In patients presenting with noncardiac chest pain, a short course (1 to 8 weeks) of

omeprazole 20 mg twice daily has been advocated.[77] In patients with asthma, antireflux medications have been shown to improve asthma symptoms and even to decrease antiasthma medication use, but were found to have little or no effect on lung function.[78] A trial of 3 months has been advocated using twice-daily proton pump inhibitor therapy for both asthma and laryngeal symptoms thought to be associated with GERD. Omeprazole doses as high as 60 mg daily have been used.[77] In patients with chronic cough, pH testing is the preferred approach for evaluation of GERD, when available.[79] Maintenance therapy is generally indicated in patients who respond to the therapeutic trial or have endoscopic evidence of reflux.

Interventional management may be indicated in selected patients not responding to medical management.

ENDOSCOPY-NEGATIVE REFLUX DISEASE

While the integrity of the esophageal mucosa is best evaluated with endoscopy, it does not confirm whether or not the patient's symptoms are related to GERD.[27] In some cases, patients with typical symptoms and increased acid exposure have no evidence of esophageal damage. Many patients with persistent severe symptoms but normal endoscopy will require therapy similar to those with positive endoscopic findings. This condition is referred to as endoscopy-negative reflux disease.[80] Patients presenting with normal esophageal mucosa on endoscopy may undergo pH testing or a therapeutic trial with a proton pump inhibitor to further confirm the diagnosis of GERD. Remember, however, that even when ambulatory pH monitoring or a therapeutic trial is used, it does not absolutely rule GERD in or out. In more serious cases, both may be necessary to confirm the diagnosis.[27]

Patients with normal endoscopy treated with omeprazole had improvement in symptoms, quality-of-life scores, and antacid use.[81] Treatment with a proton pump inhibitor is more effective than treatment with an H_2-receptor antagonist in these patients, as demonstrated by several clinical trials.[82,83]

PEDIATRIC PATIENTS WITH GERD

Gastroesophageal reflux occurs in approximately 18% of the infant population. Most have physiologic reflux with no clinical consequence.[84] Complications, although rare, include distal esophagitis, failure to thrive, esophageal peptic strictures, BE, and pulmonary disease.[85] Chronic vomiting associated with gastroesophageal reflux must be distinguished from other causes such as neurologic, metabolic, eating, and rumination disorders. Developmental immaturity of the LES is one suspected cause of gastroesophageal reflux in infants.[85] Like adults, transient LES relaxations seem to be the most common cause of gastroesophageal reflux in children. Other causes include impaired luminal clearance of gastric acid, neurologic impairment, and type of infant formula. Uncomplicated gastroesophageal reflux usually resolves without incident by 12 to 18 months of life, and usually responds to supportive therapy, including dietary adjustments, postural management, and reassurance for the parents.[85] Thickened feedings may be useful in milder cases. Smaller, more frequent feedings may also be beneficial. If there is no improvement, medical therapy may be indicated. Combined use of a prokinetic agent and an acid-suppressing agent seems to work the fastest.[85] Unfortunately, there is no longer a readily available prokinetic agent without major problems. H_2-receptor antagonists are commonly used. A dose of ranitidine 2 mg/kg twice daily is effective.[85]

The use of proton pump inhibitors is becoming more common in pediatrics. Lansoprazole recently received FDA approval for treating symptomatic and erosive GERD in pediatric patients <1 year old. A dose of 15 mg once daily is recommended for children weighing ≤30 kg, and a dose of 30 mg once daily is recommended for those weighing >30 kg. While not FDA approved for use in children, there is evidence supporting the effectiveness of omeprazole in treating children with GERD. A common dose for treating esophagitis is 1 mg/kg per day (divided once or twice daily).[86] While no major adverse events have been noted in children receiving proton pump inhibitors for up to 7 years, the relative safety of prolonged proton pump inhibitor use in children remains unknown.[86] There are no

data involving the other proton pump inhibitors in the treatment of GERD.

ELDERLY PATIENTS WITH GERD

Many elderly patients have decreased host defense mechanisms such as saliva production. More aggressive therapy with a proton pump inhibitor may be warranted in patients with symptomatic GERD in patients older than 60 years of age.[87] Often these patients do not seek medical attention because they feel their symptoms are part of the normal aging process. They may present with atypical symptoms such as chest pain, asthma, hoarseness, coughing, wheezing, poor dentition, or jaw pain. Decreased GI motility is a common problem in elderly patients. Unfortunately, there are no good prokinetic agents available to these patients.

Cisapride is not available for general use and elderly patients are especially sensitive to the central nervous system effects of metoclopramide. They may also be sensitive to the central nervous system effects of H_2-receptor antagonists. Proton pump inhibitors appear to be the most useful treatment modality because they have superior efficacy and are dosed once daily, which is beneficial in all patients, but is especially beneficial in the elderly.

PHARMACOECONOMIC CONSIDERATIONS

In addition to the traditional clinical end points that demonstrate that a certain therapy is effective, we must also evaluate the cost-effectiveness of the therapy in relation to predicted outcomes and its effects on quality of life.[2] For GERD, one must consider the primary goals of treatment: to relieve symptoms, to heal injury, to prevent recurrence, and to prevent complications. These factors must be evaluated separately, because different costs are associated with achieving each end point. For example, patients with complications associated with GERD, such as strictures, would be more likely to use medical resources as a consequence of revisits and diagnostic tests.[2] Although effects on quality of life may be difficult to evaluate when your goal is preventing recurrence,[2] untreated GERD has a more negative impact on psychological well-being than untreated hypertension, mild heart failure, angina pectoris, or menopause.[4] Improving a patient's quality of life is a measure of treatment success and may help decide which therapy a patient receives.[2]

The proton pump inhibitors are generally more expensive than the H_2-receptor antagonists or prokinetic agents. This is likely to be less of an issue now that omeprazole has become generically available and is also available over the counter. However, the most expensive therapy is the one that is ineffective.[2] This means that if the H_2-receptor antagonist does not accomplish the treatment goals, then it costs more because the patient must be retreated.

Patient compliance is another factor that will affect the outcome of drug therapy. Drug regimens that are easily managed will improve compliance, and therefore outcome for the patient. This can especially be a problem in patients who require high-dose therapy with H_2-receptor antagonists. Not only is the patient required to take the drug more often in higher doses, but there is also increased expense associated with such regimens. The patient may be unable to afford the drug. Choosing a drug that is least expensive and provides the greatest benefit related to dosing interval and number of tablets taken is the optimal regimen. Studies comparing various treatment strategies for GERD show that proton pump inhibitors are more cost effective than H_2-receptor antagonists, especially in patients with moderate to severe disease.[88–90]

Decision analysis has been used to evaluate the cost effectiveness of phase I therapy or phase I therapy combined with omeprazole 20 mg daily or ranitidine 150 mg twice daily for patients with persistent symptomatic GERD who failed phase I therapy. A complex model that evaluated the influence of empiric versus definitive therapy, compliance, and efficacy of the three treatment regimens was employed. Although the retail cost of omeprazole was highest among the treatments evaluated, it was the most cost-effective strategy and was associated with the lowest overall cost. Studies also show that proton pump inhibitors improve quality-of-life measures in symptomatic patients with erosive esophagitis.[91] Additional studies are needed to evaluate the impact of various treatment regimens on quality-of-life issues, cost, and to compare long-term medical management with antireflux surgery and endoluminal approaches. At least one study showed that proton pump inhibitors were equally effective to antireflux surgery and slightly more cost effective at 5 years. However, the costs were similar after 10 years.[92]

EVALUATION OF THERAPEUTIC OUTCOMES

❾ The long-term benefits of treatment are difficult to assess because of the limited information known about the epidemiology and natural history of GERD. Therefore successful outcomes are generally measured in terms of three separate end points: (a) relieving symptoms, (b) healing the injured mucosa, and (c) preventing complications.

The short-term goal of therapy is to relieve symptoms such as heartburn and regurgitation to the point at which they do not impair the patient's quality of life. Patients should be educated regarding lifestyle modifications that should be adhered to throughout the course of therapy including smoking cessation, weight loss, raising the head of the bed, eating smaller meals, and avoiding eating prior to bedtime. Patients should also be instructed to avoid foods that aggravate GERD symptoms, such as fat and chocolate. In addition, the patient's drug profile should be reviewed to identify medications that may contribute to GERD symptoms. These agents should be avoided if possible. Table 32–6 has recommendations for providing pharmaceutical care to patients with GERD.

The clinician should take an active role in educating the patient about potential adverse effects and drug interactions that may occur with drug therapy. The frequency and severity of symptoms should be monitored and patients should be counseled on symptoms that suggest the presence of complications requiring immediate medical attention, such as dysphagia or odynophagia. Patients with persistent symptoms should be evaluated for the presence of strictures or other complications. Patients should also be monitored for the presence of atypical symptoms such as cough, nonallergic asthma, or chest pain. These symptoms require further diagnostic evaluation. Long-term maintenance treatment is indicated in patients who have strictures because they commonly recur if esophagitis is not treated.[93]

The second goal is to heal the injured mucosa. Again, lifestyle modifications and the importance of complying with the therapeutic regimen chosen to heal the mucosa should be stressed. Patients should be educated about the risk of relapse and the need for long-term maintenance therapy to prevent recurrence or complications.

The final, more long-term goal of therapy is to decrease the risk of complications (esophagitis, strictures, and BE). A small subset of patients may continue to fail treatment despite therapy with high doses of H_2-receptor antagonists or omeprazole. Maintenance therapy with standard to higher doses of antisecretory agents may be indicated in these acid hypersecreters, because severe esophagitis that is not

TABLE 32–6. Recommendations for Providing Pharmaceutical Care to Patients with GERD

1. Assess the patient's symptoms to determine if patient-directed therapy is appropriate or whether they should be evaluated by a physician. Determine the type of symptoms, frequency, and exacerbating factors. Refer any patient with complicated or atypical symptoms to a physician for further diagnostic work-up.
2. Obtain a thorough history of prescription, nonprescription, and natural drug product use.
3. Counsel the patient on lifestyle modifications that will improve symptoms. These include avoiding foods and medications that worsen GERD, avoiding tight-fitting clothes, eating smaller meals, raising the head of the bed, losing weight, and avoiding tobacco use.
4. Recommend appropriate drug therapy based on patient presentation. Proton pump inhibitors are the drugs of choice for patients with moderate to severe symptoms.
5. Develop a plan to assess effectiveness of acid-suppressing therapy after an appropriate amount of time (8–16 weeks). Recommend alternative therapy if necessary.
6. Assess improvement in quality-of-life measures such as physical, psychological, and social functioning and well-being.
7. Evaluate the patient for the presence of adverse drug reactions, drug allergies, and drug interactions.
8. Stress the importance of compliance with the therapeutic regimen, including lifestyle modifications. Recommend a therapeutic regimen that is easy for the patient to accomplish.
9. Provide patient education with regard to disease state, lifestyle modifications, and drug therapy. Patients should be counseled on:
   - What causes GERD and what things to avoid (see #3)
   - When to take their medications
   - What potential adverse effects may occur
   - Which drugs may interact with their therapy
   - What warning signs they should report to their physician (dysphagia, odynophagia, unexplained weight loss, or bleeding)

adequately treated may lead to BE and its associated risk of adenocarcinoma. Unfortunately, data are lacking that show that effective treatment of esophagitis decreases the risk of developing adenocarcinoma in patients with BE. Patients should be monitored for the presence of continual pain, dysphagia, or odynophagia.

CONCLUSIONS

Gastroesophageal reflux disease is a common entity that classically presents as heartburn. The pathophysiology of reflux is complex, involving both aggressive factors (acid, pepsin, bile acids, pancreatic enzymes, and prostaglandins) and defense mechanisms (anatomic factors, LES pressure, esophageal clearance, and gastric emptying). Therapeutic modalities are designed to minimize the aggressive factors and/or augment defense mechanisms. The pharmacologic critical elements outlined should be considered when evaluating and treating a patient with GERD.

ABBREVIATIONS

BE: Barrett's esophagus
ENRD: endoscopy-negative reflux disease
GERD: gastroesophageal reflux disease
LES: lower esophageal sphincter
NERD: nonerosive reflux disease

REFERENCES

1. Kahrilas PJ. Gastroesophageal reflux disease. JAMA 1996;276:983–988.
2. Johnson DA. Medical therapy of GERD: Current state of the art. Hosp Pract (Off Ed) 1996;31:135–148.
3. Spechler SJ. Epidemiology and natural history of gastro-oesophageal reflux disease. Digestion 1992;51(Suppl 1):24–29.
4. Dimenas E. Methodological aspects of evaluation of quality of life in upper gastrointestinal diseases. Scand J Gastroenterol 1993;28:18–21.
5. The Gallup Organization. A Gallup Organization National Survey: HB Across America. Princeton, 1988, 2000.
6. DeVault KR, Castell DO (for the Practice Parameters Committee of the American College of Gastroenterology). Guidelines for the diagnosis and treatment of gastroesophageal reflux disease. Arch Intern Med 1995;155:2165–2173.
7. Richter JE. Severe reflux esophagitis. Gastrointest Endosc Clin North Am 1994;4:677–698.
8. Kitchin LI, Castell DO. Rationale and efficacy of conservative therapy for gastroesophageal reflux disease. Arch Intern Med 1991;151:448–454.
9. Fennerty MB, Castell D, Fendrick AM, et al. The diagnosis and treatment of gastroesophageal reflux disease in a managed care environment. Suggested disease management guidelines. Arch Intern Med 1996;156:477–484.
10. Orenstein SR. Gastroesophageal reflux disease. Semin Gastrointest Dis 1994;5:2–14.
11. Krueger KJ. Changing clinical perspectives toward gastroesophageal reflux. South Med J 1996;89:548–550. Editorial.
12. Cameron AJ, Kamalh PS, Carpenter HA. Prevalence of Barrett esophagus and intestinal metaplasia at the esophagogastric junction. Gastroenterology 1997;112:A82.
13. Lagergren J, Bergstrom R, Lindgren A, Nyren O. Symptomatic gastroesophageal reflux as a risk factor for esophageal adenocarcinoma. N Engl J Med 1999;340:825–831.
14. Lambert R. Current practices and future perspectives in the management of gastroesophageal reflux disease. Aliment Pharmacol Ther 1997;11:661–662.
15. Weinberg DS, Kadish SL. The diagnosis and management of gastroesophageal reflux disease. Med Clin North Am 1996;80:411–429.
16. Castell DO. Long-term management of GERD: The pill, the knife or the endoscopes? Gastrointest Endosc 1994;40:252–253.
17. Kahrilas P. Hiatal hernia. Program and abstracts of Digestive Disease Week; 2000 (May); San Diego, California. Session 521.
18. Smith C. Gastroesophageal reflux disease. US Pharmacist 1999;24:77–86.
19. Bozymski EM. Pathophysiology and diagnosis of gastroesophageal reflux disease. Am J Hosp Pharm 1993;50(Suppl 1):S4–S6.
20. Goldstein JL, Schlesinger PK, Mozwecz HL, et al. Esophageal mucosal resistance: A factor in esophagitis. Gastroenterol Clin North Am 1990;19:565–585.
21. McCallum RW. Gastric emptying in gastroesophageal reflux and the therapeutic role of prokinetic agents. Gastroenterol Clin North Am 1990;19:551–564.
22. Fein M. Duodenogastroesophageal reflux parallels acid and not alkaline exposure in the esophagus and contributes to complications of reflux disease. Am J Gastroenterol 1996;91:1662–1663.
23. Dent J. Roles of gastric acid and pH in the pathogenesis of gastroesophageal reflux disease. Scand J Gastroenterol 1994;29(Suppl 201):55–61.
24. Bell NJV, Burger D, Howden CW, et al. Appropriate acid suppression for the management of gastro-oesophageal reflux disease. Digestion 1992;51(Suppl 1):59–67.
25. Kiljander TO, Salomaa ER, Hietanen EK, et al. Gastroesophageal reflux in asthmatics: A double-blind, placebo controlled crossover study with omeprazole. Chest 1999;116:1257–1264.
26. Simpson WG. Gastroesophageal reflux disease and asthma. Diagnosis and management. Arch Intern Med 1995;155:798–803.
27. DeVault KR, Castell DO and the practice parameters committee of the American College of Gastroenterology. Updated guidelines for the diagnosis and treatment of gastroesophageal reflux disease. Am J Gastroenterol 1999;94:1434–1442.
28. Johnnson F, Weywadt L, Sonhaug JN, et al. One-week omeprazole treatment in the diagnosis of gastro-oesophageal reflux disease. Scand J Gastroenterol 1998;33:15–20.
29. Schenk BE, Kuipers EJ, Klinkenberg-Knol EC, et al. Omeprazole as a diagnostic tool in gastroesophageal reflux disease. Am J Gastroenterol 1997;92:1997–2000.
30. Schindlbeck NE, Klauser AG, Voderrholzer WA, Muller-Lissner SA. Empiric therapy for gastroesophageal reflux disease. Arch Intern Med 1995;155:1808–1812.
31. Ofman JJ, Gralnek IM, Udani J, et al. The cost-effectiveness of the omeprazole test in patients with noncardiac chest pain. Am J Med 1999;107:219–227.
32. Fass R, Fennerty MB, Ofman JJ, et al. The clinical and economic value of a short course of omeprazole in patients with noncardiac chest pain. Gastroenterology 1998;115:42–49.
33. Wo JM, Grist WJ, Gussack G, et al. Empiric trial of high-dose omeprazole in patients with posterior laryngitis: A prospective study. Am J Gastroenterol 1997;12:2160–2165.
34. Savary M, Miller G. The esophagus. In: Gassmann SA, ed. Handbook and Atlas of Endoscopy. Verlag Solothurn, Switzerland, 1978.
35. Welage LS, Berardi RR. Evaluation of omeprazole, lansoprazole, pantoprazole, and rabeprazole in the treatment of acid-related disorders. J Am Pharm Assoc 2000;40:52–62.
36. Richter JE, Castell DO. Drugs, foods and other substances in the cause and treatment of reflux esophagitis. Med Clin North Am 1981;65:1223–1234.
37. Locke GR, Talley NJ, Fett SL, et al. Risk factors associated with symptoms of gastroesophageal reflux. Am J Med 1999;106:642–649.
38. Anonymous. Guideline for the surgical treatment of gastroesophageal reflux disease (GERD). Surg Endosc 1998;12:186–188.
39. Lundell L, Dalenvack J, Hattlevakk J, et al. Omeprazole or antireflux surgery in the long-term management of gastroesophageal reflux disease: Results of a multicentre, randomized, clinical trial. Gastroenterology 1998;114:A207.
40. Johnson DA. Endoscopic therapy for GERD—baking, sewing, or stuffing: An evidence-based perspective. Rev Gastroenterol Disord 2003;3:142–149.
41. Washington N, Steele RJ, Jackson SJ, et al. Patterns of food and acid reflux in patients with low-grade oesophagitis—The role of an antireflux agent. Aliment Pharmacol Ther 1998;12:53–58.
42. Chevrel B. A comparative crossover study on the treatment of heartburn and epigastric pain: Liquid Gaviscon and a magnesium-aluminum antacid gel. J Med Res 1980;8:300–302.
43. Graham DY, Lanza F, Dorsch ER. Symptomatic reflux esophagitis: A double-blind controlled comparison of antacids and alginate. Curr Ther Res 1977;22:653–658.
44. Welage LS, Berardi RB. Drug interactions with antiulcer agents: Considerations in the treatment of acid-peptic disease. J Pharm Pract 1994;7:177–195.
45. Horn J. The proton-pump inhibitors: Similarities and differences. Clin Ther 2000;22:266–280.
46. Blum RA, Shi HK, Greski-Rose PA, et al. The comparative effects of lansoprazole, omeprazole and ranitidine in suppressing gastric acid secretion. Clin Ther 1997;19:1013–1023.
47. Tolman KG, Sanders SW, Buchi KN, et al. The effects of oral doses of lansoprazole and omeprazole on gastric pH. J Clin Gastroenterol 1997;24:65–70.
48. Williams MP, Sercombe J, Hamilton MI, et al. A placebo-controlled trial to assess the effects of 8 days of dosing with rabeprazole versus omeprazole on 24-h intragastric acidity and plasma gastrin concentrations in young healthy male subjects. Aliment Pharmacol Ther 1998;12:1079–1089.
49. Robinson M, Maton PN, Rodriguez S, et al. Effects of oral rabeprazole on oesophageal and gastric pH in patients with gastro-oesophageal reflux disease. Aliment Pharmacol Ther 1997;11:973–980.
50. Lind T, Kyleback A, Rydberg L, et al. Esomeprazole provides improved acid control vs omeprazole in patients with symptoms of GERD. Aliment Pharmacol Ther 2000;14:861–867.

51. Chiba N, De Cara CJ, Wilkinson JM, Hunt RH. Speed of healing and symptom relief in grade II to IV gastro-oesophageal reflux disease: A meta-analysis. Gastroenterology 1997;112:1798–1810.

52. Festen HP, Schenk E, Tan G, et al. Omeprazole versus high-dose ranitidine in mild gastroesophageal reflux disease: Short- and long-term treatment. The Dutch Reflux Study Group. Am J Gastroenterol 1999;94:931–936.

53. Castell DO, Richter JE, Robinson MJ, et al. Efficacy and safety of lansoprazole in the treatment of erosive esophagitis. Am J Gastroenterol 1996;91:1749–1757.

54. Mulder CJ, Dekker W, Gerretsen M. Lansoprazole 30 mg versus omeprazole 40 mg in the treatment of reflux oesophagitis grad II, III and IV (a Dutch multicentre trial). Dutch Study Group. Eur J Gastroenterol Hepatol 1996;8:1101–1106.

55. Kahrilas PJ, Falk GW, Johnson DA, et al. Esomeprazole improves healing and symptom resolution as compared with omeprazole in reflux oesophagitis patients: A randomized controlled trial. Aliment Pharmacol Ther 2000;14:1249–1258.

56. Dekkers CP, Beker JA, Thjodleifsson B, et al. Double-blind, placebo-controlled comparison of rabeprazole 20 mg vs omeprazole 20 mg in the treatment of erosive or ulcerative gastro-oesophageal reflux disease. The European Rabeprazole Study Group. Aliment Pharmacol Ther 1999;13:49–57.

57. Mossner J, Holscher AH, Herz R, et al. A double-blind study of pantoprazole and omeprazole in the treatment of reflux oesophagitis: A multicentre trial. Aliment Pharmacol Ther 1995;9:321–326.

58. Klinkenberg-Knol EC, Festen HPM, Jansen JBMJ, et al. Long-term treatment with omeprazole for refractory reflux esophagitis: Efficacy and safety. Ann Intern Med 1994;121:161–167.

59. Sampliner RE. Effect of up to 3 years of high dose lansoprazole on Barrett esophagus. Am J Gastroenterol 1994;89:1844–1848.

60. Peters FT, Ganesh S, Kuipers EJ, et al. Endoscopic regression of Barrett oesophagus during omeprazole treatment: A randomised double blind study. Gut 1999;45:489–494.

61. Sampliner RE, Camargo E. Normalization of esophageal pH with high-dose proton pump inhibitor therapy does not result in regression of Barrett esophagus. Am J Gastroenterol 1997;92:582–585.

62. Richardson P, Hawkey CJ, Stack WA. Proton pump inhibitors. Pharmacology and rationale for use in gastrointestinal disorders. Drugs 1998;56:307–335.

63. Pace F, Lazzaroni M, Bianchi-Porro G. Failure of sucralfate in the treatment of refractory esophagitis vs. high dose famotidine: An endoscopic study. Scand J Gastroenterol 1991;26:491–494.

64. Hetzel DJ, Dent J, Reed WD, et al. Healing and relapse of severe peptic esophagitis after treatment with omeprazole. Gastroenterology 1988;95:903–912.

65. Robinson M, Lanza F, Avner D, Haber M. Effective maintenance therapy of reflux esophagitis with low dose lansoprazole: A randomized, double blind placebo-controlled trial. Ann Intern Med 1996;124:859–867.

66. Vigneri S, Termini R, Leandro G, et al. A comparison of five maintenance therapies for reflux esophagitis. N Engl J Med 1995;333:1106–1110.

67. Talley NJ, Lauritsen K, Tunturi-Hihnala H, et al. Esomeprazole 20 mg maintains symptom control in endoscopy-negative GERD: A randomized placebo-controlled trial of on-demand therapy for 6 months. Gastroenterology 2000;118(4 Pt 2):A21. Abstract 348.

68. Talley NJ, Venables TL, Green JRB, et al. Esomeprazole 40 mg and 20 mg is efficacious in the long-term management of patients with endoscopy-negative GERD: A placebo-controlled trial of on-demand therapy for 6 months. Gastroenterology 2000;118(4 Pt 2):A658. Abstract 3608.

69. Gough AL, Long RG, Cooper BT. Lansoprazole versus ranitidine in the maintenance of reflux oesophagitis. Aliment Pharmacol Ther 1996;10:529–539.

70. Vakil NB, Shaker R, Hwang C, et al. Esomeprazole is effective as maintenance therapy in GERD patients with healed erosive esophagitis (EE). Gastroenterology 2000;118(4 Pt 2):A22.

71. Johnson DA, Benjamin SB, Whipple J, et al. Efficacy and safety of esomeprazole as maintenance therapy in GERD patients with healed erosive esophagitis (EE). Gastroenterology 2000;118(4 Pt 2):A17. Abstract 330.

72. Dent J, Yeomans ND, Mackinnon M, et al. Omeprazole vs ranitidine for prevention of relapse in reflux oesophagitis: A controlled double blind trial of their efficacy and safety. Gut 1994;35:590–598.

73. Garrett WR. Considerations for long-term use of proton-pump inhibitors. Am J Health Syst Pharm 1998;55:2268–2279.

74. Kuipers EJ, Lundell L, Klinkenberg-Knol EC, et al. Atrophic gastritis and Helicobacter pylori infection in patients with reflux esophagitis treated with omeprazole or fundoplication. N Engl J Med 1996;334:1018–1022.

75. O'Connor HJ. Helicobacter pylori and gastro-oesophageal reflux disease—Clinical implications and management. Aliment Pharmacol Ther 1999;13:117–127.

76. Anonymous. Proton pump inhibitor relabeling for cancer risk not warranted. FD & C Report 1996;58(Nov 1):T &G 1–2.

77. DeVault KR. Overview of therapy for extraesophageal manifestations of gastroesophageal reflux disease. Am J Gastroenterol 2000;95:S39–S44.

78. Field SK, Sutherland LR. Does medical antireflux therapy improve asthma in asthmatics with gastroesophageal reflux? A critical review of the literature. Chest 1998;114:275–283.

79. Irwin RS, Boulet L-P, Cloutier MM, et al. Managing cough as a defense mechanism and a symptom: A consensus panel report of the American College of Chest Physicians. Chest 1998;114(Suppl):133S–181S.

80. Van Pinxteren B, Numans ME, Ponis PA, Lau J. Short-term treatment with proton pump inhibitors, H2-receptor antagonists and prokinetics for gastro-oesophageal reflux disease-like symptoms and endoscopy negative reflux disease. Cochrane Database Syst Rev 2000;CD002095:1–27.

81. Watson RG, Tham TC, Johnston BT, et al. Double-blind cross-over placebo-controlled study of omeprazole in the treatment of patients with reflux symptoms and physiological levels of acid reflux—The sensitive esophagus. Gut 1997;40:587–590.

82. Venables TL, Newland RD, Patel AC, et al. Omeprazole 10 milligrams once daily, omeprazole 20 milligrams once daily, or ranitidine 150 milligrams twice daily, evaluated as initial therapy for the relief of symptoms of gastro-oesophageal reflux disease in general practice. Scand J Gastroenterol 1997;32:965–973.

83. Bate CM, Green JR, Axon AT, et al. Omeprazole is more effective than cimetidine for the relief of all grades of gastro-oesophageal reflux disease-associated heartburn, irrespective of the presence or absence of endoscopic oesophagitis. Aliment Pharmacol Ther 1997;11:755–763.

84. Vandenplas Y, Belli D, Benhamou P-H, et al. Current concepts and issues in the management of regurgitation in infants: A reappraisal. Management guidelines from a working party. Acta Paediatr 1996;85:531–534.

85. Faubion WA, Zein NN. Gastroesophageal reflux in infants and children. Mayo Clin Proc 1998;73:166–173.

86. Patel AS, Pohl JF, Easley DJ. Proton pump inhibitors in pediatrics. Pediatr Rev 2003;24:12–5.

87. Katz PO. Gastroesophageal reflux disease. J Am Geriatr Soc 1998;46:1558–1565.

88. Hillman AL, Bloom BS, Fendrick AM, et al. Cost and quality effects of alternative treatments for persistent gastroesophageal reflux disease. Arch Intern Med 1992;152:1467–1472.

89. Marks RD, Richter JE, Rizzo J, et al. Omeprazole versus H2 receptor antagonists in treating patients with peptic stricture and esophagitis. Gastroenterology 1994;106:907–915.

90. Harris RA, Kuppermann M, Richter JE. Proton pump inhibitors or histamine-2 receptor antagonists for the prevention of erosive reflux esophagitis: A cost-effectiveness analysis. Am J Gastroenterol 1997;92:2179–2189.

91. Revicki D, Wood M, Maton PM, et al. The impact of gastroesophageal reflux disease on health-related quality of life. Am J Med 1998;104:252–258.

92. Heudebert GR, Marks R, Wilcox CM, et al. Choice of long-term strategy for the management of patients with severe esophagitis: A cost-utility analysis. Gastroenterology 1997;112:1078–1086.

93. Dent J. Long-term aims of treatment of reflux disease, and the role of non-drug measures. Digestion 1992;51(Suppl 1):30–34.

33
PEPTIC ULCER DISEASE

Rosemary R. Berardi and Lynda S. Welage

Learning Objectives and other resources can be found at *www.pharmacotherapyonline.com.*

KEY CONCEPTS

1. Patients with peptic ulcer disease should reduce psychological stress, cigarette smoking, and nonsteroidal anti-inflammatory drug (NSAID) use, and should avoid foods and beverages that exacerbate ulcer symptoms.

2. Eradication is recommended for all *Helicobacter pylori* (HP)–positive patients with an active ulcer, a documented history of a prior ulcer, or a history of ulcer-related complications.

3. Treatment with a conventional antiulcer drug (H_2-receptor antagonist, proton pump inhibitor, or sucralfate) may be an alternative to HP eradication, but is discouraged because of the high rate of ulcer recurrence and ulcer-related complications. Combining conventional antiulcer drugs adds to treatment costs without enhancing efficacy.

4. Maintenance therapy with a low-dose H_2-receptor antagonist or proton pump inhibitor is only indicated for high-risk patients who fail HP eradication, patients with severe complications, or those with HP-negative ulcers.

5. The selection of an HP eradication regimen should be based on efficacy, safety, antibiotic resistance, cost, and the likelihood of compliance. Treatment should be initiated with a proton pump inhibitor–based three-drug regimen. If a second course of HP therapy is required, the regimen should contain different antibiotics.

6. Standard proton pump inhibitor dosages reduce the risk of NSAID-related gastric and duodenal ulcers and are at least as effective as misoprostol cotherapy. Standard-dose H_2-receptor antagonists reduce the risk of NSAID-related duodenal ulcer, but higher dosages are needed to reduce the risk of gastric ulcer.

7. Standard dosages of a proton pump inhibitor and a nonselective NSAID appear to be as effective as a selective cyclooxygenase-2 (COX-2) inhibitor in reducing the risk of NSAID-induced ulcers and upper GI complications.

8. The eradication of HP improves clinical outcomes and decreases the use of health care resources when compared to conventional antisecretory therapy. Misoprostol cotherapy, proton pump inhibitor cotherapy, or switching to a selective COX-2 inhibitor is cost effective in patients with the highest risk for NSAID-related ulcers and upper GI complications.

9. Patients with peptic ulcer disease, especially those receiving HP eradication or misoprostol cotherapy, require patient education regarding their disease and drug treatment to successfully achieve a positive therapeutic outcome.

10. Patients with peptic ulcer disease who develop recurrent ulcer signs or symptoms of GI bleeding or perforation should be referred to a specialist. Assess reasons for therapeutic failure, including noncompliance to the drug regimen, antibiotic resistance (HP eradication), heavy smoking, NSAID use, and the need for HP eradication in a patient on conventional antiulcer medications.

Acid-related diseases (gastritis, erosions, and peptic ulcer) of the upper gastrointestinal (GI) tract require gastric acid for their formation.[1–4] Peptic ulcer disease (PUD) differs from gastritis and erosions in that ulcers typically extend deeper into the muscularis mucosa.[1] There are three common forms of peptic ulcers: *Helicobacter pylori* (HP)–associated, nonsteroidal anti-inflammatory drug (NSAID)–induced, and stress ulcers (Table 33–1). The term "stress-related mucosal damage" (SRMD) is preferred to stress ulcer or stress gastritis, because the mucosal lesions range from superficial gastritis and erosions to deep ulcers.

Chronic peptic ulcers vary in etiology, clinical presentation, and tendency to recur (see Table 33–1). HP-associated and NSAID-induced ulcers develop most often in the stomach and duodenum of ambulatory patients (Fig. 33–1). Occasionally, ulcers develop in the esophagus, jejunum, ileum, or colon. Peptic ulcers are also associated with Zollinger-Ellison syndrome (ZES), radiation, chemotherapy, and vascular insufficiency (Table 33–2).[1,4] In contrast, acute ulcers (SRMD) occur primarily in the stomach in critically ill hospitalized patients (see Table 33–1). This chapter focuses on chronic PUD associated with HP and NSAIDs. A brief discussion of ZES and upper GI bleeding related to PUD and SRMD is included.

The natural course of chronic PUD is characterized by frequent ulcer recurrence. Approximately 60% to 100% of ulcers recur within 1 year of initial ulcer healing with conventional antiulcer regimens.[1] The most important factors that influence ulcer recurrence are HP infection and NSAID use. Other factors include gastric acid hypersecretion, cigarette smoking, alcohol use, a long duration of PUD, ulcer-related complications, and patient noncompliance. The cause of ulcer recurrence is most likely multifactorial.

TABLE 33–1. Comparison of Common Forms of Peptic Ulcer

Characteristic	*H. pylori*–induced	NSAID-induced	SRMD
Condition	Chronic	Chronic	Acute
Site of damage	Duodenum > stomach	Stomach > duodenum	Stomach > duodenum
Intragastric pH	More dependent	Less dependent	Less dependent
Symptoms	Usually epigastric pain	Often asymptomatic	Asymptomatic
Ulcer depth	Superficial	Deep	Most superficial
GI bleeding	Less severe, single vessel	More severe, single vessel	More severe, superficial mucosal capillaries

H. pylori, Helicobacter pylori; NSAID, nonsteroidal anti-inflammatory drug; SRMD, stress-related mucosal damage.

EPIDEMIOLOGY

Approximately 10% of Americans develop chronic PUD during their lifetime.[1] The incidence varies with ulcer type, age, gender, and geographic location. Race, occupation, genetic predisposition, and societal factors may play a minor role in ulcer pathogenesis, but are attenuated by the importance of HP infection and NSAID use. The prevalence of PUD in the United States has shifted from predominance in men to nearly comparable prevalence in men and women. Recent trends suggest a declining rate for younger men and an increasing rate for older women.[1] Factors that have influenced these trends include the declining smoking rates in younger men and the increased use of NSAIDs in older adults.

Since 1960, ulcer-related physician visits, hospitalizations, operations, and deaths have declined in the United States by more than 50%, primarily because of decreased rates of PUD among men.[1] The decline in hospitalizations has resulted from a reduction in hospital admissions for uncomplicated duodenal ulcer. However, hospitalizations of older adults for ulcer-related complications (bleeding and perforation) have increased.[1] Although the overall mortality from PUD has decreased, death rates have increased in patients older than 75 years of age, most likely a result of increased consumption of NSAIDs and an aging population. Patients with gastric ulcer have a higher mortality rate than those with duodenal ulcer because gastric ulcer is more prevalent in older individuals. Despite these trends, PUD remains one of the most common GI diseases, resulting in impaired quality of life, work loss, and high-cost medical care. To date, H_2-receptor antagonists (H_2RAs), proton pump inhibitors (PPIs), and drugs that promote mucosal defense have not altered PUD complication rates.[1]

ETIOLOGY AND RISK FACTORS

Most peptic ulcers occur in the presence of acid and pepsin when HP, NSAIDs, or other factors (see Table 33–2) disrupt normal mucosal defense and healing mechanisms.[1] Hypersecretion of acid is the primary pathogenic mechanism in hypersecretory states such as ZES.[4] Ulcer location is related to a number of etiologic factors. Benign gastric ulcers can occur anywhere in the stomach, although most are located on the lesser curvature, just distal to the junction of the antral and acid-secreting mucosa (see Fig. 33–1). Most duodenal ulcers occur in the first part of the duodenum (duodenal bulb).

HELICOBACTER PYLORI

Helicobacter pylori infection causes chronic gastritis in all infected individuals and is causally linked to PUD, gastric cancer, and mucosa-associated lymphoid tissue (MALT) lymphoma (Fig. 33–2).[1,5–7] However, only a small number of infected individuals will develop symptomatic PUD (about 20%) or gastric cancer (less than 1%).[1,6] The pattern and distribution of gastritis correlates strongly with the risk of a specific gastrointestinal disorder. The development of atrophic gastritis and gastric cancer is a slow process that occurs over 20 to 40 years. Serologic studies confirm an association between HP and gastric cancer.[1,6] Supportive evidence for PUD is based on the fact that most non-NSAID ulcers are infected with HP, and that HP eradication markedly decreases ulcer recurrence.[5,6] Host-specific cofactors and HP strain variability play an important role in the pathogenesis of PUD and gastric cancer.[5–7] Although an association between HP and PUD bleeding is less clear, eradication of HP decreases recurrent bleeding.[8] No specific link has been established between HP and dyspepsia, nonulcer dyspepsia (NUD), or gastroesophageal reflux disease.[9–11]

TABLE 33–2. Potential Causes of Peptic Ulcer

Common causes
  Helicobacter pylori infection
  Nonsteroidal anti-inflammatory drugs
  Critical illness (stress-related mucosal damage)
Uncommon causes
  Hypersecretion of gastric acid (e.g., Zollinger-Ellison syndrome)
  Viral infections (e.g., cytomegalovirus)
  Vascular insufficiency (crack cocaine–associated)
  Radiation
  Chemotherapy (e.g., hepatic artery infusions)
  Rare genetic subtypes
  Idiopathic

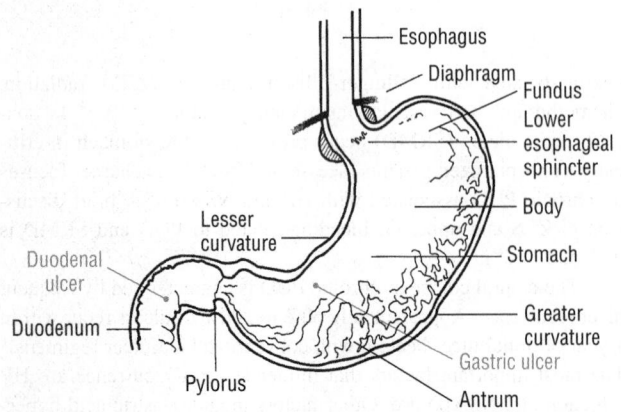

FIGURE 33–1. Anatomic structure of the stomach and duodenum and most common locations of gastric and duodenal ulcers.

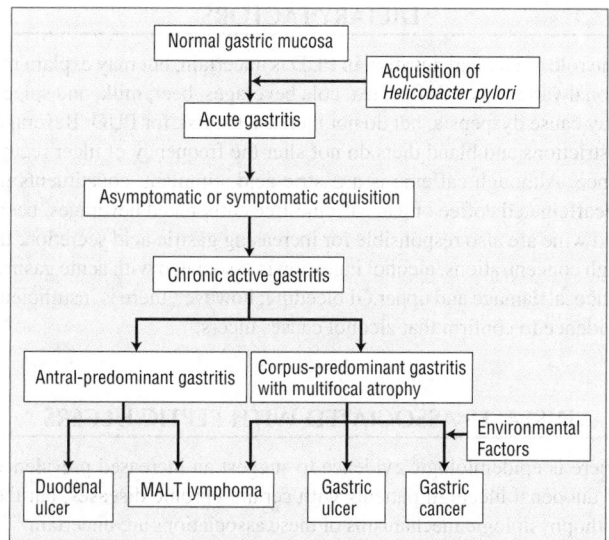

FIGURE 33–2. The natural history of *Helicobacter pylori* infection in the pathogenesis of gastric ulcer and duodenal ulcer, mucosa-associated lymphoid tissue (MALT) lymphoma, and gastric cancer.

Approximately 50% of the world's population is colonized by HP.[6] The prevalence of HP varies by geographic location, socioeconomic conditions, ethnicity, and age. In developing countries, HP prevalence exceeds 80% in adults and correlates with lower socioeconomic conditions.[5] In industrialized countries, the prevalence of HP in adults is between 20% and 50%.[5] The prevalence of HP in the United States is 30% to 40%, but remains higher in ethnic groups such as African and Latin Americans.[6] There is a decreasing frequency of infection, especially in regions with improving sanitation and socioeconomic conditions.[6] In developed countries, there is an increased HP prevalence with age.[1,6] However, this reflects a more intense transmission when older generations were children, as younger generations have been less likely to acquire the infection. Infection rates do not differ with gender or smoking status.

HP is transmitted person-to-person by three different pathways; fecal-oral, oral-oral, and iatrogenic.[1,6] Transmission of the organism is thought to occur by the fecal-oral route, either directly from an infected person, or indirectly from fecal-contaminated water or food.[1] Members of the same household are likely to become infected when someone in the same household is infected.[1] Risk factors include crowded living conditions, a large number of children, unclean water, and consumption of raw vegetables.[6] Transmission by the oral-oral route has been postulated because HP has been isolated from the oral cavity.[6] Transmission of HP can occur iatrogenically when infected instruments such as endoscopes are used.[1]

NONSTEROIDAL ANTI-INFLAMMATORY DRUGS

NSAIDs are one of the most widely prescribed classes of medications in the United States, particularly in individuals 60 years of age and older.[1] There is overwhelming evidence linking chronic nonselective NSAID (including aspirin) use to a variety of GI tract injuries (Table 33–3).[1,12–14] Subepithelial gastric hemorrhages occur within 15 to 30 minutes of ingestion, and progress to gastric erosions with continued ingestion.[1,12] These lesions heal within a few days with continued NSAID use and do not lead to GI complications. Gastroduodenal ulcers occur in 15% to 30% of regular NSAID users and may develop

TABLE 33–3. Selected Nonsteroidal Anti-Inflammatory Drugs (NSAIDs) and Cyclooxygenase-2 (COX-2) Inhibitors

Nonsalicylates
  Nonselective (traditional) NSAIDs: indomethacin, piroxicam, ibuprofen, naproxen, sulindac, ketoprofen, ketorolac, flurbiprofen, diclofenac
  Partially selective NSAIDs: etodolac, nabumetone, meloxicam
  Selective COX-2 inhibitors: celecoxib, valdecoxib
Salicylates
  Acetylated: aspirin
  Nonacetylated: salsalate, trisalicylate

within a week or with continued treatment (6 months or longer).[12] Gastric ulcers are most common, occur primarily in the antrum (see Fig. 33–1), and are of greater concern than erosions because of their potential to bleed or perforate (see Table 33–1). NSAID-induced ulcers may occur in the esophagus and colon, but are less common.[1,15] Each year, nonselective NSAIDs account for at least 16,500 deaths and 107,000 hospitalizations in the United States.[1,14] Clinically important upper GI events occur in 3% to 4.5% of arthritis patients taking NSAIDs, and 1.5% have a serious complication (major GI bleeding, perforation, or obstruction).[12]

The risk factors for NSAID-induced ulcers and GI-related complications are presented in Table 33–4. Combinations of factors confer an additive risk. The risk of NSAID complications is increased as much as 14-fold in patients with a previous history of an ulcer or ulcer-related bleeding.[1] Advanced age is an independent risk factor and increases linearly with the age of the patient.[1] The high incidence of ulcer complications in older individuals may be explained by age-related changes in gastric mucosal defense. The risk for NSAID-induced ulcers and complications is dose related, although both can occur with low dosages of nonprescription NSAIDs and the low dosages of aspirin taken for cardioprotective purposes (81 to 325 mg/day).[1,12–14,16,17] The use of corticosteroids alone does not increase the risk of ulcer or complications, but ulcer risk is

TABLE 33–4. Risk Factors for Nonsteroidal Anti-Inflammatory Drug (NSAID)-Induced Ulcers and Upper Gastrointestinal Complications[a]

Established risk factors
  Age over 60 years
  Previous peptic ulcer disease
  Previous upper GI bleeding
  Concomitant corticosteroid therapy
  High-dose and multiple NSAID use
  Concomitant anticoagulant use or coagulopathy
  Chronic major organ impairment (e.g., cardiovascular disease)
Possible risk factors
  NSAID-related dyspepsia
  Duration of NSAID use
  Helicobacter pylori infection
  Rheumatoid arthritis (extent of disability)
Questionable risk factors
  Cigarette smoking
  Alcohol consumption

[a]Combinations of risk factors are additive.
Compiled from Del Valle et al,[1] Suerbaum and Michetti,[5] Laine,[12] and Gleeson and Davis.[15]

increased twofold in corticosteroid users who are also taking concurrent NSAIDs.[1] The use of low-dose aspirin in combination with another NSAID increases the risk of upper GI complications to a greater extent than the use of either drug alone.[1,17] The risk of bleeding is markedly increased when NSAIDs are used in combination with anticoagulants.[1] NSAID-related dyspepsia that is not relieved by antiulcer medications may indicate an ulcer or ulcer complication, but dyspepsia does not correlate directly with mucosal injury or clinical events. Whether HP infection is a risk factor for NSAID-induced ulcers remains controversial.[18–20] Most evidence indicates that both HP and NSAIDs are independent risk factors and that HP does not potentiate the risk of ulcer formation in NSAID users.[18] However, recent data suggest that HP may potentiate the effects of NSAIDs and low-dose aspirin with regard to ulcer bleeding.[19,20] Cigarette smoking and alcohol ingestion contribute to increased ulcer risk but do not appear to be independent factors.[1]

There is little evidence to support clinically important differences with regard to the frequency of ulcers and upper GI complications among most available nonaspirin, nonselective NSAIDs (see Table 33–3) when used in equipotent anti-inflammatory dosages.[1] However, the nonacetylated salicylates (e.g., salsalate) and newer NSAIDs (e.g., etodolac, nabumetone, and meloxicam) may be associated with a decreased incidence of GI toxicity.[1,21,22] NSAIDs that selectively inhibit cyclooxygenase-2 (COX-2) decrease the incidence of gastroduodenal ulcers and related GI complications when compared to the nonselective NSAIDs.[21,22] The use of buffered or enteric-coated aspirin confers no added protection from ulcer or GI complications.[23]

CIGARETTE SMOKING

There is epidemiologic evidence that links cigarette smoking to PUD, impaired ulcer healing, and ulcer-related GI complications.[1] The risk is proportional to the number of cigarettes smoked and is modest when fewer than 10 cigarettes are smoked per day. Smoking does not increase ulcer recurrence after HP eradication. Death rates are higher among patients who smoke than among nonsmoking patients, although it is not known whether the increase in mortality reflects PUD or the cardiac and pulmonary sequelae of smoking. The exact mechanism by which cigarette smoking contributes to PUD remains unclear. Possible mechanisms include delayed gastric emptying of solids and liquids, inhibition of pancreatic bicarbonate secretion, promotion of duodenogastric reflux, and reduction in mucosal prostaglandin (PG) production. Although smoking increases gastric acid secretion, this effect is not consistent. It is uncertain whether nicotine or other components of smoke are responsible for these physiologic alterations. Cigarette smoking may provide a favorable milieu for HP infection.

PSYCHOLOGICAL STRESS

The importance of psychological factors in the pathogenesis of PUD remains controversial.[1] Clinical observation suggests that ulcer patients are adversely affected by stressful life events. However, results from controlled trials are conflicting and have failed to document a cause-and-effect relationship.[1] It is possible that emotional stress induces behavioral risks such as smoking and the use of NSAIDs, or alters the inflammatory response or resistance to HP infection. The role of stress and how it affects PUD is complex and probably multifactorial.

DIETARY FACTORS

The role of diet and nutrition in PUD is uncertain, but may explain regional variations.[1] Coffee, tea, cola beverages, beer, milk, and spices may cause dyspepsia, but do not increase the risk for PUD. Beverage restrictions and bland diets do not alter the frequency of ulcer recurrence. Although caffeine is a gastric acid stimulant, constituents in decaffeinated coffee or tea, caffeine-free carbonated beverages, beer, and wine are also responsible for increasing gastric acid secretion. In high concentrations, alcohol ingestion is associated with acute gastric mucosal damage and upper GI bleeding; however, there is insufficient evidence to confirm that alcohol causes ulcers.

DISEASES ASSOCIATED WITH PEPTIC ULCERS

There is epidemiologic evidence to suggest an increased prevalence of duodenal ulcers in patients with certain chronic diseases, but the pathophysiologic mechanisms of these associations are uncertain.[1] A strong association exists in patients with systemic mastocytosis, multiple endocrine neoplasia type 1, chronic pulmonary diseases, chronic renal failure, kidney stones, hepatic cirrhosis, and α_1-antitrypsin deficiency. An association may exist in patients with cystic fibrosis, chronic pancreatitis, Crohn's disease, coronary artery disease, polycythemia vera, and hyperparathyroidism.

PATHOPHYSIOLOGY

Gastric and duodenal ulcers occur because of an imbalance between aggressive factors (gastric acid and pepsin) and mechanisms that maintain mucosal integrity (mucosal defense and repair).

GASTRIC ACID AND PEPSIN

The potential for producing mucosal damage is related to the secretion of gastric (hydrochloric) acid and pepsin. Hydrochloric acid is secreted by the parietal cells, which contain receptors for histamine, gastrin, and acetylcholine. Acid (as well as HP infection and NSAID use) is an independent factor that contributes to the disruption of mucosal integrity. Increased acid secretion has been observed in patients with duodenal ulcers and may be a consequence of HP infection.[24,25] Patients with ZES (described later in the chapter) have gastric acid hypersecretion resulting from a gastrin-producing tumor.[4] Patients with gastric ulcer usually have normal or reduced rates of acid secretion (hypochlorhydria).

Acid secretion is expressed as the amount of acid secreted under basal or fasting conditions, basal acid output (BAO); after maximal stimulation, maximal acid output (MAO); or in response to a meal.[24] Basal, maximal, and meal-stimulated acid secretion varies according to time of day and the individual's psychological state, age, gender, and health status. The BAO follows a circadian rhythm, with the highest acid secretion occurring at night and the lowest in the morning. An increase in the BAO:MAO ratio suggests a basal hypersecretory state such as ZES. A review of gastric acid secretion and its regulation can be found elsewhere.[24]

Pepsinogen, the inactive precursor of pepsin, is secreted by the chief cells located in the gastric fundus (see Fig. 33–1). Pepsin is activated by acid pH (optimal pH of 1.8 to 3.5), inactivated reversibly at pH 4, and irreversibly destroyed at pH 7. Pepsin appears to play a role in the proteolytic activity involved in ulcer formation.[24]

MUCOSAL DEFENSE AND REPAIR

Mucosal defense and repair mechanisms protect the gastroduodenal mucosa from noxious endogenous and exogenous substances.[1] Mucosal defense mechanisms include mucus and bicarbonate secretion, intrinsic epithelial cell defense, and mucosal blood flow.[1,25] The viscous nature and near-neutral pH of the mucus-bicarbonate barrier protect the stomach from the acidic contents in the gastric lumen. Mucosal repair after injury is related to epithelial cell restitution, growth, and regeneration. The maintenance of mucosal integrity and repair is mediated by the production of endogenous prostaglandins. The term *cytoprotection* is often used to describe this process, but *mucosal defense* and *mucosal protection* are more accurate terms, as prostaglandins prevent deep mucosal injury and not superficial damage to individual cells. Gastric hyperemia and increased prostaglandin synthesis characterize adaptive cytoprotection, the short-term adaptation of mucosal cells to mild topical irritants. This phenomenon enables the stomach to initially withstand the damaging effects of irritants. Alterations in mucosal defense that are induced by HP or NSAIDs are the most important cofactors in the formation of peptic ulcers.

HELICOBACTER PYLORI

Helicobacter pylori is a spiral-shaped, pH-sensitive, gram-negative, microaerophilic bacterium that resides between the mucus layer and surface epithelial cells in the stomach, or any location where gastric-type epithelium is found.[1,5,6] The combination of its spiral shape and flagellum permits it to move from the lumen of the stomach, where the pH is low, to the mucus layer, where the local pH is neutral. The acute infection is accompanied by transient hypochlorhydria, which permits the organism to survive in the acidic gastric juice.[25] The exact method by which HP initially induces hypochlorhydria is unclear. One theory is that HP produces large amounts of urease, which hydrolyzes urea in the gastric juice and converts it to ammonia and carbon dioxide.[5,6] The local buffering effect of ammonia creates a neutral microenvironment within and surrounding the bacterium, which protects it from the lethal effect of acid.[6] HP also produces acid-inhibitory proteins, which allows it to adapt to the low-pH environment of the stomach.[25] HP attaches to gastric-type epithelium by adherence pedestals, which prevent the organism from being shed during cell turnover and mucus secretion. Colonization of the corpus (body) of the stomach is associated with gastric ulcer (see Fig. 33–2). Antral organisms are hypothesized to colonize gastric metaplastic tissue (which is thought to arise secondary to changes in acid or bicarbonate secretion, products of HP, or host inflammatory responses) in the duodenal bulb, leading to duodenal ulcer.[1]

A number of bacterial and host factors contribute to the ability of HP to cause gastroduodenal mucosal injury. Pathogenic mechanisms include: (a) direct mucosal damage, (b) alterations in the host immune/inflammatory response, and (c) hypergastrinemia leading to increased acid secretion.[1,5] In addition, HP enhances the carcinogenic conversion of susceptible gastric epithelial cells.[6,7]

Direct mucosal damage is produced by virulence factors (vacuolating cytotoxin, cytotoxin-associated gene protein, and growth-inhibitory factor), elaborating bacterial enzymes (lipases, proteases, and urease), and adherence.[1,5] About 50% of HP strains produce a protein toxin (Vac A) that is responsible for cellular vacuole formation. Strains with cytotoxin-associated gene (cagA) protein are associated with duodenal ulcer, atrophic gastritis, and gastric cancer.[1,5,7] Lipases and proteases degrade gastric mucus, ammonia produced by urease may be toxic to gastric epithelial cells, and bacterial adherence enhances the uptake of toxins into gastric epithelial cells. HP infection

alters the host inflammatory response and damages epithelial cells directly by cell-mediated immune mechanisms, or indirectly by activated neutrophils or macrophages attempting to phagocytose bacteria or bacterial products.[1,5] HP infection may increase gastric acid secretion in patients with duodenal ulcer, or diminish acid output in patients with gastric cancer.[1] Antral-predominant infection is associated with hypergastrinemia and increased gastric acid secretion. Responsible mechanisms include cytokines, such as tumor necrosis factor-α released in HP gastritis; products of HP, such as ammonia; and diminished expression of somatostatin. Why somatostatin is diminished is unclear, but cytokines may be involved.[1] Corpus (body)-predominant infection promotes gastric atrophy and decreases acid output.[1,6,7]

NONSTEROIDAL ANTI-INFLAMMATORY DRUGS

Nonselective NSAIDs including aspirin (see Table 33–3) cause gastric mucosal damage by two important mechanisms: (a) direct or topical irritation of the gastric epithelium and (b) systemic inhibition of endogenous mucosal prostaglandin synthesis.[1,13,14] Although the initial injury is initiated topically by the acidic properties of many of the NSAIDs, systemic inhibition of the protective prostaglandins plays the predominant role in the development of gastric ulcer.[1,13,14] Cyclooxygenase (COX) is the rate-limiting enzyme in the conversion of arachidonic acid to prostaglandins and is inhibited by NSAIDs (Fig. 33–3).

Two similar COX isoforms have been identified: cyclooxygenase-1 (COX-1) is found in most body tissue, including the stomach, kidney, intestine, and platelets; cyclooxygenase-2 (COX-2) is undetectable in most tissues under normal physiologic conditions, but its expression can be induced during acute inflammation and arthritis (Fig. 33–4).[13,14] COX-1 produces protective prostaglandins that regulate physiologic processes such as GI mucosal integrity, platelet homeostasis, and renal function. COX-2 is induced (upregulated) by inflammatory stimuli such as cytokines, and produces prostaglandins involved with inflammation, fever, and pain. COX-2 is also constitutively expressed in organs such as the brain, kidney, and reproductive tract. Adverse effects (e.g., GI toxicity or renal toxicity) of NSAIDs are associated with the inhibition of COX-1, whereas anti-inflammatory actions result from NSAID inhibition of COX-2.[13,14] Nonselective NSAIDs including aspirin (see Table 33–3) inhibit both COX-1 and COX-2 to varying degrees.[1,13,14] Aspirin irreversibly inhibits platelet COX-1 for as long as 18 hours, resulting in decreased platelet aggregation and prolonged

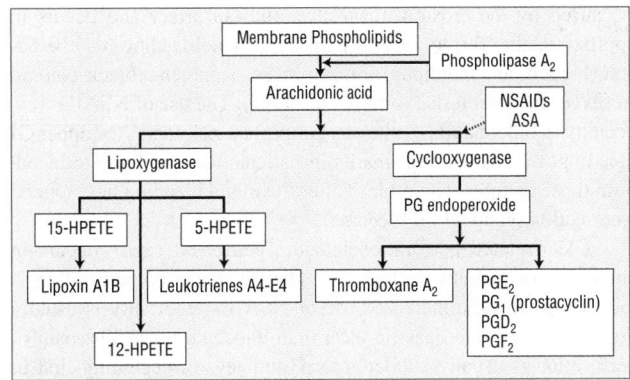

FIGURE 33–3. Metabolism of arachidonic acid after its release from membrane phospholipids. ASA, aspirin; HPETE, hydroperoxyeicosatetraenoic acid; NSAIDs, nonsteroidal antiinflammatory drugs; PG, prostaglandin. Broken arrow indicates inhibitory effects.

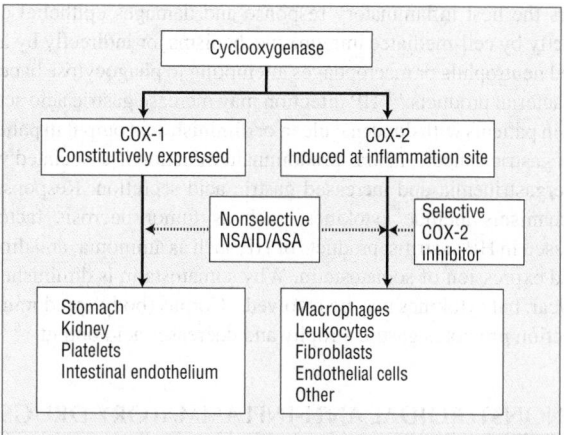

FIGURE 33–4. Tissue distribution and actions of cyclooxygenase (COX) isoenzymes. Nonselective nonsteroidal anti-inflammatory drugs (NSAIDs) including aspirin (ASA) inhibit COX-1 and COX-2 to varying degrees; COX-2 inhibitors inhibit only COX-2. Broken arrow indicates inhibitory effects.

bleeding times, which may potentiate upper and lower GI bleeding.[1] Similar effects are observed with the nonselective NSAIDs.

A number of other mechanisms may contribute to the development of NSAID-induced mucosal injury. Neutrophil adherence may damage the vascular endothelium and may lead to a reduction in mucosal blood flow, or may liberate oxygen-derived free radicals and proteases. Leukotrienes, products of lipoxygenase metabolism, are inflammatory substances that may contribute to mucosal injury through stimulatory effects on neutrophil adherence (see Fig. 33–3).

Topical irritant properties are predominantly associated with acidic NSAIDs (e.g., aspirin) and their ability to decrease the hydrophobicity of the mucous gel layer in the gastric mucosa.[1,13,14] Most nonaspirin NSAIDs have topical irritant effects, but aspirin appears to be the most damaging. Although NSAID prodrugs, enteric-coated aspirin tablets, salicylate derivatives, and parenteral or rectal preparations are associated with less-acute topical gastric mucosal injury, they can cause ulcers and related GI complications as a result of their systemic inhibition of endogenous PGs.

COMPLICATIONS

Upper GI bleeding, perforation, and obstruction occur with HP-associated and NSAID-induced ulcers and constitute the most serious, life-threatening complications of chronic PUD.[1,2,26] Bleeding is caused by the erosion of an ulcer into an artery and occurs in approximately 10% to 15% of patients.[1,2] The bleeding may be occult (hidden) and insidious, or may present as melena (black-colored stools) or hematemesis (vomiting of blood). The use of NSAIDs (especially in older adults) is the most important risk factor for upper GI bleeding. Deaths occur primarily in patients who continue to bleed, or in those patients who rebleed after the initial bleeding has stopped (see section on upper GI bleeding).

Ulcer-related perforation into the peritoneal cavity occurs in about 7% of patients with PUD.[1] The incidence of perforation is increasing with the increased use of NSAIDs. Mortality is usually higher for perforated gastric ulcer than duodenal ulcer. The pain of perforation is usually sudden, sharp, and severe, beginning first in the epigastrium, but quickly spreading over the entire abdomen. Most patients experience ulcer symptoms prior to perforation. However, older patients who experience perforation in association with NSAID use may be asymptomatic. Penetration occurs when an ulcer burrows

into an adjacent structure (pancreas, biliary tract, or liver) rather than opening freely into a cavity.

Gastric outlet obstruction occurs in about 2% of patients with peptic ulcers.[1] Mechanical obstruction is caused by scarring or edema of the duodenal bulb or pyloric channel and can lead to gastric retention. Symptoms usually occur over several months and include early satiety, bloating, anorexia, nausea, vomiting, and weight loss. Perforation, penetration, and gastric outlet obstruction occur most often in patients with long-standing PUD.

Treatment of PUD has improved so dramatically that even the most virulent ulcers can be managed with medication. Intractability to drug therapy is now an infrequent manifestation of PUD and an infrequent indication for surgery.

CLINICAL PRESENTATION

SIGNS AND SYMPTOMS

The clinical presentation of PUD varies depending on the severity of abdominal pain and the presence of complications (Table 33–5).[1]

TABLE 33–5. Presentation of Chronic Peptic Ulcer Disease

General
- Mild epigastric pain or acute life-threatening upper gastrointestinal complications

Symptoms
- Abdominal pain that is often epigastric and described as burning, but may present as vague discomfort, abdominal fullness, or cramping
- A typical nocturnal pain that awakens the patient from sleep (especially between 12 AM and 3 AM)
- The severity of ulcer pain varies from patient to patient, and may be seasonal, occurring more frequently in the spring or fall; episodes of discomfort usually occur in clusters lasting up to a few weeks followed by a pain-free period or remission lasting from weeks to years
- Changes in the character of the pain may suggest the presence of complications
- Heartburn, belching, and bloating often accompany the pain
- Nausea, vomiting, and anorexia, are more common in patients with gastric ulcer than with duodenal ulcer, but may also be signs of an ulcer-related complication

Signs
- Weight loss associated with nausea, vomiting, and anorexia
- Complications, including ulcer bleeding, perforation, penetration, or obstruction

Laboratory tests
- Gastric acid secretory studies
- Fasting serum gastrin concentrations are only recommended for patients unresponsive to therapy, or for those in whom hypersecretory diseases are suspected
- The hematocrit and hemoglobin are low with bleeding, and stool hemoccult tests are positive
- Tests for *Helicobacter pylori* (see Table 33–6)

Other diagnostic tests
- Fiberoptic upper endoscopy (esophagogastroduodenoscopy) detects more than 90% of peptic ulcers and permits direct inspection, biopsy, visualization of superficial erosions, and sites of active bleeding
- Routine single-barium contrast techniques detect 30% of peptic ulcers; optimal double-contrast radiography detects 60% to 80% of ulcers

Ulcer-related pain in duodenal ulcer often occurs 1 to 3 hours after meals and is usually relieved by food, but this is variable. In gastric ulcer, food may precipitate or accentuate ulcer pain. Antacids usually provide immediate pain relief in most ulcer patients. The abdominal pain usually diminishes or disappears during treatment; however, recurrence of pain after healing often suggests an unhealed or recurrent ulcer.

Abdominal pain does not always correlate with the presence or absence of acid or an ulcer. Asymptomatic patients may have an ulcer at endoscopy, and patients with endoscopically proven healed ulcers may have persistent symptoms. Many patients, particularly older adults, with an NSAID-induced ulcer-related complication may not have prior abdominal symptoms. The reasons for this are unclear, but may relate to the analgesic effect of the NSAID or differences in the way older individuals perceive pain.

Dyspepsia may or may not be associated with an ulcer, and in itself is of little clinical value when trying to identify subsets of patients who are most likely to have an ulcer. As many as 50% of patients who take NSAIDs report having dyspepsia.[14] Patients with dyspeptic symptoms may have either uninvestigated (no upper endoscopy) dyspepsia or investigated (underwent upper endoscopy) dyspepsia. If an ulcer is not confirmed in a patient with ulcer-like symptoms at the time of endoscopy, the disorder is referred to as nonulcer dyspepsia.[3]

Ulcer-like symptoms may also occur in the absence of peptic ulceration in association with HP gastritis or duodenitis.

DIAGNOSIS

Routine laboratory tests are not helpful in establishing the diagnosis of uncomplicated PUD (see Table 33–5).[1]

TESTS FOR *HELICOBACTER PYLORI*

The diagnosis of HP infection can be made using endoscopic or nonendoscopic tests (Table 33–6).[1,5,27] The tests that require upper endoscopy are more expensive, uncomfortable, and require a mucosal biopsy for histology, culture, or detection of urease activity. Recommendations to maximize the diagnostic yield include taking at least three tissue samples from specific areas of the stomach, as patchy distribution of HP infection can lead to false-negative results. Because certain medications may decrease the sensitivity of these tests, antibiotics and bismuth salts should be withheld for 4 weeks and PPIs for 1 to 2 weeks prior to endoscopic testing.

The nonendoscopic tests (see Table 33–6) include serologic antibody detection tests, the urea breath test (UBT), and the stool antigen

TABLE 33–6. Tests for Detection of *Helicobacter pylori*

Test	Description	Comments
Endoscopic tests		
Histology	Microbiologic examination using various stains	Gold standard; >95% sensitive and specific; permits classification of gastritis; results are not immediate; not recommended for initial diagnosis; tests for active HP infection; antibiotics, bismuth, and PPIs may cause false-negative results
Culture	Culture of biopsy	Enables sensitivity testing to determine appropriate treatment or antibiotic resistance; 100% specific; results are not immediate; not recommended for initial diagnosis, but may be used after failure of second-line treatment; tests for active HP infection; antibiotics, bismuth, and PPIs may cause false-negative results
Biopsy (rapid) urease	HP urease generates ammonia, which causes a color change	Test of choice at endoscopy; >90% sensitive and specific; easily performed; rapid results (usually within 24 hours); tests for active HP infection; antibiotics, bismuth, and PPIs may cause false-negative results; test may yield false-negatives in active ulcer bleeding; available as gel tests, paper tests, and tablets
Nonendoscopic tests		
Antibody detection (laboratory-based)	Detects antibodies to HP in serum; in the U.S., only FDA-approved anti-HP IgG antibody should be used	Quantitative; less sensitive and specific than endoscopic tests; more accurate than in-office or near-patient tests; unable to determine if antibody is related to active or cured infection; antibody titers vary markedly between individuals and take 6 months to 1 year to return to the uninfected range; not affected by PPIs or bismuth; antibiotics given for unrelated indications may cure the infection but antibody test will remain positive
Antibody detection (can be performed in office or near patient)	Detects IgG antibodies to HP in whole blood or fingerstick	Qualitative; quick (within 15 minutes); unable to determine if antibody is related to active or cured infection; most patients remain seropositive for at least 6 months to 1 year post HP eradication; not affected by PPIs, bismuth, or antibiotics
Urea breath test	HP urease breaks down ingested labeled C-urea, patient exhales labeled CO_2	Tests for active HP infection; 95% sensitive and specific; results take about 2 days; antibiotics, bismuth, PPIs, and H_2RAs may cause false-negative results; withhold PPIs or H_2RAs (1 to 2 weeks) and bismuth or antibiotics (2 to 4 weeks) before testing; may be used posttreatment to confirm eradication
Stool antigen	Identifies HP antigen in stool, leading to color change that can be detected visually or by spectrophotometer	Tests for active HP infection; sensitivity and specificity comparable to urea breath test when used for initial diagnosis; antibiotics, bismuth, and PPIs may cause false-negative results, but to a lesser extent than with the urea breath test; may be used posttreatment to confirm eradication

HP, *Helicobacter pylori*; H_2RA, H_2-receptor antagonist; PPI, proton pump inhibitor.
Compiled from Del Valle et al,[1] Suerbaum and Michetti,[5] Vaira et al,[27] Oderda et al,[28] and Bilardi et al.[29]

test.[1,5,27–29] These tests are more convenient and less expensive than the endoscopic tests. Serologic tests are of limited use in evaluating posttreatment eradication and are not reliable in young children.[1,5,27] The UBT is based on HP urease activity. The [13]carbon (nonradioactive isotope) and [14]carbon (radioactive isotope) tests require that the patient ingest radiolabeled urea, which is then hydrolyzed by HP (if present in the stomach) to ammonia and radiolabeled bicarbonate. The radiolabeled bicarbonate is absorbed in the blood and excreted in the breath. A mass spectrometer is used to detect [13]carbon, whereas[14] carbon is measured using a scintillation counter. The stool antigen test is approved by the Food and Drug Administration (FDA), but availability in the United States is limited. It is less expensive and easier to perform than the UBT, and may be useful in children.[28] Although comparable to the UBT in the initial detection of HP, the stool antigen test is less accurate when used to confirm HP eradication posttreatment.[29] Salivary and urine antibody tests are under investigation.[1,27]

Testing for HP is only recommended if eradication therapy is considered. If endoscopy is not planned, serologic antibody testing is a reasonable choice to determine HP status. Posttreatment evaluation to confirm eradication is unnecessary in most patients with PUD unless they have recurrent symptoms, complicated ulcer, MALT lymphoma, or gastric cancer.[1] The UBT is the preferred nonendoscopic method to verify HP eradication after treatment. To avoid confusing bacterial suppression with eradication, the UBT must be delayed at least 4 weeks after the completion of treatment. The term "eradication" or "cure" is used when posttreatment tests conducted 4 weeks after the end of treatment do not detect the organism. Quantitative antibody tests are considered impractical for posttreatment eradication as antibody titers remain elevated for long periods of time.

IMAGING AND ENDOSCOPY

The diagnosis of PUD depends on visualizing the ulcer crater either by upper GI radiography or endoscopy (see Table 33–5).[1] Because of its lower cost, greater availability, and greater safety, many physicians believe that radiography should be the initial diagnostic procedure in patients with suspected uncomplicated PUD. If complications are thought to exist, or if an accurate diagnosis is warranted, upper endoscopy is the diagnostic procedure of choice. If a gastric ulcer is found on radiography, malignancy should be excluded by direct endoscopic visualization and histology.

CLINICAL COURSE AND PROGNOSIS

The natural history of PUD is characterized by periods of exacerbations and remissions.[1] Ulcer pain is usually recognizable and episodic, but symptoms are variable, especially in older adults and in patients taking NSAIDs. Antiulcer medications, including the H$_2$RAs, PPIs, and sucralfate, relieve symptoms, accelerate ulcer healing, and prevent ulcers from recurring, but they do not cure the disease. Both duodenal ulcers and gastric ulcers recur unless the underlying cause (HP or NSAID) is removed. Successful HP eradication markedly decreases ulcer recurrence and complications. Prophylactic therapy or COX-2 inhibitors dramatically decrease the risk for ulcers and ulcer-related complications in high-risk patients taking NSAIDs. About 20% of patients with chronic PUD experience upper GI bleeding, perforation, or obstruction. Mortality in patients with gastric ulcer is slightly higher than in duodenal ulcer and the general population. The lifetime risk of gastric adenocarcinoma in HP-infected patients is less than 1%.[1,6]

▶ TREATMENT: Peptic Ulcer Disease

▨ DESIRED OUTCOME

The treatment of chronic PUD varies depending on the etiology of the ulcer (HP or NSAID), whether the ulcer is initial or recurrent, and whether complications have occurred (Fig. 33–5). Overall treatment is aimed at relieving ulcer pain, healing the ulcer, preventing ulcer recurrence, and reducing ulcer-related complications. The goal of therapy in HP-positive patients with an active ulcer, a previously documented ulcer, or a history of an ulcer-related complication, is to eradicate HP, heal the ulcer, and cure the disease. Successful eradication heals ulcers and reduces the risk of recurrence to less than 10% at 1 year.[1] The goal of therapy in a patient with a NSAID-induced ulcer is to heal the ulcer as rapidly as possible. Patients at high risk of developing NSAID ulcers should be switched to a COX-2 inhibitor or receive prophylactic drug cotherapy to reduce ulcer risk and ulcer-related complications. When possible, the most cost-effective drug regimen should be utilized.

▨ GENERAL APPROACH TO TREATMENT

The treatment of PUD centers on the eradication of HP in HP-positive patients and reducing the risk of NSAID-induced ulcers and ulcer-related complications. Drug regimens containing antimicrobials such as clarithromycin, metronidazole, amoxicillin, and bismuth salts and antisecretory drugs such as the PPIs or H$_2$RAs are used to relieve ulcer symptoms, heal the ulcer, and eradicate HP infection. Successful eradication will alter the natural history of PUD and cure the disease. PPIs, H$_2$RAs, and sucralfate are used to heal HP-negative NSAID-induced ulcers, but ulcer recurrence is likely in high-risk patients if the NSAID is continued. Prophylactic cotherapy with a PPI or misoprostol is used to decrease the risk of an ulcer and upper GI complications in patients taking nonselective NSAIDs. COX-2 inhibitors are often used in place of a nonselective NSAID to reduce the risk of ulcers and complications.

Dietary modifications may be important for some patients, especially those who are unable to tolerate certain foods and beverages. Lifestyle modifications such as reducing stress and decreasing or stopping cigarette smoking is often encouraged. Some patients may require radiographic or endoscopic procedures for a definitive diagnosis or for complications such as bleeding. Surgery may be necessary in patients with ulcer-related bleeding or other complications such as perforation.

▨ NONPHARMACOLOGIC THERAPY

◀ Patients with PUD should eliminate or reduce psychological stress, cigarette smoking, and the use of nonselective NSAIDs (including aspirin). Although there is no "antiulcer diet," the patient should avoid foods and beverages (e.g., spicy foods, caffeine, and alcohol) that cause dyspepsia or that exacerbate ulcer symptoms. If possible, alternative agents such as acetaminophen, nonacetylated

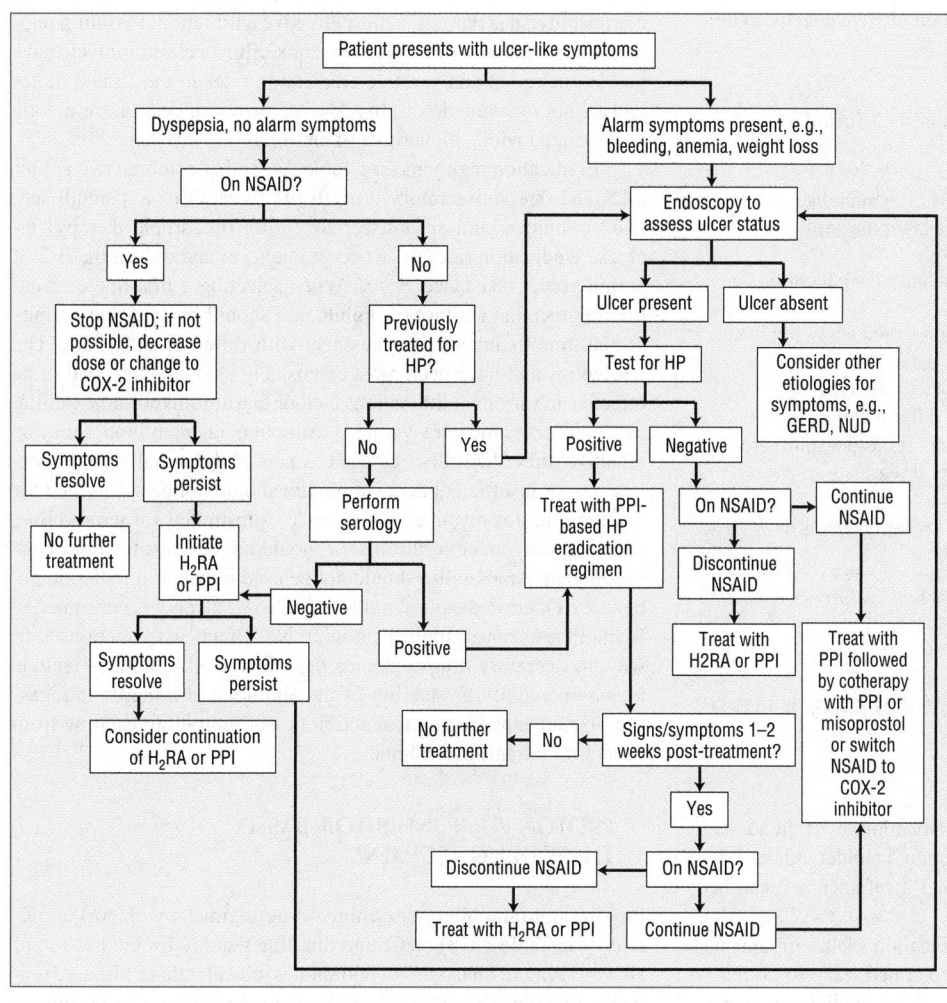

FIGURE 33–5. Algorithm: Guidelines for the evaluation and management of a patient who presents with dyspeptic or ulcer-like symptoms. COX-2, cyclooxygenase-2; GERD, gastroesophageal reflux disease; HP, *Helicobacter pylori*; H$_2$-RA, H$_2$-receptor antagonist; PPI, proton pump inhibitor; NSAID, nonsteroidal anti-inflammatory drug; NUD, nonulcer dyspepsia.

salicylate (e.g., salsalate), or COX-2 inhibitors should be used for relief of pain.

Elective surgery for PUD is rarely performed today because of highly effective medical management such as the eradication of HP and the use of potent acid inhibitors.[30] A subset of patients, however, may require emergency surgery for bleeding, perforation, or obstruction. In the past, surgical procedures were performed for medical treatment failures and included vagotomy with pyloroplasty or vagotomy with antrectomy.[30] Vagotomy (truncal, selective, or parietal cell) inhibits vagal stimulation of gastric acid. A truncal or selective vagotomy frequently results in postoperative gastric dysfunction and requires a pyloroplasty or antrectomy to facilitate gastric drainage. When an antrectomy is performed, the remaining stomach is anastomosed with the duodenum (Billroth I) or with the jejunum (Billroth II). A vagotomy is unnecessary when an antrectomy is performed for gastric ulcer. The postoperative consequences associated with these procedures include postvagotomy diarrhea, dumping syndrome, anemia, and recurrent ulceration.

■ PHARMACOLOGIC THERAPY

■ RECOMMENDATIONS

Guidelines for the eradication of infection in HP-positive individuals are presented in Table 33–7. Recommended HP

eradication regimens are presented in Table 33–8. First-line therapy should be initiated with a PPI-based three-drug regimen for a minimum of 7 days, but preferably 10 to 14 days. If a second course of treatment is required, the PPI-based three-drug regimen should contain different antibiotics or a four-drug regimen with bismuth subsalicylate, metronidazole, tetracycline, and a PPI should be used. Treatment with a conventional antiulcer drug (H$_2$RA, PPI, or sucralfate) is an alternative to HP eradication, but is discouraged because of the high rate of ulcer recurrence and ulcer-related complications associated with these regimens. Concomitant therapy (e.g., an H$_2$RA and sucralfate or an H$_2$RA and a PPI) is not recommended because it adds to drug costs without enhancing efficacy. Maintenance therapy with a PPI or H$_2$RA is recommended for high-risk patients with ulcer complications, patients who fail eradication, or those with HP-negative ulcers.

Patients with NSAID-induced ulcers should be tested to determine their HP status. If HP-positive, treatment should be initiated with a PPI-based three-drug eradication regimen. If HP-negative, the NSAID should be discontinued and the patient treated with either a PPI, H$_2$RA, or sucralfate. If the NSAID must be continued, treatment should be initiated with a PPI (if HP-negative) or with a PPI-based three-drug eradication regimen (if HP-positive). Prophylactic cotherapy with a PPI or misoprostol or switching to a selective COX-2 inhibitor is recommended for patients at risk of developing ulcer-related upper GI complications (see Table 33–4). PPI cotherapy should be considered in high-risk patients taking a COX-2 inhibitor.

TABLE 33–7. Guidelines for the Eradication of *Helicobacter pylori* (HP) Infection in HP-Positive Individuals

Strongly recommended
- Gastric and duodenal ulcer (active or inactive), including complicated ulcers, and following gastric surgery for peptic ulcer
- Mucosa-associated lymphoid tissue (MALT) lymphoma
- Atrophic changes in the gastric mucosa (atrophic gastritis)
- Following resection of gastric cancer
- Infected patients who are first-degree relatives of patients with gastric cancer
- Infected patients who are aware and concerned about the risks of infection

Recommended
- Use of nonsteroidal anti-inflammatory drugs (HP infection and the use of nonsteroidal anti-inflammatory drugs or aspirin are independent risk factors for peptic ulcer disease)
- Nonulcer dyspepsia
- Patients with gastroesophageal reflux disease receiving long-term proton pump inhibitor therapy

Compiled from Del Valle et al,[1] Suerbaum and Michetti,[5] Malfertheiner et al,[36] and Qasim and O'Morain.[37]

▤ TREATMENT OF *HELICOBACTER PYLORI*–ASSOCIATED ULCERS

The following discussion focuses on the eradication of HP in adults. Guidelines for the treatment of HP infection in older adults,[31,32] children,[33,34] and patients with chronic renal insufficiency[35] can be found elsewhere.

◄⑤ The goal of HP drug therapy is eradication of the organism. Treatment should be effective, well-tolerated, easy to comply with, and cost-effective. HP regimens should have eradication (cure) rates of at least 80% based on intention-to-treat analysis, or at least 90% based on per protocol analysis, and should minimize the potential for antimicrobial resistance.[1,5,36,37] The use of a single antibiotic, bismuth salt, or antiulcer drug does not achieve this goal.[1,5] However, clarithromycin is the single most effective antibiotic.[1] Two-drug regimens that combine a PPI and either amoxicillin or clarithromycin have yielded marginal and variable eradication rates in the United States and are not recommended.[1,5] In addition, the use of only one antibiotic is associated with a higher rate of antimicrobial resistance.[38]

Eradication regimens (see Table 33–8) that combine two antibiotics and one antisecretory drug (triple therapy) or a bismuth salt, two antibiotics, and an antisecretory drug (quadruple therapy) increase eradication rates to an acceptable level and reduce the risk of antimicrobial resistance.[1,5,36,38] When selecting a first-line eradication regimen, an antibiotic combination should be used that permits second-line treatment (if necessary) with different antibiotics. The antibiotics that have been most extensively studied and found to be effective in various combinations include clarithromycin, amoxicillin, metronidazole, and tetracycline.[1,5] Although other antibiotics may be effective, they should not be used as part of the initial HP regimen. Because of insufficient data, ampicillin should not be substituted for amoxicillin, doxycycline should not be substituted for tetracycline, and azithromycin or erythromycin should not be substituted for clarithromycin. Amoxicillin should not be used in penicillin-allergic patients and metronidazole should be avoided if alcohol is consumed.[36] Bismuth salts have a topical antimicrobial effect.[1] Explanations as to why antisecretory drugs enhance the efficacy of antibiotics include increased activity or stability of the antibiotic at a higher intragastric pH and enhanced topical antibiotic concentration resulting from decreased intragastric volume.

▤ PROTON PUMP INHIBITOR–BASED THREE-DRUG REGIMENS

Proton pump inhibitor–based three-drug regimens with two antibiotics (see Table 33–8) constitute first-line therapy for eradication of HP.[1,5,36] A meta-analysis[39] of 666 studies indicates that PPI-based regimens that combine clarithromycin and amoxicillin, clarithromycin and metronidazole, or amoxicillin and metronidazole yield similar eradication rates (78.9% to 82.8%) using intent-to-treat analysis; however, other studies suggest that the amoxicillin-metronidazole combination is less effective.[1] Eradication rates were improved when the

TABLE 33–8. Drug Regimens to Eradicate *Helicobacter Pylori* [a]

Drug #1	Drug #2	Drug #3	Drug #4
Proton pump inhibitor–based three-drug regimens			
Omeprazole 20 mg twice daily **or** lansoprazole 30 mg twice daily **or** pantoprazole 40 mg twice daily **or** esomeprazole 40 mg daily **or** rabeprazole 20 mg daily	Clarithromycin 500 mg twice daily	Amoxicillin 1 g twice daily **or** metronidazole 500 mg twice daily	
Bismuth-based four-drug regimens [b]			
Omeprazole 40 mg twice daily **or** lansoprazole 30 mg twice daily **or** pantoprazole 40 mg twice daily **or** esomeprazole 40 mg daily **or** rabeprazole 20 mg daily **or** Standard ulcer-healing dosages of an H₂-receptor antagonist taken for 4–6 weeks (see Table 33–9)	Bismuth subsalicylate 525 mg four times daily	Metronidazole 250–500 mg four times daily	Tetracycline 500 mg four times daily **or** amoxicillin 500 mg four times daily, or, clarithromycin 250–500 mg four times daily

[a]Although treatment is minimally effective if used for 7 days, 10–14 days of treatment is recommended. The antisecretory drug may be continued beyond antimicrobial treatment in the presence of an active ulcer.
[b]In the setting of an active ulcer, acid suppression is added to hasten pain relief.

clarithromycin dose was increased to 1.5 g/day, but increasing the dosage of the other antibiotics did not increase eradication rates.[39] Most clinicians prefer to initiate triple therapy with clarithromycin and amoxicillin rather than clarithromycin and metronidazole. Reserving metronidazole as an alternative or second-line agent leaves an effective back-up agent and reduces exposure and adverse effects from metronidazole. Alternatively, the PPI-clarithromycin-metronidazole regimen is an excellent alternative in penicillin-allergic patients (see Table 33–8).

An initial 7-day course of therapy provides minimally acceptable eradication rates and has been approved by the FDA and is recommended in Europe.[1,5] The duration of therapy, however, remains controversial in the United States, as longer treatment periods (10-day and 14-day) favor higher eradication rates and are less likely to be associated with antimicrobial resistance.[1,5,38,40] One meta-analysis reports a 7% to 9% increase in eradication rates with a 14-day treatment regimen when compared to a 7-day regimen.[40] A number of other antibiotics and antibiotic combinations have been evaluated as part of the PPI-based three-drug regimen with varying degrees of success.[1,5,41]

The PPI is an integral part of the three-drug regimen and should be taken 15 to 30 minutes before a meal (see section on PPIs) along with the two antibiotics (see Table 33–8). Although gastric acid inhibition is necessary to influence HP eradication rates, the specific level of inhibition remains unknown. A single daily dose of a PPI may be less effective than a double dose when used as part of a triple-therapy HP eradication regimen.[42] Substitution of one PPI for another is acceptable and does not appear to enhance or diminish HP eradication.[43] An H_2RA should not be substituted for a PPI, as better eradication rates have been demonstrated with a PPI.[44]

CLINICAL CONTROVERSY

Some clinicians favor an initial 7-day HP regimen, while others favor a 10-day or 14-day treatment course. The duration of therapy is controversial, as shorter periods may enhance compliance, but longer treatment periods in compliant patients favor higher eradication rates and are less likely to be associated with antimicrobial resistance. Patients receiving a second course of therapy after an unsuccessful eradication should receive treatment for 14 days.

BISMUTH-BASED FOUR-DRUG REGIMENS

The bismuth-based four-drug regimens presented in Table 33–8 were originally used as first-line therapy to eradicate HP. Eradication rates for a 14-day regimen containing bismuth, metronidazole, tetracycline, and an H_2-receptor antagonist are similar to those achieved with PPI-based triple therapy.[1,5,45] Increasing the duration of treatment to 1 month does not substantially increase eradication. Substitution of amoxicillin for tetracycline lowers the eradication rate and is usually not recommended.[1,45] Substitution of clarithromycin 250 to 500 mg four times a day for tetracycline yields similar results, but increases adverse effects. The antisecretory drug is also used to hasten pain relief in patients with an active ulcer. Although the original bismuth-based four-drug regimen is effective and inexpensive, it is associated with frequent adverse effects and poor compliance. A capsule containing bismuth, metronidazole, and tetracycline is under investigation.

First-line treatment with quadruple therapy using a PPI (with bismuth, metronidazole, and tetracycline) in place of the H_2RA achieves similar eradication rates as those of PPI-based triple therapy and permits a shorter treatment duration (7 days).[1,45] Although evidence supports the efficacy of bismuth-based quadruple therapy as first-line treatment, it is often recommended as second-line treatment when a clarithromycin-amoxicillin regimen is used initially (see section on eradication regimens after initial treatment failure). All medications except the PPI (see section on PPIs) should be taken with meals and at bedtime.

ERADICATION REGIMENS AFTER INITIAL TREATMENT FAILURE

HP eradication is often more difficult after initial treatment fails and eradication rates are extremely variable.[5,37] Because there are limited data on second attempts to eradicate HP, treatment failures should be handled on a case-by-case basis. Failure of first- and second-line regimens in primary care requires referral to a specialist.

Second-line empiric treatment should: utilize antibiotics that were not previously used during initial therapy; use antibiotics that do not have resistance problems; use a drug that has a topical effect such as bismuth; and the duration of treatment should be extended 10 to 14 days.[46] Thus after unsuccessful initial treatment with a PPI-amoxicillin-clarithromycin regimen, empiric second-line therapy should be instituted with bismuth subsalicylate, metronidazole, tetracycline, and a PPI for 10 to 14 days (see Table 33–8).[5,46,47] When metronidazole resistance is suspected, metronidazole may be replaced by furazolidone (100 mg four times a day) in either the proton pump inhibitor-based three-drug regimen or the bismuth-based four-drug regimen.[46] When furazolidone is used, patients should be counseled not to ingest alcohol or monoamine oxidase inhibitors.[1] Other successful second-line regimens are discussed elsewhere.[46,47]

FACTORS THAT CONTRIBUTE TO UNSUCCESSFUL ERADICATION

Factors that contribute to unsuccessful eradication include poor patient compliance, resistant organisms, low intragastric pH, and a high bacterial load.[37,38,46,48] Poor patient compliance is an important factor influencing successful therapy. Compliance decreases with multiple medications, increased frequency of administration, increased length of treatment, intolerable adverse effects, and costly drug regimens. Although a longer treatment duration may contribute to noncompliance, missed doses in a 7-day regimen may also lead to failed eradication.[46] Tolerability varies with different regimens. Metronidazole-containing regimens increase the frequency of adverse effects (especially when the dose is >1 g/day). Other common adverse effects include taste disturbances (metronidazole and clarithromycin), nausea, vomiting, abdominal pain, and diarrhea. Antibiotic-associated colitis, a serious complication, occurs occasionally. Oral thrush and vaginal candidiasis may also occur.

An important determinant of successful HP eradication therapy is the presence of preexisting antimicrobial resistance.[1,37,38,46,49] Metronidazole resistance is most common (10% to 60%), but varies depending on prior antibiotic exposure and geographic region.[1,37,38,49] The clinical importance of metronidazole resistance in eradicating HP remains uncertain, as the synergistic effect of combining metronidazole with other antibiotics appears to render resistance to metronidazole less important. Primary resistance to clarithromycin is lower (10% to 15%) than with metronidazole, but it is more likely to affect

TABLE 33–9. Oral Drug Regimens Used to Heal Peptic Ulcers or Maintain Ulcer Healing

Drug	Duodenal or Gastric Ulcer Healing (mg/dose)	Maintenance of Duodenal or Gastric Ulcer Healing (mg/dose)
Proton pump inhibitors		
Omeprazole	20–40 daily	20–40 daily
Lansoprazole	15–30 daily	15–30 daily
Rabeprazole	20 daily	20 daily
Pantoprazole	40 daily	40 daily
Esomeprazole	20–40 daily	20–40 daily
H₂-receptor antagonists		
Cimetidine	300 four times daily 400 twice daily 800 at bedtime	400–800 at bedtime
Famotidine	20 twice daily 40 at bedtime	20–40 at bedtime
Nizatidine	150 twice daily 300 at bedtime	150–300 at bedtime
Ranitidine	150 twice daily 300 at bedtime	150–300 at bedtime
Promote mucosal defense		
Sucralfate (g/dose)	1 four times daily 2 twice daily	1–2 twice daily 1 four times daily

the clinical outcome.[1,38,46] Secondary resistance occurs in up to two-thirds of treatment failures. Resistance to tetracycline and amoxicillin is uncommon.[1] Resistance to bismuth has not been reported. The role of antibiotic sensitivity testing before initiating HP treatment has not been established.

TREATMENT OF NSAID-INDUCED ULCERS

Nonselective NSAIDs should be discontinued (when possible) if an active ulcer is confirmed. If the NSAID is stopped, most uncomplicated ulcers will heal with standard regimens of an H₂-receptor antagonist, PPI, or sucralfate (Table 33–9).[1,12,14] PPIs are usually preferred because they provide more rapid ulcer healing than H₂RAs or sucralfate. If the NSAID must be continued in a patient despite ulceration, consideration should be given to reducing the NSAID dose, or switching to acetaminophen, a nonacetylated salicylate, a partially selective COX-2 inhibitor, or a selective COX-2 inhibitor (see Table 33–3). The PPIs are the drugs of choice when the NSAID must be continued, as potent acid suppression is required to accelerate ulcer healing.[1,12,14] H₂RAs are less effective in the presence of continued NSAID use; sucralfate does not appear to be effective. If HP is present, treatment should be initiated with an eradication regimen that contains a PPI.[1,12–14]

STRATEGIES TO REDUCE THE RISK OF NSAID-INDUCED ULCERS AND ULCER-RELATED UPPER GI COMPLICATIONS

A number of strategies are used to reduce the risk of NSAID-related ulcers and GI complications. Strategies aimed at reducing the topical irritant effects of nonselective NSAIDs—prodrugs, slow-release formulations, and enteric-coated products—do not prevent ulcers or GI complications such as bleeding or perforation. Medical cotherapy with misoprostol or a PPI decreases the risk of ulcers and GI complications in high-risk patients (see Table 33–3).[1,12–14,21,50,51]

Switching to a selective COX-2 inhibitor also decreases ulcer risk and complications.[1,12–14,21,50–52]

MISOPROSTOL COTHERAPY WITH A NONSELECTIVE NSAID

Misoprostol, 200 mcg four times a day, markedly reduces the risk of NSAID-induced gastric ulcer, duodenal ulcer, and ulcer-related GI complications, but diarrhea and abdominal cramping limit its use.[12–14,21] Because a dosage of 200 mcg three times a day is comparable in efficacy to 800 mcg/day, the lower dosage should be considered in patients unable to tolerate the higher dose.[1,12–14] Reducing the misoprostol dosage to 400 mcg/day or less to minimize diarrhea may compromise its prophylactic effects. A fixed combination of misoprostol 200 mcg and diclofenac (50 mg or 75 mg) is available and may enhance compliance, but the flexibility to individualize drug dosage is lost. A large double-blind clinical trial in rheumatoid arthritis patients receiving misoprostol 200 mcg four times a day provides the most compelling evidence that serious upper GI complications can be prevented, especially in high-risk patients.[53] However, the reduction in complications was less than the prevention of endoscopic lesions, indicating that it is not appropriate to extrapolate from ulcer prevention to a reduction in GI complications.

H₂-RECEPTOR ANTAGONIST COTHERAPY WITH A NONSELECTIVE NSAID

Standard H₂-receptor antagonist dosages (e.g., famotidine 40 mg/day) are effective in reducing the risk of NSAID-induced duodenal ulcer, but not gastric ulcer (the most frequent type of ulcer associated with NSAIDs).[1,12–14,21] Therefore standard H₂RA dosages should not be used as cotherapy with a nonselective NSAID for prophylaxis. There is evidence that higher dosages (e.g., famotidine 40 mg twice daily, ranitidine 300 mg twice daily) reduce the risk for gastric ulcer and duodenal ulcer.[1,21] However, there are no studies that have evaluated whether higher H₂RA dosages reduce the risk of ulcer-related upper

GI complications. The H$_2$RAs may be used when necessary to relieve NSAID-related dyspepsia.

PROTON PUMP INHIBITOR COTHERAPY WITH A NONSELECTIVE NSAID

Standard PPI dosages (e.g., omeprazole 20 mg/day and lansoprazole 30 mg/day) reduce the risk of NSAID-induced gastric ulcer and duodenal ulcer.[1,12–14,21] In a large comparative multicenter trial, omeprazole 20 mg/day was superior to ranitidine 150 mg twice daily in preventing NSAID-induced gastroduodenal ulcers.[54] Two randomized controlled trials have compared PPIs with misoprostol and placebo. In the first study,[55] omeprazole 20 mg/day was as effective as misoprostol 400 mcg/day in reducing the incidence of gastric ulcer; however, if a higher dosage of misoprostol had been used it might have been more effective. In the second study of HP-negative NSAID-users with a history of gastric ulcer,[56] misoprostol 800 mcg/day was more effective than lansoprazole (15 mg or 30 mg/day) and placebo. When withdrawals from the study (primarily related to the side effects of misoprostol) were regarded as "treatment failures," lansoprazole and full-dose misoprostol were considered clinically equivalent. Although there are no large clinical studies to prove that PPIs decrease the risk for NSAID-related upper GI complications, two small studies have reported a reduction in serious upper GI complications in patients with a history of upper GI bleeding.[57,58] Proton pump inhibitor cotherapy is considered an alternative to misoprostol in high-risk patients taking nonselective NSAIDs (including low-dose aspirin).

SELECTIVE COX-2 INHIBITORS

Of the oral selective COX-2 inhibitors now available in the U.S. (see Table 33–3) only celecoxib was investigated in arthritic patients, in a large, long-term, randomized controlled trial (named CLASS), that was specifically designed to evaluate upper gastrointestinal complications versus nonselective NSAIDs.[59,60] Patients in the CLASS trial, were permitted to take low-dose aspirin for cardioprotection.[59] The initial analysis of the CLASS trial indicated that, when compared to nonselective NSAIDs, celecoxib had 50% fewer symptomatic ulcers and serious upper GI complications in patients not taking concomitant low-dose aspirin. However, in the CLASS trial, these benefits were negated in the aspirin users. Although a systematic review[61] of celecoxib found that it is safer than nonselective NSAIDs, a re-evaluation of the CLASS data by the FDA concluded that celecoxib does not have a GI safety advantage over nonselective NSAIDs.[21,52] The manufacturer of celecoxib argued (and the FDA acknowledged) that confounding factors in study design, including the use of low-dose aspirin, account for these discrepant results. Concerns about the cardiovascular safety of selective COX-2 inhibitors (e.g., thrombotic events and myocardial infarction) have arisen.[21,52,60] GI effects such as dyspepsia and abdominal pain, fluid retention, hypertension, and renal toxicity can also occur with the COX-2 inhibitors.[21,52]

Two small comparative trials in HP-negative patients with histories of NSAID-related ulcer complications suggested that a standard dosage of a PPI and a nonselective NSAID have a GI safety profile similar to that observed with a selective COX-2 inhibitor.[62,63] However, the comparative benefits and cost effectiveness of these regimens remain controversial. Cotherapy with a PPI and a selective COX-2 inhibitor should be considered in patients with multiple or life-threatening risk factors.[1]

CONVENTIONAL TREATMENT OF ACTIVE DUODENAL AND GASTRIC ULCERS AND LONG-TERM MAINTENANCE OF ULCER HEALING

Conventional treatment with standard dosages of H$_2$-receptor antagonists or sucralfate relieves ulcer symptoms and heals the majority of gastric and duodenal ulcers in 6 to 8 weeks (see Table 33–9).[1,64] Proton pump inhibitors provide comparable ulcer healing rates over a shorter treatment period (4 weeks).[1,64] A higher daily dose or a longer treatment duration is sometimes needed to heal larger gastric ulcers. Antacids, although effective, are not used as single agents to heal ulcers because of the high volume and frequent doses required (100 to 144 mEq of acid-neutralizing capacity 1 hour and 3 hours after meals and at bedtime), as well as associated adverse effects.[1] When conventional antiulcer therapy is discontinued after ulcer healing, most HP-positive patients develop a recurrent ulcer within 1 year.[1,5]

Continuous antiulcer therapy (see Table 33–9) is aimed at the long-term maintenance of ulcer healing and at preventing ulcer-related complications. Because HP eradication dramatically decreases ulcer recurrence ($<10\%$ at 1 year), continuous maintenance therapy has become largely obsolete.[1] However, maintenance therapy may be indicated for patients who have a history of ulcer-related complications, a healed refractory ulcer, failed HP eradication therapy, or who are heavy smokers or NSAID users. Long-term maintenance therapy with an H$_2$RA, PPI, or sucralfate is safe, but sucralfate should be avoided in renal impairment.

TREATMENT OF REFRACTORY ULCERS

Ulcers are considered refractory to therapy when symptoms, ulcers, or both persist beyond 8 weeks (duodenal ulcer) or 12 weeks (gastric ulcer) despite conventional treatment, or when several courses of HP eradication fail.[1] Poor patient compliance, antimicrobial resistance, cigarette smoking, NSAID use, gastric acid hypersecretion, or tolerance to the antisecretory effects of an H$_2$RA (see section on antiulcer agents) may contribute to refractory PUD. Patients with refractory ulcers should undergo upper endoscopy to confirm a nonhealing ulcer, exclude malignancy, and assess HP status. HP-positive patients should receive eradication therapy (see section on treatment of HP-associated ulcers). In HP-negative patients, higher PPI dosages (e.g., omeprazole 40 mg/day) heal the majority of ulcers.[1] Continuous treatment with a PPI is often necessary to maintain healing, as refractory ulcers typically recur when therapy is discontinued or the dose is reduced. Switching from one PPI to another is not beneficial. Patients with refractory gastric ulcer may require surgery because of the fear of malignancy.

ANTIULCER AGENTS

A comprehensive review of the pharmacology, pharmacokinetics, pharmacodynamics, efficacy, drug interactions, and tolerability of the antiulcer agents can be found elsewhere.[1]

PROTON PUMP INHIBITORS

The PPIs (omeprazole, esomeprazole, lansoprazole, rabeprazole, and pantoprazole) dose-dependently inhibit basal and stimulated gastric acid secretion.[1,64–71] When PPI therapy is initiated, the degree of acid suppression increases over the first 3 to 4 days of therapy, as more and more proton pumps are inhibited. Upon discontinuation of therapy, full restoration of acid secretion takes 3 to 5 days.[66] Because PPIs inhibit only those proton pumps that are actively secreting acid, they are most effective when taken 15 to 30 minutes before meals.[64,72]

The PPIs are formulated as enteric-coated pH-sensitive granules contained in gelatin capsules (omeprazole, esomeprazole, and lansoprazole), powders (lansoprazole), rapidly disintegrating tablets (lansoprazole), or as enteric-coated tablets (rabeprazole, pantoprazole and nonprescription omeprazole). Available intravenous products include pantoprazole, lansoprazole, and esomeprazole (pending FDA approval at time of application).[64,73] The pH-sensitive enteric coating prevents degradation and premature protonation of the drug in stomach acid. The enteric coating dissolves in the duodenum at pH values above 6 and then the drug is systemically absorbed. The granules may be removed from the capsule and administered in acidic juices (e.g., orange or apple) by mouth, nasogastric tube, or gastrostomy tube; they can be sprinkled on applesauce; or a suspension can be prepared for nasogastric/nasoduodenal use by dissolving the granules in an 8.4% solution of sodium bicarbonate.[64,74,75] Esomeprazole granules may be administered with water via a nasogastric tube.[75]

All five PPIs provide similar ulcer-healing rates, maintenance of ulcer-healing rates, and relief of ulcer symptoms when used in recommended dosages (see Table 33–8).[1,65–70] When higher dosages are indicated, the daily dose should be divided in order to obtain better 24-hour pH control.[66] A dosage reduction is not necessary in renal impairment or older adults, but should be considered in severe hepatic disease.[1,71]

The short-term (<12 weeks) adverse effects of all five PPIs are similar and not unlike those observed with the H_2RAs (see the section on H_2RAs).[1,64] Because PPIs increase intragastric pH, they may alter the bioavailability of orally administered drugs, such as ketoconazole, digoxin, or pH-dependent dosage forms.[1,66] Omeprazole and esomeprazole selectively inhibit hepatic cytochrome P450 (CYP450) isoenzyme 2C19 and decrease the elimination of phenytoin, diazepam, and R-warfarin.[1,64,66] Lansoprazole produces a slight

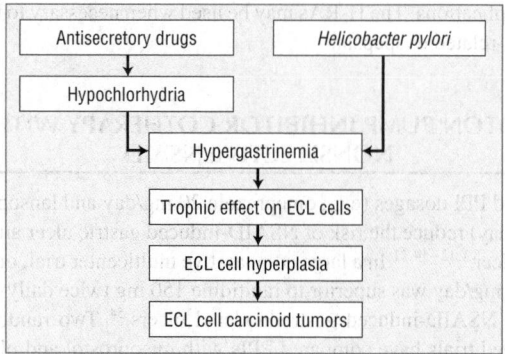

FIGURE 33–6. The gastrin hypothesis suggests that prolonged hypergastrinemia results in hyperplasia of the enterochromaffin-like (ECL) cells of the gastric fundus. The trophic influence of gastrin may be a risk factor for ECL cell carcinoid tumor formation.

increase in the metabolism of theophylline, presumably by inducing CYP1A.[1,64,66] Rabeprazole, and pantoprazole do not significantly affect CYP metabolism and thus have a lower potential for CYP-mediated drug interactions.[1,66]

Consequences of Prolonged Hypochlorhydria

All PPIs dose-dependently increase serum gastrin concentrations approximately two- to fourfold as a function of their potent acid-inhibitory effect (Fig. 33–6).[1,76] Fasting gastrin elevations are usually within the normal range and return to baseline within 1 month of discontinuing the drug. A consequence of hypergastrinemia is its trophic effect on enterochromaffin-like (ECL) cells in the gastric epithelium, which has been associated with the development of gastric carcinoid tumors in female rats. In humans, use of PPIs may lead to ECL hyperplasia; however, there has been no evidence that these changes result in dysplasia, carcinoid tumors, or gastric adenocarcinoma.[1,76] Long-term PPI therapy in HP-positive patients has been associated with progressive atrophic gastritis of the gastric body.[1,76] At this time there is inadequate evidence to link the long-term use of PPIs with gastric cancer in HP-positive patients or to support an association between PPIs, colonic polyps, and colorectal cancer.[1] Although bacterial overgrowth occurs in the stomach as a consequence of hypochlorhydria and may lead to carcinogenic N-nitroso compounds in animals, it is unlikely to result in significant gastric nitrosation in humans.[1,76] A decrease in vitamin B_{12} was reported in patients receiving long-term PPI therapy, but it is not a major concern.[76]

H_2-RECEPTOR ANTAGONISTS

Ulcer healing is comparable among H_2RAs (cimetidine, famotidine, nizatidine, and ranitidine) with equipotent multiple daily doses or a single full dose given after dinner or at bedtime (see Table 33–9), but tolerance to their antisecretory effect may occur. Twice-daily administration suppresses daytime acid and benefits patients with daytime ulcer pain. Cigarette smokers may require higher doses or a longer duration of treatment. H_2-receptor antagonists are eliminated renally and therefore a dosage reduction is recommended in patients with moderate to severe renal failure.

The short- and long-term safety of all four H_2RAs is similar.[1] Thrombocytopenia, the most common hematologic effect, is reversible and occurs with all four H_2RAs. However, the propensity for H_2RAs to cause thrombocytopenia is likely overestimated.[1,77] Cimetidine inhibits several CYP450 isoenzymes, resulting in numerous drug interactions (e.g., theophylline, lidocaine, phenytoin, and warfarin).[1] Ranitidine binds less avidly to hepatic CYP450 isoenzymes than does cimetidine, and thus has less potential for drug interactions. Famotidine and nizatidine do not interact with drugs metabolized by hepatic CYP450 isoenzymes. Because the H_2RAs decrease acid secretion and increase intragastric pH, they may alter the bioavailability of orally administered drugs such as ketoconazole or pH-dependent dosage forms. The effect of cimetidine, ranitidine, and nizatidine (but not famotidine) on serum alcohol is unlikely to be clinically important.[78]

SUCRALFATE

Sucralfate should be taken on an empty stomach to prevent binding to dietary protein and phosphate. Deterrents to its use include multiple doses per day, large tablet size, and the need to separate the drug from meals and potentially interacting medications. Adverse effects are minor and occur in less than 5% of patients. Constipation is most common and develops in about 3% of patients.[1] Nausea, dry mouth, dizziness, and a metallic taste occur infrequently. Seizures may occur in dialysis patients who are also receiving aluminum-containing antacids. Hypophosphatemia may develop with long-term treatment (see section on antacids). Gastric bezoar formation has been reported. The concomitant use of sucralfate with oral fluoroquinolones, phenytoin, digoxin, theophylline, quinidine, amitriptyline, warfarin, and ketoconazole may reduce their bioavailability.[1,79] The interaction is often minimized by giving the interacting drug at least 2 hours before sucralfate. Alternative antiulcer therapy may be warranted in patients taking oral fluoroquinolones.

PROSTAGLANDINS

Misoprostol, a synthetic prostaglandin E_1 analog, moderately inhibits acid secretion and enhances mucosal defense.[1] Antisecretory effects are dose-dependent over the range of 50 mcg to 200 mcg; cytoprotective effects occur in humans at doses of greater than 200 mcg. Because protective effects occur at higher doses, it is difficult to establish the protective effect independent of the antisecretory action. Although not recommended in the United States, a dose of 200 mcg four times daily or 400 mcg twice daily heals duodenal ulcers and gastric ulcers comparable to standard H_2RA or sucralfate regimens.[1]

Diarrhea, the most troublesome adverse effect, is dose dependent and develops in 10% to 30% of patients.[1] Abdominal cramping, nausea, flatulence, and headache typically accompany the diarrhea. Taking the drug with or after meals and at bedtime may minimize the diarrhea. Antacids (other than magnesium) may be taken with misoprostol when needed for abdominal pain. Misoprostol is uterotropic and produces uterine contractions that may endanger pregnancy; therefore the drug is contraindicated in pregnant women. If misoprostol is prescribed to women in their childbearing years, use of adequate contraceptive measures must be confirmed and a negative serum pregnancy test should be documented within 2 weeks of initiating treatment. Patients should be counseled about the GI effects and the need to avoid magnesium antacids, as they may increase the propensity for GI adverse effects. Young women should be warned about the importance of adequate contraception.

BISMUTH PREPARATIONS

Bismuth subsalicylate is currently the only available bismuth salt in the United States.[1] Possible ulcer-healing mechanisms include an antibacterial effect, a local gastroprotective effect, and stimulation of endogenous prostaglandins. Bismuth salts do not inhibit or neutralize acid. Bismuth subsalicylate is regarded as safe and has few adverse effects when taken in recommended dosages. Because renal insufficiency may decrease bismuth elimination, bismuth salts should be used with caution in older patients and in renal failure. Bismuth subsalicylate may cause salicylate sensitivity or bleeding disorders, and should be used with caution in patients receiving concurrent salicylate therapy. Patients should be advised that bismuth salts may impart a black color to the stool and possibly the tongue (liquid preparations).

ANTACIDS

Antacids neutralize gastric acid, inactivate pepsin, and bind bile salts. Aluminum-containing antacids also suppress HP and enhance mucosal defense.[1,80,81] GI adverse effects are most common with antacids and are dose dependent.[1,81] Magnesium salts cause an osmotic diarrhea, whereas aluminum salts cause constipation. Diarrhea usually predominates with magnesium/aluminum preparations. Aluminum-containing antacids (except aluminum phosphate) form insoluble salts with dietary phosphorus and interfere with phosphorus absorption.[1] Hypophosphatemia occurs most often in patients with low dietary phosphate intake (e.g., malnutrition or alcoholism). Combined treatment with sucralfate may amplify the hypophosphatemia and the potential for aluminum toxicity (see section on sucralfate).

Magnesium-containing antacids should not be used in patients with a creatinine clearance of less than 30 mL/min because magnesium excretion is impaired.[81] Hypercalcemia may occur in patients with normal renal function taking more than 20 g/day of calcium carbonate, and in renal failure patients taking more than 4 g/day. The milk-alkali syndrome (hypercalcemia, alkalosis, renal stones, increased blood urea nitrogen, and increased serum creatinine concentration) occurs with high calcium intake in patients with systemic alkalosis produced by either ingestion of absorbable antacids (sodium bicarbonate) or prolonged vomiting. Antacids may alter the absorption and excretion of drugs when administered concomitantly.[1,79,81] Important interactions may occur when antacids are administered with iron supplements, tetracycline, warfarin, digoxin, quinidine, isoniazid, ketoconazole, or the fluoroquinolones. Most interactions can be avoided by separating the antacid from the oral drug by 2 hours.

PHARMACOECONOMIC CONSIDERATIONS

❽ The eradication of HP improves clinical outcomes and decreases the use of health care resources when compared to conventional antisecretory therapy.[82] Thus the costs of continued treatment and recurrence far outweigh the cost of HP drug regimens. The cost effectiveness of misoprostol cotherapy is greatest in patients with the highest risk for NSAID-related GI complications.[83] The use of a PPI with a nonselective NSAID or switching to a selective COX-2 inhibitor has also been reported to be cost effective in high-risk patients.[84] However, the comparative cost effectiveness of these regimens requires further study. Whether cotherapy with a high-dose H_2RA is cost effective remains to be determined.

Recommendations for treating and monitoring patients with PUD are presented in Table 33–10. Relief of epigastric pain should be monitored throughout the course of treatment in patients with either HP- or NSAID-induced ulcers. Ulcer pain typically resolves in a few days when NSAIDs are discontinued and within 7 days upon initiation of antiulcer therapy. Most patients with uncomplicated PUD will be symptom free after treatment with any one of the recommended antiulcer regimens. The persistence, or redevelopment, of symptoms after several weeks of treatment suggests failure of ulcer healing or HP eradication, or an alternative diagnosis such as gastroesophageal reflux disease. The majority of patients with

uncomplicated HP-positive ulcers do not require confirmation of ulcer healing or HP eradication. When endoscopy is not indicated, the urea breath test is the preferred test to confirm HP eradication. Patient compliance should be assessed in patients who fail therapy.

High-risk patients on NSAIDs should be closely monitored for signs or symptoms of bleeding, obstruction, penetration, or perforation. Patients who remain symptomatic, have recurrent attacks, or who have ulcer-related complications should be referred to a specialist. Follow-up endoscopy can be justified in patients with frequent symptomatic recurrence, refractory disease, complications, or suspected hypersecretory states.

TABLE 33–10. Recommendations for Treating and Monitoring Patients with _Helicobacter pylori_ (HP)-Associated and Nonsteroidal Anti-inflammatory Drug (NSAID)-Induced Ulcers

Helicobacter pylori–associated ulcer
1. Recommend drug treatment as presented in the chapter text.
2. Assess patient allergies to determine if allergic to penicillin (or other antibiotics) so that drug regimens that contain penicillin (or other antibiotics) can be avoided. Avoid regimens that contain tetracycline in children.
3. Assess patient use of alcohol or alcohol-containing products with metronidazole and oral birth control medications with antibiotics and counsel appropriately.
4. Assess likelihood of noncompliance to the drug regimen as a cause of treatment failure.
5. Recommend a different antibiotic combination if HP eradication fails and a second treatment is planned.
6. Inform the patient of change in stool color when bismuth salicylate is included in an HP eradication regimen.
7. Assess and monitor patients for potential adverse effects, especially those associated with metronidazole, clarithromycin, and amoxicillin.
8. Assess and monitor patients for potential drug interactions, especially those receiving metronidazole, clarithromycin, and cimetidine.
9. Monitor patients for salicylate toxicity, especially in patients receiving cotherapy with other salicylates, anticoagulants, or in patients with renal failure.
10. Provide patient education to patients who are receiving HP eradication therapy, including why antibiotic and antiulcer combinations are used, when and how to take medications, adverse effects, alarm symptoms, when to contact their health care provider, and the importance of compliance to drug treatment.

NSAID-induced ulcer
1. Recommend drug treatment as presented in the chapter text.
2. Assess risk factors for NSAID-induced ulcers and ulcer-related complications, and when indicated recommend appropriate strategies for reducing ulcer risk.
3. Recommend eradication treatment for HP-positive patients taking NSAIDs.
4. Monitor patients for signs and symptoms of NSAID-related upper GI complications.
5. Assess and monitor patients for potential drug interactions and adverse effects (especially misoprostol).
6. Provide patient education to patients at risk of NSAID-induced ulcers or GI-related complications, including why cotherapy is used with nonselective NSAIDs, when and how to take medications, adverse effects, alarm symptoms, when to contact their health care provider, and the importance of compliance to drug treatment.

ZOLLINGER-ELLISON SYNDROME

ZES is characterized by gastric acid hypersecretion and recurrent peptic ulceration that results from a gastrin-producing tumor (gastrinoma).[4,85] In the United States, ZES accounts for 0.1% to 1% of patients with duodenal ulcer; however, this may be an underestimation of the true incidence because of the heterogeneity of clinical manifestations.[4] Gastrinomas are classified as those associated with multiple endocrine neoplasia type 1 (MEN 1) or sporadic tumors, which have a greater tendency to behave as malignant tumors. More than 90% of gastrinomas are located in the region of the pancreas, the most common site being the duodenum. Malignant gastrinomas occur in 30% to 50% of patients, with metastases to regional lymph nodes, liver, spleen, and bone.

A diagnosis of ZES should be considered in patients with multiple ulcers and recurrent or refractory PUD, often accompanied by esophagitis or ulcer complications.[4,86] Ulcers occur most often in the duodenum, but may involve the stomach or jejunum. Diarrhea occurs in 30% to 50% of patients and results from high concentrations of acid that overwhelm the duodenum's buffering capacity and damage the mucosa.[4] Intraluminal acid causes steatorrhea by inactivating pancreatic lipase and precipitating bile acids. Vitamin B_{12} malabsorption may result from reduced intrinsic factor activity. Patients may have other symptoms when the parathyroid, pituitary, thyroid, or adrenal glands are involved. The diagnosis is established in patients with a basal acid output (BAO) greater than 15 mEq/h (without prior gastric surgery) and when the fasting serum gastrin is higher than 1000 pg/mL.[4,85] Location of the tumor is essential as early surgical resection prior to liver metastases is often curative.[4,86,87] Unfortunately, effective medical therapy may delay the recognition of the disease and adversely influence outcome. The widespread use of PPIs, although effective in reducing symptoms, may mask the clinical presentation and complicate the diagnosis.[4,86] In addition, PPIs can cause hypergastrinemia, which may further complicate the diagnosis of ZES.[86]

Treatment is based on the presence or absence of peptic ulcers, esophagitis, diarrhea, and a gastrinoma, which may be malignant. The PPIs are the oral drugs of choice for managing gastric acid hypersecretion. Treatment should be instituted with omeprazole 60 mg/day (or an equivalent dose of esomeprazole, lansoprazole, rabeprazole, or pantoprazole) and should be adjusted to individual patient response.[4,64,85] Dividing the daily dose and giving the PPI every 8 to 12 hours is most effective in controlling acid output and relieving symptoms. Although doses as high as 360 mg/day of omeprazole have been administered, an average dose of 60 to 80 mg/day (40 to 80 mg/day of esomeprazole or rabeprazole; 30 to 90 mg/day of lansoprazole; or 40 to 120 mg/day of pantoprazole) reduces basal acid output to target levels. Patients should be evaluated every 6 to 12 months and the PPI dose adjusted accordingly. A gradual reduction in PPI dose is recommended after the initial dose required for adequate control of gastric acid hypersecretion is achieved.[4] Intravenous pantoprazole in dosages of 80 mg every 8 to 12 hours is safe and effective for rapid and prolonged acid suppression in patients unable to take oral PPIs.[69]

Octreotide directly inhibits gastric acid secretion and the release of gastrin.[4] Although a subcutaneous dose of 100 to 250 mcg three times a day substantially reduces gastric acid secretion, octreotide is not considered first-line treatment. The long-acting repeatable octreotide formulation is efficacious in patients with gastrointestinal neuroendocrine tumors.[88] However, it is important to demonstrate that the patient tolerates octreotide prior to converting to the long-acting product. An initial dose of 20 mg intramuscularly once monthly is subsequently titrated based on response. Patients with metastatic gastrinoma require tumor resection or treatment with chemotherapeutic agents.

UPPER GASTROINTESTINAL BLEEDING

Upper GI bleeding occurs in approximately 100 cases per 100,000 adults annually.[89] Despite a decreased incidence of PUD and improvements in the management of upper GI bleeding, the mortality rate associated with acute hemorrhage remains about 7%. Upper GI bleeding can be broadly categorized as variceal or nonvariceal bleeding. Two common types of nonvariceal bleeding are bleeding from chronic peptic ulcers and bleeding from SRMD (stress gastritis, stress ulcer, or stress erosions), both of which are acid-peptic complications.[2,89] The presentation and pathophysiology of these two conditions are somewhat different, as bleeding associated with chronic PUD usually precedes hospital admission, whereas bleeding associated with SRMD develops in severely ill patients during hospitalization.[1,90]

The underlying pathophysiology of bleeding from a peptic ulcer or from SRMD is similar in that impaired mucosal defense in the presence of gastric acid and pepsin leads to mucosal damage. In chronic PUD, HP infection and NSAID use are the most important etiologic factors, whereas the primary pathogenic factor in SRMD is thought to be mucosal ischemia resulting from reduced gastric blood flow. In contrast to chronic PUD, stress-related mucosal lesions are characteristically asymptomatic, multiple, located in the proximal stomach, and are unlikely to perforate (see Table 33–1). Bleeding from SRMD occurs from superficial mucosal capillaries, whereas bleeding associated with chronic PUD usually results from a single vessel. The mortality rate associated with stress-related mucosal bleeding (SRMB) approximates 50% and is related to the underlying severity of the patient population.[91] In contrast, the mortality associated with chronic PUD-related bleeding is about 10%, but can increase dramatically in selected patient populations.[89,92] Although the initial management of acute upper GI bleeding focuses on aggressive resuscitative measures and ensuring hemodynamic stability, and is the same for both PUD-related bleeding and SRMB, the medical management of each condition is distinctly different.[89,90,92]

PEPTIC ULCER–RELATED BLEEDING

The degree of risk must be assessed to determine how aggressively to treat the patient with chronic PUD-related bleeding.[89,92] Patients greater than 60 years of age, with comorbid conditions, low systolic blood pressure, high transfusion requirements, shock, ongoing blood loss, prolonged prothrombin time, and erratic mental status generally have poorer prognoses and usually require more aggressive intervention including admission to an intensive care unit (ICU). Diagnostic endoscopy is usually performed to identify the source of the bleeding, assess the potential risk for rebleeding, and if appropriate, therapeutic interventions are employed to promote hemostasis.[2,89,93] Several endoscopic treatment approaches (e.g., thermocoagulation, laser therapy, injection sclerotherapy, hemoclipping, and ligation) can be utilized. The appearance of the ulcer at the time of endoscopy is a prognostic indicator for the risk of rebleeding.[89,92] Clean-based ulcers are most commonly seen and are associated with a low risk of rebleeding. In most cases, these patients can be immediately discharged after endoscopy on antiulcer therapy. Patients with an adherent clot overlying the ulcer base are at intermediate risk of rebleeding. Patients with a visible vessel or active bleeding are at high risk of rebleeding, and must be carefully managed, as rebleeding increases the mortality rate 10-fold.

Antisecretory therapy is often used as adjuvant therapy to prevent PUD rebleeding in high-risk patients because acid impairs clot stability. H_2-receptor antagonists are ineffective in preventing PUD rebleeding because they do not achieve an intragastric pH of 6 (which is needed to promote clot stability), and tolerance to their antisecretory effect develops rapidly.[89,93–95] In contrast, high-dose continuous intravenous infusions of a PPI (omeprazole 80 mg loading dose, followed by 8 mg/h for 3 days) are effective in reducing the risk of rebleeding in patients who have undergone endoscopy hemostasis.[89,93,95–97] Although therapy with the PPI may be started prior to endoscopic intervention, one study indicates that the combination of therapeutic endoscopy and a high-dose PPI continuous intravenous infusion is more beneficial than either strategy alone.[97] Studies that assessed the efficacy of intermittent intravenous infusions of omeprazole have generally shown poor results and are not recommended to reduce the risk of PUD rebleeding.[89,95] A limited number of studies demonstrate the efficacy of high-dose oral therapy (omeprazole 80 mg/day for 5 days) in preventing PUD rebleeding.[89,98,99] The risk of rebleeding is greatest within the first 72 hours (especially the first 24 hours) and it is during this time that antisecretory therapy to prevent rebleeding in high-risk patients should be employed.[96] Subsequently, the patient's underlying PUD should be evaluated and treated.

Patients with upper GI bleeding should be tested for HP at the time of endoscopy (see section on tests for HP). However, tests are associated with an increased rate of false-negatives when obtained during acute bleeding episodes.[93] If the initial results are negative, a confirmatory test should be performed following the acute bleeding episode. There is no rationale for using intravenous therapy to eradicate HP. Ulcer treatment, including HP eradication, if appropriate, should be initiated after the acute bleeding episode (see sections on treatment of HP-associated ulcers and treatment of NSAID-induced ulcers).

STRESS-RELATED MUCOSAL BLEEDING

More than 75% of critically ill patients develop SRMD within 24 hours of admission to an ICU, but the incidence of clinically significant SRMB is considered to be in the range of 2% to 6%.[90,100,101] Clinically significant bleeding increases the length of ICU stay by approximately 4 to 8 days, results in excessive health care costs, and is associated with an increased mortality rate.[102] Thus attempts to prevent SRMB are warranted in high-risk patients. Prophylactic therapy to prevent bleeding is most effective if initiated early in the patient's course.

Patients at risk for SRMB include those with respiratory failure (need for mechanical ventilation for >48 hours), coagulopathy, hypotension, sepsis, hepatic failure, acute renal failure, multiple trauma, severe burns (>35% of body surface area), head injury, traumatic spinal cord injury, major surgery, or history of GI bleeding.[90,91,100]

Although the relative importance of the various risk factors remains controversial, most clinicians concur that patients with respiratory failure (mechanical ventilation for >48 hours) or coagulopathy should receive prophylaxis, as these two factors were shown to be independent risk factors in a large observational study.[91] In the absence of these two risk factors, some clinicians only use prophylaxis in patients who have two of the aforementioned risk factors.[90] Although exactly who should receive prophylaxis remains controversial, not all patients in a hospital or ICU are at increased risk of SRMB. A cost-effective approach is to target prophylactic therapy at high-risk patients.

Prevention of SRMB includes resuscitative measures which restore mucosal blood.[90] Although the benefits of enteral nutrition to patient outcome (e.g., improved nutritional status enhances mucosal integrity) are of overall clinical importance, its precise role as a sole modality to prevent SRMB remains controversial.[103] Therapeutic options for the prevention of SRMB include antacids (which are of historical interest, as they are no longer used because of cumbersome dosage schedules and side effects), antisecretory drugs (H$_2$RAs and PPIs), and sucralfate, a mucosal protectant.[90,104] Cimetidine, given as a continuous intravenous infusion, is the only regimen that is FDA-labeled for the prevention of SRMB. However, in clinical practice, intermittent intravenous H$_2$RAs are more commonly used.

H$_2$-receptor antagonists are preferred for prophylaxis of SRMB. A large landmark study demonstrated that intravenous ranitidine was superior to oral sucralfate in preventing SRMB.[101] Moreover, ranitidine did not increase the risk for nosocomial pneumonia, as the incidence of pneumonia was no different between the two treatment groups. In itself, critical illness places the patient at risk for nosocomial pneumonia. Also there are potential problems associated with sucralfate therapy (e.g., constipation, clogging tubes, hypophosphatemia, and drug interactions).[104]

Proton pump inhibitors should only be used as alternatives to H$_2$RAs or sucralfate for preventing SRMB, as their superiority has not been firmly established.[105] Only a limited number of studies have evaluated their effectiveness.[95,105,106] Only one published randomized controlled trial has demonstrated that omeprazole (40 mg/day oral or nasogastric) is superior to ranitidine (150 mg/day intravenous) in preventing SRMB.[106] Although the superiority of omeprazole may be related to its greater antisecretory potency, the possibility of study bias exists, as the population that received ranitidine was at greater risk for SRMB. The optimal dosage of the various intravenous PPIs as well as the preferred route of administration for this indication remains to be defined.

Improvement in the patient's overall medical condition (discharge from the ICU, extubation, and oral intake) suggests that prophylactic therapy can be discontinued. If a patient develops clinically significant bleeding, endoscopic evaluation of the GI tract is indicated along with aggressive drug therapy.

CONCLUSIONS

The eradication of HP infection has dramatically changed the way in which chronic PUD is treated. Although substantial progress has been made, there is still no ideal treatment, and much of what has been learned has not yet been instilled into clinical practice. The widespread use of NSAIDs and their associated GI complications remains a major concern, especially in older adults. Cotherapy with misoprostol or a PPI, or switching to a selective COX-2 inhibitor reduces NSAID-related GI events, but studies are needed to determine their comparative cost effectiveness.

ABBREVIATIONS

BAO: basal acid output
COX-1: cyclooxygenase-1
COX-2: cyclooxygenase-2
CYP450: cytochrome P450
ECL: enterochromaffin-like
HP: *Helicobacter pylori*
H$_2$RA: histamine-2 receptor antagonist
ICU: intensive care unit
MALT: mucosa-associated lymphoid tissue
MAO: maximal acid output
NSAID: nonsteroidal antiinflammatory drug
NUD: nonulcer dyspepsia
PG: prostaglandin
PPI: proton pump inhibitor
PUD: peptic ulcer disease
SRMB: stress-related mucosal bleeding
SRMD: stress-related mucosal damage
UBT: urea breath test
ZES: Zollinger-Ellison syndrome

Review Questions and other resources can be found at *www.pharmacotherapyonline.com*.

REFERENCES

1. Del Valle J, Chey WD, Scheiman JM, et al. Acid peptic disorders. In: Yamada T, Aplers DH, Kaplowitz N, et al, eds. Textbook of Gastroenterology, 4th ed. Philadelphia, Lippincott Williams & Wilkins, 2003:1321–1376.
2. Elta GH. Approach to the patient with gross gastrointestinal bleeding. In: Yamada T, Aplers DH, Kaplowitz N, et al, eds. Textbook of Gastroenterology, 4th ed. Philadelphia, Lippincott Williams & Wilkins, 2003:698–723.
3. Talley NJ, Holtmann G. Approach to the patient with dyspepsia and related functional gastrointestinal complaints. In: Yamada T, Aplers DH, Kaplowitz N, et al, eds. Textbook of Gastroenterology, 4th ed. Philadelphia, Lippincott Williams & Wilkins, 2003:655–677.
4. Del Valle J, Scheiman JM. Zollinger-Ellison syndrome. In: Yamada T, Aplers DH, Kaplowitz N, et al, eds. Textbook of Gastroenterology, 4th ed. Philadelphia, Lippincott Williams & Wilkins, 2003:1377–1394.
5. Suerbaum S, Michetti P. *Helicobacter pylori* infection. N Engl J Med 2002;347:1175–1186.
6. Go MF. Review article: Natural history and epidemiology of *Helicobacter pylori* infection. Aliment Pharmacol Ther 2002;16(Suppl 1):3–15.
7. Peterson WL. Review article: *Helicobacter pylori* and gastric adenocarcinoma. Aliment Pharmacol Ther 2002;16:(Suppl 1):40–46.
8. Van Leerdam ME, Tytgat GNJ. *Helicobacter pylori* infection in peptic ulcer haemorrhage. Aliment Pharmacol Ther 2002;16:(Suppl 1):66–78.
9. Fennerty MB. Review article: *Helicobacter pylori* and uninvestigated dyspepsia. Aliment Pharmacol Ther 2002;16(Suppl 1):52–57.
10. Talley NJ, Quan C. Review article: *Helicobacter pylori* and nonulcer dyspepsia. Aliment Pharmacol Ther 2002;16(Suppl 1):58–65.
11. Vakil NB. Review article: Gastro-oesophageal reflux disease and *Helicobacter pylori* infection. Aliment Pharmacol Ther 2002;16 (Suppl 1):47–51.
12. Laine L. Approaches to nonsteroidal anti-inflammatory drug use in the high-risk patient. Gastroenterology 2001;120:594–606.
13. Hawkey CJ. Nonsteroidal anti-inflammatory drug gastropathy. Gastroenterology 2000;119:521–535.
14. Wolfe MM, Lichtenstein DR, Singh G. Gastrointestinal toxicity of nonsteroidal antiinflammatory drugs. N Engl J Med 1999;340:1888–1899.

15. Gleeson MH, Davis AJM. Non-steroidal anti-inflammatory drugs, aspirin and newly diagnosed colitis: A case-control study. Aliment Pharmacol Ther 2003;17:817–825.

16. Derry S, Loke YK. Risk of gastrointestinal hemorrhage with long-term use of aspirin: Meta-analysis. BMJ 2000;321:1183–1187.

17. Sorensen HT, Mellemkjaer L, Blot WJ, et al. Risk of upper gastrointestinal bleeding associated with use of low-dose aspirin. Am J Gastroenterol 2000;95:2218–2224.

18. Laine L. Review article: The effect of Helicobacter pylori infection on nonsteroidal anti-inflammatory drug-induced upper gastrointestinal tract injury. Aliment Phamacol Ther 2002;16(Suppl 1):34–39.

19. Huang JQ, Sridhar S, Hunt RH. Role of Helicobacter pylori infection and nonsteroidal anti-inflammatory drugs in peptic ulcer disease: A meta-analysis. Lancet 2002;369:14–22.

20. Lanas A, Fuentes J, Benito R, et al. Helicobacter pylori increases the risk of upper gastrointestinal bleeding in patients taking low-dose aspirin. Aliment Phamacol Ther 2002;16:779–786.

21. Micklewright R, Lane S, Linley W, et al. Review article: NSAIDs, gastroprotection and cyclo-oxygenase-II-selective inhibitors. Aliment Pharmacol Ther 2003;17:321–332.

22. Warner TD, Giuliano F, Vojnovic I, et al. Nonsteroid drug selectivities for cyclo-oxygenase-1 rather than cyclo-oxygenase-2 are associated with human gastrointestinal toxicity: A full in vitro analysis. Proc Natl Acad Sci USA 1999;96:7563–7568.

23. Kelly JP, Kaufman DW, Jurgelon JM, et al. Risk of aspirin-associated major upper gastrointestinal bleeding with enteric-coated or buffered product. Lancet 1996;348:1413–1416.

24. Del Valle J, Todisco A. Gastric secretion. In: Yamada T, Aplers DH, Kaplowitz N, et al, eds. Textbook of Gastroenterology, 4th ed. Philadelphia, Lippincott Williams & Wilkins, 2003:266–307.

25. Sachs G, Shin M, Munson K, et al. The control of gastric acid and Helicobacter pylori eradication. Aliment Pharmacol Ther 2000;14:1383–1401.

26. Hernandez-Diaz S, Rodriguez LA. Association between nonsteroidal anti-inflammatory drugs and upper gastrointestinal tract bleeding/perforation: An overview of epidemiologic studies published in the 1990s. Arch Intern Med 2000;160:2093–2099.

27. Vaira D, Gatta L, Ricci C, et al. Review article: Diagnosis of Helicobacter pylori infection. Aliment Pharmacol Ther 2002;16(Suppl 1):16–23.

28. Oderda G, Rapa A, Marinello D, et al. Usefulness of Helicobacter pylori stool antigen test to monitor response to eradication treatment in children. Aliment Pharmacol Ther 2001;15:203–206.

29. Bilardi C, Biagini R, Dulbecco P, et al. Stool antigen assay (HpSA) is less reliable than urea breath test for post-treatment diagnosis of Helicobacter pylori infection. Aliment Pharmacol Ther 2002;16:1733–1738.

30. Seymour NE, Andersen DK. Surgery for peptic ulcer disease and postgastrectomy syndromes. In: Yamada T, Aplers DH, Kaplowitz N, et al, eds. Textbook of Gastroenterology, 4th ed. Philadelphia, Lippincott Williams & Wilkins, 2003:1441–1454.

31. Pilotto A, Malfertheiner P. Review article: An approach to Helicobacter pylori infection in the elderly. Aliment Pharmacol Ther 2002;16:683–691.

32. Anderson J, Gonzalez J. H. pylori infection: Review of the guideline for diagnosis and treatment. Geriatrics 2000;55:44–49.

33. Drumm B, Koletzko S, Oderda G. Helicobacter pylori infection in children: A consensus statement. J Pediatr Gastroenterol Nutr 2000;30:207–213.

34. Oderda G, Rapa A, Bona G. A systematic review of Helicobacter pylori eradication treatment schedules in children. Aliment Pharmacol Ther 2000;14(Suppl 3):59–66.

35. Sheu BS, Huang JJ, Yang HB, et al. The selection of triple therapy for Helicobacter pylori eradication in chronic renal insufficiency. Aliment Pharmacol Ther 2003;17:1283–1290.

36. Malfertheiner P, Megraud F, O'Morain C, et al. Current concepts in the management of Helicobacter pylori infection—The Maastricht 2-2000 Consensus Report. Aliment Pharmacol Ther 2002;16:167–180.

37. Qasim A, O'Morain CA. Review article: Treatment of Helicobacter pylori infection and factors influencing eradication. Aliment Pharmacol Ther 2002;16(Suppl 1):24–30.

38. Meyer JM, Silliman NP, Wang W, et al. Risk factors for Helicobacter pylori resistance in the United States; the surveillance of H. pylori antimicrobial resistance partnership (SHARP) study, 1993–1999. Ann Intern Med 2002;136:13–20.

39. Laheij RJ, Rossum LG, Janser JB, et al. Evaluation of treatment regimens to cure Helicobacter pylori infection—a meta-analysis. Aliment Pharmacol Ther 1999;13:857–864.

40. Calvet X, Garcia N, Lopez T, et al. A meta-analysis of short versus long therapy with a proton pump inhibitor, clarithromycin and either metronidazole or amoxycillin for treating Helicobacter pylori infection. Aliment Pharmacol Ther 2000;14:603–609.

41. Chey WE, Fisher L, Barnett J, et al. Low-versus high-dose azithromycin triple therapy for Helicobacter pylori infection. Aliment Pharmacol Ther 1998;12:1263–1267.

42. Vallve M, Vergara M, Gisbert JP, et al. Single vs. double dose of a proton pump inhibitor in triple therapy for Helicobacter pylori eradication: A meta-analysis. Aliment Pharmacol Ther 2002;16:1149–1156.

43. Vergara M, Vallve M, Gisbert JP, et al. Meta-analysis: Comparative efficacy of different proton-pump inhibitors in triple therapy for Helicobacter pylori eradication. Aliment Pharmacol Ther 2003;18:647–654.

44. Gisbert JP, Khorrami S, Calvet X, et al. Meta-analysis: Proton pump inhibitors vs. H_2-receptor antagonists—their efficacy with antibiotics in Helicobacter pylori eradication. Aliment Pharmacol Ther 2002;18:757–766.

45. Gene E, Calvet X, Azagra R, et al. Triple vs quadruple therapy for treating Helicobacter pylori infection: A meta-analysis. Aliment Pharmacol Ther 2003;17:1137–1143.

46. Megraud F, Lamouliatte H. Review article: The treatment of refractory Helicobacter pylori infection. Aliment Pharmacol Ther 2003;17:1333–1343.

47. Gisbert JP, Pajares JM. Review article: Helicobacter pylori "rescue" regimen when proton pump inhibitor-based triple therapies fail. Aliment Pharmacol Ther 2002;16:1047–1057.

48. Lee M, Kemp JA, Canning A, et al. A randomized controlled trial of an enhanced patient compliance program for Helicobacter pylori therapy. Arch Intern Med 1999;159:2312–2316.

49. Van Der Wouden EJ, Thijs JC, Van Zwet AA, et al. Nitroimidazole resistance in Helicobacter pylori. Aliment Pharmacol Ther 2000;14:7–14.

50. Chan FKL, Leung WK. Peptic ulcer disease. Lancet 2002;360:933–941.

51. Fennerty MB. NSAID-related gastrointestinal injury: Evidence-based approach to a preventable complication. Postgrad Med 2001;110:87–94.

52. Fitzgerald GA, Patrono C. Coxibs, selective inhibitors of cyclooxygenase-2. N Engl J Med 2002;345:433–442.

53. Silverstein FE, Graham DY, Senior JR, et al. Misoprostol reduces serious gastrointestinal complications in patients with rheumatoid arthritis receiving nonsteroidal anti-inflammatory drugs: A randomized, double-blind, placebo-controlled trial. Ann Intern Med 1995;123:241–249.

54. Yeomans ND, Tulassay Z, Juhasz L, et al. A comparison of omeprazole with ranitidine for ulcers associated with nonsteroidal antiinflammatory drugs. N Engl J Med 1998;338:719–726.

55. Hawkey CJ, Karrasch JA, Szcepanski L, et al. Omeprazole compared with misoprostol for ulcers associated with nonsteroidal anti-inflammatory drugs. N Engl J Med 1998;338:727–734.

56. Graham DY, Agrawal NM, Campbell DR, et al. Ulcer prevention in long-term users of nonsteroidal anti-inflammatory drugs: Results of a double-blind, randomized, multicenter, active- and placebo-controlled study of misoprostol vs lansoprazole. Arch Intern Med 2002;152:169–175.

57. Chan PKI, Chung SCS, Suen BY, et al. Preventing recurrence of upper gastrointestinal bleeding in patients with Helicobacter pylori infection who are taking low-dose aspirin or naproxen. N Engl J Med 2001;344:967–973.

58. Lai KC, Lam SK, Chu KM, et al. Lansoprazole for the prevention of recurrences of upper gastrointestinal complications from long-term low-dose aspirin use. N Engl J Med 2002;346:2033–2038.

59. Silverstein F, Faich G, Goldstein JL, et al. Gastrointestinal toxicity with celecoxib vs nonsteroidal antiinflammatory drugs for osteoarthritis and rheumatoid arthritis. The CLASS study: A randomized controlled trial. JAMA 2000;284:1247–1255.

60. Bombardier C, Laine L, Reicin A, et al. Comparison of upper intestinal toxicity of rofecoxib and naproxen in patients with rheumatoid arthritis. VIGOR Study Group. N Engl J Med 2000;343:1520–1528.

61. Deeks JJ, Smith LA, Bradley MD. Efficacy, tolerability, and upper gastrointestinal safety of celecoxib for treatment of osteoarthritis and rheumatoid arthritis: Systematic review of randomized controlled trials. BMJ 2002;325:619–626.

62. Chan FD, Huang LC, Suen BY, et al. Celecoxib versus diclofenac and omeprazole in reducing the risk of recurrent ulcer bleeding in patients with arthritis. N Engl J Med 2002;347:2104–2111.

63. Lai KC, Chu KM, Hui WM, et al. COX-2 inhibitor compared with proton pump inhibitor in the prevention of recurrent ulcer complications in high-risk patients taking NSAIDs. Gastroenterology 2001;120:A104. Abstract.

64. Welage LS, Berardi RR. Evaluation of omeprazole, lansoprazole, pantoprazole, and rabeprazole in the treatment of acid-related diseases. J Am Pharm Assoc 2000;40:52–62.

65. Richardson P, Hawkey CJ, Stack WA. Proton pump inhibitors: Pharmacology and rationale for use in gastrointestinal disorders. Drugs 1998;56:307–335.

66. Welage L. Pharmacologic properties of proton pump inhibitors. Pharmacotherapy 2003;23(10 Pt 2):74S–80S.

67. Matheson AJ, Jarvis B. Lansoprazole: An update of its place in the management of acid-related disorders. Drugs 2001;61:1801–1833.

68. Scott LJ, Dunn CJ, Mallarkey G, et al. Esomeprazole: A review of its use in the management of acid-related disorders. Drugs 2002;62:1503–1538.

69. Cheer SM, Prakash A, Faulds D, et al. Pantoprazole: An update of its pharmacological properties and therapeutic use in the management of acid related disorders. Drugs 2003;63:101–132.

70. Carswell CI, Goa KL. Rabeprazole: An update of its use in acid related disorders. Drugs 2001;61:2327–2356.

71. Stedman CAM, Barclay ML. Review article: Comparison of the pharmacokinetics, acid suppression and efficacy of proton pump inhibitors. Aliment Pharmacol Ther 2000;14:963–978.

72. Hatlebakk JG, Katz PO, Camacho-Lobato L, et al. Proton pump inhibitors: Better acid suppression when taken before a meal than without a meal. Aliment Pharmacol Ther 2000;14:1267–1272.

73. Baldi F, Malfertheiner P. Lansoprazole fast disintegrating tablet: A new formulation for an established proton pump inhibitor. Digestion 2003;67:1–5.

74. Sharma VK. Comparison of 24-hour intragastric pH using four liquid formulations of lansoprazole and omeprazole. Am J Health-Syst Pharm 1999;(Suppl 4):518–521.

75. Sostek MB, Chen Y, Skammer W, et al. Esomeprazole administered through a nasogastric tube provides bioavailability similar to oral dosing. Aliment Pharmacol Ther 2003;18:581–586.

76. Laine L, Ahnen D, McClain C, et al. Review article: Potential gastrointestinal effects of long term acid suppression with proton pump inhibitors. Aliment Pharmacol Ther 2000;14:651–668.

77. Wade EE, Rebuck JA, Healey MA, et al. H$_2$ antagonist-induced thrombocytopenia: Is this a real phenomenon? Intensive Care Med 2002;28:459–465.

78. Monroe ML, Doering PL. Effect of common over the counter medications on blood alcohol levels. Ann Pharmacother 2001;35:918–924.

79. Welage LS, Berardi RR. Drug interactions with antiulcer agents: Considerations in the treatment of acid-peptic disease. J Pharm Pract 1994;VII:177–195.

80. Kamiya S, Yamaguchi H, Osaki T, et al. Effect of an aluminum hydroxide-magnesium hydroxide combination drug on adhesion, IL-8 inducibility, and expression of HSP60 by Helicobacter pylori. Scand J Gastroenterol 1999;34:663–670.

81. Maton PN, Burton ME. Antacids revisited: A review of their clinical pharmacology and recommended therapeutic use. Drugs 1999;57:855–870.

82. Sonnenberg A, Schwartz JS, Cutler AF, et al. Cost savings in duodenal ulcer therapy through Helicobacter pylori eradication compared with conventional therapies: Results of a randomized, double-blind, multicenter trial. Arch Intern Med 1998;158:852–860.

83. Maetzel A, Ferraz MB, Bombardier C. The cost-effectiveness of misoprostol in preventing serious gastrointestinal events associated with the use of nonsteroidal anti-inflammatory drugs. Arthritis Rheum 1998;41:16–25.

84. El-Serag HP, Graham DY, Richardson P, et al. Prevention of complicated ulcer disease among chronic users of nonsteroidal antiinflammatory drugs: The use of a nomogram in cost-effectiveness analysis. Arch Intern Med 2002;162:2105–2110.

85. Hirschowitz BI. Zollinger-Ellison syndrome: Pathogenesis, diagnosis, and management. Am J Gastroenterol 1997;92(Suppl 4):44S–50S.

86. Corleto VD, Annibale B, Gibril F, et al. Does the widespread use of proton pump inhibitors mask, complicate and/or delay the diagnosis of Zollinger-Ellison syndrome? Aliment Pharmacol Ther 2001;15:1555–1561.

87. Fu F, Venzon DJ, Serrano J, et al. Prospective study of the clinical course, prognostic factors, causes of death and survival in patients with long-standing Zollinger-Ellison syndrome. J Clin Oncol 1999;17:615–630.

88. Tomassetti P, Migliori M, Corinaldesi R, Gullo L. Treatment of gastroenteropancreatic neuroendocrine tumors with octreotide LAR. Aliment Pharmacol Ther 2000;14:557–560.

89. Barkun AN, Coceram AW, Plourde V, Fedorak RN. Review article: Acid suppression in non-variceal acute upper gastrointestinal bleeding. Aliment Pharmacol Ther 1999;13:1565–1584.

90. American Society of Health-System Pharmacists Therapeutic Guidelines on Stress Ulcer Prophylaxis. Am J Health Syst Pharm 1999;56:347–379.

91. Cook DJ, Fuller HD, Guyatt GH, et al. Risk factors for gastrointestinal bleeding in critically ill patients. N Engl J Med 1994;330:377–381.

92. Laine L, Peterson WL. Bleeding peptic ulcer. N Engl J Med 1994;331:717–727.

93. Barkun A, Bardou M, Marshall JK. Consensus recommendations for managing patients with nonvariceal upper gastrointestinal bleeding. Ann Intern Med 2003;139:843–857.

94. Levine JE, Leontiadis GI, Sharma VK, Howden CW. Meta-analysis: The efficacy of intravenous H2-receptor antagonists in bleeding peptic ulcer. Aliment Pharmacol Ther 2002;16:1137–1142.

95. Van Leerdam ME, Rauws EAJ. The role of acid suppressants in upper gastrointestinal ulcer bleeding. Best Pract Res Clin Gastroenterol 2001;15:463–475.

96. Lau JYW, Sung JJY, Lee KKC, et al. Effect of intravenous omeprazole on recurrent bleeding after endoscopic treatment of bleeding peptic ulcers. N Engl J Med 2000;343:310–316.

97. Sung JJY, Chan FKL, Lau JYW. The effect of endoscopic therapy in patients receiving omeprazole for bleeding ulcers with nonbleeding visible vessels or adherent clots. Ann Intern Med 2003;139:237–243.

98. Javid G, Masoodi I, Zargar SA, et al. Omeprazole as adjuvant therapy to endoscopic combination injection sclerotherapy for treating bleeding peptic ulcer. Am J Med 2001;111:280–284.

99. Kaviani MJ, Hashemi MR, Kazemifar AR, et al. Effect of oral omeprazole in reducing re-bleeding in bleeding peptic ulcers: A prospective, double-blind, randomized, clinical trial. Aliment Pharmacol Ther 2003;17:211–216.

100. Cook D, Heyland D, Griffith L, et al. Risk factors for clinically important upper gastrointestinal bleeding in patients requiring mechanical ventilation. Crit Care Med 1999;27:2812–2817.

101. Cook D, Guyatt G, Marshall J, et al. A comparison of sucralfate and ranitidine for the prevention of upper gastrointestinal bleeding in patients requiring mechanical ventilation. N Engl J Med 1998;338:791–797.

102. Cook DJ, Griffith LE, Walter SD, et al. The attributable mortality and length of intensive care unit stay of clinically important gastrointestinal bleeding in critically ill patients. Crit Care 2001;5:368–375.

103. MacLaren R, Jarvis CL, Fish DN. Use of enteral nutrition for stress ulcer prophylaxis. Ann Pharmacother 2001;35:1614–1623.

104. Lam NP, Le PDT, Crawford SY, et al. National survey of stress ulcer prophylaxis. Crit Care Med 1999;27:98–103.

105. Jung R, MacLaren R. Proton-pump inhibitors for stress ulcer prophylaxis in critically ill patients. Ann Pharmacother 2002;36:1929–1937.

106. Levy MJ, Seelig CB, et al. Comparison of omeprazole and ranitidine for stress ulcer prophylaxis. Dig Dis Sci 1997;42:1255–1259.

34

INFLAMMATORY BOWEL DISEASE

Joseph T. DiPiro and Robert R. Schade

Learning Objectives and other resources can be found at *www.pharmacotherapyonline.com.*

KEY CONCEPTS

◀1 The exact cause of inflammatory bowel disease (IBD) is unknown, although there are components that appear to be infectious and other components that suggest immune dysregulation. Genetic variations explain some of the increased risk of disease occurrence.

◀2 Ulcerative colitis is confined to the rectum and colon, causes continuous lesions, and affects primarily the mucosa and the submucosa. Crohn's disease can involve any part of the GI tract, often causes discontinuous (skip) lesions, and is a transmural process that can result in fistulas, perforations, or strictures.

◀3 Common complications of IBD include rectal fissures, fistulas (Crohn's disease), perirectal abscess (ulcerative colitis), and colon cancer, in addition to hepatobiliary complications, arthritis, uveitis, skin lesions (including erythema nodosum and pyoderma gangrenosum), and aphthous ulcerations of the mouth.

◀4 The severity of ulcerative colitis may be assessed by factors such as stool frequency, presence of blood in stool, fever, pulse, hemoglobin, erythrocyte sedimentation rate, C-reactive protein, abdominal tenderness, and radiologic or endoscopic findings. The severity of Crohn's disease can be assessed by the Crohn's disease activity index, which includes stool frequency, presence of blood in stool, endoscopic appearance, and physician's global assessment.

◀5 The goals of treatment of IBD are resolution of acute inflammation and complications, alleviation of systemic manifestations, maintenance of remission, and in some patients, surgical palliation or cure.

◀6 The first-line of treatment for mild to moderate ulcerative colitis or Crohn's colitis consists of oral sulfasalazine or mesalamine; mesalamine or steroid enemas may be used for rectosigmoid disease. Delayed-release oral formulations of mesalamine may be used for Crohn's ileitis.

◀7 Corticosteroids are often required for acute ulcerative colitis or Crohn's disease. The duration of steroid use should be minimized and the dose tapered gradually over 3 to 4 weeks.

◀8 Intravenous continuous infusion of cyclosporine is effective in treating severe colitis that is refractory to steroids.

◀9 Sulfasalazine and mesalamine derivatives can prevent recurrence of acute disease in many patients, while steroids are ineffective for this purpose.

◀10 Other drugs that are useful for treatment of Crohn's disease include metronidazole (for perineal disease), azathioprine or mercaptopurine (for inadequate response or to reduce steroid dosage), cyclosporine (for refractory disease), and infliximab for refractory or fistulizing disease.

There are two forms of idiopathic inflammatory bowel disease (IBD): (a) ulcerative colitis, a mucosal inflammatory condition confined to the rectum and colon; and (b) Crohn's disease, a transmural inflammation of the gastrointestinal tract that can affect any part, from the mouth to the anus. The etiologies of both conditions are unknown, but they may have some common pathogenetic mechanisms.

EPIDEMIOLOGY

At least 1 million Americans are believed to have IBD, with 15,000 to 30,000 new cases diagnosed annually.[1] Crohn's disease has a reported incidence of 3.6 to 8.8 per 100,000 persons in the United States and a prevalence of 20 to 40 per 100,000 people.[2] The rates of IBD are highest in Scandinavia, Great Britain, and North America.[3] The incidence of Crohn's disease varies considerably among studies, but

has clearly increased dramatically over the last 3 or 4 decades.[3,4] Ulcerative colitis incidence ranges from 3 to 15 cases per 100,000 persons per year among the white population with a prevalence of 80 to 120 per 100,000.[2] The incidence of ulcerative colitis has remained relatively constant over many years.[3,4] Although most epidemiologic studies combine ulcerative proctitis with ulcerative colitis, from 17% to 49% of cases are proctitis.

Both sexes are affected equally with inflammatory bowel disease,[1,2] although some studies show slightly greater numbers of women with Crohn's disease and males with ulcerative colitis.[6,7] Ulcerative colitis and Crohn's disease have bimodal distributions in age of initial presentation. The peak incidence occurs in the second or third decades of life, with a second peak occurring between 50 and 80 years of age.[4] A significantly increased incidence of ulcerative colitis (four to five times normal) has been observed in Ashkenazi Jews, while blacks and Asians have a relatively low incidence of occurrence.[5]

TABLE 34–1. Proposed Etiologies for Inflammatory Bowel Disease

Infectious agents
   Viruses (e.g., measles)
   L-Forms of bacteria
   Mycobacteria
   Chlamydia
Genetics
   Metabolic defects
   Connective tissue disorders
Environmental Factors
   Diet
   Smoking (Crohn's disease)
Immune defects
   Altered host suceptibility
   Immune-mediated mucosal damage
Psychologic factors
   Stress
   Emotional or physical trauma
   Occupation

ETIOLOGY

Although the exact etiology of ulcerative colitis and Crohn's disease is unknown, similar factors are believed responsible for both conditions (Table 34–1). The major theories of the cause of IBD involve a combination of infectious, genetic, and immunologic factors.[8] The inflammatory response with IBD may indicate abnormal regulation of the normal immune response or an autoimmune reaction to self-antigens. The microflora of the gastrointestinal tract may provide an environmental trigger to activate inflammation.[9] Crohn's disease has been described as "a disorder mediated by T lymphocytes which arises in genetically susceptible individuals as a result of a breakdown in the regulatory constraints on mucosal immune responses to enteric bacteria."[10]

INFECTIOUS FACTORS

Microorganisms are a likely factor in the initiation of inflammation in IBD.[11] However, no definitive infectious cause of IBD has been found, even though the presentation is similar to that caused by some invasive microbial pathogens. Patients with inflammatory bowel diseases have increased numbers of surface-adherent and intracellular bacteria.[12] IBD may involve a loss of tolerance toward normal bacterial flora.[13]

Suspect infectious agents include the measles virus, protozoans, mycobacteria, and other bacteria. Also, certain strains of bacteria produce toxins (necrotoxins, hemolysins, and enterotoxins) that cause mucosal damage. Bacteria elaborate peptides (e.g., formyl-methionyl-leucyl-phenylalanine) that have chemotactic properties and that cause an influx of inflammatory cells with subsequent release of inflammatory mediators and tissue destruction. Microbes may elaborate superantigens, which are capable of global T-lymphocyte stimulation and subsequent inflammatory response.[11] Through luminal exposure to potent nonspecific stimulatory bacterial products, the state of activation of the immune system pathways may be upregulated.[14] As many as 70% of patients with Crohn's disease have circulating antibody to *Saccharomyces cerevisiae*, but this may not be a disease mechanism.[15]

GENETIC FACTORS

Genetic factors predispose patients to inflammatory bowel diseases, particularly Crohn's disease. In studies of monozygotic twins, there has been a high concordance rate, with both individuals of the pair having an IBD (particularly Crohn's disease). Also, first-degree relatives of patients with IBD had a 13-fold increase in the risk of disease.[16] Other investigators have observed genetic markers that are found more frequently in those with IBD (particularly major histocompatability complex, HLA-DR2 for ulcerative colitis and HLA-A2 for Crohn's disease).[3] Multiple genes have been associated with IBDs; however, the nature of the gene products has not been established.

IMMUNOLOGIC MECHANISMS

The immunologic basis of IBD is supported by a number of observations.[9] First is the pathology of the lesions. With Crohn's disease, the bowel wall is infiltrated with lymphocytes, plasma cells, mast cells, macrophages, and neutrophils. Similar infiltration has been observed in the mucosal layer of the colon in patients with ulcerative colitis. Inflammation in IBDs is maintained by an influx of leukocytes from the vascular system into sites of active disease. This influx is promoted by expression of adhesion molecules (such as alpha-4 integrins) on the surface of endothelial cells in the microvasculature in the area of inflammation.[12] Second, many of the systemic manifestations of IBD have an immunologic etiology (e.g., arthritis or uveitis). Finally, IBD is responsive to immunosuppressive drugs (e.g., corticosteroids and azathioprine).

The immune theory of IBD assumes that IBD is caused by an inappropriate reaction of the immune system. This may involve an immunodeficiency, such as a defect in cell-mediated immunity or of macrophages or neutrophils. Autoimmunity may be involved. Also, oxidant injury in colon epithelial crypt cells can be demonstrated from inflamed mucosa of patients with IBD.[17]

Potential immunologic mechanisms include both autoimmune and nonautoimmune phenomena.[11] Autoimmunity may be directed against mucosal epithelial cells or against neutrophil cytoplasmic elements. Some patients with IBD have abnormal structural features for colonic epithelial cells even in the absence of active disease. Autoantibodies to these structures have been reported. Also, antineutrophil cytoplasmic antibodies are found in a high percentage of patients with ulcerative colitis (70%) and much less frequently with Crohn's disease.[12] Presence of antineutrophil cytoplasmic antibodies in left-sided ulcerative colitis is associated with resistance to medical therapy.[18] Dysregulation of cytokines is a component of IBD. Specifically, Th_1 cytokine activity (which enhances cell-mediated immunity and suppresses humoral immunity) is excessive with Crohn's disease, whereas Th_2 cytokine activity (which inhibits cell-mediated immunity and enhances humoral immunity) is excessive with ulcerative colitis.[19] The result is that patients have inappropriate T-cell responses to antigens from their own intestinal microflora.[19] Expression of interferon-γ (a Th_1 cytokine) in intestinal mucosa of diseased patients is increased, while interleukin-4 (a Th_2 cytokine) is reduced.[20–22]

Tumor necrosis factor-α (TNF-α) is a pivotal proinflammatory cytokine in Crohn's disease. TNF-α can recruit inflammatory cells to inflamed tissues, activate coagulation, and promote the formation of granulomas. Production of TNF-α is increased in the mucosa and intestinal lumen of patients with Crohn's disease.[23] Eicosanoids such as leukotriene B_4 are increased in rectal dialysates and tissues of IBD patients and are related to disease activity. Leukotriene B_4 enhances neutrophil adherence to vascular endothelium and acts as a neutrophil chemoattractant. These findings have led to the consideration of leukotriene inhibitor strategies for therapy.

PSYCHOLOGICAL FACTORS

Mental health changes appear to correlate with remissions and exacerbations, especially of ulcerative colitis, but psychological factors overall are not thought to be an etiologic factor. There is a weak association between the number of stressful events experienced and the time to relapse of ulcerative colitis.[24]

DIET, SMOKING, AND NSAID USE

Changes in diet by people in industrialized countries where Crohn's disease is more common have not been consistently associated with the disease. Studies of increased intake of refined sugars or chemical food additives and reduced fiber intake have provided conflicting results regarding risk for Crohn's disease.

Smoking plays an important but contrasting role in ulcerative colitis and Crohn's disease. Smoking is protective for ulcerative colitis.[12] The risk of developing ulcerative colitis in smokers is about 40% of that in nonsmokers.[25] Clinical relapses are associated with smoking cessation, and nicotine transdermal administration has been effective in improving symptoms in patients with ulcerative colitis.[26,27] In contrast, smoking is associated with a twofold increased frequency of Crohn's disease.[3] Crohn's disease patients who stop smoking have a more benign course than patients who continue smoking.[28] The mechanisms of these differing effects have not been identified.

Use of nonsteroidal anti-inflammatory drugs (NSAIDs) can trigger disease occurrence or lead to disease flares.[12,29] The effect of NSAIDs to inhibit prostaglandin production through cyclooxygenase inhibition may impair mucosal barrier protective mechanisms. The increased risk seems to be present for cyclooxygenase-2 inhibitors as well as cyclooxygenase-1 inhibitors.

PATHOPHYSIOLOGY

Ulcerative colitis and Crohn's disease differ in two general respects: anatomic sites and depth of involvement within the bowel wall. There is, however, overlap between the two conditions, with a small fraction of patients showing features of both diseases. Confusion can occur, particularly when the inflammatory process is limited to the colon. Table 34–2 compares pathologic and clinical findings of the two diseases.

ULCERATIVE COLITIS

Ulcerative colitis is confined to the rectum and colon, and affects the mucosa and the submucosa. In some instances, a short segment of terminal ileum may be inflamed; this is referred to as *backwash ileitis*. Unlike Crohn's disease, the deeper longitudinal muscular layers, serosa, and regional lymph nodes are not usually involved.[6] Fistulas, perforation, or obstruction are uncommon because inflammation is usually confined to the mucosa and submucosa.

The primary lesion of ulcerative colitis occurs in the crypts of the mucosa (crypts of Lieberkuhn) in the form of a crypt abscess. Here, frank necrosis of the epithelium occurs; it is usually visible only with microscopy, but may be seen grossly when coalescence of ulcers occurs. Extension and coalescence ulcers may surround areas of uninvolved mucosa. These islands of mucosa are called *pseudopolyps*.

TABLE 34–2. Comparison of the Clinical and Pathologic Features of Crohn's Disease and Ulcerative Colitis

Feature	Crohn's Disease	Ulcerative Colitis
Clinical		
Malaise, fever	Common	Uncommon
Rectal bleeding	Common	Common
Abdominal tenderness	Common	May be present
Abdominal mass	Common	Absent
Abdominal pain	Common	Unusual
Abdominal wall and internal fistulas	Common	Absent
Distribution	Discontinuous	Continuous
Aphthous or linear ulcers	Common	Rare
Pathologic		
Rectal involvement	Rare	Common
Ileal involvement	Very common	Rare
Strictures	Common	Rare
Fistulas	Common	Rare
Transmural involvement	Common	Rare
Crypt abscesses	Rare	Very common
Granulomas	Common	Rare
Linear clefts	Common	Rare
Cobblestone appearance	Common	Absent

Other typical ulceration patterns include a "collar-button ulcer," which results from extensive submucosal undermining at the ulcer edge.[6] The extensive mucosal damage seen in ulcerative colitis can result in significant diarrhea and bleeding, although a small percentage of patients experience constipation.

Ulcerative colitis can be accompanied by complications that may be local (involving the colon or rectum) or systemic (not directly associated with the colon). With either type the complications may be mild, serious, or even life threatening. Local complications occur in the majority of ulcerative colitis patients. Relatively minor complications include hemorrhoids, anal fissures, or perirectal abscesses, and are more likely to be present during active colitis. Enteroenteric fistulas are rare.

A major complication is toxic megacolon, which is a segmental or total colonic distension of >6 cm with acute colitis and signs of systemic toxicity.[30] It is a severe condition that occurs in up to 7.9% of ulcerative colitis patients admitted to hospitals and results in death rates up to 50%. With toxic megacolon, ulceration extends below the submucosa, sometimes even reaching the serosa. Vasculitis, swelling of the vascular endothelium, and thrombosis of small arteries occurs; involvement of the muscularis propria causes loss of colonic tone, which leads to dilatation and potential perforation.[6] The patient with toxic megacolon usually has a high fever, tachycardia, distended abdomen, and elevated white blood cell count, and a dilated colon is observed on x-ray. Colonic perforation, however, may occur with or without toxic megacolon and is a greater risk with the first attack. Another infrequent major local complication is massive colonic hemorrhage. Colonic stricture, sometimes with clinical obstruction, may also complicate long-standing ulcerative colitis.

The risk of colonic carcinoma is much greater in patients with ulcerative colitis as compared to the general population. The risk of colon cancer begins to increase 10 to 15 years after the diagnosis of ulcerative colitis. The absolute risk may be as high as 30% 35 years after diagnosis, and as high as 49% for patients who have a long history of disease and who were less than 15 years of age at the time of diagnosis.

The inflammatory response seen in IBD has also been blamed for the systemic complications seen in both Crohn's disease and ulcerative colitis. The systemic extraintestinal complications of ulcerative colitis are summarized in the next section.

HEPATOBILIARY COMPLICATIONS

Approximately 11% of patients with ulcerative colitis are reported to have hepatobiliary complications with frequencies ranging from 5% to 95% in IBD patients overall.[31,32] Hepatic complications include fatty liver, pericholangitis, chronic active hepatitis, and cirrhosis. Biliary complications include sclerosing cholangitis, cholangiocarcinoma, and gallstones.

Fatty infiltration of the liver may be a result of malabsorption, protein-losing enteropathy, or concomitant steroid use. The most common hepatic complication is pericholangitis (acute inflammation surrounding the intrahepatic portal venules, bile ducts, and lymphatics), which occurs in up to one-third of ulcerative colitis patients. This is associated with progressive fibrosis of intrahepatic and extrahepatic bile ducts in a small percentage of ulcerative colitis patients, and is referred to as primary sclerosing cholangitis. Cirrhosis may be a sequela of cholangitis or of chronic active hepatitis. Often the severity of hepatic disease does not correlate with gastrointestinal disease activity.

Gallstones occur commonly in patients with Crohn's disease (particularly with terminal ileal disease) and may be related to bile salt malabsorption. Also, cholangiocarcinoma occurs 10 to 20 times more frequently in IBD patients as compared to the general population.[31]

JOINT COMPLICATIONS

Arthritis commonly occurs in IBD patients and is typically asymmetric (unlike rheumatoid arthritis) and migratory, involving one or a few usually large joints. The joints most often affected, in decreasing frequency, are the knees, hips, ankles, wrists, and elbows. Sacroiliitis also occurs commonly. Arthritis associated with ulcerative colitis is generally related to the severity of colonic disease, and resolution without recurrence is seen with proctocolectomy. Also, arthritis in this setting is different from rheumatoid arthritis in that rheumatoid factors are generally not detected. It is nondeforming and nondestructive, even after multiple episodes.

Another potential joint complication is ankylosing spondylitis, which is often unresponsive to treatment. The incidence of ankylosing spondylitis in patients with ulcerative colitis is 30 times that of the general population and occurs most commonly in patients with the HLA-B27 phenotype.

OCULAR COMPLICATIONS

Ocular complications including iritis, uveitis, episcleritis, and conjunctivitis occur in up to 10% of patients with IBD. The most commonly reported symptoms with iritis and uveitis include blurred vision, eye pain, and photophobia. Episcleritis is associated with scleral injection, burning, and increased secretions. These complications may parallel the severity of intestinal disease, and recurrence after colectomy with ulcerative colitis is uncommon.

DERMATOLOGIC AND MUCOSAL COMPLICATIONS

Skin and mucosal lesions associated with IBD include erythema nodosum, pyoderma gangrenosum, and aphthous ulceration. Five to ten percent of IBD patients experience dermatologic or mucosal complications.[33]

Raised, red, tender nodules that vary in size from 1 cm to several centimeters are manifestations of erythema nodosum. They are typically found on the tibial surfaces of the legs and arms. These lesions are more commonly observed in Crohn's disease patients and are noted to correlate with disease severity.

Pyoderma gangrenosum occurs more commonly in patients with ulcerative colitis (1% to 5% incidence) and is characterized by discrete skin ulcerations that have a necrotic center and a violaceous color of the surrounding skin.[33] They can be seen on any part of the body but are more commonly found on the lower extremities.

Oral lesions are found in 6% to 20% of patients with Crohn's disease and 8% of patients with ulcerative colitis.[33] The most common lesion is aphthous stomatitis, seen with Crohn's disease. The severity of these lesions tends to parallel GI disease.

CROHN'S DISEASE

Crohn's disease is best characterized as a transmural inflammatory process. The terminal ileum is the most common site of the disorder, but it may occur in any part of the GI tract from mouth to anus. About two-thirds of patients have some colonic involvement, and 15% to 25% of patients have only colonic disease.[11] Patients often have normal bowel separating segments of diseased bowel; that is, the disease is discontinuous.

Regardless of the site, bowel wall injury is extensive and the intestinal lumen is often narrowed. The mesentery first becomes thickened and edematous and then fibrotic. Ulcers tend to be deep and elongated and extend along the longitudinal axis of the bowel, at least into the submucosa. The "cobblestone" appearance of the bowel wall results from deep mucosal ulceration intermingled with nodular submucosal thickening.

Complications of Crohn's disease may involve the intestinal tract or organs unrelated to it. Small bowel stricture and subsequent obstruction is a complication that may require surgery. Fistula formation is common and occurs much more frequently than with ulcerative colitis.[11] Fistulae often occur in the areas of worst inflammation, where loops of bowel have become matted together by fibrous adhesions. Fistulae may connect a segment of the GI tract to skin (enterocutaneous fistula), two segments of the GI tract (enteroenteric fistula), or the intestinal tract with the bladder (enterovesicular fistula) or vagina. Crohn's disease fistulae or abscesses associated with them frequently require surgical treatment.

Bleeding with Crohn's disease is usually not as severe as with ulcerative colitis, although patients with Crohn's disease may have hypochromic anemia. Also, as with ulcerative colitis, the risk of carcinoma is increased but not as greatly as with ulcerative colitis.

Systemic complications of Crohn's disease are common, and similar to those found with ulcerative colitis. Arthritis, iritis, skin lesions, and liver disease often accompany Crohn's disease. Renal stones occur in up to 10% of patients with Crohn's disease (less frequently with ulcerative colitis) and are caused by fat malabsorption, which allows for greater oxalate absorption and formation of calcium oxalate stones. Gallstones also occur with greater frequency in patients with ileitis, possibly because of bile acid malabsorption at the terminal ileum.

Nutritional deficiencies are common with Crohn's disease.[34] Reported frequencies of various nutritional parameters are: weight loss, 40% to 80%; growth failure in children, 15% to 88%; iron deficiency anemia, 25% to 50%; vitamin B_{12} deficiency, 20% to 37%; folate deficiency, 13% to 37%; hypoalbuminemia, 25% to 76%; hypokalemia, 33%; and osteomalacia, 36%. There are usually decreased fat stores and lean tissue. Growth failure in children may be associated with hypozincemia.

CLINICAL PRESENTATION

The patterns of clinical presentation of IBD can vary widely. Patients may have a single acute episode that resolves and does not recur, but most patients experience acute exacerbations after periods of remission. With more severe disease, prolonged illness may occur.

ULCERATIVE COLITIS

Although a typical clinical picture of ulcerative colitis can be described, there is a wide range of presentation, from mild abdominal cramping with frequent small-volume bowel movements to profuse diarrhea (Table 34–3). Most patients with ulcerative colitis experience intermittent bouts of illness after varying intervals with no symptoms. Only a small percentage of patients have continuous unremitting symptoms or have a single acute attack with no subsequent symptoms. Complex disease classifications are generally not used in clinical practice for ulcerative colitis. The arbitrarily determined distinctions of mild, moderate, and severe disease activity are generally used, and these are determined largely by clinical signs and symptoms.[6]

Mild—Fewer than four stools daily, with or without blood, with no systemic disturbance and a normal erythrocyte sedimentation rate (ESR).

Moderate—More than four stools per day but with minimal systemic disturbance.

Severe—More than six stools per day with blood, with evidence of systemic disturbance as shown by fever, tachycardia, anemia, or ESR of >30.

It is also important to determine disease extent; that is, which part of the colon is involved—rectum, descending colon only, or the entire colon.

TABLE 34–3. Clinical Presentation of Ulcerative Colitis

Signs and symptoms
- Abdominal cramping
- Frequent bowel movements, often with blood in the stool
- Weight loss
- Fever and tachycardia in severe disease
- Blurred vision, eye pain, and photophobia with ocular involvement
- Arthritis
- Raised, red, tender nodules that vary in size from 1 cm to several centimeters

Physical examination
- Hemorrhoids, anal fissures, or perirectal abscesses may be present
- Iritis, uveitis, episcleritis, and conjunctivitis with ocular involvement
- Dermatologic findings with erythema nodosum, pyoderma gangrenosum, or aphthous ulceration

Laboratory tests
- Decreased hematocrit/hemoglobin
- Increased erythrocyte sedimentation rate
- Leukocytosis and hypoalbuminemia with severe disease

Two-thirds of patients with ulcerative colitis have mild disease, which almost always starts in the rectum. Occasionally, the mild form may progress to severe disease, which may be called "fulminant" if it occurs acutely. Systemic signs and symptoms of the disease (e.g., arthritis, uveitis, or pyoderma gangrenosum) may be present in these patients, and in fact may be the reason the patient seeks medical attention. Patients with mild disease are believed to be at lower risk of colon cancer. Moderate disease is observed in one-fourth of patients.

With severe disease, the patient is usually found to be in acute distress, has profuse bloody diarrhea, and often has a high fever with leukocytosis and hypoalbuminemia. Often, the patient is dehydrated, and therefore may be tachycardic and hypotensive. This presentation may have a sudden onset with rapid progression.

The diagnosis of ulcerative colitis is made on clinical suspicion and confirmed by biopsy, stool examinations, sigmoidoscopy or colonoscopy, or barium radiographic contrast studies. The presence of extracolonic manifestations such as arthritis, uveitis, and pyoderma gangrenosum may also aid in establishing the diagnosis.

CROHN'S DISEASE

As with ulcerative colitis, the presentation of Crohn's disease is highly variable. A single episode may not be followed by further episodes, or the patient may experience continuous, unremitting disease. The time between the onset of complaints and the initial diagnosis may be as long as 3 years. The patient typically presents with diarrhea and abdominal pain. Hematochezia occurs in about one-half of the patients with colonic involvement and much less frequently when there is no colonic involvement. Commonly, a patient may first present with a perirectal or perianal lesion (Table 34–4). The diagnosis should also be suspected in children with growth retardation, especially with abdominal complaints.

The course of Crohn's disease is characterized by periods of remission and exacerbation. Some patients may be free of symptoms for years, while others experience chronic problems in spite of medical therapy. Nearly all patients have a recurrence of Crohn's disease within 10 years of the initial episode.[17] As with ulcerative colitis, the diagnosis of Crohn's disease involves a thorough evaluation using laboratory, endoscopic, and radiologic testing to detect the extent and characteristic features of the disease. Because of similarities that may exist between ulcerative colitis and Crohn's disease confined to the colon, a definitive diagnosis cannot be made in up to 15% of cases, even with pathologic specimens in hand. Small bowel involvement and strictures detected on radiographs are characteristic of Crohn's disease.

TABLE 34–4. Clinical Presentation of Crohn's Disease

Signs and symptoms
- Malaise and fever
- Abdominal pain
- Frequent bowel movements
- Hemotachezia
- Fistula
- Weight loss
- Arthritis

Physical examination
- Abdominal mass and tenderness
- Perianal fissure or fistula

Laboratory tests
- Increased white blood cell count and erythrocyte sedimentation rate

▶ TREATMENT: Inflammatory Bowel Disease

▦ DESIRED OUTCOME

◀5 To treat IBD properly, the clinician must have a clear concept of realistic therapeutic goals for each patient. These goals may relate to resolution of acute inflammatory processes, resolution of attendant complications (e.g., fistulas and abscesses), alleviation of systemic manifestations (e.g., arthritis), maintenance of remission from acute inflammation, or surgical palliation or cure. The approach to the therapeutic regimen differs considerably with varying goals as well as with the two diseases, ulcerative colitis and Crohn's disease.

When determining goals of therapy and selecting therapeutic regimens it is important to understand the natural history of IBD.[35] Some cases of acute ulcerative colitis are self-limited. With mild to moderate acute colitis without systemic symptoms, 20% of patients may experience spontaneous improvement in their disease within a few weeks; however, a small percentage of patients may go on to experience more serious disease. With severe colitis, improvement without treatment cannot be expected. For instance, the response to medical management of toxic megacolon is variable and emergent colectomy may be required. When remission of ulcerative colitis is achieved, it is likely to last at least 1 year with medical therapy. In the absence of medical therapy, one-half to two-thirds of patients are likely to relapse within 9 months.[35] In some reports, remission rates with placebo have approached those found with active treatment.

A considerable number of patients with active Crohn's disease may achieve at least temporary remission without drug therapy. In two large trials, 26% and 42% of ambulatory patients on placebo achieved remission.[36,37] Once remission is achieved, two-thirds to three-fourths of patients remain in remission up to 2 years without drug therapy.[35] The implication of these data is that up to 40% of patients with active Crohn's disease improve in 3 to 4 months with observation alone, and that most patients remain in remission for prolonged periods without medical intervention. These observations apply more to mild or moderate disease than to severe disease.

▦ GENERAL APPROACH TO TREATMENT

◀6 Treatment of IBD centers on agents used to relieve the inflammatory process. Salicylates, corticosteroids, antimicrobials, and immunosuppressive agents such as azathioprine and mercaptopurine are commonly used to treat active disease, and for some agents, to lengthen the time of disease remission.

In addition to the use of drugs, surgical procedures are sometimes performed when active disease is inadequately controlled or when the required drug dosages pose an unacceptable risk of adverse effects. For most patients with IBD, nutritional considerations are also important, because these patients are often malnourished. Finally, a variety of therapies may be used to address complications or symptoms of IBD. For example, antidiarrheals may be used in some patients, although these are generally to be avoided in severe ulcerative colitis because they may contribute to the development of toxic colonic dilatation. Antimicrobial agents may be used in conjunction with drainage when abscesses are present. Iron may be required, particularly with ulcerative colitis, where blood loss from the colon can be significant.

▦ NONPHARMACOLOGIC THERAPY

▦ NUTRITIONAL SUPPORT

Proper nutritional support is an important aspect of the treatment of patients with IBD, not because specific types of diets are useful in alleviating the inflammatory conditions, but because patients with moderate to severe disease are often malnourished either because the inflammatory process results in significant malabsorption or maldigestion, or because of the catabolic effects of the disease process. Malabsorption may occur in the patient with Crohn's disease with inflammatory involvement of the small bowel, where many nutrients are absorbed, as well as in patients who have undergone multiple small bowel resections with subsequent reduction in absorptive surface ("short gut"). Maldigestion can occur if there is a bile salt deficiency in the gut.

Many specific diets have been tried to improve the condition of patients with IBD, but none has gained widespread acceptance. With each individual it is helpful to eliminate specific foods that exacerbate symptoms. This elimination process must be conducted cautiously, as patients have been known to exclude a wide range of nutritious products without adequate justification. Some patients with IBD, although not the majority, have lactase deficiency; therefore diarrhea may be associated with milk intake. In these patients, avoidance of milk or supplementation with lactase generally improves the patient's symptoms.

The nutritional needs of the majority of patients can be adequately addressed with enteral supplementation.[38] Patients who have severe disease may require a course of parenteral nutrition to attain a reasonable nutritional status or in preparation for surgery. In severe acute ulcerative colitis, enteral nutrition resulted in a significantly greater increase in serum albumin, fewer adverse effects related to the nutritional regimen, and fewer postoperative infections, as compared to isocaloric, isonitrogenous parenteral nutrition.[39] The regimens were similar with regard to remission rate and the need for colectomy.[39] Consideration should be given to lipid administration for its caloric value, as well as in recognition of depleted peripheral fat stores in many IBD patients and the greater potential for fatty acid deficiency.

Parenteral nutrition is an important component of the treatment of severe Crohn's disease or ulcerative colitis. The use of parenteral nutrition allows complete bowel rest in patients with severe ulcerative colitis, which may alter the need for proctocolectomy. Parenteral nutrition has also been valuable in Crohn's disease, because remission may be achieved with parenteral nutrition in about 50% of patients.[40] In some patients, the disease may worsen when parenteral nutrition is stopped. Patients with enterocutaneous fistulas of various etiologies benefit from parenteral nutrition.[40] Parenteral nutrition may also be valuable in children or adolescents with growth retardation associated with Crohn's disease, but surgery is often necessary with severe disease. Finally, when possible, home parenteral nutrition should be used for patients requiring long-term therapy, particularly those with "short gut" as a consequence of surgical resection.

There is a growing interest in using probiotic approaches for IBD. Probiotics involves the reestablishment of normal bacterial flora within the gut by oral administration of live bacteria such as nonpathogenic *Escherichia coli*, bifidobacteria, lactobacilli, or *Streptococcus thermophilus*. Probiotic formulations have been effective in maintaining remission in ulcerative colitis.[41–43]

SURGERY

Surgical procedures have an established place in the treatment of IBD. Although surgery (proctocolectomy) is curative for ulcerative colitis, this is not the case for Crohn's disease. Surgical procedures involve resection of segments of intestine that are affected, as well as correction of complications (e.g., fistulas) or drainage of abscesses.

For ulcerative colitis, colectomy may be necessary when the patient has disease uncontrolled by maximum medical therapy or when there are complications of the disease such as colonic perforation, toxic dilatation (megacolon), uncontrolled colonic hemorrhage, or colonic strictures. Colectomy may be indicated in patients with long-standing disease (greater than 8 to 10 years), as a prophylactic measure against the development of cancer, and in patients with premalignant changes (severe dysplasia) on surveillance mucosal biopsies. The most common surgical procedures include proctocolectomy, after which the patient is left with a permanent ileostomy, and abdominal colectomy, with removal of the mucosa of the rectum and anastomosis of an ileal pouch to the anus (ileoanal pull-through). The risk from surgery in these patients is relatively low if the operations are performed on a nonemergent basis.

The indications for surgery with Crohn's disease are not as well established as for ulcerative colitis, and surgery is usually reserved for the complications of the disease. A recognized problem with intestinal resection for Crohn's disease is the high recurrence rate. Surgery may be appropriate in well-selected patients who have severe or incapacitating disease or obstruction in spite of aggressive medical management. The surgical procedures performed include resections of the major intestinal areas of involvement. In some patients with severe rectal or perineal disease, diversion of the fecal stream is performed with a colostomy. Other indications for surgery include the finding of colon cancer, an inflammatory mass, or intestinal perforations.

PHARMACOLOGIC THERAPY

Drug therapy plays an integral part in the overall treatment of IBD. None of the drugs used for IBD is curative; at best they serve to control the disease process. Therefore a reasonable goal of drug therapy is resolution of disease symptoms such that the patient can carry on normal daily functions. The major types of drug therapy used in IBD include aminosalicylates, corticosteroids, immunosuppressive agents (azathioprine, mercaptopurine, cyclosporine, and methotrexate), antimicrobials (metronidazole and ciprofloxacin), and agents to inhibit TNF-α (anti-TNF-α antibodies).

Sulfasalazine, an agent that combines a sulfonamide (sulfapyridine) antibiotic and mesalamine (5-aminosalicylic acid) in the same molecule, has been used for many years to treat IBD but was originally intended to treat arthritis. Sulfasalazine is cleaved by gut bacteria in the colon to sulfapyridine (which is mostly absorbed and excreted in the urine) and mesalamine (which mostly remains in the colon and is excreted in stool).[44]

The active component of sulfasalazine is mesalamine.[44] The mechanism of action of mesalamine is not well understood. Cyclooxygenase or lipoxygenase inhibition alone do not account for the agent's effects. Aminosalicylates may block production of prostaglandins and leukotrienes, inhibit bacterial peptide-induced neutrophil chemotaxis and adenosine-induced secretion, scavenge reactive oxygen metabolites, and inhibit activation of the nuclear regulatory factor NF-κB.[12]

Because the mechanism of action of sulfasalazine is not related to the sulfapyridine component, and since sulfapyridine is believed to be responsible for many of the adverse reactions to sulfasalazine, mesalamine alone can be used. Mesalamine can be used topically as an enema for the treatment of proctitis, or given orally in slow-release formulations that deliver mesalamine to the small intestine and colon (Table 34–5 and Fig. 34–1). Slow-release oral formulations of mesalamine such as Pentasa release mesalamine from the duodenum to the ileum, with about 75% of the drug passing into the colon.[45] Olsalazine is a dimer of two 5-aminosalicylate molecules linked by an azo bond. Mesalamine is released in the colon after colonic bacteria cleave olsalazine. Balsalazide is a mesalamine prodrug that is enzymatically cleaved in the colon to produce mesalamine. The recommended daily doses of the oral mesalamine derivatives are intended to approximate the molar equivalent of mesalamine present in 4 g of sulfasalazine. At present, sulfasalazine is used in preference to oral mesalamine derivatives, mainly because it costs much less. However, it is not tolerated as well as the mesalamine alternatives. Because the oral mesalamine formulations are coated tablets or granules, they should not be crushed or chewed.

Corticosteroids and adrenocorticotropic hormone have been widely used for the treatment of ulcerative colitis and Crohn's disease, given parenterally, orally, or rectally. Corticosteroids are believed to modulate the immune system and inhibit production of cytokines and mediators. It is not clear whether the most important steroid effects are systemic or local (mucosal). Budesonide is a corticosteroid that is administered orally in a controlled-release formulation. The drug undergoes extensive first-pass metabolism, so systemic exposure is thought to be minimized. Immunosuppressive agents such as azathioprine, mercaptopurine (a metabolite of azathioprine), methotrexate, or cyclosporine are sometimes used for the treatment of IBD.[46]

TABLE 34–5. Mesalamine Derivatives for Treatment of Inflammatory Bowel Disease

Product	Trade Name(s)	Formulation	Dose/Day	Site of Action
Sulfasalazine	Azulfidine	Tablet	4–6 g	Colon
Mesalamine	Rowasa, Salofalk, Claversal, Pentasa	Enema	1–4 g	Rectum, terminal colon
	Asacol	Mesalamine tablet coated with Eudragit-S (delayed-release acrylic resin)	2.4–4.8 g	Distal ileum and colon
	Pentasa	Mesalamine capsules encapsulated in ethylcellulose microgranules	2–4 g	Small bowel and colon
Olsalazine	Dipentum	Dimer of 5-aminosalicylic acid oral capsule	1.5–3 g	Colon
Balsalazide	Colazal	Capsule	6.75 g	Colon

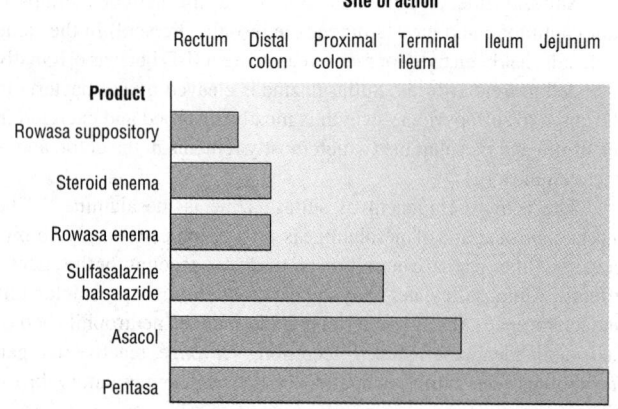

Site of action

Product	Rectum	Distal colon	Proximal colon	Terminal ileum	Ileum	Jejunum
Rowasa suppository						
Steroid enema						
Rowasa enema						
Sulfasalazine balsalazide						
Asacol						
Pentasa						

FIGURE 34–1. Site of activity of various agents used to treat inflammatory bowel disease.

Azathioprine and mercaptopurine are effective for long-term treatment of Crohn's disease and ulcerative colitis.[47] These agents are generally reserved for patients who are refractory to steroids, and they may be associated with serious adverse effects such as lymphomas, pancreatitis, or nephrotoxicity. They are usually used in conjunction with mesalamine derivatives and/or steroids, and must be used for long periods of time (from a few weeks up to 6 months) before benefits may be observed.[48] Remission can be prolonged by azathioprine in steroid-dependent patients with ulcerative colitis.[49] Cyclosporine

has also been of short-term benefit in treatment of acute, severe ulcerative colitis when used in a continuous intravenous infusion. Oral doses are ineffective. The agent poses a risk of nephrotoxicity and neurotoxicity. Methotrexate given 15 to 25 mg intramuscularly once weekly is useful for treatment and maintenance of Crohn's disease but not ulcerative colitis.

Antimicrobial agents, particularly metronidazole, are frequently used in attempts to control Crohn's disease but are not useful in ulcerative colitis. Metronidazole is of value in some patients with active Crohn's disease, particularly involving the perineal area or fistulas.[50] The mechanism of metronidazole's effect on Crohn's disease has not been determined but is theorized to relate to interruption of a bacterial role in the inflammatory process. Ciprofloxacin has also been used for treatment of IBD.

Infliximab is an IgG$_1$ chimeric monoclonal antibody that binds TNF-α and inhibits its inflammatory effect in the gut. The agent is useful for steroid-dependent or fistulizing disease, but the cost far exceeds that of other regimens.

ULCERATIVE COLITIS

Mild to Moderate Disease

Most patients with active ulcerative colitis have mild to moderate disease and do not require parenteral medications (Fig. 34–2). The first line of drug therapy for these patients is oral sulfasalazine or an oral mesalamine derivative, or topical mesalamine or steroids for distal

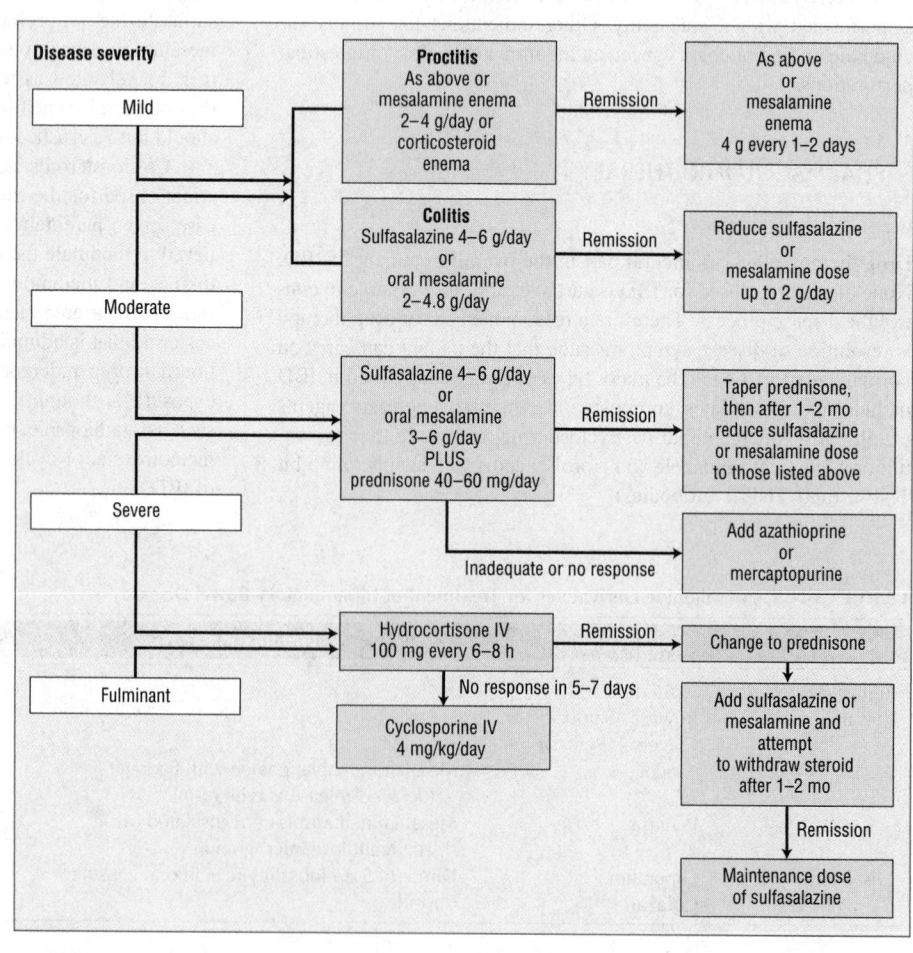

FIGURE 34–2. Treatment approaches for ulcerative colitis.

disease.[51] When given orally, usually 4 g/day, and up to 8 g/day, of sulfasalazine is required to attain control of active inflammation. There does not appear to be an increased rate of response with increased dosage over 4 g/day, although side effects increase. Even with the use of adequate doses, patient improvement usually takes 2 to 3 weeks, and sometimes longer. The dosage of sulfasalazine that can be given is usually limited by the patient's tolerance of the agent; most adverse effects of sulfasalazine are dose related (GI disturbances, headache, and arthralgia).[48] Sulfasalazine therapy should be instituted at 500 mg/day and increased every few days up to 4 g/day or the maximum tolerated. It should not be used in patients with allergy to sulfa drugs.

Oral mesalamine derivatives (such as those listed in Table 34–5) are reasonable alternatives to sulfasalazine for treatment of ulcerative colitis. These agents are clearly more effective than placebo but no more effective than sulfasalalzine. However, mesalamine preparations are better tolerated.[52] For many patients the dose of mesalamine can be increased without an increase in adverse effects. The majority of patients intolerant to sulfasalazine should tolerate one of the other oral mesalamine derivatives. While the dosage range for Pentasa is 2 to 4 g/day, 4 g/day appears to be more effective.[53] Olsalazine (a dimer of 5-aminosalicylic acid that is given orally) is effective for treatment of mild to moderate ulcerative colitis. However, of patients taking olsalazine, 15% to 25% experience severe diarrhea, often necessitating discontinuation of the drug. This results from a direct osmotic effect of the drug to induce small bowel fluid secretion. For this reason it is not the drug of first choice. Balsalazide is another mesalamine derivative that is effective for treatment of mild to moderate ulcerative colitis.[54] For patients with distal disease, combination therapy of oral mesalamine derivatives and topical (enema) mesalamine therapy may be beneficial for induction of remission as well as for maintenance.[12,55]

Steroids have a place in the treatment of moderate to severe ulcerative colitis that is unresponsive to maximal doses of oral and topical mesalamine derivatives. Oral steroids (usually up to 1 mg/kg per day of prednisone equivalent) may be used for patients who do not have an adequate response to sulfasalazine or mesalamine. Overall, steroids and sulfasalazine appear to be equally efficacious; however, the response to steroids may be evident sooner. Oral steroids should not be used as initial therapy for mild to moderate ulcerative colitis, mainly because of the known risks of steroid use. If steroids are used to attain remission, tapered drug withdrawal should be accomplished to minimize long-term steroid exposure.

Rectally administered steroids or mesalamine can be used as initial therapy for patients with ulcerative proctitis or distal colitis. Rectal agents are also beneficial for treatment of tenesmus. With these agents, local actions are believed to be responsible for drug effects. Rectal steroids are effective in the treatment of active, distal ulcerative colitis. However, rectal mesalamine is more effective than rectal steroids for inducing remission.[56,57]

CLINICAL CONTROVERSY

The choice of rectally administered steroid is a subject of debate, as there is varying potential for systemic steroid absorption with different products. Although many steroids have been administered rectally, certain agents such as betamethasone-17-valerate, beclomethasone dipropionate, prednisolone metasulfobenzoate, prednisolone-21-phosphate, and budesonide have been used in attempts to reduce systemic steroid effects. Systemic side effects may be the least severe with beclomethasone dipropionate, because

the gut wall and liver rapidly metabolize this agent.[56] Most patients do not experience adrenal suppression from rectal steroids. The use of rectal steroids may often result in reduction of the required oral dose.

Nicotine has been proposed as a treatment for ulcerative colitis (but not as a treatment for Crohn's disease) based on the observation of the onset of a flare of ulcerative colitis after smoking cessation in some individuals. When used in the highest tolerated dose, transdermal nicotine improved symptoms of patients with mild to moderate active ulcerative colitis.[58]

Severe or Intractable Disease

Patients with uncontrolled severe colitis or who have incapacitating symptoms require hospitalization for effective management. Under these conditions, patients generally receive nothing by mouth to put the bowel at rest. Most medication is given by the parenteral route. With severe colitis, there is a much greater reliance on parenteral steroids (intravenous hydrocortisone) and surgical procedures. Sulfasalazine or mesalamine derivatives are not beneficial for treatment of severe colitis because of rapid elimination of these agents from the colon with diarrhea, thereby not allowing sufficient time for gut bacteria to cleave the molecules. Overall it is difficult to evaluate drugs in this setting, because patients with severe disease almost always receive additional medications including steroids.

Steroids have been valuable in the treatment of severe disease because the use of these agents may allow some patients to avoid colectomy. A trial of steroids is warranted in most patients before proceeding to colectomy, unless the condition is grave or rapidly deteriorating. The dose of steroid generally used is 1 mg/kg of prednisone equivalent daily (up to 60 mg/day), although some patients may require much less or much more for satisfactory control. With higher doses, however, steroid side effects may limit drug benefits. The length of the medical trial before consideration of surgery is open to debate. Steroids increase surgical risk, particularly infectious risk, if an operation is required later. After a colectomy is performed, steroids should no longer be required for the disease; however, they must be withdrawn gradually (usually over 3 to 4 weeks) to avoid hypoadrenal crisis due to adrenal suppression.

Patients who are unresponsive to parenteral corticosteroids after 7 to 10 days should receive cyclosporine by intravenous infusion. Most hospitalized patients who are unresponsive to corticosteroids will respond to cyclosporine.[59–61] Continuous intravenous infusion of cyclosporine (4 mg/kg per day) was rapidly effective in steroid-resistant acute severe ulcerative colitis and reduced the need for emergent colectomy.[62] Intravenous cyclosporine has been recommended as an alternative to steroids in patients with severe attacks of ulcerative colitis (fulminant colitis).[63] Patients who are controlled on intravenous cyclosporine can then be switched to an oral cyclosporine taper regimen.

Maintenance of Remission

After remission from active disease is achieved, the goal of therapy is to maintain remission. The major agents used for maintenance of remission are sulfasalazine and the mesalamine derivatives; steroids do not have a role. The value of sulfasalazine in preventing recurrences has been documented in placebo-controlled trials.

One-fourth of patients taking sulfasalazine (2 g/day) had a relapse within 1 year, while three-fourths of patients taking placebo had a relapse.[64]

Mesalamine preparations and olsalazine are effective for maintaining remission. A meta-analysis of trials concluded that mesalalmine was more effective than placebo, but not as effective as sulfasalazine for maintaining remission.[65]

CLINICAL CONTROVERSY

A major question about the use of sulfasalazine for maintenance of remission with ulcerative colitis is the duration of the preventive regimen. Maintenance of remission has been well documented up to 1 year and may last as long as 3 years. The efficacy of sulfasalazine appears to be related to the dose administered, up to a point. Although 4 g/day has a lower recurrence rate than 2 g or 1 g, a 4-g dose will result in intolerable side effects in about one-fourth of patients. Therefore 2 g/day is recommended.

Steroids do not have a role in the maintenance of remission with ulcerative colitis because they are ineffective.[48] Steroids should be gradually withdrawn after remission is induced (over 3 to 4 weeks). If they are continued, the patient will be exposed to steroid side effects without likelihood of benefits. For patients who require chronic steroid use (>20 mg/day), there is a strong justification for alternative therapies or colectomy. Azathioprine is effective in preventing relapse of ulcerative colitis for periods of up to 2 years.[66] However, 3 to 6 months may be required before beneficial effects are noted. Oral azathioprine also maintains long-term remission after IV cyclosporine induction.[67]

CROHN'S DISEASE

Management of Crohn's disease often proves more difficult than management of ulcerative colitis, partly because of the greater complexity of presentation with Crohn's disease (Fig. 34–3). The disease may involve any segment of the GI tract, from mouth to anus, and may involve other visceral structures and soft tissues through fistulization. There is a greater reliance on drug therapy with Crohn's disease, because resection of all involved intestine may not be possible and disease recurrence after surgery is common.

Active Crohn's Disease

The goal of treatment for active Crohn's disease is to achieve remission; however, in many patients, reduction of symptoms so the patient may carry out normal activities, or reduction of the steroid dose required for control, is a significant accomplishment. In the majority of patients, active Crohn's disease is treated with sulfasalazine, mesalamine derivatives, or steroids, although azathioprine, mercaptopurine, methotrexate, or metronidazole are frequently used.

The role of sulfasalazine in the treatment of active Crohn's disease is not as well established as its role in the treatment of ulcerative colitis. Sulfasalazine is more effective when Crohn's disease involves the colon.[36] In these circumstances, sulfasalazine is as effective as prednisone.[36,68] A trial of sulfasalazine or an oral mesalamine derivative should be initiated in patients with mild to moderate Crohn's disease, particularly when the colon is involved.

Mesalamine products such as Pentasa or Asacol, that release mesalamine in the small bowel, are more effective than sulfasalazine for ileal involvement. In a trial of 310 patients with active Crohn's disease, Pentasa alone was more effective than placebo in achieving remission in a 16-week trial (43% vs. 18%, respectively).[69] This beneficial effect was dose dependent and greatest with a dose of 4 g/day. A course of steroids is appropriate in patients who cannot be controlled with mesalamine. However, when a patient is maintained on steroids, there appears to be no benefit from the addition of sulfasalazine.

Steroids are frequently used for the treatment of active Crohn's disease, particularly with more severe presentations. In the National Cooperative Crohn's Disease Study,[36] prednisone was more effective than placebo in achieving remission (60% remission rate after 17 weeks vs. a 30% remission rate for placebo). In this trial, the prednisone doses were 0.25 mg/kg per day for mild disease,

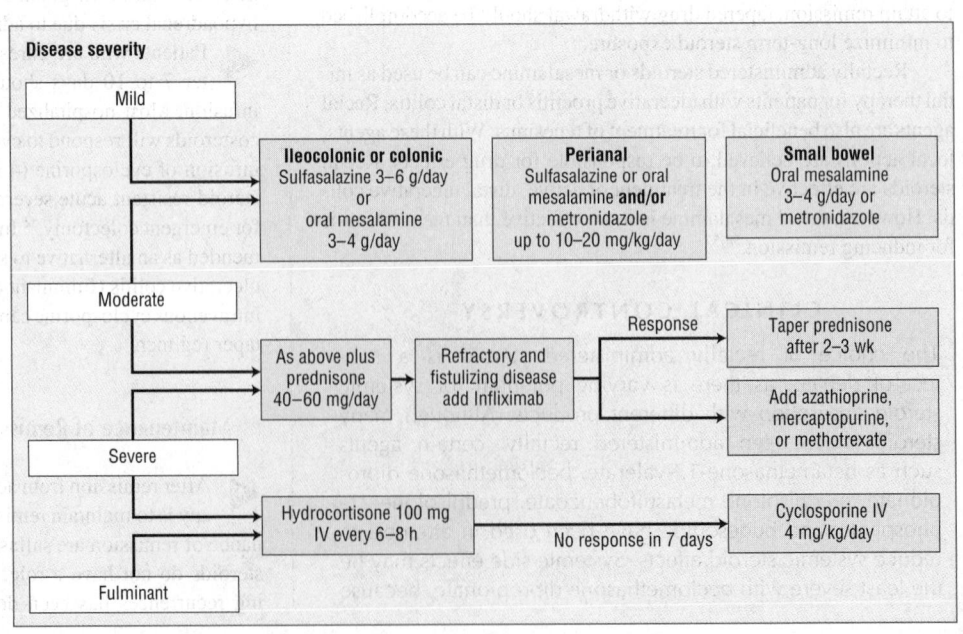

FIGURE 34–3. Treatment approaches for Crohn's disease.

0.5 mg/kg per day for moderate disease, and 0.75 mg/kg per day for severe disease. Prednisone was effective for disease limited to the small bowel. The major limitation of steroids is the risk of adverse effects with long-term use.

Steroids are preferred for treatment of severe Crohn's disease, mainly because these agents can be given parenterally and response to therapy may occur sooner than with other agents. However, once remission is achieved, it is difficult to reduce the steroid dosage without a flare of active disease.

Metronidazole (given orally up to 20 mg/kg per day in divided doses) may be useful in some patients with Crohn's disease, particularly in patients with colonic involvement, or in those patients with perineal disease.[50] For most patients, metronidazole would be added to a mesalamine product, or steroid therapy when those agents alone are not effective. The role for metronidazole is not fully defined. It may deserve a trial as adjunctive therapy for patients with colonic or perineal disease, where satisfactory control of Crohn's disease is not gained with first-line agents, or in attempts to reduce steroid dosage.[70] Ciprofloxacin has gained attention as an alternative to metronidazole and appears to be effective.[71]

The immunosuppressive agents (azathioprine and mercaptopurine) are generally limited to use in patients not achieving adequate response to standard medical therapy, or to reduce steroid doses when high steroid doses are required. Azathioprine and mercaptopurine demonstrated long-term benefits in patients with Crohn's disease.[47] The usual doses of azathioprine are 2 to 2.5 mg/kg per day, and for mercaptopurine 1 to 1.5 mg/kg per day. They are begun at 50 mg/day and increased at 2-week intervals while monitoring white blood cell and platelet counts. Treatment with azathioprine may need to be continued for up to 6 months to observe a response.[48] In one trial of patients already receiving sulfasalazine or prednisone, mercaptopurine decreased steroid requirement and healed fistulas. One problem noted with mercaptopurine was that more than 3 months was required to observe a response in 32% of patients. In a report of 20 years of experience with 148 patients, mercaptopurine (50 mg/day, mean 34 months) was judged effective for reduction of steroid dosage or elimination of the need for steroids, healing of fistulas and abscesses, and healing of Crohn's disease of the stomach and duodenum.[72] Some investigators have suggested that azathioprine or mercaptopurine should be started earlier in the course of treatment than has been traditional.

Clinical response to mercaptopurine is related to whole-blood concentrations of the metabolite 6-thioguanine, and hepatotoxicity is correlated with another metabolite, 6-methylmercaptopurine.[73] Metabolic inactivation of azathioprine and mercaptopurine occurs by thiopurine S-methyltransferase, which exhibits genetic polymorphism. Enzyme-deficient patients are at greater risk of bone marrow suppression from these agents.[74,75] Determination of enzyme activity may be necessary to determine which patients require lower doses of these agents.

Cyclosporine is not recommended for treatment of Crohn's disease except for patients with symptomatic and severe perianal or cutaneous fistulas.[12] Approximately 80% of patients with refractory fistulas responded to intravenous cyclosporine (4 mg/kg per day) within a mean of 7.9 days.[76] The dose of cyclosporine is important in determining efficacy. An oral dose of 5 mg/kg per day was ineffective,[77] whereas 7.9 mg/kg per day was effective.[78] However, toxic effects limit application of the higher dosage. At present, the therapeutic blood or plasma concentration range for cyclosporine has not been established for Crohn's disease, but whole-blood trough concentrations of 200 to 800 ng/mL (by monoclonal radioimmunoassay) or 200 to 400 ng/mL (by high-performance liquid chromatography) have been recommended.[3] When using cyclosporine, however, clinicians should

recognize the accompanying long-term risk of renal toxicity as well as the potential for drug interactions.

Methotrexate given as a weekly injection of 5 to 25 mg has demonstrated efficacy for induction of remission in Crohn's disease as well as for maintenance therapy.[79,80] It is also useful for corticosteroid-sparing effects.[81,82] While there are risks of bone marrow suppression, hepatotoxicity, and pulmonary toxicity, low-dose methotrexate appears relatively safe.[79]

Infliximab is approved for treating refractory or fistulizing Crohn's disease. A 5 mg/kg single infusion of infliximab resulted in clinical improvement in 80% of patients with chronic Crohn's disease who were receiving steroids.[83] The benefit lasted 8 to 12 weeks with reinfusion producing a sustained response. Infliximab also significantly reduced fistula drainage. Additional studies have demonstrated the effectiveness of long-term use (10 mg/kg every 8 weeks for 32 weeks).[84] Patients who receive infliximab often develop antibodies to infliximab, which can result in infusion reactions and loss of response to the drug. Administration of a second dose within 8 weeks of the first dose and concurrent administration of hydrocortisone (200 mg intravenously) significantly reduced antibody formation.[85,86] Smoking reduces the response to infliximab, both the percentage of patients responding (73% in nonsmokers and 22% in smokers) and the duration of response.[87]

Maintenance of Remission

Prevention of recurrence of disease is clearly more difficult with Crohn's disease than with ulcerative colitis. There is evidence that some agents, particularly sulfasalazine and oral mesalamine derivatives, are effective in preventing acute recurrences in quiescent Crohn's disease.[88] The support for sulfasalazine has been largely anecdotal;[88] however, a trial of 232 patients demonstrated a lower relapse rate compared with placebo for up to 2 years when given 3 g/day.[89]

There is support for the use of oral mesalamine derivatives for maintenance of symptomatic remission. On average, oral mesalamine derivatives decrease recurrence rates by 40% as compared to placebo in long-term studies.[77] In one trial of 161 patients in remission, 2 g/day of mesalamine (Pentasa) for 2 years resulted in a significantly reduced relapse rate when begun within 3 months of achieving remission.[90] In another trial of mesalamine (Asacol), 125 patients received 2.4 g/day or placebo for 12 months, resulting in a significantly reduced relapse rate with Asacol.[91] Steroids also have no place in the prevention of recurrence of Crohn's disease; these agents do not appear to alter the long-term course of the disease. However, a study of oral budesonide 6 mg/day demonstrated prolongation of time to relapse in ileal and ileocecal disease.[92]

Azathioprine, mercaptopurine, and methotrexate are useful in some patients to maintain remission. Although the published data are inconsistent, there is evidence to suggest that azathioprine and mercaptopurine are effective in maintaining remission in Crohn's disease and are documented to increase quality-adjusted life expectancy.[48,49,93] Low-dose methotrexate (15 mg intramuscularly once weekly) is also effective in maintaining remission.[94] These agents should be reserved for patients who cannot tolerate the dosages of steroids required to control their disease and who are not good surgical candidates.

Infliximab infusion given every 8 weeks is more effective than placebo in maintaining remission in patients who initially respond to infliximab for active Crohn's disease. It can be administered 5 or 20 mg/kg every 8 weeks.[95]

SELECTED COMPLICATIONS

TOXIC MEGACOLON

The treatment required for toxic megacolon includes general supportive measures to maintain vital functions, consideration for early surgical intervention, and drugs (steroids, cyclosporine, and antimicrobials). Aggressive fluid and electrolyte management is required for dehydration. Fluids and electrolytes may be lost through vomiting, diarrhea, and nasogastric intubation, as well as through fluid accumulation in the bowel. When the patient has lost significant amounts of blood (through the rectum), blood replacement is also necessary. Opiates and anticholinergics should be discontinued because these agents enhance colonic dilatation, thereby increasing the risk of bowel perforation. Broad-spectrum antimicrobials that include coverage for gram-negative bacilli and intestinal anaerobes should be used.

Steroids in high dosages should be administered intravenously to reduce acute inflammation. Doses as high as 2 mg/kg per day of prednisone equivalent have been recommended (generally administered as hydrocortisone).[6] The duration of steroid administration is not certain; however, most clinicians continue the high-dose steroids for up to 2 weeks after improvement is observed, and then reduce the dosage (approximately 0.5 to 1 mg/kg per day) for a few additional weeks. Antimicrobial regimens that are effective against enteric aerobes and anaerobes (e.g., an aminoglycoside with clindamycin or metronidazole, imipenem, or an extended-spectrum penicillin with β-lactamase inhibitor) should be administered from the time of diagnosis and continued until patient improvement is assured. The duration of the antimicrobial regimen (often 2 to 3 weeks) should be determined with consideration that there may be significant intra-abdominal contamination with signs and symptoms hidden by steroid effects.

Emergent surgical intervention, mainly an abdominal colectomy with formation of an ileostomy, is an important consideration in patients with toxic megacolon and prevents death in some patients. In most cases in which colectomy is performed in the face of toxic megacolon, there is a significant risk of operative complications, including postoperative infection.

SYSTEMIC MANIFESTATIONS

The common systemic manifestations of IBD include arthritis, anemia, skin manifestations such as erythema nodosum and pyoderma gangrenosum, uveitis, and liver disease. These problems may be related to the inflammatory process. For some of these manifestations specific therapies can be instituted, whereas for others the treatment that is used for the GI inflammatory process also addresses the systemic manifestations.

Anemia occurs when there is significant blood loss from the GI tract. If the patient can consume oral medication, ferrous sulfate should be administered. If the patient is unable to take oral medication and the patient's hematocrit is sufficiently low, blood transfusions or intravenous iron infusions may be required. Anemia may also be related to malabsorption of vitamin B_{12} or folic acid, so these may also be required.

There are no consistently recommended therapies for liver disease, skin manifestations, or uveitis associated with IBD. Some reports suggest that these manifestations are worse during exacerbations of the intestinal disease and that measures improving intestinal disease will improve these systemic manifestations. Unfortunately, this association has not been demonstrated consistently. Liver transplantation is being used more frequently for definitive treatment of primary sclerosing cholangitis. For arthritis associated with IBD, aspirin or another NSAID may be beneficial, as might be steroids.

SPECIAL CONSIDERATIONS

PREGNANCY

Either the occurrence or consideration of pregnancy may cause significant concerns in the patient with IBD. Patients with IBD do not appear to be less fertile than women in general.[6,96] The rate of normal childbirth is similar to that for healthy populations. Some studies have noted a greater risk of spontaneous abortions in patients with IBD. Also, there is a greater incidence of low birth weight infants in mothers with chronic idiopathic ulcerative colitis.[97] Pregnancy does not affect the course of IBD. Patients who are pregnant experience recurrence rates similar to those of nonpregnant females. Also, there is no justification for therapeutic abortion with IBD because termination of the pregnancy has not been observed to improve the disease. There is also unfounded concern that the drugs required to treat IBD may be teratogenic.

Steroids and sulfasalazine should be administered during pregnancy with the same guidelines that would be applied to the nonpregnant patient.[6,97] Steroids given systemically do not appear to be detrimental to the fetus. Sulfasalazine is generally well tolerated; however, there has been suggestion of increased frequency of congenital abnormalities when it is given during pregnancy.[98] Interestingly, sulfasalazine has also been reported to cause decreased sperm counts and reduced fertility in males.[99] This effect is reversible on discontinuation of the drug, and it is not reported with mesalamine. Immunosuppressive drugs (azathioprine and mercaptopurine) may be associated with fetal deformities in humans; however, they have been used without detriment in some patients.[96] Metronidazole should not be used in those contemplating pregnancy, as it may be teratogenic.

Overall, drug therapy for IBD is not a contraindication for pregnancy, and most pregnancies are well managed in patients with these diseases. The indications for medical and surgical treatment are similar to those in the nonpregnant patient. If a patient has an initial bout of IBD during pregnancy, a standard approach to treatment should be initiated.

Recommendations for the use of drugs in nursing mothers vary. Although prednisone and prednisolone can be detected in breast milk, breast-feeding is believed to be safe for the infant when low doses of prednisone are used.[100] Sulfasalazine does not pose a risk of kernicterus, as levels of sulfapyridine in breast milk are low or undetectable. Metronidazole should not be given to nursing mothers because it is excreted into breast milk.[100]

ADVERSE DRUG EFFECTS

Drug intolerance often limits the usefulness of agents used to treat IBD. Many patients receiving sulfasalazine, mesalamine, corticosteroids, metronidazole, azathioprine, mercaptopurine, or infliximab experience some undesired effects. In some cases, these adverse effects can be significant and require discontinuation of the therapy. Knowledge of the common or important adverse reactions will assist in avoiding or minimizing their effects.

Sulfasalazine is often associated with adverse drug effects and these effects may be classified as either dose related or idiosyncratic. Dose-related side effects usually include GI disturbances such as nausea, vomiting, diarrhea, or anorexia, but may also include headache and arthralgia. These adverse reactions tend to occur more commonly on initiation of therapy and decrease in frequency as therapy is continued. Patients may experience these adverse effects at the commonly used dosages. One approach to the management of these reactions is to discontinue the agent for a short period and then reinstitute therapy at a reduced dosage. The sulfapyridine portion of the sulfasalazine molecule is believed to be responsible for much of the sulfasalazine toxicity.[101] Folic acid absorption is impaired by sulfasalazine, which may lead to anemia. Patients receiving sulfasalazine should receive oral folic acid supplementation.

Adverse effects that are not dose related most commonly include rash, fever, or hepatotoxicity, as well as relatively uncommon but serious reactions such as bone marrow suppression, thrombocytopenia, pancreatitis, and hepatitis. For most patients with idiosyncratic reactions, sulfasalazine must be discontinued. In some patients who have experienced allergic reactions to sulfasalazine, a desensitization procedure can be instituted. By gradually increasing sulfasalazine dosage over weeks to months, patient tolerance has been improved.[102] Most of the idiosyncratic reactions observed with sulfasalazine are similar to those with the class of sulfonamides in general.

Oral mesalamine derivatives may impose a lower frequency of adverse effects as compared to sulfasalazine.[52] Up to 80% to 90% of patients who are intolerant to sulfasalazine will tolerate oral mesalamine derivatives.[101] Olsalazine, however, may frequently (in as many as 25% of patients) cause watery diarrhea, sometimes requiring drug discontinuation.[103]

Adverse reactions to corticosteroids are well recognized and may occur when corticosteroids are used for any indication. However, there is a greater potential for adverse effects when corticosteroids are used for the treatment of IBD because high doses must often be used for extended periods. In the National Cooperative Crohn's Disease Study, half of patients receiving high-dose steroid therapy experienced side effects, as did one-third of the patients on the lower-dose regimens for maintenance.[36] The well-appreciated adverse effects of corticosteroids include hyperglycemia, hypertension, osteoporosis, acne, fluid retention, electrolyte disturbances, myopathies, muscle wasting, increased appetite, psychosis, and reduced resistance to infection. In addition, corticosteroid use may cause adrenocortical suppression. To minimize corticosteroid effects, clinicians have used alternate-day steroid therapy; however, some patients do not do well on the days when no steroid is given. For most patients a single daily corticosteroid dose suffices, and divided daily doses are unnecessary. Another problem with corticosteroids is adrenal insufficiency after abrupt steroid withdrawal. Patients sometimes discontinue prescribed medications when they feel better.

Immunosuppressants such as azathioprine and mercaptopurine have a significant potential for adverse reactions. Azathioprine causes bone marrow suppression and has been associated with lymphomas (in renal transplant patients), skin cancer, and pancreatitis (about 3% of patients). Some investigators believe that induction of leukopenia may be necessary for therapeutic effect.[104,105] Mercaptopurine causes adverse reactions similarly to azathioprine; however, there are fewer reports of lymphomas with this agent. In one cohort of IBD patients, adverse effects from mercaptopurine were as follows: pancreatitis, 1.2%; allergic reactions, 3.9%, significant leukopenia, 11.5%; and infectious complications, 14%.[106] Ten percent of patients who received azathioprine or mercaptopurine required discontinuation of treatment because of adverse effects.[107] Allopurinol inhibits the metabolism of mercaptopurine, and a dosage reduction of the latter is required when the two are used in combination.

Myelosuppression resulting in leukopenia from azathioprine and mercaptopurine is related to a deficiency of thiopurine S-

methyltransferase (TPMT) due to excessive accumulation of toxic metabolites.[108] Approximately 0.1% of people are homozygous for a nonfunctional TPMT gene, which causes TPMT deficiency. These patients have a much greater risk of toxicity, and should not receive either drug. Heterozygous patients have an increased risk of toxicity and may receive either drug with careful monitoring of white blood cell counts.

Most patients receiving metronidazole for Crohn's disease tolerate the agent fairly well; however, mild adverse effects occur frequently. They commonly include paresthesias and reversible peripheral neuropathy, metallic taste, urticaria, and glossitis.[51] Other effects include a disulfiram-like reaction if alcohol is ingested in conjunction.

Infliximab has been related to adverse effects such as infusion reactions, serum sickness, sepsis, and reactivation of tuberculosis. Infusion reactions and serum sickness relate to the immune response to foreign protein. Patients often develop anti-infliximab antibodies with multiple infusions. Serum sickness has occurred in patients who received infliximab doses separated by a long period of time. Sepsis and tuberculosis may occur because of the inhibition of TNF-protective mechanisms.

EVALUATION OF THERAPEUTIC OUTCOMES

The success of therapeutic regimens to treat IBD can be measured by patient-reported complaints, signs, and symptoms; by direct physician examination (including endoscopy); by history and physical examination; by selected laboratory tests; and by quality-of-life measures. Evaluation of IBD severity is difficult because much of the assessment is subjective. To create more objective measures, disease rating scales or indices have been created. The Crohn's Disease Activity Index is a commonly used scale, particularly for evaluation of patients during clinical trials.[109] The scale incorporates eight elements: (1) number of stools in the past 7 days; (2) sum of abdominal pain ratings from the past 7 days; (3) rating of general well-being in the past 7 days; (4) use of antidiarrheals; (5) body weight; (6) hematocrit; (7) finding of abdominal mass; and (8) a sum of symptoms present in the past week. Elements of this index provide a guide for those measures that may be useful in assessing the effectiveness of treatment regimens.

Standardized assessment tools have also been constructed for ulcerative colitis.[110] Elements in these scales include (1) stool frequency; (2) presence of blood in the stool; (3) mucosal appearance (from endoscopy); and (4) physician's global assessment based on physical examination, endoscopy, and laboratory data.

Additional studies that are often useful include direct endoscopic examination of affected areas and/or radiocontrast studies. For patients with acute disease, assessment of fluid and electrolyte status is important, because these may be lost during diarrheal episodes. Other laboratory tests, such as serum albumin, transferrin, or other markers of visceral protein status, as well as markers of inflammation (erythrocyte sedimentation rate) may be used.

Assessment of the IBD patient must include consideration of adverse drug effects. Because many of the agents used have a relatively high probability of causing adverse effects, particularly corticosteroids and other immunosuppressive agents, patient assessment should include collection of history and physical and laboratory data that are necessary to prevent or recognize adverse drug effects.

Finally, a patient quality-of-life assessment should be performed regularly.[111] Agents that appear clinically equivalent may differ substantially in resulting quality of life. Inquiry should be made regarding general well-being, emotional function, and social function. Social function may include assessment of the ability to perform routine daily functions, maintain occupational activities, sexual function, and recreation.

Quality-of-life studies have been conducted with infliximab. To balance the exceptionally high cost of this therapy, Crohn's disease patients who receive infliximab have improved quality of life, fewer emergency room visits, a reduced requirement for surgery, and are more likely to be employed.[112,113]

ABBREVIATIONS

ESR: erythrocyte sedimentation rate
IBD: inflammatory bowel disease
NSAID: nonsteroidal anti-inflammatory drug
TPMT: thiopurine S-methyltransferase
TNF-α: tumor necrosis factor-alpha

Review Questions and other resources can be found at *www.pharmacotherapyonline.com.*

REFERENCES

1. Kraft SC. Modern clinical aspects of inflammatory bowel disease. Radiol Clin North Am 1987;25:213–224.
2. Feldman M: Sleisenger and Fordtran's Gastrointestinal and Liver Disease, 7th ed. Elsevier, New York, 2002.
3. Andres PG, Friedman LS. Inflammatory bowel disease. Epidemiology and the natural causes of inflammatory bowel disease. Gastroenterol Clinics 1999;28:255–281.
4. Sandler RS. Epidemiology of inflammatory bowel disease. In: Targan SR, Shanahan F, eds. Inflammatory Bowel Disease: From Bench to Bedside. Baltimore, Williams & Wilkins, 1994:5–30.
5. Whelan G. Epidemiology of inflammatory bowel disease. Med Clin North Am 1990;74:1–12.
6. Jewell DP. Ulcerative colitis. In: Feldman M, Scharcchmidt BF, Sleisenger MH, Klein S, eds. Sleisenger & Fordtran's Gastrointestinal and Liver Disease, 6th ed. Orlando, FL, Saunders, 1998:1735–1761.
7. Russel MG, Stockbtugger RW. Epidemiology of inflammatory bowel disease. Scand J Gastroenterol 1996;31:417–427.
8. Pavli P, Cavanaugh J, Grimm M. Inflammatory bowel disease: Germs or genes? Lancet 1996;347:1198.
9. Kagnoff MF. Immunology and inflammation of the gastrointestinal tract. In: Feldman M, Scharcchmidt BF, Sleisenger MH, Klein S, eds. Sleisenger & Fordtran's Gastrointestinal and Liver Disease, 6th ed. Orlando, FL, Saunders, 1998:38–39.
10. Shanahan F. Crohn's disease. Lancet 2003;359:62–69.
11. Shanahan F. Pathogenesis of ulcerative colitis. Lancet 1993;342:407–411.
12. Podolsky DK. Inflammatory bowel disease. N Engl J Med 2002;347:417–429.
13. Farrell RJ, Peppercorn MA. Ulcerative colitis. Lancet 2002;359:331–340.
14. MacDermott RP. Alterations of the mucosal immune system in inflammatory bowel disease. J Gastroenterol 1996;31:907–916.
15. Sendid B, Colombel J, Jacquinot P, et al. Specific antibody responses to oligomannosidic epitopes in Crohn's disease. Clin Diagn Lab Immunol 1996;3:219–226.
16. Peters M, Nevens H, Baert F, et al. Familial aggregation in Crohn's disease: Increased age-adjusted risk and concordance in clinical characteristics. Gastroenterology 1996;111:597.
17. McKenzie SJ, Baker MS, Buffington GD, Doe WF. Evidence of oxidant-induced injury to epithelial cells during inflammatory bowel disease. J Clin Invest 1996;98:136–141.
18. Sandborn WJ, Landers CJ, Tremaine WJ, Targan BR. Association of antineutrophil cytoplasmic antibodies with resistance to treatment of left-sided ulcerative colitis: Results of a pilot study. Mayo Clin Proc 1996;71:431–436.
19. Blumberg RS, Strober W. Prospects for research in inflammatory bowel disease. JAMA 2001;285:643–647.
20. Nielsen OH, Koppen T, Rudiger N, et al. Involvement of interleukin-4 and -10 in inflammatory bowel disease. Dig Dis Sci 1996;41:1786–1793.
21. Parronchi P, Romagnani P, Annunziato F, et al. Type 1 T-helper cell predominance and interleukin-12 expression in the gut of patients with Crohn's disease. Am J Pathol 1997;150:823–832.
22. Niesser M, Volk BA. Altered Th1/Th2 cytokine profiles in the intestinal mucosa of patients with inflammatory bowel disease as assessed by quantitative reversed transcribed polymerase chain reaction (RT-PCR). Clin Exp Immunol 1995;101:428–435.
23. Van Deventer SJH. Tumor necrosis factor and Crohn's disease. Gut 1997;40:443–448.
24. Bitton A, Sewitch MJ, Peppercorn MA, et al. Psychosocial determinants of relapse in ulcerative colitis: A longitudinal study. Am J Gastroenterol 2003;98:2112–2115.
25. Talala AH, Drossman DP. Psychosocial factors in inflammatory bowel disease. Gastroenterol Clin North Am 1995;24:699–716.
26. Pullan RD, Rhodes J, Ganesh S, et al. Transdermal nicotine for active ulcerative colitis. N Engl J Med 1994;330:811–815.
27. Sandborn WJ, Tremaine WJ, Offord KP, et al. Transdermal nicotine for mildly to moderately active ulcerative colitis. Ann Intern Med 1997;126:364–371.
28. Cosnes J, Beaugerie L, Carbonnel F, Gendre JP. Smoking cessation and the course of Crohn's disease: An intervention study. Gastroenterology 2001;120:1093–1099.
29. Evans JM, McMahon AD, Murray FE, et al. Non-steroidal anti-inflammatory drugs are associated with emergency admission to hospital for colitis due to inflammatory bowel disease. Gut 1997;40:619–622.
30. Gan SI, Beck PL. A new look at toxic megacolon: An update and review of incidence, etiology, pathogenesis, and management. Am J Gastroenterol 2003;98:2363–2371.
31. Monsen V, Sorstad J, Hellers G, et al. Extracolonic diagnosis in ulcerative colitis: An epidemiologic study. Am J Gastroenterol 1990;85:711–716.
32. Harmatz A. Hepatobiliary manifestations of inflammatory bowel disease. Med Clin North Am 1994;78:1387–1398.
33. Rankin GB. Extraintestinal and systemic manifestations of inflammatory bowel disease. Med Clin North Am 1990;74:39–50.
34. O'Keefe SJD, Rosser BG. Nutrition and inflammatory bowel disease. In: Targan SR, Shanahan F, eds. Inflammatory Bowel Disease: From Bench to Bedside. Baltimore, Williams & Wilkins, 1994:461–477.
35. Janowicz HD. The "natural history" of inflammatory bowel disease and therapeutic decisions. Am J Gastroenterol 1987;82:498–503.
36. Summers RW, Switz DM, Sessions JT, et al. National Cooperative Crohn's Disease Study: Results of drug treatment. Gastroenterology 1979;77:847–869.
37. Malchow H, Ewe K, Brandes JW, et al. European Cooperative Crohn's Disease Study (ECCDS): Results of drug treatment. Gastroenterology 1984;86:249–266.
38. Wu S, Craig RM. Intense nutritional support in inflammatory bowel disease. Dig Dis Sci 1995;40:843–852.
39. Gonzalez-Huix F, Fernandez-Banares F, Esteve-Comas M, et al. Enteral versus parenteral nutrition as adjunct therapy in acute ulcerative colitis. Am J Gastroenterol 1993;88:227–232.
40. Lewis JD, Fisher RL. Nutritional support in inflammatory bowel disease. Med Clin North Am 1994;78:1443–1456.
41. Rembacken BJ, Snelling AM, Hawkey PM, et al. Non-pathogenic *Escherichia coli* versus mesalamine for the treatment of ulcerative colitis. Lancet 1999;354:635–639.
42. Kruis W, Schutz E, Fric P, et al. Double-blind comparison of an oral *Escherichia coli* preparation and mesalamine in maintaining remission of ulcerative colitis. Aliment Pharmacol Ther 1997;11:853–858.
43. Venturi A, Gionchetti P, Rizzello F, et al. Impact on the composition of the fecal flora by a new probiotic: Preliminary data on maintenance

treatment of patients with ulcerative colitis. Aliment Pharmacol Ther 1999;13:1103–1109.

44. Klotz U, Maier K, Fischer C, et al. Therapeutic efficacy of sulfasalazine and its metabolites in patients with ulcerative colitis and Crohn's disease. N Engl J Med 1980;303:1499–1502.

45. DeVos M. Clinical pharmacokinetics of slow release mesalamine. Clin Pharmacokinetics 2000;39:85–97.

46. Sandborn WJ. A review of immune modifier therapy for inflammatory bowel disease: Azathioprine, 6-mercaptopurine, cyclosporine. Am J Gastroenterol 1996;91:423–433.

47. Pearson DC, May GR, Fick GH, et al. Azathioprine and 6-mercaptopurine in Crohn's disease: A meta analysis. Ann Intern Med 1995;123:134–142.

48. Hanauer SB, Baert F. Medical therapy of inflammatory bowel disease. Med Clin North Am 1994;78:1413–1426.

49. Paoluzi OA, Pica R, Marcheggiano A, et al. Azathioprine or methotrexate in the treatment of patients with steroid-dependent or steroid-resistant ulcerative colitis: Results of an open-label study on efficacy and tolerability in inducing and maintaining remission. Aliment Pharmacol Ther 2003;17:479–480.

50. Sutherland L, Singleton J, Sessions J, et al. Double-blind, placebo controlled trial of metronidazole in Crohn's disease. Gut 1991;32:1071–1075.

51. Kornbluth A, Sachar DB. Ulcerative colitis practice guidelines in adults. Am J Gastroenterol 1997;92:204–211.

52. Sutherland L, MacDonald JK. Oral 5-aminosalicylic acid for induction of remission in ulcerative colitis. Cochrane Database Syst Rev 2003;3:CD000543.

53. Clemett D, Markham A. Prolonged-release mesalamine: a review of its therapeutic potential in ulcerative colitis and Crohn's disease. Drugs 2000;59:929–956.

54. Pruitt R, Hanson J, Safdi M, et al. Balsalazide is superior to mesalamine in the time to improvement of signs and symptoms of acute mild-to-moderate ulcerative colitis. Am J Gastroenterol 2002;97:3078–3086.

55. D'Albasio G, Pacini F, Camarri E, et al. Combined therapy with 5-aminosalicylic acid tablets and enemas for maintaining remission in ulcerative colitis: A randomized double-blind study. Am J Gastroenterol 1997;92:1143–1147.

56. Marshall JK, Irvine EJ. Rectal corticosteroids versus alternative treatments in ulcerative colitis: A meta-analysis. Gut 1997;40:775–781.

57. Lee FI, Jewell DP, Mani V, et al. A randomized trial comparing mesalamine and prednisone foam enemas in patients with acute distal ulcerative colitis. Gut 1996;38:229–233.

58. Sandborn WJ, Tremaine WJ, Offord KP, et al. Transdermal nicotine for mild to moderately active ulcerative colitis. A randomized, double-blind, placebo controlled trial. Ann Intern Med 1997;126:364–371.

59. Sandborn WJ, Tremaine WJ. Cyclosporine treatment of inflammatory bowel disease. Mayo Clin Proc 1992;67:981–990.

60. Present DH, Lichtiger S. Efficacy of cyclosporine in treatment of fistula of Crohn's disease. Dig Dis Sci 1994;39:374–380.

61. Carbonnel F, Boruchowicz A, Duclos B, et al. Intravenous cyclosporine in attacks of ulcerative colitis: Short-term and long-term responses. Dig Dis Sci 1996;41:2471–2476.

62. Lichtiger S, Present DH, Kornbluth A, et al. Cyclosporine in severe ulcerative colitis refractory to steroid therapy. N Engl J Med 1994;330:1841–1845.

63. D'Haens G, Lemmens L, Geboes K, et al. Intravenous cyclosporine versus corticosteroids as single therapy for severe attacks of ulcerative colitis. Gastroenterology 2001;120:1323–1329.

64. Misiewicz JJ, Lennard-Jones JE, Connell AM, et al. Controlled trial of sulphasalazine in maintenance therapy for ulcerative colitis. Lancet 1965;1:185–188.

65. Sutherland L, Roth D, Beck P, et al. Oral 5-aminosalicylic acid for maintenance of remission in ulcerative colitis. Cochrane Database Syst Rev 2002;4:CD000544.

66. Hawthorne AB, Logan RFA, Hawkey CJ. Randomized controlled trial of azathioprine withdrawal in ulcerative colitis. BMJ 1992;305:20–22.

67. Fernandez-Banares F, Bertran X, Esteve-Comas M, et al. Azathioprine is useful in maintaining long-term remission induced by intravenous cyclosporine in steroid-refractory severe ulcerative colitis. Am J Gastroenterol 1996;91:2498–2499.

68. Salomon P, Kornbluth A, Aisenberg J, et al. How effective are current therapies for Crohn's disease? A meta-analysis. Am J Gastroenterol 1992;14:211–215.

69. Singleton JW, Hanauer SB, Gitnick GL, et al. Mesalamine capsules for the treatment of active Crohn's disease: Results of a 16-week trial. Gastroenterology 1993;104:1293–1301.

70. Ewe K, Press AG, Singe CC, et al. Azathioprine combined with prednisolone or monotherapy with prednisolone in active Crohn's disease. Gastroenterology 1993;105:367–372.

71. Colombrel JF, Lemann M, Bouhnik Y, et al. A controlled trial comparing ciprofloxacin with mesalamine for the treatment of active Crohn's disease. Gastroenterology 1997;112:A951.

72. Korelitz BI, Adler DJ, Mendelsohn RA, Sacknoff AL. Long-term experience with 6-mercaptopurine in the treatment of Crohn's disease. Am J Gastroenterol 1993;88:1198–1205.

73. Dubinsky MC, Lamothe S, Yang HY, et al. Pharmacogenomics and metabolite measurement for 6-mercaptopurine therapy in inflammatory bowel disease. Gastroenterology 2000;18:705–713.

74. Yates CR, Krnetski EY, Loennechen T, et al. Molecular diagnosis of thiopurine S-methyltransferase deficiency: Genetic basis for azathioprine and mercaptopurine intolerance. Ann Intern Med 1997;126:608–614.

75. Colombel JF, Ferrari N, Debuysere H, et al. Genotypic analysis of thiopurine S-methyltransferase in patients with Crohn's disease and severe myelosuppression during azathioprine therapy. Gastroenterology 2000;118:1025–1030.

76. Hanauer SB, Smith MB. Rapid closure of Crohn's disease fistulas with continuous intravenous cyclosporin A. Am J Gastroenterol 1993;88:646–649.

77. Stark ME, Tremaine WJ. Maintenance of symptomatic remission in patients with Crohn's disease. Mayo Clin Proc 1993;68:1183–1190.

78. Brynskov J, Freund L, Rasmussen SN, et al. A placebo-controlled, double-blind, randomized trial of cyclosporine therapy in active chronic Crohn's disease. N Engl J Med 1989;321:845–850.

79. Schroder O, Stein J. Low dose methotrexate in inflammatory bowel disease: current status and future directions. Am J Gastroenterol 2003;98:530–537.

80. Vandell AG, DiPiro JT. Low-dose methotrexate for treatment and maintenance of remission in patients with inflammatory bowel disease. Pharmacotherapy 2002;22:613–620.

81. Feagan BG, Rochon J, Fedorak RN, et al. Methotrexate for the treatment of Crohn's disease. N Engl J Med 1995;332:292–297.

82. Egan LJ, Sandborn WJ. Methotrexate for inflammatory bowel disease: Pharmacology and preliminary results. Mayo Clin Proc 1996;71:69–80.

83. Targan SR, Hanauer SB, van Deventer SJ, et al. A short-term study of chimeric monoclonal antibody to CA2 to tumor necrosis factor alpha for Crohn's disease. N Engl J Med 1997;337:1029–1035.

84. Rutgeerts P, D'Haens G, Targan S, et al. Efficacy and safety of retreatment with anti-tumor necrosis factor antibody (infliximab) to maintain remission in Crohn's disease. Gastroenterology 1999;117:761–769.

85. Farrell RJ, Alsahi M, Jeen YT, et al. Intravenous hydrocortisone premedication reduces antibodies to infliximab in Crohn's disease: a randomized controlled trial. Gastroenterology 2003;124:917–924.

86. Baert F, Noman M, Vermeire S, et al. Influence of immunogenicity on the long-term efficacy of infliximab in Crohn's disease. N Engl J Med 2003;348:601–608.

87. Parsi MA, Achkar JP, Richardson S, et al. Predictors of response to infliximab in patients with Crohn's disease. Gastroenterology 2002;123:707–713.

88. Goldstein F. Maintenance treatment for Crohn's disease: Has the time arrived? Am J Gastroenterol 1992;87:551–556.

89. Ewe K, Herfarth C, Malchow H, Jesdinsky HJ. Postoperative recurrence of Crohn's disease in relation to radicality of operation and sulfasalazine prophylaxis: A multicenter trial. Digestion 1989;42:224–232.

90. Gendre JP, Mary JY, Florent C, et al. Oral mesalamine (Pentasa) as maintenance treatment in Crohn's disease: A multicenter placebo-controlled study. Gastroenterology 1993;104:435–439.

91. Prantera C, Pallone F, Brunetti G, et al. Oral 5-aminosalicylic acid (Asacol) in the maintenance treatment of Crohn's disease. Gastroenterology 1992;103:363–368.

92. Lofberg R, Rutgeerts P, Malchow H. Budesonide prolongs time to relapse in ileal and ileocecal Crohn's disease. A placebo controlled, one-year study. Gut 1996;39:82–86.

93. Lewis JD, Schwatrz JS, Lichtenstein GR. Azathioprine for maintenance of remission in Crohn's disease: Benefits outweigh the risk of lymphoma. Gastroenterology 2000;118:1018–1024.

94. Feagan BG, Fedorak RN, Irvine EJ, et al. A comparison of methotrexate with placebo for the maintenance of remission in Crohn's disease. North America's Crohn's Study Group. N Engl J Med 2000;342:1627–1632.

95. Hanauer SB, Feagan BG, Lichtenstein GR, et al. Maintenance infliximab for Crohn's disease: the ACCENTS I randomized trial. Lancet 2002;359:1541–1549.

96. Hanan IM. Inflammatory bowel disease in the pregnant woman. Compr Ther 1993;19:91–95.

97. Schade RR, Van Thiel DH, Gavaler JS. Chronic idiopathic ulcerative colitis: Pregnancy and fetal outcome. Dig Dis Sci 1984;29:614–619.

98. Willoughby CP, Truelove SC. Ulcerative colitis and pregnancy. Gut 1980;21:469–474.

99. Toovey S, Hudson E, Hendry WF, et al. Sulfasalazine and male infertility: Reversibility and possible mechanism. Gut 1981;22:445–451.

100. Farraye FA. Pregnancy and nursing. In: Peppercorn MA, ed. Therapy of Inflammatory Bowel Disease. New York, Marcel Dekker, 1990.

101. Ardizzone S, Porro GB. Comparative tolerability of therapies for ulcerative colitis. Drug Saf 2002;25:561–582.

102. Korelitz BI, Present DH, Rubin PH, et al. Desensitization to sulfasalazine after hypersensitivity reactions in patients with inflammatory bowel disease. J Clin Gastroenterol 1984;6:27–31.

103. Zinberg J, Molinas S, Das KM. Double-blind placebo-controlled study of olsalazine in the treatment of ulcerative colitis. Am J Gastroenterol 1990;85:562–566.

104. Haber CJ, Meltzer SJ, Present DH, et al. Nature and course of pancreatitis caused by 6-mercaptopurine in the treatment of inflammatory bowel disease. Gastroenterology 1986;91:982–986.

105. Colonna T, Korelitz BI. The role of leukopenia in the 6-mercaptopurine-induced remission of refractory Crohn's disease. Am J Gastroenterol 1994;89:362–366.

106. Warman JI, Korelitz BI, Fleisher MR, Janardhanam R. Cumulative experience with short- and long-term toxicity to 6-mercaptopurine in the treatment of Crohn's disease and ulcerative colitis. J Clin Gastroenterol 2003;37:220–225.

107. O'Brien JJ, Bayless TM, Bayless JA. Use of azathioprine or 6-mercaptopurine in the treatment of Crohn's disease. Gastroenterology 1991;101:39–46.

108. Lennard L. TPMT in the treatment of Crohn's disease with azathioprine. Gut 2002;51:143–146.

109. Best WR, Becktel JM, Singleton JW, et al. Development of a Crohn's disease activity index. Gastroenterology 1976;70:439–444.

110. Sanborn WJ, Tremaine WJ, Schroeder KW, et al. Cyclosporine enemas for treatment-resistant, mildly to moderately active, left sided ulcerative colitis. Am J Gastroenterol 1993;88:640–645.

111. Irvine EJ, Zhou Q, Thompson AK. The short inflammatory bowel disease questionnaire: A quality of life instrument for community physicians managing inflammatory bowel disease. CERPT investigators. Canadian Crohn's relapse prevention trial. Am J Gastroenterol 1996;91:1571–1578.

112. Lichtenstein GR, Yan S, Balla M, Hanauer S. Remission in patients with Crohn's disease is associated with improvement in employment and quality of life and a decrease in hospitalizations and surgeries. Am J Gastroenterol 2004;99:91–96.

113. Rubenstein JH, Chong RY, Cohen RD. Infliximab decreases resource use among patients with Crohn's disease. J Clin Gastroenterol 2002;35:151–156.

35

NAUSEA AND VOMITING

Cecily V. DiPiro and A. Thomas Taylor

Learning Objectives and other resources can be found at *www.pharmacotherapyonline.com.*

KEY CONCEPTS

◀1 Nausea and vomiting may be a part of the symptom complex for a variety of gastrointestinal, cardiovascular, infectious, neurologic, metabolic, or psychogenic processes.

◀2 Nausea and vomiting may be caused by a variety of medications or other noxious agents.

◀3 The overall goal of treatment should be to prevent or eliminate nausea and vomiting regardless of etiology.

◀4 Treatment options for nausea and vomiting include drug and nondrug modalities.

◀5 The primary goal with chemotherapy-induced nausea and vomiting (CINV) is to *prevent* nausea and/or vomiting.

Optimal control of acute nausea and vomiting positively impacts the incidence and control of delayed and anticipatory nausea and vomiting.

◀6 The emetogenic potential of the chemotherapeutic regimen is the primary factor to consider when selecting prophylactic antiemetics for CINV.

◀7 Patients at high risk of vomiting should receive prophylactic antiemetics for postoperative nausea and vomiting (PONV).

◀8 Patients receiving single-exposure, high-dose radiation therapy to the upper abdomen or receiving total or hemibody irradiation should receive prophylactic antiemetics for radiation-induced nausea and vomiting (RINV).

Nausea and vomiting are common complaints among many individuals with gastrointestinal (GI) disorders. However, because of the variable etiologies of these problems, management may be quite simple or detailed and complex, essentially innocuous or associated with therapy-induced adverse reactions. This chapter provides an overview of nausea and vomiting, two multifaceted problems.

Nausea is usually defined as the inclination to vomit or as a feeling in the throat or epigastric region alerting an individual that vomiting is imminent. Vomiting is defined as the ejection or expulsion of gastric contents through the mouth and is often a forceful event. Either condition may occur transiently with no other associated signs or symptoms; however, these conditions also may be only part of a more complex clinical presentation.

ETIOLOGY

◀1 Nausea and vomiting may be associated with a variety of clinical presentations. In addition to GI diseases, either or both may accompany cardiovascular, infectious, neurologic, or metabolic disease processes. Nausea and vomiting may be a feature of such conditions as pregnancy or may follow operative procedures or administration of certain medications such as those used in cancer chemotherapy. Psychogenic etiologies of these symptoms may be present, especially in young women with an underlying emotional disturbance. Anticipatory etiologies may be involved, such as in patients who have previously received cytotoxic chemotherapy. Specific etiologies associated with nausea and vomiting are presented in Table 35–1.[1]

In addition to identifying conditions associated with nausea and vomiting, it is important to address the specific causative medical

problems. For example, nausea and vomiting may occur in as many as 70% of patients with inferior myocardial infarction or diabetic ketoacidosis. Eighty to ninety percent of patients with an Addisonian crisis, acute pancreatitis, or acute appendicitis may present with nausea and vomiting.

The etiology of nausea and vomiting may vary with the age of the patient. For example, vomiting in the newborn during the first day of life suggests upper digestive tract obstruction or an increase in intracranial pressure. Other illnesses associated with vomiting in children include pyloric stenosis, duodenal ulcer, stress ulcer, adrenal insufficiency, septicemia, or diseases of the pancreas, liver, or biliary tree. Also, the hepatocellular failure seen in Reye's syndrome may lead to profound cerebral edema followed by persistent emesis. A common etiology of vomiting in children is viral gastroenteritis caused by rotavirus. Vomiting in infants may be associated with something as simple as overfeeding, rapid feeding, inadequate burping, or lying down too soon after feeding. It should be recognized that these types of vomiting are usually indicative of minor problems and may be altered by changing the approach to feeding.

◀2 Drug-induced nausea and vomiting are of particular concern, especially with the increasing number of patients receiving cytotoxic treatment and the number of agents implicated. Included in Table 35–2 are specific cytotoxic agents categorized by their emetogenic potential. Although some agents may have greater emetogenic potential than others, combinations of agents, high doses, clinical settings, psychological conditions, prior treatment experiences, and unusual stimulus of sight, smell, or taste may alter a patient's response to drug treatment. In this setting, nausea and vomiting may be unavoidable and potentially devastating to the patient's desire to continue treatment. Indeed, some patients experience these problems so

TABLE 35–1. Specific Etiologies of Nausea and Vomiting

Gastrointestinal Mechanisms	**Neurologic Processes**
Mechanical gastric outlet obstruction	Midline cerebellar hemorrhage
Peptic ulcer disease	Increased intracranial pressure
Gastric carcinoma	Migraine headache
Pancreatic disease	Vestibular disorders
Motility disorders	Head trauma
Gastroparesis	**Metabolic Disorders**
Drug-induced gastric stasis	Diabetes mellitus (diabetic ketoacidosis)
Chronic intestinal pseudo-obstruction	Addison's disease
Postviral gastroenteritis	Renal disease (uremia)
Irritable bowel syndrome	**Psychogenic Causes**
Postgastric surgery	Self-induced
Idiopathic gastric stasis	Anticipatory
Anorexia nervosa	**Therapy-induced Causes**
Intra-abdominal emergencies	Cytotoxic chemotherapy
Intestinal obstruction	Radiation therapy
Acute pancreatitis	Theophylline preparations (intolerance, toxic)
Acute pyelonephritis	Anticonvulsant preparations (toxic)
Acute cholecystitis	Digitalis preparations (toxic)
Acute cholangitis	Opiates
Acute viral hepatitis	Amphotericin B
Acute gastroenteritis	Antibiotics
Viral gastroenteritis	**Drug Withdrawal**
Salmonellosis	Opiates
Shigellosis	Benzodiazepines
Staphylococcal gastroenteritis (enterotoxins)	**Miscellaneous Causes**
Cardiovascular Diseases	Pregnancy
Acute myocardial infarction	Any swallowed irritant (foods, drugs)
Congestive heart failure	Noxious odors
Shock and circulatory collapse	Operative procedures

From Hanson and McCallum.[1]

intensely that chemotherapy is postponed or discontinued. In addition to the emetogenic potential of various cytotoxic regimens, a variety of other common etiologies have been proposed for the development of nausea and vomiting in cancer patients. These are presented in Table 35–3.[2]

PATHOPHYSIOLOGY

The three consecutive phases of emesis include nausea, retching, and vomiting. Nausea, the imminent need to vomit, is associated with gastric stasis and may be considered a separate and singular symptom. Retching is the labored movement of abdominal and thoracic muscles before vomiting. The final phase of emesis is vomiting, the forceful expulsion of gastric contents caused by GI retroperistalsis. The act of vomiting requires the coordinated contractions of the abdominal muscles, pylorus, and antrum, a raised gastric cardia, diminished lower esophageal sphincter pressure, and esophageal dilatation.[3] Vomiting should not be confused with regurgitation, an act in which the gastric or esophageal contents rise to the pharynx because of pressure differences caused by, for example, an incompetent lower esophageal sphincter. Accompanying autonomic symptoms of pallor, tachycardia, and diaphoresis account for many of the distressing feelings associated with emesis.

Vomiting is triggered by afferent impulses to the vomiting center, a nucleus of cells in the medulla. Impulses are received from sensory centers, such as the chemoreceptor trigger zone (CTZ), cerebral cortex, and visceral afferents from the pharynx and GI tract.

When excited, afferent impulses are integrated by the vomiting center, resulting in efferent impulses to the salivation center, respiratory center, and the pharyngeal, GI, and abdominal muscles, leading to vomiting.

The CTZ, located in the area postrema of the fourth ventricle of the brain, is a major chemosensory organ for emesis and is usually associated with chemically induced vomiting. Because of its location, blood-borne and cerebrospinal fluid toxins have easy access to the CTZ. Therefore cytotoxic agents stimulate primarily this area rather than the cerebral cortex and visceral afferents. Similarly, pregnancy-associated vomiting probably occurs through stimulation of the CTZ.

Numerous neurotransmitter receptors are located in the vomiting center, CTZ, and GI tract. Examples of such receptors include cholinergic and histaminic, dopaminergic, opiate, serotonergic, neurokinin, and benzodiazepine receptors. Chemotherapeutic agents, their metabolites, or other emetic compounds theoretically trigger the process of emesis through stimulation of one or more of these receptors. Effective antiemetics are able to antagonize or block the emetogenic receptors.

CLINICAL PRESENTATION

Because it is impossible to discuss all clinical settings in which the presence of nausea and vomiting might be a pertinent finding, these processes are presented in Table 35–4 as they might occur together and also as *simple* or *complex* in presentation.

TABLE 35–2. Emetogenicity of Chemotherapeutic Agents

Level 1 (less than 10% frequency)
Androgens
Bleomycin
Busulfan (oral <4 mg/kg per day)
Capecitabine (oral)
Chlorambucil (oral)
Cladribine
Corticosteroids
Doxorubicin (liposomal)
Fludarabine
Hydroxyurea
Interferon
Melphalan (oral)
Mercaptopurine
Methotrexate ($\leq$50 mg/m^2)
Thioguanine (oral)
Tretinoin
Vinblastine
Vincristine
Vinorelbine

Level 2 (10%–30% frequency)
Asparaginase
Cytarabine (<1 g/m^2)
Docetaxel
Doxorubicin HCl (<20 mg/m^2)
Etoposide
Fluorouracil (<1 g/m^2)
Gemcitabine
Methotrexate (>50 mg/m^2; <250 mg/m^2)
Mitomycin
Paclitaxel
Teniposide
Thiotepa
Topotecan

Level 3 (30%–60% frequency)
Aldesleukin
Cyclophosphamide (IV, $\leq$750 mg/m^2)
Dactinomycin ($\leq$1.5 mg/m^2)
Doxorubicin HCl (20–60 mg/m^2)
Epirubicin HCl ($\leq$90 mg/m^2)
Idarubicin
Ifosfamide
Methotrexate (250–1000 mg/m^2)
Mitoxantrone ($\leq$15 mg/m^2)

Level 4 (60%–90% frequency)
Carboplatin
Carmustine (<250 mg/m^2)
Cisplatin (<50 mg/m^2)
Cyclophosphamide (>750 mg/m^2 to $\leq$1500 mg/m^2)
Cytarabine ($\geq$1 g/m^2)
Dactinomycin (>1.5 mg/m^2)
Doxorubicin HCl (>60 mg/m^2)
Irinotecan
Melphalan (IV)
Methotrexate (>1 g/m^2)
Mitoxantrone (>15 mg/m^2)
Oxaliplatin
Procarbazine (oral)

Level 5 (>90% frequency)
Carmustine (>250 mg/m^2)
Cisplatin (>50 mg/m^2)
Cyclophosphamide (>1500 mg/m^2)
Dacarbazine ($\geq$500 mg/m^2)
Lomustine (>60 mg/m^2)
Mechlorethamine
Pentostatin
Streptozocin

Adapted from Hesketh et al.[34]

TABLE 35–3. Nonchemotherapy Etiologies of Nausea and Vomiting in Cancer Patients

Fluid and electrolyte abnormalities
　Hypercalcemia
　Volume depletion
　Water intoxication
　Adrenocortical insufficiency
Drug-induced
　Opiates
　Antibiotics
Gastrointestinal obstruction
Increased intracranial pressure
Peritonitis
Metastases
　Brain
　Meninges
　Hepatic
Uremia
Infections (septicemia, local)
Radiation therapy

From Frytak and Moertel.[2]

TABLE 35–4. Presentation of Nausea and Vomiting

General
Depending on severity of symptoms, patients may present in mild to severe distress

Symptoms
Simple: Self-limiting, resolves spontaneously and requires only symptomatic therapy
Complex: Not relieved after administration of antiemetics; progressive deterioration of patient secondary to fluid-electrolyte imbalances; usually associated with noxious agents or psychogenic events

Signs
Simple: Patient complaint of queasiness or discomfort
Complex: Weight loss; fever; abdominal pain

Laboratory tests
Simple: None
Complex: Serum electrolyte concentrations; upper/lower GI evaluation

Other information
Fluid input and output
Medication history
Recent history of behavioral or visual changes, headache, pain, or stress
Family history positive for psychogenic vomiting

► TREATMENT: Nausea and Vomiting

DESIRED OUTCOME

③ The overall goal of antiemetic therapy is to prevent or to eliminate nausea and vomiting. This should be accomplished without adverse effects or with clinically acceptable adverse effects. Although this goal may be accomplished easily in patients with simple nausea and vomiting, patients with more complex problems require greater assistance. In addition to these clinical goals, appropriate cost issues should be considered, particularly in the management of chemotherapy-induced and postoperative nausea and vomiting.

GENERAL APPROACH TO TREATMENT

④ Treatment options for nausea and vomiting include drug and nondrug modalities. The treatment of nausea and vomiting is quite varied depending on the associated medical situation. Even though a number of potentially effective measures are available, most patients receive a medication at some point in their care. For simple nausea and vomiting, patients may choose to do nothing or to select from a variety of nonprescription drugs. As symptoms become worse or are associated with more serious medical problems, patients are more likely to benefit from prescription antiemetic drugs. When prescribed according to reliable clinical information, these agents often provide acceptable relief. However, some patients will never be totally free of symptoms. This lack of relief is most disabling to the patient when it is associated with an unresolved medical problem or when the necessary therapy for this condition is the cause of the nausea or vomiting, as in the case of patients receiving emetogenic chemotherapy.

NONPHARMACOLOGIC MANAGEMENT

Nonpharmacologic management of nausea and vomiting may include a variety of dietary, physical, or psychological changes consistent with the etiology of symptoms. For patients with simple complaints, perhaps resulting from excessive or disagreeable food or beverage consumption, avoidance or moderation in dietary intake may be preferable. Patients suffering symptoms of systemic illness may improve dramatically as their underlying condition resolves. Finally, patients in whom these symptoms result from labyrinthine changes produced by motion may benefit quickly by assuming a stable physical position.

Cancer patients undergoing chemotherapy may experience nausea and/or vomiting despite receiving prophylactic antiemetics. The fact that anticipatory side effects rarely occur unless the patient has previously experienced posttreatment nausea or vomiting suggests that the mechanism for anticipatory nausea and vomiting is a learned process involving elements of classic conditioning.[4] This conditioning model may also be important in understanding the development of pregnancy-related nausea. Nonpharmacologic interventions are classified as behavioral interventions and include relaxation, biofeedback, self-hypnosis, cognitive distraction, guided imagery, and systematic desensitization.[5–7]

The management of psychogenic vomiting is greatly dependent on psychological intervention. However, because the underlying problems are so complex and intertwined in personal relationships, psychological therapy may require lengthy, in-depth treatment. Pharmacologic therapy offers only minimal benefit in these patients. Surgery, such as gastroenterostomy, is of no value.

PHARMACOLOGIC THERAPY

④ Although many approaches to the treatment of nausea and vomiting have been suggested, antiemetic drugs (nonprescription and prescription) are most often recommended. These agents represent a variety of pharmacologic and chemical classes, as well as dosage regimens and routes of administration. With so many treatment possibilities available, factors that enable the clinician to discriminate among various choices must be recognized. These factors include (a) the suspected etiology of the symptoms; (b) the frequency, duration, and severity of the episodes; (c) the ability of the patient to use oral, rectal, injectable, or transdermal medications; and (d) the success of previous antiemetic medications. Information concerning commonly available antiemetic preparations is given in Table 35–5.

The treatment of simple nausea and vomiting usually requires minimal therapy. For these symptoms, patients may choose from a lengthy list of nonprescription products. Both nonprescription and prescription drugs useful in the treatment of simple nausea and vomiting are usually effective in small, infrequently administered doses. Side effects and toxic effects in these settings are also usually minimal. Although suitable for occasional simple nausea and vomiting, nonprescription agents are often abandoned by the patient as symptoms continue or become progressively worse. As the patient's condition warrants, prescription medications may be chosen, either as single-agent therapy or in combination.

The management of complex nausea and vomiting, for example, in patients receiving cytotoxic chemotherapy, may require combination therapy. In combination regimens, agents are prescribed in small-to-moderate dosages, achieving symptomatic control through different pharmacologic mechanisms while avoiding the untoward effects caused by high doses.

ANTACIDS

Patients who are experiencing simple nausea and vomiting may use various antacids. In this setting, single or combination nonprescription antacid products, especially those containing magnesium hydroxide, aluminum hydroxide, and/or calcium carbonate, may provide sufficient relief, primarily through gastric acid neutralization.

Common antacid regimens for the relief of acute or intermittent nausea and vomiting include one or more small doses of single- or multiple-agent products. Depending on dose, common products usually supply sufficient ingredients to allow a range of approximately 40 to 180 mEq of acid-neutralizing capacity.[8–10] Potential adverse effects from antacids are usually related to the presence of magnesium, aluminum, or calcium salts. Specifically, osmotic diarrhea from magnesium and constipation from aluminum or calcium salts may be of concern to patients, particularly those self-medicating with high or frequently administered antacid doses. Generally, however, when

TABLE 35–5. Common Antiemetic Preparations and Adult Dosage Regimens

Drug	Adult Dosage Regimen	Dosage Form/Route	Availability
Antacids			
Antacids (various)	15–30 mL every 2–4 h prn	Liquid	OTC
Histamine H₂ Antagonists			
Cimetidine (Tagamet HB)	200 mg twice daily prn	Tab	OTC
Famotidine (Pepcid AC)	10 mg twice daily prn	Tab	OTC
Nizatidine (Axid AR)	75 mg twice daily prn	Tab	OTC
Ranitidine (Zantac 75)	75 mg twice daily prn	Tab	OTC
Antihistaminic-Anticholinergic Agents			
Buclizine (Bucladin-S)	50 mg twice daily	Tab	Rx
Cyclizine (Marezine)	50 mg every 4–6 h prn	Tab, IM	Rx/OTC
Dimenhydrinate (Dramamine)	50–100 mg every 4–6 h prn	Tab, Chew tab, cap, liquid, IM, IV	Rx/OTC
Diphenhydramine (Benadryl)	10–50 mg every 4–6 h prn	Tab, cap, liquid, IM, IV	Rx/OTC
Hydroxyzine (Vistril, Atarax)	25–100 mg every 6 h prn	Tab, cap, liquid, IM	Rx
Meclizine (Bonine, Antivert)	25–50 mg every 24 h prn	Tab, chew tab, cap	Rx/OTC
Pyrilamine (Nisaval)	25–50 mg 3 to 4 times daily	Tab	Rx/OTC
Scopolamine (Transderm Scop)	0.5 mg every 72 h prn	Transdermal patch	Rx
Trimethobenzamide (Tigan)	200–250 mg 3 to 4 times daily prn	Cap, IM, supp	Rx
Phenothiazines			
Chlorpromazine (Thorazine)	10–25 mg every 4–6 h prn	SR, cap, tab, liquid, IM, IV	Rx
	50–100 mg every 6–8 h prn	Supp	Rx
Prochlorperazine (Compazine)	5–10 mg 3 to 4 times daily prn	SR, cap, tab, liquid IM, IV	Rx
	25 mg twice daily prn	Supp	Rx
Promazine (Sparine)	25–50 mg every 4–6 h prn	Tab, IM	Rx
Promethazine (Phenergan)	12.5–25 mg every 4–6 h prn	Tab, liquid, IM, IV, supp	Rx
Thiethylperazine (Torecan)	10 mg 3 times daily	Tab, IM, supp	Rx
Cannabinoids			
Dronabinol (Marinol)	5–7.5 mg/m² every 2–4 h prn	Cap	Rx (C-II)
Nabilone (Cesamet)	1–2 mg 2 to 3 times daily prn	Cap	Rx (C-II)
Butyrophenones			
Haloperidol (Haldol)	1–5 mg every 12 h prn	Tab, liquid, IM, IV	Rx
Droperidol (Inapsine)[a]	2.5–5 mg every 4–6 h prn	IM, IV	Rx
Corticosteroids			
Dexamethasone-(Decadron) for CINV	10 mg prior to chemotherapy, repeat with 4–8 mg every 6 h for total of 4 doses	IV	Rx
Methylprednisolone (Solu-Medrol)	125–500 mg every 6 h for total of 4 doses	IV	Rx
Benzodiazepines			
Lorazepam (Ativan)	0.5–2 mg prior to chemotherapy	IV	Rx (C-IV)
Substance P/Neurokinin₁ Receptor Inhibitor			
Aprepitant (Emend)	125 mg on day 1, 1 hour prior to chemotherapy, 80 mg on days 2 and 3	Cap	Rx
Selective Serotonin Antagonists for CINV[b]			
Dolasetron (Anzemet)	1.8 mg/kg 30 min prior to chemotherapy (undiluted, up to 100 mg over 30 min, or diluted, over 30 min)	IV	Rx
	OR		
	100 mg within 1 h before chemotherapy	Tab	Rx
Granisetron (Kytril)	10 mcg/kg prior to chemotherapy (diluted, infuse over 5 min or undiluted over 30 seconds)	IV	Rx
	OR		
	1 mg up to 1 h prior to chemotherapy and 1 mg 12 h after the first dose, or, 2 mg up to 1 h prior to chemotherapy	Tab	Rx
Ondansetron (Zofran)	32 mg prior to chemotherapy as a single dose (diluted, give over 15 min), or 0.15 mg/kg prior to chemotherapy, repeat at 4 and 8 h	IV	Rx
	OR		
	8 mg 30 min prior to chemotherapy, repeat at 4 and 8 h and every 12 h for 1–2 days after chemotherapy completion	Tab	Rx

TABLE 35–5. (continued)

Drug	Adult Dosage Regimen	Dosage Form/Route	Availability
Palonestron (Aloxi)	0.25 mg 30 min prior to chemotherapy (undiluted over 30 seconds; do not repeat within 7 days)	IV	Rx
Miscellaneous Agents			
Metoclopramide (Reglan), for CINV	1–2 mg/kg every 2 h × 2, then every 3 h × 3	IV	Rx
Metoclopramide (Reglan), for PONV	10–20 mg about 10 min prior to anesthesia	IV	Rx
Metoclopramide (Reglan), for delayed CINV	0.5 mg/kg or 20 mg every 6 h prn, days 2 to 4	Tab	Rx

[a]See text for current warnings.
[b]See Table 35–7 for PONV dosing.
C-II, C-IV = controlled substance schedule 2 and 4, respectively; cap, capsule; chew tab, chewable tablet; CINV, chemotherapy-induced nausea and vomiting; liquid, oral syrup, concentrate, or suspension; OTC, over the counter; PONV, postoperative nausea and vomiting; Rx, prescription; SR cap, sustained-release capsule; supp, rectal suppository; tab, tablet.

used occasionally for acute episodic relief of nausea and vomiting, antacids do not produce serious toxicities.

H₂-RECEPTOR ANTAGONISTS

Patients may use histamine₂-receptor antagonists in low doses to manage simple nausea and vomiting associated with heartburn or gastroesophageal reflux. Individual dosages of cimetidine 200 mg, famotidine 10 mg, nizatidine 75 mg, or ranitidine 75 mg may be used for brief periods. Except for potential drug interactions with cimetidine, these agents cause few side effects when used for episodic relief.

ANTIHISTAMINE-ANTICHOLINERGIC DRUGS

Antiemetic drugs from the antihistaminic-anticholinergic category appear to interrupt various visceral afferent pathways that stimulate nausea and vomiting and may be appropriate in the treatment of simple nausea and vomiting. Adverse reactions that may be apparent with the use of the antihistaminic-anticholinergic agents primarily include drowsiness, confusion, blurred vision, dry mouth, and urinary retention, and possibly tachycardia, particularly in elderly patients. Also, as doses are increased or are more frequently administered, patients with narrow-angle glaucoma, prostatic hyperplasia, or asthma are at greater risk of complications from the anticholinergic effects of these drugs.

PHENOTHIAZINES

Historically, phenothiazines have been the most widely prescribed antiemetic agents. These agents appear to block dopamine receptors, most likely in the CTZ. Phenothiazines are marketed in an array of dosage forms, none of which appears to be more efficacious than another. These agents may be most practical for long-term treatment and are inexpensive in comparison with newer drugs. Rectal administration is a reasonable alternative in patients in whom oral or parenteral administration is not feasible. In an open-label, randomized, crossover comparison between promethazine in oral syrup and rectal suppositories, the pharmacokinetics were highly variable, but in general the suppositories produced a lower maximum concentration and a later time of maximum concentration than the oral syrup.[11]

Phenothiazines are most useful in patients with simple nausea and vomiting or in those receiving mildly emetogenic doses of chemotherapy. Intravenous prochlorperazine provides quicker and more complete relief with less drowsiness than intravenous promethazine in adult patients treated in an emergency department for nausea and vomiting associated with uncomplicated gastritis or gastroenteritis.[12] There are numerous potential side effects with these medications, including extrapyramidal reactions, hypersensitivity reactions with possible liver dysfunction, bone marrow aplasia, and excessive sedation.

BUTYROPHENONES

Two butyrophenone compounds that have antiemetic activity are haloperidol and its congener droperidol. Each agent blocks dopaminergic stimulation of the CTZ. Although each agent is effective in relieving nausea and vomiting, haloperidol is not considered first-line therapy, although it has been used in palliative care situations.[13] After 30 years of clinical use, a "black box" warning was recently added to the labeling for droperidol stating that QT prolongation and/or torsades de pointes have been reported in patients receiving droperidol at doses at or below recommended doses. Some of these cases occurred in patients with no known risk factors for QT prolongation and have been fatal. The warning recommends that droperidol should be reserved for use in the treatment of patients who fail to show an acceptable response to other adequate treatments and that all patients should undergo a 12-lead electrocardiogram prior to administration of droperidol, followed by cardiac monitoring for 2 to 3 hours postadministration.[14] As a result of this change in labeling, the clinical use of droperidol has effectively ceased. After review of the cases, several authors have questioned the justification of this warning.[15,16]

CORTICOSTEROIDS

Corticosteroids have demonstrated antiemetic efficacy since the initial recognition that patients receiving prednisone as part of their Hodgkin's disease protocol appeared to develop less nausea and vomiting than those patients treated with protocols that excluded this agent. Other corticosteroids showing antiemetic efficacy include methylprednisolone and dexamethasone.

Dexamethasone has been used successfully in the management of chemotherapy-induced and postoperative nausea and vomiting, either as a single agent or in combination with selective serotonin receptor inhibitors (SSRIs). For chemotherapy-induced nausea and vomiting, dexamethasone has demonstrated efficacy in the prevention of both cisplatin-induced acute emesis[17] and delayed nausea and vomiting associated with moderately emetogenic chemotherapy.[18] For patients with simple nausea and vomiting, steroids are not indicated and may be associated with unacceptable risks.

METOCLOPRAMIDE

Metoclopramide, procainamide's congener, provides significant antiemetic effects by blocking the dopaminergic receptors centrally in the CTZ. Peripherally, metoclopramide increases lower esophageal sphincter tone, aids gastric emptying, and accelerates transit through the small bowel, possibly through the release of acetylcholine. Metoclopramide is used for its antiemetic properties in patients with diabetic gastroparesis and as a component of multiagent therapy for prophylaxis of delayed nausea and vomiting associated with chemotherapy administration. Its use as prophylaxis for acute chemotherapy-induced nausea and vomiting was supplanted by the introduction of the SSRIs in the early 1990s. These agents have greater efficacy and decreased toxicity compared with metoclopramide in patients receiving cisplatin-based regimens.[19–21]

CANNABINOIDS

Thirty randomized, controlled trials from 1975 to 1996 were analyzed to quantify the antiemetic efficacy and adverse effects of cannabis when given to 1366 patients receiving chemotherapy.[22] Oral nabilone, oral dronabinol, and intramuscular levonantradol were compared with conventional antiemetics (prochlorperazine, metoclopramide, chlorpromazine, thiethylperazine, haloperidol, domperidone, and alizapride) or placebo. Across all trials, cannabinoids were slightly more effective than active comparators and placebo when the chemotherapy regimen was of moderate emetogenic potential, and patients preferred them. No dose-response relationships were evident to the authors. The cannabinoids were also more toxic; side effects included euphoria, drowsiness, sedation, somnolence, dysphoria, depression, hallucinations, and paranoia. The efficacy of cannabinoids as compared to SSRIs has not been studied. Use of these agents should be considered when other regimens do not provide desired efficacy.

SUBSTANCE P/NEUROKININ 1 RECEPTOR ANTAGONISTS

Substance P is a peptide neurotransmitter in the neurokinin (NK) family whose preferred receptor is the NK_1 receptor.[23] The acute phase of CINV is believed to be mediated by both serotonin and substance P, whereas substance P is believed to be the primary mediator of the delayed phase. NK_1 antagonists administered as part of a multiple-drug regimen with a SSRI and a corticosteroid improved protection from both acute and delayed emesis.[24–26] Aprepitant is the first approved substance P/NK_1 receptor antagonist. In two placebo-controlled, randomized trials, patients receiving high-dose cisplatin-based chemotherapy received IV ondansetron on day 1 plus oral dexamethasone on days 1 through 4 with or without oral aprepitant on days 1, 2, and 3. The aprepitant regimen provided significantly superior control of emesis in the overall study period as well as in separate analyses of the acute and delayed phases.[27,28]

Aprepitant has the potential for numerous drug interactions because it is a substrate, moderate inhibitor, and an inducer of cytochrome isoenzyme CYP3A4 and an inducer of CYP2C9. Aprepitant can increase serum concentrations of many drugs metabolized by CYP3A4, including docetaxel, paclitaxel, etoposide, irinotecan, ifosfamide, imatinib, vinorelbine, vincristine, and vinblastine. In clinical studies, aprepitant was concomitantly administered with etoposide, vinorelbine, or paclitaxel, with no adjustment in the doses of these agents to account for potential drug interactions. The efficacy of oral contraceptives may be reduced. Concomitant administration with warfarin may result in a clinically significant decrease in the International Normalized Ratio.[29] The dose of oral dexamethasone should be reduced 50% when coadministered with aprepitant, due to the 2.2-fold increase in observed area under the plasma-concentration-versus-time curve.[30] Aprepitant is not indicated for use in children.

SELECTIVE SEROTONIN RECEPTOR INHIBITORS

SSRIs block presynaptic serotonin receptors on sensory vagal fibers in the gut wall, effectively blocking the acute phase of CINV. These agents do not completely block the acute phase of CINV and are less efficacious in preventing the delayed phase, but they are the standard of care in the management of chemotherapy-induced, radiation-induced, and postoperative nausea and vomiting. Issues involved in the use of dolasetron, granisetron, ondansetron, and palonosetron are reviewed in detail in the sections that follow. The most common side effects associated with these agents are constipation, headache, and asthenia. Safety and efficacy in children less than 2 years old have not been established.

CHEMOTHERAPY-INDUCED NAUSEA AND VOMITING

CINV can be classified as anticipatory, acute, or delayed. As defined earlier, anticipatory nausea and vomiting is a conditioned response linked to experiencing poor emetic control with previously administered chemotherapy.[4] The anxiolytic and amnestic properties of lorazepam 1 to 2 mg given orally the evening before and the morning of chemotherapy may help prevent anticipatory nausea and vomiting, but efficacy has not been demonstrated in large, randomized trials.[31] Use of the most appropriate antiemetic regimen to prevent acute and delayed nausea and vomiting, beginning with the first cycle of chemotherapy, is recommended to prevent future development of anticipatory nausea and vomiting.[32]

Nausea and vomiting that occurs within 24 hours of chemotherapy administration is defined as acute, whereas when it starts more than 24 hours after chemotherapy administration, it is defined as delayed. The primary goal with CINV is to *prevent* nausea and/or vomiting; optimal control of acute nausea and vomiting positively impacts the incidence and control of delayed and anticipatory nausea and vomiting. Clinical practice guidelines for the use of antiemetics in CINV have been published.[31–33] Despite the availability of nationally recommended guidelines, individual practice varies from one institution to the next. Product availability and recommended doses are institution-specific and may vary considerably from the doses listed in Table 35–5.

Factors to consider when selecting an antiemetic for CINV include:

- The emetogenic potential of the chemotherapy agent or regimen (see Table 35–2).
- Patient-specific factors.
- Patterns of emesis after administration of specific chemotherapy agents or regimens.

▦ Prophylaxis of CINV (Adapted from Reference 31; Used with Permission)

◀**6** ▦ *Recommendation 1.* The emetogenic potential of the chemotherapeutic agent (see Table 35–2) is the primary factor to consider when deciding whether to administer prophylactic agents and which antiemetic(s) to select. When combination therapy is prescribed, the most highly emetogenic agent in the combination should be identified, and the contribution of other agents should be considered by using the following rules:[34]

- Level 1 agents do not contribute to the emetogenicity of a given regimen.
- Adding one or more level 2 agents increases emetogenicity of the combination by one level greater than the most emetogenic agent in the combination.
- Adding level 3 and 4 agents increases emetogenicity of the combination by one level per agent.

Originally developed for adult patients, these guidelines should be used cautiously in pediatric patients; however, the information is considered generally applicable to children receiving chemotherapy.

▦ *Recommendation 2.* Adult and pediatric patients receiving chemotherapeutic agent(s) with emetogenic potential classified as level 2 through 5 should receive prophylaxis against nausea and vomiting each day on which chemotherapy is given. Antiemetic prophylaxis is not required for level 1 agents.

- Adult and pediatric patients receiving level 2 regimens can receive a corticosteroid alone for prophylaxis. Prochlorperazine is also an option for adults.
- Adult and pediatric patients receiving level 3 through 5 regimens should receive a corticosteroid in combination with a SSRI.
- Orally and intravenously administered antiemetics are generally equivalent in efficacy and safety for both adult and pediatric patients. The decision as to which formulation to use should be based on patient-specific factors and cost.
- The decision as to which SSRI to use should be based on the acquisition cost of comparable doses. Dosage recommendations for adult and pediatric patients differ.

At the time the American Society of Health-System Pharmacists (ASHP) guidelines were published, the safety and efficacy of ondansetron, granisetron, and dolasetron for prophylaxis of CINV in adult and pediatric patients receiving moderately emetogenic or highly emetogenic chemotherapeutic regimens were supported by more than 50 clinical studies. The superior efficacy and safety of this class of agents over metoclopramide, with or without dexamethasone, in CINV prophylaxis have been demonstrated in numerous studies. When used in comparable dosage regimens, the choice of whether to use ondansetron, granisetron, or dolasetron should be based primarily on acquisition costs. The oral route of administration is preferred.[35,36]

The efficacy of ondansetron, granisetron, and dolasetron for the prophylaxis of moderately or highly emetogenic chemotherapy regimens is enhanced when used in combination with dexamethasone.

▦ Treatment of CINV

▦ *Recommendation 3.* All patients receiving chemotherapy should have antiemetics available on as-needed basis for rescue of breakthrough nausea and vomiting. Chlorpromazine, prochlorperazine, methylprednisolone, lorazepam, metoclopramide, dexamethasone, and dronabinol are available for adult patients. Chlorpromazine, lorazepam, and methylprednisolone (or dexamethasone) are recommended for pediatric patients. The choice of agent should be based on patient-specific factors, including potential adverse reactions, and cost. Granisetron, dolasetron, and ondansetron are effective in the treatment of breakthrough nausea and vomiting, but they are not superior to conventional, less expensive antiemetics.

▦ Prophylaxis of Delayed CINV

▦ *Recommendation 4.* For the prevention of delayed emesis after cisplatin therapy in adults, dexamethasone with metoclopramide or a SSRI is recommended. The choice of agent should be based on patient-specific factors and cost. For delayed emesis after cyclophosphamide, doxorubicin, or carboplatin therapy, a SSRI with dexamethasone is recommended. In pediatric patients, chlorpromazine, lorazepam, or a SSRI can be used in combination with a corticosteroid.

Since the publication of the ASHP and American Society of Clinical Oncologists (ASCO) clinical guidelines,[31,32] two new agents have been released, aprepitant (Emend) and palonestron (Aloxi). Aprepitant has been studied in combination with ondansetron and dexamethasone for the prophylaxis of acute and delayed nausea and vomiting associated with highly emetogenic chemotherapy, including high-dose cisplatin. The National Comprehensive Cancer Network (NCCN) guidelines[33] also include aprepitant in their guidelines for moderately emetogenic chemotherapy regimens. Palonestron, an injectable SSRI with a prolonged serum half-life and higher receptor binding affinity, is indicated for the prophylaxis of both *acute* nausea and vomiting associated with moderately and highly emetogenic chemotherapy regimens, and *delayed* nausea and vomiting associated with moderately emetogenic chemotherapy. Palonestron 0.25 mg is administered IV over 30 minutes prior to chemotherapy and should not be repeated within 7 days.[37] It has not been approved for use in children. Two Phase III trials support the labeled indications.[38,39] Although proven safe and efficacious, the design of the trials for these two new agents raises many questions and their eventual place in therapy, and inclusion in clinical practice guidelines, remains to be determined.

CLINICAL CONTROVERSY

Current published information describes the experience with aprepitant in highly emetogenic cisplatin-based chemotherapy regimens. The NCCN has also included aprepitant for prophylaxis of nausea and vomiting induced by moderately emetogenic chemotherapy regimens.[33] This recommendation is not supported by the current literature and has been questioned by clinicians.

▦ POSTOPERATIVE NAUSEA AND VOMITING

One of the most common complications of surgery is postoperative nausea and vomiting (PONV). Most patients undergoing an operative procedure do not require preoperative prophylactic antiemetic therapy and universal PONV prophylaxis is not cost effective. Consensus therapeutic guidelines for the prophylaxis and treatment of PONV have recently been published.[31,40] Factors to be considered for PONV

TABLE 35–6. Risk Factors for PONV

Patient-specific factors
  Female gender
  Nonsmoking status
  History of motion sickness/PONV
Anesthetic risk factors
  Use of volatile anesthetics
  Nitrous oxide
  Use of opioids (intraoperative or postoperative)
Surgical risk factors
  Duration of surgery
  Operative procedure (intra-abdominal, ear-nose-throat, major gynecologic, orthopedic, or laparoscopic)

PONV, postoperative nausea and vomiting.

prophylaxis and treatment include: risk factors, potential morbidity, potential adverse events associated with various antiemetics, efficacy of antiemetics, and costs. Risk factors for PONV are summarized in Table 35–6. The incidence of PONV can be significantly decreased by reducing baseline risk factors among patients at highest risk whenever clinically practical. Strategies to reduce baseline risk include use of regional anesthesia, propofol, supplemental oxygen, and hydration, as well as avoiding nitrous oxide, volatile anesthetics, and opioids.

Prophylaxis of PONV

❼ Although the optimal management of PONV is not known, patients at high risk of vomiting should receive prophylactic antiemetics for PONV. In addition to likely lack of benefit from prophylaxis, patients at low risk for PONV may potentially experience adverse reactions from the medications. Doses for prophylactic antiemetics are summarized in Table 35–7. The consensus panel determined that there is no difference in the efficacy and safety profiles of the SSRIs in the prophylaxis of PONV, and that these drugs are most effective when given at the end of surgery. Furthermore, the panel agreed that with equivalent efficacy and safety profiles, acquisition cost was the primary factor that differentiated the SSRIs from each other.[40]

Dexamethasone is an effective prophylactic agent when administered either alone or in combination with other antiemetic drugs before the induction of anesthesia.[41] Droperidol has been one of the most effective agents for PONV prophylaxis. At a dose of 1.25 mg IV, it was more effective and much less costly than combination therapy with ondansetron 4 mg IV and droperidol 0.625 mg IV.[42] As discussed earlier, the recent FDA black box warning has effectively removed droperidol from clinical use. As a result of conflicting data,

clinicians do not agree on the role of metoclopramide as a prophylactic agent for PONV. Although effective, the use of phenothiazines in ambulatory surgery is limited due to predictable side effects including sedation, dry mouth, and dizziness. Transdermal scopolamine is an effective prophylactic agent for PONV, but its use is limited by the 2- to 4-hour delay in onset of effect in addition to age-related concerns and medical contraindications.[43,44] Combination therapy is superior to monotherapy, but optimal dosing of agents used in combination as prophylaxis of PONV has not been determined.[45,46]

Treatment of PONV

When PONV occurs in a patient who did not receive prophylaxis or who only received prophylactic dexamethasone, treatment with a SSRI is indicated. Typical adult treatment doses of SSRIs are as follows: dolasetron 12.5 mg, granisetron 0.1 mg, and ondansetron 1 mg.[47] If prophylaxis with a SSRI is not protective, a treatment dose of a SSRI is not recommended within the first 6 hours after surgery due to lack of proven efficacy.[48] Patients who experience PONV after receiving prophylactic treatment with a SSRI plus dexamethasone should receive a rescue dose from a different drug class such as a phenothiazine or droperidol.[49] If more than 6 hours has elapsed between the administration of a prophylactic dose of a SSRI and an episode of PONV, a treatment or prophylaxis dose of a SSRI or droperidol can be administered, but the optimal readministration dose and interval for these two agents have not been determined.

CLINICAL CONTROVERSY

Is the lower dose of droperidol used for PONV safer than a higher dose? Several authors have reviewed the cases used by the FDA as justification for the black box warning. One author has hypothesized that droperidol is more hazardous in the presence of acute psychosis, making the acutely psychotic, severely agitated patient at higher risk of dysrhythmia than the typical perioperative patient receiving a dose of 1.25 mg or less.[15]

RADIATION-INDUCED NAUSEA AND VOMITING

Nausea and vomiting associated with radiation therapy is not well understood. It is neither as predictable nor as severe as CINV, and many patients receiving radiation therapy will not experience nausea or vomiting. Risk factors associated with the development of RINV include the site of radiation, the dose, dose rate, and field size. ❽ Patients receiving single-exposure, high-dose radiation therapy

---

TABLE 35–7. Recommended Prophylactic Doses of Antiemetics for PONV

Drug	Adult Dose (IV)	Pediatric Dose (IV)	Timing of Dose[a]
Dolasetron	12.5 mg	350 mcg/kg up to 12.5 mg	At end of surgery
Granisetron	0.35–1 mg		At end of surgery
Ondansetron	4–8 mg	50–100 mcg/kg up to 4 mg	At end of surgery
Dexamethasone	5–10 mg	150 mcg/kg up to 8 mg	Before induction
Droperidol	0.625–1.25 mg	50–70 mcg/kg up to 1.25 mg	At end of surgery
Dimenhydrinate	1–2 mg/kg	0.5 mg/kg	

[a]Based on recommendations from consensus guidelines; may differ from manufacturer's recommendations.
PONV, postoperative nausea and vomiting.
From Gan et al.[40]

to the upper abdomen, or total or hemibody irradiation should receive prophylactic antiemetics for RINV.

Prophylaxis of RINV

The ASHP Therapeutic Guidelines[31] and the ASCO antiemetic practice guidelines[32] recommend preventive therapy in patients receiving total or hemibody irradiation or single-exposure, high-dose radiation therapy to the upper abdomen. The efficacy of oral granisetron 2 mg and ondansetron 8 mg was demonstrated in 34 patients undergoing hyperfractionated total body irradiation.[50] Patients undergoing radiation therapy procedures with low to intermediate risk of nausea or vomiting should receive a SSRI or a dopamine receptor antagonist prior to each fraction.[32]

Treatment of RINV

Patients who experience nausea and vomiting after radiation therapy should receive prochlorperazine, metoclopramide, or thiethylperazine as rescue agents, and then receive prophylactic treatment with a SSRI prior to subsequent radiation treatment.[31]

DISORDERS OF BALANCE

A variety of clinical conditions may be associated with vertigo and dizziness. The etiology of these complaints may include diseases that are infectious, postinfectious, demyelinative, vascular, neoplastic, degenerative, traumatic, toxic, psychogenic, or idiopathic. Therefore symptoms of imbalance or imbalance perceived by the patient present a particular clinical challenge. Whether associated with a minor or complex disorder, motion sickness may be associated with nausea and vomiting.

Although much progress has been made in the management of other illnesses associated with emesis, motion sickness represents an area in which newer agents have provided little benefit. Beneficial therapy for patients in this setting can most reliably be found among the antihistaminic-anticholinergic agents. However, their precise mechanisms of action are unknown to date. Neither the antihistaminic nor the anticholinergic potency appears to correlate well with the ability of these agents to prevent or treat the nausea and vomiting associated with motion sickness. When used for their depressant effects on labyrinth excitability, these agents produce variable efficacy and safety profiles. Oral regimens of antihistaminic-anticholinergic agents given one to several times each day may be effective, especially when the first dose is administered prior to motion.

The utility of scopolamine in preventing motion sickness was enhanced with the development of the transdermal system that increased patient satisfaction and decreased untoward side effects. The efficacy of transdermal scopolamine, oral meclizine, and placebo in protection against motion sickness was compared in a double-blind crossover study in 36 healthy subjects. Transdermal applications were made and tablets were taken at least 12 and 2 hours before exposure to three 90-minute periods in a ship-motion simulator. Transdermal scopolamine provided better protection than placebo or meclizine, with dryness of mouth more frequently reported in the transdermal scopolamine subjects.[51]

ANTIEMETIC USE DURING PREGNANCY

More than one-half of pregnant women experience nausea and vomiting to some degree during the first trimester of pregnancy (nausea and vomiting of pregnancy; NVP). Teratogenicity is a major consideration for the use of antiemetic drugs during pregnancy and is the primary factor that guides drug selection. A large body of evidence suggests that the histamine$_1$-receptor antagonists (dimenhydrinate, diphenhydramine, doxylamine, hydroxyzine, and meclizine) have no human teratogenic potential[52] and are effective in reducing treatment failure.[53] Whether used alone or in combination with doxylamine, pyridoxine has not been found to be teratogenic and significantly decreases the nausea score.[54,55] Other commonly prescribed agents that are effective and not teratogenic include the phenothiazines prochlorperazine and promethazine.[53] Studies using the SSRIs in NVP are limited. In a randomized controlled trial of 15 patients exposed during the first trimester to intravenous ondansetron versus promethazine for treatment of severe NVP, ondansetron was no more beneficial than promethazine with respect to the following outcome measures: severity of nausea, daily weight gain, days requiring hospitalization, treatment failures, and voluntary use of the drug.[56] The limited safety data for ondansetron does not allow it to be recommended as first-line therapy. Nonpharmacologic interventions for NVP include ginger[57] and acupuncture, although safety and efficacy trials for acupuncture are lacking.

Although many women experience nausea and vomiting during pregnancy, less than 1% develop hyperemesis gravidarum, a serious condition marked by severe physical symptoms and/or medical complications. The etiology of hyperemesis gravidarum is not well understood. In its most severe state, hyperemesis gravidarum may result in volume contraction, starvation, and electrolyte abnormalities. Other clinical strategies include attention to fluid and electrolyte management, the use of vitamin supplements, reduced intake of dietary fats with increased intake of carbohydrates, and methods aimed at reducing psychosomatic complaints.[58]

ANTIEMETIC USE IN CHILDREN

As discussed previously, the safety and efficacy of SSRIs have been established in pediatric patients receiving chemotherapy. Their side effect profile has promoted their use in children. The best doses or dosing strategies for children (by age, weight, or body surface area) have not been clearly established. Due to the lack of comparative trials in children, the ASCO antiemetic guidelines recommend that clinicians follow the adult guidelines with dosage adjustments for the pediatric population, with the exception that dopamine receptor antagonists should be avoided because of their potential for dystonic reactions.[32] Corticosteroids are often used in combination with SSRIs as prophylaxis for CINV.

For nausea and vomiting associated with pediatric gastroenteritis, there is greater emphasis on rehydration measures than on pharmacologic intervention. Only two prospective studies have been published on the safety or efficacy of antiemetics in pediatric gastroenteritis since 1966.[59,60] A recent survey of physicians revealed that promethazine suppositories were the most commonly prescribed antiemetic for pediatric gastroenteritis, despite the lack of prospective trials for this agent.[61]

PHARMACOECONOMIC CONSIDERATIONS

There are many important variables to consider when attempting to document the overall costs of using a medication in a particular medical situation. Medication costs alone cannot begin to explain the true pharmacoeconomic outcome associated with the use of antiemetic drugs. For example, the costs associated with an unexpected hospital admission because of vomiting after an outpatient surgical procedure quickly offset the savings related to the selection of an inexpensive antiemetic drug. In this and other similar situations, it is economically and clinically important to develop antiemetic protocols based on appropriate decision analysis and clinical outcomes in order to optimize drug product selection. The clinical practice guidelines that have been previously described are valuable tools when developing institution-specific antiemetic protocols. The availability of new, more expensive agents will only increase the costs associated with the prophylaxis of CINV. The need to control antiemetic costs for hospitals is universal and formulary management strategies have been described.[62]

EVALUATION OF THERAPEUTIC OUTCOMES

In accordance with the information presented concerning age and clinical condition, individualized therapy is possible through drug selection and dosage adjustment. Monitoring criteria for drug therapy should include the subjective assessment of the patient's severity of nausea, as well as objective parameters, such as changes in patient weight, the number of vomiting episodes each day, the volume of vomitus lost, and evaluation of fluid, acid-base balance, and electrolyte status, with particular attention to serum sodium, potassium, and chloride concentrations. In addition, evaluation of renal function may become important, particularly in patients with volume contraction and progressive electrolyte disturbances. Specific parameters include daily urine volume, urine specific gravity, and urine electrolyte concentrations. Physical assessment of patients should include evaluation of mucous membranes and skin turgor, because dryness of these tissues may be indicative of significant volume loss.

ABBREVIATIONS

ASCO: American Society of Clinical Oncology
ASHP: American Society of Health-System Pharmacists
CINV: chemotherapy-induced nausea and vomiting
CTZ: chemoreceptor trigger zone
NCCN: National Comprehensive Cancer Network
NK_1: neurokinin$_1$
NVP: nausea and vomiting of pregnancy
PONV: postoperative nausea and vomiting
RINV: radiation-induced nausea and vomiting
SSRI: selective serotonin receptor inhibitor

Review Questions and other resources can be found at *www.pharmacotherapyonline.com.*

REFERENCES

1. Hanson JS, McCallum RW. The diagnosis and management of nausea and vomiting: A review. Am J Gastroenterol 1985;80:210–218.
2. Frytak S, Moertel CG. Management of nausea and vomiting in the cancer patient. JAMA 1981;245:393–396.
3. Lee M. Nausea and vomiting. In: Feldman M, ed. Sleisenger and Fordtran's Gastrointestinal and Liver Disease: Pathophysiology/Diagnosis/Management. St. Louis, Elsevier, 2002:119–130.
4. Montgomery GH, Bovbjerg DH. The development of anticipatory nausea in patients receiving adjuvant chemotherapy for breast cancer. Physiol Behav 1997;61:737–741.
5. Morrow GR, Morrell C. Behavioral treatment for the anticipatory nausea and vomiting induced by cancer chemotherapy. N Engl J Med 1982;307:1476–1480.
6. King CR. Nonpharmacologic management of chemotherapy-induced nausea and vomiting. Oncol Nurs Forum 1997;24:S41–S48.
7. Matteson S, Roscoe J, Hickok J, Morrow GR. The role of behavioral conditioning in the development of nausea. Am J Obstet Gynecol 2002;186:S239–S243.
8. Dutro MP, Amerson AB. Comparison of liquid antacids. N Engl J Med 1980;302:967–971.
9. Fordtran JS, Morawski S, Richardson C. In vitro and in vivo evaluation of antacids. N Engl J Med 1973;288:923–928.
10. Seipler JK, Mahakian K, Trudeau WT. Current concepts in clinical therapeutics: Peptic ulcer disease. Clin Pharm 1986;5:128–142.
11. Strenkoski-Nix L, Ermer J, DeCleene S, et al. Pharmacokinetics of promethazine hydrochloride after administration of rectal suppositories and oral syrup to healthy subjects. Am J Health-Syst Pharm 2000;57:1499–1505.
12. Ernst A, Weiss SJ, Park S, et al. Prochlorperazine versus promethazine for uncomplicated nausea and vomiting in the emergency department: A randomized, double-blind clinical trial. Ann Emerg Med 2000;36:89–94.
13. Critchley P, Plach N, Grantham M, et al. Efficacy of haloperidol in the treatment of nausea and vomiting in the palliative patient: A systematic review. J Pain Symptom Manage 2001;22:631–634.
14. www.fda.gov/medwatch/SAFETY/2001/inapsine.htm
15. Dershwitz M. Droperidol: Should the black box be light gray? J Clin Anesth 2002;14:598–603.
16. Kao LK, Kirk, MA, Evers SJ, Rosenfeld SH. Droperidol, QT prolongation and sudden death: What is the evidence? Ann Emerg Med 2003;41:546–558.
17. Italian Group for Antiemetic Research. Double-blind, dose-finding study of four intravenous doses of dexamethasone in the prevention of cisplatin-induced acute emesis. J Clin Oncol 1998;16:2937–2942.
18. Dexamethasone alone or in combination with ondansetron for the prevention of delayed nausea and vomiting induced by chemotherapy: Italian Group for Antiemetic Research. N Engl J Med 2000;342:1554–1559.
19. De Mulder PH, Seynaeve C, Vermorken JB, et al. Ondansetron compared with high-dose metoclopramide in prophylaxis of acute and delayed cisplatin-induced nausea and vomiting: A multicenter, randomized, double-blind, crossover study. Ann Intern Med 1990;113:834–840.
20. Heron JF, Goedhals L, Jordaan JP, et al. Oral granisetron alone and in combination with dexamethasone: A double-blind randomized comparison against high-dose metoclopramide plus dexamethasone in prevention of cisplatin-induced emesis. Ann Oncol 1994;5:579–584.
21. Chevallier B, Cappelaere P, Splinter T, et al. A double-blind, multicenter comparison of intravenous dolasetron mesylate and metoclopramide in the prevention of nausea and vomiting in cancer patients receiving high-dose cisplatin chemotherapy. Support Care Cancer 1997;5:22–30.
22. Tramer MR, Carroll D, Campbell FA, et al. Cannabinoids for control of chemotherapy induced nausea and vomiting: Quantitative systematic review. BMJ 2001;323:1–8.
23. Stahl SM. The ups and downs of novel antiemetic drugs, Part 1: Substance P, 5-HT, and the neuropharmacology of vomiting. J Clin Psychol 2003;64:498–499.
24. Kris MG, Radford JE, Pizzo BA, et al. Use of a NK-1 receptor antagonist to prevent delayed emesis following cisplatin. J Natl Cancer Inst 1997;89:53–54.
25. Hesketh PJ, Gralla RJ, Webb RT, et al. Randomized phase II study of the neurokinin 1 receptor antagonist CJ-11,974 in the control of cisplatin-induced emesis. J Clin Oncol 1999;17:338–343.

26. Navari RM, Reinhardt RR, Gralla RJ, et al. Reduction of cisplatin-induced emesis by a selective neurokinin-1-receptor antagonist. N Engl J Med 1999;340:190–195.

27. Poli-Bigelli S, Rodrigues-Pereira J, Carides AD, et al. Addition of the neurokinin 1 receptor antagonist aprepitant to standard antiemetic therapy improves control of chemotherapy-induced nausea and vomiting. Results from a randomized, double-blind, placebo-controlled trial in Latin America. Cancer 2003;97:3090–3098.

28. Hesketh PJ, Grunbert SM, Gralla RJ, et al. The oral neurokinin-1 antagonist aprepitant for the prevention of chemotherapy-induced nausea and vomiting: A multinational, randomized, double-blind, placebo-controlled trial in patients receiving high-dose cisplatin—The aprepitant protocol 052 study group. J Clin Oncol 2003;21:4112–4119.

29. Emend [package insert]. Whitehouse Station, NJ, Merck & Co, March 2003.

30. McCrea JB, Majumdar AK, Goldberg MR, et al. Effects of the neurokinin-1 receptor antagonist aprepitant on the pharmacokinetics of dexamethasone and methylprednisolone. Clin Pharmacol Ther 2003;74:17–24.

31. American Society of Health-System Pharmacists (ASHP) Therapeutic Guidelines on the Pharmacologic Management of Nausea and Vomiting in Adult and Pediatric Patients Receiving Chemotherapy or Radiation Therapy or Undergoing Surgery. Am J Health-Syst Pharm 1999;56:729–764.

32. Gralla RJ, Osoba D, Kris MG, et al. Recommendations for the use of antiemetics:evidence-based, clinical practice guidelines. American Society of Clinical Oncology. J Clin Oncol 1999;17:2971–2994.

33. National Comprehensive Cancer Network. Clinical Practice Guidelines in Oncology. Antiemesis Version 2.2003. Available at http://www.nccn.org/professionals/physician_gls/default.asp. Accessed December 1, 2003.

34. Hesketh PJ, Kris MG, Grunberg SM, et al. Proposal for classifying the acute emetogenicity of cancer chemotherapy. J Clin Oncol 1997;15:103–109.

35. Lindley C, Blower P. Oral serotonin type 3-receptor antagonists for prevention of chemotherapy-induced emesis. Am J Health-Syst Pharm 2000;57:1685–1697.

36. Walker PC, Biglin KE, Constance TD, et al. Promoting the use of oral ondansetron in children receiving cancer chemotherapy. Am J Health-Syst Pharm 2001;58:598–602.

37. Aloxi [package insert]. Bloomington, MI, MGI PHARMA Inc., July 2003.

38. Eisenberg P, Figueroa-Vadillo J, Zamora R, et al. Improved prevention of moderately emetogenic chemotherapy-induced nausea and vomiting with palonosetron, a pharmacologically novel 5-HT3 receptor antagonist: Results of a phase III, single-dose trial versus dolasetron. Cancer 2003;98:2473–2482.

39. Gralla R, Lichinitser M, Van Der Vegt S, et al. Palonosetron improves prevention of chemotherapy-induced nausea and vomiting following moderately emetogenic chemotherapy: Results of a double-blind randomized phase III trial comparing single doses of palonosetron with ondansetron. Ann Oncol 2003;14:1570–1577.

40. Gan TJ, Meyer T, Apfel CC, et al. Consensus guidelines for managing postoperative nausea and vomiting. Anesth Analg 2003;97:62–71.

41. Wang JJ, Ho ST, Tzeng JI, Tang CS. The effect of timing of dexamethasone administration on its efficacy as a prophylactic antiemetic for postoperative nausea and vomiting. Anesth Analg 2000;91:136–139.

42. Hill RP, Lubarsky DA, Phillips-Bute B, et al. Cost-effectiveness of prophylactic antiemetic therapy with ondansetron, droperidol or placebo. Anesthesiology 2000;92:958–967.

43. Kranke P, Morin AM, Roewer N, et al. The efficacy and safety of transdermal scopolamine for the prevention of postoperative nausea and vomiting: A quantitative systematic review. Anesth Analg 2002;95:133–143.

44. Bailey PL, Streisand JB, Pace NL, et al. Transdermal scopolamine reduces nausea and vomiting after outpatient laparoscopy. Anesthesiology 1990;72:977–980.

45. Habib AS, Gan TJ. Combination therapy for postoperative nausea and vomiting: A more effective prophylaxis? Ambulatory Surg 2001;9:59–71.

46. Eberhart LH, Morin AM, Bothner U, Georgieff M. Droperidol and 5-HT3-receptor antagonists alone or in combination, for prophylaxis of postoperative nausea and vomiting: A meta-analysis of randomized controlled trials. Acta Anaesthesiol Scand 2000;44:1252–1257.

47. Tramer M, Moore RA, Reynolds DJM, McQuay HJ. A quantitative systematic review of ondansetron in treatment of established postoperative nausea and vomiting. BMJ 1997;314:1088–1092.

48. Kovac AL, O'Connor TA, Pearman MH, et al. Efficacy of repeat intravenous dosing of ondansetron in controlling postoperative nausea and vomiting: A randomized, double-blind, placebo-controlled multicenter trial. J Clin Anesth 1999;11:453–459.

49. Kreisler NS, Spiekermann BF, Ascari CM, et al. Small-dose droperidol effectively reduces nausea in a general surgical adult patient population. Anesth Analg 2000;91:1256–1261.

50. Spitzer TR, Friedman CJ, Bushnell W, et al. Double-blind, randomized, parallel-group study on the efficacy and safety of oral granisetron and oral ondansetron in the prophylaxis of nausea and vomiting in patients receiving hyperfractionated total body irradiation. Bone Marrow Transplant 2000;26:203–210.

51. Dahl E, Offer-Ohlsen D, Lillevold PE, Sandvik L. Transdermal scopolamine, oral meclizine, and placebo in motion sickness. Clin Pharmacol Ther 1984;36:116–120.

52. Schatz M, Petitti D. Antihistamines and pregnancy. Ann Allergy Asthma Immunol 1997;78:157–159.

53. Mazzotta P, Magee LA. A risk-benefit assessment of pharmacological and nonpharmacological treatments for nausea and vomiting of pregnancy. Drugs 2000;59:781–800.

54. Sahakian V, Rouse D, Sipes S, et al. Vitamin B_6 is effective therapy for nausea and vomiting of pregnancy: A randomized, double-blind placebo-controlled study. Obstet Gynecol 1991;78:33–36.

55. Vutyavanich T, Wongtra-ngan S, Ruangsri R. Pyridoxine for nausea and vomiting of pregnancy: A randomized, double-blind, placebo-controlled trial. Am J Obstet Gynecol 1995;173:881–884.

56. Sullivan CA, Johnson CA, Roach H, Martin RW, et al. A pilot study of intravenous ondansetron for hyperemesis gravidarum. Am J Obstet Gynecol 1996;174:1565–1568.

57. Portnoi G, Chng LA, Karimi-Tabesh L, et al. Prospective comparative study of the safety and effectiveness of ginger for the treatment of nausea and vomiting in pregnancy. Am J Obstet Gynecol 2003;189:1374–1377.

58. Quinlan JD, Hill DA. Nausea and vomiting of pregnancy. Am Fam Physician 2003;68:121–128.

59. Ginsburg CM, Clahsen J. Evaluation of trimethobenzamide hydrochloride (Tigan) suppositories for treatment of nausea and vomiting in children. J Pediatr 1980;96:767–769.

60. Cubeddu LX, Trujillo LM, Talmaciu I, et al. Antiemetic activity of ondansetron in acute gastroenteritis. Aliment Pharmacol Ther 1997;11:185–191.

61. Kwon KT, Rudkin SE, Langdorf MI. Antiemetic use in pediatric gastroenteritis: A national survey of emergency physicians, pediatricians, and pediatric emergency physicians. Clin Pediatr 2002;41:641–652.

62. Lucarelli CD. Formulary management strategies for type 3 serotonin receptor antagonists. Am J Health-Syst Pharm 2003;60:S4–S11.

36

DIARRHEA, CONSTIPATION, AND IRRITABLE BOWEL SYNDROME

William J. Spruill and William E. Wade

Learning Objectives and other resources can be found at *www.pharmacotherapyonline.com.*

KEY CONCEPTS

❶ Diarrhea is caused by many viral and bacterial organisms. It is most often a minor discomfort, not life-threatening, and usually self-limited.

❷ The four pathophysiologic mechanisms of diarrhea have been linked to the four broad diarrheal groups, which are secretory, osmotic, exudative, and altered intestinal transit. The three mechanisms by which absorption occurs from the intestines are active transport, diffusion, and solvent drag.

❸ Management of diarrhea focuses on preventing excessive water and electrolyte losses, dietary care, relieving symptoms, treating curable causes, and treating secondary disorders.

❹ Bismuth subsalicylate is marketed for indigestion, relieving abdominal cramps, and controlling diarrhea, including traveler's diarrhea, but contains multiple components that might be toxic if given excessively.

❺ Underlying causes of constipation should be identified when possible and corrective measures taken (e.g., alter-

ation of diet or treatment of diseases such as hypothyroidism).

❻ The foundation of treatment of constipation is dietary fiber or bulk-forming laxatives that provide 10 to 15 g/day of raw fiber.

❼ Irritable bowel syndrome is one of the most common gastrointestinal disorders, and is characterized by lower abdominal pain, disturbed defecation, and bloating. Many nongastrointestinal manifestations also exist with IBS. Recent studies have found that visceral hypersensitivity is a major culprit in the pathophysiology of the disease.

❽ Diarrhea-predominant IBS should be managed by dietary modification and drugs such as loperamide when diet changes alone are insufficient to control symptoms.

❾ Several drug classes are involved in the treatment of the pain associated with IBS, including tricyclic compounds and the gut-selective calcium channel blockers.

DIARRHEA

Diarrhea is a troublesome discomfort that affects most individuals in the United States at some point in their lives. Usually diarrheal episodes begin abruptly and subside within 1 or 2 days without treatment. This chapter focuses primarily on noninfectious diarrhea, with only minor reference to infectious diarrhea (see Chap. 111 on gastrointestinal infections). Diarrhea is often a symptom of a systemic disease and not all possible causes of diarrhea are discussed in this chapter.

To understand diarrhea, one must have a reasonable definition of the condition; unfortunately, the literature is extremely variable on this. Simply put, diarrhea is an increased frequency and decreased consistency of fecal discharge as compared to an individual's normal bowel pattern. Frequency and consistency are variable within and between individuals. For example, some individuals defecate as often as three times per day, whereas others defecate only two or three times per week. A Western diet usually produces a daily stool weighing between 100 and 300 g, depending on the amount of nonabsorbable materials (mainly carbohydrates) consumed. Patients with serious diarrhea may have a daily stool weight in excess of 300 g; however, a

subset of patients experience frequent small, watery passages. Additionally, vegetable fiber-rich diets, such as those consumed in some Eastern cultures such as those in Africa, produce stools weighing more than 300 g/day.

Diarrhea may be associated with a specific disease of the intestines or secondary to a disease outside the intestines. For instance, bacillary dysentery directly affects the gut, whereas diabetes mellitus causes neuropathic diarrheal episodes. Furthermore, diarrhea can be considered as acute or chronic disease. Infectious diarrhea is often acute; diabetic diarrhea is chronic. Whether acute or chronic, diarrhea has the same pathophysiologic causes that help identification of specific treatments.

EPIDEMIOLOGY

The epidemiology of diarrhea varies in developed versus developing countries.[1-3] In the United States, diarrheal illnesses are usually not reported to the Centers for Disease Control and Prevention (CDC) unless associated with an outbreak or an unusual organism or condition. For example, the acquired immune deficiency syndrome (AIDS) has been identified with protracted diarrheal illness. Diarrhea is a major problem in day care centers and nursing homes, probably because early childhood and senescence plus environmental conditions are risk factors. However, an exact epidemiologic profile in the United States is not available through the CDC or published literature.

◀ Viral and bacterial organisms account for most episodes of infectious diarrhea. Common causative bacterial organisms include *Shigella, Salmonella, Campylobacter, Staphylococcus,* and *Escherichia coli.* Food-borne bacterial infection is a major concern, as several major food poisoning episodes have occurred that were traced to poor sanitary conditions in meat-processing plants. Acute viral infections are attributed mostly to the Norwalk and rotavirus groups.

In developing countries, diarrhea is a leading cause of illness and death in children.[4] Moreover, diarrhea produces an economic burden because of costs related to hospitalization and loss of productivity. Approximately 1.3 billion episodes occur annually and 4 million deaths result from diarrhea in these countries. Factors associated with these findings include poor sanitation, poor nutrition, and age less than 5 years. Children in underdeveloped countries experience an average of three episodes of diarrhea each year (e.g., 2.7 diarrhea episodes/person/year in Latin America) as compared to 1 episode/person/year in the United States and Western Europe.

PHYSIOLOGY

In the fasting state, 9 L of fluid enters the proximal small intestine each day. Of this fluid, 2 L are ingested through diet, while the remainder consists of internal secretions. Because of meal content, duodenal chyme is usually hypertonic. When chyme reaches the ileum, the osmolality adjusts to that of plasma, with most dietary fat, carbohydrate, and protein being absorbed. The volume of ileal chyme decreases to about 1 L/day upon entering the colon, which is further reduced by colonic absorption to 100 mL daily. If the small intestine water absorption capacity is exceeded, chyme overloads the colon, resulting in diarrhea. In humans, the colon absorptive capacity is about 5 L daily. Colonic fluid transport is critical to water and electrolyte balance.

Absorption from the intestines back into the blood occurs by three mechanisms: active transport, diffusion, and solvent drag. Active transport and diffusion are the mechanisms of sodium transport. Because of the high luminal sodium concentration (142 mEq/L), sodium diffuses from the sodium-rich gut into epithelial cells, where it is actively pumped into the blood and exchanged with chloride to maintain an isoelectric condition across the epithelial membrane.

Hydrogen ions are transported by an indirect mechanism in the upper small intestine. As sodium is absorbed, hydrogen ions are secreted into the gut. Hydrogen ions then combine with bicarbonate ions to form carbonic acid, which then dissociates into carbon dioxide and water. Carbon dioxide readily diffuses into the blood for expiration through the lung. The water remains in the chyme.

Paracellular pathways are major routes of ion movement. As ions, monosaccharides, and amino acids are actively transported, an osmotic pressure is created, drawing water and electrolytes across the intestinal wall. This pathway accounts for significant amounts of ion transport, especially sodium. Sodium plays an important role in stimulating glucose absorption. Glucose and amino acids are actively transported into the blood via a sodium dependent cotransport mechanism. Cotransport absorption mechanisms of glucose-sodium and amino acid-sodium are extremely important for treating diarrhea.

Gut motility influences absorption and secretion. The amount of time in which luminal content is in contact with the epithelium is under neural and hormonal control. Neurohormonal substances, such as angiotensin, vasopressin, glucocorticoid, and aldosterone, and neurotransmitters also regulate ion transport.

PATHOPHYSIOLOGY

◀ Four general pathophysiologic mechanisms disrupt water and electrolyte balance, leading to diarrhea, and are the basis of diagnosis and therapy. These are (a) a change in active ion transport by either decreased sodium absorption or increased chloride secretion; (b) change in intestinal motility; (c) increase in luminal osmolarity; and (d) increase in tissue hydrostatic pressure. These mechanisms have been related to four broad clinical diarrheal groups: secretory, osmotic, exudative, and altered intestinal transit.

Secretory diarrhea occurs when a stimulating substance either increases secretion or decreases absorption of large amounts of water and electrolytes. Substances that cause excess secretion include vasoactive intestinal peptide (VIP) from a pancreatic tumor, unabsorbed dietary fat in steatorrhea, laxatives, hormones (such as secretin), bacterial toxins, and excessive bile salts. Many of these agents stimulate intracellular cyclic adenosine monophosphate and inhibit Na^+/K^+-ATPase, leading to increased secretion. Also, many of these mediators inhibit ion absorption simultaneously. Clinically, secretory diarrhea is recognized by large stool volumes (>1 L/day) with normal ionic contents and osmolality approximately equal to plasma. Fasting does not alter the stool volume in these patients.

Poorly absorbed substances retain intestinal fluids, resulting in osmotic diarrhea. This process occurs with malabsorption syndromes, lactose intolerance, administration of divalent ions (e.g., magnesium-containing antacids), or consumption of poorly soluble carbohydrate (e.g., lactulose). As a poorly soluble solute is transported, the gut adjusts the osmolality to that of plasma; in so doing, water and electrolytes flux into the lumen. Clinically, osmotic diarrhea is distinguishable from other types, as it ceases if the patient resorts to a fasting state.

Inflammatory diseases of the gastrointestinal tract discharge mucus, serum proteins, and blood into the gut. Sometimes bowel movements consist only of mucus, exudate, and blood. Exudative diarrhea probably affects other absorptive, secretory, or motility functions to account for the large stool volume associated with this disorder.

Altered intestinal motility produces diarrhea by three mechanisms: reduction of contact time in the small intestine, premature emptying of the colon, and bacterial overgrowth. Chyme must be exposed to intestinal epithelium for a sufficient time period to enable normal absorption and secretion processes to occur. If this contact time decreases, diarrhea results. Intestinal resection or bypass surgery and drugs (such as metoclopramide) cause this type of diarrhea. On the other hand, an increased time of exposure allows fecal bacteria overgrowth. A characteristic small intestine diarrheal pattern is rapid, small, coupling bursts of waves. These waves are inefficient, do not allow absorption, and rapidly dump chyme into the colon. Once in the colon, chyme exceeds the colonic capability to absorb water.

ETIOLOGIC EXAMINATION OF THE STOOL

Stool characteristics are important in assessing the etiology of diarrhea. A description of the frequency, volume, consistency, and color provides diagnostic clues. For instance, diarrhea starting in the small intestine produces a copious, watery or fatty (greasy), and foul-smelling stool; contains undigested food particles; and is usually free from gross blood. Colonic diarrhea appears as small, pasty, and sometimes bloody or mucoid movements. Rectal tenesmus with flatus accompanies large intestinal diarrhea.

TABLE 36–1. Clinical Presentation of Diarrhea

General
- Usually, acute diarrheal episodes subside within 72 hours of onset, whereas chronic diarrhea involves frequent attacks over extended time periods.

Signs and symptoms
- Abrupt onset of nausea, vomiting, abdominal pain, headache, fever, chills, and malaise.
- Bowel movements are frequent and never bloody, and diarrhea lasts 12 to 60 hours.
- Intermittent periumbilical or lower right quadrant pain with cramps and audible bowel sounds is characteristic of small intestinal disease.
- When pain is present in large intestinal diarrhea, it is a gripping, aching sensation with tenesmus (straining, ineffective and painful stooling). Pain localizes to the hypogastric region, right or left lower quadrant, or sacral region.
- In chronic diarrhea, a history of previous bouts, weight loss, anorexia, and chronic weakness are important findings.

Physical examination
- Typically demonstrates hyperperistalsis with borborygmi and generalized or local tenderness.

Laboratory tests
- Stool analysis studies include examination for microorganisms, blood, mucus, fat, osmolality, pH, electrolyte and mineral concentration, and cultures.
- Stool test kits are useful for detecting gastrointestinal viruses, particularly rotavirus.
- Antibody serologic testing shows rising titers over a 3- to 6-day period, but this test is not practical and is nonspecific.
- Occasionally, total daily stool volume is also determined.
- Direct endoscopic visualization and biopsy of the colon may be undertaken to assess for the presence of conditions such as colitis or cancer.
- Radiographic studies are helpful in neoplastic and inflammatory conditions.

TABLE 36–2. Drugs Causing Diarrhea

Laxatives
Antacids containing magnesium
Antineoplastics
Auranofin (gold salt)
Antibiotics
   Clindamycin
   Tetracyclines
   Sulfonamides
   Any broad-spectrum antibiotic
Antihypertensives
   Reserpine
   Guanethidine
   Methyldopa
   Guanabenz
   Guanadrel
Cholinergics
   Bethanechol
   Neostigmine
Cardiac agents
   Quinidine
   Digitalis
   Digoxin
Nonsteroidal anti-inflammatory drugs
Prostaglandins
Colchicine

history is extremely important in identifying drug-induced diarrhea. Many agents, including antibiotics and other drugs, cause diarrhea, or less commonly, pseudomembranous colitis. Self-inflicted laxative abuse for weight loss is popular. Neurotic or psychotic behavior leads to laxative abuse. Drug side effects (e.g., quinidine side effects) often present as diarrhea.

Most acute diarrhea is self-limiting, subsiding within 72 hours. However, infants, young children, the elderly, and debilitated persons are at risk for morbid and mortal events in prolonged or voluminous diarrhea. These groups are at risk for water, electrolyte, and acid-base disturbances, and potentially cardiovascular collapse and death. The prognosis for chronic diarrhea depends on the cause; for example, diarrhea secondary to diabetes mellitus waxes and wanes throughout life.

CLINICAL PRESENTATION

Table 36–1 outlines the clinical presentation of diarrhea while Table 36–2 shows common drug-induced causes of diarrhea. A medication

▶ **TREATMENT: Diarrhea**

▇ PREVENTION

Acute viral diarrheal illness often occurs in day care centers and nursing homes. As person-to-person contact is the mechanism by which viral disease spreads, isolation techniques must be initiated. For bacterial, parasite, and protozoal infections, strict food handling, sanitation, water, and other environmental hygiene practices can prevent transmission. If diarrhea is secondary to another illness, controlling the primary condition is necessary. Antibiotics and bismuth subsalicylate are advocated to prevent traveler's diarrhea, in conjunction with treatment of drinking water and caution with consumption of fresh vegetables.

▇ DESIRED OUTCOME

◀ If prevention is not successful and diarrhea occurs, therapeutic goals are to (a) manage the diet;(b) prevent excessive water, elec-

trolyte, and acid-base disturbances; (c) provide symptomatic relief; (d) treat curable causes; and (e) manage secondary disorders causing diarrhea (Figs. 36–1 and 36–2).

Clinicians must clearly understand that diarrhea, like a cough, may be a body defense mechanism for ridding itself of harmful substances or pathogens. The correct therapeutic response is not necessarily to stop diarrhea at all costs.

▇ NONPHARMACOLOGIC MANAGEMENT

Dietary management is a first priority in the treatment of diarrhea. Most clinicians recommend discontinuing consumption of solid foods and dairy products for 24 hours. However, fasting is of questionable value, as this treatment modality has not been extensively studied. In osmotic diarrhea, these maneuvers control the problem. If the mechanism is secretory, diarrhea persists. For patients experiencing

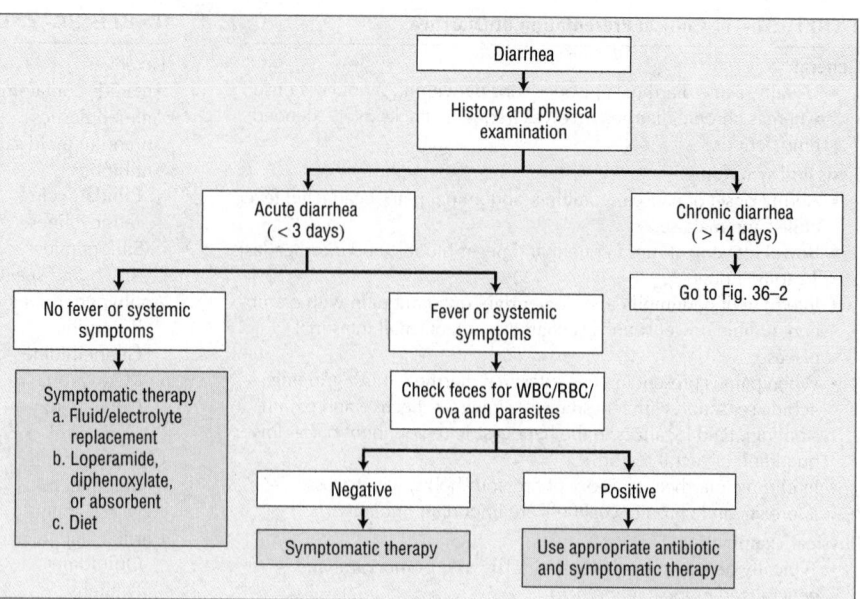

FIGURE 36–1. Recommendations for treating acute diarrhea. Follow these steps: (1) Perform a complete history and physical examination. (2) Is the diarrhea acute or chronic? If chronic diarrhea, go to Fig. 36–2. (3) If acute diarrhea, check for fever and/or systemic signs and symptoms (i.e., toxic patient). If systemic illness (fever, anorexia, or volume depletion), check for an infectious source. If positive for infectious diarrhea, use appropriate antibiotic/anthelmintic drug and symptomatic therapy. If negative for infectious cause, use only symptomatic treatment. (4) If no systemic findings, then use symptomatic therapy based on severity of volume depletion, oral or parenteral fluid/electrolytes, antidiarrheal agents (see Table 36–4), and diet.

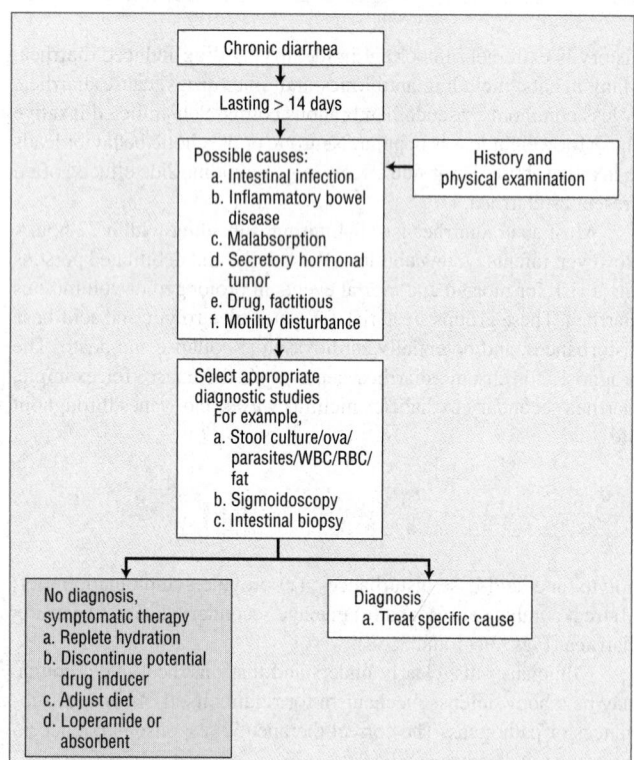

FIGURE 36–2. Recommendations for treating chronic diarrhea. Follow these steps: (1) Perform a careful history and physical examination. (2) The possible causes of chronic diarrhea are many. These can be classified into intestinal infections (bacterial or protozoal), inflammatory disease (Crohn's disease or ulcerative colitis), malabsorption (lactose intolerance), secretory hormonal tumor (intestinal carcinoid tumor or VIPoma), drug (antacid), factitious (laxative abuse), or motility disturbance (diabetes mellitus, irritable bowel syndrome, or hyperthyroidism). (3) If the diagnosis is uncertain, selected appropriate diagnostic studies should be ordered. (4) Once diagnosed, treatment is planned for the underlying cause with symptomatic antidiarrheal therapy. (5) If no specific cause can be identified, symptomatic therapy is prescribed.

nausea and/or vomiting, a mild, digestible low-residue diet should be administered for 24 hours. If vomiting is present and uncontrollable with antiemetics (see Chap. 35 on nausea and vomiting), nothing is taken by mouth. As bowel movements decrease, a bland diet is begun.

Feeding should continue in children with acute bacterial diarrhea. Fed children have less morbidity and mortality, whether or not they receive oral rehydration fluids. Studies are not available in the elderly or in other high-risk groups to determine the value of continued feeding in bacterial diarrhea.

■ WATER AND ELECTROLYTES

Rehydration and maintenance of water and electrolytes are primary treatment goals until the diarrheal episode ends. If the patient is volume depleted, rehydration should be directed at replacing water and electrolytes to normal body composition. Then water and electrolyte composition are maintained by replacing losses. Many patients will not develop volume depletion and therefore will only require maintenance fluid and electrolyte therapy. Parenteral and enteral routes may be used for supplying water and electrolytes. If vomiting and dehydration are not severe, enteral feeding is the less costly and preferred method. In the United States, many commercial oral rehydration preparations are available (Table 36–3).

Because of concerns about hypernatremia, physicians continue to hospitalize and intravenously correct fluid and electrolyte deficits in severe dehydration. Oral solutions are strongly recommended.[5,6] In developing countries, the World Health Organization Oral Rehydration Solution (WHO-ORS) saves the lives of millions of children annually.

During diarrhea, the small intestine retains its ability to actively transport monosaccharides such as glucose. Glucose actively carries sodium with water and other electrolytes. Because the WHO-ORS has a high sodium concentration, U.S. physicians have been reluctant to use it in well-nourished children. Yet controlled comparative studies describe more favorable results with the WHO-ORS than with parenteral fluids.[7] Amino acids promote sodium transport and act as

TABLE 36–3. Oral Rehydration Solutions

	WHO-ORS[a]	Pedialyte[b] (Ross)	Rehydralyte[b] (Ross)	Infalyte (Mead Johnson)	Resol[b] (Wyeth)
Osmolality (mOsm/L)	333	249	304	200	269
Carbohydrates[b] (g/L)	20	25	25	30[c]	20
Calories (cal/L)	85	100	100	126	80
Electrolytes (mEq/L)					
Sodium	90	45	75	50	50
Potassium	20	20	20	25	20
Chloride	80	35	65	45	50
Citrate	—	30	30	34	34
Bicarbonate	30	—	—	—	—
Calcium	—	—	—	—	4
Magnesium	—	—	—	—	4
Sulfate	—	—	—	—	—
Phosphate	—	—	—	—	5

[a]World Health Organization Oral Rehydration Solution.
[b]Carbohydrate is glucose.
[c]Rice syrup solids are carbohydrate source.

an antisecretory agent. Researchers have added glycine to ORS in an attempt to create a "super-ORS." Reports, however, are disappointing, because glycine causes an osmotic diarrhea and diuresis in experimental concentrations.

Rice-based oral solution is a hyposmotically active substrate that elutes glucose without increasing stool or urine outflows. Pizarro and associates[7] reported effective rehydration of infants with acute diarrhea using a rice-based solution. They also reported decreased stool output and greater absorption and retention of fluid and electrolytes. In summary, oral rehydration solution is a lifesaving treatment for millions afflicted in developing countries. Acceptance in developed countries is less enthusiastic; however, the advantage of this product in reducing hospitalizations may prove its use as a cost-effective alternative, saving millions of dollars in health care expenditures.

PHARMACOLOGIC THERAPY

Various drugs have been used to treat diarrheal attacks (Table 36–4). These drugs are grouped into several categories: antimotility, adsorbents, antisecretory compounds, antibiotics, enzymes, and intestinal microflora. Usually these drugs are not curative but palliative.

OPIATES AND THEIR DERIVATIVES

Opiates and opioid derivatives (a) delay the transit of intraluminal contents or (b) increase gut capacity, prolonging contact and absorption. Enkephalins, endogenous opioid substances, regulate fluid movement across the mucosa by stimulating absorptive processes. Limitations to the use of opiates include an addiction potential (a real concern with long-term use) and worsening of diarrhea in selected infectious diarrhea.

Most opiates act through peripheral and central mechanisms with the exception of loperamide, which acts only peripherally. Loperamide is antisecretory; it inhibits the calcium-binding protein calmodulin, controlling chloride secretion. Loperamide, available as 2-mg capsules or 1 mg/5 mL solution (both are nonprescription

products), is suggested for managing acute and chronic diarrhea. The usual adult dose is initially 4 mg orally, followed by 2 mg after each loose stool, up to 16 mg/day. Used correctly, this agent has rare side effects such as dizziness and constipation. If the diarrhea is concurrent with a high fever or bloody stool, the patient should be referred to a physician. Also, diarrhea lasting 48 hours beyond initiating loperamide warrants medical attention. Loperamide can also be used in traveler's diarrhea. It is comparable to bismuth subsalicylate for treatment of this disorder.[8]

Diphenoxylate is available as 2.5-mg tablets and as a 2.5 mg/5 mL solution. A small amount of atropine (0.025 mg) is included to discourage abuse. In adults, when taken as 2.5 to 5 mg three or four times daily, not to exceed a 20-mg total daily dose, diphenoxylate is rarely toxic. Some patients may complain of atropinism (blurred vision, dry mouth, and urinary hesitancy). Like loperamide, it should not be used in patients at risk of bacterial enteritis with *Escherichia coli, Shigella,* or *Salmonella.*

Difenoxin, a diphenoxylate derivative, is also combined with atropine and has the same uses, precautions, and side effects. Marketed as 1-mg tablet, the adult dosage is 2 mg initially followed by 1 mg after each loose stool, not to exceed 8 mg/day.

Paregoric, tincture of opium, is marketed as a 2 mg/5 mL solution and is indicated for managing both acute and chronic diarrhea. It is not widely prescribed today because of its abuse potential.

ADSORBENTS

Adsorbents are used for symptomatic relief. These products, many not requiring a prescription, are nontoxic, but their effectiveness remains unproven. Adsorbents are nonspecific in their action; they adsorb nutrients, toxins, drugs, and digestive juices. Coadministration with other drugs reduces their bioavailability. The Food and Drug Administration over-the-counter review panel recommends only polycarbophil as an effective adsorbent.

Polycarbophil absorbs 60 times its weight in water and can be used to treat both diarrhea and constipation. It is a nonprescription product and is sold as 500-mg chewable tablets. This hydrophilic nonabsorbable product is safe and may be taken four times daily, up to 6 g/day in adults.

TABLE 36–4. Selected Antidiarrheal Preparations

	Dose Form	Adult Dose
Antimotility		
Diphenoxylate	2.5 mg/tablet	5 mg four times daily; do not exceed 20 mg/day
	2.5 mg/5 mL	
Loperamide	2 mg/capsule	Initially 4 mg, then 2 mg after each loose stool; do not exceed 16 mg/day
	1 mg/5 mL	
Paregoric	2 mg/5 mL (morphine)	5–10 mL 1–4 times daily
Opium tincture	5 mg/mL (morphine)	0.6 mL four times daily
Difenoxin	1 mg/tablet	Two tablets, then one tablet after each loose stool; up to 8 tablets/day
Adsorbents		
Kaolin–pectin mixture	5.7 g kaolin + 130.2 mg pectin/30 mL	30–120 mL after each loose stool
Polycarbophil	500 mg/tablet	Chew 2 tablets four times daily or after each loose stool; do not exceed 12 tablets/day
Attapulgite	750 mg/15 mL	1200–1500 mg after each loose bowel movement or every 2 hours; up to 9000 mg/day
	300 mg/7.5 mL	
	750 mg/tablet	
	600 mg/tablet	
	300 mg/tablet	
Antisecretory		
Bismuth subsalicylate	1050 mg/30 mL	Two tablets or 30 mL every 30 min to 1 h as needed up to 8 doses/day
	262 mg/15 mL	
	524 mg/15 mL	
	262 mg/tablet	
Enzymes (lactase)	1250 neutral lactase units/4 drops	3–4 drops taken with milk or dairy product
	3300 FCC lactase units per tablet	1 or 2 tablets as above
Bacterial replacement (*Lactobacillus acidophilus, Lactobacillus bulgaricus*)		2 tablets or 1 granule packet 3 to 4 times daily; give with milk, juice, or water
Octreotide	0.05 mg/mL	Initial: 50 mcg subcutaneously
	0.1 mg/mL	1–2 times per day and titrate dose based on indication up to 600 mcg/day in 2–4 divided doses
	0.5 mg/mL	

ANTISECRETORY AGENTS

Bismuth subsalicylate appears to have antisecretory, antiinflammatory, and antibacterial effects. As a nonprescription product, it is marketed for indigestion, relieving abdominal cramps, and controlling diarrhea, including traveler's diarrhea. Bismuth subsalicylate dosage strengths are 262-mg chewable tablets, 262 mg/5 mL liquid, and 524 mg/15 mL liquid. The usual adult dose is 2 tablets or 30 mL every 30 minutes to 1 hour up to 8 doses per day.

Bismuth subsalicylate contains multiple components that might be toxic if given excessively to prevent or treat diarrhea. For instance, an active ingredient is salicylate, which may interact with anticoagulants or may produce salicylism (tinnitus, nausea, and vomiting). Bismuth reduces tetracycline absorption and may interfere with select gastrointestinal radiographic studies. Patients may complain of a darkening of the tongue and stools with repeat administration. Salicylate can induce gout attacks in susceptible individuals.

Bismuth subsalicylate suspension has been evaluated in the treatment of secretory diarrhea of infectious etiology as well. In a dose of 30 mL every 30 minutes for eight doses, unformed stools decrease in the first 24 hours. Bismuth subsalicylate may also be effective in preventing traveler's diarrhea.

Octreotide, a synthetic octapeptide analog of endogenous somatostatin, is prescribed for the symptomatic treatment of carcinoid tumors and vasoactive intestinal peptide–secreting tumors (VIPomas).[9] Metastatic intestinal carcinoid tumors secrete excessive amounts of vasoactive substances, including histamine, bradykinin, serotonin, and prostaglandins. Primary carcinoid tumors occur throughout the gastrointestinal tract, with most in the ileum. Predominant signs and symptoms experienced by patients with these tumors are attributable to excessive concentrations of 5-hydroxytryptophan and serotonin. The totality of their clinical effects is termed the *carcinoid syndrome*. Paroxysmal vasomotor attacks characterize carcinoid syndrome, most notably sudden red to purple flushing of the face and neck. These attacks are often caused by emotional outbursts or by ingestion of food or alcohol. Some patients have a violent, watery diarrhea with abdominal cramping. Initially, diarrhea might be managed with various agents such as codeine, diphenoxylate, cyproheptadine, methysergide, phenoxybenzamine, or methyldopa. Recently, octreotide has become the drug of choice.

Octreotide blocks the release of serotonin and many other active peptides and has been effective in controlling diarrhea and flushing. It is reported to have direct inhibitory effects on intestinal secretion and stimulatory effects on intestinal absorption. Non–gastrin-secreting adenomas of the pancreas are tumors associated with profuse watery diarrhea. This condition has been referred to as Verner-Morrison syndrome, WDHA (watery diarrhea, hypokalemia, and achlorhydria) syndrome, pancreatic cholera, watery diarrhea syndrome, and VIPoma. Excessive secretion of VIP from a retroperitoneal or pancreatic tumor produces most of the clinical features. Excessive VIP is isolated in about half of patients, along with numerous other peptide hormones (peptide histidine methionine [PHM], serotonin, somatostatin, gastrin, and glucagon). Surgical tumor dissection is the treatment of choice. In nonsurgical candidates, the profuse watery diarrhea and other symptoms commonly encountered are managed with octreotide.

The dose of octreotide varies with the indication, disease severity, and patient response.[9] For managing diarrhea and flushing associated with carcinoid tumors in adults, the initial dosage range is 100 to 600 mcg/day in two to four divided doses subcutaneously for 2 weeks. For controlling secretory diarrhea of VIPomas, the dosage range is 200 to 300 mcg/day in two to four divided doses for 2 weeks. Some patients may require higher doses for symptomatic control. Patients responding to these initial doses may be switched to Sandostatin LAR Depot, a long-acting octreotide formulation. This product consists of microspheres containing the drug. Initial doses consist of 20 mg given intramuscularly intragluteally at 4-week intervals for 2 months. It is recommended that during the first 2 weeks of therapy the short-acting formulation also be administered subcutaneously. At the end of 2 months, patients with good symptom control may have the dose reduced to 10 mg every 4 weeks, while those without sufficient symptom control may have the dose increased to 30 mg every 4 weeks. For patients experiencing recurrence of symptoms on the 10-mg dose, dosage adjustment to 20 mg should be made. It is not uncommon for patients with carcinoid tumors or VIPomas to experience periodic exacerbation of symptoms. Subcutaneous octreotide for several days should be reinstituted in these individuals. In so-called carcinoid crisis, octreotide is given as an intravenous infusion at 50 mcg/h for 8 to 24 hours.

Because octreotide inhibits many other gastrointestinal hormones, it has a variety of intestinal side effects. With prolonged use, gallbladder and biliary tract complications such as cholelithiasis have been reported. About 5% to 10% of patients complain of nausea, diarrhea, and abdominal pain. Local injection pain occurs with about an 8% incidence. With high doses, octreotide may reduce dietary fat absorption, leading to steatorrhea.

Two other somatostatin analogs, lanreotide and vapreotide, have been studied.[10] Lanreotide is indicated for patients with carcinoid tumors in a dose of 30 mg intramuscularly (as a depot) every 14 days. If necessary the dose can be increased to 30 mg intramuscular every 7 to 10 days. Vapreotide is an orphan drug that is indicated for pancreatic and gastrointestinal fistulas.

MISCELLANEOUS PRODUCTS

Lactobacillus preparations replace colonic microflora. This supposedly restores normal intestinal function and suppresses the growth of pathogenic microorganisms. However, a dairy product diet containing 200 to 400 g of lactose or dextrin is equally effective in producing recolonization of normal flora. The dosage varies depending on the brand used and lactobacillus preparations should be administered with milk, juice, water, or cereal. Intestinal flatus is the primary patient complaint experienced with this modality.

Anticholinergic drugs such as atropine block vagal tone and prolong gut transit time. Drugs with anticholinergic properties are present in many nonprescription products. Their value in controlling diarrhea is questionable and limited due to side effects. To stop diarrhea, clinicians have been falsely taught to dose anticholinergics until they decrease salivary and sweat secretion. Angle-closure glaucoma, selected heart diseases, and obstructive uropathies are relative contraindications to the use of anticholinergic agents.

Lactase enzyme products are helpful for patients experiencing diarrhea secondary to lactose intolerance. Lactase is required for

carbohydrate digestion. When a patient lacks this enzyme, eating dairy products causes an osmotic diarrhea. Several products are available for use each time a dairy product, especially milk or ice cream, is consumed.

CLINICAL CONTROVERSY

Long-term use of oral opiates is not routinely recommended for several pharmacologic reasons. Some opioids such as morphine and codeine have the tendency to cause constipation by slowing down the peristaltic action of the bowels, which can also result in a functional ileus. This effect can be minimized by administering laxatives and/or stool softeners in patients who require longer-term opiate therapy. Prokinetic agents may also be helpful in treating opiate-related constipation.

INVESTIGATIONAL DRUGS

Many experimental drugs have been used to control diarrhea. Phenothiazines, β-blockers, nonsteroidal anti-inflammatory drugs, calcium channel blockers, and α-adrenergic agonists are only a few agents under investigation in either animals or humans. Nifalatide is an enkephalin analog that delays the onset of castor oil–induced diarrhea and decreases stool frequency. Dizziness and dry mouth are frequent side effects. Enkephalinase inhibitors (e.g., acetorphan or racecadotril) are other therapeutic options that reduce hypersecretion of water and electrolytes into the intestinal lumen. Prostaglandin inhibitors, aspirin and its analogs, and indomethacin are safe and effective in childhood gastroenteritis; studies in animals support indomethacin use in enteropathogen secretory states such as *Vibrio cholerae* infection.

Vaccines are a new therapeutic frontier in controlling infectious diarrheas, especially in developing countries.[11,12] Cholera vaccine, which is available in the United States in the parenteral form of whole-cell inactivated bacteria, yields some protection but is not totally effective and does not prevent transmission. However, live oral vaccine is thought to be protective against *V. cholerae*. Oral *Shigella* vaccine, although effective under field conditions, requires five doses and repeat booster doses, thereby limiting its practicality for use in developing nations. With about 1,500 serotypes for *Salmonella*, a vaccine is not currently available. There are three parenteral typhoid vaccine formulations available in the United States. In addition, an oral vaccine of *S. typhi* (Tyza) is now available and is administered in 4 doses on days 1, 3, 5, and 7, to be completed at least 1 week before exposure. Rotavirus vaccine is effective in infants and children, and is administered as a three–oral dose sequence.

EVALUATION OF THERAPEUTIC OUTCOMES

GENERAL OUTCOMES MEASURES

Therapeutic outcomes are directed toward key symptoms, signs, and laboratory studies. Constitutional symptoms usually improve within 24 to 72 hours. Monitoring for changes in the frequency and character of bowel movements on a daily basis in conjunction with vital signs and improvement in appetite are of utmost importance. Also, the clinician needs to monitor body weight, serum osmolality, serum electrolytes, complete blood cell counts, urinalysis, and culture results (if appropriate).

ACUTE DIARRHEA

Most patients with acute diarrhea experience mild to moderate distress. In the absence of moderate to severe dehydration, high fever, and blood or mucus in the stool, this illness is usually self-limiting within 3 to 7 days. Mild to moderate acute diarrhea is usually managed on an outpatient basis with oral rehydration, symptomatic treatment, and diet. Elderly persons with chronic illness and infants may require hospitalization for parenteral rehydration and close monitoring.

SEVERE DIARRHEA

In the urgent/emergent situation, restoration of the patient's volume status is the most important outcome. Toxic patients (fever, dehydration, hematochezia, or hypotension) require hospitalization, intravenous fluids and electrolyte administration, and empiric antibiotic therapy while awaiting culture and sensitivity results. With timely management, these patients usually recover within a few days.

CONSTIPATION

Constipation is a commonly encountered medical condition in the United States for which many patients initiate self-treatment. One reason constipation continues to be a frequent problem in this country is lack of adequate dietary fiber. Another unfortunate problem is that many people have misconceptions about normal bowel function, and think that daily bowel movements are required for health and well being. Others believe that the lack of a daily bowel movement contributes to the accumulation of toxic substances or is associated with various somatic complaints. These misconceptions often lead to the inappropriate use of laxatives by the general public.

Constipation does not have a single, generally agreed upon definition. When using the term, the lay public or health care professional may be referring to several difficult-to-quantify variables: bowel movement frequency, stool size or consistency, and such symptoms as the sensation of incomplete defecation. Stool frequency is most often used to describe constipation; however, the frequency of bowel movements used to define constipation is not well established.

Normal people pass at least three stools per week. Some of the definitions of constipation used in clinical studies include (a) less than three stools per week for women and five stools per week for men despite a high-residue diet, or a period of more than 3 days without a bowel movement; (b) straining at stool greater than 25% of the time and/or two or fewer stools per week; or (c) straining at defecation and less than one stool daily with minimal effort. These varying definitions demonstrate the difficulty in characterizing this problem.

An international committee defined and classified constipation on the basis of stool frequency, consistency, and difficulty of defecation.[13,14] Functional constipation is defined as two or more of the following complaints present for at least 12 months in the absence of laxative use: (a) straining at least 25% of the time; (b) lumpy or hard stools at least 25% of the time; (c) a feeling of incomplete evacuation at least 25% of the time; or (d) two or fewer bowel movements in a week. Rectal outlet delay is defined as anal blockage more than 25% of the time and prolonged defecation or manual disimpaction when necessary.

EPIDEMIOLOGY

As many as 40% of patients older than 65 years of age report experiencing constipation.[15] The results from 42,375 participants of the National Health Interview Survey on Digestive Disorders demonstrated that there is not an age-related increased incidence of infrequent bowel movements; however, there is an age-related increased incidence of laxative use.[16] The frequency of subjects reporting two or fewer bowel movements per week was 5.9% for those younger than 40 years of age; 3.8% for subjects 60 to 69 years of age; and 6.3% for subjects older than 80 years of age. In a prospective study of 3166 people

older than 65 years of age in a Florida community,[17] 26% of women and 15.8% of men reported recurrent constipation. Factors found to correlate with self-reported constipation were age, sex (higher frequency in females), total number of drugs taken, abdominal pain, and hemorrhoids.

PATHOPHYSIOLOGY

Constipation is not a disease, but a symptom of an underlying disease or problem. Approaches to the treatment of constipation should begin with attempts to determine its cause. Disorders of the GI tract (irritable bowel syndrome or diverticulitis), metabolic disorders (diabetes), or endocrine disorders (hypothyroidism) may be involved. Constipation commonly results from a diet low in fiber or from use of constipating drugs such as opiates. Finally, it is believed that constipation may sometimes be psychogenic in origin.[18] Each of these causes is discussed in the following sections.

Constipation is a frequently reported problem in the elderly, probably the result of improper diets (low in fiber and liquids), diminished abdominal wall muscular strength, and possibly diminished physical activity. However, as previously stated, the frequency of bowel movements is not decreased with normal aging. In addition, diseases that may cause constipation, such as colon cancer and diverticulitis, are more common with increasing age. Table 36–5 lists common causes of constipation in specific disease states.

DRUG-INDUCED CONSTIPATION

Use of drugs that inhibit the neurologic or muscular function of the GI tract, particularly the colon, may result in constipation (Table 36–6). The majority of cases of drug-induced constipation are caused by opiates, various agents with anticholinergic properties, and antacids containing aluminum or calcium. With most of the agents listed in Table 36–6, the inhibitory effects on bowel function are dose dependent, with larger doses clearly causing constipation more frequently.

Opiates have effects on all segments of the bowel, but effects are most pronounced on the colon. The major mechanism by which opiates produce constipation has been proposed to be prolongation of intestinal transit time by causing spastic, nonpropulsive contractions. An additional contributory mechanism may be an increase in electrolyte absorption.

All opiate derivatives are associated with constipation, but the degree of intestinal inhibitory effects seems to differ between agents. Orally administered opiates appear to have greater inhibitory effects than parenterally administered products. Orally administered enkephalins (endogenous opiate-like polypeptides) are recognized to have antimotility properties.

TABLE 36–5. Possible Causes of Constipation

Conditions	Possible Causes
GI disorders	Irritable bowel syndrome
	Diverticulitis
	Upper GI tract diseases
	Anal and rectal diseases
	Hemorrhoids
	Anal fissures
	Ulcerative proctitis
	Tumors
	Hernia
	Volvulus of the bowel
	Syphilis
	Tuberculosis
	Helminthic infections
	Lymphogranuloma venereum
	Hirschsprung's disease
Metabolic and endocrine disorders	Diabetes mellitus with neuropathy
	Hypothyroidism
	Panhypopituitarism
	Pheochromocytoma
	Hypercalcemia
	Enteric glucagon excess
Pregnancy	Depressed gut motility
	Increased fluid absorption from colon
	Decreased physical activity
	Dietary changes
	Inadequate fluid intake
	Low dietary fiber
	Use of iron salts
Neurogenic causes	CNS diseases
	Trauma to the brain (particularly the medulla)
	Spinal cord injury
	CNS tumors
	Cerebrovascular accidents
	Parkinson's disease
Psychogenic causes	Ignoring or postponing urge to defecate
	Psychiatric diseases
Drug-induced	See Table 36–6

TABLE 36–6. Drugs Causing Constipation

Analgesics
    Inhibitors of prostaglandin synthesis
    Opiates
Anticholinergics
    Antihistamines
    Antiparkinsonian agents (e.g., benztropine or trihexaphenidyl)
    Phenothiazines
    Tricyclic antidepressants
Antacids containing calcium carbonate or aluminum hydroxide
Barium sulfate
Calcium channel blockers
Clonidine
Diuretics (non–potassium-sparing)
Ganglionic blockers
Iron preparations
Muscle blockers (D-tubocurarine, succinylcholine)
Nonsteroidal anti-inflammatory agents
Polystyrene sodium sulfonate

TABLE 36–7. Clinical Presentation of Constipation

Signs and symptoms
- It is important to ascertain whether the patient perceives the problem as infrequent bowel movements, stools of insufficient size, a feeling of fullness, or difficulty and pain on passing stool.
- Signs and symptoms include hard, small or dry stools, bloated stomach, cramping abdominal pain and discomfort, straining or grunting, sensation of blockade, fatigue, headache, and nausea and vomiting.

Laboratory tests
- A series of examinations, including proctoscopy, sigmoidoscopy, colonoscopy, or barium enema, may be necessary to determine the presence of colorectal pathology.
- Thyroid function studies may be performed to determine the presence of metabolic or endocrine disorders.
- With laxative abuse, fluid and electrolyte imbalances (most commonly hypokalemia), protein-losing gastroenteropathy with hypoalbuminemia may be present.

Agents with anticholinergic properties inhibit bowel function by parasympatholytic actions on innervation to many regions of the GI tract, particularly the colon and rectum. Many types of drugs possess anticholinergic action, and these agents are used commonly in both hospitalized and nonhospitalized patients. One study demonstrated that amitriptyline, diphenhydramine, and thioridazine use were associated with laxative needs in 800 nursing home patients.[15]

In patients older than 65 years of age, drugs that correlate most often with constipation are anticholinergics, aspirin, furosemide, ni- troglycerin, and amitriptyline.[22] Serum chloride and aspartate amino- transferase, as well as alcohol consumption, are negatively related to constipation.

CLINICAL PRESENTATION

Table 36–7 shows the general clinical presentation of constipation.

▶ TREATMENT: Constipation

▬ GENERAL APPROACH TO TREATMENT

The patient should be asked about the frequency of bowel movements and the chronicity of constipation. Constipation occurring recently in an adult may indicate significant colon pathology such as malignancy; constipation present since early infancy may be indicative of neuro- logic disorders. The patient also should be carefully questioned about usual diet and laxative regimens. Does the patient have a diet con- sistently deficient in high-fiber items and containing mainly highly refined foods? What laxatives or cathartics has the patient used to at- tempt relief of constipation? The patient should be questioned about other concurrent medications, with interest focused on agents that might cause constipation.

For most patients complaining of constipation, a thorough phys- ical examination is not required after it is established that constipation

TABLE 36–8. Constipation Treatment Algorithm

History
- Stool frequency
- Stool consistency
- Difficulty of defecation

Possible causes
- Diet deficient in high-fiber items and consisting mainly of highly refined foods
- GI disorders
- Metabolic and endocrine disorders
- Pregnancy
- Neurogenic
- Psychogenic
- Drug-Induced
- Laxative abusers

Symptoms seen with chronic constipation
- Fluid and electrolyte imbalances (hypokalemia)
- Protein-losing gastroenteropathy with hypoalbuminemia
- Syndromes resembling colitis

Select appropriate diagnostic studies
- Protoscopy
- Sigmoidoscopy
- Colonoscopy
- Barium enema

Diagnosis
1. Treat specific cause
2. No diagnosis, symptomatic therapy
   A. Bulk-forming agents
   B. Dietary modification
   C. Alter lifestyle (exercise)
   D. Increase fluid intake
   E. Discontinue potential drug inducer

(a) is not a chronic problem, (b) is not accompanied by signs of significant GI disease (e.g., rectal bleeding or anemia), and (c) does not cause severe discomfort. In these circumstances, the patient may be referred directly to the first-line therapies for constipation described in the next section (mainly bulk-forming laxatives and dietary fiber with occasional use of saline or stimulant laxatives). Table 36–8 presents a general treatment algorithm for the management of constipation.

The proper management of constipation requires a number of different modalities; however, the basis for therapy should be dietary modification. The major dietary change should be an increase in the amount of fiber consumed daily. In addition to dietary management, patients should be encouraged to alter other aspects of their lifestyles if necessary. Important considerations are to encourage patients to exercise (achieved even by brisk walking after dinner) and to adjust bowel habits so that a regular and adequate time is made to respond to the urge to defecate. Another general measure is to increase fluid intake. This is generally recommended and believed beneficial, although there is little objective evidence to support this measure.

If an underlying disease is recognized as the cause of constipation, attempts should be made to correct it. GI malignancies may be removed via surgical resection. Endocrine and metabolic derangements should be corrected by the appropriate methods. For example, when hypothyroidism is the cause of constipation, cautious institution of thyroid-replacement therapy is the most important treatment measure.

As discussed earlier, many drug substances may cause constipation. If a patient is consuming medications well known to cause constipation, consideration should be given to alternative agents. For some medications (e.g., antacids), nonconstipating alternatives exist. If no reasonable alternatives exist to the medication thought to be responsible for constipation, consideration should be given to lowering the dose. If a patient must remain on constipating medications, then more attention must be given to general measures for prevention of constipation, as discussed in the next section.

NONPHARMACOLOGIC THERAPY

DIETARY MODIFICATION AND BULK-FORMING AGENTS

The most important aspect of therapy for constipation for the majority of patients is dietary modification to increase the amount of fiber consumed. Fiber, the portion of vegetable matter not digested in the human GI tract, increases stool bulk, retention of stool water, and rate of transit of stool through the intestine. The result of fiber therapy is an increased frequency of defecation. Also, fiber decreases intraluminal pressures in the colon and rectum, which is thought to be beneficial for diverticular disease and for irritable bowel syndrome. The specific physiologic effects of fiber are not well understood. Patients should be advised to include at least 10 g of crude fiber in their daily diets.[19] Fruits, vegetables, and cereals have the highest fiber content. Bran, a by-product of milling of wheat, is often added to foods to increase fiber content. Raw bran is generally 40% fiber. Medicinal products, often called "bulk-forming agents," such as psyllium hydrophilic colloids, methylcellulose, or polycarbophil, have properties similar to those of dietary fiber and may be taken as tablets, powders, or granules (Table 36–9). A trial of dietary modification with high-fiber content should be continued for at least 1 month before effects on bowel function are determined. Most patients begin to notice effects on bowel

TABLE 36–9. Dosage Recommendations for Laxatives and Cathartics

Agent	Recommended Dose
Agents that cause softening of feces in 1–3 days	
Bulk-forming agents	
Methylcellulose	4–6 g/day
Polycarbophil	4–6 g/day
Psyllium	Varies with product
Emollients	
Docusate sodium	50–360 mg/day
Docusate calcium	50–360 mg/day
Docusate potassium	100–300 mg/day
Lactulose	15–30 mL orally
Sorbitol	30–50 g/day orally
Mineral oil	15–30 mL orally
Agents that result in soft or semifluid stool in 6–12 h	
Bisacodyl (oral)	5–15 mg orally
Phenolphthalein	30–270 mg orally
Cascara sagrada	Dose varies with formulation
Senna	Dose varies with formulation
Magnesium sulfate (low dose)	<10 g orally
Agents that cause watery evacuation in 1–6 h	
Magnesium citrate	18 g 300 mL water
Magnesium hydroxide	2.4–4.8 g orally
Magnesium sulfate (high dose)	10–30 g orally
Sodium phosphates	Varies with salt used
Bisacodyl	10 mg rectally
Polyethylene glycol-electrolyte preparations	4 L

function 3 to 5 days after beginning a high-fiber diet, but some patients may require a considerably longer period of time. Patients should be cautioned that abdominal distention and flatus may be particularly troublesome in the first few weeks of fiber therapy, particularly with high bran consumption. In most cases these problems resolve with continued use.

Bulk-forming laxatives have few adverse effects. The only major caution in the use of bulk-forming laxatives is that obstruction of the esophagus, stomach, small intestine, and colon has been reported when the agents have been consumed without sufficient fluid or in patients with intestinal stenosis.

SURGERY

In a small percentage of patients presenting with complaints of constipation, surgical procedures are necessary due to the presence of colonic malignancies or GI obstruction from a number of other causes. In each case, the involved segment of intestine may be resected or revised. Surgery may be required in some endocrine disorders causing constipation, such as pheochromocytoma, which requires removal of a tumor.

BIOFEEDBACK

The majority of patients with constipation related to pelvic floor dysfunction can benefit from electromyogram-guided biofeedback therapy.[19] The value of biofeedback in children with chronic constipation has not been well demonstrated.[20]

PHARMACOLOGIC THERAPY

DRUG REGIMENS OF CHOICE

Treatment and prevention of constipation should consist of bulk-forming agents in addition to dietary modifications that increase dietary fiber.[23] A variety of products are available that provide adequate bulk. Whichever agent is chosen, it should be used daily and continued indefinitely in most patients, particularly those with chronic constipation. Bulk-forming agents available in combination with diphenylmethane or anthraquinone derivatives should not be used on a routine basis.

For most persons with acute constipation, infrequent use (less than every few weeks) of laxative products is acceptable. Acute constipation may be relieved by the use of a tap-water enema or a glycerin suppository; if neither is effective, the use of oral sorbitol, low doses of diphenylmethane or anthraquinone laxatives, or saline laxatives (e.g., milk of magnesia) may provide relief. If laxative treatment is required for longer than 1 week, the person should be advised to consult a physician to determine if there is an underlying cause of constipation that requires treatment with other modalities.

For some bedridden or geriatric patients, or others with chronic constipation, bulk-forming laxatives remain the first line of treatment, but the use of more potent laxatives may be required relatively frequently. Fiber should be avoided in bedridden patients who are cognitively impaired.[19] When other than bulk-forming laxatives are used, they should be administered in the lowest effective dose and as infrequently as possible to maintain regular bowel function (more than three stools per week). Agents that may be used in these situations include diphenylmethane and anthraquinone derivatives, milk of magnesia, and sorbitol or lactulose. Mineral oil should be avoided,

particularly in bedridden patients, because of the risk of aspiration and lipoid pneumonia. Some patients with chronic constipation may present with fecal impactions. Before vigorous oral laxatives can be used, the impaction needs to be removed using mechanical methods, including tap water or saline enemas and digital extraction.

In the hospitalized patient without GI disease, constipation may be related to the use of general anesthesia and/or opiate substances. Most orally or rectally administered laxatives may be used in these situations. For prompt initiation of bowel evacuation, either a tap-water enema, glycerin suppository, or oral milk of magnesia are recommended.

With infants and children, constipation may occur commonly. In patients with persistent problems, the underlying etiology may be neurologic, metabolic, or secondary to anatomic abnormalities. Management of constipation in this age group should consist of dietary modification with an emphasis on high-fiber foods.

For acute constipation in most age groups, a tap-water enema or glycerin suppository may be helpful. Occasional use of milk of magnesia or an anthraquinone laxative in low doses is justified as well.

DRUG CLASSES

The traditional classification system for laxatives and cathartics by suspected mode of action is not very useful, as this is not clearly understood for many agents. In general, most of these products induce bowel evacuation by one or more of the mechanisms associated with the etiology of diarrhea, including active electrolyte secretion, decreased water and electrolyte absorption, increased intraluminal osmolarity, and increased hydrostatic pressure in the gut. Laxatives convert the intestine from primarily an organ that absorbs water and electrolytes to an organ that secretes these substances.

The various classes of laxatives are discussed in this section. These agents are divided into three general classifications: (a) those causing softening of feces in 1 to 3 days (bulk-forming laxatives, docusates, and lactulose); (b) those that result in soft or semifluid stool in 6 to 12 hours (diphenylmethane derivatives and anthraquinone derivatives); and (c) those causing water evacuation in 1 to 6 hours (saline cathartics, castor oil, and polyethylene glycol-electrolyte lavage solution).

EMOLLIENT LAXATIVES

Emollient laxatives are surfactant agents, docusate in its various salts, which work by facilitating mixing of aqueous and fatty materials within the intestinal tract. They may increase water and electrolyte secretion in the small and large bowel. These products are generally given orally, although docusate potassium has also been used rectally. These products result in a softening of stools within 1 to 3 days of therapy.

Emollient laxatives are ineffective in treating constipation, but are used mainly to prevent this condition. They may be helpful in situations in which straining at stool should be avoided, such as after recovery from myocardial infarction, with acute perianal disease, or after rectal surgery. It is unlikely that these agents would be very effective in preventing constipation if major causative factors (e.g., heavy opiate use, uncorrected pathology, or inadequate dietary fiber) are not concurrently addressed.

Although docusates are generally safe, a few adverse effects have been noted. They may increase the intestinal absorption of agents administered concurrently and alter toxic potential.

LUBRICANTS

Mineral oil is the only lubricant laxative in routine use. This agent, obtained from petroleum refining, acts by coating stool and allowing for easier passage. It inhibits colonic absorption of water, thereby increasing stool weight and decreasing stool transit time. Mineral oil may be given orally or rectally in a dose of 15 to 45 mL. Generally, the effect on bowel function is noted after 2 or 3 days of use.

Mineral oil is helpful in situations similar to those suggested for docusates: to maintain a soft stool and to avoid straining for relatively short periods of time (a few days to 2 weeks); however, it possesses a much greater potential for adverse effects and its routine use should be discouraged. Mineral oil may be absorbed systemically and can cause a foreign-body reaction in lymphoid tissue. Also, in debilitated or recumbent patients, mineral oil may be aspirated, causing lipoid pneumonia.[21] Mineral oil may decrease the absorption of fat-soluble vitamins (A, D, E, and K) with chronic use by causing retention in the GI tract. Finally, even when given orally, mineral oil may leak from the anal sphincter, causing pruritus and soiling of clothing.

LACTULOSE AND SORBITOL

Lactulose is a disaccharide that is used orally or rectally. It is metabolized by colonic bacteria to low-molecular-weight acids, resulting in an osmotic effect whereby fluid is retained in the colon.[22] The fluid retained in the colon lowers the pH and increases colonic peristalsis. Lactulose is generally not recommended as a first-line agent for the treatment of constipation because it is costly and not necessarily more effective than such agents as sorbitol or milk of magnesia. It may be justified as an alternative for acute constipation, and has been particularly useful in elderly patients. Occasionally, the use of lactulose may result in flatulence, cramps, diarrhea, and electrolyte imbalances.[27] Sorbitol, a monosaccharide, exerts its effect by osmotic action and has been recommended as a primary agent in the treatment of functional constipation in cognitively intact patients.[19] It is as effective as lactulose and much less expensive.

DIPHENYLMETHANE DERIVATIVES

The two commonly used diphenylmethane derivatives are bisacodyl and phenolphthalein. Bisacodyl exerts its therapeutic effect by stimulating the mucosal nerve plexus of the colon. Phenolphthalein is thought to inhibit active glucose and sodium absorption, resulting in fluid accumulation in the colon by osmotic action. With both of these agents, significant interpatient variability exists with dosing. A dose that causes no effect in one patient may result in excessive cramping and fluid evacuation in others. With phenolphthalein, a small portion of the dose undergoes enterohepatic recirculation, which may result in a prolonged laxative action.

These agents are not recommended for regular daily use. Their use is acceptable intermittently (every few weeks) to treat constipation or as a bowel preparation before diagnostic procedures in which cleansing of the colon is necessary. These agents may sometimes cause severe abdominal cramping as well as significant fluid and electrolyte imbalances with chronic use. They should not be used for patients in whom appendicitis is a possibility (perforation of the appendix may result) or during pregnancy or lactation. Finally, patients using phenolphthalein-containing laxatives should be cautioned that their urine might turn pink.

ANTHRAQUINONE DERIVATIVES

Anthraquinone derivatives include cascara sagrada, sennosides, and casanthrol. Gut bacteria metabolizes these agents to their active compounds, but the exact mechanisms of action are not understood. Effects are limited to the colon, and stimulation of Auerbach's plexus may be involved. Recommendations for the use of these agents are similar to those for the diphenylmethane derivatives. In most cases, intermittent use is acceptable; daily use should be strongly discouraged.

Most of the concerns with the use of diphenylmethane derivatives apply to the anthraquinone derivatives. In addition, the anthraquinone derivatives may cause melanosis coli, an accumulation of dark pigment, mainly in the cecum and rectum, that is evident after 4 to 13 months of use. A pathologic effect of melanosis coli has not been demonstrated, and it appears to be reversible after anthraquinones have been discontinued for 3 to 6 months.

SALINE CATHARTICS

Saline cathartics are composed of relatively poorly absorbed ions such as magnesium, sulfate, phosphate, and citrate, which produce their effects primarily by osmotic action in retaining fluid in the GI tract. Magnesium stimulates the secretion of cholecystokinin, a hormone that causes stimulation of bowel motility and fluid secretion. These agents may be given orally or rectally. A bowel movement may result within a few hours after oral doses and in 1 hour or less after rectal administration.

These agents should be used primarily for acute evacuation of the bowel, which may be necessary before diagnostic examinations, after poisonings, and in conjunction with some anthelmintics to eliminate parasites. Such agents as milk of magnesia (an 8% suspension of magnesium hydroxide) may be used occasionally (every few weeks) to treat constipation in otherwise healthy adults. Saline cathartics should not be used on a routine basis. The enema formulations of these agents may be useful in fecal impactions.

As with most laxatives, these agents may cause fluid and electrolyte depletion. Also, magnesium or sodium accumulation may occur when magnesium-containing cathartics are used in patients with renal dysfunction or when sodium phosphate is used in patients with congestive heart failure.

CASTOR OIL

Castor oil is metabolized in the GI tract to an active compound, ricinoleic acid, which stimulates secretory processes, decreases glucose absorption, and promotes intestinal motility, primarily in the small intestine. Castor oil usually results in a bowel movement within 1 to 3 hours of administration. Because the agent has such a strong purgative action, it should not be used for the routine treatment of constipation.

GLYCERIN

Glycerin is usually administered as a 3-g suppository and exerts its effect by osmotic action in the rectum. As with most agents given as suppositories, the onset of action is usually less than 30 minutes. Glycerin is considered a very safe laxative, although it may occasionally cause rectal irritation. Its use is acceptable on an intermittent basis for constipation, particularly in children.

POLYETHYLENE GLYCOL-ELECTROLYTE LAVAGE SOLUTION

Whole-bowel irrigation with polyethylene glycol-electrolyte lavage solution (PEG-ELS) has become popular for colon cleansing before diagnostic procedures or colorectal operations.

Four liters of this solution is administered over 3 hours to obtain complete evacuation of the GI tract. The solution is not recommended for the routine treatment of constipation and its use should be avoided in patients with intestinal obstruction.

OTHER AGENTS

Tap-water enemas may be used to treat simple constipation. The administration of 200 mL of tap water by enema to an adult often results in a bowel movement within 30 minutes. Soap-suds enemas are no longer recommended as their use may result in proctitis or colitis.

PREVENTION

For certain groups of patients, such as those recovering from myocardial infarction or rectal surgery, straining at defecation is to be avoided. The basis of preventive therapy in these patients should be bulk-forming laxatives. Additionally, the use of docusate is popular, although its effectiveness is debated. In pregnant patients, constipation may result because of alterations in anatomy or iron supplementation. As described earlier, bulk-forming laxatives and docusates should be the first line of prevention.

LAXATIVE ABUSE SYNDROME

Misconceptions about normal bowel patterns and the effect of laxatives have contributed to a syndrome of laxative abuse that is relatively common in the United States. The availability of laxatives as chocolates or gums conveys to the public that the use of these agents is without adverse consequences. Abuse of laxatives has occurred traditionally in persons trying to maintain daily bowel function, but more recently has extended to others who use laxatives for the purpose of controlling weight. In either case, the consistent abuse of strong laxatives and cathartics may lead to serious illness.

Laxative abuse for the purpose of maintaining daily bowel function begins with misconceptions about the frequency, quantity, or consistency of stools. With the use of strong purgatives, the colon may be so thoroughly cleansed that a bowel movement may not occur normally until a few days later. This delay reinforces the need for more purgatives and the cycle of laxative dependence is begun. Eventually the patient may require daily laxatives to maintain bowel function.

The laxative abuser may present with contradictory findings of diarrhea and weight loss. In addition, long-term abusers of laxatives tend to have vomiting, abdominal pain, lassitude, weakness, thirst, edema, and bone pain (caused by osteomalacia). With prolonged use of laxatives a number of serious illnesses may arise. These include fluid and electrolyte imbalances (including acid-base imbalances and hypokalemia), protein-losing gastroenteropathy with hypoalbuminemia, and syndromes resembling colitis.

The determination of laxative abuse syndrome can be difficult because many laxative abusers vigorously deny laxative use. Middle-aged women tend to be the most common laxative abusers. The chronic laxative abuse problem should be addressed by a combination of measures, including psychiatric evaluation, dietary modification with reliance on bulk-forming laxatives, and specific guidelines to the patient for the withdrawal of stimulant laxatives.

A variation of laxative abuse is seen in persons who use them as a means of weight loss. It appears from the medical literature and daily news sources that this type of abuse is on the increase. Treatment of patients who abuse laxatives in this way has proven very difficult.

EVALUATION OF THERAPEUTIC OUTCOMES

The ultimate goal of treatment for constipation is alteration of lifestyle (particularly diet) to prevent further episodes of constipation. Short-term goals include alleviation of acute constipation with relief from symptoms. For patients with chronic constipation, the goals are more long-term and include use of proper diet and decreased reliance on laxatives. Effective treatment of constipation requires the patient to become more knowledgeable about the causes of constipation, proper diet, and appropriate use of laxatives.

IRRITABLE BOWEL SYNDROME

Irritable bowel syndrome (IBS) is one of the most common gastrointestinal disorders encountered in clinical practice, affecting as many as 20% of adults, and is more common in women. This latter point is probably a consequence of women being more likely than men to report their symptoms to the medical community. Although a benign disorder, IBS is chronic and recurring in nature.

PATHOPHYSIOLOGY

Although the exact pathophysiologic abnormalities with IBS are still being actively investigated, it is currently thought that IBS results from altered somatovisceral and motor dysfunction of the intestine from a variety of causes. Abnormal central nervous system processing of afferent signals may lead to visceral hypersensitivity, with the specific nerve pathway affected determining the exact symptomatology expressed. This visceral hypersensitivity is a neuroenteric phenomenon that is independent of motility and psychological disturbances.[23] Factors known to contribute to these alterations include genetics, motility factors, inflammation, colonic infections, mechanical irritation to local nerves, and psychological factors.

SEROTONIN-TYPE RECEPTORS

The enteric nervous system contains a significant percentage of the body's 5-hydroxytryptamine (serotonin, 5-HT).[24] Two types of serotonin exists within the gut: serotonin type 3 (HT_3) and serotonin type 4 (HT_4), which are responsible for secretion, sensitization, and motility.[25] Previous studies show that there is an increase in the postprandial levels of 5-HT in those who suffer from diarrhea-predominant IBS when compared with nonsufferers.[24] Therefore stimulation and antagonism of these serotonin receptors has become a focused area for research on new drug therapies for both diarrhea- and constipation-predominant disease.

TABLE 36–10. Clinical Presentation of IBS

Signs and symptoms
- Lower abdominal pain
- Abdominal bloating and distention
- Diarrhea symptoms, >3 stools/day
- Extreme urgency
- Mucus passage
- Constipation symptoms, <3 stools/wk, straining, incomplete evacuation
- Psychological symptoms such as depression and anxiety

Nongastrointestinal symptoms
- Urinary symptoms
- Fatigue
- Dyspareunia

Other concurrent conditions
- Fibromyalgia
- Functional dyspepsia
- Chronic fatigue syndrome

Reduced health-related quality of life

TABLE 36–11. Symptom-Based Criteria for IBS

The Manning Criteria[23]
Chronic or recurrent abdominal pain for at least 6 months and two or more of the following:
1. Abdominal pain relieved with defecation
2. Abdominal pain associated with more frequent stools
3. Abdominal pain associated with looser stools
4. Abdominal distention
5. Feeling of incomplete evacuation after defecation
6. Mucus in stools

Rome II diagnostic criteria for IBS[26]
At least 12 weeks, which need not be consecutive, in the preceeding 12 months, of abdominal discomfort or pain that has two of three features:
1. Relieved with defecation; and/or
2. Onset associated with a change in frequency of stool; and/or
3. Onset associated with a change in form (appearance) of stool

CLINICAL PRESENTATION

Irritable bowel syndrome presents as either diarrhea-predominant or constipation-predominant disease and can be defined as lower abdominal pain, disturbed defecation (constipation, diarrhea, or an alternating pattern of both), and bloating in the absence of structural or biochemical factors that might explain these symptoms (Table 36–10).

In the past, diagnosis of IBS was based upon identification of the primary complaints of the patient and excluding other medical conditions having a similar clinical presentation. Currently, the diagnosis of IBS is based upon the use of either the symptom-based Manning[23] or Rome II[26] criteria outlined in Table 36–11.

Additional diagnostic steps that can be taken include sigmoidoscopy or colonoscopy; examination of the stool for occult blood and ova and parasites; complete blood cell count; erythrocyte sedimentation rate; and serum electrolytes. In some cases, radiographic imaging studies, such as computed tomography scans or barium swallows or enemas, may also be necessary if the findings of the above assessment are not typical for IBS.[28]

▶ TREATMENT: Irritable Bowel Syndrome

▓ GENERAL APPROACH TO TREATMENT

The treatment approach to IBS is based upon the predominant symptoms and their severity (Fig. 36–3). Milder, less frequent episodes can be managed with dietary restrictions and a higher-fiber diet with addition of bulk-forming laxatives if necessary. More persistent disease may require prn use of various antispasmodic or antidiarrheal agents such as loperamide. Lastly, the severest forms of this disease may call for pharmacologic agents directed specifically at the underlying neurohormonal imbalance, such as the 5-HT$_4$ agonists such as tegaserod or the 5-HT$_3$ receptor antagonists such as alosetron.

CLINICAL CONTROVERSY

The newer serotonin receptor agonists and antagonists tegaserod and alosetron act on GI-specific serotonin receptors to treat constipation-predominant and diarrhea-predominant IBS, respectively. However, both drugs are currently only indicated for women. Efficacy and safety in men has not been established because the initial manufacturer's sponsored clinical trials contained insufficient numbers of men with IBS to provide the necessary statistical power to prove efficacy and safety. Ongoing studies should determine if these drugs are indicated in men.

Alosetron was withdrawn from the U.S. market in 2000 due to serious adverse effects including severe constipation and ischemic colitis that did not appear in the initial clinical trials. Its use is now limited to an FDA-approved restricted use program in lower initial doses, and requires extensive postmarketing surveillance. Results of these trials are necessary to definitively determine alosetron's true safety profile, especially with regard to its association with or causation of fatal ischemic colitis.

▓ CONSTIPATION-PREDOMINANT DISEASE

In the constipation-predominant patient, dietary fiber may be beneficial. Patients should be instructed to begin with 1 tablespoonful of fiber with 1 meal daily and gradually increase the dose to include fiber with 2 and 3 meals a day until the desired outcome is achieved. Endpoints that the patient should aim for include bulkier and more easily passed stools. For patients unable to tolerate dietary bran, bulking agents such as psyllium may be substituted.[27] Laxative use is not encouraged in these patients, and it should only be used in the smallest dose for the least amount of time in cases of severe constipation.

The 5-HT$_4$ agonist tegaserod is the first therapy approved by the FDA specifically for the treatment of constipation-predominant

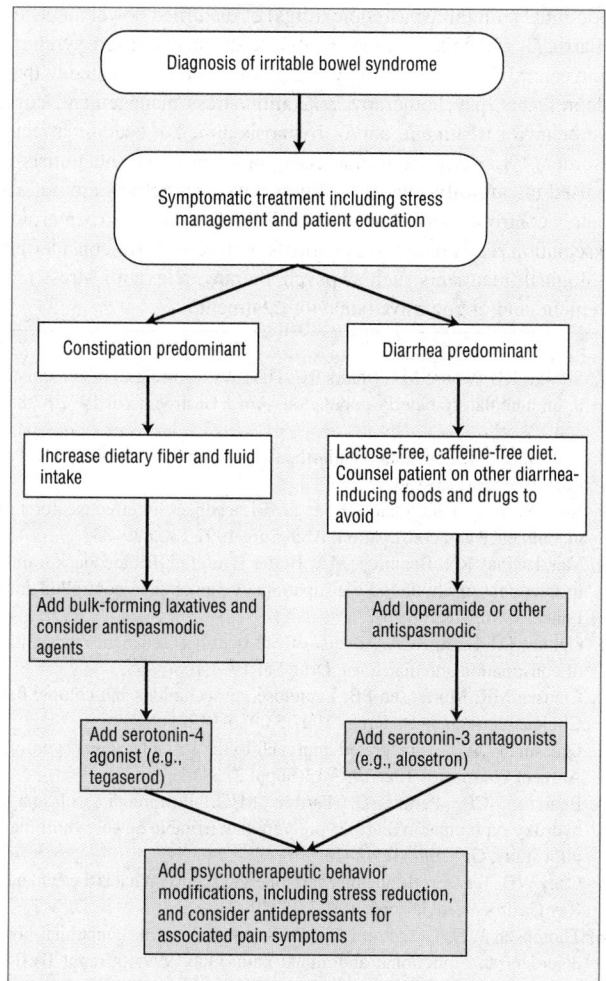

FIGURE 36–3. A general stepwise approach to the management of both constipation- and diarrhea-predominant irritable bowel syndrome.

IBS.[28] Tegaserod is a serotonin derivative that activates 5-HT$_4$ receptors on the neurons in the gastrointestinal tract, increasing GI motility and decreasing visceral sensations. It is approved as 2-mg or 6-mg doses given twice daily 30 minutes prior to a meal with water for up to 12 weeks.[29] Stimulation of the 5-HT$_4$ receptors by tegaserod increases gastric secretions and promotes motility, with improvement in symptoms generally occurring within the first week of therapy. Currently this therapy is only approved for use in women, as efficacy and safety in men has not been established due to inadequate numbers of men enrolled in clinical trials to date.[30] In addition, length of effective therapy has only been approved for 12 weeks.[37] However, recent evidence suggests that tegaserod may provide safe and effective therapy for up to 12 months.[30] Diarrhea was the most common adverse effect, resulting in drug discontinuation in 1.6% of study subjects.

DIARRHEA-PREDOMINANT DISEASE

For patients in whom diarrhea is the primary complaint, avoidance of certain food products may be necessary. Caffeine, alcohol, and artificial sweeteners (sorbitol, fructose, and mannitol) are known to irritate the gut and produce a laxative effect. Lactose

intolerance should be considered in certain patients; however, the prevalence of this condition may be exaggerated.

Herbal medicines or teas often contain senna, which may produce diarrhea. In patients with disease persistence following dietary modification, loperamide may be used for episodic management of urgent diarrhea, or in situations in which the patient wishes to avoid the possibility of an acute onset of symptoms.[29] This drug decreases intestinal transit, enhances water and electrolyte absorption, and strengthens rectal sphincter tone. Some patients may require continuous therapy, and careful dosage titration can usually be undertaken to prevent the development of constipation. Cholestyramine may be useful in patients with diarrhea related to idiopathic bile acid malabsorption or following cholecystectomy.[28]

Diarrhea-predominant IBS caused by excessive stimulation of the 5-HT$_3$ receptor can be relieved by the drug alosetron. Alosetron was the first truly effective treatment for diarrhea-predominant IBS. However, in November 2000 it was voluntarily withdrawn from the market due to severe GI adverse effects, including 113 reported cases of serious constipation and 8 cases of possible ischemic colitis and death. This decision was met with a great public outcry, as many who had suffered for years had experienced relief for the first time. Because this drug was highly effective in many patients, the FDA approved restricted use of alosetron in June 2002. Alosetron is now available via an FDA-approved restricted use program in conjunction with GlaxoSmithKline as detailed at http://www.lotronex.com. It is now indicated, in lower initial doses of 1 mg daily, for women with diarrhea-predominant symptoms of greater than 6 months' duration that are not relieved by conventional therapy. Health care providers must utilize extreme caution in therapy with this drug, and must follow strict FDA-mandated guidelines.

PAIN IN IBS

Select patients with IBS suffer significant pain associated with their disease. Data supporting the use of antispasmodic agents in these patients are conflicting.[31,32] In these cases, a trial of low-dose antidepressant therapy is indicated, especially if pain is associated with eating. Both tricyclic antidepressants and serotonin reuptake inhibitors produce analgesia, and may relieve depressive symptoms if present. Preprandial doses of drugs containing anticholinergic properties may suppress pain (and/or diarrhea) associated with an overactive postprandial gastrocolonic response. Tricyclic antidepressants should be avoided in patients with pain and constipation. In addition, psychotherapy, including cognitive behavioral therapy, relaxation therapy, and hypnotherapy have been shown to decrease IBS symptoms.[33]

DRUG CLASSES CURRENTLY UNDER INVESTIGATION FOR THE TREATMENT OF IBS

Numerous agents are currently undergoing investigation for the management of IBS.[33] Selective blockade of the muscarinic M$_3$ receptors as well as β_3-adrenoceptor agonists have been shown to alter gut motility without affecting the cardiovascular system.[34] However, two recently tested compounds, zamifenacin and darifenacin have shown limited efficacy to date.[35]

Other compounds being evaluated include neurokinin 1 and neurokinin 3 receptor antagonists, gut-selective calcium channel blockers, cholecystokinin A receptor antagonists, and agents capable of stimulating motilin receptors (motilinomimetics).[36]

■ EVALUATION OF THERAPEUTIC OUTCOMES

IBS is usually classified as constipation-predominant, diarrhea-predominant, or IBS with abdominal pain and bloating. Therapeutic goals in IBS should focus on the patient's primary complaint. Dietary and drug therapy goals should focus on end-organ treatment to relieve abdominal pain (antispasmodic drugs) or disturbed bowel habits (antidiarrheals and bulk-forming agents). Additionally, severe symptoms from central nervous system dysregulation should be treated with antidepressants, psychotherapy, relaxation/stress management, cognitive behavior treatment, and/or hypnosis aimed at specific affective disorders.[36] Lastly, the serotonin receptor agonists and antagonists can be used in carefully selected patients whose symptoms are not adequately controlled with other agents. The American Gastroenterology Association recommends that patients with severe IBS consider psychological treatments such as psychotherapy, relaxation/stress management, and/or cognitive behavior treatment.

ABBREVIATIONS

HT: serotonin
IBS: irritable bowel syndrome
ORS: oral rehydration solution
PEG-ELS: polyethylene glycol-electrolyte lavage solution
PHM: peptide histidine methionine
VIP: vasoactive intestinal peptide

Review Questions and other resources can be found at *www.pharmacotherapyonline.com*.

REFERENCES

1. DuPont HL. Diarrheal diseases in the developing world. Infect Dis Clin North Am 1995;9:313–324.
2. Feldman R, Banatvala N. The frequency of culturing stools from adults with diarrhea in Great Britain. Epidemiol Infect 1994;113:41–44.
3. Everhart JE, ed. Digestive Disease in the United States: Epidemiology and Impact. NIH Publication 94-1447. Bethesda, MD, National Institutes of Health, 1994.
4. Prado V, O'Ryan ML. Acute gastroenteritis in Latin America. Infect Dis Clin North Am 1994;8:77–106.
5. The AGA technical review on the evaluation and management of chronic diarrhea. Gastroenterology 1999;116:1464–1486.
6. Mahalanabis D. Current status of oral rehydration as a strategy for the control of diarrheal diseases. Indian J Med Res 1996;104:115–124.
7. Pizarro D, Posada G, Sandi L, et al. Rice-based electrolyte solutions for the management of infantile diarrhea. N Engl J Med 1991;324:518–521.
8. Ansdell VE, Ericsson CD. Prevention and empiric treatment of traveler's diarrhea. Med Clin North Am 1999;83:945–973.
9. Harris AG, O'Dorisio TM, Woltering EA, et al. Consensus statement: Octreotide dose titration in secretory diarrhea. Diarrhea Management Conference. Dig Dis Sci 1995;40:1464–1473.
10. Ruszniewski P, Ducreux M, Chayvialle J, et al. Treatment of the carcinoid syndrome with the long-acting somatostatin analogue lanreotide: A prospective study of 39 patients. Gut 1996;39:279–283.
11. Thompsom RF, Bass DM, Hoffman SL. Travel vaccine. Infect Dis Clin North Am 1999;13:149–167.
12. Tacket CO, Kotloff KL, Losonsky G, et al. Volunteer studies investigating the safety and efficacy of live oral El Tor Vibrio cholerae O1 vaccine strain CVD 111. Am J Trop Med Hyg 1997;56:533–547.
13. Koch A, Volderholzer WA, Klauser AG, et al. Symptoms in chronic constipation. Dis Colon Rectum 1997;40:902–906.
14. Romero Y, Evans J, Fleming KC, Phillips SF. Constipation and fecal incontinence in the elderly population. Mayo Clin Proc 1996;71:81–92.
15. Talley NJ, Fleming KC, Evans JM, et al. Constipation in an elderly community. A study of prevalence and potential risk factors. Am J Gastroenterol 1996;91:19–25.
16. Harari D, Gurwith JH, Avorn J, et al. Bowel habit in relation to age and gender. Findings from the National Health Survey and clinical implications. Arch Intern Med 1996;156:315–320.
17. Stewart RB, Moore MT, Marks RG, Hale WE. Correlates of constipation in an ambulatory elderly population. Am J Gastroenterol 1992;87:859–864.
18. Browning SM. Constipation, diarrhea and irritable bowel syndrome. Prim Care 1999;26:113–136.
19. Ko CY, Tong J, Lehman RE, et al. Biofeedback is effective for fecal incontinence and constipation. Arch Surg 1997;132:829–833.
20. Van der Plas RN, Benninga MA, Buller HA, et al. Biofeedback training in treatment of childhood constipation: A randomized controlled study. Lancet 1996;348:766–767.
21. Gattuso JM, Kamm MA. Adverse effects of drugs used in the management of constipation and diarrhoea. Drug Saf 1994;10:47–65.
22. Clausen MR, Mortensen PB. Lactulose, disaccharides and colonic flora. Clinical consequences. Drugs 1997;53:930–942.
23. Drossman DA. An integrated approach to the irritable bowel syndrome. Aliment Pharmacol Ther 1999;13(Suppl 2):3–14.
24. Bearcroft CP, Perrett D, Farthin MJG. Postprandial plasma 5-hydroxytryptamine in diarrhea predominant irritable bowel syndrome: A pilot study. Gut 1988;42:42–46.
25. Chey WD. Tegaserod and other serotonergic agents: What is the evidence? Rev Gastroenterol Disord 2003;3:35–40.
26. Thompson WG, Longstreth GF, Drossman DA, et al. Functional bowel disorders and functional abdominal pain. Gut 1999;45(Suppl II):II43–II47.
27. Thompson WG. Irritable bowel syndrome: A management strategy. Baillieres Best Pract Res Clin Gastroenterol 1999;13:453–460.
28. Camilleri M. Tegasarod. Aliment Pharmacol Ther 2001;15:277–289.
29. Tougas G, Snape WJ, Otten MH, et al. Long-term safety of tegaserod in patients with constipation-predominant irritable bowel syndrome. Aliment Pharmacol Ther 2002;16:1701–1708.
30. Muller-Lissner SA, Fumagalli I, Bardhan KD, et al. Tegaserod, a 5-HT4 receptor partial agonist, relieves symptoms in irritable bowel syndrome patients with abdominal pain, bloating and constipation. Aliment Pharmacol Ther 2001;15:1655–1666.
31. Scarpignato C, Pelosini I. Management of irritable bowel syndrome: Novel approaches to the pharmacology of gut motility. Can J Gastroenterol 1999;13(Suppl):50A–65A.
32. Jailwala K, Imperiale TF, Kroenke K. Pharmacologic treatment of the irritable bowel syndrome: A systematic review of randomized, controlled trials. Ann Intern Med 2000;133:136–147.
33. Heymann-Monnikes I, Arnold R, Florin I, et al. The combination of medical treatment plus multicomponent behavior therapy is superior to medical treatment alone in the therapy of irritable bowel syndrome. Am J Gastroenterol 2000;95:981–994.
34. Mertz H. Irritable bowel syndrome. N Engl J Med 2003;349:2136–2146.
35. Talley NJ. Pharmacologic treatment for the irritable bowel syndrome. Am J Gastroenterol 2003;98:750–758.
36. Drossman DA, Whitehead WE, Camilleri M. Irritable bowel syndrome: A technical review for practice guideline development. Gastroenterology 1997;112:2120–2137.
37. Kim HJ, Camilleri M, McKinzie S, et al. A randomized controlled trial of a probiotic, VSL#3, on gut transit and symptoms in diarrhea-predominant irritable bowel syndrome. Aliment Pharmacol Ther 2003;17:895–904.

37

PORTAL HYPERTENSION AND CIRRHOSIS

Edward G. Timm and James J. Stragand

Learning Objectives and other resources can be found at *www.pharmacotherapyonline.com.*

KEY CONCEPTS

❶ Cirrhosis is a severe, chronic, irreversible disease associated with significant morbidity and mortality. However, the progression of cirrhosis secondary to alcohol abuse can be interrupted by abstinence. It is therefore imperative for the clinician to educate and support abstinence from alcohol as part of the overall treatment strategy of the underlying liver disease.

❷ Patients with cirrhosis and portal hypertension should be considered for endoscopic screening, and patients with large varices should receive primary prophylaxis with β-adrenergic blockade therapy.

❸ When nonselective β-adrenergic blocker therapy is used to prevent rebleeding, it is essential that the dose be titrated to achieve a heart rate goal of 60 bpm or a heart rate that is 25% lower than the baseline heart rate.

❹ Octreotide is the preferred vasoactive agent employed in the medical management of variceal bleeding. Vasopressin

can no longer be recommended as a first-line agent because of its significant adverse effect profile. Endoscopy employing endoscopic band ligation or endoscopic injection sclerotherapy is the primary therapeutic tool in the management of acute variceal bleeding.

❺ The combination of spironolactone and furosemide is now the recommended initial diuretic therapy for patients with ascites.

❻ All patients who have survived an episode of spontaneous bacterial peritonitis should receive long-term antibiotic prophylaxis.

❼ The mainstay of therapy of hepatic encephalopathy involves therapy to lower blood ammonia concentrations, and includes diet therapy, lactulose, and antibiotics alone or in combination with lactulose.

Many chronic inflammatory diseases of the liver result in diffuse hepatocyte necrosis, cellular regeneration, and replacement with nodular fibrous tissue. As the number of functioning hepatocytes diminishes and fibrous tissue accumulates, a constellation of signs and symptoms develop that is collectively termed *cirrhosis*. The term cirrhosis is derived from the Greek *kirrhos* meaning orange-colored, and refers to the yellow-orange hue of the liver seen by the pathologist or surgeon. Histologically, cirrhosis is defined as a diffuse process characterized by fibrosis and a conversion of the normal hepatic architecture into structurally abnormal nodules.[1] Regardless of the mechanism of injury, the end result is the destruction of hepatocytes and their replacement with fibrous tissue. As fibrotic tissue replaces normal hepatic parenchyma, resistance to blood flow results in the clinical problems of portal hypertension and the development of varices and ascites. Hepatocyte loss and intrahepatic shunting of blood results in diminished metabolic and synthetic function, which leads to hepatic encephalopathy and coagulopathy.

❶ While cirrhosis has many causes (Table 37–1), in the United States excessive alcohol intake and chronic viral hepatitis (types B and C) are the most common causes.[2,3] A breakdown of the indications for liver transplantation (Table 37–2) provides an estimate of the clinical frequency for each of the potential causes of cirrhosis, as transplant represents the definitive therapeutic strategy for cirrhosis.[2] These data underestimate alcoholic liver disease, as these patients are often not considered suitable transplant candidates.

This chapter elucidates the pathophysiology of cirrhosis and the resultant effects on human anatomy and physiology. Treatment strategies for managing the most commonly encountered clinical complications of cirrhosis are discussed.

EPIDEMIOLOGY

Cirrhosis affects 3.6 per 1000 adults in the United States and is responsible for 26,000 deaths per year.[3] Chronic liver disease represents the fourth leading cause of deaths among all races and sexes in the 45- to 54-year-old age group, exceeded only by malignancy, heart disease, and accidents.[4] Acute variceal bleeding and spontaneous bacterial peritonitis are among the immediately life-threatening complications of cirrhosis. Associated conditions causing significant morbidity include ascites and hepatic encephalopathy. Approximately 50% of patients with cirrhosis who develop ascites die within 2 years of diagnosis.[5]

PATHOPHYSIOLOGY OF CIRRHOSIS

Any discussion of cirrhosis must be based on a firm understanding of hepatic anatomy and vascular supply. Conceptually, the liver can be thought of as an elaborate blood filtration system receiving blood

TABLE 37–1. Etiology of Cirrhosis

Category	Example
Drugs and toxins	Alcohol, methotrexate, isoniazid, methyldopa, organic hydrocarbons
Infections	Viral hepatitis (types B and C), schistosomiasis
Immune-mediated	Primary biliary cirrhosis, autoimmune hepatitis, primary sclerosing cholangitis
Metabolic	Hemochromatosis, porphyria, α_1-antitrypsin deficiency, Wilson's disease
Biliary obstruction	Cystic fibrosis, atresia, strictures, gallstones
Cardiovascular	Chronic right heart failure, Budd-Chiari syndrome, veno-occlusive disease
Cryptogenic	Unknown
Other	Nonalcoholic steatohepatitis, sarcoidosis, gastric bypass

From Williams and Iredale.[1]

from the portal vein and the hepatic artery (Fig. 37–1). Blood enters the liver via the portal triad and drains through the hepatic lobule, the smallest functional unit of this filtration system (Fig. 37–2), and into the central vein. The hepatic lobule is hexagonal in shape, at the angles of which are the sites of the portal triads, which contain the smallest branches of the portal vein and hepatic artery, as well as the bile and lymphatic ducts. Within the lobule, individual hepatocytes are arranged in plates, radiating from the periphery to a central vein. The hepatic lobule can be subdivided into functional zones based on relative oxygen supply. The hepatic artery supplies oxygen-rich blood to the portal triad.[6,7] Hepatocytes at the periphery therefore receive a higher level of oxygen than the cells near the central vein.

Arterial and venous blood from the portal triad passes through the hepatic lobules to the central veins via the hepatic sinusoids. After passing through the hepatic lobules, blood collects in the central veins, which ultimately coalesce into the hepatic veins, which then enter the inferior vena cava.

In areas of hepatocellular injury, regardless of the nature of the inciting agent, stellate cells, normally involved in the storage of retinoids like vitamin A, become activated, lose their retinoids, and develop features of fibroblasts. They then become a major source of the collagen and other matrix proteins that proliferate during fibrosis.[9,10] The progressive deposition of fibrous material within the sinusoids disrupts the normal blood flow through the hepatic lobule. As fibrous tissue accumulates, resistance to portal blood flow increases, resulting

TABLE 37–2. Indications for Liver Transplant: United Network Organ Sharing Registry, 1994

Disease	Frequency (%)
Alcohol	23
Hepatitis C	22.4
Cryptogenic	11
Primary biliary cirrhosis	9.4
Primary sclerosing cholangitis	8.3
Acute hepatic failure	6
Autoimmune hepatitis	5.8
Hepatitis B (chronic)	3.2
Hepatocellular cancer	2.9
Hemochromatosis	1.1
Hepatitis B (acute)	0.9
Budd-Chiari syndrome	0.7
Other	5.3

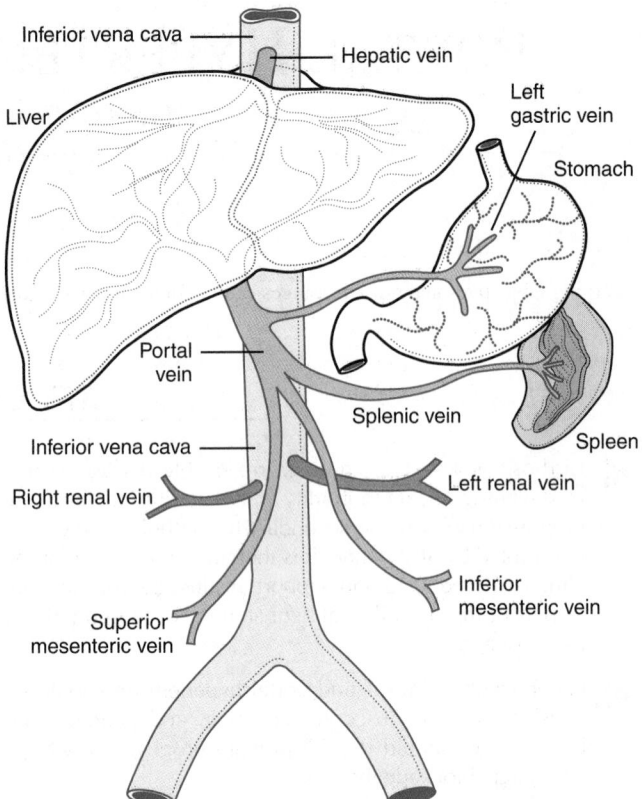

FIGURE 37–1. The portal venous system.

in persistent and progressive elevations in portal blood pressures, or portal hypertension (PHT). Normal portal venous pressure is 5 to 10 mm Hg.[11] Clinically significant PHT exists when the portal venous pressure increases to a point where it is 10 mm Hg greater than the pressure within the inferior vena cava.[11]

There is also evidence that there are changes in the vasodilatory and vasoconstricting mediators that regulate the hepatic sinusoidal blood flow.[8] A decrease in the production of nitric oxide, which acts as a vasodilator, and a increase in the levels of the vasoconstrictor endothelin combine to increase the resistance to blood flow. Concurrently, there also appears to be an increase in the blood flow to the splanchnic vasculature through a nitric oxide–mediated effect on the splanchnic arteriole. These physiologic changes are the target of the pharmacologic approach to therapy.

In summary, cirrhosis results in elevation of portal blood pressure because of fibrotic changes within the hepatic sinusoids, changes in the levels of vasodilatory and vasoconstrictor mediators, and an increase in blood flow to the splanchnic vasculature.

ANATOMIC AND PHYSIOLOGIC EFFECTS OF CIRRHOSIS

Cirrhosis and the pathophysiologic abnormalities that cause it result in the commonly encountered problems of ascites, portal hypertension and esophageal varices, hepatic encephalopathy, and coagulation disorders. Other less commonly seen problems in patients with cirrhosis include hepatorenal syndrome, hepatopulmonary syndrome, and endocrine dysfunction, and these are discussed in the section dealing with management of complications.

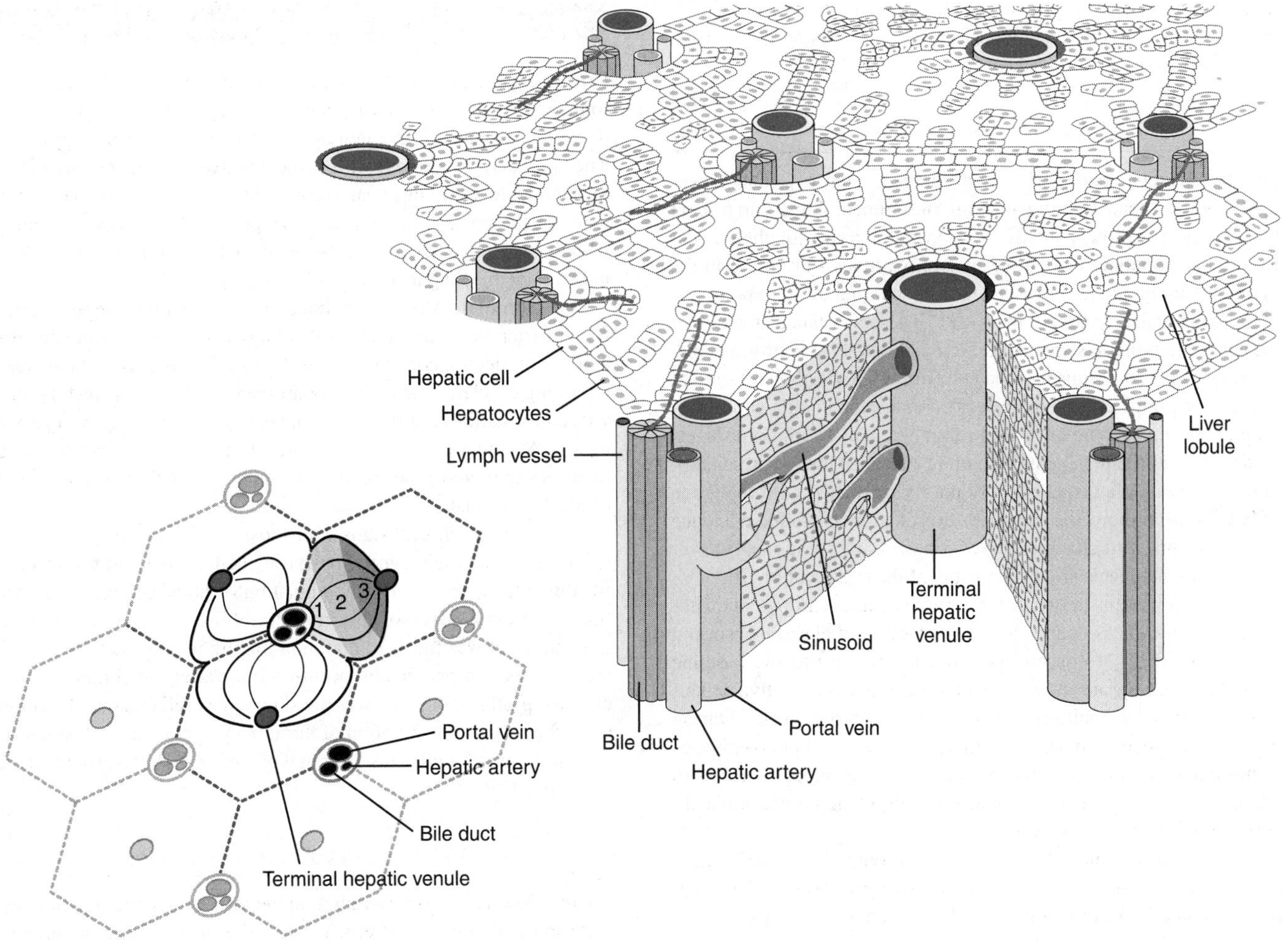

Hepatic cell
Hepatocytes
Lymph vessel
Liver lobule
Terminal hepatic venule
Sinusoid
Bile duct
Portal vein
Hepatic artery
Portal vein
Hepatic artery
Bile duct
Terminal hepatic venule

FIGURE 37–2. The hepatic lobule.

ASCITES

Ascites, from the Greek *askos* meaning waterbag or wineskin, is the pathologic accumulation of lymph fluid within the peritoneal cavity. It is one of the earliest and most common presentations of cirrhosis.[13] More than one-half of cirrhotic patients develop ascites within 10 years of diagnosis.[14] The mechanism for the development of ascites is not completely understood. The most current unifying theory involves the development of PHT in conjunction with systemic arterial vasodilation.[13,15–17] The progressive vasodilation then leads to the activation of the baroreceptors in the kidney and an activation of the renin-angiotensin system, with sodium and water retention (Fig. 37–3). The net effect of these changes is plasma volume expansion and the translocation of lymph fluid from the hepatic sinusoids and splanchnic capillaries into the peritoneal cavity.[13,17]

PORTAL HYPERTENSION AND VARICES

The most important clinical sequelae of PHT are the development of varices or alternative routes of blood flow from the portal to the systemic circulation, bypassing the liver (see Fig. 37–1). Varices decompress the portal venous system and return blood to the systemic circulation. Varices can occur at any level of the GI tract; however, the route with the most clinical significance is through the left gastric vein with the development of esophageal varices. Patients with cirrhosis are at risk for variceal bleeding when portal venous pressure is

12 mm Hg greater than vena cava pressure.[11] Hemorrhage from varices occurs in 25% to 40% of patients with cirrhosis, and each episode of bleeding carries a 5% to 50% risk of death.[19] Rebleeding can occur in as many as 60% to 70% of patients within 1 year.[20] The risk of bleeding from esophageal varices is related to the tension on the variceal wall, which in turn is related to portal vein pressure and ultimately to the degree of cirrhosis.[11] It should be apparent from this

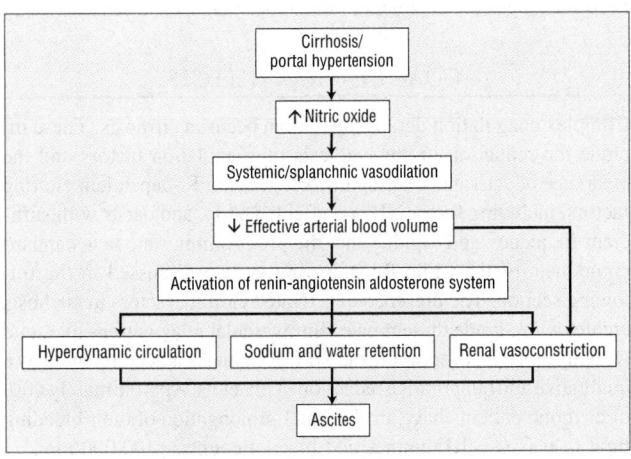

FIGURE 37–3. Pathogenesis of ascites.

understanding that the primary strategy for the treatment of esophageal varices is the reduction of portal hypertension by pharmacologic and surgical approaches.

HEPATIC ENCEPHALOPATHY

Hepatic encephalopathy (HE) is a complex neuropsychiatric syndrome with a broad spectrum of symptoms of neurologic impairment that occurs in cirrhotic patients.[18] The symptoms are thought to result from an accumulation of gut-derived nitrogenous substances in the systemic circulation as a consequence of shunting through portosystemic collaterals, bypassing the liver.[19] These substances then enter the central nervous system and result in alterations of neurotransmission that affect consciousness and behavior.[18] This is often referred to as the "gut-brain" connection. Elevated arterial ammonia concentrations are the most commonly cited causative agent, as ammonia levels tend to be elevated in patients with more advanced liver insufficiency. However, ammonia levels are only poorly correlated with the grade of HE.[20] Furthermore, the administration of ammonia failed to induce HE in patients with cirrhosis.[21] Nevertheless, interventions to lower blood ammonia levels are the mainstay of the treatment of HE.

HE can present in one of three forms: acute, chronic, and subclinical. Acute HE is defined as a distinct event of altered sensorium lasting <4 weeks, followed by complete recovery to the baseline mental status. Chronic encephalopathy is defined as cognitive or neuropsychiatric abnormalities that persist for at least 4 weeks. During this time, the severity of the abnormalities fluctuates, but no episodes of normal mentation are noted. Subclinical encephalopathy refers to subtle alterations in neuropsychiatric function that are not clinically apparent without special testing.[19]

The clinical manifestations of HE can range from subtle mental status abnormalities, detectable only with psychological testing, to deep coma.[21] Additionally, different classifications or patterns of HE can also be described. HE is seen in two broad clinical settings, acute fulminant liver failure and chronic liver failure. In patients with chronic liver failure, HE occurs in three patterns, acute, chronic, and subclinical.[17,19]

HE associated with acute fulminant liver failure has a rapid onset and a short prodrome, and patients can progress from drowsiness to delirium, convulsions, and finally to coma in as shortly as 24 hours. The prognosis in these cases is dismal.[21] This pattern of HE usually has no known precipitating factors, and patients who survive the acute insult have an excellent long-term prognosis. HE associated with chronic liver failure has a gradual onset, is commonly associated with known precipitating factors, and has a poor prognosis with the need for long-term treatment of the underlying liver disease.[19]

COAGULATION DEFECTS

Complex coagulation derangements can occur in cirrhosis. These include the reduction in the synthesis of coagulation factors and the clearance of activated clotting factors. Vitamin K–dependent clotting factors, including factor VII, are affected early, and occur with sufficient frequency and rapidity that the prothrombin time is a standard component of the Child-Pugh scoring system discussed in the following section. The presence of activated clotting factors in cirrhosis creates a low-grade disseminated intravascular coagulation–like state with fibrinolysis. In addition, the PHT of cirrhosis is accompanied by a qualitative and quantitative reduction in platelets. Approximately 40% of cirrhotic patients have an abnormal prolongation of their bleeding time to values >10 minutes and platelet counts <100,000/mm.[3,22] The net effect of these events is the development of bleeding diathesis.

CLINICAL PRESENTATION

Cirrhotic patients may present in a variety of ways, from asymptomatic patients with abnormal laboratory tests noted on routine blood donation, to acute life-threatening hemorrhage in an emergency room. The approach to a patient with suspected liver disease begins with a through history and physical exam. Table 37–3 describes the prevalence of the presenting signs and symptoms of cirrhosis.[23] Clinical jaundice is often a late manifestation of cirrhosis and its absence does not exclude the diagnosis.

A thorough history of alcohol or drug use, with the input of family and friends is important, as the patient often underestimates the amount of alcohol consumed. Family history can also provide clues regarding problems such as hemochromatosis. The social history provides information regarding potential occupational exposures to toxic agents. A history of acute pain and fever may indicate an obstructive process due to gallstones or an inflammatory condition such as viral or alcoholic hepatitis.

The classic clinical signs of cirrhosis, such as palmar erythema, spider angiomata, and gynecomastia, are neither sensitive nor specific for this disease.[12,23] Only a combination of physical and laboratory findings provides a reasonable indicator of liver disease. A decreased albumin level was the most common finding in patients with cirrhosis, but was nonspecific and occurred in a variety of conditions. An elevated prothrombin time was the single most reliable manifestation of cirrhosis. The combination of thrombocytopenia, encephalopathy, and ascites was found in just over half of cirrhotics, but had the highest predictive value.[19]

LABORATORY ABNORMALITIES

There are no laboratory or radiographic tests of hepatic function despite the commonly ordered *liver function tests*. These commonly measured markers are substances produced by the liver and released into the bloodstream during hepatocellular injury, and are more correctly termed *liver dysfunction tests*. True liver function tests that assess the ability of the liver to eliminate substances that undergo hepatic metabolism, such as the ^{14}C-aminopyrine breath test, are limited by complexity and availability.

Routine liver tests include alkaline phosphatase, bilirubin, aspartate transaminase (AST), alanine transaminase (ALT), and γ-glutamyl transpeptidase (GGT). Additional markers of hepatic synthetic activity include albumin and prothrombin time. Liver function tests are

TABLE 37–3. Clinical Presentation of Cirrhosis

Signs and symptoms (percent of patients)[a]
  Fatigue (65%), pruritus (55%)
  Hyperpigmentation (25%), jaundice (10%)
  Hepatomegaly (25%), splenomegaly (15%)
  Palmar erythema, spider angiomata, gynecomastia
  Ascites, edema, pleural effusion, and respiratory difficulties
  Malaise, anorexia, and weight loss
  Encephalopathy
Laboratory tests
  Hypoalbuminemia
  Elevated prothrombin time
  Thrombocytopenia
  Elevated alkaline phosphatase
  Elevated aspartate transaminase (AST), alanine transaminase (ALT), and γ-glutamyl transpeptidase (GGT)

[a] From Talwalkar and Lindor.[23]

often the first step in the evaluation of patients who present with symptoms or signs suggestive of cirrhosis. Liver function tests will typically be elevated in chronic inflammatory liver disease such as hepatitis C, but may be normal in patients with a previous toxic exposure or resolved infectious process such as hepatitis B. The individual liver tests are discussed in more detail in Chap. 31, on evaluation of the gastrointestinal tract.

The use of liver function tests in the diagnosis and management of cirrhosis is discussed in the following sections. It may be useful to group the tests into two broad categories: markers of hepatocyte damage such as the transaminases; and markers of hepatocellular synthetic function, prothrombin time and albumin.

AMINOTRANSFERASES

The aminotransferases, AST and ALT, are enzymes located in the cytoplasm of hepatocytes and their levels will be elevated with hepatocellular injury. The degree of elevation of the aminotransferases is helpful in suggesting possible etiologies. The highest levels (>20-fold increase above normal) are typically seen in acute viral, drug-induced, or ischemic events associated with circulatory catastrophes. Alcoholic liver disease rarely presents with ALT values >500 units/L, and higher values should alert the clinician to complicating problems.[20]

The ratio of AST to ALT also provides information in patients with suspected alcoholic liver disease. Seventy percent of patients with alcoholic liver disease had ratios greater than 2, compared to 4% of patients with viral hepatitis.[24]

ALKALINE PHOSPHATASE AND GAMMA-GLUTAMYL TRANSPEPTIDASE

Elevated levels of alkaline phosphatase and GGT occur with obstructive disorders that disrupt the flow of bile from the hepatocytes to the bile ductules, or from the biliary tree to the intestines. Examples of the former include primary biliary cirrhosis and drug-induced cholestasis; examples of the latter include gallstone disease and malignancies of the pancreas and bile ducts. In liver disease, the levels of GGT correlate well with elevations of the alkaline phosphatase, and their combination is a sensitive and specific marker for biliary tract disease.[22]

CHILD-PUGH CLASSIFICATION

The Child-Pugh classification system has gained widespread acceptance as a means of quantifying the myriad effects of the cirrhotic process on the laboratory and clinical manifestations of this disease.[28] The system employs a combination of physical and laboratory findings (Table 37–4). This classification system is important because it is used to assess and define the severity of the cirrhosis, and as a predictor for patient survival, surgical outcome, and risk of variceal bleeding.

TABLE 37–4. Criteria and Scoring for the Child-Pugh Grading of Chronic Liver Disease

Score	1	2	3
Bilirubin (mg/dL)	1–2	2–3	>3
Albumin (mg/dL)	>3.5	2.8–3.5	<2.8
Ascites	None	Mild	Moderate
Encephalopathy (grade)	None	1 and 2	3 and 4
Prothrombin time (seconds prolonged)	1–4	4–6	>6

Grade A, <7 points; grade B, 7–9 points; grade C, 10–15 points.

TABLE 37–5. Etiology of Hyperbilirubinemia

Etiology	Diagnosis
Unconjugated bilirubin	
Excessive production	Hemolysis
Immature enzyme systems	Jaundice of newborn
	Jaundice of prematurity
Inherited defects	Gilbert syndrome
	Crigler-Najjar syndrome
Drug effects	
Conjugated bilirubin	
Impaired intrahepatic excretion	
Hepatocellular disease	Hepatitis, cirrhosis, drugs
Intrahepatic cholestasis	Drugs, pregnancy
Congenital	Dubin-Johnson syndrome
	Rotor's syndrome
Obstruction	
Extrahepatic	Calculus, stricture, neoplasm
Intrahepatic	Sclerosing cholangitis, cirrhosis, neoplasm

BILIRUBIN

Bilirubin is a breakdown product of hemoglobin derived from senescent red blood cells. Elevations of the serum bilirubin are common in end-stage liver disease and obstruction of the common bile duct due to gallstones or malignancy; however, there are other causes of an elevated bilirubin (Table 37–5).

When cirrhosis has been established, the degree of bilirubin elevation has prognostic significance and is used as a component of the Child-Pugh scoring system for quantifying the degree of cirrhosis.

Figure 37–4 describes a general algorithm for the interpretation of liver function tests. The algorithm first separates the tests into two categories based on the underlying pathology (pattern of elevations): obstructive (alkaline phosphatase, GGT, and bilirubin) versus hepatocellular (AST and ALT). If a hepatocellular pattern predominates, the magnitude of elevation provides diagnostic assistance. If the degree of elevation is >20 times normal, the etiology is likely a result of drugs or other toxins, ischemia, or acute viral hepatitis. Elevations <20 times normal have a broad differential. Unfortunately, most liver

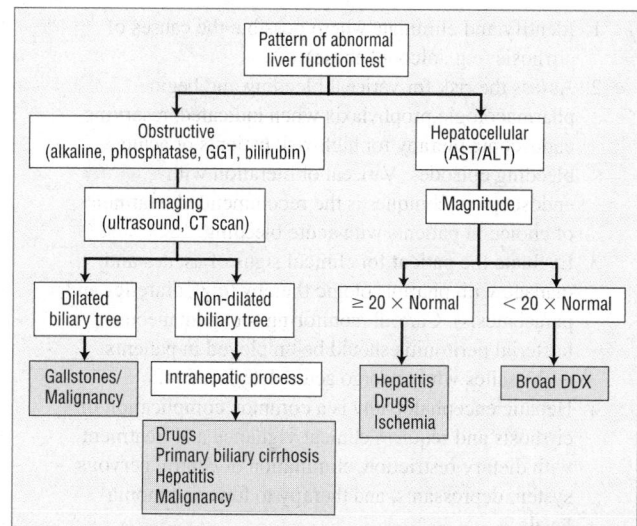

FIGURE 37–4. Interpretation of liver function tests.

enzyme abnormalities will fall into a mixed pattern, providing limited diagnostic assistance.

ALBUMIN AND COAGULATION FACTORS

These proteins are markers of hepatic synthetic activity and are therefore used to estimate the level of functioning hepatocytes in cirrhosis. They are employed in the Child-Pugh scoring system for liver disease. Albumin levels can be affected by a number of factors, including the patient's nutritional status, acute illnesses, which result in redistribution of albumin, and protein losses from renal and intestinal sources.

The liver synthesizes coagulation factors I, II, V, VII, IX, and X.[20] The prothrombin time is prolonged when any of these factors are absent. In acute liver disease the prothrombin time can be used as an outcome measurement in acetaminophen overdose and acute alcoholic hepatitis.[25] In chronic liver disease, the prothrombin time is employed as a marker of decreased synthetic capacity.

THROMBOCYTOPENIA

Thrombocytopenia is a relatively common feature in both acute and chronic liver disease and is proportional to the extent of liver disease.[26] The etiology of thrombocytopenia in liver disease is multifactorial, but involves primarily hypersplenism with pooling of platelets, immune-mediated destruction, and the inability of the bone marrow to compensate for the accelerated removal. The bone marrow depression may be related to alcohol, drugs, and nutritional deficiencies associated with the cirrhotic process.[27]

ENDOSCOPIC AND RADIOGRAPHIC ABNORMALITIES

The use of imaging techniques can provide useful information regarding the presence of liver disease and portal hypertension. The modality chosen is often determined by the clinical presentation. Examples include the use of ultrasound for the detection of gallstones and biliary duct abnormalities in patients presenting with acute pain and jaundice, or endoscopic retrograde cholangiopancreatography (ERCP) for patients with known choledocholithiasis. Upper endoscopy can be employed to detect the presence of esophageal or gastric varices as an indicator of portal hypertension. Computed tomography is a sensitive means of detecting hepatic metastases and is used for directing liver biopsy.

LIVER BIOPSY

Liver biopsy plays a central role in the diagnosis and staging of liver disease; however, for the diagnosis of cirrhosis, percutaneous liver biopsy has a significant false-negative rate because of the presence of regenerating nodules within the liver.

MANAGEMENT OF THE COMPLICATIONS OF CIRRHOSIS

The major complications of cirrhosis that require therapeutic intervention include:

- Portal hypertension and variceal bleeding
- Ascites and spontaneous bacterial peritonitis
- Hepatic encephalopathy
- Other systemic complications

▶ TREATMENT: Cirrhosis

▦ GENERAL APPROACHES TO TREATMENT

As is discussed below, the clinical manifestations of cirrhosis are protean and it is difficult to provide overall management guidelines. General approaches to therapy should include:

1. Identify and eliminate where possible the causes of cirrhosis (e.g., alcohol abuse).
2. Assess the risk for variceal bleeding and begin pharmacologic prophylaxis when indicated, reserving endoscopic therapy for high-risk patients or acute bleeding episodes. Variceal obliteration with endoscopic techniques is the recommended treatment of choice in patients with acute bleeding.
3. Evaluate the patient for clinical signs of ascites and manage with pharmacologic therapy (e.g., diuretics and paracentesis). Careful monitoring for spontaneous bacterial peritonitis should be employed in patients with ascites who undergo acute deterioration.
4. Hepatic encephalopathy is a common complication of cirrhosis and requires clinical vigilance and treatment with dietary restriction, elimination of central nervous system depressants, and therapy to lower ammonia levels.

5. Frequent monitoring for signs of hepatorenal syndrome, pulmonary insufficiency, and endocrine dysfunction is necessary.

▦ DESIRED OUTCOMES

The desired therapeutic outcomes can be viewed in two categories: *resolution of acute complications*, such as tamponade of bleeding and resolution of hemodynamic instability for an episode of acute variceal hemorrhage; and *prevention of complications*, through lowering of portal pressure with medical therapy using β-adrenergic blocker therapy, or supporting abstinence from alcohol. Treatment endpoints and desired therapeutic outcomes are presented for each of the recommended therapies discussed.

▦ PORTAL HYPERTENSION AND VARICEAL BLEEDING

The propensity of esophageal varices to bleed when a threshold pressure is exceeded is a potentially life-threatening complication of cirrhosis. Mortality after the first variceal bleed ranges from 5% to 50% and is dependent upon the severity of the underlying liver disease.[12] Cirrhotic patients who have experienced their first episode of variceal bleeding have an approximately 60% to 70% risk of rebleeding.[12] The Child-Pugh scoring system is a predictor for rebleeding and mortality.

MANAGEMENT OF PORTAL HYPERTENSION AND VARICEAL BLEEDING

The management of varices involves three strategies: (a) primary prophylaxis (prevention of the first bleeding episode); (b) treatment of acute variceal hemorrhage; and (c) secondary prophylaxis, prevention of rebleeding in patients who have previously bled.[29,30]

Primary Prophylaxis

β-Adrenergic Blockade.
The mainstay of primary prophylaxis is the use of nonselective β-adrenergic blocking agents such as propranolol or nadolol. These agents reduce cardiac output via blockade of the β_1 cardiac receptors and the blockade of the adrenergic dilatory tone of the mesenteric arterioles, resulting in unopposed α-adrenergic–mediated vasoconstriction. The net effect is the decreased blood flow to the mesenteric vascular system and decreased portal vein pressure.[29]

A meta-analysis of nine randomized controlled trials evaluating the effectiveness of either propranolol or nadolol as primary prophylaxis demonstrated effectiveness in the prevention of bleeding and a trend toward a reduction in mortality.[30–34] The average reduction in the incidence of initial bleeding achieved by nonselective β-adrenergic blockade is approximately 25%.[34] β-Blockade was effective irrespective of the presence of ascites and variceal size, and another study suggested that patients with a higher risk for bleeding, larger varices, or any size varices with a portal pressure >12 mm Hg, are the best candidates for prophylactic β-adrenergic blocker therapy.[34] β-Adrenergic blocker therapy should be lifelong unless it is not tolerated, because bleeding can occur when β-blocker therapy is abruptly discontinued.[35]

CLINICAL CONTROVERSY: THE USE OF NITRATES

Nitrates are known to cause smooth muscle vasodilation and to reduce portal pressures; however, the role of nitrates in primary prophylaxis is controversial. Isosorbide-5-mononitrate was compared with propranolol for primary prophylaxis in cirrhosis.[36] Equivalent reductions in bleeding were reported, but short-term survival was improved with isosorbide therapy. This report was met with great enthusiasm because it offered an effective alternative for patients who did not tolerate β-adrenergic blockers. Follow-up on the patients in the study was continued for up to 7 years with the finding that the early mortality benefit was lost. In fact, the use of isosorbide-5-mononitrate resulted in higher long-term mortality than propranolol in patients >50 years of age.[37] These findings are not entirely surprising because it was appreciated that a potential existed for nitrates to increase portal blood flow and consequently portal pressure by enhancing nitric oxide–mediated vasodilation of the mesenteric vasculature. Considering that vasodilation in liver disease is the hemodynamic expression of liver failure and is a prognostic indicator of morbidity and mortality, this may explain, at least in part, the negative effects on long-term survival.[38]

Another therapeutic issue arises because β-adrenergic blockers alone do not adequately lower portal pressure in all patients. A number of trials have shown that the combination of nitrates and β-adrenergic blockers is superior to β-adrenergic blockers alone in lowering portal pressures.[38] β-Adrenergic blocker therapy may suppress the neurohormonal activation associated with the relative hypovolemia induced by the vasodilation from the nitrate therapy and thereby minimize its detrimental effects.[32] With such disparate study findings the role of nitrates in primary prophylaxis is controversial and firm recommendations are difficult. Nevertheless, for patients with an inadequate response to β-adrenergic blockers alone, a long-acting nitrovasodilator should be added to try to achieve adequate lowering of portal pressure. For patients with contraindications or intolerance to β-adrenergic blockers, treatment decisions are uncertain. Groszmann suggests that nitrates can probably be used safely in this situation in younger patients who have well-compensated cirrhosis.[38]

Treatment Recommendations: Variceal Bleeding-Primary Prophylaxis

All patients with cirrhosis and portal hypertension should be considered for endoscopic screening, and patients with large varices should receive primary prophylaxis with β-adrenergic blockers. Initiate therapy with oral propranolol 10 mg three times daily or nadolol 20 mg once daily and titrate to a reduction in the resting heart rate of 20% to 25%, an absolute heart rate of 55 to 60 beats per minute (bpm), or the development of adverse effects. Patients with contraindications or intolerance to β-adrenergic blockers should be considered for trials of alternative prophylactic therapy.[39] Nitrates may be considered for these patients provided they are younger than 50 years of age and have well-compensated cirrhosis. Initiate therapy with isosorbide-5-mononitrate 20 mg orally twice daily and increase to 20 mg three times a day after 1 week if tolerated. Combination therapy with β-blockers and nitrates is recommended for patients with an inadequate lowering of portal pressure in response to β-adrenergic blockers alone. Currently, no evidence supports the use of sclerotherapy, band ligation, surgical shunting, or transjugular intrahepatic portosystemic shunt (TIPS) as primary prophylaxis.[31,39] However, one recent study comparing variceal band ligation versus β-blockers as a primary prophylaxis did show a decreased rate of bleeding at 1 year in the banding group.[40]

ACUTE VARICEAL HEMORRHAGE

Variceal hemorrhage typically presents with hematemesis or melena. Important risk factors include active alcohol abuse, use of nonsteroidal anti-inflammatory agents or aspirin, or previous variceal hemorrhage.[39] It is important to note, however, that variceal bleeding secondary to portal hypertension can occur in patients without signs of liver disease; for example, in patients with portal vein thrombosis. The initial assessment should determine the severity of the bleeding, severity of other organ dysfunction, and the severity of the liver disease. The Child-Pugh scoring system (see Table 37–4) is the most reliable means of assessing the severity of chronic liver disease.[39]

MANAGEMENT OF ACUTE VARICEAL HEMORRHAGE

Initial treatment goals include: (a) adequate fluid resuscitation; (b) correction of coagulopathy and thrombocytopenia; (c) control of bleeding; (d) prevention of rebleeding; and (e) preservation of liver function. Prompt stabilization and aggressive fluid resuscitation of patients with active bleeding is followed by endoscopic examination. General resuscitation measures should be applied in the initial management of variceal hemorrhage. Airway management is critical in patients with variceal hemorrhage because of depressed reflexes and/or combative behavior associated with drug and alcohol use. The endoscopic approach to bleeding also requires a quiet and cooperative patient, and elective intubation for airway control and adequate sedation is often necessary. Clinical practice guidelines approved by the American College of Gastroenterology recommend esophagogastroduodenoscopy (EGD) employing endoscopic injection sclerotherapy (EIS) or endoscopic band ligation (EBL) of varices as the primary diagnostic and treatment strategy for upper GI tract hemorrhage secondary to portal hypertension and varices.[41]

Fluid resuscitation involves colloids initially and subsequent blood products after blood bank matching procedures are completed. Packed red blood cells, fresh frozen plasma, and platelets may be employed both as volume expanders and corrective therapy for underlying clotting abnormalities. Vasoactive drug therapy (somatostatin, octreotide, or terlipressin) to stop or slow bleeding is routinely employed early in patient management to allow stabilization of the patient and to permit endoscopy to proceed under more favorable conditions. Antibiotic therapy to prevent sepsis should also be implemented early, especially for patients with signs of infection or ascites. Figure 37–5 presents an algorithm for the management of variceal hemorrhage.

DRUG THERAPY

Drug therapy for acute variceal bleeding is based on the principle that it is possible to reduce portal, and consequently variceal, pressure by reducing portal vein blood flow via splanchnic vasoconstriction.[42] Drugs employed to manage acute variceal bleeding include octreotide or somatostatin, vasopressin, and terlipressin (triglycyl-lysine vasopressin).

Somatostatin and Octreotide

Somatostatin is a naturally occurring 14-amino acid peptide and octreotide is a synthetic octapeptide analog that is significantly more potent than native somatostatin. Octreotide shares four amino acids with somatostatin and these moieties are responsible for its pharmacologic activity. Somatostatin increases vascular tone in the gastrointestinal tract by inhibiting vasodilatory peptides such as vasoactive intestinal peptide, producing mesenteric vasoconstriction.[43] Both somatostatin and octreotide are widely used in the treatment of variceal hemorrhage because of their reported ability to decrease splanchnic blood flow, and thereby reduce portal and variceal pressures, without significant adverse effects.[30,39] Unlike vasopressin, systemic vasoconstriction and elevations in blood pressure are not seen because the vasoconstriction that occurs with somatostatin and octreotide is selective for the mesenteric circulation. Other reports, however, have failed to demonstrate reductions in gastric mucosal blood flow or intravariceal pressure.[39] Consequently, the precise mechanism of action by which these agents may beneficially impact variceal bleeding still remains unclear.[44] Placebo-controlled clinical trials found somatostatin to be no more effective than placebo, whereas other studies show a clear benefit with somatostatin.[45–47] A meta-analysis of clinical trials comparing somatostatin and octreotide with vasopressin or terlipressin has demonstrated equivalent efficacy, but the side effect profile of somatostatin and octreotide was superior to vasopressin.[48] This analysis also reported that somatostatin was more effective in achieving initial and sustained control of bleeding.

Vasopressin (also known as antidiuretic hormone) is a potent, nonselective vasoconstrictor that has been recommended for many

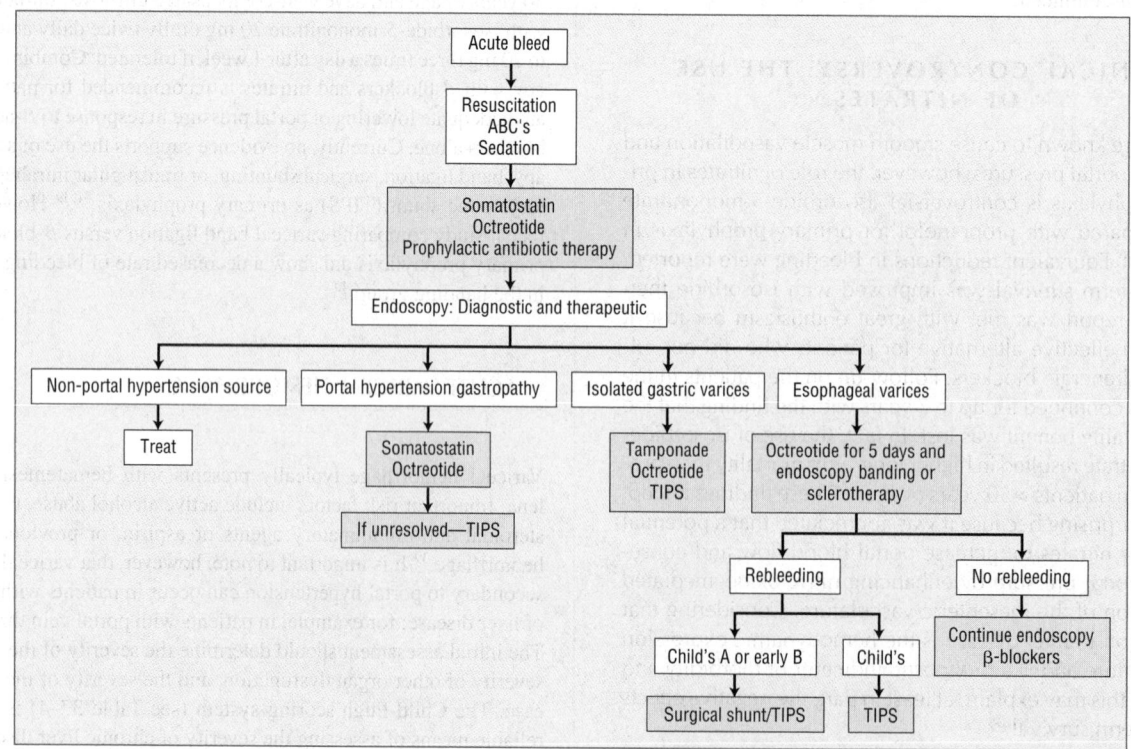

FIGURE 37–5. Management of acute variceal hemorrhage.

years for the management of acute variceal bleeding. Vasopressin reduces portal pressure by causing splanchnic vasoconstriction, which reduces splanchnic blood flow. Unfortunately, the vasoconstrictive effects of vasopressin are nonselective—the vasoconstriction produced is not restricted to the splanchnic vascular bed. Potent systemic vasoconstriction occurs in the coronary and mesenteric circulation as well, resulting in hypertension, severe headaches, coronary ischemia, myocardial infarction, and arrhythmias. A meta-analysis of 15 randomized controlled clinical trials of vasopressin for variceal hemorrhage demonstrated that vasopressin was significantly more effective than no treatment; however, control of hemorrhage was achieved in only 50% of the bleeding episodes.[48] Adverse effects were reported in 45% of patients, and vasopressin was discontinued in 25% of patients secondary to adverse effects. To minimize adverse effects associated with the peripheral vasoconstriction secondary to vasopressin, and to further lower portal pressure, the combination of vasopressin and intravenous nitroglycerin has been evaluated.[13] The combination trended toward improved control of hemorrhage with reduced side effects when compared to vasopressin alone. However, with the recent addition of safer and equally effective treatment alternatives, vasopressin, alone or combined with nitroglycerin, can no longer be recommended as first-line therapy for the management of variceal hemorrhage.[39]

Terlipressin (Glypressin), triglycyl-lysine vasopressin, is a synthetic prodrug of vasopressin with intrinsic vasoconstrictor activity that was developed in an attempt to provide an analogue of vasopressin with lower toxicity. The glycl residues are enzymatically cleaved in vivo, resulting in the slow conversion into lysine vasopressin. This process results in the availability of lysine vasopressin with a longer half-life, permitting bolus dosing every 4 hours.[39] In a number of unblinded clinical trials, terlipressin was associated with a significantly lower rate of adverse effects as compared to vasopressin alone, or as compared to vasopressin combined with nitroglycerin.[45] Terlipressin produces a marked and sustained reduction in portal pressures. This prolonged biologic effect allows intravenous administration as an intermittent infusion every 4 hours, whereas somatostatin requires administration as a continuous intravenous infusion.[49] In clinical trials that have been criticized for small sample size and unclear timing of treatments, terlipressin has demonstrated a beneficial effect on the control of bleeding compared with placebo, and is the only drug that has been shown to reduce mortality.[39] Terlipressin, the preferred drug in Europe for acute variceal bleeding, is not currently available in the United States.

Cirrhotic patients with active bleeding are at high risk of infection and sepsis secondary to aspiration, the placement of multiple intravascular access devices, sclerotherapy, translocation, and defects in humoral and cellular immunity.[39] Prophylactic antibiotic therapy to reduce the risk of sepsis during episodes of bleeding is reported to decrease the incidence of rebleeding and to increase short-term survival.[50] All patients with variceal hemorrhage should be screened for infection and pan-cultured. Patients should be evaluated at admission and observed throughout therapy for signs and symptoms of spontaneous bacterial peritonitis.[31]

ENDOSCOPIC INTERVENTIONS: SCLEROTHERAPY AND BAND LIGATION

The American College of Gastroenterology published clinical practice guidelines in 1997 recommending EGD employing EIS or EBL of varices as the primary diagnostic and treatment strategy for upper GI tract hemorrhage secondary to portal hypertension and varices.[41] EIS involves injection of 1 to 4 mL of a sclerosing agent into the lumen

of the varices to tamponade blood flow. EBL consists of placement of rubber bands around the varix through a clear plastic channel attached to the end of the endoscope. After the rubber bands are in place, the varix will slough off after 48 to 72 hours. Endoscopic approaches can successfully stop bleeding in up to 95% of cases, but rebleeding may occur in 50% of cases. A recent meta-analysis of comparative clinical trials found both techniques equally effective in controlling acute variceal bleeding, but indicated that EBL was superior to EIS in reducing the rebleeding rate, and that EBL was associated with fewer posttreatment complications.[39] Sclerosing agents employed in EIS include ethanolamine, sodium tetradecyl sulfate, polidocanol, and sodium morrhuate. There are no data establishing clinical superiority of any of the sclerosants.[51]

Eight published clinical trials have compared endoscopic sclerotherapy with vasoactive drug therapy for active variceal bleeding. Drug treatment controlled bleeding in 58% to 95% of cases, and sclerotherapy controlled bleeding in 68% to 94% of cases. Rebleeding was slightly less common in patients receiving sclerotherapy, and sclerotherapy was associated with a lower mortality rate. Clinical trials of sclerotherapy plus vasoactive drugs versus sclerotherapy alone show a significant advantage for combination therapy; however, there was no beneficial effect on mortality.[39]

INTERVENTIONAL AND SURGICAL TREATMENT APPROACHES

If standard therapy fails to control bleeding (after two failed endoscopic procedures, further attempts are unlikely to be of benefit) a salvage procedure, such as balloon tamponade, TIPS, or surgical shunting is necessary. Sengstaken-Blakemore tubes are balloon devices designed to tamponade gastric and esophageal varices that can be effective in 70% to 90% of cases of variceal bleeding.[39] However, these devices have a 10% to 30% complication rate and will be ineffective if the bleeding source is nonvariceal, a situation which occurs in 10% to 50% of patients with portal hypertension.[39] Balloon tamponade should be reserved as a temporizing measure until a TIPS procedure or surgical shunt can be performed.[31]

The development of the TIPS provided a major improvement in the management of refractory or severe cases of esophagogastric variceal bleeding and other complications of portal hypertension.[52] The TIPS procedure involves the placement of one or more stents between the hepatic vein and the portal vein (Fig. 37–6). This procedure is widely used because it provides an effective decompressive shunt without laparotomy, and can be employed regardless of Child-Pugh score. Survival rates with TIPS in patients refractory to endoscopic treatment are comparable to rates achieved with portacaval

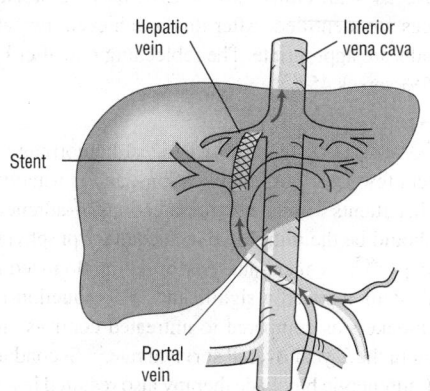

FIGURE 37–6. Transjugular intrahepatic portosystemic shunt (TIPS).

shunts.[39] Patients undergoing TIPS experience a 30% incidence of encephalopathy, and approximately 50% of shunts malfunction.[31]

Various surgical shunts have been developed and are effective for the prevention of recurrent variceal hemorrhage in patients refractory to β-adrenergic blockade and endoscopy.[31]

TREATMENT RECOMMENDATIONS: VARICEAL HEMORRHAGE

Patients require prompt resuscitation with colloids and blood products to correct intravascular losses and to reverse existing coagulopathies. Drug therapy with octreotide or somatostatin should be initiated early to control bleeding and facilitate diagnostic and therapeutic endoscopy. Based on availability octreotide is preferred. Therapy is initiated with an IV bolus of 50 to 100 mcg and is followed by a continuous infusion of 25 mcg/h, up to a maximum rate of 50 mcg/h. Monitor patients for hypo- or hyperglycemia, especially patients with diabetes, and assess for cardiac conduction abnormalities. Vasopressin is no longer recommended for control of variceal bleeding. Endoscopy employing EBL or EIS is the primary therapeutic tool in the management of acute variceal bleeding.[30,39,53] Antibiotic prophylaxis is recommended if ascites is present and EIS is planned. Appropriate choices include a third-generation cephalosporin (e.g., ceftazidime or ceftriaxone), a penicillin/β-lactamase inhibitor combination (e.g., piperacillin-tazobactam), or a fluoroquinolone (e.g., ofloxacin). Surgical shunts and TIPS are employed as salvage therapy in patients who have failed repeated endoscopy and vasoactive drug therapy.

Secondary Prophylaxis: Prevention of Rebleeding

Because the risk of rebleeding after initial control of variceal hemorrhage can approach 80%, and rebleeding significantly increases the risk of death, it is inappropriate to simply observe patients for evidence of further bleeding. Traditionally, pharmacologic therapy using β-adrenergic blockers was recommended as the initial approach for prevention of rebleeding. A major shift in therapy is underway; endoscopic therapy using EBL or EIS, repeated at regular intervals with the goal of obliteration of varices, is emerging as the preferred treatment option. Alternatives for the secondary prevention of rebleeding include surgical or interventional shunting.

The objective of both EIS and EBL in prevention of rebleeding is the obliteration of esophageal varices. The majority of rebleeding occurs in the interval between the primary endoscopic session and the time to complete obliteration. Therefore the patient should have repeat endoscopy with either EIS or EBL every 2 weeks until no further varices are identified. After this is achieved, repeat exams at 3 and 6 months are appropriate. The rebleeding rate after EBL is less than EIS, 27% versus 45%.[54]

Drug Therapy. Drug therapy of variceal hemorrhage is less expensive, offers fewer serious complications, and is usually preferred by patients. In patients without contraindications, β-adrenergic blocking agents should be the initial step in secondary prophylaxis, along with endoscopy.[39,54] A meta-analysis of 11 randomized controlled clinical trials demonstrated a significant 21% reduction in rebleeding with β-blockers as compared to untreated controls, and a 5.4% improvement in the 2-year overall survival rate.[55] Secondary prophylaxis with β-adrenergic blockade therapy also resulted in a significant

7.4% reduction in death as a consequence of rebleeding. Propranolol was used in 10 trials; nadolol was used in one trial. Patients treated with β-adrenergic blocking agents experienced significantly more adverse events, 22% versus 9% compared to untreated controls,[55] with 5.7% requiring discontinuation of β-adrenergic blockade therapy.

When considering the benefits associated with β-adrenergic blockers, it is important to appreciate that approximately 25% of cirrhotic patients either have contraindications or exhibit intolerance to β-adrenergic blockers, and portal pressures are not adequately lowered in all patients treated with β-adrenergic blockade.[56] Use of a long-acting β-blocker (such as nadolol) is usually recommended to improve compliance, and gradual, individualized dose escalation may help to minimize side effects. Ideally, portal pressure monitoring can help to assess the response to β-adrenergic blocker therapy and identify nonresponders earlier in the treatment course. This is important because patients with sinusoidal portal hypertension (the type encountered in cirrhosis) do not bleed when the hepatic venous pressure gradient is <12 mm Hg. Also, protection against rebleeding has been demonstrated when the hepatic venous pressure gradient is reduced by 20%.[57] However, the procedure for measuring portal pressures is invasive, expensive, and not available in most facilities. In addition, the cost-effectiveness of this approach (baseline and posttherapy) has not been compared with simply monitoring heart rate reduction with β-blockers.[58] For patients who fail to achieve sufficient reductions in portal pressure with β-blocker therapy alone, combination therapy with nitrates or spironolactone may more effectively lower portal pressures.[59] However, combination therapy for secondary prophylaxis has not been evaluated in randomized clinical trials.

Comparisons of β-adrenergic blocker therapy alone with EIS suggest that less variceal rebleeding is seen with EIS, but this benefit is offset by an increase in complications.[39,54] A recent study comparing nadolol plus isosorbide mononitrate with EIS suggested that combined drug therapy offered substantial advantages over EIS.[60] Rebleeding was significantly less common with nadolol and isosorbide mononitrate, and treatment-associated complications occurred significantly less often as well. However, because EBL is now increasingly preferred over EIS for secondary prophylaxis due to superior efficacy and safety, data from comparative trials with medical therapy are needed. In one series the rebleeding rate for EBL was superior to standard medical therapy.[61]

Shunting. When drug therapy and endoscopy fail, alternatives include TIPS placement or shunt surgery. Regular documentation of patency and the requirement of repeat procedures make it an unsuitable long-term solution. In patients with well-compensated hepatic function (Child-Pugh grade A or B) surgical shunting is an excellent option.

Treatment Recommendations: Secondary Prophylaxis

The preferred initial approach is currently unsettled and may depend on local experience and expertise.[54] Endoscopic therapy using either EIS or EBL and pharmacologic therapy are both effective in reducing the risk of rebleeding. As a consequence of decreased complications, bleeding, and possibly mortality, EBL has emerged as the endoscopic treatment of choice.[39,54] Either approach alone or the combination of endoscopy with pharmacologic therapy can be considered appropriate initial therapy. Pharmacologic therapy should be initiated with a nonselective β-blocker such as propranolol 20 mg three times a day, or nadolol at a dose of 20 to 40 mg once daily, and titrated weekly to achieve a goal heart rate of 55 to 60 bpm or a heart rate that is 25%

lower than the baseline heart rate. Assessment of portal pressures can identify nonresponders for whom combination therapy with β-blockers and nitrates or spironolactone may be attempted to achieve portal pressure gradients <12 mm Hg. Monitor patients for evidence of heart failure, bronchospasm, and glucose intolerance, particularly hypoglycemia in patients with insulin-dependent diabetes.

ASCITES AND SPONTANEOUS BACTERIAL PERITONITIS

Patients with cirrhosis fail to maintain normal extracellular fluid volumes secondary to abnormal sodium and fluid retention and an impaired capacity to eliminate water.[13] Patients usually present with ascites, edema, or both, and most commonly complain of discomfort from abdominal or leg swelling, respiratory difficulties, malaise, anorexia, and weight loss. The development of ascites in patients with cirrhosis is an indication of advanced liver disease and is a poor prognostic sign. Treatment goals for patients with ascites include prevention of serious complications (spontaneous bacterial peritonitis and rupture of an umbilical hernia) and improving the patient's sense of well-being and quality of life by minimizing respiratory difficulties, loss of appetite, and discomfort from abdominal distention or leg swelling.[62] Treatment of ascites is expected to have little effect on survival, however. Pleural effusions are common, and in some cases can be the primary manifestation of the fluid retention. Work-up includes a history and physical exam, laboratory tests to assess liver function, abdominal ultrasound to rule out hepatocellular carcinoma, endoscopy to evaluate esophageal and gastric varices, abdominal paracentesis with analysis of ascitic fluid, and a complete evaluation of circulatory and renal function. Treatment of ascites has risks. Depending on the treatment approach and the goals selected, significant adverse reactions can occur, including electrolyte disturbances, acid-base abnormalities, hepatic encephalopathy, hypovolemia, and renal insufficiency.

Spontaneous bacterial peritonitis (SBP), infection of preexisting ascitic fluid, in the absence of any evidence of a primary intra-abdominal source of infection, is a common complication in patients with ascites, developing in 10% to 25% of patients followed prospectively for at least 1 year.[13] The incidence of SBP is substantially higher in patients with ascitic fluid protein levels <1 g/dL and with serum bilirubin levels above 2.5 mg/dL.[63] Because the antibacterial activity of ascitic fluid is proportional to the level of ascitic fluid protein, patients with low ascitic fluid protein levels are at increased risk of SBP. The pathogenesis of SBP is unknown, but presumably results from hematogenous seeding (cirrhosis permits enteric organisms direct access to the bloodstream via the portosystemic collaterals) of the ascitic fluid that offers a favorable growth medium.[64] Consequently, most episodes of SBP are caused by gram-negative Enterobacteriaceae, with *Escherichia coli* most commonly isolated. The clinical presentation of SBP can vary from patients who present with all of the signs and symptoms of peritonitis, including fever, leukocytosis, abdominal pain, hypoactive or absent bowel sounds, and rebound tenderness, to those patients who have no signs or symptoms at all. For this reason, a diagnostic paracentesis with analysis of ascitic fluid should be performed in all patients admitted with ascites or in patients with cirrhosis who suddenly deteriorate.[5,13] Spontaneous bacterial peritonitis is diagnosed when ascitic fluid cell counts show an absolute polymorphonuclear (PMN) leukocyte count of $\geq$250 cells/mm³, a positive ascitic fluid culture is obtained, or a patient with cirrhotic ascites presents with convincing signs or symptoms of infection.[64]

MANAGEMENT OF ASCITES AND SPONTANEOUS BACTERIAL PERITONITIS

The following treatment guidelines for the management of adult patients with ascites and spontaneous bacterial peritonitis were developed and approved by the Practice Guidelines Committee of the American Association for the Study of Liver Diseases (AASLD).[5]

Ascites

In adult patients with new-onset ascites as determined by physical exam or radiographic studies, abdominal paracentesis should be performed and ascitic fluid analysis should include a cell count with differential and a serum-ascites albumin gradient (SAG). If infection is suspected, ascitic fluid cultures should be obtained at the time of the paracentesis. The SAG can accurately determine whether ascites is a result of portal hypertension or another process. If the SAG is >1.1 g/dL, portal hypertension is present with 97% accuracy.[5] If the SAG is <1.1 g/dL, with similar certainty the patient does not have portal hypertension. This is important because patients without portal hypertension will not respond to salt restriction and diuretics. The treatment of ascites secondary to portal hypertension is relatively straightforward and includes abstinence from alcohol, sodium restriction, and diuretics. This strategy is effective in approximately 90% of patients. Fifteen percent of patients will respond to dietary sodium restriction alone, and an additional 75% of patients will respond to the addition of diuretics.[65]

Abstinence from alcohol is an essential element of the overall treatment strategy. Abstinence from alcohol can result in improvement of the reversible component of alcoholic liver disease and normalize portal pressures in some patients.[5] Even in those patients with cirrhosis from another cause (e.g., autoimmune hepatitis) abstinence from alcohol can reverse alcohol-related effects and result in substantial improvement of the underlying liver disease. Patients with cirrhosis not caused by alcohol have less reversible liver disease, and by the time ascites is present, given the poor prognosis these patients may be best managed with liver transplantation rather than protracted medical therapy.[5]

Beyond avoidance of alcohol, the primary treatment is salt restriction and oral diuretic therapy. Achieving the desired fluid losses in patients with ascites caused by portal hypertension is directly related to sodium balance, not fluid restriction.[66] To monitor these patients, evaluation of urinary sodium excretion, utilizing a 24-hour urine collection, is recommended.[5] However, severe hyponatremia, serum sodium <120 mEq/L, does warrant fluid restriction; rapid correction of asymptomatic hyponatremia (patients with cirrhosis usually are not symptomatic until their serum sodium concentrations are <110 mEq/L) is not recommended.

Diuretic Therapy

The AASLD practice guidelines recommend that diuretic therapy be initiated with the combination of spironolactone and furosemide. Spironolactone alone was commonly recommended for initial therapy, but clinical trials have demonstrated a 14-day delay in the onset of action, as well as the development hyperkalemia when spironolactone is used alone.[67] Administering spironolactone in single daily doses is justified based on its pharmacokinetics and helps to improve patient compliance.[67] If tense ascites is present, paracentesis should be performed prior to institution of diuretic therapy and salt restriction.[5] For patients who respond to diuretic therapy, this approach is preferred over the use of serial paracenteses.[68] In patients with refractory ascites, serial paracenteses may be employed as needed. Albumin infusion postparacentesis is controversial but should be employed for volumes exceeding 5 L.[68] Laboratory tests for renal function and electrolytes need to be monitored during therapy. Liver transplantation should be considered in patients with refractory ascites. For patients who are not transplant candidates and who fail repeated paracentesis because of loculated ascites, TIPS or peritoneal venous shunts may be considered. Both of these procedures have significant complication rates and are not recommended for the routine treatment of ascites.[5]

Spontaneous Bacterial Peritonitis

Patients with documented or suspected SBP should receive broad-spectrum antibiotic therapy, which must adequately cover the three most commonly encountered pathogens: *Escherichia coli*, *Klebsiella pneumoniae*, and *Streptococcus pneumoniae*.[5,68] Delaying antibiotic therapy while awaiting evidence of a positive ascitic fluid culture is not recommended and can result in overwhelming infection and death.[5] In some patients, signs and symptoms of infection are present at the bacterascites stage (i.e., signs and symptoms present before the PMN count in the ascitic fluid is elevated[69]). In these patients, signs and symptoms of infection justify empiric antibiotic therapy, regardless of the PMN count in the ascitic fluid.[69]

Cefotaxime or a similar third-generation cephalosporin are considered the drugs of choice.[5] Cefotaxime is more effective than aztreonam or the combination of ampicillin and tobramycin.[13] Fluoroquinolone antibiotics provide good activity against the usual pathogens encountered in SBP, excellent oral bioavailability, and high penetration into ascitic fluid. Ofloxacin 400 mg every 12 hours administered orally is equivalent to intravenous cefotaxime in terms of resolution of infection as well as survival.[70] For many patients, oral ofloxacin therapy offers a simple, cost-effective alternative to intravenous therapy with third-generation cephalosporins. However, intravenous therapy with an agent such as cefotaxime is preferred for severely ill patients, or for patients with gastrointestinal hemorrhage or ileus, because oral bioavailability may be compromised.[69] Antibiotic therapy should be continued until all signs of infection have resolved and the ascitic fluid PMN count decreases below 250/mm^3.[69] However, in patients who respond clinically to antibiotics, routine follow-up paracentesis is not necessary. A 5-day course of antibiotic therapy was reported to be as efficacious as 10 days of therapy in a randomized trial involving 100 patients with SBP.[69]

Secondary bacterial peritonitis, ascitic fluid infection caused by a treatable intra-abdominal source, can masquerade as SBP and should be considered when multiple or atypical organisms are cultured, a very high ascitic fluid PMN count is seen, or in patients who fail to respond to appropriate antibiotic therapy. Uncomplicated SBP usually responds rapidly to appropriate therapy and the 48-hour PMN count, if obtained, is predictably lower than the initial count.[64] In this setting a follow-up paracentesis revealing a PMN count that continues to rise despite antibiotic therapy can be helpful in detecting secondary peritonitis.[5]

Antibiotic therapy for the *prevention* of SBP should be considered in all patients at high risk for this complication, including those who have experienced a prior episode of SBP or variceal hemorrhage, and those with low-protein ascites (<1 g/dL). Norfloxacin

400 mg intravenously once daily, or 400 mg every 12 hours orally or by nasogastric tube; ofloxacin 400 mg intravenously once daily; or the combination of ciprofloxacin and amoxicillin-clavulanic acid markedly reduces the risk of SBP as compared to untreated patients in these high-risk groups.[68] Long-term norfloxacin, 400 mg orally once daily, reduces the risk of recurrent SBP from 70% to 20% at 1 year, primarily by reducing the incidence of SBP caused by gram-negative bacilli from 60% to 3%.[71] However, antibiotic prophylaxis does not prolong survival and it selects resistant organisms that may subsequently cause SBP.[68,72] Fortunately, episodes of SBP caused by resistant organisms are uncommon.[73] Prolonged therapy with ciprofloxacin is a risk factor for fungal infections in patients subsequently undergoing liver transplantation.[68] Intermittent prophylactic strategies, including ciprofloxacin 750 mg orally once a week, trimethoprim-sulfamethoxazole 1 DS tablet five times a week, or inpatient norfloxacin with discontinuation at discharge, are effective and may be less likely to select resistant organisms.[5,68,74]

TREATMENT RECOMMENDATIONS: ASCITES AND SPONTANEOUS BACTERIAL PERITONITIS

Adult patients admitted to the hospital with new-onset ascites should have an abdominal paracentesis performed to establish the serum-ascites albumin gradient, the ascitic fluid PMN count, and to obtain ascitic fluid cultures. Patients who drink alcohol should be strongly discouraged from further alcohol use. Sodium restriction to 2000 mg/day, together with spironolactone and furosemide, is the mainstay of therapy. Diuretic therapy should be initiated with single morning doses of spironolactone 100 mg and furosemide 40 mg administered orally with the goal of a 0.5-kg maximum daily weight loss. Titrate diuretic therapy using the 100 mg:40 mg ratio, to a maximum daily dose of 400 mg spironolactone and 160 mg furosemide. This combination ratio is used because it usually maintains normokalemia. Fluid restriction, unless the serum sodium is <120 mEq/L, and bed rest are not recommended. Monitor urinary sodium excretion using a 24-hour urine collection, and monitor serum potassium and renal function frequently. Avoid rapid correction of asymptomatic hyponatremia in patients with cirrhosis. If tense ascites is present, a 4- to 6-L paracentesis should be performed prior to institution of diuretic therapy and salt restriction. For patients who respond to diuretic therapy this approach is preferred over the use of serial paracenteses. Discontinue diuretic therapy in patients who experience encephalopathy, severe hyponatremia (serum sodium <120 mEq/L) despite fluid restriction, or renal insufficiency (serum creatinine >2 mg/dL). Serial paracenteses may be considered for patients with refractory ascites with albumin infusion postparacentesis when volumes exceeding 5 L are removed.

Patients with documented SBP, positive ascitic fluid cultures, or ascitic fluid PMN count ≥250 cells/mm,^{3} regardless of symptoms, should receive broad-spectrum empiric antibiotic therapy with cefotaxime 2 g every 8 hours, or a similar third-generation cephalosporin. Patients with ascitic fluid PMN counts <250 cells/mm^3, but with signs and symptoms of infection (abdominal pain, tenderness, fever, encephalopathy, renal failure, acidosis, or peripheral leukocytosis), should also receive empiric antibiotic treatment with cefotaxime 2 g every 8 hours, or a similar third-generation cephalosporin. Outpatient oral therapy of SBP with fluoroquinolones or amoxicillin-clavulanic acid awaits further clinical trials. Short-term inpatient quinolone therapy should be considered for the prevention of SBP in patients with low-protein ascites (<1 g/dL), variceal hemorrhage, or prior SBP.

TABLE 37–6. Grading System for Hepatic Encephalopathy

Grade	Level of Consciousness	Personality/Intellect	Neurologic Abnormalities	EEG Abnormalities
0	Normal	Normal	None	None
Subclinical	Normal	Normal	Psychological only	None
1	Inverted sleep patterns/ restless	Forgetful, mild confusion, agitation, irritable	Tremor, apraxia, incoordination, impaired handwriting	Triphasic waves (5 cycles/s)
2	Lethargic, slow responses	Disorientation for time, amnesia, decreased inhibitions, inappropriate behavior	Asterixis, dysarthria, ataxia, hypoactive reflexes	Triphasic waves (5 cycles/s)
3	Somnolent but rousable, confused	Disorientation for place, aggressive	Asterixis, hyperactive reflexes, Babinski's sign, muscle rigidity	Triphasic waves (5 cycles/s)
4	Coma/unrousable	None	Decerebrate	Delta activity, (2–3 cycles/s)

 All patients who have survived an episode of SBP should receive long-term antibiotic prophylaxis.[5]

HEPATIC ENCEPHALOPATHY

Although management strategies are similar for both acute and chronic HE, the urgency of treatment interventions and goals of therapy are different.[21] Patients with subclinical HE often experience only minor motor and attentional deficits and compensate on their own without the need for therapy. Those with more significant deficits that impact activities of daily living can benefit from intervention.[19]

The prevalence of clinically apparent HE is unknown; however, between 50% and 80% of patients with cirrhosis demonstrate neurologic dysfunction by electroencephalography or by psychological testing.[75] To determine the severity of HE, a grading system that relates neurologic and neuromuscular signs can be used (Table 37–6). The pathogenesis of HE is unknown. It is believed to be a multifactorial metabolic/neurophysiologic abnormality.[19,21]

TABLE 37–7. Portosystemic Encephalopathy: Precipitating Factors and Therapy

Factor	Therapy Alternatives
Gastrointestinal bleeding	
Variceal	Band ligation/sclerotherapy
	Octreotide
Nonvariceal	Endoscopic therapy
	Proton pump inhibitors
Infection/sepsis	Antibiotics
	Paracentesis
Electrolyte abnormalities	Discontinue diuretics
	Fluid and electrolyte replacement
Sedative ingestion	Discontinue sedatives/tranquilizers
	Consider reversal (flumazenil/ naloxone)
Dietary excesses	Limit daily protein
	Lactulose
Constipation	Cathartics
	Bowel cleansing/enema
Renal insufficiency	Discontinue diuretics
	Discontinue NSAIDs, nephrotoxic antibiotics
	Fluid resuscitation

MANAGEMENT OF HEPATIC ENCEPHALOPATHY

Acute HE usually develops in a clinically stable cirrhotic patient as the result of an acute precipitating event.[19] Table 36–7 lists the most commonly encountered precipitating factors and suggests general treatment alternatives. Chronic HE, by definition, occurs and persists in the absence of precipitating factors. It can occur in patients who have undergone a TIPS procedure or surgical shunting or in patients with advanced cirrhosis. Patients with acute HE have potentially reversible causes of their encephalopathy, whereas patients with chronic HE usually do not. Nevertheless, the mediators of the encephalopathy are the same, justifying similar treatment strategies. The major difference is the need for urgent inpatient intervention for management of the precipitating event in acute HE, and the expectation for normal mentation after recovery. Patients with chronic HE typically exhibit a high prevalence of chronically abnormal mentation.[75]

Table 37–8 describes the treatment goals for patients with HE and contrasts the differences between acute and chronic HE. The general approach to the management of HE is to first identify and treat any precipitating factors, which often results in prompt resolution of the encephalopathy. The development of mental status changes in cirrhosis is associated with increased morbidity and mortality.[19] However, universal treatment of patients with subclinical HE is not recommended because the consequences of motor and attention deficits are considered minor, and prevention of progression to more severe HE has not been studied.[19]

Treatment approaches for HE evolve from the various hypotheses advanced to explain the pathogenesis of HE and include: (a) reducing ammonia blood concentrations by dietary restrictions and drug therapy aimed at inhibiting ammonia production or enhancing its removal; (b) inhibition of the γ-aminobutyric acid

TABLE 37–8. Treatment Goals: Acute and Chronic HE

Acute HE	Chronic HE
Control precipitating factor	Reverse encephalopathy
Reverse encephalopathy	Avoid recurrence
Hospital/inpatient therapy	Home/outpatient therapy
Maintain fluid and hemodynamic support	Manage persistent neuropsychiatric abnormalities
	Manage chronic liver disease
Expect normal mentation after recovery	High prevalence of abnormal mentation after recovery

(GABA)-benzodiazepine receptors by flumazenil; and (c) inhibition of false neurotransmitters by optimizing amino acid balance.[17,19]

Hyperammonemia

Despite criticisms of the ammonia hypothesis, treatment interventions to reduce ammonia blood concentrations are beneficial in patients with HE.[19] Decreasing ammonia blood concentrations by limiting its availability and production, or by enhancing its metabolism, remains a mainstay of therapy for patients with both acute and chronic HE.[19]

Decreasing ammonia blood concentrations can be attempted by reducing ammonia production or by decreasing the availability of ammonia in the colon. Limiting dietary protein acutely usually results in a lowering of ammonia concentrations and improvement in HE.

Guidelines for nutritional support of patients with liver disease have been published by the European Society for Parenteral and Enteral Nutrition. Protein is added back to the diet initially with 0.5 to 0.6 g/kg per day and advanced by 0.25 to 0.5 g/kg per day every 3 to 5 days until a target of 1 to 1.5 g/kg per day is reached or progression of HE occurs.[76] Vegetable-source protein may be preferable to animal-source protein because it contains fewer aromatic amino acids, which are implicated in generating false neurotransmitters (see below). Also, the higher fiber content of vegetable protein increases colonic transit time and lowers colonic pH secondary to its fermentation by colonic bacteria.[76] In patients with chronic HE, dietary therapy with restricted protein should be used in an attempt to prevent malnutrition and prevent exacerbation of HE. Protein intolerance is a common problem in patients with chronic liver disease and HE.[19,77] Bowel cleansing using cathartics or lactulose enemas (see below) results in rapid removal of ammonia substrate from the colon.

The use of lactulose, a nonabsorbable disaccharide, (and lactitol, not available in the United States) is standard therapy for both acute and chronic HE.[19,78] Lactulose, when administered orally, passes through the gastrointestinal tract and reaches the colon unchanged. For patients unable to take lactulose orally or via tube administration it may be administered as an enema. In the colon, lactulose lowers colonic pH and exerts a cathartic effect. Fermentation of lactulose by bacteria present in the colon results in the production of organic acids, decreasing colonic pH to approximately 5.[17]

Urease-producing bacteria metabolize dietary protein and endogenous protein substrates (epithelial cells), producing ammonia. Acidification of the colon inhibits the viability of these urease-producing bacteria (and may promote the growth of non–urease-producing lactobacilli) decreasing the absorption of ammonia. Acidification also enhances the net movement of ammonia from the blood into the bowel.[17] The cathartic effect of lactulose then eliminates the ammonia and protein substrates, inhibiting ammonia production.[78] More than 30 clinical trials have demonstrated the efficacy of lactulose in the management of acute HE, and more than 20 studies support its use in chronic HE.[23] Clinical improvement is noted in approximately 86% of patients with acute HE, and in approximately 77% of patients with chronic HE.

Inhibiting the activity of urease-producing bacteria by using neomycin, metronidazole, or vancomycin can decrease production of ammonia.[17] Neomycin at doses of 2 to 8 g daily in divided oral doses results in clinical improvement in as many as 80% of patients.[77] At these doses, however, absorption is 1% to 5% and can result in irreversible ototoxicity and nephrotoxicity.[79] As such, even though efficacy is equivalent to lactulose, neomycin should not be first-line therapy. Metronidazole produces response rates similar to neomycin, but side effects, particularly gastrointestinal, limit its use.[17] In patients

with an inadequate response to lactulose alone, combination therapy with neomycin may provide additive effects and improved clinical response.[17]

Decreasing ammonia production by replacement of urease-producing bacteria in the colon with non–urease-producing strains has been attempted with the oral administration of *Lactobacillus acidophilus* and *Enterococcus faecium*.[80] The data supporting this therapy are limited, especially for patients with acute HE. However, for patients with less severe HE, *Enterococcus faecium* was as effective as lactulose, treatment effects persisted during drug-free periods, and no adverse effects were reported.[80] Ammonia generated by *H. pylori* in the stomach has been associated with precipitating or worsening HE in patients with cirrhosis.[81] Routine eradication of *H. pylori* is recommended in patients with cirrhosis and a history of HE.[17,19]

Enhancing ammonia removal by stimulating its detoxification by supporting alternative metabolic pathways can reduce blood ammonia concentrations. Centrizonal periportal hepatocytes responsible for ammonia metabolism via ureagenesis are impaired in patients with cirrhosis.[82] L-Ornithine L-aspartate enhances ureagenesis and results in reductions in ammonia concentrations and clinical benefits in patients with grade 1 and grade 2 HE. Clinical response rates similar to those of lactulose were reported in one trial involving patients with chronic HE.[83] Studies in patients with more severe HE are needed.

Zinc deficiency is common in patients with cirrhosis and has been reported to cause overt HE.[84] Zinc is a required cofactor for ammonia metabolism; two of the five metabolic pathways are zinc dependent. Both supportive and nonsupportive studies evaluating the efficacy of zinc replacement have been published.[17] In a controlled trial in cirrhotic patients with mild HE, the administration of zinc sulfate 600 mg/day for 3 months resulted in increased urea formation and lower ammonia levels, along with improvement in psychological test scores.[85] Zinc supplementation is recommended for long-term management in patients with cirrhosis who are zinc deficient.[17,19]

Inhibition of γ-Aminobutyric Acid-Benzodiazepine Receptors

The GABA-receptor complex, the primary inhibitory neural network within the central nervous system, is associated with HE.[17,19] This receptor complex is composed of a GABA-binding site, and a benzodiazepine receptor site, which mediate chloride conductance. Based on evidence of an increase in benzodiazepine receptor ligands in patients with hepatic encephalopathy, flumazenil has been evaluated in uncontrolled studies and has demonstrated significant clinical improvement, with one case report documenting long-term benefit.[86] In these reports, discontinuation of flumazenil resulted in prompt clinical deterioration.

Among five prospective, placebo-controlled trials, three reported benefit with flumazenil, whereas two found no difference when compared to placebo. With dosages of 0.2 to 15 mg IV, response rates were variable, ranging from 17% to 78%; improvements, however, were often transient.[87] Flumazenil, which is only available in an intravenous dosage form, may be considered for short-term therapy in refractory patients, but cannot be recommended for routine clinical use.

CLINICAL CONTROVERSY: USE OF BRANCHED-CHAIN AMINO ACIDS

A great deal of controversy surrounds the issue of whether or not exogenous protein rich in branched-chain amino acids

(BCAAs) is superior to standard protein solutions that are higher in aromatic amino acids (AAAs).[19] Metabolism of AAAs into false neurotransmitters that penetrate the blood-brain barrier (which itself may be perturbed in patients with HE) has been implicated as a cause of HE.[88] A number of clinical trials have evaluated the use of BCAAs in the treatment of HE, with conflicting results. Reviews of these trials have also arrived at different conclusions.[19,88,89] BCAAs may have a role in the malnourished patient with cirrhosis who is intolerant of protein supplementation, but the current data do not justify routine use of BCAAs for the treatment of HE.[19] Impairment of dopaminergic transmission has also been proposed to cause HE, but trials with bromocriptine and levodopa failed to provide any benefit and are not recommended.[17]

■ TREATMENT RECOMMENDATIONS: HEPATIC ENCEPHALOPATHY

Treatment recommendations depend on the type of HE being managed, acute HE, chronic HE, or subclinical HE. The general approach to the management of HE is to first identify patients with acute HE and then to provide aggressive management of any precipitating events (see Table 36–7). When the precipitating event has been discovered and appropriate therapy initiated, then steps to rapidly reverse the encephalopathy should be implemented. Remember that the altered sensorium associated with HE itself is associated with increased morbidity and mortality.

The mainstay of therapy of HE involves measures to lower blood ammonia concentrations, and includes diet therapy, lactulose, and antibiotics, alone or in combination with lactulose. Other adjunctive therapies include zinc replacement.

In patients with acute HE, protein is withheld or limited to 10 to 20 g/day while maintaining the total caloric intake, until the clinical situation improves. Titrate protein based on tolerance, increasing intake in increments of 10 to 20 g/day every 3 to 5 days to a total of 0.8 to 1 g/kg per day. In patients with chronic HE, restrict protein to 40 g/day. Consider the addition of dietary fiber to animal-source protein diets.

In acute HE, lactulose is initiated at a dose of 45 mL orally every hour (or by retention enema, 300 mL lactulose syrup in 700 mL water, held for 30 to 60 minutes) until catharsis begins. The dose is then decreased to 15 to 45 mL orally every 8 to 12 hours (enemas every 6 to 8 hours) and titrated to produce two to four soft, acidic stools per day. In patients with chronic HE, lactulose may be initiated at a dose of 30 to 60 mL/day with titration to the same endpoint. Monitor electrolytes periodically, follow patients for changes in mental status, and titrate to the number of stools as above.

Antibiotic therapy with either metronidazole or neomycin is reserved for patients who have not responded to diet and lactulose therapy, where the combination may provide additive effects and improved clinical response. Zinc supplementation at a dose of 600 mg/day is recommended for long-term management in patients with cirrhosis who are zinc deficient.

Other adjunctive therapies that may be considered for patients refractory to standard therapy include eradication of *H. pylori* in patients with cirrhosis and a history of HE, administration of *Lactobacillus acidophilus,* L-ornithine L-aspartate, or flumazenil 0.2 mg up to 15 mg IV. Universal treatment of patients with subclinical HE is not recommended; however, therapy to improve performance of daily activities, or in patients with more significant deficits, may be considered with close monitoring for adverse effects. Finally, supportive measures to manage the underlying liver failure need to be implemented.

■ SYSTEMIC COMPLICATIONS

In addition to the more common complications of chronic liver disease discussed above, a number of other complications can occur, including hepatorenal syndrome, hepatopulmonary syndrome, coagulation disorders, and endocrine dysfunction.

Hepatorenal syndrome, functional renal failure in the setting of cirrhosis in the absence of intrinsic renal disease, occurs in patients with cirrhosis as a result of intense vasoconstriction within the renal cortical vasculature. It is common and develops in approximately 40% of patients with cirrhosis and ascites within 5 years.[92] The resultant reduction in blood supply to the kidneys causes avid sodium retention and oliguria. The vasoconstriction that occurs in the kidneys is in stark contrast to the state of systemic vasodilation that is characteristic of chronic liver failure.[90] The pathophysiologic mechanism responsible for these effects is unknown, but is linked to the systemic vasodilation, hypovolemia, and hyperkinetic circulation seen in chronic liver failure.[91,92]

Management of hepatorenal syndrome consists of excluding all other potential nephrotoxins such as nonsteroidal anti-inflammatory agents and aminoglycosides, and assessment for prerenal azotemia secondary to overaggressive diuretic use. Withholding diuretic therapy and administering a fluid challenge has been recommended for early diagnosis and therapy.[90] Case reports describe successful resolution of hepatorenal syndrome with low-dose dopamine (3 to 5 mcg/kg per minute intravenously) and the combination of dopamine and norepinephrine.[92] Liver transplantation, which if successful results in full recovery of renal function, remains the treatment of choice for refractory hepatorenal syndrome.

Hepatopulmonary syndrome affects 20% to 40% of patients with cirrhosis, and is characterized by alterations in lung mechanics caused by ascites and by intrapulmonary shunting and gas exchange.[92] These patients present with profound fatigue and dyspnea. In the absence of intrinsic cardiopulmonary disease, cirrhotic patients with these findings should be evaluated for hepatopulmonary syndrome. Physical findings of tense ascites or pleural effusions not associated with pulmonary parenchymal disease are suggestive of hepatopulmonary syndrome. A prompt resolution of symptoms after large-volume paracentesis is characteristic.[92] Long-term management requires control of ascites (see management of ascites, discussed earlier), supportive therapy with supplemental oxygen, and optimizing fluid status. The prognosis for these patients is poor. Ultimately, liver transplantation offers the best chance for long-term recovery.

Coagulation disorders are common in patients with chronic liver disease. These disorders increase the risk of bleeding and tend to become more profound as the liver failure becomes more severe. Correction of the coagulopathy is essential for patients actively bleeding (see management of variceal hemorrhage, discussed earlier), but is not required for patients who present with only minor symptoms such as bruising or nose bleeds and who are not actively bleeding. The pathophysiology of the coagulopathy is complex and involves abnormalities of platelet function, clotting factor deficiencies, and fibrinolysis.[93] Acute therapy involves platelet transfusions for thrombocytopenia, and fresh frozen plasma for prolongation of the prothrombin time because of clotting factor deficiencies. Long-term management of cirrhotic patients with identified coagulopathies is supportive for the management of the underlying cause of cirrhosis; for example, encouraging abstinence from alcohol.

The presence of cirrhosis can produce abnormal regulation and function of multiple endocrine systems.[92] Most common are feminization and hypogonadism, and hypothyroidism. Cirrhosis perturbs the hypothalamic-pituitary-axis, which is required for normal regulation of sex and thyroid hormones. In men with cirrhosis, testosterone levels are depressed, while estrogen levels are increased. The clinical manifestations of these changes include loss of libido, muscle wasting, and gynecomastia. These clinical findings are commonly seen and have been reported to occur in up to 60% of cirrhotic patients.[92] In women, feminization changes are less well studied. Alcohol use complicates and can worsen sex hormone abnormalities.

Both central and peripheral defects in thyroid secretion are noted in patients with cirrhosis. Alcohol plays a major role with direct toxic effects on the thyroid gland. Management includes thyroid hormone replacement for hypothyroidism with the usual doses (levothyroxine 50 to 100 mcg/day) and testosterone replacement (testosterone 200 mg three times daily) may be attempted to improve libido, well-being, and gynecomastia. Routine hormone replacement has not been shown to impact survival or disease progression.[92]

LIVER TRANSPLANTATION

The complications seen in patients with chronic liver disease are essentially functional as a secondary effect of the circulatory and metabolic changes that accompany liver failure. Consequently, liver transplantation is the only treatment that can offer a cure for complications of end-stage cirrhosis. However, patient selection, evaluation, and pre- and postsurgical management are beyond the scope of this review. Refer to Chap. 87 on transplantation.

PHARMACOKINETIC AND PHARMACODYNAMIC CHANGES IN LIVER FAILURE

The liver plays a major role in the absorption, biotransformation, and elimination of many drugs. In addition, patients with cirrhosis may exhibit pharmacodynamic changes with increased sensitivity to the effects of certain drugs.[94] These pharmacodynamic changes are separate and distinct from the enhancement of drug effects seen in these patients as a result of the altered serum concentrations of both total and free drug that occur because of the pharmacokinetic changes in these patients. Hepatic drug clearance is primarily dependent upon protein binding, hepatic blood flow, and intrinsic hepatic metabolic activity.[95] The pathophysiologic changes that occur in patients with cirrhosis, including reduced liver blood flow, altered microcirculatory distribution of blood flow within the liver, diminished metabolic and synthetic function, and changes in the endothelial lining of the sinusoids, can have a significant impact on each of these factors. The consequence of these changes is a reduction in intrinsic metabolic activity, a reduction in the delivery of blood to the liver that decreases clearance and prolongs half-life, and a reduction in the degree of protein binding that increases the fraction of unbound drug in the serum. Finally, patients with cirrhosis frequently accumulate large amounts of interstitial fluid resulting in substantial changes in the volume of distribution, which also prolongs drug half-life. These changes occur most commonly in combination in patients with cirrhosis and are dynamic throughout the disease course. The effect that these changes will have depends on the drug and the type of biotransformation that the drug undergoes.

Drugs with a high extraction ratio (high-extraction drugs) are dependent on blood flow for metabolism and the rate of metabolism will be sensitive to changes in blood flow. Drugs with a low extraction ratio (low-extraction drugs) are dependent on intrinsic metabolic activity for metabolism and the rate of metabolism will reflect changes in intrinsic clearance.[95] Furthermore, hepatic biotransformation involves two types of metabolic processes: phase I reactions and phase II reactions. Phase I reactions involve the cytochrome P450 system and include hydrolysis, oxidation, dealkylation, and reduction reactions. Phase II reactions involve conjugation of the drug with an endogenous molecule such as sulfate or an amino acid, rendering it more water soluble and enhancing its elimination. Drugs metabolized by phase I reactions, especially oxidation, tend to be significantly impaired in patients with cirrhosis, whereas drugs eliminated by conjugation are relatively unaffected.[96]

The variability and complexity of the interaction between the extent and severity of liver disease and individual characteristics of the drug makes it very difficult to predict the degree of pharmacokinetic perturbation in an individual patient. Unfortunately, there are no sensitive and specific clinical or biochemical markers that allow us to quantify the extent of liver insufficiency or the degree of metabolic activity. In addition, renal insufficiency and alterations that commonly accompany cirrhosis further complicate empiric dosing recommendations in these patients.[92] Most of the studies conducted to assess the effects of liver disease on pharmacokinetics have included only patients with Child-Pugh grades of A (mild cirrhosis) or B (moderate cirrhosis).[95] Dosing recommendations are most commonly nonspecific, with recommendations labeled for patients with mild to moderate liver impairment. Dosing information for patients with more severe liver impairment is not available. As a result, when patients with cirrhosis require therapy with drugs that undergo hepatic metabolism (e.g., benzodiazepines), monitoring response to therapy and anticipating drug accumulation and enhanced effects is essential. In the case of benzodiazepines, selection of an agent such as lorazepam, an intermediate-acting agent that is metabolized via conjugation and has no active metabolites, is easier to monitor than a drug such as diazepam, a long-acting benzodiazepine that is oxidized in the liver and has an active metabolite with a long half-life of its own.

A number of publications provide up-to-date analyses of the pharmacokinetic and pharmacodynamic considerations in patients with liver disease and provide the most recent data on individual drug-dosing recommendations.[97–99]

PHARMACOECONOMIC CONSIDERATIONS

Cost-benefit and cost-effectiveness analysis were highlighted as shortcomings of clinical trials in the field of cirrhosis.[53] However, a number of issues relating to drug therapy of cirrhosis have been studied. The cost-effectiveness of long-term antibiotic prophylaxis for the prevention of SBP, especially for high-risk patients as determined by simple laboratory analysis (serum bilirubin and ascitic fluid protein levels) was found to provide significant cost savings.[100] In a comparison of propranolol, sclerotherapy, and shunt surgery for prophylaxis against the first variceal bleed, propranolol was the only cost-effective alternative.[101] Because treatment approaches for patients with cirrhosis can range from supportive medical therapy, to repeated endoscopic procedures with serious complications, to liver transplantation, the need for application of economic analysis is obvious. Of critical

TABLE 37–9. Management Approach and Outcome Assessments

Complication	Treatment Approach	Monitoring Parameter	Outcome Assessment
Ascites	Diet, diuretics, paracentesis, TIPS	Daily assessment of weight	Prevent or eliminate ascites and its secondary complications
Spontaneous bacterial peritonitis	Antibiotic therapy, prophylaxis if undergoing paracentesis	Evidence of clinical deterioration (e.g., abdominal pain, fever, anorexia, malaise, fatigue)	Prevent/treat infection to decrease mortality
Variceal bleeding	Pharmacologic prophylaxis	Child-Pugh score, endoscopy, CBC	Appropriate reduction in heart rate and portal pressure
	Endoscopy, vasoactive drug therapy (octreotide), sclerotherapy, volume resuscitation, pharmacologic prophylaxis	CBC, evidence of overt bleeding	Acute: control acute bleed Chronic: variceal obliteration, reduce portal pressures
Coagulation disorders	Blood products (PPF, platelets), vitamin K	CBC, prothrombin time, platelet count	Normalize PT time, maintain/improve hemostasis
Hepatic encephalopathy	Ammonia reduction (lactulose, cathartics), elimination of drugs causing CNS depression, limit excess protein in diet	Grade of encephalopathy, EEG, psychological testing, mental status changes, concurrent drug therapy	Maintain functional capacity, prevent hospitalization for encephalopathy, decrease ammonia levels, provide adequate nutrition
Hepatorenal syndrome	Eliminate concurrent nephrotoxins (NSAIDs), decrease or discontinue diuretics, volume resuscitation, liver transplantation	Serum and urine electrolytes, concurrent drug therapy	Prevent progressive renal injury by preventing dehydration and avoiding other nephrotoxins Liver transplantation for refractory hepatorenal syndrome
Hepatopulmonary syndrome	Paracentesis, O$_2$ therapy	Dyspnea, presence of ascites	Acute: relief of dyspnea and hypoxia Chronic: manage ascites as above

CBC, complete blood cell count; CNS, central nervous system; EEG, electroencephalogram; PT, prothrombin time; NSAID, nonsteroidal anti-inflammatory drug; PPF, plasma protein fraction; TIPS, transjugular intrahepatic portosystemic shunt.

importance to this question is when in the course of chronic liver disease are the various treatment interventions employed. Should liver transplantation be attempted earlier, avoiding most if not all of the complications discussed in this chapter, and would it prove to be the most cost-effective approach?

EVALUATION OF THERAPEUTIC OUTCOMES

Table 37–9 summarizes the management approach for patients with cirrhosis, including monitoring parameters and therapeutic outcomes. Cirrhosis is generally a chronic progressive disease that requires aggressive medical management to prevent or delay common complications. Table 37–9 lists monitoring criteria that need to be carefully followed in order to achieve the maximum benefit from the medical therapies employed and prevent adverse effects. A therapeutic plan including therapeutic endpoints for each medical and diet therapy needs to be developed and discussed with the patient.

ABBREVIATIONS

AAA: aromatic amino acid
AASLD: American Association for the Study of Liver Diseases
ALT: alanine transaminase
AST: aspartate transaminase
BCAA: branched-chain amino acid
EBL: endoscopic band ligation
EGD: esophagogastroduodenoscopy
EIS: endoscopic injection sclerotherapy
ERCP: endoscopic retrograde cholangiopancreatography
GABA: γ-aminobutyric acid

GGT: γ-glutamyl transpeptidase
HE: hepatic encephalopathy
PHT: portal hypertension
PMN: polymorphonuclear leukocyte
SAG: serum-ascites albumin gradient
SBP: spontaneous bacterial peritonitis
TIPS: transjugular intrahepatic portosystemic shunt

Review Questions and other resources can be found at *www.pharmacotherapyonline.com.*

REFERENCES

1. Williams EJ, Iredale JP. Liver cirrhosis. Postgrad Med J 1998;74:193–202.
2. Bell SH, Beringer KC, Detre KM. An update on liver transplant in the US: Recipient characteristics and outcomes. In: Cecka JM, Teraski PL, eds. Clinical Transplants. Los Angeles, UCLA Tissue Type Labs, 1995:??–??.
3. Hoyert DL, Arias E, Smith BL, et al. Deaths; final data for 1999. National Vital Statistics Reports 2001;49:1–113.
4. Anderson RN, Smith BL. Deaths: Leading causes for 2001. National Vital Statistics Reports 2003;52:1–85.
5. Runyon BA. American Association for the Study of Liver Diseases (AASLD) Practice Guidelines: Management of adult patients with ascites caused by cirrhosis. Hepatology 1998;27:264–272.
6. Rappaport AM. The structural and functional units in the human liver (liver acinus). Microvasc Res 1973;6:212–218.
7. Jungermann K, Kietzmann T. Zonation of parenchymal and non-parenchymal metabolism in the liver. Annu Rev Nutr 1996;16:179–203.
8. Shah V. Cellular and molecular basis of portal hypertension. Clin Liver Dis 2001;5:629–644.
9. Albanis E, Friedman SL. Hepatic fibrosis: Pathogenesis and principles of therapy. Clin Liver Dis 2001;5:315–334.

10. Alcolado R, Arthur MJP, Iredale JP. Pathogenesis of liver fibrosis. Clin Sci 1997;92:103–112.

11. DeFranchis R. Updating consensus in portal hypertension. Report of the Baveno III consensus workshop on definitions, methodology and therapeutic strategies in portal hypertension. J Hepatol 2000;33:846–852.

12. DeFranchis R, Primigrani M. Natural history of portal hypertension in patients with cirrhosis. Clin Liver Dis 2001;5:645–663.

13. Cadenas A, Bataller R, Qarroyo V. Mechanisms of ascites formation. Clin Liver Dis 2000;4:447–465.

14. Gines P, Quintero E, Arroyo V, et al. Compensated cirrhosis: Natural history and prognostic factors. Hepatology 1987;7:122–128.

15. Gines P, Fernandez-Esparrach G, Arroyo V, et al. Pathogenesis of ascites in cirrhosis. Semin Liver Dis 1997;17:175–189.

16. Bosch J. Prevention of variceal rebleeding: Endoscopes, drugs and more. Hepatology 2000;32:660–662.

17. Riordan SM, Williams R. Treatment of hepatic encephalopathy. N Engl J Med 1997;337:473–479.

18. Butterworth RF. The neurobiology of hepatic encephalopathy. Semin Liver Dis 1996;16:235–244.

19. Blei AT, Cordoba J. Hepatic encephalopathy. Am J Gastroenterol 2001;96:1968–1976.

20. Friedman LS, Martin P, Munoz J. Liver function tests and the objective evaluation of the patient with liver disease. In: Zakim D, Boyer TD, eds. Hepatology: A Textbook of Liver Disease, 3rd ed. Philadelphia, Saunders, 1996:764–788.

21. Eichler M, Bessman SP. A double blind study of the effect of ammonium infusion on psychological functioning in cirrhotic patients. J Nerv Ment Dis 1962;134:539–562.

22. Chopra S, Griffen PH. Laboratory tests and diagnostic procedures in evaluation of liver disease. Am J Med 1985;79:221–230.

23. Talwalkar JA, Lindor KD. Primary biliary cirrhosis. Lancet 2003;362:53–61.

24. Cohen JA, Kaplan MM. The SGOT/SGPT ratio—an indicator of alcoholic disease. Dig Dis Sci 1979;24:835–838.

25. Clark R, Rake MO, Flute PT, et al. Coagulation abnormalities in acute liver failure: Pathogenetic and therapeutic implications. Scand J Gastroenterol 1973;19(Suppl):63–69.

26. de Noronha R, Taylor BA, Wild G, et al. Inter-relationships between platelet count, platelet IgG, serum IgG, immune complexes and the severity of liver disease. Clin Lab Haematol 1991;13:127–135.

27. Aoki Y, Hirai K, Tanikawa K. Mechanism of thrombocytopenia in liver cirrhosis: Kinetics of indium-111 tropeolin-labeled platelets. Eur J Nucl Med 1993;20:123–129.

28. Pugh RNH, Murray-Lyon IM, Dawson JL, et al. Transection of the oesophagus for bleeding oesophagus varices. Br J Surg 1973;60:646–649.

29. D'Amico G, Pagliaro L, Bosch J. Pharmacologic treatment of portal hypertension: An evidence based approach. Semin Liver Dis 1999;19:475–505.

30. D'Amico G, Pagliaro, L, Bosch J. The treatment of portal hypertension. A meta-analytic review. Hepatology 1995;22:332–354.

31. Sharara AJ, Rockey OC. Gastroesophageal variceal hemorrhage. N Engl J Med 2001;345:669–681.

32. Lebrec D, Nouel O, Corbic M, et al. Propranolol—A medical treatment for portal hypertension? Lancet 1980;2:180–182.

33. Bosch J, Mastai R, Kravetz D, et al. Effects of propranolol on azygos venous blood flow and hepatic and systemic hemodynamics in cirrhosis. Hepatology 1984;6:1200–1205.

34. Pagliaro L, D'Amico G, Sorensen TA, et al. Prevention of first bleeding in cirrhosis: A meta-analysis of randomized trials of nonsurgical treatment. Ann Intern Med 1992;117:59–70.

35. Grace ND. Management of portal hypertension. Gastroenterologist 1993;1:39–58.

36. Angelico M, Carli C, Piatr C, et al. Isosorbide-5-mononitrate versus propranolol in the prevention of first bleeding in cirrhosis. Gastroenterology 1993;104:1460–1465.

37. Angelico M, Carli C, Piatr C, et al. Effects of isosorbide-5-mononitrate

38. Groszmann RJ. β-Adrenergic blockers and nitrovasodilators for the treatment of portal hypertension: The good, the bad, and the ugly. Gastroenterology 1997;113:1794–1797.

39. Patch D, Burroughs AK. Variceal hemorrhage. In: Cohen S, Davis GL, Gianella RA, et al, eds. Therapy of Digestive Disorders: A Companion to Sleisenger and Fordtran's Gastrointestinal and Liver Disease. Philadelphia, Saunders, 2000:355–372.

40. Sarin SK, Lamba GS, Kumar M, et al. Comparison of endoscopic ligation and propranolol for the primary prevention of variceal bleeding. N Engl J Med 1999;340:988–993.

41. Grace ND. Diagnosis and treatment of gastrointestinal bleeding secondary to portal hypertension [practice guidelines]. Am J Gastroenterol 1997;92:1082–1091.

42. Groszmann RJ, deFranchis R. Portal hypertension. In: Schiff ER, Sorrell MF, Maddrey WC, eds. Schiff's Diseases of the Liver, 8th ed. Philadelphia, Lippincott-Raven, 1999:387–442.

43. Lamberts S, Van Der Lely A, De Herder W, Hofland L. Octreotide. N Engl J Med 1996;4:246–254.

44. Bosch J, Kravetz D, Rodes J. Effects of somatostatin on hepatic and systemic hemodynamics in patients with cirrhosis of the liver. Comparison with vasopressin. Gastroenterology 1981;80:518–525.

45. Valenzuela JE, Schubert T, Fogel MR, et al. A multicenter, randomized, double-blind trial of somatostatin in the management of acute hemorrhage from esophageal varices. Hepatology 1989;10:958–961.

46. Burroughs AK, McCormick PA, Hughes MD, et al. Randomized, double-blind, placebo-controlled trial of somatostatin for variceal bleeding. Gastroenterology 1990;99:1388–1395.

47. Gotzsche PC, Gjorup I, Bonnen H, et al. Somatostatin vs placebo in bleeding oesophageal varices: Randomized trial and meta-analysis. BMJ 1995;310:1495–1498.

48. Imperiale TF, Teran JC, McCullough AJ. A meta-analysis of somatostatin vs vasopressin in the treatment of acute esophageal variceal hemorrhage. Gastroenterology 1995;109:1289–1294.

49. Feu F, Del Arbol LR, Banares R, et al. Double-blind randomized controlled trial comparing trelipressin and somatostatin for acute variceal hemorrhage. Gastroenterology 1996;111:1291–1299.

50. Goulis J, Armonis A, Patch D, et al. Bacterial infection is independently associated with failure to control bleeding and early rebleeding in cirrhotic patients with gastrointestinal hemorrhage. Hepatology 1998;27:1207–1212.

51. Sarin SK, Kumar A. Sclerosants for variceal sclerotherapy: A critical appraisal. Am J Gastroenterol 1990;85:641–649.

52. Richter GM, Noeldge G, Palmaz JC. The transjugular intrahepatic portosystemic stent-shunt (TIPSS): Experience results of a pilot study. Cardiovasc Intervent Radiol 1990;13:200–207.

53. Grace ND, Groszman RJ, Garcia-Tsao G, et al. Portal hypertension and variceal bleeding: An AASLD single topic symposium. Hepatology 1998;28:868–880.

54. Bass KM, Somberg KA. Portal hypertension and gastrointestinal bleeding. In: Feldman M, Scharschmidt BF, Sleisenger MH, eds. Sleisenger and Fordtran's Gastrointestinal and Liver Disease: Pathophysiology/Diagnosis/Treatment, 6th ed. Philadelphia, Saunders, 1998:1284–1309.

55. Bernard B, LeBrec D, Mathurin P, et al. Beta-adrenergic antagonists in the prevention of gastrointestinal rebleeding in patients with cirrhosis: A meta-analysis. Hepatology 1997;25:63–70.

56. Garcia-Pagan JC, Feu F, Bosch J. Enhancement of portal pressure reduction by the association of isosorbide-5-mononitrate to propranolol administration in patients with cirrhosis. Hepatology 1990;11:230–238.

57. Feu F, Garcia-Pagan JC, Boscj J. Relation between portal pressure response to pharmacotherapy and risk of recurrent variceal hemorrhage in patients with cirrhosis. Lancet 1995;346:1056–1059.

58. Patch D, Sabin CA, Gerunda G, et al. A randomized controlled trial of medical therapy versus endoscopic ligation for the prevention of variceal rebleeding in patients with cirrhosis. Gastroenterology 2002;123:1013–1019.

compared with propranolol on first bleeding and long-term survival in cirrhosis. Gastroenterology 1997;113:1632–1639.

59. Nevens F, Lijnene P, VanBilloen H, Fevery J. The effect of long-term treatment with spironolactone on variceal pressure in patients with portal hypertension without ascites. Hepatology 1996;23:1047–1052.

60. Villanueva C, Balanzo J, Novella MT, et al. Nadolol plus isosorbide mononitrate compared with sclerotherapy for the prevention of variceal bleeding. N Engl J Med 1996;334:1624–1629.

61. Chen CY, Chang TT, Lin EY, et al. Endoscopic variceal ligation versus conservative treatment for patients with hepatocellular carcinoma and bleeding esophageal varices. Gastrointest Endosc 1995;42:535–539.

62. Strauss RM, Boyer TD. Diagnosis and management of cirrhotic ascites. In: Zakim D, Boyer TD, eds. Hepatology: A Textbook of Liver Disease, 3rd ed. Philadelphia, Saunders, 1996:764–788.

63. Llach J, Rimola A, Navasa M, et al. Incidence and predictive factors of first episode of spontaneous bacterial peritonitis in cirrhosis with ascites: Relevance of ascitic fluid protein concentration. Hepatology 1992;16:724–727.

64. Guarner C, Runyon BA. Spontaneous bacterial peritonitis: Pathogenesis, diagnosis, and treatment. Gastroenterologist 1995;3:311–328.

65. Zervos EE, Rosemurgy AS. Management of medically refractory ascites. Am J Surg 2001;181:256–264.

66. Eisenmenger WJ, Ahrens EH, Blondheim SH, Kunkel HG. The effect of rigid sodium restriction in patients with cirrhosis of the liver and ascites. J Lab Clin Med 1949;34:1029–1038.

67. Sungalia I, Bartle WR, Walker SE, et al. Spironolactone pharmacokinetics and pharmacodynamics in patients with cirrhotic ascites. Gastroenterology 1992;102;1680–1685.

68. Runyon B. Ascites and spontaneous bacterial peritonitis. In: Feldman M, Scharschmidt BF, Sleisenger MH, eds. Sleisenger and Fordtran's Gastrointestinal and Liver Disease: Pathophysiology/Diagnosis/Treatment, 6th ed. Philadelphia, Saunders, 1998:1310–1333.

69. Runyon B. Monomicrobial nonneutrocytic bacterascites: A variant of spontaneous bacterial peritonitis. Hepatology 1990;12:710–715.

70. Navasa M, Follo A, Llovet JM, et al. Randomized, comparative study of oral ofloxacin versus intravenous cefotaxime in spontaneous bacterial peritonitis. Gastroenterology 1996;111:1011–1017.

71. Gines P, Rimola A, Planas R, et al. Norfloxacin prevents spontaneous bacterial peritonitis recurrence in cirrhosis: Results of a double-blind, placebo-controlled trial. Hepatology 1990;12:716–724.

72. Dupeyron C, Mangeney N, Sedrati L, et al. Rapid emergence of quinolone resistance in cirrhotic patients treated with norfloxacin to prevent spontaneous bacterial peritonitis. Antimicrob Agents Chemother 1994;38:340–344.

73. Llovet J, Rodriguez-Iglesias P, Moitinho E, et al. Spontaneous bacterial peritonitis in patients with cirrhosis undergoing selective intestinal decontamination. A retrospective study of 229 spontaneous bacterial peritonitis episodes. J Hepatol 1997;26:88–95.

74. Novella M, Sola R, Soriano G, et al. Continuous versus inpatient prophylaxis of the first episode of spontaneous bacterial peritonitis with norfloxacin. Hepatology 1997;25:532–536.

75. Gitlin N, Lewis DC, Hinkley L. The diagnosis and prevalence of subclinical hepatic encephalopathy in apparently healthy, ambulant, non-shunted patients with cirrhosis. J Hepatol 1986;3:75–82.

76. Plauth M, Merli M, Kondrup J, et al. European Society for Parenteral and Enteral Nutrition (ESPEN) guidelines for nutrition in liver disease and transplantation. Clin Nutr 1997;16:43–55.

77. Mizock BA. Nutritional support in hepatic encephalopathy. Nutrition 1999;15:220–228.

78. Clausen MR, Mortensen PB. Lactulose, disaccharides and colonic floras: Clinical consequences. Drugs 1997;53:930–942.

79. Kunin CM, Chalmers TC, Leevy CM, et al. Absorption of orally administered neomycin and kanamycin with special reference to patients with severe hepatic and renal disease. N Engl J Med 1960;262:380–385.

80. Loguercio C, Abbiati R, Rinaldi M, et al. Long-term effects of Enterococcus faecium SF-68 versus lactulose in the treatment of patients with cirrhosis and grade 1–2 hepatic encephalopathy. J Hepatol 1995;23:39–46.

81. Ito S, Miyaji H, Azuma T, et al. Hyperammonemia and Helicobacter pylori. Lancet 1995;346:124–125.

82. Stoll B, McNeilly S, Buscher HP, Haussinger D. Functional hepatocyte heterogeneity in glutamate, aspartate and α-ketoglutarate uptake: A histoautoradiographical study. Hepatology 1991;13:247–253.

83. Kircheis G, Nilius R, Held C, et al. Therapeutic efficacy of L-ornithine L-aspartate infusions in patients with cirrhosis and hepatic encephalopathy: Results of a placebo-controlled, double-blind study. Hepatology 1997;25:1351–1360.

84. Van der Rijt CC, Schlam SW, et al. Overt hepatic encephalopathy precipitated by zinc deficiency. Gastroenterology 1991;100:1114–1118.

85. Marchesini G, Fabbri A, Bianchi G, et al. Zinc supplementation and amino acid-nitrogen metabolism in patients with advanced cirrhosis. Hepatology 1996;23:1084–1092.

86. Ferenci P, Grimm G, Meryn S. Successful long-term treatment of portal-systemic encephalopathy by the benzodiazepine antagonist flumazenil. Gastroenterology 1989;96:240–243.

87. Als-Nielsen B, Kjaergard LL, Gluud C. Benzodiazepine receptor antagonists for acute and chronic hepatic encephalopathy. Cochrane Database Syst Rev 2001;4:CD002798.

88. Als-Nielsen B, Koretz RL, Kjaergard LL, Gluud C. Branched-chain amino acids for hepatic encephalopathy. Cochrane Database Syst Rev 2003;2:CD001939.

89. Nompleggi DJ, Bonkovsky HL. Nutritional supplementation in chronic liver disease: An analytical review. Hepatology 1994;19:518–533.

90. Arroyo V, Gines P, Gerbes A. Definition and diagnostic criteria of refractory ascites and hepatorenal syndrome. Hepatology 1996;23;164–176.

91. Badalamenti S, Graziani D, Salerno F, Ponticelli C. Hepatorenal syndrome: New perspectives in pathogenesis and treatment. Arch Intern Med 1993;153:1957–1967.

92. Fitz G. Systemic complications of liver disease. In: Feldman M, Scharsshmidt BF, Sleisinger MH, eds. Sleisinger and Fordtran's Gastrointestinal and Liver Disease: Pathophysiology/Diagnosis/Management, 6th ed. Philadelphia, Saunders, 1999:1284–1309.

93. Mammen EF. Coagulation defects in liver disease. Med Clin North Am 1994:78:545–554.

94. Morgan DJ, McLean AJ. Clinical pharmacokinetic and pharmacodynamic consideration in patients with liver disease. Clin Pharmacokinet 1995;29:370–391.

95. Westphal JF, Brogard JM. Drug administration in chronic liver disease. Drug Saf 1997;1:47–73.

96. Reidenberg MM, Breckenridge A. Drugs and the liver. Clin Pharmacol Ther 1998;64;353–354.

97. Pacifici GM, Viani A, Franchi M, et al. Conjugation pathways in liver disease. Br J Clin Pharmacol 1990;30:427–435.

98. Rodighiero V. Effects of liver disease on pharmacokinetics: An update. Clin Pharmacokinet 1999;37:399–431.

99. Sokol SI, Cheng A, Frishman WH, Kaza CS. Cardiovascular drug therapy in patients with hepatic diseases and patients with congestive heart failure. J Clin Pharmacol 2000;40:11–30.

100. Das A. A cost analysis of long-term antibiotic prophylaxis for spontaneous bacterial peritonitis in cirrhosis. Am J Gastroenterol 1998;93:1895–1900.

101. Teran JC, Imperiale TF, Mullen KD, et al. Primary prophylaxis of variceal bleeding in cirrhosis: A cost-effectiveness analysis. Gastroenterology 1997;112:473–482.

38

DRUG-INDUCED LIVER DISEASE

William R. Kirchain and Mark A. Gil

Learning Objectives and other resources can be found at *www.pharmacotherapyonline.com.*

KEY CONCEPTS

◀1 Drug-induced liver disease occurs as several different clinical presentations: idiosyncratic reactions, allergic hepatitis, toxic hepatitis, chronic active toxic hepatitis, toxic cirrhosis, and liver vascular disorders.

◀2 The mechanisms of drug-induced liver disease are diverse, representing many phases of biotransformation, and are susceptible to genetic polymorphism.

◀3 The assessment of a possible liver injury due to drugs should include what is known in the literature, the timing involved,

the clinical course, and always an exploration for pre-existing conditions that may have encouraged the lesion's development.

◀4 Liver enzyme assays can help determine if a particular type of liver damage is present.

◀5 Monitoring for drug-induced liver disease must be tailored to the drug and the patient's potential risk factors.

The number of drugs associated with adverse reactions involving the liver is extensive.[1] One of the more common reasons for the withdrawal of a drug from the marketplace is an elevation of liver enzymes.[2] Alcohol-induced liver disease is the most common type of drug-induced liver disease. All other drugs together account for less than 10% of patients hospitalized for elevated liver enzymes.[3] In approximately 75% of these cases liver transplantation is ultimately required for patient survival.[2] The liver's function affects almost every other organ system in the body. It is important to know the patterns of drug-related pathology in order to assess adverse reactions when they occur. It is also important to understand how and when to monitor for these reactions.

PATTERNS OF DRUG-INDUCED LIVER DISEASE

IDIOSYNCRATIC REACTIONS

◀2 For some drugs, a genetic or acquired abnormality must exist in a particular metabolic pathway for a toxic reaction to take place (Fig. 38–1).[2] In other cases, the reactions are typically associated with a drug concentration and often respond to simply lowering the dose of the drug. Idiosyncratic reactions tend to occur without association to particular blood concentrations or specifically identified metabolic abnormalities. For example, sulfonylureas like glipizide and antibiotics like ciprofloxacin have caused severe liver disease, resulting in the need for transplantation in a very small group of patients.[4,5] Idiosyncratic reactions are rare and are sometimes described as liver hypersensitivity to a drug.

ALLERGIC HEPATITIS

◀1 Allergic reactions in the liver can be caused by many drugs and result in many different kinds of hepatic damage. Trimethoprim-sulfamethoxazole and penicillinase-resistant penicillins such as

dicloxacillin induce a reaction typical of hepatic hypersensitivity in a few patients. The reaction usually develops within 4 weeks of the start of therapy.[6,7] It is marked by fever, pruritus, rash, eosinophilia, arthritis, and hemolytic anemia. The formation of granulomas within the liver is often seen on biopsy.[8] The reaction reverses with discontinued therapy and reappears upon rechallenge. Most antibiotics have been associated with this type of reaction, including the fluoroquinolones, macrolides, and β-lactams.[3] Allopurinol also has been associated with a number of reports of hypersensitivity reactions involving the liver. The onset of symptoms is 1 to 6 weeks after initiation of therapy. The incidence, like all the allergic liver reactions, is low, estimated at less than 1%. The clinical presentation includes eosinophilia, fever, rash, and arthritis, as previously mentioned. The biopsy may show a pattern of fibrin-ring granulomas similar to those seen in Q fever.[9]

TOXIC HEPATITIS

◀1 Toxic reactions are predictable, often dose-related effects in the liver due to specific agents. When taken in overdose, acetaminophen becomes bioactivated to a toxic intermediate known as *N*-acetyl-*p*-benzoquinone imine (NAPQI). NAPQI is very reactive, with a high affinity for sulfhydryl groups. The amino acid glutathione provides a ready source of available sulfhydryl groups within the hepatocyte. When the liver's glutathione stores are depleted and there are no longer sulfhydryl groups available to detoxify this metabolite, it begins to react directly with the hepatocyte (see Fig. 38–1). Replenishing the liver's sulfhydryl capacity through the administration of N-acetylcysteine early after ingestion of the overdose halts this process.[10] Acetaminophen's toxicity occurs in four stages.[11] During the first hours after ingestion, some patients report mild symptoms of nausea and vomiting, but no elevations of the commonly measured liver enzymes are seen. Not for 40 to 50 hours after ingestion do elevations in the liver enzymes begin.[11]

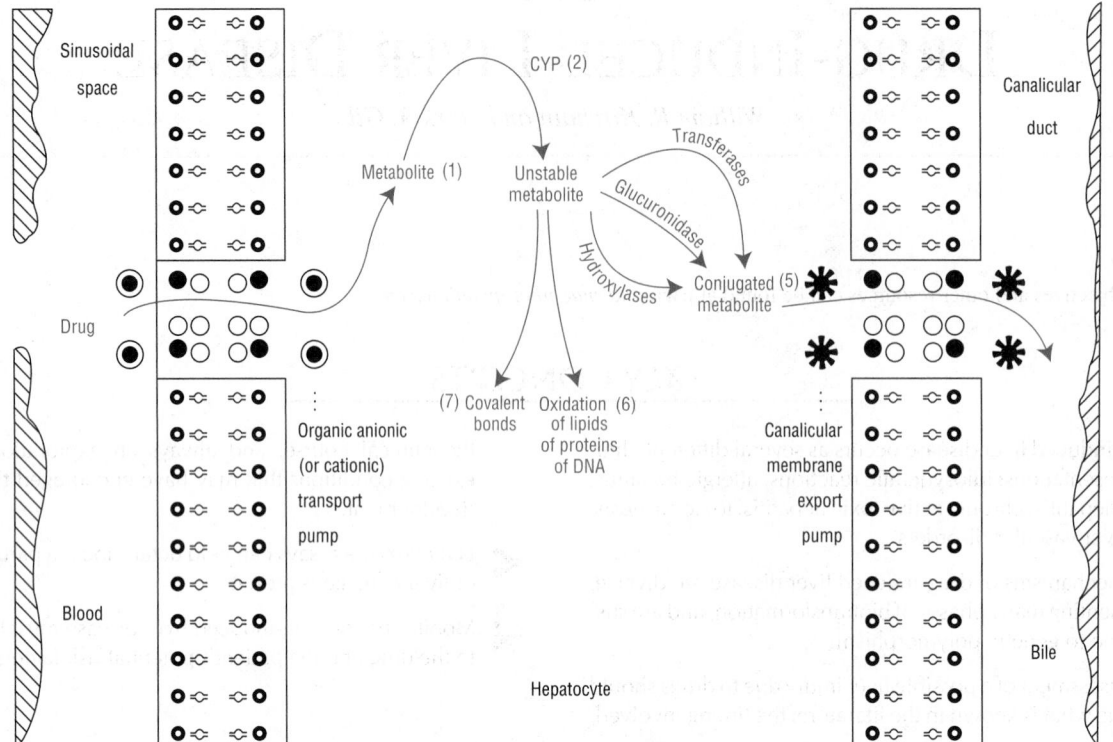

FIGURE 38–1. A general diagram of biotransformation. (1) The drug is actively transported into the hepatocyte by the organic anion transport pump, a transmembrane protein. (2) The metabolite (drug) interacts with one of a number of enzymes, the most common being CYP3A4. The CYPx family of phase I enzymes are regulated by the complementary DNA xenobiotic receptor. The xenobiotic receptor is in turn upregulated by other drugs, changes in cholesterol catabolism, and bile acids. (3) The immediate result of the action of the phase I enzyme is the production of an unstable metabolite. (4) The unstable metabolite then reacts with glucuronidase, various transferases, or hydroxylases to form a conjugated metabolite. The efficacy of these enzymes is affected by the patient's nutritional state and genetic polymorphism, leading to variations in individual risk for toxicity. (5) The conjugated metabolite is removed from the hepatocyte by the canalicular membrane export pump, one of a large family of membrane proteins (other members of this family pump conjugated metabolites back into the blood for excretion by the kidney). These proteins are subject to genetic polymorphism as well, again leading to some patients having an increased risk for toxicity. (6) If unable to form a conjugate, the unstable metabolite can participate in oxidative reactions that damage lipids, proteins, or even DNA. (7) Alternatively the unstable metabolite may form damaging covalent bonds with available anions or cations.

Reye's syndrome is an aggressive form of toxic hepatitis often associated with aspirin use in children. Valproate toxicity can also present in this pattern. Early in the process of Reye's syndrome, mitochondrial dysfunction leads to the depletion of acyl coenzyme A and carnitine. Fatty acids accumulate and gluconeogenesis is impaired, resulting in hypoglycemia. A concurrent disruption of the urea cycle occurs, leading to a decrease in the removal of ammonia and a slowing of protein use. A threefold rise in the blood ammonia level and an increase in the prothrombin time are common findings. In advanced stages of Reye's syndrome, many patients develop intracranial hypertension that can be life threatening and refractory to therapy.[12,13]

CHRONIC ACTIVE TOXIC HEPATITIS

Dantrolene, isoniazid, phenytoin, nitrofurantoin, and trazodone have been reported in association with a type of autoimmune-mediated disease in the liver.[14,15] Patients experience periods of symptomatic hepatitis followed by periods of convalescence, only to repeat the experience months later. It is a progressive disease with a high mortality rate and is more common in females than males. Antinuclear antibodies appear in most patients. These drugs appear to form

antiorganelle antibodies.[16] The exact identification of a causative agent is sometimes difficult since diagnosis requires multiple episodes occurring long after exposure to the offending drug.

TOXIC CIRRHOSIS

The scarring effect of hepatitis in the liver leads to the development of cirrhosis. Some drugs tend to cause such a mild case of hepatitis that it may not be detected. Mild hepatitis can be easily mistaken for a more routine generalized viral infection. If the offending drug or agent is not discontinued, this damage will continue to progress. The patient eventually presents not with hepatitis, but with cirrhosis. Methotrexate causes periportal fibrosis in most patients who experience hepatotoxicity.

The lesion results from the action of a bioactivated metabolite produced by cytochrome P450.[17] This process has most commonly been noted in patients treated for psoriasis and arthritis. The extent of damage can be reduced or controlled by increasing the dosage interval to once weekly or by routine use of folic acid supplements.[18] Vitamin A is normally stored in liver cells, and causes significant hypertrophy and fibrosis when taken for long periods in high doses. Hepatomegaly is a common finding, along with ascites and portal hypertension. In patients with vitamin A toxicity, gingivitis and dry skin are also very common. This is accelerated by ethanol, which competes with retinol for aldehyde dehydrogenase.[19]

LIVER VASCULAR DISORDERS

Focal lesions in hepatic venules, sinusoids, and portal veins occur with various drugs. The most commonly associated drugs are the cytotoxic agents used to treat cancer, the pyrrolizidine alkaloids, and the sex hormones. A centralized necrosis often follows and can result in cirrhosis. Azathioprine and herbal teas that contain comfrey (a source of pyrrolizidine alkaloids) are associated with the development of veno-occlusive disease. The exact incidence is rare and may be dose related.[3] Peliosis hepatitis is a rare type of hepatic vascular lesion that can be seen as both an acute and a chronic disease. The liver develops large, blood-filled lacunae within the parenchyma. Rupture of the lacunae can lead to severe peritoneal hemorrhage. Peliosis hepatitis has been associated with exposure of the liver to androgens, estrogens, tamoxifen, azathioprine, and danazol. Androgens with a methyl alkylation at the 17 carbon position of the testosterone structure are the most frequently reported agents that cause peliosis hepatitis, usually after at least 6 months of therapy.[20]

MECHANISMS OF DRUG-INDUCED LIVER DISEASE

CENTROLOBULAR NECROSIS

Centrolobular necrosis is often a dose-related, predictable reaction secondary to drugs such as acetaminophen; however, it also can be associated with idiosyncratic reactions, such as those caused by halothane. Also called *direct* or *metabolite-related hepatotoxicity*, centrolobular necrosis is usually the result of the production of a toxic metabolite (see Fig. 38–1). The damage spreads outward from the middle of a lobe of the liver.

Patients suffering from centrolobular necrosis tend to present in one of two ways, depending on the extent of necrosis. Mild drug reactions, involving only small amounts of parenchymal tissue, may be detected as asymptomatic elevations in the serum transaminases. If the reaction is diagnosed at this stage, most of these patients will recover with minimal cirrhosis and thus minimal chronic liver impairment. More severe forms of centrolobular necrosis are accompanied by nausea, vomiting, upper abdominal pain, and jaundice.[15,21]

STEATOHEPATITIS

Steatohepatitis (also known as steatonecrosis) is a specialized type of acute necrosis resulting from the accumulation of fatty acids in the hepatocyte. Drugs or their metabolites that cause steatonecrosis do so by affecting fatty-acid oxidation within the mitochondria of the hepatocyte (see Fig. 38–1). Hepatic vesicles become engorged with fatty acids, eventually disrupting the homeostasis of the hepatocyte. The liver biopsy is marked by a massive infiltration by polymorphonuclear leukocytes, degeneration of the hepatocytes, and the presence of Mallory bodies.[3]

Alcohol is the drug that most commonly produces steatonecrotic changes in the liver. When alcohol is converted into acetaldehyde, the synthesis of fatty acids is increased.[19,22] When the hepatocyte has become completely engorged with microvesicular fat, it often breaks open, spilling into the blood. If enough hepatocytes break open, an inflammatory response begins. If the offending agent is withdrawn before significant numbers of hepatocytes become necrotic, the process is completely reversible without long-term sequelae. In nonalcoholic steatohepatitis the same endpoint is often achieved through oxidation of lipid peroxidases.[23]

Tetracycline produces steatohepatitis and steatosis.[24] The lesions are characterized by large vesicles of fat found diffused throughout the liver. The development of this reaction is related to the high concentrations achieved when tetracycline is given intravenously and in doses greater than 1.5 g/day. The mortality of tetracycline steatohepatitis is very high (70% to 80%), and those who do survive often develop cirrhosis. Sodium valproate also can produce steatonecrosis through the process of bioactivation. Cytochrome P450 converts valproate to D-4-valproic acid, a potent inducer of microvesicular fat accumulation.[25]

Patients experiencing steatohepatitis may present with abdominal fullness or pain as their only complaint. Patients with more severe steatonecrosis will present with all the symptoms characteristic of alcoholic hepatitis such as nausea, vomiting, steatorrhea, abdominal pain, pruritus, and fatigue.

PHOSPHOLIPIDOSIS

Phospholipidosis is the accumulation of phospholipids instead of fatty acids. The phospholipids usually engorge the lysosomal bodies of the hepatocyte.[26] Amiodarone has been associated with this reaction. Patients treated with amiodarone who develop overt hepatic disease tend to have received higher doses of the drug. These patients also have higher amiodarone to N-desethyl-amiodarone ratios, indicating a greater accumulation of the parent compound. Amiodarone and its major metabolite N-desethyl-amiodarone remain in the liver of all patients for several months after therapy is stopped. Usually the phospholipidosis develops in patients treated for more than 1 year. The patient can present with either elevated transaminases or hepatomegaly; jaundice is rare.[3,27]

GENERALIZED HEPATOCELLULAR NECROSIS

Generalized hepatocellular necrosis mimics the changes associated with the more common viral hepatitis. The onset of symptoms is usually delayed as much as a week or more after exposure to toxin. Bioactivation is often important for toxic hepatitis to develop, but may not be the immediate cause of damage. Many drugs that are associated with toxic hepatitis produce metabolites that are not inherently toxic to the liver. Instead, they act as haptens, binding to specific cell proteins and inducing an autoimmune reaction (see Fig. 38–1).[16]

The rate of bioactivation can vary between males and females and between individuals of the same sex.[28,29] The cytochrome P450 system (CYP) tends to metabolize lipophilic substrates which are actively pumped into the hepatocyte by an organic anion (or cation) transporting protein. The CYP subspecies 1A, 2B, 3A, and 4A are regulated by the highly inducible xenobiotic receptor on complementary DNA. The receptor is found in the liver, and to a lesser extent in the cells lining the intestinal tract, and is responsible for cholesterol catabolism and bile acid homeostasis. The activity of this receptor is subject to genetic polymorphism as well. This results in a wide variation in the sensitivity of the population to generalized hepatocellular necrosis and other forms of hepatic damage.[23,30]

The long-term administration of isoniazid can lead to hepatic dysfunction in 10% to 20% of those receiving the drug. Yet severe toxic hepatitis develops in only 1% or less of this population.[31] The

N-acetyltransferase 2 (NAT2) genotype appears to play a role in determining a patient's relative risk. In one study, patients with the slow-type NAT2 genotype had a 28-fold greater risk of developing serum aminotransferase elevations than did patients with the fast-type NAT2 genotype.[32] Isoniazid is metabolized by several pathways, acetylation being the major pathway. It is acetylated to acetylisoniazid, which, in turn, is hydrolyzed to acetylhydrazine.[33] The acetylhydrazine, and to a lesser extent the acetylisoniazid, are directly toxic to the cellular proteins in the hepatocyte, but rapid acetylators also detoxify acetylhydrazine very rapidly, converting it to diacetylhydrazine (a nontoxic metabolite).

Ketoconazole produces generalized hepatocellular necrosis or milder forms of hepatic dysfunction in 1% to 2% of patients treated for fungal infections. This reaction is fatal in high numbers of patients infected with the human immunodeficiency virus. The onset is usually early in therapy, although it can be delayed until several months into therapy. In immune-compromised patients in whom ketoconazole is used for long periods of time, special care should be taken to watch for changes in liver function.[34]

CHOLESTATIC JAUNDICE

Cholestatic jaundice, or cholestasis, can be classified by the area of the bile canalicular or ductal system that is impaired. Canalicular cholestasis is very often associated with long-term high-dose estrogen therapy. Clinically, these patients are often asymptomatic and present with mild to moderate elevations of serum bilirubin.[35] An intravenous form of vitamin E, α-tocopherol acetate, causes cholestatic jaundice primarily involving the canalicular duct in premature infants. The incidence of this reaction in those receiving this formulation was high (>10%) and the mortality even higher (>50%).[36] Hepatocellular cholestasis is a much more serious form of cholestatic jaundice that involves both the parenchyma and bile canalicular cells.

The administration of total parenteral nutrition for periods greater than 1 week induces cholestatic changes and nonspecific enzyme elevations in some patients. Patients with low serum albumin concentrations may be at greater risk than patients with normal serum albumin concentrations.[3] This reaction also has been reported to occur rarely with sulfonamides, sulfonylureas, erythromycin estolate and ethylsuccinate, captopril, lisinopril, and other phenothiazines.[6]

MIXED HEPATOCELLULAR NECROSIS AND CHOLESTATIC DISEASE

Patients infrequently present with a purely hepatocellular necrosis or cholestatic damage, but rather with a mixed picture of damage. Flutamide causes a mix of lesions that appear at or about the forty-eighth week of treatment.[37] Niacin in doses greater than 3 g/day, or in doses greater than 1 g/day of sustained-release formulations, causes the same mixed pattern of damage.[38] These patients often present with only a few signs or symptoms at first, but can progress rapidly to fulminant hepatic failure. Additionally, niacin-induced and other drug-induced mixed hepatocellular disease can be misinterpreted as hepatobiliary cancers.[39]

NEOPLASTIC DISEASE

A large body of the current literature on adverse reactions and the liver addresses the development of neoplasms following drug therapy. Both carcinoma- and sarcoma-like lesions have been identified. Fortunately, hepatic tumors associated with drug therapy are usually benign and remit when drug therapy is discontinued. Except in rare instances, these lesions are associated with long-term exposure to the offend-

ing agent.[40] Androgens, estrogens, and other hormonal-related agents are the most frequently associated causes of neoplastic disease. The model for drug-induced hepatic cancer is polyvinyl chloride exposure. Used in the production of many types of plastic products, polyvinyl chloride induces angiosarcoma in exposed workers after as few as 3 years of exposure.[41]

ASSESSMENT

The best and most important technique for assessing and monitoring drug-induced liver disease is the patient's history. Questions addressing the patient's drug use along with a thorough review of systems are essential. The use of a protocol, such as that proposed by Danan and Benichou, can significantly improve the accuracy of the assessment (Table 38–1).[42] The use of drugs for recreational purposes must not be overlooked. Cocaine has been directly linked to liver disease.[43] Ecstasy, the street name of methylenedioxymethamphetamine, has induced fulminant hepatitis which has led to death in some cases.[44] The more pervasive impact of street drugs on the incidence of hepatic disease is the concomitant injection or ingestion of adulterants. Many of these adulterants are either directly toxic or serve to enhance the toxicity of the drug.

It is also good to try to determine nondrug hepatic disease risk. Arsenic, for example, is known to induce both acute and chronic hepatic reactions. Arsenic in low concentrations is found in insect-resistant lumber.[45] Following Occupational Safety and Health Administration guidelines should decrease the danger of using these products, but will not eliminate it. Even if exposure to an environmental toxin in and of itself does not produce a hepatic reaction, it may predispose a patient to a hepatic reaction when a drug is added. Table 38–2 lists some of the more common hepatic toxins found in occupational or environmental exposures that can add to a patient's risk for developing a hepatic lesion.[45]

A person's use of alternative medicine must be solicited. Many herbal remedies were once wisely abandoned because of their common adverse reactions. Comfrey tea is a common cause of hepatocellular damage. As in the case of the Chinese remedy jin bu huan, or as in the case of the more elegantly presented chaparral capsules containing grease wood leaves, the end of therapy with these types of agents is occasionally severe disability or death from fulminant hepatic failure.[46] Pennyroyal oil, maragosa oil, and clove oil cause a dose-related hepatotoxicity.[46]

The nutritional status of a patient can be as important to the development of a drug-induced liver disease as the hepatotoxin itself.[47] Patients who are malnourished because of illness or long-term alcohol abuse make up the most troublesome group.[48] Low serum levels of vitamins E and C along with lutein and the α- and β-carotenes are associated with asymptomatic elevations in transaminases. Conversely, high serum iron, transferrin, and selenium levels are also associated with asymptomatic elevations of transaminases.[49]

All potential drug reactions should be judged as to the timing of the reaction versus drug administration, pharmacokinetic considerations, the information in the literature records about previous reactions, the inclusion of alternative nondrug causes, and close clinical observation when the drug in question is stopped. It is also important to keep in mind that most elevations in liver enzymes will not be associated with a drug. In a study of all patients admitted to a hospital in the United Kingdom with elevated liver transaminase, only 9% cases involved a drug other than alcohol as the possible cause.[3] In all cases, titers of serum antibodies to hepatitis A, B, and C should be drawn. Even in cases in which the drug is absolutely targeted as the cause, viral hepatitis may be a complication.

TABLE 38–1. An Approach to Evaluating a Suspected Hepatotoxic Reaction Using a Clinical Diagnostic Scale

Patient presents with elevated liver enzymes	Score	Component subscore
Literature		
Literature supports this drug (drug combination) and pattern of liver enzyme elevation	+2	
No literature supports this, but the drug has been on the market less than 5 years	+0	____
No literature supports this and the drug has been on the market for 5 years or more	−3	
Alternative causes		
Alternative causes (i.e., viral, alcohol, etc.) are completely ruled out	+3	
Alternative causes are partially ruled out	+0	____
Alternative causes cannot be ruled out and are possible or even probable	−1	
Presentation		
The presentation includes 4 or more extrahepatic (fever, malaise, etc.) symptoms	+3	
The presentation includes 2–3 extrahepatic symptoms	+2	____
The presentation includes only 1 identifiable extrahepatic symptom	+1	
The presentation is essentially a laboratory abnormality, with no extrahepatic symptoms	+0	
Temporality		
Temporality: Initiation of drug therapy to onset is 4–56 days	+3	
Temporality: Initiation of drug therapy to onset is <4 or >56 days	+1	
Temporality: Discontinuance of therapy to onset is 0–7 days	+3	____
Temporality: Discontinuance of therapy to onset is 8–15 days	+0	
Temporality: Discontinuance of therapy to onset is >15 days	−1	
Rechallenge		
Rechallenge was positive	+3	
Rechallenge was negative or not attempted	+0	____
Total Score		____

The likelihood that this presentation is an adverse reaction in the liver increases linearly with an increasing score. The maximum score is 14, and scores below 7 are associated with an ever decreasing likelihood that the drug or drug combination in question caused the problem. This approach is not designed for the assessment of hepatic cancers or cirrhotic conditions.

Often there is no good clinical test available to determine the exact type of hepatic lesion, short of liver biopsy. There are certain patterns of enzyme elevation that have been identified and can be helpful (Table 38–3).[50,51] The specificity of any serum enzyme depends on the distribution of that enzyme in the body. Alkaline phosphatase is found in the bile duct epithelium, bone, and intestinal and kidney cells. 5'-Nucleotidase is more specific for hepatic disease than alkaline phosphatase, because most of the body's store of 5'-nucleotidase is in the liver. Glutamate dehydrogenase is a good indicator of centrolobular necrosis because it is found primarily in centrolobular mitochondria. Most hepatic cells have extremely high concentrations of transaminases. Aspartate aminotransferase (AST) and alanine aminotransferase (ALT) are commonly measured. Because of their high concentrations and easy liberation from the hepatocyte cytoplasm, AST and ALT are very sensitive indicators of necrotic lesions within the liver. After an acute hepatic lesion is established, it may take weeks for these concentrations to return to normal.[51]

Serum bilirubin concentration is a sensitive indicator of most hepatic lesions and has significant prognostic value. High peak bilirubin concentrations are associated with poor survival. Other important findings that indicate poor survival are a peak prothrombin time greater than 40 seconds, elevated serum creatinine, and low arterial pH. The presence of encephalopathy or prolonged jaundice are not good signs for the survival of the patient and are strong indicators for transplantation.[52]

Bilirubin concentrations and serum enzyme elevations give a static picture of the liver's condition and are not good indicators of hepatic function. Clinically available tests to predict hepatic function include measurement of serum proteins (albumin or transferrin). As a hepatic function decreases, serum protein concentrations in the body decrease at a rate determined by each protein's own elimination rate. Overhydration and starvation can also decrease serum protein concentrations. Changes in the prothrombin time often occur earlier than the changes in albumin or transferrin. The response of the prothrombin

TABLE 38–2. Environmental Hepatotoxins and Associated Occupations at Risk for Exposure

Hepatotoxin	Associated Occupations at Risk for Exposure
Arsenic	Chemical plant, construction, agricultural workers
Carbon tetrachloride	Chemical plant workers, laboratory technicians
Copper	Plumbers, outdoor sculpture artists, copper foundry workers
Dimethylforamide	Chemical plant workers, laboratory technicians
2,4-Dichlorophenoxyacetic acid	Horticulturists
Fluorine	Chemical plant workers, laboratory technicians
Toluene	Chemical plant, agricultural workers, laboratory technicians
Trichloroethylene	Printers, dye workers, cleaners, laboratory technicians
Vinyl chloride	Plastics plant workers, also found as a river pollutant

TABLE 38–3. Relative Patterns of Hepatic Enzyme Elevation versus Type of Hepatic Lesion

Enzyme	Abbreviations	Necrotic	Cholestatic	Chronic
Alkaline phosphatase	Alk Phos, AP	↑	↑↑↑	↑
5′-Nucleotidase	5-NC, 5NC	↑	↑↑↑	↑
γ-Glutamyltransferase	GGT, GGTP	↑	↑↑↑	↑↑
Aspartate aminotransferase	AST, SGOT	↑↑↑	↑	↑↑
Alanine aminotransferase	ALT, SGPT	↑↑↑	↑	↑↑
Lactate dehydrogenase	LDH	↑↑↑	↑	↑

↑, <100% of normal; ↑↑, >100% of normal; ↑↑↑, >200% of normal.

time to the administration of 10 mg of parenteral vitamin K is often used to differentiate between hepatic and extrahepatic disease.

MEASUREMENT OF LIVER FUNCTION

A good compound for a liver function test would theoretically be (a) nontoxic and lacking any pharmacologic effect; (b) either rapidly and completely absorbed orally or easily administered via a peripheral vein; (c) eliminated only by the liver; and (d) easily measured (drug and its metabolite) in blood, saliva, or urine.[53]

Several tests are used in research settings and in liver transplant patients to indicate liver function. Tests such as sulfobromophthalein, indocyanine green, or sorbitol measure qualities of hepatic clearance. There are also a few drugs that have been used to test liver function. Sorbitol's advantage over indocyanine green is a much lower incidence of allergic reactions. It is partially cleared by the kidney, and urine levels must also be determined during the test.[54] A good estimate of hepatic clearance can be obtained by serial blood levels of a variety of hepatically eliminated drugs if an assay is locally available. Ultrasound and CT imaging can be used on a periodic basis to monitor for the development of fibrosis or vascular lesions in the liver and for hepatocellular carcinomas.[55]

If a liver biopsy has been performed, the injury should be classified by the histologic findings. In cases in which there is no biopsy, the pattern of liver enzyme elevation can estimate the type of injury. Hepatocellular injuries are marked by elevations in transaminase that are at least two times normal. If the alkaline phosphatase is also elevated, then a hepatocellular lesion is still suspected when the elevation of ALT is notably higher than the elevation of alkaline phosphatase. If the magnitude of elevation is nearly equal between ALT and alkaline phosphatase, then the lesion is likely cholestatic.

A liver injury is acute if it lasts less than 3 months, and it is considered chronic after 3 months of consistent symptoms or enzyme elevation. A liver injury is severe if the patient has marked jaundice, if the prothrombin time does not improve by more than 50% after the administration of vitamin K, or if encephalopathy is detectable. If an acute liver injury progresses from normal to severe in a matter of a few days or weeks, it is considered fulminant.[56]

MONITORING

⑤ The serum transaminases AST and ALT are the most commonly used transaminases in the clinical setting. There are often no set rules available for a particular drug. The general guidelines found in Table 38–4 can help in determining a monitoring schedule for drugs where no prior recommendations are published. Concentrations of these enzymes should be obtained about every 4 weeks, depending on the reported characteristics of the reaction in question. Methotrexate should be monitored every 4 weeks, because toxicity usually develops over a period of several weeks to months.[57] In addition, some recommend that sulfobromophthalein or indocyanine-green excretion

TABLE 38–4. An Approach to Determining a Drug Monitoring Plan to Detect Hepatotoxicity

The patient is to be started on a drug that may cause a hepatotoxic reaction
↓
Is the patient pregnant?
Is the patient over 60 years old?
Is the patient exposed to an environmental hepatotoxin at work or at home?
Is the patient drinking more than 1 alcoholic beverage per day or binging on weekends?
Is the patient using any injected recreational drug?
Is the patient using herbal remedies or tisanes that are associated with hepatic damage?
Is the patient's diet deficient in magnesium, vitamin E, vitamin C, or α- or β-carotenes?
Is the patient's diet excessive in vitamin A, iron, or selenium?
Does the patient have hypertriglyceridemia or type 2 diabetes mellitus?
Does the patient have juvenile arthritis or systemic lupus erythematosus?
Is the patient HIV-positive, have AIDS, or are they on reverse transcriptase inhibitors?
Does the patient have chronic or chronic remitting viral hepatitis (hepatitis B or C)?
↓
Draw a baseline set of blood samples for liver enzymes, bilirubin, albumin, and transferrin before beginning the drug
↓
Does the patient have more than two risk factors?
Is the drug identified as one that may cause a predictable hepatotoxic reaction?[a]

↓ Yes   ↓ No
Redraw liver enzymes every 60–90 days depending on the drug for the first year   Redraw liver enzymes if other signs or symptoms manifest

If no toxicity is manifested during the first year of therapy, then redraw liver enzymes every 6–12 months; assess liver for cirrhosis every 1–2 years by ultrasound and every 4–6 years by CT or MRI scan; biopsy as directed by other findings

[a]A drug can become a predictable risk if it is administered concurrently with another drug or food that is known to induce or inhibit its metabolism.

studies be performed on a regular basis and that patients treated for very long periods of time should have a liver biopsy performed every 12 months.[58]

ABBREVIATIONS

ALT: alanine aminotransferase
AST: aspartate aminotransferase
CYP: cytochrome P450 liver enzyme system
NAPQI: *N*-acetyl-*p*-benzoquinone imine
NAT2: N-acetyltransferase 2 genotype

Review Questions and other resources can be found at *www.pharmacotherapyonline.com.*

REFERENCES

1. Biour M, Jaillon PJ. [Drug-induced hepatic diseases]. Pathol Biol (Paris) 1999;47:928–937.
2. Lee W. Drug-induced hepatotoxicity. N Engl J Med 2003;349:474–485.
3. Lewis J. Drug-induced liver disease. Med Clin North Am 2000;84:1275–1311.
4. Dourakis SP, Tzemanakis E, Sinani C, et al. Gliclazide-induced acute hepatitis. Eur J Gastroenterol Hepatol 2000;12:119–121.
5. Villeneuve JP, Davies C, Cote JJ. Suspected ciprofloxacin-induced hepatotoxicity. Ann Pharmacother 1995;29:257–259.
6. Olsson R, Wiholm BE, Sand C, et al. Liver damage from flucloxacillin, cloxacillin and dicloxacillin. J Hepatol 1992;15:154–161.
7. Lindgren A, Olsson R. Liver reactions from trimethoprim. J Intern Med 1994;236:281–284.
8. Pohl LR. Drug-induced allergic hepatitis. Semin Liver Dis 1990;10:305–315.
9. Vanderstigel M, Zafrani ES, Deyone JL, et al. Allopurinol hypersensitivity syndrome as a cause of hepatic fibrin granulomas. Gastroenterology 1986;90:188–190.
10. Buckley NA, Whyte IM, O'Connell DL, Dawson AHJ. Oral or intravenous N-acetylcysteine: Which is the treatment of choice for acetaminophen (paracetamol) poisoning? J Toxicol Clin Toxicol 1999;37:759–767.
11. Black M. Acetaminophen hepatotoxicity. Gastroenterology 1980;78:382–392.
12. Belay ED, Bresee JS, Holman RC, et al. Reye's syndrome in the United States from 1981 through 1997 [see comments]. N Engl J Med 1999;340:1377–1382.
13. Monto AS. The disappearance of Reye's syndrome—a public health triumph [editorial; comment] [see comments]. N Engl J Med 1999;340:1423–1424.
14. Lee WM. Drug-induced hepatotoxicity. N Engl J Med 1995;333:1118–1127.
15. Fernandes NF, Martin RR, Schenker S. Trazodone-induced hepatotoxicity: A case report with comments on drug-induced hepatotoxicity. Am J Gastroenterol 2000;95:532–535.
16. Beane PH, Bourdi M. Autoantibodies against cytochrome P450 in drug-induced autoimmune hepatitis. Ann NY Acad Sci 1993;685:641–645.
17. Hashkes PJ, Balistreri WF, Bove KE, et al. The relationship of hepatotoxic risk factors and liver histology in methotrexate therapy for juvenile rheumatoid arthritis. J Pediatr 1999;134:47–52.
18. Leonard PA, Clegg DO, Carson CC, et al. Low dose pulse methotrexate in rheumatoid arthritis: An 8-year experience with hepatotoxicity. Clin Rheumatol 1987;6:575–582.
19. Leo MA, Lieber CSJ. Alcohol, vitamin A, and beta-carotene: adverse interactions, including hepatotoxicity and carcinogenicity. Am J Clin Nutr 1999;69:1071–1085.
20. Soe KL, Soe M, Gluud CN. [Liver pathology associated with anabolic androgenic steroids]. Ugeskr Laeger 1994;156:2585–2588.
21. Fontana RJ, McCashland TM, Benner KG, et al. Acute liver failure associated with prolonged use of bromfenac leading to liver transplantation. The Acute Liver Failure Study Group. Liver Transpl Surg 1999;5:480–484.
22. Agarwal DP, Goedde HW. Human aldehyde dehydrogenases: Their role in alcoholism. Alcohol 1989;6:517–523.
23. Bohan A, Boyer J. Mechanisms of hepatic transport of drugs: Implications for cholestatic drug reactions. Semin Liver Dis 2002;22:123–136.
24. Lee WM. Acute hepatic failure. N Engl J Med 1993;329:1862–1872.
25. Konig SA, Schenk M, Sick C, et al. Fatal liver failure associated with valproate therapy in a patient with Friedreich's disease: Review of valproate hepatotoxicity in adults. Epilepsia 1999;40:1036–1040.
26. Lullman H, Lullman R, Wasserman O. Drug-induced phospholipoidosis, II. Tissue distribution of the amphiphilic drug chlorphentermine. CRC Crit Drug Rev Toxicol 1975;4:185–218.
27. Chang CC, Petrelli M, Tomashefski JF Jr., McCullough AJJ. Severe intrahepatic cholestasis caused by amiodarone toxicity after withdrawal of the drug: A case report and review of the literature. Arch Pathol Lab Med 1999;123:251–256.
28. Evans WE, Relling MV. Pharmacogenomics: Translating functional genomics into rational therapeutics. Science 1999;286:487–491.
29. Hunt CM, Westerkam WR, Stave GM. Effect of age and gender on the activity of human hepatic CYP3A. Biochem Pharmacol 1992;44:275–283.
30. Liddle C, Goodwin B. Regulation of hepatic drug metabolism: Role of nuclear receptors PXR and CAR. Semin Liver Dis 2002;22:115–122.
31. Tsagaropoou-Stinga H, Mataki-Emmanouilidon R, Karida-Kavalioti S, et al. Hepatotoxic reactions in children with severe tuberculosis treated with isoniazid-rifampin. Pediatr Infect Dis 1985;4:270–273.
32. Ohno M, Yamaguchi I, Yamamoto I, et al. Slow N-acetyltransferase 2 genotype affects the incidence of isoniazid and rifampicin-induced hepatotoxicity. Int J Tuberc Lung Dis 2000;4:256–261.
33. Kergueris MF, Bourin M, Larousse C. Pharmacokinetics of isoniazid: Influence of age. Eur J Clin Pharm 1986;30:335–340.
34. Van Puijenbroek EP, Metselaar HJ, Berghuis PH, et al. [Acute hepatocytic necrosis during ketoconazole therapy for treatment of onychomycosis. National Foundation for Registry and Evaluation of Adverse Effects.] Ned Tijdschr Geneeskd 1998;142:2416–2418.
35. Foitl DR, Hyman G, Leftowitch JH. Jaundice and intrahepatic cholestasis following high-dose megesterol acetate for breast cancer. Cancer 1989;63:438–439.
36. Lorch V, Murphy D, Hoersten L, et al. Unusual syndrome among premature infants: Associated with a new intravenous vitamin E product. Pediatrics 1985;75:598–601.
37. Cetin M, Demirci D, Unal A, et al. Frequency of flutamide induced hepatotoxicity in patients with prostate carcinoma. Hum Exp Toxicol 1999;18:137–140.
38. Rader JI, Calvert RJ, Hathcock JN. Hepatic toxicity of unmodified and time-release preparations of niacin. Am J Med 1992;92:77–81.
39. Kristensen T, Olcott EWJ. Effects of niacin therapy that simulate neoplasia: Hepatic steatosis with concurrent hepatic dysfunction. J Comput Assist Tomogr 1999;23:314–317.
40. Lee FI, Smith PM, Bennett B, Williams DMJ. Occupationally related angiosarcoma of the liver in the United Kingdom 1972–1994. Gut 1996;39:312–318.
41. Anonymous. Epidemiologic notes and reports: Angiosarcoma of the liver among polyvinyl chloride workers—Kentucky. Morb Mortal Wkly Rep 1997;46:99–101.
42. Danan G, Benichou C. Causality assessment of adverse reactions to drugs—I. A novel method based on the conclusions of international consensus meetings: Application to drug-induced liver injuries. J Clin Epidemiol 1993;46:1323–1330.
43. Van Thiel DH, Perper JA. Hepatotoxicity associated with cocaine abuse. Recent Dev Alcohol 1992;10:335–341.
44. Jones AL, Simpson KJJ. Review article: Mechanisms and management of hepatotoxicity in ecstasy (MDMA) and amphetamine intoxications. Aliment Pharmacol Ther 1999;13:129–133.
45. Wang JS, Groopman JD. Toxic liver disorders. In: Rom WN, ed. Environmental and Occupational Medicine, 3rd ed. Philadelphia, Lippincott-Raven, 1998:831–840.

46. Steadman C. Herbal hepatotoxicity. Semin Liver Dis 2002;22:195–206.

47. Wolf R, Strecker M. Endogenous and exogenous factors modifying the activity of human liver cytochrome P-450 enzymes. Exp Toxicol Pathol 1992;44:263–271.

48. Seef LB, Cuccherin BA, Zimmerman HJ, et al. Acetaminophen hepatotoxicity in alcoholics: A therapeutic misadventure. Ann Intern Med 1986;104:399–404.

49. Ruhl CE, Everhart JE. Relation of elevated serum alanine aminotransferase activity with iron and antioxidant levels in the United States. Gastroenterology 2003;124:1821–1829.

50. Whitehead MW, Haukes ND, Hainesworth I, Kingham JGC. A prospective study of causes of notably raised aspartate aminotransferase of liver origin. Gut 1999;45:129–133.

51. Choppa S, Griffin PH. Laboratory tests and diagnostic procedures in evaluation of liver disease. Am J Med 1985;79:221–230.

52. O'Grady JG, Alexander GJM, Hayllar KM, Williams R. Early indicators of prognosis in fulminant hepatic failure. Gastroenterology 1989;97: 439–445.

53. Barstow L, Smith RE. Liver function assessment by drug metabolism. Pharmacotherapy 1990;10:280–288.

54. Zech J, Lange H, Bosch J, et al. Steady-state extrarenal sorbitol clearance as a measure of hepatic plasma flow. Gastroenterology 1988;95: 749–759.

55. Mathieu D, Kobeiter H, Maison P, et al. Oral contraceptive use and focal nodular hyperplasia of the liver. Gastroenterology 2000;118:560–564.

56. Anonymous. Standardization of definitions and criteria of causality assessment of adverse drug reactions, drug-induced liver disorders: Report of an international consensus meeting. Int J Clin Pharmacol Ther Toxicol 1990;28:317–322.

57. Newman M, Auerbach R, Feiner H, et al. The role of liver biopsies in psoriatic patients receiving long-term methotrexate treatment: Improvement in liver abnormalities after cessation of treatment. Arch Dermatol 1989;125:1218–1224.

58. O'Connor GT, Olmstead EM, Sug K, et al. Detection of hepatotoxicity associated with methotrexate therapy for psoriasis. Arch Dermatol 1989;125:1209–1217.

39

PANCREATITIS

Rosemary R. Berardi and Patricia A. Montgomery

Learning Objectives and other resources can be found at *www.pharmacotherapyonline.com.*

KEY CONCEPTS

ACUTE PANCREATITIS

1 Patients with severe acute pancreatitis require early and aggressive intravenous fluid resuscitation.

2 Treatment of pancreatitis requires that if at all possible, medications that may potentially cause pancreatitis should be discontinued.

3 Use parenteral narcotic analgesics to control abdominal pain. Despite some theoretical advantages, meperidine is not recommended as a first-line agent because of dosing limitations and the risk for seizures in patients with renal failure.

4 Octreotide may be used in severe acute pancreatitis, but its efficacy in decreasing mortality remains uncertain.

5 Antibiotics should not be used in the absence of signs of infection except in patients with severe acute pancreatitis when pancreatic necrosis is present.

CHRONIC PANCREATITIS

6 Abstinence from alcohol is an important factor in preventing abdominal pain in the early stages of alcohol-induced chronic pancreatitis.

7 Initiate pain control with non-narcotic analgesics such as acetaminophen, nonsteroidal anti-inflammatory agents, or selective cyclooxygenase-2 inhibitors. The dose and frequency of administration should be increased before the patient is switched to a narcotic. Parenteral narcotics should be reserved for patients with severe pain that is unresponsive to oral agents. Patients with frequent or constant pain should receive the lowest effective analgesic dose scheduled around the clock.

8 A trial of pancreatic enzymes and acid suppression with either an H_2-receptor antagonist or proton pump inhibitor should be attempted in patients with mild to moderate disease.

9 Pancreatic enzyme supplementation and a reduction of dietary fat are used to treat malabsorption and steatorrhea. An initial lipase dose of about 30,000 international units should be given with each meal.

10 Symptomatic patients whose steatorrhea is not corrected by pancreatic enzyme supplementation and a reduction in dietary fat may benefit from the addition of an H_2-receptor antagonist or a proton pump inhibitor. An H_2-receptor antagonist should be used before trying a proton pump inhibitor.

Pancreatitis is defined as an acute or chronic inflammation of the pancreas with variable involvement of peripancreatic tissues and remote organs.[1] Acute pancreatitis (AP) is characterized by severe pain in the upper abdomen and elevations of pancreatic enzymes in the blood.[2] AP may be mild or severe based on clinical findings, laboratory tests, and diagnostic imaging studies. Mild AP is usually not associated with complications or organ dysfunction and recovery is uneventful. Severe AP is associated with impaired pancreatic function, local and systemic complications, and increased mortality. About 10% to 15% of patients develop a systemic inflammatory response syndrome and multiple organ failure.[1] Mortality, however, has decreased over the past 20 years, due in part to improved diagnosis, advances in antibiotic therapy, advances in intensive care medical management, and improved nutritional support.[3] Although exocrine and endocrine pancreatic function may remain impaired for variable periods after an attack, AP rarely progresses to chronic pancreatitis.[2,4–6]

Chronic pancreatitis (CP) is characterized by permanent damage to pancreatic structure and function because of progressive inflammation and long-standing pancreatic injury.[1,7–10] In the early stages of the disease, recurrent acute symptomatic exacerbations resemble attacks of AP and may not be distinguishable. Most patients with CP have periods of intractable upper abdominal pain, which is the dominant feature. Progressive pancreatic exocrine and endocrine insufficiency leads to maldigestion and diabetes mellitus. CP patients are at an increased risk of developing pancreatic cancer.[7,8] Patients with AP and CP suffer from many of the same complications.

EPIDEMIOLOGY

The prevalence of pancreatitis varies widely with geographic area, etiologic factors (e.g., alcohol consumption), and environmental or hereditary factors. The overall prevalence of AP in males and females in the United States is estimated to be less than 1%, whereas the prevalence of CP is 0.05% in males and 0.01% in females.[8] The reported prevalence of AP and CP most likely underestimates the true spectrum of these diseases.[8] Alcoholic CP is more common in men and has a peak incidence between 35 and 45 years of age. Blacks are two to three times more likely than whites to be hospitalized for CP than for alcoholic cirrhosis, but the underlying genetic factor remains elusive.[8]

PHYSIOLOGY OF EXOCRINE PANCREATIC SECRETION

The pancreas possesses both endocrine and exocrine functions. The islets of Langerhans, which contain the cells of the endocrine pancreas, secrete insulin, glucagon, somatostatin, and other polypeptide hormones. The exocrine pancreas is composed of acini that secrete about 1 to 2 L/day of isotonic fluid that contains water, electrolytes, and pancreatic enzymes necessary for digestion. Bicarbonate is secreted primarily by the centroacinar (ductular) cells, and is the principal ion of physiologic importance. Pancreatic juice is delivered to the duodenum via the pancreatic ducts (Fig. 39–1) where the alkaline secretion (pH about 8.3) neutralizes gastric acid and provides an appropriate pH for maintaining the activity of pancreatic enzymes.[11]

The major pancreatic exocrine enzyme groups are:

- Proteolytic: trypsinogen, chymotrypsinogen, procarboxypeptidase, and proelastase
- Amylolytic: amylase
- Lipolytic: lipase, prophospholipase A_2, and carboxylesterase lipase
- Nucleolytic: ribonuclease
- Other: trypsin inhibitor and colipase

The proteolytic enzymes are synthesized within the acinar cells and secreted as zymogens (inactive enzymes), which are activated in the lumen of the duodenum. Enterokinase secreted by the duodenal mucosa converts trypsinogen to trypsin, which then activates all other proteolytic zymogens. Two important mechanisms protect the pancreas from the potential degradative action of its own digestive enzymes. The synthesis of proteolytic enzymes as zymogens requires extrapancreatic trigger enzymes for activation. In addition, pancreatic juice contains a low concentration of trypsin inhibitor, which inactivates trypsin and partially inhibits chymotrypsin. Proteolytic activity in the intestinal lumen is not inhibited because the concentration is minimal. Lipase, amylase, and ribonuclease are secreted by the acinar cells in their active form. Colipase facilitates the action of lipase by binding to the bile salt-lipid surface and lowering the optimum pH of lipase from 8.5 to 6.5, the normal luminal pH in the duodenum.[11]

The regulation of exocrine pancreatic secretion is complex and depends on stimulatory and inhibitory factors exerted through hormonal and neuronal mechanisms. Two hormones, secretin (SC) and cholecystokinin (CCK), play an important role in mediating postprandial pancreatic secretion and have synergistic effects: SC stimulates ductular cells to increase water and bicarbonate; CCK stimulates acinar cells to secrete a juice that is low in volume and bicarbonate, but rich in enzyme content. The release of SC from the intestinal mucosa is pH dependent and occurs when the duodenal pH is approximately 4.5. Below this pH, titratable acid in the duodenum governs pancreatic bicarbonate output. Although the postprandial release of SC is small, nonacid factors such as products of fat digestion and bile can also stimulate SC release. The release of CCK from the small intestine depends on the presence of fatty acids and amino acids in the duodenum. Vasoactive intestinal polypeptide is structurally similar to SC and exhibits weak secretin-like effects on exocrine pancreatic secretion. Gastrointestinal peptides such as somatostatin inhibit enzyme secretion by modulating cholinergic transmission. Intestinal serotonin (5-hydroxytryptamine) is released in response to a number of stimuli, including duodenal acidification, and may play a role in postprandial pancreatic secretion.[11]

There are three phases of pancreatic exocrine secretion: cephalic, gastric, and intestinal. In the fasted state, basal secretion occurs at a low rate; output fluctuates in cycles with the interdigestive migrating motor complex (IMMC), so that peak secretions occur during phase III of the IMMC.[11] The cephalic phase is stimulated by the sight and smell of food and is mediated by vagal pathways. Gastric distention and the rate of gastric emptying stimulate an increase in enzyme-rich pancreatic fluid. In the intestinal phase, chyme and acid stimulate pancreatic secretion through the release of SC and CCK. A more in-depth discussion of pancreatic physiology can be found elsewhere.[11]

ACUTE PANCREATITIS

AP varies from mild disease, which is usually self-limiting, to severe disease, in which the severity of the attack correlates with the degree of pancreatic involvement and complications. The morphologic appearance of the pancreas and surrounding tissue ranges from interstitial edema and inflammatory cells (interstitial pancreatitis) to pancreatic and extrapancreatic necrosis (necrotizing pancreatitis), which has a higher risk of infection, organ failure, and mortality.[2,4] The rupture of blood vessels within or around the pancreas may lead to a collection of blood in the retroperitoneal spaces.

ETIOLOGY

The etiologic risk factors associated with AP are presented in Table 39–1. Gallstones account for more than 90% of cases worldwide.[1] Although alcohol abuse is often cited as the next most common cause, it is controversial as to whether acute alcoholic pancreatitis occurs in the absence of underlying chronic pancreatic damage. In some patients, a cause cannot be determined (idiopathic pancreatitis). Pregnancy is not considered a cause of AP because pregnant women develop pancreatitis as a result of coincident processes, most commonly cholelithiasis. AP occurs in 5% to 7% of patients who have undergone endoscopic retrograde cholangiopancreatography (ERCP).[12]

MEDICATIONS

Many medications have been implicated in AP, but a causal association is difficult to confirm because ethical and practical considerations prevent rechallenge with the suspected agent.[4,13–36] Table 39–2 lists medications according to their certainty of causing AP. A "definite" association implies a temporal relationship of drug administration to

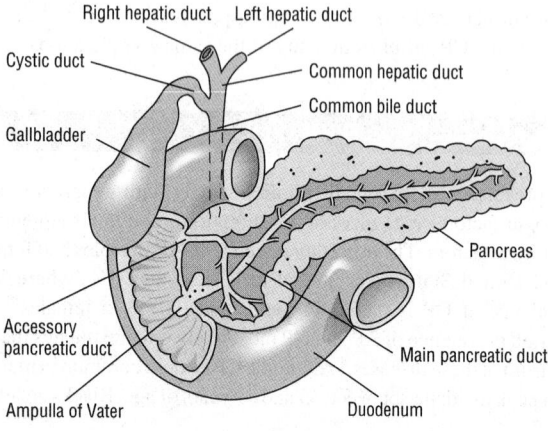

FIGURE 39–1. Anatomic structure of the pancreas and biliary tract.

TABLE 39–1. Etiologic Risk Factors Associated with Acute Pancreatitis

Structural	Gallstone disease, sphincter of Oddi dysfunction, pancreas divisum, pancreatic tumors
Toxins	Alcohol (ethanol) consumption, scorpion venom, organophosphorus insecticides
Infectious	Bacterial, viral (including AIDS), parasitic
Metabolic	Genetic hypertriglyceridemia, chronic hypercalcemia
Medications	See Table 39–2 for specific drugs
Trauma	Abdominal trauma, postoperative pancreatitis, ERCP
Vascular	Vasculitis, atherosclerosis, cholesterol emboli, coronary bypass surgery
Other etiologies	Congenital, idiopathic, hereditary (trypsinogen gene mutations), cystic fibrosis, inflammatory bowel disease, peptic ulcer disease, solid organ transplantation (liver, kidney, heart), refeeding

AIDS, acquired immune deficiency syndrome; ERCP, endoscopic retrograde cholangiopancreatography.
Compiled from Mitchell et al,[1] Topazian and Gorelick,[2] and Grendell.[4]

abdominal pain and hyperamylasemia, or to a positive response to rechallenge with the offending agent. Suggestive evidence exists for medications with a "probable" association, whereas evidence is inadequate or contradictory for drugs having a "possible" association. Certain medications, such as proton pump inhibitors and histamine₂-receptor antagonists, may be initiated in response to early symptoms of unrecognized pancreatitis. This may have led to erroneously attributing the pancreatitis to these medications.[36] Allergic reactions (e.g., urticaria) usually do not accompany drug-induced AP.

The pathogenesis of drug-induced pancreatitis does not appear to differ from other causes of AP. Exactly how medications induce AP is unknown, but postulated mechanisms include immune-mediated inflammatory response, direct cellular toxicity, pancreatic duct

constriction, arteriolar thrombosis, and metabolic effects. It is possible that thiazide diuretics lead to hypotension and pancreatic ischemia. Combination therapy with several medications has also been reported to cause AP.[26–28] Although AP is an infrequent complication of drug therapy, it is prudent to withdraw medication when an association is suspected. Discussion of the specific medications associated with AP can be found elsewhere.[13–36]

PATHOPHYSIOLOGY

The pathophysiology of AP is based on events that initiate the injury and secondary events that establish and perpetuate the injury (Fig. 39–2). The premature activation of pancreatic zymogens within the acinar cells, pancreatic ischemia, or pancreatic duct obstruction initiates AP and leads to a series of secondary events that determine the duration and severity of the injury. Trypsinogen autoactivation and trypsinogen activation by the lysosomal enzyme cathepsin B account for the intracellular activation of trypsinogen and the zymogen cascade.[1,2] Hereditary abnormalities in pathways that protect the pancreas from autodigestion are also associated with an increased risk of pancreatitis.[1] The release of active pancreatic enzymes directly causes local or distant tissue damage, or may enhance inflammation by activating the alternate complement pathway. Trypsin digests cell membranes and leads to the activation of other enzymes within the pancreas. Lipase damages the fat cells, producing noxious substances that cause further pancreatic and peripancreatic injury. The release of cytokines by the acinar cell or the inflammatory cells directly injures the acinar cell and enhances the inflammatory response.[37,38] Injured acinar cells liberate chemoattractants that attract neutrophils, macrophages, and other cells to the area of inflammation. Vascular damage and ischemia causes the release of kinins, which makes capillary walls permeable and promotes tissue edema. The release of damaging oxygen-free radicals appears to correlate with the severity of pancreatic injury.[2] Pancreatic infection may result from increased intestinal permeability and translocation of colonic bacteria.

TABLE 39–2. Medications Associated with Acute Pancreatitis

Definite Association	Probable Association	Possible Association	
5-Aminosalicylic acid	Ampicillin	Acetaminophen	Ibuprofen
Asparaginase	Angiotensin-converting	Amiodarone	Indomethacin
Azathioprine	enzyme inhibitors	Amoxapine	Interleukin-2
Didanosine	Bumetamide	Angiotensin II	Isoniazid
Estrogens	Calcium	receptor antagonists	Isotretinoin
Furosemide	Chlorthalidone	Carbamazepine	Ketoprofen
Mercaptopurine	Cimetidine	Cholestyramine	Ketorolac
Methyldopa	Cisplatin	Clarithromycin	Lipid emulsion
Metronidazole	Clozapine	Clonidine	Mefenamic acid
Pentamidine	Corticosteroids	Cyclosporine	Metolazone
Sulfonamides	Cytarabine	Cyproheptadine	Nitrofurantoin
Sulindac	Ethacrynic acid	Danazol	Octreotide
Tetracycline	Ifosfamide	Diazoxide	Ondansetron
Thiazides	Interferon alfa-2b	Diphenoxylate	Opiates
Valproic acid/salts	Losartan	Ergotamine	Oxyphenbutazone
	Meglumine antimoniate	Erythromycin	Paclitaxel
	Piroxicam	Famciclovir	Penicillin
	Procainamide	Glyburide	Propoxyphene
	Salicylates	Gold therapy	Ranitidine
	Sodium stibogluconate	Graniestron	Tryptophan
	Zalcitabine	Hepatitis A vaccination	Warfarin

Compiled from Grendell,[4] Eland et al,[13] McArthur,[14] Eland et al,[15] Gershon and Olshaker,[16] Maringhini et al,[17] Izaeli et al,[18] Liviu et al,[19] Goffin et al,[20] Hoff et al,[21] Rodier et al,[22] Balasch et al,[23] Domingo et al,[24] Torrus et al,[25] Abdul-Ghaffar and El-Sonbaty,[26] Stricker et al,[27] McDonald et al,[28] Sammett et al,[29] Goyal and Goyal,[30] Haviv et al,[31] Eland et al,[32] Birck et al,[33] Fisher and Bassett,[34] Blomgren et al,[35] and Blomgren et al.[36]

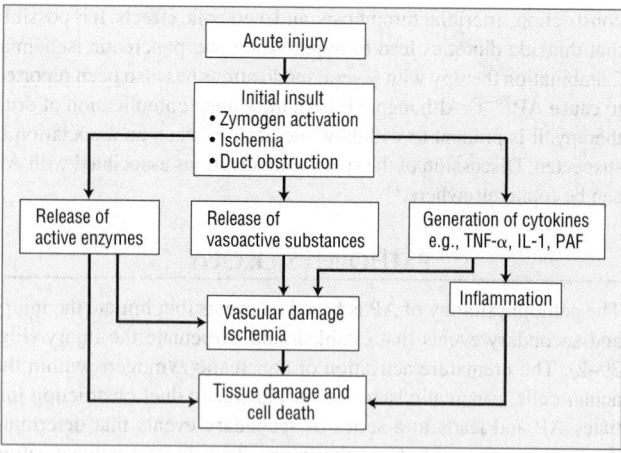

FIGURE 39–2. Pathophysiology of acute pancreatitis: initiating and secondary events. PAF, platelet-activating factor; TNF-α, tumor necrosis factor-α; IL-1β, interleukin-1β; IL-6, interleukin-6; IL-8, interleukin-8.

COMPLICATIONS

Local complications—including acute fluid collection, pancreatic necrosis, abscess, and pseudocyst (collection of pancreatic juice and tissue debris enclosed by a wall of fibrous or granulation tissue)—develop about 4 to 6 weeks after the initial attack. Pancreatic abscess is usually a secondary infection of necrotic tissue or pseudocysts and correlates with the severity of the pancreatitis. Most deaths result from infected necrosis and sepsis.[2,4] Pancreatic ascites occurs when pancreatic secretions spread throughout the peritoneal cavity. Systemic complications include cardiovascular, renal, pulmonary, metabolic, hemorrhagic, and central nervous system abnormalities.[2] Of the early complications, shock is the main cause of death. Hypotension results from hypovolemia, hypoalbuminemia, the release of kinins, and sepsis. Renal complications are usually caused by hypovolemia. Pulmonary complications develop when fluid accumulates within the pleural space and compresses the lung and the acute respiratory distress syndrome (ARDS) restricts gas exchange. The most common cause of hypoxemia in patients with AP is ARDS. Pleural effusions occur in 4% to 17% of patients with AP and occur more frequently on the left.[2] Gastrointestinal bleeding occurs secondary to numerous causes including rupture of a pseudocyst. Severe AP is associated with confusion and coma.

CLINICAL PRESENTATION

SIGNS AND SYMPTOMS

The clinical presentation of AP varies depending on the severity of the inflammatory process and whether damage is confined to the pancreas or involves contiguous organs (Table 39–3).[2,5]

DIAGNOSIS

The definitive diagnosis of AP is surgical examination of the pancreas or pancreatic histology. In the absence of these procedures, the

TABLE 39–3. Presentation of Acute Pancreatitis

General
- The patient may have acute mild symptoms or present with a severe acute attack with life-threatening complications.

Symptoms
- The patient may present initially with moderate abdominal discomfort to excruciating pain, shock, and respiratory distress.
- Abdominal pain occurs in 95% of patients and is usually epigastric, often radiating to either of the upper quadrants or the back. The onset is usually sudden and the intensity is often described as "knife-like" or "boring." The pain tends to be steady and persists for several days. Repositioning the patient relieves very little of the pain.
- Nausea and vomiting occur in 85% of patients and usually follows the onset of abdominal pain.

Signs
- Marked epigastric tenderness, abdominal distention, hypotension, and low-grade fever are observed with widespread pancreatic inflammation and necrosis.
- In severe disease, bowel sounds are diminished or absent; dyspnea and tachypnea are signs of acute respiratory complications.

Laboratory tests
- Leukocytosis, hyperglycemia, hypoalbuminemia, and mild hyperbilirubinemia may be present, as well as elevations in serum alkaline phosphatase and liver transaminases.
- Dehydration leads to hemoconcentration with elevated hemoglobin, hematocrit, blood urea nitrogen, and serum creatinine concentrations.
- The total serum calcium is usually normal initially, but hypocalcemia out of proportion to the hypoalbuminemia may develop. Marked hypocalcemia is an indication of severe necrosis and a poor prognostic sign.
- Thrombocytopenia and a prolongation in the prothrombin time are seen in some patients with severe AP.
- C-reactive protein is elevated by 48 hours after the onset of symptoms and may be useful in differentiating between mild and severe pancreatitis.

Markers of pancreatic injury
- The serum amylase concentration usually rises within 4 to 8 hours of the initial attack, peaks at 24 hours, and returns to normal over the next 8 to 14 days. Persistent elevations suggest extensive pancreatic necrosis and related complications.
- Serum lipase is specific to the pancreas and concentrations are usually elevated. Because of its longer half-life, elevations of serum lipase can be detected after the serum amylase has returned to normal.

Other diagnostic tests
- The Acute Physiology and Chronic Health Evaluation (APACHE) II score should be calculated upon admission. After 48 hours, use either the APACHE II or Ranson's criteria.
- Contrast-enhanced computed tomography distinguishes interstitial from necrotizing pancreatitis, but does not distinguish between fat necrosis and acute fluid collection.
- Endoscopic retrograde cholangiopancreatography is used to visualize and remove bile duct stones in patients with gallstone pancreatitis.

TABLE 39–4. Prognostic Indicators for Severe Acute Pancreatitis

Prognostic Factor	Criterion
Ranson's criteria	
On admission	
Age (y)	>55
White cell count/mm^3	>16,000
Glucose (mg/dL)	>200
Lactic dehydrogenase (international units/L)	>350
Aspartate aminotransferase (units/L)	>250
Within 48 hours	
Decrease in hematocrit (% points)	>10
Increase in blood urea nitrogen (mg/dL)	>5
Calcium (mg/dL)	<8
Partial pressure of oxygen (mm Hg)	<60
Base deficit (mmol/L)	>4
Estimated fluid deficit (L)	>6
Additional criteria	
Organ failure (shock)	
Systolic blood pressure (mm Hg)	<90
Pulmonary insufficiency (mm Hg)	≤60
Renal failure [creatinine (mg/dL)]	>2
Gastrointestinal bleeding (mL/24 h)	>500
Local complications	
Pseudocyst	
Necrosis	
Abscess	

Compiled from Topazian and Gorelick,[2] Grendell,[4] Dervenis et al,[5] and Banks.[6]

diagnosis depends on the recognition of an etiologic factor, the clinical signs and symptoms, abnormal laboratory tests, and imaging techniques that predict the severity of the disease. In most patients, the diagnosis of AP is based on the clinical presentation, an elevated serum amylase or lipase, and the results of either computed tomography (CT) or an ultrasound of the pancreas.[1,2] Evaluation of the patient with recurrent AP requires systematic identification and elimination of correctable inciting factors.[39]

Prognostic Indicators of Disease Severity

Patients should be categorized into either prognostically mild or severe disease using any one of a number of validated multiple-factor scoring systems (Table 39–4).[2,4–6] Two widely used measures include Ranson's criteria and the Acute Physiology and Chronic Health Evaluation (APACHE II). The APACHE II (≥8 points) system is more sensitive and specific than Ranson's criteria (≥3 criteria), but it is also more complex.[2,6] The APACHE II system uses 14 indicators of physiological and biochemical function that can be readily calculated upon admission to an intensive care unit. Ranson's criteria includes 11 variables that must be monitored at the time of admission and during the initial 48 hours of hospitalization. Patients with fewer than three Ranson criteria have a mortality rate of less than 1%, while

those with six or more have a 100% mortality rate.[2,5] Some modifications of Ranson's criteria have dropped the base deficit and fluid requirements, while others have added obesity as an independent risk factor.[2] Additional criteria enhance the predictability of these scoring systems (see Table 39–4).

Laboratory Tests

Laboratory test results vary depending on the severity of the inflammatory process, whether damage is confined to the pancreas or involves contiguous organs, and the time course from the onset of the acute attack (see Table 39–3). Serum concentrations of proinflammatory cytokines such as tumor necrosis factor-α and interleukin-6 are markers of disease severity, but elevations are not specific for pancreatitis and the tests are not widely available.[37,38]

Markers of Pancreatic Injury. Serum amylase and lipase are most widely used to detect elevations of pancreatic enzymes in AP, but elevations do not necessarily correlate with either the etiology or severity of the disease (see Table 39–3). In addition, many nonpancreatic diseases may be associated with hyperamylasemia, including salivary, renal, hepatobiliary, metabolic, female reproductive tract, and neoplastic diseases.[2] Pancreatic isoamylase studies assist in determining the origin of elevated serum amylase concentrations, but are not useful for the diagnosis of AP because the diseases that simulate pancreatitis cause pancreatic rather than nonpancreatic amylase concentration to rise. Newer markers (e.g., urinary trypsinogen activation peptide) provide both diagnostic and prognostic information, but are not routinely used in practice. A number of other tests have been used to detect pancreatic enzymes in the serum (e.g., elastase) and urine (e.g., amylase), but most of these are not considered useful in the diagnosis of AP.[1,2]

Imaging

A number of radiologic imaging techniques reveal pancreatic abnormalities during the disease course (see Table 39–3). Although no single imaging technique provides a positive diagnosis for AP, CT is considered the gold standard.

CLINICAL COURSE AND PROGNOSIS

The majority of patients with mild AP recover uneventfully. Mortality increases with unfavorable early prognostic signs, organ failure, and local complications. The mortality of patients with infected pancreatic necrosis approximates 30% and is higher than in sterile necrotizing pancreatitis or interstitial pancreatitis.[2,4–6] Mortality rates are also influenced by the etiology, as patients with idiopathic or postoperative AP have higher mortality rates than those with gallstone- or alcoholic-induced disease. Mortality is higher during the first or second attacks than during recurrent acute episodes. Death during the first few days often results from systemic complications. When death occurs after this period, it is usually associated with local complications.

▶ TREATMENT: Acute Pancreatitis

■ DESIRED OUTCOME

Treatment of AP is aimed at relieving abdominal pain, replacing fluids, minimizing systemic complications, and preventing pancreatic necrosis and infection. Management varies depending on the severity

of the attack (see Table 39–4; Fig. 39–3). In patients with mild AP, the disease is usually self-limiting and subsides spontaneously within 2 to 7 days of the initiation of supportive care and the reduction of pancreatic secretions. Patients with severe AP typically follow a more fulminant course and should be treated aggressively and monitored closely.

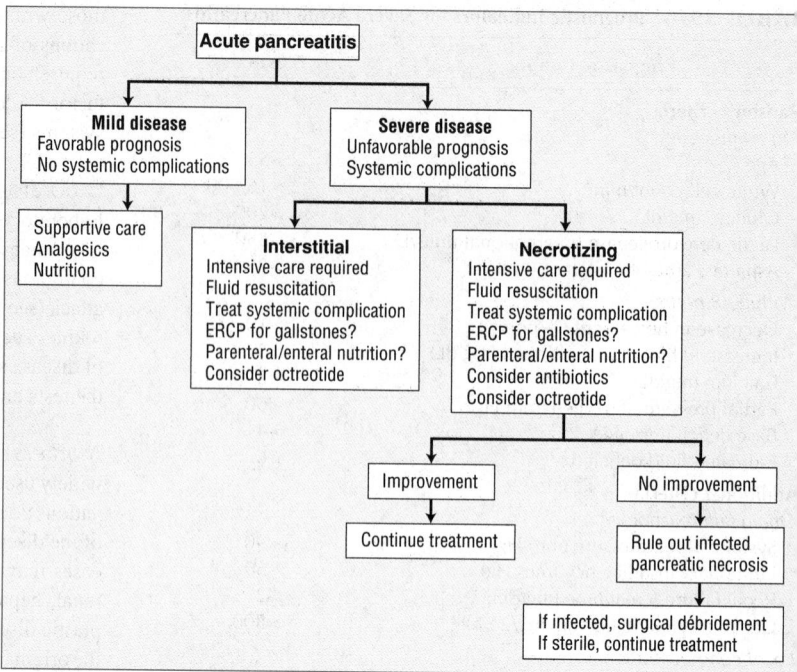

FIGURE 39–3. Algorithm of guidelines for evaluation and treatment of acute pancreatitis. ERCP, endoscopic retrograde cholangiopancreatography.

GENERAL APPROACH TO TREATMENT

All patients with AP should receive supportive care, including effective pain control, fluid resuscitation, and nutritional support. However, initial treatment usually involves withholding foods or liquids in order to minimize exocrine stimulation of the pancreas. The use of nasogastric aspiration offers no clear advantage in patients with mild AP, but is beneficial in patients with profound pain, severe disease, paralytic ileus, and intractable vomiting.[2,4]

Patients predicted to follow a severe course will require treatment of any cardiovascular, respiratory, renal, and metabolic complications. Aggressive fluid resuscitation is essential to correct intravascular volume. The prognosis of the patient often depends on the rapidity and adequacy of volume restoration, as large quantities of fluid are sequestered within the peritoneal and retroperitoneal spaces. Vasodilation from the anti-inflammatory response, vomiting, and nasogastric suction contribute to hypovolemia and fluid and electrolyte losses. Intravenous colloids may be required to maintain intravascular volume and blood pressure because fluid losses are rich in protein. Patients with pancreatitis and systemic inflammatory response syndrome may benefit from treatment with drotrecogin alfa. Intravenous potassium, calcium, and magnesium are used to correct deficiency states. Insulin is used to treat hyperglycemia. Local complications resolve as the inflammatory process subsides; however, patients with necrotizing pancreatitis may require antibiotics and surgical intervention.

NONPHARMACOLOGIC THERAPY

Patients with mild AP can begin oral feeding within several days of the onset of pain.[1] In severe disease, nutritional deficits develop rapidly and are complicated by tissue necrosis, organ failure, and surgery. Enteral or parenteral nutrition should be initiated if it is anticipated that oral nutrition will be withheld for more than 1 week, as nutritional depletion can impair recovery and increase the risk of complications.[6] Although total parenteral nutrition is very effective in critically ill patients, it can cause serious problems such as catheter sepsis and hyperglycemia.[40] In the past, there was concern that enteral feeding would stimulate pancreatic enzyme secretion and exacerbate the underlying disease. However, studies in patients with pancreatitis have demonstrated that the stimulatory effect of nutrients is minimized if administered distally into the jejunum.[40] Results of clinical trials in patients with AP confirm that jejunal feedings are safer and less expensive than parenteral nutrition.[40–42]

Enteral feedings may also prevent infection by decreasing translocation of bacteria across the gut wall.[43] Preliminary data suggest that probiotics such as lactobacillus (along with a fiber supplement) may reduce bacterial translocation and possibly decrease pancreatic necrosis and abscess.[44] If enteral feeding is not possible, total parenteral nutrition (TPN) should be implemented before protein and calorie depletion becomes advanced. Intravenous lipids should not be withheld unless the serum triglyceride concentration is greater than 500 mg/dL.[2,6] At present, there is no clear evidence that nutritional support alters outcome in most patients with AP unless malnutrition exists.[42]

Removal of an underlying biliary tract gallstone with ERCP or surgery usually resolves AP and reduces the risk of recurrence. Surgery may be indicated in AP to treat pseudocyst, pancreatic abscess, and to drain the pancreatic bed if hemorrhagic or necrotic material is present.

PHARMACOLOGIC THERAPY

RECOMMENDATIONS

Patients with AP should receive aggressive supportive care, including effective pain control, fluid resuscitation, and nutritional support. When possible, discontinue medications listed in Table 39–2. Antisecretory drugs may be used to prevent stress-related mucosal bleeding. Octreotide may be tried in severe AP, but its efficacy remains uncertain (see Fig. 39–3). Antibiotics should not be used in the absence of signs of infection except in patients with biliary tract gallstones, or in severe AP when pancreatic necrosis or abscess is likely. Patients with life-threatening complications require additional intensive medical therapy or surgery.

RELIEF OF ABDOMINAL PAIN

Analgesics are administered to reduce the severity of abdominal pain. The most important factors to consider in selecting an analgesic are efficacy and safety. Although the administration of some narcotics is associated with mild and transient increases in serum amylase and lipase, these effects are not deleterious to the patient. In the past, treatment was usually initiated with parenteral meperidine (50 to 100 mg every 3 to 4 hours) because it does not cause pancreatitis or significantly alter the function of the sphincter of Oddi.[4,45] Today many hospitals have either restricted or eliminated the use of meperidine because it is not as effective as other narcotics and because it is contraindicated in patients with renal failure. Because meperidine is less effective than other narcotics in relieving pain, higher and more frequent daily dosages are generally required. Most importantly, active metabolites of meperidine accumulate in patients with renal impairment and may cause seizures or psychosis. The maximum recommended parenteral dose of meperidine is 600 mg/day in patients with normal renal function, but it should not be used in patients with renal failure.

Parenteral morphine is often recommended for pain control, but its use in AP is sometimes avoided because it can cause spasm of the sphincter of Oddi, increases in serum amylase, and rarely pancreatitis.[2] Although not as well-studied, hydromorphone is often preferred because it has a longer half-life than meperidine and can be given parenterally by a patient-controlled analgesia pump. Patient-controlled analgesia should be considered in patients who require frequent narcotic dosing (e.g., every 2 to 3 hours) and usually achieves adequate pain control. Dosing should be monitored carefully and adjusted daily. There is no evidence that antisecretory drugs (such as H_2-receptor antagonists or proton pump inhibitors) prevent an exacerbation of abdominal pain.[6]

LIMITATION OF SYSTEMIC COMPLICATIONS AND PREVENTION OF PANCREATIC NECROSIS

Vigorous fluid resuscitation and support of respiratory, renal, cardiovascular, and hepatobiliary function may limit systemic complications.[2,46–48] However, there is no proven method to prevent these complications.[6] While hemoconcentration (decreased intravascular volume) is strongly associated with pancreatic necrosis, it is not clear whether aggressive fluid resuscitation alone during the first 24 hours can prevent pancreatic necrosis.[49] Procedures such as ERCP, hypothermia, nasogastric suction, pancreatic irradiation, peritoneal lavage, and thoracic duct drainage remain unproven.[2,6]

A number of drugs have been investigated to determine their efficacy in limiting the severity of AP by either directly or indirectly reducing pancreatic secretion, inhibiting the action of circulating inflammatory mediators, or increasing pancreatic microcirculation. The use of parenteral H_2-receptor antagonists or proton pump inhibitors is no more effective than nasogastric suction to diminish pancreatic exocrine secretion. Corticosteroids are not helpful in limiting systemic complications and altering the course of the disease.[47] Clinical studies with protease inhibitors such as aprotinin and gabexate fail to reduce mortality in AP.[46–48] However, the results of two meta-analyses and a multicenter comparative study with gabexate demonstrate a decrease in complications.[2,50] Clinical trials fail to demonstrate a decrease in mortality with lexipafant, a platelet-activating

factor antagonist.[47] Low-molecular-weight dextran increases pancreatic microcirculation in experimental animal models, but its efficacy in preventing pancreatic necrosis in humans requires further study.[51] Conflicting or inconclusive data exist regarding the efficacy of antioxidants, glucagon, calcitonin, atropine, α-aminocaproic acid, 5-fluorouracil, and indomethacin.[48]

Somatostatin and Octreotide

The use of somatostatin and its synthetic analog octreotide in severe AP may reduce mortality, but does not appear to decrease complication rates.[2,52] Although these agents are potent inhibitors of pancreatic enzyme secretion, they may have detrimental effects in patients with AP because they may increase sphincter of Oddi pressure and decrease splanchnic blood flow.[47] Many of the studies that evaluated the efficacy of somatostatin and octreotide in AP have yielded conflicting results. Most of these studies had small numbers of patients, were not placebo-controlled, and included patients with mild disease. Preliminary results of a randomized, open-label trial in severe AP indicates that octreotide 0.1 mg subcutaneously every 8 hours decreased mortality, sepsis, and length of hospital stay.[53] In a study using higher dosages (0.5 mcg/kg per hour given by continuous intravenous infusion), octreotide provided a more pronounced decrease in serum amylase, greater improvement in pancreatic edema, and earlier return to oral intake than controls.[54] Until there is evidence to support its efficacy in patients with mild disease, the use of octreotide should be limited to patients with severe AP, as it may decrease mortality and possibly the length of hospital stay.

CLINICAL CONTROVERSY

Some clinicians believe that octreotide should be used to decrease pancreatic secretions in patients with AP, while others believe that this is unnecessary. Octreotide should only be used in patients with severe AP.

PREVENTION OF INFECTION

Patients with severe AP complicated by necrosis should receive prophylactic treatment with a broad-spectrum antibiotic (Fig. 39–4).[1,2,55] Pancreatic infections occur in about 30% of patients who have greater than 30% necrosis and account for 80% of the deaths associated with AP.[46] However, the use of antibiotics in patients without definite proof of an infection remains controversial. Prophylactic antibiotics do not offer any benefit in mild AP or those who do not have necrosis.

Early clinical trials showed no benefit from antibiotic prophylaxis, but studies were flawed, as they included patients with all degrees of disease severity and did not have a sufficient number of patients with severe necrotizing AP.[1,47] In addition, the studies utilized ampicillin, which does not penetrate well into pancreatic tissue.[47] Imipenem-cilastatin, metronidazole, cefotaxime, piperacillin, mezlocillin, ofloxacin, and ciprofloxacin all achieve satisfactory bactericidal tissue concentrations, whereas aminoglycosides have poor penetration.[46,47] However, the importance of antibiotic penetration into pancreatic tissue has been debated, as it is the peripancreatic retroperitoneal necrotic fat and debris, not the pancreas itself, that becomes infected.

At present there is sufficient evidence to recommend that patients with severe acute necrotizing pancreatitis should receive antibiotic prophylaxis as soon as possible after diagnosis. Three

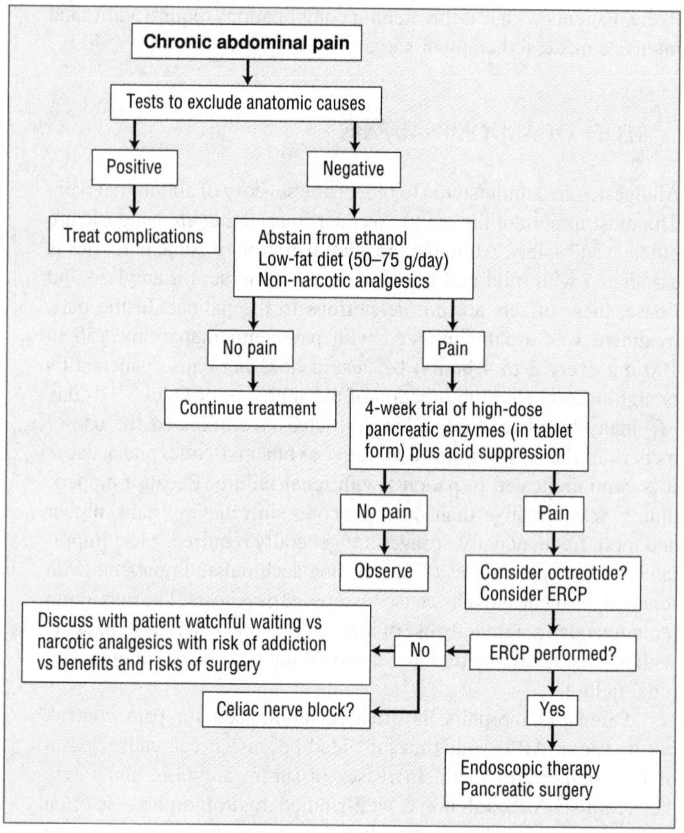

FIGURE 39–4. Algorithm of guidelines for the treatment of chronic abdominal pain in chronic pancreatitis. ERCP, endoscopic retrograde cholangiopancreatography.

randomized clinical trials have compared antibiotic prophylaxis with no antibiotics in patients with acute necrotizing pancreatitis, with varying results.[56–58] In one study, prophylaxis with cefuroxime 4 to 5 g/day lowered mortality, length of hospital stay, and the overall infection rate, but a decrease in the total number of infections was attributed to fewer urinary tract infections in the antibiotic group.[56] In contrast, prophylaxis with either ceftazidime, amikacin, and metronidazole or imipenem-cilastatin decreased the incidence of sepsis and reduced the length of stay, but had no effect on mortality.[57,58] Despite differences among the studies, the results of two meta-analyses conclude that prophylaxis with broad-spectrum antibiotics decreases sepsis and mortality in patients with severe AP and necrosis.[59,60] In a randomized comparison of perfloxacin and imipenem-cilastatin, pancreatic sepsis was reduced in the imipenem group, but mortality did not differ between groups.[61] Selective gut decontamination may be of benefit, but randomized controlled trials are needed to confirm its effectiveness when compared to parenteral antibiotic prophylaxis.[1,2,47] Because the source of bacterial contamination is most likely the colon, the choice of antibiotic should be broad-spectrum, covering the range of enteric aerobic gram-negative bacilli and anaerobic microorganisms. Treatment should be initiated within the first 48 hours and continued for 2 to 3 weeks. Imipenem-cilastatin (500 mg every 8 hours) is probably the most effective agent, but a quinolone (such as ciprofloxacin or levofloxacin) with metronidazole should be considered for the penicillin-allergic patient.[1,47]

Antibiotic prophylaxis is not always effective in eliminating the risk of infected pancreatic necrosis. Widespread use of antibiotics may lead to multiresistant bacterial and fungal infections, thus worsening the course of the disease. There appears to be a shift toward gram-positive infections (primarily enterococci and staphylococci) in AP patients who receive antibiotic prophylaxis as compared to

earlier studies when patients did not receive antibiotic prophylaxis.[62] The use of prophylactic antibiotics may also alter the bacteriology of infected necrosis and is associated with an increase in the incidence of fungal and β-lactam–resistant gram-positive organisms.[63] The rise in fungal infections has led some clinicians to consider the addition of an antifungal agent to the prophylactic regimen.[64] Although fluconazole demonstrated adequate penetration of pancreatic tissue, there is no evidence to support its efficacy in the prophylaxis of pancreatic fungal infections in patients with acute necrotizing pancreatitis.

CLINICAL CONTROVERSY

Some clinicians believe that antibiotic prophylaxis is necessary in patients with severe AP in order to prevent pancreatic infection, while others believe that this practice is unnecessary. Antibiotic use in AP remains controversial in patients without definite proof of an infection. Patients with severe AP complicated by necrosis should receive prophylactic treatment with a broad-spectrum antibiotic.

■ POST-ERCP PANCREATITIS

The clinical characteristics of post-ERCP pancreatitis are similar to those of AP from other causes. In most cases the pancreatitis is mild and resolves in several days. Pretreatment with octreotide, calcium channel blockers, and aprotinin has been disappointing, but somatostatin and gabexate have shown some benefit.[1,66] To date, there have not been any studies to evaluate the cost effectiveness of prophylactic therapy.

CHRONIC PANCREATITIS

CP is an inflammatory condition that usually results in functional and structural damage to the pancreas. In most patients CP is progressive and loss of pancreatic function is irreversible. Permanent destruction of pancreatic tissue usually leads to exocrine and endocrine insufficiency.[7-10] Cystic fibrosis may be associated with pancreatic exocrine insufficiency in children and is discussed in Chap. 30.

ETIOLOGY

Etiologic risk factors associated with CP are identified in Table 39–5. Prolonged alcohol consumption accounts for 70% of all cases in the United States, about 20% are idiopathic, and the remaining 10% constitute other less frequent causes.[7-10] Recent evidence suggests that there is a strong association between cigarette smoking and CP.[7,8] Autoimmune pancreatitis may be isolated or occur in association with immune-mediated disorders. Although cholelithiasis may coexist with CP, gallstones rarely lead to chronic disease.

PATHOPHYSIOLOGY

The exact mechanism by which alcohol causes CP is uncertain. It appears that alcohol-induced pancreatitis progresses from inflammation to cellular necrosis, and that fibrosis occurs over time. Chronic alcoholism results in a number of changes in pancreatic fluid that creates an environment for the formation of intraductal protein plugs that block small ductules.[7] Blockage of the ductules produces progressive structural damage in the ducts and the acinar tissue. Calcium complexes to the protein plugs, first in the small ductules and then in the main pancreatic duct (see Fig. 39–1), eventually resulting in injury and destruction of pancreatic tissue. Other theories have been hypothesized, all of which lead to pancreatic destruction and insufficiency.[7]

The pathogenesis of the abdominal pain associated with CP is multifactorial and related in part to increased intraductal pressure secondary to continued pancreatic secretion, pancreatic inflammation, and abnormalities involving pancreatic nerves. Malabsorption of protein and fat occurs when the capacity for enzyme secretion is reduced by 90%.[7] Lipase secretion decreases more rapidly than the proteolytic enzymes. Bicarbonate secretion may be decreased, leading to a duodenal pH of less than 4.[7] A minority of patients develop

TABLE 39–5. Etiologic Risk Factors Associated with Chronic Pancreatitis

Toxic	Alcohol (ethanol), tobacco, organotin compounds (e.g., di-*n*-butyltin dichloride)
Metabolic	Chronic hypercalcemia associated with hyperparathyroidism, chronic hypertriglyceridemia (controversial), chronic renal failure
Obstructive	Pancreas divisum, pancreatic duct obstruction (e.g., tumor), sphincter of Oddi (controversial)
Idiopathic	Tropical pancreatitis
Genetic	Autosomal dominant, autosomal recessive/modifier genes (e.g., cystic fibrosis)
Autoimmune	Isolated autoimmune, syndromic autoimmune (e.g., Sjögren syndrome, inflammatory bowel disease, primary biliary cirrhosis)
Other etiologies	Postirradiation, postnecrotic pancreatitis, vascular diseases

Compiled from Owyang,[7] Etemad and Whitcomb,[8] Toskes,[9] and Steer et al.[10]

complications, including pancreatic pseudocyst, abscess, and ascites or common bile duct obstruction, leading to cholangitis or secondary biliary cirrhosis. Bleeding is associated with a variety of causes.

CLINICAL PRESENTATION

SIGNS AND SYMPTOMS

The clinical presentation of CP varies depending on the etiology of the disease, the severity of the inflammatory process, and the extent of irreversible damage to the pancreas (Table 39–6).[7-10] The classic features of CP are abdominal pain, malabsorption, weight loss, and diabetes. Most alcoholic patients have chronic pain, while others have intermittent attacks or painless pancreatitis. Abstinence from ethanol may provide relief from pain, but does not prevent exocrine

TABLE 39–6. Presentation of Chronic Pancreatitis

General
- The patient may appear well-nourished or have coexistent signs of malnutrition and chronic alcoholic liver disease.

Symptoms
- Dull epigastric or abdominal pain that radiates to the back is seen. Pain is the most prominent clinical feature and may be either consistent or episodic.
- Characteristically the pain is deep-seated, positional, frequently nocturnal, and unresponsive to medication. The intensity of the pain varies from mild to severe, and does not usually correlate directly with the inflammatory process or other physical findings. Severe attacks last from several days to several weeks and may be aggravated by eating.
- Nausea and vomiting often accompany the pain.

Signs
- Steatorrhea (excessive loss of fat in the feces) and azotorrhea (excessive loss of protein in the feces) are seen in most patients. Steatorrhea is often associated with diarrhea and bloating.
- Weight loss may be seen.
- About 50% of patients with advanced pancreatic insufficiency present with vitamin B_{12} malabsorption.
- Jaundice occurs in about 10% of patients.
- Pancreatic diabetes is usually a late manifestation that is commonly associated with pancreatic calcification. Ketoacidosis, vascular complications, and nephropathy are uncommon with this form of diabetes.
- Neuropathy is sometimes seen.
- Complications, including pancreatic pseudocysts, pleural effusions, and ascites, may be detected on physical examination.

Laboratory tests
- The white blood cell count, fluids, and electrolytes usually remain normal unless fluids and electrolytes are lost as a result of vomiting and diarrhea.
- Serum amylase and lipase concentrations usually remain normal unless the pancreatic duct is blocked or a pseudocyst is present.

Other diagnostic tests
- Malabsorption of fat can be detected by Sudan staining of the feces or by a 72-hour quantitative measurement of fecal fat.
- Ultrasound is the simplest and least expensive of the imaging techniques. Abdominal computed tomography is often used in patients who have a negative or unsatisfactory ultrasound examination.
- Endoscopic retrograde cholangiopancreatography is the most sensitive and specific test for the diagnosis of CP. However, because it is expensive and is associated with complications, it is reserved for patients for whom the diagnosis cannot be established by imaging techniques.

dysfunction.[7,10] The course of pain is unpredictable, but it frequently lessens as pancreatic insufficiency progresses.[67]

DIAGNOSIS

Most patients with CP have a history of heavy alcohol use and attacks of recurrent upper abdominal pain. The classic triad of calcification, steatorrhea, and diabetes usually confirms the diagnosis.[7,10] Surgical biopsy of pancreatic tissue through laparoscopy or laparotomy is the gold standard for confirming the diagnosis of CP.[7] In the absence of histologic samples, imaging techniques (see Table 39–6) are helpful in detecting calcification of the pancreas, other causes of pain (ductal obstruction secondary to stones, strictures, or pseudocysts), and in differentiating CP from pancreatic cancer. Direct tests of pancreatic exocrine function involve the collection of pancreatic fluid after stimulation with exogenous hormones such as secretin or cholecystokinin. These functional tests are not diagnostic of CP, but serve as a sign of CP and a measure of the severity of injury.[7,8] Because these tests are complicated and require intubation and special collection techniques, they are not routinely performed.

CLINICAL COURSE AND PROGNOSIS

Patients with alcoholic CP usually present with an initial acute attack followed by successive attacks that are slower to resolve. Continued alcohol use leads to chronic abdominal pain and progressive exocrine and endocrine insufficiency. In about 50% of patients, the pain diminishes 5 to 10 years after the onset of symptoms.[68] Steatorrhea, calcification, and diabetes usually develop after 10 to 20 years of heavy ethanol ingestion. Most patients present with varying degrees of pain, malnutrition, and glucose intolerance. The mortality rate of CP is approximately 50% within 20 to 25 years of the diagnosis.[10] About 15% to 20% actually die of complications associated with acute attacks. Most deaths occur as a consequence of malnutrition, infection, or ethanol, narcotic, and tobacco use. The clinical course of idiopathic CP is more favorable than that of alcoholic pancreatitis.[7,8]

► TREATMENT: Chronic Pancreatitis

■ DESIRED OUTCOME

The treatment of uncomplicated CP is aimed primarily at the control of chronic abdominal pain (see Fig. 39–4) and the correction of malabsorption with pancreatic enzymes (Fig. 39–5). Diabetes associated with CP may require exogenous insulin.

■ GENERAL APPROACH TO TREATMENT

The majority of patients with alcohol-related CP require pain control and pancreatic enzyme supplementation.[7,9,10,68–71] Avoidance of alcohol usually decreases pain, but oral analgesics remain the cornerstone of therapy. Non-narcotic analgesics such as acetaminophen, nonsteroidal anti-inflammatory drugs (NSAIDs), selective cyclooxygenase-2 (COX-2) inhibitors, or tramadol should be tried initially. The dose and frequency of administration should be increased before the patient is switched to a narcotic. Patients unresponsive to non-narcotic analgesics should be given a trial of pancreatic enzymes prior to using narcotics. Narcotics are required for patients with severe pain. Specific endoscopic or surgical procedures may be necessary in patients refractory to drug therapy. Patients with malabsorption require pancreatic enzymes to reduce steatorrhea and azotorrhea. Most patients achieve satisfactory results with standard-dosage regimens. In patients who remain symptomatic, dietary fat should be reduced. Consideration may also be given to increasing the pancreatic

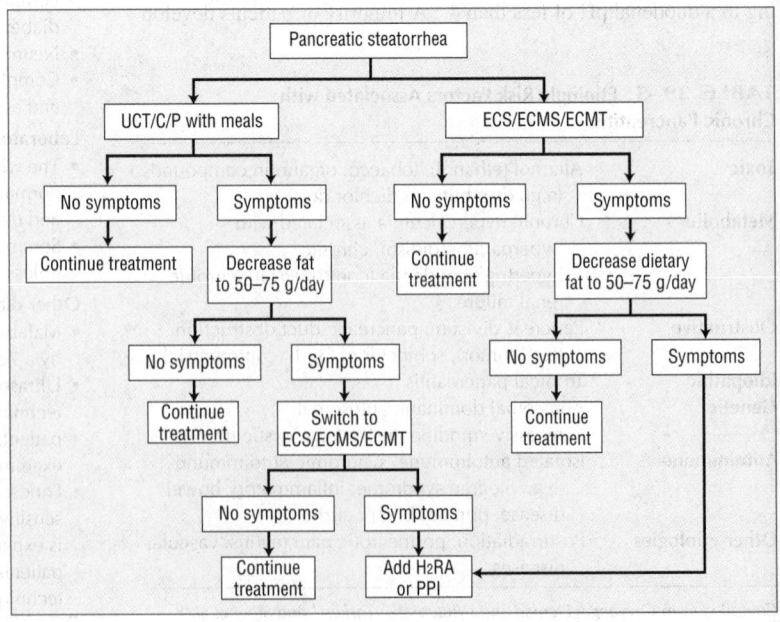

FIGURE 39–5. Algorithm of guidelines for the treatment of pancreatic steatorrhea in chronic pancreatitis. UCT, uncoated tablet; C, capsule; P, powder; ECS, enteric-coated sphere; ECMS, enteric-coated microsphere; ECMT, enteric-coated microtablet; H₂RA, H₂-receptor antagonist; PPI, proton pump inhibitor.

enzyme dose or switching from an uncoated tablet to a microencapsulated enteric-coated dosage form. The addition of an antisecretory drug should be reserved for those patients who do not respond to these maneuvers or who have documented low duodenal pH levels.

NONPHARMACOLOGIC THERAPY

6 Abstinence from alcohol is the most important factor in preventing abdominal pain in the early stages of alcoholic CP, although reports of the effect of abstinence from alcohol have varied.[7,19,68] Small and frequent meals (six meals per day) and a diet restricted in fat (50 to 75 g/day) are recommended to minimize postprandial pancreatic secretion and resulting pain.[71] Parenteral or enteral nutrition (elemental diets) may be necessary, especially if the patient is chronically debilitated, and these nutritional approaches are less likely than oral ingestion of ordinary food to simulate pancreatic secretion, as stimulation of the pancreas is of some concern in that it may contribute to pain.[41]

In some patients pain may be associated with pseudocysts, peptic ulcer, cholelithiasis, biliary or duodenal obstruction, or pancreatic cancer, and if detected may be amenable to other forms of treatment (see Fig. 39–4), including endoscopic procedures such as sphincterotomy, pancreatic duct stenting, and lithotriptic destruction of pancreatic calculi.[7,10,68,72] The most common indication for surgery is abdominal pain that is refractory to medical therapy. Surgical procedures that alleviate pain include a subtotal pancreatectomy, decompression of the main pancreatic duct, or interruption of the splanchnic nerves.[7,10,68,72] Although the pain may diminish as the gland deteriorates, it is unreasonable that a patient wait years for spontaneous relief. A percutaneous injection of a corticosteroid or local anesthetic into the celiac ganglion (celiac nerve block) may be attempted. Unfortunately, pain relief obtained by this procedure lasts only a few months, and repeated treatments are not as effective.[68,72,73]

PHARMACOLOGIC THERAPY

RECOMMENDATIONS

Pain management should begin with non-narcotic analgesics such as acetaminophen, NSAIDs, or selective COX-2 inhibitors (see Fig. 39–4). If pain persists, the response to exogenous pancreatic enzymes should be evaluated in patients with mild to moderate CP. If these measures fail, an oral narcotic should be added to the drug regimen. Parenteral narcotics should be reserved for patients with severe pain that is unresponsive to oral analgesics. Non-narcotic modulators of chronic pain should be considered in patients with difficult-to-manage pain.

Most patients with malabsorption will require pancreatic enzyme supplementation and a reduction in dietary fat in order to achieve satisfactory nutritional status and become relatively asymptomatic. An initial prandial dose of 30,000 international units of lipase (uncoated tablet, capsule, or powder) is recommended to be given with each meal (see Fig. 34–5). Alternatively, the use of microencapsulated enteric-coated dosage forms may be used. The total daily lipase dose should be titrated to reduce steatorrhea. In some patients a reduction in dietary fat may be necessary. The addition of an antisecretory drug should be reserved for patients resistant to enzyme therapy (see Fig. 39–5). If these measures are ineffective, documentation of the diagnosis and exclusion of other diseases should be undertaken.

RELIEF OF CHRONIC ABDOMINAL PAIN

Analgesics

7 Non-narcotic analgesics such as acetaminophen, NSAIDs, or selective COX-2 inhibitors should be given before meals to prevent postprandial exacerbation of pain (Table 39–7).[7,9,69–72] Treatment should be individualized and should begin with the lowest effective dose. The dosage regimen should be maximized before switching to narcotic alternatives. Analgesics should be scheduled around the clock, because they may be more effective and the total amount of medication required over 24 hours may be less. If the non-narcotic analgesic is ineffective, consideration should be given to using tramadol or adding a low-dose narcotic to the regimen (e.g., acetaminophen and codeine). Severe pain relief necessitates the use of opiate analgesics. Narcotics should not be withheld because of the risk of inducing addiction. Oral agents should be used before parenteral narcotics are administered. Non-narcotic modulators of chronic pain such as selective serotonin reuptake inhibitors (e.g., paroxetine) or tricyclic antidepressants should be considered in difficult-to-manage patients.[1,72] Tricyclic antidepressants are useful adjuncts, as they not only treat depression, but have a direct effect on pain and potentiate the effect of opioid narcotics.[72] Referral to a dedicated pain clinic should be considered when available.

Pancreatic Enzymes

8 The use of pancreatic enzymes to relieve pain remains controversial (see Table 39–7). Results from clinical trials are conflicting, especially when non–enteric-coated preparations were compared to enteric-coated enzyme products.[7,69–72,74,75] The administration of non–enteric-coated pancreatic enzymes early in the course of the disease may afford pain relief by suppressing pancreatic enzyme secretion through a negative feedback mechanism involving proteases present in the duodenum. Effective enzyme therapy should reduce pancreatic stimulation, diminish intraductal pressure, and decrease pain. Possible reasons for failure of enzymes to relieve abdominal pain include insufficient concentrations of trypsin in the pancreatic enzyme preparation, a delayed release of trypsin from pH-dependent dosage forms, and gastric acid inactivation or proteolytic destruction of trypsin.[7,72,74,75] Suppression of gastric acid with an antisecretory drug is recommended, as it reduces the degradation of proteases in the stomach.[7,69] Beneficial effects occur in a subset of individuals, primarily those with mild to moderate disease and in patients with a nonalcoholic etiology.[7,9,68,72]

CLINICAL CONTROVERSY

Some clinicians believe that pancreatic enzyme supplementation should be used to relieve mild to moderate abdominal pain, while others believe that these agents are ineffective. A trial of pancreatic enzyme supplementation should be given before initiating treatment with narcotics.

Other Agents

A number of other agents, including octreotide, allopurinol, and antioxidant therapy (e.g., organic selenium, vitamin E, vitamin C, or β-carotene), have been investigated for the purposes of relieving pain in chronic pancreatitis.[7,9,68] There is insufficient evidence to support the use of these agents.

TABLE 39–7. Guidelines for the Pharmacologic Treatment of Chronic Pancreatitis

Treatment of chronic pain (oral drug regimens)

Non-narcotic

- Acetaminophen: Dosage should be limited to 500 mg four times a day if patient drinks more than two alcoholic beverages per day; increased risk of hepatotoxicity, especially in chronic heavy alcohol use
- Nonsteroidal anti-inflammatory drugs (NSAIDs): Standard dosage regimens of aspirin or traditional NSAIDs (e.g., ibuprofen); selective cyclooxygenase-2 (COX-2) inhibitors should be used in patients at risk for upper GI bleeding; use with caution in renal insufficiency
- Tramadol: 50–100 mg every 4–6 hours not to exceed 400 mg/day; has narcotic-like effect; contraindicated in alcohol or hypnotic intoxication; drug interactions; expensive
- Consider use of selective serotonin reuptake inhibitors (e.g., paroxetine) or tricyclic antidepressants in difficult-to-manage patients

Narcotics

- Codeine 30–60 mg every 6 h; hydrocodone 5–10 mg every 4–6 h; oxycodone 5–10 mg every 6 h; fentanyl patch 25–100 mcg/h; pentazocine 25–50 mg every 4–6 h; propoxyphene 65 mg every 4–6 h not to exceed 390 mg/day; methadone 2.5–10 mg every 4–6 h; morphine sulfate (extended-release) 30–60 mg every 8–12 h; hydromorphone 2–4 mg every 4–6 h
- Risk of potentiation with alcohol; impaired respiration; constipation; hypotension
- Dosing is usually based on providing continuous pain relief; consider combining narcotic with acetaminophen, NSAIDs, or selective COX-2 inhibitors; narcotic dependence is common; narcotic abuse is a concern in alcoholics; tolerance to narcotics may develop

Pancreatic enzymes

- Requires that high doses of proteases be delivered to the duodenum for relief of pain; non–enteric-coated pancreatic enzymes are recommended and should be taken with each meal and at night if needed; recommend name brands with proven efficacy and safety, as generic products have been associated with treatment failure; add H_2-receptor antagonist or proton pump inhibitor
- Viokase-8 tablets or Ku-Zyme HP capsules: 6–8 with each meal (see Table 39–8); acid suppression adds to cost
- May cause nausea, cramping, hyperuricemia; hypersensitivity to pork protein

Treatment of maldigestion and steatorrhea

Non–enteric-coated pancreatic enzymes

- Viokase-8 tablets or Ku-Zyme HP capsules, 6–8 with each meal and at bedtime if needed (see Table 39–8)
- May cause nausea, cramping, hyperuricemia; hypersensitivity to pork protein
- Addition of antisecretory drug (H_2-receptor antagonist or proton pump inhibitor) may increase efficacy, but will also increase cost

Enteric-coated pancreatic enzymes

- Enteric-coated spheres, microspheres, and microtablets are available (see Table 39–8)
- May cause nausea, cramping, hyperuricemia; hypersensitivity to pork protein
- Fibrosing colonopathy has occurred in children using preparations that contain the methacrylic acid copolymer coating
- Usually requires fewer capsules or tablets per meal; compliance issues
- Does not usually require additional antisecretory agents; may be less expensive than non–enteric-coated plus H_2-receptor antagonist or proton pump inhibitor

Antisecretory drugs

- May improve enzyme treatment of abdominal pain or steatorrhea
- Proton pump inhibitors may be more effective than H_2-receptor antagonists, but they are also more costly

Compiled from Owyang,[7] Toskes,[9] Amann,[69] Whitcomb et al,[70] American Gastroenterological Association,[71] Conwell and Zuccaro,[72] Brown et al,[74] Mossner,[75] Greenberger,[76] Keller and Layer,[77] and Layer et al.[78]

TREATMENT OF MALABSORPTION

Malabsorption requires treatment when steatorrhea is documented (>7 g of fat in the feces per 24 hours while on a diet of 100 g/day of fat) and persistent weight loss occurs despite efforts to correct it. The combination of pancreatic enzymes (lipase, amylase, and protease) and a reduction in dietary fat (to <25 g/meal) enhances the patient's nutritional status and reduces (but does not totally correct) steatorrhea. The success of a pancreatic enzyme preparation requires that it contain a high concentration of lipase and proteases, be enteric-coated to avoid destruction by gastric acid, and be the appropriate size to permit efficient delivery of the enzymes to the small intestine.[7,76–79] A critical amount of enzymes must be delivered to the duodenum in sufficient concentrations for digestion to occur. The maximal delivery of pancreatic lipase following a meal is approximately 140,000 international units per hour for 4 hours.[7] Malabsorption is minimized if the concentration of enzymes delivered to the duodenum is at least 5% of normal maximal enzyme output. This requires that about 30,000 international units of lipase and 10,000 international units of trypsin be delivered during the 4-hour postprandial period.[7,76] In many cases the lipase dose will need to be increased (up to a maximum of 75,000 international units) because of insufficient lipolytic activity.[77] Most exogenous lipase is rapidly and irreversibly destroyed at an intragastric pH below 4.[7,76–79] Enteric-coating is an effective way to protect the acid-labile enzymes, but the enzymes must be emptied from the stomach at the same rate as the ingested food and released in the duodenum. The polymer used to coat the enzyme is pH-dependent and dissolves in the duodenum at a pH of >5, where the enzymes are released.[7,76] If an intragastric pH of <4 prevails, the enteric-coating will remain intact and the enzymes will be released in the upper portion of the small intestine. A duodenal pH of <4 may prolong dissolution of the enteric coating and release of the enzymes. The size of the enteric-coated enzyme preparation influences the timing of enzyme delivery to the duodenum.[7,76,80,81] Microencapsulated enteric-coated preparations with a microcapsular diameter of about 1.4 mm empty from the stomach in synchrony with food and mix effectively with intestinal chyme.[7,76] Large enteric-coated tablets and some microspheres (microcapsular diameter >2 mm) do not empty at the same rate as stomach contents, and thus are not as effective in treating steatorrhea.

Pancreatic Enzyme Supplements

Oral pancreatic enzyme supplements are available as a powder, uncoated or coated tablet, capsule, enteric-coated sphere (ECS) and microsphere (ECMS), or enteric-coated microtablet (ECMT) encased in a cellulose or gelatin capsule (Table 39–8). Recommended dosages of microencapsulated enteric-coated products are not necessarily more effective than recommended dosages of the non–enteric-coated enzyme preparations.[7,76] This is because a lesser quantity of lipase is usually administered at each meal with the enteric-coated preparations.

Thus the most important determinant in reducing steatorrhea is the total amount of active lipase that reaches the duodenum and empties with the meal. Generic pancreatic enzyme preparations have been associated with treatment failures when substituted for brand-name products.[83]

Pancreatic enzyme supplements differ in enzyme content and activity, bioavailability, clinical efficacy, patient acceptance, and cost. Compliance is often a problem because of the number of tablets or capsules required per dose, the need to take them with each meal or snack, and the cost of pancreatic enzyme therapy. Consideration should be given to selecting a product that contains higher lipase activity (see Table 39–8) so that fewer tablets or capsules are required. However, reports of colonic strictures and intestinal obstruction in cystic fibrosis patients taking high-dose pancreatic enzymes (>20,000 international units lipase per capsule) have led to their withdrawal from the market in the United States.[7,69,82] Pancreatic enzymes contain nucleic acids, and when given in high therapeutic doses, they have been associated with hyperuricosuria, hyperuricemia, and kidney stones.[7,69,70] Impaired folic acid absorption by oral pancreatic enzymes may lead to folic acid deficiency. Gastrointestinal side effects appear to be dose-related, but occur less frequently with the enteric-coated products. Sensitization and allergic reactions are uncommon but may occur in patients taking the powder.

Adjuncts to Enzyme Therapy

The concurrent use of antisecretory drugs may improve the efficacy of pancreatic enzyme supplementation.[7,76] The beneficial effects of an H_2-receptor antagonist or proton pump inhibitor result from

TABLE 39–8. Frequently Used Pancreatic Enzyme Preparations

Product	Dosage Form	Enzyme Content (Units)[a]		
		Lipase	Amylase	Protease
Creon-10	ECMS	10,000	33,200	37,500
Creon-20	ECMS	20,000	66,400	75,000
Ku-Zyme HP	C	8000	30,000	30,000
Lipram-CR10	ECMS	10,000	33,200	37,500
Lipram-PN16	ECMS	16,000	48,000	48,000
Lipram-CR20	ECMS	20,000	66,400	75,000
Lipram-PN20	ECMS	20,000	56,000	44,000
Lipram-UL12	ECMS	12,000	39,000	39,000
Lipram-PN10	ECMS	10,000	30,000	30,000
Lipram-UL18	ECMS	18,000	58,500	58,500
Lipram-UL20	ECMS	20,000	65,000	65,000
Pancrease	ECMS	4500	20,000	25,000
Pancrease MT-4	ECMT	4000	12,000	12,000
Pancrease MT-10	ECMT	10,000	30,000	30,000
Pancrease MT-16	ECMT	16,000	48,000	48,000
Pancrease MT-20	ECMT	20,000	56,000	44,000
Ultrase MT 12	ECMT	12,000	39,000	39,000
Ultrase MT 18	ECMT	18,000	58,500	58,500
Ultrase MT 20	ECMT	20,000	65,000	65,000
Viokase[b]	P	16,800	70,000	70,000
Viokase 8	UCT	8000	30,000	30,000
Viokase 16	UCT	16,000	60,000	60,000

[a]All listed products contain pancrealipase. Pancrealipase contains not less than 24 USP units of lipase activity, not less than 100 USP units of amylase activity, and not less than 100 USP units of protease activity per milligram.
[b]Units of 0.7 g of powder.
C, powder encased in a cellulose capsule; ECS, enteric-coated sphere encased in a cellulose capsule; ECMS, enteric-coated microspheres encased in a cellulose or gelatin capsule; ECMT, enteric-coated microtablets encased in a cellulose capsule; UCT, uncoated tablet; P, powder.

both an increase in pH and a decrease in intragastric volume.[7,84] These agents should maintain luminal gastric and duodenal pH above 4 and enhance lipase activity. Increased duodenal pH also prevents bile acid precipitation, increasing fatty acid solubility. Antacids appear to have little or no added effect in reducing steatorrhea.[7] Symptomatic ◀10 patients whose steatorrhea is not corrected by enzyme replacement therapy and a reduction in dietary fat may benefit from the addition of an H_2-receptor antagonist. A proton pump inhibitor should be considered in patients who fail to benefit from the addition of an H_2-receptor antagonist. The additional cost of antisecretory therapy and the potential for adverse effects and drug interactions should be considered.

PHARMACOECONOMIC CONSIDERATIONS

The pharmacoeconomic issues associated with the medical treatment of AP and CP have not been extensively examined. Aggressive medical and surgical care decreases mortality in AP, but the overall cost effectiveness of a specific treatment is unknown. The relief of abdominal pain in AP and CP, as well as pancreatic enzyme supplementation in patients with CP, improves quality of life and nutritional status. Although the efficacy of octreotide in AP remains uncertain, its use in severe AP is reasonable and potentially cost effective. Antibiotic prophylaxis of targeted patients may reduce mortality and length of hospital stay, but pharmacoeconomic studies have not confirmed this suspicion. However, a reduction in the length of stay could offset the cost of antibiotic therapy.

In some cases, medications that cost more may be more cost effective. This is particularly true with pancreatic enzymes and the microencapsulated enteric-coated dosage forms. These latter products may cost more per unit, but they offer greater patient acceptance and compliance when compared to uncoated tablets. In addition, when cost is based on the total number of tablets or capsules per day, rather than the cost of a single tablet or capsule, the high-potency preparations are usually similar in price to the uncoated products. The addition of an H_2-receptor antagonist or proton pump inhibitor may actually be cost effective for patients who are not adequately controlled on maximal enzyme therapy.

EVALUATION OF THERAPEUTIC OUTCOMES

ACUTE PANCREATITIS

In patients with mild AP, pain control, fluid and electrolyte status, and nutrition should be assessed periodically, depending on the degree of abdominal pain and fluid loss. Patients with severe AP should be transferred to an intensive care unit for close monitoring of vital signs, prothrombin time, fluid and electrolyte status, white blood cell count, blood glucose, lactic dehydrogenase, aspartate aminotransferase, serum albumin, hematocrit, blood urea nitrogen, and serum creatinine. Continuous hemodynamic and arterial blood gas monitoring is essential. Serum lipase, amylase, and bilirubin require less frequent monitoring. The patient should be monitored for signs of infection, relief of abdominal pain, and adequate nutritional status. Therapeutic outcome depends on the severity of the acute attack, medical management (which is primarily supportive), and prevention or treatment of infection. Despite appropriate supportive therapy, deterioration of respiratory, renal, and cardiovascular function may lead to death.

CHRONIC PANCREATITIS

The severity and frequency of abdominal pain should be assessed periodically in order to determine the efficacy of the patient's pain control regimen. Most patients with abdominal pain can be adequately controlled with acetaminophen, NSAIDs, or selective COX-2 inhibitors. A trial of pancreatic enzymes and either an H_2-receptor antagonist or proton pump inhibitor may relieve pain in patients with mild to moderate disease. Patients with severe pain will require narcotics. In these patients, pain should be monitored daily and medications adjusted accordingly. Some patients will require endoscopic therapy or pancreatic surgery.

The effectiveness of pancreatic enzyme supplementation in treating malabsorption is measured by improvement in body weight and stool consistency or frequency. The 72-hour stool test for fecal fat may be used when there is concern regarding the adequacy of treatment. Serum uric acid and folic acid concentrations should be monitored yearly in patients prone to hyperuricemia or folic acid deficiency. Blood glucose must be closely monitored in the diabetic patient.

Therapeutic outcome depends in part on the ability of the patient to discontinue alcohol and tobacco use and to maintain adequate nutrition. Pain control and pancreatic enzyme supplementation are important therapeutic measures that contribute to the patient's quality of life. A small number of patients die from complications associated with an acute attack.

CONCLUSIONS

Important advances have been made in recent years regarding our understanding of acute and chronic pancreatitis, especially as it relates to genetics, pathogenesis, and the natural history of the diseases. Although there has been a reduction in the mortality of patients with severe AP, controversy remains regarding the use of antibiotic prophylaxis. Patients with CP now benefit from improved strategies for managing pain and treating malabsorption. In the future, new and improved diagnostic techniques and medical treatments will replace many of the procedures and drugs we use today.

ABBREVIATIONS

AP: acute pancreatitis
ARDS: acute respiratory distress syndrome
CCK: cholecystokinin
COX-2: cyclooxygenase-2
CP: chronic pancreatitis
ERCP: endoscopic retrograde cholangiopancreatography
IMMC: interdigestive migrating motor complex
NSAID: nonsteroidal anti-inflammatory drug

Review Questions and other resources can be found at *www.pharmacotherapyonline.com.*

REFERENCES

1. Mitchell RMS, Byrne MF, Baillie J. Pancreatitis. Lancet 2003;361:1447–1455.
2. Topazian M, Gorelick FS. Acute pancreatitis. In: Yamada T, Aplers DH, Kaplowitz N, et al, eds. Textbook of Gastroenterology, 4th ed. Philadelphia, Lippincott Williams & Wilkins, 2003:2026–2061.

3. Bank S, Singh P, Pooran N, et al. Evaluation of factors that have reduced mortality from acute pancreatitis over the past 20 years. J Clin Gastroenterol 2002;35:50–60.

4. Grendell JH. Acute pancreatitis. Clin Perspect Gastroenterol 2000;3: 327–333.

5. Dervenis C, Johnson CD, Bassi C, et al. Diagnosis, objective assessment of severity, and management of acute pancreatitis. Int J Pancreatol 1999;25:195–220.

6. Banks PA. Practice guidelines in acute pancreatitis. Am J Gastroenterol 1997;92:377–386.

7. Owyang C. Chronic pancreatitis. In: Yamada T, Aplers DH, Kaplowitz N, et al, eds. Textbook of Gastroenterology, 4th ed. Philadelphia, Lippincott Williams & Wilkins, 2003:2061–2090.

8. Etemad B, Whitcomb DC. Chronic pancreatitis: Diagnosis, classification and new genetic developments. Gastroenterology 2001;120:682–707.

9. Toskes PP. Update on diagnosis and management of chronic pancreatitis. Curr Gastroenterol Rep 1999;1:145–153.

10. Steer ML, Waxman I, Freedman S. Chronic pancreatitis. N Engl J Med 1995;332:1482–1490.

11. Owyang C, Williams JA. Pancreatic secretion. In: Yamada T, Aplers DH, Kaplowitz N, et al, eds. Textbook of Gastroenterology, 4th ed. Philadelphia, Lippincott Williams & Wilkins, 2003:340–366.

12. Cohen S, Bacon BR, Berline JA, et al. National Institutes of Health State-of-the-Science Conference Statement: ERCP for diagnosis and therapy, January 14–16, 2002. Gastrointest Endosc 2002;56:803–809.

13. Eland IA, van Puijenbroek EP, Sturkenboom MJCM, et al. Drug-associated acute pancreatitis: Twenty-one years of spontaneous reporting in the Netherlands. Am J Gastroenterol 1999;94:2417–2422.

14. McArthur KE. Review article: Drug-induced pancreatitis. Aliment Pharmacol Ther 1996;10:23–38.

15. Eland IA, Rasch MC, Sturkenboom MJCM, et al. Acute pancreatitis attributed to the use of interferon alfa-2b. Gastroenterology 2000;119:230–233.

16. Gershon T, Olshaker J. Acute pancreatitis following lisinopril rechallenge. Am J Emerg Med 1998;16:523–524.

17. Maringhini A, Termini A, Patti R, et al. Enalapril-associated acute pancreatitis: Recurrence after rechallenge. Am J Gastroenterol 1997;92:166–167.

18. Izaeli S, Adamson PC, Blaney SM, et al. Acute pancreatitis after ifosfamide therapy. Cancer 1994;74:1627–1628.

19. Liviu L, Yair L, Yehuda S. Pancreatitis induced by clarithromycin. Ann Intern Med 1996;125:701 [Letter].

20. Goffin E, Horsmans Y, Pirson Y, et al. Acute necrotic-hemorrhagic pancreatitis after famciclovir prescription. Transplantation 1995;59:1218–1219.

21. Hoff PM, Valero V, Holmes FA, et al. Paclitaxel-induced pancreatitis: A case report. J Natl Cancer Inst 1997;89:91–92 [Letter].

22. Rodier JM, Pujade-Lauraine E, Batel-Copel L, et al. Granisetron-induced acute pancreatitis. J Cancer Res Clin Oncol 1996;122:132–133 [Letter].

23. Balasch J, Martinez-Romain S, Carreras J, et al. Acute pancreatitis associated with danazol treatment for endometriosis. Hum Reprod 1994;9:1163–1165.

24. Domingo P, Ferrer S, Kolle S, et al. Acute pancreatitis associated with sodium stibogluconate treatment in a patient with human immunodeficiency virus. Arch Intern Med 1996;156:1029–1032 [Letter].

25. Torrus D, Massa B, Boix V, et al. Meglumine antimonate-induced pancreatitis. Am J Gastroenterol 1996;91:820–821 [Letter].

26. Abdul-Ghaffar N, El-Sonbaty MR. Pancreatitis and rhabdomyolysis associated with lovastatin-gemfibrozil therapy. J Clin Gastroenterol 1995;21:340–341.

27. Stricker R, Man K, Bouvier D, et al. Pancreatorenal syndrome associated with combination antiretroviral therapy in HIV infection. Lancet 1997;349:1745–1746.

28. McDornald KB, Garbor BG, Perreault MM. Pancreatitis associated with simvastatin plus fenofibrate. Ann Pharmacother 2002;36:275–279.

29. Sammett D, Greben C, Sayeed-Shah U. Acute pancreatitis caused by penicillin. Dig Dis Sci 1998;43:1778–1783.

30. Goyal SB, Goyal R. Ketorolac tromethamine-induced acute pancreatitis. Arch Intern Med 1998;158:411 [Letter].

31. Haviv YS, Sharkia M, Galun E, et al. Pancreatitis following hepatitis A vaccination. Eur J Med Res 2000;5:229–230.

32. Eland IA, Alvarez CH, Stricker BHCH, et al. The risk of acute pancreatitis associated with acid-suppressing drugs. Br J Clin Pharmacol 2000;49:473–478.

33. Birck R, Keim V, Fiedler F, vander Woude FJ, et al. Pancreatitis after losartan. Lancet 1998;351:1178 [Letter].

34. Fisher AA, Bassett ML. Acute pancreatitis associated with angiotensin II receptor antagonists. Ann Pharmacother 2002;36:1883–1886.

35. Blomgren KB, Sundstrom A, Steineck G, et al. Obesity and treatment of diabetes with glyburide may both be risk factors for acute pancreatitis. Diabetes Care 2002;25:298–302.

36. Blomgren KB, Sundström A, Steineck G, et al. A Swedish case-control network for studies of drug-induced morbidity—acute pancreatitis. Eur J Clin Pharmacol 2002;58:275–283.

37. Mayer J, Rau B, Gansauge F, et al. Inflammatory mediators in human acute pancreatitis: Clinical and pathophysiological implications. Gut 2000;47:546–552.

38. Riche FD, Cholley BO, Laisne MJC, et al. Inflammatory cytokines, C reactive protein, and procalcitonin as early predictors of necrosis infection in acute necrotizing pancreatitis. Surgery 2003;133:257–262.

39. Somogyi L, Martin SP, Venkatesan T, et al. Recurrent acute pancreatitis: An algorithmic approach to identification and elimination of inciting factors. Gastroenterology 2001;120:708–717.

40. Abou-Assi S, Craig K, O'Keefe SJD, et al. Hypocaloric jejunal feeding is better than total parenteral nutrition in acute pancreatitis: Results of a randomized comparative study. Am J Gastroenterol 2002;97:2255–2262.

41. Scolapio J, Malhi-Chowla N, Ukleja A. Nutrition supplementation in patients with acute and chronic pancreatitis. Gastroenterol Clin North Am 1999;28:695–707.

42. Lobo DN, Memon MA, Allison SP, et al. Evolution of nutritional support in acute pancreatitis. Br J Surg 2000;87:695–707.

43. Kotani J, Usami M, Nomura H, et al. Enteral nutrition prevents bacterial translocation but does not improve survival during acute pancreatitis. Arch Surg 1999;134:287–292.

44. Oláh A, Issekutz Á, Gamal ME, et al. Randomized clinical trial of specific lactobacillus and fiber supplement to early enteral nutrition in patients with acute pancreatitis. Br J Surg 2002;89:1103–1107.

45. Isenhower HL, Mueller BA. Selection of narcotic analgesics for pain associated with pancreatitis. Am J Health-Syst Pharm 1998;55:480–486.

46. Yousaf M, McCallion K, Daimond T. Management of severe acute pancreatitis. Br J Surg 2003;90:407–420.

47. Norton ID, Clain JE. Optimizing outcomes in acute pancreatitis. Drugs 2001;61:1581–1591.

48. Ulrich CD. Medical management of acute pancreatitis: Strategies, reality, and potential. Curr Gastroenterol Rep 2000;2:115–119.

49. Brown A, Ballargeon JD, Hughes MD, et al. Can fluid resuscitation prevent pancreatic necrosis in severe acute pancreatitis? Pancreatology 2002;2:104–107.

50. Pezzilli R, Miglioli M. Multicentre comparative study of two schedules of gabexate mesilate in the treatment of acute pancreatitis. Dig Liver Dis 2001;33:49–77.

51. Holtz HG, Schmidt J, Ryschich EW, et al. Isovolemic hemodilution with dextran prevents contrast medium-induced impairment of pancreatic microcirculation in necrotizing pancreatitis of the rat. Am J Surg 1995;169:161–166.

52. Andriulli A, Leandro G, Clemente R, et al. Meta-analysis of somatostatin, octreotide and gabexate mesilate in the therapy of acute pancreatitis. Aliment Pharmacol Ther 1998;12:237–245.

53. Paran H, Mayo A, Paran D. Octreotide treatment in patients with severe acute pancreatitis. Dig Dis Sci 2000;45:2247–2251.

54. Karakoyunlar O, Sivrel E, Tanir N, et al. High-dose octreotide in the management of acute pancreatitis. Hepatogastroenterology 1999;46:1968–1971.

55. Kramer KM, Levy H. Prophylactic antibiotics for severe AP: The beginning of an era. Pharmacotherapy 1999;19:592–602.

56. Sainio V, Kemppainen P, Poulallainen P, et al. Early antibiotic treatment in acute necrotizing pancreatitis. Lancet 1995;346:663–667.

57. Pederzoli P, Bassi C, Vesentini S, et al. A randomized multicenter clinical trial of antibiotic prophylaxis with imipenem. Surg Gynecol Obstet 1993;176:480–483.

58. Delcenserie R, Yzet T, Ducroix JP. Prophylactic antibiotics in treatment of severe acute alcoholic pancreatitis. Pancreas 1996;13:198–201.

59. Golub R, Siddiai F, Pohl D. Role of antibiotics in acute pancreatitis: A meta-analysis. J Gastrointest Surg 1998;2:496–503

60. Sharma VK, Howden CW. Prophylactic antibiotic administration reduces sepsis and mortality in acute necrotizing pancreatitis: A meta-analysis. Pancreas 2001;22:1–4.

61. Bassi C, Falconi M, Talamini G, et al. Controlled clinical trial of pefloxacin versus imipenem in severe acute pancreatitis. Gastroenterology 1998;115:1513–1517.

62. Gloor B, Muller CA, Worni M, et al. Pancreatic infection in severe pancreatitis: The role of fungus and multiresistant organisms. Arch Surg 2001;136:592–596.

63. Howard TJ, Temple MB. Prophylactic antibiotics alter the bacteriology of infected necrosis in severe acute pancreatitis. J Am Coll Surg 2002:195:759–767.

64. Butturini G, Salvia R, Bettini M, et al. Infection prevention in necrotizing pancreatitis: An old challenge with new perspectives. J Hosp Infect 2001;49:4–8.

65. Shrikhande S, Friess H, Issenegger C. Fluconazole penetration into the pancreas. Antimicrob Agents Chemother 2000;44:2569–2571.

66. Poon RTP, Fan ST. Antisecretory agents for prevention of post-ERCP pancreatitis: Rationale for use and clinical results. J Pancreas 2003;4:233–240.

67. Ammann RW, Muelihaupt B, Zurich Pancreatitis Study Group. The natural history of pain in alcoholic chronic pancreatitis. Gastroenterology 1999;116:1132–1140.

68. Warshaw A, Banks PA, Fernandez-del C. American Gastroenterological Association technical review: Treatment of pain in chronic pancreatitis. Gastroenterology 1998;115:765–776.

69. Amann ST. Chronic pancreatitis. Curr Treat Option Gastroenterol 1999;2:401–408.

70. Whitcomb D, Pfutzer RH, Slivka A. Alcoholic chronic pancreatitis. Curr Treat Option Gastroenterol 1999;2:273–282.

71. American Gastroenterological Association Medical Position Statement: Treatment of pain in chronic pancreatitis. Gastroenterology 1998;155:763–764.

72. Conwell DL, Zuccaro G. Pain management in chronic pancreatitis. Curr Treat Option Gastroenterol 1999;2:295–304.

73. Bhutani MS, Pasricha PJ. Neurolytic approaches for the treatment of pain in patients with chronic pancreatitis. Curr Treat Option Gastroenterol 2003;6:375–379.

74. Brown A, Hughes M, Tenner S, et al. Does pancreatic enzyme supplementation reduce pain in patients with chronic pancreatitis: A meta-analysis. Am J Gastroenterol 1997;92:2032–2035.

75. Mossner J. Palliation of pain in chronic pancreatitis: Use of enzymes. Surg Clin North Am 1999;79:861–872.

76. Greenberger NJ. Enzymatic therapy in patients with chronic pancreatitis. Gastroenterol Clin North Am 1999;28:687–693.

77. Keller J, Layer P. Pancreatic enzyme supplementation therapy. Curr Treat Option Gastroenterol 2003;6:369–374.

78. Layer P, Keller J, Lankich PG. Pancreatic enzyme replacement therapy. Curr Gastroenterol Rep 2001;3:101–108.

79. Apte MN, Keogh GW, Wilson JS. Chronic pancreatitis: Complications and management. J Clin Gastroenterol 1999;29:225–240.

80. Bruno MJ, Borm JJ, Hock FJ, et al. Gastric transit and pharmacodynamics of a two-millimeter enteric-coated pancreatin microsphere preparation in patients with chronic pancreatitis. Dig Dis Sci 1998;43:203–213.

81. Halm U, Loser C, Lohr M, et al. A double-blind randomized, multicentre, crossover study to prove equivalence of pancreatin minimicrospheres versus microspheres in exocrine pancreatic insufficiency. Aliment Pharmacol Ther 1999;13:951–957.

82. Littlewood JM. Update on intestinal strictures. J R Soc Med 1999;92(Suppl 37):41–49.

83. Hendeles L, Hochhaus G, Kazerounian S. Generic and alternative brand-name pharmaceutical equivalent: Select with caution. Am J Hosp Pharm 1993;50:323–329.

84. Bruno MJ, Rauws EAJ, Hoek FJ, et al. Comparative effects of adjuvant cimetidine and omeprazole during pancreatic enzyme replacement therapy. Dig Dis Sci 1994;39:988–992.

40

VIRAL HEPATITIS

Manjunath P. Pai, Renee-Claude Mercier, and Marsha A. Raebel

Learning Objectives and other resources can be found at *www.pharmacotherapyonline.com.*

KEY CONCEPTS

1 Hepatitis A is transmitted via the fecal-oral route. Conditions in which transmission is more likely to occur include travel to countries with high rates of hepatitis A, poor conditions and hygiene, and overcrowded areas.

2 Hepatitis A causes an acute illness and does not lead to chronic liver disease. The infection can be divided into three stages: incubation, acute hepatitis, and convalescence. The disease is typically self-limited and rarely progresses to liver failure.

3 Treatment of acute hepatitis A infection is primarily supportive, as pharmacologic treatment with antiviral agents is of no benefit.

4 Hepatitis B virus can cause both an acute and chronic illness and is more difficult to clear if acquired as an infant compared to acquisition as an adult.

5 The choice of first-line therapy for hepatitis B virus when comparing interferon-α2b and lamivudine is controversial. The duration of interferon-α2b therapy is finite (16 to 52 weeks) relative to lamivudine (52 weeks or longer) for chronic hepatitis B, but is associated with significant side effects.

6 Long-term therapy with lamivudine is associated with the development of hepatitis B virus strains that are resistant to this agent. Although the impact of developing lamivudine-resistant hepatitis B virus is not known, adefovir may be used to treat these resistant strains.

7 All infants should be immunized against hepatitis B. Older children and adults in high-risk groups who have not been previously immunized should also receive the vaccine.

8 Hepatitis C is a significant public health problem associated primarily with illicit injection drug use in the United States.

9 No vaccines exist for the prevention of hepatitis C compared to the individual and combined vaccines that are available for the prevention of hepatitis A and B.

10 The availability of pegylated versions of interferon has allowed for less frequent dosing and better therapeutic response in chronic hepatitis C. However, therapeutic response of patients with chronic hepatitis C to combination pegylated interferon-α and ribavirin therapy is expected in less than half of treated patients with genotype 1.

Hepatitis is a major cause of morbidity and mortality in the United States. *Viral hepatitis* refers to the clinically important hepatotrophic viruses responsible for hepatitis A (HAV), hepatitis B (HBV), hepatitis C (HCV), delta hepatitis, and hepatitis E. Hepatitis G virus has also been described; however, its role in clinical illness is still not clear. Viral hepatitis has acute, fulminant, and chronic clinical forms, defined by duration or severity of infection. The clinical, biochemical, immunoserologic, and histologic features of viral hepatitis follow similar patterns regardless of the virus responsible for the patient's illness. Hepatocellular response to injury and the resulting physical signs and symptoms are nonspecific.

HAV is primarily responsible for acute hepatitis. It is most often linked to sporadic events of contaminated food in the United States and to international travel, and is usually a self-limited disease. HBV and HCV are primarily responsible for the development of chronic hepatitis, cirrhosis, and hepatocellular carcinoma. Immunomodulatory therapy and direct antiviral agents have been developed for both HBV and HCV. These therapeutic modalities require long courses of therapy and are associated with limited success. This chapter will focus on the pathophysiology, clinical course, and management of these three primary causes of viral hepatitis, namely HAV, HBV, and HCV.

HEPATITIS A VIRUS

HAV has been associated with significant morbidity and occasional mortality for centuries as a known cause of acute hepatitis.[1] Despite the availability of an effective vaccine against HAV, hepatitis A continues to be one of the most frequently reported vaccine-preventable diseases in the United States.[2] Epidemiologic data in the United States from 1997 estimated that hepatitis A infections were responsible for 255 deaths, approximately 2.5 million days of symptomatic illness, 829,000 working days lost, and costs in the range of 330 to 580 million dollars.[3]

EPIDEMIOLOGY AND ETIOLOGY

HAV causes both epidemics and sporadic infections. Both are related to overcrowded conditions and person-to-person spread or ingestion 1 of contaminated food or water. HAV is transmitted by the fecal-oral route. The incidence of HAV correlates directly with poor sanitary conditions and hygienic practices.[4] For international travelers, longer lengths of stay in a country with a high rate of hepatitis A also correlates with increased risk. In the United States, groups at increased risk of HAV, in addition to travelers, include men who have sex with men, injecting drug users, and persons working with nonhuman primates.[2]

HAV infection in the United States occurs primarily from person-to-person transmission in communitywide outbreaks, in lower socioeconomic groups, and in sporadic common-source outbreaks (outbreaks in which all infected patients contract the infection from a single person or source).[2] Children between the ages of 5 and 14 years are more likely to be involved in communitywide outbreaks, whereas common-source outbreaks primarily involve young adults. Both children and young adults can be infected from common-source outbreaks at day care centers.[4] HAV infection in children is often asymptomatic or unrecognized. Therefore, children serve as an important source for transmitting the infection to others.[2] Rarely, HAV is transmitted by transfusion of contaminated blood products collected while the donor is viremic with HAV.[2] Cases of HAV associated with parenteral drug abuse are increasing.[5]

HAV are small, nonenveloped, single-stranded ribonucleic acid (RNA) viruses belonging to the *Hepatovirus* genus of the Picornaviridae. Four genotypes are known to infect humans. Most infections are caused by strains from either genotype I or III, although the genotypes do not appear to confer important biological differences.[6]

PATHOPHYSIOLOGY

HAV usually causes a self-limiting disease with a low case-fatality rate. The disease is a systemic viral infection of up to (but not exceeding) 6 months in duration, producing inflammatory necrosis of the liver. The natural history of the infection is divided into three stages based on viral serologic markers: incubation, acute hepatitis, and convalescence. Incubation begins shortly after parenteral or oral inoculation with the virus. After the virus reaches the circulation, infective virions accumulate in hepatic sinusoids and are internalized by the hepatocytes. HAV replication occurs exclusively in the hepatocytes and gastrointestinal epithelial cells.[6] Viral antigens are found in the hepatocyte cytoplasm during incubation. They are subsequently shed into bile and feces. The largest concentration of viral particles is found in stool specimens during the 1 to 2 weeks preceding clinical illness or elevation of liver enzymes. Infected persons are at peak infectivity at this time.[2] Viral shedding declines as clinical symptoms appear. During the incubation stage, the host is asymptomatic.

Acute hepatitis begins with a preicteric phase (before the onset of jaundice), which parallels initiation of the host immune response and occurs before significant liver cell injury. The preicteric phase is frequently associated with nonspecific influenza-like symptoms consisting of anorexia, nausea, fatigue, and malaise.[6] Most patients with acute viral hepatitis develop only a few mild symptoms and minimal hepatocyte damage. This mild disease is called *acute anicteric hepatitis*. The minimal degree of liver cell damage is reflected by mild elevations of serum bilirubin, γ-globulin, and hepatic transaminase (alanine transaminase [ALT], aspartate transaminase [AST]) values to about twice normal. Subsets of patients experience enough hepatocyte destruction to produce significant liver dysfunction characterized by interruption of bilirubin metabolism and flow. This results in clinical jaundice and acute icteric hepatitis. Icteric hepatitis is generally accompanied by fever, right upper quadrant abdominal pain, nausea, vomiting, dark urine, acholic (light colored) stools, and worsening of systemic symptoms. Clinical symptoms are accompanied by elevations of the serum bilirubin, γ-globulin, and hepatic transaminases from 4 to 10 times above normal. Most patients with either acute anicteric or icteric hepatitis go through the convalescence stage

to complete recovery without developing complications or chronic sequelae.

Liver injury is immune mediated with cytolytic T cells maintaining the primary role in cell destruction.[6] Death of hepatocytes results in viral elimination and eventual resolution of the clinical illness. Viremia begins soon after infection and continues throughout the time liver enzymes are elevated.[2] The host antibody response to HAV initially appears as the viral particles begin to disappear from stool. Like most host antibody responses, antibodies of the IgM class appear first and imply recent infection. IgM anti-HAV usually is detectable 5 to 10 days before symptoms appear. After 2 to 6 months, the IgM antibodies are replaced with IgG antibodies, which usually persist throughout life and confer immunity to HAV.[2] Patients who receive immunoglobulin will have low titers of anti-HAV for several weeks after inoculation.[2] Patients who receive hepatitis A vaccine will also have anti-HAV.[2]

CLINICAL PRESENTATION

Hepatitis A infection usually results in an acute, self-limited disease that rarely leads to fulminant hepatic failure. The clinical features of acute hepatitis A are summarized in Table 40–1. After an average incubation period of 28 days, with a range of 15 to 50 days, symptomatic individuals will experience an abrupt onset of anorexia, nausea, vomiting, malaise, fever, headache, and right upper quadrant abdominal pain.[2] Patients with underlying liver disease such as chronic hepatitis C infection are more likely to develop fulminant hepatic failure.[7] Clinical symptoms also vary with age. Children younger than 6 years old are usually asymptomatic or have a mild influenza-like illness without clinical jaundice.[2] In contrast, more than 70% of infected adults and older children display the characteristic clinical syndrome of acute hepatitis with elevated hepatic transaminase levels and jaundice.[2]

The vast majority of people who become ill with HAV completely recover. HAV infection usually produces a self-limited illness that lasts less than 2 months, although 10% to 15% of patients exhibit a cholestatic illness with predominant elevations of alkaline phosphatase, γ-glutamyl transferase, and total bilirubin that continues or is relapsing for up to 6 months.[2] Pruritus is often a major complaint

TABLE 40–1. Clinical Presentation of Acute Hepatitis A

Signs and symptoms
- The preicteric phase brings nonspecific influenza-like symptoms consisting of anorexia, nausea, fatigue, and malaise
- Abrupt onset of anorexia, nausea, vomiting, malaise, fever, headache, and right upper quadrant abdominal pain with acute illness
- Icteric hepatitis is generally accompanied by dark urine, acholic (light-colored) stools, and worsening of systemic symptoms
- Pruritus is often a major complaint of icteric patients

Physical examination
- Icteric sclera, skin, and secretions
- Mild weight loss of 2 to 5 kg
- Hepatomegaly

Laboratory tests
- Positive serum IgM anti-HAV
- Mild elevations of serum bilirubin, γ-globulin, and hepatic transaminase (alanine transaminase [ALT], and aspartate transaminase [AST]) values to about twice normal in acute anicteric disease
- Elevations of alkaline phosphatase, γ-glutamyl transferase, and total bilirubin in patients with cholestatic illness

of these patients.[5] A relapse is rarely associated with extrahepatic manifestations such as cryoglobulinemia, arthritis, and vasculitis. No cases of a chronic carrier state or chronic hepatitis have been reported.

The gold standard method of diagnosis of an acute HAV infection involves detection of serum IgM anti-HAV that becomes positive at the onset of symptoms. The antibody peaks during the early phase of convalescence and remains positive for 4 to 6 months after the onset of the disease. In addition to the presence of antibody, the diagnosis is based on the clinical suspicion, characteristic symptoms, and elevated aminotransferases and bilirubin. HAV infection cannot be differentiated from other types of viral hepatitis by clinical or epidemiologic features.[2]

▶ TREATMENT: Hepatitis A Virus Infection

▨ DESIRED OUTCOME

The ultimate goal in treating acute viral hepatitis is to return the individual to the previous state of health. Intermediate goals while the individual is acutely symptomatic and infectious include decreasing morbidity and acute mortality, normalizing aminotransferases (to stop hepatic inflammation), stopping viral replication in the host, and ultimately eradicating the virus.

▨ GENERAL APPROACH TO THERAPY

Management of acute HAV infection is primarily supportive, as the disease is usually self-limited and the majority of patients infected with HAV will have full clinical and biochemical recovery within 12 weeks.[6] General measures include a healthy diet, rest, maintaining fluid balance, and avoiding hepatotoxic drugs and alcohol. Special diets are of no benefit. Management includes laboratory tests (International Normalized Ratio and liver function tests) aimed at identifying the group of patients at risk of developing fulminant liver failure. Hospitalization is necessary only for those who have prolonged vomiting, coagulation defects, or fulminant hepatitis.

▨ PHARMACOLOGIC THERAPY

Pharmacologic agents offer no clear benefit in the treatment of patients infected with HAV. Corticosteroids have been used in patients with acute HAV when cholestatic hepatitis or fulminant hepatic failure is evident. However, controlled trials have failed to demonstrate any benefit and in some cases the use of corticosteroids may worsen clinical outcomes.[8]

▨ FULMINANT HEPATITIS (ACUTE LIVER FAILURE)

Liver injury that results in fulminant hepatic necrosis and acute liver failure is relatively rare. When it occurs, death results in days or weeks in nearly 80% of cases.[9] Any potential hepatotoxic agent (e.g., acetaminophen) can be responsible, although viral hepatitis is the most common cause worldwide, especially HBV (1% of patients with acute hepatitis B develop fulminant hepatitis).[9–11] Fulminant hepatitis caused by HAV occasionally occurs; acute liver failure caused by HCV is rare.[9]

Patients with fulminant hepatic necrosis typically develop signs and symptoms of viral hepatitis, and then rapidly develop evidence of hepatic failure. The clinical syndrome is usually a 1- to 3-week course of hepatic failure and encephalopathy with coma developing within 8 weeks of the onset of acute hepatitis. Hyperexcitability, insomnia, somnolence, irritability, and impaired mental status are evidence of impending hepatic failure. Ominous signs include a rapid decrease in liver size, a rapid decline in aminotransferase levels, prolonged International Normalized Ratio or prothrombin time, and hypoglycemia. Manifestations of hepatic failure include metabolic encephalopathy, coma, coagulation defects, ascites, and edema. In fulminant liver failure, complications include gastrointestinal hemorrhage, sepsis, cerebral edema, renal failure, lactic acidosis, and disseminated coagulopathy, with death resulting from bleeding, cerebral edema, hypoglycemia, infection, and/or multisystem organ failure.[9]

Prompt referral for liver transplantation is the therapy of choice for most patients with fulminant hepatic failure.[9] Transplantation should be considered in all cases in which the patient demonstrates progressive clinical deterioration (encephalopathy, hypoglycemia, metabolic acidosis, renal failure, and coagulation defects).[11] Patients should be transferred at the first sign of altered mental status, because these patients often worsen very rapidly. One-year survival rates with liver transplantation for fulminant hepatitis are 50% to 80% (as compared to <20% with medical management alone).[11]

There is no specific medical treatment for fulminant hepatic failure. The goal of medical management is to support organ function in the interim until the liver recovers or a donor organ is available.[11] Management therefore focuses on recognition coupled with prevention and aggressive management of complications. Cerebral edema occurs in 75% to 80% of cases that progress to grade IV encephalopathy, and is the leading cause of death in these patients.[11] Management includes intracranial pressure monitoring and administration of mannitol (0.3 to 1 g/kg body weight as a 20% solution administered intravenously over 20 minutes) when intracranial pressure increases above 20 mm Hg.[11] Pentobarbital lowers intracranial pressure, but it also can cause severe hypotension, and its use is limited to cases with elevated intracranial pressure that is unresponsive to mannitol and with good cerebral blood flow.[11] Corticosteroids and hyperventilation are of little value in cerebral edema related to acute liver failure.[11] Fresh frozen plasma should be administered for bleeding, histamine$_2$-blocker therapy should be given to prevent GI bleeding, and aggressive antibiotic therapy should be used for infections. Renal replacement therapy is used for acute renal failure, while fluid replacement (with pulmonary artery wedge pressure and cardiac output monitoring) and vasopressors provide circulatory support.[11] Metabolic abnormalities (e.g., hypoglycemia) should be treated with standard metabolic support. For further information on medical therapy, drug dosing, and adverse effects, the reader is referred to the corresponding topics in appropriate chapters of this textbook. New treatment options being evaluated include artificial liver support systems and hepatocyte transplantation. These options are at an early stage of development and further controlled clinical trials are needed to determine safety and efficacy.[11]

PREVENTION OF HEPATITIS A

GENERAL APPROACH TO PREVENTION OF HEPATITIS A

Highly effective inactivated vaccines against HAV have been available in the United States since 1995. These vaccines can substantially lower the incidence of HAV infection, and potentially even eradicate the disease.[2] The most effective means of achieving control of HAV infection is to vaccinate all children by incorporating hepatitis A vaccination into routine childhood immunizations. However, a vaccine formulation is currently not available for children younger than 2 years old. Until routine infant vaccination is feasible, the vaccination strategy in the United States includes vaccinating: (a) children in states, counties, and communities with consistently elevated rates of hepatitis A; (b) persons in groups at increased risk for HAV infection, such as international travelers; and (c) persons at risk of adverse outcomes, such as persons with chronic liver disease.[2]

Even though effective active and passive immunity agents are available for HAV, the importance of avoiding exposure cannot be overemphasized. The most important measures to avoid exposure include good hand-washing techniques and good personal hygiene practices. Travelers can minimize risk by avoiding uncooked shellfish, uncooked fruits and vegetables, and by avoiding drinking water (and other beverages with ice) of unknown purity. If exposure occurs, postexposure prophylaxis is with immune globulin injection.

Immunoglobulin to Prevent Hepatitis A

Immunoglobulin (Ig) provides protection against HAV by passive transfer of concentrated antibodies (immunoglobulins) against HAV (anti-HAV). Ig is effective in modifying the course and preventing the spread of HAV in 85% or more of exposures when used within 2 weeks following the exposure.[2] Pregnancy and lactation are not contraindications to receiving Ig; however, when Ig is administered to pregnant women or infants, thimerosal-free preparations should be used.[2] Both Ig given intramuscularly and Ig for intravenous administration contain anti-HAV, but only the intramuscular formulation is used for prevention of HAV infection.[2]

International travelers are the major group receiving preexposure prophylaxis with Ig. Ig is recommended for susceptible persons traveling to developing countries. A single dose of Ig of 0.02 mL/kg IM (in the deltoid or gluteus muscle) is recommended if travel is for less than 3 months. For lengthy stays, 0.06 mL/kg IM should be given every 3 to 5 months.[2] Dosing is the same for adults and children. The concentrations of anti-HAV achieved after administration of Ig (or after active vaccination) are 10 to 100 times lower than those achieved after natural infection and are often below the limits of detection for commercial assays.[2]

The availability of an effective hepatitis A vaccine has reduced the use of Ig in travelers. However, Ig is less expensive than vaccination, and remains an alternative for the traveler who does not need long-term protection. If the interval between the first dose of the hepatitis A vaccine and travel is less than 2 weeks, administration of Ig should be considered to provide passive immunity during the interval before active vaccine-induced immunity develops. In this situation, the lower dose of Ig is used. The postexposure prophylactic benefit from Ig is greatest early in the incubation period and is of no benefit more than 2 weeks after exposure.[2] In most situations, serologic screening of contacts for anti-HAV is not recommended before Ig administration because screening is costly and delays prophylaxis. A single Ig dose of 0.02 mL/kg IM is used for postexposure prophylaxis. Again, the dose is the same for adults and children. People who have been given one dose of hepatitis A vaccine at least 1 month before exposure do not need Ig.

Ig should be given to previously unvaccinated people who have had (a) close personal contact with a person who has hepatitis A; (b) all staff and attendees of day care centers when hepatitis A is documented; (c) common-source exposures (other food handlers at locations where a food handler has hepatitis A; patrons, if the infected food handler handled food and had diarrhea or poor hygienic practices); (d) classroom contacts of an index case patient; and (e) schools, hospitals, and work settings at which close contact occurs with index patients.[2]

Serious adverse events with Ig are rare. Anaphylaxis has been reported in individuals with IgA deficiency who have received repeated doses of Ig.[2]

Hepatitis A vaccine can be given concomitantly with Ig; however, the antibody titer obtained is lower (but still protective) than when the vaccine is given alone. Ig can interfere with the response to measles, mumps, rubella (MMR), and varicella vaccines.[2] Administration of MMR vaccine should be delayed for at least 3 months after administration of Ig (5 months for varicella vaccine).[2] Conversely, Ig should not be administered within 2 weeks after the administration of MMR (3 weeks for varicella vaccine), unless the benefits of Ig clearly outweigh the benefits of vaccination. If Ig is administered within 2 weeks after administration of MMR (3 weeks for varicella vaccine), the person should be revaccinated—but no sooner than 3 months (5 months for varicella) after Ig.[2]

Vaccines to Prevent Hepatitis A

Inactivated HAV vaccines, Havrix (SmithKline Beecham) and Vaqta (Merck) both demonstrate protective efficacy in 94% to 100% of vaccinees within 1 month after primary vaccination.[12,13] When a booster dose is given 6 or more months later, essentially 100% of recipients develop high antibody levels. Both vaccines are indicated for immunization of individuals 2 years of age or older. Groups recommended for preexposure protection against HAV with hepatitis A vaccine are shown in Table 40–2. Hepatitis A vaccine is useful in preventing secondary infection in household contacts of primary cases of HAV infection.[14] However, no recommendations exist for use of hepatitis A vaccine for postexposure protection.

The two vaccine products have different formulations and the dosing differs according to the person's age. Table 40–3 lists the approved dosing for these vaccines. The primary vaccination is a single dose, with a booster dose 6 to 12 months later for children and adults. Both vaccines are injected intramuscularly into the deltoid muscle. The primary immunization should be given at least 2 weeks (preferably 4 weeks) prior to expected exposure to HAV. The vaccine can be given at the same time as many other vaccines (diphtheria, tetanus, live or inactivated polio, oral and injectable typhoid, cholera, Japanese encephalitis, rabies, yellow fever, and hepatitis B) without interfering with the immune responses. If one dose is given with one brand and the other dose given with the other brand, protective antibody levels do not differ;[2] the two brands are interchangeable. As with other inactivated vaccines, hepatitis A vaccine can be administered to immunocompromised persons.

To date, the vaccines are known to have protective levels of anti-HAV for at least 5 to 8 years.[2,14] Based on kinetic models of antibody decline, protective anti-HAV levels should be present for 20 years to life.[2] The vaccine is safe. Side effects include local reactions at the injection site (soreness, induration, redness, and swelling) and headache.[2] Finally, the recent development of a multivalent combination vaccine against both HAV and HBV (Twinrix) provides a more rapid method of vaccinating individuals at risk for both diseases. The

TABLE 40–2. Groups at Increased Risk of Hepatitis A and Recommended for Preexposure Hepatitis A Vaccination

Children living in states, counties, or communities where rates of hepatitis A are at least twice the national average (≥20 cases per 100,000 population). For 1987–1997, these states included Arizona, Alaska, Oregon, New Mexico, Utah, Washington, Oklahoma, South Dakota, Idaho, Nevada, and California.

Children living in states, counties, or communities where rates of hepatitis A are greater than the national average but lower than twice the national average should be considered for routine vaccination (≥10 cases but <20 cases per 100,000 population). For 1987–1997, these states included Missouri, Texas, Colorado, Arkansas, Montana, and Wyoming.

Persons traveling to or working in countries that have high or intermediate endemicity of infection.[a]

Men who have sex with men.

Illegal-drug users.

Persons who have occupational risk for infection (e.g., persons who work with HAV-infected primates or HAV in a research laboratory setting).

Persons who have clotting-factor disorders.

Persons who have chronic liver disease (e.g., persons with chronic liver disease caused by hepatitis B or C and persons awaiting liver transplants).

[a]Travelers to Canada, Western Europe, Japan, Australia, or New Zealand are at no greater risk for HAV infection than they are while in the United States. All other travelers should be assessed for hepatitis A risk.
From Centers for Disease Control.[2]

vaccine can be administered on days 0, 7, and 21 to provide 99% and 82% immunity against HAV and HBV within 1 month, respectively. Immunity rises to 100% for both HAV and HBV within 13 months of the end of the vaccination regimen.[15]

ECONOMIC CONSIDERATIONS IN PREVENTION OF HEPATITIS A

Vaccination against HAV without prior screening is only cost-saving for groups of young adults who are exposed to a relatively high risk of HAV infection; for example, in communities with high rates of HAV.[2,16,17] Prior screening for HAV antibodies can only be recommended from a cost-effectiveness point of view at expected levels of natural immunity exceeding 35% (moderately endemic countries or in older travelers).[13,14] Passive immunization remains the most cost-effective option for occasional short-duration travel to highly

TABLE 40–3. Recommended Dosing of Havrix and Vaqta

Vaccine	Vaccinee's Age (years)	Dose	Volume (mL)	Number Doses	Schedule (months)[b]
Havrix	2 to 18	720 ELISA units[a]	0.5	2	0, 6–12
	>18	1440 ELISA units	1	2	0, 6–12
Vaqta	2 to 17	25 Units	0.5	2	0, 6–18
	>17	50 Units	1	2	0, 6

[a]Havrix previously was also available as 360 ELISA units per dose. This formulation was administered as a three-dose schedule for persons 2 to 18 years of age. It is no longer available.
[b]0 months represents the timing of the initial dose; subsequent numbers represent months after the initial dose.
From Centers for Disease Control.[2]

endemic areas. Vaccination is cost effective for individuals who are likely to spend several or prolonged periods in highly endemic countries. On average, vaccination of the U.S. general public is unlikely to be cost-saving, as the cost per infection prevented can be several thousands of dollars.[16,17] In contrast, vaccination programs targeted to patients at risk for developing hepatitis may be cost effective. For example, substitution of HBV vaccination programs in sexually transmitted disease clinics serving a million patients with a combined HAV/HBV vaccine was anticipated to prevent 2263 occult HAV infections and cost $13,397 per quality-adjusted life year (QALY) gained.[18] Similarly, targeted vaccination of patients with chronic HCV with HAV vaccination has been deemed cost-effective.[19]

HEPATITIS B VIRUS

Worldwide, over 400 million people are infected with some form of chronic HBV. HBV is a leading cause of chronic hepatitis, cirrhosis, and hepatocellular carcinoma. The economic consequences of infection with HBV are staggering. Primary prevention through universal vaccination of neonates and adolescents is likely to have the largest impact on curtailing this disease.[20]

EPIDEMIOLOGY

HBV infection is a worldwide public health problem. The prevalence of HBV infection varies in different geographic areas of the world, with carrier rates ranging from 0.1% to 15%.[20] A review of National Health and Nutrition Examination Survey (NHANES) II (1976–1980) and NHANES III (1988–1994) reported a 5.5% prevalence of HBV infection in the United States.[21] Black participants had the highest prevalence (12.8%) compared to whites and Hispanics (3% to 5%).[21] In highly endemic areas (China, Southeast Asia, the Middle East, and parts of Africa and South America), HBV spread is predominantly by mother-to-infant perinatal transmission and by child-to-child transmission. In highly endemic areas high rates of chronic viral carriage and virus-associated primary hepatocellular carcinoma are seen. In parts of the world in which the endemicity of HBV is relatively low (North America, Australia, Western Europe, and temperate South America), the chronic viral carriage rate is correspondingly low, mother-to-infant transmission is relatively uncommon, and HBV transmission occurs either through intimate contact or parenterally. High-risk groups in low endemic areas include intravenous drug abusers, multitransfused patients, health care providers, male homosexuals, heterosexual partners of HBV-infected people, and heterosexual partners of human immunodeficiency virus (HIV)–infected individuals.[20] Transmission of HBV in the United States occurs predominantly through contact with infected blood products or body secretions (e.g., saliva, vaginal fluids, and semen). The routine practice of screening blood donors for hepatitis B surface antigen (HBsAg) has essentially eliminated HBV as a cause of posttransfusion hepatitis. However, products or concentrates of blood such as clotting factors can remain infective despite prescreening for HBsAg. Excluding cases resulting from clotting factor concentrates, most blood-borne HBV transmissions are a consequence of accidental inoculation by health care workers or the sharing of needles by intravenous drug abusers (percutaneous exposure).[20] The chief obstacles to eradication of HBV include the carrier state and infections in utero, neither of which is preventable. Individuals who acquire HBV as children (postnatally) have a very high rate of becoming chronic HBsAg carriers.[32] A small percentage of these children develop complications such as cirrhosis or hepatocellular carcinoma within

20 years of being infected.[22] Unfortunately, for infants who acquire HBV in utero, progression to chronic liver disease occurs in about 90% of cases. Immunization of neonates and adolescents is now the current standard of care in the United States; however, only half of the world's countries have such a policy in place.[23]

ETIOLOGY

HBV is the smallest known deoxyribonucleic acid (DNA) virus, with roughly 3200 base pairs in its genome.[24] It is an enveloped, double-stranded DNA virus belonging to the Hepadnaviridae family. This family of viruses replicates in the liver and cause hepatic dysfunction cycles that ultimately lead to chronic hepatitis, cirrhosis, and hepatocellular carcinoma. A small spherical and tubular particle known as HBsAg can be found circulating in the bloodstream of infected patients. The viral core contains a single molecule of partially double-stranded DNA referred to as the *HBV core antigen* (HBcAg). A DNA polymerase viral peptide is also found in the core and is referred to as the *HBV e antigen* (HBeAg).[24] Clearance of HBV is highly dependent on expression of HBeAg, which when expressed on the hepatocellular surface induces a potent immunologic response. A lack of HBeAg expression in certain precore mutants results in more aggressive hepatic disease which is resistant to interferon-α (IFN-α) therapy and a higher probability of graft failure after liver transplantation.[25] In addition, HBV has been classified into seven genotypes (A through G) with geographic variance in distribution of these genotypes; specifically, genotype A, which is predominantly found in North America, compared to genotypes B and C, which are found in Southeast Asia. HBV genotype C has been associated with more active necroinflammation in the liver compared to genotype B. The role of other HBV genotypes on the natural history of HBV is not well characterized.[26]

PATHOPHYSIOLOGY

HBV is not directly cytopathic; instead liver injury is immune related, and T lymphocytes are important for both the host cellular and humoral responses.[27] Recovery from acute HBV infection depends on both B-cell and T-cell responses. B-cell–dependent antibodies are produced to presurface and surface antigens. Cytotoxic T lymphocyte response is mounted against multiple epitopes in the HBV envelope, nucleocapsid, and polymerase regions.[27] Cytotoxic T lymphocyte–mediated lysis of infected hepatic cells occurs, resulting in liver injury. Immune clearance of virus is often accompanied by worsening liver disease, known as a flare. An extreme example of this is seen in fulminant hepatitis B, when there is often no evidence

of HBV replication when the patient presents—the virus has been rapidly and aggressively cleared by the infected individual's immune system. Immune-mediated viral clearance can also occur through non-cytolytic pathways via cytokine release.[27] In contrast, development of chronic HBV is hypothesized to be a function of poor cytotoxic T-lymphocyte response to viral antigens.

HBV is not considered a cytopathic virus; in certain circumstances, however, it can cause direct cytotoxic liver injury. Direct cytopathic liver injury can occur when the viral load is very high, as in the rare fibrosing cholestatic hepatitis.[27] After the HBV enters the vascular compartment, it migrates to the liver, where primary replication occurs. The incubation period of HBV is 1 to 6 months—much longer than HAV.[27] HBV replication occurs in liver cell nuclei, with HBsAg produced in the cell cytoplasm and expressed on the cell surface. These particles are also found circulating in the plasma of patients with acute HBV, the chronic carrier state, and chronic HBV infection.[27]

In acute HBV infection, serologic markers proceed in sequence from the development of HBsAg followed by HBeAg (30 to 60 days prior to onset of clinical symptoms) through to the appearance of anti-HBs in late convalescence (Table 40–4).[20] Antibody to HBsAg (anti-HBs) is initially detected as the concentration of HBsAg in plasma wanes (but is probably present much earlier than detected by standard serologic assays). The presence of anti-HBs without HBsAg indicates protective immunity (see Table 40–4).[20] Other antigen markers of HBV infection include pre-Surface1 and pre-Surface2 for the envelope, and the functional X protein. These markers are not routinely used clinically. Anti-HBc, the antibody directed against HbcAg, is first detected shortly after the onset of acute cellular injury (see Table 40–4). Anti-HBc is initially of the IgM class and signifies acute HBV infection. IgG-class anti-HBc antibodies become detectable several months following the acute HBV infection and persist along with HBs antibody for life. Anti-HBc is detectable in essentially all patients who have been exposed to HBV.[20] The presence of plasma anti-HBc IgG antibodies signifies prior infection, but it is not protective (see Table 40–4).[20,28]

HBeAg is a protein subunit of the viral core detected in plasma immediately prior to or at the onset of hepatocyte injury and correlates with a high degree of infectivity. In contrast, the presence of antigen against HBe (anti-HBe) correlates with a very low degree of infectivity and portends complete recovery. Anti-HBe becomes detectable either immediately after the peak of liver injury or in early convalescence, and can persist for years. HBV may also play an indirect role in the malignant transformation of hepatocytes through mechanisms related to expression of viral surface markers with oncogenic potential or through integration of viral DNA into the cell.[28]

TABLE 40–4. Interpretation of the Laboratory Profile in Hepatitis B Virus (HBV) Infection

Pattern	Is Patient Infectious?	HBsAg	HBeAg	Anti-HBc Total	Anti-HBs	Anti-HBe
Not infected/early incubation	No	−	−	−	−	−
Early acute HBV infection	Yes	+	−	−	−	−
Acute HBV infection	Yes	+	+	+	−	−
Chronic HBV infection[a]	Yes	+	+/−	+	−	−
Resolved infection	No	−	−	+	+	+
"Window" period following acute HBV infection	No	−	−	+	−	+

[a]Patient should be evaluated for complications of chronic infection such as cirrhosis and hepatocellular carcinoma.
anti-HBc, antibody to HbcAg; anti-Hbe, antibody to HbeAg; anti-HBs, antibody to HbsAg; HBcAg, hepatitis B core antigen; HbeAg, hepatitis B e antigen; HBsAg: hepatitis B surface antigen.
From Lee.[10]

CLINICAL PRESENTATION

ACUTE HEPATITIS B

The clinical course of HBV infection and the associated clinical features cannot be differentiated from other types of viral hepatitis based on symptoms. The duration of incubation is highly dependent on age and can vary between 6 and 24 weeks. Infants do not develop any symptoms and children between the ages of 1 and 5 years are asymptomatic in 85% to 95% of the cases.[29] Symptomatic infections vary in severity and include fever, anorexia, nausea, vomiting, jaundice, dark urine, clay-colored or pale stools, and abdominal pain. Extrahepatic manifestations of HBV infection rarely occur and may include skin rash, arthralgias, and arthritis. Hepatic failure occurs rarely, with a case fatality rate of 0.4%.[30]

Acute HBV infection is diagnosed by the presence of anti-HBc IgM (see Table 40–4). There are periods during the course of acute HBV infection when specific serologic markers are absent; the lack of such markers complicates diagnosis. These "window" periods can be seen in the early incubation phase when HBsAg and HBeAg are not detectable despite the presence of ongoing viral replication, and early in convalescence when these two antigens are cleared prior to the appearance of anti-HBs antibody. Markers of HBV replication (HBV DNA and DNA polymerase) are sensitive indicators, and are occasionally obtained when a patient is suspected to be in the serologic window period. Low levels of HBV DNA can be detected in peripheral mononuclear cells and livers of patients several years after recovery from acute HBV. These data indicate that HBV is not eradicated in these patients and can be reactivated when their immune systems are suppressed.[29]

CHRONIC HEPATITIS B

The presence of HBsAg in serum for at least 6 months or the presence of HBsAg and the absence of anti-HBc IgM meets the definition of chronic HBV infection. In addition, the presence of HBV DNA greater than 10^5 copies/mL and persistent or intermittent elevation in AST/ALT levels meet the diagnostic criteria for HBV.[30] Risks associated with development of chronic HBV include the presence of renal failure, diabetes, or HIV.[31] The probability of developing chronic HBV is inversely proportional to age; infants have a 90% risk while adolescents and adults have ~10% risk. Patients who develop chronic HBV are subsequently predisposed to developing chronic liver disease, cirrhosis, and hepatocellular carcinoma (HCC). The clinical presentation of chronic HBV is summarized in Table 40–5. Progression from chronic HBV to HCC is also age dependent, with prospective studies indicating a 25% risk in patients who acquire the disease as infants, compared to a 15% risk if contracted as

an adolescent.[29] In addition, very high HBV DNA levels, normal ALT, and the presence of HBeAg characterize chronic HBV acquired through perinatal transmission. This immune-tolerant phase can last for 10 to 30 years, allowing for individuals with perinatal acquisition to be infectious in their adulthood and perpetuate vertical transmission of the disease. In contrast, children and adults who acquire chronic HBV infection present in the immune-clearance phase, which is marked by clearance of HBeAg, in 70% of cases within 10 years. Most patients who seroconvert remain HBeAg-negative and anti-HBe–positive with normal ALT and low HBV DNA, and are considered to be in an "inactive carrier state."[29]

Liver biopsies performed in patients with chronic HBV infection are classified as chronic persistent hepatitis, chronic active hepatitis, and cirrhosis.[33] Histologic results do not correlate with symptoms and often patients are asymptomatic until the development of cirrhosis.[34] Cirrhosis is manifested by interlacing strands of fibrous tissue with nodules of regenerating cells resulting in a characteristic small and knobby-appearing liver. This form of injury is irreversible and can be exacerbated by heavy alcohol consumption and concomitant infection with HCV or HIV.[35] Hepatic decompensation as a result of cirrhosis includes ascites, jaundice, variceal bleeding, and hepatic encephalopathy. The 5-year risk of decompensation after the development of cirrhosis is estimated to be 20%.[26]

TABLE 40–5. Clinical Presentation of Chronic Hepatitis B[a]

Signs and symptoms
- Easy fatigability, anxiety, anorexia, and malaise
- Ascites, jaundice, variceal bleeding, and hepatic encephalopathy can manifest with liver decompensation
- Hepatic encephalopathy is associated with hyperexcitability, impaired mentation, confusion, obtundation, and eventually coma
- Vomiting and seizures

Physical examination
- Icteric sclera, skin, and secretions
- Decreased bowel sounds, increased abdominal girth, and detectable fluid wave
- Asterixis
- Spider angiomata

Laboratory tests
- Presence of hepatitis B surface antigen for at least 6 months
- Intermittent elevations of hepatic transaminase (alanine transaminase [ALT] and aspartate transaminase [AST]) and hepatitis B virus DNA greater than 10^5 copies/mL
- Liver biopsies for pathologic classification as chronic persistent hepatitis, chronic active hepatitis, or cirrhosis

[a]Chronic hepatitis B can be present even without all the signs, symptoms, and physical examination findings listed being apparent.

▶ TREATMENT: Hepatitis B Virus Infection

▨ DESIRED OUTCOME

No specific therapy is available for the management of acute HBV infection. Development of fulminant hepatitis secondary to acute HBV is rare and is managed with supportive care (see section on fulminant hepatitis). The long-term complications of chronic HBV include development of cirrhosis, liver failure, and HCC. The key goal of therapy for chronic HBV is to eradicate or permanently suppress HBV. The short-term objective is to limit hepatic inflammation and to reduce

the risk of fibrosis and/or decompensation. The longitudinal goal is to prevent transaminase flares and the development of long-term complications, as well as to prolong survival. Loss of HBeAg, either spontaneously or with pharmacologic therapy, is independently associated with improved survival in patients with chronic HBV. Thus HBeAg loss and development of anti-HBeAg is a critical outcome measure in patients with chronic HBV. In addition, durability of specific pharmacologic therapy for maintenance of HBeAg seroconversion is also important. Therapeutic strategies include the use of immunomodulators such as α-interferons and nucleoside analogs. Prevention of HBV resistance to nucleoside analogs during therapy is vital for adequate management of these patients.

GENERAL APPROACH TO TREATMENT

Acquisition of HBV within the first 5 years of life is associated with a higher risk for development of cirrhosis.[26] Consequently, early treatment of infants and children should be attempted, given that clearance of HBsAg rarely occurs spontaneously in this group. Spontaneous clearance of HBeAg occurs at a rate of approximately 10% per year in older groups.[36] Individuals with long-standing disease with hepatic inflammation are likely to be poor responders to therapy and require the most intensive management.

Numerous pharmacologic agents with varying modes of action are in clinical development. Three agents are currently approved for use in the United States by the Food and Drug Administration and include interferon-α2b (IFN-α2b), lamivudine, and adefovir dipivoxil.[37] No drug therapy is recommended for patients with normal ALT values because this group responds poorly to therapy. Instead quarterly to biannual follow-up of these patients for HCC surveillance and ALT assessment should be considered. Patients with persistent ALT levels greater than twice the upper limit of normal should be considered for treatment. Patients with rising ALT levels, specifically rising to greater than five times the upper limit of normal, are considered to be having an exacerbation. Lamivudine therapy should be used for exacerbations because it has a rapid onset of effect. In contrast, IFN-α2b onset of action may not be rapid enough to prevent hepatic decompensation.[38]

Therapeutic choice between lamivudine and interferon is more controversial for patients who are HBeAg-positive with ALT levels two to five times the upper limit of normal. Notably, the relative risk of relapse after HBeAg seroconversion with lamivudine therapy is about four times higher than with an α-interferon–containing regimen.[39] The decision to treat individuals is ultimately a function of disease severity, history of flares, hepatic function, drug cost, side-effect profile, and patient choice. The long-term effects of IFN-α2b are better known than those of lamivudine. In addition, extending the duration of lamivudine therapy with the intent to improve response risks development of resistant HBV mutations. The availability of adefovir dipivoxil is promising as rescue therapy after lamivudine because it is active against both wild-type and select mutants of HBV. However, well-controlled comparative trails of lamivudine to adefovir dipivoxil are not available. The role of combination therapy has yielded conflicting results and requires further evaluation.[38,40]

NONPHARMACOLOGIC THERAPY

About 75% of the 400 million people with chronic HBV live in Asia. Herbal medication use is a common therapeutic modality in many parts of the world and has been studied extensively in China. A meta-analysis of over 500 papers, including randomized controlled trials, concluded that existing studies were of poor quality, limiting the definitive interpretation of results.[41] However, the meta-analysis did identify that bufotoxin and kurorinone were associated with increased seroconversion of HBeAg and clearance of HBV DNA. Further evaluation of these active components as a possible therapeutic alternative is warranted, but they are not currently being recommended for routine use.

PHARMACOLOGIC THERAPY

Patients considered for treatment are those who are HBsAg-positive for greater than 6 months with persistent elevations in serum aminotransferases, detectable markers of viral replication (HBeAg and HBV DNA) in serum, and signs of chronic hepatitis on liver biopsy. Although symptomatic patients are more apt to seek medical attention and to have these irregularities discovered, symptoms alone are not a basis for treatment. To be treated with IFN-α, patients should not have decompensated liver disease or any specific contraindications to the therapy being considered.

Current strategies to eradicate HBV include the use of antiviral agents that alter viral replication or immunomodulatory agents that modify the host immune response. IFN-α2b (Intron A) was approved by the FDA for use in chronic HBV in 1992. IFN-α2b monotherapy now is used only in selected subgroups of patients with HBV. Lamivudine (Epivir-HBV) was approved for use in chronic HBV in 1998, and has broader indications for use, but questions remain regarding optimal duration of use and management of resistant viruses. Adefovir dipivoxil (Hepsera) was approved for use in chronic HBV, including lamivudine-resistant HBV, in 2002. End points of therapy for HBV include disappearance of HBV DNA and elimination of HBeAg (virologic response), resolution of elevated aminotransferases (biochemical response), and improvement of liver histology.[38] HBeAg seroconversion, an even stricter marker of viral response, denotes the loss of both HBeAg and HBV DNA and the appearance of anti-HBe. Loss of HBsAg can occur even years after completion of therapy.

FIRST-LINE THERAPY

The American Association for the Study of Liver Diseases (AASLD) has published its guidelines for the management of chronic HBV.[32] In addition, the Asian Pacific Association for the Study of the Liver (APASL) has updated a consensus statement on the management of chronic HBV.[38] The choice of first-line therapy between IFN-α2b and lamivudine is dependent on the categorization of specific patient populations by HBeAg positivity and ALT level. As stated earlier, factors such as disease severity, history of flares, hepatic function, drug cost, side-effect profile, and patient choice ultimately drive drug selection.

In patients with chronic HBV who are HBeAg-positive and have intermittent or persistent elevation of ALT, either interferon or lamivudine may be used as first-line therapy. Lamivudine should be selected in patients at risk for decompensation given its rapidity of onset. A meta-analysis of 15 randomized controlled trials demonstrated that 33% of patients had loss of HBeAg with 12 to 24 weeks of therapy with IFN-α2b compared to 12% in controls.[42] Pretreatment ALT levels of greater than 100 international units per liter and low HBV DNA levels (<200 copies/mL) were predictive of improved response to interferon-α. Similarly, these parameters predict response to lamivudine therapy. Three randomized controlled trials evaluating lamivudine for a similar patient population have demonstrated a loss of HBeAg in up to 32% of patients treated for 52 weeks.[43-45] Consequently, current guidelines do not specifically favor one agent over the other due to a lack of distinct differences in efficacy. The choice of lamivudine or interferon-α is a function of assessing the limitation of each agent. IFN-α2b is advantageous because its use follows a defined course of therapy and it lacks susceptibility to resistant HBV mutants, but it is limited by its cost and side-effect profile. In addition, IFN-α2b

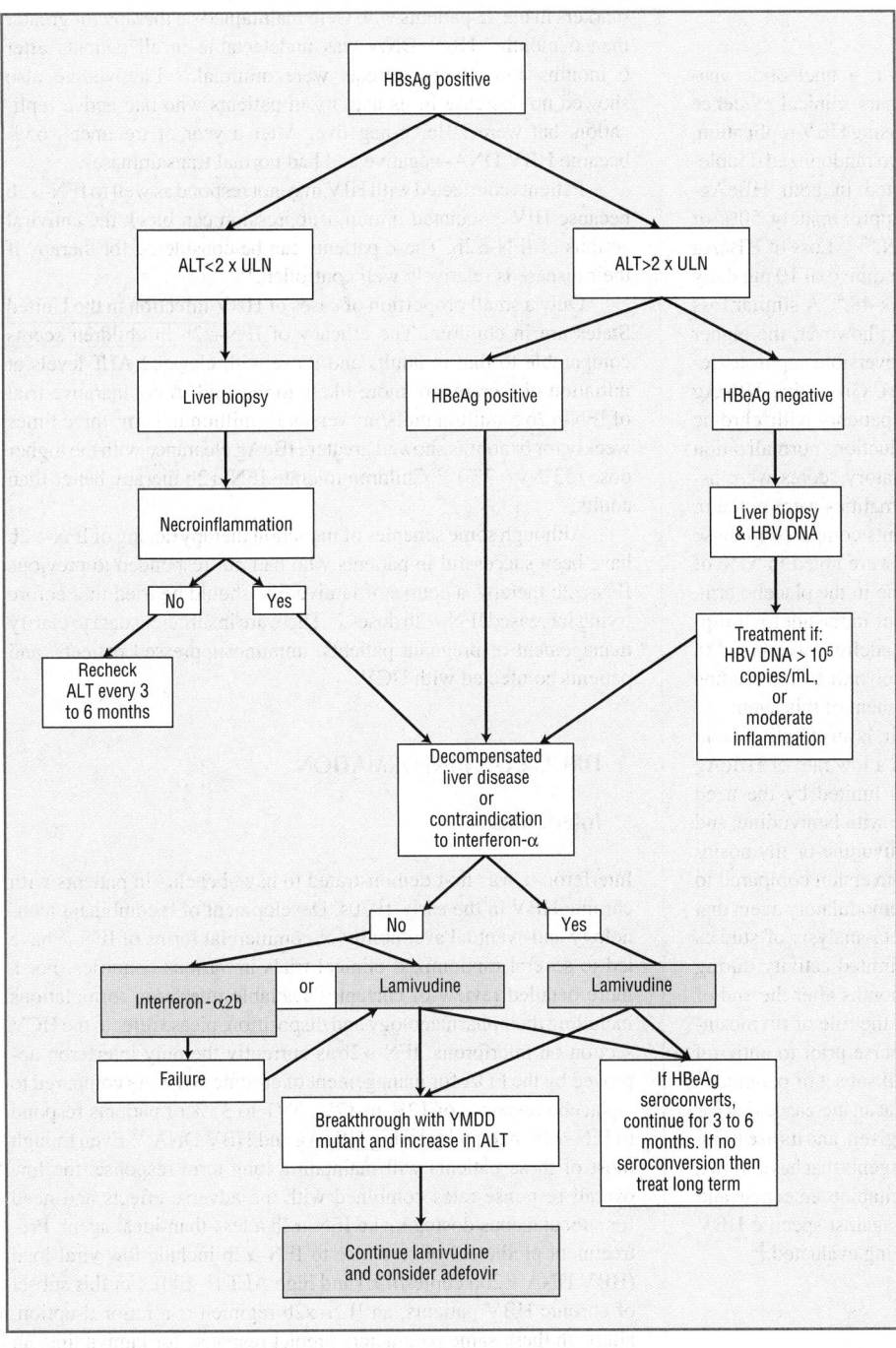

FIGURE 40–1. Treatment algorithm for the management of patients with chronic hepatitis B virus infection. ALT, alanine transaminase; HBeAg, hepatitis B e antigen; ULN, upper limit of normal.

cannot be used in patients with decompensated cirrhosis. Lamivudine is better tolerated but does not sustain a durable response and may be affected by resistant HBV mutants. Specific recommendations from the AASLD and APASL are summarized as follows and apply to both adults and children (Fig. 40–1).

1. Patients with HBeAg-positive chronic HBV:
   ALT >2 times the upper limit of normal (ULN) or moderate to severe hepatitis on biopsy: Treatment may be initiated with either lamivudine or interferon-α

   ALT >2 times ULN: Treatment with lamivudine or interferon-α should be limited to patients with significant necroinflammation on liver biopsy. Patients should have their ALT assessed every 3 to 6 months.

2. Patients with HBeAg-negative chronic HBV: Only patients with ALT >2 times ULN, HBV DNA >10^5 copies/mL, or moderate to severe hepatitis on biopsy should be considered for treatment with lamivudine or interferon-α.

3. Patients who fail to respond to a course of interferon-α and have ALT >2 times ULN, HBV DNA >10^5 copies/mL, or moderate to severe hepatitis on biopsy may be treated with a course of lamivudine.

4. Patients with decompensated cirrhosis: Interferon-α should not be used and lamivudine may be considered in these patients.

5. Patients in an inactive HBsAg carrier state: No treatment is indicated.

ALTERNATIVE DRUG TREATMENTS

Adefovir dipivoxil is the prodrug of adefovir, a nucleotide analog active against HBV. In vitro and preliminary clinical evidence demonstrate that adefovir is effective in suppressing HBV replication, including lamivudine-resistant mutants. Two randomized double-blind placebo-controlled trials were conducted in both HBeAg-positive and HBeAg-negative patients with approximately 50% of cases with ALT levels greater than 2 times ULN.[46,47] Loss of HBeAg was noted in 24% of patients receiving adefovir dipivoxil 10 mg daily compared to 11% in the placebo group at week 48.[47] A similar loss was noted with adefovir dipivoxil 30 mg daily; however, the higher dose was associated with an 8% incidence of reversible nephrotoxicity ($\geq$0.5 mg/dL increase in serum creatinine). Given that HBeAg loss cannot be assessed in HBeAg-negative patients with chronic HBV, other endpoints such as HBV DNA reduction, normalization of ALT, and changes in liver biopsy inflammatory scores were assessed. Improvement in histologic liver abnormalities were noted in twice as many adefovir dipivoxil–treated patients compared to those on placebo.[46] Undetectable HBV DNA levels were noted in 51% of patients on adefovir dipivoxil compared to none in the placebo arm. ALT normalization was also significantly higher in the adefovir dipivoxil group. No development of resistance to adefovir was noted in these trials. Comparative trials of adefovir dipivoxil to lamivudine have not been conducted to ascertain the placement of this agent.

Famciclovir, an oral prodrug of penciclovir, is an effective agent for suppression of HBV, but is associated with a low rate of HBeAg clearance compared to lamivudine. Its use is limited by the need for thrice-daily administration, cross-resistance with lamivudine, and low efficacy.[48] Combination therapy with lamivudine or thymosin-α_1 is associated with improved HBeAg seroconversion compared to famciclovir alone.[49] Thymosin-α_1 is an immunomodulatory agent that enhances the activity of T-helper$_1$ cells. A meta-analysis of studies evaluating thymosin-α_1 indicated that it has limited activity during therapy, but induces a virologic response 12 months after the end of therapy.[50] More data are necessary to evaluate the role of thymosin-α_1. Prednisone administration as a tapering course prior to antiviral therapy has been found to be beneficial in small subset of patients.[51] However, patients with underlying cirrhosis are at an increased risk for fatal exacerbations when prednisone priming is given, and its use is not recommended in these patients. Other antiviral agents that have shown promising results in clinical trials include emtricitabine, entecavir, and clevudine.[38] In addition, therapeutic vaccines against specific HBV epitopes and proinflammatory cytokines are being evaluated.[52]

SPECIAL POPULATIONS

In contrast to IFN-α2b with its significant adverse side-effect profile, almost all patients are candidates for lamivudine therapy. Patient groups in which lamivudine has shown benefit include various transplant patients, those with decompensated cirrhosis, and patients with HBV mutants with mutations in the precore region of the viral genome who present as HBeAg-negative and HBV DNA-positive.

Patients with normal aminotransferase levels should not be treated. Monitoring of this group, with treatment if disease progresses, is more advantageous than treatment, because many of these patients will not have progression of liver disease, while therapy is associated with cost and adverse event risk.

Whereas the use of IFN-α2b is discouraged in patients with decompensated cirrhosis, an open trial of 35 such patients with lamivudine demonstrated significant benefit in laboratory and clinical markers in the 23 patients who were maintained on therapy for greater than 6 months. HBV DNA was undetectable in all patients after 6 months and adverse effects were minimal.[53] Lamivudine also showed no decrease in its activity in patients who had active replication, but were HBeAg-negative. After a year of treatment, 65% became HBV DNA–negative and had normal transaminases.

Patients coinfected with HIV may not respond as well to IFN-α2b because HIV-associated immunosuppression can block the antiviral actions of IFN-α2b. These patients can be considered for therapy if their disease is relatively well controlled.[54]

Only a small proportion of cases of HBV infection in the United States are in children. The efficacy of IFN-α2b in children seems comparable to that in adults and those with elevated ALT levels at initiation of therapy are more likely to respond. A comparative trial of IFN-α2b 5 million units/m^2 versus 10 million inits/m^2 three times weekly for 6 months showed greater HBeAg clearance with the higher dose (53% vs. 7%).[55] Children tolerate IFN-α2b therapy better than adults.

Although some schemes of induction therapy dosing of IFN-α2b have been successful in patients who had not responded to previous IFN-α2b therapy, a course of lamivudine should be tried first before trying increased IFN-α2b doses.[56] There are insufficient data to clarify management of pregnant patients, immunosuppressed patients, and patients coinfected with HCV.

DRUG CLASS INFORMATION

Interferons

Interferon-α was first demonstrated to have benefits in patients with chronic HBV in the early 1970s. Development of recombinant technology and eventual availability of commercial forms of IFN-α have led to several randomized clinical trials in various countries. For a more detailed review of currently available interferon formulations including their pharmacology and disposition, please refer to the HCV section on interferons. IFN-α2b is currently the only interferon approved by the FDA for management of chronic HBV. As compared to a placebo response of 12% to 17%, 33% to 37% of patients respond to IFN-α2b therapy by losing HBeAg and HBV DNA.[42] Even though most of these patients will maintain a long-term response, the low overall response rates combined with the adverse effects and need for subcutaneous dosing make IFN-α2b a less-than-ideal agent. Pretreatment predictors of response to IFN-α2b include low viral load (HBV DNA <200 copies/mL) and high ALT (>100). For this subset of chronic HBV patients, an IFN-α2b regimen is a rational option, although these same parameters predict response for lamivudine, an alternative agent.

Resolution of HBV viremia with IFN-α2b is associated with a transient exacerbation of the hepatitis, marked by a rise in serum ALT levels during the second or third month of therapy. Although IFN-α2b may have direct antiviral effects, this flare is related to immunomodulatory effects resulting in an increased host response (Fig. 40–2). In patients who respond to interferon, HBV DNA levels decrease within days of starting therapy. After 8 to 12 weeks, ALT levels increase, and the patient loses HBV DNA and HBeAg. ALT levels then normalize, and the patient develops anti-HBe.[29] Without the flare, loss of viral replication rarely occurs. Patients infected with precore HBV mutants that prevent HBeAg expression (HBeAg-negative and HBV DNA–positive) are less likely to respond to IFN-α therapy and have a higher rate of relapse upon discontinuation.[37] About 10% of the responders to IFN-α therapy also clear HBsAg in the first year, and although

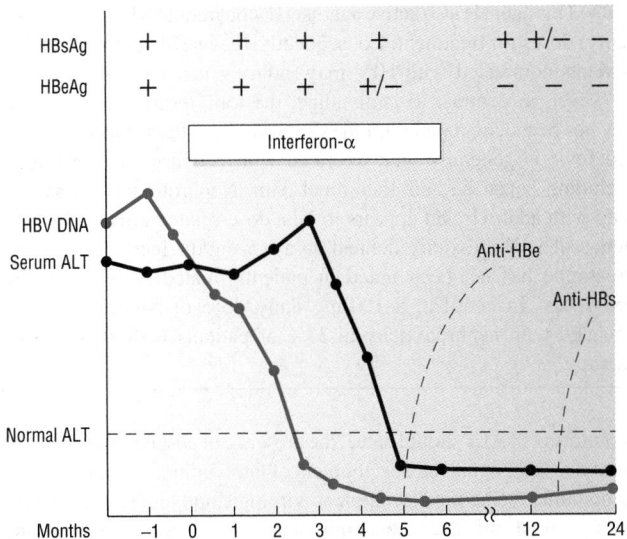

| HBsAg | + | | + | + | + | | + | +/− | − |
| HBeAg | + | | + | + | +/− | | − | − | − |

Interferon-α

HBV DNA
Serum ALT

Anti-HBe

Anti-HBs

Normal ALT

Months   −1   0   1   2   3   4   5   6   12   24

FIGURE 40–2. Typical sustained response to IFN-γ in a patient with chronic hepatitis B. ALT, alanine transaminase; Anti-HBe, antibody to hepatitis B e antigen; Anti-HBs, antibody to hepatitis B surface antigen; HBeAg, hepatitis B e antigen; HBsAg, hepatitis B surface antigen.

biochemical and histologic responses also occur, they are more frequent in the group responding virologically. Long-term follow-up of patients treated with IFN-α has shown that response is sustained in about 90% of patients at least 5 years after therapy, and that a distinct survival benefit is present in those who have a virologic response.

IFN-α2b should be administered by subcutaneous injection as 5 million units daily or 10 million units thrice weekly in adults. In children, thrice-weekly subcutaneous injections of 6 million units/m² to a maximum of 10 million units per dose is recommended. Patients with HBV who are HBeAg-positive should be treated for 16 weeks, while HBeAg-negative patients should be treated for 12 months.[26] Administration of interferon is associated with significant side effects, which diminish with continued treatment. Flu-like symptoms such as fevers, chills, and myalgias should be expected during the first month of therapy, typically several hours after administration. Consequently administration of IFN-α2b at bedtime along with a nonsteroidal anti-inflammatory agent improves tolerability. Pegylated formulations of interferon (see discussion in HCV section) are likely to be more tolerable but have not been studied sufficiently in patients with HBV. Additional adverse events associated with long-term IFN-α therapy include cytopenia, alopecia, thyroid dysfunction, and depression. Depression is a very common complication of IFN-α therapy, especially during the last third to fourth month of therapy. A high index for suspicion for the mental well being of patients should be maintained, as suicides have been linked to IFN-α therapy.[57]

Lamivudine

Lamivudine (Epivir-HBV, 3TC) is a nucleoside analog that competitively inhibits viral reverse transcriptase and terminates proviral DNA chain extension. Because it does not affect host response, it suppresses viral replication but does not directly eliminate the virus from the hepatocytes. Its efficacy is also not associated with, or dependent upon, the flare response seen with interferon. Like IFN-α2b though, lamivudine demonstrates higher response rates in patients with elevated transaminases (ALT >100) and lower viral loads.[58]

Two double-blind randomized controlled trials in adults compared lamivudine 100 mg by mouth daily for 52 weeks versus placebo in previously untreated patients.[43,44] The results are comparable except that one trial in Asia had a higher biochemical response in both treatment and placebo groups.[44] Both trials demonstrated significant histologic, virologic, and biochemical responses with lamivudine. Lamivudine also prevented histologic worsening or the development of hepatic fibrosis. The results of the Asian trial are especially impressive because it was previously thought that this was a difficult population to treat because of acquisition of disease at an early age.[44] Long-term outcomes are not proven, but the results of these trials are encouraging. Of note, the 32% rate of HBeAg loss in the American trial is similar to the response demonstrated with IFN-α2b.

Upon discontinuation of lamivudine HBV DNA tends to rebound, but to levels less than the original baseline. Virologic responses were maintained in about 75% of lamivudine-treated patients 16 weeks posttherapy. Treatment beyond 1 year increases the rate of HBeAg loss and slows the rate and extent of HBV DNA return. However, extending the duration of therapy would be associated with a possible increase in adverse effects, increased cost, and increased development of resistance to lamivudine. But a recent pilot study evaluating a 3-year lamivudine regimen in 16 patients noted histologic improvement despite development of lamivudine-resistant mutants and virologic breakthrough.[59]

Mutations in regions of reverse transcriptase, primarily the YMDD locus, confer resistance against lamivudine. These mutations occur after about 6 months of lamivudine therapy, are usually accompanied by increases in ALT and HBV DNA, and are more common in patients with elevated baseline viral loads. In the two lamivudine trials, the incidence of these mutations was 14% and 32%, respectively, after 1 year of therapy.[43,44] It is thought that the mutant viruses are relatively less harmful because they are not able to replicate as effectively, but the mutants are replaced by wild-type virus upon treatment discontinuation. Despite the development of resistance, with continued lamivudine therapy the ALT and HBV DNA often remain below baseline levels and some patients may still convert from a HBeAg-positive state.

In the foregoing studies, one reported no association between treatment and transaminase level changes, whereas the other reported posttreatment levels greater than three times baseline in 25% of the treatment group, compared to 8% in the placebo group. A different cohort of 55 patients had much a higher mutation rate (58% after 2 years of lamivudine therapy), with 13 patients (24%) experiencing an ALT spike over 10 times the normal range, and 3 patients (5%) demonstrating hepatic decompensation during the flare.[60,61]

Lamivudine has a much less toxic adverse effect profile than IFN-α2b, with serious side effects occurring at rates similar to those of placebo.[58] The most commonly reported are fatigue, nausea and vomiting, headache, cough, and diarrhea. It is administered as a tablet or oral suspension at a dose of 100 mg orally once daily. Lamivudine is well absorbed and has renal elimination, requiring dosage adjustment if the creatinine clearance is <50 mL/min. Response to lamivudine is more rapid than that of IFN-α2b, with HBV DNA levels decreasing by 97% after 2 weeks of therapy, and it has demonstrated success in patient subgroups that typically do not respond to interferons.

In summary, lamivudine is more convenient, has fewer adverse effects, and demonstrates at least comparable virologic, histologic, and biochemical activity compared to IFN-α2b. The optimal duration of therapy with lamivudine is not known, especially considering that the correct course of action when resistance occurs is still unknown. With little comparative data, one is left to choose between a relatively short course of an injectable agent with demonstrated adverse effects but documented long-term outcomes, versus a well-tolerated oral agent with activity across a greater spectrum of patients, but whose long-term effects and optimal duration of therapy are unknown.

Adefovir Dipivoxil

Adefovir is a nucleotide analog of deoxyadenosine monophosphate that is active against retroviruses (like HIV), herpes viruses, and hepadnaviruses. Adefovir dipivoxil 10 mg by mouth once daily for 48 weeks has been approved for use in adult patients with chronic HBV who are either treatment naïve or have lamivudine-resistant

PHARMACOECONOMIC CONSIDERATIONS

Treatment of chronic HBV in patients with favorable predictors of response is cost effective, especially among younger individuals. The direct cost of management of chronic HBV with IFN-α2b would be approximately $7,500 and $25,000 for a 16-week and 12-month course, respectively.[63] In contrast the annual cost of lamivudine and adefovir would be approximately $2,000 and $6,400, respectively.[63] However, acquisition cost alone cannot be used to evaluate the expected value of using each agent. Using data from a meta-analysis of nine trials with 552 chronic HBV patients, IFN-α2b treatment would increase life expectancy by 3.1 years and decrease lifetime costs by more than $2,100.[64] A more recent comparative evaluation of the cost per additional HBeAg seroconversion was estimated to be $12,703 with lamivudine compared to $39,922 with IFN-$\alpha$2b.[65] However, this assessment included a decision tree model limited to 1 year of evaluation and so did not take into account the relapse rates post lamivudine discontinuation. Pharmacoeconomic analyses of the impact of adefovir have not been published. Given that lamivudine resistance emerges in 15% to 30% of persons treated in the first year, it is likely that future regimens may include either early combination regimens of adefovir and lamivudine, or a stepwise approach. Future pharmacoeconomic analyses must compare the cost-effectiveness of IFN-α2b to potential combination regimens of adefovir and lamivudine.

CLINICAL CONTROVERSIES

Some clinicians believe that adefovir should be used as first-line therapy or at least in combination with lamivudine to prevent development of YMDD mutants. However, others argue that adefovir should be used after the development of breakthrough YMDD mutants during lamivudine therapy.

The impact of HBeAg clearance and seroconversion on the long-term outcome of patients is not clearly defined. Some clinicians would argue that the true impact of therapy may be limited given that hepatocellular carcinoma may develop in patients even after many years of serologic recovery.

EVALUATION OF THERAPEUTIC OUTCOMES

HBeAg, HBsAg, and HBV DNA should all be measured at the start of therapy, at the end of therapy, and 6 months thereafter. Aminotransferases are measured at monthly intervals in conjunction with clinical monitoring for possible decompensation (development of ascites, encephalopathy, and esophageal varices). The monthly

HBV. This agent is also active against HIV but requires higher (125 mg daily) doses for treatment. Consequently, the use of adefovir in HBV patients coinfected with HIV may induce antiretroviral resistance. However, in contrast to lamivudine, the long-term use of adefovir has not been associated with the development of resistance in HBV. Adefovir is generally well tolerated with primary adverse effects including headache and abdominal pain. Nephrotoxicity is associated with adefovir and appears to be a dose-related effect. The incidence of nephrotoxicity defined as a 0.5-mg/dL increase in serum creatinine has not been noted in patients treated with 10 mg for 48 weeks. In contrast, a 120-mg daily dose of adefovir was associated with nephrotoxicity in 35% of patients with 48 weeks of therapy.[62]

monitoring of ALT should detect the presence or absence of a flare, and may also help signal the development of lamivudine resistance. When lamivudine therapy is discontinued virologic and biochemical monitoring should still occur at 6 months posttherapy.[58] Similar monitoring parameters apply with the use of adefovir, with the added provision of routine renal function assessment.[62]

Baseline and ongoing monitoring of IFN-α toxicity includes complete blood counts with platelets weekly during the first 2 weeks of therapy and monthly thereafter. Thyroid tests should be checked at baseline and every 3 to 6 months during treatment. Patients should be asked about their level of performance, mood changes, ability to concentrate, and symptoms.[57]

PREVENTION OF HEPATITIS B

GENERAL APPROACH TO PREVENTION

The two types of products available for prevention of hepatitis B infection include hepatitis B vaccine (provides long-lasting active immunity) and hepatitis B immunoglobulin (HBIg; provides temporary passive immunity).[66] The vaccine is used in preexposure prophylaxis. It is also used in postexposure prophylaxis in combination with HBIg. Vaccination is the most effective method for preventing hepatitis B (Tables 40–6, 40–7, 40–8, and 40–9).[66,67]

HBIg and Ig to Prevent Hepatitis B

HBIg is used only in postexposure prophylaxis. Postexposure prophylaxis for HBV is recommended for perinatal exposure, sexual exposure to HBsAg-positive persons, percutaneous or permucosal exposure to HBsAg-positive blood, and exposure of an infant to a caregiver who has acute hepatitis B (see Table 40–7).[66] HBIg is given to immunocompromised patients for the same indications and in the same doses as immunocompetent individuals.[66] The recommended dose is 0.06 mL/kg administered intramuscularly. Guidelines for use are listed in Tables 40–6 and 40–7.[66]

Use of Ig for prophylaxis of HBV infection is only recommended when HBIg is not available. Ig contains anti-HBs in titers of 1:100 to 1:1000, in comparison to the 1:100,000 or greater anti-HBs titer found in HBIg. Ig and HBIg available in the United States do not transmit HBV, HIV, or other viruses.

Vaccines to Prevent Hepatitis B

The comprehensive vaccination strategy in the United States targets interruption of transmission at all age groups through routine infant immunization, continued vaccination of high-risk older adolescents and adults (e.g., HIV-infected individuals), routine screening of pregnant women for HBsAg, and vaccination of all

TABLE 40–6. Recommended Schedule of Immunoprophylaxis to Prevent Perinatal or Sexual Transmission of HBV Infection

Vaccine Recipient	Immunoprophylaxis	Timing
Infant born to HBsAg-positive mother	Vaccine dose 1	Within 12 hours of birth
	HBIg (0.5 mL intramuscularly at a site different from that used for the vaccine)	Within 12 hours of birth
	Vaccine doses 2 and 3	Usual schedule
Infant born to mother not screened for HBsAg	Vaccine dose 1[a]	Within 12 hours of birth
	HBIg (0.5 mL intramuscularly at a site different from that used for the vaccine)	If mother is found to be HBsAg-positive, administer dose to infant as soon as possible, but no later than 1 week after birth
	Vaccine doses 2 and 3[a]	Usual schedule
Sexual exposure	HBIg (0.06 mL/kg intramuscularly at a site different from that used for the vaccine)	Single dose within 14 days of sexual contact
	Vaccine dose 1	At time of HBIg treatment
	Vaccine doses 2 and 3	Usual schedule

[a]The first dose of vaccine is the same as that for the infant of an HBsAg-positive mother. If the mother is found to be HBsAg-positive, that dose is continued. If the mother is found to be HBsAg-negative, the remaining vaccine doses are those appropriate for other infants and children.

HBIg, hepatitis B immunoglobulin; HBsAg: hepatitis B surface antigen. From Centers for Disease Control and Prevention. Protection against viral hepatitis: Recommendations of the Immunization Practices Advisory Committee (ACIP). Morb Mortal Wkly Rep 1990;39:1–26; Centers for Disease Control and Prevention.

Recommendations of the Advisory Committee on Immunization Practices: Use of vaccines and immune globulins in persons with altered immunocompetence. Morb Mortal Wkly Rep 1993;42(RR-4):1–18; and Centers for Disease Control and Prevention. Hepatitis B virus: A comprehensive strategy for eliminating transmission in the United States through universal childhood vaccination. Morb Mortal Wkly Rep 1991;40(RR-13):1–25.

TABLE 40–7. Recommendations for Hepatitis B Prophylaxis Following Percutaneous or Permucosal Exposure

Vaccination Status of Exposed Person	Treatment According to HBsAg Status of Source		
	HBsAg-Positive	HBsAg-Negative	Source Not Tested or Unknown
Unvaccinated	HBIg (one dose of 0.06 mL/kg IM), plus initiate vaccine[a]	Initiative vaccine[a]	Initiate vaccine[a]
Previously vaccinated, known responder	Test exposed person for anti-HBs level	No treatment	No treatment
	If adequate,[b] no treatment		
	If inadequate or titer unknown, I vaccine booster dose		
Previously vaccinated, known nonresponder	HBIg (two doses 1 month apart) or HBIg one dose, plus dose of vaccine	No treatment	If known high-risk source, may treat as if source were HBsAg-positive
Previously vaccinated, response unknown	Test exposed person for anti-HBs level	No treatment	Test exposed for anti-HBs level
	If inadequate,[b] HBIg one dose, plus one vaccine booster dose		If inadequate,[b] vaccine booster dose
	If adequate, no treatment		If adequate, no treatment
	If titer unknown, one vaccine booster dose		

[a]Vaccine dosage is given in Table 40–8.
[b]Adequate anti-HBs is ≥ 10 milli-international units per milliliter by radioimmunoassay or enzyme immunoassay.
anti-HBs, antibody to HBsAg; HBIg, hepatitis B immunoglobulin; HBsAg, hepatitis B surface antigen.
From Centers for Disease Control and Prevention. Protection against viral hepatitis:
Recommendations of the Immunization Practices Advisory Committee (ACIP). Morb Mortal Wkly Rep 1990;391–26, Centers for Disease Control and Prevention. Recommendations of the Advisory Committee on Immunization Practices: Use of vaccines and immune globulins in persons with altered immunocompetence. Morb Mortal Wkly Rep 1993;42(RR-4);1–18, and Centers for Diseases Control and Prevention. Hepatitis B virus: A comprehensive strategy for eliminating transmission in the United States through universal childhood vaccination. Morb Mortal Wkly Rep 1991;40(RR-13):1–25.

TABLE 40–8. Recommended Doses and Schedules of Currently Licensed Hepatitis B Vaccines

Group	Vaccine		
	Recombivax HB[a] dose, mcg (mL)	Engerix-B[a,b] dose, mcg (mL)	Comvax[c] dose, mcg (mL)
Infants of HBsAg-positive mothers	5 (0.5)	10 (0.5)	Not indicated
All other infants, children and adolescents ≤19 years of age	5 (0.5)[d]	10 (0.5)	5 (0.5)[e]
Adults age 20 years and older	10 (1)	20 (1)	Not indicated
Dialysis patients and other immunocompromised persons	40 (1)[f]	40 (2)[g,h]	Not indicated

[a]Usual schedules: Infants: Three doses given at birth, at 1 to 2 months, and at 6 to 18 months of age; or, for infants, with other routine immunizations at 1 to 2 months, 4 months, and 6 to 18 months of age. Older children and adults: Three doses given at 0–, 2–, and 6-month or, at 0–, 2–, and 4-month intervals. Higher titers of HBsAg are achieved with the last two doses of vaccine being spaced at least 4 months apart.
[b]Alternative approved schedule: Four doses, one given at 0, then one each given at 1-, 2-, and 12-month intervals.
HBsAg, hepatitis B surface antigen.
[c]Contains 5 mcg 0.5 mL HBsAg and 7.5 mcg *Haemophilus influenzae* type B purified capsular polysaccharide fragments conjugated to 125 mcg *Neisseria meningitidis* outer membrane protein complex.
[d]An alternate two-dose schedule can be used for adolescents aged 11 to 15 years. If the two-dose schedule is used, the adult dose (1 mL containing 10 mcg of HBsAg) is administered with the second dose given 4 to 6 months after the first dose.
[e]Usually given at 2, 4 and 12 to 15 months of age. Comvax is not used when immunizing older children or adolescents.
[f]Special formulation for dialysis patients.
[g]Two 1-mL doses given at different sites.
[h]Four-dose schedule recommended at 0 then at 1-, 2-, 6-month intervals.

unvaccinated children ages 0 to 18 years of age (see Tables 40–8 and 40–9).[67] Several states have laws mandating hepatitis B immunization prior to entry into kindergarten or middle school.

In countries where the risk of hepatitis B is relatively low, such as the United States, determining who to vaccinate prior to exposure depends on the risk of infection in that group and the relative cost of pretesting versus the cost of vaccination. Everyone in high-risk low-prevalence groups (such as health care professionals in training) can be vaccinated without screening.[67] To comply with federal guidelines, employers offer health care workers with potential exposure to blood hepatitis B vaccination at no cost.

In addition to vaccinating health care workers against hepatitis B, other infection control practices are important in preventing transmission of the virus because up to 10% of people do not develop an adequate antibody response to the vaccine. The most important infection control measure is the use of universal precautions. These precautions prevent exposure to blood and blood-derived body fluids via use of a variety of barrier precautions, measures to prevent needlesticks, environmental control measures, and good hand-washing techniques. However, if a worker is exposed to material that potentially contains HBV, recommendations for percutaneous exposure to HBV should be followed (see Table 40–7).[66]

The two recombinant hepatitis B vaccine products available in the United States (Recombivax HB, Merck; Engerix-B, SmithKline Beecham) have comparable immune responses and safety profiles.[66] The vaccines contain 5 to 40 mcg HBsAg protein per milliliter adsorbed onto aluminum. Neither brand of hepatitis B vaccine contains thimerosal. The recent availability of a combined HAV and HBV vaccine allows for a more accelerated schedule for immunization. For a more detailed comparison of the potential vaccination schedules refer to the cited reference.[15] These vaccines are some of the safest available.[68] Side effects of the vaccine are soreness at the injection site, headache, fatigue, irritability, and fever. The number of patients experiencing adverse reactions decreases with each vaccine dose, and adverse reactions are less common in infants and children than in adults. There is no association between Guillain-Barré syndrome and the recombinant vaccine, and the vaccine does not transmit HIV. The hepatitis B vaccine is contraindicated for patients with anaphylaxis to

TABLE 40–9. Groups Recommended for Preexposure Hepatitis B Vaccination

All infants via routine infant vaccination
Unvaccinated 11- to 12-year-old children
Unvaccinated children ages <11 years of age who are Pacific Islanders of who reside in households of first-generation immigrants from countries where HBV is of high or intermediate endemicity
Health care and public safety workers who have occupational exposure to blood
HIV-infected individuals
Injection drug users
Heterosexual individuals who have had more than one sexual partner in the previous 6 months and/or those with a recent episode of a sexually transmitted disease
Sexually active homosexual or bisexual males
Hemodialysis patients
Recipients of certain blood products (i.e., patients with hemophilia and other clotting disorders)
Clients and staff of institutions for the developmentally disabled
Household, sexual, and blood exposure contacts of either HBsAg-positive persons or those with acute HBV infection
Household contacts of adoptees from countries where HBV is highly endemic
Populations where HBV is highly endemic (e.g., Alaskan Eskimos)
Inmates of long-term correctional facilities
International travelers to highly endemic HBV regions for >6 months and who have close contact with the local population; also short-term travelers who have contact with blood, or sexual contact with residents in high- or intermediate-risk areas
Unvaccinated infants under 12 months of age exposed to acute HBV infection through primary caregiver

HBsAg, hepatitis B surface antigen; HBV, hepatitis B virus; HIV, human immunodeficiency virus.
From Centers for Disease Control and Prevention. Protection against viral hepatitis: Recommendations of the Immunization Practices Advisory Committee (ACIP). Morb Mortal Wkly Rep 1990;39:1–26 and Centers for Disease Control and Prevention. 1999 USPHS/IDSA guidelines for the prevention of opportunistic infections in persons infected with human immunodeficiency virus. Morb Mortal Wkly Rep 1999;48(RR-10):1–66.

common baker's yeast. Hepatitis B vaccines are inactivated and can be simultaneously administered with other vaccines.[68] Breast-fed infants can be vaccinated with hepatitis B vaccine, as can immunocompromised infants and children.[66] The vaccine can be given to pregnant and lactating women. In the last several years, a small number of claims of serious adverse effects after hepatitis B vaccine administration have occurred. Complaints cover a spectrum of autoimmune and nervous system disorders such as rheumatoid arthritis, optic neuritis, and neurodegenerative disorders similar to multiple sclerosis. Public health officials are confident the vaccine is safe, but because claims of vaccine-induced injury are likely to continue, several epidemiologic studies are underway to evaluate association. Millions of people receive hepatitis B vaccine each year, and some will blame the vaccine for any adverse event that is temporally related to vaccine administration.[68]

HEPATITIS C VIRUS

◀**8** Chronic hepatitis as a consequence of HCV has reached epidemic proportions worldwide. The indolent course of HCV, which is primarily asymptomatic, has contributed to its transmission. ◀**9** The lack of an in vitro model and its mutability has prevented the development of a prevention strategy through vaccination. Therapeutic agents against HCV have provided limited success and have been tempered by their significant adverse event profiles.

EPIDEMIOLOGY

◀**8** HCV is found worldwide and is transmitted primarily through injecting drug use and contaminated blood products. In the United States, HCV is the most common chronic blood-borne infection—40% of chronic liver disease is related to HCV, and an estimated 8,000 to 10,000 HCV-related deaths occur per year.[69,70] NHANES completed the largest population-based household survey to date from 1988 to 1994.[71] This survey revealed that 3.9 million persons (1.8% of the general population) were infected with HCV and 2.7 million Americans from this group were estimated to have chronic disease. However, this survey did not include data from homeless and incarcerated persons known to have a higher risk for HCV infection.[72,73] Currently, persons in their third and fourth decades of life have the highest prevalence of acute HCV, while chronic HCV has the highest prevalence rates in persons in the fifth and sixth decades of life.[70,74] Given that most patients with chronic HCV have yet to be diagnosed, a fourfold increase in the number of adults diagnosed with HCV is projected between 1990 and 2015.[75]

Injecting drug use now accounts for about 60% of new HCV cases in the United States.[70] Thirty percent of people with HCV report sexual, hemodialysis, household, occupational, or perinatal exposure.[70] No recognized source of exposure can be determined for the remaining 10% of HCV infections. Other potential methods of transmitting HCV infection include contact with other instruments capable of penetrating the skin or mucous membranes, such as shared contaminated razors, intranasal cocaine ("snorting") use, tattooing, and body piercing. Snorting cocaine with heroin is associated with nasal ulceration and bleeding thought to promote transmission of HCV.[76] Perinatal transmission rates of HCV are very low (<6%), increase with increasing maternal viral load, and are higher when the mother is coinfected with HIV.[70,77] The virus is inefficiently spread by sexual contact. In studies of long-term spouses of patients with chronic HCV and no other risk factors, HCV infection prevalence is about 1.5%.[70] Transmission of HCV is higher in those with high-risk sexual practices.[70] Homosexual men do not have a higher risk for HCV acquisition even when they have a higher number of sexual partners.[78]

ETIOLOGY

HCV is a enveloped, spherical, single-stranded RNA virus that belongs to the Flaviviridae family.[79] There are six known genotypes (numbered 1 through 6) and greater than 50 subtypes (designated by letter: 1a, 1b, and so forth) of HCV.[79] Genotype 1b often results in the ◀**10** most aggressive form of liver disease, is resistant to interferon therapy, and is associated with a worse prognosis posttransplantation.[80] Frequent errors in RNA transcription coupled with mutations driven by host immunologic pressure lead to generation of extensive genetic heterogeneity. This ability of HCV to change rapidly to host pressure permits the ultimate development of chronic infection.[79,80]

PATHOPHYSIOLOGY

After HCV gains access to the host, the virus enters hepatocytes. The virus then uncoats and releases the genome to begin replication. The viral genome serves as a template for translation of the polyprotein. The processed nonstructural protein forms a complex with the genome and begins synthesis for the negative strand. The negative strand functions as the template for synthesis of the positive strand. The RNA intermediate matures and interacts with the envelope and core proteins to assemble into new virus. Most of the replicative processes are not clearly understood.[81]

In comparison to other viruses, HCV is more likely to cause clinically chronic silent infection in immunocompetent people. HCV accomplishes this despite active humoral and cellular immune responses that are generally targeted against all viral proteins. In acute HCV infection, specific T-cell receptors are activated and HCV-specific helper T cells assist with activation, differentiation, and induction of B cells, as well as stimulating virus-specific cytotoxic T cells.[81] These effects are mediated by various immunoregulatory cytokines. CD8+ cytotoxic T cells recognize HCV peptides synthesized in infected cells, with resulting lysis of the infected cells.[81] Both the strength and quality of helper T-cell and cytotoxic T-cell responses appear to differ between patients who recover and those who develop chronic HCV infection. HCV elicits only a weak T-cell response in patients who develop chronic infection.[81] Individuals who clear HCV have a stronger type 1 T-helper response that upregulates cellular immunity. The reasons for this are unclear, but are unrelated to general immune tolerance or immunosuppression.

Virus-specific antibodies interfere with viral entry into host cells and opsonize the virus for elimination by macrophages; however, they cannot eliminate the virus from infected cells. In addition, the humoral immune response can select HCV variants with sequence changes that allow escape from antibody recognition.[81] Antibodies to one genotype confer no resistance to another genotype. As a consequence of these factors, HCV is able to escape immune surveillance and establish persistent infection more readily. These characteristics of HCV also contribute to poor interferon response and make it difficult to develop a vaccine. Furthermore, the absence of an in vitro cell culture system has limited studies designed to screen newer antiviral compounds.

HCV is found in both serum and in an intracellular reservoir. Whereas the half-life of HCV in serum is only hours, HCV in the infected cell can have a half-life between 2 and 70 days.[82] HCV production can occur in infected cells at a rate of $>3.7 \times 10^{11}$ virions per day. Therefore therapy may have to be targeted to eradication of HCV-infected cells or administered for prolonged periods.

CLINICAL PRESENTATION

ACUTE HEPATITIS C

Patients with acute hepatitis C are often asymptomatic, but they may have malaise, anorexia, and jaundice, which occur in up to 25% of cases.[83] The mean incubation period of HCV is 50 days and viremia can be detected within 3 weeks of initial exposure. Hepatic transaminase values, specifically serum ALT, can be elevated within 4 to 12 weeks of exposure.[83] Acute hepatitis C can be associated with severe symptoms, but fulminant disease is rare.[83] Coinfection with HIV and a history of chronic alcohol consumption are associated with more severe disease during acute HCV infection.[84] An important feature of hepatitis C infection is that up to 70% of cases develop chronic hepatitis.[84] Of note, patients with asymptomatic acute HCV infection may be more likely to develop chronic HCV.[85]

Several diagnostic tests are available to detect acute HCV infection through detection of antibodies or viral target amplification.[86] Antibody detection methods include enzyme immunoassay (EIA) and the recombinant immunoblot assay (RIBA). Specific antibodies to HCV by EIA are positive in only 50% to 70% of patients during the initial onset of symptoms, but 90% of patients have HCV antibodies after 3 months. A number of viral antigens are included in the current version of EIA, resulting in a 99% sensitivity and specificity for detection of HCV antibodies in immunocompetent patients.[86] Patients with autoimmune disorders may have a false-positive EIA and no detectable HCV RNA, in which case the RIBA may be used as a supplemental test to rule out HCV. Viral target amplification techniques are used to detect HCV RNA either qualitatively or quantitatively. Qualitative tests are more sensitive with a detection limit of up to 100 copies/mL and should be reserved to determine spontaneous clearance of acute infection.[86] Spontaneous clearance of HCV can occur in 50% of patients within 3 months of the acute onset of symptoms.[85]

CHRONIC HEPATITIS C

Most patients with HCV remain asymptomatic until the development of progressive liver fibrosis leading to cirrhosis, end-stage liver disease, and HCC.[84] Current estimates indicate that 10% to 30% of patients with HCV infection develop cirrhosis, and 1% to 5% develop hepatocellular carcinoma.[83] If an HCV patient is symptomatic, fatigue, malaise, anorexia, and weight loss are common. Many patients have a history of jaundice. On physical examination, hepatomegaly is usually present, but the stigmata of chronic liver disease (spider nevi, splenomegaly, palmar erythema, testicular atrophy, and caput medusae) are generally absent until late in the disease course. Mild but persistent elevations of the serum aminotransferases, bilirubin, and γ-globulin levels can be seen. Physical symptoms do not correlate well with the severity of liver injury. The diagnosis of HCV is made by detecting anti-HCV via EIA, with confirmatory RIBA testing reserved for low-risk populations to exclude potential false-positive EIA results.[84]

In chronic hepatitis C, there is frequently little clinical evidence that the disease is progressing. The patient is asymptomatic, yet viral RNA remains positive, and if a liver biopsy is performed it demonstrates ongoing liver injury and progressive histologic changes. To assess chronic HCV, liver biopsy is the only reliable indicator of disease progression.[83,84] Importantly, a liver biopsy contributes information on the possible interplay between steatosis and concurrent alcoholic liver disease toward the progression of chronic hepatitis C to cirrhosis. Serum transaminases are prone to fluctuation and can even normalize, confounding the diagnosis. Unfortunately, the patient can be on an insidious course that progresses to complications after a period of years to decades. It is not uncommon for a patient to present to a physician with cirrhosis or portal hypertension secondary to HCV infection that occurred years to decades prior, yet the patient may have had few or no clinical signs or symptoms during the intervening years. HCC may present as a nonspecific right upper quadrant pain in patients with cirrhosis. Specific screening guidelines have not been validated to predict the development of HCC. Hepatic ultrasound is more sensitive for the diagnosis of HCC compared to serum α-fetoprotein concentrations.[87] Diagnostic procedures for the evaluation of HCC should be reserved for patients with cirrhosis, as the development of this disease is very rare in noncirrhotic patients.

A variety of rare extrahepatic clinical syndromes have been associated with chronic HCV infection.[88] These syndromes include cryoglobulinemia, cutaneous vasculitis, renal disease, neuropathy, lymphoma, and Sjögren's syndrome. Cryoglobulinemia involves the presence of circulating immunoglobulins that reversibly precipitate at $\leq 37°C$. These cryoglobulins can precipitate in small blood vessels and induce a vasculitis. The cutaneous manifestation typically includes a palpable purpura in the lower extremities, and is diagnosed as a leukocytoclastic vasculitis on biopsy of the lesions.[88] Renal disease typically manifests as nephrotic syndrome with pathology consistent with membranoproliferative glomerulonephritis.

Peripheral neuropathy is the most common neurologic symptom in patients with HCV. Sensory loss may manifest bilaterally or may affect multiple isolated nerves. HCV-related non-Hodgkin's lymphoma is the most common lymphoproliferative disorder recognized in patients with HCV. Interestingly, extranodal involvement in the liver and salivary glands may be 3 to 4 times higher in patients with HCV versus non–HCV-infected patients with non-Hodgkin's lymphoma.[88] Finally, symptoms of Sjögren's syndrome such as xerostomia and xerophthalmia may occur in up to 10% of patients with HCV. HCV-associated Sjögren's syndrome appears to affect women more than men. Interferon therapy with ribavirin has been reported to have beneficial effects on these extrahepatic manifestations, with the exception of neuropathy and Sjögren's syndrome.[88]

▶ TREATMENT: Hepatitis C Virus Infection

▪ DESIRED OUTCOME

The ultimate goal in treating acute HCV is to return the individual to the previous state of health, and prevent the development of chronic infection. Intermediate goals, while the individual is acutely symptomatic and infectious, include decreasing morbidity and acute mortality, minimizing the chance that the infected person is infecting others, normalizing aminotransferases (cease hepatic inflammation), stopping viral replication in the host, and ultimately eradicating the virus. The goal of treatment is to prevent the morbidity and mortality associated with end-stage liver disease by eradicating HCV. Effective treatment of chronic viral hepatitis should also increase the quality of life and prevent infected patients from serving as reservoirs of infection. Because the complications of chronic hepatitis may take decades to manifest, clinical trials primarily use outcomes of virologic response (clearance of virus), biochemical response (return of transaminases to normal levels), and histologic response as surrogate markers for decreased risk of cirrhosis, HCC, or death. Long-term outcome studies show that the response to therapy can be maintained for years and that progression of liver disease can be halted. Even regression of fibrosis, once thought to be irreversible, is possible.[83] Sustained virologic or biochemical response is also associated with a reduced risk of HCC.

GENERAL APPROACH TO TREATMENT

Management of acute HCV is primarily supportive. General measures include a healthy diet, rest, maintaining fluid balance, and avoiding hepatotoxic drugs and alcohol. Hospitalization is sometimes required in patients with prolonged vomiting, coagulation defects, or fulminant hepatitis. Upon the diagnosis of chronic viral hepatitis, the patient should be informed about the disease risks and a program of regular monitoring established. Depending upon where in the course of infection the disease is diagnosed, monitoring for progression is important for selection of patients for pharmacologic treatment, because many more patients die with chronic viral hepatitis than from it. The relative benefits of pharmacologic therapy and their attendant adverse effects and risks need to be discussed as well.

NONPHARMACOLOGIC THERAPY

Liver transplantation is currently the only definitive therapy for the management of hepatic failure. However, transplants cannot be performed in all patients that require them due to the shortage of cadaveric organs. Consequently, the use of liver support systems can provide specific liver functions until an orthotopic liver transplantation is performed. The molecular adsorbents recycling system is a novel technologic system that uses albumin to remove water-soluble and albumin-bound toxins such as bile acid and bilirubin from the bloodstream. This liver dialysis system improves the maintenance of electrolytes, acid-base and fluid balance, glucose concentrations, and removes ammonia. The system benefits patients with liver failure who have renal complications as well. Prospective trials evaluating the efficacy and cost-effectiveness of the molecular adsorbents recycling system versus standard care are currently being completed.[89]

PHARMACOLOGIC THERAPY

Patients seropositive for HCV with elevated ALT and inflammation on liver biopsy are candidates for antiviral therapy. A more difficult treatment decision occurs when a patient has elevated ALT, but the histologic changes are mild. In that situation the patient may be closely monitored and treatment withheld. Because relapse frequently occurs shortly after IFN-α monotherapy is stopped, response to HCV treatment is broken into three general categories:

Response: Reduction of HCV RNA to undetectable levels and normalization of ALT during treatment and 6 months after completion of therapy

Nonresponse: HCV RNA remains detectable or ALT fails to normalize during the course of therapy

Relapse: HCV RNA becomes undetectable and ALT normalizes during treatment, but either ALT or HCV RNA re-emerge in the 6 months after therapy

Occasionally, different time points are used to record results as end-of-therapy responses or as sustained virologic response (SVR; at least 6 months after therapy). SVR has been acknowledged as the best predictor of a long-term clinical outcome.

The National Institutes of Health consensus panel published recommendations on the management of HCV infection in 2003.[90] Combination therapy has been recognized to be better than monotherapy. In addition, many of the early treatment recommendations have been supplanted by comparative data showing the superiority of pegylated interferon therapy in conjunction with ribavirin. The duration of therapy has now become a function of the specific genotype of HCV. A review of the published guidelines and the data supporting these recommendations are presented below.

FIRST-LINE THERAPY

The pharmacologic management of acute HCV is confounded by limitations in the ability to recognize the infection in mainly asymptomatic patients. Trials evaluating the role of interferon therapy included small sample sizes and used heterogeneous end-points to evaluate outcomes. Despite these limitations, SVRs in the range of 83% to 100% have been reported with IFN-α monotherapy in small uncontrolled trials, suggesting the potential advantages of early therapy.[90] However, the timing, type of regimen, and duration of therapy remain undefined. The management of treatment-naïve patients with chronic HCV is better defined with recent large randomized controlled trials comparing pegylated interferon plus ribavirin to interferon and ribavirin.[91,92]

Interferon is an immunomodulatory protein that works by binding to specific cell surface receptors that stimulate a host of gene transcriptions to prevent de novo infection in hepatocytes. In addition, IFN-α is thought to reduce HCV heterogeneity while stimulating proinflammatory systems to help increase viral eradication. Interferon is commercially available as IFN-α2a, IFN-α2b, pegylated versions of both products, and as IFN alfacon-1. The process of pegylation includes the attachment of inert polyethylene glycol to protein, resulting in an increase in net molecular size. This decreases the rate of subcutaneous absorption, decreases systemic clearance, increases exposure, and thus allows less frequent administration of the product. Ribavirin is a guanosine nucleotide analog that inhibits viral replication and works synergistically with IFN-α.[93]

The pegylated forms of IFN-α2a and IFN-α2b have distinct pharmacokinetic profiles. Both forms have been compared to monotherapy, in combination with ribavirin, and against IFN-α2b plus ribavirin. However, pegylated IFN-α2a has not been directly studied against pegylated IFN-α2b. These trials excluded patients with comorbid conditions such as HIV infection, autoimmune disorders, preexisting psychiatric illness, cytopathies, and patients with decompensated liver disease. In general, both pegylated IFN-α products plus ribavirin were more effective than IFN-α plus ribavirin or pegylated IFN-α alone. Patients with HCV genotype 1 demonstrated an SVR in about 40% of cases, while close to 80% of patients with HCV genotypes 2 and 3 had an SVR. In addition, patients with lower baseline HCV RNA levels, less fibrosis on liver biopsy, and a lower body surface area or weight were more likely to have a successful clinical outcome. A 24-week course of pegylated IFN-α plus ribavirin results in similar outcomes to a 48-week course for patients with HCV genotypes 2 and 3. However, a 48-week course of therapy results in a higher response rate than 24 weeks of therapy in patients with HCV genotype 1. In addition, 800 mg of ribavirin daily is sufficient for management of patients with genotypes 2 and 3, but a higher dose of 1000 to 1200 mg daily is required for patients with HCV genotype 1.[89]

ALTERNATIVE DRUG TREATMENTS

Current therapeutic options for chronic hepatitis C are limited to ribavirin, IFN-α, IFN alfacon-1, and pegylated IFN-α. As stated, monotherapy is inferior in attaining SVR compared to combination therapy. However, combination therapy with ribavirin may be limited by its contraindication for men whose female partners are pregnant, patients with hemoglobinopathies like sickle cell anemia, or known hypersensitivity to this agent. Consequently monotherapy with pegylated IFN-α may be considered. This is especially true in patients with HCV genotypes 2 and 3, in whom SVR was achieved in 45% of patients managed with pegylated IFN-α2a for 48 weeks. However, the same regimen was associated with an SVR in only 21% of patients with HCV genotype 1. Ribavirin monotherapy using doses of 600 to 1200 mg daily has demonstrated a reduction in necroinflammation. However, patients treated with such a regimen do not achieve an undetectable HCV RNA level, and these levels usually rebound to baseline upon completion of therapy.

The preclinical evaluation of new antivirals is hindered by a lack of animal models of HCV infection. Development of novel interferons and delivery systems, nucleoside analogues with reduced hemolytic potential compared with ribavirin, and inosine 5' monophosphate dehydrogenase inhibitors are being studied as adjunctive therapy to interferon-α–based regimens. In addition, compounds that inhibit specific HCV enzymes like serine proteases, RNA polymerase, and helicase are being evaluated. Prevention of disease progression through the use of antifibrotic agents in patients in whom HCV RNA cannot be eradicated is in development. The safety and efficacy of these newer therapies are currently being investigated, and is it likely that these treatment modalities will not be available for at least 3 to 5 years.[94] Herbal medications for the management of HCV were recently systematically reviewed, but none of the 14 tested agents demonstrated benefit.[95]

SPECIAL POPULATIONS

The strict inclusion and exclusion criteria in most studies to date would exclude more than half of all HCV-infected patients.[96] Patients with mild liver disease and normal ALT levels are less likely to progress to cirrhosis. Consequently the role of HCV therapy remains controversial. Some experts believe documentation of disease progression through liver biopsies should serve as the impetus for therapy. However, decisions to treat in such populations should be driven by the patient's desire to eradicate HCV or their unwillingness to undergo sequential liver biopsies to assess progression.

Children and adolescents with chronic HCV are likely to be asymptomatic. Pegylated IFN-α has not been studied in children, and most studies evaluating IFN-α have been uncontrolled with small sample sizes. These studies have demonstrated a better response in children compared to adults receiving IFN-α monotherapy, with SVR rates of 26% with HCV genotype 1 and 70% with genotypes 2 and 3.[90]

Active illicit injection drug use should not be used to exclude patients from receiving HCV therapy and should be assessed on an individual basis. This is critically important given that this group of patients represents the majority of new cases of HCV in the United States, and treatment may reduce potential transmission. However, data are limited when evaluating the role of HCV therapy in patients with active illicit drug use who are not in a drug treatment program. Use of substance abuse programs such as methadone treatment centers should be encouraged to help reduce risky behaviors.

Coinfection with HIV is common in patients with HCV given the shared risk factors for transmission. Patients coinfected with these viruses have a more accelerated progression of their HCV disease. Most trials to date have excluded patients with HIV or limited them to patients with stable HIV infection. Combination therapy using ribavirin is considered to be superior; however, enhancement of antiretroviral adverse events such as lactic acidosis limits therapy. Concurrent use of ribavirin therapy with didanosine, stavudine, or zidovudine is relatively contraindicated.[93]

Obesity has been recognized as a poor prognostic variable for outcomes associated with therapy for chronic HCV. Patients with a body mass index of >30 kg/m^2 had a 77% lower chance of response to therapy compared to overweight and normal-weight patients.[97] The exact mechanism of this interaction between weight and effect is not known. However, the natural progression of disease may be faster in obese patients and may be related to nonalcoholic steatohepatitis.[98,99]

DRUG CLASS INFORMATION

Interferons

Three FDA approved IFN-α preparations are currently available in the United States and include IFN-α2a (Roferon-A), IFN-α2b (Intron A), and IFN alfacon-1 (Infergen). IFN-α2a and IFN-α2b are naturally occurring cytokines that have been manufactured using human recombinant techniques in *Escherichia coli*.[100] In contrast, IFN alfacon-1 is a non–naturally occurring type 1 interferon also produced using human recombinant techniques, but it has a tenfold higher affinity for cell surface receptors.[100] Despite this theoretical higher activity, IFN alfacon-1 has not been found to be superior to IFN-α2b. The mechanism of action of these interferons includes activation of tyrosine kinases that upregulate production of several gene products like 2'-5' oligoadenylate synthetase, β_2-microglobulin, neopterin, and p68 kinases. These gene products are responsible for the immunomodulatory, antiviral, and antiproliferative properties of these agents. All of these products have to be administered subcutaneously three times a week. The dosage of 3 to 5 million units of IFN-α2a and IFN-α2b corresponds to 9- to 15-mcg doses of IFN alfacon-1. The expected rate of SVR response of these products is less than 20% when monotherapy is employed for 24 weeks. Flu-like symptoms such as headache, fatigue, and chills occur in more than two thirds of patients. Psychiatric adverse events such as nervousness and depression and hematologic toxicities such as neutropenia occur in almost a third of patients.[101]

Pegylated Interferons

Peginterferon-α2a (Pegasys) and peginterferon-α2b (PEG-Intron) are FDA approved for use as monotherapy and in combination with ribavirin for the treatment of chronic HCV in patients with compensated liver disease who are interferon-treatment–naïve. Their mechanism of action is similar to that of IFN-α, but they offer the advantage of higher and sustained concentrations compared to their nonpegylated versions.[93] The size and branching of the polyethylene glycol structure affects tissue distribution and elimination of the parent compound. The polyethylene glycol moiety with peginterferon-α2a is

TABLE 40–10. Side Effects of Interferon-α

Early (in First 2 Weeks of Therapy)	Hematologic	Neuropsychiatric	Autoimmune	Miscellaneous
Fever	Neutropenia	Irritability	Development of	Chronic fatigue
Chills	Thrombocytopenia	Mood lability	autoantibodies	Infections
Myalgias	Anemia	Depression	Hepatitis	Increased sleep
Fatigue		Tearfulness	Thyroid dysfunction	requirement
Malaise		Delirium	Thyroiditis	Anorexia
Nausea		Paresthesias	Arthropathy	Weight loss
Sleep disturbance		Seizures	Type I diabetes mellitus	Myalgias
Abdominal pain		Psychosis	Exacerbation of psoriasis or	Low-grade fevers
			lichen planus	
Diarrhea			Exacerbation of other	Decreased libido
Headache			autoimmune phenomena	Alopecia
Appetite changes				Hypertriglyceridemia
				Irritability
				Anxiety
				Depression
				Attention span deficits

Absolute contraindications to use of interferon include current or past psychosis or severe depression, neutropenia or thrombocytopenia, organ transplant (except liver), symptomatic heart disease, decompensated cirrhosis, and uncontrolled seizures. Relative contraindications to interferon include uncontrolled diabetes and autoimmune disorders.

approximately twice the size of that of peginterferon-α2b. Consequently the elimination half-life of peginterferon-α2a and peginterferon-α2b are 80 and 40 hours, respectively. This extension in half-life is in stark contrast to the nonpegylated interferons, which have a half-life of ∼5 hours. Peginterferon-α2a should be administered as a 180-mcg dose subcutaneously once weekly for 48 weeks. In contrast, peginterferon-α2b follows a weight-based dosing strategy of 1.5 mcg/kg subcutaneously for 1 year. Other pharmaceutical differences include a requirement for reconstitution of lyophilized peginterferon-α2b prior to administration, and a requirement for refrigeration for storage of peginterferon-α2a. In addition, peginterferon-α2a contains benzyl alcohol and so its use is contraindicated in neonates and infants. The adverse event profile of both agents is comparable to their respective nonpegylated versions. A summary of the incidence of specific adverse events is displayed in Table 40–10. Interferons can significantly decrease the clearance of theophylline, resulting in an increased area under the plasma concentration-versus-time curve. Caution should be used when α-interferons are initiated in patients on theophylline, as they are likely to require dosage reductions based on therapeutic drug monitoring.[101]

Ribavirin

Ribavirin is a synthetic nucleoside antagonist that is administered orally in combination with α-interferons. Ribavirin has limited utility as monotherapy and should be administered twice daily with food when used in combination with α-interferons. Ribavirin is currently available in two 200-mg oral formulations, as a capsule (Rebetol) and as a tablet (Copegus). When ribavirin is used with peginterferon-α2a for patients with HCV genotype 1, it is dosed as 400 mg orally every morning and 600 mg orally every evening in patients up to 75 kg, and 600 mg orally twice daily for patients weighing more than 75 kg. For patients with genotypes 2 and 3 ribavirin is administered 400 mg orally twice daily when administered with peginterferon-α2b or peginterferon-α2a. Hemolytic anemia is a common complication of ribavirin therapy. Dosage reductions of ribavirin are recommended for changes in hemoglobin values when used in combination with peginterferon-α2a. In general, the combination of ribavirin with α-interferons is associated with numerous adverse events to multiple organ systems, and these should be discussed with patients prior to initiation of therapy.[101]

PHARMACOECONOMIC CONSIDERATIONS

Ten to thirty percent of patients progress to cirrhosis after 30 years. Most individuals with chronic HCV in the United States are between the ages of 30 and 49 years and have yet to manifest sequelae of the disease. As a result, the impact of HCV on future health care costs is anticipated to be high. Unfortunately, clinical decisions to treat individual patients are confounded by the inconsistent progression and a lack of ability to predict clinical deterioration. Therapy with pegylated interferons and ribavirin can be very expensive and associated with serious adverse events. Consequently, assessing the cost, benefits, and cost-effectiveness of the various therapies is vital.

The cost of medications based on average wholesale prices with the use of a pegylated interferon plus ribavirin is approximately $30,000 for a 48-week course of therapy.[63] The cost of using nonpegylated interferon plus ribavirin is approximately $15,000 to $20,000.[63]

Assuming conservatively that 10% of all chronic hepatitis C patients (2.7 million) were eligible for therapy in the United States, with 70% of patients having HCV genotype 1, the estimated cost for the pharmaceuticals alone would be approximately $4 billion. However, the cost of not treating HCV could lead to future costs associated with hospitalizations related to ascites, cirrhosis, variceal hemorrhage, HCC, and liver transplantation.

A recent pharmacoeconomic analysis to examine the clinical benefits and cost-effectiveness of newer treatments for chronic HCV infection evaluated the incremental cost-effectiveness of using peginterferon-α2b plus ribavirin compared to IFN-α2b plus ribavirin, and monotherapy regimens of both interferons.[102] The incremental cost per quality-adjusted life year (QALY) saved for combination therapy with peginterferon-α2b compared to standard therapy was $36,000 and $55,000 for men and women with HCV genotype 1, respectively. A QALY is defined as a patient's desire for a year of life at a diminished state of health compared with life at an optimal state of health. The use of the QALY as a measure helps create a uniform set of values that can be applied to cost-effectiveness data from heterogeneous patient groups. Interpretation of data defining cost per QALY is further hampered by a lack of a standard benchmark to define when a therapeutic regimen should or should not be used. Historically, a cost-effectiveness threshold of $\leq$\$50,000 has been used to define a cost-effective regimen, but this remains controversial when applied clinically. The QALY gains ranged from 0.6 months with IFN-α2b monotherapy to 6 months with combination peginterferon-α2b and ribavirin therapy in men.

The key points of contention when evaluating any pharmacoeconomic analysis are the basic underlying assumptions. A lack of clear understanding of the natural course of chronic HCV, including the probability of progression, impairs such studies. For the time being, patient selection on the basis of predictors of response coupled with informed patient decision making regarding benefits and risks is appropriate.

CLINICAL CONTROVERSIES

Clinicians argue that a noninvasive dynamic measure of hepatic fibrosis is necessary given that the probability of progression of chronic HCV is unclear. Others argue that the development of such tests will still not predict when to initiate therapy.

The role of long-term continuous therapy with peginterferon alone or in combination with ribavirin is unknown. Some clinicians believe that long-term combination therapy may improve clinical outcomes in select nonresponders.

EVALUATION OF THERAPEUTIC OUTCOMES

To carry out the plans outlined above requires that viral genotyping be performed at baseline, with a viral load being assessed if the patient has HCV genotype 1. Before treatment, all patients should have a viral genotype performed, have thyroid function assessed, and women should have a negative pregnancy test. Liver biopsy is a useful test to evaluate the stage of fibrosis and may aid with the decision of when to initiate or defer therapy. The value of a pretreatment liver biopsy in patients with HCV genotypes 2 and 3 is limited given that antiviral therapy may lead to a favorable response in up to 80% of patients.[90]

During treatment, a complete blood count with platelets should be performed weekly for the first 4 weeks and monthly thereafter. Thyroid tests should be checked every 3 to 6 months during treatment and 6 months after.[101] HCV RNA should be evaluated at baseline and 12 weeks of combination therapy, and additionally depending on the intended duration. This is because early virologic response, defined as a minimum two $\log_{10}$ reduction in the viral load in the first 12 weeks of therapy, is predictive of SVR in patients with HCV genotype 1. Consequently, patients without an early virologic response should have their treatment discontinued to reduce cost and prevent unnecessary adverse events.[90] Aminotransferase and qualitative HCV RNA should be performed at the end of therapy and 6 and 18 months after the cessation of therapy. Follow-up biopsy is not indicated. In patients with established or suspected cirrhosis, screening for HCC with abdominal ultrasound and serum α-fetoprotein is recommended.[90] However, neither the time frame nor cost-effectiveness of such screening has been defined. For patients not started on therapy because of mild histologic disease or normal ALT, liver biopsy should be repeated in 4 to 5 years and ALT at 6-month intervals, respectively.

The side effects of α-interferons occur frequently enough that the patient should be informed about them before treatment begins (see Table 40–10). Many side effects are dose related. The most common and predictable effects are influenza-like and can be counteracted by premedication with a single dose of acetaminophen around the time of injection. Severity decreases with subsequent injections and usually abates in 1 to 2 weeks.[101] Later common adverse effects are fatigue, malaise, and cognitive changes.

Because α-interferon therapy can exacerbate autoimmune disorders, it is important to exclude autoimmune diagnoses before initiating therapy. Thrombocytopenia and granulocytopenia are more common in patients with cirrhosis and hypersplenism. The psychiatric complications are especially severe in those with severe liver disease, occur in up to 20% of patients, and are the most common dose-limiting side effects. Therapy should be discontinued if serious complications occur. The dose of α-interferon must be reduced in 10% to 40% of patients. Treatment must be discontinued because of adverse effects in 5% to 10% of patients. For many patients, reassurance that the side effects are therapy related, not severe, and will disappear when therapy is stopped is sufficient. It is always important to reassure both patient and family, especially when psychiatric side effects are evident. These points are critical given that patient adherence is crucial to the ultimate success of HCV treatment.[101]

Ongoing monitoring of α-interferon toxicity includes weekly complete blood counts during the first 2 weeks of therapy and monthly thereafter. Patients should be asked about level of performance, mood changes, ability to concentrate, and symptoms. The dose of α-interferon should be decreased by 50% if any of the following develop: fatigue that interferes with the daily routine, serious mood changes, daily nausea with occasional vomiting, granulocytopenia ($<750/mm^3$), and/or thrombocytopenia ($<50,000/mm^3$). Interferon should be immediately discontinued if fatigue is so severe that it requires bed rest, vomiting occurs more than twice daily, or if profound granulocytopenia ($<500/mm^3$) or thrombocytopenia ($<30,000/mm^3$) occurs.[101]

PREVENTION OF HCV INFECTION

No vaccine for hepatitis C is available. Vaccine development for HCV is difficult because of the extensive genomic variability of the virus, viral mutants, and the lack of efficacy of serum antibodies. Current recommendations for prevention of HCV include universal precautions for the prevention of blood-borne infections, and anti-HCV screening of blood, organ, and tissue donors. Screening of blood donors has virtually eliminated HCV transmission through blood and blood products. Programs that focus on reducing HIV transmission are also likely to decrease transmission of HCV in high-risk groups. No clear policy for counseling women of childbearing age exists.

Benefit associated with identification of HCV infections in health care workers is limited. However, the CDC, in collaboration with the Hospital Infection Control Practices Advisory Committee, recommends that health care institutions consider implementing policies and procedures for follow-up for HCV infection after percutaneous or permucosal exposures to blood.[66,69] Follow-up should include testing the source for anti-HCV; baseline and 6-month follow-up testing for anti-HCV and AST for the person exposed to an anti-HCV–positive source; confirmation by supplemental anti-HCV testing of all anti-HCV–reactive results; and education of health care workers about blood-borne infections. Postexposure prophylaxis with Ig or interferon is not recommended. There are no specific recommendations for HCV immune prophylaxis for exposed individuals. Prophylaxis with Ig after needlestick exposure to hepatitis C is not recommended.[66]

ABBREVIATIONS

AASLD: American Association for the Study of Liver Diseases
ALT: alanine transaminase
anti-HBc: antibody to HbcAg
anti-HBe: antibody to HBeAg
anti-HBs: antibody to HBsAg
APASL: Asian Pacific Association for the Study of the Liver
AST: aspartate transaminase
EIA: enzyme immunoassay
HAV: hepatitis A virus
HBcAg: hepatitis B core antigen
HBeAg: hepatitis B e antigen
HBIg: hepatitis B immunoglobulin
HBsAg: hepatitis B surface antigen
HBV: hepatitis B virus
HCC: hepatocellular carcinoma
HCV: hepatitis C virus
HIV: human immunodeficiency virus
IFN-α: interferon-α
IFN-α2b: interferon-α2b
IFN-γ: interferon-γ
Ig: immunoglobulin
MMR: measles, mumps, rubella vaccine
NHANES: National Health and Nutrition Examination Survey
QALY: quality-adjusted life year
RIBA: recombinant immunoblot assay
SVR: sustained virologic response

Review Questions and other resources can be found at *www.pharmacotherapyonline.com.*

REFERENCES

1. World Health Organization position paper: Hepatitis A vaccines. Wkly Epidemiol Rec 2000;(Feb 4)5:38–44.
2. Centers for Disease Control and Prevention. Prevention of hepatitis A through active or passive immunization: Recommendations of the Advisory Committee on Immunization Practices (ACIP). MMWR Morb Mortal Wkly Rep 1999;48(RR-12):1–37.
3. Berge JJ, Drennan DP, Jacobs RJ, et al. The cost of hepatitis A infections in American adolescents and adults in 1997. Hepatology 2000;31:469–473.
4. Koopmans M, von Bonsdorff CH, Vinje J, et al. Foodborne viruses. FEMS Microbiol Rev 2002;26:187–205.
5. O'Donovan D, Cooke RP, Joce R, et al. An outbreak of hepatitis A amongst injecting drug users. Epidemiol Infect 2001;127:469–473.
6. Cuthbert JA. Hepatitis A: Old and new. Clin Microbiol Rev 2001;14:38–58.
7. Vento S, Garofano T, Renzini C, et al. Fulminant hepatitis associated with hepatitis A virus superinfection in patients with chronic hepatitis C. N Engl J Med 1998;338:286–290.
8. Gregory PB, Knauer CM, Kempson RL, Miller R. Steroid therapy in severe viral hepatitis. A double-blind, randomized trial of methylprednisolone versus placebo. N Engl J Med 1976;294:681–687.
9. Pappas SC. Fulminant viral hepatitis. Gastroenterol Clin North Am 1995;24:161–173.
10. Lee WM. Hepatitis B virus infection. N Engl J Med 1997;24:1733–1745.
11. Plevris JN, Schina M, Hayes PC. Review article: The management of acute liver failure. Aliment Pharmacol Ther 1998;12:405–418.
12. Werzberger A, Mensch B, Kuter B, et al. A controlled trial of a formalin-inactivated hepatitis A vaccine in healthy children. N Engl J Med 1992;327:453–457.
13. Bell BP. Hepatitis A vaccine. Semin Pediatr Infect Dis 2002;13:165–173.
14. Sagliocca L, Amoroso P, Stroffolini T, et al. Efficacy of hepatitis A vaccine in prevention of secondary hepatitis A infection: A randomised trial. Lancet 1999;353:1136–1139.
15. Zuckerman J. The place of accelerated schedules for hepatitis A and B vaccinations. Drugs 2003;63:1779–1784.
16. Rosenthal P. Cost-effectiveness of hepatitis A vaccination in children, adolescents, and adults. Hepatology 2003;37:44–51.
17. Beutels P, Edmunds WJ, Antonanzas F, et al. Economic evaluation of vaccination programmes: A consensus statement focusing on viral hepatitis. Pharmacoeconomics 2002;20:1–7.
18. Jacobs RJ, Meyerhoff AS. Cost-effectiveness of hepatitis A/B vaccine versus hepatitis B vaccine in public sexually transmitted disease clinics. Sex Transm Dis 2003;30:859–865.
19. Arguedas MR, Heudebert GR, Fallon MB, Stinnett AA. The cost-effectiveness of hepatitis A vaccination in patients with chronic hepatitis C viral infection in the United States. Am J Gastroenterol 2002;97:721–728.
20. Lee WM. Hepatitis B virus infection. N Engl J Med 1997;24:1733–1745.
21. McQuillan GM, Coleman PJ, Kruszon-Moran D, Moyer LA, et al. Prevalence of hepatitis B virus infection in the United States: The National Health and Nutrition Examination Surveys, 1976 through 1994. Am J Public Health 1999;89:14–18.
22. Broderick AL, Jonas MM. Hepatitis B in children. Semin Liver Dis 2003;23:59–68.
23. Alter MJ. Epidemiology and prevention of hepatitis B. Semin Liver Dis 2003;23:39–46.
24. Mahoney FJ. Update on diagnosis, management, and prevention of hepatitis B virus infection. Clin Microbiol Rev 1999;12:351–366.
25. Angus PW, Locarnini SA, McCaughan GW, et al. Hepatitis B virus pre-core mutant infection is associated with severe recurrent disease after liver transplantation. Hepatology 1995;21:14–18.
26. Huang MA, Lok ASF. Natural history of hepatitis B and outcomes after liver transplantation. Clin Liver Dis 2003;7:521–536.
27. Lok ASF. Hepatitis B infection: Pathogenesis and management. J Hepatol 2000;32(Suppl):89–97.
28. Rapicetta M, Ferrari C, Levrero M. Viral determinants and host immune responses in the pathogenesis of HBV infection. J Med Virol 2002;67:454–457.
29. Fattovich G. Natural history and prognosis of hepatitis B. Semin Liver Dis 2003;23:47–58.
30. Bianco E, Stroffolini T, Spada E, et al. Case fatality rate of acute viral hepatitis in Italy: 1995–2000. An update. Dig Liver Dis 2003;35:404–408.
31. Lok AS, Heathcote EJ, Hoofnagle JH. Management of hepatitis B: 2000—summary of a workshop. Gastroenterology 2001;120:1828–1853.
32. Lok ASF, McMahon BJ. Chronic hepatitis B. Hepatology 2001;34:1225–1241.
33. Myers RP, Tainturier MH, Ratziu V, et al. Prediction of liver histological lesions with biochemical markers in patients with chronic hepatitis B. J Hepatol 2003;39:222–230.
34. Rozario R, Ramakrishna B. Histopathological study of chronic hepatitis B and C: A comparison of two scoring systems. J Hepatol 2003;38:223–229.
35. Ikeda K, Saitoh S, Suzuki Y. Disease progression and hepatocellular carcinogenesis in patients with chronic viral hepatitis: A prospective observation of 2215 patients. J Hepatol 1998;28:930–938.
36. Chu CM. Natural history of chronic hepatitis B virus infection in adults with emphasis on the occurrence of cirrhosis and hepatocellular carcinoma. J Gastroenterol Hepatol 2000;15(Suppl):E25–E30.
37. Lagget M, Rizzetto M. Current pharmacotherapy for the treatment of chronic hepatitis B. Expert Opin Pharmacother 2003;4:1821–1827.
38. Liaw YF, Leung N, Guan R, et al. Asian-Pacific consensus statement on the management of chronic hepatitis B: An update. J Gastroenterol Hepatol 2003;18:239–245.
39. van Nunen AB, Hansen BE, Suh DJ. Durability of HBeAg seroconversion following antiviral therapy for chronic hepatitis B: Relation to type

of therapy and pretreatment serum hepatitis B virus DNA and alanine aminotransferase. Gut 2003;52:420–424.

40. Yalcin K, Degertekin H, Yildiz F, Celik Y. Comparison of 12-month courses of interferon-alpha-2b-lamivudine combination therapy and interferon-alpha-2b monotherapy among patients with untreated chronic hepatitis B. Clin Infect Dis 2003;36:1516–1522.

41. McCulloch M, Broffman M, Gao J, Colford JM Jr. Chinese herbal medicine and interferon in the treatment of chronic hepatitis B: A meta-analysis of randomized, controlled trials. Am J Public Health 2002;92:1619–1628.

42. Wong DK, Cheung AM, O'Rourke K, et al. Effect of alpha-interferon treatment in patients with hepatitis B e antigen-positive chronic hepatitis B. A meta-analysis. Ann Intern Med 1993;119:312–323.

43. Dienstag JL, Schiff ER, Wright TL, et al. Lamivudine as initial treatment for chronic hepatitis B in the United States. N Engl J Med 1999;341:1256–1263.

44. Lai CL, Chien RN, Leung NW, et al. A one-year trial of lamivudine for chronic hepatitis B. Asia Hepatitis Lamivudine Study Group. N Engl J Med 1998;339:61–68.

45. Jonas MM, Kelley DA, Mizerski J, et al. Clinical trial of lamivudine in children with chronic hepatitis B. N Engl J Med 2002;346:1706–1713.

46. Hadziyannis SJ, Tassopoulos NC, Heathcote EJ, et al. Adefovir dipivoxil for the treatment of hepatitis B e antigen-negative chronic hepatitis B. N Engl J Med 2003;348:800–807.

47. Marcellin P, Chang TT, Lim SG, et al. Adefovir dipivoxil for the treatment of hepatitis B e antigen-positive chronic hepatitis B. N Engl J Med 2003;348:808–816.

48. Papatheodoridis GV, Dimou E, Papadimitropoulos V. Nucleoside analogues for chronic hepatitis B: Antiviral efficacy and viral resistance. Am J Gastroenterol 2002;97:1618–1628.

49. Lau GKK, Nanji A, Hov J, et al. Thymosin-alpha1 and famcyclovir combination therapy activate T-cell response in patients with chronic hepatitis B virus infection in immune-tolerant phase. J Viral Hepatol 2002;9:280–287.

50. Chan HL, Tang JL, Tam W, Sung JJ. The efficacy of thymosin in the treatment of chronic hepatitis B virus infection: A meta-analysis. Aliment Pharmacol Ther 2001;15:1899–1905.

51. Krogsgaard K, Marcellin P, Trepo C, et al. Prednisolone withdrawal therapy enhances the effect of human lymphoblastoid interferon in chronic hepatitis B. INTERPRED Trial Group. J Hepatol 1996;25:803–813.

52. Karayiannis P. Hepatitis B virus: Old, new and future approaches to antiviral treatment. J Antimicrob Chemother 2003;51:761–785.

53. Villeneuve JP, Condreay LD, Willems B, et al. Lamivudine treatment for decompensated cirrhosis resulting from chronic hepatitis B. Hepatology 2000;31:207–210.

54. Rockstroh JK. Management of hepatitis B and C in HIV co-infected patients. J Acquir Immune Defic Syndr 2003;34(Suppl 1):S59–S65.

55. Figen G, Nurten K, Hasan O, Aysel Y. Comparison of standard and high dosage recombinant interferon-alpha 2b for treatment of children with chronic hepatitis B infection. Pediatr Infect Dis J 2000;19:52–56.

56. Carreno C, Marcellin P, Hadziyannis S, et al. Retreatment of chronic hepatitis B e antigen-positive patients with recombinant interferon alpha-2a. Hepatology 1999;29:277–282.

57. Kirkwood JM, Bender C, Agarwala S, et al. Mechanisms and management of toxicities associated with high-dose interferon alfa-2b therapy. J Clin Oncol 2002;20:3703–3718.

58. Jarvis B, Faulds D. Lamivudine. A review of its therapeutic potential in chronic hepatitis B. Drugs 1999;58:101–141.

59. Suzuki Y, Arase Y, Ikeda K, et al. Histological improvements after a three-year lamivudine therapy in patients with chronic hepatitis B in whom YMDD mutants did not or did develop. Intervirology 2003;46:164–170.

60. Liaw YF, Chien RW, Yeh CT, et al. Acute exacerbation and hepatitis B clearance after emergence of YMDD motif mutation during lamivudine therapy. Hepatology 1999;30:567–572.

61. Malik AH, Lee WM. Hepatitis B therapy: The plot thickens. Hepatology 1999;30:579–581.

62. Dando T, Plosker G. Adefovir dipivoxil: A review of its use in chronic hepatitis B. Drugs 2003;63:2215–2234.

63. 2003 Drug Topics Red Book. Montvale, NJ, Medical Economics, 2003.

64. Wong JB, Koff RS, Tine F, Pauker SG. Cost-effectiveness of interferon-alpha 2b treatment of hepatitis B e antigen-positive chronic hepatitis B. Ann Intern Med 1995;122:664–675.

65. Brooks EA, Lacey LF, Payne SL, Miller DW. Economic evaluation of lamivudine compared with interferon-alpha in the treatment of chronic hepatitis B in the United States. Am J Manag Care 2001;7:677–682.

66. United States Public Health Service. Updated U.S. Public Health Service Guidelines for the Management of Occupational Exposures to HBV, HCV, and HIV and Recommendations for Postexposure Prophylaxis. MMWR Recomm Rep 2001;50(RR-11):1–52.

67. Keating GM, Noble S. Recombinant hepatitis B vaccine (Engerix-B): A review of its immunogenicity and protective efficacy against hepatitis B. Drugs 2003;63:1021–1051.

68. Duclos P. Safety of immunisation and adverse events following vaccination against hepatitis B. Expert Opin Drug Saf 2003;2:225–231.

69. Centers for Disease Control and Prevention. Recommendations for prevention and control of hepatitis C (HCV) infection and HCV-related chronic disease. MMWR Morb Mortal Wkly Rep 1998;47(RR-19):1–39.

70. Williams I. Epidemiology of hepatitis C in the United States. Am J Med 1999;107(6B):2S–9S.

71. Alter MJ, Kruszon-Moran D, Nainan OV, et al. The prevalence of hepatitis C virus infection in the United States, 1988 through 1994. N Engl J Med 1999;341:556–562.

72. Baillargeon J, Wu H, Kelley MJ, et al. Hepatitis C seroprevalence among newly incarcerated inmates in the Texas correctional system. Public Health 2003;117:43–48.

73. Desai RA, Rosenheck RA, Agnello V. Prevalence of hepatitis C virus infection in a sample of homeless veterans. Soc Psychiatry Psychiatr Epidemiol 2003;38:396–401.

74. World Health Organisation. Hepatitis C: Global prevalence. Wkly Epidemiol Rec 1997;72:341–344.

75. Kim WR. The burden of hepatitis C in the United States. Hepatology 2002;36(5 Suppl 1):S30–S34.

76. Koblin BA, Factor SH, Wu Y, Vlahov D. Hepatitis C virus infection among noninjecting drug users in New York City. J Med Virol 2003;70:387–390.

77. Zanetti AR, Tanzi E, Newell ML. Mother-to-infant transmission of hepatitis C virus. J Hepatol Suppl 1999;31:96–100.

78. Melbye M, Biggar RJ, Wantzin P, et al. Sexual transmission of hepatitis C virus: Cohort study (1981-9) among European homosexual men. BMJ 1990;301:210–212.

79. Simmonds P, Alberti A, Alter HJ, et al. A proposed system for the nomenclature of hepatitis C viral genotypes. Hepatology 1994;19:1321–1324.

80. Heintges T, Wands JR. Hepatitis C virus: Epidemiology and transmission. Hepatology 1997;26:521–526.

81. Liang TJ, Rehermann B, Seeff LB, Hoofnagle JH. NIH Conference: Pathogenesis, natural history, treatment, and prevention of hepatitis C. Ann Intern Med 2000;132:296–305.

82. Malnick SDH, Beergabel M, Lurie Y. Treatment of chronic hepatitis C virus infection. Ann Pharmacother 2000;34:1156–1164.

83. Zoulim F, Chevallier M, Maynard M, Trepo C. Clinical consequences of hepatitis C virus infection. Rev Med Virol 2003;13:57–68.

84. Amarapurkar D. Natural history of hepatitis C virus infection. J Gastroenterol Hepatol 2000;15(Suppl):E105–E110.

85. Gerlach JT, Diepolder HM, Zachoval R, et al. Acute hepatitis C: High rate of both spontaneous and treatment-induced viral clearance. Gastroenterology 2003;125:80–88.

86. Pawlotsky JM. Use and interpretation of hepatitis C virus diagnostic assays. Clin Liver Dis 2003;7:127–137.

87. Gupta S, Bent S, Kohlwes J. Test characteristics of alpha-fetoprotein for detecting hepatocellular carcinoma in patients with hepatitis C. A systematic review and critical analysis. Ann Intern Med 2003;139:46–50.

88. Mayo MJ. Extrahepatic manifestations of hepatitis C infection. Am J Med Sci 2003;325:135–148.

89. Stange J, Hassanein TI, Mehta R, et al. The molecular adsorbents recycling system as a liver support system based on albumin dialysis: a summary of preclinical investigations, prospective, randomized,

controlled clinical trial, and clinical experience from 19 centers. Artif Organs 2002;26:103–110.

90. Seeff LB, Hoofnagle JH. **Appendix:** National Institutes of Health Consensus Development Conference Management of Hepatitis C 2002. Clin Liver Dis 2003;7:261–287.

91. Manns MP, McHutchison JG, Gordon SC, et al. Peginterferon alfa-2b plus ribavirin compared with interferon alfa-2b plus ribavirin for initial treatment of chronic hepatitis C: A randomised trial. Lancet 2001;358:958–965.

92. Fried MW, Shiffman ML, Reddy KR, et al. Peginterferon alfa-2a plus ribavirin for chronic hepatitis C virus infection. N Engl J Med 2002;347:975–982.

93. Baker DE. Pegylated interferon plus ribavirin for the treatment of chronic hepatitis C. Rev Gastroenterol Disord 2003;3:93–109.

94. McHutchison JG, Patel K. Future therapy of hepatitis C. Hepatology 2002;36(5 Suppl 1):S245–S252.

95. Liu J, Manheimer E, Tsutani K, Gluud C. Medicinal herbs for hepatitis C virus infection: A Cochrane hepatobiliary systematic review of randomized trials. Am J Gastroenterol 2003;98:538–544.

96. Strader DB. Understudied populations with hepatitis C. Hepatology 2002;36(5 Suppl 1):S226–S236.

97. Bressler BL, Guindi M, Tomlinson G, Heathcote J. High body mass index is an independent risk factor for nonresponse to antiviral treatment in chronic hepatitis C. Hepatology 2003;38:639–644.

98. Ortiz V, Berenguer M, Rayon JM, et al. Contribution of obesity to hepatitis C-related fibrosis progression. Am J Gastroenterol 2002;97:2408–2814.

99. Monto A, Alonzo J, Watson JJ, et al. Steatosis in chronic hepatitis C: Relative contributions of obesity, diabetes mellitus, and alcohol. Hepatology 2002;36:729–736.

100. Melian EB, Plosker GL. Interferon alfacon-1: A review of its pharmacology and therapeutic efficacy in the treatment of chronic hepatitis C. Drugs 2001;61:1661–1691.

101. Fried MW. Side effects of therapy of hepatitis C and their management. Hepatology 2002;36(5 Suppl 1):S237–S244.

102. Salomon JA, Weinstein MC, Hammitt JK, Goldie SJ. Cost-effectiveness of treatment for chronic hepatitis C infection in an evolving patient population. JAMA 2003;290:228–237.

41

QUANTIFICATION OF RENAL FUNCTION

Thomas C. Dowling and Thomas J. Comstock

Learning Objectives and other resources can be found at *www.pharmacotherapyonline.com.*

KEY CONCEPTS

❶ For patients with chronic kidney disease (CKD) the stage of disease should be determined based on the level of kidney function, independent of etiology, according to the National Kidney Foundation Kidney Disease Outcomes Quality Initiative (NKF K/DOQI) CKD classification system.

❷ Persistent proteinuria indicates the presence of CKD.

❸ Semiquantitative methods of urine protein excretion, such as the spot urine albumin:creatinine ratio, are recommended for determining the severity of CKD and monitoring the rate of disease progression.

❹ The glomerular filtration rate (GFR) is the single best indicator of overall renal function.

❺ Measurement of the GFR is ideally performed using the exogenous administration of inulin, iothalamate, or radioisotope techniques such as ^{99m}Tc-DTPA.

❻ Measurement of creatinine clearance is not routinely recommended; however pretreatment with cimetidine improves the accuracy of this estimate of GFR.

❼ Equations to estimate creatinine clearance or GFR are commonly used in ambulatory and inpatient settings, and incorporate patient demographic variables such as serum creatinine, age, gender, weight, and ethnicity.

❽ Longitudinal assessment of kidney function is important for monitoring the efficacy of therapeutic interventions, such as angiotensin-converting enzyme inhibitors (ACEIs) and angiotensin receptor blockers, that are intended to slow the progression of kidney disease.

❾ The serum creatinine concentration (S_{cr}) or the reciprocal of S_{cr} versus time should be used with caution to estimate the rate of decline in renal function in CKD patients, as these indices do not consider patient age, lean body mass, gender, diet, concomitant diseases and drug therapy, circadian rhythm, stability of kidney function, tubular secretion of creatinine, or analytic method.

❿ Qualitative assessments of renal function, such as x-ray, computed tomography, magnetic resonance imaging, sonography, and biopsy, are useful for determining the etiology and structural aspects of kidney disease.

It is estimated that nearly 20 million people in the United States have impaired renal function, and in most cases the disease is undiagnosed. Evaluation of renal function is an important part of pharmaceutical care that can be performed in clinical and research settings using both qualitative and quantitative methods. Estimation of creatinine clearance is often considered the clinical standard for assessment of renal function. Other tests, such as the urinalysis, radiographic procedures, and biopsy, are also valuable tools in the assessment of renal disease, and these qualitative assessments are useful for determining the pathology and etiology of kidney disease. The urinalysis, for example, may give clues to the primary location, such as glomerular or tubular, of the renal disease. Follow-up studies such as imaging procedures or kidney biopsy may then further differentiate the specific cause, thereby pointing to the appropriate therapeutic intervention.

❶ Quantitative indices such as creatinine clearance or glomerular filtration rate (GFR) are most useful for determining the degree of renal insufficiency and stage of chronic kidney disease (CKD) in accordance with the National Kidney Foundation (NKF) classification system. These indices can also be used to measure changes in

function that may occur as a result of disease progression, therapeutic intervention, or toxic insult.[1] Moreover, the design of dosage regimens for drugs eliminated by the kidneys is also dependent on the availability of a quantitative measure of kidney function.

Renal "function" includes the processes of filtration, secretion, and reabsorption, as well as endocrine and metabolic functions. Alterations of all five renal functions, whether declining or improving, have been associated primarily with GFR. This chapter critically evaluates the various methods that can be used for the quantitative assessment of kidney function (Table 41–1). Where appropriate, discussion regarding the qualitative assessment of kidney function is also presented, including specialized tests such as kidney biopsy.

EXCRETORY FUNCTION

The most important contribution of the kidney to overall maintenance of body homeostasis is the urinary excretion of water, endogenous

TABLE 41–1. Markers of Renal Function

Renal plasma/blood flow	p-Aminohippurate (PAH)
	^{131}I-Orthoiodohippurate (^{131}I-OIH)
	^{99m}Tc-mercaptoacetyltriglycine
	(^{99m}Tc-MAG3)
Glomerular filtration rate	Inulin, sinistrin
	Iothalamate
	Iohexol
	^{99m}Tc-diethylenetriaminepentaacetic acid
	(^{99m}Tc-DTPA)
	^{125}I-Iothalamate
	Creatinine
	Cystatin C
Tubular function	p-Aminohippurate
	N-1-Methylnicotinamide (NMN)
	Tetraethylammonium (TEA)
	β_2-Microglobulin
	Retinol-binding protein (RBP)
	Protein HC (α_1-microglobulin)
	N-Acetylglucosaminidase (NAG)
	Alanine aminopeptidase (AAP)
	Adenosine binding protein (ABP)

substances, and toxins. Through the combined processes of glomerular filtration, tubular secretion, and tubular reabsorption, the nephron, as the functional unit of the kidney, maintains balance between input and output of water and solutes from the body. Thus the kidney is the key organ responsible for maintenance of homeostasis. This is represented as:

$$\text{Rate of excretion} = \text{rate of filtration} + \text{rate of secretion}$$
$$- \text{rate of reabsorption}$$

FILTRATION

Glomerular filtration occurs through the passive diffusion of water and low-molecular-weight ions and molecules across the glomerular-capillary membrane into Bowman's capsule and the proximal tubule (Fig. 41–1). Because most proteins are too large to be substantially filtered (>60 kDa), or their filtration is impeded by the electronegative charge of the glomerulus, compounds presented to the glomerulus in the protein-bound state are not filtered and enter the peritubular circulation.

SECRETION

Secretion occurs primarily along the proximal tubule and facilitates elimination of compounds from the plasma into the tubular lumen via active transport. Highly efficient anionic and cationic transport systems for a wide range of endogenous and exogenous substances yield renal clearance values that greatly exceed the GFR. Examples include probenecid, p-aminohippurate (PAH), and penicillin as anions; and creatinine, cimetidine, and procainamide as cations.[2] These systems are not mutually exclusive, as probenecid has been observed to compete with the tubular secretion of cimetidine.[3] Other transport pathways, such as P-glycoprotein (P-gp) and multidrug resistance protein (MRP), are distributed in tissues including kidney, liver, jejunum, colon, and brain. These efflux proteins are being recognized as an important element in drug elimination by the kidneys.[4] For example, P-gp is located on the apical membrane of the proximal tubule and

may play an important role in the renal elimination of a wide range of drugs such as cimetidine, digoxin, and procainamide. Blockade of P-gp could result in decreased renal elimination of such compounds, leading to an increased drug exposure. Verapamil, cyclosporine, and the P-gp–specific inhibitor PSC 833 all reduce the activity of this tubular transport mechanism.[5] Further investigations into the exact role of the P-gp and MRP efflux pathways on drug elimination are presently underway.

Measurement of GFR may not be an appropriate assessment for the prediction of renal clearance of a drug that undergoes active tubular secretion, or for a drug that is extensively reabsorbed. As an example, Hori and associates[6,7] demonstrated that the postfiltration renal handling of ampicillin, which is secreted, and cephalexin, which is secreted and reabsorbed, remained normal in patients with renal failure caused by glomerulonephritis, but was reduced in patients with renal failure associated with tubular dysfunction. They concluded that dosage adjustment based on creatinine clearance would be inappropriate for drugs eliminated by tubular secretion. Maiza and Daley-Yates[8] observed glomerulotubular imbalance in experimentally induced renal failure in rats based on differential effects on inulin (an index of filtration), PAH (an index of anionic secretion), and N-1-methylnicotinamide clearance (an index of cationic secretion). Using an experimental nephrotoxic (uranyl nitrate) acute renal failure rat model, Lin and Lin[9] and Gloff and Benet[10] demonstrated differential handling of tetraethylammonium (TEA) bromide and PAH, with greater impairment of tubular secretion than of GFR. Lin and Lin[9] further studied an ischemic acute renal failure model (glycerol) and showed a parallel decline of secretion and GFR for TEA, whereas secretion of PAH decreased at a greater rate than did GFR. These results support the hypothesis that the integrity of different pathways for elimination of compounds may be dependent on the mode of injury as well as the chemical characteristics of the compound. Thus the kidney should not be considered as a single homogeneously functioning organ, but one with several different discrete functions. It is thus analogous to the liver, in which the multiple metabolic pathways may be impaired to variable degrees, depending on the type of injury or disease. Despite these observations, the clinical impact of the findings has not been fully evaluated.

REABSORPTION

Reabsorption of water and solutes occurs throughout the nephron, whereas drug reabsorption occurs predominantly along the distal tubule and collecting tubules. Urine flow rate and physicochemical characteristics of the molecule influence these processes. Highly ionized compounds are not reabsorbed unless pH changes within the urine increase the fraction that is un-ionized, so that reabsorption may be facilitated.

INTACT NEPHRON HYPOTHESIS

The homeostasis afforded by the kidneys is affected by catecholamines, prostaglandins, renin, antidiuretic hormone, natriuretic hormone, and the number of functioning nephrons. The "intact nephron hypothesis" described by Bricker,[11] which was first published more than 30 years ago, proposes that kidney function of patients with renal disease is the net result of a reduced number of appropriately functioning nephrons. As the number of nephrons is reduced from the initial complement of 2 million, those that are unaffected compensate for those that are damaged by disease or toxic

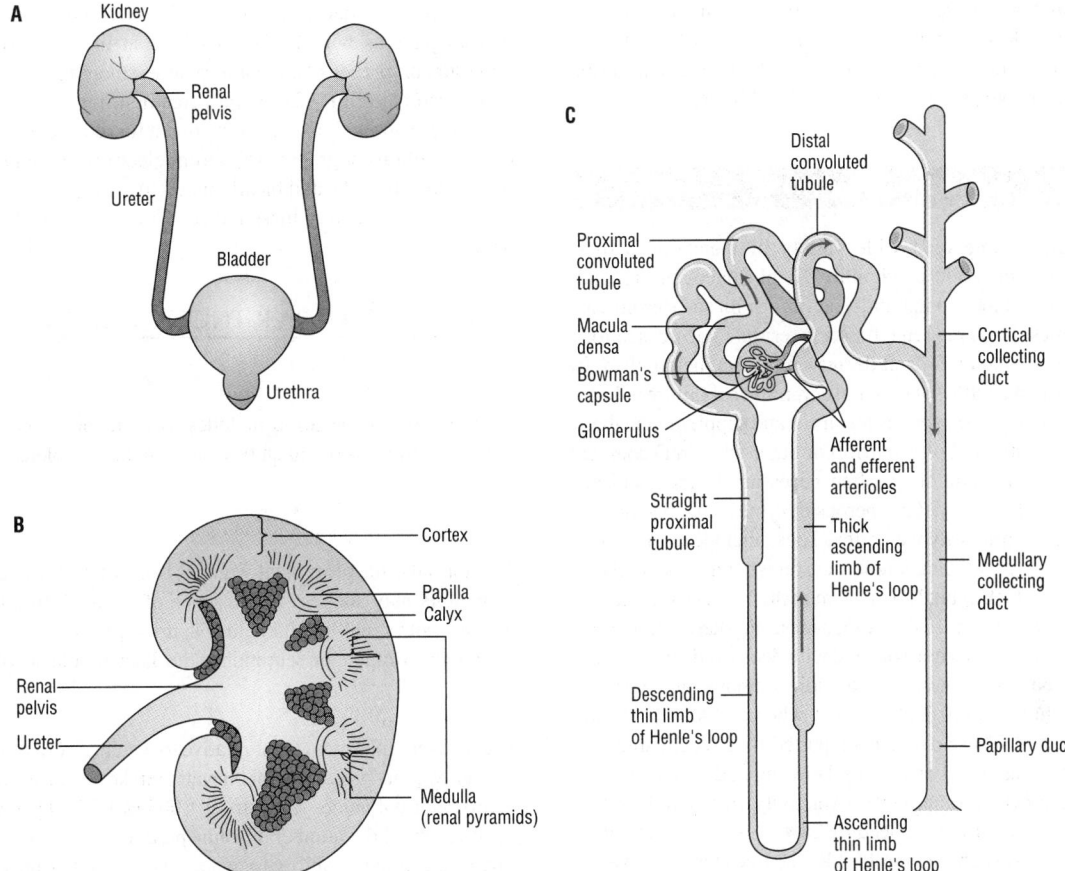

FIGURE 41-1. Structures of the (*A*) urinary system, (*B*) kidney, and (*C*) nephron, which is the functional unit of the kidney.

insult. The cornerstone of this hypothesis is that glomerulotubular balance is maintained, such that those nephrons capable of functioning will continue to perform in an appropriate fashion. As GFR declines, tubular reabsorption must decrease to allow for elimination of the solute load. Single nephron GFR (SNGFR) increases in the remaining nephrons, whereas the whole-kidney GFR represents the sum of the SNGFR of the remaining functional nephrons. Based on this, one would presume that a measure of one component of nephron function could be used as an estimate of all renal functions. This, indeed, has been and remains our clinical approach.

FILTRATION CAPACITY

It is recognized that GFR is dependent on numerous factors, one of which is protein load. Bosch[12] suggested that an appropriate measure of renal function should reflect the "filtration capacity" of the kidney, and not the "resting GFR." Subjects with normal renal function administered an oral or intravenous protein load prior to measurement of GFR have increased their GFR by as much as 50%.[12] As renal function declines, the kidneys compensate by increasing SNGFR. The renal reserve, the maximal degree by which GFR can be increased, usually declines and thus may be a complementary measure of renal function for these patients.

Quantification of renal function is not only an important diagnostic index, but it also serves as an important parameter for monitoring therapy directed at the etiology of the diminished function itself,

thereby allowing for objective measurement of the success or failure of treatment. Measurement of renal function also serves as a useful indicator of the ability of the kidneys to eliminate drugs from the body. Furthermore, alterations of drug distribution and metabolism are associated with the degree of renal function. See Chap. 48 for a discussion of pharmacokinetic changes in renal disease. Although several indices have been used for the quantification of renal function in the research setting, GFR, and more specifically creatinine clearance, are the primary markers of renal function in the clinical arena.[13–15]

ENDOCRINE FUNCTION

The kidney synthesizes and secretes many important hormones involved in maintaining homeostasis. Secretion of renin by the cells of the juxtaglomerular apparatus and production and metabolism of prostaglandins and kinins are among the kidney's endocrine functions. In response to decreased oxygen tension in the blood, erythropoietin (EPO) is produced and secreted by peritubular fibroblasts. Because these functions are related to renal mass, decreased endocrine activity is associated with the loss of viable EPO-producing cells. In the presence of nephropathy, secretion of EPO is impaired, leading to reduced red blood cell mass formation, normocytic anemia, and symptoms of reduced oxygen delivery to tissues such as fatigue, dyspnea, and angina (see Chap. 44). Renal anemia is clearly associated with comorbidities such as left ventricular hypertrophy, which is present in nearly 40% of CKD patients.[16] Here, renal hypoxia leads to the release of hypoxia-induced factors that cause EPO gene activation, tubular necrosis, apoptosis, or sublethal renal cell injury.[17]

METABOLIC FUNCTION

The kidneys are capable of a wide variety of metabolic activities, including the activation of vitamin D_3, gluconeogenesis, and metabolism of endogenous compounds such as insulin and steroids, as well as xenobiotics. Impaired renal function results in decreased formation of activated vitamin D_3 and decreased insulin metabolism. It is common for patients with diabetes and chronic renal failure to have reduced requirements for exogenous insulin,[18] and supplemental therapy with activated vitamin D_3 (calcitriol) or other vitamin D analogs (paricalcitol or doxercalciferol) is often necessary in the management of renal osteodystrophy.[19] Numerous enzymes have been identified in the kidneys, primarily the cortex. These include cytochrome P450, N-acetyltransferase, glutathione transferase, renal peptidases, and others.[20] The cytochrome P450 system in the kidneys is as active as that in the liver, when corrected for organ mass. Furthermore, the accumulation of uremic toxins is associated with decreased cytochrome activity for selected isoenzymes. In vitro studies demonstrate impaired function of cytochrome P450 3A4 and 2C9, whereas 1A2, 2C19, and 2D6 are not affected. These data are supported by a recent study in patients with end-stage renal disease by Dowling and colleagues. In this study hepatic cytochrome P450 3A activity (measured by the erythromycin breath test) was reduced by 28% ($p < 0.05$) compared to that of healthy age-matched controls.[21] Reversible metabolism may also be affected by renal disease when normal enzyme function is disrupted. This has been observed with clofibrate,[22] and may apply to other compounds eliminated by the same route, such as ketoprofen.[23] See Chap. 48 for a more detailed discussion.

QUALITATIVE AND SEMIQUANTITATIVE INDICES OF KIDNEY FUNCTION

Patients who develop renal disease remain relatively asymptomatic until impairment has progressed to the point that systemic manifestations and/or secondary complications become evident (Table 41–2).

Diabetes mellitus and hypertension are the two most common causes of end-stage kidney disease (ESKD), and as renal function declines, patients may experience development or exacerbation of hypertension, edema, electrolyte abnormalities, anemia, or other com-plications (see Chaps. 43 and 44). The NKF currently recommends that all patients with CKD, and those at increased risk for CKD, undergo comprehensive laboratory assessment for: (1) serum creatinine to estimate GFR, (2) albumin:creatinine ratio in a spot urine specimen, (3) examination of urine sediment for red and white blood cells, (4) renal ultrasonography, (5) serum electrolytes including sodium, potassium, chloride, and bicarbonate, (6) urine pH, and (7) urine specific gravity.[24] Each of these indices will be discussed in more detail below.

LABORATORY EVIDENCE FOR KIDNEY DISEASE

URINALYSIS

Examination of the urine includes assessment of its chemical and physical composition, most of which can be completed with dipstick testing.

pH

The normal urine pH typically ranges from 4.5 to 7.8, and an elevation above this may suggest the presence of urea-splitting bacteria.[25] In patients with renal tubular acidosis, urine pH is usually >5.5 due to impaired hydrogen ion secretion in the distal tubule or collecting duct.

Specific Gravity

The measure of urine weight relative to water ($H_2O = 1.00$) is its specific gravity and is dependent on water intake and urine-concentrating ability. Normal values range from 1.003 to 1.030. Osmolality, which is a measure of the number of solute particles, is a more accurate measure of the kidney's ability to make concentrated urine. Generally the two values are correlated; however, when large quantities of heavier molecules such as glucose are in the urine, the specific gravity may be elevated relative to the osmolality. These values are used in the assessment of urine concentrating ability and are most informative when interpreted along with the hydration status of the patient and plasma osmolality.[25]

Glucose

Glucose is normally absent in the urine, because the kidney normally completely reabsorbs all the glucose filtered at the glomerulus. In patients with plasma glucose concentrations that exceed the maximum threshold for glucose reabsorption (~180 mg/dL), glucosuria will be present. In the past, patients with diabetes mellitus would use the urine glucose level as a guide to insulin therapy. However, fingerstick methods for direct blood glucose measurements have now

TABLE 41–2. Presentation of Chronic Kidney Disease (CKD)

	Early CKD (Stages 1–2)	Late CKD (Stages 3–4)
General	The patient may not appear in distress	Patient may have edema
Symptoms	Not likely present	The patient may have fatigue, malaise, pruritus, nausea
Signs	Not likely present	May present with fluid retention, anemia, dyspnea, reduced urine output
Laboratory tests	Microalbuminuria	Persistent proteinuria
	Mildly-elevated S_{cr} and BUN	Reduced GFR or CL_{cr}
		Abnormal urinalysis
		Renal ultrasound shows reduced kidney mass

BUN, blood urea nitrogen; CL_{cr}, creatinine clearance; GFR, glomerular filtration rate; S_{cr}, serum creatinine concentration.

replaced the urine tests as a guide to therapy in most clinical settings.[26] Urine glucose testing still remains a valuable tool for the detection of diabetes.

Ketones

Acetoacetate and acetone are excreted in patients with diabetic ketoacidosis. They are also produced under conditions of fasting or starvation.

Nitrite

Nitrite is formed by conversion from nitrate by urinary bacteria. The presence of nitrite may indicate that the patient has a urinary tract infection.

Leukocyte Esterase

Leukocyte esterase is released from lysed granulocytes in the urine; its presence is suggestive of urinary tract infection. If the processing of the urine sample is delayed, a false-positive leukocyte esterase may be reported if the sample is contaminated.

Heme

The heme test indicates the presence of hemoglobin or myoglobin. A positive test without the presence of red blood cells suggests either red cell hemolysis or rhabdomyolysis.[25]

Protein or Albumin

Persistent proteinuria is now considered the principal marker of kidney damage.[24,25] Evaluation of proteinuria is needed to characterize the severity of CKD and to monitor the rate of disease progression. Under normal conditions, large quantities of plasma proteins pass through the glomerular capillaries but do not enter the urinary space. These proteins are retained by the glomerulus due to charge and size selectivity, preventing filtration of large proteins (>40 kDa) such as albumin and globulins. Smaller proteins (<20 kDa) pass across the capillary wall but are readily reabsorbed by the proximal tubule. Most healthy individuals excrete between 30 and 150 mg/day of total protein, consisting of approximately 30 mg/day of albumin. The remainder of the protein in the urine is secreted by the tubules (Tamm-Horsfall, IgA, and urokinase), or filtered by the glomerulus such as β_2-microglobulin, apoproteins, enzymes, and peptide hormones. Increased excretion of these low-molecular-weight proteins is considered a sensitive marker of tubulointerstitial disease.

Historically, the sulfosalicylic acid test was used as a crude measure of proteinuria. This test can be performed by adding five drops of 20% sulfosalicylic acid to 3 mL of urine in one test tube. The specimen tube is then visually compared with a tube of untreated urine held against a dark background, with the presence of turbidity indicating proteinuria.

More recently, dipstick tests to measure total protein and albumin have been developed to provide a semiquantitative measure of daily urine protein excretion. Here, urine proteins react with an indicator dye–impregnated test strip yielding a color change from yellow (negative) to green. False-positive results can occur in the presence of alkaline urine (pH >7.5), when the dipstick is immersed too long; in highly concentrated urine; with gross hematuria; in the presence of drugs such as penicillin, sulfonamides or tolbutamide; and with pus, semen, or vaginal secretions. False-negative results occur with dilute urine (specific gravity <1.015) and when proteinuria is caused by nonalbumin or low-molecular-weight proteins such as heavy or light chains or Bence Jones proteins. The results of most urine protein dipsticks are graded as negative (<10 mg/dL), trace (10 to 20 mg/dL), 1 + (30 mg/dL), 2 + (100 mg/dL), 3 + (300 mg/dL) or 4 + (>1,000

mg/dL). Portable desktop analyzers such as the Chemstrip 101 Urine Analyzer and Clinitek 50 Urine Chemistry Analyzer can also be used as an alternative to visual urinalysis test-strip evaluation.

All patients with CKD and those with risk factors should be tested for albuminuria using an albumin-specific dipstick test. Since most dipstick methods are not specific for albumin, newer tests for microalbuminuria (30 to 300 mg/day) should be employed.[27] Microalbuminuria test strips, such as the Chemstrip Micral-Test II strip, are optically read immunoassay-based methods. Here, the test strip is dipped into a urine sample and albumin present in the sample binds to gold-labeled antibodies. The detection field assumes a color ranging from white (0 mg/L) to red (100 mg/L).

In patients with a positive protein or albumin dipstick test, a 24-hour urine collection with measurement of albumin excretion can be used to further define the degree of proteinuria.

CLINICAL CONTROVERSY

In the past, measurement of the urinary protein excretion rate was accomplished using a 24-hour urine collection in patients at risk for CKD. Use of an untimed "spot" urine sample with either an albumin-specific dipstick or measurement of albumin:creatinine ratio is now recommended by some because it is more convenient than the extended-interval urine collection.

The 24-hour collection requires patient compliance and is being replaced by a similarly accurate but less cumbersome ratio of protein or albumin (mg) to creatinine (g) obtained from an untimed (spot) urine specimen.[28,29] The ratio is used to correct for changes in urine volume since creatinine production per day is constant in those with stable kidney function. The normal ratio is <30 mg albumin or 200 mg protein per gram of creatinine in the urine, with values between 30 and 300 mg albumin:1 g creatinine considered to be in the microalbuminuria range.[30] Positive test results should be confirmed, particularly in patients without an underlying cause for renal disease, such as diabetes or hypertension. Ruggenenti and associates[31] observed a positive correlation between the degree of proteinuria (using the spot morning protein:creatinine ratio) and rate of progression of renal disease in patients with nondiabetic chronic renal disease. For continued monitoring of proteinuria in CKD patients, the albumin:creatinine ratio is recommended. In patients with clinical proteinuria (albumin:creatinine ratio >500 mg/g), the protein:creatinine ratio can be used.

Microscopic Analysis of Urine

Formed elements that may be detected in the urine include erythrocytes and leukocytes, casts, and crystals. An important consideration in the assessment of hematuria is whether the cells are of renal origin. More than two cells per high-power field is abnormal, and dysmorphic cells suggest renal parenchymal origin, either because of damage as they pass through the glomerulus, or during exposure to the varying osmotic environment of the tubular lumen. White blood cells may be present in the urine in association with infection or inflammatory conditions, such as interstitial nephritis, and more than one cell per high-power field may be considered abnormal. For both red and white cells, contamination of the sample should also be considered, such as during menses or with inadequate sample collection. *Casts* are cylindrical forms composed of protein, with or without cells that take the shape of the collecting tubules, where they are formed. Casts without cells are called *hyaline casts* and consist of the Tamm-Horsfall mucoprotein secreted by the renal tubules. They are nonspecific and may appear in concentrated urine. In the presence of red or white blood cells, casts may be formed that include the cells, indicating that the cells were of renal origin. Solubility of the Tamm-Horsfall protein is increased as urine pH rises; therefore sample collection for casts should occur with the first morning void when the urine is most acidic. Otherwise casts may dissolve and elude detection.[25,32]

A variety of crystals may be present in the urine, including uric acid, calcium oxalate, calcium phosphate, calcium magnesium ammonium pyrophosphate, and cystine. Many of these have a unique crystalline form which permits them to be identified with microscopy.

SERUM OR BLOOD UREA NITROGEN

Amino acids metabolized to ammonia are subsequently converted in the liver to form urea, the production of which is dependent on protein availability (diet) and hepatic function. Renal handling of urea includes glomerular filtration followed by reabsorption of up to 50% of the filtered load in the proximal tubule. As urea is able to cross cell membranes by passive diffusion, its reabsorption rate is variable and dependent on the reabsorption of water. The excretion of urea may therefore be decreased under conditions of water conservation by the kidneys, although the GFR may be reduced only slightly. This condition is evident when a patient exhibits prerenal azotemia, or a greater increase in the blood urea nitrogen (BUN) than the serum creatinine. The normal BUN:creatinine ratio is 10 to 15:1, and an elevated ratio is suggestive of a decreased effective circulating volume, which stimulates increased water, and hence urea reabsorption.[21] Creatinine is not reabsorbed to any significant extent by the kidneys. Despite these limitations, the BUN is often used as a simple screening tool for the detection of renal dysfunction, but particularly in combination with the serum creatinine concentration.

SERUM CREATININE

Creatinine is the standard laboratory marker for the detection of kidney disease. The third National Health and Nutrition Examination Survey revealed a mean serum creatinine of 0.96 mg/dL in women, and 1.16 mg/dL in men in the United States.[33] Values were lower among Mexican-Americans and higher among non-Hispanic blacks. For all groups the serum creatinine increased with age. The report also noted that among noninstitutionalized adults, 10.9 million have a serum creatinine greater than 1.5 mg/dL, 3 million have a serum creatinine greater than 1.7 mg/dL, and 0.8 million have a serum creatinine >2 mg/dL. While the serum creatinine concentration alone is not an optimal measure of kidney function, it is often used as a marker for referral. There is presently no accepted single standard for an "abnormal" serum creatinine, as it is gender, race, and age dependent.

The concentration of creatinine in serum is a function of creatinine production and renal excretion. Creatinine is a product of creatine metabolism from muscle; therefore its production is directly dependent on muscle mass. At steady state, the "normal" serum creatinine concentration is approximately 0.5 to 1.5 mg/dL for males and females.[25] Creatinine is eliminated primarily by glomerular filtration, and as GFR declines, the serum creatinine concentration rises (Fig. 41–2).

Several methods may be used for the determination of the serum creatinine concentration, most of which are based on the nonspecific Jaffé reaction, a colorimetric method based on the reaction of creatinine with alkaline picrate. This nonspecific method also reacts with noncreatinine chromogens in the serum, which may result in a falsely high Jaffé serum creatinine concentration.[25] The noncreatinine chromogens are not present in the urine in sufficient quantities to interfere

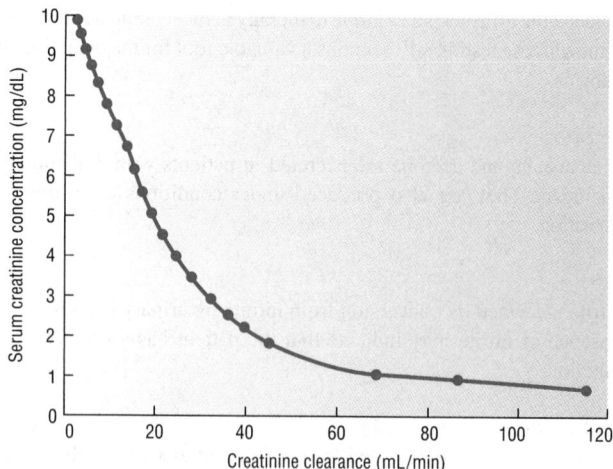

FIGURE 41–2. Relationship between serum creatinine and creatinine clearance.

with the creatinine measurement, which will be severalfold greater than the serum concentration. The impact of this interference is seen with the creatinine clearance (CL_{cr}) calculation:

$$CL_{cr} = (U_{cr} \times V)/(S_{cr} \times t)$$

where U_{cr} = urine creatinine concentration, V = urine volume, S_{cr} = serum creatinine concentration, and t = duration of the urine collection.

This "normal" interference results in an increase in the serum creatinine concentration of approximately 10%, and thereby the creatinine clearance would underestimate the GFR by 10%. In subjects with normal renal function, this tends to counterbalance the effect of the contribution of tubular secretion of creatinine, which increases urine creatinine by nearly 10%. Thus CL_{cr} may serve as a good measure of GFR in subjects with normal renal function. However, this false increase in serum creatinine becomes less noticeable as the true creatinine concentration rises, due to the increasing contribution of tubular secretion to the renal clearance of creatinine.[34] This becomes important when kidney function is reduced to less than 50% of normal.

Diabetic ketoacidosis may produce increased concentrations of acetoacetate, which serves as a chromophore in the Jaffé reaction, thereby increasing the serum creatinine concentration.[25] Other substances in the serum that affect this reaction include glucose, protein, pyruvate, fructose, uric acid, and ascorbic acid (Table 41–3).[25] In

TABLE 41–3. Factors That May Alter Creatinine Clearance Determinations

Analytical	Physiologic
Acetoacetate	Age, weight, gender
Ascorbic acid	Diet
Cephalosporins (cephalothin, cefazolin, cephalexin, cefoxitin, cefaclor, cephradine)	Diurnal variation
	Drugs (cimetidine, trimethoprim, probenecid)
Dobutamine	Exercise
Dopamine	
5-Flucytosine	
Fructose	
Glucose	
Protein	
Pyruvate	
Uric acid	

addition, some cephalosporin antibiotics are associated with a false increase in the serum creatinine concentration, including cephalothin, cefazolin, cephalexin, cefoxitin, cefaclor, and cephradine,[35] whereas other antibiotics such as the fluoroquinolones (ciprofloxacin, fleroxacin, lomefloxacin, ofloxacin, levofloxacin, sparfloxacin, and temafloxacin) do not produce a false elevation in serum creatinine.[36] The degree of interference is dependent on the serum concentration of the antibiotic, so blood samples for creatinine should be obtained when the antibiotic concentration is lowest (at the end of a dosing interval). These interferences are not observed when the serum creatinine is measured using an enzymatic technique. The antifungal agent 5-flucytosine causes an increase in the serum creatinine when measured using the Ektachem enzymatic system, but does not interact with the Jaffé method.[37] Daly and associates[38] reported a false-negative effect of dobutamine and dopamine on the serum creatinine value when measured using the Ektachem system. The interference is concentration dependent, and results in a 10% to 100% decrease of the serum creatinine concentration. The authors hypothesized that both drugs compete with the chromogenic dye for oxidation by hydrogen peroxide in a concentration-dependent manner. The problem is most evident when blood samples are contaminated with residual IV solution containing the interfering drug. These differences emphasize the need to standardize a method within the research or clinic setting, and to be aware of methods employed in the laboratory for the determination of creatinine concentrations.

Other compounds are known to interfere with the serum creatinine concentration through inhibition of the active tubular secretion of creatinine. Among these are cimetidine and trimethoprim, which compete for creatinine secretion by the cationic transport system.[25] Both trimethoprim and cimetidine demonstrate dose dependency with respect to competition with creatinine for secretion. Ranitidine, an H_2-receptor antagonist similar to cimetidine, was evaluated for its effect on creatinine clearance in 10 healthy subjects. There was no effect following single doses of 300 or 1200 mg as determined by the ratio of CL_{cr} to inulin clearance (CL).[39] Cimetidine, given as a single 400-mg dose in six of the same subjects, resulted in a reduction of the ratio of CL_{cr} to CL inulin from 1.30 to 1.03, without any change in CL inulin.

The serum creatinine concentration is dependent on the "input" function, or formation rate, and "output" function, or elimination rate. Its formation rate depends on the zero-order production from creatine metabolism, as well as input from other sources such as dietary intake.[40] Creatine metabolism is directly proportional to muscle mass; therefore individuals with more muscle mass have a higher serum creatinine concentration at any given degree of kidney function than those with less muscle mass. Exercise is associated with an increase of approximately 10% in the serum creatinine concentration. As the result of minimal muscle mass patients who are cachectic will have very low serum creatinine concentrations, as do those with spinal cord injuries.[41] Elderly patients and those with poor nutrition may also have low serum creatinine concentrations (<1 mg/dL) secondary to decreased muscle mass. Other factors that influence the serum creatinine concentration include the dietary intake of creatine. During the cooking of meat, some creatine is converted to creatinine, which is rapidly absorbed following ingestion.

Serum creatinine concentrations may rise as much as 50% within 2 hours of a meat meal and remain elevated for as long as 8 to 24 hours.[40] Ingestion of creatine as an ergogenic dietary supplement is currently popular. There are conflicting reports on the effect of creatine ingestion on the serum creatinine concentration. Poortsmans and Francaux[42] evaluated a short-term regimen of 20 g creatine per day for 5 days in healthy subjects, and reported no significant change

in the serum creatinine, creatinine excretion rate, or creatinine clearance. Robinson and associates,[43] however, reported a 25% to 40% increase in the serum creatinine concentration after ingestion of 20 g creatine per day for either 5 days or 8 weeks. The renal excretion rate of creatinine was not measured. The issue of whether creatine ingestion adversely affects kidney function was studied by Edmonds and coworkers.[44] They noted that creatine supplementation led to an increase in renal disease progression in a rat model for renal cystic disease, suggesting that creatine supplementation may be a risk factor in patients with preexisting renal disease. These conditions present a problem only when a single serum creatinine concentration is used to represent the entire 24-hour collection period, which is usually the case. An alternative is to obtain multiple samples and calculate the area under the serum concentration time curve and divide this by the collection time interval to obtain the average plasma creatinine concentration. This is rarely done in clinical practice, but points out the need to question patients regarding dietary intake for the 24 hours preceding the measurement of CL_{cr}.

Diurnal variation in serum creatinine concentration may also affect the accuracy of the CL_{cr} determination. Although the fluctuation is minimal, the observed peak plasma creatinine concentration generally occurs at approximately 7:00 PM, whereas the nadir is in the morning. To minimize this effect, the CL_{cr} is usually measured over a 24-hour period with the plasma creatinine obtained in the morning, as long as the patient has stable kidney function. Collection of urine remains a limiting factor in the 24-hour CL_{cr} because of incomplete collections and interconversion between creatinine and creatine that can occur if the urine is not maintained at a pH <6.

CYSTATIN C

The newest endogenous marker of renal function to be proposed is serum cystatin C, a 132-amino-acid (13.3-kDa) cysteine protease inhibitor. It is produced by all nucleated cells of the body and serum concentrations appear to be independent of gender, age, body mass, nutritional status, and acute inflammatory conditions.[45–47] Although it is freely filtered at the glomerulus, like other low-molecular-weight proteins it undergoes reabsorption and catabolism in the proximal tubule. Originally used in Europe, it has been recommended as a test of kidney function due to findings that serum concentrations were significantly correlated with GFR as well as serum creatinine.[45–47] The recent development of an automated immunoassay technique has led to suggested reference ranges of 0.70 to 1.38 mg/L in children over 1 year of age, and 0.54 to 1.21 mg/L in adults.[47] It may be a more sensitive indicator of reduced renal function than creatinine, so cystatin C may have future clinical utility in the assessment of renal function.[46,47] However, comparison of ^{125}I-iothalamate with serum creatinine and cystatin C showed that the serum creatinine began to increase when the GFR was 75 mL/min per 1.73 m^2 as compared to 88 mL/min per 1.73 m^2 for cystatin C.[45] Keevil and associates[48] reported that serum cystatin C had greater intra-individual variability than serum creatinine in healthy individuals, which may limit its use in longitudinal evaluations of renal function. In patients being treated for malignant disease, Page and coworkers[49] reported increased concentrations that were independent of CL_{cr}. In pediatric and adult renal transplant recipients, cystatin C concentrations were independent of GFR and weakly associated with measured creatinine clearance, possibly due to formation of cystatin-immunoglobulin complexes or reduced tubular catabolism.[50,51] These mixed observations suggest that cystatin C requires further evaluation in populations such as pediatrics, renal transplant, and CKD before it is accepted as a routine marker for renal function.

MEASUREMENT OF KIDNEY FUNCTION

The gold standard for the quantitative measure of kidney function is the GFR. However, protein intake such as oral protein loading or an infusion of amino acid solution may increase GFR.[12] As a result, inter- and intrasubject variability must be considered when it is used as a longitudinal marker of renal function. Dietary protein intake has been demonstrated to correlate with GFR in healthy subjects. Brändle and colleagues[52] evaluated renal function in four groups of healthy volunteers, each ingesting a diet controlled for protein over a 4-month period. The GFR was nonlinearly related to the urine nitrogen excretion, with an observed maximum of 181.7 mL/min at a urinary nitrogen excretion rate of 20 g/day, or 125 g/day protein intake. Subjects who are vegetarian will have a low GFR because of reduced dietary protein intake.

CLINICAL CONTROVERSY

Estimation of creatinine clearance in vegetarians is controversial. Some clinicians advocate use of the 24-hour creatinine clearance in these patients since this method is based on the renal clearance of creatinine. The six-variable Modification of Diet in Renal Disease (MDRD) study equation (see below), which incorporates nutritional parameters such as BUN and albumin, has been suggested as an alternative approach.

When challenged with a protein load, these same subjects are able to increase their GFR to the normal range.[12] Findings from the Nurses' Health Study[53] indicate that longitudinal changes in GFR are independent of the source of protein (nondairy animal, dairy, or vegetable) in women with normal renal function. However, women with mild renal insufficiency (GFR 71 ± 7 mL/min) who consumed the highest amount of protein (93 g/day) had a threefold greater risk of a ≥15-mL/min decline in GFR compared to the lowest protein-consuming group (60 g/day), and rates of decline were highest in those consuming nondairy animal protein. The increased GFR following a protein load is the result of renal vasodilation accompanied by increased renal plasma flow. The exact mechanism of the renal response to protein is not known, but it may be related to extrarenal factors such as glucagon, prostaglandins, and angiotensin II, or intrarenal mechanisms such as tubular transport and tubuloglomerular feedback.[54,55] Despite the evidence of a "renal reserve," standardized evaluation techniques have not been developed. Therefore assessment of the standard GFR measurement must consider the dietary protein status of the patient at the time of the study.

MEASUREMENT OF GLOMERULAR FILTRATION RATE

The GFR remains the single best index of functioning renal mass. As renal mass declines in the presence of age-related loss of nephrons or coexisting disease states such as hypertension or diabetes, there is a progressive decline in GFR. The GFR can be used to predict the time to onset of ESKD as well as the risk of complications of chronic kidney disease. Furthermore, accurate assessment of GFR in clinical practice allows proper dosing of drugs excreted renally in order to maximize therapeutic efficacy and avoid potential drug toxicity.

The GFR is expressed as the volume of plasma filtered across the glomerulus per unit time. The most commonly reported range of normal GFR values is 100 to 140 mL/min. For example, if the normal renal blood flow (RBF) were approximately 1 L/min, plasma volume was 60% of blood volume, and filtration fraction across the glomerulus was 20%, then the normal GFR would be approximately 120 mL/min.

Since GFR cannot be measured directly, clearance methods involving substances that freely diffuse across the glomerulus and into Bowman's capsule without additional clearance by tubular secretion or reduction by reabsorption are required. Additionally, the substance should not be susceptible to metabolism within renal tissues and should not alter renal function. Given these conditions, the GFR is equivalent to the renal clearance of the solute marker:

$$\text{GFR} = \text{renal CL} = (A_e)/\text{AUC}_{0-t}$$

where renal CL is renal clearance of the marker; A_e is the amount of marker excreted in a specified period of time, t; and AUC_{0-t} is the area under the plasma concentration time curve of the marker.

Under steady-state conditions, the expression simplifies to:

$$\text{GFR} = \text{renal CL} = (A_e)/[(C_{ss}) \times t]$$

where C_{ss} is the steady-state plasma concentration of the marker.

The GFR marker is most often administered as a combination of an IV loading dose and a continuous infusion. Here a loading dose is administered followed by a maintenance infusion designed to achieve the desired target plasma concentration. Following a 60-minute equilibration period, sequential measurements of clearance are made over three periods of 30 to 60 minutes each. Urine is collected, and blood samples bracket each collection period. It is necessary to maintain adequate hydration during the test because GFR is dependent on renal blood flow, and hydration assures adequate urine output during the procedure. A relatively constant urine flow will decrease the variability among repeated measurements, and should be within the range of 1 to 10 mL/min. An initial water load of 10 to 15 mL/kg body weight will usually initiate a diuresis, and additional water equal to 50% to 70% of urine output during the previous interval should be given orally or intravenously to maintain urinary output. It is essential to ensure complete bladder emptying to minimize variability of results. Alternative clearance calculation methods should be employed for patients with benign prostatic hypertrophy and neurogenic bladder.

This continuous infusion method can also be employed without urine collection, and plasma clearance is then calculated as CL = infusion rate/C_{ss}. Requirements of this method include steady-state plasma concentrations and accurate measurement of infusate concentrations. Plasma clearance can also be determined following a single-dose intravenous injection with multiple samples of blood taken to estimate the area under the curve ($\text{AUC}_{0-\infty}$). Here clearance is calculated as CL = dose/AUC. These plasma clearance methods commonly yield clearance values 10% to 15% higher than urine collection methods.[56,57]

Several markers have been used for the measurement of GFR and include both exogenous and endogenous compounds. Those administered as exogenous agents, such as inulin, iothalamate, iohexol, and radioisotopes, require specialized administration techniques and detection methods for the quantitation of function, but generally provide a more accurate measure of GFR. Methods that employ endogenous compounds such as creatinine require less technical expertise, but produce results with greater variability.[35] The marker of choice depends on the purpose and cost of the test; research protocols will generally use more accurate tests than those used in clinical settings (Table 41–4).

TABLE 41-4. Sensitivity and Clinical Utility of Renal Function Tests

	Accuracy	Clinical Utility	Cost
Inulin clearance	++++	+	$$$$
Radiolabeled markers	+++	+	$$$
Nonisotopic contrast agents	+++	++	$$$
Creatinine clearance	++	+++	$$
Serum creatinine	+	++++	$

+, least acceptable; ++, adequate; +++, better; ++++, best.

INULIN CLEARANCE

Inulin is a relatively large molecule (5200 daltons) and has the necessary characteristics to serve as a marker for the measurement of GFR. Inulin is a fructose polysaccharide obtained from the tubers of the Jerusalem artichoke, dahlia, and chicory plants. It is not bound to plasma proteins, is freely filtered at the glomerulus, is not secreted or reabsorbed, and is not metabolized by the kidney.[35] The volume of distribution of inulin approximates extracellular volume, or 20% of ideal body weight. Because it is eliminated by glomerular filtration, its elimination half-life is dependent on renal function and is approximately 1.3 hours in subjects with normal renal function. Measurement of plasma and urine inulin concentrations using high-performance liquid chromatography (HPLC) was recently described. Glucose and drugs commonly administered to patients with renal disease, including corticosteroids, calcitriol, azathioprine, nifedipine, and atenolol, did not interfere with the assay.[58] Sinistrin, another polyfructosan, is handled in the same fashion as inulin in humans. It is filtered at the glomerulus and not secreted or reabsorbed to any significant extent. It is a naturally occurring substance derived from the root of the North African vegetable red squill, *Urginea maritima*. Its primary difference from inulin is its greater degree of water solubility. Whereas inulin must be boiled to solubilize it, sinistrin is soluble at room temperature. Assay methods for sinistrin have been described using enzymatic procedures, as well as HPLC.[59-61]

IOTHALAMATE CLEARANCE

Alternatives have been sought for inulin as a marker for GFR because of the problems of intermittent availability, high cost, sample preparation, and assay variability. Iothalamate is an iodine-containing radiocontrast agent that is available in both radiolabeled (125I) and nonradiolabeled forms. This agent is handled in a manner similar to that of inulin, and appears to be freely filtered at the glomerulus but does not undergo substantial tubular secretion or reabsorption.[25] The nonradiolabeled form is most widely used to measure GFR in ambulatory and research settings, and can safely be administered by IV bolus, continuous infusion, or subcutaneous injection with minimal biohazardous waste.[62] Plasma and urine iothalamate concentrations can be measured using HPLC methods.[63] Plasma iothalamate clearance methods that do not require urine collections have been shown to be highly correlated with iothalamate renal clearance, with a positive bias of approximately 10 mL/min. Here, corrected plasma clearance provided a good estimate of GFR that is well suited for longitudinal evaluations of renal function.[64]

IOHEXOL CLEARANCE

Iohexol, a nonionic, low osmolar, iodinated contrast agent, has also been used for the determination of GFR. It is eliminated almost entirely by glomerular filtration, and plasma and renal clearance values are similar.[65] Rocco and associates[66] compared iohexol plasma clearance with 125I-iothalamate renal clearance and demonstrated a strong correlation ($r = 0.95$) between the two tests: CL iohexol = 0.90 CL iothalamate + 6.8 mL/min. The plasma iohexol assay was performed using a reverse-phase HPLC method. Lundqvist and colleagues[67] evaluated a single-sample plasma clearance calculation method using iohexol compared to 51Cr-ethylenediaminetetraacetic acid (EDTA) and demonstrated similar results ($r = 0.918$). These data support iohexol as a suitable alternative marker for the measurement of GFR. Following iohexol administration, a single plasma sample can be used to quantify renal function, provided sufficient time has elapsed since injection in patients with a reduced GFR—more than 24 hours if GFR is less than 20 mL/min.[65] Iohexol has also been assessed for potential renal toxicity in a population of 100 patients, 63 of whom had renal insufficiency. There were no significant changes in renal function as assessed by the serum creatinine concentration and urine protein excretion for up to 1 week after the study.[68]

RADIOLABELED MARKERS

The GFR has also been quantified using radiolabeled markers, such as 125I-iothalamate (614 daltons, radioactive half-life of 60 days), 99mTc-diethylenetriamine pentaacetic acid (DTPA, 393 daltons, radioactive half-life of 6.03 hours), and 51Cr-EDTA (292 daltons, radioactive half-life of 27 days).[69] These relatively small molecules are minimally bound to plasma proteins and do not undergo tubular secretion or reabsorption to any significant degree. 125I-iothalamate and 99mTc-DTPA are used in the United States, whereas 51Cr-EDTA is used extensively in Europe. An advantage of using radiolabeled markers relates to their diagnostic ability to determine the individual contribution to overall renal function of each kidney.[70] Various protocols exist for the administration of these markers and subsequent determination of GFR using both plasma and renal clearance methods. The nonrenal clearance of these agents appears to be low (3 to 8 mL/min), suggesting that plasma clearance is an acceptable technique except in patients with severe renal insufficiency (GFR <30 mL/min). Indeed, high correlations between renal clearance among radiolabeled markers has been demonstrated.[63,64] Morton and coworkers[71] recently demonstrated that 99mTc-DTPA plasma clearance and 131I-iothalamate renal clearance were highly correlated in patients with clearance values >20 mL/min: CL DTPA = 0.943 CL iothalamate + 1.12 mL/min ($r = 0.983$). Although total radioactive exposure to patients is usually minimal, disadvantages of using radiolabeled markers include the requirement for radiation safety oversight and biohazard waste disposal.

ESTIMATION OF GFR

A series of equations proposed by Levey and associates[72] may be used to estimate GFR in selected patient populations.

These equations were derived from multiple regression analysis of data obtained from patients enrolled in part of the Modification of Diet in Renal Disease Study (MDRD). Of the 1628 patients enrolled in the baseline phase of the study (mean GFR = 40 mL/min per 1.73 m^2), 1070 were randomly assigned to a training sample, with the remaining 558 included in the validation sample. The initial regression model yielded the following six-variable equation:

$$GFR = 170 \times (Pl_{cr})^{-0.999} \times [Age]^{-0.176} \times [0.762 \text{ if patient is female}]$$
$$\times [1.180 \text{ if patient is black}] \times [SUN]^{-0.170} \times [Alb]^{0.318}$$

where Pl_{cr} = plasma creatinine, SUN = serum urea nitrogen concentration, and Alb = serum albumin concentration. Comparison of various prediction equations showed that the new equation (r = 0.95) provided a more precise estimate of GFR than measured CL_{cr} (r = 0.93) or the CG method (r = 0.92) in the MDRD population. More recent analysis has shown mixed results. In renal transplant patients with severe renal insufficiency ($CL_{cr} < 30$ mL/min per 1.73 m^2), the MDRD equation was highly correlated with mean CL_{cr} and urea clearances, less biased, and more precise than CG.[73] However, this equation was less accurate than CG in healthy subjects, diabetic patients with normal GFRs (88 to 182 mL/min per 1.73m^2), and healthy potential kidney donors.[74,75] In cirrhotic patients being evaluated for liver transplant (GFR 58 ± 5.1 mL/min per 1.73 m^2) both the MDRD and CG equations significantly overestimated GFR by 30% to 50%, and were imprecise estimates of GFR in liver disease patients before and after liver transplantation.[76,77] In a small study of elderly subjects (age > 68 years) with mild to moderate CKD (GFR 53 ± 18 mL/min per 1.73 m^2), the MDRD equation was slightly positively biased compared to CG (8% vs.–10%), but precision was similar between methods relative to measured GFR. Beddhu and associates[78] reported that the MDRD equation, like the CG method, is dependent on creatinine production and is susceptible to bias in malnourished patients with ESRD.

CLINICAL CONTROVERSY

The MDRD equation was derived from a study evaluating GFR in patients with CKD (GFR <90 mL/min). Some practitioners are advocating the use of this equation in patients without CKD, although it appears to have a weaker correlation with GFR than the Cockcroft-Gault equation. Therefore current evidence suggests that the MDRD equation should be reserved for patients with GFR <90 mL/min.

Recently,[24] a modified four-variable version of the original MDRD equation has been proposed for predicting GFR:

$$GFR = 186 \times (Pl_{cr})^{-1.154} \times (Age)^{-0.203} \times (0.742 \text{ if patient is female})$$
$$\times (1.210 \text{ if patient is black})$$

This equation, based on plasma creatinine, age, sex, and race, has been validated in the MDRD study sample, and is now recommended by the NKF for estimating GFR in patients with CKD and a GFR <90 mL/min per 1.73 m^2 in the updated NKF K/DOQI guidelines. The accuracy of these MDRD equations in estimating GFR in individuals with normal renal function; those with diabetes; pediatric, elderly, and obese patients; and for drug dosage adjustment requires further evaluation.

CLINICAL CONTROVERSY

Drug dose individualization is often required in patients with CKD. The drug product label typically includes a dose adjustment table based on the patient's estimated CL_{cr} using the Cockcroft-Gault method. Although some hospital laboratories are now reporting MDRD GFR values (see below), its use for drug dose adjustments for the present time has not been evaluated.

MEASURED CREATININE CLEARANCE

Despite the common use of a measured (24-hour) CL_{cr} to estimate GFR, it remains a controversial measurement. Short-duration witnessed CL_{cr} correlates with iothalamate clearance performed using the single-injection technique. In a multicenter study[79] of 136 patients with type I diabetic nephropathy, GFR was assessed using duplicate serum creatinine and 24-hour urine collection, the mean of four iothalamate clearance periods by single-injection technique during water diuresis, and CL_{cr}. CL_{cr} was also estimated for each patient using the Cockcroft-Gault method,[80] corrected for weight and gender. The simultaneous iothalamate and CL_{cr} were 78 ± 35 and 86 ± 35 mL/min, respectively, while the separate 24-hour CL_{cr} was 75 ± 33 mL/min. The Cockcroft-Gault estimate was 79 ± 29 mL/min. Using CL iothalamate as the standard, the correlation coefficient values for the simultaneous CL_{cr}, 24-hour CL_{cr}, and Cockcroft-Gault CL_{cr} were 0.90, 0.70, and 0.82, respectively, indicating increased variability with the 24-hour clearance determination. It was not stated whether the 24-hour CL_{cr} measurements were performed as inpatient or ambulatory procedures.[79] In a selected group of 110 patients, measurement of a 4-hour CL_{cr} during water diuresis provided the best estimate of the GFR as determined by the CL iothalamate. Furthermore, the ratio of CL_{cr} to CL iothalamate did not appear to increase as the GFR decreased. These data suggest that a short collection period with a water diuresis may be the best method for estimation of GFR by creatinine clearance.[79]

Creatinine is eliminated by both glomerular filtration and tubular secretion. Tubular secretion augments the filtered creatinine by about 10% in subjects with normal kidney function. If the nonspecific Jaffé reaction is used, which overestimates the serum creatinine concentration by about 10% because of the noncreatinine chromogens, then the creatinine clearance is a very good measure of GFR in patients with normal kidney function. Tubular secretion, however, increases to as much as 100% in patients with renal insufficiency.[34] As renal impairment develops, the remaining nephrons hypertrophy, and the degree of tubular secretion decreases disproportionately (less than) to the decrease in filtration. The result is an overestimation of creatinine clearance as a function of GFR assessed by using inulin clearance. Bauer and associates[34] assessed creatinine clearance as a function of inulin clearance in 123 subjects with various degrees of kidney function. Using a specific assay for the measurement of creatinine, the ratio of CL_{cr} exceeded CL inulin by 14%, which suggested that 14% of the creatinine was eliminated by secretion. The CL_{cr}:CL inulin ratio in subjects with mild impairment was 1.20; for moderate impairment, it was 1.87; and for severe impairment, it was 2.32. Thus creatinine clearance is a poor indicator of GFR in patients with moderate to severe renal insufficiency.

Creatinine is secreted via the organic cationic pathway, which can be blocked by the coadministration of drugs that compete for the same secretory path, such as cimetidine and trimethoprim. Shemesh and colleagues[81] studied the effect of an infusion of cimetidine on the tubular secretion of creatinine. The ratio of CL_{cr}:CL inulin was reduced from 1.67 ± 0.10 to 1.16 ± 0.06 within 80 minutes of the start of the cimetidine infusion with no effect on CL inulin. Roubenoff and coworkers[82] evaluated the potential role of oral cimetidine to improve the accuracy and precision of creatinine clearance as an indicator of GFR. Thirteen patients with lupus nephritis and 24-hour CL_{cr} ranging from 24 to 115.3 mL/min were given 400 mg of cimetidine orally 4 times daily for 2 days before and during a 24-hour CL_{cr} determination. A simultaneous 4-hour ^{99m}Tc-DTPA and CL_{cr} were also determined. Cimetidine reduced the CL_{cr}:CL DTPA ratio from 1.33 with placebo to 1.07 with cimetidine treatment ($p < .05$). No adverse effects were observed from the 2-day cimetidine treatment. Zaltzman and associates[83] administered cimetidine, 800 mg as a single dose, 1 hour prior to a 3-hour timed collection for creatinine and ^{125}I-iothalamate clearances. The CL_{cr}:CL iothalamate ratio was reduced from 1.53 ± 1.02 to 1.12 ± 0.02, and the authors suggest that this method effectively inhibited the tubular secretion of creatinine. Van Acker and coworkers[84] demonstrated similar results using multiple doses, although they noted a dose dependency in the effect of cimetidine; subjects with higher renal cimetidine clearance required larger cimetidine doses for complete blockade of creatinine tubular secretion. A single oral dose of cimetidine, 800 mg, should provide adequate blockade of creatinine secretion to improve the use of the creatinine clearance measurement to estimate GFR.

ESTIMATION OF CREATININE CLEARANCE

Several investigators have developed mathematical relationships between various patient factors as a means to estimate CL_{cr} when urine is unavailable (Table 41–5). These factors include age, gender, weight, and serum creatinine concentration. Perhaps the most widely used of these estimators is the one developed by Cockcroft and Gault,[80] which identified age and body mass as factors that significantly improved the estimate of CL_{cr}. Their relationship was based on

observations of 249 male patients with stable kidney function whose 24-hour creatinine excretion was >10 mg/kg, except for 23 patients who were included because their 24-hour urine volume was >500 mL. Creatinine clearance ranged from 11 mL/min to normal. Creatinine production (P_{cr}, in mg/kg per day) and excretion significantly decreased with increasing age for males ($P_{cr} = 28-[0.2 \times age]$) and females ($P_{cr} = 0.8 \times P_{cr}$ males). Based on the usual CL_{cr} formula and the relationship of creatinine excretion to age, they derived the following formula to estimate CL_{cr}:

$$CL_{cr} \, (mL/min) = [(140 - age) \times ABW]/(S_{cr} \times 72)$$

where age is expressed in years, S_{cr} is the serum creatinine in mg/dL, and ABW is the actual body weight in kg. For females, the result is multiplied by 0.85. For individuals weighing more than 30% above their ideal body weight (IBW), it is recommended that IBW be used in place of ABW,[85] where:

$$IBW \, (kg, males) = 50 + 2.3 \, (height \, in \, inches > 60)$$

$$IBW \, (kg, females) = 45 + 2.3 \, (height \, in \, inches > 60)$$

An alternative approach for estimating CL_{cr} (mL/min) in obese patients is the Salazar-Corcoran equation:[86]

$$Men: CL_{cr} = [(137 - age)] \times [(0.285 \times ABW)$$
$$+ (12.1 \times height^2)]/(51 \times S_{cr})$$

$$Women: CL_{cr} = [(146 - age)] \times [(0.287 \times ABW)$$
$$+ (9.74 \times height^2)]/(60 \times S_{cr})$$

where ABW is actual body weight in kilograms, and height is the height in meters. This equation has been shown to be unbiased and superior to the CG equation in obese individuals.[85,86]

Luke and associates[87] evaluated the ability of the CG method and four other methods to predict CL_{cr}, with inulin clearance being considered the standard measure of GFR. Simultaneous inulin and creatinine clearances, and a 24-hour ambulatory CL_{cr} were conducted in 109 patients. The simultaneously determined inulin and creatinine clearances correlated best ($r = 0.92$), and the CL_{cr} overestimated CL inulin by approximately 15% due to tubular secretion of creatinine. The correlation coefficient between CL inulin and 24-hour ambulatory CL_{cr} was 0.71. For the five calculated clearances, CG and the Mawer[88] method correlated the best with inulin clearance. The CG method showed a linear relationship with CL inulin equal to 1.121 of CL_{cr} plus 20.6 mL/min ($r = 0.81$), whereas for Mawer the relationship was CL inulin equal to 1.051 of CL_{cr} plus 18.3 mL/min ($r = 0.81$). The calculated CL_{cr} values from CG and Mawer both appeared to correlate well with the ambulatory and 4-hour CL_{cr}, but the regressions were not reported. Based on their findings, Luke and associates[87] propose continued use of the CG or Mawer method for rapid estimation of CL_{cr} in patients with stable kidney function. The other methods, of Jelliffe[89,90] and of Hull and colleagues,[91] consistently underestimated the CL_{cr}. As kidney function declined, there was an increase in the fraction of creatinine eliminated by secretion as measured by the CL_{cr}:CL inulin ratio, consistent with earlier reports. This limitation should be taken into consideration when attempting to use CL_{cr} for the estimation of renal function and the individualization of drug dosage regimens. Gault and coworkers[92] also evaluated the performance of the CG estimator of renal function compared with inulin and ^{99m}Tc-DTPA. Except for conditions of unstable kidney function, it performed similarly to the 24-hour creatinine clearance method.

TABLE 41–5. Equations for the Estimation of Creatinine Clearance in Adults with Stable Renal Function

Cockcroft and Gault[80]	Men: $CL_{cr} = (140 - age) \, ABW/(S_{cr} \times 72)$ Women: $CL_{cr} \times 0.85$
Jelliffe[89]	Men: $CL_{cr} = (100/S_{cr}) - 12$ Women: $CL_{cr} = (80/S_{cr}) - 7$
Jelliffe[90]	Men: $CL_{cr} = 98 - [0.8 \, (age - 20)]/S_{cr}$ Women: $CL_{cr} \times 0.9$
Mawer et al[88]	Men: IBW $[29.3 - (0.203 \times age)]$ $[1 - (0.03 \times S_{cr})]/(14.4 \times S_{cr})$ Women: IBW $[25.3 - (0.175 \times age)]$ $[1 - (0.03 \times S_{cr})]/(14.4 \times S_{cr})$
Hull et al[91]	Men: $CL_{cr} = [(145 - age)/S_{cr}] - 3$ Women: $CL_{cr} \times 0.85$
Levey et al (MDRD)[72]	GFR $= 170 \times (S_{cr})^{-0.999} \times (age)^{-0.176} \times$ $[0.762 \, if \, patient \, is \, female] \times [1.180 \, if$ patient is black] $\times [SUN]^{-0.170} \times [Alb]^{0.318}$
Levey et al (MDRD)[24]	GFR $= 186 \times (S_{cr})^{-1.154} \times (Age)^{-0.203} \times$ $(0.742 \, if \, patient \, is \, female) \times (1.210 \, if$ patient is black)

Alb, serum albumin concentration (g/dL); CL_{cr}, creatinine clearance in mL/min; IBW, ideal body weight (kg); S_{cr}, serum or plasma creatinine (mg/dL); SUN, serum urea nitrogen concentration (mg/dL).

Patients undergoing screening for participation in the African-American Study of Kidney Disease and Hypertension were evaluated for kidney function based on an estimated CL_{cr} compared with the simultaneous CL_{cr} and ^{125}I-iothalamate, and 24-hour CL_{cr}.[93] The simultaneous CL_{cr} provided the best estimate of GFR. The CG method was the preferred method for estimation of GFR, based on performance and ease of use. This method was noted to underestimate the GFR by 9%, perhaps because of the increased excretion rate of creatinine by black patients.[93,94]

Administration of cimetidine has also resulted in improved performance of CG to predict GFR. Ixkes and associates[95] gave patients three 800-mg doses of cimetidine in 24 hours, and measured creatinine plasma levels from 3 to 7 hours following the final dose. During this 4-hour period, the CL iothalamate was used to measure the GFR. The CG calculations were performed with the plasma creatinine measurement 3 hours after the last dose of cimetidine. The ratio of the CG-estimated CL_{cr}:CL iothalamate decreased from 1.28 ± 0.21 to 0.98 ± 0.11 in the presence of cimetidine.

SPECIAL POPULATIONS

Assessment of Renal Function In Liver Disease

CL_{cr} estimation in patients with liver disease is problematic. Orlando and coworkers[96] evaluated 10 healthy subjects, 10 patients with mild liver disease, and 10 with severe liver disease, and observed a measured CL_{cr}:CL inulin ratio of 1.05, 1.03, and 1.04 for each group, respectively. However, when the CL_{cr} of patients with severe liver disease was estimated using the CG equation the resultant ratio (CL_{cr} using CG:CL inulin) was 1.23. Lam and associates[97] likewise noted an overprediction by CG of the measured CL_{cr} in patients with severe disease, by 40% to 100%.

Studies of renal function in patients with severe hepatic disease and concomitant renal disease confirm the earlier observations of Hull and colleagues[91] and Caregaro and associates,[98] who reported that measured CL_{cr} overestimated GFR by 50% in patients with hepatic disease, likely due to increased tubular secretion of creatinine. DeSanto and coworkers[99] studied 19 patients with mild liver disease whose inulin and creatinine clearances were 90 ± 4.4 and 122 ± 7 mL/min per 1.73 m^2, respectively. The degree of overestimation of GFR by creatinine clearance was inversely correlated with GFR ($r = 0.452$; $p < .04$). Thus measurement of renal function in patients with hepatic disease should be performed by using a method that is specific for glomerular filtration, not creatinine clearance.

Other Special Populations

Davis and Chandler[100] confirmed the accuracy of the CG equation to predict CL_{cr} in trauma patients with stable kidney function, and Thakur and colleagues[41] demonstrated its successful utility in 42 paraplegic subjects. Renal transplant recipients are frequently monitored for renal function, as numerous complications may occur during the life of the allograft. Goerdt and associates[101] assessed the bias and precision with which several nomographic methods predicted GFR (iohexol clearance) in 127 transplant patients with stable kidney function. The CG method performed poorly, overestimating iohexol clearance. This is expected, as iohexol clearance provides a true measure of GFR, whereas the CG CL_{cr} estimate is falsely high because of the tubular secretion of creatinine. Schuck and coworkers[102] compared the CG method with CL sinistrin, an accurate measure of GFR. The clearance of sinistrin was significantly overestimated by the CG method. These investigators noted significant variability in CG estimates of GFR and concluded that it was an unreliable predictor of

GFR in this patient population. Huang and associates[103] reported the inability of several CL_{cr} equations to predict renal function in hospitalized patients with advanced human immunodeficiency virus disease. All methods, including CG, Jelliffe, and Mawer, overestimated the measured 24-hour CL_{cr}. The reasons for the poor predictability of these methods is unclear, although 24-hour collection methods often yield highly variable results because of inadequate urine collection.

Renal function assessment during pregnancy is usually performed using a 24-hour creatinine clearance determination. Quadri and colleagues[104] evaluated the CG method during each trimester in 34 pregnant women and compared these estimates with the measured 24-hour CL_{cr}. Prepregnancy weights were used throughout the study for the CG method, and results correlated well with those for the measured clearance ($r^2 = 0.76$). The maximal CL_{cr} occurred during the second trimester for both methods.

Unstable Renal Function

Patients with unstable kidney function present a unique situation because serum creatinine values are changing, and steady state cannot be assumed when estimating CL_{cr}. It can take several days for serum creatinine values to reach steady state in early acute renal failure, but this time can be reduced when renal function is improving. In patients with previously normal renal function, a change in the serum creatinine concentration of more than 50% over a period of 1 day is suggestive of unstable renal function. In patients with preexisting CKD ($S_{cr} > 2$ mg/dL), an increase in serum creatinine of more than 1.0 mg/dL over a 24- to 48-hour period indicates the presence of acute renal failure. Table 41–6 lists several equations that are commonly used to estimate CL_{cr} in patients with acute renal failure.[105–107] However, a rigorous evaluation of the accuracy and precision of each of these proposed methods is lacking, in part due to the absence of measured creatinine clearance and inability to accurately measure GFR in the acute care setting. The equation proposed by Jelliffe is a revised dynamic model of creatinine kinetics based on theoretical estimates of creatinine production and adjusted for age and changes in serum creatinine. However, its ability to predict changes in drug clearance (and dose adjustments) has not been evaluated. In the acute setting, factors previously discussed that may alter the serum creatinine concentration must be evaluated to avoid misinterpretation. It is ultimately most important to recognize that renal function in patients with acute renal failure is generally markedly lower than one would estimate using steady-state methods.

CLINICAL CONTROVERSY

Serum creatinine values can fluctuate widely in patients with unstable renal function. Although some practitioners advocate use of the Cockcroft-Gault equation using the highest of the two serum creatinine values, most recommend calculation of CL_{cr} using either the Brater or Jelliffe equations.

Inappropriate use of the Cockcroft-Gault equation can significantly overestimate the value of CL_{cr} when compared to equations that are designed to account for changes in serum creatinine in patients with unstable renal function. Table 41–7 illustrates the variability in the CL_{cr} values when three different equations are used to estimate CL_{cr} in patients with decreasing or improving renal function.

Kidney Function in Children

Kidney function in the neonate is difficult to assess because of difficulty in urine and blood collection, the frequent presence of a

TABLE 41–6. Equations for the Estimation of Creatinine Clearance in Adults with Unstable Renal Function

Reference	Units	Equations Males	Equations Females
Jelliffe[105]	mL/min per 1.73 m²	$E^{ss} = wt^a[29.3 - 0.203\,(age)]$ $E^{ss}_{corr} = E^{ss}[1.035 - 0.0337\,(S_{cr})]$ $E = E^{ss}_{corr} - \dfrac{[4wt^a(S_{cr_2} - S_{cr_1})]}{\Delta t\,day}$ $CL_{cr} = \dfrac{E}{14.4(S_{cr})}$	$E^{ss} = wt^a[25.1 - 0.175\,(age)]$ $E^{ss}_{corr} = E^{ss}[1.035 - 0.0337\,(Scr)]$ $E = E^{ss}_{corr} - \dfrac{[4wt^a(S_{cr_2} - S_{cr_1})]}{\Delta t\,day}$ $CL_{cr} = \dfrac{E}{14.4(S_{cr})}$
Chiou et al[106]	mL/min	$V_d = 0.6\,L\,(wt^a)$ $CL_{cr} = \dfrac{2[28 - 0.2\,(age)]}{14.4(S_{cr_1} + S_{cr_2})}$ $+ \dfrac{2[V_d(S_{cr_1} - S_{cr_2})]}{(S_{cr_1} + S_{cr_2})\,\Delta t\,min} - [CrCl^{NR} \times wt^a]$	$V_d = 0.6\,L\,(wt^a)$ $CL_{cr} = \dfrac{2\,wt^a[22.4 - 0.16\,(age)]}{14.4(S_{cr_1} + S_{cr_2})}$ $+ \dfrac{2[V_d(S_{cr_1} - S_{cr_2})]}{(S_{cr_1} + S_{cr_2})\,\Delta t\,min} - [CrCl^{NR} \times wt^a]$
Brater[107]	mL/min per 70 kg	$CL_{cr} = \dfrac{[293 - 2.03\,(age)] \times [1.035 - 0.01685\,(S_{cr_1} + S_{cr_2})]}{(S_{cr_1} + S_{cr_2})}$ $+ \dfrac{49(S_{cr_1} - S_{cr_2})}{(S_{cr_1} + S_{cr_2})\Delta t\,day}$	$CL_{cr} = $ Male value $\times\ 0.86$

[a]Use ideal body weight (IBW) if weight >30% above IBW.
CL_{cr}, creatinine clearance; $CrCl^{NR}$, nonrenal clearance of creatinine = 0.048 mL/min per kg; E, creatinine excretion; E^{ss}, steady-state creatinine excretion; E^{ss}_{corr}, corrected steady-state creatinine excretion; Δt day, time in days between S_{cr_1} and S_{cr_2}; Δt min, time in minutes between S_{cr_1} and S_{cr_2}; S_{cr_1}, first serum creatinine value; S_{cr_2}, second serum creatinine value; V_d, volume of distribution.

TABLE 41–7. Estimation of Creatinine Clearance in Patients with Acute Renal Failure

A patient with worsening renal function:
JR is a 50-year-old male (70 kg, BSA 1.73m²), admitted to the ICU following an automobile accident. His renal function was normal prior to admission; however, his serum creatinine has increased from 0.6 mg/dL to 3 mg/dL in the past 24 hours.

Authors	CL_{cr}	Assumptions
1. Jelliffe[105]	21.9 mL/min per 1.73m²	$E^{ss} = 1341.2$ mg/day $E^{ss}_{corr} = 1241$ mg/day $S_{cr} = 1.8$ mg/dL $S_{cr_1} = 0.6$ mg/dL $S_{cr_2} = 3$ mg/dL $\Delta t = 1$ day Wt = 70 kg
2. Brater[107]	19.1 mL/min	$S_{cr_1} = 0.6$ mg/dL $S_{cr_2} = 3$ mg/dL $\Delta t = 1$ day
3. Cockcroft-Gault[80]	29.2 mL/min	$S_{cr} = 3$ mg/dL Wt = 70 kg

A patient with improving renal function:
JR has been in the ICU for 1 week, and his status is improving. His serum creatinine has decreased from 3.0 mg/dL to 1.0 mg/dL in the past 24 hours.

Authors	CL_{cr}	Assumptions
1. Jelliffe[105]	64.5 mL/min per 1.73m²	$E^{ss} = 1341.2$ mg/day $E^{ss}_{corr} = 1297.7$ mg/day $S_{cr} = 2$ mg/dL $S_{cr_1} = 3$ mg/dL $S_{cr_2} = 1$ mg/dL $\Delta t = 1$ day Wt = 70 kg
2. Brater[107]	78.7 mL/min	$S_{cr_1} = 3$ mg/dL $S_{cr_2} = 1$ mg/dL $\Delta t = 1$ day
3. Cockcroft-Gault[80]	87.5 mL/min	$S_{cr} = 1$ mg/dL Wt = 70 kg

BSA, body surface area; CL_{cr}, creatinine clearance; E^{ss}, steady-state creatinine excretion; E^{ss}_{corr}, corrected steady-state creatinine excretion; Δt, time between S_{cr_1} and S_{cr_2}; S_{cr_1}, first serum creatinine level; S_{cr_2}, second serum creatinine level; Wt, weight.

non–steady-state serum creatinine, and disparity between development of glomerular and tubular function. Preterm infants demonstrate significantly reduced GFR prior to 34 weeks, which rapidly increases and becomes similar to that of term infants within the first week of life.[108] Evaluation of GFR in preterm infants on day 3 of life, using an inulin infusion, failed to identify a relationship between patient weight and GFR. However, gestational age, which ranged from 23.4 to 36.9 weeks (mean 30.2 weeks), correlated with both GFR and the reciprocal of serum creatinine. The inulin clearance increased from 0.67 to 0.85 mL/min in those with gestational age <28 weeks versus those of 32 to 37 weeks of age, while S_{cr} decreased from 1.05 to 0.73 mg/dL, respectively. Creatinine was measured using a specific enzymatic method to avoid interference from bilirubin or drugs.[109] Creatinine clearance has also been evaluated in infants less than 1 week of age, and values of 17.8 mL/min per 1.73 m^2 on day 1 increased to 36.4 mL/min per 1.73 m^2 by day 6.[110] In light of these rapid changes in GFR, estimation of GFR is not recommended for infants less than 1 week of age. Kidney function expressed as GFR standardized to body surface area increases with age and stabilizes at approximately 1 year. In older children, GFR is best assessed using standard measurement techniques for GFR. Subcutaneous administration of ^{125}I-iothalamate has been effectively used to measure GFR in children ranging in age from 1 to 20 years.[111]

Estimation of CL_{cr} as described by Schwartz and colleagues[112] is dependent on the child's age and length:

$$GFR = [length (cm) \times k]/S_{cr}$$

where k is defined by age group: infant (1 to 52 weeks) = 0.45; child (1 to 13 years) = 0.55; adolescent male = 0.7; and adolescent female = 0.55.

Subsequent studies verified these relationships in children with normal renal function or mild renal impairment. However, variability increases at clearance values <50 mL/min. Al-Harbi and Lireman[113] reported a good correlation of the predicted CL_{cr} with measured 4-hour CL_{cr} and ^{99m}Tc-DTPA ($r = 0.75$) in 48 pediatric renal allograft recipients aged 3 to 19 years. However, predictive performance measures of bias and precision were not reported. Fong and associates[114] evaluated the method in critically ill children (mean age 5.6 years; range 0.1 to 20.8 years), and concluded that the method significantly overestimated the measured CL_{cr} (bias = 45%). Pierrat and colleagues recently compared the MDRD, Schwartz, and CG equations in children aged 3 to 19 years. In children <12 years, the Schwartz and MDRD equations were significantly more biased than CG, and CG provided the best prediction of GFR in children >12 years of age.[115] Dose adjustments and other therapeutic decisions based on kidney function warrant appropriate measures of renal status to avoid incorrect decisions. The results of these investigations suggest that further studies will be needed to clarify the value of these predictive methods.

Kidney Function in the Elderly

Cross-sectional studies demonstrate decreased GFR as a function of age when GFR is measured as inulin, iothalamate, or creatinine clearance.[80,116] The Baltimore Longitudinal Study on Aging,[117] an evaluation of 254 normal healthy subjects, revealed that creatinine clearance decreases at the rate of approximately 0.75 mL/min per 1.73 m^2 per year beginning at the fourth decade of life. These subjects were evaluated prospectively for up to 23 years. Interestingly, approximately one-third of the subjects showed no change in renal function from their baseline value, and a small number showed an increased clearance. These changes may be due to normal physio-

logic changes or to subclinical insults to the kidneys that initiate the events leading to chronic progressive loss of renal function. Fliser and coworkers[118] studied renal functional reserve in healthy young (23 to 32 years) and elderly (61 to 82 years) volunteers using an amino acid infusion technique. Inulin clearance was used as the measure of GFR, which increased 16% in young and 17% in elderly subjects following the infusion. Renal functional reserve thus appears to be maintained in healthy elderly individuals.

Interpretation of the serum creatinine concentration alone is difficult in the elderly patient because of the decreased muscle mass and resultant lower production rate of creatinine. Thus the serum creatinine often remains within the normal range despite a reduction in the number of functional nephrons. As renal function declines, the kidneys excrete a larger fraction of creatinine. This perpetuates the "normal" serum creatinine. The CG formula[80] can be used to estimate the CL_{cr} of elderly patients. Smythe and associates[119] estimated CL_{cr} in 23 patients >60 years of age using seven different methods, and compared the results to a measured 24-hour CL_{cr} determination. Estimations were performed with the actual serum creatinine concentration and also with the serum creatinine rounded up to 1.0 mg/dL if the actual value was <1 mg/dL. Rounding the serum creatinine to 1 mg/dL resulted in a significantly lower (bias = 28.8 mL/min) estimate of GFR, as compared with the actual clearance, than when the unadjusted serum creatinine (bias = 2.3 mL/min) was used. These data strongly suggest that one should not arbitrarily fix the serum creatinine concentration in elderly patients at 1 mg/dL. An alternative to the estimation of GFR or a 24-hour clearance determination is a 4-hour clearance performed during water diuresis.[79] This correlated with the inulin clearance as well as an inpatient 24-hour CL_{cr}. However, one must be aware of the potential risk of hyponatremia in the geriatric patient who is unable to tolerate an oral water load, as well as the need for complete bladder emptying to ensure accurate results. O'Connell and associates[120] assessed the accuracy of 2- and 8-hour urine collections compared with 24-hour creatinine clearance determinations in 45 hospitalized patients >65 years old with indwelling urethral catheters. Single, timed urine collections for CL_{cr} showed minimal bias with the 8-hour collection as compared with the 24-hour value, whereas the 2-hour determination was both biased and imprecise. Unfortunately, the amount of residual urine was not determined, the bladder was not rinsed at each collection period, and the mean urine flow was low at 1.23 mL/min; all of these factors may have negatively affected the results of the 2-hour collection.

ASSESSMENT OF PROGRESSION

Chronic kidney disease (see Chap. 43) will eventually lead to ESKD (see Chap. 44), necessitating dialysis or transplantation for survival (see Chaps. 45 and 87). The rate of progression can be slowed and in some cases halted through dietary modification and blood pressure control, angiotensin-converting enzyme (ACE) inhibitor or angiotensin receptor blocker therapy, and improved glucose control in patients with type I diabetes mellitus (see Chap. 43). The efficacy of these interventions is optimally assessed with serial measurements of accurate and sensitive indices of GFR such as iohexol, iothalamate, or radioisotope clearances.[121]

Alternatively, use of newer methods to estimate GFR, such as the MDRD equation, or the linear decline in the reciprocal of the serum creatinine concentration as a function of time, are simple clinical tools that can be used to evaluate the rate of progression of renal disease, and to predict the time when dialysis will be needed.[33] Under

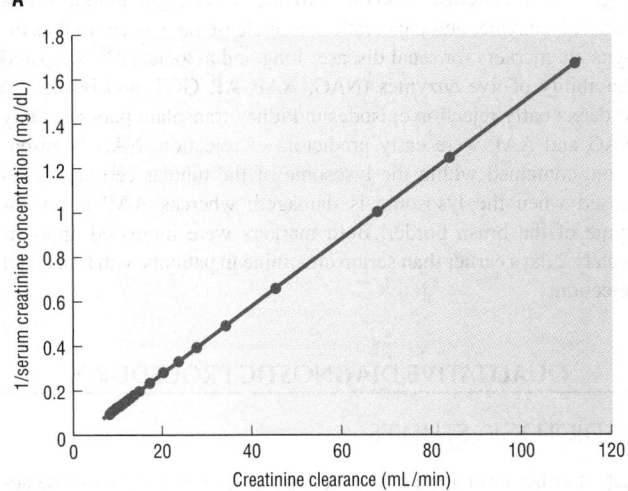

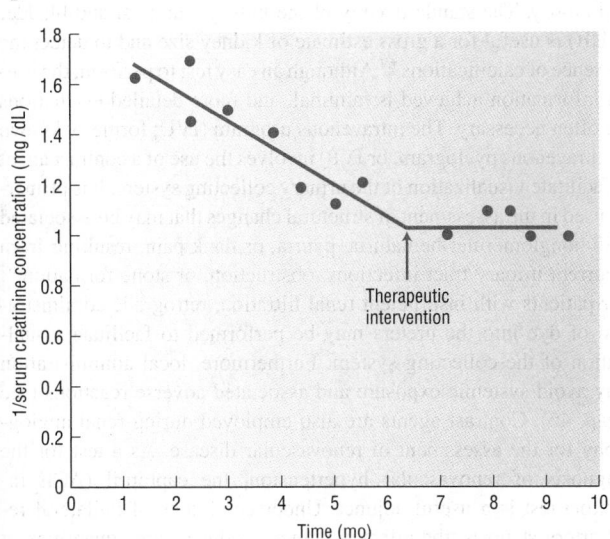

FIGURE 41–3. Linear relationship between 1/serum creatinine concentration and creatinine clearance (*A*) and 1/serum creatinine concentration as a function of time in a hypothetical patient with progressive renal impairment (*B*). The arrow indicates a change in the rate of progression, which may be related to a therapeutic intervention.

steady-state conditions, the formation rate of creatinine equals the elimination rate (R), and CL_{cr} is inversely related to S_{cr} as:

$$S_{cr} = R/CL_{cr}$$

The reciprocal relationship between S_{cr} and CL_{cr} is then expressed as:

$$1/S_{cr} = 1/R \times CL_{cr}$$

As renal function declines, the reciprocal of the serum creatinine concentration decreases as a linear function of the CL_{cr}, and the slope of the relationship is the reciprocal of the elimination rate of creatinine (Fig. 41–3A). Clinicians can use the reciprocal serum creatinine plotted as a function of time as a prognostic tool to predict when dialysis may be needed (when $1/S_{cr} \sim 0.1$), or as a marker for evaluating the success of therapeutic interventions to alter the rate of decline in renal function (Fig. 41–3B). Several factors, such as changes in

dietary intake of creatinine and decreased muscle mass, which are associated with a reduction in the production of creatinine, may alter the utility of the relationship. Furthermore, if tubular secretion increases in response to nephron hypertrophy disproportionately to filtration, or if nonrenal routes of elimination of creatinine such as metabolism by intestinal bacteria become more important, then changes in the slope of the reciprocal creatinine versus time relationship may be altered. It is most important to be aware of the limitations of serum creatinine measurement and to realize that it is not an adequate test to detect early chronic renal disease or to precisely estimate the rate of progression.

Although not a quantitative measure of renal function, urinary microalbuminuria has been identified as an early marker of renal disease in patients with diabetic nephropathy[122] and numerous other conditions, such as hypertension and obesity.[15,123,124] Patients with microalbuminuria (30 to 300 mg/day) on at least two occasions or overt albuminuria (>300 mg/day) should begin to receive pharmacotherapy. For children, microalbuminuria is considered present if albumin excretion exceeds 0.36 mg/kg per day, and overt albuminuria has been defined as an excretion rate that exceeds 4 mg/kg per day. The urinary albumin:creatinine ratio is also an accurate predictor of 24-hour proteinuria, a marker of renal disease. Guidelines for monitoring indicate that a urine albumin:creatinine ratio of >30 mg/g places the patient at increased risk of developing diabetic nephropathy and is an indication for the initiation of pharmacotherapeutic intervention.[30] Microalbuminuria has also been suggested as a risk factor for renal dysfunction among patients with essential hypertension.[125]

MEASUREMENT OF RENAL PLASMA AND BLOOD FLOW

Measurement of renal plasma and blood flow is usually reserved for research settings to evaluate hemodynamic changes related to disease or drug therapy. The kidneys receive approximately 20% of cardiac output and representative values of renal blood flow in men and women of about 1200 ± 250 and 1000 ± 180 mL/min per 1.73 m² have been reported, respectively.[126] Renal plasma flow (RPF) can be estimated to be 60% of renal blood flow if it is assumed that the average hematocrit is 40%.

PAH is an organic anion that has been used extensively for the quantitation of renal plasma flow. PAH is approximately 17% bound to plasma proteins and is eliminated extensively by active tubular secretion. Because PAH elimination is active, saturation of the transport processes have historically been anticipated, at concentrations of PAH in plasma above 10 to 20 mg/L.[44] Recently, Dowling and associates[127] used a sequential infusion technique and only observed concentration-dependent renal clearance of PAH at concentrations above 100 mg/dL. Furthermore, PAH is also metabolized, possibly within the kidney, to *N*-acetyl-PAH, and the analytical method must be able to differentiate the parent compound from the metabolite if one desires to obtain an accurate assessment of RPF.[63] Prescott and coworkers[128] noted that the renal clearance of PAH alone decreases at low plasma concentrations, while the clearance of the acetyl metabolite increases. Further studies are necessary to evaluate the mechanisms and significance of these findings. The extraction ratio (ER) for PAH is 70% to 90% at plasma concentrations of 10 to 20 mg/L, hence the term "effective" renal plasma flow (ERPF) has been used when the clearance of PAH is not corrected for the extraction ratio or if it is assumed to be 1.[2] Normal values for ERPF are about 650 ± 160 mL/min for men and 600 ± 150 mL/min for women.[126] Children will reach normalized adult values by 3 years of age, and ERPF will begin to decline as a function of age after 30 years, reaching about one-half of its peak value by 90 years of age. The method for calculation of ERPF is based on the relationship between organ clearance, ER, and flow:

$$ERPF = renal\ PAH\ CL = RPF \times ER$$

Effective renal blood flow (ERBF) can be estimated from ERPF by assuming the extraction ratio is 1 and correcting for the red blood cell volume of the blood (Hct, hematocrit):

$$ERBF = ERPF/(1 - Hct)$$

ERPF can also be measured using the radioisotopes ^{131}I-orthoiodo-hippurate or ^{99m}Tc-mercaptoacetyltriglycine.[129] One important advantage of this method is its ability to measure ERPF in total or for each kidney independently, as well as its ability to produce renal images. Russell and Dubovsky,[130] using a single-injection technique, compared clearance methods with and without urine collection and showed similar results with each method.

QUANTITATIVE AND SEMIQUANTITATIVE ASSESSMENT OF TUBULAR FUNCTION

Although GFR is perhaps the best overall indicator of renal function, it may not be reflective of tubular function; either secretory capacity or cellular function.[131] Tubular secretory function can be assessed by measuring PAH transport as the prototype marker of the organic anion secretory system. N-1-Methylnicotinamide (NMN) and tetraethylammonium (TEA) are prototype compounds secreted by the cationic transport system and may be used as markers of cationic secretory capacity.[2,132] Studies with NMN suggested its use to assess the effects of selected renal diseases on drug handling by the kidneys.[133] Dowling and colleagues[127] explored the utility of famotidine as a marker for cationic transport, but were unable to demonstrate saturation, perhaps due to contribution from other secretory pathways such as p-glycoprotein. It should be recognized that these transport systems are not necessarily mutually exclusive. Indeed, probenecid, which is secreted by the anionic pathway, inhibits the secretion of cationic compounds. Quantitative measures of tubular transport capacity are currently limited primarily to the research setting.

Other measures of tubular function are less specific and are regarded primarily as indices of damage within the nephron.[134] Schentag and Plaut[131] demonstrated a delay in the increase of serum creatinine following aminoglycoside toxicity when compared to markers for tubular damage such as the low-molecular-weight protein β_2-microglobulin (11.8 kDa) and urinary enzymes. The rise in β_2-microglobulin is related to an early functional defect in the proximal tubular cell. This is followed by a rise in the excretion of enzymes released as a result of structural damage to the cells, and finally, by the formation and excretion of cellular casts. Other low-molecular-weight proteins used as markers of tubular function include retinol-binding protein (21 kDa) and protein HC (also known as α_1-microglobulin, 27 kDa).[134] These proteins are normally freely filtered at the glomerulus and then completely reabsorbed by the proximal tubule. Increases in their excretion are thus suggestive of tubular dysfunction but are not diagnostic, as an increased production rate or GFR of less than 30 mL/min may lead to increased excretion. In both cases, the maximal reabsorptive capacity may be exceeded, leading to net excretion of the protein. Retinol-binding protein and protein HC are elevated with tubular damage and may be more appropriate markers than β_2-microglobulin.

Numerous urinary enzymes such as N-acetylglucosaminidase (NAG), alanine aminopeptidase (AAP), alkaline phosphatase (AP), γ-glutamyltransferase (GGT), pyruvate kinase, glutathione transferase, lysozyme, and pancreatic ribonuclease have been used as diagnostic markers for renal disease. Jung and associates[135] compared the ability of five enzymes (NAG, AAP, AP, GGT, and lysozyme) to detect early rejection episodes in kidney transplant patients. Only NAG and AAP were early predictors of rejection. NAG is an enzyme contained within the lysosome of the tubular cell and is released when the lysosome is damaged, whereas AAP is an enzyme of the brush border. Both markers were increased approximately 2 days earlier than serum creatinine in patients with transplant rejection.

QUALITATIVE DIAGNOSTIC PROCEDURES

RADIOLOGIC STUDIES

Further evaluation of the etiology of kidney disease can be accomplished using several qualitative diagnostic techniques, including radiography, ultrasound, magnetic resonance imaging (MRI), and biopsy. The standard x-ray of the kidneys, ureters, and bladder (KUB) is useful for a gross estimate of kidney size and to detect the presence of calcifications.[69] Although an easy test to perform, the useful information achieved is minimal, and more detailed evaluations are often necessary. The intravenous urogram (IVU; formerly known as intravenous pyelogram, or IVP) involves the use of a contrast agent to facilitate visualization of the urinary collecting system. It is primarily used in the assessment of structural changes that may be associated with nonglomerular hematuria, pyuria, or flank pain, resulting from recurrent urinary tract infections, obstruction, or stone formation.[69] For patients with insufficient renal filtration, retrograde administration of dye into the ureters may be performed to facilitate visualization of the collecting system. Furthermore, local administration may avoid systemic exposure and associated adverse reactions (see Chap. 46). Contrast agents are also employed during renal angiography for the assessment of renovascular disease. As a test for the diagnosis of renovascular hypertension, the captopril (ACE inhibitor) test is a useful adjunct. Under conditions of unilateral renal artery stenosis, the affected kidney produces large quantities of angiotensin II, which vasoconstricts the efferent arteriole to maintain GFR. The administration of an ACE inhibitor results in reduced uptake of the contrast agent because perfusion of the affected kidney decreases. This occurs as a result of decreased efferent arteriolar vasoconstriction. For patients with bilateral disease, a decrease in uptake is observed in both kidneys.[136] Computed tomography (CT) is a cross-sectional anatomic imaging procedure based on x-ray data. The procedure is frequently performed with contrast to enhance imaging. Spiral, or helical, CT, a more recent technique, provides visual three-dimensional reconstruction of tissues. CT is performed as a test for the evaluation of obstructive uropathy, malignancy, and infections of the kidney.

RENAL ULTRASOUND

Ultrasound uses sound waves to generate a two-dimensional image. The echogenicity of the kidney is compared with that of an adjacent organ—liver on the right and spleen on the left—with an increased echogenicity indicating an abnormal finding. Ultrasonography can distinguish the renal pyramids, medulla, and cortex, and abnormalities in structure, such as occurs with obstruction. Renal ultrasound is also used as a guide for site localization during percutaneous kidney biopsy.

MAGNETIC RESONANCE IMAGING

The MRI is based on aligning hydrogen nuclei in the body with the use of a powerful magnet and applying radiofrequency pulses. The signals emitted by the hydrogen nuclei during realignment on repeated pulses allows for generation of the tissue image. Realignment times can also be altered with the use of contrast agents (e.g., gadolinium or gadopentetate), leading to increased signal intensity and improved imaging. MRI is useful for the assessment of obstruction, malignancy, and renovascular lesions. The relative advantages and limitations of these procedures are discussed in more detail in several recent reviews.[69,137,138]

BIOPSY

Renal biopsy is used in several conditions to facilitate diagnosis when clinical, laboratory, and imaging findings prove inconclusive. Proteinuria and hematuria are both associated with renal parenchymal disease. When less-invasive studies are unsuccessful in differentiating the cause and the possible causes have different therapeutic approaches, biopsy may be indicated. Functional status of the kidney is not assessed with biopsy, and severity of disease and progression is best measured using the quantitative tests discussed above. Contraindications to renal biopsy include a solitary kidney, severe hypertension, bleeding disorder, severe anemia, cystic kidney, and hydronephrosis, among others. Complications resulting from biopsy primarily include hematuria, which may last for several days, and perirenal hematoma.[25]

CONCLUSION

The prevalence of kidney disease has increased dramatically over the past decade, indicating a need for early classification and monitoring of renal function in CKD patients. Renal function can be evaluated in clinical settings using estimated or measured creatinine clearance, estimated GFR, and measurement of urinary protein excretion. Accurate measurement of GFR using exogenous administration of inulin, iothalamate, or radioisotope techniques such as ^{99m}Tc-DTPA is required in research settings to assess drug therapy outcomes and progression of disease. Use of qualitative assessments of renal function, such as x-ray, CT, MRI, sonography, and biopsy, can help to determine the underlying cause of kidney disease. The clinical pharmacist can have an important role in the care of CKD patients, including renal function assessment, dose individualization, drug therapy monitoring, and evaluation of therapeutic outcomes.

ABBREVIATIONS

AAP: alanine aminopeptidase
ABW: actual body weight
ACE: angiotensin-converting enzyme
Alb: serum albumin concentration
AP: alkaline phosphatase
CG: Cockcroft-Gault (method of calculating CL_{cr})
CKD: chronic kidney disease
CL: clearance
CL_{cr}: creatinine clearance
DTPA: diethylenetriamine pentaacetic acid
EDTA: ethylenediaminetetraacetic acid
EPO: erythropoietin

ER: extraction ratio
ERBF: effective renal blood flow
ERPF: effective renal plasma flow
ESRD: end-stage renal disease
GFR: glomerular filtration rate
GGT: γ-glutamyltransferase
HPLC: high-performance liquid chromatography
IBW: ideal body weight
IVU: intravenous urogram
KUB: kidneys, ureters, and bladder (radiograph)
MDRD: Modification of Diet in Renal Disease (study)
MRP: multidrug resistance protein
NAG: N-acetylglucosaminidase
NKF K/DOQI: National Kidney Foundation Kidney Disease Outcomes Quality Initiative
NMN: N-1-methylnicotinamide
PAH: p-aminohippurate
P_{cr}: creatinine production rate
Pl_{cr}: plasma creatinine level
P-gp: P-glycoprotein
RBF: renal blood flow
RPF: renal plasma flow
S_{cr}: serum creatinine concentration
SNGFR: single nephron glomerular filtration rate
SUN: serum urea nitrogen (concentration)
TEA: tetraethylammonium

Review Questions and other resources can be found at *www.pharmacotherapyonline.com*.

REFERENCES

1. Campens D, Buntinx F. Selecting the best renal function tests. Int J Technol Assess Health Care 1997;13:343–356.
2. Sica DA, Schoolwerth AC. Renal handling of organic anions and cations: Excretion of uric acid. In: Brenner BM, ed. Brenner and Rector's The Kidney, 6th ed. Philadelphia, WB Saunders, 2000:680–700.
3. Hsyu PH, Gisclon LG, Hui AC, Giacomini KM. Interactions of organic anions with the organic cation transporter in renal brush-border membrane vesicles. Am J Physiol 1988;254:F56–F61.
4. Bendayan R. Renal drug transport: A review. Pharmacotherapy 1996;16:971–985.
5. Sikic BI. Pharmacologic approaches to reversing multidrug resistance. Semin Hematol 1997;34:40–47.
6. Hori R, Okumura K, Kamiya A, et al. Ampicillin and cephalexin in renal insufficiency. Clin Pharmacol Ther 1983;34:792–798.
7. Hori R, Okumura K, Nihira H. A new dosing regimen in renal insufficiency: Application to cephalexin. Clin Pharmacol Ther 1985;38:290–295.
8. Maiza A, Daley-Yates PT. The clearance of drugs in different types of renal disease. Ren Fail 1988;11:67 (Abstract).
9. Lin JH, Lin T. Renal handling of drugs in renal failure. I. Differential effects of uranyl nitrate- and glycerol-induced acute renal failure on renal excretion of TEAB and PAH in rats. J Pharmacol Exp Ther 1988;246:896–901.
10. Gloff CA, Benet LZ. Differential effects of the degree of renal damage on p-aminohippuric acid and inulin clearances in rats. J Pharmacokinet Biopharm 1989;17:169–177.
11. Bricker NS. On the meaning of the intact nephron hypothesis. Am J Med 1969;46:1–11.
12. Bosch JP. Renal reserve. A functional view of glomerular filtration rate. Semin Nephrol 1995;15:381–385.
13. Gaspari F, Perico N, Remuzzi G. Measurement of glomerular filtration rate. Kidney Int Suppl 1997;63:S151–S154.

14. Walser M. Assessing renal function from creatinine measurements in adults with chronic renal failure. Am J Kidney Dis 1998;32:23–31.

15. Rahn KH, Heidenreich S, Bruckner D. How to assess glomerular filtration and damage in humans. J Hypertens 1999;17:309–317.

16. Levin A, Singer J, Thompson CR, et al. Prevalent left ventricular hypertrophy in the predialysis population: Identifying opportunities for intervention. Am J Kidney Dis 1996;27:347–354.

17. Lacombe C, Mayeux P. The molecular biology of erythropoietin. Nephrol Dial Transplant 1999;14(Suppl 2):22–28.

18. Alvestrand A. Carbohydrate and insulin metabolism in renal failure. Kidney Int Suppl 1997;62:S48–S52.

19. Martin KJ, Olgaard K, Coburn JW, et al. Diagnosis, assessment, and treatment of bone turnover abnormalities in renal osteodystrophy. Am J Kidney Dis 2004;43:558–565.

20. Nolin TD, Frye RF, Matzke GR. Hepatic drug metabolism and transport in the presence of kidney disease. Am J Kidney Dis 2003;42:906–925.

21. Dowling TC, Briglia AE, Fink JC, et al. Characterization of hepatic cytochrome P450 3A (CYP3A) activity in ESRD patients. Clin Pharmacol Ther 2003;73:427–434.

22. Meffin PJ, Zilm DM, Veenendaal JR. Reduced clofibric acid clearance in renal dysfunction is due to a futile cycle. J Pharmacol Exp Ther 1983;227:732–738.

23. Verbeeck RK, Wallace SM, Loewen GR. Reduced elimination of ketoprofen in the elderly is not necessarily due to impairment of glucuronidation. Br J Clin Pharmacol 1984;17:783–784.

24. Levey AS, Coresh J, Balk E, et al. National Kidney Foundation practice guidelines for chronic kidney disease: Evaluation, classification, and stratification. Ann Intern Med 2003;139:137–147.

25. Kasiske BL, Keane WF. Laboratory assessment of renal disease: Clearance, urinalysis, and renal biopsy. In: Brenner BM, ed. Brenner and Rector's The Kidney, 6th ed. Philadelphia, WB Saunders, 2000:1129–1170.

26. Goldstein DE, Little RR. Monitoring glycemia in diabetes. Short-term assessment. Endocrinol Metab Clin North Am 1997;26:475–486.

27. Pugia MJ, Lott JA, Clark LW, et al. Comparison of urine dipsticks with quantitative methods for microalbuminuria. Eur J Clin Chem Clin Biochem 1997;35:693–700.

28. Newman DJ, Pugia MJ, Lott JA, et al. Urinary protein and albumin excretion corrected by creatinine and specific gravity. Clin Chim Acta 2000;294:139–155.

29. Parsons M, Newman DJ, Pugia M, et al. Performance of a reagent strip device for quantitation of the urine albumin:creatinine ratio in a point of care setting. Clin Nephrol 1999;51:220–227.

30. Keane WF, Eknoyan G. Proteinuria, albuminuria, risk, assessment, detection, elimination (PARADE): A position paper of the National Kidney Foundation. Am J Kidney Dis 1999;33:1004–1010.

31. Ruggenenti P, Gaspari F, Perna A, Remuzzi G. Cross-sectional longitudinal study of spot morning urine protein:creatinine ratio, 24-hour urine protein excretion rate, glomerular filtration rate, and end stage renal failure in chronic renal disease in patients without diabetes. BMJ 1998;316:504–509.

32. Rose BD, Renneke HG. Renal Pathophysiology—The Essentials. Baltimore, Williams & Wilkins, 1994.

33. Jones CA, McQuillan GM, Kusek JW, et al. Serum creatinine levels in the U.S. population: Third National Health and Nutrition Examination Survey. Am J Kidney Dis 1998;32:992–999.

34. Bauer JH, Brooks CS, Burch RN. Clinical appraisal of creatinine clearance as a measurement of glomerular filtration rate. Am J Kidney Dis 1982;2:337–346.

35. Green AJE, Halloran SP, Mould GP, et al. Interference by newer cephalosporins in current methods for measuring creatinine. Clin Chem 1990;36:2139–2140.

36. Massoomi F, Matthews HG III, Destache CJ. Effect of seven fluoroquinolones on the determination of serum creatinine by the picric acid and enzymatic methods. Ann Pharmacother 1993;27:586–588.

37. Young DS, ed. Effects of Drugs on Clinical Laboratory Tests, 4th ed. Washington, American Association of Clinical Chemistry (AACC) Press, 1995:3.190–3.211.

38. Daly TM, Kempe KC, Scott MG, et al. "Bouncing" creatinine levels. N Engl J Med 1996;334:1749–1750 (Letter).

39. van den Berg JG, Koopman MG, Arisz L. Ranitidine has no influence on tubular creatinine secretion. Nephron 1996;74:705–708.

40. Mayersohn M, Conrad KA, Achari R. The influence of a cooked meat meal on creatinine plasma concentration and creatinine clearance. Br J Clin Pharmacol 1983;15:227–230.

41. Thakur V, Reisin E, Solomonow M, et al. Accuracy of formula-derived creatinine clearance in paraplegic subjects. Clin Nephrol 1997;47:237–242.

42. Poortsmans JR, Francaux M. Long-term oral creatine supplementation does not impair renal function in healthy athletes. Med Sci Sports Exerc 1999;31:1108–1110.

43. Robinson TM, Sewell DA, Casey A, et al. Dietary creatine supplementation does not affect some haematological indices, or indices of muscle damage and renal function. Br J Sports Med 2000;34:284–288.

44. Edmunds JW, Jayapalan S, DiMarco NM, et al. Creatine supplementation increases renal disease progression in Han:SPRD-cy rats. Am J Kidney Dis 2001;37:73–78.

45. Coll E, Botey A, Alvarez L, et al. Serum cystatin C as a new marker for noninvasive estimation of glomerular filtration rate and as a marker for early renal impairment. Am J Kidney Dis 2000;36:29–34.

46. Price CP, Finney H. Developments in the assessment of glomerular filtration rate. Clin Chim Acta 2000;297:55–66.

47. Randers E, Erlandsen EJ. Serum cystatin C as an endogenous marker of the renal function—A review. Clin Chem Lab Med 1999;37:389–395.

48. Keevil BG, Kilpatrick ES, Nichols SP, Maylor PW. Biological variation of cystatin C: Implications for the assessment of glomerular filtration rate. Clin Chem 1998;44:1535–1539.

49. Page MK, Bükki B, Luppa P, Neumeier D. Clinical value of cystatin C determination. Clin Chim Acta 2000;297:67–72.

50. Bokenkamp A, Domanetzki M, Zinck R, et al. Cystatin C serum concentrations underestimate glomerular filtration rate in renal transplant recipients. Clin Chem 1999;45:1866–1868.

51. Akbas SH, Yavuz A, Tuncer M, et al. Serum cystatin C as an index of renal function in kidney transplant patients. Transplant Proc 2004;36:99–101.

52. Brändle E, Sieberth HG, Hautman RE. Effect of chronic dietary protein intake on the renal function in healthy subjects. Eur J Clin Nutr 1996;50:734–740.

53. Knight EL, Stampfer MJ, Hankinson SE, et al. The impact of protein intake on renal function decline in women with normal renal function or mild renal insufficiency. Ann Intern Med 2003;138:460–467.

54. Brenner BM, Lawler EV, Mackenzie HS. The hyperfiltration theory: A paradigm shift in nephrology. Kidney Int 1996;49:1774–1777.

55. Woods LL. Intrarenal mechanisms of renal reserve. Semin Nephrol 1995;15:386–395.

56. Dowling TC, Frye RF, Fraley DS, Matzke GR. Comparison of iothalamate clearance methods for measuring GFR. Pharmacotherapy 1999;19:943–950.

57. Florijn KW, Barendregt JNM, Lentjes EGWM, et al. Glomerular filtration rate measurement by "single-shot" injection of inulin. Kidney Int 1994;46:252–259.

58. Soper CPR, Bending MR, Barron JL. An automated enzymatic inulin assay, capable of full sinistrin hydrolysis. Eur J Clin Chem Clin Biochem 1995;33:497–501.

59. Dall'Amico R, Montini G, Pisanello L, et al. Determination of inulin in plasma and urine by reverse-phase high-performance liquid chromatography. J Chromatogr B Biomed Appl 1995;672:155–159.

60. Buclin T, Pechère-Bertschi A, Sáechaud R, et al. Sinistrin clearance for determination of glomerular filtration rate: A reappraisal of various approaches using a new analytical method. J Clin Pharmacol 1997;37:679–692.

61. Ruiz R, Cordova MA, Sierra M, et al. Automated sinistrin measurement. Clin Biochem 1997;30:501–504.

62. Agarwal R. Ambulatory GFR measurement with cold iothalamate in adults with chronic kidney disease. Am J Kidney Dis 2003;41:752–759.

63. Dowling TC, Frye RF, Zemaitis MA. Simultaneous determination of p-aminohippuric acid, acetyl-p-aminohippuric acid and iothalamate in human plasma and urine by high-performance liquid chromatography. J Chromatogr B Biomed Sci Appl 1998;716:305–313.

64. Dowling TC, Frye RF, Fraley DS, Matzke GR. Comparison of iothalamate clearance methods for measuring GFR. Pharmacotherapy 1999; 19:943–950.

65. Frennby B, Sterner G, Almán T, et al. The use of iohexol clearance to determine GFR in patients with severe chronic renal failure—A comparison between different clearance techniques. Clin Nephrol 1995;43:35–46.

66. Rocco MV, Buckalew VM Jr, Moore LC, Shihabi ZK. Measurement of glomerular filtration rate using nonradioactive iohexol: Comparison of two one-compartment models. Am J Nephrol 1996;16:138–143.

67. Lundqvist S, Hietala S-O, Groth S, Sjdin J-G. Evaluation of single sample clearance calculations in 903 patients. A comparison of multiple and single sample techniques. Acta Radiol 1997;38:68–72.

68. Lundqvist S, Holmberg G, Jakobsson G, et al. Assessment of possible nephrotoxicity from iohexol in patients with normal and impaired renal function. Acta Radiol 1998;39:362–367.

69. Hricak H, Meux M, Reddy GP. Radiologic assessment of the kidney. In: Brenner BM, ed. Brenner and Rector's The Kidney, 6th ed. Philadelphia, WB Saunders, 2000:1171–1200.

70. Frennby B, Almén T, Lilja B, et al. Determination of the relative glomerular filtration rate of each kidney in man. Acta Radiol 1995;36: 410–417.

71. Morton K, Pisani DE, Whiting JH Jr, et al. Determination of glomerular filtration rate using technitium-99m-DTPA with differing degrees of renal function. J Nucl Med Technol 1997;25:110–114.

72. Levey AS, Bosch JP, Lewis JB, et al. A more accurate method to estimate glomerular filtration rate from serum creatinine: A new prediction equation. Ann Intern Med 1999;130:461–470.

73. Rodrigo E, Fernandez-Fresnedo G, Ruiz JC, et al. Assessment of glomerular filtration rate in transplant recipients with severe renal insufficiency by Nankivell, Modification of Diet in Renal Disease (MDRD), and Cockroft-Gault equations. Transplant Proc 2003;35:1671–1672.

74. Vervoort G, Willems HL, Wetzels JF. Assessment of glomerular filtration rate in healthy subjects and normoalbuminuric diabetic patients: Validity of a new (MDRD) prediction equation. Nephrol Dial Transplant 2002;17:1909–1913.

75. Rule AD, Gussak HM, Pond GR, et al. Measured and estimated GFR in healthy potential kidney donors. Am J Kidney Dis 2004;43:112–119.

76. Skluzacek PA, Szewc RG, Nolan CR, et al. Prediction of GFR in liver transplant candidates. Am J Kidney Dis 2003;42:1169–1176.

77. Gonwa TA, Jennings L, Mai ML, et al. Estimation of glomerular filtration rates before and after orthotopic liver transplantation: Evaluation of current equations. Liver Transpl 2004;10:301–309.

78. Beddhu S, Samore MH, Roberts MS, et al. Creatinine production, nutrition, and glomerular filtration rate estimation. J Am Soc Nephrol 2003; 14:1000–1005.

79. Lemann J, Bidani AK, Bain RP, et al. Use of the serum creatinine to estimate glomerular filtration rate in health and early diabetic nephropathy. Am J Kidney Dis 1990;16:236–243.

80. Cockroft DW, Gault MH. Prediction of creatinine clearance from serum creatinine. Nephron 1976;16:31–41.

81. Shemesh O, Golbetz H, Kriss JP, et al. Limitations of creatinine as a filtration marker in glomerulopathic patients. Kidney Int 1985;28:830–838.

82. Roubenoff R, Drew H, Moyer M, et al. Oral cimetidine improves the accuracy and precision of creatinine clearance in lupus nephritis. Ann Intern Med 1990;113:501–506.

83. Zaltzman JS, Whiteside C, Cattran D, et al. Accurate measurement of impaired glomerular filtration using single-dose oral cimetidine. Am J Kidney Dis 1996;27:504–511.

84. Van Acker BAC, Koomen GCM, Koopman MG, et al. Creatinine clearance during cimetidine administration for measurement of glomerular filtration rate. Lancet 1992;340:1326–1329.

85. Spinler SA, Nawarskas JJ, Boyce EG, et al. Predictive performance of ten equations for estimating creatinine clearance in cardiac patients. Iohexol Cooperative Study Group. Ann Pharmacother 1998;32:1275–1283.

86. Salazar DE, Corcoran GB. Predicting creatinine clearance and renal drug clearance in obese patients from estimated fat-free body mass. Am J Med 1988;84:1053–1060.

87. Luke DR, Halstenson CE, Opsahl JA, et al. Validity of creatinine clearance estimates in the assessment of renal function. Clin Pharmacol Ther 1990;48:503–508.

88. Mawer CE, Knowles BR, Lucas SB, et al. Computer-assisted prescribing of kanamycin for patients with renal insufficiency. Lancet 1972;1:12–15.

89. Jelliffe RW. Estimation of creatinine clearance when urine cannot be collected. Lancet 1971;1:975–976.

90. Jelliffe RW. Creatinine clearance: Bedside estimate. Ann Intern Med 1973;79:604–605.

91. Hull JH, Hak LJ, Koch GC, et al. Influence of range of renal function and liver disease on predictability of creatinine clearance. Clin Pharmacol Ther 1981;29:516–521.

92. Gault MH, Longerich LL, Harnett JD, et al. Predicting glomerular function from adjusted serum creatinine. Nephron 1992;62:249–256.

93. Coresh J, Toto RD, Kirk KA, et al. Creatinine clearance as a measure of GFR in screens for the African-American study of kidney disease. Am J Kidney Dis 1998;32:32–42.

94. Goldwasser P, Aboul-Magd A, Maru M. Race and creatinine excretion in chronic renal insufficiency. Am J Kidney Dis 1997;30:16–22.

95. Ixkes MCJ, Koopman MG, van Acker BAC, et al. Cimetidine improves GFR-estimation by the Cockcroft-Gault formula. Clin Nephrol 1997; 47:229–236.

96. Orlando R, Floreani M, Padrini R, Palatini P. Evaluation of measured and calculated creatinine clearances as glomerular filtration markers in different stages of liver cirrhosis. Clin Nephrol 1999;51:341–347.

97. Lam NP, Sperelakis R, Kuk J, et al. Rapid estimation of creatinine clearances in patients with liver dysfunction. Dig Dis Sci 1999;44:1222–1227.

98. Caregaro L, Menon F, Angeli P, et al. Limitations of serum creatinine level and creatinine clearance as filtration markers in cirrhosis. Arch Intern Med 1994;154:201–205.

99. DeSanto NG, Anastasio P, Loguercio C, et al. Creatinine clearance: An inadequate marker of renal filtration in patients with early posthepatitic cirrhosis (Child A) without fluid retention and muscle wasting. Nephron 1995;70:421–424.

100. Davis GA, Chandler MHH. Comparison of creatinine clearance estimation methods in patients with trauma. Am J Health Syst Pharm 1996;53: 1028–1032.

101. Goerdt PJ, Heim-Duthoy KL, Macres M, Swan SK. Predictive performance of renal function equations in renal allografts. Br J Clin Pharmacol 1997;44:261–265.

102. Schuck O, Teplan V, Vitko S, et al. Predicting glomerular function from adjusted serum creatinine in renal transplant patients. Int J Clin Pharmacol Ther 1997;35:33–37.

103. Huang E, Hewitt R, Shelton M, Morse GD. Comparison of measured and estimated creatinine clearance in patients with advanced HIV disease. Pharmcotherapy 1996;16:222–229.

104. Quadri KHM, Bernardini J, Greenberg A, et al. Assessment of renal function during pregnancy using a random urine protein to creatinine ratio and Cockcroft-Gault formula. Am J Kidney Dis 1994;24: 416–420.

105. Jelliffe RW. Estimation of creatinine clearance in patients with unstable renal function, without a urine specimen. Am J Nephrol 2002;22: 320–324.

106. Chiou WL, Hsu FH. A new simple rapid method to monitor renal function based on pharmacokinetic considerations of endogenous creatinine. Res Commun Chem Pathol Pharmacol 1975;10:315–330.

107. Brater DC. Drug Use in Renal Disease. Balgowlah, Australia, ADIS Health Science Press, 1983:22–56.

108. Arant BS Jr. Developmental patterns of renal functional maturation compared in the human neonate. J Pediatr 1978;92:705–712.

109. van den Anker, de Groot R, Broerse HM, et al. Assessment of glomerular filtration rate in preterm infants by serum creatinine: Comparison with inulin clearance. Pediatrics 1995;96:1156–1158.

110. Sertel H, Scopes J. Rates of creatinine clearance in babies less than one week of age. Arch Dis Child 1973;48:717–720.

111. Bajaj G, Alexander SR, Browne R, et al. [125]Iodine-iothalamate clearance in children. A simple method to measure glomerular filtration. Pediatr Nephrol 1996;10:25–28.

112. Schwartz GJ, Brion LP, Spitzer A. The use of plasma creatinine concentration for estimating glomerular filtration rate in infants, children, and adolescents. Pediatr Clin North Am 1987;34:571–590.

113. Al-Harbi N, Lireman D. Comparison of three different methods of estimating the glomerular filtration rate in children after renal transplantation. Am J Nephrol 1997;17:68–71.

114. Fong J, Johnston S, Valentino T, Notterman D. Length/serum creatinine ratio does not predict measured creatinine clearance in critically ill children. Clin Pharmacol Ther 1995;58:192–197.

115. Pierrat A, Gravier E, Saunders C, et al. Predicting GFR in children and adults: a comparison of the Cockcroft-Gault, Schwartz, and modification of diet in renal disease formulas. Kidney Int 2003;64:1425–1436.

116. Lindeman RD, Tobin J, Shrock NW. Longitudinal studies on the rate of decline in renal function with age. J Am Geriatr Soc 1985;33:278–281.

117. Lindeman RD. Assessment of renal function in the old. Clin Lab Med 1993;13:269–277.

118. Fliser D, Ritz E, Franek E. Renal reserve in the elderly. Semin Nephrol 1995;15:463–467.

119. Smythe M, Hoffman J, Kizy K, et al. Estimating creatinine clearance in elderly patients with low serum creatinine concentrations. Am J Hosp Pharm 1994;51:198–204.

120. O'Connell MB, Wong MO, Bannick-Mohrland SD, et al. Accuracy of 2- and 8-hour urine collections for measuring creatinine clearance in the hospitalized elderly. Pharmacother 1993;13:135–142.

121. Agodoa L, Eknoyan G, Ingelfinger J, et al. Assessment of structure and function in progressive renal disease. Kidney Int Suppl 1997;63:S144–S150.

122. Rossing P, Astrup A-S, Smidt UM, et al. Monitoring kidney function in diabetic nephropathy. Diabetologia 1994;37:708–712.

123. Valensi P, Assayag M, Busby M, et al. Microalbuminuria in obese patients with or without hypertension. Int J Obes Relat Metab Disord 1996;20:574–579.

124. Berrut G, Bouhanick B, Fabbri P, et al. Microalbuminuria as a predictor of a drop in glomerular filtration rate in subjects with non-insulin-dependent diabetes mellitus and hypertension. Clin Nephrol 1997;48:92–97.

125. Mimran A, Ribstein J, DuCailar G. Is microalbuminuria a marker of early intrarenal vascular dysfunction in essential hypertension? Hypertension 1994;23:1018–1021.

126. Dworkin LD, Sun AM, Brenner BM. The renal circulations. In: Brenner BM, ed. Brenner and Rector's The Kidney, 6th ed. Philadelphia, WB Saunders, 2000:277–318.

127. Dowling TC, Frye RF, Fraley DS, Matzke GR. Characterization of tubular functional capacity in humans using para-aminohippurate and famotidine. Kidney Int 2001;59:295–303.

128. Prescott LF, Freestone S, McAuslane JAN. The concentration-dependent disposition of intravenous p-aminohippurate in subjects with normal and impaired renal function. Br J Clin Pharmacol 1993;35:20–29.

129. Taylor A, Manatunga A, Morton K, et al. Multicenter trial validation of a camera-based method to measure Tc-99m mercaptoacetyltriglycine, or Tc-99m MAG3, clearance. Radiology 1997;204:47–54.

130. Russell CD, Dubovsky EV. Comparison of single-injection multisample renal clearance methods with and without urine collection. J Nucl Med 1995;36:603–606.

131. Schentag JJ, Plaut ME. Patterns of urinary β2-microglobulin excretion by patients treated with aminoglycosides. Kidney Int 1980;17:654–661.

132. Nassseri K, Daley-Yates PT. A comparison of N-1-methylnicotinamide clearance with 5 other markers of renal function in models of acute and chronic renal failure. Toxicol Lett 1990;53:243–245.

133. Maiza A, Daley-Yates PT. Estimation of the renal clearance of drugs using endogenous N-1-methylnicotinamide. Toxicol Lett 1990;53:231–235.

134. Jung K. Urinary enzymes and low-molecular-weight proteins as markers of tubular dysfunction. Kidney Int Suppl 1994;47:S29–S33.

135. Jung K, Diego J, Strobelt V, et al. Diagnostic significance of some urinary enzymes for detecting acute rejection crises in renal transplant recipients: Alanine aminopeptidase, alkaline phosphatase, gamma-glutamyl transferase, N-acetyl-beta-glucosaminidase, and lysozyme. Clin Chem 1986;32:1807–1811.

136. Taylor A, Nally JV. Clinical applications of renal scintigraphy. Am J Roentgenol 1995;164:31–41.

137. Mindell HJ, Fairbank JT. Renal imaging techniques. In: Greenberg A, ed. Primer on Kidney Diseases, 2nd ed. San Diego, Academic Press, 1998:47–53.

138. Lerman LO, Rodriguez-Porcel M, Romero JC. The development of x-ray imaging to study renal function. Kidney Int 1999;55:400–416.

42

ACUTE RENAL FAILURE

Bruce A. Mueller

Learning Objectives and other resources can be found at *www.pharmacotherapyonline.com.*

KEY CONCEPTS

1 Identify acute renal failure (ARF) early and eliminate its cause to avoid the spread of damage.

2 Prevention is key; little can be done for established acute renal failure.

3 In situations in which development of ARF is likely, patients should receive therapy to prevent occurrence or reduce its severity. These situations include: diabetes mellitus, chronic kidney disease, the elderly, radiocontrast dye administration, and ICU patients. Some preventive thera-

pies include: glucose control, sodium loading, and use of L-carnitine.

4 Avoid nephrotoxins as much as possible.

5 Once the cause of ARF is identified and is eliminated, supportive therapy is the only remaining option, as we cannot hasten recovery of established ARF. Supportive therapies include: renal replacement therapies, nutritional support, avoidance of nephrotoxins, and aggressive fluid management.

The development of acute renal failure (ARF) presents a difficult challenge to the clinician. It has widely varying causes, and unlike other cases of organ failure such as neurologic or cardiovascular failure, the onset of ARF is often silent. In the ambulatory setting, patients may not notice ARF symptoms for days or weeks. Clinical and laboratory markers of its presence can be subtle and are often overlooked. Despite its often insidious presentation, ARF can be one of the most serious consequences that can occur, especially in a hospitalized patient.

Renal replacement therapies (RRTs) like hemodialysis, peritoneal dialysis, and other related treatments have been available for decades, but have not resulted in dramatic improvements in patient outcomes. RRT can help patient management by normalizing blood electrolyte values, augmenting waste product removal, and maintaining fluid balance. Despite the supportive care that RRT offers, development of ARF is frequently a catastrophic event.

DEFINITION OF ARF

A unifying definition of ARF does not exist. Clinicians disagree about when to make the diagnosis and published epidemiologic studies use different definitions in nearly every study.[1] Nonetheless, most use some combination of absolute serum creatinine value and a change in serum creatinine value or daily urine output as criteria for making the diagnosis.[2,3] In general, these studies typically view ARF as being a condition in which a previously normal serum creatinine rises by 0.5 mg/dL, or an absolute increase in serum creatinine of >1 mg/dL in a patient with previous chronic kidney disease (CKD). Clinicians must recognize that serum creatinine, while simple to measure, is not a very sensitive laboratory test. For example, a patient with an acute event that reduces the glomerular filtration rate (GFR) to zero will have no immediate change in serum creatinine. Depending on the creatinine generation rate and fluid status of the patient,

it may take days before serum creatinine values meet the threshold of a rise of 0.5 mg/dL. This may delay recognizing that ARF has occurred.[4]

ARF CLASSIFICATION

In the clinical setting, ARF is classified in a variety of ways. Classifying ARF by daily urine output can be useful. Anuria is defined as a urine output of <50 mL/d, oliguria is when the daily urine output is 50 to 450 mL/d, and nonoliguria occurs when the patient can make >450 mL of urine per day. This simplistic approach actually is quite useful in determining prognosis. Hospitalized anuric or oliguric patients have significantly higher mortality rates than similar ARF patients with nonoliguria.[5] Surviving oliguric ARF patients are also less likely to ever fully recover their renal function compared to nonoliguric patients.[6] Clinically, the nonoliguric patient is easier to manage than the oliguric patient because of reduced concerns about fluid overload. Consequently, knowledge of something as simple as the amount of urine produced per day can yield important information for the clinician.

EPIDEMIOLOGY

ARF is a common condition in the general population, with an annual incidence of approximately 200 cases per million population per year.[2] The incidence rate is higher in hospitalized patients, 5% of whom may require RRT (Table 42–1).[7] The highest incidence of ARF is in hospitalized patients in the intensive care unit. Depending on the definition used, ARF develops in 2% to 25% of patients in intensive care units.[8–10]

TABLE 42–1. Incidence and Outcomes of Acute Renal Failure (ARF) Relative to Where It Occurs

	Community-Acquired	Hospital-Acquired	ICU-Acquired
Incidence	Low (<1%)	Moderate (2–5%)	High (6–23%)
Cause	Single	Single or multiple	Multifactorial
Overall survival rate	70–95%	30–50%	10–30%
Worsened outcome if:	RRT required	RRT required	Intrinsic renal disease
	Poor preadmission health	Poor preadmission health	Ischemic cause
	Other failed organ systems	Ischemic ARF cause	Septic
		Other failed organ systems	RRT required
			Poor preadmission health
			Other failed organ systems
Better outcome if:	Nonoliguric	Nonoliguric	Prerenal cause
		Nephrotoxic cause	Postrenal cause
			Nonoliguric
			Nephrotoxic cause
			Hyperglycemia prevented

Many patient-specific factors cause a predisposition to the development of ARF. In nonhospitalized patients, ARF is often drug-induced. Common causes of drug-induced ARF include nonprescription nonsteroidal anti-inflammatory drugs (NSAIDs), prompting the FDA to convene an advisory committee to re-examine labeling of these products.[11] This drug class alone may be responsible for 500,000 to 2,500,000 cases of nephrotoxicity in the United States per year.[12] More information on drug-induced ARF can be found in Chap. 46.

Preexisting CKD has been associated with a threefold increased risk of ARF in patients requiring intravenous contrast dye during cardiac catheterization.[13] In patients without preexisting kidney disease who require cardiac catheterization, the development of ARF leads to similarly lethal results. These ARF patients who require dialysis have a ninefold higher 1-year mortality rate and a threefold higher rate of myocardial infarction than cardiac catheterization patients who do not require dialysis.[14] Indeed, it has been suggested that the most important risk factors for development of ARF are present when the patient is admitted to the hospital.[8] Many studies have reported that hospitalized patients at risk for development of ARF are more likely to have preexisting renal disease, heart failure, or other organ system failure, infection at admission to the hospital, poor nutritional status, and age >65 years than those not developing ARF.[8,14–15]

Few factors that clinicians can control are associated with ARF development. However, one of these factors that may be under control of prescribers is that of nephrotoxin exposure to the patient. For example, higher cumulative doses of intravenous contrast dye are directly related to the risk of developing ARF in patients receiving cardiac catheterization.[14] This risk can be ameliorated by avoidance of nephrotoxins in patients at high risk of ARF development, or by dosing unavoidable nephrotoxins like aminoglycosides in ways documented to reduce ARF development.[16] Additionally, clinicians can exert tighter control of serum glucose using insulin, and by doing so can reduce the rate of ARF development.[17]

One series reported that 5% of all patients admitted to an intensive care unit will require some RRT due to ARF.[10] The mortality rate for these patients is remarkably higher than ICU patients not requiring RRT, even when severity of illness and other factors are controlled for (63% vs. 15%).[10] The cause for this increase in mortality rates due to ARF does not appear to be solely related to the absence of renal function. Patients admitted to the ICU with CKD have significantly lower mortality rates than patients who are admitted to the ICU with ARF or who develop ARF in the ICU.[18]

OUTCOMES

The development of ARF is one of the most serious events that can happen to a hospitalized patient, regardless of the reason for hospitalization. In patients admitted for cardiac surgery, the mortality risk is seven- to eightfold higher if the patient develops ARF.[19] Patients who develop ARF following administration of intravenous radiocontrast dye and requiring dialysis have twice the mortality rate of similar patients receiving radiocontrast dye who do not experience an increase in their serum creatinine values.[13]

The outcome of a patient with ARF predominantly depends on the cause of the condition. In general, higher mortality rates are seen in conditions that result in hypoxia to the kidney causing acute tubular necrosis (ATN; 60%) or cortical necrosis (100%) compared to the lower mortality associated with autoimmune ARF causes like glomerulonephritis (9% to 25%), vasculitis (45%), or interstitial nephritis (13%).[2] Similarly, postrenal causes like obstructive ARF tend to have lower mortality rates (27%), ostensibly because these obstructions can be surgically repaired before permanent damage can be done to the kidney. Other patient factors influence ARF outcomes. Understandably, those patients with higher severity of illness have higher mortality rates than those who do not.[18] Critically ill patients with ARF due to sepsis have mortality rates that are significantly higher than those of patients who develop ARF for other reasons (74% vs. 45%).[20]

ETIOLOGY

The classification of ARF into broad categories based on the precipitating factors facilitates the diagnosis and management of patients presenting with this disorder (Table 42–2). Traditionally, the causes of ARF have been categorized into prerenal azotemia (resulting from decreased renal perfusion), acute intrinsic renal failure (resulting from structural damage to the kidney), and postrenal obstruction (obstruction of urine flow from the kidney out of the body). The addition of the category "functional ARF" aids in the understanding of the pathophysiology of ARF. This category is the result of hemodynamic changes at the level of the glomerulus without decreased perfusion of the kidney or structural damage to it.

The cause of ARF strongly influences patient outcome.[2] Kidneys that are not perfused with blood for prolonged periods will develop

TABLE 42–2. Classification of Acute Renal Failure

Category	Classification of Acute Renal Failure	Differential Diagnosis

Prerenal renal failure	Systemic hypoperfusion	Intravascular volume depletion
		  Dehydration
		  Hemorrhage
		  CHF
		  Liver disease
		  Nephrotic syndrome
		  Overdiuresis

	Isolated renal hypoperfusion	Bilateral renal artery stenosis (unilateral renal artery stenosis in solitary kidney)
		Emboli
		  Cholesterol
		  Thrombotic

Functional acute renal failure		Medications
		  Cyclosporine
		  ACEIs
		  NSAIDs
		  Hypercalcemia
		  Hepatorenal syndrome

Acute intrinsic renal failure	Vascular	Vasculitis
		  Polyarteritis nodosa
		  Thrombotic thrombocytopenic purpura
		  Hemolytic uremic syndrome
		Emboli
		  Cholesterol
		  Thrombotic

	Glomerular	Systemic lupus erythematosus Poststreptococcal glomerulonephritis Antiglomerular basement membrane disease

	Acute tubular necrosis	Ischemic
		  Hypotension
		  Vasoconstriction
		Exogenous toxins
		  Contrast dye
		  Heavy metals
		  Drugs (amphotericin B, aminoglycosides, etc.)
		Endogenous toxins
		  Myoglobin
		  Hemoglobin

	Acute interstitial nephritis	Drugs
		  Penicillins
		  Ciprofloxacin
		  Sulfonamides
		Infection
		  Streptococcal

Postrenal renal failure (obstruction)	Bladder outlet obstruction	Prostatic hypertrophy Improperly placed bladder catheter
	Ureteral (bilateral or unilateral with solitary functioning kidney)	Cervical cancer Retroperitoneal fibrosis

	Renal pelvis or tubules	Crystal deposition
		  Oxalate
		  Indinavir
		  Sulfonamides
		  Acyclovir
		  Tumor lysis syndrome

cortical necrosis and this condition is uniformly fatal. In contrast, ARF due to postrenal causes like obstruction have much lower mortality rates.[2] Consequently, rapid diagnosis of the etiology of ARF is essential so that renal perfusion can be corrected and other causes of ARF eliminated.

PRERENAL AZOTEMIA

Prerenal ARF results from hypoperfusion of the renal parenchyma, with or without systemic arterial hypotension. Renal hypoperfusion with systemic arterial hypotension may be caused by a decline in intravascular volume (e.g., hemorrhage or dehydration) or a decline in effective blood volume (i.e., the blood volume perceived by the arterial baroreceptors). Examples of disease states in which there is a decline in effective blood volume without a decrease in intravascular volume include congestive heart failure (CHF) and liver failure. Because the kidney is initially undamaged, the urinalysis will be normal. Eventually, the fractional excretion of sodium will be low, reflecting an increase in the concentrations of the sodium-retentive hormones renin, angiotensin, and aldosterone. Urinary solutes will be concentrated as a result of the increased circulating levels of antidiuretic hormone that is released in response to the diminished arterial blood pressure.

Renal hypoperfusion without systemic hypotension most commonly results from bilateral renal artery occlusion, or unilateral occlusion in a patient with a single functioning kidney. In these conditions, the sodium-retentive hormones are activated by the decline in renal parenchymal perfusion. However, systemic arterial blood pressure is usually elevated, leading to an inhibition of antidiuretic hormone release. Consequently, the urinary indices will reflect enhanced sodium reabsorption (i.e., a low fractional excretion of sodium), but the urinary solutes may not be maximally concentrated.

FUNCTIONAL ACUTE RENAL FAILURE

Functional ARF refers to those entities that result in a decline in glomerular ultrafiltrate production secondary to a reduced glomerular hydrostatic pressure without damage to the kidney itself. The decline in glomerular hydrostatic pressure is a direct consequence of changes in glomerular afferent (vasoconstriction) and efferent (vasodilation) arteriolar circumference. These clinical conditions most commonly occur in individuals who have reduced effective blood volume (e.g., CHF, cirrhosis, severe pulmonary disease, or hypoalbuminemia) or renovascular disease (e.g., renal artery stenosis), and cannot compensate for changes in afferent or efferent arteriolar tone. Examples of disorders that result in afferent arteriolar vasoconstriction (and an increase in afferent arteriolar resistance) include hypercalcemia and the administration of certain medications (e.g., Cyclosporine and NSAIDs). A decrease in efferent arteriolar resistance usually results from the administration of an angiotensin-converting enzyme inhibitor (ACEI) or angiotensin II receptor antagonist. With correction of the underlying pathologic process or discontinuation of the responsible medication, renal function rapidly returns to baseline. The hepatorenal syndrome is included in this classification scheme since the kidney itself is not damaged and there is intense afferent arteriolar vasoconstriction leading to a decline in glomerular filtration. In all the above conditions, the urinalysis is no different from its baseline state and the urinary indices suggest prerenal azotemia.

This syndrome of functional ARF is very common in individuals with CHF who receive an ACEI in an attempt to improve left ventricular function. The decline in efferent arteriolar resistance resulting from the inhibition of angiotensin II occurs rapidly. Therefore, if the dose of the ACEI is increased too rapidly, there will be a decline in glomerular ultrafiltrate production with a concomitant rise in the serum creatinine, leading to functional ARF. If the increase in the serum creatinine is not too severe (usually <1 mg/dL) the medication can be continued. Renal function should gradually improve as renal parenchymal perfusion pressure increases with improvement in left ventricular function.

ACUTE INTRINSIC RENAL FAILURE

Acute intrinsic renal failure results from damage to the kidney itself. Conceptually, acute intrinsic renal failure can best be understood in terms of the structures within the kidney: the small blood vessels, the

glomeruli, renal tubules, and interstitium. Renal failure secondary to small vessel vasculitis [e.g., polyarteritis nodosa, hemolytic uremic syndrome (HUS), or malignant hypertension] or cholesterol emboli can present with relatively normal urinary sediment since at least initially, the glomerulus and tubules are not damaged. When renal failure results from small vessel vasculitis, the vasculitic process is rarely confined to the kidney. A careful search for diagnostic clues suggesting other organ system involvement usually provides evidence of the diffuse nature of these disease processes.

Acute glomerular inflammation (acute glomerulonephritis) can result from a variety of precipitating causes (systemic lupus erythematosus and antiglomerular basement membrane disease, among others) (see Chap. 47). In these disorders the urinalysis usually reveals the presence of heavy proteinuria (>3 g urinary protein per 24-hour collection period) and hemoglobinuria. Microscopic analysis of the urinary sediment frequently shows numerous red blood cells (RBCs) and RBC casts, the latter being considered diagnostic for glomerulonephritis. In the early stages of the illness, the fractional excretion of sodium is less than 1 because tubular function is still intact. However, as renal failure becomes more established, the fractional excretion of sodium may increase.

The renal tubules are susceptible to a variety of insults. The tubules contained within the medulla of the kidney are particularly at risk from ischemic injury, as this portion of the kidney is very metabolically active, and thus has a high oxygen requirement. Severe hypotension or the administration of vasoconstricting drugs preferentially affects the tubules more than any other portion of the kidney. In addition, exogenous toxic substances (e.g., contrast agents, heavy metals, and pharmacologic agents such as aminoglycosides, amphotericin B, and foscarnet) and endogenous toxins (e.g., myoglobin, hemoglobin, and uric acid) may cause tubular injury. Once tubular cells die, they slough off into the tubular lumen, forming casts causing increased tubular pressures and reduced glomerular filtration.[21] Regardless of the etiology, tubular injury leads to a loss of urine concentrating ability, defective distal sodium reabsorption, and a reduction in the GFR. The etiology of acute intrinsic renal failure secondary to tubular injury (referred to as acute tubular necrosis or ischemic ARF) is usually discernible by reviewing the patient's history and medication list. The urinalysis suggests tubular injury by the presence of coarse "dirty brown" casts. RBCs and RBC casts are only rarely seen. The urinary indices suggest intrinsic renal dysfunction (i.e., high fractional excretion of sodium, urine osmolality equal to plasma osmolality, and a low urine creatinine:serum creatinine ratio).

The therapeutic approach for the management of ATN secondary to ischemia of the kidneys is changing. Historically, clinicians viewed ischemic ARF as a one-time event that resulted in tubular death. During this time the patient should be supported until renal function recovers. The new model for ischemic ARF is much like that used in treatment of myocardial infarction and stroke. Now, in addition to an initiation phase, when the patient experiences a hypoxic insult, an extension phase has been hypothesized.[22] Similar to what is postulated to occur during a myocardial infarction, in the kidney continued hypoxia after the original ischemic event results in an inflammatory response that further damages the kidney. More renal tubular epithelial cells are damaged and die, particularly in the corticomedullary junction. Cytokine release further increases the inflammation. Renal perfusion becomes less organized, as renal vasodilation and vasoconstriction are not occurring efficiently, and the area of injury grows. All of this occurs in the first 24 hours after the initial insult.[22] New therapies will address the development of ATN and stop the extension phase as early as possible by blocking the pathways that cause inflammation after the initial insult.[23]

The interstitium of the kidney is also susceptible to injury from a variety of causes. Although acute interstitial nephritis is most commonly caused by medications (see Chap. 46), infections (e.g., streptococcal, leptospirosis, hantavirus, and human immunodeficiency virus), selected autoimmune disorders (systemic lupus erythematosus or mixed connective tissue disease) also may produce a similar syndrome. The presence of white blood cells (WBCs), WBC casts, and coarse granular casts in the urine all suggest interstitial inflammation. The presence of eosinophilia and eosinophiluria also strongly suggest the presence of an interstitial nephritis. Occasionally low to moderate proteinuria can be seen on urinalysis.

POSTRENAL OBSTRUCTION

ARF resulting from obstruction may occur at any level within the urinary system from renal tubule to urethra. However, to cause ARF, the obstructing process must involve both kidneys, or one kidney in a patient with a single functioning kidney. Bladder outlet obstruction is the most common cause of obstructive uropathy. Crystal deposition within the tubules (e.g., secondary to uric acid, oxalate, acyclovir, sulfonamide, indinavir, or methotrexate), and ureteral obstruction (e.g., secondary to shed renal papilla or calculi) are infrequent causes of obstructive ARF. Crystal-induced ARF is often seen in patients who have severe volume contraction or who are receiving large doses of a drug with relatively low solubility. In these cases, patients do not have sufficient urine volume to keep the crystals from coming out of solution in the urine.[24] The onset of acute anuria in the absence of a catastrophic event should suggest acute urinary tract obstruction. However, the development of ARF in a hospitalized patient admitted with normal renal function is rarely secondary to obstruction unless an indwelling urinary catheter has been misplaced. When the obstructing process (e.g., prostatic hypertrophy or cervical cancer) is gradual and incomplete, the patient may present with complaints of decreased force of the urinary stream and polyuria.

PATHOPHYSIOLOGY

A basic knowledge of renal function facilitates the understanding of how ARF manifests itself clinically. The most logical approach to understanding renal function is to divide the kidney into its four basic component parts: the vasculature, the glomeruli, the tubules, and the interstitium surrounding the other three component parts.

RENAL VASCULATURE

The kidney is a highly vascular organ with blood vessels ranging from the very large (renal arteries) to the very small capillaries providing blood to each individual glomerulus. Obstruction of the renal artery will result in an increase in serum creatinine, hematuria, and proteinuria, but obstruction of smaller vessels will only cause infarction of the downstream parenchyma. If this area is small, no change in serum creatinine will occur.

Smaller vessels may be obstructed with cholesterol emboli, vascular lesions, or platelet plugs, all of which will present as isolated decreased perfusion of the glomeruli. The serum creatinine frequently is increased since the lesions are usually diffuse. However, the urinalysis most commonly will be normal since the kidney itself is not ischemic and the glomeruli are not involved. The urinary indices suggest prerenal azotemia (i.e., a low urine sodium concentration and a low fractional excretion of sodium) in the absence of systemic hypotension or a decrease in effective blood volume. The urine volume may or may not be diminished. However, the onset of oliguria secondary to diffuse arterial lesions within the kidney, such as that which occurs with hemolytic uremia syndrome, denotes a poor chance for salvage of renal function.

GLOMERULI

The glomerulus consists of an enlargement of the proximal end of the renal tubule to incorporate a vascular tuft connecting the afferent and efferent arterioles (Fig. 42–1). The production of glomerular ultrafiltrate is predominantly dependent on the transcapillary hydrostatic pressure (dictated by the afferent and efferent arteriolar resistance) and the glomerular surface area. Afferent arteriolar tone is determined primarily by the local levels of angiotensin II (which induces vasoconstriction) and prostaglandins (which induce vasodilation). Efferent arteriolar tone is predominantly determined by the local concentration of angiotensin II.

Pathophysiologic processes and medications that result in alterations of the afferent and efferent arteriolar tone (i.e., systemic hypotension, hypercalcemia, or use of ACEIs, angiotensin II receptor blockers, or NSAIDs) reduce glomerular ultrafiltrate production as a result of a decrease in glomerular hydrostatic pressure. Under these conditions, the serum creatinine will rise, the urine sediment will be normal, and the urine indices will suggest prerenal azotemia. However, the urinary solutes may or may not be maximally concentrated, depending on the circulating level of antidiuretic hormone that is necessary to maximally concentrate the urine. Damage to the glomerular capillary tuft (e.g., acute glomerulonephritis) results in a decline in the production of glomerular ultrafiltrate as a result of a decrease in glomerular capillary surface area. Under these conditions the serum creatinine rises and the urinalysis is significant for hematuria and proteinuria because of the increased permeability of the damaged glomerular capillaries. Proteinuria exceeding 3 g/day is often referred to as nephrotic range proteinuria. Prolonged heavy proteinuria secondary to glomerular damage may result in the nephrotic syndrome.

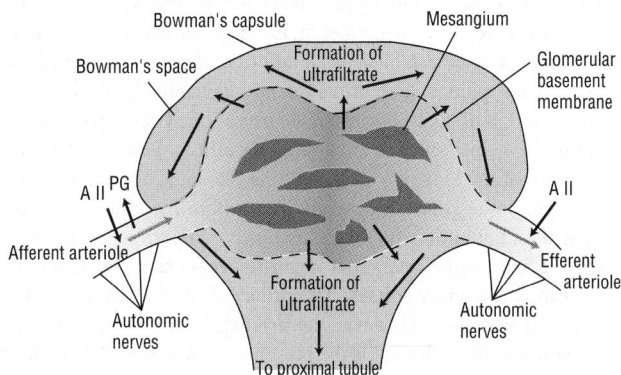

FIGURE 42–1. The formation of glomerular ultrafiltrate is dependent on the surface area of the glomerular capillaries, their permeability, and the net hydrostatic pressure across the capillary wall. As the glomerular capillary surface area increases secondary to mesangial cell relaxation, the formation of glomerular ultrafiltrate is increased. An increase or decrease in glomerular hydrostatic pressure results in either an increase or decrease in glomerular ultrafiltrate production. Afferent arteriolar vasoconstriction (which is primarily mediated by angiotensin II) or vasodilation (primarily mediated by prostaglandins) can result in a decrease or increase, respectively, in hydrostatic pressure across the capillary. Efferent arteriolar vasoconstriction (primarily mediated by angiotensin II) results in an increase in glomerular hydrostatic pressure. Under conditions in which renal blood flow is diminished, the kidney maintains glomerular ultrafiltration by vasodilating the afferent and vasoconstricting the efferent arterioles. Medications that may interfere with these processes might result in an abrupt decline in glomerular filtration.

RENAL TUBULES

Under normal conditions, approximately 180 L of glomerular ultrafiltrate are produced per day, the vast majority of which must be reabsorbed by the renal tubules to maintain homeostasis. Clinically, the renal tubule can be divided into three major sections: the proximal tubule, Henle's loop, and the distal nephron, which includes the distal tubule, the cortical collecting tubule, and the medullary collecting ducts. In the proximal tubule, approximately 60% to 70% of the filtered load of water and solute is isovolemically reabsorbed, as is the vast majority of filtered amino acids, glucose, and bicarbonate.

In addition to its other functions, Henle's loop is responsible for a significant portion of the total reabsorption of potassium, calcium, and magnesium, as well as for generating the osmotic gradient within the kidney that is necessary for the concentration of urinary solutes. Damage to this portion of the nephron results in wasting of potassium and magnesium by the kidney and an inability of the kidney to concentrate the urine. The medullary portions of Henle's loop are very sensitive to ischemia secondary to hypoperfusion. Consequently, in severe prerenal azotemia with renal hypoperfusion, there may be a loss of urinary concentrating ability despite the continued presence of a low urinary sodium concentration and a low fractional excretion of sodium.

Major functions of the distal nephron include the regeneration of bicarbonate, the excretion of acid (hydrogen ion), the secretion of potassium, and the reabsorption of water. Damage to this portion of the nephron may present as significant acidemia and either hypo- or hyperkalemia, depending on the mechanism of injury. For example, amphotericin B produces small pores in the luminal membrane of distal tubular cells. These pores allow small molecules such as potassium to leak out; the molecules are then wasted in the urine. Consequently, amphotericin B nephrotoxicity is characterized by hypokalemia secondary to renal potassium wasting. ATN is associated with urinary sediment characterized by the presence of tubular cells, coarse granular casts, and rarely, RBC casts.

INTERSTITIUM

The interstitium of the kidney provides the structural support for the kidney and serves to provide the environment in which concentrating gradients can be established. In addition, the interstitium of the kidney plays a major role in urinary ammonia handling. To facilitate the regeneration of bicarbonate and the excretion of acid by the distal nephron, the kidney utilizes ammonia as a urinary buffer. When the interstitium of the kidney is damaged (e.g., in acute allergic interstitial nephritis), the concentrating gradient within the kidney may be dissipated and ammonia handling disrupted. Consequently, patients presenting with acute interstitial nephritis frequently are unable to concentrate the urinary solutes. The urinalysis may show mild proteinuria and hematuria. However, the striking finding on microscopic examination of the sediment is the presence of numerous WBCs and WBC casts.

Rapid diagnosis is essential in the treatment of ARF in order to prevent extension of renal damage. The cause of most cases of ARF can be diagnosed from relatively few laboratory tests in conjunction with a good history and physical exam.

HISTORY

The diagnostic approach to the patient with ARF differs depending on the clinical setting in which the kidneys fail. For patients who present to the outpatient clinic or hospital with an elevated serum creatinine, the first objective is to determine if the renal failure is acute or chronic. A past medical history of renal disease or chronic conditions such as poorly controlled hypertension or diabetes mellitus, previous laboratory data documenting the presence of proteinuria or an elevated serum creatinine, and the finding of bilateral small kidneys on renal ultrasonography all suggest the presence of severe and chronic kidney disease.

For patients who do not have the above findings, their renal failure should be considered acute until proven otherwise. In these individuals, a careful review of their recent medications, including nonprescription, complementary, and alternative medications is mandatory. Special attention should be focused on diuretics, NSAIDs, antihypertensives, and any recent additions or changes in the patient's medications.

The patient's recent history can usually provide an indication of when the onset of renal dysfunction began. Frequently, patients may notice a change in their voiding habits with an increase in urinary frequency or nocturia, both suggesting a urinary concentrating defect. A decrease in the force of the urinary stream may suggest an obstruction. The presence of cola-colored urine, indicating the presence of blood in the urine, is common in acute glomerulonephritis. If the accompanying proteinuria is severe, the patient may note excessive foaming of the urine in the toilet. The onset of bilateral flank pain may suggest swelling of the kidneys secondary to either acute glomerulonephritis or acute interstitial nephritis. The onset of severe headaches may suggest the development of hypertension as a result of ARF. A recent increase in the patient's weight or complaints of tight-fitting rings secondary to salt and water retention also may be helpful in defining the onset of renal failure.

For patients who develop ARF while hospitalized, a review of the laboratory data is usually sufficient to define the onset of ARF. However, significant renal injury can occur prior to an increase in the serum creatinine. Consequently, clinicians must pay careful attention to subtle changes in the patient's weight, blood pressure, and urine output if they are to diagnose the onset of ARF. In addition to its prognostic significance, changes in urine output may be helpful in diagnosing the type of renal dysfunction that is present. Acute anuria is secondary to either complete urinary obstruction or a catastrophic event (e.g., shock, HUS, or acute cortical necrosis). Initial presentation with oliguria suggests prerenal azotemia, functional ARF, or acute intrinsic renal failure. Nonoliguric renal failure usually results from acute intrinsic renal failure or incomplete urinary obstruction.

CLINICAL PRESENTATION OF ACUTE RENAL FAILURE

GENERAL
Outpatients often are not in acute distress; hospitalized patients may develop ARF after a catastrophic event

SYMPTOMS
Outpatient: Change in urinary habits, weight gain, or flank pain
Inpatient: Typically ARF is noticed by clinicians before it is noticed by the patient

SIGNS
Patient may have edema; urine may be colored or foamy. Vital signs may indicate orthostatic hypotension in volume-depleted patients

LABORATORY TESTS
Urine and blood chemistries may determine prerenal cause complete blood cell count (CBC) and differential rules out infectious causes

Urine microscopy may reveal casts, WBCs, RBCs, and eosinophils

OTHER DIAGNOSTIC TESTS

Renal ultrasound or cystoscopy may be needed to rule out obstruction; renal biopsy reserved for difficult diagnoses

PHYSICAL EXAMINATION

A physical examination, including assessment of the patient's volume and hemodynamic status, is the next step in evaluating individuals with ARF. Common physical findings in patients with ARF are listed in Table 42–3. The physical exam should be thorough, as clues regarding etiology can come from anywhere from the patient's head (eye exam) to toe (evidence of dependent edema).

LABORATORY TESTS AND INTERPRETATION

Chapter 41 describes the use of serum creatinine as a determinant of renal function. As stated earlier, many clinicians do not agree on the definition of ARF based on specific changes in serum creatinine

values. The difficulty of using serum creatinine as a diagnostic laboratory test for hospitalized patients with ischemic ARF is that it is too insensitive to rapid changes in glomerular filtration rates. An abrupt cessation in glomerular filtration will not yield an immediate measurable change in serum creatinine. Reasons for this include: creatinine generation is relatively slow, lab tests are not very sensitive to small changes, and because fluid retention in renal failure dilutes the retained serum creatinine.[4] By the time serum creatinine elevates enough to be noticed, the extension phase of ischemic ARF is complete.[22] "Correction" of serum creatinine values for hypervolemic patients with ARF has been suggested for earlier detection of ARF in at-risk patients.[4]

Selected blood tests in addition to blood urea nitrogen (BUN) and serum creatinine can have value in the management of the patient with ARF. For example, infectious causes of ARF can be ruled out using a CBC with differential. Serum electrolyte values are likely to be abnormal, and particular attention should be paid to serum potassium and phosphorus values, which can be elevated and cause life-threatening conditions.

Given the limited usefulness of solely using blood markers like creatinine or BUN to diagnose ARF, urinalysis should be performed. Urinalysis is an essential battery of tests when the clinician is attempting to determine the cause of renal failure. The finding of a high urinary

TABLE 42–3. Physical Examination Findings in Acute Renal Failure

Physical Examination Finding	Possible Diagnosis	Category of Acute Renal Failure
Vital signs		
Orthostatic hypotension	Volume depletion	Prerenal azotemia
Febrile	Sepsis	Acute intrinsic
Skin		
Tenting	Volume depletion	Prerenal azotemia
Rash	Hypersensitivity reaction	Acute interstitial nephritis
Petechiae	Thrombotic thrombocytopenic purpura	Acute intrinsic renal failure—vasculitis
	Hemolytic uremic syndrome	
	Sepsis	Acute intrinsic
Splinter hemorrhages	Endocarditis	Intrinsic renal failure—glomerulonephritis
Janeway lesions		
Osler's nodes		
Edema	Total body volume overload	Suggests prerenal azotemia unlikely
HEENT		
Hollenhorst plaque	Cholesterol emboli	Acute intrinsic renal failure—vascular
Roth spots	Endocarditis	Acute intrinsic renal failure—acute glomerulonephritis
Heart		
S$_3$ heart sound	Congestive heart failure	Prerenal azotemia
New murmur (particularly diastolic murmurs)	Endocarditis	Acute intrinsic renal failure—acute glomerulonephritis
Lung		
Rales	Pulmonary edema with volume overload or left ventricular dysfunction	Suggests prerenal azotemia unlikely
Abdomen		
Renal artery bruit	Renal artery stenosis	Prerenal azotemia
Ascites	Liver failure or right heart failure	Prerenal azotemia
Bladder distention	Bladder outlet obstruction	Hepatorenal syndrome
		Postobstruction renal failure
Genitourinary		
Prostatic enlargement	Prostatic hypertrophy or cancer	Postobstruction renal failure
Gynecologic		
Abnormal bimanual examination	Possible bilateral ureteral obstruction or cervical cancer	Postobstruction renal failure

CHF, congestive heart failure; HEENT, head, eyes, ears, nose, and throat.

TABLE 42–4. Diagnostic Parameters for Differentiating Causes of Acute Renal Failure

Laboratory Test	Prerenal Azotemia	Acute Intrinsic Renal Failure	Postrenal Obstruction
Urine sediment	Normal	Casts, cellular debris	Cellular debris
Urinary RBC	None	2 – 4+	Variable
Urinary WBC	None	2 – 4+	1+
Urine sodium	<20	>40	>40
FE$_{Na}$ (%)	<1	>2	Variable
Urine/serum osmolality	>1.5	<1.3	<1.5
Urine/serum creatinine	>40:1	<20:1	<20:1
BUN/S$_{Cr}$	>20	15	15

Common laboratory tests are used to classify the cause of acute renal failure. Functional acute renal failure, which is not included in this table, would have laboratory values similar to those seen in prerenal azotemia. However, the urine osmolality to plasma osmolality ratios may not exceed 1.5 depending on the circulating levels of antidiuretic hormone. The laboratory results listed under acute intrinsic renal failure are those seen in acute tubular necrosis, the most common cause of acute intrinsic renal failure.

BUN, blood urea nitrogen; FE$_{Na}$, fractional excretion of sodium; S$_{Cr}$, serum creatinine; RBC, red blood cell; WBC, white blood cell.

specific gravity, in the absence of glucosuria or mannitol administration, suggests an intact urinary concentrating mechanism, and that the cause is likely prerenal azotemia or functional ARF. The presence of proteinuria and hematuria indicate glomerular injury. Microscopic examination of the urine also is helpful in determining the cause of ARF. Benign urine sediment suggests prerenal azotemia, functional ARF, or urinary obstruction. The presence of RBCs and RBC casts indicates a glomerular injury. The finding of WBCs and WBC casts results from interstitial inflammation (i.e., interstitial nephritis), which can be secondary to an allergic, granulomatous, or infectious process.

Simultaneous measurement of serum and urinary chemistries is often helpful in determining the etiology of ARF (Table 42–4). From these values a fractional excretion of sodium from urinary and plasma creatinine and sodium concentrations can be calculated. The equation for the calculation of the fractional excretion of sodium (FE$_{Na}$) is:

$$FE_{Na} = (\text{excreted Na/filtered Na}) \cdot 100$$

$$= (U_{vol} \cdot U_{Na})/(GFR \cdot P_{Na}) \cdot 100$$

where

$$GFR = (U_{vol} \cdot U_{Cr})/(P_{Cr} \cdot t)$$

Thus:

$$FE_{Na} = (U_{Na} \cdot P_{Cr} \cdot 100)/(U_{Cr} \cdot P_{Na})$$

where U$_{vol}$ is urine volume; U$_{Cr}$ is urine creatinine; U$_{Na}$ is urine sodium; P$_{Cr}$ is plasma creatinine; P$_{Na}$ is plasma sodium; GFR is the glomerular filtration rate; and t is the time period over which the urine is collected.

The fractional excretion of sodium calculation from plasma and urinary chemistry values is used to differentiate the cause of ARF. A low urinary sodium concentration and low fractional excretion of sodium (<1%) in a patient with oliguria suggest that there is stimulation of the sodium-retentive mechanisms in the kidney and that tubular function is intact. These findings are most characteristic of prerenal azotemia or functional ARF. Inability to concentrate urine results in a high fractional excretion of sodium (>2%), suggesting tubular damage as is seen with ATN. Diagnosing the type of ARF using fractional excretion of sodium is not absolute, as there are some causes that can be associated with a low fractional excretion of sodium (e.g., contrast nephropathy, myoglobinuria, and interstitial nephritis). Highly concentrated urine (>500 mOsm/L) suggests stimulation of antidiuretic hormone and intact tubular function. These findings are consistent with prerenal azotemia. Diuretic use limits the utility of the fractional excretion of sodium calculation by increasing natriuresis, even in hypovolemic patients.

DIAGNOSTIC PROCEDURES

Renal ultrasound is rarely helpful in determining the cause of ARF in a hospitalized patient who previously had normal renal function; however, for the outpatient who presents with renal failure, the renal ultrasound is instrumental in determining whether the renal failure is acute or chronic and whether or not obstruction is present. A plain film radiograph of the abdomen may be useful in documenting the presence of two kidneys and in checking for renal stones. If the possibility of renal artery obstruction exists, a radioisotope scan or renal angiography may be required. Intravenous pyelography is rarely used in the diagnostic work-up of ARF. Cystoscopy with retrograde pyelography may be helpful if the possibility of obstruction exists. If insertion of a urinary catheter into the patient's bladder after the patient has voided does not yield a large volume of urine (>500 mL), then one can usually exclude postrenal obstruction as the cause of ARF. If a large volume of urine remains after the patient has voided, or if the patient is unable to void, urinary catheter placement into the bladder may result in alleviation of symptoms if the obstruction is somewhere between the bladder to the urethral opening.

If the etiology of the ARF is unclear despite a careful history, physical examination, and appropriate diagnostic tests, percutaneous renal biopsy may be indicated. Renal biopsy is associated with some risk (primarily bleeding) and should only be performed in those few patients who meet criteria for biopsy. However, in cases in whom the cause of ARF is not evident, renal biopsies are useful in determining the cause in more than 90% of patients.[25]

▶ PREVENTION AND TREATMENT: Acute Renal Failure

■ DESIRED OUTCOME

Given the dismal outcomes of patients with ARF, prevention is critical. In many cases, the risk of ARF development is known and is predictable. For example, when patients with risk factors for ARF development are scheduled to receive radiocontrast dye or sur-

gery that will stop blood flow to the kidneys, the clinician knows that ARF may develop. In these cases preventive measures must be taken. Fortunately many therapeutic maneuvers have been identified that can reduce the risk of ARF development in these situations. Consequently the goals of treatment are (1) to prevent ARF, but if ARF develops, (2) avoid or minimize further renal insults that would delay recovery, and (3) provide supportive measures until kidney function returns.

GENERAL APPROACH TO TREATMENT

The general approach to the treatment of established ARF is dependent on the setting in which it develops. In the community setting, the first goal is to remove the causative agent (drugs or nephrotoxins) if possible. If the cause is immune-related, as may be the case with interstitial nephritis or glomerulonephritis, a rapid diagnosis must be made to begin appropriate immunologic therapy (usually corticosteroids). In the hospital setting, nephrotoxic agents should be discontinued and prerenal causes must be ruled out. Renal perfusion should be optimized to stop extension of any ischemic processes. This typically means a fluid challenge with close watch of the patient's vital signs and urine output. Care must be taken not to fluid overload a patient with absent kidney function. Once renal failure is established and the cause is known, supportive care is all that can be provided. Renal replacement therapy is provided to maintain fluid and electrolyte balance while removing accumulating waste products. All further insults to the kidney must be prevented so the slow process of renal recovery can begin. In the case of ATN, this typically occurs within 10 to 14 days. Longer courses of ARF can occur if the kidney is exposed to repeated insults.

PREVENTION OF ARF

❸ The therapies used to prevent ARF are much different than those used to treat established ARF; consequently preventive therapies will be reviewed first and treatment options will follow. Given the dismal outcome of patients with ARF, numerous regimens have been tried to prevent the development of ARF in patients who will be receiving known nephrotoxins. Typically, these interventions are made prior to administration of nephrotoxins like radiocontrast dye, or prior to surgical procedures that will restrict blood flow to the kidneys for extended periods. Because the timing of the renal insult is known, this setting is ideal for conducting clinical studies into ARF prevention. Unfortunately the list of interventions that do not prevent ARF in this setting is longer than the list of those that do. Table 42–5 lists some of the interventions that have been studied to prevent ARF.

NONPHARMACOLOGIC

In situations in which administration of a nephrotoxin cannot be avoided, such as when radiocontrast dye is to be administered, nonpharmacologic therapies can be employed to prevent ARF. The key to nonpharmacologic ARF prevention is the elimination of the patient's risk factors to the degree that is possible. The best-studied examples of this are the interventions used to maximize renal perfusion when radiocontrast dye is administered. Adequate hydration and sodium loading prior to radiocontrast dye administration have been shown to be beneficial therapies. A trial comparing infusions of 0.9% NaCl or 5% dextrose with 0.45% NaCl administered prior to radiocontrast dye infusion conclusively demonstrated that the normal saline was superior in preventing ARF.[26] The intravenous solution infusion rate used in this study was 1 mL/kg per hour beginning the morning that the radiocontrast dye was going to be given, and all subjects were encouraged to drink fluids liberally as well. The benefits of 0.9% NaCl infusions have been found in similar studies,[27] suggesting this regimen should be used in all at-risk patients who can tolerate the sodium and fluid load.

Preventive Dialysis

A novel approach to reducing the incidence of nephrotoxicity associated with radiocontrast dye administration is to provide RRT prophylactically to patients at high risk. Hemofiltration provided prior to and 24 hours after dye administration resulted in significantly reduced mortality rates and a reduced need for dialysis.[28] In contrast, the use of hemodialysis within an hour of contrast dye infusion did not yield an improvement in nephrotoxicity rates, possibly because the toxicity due to dye occurs within minutes of its administration.[29]

PHARMACOLOGIC

❹ One of the simplest ways to prevent acute nephrotoxicity is to avoid the use of nephrotoxic agents when possible. If

TABLE 42–5. Evidence of Benefit of Prophylactic Therapies for the Prevention of Acute Renal Failure Due to Nephrotoxin Exposure

Intervention	Evidence for Prevention of Nephrotoxicity	Situations in Which Intervention Documented to be Effective
Hydration (sodium loading)	Y	Prior to amphotericin or contrast dye administration; tumor lysis syndrome prevention
Mannitol	N	
Loop diuretics	N	
Dopamine	N	
Calcium channel blockers	+/−	Recipient should receive drug prior to transplantation and when kidney is stored in solution containing drug. Not useful for preventing contrast dye nephropathy.
Theophylline	Y	Prior to contrast dye administration
Acetylcysteine	Y	Prior to contrast dye administration
Fenoldopam	N	
Insulin (to maintain serum glucose of 80–110 mg/dL)	Y	Critically ill patients

Y, some evidence exists for benefit; +/−, evidence equivocal; N, evidence suggests no benefit.

nephrotoxic agents cannot be avoided, there may be ways to administer them in a manner that reduces their nephrotoxic potential. A good example of this is the use of amphotericin B to treat fungal infections. Amphotericin is a highly nephrotoxic agent, causing ARF in approximately 30% of patients who receive it.[30] However, there are many infections for which no good alternative treatment exists. The nephrotoxic potential of amphotericin B deoxycholate can be reduced significantly simply by slowing the infusion rate from a standard 4-hour infusion to a slower 24-hour infusion of the same dose.[31] In a patient with risk factors for the development of ARF, liposomal forms of amphotericin B can be used. These liposomal formulations are more expensive, but cause a lower incidence of kidney damage.[32]

Given the dismal outcome of established ARF, many drugs have been investigated for its prevention. Surprisingly, many of these interventions have been found to be of no benefit. Low doses of dopamine (≤2 mcg/kg per minute) increase renal blood flow and might be expected to increase GFR. Theoretically, this might be considered beneficial, as an enhanced GFR might flush nephrotoxins from the tubules, minimizing their toxicity. Furthermore, loop diuretics may decrease tubular oxygen consumption by reducing solute reabsorption.[33] Despite these theoretical suggestions that loop diuretics and dopamine might be useful in ARF prevention, controlled studies do not support these theories. In a blinded and randomized trial conducted in patients undergoing cardiac surgery, dopamine 2 mcg/kg per minute, furosemide 0.5 mcg/kg per minute, and a 0.9% NaCl placebo given at initiation of surgery were compared to determine whether any of the these interventions would be beneficial.[34] Postoperative increases in serum creatinine occurred significantly more often in the furosemide-treated subjects than in the other two groups. Dopamine afforded no benefit compared to the sodium chloride infusion, and therefore should not be used routinely in this manner.

The use of diuretics to prevent nephrotoxicity may actually result in intravascular depletion, a prerenal state, and an exacerbation of ARF. A trial of forced diuresis, in which mannitol, furosemide, and/or dopamine were given, and resultant urinary losses were replaced with intravenous solutions found that diuretic use resulted in little benefit compared to IV solutions given alone.[35] Interestingly, these investigators noted that patients that were unable to produce much urine despite diuretic administration were more likely to develop ARF than patients who did respond to diuretics. While this unresponsiveness to diuretics might simply be an indication of preexisting kidney damage, similar reports have linked diuretic unresponsiveness to increased mortality rates in critically ill patients with ARF.[6]

CLINICAL CONTROVERSIES

Despite the fact that most studies do not show improved patient outcomes with its use, low-dose dopamine continues to be commonly used. The risks associated with dopamine use (extravasation and the potential for significant dosing errors) suggest that it should usually be avoided.

Giving low-dose dopamine infusions (≤2 mcg/kg per minute) for the prevention of ARF is a surprisingly common practice given the paucity of data to support its use. While most studies do report an increase in urine output when low-dose dopamine is administered, almost none report that this practice yields a benefit to the patient. A meta-analysis of all low-dose dopamine studies conducted from 1966 to 2000 concluded that low-dose dopamine does not prevent ARF and its use could not be justified.[36]

Fenoldopam

Fenoldopam is a selective dopamine-1 receptor agonist that has been investigated for its ability to prevent radiocontrast dye nephropathy. Originally approved for use as an intravenous antihypertensive agent, fenoldopam reduces systemic blood pressure while preserving renal blood flow, it appears to have salutary properties for the prevention of drug-induced nephrotoxicity. A large, multicenter, randomized, placebo-controlled trial of fenoldopam use to prevent radiocontrast dye nephropathy in patients with CKD found that fenoldopam provided no benefit.[37] The disappointing results of this trial and that of the dopamine studies suggest that dopaminergic manipulation of the kidney is not likely to work as a preventive measure for nephrotoxicity (see Chap. 46).

Acetylcysteine

Pretreatment with oral acetylcysteine, (also called n-acetylcysteine), 600 mg twice daily on the day before and the day of radiocontrast dye administration has been documented to lower the rate of ARF in patients with pre-existing CKD.[38–39] The mechanism for acetylcysteine's ability to reduce the incidence of radiocontrast dye nephrotoxicity is not fully elucidated, but likely is due to its antioxidant effects. Given the consistent findings of its efficacy and its relatively low cost, acetylcysteine should be given to all patients at risk for radiocontrast dye nephrotoxicity.

Many other drugs have been investigated for the prevention of ARF, with varying degrees of success.[33] A few of these agents bear mentioning. Theophylline 200 mg infused 30 minutes before contrast dye administration resulted in a fivefold decrease in nephropathy compared to a placebo infusion in high-risk patients.[40] Despite this finding and for reasons that are unclear, most centers typically do not use this intervention to prevent contrast dye nephropathy. Calcium antagonists have shown promise in reducing ATN in kidneys that are transplanted,[41] but their utility is limited in other clinical settings due to their hypotensive effects.

Glycemic Control

Perhaps the most promising agent for the prevention of hospital-acquired ARF is a very old drug, but its use in the prevention of ARF is a very new finding. Van den Berghe and associates randomized patients in a surgical ICU to receive standard control (<200 mg/dL) or intensive glucose control measures (goal blood glucose concentrations of 80 to 110 mg/dL).[42] Tight blood glucose resulted in significant improvements in mortality and a 41% reduction in the development of ARF. It appears that while it was blood glucose control that caused the mortality benefit, the reduction in ARF may have been due to the total dose of insulin used to treat the patient, suggesting a direct protective effect of insulin.[17] Strict glycemic control is recognized as an important goal for outpatient diabetics;[43] however, intensive insulin therapy will likely also become the standard of care for all critically ill patients to prevent ARF and improve mortality.

TREATMENT OF ESTABLISHED ARF

Once the kidney has been damaged by an initial insult (reduced perfusion, nephrotoxins, etc.), initial therapies should be directed to eliminate further harm to the kidney, thus preventing extension of the injury.[22] The time to recovery from ARF is determined from the most recent insult to the kidney, not the first insult. Hospitalized patients with ARF are at risk for repeated episodes of kidney damage through nephrotoxic agents and hypotensive episodes, among other problems. These increased risks coupled with the fact that no drugs have been found to accelerate ARF recovery change the way clinicians approach the ARF patient. Patients with established ARF should be viewed as patients who should be supported and protected through the period of ARF rather than as patients who will respond to therapies designed to hasten renal recovery.

NONPHARMACOLOGIC THERAPY

Supportive care goals for the critically ill patient with ARF include aggressive fluid management. Cardiac output and blood pressure must be supported to allow for adequate tissue perfusion. However, a fine balance must be struck in this regard. For example, fluids must be typically restricted in anuric and oliguric patients unless the patient is hypovolemic or is able to achieve fluid balance via renal replacement therapy. If fluid intake is not minimized, edema rapidly occurs, especially in hypoalbuminemic patients. In contrast, vasopressors like dopamine ≥ 2 mcg/kg per minute or norepinephrine are used to maintain adequate tissue perfusion, but may also induce kidney hypoxia via a reduction in renal blood flow. Consequently, Swan-Ganz monitoring is essential for critically ill patients.

Another related supportive care issue is electrolyte management. Hyperkalemia, hypermagnesemia, and hyperphosphatemia are common electrolyte disorders in patients with ARF who are unable to use their kidneys to maintain electrolyte balance. This is generally not a serious concern in patients who are achieving electrolyte control via RRT, but electrolytes should be monitored closely in all patients with ARF.

Renal replacement therapies are the most common nonpharmacologic treatment that patients with ARF receive. Absolute indications for starting RRT in an ARF patient do not exist, but some general guidelines for therapy initiation do exist (Table 42–6). Renal replacement therapies come in two different forms, intermittent therapies like hemodialysis, and continuous RRTs like continuous hemofiltration or peritoneal dialysis. A more detailed explanation of these therapies appears in Chap. 45. The choice of whether continuous therapies or intermittent RRTs are used is a matter of debate and is usually determined by physician preference and the resources available at the hospital.

The merits of intermittent hemodialysis are many. Hemodialysis machines usually are available at hospitals and health care workers are familiar with their use. Hemodialysis treatments usually last 3 to 4 hours, so they can be done during work hours when hospitals are best staffed. The disadvantages of intermittent hemodialysis are also numerous. Venous dialysis access can be difficult in hypotensive patients with ARF. Because intermittent hemodialysis only runs for a few hours per day, large amounts of fluid must be removed in a relatively short period of time in volume-overloaded patients. This can result in hypotension that may delay the recovery from ARF. If hemodialysis is carefully monitored and hypotension avoided, better patient outcomes can be achieved.[44] Patients with CKD can achieve adequate solute and volume control with thrice weekly dialysis, but hypercatabolic, fluid-overloaded patients with ARF may require daily hemodialysis treatments.[45]

In contrast, continuous RRTs have a different set of advantages and disadvantages.[46] Typically peritoneal dialysis does not provide enough solute and fluid control for hypercatabolic patients with ARF. The exception to this rule may be in the treatment of small children, who have a larger peritoneal membrane surface area to body weight ratio than do adults. This larger ratio may allow for enough clearance for peritoneal dialysis to be used in these children. Other than in this pediatric scenario, continuous renal replacement therapy (CRRT) is performed as continuous hemodialysis, continuous hemofiltration, or a combination of the two. Disadvantages of CRRT are that not all hospitals have the special machinery necessary to conduct these treatments, they require intensive nursing care around the clock, they are more expensive because of the custom intravenous and dialysis fluids used, and less is known about drug dosing in these therapies. The main advantage of CRRT is that the continuous nature of these therapies allows for a more gradual removal of solutes and fluid that is better tolerated by critically ill patients. Raw comparisons of patient outcome when treated with intermittent hemodialysis versus CRRT typically show a higher mortality rate with the continuous therapies.[47] However, patients treated with continuous therapies are almost always more critically ill than those treated by intermittent hemodialysis. The reason for this selection bias is that the sickest patients are unable to tolerate intermittent hemodialysis; consequently comparisons of outcome must control for illness severity. It appears that patient outcome, once adjusted for severity of illness, is no different between intermittent and continuous therapies, and patients who are intolerant of intermittent dialysis may do quite well with continuous therapies.[48]

CLINICAL CONTROVERSY

Some clinicians believe that CRRTs are preferable to intermittent hemodialysis because they provide more consistent fluid and waste product removal. Others suggest that intermittent hemodialysis is preferable because nursing and medical staff are more familiar with its use and round-the-clock nursing is not needed.

Continuous renal replacement therapies are becoming more commonly used for critically ill patients with ARF. Continuous renal replacement therapy operating for 24 hours a day means that more RRT can be given per week than can be accomplished with the thrice-weekly hemodialysis treatments used in patients with CKD. This has influenced how dialysis is prescribed in the ICU for hypercatabolic patients with ARF. Intermittent hemodialysis administered daily has been associated with improved survival and faster resolution of ARF compared to dialysis given every other day.[49] Daily dosing of dialysis presents challenges to clinicians prescribing drug and nutrition therapy, as most of these dosing guidelines are based on thrice-weekly dialysis, and application of these guidelines may yield inappropriate dosing.

TABLE 42–6. The AEIOUs That Describe the Indications for Renal Replacement Therapy

Indication for Renal Replacement Therapy	Clinical Setting
A Acid-base abnormalities	Metabolic acidosis resulting from the accumulation of organic and inorganic acids
E Electrolyte imbalance	Hyperkalemia, hypermagnesemia
I Intoxications	Salicylates, lithium, methanol, ethylene glycol, theophylline, phenobarbital
O fluid Overload	Postoperative fluid gain
U Uremia	High catabolism of acute renal failure

Modifications to standard intermittent dialysis techniques have been made to try to take advantage of the higher overall doses of renal replacement that can be obtained with CRRT. Some have made a hybrid between intermittent dialysis and continuous therapies. These hybrid therapies have a variety of names, with the two most common being sustained low-efficiency dialysis[50] and extended daily dialysis.[51] These therapies use standard hemodialysis machines with the blood and dialysate flows slowed down, and they are run for extended periods compared to intermittent hemodialysis. Proposed advantages of these therapies are that no new machinery is needed, and that therapy can be given for 8 to 12 hours per day, allowing for gradual fluid removal. These therapies do not require 24 hour-a-day nursing supervision, yet deliver plenty of urea and waste product removal. The main negative of these hybrid therapies is that while they yield large amounts of urea clearance, drug clearance changes every time the dialysis machine is turned on and off. This makes drug dosing difficult to manage.[52] Very few pharmacokinetic studies have been conducted with these hybrid therapies.[53]

One aspect of RRT that is overlooked by most clinicians is which hemodialyzer or hemofilter is used during the treatment. The material used to make the membranes of hemodialyzers (for hemodialysis) and hemofilters (for hemofiltration) varies by manufacturer, and recent evidence suggests that which membrane material is used may influence the outcomes of patients with ARF. When blood comes into contact with these membranes, the complement cascade is activated, resulting in an immune reaction. Each type of membrane induces complement to a different degree. Those that cause less of a complement cascade are termed "biocompatible," while membranes that induce a large reaction are considered "bioincompatible." Bio-compatible membranes tend to be made of newer, more expensive, synthetic materials and usually have larger pores in them. Bioincompatible membranes are usually made of cellulosic materials and have relatively small pores. The use of biocompatible membranes has been associated with slightly better patient outcomes than the use of more complement-activating membranes.[54–55]

PHARMACOLOGIC THERAPY

The use of drug therapy in patients with ARF to accelerate the recovery of renal function has been a dream of clinicians for years. To date, no drug therapy has ever been documented to do this. Many agents have looked promising in animal trials, only to be found ineffective in human trials. The list of drugs that have been investigated and shown no benefit is long.[56] In recent years thyroxine,[57] dopamine,[58] and loop diuretics[6] have all been documented to either be of no help or to worsen patient outcomes. For example, loop diuretic use in patients with ARF was associated with a 77% increase in mortality or nonrecovery of renal function compared to patients who did not receive loop diuretics.[6] These findings may be explained by the fact that sicker, fluid-overloaded patients may be more likely to receive diuretics, nonetheless no benefit to loop diuretic use could be found in any subanalysis. Consequently, loop diuretic use should be reserved for fluid-overloaded patients who make adequate urine in response to diuretics to merit their use.

In fluid-overloaded nonoliguric patients, diuretics can facilitate patient management (Fig. 42–2). Prevention of pulmonary edema is an important goal, and it is preferable that this be accomplished

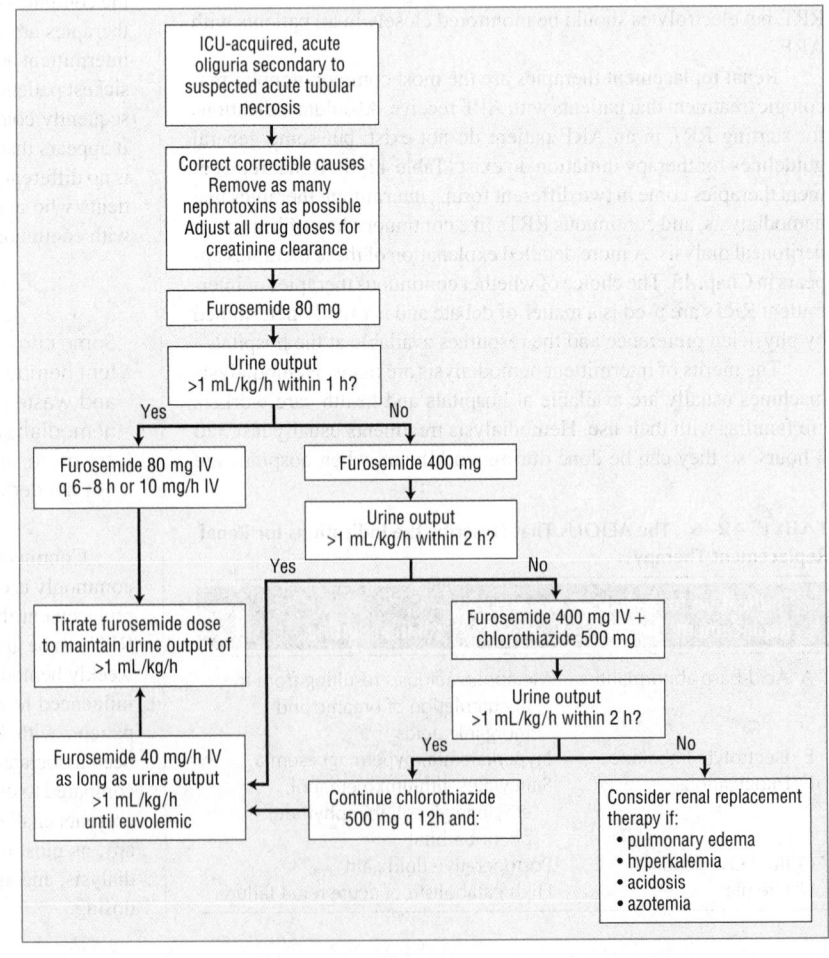

FIGURE 42–2. Suggested treatment algorithm for ICU-acquired oliguric acute renal failure resulting from acute tubular necrosis.

with diuretics instead of more invasive RRTs, despite the previously mentioned finding that diuretic use may be associated with a worse outcome.[6] The most effective drugs in causing diuresis in the ARF setting are mannitol and the loop diuretics. These two therapies have distinct advantages and disadvantages. Mannitol, which works as an osmotic diuretic, can only be given parenterally. A typical starting dose is mannitol (20%) 12.5 to 25 g infused intravenously over 3 to 5 minutes. It has little nonrenal clearance, so when given to anuric or oliguric patients, mannitol will remain in the patient, potentially causing a hyperosmolar state. Additionally mannitol may cause ARF itself, so its use in ARF must be monitored carefully by measuring urine output and serum electrolytes and osmolality.[59] Due to these limitations of mannitol, some have recommended that it be reserved for its nondiuretic uses, like management of cerebral edema.[60]

CLINICAL CONTROVERSIES

In edematous patients, occasionally a clinician will suggest infusing albumin to provide intravascular oncotic pressure to mobilize fluid back into the intravascular space, and then administering loop diuretics to remove this fluid. Studies on the merits and costs of this combination have had mixed results.

Furosemide, bumetanide, torsemide, and ethacrynic acid are the most frequently used loop diuretics in patients with ARF. Ethacrynic acid is reserved for patients who are allergic to sulfa compounds. Furosemide is the most commonly used loop diuretic because of its lower cost, availability in oral and parenteral forms, and good safety and efficacy profiles. A disadvantage with furosemide is its variable oral bioavailability in many patients. Consequently, initial furosemide doses (usually 40 to 80 mg) are usually administered intravenously to assess whether the patient will respond. Torsemide and bumetanide have better oral bioavailability than furosemide. Torsemide has a longer duration of activity than the other loop diuretics which allows for less frequent administration but also may make it more difficult to titrate the dose. Loop diuretics should all work equally well in a given patient provided that they are administered in equipotent doses parenterally so that bioavailability issues are obviated. In a patient who is unresponsive to aggressive loop diuretic dosing, switching to another loop diuretic is unlikely to be beneficial. In the outpatient setting, torsemide may be preferred because it can be administered once daily, and because of its relatively better oral bioavailability than furosemide.

Diuretic Resistance

Inability to respond to administered diuretics is common in ARF and is associated with a poor patient outcome.[6] An effective technique to overcome diuretic resistance is to give loop diuretics via continuous infusions instead of intermittent boluses. Less natriuresis occurs when equal doses of loop diuretics are given as a bolus instead of as a continuous infusion. Furthermore, adverse reactions from loop diuretics (myalgias and hearing loss) occur less frequently in patients receiving continuous infusion compared to those receiving intermittent boluses, ostensibly because lower serum concentrations are attained. However, these adverse effects still may occur with continuous infusion loop diuretics and should be monitored.[61] The finding that the continuous infusions of loop diuretics have efficacy that is at least as good as intermittent bolus dosing, with fewer adverse effects, appears to be consistent for all agents, including furosemide,[62] bumetanide,[63] and torsemide.[64] When continuous loop diuretic infusion is used, an initial loading dose is given (equivalent to furosemide 40 to 80 mg) prior to the initiation of the continuous infusion at a dose of 10 to 20 mg/hour of furosemide or its equivalent. Patients with low creatinine clearances have much lower rates of diuretic secretion into the tubular fluid; consequently, higher doses are generally used in patients with renal insufficiency.[60]

Diuretic resistance may occur simply because excessive sodium intake overrides the ability of the diuretics to eliminate sodium. Other reasons exist for diuretic resistance in this population. Patients with ATN have a reduced number of functioning nephrons on which the diuretic may exert its action. Other clinical states like glomerulonephritis are associated with heavy proteinuria. Intraluminal loop diuretics cannot exert their effect in the loop of Henle because they are extensively bound to the protein present in the urine. Still other patients may have reduced bioavailability of oral furosemide. Possible therapeutic options to counteract each form of diuretic resistance are presented in Table 42–7. Combination therapy of loop diuretics plus a diuretic from a different pharmacologic class can be an effective tool in the setting of ARF.[65] Loop diuretics increase the delivery of sodium chloride to the distal convoluted tubule and collecting duct. With time, these areas of the nephron compensate for the activity of the loop diuretic and increase sodium and chloride resorption. Diuretics that work at the

TABLE 42–7. Common Causes of Diuretic Resistance in Patients with Acute Renal Failure and the Measures Used to Counteract Them

Causes of Diuretic Resistance	Potential Therapeutic Solutions
Excessive sodium intake (sources may be dietary, IV fluids, and drugs)	Remove sodium from nutritional sources and medications
Inadequate diuretic dose or inappropriate regimen	Increase dose, use continuous infusion or combination therapy
Reduced oral bioavailability (usually furosemide)	Use parenteral therapy; switch to oral torsemide or bumetanide
Nephrotic syndrome (loop diuretic protein binding in tubule lumen)	Increase dose, switch diuretics, use combination therapy
Reduced renal blood flow	
Drugs (NSAIDs ACEIs, vasodilators)	Discontinue these drugs if possible
Hypotension	Intravascular volume expansion and/or vasopressors
Intravascular depletion	Intravascular volume expansion
Increased sodium resorption	
Nephron adaptation to chronic diuretic therapy	Combination diuretic therapy, sodium restriction
NSAID use	Discontinue NSAID
Congestive heart failure	Treat the CHF, increase diuretic dose, switch to better absorbed loop diuretic
Cirrhosis	High-volume paracentesis
Acute tubular necrosis	Higher dose of diuretic, diuretic combination therapy, add low-dose dopamine

distal convoluted tubule (thiazides) or the collecting duct (amiloride, triamterene, and spironolactone) may have a synergistic effect when administered with loop diuretics by blocking the compensatory increase in sodium and chloride resorption. The combination of loop diuretics and usual doses of thiazide diuretics may be effective in renal disease despite the accumulation of endogenous organic acids in renal disease that blocks the transport of loop diuretics into the lumen. If oral thiazides cannot be given to the patient, chlorothiazide can be administered parenterally.

Several drug combinations with loop diuretics have been investigated, including the addition of one or more of the following: theophylline, acetazolamide, spironolactone, thiazides, or metolazone.[65] Of these combinations, metolazone is used most frequently with furosemide. Metolazone, unlike other thiazides, produces effective diuresis at a GFR below 20 mL/minute. This combination of metolazone and a loop diuretic has been used successfully in the management of fluid overload in patients with CHF, cirrhosis, and nephrotic syndrome. Additionally, this combination has been found to be efficacious in pediatric patients as well as adults.[66] The combination of mannitol plus intravenous loop diuretics is used by some practitioners,[67] but no convincing evidence of the superiority of this combination regimen to conventional dosing of either diuretic alone exists.

NUTRITIONAL INTERVENTIONS

While most drug therapy has yet to show benefit in patients with ARF, certain nutritional interventions may be useful. Pre-existing nutrition status has been shown to be a strong predictor of outcomes in patients with ARF.[15] The use of enteral nutrition in patients with ARF in ICUs has been associated with an improvement in outcomes.[10] Parenteral nutrition did not show the same benefit and some have questioned whether parenteral nutrition should ever be used in this population.[68]

The most common interventions that must be made when treating patients with ARF involve fluid and electrolyte management. Most patients with ARF are fluid overloaded, and fluids must be restricted. This means maximally concentrated drug infusions and nutrition solutions. So-called "keep vein open" or maintenance intravenous infusions should be halted unless the patient is euvolemic or is receiving renal replacement solution that is able to maintain fluid balance.

The most common electrolyte disorder in ARF is hyperkalemia. Life-threatening cardiac arrhythmias may occur from hyperkalemia, so potassium restriction is essential. The treatment of hyperkalemia is discussed in Chap. 50. Typically no potassium should be added to parenteral solutions unless hypokalemia is documented. Patients receiving enteral nutrition should be limited to a 3-g potassium diet. Serum potassium concentrations should be monitored daily, even in patients receiving RRT. Some centers add no potassium to their CRRT solutions and hypokalemia can result with prolonged therapy.

Sodium restriction is also a necessary intervention. A diet with 3 g of sodium per day is usually a reasonable place to start. Ingestion of too much sodium is a common reason diuretic therapy fails. Clinicians should be vigilant about sources of sodium. For example, 1 L of 0.9% NaCl yields 154 mEq of sodium, or 3.5 g. Sodium is usually restricted even in patients who are receiving RRT. In continuous and intermittent RRTs there usually is no worry about hyponatremia developing because these therapies will incorporate isonatremic (135 to 140 mEq/L of sodium) solutions as dialysate or ultrafiltrate replacement solutions. Serum sodium concentrations should be monitored daily.

Other electrolytes that require monitoring include magnesium and phosphorus. Both are eliminated by the kidneys and are not removed efficiently by dialysis. Typically their dietary intake is restricted, but in patients receiving prolonged renal replacement, deficiency states can occur, particularly in pediatric patients due to their reduced body stores. Hypophosphatemia can also occur in these critically ill patients as a result of the refeeding syndrome, in which nutritional supplementation is instituted after the patient goes a long period of time without being fed. Nonetheless, in initial ARF, hyperphosphatemia is more likely. Patients who also have significant tissue destruction (trauma, rhabdomyolysis, tumor lysis syndrome, or sepsis) may have significant phosphorus released from the destroyed tissue. Treatment of the hyperphosphatemic state can include RRT; however, for patients not receiving these therapies, oral phosphate-binding antacids or sevelamer can be administered (see Chap. 44). In hyperphosphatemic patients, calcium-containing antacids are often avoided to prevent precipitation of calcium phosphate in the soft tissues. A common guideline is to maintain the calcium-phosphate product <55 in those with CKD. The calcium-phosphate product is calculated by multiplying the serum calcium (in milligrams per deciliter) by the serum phosphorus (also in milligrams per deciliter). When this product is above 55, sevelamer or aluminum-containing antacids are used, and once the phosphorus is better controlled, calcium-containing antacids can be used.

In contrast to the patient with CKD, the calcium balance is usually not an important issue for the ARF patient due to the limited duration of the illness. One exception to this is in patients receiving continuous RRT that is anticoagulated with citrate. Citrate binds to serum calcium and without calcium, blood cannot form a clot. Citrate is typically infused as blood leaves the body. A calcium infusion must be administered either at the end of the extracorporeal circuit or centrally to provide sufficient unbound calcium to the patient. Insufficient calcium infusions will result in hypocalcemia, arrhythmias, and even death, so frequent monitoring of unbound serum calcium concentrations is essential.

Other nutrition goals for ARF are patient-specific. It may be necessary to limit fluid intake in severely volume-overloaded patients even though this means restricting parenteral or enteral nutrition. Septic patients with ARF usually are hypercatabolic. The net protein catabolism results in rapidly rising BUN and serum creatinine values. The normalized protein catabolic rate has been reported to be 1.75 g/kg per day, but this value varies widely with each patient.[69] Most patients with ARF cannot tolerate the amount of fluid required to replace catabolized protein unless they are receiving continuous RRT or daily hemodialysis to remove excess volume.

Another nutritional consideration for patients receiving CRRT is the amount of heat each patient loses from the extracorporeal blood circuit and from receipt of room-temperature intravenous ultrafiltrate replacement solutions. Hypothermia occurs in up to half of all patients who receive CRRT, ostensibly because their body heat is radiated away as blood goes through the CRRT circuit.[70] The energy loss of continuous hemofiltration has been estimated to be almost 800 kcal/day when blood flow is 120 mL/minute and 23 mL/minute of ultrafiltrate is formed.[71] Most of this heat loss can be attenuated by warming the intravenous ultrafiltrate replacement solution.[71] However, most hospitals are unable to heat intravenous solutions as they are infused, so recognition of this large source of energy loss is necessary for the clinician ordering the nutrition prescription.

PUBLISHED GUIDELINES OR TREATMENT PROTOCOLS

Standards for the treatment of patients with CKD have been in place for many years as a result of the National Kidney Foundation's Kidney/Dialysis Outcomes Quality Initiative, begun in 1997. Only recently has a similar initiative been started for patients with ARF. The ADQI (Acute Dialysis Quality Initiative) was started by a group of interested physicians and is officially endorsed by the American Society of Nephrology and the Society of Critical Care Medicine. The goal of this group is to develop evidence-based treatment recommendations for patients with ARF. Seven areas of practice have been targeted by ADQI. They are (1) Definitions/Nomenclature; (2) Patient Selection; (3) Solute Control (Treatment Dose); (4) Membranes; (5) Operational Characteristics (Convection/Diffusion); (6) Fluid Management/Composition; and (7) Anticoagulation/Access. As these guidelines are developed, they will be published in nephrology journals and at the ADQI website (www.adqi.net).

PHARMACOKINETIC CONSIDERATIONS

Patients with ARF present some interesting pharmacokinetic challenges. Some of these challenges are obvious by simply looking at the patient. Edema is a common finding in patients with ARF, and this can influence the volume of distribution of many drugs, particularly those with relatively small volumes of distribution and those that are water soluble. CRRT can rapidly remove excess fluid from edematous patients, thereby changing the volume of distribution of these drugs fairly rapidly. A dose that provides the desired serum concentration on one day may be inappropriate only a few days later if the patient's fluid status changes dramatically. Another readily apparent factor that changes drug dosing is the type of RRT used in the patient. Drug clearances attained by intermittent hemodialysis, CRRTs, and hybrid RRTs all differ from each other and must be added to any endogenous drug clearance that the patient generates.[52]

A pharmacokinetic change in ARF that is not evident by examining the patient is the change in hepatic drug metabolism and drug transport that occurs. Altered cytochrome P450 enzyme activity has been demonstrated in patients with CKD in many instances.[72] Patients with ARF likely also have changes in nonrenal clearance of drugs, but controlled studies are difficult to conduct in this population. Evidence suggests that vancomycin[73] and imipenem[74] nonrenal clearances are reduced in patients with ARF compared to normal values. As ARF persists, these nonrenal clearances approach those observed in patients with CKD.[73-74] The nonrenal clearance of these drugs is less than that of normals but higher than that observed in CKD, consequently imipenem and vancomycin doses in patients with ARF likely should fall somewhere in between the doses recommended for patients with normal renal function and doses recommended for CKD. Application of doses derived from studies in patients with CKD will result in underdosing of these agents.

PHARMACOECONOMIC CONSIDERATIONS

ARF is a large burden on the health care system. Much of this cost is due to the fact that many of these patients are in intensive care units where daily costs are high. It has been estimated that the average total hospital cost of a patient with ARF who requires RRT is approximately $50,000.[9] Most patients surviving ARF recover life-sustaining renal function, but the 3% that do not recover renal function[2] continue to incur the costs of a lifetime of dialysis therapy or kidney transplantation. Nonetheless, even in patients who required RRT for their ARF, the quality of life of survivors has been reported to be good.[9]

Medical intervention costs can be normalized to assess total costs using quality-adjusted life years (QALYs) gained by the intervention. The use of a QALY approach to treatment of critically ill patients with ARF indicates that treating these patients is very expensive relative to other common medical interventions.[7] For example, using 2001 cost values, the treatment of critically ill ARF patients cost per QALY was $168,711, compared to treatment of acute myocardial infarction cost per QALY of $45,000, and the routine treatment of hypertension cost per QALY of $31,321.[3] A typical cost per QALY of <$100,000 is considered to be cost effective. While nobody is suggesting that serious ARF not be treated, it is clear that research needs to be done to improve the ARF survival rate to reduce this cost per QALY. Furthermore, it underscores the need to prevent the occurrence of ARF in the first place.

EVALUATION OF THERAPEUTIC OUTCOMES

MONITORING OF THE PHARMACEUTICAL CARE PLAN (INCLUDING SPECIFIC PARAMETERS AND FREQUENCY OF MONITORING)

Vigilant monitoring of patients with ARF is essential, particularly in those who are critically ill (Table 42–8). Once the laboratory-based tests (urinalysis, fractional excretion of sodium calculations, etc.) have been conducted to diagnose the cause of ARF, they usually do not have to be repeated. In established ARF, daily measurements

TABLE 42–8. Key Monitoring Parameters for Patients with Established Acute Renal Failure

Parameter	Frequency
Fluid ins/outs	Every shift
Patient weight	Daily
Vital signs	Every shift
Blood cultures and sensitivities	Check for results daily; obtain more when clinical signs of infection present
Blood chemistries	
Sodium, potassium, chloride, bicarbonate, calcium, phosphate, magnesium	Daily
BUN/S$_{Cr}$	Daily
Albumin	Once or twice weekly
Complete blood cell count with white cell differential	Daily
Drugs and their dosing regimens	Daily
Nutritional regimen	Daily
Blood glucose	Every shift for critically ill patients
Serum concentration data for drugs	After regimen changes and after RRT has been instituted
Times of administered doses	Daily
Doses relative to administration of RRT	Daily
Urinalysis	
Calculate measured creatinine clearance	Every time measured urine collection performed
Calculate fractional excretion of sodium	Every time measured urine collection performed
Plans for renal replacement	Daily
Invasive monitoring parameters	As indicated
Swan-Ganz readings	Every shift

of urine output, fluid intake, and weight should be performed. Vital signs should be monitored at least daily, more often if patient acuity of illness is high. Daily blood tests for electrolytes, BUN, and serum creatinine, and a CBC should be considered routine for hospitalized patients. Therapeutic drug monitoring should be performed for drugs that can be measured by the hospital laboratory. If results from these serum drug concentrations cannot be turned around in a timely fashion (<24 h) to the patient's care team, then their value is limited. Therapeutic drug monitoring should be conducted more often in patients with ARF than what is done routinely for other patients because of their dynamic status (changing volume status, changing renal function, and RRTs). Swan-Ganz monitoring should be performed in critically ill patients when feasible. Obviously other laboratory tests should be conducted as the patient's status dictates.

ABBREVIATIONS

ACEI: angiotensin-converting enzyme inhibitor
ADQI: Acute Dialysis Quality Initiative
ARF: acute renal failure
ATN: acute tubular necrosis
BUN: blood urea nitrogen
CBC: complete blood cell count
CHF: congestive heart failure
CKD: chronic kidney disease
CRRT: continuous renal replacement therapy
FE_{Na}: fractional excretion of sodium
GFR: glomerular filtration rate
HUS: hemolytic uremic syndrome
NSAID: nonsteroidal anti-inflammatory drug
QALY: quality-adjusted life year
RBC: red blood cell
RRT: renal replacement therapy
WBC: white blood cell

Review Questions and other resources can be found at *www.pharmacotherapyonline.com*.

REFERENCES

1. Mehta RL. Outcomes research in acute renal failure. Semin Nephrol 2003;23:283–294.
2. Liaño F, Pascual J. Epidemiology of acute renal failure: a prospective, multicenter, community-based study. Madrid Acute Renal Failure Study Group. Kidney Int 1996;50:811–818.
3. Pruchnicki MC, Dasta JF. Acute renal failure in hospitalized patients: Part I. Ann Pharmacother 2002;36:1261–1267.
4. Mehta RL, McDonald B, Gabbai F, et al. Nephrology consultation in acute renal failure: does timing matter? Am J Med 2002;113:456–461.
5. Sural S, Sharma RK, Singhal M, et al. Etiology, prognosis, and outcome of post-operative acute renal failure. Ren Fail 2000;22:87–97.
6. Mehta RL, Pascual MT, Soronko S, Chertow GM. Diuretics, mortality, and nonrecovery in acute renal failure. JAMA 2002;288:2547–2553.
7. Hamel MB, Phillips RS, Davis RB, et al. Outcomes and cost-effectiveness of initiating dialysis and continuing aggressive care in seriously ill hospitalized adults. Ann Intern Med 1997;127;195–202.
8. de Mendonca A, Vincent JL, Suter PM, et al. Acute renal failure in the ICU : risk factors and outcome evaluated by SOFA score. Intensive Care Med 2000;26:915–921.
9. Korkeila M, Ruokonen E, Takala J. Costs of care, long-term prognosis and quality of life in patients requiring renal replacement therapy during intensive care. Intensive Care Med 2000;26:1824–1831.
10. Metnitz PGH, Krenn CG, Steitzer H, et al. Effect of acute renal failure requiring renal replacement therapy on outcome in critically ill patients. Crit Care Med 2002;30:2051–2058.
11. Food and Drug Administration Nonprescription Drugs Advisory Committee Meeting convened September 19–20, 2002, Silver Spring, MD.
12. Whelton A. Nephrotoxicity of nonsteroidal anti-inflammatory drugs: physiologic foundations and clinical implications. Am J Med 1999;106:13S–24S.
13. Gruberg L, Mintz GS, Mehran R, et al. The prognostic implications of further renal function deterioration within 48 h of interventional coronary procedures in patients with pre-existent chronic renal insufficiency. J Am Coll Cardiol 2000;36:1542–1548.
14. Gruberg L, Mehran R, Dangas G, et al. Acute renal failure requiring dialysis after percutaneous coronary interventions. Catheter Cardiovasc Interv 2001;52:409–416.
15. Fiaccadori E, Lombardi M, Leonardi S, et al. Prevalence and clinical outcome associated with preexisting malnutrition in acute renal failure: a prospective cohort study. J Am Soc Nephrol 1999;10:581–591.
16. Barza M, Ioannidis JP, Cappelleri JC, Lau J. Single or multiple daily doses of aminoglycosides: a meta-analysis. BMJ 1996;312:338–345.
17. Van den Berghe G, Wouters PJ, Bouillon R, et al. Outcome benefit of intensive insulin therapy in the critically ill: Insulin dose versus glycemic control. Crit Care Med 2003;31:359–366.
18. Clermont G, Acker CG, Angus DC, et al. Renal failure in the ICU: comparison of the impact of acute renal failure and end-stage renal disease on ICU outcomes. Kidney Int 2002;62:986–996.
19. Chertow GM, Levy EM, Hammermeister KE, et al. Independent association between acute renal failure and mortality following cardiac surgery. Am J Med 1998;104:343–348.
20. Neveu H, Kleinknecht D, Brivet F, et al. Prognostic factors in acute renal failure due to sepsis. Results of a prospective multicentre study. Nephrol Dial Transplant 1996;11:293–299.
21. Kelly KJ, Molitoris BA. Acute renal failure in the new millennium: Time to consider combination therapy. Semin Nephrol 2000;20:4–19.
22. Sutton TA, Fisher CJ, Molitoris BA. Microvascular endothelial injury and dysfunction during ischemic acute renal failure. Kidney Int 2002;62:1539–1549.
23. Molitoris BA. Transitioning to therapy in ischemic acute renal failure. J Am Soc Nephrol 2003;14:265–267.
24. Perazella MA. Crystal-induced acute renal failure. Am J Med 1999;106:459–465.
25. Haas M, Spargo BH, Wit EJC, Meehan SM. Etiologies and outcome of acute renal insufficiency in older adults: A renal biopsy study of 259 cases. Am J Kidney Dis 2000;35:433–447.
26. Mueller C, Buerkle G, Buettner HJ. Prevention of contrast media-associated nephropathy. Arch Intern Med 2002;162;329–336.
27. Solomon R, Werner C, Mann D, et al. Effects of saline, mannitol, and furosemide to prevent acute decreases in renal function induced by radiocontrast agents. N Engl J Med 1994;331:1416–1420.
28. Marenzi G, Marana I, Lauri G, et al. The prevention of radiocontrast-agent-induced nephropathy by hemofiltration. N Engl J Med 2003;349:1333–1340.
29. Huber W, Jeschke B, Kreymann B, et al. Haemodialysis for the prevention of contrast-induced nephropathy. Invest Radiol 2002;37:471–481.
30. Bates DW, Su L, Yu DT, et al. Mortality and costs of acute renal failure associated with amphotericin B therapy. Clin Infect Dis 2001;32:686–693.
31. Eriksson U, Seifert B, Schaffner A. Comparison of effects of amphotericin B deoxycholate infused over 4 or 24 hours: randomized controlled trial. BMJ 2001;322:1–6.
32. Walsh TJ, Finberg RW, Arndt C, et al. Liposomal amphotericin B for empirical therapy in patients with persistent fever and neutropenia. N Engl J Med 1999;340:764–771.
33. Ronco C, Bellomo R. Prevention of acute renal failure in the critically ill. Nephron Clin Pract 2003;93:c13–c20.
34. Lassnigg A, Donner E, Grubhofer G, et al. Lack of renoprotective effects of dopamine and furosemide during cardiac surgery. J Am Soc Nephrol 2000;11:97–104.
35. Stevens MA, McCullough PA, Tobin KJ, et al. A prospective randomized

trial of prevention measures in patients at high risk for contrast nephropathy. J Am Coll Cardiol 1999;33:403–411.

36. Kellum J, Decker JM. Use of dopamine in acute renal failure: a meta-analysis. Crit Care Med 2001;29:1526–1531.

37. Stone GW, McCollough PA, Tumlin JA, et al. Fenoldopam mesylate for the prevention of contrast-induced nephropathy. JAMA 2003;290:2284–2292.

38. Tepel M, van der Giet M, Schwarzfeld C, et al. Prevention of radiographic-contrast-agent-induced reductions in renal function by acetylcysteine. N Engl J Med 2000;343:180–184.

39. Raven QL, Walton T, Howe AM, Macon EJ. Role of acetylcysteine in the prevention of contrast-media-induced nephrotoxicity. Am J Health-Syst Pharm 2003;60:2232–2235.

40. Huber W, Schipek C, Ilgmann K, et al. Effectiveness of theophylline prophylaxis of renal impairment after coronary angiography in patients with chronic renal insufficiency. Am J Cardiol 2003;91:1157–1162.

41. Wagner K, Albrecht S, Neumeayer HH. Prevention of post-transplant acute tubular necrosis by the calcium antagonist diltiazem: a prospective randomized study. Am J Nephrol 1987;7:287–291.

42. Van den Berghe G, Wouters P, Weekers F, et al. Intensive insulin therapy in critically ill patients. N Engl J Med 2001;345:1359–1367.

43. ASHP Commission on Therapeutics. ASHP therapeutic position statement on strict glycemic control in patients with diabetes. Am J Health-Syst Pharm 2003;60:2357–2362.

44. Schortgen F, Soubrier N, Delclaux C, et al. Hemodynamic tolerance of intermittent hemodialysis in critically ill patients. Am J Respir Crit Care Med 2000;162:197–202.

45. Clark WR, Mueller BA, Kraus MA, et al. Extracorporeal therapy requirements for patients with acute renal failure. J Am Soc Nephrol 1997;8:804–812.

46. Ronco C, Bellomo R, Kellum JA. Continuous renal replacement therapy: opinions and evidence. Adv Ren Replace Ther 2002;9:229–244.

47. Tonelli M, Manns B, Feller-Kopman D. Acute renal failure in the intensive care unit: a systematic review of the impact of dialytic modality on mortality and renal recovery. Am J Kidney Dis 2002;40:875–885.

48. Swartz RD, Messana JM, Orzol S, Port FK. Comparing continuous hemofiltration with hemodialysis in patients with severe acute renal failure. Am J Kidney Dis 1999;34:424–432.

49. Schiffl H, Lang SM, Fischer R. Daily hemodialysis and the outcome of acute renal failure. N Engl J Med 2002;346:305–310.

50. Marshall MR, Golper TA, Shaver MJ, et al. Urea kinetics during sustained low-efficiency dialysis in critically ill patients requiring renal replacement therapy. Am J Kidney Dis 2002;39:556–570.

51. Kumar VA, Craig M, Depner TA, et al. Extended daily dialysis: a new approach to renal replacement for acute renal failure in the intensive care unit. Am J Kidney Dis 2000;36:294–300.

52. Mueller BA, Pasko DA, Sowinski KM. Higher renal replacement therapy dose delivery influences on drug therapy. Artif Organs 2003;27:808–814.

53. Manley HJ, Bailie GR, McClaran ML, Bender WL. Gentamicin pharmacokinetics during slow daily home hemodialysis. Kidney Int 2003;63:1072–1078.

54. Jaber BL, Lau J, Schmid CH, et al. Effect of biocompatibility of hemodialysis membranes on mortality in acute renal failure: a meta-analysis. Clin Nephrol 2002;57:274–282.

55. Subramanian S, Venkataraman R, Kellum JA: Influence of dialysis membranes on outcomes in acute renal failure: a meta-analysis. Kidney Int 2002;62:1819–1823.

56. Pruchnicki MC, Dasta JF. Acute renal failure in hospitalized patients: part II. Ann Pharmacother 2002;36:1430–1442.

57. Acker CG, Singh AR, Flick RP. A trial of thyroxine in acute renal failure. Kidney Int 2000;57:293–298.

58. ANZICS Clinical Trials Group. Low-dose dopamine in patients with early renal dysfunction: a placebo-controlled randomised trial. Lancet 2000;356:2139–2143.

59. Better OS, Rubinstein I, Winaver JM, Knochel JP. Mannitol therapy revisited. Kidney Int 1997;51:886–894.

60. Brater DC. Diuretic therapy. N Engl J Med 1998;339:387–395.

61. Howard PA, Dunn MI. Severe musculoskeletal symptoms during continuous infusion of bumetanide. Chest 1997;111:359–364.

62. Schuller D, Lynch JP, Fine D. Protocol-guided diuretic management: comparison of furosemide by continuous infusion and intermittent bolus. Crit Care Med 1997;25:1969–1975.

63. Rudy DW, Voelker JR, Greene PK, et al. Loop diuretics for chronic renal insufficiency: a continuous is more efficacious than bolus therapy. Ann Intern Med 1991;115:360–366.

64. Kramer WG, Smith WB, Ferguson J, et al. Pharmacodynamics of torsemide administered as an intravenous injection and as a continuous infusion to patients with congestive heart failure. J Clin Pharmacol 1996;36:265–270.

65. Ellison DH. Diuretic resistance: Physiology and therapeutics. Semin Nephrol 1999;19:581–597.

66. Segar JL, Chemtob S, Bell EF. Changes in body water compartments with diuretic therapy in infants with chronic lung disease. Early Hum Dev 1997;48:99–107.

67. Sirivella S, Gielchinsky I, Parsonnet V. Mannitol, furosemide, and dopamine infusion in postoperative renal failure complicating cardiac surgery. Ann Thorac Surg 2000;69:501–506.

68. Koretz RL. Does nutritional intervention in protein-energy malnutrition improve morbidity or mortality? J Renal Nutr 1999;9:119–121.

69. Leblanc M, Garred LJ, Cardinal J, et al. Catabolism in critical illness: estimation from urea nitrogen appearance and creatinine production during continuous renal replacement therapy. Am J Kidney Dis 1998;32:444–453.

70. Yagi N, Leblanc M, Sakai K, et al. Cooling effect of continuous renal replacement therapy in critically ill patients. Am J Kidney Dis 1998;32:1023–1030.

71. Manns M, Maurer E, Steinbach B, Evering HG. Thermal energy balance during in vitro continuous veno-venous hemofiltration. ASAIO J 1998;44:M601–M605.

72. Nolin TD, Frye RF, Matzke GR. Hepatic drug metabolism and transport in patients with kidney disease. Am J Kidney Dis 2003;42:906–225.

73. Macias WL, Mueller BA, Scarim SK, et al. Continuous venovenous hemofiltration: An alternative to continuous arteriovenous hemofiltration and hemodiafiltration in acute renal failure. Am J Kidney Dis 1991;18:451–458.

74. Mueller BA, Scarim SK, Macias WL. Comparison of imipenem pharmacokinetics in patients with acute or chronic renal failure treated with continuous hemofiltration. Am J Kidney Dis 1993;21:172–179.

43

CHRONIC KIDNEY DISEASE: PROGRESSION-MODIFYING THERAPIES

Melanie S. Joy, Abhijit Kshirsagar, and James Paparello

Learning Objectives and other resources can be found at *www.pharmacotherapyonline.com.*

KEY CONCEPTS

◀1 The prevalence of chronic kidney disease (CKD) is estimated at nearly 19 million people in the United States.

◀2 Since the development of CKD is a complex phenomenon, the Kidney Disease Outcomes Quality Initiative (K/DOQI) has recommended categorizing risk factors associated with CKD as susceptibility, initiation, and progression factors.

◀3 The most common initiation risk factors are diabetes mellitus, hypertension, glomerulonephritis, and polycystic kidney disease.

◀4 The most important progression risk factors include proteinuria, uncontrolled blood pressure, and for diabetic patients, glycemic control.

◀5 Reduction of kidney mass, development of glomerular hypertension, and intratubular proteinuria are key mechanisms responsible for the progression of chronic kidney disease.

◀6 CKD is classified into five stages based on the presence of proteinuria and/or glomerular filtration rate, with 1 being the mildest form and 5 being the most severe.

◀7 It is critical to determine the glomerular filtration rate rather than just measuring the serum creatinine, since glomerular filtration is a more consistent marker of renal function in most clinical settings.

◀8 The classic symptoms of stage 5 CKD are asterixis, pruritus, dysgeusia, nausea, vomiting, anorexia, and bleeding.

◀9 Optimization of blood glucose and hypertension control are integral in limiting the rate of CKD progression.

◀10 The cornerstones of pharmacologic treatment to limit progressive kidney disease are angiotensin-converting enzyme inhibitors (ACEIs) and angiotensin receptor blockers (ARBs).

◀11 Diabetic patients with or without hypertension who demonstrate persistent microalbuminuria despite intensive insulin therapy should have their ACEI or ARB dose titrated to achieve maximal suppression of urinary albumin excretion to halt or slow CKD progression.

◀12 Supportive therapies that may help to improve the quality of life and slow the rate of progression of CKD include dietary protein restriction, lipid lowering medications, smoking cessation, and anemia management.

Under normal conditions each of the two million nephrons of the kidney work in an organized approach to filter, reabsorb, and excrete various solutes and water. The kidney is a primary regulator of sodium and water as well as acid-base homeostasis. The kidney also produces hormones necessary for red blood cell synthesis and calcium homeostasis. Impairment of normal kidney function is often referred to as renal insufficiency. Based on the time course of development, renal insufficiency has historically been divided into two broad categories. Acute renal failure (ARF) refers to the rapid loss of renal function over days to weeks. Chronic kidney disease (CKD)[a], also called chronic renal insufficiency (CRI) by some, is defined as a progressive loss of function occurring over several months to years, and is characterized by the gradual replacement of normal kidney architecture with interstitial fibrosis. Progressive kidney disease or nephropathy is generally synonymous with CKD, and the two phrases are often used interchangeably.

The working group of the National Kidney Foundation's Kidney Dialysis Outcomes and Quality Initiative (K/DOQI) has recently developed a new scheme to classify CKD based on the presence of kidney damage, structural or functional, for ≥3 months, with or without decreased glomerular filtration rate (GFR) from normal values of ~120 mL/min.[1] CKD is further categorized by the level of kidney function (as defined by GFR) into stages 1 through 5.[1] Although these stages are defined later in this chapter, it is necessary to denote at this point that Stage 5 was previously referred to as end-stage renal disease (ESRD) or end-stage kidney disease (ESKD).

EPIDEMIOLOGY OF CKD

The epidemiology of Stage 5 CKD has been well documented through the efforts of the United States Renal Data System (USRDS), a national data system that collects, analyzes, and distributes information

---

[a]*TheExecutive Committee of the Kidney Dialysis Outcomes Initiative (KDOQI) has recentlyrecommended that* CKD *replace chronic renal insufficiency (CRI).* CRI *does not usethe word kidney, and thus may be obtuse/obscure to the lay population.*

about ESKD in the United States.[2] Information on the epidemiology of the earlier stages of CKD is less well characterized. In the United States alone, there are several major epidemiologic studies currently in progress or in development to elucidate the natural history of CKD, its progression, and concurrent morbidities. Another study targets individuals with polycystic kidney disease,[3] while another study targets African-Americans with hypertensive nephrosclerosis.[4] The Chronic Renal Insufficiency Cohort study[5] and an Amgen-sponsored study (Stride Registry) are investigating progressive CKD and its relationship with comorbid cardiovascular disease. The National Kidney Foundation has recognized the importance of early detection and has initiated the Kidney Early Evaluation Program,[6] to identify, educate, and provide free screening for people at increased risk of developing kidney disease. Furthermore, U.S. governmental agencies have targeted CKD as one of 28 major focus areas for improvement by the year 2010, as set forth in the Healthy People 2010 document.[7] Over the next decade, as a result of these initiatives our understanding of the epidemiology, pathophysiology, and management of mild (Stage 1) to moderate (Stage 4) CKD will undoubtedly increase.

CKD has been described as a silent epidemic[8] and is a worldwide public health problem.[9] Three different national surveys have estimated that the prevalence of CKD is at least 5% of the adult population when using a serum creatinine concentration of greater than 1.2 to 1.5 mg/dL as the definition.[10–12] The most representative of these studies, the Third National Health and Nutritional Examination Survey (NHANES III)[10] projected that at least 10.9 million people had a decreased level of kidney function as evidenced by serum creatinine concentration ($\geq$1.5 mg/dL). The NHANES III analysis also revealed that the prevalence of CKD was significantly associated with age, race, gender, and hypertension; the prevalence of CKD was higher in those of advanced age, black race, male gender, and a diagnosis of hypertension.

Prevalence estimates were revised upwards in 2002 based on the inclusion of the presence of albuminuria in addition to increased serum creatinine in the definition of CKD, and by incorporating adjustments for age, gender, and race into the calculations of GFR.[1] The working group of K/DOQI estimated that CKD affected 10.9% of the adults ($\geq$20 years old) population in the United States. This translates into an astonishing 19 million individuals (Fig. 43–1). Worldwide figures on prevalence are not available, but if one extrapolates the prevalence estimates from the U.S. population to the entire world population, it would exceed 100 million individuals. The prevalence

of CKD is thus similar to that of conditions such as hypertension, diabetes mellitus, and cardiovascular disease. However, financial and societal costs of the care of individuals with CKD, especially those individuals with the latter stages, are disproportionately high. ESKD beneficiaries accounted for 0.5% of the total Medicare population, yet received 5% of all Medicare expenditures.[13] Annualized expenditures per beneficiary ranged from $36,000 for those 24 years of age and younger to $51,000 for those 75 years and older.[13] These costs for the care of advanced CKD are estimated to increase dramatically over the next decade, reaching an estimated $28 billion dollars by the year 2010 for Medicare alone.[14]

Incidence estimates of CKD have generally been extrapolated from the USRDS.[2] The four most common medical conditions associated with incident Stage 5 CKD are diabetes mellitus, hypertension, glomerulonephritis, and polycystic kidney disease. The respective incidence rates for these conditions are: 150 cases/million, 80 cases/million, 22 cases/million, and 5 cases/million.[2] Much like the prevalence data, the estimates of incident Stage 5 cases are also greatly increased in the presence of advanced age and black race.[2] For example, the rate of Stage 5 CKD is fourfold higher for African-Americans as compared to Caucasians.[2]

It is often assumed that all early stages of CKD progress continuously towards Stage 5. Thus information on risk factors obtained from USRDS data are assumed to be generalizable to all stages of CKD. The validity of this approach to projecting future incidence data has not been tested. Further complicating these issues is the fact that the development and progression of the early stages of CKD is a complex phenomenon.[15] The risk factors associated with CKD are numerous and varied and many of these are not those one would traditionally consider as having a direct influence on the causal pathway. The working group of K/DOQI has recommended categorizing CKD risk factors as *susceptibility* factors, *initiation* factors, or *progression* factors[9] to help clinicians stratify the overall risks of individual patients (Table 43–1).[9]

ETIOLOGY

SUSCEPTIBILITY FACTORS

Individuals with susceptibility factors have an increased risk for the development of kidney disease, although these risk factors have not been proven to directly cause kidney damage. These factors include

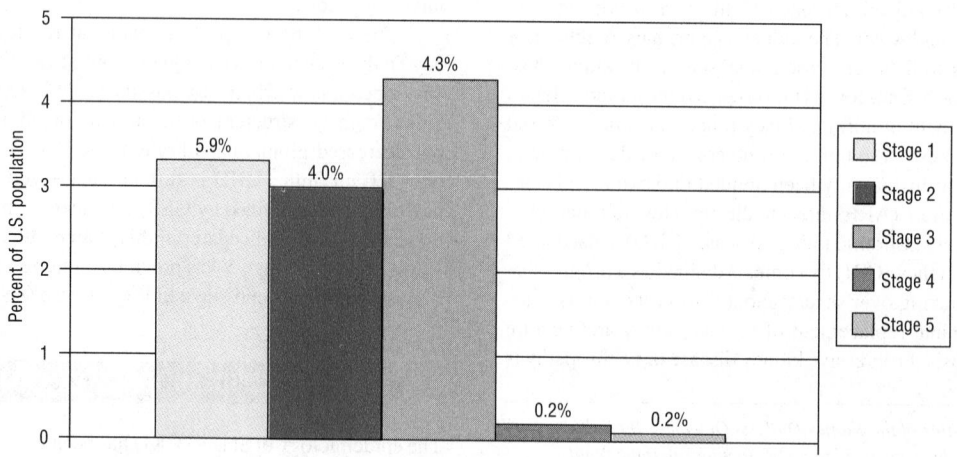

FIGURE 43–1. Prevalence of CKD by stage among those residing in the United States. Adapted from National Kidney Foundation.[1]

TABLE 43–1. Risk Factors Associated with Chronic Kidney Disease

Risk Factor	Key Studies
Susceptibility	
• Advanced age	Lindeman et al,[17] Goetz et al[71]
• Reduced kidney mass and low birth weight	Lackland et al[24]
• Racial/ethnic minority	Tierney et al,[21] Rostand et al,[22] Perry et al[23]
• Family history	Freedman et al,[25] FIND Research Group[26]
• Low income or education	Byrne et al[19] Perneger et al[20]
• Systemic inflammation	Kshirsagar et al,[27] Erlinger et al[28]
• Dyslipidemia	Muntner et al[29] Schaeffner et al[30]
Initiation	
• Diabetes mellitus	Hasslacher et al,[32] Brancati et al,[34] Fabre et al[168]
• Hypertension	Coresh et al,[38] Perneger et al,[39] Klag et al[40]
• Autoimmune disease	
• Polycystic kidney disease	Gabow et al[169]
• Drug toxicity	McLaughlin et al,[170] Walsh et al[171]
Progression	
• Glycemia (among diabetic patients)	Reichard et al,[60] DCCT Research Group[61]
• Elevated blood pressure	Klahr et al,[49] Jafar et al, Bakris,[56] UKPDS Group,[57] UKPDS Group,[58] Bakris[59]
• Proteinuria	Keane et al,[48] Klahr,[49] Jafar et al[50]
• Smoking	Orth et al,[63] Orth et al[72]

sociodemographic risk factors, such as advanced age,[16–18] low income or education,[19,20] and racial or ethnic minority status,[21–23] as well as reduction in kidney mass, low birth weight,[24] and family history of CKD.[25,26] Novel susceptibility factors that have been proposed include systemic inflammation[27,28] and dyslipidemia.[29,30] Most of these susceptibility factors are not necessarily modifiable by pharmacologic or lifestyle interventions, but rather help to identify potential populations to target screening programs for the presence of CKD.

INITIATION FACTORS

Initiation factors are factors or conditions that directly initiate kidney damage, and are modifiable by pharmacologic therapy. These factors include diabetes mellitus, hypertension, autoimmune diseases, polycystic kidney disease, systemic infections, urinary tract infections, urinary stones, lower urinary tract obstructions, and drug toxicity. Since diabetes mellitus, hypertension, and glomerular diseases are respectively the first, second, and third most common causes for CKD in the U.S., the following discussion focuses on these three conditions.

DIABETES MELLITUS

Individuals with type 1 diabetes mellitus have a 40% lifetime risk of developing CKD,[31] while individuals with type 2 diabetes mellitus have a 50% lifetime risk.[32] Given the greater prevalence of type 2 diabetes mellitus compared to type 1, generally a 10:1 ratio in most countries,[33] the majority of CKD from diabetes would be among individuals with type 2 disease. Importantly, although not all individuals with diabetic nephropathy progress to Stage 5 CKD, the lifetime risk is considerable. A recent prospective study of over 300,000 individuals,

screened from the Multiple Risk Factor Intervention Trial (MRFIT), estimated that approximately 3% of individuals with diabetes mellitus will develop Stage 5 CKD during their life.[34] Thus diabetics have a 12-fold greater relative risk of developing Stage 5 CKD than someone without diabetes mellitus. The presence of diabetes mellitus also increased the risk of Stage 5 CKD from nondiabetic causes of renal failure as well, suggesting at least an additive effect of concomitant diseases.

HYPERTENSION

The presence of hypertension also increases the risk of CKD. The data are less clear than with diabetes mellitus because the kidney has a fundamental role in the development and modulation of high blood pressure.[35–37] The interpretation of epidemiologic studies regarding the presence of high blood pressure and the risk of progressive kidney disease may be limited by reverse causation. Hypertension generally develops concomitantly with progressive kidney disease. For example, at a GFR of 90 mL/min per 1.73m^2, 40% of individuals have hypertension; at a GFR of 60 mL/min per 1.73 m^2, 55% have hypertension; and at a GFR of 30 mL/min per 1.73m^2, over 75% have hypertension.[1] Furthermore, an analysis of the NHANES III survey demonstrated that elevated serum creatinine, defined as $\geq$1.6 mg/dL for men and $\geq$1.4 mg/dL for women, was more common in persons with hypertension (9.1%) than in persons without hypertension (1.1%).[38] A landmark prospective study of individuals with normal kidney function at baseline[39] showed that elevated levels of blood pressure are a risk factor for the development of early CKD. In another analysis of the MRFIT cohort, the overall lifetime risk of developing Stage 5 CKD for individuals with hypertension was 5.6%.[40] The risk varied dramatically by level of blood pressure, from 0.33% at stage 1 hypertension (systolic blood pressure 140 to 150 mm Hg and/or diastolic blood pressure 90 to 100 mm Hg) to 4.5% for systolic blood pressure levels greater than 180 mm Hg or diastolic blood pressure levels greater than 110 mm Hg[40] over a follow-up period of approximately 16 years.

GLOMERULONEPHRITIS

Glomerular diseases are another important category of initiation factors for CKD. The epidemiology and pathophysiology of glomerular diseases are variable and thus all diseases cannot be lumped into one disease category. Some conditions, such as Goodpasture's disease or Wegener's granulomatosis, progress rapidly to stage 5 CKD, and thus may best be categorized as causes of ARF. Other conditions, such as IgA nephropathy, membranous nephropathy, focal segmental glomerulosclerosis, lupus nephritis, and others, are more indolent diseases, and are considered causes of CKD (see Chap. 47). The chronic nephritides progress at variable rates, with the loss of GFR ranging from 1.4 to 9.5 mL/min per year.[41–44]

PROGRESSION FACTORS

Progression risk factors are those that cause a worsening of kidney damage, and are associated with a faster decline in kidney function after initiation of kidney damage. The most important predictors of progressive CKD are the persistence of underlying initiation diseases (e.g., diabetes mellitus, hypertension, glomerulonephritis, and polycystic kidney disease), and the progression factors such as proteinuria, elevated blood pressure, and smoking.

PROTEINURIA

Numerous studies have documented the importance of proteinuria in the progression of both diabetic[45-48] and nondiabetic[49,50] kidney disease. These studies are not what one would term primary cohort studies, such as the Atherosclerosis Risk in Communities Study,[51] but rather are secondary analyses of intervention trials. Nevertheless, these studies have provided valuable information. In diabetic kidney disease (types 1 and 2), several studies have demonstrated that an albumin excretion rate >30 mg/24 hours strongly predicted the development of overt nephropathy and subsequent loss of kidney function.[45-47,52] In nondiabetic kidney disease, the Modification of Diet in Renal Disease (MDRD) study, a landmark trial examining the effect of oral protein restriction on the progression of CKD among individuals with advanced CKD, demonstrated that a patient's baseline level of proteinuria strongly predicted the loss of GFR.[49] Furthermore, the level of proteinuria significantly altered the effectiveness of blood pressure control with antihypertensive agents; specifically, individuals with the highest levels of baseline proteinuria benefited the most from reduction of blood pressure. Recently, data from a large cohort of over 1800 individuals with varying stages of CKD demonstrated a strong, graded risk for progressive CKD; each 1.0 g/day increase in urinary protein excretion increased the risk of progression fivefold.[50] Figure 43–2 shows the relationship between systolic blood pressure and relative risk of CKD progression at proteinuria levels of greater than and less than 1 g/day.[53] Interestingly, this cohort included individuals with various primary etiologies of kidney disease, including hypertensive nephrosclerosis, polycystic kidney disease, tubulointerstitial disease, and others. Physiologically, the data demonstrating the role of proteinuria in progressive kidney disease makes sense for conditions associated primarily with glomerular damage, such as diabetes mellitus, and a host of traditional glomerulonephritides. Intuitively, it is not clear why proteinuria should predict progressive loss of renal function in conditions under which the primary pathophysiologic insult is vascular (hypertension) or interstitial (polycystic kidney disease or chronic reflux). It is possible that an unknown secondary insult may trigger the development of proteinuria in these conditions, and then lead to the progressive loss of renal function.

HYPERTENSION

The treatment and control of hypertension can delay the progression of CKD.[49,50,54-58] Bakris and colleagues demonstrated a direct correlation between the level of achieved blood pressure and preservation of

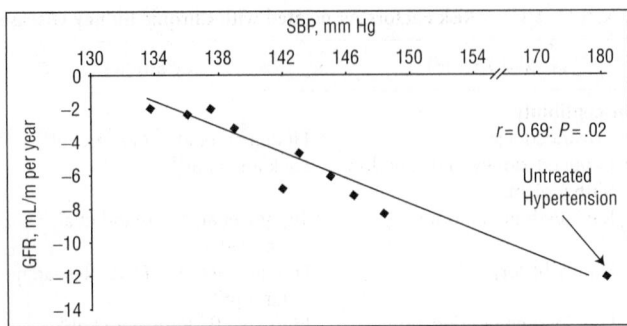

FIGURE 43–3. Rates of decline in glomerular filtration rate (GFR) vs the systolic blood pressure (SBP) in studies extending for 3 years or more in patients with type 2 diabetes mellitus nephropathy. From Bakris,[59] with permission.

kidney function.[59] The analysis included 10 studies in which patients were treated with various antihypertensive agents. Each study measured the change in GFR during the study period. Bakris demonstrated an inverse linear relationship between the average attained blood pressure at study completion and average GFR—lower mean arterial blood pressure resulted in a lower average decline in GFR. Thus a systolic blood pressure of 180 mm Hg was associated with a decline in GFR of 14 mL/min per year, whereas a systolic blood pressure of 135 mm Hg was associated with a decline of GFR of only 2 mL/min per year (Fig. 43–3).[59] Though the analysis was conducted among patients with diabetic kidney disease, the results may be extrapolated to individuals with nondiabetic kidney disease.

DIABETES MELLITUS

Hyperglycemia is another initiation and progression risk factor in CKD. Two large prospective studies that showed the benefits of blood glucose control were reported in the early 1990s,[60,61] and a few years later two British studies[54,55] confirmed these results. The 1441 patients with type I diabetes mellitus enrolled in the Diabetes Control and Complications Trial (DCCT) were randomized to conventional blood glucose control or to intensive control. Conventional control consisted of up to two insulin injections per day and no goal hemoglobin A_{1c}. However, intensive control consisted of administration of insulin three or more times daily by injection or by external pump to achieve a hemoglobin $A_{1c} \leq 6.05\%$. Roughly half of the patients had mild retinopathy, a marker for microvascular complications, at study entry. Primary prevention was defined as a reduction in new occurrence of retinopathy among patients with no baseline retinopathy, and secondary prevention was defined as a reduction of new cases of retinopathy among individuals with retinopathy. A primary risk reduction of 76% and secondary risk reduction of 54% were noted with intensive control. The intensive therapy was associated with a 39% risk reduction for the development of "microalbuminuria" (urinary albumin excretion ≥ 40 mg/day), and a 54% reduction in the development of "frank albuminuria" (urinary albumin excretion ≥ 300 mg/day) compared to conventional therapy.

SMOKING

Multiple studies support a relationship between smoking and the initiation and progression of CKD in those with type 1 and type II diabetes.[62-64] Smoking has been suggested to increase the rate of progression in type 1 and type 2 diabetes by approximately twofold.[65] In diabetics, "cigarette pack years" was an independent predictive factor for progression.[66] Smoking has also been associated with renal

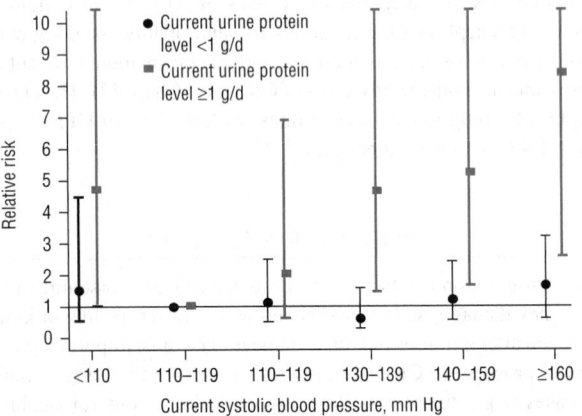

FIGURE 43–2. Relative risk for kidney disease progression based on current level of systolic blood pressure and current urine protein excretion. From Jafar,[53] with permission.

insufficiency in a study of severe essential hypertension[67] and in African-American patients with hypertension.[68] A few prospective studies have demonstrated an association between smoking and microalbuminuria and the development of stage 5 CKD.[69–71] Smoking has also been identified as a risk factor for progression in patients with IgA nephropathy, polycystic kidney disease, and systemic lupus erythematosus.[72,73]

HYPERLIPIDEMIA

Although the data are not conclusive, hyperlipidemia has been associated as a susceptibility factor for CKD in both animal and human studies.[74] The use of lipid-lowering agents in some animal models has been found to decrease the extent of glomerular injury when both underlying renal disease and hyperlipidemia are present.[75] Therefore the correction of lipid abnormalities in patients with CKD was proposed to have a beneficial effect on the rate of progression of the disease. CKD with or without nephrotic syndrome is frequently accompanied by abnormalities in lipoprotein metabolism. The prevalence of hyperlipidemia appears to increase as kidney function declines and with the presence of the nephrotic syndrome.[76]

In patients with renal insufficiency and urinary protein excretion greater than 3 g/day, the major lipid abnormalities are elevations of plasma total and low density lipoprotein cholesterol (prevalence 85% to 90%), with approximately 50% of patients experiencing a low level (<35 mg/dL) of high density lipoprotein (HDL) cholesterol, and 60% of patients showing triglyceride concentrations greater than 200 mg/dL.[76]

PATHOPHYSIOLOGY

5 The various etiologic factors actually damage the kidney in a heterogenous manner. For example, the key structural lesion in dia-

betic nephropathy is glomerular mesangial expansion. In hypertensive nephrosclerosis, it is hyalinosis of the kidney's arterioles, and in polycystic kidney disease it is the development and growth of renal cysts. A variety of morphologic glomerular changes have been noted to occur, depending on the primary diagnosis of the glomerulonephritis.

The majority of progressive nephropathies share a final common pathway to irreversible renal parenchymal damage and ESKD[77,78] (Fig. 43–4). The key elements of this pathway are: (1) loss of nephron mass; (2) glomerular capillary hypertension; and (3) proteinuria.

The presence of or exposure to the initiation risk factors results in loss of nephron mass. The remaining nephrons hypertrophy to compensate for the loss of renal function and nephron mass.[79] Initially this compensatory hypertrophy may be adaptive. Yet over time the hypertrophy often becomes maladaptive and leads to the development of glomerular hypertension, possibly mediated by angiotensin II.[80,81] Angiotensin II, a potent vasoconstrictor of both the afferent and efferent arterioles, preferentially affects the efferent arterioles, leading to increased pressure within the glomerular capillaries. The development of intraglomerular hypertension generally correlates with the development of systemic arterial hypertension. Animal studies have demonstrated that high intraglomerular capillary pressure impairs the size-selective function of the glomerular permeability barrier, and results in albuminuria and proteinuria.[82,83]

The resultant proteinuria is thought to accelerate the progressive loss of nephrons due to direct cellular damage. The filtered proteins consist of albumin, transferrin, complement factors, immunoglobulins, cytokines, and angiotensin II, which have varying molecular weights. Numerous studies have demonstrated that the presence of these proteins in the renal tubule activate tubular cells which leads to the upregulated production of inflammatory and vasoactive cytokines, such as endothelin, monocyte chemoattractant protein (MCP-1), and RANTES (regulated upon activation, normal T-cell expressed and secreted).[77,84–87] Accumulating evidence now suggests

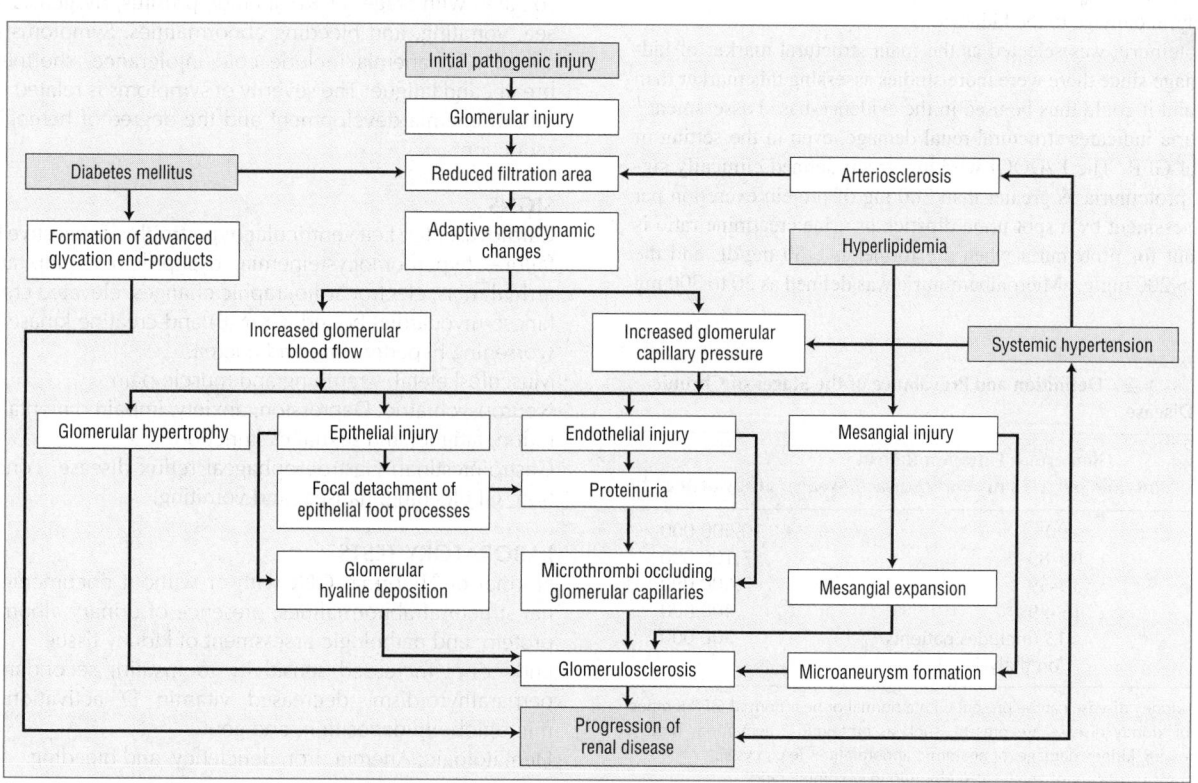

FIGURE 43–4. Proposed mechanisms for progression of renal disease.

that intratubular complement activation may be the key mechanism of damage in the progressive proteinuric nephropathies.[88–90] Proteinuria is associated with the activation of complement components on the apical membrane of proximal tubules.[91] These events eventually lead to scarring of the interstitium, and the progressive loss of structural nephron units, and ultimately function (reduced GFR).

ASSESSMENT FOR CKD

As CKD presentation is often asymptomatic, recommended screening studies include serum creatinine measurement, urinalysis, and/or imaging studies of the kidneys. Diabetes, hypertension, genitourinary abnormalities, and autoimmune diseases represent some of the more common conditions associated with kidney disease. People who are older or those who have a family history of kidney disease should also be screened. If the serum creatinine is elevated, or more appropriately the GFR decreases, or if there are abnormalities in the urinalysis or imaging studies, an evaluation for CKD should be performed.[1]

The rate of loss of GFR is difficult to assign to each case of progressive CKD, as this can vary by treatment responsiveness, compliance with therapies, and the underlying disease process. Recognizing the variable course of CKD and the need to denote the particular stage of the disease, the K/DOQI classification system was developed. The classification system divides CKD into five stages, with each increasing number indicating a more advanced stage of the disease, as defined by a declining GFR[1] (Table 43–2). Although the stages are defined functionally by the GFR, the classification system also accounts for structural evidence of kidney damage. The use of GFR versus serum creatinine to define the stages of CKD was chosen since the serum creatinine is an inaccurate index of GFR, and there is marked variability in GFR between subjects with similar serum creatinine values (see Chap. 41). A patient can be diagnosed with CKD despite a GFR of >90 mL/min per 1.73m^2 if there is evidence of structural damage to the kidneys.

Proteinuria was selected as the main structural marker of kidney damage since there were more studies assessing this marker than others, and it could thus be used in the evidence-based assessment.[1] Proteinuria indicates structural renal damage, even in the setting of a normal GFR. The K/DOQI working group defined clinically significant proteinuria as greater than 300 mg of protein excretion per day. Assessment by a spot urine dipstick or urine:creatinine ratio is significant for proteinuria when the former is >30 mg/dL and the latter is >200 mg/g.[1] Microalbuminuria was defined as 30 to 300 mg

of albumin in a 24-hour urine collection. Assessment by a spot urine dipstick or urine:creatinine ratio is significant for microalbuminuria when the former is >3 mg/dL and the latter is between 17 and 250 mg/g and 25 to 355 mg/g for men and women, respectively.[1] The spot protein/albumin:creatinine ratio on a random urine sample (preferably a morning sample) allows a clinician to easily screen for microalbuminuria or proteinuria without the cumbersome process of having the patient collect a 24-hour urine collection. Table 43–3 summarizes the clinical tools that are available to detect and interpret protein in the urine. Renal biopsy and/or ultrasound are common assessment tools for specific or gross structural abnormalities associated with kidney dysfunction. Structural abnormalities of the kidney can also be evidenced by pathologic abnormalities in biopsy specimens, abnormal imaging studies, or abnormalities in the urine sediment, such as hematuria.[1] Representative examples of kidney damage found on biopsy from patients with hypertension and diabetes mellitus are depicted in Fig. 43–5.

CLINICAL PRESENTATION OF CHRONIC KIDNEY DISEASE

GENERAL
CKD development and progression is typically insidious in onset, often with the absence of any noticeable symptoms. At a minimum, the diagnosis of CKD requires measurement of serum creatinine, calculation of GFR and assessment of a urinalysis for urinary microalbumin or total protein. The diagnosis of Stages 3, 4, and 5 CKD requires the work-up for other common complications including anemia, cardiovascular risks, metabolic bone disease, malnutrition, and disorders of fluids and electrolytes.

SYMPTOMS
Symptoms are generally absent in CKD Stages 1 and 2, and may be minimal during Stages 3 and 4. Classic symptoms associated with Stage 5 CKD include pruritus, dysgeusia, nausea, vomiting, and bleeding abnormalities. Symptoms associated with anemia include cold intolerance, shortness of breath, and fatigue. The severity of symptoms is related to the rate of anemia development and the degree of hemoglobin reduction.

SIGNS
Cardiovascular: Left ventricular hypertrophy, congestive heart failure, hyperhomocysteinemia, dyslipidemia, palpitations, arrhythmias, electrocardiographic changes, elevated creatine kinase-myocardial bound (CK-MB) and creatine kinase (CK), worsening hypertension, and edema.
Musculoskeletal: Cramping and muscle pain.
Neuropsychiatric: Depression, anxiety, impaired mental cognition, fatigue, and sexual dysfunction.
Gastrointestinal: Gastroesophageal reflux disease, constipation, GI bleeding, nausea, and vomiting.

LABORATORY TESTS
Normal or abnormal GFR with or without documented renal structural abnormalities; presence of urinary albumin or protein; and pathologic assessment of kidney tissue.
Endocrine: Increased sensitivity to insulin, secondary hyperparathyroidism, decreased vitamin D activation, β_2-microglobulin deposition, and gout.
Hematologic: Anemia, iron deficiency, and bleeding.

TABLE 43–2. Definition and Prevalance of the Stages of Chronic Kidney Disease

Stage	Glomerular Filtration Rate in mL/min per 1.73 m^2 Body Surface Area	Prevalence^b
1	≥90^a	10,500,000
2	60–89	7,100,000
3	30–59	7,600,000
4	15–29	400,000
5	<15 (includes patients on dialysis)	300,000

^{a}Chronic kidney disease can be present with a normal or near normal GFR if other markers of kidney disease are present, such as proteinuria, hematuria, biopsy results showing kidney damage, or anatomic abnormalities (e.g., cysts).
^{b}Based on measurement of an elevated albumin to creatinine ratio.

TABLE 43–3. Quantification of Proteinuria by Various Methods

Category	24-Hour Collection	Spot Collection: Protein:Creatinine Ratio	Spot Collection: Albumin:Creatinine Ratio	Timed Collection
	Unit: Milligrams of Protein or Albumin (per 24-Hour Period)	Unit: Milligrams of Protein per Gram of Creatinine	Unit: Micrograms of Albumin per Milligram of Creatinine[a]	Unit: Micrograms of Protein per Minute[b]
Normal	<300 mg/day protein or <30 mg/day albumin	<200 mg/g	<30 mcg/mg	<20 mcg/min
Microalbuminuria	30–300 mg/day (of albumin)	Not applicable	30–299 mcg/mg	20–199 mcg/min
Clinical proteinuria or albuminuria	≥300 mg/day of protein or albumin	>200 mg/g	≥300 mcg/mg	≥200 mcg/min

[a]Micrograms of albumin per milligram of creatinine is equal, as a ratio, to milligrams of albumin per gram of creatinine. The National Kidney Foundation recommendations cite gender differences for values of spot albumin:creatinine ratios that are not included here.
[b]If one converts the rate of micrograms per minute to milligrams per day by multiplying by 1440 minutes in a day, the values obtained are very near those listed under the 24-hour collection column of milligrams per day of albumin, as expected.

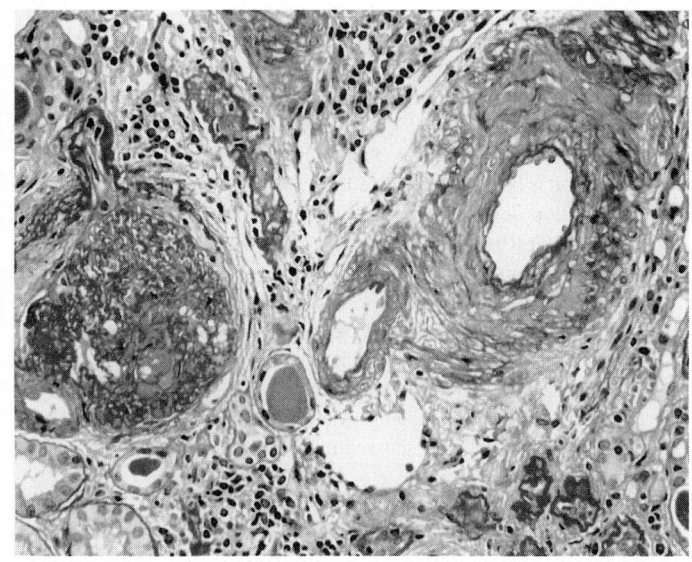

A

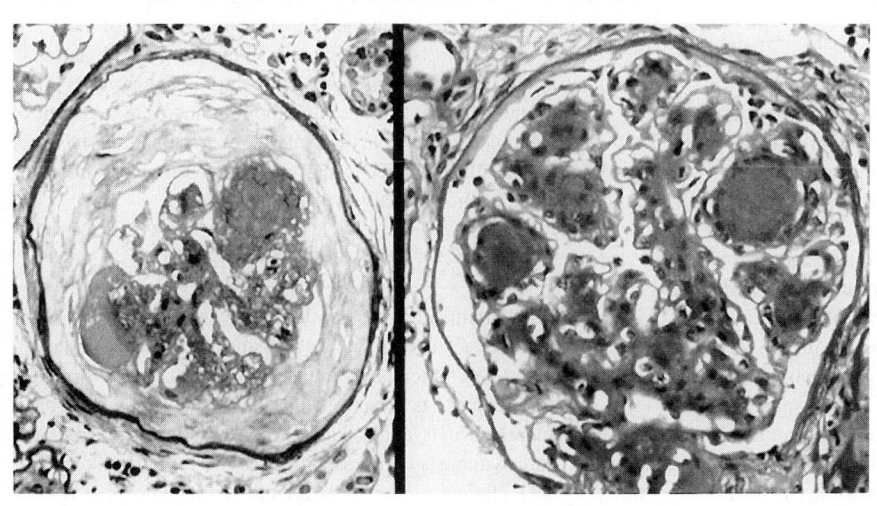

B

FIGURE 43–5. A. Advanced hypertensive arterio-nephrosclerosis with global sclerosis of a glomerulus on the left and marked sclerosis in the wall of an artery on the upper right. In the background is interstitial fibrosis, tubular atrophy, and chronic inflammation (PAS stain) **B.** Active (left) and advanced (right) glomerular injury caused by diabetic glomerulosclerosis. The glomerulus on the left shows marked increase in mesangial collagenous matrix, resulting in nodule formation. The glomerulus on the right shows advanced global sclerosis that has obliterated most normal glomerular structures. (PAS stain)

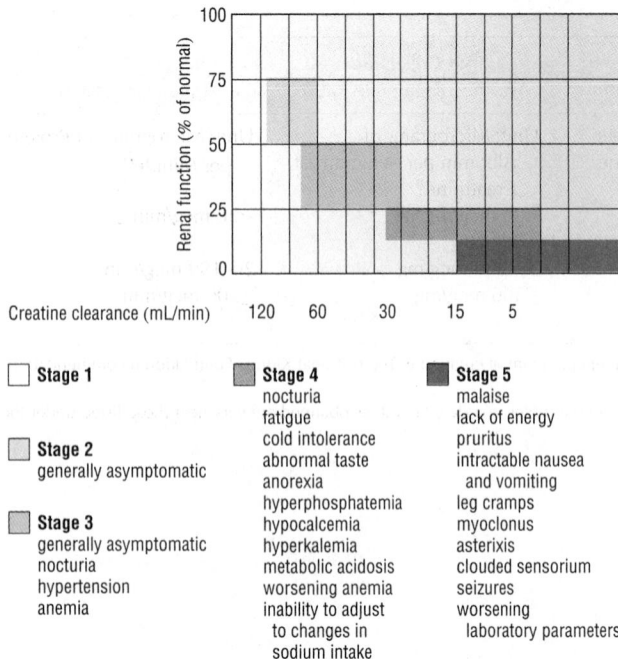

FIGURE 43–6. Staging of CKD.

Stage 1

Stage 2
generally asymptomatic

Stage 3
generally asymptomatic
nocturia
hypertension
anemia

Stage 4
nocturia
fatigue
cold intolerance
abnormal taste
anorexia
hyperphosphatemia
hypocalcemia
hyperkalemia
metabolic acidosis
worsening anemia
inability to adjust
  to changes in
  sodium intake

Stage 5
malaise
lack of energy
pruritus
intractable nausea
  and vomiting
leg cramps
myoclonus
asterixis
clouded sensorium
seizures
worsening
  laboratory parameters

⑦ Patients with Stage 1 or 2 kidney disease usually do not have any symptoms, and metabolic derangements such as acidosis, anemia, and bone disease are rarely present. Impairment of kidney function may not be recognized in the early stages of CKD, since in addition to the patient being asymptomatic, there is a lack of concomitant complications from the mildly decreased GFR, and the serum creatinine may be only slightly elevated.

⑧ The development and early stages of CKD is often clinically silent, and is usually not routinely detected unless the clinician is prudently evaluating for its presence. The classic symptoms of kidney failure are asterixis, pruritus, dysgeusia, nausea, vomiting, anorexia, encephalopathy, and bleeding. Many of these symptoms only appear when the patient has Stage 4 or 5 disease (see Chap. 44) and are therefore not useful in detecting CKD in the earlier stages (Fig. 43–6).

Signs and symptoms associated with CKD become more prevalent in Stages 3, 4, and 5. Anemia, abnormalities of calcium and phosphorus metabolism (and therefore secondary hyperparathyroidism), malnutrition, and fluid and electrolyte abnormalities become more common as kidney function deteriorates (see Chap. 44).

ANEMIA

The kidneys are responsible for secreting 90% of the endogenous hormone erythropoietin, and hence declining kidney function can lead to a reduction in the serum concentration. The consequence of reduced erythropoietin is the development of anemia. The prevalence of anemia at specific stages of CKD is difficult to ascertain, as there are limited data available correlating GFR to anemia, and there are various definitions that are used.[1] Although anemia can appear early in CKD, its prevalence has been estimated to be between 1% and 30% if anemia is defined as a hemoglobin of <12 g/dL in patients with a GFR of >80 mL/min per 1.73 m^2.[92] The true prevalence rate estimation is further complicated by the fact that covariates such as ethnicity, age, and gender can also contribute. Anemia, when defined by a hemoglobin of <13 g/dL, was found to increase in prevalence at Stage 3 CKD and become even more prevalent into Stages 4 and 5.[1] Anemia can lead to

symptoms of fatigue, decreased energy level, and shortness of breath. However, mild anemia, especially when present for a prolonged time period, can be asymptomatic. The K/DOQI guidelines recommend evaluating hemoglobin levels in all patients with CKD, noting the increase in anemia prevalence beginning with Stage 3.[93] The treatment of anemia can improve or resolve symptoms and may help to stabilize kidney function.[94] The management of anemia in CKD is discussed in Chap. 44.

CARDIOVASCULAR DISEASE

Monitoring for the presence or development of cardiovascular disease in patients with CKD is of utmost importance due to the recognized high rate of cardiovascular morbidity and mortality in these patients. Patients with CKD have been found to have 16% to 37% of the life expectancy of a matched population without kidney disease.[95] It has been suggested that a higher proportion of patients with Stages 3 and 4 CKD will actually die from cardiovascular causes than will progress to requiring dialysis therapy. Appropriate traditional and nontraditional cardiovascular risk factor assessments are necessary in the evaluation of the patient with CKD. Guidelines concerning evaluation, monitoring, and treatment for cardiovascular diseases in patients with CKD are currently being written.

METABOLIC BONE DISEASE

There is a high prevalence of abnormalities in calcium and phosphorus metabolism in Stage 5 CKD. However, since these abnormalities can and do occur in Stages 3 and 4, the clinician should monitor all patients. It is often unrecognized that secondary hyperparathyroidism can develop despite normal serum calcium and phosphorus levels, when the GFR is 80 mL/min per 1.73 m^2 or below.[96] Thus the clinician should not overlook the possibility of an elevated parathyroid hormone concentration. The calcium, phosphorus, and parathyroid hormone should be evaluated beginning in Stage 3 to evaluate for secondary hyperparathyroidism and serve to limit the manifestations on bone.[97] Additional systemic benefits such as cardiovascular risk reduction are currently being evaluated. The management of bone disease due to CKD is discussed in Chap. 44.

MALNUTRITION

Anorexia and malnutrition are complications of CKD. Although there are limited data defining at exactly which stage malnutrition develops, the K/DOQI guidelines recommend evaluating for signs of malnutrition when the GFR is <60 mL/min per 1.73 m^2 (Stages 3, 4, and 5).[98] An investigation for malnutrition should include a dietary assessment for protein and calorie intake, serum albumin, and/or assessment of protein appearance in the urine (as a marker of protein intake). Proper nutritional counseling in CKD can prevent malnutrition from occurring as patients approach dialysis (Stage 5).[1]

FLUID AND ELECTROLYTE DISORDERS

Elevations in sodium and potassium often are associated with Stages 4 and 5 CKD (see Chaps. 49 and 50). Disturbances in volume management due to CKD often occur in those with reduced levels of GFR or if structural damage is present. Other than in nephrotic syndrome, the fluid and electrolyte abnormalities of CKD can occur gradually and therefore without symptoms. Similarly to the other complications of CKD, clinicians must be aware that derangements in volume and electrolytes can occur at any stage of the disease process. Clinicians should evaluate for electrolyte abnormalities at regular intervals, with the frequency dictated by the stage of CKD and history of these abnormalities. It is common for clinicians to evaluate Stage 3 and 4 CKD patients every 3 to 4 months and Stage 5 patients every 1 to 2 months. Evaluation should include an adequate patient history in order to assess for shortness of breath or edema, signs of crackles on lung exam, and increased jugular venous pressure.

▶ TREATMENT: Diabetic Chronic Kidney Disease

DESIRED OUTCOME

The primary goal is to increase the identification of patients at risk so that appropriate interventions can be initiated early in the course of the disease. Nonpharmacologic and pharmacologic interventions are available to slow or halt the rate of CKD progression and thereby decrease the incidence and prevalence of ESKD.

NONPHARMACOLOGIC THERAPY

DIETARY PROTEIN RESTRICTION

Studies in animals with experimental kidney disease, over 20 years ago suggested that dietary protein restriction may result on a reduction in the rate of progression of renal function decline.[99] Various deleterious effects of proteinuria on the kidney have been suggested, including damage to the filtration barrier, and increased delivery of iron, complement, and lipids to the tubules. Patients with nephrotic syndrome are likely at high risk for protein-associated kidney damage due to the higher protein content in the filtered urine secondary to glomerular structural damage. The MDRD study was a large, randomized controlled study that showed a benefit to dietary protein restriction.[49,100] The MDRD study included no type 1 diabetics, and only a few type 2 diabetics who were not receiving insulin. Subjects who were defined as having moderate renal insufficiency (GFR of 25 to 55 mL/min per 1.73 m^2) were randomized into one of four groups stratified by a goal dietary protein intake and mean arterial blood pressure (MAP): usual or low-protein diet (1.3 g/kg per day vs. 0.58 g/kg per day) and usual or low MAP goal (107 mm Hg vs. 92 mm Hg). Subjects who were defined as having severe renal insufficiency (GFR 13 to 24 mL/min per 1.73 m^2) were also randomized to one of four groups: a low-protein diet (0.58/kg/day) or a very-low-protein diet (0.28 g/kg/day), along with a keto-amino acid supplement with a usual or low MAP goal as defined above. Follow-up measurements included monthly 24-hour urea excretion and blood pressure measurements, dietary records every 3 months, and GFR at months 2, 4, and then every 4 months for the 2- to 3-year study period. Although protein restriction failed to show a statistical benefit after 3 years of follow-up in any of the groups, these results are complicated by the fact that 24% of the subjects had a diagnosis of polycystic kidney disease (a disease that is not glomerular in origin), which may have reduced the ability to see the benefit of dietary protein and blood pressure interventions (interventions hypothesized to result from alterations at the level of the glomerulus).

In order to define the association between dietary protein restriction and CKD progression, two meta-analyses (comprised of several smaller studies) evaluated the effect of dietary protein restriction in diabetic and nondiabetic kidney diseases.[101,102] The larger study, comprising over 1000 patients (who were predominantly nondiabetic) from 13 randomized controlled trials, found a weak association between dietary protein restriction and reduction in the rate of kidney disease progression.[102] An analysis of the diabetic group from this study and the diabetic population from the meta-analysis by Pedrini and associates, showed a greater benefit from dietary protein restriction.[101] The level of protein restriction ranged from 0.5 to 0.85 g/kg per day in the meta-analysis comprised of diabetics.[101] These data suggest a preferential benefit from dietary protein restriction in the diabetic patient population. One recent study employing nutrition counseling in diabetics suggested that patients are generally noncompliant to long-term low-protein diets outside of a regimented study design, and thus this intervention is not likely to be effective long term.[103]

The National Kidney Foundation's K/DOQI guidelines for nutrition in patients with CKD recommend a dietary protein intake of 0.6 g/kg per day for patients with a GFR <25 mL/min.[98] Titration of protein intake up to 0.75 g/kg per day is suggested for patients who cannot achieve or maintain adequate nutritional status with the lower-protein (0.6 g/kg per day) diet.[98]

PHARMACOLOGIC THERAPY

Intensive Insulin Therapy

The Diabetes Control and Complications Trial (DCCT) is considered to be the landmark study showing the positive long-term benefits of intensive insulin therapy (IIT).[61] IIT was defined as the administration of insulin three or more times daily by injection or by external pump to achieve preprandial and postprandial blood glucose values of 70 to 120 mg/dL and <180 mg/dL, respectively. IIT reduced the incidence of microalbuminuria and albuminuria as compared to standard therapy in both the primary prevention and secondary prevention groups, as described previously.[61] However, IIT was associated with a higher incidence of hypoglycemic reactions (at least one episode of hypoglycemia in 65% of patients, as compared to 35% in the standard treatment group).[61] The positive renal outcomes from this trial may be difficult to reproduce in routine clinical practice since many poorly controlled type 1 diabetic patients may be reluctant to comply with IIT because they fear the risk of hypoglycemia.[104]

A meta-analysis of 16 clinical studies showed a benefit of intensive blood glucose control in patients with type 1 diabetes as evidenced by a reduction in the frequency, severity, and a delay in the development or progression of diabetic complications including nephropathy.[105] The Epidemiology of Diabetes Interventions and Complications study, which observed the DCCT subjects for an additional 4 years while they were receiving care from primary physicians, showed a continued benefit of IIT on the risk of nephropathy as defined by the development of microalbuminuria (53% odds ratio reduction in microalbuminuria).[106]

Optimize Hypertension Control

The Seventh Joint National Committee on Prevention, Detection, Evaluation, and Treatment of High Blood Pressure recommends a goal blood pressure of <130/80 mm Hg for patients with kidney disease.[107] Although these are the goals set forth by the Joint National Committee, any reduction in blood pressure may be deemed beneficial. The UK Prospective Diabetes Study revealed that tight blood pressure control (with captopril or atenolol) to 144/82 mm Hg versus 154/87 mm Hg in the other group conferred reductions of 24% in diabetes-related end points, 32% in deaths related to diabetes, 44% in strokes, and 37% in microvascular end points.[57] The effect of a rigorous blood pressure goal (MAP of ≤92 mm Hg) on proteinuria and progression of kidney disease in type 1 diabetics leads to a decrease in proteinuria.[108] To achieve these goal blood pressures, three or more different blood pressure medications are likely to be required.[109] Figure 43–7 depicts the proposed algorithm for the management of hypertension in people with CKD and diabetes. Chapter 13 reviews the individual agents and proposed doses for optimal management of hypertension.

Elevated blood pressure is more difficult to control in patients with CKD than those with normal kidney function. Patients diagnosed with both hypertension and diabetes mellitus have been estimated to have up to a sixfold higher risk of developing ESKD than do those patients with diabetes mellitus alone.[109] Adequate blood pressure control can reduce the rate of decline in GFR and the degree of albuminuria in hypertensive type 1 or type 2 diabetics.[109] Although interventions that reduce blood pressure have historically shown reductions in urinary albumin and protein excretion, the angiotensin-converting enzyme inhibitors (ACEIs) were the first agents shown to reduce glomerular capillary pressure and volume, which in animal models and human studies have resulted in preservation of renal function.[110–112] Table 43–4 summarizes the documented effects of the various available antihypertensive agents on renal blood flow and GFR.[113,114]

Several studies have confirmed the beneficial effects of ACEIs on renal function in diabetics as well as nondiabetics. The results of the key (>100 evaluated subjects) studies in diabetics are presented in Table 43–5.[115–121] These studies were conducted over a time frame of 2 to 6 years and thus were likely long enough in duration to

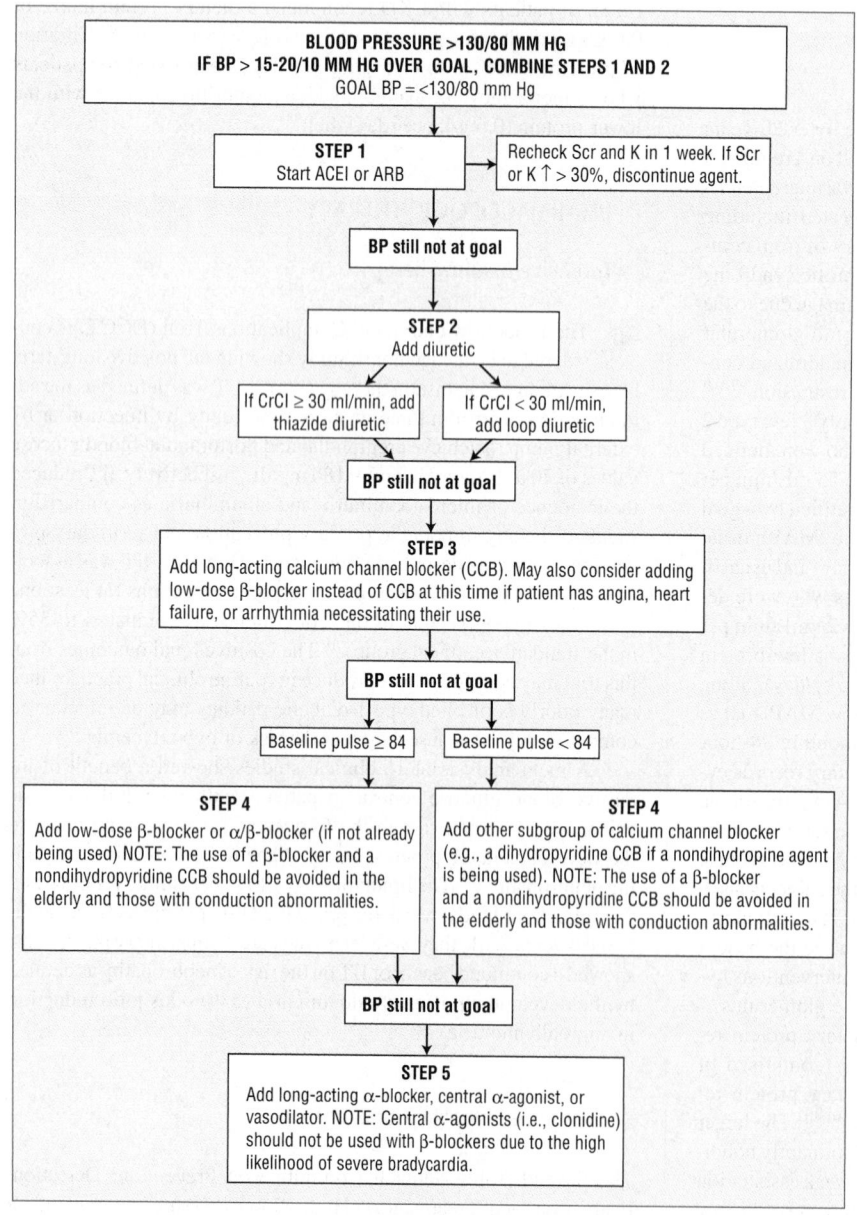

FIGURE 43–7. Hypertension management algorithm for patients with CKD. Dosage adjustments should be made every 2 to 4 weeks as needed. The dose of one agent should be maximized before another is added. Adapted from Bakris,[109] with permission.

TABLE 43–4. Effects of Antihypertensive Agents on Renal Blood Flow (RBF) and Glomerular Filtration Rate (GFR)

Antihypertensive Agent	Mechanism of Action	Effects on Renal Hemodynamics
Diuretics	Sodium and volume depletion	Decrease in GFR and RBF
	↑Vasodilatory prostaglandin levels (IV loop diuretics)	Increase in RBF
	Renal vasoconstriction (IV thiazide diuretics)	Decrease in GFR and RBF
β-Adrenergic blockers	↓ Cardiac output	Decrease in GFR and RBF
	↑ Renal vascular resistance (nonselective agents)	Decrease in GFR and RBF
	↓ Renal vascular resistance (β_1-selective agents)	No change in GFR and RBF
Centrally acting antiadrenergic drugs	↓ Renal vascular resistance (methyldopa)	No change in GFR and RBF
	↓ Renal perfusion pressure (clonidine, α_2-adrenergic agonist)	Decrease in GFR and RBF
Peripherally acting antiadrenergic drugs	Direct vasodilation (postsynaptic α_1-adrenoreceptor blocking agents)	No change in GFR and RBF
Direct vasodilator agents	↓ Renal vascular resistance (hydralazine, minoxidil)	Increase in RBF and no effect on GFR
	Arterial vasodilation plus dilatation of venous capacitance vessels (nitroprusside)	Decrease in GFR and RBF (acute effect)
Angiotensin-converting enzyme inhibitors/angiotensin-II receptor blockers	Dilation of the efferent arteriole	Decrease in GFR and no change in RBF
Calcium channel blockers	↓ Renal vascular resistance by vasodilation of afferent arterioles (hypertensive patients)	Increase in RBF and no change in GFR

TABLE 43–5. Summary of Angiotensin-Converting Enzyme Inhibitor Studies in Diabetic Patients

Drug, Dose and Study Design	Baseline Renal Characteristics	Number of Subjects and Disease	Study Duration	Outcome	Reference and Study Name
Captopril 25 mg three times a day; randomized, placebo-controlled trial	UPE≥500 mg/day, S_{Cr}≤2.5 mg/dL	409 Type 1 DM	3 years	Risk reduction of doubling S_{Cr} was 48% with captopril treatment; subanalysis showed a larger risk reduction with more elevated S_{Cr} (76% when the S_{Cr} was 2 g/dL)	Lewis et al[115]
Enalapril once daily; randomized, placebo-controlled trial	Normotensive, UAE 20–200 mcg/min	103 Type 2 DM	5 years	Risk reduction of 66.7% for progression to clinical albuminuria with enalapril	Ahmad et al[116]
Enalapril 10 mg once daily; randomized, placebo-controlled trial	Normotensive, UAE≤30 mg/day	156 Type 2 DM	6 years	Risk reduction of 12.5% for microalbuminuria with enalapril treatment; GFR reductions were two times greater in the placebo treated patients at 6 years.	Ravid et al[117]
Lisinopril 10 mg once daily with titration to BP; placebo-controlled trial	Normotensive patients either normoalbuminuria or microalbuminuria	530 Type 1 DM	2 years	18.8% lower UPE with lisinopril treatment; greater treatment effect in those with baseline microalbuminuria (34.2 mcg/min vs. 1 mcg/min)	EUCLID Study Group[118]
Ramipril 10 mg once daily; randomized, placebo-controlled trial	Normoalbuminuria or microalbuminuria	3577 Type 2 DM	4.5 years	Ramipril lowered risk of overt nephropathy with and without baseline microalbuminuria (relative risk of 0.8); lower UP:Cr at 1 and 4.5 years with ramipril treatment	HOPE and MICROHOPE[119]
Captopril 50 mg twice a day; randomized, placebo-controlled trial	Normotensive patients with microalbuminuria	143 Type 1 DM	2 years	Risk reduction of 67.8% for clinical proteinuria with captopril treatment; GFR reductions of 7.9 mL/min per 1.73 m^2 per year in placebo while stable in captopril group	North American Microalbuminuria Study Group[120]
Enalapril 5 mg once daily, titrated to BP; placebo-controlled trial	Hypertensive, GFR of 30–100 mL/min per 1.73 m^2	121 Type 2 DM	3 years	Clinical albuminuria progression in 7% of enalapril vs. 21% of placebo group; enalapril therapy preserved GFR, while placebo treatment resulted in a loss of 0.33 mL/min per 1.73 m^2 per month	Lebovitz et al[121]

BP, blood pressure; DM, diabetes mellitus; GFR, glomerular filtration rate; S_{Cr}, serum creatinine; UP:Cr, urinary protein:creatinine ratio; UPE, urinary protein excretion; UAE, urinary albumin excretion.

adequately assess the proposed outcomes. Various ACEIs and dosages were assessed in both type 1 and type 2 diabetic subjects. Patients with various severity levels of nephropathy were represented, from normoalbuminuria with risk of renal function decline to patients with severe levels of albuminuria/proteinuria and reductions in GFR. The outcomes consistently support the role of ACEI therapy in the management of CKD.

⟨10⟩ The results of a meta-analysis serves to confirm the beneficial effects demonstrated in several of the small and large randomized controlled studies that evaluated the effects of ACEI therapy on diabetic nephropathy. Progression to proteinuria was reduced by 65% in patients with diabetes mellitus and microalbuminuria, and progression of nephropathy (doubling of serum creatinine) was reduced by 40% in patients with overt proteinuria (comprised of 30% diabetics and 70% nondiabetics) (Fig. 43–8).[122] The meta-analysis, in addition to the available single studies, provide strong support for the use of ACEIs in diabetic patients with or without hypertension.

⟨11⟩ Although a variety of individual ACEIs and doses have been evaluated, there is no consensus regarding the optimal agent, or the starting or maximum dosages to achieve optimal levels of proteinuria reduction. The reason for this lack of consensus is due to the design of the studies, whereby there was assessment of only one ACEI versus a placebo and fixed doses were generally administered. Hence comparative information between the individual ACEIs or variations in proteinuric response relative to dosage titration is sparse. The meta-

analysis referred to previously, however, demonstrated homogeneity among the ACEIs that were included, suggesting that no one agent is superior to the other agents.[122] In patients with hypertension, the primary goal is to optimally treat the blood pressure to target, and the secondary goal is to minimize proteinuria. For normotensive patients with microalbuminuria, one should titrate the ACEI to reduce the microalbuminuria. The hypertensive ceiling effect noted for ACEI therapy and dosage titration has not been confirmed for treatment to lower urinary protein restriction. However, patients with hypertension and proteinuria can still exhibit side effects associated with blood pressure lowering, and hence dosages should be titrated to the maximal level of proteinuria reduction without reducing the blood pressure to a level associated with adverse events. Patients should be initiated on the lowest possible dose of ACEI and titrated to blood pressure control and proteinuria reduction.

The angiotensin II receptor blockers (ARBs) have been investigated and show favorable results in slowing the progression of diabetic kidney disease. Data from several studies (that included at least 100 patients) evaluating ARB efficacy in type 2 diabetes are summarized in Table 43–6.[123–126] All patients in these trials had at least a level of proteinuria consistent with microalbuminuria and all were hypertensive. With the exception of one, the studies were of a sufficiently long enough duration to determine the beneficial effects of ARBs on nephropathy. Of note, the beneficial effect of actually delaying the onset of diabetic nephropathy was significant in type 2 patients who received irbesartan 300 mg daily for up to 2 years.[124] A similar trend (although not statistically significant) was observed in those subjects who received a lower dose of irbesartan (150 mg daily). Although renal benefits of ARBs have been observed in these type 2 diabetic subjects, no differences in death between losartan and placebo-treated subjects were shown. The ELITE study (which assessed losartan versus captopril in diabetics and nondiabetics) showed comparable renal benefits of both ARBs and ACEIs in a population of heart failure patients.[127] Currently, the data show efficacy of both ACEIs and ARBs in type 2 diabetes, while only ACEIs have been adequately evaluated in patients with type 1 diabetes. Thus, until head-to-head trials with these agents are assessed, they should not be considered interchangeable in all forms of diabetes.[128]

Since ACEIs and ARBs have demonstrated efficacy in patients with diabetes, the possibility of using both agents in type 2 diabetics has been investigated.[129] This short-term (12 to 24 weeks) study evaluated lisinopril (20 mg once daily) and candesartan (16 mg once daily) versus the combination in 199 patients. The reduction of urinary albumin:creatinine ratios were greater with combination therapy (50%) than either lisinopril (39%) or candesartan (24%) alone. Blood pressure reduction, however, was also significantly greater in the combination therapy patients. Thus it is not clear if the combination produced an enhanced antiproteinuric effect or if the reduction in the albumin: creatinine ratio could be attributable to the greater reduction in blood pressure.[129]

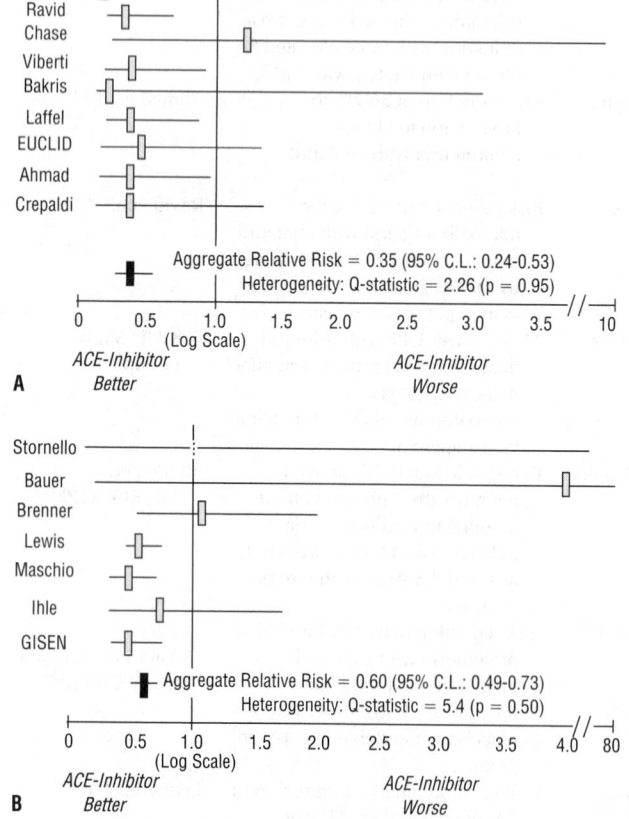

FIGURE 43–8. A. Relative risk for developing microalbuminuria with 95% confidence intervals (CIs) in each study, and the aggregate relative risk with 95% CIs for all studies (N = 642 with diabetes). B. Relative risk for doubling serum creatinine concentration or development of ESRD with 95% CIs in each study, and aggregate relative risk with 95% CIs for all studies (N = 1,277; 479 with diabetes). From Kshirsagar,[122] with permission.

CLINICAL CONTROVERSY

Some clinicians believe that ACEI and ARB medications should be titrated to achieve tight blood pressure control and that this will automatically result in optimal proteinuria reduction.

Some calcium channel blockers have been shown to decrease glomerular injury without negatively changing renal hemodynamics.[111] The postulated mechanisms for this decrease in renal injury

TABLE 43–6. Summary of Angiotensin Receptor Blocker Studies in Diabetic Patients

Drug, Dose, and Study Design	Baseline Characteristics	Number of Subjects and Disease	Duration	Outcomes	Reference and Study Name
Irbesartan 300 mg once daily; amlodipine 10 mg once daily, randomized, placebo-controlled trial	Hypertensive, UPE ≥900 mg/day	1715 Type 2 DM	2.6 years	Irbesartan therapy resulted in a 20% (for placebo) and 23% (for amlodipine) risk reduction in primary composite end point of doubling of S_{Cr}, development of ESKD, or death	Lewis et al[123]
Irbesartan 150 mg once daily; irbesartan 300 mg once daily; randomized, placebo-controlled trial	Hypertensive, AER of 20–200 mcg/min	590 Type 2 DM	2 years	Irbesartan 150 mg resulted in a 24% reduction in UAE; irbesartan 300 mg resulted in a 38% reduction in UAE; placebo resulted in a 2% decrease; hazard ratio for diabetic nephropathy was 0.56 and 0.32 in the 150-mg and 300-mg irbesartan groups, respectively	Parving et al[124]
Losartan 50–100 mg once daily; randomized placebo-controlled trial	Hypertensive, UA:U$_{Cr}$ of at least 300 and S_{Cr} 1.3–3 mg/dL	1513 Type 2 DM	3.4 years	Losartan therapy resulted in a 16% risk reduction of primary composite end point of doubling of S_{Cr}, ESKD, or death; level of proteinuria declined by 35% with losartan therapy	Brenner et al[125]
Irbesartan 150 mg twice a day; randomized, placebo-controlled trial, crossover study	Hypertensive and normotensive, microalbuminuria	128 Type 2 DM	120 days	Irbesartan had a beneficial effect on reducing AER in both hypertensive and normotensive patients with type 2 diabetes	Sasso et al[126]

AER, albumin excretion rate; DM, diabetes mellitus; ESKD, end-stage kidney disease; S_{Cr}, serum creatinine; UAE, urinary albumin excretion; UA:U$_{Cr}$, urinary albumin:urinary creatinine ratio; UPE, urinary protein excretion.

include suppression of glomerular hypertrophy, inhibition of platelet aggregation, and decreased salt accumulation.[111] Although the data regarding dihydropyridine calcium channel blockers do not suggest any beneficial effects beyond those attributable to reducing blood pressure, there is some suggestion that the nondihydropyridine agents (diltiazem and verapamil) may have beneficial effects on proteinuria that are similar to those of ACEIs.[130–132] A few studies have suggested that the efficacy of combination therapy with ACEIs and nondihydropyridine calcium channel blockers may be superior in terms of proteinuria reduction than the use of either agent alone.[133]

▶ TREATMENT: Nondiabetic Chronic Kidney Disease

▪ NUTRITIONAL MANAGEMENT

The MDRD study was the largest prospective trial that evaluated the influence of dietary protein and phosphorus restriction on the progression of CKD in a population of patients that consisted mostly of nondiabetics.[49,100] A secondary analysis of the MDRD study was conducted and revealed that in those patients with a GFR of less than 25 mL/min per 1.73 m^2, a protein intake of 0.6 g/kg per day was significantly associated with a decreased rate of progressive renal disease.[100] In addition, this analysis showed that the rate of progression to ESKD was significantly reduced by 41% for each 0.2 g/kg per day reduction in dietary protein intake. The discrepancy in results between the primary and secondary analyses can be explained by the different statistical methods used in each of the two analyses, in that the later analysis evaluated participants who were actually compliant with their dietary prescription. Based on these findings, the K/DOQI has advocated a dietary protein intake of 0.6 mg/kg per day in patients with a GFR <25 mL/min per 1.73m^2.[98]

Two meta-analyses of randomized clinical trials reported that reducing protein intake in nondiabetic patients with CKD could delay the time to onset and reduce the occurrence of ESKD by approximately 40%.[108,134] Another meta-analysis reported a reduction in the rate of GFR decline of 0.53 mL/min per year after the addition of a low-protein diet.[102] The suggested benefit of dietary protein restriction in patients without diabetes offers another interventional strategy to reduce the rate of CKD progression. The benefits of dietary protein restriction need to be weighed against the potential adverse event of protein malnutrition and related sequelae including increased morbidity and mortality.

▪ PHARMACOLOGIC THERAPY

▪ ANTIHYPERTENSIVE AGENTS

Reduction of blood pressure is key to decreasing cardiovascular and renal sequelae. However, antihypertensive agents are not equal in their ability to preserve kidney function despite similar efficacy in terms of blood pressure reduction. As precipitous reductions in blood pressure may be deleterious to kidney function in patients with underlying renal impairment, blood pressure targets in these patients should be

TABLE 43–7. Summary of Studies with Angiotensin-Converting Enzyme Inhibitors in Patients without Diabetes

Drug, Dose and Study Design	Baseline Characteristics	Number of Subjects and Disease	Duration	Outcomes	Reference and Study Name
Benazepril 10 mg once daily; randomized, placebo-controlled trial	Mild (46–60 mL/min GFR) and moderate (30–45 mL/min GFR) renal insufficiency	583 Patients with various renal disorders including diabetes mellitus	3 years	Benazepril afforded a 53% risk reduction in primary end point of doubling of S_{Cr} or requirement for dialysis; 71% and 46% risk reductions in the mild and moderate renal insufficiency groups, respectively.	Maschio et al;[136]
Ramipril 2.5 mg once daily and titrated to BP; randomized, placebo-controlled trial	GFR 20–70 mL/min per 1.73 m², UPE ≥1 g/day	352 Proteinuric patients	5 years	Rate of loss of GFR was 0.89 mL/min per month in placebo versus 0.39 mL/min per month in ramipril group; twice the numbers of patients receiving placebo vs. ramipril reached primary composite end point of doubling of S_{Cr} or ESKD	The GISEN Group[137]
Enalapril 20 mg once daily vs. losartan 50 mg one daily; randomized trial	Proteinuria	93 Hypertensives	12 weeks	UP:Cr was reduced by 43% in losartan group vs. 23% in enalapril group ($p = 0.05$)	Nielsen et al[138]
Enalapril 5–40 mg daily vs. other antihypertensive agents; randomized, controlled trial	UPE ≥0.5 g/day, S_{Cr} ≤1.5 mg/dL	44 IgAN patients	7 years	Renal survival was significantly better in the enalapril group (100%) versus the other antihypertensive group (70%) after 4 years, and 92% vs. 55% respectively, after 7 years; proteinuria significantly decreased in the enalapril group, whereas it tended to increase in the control group	Praga et al[139]
Ramipril 1.25–5 mg daily vs. conventional therapy; randomized controlled trial	Proteinuria 1–3 g/day	186 Chronic nephropathies	31 months	Progression to ESKD was half as common in the ramipril group; patients with GFR ≤45 mL/min per 1.73 m² and proteinuria ≥1.5 g/24 hours had the greatest benefit from ramipril therapy	Ruggenenti et al[140]

ESKD, end-stage kidney disease; GFR, glomerular filtration rate; IgAN, Ig A nephropathy; S_{Cr}, serum creatinine; UP:Cr, urinary protein:creatinine ratio; UPE, urinary protein excretion.

achieved over several weeks to allow the kidney to adapt to reduced perfusion pressures.[107] Typically there is an acute but sustained reduction in GFR of about 25% to 30% within 3 to 7 days after initiation of ACEI therapy, due to a reduction in intraglomerular pressure.[135] If the serum creatinine increases by more than 0.5 mg/dL and is sustained after ACEI therapy initiation or dosage increase, the patient may require therapy discontinuation due to drug-induced acute renal failure. It is necessary to realize that although ACEI therapy may be effective in reducing the rate of nephropathy, one needs to consider the projected benefit in terms of clinical improvement when the baseline GFR is already too far progressed, propensity for hyperkalemia exists, and potential for acute GFR reduction exists in patients who already have compromised GFR.

CLINICAL CONTROVERSY

Some clinicians fail to prescribe ACEI or ARB medications when the GFR is less than 20 to 30 mL/min per 1.73m² due to fear of the patient developing a further elevation in serum creatinine.

Several short- and long-term clinical trials (that evaluated at least 40 patients) assessed the effect of ACEIs on renal function in patients without diabetes, and these are summarized in Table 43–7.[136–140] These studies vary in length from 12 weeks to 7 years. Also, the numbers of subjects enrolled in the studies are generally smaller than those studies that evaluated diabetic individuals. Since these patients had forms of nephropathy that are often associated with significant proteinuria, they tended to have more proteinuria and more severe reductions in GFR as compared to the diabetic populations in which ACEI therapy was evaluated. Significant reductions in terms of the risk of doubling serum creatinine or requirement for dialysis or reductions in proteinuria were demonstrated for patients receiving the ACEIs. Ramipril (1.25 to 5 mg daily) reduced proteinuria and the rate of GFR decline to a greater extent than that expected from blood pressure reduction alone.[137] The proteinuria reduction was greatest in those patients with the highest baseline levels. A limitation of this study was that the additional antihypertensive agents that were administered to study participants were not specified. A subsequent study by the same group of investigators in patients with less proteinuria revealed similar beneficial effects and found that the relative risk of

TABLE 43–8. Summary of Studies with Angiotensin Receptor Blockers in Patients without Diabetes

Drug, Dose, and Study Design	Baseline Characteristics	Number of Subjects and Disease	Duration	Outcomes	Reference
Losartan 50 mg once daily vs. control	Normotensive, proteinuria	23 FSGS patients	1 year	Proteinuria decreased 47% in the losartan group at 1 year, while there was a significant increase in proteinuria in the control group; total serum protein and albumin concentrations also increased in the losartan group; cholesterol levels of the losartan group were significantly reduced	Usta et al[142]
Losartan 25 mg once daily vs. enalapril 10 mg once daily; randomized, controlled trial	GFR 36–93 mL/min	34 Primary glomerulonephritis	3 months	Proteinuria reduced 25% vs. 45% in losartan and enalapril groups, respectively; significant decline in GFR in enalapril group and no change in losartan group	Tylicki et al[143]

FSGS, focal segmental glomerulosclerosis; GFR, glomerular filtration rate; UPE, urinary protein excretion.

developing ESKD was 2.3 times higher with conventional therapy plus placebo than for ramipril therapy.[140] The results of these studies and a meta-analysis revealed that ACEIs conferred a 40% reduction in the risk of developing ESKD or doubling of serum creatinine in patients with overt proteinuria (>300 mg protein/24 hours) and renal disease of various etiologies (about 50% diabetic patients; see Fig. 43–8).[122]

Since the clearance of all ACEIs (with the exception of fosinopril) is reduced in CKD, it is prudent to commence therapy at lower initial doses and then later titrate to achieve the optimal therapeutic effects.[141] The antiproteinuric effects of ACEIs are not necessarily attained at the same doses as the antihypertensive effects. Thus patients who have reached their blood pressure goals may require further dosage adjustments to achieve maximal reductions in urinary protein excretion. Serum potassium needs to be monitored when initiating therapy with ACEIs, especially when patients are concurrently receiving drugs that may increase the risk of hyperkalemia, such as nonsteroidal anti-inflammatory agents.

The ARBs, although evaluated to a lesser extent, appear to have similar efficacy in terms of renal protection in patients with several forms of glomerulonephritis (Table 43–8).[142,143] Proteinuria reduction on the order of 25% to 47% was shown with ARB therapy. It is necessary to note that these studies employed much smaller numbers of patients and follow-up was of shorter duration than many evaluations of diabetic patients. Despite these limitations, most clinicians use either ACEI or ARB therapy as the standard of care in patients with glomerulonephritis and proteinuria. The combination of ARBs with ACEIs has been proposed and preliminary data suggest that this approach is safe and results in a greater decrease in proteinuria than that seen with either agent alone.[144] A recent study prospectively evaluated losartan 100 mg daily or trandolapril 3 mg daily or the combination of the two in 336 patients with nondiabetic kidney diseases. The primary end point, time to doubling of serum creatinine or ESKD was observed in 11% of combination therapy patients and 23% in each of the single-agent treatment groups.[145]

The calcium channel blockers also effective treatments for hypertension in patients with CKD but without diabetes. However, as was mentioned previously, only the nondihydropyridine CCBs have data suggesting a reduction in the rate of decline of renal function.[130,146] There are currently no data to suggest that higher doses of nondihydropyridine CCBs are needed to elicit a reduction in proteinuria as compared to a reduction in blood pressure.

Although diuretics are commonly used to treat fluid overload and hypertension in patients with CKD, there are no compelling data to suggest any renal protection in terms of proteinuria regression or progression. The use of diuretics for managing volume overload is addressed in Chap. 49. Other available antihypertensive agents are used to control blood pressure in patients with kidney disease. The selection of individual agents and dosage to manage blood pressure in patients with CKD is quite similar to that for patients without kidney disease. One must consider the need for dosage reductions due to CKD and/or supplemental doses due to dialysis removal for selected agents such as the hydrophilic β-blockers nadolol, acebutolol, and atenolol.

Regardless of the treatment regimen, hypertension should be treated to the currently accepted targets in patients with CKD. If proteinuria is present, the use of ACEIs, ARBs, and possibly nondihydropyridine CCBs may be superior to conventional agents in decreasing proteinuria and glomerular hypertension.

OTHER INTERVENTIONS TO LIMIT DISEASE PROGRESSION

HYPERLIPIDEMIA TREATMENT

Supportive therapies such as lipid-lowering regimens, smoking cessation, and anemia management may also slow the progression of CKD. Although several drugs are available for lipid lowering, the 3-hydroxy-3-methylglutaryl coenzyme A (HMG-CoA) reductase inhibitors and gemfibrozil have been used most frequently in dyslipidemic patients with CKD with and without proteinuria.[76] While the primary goal of treatment is to adequately reduce the elevations in lipid parameters in order to decrease one's risk for progressive atherosclerotic cardiovascular disease, a secondary goal of treatment is a reduction in proteinuria and renal function decline. A meta-analysis examined various hypolipidemic modalities including carnitine, fish oil, low-molecular-weight heparins, and exercise, in order to determine their lipid-lowering efficacy in patients with nephrotic syndrome and CKD.[147] These data suggest a consideration of less common therapeutic approaches to lipid lowering in patients in whom contraindications to specific first-line therapies exist. The National Cholesterol Education Program III and K/DOQI guidelines as well as Chapter 21 should be consulted for a thorough review of lipid reduction and cardiovascular disease in patients with CKD.[148,149]

A meta-analysis of 13 prospective controlled trials did conclude that lipid-lowering therapies may decrease proteinuria and slow the rate of GFR decline (by a 0.156-mL/min-per-month).[150] It has been suggested that HMG-CoA reductase inhibitors may have some other advantages that may help to reduce kidney disease progression in addition to lipid reduction, such as reduction of monocyte infiltration, mesangial cell proliferation, mesangial matrix expansion, and tubulointerstitial inflammation and fibrosis.[151]

SMOKING CESSATION

Although the adverse cardiovascular disease risks of smoking have been documented, it has only been in the last decade that information has been published regarding the effects of smoking on the progression of CKD. Although the exact physiologic effects of smoking on kidney function have not been fully elucidated, smoking can result in several acute changes, including a drop in GFR and a corresponding increase in heart rate and blood pressure, likely secondary to nicotine.[152] Nicotine has also been shown to cause an increase in urinary albumin excretion.[65,152] Although the effectiveness of smoking cessation on limiting progressive CKD has not been prospectively evaluated, one recent study suggested that smoking cessation resulted in a protective effect against proteinuria and reduced GFR.[153] Based on the evolving data concerning the detrimental effects of smoking on the kidney, it is prudent to educate patients regarding this risk, and institute appropriate therapeutic options institute for smoking cessation as discussed in Chapter 65.

ANEMIA TREATMENT

Prolonged anemia has been associated with left ventricular hypertrophy and even heart failure, but only approximately 15% to 23% of anemic CKD patients receive therapy prior to the initiation of dialysis.[95,154] The cardiovascular sequelae of anemia in patients with kidney disease and a management algorithm is presented in Chapter 44. The presence of anemia may actually be associated with an increased rate of CKD progression.[155] Researchers have coined the phrase "cardio-renal anemia syndrome" to describe the interrelated aspects of anemia, congestive heart failure (CHF), and CKD.[155] It has been hypothesized that by actively treating CHF and anemia, the progression of both CHF and CKD can be reduced.[156,157] A recent study in renal transplant recipients showed an absence of loss of renal function in newly anemic patients who had erythropoietin therapy initiated, while there was a reduction in the loss of renal function in patients who had anemia for a short time period and subsequently received therapy with erythropoietin.[158] The other finding of this study was that of longer renal graft survival in erythropoietin-treated patients. These data support further study of the potential role of anemia management in reducing renal function decline. Tissue hypoxia associated with anemia may be a stimulus for continued renal injury in those with Stages 3 to 5 CKD. In addition, anemia-related alterations of renal sympathetic nerve activity and related increases in oxidative stress have been reported.[159]

PHARMACOECONOMIC CONSIDERATIONS

There have been a few evaluations of the potential pharmacoeconomic impact of screening for microalbuminuria and the subsequent initiation of various pharmacotherapeutic regimens in type 1 diabetic patients.[160,161] According to one study, the historical standard approach to proteinuria reduction was considered to be treatment with hydrochlorothiazide at the time of hypertension diagnosis, while the newer treatment approach assumed three different screening and treatment strategies with ACEIs. The results from this evaluation suggested that with early screening and treatment of persistent microalbuminuria with ACEIs, it is possible to realize a cost-effectiveness ratio of $7,900 to $16,500 per year of life saved. This ratio is similar to the cost effectiveness associated with treating hypertension in the general population. A similar cost-effectiveness analysis using different strategies but the same basic model was also performed,[161] and projected that treating all patients with an ACEI 5 years after the diagnosis of diabetes was as cost effective as annual screening for microalbuminuria beginning 5 years after diagnosis, with the initiation of an ACEI when and if persistent microalbuminuria was detected. The DCCT Research Group evaluated the cost effectiveness of intensive insulin therapy as compared with conventional diabetes treatment.[162] The analysis demonstrated that implementing intensive insulin therapy would result in an incremental cost per year of life gained of $28,661, which represents a good value to the health care system. Overall, it appears that aggressive insulin therapy, as well as treatment with ACEIs when persistent microalbuminuria is identified, reduces complications, improves quality of life by preserving renal function, and ultimately increases length of life at reasonable costs to society. The results of these simulated analyses remain to be prospectively confirmed.

The UK Prospective Diabetes Study also included a cost-effectiveness study that compared tight blood pressure control (ACEI and β-blocker therapy) with less-tight blood pressure control. The main outcomes included use of health care resources and the time free from diabetes-related end points. The investigators concluded that tight blood pressure control in patients with type 2 diabetes and hypertension produced a positive cost-effectiveness ratio with regard to reducing the cost of complications and increasing the interval without complications.[163] A recent study concluded that all middle-aged patients with newly diagnosed type 2 diabetes should be treated with an ACEI rather than be screened for microalbuminuria and then treated.[164] They determined that this treatment method would provide additional benefit with only a modest increase in cost.

EVALUATION OF THERAPEUTIC OUTCOMES

DIABETICS

Based on the available clinical and experimental data, pharmacologic interventions can help to limit the progression of CKD in diabetic patients. Figure 43–9 summarizes these interventions in the form of an algorithm.[165] All patients with type 1 diabetes of more than 5 years' duration and all type 2 diabetics should be screened yearly for microalbuminuria (annual urinary albumin excretion or urinary albumin:creatinine ratio).[52] Blood glucose should be maintained within or close to the normal range by frequent insulin injections or by use

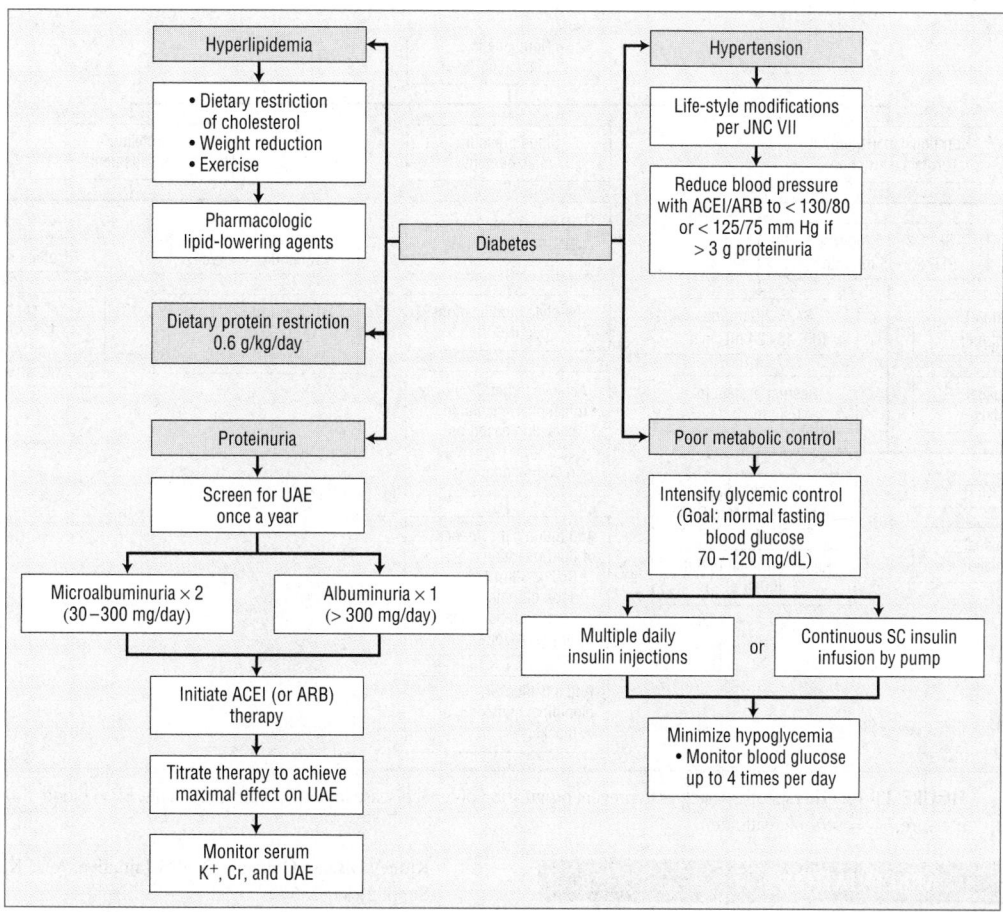

FIGURE 43–9. Therapeutic strategies to prevent progression of renal disease in diabetic individuals. UAE = urinary albumin excretion; SC = subcutaneous; JNC VII = the seventh report of the Joint National Committee on Prevention, Detection, Evaluation, and Treatment of High Blood Pressure.

of an insulin pump, while minimizing the risk of hypoglycemia by frequent blood glucose monitoring. ACEI therapy should be initiated in normotensive and hypertensive type 1 or type 2 diabetic patients with persistent microalbuminuria (30 to 300 mg/day) or overt albuminuria (>300 mg/day). ACEIs should be titrated every 1 to 3 months to achieve a maximal reduction in urinary albumin excretion. Within 1 week of initiating or increasing the dose of an ACEI, serum creatinine and potassium should be evaluated to detect abrupt reductions in GFR or development of hyperkalemia. ARBs should be considered as another first-line therapy in type 2 diabetic patients for the reduction of persistent proteinuria or albuminuria. A nondihydropyridine CCB may be an effective secondary alternative agent in patients who are unable to tolerate either an ACEI or an ARB. Preliminary data suggest that the combination of an ACEI with an ARB may result in a greater reduction in proteinuria or albuminuria than either agent alone, and thus may be a therapeutic alternative in patients who are not maximally responding to single-agent therapy.

NONDIABETIC PATIENTS

Figure 43–10 summarizes therapeutic interventions for nondiabetic patients with CKD. Nutritional management should be monitored frequently, regardless of the amount of protein intake prescribed, to avoid malnutrition. Based on the results of the MDRD study, a low-protein diet is of variable benefit in patients with moderate kidney dysfunction (GFR 25 to 55 mL/min per 1.73 m²). Therefore it is probably reasonable to prescribe a standard protein diet unless the patient develops rapid progression of their kidney disease.[165] For patients with moderate kidney dysfunction, as defined by the MDRD study as a GFR of 13 to 24 mL/min per 1.73 m², a low-protein diet of 0.6 g/kg per day may reduce the rate of decline in kidney function, time to reach ESKD, and onset of uremic symptoms.[100]

Blood pressure control should target normotensive levels (<130/80 mm Hg in nonproteinuric patients and <125/75 in proteinuric patients).[166] In patients with proteinuria above 3 g/day and CKD, an ACEI or ARB should be considered as first-line therapy. Hyperlipidemia should also be managed due to some studies that have associated lipid abnormalities with CKD progression.

As renal function approaches Stage 4 and the progression-limiting strategies have been or are all being applied, the patient should begin to get prepared for the eventuality of renal replacement therapy. Hemodialysis, peritoneal dialysis, and renal transplantation options need to be discussed (see Chaps. 45 and 87). Early referral to a nephrologist or other clinician specializing in the care of patients with progressive CKD may allow the proper dialysis access to be placed, dialysis to be initiated before adverse effects of uremia develop, and may also enable the identification and treatment of the complications of anemia and of calcium and phosphorus abnormalities.[167]

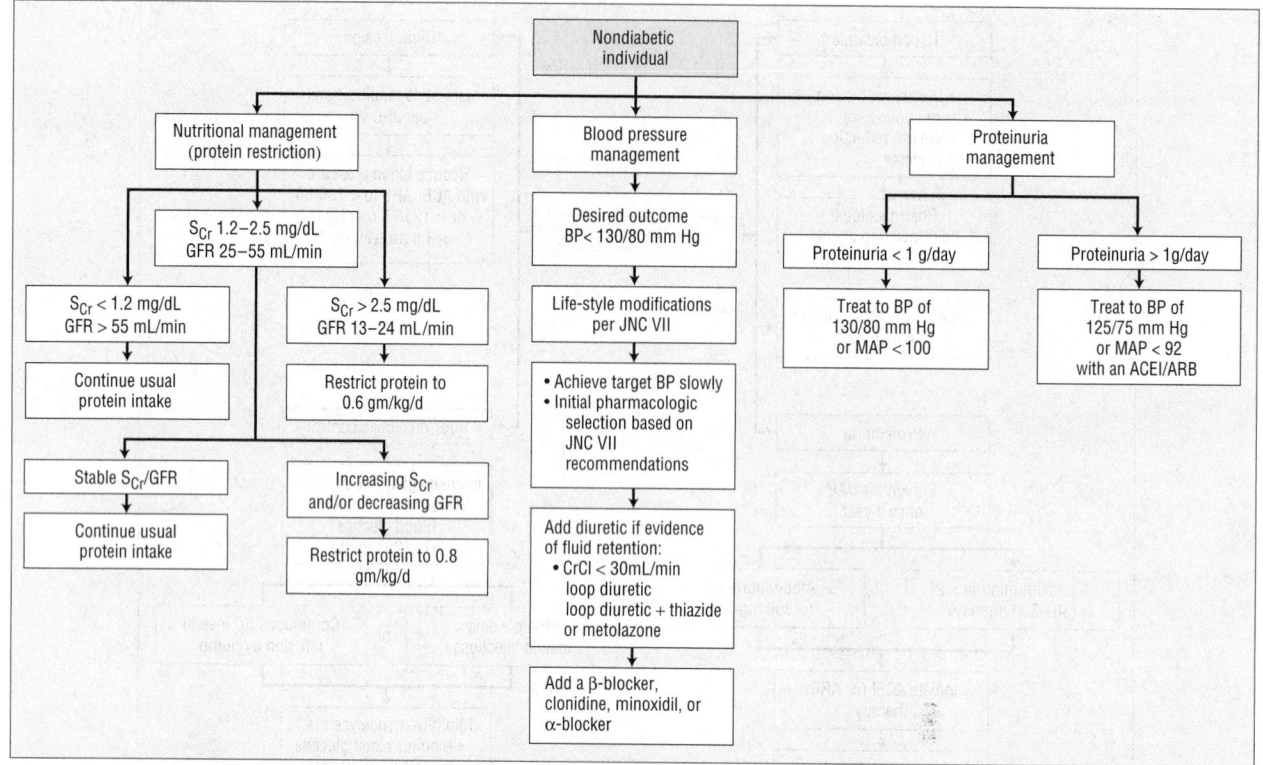

FIGURE 43–10. Therapeutic strategies to prevent progression of renal disease in nondiabetic individuals. BP = blood pressure; S_{Cr} = serum creatinine.

ABBREVIATIONS

ACEI: angiotensin-converting enzyme inhibitor
ARB: angiotensin receptor blocker
ARF: acute renal failure
CCB: calcium channel blocker
CHF: congestive heart failure
CKD: chronic kidney disease
CRI: chronic renal insufficiency
DCCT: Diabetes Control and Complications Trial
ESKD: end-stage kidney disease
ESRD: end-stage renal disease
GFR: glomerular filtration rate
HMG-CoA: 3-hydroxy-3-methylglutaryl coenzyme A (reductase)
IIT: intensive insulin therapy
K/DOQI: Kidney Dialysis Outcomes and Quality Initiative
MAP: mean arterial blood pressure
MDRD: Modification of Diet in Renal Disease
MRFIT: Multiple Risk Factor Intervention Trial
NHANES III: Third National Health and Nutritional Examination Survey
RANTES: regulated upon activation, normal T-cell expressed and secreted
USRDS: United States Renal Data Service

Review Questions and other resources can be found at *www.pharmacotherapyonline.com.*

REFERENCES

1. National Kidney Foundation. K/DOQI clinical practice guidelines for chronic kidney disease: evaluation, classification, and stratification. Kidney Disease Outcome Quality Initiative. Am J Kidney Dis 2002;39(2 Suppl 2):S1–266.
2. U.S. Renal Data System 2003 Annual Data Report. Bethesda, MD, National Institutes of Health, National Institute of Diabetes and Digestive and Kidney Disease, 2003.
3. http://www.niddk.nih.gov/fund/divisions/kuh/kdcsi/halt-pkd.pdf. Accessed on December 5, 2003.
4. Gassman JJ, Greene T, Wright JT Jr., et al. Design and statistical aspects of the African American Study of Kidney Disease and Hypertension (AASK). J Am Soc Nephrol 2003;14(7 Suppl 2):S154–165.
5. Feldman HI, Appel LJ, Chertow GM, et al. The Chronic Renal Insufficiency Cohort (CRIC) Study: Design and Methods. J Am Soc Nephrol 2003;14(7 Suppl 2):S148–153.
6. Ohmit SE, Flack JM, Peters RM, et al. Longitudinal study of the National Kidney Foundation's (NKF) Kidney Early Evaluation Program (KEEP). J Am Soc Nephrol 2003;14(7 Suppl 2): S117–121.
7. U.S. Department of Health and Human Services, Healthy People 2010. U.S. Government Printing Office, 2000.
8. Pereira BJ. Introduction: new perspectives in chronic renal insufficiency. Am J Kidney Dis 2000;36(6 Suppl 3):S1–3.
9. Levey AS, Coresh J, Balk E, et al. National Kidney Foundation practice guidelines for chronic kidney disease: evaluation, classification, and stratification. Ann Intern Med 2003;139:137–147.
10. Jones CA, McQuillan GM, Kusek JW, et al. Serum creatinine levels in the US population: third National Health and Nutrition Examination Survey. Am J Kidney Dis 1998;32:992–999.
11. Culleton BF, Larson MG, Evans JC, et al. Prevalence and correlates of elevated serum creatinine levels: the Framingham Heart Study. Arch Intern Med 1999;159:1785–1790.
12. Nissenson AR, Pereira BJ, Collins AJ, Steinberg EP. Prevalence and characteristics of individuals with chronic kidney disease in a large health maintenance organization. Am J Kidney Dis 2001;37:1177–1183.
13. Rettig RA. The social contract and the treatment of permanent kidney failure. JAMA 1996;275:1123–1126.
14. U.S. Renal Data System (USRDS). USRDS 2001 Annual Data Report.

Bethesda, MD, National Institutes of Health, National Institute of Diabetes and Digestive and Kidney Disease, 2001.

15. McClellan WM, Flanders WD. Risk factors for progressive chronic kidney disease. J Am Soc Nephrol 2003;14(7 Suppl 2):S65–70.

16. Davies SN. Age changes in glomerular filtration rate, effective renal plasma flow, and tubular excretory capacity in adult males. J Clin Invest 1950;29:496–507.

17. Lindeman RD, Tobin J, Shock NW. Longitudinal studies on the rate of decline in renal function with age. J Am Geriatr Soc 1985;33:278–285.

18. Rowe JW, Andres R, Tobin JD, et al. The effect of age on creatinine clearance in men: a cross-sectional and longitudinal study. J Gerontol 1976;31:155–163.

19. Byrne C, Nedelman J, Luke RG. Race, socioeconomic status, and the development of end-stage renal disease. Am J Kidney Dis 1994;23:16–22.

20. Perneger TV, Whelton PK, Klag MJ. Race and end-stage renal disease. Socioeconomic status and access to health care as mediating factors. Arch Intern Med 1995;155):1201–1208.

21. Tierney WM, Harris LE, Copley JB, Luft FC. Effect of hypertension and type II diabetes on renal function in an urban population. Am J Hypertens 1990;3:69–75.

22. Rostand SG. US minority groups and end-stage renal disease: a disproportionate share. Am J Kidney Dis 1992;19:411–413.

23. Perry HM Jr., Miller JP, Fornoff JR, et al. Early predictors of 15-year end-stage renal disease in hypertensive patients. Hypertension 1995;25(4 Pt 1):587–594.

24. Lackland DT, Bendall HE, Osmond C, et al. Low birth weights contribute to high rates of early-onset chronic renal failure in the Southeastern United States. Arch Intern Med 2000;160:1472–1476.

25. Freedman BI, Bowden DW, Rich SS, Appel RG. Genetic initiation of hypertensive and diabetic nephropathy. Am J Hypertens 1998;11:251–257.

26. The Family Investigation of Nephropathy and Diabetes (FIND) Research Group. Genetic determinants of diabetic nephropathy: The family investigation of nephropathy and diabetes (FIND). J Am Soc Nephrol 2003;14(7 Suppl 2):S202–204.

27. Kshirsagar AV, Elter J, Beck J, et al. Periodontal disease is associated with moderate renal insufficiency in a general population sample. J Am Soc Nephrol 2001;12:218 (Abstract).

28. Erlinger TP, Tarver-Carr ME, Powe NR, et al. Leukocytosis, hypoalbuminemia, and the risk for chronic kidney disease in US adults. Am J Kidney Dis 2003;42:256–263.

29. Muntner P, Coresh J, Smith J, et al. Plasma lipids and risk of developing renal dysfunction: the atherosclerosis risk in communities study. Kidney Int 2000;58:293–301.

30. Schaeffner ES, Kurth T, Curhan GC, et al. Cholesterol and the risk of renal dysfunction in apparently healthy men. J Am Soc Nephrol 2003;14:2084–2091.

31. Favre L, Glasson P, Vallotton MB. Reversible acute renal failure from combined triamterene and indomethacin: a study in healthy subjects. Ann Intern Med 1982;96:317–320.

32. Hasslacher C, Ritz E, Wahl P, Michael C. Similar risks of nephropathy in patients with type I or type II diabetes mellitus. Nephrol Dial Transplant 1989;4:859–863.

33. Ritz E, Orth SR. Nephropathy in patients with type 2 diabetes mellitus. N Engl J Med 1999;341:1127–1133.

34. Brancati FL, Whelton PK, Randall BL, et al. Risk of end-stage renal disease in diabetes mellitus: a prospective cohort study of men screened for MRFIT. Multiple Risk Factor Intervention Trial. JAMA 1997;278:2069–2074.

35. Cowley AW Jr, Roman RJ. The role of the kidney in hypertension. JAMA 1996;275:1581–1589.

36. Guyton AC, Coleman TG, Cowley AV Jr., et al. Arterial pressure regulation. Overriding dominance of the kidneys in long-term regulation and in hypertension. Am J Med 1972;52:584–594.

37. Goldblatt H, Hanzal RF, Summerville WW. Studies on experimental hypertension. 1. The production of persistent elevation of systolic blood pressure by means of renal ischemia. J Exp Med 1934;59:347–379.

38. Coresh J, Wei GL, McQuillan G, et al. Prevalence of high blood pressure and elevated serum creatinine level in the United States: findings from the third National Health and Nutrition Examination Survey (1988–1994). Arch Intern Med 2001;161:1207–1216.

39. Perneger TV, Nieto FJ, Whelton PK, et al. A prospective study of blood pressure and serum creatinine. Results from the 'Clue' Study and the ARIC Study. JAMA 1993;269:488–493.

40. Klag MJ, Whelton PK, Randall BL, et al. Blood pressure and end-stage renal disease in men. N Engl J Med 1996;334:13–18.

41. Rekola S, Bergstrand A, Bucht H. Deterioration of GFR in IgA nephropathy as measured by 51Cr-EDTA clearance. Kidney Int 1991;40:1050–1054.

42. Pei Y, Cattran D, Greenwood C. Predicting chronic renal insufficiency in idiopathic membranous glomerulonephritis. Kidney Int 1992;42:960–966.

43. Hannedouche T, Chauveau P, Kalou F, et al. Factors affecting progression in advanced chronic renal failure. Clin Nephrol 1993;39:312–320.

44. Massy Z, Khoa T, Lacour B, et al. Dyslipidemia and the progression of renal disease in chronic renal failure patients. Nephrol Dial Transplant 1999;14:2392–2397.

45. Viberti G, Hill R, Jarrett RJ, et al. Microalbuminuria as a predictor of clinical nephropathy in insulin-dependent diabetes mellitus. Lancet 1982;1:1430–1432.

46. Mogensen C, Christensen CK. Predicting diabetic nephropathy in insulin-dependent patients. N Engl J Med 1984;311:89–93.

47. Wirta O, Pasternack A, Mustonen J, et al. Albumin excretion rate and its relation to kidney disease in non-insulin-dependent diabetes mellitus. J Intern Med 1995;237:367–373.

48. Keane WF, Brenner BM, De Zeeuw D, et al. The risk of developing end-stage renal disease in patients with type 2 diabetes and nephropathy: the RENAAL study. Kidney Int 2003;63:1499–1507.

49. Klahr S, Levey AS, Beck GJ, et al. The effects of dietary protein restriction and blood-pressure control on the progression of chronic renal disease. Modification of Diet in Renal Disease Study Group. N Engl J Med 1994;330:877–884.

50. Jafar TH, Stark PC, Schmid CH, et al. Proteinuria as a modifiable risk factor for the progression of non-diabetic renal disease. Kidney Int 2001;60:1131–1140.

51. The Atherosclerosis Risk in Communities (ARIC) Study: design and objectives. The ARIC investigators. Am J Epidemiol 1989;129:687–702.

52. Keane WF. Proteinuria: its clinical importance and role in progressive renal disease. Am J Kidney Dis 2000;35(4 Suppl 1):S97–105.

53. Jafar TH, Stark PC, Schmid CH, et al. Progression of chronic kidney disease: the role of blood pressure control, proteinuria, and angiotensin-converting enzyme inhibition: a patient-level meta-analysis. Ann Intern Med 2003;139:244–252.

54. Intensive blood-glucose control with sulphonylureas or insulin compared with conventional treatment and risk of complications in patients with type 2 diabetes (UKPDS 33). UK Prospective Diabetes Study (UKPDS) Group. Lancet 1998;352:837–853.

55. Effect of intensive blood-glucose control with metformin on complications in overweight patients with type 2 diabetes (UKPDS 34). UK Prospective Diabetes Study (UKPDS) Group. Lancet 1998;352:854–865.

56. Bakris GL. Treatment of stage I hypertension and development of renal dysfunction. J Hum Hypertens 2001;15:81–84.

57. Tight blood pressure control and risk of macrovascular and microvascular complications in type 2 diabetes: UKPDS 38. UK Prospective Diabetes Study Group. BMJ 1998;317:703–713.

58. Efficacy of atenolol and captopril in reducing risk of macrovascular and microvascular complications in type 2 diabetes: UKPDS 39. UK Prospective Diabetes Study Group. BMJ 1998;317:713–720.

59. Bakris GL. A practical approach to achieving recommended blood pressure goals in diabetic patients. Arch Intern Med 2001;161:2661–2667.

60. Reichard P, Nilsson BY, Rosenqvist U. The effect of long-term intensified insulin treatment on the development of microvascular complications of diabetes mellitus. N Engl J Med 1993;329:304–309.

61. The Diabetes Control and Complications Trial (DCCT) Research Group. The effect of intensive treatment of diabetes on the development and progression of long-term complications in insulin-dependent diabetes mellitus. N Engl J Med 1993;329:977–986.

62. Muhlhauser I, Bender R, Bott U, et al. Cigarette smoking and progression of retinopathy and nephropathy in type 1 diabetes. Diabet Med 1996;13:536–543.

63. Orth SR, Ritz E, Schrier RW. The renal risks of smoking. Kidney Int 1997;51:1669–1677.

64. Holl RW, Grabert M, Heinze E, Debatin KM. Objective assessment of smoking habits by urinary cotinine measurement in adolescents and young adults with type 1 diabetes. Reliability of reported cigarette consumption and relationship to urinary albumin excretion. Diabetes Care 1998;21:787–791.

65. Ritz E, Benck U, Franek E, et al. Effects of smoking on renal hemodynamics in healthy volunteers and in patients with glomerular disease. J Am Soc Nephrol 1998;9:1798–1804.

66. Sawicki PT, Didjurgeit U, Muhlhauser I, et al. Smoking is associated with progression of diabetic nephropathy. Diabetes Care 1994;17:126–131.

67. Regalado M, Yang S, Wesson DE. Cigarette smoking is associated with augmented progression of renal insufficiency in severe essential hypertension. Am J Kidney Dis 2000;35:687–694.

68. Bakris G, Rahman M, Lea J, et al. Associations between cardiovascular risk factors and glomerular filtration rate at baseline in the African American Study of Kidney Disease (AASK) trial. J Am Soc Nephrol 1998;10:A0717.

69. Whelton P K. The evolving epidemic of cardiovascular and renal diseases: a worldwide challenge. Curr Opin Nephrol Hypertens 1995;4:215–217.

70. Haroun MK, Jaar BG, Hoffman SC, et al. Risk factors for chronic kidney disease: a prospective study of 23,534 men and women in Washington county, Maryland. J Am Soc Nephrol 2003;14:2934–2941.

71. Goetz FC, Jacobs DR Jr., Chavers B, et al. Risk factors for kidney damage in the adult population of Wadena, Minnesota. A prospective study. Am J Epidemiol 1997;145:91–102.

72. Orth SR, Stockmann A, Conradt C, et al. Smoking as a risk factor for end-stage renal failure in men with primary renal disease. Kidney Int 1998;54:926–931.

73. Chapman AB, Johnson AM, Gabow PA, Schrier RW. Overt proteinuria and microalbuminuria in autosomal dominant polycystic kidney disease. J Am Soc Nephrol 1994;5:1349–1354.

74. Mackenzie HS, Brenner BM. Current strategies for retarding progression of renal disease. Am J Kidney Dis 1998;31:161–170.

75. Walker WG. Relation of lipid abnormalities to progression of renal damage in essential hypertension, insulin-dependent and non insulin-dependent diabetes mellitus. Miner Electrolyte Metab 1993;19:137–143.

76. Kasiske BL. Hyperlipidemia in patients with chronic renal disease. Am J Kidney Dis 1998;32(5 Suppl 3):S142–156.

77. Remuzzi G, Bertani T. Pathophysiology of progressive nephropathies. N Engl J Med 1998;339:1448–1456.

78. Remuzzi G, Ruggenenti P, Perico N. Chronic renal diseases: renoprotective benefits of renin-angiotensin system inhibition. Ann Intern Med 2002;136:604–615.

79. Platt R. Structural and functional adaptation in renal failure. Br Med J 1952;1:1372–1377.

80. Hostetter TH, Olson JL, Rennke HG, et al. Hyperfiltration in remnant nephrons: a potentially adverse response to renal ablation. Am J Physiol 1981;241:F85–93.

81. Brenner BM, Meyer TW, Hostetter TH. Dietary protein intake and the progressive nature of kidney disease: the role of hemodynamically mediated glomerular injury in the pathogenesis of progressive glomerular sclerosis in aging, renal ablation, and intrinsic renal disease. N Engl J Med 1982;307:652–659.

82. Yoshioka T, Mitarai T, Kon V, et al. Role for angiotensin II in an overt functional proteinuria. Kidney Int 1986;30:538–545.

83. Yoshioka T, Rennke HG, Salant DJ, et al. Role of abnormally high transmural pressure in the permselectivity defect of glomerular capillary wall: a study in early passive Heymann nephritis. Circ Res 1987;61:531–538.

84. Park CH, Maack T. Albumin absorption and catabolism by isolated perfused proximal convoluted tubules of the rabbit. J Clin Invest 1984;73:767–777.

85. Zoja C, Morigi M, Figliuzzi M, et al. Proximal tubular cell synthesis and secretion of endothelin-1 on challenge with albumin and other proteins. Am J Kidney Dis 1995;26:934–941.

86. Wang Y, Chen J, Chen L, et al. Induction of monocyte chemoattractant protein-1 in proximal tubule cells by urinary protein. J Am Soc Nephrol 1997;8:1537–1545.

87. Zoja C, Donadelli R, Colleoni S, et al. Protein overload stimulates RANTES production by proximal tubular cells depending on NF-kappa B activation. Kidney Int 1998;53:1608–1615.

88. Morita Y, Nomura A, Yuzawa Y, et al. The role of complement in the pathogenesis of tubulointerstitial lesions in rat mesangial proliferative glomerulonephritis. J Am Soc Nephrol 1997;8:1363–1372.

89. Nangaku M, Pippin J, Couser WG. Complement membrane attack complex (C5b-9) mediates interstitial disease in experimental nephrotic syndrome. J Am Soc Nephrol 1999;10:2323–2331.

90. Morita Y, Ikeguchi H, Nakamura J, et al. Complement activation products in the urine from proteinuric patients. J Am Soc Nephrol 2000;11:700–707.

91. Nath KA, Hostetter MK, Hostetter TH. Pathophysiology of chronic tubulo-interstitial disease in rats. Interactions of dietary acid load, ammonia, and complement component C3. J Clin Invest 1985;76:667–675.

92. Hsu CY, McCulloch CE, Curhan GC. Epidemiology of anemia associated with chronic renal insufficiency among adults in the United States: results from the Third National Health and Nutrition Examination Survey. J Am Soc Nephrol 2002;13:504–510.

93. IV. NKF-K/DOQI Clinical Practice Guidelines for Anemia of Chronic Kidney Disease: update 2000. Am J Kidney Dis 2001;37(1 Suppl 1): S182–238.

94. Jungers P, Choukroun G, Oualim Z, et al. Beneficial influence of recombinant human erythropoietin therapy on the rate of progression of chronic renal failure in predialysis patients. Nephrol Dial Transplant 2001;16:307–312.

95. Obrador GT, Ruthazer R, Arora P, et al. Prevalence of and factors associated with suboptimal care before initiation of dialysis in the United States. J Am Soc Nephrol 1999;10:1793–1800.

96. Martinez I, Saracho R, Montenegro J, Llach F. The importance of dietary calcium and phosphorus in the secondary hyperparathyroidism of patients with early renal failure. Am J Kidney Dis 1997;29:496–502.

97. National Kidney Foundation. K/DOQI clinical practice guidelines for bone metabolism and disease in chronic kidney disease. Am J Kidney Dis 2003;42(Suppl 3):S1–S202.

98. Kopple JD. National Kidney Foundation K/DOQI clinical practice guidelines for nutrition in chronic renal failure. Am J Kidney Dis 2001;37(1 Suppl 2):S66–70.

99. Brenner BM. Hemodynamically mediated glomerular injury and the progressive nature of kidney disease. Kidney Int 1983;23:647–655.

100. Levey AS, Adler S, Caggiula AW, et al. Effects of dietary protein restriction on the progression of advanced renal disease in the Modification of Diet in Renal Disease Study. Am J Kidney Dis 1996;27:652–663.

101. Pedrini MT, Levey AS, Lau J, et al. The effect of dietary protein restriction on the progression of diabetic and nondiabetic renal diseases: a meta-analysis. Ann Intern Med 1996;124:627–632.

102. Kasiske BL, Lakatua JD, Ma JZ, Louis TA. A meta-analysis of the effects of dietary protein restriction on the rate of decline in renal function. Am J Kidney Dis 1998;31:954–961.

103. Pijls LT, De Vries H, Van Eijk JT, Donker AJ. Protein restriction, glomerular filtration rate and albuminuria in patients with type 2 diabetes mellitus: a randomized trial. Eur J Clin Nutr 2002;56:1200–1207.

104. Gautier JF, Beressi JP, Leblanc H, et al. Are the implications of the Diabetes Control and Complications Trial (DCCT) feasible in daily clinical practice? Diabetes Metab 1996;22:415–419.

105. Wang PH, Lau J, Chalmers TC. Meta-analysis of effects of intensive blood-glucose control on late complications of type I diabetes. Lancet 1993;341:1306–1309.

106. Retinopathy and nephropathy in patients with type 1 diabetes four years

after a trial of intensive therapy. The Diabetes Control and Complications Trial/Epidemiology of Diabetes Interventions and Complications Research Group. N Engl J Med 2000;342:381–389.

107. Chobanian AV, Bakris GL, Black HR, et al. Seventh report of the Joint National Committee on Prevention, Detection, Evaluation, and Treatment of High Blood Pressure. Hypertension 2003;42:1206–1252.

108. Lewis JB, Berl T, Bain RP, et al. Effect of intensive blood pressure control on the course of type 1 diabetic nephropathy. Collaborative Study Group. Am J Kidney Dis 1999;34:809–817.

109. Bakris GL, Williams M, Dworkin L, et al. Preserving renal function in adults with hypertension and diabetes: a consensus approach. National Kidney Foundation Hypertension and Diabetes Executive Committees Working Group. Am J Kidney Dis 2000;36:646–661.

110. Parving HH. Impact of blood pressure and antihypertensive treatment on incipient and overt nephropathy, retinopathy, and endothelial permeability in diabetes mellitus. Diabetes Care 1991;14:260–269.

111. Dworkin LD, Benstein JA, Parker M, et al. Calcium antagonists and converting enzyme inhibitors reduce renal injury by different mechanisms. Kidney Int 1993;43:808–814.

112. Kasiske BL, Kalil RS, Ma JZ, et al. Effect of antihypertensive therapy on the kidney in patients with diabetes: a meta-regression analysis. Ann Intern Med 1993;118:129–138.

113. Schlueter WA, Batlle DC. Renal effects of antihypertensive drugs. Drugs 1989;37:900–925.

114. Risler T, Kramer B, Muller GA. The efficacy of diuretics in acute and chronic renal failure. Focus on torasemide. Drugs 1991;41(Suppl 3):69–79.

115. Lewis EJ, Hunsicker LG, Bain RP, Rohde RD. The effect of angiotensin-converting-enzyme inhibition on diabetic nephropathy. The Collaborative Study Group. N Engl J Med 1993;329:1456–1462.

116. Ahmad J, Siddiqui MA, Ahmad H. Effective postponement of diabetic nephropathy with enalapril in normotensive type 2 diabetic patients with microalbuminuria. Diabetes Care 1997;20:1576–1581.

117. Ravid M, Brosh D, Levi Z, et al. Use of enalapril to attenuate decline in renal function in normotensive, normoalbuminuric patients with type 2 diabetes mellitus. A randomized, controlled trial. Ann Intern Med 1998;128(12 Pt 1):982–988.

118. Randomised placebo-controlled trial of lisinopril in normotensive patients with insulin-dependent diabetes and normoalbuminuria or microalbuminuria. The EUCLID Study Group. Lancet 1997;349:1787–1792.

119. Effects of ramipril on cardiovascular and microvascular outcomes in people with diabetes mellitus: results of the HOPE study and MICRO-HOPE substudy. Heart Outcomes Prevention Evaluation Study Investigators. Lancet 2000;355:253–259.

120. Laffel LM, McGill JB, Gans DJ. The beneficial effect of angiotensin-converting enzyme inhibition with captopril on diabetic nephropathy in normotensive IDDM patients with microalbuminuria. North American Microalbuminuria Study Group. Am J Med 1995;99:497–504.

121. Lebovitz HE, Wiegmann TB, Cnaan A, et al. Renal protective effects of enalapril in hypertensive NIDDM: role of baseline albuminuria. *Kidney Int Suppl* 1994;45:S150–155.

122. Kshirsagar AV, Joy MS, Hogan SL, et al. Effect of ACE inhibitors in diabetic and nondiabetic chronic renal disease: a systematic overview of randomized placebo-controlled trials. Am J Kidney Dis 2000;35:695–707.

123. Lewis EJ, Hunsicker LG, Clarke WR, et al. Renoprotective effect of the angiotensin-receptor antagonist irbesartan in patients with nephropathy due to type 2 diabetes. N Engl J Med 2001;345:851–860.

124. Parving HH, Lehnert H, Brochner-Mortensen J, et al. The effect of irbesartan on the development of diabetic nephropathy in patients with type 2 diabetes. N Engl J Med 2001;345:870–878.

125. Brenner BM, Cooper ME, De Zeeuw D, et al. Effects of losartan on renal and cardiovascular outcomes in patients with type 2 diabetes and nephropathy. N Engl J Med 2001;345:861–869.

126. Sasso FC, Carbonara O, Persico M, et al. Irbesartan reduces the albumin excretion rate in microalbuminuric type 2 diabetic patients independently of hypertension: a randomized double-blind placebo-controlled crossover study. Diabetes Care 2002;25:1909–1913.

127. Pitt B, Segal R, Martinez FA, et al. Randomised trial of losartan versus captopril in patients over 65 with heart failure (Evaluation of Losartan in the Elderly Study, ELITE). Lancet 1997;349:747–752.

128. Hostetter TH. Prevention of end-stage renal disease due to type 2 diabetes. N Engl J Med 2001;345:910–912.

129. Mogensen CE, Neldam S, Tikkanen I, et al. Randomised controlled trial of dual blockade of renin-angiotensin system in patients with hypertension, microalbuminuria, and non-insulin dependent diabetes: the candesartan and lisinopril microalbuminuria (CALM) study. BMJ 2000;321:1440–1444.

130. Maki DD, Ma JZ, Louis TA, Kasiske BL. Long-term effects of antihypertensive agents on proteinuria and renal function. Arch Intern Med 1995;155:1073–1080.

131. Weidmann P, Schneider M, Bohlen L. Therapeutic efficacy of different antihypertensive drugs in human diabetic nephropathy: an updated meta-analysis. Nephrol Dial Transplant 1995;10(Suppl 9):39–45.

132. Bakris GL, Copley JB, Vicknair N, et al. Calcium channel blockers versus other antihypertensive therapies on progression of NIDDM associated nephropathy. Kidney Int 1996;50:1641–1650.

133. Epstein M. Effects of ACE inhibitors and calcium antagonists on progression of chronic renal disease. *Blood Press Suppl* 1995;2:108–112.

134. Fouque D, Laville M, Boissel JP, et al. Controlled low protein diets in chronic renal insufficiency: meta-analysis. BMJ 1992;304:216–220.

135. Apperloo AJ, De Zeeuw D, De Jong PE. A short-term antihypertensive treatment-induced fall in glomerular filtration rate predicts long-term stability of renal function. Kidney Int 1997;51:793–797.

136. Maschio G, Alberti D, Janin G, et al. Effect of the angiotensin-converting-enzyme inhibitor benazepril on the progression of chronic renal insufficiency. The Angiotensin-Converting-Enzyme Inhibition in Progressive Renal Insufficiency Study Group. N Engl J Med 1996;334:939–945.

137. Randomised placebo-controlled trial of effect of ramipril on decline in glomerular filtration rate and risk of terminal renal failure in proteinuric, non-diabetic nephropathy. The GISEN Group (Gruppo Italiano di Studi Epidemiologici in Nefrologia). Lancet 1997;349:1857–1863.

138. Nielsen S, Dollerup J, Nielsen B, et al. Losartan reduces albuminuria in patients with essential hypertension. An enalapril controlled 3 months study. Nephrol Dial Transplant 1997;12(Suppl 2):19–23.

139. Praga M, Gutierrez E, Gonzalez E, et al. Treatment of IgA nephropathy with ACE inhibitors: a randomized and controlled trial. J Am Soc Nephrol 2003;14:1578–1583.

140. Ruggenenti P, Perna A, Gherardi G, et al. Renoprotective properties of ACE-inhibition in non-diabetic nephropathies with non-nephrotic proteinuria. Lancet 1999;354:359–364.

141. Sica DA, Gehr TW. The pharmacokinetics of angiotensin-converting enzyme inhibitors in end-stage renal disease. Semin Dialysis 1994;7:205–213.

142. Usta M, Ersoy A, Dilek K, et al. Efficacy of losartan in patients with primary focal segmental glomerulosclerosis resistant to immunosuppressive treatment. J Intern Med 2003;253:329–334.

143. Tylicki L, Rutkowski P, Renke M, Rutkowski B. Renoprotective effect of small doses of losartan and enalapril in patients with primary glomerulonephritis. Short-term observation. Am J Nephrol 2002;22:356–362.

144. Ruilope LM. Is it wise to combine an ACE inhibitor and an angiotensin receptor antagonist? Nephrol Dial Transplant 1999;14:2855–2856.

145. Nakao N, Yoshimura A, Morita H, et al. Combination treatment of angiotensin-II receptor blocker and angiotensin-converting-enzyme inhibitor in non-diabetic renal disease (COOPERATE): a randomised controlled trial. Lancet 2003;361:117–124.

146. Tarif N, Bakris GL. Preservation of renal function: the spectrum of effects by calcium-channel blockers. Nephrol Dial Transplant 1997;12:2244–2250.

147. Massy ZA, Ma JZ, Louis TA, Kasiske BL. Lipid-lowering therapy in patients with renal disease. Kidney Int 1995;48:188–198.

148. Executive Summary of The Third Report of The National Cholesterol Education Program (NCEP) Expert Panel on Detection, Evaluation, And Treatment of High Blood Cholesterol In Adults (Adult Treatment Panel III). JAMA 2001;285:2486–2497.

149. National Kidney Foundation. K/DOQI clinical practice guidelines for managing dyslipidemias in chronic kidney disease. Am J Kidney Dis 2003;41:S1–S92.

150. Fried LF, Orchard TJ, Kasiske BL. Effect of lipid reduction on the progression of renal disease: a meta-analysis. Kidney Int 2001;59:260–269.

151. Oda H, Keane WF. Recent advances in statins and the kidney. Kidney Int Suppl 1999;71:S2–5.

152. Halimi JM, Mimran A. Renal effects of smoking: potential mechanisms and perspectives. Nephrol Dial Transplant 2000;15:938–940.

153. Pinto-Sietsma SJ, Mulder J, Janssen WM, et al. Smoking is related to albuminuria and abnormal renal function in nondiabetic persons. Ann Intern Med 2000;133:585–591.

154. Collins AJ. Anaemia management prior to dialysis: cardiovascular and cost-benefit observations. Nephrol Dial Transplant 2003;18(Suppl 2):ii2–6.

155. Silverberg D, Wexler D, Blum M, et al. The cardio-renal anaemia syndrome: does it exist? Nephrol Dial Transplant 2003;18(Suppl 8):viii7–12.

156. Silverberg DS, Wexler D, Blum M, et al. The correction of anemia in severe resistant heart failure with erythropoietin and intravenous iron prevents the progression of both the heart and the renal failure and markedly reduces hospitalization. Clin Nephrol 2002;58(Suppl 1):S37–45.

157. Silverberg DS, Wexler D, Blum M, et al. Effect of correction of anemia with erythropoietin and intravenous iron in resistant heart failure in octogenarians. Isr Med Assoc J 2003;5:337–339.

158. Becker BN, Becker YT, Leverson GE, Heisey DM. Erythropoietin therapy may retard progression in chronic renal transplant dysfunction. Nephrol Dial Transplant 2002;17:1667–1673.

159. Deicher R, Horl WH. Anaemia as a risk factor for the progression of chronic kidney disease. Curr Opin Nephrol Hypertens 2003;12:139–143.

160. Siegel JE, Krolewski AS, Warram JH, Weinstein MC. Cost-effectiveness of screening and early treatment of nephropathy in patients with insulin-dependent diabetes mellitus. J Am Soc Nephrol 1992;3(4 Suppl):S111–119.

161. Kiberd BA, Jindal KK. Routine treatment of insulin-dependent diabetic patients with ACE inhibitors to prevent renal failure: an economic evaluation. Am J Kidney Dis 1998;31:49–54.

162. Lifetime benefits and costs of intensive therapy as practiced in the diabetes control and complications trial. The Diabetes Control and Complications Trial Research Group. JAMA 1996;276:1409–1415.

163. Cost effectiveness analysis of improved blood pressure control in hypertensive patients with type 2 diabetes: UKPDS 40. UK Prospective Diabetes Study Group. BMJ 1998;317:720–726.

164. Golan L, Birkmeyer JD, Welch HG. The cost-effectiveness of treating all patients with type 2 diabetes with angiotensin-converting enzyme inhibitors. Ann Intern Med 1999;131:660–667.

165. Jacobson HR, Striker GE. Report on a workshop to develop management recommendations for the prevention of progression in chronic renal disease. Am J Kidney Dis 1995;25:103–106.

166. The sixth report of the Joint National Committee on prevention, detection, evaluation, and treatment of high blood pressure. Arch Intern Med 1997;157:2413–2446.

167. Eknoyan G, Levin N. NKF-K/DOQI Clinical Practice Guidelines: Update 2000. Foreword. Am J Kidney Dis 2001;37(1 Suppl):S5–6.

168. Fabre J, Balant LP, Dayer PG, et al. The kidney in maturity onset diabetes mellitus: a clinical study of 510 patients. Kidney Int 1982;21:730–738.

169. Gabow PA, Johnson AM, Kaehny WD, et al. Factors affecting the progression of renal disease in autosomal-dominant polycystic kidney disease. Kidney Int 1992;41:1311–1319.

170. McLaughlin JK, Lipworth L, Chow WH, Blot WJ. Analgesic use and chronic renal failure: a critical review of the epidemiologic literature. Kidney Int 1998;54:679–686.

171. Walsh TJ, Finberg RW, Arndt C, et al. Liposomal amphotericin B for empirical therapy in patients with persistent fever and neutropenia. National Institute of Allergy and Infectious Diseases Mycoses Study Group. N Engl J Med 1999;340:764–771.

44

CHRONIC KIDNEY DISEASE: THERAPEUTIC APPROACH FOR THE MANAGEMENT OF COMPLICATIONS

Joanna Q. Hudson and Kunal Chaudhary

Learning Objectives and other resources can be found at *www.pharmacotherapyonline.com.*

KEY CONCEPTS

◀1 The number of patients with chronic kidney disease (CKD) is increasing, with a doubling in the number of patients with Stage 5 CKD expected by 2010.

◀2 Common complications of Stages 3 to 5 CKD include anemia, hyperphosphatemia, secondary hyperparathyroidism, fluid and electrolyte abnormalities, metabolic acidosis, and malnutrition.

◀3 Cardiovascular complications are prevalent in the chronic kidney disease population and are the leading cause of mortality in patients with Stage 5 disease.

◀4 The management of CKD and the associated secondary complications should be initiated in patients with Stages 1 through 4 CKD, prior to development of end-stage renal disease (Stage 5 CKD).

◀5 Guidelines by the National Kidney Foundation-Kidney Disease Outcomes Quality Initiative (NKF-K/DOQI) should be used as a basis for the work-up of chronic kidney disease and the design of appropriate therapy for associated complications.

◀6 Patient education plays a critical role in the appropriate management of CKD and related complications. A multi-

disciplinary team structure is a rational approach to provide this education and effectively design and implement the extensive nonpharmacologic and pharmacologic interventions required.

◀7 Anemia is the most common complication of CKD and can lead to cardiovascular disease. It is primarily due to a deficiency in the production of endogenous erythropoietin by the kidney.

◀8 Management of anemia includes administration of erythropoietic agents (epoetin alfa and darbepoetin alfa) and regular iron supplementation (oral and/or intravenous administration) to achieve a target hemoglobin of 11 to 12 g/dL and a hematocrit of 33% to 36%, and to potentially prevent the development of left ventricular hypertrophy.

◀9 Hyperphosphatemia, changes in calcium homeostasis, and secondary hyperparathyroidism are common in patients with CKD and contribute to extravascular calcifications and an increased risk of cardiovascular mortality.

◀10 Management of hyperphosphatemia, calcium balance, and secondary hyperparathyroidism includes dietary phosphorus restriction, use of phosphate binding agents, and vitamin D therapy.

The clinical syndrome that develops insidiously as kidney function declines begins with nonspecific symptoms such as nausea and vomiting, which become progressively worse as the glomerular filtration rate (GFR) drops below 15 mL/min. It is at this stage that renal replacement therapy, either dialysis (see Chap. 45) or transplantation (see Chap. 87), is indicated to remove uremic toxins and to maintain hemodynamic stability. The patient with Stage 5 CKD requiring chronic dialysis or renal transplantation for relief of uremic symptoms is said to have end-stage renal disease (ESRD) or end-stage kidney disease (ESKD). Use of the term ESKD in this chapter will refer specifically to patients receiving chronic dialysis.

The staging system for CKD is designed to trigger implementation of appropriate interventions to delay progression of CKD, as discussed in the previous chapter, and to manage the complications

of CKD, which include anemia and secondary hyperparathyroidism, among others. Comorbidities such as cardiovascular disease are also common in patients with CKD and require early and aggressive intervention.[1] Many of these complications are unrecognized or are inappropriately managed, and for many patients may lead to premature mortality or a poor prognosis by the time they reach ESKD.[2,3] In this chapter we discuss the pathophysiology and pharmacotherapeutic management of the complications and comorbidities that are frequently seen in patients with Stages 3 through 5 CKD, with a particular focus on the ESKD population. Specifically, the etiology, epidemiology, clinical presentation, treatment, economic considerations, and monitoring parameters for anemia, secondary hyperparathyroidism, renal osteodystrophy, and metabolic acidosis are addressed in this chapter.

EPIDEMIOLOGY

◀ It is estimated that 19 million people in the United States have CKD, 8 million of whom have a GFR <60 mL/min per 1.73 m² (Stage 3, 4, or 5) based on data derived from the third National Health and Nutrition Examination Survey.[3-5] In 2001 a total of 96,295 new cases of ESKD were reported and the prevalence as of the end of 2001 was 406,081, including 292,215 patients on dialysis and 113,866 with a functioning kidney posttransplant.[3] Incidence rates are higher in blacks (fourfold higher), Native Americans (threefold higher), and Hispanics (twofold higher) compared to whites, a trend that has persisted over the last decade. Incidence rates have increased during this time period most notably in patients aged 65 and older. While the overall number of patients with ESKD is already substantial, it is projected that by the year 2010 the number will exceed 660,000, and by 2030 there will be 2.2 million patients with the disease: 1.3 million due to diabetes and 945,000 with other primary causes for their kidney disease.[3]

Compared to the general Medicare population, CKD patients in the earlier stages of the disease (i.e., Stages 1 through 4 CKD) have twice the risk of death.[3] These patients are also 5 to 10 times more likely to die primarily due to cardiovascular disease before they reach ESKD.[3] One of the most striking observations is the decreased prevalence between Stage 3 (7.6 million patients) and Stage 4 (400,000 patients) CKD.[5] While one would like to think that this decrease in prevalence is due to delaying the progression to Stage 4, the data indicate that this difference is due largely to the fact that many patients die before progressing to Stage 4 CKD. Dialysis patients have the highest risk of death, up to four times higher than comparable patients age 65 or older without kidney disease.[3] Associated predictors of mortality at the start of dialysis include a lower estimated GFR, decreased serum albumin, and the presence of comorbidities such as diabetes and cardiovascular disease.[2] Lower hemoglobin levels and body mass index are also associated with increased mortality, although there is some variation in the effect of body mass index according to race.

The incidence of treated ESKD is increasing worldwide; however, the United States has one of the highest incidence rates along with Japan and Taiwan when compared to other countries.[3] The United States also has one of the highest prevalence rates of treated ESKD and the highest percentage of ESKD patients with diabetes as the primary cause of their disease. Differences in rates of treated cases of ESKD among countries are dependent to a large extent on the economic conditions and health care delivery systems within each country.

ETIOLOGY

Many clinical conditions and diseases lead to progressive kidney damage and ESKD. A detailed discussion of the pathophysiology and management of progressive CKD is presented in Chap. 43. Diabetes mellitus continues to be the leading cause of CKD and ultimately ESKD in the United States.[3] The incidence rate of ESKD attributed to diabetes has doubled while the prevalence has more than tripled in the last 10 years. The incidence of diabetes as the primary cause of ESKD in the year 2001 was 43% in non-Hispanics, 64% in Mexican Hispanics, and 55% in Hispanics of other origin.[3] Diabetes is also a common primary and secondary cause of ESKD in Native Americans. Approximately 80% of Native Americans alive 1 year after diagnosis of ESKD had diabetes, classified as either a primary cause of ESKD or a comorbid condition.

Rates of ESKD due to hypertension, the second leading cause of ESKD in the United States, grew almost 50% in the last decade, with

incidence rates in the black population well above those of other racial groups.[3] Glomerulonephritis, the third leading cause of ESKD in the United States, includes a wide variety of glomerular lesions caused by immunologic, vascular, and other idiopathic diseases. While other diseases and conditions such as cystic kidney disease, IgA nephropathy, Wegener's granulomatosis, systemic lupus erythematosus, vascular diseases, and acquired immunodeficiency syndrome (AIDS) nephropathy account for fewer cases of ESKD compared to diabetes and hypertension, the number of patients developing ESKD secondary to these conditions has increased dramatically in the last decade.[3] The increase in the incidence of AIDS nephropathy was most dramatic between 1991 and 1995, but has since stabilized. While it is encouraging that the incidence has stabilized, it is concerning that the incidence has not dropped in parallel with the decline in incidence of opportunistic infections observed in this population since the introduction of antiretroviral therapy.

PATHOPHYSIOLOGY

Progression of CKD to ESKD occurs over months to years in the majority of cases with the precise mechanism of kidney damage dependent on the etiology of the disease (see Chap. 43). However, the consequences and complications of marked reductions in kidney function are fairly uniform irrespective of the etiology.

No single toxin is responsible for all of the signs and symptoms of uremia observed in patients with Stage 4 or 5 CKD (Table 44–1). Accumulation of these known and potential toxins may be the result of increased secretion of biologically active substances such as parathyroid hormone (PTH) and atrial natriuretic peptide, which are overproduced as part of the adaptation to the loss of renal mass; decreased clearance of endogenous substances normally metabolized by the kidney, such as PTH, gastrin, growth hormone, glucagon, somatostatin, prolactin, calcitonin, and insulin; and/or decreased clearance of metabolic by-products of protein metabolism. The clinical manifestations of a build-up of these uremic toxins ultimately result in altered organ, immune, and other bodily functions and lead to secondary complications.[6]

TABLE 44–1. Potential Uremic Toxins

Acetoin	Indoles
Acids	Indoxyl sulfate
Aliphatic amines	Insulin
α_2-Glycoprotein	Lipochromes
Amino acids	Lysozyme
Aromatic amines	Mannitol
β_1-Microglobulin	Methylguanidine
β_2-Microglobulin	Middle molecules
2,3 Butylene	Myoinositol
Calcitonin	Natriuretic hormone
Chemotaxis-inhibiting protein	Oxalic acid
Creatinine	Parathyroid hormone
Cyanate	P-cresol
Cyclic adenosine monophosphate	Phenols
Degranulation-inhibiting proteins	Potassium
Gastric inhibitory peptide	Prolactin
Gastrin	Pyridine derivatives
Glucagon	Renin
Glucuronic acid	Retinol-binding protein
Growth hormone	Ribonuclease
Granulocyte-inhibitory proteins	Urea
Guanidines	Uric acid
Hippuric acid	
Human pancreatic polypeptide	

Anemia of CKD, secondary hyperparathyroidism, altered fluid and electrolyte homeostasis, metabolic acidosis, and nutritional abnormalities are all associated with a substantial decline in GFR. Reduced production of erythropoietin by the progenitor cells of the kidney is the primary cause of anemia of CKD. The decline in hemoglobin is generally observed as GFR falls below 60 mL/min and becomes more severe as GFR decreases further.[7] Secondary hyperparathyroidism occurs in response to the metabolic abnormalities of CKD; hyperphosphatemia in conjunction with a decrease in conversion of vitamin D to its active form (calcitriol) within the kidney leads to hypocalcemia, the primary stimulus for release of PTH.[8] If inappropriately managed, secondary hyperparathyroidism can lead to "renal osteodystrophy." Management of these complications based on the patient's stage of CKD is discussed later in this chapter.

Fluid and electrolyte disorders and metabolic acidosis are primarily the result of altered transport mechanisms within the kidney and decreased elimination of solutes (see Chaps. 49, 50, and 51). Malnutrition may also occur as dietary changes such as phosphorus restriction are implemented. Foods high in phosphorus are generally also high in protein; therefore restriction of these protein sources contributes to malnutrition. Malnutrition may also develop due to decreased appetite in those with severe kidney disease. The likelihood of developing these secondary complications and comorbidities increases as GFR declines.

Patients with CKD are at increased risk of cardiovascular disease, independent of the etiology of their kidney disease. While a clearly unique pathogenesis of cardiovascular disease specific to CKD has not been identified, it is known that manifestations of kidney disease are contributory. Risk factors for cardiovascular disease in this population include hemodynamic and metabolic abnormalities, as well as hypertension, dyslipidemia, elevated homocysteine levels, anemia, hyperparathyroidism, malnutrition, and oxidative stress.[9] Hypertension induced by volume expansion and increased systemic vascular resistance increases myocardial work and contributes to development of left ventricular hypertrophy (LVH). Hyperlipidemia may enhance atherogenesis, while some uremic toxins can decrease myocardial contractility. In addition, uremic toxins can induce pericarditis, a potentially fatal complication. Currently, measures to screen this high-risk population for cardiovascular risk factors are not routine.[1,10]

While an understanding of the mechanisms of progression and measures to delay progression is essential and should be a focus of primary care clinicians, those who provide care for patients with Stage 4 and 5 CKD must also have a clear understanding of the pathogenesis and management strategies for secondary complications and comorbidities to improve the quality of care and patient outcomes.

CLINICAL PRESENTATION

Every major organ system is affected by CKD, particularly once patients develop ESKD. At the time of referral to a nephrologist patients may present with some, but rarely all, of the signs and symptoms associated with uremia and secondary complications of CKD, unless they are in the more advanced stages of the disease (Stage 4 or 5 CKD).

CLINICAL PRESENTATION OF CHRONIC KIDNEY DISEASE

Patient may appear healthy by observation alone. If in the later stages of CKD, signs and symptoms of uremia and secondary complications may be apparent.

SYMPTOMS

May present with uremic symptoms[a] (fatigue, weakness, shortness of breath, mental confusion, nausea and vomiting, bleeding, and loss of appetite), as well as itching, cold intolerance, weight gain, and peripheral neuropathies.

SIGNS

Edema, changes in urine output[a] (volume and consistency), "foaming" of urine (indicative of proteinuria), and abdominal distension.

LABORATORY TESTS

Increased serum creatinine, increased BUN, decreased creatinine clearance, hyperkalemia,[a] decreased bicarbonate (metabolic acidosis)[b], decreased hemoglobin/hematocrit (anemia),[b] low iron stores (iron deficiency),[b] elevated phosphorus,[b] abnormal calcium[b] (low in early stages of CKD; may be elevated in Stage 5 CKD), decreased vitamin D levels, elevated PTH,[b] decreased albumin (malnutrition),[b] blood pressure may be elevated (hypertension is a common cause and result of CKD), hyperglycemia (uncontrolled diabetes as a cause of CKD), hypoglycemia (from decreased degradation of insulin with impaired kidney function or poor oral intake), increased low-density lipoprotein and triglycerides, may be hemoccult-positive if GI bleeding occurs secondary to uremia, and hypothyroidism (increased T_4 levels).

OTHER DIAGNOSTIC TESTS

Left ventricular hypertrophy may be observed, as well as increased homocysteine levels and increased C-reactive protein.

[a]Most likely to be seen at more advanced stages of CKD (i.e., Stages 4 and 5).
[b]Common secondary complication of CKD.

The subjective and objective findings of CKD that may be present in an individual are dependent on the severity of disease (i.e., stage of CKD). It is also apparent that management of CKD will likely require the treatment of multiple secondary complications. Damage to the kidney thus has detrimental consequences on many other organ systems, which often go unrecognized or are inappropriately managed.

▶ TREATMENT: Chronic Kidney Disease

■ DESIRED OUTCOME

Once a patient is diagnosed with CKD, implementation of therapy to address the primary cause (e.g., diabetes, hypertension, or glomerulonephritis) and potentially delay progression is a priority (see Chap. 43). When patients reach Stage 4, progression to Stage 5 is almost inevitable, although the process may be slowed if appropriate therapy is initiated. It is during Stage 4 CKD that plans for renal replacement therapy (hemodialysis or peritoneal dialysis) need to be made, and patients educated on dialysis modalities and options for transplantation if they are good candidates.

◄4 Regardless of the stage of CKD at which the patient presents, the management of secondary complications (e.g., anemia and secondary hyperparathyroidism) and comorbid conditions including diabetes and cardiovascular complications is critical. Historically these conditions have not been appropriately managed.[11,12] Late referral to a nephrologist may account for this poor management; however, even in ideal clinical environments these conditions are not always aggressively treated. Appropriate management of anemia and malnutrition improve the prognosis for Stage 5 patients in their first year on dialysis, the time period historically associated with the highest mortality rate.[13,14]

GENERAL APPROACH TO PATIENT CARE

◄5 Interventions to slow or halt progression in patients with Stage 1 through 3 CKD are critically reviewed in Chap. 43. Once a patient reaches Stage 4 or 5 CKD, one of the most important approaches to treatment is early identification of secondary complications and appropriate management based on available guidelines. Guidelines for the work-up and treatment of CKD and its complications are available from the National Kidney Foundation-Kidney Disease Outcomes Quality Initiative (NKF-K/DOQI).[5,15–19] Unfortunately, laboratory data to diagnose such complications, including anemia and secondary hyperparathyroidism (e.g., iron studies and PTH levels), are often not evaluated until the patient has reached Stage 5 CKD.

Another important consideration in patients with CKD is the avoidance of nephrotoxic agents (see Chap. 46). Chronic use of nonsteroidal anti-inflammatory drugs and cyclooxygenase-2 inhibitors should be minimized or avoided when possible. Patients should be instructed on all brand and generic names of these classes of medications to reduce the risk of exposure. Appropriate measures should also be taken for hospitalized patients to decrease the risk of nephrotoxicity from radiocontrast agents (for procedures requiring such dyes), and antibiotics such as aminoglycosides, as well as from nonsteroidal anti-inflammatory drugs and angiotensin-converting enzyme inhibitors (ACEIs) (see Chaps. 42 and 46). Drug dosing guidelines based on the degree of kidney function should also be implemented, and a complete medication history of prescription and over-the-counter medications as well as herbals and nutritional supplements should be obtained and routinely updated.

◄6 Appropriate management of secondary complications of CKD usually involves a multidisciplinary approach to manage the nonpharmacologic and pharmacologic interventions, dietary education, and social/financial concerns. The typical team includes physicians (primary care physicians and nephrologists), nurses, dietitians, and social workers in outpatient dialysis facilities. In some outpatient dialysis centers pharmacists are also active members of the care team, although this is more common in institutionalized environments. Patient education for the population with CKD, particularly those with Stage 3, 4, and 5 disease, by all clinicians cannot be overemphasized.

FLUID AND ELECTROLYTE ABNORMALITIES

Maintenance of fluid volume, osmolarity, electrolyte balance, and acid-base status are all regulated in large part by the kidney. Homeostasis of sodium, potassium, chloride, calcium, magnesium, and phosphorus is altered due to changes in urinary excretion that occur in patients with impaired kidney function. A comprehensive discussion of fluid and electrolyte disorders and treatment options is presented in Chaps. 49, 50, and 51; the pathophysiology and therapeutics of these disorders in CKD patients are highlighted here.

ETIOLOGY

Sodium and Water Balance

In persons with normal kidney function, sodium balance is maintained at a sodium intake of 120 to 150 mEq/day. The fractional excretion of sodium (FE_{Na}) is approximately 1% to 3%. Water balance is also maintained, with a normal range of urinary osmolality of 50 to 1200 mOsm/L. In patients with severe CKD (Stages 4 and 5), sodium balance is achieved, but results in a volume-expanded state. FE_{Na} may increase to as much as 10% to 20%, possibly due to increased concentrations of atrial natriuretic peptide.[20] An osmotic diuresis occurs with an increase in FE_{Na} leading to obligatory water losses and impairment in the kidney's ability to dilute or concentrate urine (urinary osmolality is often fixed at that of plasma or approximately 300 mOsm/L). Nocturia is present relatively early in the course of CKD (Stage 3) secondary to the defect in urinary concentrating ability. Total renal sodium excretion decreases despite an increase in sodium excretion by remaining nephrons. Volume overload with pulmonary edema can result, but the most common manifestation of increased intravascular volume is systemic hypertension.[20]

Potassium Homeostasis

The kidneys normally excrete 90% to 95% of the daily potassium dietary load, predominantly via distal tubular secretion. The fractional excretion of potassium (FE_K) is approximately 25%. Normally only 5% to 10% of ingested potassium is excreted through the gut. Potassium homeostasis is also maintained by shifting extracellular potassium intracellularly immediately following ingestion of a potassium load. In patients with CKD, potassium balance is maintained by an increase in distal tubular potassium secretion in which aldosterone plays an important role; FE_K can increase to as high as five times normal. Thus the serum potassium concentration is usually maintained in the normal range until the patient reaches Stage 5 CKD (GFR <15 mL/min per 1.73 m² body surface area), at which point hyperkalemia is likely to develop. A significant increase in potassium secretion by the colon also contributes to the maintenance of potassium balance, but this adaptation cannot compensate fully for the decrease in renal potassium excretion.

DESIRED OUTCOME

Sodium and Water Balance

The goal in managing sodium and water balance is to maintain a normal serum sodium concentration while preventing fluid overload or volume depletion (i.e., maintaining hemodynamic stability). By achieving these goals, the risk of developing hypertension secondary to volume overload is also reduced, although hypertension is already present in many patients with Stage 3 to 4 CKD.

Potassium Homeostasis

The acute goal is to prevent the adverse consequences of hyperkalemia, particularly cardiac effects, and the chronic goal is to maintain potassium concentrations of approximately 4.5 to 6 mEq/L. The contribution of dialysis modalities to potassium homeostasis in patients with Stage 5 CKD must also be considered (see Chaps. 45 and 50).

PATIENT EVALUATION

Sodium and Water Balance

Edema is a common manifestation of volume overload and extracellular fluid volume expansion. Clinicians should evaluate patients for signs and symptoms of volume overload (e.g., pitting edema, rales, ascites, shortness of breath, and increased weight). Blood pressure monitoring in the clinic setting and at home if feasible to detect hypertension is also warranted. As kidney disease progresses dietary intervention and diuretic therapy (based on the degree of kidney function) will likely become necessary.

Potassium Homeostasis

In addition to CKD as a risk factor, other contributing factors should also be considered. This includes exposure to potassium-sparing diuretics; β-blockers, which work predominantly via β_2-antagonistic effects to interfere with the extrarenal translocation of potassium into cells; and ACEIs, which may cause hyperkalemia by reducing aldosterone production. Polycitra, used for the treatment of metabolic acidosis, contains potassium citrate and should not be prescribed for patients with severe CKD. If hyperkalemia develops, management options are based on the degree to which potassium is elevated (see Chap. 50).

NONPHARMACOLOGIC THERAPY

Sodium and Water Balance

The ability of the kidney to adjust to abrupt changes in sodium intake is greatly diminished in patients with severe CKD. Sodium restriction beyond a no-added-salt diet should not be recommended except in the face of hypertension or edema. The kidney maintains the ability to lower urinary sodium content to essentially zero, but this can only be accomplished by very gradual sodium restriction over a period of several days. Hospitalized patients should not routinely be sodium restricted because they have adapted to their outpatient intake. Negative sodium balance and its resultant volume contraction can result in decreased perfusion to the kidney and a subsequent further decline in GFR. Saline-containing IV solutions should be used cautiously in patients with CKD because the kidney's ability to excrete a salt load is impaired and such patients are prone to volume overload. Sodium retention and volume expansion contribute to hypertension in many patients with severe CKD, and diuretic therapy or dialysis may be necessary for control of edema or blood pressure.

Fluid restriction is generally unnecessary provided sodium intake is controlled, although fluid intake between dialysis sessions is generally limited for hemodialysis patients. An intact thirst mechanism maintains total body water and effective plasma osmolality near normal. Since urine volume is relatively fixed at approximately 2 L/day, fluid restriction below this amount should be avoided. Large amounts of free water administered orally or as IV fluid may induce hyponatremia and volume overload. When the patient develops ESKD, dialysis (specifically ultrafiltration) or a kidney transplant becomes necessary to maintain normovolemia.

Potassium Homeostasis

Hyperkalemia is more common in patients with Stage 5 CKD; therefore the discussion of treatment options focuses on interventions in this population. The majority of patients can be managed with a dietary potassium restriction of 50 to 80 mEq/day and alterations in dialysate potassium concentrations for patients receiving hemodialysis or peritoneal dialysis. Hyperkalemia is less common, however, in the peritoneal dialysis population due to differences in potassium transport. Constipation in patients with CKD can interfere with colonic potassium excretion; therefore a good bowel regimen is important. For severe hyperkalemia hemodialysis is often required using a low-potassium dialysate bath (see Chap. 50).

PHARMACOLOGIC THERAPY

Sodium and Water Balance

Diuretic therapy is often necessary to prevent edema from volume overload and prevent the associated symptoms. Loop diuretics, particularly when administered by continuous infusion, increase urine volume and renal sodium excretion. A combination of a loop diuretic along with a thiazide diuretic (such as hydrochlorothiazide or metolazone) can result in a profound excretion of sodium and water. Alone, thiazide diuretics are ineffective in patients with a GFR below 30 mL/min (see Chap. 49).

Potassium Homeostasis

The definitive treatment of severe hyperkalemia in ESKD is hemodialysis. In reality, there is often a delay between diagnosis of hyperkalemia and institution of dialysis, which necessitates the use of other temporizing measures, such as IV calcium gluconate, insulin and glucose, nebulized albuterol, and sodium polystyrene sulfonate (see Chap. 50). Unfortunately, shifting potassium into the intracellular fluid compartment with insulin and glucose or with albuterol makes removal of potassium via dialysis more difficult. Multiple dialysis sessions may be necessary following potassium redistribution to the extracellular space. Sodium polystyrene sulfonate (with sorbitol), a potassium-sodium exchange resin, can be given orally in doses of 15 to 30 g to increase potassium excretion via the ileum and colon. Lastly, sodium bicarbonate therapy is no longer advocated in the treatment of ESKD hyperkalemia unless severe metabolic acidosis is also present, because the potassium-lowering effect is unreliable. Loop diuretics, a standard pharmacologic treatment option for hyperkalemia, are not effective in patients with severe CKD.

CLINICAL CONTROVERSY

Low-dose spironolactone has been shown to decrease cardiovascular mortality in patients with severe heart failure. However, since spironolactone contributes to hyperkalemia, this agent should not be used in patients with Stage 4 or 5 CKD. New studies will be required before concluding that spironolactone administration is safe in the chronic hemodialysis population to reap the potential cardiovascular benefits.

▪ EVALUATION OF THERAPEUTIC OUTCOMES

Monitoring of volume status and serum electrolyte levels should be done at each follow-up visit in patients with Stages 4 or 5 CKD, particularly given the risk and detrimental consequences of volume overload (e.g., hypertension and pulmonary edema) and hyperkalemia (e.g., arrhythmias). Changes in volume status may warrant a change in diuretic therapy or dialysis regimens required to maintain hemodynamic stability. Patients should be educated on modifications in dietary intake and self-evaluation for signs and symptoms of edema.

▪ TREATMENT OF ANEMIA OF CKD

◄ The primary cause of anemia in CKD patients is a decrease in production of the hormone erythropoietin (EPO) by the progenitor cells of the kidney, where 90% of production typically occurs. Plasma concentrations of EPO increase exponentially in individuals with normal kidney function as hematocrit declines (i.e., in response to decreased oxygenation). In contrast, there is no correlation between the degree of anemia and EPO concentrations in anemic dialysis patients because they are unable to increase production of EPO in response to hypoxia.[21] The result is a normochromic, normocytic anemia. Additional factors contributing to the development of anemia of CKD are the decreased red cell life span in the presence of uremia (from the normal of 120 days to approximately 60 days in Stage 5 CKD), iron deficiency, blood loss from regular laboratory testing, and blood loss with hemodialysis for patients requiring this modality of renal replacement therapy. Iron deficiency is the primary cause of resistance to therapy with erythropoietic agents (i.e., epoetin alfa or darbepoetin alfa).

Despite the fact that its etiology is well known, anemia of CKD often goes unrecognized and is not appropriately managed in many patients prior to the development of Stage 5 CKD.[22,23] Lack of attention to the disorder, problems with payment for drug therapy by third-party payers, and the logistics of maintaining the regular follow-up necessary for therapy with erythropoietic agents contribute to this poor management. The effects of anemia and decreased oxygen delivery on other comorbid conditions, including the development of LVH, must also be considered given the burden of cardiovascular complications in this population.[24] The negative effects of anemia on quality of life are also important from a patient perspective and a compelling reason for early and aggressive treatment.[23,25]

▪ DESIRED OUTCOME

The desired outcomes are to increase oxygen-carrying capacity and thereby decrease dyspnea, orthopnea, and fatigue,[15] and to prevent long-term consequences such as LVH and associated mortality. The NKF-K/DOQI guidelines include specific targets for hemoglobin/hematocrit; folate, vitamin B_{12}, and iron indices; and recommendations for appropriate use of erythropoietic agents and iron supplements. The hemoglobin concentration (Hgb) is the preferred monitoring parameter since hematocrit (Hct) fluctuates with volume status and may be falsely elevated if a blood sample has been stored for a prolonged period of time. The target Hgb in patients treated for anemia of CKD is 11 to 12 g/dL (Hct 33% to 36%). These values are less than "the normal values" in patients without kidney disease due to the lack of compelling evidence to warrant targeting normal values in the population with CKD and limitations of the existing reimbursement structure for erythropoietic therapy. Although a higher mortality rate for dialysis patients with Hgb/Hct values above the target ranges has been reported, particularly in patients with cardiac disorders,[26] beneficial effects of increasing Hct up to 39% have been shown, including improvements in cardiac function, cognitive ability, and quality of life.[27] Thus it is unclear whether the current target ranges for Hgb/Hct are appropriate for all patients with anemia of CKD.[28] Until further evidence is available, the current target range recommended in the K/DOQI guidelines should be considered the standard of therapy.[15]

Iron indices that should be monitored include the transferrin saturation (TSat), an indicator of iron immediately available for delivery to the bone marrow, and serum ferritin, an indirect measure of storage iron. Transferrin is the carrier protein for iron; therefore the degree of saturation of this protein with iron is a measure of the iron that is most readily available for delivery to the bone marrow. As a protein, transferrin may be affected by nutritional status. Serum ferritin is an acute-phase reactant, and as such may be elevated under certain inflammatory conditions, giving a false indication of storage iron. The reticulocyte hemoglobin content has also proven reliable in assessing iron status and may be evaluated if reliable laboratory methods are available.[29] Currently, the TSat and serum ferritin are recommended as the most sensitive and specific indices of iron deficiency in the CKD population.[15] The target levels to achieve prior to initiation of erythropoietic therapy and to maintain during therapy are a TSat of 20% to 50% and a serum ferritin of 100 to 800 ng/mL.[15] These ranges are advocated to maintain adequate iron for red blood cell production (erythropoiesis) yet minimize the risk of iron overload.

The potential benefits of anemia management on cardiovascular risk reduction are currently being investigated in trials such as the Cardiovascular risk Reduction by Early Anaemia Treatment with Epoetin beta (CREATE) trial, in which different Hgb goals are being targeted in anemic patients with Stages 3 and 4 CKD.[30] While retrospective evaluations suggest that active interventions for anemia of CKD are beneficial, if cardiovascular outcomes are improved in prospective trials, earlier and more aggressive therapy will clearly be warranted.[13]

▪ PATIENT EVALUATION

Patients with CKD should be evaluated for anemia when the GFR falls below 60 mL/min (Stage 3 CKD). If the Hgb is less than 11 g/dL in premenopausal females or less than 12 g/dL in males and postmenopausal females, a complete work-up for anemia of CKD should be done.[15] This includes evaluation of other causes of anemia such as bleeding, deficiencies in vitamin B_{12} or folate, or other disease states that contribute to anemia, including human immunodeficiency virus infection and malignancies (see Chap. 99). As the primary cause of resistance to therapy for anemia of CKD, iron deficiency must be considered. Red blood cell indices and iron indices should be measured, including the red blood cell count, reticulocyte count, mean corpuscular volume (MCV), serum iron, total iron binding capacity (TIBC), and serum ferritin. A stool guaiac test should also be performed to rule out GI bleeding. Iron deficiency manifests as a microcytic anemia, as observed by a low MCV, while deficiencies in vitamin B_{12} and folate appear as a macrocytic anemia, with an increase in MCV. The TSat is calculated as ([serum iron/TIBC] × 100). If the TSat and serum ferritin values are below the desired range, iron supplementation is warranted prior to starting erythropoietic therapy. If all other causes of anemia are ruled out and the anemia persists despite iron supplementation, patients should be treated with erythropoietic agents, either epoetin alfa or darbepoetin alfa. The need for iron supplementation is based on iron status, but in general is required by most patients with anemia of CKD due to the increased demand as the result of the stimulation of the production rate of red blood cells.

As CKD worsens, a progressive decline in Hgb/Hct despite erythropoietic therapy may be observed. Therefore regular follow-up of Hgb/Hct and iron status is warranted to ensure the desired outcomes are met and to make necessary dose adjustments in erythropoietic and iron therapy (see section on evaluation of therapeutic outcomes).

NONPHARMACOLOGIC THERAPY

Nonpharmacologic therapy for anemia of CKD includes maintaining adequate dietary intake of iron. A relatively small amount of dietary iron, approximately 1 to 2 mg (or approximately 10%), is absorbed each day, primarily in the duodenum. While there is some debate as to whether GI absorption of iron is significantly altered in patients with severe CKD, it is clear that oral intake from dietary sources alone is generally not sufficient to meet the increased iron requirements that are necessitated by the initiation of erythropoietic therapy.[15,31]

PHARMACOLOGIC THERAPY

Pharmacologic therapy for anemia of CKD includes chronic erythropoietic therapy to correct erythropoietin deficiency and iron supplementation to correct and prevent iron deficiency caused by ongoing blood loss and increased iron demands associated with the initiation of erythropoietic therapy (Figs. 44–1 and 44–2).

RBC transfusions and androgen therapy are currently third-line treatment options for anemia of CKD. RBC transfusions carry many risks and therefore should only be used in select situations such as acute management of symptomatic anemia, following significant acute blood loss, and prior to surgical procedures that carry a high risk of blood loss. Androgen therapy was used extensively before availability of erythropoietic agents; however, today there is not ample evidence to support use of androgens alone over erythropoietic agents.[32] The risks of liver toxicity, malignancy, virilization in females, and hypertriglyceridemia outweigh the benefits of androgen therapy in most individuals.[32] L-carnitine supplementation has also been studied as adjunctive treatment of anemia associated with kidney disease.[33] There may in fact be some changes in erythropoiesis that

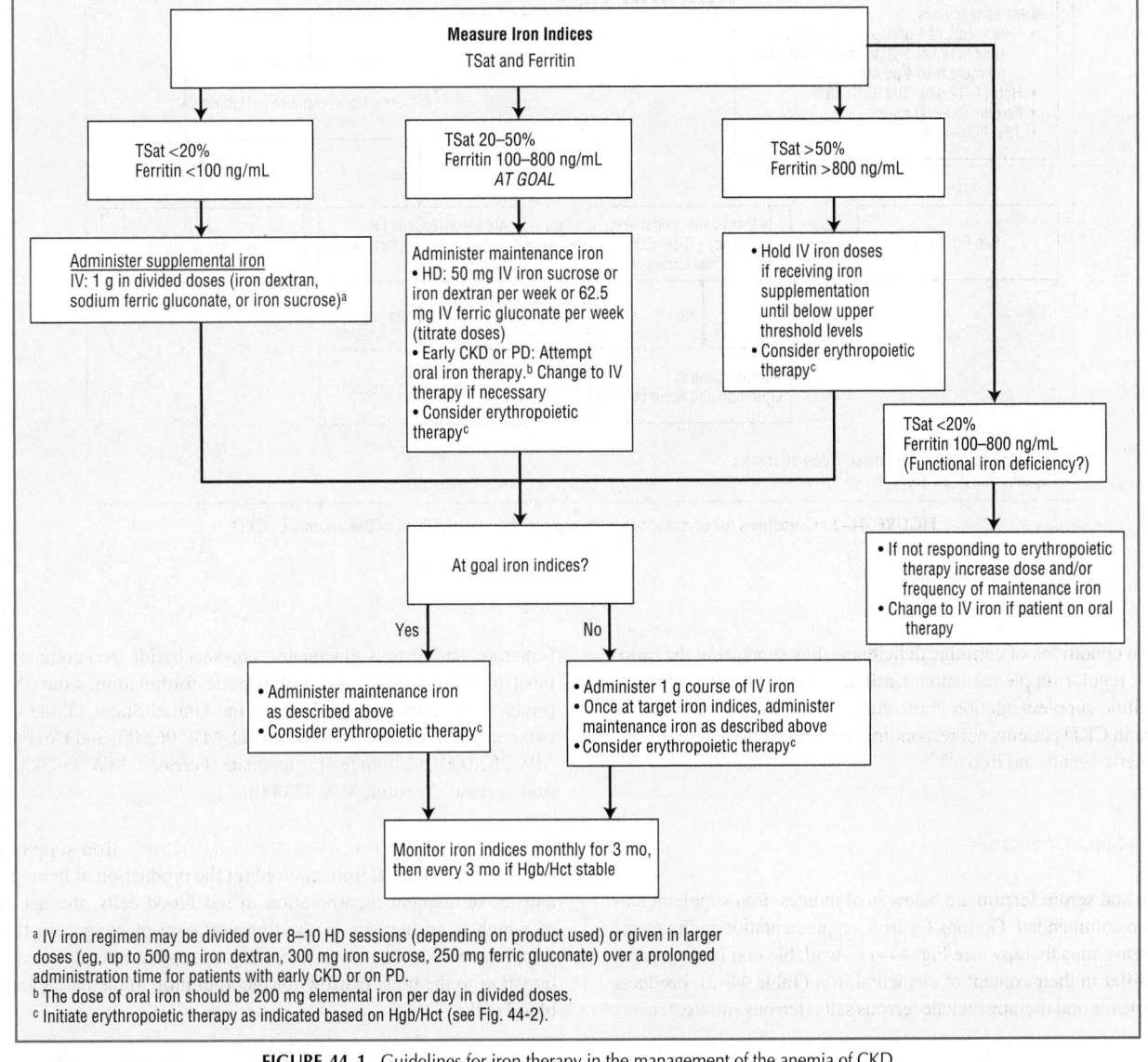

FIGURE 44–1. Guidelines for iron therapy in the management of the anemia of CKD.

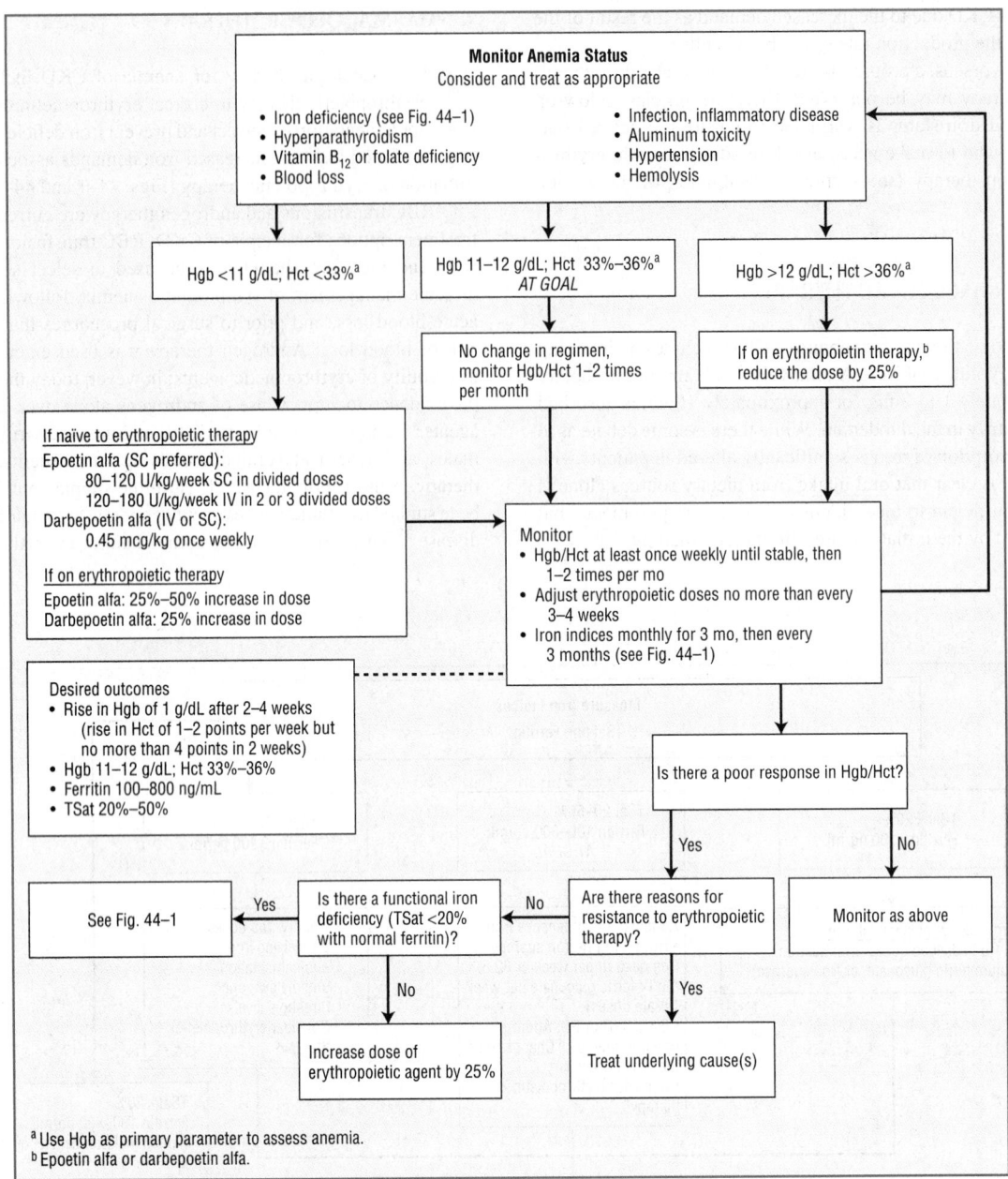

Monitor Anemia Status
Consider and treat as appropriate

- Iron deficiency (see Fig. 44–1)
- Hyperparathyroidism
- Vitamin B_{12} or folate deficiency
- Blood loss

- Infection, inflammatory disease
- Aluminum toxicity
- Hypertension
- Hemolysis

Hgb <11 g/dL; Hct <33%[a]

Hgb 11–12 g/dL; Hct 33%–36%[a]
AT GOAL

Hgb >12 g/dL; Hct >36%[a]

No change in regimen, monitor Hgb/Hct 1–2 times per month

If on erythropoietin therapy,[b] reduce the dose by 25%

If naïve to erythropoietic therapy
Epoetin alfa (SC preferred):
    80–120 U/kg/week SC in divided doses
    120–180 U/kg/week IV in 2 or 3 divided doses
Darbepoetin alfa (IV or SC):
    0.45 mcg/kg once weekly

If on erythropoietic therapy
Epoetin alfa: 25%–50% increase in dose
Darbepoetin alfa: 25% increase in dose

Monitor
- Hgb/Hct at least once weekly until stable, then 1–2 times per mo
- Adjust erythropoietic doses no more than every 3–4 weeks
- Iron indices monthly for 3 mo, then every 3 months (see Fig. 44–1)

Desired outcomes
- Rise in Hgb of 1 g/dL after 2–4 weeks (rise in Hct of 1–2 points per week but no more than 4 points in 2 weeks)
- Hgb 11–12 g/dL; Hct 33%–36%
- Ferritin 100–800 ng/mL
- TSat 20%–50%

Is there a poor response in Hgb/Hct?

Yes   No

See Fig. 44–1

Yes

Is there a functional iron deficiency (TSat <20% with normal ferritin)?

No

Are there reasons for resistance to erythropoietic therapy?

Monitor as above

No

Yes

Increase dose of erythropoietic agent by 25%

Treat underlying cause(s)

[a] Use Hgb as primary parameter to assess anemia.
[b] Epoetin alfa or darbepoetin alfa.

FIGURE 44–2. Guidelines for erythropoietic therapy in the management of the anemia of CKD.

occur in conditions of carnitine deficiency, thus supporting the rationale for regular supplementation. Until this association is confirmed, L-carnitine supplementation is recommended only for treatment of anemia in CKD patients not responding to standard therapy (i.e., erythropoietic agents and iron).[16,33]

■ Iron Supplementation

If TSat and serum ferritin are below goal indices, iron supplementation is recommended. Options for iron supplementation include oral and intravenous therapy (see Fig. 44–1). Available oral iron preparations differ in their content of elemental iron (Table 44–2). Products available for oral therapy include ferrous salts (ferrous sulfate, ferrous fumarate, and ferrous gluconate), polysaccharide iron complex, and most recently a heme iron polypeptide formulation. Four IV iron products are currently available in the United States (Table 44–3): two composed of iron dextran (InFeD, MW 96,000; and DexFerrum, MW 267,000), sodium ferric gluconate (Ferrlecit, MW 350,000), and iron sucrose (Venofer, MW 43,000).

■ *Pharmacology and Mechanism of Action.* Iron supplements provide the elemental iron required for the production of hemoglobin and its subsequent incorporation in red blood cells, the net result of which is an increase in the transportation of oxygen to tissues. Supplementation of iron is necessary to replete iron stores and for transport to the bone marrow for incorporation immediately into red blood cells.

TABLE 44–2. Oral Iron Preparations

Iron Product	Common Agents and Available Units	Amount of Elemental Iron per Unit	Number of Units Per Day[a]
Ferrous sulfate	Fer-In-Sol (75 mg/0.6 mL)	75 mg	2–3
	Feosol (200 mg)	50 mg	4
	Ferrous sulfate, various preparations (325 mg)	65 mg	3–4
	Slow FE (160 mg)	50 mg	4
Ferrous fumarate	Ferrous fumarate, various preparations (300 mg)	99 mg	2
	Femiron (20 mg)	20 mg	10
	Nephro-Fer (350 mg)	115 mg	2
	Vitron-C (65–125 mg)	65 mg	3
Ferrous gluconate	Ferrous gluconate, various (325 mg)	36 mg	6
	Fergon (240 mg)	27 mg	6
Polysaccharide iron	Hytinic (150 mg)	150	1–2
	Niferex (50 mg)	50 mg	4
Heme iron polypeptide	Proferrin-ES (12 mg)	12 mg	17

[a]Number of units per day depends on the amount of elemental iron per unit; must give 200 mg elemental iron per day.

Pharmacokinetics.

Approximately 10% of iron administered orally is absorbed in the duodenum and upper jejunum. Absorption of iron is decreased by food and achlorhydria. In patients with iron deficiency GI absorption may be increased, up to 25% to 30%; however, this adaptive response may be impaired in patients with kidney disease.[15] The heme form of oral iron binds to a different receptor in the GI tract than nonheme iron, is absorbed to a greater extent, and may be better tolerated.[34] Some oral iron formulations also include ascorbic acid to enhance iron absorption. While there is an association between ascorbic acid intake and oxalate formation, this association is generally not observed at doses of ascorbic acid contained in these iron formulations.[35]

Intravenous iron preparations differ in the composition of the complex to which elemental iron is bound. These differences affect the rate of dissociation of iron from the complex to the reticuloendothelial system and subsequent storage as ferritin. Iron sucrose is also delivered directly to transferrin. The half-life of these formulations also differ: ferric gluconate 1 hour, iron sucrose 6 hours, and iron dextran 40 to 60 hours. However, there is minimal to no correlation between the pharmacokinetics of these formulations and their pharmacodynamic effects.[36]

Efficacy.

While supplementation using oral preparations may seem more practical than IV administration, oral iron therapy is lim-ited by poor absorption and is often inadequate to achieve goal iron indices. This is particularly true for patients with ESKD, who may have higher iron needs due to chronic blood loss associated with hemodialysis.[15] Oral iron supplementation is more convenient for patients who do not have regular IV access, including patients with Stages 3 and 4 CKD and those receiving peritoneal dialysis. Even these patients, however, are likely to require IV iron supplementation periodically to meet iron needs and correct absolute iron deficiency.[31] Success of oral therapy is also limited by noncompliance due to side effects, primarily GI in nature, and the frequency of administration (up to three times per day).

Intravenous iron therapy is an effective means to prevent iron deficiency and maintain adequate iron status for erythropoiesis. Parenteral iron improves the responsiveness to erythropoietic therapy and reduces the dose required to achieve and maintain the target Hgb/Hct.[37,38] Iron administration in patients with what is known as a functional iron deficiency is more questionable. Functional iron deficiency is characterized by a low TSat (<20%) in the presence of a normal or elevated serum ferritin. In other words, there may appear to be adequate storage iron, but iron is not being carried by transferrin to the bone marrow for red blood cell production. If the Hgb is less than the target of 11 g/dL, under these conditions a trial of IV iron therapy may be warranted. Iron supplementation alone may improve Hgb/Hct and may

TABLE 44–3. Intravenous Iron Preparations[a]

Iron Compounds	Brand Name	Availability	Warnings	Need for Test Dose	Dose Ranges[b]
Iron dextran[c]	InFeD	50 mg/mL	Black box	Yes	25–1000 mg
	DexFerrum	50 mg/mL	Black box	Yes	25–1000 mg
Sodium ferric gluconate[d]	Ferrlecit	62.5 mg/5 mL	General	No	62.5–1000 mg
Iron sucrose[e]	Venofer	100 mg/5 mL	General	No	25–1000 mg

[a]All products may be administered IV push (small doses only).
[b]Maintenance regimens range from 25–100 mg weekly. Larger doses should be administered in divided doses or over a prolonged dosing interval.
[c]Supplied in 2-mL single-dose vials containing 50 mg of elemental iron per milliliter.
[d]Available in colorless glass ampules containing 62.5 mg elemental iron in 5 mL (12.5 mg/mL). The 125-mg dose may be diluted in 100 mL of 0.9% sodium chloride administered IV over 1 hour, or administered undiluted as an IV injection at a rate of up to 12.5 mg/min.
[e]Supplied in 5-mL single-dose vials containing 100 mg elemental iron (20 mg/mL). The 100-mg dose may be diluted in 100 mL of 0.9% sodium chloride administered IV over at least 15 minutes, or administered undiluted by slow IV injection at a rate of 20 mg/min.

lead to improved erythropoiesis at reduced doses of erythropoietic therapy.[37]

To avoid errors in evaluating iron status, clinicians should wait at least 2 weeks after a loading dose regimen of IV iron to re-assess iron indices; however, iron indices can be evaluated after 1 week if the patient is receiving regular maintenance doses of iron (e.g., 25 to 125 mg/wk).[37,39]

▓ *Adverse Effects.* Adverse effects of oral iron, including constipation, nausea, and abdominal cramping, increase as the dose is escalated and may be present in over 50% of those receiving 200 mg of elemental iron per day. These untoward effects often discourage patients from taking these medications on a chronic basis. Some of these GI side effects can be minimized if oral iron products are taken with food; however, food may decrease absorption of oral iron. Therefore it is generally recommended that iron be taken on an empty stomach.

Adverse effects of IV iron include allergic reactions, hypotension, dizziness, dyspnea, headaches, lower back pain, arthralgia, syncope, and arthritis. Some of these reactions, in particular hypotension, can be minimized by decreasing the dose or rate of infusion of iron. The most concerning potential consequence of IV iron administration is anaphylaxis. Anaphylactoid reactions to iron dextran have been reported in up to 1.8% of patients, with serious reactions including respiratory complications and cardiovascular collapse occurring in approximately 0.6%.[40] Such reactions are believed to be due in part to antibody formation to the dextran component. Adverse reactions have been reported more frequently in those receiving DexFerrum compared to InFeD; a two- to eightfold increase in the incidence was noted with DexFerrum.[41] Such differences were particularly influential in product selection prior to the availability of sodium ferric gluconate and iron sucrose. These IV iron formulations have a better safety record than either of the iron dextran products, based on their history of use in Europe over the last four decades and recent data in the United States since these products were approved.[42,43] Sodium ferric gluconate and iron sucrose do not require a test dose prior to administration of the full dose, unlike iron dextran, which requires a 25-mg test dose to reduce the risk of anaphylactic reactions. As a precaution with all IV preparations, patients should be observed during and immediately following administration for any adverse reactions.

Administration of IV iron also introduces a risk of iron overload. Deposition of excess iron may affect several organ systems, leading to hepatic, pancreatic, and cardiac dysfunction. Bone marrow biopsy provides the most definitive diagnosis of iron overload, but since it is an extremely invasive procedure, it is not widely employed in most clinical settings. Maintaining serum ferritin and TSat below the upper threshold values associated with iron overload is the most reasonable approach to minimize the risk of iron toxicity. The challenge is in defining these upper limits, particularly for serum ferritin which may be elevated in inflammatory conditions and not reflective of true iron stores in such situations. Currently the K/DOQI guidelines recommend not to exceed a serum ferritin of 800 ng/mL and a TSat of 50%.[15] If these limits are exceeded, maintenance IV iron therapy should be discontinued, until TSat and serum ferritin levels fall below 50% and 800 ng/mL, respectively. If symptomatic overload does occur, deferoxamine (Desferal) or phlebotomy may be necessary.

The safety and efficacy of high-dose IV iron regimens have been evaluated to determine the most cost-effective and efficacious dosing strategies. Iron dextran has been safely administered in total dose infusions ranging from 400 mg to 2 g to dialysis patients.[44] Similar high-dose regimens of 500 mg have also been safely administered to patients with Stages 3 and 4 CKD.[45] While such iron dextran regimens have been safely administered, it is important to consider that with the information available today on the safety profile of sodium ferric gluconate and iron sucrose, many clinicians would consider these newer agents as first-line therapy. Sodium ferric gluconate has been safely administered at doses of 250 mg infused over 1 hour (4.2 mg/min).[46] In this same evaluation there were 19 doses of greater than 250 mg administered; one dose of 312.5 mg, fourteen doses of 375 mg, and four doses of 500 mg, with infusion rates varying from 1.22 mg/min to 25 mg/min. No serious adverse events were reported, although nonserious events such as pruritus did occur in 4 of the 144 patients who received the 250-mg dose. Additional studies evaluating higher doses of sodium ferric gluconate are ongoing in the early CKD and dialysis populations. Doses in these higher ranges should not be adopted as standard of care until further safety data become available. If doses higher than those currently approved are used in practice, they should be administered over a prolonged time period (at least 2 hours) and should not exceed 250 mg, based on the limited evidence available. Iron sucrose at doses of up to 500 mg administered over 3 hours on consecutive days has been successful in maintaining iron stores without causing serious adverse events.[47] When administered over a shorter time period this same dose was associated with dizziness, hypotension, and nausea.[48] In this same evaluation the administration of lower doses of 200 to 300 mg given over 2 hours resulted in fewer adverse events.

Although there have been conflicting reports, most clinicians believe that exposure to iron may contribute to the risk of bacterial infection since iron is used by microorganisms for metabolic functions.[49,50] The association of IV iron with oxidative stress, acceleration of atherosclerosis, and other cardiovascular conditions has also been suggested.[51] These potential long-term risks of IV iron therapy are not clearly defined and there are no data that unequivocally confirm that aggressive use of IV iron in CKD patients treated with erythropoietic therapy increases patient morbidity or mortality.[37]

▓ *Drug-Drug and Drug-Food Interactions.* Drugs commonly used in the CKD population that may decrease absorption of oral iron include calcium preparations and antacids. Oral iron may also decrease the absorption of quinolone antibiotics. Medications that increase gastric pH such as H_2-antagonists and proton pump inhibitors may also decrease iron absorption since iron absorption in the duodenum is maximized at an acidic pH.

▓ *Dosing and Administration.* If oral therapy is initiated, the recommended dose is 200 mg of elemental iron per day. Patients must generally take two to three pills per day to receive the recommended dose of elemental iron (see Table 44–2). Correction of absolute iron deficiency (TSat <20%, serum ferritin <100 ng/mL) generally requires administration of at least 1 g of IV iron. For the hemodialysis population typical dosing regimens are 100 mg as iron dextran or iron sucrose over 10 dialysis sessions, or 125 mg of sodium ferric gluconate over 8 dialysis sessions (see Table 44–3).[15,42,43] These regimens are FDA-approved and reduce the risk of adverse reactions to IV iron therapy.

Administration of 1 g of IV iron is reasonable to initially replete patients with an absolute iron deficiency (TSat <20%, serum ferritin <100 ng/mL); however, many patients become iron deficient quickly without ongoing iron supplementation. There is sufficient evidence to support use of maintenance doses of IV iron (e.g., iron sucrose or iron dextran 25 to 100 mg/wk; sodium ferric gluconate 62.5 to 125 mg/wk), particularly in hemodialysis patients.[15,52]

Erythropoietic Therapy

Pharmacology and Mechanism of Action. Erythropoietic growth factors are required to stimulate division and differentiation of erythroid progenitor cells and induce the release of reticulocytes from the bone marrow to the bloodstream where they mature into erythrocytes (red blood cells). Available erythropoietic agents include epoetin alfa (distributed as Epogen by Amgen, Inc., Thousand Oaks, CA; and Procrit by Ortho Biotech, Johnson & Johnson, Raritan, NJ) and darbepoetin alfa (Aranesp by Amgen, Inc.). Epoetin beta is available outside the United States. These agents are glycoproteins manufactured by recombinant DNA technology that have the same biological activity as endogenous erythropoietin. The amino acid sequence of epoetin alfa is identical to the endogenous protein; however, the carbohydrate structure differs. Since 1989, epoetin alfa has been the mainstay of therapy for anemia of CKD and substantially reduced the percentage of patients dependent on transfusions for management of anemia. Darbepoetin alfa was approved for treatment of anemia of CKD in September 2001.[53] Darbepoetin alfa differs from epoetin alfa by the addition of two N-linked carbohydrate side chains. This change in structure increases the sialic acid content of darbepoetin compared with epoetin alfa, resulting in a higher molecular weight (~38,000 daltons for darbepoetin compared with 30,400 daltons for epoetin alfa).[54]

Pharmacokinetics and Pharmacodynamics. Epoetin alfa may be administered by either the IV or subcutaneous (SC) routes. Although bioavailability with SC administration is poor (approximately 20%), the low peak serum concentrations and the prolonged half-life (approximately 24 hours as compared to 8.5 hours IV)[55,56] yield a Hgb/Hct response that is at least as good or better than that attained with IV administration.[57] This enhanced efficacy is presumed to be caused by a more prolonged physiologic stimulation of erythroid precursors. Darbepoetin alfa has a longer half-life and prolonged biological activity compared with epoetin alfa (darbepoetin alfa 25.3 h [IV], 48.8 h [SC]) due to the increased sialic acid content.[55,56]

The pharmacodynamic profile of epoetin and darbepoetin are important to consider when evaluating response to therapy. These erythropoietic agents stimulate erythropoiesis, and therefore increase the red blood cell production rate. Patients with Stages 4 and 5 CKD also have a shorter red blood cell life span compared to patients with normal kidney function (64 days in contrast to 120 days in normal subjects). When the red cell production rate equals the destruction rate, as determined by the red cell life span, steady state is achieved. The challenge is in determining the appropriate dosing regimen of erythropoietic therapy to maintain the target Hgb of 11 to 12 g/dL (Hct 33% to 36%). Figure 44–3 illustrates the Hct response to the pharmacodynamic effect of epoetin (an increase in Hct). Prior to starting epoetin, the baseline Hct is constant, demonstrating that RBC production is at steady state (the rate at which RBCs are being produced equals the rate at which they are leaving the circulation). Although the Hct may begin to rise shortly following epoetin initiation as the result of demargination of reticulocytes, it takes approximately 10 days before erythrocyte progenitor cells mature and begin to be continuously released into the circulation at an increased rate. The Hct continues to increase until the life span of the cells stimulated by epoetin or darbepoetin is reached (mean 2 months; range 1 to 4 months) and a new steady state is achieved. For this reason it is important to evaluate response over several weeks as opposed to making changes to the dosing regimen prematurely.

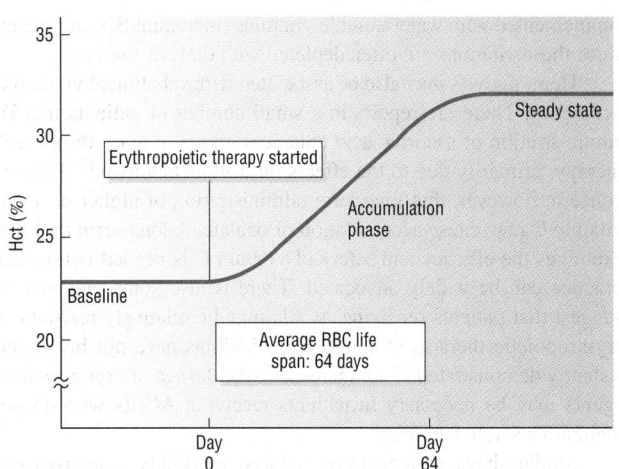

FIGURE 44–3. Pharmacodynamic effect of epoetin or darbepoetin on hematocrit (Hct).

Efficacy. Subcutaneous administration is preferable for chronic ambulatory peritoneal dialysis patients and those in the earlier stages of CKD because these patients do not usually have regular IV access. This route of administration is also recommended for most hemodialysis patients since the dose required to achieve and maintain target Hgb/Hct is lower by 15% to 50% than that associated with the intravenous route of administration.[15,58] For many hemodialysis patients, however, IV therapy continues to be the predominant method of administration due to convenient IV access during the procedure. Comparison of weekly SC epoetin dosing with dosing three times per week in peritoneal dialysis patients showed weekly dosing to be effective in maintaining Hgb/Hct, albeit at a higher total weekly dose.[59] Similar evaluations of less frequent dosing of epoetin in the CKD population are ongoing. Figures 44–1 and 44–2 provide an algorithmic approach to management of anemia using erythropoietic agents and iron therapy in patients with CKD.

The prolonged half-life of darbepoetin offers the advantage of less frequent dosing, starting at once-a-week or once-every-other-week when given IV or SC.[60,61] This is of particular benefit in patients with early CKD and the peritoneal dialysis population, who are not seen in the clinic as often. Prolonged dosing intervals, as infrequent as once every 3 to 4 weeks, have also been effective in maintaining target Hgb/Hct in some dialysis patients.[62]

Iron deficiency is the most common cause of resistance to erythropoietic therapy.[15] Evaluation and treatment of iron deficiency should occur prior to initiation of erythropoietic therapy as previously discussed (see Figs. 44–1 and 44–2). Inflammation (localized or systemic infection, active inflammatory disease, or surgical trauma) is associated with defective iron utilization known as reticuloendothelial block. Reticuloendothelial block is characterized by a reduction in iron delivery from body stores to the bone marrow, and is generally refractory to iron therapy. Failure to respond to erythropoietic therapy requires evaluation of other factors causing resistance, such as infection, inflammation, chronic blood loss, aluminum toxicity, hemoglobinopathies, malnutrition, and hyperparathyroidism.[15] Erythropoietic therapy may be continued in the infected or postoperative patient, although increased doses are often required to maintain or slow the rate of decline in Hgb/Hct. Deficiencies in folate and vitamin B$_{12}$ should also be considered as potential causes of resistance to erythropoietic therapy, as both are essential for optimal erythropoiesis. Patients on hemodialysis or peritoneal dialysis should be routinely supplemented with water-soluble vitamins (including B_{12} and folate) since these vitamins are often depleted with dialysis therapy.

Hemodialysis may also be associated with subclinical vitamin C deficiency. There are reports in a small number of patients that IV administration of ascorbic acid enhances response to erythropoietic therapy, primarily due to the effects on iron metabolism.[63] There is concern, however, that long-term administration of higher doses of vitamin C may cause accumulation of oxalate. A long-term trial that examines the efficacy and safety of vitamin C is needed before this practice can be widely advocated. There is also some evidence to suggest that patients receiving ACEIs may be relatively resistant to erythropoietic therapy, although these findings have not been consistently demonstrated.[64] An increase in the dosage of erythropoietic agents may be necessary in patients receiving ACEIs who do not maintain a stable Hgb/Hct.

Studies have demonstrated reduced morbidity, increased exercise capacity and tolerance, and enhanced quality of life when erythropoietic therapy was initiated, iron stores maintained, and target Hgb attained.[15,27] Data also suggest a stabilization or regression of LVH in patients with early kidney disease and in those with ESRD when anemia is successfully treated.[65,66] Preventing the development of LVH is one of the desired outcomes of anemia management. Thus these findings which demonstrate regression of LVH at increased Hgb levels support more aggressive management of anemia in the early stages of CKD. Whether there is an optimal Hgb target to prevent development of LVH remains to be determined. In a 2-year study no difference in left ventricular mass index was observed for patients with Stages 3 or 4 CKD maintained at a Hgb of 9 to 10 g/dL versus 12 to 13 g/dL.[67] Given these observations of a relationship between anemia and LVH, additional prospective studies addressing this question will be needed to resolve the controversy.

■ *Adverse Effects.* Epoetin alfa and darbepoetin alfa are generally well tolerated; however, hypertension is the most common adverse event reported.[15,53] Protocols established in some clinical settings, primarily in outpatient dialysis clinics, sometimes recommend withholding erythropoietic therapy based on the degree of elevation in blood pressure. This practice on a routine basis is not rational given the benefits of maintaining the target Hgb and the availability of more practical measures to control blood pressure. K/DOQI guidelines for anemia recommend withholding erythropoietic therapy only when hypertension is refractory to aggressive blood pressure management approaches such as pharmacologic therapy and dialysis.[15] Of interest is the fact that epoetin doses were 5.5% higher in dialysis patients with hypertension compared to patients without high blood pressure.[3] Seizures have occurred in patients treated with epoetin; however, the incidence does not appear to be increased over the baseline levels seen in placebo control groups. Vascular access thrombosis may be more frequent during epoetin therapy, but this finding has not been supported to the extent necessary to advocate increased monitoring for this effect.[15]

Neutralizing antibodies to epoetin have been identified in a small number (less than 200) of patients treated with either epoetin alfa or epoetin beta.[68] These patients developed an absolute resistance to epoetin therapy which relegates them to intermittent blood transfusions as the primary therapeutic option. Cases have been reported, primarily with one epoetin alfa product manufactured outside the United States, Eprex (Johnson & Johnson, Manati, Puerto Rico), and have occurred in parallel with the increase in SC administration. Although the case reports are relatively few in number, clinicians should be aware of this thus far rare phenomenon in patients resistant to erythropoietic

therapy. Patients who develop antierythropoietin antibodies should not receive other erythropoietic agents, as cross-reactivity has been demonstrated.

■ *Drug-Drug Interactions.* No significant drug interactions have been reported with the available erythropoietic agents.

■ *Dosing and Administration.* Starting doses of epoetin alfa are 80 to 120 units/kg per week for SC administration and 120 to 180 units/kg per week for IV administration divided in two to three doses per week (typically three times per week for hemodialysis patients receiving IV therapy). If a patient is converted from IV to SC epoetin and is not at the target Hgb/Hct, the weekly SC dose should remain the same as the IV dose. If they have achieved the target Hgb/Hct a one-third reduction in dose is appropriate.[15] The starting dose of darbepoetin alfa in patients not previously receiving erythropoietic therapy is 0.45 mcg/kg IV or SC administered once weekly.[53] A conversion table is available for patients who are to be switched from epoetin alfa (units per week) to darbepoetin alfa (micrograms per week) (Table 44–4).

Currently two formulations of epoetin alfa are available: a single-dose, preservative-free solution (2000-, 3000-, 4000-, 10,000-, and 40,000-unit/mL vials) and a multidose, preserved solution (10,000- and 20,000-unit/mL vials). A clinical trial comparing these two formulations in terms of pain intensity after SC administration found that the multiple-dose formulation was associated with less stinging, although several patients did not experience pain with the single-dose preparation.[69] Darbepoetin alfa is available in two solutions, a polysorbate solution and an albumin solution, supplied as single-dose vials (25-, 40-, 60-, 100-, and 200-mg/mL vials containing polysorbate) and (25-, 40-, 60-, 100-, 150-, 200-, 300-, and 500-mg/mL vials containing albumin), respectively.[53]

Generally the response to erythropoietic therapy should be evaluated over at least 2 to 4 weeks before a change in the dose of epoetin alfa or darbepoetin alfa is made. If the change in Hgb is <1 g/dL (Hct less than 2% to 3%), over this time interval the dose of erythropoietic agent should be increased by 50% for epoetin alfa or 25% for darbepoetin alfa. If the change in Hgb is >2 to 3 g/dL (Hct greater than 6% to 8%) the dose of epoetin alfa or darbepoetin alfa should be reduced by 25%.

TABLE 44–4. Estimated Darbepoetin Alfa Starting Doses Based on Previous Epoetin Alfa Dose

Previous Weekly Epoetin Alfa Dose[a,b] (units/week)	Weekly Darbepoetin Alfa Dose (mcg/week)
<2,500	6.25
2,500 to 4,999	12.50
5,000 to 10,999	25.00
11,000 to 17,999	40.00
18,000 to 33,999	60.00
34,000 to 89,999	100.00
≥90,000	200.00

[a]Darbepoetin alfa should be administered weekly for patients receiving epoetin alfa two or three times per week and every other week for patients receiving epoetin alfa once per week.

[b]For patients requiring darbepoetin alfa every other week, the weekly dose of epoetin alfa should be multiplied by two and this dose used in the conversion chart to determine the appropriate darbepoetin alfa dose.

From darbepoetin package insert.[53]

PHARMACOECONOMIC CONSIDERATIONS

Pharmacoeconomic considerations in the management of anemia of CKD relate primarily to the costs associated with erythropoietic agents and the increased use of IV iron to sustain erythropoiesis. Over the last decade there has been a steady rise in cost associated with the provision of epoetin and IV iron for the dialysis population: the cost to Medicare has stabilized at just over $1 billion per year during the last 2 to 3 years.[3] Cost advantages can be realized, however, from the benefits associated with appropriate management of anemia, including fewer days of hospitalization, decreased mortality, and increased transplant success.[3,27] Implementation of maintenance IV iron therapy, as well as SC administration of epoetin, also has the potential to reduce Medicare cost for anemia management. Current Medicare reimbursement rates for epoetin and IV iron produce profits of 12% and 45%, respectively for most dialysis programs, and thus there is little incentive to minimize the use of either agent. In the case of iron therapy, IV iron is reimbursable by Medicare, whereas oral iron is either paid for by the patient out-of-pocket or by secondary insurers (usually with a copayment). Capitation of payments for medications such as erythropoietic agents and IV iron therapy may force the dialysis community to change their clinical practices and thereby optimize their utilization.

Considerations are a bit different in patients with early CKD since Medicare does not cover medication costs for this population. The lack of payment is a deterrent to timely implementation of therapy and likely contributes to the development of secondary complications such as anemia. A recent pharmacoeconomic consideration in the CKD population is whether the addition of darbepoetin alfa offers a financial incentive in addition to advantages of less frequent dosing from a patient's perspective. As use of darbepoetin has become more widespread and the costs more stable, clinicians involved in the care of this patient population are beginning to consider economic factors that influence selection of erythropoietic therapy.[70]

CLINICAL CONTROVERSY

Some clinicians advocate discontinuing IV iron therapy when patients are actively infected. This applies also to erythropoietic therapy if it is believed that the patient will not respond (i.e., they are resistant to therapy because of the inflammatory process).

EVALUATION OF THERAPEUTIC OUTCOMES

An algorithmic approach to patient evaluation and treatment with iron and erythropoietic therapies in adults is depicted in Figs. 44–1 and 44–2. Iron status should be assessed every month for patients started on erythropoietic therapy who are not concurrently receiving iron and every 3 months for patients receiving iron until a stable Hgb/Hct has been achieved. Once at the goal Hgb/Hct, iron indices should be measured every 3 months to determine the need for iron supplementation or any adjustments in the current regimen.[15] Hgb/Hct should be monitored every 1 to 2 weeks after initiation of erythropoietic therapy or following a dose change until stable. Once stable, the Hgb should be monitored every 2 to 4 weeks. An inadequate response to epoetin alfa therapy is defined as failure to achieve target Hgb/Hct in iron-replete patients when an adequate dose (usually 450 units/kg per week IV or 300 units/kg per week SC) has been administered for 4 to 6 months, or failure to maintain target Hgb/Hct subsequently at that dose.[15]

SECONDARY HYPERPARATHYROIDISM AND RENAL OSTEODYSTROPHY

Calcium and phosphorus balance is mediated through the complex interplay of hormones and their effects on bone, the GI tract, kidney, and parathyroid gland. What begins as relatively minor imbalances in phosphorus and calcium homeostasis leads to secondary hyperparathyroidism (sHPT) in the short term and ultimately renal osteodystrophy (ROD) if these metabolic abnormalities are not corrected.

As kidney function declines there is a decrease in phosphorus elimination which results in hyperphosphatemia and a reciprocal decrease in serum calcium concentration. Hypocalcemia is the primary stimulus for release of PTH by the parathyroid glands, the effects of which are mediated by the interaction of ionized calcium with the calcium-sensing receptor on the chief cells of the parathyroid gland. Hyperphosphatemia also increases PTH synthesis and release through its direct effects on the parathyroid gland and production of prepro-PTH messenger RNA.[71] In an attempt to normalize ionized calcium, PTH decreases phosphorus reabsorption and increases calcium reabsorption by the proximal tubules of the kidney (at least until the GFR falls to less than approximately 30 mL/min), and also increases calcium mobilization from bone. The result is a correction in calcium and phosphorus, at least in the early stages of CKD; however, this occurs at the expense of an elevated PTH ("the trade-off hypothesis"). The increase in PTH is most notable when GFR is <60 mL/min per 1.73 m² (Stage 3 CKD) and worsens as kidney function declines further.

Active vitamin D (1,25-dihydroxyvitamin D_3 or calcitriol) promotes increased intestinal absorption of calcium which helps to normalize ionized calcium. Calcitriol also works directly on the parathyroid gland to suppress PTH production. The enzyme 1-α-hydroxylase is responsible for the final hydroxylation and conversion of the vitamin D precursor, 25-hydroxyvitamin D, to the active form in the kidney. As kidney disease progresses this conversion is impaired and vitamin D deficiency results. Calcitriol levels have been shown to decrease significantly before there is a perceptible rise in PTH in CKD patients.[72] Other differences in vitamin D metabolism observed in patients with CKD that lead to deficiencies in the 25-hydroxyvitamin D precursor include decreased dermal synthesis of vitamin D, decreased exposure to sunlight, and reduced dietary intake of vitamin D.[18] Although 1,25-dihydroxyvitamin D_3 is the most potent form, 25-hydroxyvitamin D is the main circulating metabolite and is considered the best functional indicator of vitamin D stores in humans. In patients with Stage 3 or Stage 4 CKD, 25-hydroxyvitamin D levels of <30 ng/mL have been associated with increased PTH.[18] As a result of such findings, evaluation of 25-hydroxyvitamin D levels is warranted in patients with Stage 3 and 4 CKD, with supplementation recommended in patients with observed deficiencies.

A multiplicity of metabolic disorders in patients with CKD contributes to worsening sHPT and the consequences associated with elevated PTH (Fig. 44–4). The continuous production of PTH by the parathyroid glands leads to parathyroid hyperplasia (nodular or diffuse). Nodular tissue demonstrates more rapid growth potential and appears to be associated with fewer vitamin D and calcium-sensing receptors, which results in resistance to the effects of calcium and vitamin D therapy and subsequent development of ROD.[8] Bone loss can be detected in patients with early stages of kidney disease and multiple types of bone lesions have been identified from bone biopsies of patients on dialysis.[73] The skeletal complications associated with ROD

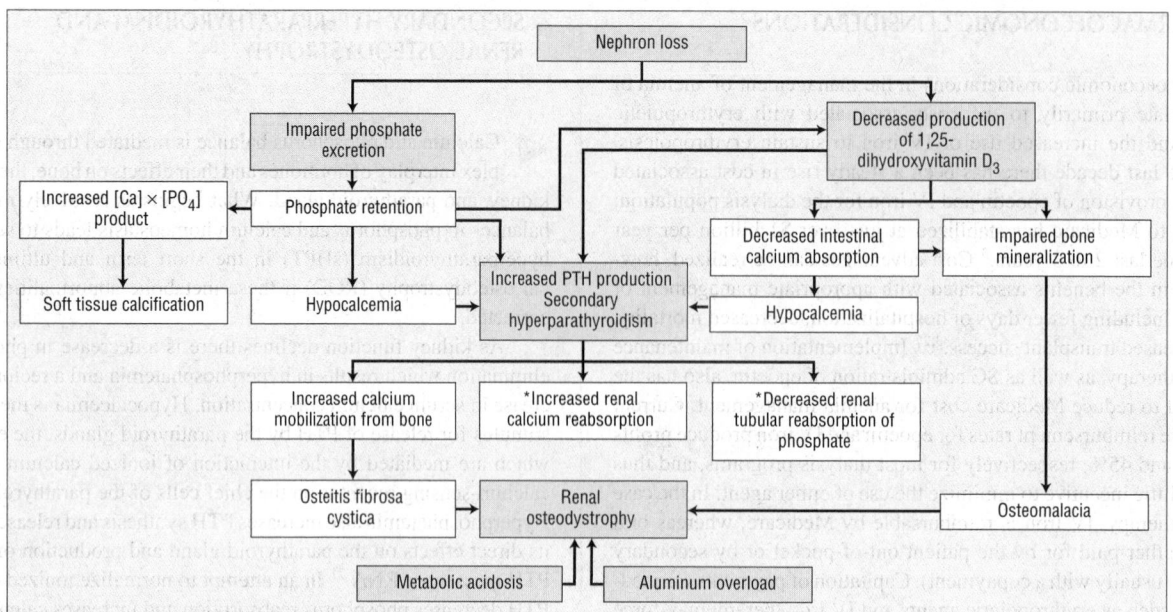

FIGURE 44–4. Pathogenesis of secondary hyperparathyroidism and renal osteodystrophy in patients with CKD. (These adaptations are lost as renal failure progresses.)

include osteitis fibrosa cystica (high bone turnover disease), osteomalacia (low bone turnover disease) and adynamic bone disease. Osteitis fibrosa cystica is characterized by areas of peritrabecular fibrosis. Dynamic measurements show a high bone formation rate, which results from high circulating concentrations of PTH. Osteomalacia was historically caused by aluminum toxicity in hemodialysis patients, a finding less common today with decreased use of aluminum-containing phosphate binders and changes in the processing of dialysate solutions to decrease aluminum absorption. Adynamic lesions are characterized by low amounts of fibrosis or osteoid tissue and low bone formation rates. The incidence of adynamic lesions has increased dramatically over the last 10 years, and may be present in as many as 50% of dialysis patients.[74] Multiple risk factors for the development of this bone disease have been identified: aluminum toxicity; high concentrations of dialysate calcium along with high doses of calcium-containing phosphate binders; aggressive management with vitamin D therapy; diabetes; and advanced age.[74] Symptoms often occur late, when significant skeletal damage has developed; therefore prevention is the key to management and controlling long-term complications.

Secondary HPT as evidenced by PTH levels >495 pg/mL in CKD patients has been associated with increased morbidity and mortality and sudden death in hemodialysis patients.[75] Other adverse consequences of sHPT include alterations in lipid metabolism, insulin secretion, resistance to erythropoietic therapy, and myocardial and skeletal muscle, as well as neurologic and immune functions.[76] An elevated calcium times phosphorus product (Ca × P) is also associated with poor outcomes, including vascular calcification, cardiovascular disease, calciphylaxis, and death.[77] In two large national cross-sectional samples of hemodialysis patients who had received dialysis for at least 1 year, elevated serum phosphorus levels and Ca × P were associated with increased risk of death.[77,78] Patients with a Ca × P >72 mg^2/dL^2 were found to have a 34% higher risk of death compared with patients with a Ca × P in the reference range of 43 to 52 mg^2/dL^2. Calcium scores, as measured by electron beam computed tomography, were significantly higher in hemodialysis patients than patients without kidney disease who had proven coronary artery disease (CAD). Intake of calcium from calcium-based binders also

appears to be a significant contributor to coronary artery calcification, even in young dialysis patients.[79] These data underscore the need to consider all the consequences of elevated PTH and Ca × P, not only ROD.

■ DESIRED OUTCOME

The overall goal of therapy is to prevent sHPT and ROD, and the detrimental consequences of these disorders, including cardiovascular and extravascular calcifications. While clinicians are becoming more aware of such consequences, efforts to improve evaluation and management in patients prior to development of more severe disease are needed. Over 50% of patients with Stage 4 CKD have abnormal bone histology despite having relatively normal PTH levels.[80] There is also need for improvement in management of metabolic disorders in dialysis patients. In a random sample of 612 hemodialysis patients, 50% had an intact PTH level more than three times the established range.[81] Hyperphosphatemia is present in about 70% of ESKD patients and 40% of these patients had values exceeding 6.5 mg/dL.[78] Data on medication use in patients with ESKD revealed that only 42% of hemodialysis and 33% of peritoneal dialysis patients were prescribed either oral (8% hemodialysis, 30% peritoneal dialysis patients) or IV (35% hemodialysis, 1% peritoneal dialysis) calcitriol, the only available vitamin D preparation at the time of data collection.[82] These evaluations show that many patients with CKD are receiving suboptimal management of their disorders of calcium, phosphorus, and PTH homeostasis.

K/DOQI guidelines for the diagnosis and management of bone disease in CKD proposed new criteria for calcium, phosphorus, Ca × P, and intact PTH (iPTH) based on the stage of CKD (Table 44–5).[18] The recommended corrected serum calcium for patients with Stage 3 or Stage 4 CKD, is within the normal range while the proposed upper range for patients with Stage 5 CKD is slightly lower than what is considered a normal total calcium. This is based on the observation of an increased risk of soft tissue and vascular calcifications in this population and the exposure to dialysate calcium.

TABLE 44–5. K/DOQI Guidelines for Calcium, Phosphorus, Calcium Phosphorus Product, and Intact Parathyroid Hormone

Parameter	Stage 3 CKD	Stage 4 CKD	Stage 5 CKD
Corrected calcium (mg/dL)	"Normal"	"Normal"	8.4–9.5
Phosphorus (mg/dL)	2.7–4.6	2.7–4.6	3.5–5.5
Ca × P (mg^2/dL^2)	<55	<55	<55
Intact PTH (pg/mL)	35–70	70–110	150–300

K/DOQI, Kidney Disease Outcomes Qualitiy Initiative.
From Eknoyan et al.[18]

It is important to note that these are calcium concentrations corrected for the degree of protein binding (i.e. corrected based on serum albumin concentration). The corrected calcium value should also used to determine the Ca × P product. Recommended serum phosphorus concentrations are 2.7 to 4.6 mg/dL, with higher concentrations acceptable in Stage 5 CKD. The proposed Ca × P of 55 mg^2/dL^2 is much lower than the historically accepted range of 65 to 70 mg^2/dL^2. The iPTH recommended for patients with Stage 4 or 5 CKD is above the normal range in order to prevent oversuppression of PTH and reduce the risk of adynamic bone disease. Serum aluminum levels should also be maintained below 20 mcg/L to minimize the risk of developing aluminum toxicity, a contributing factor to bone disease.[18]

PATIENT EVALUATION

Bone mineral density and serum calcium and calcitriol concentrations decrease progressively, while serum PTH, osteocalcin, bone-specific alkaline phosphatase, and phosphorus concentrations increase as GFR declines.[73] Evaluation of bone histology may be warranted in patients with severe sHPT or in Stage 4 or 5 CKD patients who develop symptoms. Bone disease can be diagnosed using iliac crest bone biopsy and bone histomorphometric analysis. Bone-mineral densitometry studies may also be used to detect bone loss in patients with CKD and are useful to follow progress after therapeutic intervention. Coronary artery calcification can be evaluated by noninvasive means using electron beam computed tomography. Invasive procedures such as coronary angiography can also be used to ascertain the degree of damage if the newer technology is not available.

Regular monitoring of serum aluminum levels should be done at least yearly and as frequently as every 3 months in patients receiving aluminum-containing phosphate binders or other aluminum-based medications, although regular use of these agents is not recommended in patients with CKD.[18] If aluminum concentrations are elevated (60 to 200 mcg/L) a deferoxamine (DFO) test should be done. The DFO infusion test is based on the concept that the amount of aluminum mobilized following a single dose of DFO is representative of the total body burden of aluminum. A dose of 5 mg/kg of DFO is administered, generally over the last hour of dialysis for hemodialysis patients. The serum aluminum level predose and 2 days postdose are compared. A change in serum aluminum concentration of ≥50 mcg/L is considered a positive test. A change of this magnitude in conjunction with a iPTH of <150 pg/mL is indicative of aluminum bone disease, which should then be confirmed by bone biopsy.[18]

PTH is secreted from the parathyroid gland as intact PTH, an 84-amino-acid peptide chain (1-84 PTH) that is biologically active, and as smaller carboxy-terminal PTH fragments.[83] Circulating levels of these fragments (e.g., 7-84 PTH) may increase substantially in patients

with CKD and have activity antagonistic to the effects to 1-84 PTH.[83] Available immunoradiometric and immunochemiluminescent assays for measurement of intact PTH such as the Nichols Institute Allegro IRMA measure not only the intact molecule, but also fragments, which may lead to overestimation of biologically active PTH. The goal iPTH based on this assay method in ESKD patients is three to five times the upper limits of normal (approximately 200 to 300 pg/mL). A new assay called the whole PTH or Bio-Intact PTH is now available that detects the full-length PTH molecule.[84] The predictive power of this newer assay and acceptable target ranges based on the stage of CKD have not been determined. The ratio of the 1-84 PTH to 7-84 PTH has also been evaluated as a tool to assess bone turnover and has been proposed as a better predictor of bone turnover than the other biochemical parameters.[85] Clinicians involved in the care of patients with CKD should become familiar with the tests used in their facilities in order to provide optimal care for their patients.

GENERAL APPROACH TO TREATMENT

ROD progresses insidiously for several years before patients become symptomatic. When symptoms such as bone pain and skeletal fractures occur, the disease is not easily amenable to treatment. Bone marrow fibrosis and decreased hematopoiesis are also consequences of severe osteitis fibrosa cystica. Therefore preventative measures should be initiated in patients in the early stages of CKD (GFR <60 mL/min).

Management of PTH, phosphorus, and calcium balance, and minimization of patient exposure to aluminum are important in preventing the development of sHPT and slowing or preventing the progression of ROD and associated consequences. Control of serum phosphorus is paramount since hyperphosphatemia is an initiating event in the development of other metabolic disturbances. Unfortunately, hyperphosphatemia is difficult to control and hypercalcemia may develop as a result of treatment with calcium-containing phosphate binders.[79] There are different considerations in management of sHPT based on the stage of CKD. Hyperphosphatemia and sHPT in patients with Stage 3 or Stage 4 CKD are often overlooked. If these patients are not evaluated early in the course of the disease, they have a higher likelihood of developing metabolic abnormalities that contribute to poor outcomes by the time they reach Stage 5 CKD. Patients with Stage 5 CKD usually require a combination of phosphate-binding medication and vitamin D therapy to slow the progression of sHPT, ROD, and cardiovascular and extravascular calcifications. Appropriate management includes all options identified for patients in earlier stages of CKD, with the exception that active vitamin D therapy is generally prescribed for a larger percentage of this population. The risks and benefits of phosphate-binding agents and the risks and benefits of vitamin D therapy must also be considered when choosing a treatment regimen (see section on pharmacologic therapy).

NONPHARMACOLOGIC THERAPY

Dietary Phosphorus Restriction

Dietary phosphorus restriction should be a first-line intervention for management of hyperphosphatemia in patients with CKD and should be initiated for most patients with Stage 3 or higher CKD. The K/DOQI guidelines recommend phosphorus restriction to 800 to 1000 mg/day when the upper levels of phosphorus are reached (see Table 44–5).[18] This recommendation also holds true for patients with iPTH levels above the recommended range, given the evidence that lowering phosphorus ingestion directly decreases PTH synthesis and secretion.[8,18] The challenge with dietary restriction of phosphorus is providing enough protein to prevent malnutrition, a common problem in the CKD population, since foods high in phosphorus are generally high in protein. Examples of foods or beverages that contain high amounts of phosphorus include meats, dairy products, dried beans, nuts, colas, peanut butter, and beer. Nutritional goals must be evaluated on an individual basis, preferably by a dietitian specializing in the care of CKD patients. Dialysis patients require a higher protein intake (1.2 to 1.3 g/kg per day) making restriction of phosphorus even more challenging. Removal of phosphorus does occur with peritoneal dialysis and hemodialysis (approximately 2 to 3 g/wk, dependent on the dialysis prescription); however, dialysis alone does not adequately control hyperphosphatemia for these patients.

One of the most common obstacles to the success of dietary restriction is patient noncompliance due to the poor palatability and inconvenience. Regular counseling by a dietitian is essential to improve patient compliance. As kidney function declines, dietary restriction alone is usually inadequate to control serum phosphorus, and phosphate-binding agents are necessary (see section on pharmacologic therapy).

Parathyroidectomy

Parathyroidectomy is the last therapeutic option for patients with sHPT. The K/DOQI guidelines for bone metabolism and disease recommend surgery only for those with persistently elevated iPTH (iPTH >800 pg/mL) associated with hypercalcemia and/or hyperphosphatemia that are refractory to medical therapy.[18] Surgical approaches include either subtotal parathyroidectomy or total parathyroidectomy with autotransplantation of parathyroid tissue to an accessible site, such as the forearm. Postoperative hypocalcemia, hypophosphatemia, and hypomagnesemia may occur because of a marked increase in bone production in relation to bone absorption ("hungry bone syndrome"). Following surgery frequent monitoring of ionized calcium is required (every 4 to 6 hours for the first 48 to 72 hours postsurgery). Ionized calcium should be maintained above 3.6 mg/dL (0.9 mmol/L) using calcium gluconate infusions if necessary. The recommended dose of calcium gluconate is 1 to 2 mg of elemental calcium per kilogram per hour, adjusted to maintain ionized calcium at 4.6 to 5.4 mg/dL (1.15 to 1.36 mmol/L). Once the ionized calcium is stable, oral therapy may be initiated with 1 to 2 g of calcium carbonate in conjunction with calcitriol in doses of up to 2 mcg per day. Adjustments in phosphate binders will also be necessary to maintain target phosphorus levels (see section on pharmacologic

therapy).[18] Treatment with supplemental calcium and vitamin D may be necessary for weeks or months.

PHARMACOLOGIC THERAPY

Phosphate Binding Agents

Pharmacology and Mechanism of Action. Drugs that bind dietary phosphorous in the GI tract form insoluble aluminum, calcium, or magnesium phosphate which is excreted in feces, thus reducing phosphorus absorption and serum phosphorus concentrations. A variety of phosphate-binding agents are available including calcium-, aluminum-, or magnesium-containing compounds and the nonelemental agent sevelamer hydrochloride (Table 44–6). Patients must be instructed to take these agents with meals to minimize absorption of phosphorus from dietary sources.

Efficacy. Oral calcium compounds are well established as first-line agents for control of both serum phosphorus and calcium concentrations, at least in the early stages of CKD when hypocalcemia is more common. Calcium carbonate and calcium acetate are the primary preparations used; calcium citrate is also available, but is not recommended since the citrate component increases aluminum absorption. The chloride salt is also not recommended since it is very astringent and unpalatable, and absorbed chloride may contribute to systemic acidosis. Calcium carbonate is marketed in a variety of dosage forms (see Table 44–6) and is relatively inexpensive. Unfortunately, many calcium carbonate products are considered food supplements and thus are not required by law to meet United States Pharmacopeia (USP) disintegration and dissolution requirements. In general, nationally advertised brands meet USP quality standards for disintegration and dissolution, but it is difficult to determine whether private label or house brands conform to these standards. Variability in gastric pH may also affect disintegration or dissolution, and thus phosphate binding efficacy.[86] Calcium carbonate is more soluble in an acidic medium, and therefore should be administered prior to meals when stomach acidity is highest. In addition, acid-suppressing agents such as ranitidine or proton pump inhibitors may reduce the phosphate-binding activity of calcium carbonate by increasing gastric pH. Calcium acetate binds approximately twice as much phosphorus as calcium carbonate at comparable doses of elemental calcium.[87] Increased binding potency limits GI calcium absorption; however, calcium acetate is more soluble, and therefore better absorbed than calcium carbonate in an alkaline pH, which may explain the similar incidence of hypercalcemia. Patients with a corrected calcium of less than 8.4 mg/dL should receive calcium carbonate or calcium acetate as a calcium supplement (with or without vitamin D therapy).

Although calcium-containing phosphate-binding agents continue to be used as first-line therapy, their chronic use may increase the risk for vascular and tissue calcification.[79] The K/DOQI guidelines now recommend that the total dose of elemental calcium provided by calcium-containing binders not exceed 1500 mg per day and the total daily intake from all sources not exceed 2000 mg.[18] This presents clinicians with a challenge for patients in whom maximum doses do not achieve the goal phosphorus or who have an elevated serum calcium. In such situations, a non–calcium-based binder alone or in combination with a calcium product may be needed. Calcium-containing binders are not recommended in dialysis patients when on two consecutive measurements the serum calcium is >10.2 mg/dL or the iPTH is <150 pg/mL.[18]

TABLE 44–6. Phosphate-Binding Agents Used in the Treatment of Hyperphosphatemia in CKD

Compound	Trade Name	Compound Content (mg)	Elemental Calcium Content (mg)	Starting Doses	Comments
Calcium carbonate[a] (40% elemental calcium)	Tums	500, 750, 1000, 1250	200, 300, 400, 500	0.5–1 g (elemental calcium) three times a day with meals	First-line agent; dissolution characteristics and phosphate binding affect may vary from product to product; try to limit daily intake of elemental calcium to 1500 mg/day
	Oscal-500	1250	500		Approximately 39 mg phosphorus bound per 1 g calcium carbonate
	Caltrate 600	1500	600		
	Nephro-Calci	1500	600		
	LiquiCal	1200	480		
	CalciChew	1250	500		
Calcium acetate (25% elemental calcium)	PhosLo	667	167	0.5–1 g (elemental calcium) three times a day with meals	First-line agent; comparable efficacy to calcium carbonate with half the dose of elemental calcium; do not exceed 1.5 mg of elemental calcium per day
					Approximately 45 mg phosphorus bound per 1 g calcium acetate
					By prescription only
Sevelamer	Renagel	400, 800	—	800 mg three times a day with meals	First-line agent; lowers LDL cholesterol
					More expensive than calcium products; preferred in patients at risk for extraskeletal calcification
Aluminum hydroxide	Alterna GEL	600 mg/5 mL	—	300–600 mg three times a day with meals	Third-line agents; do not use concurrently with citrate-containing products
	Amphojel	300, 600 (tablet) 320 mg/ 5 mL (suspension)			Reserve for short-term use (4 weeks) in patients with hyperphosphatemia not responding to other binders
	Alu-Cap	400			
Aluminum carbonate	Basaljel	500 (tablet, capsule) 400 mg/5 mL (suspension)		450–500 mg three times a day with meals	Same as for aluminum hydroxide
Magnesium carbonate	Mag-Carb	70 mg capsule	—	70 mg three times a day with meals	Third-line agent; diarrhea common; monitor serum magnesium
Magnesium hydroxide	Milk of magnesia	300, 600 (tablet) 400 mg/5 mL, 800 mg/5 mL (suspension)	—	300–400 mg three times a day with meals	Same as for magnesium carbonate
Magnesium carbonate/ calcium carbonate	MagneBind 200	200 mg	160	200 mg three times a day with meals (based on magnesium content)	Same as for calcium carbonate and magnesium carbonate

[a]Multiple preparations available which are not listed.
LDL, low-density lipoprotein.

Sevelamer hydrochloride is a nonabsorbable hydrogel phosphate-binding agent which does not contain aluminum, calcium, or magnesium.[88] The dosage needed to control serum phosphorus concentrations may be as high as 6.3 g/day.[88] Sevelamer also significantly lowers low-density lipoprotein (LDL) cholesterol and resulted in an elevation in high-density lipoprotein (HDL) by a mean of 30% and 18%, respectively. This is an added beneficial effect in a population at risk for cardiovascular events. Recent evidence has shown a decreased rate of vascular calcification in hemodialysis patients receiving this agent relative to those prescribed calcium-containing binders.[89] Sevelamer is now recommended as primary therapy in dialysis patients with severe vascular or soft tissue

calcifications, and may also be used as a first-line phosphate-binding agent in patients with Stage 5 CKD.[18] The cost of sevelamer may be a limiting factor for some patients.

Aluminum salts were widely used in the 1980s as phosphate-binding agents because of their high binding potency. They should be considered as third-line agents now and be reserved for acute treatment of severe hyperphosphatemia or used at low doses in combination with either calcium-containing binding agents or sevelamer hydrochloride in cases of hyperphosphatemia that is not responding to therapy with a single agent. The duration of aluminum therapy should be limited to 4 weeks.[18] Magnesium-containing antacids are also effective phosphate binders and may decrease the amount of calcium-containing binders necessary for control of phosphorus. Their use may be limited by the frequent occurrence of GI side effects. Other phosphate binders being investigated include lanthanum carbonate, an agent that has demonstrated significant efficacy as measured by decreases in phosphorus, Ca × P, and PTH when compared with placebo.[90] Ferric salts have been shown to bind with intestinal phosphorus in animal and human studies, although the clinical application of these results needs to be confirmed in subsequent clinical trials.[91]

Adverse Effects. Adverse effects of calcium-containing phosphate binders are generally limited to GI side effects including constipation, diarrhea, nausea, vomiting, and abdominal pain. The risk of hypercalcemia is also a concern and may necessitate restriction of calcium intake from the combination of calcium-containing binders and dietary intake. Aluminum binders can no longer be recommended as first-line therapy because of the CNS toxicity and the worsening of anemia associated with aluminum accumulation. While an effective phosphate binder, use of magnesium is often limited by side effects including diarrhea, abdominal cramps, hypermagnesemia, and hyperkalemia.

Drug-Drug and Drug-Food Interactions. Calcium-containing phosphate-binding agents interfere with the absorption of several other oral medications that are commonly prescribed for CKD patients, including oral iron and zinc and quinolone antibiotics. Data regarding drug interactions with sevelamer are limited; however, in recent evaluations no drug interactions with digoxin, warfarin, metoprolol, or enalapril were observed.[92,93] Many phosphate binders are marketed as antacids or calcium supplements and often CKD patients do not know why they have been prescribed these agents. Regular patient counseling by a pharmacist is essential to enhance compliance and minimize the potential for drug interactions.

Dosing and Administration. Starting doses of phosphate binding agents are listed in Table 44–6. Doses should be titrated to achieve the recommended serum phosphorus concentrations yet avoid complications such as hypercalcemia.

Vitamin D Therapy

Vitamin D compounds include ergocalciferol (vitamin D_2) and cholecalcifediol (vitamin D_3) that must be converted to the active form in the kidney. Calcitriol (1,25-dihydroxyvitamin D_3) is the most active form of vitamin D and is available as an oral formulation (Rocaltrol) as well as an IV formulation (Calcijex). The currently available vitamin D analogs include paricalcitol (19-nor-1,25-dihydroxyvitamin D_2; Zemplar), doxercalciferol (1-α-hydroxyvitamin D_2; Hectorol) and 1-α-hydroxyvitamin D_3 (alfacalcidol, not available in the United States). Calcitriol or one of the vitamin D analogs is required for patients with severe kidney disease since these agents do not require conversion by the kidney to the most biologically active form.

Pharmacology and Mechanism of Action. Active vitamin D suppresses PTH secretion by stimulating absorption of serum calcium (and phosphorus) by intestinal cells and through direct activity on the parathyroid gland to decrease PTH synthesis. As a result, the serum calcium concentration is raised and the parathyroid glands decrease the rate of secretion and formation of PTH. The set point for calcium (i.e., the calcium concentration at which PTH secretion is decreased by 50%), which is generally raised in sHPT, is lowered when active vitamin D therapy is initiated. This indicates that a lower ionized calcium concentration is effective at suppressing secretion of PTH. All of these actions are mediated by the interaction of vitamin D with vitamin D receptors (VDRs) which are located in many organs, including the parathyroid gland, GI tract, and kidney.[94] Calcitriol also upregulates VDRs, which ultimately may reduce parathyroid hyperplasia. Unfortunately, the enhanced GI absorption of calcium and phosphorus with calcitriol therapy frequently leads to hypercalcemia and hyperphosphatemia. There is also evidence that hyperphosphatemia results in resistance to the PTH-suppressing effects of vitamin D analogs and directly stimulates PTH release. These actions contribute to the increase in the Ca × P product, which can lead to soft-tissue and vascular calcification.[78,79] Therefore control of calcium and phosphorus must be achieved before vitamin D therapy is initiated.

The unique interactions of vitamin D with the VDRs have been a focus of research and have led to the development of vitamin D analogs, which vary in their affinity for this receptor and thus may result in less hypercalcemia, while retaining the positive physiologic actions on bone and parathyroid tissue.[94] Paricalcitol and doxercalciferol are D_2 compounds which effectively lower PTH in dialysis patients.[95,96] Paricalcitol differs from calcitriol by the absence of the exocyclic carbon 19 and the fact that it is a vitamin D_2 derivative. Currently this analog is available only for IV administration; however, an oral formulation is in development. Doxercalciferol, in contrast to calcitriol and paricalcitol, is a prohormone that needs to be hydroxylated in the liver to its active 1,25-dihydroxyvitamin D_2 product. Doxercalciferol is available for both IV and oral administration.

Pharmacokinetics. Calcitriol can be administered orally as well as by IV injection. Oral absorption occurs rapidly; therefore oral and IV therapies are both reasonable options for treatment of sHPT. While historically a topic of controversy, a review of the available literature has led to the conclusion that intermittent IV administration of calcitriol is more effective than daily oral calcitriol for sHPT.[18] Paricalcitol is administered intravenously and its half-life is similar to that of calcitriol (up to 30 hours). Doxercalciferol as a prodrug has a slightly prolonged half-life of 45 hours, although this difference is not of clinical significance.

Efficacy. Administration of calcitriol by either the oral or IV route may be based on conventional dosing (usually 0.25 to 0.5 mcg/day) or pulse dosing (0.5 to 2 mcg two to three times per week). Logistically, IV dosing is more practical in hemodialysis patients, while oral therapy is more practical for those with Stage 1 through 4 CKD and peritoneal dialysis patients. Conventional daily oral doses of calcitriol (0.25 mcg) may be more frequently associated with hypercalcemia and hyperphosphatemia, since VDRs are located in intestinal mucosa where direct stimulation can occur. Effects such as this reinforce the importance of regular monitoring of calcium and phosphorus.

When administered at doses ten times that of calcitriol and at a dose equivalent to doxercalciferol, paricalcitol has been less frequently associated with hypercalcemia in animal studies and in human trials.[97,98] Doxercalciferol has also been associated with a lower incidence of hypercalcemia.[96] While hypercalcemia is less likely, based on differences in selectivity of these analogs for the VDRs, elevated calcium concentrations have been observed with these agents in patients with ESKD. However, some of these cases were associated with excessive dosing of these agents and oversuppression of PTH, a condition more likely to promote hypercalcemia.[99] Limited data are available regarding the use of vitamin D analogs in patients with

TABLE 44-7. Dosing Recommendations for Vitamin D in Patients with Stage 3 and 4 CKD

Definition	Serum 25(OH)D[a] (ng/mL)	Dose of Ergocalciferol[b]
Severe vitamin D deficiency	<5	50,000 international units/wk PO × 12 weeks, then monthly × 6 months or 500,000 international units as a single IM dose
Mild vitamin D deficiency	5–15	50,000 international units/wk PO × 4 weeks, then monthly × 6 months
Vitamin D insufficiency	16–30	50,000 international units/month PO × 6 months

[a]25 (OH) D, 25 hydroxyvitamin D.
[b]25 (OH) D levels should be measured following the 6-month course of therapy for patients with mild and severe vitamin D deficiency.
From Eknoyan et al.[18]

early CKD; doxercalciferol has been shown to reduce PTH in this population.[100] Clinical trials are ongoing to evaluate an oral formulation of paricalcitol in patients with Stage 3 and 4 CKD.

Although comparisons between vitamin D analogs are relatively limited, fewer cases of hyperphosphatemia have been reported with paricalcitol than calcitriol. While the degree of suppression of PTH was similar with both agents, a trend toward a more rapid suppression of PTH was seen in paricalcitol-treated patients.[101] An improvement in 3-year survival in a large dialysis population receiving paricalcitol was also recently noted compared with a historic cohort that received calcitriol.[102] These findings are encouraging, but will require confirmation in prospective randomized trials.

Adverse Effects. While all agents are effective in suppressing PTH levels, they differ in the degree to which they cause other metabolic abnormalities. Adverse effects of note with vitamin D therapy in patients treated for sHPT include hypercalcemia and hyperphosphatemia. Differences in calcitriol and vitamin D analogs have been demonstrated in animal studies and in clinical trials evaluating the effect on reduction of PTH while minimizing the risk of these adverse consequences.

Drug-Drug and Drug-Food Interactions. Cholestyramine may reduce the absorption of orally administered calcitriol and doxercalciferol. No other significant interactions have been reported.

Dosing and Administration. Recommendations for vitamin D therapy differ based on the stage of CKD.[18] Changes in vitamin D metabolism may lead to deficiencies in vitamin D precursors in patients with Stage 3 or 4 CKD. Therefore 25-hydroxyvitamin D levels should be measured in patients with PTH values above the upper recommended ranges of 70 pg/mL or 110 pg/mL for Stage 3 and 4 CKD, respectively (see Table 44–5). If the 25-hydryoxyvitamin D level is less than 30 ng/mL, a vitamin D precursor (e.g., ergocalciferol) is recommended (Table 44–7).[18] To prevent vitamin D insufficiency, doses of 600 to 800 units per day of ergocalciferol are recommended. According to the guidelines, active vitamin D or an analog should be administered orally (e.g., as oral calcitriol or doxercalciferol) when PTH remains elevated despite adequate 25-hydroxyvitamin D levels.

Active vitamin D therapy should be initiated in patients with Stage 3 or 4 CKD with oral calcitriol 0.25 mcg per day or oral doxercalciferol 2.5 mcg three times per week. Prior to starting therapy the serum calcium and phosphorus should be well controlled (serum calcium <9.5 mg/dL and phosphorus <4.6 mg/dL) to minimize the risk of hypercalcemia and an elevated Ca × P. In patients with Stage 5 CKD there is a clearly defined role for treatment with active vitamin D or a vitamin D analog since the conversion of precursors to active vitamin D is impaired. Dosing recommendations based on PTH are provided in Table 44–8. Serum calcium and Ca × P should be monitored regularly while the patient is receiving therapy.[18]

TABLE 44-8. Dosing Recommendations for Vitamin D in Patients with Stage 5 CKD on Hemodialysis (HD)[a]

PTH (pg/mL)	IV and PO Calcitriol Dose per HD	IV Paricalcitol Dose per HD	PO and IV Doxercalciferol Dose per HD
300–600[b]	0.5–1.5 mcg PO or IV	2.5–5 mcg	5 mcg PO 2 mcg IV
600–1000[b]	1–4 mcg PO 1–3 mcg IV	6–10 mcg	5–10 mcg PO 2–4 mcg IV
>1000[c]	3–7 mcg PO 3–5 mcg IV	10–15 mcg	10–20 mcg PO 4–8 mcg IV

[a]Peritoneal dialysis patients may be treated with PO doses of calcitriol (0.5–1.0 mcg) or doxercalciferol (2.5–5 mcg) two or three times weekly. May also use PO calcitriol at 0.25 mcg daily.
[b]If serum calcium <9.5 mg/dL, phosphorus <5.5 mg/dL, and Ca × P <55 mg²/dL².
[c]If serum calcium <10 mg/dL, phosphorus <5.5 mg/dL, and Ca × P <55 mg²/dL².
PTH, parathyroid hormone.
From Eknoyan et al.[18]

The recommended starting dose in patients with ESKD is calcitriol 0.5 to 1.5 mcg IV or paricalcitol 0.04 to 0.08 mcg/kg IV (range, 2.5 to 5 mcg) with each dialysis session, based on the level of PTH.[18] Dose adjustments should be made every 2 to 4 weeks based on PTH concentrations. For patients who need to be converted from calcitriol to paricalcitol, a dosing conversion ratio of 1:4 of IV calcitriol to paricalcitol has been proposed; however, some suggest a ratio of 1:3 to avoid oversuppression of PTH.[18,103] Starting doses of paricalcitol have also been dosed based on initial PTH levels (PTH/80).[104] The recommended starting dose of doxercalciferol in ESKD patients is 2 mcg IV or 5 mcg administered orally three times per week, with dosing titration based on changes in PTH.[18]

Calcimimetics

Pharmacology and Mechanism of Action.

Cinacalcet hydrochloride (Sensipar) is a calcimimetic agent recently approved for treatment of sHPT in ESKD patients and for treatment of hypercalcemia in patients with parathyroid carcinoma. Cinacalcet is the first agent in this class to receive FDA approval. This compound acts on the calcium-sensing receptor on the surface of the chief cell of the parathyroid gland to mimic the effect of extracellular ionized calcium and increase the sensitivity of the calcium-sensing receptor to calcium, subsequently reducing PTH secretion.

Pharmacokinetics.

The maximum plasma concentration of cinacalcet is achieved in approximately 2 to 6 hours following oral administration. The half-life is approximately 30 to 40 hours. Cinacalcet has a large volume of distribution (approximately 1000 L), and is 93% to 97% bound to plasma proteins, both characteristics indicating that removal by dialysis is negligible. Cinacalcet is metabolized by the liver, specifically by the cytochrome P450 isoenzymes CYP3A4, CYP2D6, and CYP1A2.[105]

Efficacy.

In placebo-controlled clinical trials conducted in dialysis patients (predominantly those receiving hemodialysis) cinacalcet significantly decreased PTH and the Ca × P product within the 6-month study period, regardless of the severity of sHPT.[106,107] The starting dose of 30 mg per day was titrated every 3 or 4 weeks to a maximum dose of 180 mg per day to achieve the target PTH of ≤250 pg/mL and avoid hypocalcemia. Approximately 66% and 93% of patients in the clinical trials were receiving concurrent vitamin D and phosphate binders, respectively. If a patient experienced symptoms of hypocalcemia or had a serum calcium <8.4 mg/dL, calcium supplements and/or calcium-based phosphate binders could be increased. If ineffective, the vitamin D dose could be increased. The median dose required to achieve the desired PTH by the end of the study period was 90 mg. The challenge to clinicians now that this agent is approved is in deciding how to most effectively use cinacalcet in conjunction with other therapies for hyperphosphatemia and sHPT.

Adverse Effects.

The most frequently reported adverse events with cinacalcet were nausea and vomiting. Although nausea and vomiting occurred more frequently with cinacalcet, these events were generally transient, mild to moderate in nature, and infrequently led to withdrawal from clinical trials.[105]

Cinacalcet lowers serum calcium and may cause hypocalcemia; therefore this agent should not be started if the serum calcium is less than the lower limit of normal, approximately 8.4 mg/dL. Serum calcium should be measured within 1 week after initiation or dose adjustment of cinacalcet. Once the maintenance dose has been established, serum calcium should be measured approximately monthly. Potential manifestations of hypocalcemia include paresthesias, myalgias, cramping, tetany, and convulsions.

Drug-Drug and Drug-Food Interactions.

Since cinacalcet is metabolized by multiple hepatic enzymes there is potential for drug interactions. Cinacalcet is also a potent inhibitor of the enzyme CYP2D6. As a result, dose adjustments of concomitant medications that are predominantly metabolized by this enzyme and have a narrow therapeutic index such as flecainide, thioridazine, vinblastine, and most tricyclic antidepressants (i.e., amitriptyline) may be required.[105]

Several agents commonly used in the CKD population have been evaluated for interactions with cinacalcet.[105] Coadministration of calcium carbonate or sevelamer did not affect the pharmacokinetics of cinacalcet. Pantoprazole did not alter the pharmacokinetics of cinacalcet HCl, an important finding since pantoprazole alters gastric pH, and the solubility of cinacalcet decreases as the gastric pH rises over 5.5. Coadministration of cinacalcet with warfarin also did not affect the pharmacokinetics of warfarin. Coadministration of cinacalcet and ketoconazole, a strong inhibitor of CYP3A4, resulted in an increase in the area under the curve and maximum concentration of 2.3 and 2.2 times, respectively. Concurrent administration of cinacalcet with amitriptyline increased amitriptyline exposure and nortriptyline (active metabolite) exposure by approximately 20% in CYP2D6-extensive metabolizers.

Food has been shown to increase absorption of cinacalcet by up to 81% compared to fasting; therefore this medication should be taken with meals to achieve the maximal effect.

Dosing and Administration.

The recommended starting oral dose of cinacalcet is 30 mg once daily. The dose should be titrated every 2 to 4 weeks to a maximum dose of 180 mg once daily to achieve the desired PTH levels and maintain near normal serum calcium concentrations. Patients with hepatic disease may require lower doses, as studies have shown a decrease in metabolism of cinacalcet in this patient population. Cinacalcet is available as a film-coated tablet containing 30, 60, or 90 mg.

PHARMACOECONOMIC CONSIDERATIONS

Pharmacoeconomic considerations in the management of sHPT and ROD include medication costs, the cost associated with laboratory procedures (e.g., monitoring of 25-hydroxyvitamin D and more frequent evaluation of iPTH in patients with Stage 3 or 4 CKD), and the medical expenditures associated with the management of cardiovascular disease and bone fractures. The pattern of vitamin D product use in U.S. dialysis units has been strongly influenced by Medicare reimbursement. Currently, IV vitamin D products are separately reimbursable expenses for dialysis programs. In fact, dialysis programs often generate significant profit from the IV administration of these agents to patients on dialysis. In contrast, oral medications such as calcitriol and doxercalciferol are more convenient for patients with Stage 3 or 4 CKD and the peritoneal dialysis population; however, these agents are not separately reimbursable, and because they must be purchased by the patient, compliance becomes an issue.

The cost:benefit ratio associated with more aggressive management of metabolic disorders (e.g., hyperphosphatemia and hypercalcemia) and sHPT has not been formally evaluated. If the associated complications such as vascular and soft tissue calcifications that may increase morbidity and hospitalizations can be significantly reduced, the additional medication costs may ultimately be of minimal consequence.

CLINICAL CONTROVERSY

Some clinicians advocate use of the Bio-Intact PTH, which detects the full-length 84–amino acid active peptide chain, as opposed to the intact PTH, which also detects active and inactive fragments. The Bio-Intact PTH/Intact PTH ratio, an index of the active fraction of PTH, has also been evaluated as a clinical monitoring tool; however, additional studies are needed to determine how values for the Bio-Intact PTH and this ratio correlate with bone formation and turnover in patients with CKD.

EVALUATION OF THERAPEUTIC OUTCOMES

The goals for treatment with dietary phosphate restriction, phosphate-binding agents, vitamin D therapy, and/or calcimimetic therapy are to prevent sHPT and subsequent ROD without inducing adynamic bone disease from oversuppression of PTH or vascular or extravascular calcifications. Regular monitoring of serum calcium, phosphorus, Ca × P, iPTH, and vitamin D status to achieve and maintain target goals is currently the most practical and effective means of achieving these outcomes.

The serum calcium, phosphorus, and iPTH levels should be measured in all patients with a GFR of less than 60 mL/min.[18] Patients with Stage 3 or Stage 4 CKD should have follow-up measurements done at least every 12 months and every 3 months, respectively. More frequent monitoring is required for Stage 5 CKD patients; monitor iPTH every 3 months and calcium and phosphorus every month. More frequent monitoring (monthly for iPTH and every 2 weeks for calcium and phosphorus) may be warranted following any change in the therapeutic interventions to correct these abnormalities.

METABOLIC ACIDOSIS

ETIOLOGY

Individuals with normal kidney function generate enough hydrogen ion to reclaim all filtered bicarbonate and to secrete approximately 1 mEq/kg per day of hydrogen ions, which are generated from the metabolism of dietary proteins (see Chap. 51). As a result they maintain a constant body fluid pH through the buffering of hydrogen ion by proteins, hemoglobin, phosphate, and especially bicarbonate. Renal ammoniagenesis and phosphate excretion buffer the urine and facilitate acid excretion. In severe CKD, all filtered bicarbonate is reclaimed, but the ability of the kidneys to synthesize ammonia is impaired. This decrease in urinary buffer results in decreased net acid excretion and continuous positive hydrogen ion balance; thus metabolic acidosis develops. A clinically significant metabolic acidosis is commonly seen when the GFR drops below 20 to 30 mL/min (Stage 4 CKD). In these patients the plasma bicarbonate concentration tends to stabilize at 15 to 20 mEq/L.

DESIRED OUTCOME

The goals of therapy for patients with CKD are to normalize the pH of the blood (pH of approximately 7.35 to 7.45) and maintain the serum bicarbonate within the normal range (22 to 28 mEq/L). In patients on hemodialysis, the goal of therapy is to maintain a predialysis or stabilized bicarbonate concentration at or above 22 mEq/L.[16]

The prevention and treatment of severe metabolic acidosis in patients with kidney disease is also important to prevent the development of renal bone disease, fatigue, decreased exercise tolerance, reduced cardiac contractility, and increased ventricular irritability. Metabolic acidosis also appears to stimulate protein catabolism, which can contribute to a negative nitrogen balance and lower albumin concentrations, as well as cause growth retardation in children.[16] Lower serum bicarbonate levels in peritoneal dialysis patients have also been associated with a higher hospitalization rate and longer hospital stays.[16] Severe acidemia (blood pH <7.1 to 7.2) suppresses myocardial contractility, predisposes patients to cardiac arrhythmias, and may lead to a decrease in total peripheral vascular resistance and blood pressure, reduced hepatic blood flow, and impaired oxygen delivery.[108]

GENERAL APPROACH TO EVALUATION AND TREATMENT

Arterial blood gases and serum electrolytes should be measured regularly in patients with CKD. These patients should also have a complete medical history and review of medications to determine if there are other potential causes of acid-base disturbances (e.g., diabetic ketoacidosis, ingestion of toxins, or GI disorders). The anion gap, indicating the differences in unmeasured anions and cations, should also be calculated (see Chap. 51). An elevated anion gap (>17 mEq/L) is often present in those with CKD due to the accumulation of organic anions, phosphates, and sulfates.

Treatment of metabolic acidosis in patients with CKD generally includes administration of bicarbonate to correct academia, the time course of which depends on the severity of the acidosis. Asymptomatic patients with mild acidosis (bicarbonate of 12 to 20 mEq/L; pH of 7.2 to 7.4) generally do not require emergent therapy and gradual correction over days to weeks is appropriate.

NONPHARMACOLOGIC THERAPY

Therapy for metabolic acidosis requires pharmacologic intervention to correct the acidemia. Treatment of other underlying disorders that may be contributory is also warranted.

PHARMACOLOGIC THERAPY

In patients with Stage 3 or higher CKD, the use of alkalinizing salts, such as sodium bicarbonate or citrate/citric acid preparations, is useful to replenish depleted body bicarbonate stores. Sodium bicarbonate tablets are manufactured in 325- and 650-mg strengths (a 650-mg tablet contains 7.7 mEq sodium and 7.7 mEq bicarbonate). Shohl's solution and Bicitra contain 1 mEq/mL of sodium and the equivalent of 1 mEq/mL of bicarbonate as sodium citrate/citric acid. Citrate is metabolized in the liver to bicarbonate, and citric acid is metabolized to CO_2 and water. Polycitra, which contains potassium citrate, (1 mEq/mL of sodium, 1 mEq/mL of potassium, and 2 mEq/mL of bicarbonate) should not be used in patients with severe CKD since hyperkalemia may result.

The replacement dose of alkali (base) needed to restore the serum bicarbonate concentration to normal (24 mEq/L) can be approximated by multiplying the volume of distribution of bicarbonate (0.5 L/kg) by the patient's body weight (in kilograms) and their base deficit (difference between the patient's serum bicarbonate value and 24 mEq/L). The calculated amount of bicarbonate replacement therapy (in milliequivalents) should be administered over several days to prevent volume overload from excessive sodium intake. After the serum bicarbonate has normalized, a maintenance regimen of bicarbonate to neutralize daily acid production may be all that is necessary (12 to 20 mEq/day in divided doses). Doses are subsequently titrated to maintain normal plasma bicarbonate concentrations. Patients with renal tubular acidosis may require higher doses of alkalinizing agents (see Chap. 51). Fluid balance should be monitored carefully because of the sodium content of these agents. Citrate-containing solutions should not be used in combination with aluminum-containing compounds because they can enhance aluminum absorption and increase the risk of aluminum intoxication. Excessive doses of alkalinizing agents may cause metabolic alkalosis, as well as lethargy or cardiac depression secondary to a decrease in ionized serum calcium concentration. Gastrointestinal distress characterized by gastric distention and flatulence is relatively common with high doses of oral sodium bicarbonate. Patients with severe acidosis (serum bicarbonate <8 mEq/L; pH <7.2) may require IV therapy (see Chap. 51).

Metabolic acidosis in both adult and pediatric patients undergoing dialysis can often be managed by using higher concentrations of bicarbonate or acetate in the dialysate (>38 mEq/L bicarbonate is safe and effective). Administration of oral bicarbonate salts as described above may also be necessary for some patients.

Tromethamine (tris-hydroxymethyl aminomethane) and Carbicarb (sodium carbonate and sodium bicarbonate) are alternative alkalinizing agents that have been evaluated for treatment of more severe acidemia. There are extremely limited data regarding their use in patients with CKD, which precludes their use in this population.[108]

EVALUATION OF THERAPEUTIC OUTCOMES

Regular monitoring of arterial blood gases and serum electrolytes are necessary to determine the effectiveness of therapy. A gradual correction is appropriate to avoid overcorrection and subsequent complications such as alkalosis and other electrolyte abnormalities (see Chap. 51). Laboratory measurement of serum bicarbonate is associated with several technical problems. Blood collection techniques, transportation, and assay methodology can affect the measured concentrations. Blood samples should not have contact with air; process delays should be avoided; and consistent analytical methods should be used with serial measurements to improve accuracy.[16]

TREATMENT OF CARDIOVASCULAR DISEASE IN CKD

Mortality secondary to cardiovascular disease is 10 to 30 times greater in dialysis patients than in the general population.[9] In addition to traditional cardiac risk factors such as diabetes, hypertension, hyperlipidemia, tobacco use, and physical inactivity, patients with kidney disease have other unique risk factors. Among these are hyperhomocysteinemia, elevated levels of C-reactive protein, increased oxidant stress, and hemodynamic overload.[109] Complications previously discussed such as anemia and metabolic disorders of CKD are also contributory. In particular, arterial vascular disease (i.e., atherosclerosis) and cardiomyopathy are the primary types of cardiovascular disorders present in the CKD population.[9] These disorders lead to development of ischemic heart disease and its manifestations including myocardial infarction. As a predominant comorbidity, cardiovascular disorders and their sequela are the leading cause of death in the ESKD population.[3,5]

ETIOLOGY AND EPIDEMIOLOGY

Hypertension

As a primary cause or a consequence of progressive loss of kidney function, hypertension is prevalent in the majority of patients with Stage 3 or 4 CKD (see Chap. 43). Approximately 80% to 90% of patients initiating dialysis are hypertensive.[110] The pathogenesis of hypertension in CKD is multifactorial, but in many hypertensive dialysis patients, fluid retention is a major contributor.[110] In addition to the general pathophysiologic mechanisms responsible for the development of hypertension, patients with ESKD may also have increased sympathetic activity, the presence of an endogenous digitalis-like substance, elevated levels of endothelin-1, erythropoietin use, hyperparathyroidism, and structural changes in the arteries (e.g., metastatic calcification) as contributing factors.[110]

Patients with ESKD also display an abnormal diurnal blood pressure rhythm as evidenced by the fact that their blood pressure does not decrease during the nighttime hours.[110] It is unclear what causes this disturbance in the diurnal rhythm, but this "nondipping" phenomenon indicates sustained elevations in blood pressure are present over a prolonged period of time when compared to the general population.

Hyperlipidemia

CKD with or without nephrotic syndrome is frequently accompanied by abnormalities in lipoprotein metabolism. It is well established that dyslipidemias cause atherosclerotic cardiovascular disease and there are many compelling reasons to aggressively treat these disorders.[111] A clear association between hypercholesterolemia, hypertriglyceridemia, or other lipoprotein changes in patients with CKD and the high incidence of cardiovascular disease has not been demonstrated in large prospective studies. However, it is likely that the same lipoprotein abnormalities that confer increased risk of cardiovascular disease in the general population would also be harmful to patients with kidney disease. A low or declining serum cholesterol in patients with ESKD is also indicative of malnutrition and is associated with increased mortality.[16] Thus a fine balance must be struck to optimize patient outcomes.

The few epidemiologic studies in CKD patients with nephrotic syndrome suggest that their relative risk of coronary death or myocardial infarction is higher than that of matched controls.[112] Similar analyses have been done in CKD patients without nephrotic syndrome and in patients on dialysis; low HDL, high triglycerides, high apolipoprotein B, and high lipoprotein (a) were all associated with a higher risk of cardiovascular disease.[112] The findings are not uniform, as hypertriglyceridemia alone has not been shown to be a strong independent risk factor for coronary heart disease in patients with normal kidney function.[111] However, hypertriglyceridemia may reduce levels of "protective" HDL, which is now classified as a major risk factor for coronary heart disease. Based on these findings and the high prevalence of atherosclerotic cardiovascular disease in patients with CKD, this population is considered to be in the highest-risk group for such cardiovascular conditions (i.e., equivalent to that of patients with known coronary heart disease).[111]

The prevalence of hyperlipidemia appears to increase as kidney function declines.[112] In patients with CKD without nephrotic syndrome, hypertriglyceridemia (plasma concentrations >200 mg/dL) is observed in approximately 40% to 50% of patients. In addition, 20% to 30% of these patients have total cholesterol levels greater than 240 mg/dL, while 10% to 45% have LDL concentrations >130 mg/dL.

Although the concentrations of LDL are not uniformly increased in patients with kidney disease, these patients appear to produce small, dense LDL particles that are more susceptible to oxidation and more atherogenic than larger LDL subfractions. Other lipoprotein abnormalities include a reduction in HDL concentrations in 25% to 30% of patients, as well as changes in apoprotein content of lipoprotein molecules.[112,113] Peripheral insulin resistance, carnitine deficiency, and hyperparathyroidism may also contribute to lipid abnormalities. For patients with CKD and a urinary protein excretion greater than 3 g/day, the major lipid abnormalities are elevation of plasma total and LDL cholesterol (prevalence 85% to 90%), with approximately 50% of patients experiencing a low HDL cholesterol (<35 mg/dL), while 60% of patients have triglyceride concentrations greater than 200 mg/dL.[112] Treatment of proteinuria resolves the hyperlipidemia in most patients with nephrotic syndrome.

DESIRED OUTCOME

Hypertension

Goals of antihypertensive therapy in patients with CKD are to lower blood pressure to target levels and reduce the risk of cardiovascular disorders. The target blood pressure in patients with ESKD is not well defined. The potential complications of decreasing diastolic blood pressures to below 80 mm Hg, as recommended for patients with Stage 1 through 4 CKD, may outweigh the benefits in this population. Thus different blood pressure goals may need to be set for individual patients based on their clinical status, age, and cardiovascular condition. A target blood pressure in ESKD patients of less than 150/90 mm Hg has been proposed to reduce the risk of associated cardiovascular disorders, yet keep patients hemodynamically stable during dialysis, when hypotension may occur as the result of volume status changes during treatment.[110] Hypertension is not adequately controlled in as many as 50% of ESKD patients, especially those with diabetes.[110]

Hyperlipidemia

Based on strong evidence of risk reduction and the benefits of lipid-lowering therapy in the general population, and the high prevalence of atherosclerotic cardiovascular disease in patients with CKD, the consensus is that CKD patients should be treated aggressively for dyslipidemia to an LDL-C goal below 100 mg/dL.[17,111] Goals for patients with Stage 5 CKD based on lipid abnormality and the appropriate course of therapy are listed in Table 44–9.

PATIENT EVALUATION

Hypertension

Patients with ESKD should have blood pressure monitored at every scheduled clinic visit (or hemodialysis session) and they should be encouraged to learn how to monitor their blood pressure while at home. These patients should also be evaluated for existing cardiovascular conditions and cardiovascular risk factors. Goals of therapy can be achieved using lifestyle modifications in conjunction with antihypertensive therapy. While these strategies are similar to those used in the general population with hypertension, certain aspects of selection of pharmacologic therapy and dietary instructions are unique to the population with CKD. Recommendations for antihypertensive therapy in patients with CKD are often extrapolated from results of studies conducted in the normal population, as CKD patients are generally excluded from these studies.

Hyperlipidemia

A complete fasting lipid profile including total cholesterol, LDL, HDL, and triglycerides should be done in all CKD patients. Lipoprotein levels may be influenced by several factors including GFR and proteinuria. It is recommended that these patients have their lipid profile assessed more frequently than in the general population in order to identify abnormalities and treat them early. In patients on hemodialysis the lipid profile should be done prior to dialysis or on nondialysis days.[17] Patients should also be evaluated for other conditions that are known to cause dyslipidemias (e.g., liver disease and hypothyroidism).

NONPHARMACOLOGIC THERAPY

Hypertension

The primary intervention for management of hypertension in patients with Stage 1, 2, and 3 CKD is sodium restriction to approximately 2 to 3 g/day. Fluid intake should be restricted in patients with volume overload, and particularly in patients on hemodialysis, who are at risk for substantial fluid accumulation between dialysis sessions. Regular dietary counseling becomes critical to the success of nonpharmacologic interventions, given the large number of lifestyle changes typically required by CKD patients. Other lifestyle modifications

TABLE 44–9. Management of Dyslipidemia in Patients with CKD

Dyslipidemia	Goal	Initial Therapy	Modification in Therapy[a]	Alternative[a]
TG ≥500 mg/dL	TG <500 mg/dL	TLC	TLC + fibrate or niacin	Fibrate or niacin
LDL 100–129 mg/dL	LDL <100 mg/dL	TLC	TLC + low-dose statin	Bile acid sequestrant or niacin
LDL ≥130 mg/dL	LDL <100 mg/dL	TLC + low-dose statin	TLC + max dose statin	Bile acid sequestrant or niacin
TG ≥200 mg/dL and non-HDL ≥130 mg/dL	Non-HDL <130 mg/dL	TLC + low-dose statin	TLC + max dose statin	Fibrate or niacin

[a]Dosing of selected agents by class: fibrate (gemfibrozil 600 mg twice a day); niacin (1.5–3 g/day of immediate-release product); statin (simvastatin 10–40 mg/day if glomerular filtration rate [GFR] <30 mL/min, 20–80 mg/day if GFR >30 mL/min); bile acid sequestrant (cholestyramine 4–16 g/day). HDL, high-density lipoprotein; LDL, low-density lipoprotein; Non-HDL, total cholesterol minus HDL cholesterol; TG, triglycerides; TLC, therapeutic lifestyle changes.
See Chap. 21 for more complete dosing information.
From K/DOQI Clinical Practice Guidelines.[17]

including regular exercise, weight loss, and smoking cessation are also recommended, but difficult to implement.

In hemodialysis patients, achievement of an individual's "dry weight" and control of total-body sodium through the dialytic process may control blood pressure (see Chap. 45). The effects of salt restriction and aggressive ultrafiltration were studied in a small number of hemodialysis patients (n = 19) over 12 months.[114] After 3 months blood pressure was controlled to <140/90 mm Hg and decreases in left ventricular mass index were observed at the end of the study period. Prolonged hemodialysis (8-hour sessions three times per week) has also been shown to maintain normal blood pressures and reduce the need for antihypertensive medications in ESKD patients.[110] A lag phenomenon in blood pressure reduction following achievement of "dry weight" was also shown in this population. Blood pressure continued to fall over several months while using the "dry-weight" method of blood pressure control.[115] However, the majority of hemodialysis programs in the United States use shorter dialysis methods (3- to 4-hour sessions three times per week).

Hyperlipidemia

In patients with elevated triglyceride levels (≥500 mg/dL) and/or LDL between 100 and 129 mg/dL, lifestyle changes are recommended (see Chap. 21). Unfortunately, most patients with CKD have already been advised to adhere to difficult dietary regimens, which may include protein, phosphorus, sodium, potassium, and fluid restrictions, as well as diabetic exchanges. Thus although diet therapy is a reasonable first-step approach, it may not be successful in many patients with CKD because of noncompliance. A dietitian who is well versed in the management of kidney disease should be consulted.

PHARMACOLOGIC THERAPY

Hypertension

Most patients with hypertension and CKD require drug regimens that include three or more antihypertensive agents to achieve target blood pressure.[116] Blood pressure reductions can be achieved with agents in all antihypertensive classes, and choice should be guided by the individual patient's concomitant disease states.

Diuretic therapy is beneficial for management of blood pressure in patients with early CKD; however, thiazide diuretics are not generally effective in patients with a GFR of <30 mL/min. Loop diuretics can be used throughout all stages of CKD. In most cases the dose must be increased as kidney function declines, to achieve a similar degree of blood pressure reduction. Patients with ESKD who have minimal to no residual renal function are especially poor responders to these agents.

Angiotensin-converting enzyme inhibitors (ACEIs) or angiotensin receptor blockers (ARBs) are the preferred agents for patients with progressive CKD. They are also effective in patients with ESKD because of the important role the renin-angiotensin axis plays in the etiology of some cases of dialysis-resistant hypertension.[110,117] ACEIs may also be of benefit since they are associated with substantial reductions in left ventricular mass in patients with ESKD.[117] Lower initial doses of these agents may be necessary since the elimination half-lives of the parent compound (captopril and lisinopril) or active metabolite (enalapril, benazepril, or ramipril) are prolonged in ESKD patients. ARBs have not been well studied in patients with ESKD. One notable difference when compared to ACEIs is that ARBs do not affect bradykinin metabolism, thus they are not expected to cause anaphylactoid reactions when used in conjunction with polyacrylonitrile dialysis membranes. Available ARBs do not require dosage adjustment for decreased kidney function and they are not effectively removed by hemodialysis.

Calcium channel blockers, particularly the dihydropyridines, which selectively lower systemic vascular resistance, also appear to be effective in the treatment of hypertension in patients with ESKD. β-Blockers may be particularly useful in hypertensive CKD patients given the beneficial effects post–myocardial infarction. Agents such as esmolol, timolol, pindolol, metoprolol, or labetalol, which are metabolized and not significantly removed by dialysis, may be easier to dose titrate than agents that are both dialyzable and extensively eliminated unchanged by the kidney (e.g., acebutolol, atenolol, bisoprolol, and nadolol). Agents requiring less frequent dosing may be used to improve patient compliance.

Use of other antihypertensive agents in the patient with CKD should be based on recommendations in the general population (see Chap. 13).[116] In the ESKD population there may be some special considerations for use of other antihypertensive therapy. Agents that act on the sympathetic nervous system, such as prazosin, terazosin, doxazosin, clonidine, guanabenz, and guanfacine, may be required in patients unresponsive to ACEIs, calcium channel blockers, or β-blocker therapy used in conjunction with adequate dialysis. Central α_2-agonists such as clonidine appear to be the safest of these agents; however, adverse effects such as dry mouth may lead to extra fluid consumption in some patients. Postsynaptic α-blockers (e.g., prazosin) are associated with postural hypotension following hemodialysis. Guanethidine and methyldopa should be avoided because of potential complications, including severe postural hypotension, severe dialysis-related hypotension, and impotence. The addition of vasodilators such as minoxidil or hydralazine may prove useful in patients resistant to combinations of the previously mentioned agents. The incidence of systemic lupus erythematosus associated with the use of hydralazine does not appear to be increased by the presence of ESKD. Minoxidil therapy may be associated with pericardial effusion and profound reflex tachycardia, which can be suppressed with either the addition of a β-blocker or a central α-adrenoreceptor agonist.

Hyperlipidemia

Management of dyslipidemia in patients with CKD should be based on the report from the National Cholesterol Education Program and the K/DOQI guidelines for dyslipidemia in patients with CKD.[17,111] If lifestyle changes are not effective in achieving goal triglyceride and LDL levels after a few months, drug therapy is warranted (see Table 44–9). Drug therapy is also recommended for those with more extreme elevations in LDL (≥130 mg/dL).

Drug classes that may prove useful in treatment of lipid disorders include: 3-hydroxy-3-methylglutaryl coenzyme A (HMG-CoA) reductase inhibitors (statins); the bile acid sequestrants; nicotinic acid; and fibric acids (gemfibrozil and clofibrate). Statins are the most effective drugs for lowering LDL and total cholesterol in patients with kidney disease (with or without nephrotic syndrome) and should generally be regarded as the drugs of first choice.[17,112] Drug therapy for hypertriglyceridemia includes a fibrate or nicotinic acid; in general fibrates are better tolerated. Statins are indicated to lower LDL to acceptable levels in CKD patients, based on efficacy and additional benefits observed in the general population, including the reduction in cardiovascular events and all-cause mortality.[17]

Several potential drug interactions and/or side effects have been observed in those CKD patients receiving antilipemic therapy. The nonselective binding activity of bile acid sequestrants may reduce absorption of corticosteroids, digoxin, thiazide diuretics, warfarin, and other commonly used medications. Myositis and myalgias, along with increased serum creatine phosphokinase (CPK), may occur in ESKD patients who use clofibrate. Determining the optimal dose of clofibrate in this patient population is difficult, as plasma protein-binding changes markedly affect free concentrations of the active metabolite, clofibric acid, which has a prolonged half-life in patients with Stage 5 CKD. Gemfibrozil may be a safer alternative, as the half-life is not altered with kidney dysfunction. Lower doses of 300 mg twice a day with close monitoring of CPK is recommended by some clinicians, based on an association of standard dose therapy with increases in CPK concentrations in dialysis patients.

Although HMG-CoA reductase inhibitors are remarkably free of adverse effects in otherwise healthy subjects, one should be cognizant of the potential myotoxic effects of these drugs, especially when administered with interacting agents including, but not limited to, azole antibiotics, cyclosporine, gemfibrozil, niacin, and in the presence of hepatic disease.[17] Patients receiving sevelamer as a phosphate binder may reap the benefits of its cholesterol-lowering effects.[118]

The best approach to the treatment of hyperlipidemia in patients with nephrotic syndrome is to induce remission of the disease (see Chap. 47), or at least to reduce urine protein excretion by aggressive treatment of concurrent hypertension and/or administration of ACEIs or ARBs.[17] Several trials have assessed the effect of L-carnitine supplementation on abnormal lipid metabolism in dialysis patients, but results have been contradictory.[119]

PHARMACOECONOMIC CONSIDERATIONS

Hypertension

Compliance and economic factors must be considered in the selection of antihypertensive therapy for CKD patients. Patients with ESKD are prescribed an average of 9 to 12 medications. Choosing agents that can be administered once or twice daily may improve patient compliance. In addition, there are now many options within some antihypertensive classes, such as calcium channel blockers, ACEIs, ARBs, and β-blockers, which allow for less frequent dosing. In most cases, no clear therapeutic advantage has been demonstrated with any particular agent within a class. Therefore selecting the least costly agent that can be administered once or twice daily is reasonable.

As more information becomes available from studies evaluating the effects of long-term therapy of hypertension on cardiovascular events in patients with ESKD, cost benefits from potentially decreasing the occurrence of such events and their comorbidities may be quantified.

Hyperlipidemia

Statin therapy for treatment of dyslipidemias has been shown to be cost-effective in patients at high risk for coronary heart disease. While this has not specifically been evaluated in patients with CKD, this population is considered in the highest-risk group for coronary heart disease and cardiovascular events. It may be reasonable at least in theory to extrapolate this information on the cost benefits of therapy to the CKD population.

CLINICAL CONTROVERSY

Currently there is no consensus on the target blood pressure for patients with ESKD. Maintaining a blood pressure of <150/90 mm Hg has been proposed to maintain hemodynamic stability, particularly in the hemodialysis patient, who has frequent shifts in volume status and is thus at high risk for hypotension during and postdialysis.

EVALUATION OF THERAPEUTIC OUTCOMES

Hypertension

Blood pressure monitoring to determine the effectiveness of therapy should be done at each visit for patients with ESKD, particularly following initiation of therapy (nonpharmacologic or pharmacologic). The importance of home monitoring becomes essential in those patients for whom dose titration and close follow-up is required. Patients on hemodialysis should have blood pressure measured before, during, and after dialysis to determine the effect of changes in their volume status on blood pressure in conjunction with medication therapy. Patients may need to adjust the time of administration of antihypertensive therapy relative to the dialysis session if hypotension during dialysis is problematic. Such decisions should be based on the pharmacokinetic profile of the antihypertensive agent in patients with ESKD. In cases when antihypertensive agents need to be discontinued, they should be withdrawn slowly. Other aspects of monitoring blood pressure and associated complications may be found in Chap. 13.

Hyperlipidemia

Patients should have their lipid profile reassessed 2 to 3 months following a change in treatment and at least annually. Periodic evaluations of cardiovascular performance and cardiovascular condition as described in Chap. 21 are also warranted in this patient population.

TREATMENT OF OTHER COMPLICATIONS OF CKD

NUTRITIONAL STATUS

Protein-energy malnutrition is very common among patients with advanced CKD (Stages 4 and 5; see Chap. 139).[16] Causes of malnutrition in these patients include inadequate food intake secondary to anorexia, altered taste sensation, intercurrent illness, and the unpalatablity of prescribed diets. Other factors such as the effect of the dialysis procedure on removal of nutrients, hypercatabolism induced by other inflammatory conditions, and blood loss are also contributory. Protein restriction as an intervention to potentially delay progression of kidney disease in patients with Stage 3 or 4 CKD may also lead to protein malnutrition by the time a patient reaches ESKD; therefore the risks vs. the benefits of this intervention must be considered on an individual basis (see Chap. 43). Hypoalbuminemia and malnutrition have a strong association to mortality in chronic dialysis patients.[16]

Patients with ESKD have increased nutritional needs relative to the general population, based on the effect of the disease state and the dialysis procedure on nutritional status. The recommended dietary protein intake in chronic hemodialysis patients is 1.2 g/kg body weight per day.[16] The recommended intake for chronic peritoneal dialysis patients is at least 1.2 to 1.3 g/kg body weight per day, based on the increased protein loss that occurs with this dialysis modality.[16] Protein requirements are higher in patients who are acutely ill (see Chap. 139). The recommended total daily energy intake in both hemodialysis and peritoneal dialysis patients is 35 kcal/kg body weight per day.[16] For peritoneal dialysis patients, this includes intake from both diet and that obtained from the glucose absorbed from peritoneal dialysate. For patients older than 60 years of age this criterion differs, since increasing age is generally associated with reduced physical activity and lean body mass. Daily energy intake for these patients is 30 to 35 kcal/kg per day.[16] Nutritional support should be considered for those patients who cannot achieve these goals with oral intake alone. Another option for nutritional supplementation in patients on hemodialysis includes interdialytic parenteral nutrition (see Chap. 139).

Vitamin requirements for ESKD patients receiving dialysis differ from those of a healthy person because of dietary modifications, kidney dysfunction, and dialysis therapy.[120] The plasma concentrations of vitamins A and E are elevated in ESKD, while those of the water-soluble vitamins (B_1, B_2, B_6, B_{12}, niacin, pantothenic acid, folic acid, biotin, and vitamin C) tend to be low in this population, in large part due to the fact that many are dialyzable. The goal for vitamin supplementation in this population should be to prevent subclinical and frank deficiency and to avoid pathology from overdosage. Special vitamin supplements have been formulated for the dialysis population, which primarily include B vitamins with C and folic acid.

Supplementation with L-carnitine has been advocated for its potential benefits in patients with ESKD including management of hypertriglyceridemia, hypercholesterolemia, and anemia.[119] In the hemodialysis population L-carnitine may improve complications of dialysis, including intradialytic arrhythmias and hypotension, low cardiac output, interdialytic and postdialytic symptoms of malaise or asthenia, general weakness or fatigue, skeletal muscle cramps, and decreased exercise capacity or low peak oxygen consumption. While some of these benefits have been demonstrated, the evidence does not strongly support routine supplementation with L-carnitine in patients with ESKD. Cost and the addition of yet another medication to the already complex regimen prescribed for many of these patients also mitigates against the routine use of this agent. The K/DOQI nutrition guidelines recommend supplementation with L-carnitine only if the disorders for which L-carnitine has shown some benefit are not responding to standard therapies.[16]

▪ UREMIC BLEEDING

Bleeding complications in patients with CKD are usually mild, but can result in major hemorrhagic events. The primary mechanisms underlying the hemostatic problem are platelet biochemical abnormalities and alterations in platelet–vessel wall interactions. Decreased platelet aggregation and adhesiveness have been shown in a number of studies.[121] Additionally, there is a decreased plasma concentration and defective binding of the large multimer of von Willebrand factor (vWF), which results in abnormal platelet–blood vessel wall interactions. Patients on hemodialysis are at even greater risk of bleeding due not only to the hemodialysis process itself, but from administration of other medications. Heparin is frequently administered during dialysis procedures to prevent clotting during dialysis. Patients at high risk for bleeding may require alternative anticoagulation procedures rather than traditional hemodialysis with systemic heparinization (see Chap. 45). In addition, dialysis patients often receive systemic anti-

coagulation (warfarin) or antiplatelet therapy (aspirin or clopidogrel) for prevention of access clotting or other cardiovascular disorders.

There are several nondialytic adjunctive therapies that may temporarily shorten the increased bleeding time observed in patients with kidney disease.[121] Cryoprecipitate is rich in factor VIII, fibrinogen, and fibronectin, and shortens bleeding time in 50% of uremic patients within 1 hour.[121] Desmopressin (1-deamino-8-D-arginine vasopressin) has minimal vasoconstrictive effects as compared to vasopressin, but effectively releases autologous factor VIII (vWF) from the endothelial lining of vessel walls. A consistent lowering of bleeding time has been observed with intravenous, subcutaneous, and intranasal routes of administration. A drawback to the use of desmopressin is tachyphylaxis with repeated doses; response may return after 3 to 4 days. This effect is felt to be caused by depletion of vWF stores following the first dose.

Administration of estrogens has also been effective as an intervention to reduce bleeding time in uremic patients, an intervention studied based on the observation that women with von Willebrand's disease improved during pregnancy.[121] The mechanism of action is unknown. Oral conjugated estrogens and low-dose transdermal patches have also been shown to be effective.[121] Side effects, which are uncommon and usually mild, include hot flashes, nausea, vomiting, hypertension, gynecomastia, and loss of libido. An increased risk of thromboembolism may result from estrogen therapy, especially with chronic use.[122]

▪ GASTROINTESTINAL DISORDERS

Anorexia, hiccups, and a metallic taste in the mouth are common as kidney disease becomes more severe. Nausea, vomiting, diarrhea, or abdominal distention may also occur. Gastric and colonic mucosal ulcerations and telangiectasias with resultant gastrointestinal bleeding are common. Ascites may develop secondary to fluid overload or peritoneal serositis.

▪ IMMUNE FUNCTION

Infectious diseases are common and result in significant morbidity and mortality in patients with ESKD.[3] Although multiple abnormalities in host defenses and an increased susceptibility to infection have been described, the causal link between these observations remains speculative. Absolute lymphopenia and impaired cell-mediated immunity are common in ESKD patients and may be caused by uremic toxins or protein-calorie malnutrition. Although plasma concentrations of IgG, IgM, and IgA are usually normal, antibody responses appear to be significantly depressed.[123] Patients requiring dialysis have many problems with vascular access which puts them at higher risk for exposure to infectious sources. The risk of infections in patients with CKD, and particularly ESKD, is an important consideration when reviewing the clinical presentation of a patient, as hospitalization rates for infection and sepsis have increased dramatically in the last 10 years.[3]

▪ PRURITUS

Despite advances in dialysis treatment, pruritus (itching) remains a problem for 60% to 90% of ESKD patients.[124] The pathogenesis of uremic pruritus is poorly understood, but has been attributed to multiple factors such as inadequate dialysis, skin dryness, secondary hyperparathyroidism, increased vitamin A and histamine plasma concentrations, and increased sensitivity to histamine. This complication of ESKD is extensively reviewed in Chap. 45.

NEUROLOGIC ABNORMALITIES

Uremic encephalopathy occurs as a result of the effects of uremia on the central nervous system and is associated with symptoms including alterations in consciousness, thinking, memory, speech, psychomotor behavior, and emotion. Sensory and motor function may be altered, particularly affecting leg nerves, resulting in leg cramps and restless leg syndrome. Uremic encephalopathy is less common because of earlier initiation of dialysis in patients with Stage 5 CKD.

Peripheral neuropathy is also common with advanced CKD and is typically indistinguishable from other types of neuropathy (e.g., diabetic neuropathy). Symptoms are often uncomfortable for the patient and prompt many clinicians to initiate pharmacologic therapy in an attempt to reduce these symptoms. Tricyclic antidepressants (e.g., amitriptyline) and anticonvulsants (e.g., phenytoin and gabapentin) may have some benefit in alleviating symptoms of neuropathy; however, risks and benefits must be considered for agents such as gabapentin, which is eliminated exclusively by the kidney and itself may cause neurologic symptoms with accumulation. Abnormalities of the autonomic nervous system that may occur with advanced CKD include postural hypotension, impotence, impaired sweating, and alterations in gastric motility.

ENDOCRINE DISORDERS

A variety of endocrine and metabolic abnormalities are common with CKD. Most patients have symptoms of hypothyroidism (low energy, cold intolerance, and constipation), but typically the levothyroxine (T_4) concentration is low and the thyroid-stimulating hormone concentration is normal.[125] Hypothermia is common; body temperatures are approximately $1°F$ lower as compared to individuals with normal kidney function. Hyperglycemia secondary to peripheral resistance to insulin can occur. Diabetic patients with CKD may present with more frequent hypoglycemic episodes because the kidney is responsible in large part for the degradation of insulin. Insulin doses often must be adjusted downward as kidney disease progresses. Primary hypogonadism as well as hypothalamic abnormalities contribute to sexual dysfunction and sterility.

ABBREVIATIONS

ACEI: angiotensin-converting enzyme inhibitor
AIDS: acquired immunodeficiency syndrome
ARB: angiotensin receptor blocker
Ca × P: calcium phosphorus product; serum calcium multiplied by serum phosphorus
CKD: chronic kidney disease
CPK: creatine phosphokinase
DFO: deferoxamine
EPO: erythropoietin
ESKD: end-stage kidney disease
ESRD: end-stage renal disease
FE_K: fractional excretion of potassium
FE_{Na}: fractional excretion of sodium
GFR: glomerular filtration rate
Hct: hematocrit
HDL: high-density lipoprotein
Hgb: hemoglobin
HMG-CoA: 3-hydroxy-3-methylglutaryl coenzyme A (reductase)
iPTH: intact parathyroid hormone
LDL: low-density lipoprotein
LVH: left ventricular hypertrophy
MCV: mean corpuscular volume
NKF-K/DOQI: National Kidney Foundation-Kidney Disease Outcomes Quality Initiative
PTH: parathyroid hormone
ROD: renal osteodystrophy
sHPT: secondary hyperparathyroidism
TIBC: total iron-binding capacity
TSat: transferrin saturation
VDR: vitamin D receptor
vWF: von Willebrand factor

Review Questions and other resources can be found at *www.pharmacotherapyonline.com.*

REFERENCES

1. Sarnak MJ. Cardiovascular complications in chronic kidney disease. Am J Kidney Dis 2003;41(5 Suppl):11–17.
2. Pereira BJ. Overcoming barriers to the early detection and treatment of chronic kidney disease and improving outcomes for end-stage renal disease. Am J Manag Care 2002;8(4 Suppl):S122–S135.
3. USRDS: The United States Renal Data System. Am J Kidney Dis 2003; 42(6 Pt 6):1–230.
4. Jones CA, et al. Serum creatinine levels in the US population: Third National Health and Nutrition Examination Survey. Am J Kidney Dis 1998;32:992–999.
5. K/DOQI clinical practice guidelines for chronic kidney disease: Evaluation, classification, and stratification. Kidney Disease Outcomes Quality Initiative. Am J Kidney Dis 2002;39(2 Suppl 2):S1–S246.
6. Ringoir S. An update on uremic toxins. Kidney Int Suppl 1997;62:S2–S4.
7. Astor BC, et al. Association of kidney function with anemia: The Third National Health and Nutrition Examination Survey (1988–1994). Arch Intern Med 2002;162:1401–1408.
8. Slatopolsky E, Brown A, Dusso A. Pathogenesis of secondary hyperparathyroidism. Kidney Int Suppl 1999;73:S14–S19.
9. Sarnak MJ, et al. Kidney disease as a risk factor for development of cardiovascular disease: A statement from the American Heart Association Councils on Kidney in Cardiovascular Disease, High Blood Pressure Research, Clinical Cardiology, and Epidemiology and Prevention. Hypertension 2003;42:1050–1065.
10. Collins AJ, et al. Chronic kidney disease and cardiovascular disease in the Medicare population. Kidney Int Suppl 2003;87:S24–S31.
11. Owen WF, Jr. Patterns of care for patients with chronic kidney disease in the United States: Dying for improvement. J Am Soc Nephrol 2003; 14(Suppl 2):S76–S80.
12. St Peter WL, et al. Chronic kidney disease: Issues and establishing programs and clinics for improved patient outcomes. Am J Kidney Dis 2003;41:903–924.
13. Collins AJ. Anaemia management prior to dialysis: Cardiovascular and cost-benefit observations. Nephrol Dial Transplant 2003;18(Suppl 2): ii2–6.
14. Biesenbach G, et al. Predialysis management and predictors for early mortality in uremic patients who die within one year after initiation of dialysis therapy. Ren Fail 2002;24:197–205.

15. NKF-K/DOQI Clinical Practice Guidelines for Anemia of Chronic Kidney Disease: Update 2000. Am J Kidney Dis 2001;37(Suppl 1): S182–S238.

16. Clinical practice guidelines for nutrition in chronic renal failure. K/DOQI, National Kidney Foundation. Am J Kidney Dis 2000; 35(Suppl 2):S1–S140.

17. K/DOQI Clinical Practice Guidelines for managing dyslipidemias in patients with chronic kidney disease. Am J Kidney Dis 2003;41(Suppl 3): S1–S91.

18. Eknoyan G, Levin A, Levin NW. Bone metabolism and disease in chronic kidney disease. Am J Kidney Dis 2003;42(Suppl 3):1–201.

19. Abosaif NY, et al. K/DOQI clinical practice guidelines on hypertension and antihypertensive agents in chronic kidney disease. Am J Kidney Dis 2004;43(Suppl 1):S1–290.

20. Shemin D, Dworkin LD. Sodium balance in renal failure. Curr Opin Nephrol Hypertens 1997;6:128–132.

21. Erslev AJ. Erythropoietin. N Engl J Med 1991;324:1339–1344.

22. Obrador GT, et al. Trends in anemia at initiation of dialysis in the United States. Kidney Int 2001;60:1875–1884.

23. Walters BA, et al. Health-related quality of life, depressive symptoms, anemia, and malnutrition at hemodialysis initiation. Am J Kidney Dis 2002;40:1185–1194.

24. Levin A. Clinical epidemiology of cardiovascular disease in chronic kidney disease prior to dialysis. Semin Dial 2003;16:101–105.

25. Ross SD, et al. The effect of anemia treatment on selected health-related quality-of-life domains: A systematic review. Clin Ther 2003;25:1786–1805.

26. Besarab A, et al. The effects of normal as compared with low hematocrit values in patients with cardiac disease who are receiving hemodialysis and epoetin. N Engl J Med 1998;339:584–590.

27. Collins AJ. Influence of target hemoglobin in dialysis patients on morbidity and mortality. Kidney Int Suppl 2002;80:44–48.

28. Stevens L, Stigant C, Levin A. Should hemoglobin be normalized in patients with chronic kidney disease? Semin Dial 2002;15:8–13.

29. Tsuchiya K, et al. Content of reticulocyte hemoglobin is a reliable tool for determining iron deficiency in dialysis patients. Clin Nephrol 2003;59:115–123.

30. Macdougall IC, Steering Committee of the CREATE trial, CREATE Study Group. CREATE: New strategies for early anaemia management in renal insufficiency. Nephrol Dial Transplant 2003;18(Suppl 2):ii13–6.

31. Van Wyck DB. Management of early renal anaemia: Diagnostic work-up, iron therapy, epoetin therapy. Nephrol Dial Transplant 2000; 15(Suppl 3):36–39.

32. Johnson CA. Use of androgens in patients with renal failure. Semin Dial 2000;13:36–39.

33. Golper TA, et al. L-carnitine treatment of anemia. Am J Kidney Dis 2003;41(Suppl 4):S27–S34.

34. Nissenson AR, et al. Clinical evaluation of heme iron polypeptide: Sustaining a response to rHuEPO in hemodialysis patients. Am J Kidney Dis 2003;42:325–330.

35. Mydlik M, et al. Oral use of iron with vitamin C in hemodialyzed patients. J Ren Nutr 2003;13:47–51.

36. Seligman P, et al. Single-dose pharmacokinetics of sodium ferric gluconate complex in iron-deficient subjects. Pharmacotherapy 2004; 24:564–573.

37. Besarab A, Kaiser JW, Frinak S. A study of parenteral iron regimens in hemodialysis patients. Am J Kidney Dis 1999;34:21–28.

38. Kato A, et al. Effect of weekly or successive iron supplementation on erythropoietin doses in patients receiving hemodialysis. Nephron 2001; 89:110–112.

39. Schaefer RM, Bahner U. Iron metabolism in rhEPO-treated hemodialysis patients. Clin Nephrol 2000;53(Suppl):S65–S68.

40. Fishbane S. Safety in iron management. Am J Kidney Dis 2003; 41(5 Suppl):18–26.

41. Fletes R, et al. Suspected iron dextran-related adverse drug events in hemodialysis patients. Am J Kidney Dis 2001;37:743–749.

42. Michael B, et al. Sodium ferric gluconate complex in hemodialysis patients: Adverse reactions compared to placebo and iron dextran. Kidney Int 2002;61:1830–1839.

43. Charytan C, et al. Efficacy and safety of iron sucrose for iron deficiency in patients with dialysis-associated anemia: North American clinical trial. Am J Kidney Dis 2001;37:300–307.

44. Auerbach M, et al. A randomized trial of three iron dextran infusion methods for anemia in EPO-treated dialysis patients. Am J Kidney Dis 1998;31:81–86.

45. Dahdah K, Patrie JT, Bolton WK. Intravenous iron dextran treatment in predialysis patients with chronic renal failure. Am J Kidney Dis 2000;36:775–782.

46. Folkert VW, et al. Chronic use of sodium ferric gluconate complex in hemodialysis patients: Safety of higher-dose (> or = 250 mg) administration. Am J Kidney Dis 2003;41:651–657.

47. Blaustein DA, et al. The safety and efficacy of an accelerated iron sucrose dosing regimen in patients with chronic kidney disease. Kidney Int Suppl 2003;87:S72–S77.

48. Chandler G, Harchowal J, Macdougall IC. Intravenous iron sucrose: Establishing a safe dose. Am J Kidney Dis 2001;38:988–991.

49. Parkkinen J, et al. Catalytically active iron and bacterial growth in serum of haemodialysis patients after i.v. iron-saccharate administration. Nephrol Dial Transplant 2000;15:1827–1834.

50. Canziani ME, et al. Risk of bacterial infection in patients under intravenous iron therapy: Dose versus length of treatment. Artif Organs 2001;25:866–869.

51. Kletzmayr J, Horl WH. Iron overload and cardiovascular complications in dialysis patients. Nephrol Dial Transplant 2002;17(Suppl 2):25–29.

52. Bolanos L, et al. Continuous intravenous sodium ferric gluconate improves efficacy in the maintenance phase of EPOrHu administration in hemodialysis patients. Am J Nephrol 2002;22:67–72.

53. Darbepoetin alfa package insert. Thousand Oaks, CA, Amgen, Inc., 2002.

54. Egrie JC, Browne JK. Development and characterization of novel erythropoiesis stimulating protein (NESP). Nephrol Dial Transplant 2001;16(Suppl 3):3–13.

55. Ateshkadi A, et al. Pharmacokinetics of intraperitoneal, intravenous, and subcutaneous recombinant human erythropoietin in patients on continuous ambulatory peritoneal dialysis. Am J Kidney Dis 1993;21:635–642.

56. Macdougall IC, et al. Pharmacokinetics of novel erythropoiesis stimulating protein compared with epoetin alfa in dialysis patients. J Am Soc Nephrol 1999;10:2392–2395.

57. McClellan WM, et al. Subcutaneous erythropoietin results in lower dose and equivalent hematocrit levels among adult hemodialysis patients: Results from the 1998 End-Stage Renal Disease Core Indicators Project. Am J Kidney Dis 2001;37:E36.

58. Kaufman JS, et al. Subcutaneous compared with intravenous epoetin in patients receiving hemodialysis. Department of Veterans Affairs Cooperative Study Group on Erythropoietin in Hemodialysis Patients. N Engl J Med 1998;339:578–583.

59. Frifelt JJ, et al. Efficacy of recombinant human erythropoietin administered subcutaneously to CAPD patients once weekly. Perit Dial Int 1996;16:594–598.

60. Vanrenterghem Y, et al. Randomized trial of darbepoetin alfa for treatment of renal anemia at a reduced dose frequency compared with rHuEPO in dialysis patients. Kidney Int 2002;62:2167–2175.

61. Suranyi MG, et al. Treatment of anemia with darbepoetin alfa administered de novo once every other week in chronic kidney disease. Am J Nephrol 2003;23:106–111.

62. Jadoul M, et al. Darbepoetin alfa administered once monthly maintains haemoglobin levels in stable dialysis patients. Nephrol Dial Transplant 2004;19:898–903.

63. Lin CL, et al. Low dose intravenous ascorbic acid for erythropoietin-hyporesponsive anemia in diabetic hemodialysis patients with iron overload. Ren Fail 2003;25:445–453.

64. Abu-Alfa AK, et al. ACE inhibitors do not induce recombinant human erythropoietin resistance in hemodialysis patients. Am J Kidney Dis 2000;35:1076–1082.

65. Hampl H, et al. Regression of left ventricular hypertrophy in hemodialysis patients is possible. Clin Nephrol 2002;58(Suppl 1):S73–S96.

66. Silverberg D. Outcomes of anaemia management in renal insufficiency and cardiac disease. Nephrol Dial Transplant 2003;18(Suppl 2):ii7–12.

67. Roger SD, et al. Effects of early and late intervention with epoetin alpha

on left ventricular mass among patients with chronic kidney disease (stage 3 or 4): Results of a randomized clinical trial. J Am Soc Nephrol 2004;15:148–156.

68. Casadevall N. Pure red cell aplasia and anti-erythropoietin antibodies in patients treated with epoetin. Nephrol Dial Transplant 2003;18(Suppl 8): viii37–41.

69. St Peter WL, Lewis MJ, Macres MG. Pain comparison after subcutaneous administration of single-dose formulation versus multidose formulation of epogen in hemodialysis patients. Am J Kidney Dis 1998;32:470–474.

70. Brophy DF, Ripley EB, Holdford DA. Pharmacoeconomic considerations in the health system management of anaemia in patients with chronic kidney disease and end stage renal disease. Expert Opin Pharmacother 2003;4:1461–1469.

71. Slatopolsky E, Dusso A, Brown AJ. The role of phosphorus in the development of secondary hyperparathyroidism and parathyroid cell proliferation in chronic renal failure. Am J Med Sci 1999;317:370–376.

72. Martinez I, et al. A deficit of calcitriol synthesis may not be the initial factor in the pathogenesis of secondary hyperparathyroidism. Nephrol Dial Transplant 1996;11(Suppl 3):22–28.

73. Rix M, et al. Bone mineral density and biochemical markers of bone turnover in patients with predialysis chronic renal failure. Kidney Int 1999;56:1084–1093.

74. Kurokawa K, Fukagawa M. Uremic bone disease: Advances over the last 30 years. J Nephrol 1999;12(Suppl 2):S63–S67.

75. Ganesh SK, et al. Association of elevated serum PO(4), Ca × PO(4) product, and parathyroid hormone with cardiac mortality risk in chronic hemodialysis patients. J Am Soc Nephrol 2001;12:2131–2138.

76. Bro S, Olgaard K. Effects of excess PTH on nonclassical target organs. Am J Kidney Dis 1997;30:606–620.

77. Block GA, et al. Association of serum phosphorus and calcium × phosphate product with mortality risk in chronic hemodialysis patients: A national study. Am J Kidney Dis 1998;31:607–617.

78. Block GA, Port FK. Re-evaluation of risks associated with hyperphosphatemia and hyperparathyroidism in dialysis patients: Recommendations for a change in management. Am J Kidney Dis 2000;35:1226–1237.

79. Goodman WG, et al. Coronary-artery calcification in young adults with end-stage renal disease who are undergoing dialysis. N Engl J Med 2000;342:1478–1483.

80. Spasovski GB, et al. Spectrum of renal bone disease in end-stage renal failure patients not yet on dialysis. Nephrol Dial Transplant 2003;18:1159–1166.

81. Salem MM. Hyperparathyroidism in the hemodialysis population: A survey of 612 patients. Am J Kidney Dis 1997;29:862–865.

82. U.S. Renal Data System. Medication use among dialysis patients in the dialysis morbidity and mortality study. USRDS 1998 Annual Data Report, National Institutes of Health, National Institute Diabetes and Digestive and Kidney Diseases, Bethesda, MD, 1998.

83. Slatopolsky E, et al. A novel mechanism for skeletal resistance in uremia. Kidney Int 2000;58:753–761.

84. Gao P, et al. Development of a novel immunoradiometric assay exclusively for biologically active whole parathyroid hormone 1-84: Implications for improvement of accurate assessment of parathyroid function. J Bone Miner Res 2001;16:605–614.

85. Monier-Faugere MC, et al. Improved assessment of bone turnover by the PTH-(1-84)/large C-PTH fragments ratio in ESRD patients. Kidney Int 2001;60:1460–1468.

86. Stamatakis MK, Alderman JM, Meyer-Stout PJ. Influence of pH on in vitro disintegration of phosphate binders. Am J Kidney Dis 1998;32: 808–812.

87. Lau AH, Kuk JM, Franson KL. Phosphate-binding capacities of calcium and aluminum formulations. Int J Artif Organs 1998;21:19–22.

88. Chertow GM, et al. Long-term effects of sevelamer hydrochloride on the calcium × phosphate product and lipid profile of haemodialysis patients. Nephrol Dial Transplant 2000;15:559.

89. Chertow GM. Slowing the progression of vascular calcification in hemodialysis. J Am Soc Nephrol 2003;14(Suppl 4):S310–S314.

90. Joy MS, Finn WF. Randomized, double-blind, placebo-controlled, dose-titration, phase III study assessing the efficacy and tolerability of lan-

thanum carbonate: A new phosphate binder for the treatment of hyperphosphatemia. Am J Kidney Dis 2003;42:96–107.

91. Bleyer AJ. Phosphate binder usage in kidney failure patients. Expert Opin Pharmacother 2003;4:941–947.

92. Burke SK, et al. Sevelamer hydrochloride (Renagel), a phosphate-binding polymer, does not alter the pharmacokinetics of two commonly used antihypertensives in healthy volunteers. J Clin Pharmacol 2001;41:199–205.

93. Burke S, et al. Sevelamer hydrochloride (Renagel), a nonabsorbed phosphate-binding polymer, does not interfere with digoxin or warfarin pharmacokinetics. J Clin Pharmacol 2001;41:193–198.

94. Slatopolsky E, Finch J, Brown A. New vitamin D analogs. Kidney Int Suppl 2003;85:S83–S87.

95. Lindberg J, et al. A long-term, multicenter study of the efficacy and safety of paricalcitol in end-stage renal disease. Clin Nephrol 2001;56:315–323.

96. Maung HM, et al. Efficacy and side effects of intermittent intravenous and oral doxercalciferol (1alpha-hydroxyvitamin D(2)) in dialysis patients with secondary hyperparathyroidism: A sequential comparison. Am J Kidney Dis 2001;37:532–543.

97. Brown AJ, Finch J, Slatopolsky E. Differential effects of 19-nor-1,25-dihydroxyvitamin D(2) and 1,25-dihydroxyvitamin D(3) on intestinal calcium and phosphate transport. J Lab Clin Med 2002;139:279–284.

98. Coyne DW, et al. Differential effects of acute administration of 19-Nor-1,25-dihydroxy-vitamin D2 and 1,25-dihydroxy-vitamin D3 on serum calcium and phosphorus in hemodialysis patients. Am J Kidney Dis 2002;40:1283–1288.

99. Martin KJ, et al. Therapy of secondary hyperparathyroidism with 19-nor-1alpha,25-dihydroxyvitamin D2. Am J Kidney Dis 1998;32(Suppl 2): S61–S66.

100. Coburn JW, et al. Doxercalciferol safely suppresses PTH levels in patients with secondary hyperparathyroidism associated with chronic kidney disease stages 3 and 4. Am J Kidney Dis 2004;43:877–890.

101. Sprague SM, et al. Paricalcitol versus calcitriol in the treatment of secondary hyperparathyroidism. Kidney Int 2003;63:1483–1490.

102. Teng M, et al. Survival of patients undergoing hemodialysis with paricalcitol or calcitriol therapy. N Engl J Med 2003;349:446–456.

103. Llach F, Yudd M. Paricalcitol in dialysis patients with calcitriol-resistant secondary hyperparathyroidism. Am J Kidney Dis 2001;38(Suppl 5): S45–S50.

104. Martin KJ, et al. Paricalcitol dosing according to body weight or severity of hyperparathyroidism: A double-blind, multicenter, randomized study. Am J Kidney Dis 2001;38(Suppl 5):S57–S63.

105. Sensipar (cinacalcet HCl) tablets package insert. Amgen Inc., Thousand Oaks, CA, 2004.

106. Quarles LD, et al. The calcimimetic AMG 073 as a potential treatment for secondary hyperparathyroidism of end-stage renal disease. J Am Soc Nephrol 2003;14:575–583.

107. Block GA, et al. Cinacalcet for secondary hyperparathyroidism in patients receiving hemodialysis. N Engl J Med 2004;350:1516–1525.

108. Kraut JA, Kurtz I. Use of base in the treatment of severe acidemic states. Am J Kidney Dis 2001;38:703–727.

109. Parfrey PS. The clinical epidemiology of cardiovascular disease in chronic kidney disease. Semin Dial 2003;16:83–84.

110. Mailloux LU, Haley WE. Hypertension in the ESRD patient: Pathophysiology, therapy, outcomes, and future directions. Am J Kidney Dis 1998;32:705–719.

111. Executive Summary of The Third Report of The National Cholesterol Education Program (NCEP) Expert Panel on Detection, Evaluation, and Treatment of High Blood Cholesterol in Adults (Adult Treatment Panel III). JAMA 2001;285:2486–2497.

112. Kasiske BL. Hyperlipidemia in patients with chronic renal disease. Am J Kidney Dis 1998;32(Suppl 3):S142–S156.

113. Prichard SS. Impact of dyslipidemia in end-stage renal disease. J Am Soc Nephrol 2003;14(Suppl 4):S315–S320.

114. Ozkahya M, et al. Impact of volume control on left ventricular hypertrophy in dialysis patients. J Nephrol 2002;15:655–660.

115. Charra B, Bergstrom J, Scribner BH. Blood pressure control in dialysis patients: Importance of the lag phenomenon. Am J Kidney Dis 1998; 32:720–724.

116. Chobanian AV, et al. Seventh Report of the Joint National Committee on Prevention, Detection, Evaluation, and Treatment of High Blood Pressure. Hypertension 2003;42:1206–1252.

117. Horl MP, Horl WH. Hemodialysis-associated hypertension: Pathophysiology and therapy. Am J Kidney Dis 2002;39:227–244.

118. Bleyer AJ, et al. A comparison of the calcium-free phosphate binder sevelamer hydrochloride with calcium acetate in the treatment of hyperphosphatemia in hemodialysis patients. Am J Kidney Dis 1999;33: 694–701.

119. Matera M, et al. History of L-carnitine: Implications for renal disease. J Ren Nutr 2003;13:2–14.

120. Makoff R. Vitamin replacement therapy in renal failure patients. Miner Electrolyte Metab 1999;25:349–351.

121. Weigert AL, Schafer AI. Uremic bleeding: Pathogenesis and therapy. Am J Med Sci 1998;316:94–104.

122. Sloand JA. Long-term therapy for uremic bleeding. Int J Artif Organs 1996;19:439–440.

123. Cohen G, Haag-Weber M, Horl WH. Immune dysfunction in uremia. Kidney Int Suppl 1997;62:S79–S82.

124. Zucker I, et al. Prevalence and characterization of uremic pruritus in patients undergoing hemodialysis: Uremic pruritus is still a major problem for patients with end-stage renal disease. J Am Acad Dermatol 2003;49:842–846.

125. Kovalik E. Endocrine manifestations of renal failure. In: Greenberg A, ed. Primer on Kidney Diseases, 2nd ed. San Diego, Academic Press, 1998: 472.

45

HEMODIALYSIS AND PERITONEAL DIALYSIS

Rowland J. Elwell and Edward F. Foote

Learning Objectives and other resources can be found at *www.pharmacotherapyonline.com.*

KEY CONCEPTS

❶ In hemodialysis, blood and dialysate are perfused on opposite sides of a semipermeable membrane. Substances are removed from the blood due to diffusion and ultrafiltration.

❷ Due to fewer complication and longer survival rates, the native arteriovenous fistula is the preferred access for hemodialysis. Venous catheters are plagued by complications such as infection and thrombosis and often deliver relatively poor blood flow rates.

❸ The *Kt/V* and urea reduction ratio are the most commonly used indicators for hemodialysis adequacy. The National Kidney Foundation's Kidney Disease Outcomes Quality Initiative has set a goal *Kt/V* of greater than 1.2 and a goal urea reduction ratio of greater than 65%.

❹ Hypotension and cramps are common intradialytic complications. Other serious complications include infection and thrombosis of the access.

❺ In peritoneal dialysis, dialysate is instilled via a permanent peritoneal catheter into the peritoneal cavity. The peritoneal

membrane lines the highly vascularized abdominal viscera and acts as the semipermeable membrane across which diffusion and ultrafiltration occur.

❻ The most common type of peritoneal dialysis is continuous ambulatory peritoneal dialysis, during which a patient manually instills 2 to 3 L of dialysate four times a day. Other types include a variety of automated systems collectively termed automated peritoneal dialysis in which some of the daily dialysate exchanges (usually the overnight exchanges) are completed using an automated device.

❼ Peritonitis is a common complication of peritoneal dialysis. Initial empiric therapy for peritonitis should include intraperitoneal administration of agents effective against both gram-positive and gram-negative organisms.

❽ Nasal carriage of *Staphylococcus aureus* is associated with an increased risk of catheter-related infections and peritonitis. Prophylaxis with intranasal mupirocin (twice a day for 5 days every month) or mupirocin (daily) at the exit site can effectively reduce *S. aureus* infections.

Hemodialysis (HD), peritoneal dialysis (PD), and kidney transplantation are the major treatment options for patients with end-stage kidney disease (ESKD) which has also been referred to as end-stage renal disease (ESRD); or kidney failure. The United States Renal Data System (USRDS)[1] reported in 2003 that there were 406,081 Americans with ESKD. Of these, 65% were treated with HD, 7% were on PD, and 28% had a functioning kidney transplant. During the period between 1997 and 2001, the prevalent HD population grew by 4.5% per year, while the PD population decreased by 4.9% per year. Although the number of kidney transplants performed during this period has risen steadily, transplantation has not kept pace with the growing incidence of ESKD. Although the use of PD has declined, dialysis remains the most common form of chronic renal replacement therapy with 72% of patients receiving either HD or PD. Based on current trends and estimated population growth, it is projected that the number of ESKD patients in the United States may reach 2.24 million by the year 2030.[1] Assuming that the proportion of patients dependent on dialysis remains constant, this population may exceed 1.6 million in 2030. For a more thorough discussion on the epidemiology of chronic kidney disease, see Chap. 43.

This chapter is a primer on the principles and practice of dialysis. The chapter focuses on HD and PD as the dialysis modalities most commonly employed in chronic renal replacement therapy (the reader

is referred to Chap. 42 for a discussion of the use of dialysis in acute renal failure). The pertinent factors involved in the appropriate initiation of dialysis are described. There is discussion and comparison of the morbidity and mortality associated with HD and PD, as these considerations may influence the dialysis method chosen by patients and clinicians. Since dialysis by either method is not a generic procedure, the variants of HD and PD are detailed. The multiple types of vascular and peritoneal access used to provide HD and PD, including various catheters and surgical techniques, are illustrated. The concept of dialysis adequacy for each modality is reviewed, and methodologies to quantify the delivered dose of dialysis are described. Finally, the clinical presentation of the common complications of both dialytic therapies are presented, along with pertinent nonpharmacologic and pharmacologic therapeutic alternatives.

MORBIDITY AND MORTALITY IN DIALYSIS

Morbidity can be grossly assessed by the number of hospitalizations per patient-year, the number of days hospitalized, or the incidence of certain complications such as cardiovascular events. Among dialysis patients, the number of hospital admissions per patient-year has remained fairly constant since 1991. However, average length of stay has decreased 17% and 21% for HD and PD patients, respectively.[1] Early comparative studies demonstrated more hospitalized days with PD (21.9 vs. 17.3 per year), but the policy at that time was for inpatient treatment of peritonitis. Because many PD infections are now treated on an outpatient basis, the number of hospital days is dramatically lower than for HD patients in some centers.[2] In fact, admissions for peritonitis have decreased 47% since 1991. Overall, hospitalizations are more frequent for whites than for blacks, and the frequency and duration increase with age in both groups. Although cardiovascular complications and infection are common, the combined category of "other," which includes vascular access problems, accounts for the greatest number of admissions and days in hospital.[1]

In recognition of the high morbidity and mortality of dialysis patients, the Centers for Medicare & Medicaid Services, at that time known as the Health Care Financing Administration, developed a series of health care quality improvement programs in 1993. Now called the ESKD Clinical Performance Measures Project, they examine markers of the quality of dialysis care (anemia management, serum albumin, vascular access for hemodialysis, and adequacy of dialysis). The 2003 report studied a sample population of 8,487 HD and 1354 PD patients.[3] The report showed that 79% of HD patients had hemoglobin values at or above the target range (11 to 12 g/dL) in 2002, compared to only 43% in 1997. Similarly, 79% of PD patients had achieved target hemoglobin values in 2002, compared to 55% in 1997. Although less dramatic, improvements in other clinical indicators were also reported. The report concluded that opportunities still exist to improve the care of U.S. dialysis patients in the areas of adequacy of dialysis, vascular access, and anemia management.

Regardless of dialysis modality, the life expectancy of U.S. dialysis patients is markedly lower than that of healthy subjects of the same age and gender. In comparison to the general population, dialysis patients have one-third to one-sixth of the expected remaining lifetime. Nonetheless, improvement has been made and the overall patient mortality rate has fallen 10% among dialysis patients since 1980. The changes in mortality rates are more impressive when dialysis vintage is examined. In patients receiving dialysis for fewer than 2 years and from 2 to 5 years, mortality rates decreased 22% and 15%, respectively, since 1980. However, in those treated for 5 years or more, mortality rates increased 7%. These changes suggest that death is occurring later in the course of dialysis therapy.[1]

Life expectancy is reduced for both HD and PD patients, but comparative mortality studies have shown inconsistent results.[4–9] Bloembergen and colleagues found that there was a 19% increase in the relative risk of death of U.S. peritoneal dialysis patients as compared to those receiving hemodialysis, and that peritoneal dialysis patients had more deaths as a result of infections, acute myocardial infarctions, other cardiac causes, and cerebrovascular diseases.[4,5] The results of two Canadian studies highlight the extent of the current controversy. Fenton and colleagues retrospectively compared mortality rates of HD and PD patients who started therapy between 1990 and 1994.[6] They reported that the mortality rate in PD patients was significantly lower than that observed in HD patients; the mortality rate ratio was 0.73 (PD:HD). This effect was most evident in the first 2 years of therapy, as demonstrated by the finding of similar 5-year survival probabilities of approximately 35%. Foley and colleagues prospectively followed a cohort of PD and HD patients who initiated dialysis therapy between 1984 and 1991.[7] They reported that there was no difference in mortality rate during the first 2 years (17.8% and 16.5% of PD and HD patients, respectively). However, after 2 years the mortality rate in the PD group was significantly greater than in the HD patients (mortality rate ratio = 1.57). These differences in outcome may be related to a wide array of factors, such as the dose of dialysis, physician bias in selection of the initial mode of therapy, patient compliance, and

unmeasured comorbidities, such as hyperlipidemia or degree of diabetic control.[8] Cardiovascular events account for 25% to 40% of deaths in HD and PD patients, whereas peritonitis is the second most common cause of mortality among peritoneal dialysis patients. Of patients leaving PD, the major reasons are death or transfer to hemodialysis because of inadequate dialysis or frequent episodes of peritonitis.[7,9] Thus the selection of the optimal therapy for a given patient must be individualized.

CLINICAL CONTROVERSY

There is much debate over which dialysis modality, hemodialysis or PD, is best in terms of morbidity and mortality. Outcomes studies have provided conflicting results. Although only 7% of U.S. patients are treated with PD, surveyed nephrologists report that as many as 45% of prevalent ESKD patients could be treated with PD.

INDICATIONS FOR DIALYSIS

Dialysis should be initiated electively rather than urgently in patients with chronic kidney disease (see Chap. 44). Because of the progressive nature of the disease, the planning for dialysis should begin once the patient's creatinine clearance (Cl_{cr}) drops below 30 mL/min per 1.73m^2.[10] Beginning the preparation process at this point allows adequate time for proper education of the patient and family and for the creation of suitable vascular or peritoneal access.

The primary criterion for initiation of dialysis is the patient's clinical status: the presence of persistent anorexia, nausea, and vomiting, especially if accompanied by weight loss, fatigue, declining serum albumin levels, uncontrolled hypertension or congestive heart failure, and neurologic deficits or pruritus. Some nephrologists use critical lab values of serum creatinine or blood urea nitrogen (BUN) as indicators of when to initiate dialysis. The National Kidney Foundation's Kidney Disease Outcomes Qualitative Initiative (NKF-K/DOQI) guidelines suggest that nondiabetic patients should be started when their Cl_{cr} is 9 to 14 mL/min per 1.73 m^2. Diabetics may need to be started earlier.[11] Table 45–1 lists the advantages and disadvantages of hemodialysis,

---

TABLE 45–1. Advantages and Disadvantages of Hemodialysis

Advantages
1. Higher solute clearance allows intermittent treatment.
2. Parameters of adequacy of dialysis are better defined and therefore underdialysis can be detected early.
3. Technique failure rate is low.
4. Even though intermittent heparinization is required, hemostasis parameters are better corrected with hemodialysis than peritoneal dialysis.
5. In-center hemodialysis enables closer monitoring of the patient.

Disadvantages
1. Requires multiple visits each week to the hemodialysis center, which translates into loss of control by the patient.
2. Disequilibrium, dialysis hypotension, and muscle cramps are common. May require months before the patient adjusts to hemodialysis.
3. Infections in hemodialysis patients may be related to the choice of membranes, the complement-activating membranes being more deleterious.
4. Vascular access is frequently associated with infection and thrombosis.
5. Decline of residual renal function is more rapid compared to peritoneal dialysis.

TABLE 45–2. Advantages and Disadvantages of Peritoneal Dialysis

Advantages

1. More hemodynamic stability (blood pressure) due to slow ultrafiltration rate.
2. Increased clearance of larger solutes, which may explain good clinical status in spite of lower urea clearance.
3. Better preservation of residual renal function.
4. Convenient intraperitoneal route of administration of drugs such as antibiotics and insulin.
5. Suitable for elderly and very young patients who may not tolerate hemodialysis well.
6. Freedom from the "machine" gives the patient a sense of independence (for continuous ambulatory peritoneal dialysis).
7. Less blood loss and iron deficiency, resulting in easier management of anemia or reduced requirements for erythropoietin and parenteral iron.
8. No systemic heparinization requirement.
9. Subcutaneous versus intravenous erythropoietin or darbepoetin is usual, which may reduce overall doses and be more physiologic.

Disadvantages

1. Protein and amino acid losses through peritoneum and reduced appetite owing to continuous glucose load and sense of abdominal fullness predispose to malnutrition.
2. Risk of peritonitis.
3. Catheter malfunction, exit site, and tunnel infection.
4. Inadequate ultrafiltration and solute dialysis in patients with a large body size, unless large volumes and frequent exchanges are employed.
5. Patient burnout and high rate of technique failure.
6. Risk of obesity with excessive glucose absorption.
7. Mechanical problems such as hernias, dialysate leaks, hemorrhoids, or back pain may occur.
8. Extensive abdominal surgery may preclude peritoneal dialysis.
9. No convenient access for intravenous iron administration.

while those for peritoneal dialysis are delineated in Table 45–2. These factors, along with the patient's concomitant diseases, preferences, and support environments, are the principal determinants of the dialysis mode they will receive. Timely initiation of dialysis in the ambulatory setting before the onset of severe complications such as pericarditis, encephalopathy, or pulmonary edema may result in significant cost savings as compared with the initiation of dialysis in an acute care environment.

HEMODIALYSIS

PRINCIPLES OF HEMODIALYSIS

Hemodialysis consists of the perfusion of blood and a physiologic salt solution on opposite sides of a semipermeable membrane. Multiple substances, such as water, urea, creatinine, uremic toxins, and drugs move from the blood into the dialysate, thus facilitating removal from the blood. Solutes are transported across the membrane by either passive diffusion or ultrafiltration. Diffusion is the movement of substances along a concentration gradient, the rate of diffusion depends on the difference between the concentrations of solute in blood and dialysate, solute characteristics, the dialyzer composition, and flow rates (blood and dialysate). Ultrafiltration is the movement of water across the membrane due to hydrostatic or osmotic pressure, and is the primary means for removal of excess body water. Convection (expressed as mL of plasma water removed per hour per mm of mercury of pressure within the dialyzer) occurs

when dissolved solutes are "dragged" across a membrane with fluid transport (as long as the pores in the dialyzer are large enough to allow them to pass). Convection can be maximized by increasing the hydrostatic pressure gradient across the dialysis membrane, or by changing to a dialyzer that is more permeable to water transport. These two processes can be controlled independently, and thus a patient's hemodialysis prescription can be individualized to attain the desired degree of solute (urea) removal and fluid balance.

HEMODIALYSIS ACCESS

Permanent access to the bloodstream for hemodialysis may be accomplished by several techniques, including creation of an arteriovenous (AV) fistula, the AV graft, and venous catheters[12,13] (Fig. 45–1). The AV fistula has the longest survival of all blood-access devices and is associated with the lowest rate of complications such as infection and thrombosis, and is therefore considered the preferred access. However, fistulas require 2 months or more for the access to dilate and thicken ("mature") as the result of the increased arterial pressure. In addition, creation of an AV fistula may be difficult in elderly patients or patients with peripheral vascular disease (particularly common in patients with diabetes). Synthetic AV grafts, usually made of polytetrafluoroethylene, are another option for permanent AV access. Polytetrafluoroethylene grafts require only 2 to 3 weeks to endothelialize before they can be routinely used. The primary disadvantages of this type of access are the shorter survival, and the fact that they have higher rates of infection and thrombosis than do AV fistulas. Cuffed, double-lumen or twin single-lumen venous catheters are now commonly used for patients in whom AV access is not an option. Venous catheters can be placed in the femoral, subclavian, or internal jugular vein. These catheters are often used in small children, diabetic patients with severe vascular disease, the morbidly obese, and those patients who have no viable sites for AV access. The cuff on the catheter stabilizes the catheter placement, reduces the incidence of infection, and prolongs the period of use from several weeks to 6 months or more. The major problem with all venous catheters is they have a shorter life span and are more prone to infection and thrombosis than permanent AV accesses. Furthermore, catheters are generally not able to provide adequate blood flow rates, which can limit the amount of dialysis delivered.

The K/DOQI guidelines suggest that the AV fistula should be the first choice of access for all eligible patients who will become dialysis dependent.[14] If creation of an AV fistula is not possible, a synthetic graft should be constructed. Unless AV access is not possible, cuffed venous catheters should not be used as a permanent dialysis access. Patients who will need dialysis for only a short period of time (i.e., acute kidney failure) generally have a venous catheter (cuffed or noncuffed) placed. The use of temporary catheters and grafts has declined since 1991, while fistula insertions have shown a modest increase. Of some concern, the most commonly placed access is permanent venous catheters.[1] The extensive use of catheters may be due to the large population of patients who are not candidates for AV access, or they are being used until permanent AV access can be accomplished. Clearly, earlier referral to nephrology and vascular surgery makes it easier to place the most appropriate access.

HEMODIALYSIS PROCEDURES

The HD system consists of an external vascular circuit through which the patient's blood is transferred in sterile polyethylene tubing to the dialysis filter or membrane (dialyzer) via a mechanical pump (Fig. 45–2). The patient's blood then passes through the dialyzer on one side of the semipermeable membrane and is returned to the

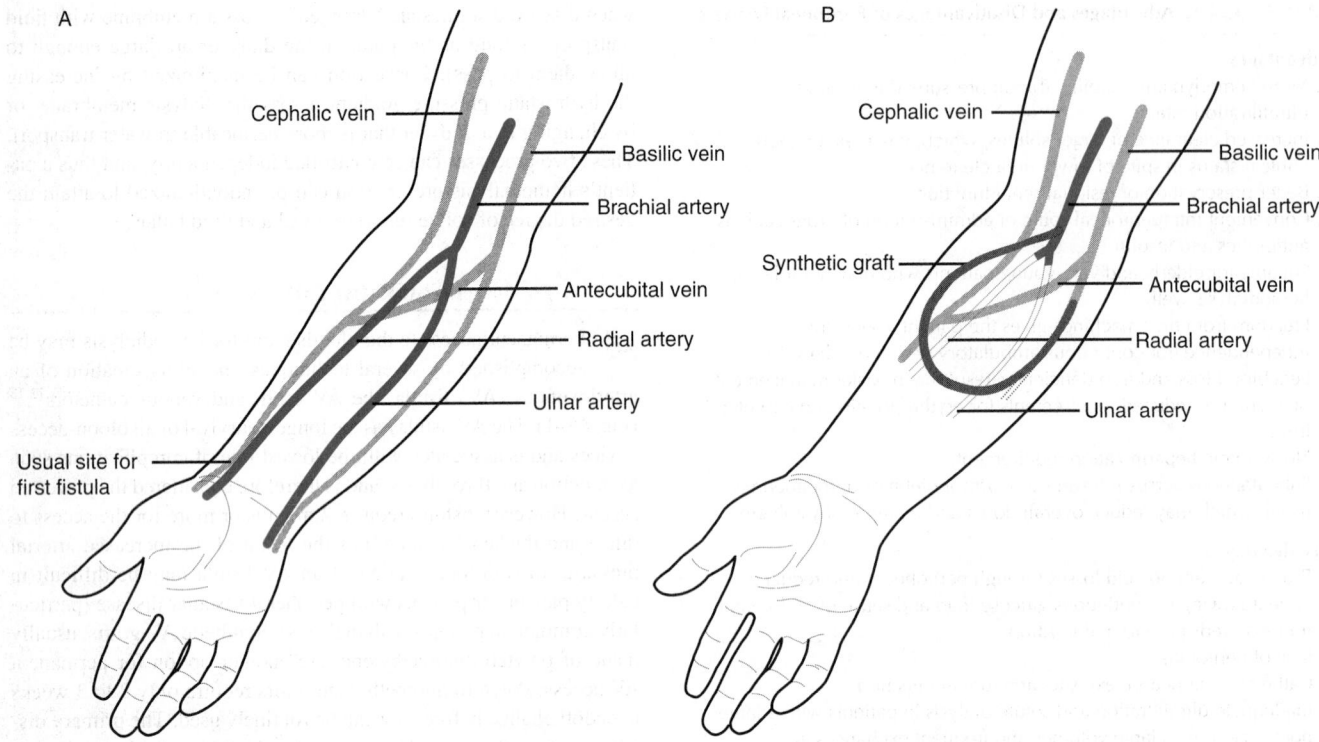

FIGURE 45–1. The predominant types of vascular access for chronic dialysis patients are (*A*) the arteriovenous fistula and (*B*) the synthetic arteriovenous forearm graft. The first primary arteriovenous fistula is usually created by the surgical anastomosis of the cephalic vein with the radial artery. The flow of blood from the higher-pressure arterial system results in hypertrophy of the vein. The most common AV graft is between the brachial artery and the basilic or cephalic vein.

patient. The dialysate solution, which consists of purified water and electrolytes, is pumped through the dialyzer countercurrent to the flow of blood on the other side of the semipermeable membrane. The dialysate circuit, unlike the vascular circuit, is not sterile and is a potential source of infection for the patient, particularly if the membrane were to rupture.

Dialysis membranes are classified as conventional (standard), high-efficiency, and high-flux. Conventional dialyzers, mostly made of cuprophane, have small pores that limit clearance to relatively small molecules such as urea and creatinine. High-efficiency membranes have large surface areas and thus have a greater ability to remove water, urea, and other small molecules from the blood. High-flux

FIGURE 45–2. In conventional or high-flux hemodialysis, the patient's blood is pumped to the dialyzer at a rate of 300 to 600 mL/min. Heparin is administered to prevent clotting in the dialyzer. The predominant dialyzers for conventional dialysis are small (0.8 to 1.5 m^2), low- to medium-flux dialyzers made of cellulose acetate, cuprophane, or hemophan. High-flux hemodialysis systems incorporate a synthetic dialyzer made of polysulfone, polyacrylonitrile, polymethylmethacrylate, or a high-flux cellulosic-based filter; for example, cellulose triacetate of variable size (0.65 to 2.1 m^2). The dialysate, which is usually bicarbonate buffered, is pumped at a rate of 500 to 1000 mL/min through the dialyzer countercurrent to the flow of blood. The rate of fluid removal from the patient is controlled by adjusting the pressure in the dialysate compartment.

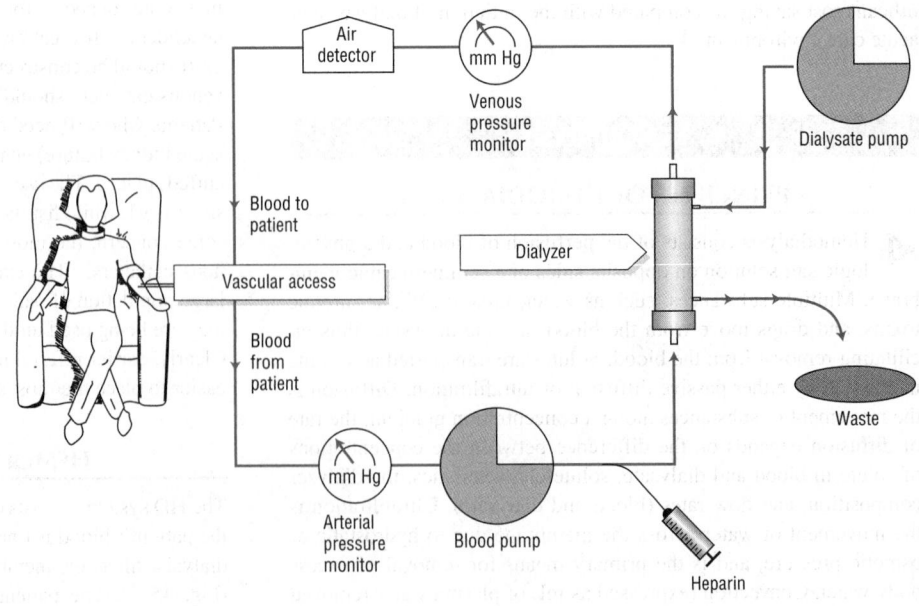

membranes have large pores that are capable of removing high-molecular-weight substances such as β_2-microglobulin and certain drugs, such as vancomycin.[15,16] The primary reason to use high-efficiency and/or high-flux membranes is that clearance of both low- and high-molecular-weight substances is much greater than with the conventional membranes, so treatment times can be shorter for any set amount of dialysis dose. The use of high-flux and high-efficiency dialysis increased significantly in the United States during the 1990s. High-efficiency and high-flux dialysis require blood flow rates greater than 400 mL/min, dialysate flow rates greater than 500 mL/min, and the use of strict controls on the rate of fluid removal. Typically these dialyzers are composed of polysulfone (PS), polymethylmethacrylate (PMMA), polyamide, cellulose triacetate, and polyacrylonitrile (PAN).[15]

Another issue relating to dialysis membranes is their ability to stimulate the immune system. If the dialysis filter membrane does not activate the complement system (C3a and C5a) when it comes in contact with the patient's blood, it is considered biocompatible. In the acute setting, the incidence of hypotension, fever, bronchoconstriction, and thrombocytopenia are lower in patients dialyzed with biocompatible filters. The most biocompatible dialyzers use a synthetic membrane of PS, PAN, or PMMA. Although not definitive, biocompatible membranes may be associated with fewer adverse events during dialysis, lower rates of hospitalization, reduced death rates, and slower declines in residual renal function.[17]

ADEQUACY OF HEMODIALYSIS

The objective of hemodialysis dosing is to prescribe and deliver the optimal dose for each individual patient, that is, the amount of therapy above which there is no cost-effective increment in the patient's quality-adjusted life expectancy. The two key goals of the prescription are to achieve the desired dry weight and the adequate removal of endogenous waste products such as urea. Dry weight is the target postdialysis weight at which the patient is normotensive and free of edema.

The desired dose of dialysis in terms of solute removal can be expressed as a urea reduction ratio (URR) or the Kt/V (pronounced "K-T-over-V"). The URR is calculated as:

$$URR = \frac{\text{Predialysis BUN} - \text{Postdialysis BUN}}{\text{Predialysis BUN}} \times 100$$

The URR is an easy calculation and thus is frequently used to measure the delivered dialysis dose. However, the URR does not account for the contribution of convective removal of urea. The Kt/V is the dialyzer clearance of urea (K) in L/h multiplied by the duration of dialysis (t) in hours, divided by the urea distribution volume of the patient (V) in liters.[18] Kt/V is a unitless parameter that quantitates the fraction of the patient's total body water that is cleared of urea during a dialysis session. Urea kinetic modeling, using special computer software, is the optimal means to determine the Kt/V. Kt/V can also be calculated by using the following equation.[19]

$$Kt/V = \ln(R - 0.008t) + [(4 - 3.5R)(UF/Wt_{\text{post}})]$$

where R is the post-BUN:pre-BUN ratio, t is the duration of dialysis in hours, and UF is the weight loss during dialysis. This equation provides the best estimate of kinetically modeled Kt/V because it considers the effect of the efficiency of the treatment as a function of the treatment time, and the convective removal of urea in the ultrafiltrate (UF/Wt).

With high-efficiency dialysis, urea clearance exceeds 180 mL/min and urea kinetics are best characterized by a two-compartment

model with a central compartment volume that increases during the time between dialysis treatments.[18] As a the result of this kinetic behavior, a marked rebound in urea concentrations is seen after dialysis, as has been described for many drugs. Because of the two-compartment behavior of urea, the timing of the posttreatment BUN sample is critical. If the sample is obtained immediately after the end of the treatment, equilibration between the two compartments is incomplete and the sample will overestimate the effect of the treatment administered. The only "true" sample is the one obtained after the two compartments have reached equilibrium. In general, complete equilibration between compartments occurs within 15 to 30 minutes after the end of the treatment; however, this approach is not clinically practical. It is possible to calculate Kt/V using a sample immediately after the treatment if appropriate corrections are made to transform that sample into an equilibrated value (eKt/V). This correction considers the urea clearance of the dialyzer used during the treatment, since the magnitude of the rebound is proportional to the efficiency of the treatment. The eKT/V is typically about 0.2 lower than the standard Kt/V, (often termed the *single pool Kt/V* [*spKt/V*]). Many computer packages, often included in newer dialysis machines, do these calculations automatically.

The K/DOQI recommends that the delivered dose of dialysis be at least a Kt/V of 1.2 (equivalent to an average URR of 65%). To achieve this goal, the recommended *target* Kt/V is 1.3. Many nephrologists believe that even greater doses of dialysis would have positive outcomes in dialysis patients, and so the average dose of dialysis has been increasing in the U.S. In 2001, the median Kt/V was 1.49.[3] The HEMO study was designed to determine the effects of high-dose dialysis and the use of high-flux hemodialysis membranes on morbidity and mortality.[20] The results of this prospective, randomized trial that assigned patients to either standard (Kt/V 1.25) or high-dose (Kt/V 1.65) dialysis with high- or low-flux membranes, revealed that the risk of death was similar in both the standard and high-dose and the low- and high-flux groups. Thus there does not appear to be any benefit in increasing the amount of dialysis above the current recommendations. As many patients in the U.S. are well above the target Kt/V range, it is unclear if a patient's dose of dialysis should actually be *decreased*. The HEMO study only enrolled patients who were on traditional three-times-weekly dialysis, thus the applicability of these findings to patients on more intensive regimens such as daily or nocturnal HD regimens that provide long, frequent dialysis remain to be determined.[21,22] Although early data indicate that these intensive HD regimens result in better blood pressure, anemia, and phosphate control,[21] currently these HD regimens are not widely utilized, in part due to Medicare reimbursement issues.

CLINICAL CONTROVERSY

It remains to be determined what type of hemodialysis is best. Intensive hemodialysis treatments (nocturnal and daily dialysis) may provide better outcomes in hemodialysis patients. Studies on the value of these regimens are currently in development.

A deficiency in delivered hemodialysis therapy may be related to patient compliance with the dialysis prescription (ending dialysis early). Other causes for a low Kt/V include low blood flow rates due to access stenosis or thrombosis, or due to the use of catheters. Adequate dialysis may not be achieved in some patients despite compliance and sufficient blood flow. For these patients there are really only two options to increase urea clearance: use a larger membrane or increase the treatment time.

COMPLICATIONS OF HEMODIALYSIS

INTRADIALYTIC COMPLICATIONS

◄4 The most common complications that occur during the hemodialysis procedure include hypotension, cramps, nausea and vomiting, headache, chest pain, back pain, and fever or chills. Table 45–3 lists these complications and the etiology with predisposing factors.[23]

Hypotension is the most common complication during HD and is primarily related to the large amount of fluid removed during typical treatments, although the other causes listed in Table 45–3 are also important.[24,25] Intradialytic hypotension is more common in the elderly and patients with diabetes. Other symptoms (nausea and cramping) are often present during acute hypotensive episodes. The replacement of acetate with bicarbonate as the dialysate buffer, the use of volumetric ultrafiltration controllers, as well as individualized dialysate sodium levels has helped reduce the incidence of hypotension. While pruritus may appear worse during the HD treatment, it is actually a complication of ESKD.

OTHER COMPLICATIONS: THROMBOSIS AND INFECTION

Thrombosis of the vascular access is a major problem in chronic HD. Although thrombosis occurs in grafts, and to a lesser extent fistulas, thrombosis associated with catheters is the most problematic and will be the focus of discussion here. Early dysfunction (less than 5 days after placement) of an HD catheter is usually associated with an intracatheter or catheter-tip thrombosis, or a malpositioned catheter. Thrombi that occur after approximately 1 week can be outside the catheter (extrinsic) or within the catheter (intrinsic). Intrinsic thrombosis is the major cause of catheter failure and can occur within the lumen of the catheter, at the tip of the catheter, or can present as a fibrin sleeve surrounding the catheter. Fibrin sleeves can obstruct the catheter and be a nidus for infection. Thrombosis is first suspected when blood cannot be aspirated from the catheter yet saline flows in freely. Catheter-related thrombosis can be diagnosed using ultrasonography, venography or computed tomography scans.[12,26,27]

Infections of the vascular access are a major problem in HD patients. The most common cause of access infection is *Staphylococcus aureus,* although other organisms can be isolated. The type of access is one of the most important risk factors for infection. AV fistulas have the lowest rate of infection followed by grafts, tunneled catheters, and temporary catheters. Catheters in general have more than a sevenfold risk of infection versus fistulas.[28,29] Catheter-related infections can be exit site, tunnel infection, and catheter-related bacteremia.[30] Patients with diabetes, immunosuppression, a history of bacteremia, and those with *S. aureus* nasal carriage are at highest risk for catheter-related bacteremia. Bacteria can seed distant sites and cause endocarditis, osteomyelitis, and septic arthritis.[31] Clinically, patients present with fever and chills. If fever and chills occur after catheter manipulation, it is highly suggestive of catheter-related bacteremia.[28,29]

DIALYZER REACTIONS

Dialyzer reactions encompass a broad range of clinical symptoms that include anaphylactic (type A) and nonspecific (type B) events.[23] In the past, these two types of reactions were considered to be part of the "first-use" syndrome because they occurred much more frequently when new, as opposed to reprocessed, dialyzers were used. Although reprocessing may reduce the incidence of type B events, it has little to no benefit for patients who experience a type A reaction.[32] The

TABLE 45–3. Common Complications during Hemodialysis

	Incidence (%)	Etiology/Predisposing Factors
Hypotension	20–30	Hypovolemia and excessive ultrafiltration Antihypertensive medications prior to dialysis Target dry weight too low Diastolic dysfunction Autonomic dysfunction Low calcium and sodium in dialysate High dialysate temperature Meal ingestion prior to dialysis
Cramps	5–20	Muscle hypoperfusion due to ultrafiltration and hypovolemia Hypotension Electrolyte imbalance Acid-base imbalance
Nausea and vomiting	5–15	Hypotension Dialyzer reaction
Headache	5	Disequilibrium syndrome Caffeine withdrawal due to dialysis removal
Chest and back pain	2–5	Unknown
Pruritus	5	Inadequate dialysis Skin dryness Secondary hyperparathyroidism Abnormal skin levels of electrolytes Histamine release Mast cell proliferation
Fever and chills	<1	Endotoxin release Infection of dialysis catheter

symptom complex associated with type A reactions is similar to a drug-induced anaphylactic reaction and may be a result of hypersensitivity to ethylene oxide (a common dialyzer sterilant), heparin, or formaldehyde and glutaraldehyde (common reuse sterilants). This type of reaction has also been associated with activation of the bradykinin system by some dialyzer membranes (especially the AN69), particularly in patients receiving angiotensin-converting enzyme inhibitors, because these agents block bradykinin inactivation.[23] A similar reaction has been reported with the use of the angiotensin receptor blocker losartan.[33] However, the mechanism is unclear, as angiotensin receptor blockers do not increase bradykinin levels. In the event of an anaphylactic reaction, the dialysis procedure should be stopped immediately. The blood in the dialysis circuit should not be returned to the patient, and resuscitative therapy with epinephrine, antihistamines, and steroids is likely to be required.

Type B reactions are more common than type A reactions, but are less severe (3 to 5 per 100 treatments vs. 5 per 100,000 treatments). Chest and back pain are the most frequently reported symptoms and may be noted within minutes of the start of dialysis or delayed (up to 1 to 2 hours). Complement activation has been suggested as the initiating event. Although no specific treatment is warranted and the patient can continue with dialysis treatment, the patient may be switched to a different dialyzer and/or put on a reprocessing program because this may minimize the occurrence of this reaction in the future.[23]

▶ TREATMENT: Hemodialysis Complications

■ HYPOTENSION

Acute management of hypotension includes placing the patient in the Trendelenburg position, decreasing the ultrafiltration rate, and/or administering normal or hypertonic saline.[23,25] Numerous nonpharmacologic and pharmacotherapeutic interventions have been used to prevent or reduce the incidence of symptomatic dialysis hypotension (Table 45–4). Randomized, blinded, prospective trials are rare and thus comparisons between therapeutic alternatives are difficult to quantify. If patients remain symptomatic after nonpharmacologic interventions, oral midodrine, an α_1-adrenergic agonist prodrug with peripheral vasoconstrictive properties may be considered. Midodrine, when administered in doses ranging from 2.5 to 25 mg prior to dialysis, has been shown to significantly increase the minimal systolic (from 93 to 97 raised to 107 to 114 mm Hg) and diastolic (from 52 to 53 raised to 58 to 59 mm Hg) blood pressures during dialysis.[34–36] Furthermore, dialysis symptoms of cramps, fatigue, dizziness, and weakness are reduced with midodrine treatment.[34] A long-term study of the benefits of midodrine found that 10 mg given 30 minutes prior to dialysis resulted in correction of hypotension over a 8-month period without any adverse events.[37] Some HD patients have chronic hypotension and experience low blood pressure even when not on dialysis. Oral midodrine given 5 mg twice daily can increase blood pressure in these patients as well.[38] It is important to note that the effects of midodrine are probably best in patients with hypotension related to autonomic dysfunction as opposed to other causes of hypotension.

Other medications have also been studied in hypotension. The intravenous administration of levocarnitine (20 mg/kg at the end of each dialysis session) reduced the number of hypotensive episodes from 17 to 7 ($p < 0.02$) in a study of 38 patients, while a placebo group demonstrated no significant benefit.[39] The high cost and fairly limited data on levocarnitine relegates this agent to a third- to fourth-line alternative. There has been some speculation that caffeine administration may decrease the incidence of dialysis-associated hypotension. Shinzato and colleagues observed a significantly lower frequency of sudden-onset hypotension (1.7 ± 1.5 times per 4 weeks in the caffeine group versus 4.4 ± 1.5 times per 4 weeks in the placebo group), but no effect on gradual-onset hypotension.[40] However, an earlier trial failed to show an effect of caffeine when patients experienced hypotension due to food ingestion.[41] Caffeine has a minimal likelihood of adverse events and can be easily administered, and thus may be considered if midodrine is ineffective.

Other drugs that may have some benefit include sertraline[42,43] and fludrocortisone.[44] These medications may be tried in individual patients with hypotension, but clearly more studies are required before they can be broadly recommended.

■ MUSCLE CRAMPS

Skeletal muscle cramps complicate 5% to 20% of hemodialysis treatments.[23] Although the pathogenesis of cramps is multifactorial, plasma volume contraction and decreased muscle perfusion caused by excessive ultrafiltration is frequently the initiating event. Although there are no comparative data regarding the efficacy of nonpharmacologic and pharmacologic therapy, the former should be the first line of treatment because the adverse consequences are minimal (Table 45–5).

Both vitamin E and quinine significantly reduce the incidence of cramps (in one study from 10.4 and 10.9 per month to 3.3 and 3.6 per month, respectively [$p < 0.0005$]).[45] Quinine is usually well tolerated,

TABLE 45–4. Management of Hypotension

Acute treatment	Place patient in Trendelenburg position
	Decrease ultrafiltration rate
	Give a 100- to 200-mL bolus of normal saline
	Give 10–20 mL of hypertonic saline (23.4%) over 3–5 min
	Give 12.5 g mannitol
Prevention	
Nonpharmacologic	Accurately set dry weight
	Use a constant ultrafiltration rate
	Keep dialysate sodium greater than serum sodium
	Use cool dialysate
	Use bicarbonate dialysate
	Avoid food before or during hemodialysis
Pharmacologic	Midodrine 2.5–10 mg orally 30 min before hemodialysis (start at 2.5 mg and titrate)
	Other options (not well studied):
	Caffeine 250 mg orally 2 hours into hemodialysis session
	Levocarnitine 20 mg/kg IV after hemodialysis
	Sertraline 50–100 mg daily
	Fludrocortisone 0.1 mg before hemodialysis

TABLE 45–5. Management of Cramps

Acute treatment	Give a 100- to 200-mL bolus of normal saline
	Give 10–20 mL of hypertonic saline (23.4%) over 3–5 min
	Give 50 mL of 50% glucose (nondiabetic patients)
Prevention	
Nonpharmacologic	Accurately set dry weight
	Keep dialysate sodium greater than serum sodium
	Stretching exercises
Pharmacologic	Give vitamin E 400 international units at bedtime
	Quinine (not recommended)
	Other options (not well studied):
	Oxazepam 5–10 mg 2 hours before hemodialysis
	Prazosin 0.25 mg orally at the start of hemodialysis

TABLE 45–6. Management of Hemodialysis Catheter Thrombosis

Nonpharmacologic therapy
Forced saline flush
Mechanical thrombectomy
Catheter stripping
Exchange of catheter over guidewire
Pharmacologic therapy
Alteplase: Instill 2 mg/2 mL per catheter port. Attempt to aspirate after 30 minutes. May repeat dose if catheter function not restored in 120 minutes. Longer durations of instillation have been used.
Reteplase: Instill 0.5 units/2 mL per catheter port

but rarely may cause temporary sight and hearing disturbances, thrombocytopenia, or gastrointestinal distress. Furthermore, it tends to increase plasma digoxin levels and may enhance the effect of warfarin. This constellation of adverse events prompted the withdrawal of quinine from the over-the-counter market in 1995. Prescription quinine can no longer be marketed for leg cramps. A recent randomized double-blind, placebo-controlled trial demonstrated that both vitamin E (400 mg) and vitamin C (250 mg) reduce the frequency of cramps in dialysis patients. The combination of these two drugs had an additive effect. Although these data further strengthen the case for vitamin E, it is unclear what role oral vitamin C would play in the U.S. since many patients are on a renal multiple vitamin that contains vitamin C (the current study restricted all vitamin products for 1 month prior to the study). Furthermore, there is some concern that oxalate, a metabolite of vitamin C, may accumulate in dialysis patients.

There have been other drugs studied in HD-related cramps. Prazosin appears to significantly reduce the incidence of cramps during hemodialysis.[46] Unfortunately, its use was associated with a significant increase in the incidence of hypotension that required therapeutic intervention during and after dialysis. A recent study by Chang and colleagues suggested that creatine might have some beneficial effects on muscle cramps in dialysis patients.[47] Ten patients with intradialytic muscle cramps were randomized to either creatine (12 mg before dialysis) or placebo. The frequency of muscle cramps decreased 60% in the creatine group, while there were no differences in the placebo group. Although serum creatinine concentrations rose in the treatment group, no side effects were noted.

Thus vitamin E appears to be the first choice among these therapeutic options due to the accumulated evidence in clinical trials and because of its fairly good safety profile.

■ THROMBOSIS

If a catheter-related thrombus is suspected, a series of saline flushes can be used to try to clear the catheter. Although this would indicate the thrombi has embolized, it is considered safe and frequently effective. Intraluminal thrombolytics are a second option and are widely used in dialysis units.[27] The thrombolytic with the most ex-

perience is urokinase, but this was withdrawn from the U.S. market in 1999 due to the risks of transmitting infectious agents. Urokinase was reintroduced in the U.S. market in 2002, but is only available as a 250,000-international unit vial (prior to 1999 there was a 5000-international unit vial specifically designed for catheter clearance). There have been a number of studies published using alteplase[48–51] and reteplase[52,53] for thrombosed hemodialysis catheters. Two studies that compared alteplase vs. urokinase suggest that alteplase might be more effective.[48,50] The initial clearance rate for both alteplase and reteplase is approximately 90%. However, there are no data available that directly compare alteplase and reteplase for management of dialysis catheter thrombosis. Alteplase (but not reteplase) is FDA approved for restoration of function to central venous catheters due to thrombosis, and is commercially available as a 2-mg vial. Therapeutic alternatives for thrombosed venous catheters are presented in Table 45–6.

TABLE 45–7. Guidelines for the Treatment of Hemodialysis Access Infections

 I. Primary Arteriovenous Fistula
   A. Treat as subacute bacterial endocarditis for 6 weeks.
   B. Initial antibiotic choice should always cover gram-positive organisms, e.g., vancomycin 20 mg/kg IV with serum concentration monitoring or cefazolin 20 mg/kg IV 3 times per week.
   C. Gram-negative coverage is indicated for patients with diabetes, HIV infection, prosthetic valves, or those receiving immunosuppressive agents, gentamicin 2 mg/kg IV with serum concentration monitoring.
 II. Synthetic Arteriovenous Grafts
   A. Local infection—empiric antibiotic coverage for gram-positive, gram-negative, and *Enterococcus*, e.g., gentamicin plus vancomycin then individualized after culture results available. Continue for 2 to 4 weeks.
   B. Extensive infection—antibiotics as above plus total resection.
   C. If access is less than 1 month old, antibiotics as above plus remove the graft.
 III. Tunneled Cuffed Catheters (Internal Jugular, Subclavians)
   A. Infection localized to catheter exit site.
     1. No drainage—topical antibiotics, e.g., mupirocin ointment.
     2. Drainage present—gram-positive antibiotic coverage, e.g., cefazolin 20 mg/kg IV 3 times per week.
   B. Bacteremia with or without systemic signs or symptoms.
     1. Gram-positive antibiotic coverage as in III A2.
     2. If symptomatic at 36 hours, remove the catheter.
     3. If stable and asymptomatic, change catheter and provide culture-specific antibiotic coverage for a minimum of 3 weeks.

◾ INFECTION

Patients who experience fever during HD should immediately have blood cultures obtained. If a temporary catheter is being used, it should be removed and the tip of the catheter cultured. Commonly used preventive approaches to catheter-related infections include minimizing use and duration of catheters, proper disinfection and sterile technique, and use of exit-site mupirocin or povidone-iodine ointment. Adoption of strict unit protocols that employ universal precautions, limit manipulation of the catheter, use disinfection with povidone-iodine, and require the use of face masks by the patient and caregiver can significantly reduce the incidence of catheter-related bacteremia.[30] Optimal approaches for the treatment of HD access–related infection have been proposed by the K/DOQI, and Table 45–7 outlines these recommendations.[14] Many clinicians also add an aminoglycoside to the regimen for empiric therapy in catheter-related bacteremia. If the isolated organism is methicillin-sensitive *S. aureus*, therapy may be changed to cefazolin (20 mg/kg, rounded to nearest 500 mg) after each dialysis session.[31,54,55]

PERITONEAL DIALYSIS

Although the concept of peritoneal lavage has been described as far back as 1744, it wasn't until 1923 that PD was first employed as an acute treatment for uremia. It was used infrequently during subsequent years until the concept of PD as a chronic therapy for ESKD was proposed in 1975. In 1978, the results of a cooperative study were published describing the successful management of nine patients with continuous ambulatory peritoneal dialysis (CAPD). Over the ensuing years the number of patients receiving CAPD increased slowly until the early 1980s. At that time, several innovations in PD delivery systems were introduced, such as improved catheters and dialysate bags. These innovations led to improved outcomes, decreased morbidity, and a corresponding increase in the use of CAPD as a viable alternative to HD for the treatment of ESKD.

Although PD use steadily increased through the 1980s and 1990s, it peaked in 1996 and there has been slow but constant decline since then. Between 1997 and 2001 the prevalent PD population has decreased at a rate of 4.9% per year.[1] Reasons for this decline are not well defined. However, it has been shown that certain patient populations may fare better on one dialysis modality compared to the other and this may be a factor.[4,6,56,57] Some patients—such as those with more hemodynamic instability (angina or hyper- or hypotension) or significant residual renal function, and perhaps patients who desire to maintain a significant degree of self-care may be better suited to PD rather than to HD. Table 45–2 shows the advantages and disadvantages of PD.

PRINCIPLES OF PERITONEAL DIALYSIS

The three basic components of dialysis—namely, a blood-filled compartment separated from a dialysate-filled compartment by a semipermeable membrane—are also used for PD. In PD, the dialysate-filled compartment is the peritoneal cavity, into which dialysate is instilled via a permanent peritoneal catheter that traverses the abdominal wall. The contiguous peritoneal membrane surrounds the peritoneal cavity. The cavity, which normally contains about 100 mL of lipid-rich lubricating fluid, can expand to a capacity of several liters. The peritoneal membrane that lines the cavity functions as the semipermeable membrane, across which diffusion and ultrafiltration occur. The membrane is classically described as a monocellular layer of mesothelial cells. However, the dialyzing membrane is also comprised of the basement membrane and underlying connective and interstitial tissue. The peritoneal membrane has a total area that approximates body surface area (about 1 to 2 m^2). Blood vessels supplying and draining the abdominal viscera, musculature, and mesentery constitute the blood-filled compartment.

Metabolic waste products (urea, creatinine, uremic toxins, and water) to be removed from blood during PD are not in intimate contact with the dialysis membrane as they are in hemodialysis, and must therefore travel a considerable distance to the dialysate-filled compartment. Unlike hemodialysis, there is no easy method to regulate blood flow to the surface of the peritoneal membrane, nor is there a countercurrent flow of blood and dialysate to increase diffusion and convection via changes in hydrostatic pressure. For these reasons, PD is a much less efficient process per unit time compared with HD, and must therefore be a virtually continuous procedure to achieve acceptable goals for clearance of metabolic waste products.

During most PD modalities, the metabolic waste clearance profile is markedly different from what is observed in HD patients. In patients treated with intermittent HD, the serum concentrations of metabolic wastes exhibit a "sawtooth" pattern over time. Because CAPD is essentially continuous, a condition similar to a steady state can occur. When the PD dose is well matched to the generation rate of metabolic waste, the serum levels of metabolic waste products fluctuate less over time. Therefore CAPD may represent a more physiologic process that is similar to endogenous renal function. Furthermore, the massive swings in body water content and high peak concentrations of uremic toxins in HD patients are less than optimal. CAPD may therefore be more beneficial for patients with cardiovascular instability.

The peritoneal membrane has different transport characteristics and permits the passage of larger-molecular-weight solutes than the older, low-flux conventional type of HD membranes. However, this difference is less marked for newer, high-flux membranes. These differences not only aid our understanding of the relative efficiency of each system in the removal of endogenous solutes, but also help us to predict the dialyzability of exogenously administered drugs.

PERITONEAL DIALYSIS ACCESS

Access to the peritoneal cavity is via the placement of an indwelling catheter. Many types are available and a typical example is shown in Fig. 45–3. Most catheters are manufactured from Silastic, which is soft, flexible, and biocompatible. A typical adult catheter is about 40 to 45 cm long, 20 to 22 cm of which are inside the peritoneal cavity. Placement of the catheter is such that the distal end lies low in a pelvic gutter. The center section of the catheter has one or two cuffs made of a porous material. This section is tunneled inside the anterior abdominal wall so that the cuffs provide mechanical support and stability to the catheter, a mechanical barrier to skin organisms, and prevent their migration along the catheter into the peritoneal cavity. The cuffs are placed at different sites surrounding the abdominal rectus muscle. The remainder of the central section of the catheter is tunneled subcutaneously before exiting the abdominal surface, usually a few centimeters below and to one side of the umbilicus.

The placement of the exit site of the catheter is one of the factors related to the development or prevention of exit-site infections and peritonitis. Many new catheters and surgical techniques for catheter placement have recently been developed. The driving forces for this

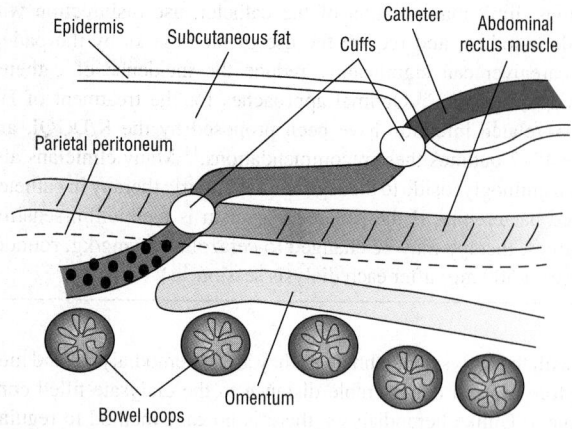

FIGURE 45–3. Diagram of the placement of a peritoneal dialysis catheter through the abdominal wall into the peritoneal cavity.

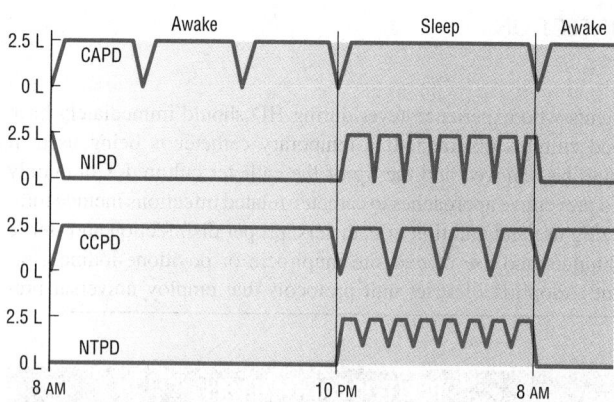

FIGURE 45–4. Comparison of peritoneal dialysis modalities. Continuous ambulatory peritoneal dialysis (CAPD). Patients perform three 2.5-L peritoneal dialysate exchanges during waking hours (8 AM to 10 PM), with each dialysate dwell lasting approximately 4 hours. Before bedtime, they perform an exchange and instill 2.5 L of dialysate overnight (10 PM to 8 AM). The following morning, the patient performs an exchange and the process begins again.

Nocturnal intermittent peritoneal dialysis (NIPD). Patients are free from performing dialysate exchanges during their waking hours (8 AM to 10 PM). Prior to bedtime, they attach their catheter to a cycling machine and receive six to eight 2.5-L exchanges of dialysate while they sleep. Each dialysate dwell time is approximately 1–2 hours. The following morning, the patient unhooks their catheters from the cycler and goes about their normal activities with an empty peritoneum.

Continuous cycling peritoneal dialysis (CCPD). Patients instill 2.5 L of dialysate into their peritoneal cavity upon waking and allow it to dwell for the remainder of their waking hours (8 AM to 10 PM). Prior to bedtime, they drain the daytime dwell and attach their catheter to a cycling machine and receive three to five dialysate exchanges while they sleep. Each dialysate dwell time is approximately 2 hours long. The following morning, a 2.5-L dwell is instilled into the peritoneal cavity and the patient carries it during waking hours (8 AM to 10 PM).

Nocturnal tidal peritoneal dialysis (NTPD). Patients are free from performing dialysate exchanges during their waking hours (8 AM to 10 PM). Prior to bedtime, they attach their catheter to a cycling machine and instill a volume of 2500 mL of dialysate into their peritoneal cavity. Six to eight exchanges of 1250 mL are carried out approximately every hour. Thus the total dialysate volume introduced into the peritoneal cavity ranges from 10–12 L per day. The following morning, the patients unhook their catheters from the cycler and go about normal activities with an empty peritoneum. (Adapted from Brophy et al.[59])

development are to enhance patient comfort and to reduce infectious risk. The external section of most peritoneal catheters ends with a Luer-lock, which can be connected to a variety of administration sets.[58] These catheters can be used immediately if necessary, provided small initial volumes are instilled; however, a maturation period of 2 to 6 weeks is preferred.

PERITONEAL DIALYSIS PROCEDURES

6 There are several types of peritoneal dialysis, of which CAPD remains the most common. Others include a variety of automated systems (collectively termed automated peritoneal dialysis [APD]), including continuous cycling PD (CCPD), nocturnal tidal PD (NTPD), and nightly intermittent PD (NIPD) (Fig. 45–4).[59] In recent years, there has been a substantial increase in the number of PD patients being treated with APD systems. APD may eventually be used to treat more patients than CAPD. The prototypic form of APD is usually a hybrid between CAPD and CCPD, in which some of the daily exchanges (usually the overnight exchanges) are completed using an automated device. All variants of PD require the placement of a dialysis solution in the peritoneal cavity, allowing it to remain in situ for some period of time (called the dwell time), removing the spent dialysate, and then repeating the process.

All forms of PD use the same dialysate solutions, which are commercially available in volumes of 1 to 3 L in flexible polyvinyl chloride plastic bags. Commercial PD solutions include varying concentrations of electrolytes, such as sodium, chloride, lactate, and calcium. In addition, these solutions usually contain dextrose in hyperosmolar concentrations, which induces ultrafiltration (removal of free water) by crystalline osmosis. Dextrose concentrations range from 1.5% to 4.25%, which provides osmolarities of 350 to 480 mOsm/L, as compared to that of serum, which is 280 mOsm/L. It should be recognized that dextrose is not the ideal osmotic agent for peritoneal dialysate because these solutions are not biocompatible with peritoneal mesothelial cells or with peritoneal leukocytes.[60] The cytotoxic effects on these cells are mediated by the osmolar load and the low pH of the solutions, as well as the presence of glucose degradation products formed during heat sterilization of these products.

Icodextrin is a glucose polymer recently introduced for use as an alternative osmotic agent in PD solutions. Icodextrin PD solution contains 7.5% icodextrin, a starch-derived glucose polymer. It has an osmolality of 282 to 286 mOsm/L, which is iso-osmolar with

serum. Icodextrin produces prolonged ultrafiltration by a mechanism resembling colloid osmosis. Icodextrin produces ultrafiltration volumes similar to those with 4.25% dextrose, but may have fewer of the metabolic effects associated with dextrose, such as hyperglycemia and weight gain. It is indicated for use during the long (8- to 16-hour) dwell of a single daily exchange in CAPD and APD patients.[61] Other osmotic agents have been used in PD solutions, including mannitol, glycerol, and amino acids, but are not in widespread use because of expense or difficulty in manufacture.

In a basic CAPD system, prewarmed dialysate is permitted to flow into the peritoneal cavity under gravity over a period of about 15 minutes. A bag of PD solution is connected to the patient's PD catheter by a length of tubing called a transfer set. The most common transfer set used is the Y transfer set. This consists of a Y-shaped piece of tubing that is attached at its stem to the patient's catheter, leaving the remaining two limbs of the Y attached to dialysate bags, one filled with fresh dialysate and the other empty. The spent dialysate from the previous dwell is drained into the empty bag, and the peritoneum is subsequently refilled from the bag containing fresh dialysate. The Y set is then disconnected and the bag containing the spent fluid, along with the empty bag that had contained fresh dialysate, is detached and discarded. The Y transfer set with the double-bag system permits both a flush-before-fill procedure and disconnection during the dwell. This minimizes the number of times a patient manipulates the catheter, thereby reducing the risk of peritonitis and catheter-related infections. A typical dwell period for daytime exchanges in CAPD is 4 to 6 hours, using one of the lower-dextrose-concentration dialysate solutions. At the end of the prescribed dwell period a new Y set is attached and the process is repeated. The process of outflow, aseptic manipulation of the administration set and catheter, and inflow requires a total time of about 30 minutes. Thus dialysis actually occurs for about 3.5 hours out of a prescribed 4-hour period. Typically a patient instills 2 to 3 L of dialysate three times during the day, and then a single exchange using a higher-dextrose-concentration dialysate for an overnight, 8 to 12 hour dwell.

The prescribed dose of dialysis may be altered by changing the number of exchanges per day, by altering the volume of each exchange, or by altering the strength of dextrose in the dialysate for some or all exchanges. Increasing any one of these variables increases the effective osmotic gradient across the peritoneum, leading to increased ultrafiltration and diffusion (solute removal). If the dwell time is extended, equilibrium may be reached, after which time there will be no further water or solute removal. Indeed after a critical period, reverse water movement may occur.

Automated PD systems have been designed for patients who are unable or unwilling to perform the necessary aseptic manipulations, and for those who require more dialysis. APD provides an automated cycler that performs the exchanges. The device is set up in the evening, and the patient attaches the peritoneal catheter to it at bedtime. The machine performs several short-dwell exchanges (usually 1 to 2 hours) during the night. This permits a long cycle-free daytime dwell of up to 12 to 14 hours. Thus APD provides an exchange profile in reverse of that in CAPD. Typical APD regimens involve total 24-hour exchanges of about 12 L, which include one or more daytime dwells.[62] This type of regimen is sometimes referred to as APD with a "wet" day. The APD variant, NIPD, has a similar theme, except that the peritoneal cavity tends to be dialysate-free during the day. This type of regimen is frequently referred to as APD with a "dry" day. A number of variants exist and depend largely on equipment availability, patient and prescriber preference, and whether the patient retains any residual renal function, which influences the quantity of dialysis prescribed (see Fig. 45–4).[59]

ADEQUACY OF PERITONEAL DIALYSIS

Like HD, the subject of PD adequacy has received considerable attention. The K/DOQI recommends the use of two criteria to assess the dose of dialysis delivered during PD: total weekly Kt/V_{urea} and total weekly Cl_{cr} (in liters per week) normalized to 1.73 m^2 body surface area.[63] Although K/DOQI recommends target values for these adequacy indices, which are discussed below, the optimal dose of PD remains undefined, and the lower threshold of dialysis dose that constitutes an acceptable risk for patient outcome has been termed "adequate dialysis."

Unfortunately, it is easier to describe inadequate PD than it is to provide a universally accepted definition of adequate PD. True PD adequacy requires the identification of an optimal dialysis dose that will result in favorable long-term outcomes, such as survival and quality of life. Compared to hemodialysis, which is used by a much larger patient population, there are few data available regarding the optimal dose of dialysis in PD. As a result, much of the work in this area has focused on establishing the minimum acceptable PD

dose, and what constitutes "adequate" versus "optimal" dialysis is controversial.

The Canada-USA cooperative study (CANUSA) evaluated 680 PD patients in 14 centers who began dialysis between 1990 and 1992.[64] Decreases of 0.1 in weekly Kt/V_{urea} or 5 L/1.73 m^2 per week in Cl_{cr} were associated with 5% to 7% increases in the risk for death. No plateau was observed. Based on this finding it would appear that the greater the urea and creatinine clearances, the greater the rate of patient survival. One criticism of the CANUSA study was that it was assumed that the renal and peritoneal contributions to Kt/V were equivalent. Interestingly, the CANUSA data were reanalyzed to assess the contribution of residual renal function to the clinical results reported in CANUSA.[65] When solute clearance was subdivided into that contributed by residual renal function and that from peritoneal clearance, the former was found to be a more significant predictor of patient survival.

More recently, the Adequacy of Peritoneal Dialysis in Mexico (ADEMEX) study evaluated the effects of increased peritoneal solute clearance on clinical outcomes in 965 CAPD patients.[66] Despite significantly greater delivered peritoneal Cl_{cr} (56.9 ± 0.48 vs. 46.1 ± 0.45) and Kt/V (2.13 ± 0.01 vs. 1.62 ± 0.01) in the intervention group compared to controls, respectively, patient 2-year survival was similar in both groups. It has been suggested that the lack of an observed difference in mortality in the ADEMEX study resulted from the inclusion of both incident and prevalent PD patients. Prevalent patients, who represented 58% of the total, have already demonstrated their tendency for better long-term survival on PD.[67]

DIALYSIS DOSE (Kt/V)

As in hemodialysis, the clearance of urea, a product of protein catabolism, is measured with Kt/V. Kt/V is a unitless value that correlates the patient's peritoneal membrane urea clearance (K) with the duration of dialysis (t) and the volume of distribution (V) of urea. Calculation of Kt/V for PD requires that the total volume of drained effluent per day be determined (this value is the volume instilled plus volume of water ultrafiltered). The dialysate to plasma (D/P) urea concentration is determined, and Kt is estimated as:

$$Kt = D/P \times \text{volume drained (L/d)}$$

The urea distribution volume (V) is determined from a nomogram based on height, weight, age, and gender, or is approximated as 0.6 L/kg. The Kt/V calculated in this way is a value per day and must be multiplied by seven and reported as a weekly value for PD patients.

The K/DOQI clinical practice guidelines recommend that in CAPD patients, weekly Kt/V values should exceed 2. For APD with a dry day and wet day, the Kt/V values should exceed 2.2 and 2.1, respectively.[63] This difference may be because of the differences in efficiency of different variants of PD in clearing small- and middle-sized molecules. One problem associated with the determination of Kt/V for PD patients is the impracticality of 24-hour collections of dialysis effluent. Abbreviated collection periods have been used, and calculations based on the first morning exchange after an overnight dwell correlated well ($r = 0.92$) with a 24-hour collection.[68]

CREATININE CLEARANCE

Weekly measured Cl_{cr} normalized to 1.73 m^2 is also used to assess adequacy of PD. The Cl_{cr} measures the removal of a product of muscle metabolism and correlates well ($r = 0.71$) with Kt/V. For CAPD patients, the total Cl_{cr} should be at least 60 L/wk per 1.73 m^2, which is approximately equivalent to a weekly Kt/V_{urea} of 1.96. For APD with a dry day or a wet day, the corresponding values are 66 and 63 L/wk per 1.73 m^2, respectively. Such values are the sum of both peritoneal and residual renal clearance and are influenced by body muscle mass.[63]

PERITONEAL EQUILIBRATION TEST

The peritoneal equilibration test (PET) is a diagnostic test designed to determine an individual PD patient's peritoneal membrane clearance and ultrafiltration characteristics. The objective of the PET is to determine which variant of PD is appropriate for an individual patient and to predict the daily dialysis requirement. The PET simultaneously determines the passage of creatinine and urea from blood to dialysate, glucose from dialysate to blood, and free water transfer across the peritoneal membrane. During a PET, simultaneous blood and dialysate samples (for determination of creatinine, urea, and glucose) are obtained at predetermined intervals during a standardized dialysate dwell. The dialysate is drained after 4 hours and the drain volume is recorded. Dialysate to plasma (D:P) ratios of creatinine and urea, and ratios of glucose in the dialysate compared to its initial concentration (D:D$_0$) are calculated. Based on these ratios, peritoneal membrane transport status is divided into four categories: high, high average, low average, or low. Based on the drain volume, the ultrafiltration rate is categorized as poor, adequate, good, or excellent. Patients with "high" membrane transport will have rapid clearance of creatinine and urea. However, they will also rapidly absorb glucose. Because the glucose concentration in the dialysate is the primary force that results in ultrafiltration, it follows that patients who have a high transport rate often have poor ultrafiltration. Conversely, patients with "low" membrane transport generally have excellent ultrafiltration but inadequate clearance of creatinine and urea. As a result, "low" transporters may be more appropriately treated with HD than PD.

CHANGING THE PD PRESCRIPTION

The K/DOQI clinical practice guidelines suggest that the adequacy of PD be assessed by using measured Kt/V and Cl$_{cr}$ three times in the first 6 months of dialysis (i.e., at months 1, 4, and 6).[63] The reasoning behind this frequency is to accurately establish a baseline creatinine and urea excretion rate. Thereafter the Kt/V and Cl$_{cr}$ should be measured every 4 months, at months 10, 14, and so on. The rationale for this is that it is imperative to detect subtle decreases in residual renal function and noncompliance and to make the necessary alterations to the prescribed PD dose to compensate for them. It is recommended that the first PET be conducted within the first month of treatment. Because solute clearance is dependent on peritoneal membrane transport properties, the guidelines also recommend that a PET be conducted within the first month of treatment. Future PET assessment is only recommended for patients with suspected changes in peritoneal membrane transport function, particularly when usual efforts to increase the PD dose are not successful.

It is important to note that residual renal function may provide a significant component of the total Kt/V and Cl$_{cr}$. Patients may commence PD with a residual Cl$_{cr_{renal}}$ of about 9 to 12 mL/min, which might equate to a Kt/V_{renal} of 0.2 to 0.4. Over a period of 1 to 2 years, residual renal function tends to progressively deteriorate to zero. Because Kt/V_{total} is the sum of Kt/V_{PD} and Kt/V_{renal}, the Kt/V_{total} will progressively diminish unless Kt/V_{PD} is increased (by increasing the prescribed dose of PD) to compensate for the reduced Kt/V_{renal}. Thus

unless Kt/V_{PD} is increased, Kt/V_{total} may diminish from 2 to 1.7 over this period of time.

This progressive loss of residual renal function is the major cause of decreased total clearance in PD patients over time. Unfortunately, the standard regimen of four 2-L exchanges per day in CAPD may provide inadequate clearances in some patients, especially larger patients. In larger patients, clearances might be maximized by adopting larger fill volumes (2.5 to 3 L), more frequent exchanges (5 to 6 per day), and the use of wet days in APD patients.[63] A wet day is a regimen that includes a prolonged dwell during the daytime, between the frequent automated nighttime exchanges.

COMPLICATIONS OF PERITONEAL DIALYSIS

Mechanical, medical, and infectious problems complicate peritoneal dialysis therapy. Mechanical complications include kinking of the catheter and inflow and outflow obstruction; excessive catheter motion at the exit site, leading to induration and possible infection and aggravation of tissues; pain from impingement of the catheter tip on the viscera; or inflow pain resulting from a jet effect of too rapid dialysate inflow.

Table 45–8 lists the numerous medical complications of PD. An average PD patient absorbs up to 60% of the dextrose in each exchange. This continuous supply of calories leads to increased adipose tissue deposition, decreased appetite, malnutrition, and altered requirements for insulin in diabetic patients. Fibrin formation in dialysate is common and can lead to obstruction of catheter outflow. Infectious complications of PD are a major cause of morbidity and mortality and are the leading cause of technique failure and transfer from PD to hemodialysis. The two predominant infectious complications are peritonitis and catheter-related infections, which include both exit-site and tunnel infections.

PERITONITIS

Some 40% to 60% of patients develop their first episode of peritonitis within 1 year of starting CAPD, although the incidence is significantly lower in APD patients.[69] Peritonitis is a major cause of catheter loss in PD patients. A statistically significant correlation between infectious complications and death rates has been reported.[70] Of patients who had more than 1 peritonitis episode per year, 0.5 to 1 episode per year, or less than 0.5 episode per year, 50% died after 3, 4, and

TABLE 45–8. Medical Complications of Peritoneal Dialysis

Cause	Complication	Treatment
Glucose load	Exacerbation of diabetes mellitus	IP insulin
Fluid overload	Exacerbation of CHF	Increase ultrafiltration
	Edema	
	Pulmonary congestion	Diuretics, if the patient has residual renal function
Electrolyte abnormalities	Hyper- and hypocalcemia	Alter dialysate calcium content
PD additives	Chemical peritonitis	Discontinue PD additives
Malnutrition	Albumin loss	Dietary changes, parenteral nutrition, discontinue PD
	Loss of amino acids	
	Muscle wasting	
	Increased adipose tissue	
Unknown	Fibrin formation in dialysate	IP heparin

years of therapy, respectively. It is important to note that these relationships are not necessarily cause and effect, because many of these patients succumb to cardiovascular events. The incidence of peritonitis is influenced by connector technology, by the composition of patient populations, and by the use of APD versus CAPD. The incidence of peritonitis for most dialysis centers in the United States is about one episode every 24 patient-months, although it may be as low as one episode every 60 patient-months.[71]

CLINICAL PRESENTATION OF PERITONEAL DIALYSIS–RELATED PERITONITIS

GENERAL
Patients generally present with abdominal pain and cloudy effluent.

SYMPTOMS
The patient may complain of abdominal tenderness, abdominal pain, fever, nausea and vomiting, and chills.

SIGNS
Cloudy dialysate effluent may be observed following exchange.
Temperature may or may not be elevated.

LABORATORY TESTS
Dialysate white blood cell count >100/mm^3, of which at least 50% are polymorphonuclear neutrophils.
Gram stain of a centrifuged dialysate specimen.

OTHER DIAGNOSTIC TESTS
Culture and sensitivity of dialysate should be obtained.

Peritonitis has several imprecise definitions, but guidelines suggest that an elevated dialysate white blood cell (WBC) count of less than 100 per microliter with at least 50% polymorphonuclear neutrophils indicates the presence of inflammation, of which peritonitis is the most likely cause.[72] A patient who presents with abdominal pain and a cloudy effluent is usually given a provisional diagnosis of peritonitis. Inherent in this definition is a number of false-positive and false-negative diagnoses, because a small percentage of patients with culture-proven peritonitis will have clear dialysate, and some patients, such as menstruating females, may have cloudy PD effluent without clinical infection.[71] Sterile culture peritonitis remains problematic; it is defined as an episode in which there is clinical suspicion of peritonitis, but for which the culture of the dialysate reveals no organisms. There are several postulates for the high incidence (up to 20% of episodes) of culture-negative peritonitis. Many peritonitis-producing organisms are slime producers and may adhere to the peritoneal membrane or to the catheter surface and be protected from exogenous antibiotics.[73] Sufficient numbers of these bacteria may proliferate to cause peritoneal membrane inflammation and clinical peritonitis, but an inadequate number may seed into the peritoneal cavity to be recovered by conventional microbiologic techniques. In addition, planktonic bacteria may be rapidly phagocytosed by peritoneal WBCs, thereby rendering them unavailable for culture.

Most of the organisms producing peritonitis adhere to the peritoneal membrane, with a relatively smaller number appearing as free-floating planktonic bacteria in dialysate. There may be as few as 10^4 planktonic organisms per milliliter of effluent. Removal of a small volume of dialysate from the bag may thus result in too few organisms to culture. Contemporary methods have increased the recovery rate of organisms and decreased the culture-negative rate. Centrifugation is currently recommended as the optimum culture method. Centrifugation of a large volume of dialysate (50 mL), resuspension of the sediment in 3 to 5 mL of sterile saline, and subsequent inoculation in culture media produces a culture-negative rate less than 5%. If centrifuge equipment is not available, blood culture bottles can be directly injected with 5 to 10 mL of dialysate effluent. However, this method results in a culture-negative rate up to 20%.[72]

The majority of infections are caused by gram-positive bacteria in CAPD, of which *Staphylococcus epidermidis* is the predominant organism.[74] There is no single predominant gram-negative organism. Together, gram-positive and gram-negative organisms account for 80% to 90% of all episodes of peritonitis, and constitute the spectrum against which initial empiric therapy is directed. In APD, there is a relative increase in the percentage of infections caused by polymicrobial and fungal organisms.

▶ TREATMENT: Peritonitis

The International Society of Peritoneal Dialysis (ISPD) Ad Hoc Advisory Committee on Peritoneal Dialysis Related Infections evaluates the diagnostic and therapeutic literature periodically. The most recent report, published in 2005, provides guidelines for the diagnosis and pharmacotherapy of PD-associated infections.[72] The 2005 ISPD guidelines reflect significant changes from the previous version and specifically address the increasing importance of dialysis center specific antibiotic selection, the effect of residual renal function on the pharmacokinetics of antibiotics, and updated recommendations regarding the use of aminoglycosides and vancomycin.

Intraperitoneal (IP) administration of antibiotics remains the preferred route over IV therapy. The guidelines provide dosing recommendations for intermittent (one large dose into one exchange per day) and continuous therapy (antibiotic addition to each exchange). In addition, dosing recommendations are modified on the basis of the patient's PD modality (CAPD or APD) and whether or not the patient has residual renal function (>100 mL/day urine output). The choice between intermittent and continuous therapies requires careful consideration for several reasons. The dialysate and serum concentrations achieved after these regimens are very different. The pharmacokinetics of intermittent intraperitoneal ceftazidime and cefazolin are well described. Single daily doses of cefazolin and ceftazidime in CAPD are effective in achieving serum concentrations greater than the minimum inhibitory concentration for sensitive organisms over 48 hours. In CAPD, it is usual to add the single daily dose into the exchange with the longest dwell, to ensure maximal bioavailability. Intermittent (once-daily) IP dosing of antibiotics is recommended for CAPD patients with peritonitis.[72] However, APD dosing strategies are different, because of the increased clearances of solutes in such systems. This appears to be particularly important for first-generation cephalosporins. The ISPD guidelines recommend continuous dosing of first generation cephalosporins due to concerns over inadequate IP drug concentration during the shorter APD dialysate dwells. With regard to residual renal function, in patients with daily urine output greater than 100 mL, the dose should be empirically increased by 25% for drugs that are renally eliminated. The ISPD dosing recommendations for IP antibiotics in CAPD and APD patients are shown in Tables 45–9 and 45–10, respectively.[72]

TABLE 45–9. Intraperitoneal Antibiotic Dosing Recommendations for CAPD Patients[72]

Drug	Intermittent (per exchange, once daily)	Continuous (mg per liter, all exchanges)
Aminoglycosides		
Amikacin*	2 mg/kg	LD 25, MD 12
Gentamicin*	0.6 mg/kg	LD 8, MD 4
Netilmicin*	0.6 mg/kg	LD 8, MD 4
Tobramycin*	0.6 mg/kg	LD 8, MD 4
Cephalosporins		
Cefazolin*	15 mg/kg	LD 500, MD 125
Cefepime*	1 g	LD 500, MD 125
Cephalothin*	15 mg/kg	LD 500, MD 125
Cephradine*	15 mg/kg	LD 500, MD 125
Ceftazidime*	1000–1500 mg	LD 500, MD 125
Ceftizoxime*	1000 mg	LD 250, MD 125
Penicillins		
Azlocillin*	ND	LD 500, MD 250
Ampicillin*	ND	MD 125
Oxacillin*	ND	MD 125
Nafcillin*	ND	MD 125
Amoxicillin*	ND	LD 250–500, MD 50
Penicillin G*	ND	LD 50,000 units, MD 25,000 units
Quinolones		
Ciprofloxacin*	ND	LD 50, MD 25
Others		
Vancomycin*	15–30 mg/kg Q5-7d	LD 1000, MD 25
Aztreonam*	ND	LD 1000, MD 250
Antifungals		
Amphotericin B	NA	1.5
Combinations		
Ampicillin/sulbactam*	2 g Q12h	LD 1000, MD 100
Imipenem/cilastatin*	1 g BID	LD 500, MD 200
Quinupristin/dalfopristin	25 mg/L in alternate bags**	

LD, loading dose in mg; MD, maintenance dose in mg; NA, not applicable; ND, no data; NA, not applicable.
* Dosing of drugs with renal clearance in patients with residual renal function (defined as more than 100 mL/day urine output) dose should be empirically increased by 25%.
** Given in conjunction with 500 mg IV twice daily.

Initial empiric therapy for peritonitis, regardless of whether a Gram stain was performed or organisms were identified, should include agents effective against both gram-positive and gram-negative organisms. Antibiotic selection should be made with consideration given to the dialysis center's and the patient's history of infecting organisms and the antibiotic sensitivity profile of the organisms. In many cases, a first-generation cephalosporin such as cefazolin in combination with a second drug that provides broader gram-negative coverage, such as ceftazidime, cefepime, or an aminoglycoside, will prove suitable. Patients with documented allergy to cephalosporin

TABLE 45–10. Intermittent Intraperitoneal Antibiotic Dosing Recommendations for APD Patients[72]

Drug	Intraperitoneal Dose
Vancomycin	Loading dose 30 mg/kg IP in long dwell, repeat dosing 15 mg/kg IP in long dwell every 3–5 days, following levels
Tobramycin	Loading dose 1.5 mg/kg IP in long dwell, then 0.5 mg/kg IP each day in long day dwell
Fluconazole	200 mg IP in one exchange per day every 24–48 h
Cefepime	1 g IP in one exchange per day

antibiotics can be treated with vancomycin and an aminoglycoside. High rates of methicillin resistance have been reported by many dialysis centers and vancomycin should be used as first-line therapy against gram-positive organisms for patients treated at these centers. Monotherapy with agents providing both gram-positive and gram-negative coverage is an alternative option. Both imipenem/cilastin and cefepime have been found to be effective in treating CAPD related peritonitis.

After culture and sensitivity results are obtained, antibiotic therapy should be adjusted appropriately (Fig. 45–5). If the patient does not show signs of clinical improvement within 72 hours after antibiotic treatment is initiated, the culture should be repeated and the patient re-evaluated. For streptococcal or enterococcal peritonitis, IP ampicillin (125 mg/L in each exchange) is the preferred treatment. For *Enterococcus*, the addition of an aminoglycoside, depending on sensitivities, may be warranted for synergy. In addition, if the *Enterococcus* is resistant to both ampicillin and vancomycin, linezolid or quinupristin/dalfopristin are recommended. However, quinupristin/dalfopristin is not effective against *E. faecalis*.

The presence of *S. aureus* warrants the use of either cefazolin or vancomycin. If the strain of *S. aureus* is methicillin resistant, then vancomycin should be used. Oral rifampin can be added if there is an inadequate clinical response, defined as continued cloudy dialysate, abdominal pain, and elevated dialysate white blood cells.

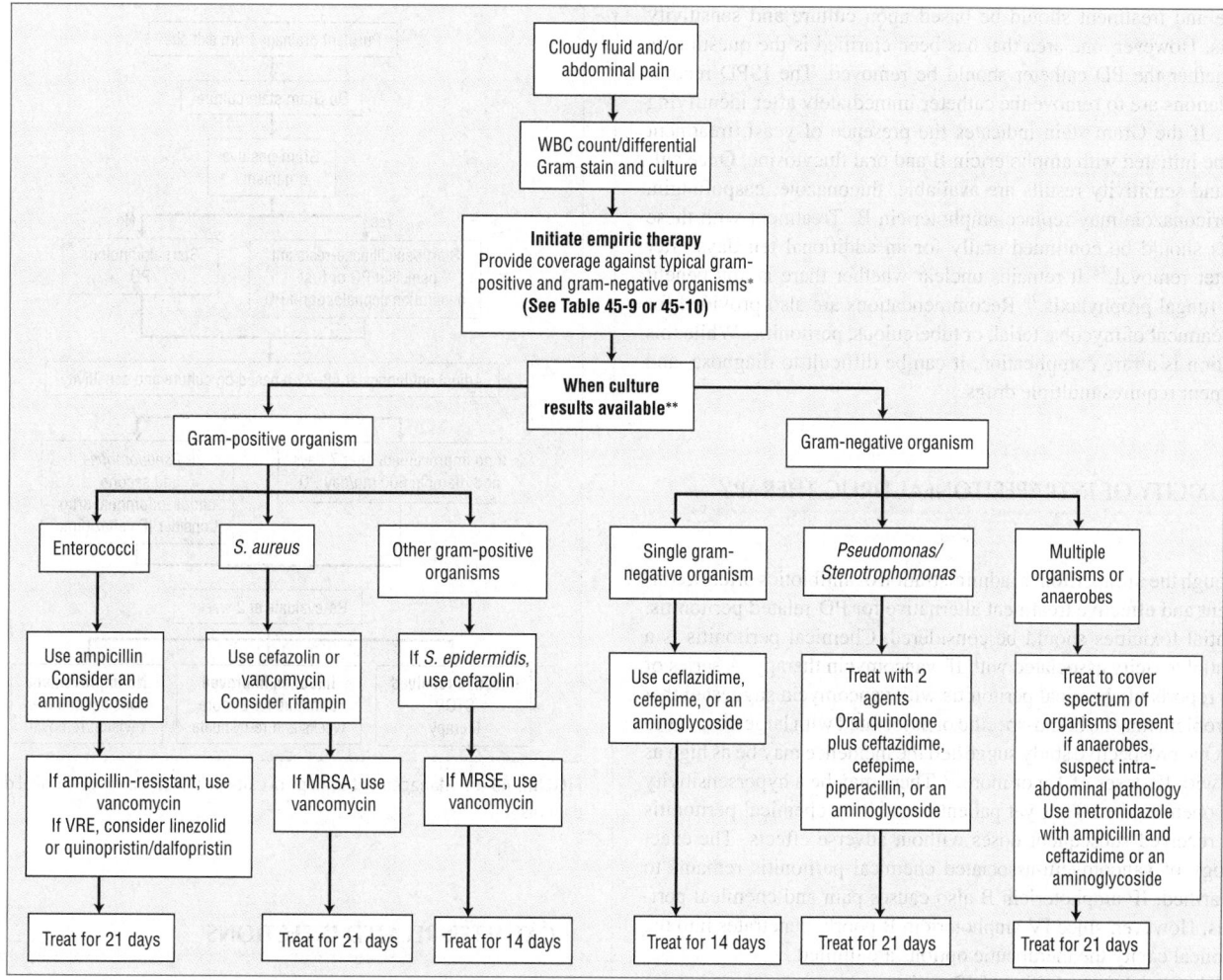

FIGURE 45–5. Pharmacotherapy recommendations for the treatment of bacterial peritonitis in PD patients.
* Choice of empiric treatment should be made based upon the dialysis center's and the patient's history of infecting organisms and their sensitivities.
** Final choice of therapy should always be guided by culture and sensitivity results.

Rifampin therapy should be limited to one week as resistance often develops with extended use. Infections with *S. aureus* or *Enterococcus* are usually more severe than other gram-positive peritonitis episodes and treatment should be continued for at least three weeks. If *S. aureus* peritonitis occurs as a result of an exit site or catheter infection with the same organism the catheter must be removed. Coagulase negative staphylococcus, especially *S. epidermidis,* is very commonly identified as the causative organism and can usually be treated by IP cefazolin alone. However, *S. epidermidis* is often reported as methicillin-resistant, in which case vancomycin should be used. Treatment should be continued for at least one week after the effluent clears and for at least 14 days total. If a single gram-negative organism, such as *E. coli, Klebsiella,* or *Proteus,* is cultured, the antibiotic should be selected based on sensitivities, safety and convenience. Based on sensitivity testing, a cephalosporin, such as ceftazidime or cefepime, or an aminoglycoside may be indicated (see Fig. 45–5). However, isolation of *Pseudomonas* or *Stenotrophomonas* should dictate the use of two concurrent agents with activity against these organisms. For *P. aeruginosa* peritonitis, an oral quinolone can be used as one of the antibiotics. Other alternatives include ceftazidime, cefepime, piperacillin, or an aminoglycoside. If catheter

infection is believed to have caused *P. aeruginosa* peritonitis, the catheter should be removed. Infections with gram-negative organisms are usually severe and treatment should be continued for at least three weeks.

In polymicrobial peritonitis, where multiple organisms are identified, treatment is directed to cover the spectrum of organisms present. If multiple enteric organisms are found, particularly in association with anaerobic bacteria, there should be suspicion of intra-abdominal pathology. When the source is believed to be the intestines, therapy should include metronidazole in combination with ampicillin and ceftazidime or an aminoglycoside. Peritonitis due to multiple gram-positive organisms is more common and can be treated based on microbial sensitivities. Treatment should be continued for at least three weeks.[72]

Fungal peritonitis is associated with a poor prognosis and high morbidity and mortality. One problem with prospective assessment of antifungal regimens is the infrequency with which these infections occur. This makes it difficult to design and implement comparative studies. Most literature about antifungal treatment is therefore retrospective or limited to reports of local experience.[75] As a result, the ISPD recommendations for treatment of fungal peritonitis are somewhat vague and treatment should be based upon culture and sensitivity results. However, one area that has been clarified is the question as to whether the PD catheter should be removed. The ISPD recommendations are to remove the catheter immediately after identifying fungi. If the Gram stain indicates the presence of yeast, treatment may be initiated with amphotericin B and oral flucytosine. Once culture and sensitivity results are available, fluconazole, caspofungin, or voriconazole may replace amphotericin B. Treatment with these agents should be continued orally for an additional ten days after catheter removal.[72] It remains unclear whether there is any benefit from fungal prophylaxis.[76] Recommendations are also provided for the treatment of mycobacterial, or tuberculous, peritonitis. While this infection is a rare complication, it can be difficult to diagnose, and treatment requires multiple drugs.

TOXICITY OF INTRAPERITONEAL DRUG THERAPY

Although the intraperitoneal administration of antibiotics offers a convenient and effective treatment alternative for PD-related peritonitis, potential toxicities should be considered. Chemical peritonitis is a potential toxicity associated with IP vancomycin therapy. A series of early reports of chemical peritonitis with vancomycin suggested that the problem may be brand-specific or associated with large doses (1 to 2 g). One prospective study suggested the incidence may be as high as 23% with IP doses of 1 g or more.[77] There may be a hypersensitivity component to the effect, yet patients exhibiting chemical peritonitis have received subsequent doses without adverse effects. The exact etiology of vancomycin-associated chemical peritonitis remains to be clarified. IP amphotericin B also causes pain and chemical peritonitis. However, since IV amphotericin B poorly penetrates into the peritoneal cavity the therapeutic options are limited.[72]

The systemic toxicities of IP regimens remain unclear, but are likely similar to those associated with IV and oral antibiotic administration. Intermittent (once daily) IP dosing of drugs, such as aminoglycosides, may reduce the risk of systemic toxicity (ototoxicity and nephrotoxicity). In the prior ISPD guidelines (2000) there was a recommendation that routine use of aminoglycosides should be avoided in patients with significant residual renal function if other antibiotic choices are available.[71] This was based on a study that showed rapid loss of residual renal function in PD patients treated with aminoglycosides.[78] However, a later study concluded that aminoglycosides do not accelerate the decline of residual renal function.[79] As a result the current ISPD guidelines state that there is not convincing evidence that short courses of aminoglycosides lead to loss of residual renal function. They also state that prolonged or repeated courses are probably not advisable if an alternative approach is possible.[72] This latter controversial recommendation was based on the opinion of the committee.

CLINICAL CONTROVERSY

The ISPD guidelines for peritonitis treatment state that patients with significant residual renal function should not receive aminoglycosides if other antibiotic choices are available. Aminoglycosides were found to increase the rate of decline in residual renal function in one study. However, another study refuted this claim. It seems reasonable to withhold aminoglycosides if appropriate alternative antibiotics are available.

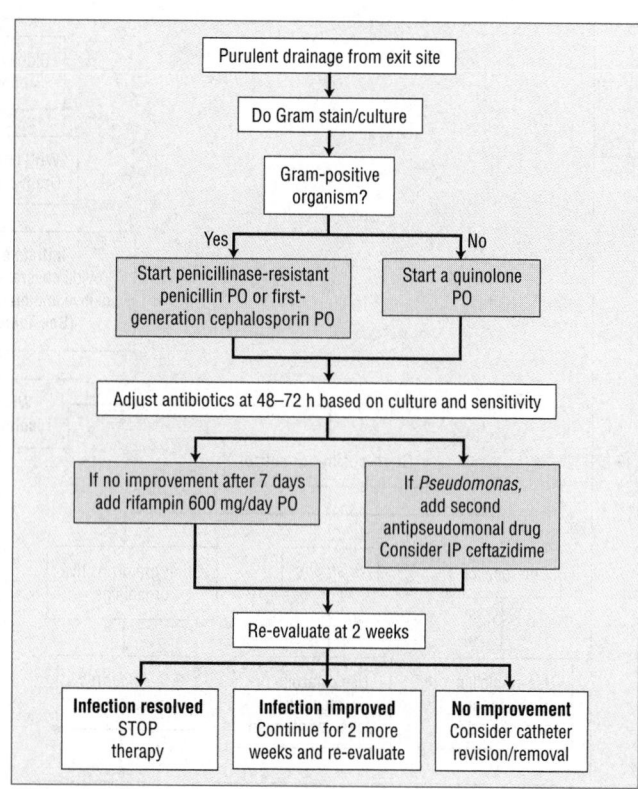

FIGURE 45–6. Management strategy of exit-site infections for peritoneal dialysis patients.

CATHETER-RELATED INFECTIONS

PD patients experience exit-site infections with an approximate incidence of one episode every 24 to 48 months. Patients with previous infections tend to have a higher incidence. The majority of exit-site infections are caused by *S. aureus*. In contrast to peritonitis, *S. epidermidis* accounts for less than 20% of exit-site infections. Although gram-negative organisms, such as *Pseudomonas,* are less common, they can result in significant morbidity.[74] The diagnostic characteristics of these infections are somewhat vague but generally include the presence of purulent drainage, with or without erythema at the catheter exit site. The risk of exit-site infections is increased severalfold in patients who are nasal carriers of *S. aureus*.[72] The use of topical antibiotics and disinfectants to treat catheter-related infections is controversial and there are few adequately controlled studies to determine the effectiveness of topical antibiotics.[80,81] Current recommendations suggest that gram-positive organisms should be treated with an oral penicillinase-resistant penicillin or first-generation cephalosporin, such as cephalexin (Fig. 45–6). Rifampin may be added if necessary, in slowly resolving or particularly severe appearing *S. aureus* infections. Vancomycin should be avoided in routine or empiric treatment of gram-positive catheter-related infections, but will be necessary for MRSA. Gram-negative organisms should be treated with oral quinolones. The effectiveness of oral quinolones may be diminished owing to the chelation drug interactions with divalent and trivalent metal ions, which are commonly taken by dialysis patients. Administration of quinolones should occur at least 2 hours prior to these drugs. In cases where *P. aeruginosa* is the pathogen, a second antipseudomonal drug should be added. IP ceftazidime may be considered.

In all cases antibiotics should be continued until the exit site appears normal and 2 to 3 weeks of therapy may be necessary. A patient with a catheter-related infection that progresses to peritonitis will usually require catheter removal.[72]

▶ TREATMENT: Prophylaxis of Peritonitis and Catheter-Related Infections

8 Attempts to prevent peritonitis and catheter-related infections have included refinement of connector system technology and the use of prophylactic antibiotic regimens and vaccines. Several studies have examined the impact of antibacterial agents as prophylaxis against both peritonitis and tunnel-related infections. Intermittent rifampin, 300 mg orally twice a day for 5 days, repeated every 3 months, appears to decrease the number of catheter-related infections, but not peritonitis. The efficacy of other antibiotic prophylaxis for peritonitis and catheter-related infections is limited. Long-term, extended-duration prophylaxis with penicillins or cephalosporins has not been shown to be effective.[71]

Nasal carriage of *S. aureus* is associated with an increased risk of catheter-related infections and peritonitis. In addition, diabetic patients and those on immunosuppressive therapy are at increased risk for *S. aureus* catheter infections. Prophylaxis with intranasal mupirocin (twice a day for 5 days every month), mupirocin (daily) at the exit site, or oral rifampin can effectively reduce *S. aureus* exit-site infections. Because of the minimal toxicity of mupirocin and the risk of rifampin resistance, mupirocin regimens are preferred.[71,72] However, it is important to note that *S. aureus* isolates with a high degree of resistance to mupirocin have been isolated from PD patients using prophylactic mupirocin at the peritoneal catheter exit site.[82] In addition, gentamicin cream applied daily to the exit site has been found to effectively reduce the incidence of both *S. aureus* and *P. aeruginosa* exit-site infection.[72]

PHARMACOKINETICS OF INTRAPERITONEAL DRUG THERAPY

The pharmacokinetics of intraperitoneal drug therapy have become more clearly defined in recent years.[83,84] Drugs may be added to dialysate to produce a local effect with limited systemic absorption. Alternatively, high systemic bioavailability may be desired for a systemic effect, or to ensure there is an adequate systemic reservoir, which would produce appropriate dialysate concentrations in subsequent drug-free exchanges (as with intermittent IP antibiotics). The primary pharmacokinetic factor that influences the bidirectional transfer of drugs is the magnitude of the ratio of systemic volume of distribution compared to the dialysate volume. The greater the ratio of the systemic volume to dialysate volume, the more readily a drug molecule will pass into the systemic circulation from the dialysate under the influence of a large concentration gradient. Conversely, drugs will more readily pass from the blood into the dialysate if the ratio of the systemic volume to the dialysate volume is small. Thus drug regimens can be manipulated depending on whether one desires adequate clearance from dialysate into blood, or into dialysate from blood.

Over the past decade, sound pharmacokinetic information has become available for a number of drugs in CAPD patients, and to a lesser extent for APD. Significant systemic bioavailability has been reported for some agents. In addition to their local effects for the management of peritonitis, as a result of their excellent systemic bioavailability, intraperitoneal antibiotics can be used to treat systemic infections.[85] Potential benefits of the intraperitoneal versus intravenous route for the management of systemic infections include use of an already existing access for administration, ability to treat infections on an outpatient basis, avoidance of costs for intravenous lines, possible avoidance of intravenous drug-related toxicities (such as thrombophlebitis and possibly redneck syndrome), and improved patient acceptance. The pharmacoeconomics of this strategy, however, remain to be carefully studied and reported.

OTHER INTRAPERITONEAL DRUG THERAPY

Possible advantages of intraperitoneal versus subcutaneous insulin include the avoidance of erratic absorption (both rate and extent of absorption), convenience, avoidance of subcutaneous injection site-related complications, and prevention of peripheral hyperinsulinemia.[86] Insulin appears to be cleared into the systemic compartment by an active transport process, or via the peritoneal lymphatics. A number of studies have demonstrated the bioavailability of intraperitoneal insulin to be about 25% to 30%, although none clearly compares the clinical effectiveness of intraperitoneal versus subcutaneous insulin in diabetes control. Insulin requirements for PD patients may be greater than in hemodialysis patients because of the continued absorption of dextrose from the peritoneal cavity. Furthermore, because of adsorption of insulin to the polyvinyl chloride bag and administration set, the intraperitoneal dose of insulin often needs to be two to three times the subcutaneous maintenance dose.

Many PD patients secrete large quantities of fibrinogen into the peritoneal cavity, which results in fibrin formation. This can lead to intraperitoneal adhesions and outflow obstruction. Intraperitoneal heparin may prevent this complication as a result of its local antifibrin effect.[87] Because standard heparin has a molecular weight of 12,000 to 15,000 daltons, it is minimally absorbed and thereby has limited systemic effects. The absorption of intraperitoneal erythropoietin has also been studied. Its bioavailability is low, but may be increased when added into a dry peritoneum.[88]

STABILITY OF INTRAPERITONEAL ADDITIVES

There have been relatively few stability studies of drug additives to peritoneal dialysate, and the majority of those completed have been for antibiotics in dextrose-containing PD solutions.[89] In dextrose solutions, most antibiotic additives appear to be stable (usually defined as retaining at least 90% of initial activity) for about 1 week if refrigerated or 1 to 2 days at room temperature. There are fewer data available regarding drug stability in icodextrin solutions. It is important to note that some studies may not be indicative of stability (i.e., they may assay total concentration of an agent, some of which may be from parent-drug degradation products and which may not therefore maintain the same degree of pharmacologic activity). Thus appropriate studies would be those that also determine the concentrations of known degradation products. Clinicians must recall that chemical stability does not imply microbiologic sterility.

CONCLUSION

Dialysis (HD and PD) remains the most widely available and commonly used means of chronic renal replacement therapy. Despite continual advances in dialysis and transplantation, kidney failure is associated with significant morbidity and mortality. Both HD and PD are associated with complications and are burdensome to affected patients. Given the lack of a true cure for kidney failure, emphasis has recently been placed on the prevention and early detection of kidney disease.[10] In light of the persistent increase in the incidence of ESKD, this approach deserves much effort and should remain a priority for the foreseeable future.

For patients with ESKD, a focus on quality of life and rehabilitation may be a valuable and viable goal toward which the nephrology community should direct its research resources. Efforts to improve the care given to dialysis patients have been admirable, but much remains to be done. The K/DOQI continues to update existing clinical practice guidelines and persists in developing additional guidelines for the treatment of other dialysis-associated disease states. Many of these guidelines offer definitive statements, such as target values for Kt/V, hemoglobin, or serum albumin levels. However, other recommendations remain rather vague. For example, it is suggested that patient quality of life and pediatric growth and development be measured, but no specific goals are cited. This is because of the lack of published literature that might indicate an appropriate goal. Given these circumstances, clinicians are not only encouraged to implement current clinical practice guidelines, but also to become involved in efforts to develop and assess alternative treatment strategies. The ultimate goal of these endeavors is to improve the care that dialysis patients receive.

ABBREVIATIONS

ADEMEX: Adequacy of Peritoneal Dialysis in Mexico (study)
APD: automated peritoneal dialysis
AV: arteriovenous
BUN: blood urea nitrogen
CANUSA: Canada-USA Peritoneal Dialysis Study Group
CAPD: continuous ambulatory peritoneal dialysis
CCPD: continuous cycling peritoneal dialysis
Cl_{cr}: creatinine clearance
HD: hemodialysis
NIPD: nightly intermittent peritoneal dialysis
NTPD: nocturnal tidal peritoneal dialysis
PD: peritoneal dialysis
PET: peritoneal equilibration test
ESKD: end-stage kidney disease
ESRD: end-stage renal disease
IP: intraperitoneal
ISPD: International Society of Peritoneal Dialysis
MRSA: methicillin-resistant *Staphylococcus aureus*
MRSE: methicillin-resistant enterococcus
NKF-K/DOQI: National Kidney Foundation Kidney Disease
   Outcomes Qualitative Initiative
PAN: polyacrylonitrile
PMMA: polymethylmethacrylate
PS: polysulfone
URR: urea reduction ratio
USRDS: United States Renal Data System
VRE: vancomycin-resistant enterococcus
WBC: white blood cell (count)

ACKNOWLEDGMENT

The authors wish to acknowledge the contributions of Gary Matzke, PharmD, FCCP, FCP and George Bailie, PharmD, PhD, FCCP to previous editions of this chapter.

Review Questions and other resources can be found at *www.pharmacotherapyonline.com.*

REFERENCES

1. U.S. Renal Data System. USRDS 2003 Annual Data Report: Atlas of End-Stage Renal Disease in the United States. Bethesda, MD, National Institutes of Health, National Institute of Diabetes and Digestive and Kidney Diseases, 2003.
2. McMurray SD, Miller J. Impact of capitation on free-standing dialysis facilities: can you survive? Am J Kidney Dis 1997;30:542–548.
3. Centers for Medicare & Medicaid Services. 2003 Annual Report, End Stage Renal Disease Clinical Performance Measures Project. Department of Health and Human Services, Centers for Medicare & Medicaid Services, Center for Beneficiary Choices, Baltimore, December 2003. Am J Kidney Dis 2003;42(Suppl 2):S1–S96.
4. Bloembergen WE, Port FK, Mauger EA, Wolfe RA. A comparison of mortality between patients treated with hemodialysis and peritoneal dialysis. J Am Soc Nephrol 1995;6:177–183.
5. Bloembergen WE, Port FK, Mauger EA, Wolfe RA. A comparison of cause of death between patients treated with hemodialysis and peritoneal dialysis. J Am Soc Nephrol 1995;6:184–191.
6. Fenton SS, Schaubel DE, Desmeules M, et al. Hemodialysis versus peritoneal dialysis: a comparison of adjusted mortality rates. Am J Kidney Dis 1997;30:334–342.
7. Foley RN, Parfrey PS, Harnett JD, et al. Mode of dialysis therapy and mortality in end-stage renal disease. J Am Soc Nephrol 1998;9:267–276.
8. Wu MS, Yu CC, Yang CW, et al. Poor pre-dialysis glycaemic control is a predictor of mortality in type II diabetic patients on maintenance haemodialysis. Nephrol Dial Transplant 1997;12:2105–2110.
9. De Fijter CW, Oe LP, Nauta JJ, et al. Clinical efficacy and morbidity associated with continuous cyclic compared with continuous ambulatory peritoneal dialysis. Ann Intern Med 1994;120:264–271.
10. Kidney Disease Outcome Quality Initiative. K/DOQI clinical practice guidelines for chronic kidney disease: evaluation, classification, and stratification. Am J Kidney Dis 2002;39:S1–246.
11. National Kidney Foundation. NKF-K/DOQI clinical practice guidelines for hemodialysis adequacy: update 2000. Am J Kidney Dis 2001;37:S7–S64.
12. Besarab A, Raja RM. Vascular access for hemodialysis. In: Daugirdas JT, Blake PG, Ing TS, eds. Handbook of Dialysis. Philadelphia, Lippincott Williams & Wilkins, 2001:67–101.
13. Vanholder R. Vascular access. Int J Artif Organs 2002;25:347–353.
14. National Kidney Foundation. NKF-K/DOQI Clinical practice guidelines for vascular access: update 2000. Am J Kidney Dis 2001;37:S137–S181.
15. Daugirdas JT, Van Stone JC, Boag JT. Hemodialysis apparatus. In: Daugirdas JT, Blake PG, Ing TS, eds. Handbook of Dialysis. Philadelphia, Lippincott Williams & Wilkins, 2001:46–66.
16. Schulman G. Clinical application of high-efficiency hemodialysis. In: Nissenson AR, Fine RN, eds. Dialysis Therapy. Philadelphia, Hanley & Belfus, 2002:205–210.
17. Biocompatibility of dialysis membranes. In: Nissenson AR, Fine RN, eds. Dialysis Therapy. Philadelphia, Hanley & Belfus, 2002:110–115.
18. Daugirdas JT, Van Stone JC. Physiologic principles and urea kinetic modeling. In: Daugirdas JT, Blake PG, Ing TS, eds. Handbook of Dialysis. Philadelphia, Lippincott Williams & Wilkins, 2001:15–45.
19. Daugirdas JT, Kjellstrand CM. Chronic hemodialysis prescription: A urea kinetic approach. In: Daugirdas JT, Blake PG, Ing TS, eds. Handbook of Dialysis. Philadelphia, Lippincott Williams & Wilkins, 2001:121–147.

20. Eknoyan G, Beck GJ, Cheung AK, et al. Effect of dialysis dose and membrane flux in maintenance hemodialysis. N Engl J Med 2002;347:2010–2019.

21. Pierratos A. Daily hemodialysis. In: Nissenson AR, Fine RN, eds. Dialysis Therapy. Philadelphia, Hanley & Belfus, 2002:134–137.

22. Kooistra MP. Frequent prolonged home haemodialysis: three old concepts, one modern solution. Nephrol Dial Transplant 2003;18:16–19.

23. Bregman H, Daugirdas JT, Ing TS. Complications during hemodialysis. In: Daugirdas JT, Blake PG, Ing TS, eds. Handbook of Dialysis. Philadelphia, Lippincott Williams & Wilkins, 2001:148–168.

24. Sherman RA. Intradialytic hypotension: an overview of recent, unresolved and overlooked issues. Semin Dial 2002;15:141–143.

25. Levin NW, Ronco C. Common clinical problems during hemodialysis. In: Nissenson AR, Fine RN, eds. Dialysis Therapy. Philadelphia, Hanley & Belfus, 2002:171–179.

26. Kaufman JL. Major complications from vascular access for chronic hemodialysis. In: Nissenson AR, Fine RN, eds. Dialysis Therapy. Philadelphia, Hanley & Belfus, 2002:31–40.

27. Beathard GA. Thrombosis associated with chronic hemodialysis vascular access: Catheters. In: Rose BD, ed. UpToDate. Wellesley, UpToDate, 2003.

28. Lentino JR, Leehey DJ. Infections. In: Daugirdas JT, Blake PG, Ing TS, eds. Handbook of Dialysis. Philadelphia, Lippincott Williams & Wilkins, 2001:495–521.

29. Piraino B. *Staphylococcus aureus* infections in dialysis patients: focus on prevention. ASAIO J 2000;46:S13–S17.

30. Beathard GA. Catheter management protocol for catheter-related bacteremia prophylaxis. Semin Dial 2003;16:403–405.

31. Oliver MJ, Schwab SJ. Temporary vascular access for hemodialysis. In: Nissenson AR, Fine RN, eds. Dialysis Therapy. Philadelphia, Hanley & Belfus, 2002:7–12.

32. Kaufman AM, Levin NW. Dialyzer reuse. In: Daugirdas JT, Blake PG, Ing TS, eds. Handbook of Dialysis. Philadelphia, Lippincott Williams & Wilkins, 2001:169–181.

33. John B, Anijeet HK, Ahmad R. Anaphylactic reaction during haemodialysis on AN69 membrane in a patient receiving angiotensin II receptor antagonist. Nephrol Dial Transplant 2001;16:1955–1956.

34. Cruz DN, Mahnensmith RL, Perazella MA. Intradialytic hypotension: is midodrine beneficial in symptomatic hemodialysis patients? Am J Kidney Dis 1997;30:772–779.

35. Flynn JJ III, Mitchell MC, Caruso FS, McElligott MA. Midodrine treatment for patients with hemodialysis hypotension. Clin Nephrol 1996;45:261–267.

36. Lim PS, Yang CC, Li HP, et al. Midodrine for the treatment of intradialytic hypotension. Nephron 1997;77:279–283.

37. Cruz DN, Mahnensmith RL, Brickel HM, Perazella MA. Midodrine is effective and safe therapy for intradialytic hypotension over 8 months of follow-up. Clin Nephrol 1998;50:101–107.

38. Lin YF, Wang JY, Denq JC, Lin SH. Midodrine improves chronic hypotension in hemodialysis patients. Am J Med Sci 2003;325:256–261.

39. Ahmad S, Robertson HT, Golper TA, et al. Multicenter trial of L-carnitine in maintenance hemodialysis patients. II. Clinical and biochemical effects. Kidney Int 1990;38:912–918.

40. Shinzato T, Miwa M, Nakai S, et al. Role of adenosine in dialysis-induced hypotension. J Am Soc Nephrol 1994;4:1987–1994.

41. Barakat MM, Nawab ZM, Yu AW, et al. Hemodynamic effects of intradialytic food ingestion and the effects of caffeine. J Am Soc Nephrol 1993;3:1813–1818.

42. Yalcin AU, Sahin G, Erol M, Bal C. Sertraline hydrochloride treatment for patients with hemodialysis hypotension. Blood Purif 2002;20:150–153.

43. Yalcin AU, Kudaiberdieva G, Sahin G, et al. Effect of sertraline hydrochloride on cardiac autonomic dysfunction in patients with hemodialysis-induced hypotension. Nephron Physiology 2003;93:21–28.

44. Perazella MA. Pharmacologic options available to treat symptomatic intradialytic hypotension. Am J Kidney Dis 2001;38:S26–S36.

45. Roca AO, Jarjoura D, Blend D, et al. Dialysis leg cramps. Efficacy of quinine versus vitamin E. ASAIO J 1992;38:M481–M485.

46. Sidhom OA, Odeh YK, Krumlovsky FA, et al. Low-dose prazosin in patients with muscle cramps during hemodialysis. Clin Pharmacol Ther 1994;56:445–451.

47. Chang CT, Wu CH, Yang CW, et al. Creatine monohydrate treatment alleviates muscle cramps associated with haemodialysis. Nephrol Dial Transplant 2002;17:1978–1981.

48. Zacharias JM, Weatherston CP, Spewak CR, Vercaigne LM. Alteplase versus urokinase for occluded hemodialysis catheters. Ann Pharmacother 2003;37:27–33.

49. Little MA, Walshe JJ. A longitudinal study of the repeated use of alteplase as therapy for tunneled hemodialysis catheter dysfunction. Am J Kidney Dis 2002;39:86–91.

50. Eyrich H, Walton T, Macon EJ, Howe A. Alteplase versus urokinase in restoring blood flow in hemodialysis-catheter thrombosis. Am J Heath Syst Pharm 2002;59:1437–1440.

51. Daeihagh P, Jordan J, Chen J, Rocco M. Efficacy of tissue plasminogen activator administration on patency of hemodialysis access catheters. Am J Kidney Dis 2000;36:75–79.

52. Hilleman DE, Dunlay RW, Packard KA. Reteplase for dysfunctional hemodialysis catheter clearance. Pharmacotherapy 2003;23:137–141.

53. Castner D. The efficacy of reteplase in the treatment of thrombosed hemodialysis venous catheters. Nephrol Nurs J 2001;28:403–404.

54. Marx MA, Frye RF, Matzke GR, Golper TA. Cefazolin as empiric therapy in hemodialysis-related infections: efficacy and blood concentrations. Am J Kidney Dis 1998;32:410–414.

55. Fogel MA, Nussbaum PB, Feintzeig ID et al. Cefazolin in chronic hemodialysis patients: a safe, effective alternative to vancomycin. Am J Kidney Dis 1998;32:401–409.

56. Vonesh EF, Moran J. Mortality in end-stage renal disease: a reassessment of differences between patients treated with hemodialysis and peritoneal dialysis. J Am Soc Nephrol 1999;10:354–365.

57. Collins AJ, Hao W, Xia H, et al. Mortality risks of peritoneal dialysis and hemodialysis. Am J Kidney Dis 1999;34:1065–1074.

58. Buoncristiani U. Continuous ambulatory peritoneal dialysis connection systems. Perit Dial Int 1993;13(Suppl 2):S139–S145.

59. Brophy DF, Mueller BA. Automated peritoneal dialysis: new implications for pharmacists. Ann Pharmacother 1997;31:756–764.

60. Krediet RT, van Westrhenen R, Zweers MM, Struijk DG. Clinical advantages of new peritoneal dialysis solutions. Nephrol Dial Transplant 2002;17(Suppl 3):16–18.

61. Frampton J, Plosker G. Icodextrin: A review of its use in peritoneal dialysis. Drugs 2003;63:2079–2105.

62. Frankenfield DL, Prowant BF, Flanigan MJ, et al. Trends in clinical indicators of care for adult peritoneal dialysis patients in the United States from 1995 to 1997. ESKD Core Indicators Workgroup. Kidney Int 1999;55:1998–2010.

63. National Kidney Foundation: NKF-K/DOQI clinical practice guidelines for peritoneal dialysis adequacy: update 2000. Am J Kidney Dis 2001;37:S65–S136.

64. Adequacy of dialysis and nutrition in continuous peritoneal dialysis: association with clinical outcomes. Canada-USA (CANUSA) Peritoneal Dialysis Study Group. J Am Soc Nephrol 1996;7:198–207.

65. Bargman JM, Thorpe KE, Churchill DN. Relative contribution of residual renal function and peritoneal clearance to adequacy of dialysis: A reanalysis of the CANUSA study. J Am Soc Nephrol 2001;12:2158–2162.

66. Paniagua R, Amato D, Vonesh E, et al. Effects of increased peritoneal clearances on mortality rates in peritoneal dialysis: ADEMEX, a Prospective, Randomized, Controlled Trial. J Am Soc Nephrol 2002;13:1307–1320.

67. Churchill DN. The ADEMEX Study: Make haste slowly. J Am Soc Nephrol 2002;13:1415–1418.

68. Dumler F, Schmidt R, Cruz C. Abbreviated method for urea kinetic modeling in continuous ambulatory peritoneal dialysis patients. Perit Dial Int 1993;13(Suppl 2):S50–S52.

69. Rodriguez-Carmona A, Perez FM, Garcia FT, et al. A comparative analysis on the incidence of peritonitis and exit-site infection in CAPD and automated peritoneal dialysis. Perit Dial Int 1999;19:253–258.

70. Maiorca R, Cancarini GC, Brunori G, et al. Morbidity and mortality of CAPD and hemodialysis. Kidney Int Suppl 1993;40: S4–15.

71. Keane WF, Bailie GR, Boeschoten E, et al. Adult peritoneal dialysis-related peritonitis treatment recommendations: 2000 update. Perit Dial Int 2000;20:396–411.

72. Piraino B, Bailie GR, Bernardini J, et al. Peritoneal dialysis related infections: 2005 update. Perit Dial Int 2005;(in press).

73. Dasgupta MK. Biofilms and infection in dialysis patients. Semin Dial 2002;15:338–346.

74. Leehey DJ, Gandhi VC, Daugirdas JT. Peritonitis and exit site infection. In: Daugirdas JT, Blake PG, Ing TS, editors. Handbook of Dialysis. Philadelphia, Lippincott Williams & Wilkins, 2001:373–398.

75. Goldie SJ, Kiernan-Tridle L, Torres C, et al. Fungal peritonitis in a large chronic peritoneal dialysis population: a report of 55 episodes. Am J Kidney Dis 1996;28:86–91.

76. Williams PF, Moncrieff N, Marriott J. No benefit in using nystatin prophylaxis against fungal peritonitis in peritoneal dialysis patients. Perit Dial Int 2000;20:352–353.

77. Wong PN, Mak SK, Lee KF, et al. A prospective study of vancomycin-(Vancoled-)induced chemical peritonitis in CAPD patients. Perit Dial Int 1997;17:202–204.

78. Shemin D, Maaz D, St Pierre D, et al. Effect of aminoglycoside use on residual renal function in peritoneal dialysis patients. Am J Kidney Dis 1999;34:14–20.

79. Baker RJ, Senior H, Clemenger M, Brown EA. Empirical aminoglycosides for peritonitis do not affect residual renal function. Am J Kidney Dis 2003;41:670–675.

80. Bernardini J, Piraino B, Holley J, et al. A randomized trial of *Staphylococcus aureus* prophylaxis in peritoneal dialysis patients: mupirocin calcium ointment 2% applied to the exit site versus cyclic oral rifampin. Am J Kidney Dis 1996;27:695–700.

81. Waite NM, Webster N, Laurel M et al. The efficacy of exit site povidone-iodine ointment in the prevention of early peritoneal dialysis-related infections. Am J Kidney Dis 1997;29:763–768.

82. Berns JS. Infection with antimicrobial-resistant microorganisms in dialysis patients. Semin Dial 2003;16:30–37.

83. Taylor CA III, Abdel-Rahman E, Zimmerman SW, Johnson CA. Clinical pharmacokinetics during continuous ambulatory peritoneal dialysis. Clin Pharmacokinet 1996;31:293–308.

84. Manley HJ, Bailie GR. Treatment of peritonitis in APD: pharmacokinetic principles. Semin Dial 2002;15:418–421.

85. Gorman T, Eisele G, Bailie GR. Intraperitoneal antibiotics effectively treat non-dialysis-related infections. Perit Dial Int 1995;15:283–284.

86. Quellhorst E. Insulin therapy during peritoneal dialysis: pros and cons of various forms of administration. J Am Soc Nephrol 2002;13(Suppl 1):S92–S96.

87. Tabata T, Shimada H, Emoto M, et al. Inhibitory effect of heparin and/or antithrombin III on intraperitoneal fibrin formation in continuous ambulatory peritoneal dialysis. Nephron 1990;56:391–395.

88. Taylor CA III, Kosorok MR, Zimmerman SW, Johnson CA. Pharmacokinetics of intraperitoneal epoetin alfa in patients on peritoneal dialysis using an 8-hour "dry dwell" dosing technique. Am J Kidney Dis 1999;34:657–662.

89. Bailie GR, Kane MP. Stability of drug additives to peritoneal dialysate. Perit Dial Int 1995;15:328–335.

46
DRUG-INDUCED KIDNEY DISEASE

Thomas D. Nolin, Jonathan Himmelfarb, and Gary R. Matzke

Learning Objectives and other resources can be found at *www.pharmacotherapyonline.com.*

KEY CONCEPTS

◀1 The initial diagnosis of drug-induced kidney disease typically involves detection of elevated serum creatinine and blood urea nitrogen, for which there is a temporal relationship between the toxicity and use of a potentially nephrotoxic drug.

◀2 Mechanisms of drug-induced kidney disease include immune-mediated toxicities (e.g., glomerulonephritis and allergic interstitial nephritis) and nonimmunologic-mediated toxicities which effect specialized characteristics of normal renal physiology.

◀3 Drug-induced kidney disease is best prevented by avoiding the use of potentially nephrotoxic agents in patients at increased risk for toxicity. However, when exposure to these drugs cannot be avoided, recognition of risk factors and specific techniques such as hydration may be used to reduce potential nephrotoxicity.

◀4 Acute tubular necrosis is the most common presentation of drug-induced kidney disease in hospitalized patients. The primary agents implicated are aminoglycosides, radiocontrast media, cisplatin, amphotericin B, foscarnet, and osmotically active agents.

◀5 Angiotensin-converting enzyme inhibitors and nonsteroidal anti-inflammatory drugs are associated with hemodynamically-mediated renal failure, the pathogenesis of which is a decrease in glomerular capillary hydrostatic pressure.

◀6 Acute allergic interstitial nephritis is the underlying cause for up to 3% of all cases of acute renal failure. Clinical manifestations of AIN typically present about 14 days after initiation of therapy and include fever, maculopapular rash, eosinophilia, pyuria, hematuria, proteinuria, and oliguria.

◀1 Drug-induced kidney disease or nephrotoxicity (DIN) is a relatively common complication of several diagnostic and therapeutic agents. It is seen in both inpatient and outpatient settings with variable presentations depending on the drug and clinical setting. Manifestations of DIN include acid-base abnormalities, electrolyte imbalances, urine sediment abnormalities, proteinuria, pyuria, and/or hematuria. However, the most common manifestation of DIN is a decline in the glomerular filtration rate (GFR), which results in a rise in the serum creatinine (S_{cr}) and blood urea nitrogen (BUN). Thus initial diagnosis of DIN typically involves detection of elevated S_{cr} and BUN, for which there is a temporal relationship between the toxicity and use of a potentially nephrotoxic drug. This is consistent with the qualitative definition of acute renal failure (ARF) or an "abrupt and sustained decrease in glomerular filtration, urine output, or both."[1] Unfortunately, numerous quantitative definitions of DIN and/or ARF based primarily on changes in the serum creatinine concentration have been published.[1,2] Thus it is difficult to ascertain the true incidence of DIN for any drug. As a result, broad ranges of incidence have been reported in various studies of the same agent. DIN is often reversible on discontinuation of the offending agent, but may also lead to acute and/or end-stage renal failure (see Chaps. 42 and 44). Many different mechanisms are involved in the pathogenesis of DIN. The development of drugs with novel mechanisms of action provides the potential for the presentation and identification of new unique nephropathies. This chapter reviews the epidemiology, pathophysiology, risk factors, and basic principles of prevention of drug-induced nephrotoxicity. Detailed discussions of these issues plus management strategies are

presented for widely used agents that have been associated with a moderate to high likelihood of DIN.

EPIDEMIOLOGY

Drug-induced nephrotoxicity occurs in all settings in which drugs are ingested or administered. It is a significant source of morbidity and mortality in the acute care hospital setting. DIN accounts for nearly 7% of all drug toxicity and from 18% to 27% of all cases of acute renal failure in hospitals.[3–5] Overall, in-hospital drug use may contribute to 35% of all cases of acute tubular necrosis (ATN), most cases of allergic interstitial nephritis (AIN), as well as to nephropathy due to alterations in renal hemodynamics and postrenal obstruction.[6] Aminoglycoside antibiotics, radiocontrast media, nonsteroidal anti-inflammatory drugs (NSAIDs), amphotericin B, and angiotensin-converting enzyme inhibitors (ACEIs) are frequently implicated.[5] Computer-guided medication dosing for hospital inpatients may improve the safety of potentially harmful drugs and minimize the occurrence of DIN in this setting.[7]

The incidence and characteristics of outpatient or community-acquired DIN are less well understood since mild toxicity is often unrecognized. However, the pharmacoepidemiology of these effects has become more important as care increasingly shifts to the outpatient setting. Although as many as 3% to 6% of hospital admissions have been attributed to adverse drug effects during outpatient therapy,[8] 20% of hospital admissions due to acute renal failure have been attributed specifically to community-acquired DIN.[9] NSAID nephrotoxicity is common and well defined, with between 1% and 5% of NSAID users developing nephrotoxicity.[10] Prescribed and over-the-counter (OTC) NSAID therapy has been associated with a fourfold-increased risk of hospitalization for acute renal failure during the first month of therapy.[11] Since more than 50 million people use NSAIDs in the United States, it is not surprising that 500,000 to 2.5 million people likely develop NSAID nephrotoxicity in this country annually.[10]

ASSESSMENT OF KIDNEY TOXICITY

Since the most common manifestation of DIN is a decline in the GFR leading to a rise in the S_{cr} and BUN, the onset of toxicity in hospitalized acutely ill patients is most often recognized by routine laboratory monitoring of the two chemistries. Decreased urine output may also be an early sign of toxicity, particularly with radiographic contrast media, NSAIDs, and ACEIs. In the outpatient setting, nephrotoxicity is often recognized by symptoms such as malaise, anorexia, vomiting, volume overload (shortness of breath or edema) or hypertension. Serum creatinine or BUN concentrations and urine collection for creatinine clearance may subsequently be measured to quantify the degree of loss of glomerular filtration. Marked intrasubject between-day variability of S_{cr} values has been noted (±20% for values within the normal range; see Chap. 41). Furthermore, they may be altered as the result of dietary changes and initiation of drug therapy, which may interfere with the assay procedure. Thus a change in S_{cr} of at least 0.5 mg/dL for subjects with a baseline S_{cr} <2 mg/dL and an increase of about 30% for those with S_{cr} >2 mg/dL, when correlated temporally with the initiation of drug therapy is a common threshold for the identification of DIN.[2,5]

Nephrotoxicity may be evidenced by alterations in renal tubular function without loss of glomerular filtration. Indicators of proximal tubular injury include metabolic acidosis with bicarbonaturia; glycosuria in the absence of hyperglycemia; and reductions in serum phosphate, uric acid, potassium, and magnesium due to increased urinary losses. Indicators of distal tubular injury include polyuria from failure to maximally concentrate urine, metabolic acidosis from impaired urinary acidification, and hyperkalemia from impaired potassium excretion. Urinary enzymes and low-molecular-weight proteins are also used as early markers of nephrotoxicity. For example, urinary excretion of the enzymes N-acetyl-βD-glucosaminidase, γ-glutamyl transpeptidase and glutathione S-transferase are markers of proximal tubular injury and have been used for the early detection of acute kidney damage in critically ill patients.[12] The transmembrane protein kidney injury molecule-1 (KIM-1) is expressed in the proximal tubule and is upregulated in patients with ischemic acute tubular necrosis, appearing in the urine within 12 hours after the ischemic insult. High urinary excretion of KIM-1 is associated with a greater than 12-fold increase in the likelihood of ATN.[13] In the future, novel biomarkers such as KIM-1 may facilitate the earlier diagnosis of nephrotoxicity and minimize the long-term consequences of this common drug-induced disorder.

PATHOPHYSIOLOGIC MECHANISMS OF NEPHROTOXIC SUSCEPTIBILITY

The kidneys are more sensitive than many other organs to drug toxicity. Immune-mediated, drug-induced nephrotoxicities include glomerulonephritis and allergic interstitial nephritis, either with or without nephrotic syndrome. The kidney is highly susceptible in part because of its large vascular surface area for exposure to circu-

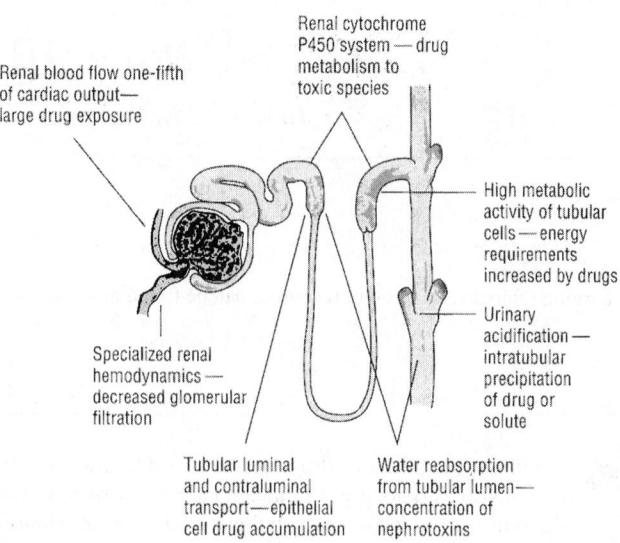

FIGURE 46–1. Mechanisms of renal susceptibility to drug toxicity. See text for discussion.

lating immune mediators and intrinsic immune function of glomerular mesangial cells and renal cytokine activation. Nonimmunologic mechanisms of DIN relate to several specialized characteristics of normal renal physiology, including regulation of blood flow, intrarenal drug metabolism, tubular transport processes, and urine concentration and acidification abilities (Fig. 46–1).

AUTOREGULATION OF RENAL BLOOD FLOW

The kidneys constitute only 0.4% of body weight, but receive 20% to 25% of resting cardiac output. This enhances the kidney's exposure to circulating drugs. Within each nephron, blood flow and pressure are regulated by glomerular afferent and efferent arterioles to maintain capillary hydrostatic pressure and glomerular filtration (Fig. 46–2). This specialized blood flow is precisely regulated by interrelations between arachidonic acid metabolites, natriuretic factors, nitric oxide, the sympathetic nervous system, the renin-angiotensin system, and the macula densa response to distal tubular solute delivery. In this unique vascular setting NSAIDs may reduce total renal blood flow,[10] radiographic contrast media may shunt intrarenal blood flow to the cortex and promote medullary ischemia,[14] osmotic diuresis secondary to mannitol therapy may reduce glomerular blood flow due to tubuloglomerular feedback,[15] and ACEIs dilate glomerular efferent arterioles and result in a decrease in glomerular filtration pressure.[16] Finally, dietary salt restriction can activate neurohumoral renal hemodynamic control systems that increase renal susceptibility to these drug nephrotoxicities.[17]

INTRARENAL DRUG METABOLISM

Multiple renal enzymes, including cytochrome P450 (CYP 450), UDP-glucuronyltransferase, and aldehyde dehydrogenase (ALDH) metabolize drugs and either protect the kidney from toxic insults or promote toxicity by transforming a drug to a nephrotoxic metabolite.[18] For instance, the chemotherapeutic agent ifosfamide undergoes hepatic metabolism to form the metabolite chloroacetaldehyde, thought to be responsible for the dose-limiting nephrotoxicity of ifosfamide observed in some patients.[19] Subsequent biotransformation and detoxification of chloroacetaldehyde via ALDH present in the renal tubules appears to play an important role in the

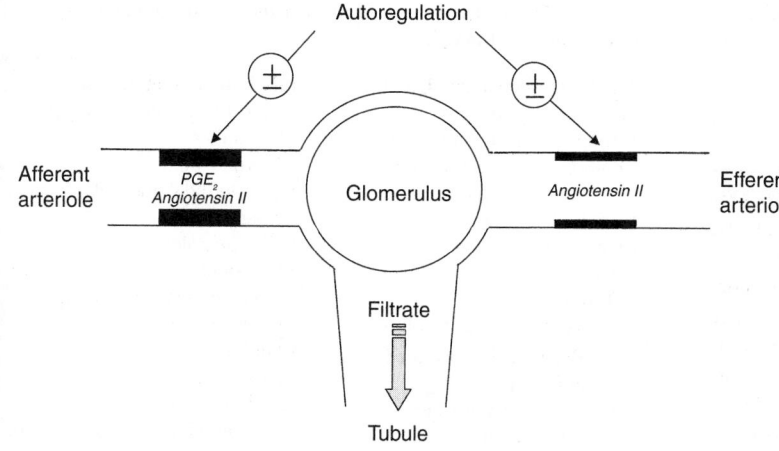

FIGURE 46–2. Normal glomerular autoregulation serves to maintain intraglomerular capillary hydrostatic pressure, glomerular filtration rate (GFR), and ultimately, urine output. This is accomplished by modulation of afferent and efferent arterioles. Afferent and efferent arteriolar vasoconstriction are primarily mediated by angiotensin II, whereas afferent vasodilation is primarily mediated by prostaglandins.

prevention of ifosfamide-induced nephrotoxicity. In contrast, oxidative metabolism of the chemotherapeutic agent cisplatin via CYP 2E1 located in the proximal tubule leads to the development of reactive oxygen intermediates which are responsible for cisplatin-induced nephrotoxicity.[20]

TUBULAR TRANSPORT PROCESSES

Tubular transport systems within the kidney, including the organic cation transporter 1 (OCT1), organic anion transporter 1 (OAT1), and P-glycoprotein (P-gp), play a vital role in the elimination of drugs and their metabolites from the body.[21–23] Proximal tubule cells are the primary site of active carrier-mediated transport of organic ions from blood to urine.[23] The concentration of drugs in the proximal tubule can thus be severalfold higher than systemic concentrations, resulting in local cytotoxicity that can eventually manifest as clinical nephrotoxicity. OAT1 has been implicated in the cellular uptake, accumulation, and nephrotoxicity of the acyclic nucleotide antivirals adefovir and cidofovir,[24] and some cephalosporin antibiotics.[25] Administration of OAT1 inhibitors such as probenecid markedly reduced cytotoxicity induced by these agents. Conversely, P-gp has been called the molecular "vacuum cleaner" due to the varied substrates it is known to pump out of cells, including anticancer agents, calcium channel blockers, steroids, digoxin, cyclosporine, and tacrolimus.[21,26] Unlike OCT1 and OAT1, overexpression of P-gp in the renal tubular cells has been shown to prevent nephrotoxicity induced by cyclosporine, and inhibition of the protein leads to toxicity.[21] Elevated intracellular drug concentrations may cause cytotoxicity as the result of impairment of mitochondrial function and decreased adenosine triphosphate synthesis, increased oxidative stress, depletion of reduced glutathione and other antioxidants, inhibition of phospholipid metabolism, or disruption of protein synthesis. Aminoglycosides, cyclosporine, and cisplatin appear to mediate nephrotoxicity by increasing the formation of superoxide ion and hydrogen peroxide, which in the presence of iron may subsequently generate hydroxyl radical, a reactive oxygen species that contributes to cellular oxidative stress and nephrotoxicity.[27]

CONCENTRATION OF SOLUTE IN THE TUBULAR LUMEN

Ninety-nine percent of the water filtered by the glomerulus is reabsorbed. Normally, 50% to 85% of water reabsorption occurs in the proximal tubule, while the remainder occurs in the descending loop

of Henle and collecting duct. Systemic volume depletion increases the degree of water reabsorption in the proximal tubule. As water reabsorption increases, the concentration of drugs increase within the tubular lumen. Thus the luminal surfaces of cells, particularly in the proximal tubule, can be exposed to higher concentrations of potential toxins and for a longer time than most other tissues in the body. This enhances binding of drugs to tubular epithelial cells and promotes active and passive transport into cells. The enhancement of aminoglycoside nephrotoxicity by systemic volume depletion is an example.[28]

HIGH ENERGY REQUIREMENTS

Renal tubular epithelial cells have high energy requirements because of active tubular transport and metabolic processes. These high energy needs are precariously supplied to medullary tubular epithelial cells, which function in a state of chronic hypoxia due to their perfusion with venous blood returning from the deep medulla. As a consequence these medullary tubular epithelial cells are especially sensitive to drugs that increase energy demands or decrease oxygen delivery, which can result in ischemic cell death. Amphotericin B–induced medullary tubular cell damage appears to result from an imbalance between increased cellular energy requirements and inadequate oxygen delivery.[29]

URINE ACIDIFICATION

Urine pH decreases to approximately 4.5 during maximal stimulation of renal tubular hydrogen ion secretion. Certain solutes can precipitate and obstruct the tubular lumen at this acid pH, particularly when urine is concentrated. For example, in the presence of a maximally acidic urine, intratubular precipitation of methotrexate may occur and result in acute renal failure.[30]

SUSCEPTIBLE PATIENT POPULATIONS

CHRONIC KIDNEY DISEASE

Chronic kidney disease develops as the result of injury to involved glomerular and tubular units while others remain relatively intact. The remaining functional nephron units develop hyperfiltering glomeruli and hyperfunctioning tubules to compensate for the damaged nephrons. These residual nephrons are more susceptible to nephrotoxic injury due to their increased energy requirements and exposure to elevated concentrations of drugs. The nephrotoxicity of radiographic contrast media in patients with chronic kidney disease is such an example.[31]

ELDERLY

Renal blood flow and GFR decline progressively with age. Progressive sclerosis of glomeruli occurs, and residual glomerular and tubular units increase function in compensation, similarly to patients with chronic kidney disease. This decline in renal function is not accompanied by a rise in the serum creatinine concentration due to the age-related decline in muscle mass and decreased creatinine generation. Older individuals are also more likely to have heart failure and hepatic insufficiency, which also reduce renal blood flow. Together, these processes predispose the elderly to an increased risk of nephrotoxicity.[32]

PRINCIPLES FOR PREVENTION OF DRUG NEPHROPATHY

❸ The primary principle for prevention of drug-induced nephrotoxicity is to avoid the use of potentially nephrotoxic agents in patients at increased risk for toxicity. However, when exposure to these drugs cannot be avoided, recognition of risk factors and specific techniques may be used to reduce potential nephrotoxicity. No generalizable risk factors are applicable to all drug classes and patient situations, since drug toxicity develops as a result of a wide range of mechanisms, from idiosyncratic hypersensitivity reactions to direct cellular toxicity. An exception is hemodynamically-mediated acute renal failure due to NSAIDs and ACEIs. Their toxicity is frequently preventable by recognizing pre-existing renal insufficiency and decreased effective renal blood flow due to volume depletion, heart failure, or liver disease.[16] Elderly patients with hypertension or heart failure may be especially sensitive to the combined use of ACEIs and NSAIDs, particularly with concurrent diuretic use.

Certain approaches to reduce drug toxicity are prudent and generally effective, for example, careful and adequate hydration to establish high renal tubular urine flow rates. However, other strategies to reduce drug toxicity are still theoretical and/or investigational and relate directly to the nephrotoxic mechanisms of the drug. For example, adefovir is a nucleotide antiviral that is actively transported by OAT1.[24] Inhibition of OAT1-mediated transport with NSAIDs minimizes accumulation of adefovir in renal proximal tubule cells and results in a reduction in toxicity.[33] Diflunisal, ketoprofen, flurbiprofen, indomethacin, naproxen, and ibuprofen were at least as effective as probenecid, a known potent inhibitor of OAT1, at preventing cytotoxicity. Antioxidants have also been shown to be protective in gentamicin-, cyclosporine-, and cisplatin-induced nephrotoxicity in experimental models.[27] Iron chelators are also protective against gentamicin toxicity.

Specific drug-induced renal structural–functional alterations constitute the remainder of this discussion under the seven broad headings listed in Table 46–1. The general orientation of these topics is in order of decreasing clinical incidence. Pathophysiologic mechanisms of nephrotoxicity will be emphasized, in addition to clinical findings, prevention, and management.

TUBULAR EPITHELIAL CELL DAMAGE

❹ Renal tubular epithelial cell damage may be caused by either direct toxic or ischemic effects of drugs. Damage localizes in

TABLE 46–1. Drug-Induced Renal Structural–Functional Alterations and Examples

Tubular epithelial cell damage
Acute tubular necrosis
- Aminoglycoside antibiotics
- Radiographic contrast media
- Cisplatin/carboplatin
- Amphotericin B
Osmotic nephrosis
- Mannitol
- Dextran
- Intravenous immunoglobulin

Hemodynamically-mediated renal failure
- Angiotensin-converting enzyme inhibitors
- Angiotensin II receptor antagonists
- Nonsteroidal anti-inflammatory drugs

Obstructive nephropathy
Intratubular obstruction
- Acyclovir
- Sulfadiazine
- Indinavir
- Foscarnet
- Methotrexate
Extrarenal obstruction
- Tricyclic antidepressants
- Indinavir
Nephrolithiasis
- Triamterene
- Indinavir

Glomerular Disease
- Gold
- Nonsteroidal anti-inflammatory drugs
- Pamidronate

Tubulointerstitial disease
Acute allergic interstitial nephritis
- Penicillins
- Ciprofloxacin
- Nonsteroidal anti-inflammatory drugs
- Omeprazole
- Furosemide
Chronic interstitial nephritis
- Cyclosporine
- Lithium
- Aristolochic acid
Papillary necrosis
- Combined phenacetin, aspirin, and caffeine analgesics

Renal vasculitis, thrombosis, and cholesterol emboli
Vasculitis and thrombosis
- Hydralazine
- Propylthiouracil
- Allopurinol
- Penicillamine
- Gemcitabine
- Mitomycin C
- Methamphetamines
Cholesterol emboli
- Warfarin
- Thrombolytic agents

Pseudo-renal failure
- Corticosteroids
- Trimethoprim
- Cimetidine

the proximal and distal tubular epithelia. This may be seen as cellular degeneration and sloughing from proximal and distal tubular basement membranes in acute tubular necrosis (ATN) or swelling and vacuolization of proximal tubular cells in osmotic nephrosis. ATN is the most common presentation of DIN in the inpatient setting. The primary agents implicated in renal tubular epithelial cell damage are aminoglycosides, radiocontrast media, cisplatin, amphotericin B, foscarnet, and osmotically-active agents such as immunoglobulins, dextrans, and mannitol.[4,34]

ACUTE TUBULAR NECROSIS

AMINOGLYCOSIDE NEPHROTOXICITY

Incidence

Nephrotoxicity has been reported in 1.7% to 58% of patients receiving aminoglycoside therapy. The large variance is in part due to the use of different definitions of toxicity, variability between agents in the class, as well as the risk factors in the study population.[35] The management of nephrotoxicity, a major contributor to the total cost of aminoglycoside therapy, was estimated to be over $4500 per case in the late 1990s.

Clinical Presentation

A gradual rise in the serum creatinine concentration and decrease in creatinine clearance after 6 to 10 days of therapy are the initial clinical manifestations of toxicity. Increased renal tubular proteinuria (β_2-microglobulin) and brush border enzymuria precede the creatinine rise by several days, but are not usually detected clinically.[28] Patients typically present with nonoliguria, maintaining urine volumes greater than 500 mL/day. Renal magnesium and potassium wasting can occur. Renal failure is usually mild if aminoglycoside therapy is stopped, but may be severe and require dialysis therapy. Aminoglycoside-associated nephropathy must be evaluated carefully since not all renal failure during a course of therapy is due to the aminoglycoside. Dehydration, sepsis, ischemia, and other nephrotoxic drugs frequently contribute.

Pathogenesis

The pathogenesis of reduced GFR in patients receiving aminoglycosides is predominantly the result of proximal tubular epithelial cell damage leading to obstruction of the tubular lumen and backleakage of the glomerular filtrate across the damaged tubular epithelium.[36] The toxicity of various aminoglycosides is related to cationic charge, which facilitates binding of filtered aminoglycosides to renal tubular epithelial cell luminal membranes. For instance, neomycin has six cationic amino groups and is the most nephrotoxic aminoglycoside, whereas streptomycin, with three groups, is least toxic. Gentamicin and tobramycin, with five amino groups, have similar and intermediate toxicity, whereas amikacin and netilmicin, with four and three amino groups, respectively, may be less toxic. Binding to tubular epithelial cells is followed by intracellular transport and concentration in lysosomes. Subsequent binding to acidic phospholipids (phosphatidylinositol) causes their aggregation and inhibits phospholipase activity.[28,36] This presents histopathologically as myeloid bodies within lysosomes of renal tubular epithelial cells. Cellular dysfunction and death may result from release of lysosomal enzymes into the cytosol, generation of reactive oxygen species, altered cellular metabolism, and alterations in cell membrane fluidity, leading to reduced activity of membrane-bound enzymes, including Na^+-K^+-ATPase, dipeptidyl peptidase IV, and neutral aminopeptidase.[28] Although binding of aminoglycosides to tubular epithelial cells is facilitated by the number of cationic groups present, inherent risks of toxicity are also a factor.

Risk Factors

Multiple risk factors for aminoglycoside nephrotoxicity have been identified. These relate to aminoglycoside dosing, synergistic toxicity in combination with other drugs, and predisposing conditions in the patient (Table 46–2). These risk factors have been consistently identified in all investigations and the reader is referred to in-depth reviews on this issue.[28,36]

Prevention

The prevention of aminoglycoside-induced nephrotoxicity has received considerable attention in recent years. Alternative antibiotics should be used whenever possible and as soon as microbial sensitivities are known. Commonly used alternatives include fluoroquinolones (e.g., ciprofloxacin or levofloxacin) and third-generation cephalosporins (e.g., ceftazidime). When aminoglycosides are necessary, the specific drug used does not appear to significantly affect the risk of nephrotoxicity, and therapy should be selected to optimize antimicrobial efficacy. Furthermore, it is imperative to avoid volume depletion, limit the total aminoglycoside dose administered, and avoid concomitant therapy with other nephrotoxic drugs.

TABLE 46–2. Potential Risk Factors for Aminoglycoside Nephrotoxicity

A. Related to aminoglycoside dosing:
    Large total cumulative dose
    Prolonged therapy
    Trough concentration exceeding 2 mg/L
    Recent previous aminoglycoside therapy
B. Related to synergistic nephrotoxicity. Aminoglycosides in combination with:
    Cyclosporine
    Amphotericin B
    Vancomycin
    Diuretics
C. Related to predisposing conditions in the patient:
    Pre-existing renal insufficiency
    Increased age
    Poor nutrition
    Shock
    Gram-negative bacteremia
    Liver disease
    Hypoalbuminemia
    Obstructive jaundice
    Dehydration
    Potassium or magnesium deficiencies

Prospective, individualized pharmacokinetic monitoring has been used for over 25 years. Although many have reported a decrease in the incidence of aminoglycoside-induced nephrotoxicity, the studies are often small and statistically underpowered. Recently Streetman and associates estimated that pharmacokinetic monitoring decreased costs associated with aminoglycoside nephrotoxicity by over $900 per patient.[37] High intermittent dosing of aminoglycosides, often called "once-daily dosing," used in combination with other antibiotics, has been intensively investigated as a practical cost-effective method to maintain antimicrobial efficacy while potentially reducing nephrotoxicity, and vestibular and ototoxicity.[28,38] Historically, high 1-hour postdose concentrations such as those obtained during once-daily dosing were thought to contribute to the renal and auditory toxicity. Recent data suggest otherwise, and in fact even calls into question the utility of monitoring peak concentrations.[38,39] Nephrotoxicity may be reduced since proximal tubular aminoglycoside uptake appears to be limited during the transient, high-peak serum concentrations due to saturation of binding sites. The achievement of low aminoglycoside concentrations for a greater proportion of the dosing interval facilitates excretion of the aminoglycoside. A recent meta-analysis suggests greater clinical efficacy and reduced nephrotoxicity with once-daily compared to standard dosing.[38] However, seriously ill, immunocompromised, renal-insufficient, and elderly patients are not ideal candidates for this approach. Prevention of nephrotoxicity may be enhanced by more discriminating selection of patients in whom aminoglycosides are used, as well as dosing based on accurate estimates of GFR, such as those provided by the Modification of Diet in Renal Disease (MDRD) equation (see Chap. 41).[40]

Management

Serum creatinine concentrations should be measured frequently (every 2 to 4 days) during therapy. Aminoglycoside use should be discontinued or the dosage regimen revised if the S_{cr} increases by >0.5 mg/dL during a course of therapy. Other nephrotoxic drugs should be discontinued if possible, and the patient should be maintained adequately hydrated and hemodynamically stable. Dialysis may be necessary, but renal failure due solely to aminoglycoside toxicity is usually reversible.

RADIOGRAPHIC CONTRAST MEDIA NEPHROTOXICITY

Incidence

Nephrotoxicity induced by radiographic contrast media is the third leading cause of hospital-acquired acute renal failure.[14] The incidence rises from <2% in patients with low risk to 40% to 50% in high-risk patients such as those with pre-existent renal insufficiency or diabetes mellitus.[14,41] The risk of contrast nephropathy increases as the number of risk factors increases, and diabetic patients with renal insufficiency have the greatest risk.[42,43]

Clinical Presentation

Toxicity ranges from transient tubular enzymuria to irreversible oliguric (urine volume <500 mL/day) renal failure requiring dialysis therapy.[31,42] Severe toxicity is most frequent in diabetic patients with pre-existent kidney disease. The typical course is an initial transient osmotic diuresis followed by tubular proteinuria and enzymuria. The serum creatinine rises and peaks between 2 and 5 days after exposure, with recovery after 4 to 10 days. Oliguria is present in about 50% of cases. Urinalysis typically reveals only hyaline and granular casts, but may also be completely bland.[43] The urine sodium concentration and fractional excretion of sodium are frequently low. Although toxicity has generally been considered to be mild and reversible, an in-hospital mortality rate of 34% has been reported in patients with contrast media–induced acute renal failure, compared to 7% in those without contrast nephrotoxicity.[42] Death was attributable to sepsis, respiratory failure, delirium, and bleeding that intensified after the onset of acute renal failure.

Pathogenesis

Contrast nephropathy appears to be due to direct tubular toxicity and renal ischemia.[31,42] Direct tubular toxicity is suggested by renal tubular enzymuria and biopsy findings of proximal tubular epithelial cell vacuolization and acute tubular necrosis. In addition to the direct toxic effects of contrast media, the nonselective proteinuria induced by contrast media may indirectly damage tubular epithelial cells. In contrast to these findings, the low urine sodium concentration and low fractional excretion of sodium frequently observed suggest preserved renal tubular function and participation of renal ischemia more than tubular toxicity. Renal ischemia may result from systemic hypotension associated with contrast injection, as well as renal vasoconstriction mediated by an imbalance of humoral agents, including prostaglandins, adenosine, atrial natriuretic peptide, nitric oxide, and endothelin.[31,42,43] Renal ischemia may also result from dehydration due to osmotic diuresis accompanying use of hyperosmolar agents (900 to 1780 mOsm/kg) and increased blood viscosity due to red blood cell crenation and aggregation.

Risk Factors

Pre-existent kidney disease, particularly diabetic nephropathy with renal insufficiency, is the major risk factor. Conditions associated with decreased renal blood flow, including congestive heart failure and dehydration, also confer risk. The presence of multiple myeloma has been considered a relative contraindication for contrast use, but the risk appears to be associated with concomitant dehydration, renal insufficiency, or hypercalcemia rather than the diagnosis itself. Both larger doses of contrast and use of older hyperosmolar contrast agents promote risk in susceptible patients.[31]

Prevention

The importance of strategies aimed at preventing radiocontrast-induced nephrotoxicity cannot be overemphasized. All patients scheduled to receive radiocontrast media should be assessed for risk factors, and the risk:benefit ratio should be considered.[44] Nephrotoxicity can be predicted in the majority of patients at risk, which justifies the use of preventative procedures with even minimal benefit.[45] High-risk patients should be identified, primarily by medical history and indication for the contrast study, but also by prestudy serum creatinine concentrations. Nephrotoxicity is best prevented in high-risk patients by using alternative imaging procedures (e.g., ultrasound, magnetic resonance imaging, and nuclear medicine scans). However, if contrast media must be used, the smallest adequate dose should be administered. Dose reduction proportional to the level of renal insufficiency may be protective, but may limit the adequacy of imaging.[44]

Low-osmolality nonionic (iohexol and iopamidol) and ionic (ioxaglate) contrast agents may be used to prevent nephrotoxicity. Standard contrast media are not reabsorbed in the kidney and cause osmotic diuresis, which contributes to the renal toxicity observed with these agents. The second generation of contrast agents have half the osmolality of standard agents, and have been associated with less toxicity, especially when used in patients with pre-existing kidney disease.[43] The incidence of contrast nephropathy in nondiabetic patients with underlying kidney disease is more than twofold higher in those receiving standard contrast agents compared to those receiving low-osmolar agents.[14] However, use of low osmolar agents does not eliminate nephrotoxicity and the preventive measures outlined below should be utilized.

CLINICAL CONTROVERSY

The true cost and benefit of using low-osmolar contrast agents to prevent nephrotoxicity is questionable because they are considerably (three to five times) more expensive than standard higher osmolar ionic agents. A cost-effective strategy may be to use low osmolar contrast agents in patients with pre-existing kidney disease, particularly those with diabetes mellitus, and standard agents in patients with normal renal function. Conversely, the low-osmolar agents cause less histamine release and may be advantageous for hemodynamically unstable patients or those with a history of hypersensitivity to contrast media.

Dehydration should be corrected before contrast administration, other nephrotoxic drugs discontinued if possible, and subsequent contrast studies appropriately timed to avoid cumulative toxicity. Hydration with isotonic saline before and after contrast administration reduces the incidence of toxicity, particularly in high-risk patients.[46] In addition to the obvious correction of dehydration, saline administration may lessen the impact of contrast-induced osmotic diuresis. Additional beneficial effects of saline prehydration may include dilution of contrast media, prevention of renal vasoconstriction leading to ischemia, and avoidance of tubular obstruction. Acetylcysteine is a thiol-containing antioxidant that may effectively reduce the risk of developing contrast nephropathy in patients with pre-existing kidney disease. Its use should be considered, along with hydration, in all patients at risk of toxicity.[47,48] Continuous venovenous hemofiltration may be an effective means of preventing contrast nephrotoxicity and is associated with improved outcomes in patients with chronic kidney disease (CKD).[49] In contrast, use of mannitol and furosemide to prevent toxicity remains controversial,[45] and recent evidence indicates that the dopamine$_1$-receptor agonist fenoldopam may not prevent contrast-induced nephropathy in CKD patients.[41]

Management

Currently there is no specific therapy available for managing established contrast nephropathy. Care is supportive with dialysis as needed in selected patients. Careful attention must be given to preventing infection and bleeding and providing respiratory support in view of the high association of these complications with death.

CISPLATIN AND CARBOPLATIN NEPHROTOXICITY

Incidence

Platin-containing compounds are important chemotherapeutic agents that frequently cause renal tubular damage.[30,50] The incidence of cisplatin nephrotoxicity was 50% to 100% in the 1980s. Subsequently, the incidence of toxicity decreased to 6% to 13%, primarily by limiting the total drug dose and reducing the rate of administration. However, when used in combination with other nephrotoxins, high-dose cisplatin continues to contribute to ARF. A 20% to 40% decline in GFR is frequently observed in patients treated with cisplatin.[50] Carboplatin, a second-generation platinum analog, is associated with a lower incidence of nephrotoxicity than cisplatin.[30]

Clinical Presentation

Nephrotoxicity manifests early during therapy as transient proximal tubular cell brush border and lysosomal enzymuria.[30] Peak serum creatinine concentrations occur approximately 10 to 12 days after initiation of therapy, with recovery by 21 days. However, renal damage can be cumulative with subsequent cycles of therapy and the serum creatinine concentration may continue to rise. Irreversible kidney disease may result. Renal magnesium wasting is common and can be accompanied by hypocalcemia and hypokalemia. Hypomagnesemia may be severe, causing seizures, neuromuscular irritability, or personality changes, and persist long after chemotherapy has ended. Hypomagnesemia results primarily from urinary losses due to renal tubular damage as well as magnesuric effects of saline hydration and diuretic therapy to prevent toxicity. Anorexia and diarrhea also contribute, due to decreased intake and increased loss of magnesium, respectively.

Pathogenesis

Proximal tubular damage appears acutely after administration of platin-containing compounds, as the result of impairment of cell energy production, possibly by binding to proximal tubular cellular proteins and sulfhydryl groups with disruption of cell enzyme activity and uncoupling of oxidative phosphorylation.[30] The initial proximal tubular damage is followed by a progressive loss of glomerular filtration and impaired distal tubular function.[50] Renal biopsies generally show sparing of glomeruli with necrosis of proximal and distal tubules and collecting ducts.

Risk Factors

Risk factors include increased age, dehydration, renal irradiation, concurrent use of aminoglycoside antibiotics, and alcohol abuse.[50]

Prevention

Toxicity is best prevented by dose reduction and decreased frequency of administration, which usually requires using the platin compounds in combination with other chemotherapeutic agents. Vigorous saline hydration is important and should be used in all patients; doses range from 1 to 4 L within 24 hours of cisplatin treatment to as high as 3 L/m^2 within 24 hours for high-dose carboplatin.[50] Although protective roles per se for furosemide or mannitol diuresis are less clear,[31] their use is often necessary to maintain volume homeostasis. Amifostine, an organic thiophosphate that is converted to an active metabolite, chelates cisplatin in normal cells and has been shown to reduce the nephrotoxicity, neurotoxicity, ototoxicity, and myelosuppression associated with cisplatin and carboplatin therapy.[51] The renoprotective effect of amifostine administration was recently demonstrated in patients receiving cisplatin/ifosfamide-based chemotherapy.[52] Amifostine fully preserved GFR in patients with solid tumors after administration of two cycles of chemotherapy compared to a 30% reduction in GFR in controls. In addition, less severe hypomagnesemia and decreased tubular damage were observed in the amifostine group. Pretreatment with amifostine should be considered in patients at risk for renal dysfunction. Promising investigational techniques have included the use of hypertonic saline to reduce tubular cisplatin uptake; reduced renal exposure by use of localized intraperitoneal administration in conjunction with systemic administration of sodium thiosulfate for those with peritoneal tumors; use of N-acetylcysteine, a sulfhydryl donor; and disulfiram metabolite diethyldithiocarbamate.[30,50] Recently the protective effect of melatonin,[53] and the ability of cisplatin-incorporated polymeric micelles to maintain antitumor activity while reducing nephrotoxicity have been demonstrated.[54]

Management

Acute renal failure due to cisplatin therapy is usually partially reversible with time and supportive care, including dialysis. Serum magnesium concentrations should be monitored frequently and hypomagnesemia corrected (see Chap. 50). Hypocalcemia and hypokalemia may be difficult to reverse until hypomagnesemia is corrected. Progressive chronic kidney disease due to cumulative toxicity may not be reversible and in some cases may require chronic dialysis support.

AMPHOTERICIN B NEPHROTOXICITY

Incidence

Amphotericin B remains the antifungal drug of choice for most systemic infections, but dose-dependent nephrotoxicity occurs to varying degrees in many patients.[55] Toxicity is seen initially with cumulative doses as low as 300 to 400 mg, and reaches an incidence of 80% when cumulative doses approach 4 g. Several liposomal amphotericin B formulations are now available. Although numerous studies demonstrate lower rates of nephrotoxicity with liposomal formulations compared to conventional amphotericin B, it is difficult to compare rates of toxicity between products and studies due to varying study populations enrolled, different doses administered, and inconsistent definitions of nephrotoxicity and methods of assessment.[56]

Clinical Presentation

Toxicity is often initially manifest by abnormalities of renal tubular function including potassium, sodium, and magnesium wasting, impaired urine concentrating ability, and distal renal tubular acidosis due to a leak of hydrogen ions back out of the tubular lumen.[57] Substantial potassium and magnesium replacement may be necessary. Renal blood flow and GFR decreases are common, and result in a rise in serum creatinine and blood urea nitrogen concentrations.

Pathogenesis

Renal pathologic findings include focal vacuolization of small arterial and arteriolar smooth muscle cells, as well as proximal and distal tubular epithelial cell damage. The mechanisms of renal dysfunction include direct tubular epithelial cell toxicity with increased tubular permeability and necrosis, as well as arterial vasoconstriction and ischemic injury.[58] Tubular membrane permeability to solutes such as sodium and potassium increases when amphotericin binds to membranes and acts as an ionophore. Renal vasoconstriction occurs by unclear mechanisms, possibly including direct effects of amphotericin B on cellular calcium fluxes and activation of vasoconstrictor prostaglandins. Overall, the combined effects of increased cell energy and oxygen requirements due to greater cell membrane permeability, and reduced cellular oxygen delivery due to renal vasoconstriction, results in renal medullary tubular epithelial cell necrosis and renal failure.[29,57]

Risk Factors

Risk factors include baseline renal insufficiency, higher average daily doses, diuretic use, volume depletion, and concomitant administration of other nephrotoxins (cyclosporine in particular).[55,57] Rapid infusions of amphotericin B have the potential to increase toxicity. A recent comparison of 24-hour continuous infusions with conventional 4-hour infusions revealed a significant reduction of toxicity, attributed to decreased "pretubular" effects (e.g., effects on renal blood flow and GFR).[59]

Prevention

Nephrotoxicity is best minimized by limiting the cumulative dose and avoiding concomitant administration of other nephrotoxins, particularly cyclosporine.[60] Additionally, providing hydration with a high sodium diet and 1 L intravenous 0.9% sodium chloride daily appears to reduce toxicity.[55] Mannitol infusion to induce an osmotic diuresis has not been protective.[57] Lastly, several liposomal amphotericin B formulations are now available and have been reported to reduce nephrotoxicity by enhancing drug delivery to sites of infection and thereby reducing exposure of mammalian cell membranes.[61,62]

CLINICAL CONTROVERSY

Many clinicians recommend using liposomal formulations of amphotericin B in all patients with pre-existing kidney disease and those at risk for developing nephrotoxicity, while others maintain that the safety and efficacy of liposomal formulations remains to be unequivocally established and their judicious use is warranted.

Management

Amphotericin nephrotoxicity is best treated by discontinuation of therapy and substitution of alternative antifungal therapy, if possible. Renal tubular dysfunction and glomerular filtration will improve gradually to some degree in most patients, but damage may be irreversible.

PENTAMIDINE NEPHROTOXICITY

Pentamidine therapy for *Pneumocystis carinii* infections is also limited by nephrotoxicity. Prospective studies have shown azotemia in 60% to 90% of treated patients.[63] Hyperkalemia, metabolic acidosis, hypomagnesemia, and hypocalcemia may also occur. Toxicity is more frequent in patients with the acquired immunodeficiency syndrome (AIDS) than in patients without this immune deficiency, and may be accentuated by concomitant amphotericin B therapy. The mechanism of toxicity is unknown, but tubular degeneration has been seen histopathologically. The primary alternative therapy for *P. carinii*, trimethoprim- sulfamethoxazole, may also cause renal dysfunction due to allergic interstitial nephritis and/or inhibition of tubular secretion of creatinine, but the incidence is lower than with pentamidine.[63]

FOSCARNET NEPHROTOXICITY

Foscarnet, an antiviral pyrophosphate analog used in AIDS and other immunosuppressed patients to treat cytomegalovirus (CMV) retinitis and life-threatening CMV infections, is a highly nephrotoxic agent. As many as 66% of patients treated with foscarnet develop renal insufficiency.[64] The mechanism appears to be complexation of foscarnet with ionized calcium and precipitation of calcium-foscarnet salt crystals in renal glomeruli causing a crystalline glomerulonephritis. The salt crystals may then secondarily precipitate in the renal tubules causing tubular necrosis. Foscarnet nephrotoxicity can be minimized by administering the appropriate dose after vigorously prehydrating the patient. Intravenous hydration provides better nephroprotection than oral hydration.[65] In addition, cidofovir and adefovir, potent nucleotide analogs administered for CMV infection in AIDS patients, have been associated with renal proximal tubular cell injury and renal failure.[16] Probenecid blocks renal tubular epithelial cell uptake of cidofovir, and when combined with saline hydration can reduce the incidence of nephrotoxicity.

OSMOTIC NEPHROSIS

Several drugs, including mannitol, low-molecular-weight dextran, and radiographic contrast media, or drug vehicles, including sucrose and propylene glycol, have been associated with vacuolization, swelling, and ultimately necrosis of proximal tubular epithelial cells with a decline in renal function.[16,66] The decline in renal function may be due to the hypertonic and osmotically active nature of these agents. Intravenous immunoglobulin solutions contain hyperosmolar sucrose and may cause osmotic nephrosis and acute renal failure, which is rapidly reversible on discontinuing therapy. Toxicity may be prevented by diluting the solution and reducing the rate of infusion. Hydroxyethylstarch, used as a plasma volume expander, has also been implicated in the development of osmotic nephrosis.[16]

Mannitol may rarely cause oligo-anuric renal failure with proximal tubular cell vacuolization on biopsy. Mechanisms include pinocytosis of mannitol into cells, causing swelling and tubular lumen obstruction.[15] Mannitol can also cause direct renal vasoconstriction or induce an osmotic diuresis with increased solute delivery to the macula densa and subsequent tubuloglomerular feedback, leading to vasoconstriction of the glomerular afferent arteriole and decreased renal blood flow. Risk factors for mannitol DIN include excessive doses, pre-existent renal insufficiency, and concomitant diuretic or cyclosporine therapy. Nephrotoxicity may be prevented by limiting the dose and avoiding dehydration and concomitant diuretic therapy. The serum mannitol concentration should be maintained <1000 mg/dL (as evidenced by an osmolal gap <55 mOsm/kg water). Patients usually recover normal renal function when elevated mannitol concentrations decrease following drug withdrawal or hemodialysis. Mannitol-induced osmotic diuresis and volume depletion could increase the nephrotoxicity of other drugs, particularly NSAIDs, ACEIs, and cyclosporine.

HEMODYNAMICALLY-MEDIATED RENAL FAILURE

5 Hemodynamically-mediated renal insufficiency results from a decrease in intraglomerular pressure. Mechanisms commonly include a decrease in renal blood flow, vasoconstriction of glomerular afferent arterioles, or vasodilation of glomerular efferent arterioles.

ANGIOTENSIN-CONVERTING ENZYME INHIBITORS AND ANGIOTENSIN II RECEPTOR BLOCKERS

INCIDENCE

The incidence of ACEI- or angiotensin II receptor blocker (ARB)-mediated renal failure has not been established. However, patients with severe atherosclerotic renal artery stenosis, those hospitalized with congestive heart failure, and those with chronic kidney disease, including diabetic nephropathy, are most likely to experience a significant decline in renal function with these agents.

CLINICAL PRESENTATION

Therapy with ACEIs and ARBs can acutely reduce GFR, manifesting as a rise in serum creatinine.[16] Importantly, a distinction must be made between a potentially detrimental reduction in GFR and a normal, predictable rise in serum creatinine. Dose-related changes in serum creatinine should be anticipated in most patients with ACEIs, based

on their pathophysiologic effects.[67,68] An increase in serum creatinine of up to 30% within 2 to 5 days of initiating therapy is an indication that the drug has begun to exert its desired pharmacologic effect.[67] The increase in creatinine usually stabilizes within 2 to 3 weeks and is usually reversible upon stopping the drug. Furthermore, an association exists between acute increases in serum creatinine of ≤30% from baseline that stabilize within the first 2 months of initiating therapy and preservation of renal function.

A reduction in GFR has been reported in the presence and absence of renal artery stenosis. The rise is often minimal in renovascular disease if only one renal artery is stenotic, but is more apparent in patients with a single kidney with renovascular disease, congestive heart failure, volume depletion, or bilateral renal small vessel disease. Up to one-third of patients with bilateral renal artery stenosis demonstrate a rise in serum creatinine >30% after starting ACEI therapy.[69]

PATHOGENESIS

The pathogenesis of ACEI- or ARB-mediated renal failure is a decrease in glomerular capillary hydrostatic pressure sufficient to reduce glomerular ultrafiltration.[4] This often occurs in settings in which glomerular afferent arteriolar blood flow is reduced and the efferent arteriole is vasoconstricted to maintain sufficient glomerular capillary hydrostatic pressure for ultrafiltration (Fig. 46–3A). ACEI or ARB therapy reduces angiotensin II synthesis or activity, respectively, thereby dilating the efferent arteriole and reducing glomerular

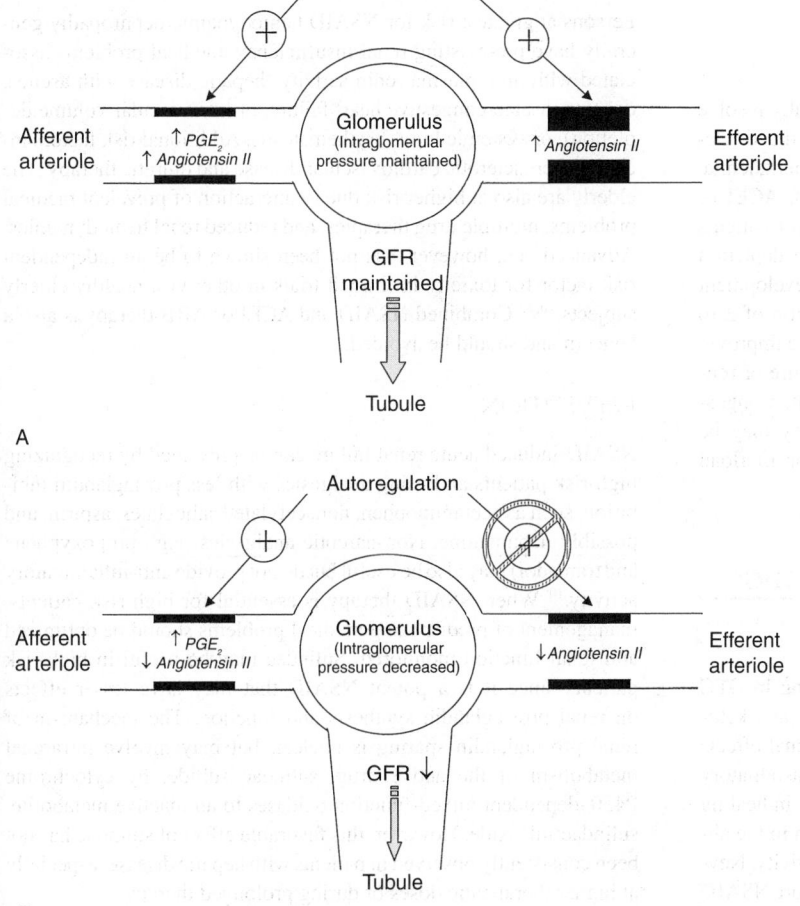

FIGURE 46–3. A. The kidney maintains GFR by dilating the afferent arteriole and constricting the efferent arteriole, specifically in response to a decrease in renal blood flow. During states of reduced blood flow, the juxtaglomerular apparatus increases renin secretion. Plasma renin converts angiotensinogen to angiotensin I, and ultimately angiotensin II (AII) by angiotensin-converting enzyme. AII constricts the afferent and efferent arterioles resulting in a net increase in intraglomerular pressure. Additionally, renal prostaglandins, prostaglandin E_2 (PGE_2) in particular, are released and induce a net dilation of the afferent arteriole, thereby improving blood flow into the glomerulus. Together these processes maintain GFR and urine output. **B.** ACE inhibitor nephropathy often occurs in the setting of reduced blood flow. When ACE inhibitor therapy (e.g., enalapril or ramipril) is initiated, the synthesis of angiotensin II is decreased, thereby preferentially dilating the efferent arteriole. This reduces outflow resistance from the glomerulus and decreases hydrostatic pressure in the glomerular capillaries, which alters Starling's forces across the glomerular capillaries to decrease intraglomerular pressure and GFR.

capillary hydrostatic pressure (Fig. 46–3*B*). This decreases glomerular ultrafiltration and GFR.

RISK FACTORS

Patients at greatest risk are those dependent on angiotensin II to maintain blood pressure and renal efferent arteriolar constriction. These include patients with hemodynamically significant renal artery stenosis, particularly bilateral stenosis, and those with decreased effective arterial renal blood flow, particularly those with congestive heart failure, volume depletion from excess diuresis or gastrointestinal fluid loss, hepatic cirrhosis with ascites, and the nephrotic syndrome.[4,69]

PREVENTION

A common strategy for at-risk patients is to initiate therapy with very low doses of a short-acting ACEI, then gradually titrate the dose upward and convert to a longer-acting agent after patient tolerance has been demonstrated. Outpatients may be started on low doses of long-acting ACEIs with gradual dose titration. Renal function and serum potassium concentrations must be monitored carefully, daily for hospitalized patients and every 2 to 3 days for outpatients. Monitoring may need to be more frequent during outpatient initiation of ACEI or ARB therapy for patients with pre-existing renal insufficiency, congestive heart failure, or suspected renovascular disease. Use of concurrent hypotensive agents and diuretics should be discouraged and dehydration avoided.[69]

MANAGEMENT

Acute decreases in renal function and hyperkalemia usually resolve over several days after ACEI or ARB therapy is discontinued. Occasional patients will require management of severe hyperkalemia, usually with sodium polystyrene sulfate (see Chap. 50). ACEI or ARB therapy may frequently be reinitiated, particularly for patients with congestive heart failure, after intravascular volume depletion has been corrected or the diuretic doses reduced. The development of mild renal insufficiency (serum creatinine concentration of 2 to 3 mg/dL) may be an acceptable trade-off for hemodynamic improvement in certain patients with severe congestive heart failure or renovascular disease not amenable to invasive management. Congestive heart failure patients with greater renal insufficiency may be best treated by substitution of hydralazine and nitrates for afterload reduction.

NONSTEROIDAL ANTI-INFLAMMATORY DRUGS

INCIDENCE

NSAIDs have an overall favorable safety profile resulting in OTC availability in the United States of ibuprofen, naproxen, and ketoprofen for short-term therapy. While potential adverse renal effects from OTC NSAIDs have been a concern, activity of vasodilatory prostaglandins is not necessary to maintain renal function in healthy individuals. NSAIDs are unlikely to impair renal function in the absence of renal ischemia or excess renal vasoconstrictor activity. Nevertheless, given the fact that 50 million U.S. citizens report NSAID use, it has been estimated that 500,000 to 2.5 million people will develop NSAID nephrotoxicity in this country annually.[10]

CLINICAL PRESENTATION

Renal failure can occur within days of initiating therapy, particularly with a short-acting NSAID such as ibuprofen.[10] Urine volume and sodium concentration are usually low, edema and/or weight gain is noticeable, and BUN, serum creatinine, and potassium are typically elevated. The urine sediment is usually unchanged from baseline, but may show granular casts.

PATHOGENESIS

NSAIDs inhibit cyclooxygenase (COX)-catalyzed prostaglandin production and impair renal function by decreasing synthesis of vasodilatory prostaglandins from arachidonic acid.[10] Renal prostaglandins are synthesized in the renal cortex and medulla by vascular endothelial and glomerular mesangial cells. Their effects are primarily local and result in renal vasodilation (particularly prostacyclin and prostaglandin E_2 [PGE_2]). They have limited activity in states of normal renal blood flow, but in states of decreased renal blood flow their synthesis is increased and they protect against renal ischemia and hypoxia by antagonizing renal vasoconstriction due to angiotensin II, norepinephrine, endothelin, and vasopressin. Administration of NSAIDs in the setting of renal ischemia and compensatory increased prostaglandin activity may thus alter the balance of activity between renal vasoconstrictors and vasodilators. This leaves the activity of renal vasoconstrictors unopposed and promotes renal ischemia with loss of glomerular filtration. This hemodynamically-mediated acute renal failure is the most common adverse renal effect of NSAIDs.

RISK FACTORS

Persons at greatest risk for NSAID hemodynamic nephropathy generally have pre-existing renal insufficiency, medical problems associated with high plasma renin activity (hepatic disease with ascites, decompensated congestive heart failure, or intravascular volume depletion), or systemic lupus erythematosus. Additional risk factors include atherosclerotic cardiovascular disease and diuretic therapy. The elderly are also at higher risk due to interaction of prevalent medical problems, multiple drug therapies, and reduced renal hemodynamics. Advanced age, however, has not been shown to be an independent risk factor for toxicity in limited trials in otherwise healthy elderly subjects.[10,70] Combined NSAID and ACEI or ARB therapy is also a concern and should be avoided.

PREVENTION

NSAID-induced acute renal failure can be prevented by recognizing high-risk patients and using analgesics with less prostaglandin inhibition, such as acetaminophen, nonacetylated salicylates, aspirin, and possibly nabumetone. Non-narcotic analgesics (e.g., propoxyphene and tramadol) may also be useful but do not provide anti-inflammatory activity.[10] When NSAID therapy is essential for high-risk patients, management of predisposing medical problems should be optimized and renal function monitored. Sulindac may be useful in high-risk patients since it is a potent NSAID that may have lesser effects on renal prostaglandin synthesis and function. The mechanism of renal prostaglandin sparing is unclear, but may involve intrarenal metabolism of the active drug, sulindac sulfide, by cytochrome P450–dependent mixed-function oxidases to an inactive metabolite, sulindac sulfoxide. However, this favorable effect of sulindac has not been consistently observed in patients with hepatic disease, especially at higher therapeutic doses or during prolonged therapy.

Traditional, nonselective NSAIDs inhibit COX-1 and COX-2, while the selective drugs meloxicam, celecoxib, and valdecoxib preferentially inhibit COX-2.[71] COX-2 inhibitors were anticipated to be beneficial in high-risk patients. However, recent data indicate they affect renal function similarly to nonselective NSAIDs and thus caution is warranted with their use, particularly in high-risk patients.[71,72]

MANAGEMENT

NSAID-induced acute renal failure is treated by discontinuation of therapy and supportive care. Renal failure may be severe, but recovery is usually rapid and dialysis is rarely necessary. Occasionally the hemodynamic insult is sufficiently severe to cause frank tubular necrosis, which can prolong recovery. The differential diagnosis of NSAID hemodynamically-mediated acute renal failure must include NSAID-induced acute interstitial nephritis, with or without the nephrotic syndrome, because steroid therapy may benefit this type of renal injury.

SULFINPYRAZONE

Sulfinpyrazone, a uricosuric congener of phenylbutazone, also causes hemodynamically-mediated acute renal failure.[73] Sulfinpyrazone inhibition of renal prostaglandin synthesis or reduction of renal kallikrein-kinin activity may imbalance renal hemodynamics, causing renal ischemia. Renal insufficiency may be transient despite continued sulfinpyrazone administration or prolonged and oliguric with a low urinary sodium concentration.

CYCLOSPORINE AND TACROLIMUS

Cyclosporine and tacrolimus have dramatically enhanced the success of solid organ transplantation. Nephrotoxicity, however, remains a major dose-limiting adverse effect of both drugs.[74] Early acute hemodynamically-mediated renal insufficiency and delayed chronic interstitial nephritis have been observed (see section on chronic interstitial nephritis later in this chapter).[75]

INCIDENCE

Historically, reversible acute renal insufficiency occurred frequently in transplant recipients during the first 6 months of cyclosporine therapy. The incidence of chronic kidney disease in nonrenal transplant patients is reported to be from 10% to 83%.[74] Recent data indicate that the 5-year risk of CKD after transplantation of a nonrenal organ ranges from 7% to 21%, depending on the type of organ transplanted. In addition, the occurrence of CKD in these patients is associated with more than a fourfold increase in the risk of death.

CLINICAL PRESENTATION

Acute renal toxicity may occur within days of initiating therapy. Serum creatinine concentration rises and creatinine clearance decreases. Hypertension, hyperkalemia, sodium avidity, and hypomagnesemia may occur. No urine sediment abnormalities are seen. Urinary enzyme excretions increase, but are not reliable indicators of toxicity. Renal biopsy reveals thickening of arterioles, mild focal glomerular sclerosis, proximal tubular epithelial cell vacuolization and atrophy, and interstitial fibrosis. Biopsy is useful to distinguish acute cyclosporine nephrotoxicity from renal allograft rejection, the latter being evidenced by cellular infiltration.[75]

Chronic toxicity typically becomes apparent after 6 to 12 months of therapy as a slowly rising serum creatinine concentration and decreased creatinine clearance. However, the rise in serum creatinine

concentration and decreased creatinine clearance may be delayed and not reflect the severity of histopathologic changes. Urinalysis reveals few red and white blood cells with low-range proteinuria. Renal biopsy shows progressive renal arteriolar hyalinosis, glomerular sclerosis, and a striped pattern of tubulointerstitial fibrosis. Biopsy cannot easily distinguish chronic cyclosporine toxicity from chronic rejection.[76]

PATHOGENESIS

A dose-related hemodynamic mechanism is likely during the initial months of therapy since renal function improves rapidly following dose reduction. Reversible vasoconstriction and injury to glomerular afferent arterioles occurs, possibly due to increased activity of vasoconstrictors, including thromboxane A_2, endothelin, and the sympathetic nervous system, or diminished activity of vasodilators, nitric oxide, or prostacyclin.[76,77] Vasoconstriction due to increased renin-angiotensin system activity may also contribute. In contrast renal arteriolar hyalinization and chronic renal ischemia as well as increased extracellular matrix synthesis appear to contribute to cyclosporine-induced chronic kidney disease.[76,77]

RISK FACTORS

Risk factors include increased age and higher initial cyclosporine dose, as well as renal graft rejection, hypotension, infection, and concomitant therapy with nephrotoxic drugs such as aminoglycosides, amphotericin B, acyclovir, NSAIDs, and radiocontrast agents, as well as drugs that inhibit cyclosporine hepatic metabolism.[75] (see Chap. 87) The high incidence of acute renal insufficiency with potential progression to chronic nephropathy has decreased with current lower-dose therapy, but concern remains for a slow, dose-dependent decline in glomerular filtration.

PREVENTION

Since acute DIN appears to be dose related, pharmacokinetic and pharmacodynamic monitoring is an important means of preventing toxicity. However, the persistent presence of therapeutic or low cyclosporine concentrations cannot preclude nephrotoxicity. Calcium channel blockers may antagonize the vasoconstrictor effect of cyclosporine by dilating glomerular afferent arterioles and preventing acute decreases in renal blood flow and glomerular filtration.[75] Lastly, decreased doses of cyclosporine or tacrolimus, primarily when used in combination with other non-nephrotoxic immunosuppressants, may minimize the risk of toxicity, but this may increase the risk of chronic rejection.

MANAGEMENT

Acute renal insufficiency usually improves with dose reduction, and treatment of contributing illness or the discontinuation of interacting drugs. Chronic kidney disease is usually irreversible, but progressive toxicity may be limited by discontinuation of cyclosporine therapy or dose reduction, with the continuation of other immunosuppressants (e.g., prednisone or azathioprine).

TRIAMTERENE

Triamterene, a potassium-sparing diuretic, has been associated with transient decreases in creatinine clearance and abnormal urinary sediment in normal subjects and hypertensive patients.[78] In combination with hydrochlorothiazide, triamterene has caused reversible acute renal failure in elderly patients. In combination with indomethacin, triamterene has induced acute renal failure in normal subjects and patients at risk for NSAID nephropathy. A hemodynamic mechanism is most likely, as suggested by the apparent increased risk for nephrotoxicity during combined triamterene and indomethacin therapy. Presumably, triamterene causes renal vasoconstriction that is counterbalanced by increased renal synthesis of vasodilatory prostaglandins. Concomitant NSAID therapy may induce renal ischemia by preventing the compensatory increase in renal prostaglandin synthesis. The implications of these observations are unclear because triamterene and NSAIDs are frequently used together without apparent nephrotoxicity.

OKT3

OKT3 therapy for the prevention and treatment of acute renal and cardiac allograft rejection is often accompanied by a rise in the serum creatinine concentration that returns toward baseline after 3 to 5 days.[77] Renal biopsy findings of mild interstitial edema or no abnormalities suggest the mechanism is increased vascular permeability due to a renal capillary leak. This renal dysfunction is believed to be part of a cytokine syndrome associated with OKT3 therapy. OKT3 causes lymphocyte activation and release of cytokines, particularly tumor necrosis factor, γ-interferon, and interleukin-2 and interleukin-6, which may induce secretion of group II secretory phospholipase A_2 as a mediator of nephrotoxicity.[79] Renal function often improves spontaneously despite continued OKT3 therapy.

OBSTRUCTIVE NEPHROPATHY

Obstructive nephropathy is the result of mechanical obstruction to urine flow following glomerular filtration. This may be due to intratubular obstruction from crystal precipitation within the tubules of the kidney or extrarenal obstruction of the ureters or bladder.[80] Pain, hematuria, and infection may precede a significant rise in serum creatinine.

RENAL TUBULAR OBSTRUCTION

Drug-induced acute renal tubular obstruction can be caused by intratubular precipitation of tissue degradation products as well as by drugs or their metabolites. Acute uric acid nephropathy following chemotherapy is the most common cause of renal failure due to obstruction by tissue degradation products. Acute oliguric or anuric renal failure develops rapidly. The diagnosis is supported by a urine uric acid:creatinine ratio greater than 1. Uric acid precipitation can be prevented by pretreatment hydration, urinary alkalinization to pH 7.0, and allopurinol.

Drug-induced rhabdomyolysis leads to intratubular precipitation of myoglobin and if severe, acute renal failure.[81] The most common cause of drug-induced rhabdomyolysis is direct myotoxicity from HMG-CoA reductase inhibitors, including lovastatin and simvastatin.[81] The risk of rhabdomyolysis is increased when this class of drugs is administered concurrently with gemfibrozil, niacin, or inhibitors of the CYP3A4 metabolic pathway (e.g., cyclosporine, erythromycin, or itraconazole). Rhabdomyolysis may also result from pressure necrosis during stupor or coma following ingestion of CNS depressants (e.g., alcohol or narcotics), or extreme neuromuscular agitation and associated metabolic demands with abuse of central

nervous system stimulants (e.g., amphetamines, cocaine, ecstasy, or phencyclidine).[81]

Intratubular precipitation of drugs (e.g., sulfonamides) or their metabolites can also cause acute renal failure.[80] Sulfadiazine when used at high doses,[80] and methotrexate and its less soluble metabolite, 7-hydroxymethotrexate,[30] may also precipitate in acidic urine and can cause oligo-anuric renal failure. Intravenous and high-dose oral acyclovir therapy for acute herpes zoster has also been associated with intratubular precipitation in dehydrated oliguric patients.[80] This can be diagnosed by the presence of birefringent needle-shaped crystals within leukocytes using polarized light microscopy. Massive administration of ascorbic acid can also result in obstruction of renal tubules with calcium oxalate crystals. Oxalate, a poorly soluble ascorbic acid metabolite, can also precipitate and worsen renal function when ascorbic acid is administered to patients with acute renal failure or the congenital nephrotic syndrome. Low-molecular-weight dextran therapy for volume expansion and rheologic effects has also caused renal failure, possibly by intratubular precipitation of filtered dextran. Triamterene may also precipitate in renal tubules and cause renal failure.[80] Foscarnet complexation with ionized calcium may result in precipitation of calcium-foscarnet salt crystals in renal glomeruli, causing primarily a crystalline glomerulonephritis. The salt crystals may then secondarily precipitate in the renal tubules causing tubular necrosis.[64]

Renal failure due to intratubular precipitation of most tissue-degradation products or drugs and their metabolites can be largely prevented and possibly treated by administering the appropriate dose after vigorously prehydrating the patient, maintaining a high urine volume and urinary alkalinization.

EXTRARENAL URINARY TRACT OBSTRUCTION

Drug therapy may also cause renal insufficiency due to lower urinary tract obstruction. Ureteral obstruction can be caused by calculi or retroperitoneal fibrosis. Bladder dysfunction with urinary outflow obstruction can result, particularly in males with prostatic hypertrophy, from anticholinergic drugs including tricyclic antidepressants and disopyramide. Bladder outlet and ureteral obstruction may result from bladder fibrosis following hemorrhagic cystitis with cyclophosphamide or ifosfamide therapy. Concurrent treatment with mesna can prevent cystitis and this complication.

NEPHROLITHIASIS

Nephrolithiasis (formation of kidney stones) does not present as classic nephrotoxicity since GFR is usually not decreased. Drug-induced nephrolithiasis represents abnormal crystal precipitation in the renal collecting system, potentially causing pain, hematuria, infection, or occasionally urinary tract obstruction with renal insufficiency.

Renal stone formation, possibly also accompanied by intratubular precipitation of crystalline material, has been a rare complication of drug therapy. Until the AIDS era, triamterene had been the drug most frequently associated with renal stone formation, with an incidence approximating 1 in 1500 users of triamterene-hydrochlorothiazide.[78] However, it has been unclear whether triamterene or its metabolites actually initiated stone formation, or are passively absorbed onto the organic matrix of pre-existing calculi. Sulfadiazine is a poorly soluble sulfonamide that has caused symptomatic acetylsulfadiazine crystalluria with stone formation and flank or back pain, hematuria, or renal insufficiency in up to 29% of patients treated with the drug.[16] A high urine volume and urinary alkalinization to pH >7.15 may be protective. Similarly, the protease inhibitor indinavir has been associated with crystalluria, dysuria, urinary frequency, back and flank pain, or nephrolithiasis in approximately 10% of AIDS patients.[82] Acute renal failure due to intratubular precipitation of crystalline indinavir and collecting system obstruction from nephrolithiasis have occurred.[16] Since indinavir is more water soluble at acidic pH, urine acidification could be protective, but is not practical. Maintaining a high urine volume may be most protective. Recently, nephrolithiasis has been reported to be a complication of the ingestion of various products containing ephedrine, norephedrine, and pseudoephedrine.[83]

GLOMERULAR DISEASE

Proteinuria with or without a decline in the GFR is a hallmark sign of glomerular injury (see Chap. 47) Several different glomerular lesions may occur, mostly by immune mechanisms rather than direct toxicity. Although drug-induced glomerular disease is uncommon, a variety of agents have been implicated.

Minimal change glomerular injury with nephrotic range proteinuria (i.e., >3.5 g/day) due to drugs is frequently accompanied by interstitial nephritis and is most common during NSAID therapy.[10,84] Ampicillin, rifampin, phenytoin, and lithium have also been implicated. The pathogenesis is unknown, but nephrotic-range proteinuria due to NSAID therapy is frequently associated with a T-lymphocytic interstitial infiltrate, suggesting disordered cell-mediated immunity. These cells may release lymphokines that increase glomerular capillary permeability to proteins. Proteinuria usually resolves rapidly after discontinuation of the offending drug, and a 3- to 4-week course of corticosteroids may help resolve the lesion.[85]

Focal segmental glomerulosclerosis (FSGS) is characterized by patchy areas of glomerular sclerosis with interstitial inflammation and fibrosis (see Chap. 47). Chronic heroin abuse is the most common drug cause of this lesion.[86] The pathogenesis is unknown but may include direct toxicity by heroin or adulterants and injury from bacterial or viral infections accompanying intravenous drug use. End-stage kidney disease (ESKD) develops in most cases. No specific therapy is available, although discontinuation of heroin use may prevent progression. FSGS is the predominant renal lesion in AIDS patients and may result from human immunodeficiency virus (HIV) infection or heroin abuse. Glomerulosclerosis due to HIV infection may be distinguished from heroin nephropathy by tubuloreticular structures in endothelial cells on electron microscopy and a more rapid course and poorer prognosis. The bisphosphonate pamidronate, commonly used to treat malignancy-associated hypercalcemia, is associated with the development of collapsing FSGS. Patients receiving either high doses or prolonged therapy are at highest risk.[87]

Membranous nephropathy, the most common drug-induced glomerular lesion, is characterized by immune complex formation along glomerular capillary loops. Gold therapy is the most common drug-induced cause.[88,89] The pathogenesis may involve damage to proximal tubule epithelium with antigen release, antibody formation, and glomerular immune complex deposition. Gold has been identified in proximal tubular cells, but not in the glomerular deposits. Genetic factors appear to be important because patients with human leukocyte antigens DR3 or B8 have increased susceptibility. Renal function is preserved and proteinuria resolves 6 to 39 months after discontinuing gold therapy.[88] Similarly, mercury found in diuretics, topical skin preparations, and industrial vapors causes membranous nephropathy.[89] NSAIDs have also caused membranous nephrotic

syndrome.[84] The prognosis appears favorable with resolution after discontinuing NSAID use.

TUBULOINTERSTITIAL DISEASE

These diseases involve the renal tubules and their surrounding interstitial tissue. The presentation may be acute and reversible with interstitial inflammatory cell infiltrates, rapid loss of renal function, and systemic symptoms; or chronic and irreversible with interstitial fibrosis, slow loss of renal function, and no systemic symptoms. Papillary necrosis, a variant of chronic interstitial nephritis, originates deep in the renal medulla and papillae.

ACUTE ALLERGIC INTERSTITIAL NEPHRITIS

INCIDENCE

Allergic interstitial nephritis (AIN) is fairly common and the underlying cause for up to 3% of all cases of acute renal failure.[85] Multiple drugs have been implicated (Table 46–3).

PENICILLINS

Clinical Presentation

Methicillin-induced allergic interstitial nephritis is the prototype for most presentations of AIN.[85] Clinical signs present approximately

TABLE 46–3. Drugs Associated with Allergic Interstitial Nephritis

Antimicrobials	Nonsteroidal anti-inflammatory drugs
Acyclovir	Aspirin
Aminoglycosides	Indomethacin
Amphotericin B	Naproxen
Aztreonam	Ibuprofen
Cephalosporins	Diflunisal
Ciprofloxacin	Piroxicam
Erythromycin	Ketoprofen
Ethambutol	Phenylbutazone
Indinavir	Diclofenac
Penicillins	Zomepirac
Rifampin	**Miscellaneous**
Sulfonamides	Acetaminophen
Tetracyclines	Allopurinol
Trimethoprim-sulfamethoxazole	Interferon-alfa
Vancomycin	Aspirin
Diuretics	Azathioprine
Acetazolamide	Captopril
Amiloride	Cimetidine
Chlorthalidone	Clofibrate
Furosemide	Cyclosporine
Triamterene	Glyburide
Thiazides	Gold
Neuropsychiatric	Methyldopa
Carbamazepine	Omeprazole
Lithium	P-aminosalicylic acid
Phenobarbital	Phenylpropanolamine
Phenytoin	Propylthiouracil
Valproic acid	Radiographic contrast media
	Ranitidine
	Sulfinpyrazone
	Warfarin sodium

14 days after initiation of therapy and include (with their approximate incidence) fever (80%), maculopapular rash (25%), eosinophilia (80%), pyuria and hematuria (90%), low-level proteinuria (90%), and oliguria (20%). Systemic hypersensitivity findings of fever, rash, eosinophilia, and eosinophiluria suggest the diagnosis, but this constellation of findings is not consistently reliable since one or more are frequently absent. Eosinophiluria, an important marker of drug-induced AIN, is frequently absent, possibly due to fragility of eosinophils in urine and inadequate laboratory methodology. Anemia, leukocytosis, and elevated IgE levels may occur. Tubular dysfunction may be manifested by acidosis, hyperkalemia, salt wasting, and concentrating defects.

NSAIDs

Clinical Presentation

NSAID-induced AIN has a different clinical presentation than that seen with most other drugs.[85] Patients are typically over age 50 (reflecting NSAID use for degenerative joint disease), the onset is delayed a mean of 6 months from initiation of therapy, and extrarenal symptoms are observed in only 10% of patients. Concomitant nephrotic syndrome (proteinuria >3.5 g/day) occurs in more than 70% of patients. Fenoprofen-allergic interstitial nephritis is considered the prototype for NSAID-induced AIN because it accounts for nearly 50% of cases.[85]

Prompt diagnosis of allergic interstitial nephritis is important since discontinuation of the offending drug may prevent irreversible renal damage. Renal biopsy is the most specific method for diagnosis but is usually not possible in acutely ill patients. Gallium-67 renal imaging is a sensitive diagnostic technique, but is nonspecific and of limited usefulness since glomerulonephritis, minimal change disease, and acute pyelonephritis also give positive scans.[90]

Pathogenesis

The pathology of AIN is a diffuse or focal interstitial infiltrate of lymphocytes, plasma cells, eosinophils, and occasional polymorphonuclear neutrophils.[85,90] Granulomas and tubular epithelial cell necrosis are relatively common with drug-induced AIN. The pathogenesis is an allergic hypersensitivity response.[90] Occasionally a humoral antibody-mediated mechanism is implicated by the presence of circulating antibody to a drug hapten–tubular basement membrane complex, low serum complement levels, and deposition of IgG and complement in the tubular basement membrane. More commonly, a cell-mediated immune mechanism is suggested by the absence of these findings and the presence of a predominantly T-lymphocyte infiltrate with an increased helper:suppressor cell ratio. In particular, NSAID interstitial nephritis involves T lymphocytes, possibly in response to altered prostaglandin synthesis.

Risk Factors

No specific risk factors have been identified because these are idiosyncratic hypersensitivity reactions. Individuals with other drug allergies may have increased risk and warrant close monitoring.

Prevention

No specific preventive measures are known due to the idiosyncratic nature of these reactions. Patients must be monitored carefully to recognize the signs and symptoms and discontinue therapy promptly.

Management

No prospective treatment trials have been reported. However, prednisone therapy in a dose of 1 mg/kg daily for 4 weeks has been used and may improve the rate and extent of renal recovery.[90]

CHRONIC INTERSTITIAL NEPHRITIS

Lithium, cyclosporine, and only a few other drugs have been reported to cause chronic interstitial nephritis, which is usually a progressive and irreversible lesion. Streptozotocin and other antineoplastic nitrosoureas also cause dose-dependent chronic interstitial disease.[30] In addition, mesalazine, 5-aminosalicylic acid, and ifosfamide may cause chronic interstitial nephritis, which usually resolves promptly when drug use is discontinued.

LITHIUM

Incidence

Several renal tubular lesions have been associated with lithium therapy; an impaired ability to concentrate urine (nephrogenic diabetes insipidus) has been seen in up to 87% of patients.[91] Acute tubular necrosis and chronic tubulointerstitial nephritis are less frequently noted, and incomplete distal renal tubular acidosis is rarely reported. The most important question regarding lithium use is whether long-term lithium therapy, with lithium concentrations maintained in the therapeutic range, causes chronic tubulointerstitial nephritis with renal insufficiency. While mild nonprogressive renal insufficiency has been reported in 10% or more of patients during long-term therapy, the role for lithium has not been established since occurrences have been infrequent and studies suggesting nephrotoxicity were frequently uncontrolled.[92] Chronic toxicity is also questioned since renal function has not declined during short- and long-term lithium therapy in studies when lithium concentrations have been maintained in the therapeutic range.

Clinical Presentation

Patients with nephrogenic diabetes insipidus often have polydipsia and polyuria (see Chap. 49). They adapt well to their urinary-concentrating defect and these concerns are usually minimal. Acute tubular necrosis is frequent in the setting of acute lithium toxicity. Urinalysis may show moderate proteinuria, a few red and white blood cells, and granular casts. Renal function usually returns to baseline values after lithium concentrations are reduced to the therapeutic range. Nephrotoxicity may develop insidiously and be recognized by rising BUN or creatinine concentrations or the onset of hypertension. The urinalysis may show mild proteinuria and a few red and white blood cells.

Pathogenesis

Impaired ability to concentrate urine is due to a dose-related decrease in collecting duct response to antidiuretic hormone. This results from impaired formation of cellular cyclic adenosine monophosphate in response to antidiuretic hormone. Lithium-induced acute renal failure occurs predominantly during episodes of acute lithium intoxication.[92] The pathogenesis includes dehydration secondary to nephrogenic diabetes insipidus, as well as direct proximal and distal tubular cell toxicity. Chronic tubulointerstitial nephritis attributed to lithium is evidenced by biopsy findings of interstitial fibrosis, focal tubular atrophy, and glomerular sclerosis.[92] The pathogenesis may involve cumulative damage from lithium-induced acute tubular necrosis. Alternatively, cumulative direct lithium toxicity may occur since duration of therapy has correlated with the decline in the GFR. Finally, some patients may have increased susceptibility to lithium toxicity. Although the reason for this is unknown, this could explain the difficulty in characterizing the nephrotoxic effects of chronic lithium therapy.

Risk Factors

The major risk factor for acute renal failure is an elevated lithium concentration, particularly in association with dehydration. Concomitant therapy with neuroleptic agents[92] may contribute. Chronic nephrotoxicity may result from cumulative damage due to repeated episodes of acute renal injury.

Prevention

Prevention of acute and chronic toxicity includes maintaining lithium concentrations as low as therapeutically possible, avoiding dehydration, and monitoring renal function. It is unknown whether progression to severe renal failure can be prevented by stopping lithium use when mild renal insufficiency is first recognized. This poses a dilemma since lithium is highly effective for affective disorders and the risks and potential benefits of discontinuing such a beneficial drug need to be carefully considered. However, if lithium therapy is continued, renal function must be monitored and therapy discontinued if it continues to decline.

Management

Symptomatic polyuria and polydipsia can be reversed by discontinuation of lithium therapy or ameliorated with amiloride or NSAIDs during continued lithium therapy[93] (see Chap. 49). Acute renal failure is usually reversible with supportive care, including dialysis to reduce toxic blood lithium concentrations. Progressive chronic interstitial nephritis is treated by discontinuation of lithium therapy, adequate hydration, and avoidance of other nephrotoxic agents.

CYCLOSPORINE

Cyclosporine causes both acute hemodynamically-mediated renal failure and chronic interstitial nephritis after 6 to 12 months of therapy. This can result in irreversible renal insufficiency and biopsy findings of arteriolar hyalinosis, glomerular sclerosis, and a striped pattern of tubulointerstitial fibrosis.[75,76] Chronic cyclosporine toxicity has become the more important of these two entities since reduced cyclosporine dosages and monitoring of drug concentrations has decreased acute toxicity. Chronic interstitial nephritis has been a major concern for therapy. The pathogenesis appears to involve sustained renal arteriolar endothelial cell injury causing chronic renal ischemia stemming from increased release of endothelin-1, decreased production of nitric acid, and increased expression of transforming growth factor-β.[94] Cyclosporine may also induce synthesis and accumulation of interstitial matrix, apparently due to increased activity of cytokines, peptide growth factors, or thromboxane. Nephrotoxicity has been dose dependent in some, but not all analyses, and occurs even following low-dose therapy. The risk of chronic interstitial kidney disease appears to be reduced in those receiving low-dose therapy.[76]

ARISTOLOCHIC ACID (CHINESE HERB NEPHROPATHY)

Incidence

In early the early 1990s, several young women with rapidly progressive kidney failure leading to ESKD were reported in Brussels, Belgium.[95] The patients had strikingly similar pathologic findings of interstitial fibrosis with tubular atrophy on renal biopsy. Further investigation revealed that all the women were patients of the same weight loss clinic and had received a weight loss treatment containing Chinese herbs. Subsequent analysis of the herb-based treatment demonstrated significant amounts of *Aristolochia fangchi* (Guang fang ji), known to contain aristolochic acid, the major alkaloid of the botanical species *Aristolochia*.[95] The term "Chinese herb nephropathy" was established and associated with aristolochic acid exposure after confirmatory renal biopsies were obtained from additional Belgian renal failure patients with prior exposure to the same Chinese herb–based treatment. Approximately 3% to 5% of patients who received the weight loss regimen developed disease, and numerous additional cases of nephropathy and ESKD associated with the use of *Aristolochia* species have been reported from around the globe.[95]

Clinical Presentation

Patients with Chinese herb nephropathy typically present with mild to moderate hypertension, mild proteinuria, glucosuria, and subacute renal failure evidenced by elevated serum creatinine concentrations.[95,96] Anemia and shrunken kidneys are also common on initial presentation. The overwhelming majority of cases reported to date have been in women. The main pathologic lesions observed in the kidneys of Chinese herb nephropathy patients are interstitial fibrosis with atrophy and destruction of tubules throughout the renal cortex. In general, the glomeruli are not affected. However, collapse of the capillaries, wrinkling of the basement membrane, and thickening of Bowman's capsule and afferent arteriolar walls are evident. These findings may suggest that the primary lesion is located in the vessel walls, which leads to renal ischemia, tubular necrosis, interstitial nephritis, and ultimately the extensive interstitial fibrosis observed. Atypical urothelial cells are also apparent. Perhaps the most remarkable feature of Chinese herb nephropathy is the rate at which it progresses. In most instances nephropathy progresses to ESKD requiring dialysis or transplantation within 6 to 24 months of exposure to aristolochic acid.[96] Several cases of malignancy have also been reported in Chinese herb nephropathy patients. An alarming 40% to 46% prevalence of urothelial transitional cell carcinoma has been observed in nephroureterectomy specimens obtained from Belgian patients who underwent renal transplantation.[97,98]

Pathogenesis

Although the precise mechanism of aristolochic acid–induced nephropathy and urothelial carcinoma is yet to be characterized, recent data indicate direct DNA damage may be the cause. The major components of aristolochic acid are metabolized to mutagenic compounds called aristolactam I and aristolactam II, respectively, which have been demonstrated to form DNA adducts in humans. Direct cellular toxicity is an unlikely mechanism of injury since the onset is delayed and progression of renal failure continues after aristolochic acid exposure.[96]

Risk Factors

Possible risk factors for the development of aristolochic acid–induced toxicity remain speculative. Over 1,700 patients were exposed to aristolochic acid in the Belgian weight loss clinic, yet only 100 patients with nephropathy have been identified.[97] Furthermore, why is this type of nephropathy not prevalent in China and other Eastern cultures, where use of *Aristolochia* species is commonplace? Possible explanations may include differences in dose and duration of use, since batch-to-batch variability in the composition of herbs in the weight loss regimen was evident. The concurrent use of other medications may also contribute. Many individuals receiving the herbal regimen were also prescribed the appetite stimulants dexfenfluramine and/or phentermine. It is possible the sympathomimetic agents induced renal ischemia which then potentiated the aristolochic acid toxicity. Lastly, interindividual differences in drug metabolism cannot be ruled out, since the aristolochic acid metabolites have been implicated in the development of toxicity.

Prevention

The primary means of preventing Chinese herb nephropathy appears to be limiting exposure to compounds containing aristolochic acids. Several countries, including the United Kingdom, Canada, Australia, and Germany have banned the use of *Aristolochia*-containing herbs.[95]

PAPILLARY NECROSIS

Papillary necrosis is a form of chronic interstitial nephritis characterized by necrosis of the renal papillae, which are the regions of the kidney where the collecting ducts enter the renal pelvis. Analgesic use is the most common cause of papillary necrosis, accounting for 36% of all cases.[99]

ANALGESIC NEPHROPATHY

Incidence

"Classic" analgesic nephropathy, characterized by chronic tubulointerstitial nephritis with papillary necrosis,[100] was initially reported in 1953 and was subsequently recognized as a worldwide public health concern. Chronic excessive consumption of combination analgesics, particularly those containing phenacetin, was believed to be the major cause and led to the removal of phenacetin and phenacetin mixtures from most world markets. It was subsequently thought, however, that abuse of contemporary analgesics, aspirin, acetaminophen, and NSAIDs, alone or in combinations, also results in analgesic nephropathy regardless of phenacetin content.[100,101] The incidence of analgesic nephropathy reported among dialysis patients in the United States, Europe, and Australia was 0.8%, 3%, and 9%, respectively.[101] This controversial issue is still being scrutinized, and a recent review of the subject suggests that currently there is insufficient evidence to associate nonphenacetin combined analgesics with nephropathy.[102]

Clinical Presentation

Analgesic nephropathy evolves insidiously over years. It is difficult to recognize and may be underdiagnosed as a cause of ESKD. The most sensitive and specific diagnostic criteria include (1) a history of chronic daily habitual analgesic ingestion (classically this equated to daily use for at least 5 years); (2) intravenous pyelography, renal ultrasound, or renal computed tomography imaging, which reveals decreased renal mass and bumpy renal contours; and (3) papillary calcifications.[101,103] Frequently, however, imaging only demonstrates chronic pyelonephritis and small kidneys with thin renal cortices and blunted calyces. Analgesics are taken most commonly for chronic headaches. Women are affected more than men. Upper gastrointestinal irritation from analgesics with blood loss leading to anemia has been characteristic. Hypertension and atherosclerotic cardiovascular disease are common. Early renal manifestations include impaired maximal urinary concentration, sterile pyuria, microscopic hematuria, and low levels of proteinuria. Urinary tract infection is common. Creatinine clearance declines slowly. Renal biopsy reveals nonspecific chronic interstitial inflammation and scarring. The incidence of lower urinary tract transitional cell carcinoma is increased with heavy phenacetin use.

Pathogenesis

Mechanisms of analgesic nephropathy remain unclear and difficult to study. This is due in part to a lack of diagnostic markers of evolving renal damage in vivo. In addition, animal models of analgesic nephropathy have been difficult to establish. The increased risk with analgesic mixtures containing phenacetin or acetaminophen and salicylates or NSAIDs is based on the following observations.[103,101] The renal lesion begins in the papillary tip as a result of accumulated toxic metabolites, decreased blood flow, and impaired cellular energy production. The metabolism of phenacetin to acetaminophen, which is then oxidized to toxic free radicals that are concentrated in the papilla, appears to be the initiating factor that causes toxicity by mechanisms analogous to acetaminophen hepatotoxicity. Toxicity is prevented by availability of reduced glutathione. However, salicylates deplete renal glutathione and thereby facilitate phenacetin and acetaminophen toxicity. In addition, renal medullary and papillary ischemia may contribute due to decreased synthesis of vasodilatory renal prostaglandins by salicylates and NSAIDs.

Risk Factors

The epidemiology of analgesic use and analgesic nephropathy continues to evolve.[102,104] The classic concept persists that risk for ESKD increases with cumulative consumption of combination analgesics, phenacetin, or acetaminophen and aspirin or NSAIDs.[101] Caffeine contained in combination analgesics may increase risk, but the role is not clear.[103] Chronic use of therapeutic doses of NSAIDs alone, but not aspirin or salicylates alone, can cause analgesic nephropathy. Case-control studies have associated high-dose acetaminophen use alone with an increased risk for ESKD. However, these associations remain inconclusive due to study design flaws and the fact that acetaminophen has been the preferentially prescribed analgesic for patients with chronic kidney disease.[102]

Prevention

Prevention has depended primarily on public health efforts to restrict the sale of phenacetin and combination analgesics. This has effectively reduced analgesic nephropathy in Australia and Europe. However, risk continues with continued availability of OTC combination analgesics containing aspirin, acetaminophen, and caffeine in the United States and throughout the world.

Individuals requiring chronic analgesic therapy may reduce risk by limiting the total dose, avoiding combined use of two or more analgesics, and maintaining good hydration to prevent renal ischemia and decrease the papillary concentration of toxic substances. Acetaminophen remains the preferred nonopiate analgesic for renal-insufficient patients.

Management

Treatment of established nephrotoxicity requires cessation of analgesic consumption. This can prevent progression and may improve renal function. Persistent surreptitious analgesic abuse should be considered if renal function continues to decline. Patients should also be monitored for associated transitional cell carcinoma of the renal pelvis, calyces, ureters, and bladder, which may present years after analgesic nephropathy is diagnosed.

RENAL VASCULITIS, THROMBOSIS, AND CHOLESTEROL EMBOLI

Systemic polyarteritis nodosa, a vasculitis with involvement of small- and medium-sized renal arteries, has been described following methamphetamine abuse.[105] Patients may have hematuria, proteinuria, renal insufficiency, and hypertension. Renal and visceral vascular aneurysms can be demonstrated by angiography. The pathogenesis may be a toxic reaction to methamphetamine or the result of associated hepatitis B infection.

Numerous medications, including mitomycin C, oral contraceptive agents, cyclosporine, tacrolimus, muromonab-CD3, antineoplastic agents, interferon, ticlopidine, clopidogrel, and quinine can cause a thrombotic microangiopathy (hemolytic uremic syndrome or thrombotic thrombocytopenic purpura) manifested by endothelial proliferation and thrombus formation in the renal and central nervous system vasculature.[106,107] The association with mitomycin C is notable since the pathogenesis appears to be a direct, dose-related toxic effect, rarely occurring in patients who receive doses <30 mg/m^2. Nephrotoxicity has occurred following chemotherapy with mitomycin C alone or with 5-fluorouracil, cisplatin, bleomycin, a vinca alkaloid, and tamoxifen.[106] Microangiopathic hemolytic anemia and thrombocytopenia are usually present. Systemic endothelial damage with multisystem organ failure has occurred. Renal failure can be severe and irreversible, although corticosteroids, antiplatelet agents, vincristine, plasma exchange, plasmapheresis, and high-dose intravenous IgG have each induced clinical improvement. Gemcitabine is a pyrimidine analog used for the treatment of various solid tumors which was recently associated with the development of hemolytic uremic syndrome, with an estimated incidence of 0.015%.[50] The drugs hydralazine, propylthiouracil, allopurinol, and penicillamine have been implicated in the development of antineutrophil cytoplasmic antibody (ANCA)-positive vasculitis.[108] Patients exposed to these drugs who subsequently develop ANCA-positive vasculitis appear to exhibit high titers of antimyeloperoxidase antibodies.

Anticoagulants and thrombolytics, particularly warfarin, can systemically embolize cholesterol particles from aortic atherosclerotic plaques to small arteries and arterioles, including renal arterioles. These agents remove or prevent thrombus formation over ulcerative plaques, causing emboli.[109] Cholesterol emboli induce an inflammatory obliterative vascular response, causing renal ischemia. Purple discoloration of the toes and mottled skin over the legs are important clinical clues.

PSEUDO-RENAL FAILURE

Pseudo-renal failure occurs when either the blood urea nitrogen (BUN) or creatinine concentration rises suggesting a decrease in renal function, despite maintenance of the GFR. The BUN concentration commonly increases without an increase in creatinine concentration during corticosteroid or tetracycline therapy. These drugs cause protein catabolism and thereby increase ureagenesis and the BUN concentration as the result of tissue breakdown. The GFR is unchanged and accurately reflected by the creatinine clearance and creatinine concentration.

Similarly, the serum creatinine concentration may rise while the BUN concentration remains unchanged by either of two mechanisms. First, drugs, including trimethoprim, cimetidine, or pyrimethamine, competitively inhibit secretion of creatinine into the proximal tubular lumen (see Chap. 41).[110] This effect is minimal during therapy in patients with normal renal function in whom the serum creatinine concentration usually remains in the normal range since tubular secretion of creatinine contributes only 5% to 10% to creatinine excretion. In contrast, in patients with CKD, the rise in serum creatinine is generally greater since tubular secretion of creatinine contributes a proportionately greater amount to urinary creatinine excretion. Ranitidine and famotidine do not inhibit tubular secretion of creatinine

at therapeutic doses.[110] Competitive inhibition of creatinine secretion has been considered useful in the evaluation of renal function since creatinine clearance usually overestimates true GFR in the presence of kidney disease. Administration of cimetidine during urine collection decreases creatinine secretion and provides a creatinine clearance value that more closely approximates true glomerular filtration, particularly in patients with renal disease (see Chap. 41). Second, several drugs, particularly cefoxitin and other cephalosporin antibiotics, can increase the serum creatinine concentration by direct interference with the enzymatic measurement of creatinine by the Jaffé method. The incidence of this effect is unknown, but it is uncommon; it is most prevalent among patients with decreased renal function. These drugs do not appear to interfere with determination of creatinine clearance.

COSTS OF DRUG-INDUCED KIDNEY DISEASE

The pharmacoeconomics of drug-induced kidney disease have not been well defined. An analysis of aminoglycoside therapy in the acute care environment for 1984 to 1985 revealed 7.3% of patients experienced nephrotoxicity. The mean additional cost for each episode of toxicity (in 1984 dollars) was $2501. The average additional cost of toxicity for each individual treated with aminoglycosides was $183.[111] Individualized pharmacokinetic monitoring efforts were recently reported to decrease costs associated with aminoglycoside nephrotoxicity by more than $900 per patient.[37] Outpatient care costs of NSAID toxicity have also been evaluated. Costs for hospital care for NSAID-induced acute hemodynamically-mediated renal failure and interstitial nephritis combined have been estimated at $990 million per year.[112] The risk of ESKD stemming from immunosuppressant-induced nephrotoxicity contributes substantially to the cost of heart transplantation.[75] The estimated cost per transplant patient was $6700 within 5 years, increasing to $14,200 within 8 years post-transplantation. Finally, patients who develop ESKD require dialysis, which typically costs more than $50,000 per year.

ABBREVIATIONS

ACEI: angiotensin-converting enzyme inhibitor
AIDS: acquired immunodeficiency syndrome
AIN: allergic interstitial nephritis
ALDH: aldehyde dehydrogenase
ANCA: antineutrophil cytoplasmic antibody
ARB: angiotensin II receptor blocker
ARF: acute renal failure
ATN: acute tubular necrosis
BUN: blood urea nitrogen
CKD: chronic kidney disease
CMV: cytomegalovirus
COX: cyclooxygenase
CYP 450: cytochrome P450
DIN: drug-induced nephrotoxicity
FSGS: focal segmental glomerulosclerosis
GFR: glomerular filtration rate
HIV: human immunodeficiency virus
KIM-1: kidney injury molecule-1
NSAID: nonsteroidal anti-inflammatory drug
OAT1: organic anion transporter 1
OCT1: organic cation transporter 1
OTC: over-the-counter
PGE$_2$: prostaglandin E$_2$

P-gp: P-glycoprotein
S_{cr}: serum creatinine

Review Questions and other resources can be found at *www.pharmacotherapyonline.com*.

REFERENCES

1. Kellum JA, Levin N, Bouman C, Lameire N. Developing a consensus classification system for acute renal failure. Curr Opin Crit Care 2002;8:509–514.
2. Mehta RL, Chertow GM. Acute renal failure definitions and classification: time for change? J Am Soc Nephrol 2003;14:2178–2187.
3. Leape LL, Brennan TA, Laird N, et al. The nature of adverse events in hospitalized patients. Results of the Harvard Medical Practice Study II. N Engl J Med 1991;324:377–384.
4. Choudhury D, Ahmed Z. Drug-induced nephrotoxicity. Med Clin North Am 1997;81:705–717.
5. Nash K, Hafeez A, Hou S. Hospital-acquired renal insufficiency. Am J Kidney Dis 2002;39:930–936.
6. Thadhani R, Pascual M, Bonventre JV. Acute renal failure. N Engl J Med 1996;334:1448–1460.
7. Chertow GM, Lee J, Kuperman GJ, et al. Guided medication dosing for inpatients with renal insufficiency. JAMA 2001;286:2839–2844.
8. Strom BL, Tugwell P. Pharmacoepidemiology: current status, prospects, and problems. Ann Intern Med 1990;113:179–181.
9. Elasy TA, Anderson RJ. Changing demography of acute renal failure. Semin Dial 1996;9:438–443.
10. Whelton A. Nephrotoxicity of nonsteroidal anti-inflammatory drugs: physiologic foundations and clinical implications. Am J Med 1999;106: 13S–24S.
11. Perez GS, Garcia Rodriguez LA, Raiford DS, et al. Nonsteroidal anti-inflammatory drugs and the risk of hospitalization for acute renal failure. Arch Intern Med 1996;156:2433–2439.
12. D'Amico G, Bazzi C. Urinary protein and enzyme excretion as markers of tubular damage. Curr Opin Nephrol Hypertens 2003;12:639–643.
13. Han WK, Bailly V, Abichandani R, et al. Kidney Injury Molecule-1 (KIM-1): a novel biomarker for human renal proximal tubule injury. Kidney Int 2002;62:237–244.
14. Waybill MM, Waybill PN. Contrast media-induced nephrotoxicity: identification of patients at risk and algorithms for prevention. J Vasc Intervent Radiol 2001;12:3–9.
15. Visweswaran P, Massin EK, Dubose TD Jr. Mannitol-induced acute renal failure. J Am Soc Nephrol 1997;8:1028–1033.
16. Perazella MA. Drug-induced renal failure: update on new medications and unique mechanisms of nephrotoxicity. Am J Med Sci 2003;325:349–362.
17. Bennett WM. Drug interactions and consequences of sodium restriction. Am J Clin Nutr 1997;65:678S–681S.
18. Lohr JW, Willsky GR, Acara MA. Renal drug metabolism. Pharmacol Rev 1998;50:107–141.
19. Dubourg L, Michoudet C, Cochat P, Baverel G. Human kidney tubules detoxify chloroacetaldehyde, a presumed nephrotoxic metabolite of ifosfamide. J Am Soc Nephrol 2001;12:1615–1623.
20. Liu H, Baliga R. Cytochrome P450 2E1 null mice provide novel protection against cisplatin-induced nephrotoxicity and apoptosis. Kidney Int 2003;63:1687–1696.
21. del Moral RG, Olmo A, Aguilar M, O'Valle F. P glycoprotein: a new mechanism to control drug-induced nephrotoxicity. Exp Nephrol 1998;6:89–97.
22. Zhang L, Brett CM, Giacomini KM. Role of organic cation transporters in drug absorption and elimination. Annu Rev Pharmacol Toxicol 1998;38:431–460.
23. Van Aubel RA, Masereeuw R, Russel FG. Molecular pharmacology of renal organic anion transporters. Am J Physiol Renal Physiol 2000;279:F216–F232.
24. Ho ES, Lin DC, Mendel DB, Cihlar T. Cytotoxicity of antiviral nucleotides adefovir and cidofovir is induced by the expression of human renal organic anion transporter 1. J Am Soc Nephrol 2000;11:383–393.
25. Takeda M, Tojo A, Sekine T, et al. Role of organic anion transporter 1 (OAT1) in cephaloridine (CER)-induced nephrotoxicity. Kidney Int 1999;56:2128–2136.
26. Yu DK. The contribution of P-glycoprotein to pharmacokinetic drug-drug interactions. J Clin Pharmacol 1999;39:1203–1211.
27. Baliga R, Ueda N, Walker PD, Shah SV. Oxidant mechanisms in toxic acute renal failure. Drug Metab Rev 1999;31:971–997.
28. Swan SK. Aminoglycoside nephrotoxicity. Semin Nephrol 1997;17:27–33.
29. Brezis M, Rosen S. Hypoxia of the renal medulla—its implications for disease. N Engl J Med 1995;332:647–655.
30. Berns JS, Ford PA. Renal toxicities of antineoplastic drugs and bone marrow transplantation. Semin Nephrol 1997;17:54–66.
31. Rudnick MR, Berns JS, Cohen RM, Goldfarb S. Contrast media-associated nephrotoxicity. Semin Nephrol 1997;17:15–26.
32. Bennett WM. Drug-related renal dysfunction in the elderly. Geriatr Nephrol Urol 1999;9:21–25.
33. Mulato AS, Ho ES, Cihlar T. Nonsteroidal anti-inflammatory drugs efficiently reduce the transport and cytotoxicity of adefovir mediated by the human renal organic anion transporter 1. J Pharmacol Exp Ther 2000;295:10–15.
34. Nolan CR, Anderson RJ. Hospital-acquired acute renal failure. J Am Soc Nephrol 1998;9:710–718.
35. Slaughter RL, Cappelletty DM. Economic impact of aminoglycoside toxicity and its prevention through therapeutic drug monitoring. Pharmacoeconomics 1998;14:385–394.
36. Mingeot-Leclercq MP, Tulkens PM. Aminoglycosides: nephrotoxicity. Antimicrob Agents Chemother 1999;43:1003–1012.
37. Streetman DS, Nafziger AN, Destache CJ, Bertino AS Jr. Individualized pharmacokinetic monitoring results in less aminoglycoside-associated nephrotoxicity and fewer associated costs. Pharmacotherapy 2001;21:443–451.
38. Freeman CD, Nicolau DP, Belliveau PP, Nightingale CH. Once-daily dosing of aminoglycosides: review and recommendations for clinical practice. J Antimicrob Chemother 1997;39:677–686.
39. McCormack JP. An emotional-based medicine approach to monitoring once-daily aminoglycosides. Pharmacotherapy 2000;20:1524–1527.
40. Levey AS, Bosch JP, Lewis JB, et al. A more accurate method to estimate glomerular filtration rate from serum creatinine: a new prediction equation. Modification of Diet in Renal Disease Study Group. Ann Intern Med 1999;130:461–470.
41. Asif A, Epstein DL, Epstein M. Dopamine-1 receptor agonist: renal effects and its potential role in the management of radiocontrast-induced nephropathy. J Clin Pharmacol 2004;44:1342–1351.
42. Solomon R. Contrast-medium-induced acute renal failure. Kidney Int 1998;53:230–242.
43. Murphy SW, Barrett BJ, Parfrey PS. Contrast nephropathy. J Am Soc Nephrol 2000;11:177–182.
44. Gerlach AT, Pickworth KK. Contrast medium-induced nephrotoxicity: pathophysiology and prevention. Pharmacotherapy 2000;20:540–548.
45. Stevens MA, McCullough PA, Tobin KJ, et al. A prospective randomized trial of prevention measures in patients at high risk for contrast nephropathy: results of the P.R.I.N.C.E. Study. Prevention of Radiocontrast Induced Nephropathy Clinical Evaluation. J Am Coll Cardiol 1999;33:403–411.
46. Mueller C, Buerkle G, Buettner HJ, et al. Prevention of contrast media-associated nephropathy: randomized comparison of 2 hydration regimens in 1620 patients undergoing coronary angioplasty. Arch Intern Med 2002;162:329–336.
47. Kay J, Chow WH, Chan TM, et al. Acetylcysteine for prevention of acute deterioration of renal function following elective coronary angiography and intervention: a randomized controlled trial. JAMA 2003;289:553–558.
48. Birck R, Krzossok S, Markowetz F, et al. Acetylcysteine for prevention of contrast nephropathy: meta-analysis. Lancet 2003;362:598–603.

49. Marenzi G, Marana I, Lauri G, et al. The prevention of radiocontrast-agent-induced nephropathy by hemofiltration. N Engl J Med 2003;349:1333–1340.

50. Kintzel PE. Anticancer drug-induced kidney disorders. Drug Saf 2001;24:19–38.

51. Koukourakis MI. Amifostine in clinical oncology: current use and future applications. Anticancer Drugs 2002;13:181–209.

52. Hartmann JT, Knop S, Fels LM, et al. The use of reduced doses of amifostine to ameliorate nephrotoxicity of cisplatin/ifosfamide-based chemotherapy in patients with solid tumors. Anticancer Drugs 2000;11:1–6.

53. Sener G, Satiroglu H, Kabasakal L, et al. The protective effect of melatonin on cisplatin nephrotoxicity. Fundam Clin Pharmacol 2000;14:553–560.

54. Mizumura Y, Matsumura Y, Hamaguchi T, et al. Cisplatin-incorporated polymeric micelles eliminate nephrotoxicity, while maintaining antitumor activity. Jpn J Cancer Res 2001;92:328–336.

55. Luber AD, Maa L, Lam M, Guglielmo BJ. Risk factors for amphotericin B-induced nephrotoxicity. J Antimicrob Chemother 1999;43:267–271.

56. Wingard JR, White MH, Anaissie E, et al. A randomized, double-blind comparative trial evaluating the safety of liposomal amphotericin B versus amphotericin B lipid complex in the empirical treatment of febrile neutropenia. L Amph/ABLC Collaborative Study Group. Clin Infect Dis 2000;31:1155–1163.

57. Sawaya BP, Briggs JP, Schnermann J. Amphotericin B nephrotoxicity: the adverse consequences of altered membrane properties. J Am Soc Nephrol 1995;6:154–164.

58. Fanos V, Cataldi L. Amphotericin B-induced nephrotoxicity: a review. J Chemother 2000;12:463–470.

59. Eriksson U, Seifert B, Schaffner A. Comparison of effects of amphotericin B deoxycholate infused over 4 or 24 hours: randomised controlled trial. BMJ 2001;322:579–582.

60. Bates DW, Su L, Yu DT, et al. Correlates of acute renal failure in patients receiving parenteral amphotericin B. Kidney Int 2001;60:1452–1459.

61. Deray G. Amphotericin B nephrotoxicity. J Antimicrob Chemother 2002;49(Suppl 1):37–41.

62. Carrigan HC, Hanf-Kristufek L. Comparison of nephrotoxicity of amphotericin B products. Clin Infect Dis 2001;32:990–991.

63. Peters BS, Carlin E, Weston RJ, et al. Adverse effects of drugs used in the management of opportunistic infections associated with HIV infection. Drug Saf 1994;10:439–454.

64. Maurice-Estepa L, Daudon M, Katlama C, et al. Identification of crystals in kidneys of AIDS patients treated with foscarnet. Am J Kidney Dis 1998;32:392–400.

65. Cheung TW, Jayaweera DT, Pearce D, et al. Safety of oral versus intravenous hydration during induction therapy with intravenous foscarnet in AIDS patients with cytomegalovirus infections. Int J STD AIDS 2000;11:640–647.

66. Yorgin PD, Theodorou AA, Al Uzri A, et al. Propylene glycol-induced proximal renal tubular cell injury. Am J Kidney Dis 1997;30:134–139.

67. Bakris GL, Weir MR. Angiotensin-converting enzyme inhibitor-associated elevations in serum creatinine: is this a cause for concern? Arch Intern Med 2000;160:685–693.

68. Reardon LC, Macpherson DS. Hyperkalemia in outpatients using angiotensin-converting enzyme inhibitors. How much should we worry? Arch Intern Med 1998;158:26–32.

69. Wynckel A, Ebikili B, Melin JP, et al. Long-term follow-up of acute renal failure caused by angiotensin converting enzyme inhibitors. Am J Hypertens 1998;11:1080–1086.

70. Solomon DH, Gurwitz JH. Toxicity of nonsteroidal anti-inflammatory drugs in the elderly: is advanced age a risk factor? Am J Med 1997;102:208–215.

71. Brater DC. Effects of nonsteroidal anti-inflammatory drugs on renal function: focus on cyclooxygenase-2-selective inhibition. Am J Med 1999;107:65S–70S.

72. Swan SK, Rudy DW, Lasseter KC, et al. Effect of cyclooxygenase-2 inhibition on renal function in elderly persons receiving a low-salt diet. A randomized, controlled trial. Ann Intern Med 2000;133:1–9.

73. Walls M, Goral S, Stone W. Acute renal failure due to sulfinpyrazone. Am J Med Sci 1998;315:319–321.

74. Ojo AO, Held PJ, Port FK, et al. Chronic renal failure after transplantation of a nonrenal organ. N Engl J Med 2003;349:931–940.

75. de Mattos AM, Olyaei AJ, Bennett WM. Nephrotoxicity of immunosuppressive drugs: long-term consequences and challenges for the future. Am J Kidney Dis 2000;35:333–346.

76. Burdmann EA, Andoh TF, Yu L, Bennett WM. Cyclosporine nephrotoxicity. Semin Nephrol 2003;23:465–476.

77. Olyaei AJ, de Mattos AM, Bennett WM. Immunosuppressant-induced nephropathy: pathophysiology, incidence and management. Drug Saf 1999;21:471–488.

78. Sica DA, Gehr TW. Triamterene and the kidney. Nephron 1989;51:454–461.

79. Wever PC, Roest RW, Wolbink-Kamp AM, et al. OKT3-induced nephrotoxicity is associated with release of group II secretory phospholipase A2. Eur J Clin Invest 1996;26:873–878.

80. Perazella MA. Crystal-induced acute renal failure. Am J Med 1999;106:459–465.

81. Vanholder R, Sever MS, Erek E, Lameire N. Rhabdomyolysis. J Am Soc Nephrol 2000;11:1553–1561.

82. Kopp JB, Miller KD, Mican JA, et al. Crystalluria and urinary tract abnormalities associated with indinavir. Ann Intern Med 1997;127:119–125.

83. Powell T, Hsu FF, Turk J, Hruska K. Ma-huang strikes again: ephedrine nephrolithiasis. Am J Kidney Dis 1998;32:153–159.

84. Ravnskov U. Glomerular, tubular and interstitial nephritis associated with non-steroidal antiinflammatory drugs. Evidence of a common mechanism. Br J Clin Pharmacol 1999;47:203–210.

85. Rossert J. Drug-induced acute interstitial nephritis. Kidney Int 2001;60:804–817.

86. D'agati V. Pathologic classification of focal segmental glomerulosclerosis. Semin Nephrol 2003;23:117–134.

87. Markowitz GS, Appel GB, Fine PL, et al. Collapsing focal segmental glomerulosclerosis following treatment with high-dose pamidronate. J Am Soc Nephrol 2001;12:1164–1172.

88. Hall CL. Gold nephropathy. Nephron 1988;50:265–272.

89. Bigazzi PE. Metals and kidney autoimmunity. Environ Health Perspect 1999;107(Suppl 5):753–765.

90. Michel DM, Kelly CJ. Acute interstitial nephritis. J Am Soc Nephrol 1998;9:506–515.

91. Markowitz GS, Radhakrishnan J, Kambham N, et al. Lithium nephrotoxicity: a progressive combined glomerular and tubulointerstitial nephropathy. J Am Soc Nephrol 2000;11:1439–1448.

92. Walker RG. Lithium nephrotoxicity. Kidney Int Suppl 1993;42:S93–S98.

93. Lam SS, Kjellstrand C. Emergency treatment of lithium-induced diabetes insipidus with nonsteroidal anti-inflammatory drugs. Ren Fail 1997;19:183–188.

94. Olyaei AJ, de Mattos AM, Bennett WM. Nephrotoxicity of immunosuppressive drugs: new insight and preventive strategies. Curr Opin Crit Care 2001;7:384–389.

95. Cosyns JP. Aristolochic acid and 'Chinese herbs nephropathy': a review of the evidence to date. Drug Saf 2003;26:33–48.

96. Reginster F, Jadoul M, van Ypersele dS. Chinese herbs nephropathy presentation, natural history and fate after transplantation. Nephrol Dial Transplant 1997;12:81–86.

97. Cosyns JP, Jadoul M, Squifflet JP, et al. Urothelial lesions in Chinese-herb nephropathy. Am J Kidney Dis 1999;33:1011–1017.

98. Nortier JL, Martinez MC, Schmeiser HH, et al. Urothelial carcinoma associated with the use of a Chinese herb (Aristolochia fangchi). N Engl J Med 2000;342:1686–1692.

99. Griffin MD, Bergstralhn EJ, Larson TS. Renal papillary necrosis—a sixteen-year clinical experience. J Am Soc Nephrol 1995;6:248–256.

100. Henrich WL, Agodoa LE, Barrett B, et al. Analgesics and the kidney: summary and recommendations to the Scientific Advisory Board of the National Kidney Foundation from an Ad Hoc Committee of the National Kidney Foundation. Am J Kidney Dis 1996;27:162–165.

101. Elseviers MM, De Broe ME. Analgesic nephropathy: is it caused by multi-analgesic abuse or single substance use? Drug Saf 1999;20:15–24.

102. Feinstein AR, Heinemann LA, Curhan GC, et al. Relationship between nonphenacetin combined analgesics and nephropathy: a review. Ad Hoc Committee of the International Study Group on Analgesics and Nephropathy. Kidney Int 2000;58:2259–2264.

103. De Broe ME, Elseviers MM. Analgesic nephropathy. N Engl J Med 1998;338:446–452.

104. Michielsen P, de Schepper P. Trends of analgesic nephropathy in two high-endemic regions with different legislation. J Am Soc Nephrol 2001; 12:550–556.

105. Cuellar ML. Drug-induced vasculitis. Curr Rheumatol Rep 2002;4: 55–59.

106. Groff JA, Kozak M, Boehmer JP, et al. Endotheliopathy: a continuum of hemolytic uremic syndrome due to mitomycin therapy. Am J Kidney Dis 1997;29:280–284.

107. Pisoni R, Ruggenenti P, Remuzzi G. Drug-induced thrombotic microangiopathy: incidence, prevention and management. Drug Saf 2001;24: 491–501.

108. Choi HK, Merkel PA, Walker AM, Niles JL. Drug-associated antineutrophil cytoplasmic antibody-positive vasculitis: prevalence among patients with high titers of antimyeloperoxidase antibodies. Arthritis Rheum 2000;43:405-413.

109. Lye WC, Cheah JS, Sinniah R. Renal cholesterol embolic disease. Case report and review of the literature. Am J Nephrol 1993;13:489–493.

110. Andreev E, Koopman M, Arisz L. A rise in plasma creatinine that is not a sign of renal failure: which drugs can be responsible? J Intern Med 1999;246:247–252.

111. Eisenberg JM, Koffer H, Glick HA, et al. What is the cost of nephrotoxicity associated with aminoglycosides? Ann Intern Med 1987;107: 900–909.

112. McGoldrick MD, Bailie GR. Nonnarcotic analgesics: prevalence and estimated economic impact of toxicities. Ann Pharmacother 1997;31: 221–227.

47

GLOMERULONEPHRITIS

Alan H. Lau

Learning Objectives and other resources can be found at *www.pharmacotherapyonline.com.*

KEY CONCEPTS

❶ Glomerulonephritis is a collection of glomerular diseases mediated by different immunologic pathogenic mechanisms, resulting in varied clinical presentation and therapeutic outcomes.

❷ The signs and symptoms associated with glomerulonephritis can be nephritic in nature, characterized by inflammatory injury, or nephrotic in nature, characterized by proteinuria.

❸ In the absence of specific and effective therapy for many types of glomerulonephritis, supportive treatments for edema, hypertension, hyperlipidemia, and intravascular thrombosis play important roles in alleviating the complications associated with the disease.

❹ To maximize therapeutic benefits and minimize drug-induced complications, patients have to be monitored closely to delineate their therapeutic responses as well as the development of any treatment-induced toxicities.

❺ Among all the types of glomerulonephritis, minimal-change nephropathy is most responsive to treatment. Steroids can induce good responses in most patients during initial treatment as well as relapse.

❻ Due to the lack of consistently effective treatment for primary focal segmental glomerular sclerosis, angiotensin-converting enzyme inhibitors or angiotensin receptor blockers are commonly used for patients with mild disease to control symptoms. Steroids and immunosuppressive agents are used only for patients with severe disease.

❼ The optimal treatment for lupus nephritis depends on the underlying lesion and disease activity, as well as the severity and duration of the clinical presentation.

❽ The treatment of poststreptococcal glomerulonephritis is mainly supportive and symptomatic. Antibiotic therapy does not prevent subsequent diseases, but may reduce the severity.

Clinical and pathologic findings associated with primary glomerular injury were first reported in the nineteenth century. The natural history of many glomerular diseases was not described until the 1950s, when percutaneous diagnostic kidney biopsy became available. The development of immunofluorescence microscopy and advances in immunopathology in the 1960s and 1970s further expanded our understanding of the antibody-related immune mechanisms that are responsible for the different types of glomerular injury. Recent advances in cell and molecular biology afford us a plethora of new information concerning the disease processes. However, the precise pathogenetic mechanisms for many glomerular diseases remain unknown and the available therapeutic regimens are still far from optimal. In the United States in 2001, glomerulonephritis was the third most common cause of end-stage kidney disease (ESKD), which is also referred to as end-stage renal disease (ESRD), accounting for about 15% of all the living ESKD patients. About 8,000 patients (8.3% of all patients) develop ESKD due to glomerulonephritis each year.[1]

This chapter provides an overview of the pathophysiologic mechanisms of glomerular injury and the clinical presentations of glomerulonephritis. The treatment approach for the common forms of glomerulonephritis are also discussed. Although diabetes mellitus and amyloidosis are important secondary causes of glomerular diseases, the scope of this chapter is limited to the primary causes of glomerulonephritis.

PATHOPHYSIOLOGY

NORMAL ANATOMY AND FUNCTION

The glomerulus, which is enclosed within the Bowman's capsule, consists of two important components: the filtration barrier and the mesangium (Fig. 47–1). Blood flow in the glomerular capillary bed is supplied by the afferent arteriole, while the efferent arterioles channel the flow leaving the glomerular tuft. The capillary wall, which serves as a filtration barrier, consists of three well-defined layers: fenestrated endothelium, glomerular basement membrane (GBM), and epithelial cells. The epithelial cells, also known as podocytes, have specialized foot processes embedded in the outer layer of the GBM. It is across this barrier that fluid flows and ultimately forms ultrafiltrate. Under normal conditions, the GBM appears to function as a compact hydrated gel of matrix proteins with a pore-like structure. The mesangium provides support for the glomerular capillaries and also modulates blood flow through the capillaries. It consists of mesangial cells embedded in an extracellular matrix.

The unique capillary bed of the glomerulus allows small nonprotein plasma constituents up to the size of inulin, which has a molecular weight of 5,200 daltons, to pass freely while excluding macromolecules equal to or larger than albumin, which has a molecular weight of 69,000 daltons (Fig. 47–2). Both the size and charge

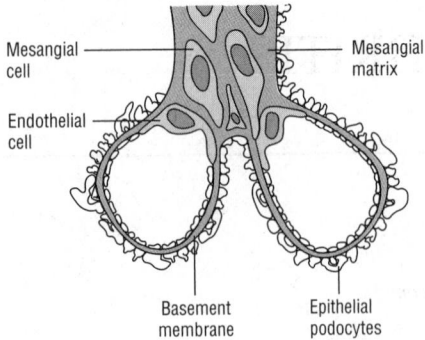

FIGURE 47-1. Microanatomy of the glomerulus.

of the molecules affect the ease of passage through the glomerular membrane. Fixed, negatively charged sites are found within the glomeruli in all three layers of the capillary wall: the endothelium, the epithelium, and the GBM. Biochemical and cytochemical studies show that the epithelial cell coat is composed of a negatively charged glycoprotein (podocalyxin), made up largely of sialic acid. The GBM contains an abundance of negatively charged sulfated glycosaminoglycans that can affect the passage of ionic molecules through the capillary wall. The movement of negatively charged molecules is restricted more than that of neutral or positively charged molecules. Different glomerular diseases affect this size- and charge-selective barrier to different extents, and glomerulopathies therefore present with varied clinical features and solute-excretion patterns.

Aside from being a barrier for solute excretion, some of the glomerular cells, such as the epithelial cells, have phagocytic function that can remove macromolecules trapped within the filtration barrier. They are also capable of synthesizing the GBM. In contrast, the mesangial cells regulate glomerular hemodynamics by responding to angiotensin II and producing prostaglandins. They also synthesize and respond to various cytokines and thus play a key role in immune-mediated glomerular diseases. There are also resident phagocytes in the mesangium. They remove macromolecules trapped in the basement membrane and move them into the urinary space. These phagocytes are involved in the development of both immune and nonimmune glomerular injury.

ETIOLOGY

The etiology of most human glomerulonephritides is unknown. However, humoral and cellular immunologic mechanisms are implicated in the pathogenesis. Abnormalities in coagulation and metabolism, as well as hereditary and vascular diseases, also contribute to glomerular damage. The histopathologic manifestations vary substantially among the different types of glomerulonephritis. An overview of the primary pathogenetic mechanisms is presented in this section, and specific abnormalities for each of the primary types of glomerulonephritis are presented in subsequent sections.

PATHOGENESIS OF GLOMERULAR INJURY AND PATHOLOGIC MANIFESTATIONS

The glomerular lesion may be diffuse (involving all glomeruli), focal (involving some but not all glomeruli), or segmental, also known as local (involving part of the individual glomerulus). The pathologic manifestations may also be described as proliferative (overgrowth of epithelium, endothelium, or mesangium), membranous (thickening of GBM), and/or sclerotic.

The glomerular capillary wall is particularly susceptible to immune-mediated injury. Antigen and antibody tend to localize in the glomerulus, probably because of its high blood flow and capillary hydrostatic pressure. Parenchymal damage can be induced as a result of humoral- and cell-mediated immune reactions (Table 47–1). Antibodies and sensitized T lymphocytes are the primary mediators of glomerular injury.[2,3]

Production of antibodies to endogenous or exogenous antigens that are recognized as foreign by the host is the first step in humoral immunologic damage to the glomerulus. Endogenous antigens may be intrinsic glomerular antigens, such as Heymann's antigen on the epithelial cell or Goodpasture's antigen on the GBM, or previously sequestered antigens, such as DNA or thyroglobulin. Exogenous antigens are most often viral, bacterial, parasitic, or fungal in origin (Table 47–2). Antineutrophil cytoplasmic autoantibodies (ANCAs), autoantibodies that react to the cytoplasmic components of neutrophils and monocytes, have been found in patients with idiopathic crescentic glomerulonephritis and also in the accompanying vasculitis.

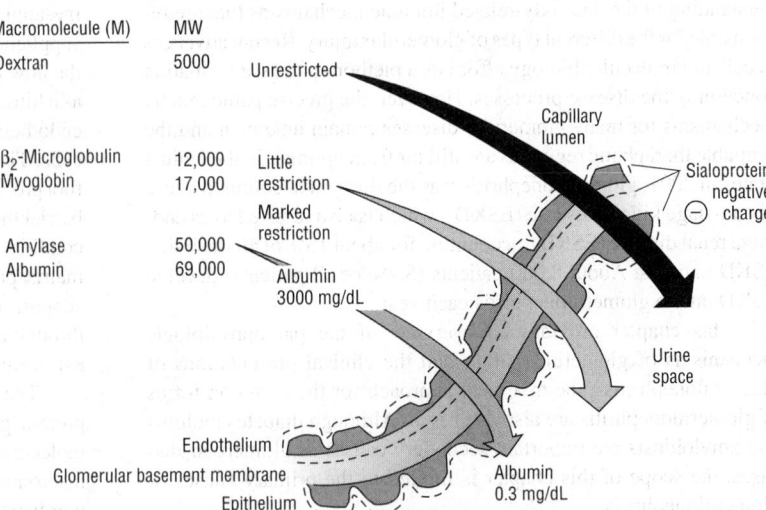

FIGURE 47-2. Movement of various macromolecules across the glomerular capillary. The fractional clearance of each macromolecule decreases as molecular weight (MW) increases. The disproportionately greater restriction of albumin movement indicates importance of factors other than size, such as negative charge of albumin. (Adapted from Hutt MP, Kelleher SP. Proteinuria and the nephrotic syndrome. In: Schrier RW, ed. Renal and Electrolyte Disorders, 3rd ed. Boston, Little, Brown, 1986: p. 568.)

TABLE 47–1. Immunologic Mechanisms of Glomerular Injury

Circulating immune complexes
In situ antigen–antibody interaction
   Intrinsic glomerular antigen; e.g., GBM antigens
   Exogenous planted antigens
Cell-mediated mechanism

GBM, glomerular basement membrane.

Classically, it was considered that complexes of antigens and antibodies were formed in the circulation and then passively entrapped in the glomerular capillary or mesangium. However, experimental data show that antibodies may combine with endogenous glomerular antigens or exogenous antigens entrapped in the glomerulus to form complexes locally, or in situ.[3] Regardless of the mechanism of formation, these antigen–antibody complexes are often localized along the capillary loop or the mesangium (see Fig. 47–1) and can be detected by immunofluorescence microscopy. The type and extent of glomerular damage is dependent on the location of the immune complex formation and the rate at which it is removed. Impaired removal facilitates the growth of the complex and thus increases the likelihood of glomerular damage.

Subsequent to antigen-antibody formation, a series of biologic events is triggered that ultimately leads to glomerular injury. Both inflammatory and noninflammatory lesions can be induced by antibody deposition. Noninflammatory lesions can be a result of noncomplement-fixing antibody binding to the glomerular epithelial cell (mechanism 1), or activation of the complement system to form the C5b-9 membrane attack complex (mechanism 2).[3] Both mechanisms can damage the glomerular epithelial cell and result in capillary wall injury and proteinuria (Fig. 47–3). Inflammatory lesions are induced by glomerular infiltration of circulating inflammatory cells such as neutrophils, monocytes/macrophages, and platelets (mechanism 3), or proliferation of resident glomerular mesangial cells (mechanism 4), resulting in GBM damage.[3] The migration of neutrophils and monocytes to the glomerular tufts is promoted by chemoattractants such as complement fragments (C3a and C5a),

TABLE 47–2. Antigens Possibly Involved in Immune-Mediated Glomerular Injury

Source of Antigen	Clinical Example
Endogenous antigens	
Released sequestered cellular antigens	DNA, thyroglobulin
Endogenous antigens modified by exogenous source	IgG modified by streptococcal neuraminidase
Tumor antigens	CEA in bronchial and other solid tumors
Intrinsic glomerular antigens	Goodpasture's syndrome
Neutrophil granule constituents	ANCA-associated glomerulonephritis
Exogenous	
Viral	Hepatitis B
Bacterial	Streptococcal organisms
Parasitic	Malaria
Fungal	Candida

CEA, carcinoembryonic antigen; ANCA, antineutrophil cytoplasmic antibody.

platelet-activating factor, interleukin-8, and monocyte chemotactic protein-1.[4] Various cytokines, chemokines, and growth factors are then released to participate in the inflammatory process.[2]

T cells sensitized to glomerular antigen, macrophages, and resident mesangial cells are important participants in cell-mediated injury. Sensitized T cells can cause glomerular hypercellularity in the absence of antibody deposition.[2–4] Cytotoxic T cells may bind with the target cells and destroy them. Alternatively, a delayed-type hypersensitivity reaction may be initiated by activated T cells through the release of lymphokines, to attract, activate, and transform monocytes into macrophages.[3] These humoral and cellular mediators, in conjunction with a host of toxic molecular entities including reactive oxygen species, proteinases, eicosanoids, and procoagulants, which are secreted by neutrophils, macrophages, platelets, and resident glomerular cells can alter the permeability, blood flow, and function of the

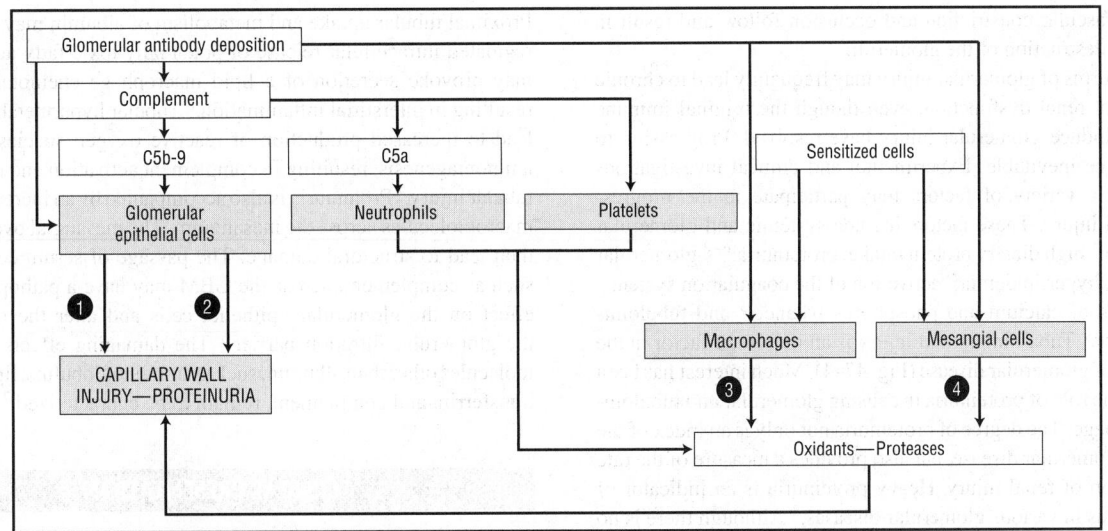

FIGURE 47–3. The major pathways of immune-mediated glomerular injury. Mechanisms 1 and 2 primarily act on the glomerular epithelial cell and result in noninflammatory lesions. Mechanisms 3 and 4 involve participation of effector cells and result in glomerular inflammation and structural damage. (Adapted from Couser.[3])

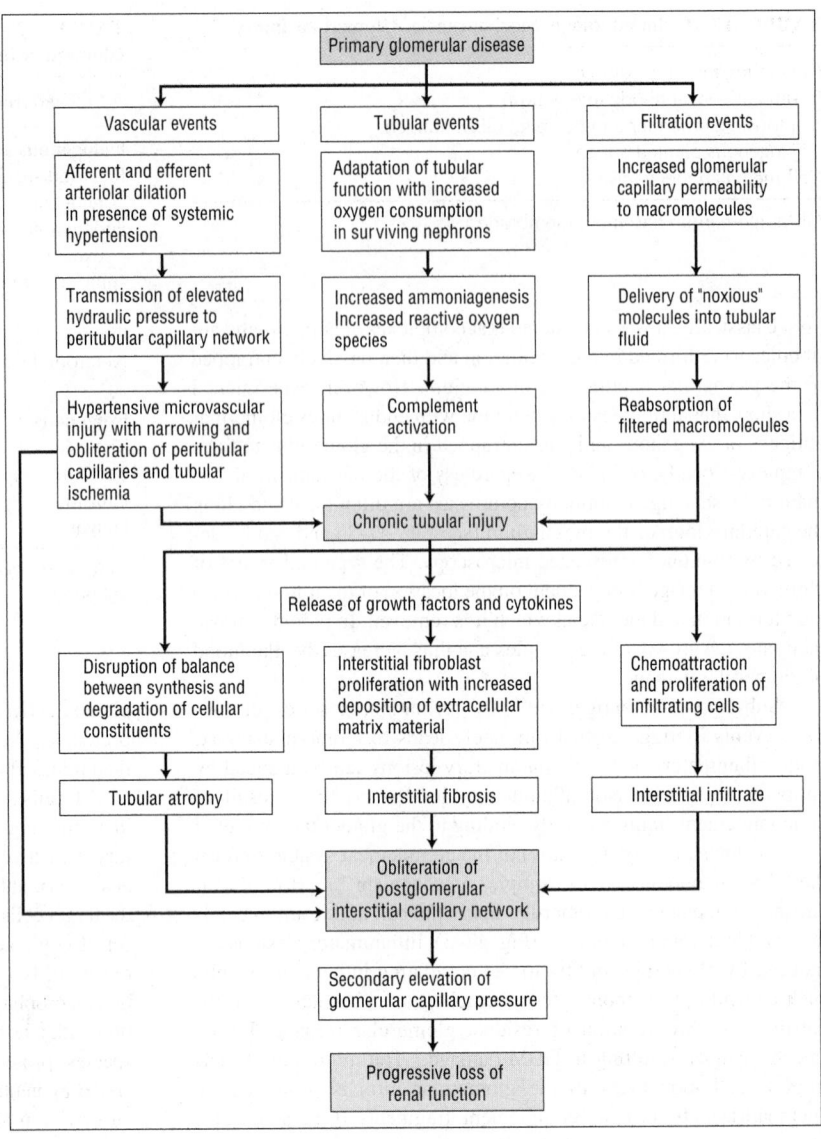

FIGURE 47–4. Proposed sequence of events leading from primary glomerular disease to progressive loss of renal function through tubulointerstitial injury. (Modified from Ong et al,[7] with permission.)

glomeruli. Vascular constriction and occlusion follow and result in the eventual destruction of the glomeruli.

Acute forms of glomerular injury may frequently lead to chronic and persistent renal dysfunction, even though the original immune factors that induce glomerular injury have resolved. Progression to ESKD may be inevitable. Experimental and clinical investigations suggest that a variety of factors may participate in the progression of renal injury. These factors include systemic and glomerular hypertension;[5] high dietary protein intake; proteinuria;[6-8] glomerular hypertrophy; hyperlipidemia;[9] activation of the coagulation system;[5] abnormalities of calcium and phosphorus balance;[5] and tubulointerstitial injury.[7] Tubulointerstitial injury is an important factor in the progression of glomerular disease (Fig. 47–4). Much interest has been focused on the role of proteinuria in causing glomerular and tubulointerstitial damage. The degree of proteinuria not only is an index of the severity of glomerular disease, but also provides a measure of the rate of progression of renal injury. Heavy proteinuria is an indicator of poor prognosis in various glomerular diseases.[8] Although there is no direct evidence to substantiate that proteinuria per se results in progression of renal impairment,[6,7] there are many possible mechanisms through which proteinuria directly or indirectly causes renal damage.

Proximal tubular uptake and metabolism of albumin may lead to unregulated intracellular release of potentially toxic fatty acids, which may provoke secretion of a lipid macrophage chemotactic factor, resulting in interstitial inflammation.[8] Tubular hypermetabolism may lead to increased production of reactive oxygen species and renal ammoniagenesis, resulting in complement activation and consequent tubular injury.[7] Proteinuria is also accompanied by an increased flux of macromolecules across the mesangium. The mesangial overload may then lead to structural damage. The passage of serum components, such as complement, across the GBM may have a pathophysiologic effect on the glomerular epithelial cells and alter the integrity of the glomerular filtration barrier.[6] The damaging effects of macromolecules other than albumin, such as immunoglobulins, lipoproteins, transferrin, and complement, remain to be characterized.[7]

CLINICAL PRESENTATION

Patients with glomerular disease may present with a nephritic or a nephrotic syndrome (Table 47–3). Nephritic syndrome reflects glomerular inflammation and frequently results in hematuria. White

TABLE 47–3. Tendencies of Glomerular Diseases to Manifest Nephrotic and Nephritic Features

	Nephrotic Features	Nephritic Features
Minimal-change nephropathy	++++	–
Membranous nephropathy	++++	+
Diabetic glomerulosclerosis	++++	+
Amyloidosis	++++	+
Focal segmental glomerulosclerosis	+++	++
Mesangioproliferative glomerulonephritis	++	++
Membranoproliferative glomerulonephritis	++	+++
Proliferative glomerulonephritis	++	+++
Acute poststreptococcal glomerulonephritis	+	++++
Crescentic glomerulonephritis[a]	+	++++

[a]Can be immune complex–mediated, antiglomerular basement membrane antibody–mediated, or associated with antineutrophil cytoplasmic autoantibodies.

cells and cellular and granular casts are commonly found in the urine. In contrast, nephrotic syndrome reflects noninflammatory injury to the glomerular structures, and results in few cells or cellular casts in the urine. Initially, there may be limited or no reduction in renal excretory function.

Hematuria occurs when red blood cells leak through the openings of the GBM. The presence of red cell casts is highly indicative of glomerulonephritis or vasculitis. The presence of dysmorphic red blood cells in the urine is suggestive of glomerular disease. The red blood cells are damaged as they pass through the openings in the GBM or the cells may sustain osmotic injury as they travel through the different osmotic environments within the lumen of the kidney tubules.

The presence of proteinuria indicates a defect of the size- and/or charge-selective barriers within the GBM. Normal urinary protein excretion is between 40 and 80 mg/day, with a maximum of 150 mg. Fewer than 20 mg of the excreted proteins are albumin. Most of the albumin that enters the glomerular filtrate is either reabsorbed or catabolized by the tubular epithelium. The dipsticks that are commonly used to identify proteinuria detect only albumin; they become positive when protein excretion is more than 300 to 500 mg/day. They are therefore unable to detect the early stages of renal injury secondary to diabetes mellitus or hypertension, which often result in microalbuminuria with urinary albumin excretion ranges between 30 and 300 mg/day. Chemstrip Micral-Test II (Boehringer Mannheim Diagnostics), a simple immunoassay on a dipstick, permits specific and semiquantitative determination of urinary albumin concentrations at five levels: 0, 10, 20, 50, and 100 mg/L. It shows no cross-reactivity with other human proteins that may possibly be present in urine. The test may be used reliably for a urine specimen that has been stored for up to 7 days at 4°C (39.2°F), and even in the presence of bacterial contamination. Another qualitative test, Micro-Bumintest (Ames), registers a positive reading when the urine albumin concentration is greater than 40 mg/L.[10]

Hypertension is a common feature in patients with glomerular diseases. Expansion of plasma volume as a result of renal salt retention is frequently the cause of hypertension, especially during acute disease. In contrast, increased activity of vasoconstrictors such as angiotensin II is often the cause in patients with chronic glomerular diseases. Scarring of the glomerulus resulting in regional ischemia is thought to be responsible for the hypertension. Activation of the sympathetic nervous system and the release of vasoconstrictor substances may also contribute.

TABLE 47–4. Evaluation of Patients Suspected of Having Glomerular Disease

Medical history
To identify symptoms of medical conditions that may cause glomerular disease:
- Diabetes mellitus
- Amyloidosis
- Systemic lupus erythematosus
- Other familial conditions associated with renal disease
To identify symptoms suggestive of nephrotic syndrome:
- Reduced appetite
- Fatigue
- Weight gain
- Edema

Medication, environmental and occupational histories
To identify possible exposure to potentially nephrotoxic drugs, toxins, or chemicals

Physical examination
To identify signs and symptoms associated with systemic diseases
- Hypertension
- Rash
- Arthritis
- Retinopathy
- Neuropathy
- Lymphadenopathy
- Hepatomegaly
- Malignancy

Laboratory evaluation
Urinalysis
- To determine nephrotic nature of gomerular disease:
  Heavy proteinuria (usually >3 g/day), or
  Lipiduria, to determine nephritic nature of glomerular disease
- Hematuria
- Pyuria
- Cellular, granular casts
Glomerular filtration rate
- To determine extent of glomerular damage
Other tests
- To identify type and etiology of glomerular disease
- Serum complement concentration
- Antinuclear and anti-DNA antibodies
- Antistreptolysin antibodies
- Circulating anti-GBM antibodies
- Cryoglobulins
Percutaneous renal biopsy
- To provide definitive diagnosis of glomerular disease

GBM, glomerular basement membrane.

NEPHRITIC SYNDROME

Glomerular bleeding resulting in hematuria is a typical finding in nephritic syndrome. Dysmorphic red cells, especially acanthocytes, are a sensitive and specific marker of glomerular bleeding. The presence of pus and cellular and granular casts in the urine is common. The extent of proteinuria is variable, typically about 1 to 3 g/day, but it may be in the nephrotic range (>3 g/day). Patients with severe nephritic glomerular injury have renal function impairment because of the reduced glomerular surface area available for filtration. The latter is a result of constriction of the capillary lumen by proliferating mesangial cells or inflammatory cells. As renal function declines, hypertension and edema may develop or pre-existing conditions may worsen.

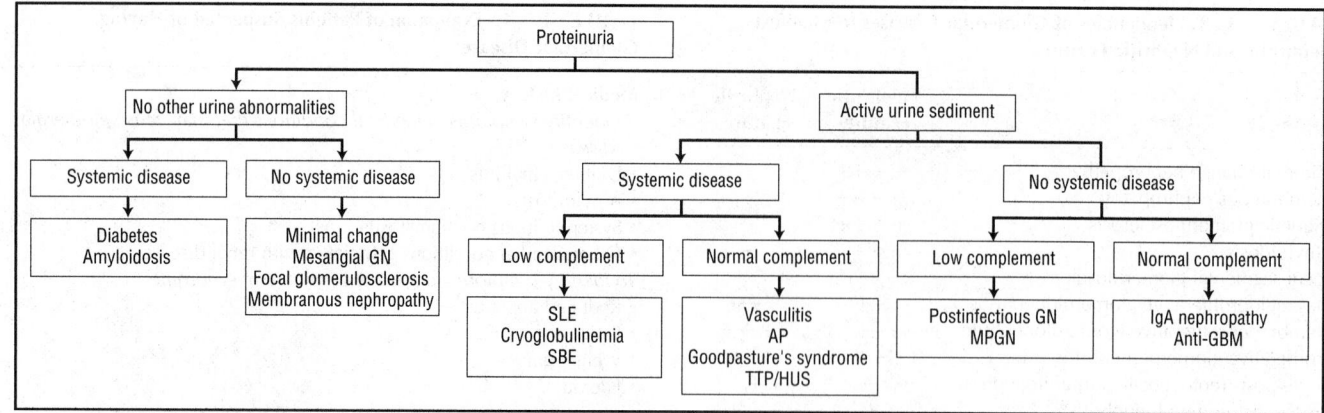

FIGURE 47–5. Clinical presentations of glomerulonephritis. AP, anaphylactoid purpura; GBM, glomerular basement membrane; GN, glomerulonephritis; HUS, hemolytic uremic syndrome; MPGN, membranoproliferative glomerulonephritis; SBE, subacute bacterial endocarditis; SLE, systemic lupus erythematosus; TTP, thrombotic thrombocytopenic purpura.

NEPHROTIC SYNDROME

Nephrotic syndrome is characterized by proteinuria greater than 3.5 g/day per 1.73 m², hypoproteinemia, edema, and hyperlipidemia. A hypercoagulable state may also be present in some patients. The syndrome may be the result of primary diseases of the glomerulus, or be associated with systemic diseases such as diabetes mellitus, lupus, amyloidosis, and preeclampsia. Hypoproteinemia, especially hypoalbuminemia, results from increased urinary loss of albumin and an increased rate of catabolism of filtered albumin by proximal tubular cells. The compensatory increase in hepatic synthesis of albumin is insufficient to replenish the protein loss, probably because of malnutrition.

Edema formation in patients with nephrotic syndrome was traditionally thought to be driven by the reduced plasma oncotic pressure secondary to hypoalbuminemia. If the oncotic pressure is low, the movement of fluid from the vascular space to the interstitial compartment results in a reduction of the plasma volume, which can trigger compensatory renal sodium and water retention through the activation of the renin-angiotensin-aldosterone axis, vasopressin, and the sympathetic nervous system (the "underfill" mechanism). However, experimental data suggest that the plasma volume is actually normal or elevated. Hypoalbuminemia may not cause edema until the serum albumin concentration is less than 2 g/dL. In addition, the transcapillary oncotic pressure gradient is not as high as previously thought because increased lymphatic flow reduces the interstitial oncotic pressure by removing protein and fluid from the interstitium, thereby reducing the transcapillary oncotic pressure gradient.[11] Thus fluid retention is likely mediated by a primary increase in sodium reabsorption at the distal nephron, which is probably caused by tubular resistance to the action of atrial natriuretic peptide (the "overflow" mechanism).[12] It is likely that both mechanisms may contribute to nephrotic edema in different patients.[12]

Although albuminuria below the nephrotic range appears to have a minor influence on serum cholesterol in patients with primary glomerular disease, daily urinary albumin excretion of greater than 3 g is associated with a significant increase in serum cholesterol concentrations.[13] Hyperlipidemia in nephrotic syndrome is characterized by elevated serum total cholesterol and triglyceride concentrations, with increased very-low-density lipoprotein (VLDL) and low-density lipoprotein (LDL) cholesterol concentrations. Although high-density lipoprotein (HDL) cholesterol concentrations are nor-

mally distributed, there is a maldistribution of HDL subtypes, with a reduction in HDL_2 and an increase in HDL_3.[14,15] Furthermore, lipoprotein (a) levels may also be increased. Oval fat bodies and fatty casts are also found in the urine. The mechanisms for nephrotic hyperlipidemia are not well defined. A reduction in plasma oncotic pressure as a result of hypoalbuminemia may stimulate hepatic synthesis of lipids and lipoproteins. The increased VLDL production and increased liver cholesterol synthesis along with a decrease in LDL receptor activity can then lead to an increase in LDL cholesterol concentrations. In addition, reduced serum albumin or the loss of a liporegulatory substance may result in reduced VLDL clearance.[14,15] Nephrotic patients with hyperlipidemia, especially those with concomitant hypertension, are presumed to have an increased risk for atherosclerotic vascular disease. Hyperlipidemia also promotes the progression of glomerular injury, as evidenced by glomerulosclerosis, mesangial expansion, and hyalinosis.[9,14]

Many patients with nephrotic syndrome have a hypercoagulable state caused by defects of several control proteins in the coagulation cascade. The concentration of the coagulation inhibitor antithrombin III is reduced because of increased loss in the urine. A reduced amount of the coagulation inhibitors proteins C and S, along with increased concentrations of factors V and VIII, increased fibrinogen concentrations, and abnormal platelet function, may also contribute to the hypercoagulable state. The net result of these alterations in coagulation is an increased risk for arterial and venous thrombosis, especially in the deep veins and renal veins. As many as 25% of patients with membranous nephropathy may have renal vein thrombosis.

DIAGNOSIS

Patients with suspected glomerular disease should have an extensive medical history obtained to identify potential systemic causes (Table 47–4). Medication, environmental, and occupational histories may also help identify possible exposure to potentially nephrotoxic agents. A carefully conducted physical examination and laboratory evaluation may reveal the presence of systemic diseases (Fig. 47–5; Table 47–5) that may contribute to the development of glomerular disease. In addition, the patient's age, gender, and ethnic background may be helpful in pinpointing the specific type of glomerular disease. Many of the conditions are more prevalent in certain age groups, although they

TABLE 47–5. Categorization of Renal Diseases Based on Serum Complement Levels

Low Serum Complement Level	Normal Syrum Complement Level
Systemic diseases	**Systemic diseases**
Systemic lupus erythematosus	Vasculitis group
Infection-related glomerulonephritis	Polyarteritis nodosa
	Hypersensitivity vasculitis
Subacute bacterial endocarditis	Wegener's granulomatosis
"Shunt" nephritis	Henoch–Schönlein purpura
Cryoglobulinemia	Goodpasture's syndrome
Primary renal diseases	**Primary renal diseases**
Acute poststreptococcal glomerulonephritis	IgA nephropathy
	Idiopathic rapidly progressive glomerulonephritis
Membranoproliferative glomerulonephritis	Idiopathic nephrotic syndrome

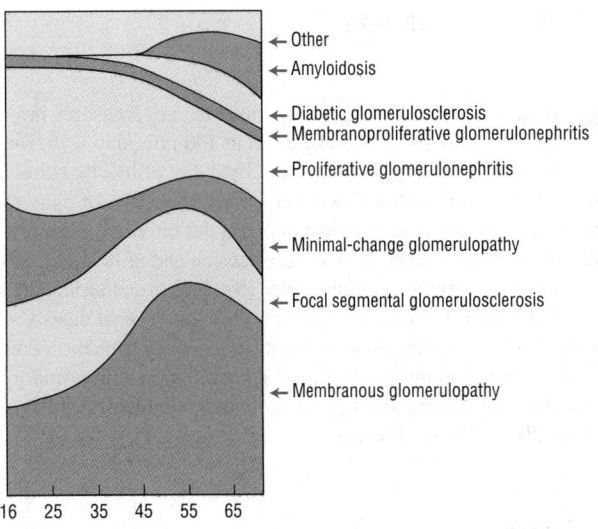

FIGURE 47–6. Frequency of various causes for nephrotic-range proteinuria (>3 g/day) relative to age in patients undergoing renal biopsy evaluation at the University of North Carolina Nephropathology Laboratory. The full vertical height of the bar represents 100% of the patients. The patients with proliferative glomerulonephritis generally presented with nephritic features in addition to the proteinuria, and included patients with lupus nephritis, IgA nephropathy, and postinfectious glomerulonephritis. (Used with permission from Jennette et al.[40])

may occur at any age. Figure 47–6 indicates the distribution of different causes of nephrotic-range proteinuria relative to the age of patients who had undergone renal biopsy.

Laboratory evaluation such as urinalysis can help differentiate the nephrotic or nephritic nature of the disease. The glomerular filtration rate (GFR) may be used to determine the extent of glomerular damage. In the early stages of the disease, the GFR may remain normal. Initial injury to the glomerulus primarily lowers the permeability coefficient (K_f) of the GBM, by reducing the surface area available for filtration and/or the unit permeability of the membrane. The reduced permeability is compensated by an elevation in the glomerular capillary hydrostatic pressure through afferent arteriolar dilation and efferent arteriolar constriction. Extensive glomerular damage may

therefore be present before a substantial reduction of total GFR is evident (Table 47–5).

Although the cause of glomerular disease may be established from clinical and laboratory evaluation, sometimes percutaneous renal biopsy may be needed to provide a definitive diagnosis.

▶ TREATMENT: Glomerulonephritis

■ GENERAL APPROACH TO TREATMENT

The management of patients with glomerulonephritis involves specific pharmacologic therapy for the glomerular disease, and supportive measures to prevent and/or treat the pathophysiologic sequelae, namely hypertension, edema, and progression of renal disease. In patients with nephrotic syndrome, supportive therapy should also address the management of extrarenal complications of heavy proteinuria, namely hypoalbuminemia, hyperlipidemia, and thromboembolism. Patients with significant proteinuria tend to have a more rapid decline of renal function. Thus reduction of proteinuria becomes critical in delaying the rate of progression towards end-stage renal disease.

Immunosuppressive agents, alone or in combination, are commonly used to alter the immune processes that are responsible for the glomerulonephritides. Corticosteroids, in addition to their immunosuppressive effect, also possess anti-inflammatory activities. They reduce the production and/or release of many substances that mediate the inflammatory process, such as prostaglandins, leukotrienes, platelet-activating factors, tumor necrosis factors (TNFs), and interleukin-1 (IL-1). Movement of leukocytes and macrophages to the site of inflammation is also inhibited. The immunosuppressive effects of corticosteroids are mediated through the inhibition of the release

of IL-1 and TNF by activated macrophages, and IL-2 by activated T cells. In addition, the actions of migration-inhibiting factor and γ-interferon are inhibited. Processing of antigens is thus affected by the presence of corticosteroids. Cytotoxic agents, such as cyclophosphamide, chlorambucil, or azathioprine, are used occasionally to treat glomerular diseases. Cyclosporine is also used to treat certain types of glomerulonephritis. It can reduce lymphokine production by activated T lymphocytes and it can decrease proteinuria by improving the permselectivity of the GBM.

Because many immune factors are implicated in the pathogenesis of glomerulonephritis, plasmapheresis may be used to remove these mediators. During the procedure, whole blood is removed from the body and centrifugation is used to separate the cellular elements from the plasma. The cells are then infused back to the patient after resuspension in saline or plasma substitute. The plasma proteins, presumably including the pathogenic immune factors, are thereby removed from the patient.

Various new experimental agents, such as etanercept and alemtuzumab, have also been used to treat glomerulonephritis.[16] Sufficient experiences are not yet available to determine their role in therapy. However, as we acquire further understanding of the pathogenic processes, innovative therapy can be developed to improve patient outcome.

■ SUPPORTIVE THERAPY

In patients with nephrotic syndrome, dietary measures involve restriction of sodium intake to 50 to 100 mEq/day,[11,17] protein intake of 0.8 to 1 g/day,[17,18] and a low-lipid diet of less than 200 mg cholesterol. Total fat should account for less than 30% of daily total calories.[17] Sodium restriction is important not only in the control of edema, but also in the control of hypertension and proteinuria. Similarly, protein restriction not only helps to reduce proteinuria, but also has a potential role in retarding the progression of renal disease. Patients should also stop smoking because a dose-dependent increase in risk for developing ESKD was observed in men with primary inflammatory (IgA glomerulonephritis) or noninflammatory (polycystic kidney disease) renal diseases.[19]

■ EDEMA

Management of nephrotic edema involves salt restriction, bedrest, and use of support stockings and diuretics. However, severe salt restriction is difficult to achieve in patients who are sodium-avid, and prolonged bedrest could predispose nephrotic patients to thromboembolism. Hence the use of a loop diuretic such as furosemide is frequently required. Although the delivery of diuretic to the kidney tubules is normal, the presence of large amounts of protein in the urine promotes drug binding, and thereby reduces the availability of the diuretic to the luminal receptor sites. In addition, reduced sodium delivery to the distal tubule secondary to decreased glomerular perfusion may also alter diuretic effectiveness. Large doses of the loop diuretic, such as 160 to 480 mg of furosemide, may be needed for patients with moderate edema (see Chap. 49). In some patients, a thiazide diuretic or metolazone may be added to enhance natriuresis.[17,20] Alternatively, continuous intravenous infusion of a loop diuretic, such as furosemide 160 to 480 mg/day, may be employed and is more effective than intermittent bolus injections in inducing urinary sodium excretion.[21] In patients with morbid edema, albumin infusion may be used to expand plasma volume and to increase diuretic delivery to the renal tubules, thus enhancing diuretic effect. However, it may precipitate congestive heart failure and may also reduce therapeutic response to steroid in minimal-change nephropathy. In patients with significant edema, the goal of treatment should be a daily loss of 1 to 2 lb of fluid until a reasonable weight has been obtained.

■ HYPERTENSION

Optimal control of hypertension in patients with glomerular disease is important in reducing both the progression of renal disease and the risk for cardiovascular disease[18,22] (see Chaps. 13 and 43). The Seventh Report of the Joint National Committee on Prevention, Detection, Evaluation, and Treatment of High Blood Pressure report recommended the target blood pressure to be 130/80 mm Hg in patients with chronic renal insufficiency defined by GFR <60 mL/min or albuminuria >300 mg/d.[23] Angiotensin-converting enzyme inhibitors (ACEIs) or angiotensin II receptor blockers (ARBs) have been shown to delay the loss of renal function in patients with diabetic and nondiabetic (primarily glomerulonephritis) renal diseases.[24] They reduce renal protein excretion and exert renoprotection through mechanisms independent of their blood pressure–lowering effects. Alternatively, nondihydropyridine calcium channel blockers (e.g., diltiazem) may have proteinuria-reduction properties and could be used as an additional agent. The dihydropyridine calcium channel blockers (e.g., nifedipine, amlodipine, or nisoldipine) can also be used to lower blood pressure, but without the benefit of urinary protein reduction.[25]

■ PROTEINURIA

Dietary protein restriction reduces proteinuria and may retard renal function deterioration. The intent-to-treat analysis of the Modification of Diet in Renal Disease study in patients with moderate renal insufficiency (GFR of 25 to 55 mL/min per 1.73 m^2), did not show that a low-protein diet was able to slow renal disease progression. However, the secondary analysis revealed that protein intake of 0.66 g/kg per day reduced the rate of GFR deterioration in patients with severe renal insufficiency, GFR of 13 to 24 mL/min per 1.73 m^2.[26] In view of the lack of definitive proof about the benefit of protein restriction on disease progression, modest protein restriction of 0.8 g/kg per day is reasonable for patients with moderate renal insufficiency. Decreasing dietary protein will also reduce the intake of phosphorus and potassium. In many instances, the potential benefits of protein restriction have to be balanced against the need for protein intake to overcome nutritional deficiencies. The patient's protein and energy intake as well as the nutritional status therefore have to be monitored adequately. For nondialyzed patients who have GFRs of less than 25 mL/min per 1.73 m^2, dietary protein intake should be reduced to 0.6 g/kg per day because it can retard the rate of renal function loss and also the time to reach end-stage renal disease.[18]

It is now recognized that patients with significant proteinuria may experience a rapid decline of GFR. In both patients with diabetic nephropathy and nondiabetic chronic renal disease, reducing proteinuria is associated with slowing of renal function loss and delaying the progression to end-stage renal failure.[27,28] The antiproteinuric effect of ACEIs is associated with a fall in filtration fraction, suggesting a reduction in intraglomerular pressure. However, an improvement of GBM permselectivity may be responsible for the long-term effect of ACEIs.[29] Such beneficial effects on proteinuria and reduction of glomerular hyperfiltration secondary to nephron loss are beyond what can be attributed by the drug's antihypertensive effects (see Chap. 43).[30,31]

Recent studies indicate that combined use of an ACEI and an ARB reduced the rate of renal function decline more than either treatment alone.[24,32] Such combination maximizes blockade of the renin-angiotensin system by counteracting the effects of angiotensin II produced by non-ACE pathways. In addition, with the blockade of the angiotensin II type 1 receptor, the angiotensin II produced by the non-ACE pathways may still act on the angiotensin II type 2 receptors, further facilitating vasodilatation.[33] Patients with IgA nephropathy seem to respond the best when they receive such combination therapy.[32] An angiotensin II receptor antagonist should therefore be added to the regimen for those patients who do not attain full and persistent remission of proteinuria with an ACEI alone.[44]

NSAIDs probably reduce proteinuria through prostaglandin E$_2$ inhibition, resulting in a reduction of intraglomerular pressure, a decrease in GFR, and also restoration of the barrier size-selectivity of the GBM.[17,29] Indomethacin and meclofenamate are the two NSAIDs that have been evaluated the most. Their antiproteinuric effect is comparable to those attained with ACEIs, and combined treatment with an ACEI results in additional proteinuria reduction.[34] However, adherence to a low-sodium diet or concurrent use of a diuretic is needed to maximize the antiproteinuric effect. Due to their potential for nephrotoxicity, especially in patients with poor renal function, long-term use of an NSAID for renoprotection is not preferred.[30]

Recently, cyclooxygenase-2 inhibitors have been shown to have proteinuria-lowering and renoprotective effects in animal models. If such beneficial effects are confirmed in humans, cyclooxygenase-2 inhibitors may become useful renoprotective agents for those patients whose low blood pressure preclude further use of drugs for ACE inhibition.[30]

HYPERLIPIDEMIA

An abnormal lipoprotein profile increases the risk of atherosclerosis and coronary heart disease in patients with nephrotic syndrome. It is therefore prudent to treat patients with persistent nephrotic syndrome and sustained dyslipidemia, especially those with high VLDL and LDL cholesterol levels in the presence of a normal or low HDL cholesterol level (see Chaps. 21 and 43). Therapy is especially needed for those with concurrent atherosclerotic cardiovascular disease, or with additional risk factors for atherosclerosis, such as smoking and hypertension.[14] Whether correction of lipoprotein abnormalities will slow the progression of renal disease as demonstrated in animal studies requires clinical confirmation.[14]

A low-fat diet is usually not sufficient to correct hyperlipoproteinemia.[9,17,35] Lipid-lowering agents are usually required. Probucol, bile acid resins, fibric acid derivatives, and hydroxymethylglutaryl coenzyme A (HMG-CoA) reductase inhibitors have been evaluated in patients with nephrotic syndrome.[14] HMG-CoA reductase inhibitors, also known as the statins such as lovastatin, pravastatin, simvastatin, and fluvastatin, are considered the treatment of choice.[9,14,17] In short-term studies, they reduce total plasma cholesterol concentration, LDL cholesterol, and total plasma triglyceride concentrations.[14] The increase in HDL cholesterol and/or decrease in atherogenic lipoprotein (a) is variable.[22] Meta-analysis showed that use of HMG-CoA reductase inhibitors resulted in the greatest and most consistent decrease in LDL cholesterol levels.[35] Recent experimental data reveal that the statins may modulate intracellular signaling systems that involve in cell proliferation, inflammation, and fibrogenic responses. As such, the statins may also have beneficial effects on the progression of renal disease.[36]

When ACEIs are used to reduce proteinuria, it is common to see an accompanying decrease in total plasma cholesterol and the lipoprotein (a) level.[26] Combined use of an ACEI with an HMG-CoA reductase inhibitor may therefore offer additional benefits in controlling nephrotic hyperlipidemia.

ANTICOAGULATION

Intravascular thrombosis is a serious and common complication of nephrotic syndrome, particularly in membranous nephropathy. Patients are at risk for developing renal vein thrombosis, pulmonary emboli, or other thromboembolic events. Although it is generally agreed that patients who have documented thromboembolic episodes should be anticoagulated with warfarin until remission of nephrotic syndrome, the use of prophylactic anticoagulation is controversial. A decision analysis study suggested that prophylactic anticoagulation is beneficial in patients with membranous nephropathy.[37] However, prospective controlled studies should be conducted to confirm these findings. Anticoagulation should also be considered in patients with increased risks for thrombosis, such as prolonged bedrest, surgery, episodes of dehydration, or use of high-dose intravenous steroids.[17] As an example, low-dose subcutaneous heparin may be given prophylactically for a limited duration in patients with severe nephrotic syndrome who are placed on bedrest. For patients with a history of

a thromboembolic episode, warfarin should be given after an initial course of standard or low-molecular-weight heparin, for as long as heavy proteinuria and hypoalbuminemia are present. The role of low-molecular-weight heparin in preventing thromboembolism is uncertain, but preliminary results are encouraging.[38]

DISEASE PROGRESSION AND TREATMENT CONSIDERATIONS

The course and prognosis of the different glomerular diseases are extremely variable and depend on the underlying etiology. In glomerular diseases with a secondary cause, such as poststreptococcal glomerulonephritis, after the initiating factor is removed, the prognosis of the renal disease is often good. In contrast, the rates of renal function deterioration among the primary glomerulonephritides vary according to the form of glomerulonephritis. The majority of patients with minimal-change disease, IgA nephropathy, and membranous nephropathy have a fairly good prognosis. However, those with focal segmental glomerulosclerosis who are resistant to therapy, as well as those with rapidly progressive glomerulonephritis who are untreated, are likely to experience rapid loss of renal function. In some instances, half of the renal function may be lost within a 3-month period. Certain glomerulonephritides, such as minimal-change nephropathy, are very responsive to treatment. In contrast, for some other types of glomerulonephritis, such as membranous proliferative glomerulonephritis, consistently effective therapy has yet to be found.

Because of the variable courses exhibited by the different glomerulonephritides, specific treatment approaches have been developed for each disease. The natural history of the glomerulonephritis has to be well delineated before a promising regimen can be evaluated, from both therapeutic and economic perspectives. Otherwise patients will be exposed to unnecessary treatment-related toxicities if they have a type of glomerulonephritis that is likely to undergo spontaneous remission. The potential therapeutic benefits of treatment regimens should always be weighed against the risks to which the patients are being exposed. It is therefore imperative to identify patients who are most likely to benefit from treatment, especially those who have other risk factors that may contribute to the deterioration of their renal function. In those instances in which satisfactory regimens are not available to treat the primary disease, appropriate supportive measures should be employed. Optimization of systemic and glomerular pressure, reducing proteinuria, and possibly controlling hyperlipidemia may all improve the long-term outcome as well as the quality of life of these patients.

TREATMENT MONITORING

Patients should be monitored closely for therapeutic response as well as the development of treatment-related toxicities. While the rate of renal function deterioration is an important indicator of the long-term success of treatment, resolution of nephrotic and nephritic signs and symptoms associated with the glomerulopathies are important short-term therapeutic targets.

Serum creatinine concentration as well as creatinine clearance should be evaluated prior to and during treatment; 24-hour urine outflow should be collected to determine the extent of proteinuria. Alternatively, the daily urine protein excretion may be estimated by the urinary total protein:creatinine concentration ratio. After establishing the correlation between the 24-hour urinary protein excretion and the protein:creatinine ratio, single random urine specimens may be used in place of a 24-hour urine collection. Blood pressure should be monitored periodically to assess the need for and also the adequacy of antihypertensive therapy. The pressures should also be evaluated in conjunction with clinical signs and symptoms of edema and fluid overload to gauge the need for volume control as well as diuretic use. For patients with nephrotic syndrome, serum lipid concentrations should be monitored. If the patient has hematuria, urinalysis and a complete blood count should be obtained. The clinician should also be aware of the patient's appetite and energy level, because these are indicators of the patient's overall state of well-being. At times, renal biopsy is needed to assess response to treatment and disease progression, to determine future treatment strategy, and to confirm the initial diagnosis.

Patients receiving cytotoxic drug treatment should be evaluated for drug-related toxicities every week during the initial treatment period. After 1 month of treatment, the frequency of monitoring may be reduced. When the patient is on long-term steroid treatment, monthly visits are often required for assessment of both efficacy and toxicities. If a favorable response is obtained after a course of treatment, the patient may be evaluated every 3 to 4 months. The patient's renal function, proteinuria, urinalysis, blood pressure, lipid profile,

and the overall state of health should be assessed during these regular follow-up visits.

OUTCOME AND ECONOMIC EVALUATION

Prospective, randomized, controlled comparative trials need to be conducted in a sizable patient population before the efficacy and economic implications of a new regimen can be established. This type of large-scale study is potentially feasible for the more common forms of glomerulonephritis, such as minimal-change disease, IgA nephropathy, and membranous nephropathy. In contrast, prospective controlled trials are difficult to conduct for the relatively uncommon glomerulonephritides such as membranous proliferative glomerulonephritis. After defining the natural history and the optimal drug regimen for each glomerulonephritis, in conjunction with the incidence of drug-induced complications, the economic implications of the individual treatment approach can be assessed. However, the optimal approaches for treating most types of glomerulonephritis have not been identified and the economic implications of the individual treatment regimens have yet to be established.

PATHOPHYSIOLOGY AND PHARMACOTHERAPY OF INDIVIDUAL GLOMERULOPATHIES

MINIMAL-CHANGE NEPHROPATHY

Minimal-change nephropathy (also termed minimal-change disease) is commonly found in children between 3 months and 6 years of age. It is one of the most common chronic diseases in childhood. In children between 1 and 4 years of age, minimal-change disease accounts for more than 90% of all cases of nephrotic syndrome. The percentage drops gradually to less than 50% after age 10 years, and only accounts for 10% to 15% of all cases of idiopathic nephrotic syndrome in adults. Secondary causes of minimal-change nephropathy have been reported with NSAIDs, lymphoproliferative disorders, lupus, and interferon-β treatment of malignant melanoma. They are responsible for up to 13% of all cases of minimal-change nephropathy in adults.

PATHOPHYSIOLOGY

Minimal-change disease is also known as "nil" disease, primarily because of the absence of definitive pathologic changes observed under light and immunofluorescence microscopy. The characteristic lesion in patients with minimal-change disease, as visualized under electron microscopy, is the spreading and fusion of the foot processes of epithelial cells over an unchanged GBM. *Lipoid nephrosis* is another term that has been used to describe this type of glomerular disease because lipids, as well as renal tubular cells, are found in the urine.

The pathogenesis of minimal-change disease is still unknown. Altered cell-mediated immunologic response, specifically T-cell dysfunction or changes in the T-cell subpopulations, is suspected to be responsible. The activated lymphocytes are thought to secrete lymphokines that reduce the production of anions in the GBM. The permeability of the GBM to plasma albumin is therefore increased through a reduction of electrostatic repulsion. The loss of anionic charges also results in fusion of the foot processes of the epithelial cells. Other conditions that involve T-cell abnormalities, such as Hodgkin's disease, T-cell lymphoma, and nephritis induced by NSAIDs, are also associated with minimal-change disease.

CLINICAL PRESENTATION

Most patients present initially with edema, frequently acute in onset, following a nonspecific upper respiratory tract infection, allergic reaction, or vaccinations, which might have activated the T lymphocytes. Nephrotic syndrome with massive proteinuria (substantially more than 40 mg/m^2 per hour for children and 3 g/day for adults), edema, hypoalbuminemia, and hyperlipidemia is common. The patient's weight may be increased dramatically because of sodium and fluid retention. Nephrotic features such as gross hematuria are uncommon. However, microscopic hematuria may be seen in up to 20% to 25% of patients. Hypertension and decreased renal function are uncommon in children but are more common in older adults.[39] In some patients, volume depletion may result in mild to moderate azotemia.

▶ TREATMENT: Minimal-Change Nephropathy

▦ PHARMACOLOGIC THERAPY

▦ STEROIDS

◀5 Minimal-change disease is the most responsive to initial treatment with corticosteroids. In children, steroid therapy is expected to reduce proteinuria in about 90% of the patients. The 10-year renal survival is greater than 95%.[40] Because of the excellent response to initial therapy with steroids and the prevalence of this

glomerular disease in children, reduction of proteinuria secondary to steroid treatment is considered diagnostic for minimal-change disease without the need for biopsy. In the International Study of Kidney Disease in Children, remission was induced, as evidenced by diuresis, loss of edema, and resolution of proteinuria, within 8 weeks of therapy in more than 93% of the 363 children.[41] Prednisone was administered at a dose of 60 mg/m^2 per day, with a maximum of 80 to 100 mg daily, in divided doses during the first 4 weeks. The dose was then reduced to 40 mg/m^2 per day, or a maximum of 60 mg daily, in divided doses for

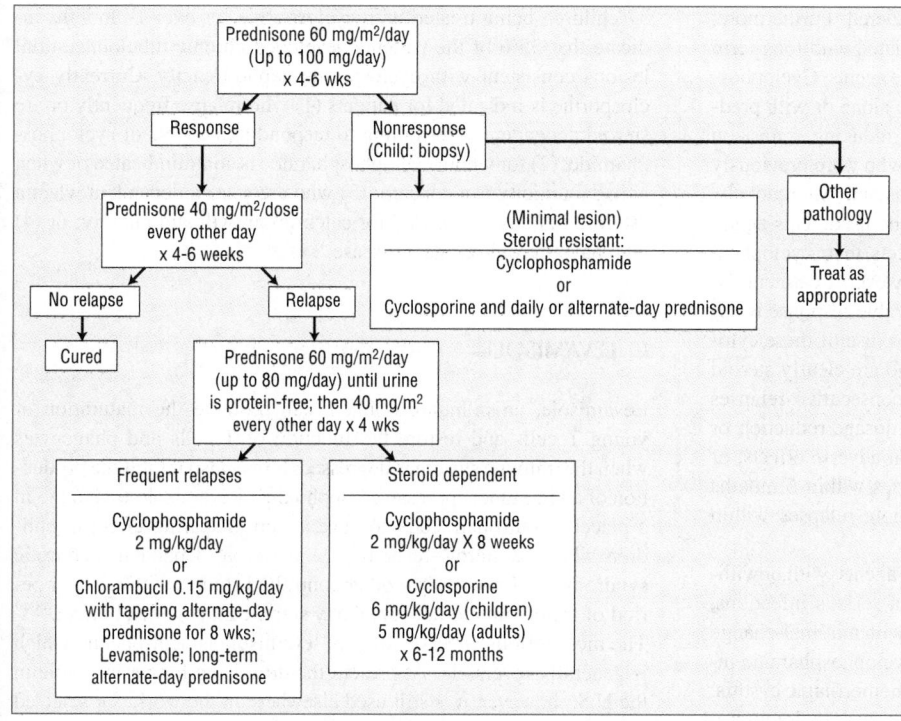

FIGURE 47–7. Treatment algorithm for minimal-change nephropathy. (Modified from Bargman.[42])

3 consecutive days every 7 days for another 4 weeks. An alternate-day dosage regimen can be used instead in the second 4 weeks, after which the prednisone dosage is tapered over several months (Fig. 47–7).[40,42] Single daily doses of prednisone, instead of multiple daily doses, may result in faster and more sustained response with less-frequent and less-severe side effects.[40] Proteinuria will disappear in 50% of patients after 1 week and in 90% of patients after 4 weeks of treatment. Studies conducted to evaluate the effectiveness of longer and shorter courses of steroid therapy for initial treatment, as well as recurrences,[42] showed that longer therapy (6 weeks of daily prednisone followed by 6 weeks of alternate-day treatment) results in lower incidence of relapse (36%) than both standard-course (4 weeks; 61%) and short-course (3 weeks; 81%) therapy. However, the cumulative doses of steroid received for the initial treatment and subsequent relapses during the entire follow-up period were no different between the long and standard courses. As a result, long-course therapy is commonly used for the initial episode, followed by short-course treatment for relapses.[43]

For adults, the dose of prednisone is 1 mg/kg per day during the initial 4 weeks with a reduction to 0.75 mg/kg per day every other day for the next 4 weeks. Proteinuria will disappear in 50% to 60% of patients after 8 weeks of treatment, and complete remission will be attained in 80% of patients after 28 weeks of therapy.[39] In some patients, 16 weeks of therapy may be needed before remission is induced.[39,41] Use of lower doses of steroids may increase relapse rate and alternate-day high-dose steroid therapy may reduce the rate of total remission.

■ Relapse

As many as 75% to 85% of the patients who respond to initial steroid therapy (steroid sensitive) will experience a relapse of proteinuria, mostly within 6 to 12 months after disease onset. However, some patients may not have the first relapse until 24 to 30 months later. The risk of relapse is affected by the duration of initial steroid therapy.[17,42]

Children who were asymptomatic with proteinuria diagnosed on a urinary screening program tend to have less frequent relapses and a more favorable clinical course.[44] In those who relapse, 50% to 65% may have steroid-responsive relapse episodes over the subsequent 3- to 5-year period. The dose and duration of steroid treatment for the relapse do not influence the subsequent rate of relapse.[17,42] The current regimen for relapse consists of 60 mg/m^2 per day, up to 80 mg/day of prednisone, until the urine is free of protein for 3 days. Four weeks of alternate-day prednisone at 40 mg/m^2 per dose will then be used.[42] Giving the initial daily doses of prednisone for 4 weeks, instead of until the urine is clear of protein may induce a more prolonged remission; however, the cumulative dose of prednisone will be doubled. Because most patients will relapse soon, it is preferred to treat until the urine is free of protein for 3 days and then proceed with the tapering regimen as described earlier.[42]

■ Frequent Relapse

About 10% to 20% of children experience three or four relapses that are responsive to steroid. However, half of these patients will relapse frequently and become steroid dependent, requiring continuous low-dose alternate-day prednisone to maintain an extended relapse-free period.[42] A small number of patients eventually develop resistance to steroids, and a biopsy done at that time often reveals another pathology such as focal segmental glomerulosclerosis. It is controversial whether minimal-change disease progresses into focal segmental glomerulosclerosis or whether the glomerulosclerosis that was present at the time of initial diagnosis was inadvertently diagnosed as minimal-change nephropathy because of tissue-sampling error during the renal biopsy.

■ CYTOTOXIC AGENTS

For patients who are steroid resistant, as well as for those patients who require large doses of steroids to sustain remission (steroid dependent), alternative therapy should be considered. Furthermore, in pediatric patients the growth inhibition associated with long-term steroid use often necessitates the use of alternative agents. Cyclophosphamide at 2 mg/kg per day for 12 weeks given alone or with prednisone (50 to 75 mg/m^2) is very effective in inducing remission and restoring steroid responsiveness in patients who were previously steroid dependent and then became steroid resistant. Alternatively, chlorambucil at 0.1 to 0.2 mg/kg per day may be used. This agent, however, is associated with more adverse effects than cyclophosphamide. Azathioprine has also been used; however, treatment for 6 to 12 months is often needed before any favorable response is apparent. Because of the risk for adverse reactions, use of these cytotoxic agents should be reserved for patients who are clearly steroid resistant, or who are steroid dependent (two consecutive relapses during therapy or relapse within 14 days after dosage reduction or termination of steroid treatment) with significant adverse effects; or for those patients who have two or more relapses within 6 months after the first episode, or who had three or more relapses within 12 months.[17]

The immunosuppressive effect of cytotoxic agents, with or without the concurrent use of steroids, can result in serious infections, which are the primary cause of death in patients with minimal-change nephropathy. Other toxicities associated with cyclophosphamide include gonadal fibrosis, which results in sterility, hemorrhagic cystitis, alopecia, and a potential to develop malignancy in those on long-term treatment. Patients on chronic steroid therapy often develop growth retardation, osteoporosis, obesity, and cataracts.[42]

■ CYCLOSPORINE

Cyclosporine has been used in adult and pediatric patients. The drug decreases lymphokine production by activated T lymphocytes and thereby reduces proteinuria by reversing the lymphokine-induced alterations in the anionic charge and permeability of the GBM to albumin. Cyclosporine can also reduce proteinuria by improving the permselectivity of the GBM.

In patients with steroid-sensitive or steroid-dependent minimal-change disease, cyclosporine induces remission in 80% to 85% of patients. However, the disease-free period is not often sustained, and relapse, which is usually not as responsive to cyclosporine retreatment, may occur as soon as the drug is tapered or discontinued.[45] The rate of relapse is also reduced when the dose tapering is gradual or when the cyclosporine treatment period is prolonged.[46] Although only 10% to 20% of patients who have steroid-resistant disease respond to cyclosporine, combination treatment with low-dose steroid may increase the effectiveness.[45] A 2-month trial treatment with cyclosporine may therefore be warranted in steroid-resistant patients. The steroid-sparing effect of cyclosporine is also useful in steroid-dependent patients, especially those who have experienced significant adverse effects.

The usual starting daily dose of cyclosporine for remission induction is 5 mg/kg for adults and 100 to 150 mg/m^2 for children. Similar dosages are used to maintain remission long term. The need to monitor cyclosporine blood concentrations is controversial. No correlation has been found between the severity of the cyclosporine-induced tubulointerstitial lesions and mean dose or trough drug concentration. The incidence of these lesions increases with the duration of treatment and cyclosporine should therefore not be given for more than 4 months in the absence of any beneficial effect.[45] Results from a recent study of

37 children being treated with cyclosporine for over 18 months indicate that 35% of the patients developed chronic tubulointerstitial lesions consistent with cyclosporine nephrotoxicity. Currently cyclosporine is indicated for patients (1) who relapse frequently or are steroid dependent, after failing to respond to a course of cyclophosphamide; (2) for whom cyclophosphamide is contraindicated or when gonadal toxicity is a concern; (3) who are steroid dependent when a "steroid holiday" is needed for catch-up growth and puberty; or (4) who have steroid-resistant disease.[42]

■ LEVAMISOLE

Levamisole, an immunostimulant, can promote the maturation of young T cells and restore the function of T cells and phagocytes when the immune system is depressed. It may also inhibit the production of an immunosuppressive lymphokine. Levamisole was found in a placebo-controlled study to have a steroid-sparing effect in children who had steroid-responsive and steroid-dependent nephrotic syndrome.[47] However, two other controlled studies with a longer period of follow-up did not reveal any significant beneficial effect.[48,49] The most serious adverse effect of levamisole is neutropenia, which is generally reversible. At present the drug is no longer available in the U.S.; however, it is still used elsewhere in the world for selected steroid-dependent patients.

■ MYCOPHENOLATE MOFETIL

Mycophenolate mofetil is an immunosuppressant that can suppress lymphocyte proliferation. It inhibits inosine monophosphate dehydrogenase, which is pivotal in de novo purine synthesis in lymphocytes. Mycophenolate mofetil, 1 to 3 g/day, has been reported to have steroid-sparing effects in patients with minimal-change disease as well as other forms of glomerulonephritis.[50,51]

■ THERAPEUTIC OUTCOMES

The long-term prognosis of most patients with minimal-change disease is good. The majority of pediatric patients will not experience any relapse of the disease 10 years after the initial onset, and most will be free of the proteinuria after puberty. In adults, an 85% to 90% survival rate is seen 10 years after disease onset. Although this condition may spontaneously remit in up to 70% of untreated adults, life-threatening complications may be associated with untreated nephrotic syndrome. Development of renal failure is uncommon in both adult and pediatric patients. Significant deterioration of renal function is observed only in those patients who are steroid resistant or steroid dependent. Because of the overall favorable outcome of the disease and the relatively uncommon progression into chronic renal failure, aggressive use of cytotoxic agents is not indicated even in most patients with frequent relapses. Toxicities associated with aggressive therapy do not justify the need to induce remission in those patients who fail to respond to steroids and the nonaggressive use of cytotoxic agents. Symptomatic therapy with diuretics to control edema, in conjunction with a low-salt diet and albumin infusion as needed for acute development of anasarca, is often a more rewarding therapeutic approach. NSAIDs and ACEIs may also be used to reduce the proteinuria.

FOCAL SEGMENTAL GLOMERULOSCLEROSIS

Focal segmental glomerulosclerosis (FSGS) is a histologic lesion that can be idiopathic (primary) or secondary to a variety of causes. Conditions such as sickle cell disease, cyanotic congenital heart disease, and morbid obesity can induce hemodynamic stress on an initially normal nephron population and result in FSGS.[52] Severe glomerular injury can also be seen in patients with nephropathy associated with heroin abuse, human immunodeficiency virus (HIV) infection and genetic mutations involving the podocin and WT1 genes.[52,53] The primary and secondary sclerotic lesions may be morphologically similar, but they represent diseases with different courses and responses to therapy.

PATHOPHYSIOLOGY

Sclerotic lesions are characteristically found in some of the glomeruli (focal) and usually involve only a portion of the glomeruli (segmental).[54] Similar to minimal-change disease, fusion of foot processes is commonly seen in those glomeruli that are not sclerotic. It is thought that both minimal-change disease and FSGS share similar pathogenetic mechanisms, with FSGS resulting in severe injury to the glomerular epithelial cells. During the early stage of FSGS, only a small number of glomeruli may have the segmental sclerotic lesion and the disease may be confined to the juxtamedullary region. If an inadequate number of glomeruli are sampled during renal biopsy, the diagnosis of FSGS may be missed, or the patient may be thought to have minimal-change disease. Resistance to steroid therapy may thus be one of the first clues that the patient indeed has FSGS rather than minimal-change disease. Alternatively, a patient may have the steroid-sensitive minimal-change disease initially, which subsequently progresses to steroid-resistant FSGS. In those patients who have cellular lesions, such as collapse of glomerular capillaries, or hypertrophy and hyperplasia of surrounding glomeruli epithelial cells, the risk for developing renal failure is increased.[55]

CLINICAL PRESENTATION

FSGS accounts for less than 15% of the cases of idiopathic nephrotic syndrome in children and about 15% to 20% in adults; however, it may account for 36% to 80% of the cases in African-Americans.[53] Almost all the patients present with proteinuria, and many of them have all the features of nephrotic syndrome.[56] The proteinuria is nonselective, containing albumin and other higher-molecular-weight proteins, and is usually less severe when compared to patients who have minimal-change disease. Hypertension, microscopic hematuria, and renal dysfunction may be seen in up to half of the patients. Reduced renal function becomes more prevalent as the disease progresses.

The presenting clinical features in nephrotic adults with minimal-change nephropathy can be indistinguishable from that of FSGS, and renal biopsy is therefore critical in the treatment of adults with nephrotic syndrome. FSGS is two to four times more common in black patients than in white patients. They tend to present with proteinuria more frequently in the nephrotic range and are more likely to experience a rapid decline in renal function.

► TREATMENT: Focal Segmental Glomerulosclerosis

PHARMACOLOGIC THERAPY

STEROIDS

Because the pathophysiology of primary FSGS is unknown, it is impossible to direct pharmacologic treatment against any specific pathologic processes. Furthermore, the treatment of FSGS remains controversial because of the lack of data from randomized, prospective, controlled trials. A course of prednisone (1 to 2 mg/kg per day) with tapering after 3 to 4 months of treatment is first used for nephrotic patients.[53,54] Urinary protein excretion and serum albumin concentration should be monitored to assess efficacy. The median time to induce complete remission is 3 months, although 5 to 9 months may be needed in some patients.[53] Of all patients 30% to 40% can be expected to attain complete remission; however, fewer patients will respond with regimens of shorter duration.[53] In general, treatment should be continued for 6 months before the patient is considered steroid resistant.[46,57]

For patients who relapse after an adequate response to the initial treatment, a second course of steroids is generally sufficient.[53] However, for those who relapse frequently, cytotoxic agents or cyclosporine are indicated.

The relatively favorable prognosis of patients who are not nephrotic does not support the use of steroids or other immunosuppressive agents. However, close follow-up and good blood pressure control with ACEIs are necessary to minimize disease progression.[54]

CYTOTOXIC AGENTS

Cytotoxic agents such as cyclophosphamide, chlorambucil, and azathioprine historically have been ineffective in the treatment of FSGS. However, Ponticelli and associates recently reported that treatment with the immunosuppressive agents chlorambucil and cyclophosphamide for more than 1 year was successful in inducing remission in those patients receiving their first treatment, as well as in those patients who did not respond initially.[58] Cyclophosphamide (2 mg/kg per day) or chlorambucil (0.1 to 0.2 mg/kg per day), when used with steroids, results in remission in more than 70% of patients.[53] The rate of relapse is also reduced. When combined with pulse methylprednisolone, these alkylating agents were reported in some trials to be effective in inducing remission in steroid-resistant patients.[43]

CYCLOSPORINE

Short-term cyclosporine therapy reduces proteinuria in many steroid-responsive patients and in some patients who are resistant to corticosteroid and cytotoxic agents.[56,57] However, more than 75% of the patients have relapse of proteinuria occurring within 2 months of tapering or drug discontinuation.[56] A prolonged period of treatment with slow tapering may result in longer periods of remission.[46] Long-term cyclosporine therapy was evaluated in 21 black and Hispanic children (who tend to have more rapid renal function deterioration than do white children) who had steroid-resistant FSGS.[59] This aggressive regimen (4 to 20 mg/kg per day for 3 to 97 months) reduced proteinuria from 6.2 to 2 g/day and the percentage of patients who developed ESKD.[59] Although histologic evidence of cyclosporine nephrotoxicity was not seen in this study, the drug was found by others to be more nephrotoxic in steroid-resistant than in steroid-responsive disease.[43] When cyclosporine was combined with low-dose prednisone for 26 weeks, the regimen was found to induce partial or complete remission of proteinuria in 70% of steroid-resistant patients. Renal function was also better preserved than treatment with steroids alone. However, the relapse rate was still high upon treatment discontinuation.[60] In a recent study, once-daily low-dose cyclosporine (mean, 4.6 mg/kg per day) was effective in inducing total and partial remission in 76% of children with minimal side effects.[61]

■ MYCOPHENOLATE MOFETIL

Mycophenolate mofetil, 1 to 3 g daily, has been used effectively in a small number of patients to reduce proteinuria and induce remission.[50] Further studies are needed to further define its role among the various treatment options.

■ SYMPTOMATIC THERAPY

Because of the lack of a consistently effective regimen for primary FSGS, many patients with mild disease are treated conservatively for symptomatic control. ACEIs and ARBs are effective in reducing proteinuria and in stabilizing renal function in patients with primary or secondary FSGS.[53] They should be used in all patients with primary glomerular diseases. The dilation of efferent arterioles by these agents reduces intraglomerular pressure, which may diminish the potential effect of glomerular hypertension on the development of FSGS.[32] The driving force for proteinuria may also be reduced without necessarily correcting the primary defect in glomerular wall permselectivity.[52] The NSAID meclofenamate is effective in reducing proteinuria in patients with steroid-resistant FSGS.[33] These favorable results have, however, not been confirmed in studies using a larger number of patients. Thus their role in the overall scheme of therapy remains to be defined. For patients with more severe disease, corticosteroids with or without immunosuppressive agents should be considered. Treatment should not be continued for more than 3 to 4 months unless the patient experiences a remission. In this case, therapy may be continued for 12 to 24 months to maintain the therapeutic response.

■ THERAPEUTIC OUTCOMES

Patients with primary FSGS are at risk for developing ESKD. For the 30% to 50% of adults and children who had attained complete remission, ESKD develops in about 10% or less of these patients at 10 years.[56,61] For those patients who are resistant to therapy, the rate of renal function deterioration to ESKD may be rapid, within 1 year, or slow, over as long as 10 to 20 years. About 50% of them develop ESKD in 10 years.[61] Those patients with severe proteinuria (> 10 to 15 g/day), high serum creatinine concentration at diagnosis, initial steroid resistance, or interstitial fibrosis on renal biopsy are likely to have a more rapid decline in renal function.[54] African-American patients may also have a higher risk. Kidney transplantation is often indicated for those patients who develop ESKD; however, FSGS has recurred in 20% to 50% of the renal allografts soon after transplantation. Children and those with severe disease or rapid progression to ESKD prior to transplantation are more likely to experience a recurrence. The proteinuria may reappear within hours after transplantation and graft failure may occur in one-third to one-half of the patients. The median time to recurrence was reported to be 14 days in one study. Although cyclosporine is ineffective in preventing the recurrence of nephrotic syndrome after transplantation, a high dose of the agent (up to 35 mg/kg per day) induces a remission of the recurrent disease. ACEIs and plasmapheresis are also used to prolong graft survival. The effectiveness of these therapies and the rapid recurrence of the disease in the transplanted kidney substantiate the possibility that a circulating humoral mediator is responsible for the nephropathy.

MEMBRANOUS NEPHROPATHY

Membranous nephropathy is the most common disorder responsible for idiopathic nephrotic syndrome in adults, accounting for about 20% to 25% of cases.[62] It is also a frequent cause of renal failure secondary to glomerulonephritis. The hallmark histologic features of membranous nephropathy are glomerular capillary wall thickening with subepithelial deposits under light and electron microscopy. Most cases are idiopathic, but about 25% of adults and 80% of children have secondary causes.[62,63] In the United States, the most common etiologies are autoimmune diseases (e.g., lupus), infection (e.g., hepatitis B), syphilis, neoplasm (e.g., carcinoma of the lung, breast, gastrointestinal tract, or kidney), and medications (e.g., organic gold, penicillamine, mercury, or captopril). Malaria and schistosomiasis are common causes in other parts of the world. De novo membranous nephropathy can also occur in the allografts of renal transplant patients. Because the response to therapy as well as the prognosis for idiopathic and secondary membranous nephropathy are different, it is important to identify any potential underlying causes for the nephropathy prior to treatment. Although this glomerular disease can occur at any age, the peak incidence is between 30 and 50 years and is especially likely in patients over 50 years old who present with nephrotic syndrome.[62]

PATHOPHYSIOLOGY

Examination of kidney tissue under light microscopy reveals normal mesangium and normocellularity. The glomerular capillary wall may be thickened in well-developed lesions. In the advanced stage, the capillary wall is markedly thickened and intramembranous deposits are found. Progressive changes in capillary lumen patency parallel those in the GBM, resulting in glomerulosclerosis with capillary collapse and tubular atrophy in end-stage membranous nephropathy. Immunofluorescence microscopy shows strong capillary wall staining of IgG and C3 on the epithelial side of the basement membrane. Antibody-mediated immune injury appears to be the main pathogenetic mechanism. The immune complex can be formed in situ or deposited from circulating immune complexes.

CLINICAL PRESENTATION

Most patients with membranous nephropathy present with heavy proteinuria exceeding 3.5 g/day. Those excreting large amounts of IgG and α_1-microglobulin, indicating more significant tubulointerstitial damage, have a lower remission rate and are more likely to progress towards renal failure.[64]

The signs and symptoms are usually insidious in onset and may consist of anorexia, malaise, edema, anasarca, or ascites, and pericardial and pleural effusions may also be present. As a result of a hypercoagulable state, pulmonary embolism may develop, but rarely results in death.[64] The incidence of renal vein thrombosis varies from 5% to 62%,[63,64] and membranous nephropathy should be suspected when there is a sudden onset of hematuria; loin pain; pulmonary embolus; fluctuating or worsening proteinuria or glomerular filtration rate; renal tubular acidosis; or an increase in leg edema. Hypertension is found in about 30% of patients and is more common in the presence of renal insufficiency or until the disease is advanced.

In addition to heavy proteinuria, urinalysis often reveals lipiduria and oval fat bodies. Microhematuria is seen in fewer than 25% of patients, and gross hematuria and red cell casts are rare. In idiopathic membranous nephropathy, the serum complement concentrations are normal. Low levels of complement should alert one to search for secondary causes, such as lupus, hepatitis B infection, or an alternative diagnosis. Similarly, antinuclear antibodies, anti-DNA antibodies, rheumatoid factor, hepatitis B serologies, and serum cryoglobulins are generally negative in idiopathic membranous nephropathy. Occult malignancy has been found in as many as 10% of elderly patients with membranous nephropathy.

The natural course of idiopathic membranous nephropathy is variable. About 25% of patients experience spontaneous remission of the disease over a mean of 5.5 years.[63] Less than 10% of the nonnephrotic patients and about one-third to one-half of the nephrotic patients will progress to end-stage renal failure over 10 to 15 years.[62] Some other patients have various degrees of renal insufficiency and persistent proteinuria. Heavy proteinuria (>10 g/day); male gender; elevated serum creatinine concentration at the time of presentation; poorly controlled hypertension; advanced age at onset of disease; non-Asian race; certain human leukocyte antigen phenotypes; and tubulointerstitial fibrosis on initial renal biopsy are associated with progressive renal disease.[62,63] Overall, patients with idiopathic membranous nephropathy have a relatively benign course. The mean 10-year survival is about 70%. Those who present with persistent nonnephrotic proteinuria seldom develop renal insufficiency and have a normal life expectancy. Fewer than 10% of patients develop a remitting and relapsing course.[63] The prognosis for secondary membranous nephropathy depends on the underlying cause. Remission occurs when the infection resolves or when the causative medication is withdrawn.

▶ TREATMENT: Membranous Nephropathy

The treatment of idiopathic membranous nephropathy is controversial and ranges from supportive therapy to immunosuppression with steroids alone, or in combination with alkylating agents. Conservative management of membranous nephropathy includes the control of edema with salt restriction and diuretics[11] and reduction of proteinuria with protein restriction and ACEIs (Fig. 47–8).[65] Management of hypertension and hyperlipidemia is required for most patients, whereas prophylactic anticoagulation, despite having benefits shown to outweigh the risks, is usually given only for patients with renal vein thrombosis or documented pulmonary embolus.[37,63]

CLINICAL CONTROVERSY

The optimal treatment for membranous nephropathy is controversial since there is no consistently effective drug regimen.

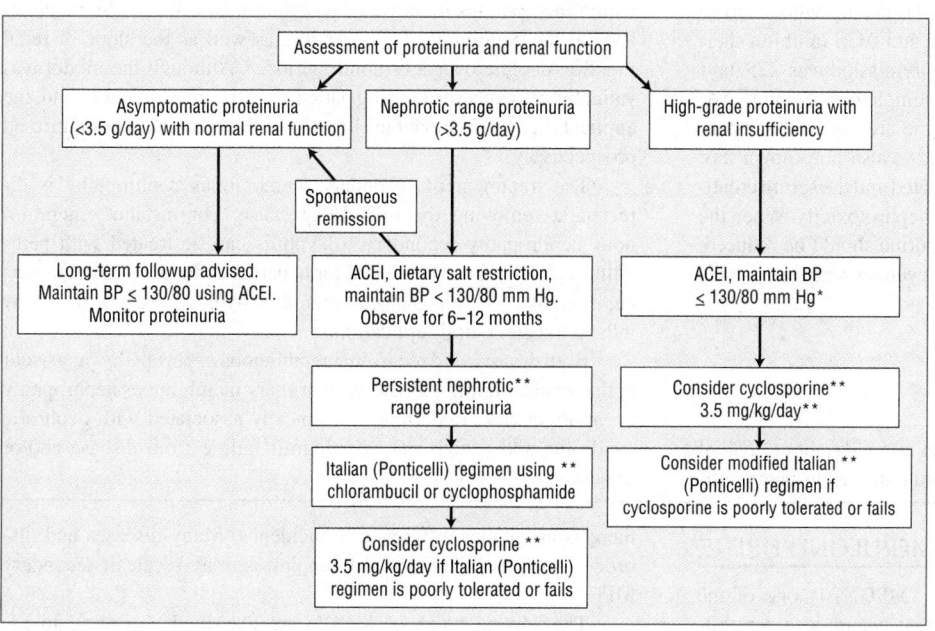

FIGURE 47–8. Treatment algorithm for idiopathic membranous nephropathy. Patients may change from one category to another during the course of follow-up. *, supported by evidence from controlled trials; ACEI, angiotensin-converting enzyme inhibitor; **, introduction of risk reduction strategies for both secondary effects of disease and adverse effects of immunotherapy. (Modified from Geddes et al.[63])

PHARMACOLOGIC THERAPY

STEROIDS

Remission of proteinuria, whether spontaneously or treatment related, may confer a good prognosis. Corticosteroids alone were ineffective in increasing the remission rate of proteinuria in all controlled trials and in preventing progression in all but one study.[63] The result of a meta-analysis also confirmed the lack of efficacy of steroids alone.

CYTOTOXIC AGENTS

Cytotoxic agents, when used in conjunction with corticosteroids, are effective in increasing the remission rate of nephrotic syndrome and reducing the frequency of ESKD at 10 years.[63,66] Ponticelli and colleagues devised such a regimen by combining intravenous methylprednisolone (1 g) for 3 days followed by oral methylprednisolone (0.4 mg/kg) for the subsequent 27 days of months 1, 3, and 5. Oral chlorambucil (0.2 mg/kg) is to be given daily in months 2, 4, and 6.[66] They also substituted cyclophosphamide (2.5 mg/kg per day) for chlorambucil, which resulted in similar rates of proteinuria remission and relapse, but with fewer serious side effects in those who received cyclophosphamide.[67]

A meta-analysis was conducted to evaluate the data from prospective trials using steroids and cytotoxic agents. The cytotoxic agents, but not steroids, were found to be effective in reducing nephrotic-range proteinuria as well as increasing the likelihood of complete or partial remission.[68]

CYCLOSPORINE

For patients with severe nephrotic syndrome who did not respond to cytotoxic therapy, cyclosporine may offer some benefits; however, the risk for cyclosporine nephrotoxicity is of concern, especially during long-term therapy. A 12-month course of cyclosporine (mean dose of 3.8 mg/kg per day) was found to reduce proteinuria as well as the rate of renal deterioration.[69] In a recent study of 41 patients who received cyclosporine, many with concurrent steroid and ACE inhibitor therapy, the median treatment time to complete remission was 225 days among the 34% of patients who attained complete remission.[70] At present, the beneficial effects of cyclosporine are not well substantiated and the optimal duration of treatment is also not known. For many patients, hypertension may be exacerbated and the serum creatinine concentration may be increased due to nephrotoxicity. When the renal function declines, the dose of cyclosporine should be reduced. In addition, proteinuria may recur when the cyclosporine treatment is stopped.

THERAPEUTIC OUTCOMES

Because spontaneous remission is common and only about 25% of patients with new-onset idiopathic membranous nephropathy ulti-

mately develop ESKD in 20 to 30 years, it is prudent not to aggressively treat all patients at the onset of the disease.[71] Patients who have a low likelihood for renal disease progression can be managed with observation and symptomatic therapy. Normalizing the blood pressure and reducing proteinuria with ACEIs is reasonable because both hypertension and proteinuria are independent risk factors for the progression of renal failure.[63] Patients with low risk for renal disease progression include children 2 to 16 years of age, adult males with proteinuria less than 2 g/day, or adult females with proteinuria less than 5 g/day and normal renal function.[72] In contrast, patients who have a high risk of developing renal failure, including those with proteinuria greater than 10 g/day with or without impaired renal function, and patients with symptomatic nephrotic syndrome with a plasma albumin of less than 2 g/dL, should be aggressively treated to induce remission.[71] An alkylating agent such as chlorambucil or cyclophosphamide, combined with steroids[71,72] or the high-dose steroid regimen used in the study by Ponticelli,[72] can be given to induce remission after considering the benefits and risks of treatment.[17,72] Recently, mycophenolate mofetil and rituximab have been shown separately to be effective in treating a small number of patients.[50,73]

When a slightly modified version of the regimen by Ponticelli (methylprednisolone plus chlorambucil) was used in patients with renal insufficiency, improvement in renal function was reported in some small, uncontrolled studies.[63] However, more than half of the patients experienced significant myelosuppression secondary to chlorambucil. When cyclophosphamide was used with steroid, beneficial effects were observed in a small case series, but not in a randomized, controlled trial.[63–68,71–74] Although the therapeutic effects of cytotoxic agents for these patients have yet to be confirmed, patients with renal insufficiency are more susceptible to immunosuppression by cytotoxic agents. Cytotoxic therapy should thus be avoided when the serum creatinine concentration at diagnosis is greater than 3 mg/dL.[72] The dose of cytotoxic agents should also be reduced in patients with renal impairment to minimize side effects.

Because aggressive treatment is not warranted for patients with mild disease and the risk of immunosuppression by cytotoxic agents is high, there has been attempt to identify, early in the course of disease, patients at high risk for progressing to ESKD. A model to predict the probability of progression to renal insufficiency has been developed which incorporates the level of proteinuria and the creatinine clearance at the beginning of observation, as well as the slope of renal function decline over a 6-month period.[75] Although the model was validated retrospectively using patient data from Italy and Finland, the applicability of this model in clinical practice remains to be confirmed prospectively.

The treatment of secondary membranous nephropathy is directed at removing the underlying cause. For instance, membranous nephropathy secondary to syphilis can be treated with penicillin. α-Interferon is beneficial for hepatitis B–induced membranous nephropathy.[76] Corticosteroids should be avoided because they may induce transient viral replication.[77]

Both de novo and recurrent membranous nephropathy may occur in the renal allograft. Patients with primary membranous nephropathy are more at risk. Recurrence is typically associated with nephrotic syndrome and a high risk of allograft failure from disease and/or rejection.

MEMBRANOPROLIFERATIVE GLOMERULONEPHRITIS

Membranoproliferative glomerulonephritis (MPGN) is one of the least-common renal morphologic entities that occurs in older children and adults. Although whites are more frequently affected,

there is no gender difference in incidence. Many diseases and disorders, such as infections and neoplasms, may result in secondary MPGN.

The several types of MPGN are classified according to the pathologic features. Type I MPGN, also known as mesangiocapillary glomerulonephritis, is characterized by diffuse thickening of glomerular capillary walls and mesangial hypercellularity. Subendothelial dense deposits that frequently contain immunoglobulins and C3 of the complement system are responsible for the capillary wall thickening. Immune complexes are therefore presumed to have a major role in the pathogenesis of type I MPGN, which is the most common type of primary, idiopathic MPGN. Hepatitis C is the most common cause of type I MPGN; other secondary etiologies may include systemic immune-complex–mediated disease (lupus), chronic infection (HIV, infected ventriculoatrial shunt, endocarditis, and malaria), chronic liver disease (hepatitis B and cirrhosis), and malignancy (lymphoma and leukemia).[78]

Type II MPGN is also known as dense-deposit disease because of the presence of dense deposits of C3 within the glomerular basement membrane, which gives rise to a ribbon-like appearance. The deposit contains C3, but without immunoglobulins. Other variants of the disease include type III MPGN, which is seen rarely and consists of subendothelial and subepithelial deposits with lamination and disruption of the lamina densa of the GBM.[79]

Type I MPGN is a slowly progressive disease that accounts for 80% of all cases of MPGN, but only 5% to 15% of all cases of nephrotic syndrome seen in pediatric and adult patients. It occurs most frequently in patients between 5 and 30 years of age, and because remissions are rare, many patients eventually develop ESKD. The renal survival is 60% to 65% at 10 years, and the presence of nephrotic syndrome, interstitial disease, and hypertension are poor prognostic indicators.[80] Type II MPGN is a more aggressive disease that constitutes about 15% of all patients with MPGN. Only 20% of patients remain stable for more than a few years and the median time before the development of ESRD is 7 years. There is an impression that the incidence of idiopathic MPGN has declined recently worldwide.

Nephrotic syndrome is the most common presenting condition and some patients may also have a nephritic component (hematuria), hypertension, and renal insufficiency. Hypocomplementemia is commonly seen.

▶ TREATMENT: Membranoproliferative Glomerulonephritis

The efficacy of corticosteroids, cyclophosphamide, antiplatelet drugs, and anticoagulants has been evaluated in patients with MPGN. In children, prednisone 40 mg/m^2 given on alternate days is effective, when compared with placebo, in reducing the decline in GFR.[81] This observation was confirmed by other uncontrolled studies.[80] Prednisone should therefore be given for 6 to 12 months to children with MPGN, proteinuria (more than 3 g/day), and/or impaired renal function.[80] Other studies suggest that this regimen may also be beneficial in children with mild proteinuria.

While the effect of steroids has not been proven in adults, antiplatelet drugs, such as dipyridamole and aspirin, as well as warfarin, were found in randomized controlled trials to reduce proteinuria, but had no effect on GFR.[80] However, an increased incidence of bleeding was observed in the treatment groups.[82] Adult patients with idiopathic MPGN, heavy proteinuria, and/or impaired renal function should be given dipyridamole or aspirin. Unfortunately, no controlled study comparing the effect of steroids with antiplatelet agents is yet available.

Cyclophosphamide and azathioprine were found to have no beneficial effect. Cyclosporine was evaluated in a limited number of patients with MPGN with some beneficial effect; however, the trials were not controlled or randomized.[83] In addition, the risks for developing adverse effects were high. Figure 47–9 presents an algorithm for treatment and follow-up.

It is difficult to conduct large-scale controlled trials for MPGN because of the low incidence of the disease. Based on the available studies, many of the drugs evaluated do not have any consistent, beneficial effect on renal function and proteinuria. Renal transplantation is an alternative; however, the recurrence rate is close to 100% for type II MPGN and is about 20% to 30% for type I MPGN. Nonetheless, fewer than 10% of the transplanted patients have graft failure as a result of recurrence.

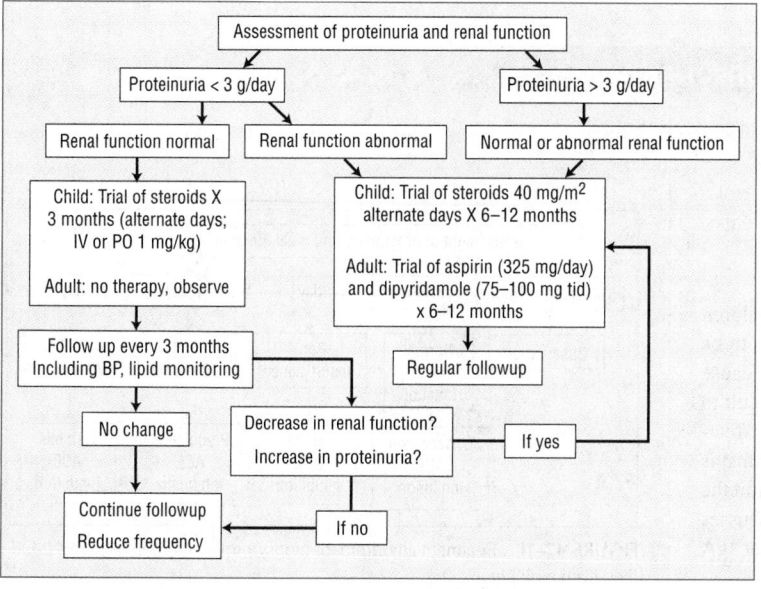

FIGURE 47–9. Treatment algorithm for membranoproliferative proliferative glomerulonephritis. (Modified from Levin.[80])

IMMUNOGLOBULIN A NEPHROPATHY

Immunoglobulin A nephropathy, also known as Berger's disease, was first described by Berger and Hinglais in France in 1968. It is now recognized to be the most common primary glomerulonephritis in the world and accounts for 10% of patients with ESRD in many countries. The prevalence among patients with glomerulonephritis or patients who had kidney biopsy varies around the world from as high as 50% in Japan and East Asia to 10% to 30% in Europe. In the United States, the overall prevalence is about 10% to 15%, but is as high as 35% among Native Americans living in New Mexico.[84] These differences in prevalence may reflect the more conservative diagnostic approach used for U.S. patients with isolated hematuria or mild proteinuria, who are generally not referred for kidney biopsy in the United States.

IgA nephropathy has a male predominance, and the disease is two to six times more common than in females, and it is more frequently seen in younger adults. It is uncommon in blacks both in the United States and in Africa.[84] IgA nephropathy was once thought to be a benign disease presenting with asymptomatic hematuria; however, it is now recognized that IgA nephropathy can present with any clinical syndrome associated with glomerular disease, and some of the patients will develop ESRD over variable periods of time.

PATHOPHYSIOLOGY

Primary IgA nephropathy an immune-complex–mediated disease in which IgA deposits and other pathologic lesions are found in kidney tissues. In contrast, Henoch-Schönlein purpura is a systemic disease that is believed to be closely linked to IgA nephropathy because they share similar immunohistologic features. Only the joints, skin, and gastrointestinal tract are affected in Henoch-Schönlein purpura. Mesangial deposition of IgA immune complex is also seen in patients with celiac disease and dermatitis herpetiformis, possibly due to an increased exposure to antigens. Patients with chronic liver disease may have IgA nephropathy because of reduced clearance of IgA immune complexes. Secondary IgA nephropathy may be present in patients with different connective tissue diseases, carcinomas, and HIV infection.

The diagnosis of IgA nephropathy can be established by immunofluorescence examination of the kidney biopsy. The hallmark feature is the dominance or codominance of IgA deposition in the mesangium. The IgA immune complex, composed of IgA antibody bound with an environmental antigen, such as a virus, bacteria, or food substances, is presumed to be deposited from the systemic circulation. Alternately, the complex may be formed in situ, with the IgA antibody bound with an endogenous antigen in the mesangium. Another theory postulates that abnormal IgA, produced in excess by B cells during upper respiratory infection, self-aggregates or causes production of autoantibodies and immune complexes, which deposit in the mesangium. In the mesangium, IgA can bind with receptors on the mesangial cells to induce proliferation and cytokine production. In addition, it can activate complement through the alternate pathway to induce glomerular damage.[85]

Conditions that stimulate the release of IgA are believed to cause IgA deposition in the mesangium. In fact, infections of the upper respiratory tract or intestinal mucosa are known to correlate with the onset or exacerbation of IgA nephropathy. IgA production is likely to be increased through antigenic stimulation of IgA-producing mucosal lymphoid tissue by microorganisms as well as ingested or inhaled substances.

CLINICAL PRESENTATION

IgA nephropathy commonly presents in the second and third decades of life, but it can occur at any age. Many of the patients have gross hematuria concurrent with an infection, most commonly pharyngitis or tonsillitis, and less often pneumonia, gastroenteritis, or urinary tract infection.[84] In contrast to the 10- to 14-day delay after the pharyngitis in poststreptococcal glomerulonephritis, the hematuria of IgA nephropathy occurs 1 to 2 days after the onset of infection symptoms. The hematuria lasts from 24 hours to a few days, and it may recur with a febrile illness months or years later. Frequently, there is persistent microscopic hematuria between episodes of gross hematuria. Proteinuria is common and sometimes it can be in the nephrotic range. In contrast, hypertension and edema that are frequent in poststreptococcal glomerulonephritis are infrequent in IgA nephropathy. Renal dysfunction is uncommon at the initial presentation; however, about 10% to 20% of the patients develop ESKD within 10 years, and 30% develop it after 20 years.[86] Hypertension, severe proteinuria, renal function impairment, old age, and the severity of histologic lesions are all predictive factors for poor long-term outcome.[85,86] The alternative, but less common, clinical presentations are asymptomatic, microscopic hematuria with variable degrees of proteinuria or nephrotic syndrome.

▶ TREATMENT: Immunoglobulin A Nephropathy

CLINICAL CONTROVERSY

The role of specific therapies for IgA nephropathy is not known since no conclusive data are available for each treatment option.

Spontaneous remission is seen in only 10% to 25% of children and 5% to 7.5% of adults. Unfortunately, no therapy is known to be consistently effective for the treatment of IgA nephropathy. Because of the slow progression of the disease to ESKD, it is very difficult to conduct trials to evaluate the long-term effectiveness of specific treatments. The lack of understanding of the pathogenetic mechanisms and the unavailability of appropriate animal models severely limit the development of rational treatment regimens. This section discusses the several therapeutic approaches that have been used to treat IgA nephropathy (Fig. 47–10).

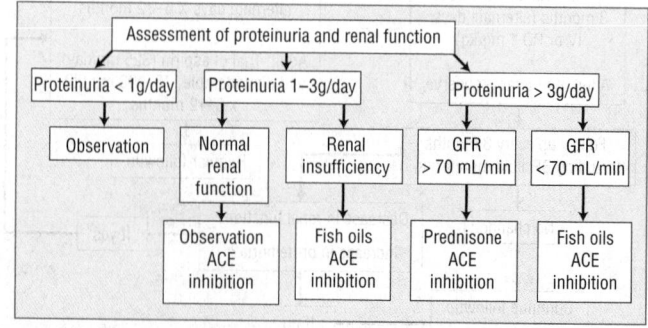

FIGURE 47–10. Treatment algorithm for biopsy-proven IgA nephropathy. (Modified from Nolin et al.[86])

REDUCTION OF IgA IMMUNE COMPLEX: LOW-GLUTEN DIET, PHENYTOIN, AND TONSILLECTOMY

Restriction of dietary gluten is effective in patients with celiac disease, but not in patients with no identifiable nephritogenic antigens. Phenytoin was evaluated because of its ability to reduce the amount of polymeric IgA in the circulation.[87] Although phenytoin reduced serum IgA concentrations and frequency of macroscopic hematuria, the glomerular lesions deteriorated in some of the patients despite treatment. Removal of the tonsils, which produce IgA_1 and may contribute to IgA nephropathy, may reduce proteinuria and hematuria; however, the beneficial effect of tonsillectomy on renal function long-term has not yet been substantiated.[88]

REDUCTION OF IgA PRODUCTION: CORTICOSTEROIDS AND IMMUNOSUPPRESSANTS

The second approach is to reduce IgA production. Corticosteroids with or without immunosuppressive agents have been evaluated in several studies. Low-dose, short-term (<3 months) therapy is not expected to yield favorable results. Patients with progressive renal failure will not generally benefit from steroid therapy. Early treatment of proteinuric patients using an intensive and prolonged regimen (IV methylprednisolone and oral prednisolone combination for 6 months) reduces proteinuria and may preserve renal function.[86,89] A meta-analysis of randomized trials reveals that heavy proteinuria (greater than 3 g/day) may be reduced by steroids and/or cytotoxic drugs in 66.7% of the patients.[90] Prednisone and azathioprine, when used together, has been found retrospectively to preserve renal function for up to 10 years in patients with significant proteinuria who had mild renal dysfunction initially.[91] The combination of cyclophosphamide, dipyridamole, and warfarin was shown to reduce proteinuria; however, renal function continued to decline on long-term follow-up.[86] Another study showed that the azathioprine, prednisolone, heparin, and warfarin combination was better than heparin and warfarin alone in preserving renal function and reducing proteinuria at 2 years.[92] However, long-term follow-up data are not yet available.

REDUCTION OF GLOMERULAR INFLAMMATION: FISH OIL

The third approach is to reduce glomerular inflammation and glomerulosclerosis induced by IgA deposits. Anti-inflammatory agents, antiplatelet drugs, and anticoagulants have been tried without success to decrease the production or action of mediators responsible for IgA immune complex–induced glomerular damage. However, the n-3 fatty acids in fish oil, which limit the production or action of cytokines and eicosanoids, delay the progression of renal failure and reduce proteinuria slightly in patients with marked proteinuria and serum creatinine concentrations less than 3 mg/dL prior to study enrollment. A meta-analysis of five controlled studies indicated that a minor, but not statistically significant, beneficial effect on renal function may be observed.[93] Donadio and colleagues recently reported that fish oil was effective in reducing renal function deterioration over a 2-year period in patients with severe disease.[94] However, reduction in proteinuria, a key cause for renal injury, was only modest. Some of the fish oil preparations are rich in cholesterol; it is therefore appropriate

to monitor the low-density lipoprotein cholesterol levels in patients receiving fish oil therapy.

ACE INHIBITION

ACE inhibitors can reduce proteinuria in patients with IgA nephropathy through their effect on the filtration barrier in the glomerular membrane.[94] Several randomized trials and a large retrospective trial demonstrated that ACEIs moderately reduced proteinuria without improving renal function.[95] Combined use of ACEIs and ARBs may have an additive effect on proteinuria reduction.[84,96] However, their effects on renal function preservation is not known.[84,97] Because hypertension is a negative prognostic indicator of IgA nephropathy and many of these patients already have left ventricular diastolic malfunction, despite being normotensive, early antihypertensive intervention with ACEIs or ARBs should be instituted.[84,85]

OTHER THERAPEUTIC APPROACHES

Patients with IgA nephropathy have abnormal production of IgA and several different immunoglobulins. High-dose immunoglobulins, initially administered intravenously followed by the intramuscular route, for over 9 months arrested the decline of renal function and reduced hematuria and proteinuria in all of the 11 patients evaluated.[97] The efficacy of this regimen must be confirmed in a larger number of patients before it is used as primary therapy.

Urokinase, danazol, dapsone, sodium cromoglycate, and plasma exchange have also been evaluated, but none is consistently effective nor shown to affect renal function.[86] Cyclosporine treatment for 12 weeks was evaluated in nine patients. Proteinuria was reduced and plasma albumin concentrations increased. However, the creatinine clearance decreased during treatment and did not return to baseline after termination of cyclosporine therapy.[98] Cyclosporine is not, therefore, indicated for patients with IgA nephropathy.

Recently, the HMG-CoA reductase inhibitor fluvastatin was reported to reduce urinary protein excretion in moderately proteinuric (0.6 to 1.6 g/day) patients who had IgA nephropathy with normal renal function.[99] Creatinine clearance remained stable during the 6-month study. Longer-term evaluation in a larger patient population will be needed to confirm the effect of this class of agents.

Mycophenolate mofetil and several new strategies are being evaluated as experimental treatments for IgA nephropathy on the premise that they may reduce IgA synthesis and mesangial uptake and/or suppress the effects of proinflammatory or profibrogenic mediators.[100]

THERAPEUTIC OUTCOMES

Normotensive patients with normal renal function, isolated microhematuria, and proteinuria less than 1 g/day should be observed closely without specific treatment.[85] Because corticosteroids reduce proteinuria, a course of alternate-day prednisone (1 mg/kg per day) with subsequent tapering is indicated for patients with proteinuria greater than 3 g/d who have good renal function (>70 mL/min).[86] The more aggressive IV or oral steroid regimen described above may also be considered, even though its efficacy has not been definitively established. For patients with a slow progressive decline in creatinine clearance (<70 mL/min), fish oil should be given. Azathioprine, mycophenolate mofetil, or dipyridamole/warfarin therapy may also be used, although the efficacy of these agents has not been established. If the patient experiences rapid GFR decline of more than 2 mL/min per month, immunoglobulin therapy may be considered despite the fact that only limited data are available. Other therapies that may be considered for these patients include pulse steroids, a cyclophosphamide/steroid combination, mycophenolate mofetil, and plasmapheresis.[85,86,98]

If the patient is hypertensive, ACEIs or ARBs should be used to control the blood pressure as well as the proteinuria. The target blood pressure should be <125/75 mm Hg. Some clinicians recommend using ACEIs or ARBs for all patients with >1 g/day proteinuria.[97] In patients with recurrent macroscopic hematuria in conjunction with tonsillitis, tonsillectomy should be considered.[86] In all of the patients,

smoking should be avoided because of the dose-dependent increase in risk for developing ESKD.[19]

Urinary protein excretion and the mean arterial blood pressure at follow-up correlate well with the progression of disease. The risk of developing end-stage renal disease is proportional to the amount of proteinuria, under the influence of ACEI and ARB therapy, after 1 year of follow-up.[101] For those patients who develop end-stage renal failure, transplantation is appropriate, especially for young adults. Recurrence of IgA mesangial deposits in the renal allograft may occur in up to 50% of patients in 5 years and be universally present at 10 years or more posttransplant, but the recurrence of clinical disease is only about 10% to 15%.[84,85] There is also no correlation between the aggressiveness of the primary disease and the rate of recurrence.[84] Immunosuppression using corticosteroids, azathioprine, and/or cyclosporine is not expected to prevent the recurrent nephropathy.

LUPUS NEPHRITIS

Glomerulonephritis is one of the most serious complications of systemic lupus erythematosus (SLE) and accounts for much of the morbidity and mortality of patients afflicted with the disease. The renal manifestations of lupus nephritis are variable and encompass a wide spectrum of histopathologic lesions.[102,103] The underlying histopathology is associated with different prognoses and responses to therapy, which cannot be predicted solely based on clinical manifestations. A renal biopsy is therefore required to assess the severity of the disease and to predict the short-term and long-term outcomes associated with therapy. Drugs, such as hydralazine and procainamide, are known to precipitate a lupus syndrome; however, they are unlikely to cause disease that affects the kidney.

PATHOPHYSIOLOGY

Immune complex deposits, whether formed in the circulation or in situ, can be found in various regions of the glomerulus, as well as the peritubular interstitium and vasculature outside the glomerulus.[103] Based on light, immunofluorescence, and electron microscopy findings, lupus nephritis can be categorized into six World Health Organization (WHO) classes: I—normal; II—mesangial; III—focal proliferative; IV—diffuse proliferative; V—membranous; and VI—advanced sclerosing.[104] In an attempt to enhance the predictive values of the histologic findings, semiquantitative assessment of active lesions and sclerotic changes are used to determine activity index and chronicity index, respectively.[103] The hallmark feature in the pathogenesis of SLE is the dysregulated production of antibodies against multiple antigens in the body.[102] The size and location of the immune complexes in the glomerulus correlate with the nature and severity

of renal injury.[103] Deposition of small numbers of stable immune complexes of intermediate size in the mesangium tends to produce less-severe inflammation in the glomerulus. The sequestration of the immune complexes in the mesangium prevents them from activating inflammatory mediators. Hence the lesion is noninflammatory in nature. In contrast, large numbers of intermediate-sized or large immune complexes results in infiltration of inflammatory cells and release of necrotizing enzymes.

CLINICAL PRESENTATION

Females have a higher risk for developing lupus, especially in the adult years. Nephritis is usually seen within the first 4 years of diagnosis of SLE, but may also be the first manifestation of the disease. The clinical presentation ranges from minimal hematuria and proteinuria to severe, rapidly progressive diffuse glomerulonephritis. Proteinuria is very common and nephrotic syndrome is seen in most patients with membranous lesions. Microscopic hematuria is almost always present, while macroscopic hematuria is rare.[104] Active urinary sediments (red cell casts, dysmorphic red cells, and hematuria) are suggestive of the diffuse proliferative lesion.[102] Hypertension is present in 25% to 45% of patients, and is associated with a worse prognosis. Other conditions found to be associated with poor prognosis include elevated serum creatinine concentration, heavy proteinuria, anemia (hematocrit <26%), black race, and disease onset during childhood or in those >60 years of age. Most patients have hypocomplementemia and increased antibody titers for anti–double-stranded DNA, particularly those with focal or diffuse proliferative lesions.[62] Serum creatinine concentration at the time of diagnosis is most predictive of short-term outcome.[103]

▶ TREATMENT: Lupus Nephritis

The treatment of lupus nephritis has evolved over the past several decades. The choice of therapy depends on the underlying lesion and the activity, as well as the chronicity indices. Acute life-threatening disease involving multiple organs requires induction treatment that can suppress the disease promptly. In contrast, long-term management of chronic indolent disease requires therapy with more acceptable side-effect profiles. Corticosteroids are the cornerstone of therapy. However, for severe lupus nephritis, primarily the diffuse proliferative type, alkylating agents may be needed to reduce or prevent the progression to ESKD.

Patients with normal renal function and less than 2 g of proteinuria usually do not require therapy, except for the management

of extrarenal lupus manifestations. The prognosis of these patients is generally good and renal biopsy can be delayed. However, close follow-up of renal function and urinalysis is required.

■ ACUTE INDUCTION TREATMENT

Patients with more than 2 g of proteinuria, deteriorating renal function, and/or active urinary sediments require a renal biopsy to define the underlying lesion and determine the activity and chronicity of disease. Those with class III or V lesions can be treated with oral steroids or 12 to 16 weeks with subsequent tapering to low doses to maintain emission. The concurrent use of an immunosuppressive agent was found in meta-analysis to be more effective in reducing the incidence of ESKD than steroid alone.[105] Patients with class IV lesions and those with class III lesions associated with subendothelial deposits and signs of severe disease activity, should be treated with pulse intravenous methylprednisolone followed by low-dose oral steroids. Cyclophosphamide is used concurrently because it is a powerful B-cell inhibitor and can suppress the resynthesis of autoantibodies to normal levels.[104] Combined use of intravenous cyclophosphamide and methylprednisolone is more effective than either agent alone in inducing remission.[106] However, the risk for adverse events, such as infection, amenorrhea, and cervical dysplasia, is increased with the cytotoxic regimens.[107]

Investigators at the National Institutes of Health have used fludarabine, which targets lymphoid cells, with cyclophosphamide.[108] Favorable results have been obtained thus far with respect to proteinuria reduction. Also being investigated is the use of immunoablative high-dose cyclophosphamide with reinfusion of autologous stem cells. Alternately, granulocyte-stimulating factor may be used without stem-cell rescue.[108]

CHRONIC MAINTENANCE TREATMENT

Oral steroid is most frequently used for maintenance treatment (prednisolone 5 to 15 mg/day or equivalent).[104] Alternate-day regimens, although not evaluated, are often used in children to minimize growth retardation. Monthly pulse IV steroids in conjunction with cyclophosphamide resulted in more sustained remission, fewer relapses, and no significant increase in side effects.[109] This combination has also been shown by meta-analysis to be more beneficial than steroid or cyclophosphamide alone.[105] Cyclophosphamide, because of its bladder and gonadal toxicity, has been given as monthly and then bimonthly intravenous injection, instead of daily administration, for up to 2 or more years. However, toxicity is still a concern. A recent trial in Europe showed that after initial lower pulse doses of IV cyclophosphamide, oral azathioprine was able to attain remission rates similar to those of higher initial pulse doses of cyclophosphamide with quarterly follow-up doses.[110]

Cyclosporine has been evaluated in a few studies with varied results. There are recent data to suggest that it may reduce proteinuria and lupus activity, stabilize renal function, and improve kidney morphology. A randomized trial is currently underway at the National Institutes of Health to evaluate its effectiveness.

Mycophenolate mofetil has been used for patients resistant to or intolerant of cyclophosphamide with good efficacy and limited side effects.[108,111] A recent controlled study indicates that it may be a better maintenance therapy option than cyclophosphamide.[112]

Other therapeutic measures that have been used for lupus nephritis include plasmapheresis, intravenous γ-globulin, fish oil, total lymphoid irradiation, and intravenous thromboxane antagonists.[113] None of these modalities was effective in controlled trials. However, plasmapheresis, in place of cyclophosphamide, was found to be effective when used with steroids in a small number of patients.[114] LJP-394, composed of four double-stranded oligodeoxynucleotides, can reduce anti-DNA antibody production and render specific B-lymphocytes unresponsive to immunogen. It may reduce renal and systemic SLE flares in a subgroup of patients whose anti-DNA antibodies are bound avidly to the compound. However, whether such beneficial effect is reproducible in other settings is questionable.[115] Anti-C5A is a monoclonal antibody that is being evaluated for membranous nephropathy and is potentially beneficial for lupus nephritis. Anti-CD40 ligand, which exerts immunosuppression by blocking communication between B and T cells, was not found to be useful because of thromboembolic complications.[116] Also being investigated is bindarit, which blocks the production of monocyte chemoattractant protein MCP-1. As a result, the inflammation in the glomeruli is reduced.[107]

TREATMENT OUTCOME

The prognosis of patients with class II disease is generally good and no specific treatment is commonly needed. In patients with class V disease, steroids alone commonly induce partial or complete remission. Immunosuppressive agents can be used for those who are not responsive to steroids. The survival of patients with class III and IV disease has improved during the last two to three decades to about 74% to 80% at 10 years.[102] Besides the judicious use of cytotoxic agents, the lower steroid dosage and better management of complications such as hypertension, infections, hyperlipidemia, and other metabolic complications of the disease have all likely contributed to the more favorable long-term outcome. Lupus patients with ESKD on dialysis fare as well as those with non–lupus-related renal disease. In those patients who received a renal transplant, the allograft outcome of patients with lupus nephritis is favorable.[117] Recurrence of lupus in the renal allograft can occur, but is usually of minor clinical importance.

RAPIDLY PROGRESSIVE GLOMERULONEPHRITIS

Rapidly progressive glomerulonephritis (RPGN) describes a clinicopathologic syndrome of rapid loss of renal function—usually a greater than 50% decrement of the glomerular filtration rate within 3 months. The predominant histologic finding of RPGN is extensive crescent formation, usually in more than 50% of the glomeruli. Hence, it is also known as crescentic glomerulonephritis. RPGN accounts for 2% to 7% of all renal biopsy findings, and is responsible for up to 5% of patients with ESKD. Although a rare disease, RPGN usually leads to renal demise within weeks or months if left untreated.

RPGN is not a single disease entity. A variety of glomerulonephritides with or without systemic diseases may present as RPGN, including anti-GBM glomerulonephritis; Goodpasture's syndrome; lupus nephritis; poststreptococcal glomerulonephritis; membranoproliferative glomerulonephritis; IgA nephropathy; polyarteritis nodosa; Wegener's granulomatosis; and idiopathic crescentic glomerulonephritis.[118] RPGN may also be found superimposed on an underlying primary glomerulopathy such as membranous nephropathy.

Besides the hallmark feature of extensive crescents, severe endocapillary proliferation and segmental necrosis can also be seen on light microscopy. Based on immunofluorescence microscopic findings, three types of primary RPGN can be identified. Type I RPGN is characterized by the linear localization of immunoglobulins, mainly IgG, along the GBM, signifying anti-GBM antibody–induced injury. Type II is defined by the coarse granular deposition of immunoglobulins and complement within the capillary walls and mesangium, denoting immune-complex–mediated injury. Type III is characterized by scanty or complete lack of immune complex deposits; therefore it is also known as pauci-immune RPGN. Circulating ANCAs are often detected in type III RPGN. This immunohistologic classification of RPGN reflects the immunopathogenesis of the different types of crescentic glomerulonephritis.

PATHOPHYSIOLOGY

Several etiologic factors are implicated as the cause of RPGN: toxins, drugs, viral and bacterial infections, neoplasms, autoimmune mechanisms, and various immunogenetic factors.[118]

Regardless of the etiology and type of RPGN, the disruption in the glomerular capillary wall seems to be the common lesion in crescentic glomerulonephritis.[118] Both humoral and cellular pathways of inflammation are responsible for the severe damage to the capillary wall. Activation of the terminal C5b-9 (membrane-attacking complex) of the complement system produces severe capillary wall injury. Both neutrophils and macrophages release proteinases and reactive oxygen species and may thereby produce severe glomerular injury. Platelets and the coagulation system are activated and result in capillary thrombosis. Fibrinogen and procoagulants that are released from ruptured capillaries may come into contact with thrombogenic tissue debris and lead to fibrinoid changes. In anti-GBM glomerulonephritis, the direct attack of the anti-GBM antibody on the noncollagenous region of the type IV collagen molecule of the GBM, is responsible for the capillary wall injury.[118] ANCAs may also play an important role in mediating the vascular injury in patients with ANCA-associated disease. The interaction of ANCAs with neutrophils and monocytes, which have been primed by concurrent infections or inflammatory processes, can lead to activation of these leukocytes and release of toxic oxygen species and lytic enzymes, resulting in vascular injury.

The disruption of the capillary wall allows movement of macrophages and other plasma constituents into Bowman's space and stimulates the formation of crescents, which are composed mainly of parietal epithelial cells, as well as macrophages and fibroblasts. Crescent formation indicates the severity of the glomerular capillary disease but not its pathogenesis. The age of crescents can serve as a marker for disease duration and the likelihood of successful therapeutic intervention.[118]

CLINICAL PRESENTATION

Among the crescentic glomerulonephritides, the pauci-immune RPGN is the most frequent, accounting for more than 50% of cases, whereas the anti-GBM antibody–mediated RPGN is the least fre-

quent, occurring in roughly 10% to 20% of patients. Of patients with type I RPGN, 60% to 70% may have concurrent pulmonary hemorrhage and Goodpasture's syndrome, which is caused by antibodies directed against the pulmonary alveolar basement membrane. Most patients with immune complex–mediated RPGN have collagen vascular disease, systemic infections, or a severe form of primary glomerular disease. Approximately 70% of patients with type III RPGN also present with evidence of systemic vasculitis, such as Wegener's granulomatosis and polyarteritis nodosa. They often have insidious onset with initial symptoms such as fatigue, fever, night sweats, and arthralgias. Other patients have only renal manifestations, and they are said to have idiopathic crescentic glomerulonephritis or renal vasculitis.[118]

The clinical presentation is dominated by progressive renal insufficiency with complaints of tea-colored urine, malaise, anorexia, low-grade fever, and migratory polyarthropathy. Mild hypertension is usually present. Uremic signs and symptoms may develop as renal function worsens. Type I RPGN is more commonly found in the third and sixth decades of life, while patients with ANCA-mediated disease tend to be older, with peak incidence occurring between 50 and 60 years of age. The age-related incidence varies among the immune complex–mediated RPGN; for example, poststreptococcal glomerulonephritis and Henoch-Schönlein purpura nephritis are more common in young children, whereas membranoproliferative glomerulonephritis is more frequently seen in older children. Urinalysis commonly shows nephritic sediments with hematuria, erythrocyte casts, and proteinuria. However, overt nephrotic syndrome is rare.

Serologic analysis is very useful in distinguishing the different types of RPGN. The detection of serum anti-GBM antibodies with the appropriate clinical presentation confirms the diagnosis of anti-GBM glomerulonephritis. More than 80% of patients with pauci-immune or idiopathic crescentic glomerulonephritis have circulating ANCAs. ANCAs are autoantibodies specific for the cytoplasmic constituents of neutrophil granules and monocyte lysosomes. Patients with ANCA-associated disease limited to renal involvement often have P-ANCA (perinuclear staining), whereas patients with Wegener's granulomatosis tend to have C-ANCA (cytoplasmic staining). Both the anti-GBM antibody and the ANCAs are absent in patients with type II RPGN. Measurements of circulating immune complexes are not useful for making a specific diagnosis, but detection of specific serum antibodies known to mediate immune complex–associated nephritis is helpful: anti-DNA antibody as a marker for lupus nephritis and elevated anti-streptolysin-O titers for poststreptococcal glomerulonephritis. The serum complement levels are normal in RPGN, although they can be low in the immune complex–mediated category.

▶ TREATMENT: Rapidly Progressive Glomerulonephritis

CLINICAL CONTROVERSY

The optimal treatment of many types of rapidly progressive glomerulonephritis is not known since it is difficult to find sufficient number of patients to conduct well designed and credible clinical trials.

Early aggressive therapy has improved the renal prognosis of patients with crescentic glomerulonephritis. The rapid deterioration of renal function and the paucity of a large number of patients make randomized controlled studies very difficult to conduct. Based on the available data, immunosuppressive therapy alone appears to be ineffective for type I RPGN, while types II and III RPGN respond well to high-dose steroid therapy.[118,119] Regardless of the type of

RPGN, poor response to therapy and an ominous renal survival are expected if the patient presents with oliguria, has a serum creatinine concentration greater than 6 or 7 mg/dL, is dialysis dependent, or has a renal biopsy showing advanced chronic parenchymal disease.[120]

◼ ANTI-GBM GLOMERULONEPHRITIS (TYPE I)

Pulse intravenous administration of corticosteroids has been used successfully to alleviate pulmonary hemorrhage, but the results are not as convincing for glomerulonephritis.[118,119] When used, the immunosuppression should be maintained for 8 weeks to prevent antibody rebound.[118] Plasmapheresis, in combination with steroids and cytotoxic agents, was found to be more beneficial than immunosuppression alone.[98,119] Plasmapheresis may confer its benefits by removing the circulating pathogenetic anti-GBM antibody, and is therefore used for 2 weeks or until the antibody disappears.[119,121] The treatment was found to be useful in treating pulmonary hemorrhage; however, the long-term benefits on renal function are unknown. Because of the rapid decline in renal function, diagnosis should be established early so that therapy can proceed without delay. When the serum creatinine concentration is 6 mg/dL or above, or the patient is oliguric or requires dialysis, the response to therapy is usually poor and the patient should be treated conservatively.[118,119] Poor response should also be expected when crescents are found in more than 85% of the glomeruli.

IMMUNE COMPLEX–MEDIATED GLOMERULONEPHRITIS (TYPE II)

The treatment of this type of RPGN varies with the underlying glomerulonephritis. Patients with postinfectious RPGN generally have a favorable prognosis even without treatment. Complete spontaneous recovery occurs in 50% of cases, whereas chronic renal failure develops in 32%.[118] Pulse doses of methylprednisolone, followed by oral prednisone and then tapering, have been shown to be beneficial in type II RPGN, with a response rate of 85% in patients with acute disease and 70% in those with more chronic disease.[119] Plasmapheresis does not appear to provide any additional benefit.[119]

ANTINEUTROPHIL CYTOPLASMIC AUTOANTIBODY (ANCA)-ASSOCIATED GLOMERULONEPHRITIS (TYPE III)

Type III RPGN has been treated successfully with pulse doses of intravenous methylprednisolone, followed by oral prednisone for 1 month and then tapering over the next 6 to 12 months.[118,119] The recognition that pauci-immune necrotizing crescentic glomerulonephritis is part of the spectrum of necrotizing vasculitides, especially with the detection of ANCAs in these patients, has led to the use of cyclophosphamide with steroids.[119] Cyclophosphamide should be given for

6 to 12 months, either orally (2 mg/kg per day) adjusted to maintain the leukocyte count between 3000 and 5000/mL, or intravenously starting at 0.5 g/m² per month and increased monthly by 0.25 g to a maximum of 1 g/m² per month.[119,122] Vigilant monitoring of the white cell count is necessary to prevent severe leukopenia. The combined use of cyclophosphamide and steroids resulted in a higher remission rate and less risk for relapse than steroids alone. This regimen is indicated even for patients with advanced disease or dialysis dependence as well as for relapse. During treatment the serum ANCA levels can be monitored to determine the efficacy of therapy. However, the precise role of ANCA monitoring is not clear.

At present, plasmapheresis is not expected to have any additional benefits for patients with mild to moderate disease who are receiving immunosuppressive therapy.[121] However, recently completed randomized studies and meta-analyses of controlled trials strongly suggest that, when used as an adjunct to immunosuppressive therapy, plasmapheresis is beneficial for patients with severe disease presenting with acute renal failure.[98] In those patients presenting with pulmonary hemorrhage, early and aggressive use of plasmapheresis has reduced substantially the nearly 50% mortality rate.[122]

Several other agents have been used to prevent recurrence of ANCA-associated diseases.[120,122] Mycophenolate mofetil has been used anecdotally with favorable results for remission maintenance. Methotrexate has also been used; however, it should not be given when the creatinine clearance is <50 mL/min. Trimethoprim-sulfamethoxazole was found to reduce ANCA-associated vasculitis, especially in the upper respiratory tract.

RENAL TRANSPLANTATION

Anti-GBM nephritis may recur in up to 55% of patients who received a renal transplant. However, only 25% of these patients showed clinical disease activity, with rare allograft failure. Because the frequency of recurrence and its severity are related to the presence of circulating anti-GBM antibody, it is recommended that transplantation should not be performed until the anti-GBM antibody is undetectable for at least 6 to 12 months.[123] The recurrence rate of ANCA-associated nephritis is 17%, with the average time to relapse from transplantation of 31 months.[124]

POSTSTREPTOCOCCAL GLOMERULONEPHRITIS

Poststreptococcal glomerulonephritis (PSGN) and glomerulonephritis caused by other infectious agents, such as bacteria, viruses, and parasites, were once common. Improved sanitation, personal hygiene, medical care, and public health measures helped to decrease the incidence of group A streptococcal infection both in the United States and other developed countries, resulting in a decline of PSGN. However, PSGN is still common in developing countries. In contrast, glomerulonephritis secondary to other infectious agents, such as hepatitis C and HIV, is seen with increasing frequency in developed countries.

It was more than 200 years ago when hematuria and proteinuria were found to be associated with epidemics of scarlet fever. Certain strains of group A streptococci were identified in the 1950s to be responsible for the glomerular disease. PSGN is now the most common form of glomerulonephritis in children, but is less common than the other types of glomerulonephritis in adults. It normally follows pharyngeal or skin infection caused by the nephritogenic strains of

group A streptococci; however, other strains of streptococci, such as group C and G, have also been reported to cause PSGN. Streptococcal pharyngitis is more common in winter and early spring, whereas skin infection is frequently found in the summer. The risk for developing acute glomerulonephritis secondary to the nephritogenic strains of bacteria is about 10% to 15% in infected patients. However, three to four times more patients may experience a subclinical form of the disease.

PATHOPHYSIOLOGY

Despite decades of research, the characteristics of the antigens responsible for the production of the nephritogenic immune complexes remain unclear. It has been postulated that the streptococcal antigens may induce changes in the glomerular components so that they become immunogenic or that autologous IgG may be altered to become antigenic. Alternately, the streptococcal antigens may induce antibodies that react with glomerular antigens. In situ immune complexes are then formed and result in a complement-mediated inflammatory response. The kinin and coagulation cascades are activated and chemotactic factors are released to recruit neutrophils and monocytes, resulting in acute glomerular lesions.

Examination of the acute PSGN kidneys reveals hypercellular glomeruli with proliferation of mesangial and endothelial cells. Infiltration of neutrophils, monocytes, and eosinophils is apparent within the capillary lumen and also in the mesangial areas. Crescent formation may be seen in patients with severe disease, and if found in more than 30% of the glomeruli, RPGN may be present concurrently.[125] The prognosis is generally poor for these patients and complete recovery is unlikely. When the tissue is examined under electron microscope, "humps," which are multiple large, discrete, electron-dense, dome-shaped deposits can be found beneath the epithelial foot processes. Immunofluorescence examination reveals diffuse granular deposits of IgG and C3 along the glomerular basement membrane and also in the mesangium.

CLINICAL PRESENTATION

PSGN is seen mostly in children aged between 5 and 15 years, with a peak incidence between ages 6 and 7 years. It is uncommon in children younger than 2 years of age and in adults older than 50 years of age. Males are twice as likely to be affected as females. The nephritis is preceded by a latent period following a streptococcal infection. The latent period is commonly 7 to 14 days for pharyngitis and 14 to 28 days for skin infection. In patients with pre-existing nephritis such as IgA nephropathy and membranoproliferative glomerulonephritis, the streptococcal infection may exacerbate the nephritis and result in hematuria.

Following the latent period, an acute nephritic syndrome develops with hematuria and edema being the most common characteristics. Gross hematuria is seen in 70% of patients, and microscopic hematuria can be found in all patients. Edema, which is often worse in the morning, is found commonly in the periorbital area and around the eyelids. Hypertension is usually mild to moderate and results from sodium and water retention; at times, it may be severe enough to cause hypertensive encephalopathy. Many patients have signs and symptoms associated with volume overload, which include dyspnea, orthopnea, and cough. In some instances, progression to overt congestive heart failure may be seen. Severe hypertension may also result in neurologic abnormalities.

Urinalysis of patients with PSGN reveals hematuria, dysmorphic red blood cells, and red cell casts. Proteinuria is common, but often not in the nephrotic range. Renal function is frequently mildly impaired and serum creatinine concentration is often normal. However, blood urea concentration may be disproportionately high.

Throat or skin culture may be positive for group A streptococci despite the latent period following the initial infection. However, antibiotic therapy may render the culture result negative. Serologic measurements of antibodies to different streptococcal antigens can confirm recent exposure to the infection. Titers that can be measured include the antistreptolysin (ASO), antistreptokinase, anti-hyaluronidase (AHase), antideoxyribonuclease B (ADNase B), and antinicotyladenine dinucleotidase (NADase).[126] In most patients with streptococcal pharyngitis, the ASO titers begin to rise about 10 to 14 days later, peak at 3 to 4 weeks, and persist for several months before decreasing. The rise in ASO titers can be reduced by antibiotic treatment and may not be seen in patients with streptococcal skin infection in whom the streptolysin may be bound to skin lipids. ADNase B and AHase titers should be used instead because they are specific and are positive in the majority of patients. The streptozyme test is a combined assay for ASO, ADNase B, NADase, and AHase. It has a high rate of false-positive and false-negative results, and the antibody levels do not correlate with nephritogenicity or disease severity. Recently, antizymogen titers were found to be the best marker to diagnose streptococcal-associated nephritis.[127] Increased availability of this test may facilitate early and accurate diagnosis of nephritis.

Serum complement levels are often decreased in patients with PSGN in whom hemolytic complement activity and C3 levels are reduced in more than 90% of the patients for 4 to 6 weeks. If the C3 level is depressed for more than 6 to 8 weeks, MPGN, lupus nephritis or glomerulonephritis related to endocarditis or occult visceral abscess should be suspected.

Renal biopsy is not normally indicated for PSGN unless the patient has severe renal dysfunction, severe proteinuria, significant hypertension, and/or prolonged oliguria, which are not typical for PSGN. If the hematuria is prolonged or proteinuria or depressed C3 level persists, renal biopsy is needed to detect other types of glomerulonephritis such as lupus, RPGN, or MPGN.

▶ TREATMENT: Poststreptococcal Glomerulonephritis

The treatment of PSGN is mainly supportive and symptomatic. Early antibiotic therapy does not prevent subsequent PSGN, but it may reduce the severity of the disease. It can, however, prevent the spread of the streptococcal infection to other family members. Antibiotic prophylaxis is not recommended because infected patients will develop long-lasting, often lifelong immunity against the strain of streptococci. Exposure to another nephritogenic strain of streptococci is possible, but unlikely.

Supportive measures, as discussed earlier in this chapter, should be used to control fluid volume and blood pressure. Because the hypertension is of the low-renin type, ACEIs and β-blockers are not expected to be useful. If the patient has crescentic disease, use of pulse steroids and/or immunosuppressive agents can be considered;[118] however, the efficacy and safety of these agents have not been established for this condition.

The acute manifestations of PSGN are normally self-limited, and more than 95% of the patients have renal function restored within 3 to 6 weeks. Diuresis usually begins 7 to 10 days after onset of the acute episode, whereas hypertension and azotemia resolve in 1 to 2 weeks. Gross hematuria lasts for 1 to 2 weeks and proteinuria usually resolves within 6 months in more than 90% of children. However, microscopic hematuria may persist for up to 2 years. In general, children have more rapid recovery than adults. Prognosis is often better when PSGN occurs during an epidemic than in cases found sporadically. Most of the children will recover fully and be free from chronic complications of PSGN if they have no pre-existing renal disorder, heavy proteinuria, or crescentic glomerular lesions, or did not require hospitalization during the acute episode.[128] In contrast, adult patients have a less favorable long-term outcome. As many as 50% of the patients had persistent proteinuria, hypertension, and renal insufficiency.[129] Some of the patients may develop end-stage renal failure.

CONCLUSIONS

A better understanding of the pathogenetic mechanisms leading to glomerular injury has improved the treatment of glomerulonephritis. However, the glomerulonephritides are a heterogeneous group of immune disorders with different clinical courses, prognoses, and responses to current immunologic and nonimmunologic therapies. The clinician should understand the natural history and prognosis of each subgroup of glomerulonephritis, the efficacy of different immunomodulating regimens in inducing disease remission and preserving renal function, and the characteristics of at-risk patients who warrant aggressive therapy. Judicious use of immunosuppressive agents with careful monitoring of their adverse effects cannot be overemphasized. In addition, treatment of the disease complications and control of factors that lead to progression of renal disease are important in reducing the morbidity and mortality of patients with glomerulonephritis.

ABBREVIATIONS

ACE: angiotensin-converting enzyme
ADNase B: antideoxyribonuclease B
AHase: antihyaluronidase
ANCA: antineutrophil cytoplasmic autoantibody
ARB: angiotensin II receptor blocker
ASO: antistreptolysin
ESRD: end-stage renal disease
GBM: glomerular basement membrane
GFR: glomerular filtration rate
FSGS: focal segmental glomerulosclerosis
HDL: high-density lipoprotein (cholesterol)
HIV: human immunodeficiency virus
HMG-CoA: hydroxymethylglutaryl coenzyme A (reductase)
IL-1: interleukin-1
IL-2: interleukin-2
LDL: low-density lipoprotein (cholesterol)
MPGN: membranoproliferative glomerulonephritis
NADase: antinicotyladenine dinucleotidase
PSGN: poststreptococcal glomerulonephritis
RPGN: rapidly progressive glomerulonephritis
SLE: systemic lupus erythematosus
TNF: tumor necrosis factor
VLDL: very-low-density lipoprotein (cholesterol)
WHO: World Health Organization

Review Questions and other resources can be found at *www.pharmacotherapyonline.com.*

REFERENCES

1. U.S. Renal Data System 2003 Annual Data Report. USRDS Coordinating Center, Minneapolis, MN, 2003. www.usrds.org
2. Schena FP, Gesualdo L, Grandaliano G, Montinaro V. Progression of renal damage in human glomerulonephritides: Is there sleight of hand in winning the game? Kidney Int 1997;52:1439–1457.
3. Couser WG. Mediation of immune glomerular injury. J Am Soc Nephrol 1990;1:13–29.
4. Remuzzi G, Zoja C, Perico N. Proinflammatory mediators of glomerular injury and mechanisms of activation of autoreactive T cells. Kidney Int Suppl 1994;44:S8–S16.
5. Ritz E, Orth S, Wennich T, et al. Systemic hypertension versus intraglomerular hypertension in progression. Kidney Int 1994;45:438–442.
6. Williams JD, Coles GA. Proteinuria: A direct cause of renal injury morbidity? Kidney Int 1994;45:443–450.
7. Ong ACM, Fine LG. Loss of glomerular function and tubulointerstitial fibrosis: Cause or effect? Kidney Int 1994;45:345–351.
8. Thomas ME, Schreiner F. Contribution of proteinuria to progressive renal injury: Consequences of tubular uptake of fatty acid bearing albumin. Am J Nephrol 1993;13:385–398.
9. Keane WF. Lipids and the kidney. Kidney Int 1994;46:910–920.
10. Kasiske BL, Keene WF. Laboratory assessment of renal disease: Clearance, urinalysis and renal biopsy. In: Brenner BM, ed. The Kidney, 5th ed. Philadelphia, WB Saunders, 1996:1137–1174.
11. Humphreys MH. Mechanisms and management of nephrotic edema. Kidney Int 1994;45:266–281.
12. Schrier RW, Fassett RG. A critique of the overfill hypothesis of sodium and water retention in the nephrotic syndrome. Kidney Int 1998;53:1111–1117.
13. Warwick GL, Fox JG, Boulton-Jones JM. The relationship between urinary albumin excretion rate and serum cholesterol in primary glomerular disease. Clin Nephrol 1994;41:135–137.
14. Wheeler DC, Bernard DB. Lipid abnormalities in the nephrotic syndrome: Causes, consequences, and treatment. Am J Kidney Dis 1994;23:331–346.
15. Kaysen GA, De Sain-van der Verlden M. New insights into lipid metabolism in the nephrotic syndrome. Kidney Int Suppl 1999;71:S18–21.
16. Nachman PH, Martin J. Developments in the immunotherapy of glomerular disease. J Pharm Prac 2002;15:472–489.
17. Ponticelli C, Passerini P. Treatment of the nephrotic syndrome associated with primary glomerulonephritis. Kidney Int 1994;46:595–604.
18. Klahr S, Levey A, Beck G, et al. The effects of dietary protein restriction and blood pressure control on the progression of chronic renal disease. N Engl J Med 1994;330:877–884.
19. Orth SR, Stockmann A, Conradt C, et al. Smoking as a risk factor for end-stage renal failure in men with primary renal disease. Kidney Int 1998;54:926–931.
20. Fliser D, Schroter M, Neubeck M. Coadministration of thiazides increases the efficacy of loop diuretics even in patients with advanced renal failure. Kidney Int 1994;46:482–488.
21. Rudy DW, Voelker JR, Greene PK, et al. Loop diuretics for chronic renal insufficiency: A continuous infusion is more efficacious than bolus therapy. Ann Intern Med 1991;115:360–366.
22. Ruggenenti P, Perna A, Gherardi G, et al. Chronic proteinuric nephropathies: Outcomes and response to treatment in a prospective cohort of 352 patients with different patterns of renal injury. Am J Kidney Dis 2000;35:1155–1165.
23. Chobanian AV, Bakris GL, Black HR, et al. The seventh report of the joint national committee on prevention, detection, evaluation and treatment of high blood pressure: The JNC 7 report. JAMA 2003;289:2560–2572.
24. Ruggenenti P, Remuzzi G. Is therapy with combined ACE inhibitor and angiotensin receptor antagonist the new gold standard of treatment for nondiabetic, chronic proteinuric nephropathies? NephSAP 2003;2:235–237.
25. Gansevoot R, Slinter W, Hemmelder M, et al. Antiproteinuric effect of blood pressure lowering agents: A meta analysis of comparative trials. Nephrol Dial Transplant 1995;10:1963–1974.
26. Levey AS, Adler S, Caggiula AW, et al. Effects of dietary protein restriction on the progression of advanced renal disease in the Modification of Diet in Renal Disease Study. Am J Kidney Dis 1996;27:652–663.
27. Peterson J, Adler S, Burkart J. Blood pressure control, proteinuria, and the progression of renal disease. Ann Intern Med 1995;123:754–762.
28. The GISEN group (Gruppo Italiano di Studi Epidemiologici in Nefrologia). Randomized placebo-controlled trial effect of ramipril on decline in glomerular filtration rate and risk of terminal renal failure in proteinuric, non-diabetic nephropathy. Lancet 1997;349:1857–1863.
29. ter Wee PM, Donker AJM. Pharmacologic manipulation of glomerular function. Kidney Int 1994;45:417–424.

30. Vogt L, Navis G, de Zeeuw D. Renoprotection: A matter of blood pressure reduction or agent-characteristics? J Am Soc Nephrol 2002;13(Supp 3):S202–S207.

31. Remuzzi A, Imberti O, Puntorieri S, et al. Dissociation between antiproteinuric and antihypertensive effect of angiotensin converting enzyme inhibitors in rats. Am J Physiol 1994;267:F1034–F1044.

32. Combination treatment of angiotensin-II receptor blocker and angiotensin-converting-enzyme inhibitor in non-diabetic renal disease (COOPERATE): A randomized controlled trial. Lancet 2003;361:117–124.

33. Taal MV, Brenner BM. Combination ACEi and ARB therapy: Additional benefit in renoprotection? Curr Opin Nephrol Hypertens 2002;11:377–381.

34. Perico N, Remuzzi A, Sangalli F, et al. The antiproteinuric antagonism in human IgA nephropathy is potentiated by indomethacin. J Am Soc Nephrol 1998;9:2308–2317.

35. Massy ZA, Ma JZ, Louis TA, Kasiske BL. Lipid-lowering therapy in patients with renal disease. Kidney Int 1995;48:188–198.

36. Oda H, Keane WF. Recent advances in statins and the kidney. Kidney Int Suppl 1999;71:S2–S5.

37. Sarasin FP, Schifferli JA. Prophylactic oral anticoagulation in nephrotic patients with idiopathic membranous nephropathy. Kidney Int 1994;45:578–585.

38. Rostoker G, Durand-Zaleski I, Petit-Phar M, et al. Prevention of thrombotic complications of the nephrotic syndrome by the low-molecular-weight heparin enoxaparin. Nephron 1995;69:20–28.

39. Nolasco F, Cameron JS, Heywood EF, et al. Adult-onset minimal-change nephrotic syndrome: A long-term follow-up. Kidney Int 1986;29:1215–1223.

40. Jennette JC, Mandal AK. The nephrotic syndrome. In: Mandal AK, Jennette JC, eds. Diagnosis and Management of Renal Disease and Hypertension, 2nd ed. Durham, NC, Carolina Academic Press, 1994:235–272.

41. A report of the International Study of Kidney Disease in Children: The primary nephrotic syndrome in children. Identification of patients with minimal change nephrotic syndrome for initial response to prednisone. J Pediatr 1981;98:561–564.

42. Bargman JM. Management of minimal lesion glomerulonephritis: Evidence-based recommendations. Kidney Int Suppl 1999;70:S3–S16.

43. Tune BM, Mendoza SA. Treatment of the idiopathic nephrotic syndrome: Regimens and outcomes in children and adults. J Am Soc Nephrol 1997;8:824–832.

44. Hiraoka M, Takeda N, Tsukahara H, et al. Favorable course of steroid-responsive nephrotic children with mild initial attack. Kidney Int 1995;47:1392–1393.

45. Niaudel P, Habib R. Cyclosporine in the treatment of idiopathic nephrosis. J Am Soc Nephrol 1994;5:1049–1056.

46. Meyrier A, Noel H, Auriche P, Gallard P, and the Collaborative Group of the Societe de Nephrologie. Long-term renal tolerance of cyclosporin A treatment in adult idiopathic nephrotic syndrome. Kidney Int 1994;45:1446–1456.

47. British Association for Paediatric Nephrology. Levamisole for corticosteroid-dependent nephrotic syndrome in childhood. Lancet 1991;337:1555–1557.

48. Weiss R. Randomized, double-blind, placebo controlled trial of levamisole for children with frequently relapsing/steroid dependent nephrotic syndrome. J Am Soc Nephrol 1993;4:289.

49. Dayal U, Dayal A, Shastry JCM, Raghupathy P. Use of levamisole in maintaining remission in steroid-sensitive nephrotic syndrome in children. Nephron 1994;66:408–412.

50. Choi MJ, Eustace JA, Gimenez LF, et al. Mycophenolate mofetil treatment for primary glomerular disease. Kidney Int 2002;61:1098–1114.

51. Day CJ, Cockwell P, Lipkin GW, et al. Mycophenolate mofetil in the treatment of resistant idiopathic nephrotic syndrome. Nephrol Dial Transplant 2002;17:2011–2013.

52. D'Agati V. The many masks of focal segmental glomerulosclerosis. Kidney Int 1994;46:1223–1241.

53. Korbet SM. Treatment of primary focal segmental glomerulosclerosis. Kidney Int 2002;62:2301–2310.

54. Korbet SM. Primary focal segmental glomerulosclerosis. J Am Soc Nephrol 1998;9:1333–1340.

55. Schwartz MM, Evans J, Bain R, Korbet SM. Focal segmental glomerulosclerosis: Prognostic implications of the cellular lesion. J Am Soc Nephrol 1999;10:1900–1907.

56. Korbet SM, Schwartz MM, Lewis EJ. Primary focal segmental glomerulosclerosis: Clinical course and response to therapy. Am J Kidney Dis 1994;23:773–783.

57. Burgess E. Management of focal segmental glomerulosclerosis: Evidence-based recommendations. Kidney Int Suppl 1999;70:S26–S32.

58. Ponticelli C, Villa M, Banfi G, et al. Can prolonged treatment improve the prognosis in adults with focal segmental glomerulosclerosis? Am J Kidney Dis 1999;34:618–625.

59. Ingulli E, Singh A, Baqi N, et al. Aggressive, long-term cyclosporine therapy for steroid-resistant focal segmental glomerulosclerosis. J Am Soc Nephrol 1995;5:1820–1825.

60. Cattran DC, Appel GB, Hebert LA, et al. A randomized trial of cyclosporine in patients with steroid-resistant focal segmental glomerulosclerosis. Kidney Int 1999;56:2220–2226.

61. Chishti AS, Sorof JM, Brewer ED, et al. Long-term treatment of focal segmental glomerulosclerosis in children with cyclosporine given as a single daily dose. Am J Kidney Dis 2001;38:754–760.

62. Wasserstein AG. Membranous glomerulonephritis. J Am Soc Nephrol 1997;8:664–674.

63. Geddes CC, Cattran DC. The treatment of idiopathic membranous nephropathy. Semin Nephrol 2000;20:299–308.

64. Bazzi C, Petrini C, Rizza V, et al. Urinary excretion of IgG and alpha(1)-microglobulin predicts clinical course better than extent of proteinuria in membranous nephropathy. Am J Kidney Dis 2001;38:240–248.

65. Rostoker G, Maadi AB, Remy P, et al. Low-dose angiotensin-converting enzyme inhibitor captopril to reduce proteinuria in adult idiopathic membranous nephropathy: A prospective study of long-term treatment. Nephrol Dial Transplant 1995;10:25–29.

66. Ponticelli C, Zucchelli P, Passerini P, et al. A 10-year follow-up of a randomized study with methylprednisolone and chlorambucil in membranous nephropathy. Kidney Int 1995;48:1600–1604.

67. Ponticelli C, Altieri P, Scolari F, et al. A randomized study comparing methylprednisolone plus chlorambucil versus methylprednisolone plus cyclophosphamide in idiopathic membranous nephropathy. J Am Soc Nephrol 1998;9:444–450.

68. Imperiale TF, Goldfarb S, Berns JS. Are cytotoxic agents beneficial in idiopathic membranous nephropathy? A meta-analysis of the controlled trials. J Am Soc Nephrol 1995;5:1553–1558.

69. Cattran DC, Greenwood C, Ritchie S, et al. A controlled trial of cyclosporine in patients with progressive membranous nephropathy. Kidney Int 1995;47:1130–1135.

70. Fritsche L, Budde K, Farber L, et al. Treatment of membranous glomerulopathy with cyclosporin A: How much patience is required? Nephrol Dial Transplant 1999;14:1036–1038.

71. Hebert LA. Therapy of membranous nephropathy: What to do after (meta) analyses. J Am Soc Nephrol 1995;5:1543–1545.

72. Piccoli A, Pillon L, Passerini P, et al. Therapy for idiopathic membranous nephropathy: Tailoring the choice by decision analysis. Kidney Int 1994;45:1193–1202.

73. Remuzzi G, Chiurchiu C, Abbate M, et al. Rituximab for idiopathic membranous nephropathy. Lancet 2002;360:923–924.

74. Branten AJ, Reichert LJ, Koene RA, et al. Oral cyclophosphamide versus chlorambucil in the treatment of patients with membranous nephropathy and renal insufficiency. QJM 1998;91:359–366.

75. Cattran DC, Pei Y, Greenwood CM, et al. Validation of a predictive model of idiopathic membranous nephropathy: Its clinical and research implications. Kidney Int 1997;51:901–907.

76. Lin CY. Treatment of hepatitis B virus-associated membranous nephropathy with recombinant alpha-interferon. Kidney Int 1995;47:225–230.

77. Lai KN, Tam JS, Lin HJ, et al. The therapeutic dilemma of the usage of corticosteroid in patients with membranous nephropathy and persistent hepatitis B virus surface antigenaemia. Nephron 1990;54:12–17.

78. Rennke HG. Secondary membranoproliferative glomerulonephritis. Kidney Int 1995;47:643–656.

79. D'Amico G, Ferrario F. Mesangiocapillary glomerulonephritis. J Am Soc Nephrol 1992;2:S159–S166.

80. Levin A. Management of membranoproliferative glomerulonephritis: Evidence-based recommendations. Kidney Int Suppl 1999;70:S41–46.

81. Tarshish P, Bernstein J, Tobin JN, et al. Treatment of mesangiocapillary glomerulonephritis with alternate-day prednisone—A report of the International Study of Kidney Disease in Children. Pediatr Nephrol 1992;6:123–130.

82. Zimmerman SW, Moorthy AV, Dreher WH, et al. Prospective trial of warfarin and dipyridamole in patients with membranoproliferative glomerulonephritis. Am J Med 1983;75:920–927.

83. Klein M, Radhakrishnan J, Appel G. Cyclosporine treatment of glomerular diseases. Annu Rev Med 1999;50:1–15.

84. Donadio JV, Grande JP. Immunoglobulin A nephropathy. N Engl J Med 2002;347:738–748.

85. Floege J, Feehally J. IgA nephropathy: recent developments. J Am Soc Nephrol 2000;11:2395–2403.

86. Nolin L, Courteau M. Management of IgA nephropathy: Evidence-based recommendations. Kidney Int Suppl 1999;70:S56–S62.

87. Egido J, Rivera F, Sancho J, et al. Phenytoin in IgA nephropathy: A long-term controlled trial. Nephron 1984;38:30–39.

88. Rasche FM, Schwarz A, Keller F. Tonsillectomy does not prevent a progressive course in IgA nephropathy. Clin Nephrol 1999;51:147–152.

89. Pozzi C, Bolasco PG, Fogazzi GB, et al. Corticosteroids in IgA nephropathy: A randomized controlled trial. Lancet 1999;353:883–887.

90. Schena FR, Montenegro M, Scivittaro V. Meta-analysis of randomized controlled trials in patients with IgA nephropathy (Berger's disease). Nephrol Dial Transplant 1990;5(Suppl 1):47–52.

91. Goumenos DS, Davlouros P, El Nahas AM, et al. Prednisolone and azathioprine in IgA nephropathy—a ten-year follow-up study. Nephron Clin Pract 2003;93:C58–C68.

92. Yoshikawa N, Ito H. Combined therapy with prednisolone, azathioprine, heparin-warfarin, and dipyridamole for paediatric patients with severe IgA nephropathy: Is it relevant for adult patients? Nephrol Dial Transplant 1999;14:1097–1099.

93. Dillon JJ. Fish oil therapy for IgA nephropathy: Efficacy and interstudy variability. J Am Soc Nephrol 1997;8:1739–1744.

94. Donadio JV, Larson TS, Bergstralh EJ, et al. A randomized trial of high-dose compared with low-dose omega-3 fatty acids in severe IgA nephropathy. J Am Soc Nephrol 2001;12:791–799.

95. Cattran DC, Greenwood C, Ritchie S. Long-term benefits of angiotensin-converting enzyme inhibitor therapy in patients with severe immunoglobulin A nephropathy: A comparison to patients receiving treatment with other antihypertensive agents and to patients receiving no therapy. Am J Kidney Dis 1994;23:247–254.

96. Russo D, Pisani A, Balletta MM, et al. Additive antiproteinuric effect of converting enzyme inhibitor and losartan in normotensive patients with IgA nephropathy. Am J Kidney Dis 1999;33:851–856.

97. Dillon JJ. Treating IgA nephropathy. J Am Soc Nephrol 2001;12:846–847.

98. Sanz-Guajardo D. Plasmapheresis in the treatment of glomerulonephritis: indications and complications. Am J Kidney Dis 2000;36:liv–lvi.

99. Buemi M, Allegra A, Corica F, et al. Effect of fluvastatin on proteinuria in patients with immunoglobulin A nephropathy. Clin Pharmacol Ther 2000;67:427–431.

100. Lai KN. Future directions in the treatment of IgA nephropathy. Nephron 2002;92:263–270.

101. Donadio JV, Bergstralh EJ, Grande JP, et al. Proteinuria patterns and their association with subsequent end-stage renal disease in IgA nephropathy. Nephrol Dial Transplant 2002;17:1197–1203.

102. Contreras G, Roth D, Pardo V, et al. Lupus nephritis: a clinical review for practicing nephrologists. Clin Nephrol 2002;57:95–107.

103. Kashgarian M. Lupus nephritis: Lessons from the path lab. Kidney Int 1994;45:928–938.

104. Cameron JS. Lupus nephritis. J Am Soc Nephrol 1999;10:413–424.

105. Bansal VK, Beto JA. Treatment of lupus nephritis: A meta-analysis of clinical trials. Am J Kidney Dis 1997;29:193–199.

106. Gourley MF, Austin HA, Scott D, et al. Methylprednisolone and cyclophosphamide, alone or in combination, in patients with lupus nephritis. A randomized, controlled trial. Ann Intern Med 1996;125:549–557.

107. Zoja C, Corna D, Benedetti G, et al. Bindarit retards renal disease and prolongs survival in murine lupus autoimmune disease. Kidney Int 1998;53:726–734.

108. Austin HA, Balow JE. Treatment of lupus nephritis. Semin Nephrol 2000;20:265–276.

109. Illei GG, Austin HA, Crane M, et al. Combination therapy with pulse cyclophosphamide plus pulse methylprednisolone improves long-term renal outcome without adding toxicity in patients with lupus nephritis. Ann Intern Med. 2001;135:248–257.

110. Houssiau FA, Vasconcelos C, D'Cruz D, et al. Immunosuppressive therapy in lupus nephritis: the Euro-Lupus Nephritis Trial, a randomized trial of low-dose versus high-dose intravenous cyclophosphamide. Arthritis Rheum 2002;46:2121–2131.

111. Mok CC, Lai KN. Mycophenolate mofetil in lupus glomerulonephritis. Am J Kidney Dis 2002;40:447–457.

112. Contreras G, Pardo V, Leclercq B, et al. Sequential therapies for proliferative lupus nephritis. N Engl J Med 2004;350:971–1046.

113. Zimmerman R, Radhakrishnan J, Valeri A, et al. Advances in the treatment of lupus nephritis. Annu Rev Med 2001;52:63–78.

114. Nakamura T, Ushiyama C, Hara M, et al. Comparative effects of plasmapheresis and intravenous cyclophosphamide on urinary podocyte excretion in patients with proliferative lupus nephritis. Clin Nephrol 2002;57:108–113.

115. Alarcon-Segovia D, Tumlin JA, Furie RA, et al. LJP 394 for the prevention of renal flare in patients with systemic lupus erythematosus: results from a randomized, double-blind, placebo-controlled study. Arthritis Rheum 2003;48:442–454.

116. Kawai T, Andrews D, Colvin RB, et al. Thromboembolic complications after treatment with monoclonal antibody against CD40 ligand. Nat Med 2000;6:114.

117. Clark WF, Jevnikar AM. Renal transplantation for end-stage renal disease caused by systemic lupus erythematosus nephritis. Semin Nephrol 1999;19:77–85.

118. Couser WG. Rapidly progressive glomerulonephritis: Classification, pathogenetic mechanisms, and therapy. Am J Kidney Dis 1988;11:449–464.

119. Bolton WK. Treatment of glomerular disease: ANCA-negative RPGN. Semin Nephrol 2000;20:244–255.

120. Jennette JC. Rapidly progressive crescentic glomerulonephritis. Kidney Int 2003;63:1164–1177.

121. Madore F, Lazarus MJ, Brady HR. Therapeutic plasma exchange in renal disease. J Am Soc Nephrol 1996;7:367–385.

122. Falk RJ, Nachman PH, Hogna SL, et al. ANCA glomerulonephritis and vasculitis: A Chapel Hill perspective. Semin Nephrol 2000;20:233–243.

123. Ramos EL, Tisher CC. Recurrent diseases in the kidney transplant. Am J Kidney Dis 1994;24:142–154.

124. Nachman PH, Segelmark M, Westman K, et al. Recurrent ANCA-associated small-vessel vasculitis after transplantation: A pooled analysis. Kidney Int 1999;56:1544–1550.

125. Couser WG, Johnson RJ. Postinfective glomerulonephritis. In: Neilson EG, Couser WG, eds. Immunologic Renal Diseases. Philadelphia, Lippincott-Raven, 1997:915–944.

126. Rodriguez-Iturbe B, Parra G. Glomerulonephritis associated with infection: Poststreptococcal glomerulonephritis. In: Massry SG, Glassock RJ, ed. Massry & Glassock's Textbook of Nephrology, 4th ed. Philadelphia, Lippincott Williams & Wilkins, 2001:667–671.

127. Parra G, Rodriguez-Iturbe B, Batsford S, et al. Antibody to streptococcal zymogen in the serum of patients with acute glomerulonephritis: a multicentric study. Kidney Int 1998;54:509–517.

128. Moudgil A, Bagga A, Fredrich R, et al. Poststreptococcal and other infection-related glomerulonephritides. In: Greenberg A, ed. Primer on Kidney Diseases, 2nd ed. San Diego, Academic Press, 1998:193–199.

129. Pinto SW, Sesso R, Vasconcelos E, et al. Follow-up of patients with epidemic poststreptococcal glomerulonephritis. Am J Kidney Dis 2001;38:249–255.

48

DRUG THERAPY INDIVIDUALIZATION FOR PATIENTS WITH RENAL INSUFFICIENCY

Reginald F. Frye and Gary R. Matzke

Learning Objectives and other resources can be found at *www.pharmacotherapyonline.com.*

KEY CONCEPTS

◀ Chronic kidney disease can affect all aspects of drug disposition, including absorption, distribution, metabolism, and elimination.

◀ Changes in protein binding induced by renal failure can alter the relationship between total drug concentration and response.

◀ In addition to the expected changes in renal drug elimination, nonrenal drug clearance (i.e., hepatic drug metabolism) may also be decreased in patients with chronic kidney disease.

◀ Individualization of a drug dosage regimen in a patient with renal disease is based on the pharmacokinetic characteristics of the drug and the patient's level of renal function.

◀ The effect of hemodialysis or chronic renal replacement therapy on drug elimination is dependent on the characteristics of the drug and the dialysis conditions.

Patients with renal insufficiency are commonly encountered in clinical practice. Indeed, it is estimated that nearly 11 million people in the United States have serum creatinine values of 1.5 mg/dL or greater and another 0.8 million have serum creatinine values of 2.0 mg/dL or greater.[1] Reductions in renal function can be associated with disease states, drug effects (e.g., drug-induced nephrotoxicity), or the result of the known age-related maturation or diminution of renal function. In children, renal function does not mature to adult values until approximately 1 year of age.[2] In older adults, age-related declines in renal function combined with the increased use of medications make this patient group particularly susceptible to adverse effects secondary to inappropriate pharmacotherapy.[3] The presence of compromised renal function in any patient age group, ranging from pediatric to geriatric, requires that the clinician understand the aspects of drug disposition that are altered in the presence of renal insufficiency and the appropriate methods to individualize drug therapy.[4,5]

Acute renal failure (ARF) and chronic kidney disease (CKD) are often accompanied by alterations in several other organ systems and results in the development of anemia, hyperparathyroidism, bleeding abnormalities, hyperlipidemia, hypertension, and changes in gastrointestinal tract integrity (see Chaps. 42 and 44). There are now many reports that document changes in the disposition of some drugs in patients with renal insufficiency as the result of changes in bioavailability,[6] protein binding,[7] distribution volume,[8] and metabolic activity.[9]

Drug therapy individualization for patients with renal insufficiency may require only a simple dose adjustment based on the fractional reduction in creatinine clearance.[10] However, the use of medications that are extensively metabolized or for which dramatic changes in protein binding and/or distribution volume have been noted may require a more complex adjustment.[8,10] Furthermore, because of the physiologic and biochemical changes associated with progressive renal insufficiency, patients may respond to a given dose or serum concentration of a drug differently than patients with normal renal function.[11]

Knowledge of basic pharmacokinetic principles combined with the drug disposition properties of a particular compound and the degree and type of pathophysiologic alterations associated with renal insufficiency makes it possible for the clinician to design an individualized therapeutic regimen. This chapter describes the influence of renal insufficiency on drug absorption, distribution, metabolism, and elimination, and provides a practical approach for drug dosage individualization for patients with ARF or CKD as well as those receiving continuous renal replacement therapy, continuous ambulatory peritoneal dialysis, or hemodialysis.

EFFECT ON DRUG ABSORPTION

◀ There is little quantitative information regarding the influence of impaired renal function on drug absorption and bioavailability. Drug bioavailability in ARF or CKD patients may be altered by several factors, including changes in gastrointestinal transit time and gastric pH; edema of the gastrointestinal tract; vomiting and diarrhea (frequent complications of severe renal insufficiency); and antacid administration. Evaluations of bioavailability are generally conducted in those with severe stable renal insufficiency, i.e. stage 5 CKD also called end-stage kidney disease (ESKD). The assessment of bioavailability in this patient population is further complicated, because most patients with severe CKD receive multiple medications, many of which cannot be discontinued during the course of a bioavailability study.

Some of the drug absorption "bioavailability" studies in ESKD patients have not provided an assessment of absolute bioavailability (i.e., they have not included intravenous administration of the drug). Rather, they have documented alterations in the peak concentration (C_{max}), time at which the peak concentration was attained (t_{max}), or in the fractional amount of drug recovered in the urine in a finite time period. Unfortunately, this limited information has been extrapolated to suggest that drug absorption is slowed and/or that the extent of absorption is reduced.[6]

The absolute bioavailability of only a few drug compounds is affected by ESKD. An increase in bioavailability as the result of a decrease in metabolism during the drug's first pass through the gastrointestinal tract and liver has been noted for some β-blockers (i.e., bufuralol, oxprenolol, propranolol, and tolamolol), dextropropoxyphene, and dihydrocodeine.[6,8] Although the bioavailability of these compounds is increased, clinical consequences (development of excessive or unexpected adverse effects) have only been demonstrated with dextropropoxyphene and dihydrocodeine. The lack of association between the pharmacokinetic profile and clinical consequences of the β-blockers may result from an alteration in the responsiveness of patients with renal disease to these agents, as has been reported with propranolol in the elderly.[3]

EFFECT ON DRUG DISTRIBUTION

The volume of distribution of many drugs may be significantly increased or decreased in patients with renal insufficiency (Table 48–1).[8,12,13] Alterations in distribution volume may result from increased or decreased protein binding; altered tissue binding; or pathophysio-

TABLE 48–1. Effect of End-Stage Kidney Disease (ESKD) on the Volume of Distribution of Selected Drugs[a]

	Normal	ESKD	Change from Normal (%)
Increased			
Amikacin	0.20	0.29	45
Azlocillin	0.21	0.28	33
Bretylium	3.58	4.48	25
Cefazolin	0.13	0.17	31
Cefonicid	0.11	0.14	27
Cefoxitin	0.16	0.26	63
Cefuroxime	0.20	0.26	30
Clofibrate	0.14	0.24	71
Cloxacillin	0.14	0.26	86
Dicloxacillin	0.08	0.18	125
Erythromycin	0.57	1.09	91
Furosemide	0.11	0.18	64
Gentamicin	0.20	0.32	60
Isoniazid	0.6	0.8	33
Minoxidil	2.6	4.9	88
Nalmefene	7.9	14.7	86
Naproxen	0.12	0.17	42
Phenytoin	0.64	1.4	119
Trimethoprim	1.36	1.83	35
Vancomycin	0.64	0.85	33
Decreased			
Chloramphenicol	0.87	0.60	−31
Digoxin	7.3	4.0	−45
Ethambutol	3.7	1.6	−57
Methicillin	0.45	0.30	−33
Pindolol	150 L	80 L	−47
Pipemidic acid	2.0	0.84	−58

[a]All data are in liters per kilogram unless otherwise stated.

TABLE 48–2. Change in Percent Unbound of Acidic Drugs in Patients with Normal Renal Function and End-Stage Kidney Disease (ESKD)

	Normal	ESKD	Change from Normal (%)
Abecarnil	4	15	275
Azlocillin	62.5	75	20
Cefazolin	16	29	81
Cefoxitin	27	59	119
Ceftriaxone	10	20	100
Clofibrate	3	9	200
Cloxacillin	5	20	300
Diazoxide	6	16	167
Dicloxacillin	3	9	200
Diflunisal	12	44	267
Doxycycline	12	28	133
Eprosartan	2	4	100
Furosemide	4	6	50
Methotrexate	57.2	63.8	12
Metolazone	5	10	100
Moxalactam	48	64	33
Naproxen	0.2	0.8	300
Pentobarbital	34	41	21
Phenylbutazone	5.5	16	191
Phenytoin	10	21.5	115
Salicylate	8	20	150
Sulfamethoxazole	34	58	71
Valproic acid	8	23	188
Warfarin	1	2	100
Zomepirac	1.3	3.8	192

logic alterations in body composition (e.g., the fractional contribution of total body water to total body weight; or they may be an artifact of the volume term used in the comparison).

Generally, the plasma protein binding of acidic drugs (e.g., warfarin and phenytoin) is decreased in those with ESKD[7,14] (Table 48–2), whereas the binding of basic drugs (e.g., quinidine and lidocaine) is usually normal or slightly decreased or increased[7,15,16] (Table 48–3). The decrease in binding of acidic drugs has been attributed to qualitative changes in the binding sites, accumulation of endogenous inhibitors of binding, and decreased concentrations of albumin. The first two of these mechanisms appear to account for most of the observed changes in binding. In addition, the high concentrations of metabolites of some compounds that accumulate in patients with ESKD may interfere with the protein binding of the parent compound.

Although the fraction of unbound drug increases in patients with renal insufficiency, a new equilibrium is established as a result of increased drug elimination/distribution such that the free concentrations remain comparable. However, total concentrations are reduced because of an increase in drug clearance. Thus the net effect of changes in protein binding is an alteration in the relationship between total drug concentration and effect. This can be illustrated with the anticonvulsant phenytoin. The protein binding of this acidic drug, which binds to albumin, is significantly reduced as a result of endogenous substances that accumulate in renal failure and compete for binding, as well as by conformational changes in albumin in CKD patients.[17] This change in protein binding alters the relationship between total phenytoin concentration and effect or toxicity. The resulting increase in unbound fraction, from the normal of 0.1 to 0.2 or more, results in increased hepatic clearance and decreased total concentrations. Thus in patients with CKD, the therapeutic range based on total phenytoin

TABLE 48–3. Change in Percent Unbound of Basic Drugs in Patients with Normal Renal Function and End-Stage Kidney Disease (ESKD)

	Normal	ESKD	Change from Normal (%)
Decreased			
Bepridil	0.3	0.1	−67
Clonidine	55.6	47.6	−14
Disopyramide	32	28	−13
Propafenone	3.4	2.4	−29
Increased			
Amphotericin B	3.5	4.1	17
Chloramphenicol	45	64	42
Clonazepam	13.9	16	15
Clorazepate	2	5	150
Diazepam	2	8	300
Fluoxetine	5.5	6.5	18
Ketoconazole	1	1.5	50
Morphine	65	71	9
Prazosin	6	10.1	68
Rosiglitazone	0.16	0.22	38
Triamterene	19	43	126

concentration (normal, 10 to 20 mcg/mL) shifts downward as the degree of renal impairment increases. The unbound concentration therapeutic range is however unchanged in the presence of renal failure.

Unbound concentration measurements provide the best means for individualizing phenytoin therapy in patients with renal insufficiency. They are however not widely available nor routinely utilized. Therefore methods have been presented to equate an observed total concentration in patients with ESKD receiving hemodialysis treatment to what would be expected in patients with normal renal function. Liponi and associates[17] suggested a method by which the total phenytoin concentration (C_m^{total}) in patients with creatinine clearance values of 10 to 24 mL/min or less than 10 mL/min can be equated to the concentration that would be observed if plasma protein concentrations and phenytoin-binding characteristics were normal. A patient's "equated" total phenytoin concentration (C_e^{total}) would thus equal:

$$C_e^{total} = \left(\frac{1}{[1] + [(nK_a)(p)]} \right) \left(C_m^{total}(10) \right)$$

where nK_a is the binding parameter based on the patient's renal function (10 to 24 mL/min = 1.5, and <10 mL/min = 1.0), and p is the measured serum albumin concentration. This methodology allows one to approximate the equivalent "total" phenytoin concentration in a patient with reduced renal function and can be used to predict dosage requirements via a standard nonlinear approach (see Chap. 5).

The principal binding protein for several basic drug compounds is α_1-acid glycoprotein, which is an acute-phase reactant with increased plasma concentrations in a wide variety of patients, including renal transplant patients and hemodialysis patients.[8] The fraction of those drugs principally bound to α_1-acid glycoprotein may be significantly increased in ESKD patients.[7] Thus patients with renal insufficiency may experience increased or decreased protein binding, depending on the principal binding protein for the drug in question.

Altered tissue binding may also affect the apparent volume of distribution of a drug. For example, the distribution volume of digoxin has been reported to be reduced by 30% to 50% from normal values in patients with renal disease.[18] It has been postulated that this reduction in the distribution volume is secondary to a decrease in tissue

binding as a result of competitive inhibition by endogenous or exogenous substances. This factor must therefore be considered when designing individualized dosage regimens. Multiple methods have been proposed to estimate the degree of reduction in digoxin's distribution volume.[18] The volume of distribution (V_D) of digoxin can be estimated as follows:

$$V_{D(liters)} = [226] + \left[\frac{(298)(CLcr)}{29.1 + CLcr} \right]$$

For a patient weighing 60 kg with a creatinine clearance (CLcr) of approximately 15 mL/min per 1.73 m^2, the volume of distribution for digoxin would be:

$$V_{D(liters)} = [226] + \left[\frac{(298)(15)}{29.1 + 15} \right] = 327 \text{ L or } 5.5 \text{ L/kg}$$

This represents a 30% reduction from the volume of distribution that would have been anticipated in a patient with normal renal function. Acidosis or the presence of digoxin-like immunoreactive substances that bind to and inhibit membrane ATPase may also contribute to this phenomenon.[19] In this situation, the absolute amount of digoxin bound to the receptor is reduced and the resultant serum digoxin concentration from any dose would be greater.

Knowledge of protein and tissue binding changes in patients with renal insufficiency is critically important in the interpretation of serum drug concentrations. Numerous investigations show that the unbound concentration of several drugs in plasma correlates more closely with the concentration of drug at the receptor site, and therefore with the pharmacologic effect, than does the total concentration of drug in plasma.[20] Because an alteration in plasma protein or tissue binding of a drug will likely alter the total drug concentration, the usual expected relationship between total drug concentration and pharmacologic response will be perturbed, but the relationship to unbound drug should not be affected.

Thus in patients with renal insufficiency, particularly those with ESKD a "normal" total drug concentration may be associated with either serious adverse reactions secondary to elevated unbound drug concentrations, or subtherapeutic responses because of an altered plasma:tissue drug concentration ratio. Therefore the monitoring of unbound drug concentrations in this patient population is suggested for those drugs that have a narrow therapeutic range, are highly protein bound (free fraction of <20%), and for which marked variability in the free fraction has been reported (e.g., phenytoin and disopyramide).

Finally, the method used to calculate the volume of distribution may be influenced by renal insufficiency. The three most commonly used volume of distribution terms are volume of the central compartment (V_c), volume of the terminal phase (V_β, V_{area}), and volume of distribution at steady state (V_{ss}). The central compartment volume is calculated as the intravenous bolus dose divided by the initial plasma concentration. V_c for many drugs approximates extracellular fluid volume and thus may be increased or decreased by shifts in this physiologic volume. Renal insufficiency, especially oliguric acute renal failure, is often accompanied by fluid overload and a resultant increased V_c due to reduced renal elimination of water and sodium. V_{area} or V_β is calculated as the total body clearance divided by the terminal elimination rate constant (k or β). This volume term represents the proportionality constant between plasma concentrations in the terminal elimination phase and the amount of drug remaining in the body. V_β is affected by both distribution characteristics, as well as by the elimination rate constant. The third volume term, the steady-state volume of distribution (V_{ss}), is calculated as (AUMC × dose)/AUC^2, where AUMC is the area under the first moment of the concentration-time curve and AUC is the area under the concentration-time curve (see Chap. 5). V_β and V_{ss} will often be similar in magnitude, with V_β being slightly larger. In situations in which V_β is much larger than V_{ss}, V_β may reflect the elimination rate more than the distribution volume. Because V_{ss} has the advantage of being independent of drug elimination, it may be the most appropriate volume term to use when one desires to compare drug distribution volumes between patients with renal insufficiency and those with normal renal function.[21]

EFFECT ON METABOLISM

A decrease in the renal elimination of drugs in patients with renal insufficiency is well appreciated and rational methods for adjusting treatment regimens on the basis of renal function are presented in this chapter. However, in addition to the expected decrease in renal drug elimination, there is increasing evidence that CKD also alters other elimination pathways, most notably cytochrome P450 (CYP450)-mediated metabolism in the liver and other organs.[9]

Initial clinical evidence supporting the notion that kidney disease affects hepatic drug metabolism included observations of reduced nonrenal clearance for several drugs in patients with renal insufficiency.[9,11] The observed reductions in nonrenal clearance were generally proportional to the reductions in glomerular filtration rate (GFR). However, the effect(s) of renal failure on nonrenal drug clearance may also depend on whether the renal failure is acute or chronic in nature. Effects observed in ARF do not appear to be as great as those observed in ESKD patients, potentially due to less accumulation of/or exposure to metabolic inhibitors.[11] The nonrenal clearance of a drug may be increased, decreased, or unaffected by renal failure, depending on the metabolic pathway(s) involved and the drug and the species (animals versus humans) investigated[22–24] (Table 48–4). In general, these studies should be interpreted with caution since concurrent drug intake, age, smoking status, and alcohol intake were often not controlled. Furthermore, the possibility of pharmacogenetic variation in drug-metabolizing enzymes (e.g., CYP450 enzymes) must be considered. Prediction of the effect of renal insufficiency on the metabolism of a particular drug is thus difficult and a general quantitative strategy to adjust treatment regimens is not available. However, some insight can be gained if one knows what particular enzyme is involved in the metabolism of the drug of interest and how the enzyme(s) is affected in the presence of renal insufficiency.

CYP450 enzymes are widely distributed throughout the body with the most abundant expression being found in the liver and intestine. CYP450 enzymes in the kidney catalyze the metabolism of a variety of chemicals and drugs with activity similar to that in the liver on an activity-per-gram-of-tissue basis, but the contribution to total metabolic activity is generally low since total kidney weight is far less than total liver weight.

Investigations of the effect of chronic renal failure on hepatic enzyme activity in animals have demonstrated reductions in some, but not all, pathways of drug metabolism.[9,25] The mechanism(s) by which chronic renal failure affects hepatic drug metabolism is not clearly known, but may relate to accumulation of endogenous inhibitors (e.g., uremic toxins) or to the fact that CKD patients exist in a chronic inflammatory state and have increased levels of oxidative stress,[26] factors known to downregulate CYP450 enzymes.[27] It has been shown in rat models of chronic renal failure that protein expression of several CYP450 enzymes, including CYP450 3A1 and CYP450 3A2 (corresponding to human CYP450 3A4), is reduced in the liver by as much as 75%. The mechanism of this decrease in protein content is reduced mRNA expression, indicating transcriptionally mediated downregulation.[25] The in vivo relevance of these effects was demonstrated in rats with chronic renal failure using enzyme-selective breath tests; the results showed that chronic renal failure has differential effects on enzyme activity with CYP450 2C11 and CYP450 3A2 being significantly reduced (by 35%), while CYP450 1A2 activity was no different from that in control animals.[28] Consistent with these observations in animals, CYP450 3A activity as measured by the erythromycin breath test was 28% lower in ESKD patients as compared to healthy controls.[29] While baseline CYP450 3A activity was lower in these patients, the increase in CYP450 3A activity observed following enzyme induction with rifampin was similar.[29] Collectively, these data indicate that chronic renal impairment has a detrimental effect on some important pathways of hepatic drug metabolism.

In addition to changes in hepatic metabolism, chronic renal failure has also been shown in animals to affect the expression and activity of CYP450 enzymes in the intestine.[30] CYP450 1A1 and CYP450 3A2 enzyme content was reduced by 43% and 71%, respectively, and corresponding mRNA levels were decreased by 32% and 36%, respectively. Although this has not been specifically evaluated in humans, an effect on intestinal metabolism may be clinically relevant for those drugs for which intestinal metabolism is known to be important (e.g., CYP450 3A substrates with low bioavailability).

Unfortunately, the effect of renal insufficiency on CYP450 enzymes has not been fully evaluated, but current data suggest a differential effect on the individual enzymes with the activity of some enzymes (e.g., CYP450 3A4 and CYP450 2C9) being reduced,[29,31] while others (e.g., CYP450 2E1) are not affected.[32] This differential effect on individual enzymes may help to explain some of the conflicting reports of whether drug metabolism is altered in the presence of renal disease. If the metabolism of a drug is known to be increased or decreased in patients with renal failure, then the dose will need to be adjusted appropriately to achieve the desired effect. If the effect of renal failure on metabolism is unknown, then the agent should be used with extreme caution.

TABLE 48–4. Effect of End-Stage Kidney Disease on Nonrenal Clearance

Decreased			
Acyclovir	Aztreonam	Bufuralol	Captopril
Cefmenoxime	Cefmetazole	Cefonicid	Cefotaxime
Cefotiam	Cefsulodin	Ceftizoxime	Cilastatin
Cimetidine	Ciprofloxacin	Cortisol	Encainide
Erythromycin	Imipenem	Isoniazid	Methylprednisolone
Metoclopramide	Moxalactam	Nicardipine	Nimodipine
Nitrendipine	Procainamide	Quinapril	Repaglinide
Verapamil	Zidovudine		
Unchanged			
Acetaminophen	Chloramphenicol	Clonidine	Codeine
Diflunisal	Indomethacin	Insulin[a]	Isradipine
Lidocaine	Morphine	Metoprolol	Nisoldipine
Nortriptyline	Pentobarbital	Propafenone	Quinidine
Theophylline	Tocainide	Tolbutamide	
Increased			
Bumetanide	Cefpiramide	Fosinopril	Nifedipine
Phenytoin	Rosiglitazone	Sulfadimidine	

[a]May be unchanged or decreased.

EFFECT OF RENAL INSUFFICIENCY ON METABOLITE ELIMINATION

Patients with severe renal insufficiency receiving chronic treatment with some agents may experience accumulation of metabolite(s) as

TABLE 48–5. Pharmacologic Activity of Selected Drug Metabolites

Parent Drug	Metabolite	Pharmacologic Activity of Metabolites
Acetaminophen	N-acetyl-p-benzo-quinoneimine	Responsible for hepatotoxicity
Allopurinol	Oxipurinol	Metabolite primarily responsible for suppression of xanthine oxidase
Azathioprine	Mercaptopurine	All of the immunosuppressive activity resides in the metabolite
Cefotaxime	Desacetyl cefotaxime	Similar antimicrobial spectrum, but one-fourth to one-tenth as potent
Chlorpropamide	2-Hydroxychlorpropamide	Similar in vitro insulin-releasing activity
Clofibrate	Chlorophenoxyisobutyric acid	Primarily responsible for hypolipidemic effect and direct muscle toxicity
Codeine	Morphine-6-glucuronide	Possibly more active than parent compound; may contribute to prolonged narcotic effect in renal failure patients
Imipramine	Desmethylimipramine	Similar antidepressant activity
Ketoprofen	Ketoprofen glucuronide	Accumulation of acyl glucuronide may worsen toxic effects (gastrointestinal disturbances and impairment of renal function)
Meperidine	Normeperidine	Less analgesic activity than parent, but more CNS-stimulatory effects
Morphine	Morphine-6-glucuronide	Possibly more active than parent compound; may contribute to prolonged narcotic effect in renal failure patients
Mycophenolic acid	Mycophenolic acid glucuronide	Lacks pharmacological activity but may be associated with dose-limiting (gastrointestinal) side effects
Procainamide	N-acetyl procainamide	Distinct antiarrhythmic activity, the mechanism of which is different from that of the parent compound
Sulfonamides	Acetylated metabolites	Devoid of antibacterial activity, but elevated concentrations are associated with increased toxicity
Theophylline	1,3-Dimethyl uric acid	Cardiotoxicity has been demonstrated
Zidovudine	Zidovudine triphosphate	Primarily responsible for antiretroviral activity

well as parent compound. Metabolites of several drugs have been reported to have significant pharmacologic and/or toxicologic activity. However, the pharmacokinetics and pharmacology of metabolites are not often fully elucidated in humans. In a sense, the patient with severe renal impairment is being exposed to a new pharmacologic entity if the serum concentrations of the metabolite exceed those reported in patients with normal renal function.

The metabolite may have pharmacologic activity similar to that of the parent drug and thus contribute significantly to clinical response; for example, oxypurinol and desacetyl cefotaxime.[33] Alternatively, the metabolite may have qualitatively dissimilar pharmacologic action; for example, normeperidine has central nervous system (CNS)-stimulatory activity that reportedly produces seizures, whereas meperidine has CNS-depressant actions.[34] Because of the multiplicity of potential interactions of compounds that are primarily metabolized, the practical consequences of metabolite accumulation are difficult to predict and are most often identified in those patients at risk by trial and error (Table 48–5).

EFFECT ON RENAL EXCRETION

Net renal clearance (CL_R) of a drug is the composite of GFR, tubular secretion, and reabsorption ($CL_R = (GFR \times f_u) + CL_{secretion} - CL_{reabsorption}$), where f_u is the fraction of the drug unbound to plasma proteins. Drug elimination by filtration occurs by a diffusion process, but tubular secretion and reabsorption are bidirectional processes that involve carrier-mediated renal transport systems.[35] Renal transport systems have been broadly classified on the basis of substrate selectivity into the anionic and cationic renal transport systems, which are responsible for the transport of a number of organic acidic and basic drugs, respectively. Renal organic anion transport is mediated by organic anion transporters, organic anion transporting polypeptides, and multidrug resistance–associated protein transporters.[35] Several drugs including β-lactam antibiotics, diuretics, and nonsteroidal anti-inflammatory drugs are eliminated by members of these transporter families. These transporters also have an essential role in the elimination of glucuronide metabolites. Organic cation transport systems mediate the reabsorption and excretion of endogenous cationic compounds and cationic drugs (e.g., cimetidine, famotidine, and quinidine). The P-glycoprotein transport system in the kidney is also involved in the secretion of cationic and hydrophobic drugs (e.g., digoxin and vinca alkaloids).[35]

Other important renal transport systems include the peptide transporters, which are involved in the uptake of peptide-like drugs including β-lactam antibiotics and angiotensin-converting enzyme inhibitors, and nucleoside transporter proteins, which are involved in uptake of nucleosides and nucleoside analogs (e.g., zidovudine and dideoxyinosine).[35]

Alterations in one or more of the three renal processes (filtration, secretion, or reabsorption) secondary to reductions in functional nephron mass may have a dramatic effect on the pharmacokinetics of a drug. A reduction in glomerular filtration rate results in a decrease in renal drug clearance. For drugs that are extensively renally secreted (CL_R >300 mL/min), the loss of filtration clearance (up to 120 mL/min) will have less of an impact than for those primarily dependent on GFR.

Although it was once thought that the mechanisms of renal elimination declined in a parallel manner in the presence of renal disease, it is now known that this may not be a valid assumption. Kamiya and associates[36] and Hori and colleagues[37] demonstrated that the type of renal disease may explain in part the differences in pharmacokinetic parameters observed among patients with similar reductions in GFR. The disposition of antibiotic agents extensively secreted by the proximal renal tubules (e.g., ampicillin and cephalexin) was altered to a greater degree in patients with tubulointerstitial disease as compared to those with primary glomerular disease. Quantitative investigations of renal handling of new drugs will be required to elucidate the relative contribution of tubular and glomerular function to renal drug clearance. The availability of these data should provide a more rational approach to dosage regimen design for those agents that undergo extensive tubular secretion or reabsorption.

In the absence of data delineating the contribution of tubular function to renal elimination, the clinical measurement or estimation of creatinine clearance remains the guiding factor for drug-dosage regimen design.[8,10] Although several methods have been proposed to estimate GFR from routinely available clinical data (see Chap. 41) the utility of a calculated GFR to guide drug dosing has not been extensively evaluated. The importance of an alteration in renal function on drug elimination thus depends on two factors: the fraction of drug normally eliminated by the kidney unchanged and the degree of renal insufficiency.

Quantitation of the patient's renal function can be accomplished by measurement of creatinine clearance or estimation based on the stable serum creatinine (see Chap. 41). Because of the time delay involved and problems in obtaining complete urine collections, measured creatinine clearance values are infrequently used for initial drug-dosage regimen design. Therefore the calculation of initial drug dosage regimens relies on the estimation of creatinine clearance (CLcr) in adults and children from such routinely available clinical data as age, gender, height, weight, and serum creatinine. These relationships are most accurate for individuals of average muscle mass for their age, weight, and height. The creatinine clearance of emaciated and obese adult patients is difficult to predict, and incorrect estimates have been obtained with most methods.

Several methods are also available for estimating creatinine clearance in adults with ARF using age, height, weight, serum creatinine, and time data (see Chap. 41). These methods have not been as rigorously validated as the equations for patients with stable renal function. However, they are one of the few methods we have to approximate renal function in this complex patient situation.

DRUG-DOSAGE REGIMEN DESIGNS

PATIENTS WITH RENAL INSUFFICIENCY

The typical steps involved in designing a dosage regimen in a patient with renal insufficiency as the result of an acute insult or CKD are listed in Table 48–6. Most dosage adjustment guidelines have proposed the use of a fixed dose or interval for patients with broad ranges of renal function.[12,38,39] For example, moderate renal insufficiency may encompass a creatinine clearance range of 30 to 50 mL/min, severe renal insufficiency is often defined as a creatinine clearance of 15 to 29 mL/min, and ESKD is defined by a creatinine clearance <15 mL/min. These categories encompass up to a 10-fold range in renal function, and thus the drug regimen may not be optimal for all patients whose renal function lies within the range.

The design of the optimal dosage regimen for patients with renal insufficiency requires an individualized assessment and is dependent on the availability of an accurate characterization of the relationship between the pharmacokinetic parameters of the drug and renal function, and an accurate assessment of the patient's renal function, CLcr. Secondary references such as the American Hospital Formulary Service Drug Information book,[38] and textbooks[13,40] and computer databases (e.g., Micromedex or Clinical Pharmacology) are excellent sources of information about a drug's pharmacokinetic characteristics in subjects with normal renal function. However, they often do not provide the explicit relationships of the kinetic parameters of interest (total body clearance, elimination rate constant, and distribution volume) with a continuous index of renal function, such as CLcr. To find this information, one may need to identify the original research study that assessed the drug's disposition, or a comprehensive review article on the class of drugs of interest. Ideally, one should be able to identify a relationship between total body clearance (CL), elimination rate constant (k), or distribution volume (V_D) with CLcr (Table 48–7). This information, along with the patient's CLcr, will enable prediction of the patient's kinetic parameters and then formulation of a therapeutic regimen to attain the desired therapeutic outcome (see Chap. 5).

If specific literature recommendations and/or the relationship of kinetic parameters to CLcr are not available, then one can estimate the kinetic parameters of the patient with the method of Rowland and Tozer,[10] provided you know the fraction of the drug that is eliminated renally unchanged (f_e) in subjects with normal renal function.[13] This approach assumes that the change in CL and k are proportional to CLcr, that renal disease does not alter the drug's metabolism, that the metabolites if formed are inactive and nontoxic, that the drug obeys first-order (linear) kinetic principles, and that it is adequately described by a one-compartment model. If these assumptions are true, then the kinetic parameter/dosage adjustment factor (Q) can be calculated as:

$$Q = 1 - [f_e(1 - KF)]$$

where KF is the ratio of the patient's CLcr to the assumed normal value of 120 mL/min. Thus for a drug that is 85% eliminated renally

TABLE 48–6. Steps to Adjust Drug Dosages for Patients with Renal Insufficiency

Step 1	Obtain history and relevant demographic/clinical information	Record demographic information, obtain past medical history including history of renal disease, and record current laboratory information (e.g., serum creatinine)
Step 2	Estimate creatinine clearance	Use equation (e.g., Cockcroft-Gault) to estimate creatinine clearance, or calculate creatinine clearance from timed urine collection
Step 3	Review current medications	Identify drugs for which individualization of the treatment regimen will be necessary
Step 4	Calculate individualized treatment regimen	Determine treatment goals (see text); calculate dosage regimen based on pharmacokinetic characteristics of the drug and the patient's renal function
Step 5	Monitoring	Monitor parameters of drug response and toxicity; monitor drugs levels if available/applicable
Step 6	Revise regimen	Adjust regimen based on drug response or change in patient status (including renal function) as warranted

TABLE 48–7. Relationship between Renal Function and Pharmacokinetic Parameters of Selected Drugs

Drug	Total Body Clearance
Acyclovir	CL = 3.37 (CLcr) + 0.41
Amikacin	CL = 0.6 (CLcr) + 9.6
Cefmetazole	CL = 1.18 (CLcr) − 0.29
Ceftazidime	CL = 1.15 (CLcr) + 10.6
Ciprofloxacin	CL = 2.83 (CLcr) + 363
Digoxin	CL = 0.88 (CLcr) + 23
Gentamicin	CL = 0.983 (CLcr)
Lithium	CL = 0.235 (CLcr)
Netilmicin	CL = 0.65 (CLcr) + 3.72
Ofloxacin	CL = 1.04 (CLcr) + 38.7
Piperacillin	CL = 1.36 (CLcr) + 1.50
Teicoplanin	CL = 7.09 (CLcr) − 16.2
Tobramycin	CL = 0.801 (CLcr)
Vancomycin	CL = 0.69 (CLcr) + 3.7

ABW, average body weight; CL, total body clearance; CLcr, creatinine clearance. Compiled from St. Peter et al,[12] Thummel et al,[13] and Murphy.[42]

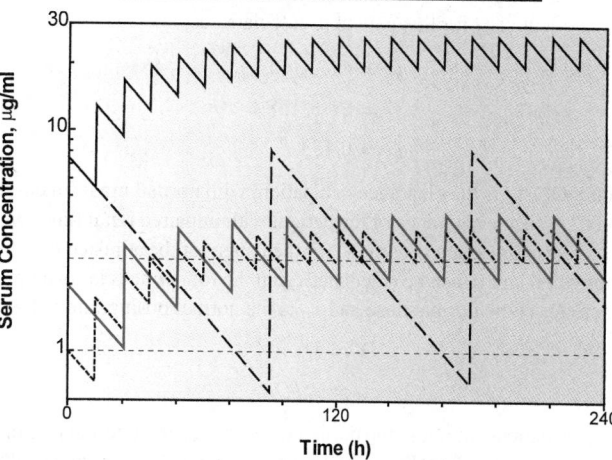

Scenario	Dose	τ	Cmax	Cmin	Cave	
A	5.0	12	27.0	19.6	22.6	——
B	0.67	12	3.6	2.6	3.0	······
C	5.0	90	8.1	0.7	3.0	– · –
D	1.33	24	4.2	2.2	3.0	– –

FIGURE 48–1. Without a change in dosage regimen, this patient would achieve excessive steady-state serum concentrations (Scenario A). Although the average steady-state concentrations (Cave) are identical, the concentration-time profile will be markedly different if one changes the dose and maintains the dosing interval (τ) constant (Scenario B), versus changing the dosing interval and maintaining the dose constant (Scenario C) or changing both (Scenario D).

unchanged in a patient who has a CLcr of 10 mL/min, the Q factor would be:

$$Q = 1 - [0.85(1 - (10/120))]$$
$$= 1 - [0.85(0.92)]$$
$$= 1 - 0.78$$
$$= 0.22$$

The estimated total body clearance for this patient would then be calculated as $CL_{PT} = CL_{norm} \times Q$, where CL_{norm} is the mean value in patients with normal renal function as reported in the literature.

After the kinetic parameters for the patient are estimated, the best method for dosage regimen adjustment should be selected. Specifically, one must determine whether the desired goal is the maintenance of a similar peak, trough, or average steady-state drug concentration. If there is a significant relationship between peak concentration and clinical response[41] (e.g., aminoglycosides) or toxicity[42] (e.g., quinidine, phenobarbital, and phenytoin), then attainment of the specific target values is critical. If, however, no specific target values for peak or trough concentrations have been reported (e.g., antihypertensive agents, benzodiazepines, and cephalosporins), then a regimen goal of attaining the same average steady-state concentration may be appropriate.

Although several methods have been proposed to attain the desired average steady-state concentration profile, the principal choices are to decrease the dose or prolong the dosing interval. If the size of the dose is reduced while the dosing interval remains unchanged, the desired average steady-state concentration will be similar; however, the peak will be lower and the trough higher (Fig. 48–1). Alternatively, if the dosing interval is increased and the dose size remains unchanged, the peak and trough concentrations in the patient with reduced renal function will be similar to those in the patient with normal renal function. This dosage adjustment method is often preferred because it is likely to yield significant cost savings as a result of a reduction in nursing and pharmacy time, as well as a reduction in the supplies associated with frequent drug administration. Finally, the dose and dosing interval may both need to be changed to attain a desired peak or trough serum concentration time profile.

Regardless of the approach chosen to adjust the dosage regimen, the first step in the process, if the relationship between the pharma-

cokinetic parameters of the drug and renal function are known, is to estimate the drug disposition parameters in the patient with renal insufficiency. The ratio (Q) of the estimated elimination rate constant or total body clearance of the patient relative to subjects with normal renal function (CLcr >120 mL/min) may then be calculated. This parameter may be used to determine the dose or dosing interval alterations necessary for the patient.

For example, the following relationship between total clearance (CL) and creatinine clearance has been reported for ganciclovir:[43]

$$CL(mL/min/1.8\,m^2) = 1.25(CLcr) + 8.57$$

Thus CL for a subject with normal renal function (CL_{norm}) would be calculated as:

$$CL_{norm} = [1.25(120)] + 8.57$$
$$CL_{mean} = 158.6\,mL/min\ per\ 1.8\,m^2$$

Clearance (CL_{fail}) for a patient with a creatinine clearance of 10 mL/min would be:

$$CL_{fail} = [1.25(10)] + 8.57$$
$$CL_{fail} = 21.1\,mL/min\ per\ 1.8\,m^2$$

Ganciclovir is commonly used in solid organ transplant patients as prophylaxis against or treatment for cytomegalovirus infection.[44] The inhibitory concentration of 50% (IC_{50}) of ganciclovir against most clinical isolates of cytomegalovirus is between 0.1 and 2.8 mcg/mL (approximately 0.4 to 11 mcmol/L).[43] Therefore trough concentrations should exceed these values, but caution is warranted since neutropenia has been associated with the attainment of ganciclovir trough concentrations exceeding 2.6 mcg/mL (10 mcmol/L).[45] Although a definitive relationship between ganciclovir concentration and either efficacy or toxicity has not been established,[43] it is standard practice to adjust the dose based on renal function. If a patient with reduced renal function received the typical ganciclovir dose for a patient with normal renal function, the predicted trough concentrations would approach 20 mcmol/L. Therefore a dosage modification in this patient is necessary to avoid potential toxicity. The dosing regimen can be modified using the ratio of the predicted clearance values. Therefore the quotient or Q for this patient is calculated as:

$$Q = CL_{fail}/CL_{norm}$$
$$Q = 21.1/158.6$$
$$Q = 0.133$$

where CL_{norm} is the clearance in a patient with normal renal function and CL_{fail} is the clearance of the patient with impaired renal function.

The maintenance dose (D_f) for the patient or the adjusted dosing interval (τ_f) may then be calculated from the following relationships, where D_n is the normal dose and τ_n is the normal dosing interval:

$$D_f = D_n \times Q$$
$$\tau_f = \tau_n/Q$$

For this patient situation, the normal dose and dosing interval of ganciclovir would be 5 mg/kg and 12 hours, respectively. If we wanted to maintain the dosing interval at 12 hours, then D_f would be calculated as:

$$D_f = (5\,\text{mg/kg}) \times (0.133) = 0.67\,\text{mg/kg}$$

This regimen would result in decreased peak and trough concentrations compared to a patient with this degree of renal insufficiency who received a normal dosage regimen (see Fig. 48–1, Scenario B). The peak concentrations would however be lower and the trough concentrations higher than those observed when a patient with normal renal function received a standard regimen.

If we want to maintain D_n and extend the dosing interval, τ_f would be calculated as:

$$\tau_f = \tau_n/Q = 12/0.133 = 90\,\text{hours}$$

This regimen would yield similar peak and trough concentrations in the renally impaired patient as in the patient with normal renal function, but there is a risk of missed doses with such an unorthodox interval (see Fig. 48–1, Scenario C). In addition, the prolonged period below the C_{ss} average concentration may be less than optimal.

Finally, a practical dosing interval (τ_p) may be selected and then a dose based on that interval can be calculated (see Fig. 48–1, Scenario D). If a dosage interval τ_f of 24 hours were selected, because in many institutions there is an increased risk of missed doses with longer dosing intervals, then the D_f would be calculated as follows:

$$D_f = [D_n \times Q \times \tau_f]/\tau_p$$
$$= [(5\,\text{mg/kg}) \times (0.133) \times (24)]/12$$
$$= 1.33\,\text{mg/kg}$$

This method would likely be most appropriate in this case; prolonged subtherapeutic concentrations are avoided and troughs are reduced from the first method. The selection of which dosage adjustment method to use to calculate an optimal regimen depends on the drug characteristics and the patient care situation. This dosage adjustment method assumes that the protein binding and volume of distribution of the drug are not significantly altered by renal insufficiency. Thus this approach cannot be used with accuracy for those drugs with demonstrated differences in these pharmacokinetic parameters.

If the volume of distribution (V_D) of a drug is significantly altered in patients with renal insufficiency or in whom one desires to attain a specific maximum or minimum concentration, the estimation of a dosage regimen becomes more complex. If the relationship between V_D and creatinine clearance has been characterized, then V_D may be estimated. If one assumes that a one-compartment linear model can describe the drug, the predicted V_D may then be used with the predicted elimination rate constant (k) of the drug to yield an adjusted dosing interval and intravenous or oral dose.

For orally administered drugs, the τ_f can be calculated as:

$$\tau_f = [(-1/k_f)(\ln[C_{min}/C_{max}])] + t_{peak}$$

and the dose can be approximated as:

$$\text{Dose}_{po} = [SFC_p^t\, V_D(k_a - k)]/[k_a\,(e^{-kt}/1 - e^{-k\tau})\,(e^{-k_a t}/1 - e^{-k_a \tau})]$$

where, S equals the salt fraction, F equals bioavailability, C_p^t equals the desired plasma concentration at time t, and k_a is the absorption rate constant. This approach allows for the individualization of a dosage regimen for attainment of specific peak and trough serum concentrations. If the drug is absorbed extremely rapidly, one can approximate the τ_f as:

$$\tau_f = (-1/k_f)(\ln[C_{min}/C_{max}])$$

and the dose as:

$$\text{Dose}_{po} = V_D \times (C_{max} - C_{min})$$

Digoxin is a frequently used oral medication for which the V_D is decreased in patients with renal insufficiency, and for which one usually desires to closely control the plasma concentration time profile. The V_D and CL_{fail} of digoxin can be estimated for a 70-kg patient with a CLcr of 12 mL/min per 1.73 m^2 as summarized by Job[18]:

$$V_D = 226 + [(298(CLcr))/(29.1 + CLcr)]$$
$$= 226 + [(298(12))/(29.1 + 12)]$$
$$= 226 + 87.0$$
$$= 313\,\text{L}$$
$$CL_{fail} = (0.88 \times CLcr) + 23\,\text{mL/min}$$
$$= 10.6 + 23$$
$$= 33.6\,\text{mL/min}$$
$$k_f = CL_{fail}/V_D$$
$$= (33.6\,\text{mL/min} \times 1440\,\text{min/d})/313\,\text{L}$$
$$= (48.3\,\text{L/d})/313\,\text{L}$$
$$= 0.154\,\text{day}^{-1}$$

The t_{peak} is generally at 2 hours, and the k_a from the literature is about 0.76 hour^{-1} or 18 day^{-1}.[13] Thus one now has all the information needed to calculate the τ_f and dose for this patient:

$$\tau_f = [(-1/k_f)(\ln[C_{min}/C_{max}])] + t_{peak}$$
$$= [(-1/0.154)(\ln[0.8/1.4])] + 2\,\text{hours}$$
$$= [(-6.49)(-0.56)] + 2\,\text{hours}$$
$$= 3.6\,\text{days} + 2\,\text{hours}$$
$$\approx 4\,\text{days}$$
$$\text{Dose}_{po} = [(1.4)(313)(18 - 0.154)]/[18(e^{-0.154(0.083)}/1 - e^{-0.154(4)})$$
$$-(e^{-18(0.083)}/1 - e^{-18(4)})]$$
$$= 0.226\,\text{mg or one 0.25 mg oral capsule every 4 days}$$

Alternately, the predicted volume of distribution and elimination rate constant or the total body clearance may be used to calculate a dose regimen that will maintain the desired average steady-state concentration of the drug (C_{ss}).

$$\text{Dose (mg/h)} = C_{SS}[(k_f \times V_D) \text{ or } (CL_f)]$$

Depending on how much variance above and below the average steady state one desires, the dosing interval may range from hourly to as infrequently as every 48 hours or longer. For example, if the calculated dose were 10 mg/h, the desired average steady-state concentration would be maintained with a dosing interval of 60 mg every 6 hours or 480 mg every 48 hours.

PATIENTS RECEIVING CONTINUOUS RENAL REPLACEMENT THERAPY

Continuous renal replacement therapy (CRRT) is used for the management of fluid overload and the removal of uremic toxins in patients with ARF and other conditions.[46] The several forms of CRRT are extensively described in Chap. 42. Which of these therapies will be optimal for a given patient is dependent on several factors, including bleeding risk, degree of hypercatabolism, acid-base balance, and experience of the health care provider.

Drug therapy individualization for the patient receiving CRRT is complicated by the fact that patients with ARF may have a higher residual nonrenal clearance of some drugs than patients with CKD who have a similar CLcr.[33,47–49] For example, the nonrenal clearance of imipenem in patients with ARF (91 mL/min) is between the values observed in CKD patients (50 mL/min) and those with normal renal function (130 mL/min).[48] This may occur because of less exposure to or accumulation of uremic by-products that may alter hepatic function. A nonrenal clearance value in a patient with ARF that is higher than anticipated based on chronic renal failure data would result in lower than expected, possibly subtherapeutic, serum concentrations. For example, in order to maintain comparable serum concentration, the imipenem dose requirement in patients with ARF would be 2,000 mg/24 hours as compared to the recommended dosage for patients with ESKD of 1,000 mg/24 hours.[48]

In addition to patient-specific differences, there are marked differences between intermittent hemodialysis and the three primary types of CRRT: continuous arteriovenous or venovenous hemofiltration (CAVH/CVVH), continuous arteriovenous or venovenous hemodialysis (CAVHD/CVVHD), and continuous arteriovenous or venovenous hemodiafiltration (CAVHDF/CVVHDF) with regard to drug removal.[46,50,51]

During CAVH/CVVH, drug removal primarily occurs via convection/ultrafiltration (the passive transport of drug molecules at the concentration at which they exist in plasma water into the ultrafiltrate). The clearance of a drug by either of these methods is thus a function of the membrane permeability for the drug, which is called the sieving coefficient (SC) and the rate of ultrafiltrate formation (UFR). The SC can be calculated as:

$$SC = (2C_{UF})/[(C_a/1 - \theta) + (C_v/1 - \theta)]$$

where C_a and C_v are the concentration of the drug in the plasma going into and returning from the filter, respectively; C_{UF} is the concentration in the ultrafiltrate; and θ is 0.0107 times the total protein concentration in plasma. The SC is often approximated by the fraction unbound (f_u) because this information may be more readily available. Thus the clearance by these two modes of CRRT can be calculated as:

$$CL_{CVVH} = UFR \times SC$$

or approximated as:

$$CL_{CVVH} = UFR \times f_u$$

Clearance of a drug by CAVHDF/CVVHDF (CL_{CAVHDF}/CL_{CVVHDF}) is generally greater than that by CAVH/CVVH, because in addition to the convection/ultrafiltration process, drug is removed by diffusion from the plasma water into the dialysate. The CL_{CVVHDF} can be mathematically approximated providing the blood flow rate is greater than 100 mL/min and the dialysate flow rate (DFR) is between 8 and 33 mL/min as:

$$CL_{CVVHDF} = (UFR \times f_u) + CL_{diffusion}$$

where $CL_{diffusion}$ is the clearance via diffusion from plasma water to the dialysate. In the clinical setting, it is not possible to separate these two components (blood flow rate and DFR) of CL_{CVVHDF}. In essence the CL_{CVVHDF} is calculated as the product of the combined ultrafiltrate and dialysate volume (V_{df}) and the concentration of the drug in this fluid (C_{df}) divided by the plasma concentration (C_p^{mid}) at the midpoint of the V_{df} collection period.

There are differences in the rate of drug removal, not only between the three primary modes of CRRT, but also within each mode.[46,49,50,52] This is a result of differences in the filter membrane composition, variable degrees of drug binding to the membrane and the permeability characteristics of the membrane.[53–56] The primary factors that influence drug clearance during CRRT are thus ultrafiltration rate, blood flow rate, and dialysate flow rate. For example, clearance in CAVH/CVVH is directly proportional to the ultrafiltration rate, whereas clearance during CAVHDF/CVVHDF, which depends on both the ultrafiltration rate and the dialysate flow rate, increases as either flow rate increases. Changes in blood flow rate generally have only a minor effect on drug clearance by any mode of CRRT. An increase in ultrafiltration flow rate (5 to 45 mL/min) and dialysate flow rate (8.3 to 33.3 mL/min) however have dramatic effects on ceftazidime clearance during CVVH and CVVHD respectively.[55] (Fig. 48-2)

An algorithmic approach for drug dosage adjustment in patients undergoing CRRT has been proposed.[46] Individualization of therapy for a patient receiving CRRT therapy is dependent on the patient's residual renal function and the clearance of the drug by the mode of

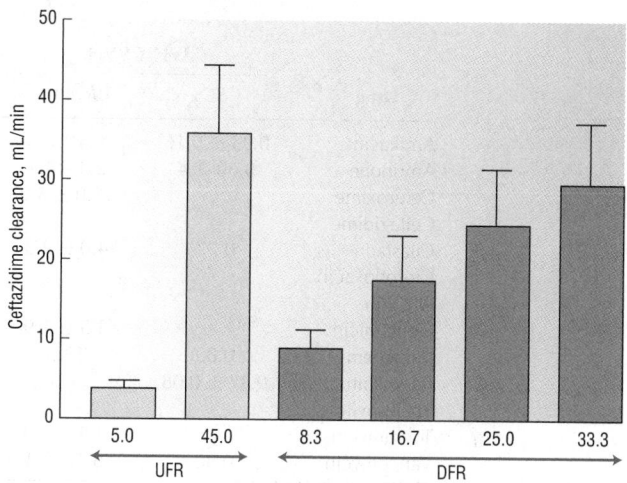

FIGURE 48-2. The effect of increasing ultrafiltration rate (UFR in milliliters per minute) and dialysate flow rate (DFR in milliliters per minute) on the clearance of ceftazidime.

TABLE 48–8. Predicted and Measured Sieving Coefficients of Selected Drugs

Drug	Predicted	Measured
Amikacin	0.95	0.88
Amphotericin	0.01	0.32–0.4
Ampicillin	0.8	0.6–0.69
Cefoperazone	0.10	0.27–0.69
Cefotaxime	0.62	0.55–1.1
Cefoxitin	0.30	0.32
Ceftazidine	0.90	0.38–0.78
Ceftriaxone	0.10	0.71–0.82
Clindamycin	0.25	0.49–0.98
Digoxin	0.75	0.96
Erythromycin	0.25	0.37
5-Fluorocytosine	0.96	0.98
Gentamicin	0.95	0.81–0.75
Imipenem	0.80	0.78
Metronidazole	0.80	0.80
Mezlocillin	0.68	0.68
Nafcillin	0.20	0.47
N-acetyl procainamide	0.80	0.92
Netilmicin	—	0.85
Oxacillin	0.05	0.02
Phenobarbital	0.60	0.86
Phenytoin	0.10	0.45
Procainamide	0.80	0.86
Theophylline	0.47	0.85
Tobramycin	0.95	0.78–0.86
Vancomycin	0.90	0.5–0.8

Adapted from Joy et al,[46] Mueller et al,[49] and Bugge.[50]

CRRT they are receiving. The patient's residual drug clearance can be predicted as described in the previous section of this chapter. The CRRT clearance can also be ascertained from published reports.[46,57,58] The SCs of frequently used drugs are summarized in Table 48–8, and the clearance of selected drugs by CAVH/CVVH or CAVHD/CVVHD is listed in Table 48–9. These data can be used to design initial dosage regimens for patients receiving CRRT.[50,52]

For example, WT is a 48-year-old, 60-kg male in ARF with a serum creatinine that has increased from 2.3 mg/dL to 7.2 mg/dL over 3 days. The residual CLcr value in this patient, calculated using the Jelliffe and Jelliffe equation for changing serum creatinine levels (see Chap. 41) is 4.8 mL/min. The consulting nephrologist recommends that CVVHDF be initiated using a Fresenius F-40 filter at blood and dialysate flow rates of 100 and 33.3 mL/min, respectively. The patient is to receive ceftazidime while on CVVHDF. The patient's residual ceftazidime clearance can be estimated using the regression equation in Table 48–7 relating CLcr and drug clearance:

$$CL_{RES} \text{ (mL/min)} = [1.15 \times (CLcr)] + 10.6$$
$$CL_{RES} = [1.15 \times (4.8)] + 10.6 = 16.1 \text{ mL/min}$$

The total clearance while on CVVHDF would be the sum of the patient's residual clearance and the ceftazidime clearance associated with CVVHDF (see Table 48–9) as follows:

$$CL_T = CL_{RES} + CL_{CVVHDF}$$
$$CL_T = 16.1 \text{ mL/min} + 15.2 \text{ mL/min} = 31.3 \text{ mL/min}$$

This patient's clearance value can be used to adjust the ceftazidime dose as described earlier. The ceftazidime clearance in a patient with normal renal function would be calculated as:

$$CL_{norm} \text{ (mL/min)} = [1.15 \times (CLcr)] + 10.6$$
$$CL_{norm} = [1.15 \times (120)] + 10.6 = 148.6 \text{ mL/min}$$

The dosage adjustment factor would then be:

$$Q = CL_{fail}/CL_{norm}$$
$$Q = 31.3/148.6 = 0.21$$

For this patient's situation, the normal regimen of ceftazidime would be 1,000 mg (D_n) every 8 hours (τ_n). If one wanted to maintain D_n and extend the dosing interval, then τ_f would be calculated as:

$$\tau_f = \tau_n/Q$$
$$\tau_f = 8 \text{ hours}/0.21$$
$$\tau_f = 38 \text{ hours, or a more practical value of 36 hours}$$

TABLE 48–9. Clearance of Selected Drugs by CAVH/CVVH and/or CAVHD/CVVHD

Drug	CAVH/CVVH SC	CAVH/CVVH Clearance	CAVHD/CVVHD SC	CAVHD/CVVHD DFR 1 L/h Clearance	CAVHD/CVVHD DFR 2 L/h Clearance
Amikacin	0.93 ± 0.16	10.1			
Amrinone	0.80–1.4	2.4–14.4			
Cefuroxime		11.0 ± 5.2	0.90 ± 0.30	14.0 ± 2.2	16.2 ± 3.4
Ceftazidime			0.86 ± 0.07	13.1 ± 1.3	15.2 ± 1.3
Cilastatin	0.77	4.0 ± 2.3	0.68 ± 0.08	10.0 ± 3.0	18.0 ± 4.0
Ciprofloxacin				16.3	19.9
Digoxin				6.4–10.0	11
Gentamicin		3.5 ± 1.9		5.2 ± 1.8	
Imipenem	0.80	13.3	1.05 ± 0.19	16.0 ± 7.0	
Phenytoin	0.37 ± 0.08	1.0		6.5	
Theophylline				14.8	
Tobramycin		3.5 ± 1.9		11.1–29	14.9
Vancomycin	0.80	6.7–13.3	0.66 ± 0.08	12.1 ± 5.7	16.6 ± 5.7

Clearance is in milliliters per minute.
DFR, dialysate flow rate; SC, sieving coefficient.
From Joy et al,[46] Mueller et al,[49] and Bugge.[50]

Therefore, this patient should receive 1,000 mg every 36 hours. If the additional clearance associated with CVVHDF (15.2 mL/min) was not considered, the calculated dosing interval would have been considerably longer, at approximately 72 hours.

PATIENTS RECEIVING CHRONIC AMBULATORY PERITONEAL DIALYSIS

Although the majority of patients with ESKD receive treatment with hemodialysis, approximately 15% of dialysis patients receive one of the multiple variants of continuous peritoneal dialysis. Peritoneal dialysis, like other dialysis modalities, has the potential to affect drug disposition; however, drug therapy individualization is often less complicated in these patients owing to the continuous nature of the procedure (see Chap. 45).

Many of the factors that are important in determining drug dialyzability for other treatment modalities pertain to peritoneal dialysis as well.[59,60] Peritoneal dialysis involves the instillation of 1 to 3 L of dialysis solution into the peritoneal cavity. Waste products and other substances, including drugs, move from the blood and surrounding tissues into the dialysis solution by means of diffusion and ultrafiltration. Factors that influence drug dialyzability in peritoneal dialysis include drug-specific characteristics such as molecular weight, solubility, degree of ionization, protein binding, and volume of distribution. The intrinsic properties of the peritoneal membrane that affect drug removal include blood flow, pore size, and peritoneal membrane surface area, which is approximately equal to the body surface area. There is an inverse relationship between peritoneal drug clearance and molecular weight, protein binding, and volume of distribution. Also, drug compounds that are ionized at physiologic pH will diffuse across the membrane more slowly than un-ionized compounds. In general, hemodialysis is more effective in removing drug substances than peritoneal dialysis such that if a drug is not removed by hemodialysis, it is not likely to be removed by peritoneal dialysis. As shown in Table 48–10, the contribution of peritoneal dialysis to total body clearance is often low, and for most drugs, markedly less than the contribution of hemodialysis. Detailed reviews of the disposition of other drugs in chronic ambulatory peritoneal dialysis patients are reported elsewhere.[8,59,60] Anti-infective agents are the most commonly studied drugs due to their primary role in the treatment of peritonitis.[61] Most other drugs can generally be dosed according to the residual renal function of the patient because additional clearance by peritoneal dialysis is so small.

CHRONIC HEMODIALYSIS PATIENTS

The number of patients with ESKD who receive chronic hemodialysis has steadily increased since the early 1970s and currently over 260,000 patients receive this life-sustaining therapy.[62] Although many new hemodialyzers have been introduced in the past 20 years and the efficiency of the hemodialysis procedure has been increased, the effect of hemodialysis on drug disposition is rarely re-evaluated after it is initially reported. Thus most of the literature probably represents an underestimation of the impact of hemodialysis on drug disposition.

The impact of hemodialysis on a patient's drug therapy is dependent on several factors, including the characteristics of each drug, the dialysis conditions, and the clinical situation for which dialysis is performed. Drug-related factors that affect dialyzability include the molecular weight, protein binding, and distribution volume of each drug.[8] The impact of distribution volume (V_D) on drug removal by dialysis is evident in the following example, in which drug A has a 10-L V_D, but drug B has a V_D of 80 L. Neither drug is bound to plasma proteins. They are exclusively eliminated unchanged by the kidney and both drugs have a molecular weight of 300 and a dialyzer clearance of 40 mL/min (2.4 L/h). The half-life in an anuric patient during dialysis [$t_{1/2} = (V_D \times 0.693)/CL$] will be markedly different for these two drugs (2.9 hours vs. 23 hours), and thus approximately 50% of drug A but only 10% of drug B will be removed during 3 hours of dialysis as a direct result of the larger distribution volume.

Prior to the mid-1980s these were the primary factors that needed to be known to assess the degree of dialyzability of a given drug, because the vast majority of dialysis filters were composed of cellulose, cellulose acetate, or regenerated cellulose (cuprophane) (see Chap. 45). These "conventional" filter materials were generally impermeable to drugs with a molecular weight over 1,000 daltons, and the clearance by hemodialysis tended to decline dramatically (by up to 60%) as molecular weight increased from 100 to 500 daltons.[63] Drugs that are small but highly protein bound are also not well dialyzed because both of the principal binding proteins, α_1-acid glycoprotein and albumin, have a very high molecular weight. Finally, those drugs that are widely distributed throughout the body are poorly removed by hemodialysis.

The dialysis prescription for the patient can also dramatically affect the degree of drug removal. The primary factors that can vary between patients are the type of hemodialysis they are prescribed, which is primarily reflected in the composition of the dialysis membrane; the filter surface area; blood and dialysate flow rates; and whether or not the dialysis unit reuses the dialysis filter. Dialysis membranes are composed of cellulose-based, semisynthetic, or synthetic materials (e.g., polysulfone, polymethylmethacrylate, or acrylonitrile). The synthetic filter materials are now available for low-, medium-, and high-flux modes of dialysis (see Chap. 45), with the principal difference between modes being in the filter pore size, which can range from 25 to greater than 60 angstroms, and the degree of water transport (ultrafiltration coefficient). The dialysis membranes used in high-flux hemodialysis have the greatest pore sizes and more closely mimic the filtration characteristics of the human kidney than the filters used to deliver conventional hemodialysis. This allows the passage of most solutes, including drugs, that have a molecular weight of 20,000 daltons or less.[63] Thus high-molecular-weight drugs such as vancomycin are likely to be removed by this mode of dialysis, although they are not by conventional dialysis.

An increase in removal has also been reported with several other drugs that have lower molecular weights (Table 48–11).[64–71] Figure 48–3 shows the plasma concentration–time profile of gentamicin in patients receiving dialysis using either a low-flux conventional

TABLE 48–10. Comparison for Selected Drugs of Residual Drug Clearance in End-Stage Kidney Disease (CL_{ESKD}) to Clearance by Continuous Ambulatory Peritoneal Dialysis (CL_{CAPD}), Intermittent Peritoneal Dialysis (CL_{IPD}), and Hemodialysis (CL_{HD})[a]

Drug	CL_{ESKD}	CL_{CAPD}	CL_{IPD}	CL_{HD}
Aztreonam	1.44	0.13	0.13	2.6
Cefazolin	0.30	0.06		2.1
Cefotaxime	7.13	0.40		1.6
Ceftazidime	0.74	0.10	0.50	2.3
Gentamicin	0.24	0.17	0.75	2.1
Mezlocillin	6.0		0.44	1.7
Pipericillin	3.90	0.22		4.4
Ticarcillin	0.96		0.43	2.0
Vancomycin	5.0	0.85		0.8

[a]All data are mean in liters per hour.
From St. Peter et al,[12] Taylor et al,[59] and Matzke.[80]

TABLE 48–11. Drug Disposition during Dialysis Depends on Filter Characteristics

Drug	Hemodialysis Clearance (mL/min)		Half-Life during Dialysis (h)	
	Conventional	*High-Flux*	*Conventional*	*High-Flux*
Ceftazidime	55–60	155[a]	3.3	1.2[a]
Cefuroxime	NR	103[b]	3.8	1.6[b]
Foscarnet	183	253[b]	NR	NR
Gentamicin	58.2	116[b]	3.0	4.3[b]
Netilmicin	46	87–109	5.0–5.2	2.9–3.4
Ranitidine	43.1	67.2[b]	5.1	2.9[b]
Vancomycin	9–21	31–60[c]	35–38	12.0[c]
		40–150[b]		4.5–11.8[b]
		72–116[d]		NR[d]

[a]Polyamide filter.
[b]Polysulfone filter.
[c]Polyacrylonitrile filter.
[d]Polymethylmethacrylate.
NR, not reported.
Adapted from Matzke.[80]

[cellulose acetate (CA170)] or a high-flux [polysulfone (F80)] dialyzer. The net result is that the patient receiving high-flux dialysis will require larger postdialysis doses relative to the patient receiving low-flux dialysis to maintain similar concentrations.

The final component of the dialysis prescription that may affect drug clearance by dialysis is whether or not the patient has authorized the unit to reuse his or her dialyzer. Currently, more than 75% of all dialysis units in the United States use this procedure to reduce the cost of chronic hemodialysis.[72] The effect of dialysis filter reuse on the clearance of endogenous molecules such as urea, creatinine, and β_2-microglobulin has been evaluated for many dialyzers.[73] A decrease in urea and creatinine clearances and an increase in β_2-microglobulin clearance was observed with some, but not all, dialyzers. Only one center has evaluated the effect of reuse on drug clearance (cefazolin, ceftazidime, tobramycin, and vancomycin) following the first and tenth use of cellulose acetate, cellulose triacetate, and polysulfone

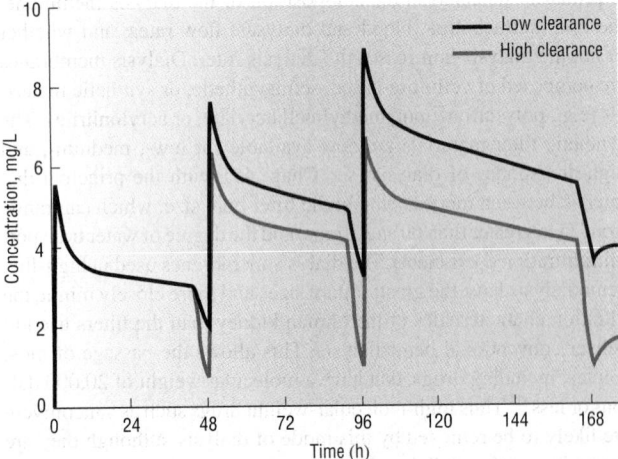

FIGURE 48–3. Clearance of gentamicin by low- and high-clearance dialyzers in patients given the same gentamicin dose after each dialysis treatment. Concentrations in the patient receiving dialysis with a low-clearance dialyzer will continue to increase, whereas concentrations in the patient receiving dialysis with the high-clearance dialyzer will be maintained at the same peak and predialysis concentrations observed after the third dose.

dialyzers.[74] No change was noted with the cellulose acetate dialyzer. Ceftazidime and vancomycin clearance decreased by up to 13% with the polysulfone filter. In contrast, significant decreases in clearance were observed with the cellulose triacetate dialyzer (24% to 43%) for all four drugs.

The impact of hemodialysis on drug therapy should thus not be viewed as a generic procedure such that a certain percentage of drug in the body is removed with each dialysis session; neither should simple "yes-no" answers on the dialyzability of drug compounds be considered sufficient information to make therapeutic decisions. Reference materials that indicate "yes-no" status regarding the dialyzability of drug compounds provide no quantification of the impact of hemodialysis, and are thus of little value to the clinician who needs to design a rational dosing regimen for a patient. Compounds considered nondialyzable with low-flux dialyzers may in fact be significantly removed by high-flux hemodialyzers. Characteristics of the dialysis prescription such as membrane composition and surface area, and blood and dialysis flow rates, are thus critical data for the design of drug dosing regimens for chronic hemodialysis patients.

The effect of hemodialysis on drug disposition can be estimated in several ways.[8] The determination of drug concentrations at the start and end of dialysis, with the subsequent calculation of the half-life during dialysis ($t_{1/2,onHD}$), has frequently been used as an index of drug removal by dialysis. Unfortunately, the $t_{1/2,onHD}$ may not be interpretable because declining plasma drug concentrations during dialysis represent elimination by the body as well as by dialysis. Furthermore, if significant rebound in drug concentrations after dialysis has been reported, the removal of drug by the dialysis procedure may be artificially high, depending on when after dialysis the concentration is determined.[75–79]

An alternative and more accurate means of assessing the effect of hemodialysis is to calculate the dialyzer clearance of the drug.[8] The dialyzer clearance (CL_D) can be calculated by several approaches. The CL^b_D from blood can be calculated as $CL_D = Q_b[(A_b - V_b)/A_b]$, where Q_b is blood flow through the dialyzer, A_b is the concentration of drug in blood going into the dialyzer, and V_b is the blood concentration of drug leaving the dialyzer. This equation is valid only if the drug concentrations are measured in whole blood and if the drug rapidly and completely distributes into red blood cells. Because drug concentrations are generally determined in plasma, the previous equation is usually modified to $CL^p_D = Q_p[(A_p - V_p)/A_p]$ where p represents plasma and Q_p is plasma flow, which equals Q_b (1 − hematocrit). This clearance calculation accurately reflects dialysis drug clearance only if the drug does not penetrate red blood cells or bind to formed blood elements.

Because of potential problems in accurately determining Q_b or Q_p, the dialysate recovery method is widely used. In addition, venous plasma concentrations may be concentrated, because plasma water is generally removed from the blood at a faster rate than drug when ultrafiltration is performed simultaneously with diffusion during dialysis.

The recovery clearance approach, the benchmark for the determination of dialyzer clearance, can be calculated as:[8]

$$CL^r_D = R/AUC_{0-t}$$

where R is the total amount of drug recovered unchanged in the dialysate and AUC_{0-t} is the area under the predialyzer plasma concentration-time curve during the period of time that the dialysate was collected. To determine the AUC_{0-t}, at least two, and preferably three to four plasma concentrations should be obtained during dialysis.

The hemodialysis clearance values reported in the literature may vary significantly depending on which of the previous methods was used to calculate CL_D. The principal reason for this is that for most medications we do not know the degree and rapidity with which the drug crosses the red blood cell membrane. Because the CL^r_D method incorporates no assumption of the degree of red blood cell permeability, it can be reliably used as the benchmark value. Comparisons of CL^p_D and CL^b_D values to the CL^r_D benchmark thus provide valuable insight to a drug's dialyzability.

The following principles may be applied to drug dosage regimen design for hemodialysis patients by using a value of CL_D that is reported in the literature.[8,12,80] Because clearance terms are additive, the total clearance during dialysis can be calculated as the sum of the patient's residual clearance during the interdialytic period (CL_{RES}) and dialyzer clearance (CL_D):

$$CL_T = CL_{RES} + CL_D$$

The half-life during the period between dialysis treatments and during dialysis can then be calculated from the following relationships using an estimate of the drug's distribution volume (V_D), which can be obtained from review articles:[8,12,80]

$$t_{1/2}, \text{offHD} = 0.693 \, [V_D/CL_{RES}]$$

$$t_{1/2}, \text{onHD} = 0.693 \, [V_D/(CL_{RES} + CL_D)]$$

Once the key pharmacokinetic parameters have been estimated/calculated, they may be used to simulate the plasma concentration-time profile of the drug for the individual patient and ascertain how much drug to administer and when. This approach to drug therapy individualization can be accomplished in a stepwise fashion assuming first-order elimination of the drug and a one-compartment model. For example, a 34-year-old male with ESKD was admitted to a hospital from the outpatient hemodialysis unit, where he experienced shaking and chills and had a temperature of 40°C (104°F). He weighed 70 kg and was 69 inches tall, had a residual CL_{cr} of 3 mL/min, and received conventional low flux dialysis for 4 hours three times a week on a CA210 cellulose acetate dialyzer. He received 140 mg of tobramycin at the end of his most recent hemodialysis treatment which end less than an hour prior to admission.

The first step is to estimate this patient's pharmacokinetic parameters of tobramycin on the basis of published population data.[12] The volume of distribution in this patient is 23.1 L (0.33 L/kg × 70 kg), and his residual total body clearance (CL_{RES}) estimated from the relationship between CL and creatinine clearance [$CL_{RES} = CL_{cr} \times 0.98$] is 3 mL/min or 0.176 L/h. The elimination rate constant can be approximated as:

$$k = CL_{RES} \div V_D$$
$$= 0.176 \, \text{L/h} \div 23.1 \, \text{L}$$
$$= 0.0076 \, \text{hr}^{-1}$$

The hemodialysis clearance of tobramycin is dependent on the dialyzer, and a value of 73 mL/min has recently been reported by Matzke and associates[67] for the CA210 dialyzer.

One now can predict what the plasma concentrations of tobramycin will be over the next 24 to 48 hours, assuming the infusion time for the drug (t') was 30 minutes. The concentration at the end of the 30-minute infusion (C_{max}) would be:

$$C_{max} = \frac{(\text{Dose}/t')1 - e^{-kt'}}{CL_{RES}}$$

$$C_{max} = \frac{(280 \, \text{mg/h})1 - e^{-(0.0076)\,0.5}}{0.176 \, \text{L/h}}$$

$$C_{max} = (1944 \, \text{mg/L}) \, (0.003) = 6.0 \, \text{mg/L}$$

The plasma concentration prior to the next dialysis session (C_{bD}), which is 44 hours away, and the concentration after dialysis (C_{aD}) can be calculated as:

$$C_{bD} = C_{max} \times e^{-(CL_{RES}/V_D) \times t}$$
$$= 6.0 \times e^{-0.0076 \times 44}$$
$$= 4.3 \, \text{mg/L}$$
$$C_{aD} = C_{bD} \times e^{-((CL_{RES} + CL_D)/V_D) \times t}$$
$$= 4.3 \times e^{-((0.176 + 4.38)/23.1) \times 4}$$
$$= 4.3 \times e^{-0.197 \times 4}$$
$$= 1.9 \, \text{mg/L}$$

On the basis of these data, no further therapy will likely be required until after the next dialysis treatment since one generally desires to have tobramycin concentrations fall below 2 mg/L before administering another dose.

During this interdialytic interval, however, several blood samples should be collected to characterize this patient's residual tobramycin clearance, distribution volume, and then the clearance of tobramycin during dialysis. Blood samples were therefore collected at the following times after the first dose:

DAY 1   7 PM (2 hours after dose)   6.5 mg/L

DAY 2   8 AM (39 hours after dose; just before dialysis)   4.1 mg/L

DAY 3   12 noon (immediately after dialysis)   2.0 mg/L

The C_{max} can be calculated by back-extrapolation to the end of the infusion as described in Chap. 5. The elimination rate during the interdialytic period (k_{ID}) and during dialysis (k_{DD}), and the V_D can be calculated as:

$$k_{ID} = (\ln C_1/C_2)/\Delta t$$
$$k_{ID} = (\ln 6.5/4.1)/37 = 0.0125/h$$
$$k_{DD} = (\ln C_2/C_3)/\Delta t$$
$$k_{DD} = (\ln 4.1/2.0)/4 = 0.179/h$$
$$V_D = \frac{\text{Dose}/t'}{k_{ID}} \frac{1 - e^{-k_{ID}t'}}{(C_{max} - C_{min}e^{-k_{ID}t'})}$$
$$V_D = \frac{140/0.5}{0.0125} \frac{1 - e^{-(0.0125)0.5}}{(6.7 - 0.0 \, e^{-(0.0125)0.5})}$$
$$V_D = \frac{134.4}{6.7} = 20 \, \text{L}$$

where Δt is the time in hours between the two measured concentrations and C_{min} is the tobramycin concentration in plasma prior to the administration of this dose.

The patient's residual clearance (CL_{RES}) of tobramycin can then be calculated as:

$$CL_{RES} = V_D \times k_{ID}$$
$$CL_{RES} = 20.0 \, \text{L} \times 0.0125 = 0.25 \, \text{L/h or } 4.2 \, \text{mL/min}$$

The dialyzer clearance (CL_D) can be calculated since one knows the total clearance during dialysis (CL_T) and CL_{RES} as:

$$CL_D = CL_T - CL_{RES}$$
$$CL_D = (k_{DD} \times V_D) - 4.2 \, \text{mL/min}$$
$$CL_D = (0.179/h \times 20.0 \, \text{L}) - 4.2 \, \text{mL/min}$$
$$CL_D = (3.6 \, \text{L/h or } 59.6 \, \text{mL/min}) - 4.2 \, \text{mL/min}$$
$$CL_D = 55.4 \, \text{mL/min}$$

This case illustrates the need for individualizing drug therapy for hemodialysis patients since this patient's V_D was 13% smaller, CL_{RES} was 42% greater, and CL_D was 25% less than the estimates based on population parameters.

The ultimate reason for measuring the plasma concentrations of aminoglycosides and several other agents is to individualize the patient's dosage regimen. Thus there remains one important step in our evaluation: the calculation of the dose this patient should receive next. The two factors that enter into this decision are the desired peak and trough concentrations and the degree of rebound in drug concentrations, after the end of dialysis. Because tobramycin concentrations have been noted to increase by about 20% within 1.5 to 2 hours after the end of hemodialysis, the trough concentration of this patient can be considered to be 2.4 mg/L (2.0 mg/L × 1.2). Although this value is higher than one might like to maintain in an individual with normal renal function, a prolonged period of almost 24 hours would be required just to have the concentration drop below 2.0 mg/L. It is frequently necessary in critically ill individuals with ESKD to redose the patient even though the postdialysis trough serum concentration is between 2 and 3 mg/L. Assuming the desired peak concentration was 7.0 mg/L, the postdialysis dose this patient would need can then be calculated using the simplified approach below, because the elimination half-life is extremely prolonged relative to the infusion time, and thus minimal drug is eliminated during the infusion period:

$$\text{Dose} = V_D \times (C_{max} - C_{min})$$
$$= 20.0\,\text{L} \times (7.0 - 2.4) = 92\,\text{mg}$$

Combination antibiotic therapy with aminoglycosides and extended-spectrum penicillins are frequently prescribed for ESKD patients to provide wider antibacterial coverage against gram-negative bacilli through a synergistic effect. The combined use may result in in vitro chemical inactivation of the aminoglycoside, leading to a loss in antibiotic activity. The rate of inactivation is related to the incubation period, temperature, presence of solutes, and β-lactam concentration.

The extent of aminoglycoside inactivation in vivo may not be clinically significant in patients with normal or slightly impaired renal function due to the short contact time. However, in patients with ESKD, subtherapeutic aminoglycoside concentrations and a decreased aminoglycoside elimination half-life have been reported. Patients will require appropriate dosage modification to maintain the desired serum concentrations. Inactivation of gentamicin and tobramycin by ticarcillin[81,82] and pipercillin[83,84] has been reported in patients receiving chronic dialysis therapy. The disposition of netilmicin and isepamicin, however, is unaffected by piperacillin administration.[83,84] No significant changes in V_D were noted for any of the aminoglycosides, and thus the inactivation clearances of netilmicin and isepamicin were significantly less than those of tobramycin and gentamicin. From these data tobramycin appears to be affected to the greatest degree, followed by gentamicin, netilmicin, and isepamicin, in descending order.

Thus the elimination of aminoglycosides in ESKD patients also receiving antipseudomonal penicillins will be increased; therefore frequent serum concentration monitoring should be performed. To minimize any in vitro inactivation of aminoglycosides that would complicate assessment of the in vivo effects, serum samples should be assayed as soon as possible after collection. If this is not possible, serum samples should be frozen (preferably at –70°C, or –94°F) until they can be assayed.

CONCLUSIONS

Subtherapeutic or supratherapeutic responses to drugs in patients with renal insufficiency are often misinterpreted and not recognized as such. The adverse outcomes associated with inappropriate drug use and dosing have not been quantified but do warrant future investigations. Sound pharmacokinetic principles as illustrated in this chapter, used in concert with reliable population pharmacokinetic estimates, should ultimately yield the optimal approach to drug dosage regimen design for patients with renal insufficiency. Individualization of therapy should be undertaken whenever clinical therapeutic monitoring tools are available.

ABBREVIATIONS

A_b: concentration of drug in blood going into the dialyzer (arterial side)

A_p: concentration of drug in plasma going into the dialyzer (arterial side)

AUC: area under the concentration-time curve

AUC_{0-t}: the area under the predialyzer plasma concentration-time curve during hemodialysis

AUMC: the area under the first moment of the concentration-time curve

C_a: concentration of the drug in the plasma going into a filter

C_{aD}: plasma concentration after dialysis

C_{ave}: average plasma concentration

CAVH: continuous arteriovenous hemofiltration

CAVHD: continuous arteriovenous hemodialysis

CAVHDF: continuous arteriovenous hemodiafiltration

C_{bD}: plasma concentration prior to the next dialysis session

C_{df}: concentration of drug in the dialysis fluid

C_e^{total}: equated total phenytoin concentration

C_m^{total}: total drug concentration measured in a patient with altered protein binding

C_{ss}: average steady-state plasma concentration

C_v: concentration of the drug in the plasma returning from a filter

CVVH: continuous venovenous hemofiltration

CVVHD: continuous venovenous hemodialysis

CVVHDF: continuous venovenous hemodiafiltration

CL: total body clearance

CL^b_D: dialyzer clearance from blood

CL_{CAVHDF}: clearance of a drug by CAVHDF

CL_{CAVH}: clearance of a drug by CAVH

CLcr: creatinine clearance

CL_{CVVHDF}: clearance of a drug by CVVHDF

CL_{CVVH}: clearance of a drug by CVVH

CL_D: dialyzer clearance

$CL_{diffusion}$: clearance via diffusion from plasma water to the dialysate

CL_{fail}: clearance of a drug in a patient with impaired renal function

CL_{norm}: clearance of a drug in patients with normal renal function

CL^p_D: dialyzer clearance from plasma

CL_{PT}: estimated total body clearance for a given patient

CL_R: net renal excretion

$CL_{reabsorption}$: tubular reabsorption

CL_{RES}: residual drug clearance in a dialysis patient

$CL_{secretion}$: tubular secretion

CL_T: total clearance while on CVVHDF

C_{max}: peak drug concentration

C_p^{mid}: plasma drug concentration at the midpoint of the dialysis session

CNS: central nervous system

CRRT: continuous renal replacement therapy

C_p^t: desired plasma concentration at time t

CYP450: cytochrome P450 enzymes

D_f: maintenance dose for a patient with renal insufficiency

DFR: dialysate flow rate

D_n: dose for a patient with normal renal function

ESKD: end-stage kidney disease

F: bioavailability

f_e: fraction of drug eliminated unchanged in the urine

f_u: fraction of drug unbound to plasma proteins

GFR: glomerular filtration rate

IC_{50}: inhibitory concentration of 50%

k_a: absorption rate constant

k: elimination rate constant

k_{DD}: elimination rate constant during dialysis

KF: ratio of the patient's creatinine clearance to the assumed normal value of 120 mL/min

k_{ID}: elimination rate constant between dialysis sessions (interdialytic)

Q: kinetic parameter/dosage adjustment factor

Q_b: blood flow through the dialyzer

Q_p: plasma flow through the dialyzer $= Q_b(1 - HCT)$

R: the total amount of drug recovered unchanged in the dialysate

S: salt form

SC: sieving coefficient

τ_f: dosing interval in a patient with renal failure

τ_p: practical dosing interval for a patient with renal failure

τ_n: dosing interval in a patient with normal renal function

θ: 0.0107 times the total protein concentration in plasma

t_{max}: time to peak drug concentration

$t_{1/2}$: half-life

$t_{1/2,onHD}$: half-life during dialysis

$t_{1/2,offHD}$: half-life off dialysis

UFR: ultrafiltrate formation

V_{area}: volume of distribution area

V_β: volume of distribution beta

V_c: volume of the central compartment

V_D: volume of distribution

V_{df}: volume of dialysate/ultrafiltrate fluid

V_{ss}: volume of distribution at steady state

Review Questions and other resources can be found at *www.pharmacotherapyonline.com.*

REFERENCES

1. Jones CA, McQuillan GM, Kusek JW, et al. Serum creatinine levels in the US population: third National Health and Nutrition Examination Survey. Am J Kidney Dis 1998;32:992–999.

2. Kearns GL, Abdel-Rahman SM, Alander SW, et al. Developmental pharmacology—drug disposition, action, and therapy in infants and children. N Engl J Med 2003;349:1157–1167.

3. Mangoni AA, Jackson SH. Age-related changes in pharmacokinetics and pharmacodynamics: basic principles and practical applications. Br J Clin Pharmacol 2004;57:6–14.

4. Hammerlein A, Derendorf H, Lowenthal DT. Pharmacokinetic and pharmacodynamic changes in the elderly. Clinical implications. Clin Pharmacokinet 1998;35:49–64.

5. Milsap RL, Jusko WJ. Pharmacokinetics in the infant. Environ Health Perspect 1994;102(Suppl 11):107–110.

6. Ritschel WA, Denson DD. Influence of disease on bioavailability.

In: Pharmacokinetics: Regulatory, Industrial, Academic Perspectives. New York, Marcel Dekker, 1995.

7. Grandison MK, Boudinot FD. Age-related changes in protein binding of drugs: implications for therapy. Clin Pharmacokinet 2000;38:271–290.

8. Matzke GR, Comstock TJ. Influence of renal disease and dialysis on pharmacokinetics. In: Applied Pharmacokinetics: Principles of Therapeutic Drug Monitoring, 4th ed. Evans WE, Schentag JJ, Burton ME (eds.). Baltimore, Lippincott Williams and Wilkins, 2005.

9. Nolin TD, Frye RF, Matzke GR. Hepatic drug metabolism and transport in patients with kidney disease. Am J Kidney Dis 2003;42:906–925.

10. Rowland M, Tozer TN. Clinical Pharmacokinetics: Concepts and Applications, 3rd ed. Philadelphia, Lea and Febiger, 1995:156–183.

11. Matzke GR, Frye RF. Drug administration in patients with renal insufficiency: minimising renal and extrarenal toxicity. Drug Saf 1997;16:205–231.

12. St. Peter WL, Halstenson CE. Pharmacologic approach in patients with renal failure. In: Chernow B, ed. The Pharmacologic Approach to the Critically Ill Patient. Baltimore, Williams & Wilkins, 1994:41–79.

13. Thummel KE, Shen DD. Design and optimization of dosage regimens: pharmacokinetic data. In: Hardman JG, Limbird LE, Goodman GA, eds. Goodman & Gilman's the Pharmacological Basis of Therapeutics, 10th ed. New York, McGraw-Hill, 2001:1917–2024.

14. Vanholder R, Van Landeshoot N, De Smet R, et al. Drug protein binding in chronic renal failure: Evaluation of nine drugs. Kidney Int 1988;33:996–1004.

15. Chan GL, Axelson JE, Price JD, et al. In vitro protein binding of propafenone in normal and uraemic human sera. Eur J Clin Pharmacol 1989;36:495–499.

16. Pritchard JF, Matzke GR, Opsahl JA, et al. Effects of hemodialysis on plasma protein binding of bepridil. J Clin Pharmacol 1995;35:137–141.

17. Liponi DF, Winter ME, Tozer TN. Renal function and therapeutic concentrations of phenytoin. Neurology 1984;34:395–397.

18. Job ML. Digoxin. In: Murphy JE, ed. Clinical Pharmacokinetics Pocket Reference, 3rd ed. Bethesda, MD, American Society of Health-System Pharmacists, 2005:153.

19. Malini PL, Strocchi E, Feliciangeli G, et al. Digitalis receptors and digoxin sensitivity in renal failure. Clin Pharm Physiol 1985;12:115–115.

20. Lam YW, Banerji S, Hatfield C, Talbert RL. Principles of drug administration in renal insufficiency. Clin Pharmacokinet 1997;32:30–57.

21. Koup J. Disease states and drug pharmacokinetics. J Clin Pharmacol 1989;29:674–679.

22. Prescott LF, Freestone S, McAuslane JA. The concentration-dependent disposition of intravenous p-aminohippurate in subjects with normal and impaired renal function. Br J Clin Pharmacol 1993;35:20–29.

23. Touchette MA, Slaughter RL. The effect of renal failure on hepatic drug clearance. Ann Pharmacother 1991;25:1214–1224.

24. Kim YG, Shin JG, Shin SG, et al. Decreased acetylation of isoniazid in chronic renal failure. Clin Pharmacol Ther 1993;54:612.

25. Leblond F, Guevin C, Demers C, et al. Downregulation of hepatic cytochrome P450 in chronic renal failure. J Am Soc Nephrol 2001;12:326–332.

26. Himmelfarb J, Stenvinkel P, Ikizler TA, Hakim RM. The elephant in uremia: oxidant stress as a unifying concept of cardiovascular disease in uremia. Kidney Int 2002;62:1524–1538.

27. Morgan ET, Li-Masters T, Cheng PY. Mechanisms of cytochrome P450 regulation by inflammatory mediators. Toxicology 2002;181–182:207–210.

28. Leblond FA, Giroux L, Villeneuve JP, Pichette V. Decreased in vivo metabolism of drugs in chronic renal failure. Drug Metab Dispos 2000;28:1317–1320.

29. Dowling TC, Briglia AE, Fink JC, et al. Characterization of hepatic cytochrome p4503A activity in patients with end-stage renal disease. Clin Pharmacol Ther 2003;73:427–434.

30. Leblond FA, Petrucci M, Dube P, et al. Downregulation of intestinal cytochrome p450 in chronic renal failure. J Am Soc Nephrol 2002;13:1579–1585.

31. Dreisbach AW, Japa S, Gebrekal AB, et al. Cytochrome P4502C9 activity in end-stage renal disease. Clin Pharmacol Ther 2003;73:475–477.

32. Nolin TD, Gastonguay MR, Bies RR, et al. Impaired 6-hydroxy-chlorzoxazone elimination in patients with kidney disease: Implication for cytochrome P450 2E1 pharmacogenetic studies. Clin Pharmacol Ther 2003;74:555–568.

33. Heinemeyer G, Link J, Weber W, et al. Clearance of ceftriaxone in critical care patients with acute renal failure. Intensive Care Med 1990;16:448–453.

34. Wolfert AI, Sica DA. Narcotic usage in renal failure. Int J Artif Organs 1988;11:411–415.

35. Lee W, Kim RB. Transporters and renal drug elimination. Annu Rev Pharmacol Toxicol 2004;44:137–166.

36. Kamiya A, Okumura K, Hori R. Quantitative investigation of renal handling of drugs in dogs with renal insufficiency. Pharm Sci 1984;74:892–896.

37. Hori R, Okumura K, Kamiya A, et al. Ampicillin and cephalexin in renal insufficiency. Clin Pharmacol Ther 1983;34:792–798.

38. McEvoy GK, Litvak K, Welsh OH, et al. American Hospital Formulary Service, Drug Information. Bethesda, MD, American Society of Hospital Pharmacists, 2001.

39. Blakey S. Dosing concepts in renal dysfunction. In: Murphy JE, ed. Clinical Pharmacokinetics Pocket Reference, 2nd ed. Bethesda, MD, American Society of Health-System Pharmacists, 2001:507–530.

40. Aronoff GR, Berns JS, Brier ME, et al. Drug Prescribing in Renal Failure: Dosing Guidelines for Adults, 4th ed. Philadelphia, American College of Physicians-American Society of Internal Medicine, 1999.

41. Craig WA. Pharmacokinetic/pharmacodynamic parameters: Rationale for antibacterial dosing of mice and men. Clin Infect Dis 1998;26:1–12.

42. Murphy JE. Clinical Pharmacokinetics Pocket Reference, 3rd ed. Bethesda, MD, American Society of Health-System Pharmacists, 2005.

43. Scott JC, Partovi N, Ensom MH. Ganciclovir in solid organ transplant recipients: Is there a role for clinical pharmacokinetic monitoring? Ther Drug Monit 2004;26:68–77.

44. Pescovitz MD, Pruett TL, Gonwa T, et al. Oral ganciclovir dosing in transplant recipients and dialysis patients based on renal function. Transplantation 1998;66:1104–1107.

45. Balfour HH. Management of cytomegalovirus disease with antiviral drugs. Rev Infect Dis 1990;12:S849–S860.

46. Joy MS, Matzke GR, Armstrong DK, et al. A primer on continuous renal replacement therapy for critically ill patients. Ann Pharmacother 1998;32:362–375.

47. Macias WL, Mueller BA, Scarim SK. Vancomycin pharmacokinetics in acute renal failure: preservation of non-renal clearance. Clin Pharmacol Ther 1991;50:688–694.

48. Tegeder I, Bremer F, Oelkers R, et al. Pharmacokinetics of imipenem-cilastatin in critically ill patients undergoing continuous venovenous hemofiltration. Antimicrob Agents Chemother 1997;41:2640–2645.

49. Mueller BA, Pasko DA, Sowinski KM. Higher renal replacement therapy dose delivery influences on drug therapy. Artif Organs 2003;27:808–814.

50. Bugge JF. Pharmacokinetics and drug dosing adjustments during continuous venovenous hemofiltration or hemodiafiltration in critically ill patients. Acta Anaesthesiol Scand 2001;45:929–934.

51. Veltri MA, Neu AM, Fivush BA, et al. Drug dosing during intermittent hemodialysis and continuous renal replacement therapy: special considerations in pediatric patients. Paediatr Drugs 2004;6:45–65.

52. Bohler J, Donauer J, Keller F. Pharmacokinetic principles during continuous renal replacement therapy: drugs and dosage. Kidney Int Suppl 1999;72:S24–28.

53. Kronfol NO, Lau AH, Barakat MM. Aminoglycoside binding to polyacrylonitrile hemofilter membranes during continuous hemofiltration. ASAIO Transactions 1987;33:300–303.

54. Joy MS, Matzke GR, Frye RF, Palevsky PM. Determinants of vancomycin clearance by CVVH and CVVHD. Am J Kidney Dis 1998;31:1019–1027.

55. Matzke GR, Frye RF, Joy MS, Palevsky PM. Determinants of ceftazidime clearance by continuous venovenous hemofiltration and continuous venovenous hemodialysis. Antimicrob Agents Chemother 2000;44:1639–1644.

56. Lau AH, Kronfol NO. Determinants of drug removal by continuous hemofiltration. Int J Artif Organs 1994;17:373–378.

57. Reetze-Bonorden P, Bohler J, Keller E. Drug dosage in patients during continuous renal replacement therapy. Clin Pharmacokinet 1993;24:362–379.

58. Bressolle F, Kinowski JM, de la Coussaye JE, et al. Clinical pharmacokinetics during continuous hemofiltration. Clin Pharmacokinet 1994;26:457–471.

59. Taylor CA, Abdel-Rahman E, Zimmerman SW, Johnson CA. Clinical pharmacokinetics during continuous ambulatory peritoneal dialysis. Clin Pharmacokinet 1996;31:293–308.

60. Manley HJ, Bailie GR. Treatment of peritonitis in APD: pharmacokinetic principles. Semin Dial 2002;15:418–421.

61. Piraino B, Bailie GR, Bernardini J et al. Peritoneal dialysis related infections: 2005 update. Perit Dial Int (in press).

62. U.S. Renal Data Systems. USRDS 2003 annual data report. Bethesda, MD, The National Institutes of Health, Institute of Diabetes and Digestive and Kidney Diseases, 2003.

63. Konstantin P. Newer membranes: cuprophane versus polysulfone versus polyacrylonitrile. In: Bosch JP, ed. Contemporary Issues in Nephrology Hemodialysis: High Efficiency Treatments, Vol. 27. New York, Churchill Livingstone, 1993:63–78.

64. Golper TA, Vincent HH, Gleason JR, Vos MC. Drug removal during high efficiency and high-flux hemodialysis. In: Bosch JP, ed. Contemporary Issues in Nephrology Hemodialysis: High Efficiency Treatments, Vol. 27. New York, Churchill Livingstone, 1993:175–209.

65. Pollard TA, Lampasona V, Mullins RE, et al. Vancomycin redistribution: Dosing recommendations following high flux hemodialysis. 1994;45:232–237.

66. Matzke GR, Palevsky PM, Frye RF. In-vitro model for ceftazidime disposition during hemodialysis with conventional and high-flux biocompatible membranes. Annual Meeting of the American Association of Pharmaceutical Scientists, Indianapolis, IN, November 2000.

67. Matzke GR, Palevsky PM, Frye RF. In-vitro model for tobramycin disposition during hemodialysis with conventional and high flux biocompatible membranes. J Am Soc Nephrol 2000;10:286A.

68. Matzke GR, Frye RF, Nolin TD. Vancomycin removal by low- and high-flux hemodialysis with polymethylmethacrylate dialyzers. J Am Soc Nephrol 1999;10:193A.

69. Amin NB, Padhi ID, Touchette MA, et al. Characterization of gentamicin pharmacokinetics in patients hemodialyzed with high-flux polysulfone membranes. Am J Kidney Dis 1999;34:222–227.

70. Tsuruoka S, Sugimoto KI, Hayasaka T, et al. Ranitidine clearance during hemodialysis with high-flux membrane: comparison of polysulfone and cellulose acetate hemodialyzers. Eur J Clin Pharmacol 2000;56:581–583.

71. Aweeka FT, Jacobson MA, Martin-Munley S, et al. Effect of renal disease and hemodialysis on foscarnet pharmacokinetics and dosing recommendations. J Acquir Immune Defic Syndr Hum Retrovirol 1999;20:348–347.

72. U.S. Renal Data Systems. USRDS 2000 Annual Data Report. Bethesda, MD, The National Institutes of Health, Institute of Diabetes and Digestive and Kidney Diseases, 2000.

73. Cheung AK, Agodoa LY, Daugirdas JT, et al. Effects of hemodialyzer reuse on clearances of urea and beta2-microglobulin. The Hemodialysis (HEMO) Study Group. J Am Soc Nephrol 1999;10:117–127.

74. Palevsky PM, Matzke GR, Frye RF. Effect of dialyzer reprocessing on the clearance of low and intermediate molecular weight solutes. J Am Soc Nephrol 2001;12:273A.

75. Barbhaiya RH, Knupp CA, Forgue ST, et al. Pharmacokinetics of cefepime in subjects with renal insufficiency. Clin Pharmacol Ther 1990;48:268–276.

76. Halstenson CE, Guay DR, Opsahl JA, et al. Disposition of cefmetazole in healthy volunteers and patients with impaired renal function. Antimicrob Agents Chemother 1990;34:519–523.

77. Matzke GR, O'Connell ME, Collins AJ, Keshaviah PR. Disposition of vancomycin during hemofiltration. Clin Pharmacol Ther 1986;40:425–430.

78. Kelloway JS, Awni WM, Lin CC, et al. Pharmacokinetics of ceftibuten-cis and its trans metabolite in healthy volunteers and in patients with chronic renal insufficiency. Antimicrob Agents Chemother 1991; 35:2267–2274.

79. Halstenson CE, Berkseth RO, Mann HJ, Matzke GR. Aminoglycoside redistribution phenomenon after hemodialysis: netilmicin and tobramycin. Int J Clin Pharmacol Ther Toxicol 1987;25:48–55.

80. Matzke GR. Status of hemodialysis of drugs in 2002. J Pharmacy Practice 2002;15:405–418.

81. Russo ME, Atkin-Thor E. Gentamicin and ticarcillin in subjects with end-stage renal disease. Clin Nephrol 1981;15:175–180.

82. Matzke GR, Luckham DR, Collins AJ, Halstenson CE. Effect of ticarcillin on gentamicin and tobramycin pharmacokinetics in a patient with end-stage renal disease. Pharmacotherapy 1984;4:158–160.

83. Halstenson CE, Wong MO, Herman CS, et al. Effect of concomitant administration of piperacillin on the dispositions of isepamicin and gentamicin in patients with end-stage renal disease. Antimicrob Agents Chemother 1992;36:1832–1836.

84. Halstenson CE, Hirata CA, Heim-Duthoy KL, et al. Effect of concomitant administration of piperacillin on the dispositions of netilmicin and tobramycin in patients with end-stage renal disease. Antimicrob Agents Chemother 1990;34:128–133.

49

DISORDERS OF SODIUM, WATER, CALCIUM, AND PHOSPHORUS HOMEOSTASIS

Melanie S. Joy and Gerald A. Hladik

Learning Objectives and other resources can be found at *www.pharmacotherapyonline.com.*

KEY CONCEPTS

1. Patients with symptomatic hyponatremia are at high risk of neurologic complications, and the serum sodium concentration in these patients should be raised 1.5 to 2 mEq/L per hour for the first 3 to 4 hours, but no more than 12 mEq/L per day to avoid cerebral demyelination.

2. In patients with the syndrome of inappropriate secretion of antidiuretic hormone and symptomatic hypotonic hyponatremia, the most efficient means of correcting the hyponatremia involves the administration of 3% saline in conjunction with a loop diuretic.

3. Patients with hypotonic hyponatremia caused by volume depletion should initially receive normal saline followed by 0.45% saline once signs of extracellular fluid volume depletion abate in order to avoid overly rapid correction of the serum sodium concentration.

4. The serum sodium concentration should be corrected at a rate of approximately 0.5 mEq/L per hour in patients with hypernatremia. The serum sodium concentration in patients who develop hypernatremia over the course of several hours (such as following hypertonic saline infusion) should be corrected at approximately 1 mEq/L per hour.

5. Patients with central diabetes insipidus should be treated with intranasal desmopressin acetate, with goals of decreasing urine volume to less than 2 L/day while maintaining the serum sodium concentration between 137 and 142 mEq/L.

6. Patients with nephrogenic diabetes insipidus should be treated by correcting the underlying cause when possible, and sodium chloride restriction in conjunction with a thiazide diuretic to decrease the extracellular fluid volume by approximately 1 to 1.5 L.

7. Patients with nephrotic syndrome commonly develop diuretic resistance. It is suggested that the impaired natriuretic response may be overcome by using higher doses to increase the delivery of free drug to the secretory site in the proximal nephron. Another approach is to use the combination of a loop diuretic with a distal diuretic.

8. Patients with cirrhosis should initially be treated with spironolactone in the absence of impaired glomerular filtration rate and hyperkalemia. Thiazides may then be added for patients with a creatinine clearance >50 mL/min. For those patients who remain diuretic resistant, a loop diuretic may replace the thiazide.

9. The fluid and electrolyte complications of diuretic therapy usually occur within the first 2 weeks of diuretic therapy, and repeated monitoring of serum chemistries is generally not necessary in the absence of a change in clinical status, diuretic dose, or dietary intake.

10. The correction of hypercalcemia includes multiple treatment modalities including hydration, diuretics, bisphosphonates, and steroids.

11. Hypophosphatemia can result from decreased gastrointestinal absorption, increased urinary excretion, and intracellular redistribution.

12. The treatment for hypophosphatemia consists of intravenous phosphate salts in doses of 0.08 to 0.64 mmol/kg for acute therapy and oral doses of 50 to 60 mmol/d for maintenance therapy.

Homeostasis of fluid and electrolytes is necessary for the body's normal physiologic functions. Disorders of sodium, water, calcium, and phosphorus are common complications of multiple acute and chronic diseases. These disorders are frequently associated with the acute care setting; however, they are clearly present in a less-severe state in the ambulatory care environment. The consequences of electrolyte disorders can range from asymptomatic to life-threatening requiring hospitalization. The maintenance of fluid and electrolyte homeostasis requires adequate functioning of feedback mechanisms, hormones, and multiple organ systems. It is necessary to understand the pathophysiology of these disorders in order to develop appropriate treatment plans.

From a pharmaceutical care perspective, disorders of electrolyte homeostasis can result from drug therapy. In addition, with some drug therapies, toxicity can be enhanced when underlying electrolyte disorders are present. Drug-induced disorders respond well to discontinuation of the offending agent(s); however, additional therapies are sometimes required to correct the disorder. This chapter reviews the etiology, classification, clinical presentation, and therapy for disorders of sodium, water, calcium, and phosphorus homeostasis.

SODIUM AND WATER HOMEOSTASIS

Two-thirds of total body water is distributed intracellularly while one-third is contained in the extracellular space.[1] Sodium and its accompanying anions, chloride and bicarbonate, comprise more than 90% of the total osmolality of the extracellular fluid (ECF), while intracellular osmolality is primarily dependent on the concentration of potassium and its accompanying anions (mostly organic and inorganic phosphates). The differential concentrations of sodium and potassium in the intra- and extracellular fluid is maintained by the Na^+-K^+-ATPase pump.[2] Most cell membranes are freely permeable to water, and thus the osmolality of intra- and extracellular body fluids is the same. Symptoms in patients with hypo- and hypernatremia are primarily related to alterations in cell volume.[3] It is therefore essential to understand the factors that cause changes in cell volume.

Solutes that cannot freely cross cell membranes, such as sodium, are referred to as effective osmoles. The concentration of effective osmoles in the ECF determines the tonicity of the ECF, which directly affects the distribution of water between the extra- and intracellular compartments.[4] Addition of an isotonic solution to the ECF will result in no change in intracellular volume because there will be no change in the effective osmolality of the ECF. Addition of a hypertonic solution to the ECF, however, will result in a decrease in cell volume, whereas addition of a hypotonic solution to the ECF will result in an increase in cell volume. Table 49–1 summarizes the composition of commonly used intravenous solutions and their respective distribution into extracellular and intracellular compartments following infusion.

Hypo- and hypernatremia are syndromes of altered tonicity and cell volume caused by changes in water balance. Thus an understanding of factors that affect tonicity and water balance is essential in order to understand the pathogenesis and evaluation of these syndromes. The serum sodium concentration is tightly regulated, and usually varies by no more than 2% to 3%. The kidney regulates water excretion through a feedback mechanism with the hypothalamus, such that the serum osmolality remains relatively constant (275 to 290 mOsm/kg) despite day-to-day variations in water intake. The serum osmolality is comprised primarily of sodium and the accompanying anions chloride and bicarbonate, and may be estimated by:

$$Sosm = (2 \times S_{Na}) + (B_{glucose}/18) + (BUN/2.8)$$

where Sosm = serum osmolality in milliosmoles per kilogram; S_{Na} = serum sodium concentration in mEq/L; $B_{glucose}$ = glucose concentration in mg/dL; and BUN = blood urea nitrogen concentration in mg/dL.[5]

Antidiuretic hormone (ADH) is released from the posterior pituitary when the plasma osmolality rises by 1% to 2% or more.[6] ADH binds to the vasopressin-2 (V2) receptors on the basolateral surface of renal tubular epithelial cells, and through a series of second messenger reactions, a water channel (aquaporin-2) is inserted into the apical tubular lumen surface of the cell.[7] Water may then pass through the cell into the peritubular capillary space, and is then reabsorbed into the systemic circulation. A rise in serum osmolality sensed in the hypothalamus results not only in ADH release, but also in stimulation of thirst. The combination of an increase in water intake and a decrease in water excretion results in a decrease in the serum osmolality and inhibition of ADH secretion once the plasma osmolality is restored to normal.

Nonosmotic release of ADH occurs when the effective arterial blood volume (EABV) decreases by approximately 5% to 10%.[8] The EABV is the vascular component of the ECF that is responsible for organ perfusion.[9] A change in the EABV promotes an afferent response from baroreceptors in the chest and neck and activation of the renin-angiotensin system, leading to synthesis of angiotensin II. Angiotensin II then stimulates both nonosmotic release of ADH and thirst. The volume stimulus overrides osmotic inhibition of ADH release, and conservation of water fosters restoration of blood pressure and EABV at the expense of hypo-osmolality.

The proper assessment of a patient with an abnormal serum sodium concentration requires recognition that the serum sodium level may bear no relationship to the ECF volume and sodium content. Hypernatremia and hyponatremia may be associated with conditions of high, low, or normal ECF sodium and volume. Abnormalities in the serum sodium concentration are thus a result of an alteration in the normal ratio between the total sodium and water content in the ECF.

HYPONATREMIA

EPIDEMIOLOGY AND ETIOLOGY

Hyponatremia (serum sodium <135 mEq/L) is the most common electrolyte abnormality in hospitalized patients, with a reported incidence of about 2.5%.[10] Brain injury results from either the acute effects of hypo-osmolality or from too rapid correction of hypo-osmolality in patients with symptomatic hyponatremia, and is associated with a 20% incidence of significant morbidity and a mortality rate as high as 25%.[11] Hyponatremia is predominantly the result of an excess of extracellular water relative to sodium because of impaired water excretion. The kidney normally has the capacity to excrete large volumes of dilute urine after ingestion of a water load. Nonosmotic

TABLE 49–1. Composition of Intravenous Replacement Solutions

Solution	Dextrose g/dL	[Na+] (mEq/L)	[C−] (mEq/L)	Tonicity	Distribution		
					% ECF	%ICF	Free Water/L
5% dextrose in water (D₅W)	5	0	0	Hypotonic	40	60	1,000 mL
0.45% saline (1/2 normal saline)	0	77	77	Hypotonic	73	37	500 mL
0.9% saline (normal saline)	0	154	154	Isotonic	100	0	0 mL
3% saline (hypertonic saline)	0	513	513	Hypertonic	100[a]	0	−2,331 mL

[a]This solution will result in osmotic removal of water from the intracellular space.

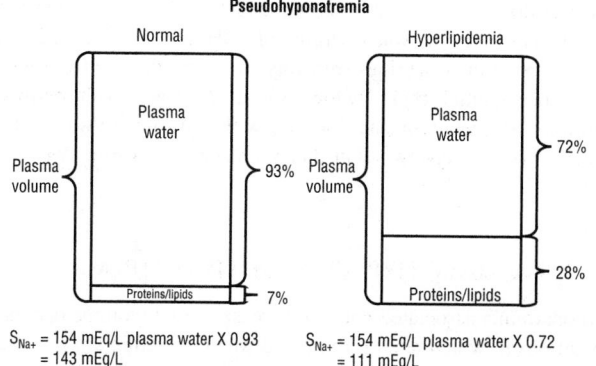

Pseudohyponatremia

S_{Na+} = 154 mEq/L plasma water X 0.93
    = 143 mEq/L

S_{Na+} = 154 mEq/L plasma water X 0.72
    = 111 mEq/L

FIGURE 49–1. Elevated lipids or proteins result in a larger discrepancy between the volume of the sample and plasma water, leading to a falsely low measurement of the serum sodium concentration when using the method of flame photometry.

release of ADH, however, can lead to retention of water and to a drop in serum sodium concentration, despite a fall in both serum and intracellular osmolality. The causes of nonosmotic release of ADH include hypovolemia; decreased EABV as seen in patients with CHF, nephrosis, and cirrhosis; and the syndrome of inappropriate secretion of ADH (SIADH). The pathophysiology, clinical features, and management of hyponatremia are detailed below.

PATHOPHYSIOLOGY

Hyponatremia in patients with normal serum osmolality may be caused by hyperlipidemia or hyperproteinemia. If serum sodium concentration is measured by flame photometry, the volume of serum is overestimated because the elevated lipids or proteins account for a greater proportion of the total volume of the sample (Fig. 49–1).[12] Because the sodium is distributed in only the water component of

serum, the measured serum sodium concentration is falsely decreased. The measurement of serum osmolality, however, is not significantly affected, leading to a discrepancy between the calculated and measured serum osmolality. Because the serum sodium level is falsely decreased, this condition has been termed *pseudohyponatremia*. This laboratory artifact is uncommon today and has been overcome with the use of ion-specific electrodes to measure the serum sodium concentration.[13]

Hyponatremia in the presence of an elevated serum osmolality suggests the presence of excess effective osmoles in the ECF. This is most frequently encountered in patients with hyperglycemia, but is also seen in patients who have received irrigation with glycine during surgery, or in patients who have been treated with osmotic diuretics such as mannitol.[14,15] The presence of glucose, glycine, or mannitol leads to diffusion of water from the cells into the extracellular compartment resulting in hyponatremia. For every 100-mg/dL rise in the serum glucose concentration, the serum sodium level decreases by 1.7 mEq/L[16] and the serum osmolality rises by 2 mOsm/kg.[17] Unmeasured osmoles should be suspected in patients with hypertonic hyponatremia when the difference between the measured and calculated osmolality, the "osmolal gap," exceeds 15 mOsm/kg.[18]

In patients with a low plasma osmolality (hypotonicity), the most important step in the diagnostic evaluation of hyponatremia is the clinical assessment of the extracellular fluid volume.[19] Categorization of patients with hypotonic hyponatremia into one of three groups (decreased, increased, or clinically normal ECF volume) is crucial in order to identify the pathophysiologic mechanisms responsible for the hyponatremia and thereby propose an appropriate treatment regimen (Fig. 49–2).

HYPOVOLEMIC HYPOTONIC HYPONATREMIA

Most patients with ECF volume contraction lose fluids that are hypotonic relative to plasma and thus may be transiently hypernatremic.

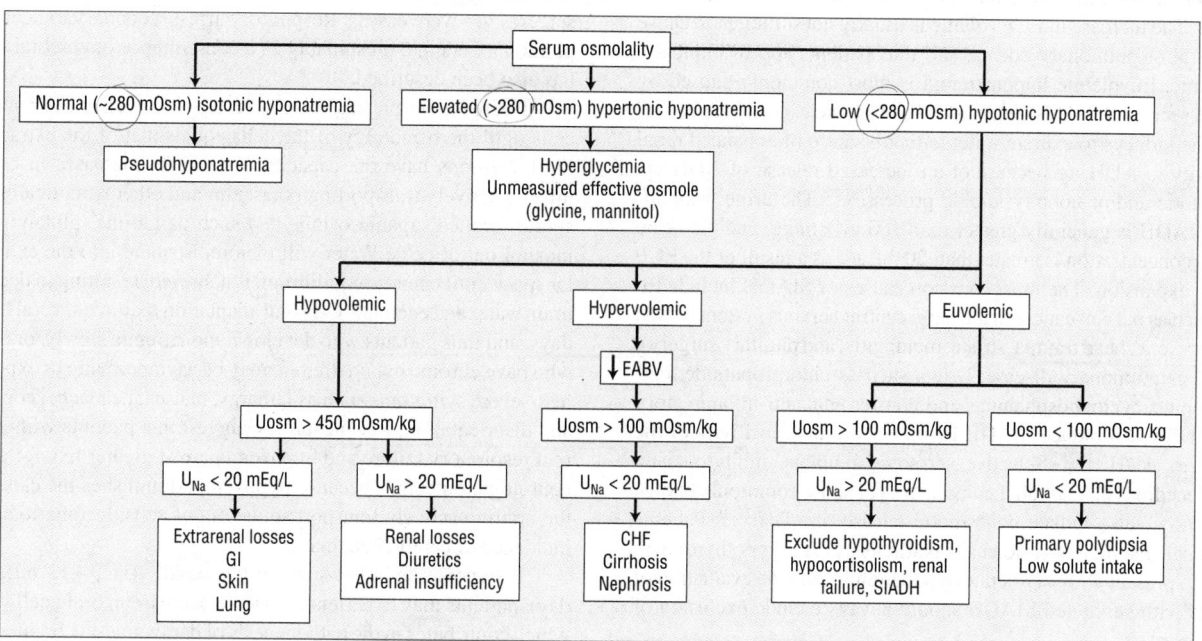

FIGURE 49–2. Diagnostic algorithm for the evaluation of hyponatremia. CHF, congestive heart failure; SIADH, syndrome of inappropriate secretion of antidiuretic hormone; U_{Na}, urine sodium concentration; Uosm, urine osmolality.

This includes patients with fluid losses caused by diarrhea, excessive sweating, and diuretics. This "transient" hypernatremic hyperosmolality results in osmotic release of ADH and stimulation of thirst. If sodium and water losses continue, more ADH is released as a result of hypovolemia. Patients who then drink water or who are given hypotonic fluids intravenously retain water and develop hyponatremia. Urine osmolality is generally greater than 450 mOsm/kg, reflecting the presence of ADH and formation of a concentrated urine.[19] The urine sodium concentration is <20 mEq/L when sodium losses are extrarenal, as in patients with diarrhea, and >20 mEq/L in patients with renal sodium losses, as occurs in the setting of diuretic use or adrenal insufficiency.[20]

Diuretic-induced hyponatremia occurs more frequently in patients treated with thiazide diuretics than in patients who are receiving loop diuretics.[21] In addition to causing extracellular volume depletion and nonosmotic stimulation of ADH, thiazides interfere with urinary dilution and water excretion by blocking tubular sodium and potassium reabsorption in the distal tubule. Water is then retained in excess of sodium by virtue of nonosmotic release of ADH and excretion of urine with a concentration of sodium and potassium that exceeds that of the plasma.

Hyponatremia occurs less commonly with loop diuretics for several reasons. First, most loop diuretics have a shorter half-life than that of thiazides, and patients can therefore replete the urinary sodium and water losses prior to taking the next dose, thereby minimizing the degree of nonosmotic ADH stimulation. Loop diuretics also interfere with both urinary dilution and concentration. The latter is disrupted through inhibition of solute transport into the medulla, which interferes with creation of the medullary osmotic gradient. Thus relatively less water is retained in the presence of ADH.

EUVOLEMIC HYPOTONIC HYPONATREMIA

normovolemic

Euvolemic hyponatremia is associated with a normal or slightly decreased ECF sodium content and increased total body water and ECF volume. The increase in ECF volume is usually not sufficient to cause peripheral or pulmonary edema, and thus patients appear clinically euvolemic. Euvolemic hyponatremia is most commonly caused by SIADH secretion. In this syndrome, water intake exceeds the capacity of the kidneys to excrete water, either because of enhanced renal sensitivity to ADH, or because of an increased release of ADH via nonosmotic and/or nonphysiologic processes.[22] The urine osmolality in SIADH is generally greater than 100 mOsm/kg, and the urine sodium concentration is greater than 20 mEq/L as a result of the ECF volume expansion. The most common causes of SIADH include tumors such as oat cell cancer of the lung, central nervous system (CNS) disorders (e.g., head trauma, stroke, meningitis, and pituitary surgery), as well as pulmonary disease. Drugs such as chlorpropamide, carbamazepine, cyclophosphamide, and nonsteroidal anti-inflammatory drugs (NSAIDs) induce SIADH by enhancing the sensitivity of the kidney to ADH.[23-26] Selective serotonin reuptake inhibitors and methylenedioxymethamphetamine, a drug of abuse commonly known as "ecstasy," also induce nonosmotic release of ADH.[27,28] Patients with renal insufficiency, adrenal insufficiency, and hypothyroidism may also present with euvolemic hyponatremia, and the evaluation of patients with suspected SIADH should always include exclusion of these disorders.

The differential diagnosis of euvolemic hypotonic hyponatremia also includes primary or psychogenic polydipsia. Patients with this disorder drink more water (usually >20 L/day) than the kidneys can excrete as solute-free water. Unlike SIADH, however, ADH is suppressed, resulting in a urine osmolality that is less than 100 mOsm/kg. The urine sodium is typically low (<15 mEq/L) as a result of urinary dilution.[29] Hyponatremia may develop with more modest water intake in patients on a very-low-solute diet, such as a sodium-free vegetarian diet.

HYPERVOLEMIC HYPOTONIC HYPONATREMIA

Hyponatremia associated with an increase in ECF volume occurs in conditions in which renal sodium and water excretion are impaired. Patients with cirrhosis, congestive heart failure, and nephrotic syndrome have an expanded ECF volume and edema, but a decreased EABV. The decreased EABV results in renal sodium retention, and eventually ECF volume expansion and edema. At the same time, there is nonosmotic release of ADH and retention of water in excess of sodium, thus perpetuating the hyponatremia.

CLINICAL PRESENTATION

Most patients with hyponatremia are asymptomatic, and the laboratory finding is often uncovered in the routine evaluation of patients presenting with symptoms attributable to another medical condition such as volume depletion or congestive heart failure.[5] Hyponatremic patients with a decreased ECF volume present with decreased skin turgor, orthostatic hypotension, and dry mucous membranes as the result of excessive losses or inadequate intake of sodium and water. Both total body water and extracellular sodium are decreased, but the sodium deficit exceeds that of water, thus accounting for the decrease in the serum sodium concentration. Patients with serum sodium values greater than 125 mEq/L are generally asymptomatic except when hyponatremia develops in less than 24 hours. The symptoms of acute hypotonic hyponatremia usually result from an increase in neuronal cell volume and consequent cerebral edema. Symptoms may range from nausea, malaise, and headache in milder cases, to coma and seizures in severe cases.[5] Respiratory arrest secondary to neurogenic pulmonary edema, presumably as a consequence of cerebral edema, has also been described.[30]

Decreases in plasma tonicity result in movement of water into cells until the osmolality of the cells equals that of the extracellular fluid. Neurons have the capacity to adapt to increases in cell volume by actively transporting potassium and other osmotically active solutes (called organic osmolytes) such as taurine, glutamine, and inositol out of cells. Water will then redistribute into the extracellular space until osmotic equilibrium is achieved, resulting in decreased brain water and edema.[31] Cerebral adaptation requires several hours to days, and thus patients who develop hyponatremia slowly, or patients who have chronic hyponatremia, may be asymptomatic or experience less-severe symptoms such as lethargy, nausea, headache, confusion, and disorientation. Recent studies suggest that patients with concurrent respiratory failure and hypoxemia are at greater risk for adverse neurologic outcomes because hypoxemia diminishes the capacity of the brain to actively transport solute out of cells, leading to a higher incidence of cerebral edema.[32]

If hyponatremia is corrected too rapidly (i.e., >12 mEq/L per day), patients may experience an acute decrease in brain cell volume, which contributes to the pathogenesis of demyelinating brain injury.[33] Patients with this complication may develop paralysis or coma 5 to 7 days after treatment.[34] Patients who have a significant degree of cerebral adaptation are at highest risk for this complication, presumably because rapid increases in plasma tonicity will result in larger decrements in cell volume.

CLINICAL PRESENTATION OF HYPONATREMIA

GENERAL

Hyponatremia is asymptomatic in most patients. The symptoms that may be seen with hyponatremia are primarily associated with concomitant volume depletion or congestive heart failure. Neurologic symptoms are related both to the severity and in particular to the rapidity of onset of the change in the plasma sodium concentration.

SYMPTOMS

The symptoms directly attributable to hyponatremia primarily occur with acute and marked reductions in the plasma sodium concentration and reflect neurologic dysfunction induced by cerebral edema.

Nausea and malaise are the earliest findings, followed by headache, lethargy, and obtundation, and eventually seizures, coma, and respiratory arrest if the plasma sodium concentration falls below 115 to 120 mEq/L.

> lessen or do away with

SIGNS

Pulmonary: Noncardiogenic pulmonary edema has been described.

Neurologic: Rapid correction of hyponatremia may result in an acute decrease in brain cell volume resulting in demyelinating brain injury.

LABORATORY TESTS

Serum sodium values lower than 135 mmol/L are present.

▶ TREATMENT: Hyponatremia

◾ DESIRED OUTCOME

The goal of treating patients with hypovolemic hypotonic hyponatremia is to correct the ECF volume deficit, which will then lead to correction of the hyponatremia and restoration of organ perfusion. The treatment goals for hypervolemic and euvolemic hypotonic patients depend on the underlying cause of the hyponatremia and whether the patient is symptomatic. Patients who develop hyponatremia rapidly have the highest risk for cerebral edema, and thus require more aggressive therapy to correct the hypotonicity. The goal for these patients is to increase the tonicity at a rate appropriate to restore and maintain cell volume as close to normal as possible. Asymptomatic patients do not require rapid correction of the serum sodium, and the treatment is dictated by the underlying etiology. In all cases the goal is to avoid a rise in the serum sodium concentration greater than 12 mEq/L in 24 hours.

◾ ACUTE SYMPTOMATIC HYPOTONIC HYPONATREMIA

◀ The patient with symptoms attributable to hypotonicity regardless of fluid status should initially be treated with either a 0.9% or a 3% concentrated solution of sodium chloride until symptoms resolve, which generally requires that the serum sodium be increased to approximately 120 mEq/L.[35] The relative concentrations of urine sodium and potassium (osmotically effective urine cations) must be compared with those of the infusate in planning a treatment regimen for patients with hypotonic hyponatremia. For the serum sodium to rise after infusion of a solution of sodium chloride, the concentration of sodium in the infusate must exceed the sum of the sodium and potassium concentration in the urine in order to effect net free water excretion.

◀ Patients with SIADH often have urinary concentrations of osmotically effective urine cations that exceed the sodium concentration of 0.9% saline (154 mEq/L), and thus patients should be preferentially treated with 3% saline (513 mEq/L). In this case use of isotonic saline carries the potential hazard of actually worsening hyponatremia.[35] The relatively high concentration of urinary sodium in patients with SIADH stems from the fact that the ECF is expanded, thus minimizing reabsorption of sodium along the nephron. When the urine osmolality exceeds 300 mOsm/kg, it is generally advisable to add an intravenous loop diuretic, not only to increase the excretion of solute-free water, but also to prevent volume overload, which may result from infusion of hypertonic saline. Intravenous furosemide, initially at a dose of 40 mg every 6 hours, is generally sufficient to prevent volume overload and to decrease the concentration of osmotically active urine cations to less than 150 mEq/L.

Patients with hypovolemic hypotonic hyponatremia, on the other hand, should be treated with normal saline because the concentration of osmotically effective urine cations is invariably less than that of isotonic saline. In contrast to patients with SIADH, sodium is avidly reabsorbed throughout the nephron when the effective circulating blood volume is decreased. Thus the urine osmolality is primarily comprised of urea, and the concentration of urine sodium is often less than 20 mEq/L.

Hypervolemic patients are particularly problematic to manage acutely because the sodium and volume required to minimize the risk of cerebral edema or seizures may worsen their already compensated hepatic, cardiac, or renal function. It is generally agreed that these patients should be treated with hypertonic saline and prompt initiation of fluid restriction. Loop diuretic therapy will also likely be required to facilitate urinary excretion of free water.

◾ DETERMINATION OF THE HYPERTONIC SALINE REGIMEN

Several methods have been developed to determine the correct volume of 3% saline to administer, but it is important to keep in mind that these formulas do not account for ongoing solute and water excretion, and only provide a rough estimate of the correct dose. The formula below is valid only for estimating the change in S_{Na} that will result from the infusion of 3% or 0.9% saline. The change in plasma sodium resulting from the infusion of 3% saline can be estimated as:[5]

$$\text{Change in } S_{Na} \text{ with 1 liter of infusate}$$
$$= [IV_{Na} - S^1_{Na}] \div (BW + IV_{vol})$$

where S_{Na}^1 = initial patient serum sodium concentration; IV_{Na} = sodium concentration of infusate; IV_{vol} = 1L of infusate; and BW = total body water (in liters), which may be estimated as a fraction of total body weight (kilograms) as follows:[36]

0.6 × Body weight for children and men <70 years old

0.5 × Body weight for men ≥70 years old and females <70 years old

0.45 × Body weight for women ≥70 years old

The serum sodium of a 50-kg 80-year-old female with SIADH presenting with confusion and a serum sodium level of 108 mEq/L, for example, should be corrected to approximately 120 mEq/L over the first 24 hours of hospitalization. The change in serum sodium of 12 mEq/L may be calculated as follows:

Change in S_{Na}^1 with 1L of infusate = (513 mEq/L − 108 mEq/L)

$$÷[(0.45 \text{ kg} × 50 \text{ kg}) + 1.0 \text{ L}]$$

$$= [405 \text{ mEq/L}] ÷ 23.5\text{L}$$

Change in S_{Na}^1 with 1L of infusate = 17 mEq/L

Because 1 L of 3% saline results in a 17 mEq/L rise in the serum sodium, one can extrapolate that each 100 mL would increase the serum sodium by 1.7 mEq/L. Thus the total dose required to achieve a change of 12 mEq/L in 24 hours will be approximately 705 mL. In the presence of symptoms, the serum sodium should be raised by approximately 1.5 mEq/L per hour over the first 2 to 4 hours (for a total of 6 mEq/L) or until the symptoms have resolved. Thus an initial infusion rate of 88 mL/h [1.5 mEq/L per hour ÷ 1.7 mEq/L per 100 mL] for the first 2 to 4 hours, followed by an infusion rate of approximately 17.5 to 22 mL/h for the next 20 to 22 hours, respectively, would be a reasonable initial treatment plan.

CLINICAL CONTROVERSY

Clinicians are often in disagreement regarding administration of 0.9% versus 3% saline in patients with symptomatic hypotonicity.

■ EVALUATION OF THERAPEUTIC OUTCOMES

Patients with symptomatic hypotonic hyponatremia should be admitted to the intensive care unit or to a highly monitored setting for close monitoring of neurologic and volume status. Serial physical examinations of the heart, lungs, and neurologic status should be performed several times over the initial 12 hours of hospitalization. The serum sodium concentration should be measured every 2 to 4 hours, and the urine osmolality, sodium, and potassium should be measured every 4 to 6 hours over the first day of therapy. The rate of administration of the infusate should then be adjusted to avoid exceeding a rise in the serum sodium greater than 12 mEq/L per day.

■ HYPOVOLEMIC HYPOTONIC HYPONATREMIA

Because this condition is rarely associated with symptoms, the desired outcomes can generally be achieved with restoration of the blood pressure to the normal range, and absence of postural changes in blood pressure or increases in the central venous pressure or pulmonary cap-

illary wedge pressure to greater than 10 cm H_2O as assessed by central venous or pulmonary artery catheter. A 0.9% solution of sodium chloride, which has a tonicity that approximates that of the ECF, should be infused to correct the volume deficit, because all of the infused solution will remain in the ECF.

ECF volume deficit (ECFVd) is dependent on the patient's weight, age, and the degree of volume depletion, and is difficult to precisely estimate. An ECFVd loss that is equal to a 10% to 15% decrease in body weight is associated with the development of postural hypotension. An ECFVd loss as low as 5%, however, can result in hyponatremia caused by nonosmotic ADH release as a result of stimulation of baroreceptors located in the chest and neck. The ECFVd of patients can be estimated as illustrated in this case: a 42-year-old male weighs 70 kg on initial examination and presents with postural hypotension and has a serum sodium of 125 mEq/L:[37]

$$ECFVd = ECFV_{norm} − ECFV_{current}$$

$$ECFVd = [TBW_{norm} × 0.6 \text{ L/kg} × 0.33]$$
$$−[TBW_{current} × 0.6 \text{ L/kg} × 0.33]$$

where TBW_{norm} is 15% greater than $TBW_{current}$:

$$ECFVd = [80.5 \text{ kg} × 0.6 \text{ L/kg} × 0.33]$$
$$−[70 \text{ kg} × 0.6 \text{ L/kg} × 0.33]$$

$$ECFVd = 15.9 \text{ L} − 13.9 \text{ L}$$

$$ECFVd = 2 \text{ L}$$

A 0.9% solution of sodium chloride is considered to be isotonic and thus is optimal to correct the volume deficit because it will remain in the ECF space (see Table 49–1).

The expected rise in the serum sodium concentration following infusion of 1 L 0.9% saline (154 mEq/L) may be estimated as:

$$\text{Change in } S_{Na} \text{ with 1 liter of infusate} = [IV_{Na} − S_{Na}^1] ÷ (BW + IV_{vol})$$

$$= [154 \text{ mEq/L} − 125 \text{ mEq/L}]$$
$$÷\{(0.6 × 70 \text{ kg}) + 1.0 \text{ L}\}$$
$$= [29 \text{ mEq/L}] ÷ 43 \text{ L}$$
$$= 0.67 \text{ mEq/L}$$

Thus the infusion of 2L of 0.9% saline will result in an increase of serum sodium of 1.34 mEq/L (2 × 0.67 mEq/L). The patient's sodium serum concentrations can thus be approximated to be 126.3 mEq/L (125 mEq/L + 1.34 mEq/L).

Because the overriding initial treatment goal is to restore vital organ perfusion, it is generally necessary to infuse 0.9% saline at 200 to 400 mL/h until hemodynamic stability is restored. The infusion rate can then be decreased to 100 to 150 mL/h such that the serum sodium level rises no more than 12 mEq/L over the initial 24 hours. Infusion of 0.9% saline at rates greater than 250 mL/h, however, should be used cautiously in patients with a history of left ventricular dysfunction or renal insufficiency. Once the ECF volume is restored, ADH secretion will cease, and a rapid water diuresis may ensue, which may potentially result in a rise in the serum sodium at a rate greater than 12 mEq/L per day. If this occurs, the infusate should be changed to 0.45% saline at a rate that approximates urine output (approximately 1.5 to 2 mL/kg per hour is a reasonable initial rate), in order to decrease the rate of rise in the serum sodium concentration.[5]

EVALUATION OF THERAPEUTIC OUTCOMES

Patients presenting with evidence of volume depletion should be re-examined frequently during the initial few hours of the resuscitation phase until hemodynamic stability is restored. Intravenous 0.9% saline should be administered judiciously in patients with a history of congestive heart failure or renal insufficiency, with frequent assessments of the cardiopulmonary examination so the infusion rate may be appropriately decreased when pulmonary congestion is detected. The serum sodium concentration should be measured every 2 to 4 hours to allow timely adjustment of the rate and composition of intravenous fluids in order to avoid a rise in the serum sodium greater than 12 mEq/L per day.

ASYMPTOMATIC EUVOLEMIC HYPOTONIC HYPONATREMIA

The treatment of SIADH always involves water restriction and correction of the underlying cause. Drugs that could be contributing should be identified and discontinued when possible. The goal is to induce negative water balance by restricting water intake to approximately 1,000 to 1,200 mL/day, such that water losses from insensible sources (skin and lung) and from obligate urine and fecal losses exceed intake. Daily insensible water losses via skin and lungs are approximately 700 mL/day, while approximately 100 to 200 mL and 1,500 mL/day is lost in stool and in urine output, respectively. Because approximately 850 mL of water per day is ingested in food, and an additional 350 mL are generated from oxidative processes, the water intake reduction should result in a negative water balance of several hundred milliliters per day.[38] Other goals include maintenance of the serum sodium level above 125 mEq/L to prevent symptoms of hypotonicity, and avoidance of iatrogenic hypo- or hypervolemia.

Patients with chronic SIADH who are unable to restrict water sufficiently to maintain the serum sodium greater than 120 to 125 mEq/L may be treated by increasing solute intake with either urea or sodium chloride and/or loop diuretics.[39] Sodium chloride or urea tablets increase the obligatory daily solute excretion, which augments the capacity for renal water excretion. The goal is to increase the daily solute intake and excretion to approximately 900 mOsm per day. Because an average diet contains approximately 600 mOsm, 9 g of sodium chloride would be required to increase the osmolar excretion to 900 mOsm/day (each 1-g sodium chloride tablet contains 17 mmol of sodium and 17 mmol of chloride). Because extracellular volume expansion is an expected adverse effect, a loop diuretic should be administered concurrently to avoid pulmonary congestion and peripheral edema. Loop diuretics also enhance water excretion by limiting the formation of the medullary concentration gradient.[40]

Other treatment options include demeclocycline therapy and investigational ADH receptor antagonists. Demeclocycline (initially 900 to 1,200 mg/day, then decreased to 600 to 900 mg/day total daily dose given in three to four divided doses), interferes with tubular ADH activity, and is yet another option for patients with chronic SIADH.[41] Because of its delayed onset of action (3 to 6 days), this agent has no role in the acute management of severe hyponatremia. It should not, however, be used in patients with liver disease or compromised fluid intake, who are at high risk for demeclocycline-induced renal tubular toxicity and acute renal failure.[42] Recently several V2 receptor antagonists of ADH have been developed. These agents competitively bind to the V2 receptor on the basolateral surface of epithelial cells in the collecting duct. Blockade of ADH binding to the V2 receptor prevents aquaporin transport to the apical surface, thereby precluding water reabsorption. Several antagonists are under investigation, and show promise for the treatment of chronic hypo-osmolal syndromes such as chronic SIADH.[43]

EVALUATION OF THERAPEUTIC OUTCOMES

The serum sodium level should be measured every 24 to 48 hours after the water restriction is initiated until it stabilizes at a concentration of greater than 125 mEq/L. A continued decline in the serum sodium level would indicate either noncompliance with the prescribed restriction or the need for a more stringent restriction. Once the serum sodium level has stabilized above 125 mEq/L, patients should then be seen every 2 to 4 weeks to assess neurologic status and to obtain serum and urine for sodium, potassium, and osmolality. Again attention should be given to volume status (i.e., blood pressure, skin turgor, and heart and lung exam), particularly in patients who are being treated with sodium chloride tablets and loop diuretics.

ASYMPTOMATIC HYPERVOLEMIC HYPOTONIC HYPONATREMIA

The goals of treatment of asymptomatic hyponatremic patients with an expanded ECF volume include minimizing rapid changes in cell volume and effecting negative water balance until the serum sodium is greater than 125 mEq/L. This entails correction of the underlying cause when possible, as well as restriction of water intake to a volume less than 1,000 to 1,200 mL/day. Dietary intake of sodium chloride should be restricted to 1,000 to 2,000 mg/day, depending on the degree of ECF volume expansion and edema.

Patients with hypervolemic hypotonic hyponatremia caused by congestive heart failure should be treated with measures that can potentially improve cardiac contractility and improve the EABV, thereby limiting the nonosmotic release of ADH. Therapeutic options include digitalis or afterload reduction with angiotensin-converting enzyme inhibitors (ACEIs) or angiotensin II receptor blockers (ARBs). Of these, only ACEIs have been shown in clinical trials to be of benefit in partially correcting hyponatremia in patients with congestive heart failure.[44] No specific ACE inhibitor offers any particular advantage for this indication, and the dose should be titrated to keep the systolic blood pressure in the 110 to 130 mm Hg range. Dose-limiting adverse effects include hyperkalemia (serum potassium >5.5 mEq/L), as well as a decline in renal function. The benefits and risks of continuing ACE inhibition must be weighed carefully in each case, but in general, an acute increase in the serum creatinine greater than 30% would require either a decrease in dose or discontinuation of the ACE inhibitor.

CLINICAL CONTROVERSY

Some clinicians regard any increase in serum creatinine in patients on ACEIs as a reason to decrease dosage or discontinue the medication.

Other potentially treatable causes of asymptomatic hyponatremia associated with an expanded ECF volume include nephrotic syndrome and cirrhosis. ACEIs may be used to decrease proteinuria in patients with nephrotic syndrome, leading to partial correction of hypoalbuminemia and to a decrease in nonosmotic release of ADH. Patients with advanced cirrhosis may benefit from placement of a transjugular intrahepatic portosystemic shunt, which can increase the EABV and thus reduce the nonosmotic release of ADH. This procedure can potentially exacerbate or precipitate hepatic encephalopathy, and should be avoided in patients with a history of encephalopathy. V2 receptor antagonists also show promise for treating hyponatremia in the setting of cirrhosis.[45]

HYPERNATREMIA

EPIDEMIOLOGY AND ETIOLOGY

Hypernatremia (serum sodium >145 mEq/L) is always associated with hypertonicity and results from a deficit of water relative to ECF sodium content. Hyperosmolar states are a potent stimulus for thirst, and therefore hypernatremia is most commonly observed in patients with an impaired thirst response or in those without access to water. Infants and comatose patients, as well as elderly or disabled patients with an impaired sensorium or functional status are therefore at highest risk for this disorder.[46] Hypernatremia occurs in approximately 0.3% to 1% of hospitalized patients.[47] Outcome generally depends on the rapidity with which the hypernatremia developed. Mortality from acute hypernatremia in children, which develops in less than 72 hours, ranges from 10% to 70%. In contrast, chronic hypernatremia in children, defined as that which develops over three or more days, has a mortality rate of 10%.[48] An acute increase in serum sodium in adults to greater than 160 mEq/L is associated with a 75% mortality rate. Adults in whom the hypernatremia developed chronically also have a high mortality in the 60% range.[49] Hypernatremia in adults is often associated with a serious underlying illness, which may contribute to the high mortality rates.

PATHOPHYSIOLOGY

Hypernatremia may result from either loss of water or hypotonic fluids, or less commonly from administration of hypertonic fluids or ingestion of sodium (Fig. 49–3). Water loss commonly occurs as a result of insensible losses (evaporative losses of water through the skin and lungs) in patients deprived of water. Hospitalized patients who are febrile or receiving mechanical ventilation are often treated with intravenous fluids containing insufficient free water to replace insensible losses. Hypernatremia may be observed in patients with hypotonic gastrointestinal losses (diarrhea or vomiting) or in patients who have been exposed to high temperatures who suffer large water losses from both sweat and insensible losses.

EVALUATION OF TREATMENT OUTCOMES

Patients should initially be evaluated on a daily basis with a thorough physical exam to assess for lung congestion, ascites, and peripheral edema. The serum sodium concentration should be measured daily until it stabilizes above 125 mEq/L following initiation of water restriction. Patients should then be assessed 1 week following discharge, and then every 2 to 4 weeks to assess compliance with the water restriction and to reassess volume status.

Patients with diabetes insipidus (DI), or those undergoing an osmotic diuresis, may also have large urinary losses of water. DI is classified as either central (characterized by deficient secretion of ADH) or nephrogenic (characterized by resistance to ADH activity). Table 49–2 summarizes the causes of DI. Patients with central DI often present with sudden onset of polyuria, whereas patients with nephrogenic DI develop polyuria more gradually.

Administration of hypertonic saline can result in hypernatremia and an expanded ECF volume. This is typically iatrogenic, and may follow administration of sodium bicarbonate, use of hypertonic saline enemas, or intrauterine injection of hypertonic saline. Rarely, patients with hyperaldosteronism spontaneously present with an expanded ECF and mild hypernatremia.[50]

CLINICAL PRESENTATION

The symptoms of hypernatremia are primarily caused by a decrease in neuronal cell volume, and may include weakness, restlessness, confusion, and coma. Hypernatremia results in movement of water from the intracellular space to the extracellular fluid. Neurons can adapt to hypertonicity in the ECF by generating intracellular organic osmolytes within 24 hours of onset. This increase in intracellular fluid tonicity then draws water into the neurons, thus limiting the decrease in cell volume. Patients with chronic hypernatremia are less likely to present with symptoms caused by this cerebral adaptation.

Hypernatremia is often associated with serious underlying illness, and thus symptoms may also be due to coexisting disorders. Patients with a history of severe diarrhea or vomiting may present with ECF volume depletion. Elderly patients deprived of water after sustaining a stroke or hip fracture often present with mental status changes and signs of ECF volume depletion. Clinically detectable extracellular fluid volume depletion, however, may not be evident until the serum sodium concentration exceeds 160 mEq/L, because these patients primarily have water loss, two-thirds of which is derived from the intracellular space. The urine is concentrated with an osmolality greater than 450 mOsm/kg as a result of both osmotic and nonosmotic release of ADH. The first step in evaluating patients with

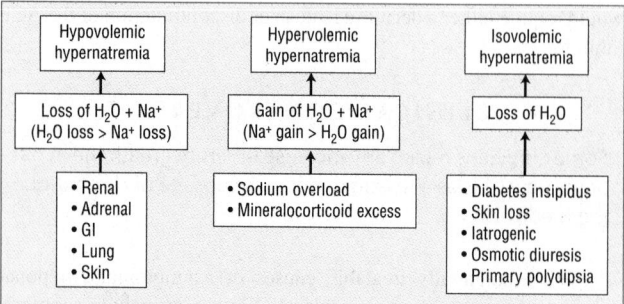

FIGURE 49–3. Common etiologies of hypernatremia.

TABLE 49–2. Causes of Diabetes Insipidus

Central DI	Nephrogenic DI
Idiopathic	Lithium toxicity
Familial	Hypercalcemia
Neurosurgery	Hypokalemia
Head trauma	Cidofavir
CNS malignancy	Foscarnet
Hypoxic encephalopathy	Inherited aquaporin-2 defect
Sheehan's syndrome	Inherited ADH-V2 recepter defect
	Demeclocycline

ADH, antidiuretic hormone; CNS, central nervous system.

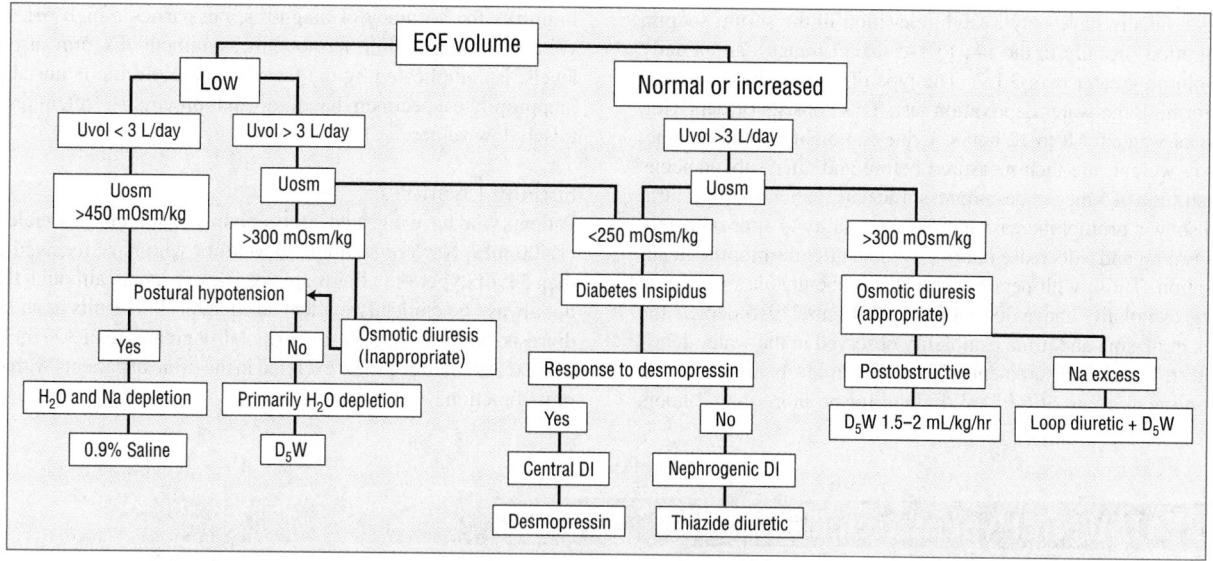

FIGURE 49–4. Diagnostic and treatment algorithm for hypernatremia. D_5W, 5% dextrose in water; ECF, extracellular fluid; H_2O, water; Na, sodium; Uosm, urine osmolality; Uvol, daily urine volume. See text for guidelines regarding calculations of infusion rates for intravenous solutions.

hypernatremia is the clinical assessment of the ECF volume, urine volume, and urine osmolality (Fig. 49–4).

Patients with a contracted ECF volume and a low urine output include those who have sustained insensible water losses that exceed intake, as well as those with extrarenal losses of hypotonic fluids. On physical exam, one should search for postural hypotension, diminished skin turgor, and delayed capillary refill. The daily urine output is typically less than 1 L.

CLINICAL PRESENTATION OF HYPERNATREMIA

GENERAL
The rise in the plasma sodium concentration and osmolality causes acute water movement from the intracellular to the extracellular fluid. In the brain this decrease in volume can cause rupture of the cerebral veins, leading to focal intracerebral and subarachnoid hemorrhages and possible irreversible neurologic damage.

SYMPTOMS
The clinical manifestations of this disorder begin with lethargy, weakness, confusion, restlessness, and irritability, and can progress to twitching, seizures, and coma. Severe symptoms usually require an acute elevation in the plasma sodium concentration to above 160 mEq/L. Values above 180 mEq/L are associated with a high mortality rate.

SIGNS
Signs of hypernatremia may include postural hypotension, diminished skin turgor, and reduced urine output.
Signs associated with chronic hypernatremia are often difficult to detect because most affected adults have underlying neurologic disease.

LABORATORY TESTS
Serum sodium levels are generally higher than 145 mEq/L.

OSMOTIC DIURESIS

Patients undergoing an osmotic diuresis generally have urine volumes greater than 3 L/day. Excessive urinary excretion of glucose, sodium, urea, or an exogenously administered solute such as mannitol, are identified either by history or by direct measurement of serum and urinary concentrations of the suspected solute. Patients with postobstructive diuresis, such as those with bladder outlet obstruction due to prostatic hypertrophy, are usually volume expanded as a result of retained excess solute due to a decline in the glomerular filtration rate (GFR).[51] The osmotic diuresis that follows alleviation of the obstruction is appropriate in that it promotes excretion of the excess retained solute. Patients with severe hyperglycemia, on the other hand, present with signs of volume depletion, and the diuresis is therefore inappropriate, further exacerbating the degree of ECF volume contraction.

Diabetes Insipidus
Patients with diabetes insipidus tend to maintain a normal ECF volume as long as they are conscious and have free access to water.

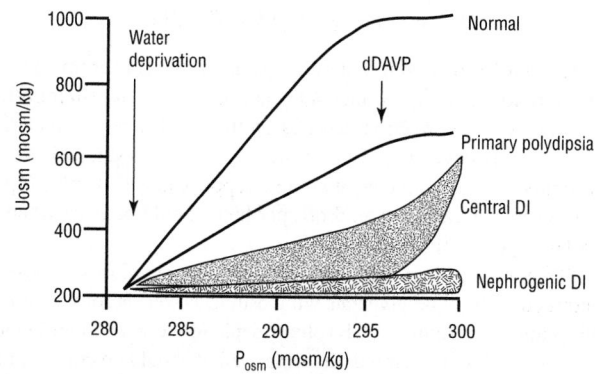

FIGURE 49–5. Water deprivation test. The change in plasma osmolality is plotted against the change in urine osmolality following water deprivation and subcutaneous administration of 5 mcg of desmopressin acetate. DI, diabetes insipidus; P_{osm}, plasma osmolality; Uosm, urine osmolality. (Adapted from Rose et al.[51])

Patients typically have only a slight elevation in the serum sodium concentration (usually in the 141 to 145 mEq/L range), and a daily urine volume greater than 3 L.[52] The type of DI may be diagnosed by performing the water deprivation test. This consists of depriving patients of water for 8 to 12 hours. Urine osmolality, urine volume, and body weight, are then measured before and after subcutaneous administration of 5 mcg of desmopressin acetate. Patients with central DI will show a prompt increase in urine osmolality to approximately 600 mOsm/kg and a decrease in urine volume after desmopressin administration. Those with nephrogenic DI will be unable to increase the urine osmolality above 300 mOsm/kg.[51] Figure 49–5 depicts the changes in plasma and urine osmolality observed in the water deprivation test. Direct measurement of vasopressin levels after infusion of 5% saline at a rate of 0.05 mL/kg/min for no more than 2 hours improves the accuracy of diagnosis, but carries a high risk of ECF volume overload.[53] Furthermore, measurement of serum vasopressin levels, is complicated by the fact that the molecule is unstable, and inappropriate specimen handling and processing often results in falsely low values.

Sodium Overload

Patients who have ingested large amounts of sodium [>4 tablespoons (1,400 mEq Na^+) of sodium chloride] or who have received greater than 5 L of hypertonic fluids are volume expanded, although this may not always be clinically evident as edema. This results in an osmotic diuresis, polyuria, and a urine osmolality greater than 300 mOsm/kg. The excess sodium will be excreted in the urine in patients with normal renal function.

▶ TREATMENT: Hypernatremia

▦ DESIRED OUTCOME

The goals in treating patients with hypernatremia include correction of the serum sodium concentration at a rate that restores and maintains cell volume as close to normal as possible, as well as normalizing the ECF volume in states of ECF volume depletion and expansion. Adequate treatment should result in the resolution of symptoms associated with hypovolemia. Careful titration of fluids and medications should minimize the adverse effects from too rapid correction. Modulation of dietary sodium intake and sodium replacement may be necessary to prevent recurrence of hypernatremia.

▦ PHARMACOLOGIC THERAPY

▦ HYPOVOLEMIC HYPERNATREMIA

◀4 Hypovolemic hypernatremia (postural hypotension, tachycardia, and decreased skin turgor) should initially be treated with 0.9% saline until hemodynamic stability is restored. An initial infusion rate of 200 to 300 mL/h will likely be appropriate for many patients. Once intravascular volume is restored, 0.45% saline or 5% dextrose in water (D_5W) can then be infused to correct the water deficit,[37] the volume of which may be estimated as:

$$\left| \text{Water Deficit} = \text{Present TBW} \times [(S_{Na}^1/140) - 1] \right|$$

where TBW = total body water; S_{Na}^1 = initial patient serum sodium concentration (in mEq/L); and 140 = normal or goal S_{Na} (in mEq/L).

The rate of correction depends on the rapidity with which the hypernatremia developed. Hypernatremia that has developed over a few hours may be corrected at a rate of approximately 1 mEq/L per hour, whereas a rate of 0.5 mEq/L per hour should be used when it has developed more slowly.[50]

Treatment of hyperglycemia-induced osmotic diuresis consists of correcting the hyperglycemia with insulin, as well as administering 0.9% saline until signs of ECF volume depletion resolve. Once hemodynamic stability is restored, the water deficit should be corrected in a manner analogous to that described for patients with hypovolemic hypernatremia above. The corrected serum sodium level should be calculated by adding 1.7 mEq/L for every 100-mg/dL rise in the serum glucose concentration before estimating the water deficit.[5]

Hypernatremia in patients undergoing a postobstructive diuresis should be treated with infusion of hypotonic fluids such as 0.45% saline at maintenance rates of approximately 1.5 mL/kg per hour. It is important to avoid the temptation to administer fluids to replace urine output on a 1 mL:1 mL volume basis, because this tends to perpetuate the diuresis.

The serum sodium concentration and fluid status should be monitored every 2 to 3 hours over the first 24 hours of admission in patients with symptomatic hypernatremia to permit appropriate adjustment in the rate of infusion of hypotonic fluids. After symptoms resolve and the serum sodium is less than 148 mEq/L, serum sodium determinations every 6 to 12 hours and fluid status assessment every 8 to 24 hours are generally sufficient to follow the course of therapy.

▦ CENTRAL DIABETES INSIPIDUS

◀5 The beginning dose of intranasal desmopressin should be 10 mcg once daily. Ultimately the dose may need to be titrated up to 10 mcg twice daily for most adults. Because of variable absorption of oral desmopressin, DI is best treated with the intranasal formulation 1-deamino-8-D-arginine vasopressin (DDAVP). Each insufflation of intranasal DDAVP delivers 10 mcg of desmopressin acetate at a concentration of 100 mcg/mL.[54] Drugs with antidiuretic properties have been successful in the management of central and nephrogenic DI (Table 49–3). They may be used as an alternative to DDAVP or adjunctively.

The desmopressin dose should be adjusted to achieve adequate urinary concentration during sleep to prevent nocturia, to result in a daily urine volume of approximately 1.5 to 2 L, and to maintain the serum sodium concentration in the 137 to 142 mEq/L range. The serum sodium concentration should be measured every 3 to 4 days during the initial dose titration period, and then every 2 to 4 months.

▦ NEPHROGENIC DIABETES INSIPIDUS

◀6 Hypercalcemia and hypokalemia should be corrected and medications that may contribute to the pathogenesis should be discontinued. One key goal in treating nephrogenic DI is to induce a mild ECFVd (1 to 1.5 L) with a thiazide diuretic and dietary sodium restriction (85 mEq Na^+ or 2,000 mg sodium chloride per day), which

TABLE 49–3. Drugs Used to Manage Central and Nephrogenic Diabetes Insipidus

Drug	Indication	Dose
Desmopressin acetate (DDAVP)	Central and nephrogenic DI	5–20 mcg intranasally every 12–24 h
Chlorpropamide	Central DI	125–250 mg orally daily
Carbamazepine	Central DI	100–300 mg orally twice a day
Clofibrate	Central DI	500 mg orally four times a day
Hydrochlorothiazide	Central and nephrogenic DI	25 mg orally every 12–24 h
Amiloride	Lithium-related nephrogenic DI	5–10 mg orally daily
Indomethacin	Central and nephrogenic DI	50 mg orally every 8–12 h

often can decrease urine volume by as much as 50% (see Table 49–3). This will increase proximal water reabsorption and therefore decrease the volume of filtrate delivered to the distal nephron, thus resulting in decreased urine volume. NSAIDs such as indomethacin at a dose of 50 mg three times a day may be used as adjunctive therapy by potentiating the activity of ADH.[55] Patients with lithium-induced nephrogenic DI may derive particular benefit from amiloride at a dose of 5 to 10 mg daily, which directly inhibits uptake of lithium from the tubular lumen into principal cells in the cortical collecting duct.[56]

CLINICAL CONTROVERSY

The use of NSAIDs or amiloride to produce mild extracellular volume depletion needs to be evaluated in terms of the risks of an increase in serum creatinine concentration.

■ EVALUATION OF TREATMENT OUTCOMES

Physical examination with attention to volume status and measurement of serum and urine sodium concentration and osmolality should be assessed every 2 to 3 months. A 24-hour urine collection to measure urine volume and sodium excretion will help guide therapy with diuretics and determine compliance with sodium restriction.

■ SODIUM OVERLOAD

Treatment of sodium overload consists of administration of loop diuretics to facilitate excretion of the excess sodium, as well as intravenous D_5W. The latter should be infused at a rate that will decrease the serum sodium at approximately 0.5 mEq/L per hour, or 1 mEq/L per hour in cases in which the hypernatremia developed rapidly over several hours.[50] The volume of infusate may be estimated as described previously. Furosemide should be administered at a dose of 20 to 40 mg intravenously every 6 hours.

The serum sodium should initially be measured every 2 to 4 hours, and the diuretic continued until signs of ECF volume overload (pulmonary congestion and edema) resolve. The serum sodium concentration can be determined every 6 to 12 hours once the serum sodium level is less than 148 mEq/L and symptoms of hypertonicity resolve.

EDEMA

The kidney responds to changes in the EABV, rather than directly sensing or measuring the sodium content of the ECF. A decline in the EABV results in decreased sodium and water excretion.[9] Under these conditions, the kidneys retain all of the water and sodium ingested until the EABV is restored to normal. An increase in dietary sodium is accompanied by an increase in water intake caused by the initial increase in serum osmolality and stimulation of thirst. The resultant increase in ECF volume augments renal perfusion, effecting a transient increase in GFR which leads to enhanced sodium filtration and excretion.[57] These homeostatic mechanisms are crucial in maintaining sodium balance, as retention of just a few milliequivalents of sodium per day can eventually lead to an expanded ECF volume and edema formation.

PATHOPHYSIOLOGY

Edema is clinically detectable in adults when the interstitial volume increases by approximately 2.5 to 3 L, which correlates with a 4- to 4.5-L increase in ECF volume, and a 500 to 600 mEq increase in ECF sodium.[58] Edema develops when excess sodium is retained either as a primary defect in renal sodium excretion, or as a response to a decrease in the EABV despite an already expanded or normal ECF volume. An increase in the capillary hydrostatic pressure because of an expansion of the ECF volume, or an increase in central venous pressure may lead to edema formation. Edema may also occur when there is an alteration in Starling forces within the capillary.[59] The Starling equation denotes the relationship between factors affecting the movement of fluid between the capillary and interstitium and is discussed in detail in Chap. 24.

An acute decompensation in myocardial contractility leads to an elevation in pulmonary venous pressure that is transmitted back to the pulmonary capillaries resulting in pulmonary edema. On a chronic basis, renal sodium and water retention due to diminished EABV leads to a rise in the ECF volume and edema formation in both peripheral and pulmonary interstitial tissues.

Edema formation in patients with nephrotic syndrome is primarily related to renal sodium and water retention. A decrease in capillary oncotic pressure does not appear to play a major role until the serum albumin concentration falls to less than 2 g/dL. This is explained by the fact that both capillary and interstitial oncotic pressure decrease proportionately above a serum albumin concentration of 2 g/dL, and thus the transcapillary oncotic gradient is not significantly altered.[60]

Patients with cirrhosis initially develop ascites as a result of an increase in the pressure in the portal circulation proximal to the diseased liver. Sequestration of fluid in the abdominal cavity (ascites) and peripheral vasodilation as a consequence of increased levels of circulating cytokines, result in a decrease in the effective circulating volume, activation of the sympathetic nervous system and secondary hyperaldosteronism. Therefore renal sodium retention leads to worsened ascites and edema.

CLINICAL PRESENTATION

Edema is usually first detected in the feet or pretibial area of ambulatory patients and in the presacral area of bed-bound individuals. Edema is described as "pitting" when a depression created by exerting pressure for several seconds over a bony prominence such as the tibia does not rapidly refill. The severity of the edema may be quantified based on the depth of the pit thusly: 1+ = 2 mm, 2+ = 4 mm, 3+ = 6 mm, and 4+ = 8 mm.

The extent of the edema should also be quantified according to the area of involvement. Pretibial edema, for example, should be quantified according to how far it extends up the lower leg (e.g., one-third up the lower leg). Pulmonary edema, defined as an increase in lung interstitial and alveolar water, is manifest as end-inspiratory rales, initially localized to the dependent portions of the lungs.

▶ TREATMENT: Edema

GENERAL APPROACH TO TREATMENT

The goals of diuretic therapy are to minimize tissue edema and thus improve organ function, as well as to relieve symptoms of edema such as dyspnea in patients with congestive heart failure (CHF) or abdominal distention in patients with ascites. It is important to emphasize that the presence of edema does not always dictate the need for instituting pharmacologic (diuretic) therapy. Only pulmonary edema requires immediate pharmacologic treatment because it is life-threatening. Other forms of edema may be treated gradually, with a comprehensive approach that includes not only diuretics, but also sodium restriction and treatment of the underlying disease state. Sodium chloride intake should generally be restricted to 1,000 to 2,000 mg/day. A slow, more judicious approach in non–life-threatening situations will help to minimize complications of diuretic therapy and excessive fluid removal. These may include impaired vital organ perfusion, azotemia, and impaired cardiac output due to a fall in the left ventricular end-diastolic filling pressure.

[handwritten: uremia (poisoning 2° to disease or poor fxn of kidneys)]

PHARMACOLOGIC THERAPY

Diuretics are the primary pharmacologic therapy for the management of edema. Patients with expanded ECF volume and edema often require therapy with diuretics when treatment of the underlying disease and daily sodium restriction are insufficient to relieve the edema. Diuretics can be categorized according to the site in the nephron where sodium reabsorption is inhibited. Loop diuretics inhibit the Na^+-K^+-$2Cl^-$ carrier in the loop of Henle. Thiazide diuretics inhibit the Na^+- Cl^- carrier in the distal tubule. Finally, potassium-sparing diuretics inhibit the sodium channel in the cortical collecting duct either directly (triamterene and amiloride), or by interfering with aldosterone activity (spironolactone and eplerenone). The efficacy of a diuretic depends on the presence of several factors, including the amount of filtered solute normally reabsorbed at the site of action, the amount of solute reabsorbed distal to the site of action, and adequate delivery of drug to the site of action in the nephron.

Loop diuretics are the most potent diuretics, as evidenced by the fact that they increase peak fractional excretion of sodium (Fe_{Na}) to 20% to 25%. Thiazide- and potassium-sparing diuretics are less potent and increase peak FeNa to 3% to 5% and 1% to 2%, respectively.[61] Although a large portion of the filtered sodium is reabsorbed in the proximal nephron, the efficacy of proximal-acting diuretics such as acetazolamide are limited by reabsorption of the excess fluid and sodium in the loop of Henle.

The effectiveness of thiazide and loop diuretics is dependent on the concentration of the drug in the tubular lumen. Diuretics are delivered to the tubular lumen of the kidney by active transport by the proximal tubular cells. Osmotic diuretics, on the other hand, are freely filtered into the tubular lumen in the proximal tubule, whereas spironolactone gains access to mineralocorticoid receptors in the cortical collecting duct through diffusion from the systemic circulation.

A threshold concentration of loop or thiazide diuretic must be delivered to the active site (e.g., loop of Henle or distal tubule) in order to achieve a natriuresis.[62] Once this concentration is achieved, further increases in diuretic dose will not elicit an increase in diuretic response. Thus a ceiling dose of diuretic is recognized. Administration of 40 mg of intravenous furosemide to a normal subject will result in excretion of 200 to 250 mEq of sodium in 3 to 4 L of urine over a 3- to 4-hour period.[62] Table 49–4 summarizes the maximal effective

TABLE 49–4. Maximal Effective Dose and Dosing Interval for Edema Management with Loop Diuretics

Diuretic	Dosing Interval	Normal	Cirrhosis	CHF	Nephrotic Syndrome	GFR 10–50 mL/min	GFR <10 mL/min
Furosemide							
IV	6–8 h	10–40 mg	40 mg	40–80 mg	120 mg	80 mg	200 mg
Oral	6–8 h	20–80 mg	80 mg	80–160 mg	240 mg	160 mg	320–400 mg
Bumetanide							
IV/Oral	6–8 h	1 mg	1 mg	2–3 mg	3 mg	2–3 mg	8–10 mg
Torsemide							
IV/Oral	24 h	15–20 mg	10–20 mg	20–50 mg	50 mg	20–50 mg	50–100 mg

CHF, congestive heart failure; GFR, glomerular filtration rate.

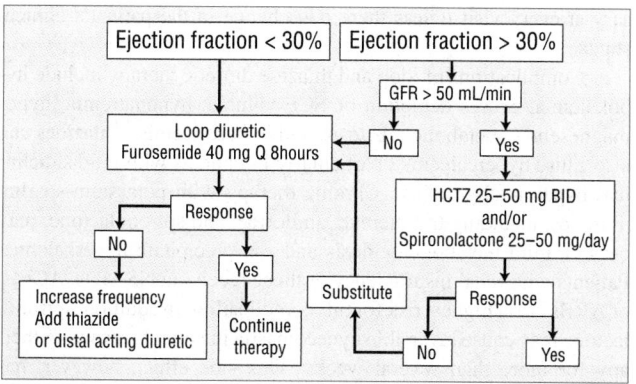

FIGURE 49–6. Therapeutic algorithm for diuretic use in patients with congestive heart failure. GFR, glomerular filtration rate; HCTZ, hydrochlorothiazide.

doses and dosing intervals for loop diuretics in patients with cirrhosis, CHF, and nephrotic syndrome, with normal and decreased glomerular filtration rates. Patients with renal insufficiency require larger doses of diuretics to achieve adequate concentration of the drug to the active site (see Chap. 42). The natriuretic response is decreased in patients with renal insufficiency because the filtered load of sodium falls proportionately as GFR declines. This may be partially overcome by dosing diuretics more frequently, as well as by using continuous infusions in critically ill hospitalized patients.[63] The latter will maintain more consistent levels of the diuretic above the threshold concentration. Patients that are diuretic resistant should be treated with both a loop and a thiazide-type diuretic. Patients with CHF and a normal GFR have impaired oral absorption of furosemide. An adequate diuresis is most readily sustained by increasing the frequency of diuretic administration (Fig. 49–6).

Diuretic resistance may be due to increased uptake of sodium in the distal tubule, impaired delivery of diuretics to the site of action, or decreased intrinsic diuretic activity. Animal studies have demonstrated binding of furosemide to albumin in the tubular lumen, which decreases the availability of the drug to the active site.[64] Human studies, however, have demonstrated that when albumin binding is inhibited by concurrent administration of sulfasoxazole, diuretic resistance persists, suggesting a decrease in intrinsic tubular sensitivity to loop diuretics.[65] This impaired natriuretic response may be overcome by using higher diuretic doses to increase the delivery of free drug to the secretory site in the nephron.[63] Combinations of loop diuretics with distally-acting diuretics are generally necessary

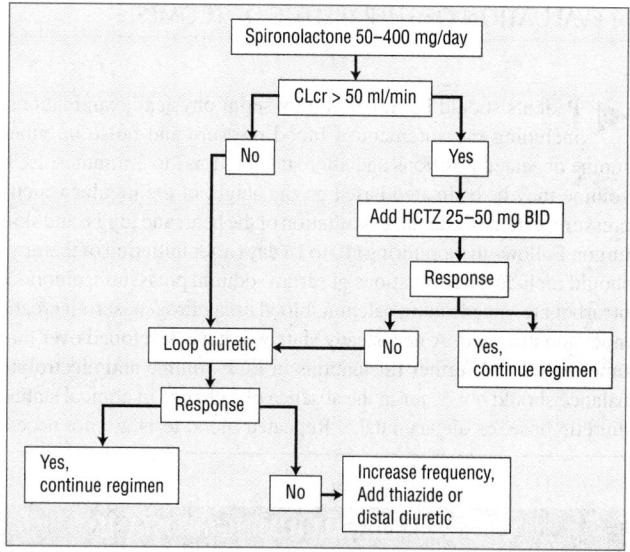

FIGURE 49–8. Therapeutic algorithm for diuretic use in patients with cirrhosis. Clcr, creatinine clearance; HCTZ, hydrochlorothiazide.

to promote a natriuresis that exceeds tubular sodium reabsorption (Fig. 49–7).

CLINICAL CONTROVERSY

Some clinicians advocate using combinations of diuretics in cases of diuretic resistance associated with nephrotic syndrome, while others prefer to use larger-than-average doses to overcome enhanced protein binding in the tubular lumen associated with proteinuria.

Secondary hyperaldosteronism plays a major role in the pathogenesis of edema in patients with cirrhosis. Therefore these patients should initially be treated with spironolactone in the absence of impaired GFR and hyperkalemia. Thiazides may then be added for patients with a creatinine clearance >50 mL/min. For those patients who remain diuretic resistant, a loop diuretic may replace the thiazide. Patients with impaired GFR (creatinine clearance of <30 mL/min) generally will require a loop diuretic, with addition of a thiazide in those who do not achieve adequate diuresis.[63] Care should be taken to avoid hypokalemia, which may precipitate hepatic encephalopathy by increasing ammoniagenesis (Fig. 49–8).[66]

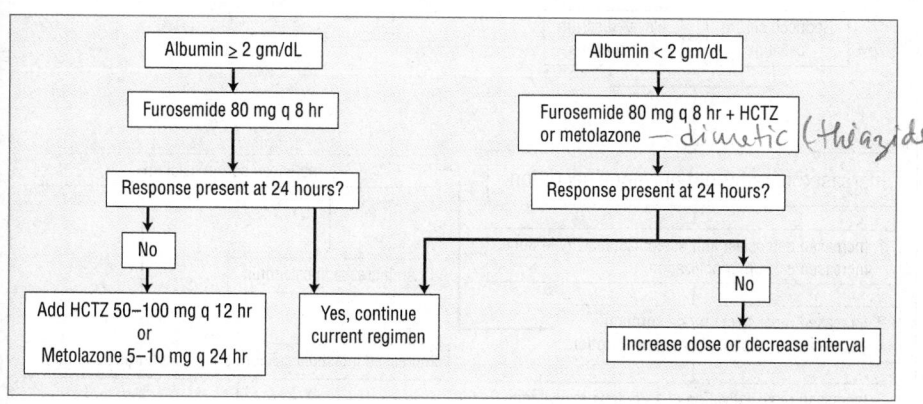

FIGURE 49–7. Therapeutic algorithm for diuretic therapy in patients with nephrotic syndrome. HCTZ, hydrochlorothiazide.

■ EVALUATION OF THERAPEUTIC OUTCOMES

Patients should be monitored by serial physical examinations, including measurement of blood pressure and pulse in either supine or seated positions and after standing for 2 to 3 minutes. ECF volume may be estimated based on the height of the jugular venous pressure, extent of edema, auscultation of the heart and lungs, and skin turgor. Follow-up monitoring (10 to 14 days after initiation of therapy) should include determinations of serum sodium, potassium, chloride, bicarbonate, magnesium, calcium, blood urea nitrogen, serum creatinine, and uric acid. A new steady state will have developed over that time period and further fluctuations in ECF volume and electrolyte balance should not occur in the absence of a change in clinical status, diuretic dose, or dietary intake. Repeated blood tests are not neces-

sary at every visit unless there is a change in the patient's clinical status.

Complications of loop and thiazide diuretic therapy include hypokalemia, excess depletion of ECF volume, hyponatremia, hypomagnesemia, metabolic alkalosis, and hyperuricemia. Thiazides can also cause hypercalcemia, particularly in patients with mild subclinical hyperparathyroidism. Chronic therapy with potassium-sparing diuretics, including triamterene, amiloride, and spironolactone, may cause a mild metabolic acidosis and can precipitate hyperkalemia. Patients with renal insufficiency or those receiving NSAIDs, ACEIs, or ARBs are at highest risk for this complication. In addition, spironolactone may cause reversible gynecomastia in patients receiving therapy for more than several weeks. This side effect, however, has not been associated with eplerenone, a newly available aldosterone antagonist.[67]

DISORDERS OF CALCIUM HOMEOSTASIS

The maintenance of physiologic calcium concentrations in the intracellular and extracellular spaces is vital for the preservation and function of cell membranes; propagation of neuromuscular activity; regulation of endocrine and exocrine secretory functions; blood coagulation cascade; platelet adhesion process; bone metabolism; muscle cell excitation/contraction coupling; and mediation of the electrophysiologic slow-channel response in cardiac and smooth-muscle tissue.

The disorders of calcium homeostasis are related to the calcium content of the extracellular fluid, which contains less than 0.5% of the total body stores of calcium. Skeletal bone contains more than 99% of total body stores of calcium.[68] ECF calcium is moderately bound to plasma proteins (46%), primarily albumin.[69] Unbound or ionized calcium is the physiologically active form and is the fraction that is homeostatically regulated.[70] Extracellular calcium, however, is most commonly measured as the total serum calcium level, which includes both bound and unbound calcium.[69] The normal total calcium serum concentration range is 8.5 to 10.5 mg/dL.[70]

The concentration of ionized calcium is closely regulated by the interactions of parathyroid hormone (PTH), phosphorus, vitamin D, and calcitonin (Fig. 49–9). Parathyroid hormone increases serum calcium concentrations by stimulating calcium release from bone, reducing renal excretion, and enhancing absorption in the gastrointestinal tract secondary to increased renal production of 1,25-

dihydroxyvitamin D_3. Vitamin D directly increases serum calcium, as well as phosphorus concentrations, by increasing gastrointestinal absorption. Indirectly, it can also lead to calcium release from bone and reduced renal excretion. Calcitonin inhibits osteoclastic bone resorption. Its plasma concentrations are increased when ionized calcium concentrations are high as the body attempts to return the calcium level to the normal range. Disruption of these homeostatic mechanisms results in the clinical manifestations of hypercalcemia or hypocalcemia.

Any factor that alters the concentration of albumin or its binding of calcium may be expected to change the fraction of total serum calcium in the ionized form. The most significant cause of changes in calcium binding to albumin is a change in extracellular fluid pH. In the presence of metabolic alkalosis the fraction of calcium bound to albumin is increased, thus reducing the plasma concentration of ionized calcium. This may result in symptomatic hypocalcemia; that is, paresthesias, muscle cramping and spasms, memory loss, and seizures.[68] Conversely, metabolic acidosis decreases calcium binding to albumin and results in increased ionized calcium. Hypoalbuminemic states are probably the most common cause of "laboratory hypocalcemia." When the albumin level is decreased, ionized calcium concentration may be normal even though total concentration is reduced. Each 1 g/dL drop in the serum albumin concentration below 4 g/dL will result in a decrease of total serum calcium concentration by 0.8 mg/dL.[68,69] This approach of calculating an albumin-adjusted calcium concentration has been found to overestimate

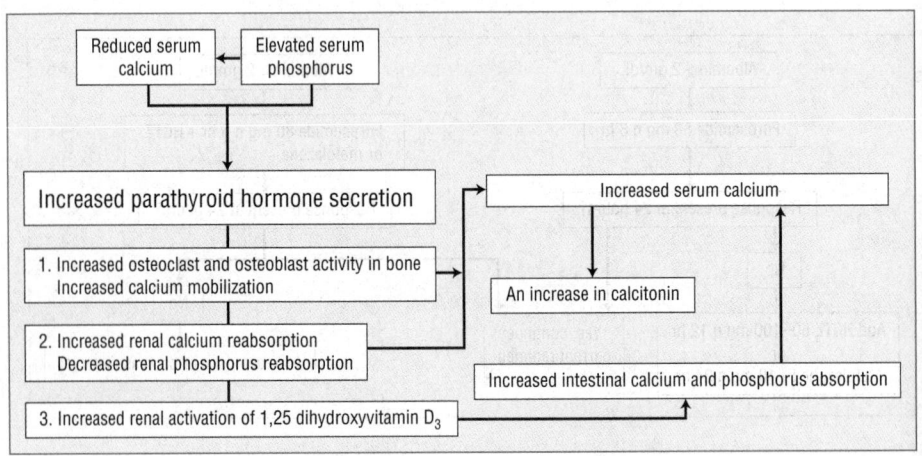

FIGURE 49–9. Homeostatic mechanisms to maintain serum calcium concentrations.

TABLE 49–5. Etiologies of Hypercalcemia

Neoplasms	Medications
Bone metastasis	Thiazides
Breast	Lithium
Multiple myeloma	Vitamin D
Lymphoma	Vitamin A
Leukemia	Calcium
Humoral induced	Aluminum/magnesium
Ovary	antacids
Kidney	Theophylline
Pheochromocytoma	Tamoxifene
Multiple endocrine	Gancyclovir
neoplasia	**Granulomatous disease**
Lung	Sarcoidosis
Head and neck	Tuberculosis
Esophagus	Cryptococcus
Cervix	Berylliosis
Lymphoproliferative disease	Histoplasmosis
Hyperparathyroidism	Coccidioidomycosis
Primary	Leprosy
Tertiary	**Endocrine disease**
Miscellaneous	Adrenal insufficiency
Immobilization	Hyperthyroidism
Paget's disease	Acromegaly
Familial hypocalciuric	
hypercalcemia	
Adolescence	
Rhabdomyolysis	

hypercalcemia and usually fails to identify hypocalcemia in critically ill patients.[71]

HYPERCALCEMIA

Hypercalcemia (total serum calcium >10.5 mg/dL) may be induced by a multitude of causes (Table 49–5). The most common causes of hypercalcemia are cancer and primary hyperparathyroidism. The incidence of primary hyperparathyroidism is approximately 270 new cases per million persons per year.[72] Hypercalcemia of cancer occurs in approximately 20% to 40% of cancer patients at some time during the course of their disease.[73] Cancer-associated hypercalcemia is predominantly encountered in hospitalized patients, while primary hyperparathyroidism accounts for the vast majority of cases in the outpatient setting.[74,75]

PATHOPHYSIOLOGY

Hypercalcemia is the result of one of three primary mechanisms: increased bone resorption, increased gastrointestinal absorption, or decreased elimination by the kidneys (see Fig. 49–9). Many tumors secrete parathyroid hormone–related protein which binds to the parathyroid hormone receptors in bone and renal tissues, leading to increased bone resorption and renal tubular reabsorption.[76] Tumors may also secrete substances such as vitamin D, transforming growth factor, interleukins, prostaglandins, interferon, tumor necrosis factor, and granulocyte-macrophage colony stimulating factor, which are associated with the development of hypercalcemia.[73] Hypercalcemia of malignancy is a common complication of squamous cell carcinomas of the lung, head, and neck, hematologic malignancies such as multiple myeloma and T-cell lymphomas, and carcinomas of ovary, kidney, bladder, and breast. The most frequent types of malignancy associated with hypercalcemia are carcinomas of the lung and breast.[69] Further-

more, up to 40% of patients with multiple myeloma may develop hypercalcemia.[75] Primary hyperparathyroidism is the most common cause of hypercalcemia in the general population. Benign parathyroid adenomas account for 80% to 85% of these cases of hyperparathyroidism, parathyroid hyperplasia accounts for 15%, and parathyroid carcinoma is the cause in less than 1% of cases.[73,74]

Other causes of hypercalcemia include medications, endocrine and granulomatous disorders, immobilization, high bone-turnover states (adolescence and Paget's disease), and rhabdomyolysis. Increased gastrointestinal absorption may be the result of excessive ingestion of vitamin D analogs, calcium supplements, and lithium. Lithium and vitamin A therapy can increase bone resorption, while increased renal tubular reabsorption of calcium can occur with thiazide and lithium therapy. Aluminum antacids prevent calcium deposition, thereby increasing serum concentrations.[77] Addison's disease, acromegaly, and thyrotoxicosis are endocrine disorders that may lead to hypercalcemia due to increased renal tubular reabsorption and increased bone resorption. Finally, the granulomatous disorders (sarcoidosis, tuberculosis, histoplasmosis, and leprosy) are associated with hypercalcemia caused by an increase in gastrointestinal absorption.[78]

CLINICAL PRESENTATION

Patients with mild to moderate hypercalcemia, that is, serum calcium concentrations of less than 13 mg/dL, may often be asymptomatic. This is usually the case in drug-induced hypercalcemia and the vast majority of patients with primary hyperparathyroidism.[74,79–80] In fact, one study noted nearly normocalcemia in approximately 20% of patients with a diagnosis of primary hyperparathyroidism, suggesting target tissue resistance to parathyroid hormone.[80] The signs and symptoms of hypercalcemia that are usually present if the total serum calcium concentration is >13 mg/dL may differ depending on the acuity of onset.[69] Hypercalcemia of malignancy usually develops quickly and is accompanied by a classic symptom complex of anorexia, nausea and vomiting, constipation, polyuria, polydipsia, and nocturia.[79] Polyuria and nocturia secondary to a urinary-concentrating defect constitute some of the most frequent renal effects of hypercalcemia.[79] Hypercalcemic crisis is characterized by an acute elevation of serum calcium to a value >15 mg/dL, acute renal insufficiency, and obtundation (inability to arouse).[79] If untreated, hypercalcemic crisis may progress to oliguric renal failure, coma, and life-threatening ventricular arrhythmias that may lead to death.[79] Complications associated with chronic hypercalcemia (hyperparathyroidism) include metastatic calcification, nephrolithiasis, and chronic renal insufficiency.[79]

Calcium and/or calcium-phosphorus complex deposition in blood vessels and multiple organs is a complication of chronic hypercalcemia and/or concomitant hyperphosphatemia and hyperparathyroidism (see Chap. 44). Calcium deposits in atherosclerotic lesions contribute to cardiac disease. Patients with renal insufficiency are especially vulnerable due to the use of calcium products as phosphate-binding agents and their higher overall risk of developing cardiovascular disease. The rate of coronary artery calcification progression was found to be 50% greater in young hemodialysis patients versus normal middle-aged adults.[81] Furthermore, patients with calcifications had higher serum phosphorus concentrations, higher calcium-phosphorus product, and higher intake of calcium-based phosphate-binding agents.[81,82] Another study showed that the intake of calcium-containing phosphate binders was solely associated with vascular calcification score.[83] Intracardiac and arterial calcifications have been found in patients with Paget's disease who have normal renal function. These calcifications were found to be five times more common than in the general population. Although usually asymptomatic, these lesions can result in heart block and valvular disease.[84]

The electrocardiographic changes associated with hypercalcemia include shortening of the QT interval and coving of the ST-T wave.[79] Very high serum calcium concentrations may cause T-wave widening, indicating a repolarization defect that may be associated with spontaneous ventricular tachyarrhythmias.[79] Hypertension and arrhythmias have occurred in the setting of hypercalcemia. Sensitivity to the pharmacologic and toxic actions of digitalis may be enhanced in the setting of hypercalcemia.[73]

Nephrolithiasis (kidney stones) and nephrocalcinosis (calcium deposits in the kidney) are the primary renal complications arising from long-standing hypercalcemia, as the result of primary hyperparathyroidism. It is estimated that hyperparathyroidism accounts for 2% to 8% of all patients with calcium stones.[85,86] Of note, in those patients with low glomerular filtration rates, the 24-hour urinary calcium will actually diminish secondary to the reduced urine flow. However, the fractional excretion of calcium may increase.[86] Sarcoidosis is the other hypercalcemic condition frequently associated with calcium stones.[85] Other causes of nephrolithiasis with calcium-containing stones include hypocitraturia, renal tubular acidosis, hyperoxaluria, and hyperuricosuria.[87,88] Stone formers who have primary hyperparathyroidism are more likely to be female, over age 50 years, and have a family history of multiple endocrine disorders.[85] High dietary sodium intake can also raise urinary calcium concentrations, thus predisposing patients to calcium stones. The proposed mechanism is a reduction in calcium reabsorption in the kidney. Although chronic renal failure can be the ultimate result of persistent stones, it is the primary cause of renal disease in <2% of the end-stage renal disease population.[89] A patient's first renal symptom is a loss of medullary concentrating ability.[85]

CLINICAL PRESENTATION OF HYPERCALCEMIA

GENERAL
The signs and symptoms of hypercalcemia depend on its level, and also on the rapidity of the onset.

SYMPTOMS
Symptoms include fatigue, weakness, anorexia, depression, anxiety, cognitive dysfunction, vague abdominal pain, and constipation. Renal symptoms can include polyuria, polydipsia, and nocturia. The extent of symptoms is related to both the degree of hypercalcemia and the rate of onset of the elevation in the serum calcium concentration. Rarely, severe hypercalcemia leads to acute pancreatitis.

SIGNS
Renal: The most important renal manifestations of hypercalcemia are nephrolithiasis; renal tubular dysfunction, particularly decreased concentrating ability; and acute and chronic renal insufficiency.

Cardiovascular: Long-standing hypercalcemia can lead to the deposition of calcium in heart valves, coronary arteries, and myocardial fibers. Hypercalcemia also directly shortens the myocardial action potential, which is reflected in a shortened QT interval and coving of the ST-T wave. Spontaneous ventricular tachyarrhythmias and elevations in blood pressure have also been reported.

Musculoskeletal: A number of rheumatologic complaints have been described in hyperparathyroidism, including gout, pseudogout, and chondrocalcinosis. The relative roles of hypercalcemia and PTH excess in these problems are not known.

Other signs: Band keratopathy, a reflection of subepithelial calcium phosphate deposits in the cornea, is a very rare finding associated with hypercalcemia. It extends as a horizontal band across the cornea in the area that is exposed between the eyelids.

LABORATORY TESTS
Serum calcium concentrations of more than 10.5 mg/dL are considered to represent hypercalcemia. Values up to 13 mg/dL suggest mild or moderate hypercalcemia, while values greater than this indicate severe hypercalcemia.

▶ TREATMENT: Hypercalcemia

▓ DESIRED OUTCOME

The indications for the treatment of acute hypercalcemia are dependent on the degree of hypercalcemia, acuity of its development, and presence or absence of symptoms. The objectives of treatment are reversal of signs and symptoms, restoration of normocalcemia, treatment of the underlying cause of hypercalcemia, and prevention of long-term consequences. Chronic hypercalcemia is usually caused by an underlying medical condition or prescribed therapies. The treatment of malignancies may help mitigate acute hypercalcemic episodes. The goals of treatment of hyperparathyroidism are to reduce serum calcium concentrations as well as to reduce long-term complications such as vascular complications, chronic renal insufficiency, and kidney stones. Medications including thiazides, lithium, antacids, and vitamins A and D need to be recognized as potential reversible causes of hypercalcemia.

▓ NONPHARMACOLOGIC THERAPY

Hypercalcemic crisis and acute symptomatic severe hypercalcemia should be considered medical emergencies and treated immediately (Fig. 49–10). These patients may require immediate-acting interventions to promptly reduce the serum calcium concentration. Hemodialysis against a zero- or low-calcium dialysate solution is considered the treatment of choice, especially in patients with impaired renal function or life-threatening hypercalcemia.[77] However, because there may be considerable delays in initiating dialysis due to the need for evaluation by a nephrologist and placement of a vascular access device, pharmacologic therapy consisting of volume expansion and enhancement of urinary calcium excretion (when not contraindicated by renal dysfunction) and/or calcitonin is usually initiated in the interim. Effective treatment of moderate to severe hypercalcemia in the absence of life-threatening symptoms begins with attention to the underlying

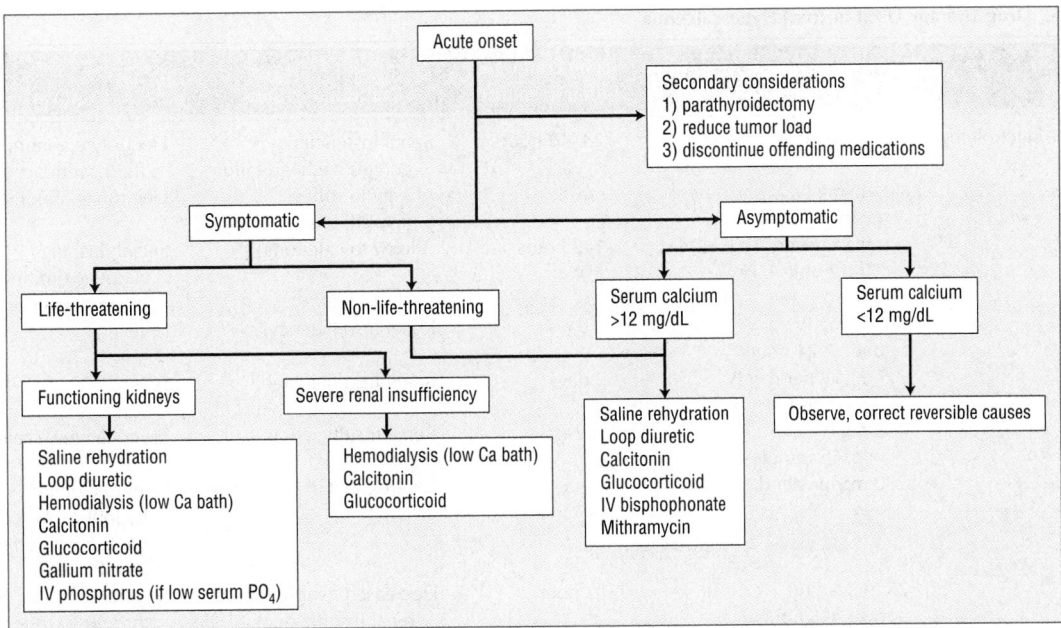

FIGURE 49-10. Pharmacotherapeutic options for the acutely hypercalcemic patient. Ca, calcium; PO₄, phosphorus.

disorder and correction of associated fluid and electrolyte abnormalities. Patients with primary hyperparathyroidism may ultimately need surgery, particularly if they have had calcium nephrolithiasis. Patients with malignancy often require reduction of tumor load to control the exogenous supply of cytokines and hormones that cause the hypercalcemia. In contrast, patients with drug-induced hypercalcemia generally respond to discontinuation of the offending agent.

CLINICAL CONTROVERSY

Although dialysis is the best method for rapidly reducing a highly elevated serum calcium, many clinicians choose a pharmacologic approach as the initial therapy.

■ PHARMACOLOGIC THERAPY

For those patients with normal to moderately impaired renal function, the cornerstone of initial treatment of hypercalcemia is volume expansion to increase urinary calcium excretion (see Table 49–6). Patients with severe renal insufficiency usually do not tolerate volume expansion; they may be initiated on therapy with calcitonin. Patients with symptomatic hypercalcemia are often dehydrated secondary to vomiting and polyuria; thus rehydration with saline-containing fluids is necessary to interrupt the stimulus for sodium and calcium reabsorption in the renal tubule.[90] Rehydration can be accomplished by the infusion of normal saline at rates of 200 to 300 mL/h, depending on concomitant conditions (primarily cardiovascular and renal) and extent of hypercalcemia. Adequacy of hydration is assessed by measuring fluid intake and output or by central venous pressure monitoring.[75,76] Loop diuretics such as furosemide (40 to 80 mg IV every 1 to 4 hours) or ethacrynic acid (for patients with sulfa allergies) may also be instituted to increase urinary calcium excretion and to minimize the development of volume overload from the administration of saline[75] (see Table 49–6). Loop diuretics such as furosemide

block calcium (and sodium) reabsorption in the thick ascending limb of the loop of Henle and augment the calciuric effect of saline alone. The importance of rehydration prior to loop diuretic use is reiterated because dehydration may lead to increased serum calcium because of enhanced proximal tubule calcium reabsorption.[69] Potassium chloride should be added to the saline solution after rehydration is accomplished to maintain normokalemia in the presence of diuretic therapy. Serum magnesium levels should also be monitored, and magnesium replacement instituted if magnesium levels begin to trend downward. Rehydration with saline and administration of furosemide can result in a decrease of 2 to 3 mg/dL in total serum calcium within 24 to 48 hours.[75]

In those patients in whom saline hydration therapy may be contraindicated (e.g., those with CHF or moderate to severe renal dysfunction), short-term therapy with calcitonin is effective in reducing serum calcium levels within hours. Calcitonin decreases serum calcium concentrations, primarily by inhibiting bone resorption. It may also reduce renal tubular reabsorption of calcium, thus promoting calciuresis. Calcitonin may be administered subcutaneously or intramuscularly (for larger volumes) in a starting dose of 4 units/kg every 12 hours, or intravenously at a rate of 10 to 12 units/h. The side effects from intravenously administered calcitonin (facial flushing, nausea, and vomiting) limit patient acceptability. Allergic reactions, although rare, do occur; therefore a test dose (intradermal injection of 0.1 mL of a 10-units/mL solution) is recommended prior to starting therapy. If marked erythema and/or wheal formation does not occur within 15 minutes after administration, therapy can begin. Calcitonin has a rapid onset of action (within 1 to 2 hours); however, the degree and extent of serum calcium level reduction are often unpredictable.[69] Calcitonin therapy is frequently associated with tachyphylaxis caused by antibody formation to foreign proteins or molecules resembling the calcitonin polypeptide.[91] The addition of corticosteroid therapy or conversion to human calcitonin increases effectiveness.[69] Subcutaneous administration of salmon calcitonin in doses of 50 to 100 international units daily or three times weekly have been prescribed in patients with Paget's disease. The intranasal formulation of calcitonin has been used in the treatment of Paget's disease, in

TABLE 49–6. Drug Therapy Used to Treat Hypercalcemia

Drug	Starting Dosage	Time Frame to Initial Response	Contraindications	Adverse Effects
0.9% saline ± electrolytes	200–300 mL/h	24–48 hours	Renal insufficiency; congestive heart failure	Electrolyte abnormalities; fluid overload
Loop diuretics	40–80 mg IV every 1–4 hours	n/a	Allergy to sulfas (use ethacrynic acid)	Electrolyte abnormalities
Calcitonin	4 units/kg every 12 h SQ/IM 10–12 units/h IV	1–2 hours	Allergy to calcitonin	Facial flushing nausea/vomiting allergic reaction
Pamidronate	30–90 mg IV over 2–24 hours	2 days	Renal insufficiency	Fever
Etidronate	7.5 mg/kg per day IV over 2 hours	2 days	Renal insufficiency	Fever
Zoledronate	4–8 mg IV over 15 minutes	1–2 days	Renal insufficiency	Fever, fatigue, skeletal pain
Gallium nitrate	200 mg/m² per day	?	Severe renal insufficiency	Nephrotoxicity; hypophosphatemia; nausea/vomiting/diarrhea; metallic taste
Mithramycin	25 mcg/kg IV over 4–6 hours	12 hours	Decreased liver function; renal insufficiency; thrombocytopenia	Nausea/vomiting; stomatitis; thrombocytopenia; nephrotoxicity; hepatotoxicity;
Glucocorticoids	40–60 mg oral prednisone equivalents	?	Serious infections; hypersensitivity	Diabetes; osteoporosis; infection

doses of 200 to 400 international units daily; unfortunately this has resulted in only mild decreases in serum calcium. The lack of significant efficacy of the synthetic intranasal formulation is a result of the lower potency and shorter duration of action as compared to salmon calcitonin.

Bisphosphonates block bone resorption very efficiently, render the hydroxyapatite crystal of bone mineral resistant to hydrolysis by phosphatases, and also inhibit osteoclast precursors from attaching to the mineralized matrix, thus blocking their transformation into mature functioning osteoclasts.[75,79,92] Pamidronate is very effective in controlling hypercalcemia associated with malignancy and slightly more effective than etidronate.[73] The usual dose of pamidronate is 30 to 90 mg as an IV infusion given over 2 to 24 hours. Pamidronate also has the advantage of single-day therapy.[75] Etidronate, when administered in doses of 7.5 mg/kg per day by slow intravenous infusion over at least 2 hours for 3 days, is effective in the therapy of hypercalcemia of malignancy.[75] Zoledronate and ibandronate are the newest high-potency bisphosphonates with demonstrated effectiveness in the treatment of hypercalcemia of malignancy. Complete response has been reported in 88.4% to 86.7% of zoledronate-versus 69.7% of pamidronate-treated patients.[93,94] Zoledronate intravenous doses of 4 to 8 mg given over 5 minutes have resulted in normalization of serum calcium concentrations.[94] Intravenous infusions of 0.02 or 0.04 mg/kg diluted in 5% dextrose (given over 20 to 50 minutes) have also been effective.[95] A similar hypocalcemic response has been noted with ibandronate in comparison to pamidronate (76.5% versus 75.8%); however, the time period to a relapse of hypercalcemia was longer with ibandronate (14 days versus 4 days), suggesting a therapeutic advantage.[96] Ibandronate is administered (diluted in 500 mL 0.9% sodium chloride) by intravenous infusion in doses of 2 mg up to 6 mg.

The onset of serum calcium concentration decline is slower with bisphosphonate therapy (concentrations begin to decline in 2 days and reach a nadir in 7 days); thus calcitonin therapy may be necessary if rapid serum level reduction is required.[75,97] Duration of normocalcemia varies, but usually does not exceed 2 to 3 weeks, depending on the severity and treatment response of the underlying malignancy.[69] The duration of response has been suggested to be longer with zoledronate (4 to 5 weeks).[95] Fever is a common side effect of intravenous bisphosphonate therapy. Data on the use of these agents for maintenance intravenous therapy are limited; however, pamidronate has demonstrated more promise than etidronate. Although oral bisphosphonates are useful for the treatment of bone turnover in Paget's disease, there are insufficient data to suggest their use for the initial treatment of hypercalcemia. The use of oral bisphosphonates for maintenance therapy in patients predisposed to hypercalcemia (malignancy) has been successful in some cases.[98] The safety of continuous bisphosphonate therapy in patients with moderate to severe renal insufficiency is currently unknown. Renal function monitoring (serum creatinine) is advised with the use of bisphosphonates, as cases of acute tubular necrosis have been reported.[99,100] Although there are no published guidelines for frequency of serum creatinine monitoring, it is advisable to evaluate serum creatinine within a week after the infusion and just prior to the next scheduled dose.

CLINICAL CONTROVERSY

Although some clinicians administer bisphosphonates to patients regardless of their degree of renal function, the FDA approved labeling states that they are contraindicated when GFR is less than 30 mL/min.

Gallium nitrate is indicated for the treatment of symptomatic hypercalcemia of malignancy not responsive to hydration therapy.[101] However, because of its adverse side-effect profile, it is generally reserved for those who fail to respond to less toxic agents. Gallium itrate inhibits bone resorption, and may be superior to calcitonin in nducing normocalcemia. It may provide a longer duration of nor-mocalcemia as compared to etidronate. The initial dose is usually a continuous IV infusion of 200 mg/m^2 per day for 5 consecutive days. Because gallium nitrate is nephrotoxic, use caution if it is coadminis-ered with other nephrotoxic drugs. Other common adverse effects in-clude hypophosphatemia, nausea, vomiting, diarrhea, hypocalcemia, and metallic taste.

Mithramycin (plicamycin) is a potent cytotoxic antibiotic that in-hibits osteoclast-mediated bone resorption and thereby reduces hyper-calcemia. Mithramycin may be administered at a dose of 25 mcg/kg via intravenous infusion over 4 to 6 hours in saline or 5% dextrose solutions. This therapy may be repeated daily for 3 to 4 days or on alternating days for 3 to 8 doses.[75,102] Serum calcium levels begin to fall within 12 hours of a mithramycin dose, with the peak effect generally occurring within 48 to 96 hours.[69,75] Single doses are usu-ally well tolerated.[102] Adverse effects of mithramycin include nausea, vomiting, stomatitis, thrombocytopenia, inhibition of platelet func-tion, and renal and hepatotoxicity.[69] Because these adverse effects are more commonly associated with multiple doses, mithramycin is usually limited to short-term therapy in patients who have not re-sponded to alternative therapies. Monitoring parameters include com-plete blood count, liver function, and renal function. Mithramycin should be avoided in patients with thrombocytopenia and liver and renal insufficiency.[75]

Glucocorticoids are usually effective in the treatment of hyper-calcemia resulting from multiple myeloma, leukemia, lymphoma, sar-coidosis, and hypervitaminoses A and D.[69,92,102] The mechanisms of glucocorticoid-induced reductions in serum calcium include reduced gastrointestinal absorption, defective vitamin D metabolism causing hypercalciuria, increased bone resorption, decreased osteoblast pro-liferation, and reduction in sex hormone (estrogen and testosterone) concentrations.[103] Daily doses of 40 to 60 mg of prednisone or the equivalent is effective.[69] The disadvantages of glucocorticoid therapy are its relatively slow onset of action and the potential for diabetes mellitus, osteoporosis, and increased susceptibility to infection.[72,91]

Finally, intravenous phosphate may rapidly reduce ionized cal-cium concentrations through the formation of insoluble calcium-phosphate salts. However, intravenous phosphate is extremely haz-ardous because extraskeletal precipitation of calcium-phosphate may result in metastatic calcification, hypotension, acute renal failure, or death.[69,81] Therefore intravenous phosphates should be reserved for the extraordinary patient with severe hypercalcemia and concomi-tant hypophosphatemia.[69] Oral phosphorus is not used chronically for the treatment of hypercalcemia because calcium-phosphate crys-tals may precipitate in the kidneys or other major organs when the calcium-phosphorus product is >50 to 60 mg^2/dL^2.[104] Serum cal-cium, phosphorus, and creatinine should be monitored closely. Oral phosphorus treatment is only indicated when there is concomitant hypophosphatemia (<2 mg/dL).

Inhibitors of prostaglandin synthesis such as indomethacin are rarely effective and thus not currently recommended. Asymptomatic patients with mild hypercalcemia may be carefully observed, espe-cially if treatment for the underlying condition (malignancy) is initi-ated. The calcimimetic agent cinacalcet HCl was recently approved for the treatment of secondary hyperparathyroidism in patients with chronic kidney disease and for its calcium-lowering effect in the man-agement of parathyroid carcinoma.[105,106] These agents bind to the calcium-sensing receptor, albeit at a different location than calcium, and increase the sensitivity for receptor activation by extracellular cal-cium. This results in reduced parathyroid hormone and serum calcium concentrations.[105,106]

A review of the use of cinacalcet HCl for secondary hyper-parathyroidism is provided in Chap. 44. Cinacalcet HCl is admin-istered at a starting dose of 30 mg given orally twice daily for the treatment of parathyroid carcinoma. The dosage is titrated every 2 to 4 weeks in 30-mg increments twice daily. The maximum approved dosage is 90 mg three to four times daily.

HYPOCALCEMIA

The incidence of hypocalcemia (total serum calcium less than 8.5 mg/dL) in intensive care unit patients ranges from 70% to 90% based on total, to 15% to 50% based on ionized calcium concentrations.[70] Hypocalcemia is more commonly seen in hospi-talized patients than in outpatients.

PATHOPHYSIOLOGY

Hypocalcemia is the result of alterations in the effect of parathyroid hormone and vitamin D on the bone, gut, and kidney (see Fig. 49–9). The primary causes of hypocalcemia are postoperative hypoparathy-roidism and vitamin D deficiency. Other causes include magnesium deficiency, thyroid surgery, medications, hypoalbuminemia, blood transfusions, peripheral blood progenitor cell harvesting, tumor ly-sis syndrome, and mutations in the calcium-sensing receptor.[107–112] Parathyroid hormone concentrations are elevated in conditions of hypocalcemia, with the exception of hypoparathyroidism and hypo-magnesemia (Fig. 49–11).[113]

A symptomatic rapid fall in serum calcium concentrations (often to values <7 mg/dL) is common in patients who have had a parathy-roidectomy or thyroidectomy. Hypocalcemia in these postsurgical pa-tients is generally transient in nature.[114] The "hungry bone syndrome" is a condition of profound hypocalcemia whereby the bone avidly in-corporates calcium and phosphorus from the blood in an attempt to recalcify bone. This is common after correction (usually surgery) of prolonged states of hyperparathyroidism and/or hyperthyroidism. Serum calcium concentrations should be monitored every 6 hours dur-ing the 24 to 48 hours following such surgeries, and pharmacologic doses of calcium may be necessary to prevent or minimize the drop in serum calcium (see the treatment discussion).

Vitamin D and its metabolites play an important role in the main-tenance of extracellular calcium concentrations and in normal skeletal structure and mineralization. Vitamin D is necessary for the optimal absorption of calcium and phosphorus. On a worldwide basis, the most common cause of hypocalcemia is nutritional vitamin D deficiency. In malnourished populations, manifestations include rickets and osteo-malacia. Nutritional vitamin D deficiency is uncommon in Western societies because of the fortification of milk with ergocalciferol.[114] The most common cause of vitamin D deficiency in Western societies is gastrointestinal disease.[79] Gastric surgery, chronic pancreatitis, small-bowel disease, intestinal resection, and bypass surgery are associated with decreased concentrations of vitamin D and its metabolites.[79] Vitamin D replacement therapy may need to be ad-ministered by the intravenous route if poor oral bioavailability is noted. Decreased production of 1,25-dihydroxyvitamin D$_3$ may oc-cur as a result of a hereditary defect resulting in vitamin D–dependent rickets. It also can occur secondary to chronic renal insufficiency if there is insufficient production of the 1-α-hydroxylase enzyme for the

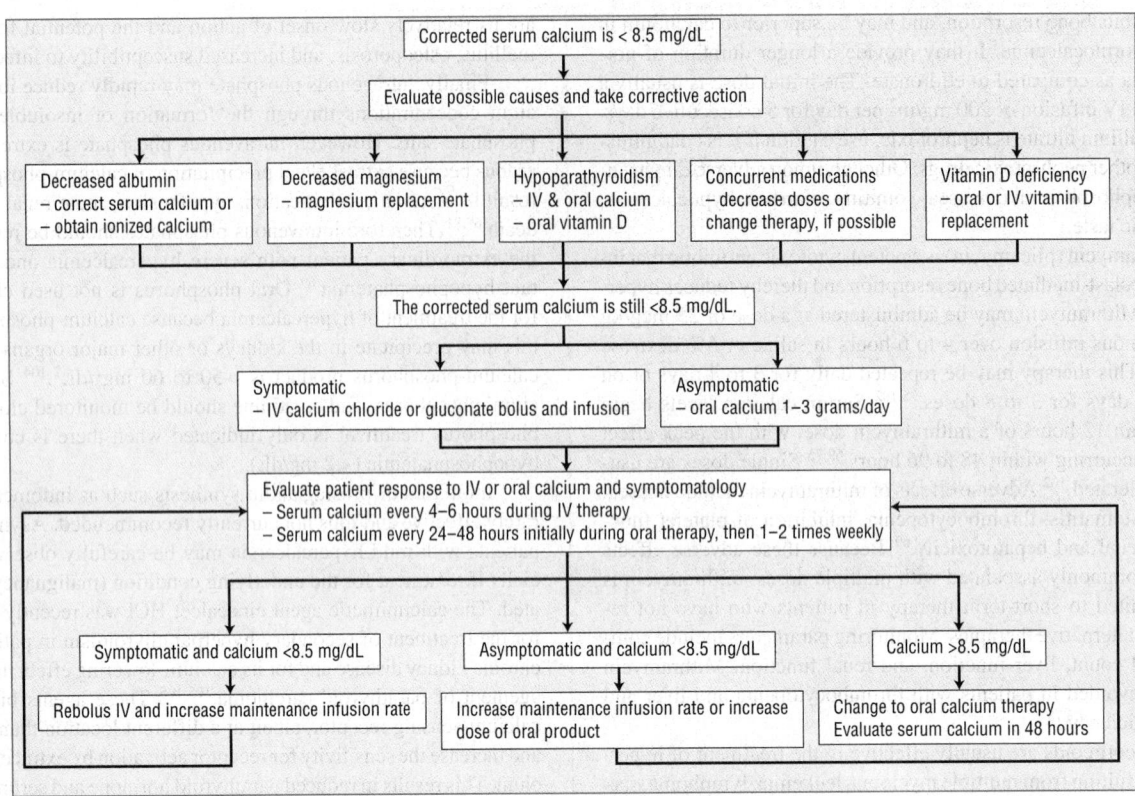

FIGURE 49–11. Hypocalcemia diagnostic and treatment algorithm.

production of the most active metabolite, 1,25-dihydroxyvitamin D_3.[115] Treatment of hypocalcemia associated with chronic kidney disease is reviewed in Chap. 44.

Hypomagnesemia of any cause may be associated with severe symptomatic hypocalcemia that is unresponsive to calcium replacement therapy (see Chap. 50). Reduced serum magnesium concentrations can impair PTH secretion and induce resistance of target organs to the actions of PTH.[107] Normalization of serum calcium concentrations in these patients is thus dependent on appropriate replacement of magnesium.

Drug-induced hypocalcemia has been reported with furosemide, calcitonin, bisphosphonates, gallium nitrate, and mithramycin. Oral phosphorus therapy, commonly used to treat patients with malabsorption syndromes caused by gastrointestinal diseases, can also result in hypocalcemia, necessitating calcium-concentration monitoring. The anticonvulsants phenobarbital and phenytoin cause hypocalcemia by increasing catabolism of vitamin D and thereby impairing calcium release from bone and reducing intestinal calcium absorption.[107] Drugs that cause hypomagnesemia (aminoglycosides, amphotericin B, cyclosporine, diuretics, foscarnet, and cisplatin) are associated with an increased risk of hypocalcemia. Chelating agents in blood (citrate) and in radiographic contrast media (ethylenediamine tetraacetate) can also cause transient hypocalcemia.[108,109,116] Other agents associated with hypocalcemia include fluoride, ketoconazole, calcimimetics, and pentamidine.[107]

Proper assessment of total serum calcium concentrations includes measurement of serum albumin concentrations. Hypoalbuminemia, which may be associated with many chronic disease states, is probably the most common cause of "laboratory hypocalcemia." Patients remain asymptomatic because the ionized fraction of serum calcium remains normal (reference range 4.4 to 5.4 mg/dL). A

corrected total serum calcium concentration can be calculated based on the measured total serum calcium and the difference between a patient's measured albumin concentration and the normative value of 4 g/dL by the following equation:

$$\text{Corrected } S_{ca}(\text{mg/dL}) = \text{measured } S_{ca}\ (\text{mg/dL}) + [0.8 \times (4.0\ \text{g/dL} - \text{measured albumin (g/dL)})]$$

CLINICAL PRESENTATION

The clinical manifestations of hypocalcemia are quite variable. The acuteness of the development of hypocalcemia plays a large role in whether or not symptoms will occur.[114] The more acute the drop in ionized calcium concentration, the more likely the patient will develop symptoms. Thus acid-base balance plays a significant role in the likelihood of the development of hypocalcemic symptoms, with alkalosis predisposing to symptom development. Concomitant hypomagnesemia, hypokalemia, hyponatremia, and additive side effects from prescribed medications also increase the likelihood of symptomatic presentation.

Hypocalcemia may manifest as neuromuscular, CNS, dermatologic, and cardiac sequelae.[79] Acute hypocalcemia is more likely to manifest as neuromuscular (paresthesias, muscle cramps, tetany, and laryngeal spasm) and cardiovascular symptoms, whereas chronic hypocalcemia often presents as CNS (depression, anxiety, memory loss, confusion, hallucinations, and tonic-clonic seizures) and dermatologic symptoms (hair loss, grooved and brittle nails, and eczema).[107] The hallmark sign of acute hypocalcemia is tetany caused by enhanced peripheral neuromuscular irritability.[79] Tetany manifests as paresthesias around the mouth and in the extremities, muscle spasms and cramps, carpopedal (hands and feet) spasms, and rarely as laryngospasm and bronchospasm.[79] Chvostek's and/or Trousseau's sign may be elicited during physical examination.[107] Chvostek's sign is elicited as twitching of facial muscles when the facial nerve is tapped anterior to the ear. Trousseau's sign is elicited by carpal spasm when a blood pressure cuff is inflated above systolic blood pressure for 3 minutes.

The cardiovascular manifestations of hypocalcemia result in electrocardiographic changes characterized by a prolonged QT interval and symptoms of decreased myocardial contractility often associated with congestive heart failure.[107] Both acute and chronic hypocalcemia may result in a reversible syndrome characterized by acute myocardial failure or refractory congestive heart failure. Other cardiovascular manifestations include arrhythmias, bradycardia, and hypotension that is unresponsive to fluid and pressor administration.[107]

CLINICAL PRESENTATION OF HYPOCALCEMIA

GENERAL

Hypocalcemia is caused in part by disorders of vitamin D or parathyroid hormone. Other causes of hypocalcemia include sepsis and disorders that result in a decrease in serum ionized calcium concentration by either binding of calcium within the vascular space or its deposition in tissues, or drug-induced causes. Parathyroidectomy or thyroidectomy are also associated with a rapid reduction in serum calcium. Malnutrition associated with vitamin D deficiency should not be overlooked as an etiology of hypocalcemia.

SYMPTOMS

The symptoms of hypocalcemia, usually associated with an acute decrease in serum calcium, include tetany, paresthesias, muscle cramps, and laryngeal spasms. Chronic hypocalcemia is usually associated with the symptoms of depression, anxiety, memory loss, confusion, seizures, hair loss, grooved and brittle nails, and eczema. Associated hypomagnesemia, hypokalemia, and hyponatremia can increase the likelihood of symptoms.

SIGNS

Neurologic: Chvostek's and/or Trousseau's signs can be elicited during physical examination. The hallmark of acute hypocalcemia is tetany, which is characterized by neuromuscular irritability including seizure potential. Extrapyramidal disorders, mainly parkinsonism but also dystonia, hemiballismus, choreoathetosis, and oculogyric crises, occur in 5% to 10% of patients with idiopathic hypoparathyroidism.

Dermatologic: The skin can be dry, puffy, and coarse. Other dermatologic manifestations may include hyperpigmentation, dermatitis and eczema, and psoriasis. Hair and skin signs including coarse, brittle, and sparse hair with patchy alopecia and brittle nails can also appear.

Ophthalmologic: Cataract development has been reported to occur with hypocalcemia.

Dental manifestations: These are usually associated with the presence of hypocalcemia in early development. Signs include dental hypoplasia, failure of tooth eruption, defective enamel and root formation, and abraded carious teeth.

Cardiovascular: Hypotension, decreased myocardial performance, and congestive heart failure have been reported. A prolonged QT interval, arrhythmias, and bradycardia may also occur.

Gastrointestinal: Steatorrhea may be associated with hypocalcemia.

Musculoskeletal: While patients with several hypocalcemic disorders have skeletal abnormalities, such findings do not appear to be direct consequences of hypocalcemia. Some patients with hypocalcemia have myopathy.

Endocrine: Hypocalcemia alone may impair insulin release. In addition, idiopathic hypoparathyroidism may be associated with polyglandular autoimmune syndromes.

LABORATORY TESTS

Serum calcium levels of less than 8.5 mg/dL are considered to represent hypocalcemia.

▶ TREATMENT: Hypocalcemia

■ DESIRED OUTCOME

The goals of therapy for patients with normal renal function are the resolution of signs and symptoms of hypocalcemia, restoration of normocalcemia, management of associated electrolyte abnormalities, and treatment of the underlying cause of hypocalcemia. The goals for patients with chronic renal insufficiency are different and are discussed in detail in Chap. 44. Asymptomatic hypocalcemia associated with hypoalbuminemia requires no treatment because ionized (physiologically active) plasma calcium concentrations are normal. Treatment of hypocalcemia is dependent on identification of the pathogenesis of the underlying disorder, acuteness of onset, and presence and severity of symptoms. Acute symptomatic hypocalcemia requires parenteral administration of soluble calcium salts (see Fig. 49–11).

■ PHARMACOLOGIC THERAPY

The initial therapeutic intervention for patients with acute symptomatic hypocalcemia is to administer 100 to 300 mg of elemental calcium intravenously over 5 to 10 minutes.[117] This may be provided by the administration of 1 g of calcium chloride (27% elemental calcium) or 2 to 3 g of calcium gluconate (9% elemental calcium). Calcium gluconate is generally preferred over calcium chloride for peripheral venous administration because calcium gluconate is less irritating to veins. Disadvantages to the use of calcium gluconate are the lower percentage of elemental calcium per volume and the less predictable, slightly smaller increase in plasma ionic calcium compared with calcium chloride. Calcium should not be infused at a rate greater than 60 mg of elemental calcium per minute because severe cardiac dysfunction may result.[117] Intravenous calcium administration should be used with caution in patients receiving digitalis glycosides, because of the possibility of cardiac arrhythmias.[70] Calcium should not be added to bicarbonate- or phosphate-containing solutions because of the possibility of precipitation. The bolus dose of calcium is only effective for 1 to 2 hours and should be followed by a continuous infusion of elemental calcium at a rate of 0.5 to 2 mg/kg per hour.[70] The calcium concentrations should be monitored every 4 to 6 hours during the intravenous infusions. The ionized calcium concentration usually normalizes within 4 hours, and the maintenance infusion rate of elemental calcium can then be decreased to 0.3 to 0.5 mg/kg per hour.[69] The maintenance infusion can be adjusted to maintain the desired concentration of calcium.

Once acute hypocalcemia is corrected by parenteral administration, further treatment modalities should be individualized according to the cause of hypocalcemia. If hypomagnesemia is present, magnesium supplementation is indicated (see Chap. 50). Asymptomatic and chronic hypocalcemia associated with hypoparathyroidism and vitamin D–deficient states may be managed by oral calcium and vitamin D supplementation (see Tables 44–6 and 44–7). Therapy is begun with 1 to 3 g/day of elemental calcium.[68] Average maintenance doses range from 2 to 8 g of elemental calcium per day in divided doses. If serum calcium does not normalize, a vitamin D preparation may need to be added.

Treatment of hypocalcemia associated with vitamin D–deficient states should be individualized. In patients with malabsorption, vitamin D requirements vary markedly, and large doses may be required. In contrast, vitamin D deficiency associated with anticonvulsant med-ication may be corrected with smaller doses of vitamin D. Oral doses of 1,25-dihydroxyvitamin D_3 usually range from 0.5 to 3 mcg daily. The usual initial oral dose of ergocalciferol is 50,000 international units daily.[117] Vitamin D doses are usually adjusted approximately every 4 weeks. The treatment of vitamin D deficiency associated with chronic renal failure generally requires the administration of 1,25-dihydroxyvitamin D_3 or another synthetic analog, such as paricalcitol or doxercalciferol. Situations in which 25-hydroxylase activity is reduced (e.g., hepatic disease) may also require treatment with calcitriol (1,25-dihydroxyvitamin D). The newer vitamin D analogs (paricalcitol and doxercalciferol) were developed to preferentially suppress PTH secretion with less effect on serum calcium concentration. Their efficacy in treating hypocalcemia may thus be less apparent. In selected cases, calcium supplementation may be required if vitamin D replacement alone is ineffective in returning calcium concentrations to normal.

Adverse effects of oral calcium and vitamin D supplementation include hypercalcemia and hypercalciuria, especially in the hypoparathyroid patient, in whom the renal calcium-sparing effect of parathyroid hormone is absent. Hypercalciuria may increase the risk of calcium stone formation and nephrolithiasis in susceptible patients. One maneuver to help prevent calcium stones is to maintain the calcium at a low normal concentration. Monitoring 24-hour urine collections for total calcium concentrations (goal <300 mg/24 h) may also minimize the occurrence of hypercalciuria. The addition of thiazide diuretics for patients at risk for stone formation may result in a reduction of both urinary calcium excretion and vitamin D requirements.[117]

DISORDERS OF PHOSPHORUS HOMEOSTASIS

Phosphorus is an essential element in phospholipid cell membranes, nucleic acids, and phosphoproteins required for mitochondrial function.[118] Phosphorus regulates the intermediary metabolism of carbohydrates, fats, and proteins. Phosphorus also regulates enzymatic reactions including glycolysis, ammoniagenesis, and the 1-hydroxylation of 25-hydroxyvitamin D_3.[118] In addition, phosphorus is required for the generation of 2,3-diphosphoglycerate (2,3-DPG) in red blood cells, which is required for normal oxygen-hemoglobin dissociation and delivery of oxygen to the tissues.[119] Phosphorus is the source of the high-energy bonds of adenosine triphosphate (ATP), thus fueling a wide variety of physiologic processes, including muscle contractility, electrolyte transport, neurologic function, and other important biochemical reactions.[118] Considering its diverse biologic importance, it is not difficult to appreciate the clinical implications of disorders of phosphorus homeostasis.

Phosphorus is present in living organisms mainly as inorganic phosphate and organic phosphate esters. Phosphorus is the major intracellular anion. The majority of intracellular phosphorus exists as organic esters, mainly 2,3-DPG, adenosine and guanosine triphosphate, and fructose 1,6-diphosphate.[118] Only a small fraction of intracellular phosphorus exists as inorganic phosphate; however, this fraction is critical because it is the source from which ATP is resynthesized.[118] The majority of inorganic phosphate is located in the extracellular space. Normal serum phosphorus concentration in the adult is 2.5 to 4.5 mg/dL. Extracellular inorganic phosphate is the prime determinant of intracellular phosphate; thus small increments in the organic phosphate pool can profoundly alter both the extracellular and intracellular phosphate pools. Metabolic disturbances (acidosis, alkalosis, and ketoacidosis), hydrogen ion shifts, and hormones (PTH, calcitonin, cortisol, and vitamin D) all can cause shifts in phosphorus concentrations. Because of these phenomena, the serum phosphorus level does not accurately reflect total body stores.[119]

The typical western diet provides a daily intake of 800 to 1,600 mg of phosphorus. Approximately 60% to 80% of this is absorbed in the gastrointestinal tract by passive and active transport (vitamin D–mediated). PTH, 1,25-dihydroxyvitamin D_3, and low-phosphate diets mediate increased absorption. Decreased absorption occurs under conditions of increased dietary intake of phosphorus and magnesium, glucocorticoid therapy, and hypothyroidism. Excretion by the kidney is the single most important regulator of steady-state serum phosphorus concentrations. Renal excretion of phosphorus is regulated by glomerular filtration and proximal tubular reabsorption by passive transport coupled to sodium (sodium-phosphate cotransport). Under normal conditions, 85% to 90% of filtered phosphate is reabsorbed, the majority in the early proximal tubule. Renal tubular reabsorption of phosphorus is inhibited by parathyroid hormone and 1,25-dihydroxyvitamin D_3.[118] Conversely, phosphorus reabsorption in the renal tubule is increased by growth hormone.[118] Internal phosphorus balance (transcellular phosphate distribution) is also of importance in the maintenance of normal serum phosphorus. The serum phosphorus level may vary by as much as 2 mg/dL throughout the day, as the result of acute changes in transcellular distribution of phosphate influenced primarily by carbohydrate intake, insulin secretion, and diurnal variation.[119]

HYPERPHOSPHATEMIA

Serum phosphorus concentration is so closely regulated by the kidneys that it is unusual for hyperphosphatemia (serum phosphorus concentration >4.5 mg/dL) to develop in patients with normal renal function. The most frequent causes of hyperphosphatemia are decreases in urinary phosphorus excretion, and increases in phosphate entrance into the extracellular fluid via either exogenous administration or endogenous intracellular phosphate release.

PATHOPHYSIOLOGY

The most common cause of hyperphosphatemia is a decrease in urinary phosphorus excretion secondary to decreased glomerular filtration rate.[120] Retention of phosphorus decreases vitamin D synthesis and induces hypocalcemia, which leads to an increase in PTH. This physiologic response inhibits further tubular reabsorption of phosphorus to correct hyperphosphatemia and normalize serum calcium concentrations. Patients with excessive exogenous phosphorus administration or endogenous intracellular phosphorus release in the setting of acute renal failure may develop profound hyperphosphatemia.[118] Severe hyperphosphatemia is commonly encountered in patients with chronic kidney disease, especially those with GFRs less than 15 mL/min per 1.73 m^2 (see Chap. 44).

Hypoparathyroidism results in increased renal tubular reabsorption of phosphorus and may result in hyperphosphatemia. Hyperphosphatemia associated with hypoparathyroidism is usually less severe than that associated with severe renal failure or excessive exogenous or endogenous introduction of phosphorus into the ECF. Hypoparathyroidism is the most important cause of increased tubular phosphorus reabsorption. Acromegaly and thyrotoxicosis may also cause hyperphosphatemia by reducing urinary phosphorus excretion.

Iatrogenic causes of hyperphosphatemia have been widely reported, and awareness of the phosphorus content of intravenous, oral, and rectally administered phosphorus-containing products can aid in its prevention. It is often recognized that large doses of phosphorus administered intravenously to treat hypercalcemia can result in severe life-threatening hyperphosphatemia. Although less-well recognized, oral and rectal administration of phosphate-containing solutions can also result in severe and life-threatening hyperphosphatemia, especially in patients with moderate and severe renal insufficiency.[120] The risk of mortality (because of sudden hypocalcemia with tetany and hyperphosphatemia) is dependent on the amount of phosphorus absorbed from the administered product; a 25% mortality rate has been observed with serum phosphorus concentrations ≥33 mg/dL.[120]

Any disorder that results in necrosis of skeletal muscle cells (i.e., rhabdomyolysis) can result in the release of large amounts of intracellular phosphorus into the systemic circulation. This condition is frequently associated with acute renal failure and thus severe hyperphosphatemia may develop due to increased endogenous phosphorus release coupled with decreased renal phosphorus excretion. Bowel infarction, malignant hyperthermia, and severe hemolysis are also conditions that may increase endogenous release of phosphorus.

Hyperphosphatemia is not uncommonly observed in patients undergoing treatment for acute leukemia and lymphomas.[121] Chemotherapeutic treatment of acute lymphoblastic leukemia may result in the release of large amounts of phosphorus into the systemic circulation secondary to lysis of lymphoblasts. Initiation of chemotherapy for Burkitt's lymphoma results in a rapid lysis of malignant cells, resulting in hyperphosphatemia, hyperuricemia, hyperkalemia, and hypocalcemia. This syndrome is commonly referred to as tumor lysis syndrome.[121]

Acid-base disorders such as lactic acidosis and diabetic ketoacidosis can release endogenous intracellular phosphorus and cause hyperphosphatemia. In one study, hyperphosphatemia was present in 94.7% of patients with diabetic ketoacidosis prior to the initiation of treatment.[122] After the institution of treatment, serum phosphorus levels decrease and patients may ultimately develop hypophosphatemia.

Medications are another cause of hyperphosphatemia. Excessive intravenous or oral administration of phosphorus is an obvious potential cause of elevated serum phosphate concentrations. Phosphate-containing enemas increase concentrations, especially in those with renal insufficiency. Intravenous or oral vitamin D therapy can increase absorption of phosphorus in the gastrointestinal tract by up to 50%. Bisphosphonate therapy is associated with increased serum phosphate concentrations. Acute phosphorus poisoning as a result of ingestion of laundry detergents is a rare and often unrecognized cause of elevated phosphate concentrations.

CLINICAL PRESENTATION

The major effects of hyperphosphatemia are related to the development of hypocalcemia (caused by phosphate inhibition of renal 1α-hydroxylase) and its related consequences, as well as vascular and organ damage resulting from the deposition of calcium-phosphate crystals. Extravascular calcification can result in band keratopathy, "red eye," pruritus, and periarticular calcification, especially in renal failure patients (see Chap. 44). In addition, soft-tissue calcifications in the conjunctiva, skin, heart, cornea, lung, gastric mucosa, and kidney have been observed, primarily in chronic renal failure patients.[118] Hyperphosphatemia associated with chronic renal disease may result in renal osteodystrophy because of overproduction of parathyroid hormone. This condition is discussed in detail in Chap. 44.

CLINICAL PRESENTATION OF HYPERPHOSPHATEMIA

GENERAL

Since the serum phosphate concentration is primarily determined by the ability of the kidneys to excrete dietary phosphate, hyperphosphatemia is uncommon in patients with normal kidney function.

SYMPTOMS

Symptoms associated with hyperphosphatemia are associated with deposition of calcium-phosphate crystals and include "red eye" and pruritus. Other symptoms are attributable to hypercalcemia.   ↳ itching

SIGNS

The elevated calcium-phosphate product results in precipitation in arteries, joints, soft tissues, and the viscera. This can result in tissue ischemia, termed *calciphylaxis*.

LABORATORY TESTS

Serum phosphate levels higher than 4.5 mg/dL represent hyperphosphatemia.

▶ TREATMENT: Hyperphosphatemia

■ DESIRED OUTCOME

The treatment of hyperphosphatemia should be directed at the correction of reversible factors, treatment of the disease states associated with its development, the management of associated signs and symptoms, management of associated electrolyte abnormalities, return of serum phosphate concentrations to the normal range, and minimize the long-term cardiovascular consequences of calcium-phosphorus deposition. It has been estimated that calcium-phosphate crystals are likely to form in vivo when the product of the serum calcium and phosphate concentrations exceeds 50 to 60 mg^2/dL^2.[104] Recent evidence suggests that the calcium-phosphorus product should be maintained at less than 55 mg^2/dL^2 to reduce cardiovascular morbidity and mortality secondary to arterial calcification.[81,104] The recently published National Kidney Foundation's Dialysis Outcomes Quality Initiative guidelines for bone metabolism and disease defines the goal calcium-phosphorus product as less than 55 mg^2/dL^2.[123] Furthermore, serum phosphorus concentrations greater than 6.5 mg/dL, but not serum calcium concentrations, are associated with increased morbidity and mortality.[104] Serum phosphorus concentrations should be maintained in the 2.7 to 4.6 mg/dL range for those with Stage 3 and 4 chronic kidney disease, while for patients in Stage 5 chronic kidney disease the goal is to maintain values between 3.5 and 5.5 mg/dL.[123]

◼ PHARMACOLOGIC THERAPY

Severe symptomatic hyperphosphatemia manifesting as hypocalcemia and tetany should be treated by the intravenous administration of calcium salts (see the discussion of hypocalcemia). Although this may seem counterintuitive in a patient with a phosphorus of 16 mg/dL and a calcium of 7 mg/dL (the calcium-phosphorus product is 112 mg^2/dL^2), correction of severe hypocalcemia is of primary importance because of the critical nature of this disorder. In general, the most effective way to treat asymptomatic chronic hyperphosphatemia is to decrease phosphate absorption in the lumen of the GI tract by the use of phosphate-binding agents.[118] Antacids containing divalent and trivalent cations (calcium, magnesium, and aluminum) or sevelamer are the agents most frequently used in the prevention and treatment of hyperphosphatemia (see Table 44–6). The recently approved phosphate binder lanthanum carbonate is another non–calcium-based product that has demonstrated efficacy and safety.[124,125] Long-term treatment with aluminum hydroxide and aluminum carbonate should be discouraged because of the association with anemia, CNS disorders, and bone disease. Short-term therapy with these agents is effective and safe. The most frequent adverse effect from phosphate-binding agents (especially calcium) is constipation. Calcium salts are the preferred phosphate-binding agents except when there is concomitant hypercalcemia. Therapy with the polymer agent (sevelamer) or lanthanum carbonate may avoid the detrimental effects associated with aluminum, magnesium, or calcium therapy. A thorough review of phosphate-binding agents is provided in Chap. 44.

CLINICAL CONTROVERSY

The selection of a phosphate binding agent is often arbitrary although it should be based on limiting the total daily intake of calcium and avoiding drug-related adverse events. The optimal therapeutic regimen may involve a combination of agents.

HYPOPHOSPHATEMIA

Mild to moderate hypophosphatemia is defined as a serum phosphorus concentration of 1 to 2 mg/dL, whereas severe hypophosphatemia is defined as a serum phosphorus concentration of less than 1 mg/dL.[126] Hypophosphatemia is found in approximately 1% to 3% of hospital admissions.[119] The incidence in hospitalized critically ill patients is 18% to 28%.[126] Unlike its severe form, mild or moderate hypophosphatemia seldom causes recognizable signs and symptoms.[121]

PATHOPHYSIOLOGY

Hypophosphatemia may be the result of decreased gastrointestinal absorption, increased urinary excretion, or extracellular to intracellular redistribution.[118] Although mild to moderate hypophosphatemia is common and can occur in inpatients and outpatients, severe hypophosphatemia is predominantly encountered in the acute care setting and can be associated with life-threatening symptoms (Table 49–7).

Phosphate-binding substances such as sucralfate, calcium carbonate, sevelamer, lanthanum carbonate and aluminum- or magnesium-containing antacids have the potential to bind large amounts of phosphorus in the gut, thereby preventing absorption. If phosphate-binding agents are ingested on a chronic basis in conjunction with a dietary phosphorus deficiency, hypophosphatemia may result.[121] Patients who are receiving long-term phosphate-binding agents, those with peptic ulcer disease or chronic renal insufficiency, and those who may be predisposed to moderate hypophosphatemia (alcoholics) are at highest risk for the development of severe hypophosphatemia. Hyperparathyroidism may cause hypophosphatemia as a result of decreased gastrointestinal absorption of dietary phosphorus.

Increased renal losses of phosphorus can occur in hyperparathyroid (primary and secondary) patients with normal renal function and those with vitamin D deficiency. Elevated parathyroid hormone levels lead to an increase in serum calcium concentrations and decreased serum phosphorus concentrations. Serum phosphorus is decreased as the result of a reduction in renal tubular reabsorption.[127] Recovery from extensive third-degree burns is associated with a marked diuretic phase associated with an impressive renal loss of phosphate.[121] This recovery may also be associated with the development of an anabolic state as stress levels decrease and nutritional therapies take effect. Because phosphorus is rapidly incorporated into the new cells, this may contribute to the severity of the hypophosphatemia. Drugs that cause increased renal elimination of phosphorus include diuretics (acetazolamide and osmotic diuretics), glucocorticoids, and sodium bicarbonate.

Rapid refeeding of malnourished patients with high-carbohydrate, high-calorie nutritional diets with inadequate amounts of supplemental phosphorus may result in severe symptomatic hypophosphatemia. This phenomenon is especially prevalent in patients with other underlying risk factors for the development of hypophosphatemia, such as alcoholism.[127] The etiology of severe hypophosphatemia associated with hyperalimentation and nutritional recovery may be separated into two phases: acute, rapid hypophosphatemia secondary to intracellular shifts of phosphorus resulting from glucose-induced insulin secretion; and the gradual decrease in serum phosphorus concentration over 5 to 10 days secondary to tissue repair in the presence of phosphorus deprivation.[128] The development of severe hypophosphatemia secondary to hyperalimentation can be prevented by the administration of 12 to 15 mmol of phosphorus per liter of hyperalimentation solution or 15 mmol per 1,000 calories of dextrose.[129] Transcellular shifts in phosphorus also occur after parathyroidectomy, causing severe hypocalcemia and hypophosphatemia because of hungry bone syndrome (deposition of phosphorus and calcium in the bone).

TABLE 49–7. Conditions Associated with the Development of Hypophosphatemia

Decreased gastrointestinal absorption
 Phosphate-binding drugs
  Sucralfate
  Calcium carbonate
  Aluminum/magnesium antacids
  Sevelamer
  Lanthanum carbonate
 Decreased dietary phosphorus intake
 Glucocorticoids
 Vitamin D deficiency/resistance
 Hypoparathyroidism
 Chronic diarrhea
 Steatorrhea
Increased urinary excretion
 Hyperparathyroidism (primary and secondary)
 Recovery from burns
 Rickets
 Malignant neoplasms
 Fanconi's syndrome
 Acute volume expansion
 Metabolic acidosis
 Renal transplantation
 Vitamin D deficiency and/or resistance
 Diuretics
  Acetazolamide
  Osmotic agents
 Glucocorticoids
 Sodium bicarbonate
Internal redistribution
 Refeeding syndrome
 Parenteral nutrition
 Parathyroidectomy (hungry bone syndrome)
 Alcoholism
 Respiratory alkalosis
 Diabetic ketoacidosis (correction)
 Dextrose solutions
 Insulin
 Catecholamines
 Anabolic steroids
 Glucagon
 Calcitonin
 Erythropoietin

Severe and prolonged respiratory alkalosis (a result of hyperventilation, pain, anxiety, and sepsis) can cause hypophosphatemia.[119] Respiratory alkalosis is thought to contribute significantly to the hypophosphatemia observed during alcohol withdrawal.[119] Although patients with diabetic ketoacidosis may present with hyperphosphatemia, the institution of therapy to correct it may cause serum phosphorus concentrations to decrease rapidly as phosphorus shifts back into the intracellular compartment. In addition, the acidosis associated with the diabetic ketoacidotic state can cause a decomposition of organic compounds inside the cell and a release of inorganic phosphorus into the plasma and subsequently into the urine.[128] The combination of intracellular phosphorus breakdown and the shift of phosphorus into cells on initiation of treatment may lead to severe hypophosphatemia. Drugs associated with transcellular shifts in phosphorus include dextrose solutions, glucagon, insulin, catecholamines, calcitonin, erythropoietic agents, and anabolic steroids.

Chronic ethanol abusers are prone to a variety of serum electrolyte disorders including hypocalcemia, hypomagnesemia,

hypokalemia, and hypophosphatemia. The etiology of hypophosphatemia in the alcoholic patient is multifactorial. Malnutrition, poor dietary intake, diarrhea, vomiting, and the use of phosphate-binding antacids may all contribute to the hypophosphatemia of alcoholism.[128] In addition, serum phosphorus concentrations may decrease after hospitalization in the alcoholic patient with the institution of dextrose-containing intravenous fluids, as a result of an intracellular shift of phosphorus.[129,130] Hyperventilation associated with the alcohol withdrawal syndrome may also contribute to the development of hypophosphatemia.[121] Alcoholic patients are particularly susceptible to the complications of hypophosphatemia such as rhabdomyolysis, which is often seen during withdrawal or refeeding.[121,130] Thus serum phosphorus concentrations should be routinely monitored in alcoholic patients.

CLINICAL PRESENTATION

The clinical manifestations of severe hypophosphatemia are diverse and may affect many organ systems (Table 49–8). It is likely that two primary biochemical abnormalities are responsible for most of the clinical manifestations of severe hypophosphatemia.[118] First, intracellular energy stores may be decreased secondary to depletion of intracellular ATP, which is dependent on inorganic intracellular phosphate. This can result in disruptions in cellular function. Second, reduced red blood cell 2,3-DPG concentrations are associated with a shift to the left of the oxyhemoglobin saturation curve. This shift is associated with a decrease in the release of oxygen to peripheral tissues (increased oxygen affinity for hemoglobin) and may result in tissue hypoxia.[118] These metabolic disorders can be seen in a wide variety of organ systems.

Neurologic (CNS) manifestations of severe hypophosphatemia result in a metabolic encephalopathy syndrome.[128] This progressive syndrome of irritability, apprehension, weakness, numbness, paresthesias, dysarthria, confusion, obtundation, seizures, and coma has been described in patients with severe hypophosphatemia.[121,127] Neuropsychiatric disturbances include apathy, delirium, hallucinations,

TABLE 49–8. Manifestations of Severe Hypophosphatemia

Neurologic	Hematologic
Irritability	Decreased 2,3-diphosphoglycerate
Apprehension	Hemolysis
Weakness	White blood cell dysfunction
Numbness	Platelet dysfunction
Paresthesias	**Bone**
Dysarthria	Osteopenia
Confusion	Osteomalacia
Obtundation	Bone pain
Seizures	**Pulmonary**
Coma	Acute respiratory failure
Apathy	Slow weaning from ventilator
Delirium	Respiratory muscle fatigue
Hallucinations	**Renal**
Paranoia	Acute tubular necrosis (rhabdomyolysis)
Peripheral neuropathy	**Cardiac**
Muscular	Congestive cardiomyopathy
Myalgia	Decreased contractility
Weakness	Arrhythmias
Rhabdomyolysis	
Dysphagia	
Ileus	

→ *neuritis assoc. w/ fever*

and paranoia. Peripheral neuropathy and symptoms resembling Guillain-Barré syndrome have also been reported.[127]

Severe hypophosphatemia may result in significant dysfunction of skeletal muscle ranging from myalgia, bone pain, and weakness, with chronic hypophosphatemia, to potentially fatal rhabdomyolysis with severe acute hypophosphatemia.[127] Laboratory evaluations can help to distinguish between chronic and acute or chronic hypophosphatemia. Elevated alkaline phosphatase, normal creatine phosphokinase, and normal to low phosphorus and calcium are present in cases of chronic hypophosphatemia. In contrast, hyperkalemia, hyperuricemia, elevated blood urea nitrogen and creatinine, hypercalcemia, and myoglobinuria are present in cases in which rhabdomyolysis complicates the acute or chronic hypophosphatemia.[127] Hypophosphatemia can result in acute respiratory failure secondary to respiratory muscle weakness and diaphragmatic contractile dysfunction. Thus frequent assessment of serum phosphorus concentration is indicated in patients at risk for respiratory failure. Likewise, adequate treatment of hypophosphatemia in respiratory failure may aid in successful weaning from the ventilator.[119] Dysphagia and ileus have also been attributed to hypophosphatemia.[119]

Cardiac muscle function has been reported to be impaired in the setting of hypophosphatemia and has resulted in congestive cardiomyopathy.[131] This has been reported in alcoholics, and postoperative and intensive care patients. A depletion in cardiac ATP stores has been hypothesized as the cause of this syndrome.[127] Arrhythmias have also been reported in patients with hypophosphatemia. Because hypophosphatemia is a potentially reversible cause of heart failure, it should be considered in patients who experience an acute deterioration in ventricular function.

Hematologic manifestations of hypophosphatemia include decreased levels of 2,3-DPG, decreased red blood cell ATP, and membrane rigidity.[118] When red blood cell ATP decreases to below 15% of normal, cells become spherocytic and rigid, and are trapped and destroyed in the spleen.[128] Therefore hemolysis may be a manifestation of severe hypophosphatemia. Reduction in ATP content of white blood cells may result in mobility, chemotaxis, phagocytosis, and bactericidal dysfunction.[121] These changes may contribute to an increased risk of infection in hypophosphatemic patients. Animal studies also demonstrate platelet abnormalities in the setting of hypophosphatemia.[127] The implications of hypophosphatemia for human platelet function, however, have not been determined.

Finally, prolonged hypophosphatemia may result in osteopenia and osteomalacia because of enhanced osteoclastic resorption of bone. Glucose intolerance from hypophosphatemia caused by tissue insensitivity to insulin has also been described.

CLINICAL PRESENTATION OF HYPOPHOSPHATEMIA

GENERAL
The manifestations of hypophosphatemia depend on the chronicity and severity of the phosphate depletion. The major conditions associated with symptomatic hypophosphatemia are chronic alcoholism, intravenous hyperalimentation without adequate phosphate supplementation, and the chronic ingestion of antacids. Severe hypophosphatemia can also be seen during treatment of diabetic ketoacidosis and with prolonged hyperventilation.

SYMPTOMS
Except for the effects on mineral metabolism, the symptoms of hypophosphatemia are due to two consequences (reduction of red cell 2,3-DPG and reduction of intracellular ATP levels), and can impact virtually all organ systems. Resulting symptoms can include irritability, apprehension, weakness, numbness, paresthesias, confusion, seizures, and coma.

SIGNS
The initial response of bone to hypophosphatemia is increased resorption and the associated release of bone calcium, contributing to hypercalciuria. Prolonged hypophosphatemia can result in rickets and osteomalacia due to decreased bone mineralization.

Neurologic: Severe hypophosphatemia can lead to a metabolic encephalopathy.

Cardiopulmonary: Impaired myocardial contractility and respiratory failure secondary to ATP depletion has been described. The reduction in cardiac output may become clinically significant, leading to congestive heart failure.

Musculoskeletal: Proximal myopathy, dysphagia, and ileus have been reported. Acute hypophosphatemia superimposed upon pre-existing severe phosphate depletion can lead to rhabdomyolysis.

Hematologic: Alterations in the hematopoietic system can also occur, resulting in hemolysis, reduction in phagocytotic and granulocyte chemotactic ability, as well as defective clot retraction and thrombocytopenia.

LABORATORY TESTS
Serum phosphate levels below 2.4 mg/dL represent hypophosphatemia.

▶ TREATMENT: Hypophosphatemia

▓ DESIRED OUTCOME

The goals of therapy are the reversal of signs and symptoms of hypophosphatemia, normalization of serum phosphorus concentrations, and management of underlying conditions. Awareness of the clinical situations in which hypophosphatemia may be anticipated (alcoholism, diabetic ketoacidosis, and parenteral nutrition) is of vital importance in preventing iatrogenic hypophosphatemia. The routine addition of phosphorus in concentrations of 12 to 15 mmol/L to intra-

venous hyperalimentation solutions is of utmost importance for the prevention of severe hypophosphatemia in hospitalized patients.

▓ PHARMACOLOGIC THERAPY

Severe (<1 mg/dL) or symptomatic hypophosphatemia should be treated with parenteral phosphorus replacement. Oral phosphorus supplementation is usually reserved for patients who are asymptomatic or who exhibit mild to moderate hypophosphatemia. Estimation of total body phosphorus deficit is difficult because phosphorus is an intracellular electrolyte. Dosage and infusion recommendations, as well as response to parenteral phosphorus replacement, are highly variable.[126] The infusion of 15 mmol of phosphorus in 250 mL 5% dextrose or 0.9% sodium chloride over 3 hours is a safe and effective treatment for severe hypophosphatemia.[126] Mean increases in serum phosphate of 0.5 to 0.8 mg/dL have been reported. Doses of 15 to 30 mmol of phosphorus can be given over 1 to 3 hours in patients without hypercalcemia (serum calcium >10.5 mg/dL).[126,132] Other authors recommend a wider dosage range of 0.08 to 0.64 mmol/kg body weight (5 to 45 mmol in a 70-kg patient) given over 4 to 12 hours.[132–134] Intravenous phosphate therapy produces the desired increase in serum phosphorus at 24 hours in 20% to 80% of patients. Response is dependent on the degree of phosphate depletion and replacement dose administered.[118] Furthermore, the initial success is often followed in 48 to 72 hours by recurrent hypophosphatemia, necessitating close monitoring of serum phosphorus and repeated administration of phosphorus products as warranted.

CLINICAL CONTROVERSY

The recommended dosage of intravenous phosphorus in conditions of severe hypophosphatemia is not well established and may range from 5 to 45 mmol of phosphorus.

Parenteral phosphorus supplementation is associated with risks of hyperphosphatemia, metastatic soft tissue deposition of calcium-phosphate product, hypomagnesemia, hypocalcemia, and hyperkalemia or hypernatremia (caused by intravenous phosphorus salt) (Table 49–9). Inappropriate administration of large doses of parenteral phosphorus over relatively short time periods has resulted in symptomatic hypocalcemia and soft-tissue calcification.[118] The rate of infusion and choice of initial dosage should therefore be based on severity of hypophosphatemia, presence of symptoms, and coexistent medical conditions. Patients should be closely monitored with frequent (every 6 hours) serum phosphorus determinations for 48 to 72 hours after starting intravenous therapy. It may be necessary to continue administration of intravenous phosphorus for several days in some patients, while other patients may be able to tolerate an

TABLE 49–9. Phosphorus Replacement Therapy

Product (Salt)	Phosphate Content
Oral therapy	
Neutra-Phos (7 mEq/packet each of Na and K)	250 mg (8 mmol)/packet
Neutra-Phos-K (14.25 mEq/packet K)	250 mg (8 mmol)/packet
K-Phos Neutral (13 mEq/tablet Na and 1.1 mEq/tablet K)	250 mg (8 mmol)/tablet
Uro-KP-Neutral (10.9 mEq/tablet Na and 1.27 mEq/tablet K)	250 mg (8 mmol)/tablet
Intravenous therapy	
Sodium PO_4 (4.0 mEq/mL Na)	3 mmol/mL
Potassium PO_4 (4.4 mEq/mL K)	3 mmol/mL

oral maintenance regimen. Monitoring should also include assessment of serum potassium, calcium, and magnesium concentrations. Hypomagnesemia secondary to intracellular shifts occurs frequently (27% to 80%) in severely hypophosphatemic patients.[126] Therapy with parenteral phosphorus should be undertaken with great caution and at reduced dosage for patients with hypercalcemia or renal dysfunction.[121,130]

Mild to moderate or asymptomatic hypophosphatemia can be treated by the administration of oral phosphorus salts in doses of 1.5 to 2 g (50 to 60 mmol) daily in divided doses (see Table 49–9). Phosphorus concentrations should be monitored daily, with the goal of correcting the reduced phosphorus concentration in approximately 7 to 10 days. The primary dose-limiting adverse effect associated with oral phosphorus replacement is the development of osmotic diarrhea. Patients with mild to moderate hypophosphatemia and moderate to severe renal insufficiency should receive reduced daily oral doses (i.e., 1 g or approximately 30 mmol of phosphorus) with careful monitoring of serum phosphorus concentration, because they are predisposed to phosphorus retention. In addition to phosphorus supplementation for hypophosphatemia, dipyridamole may decrease renal phosphate leaking and increase serum phosphorus. Doses of 75 mg four times daily have resulted in increases in serum 1,25-dihydroxyvitamin D_3 and decreases in serum calcium and urolithiasis events.[135]

CONCLUSIONS

Clinicians play an integral part in the management of fluid and electrolyte abnormalities; initially they should review the patient's medication history to determine if any of the patient's current drug therapy may have contributed to the existing abnormalities. They should also carefully evaluate all drug therapy options to reduce the risk of developing new electrolyte problems and to optimize the outcome of the current management plan. This proactive interventional approach will facilitate the management of mild disorders in the community and may reduce the need for hospitalization.

ABBREVIATIONS

ACEI: angiotensin-converting enzyme inhibitor
ADH: antidiuretic hormone
ATP: adenosine triphosphate
BUN: blood urea nitrogen

CHF: congestive heart failure
CNS: central nervous system
DDAVP: 1-deamino-8-D-arginine vasopressin
2,3-DPG: 2,3-diphosphoglycerate
D_5W: 5% dextrose in water
DI: diabetes insipidus
EABV: effective arterial blood volume
ECF: extracellular fluid
ECFVd: extracellular fluid volume deficit
$ECFV_{current}$: current extracellular fluid volume
$ECFV_{norm}$: normal extracellular fluid volume
FeNa: fractional excretion of sodium
GFR: glomerular filtration rate
IV_{Na}: sodium concentration of infusate
IV_{vol}: volume of infusate
NSAID: nonsteroidal anti-inflammatory drug
PTH: parathyroid hormone
S_{ca}: serum calcium
S_{Na}^1: initial patient serum sodium concentration

SIADH: syndrome of inappropriate secretion of antidiuretic
  hormone
TBW: total body water
$TBW_{current}$: current total body water
TBW_{norm}: normal total body water
V2: vasopressin-2

Review Questions and other resources can be found at
www.pharmacotherapyonline.com.

REFERENCES

1. Berl T, Robertson GL. Pathophysiology of water metabolism. In: Brenner BM, ed. The Kidney, 6th ed. Philadelphia, WB Saunders, 2000: 866–924.
2. Andreoli TE. Water: Normal balance, hyponatremia, and hypernatremia. Ren Fail 2000;2:711–735.
3. McManus ML, Churchwell KB, Strange K. Regulation of cell volume in health and disease. N Engl J Med 1995;333:1260–1266.
4. Gennari FJ. Serum osmolality: Uses and limitations. N Engl J Med 1984;310:102–105.
5. Androgué HJ, Madias NE. Hyponatremia. N Engl J Med 2000;342:1581–1589.
6. Baylis PH. Osmoregulation and control of vasopressin secretion in healthy adults. Am J Physiol 1987;253(5 pt 2):R671–R678.
7. Deen PM, Verdijk MA, Knoers NV, et al. Requirement of human renal water channel aquaphorin-2 for vasopressin-dependent concentration of urine. Science 1994;264:92–95.
8. Bourque CW, Oliet SH, Richard D. Osmoreceptors, osmoreception, and osmoregulation. Front Neuroendocrinol 1994;15:231–274.
9. Skorecki KL, Brenner BM. Body fluid homeostasis. A contemporary overview. Am J Med 1981;70:77–88.
10. Anderson RJ. Hospital-associated hyponatremia. Kidney Int 1986;29:1237–1247.
11. Nzerue CM, Baffoe-Bonnie H, You W, et al. Predictors of outcome in hospitalized patients with severe hyponatremia. J Natl Med Assoc 2003;95:335–343.
12. Oster JR, Singer I. Hyponatremia, hyposmolality, and hypotonicity: Tables and fables. Arch Intern Med 1999;159:333–336.
13. Maas AHJ, Siggard-Andersen O, Weisberg HF, Zijlstra WG. Ion-selective electrodes for sodium and potassium: A new problem of what is measured and what should be reported. Clin Chem 1985;31:482–485.
14. Star RA. Hyperosmolar states. Am J Med Sci 1990;300:402–412.
15. Agarwal R, Emmett M. The post-transurethral resection of prostate syndrome: Therapeutic proposals. Am J Kidney Dis 1994;24:108–111.
16. Arieff AI. Management of hyponatremia. Br Med J 1993;307:305–308.
17. Aabakken L, Johansen KS, Rydningen EB, et al. Osmolal and anion gaps in patients admitted to an emergency medical department. Hum Exp Toxicol 1994;13:131–134.
18. Arieff AI, DeFronzo RA. Disorders of sodium metabolism—hyponatremia. In: Arieff AI, DeFronza RA, eds. Fluid, Electrolyte, and Acid-Base Disorders, 2nd ed. New York, Churchill Livingstone, 1995: 255–303.
19. Sterns RH, Narins RG. Hypernatremia and hyponatremia: Pathophysiology, diagnosis, and therapy. In: Androgué HJ, ed. Contemporary Management in Critical Care, Vol. 1, No. 2. Acid-Base and Electrolyte Disorders. New York, Churchill Livingstone, 1991:161–191.
20. Kamel KS, Ethier JH, Richardson RM, et al. Urine electrolytes and osmolality: When and how to use them. Am J Nephrol 1990;10:89–102.
21. Jolobe OM. Diuretic-induced hyponatraemia in elderly hypertensive women. J Hum Hypertens 2003;17:151.
22. Smith DM, McKenna K, Thompson CJ. Hyponatraemia. Clin Endocrinol 2000;52:667–678.
23. Hensen J, Haenelt M, Gross P. Water retention after oral chlorpropamide is associated with an increase in renal papillary arginine vasopressin receptors. Eur J Endocrinol 1995;132:459–464.
24. Kamiyama T, Iseki K, Kawazoe N, et al. Carbamazepine-induced hyponatremia in a patient with partial central diabetes insipidus. Nephron 1993;64:142–145.
25. Bressler RB, Huston DP. Water intoxication following moderate dose intravenous cyclophosphamide. Arch Intern Med 1985;145:548.
26. Rault RM. Case report: hyponatremia associated with nonsteroidal anti-inflammatory drugs. Am J Med Sci 1993;305:318–320.
27. Liv BA, Mittman N, Knowles SR, Shear NH. Hyponatremia and the syndrome of inappropriate secretion of antidiuretic hormone associated with the use of selective serotonin reuptake inhibitors: A review of spontaneous reports. Can Med Assoc J 1996;155:519–527.
28. Holden R, Jackson MA. Near-fatal hyponatremic coma due to vasopressin over-secretion after "ecstasy" (3,4-MDMA). Lancet 1996;347:1052.
29. Hairprasad MK, Eisinger RP, Nadler IM, et al. Hyponatremia in psychogenic polydipsia. Arch Intern Med 1980;140:1639–1642.
30. Ayus JC, Arieff AI. Pulmonary complications of hyponatremic encephalopathy—Non-cardiogenic pulmonary edema and hypercapnic respiratory failure. Chest 1995;107:517–521.
31. Verbalis JG, Gullans SR. Hyponatremia causes large sustained reductions in brain content of multiple organic osmolytes in rats. Brain Res 1991;567:274–282.
32. Ayus JC, Arieff AI. Chronic hyponatremic encephalopathy in postmenopausal women—Association of therapies with morbidity and mortality. JAMA 1999;281:2299–2304.
33. Sterns RH. Severe symptomatic hyponatremia: Treatment and outcome: A study of 64 cases. Ann Intern Med 1987;107:656–664.
34. Sterns RH, Riggs JE, Schochet SS Jr. Osmotic demyelination syndrome following correction of hyponatremia. N Engl J Med 1986;314:1535–1542.
35. Decaux G, Soupart A. Treatment of symptomatic hyponatremia. Am J Med Sci 2003;326:25–30.
36. Fanestil DD, Moore FD. Compartmentation of body water. In: Narins RG, ed. Maxwell and Kleeman's Fluid and Electrolyte Metabolism, 5th ed. New York, McGraw-Hill, 1994:1–20.
37. Mange K, Matsuura D, Cizman B, et al. Language guiding therapy: The case of dehydration versus volume depletion. Ann Intern Med 1997;127:848–853.
38. Inadomi DW, Kopple JD. Fluid and electrolyte complications in total parenteral nutrition. In: Narins RG, ed. Maxwell and Kleeman's Fluid and Electrolyte Metabolism, 5th ed. New York, McGraw-Hill, 1994:1446–1447.
39. Lauriat SM, Berl T. The hyponatremic patient: Practical focus on therapy. J Am Soc Nephrol 1997;8:1599–1607.
40. Decaux G, Waterlot Y, Genette F, Mockel J. Treatment of the syndrome of inappropriate secretion of antidiuretic hormone with furosemide. N Engl J Med 1981;304:329–330.
41. Verbalis JG. Hyponatremia and hyposmolar disorders. In: Greenberg A, ed. Primer on Kidney Diseases, 2nd ed. San Diego, CA, Academic Press, 1998:57–63.
42. Curtis NJ, van Heyningen C, Turner JJ. Irreversible nephrotoxicity from demeclocycline in the treatment of hyponatremia. Age Ageing 2002;31:151-152.
43. Saito T, Ishikawa S, Abe K, et al. Acute aquaresis by the nonpeptide arginine vasopressin (AVP) antagonist OPC-31260 improves hyponatremia in patients with syndrome of inappropriate secretion of antidiuretic hormone (SIADH). J Clin Endocrinol Metab 1997;82:1054–1057.
44. Elisaf M, Theodorou J, Pappas C, Siamopoulos K. Successful treatment of hyponatremia with angiotensin-converting enzyme inhibitors in patients with congestive heart failure. Cardiology 1995;86:477–480.
45. Gerbes AL, Gulberg V, Gines P, et al. Therapy of hyponatremia in cirrhosis with a vasopressin receptor antagonist: a randomized double-blind multicenter trial. Gastroenterology 2003;124:933–939.
46. Oh MS, Carroll HJ. Regulation of intracellular and extracellular volume. In: Arieff AI, DeFronzo RA, eds. Fluid, Electrolyte, and Acid-Base Balance Disorders, 2nd ed. New York, Churchill Livingstone, 1995:1–28.
47. Fried LF, Palevsky PM. Hyponatremia and hypernatremia. Med Clin North Am 1997;81:585–609.

48. Moritz ML, Ayus JC. The changing pattern of hypernatremia in hospitalized children. Pediatrics 1999;104:435–439.

49. Oh MS, Carroll HJ. Disorders of sodium metabolism: Hypernatremia and hyponatremia. Crit Care Med 1992;20:94–103.

50. Androgué HJ, Madias NE. Hypernatremia. N Engl J Med 2000;342: 1493–1499.

51. Rose BD, Post TW. Hyperosmolar states—Hypernatremia. In: Rose BD, Post TW, eds. Clinical Physiology of Acid-Base and Electrolyte Disorders, 5th ed. New York, McGraw-Hill, 2001:746–793.

52. Andreoli TE. The polyuric syndromes. Nephrol Dial Transplant 2001;16(Suppl 6):10–12.

53. Zerbe RL, Robertson GL. A comparison of plasma vasopressin measurements with a standard indirect test in the differential diagnosis of polyuria. N Engl J Med 1981;304:1539–1546.

54. Physicians Desk Reference, 55th ed. Montvale, NJ, 2001:702–704.

55. Monnens L, Jonkman A, Thomas C. Response to indomethacin and hydrochlorothiazide in nephrogenic diabetes insipidus. Clin Sci 1984;66:709–715.

56. Battle DC, Von Riotte AB, Gaviria M, Grupp M. Amelioration of polyuria by amiloride in patients receiving long-term lithium therapy. N Engl J Med 1985;312:408–414.

57. Bonventre JV, Leaf A. Sodium homeostasis: Steady states without a setpoint. Kidney Int 1982;21:880–883.

58. Rose BD. Clinical Physiology of Acid-Base and Electrolyte Disorders, 5th ed. New York, McGraw-Hill, 2001:478.

59. Taylor AE. Capillary fluid filtration: Starling forces and lymph flow. Circ Res 1981;49:557–575.

60. Schrier RW. Pathogenesis of sodium and water retention in high-output and low-output cardiac failure, nephrotic syndrome, cirrhosis, and pregnancy. N Engl J Med 1988;319:1127–1134.

61. Rose BD. Diuretics. Kidney Int 1991;39:336–352.

62. Brater DC. Diuretic therapy. N Engl J Med 1998;339:387–395.

63. Rudy DW, Voelker JR, Greene PK, et al. Loop diuretics for chronic renal insufficiency: A continuous infusion is more efficacious than bolus therapy. Ann Intern Med 1991;115:360–366.

64. Kirchner KA, Voelker JR, Brater DC. Intratubular albumin blunts the response to furosemide—A mechanism for diuretic resistance in the nephrotic syndrome. J Pharmacol Exp Ther 1990;252:1097–1101.

65. Agarwal R, Gorski JC, Sundblad K, Brater DC. Urinary protein binding does not affect response to furosemide in patients with nephrotic syndrome. J Am Soc Nephrol 2000;11:1100–1105.

66. Weiner ID, Wingo CS. Hypokalemia—Consequences, causes, and correction. J Am Soc Nephrol 1997;8:1179–1188.

67. Liew D, Martin J, Krum H. Eplerenone. Pharmacia. Curr Opin Investig Drugs 2003;4:316–322.

68. Reber PM, Heath H III. Hypocalcemic emergencies. Med Clin North Am 1995;79:93–106.

69. Nussbaum SR. Pathophysiology and management of severe hypercalcemia. Endocrinol Metab Clin North Am 1993;22:343–362.

70. Zaloga GP. Hypocalcemia in critically ill patients. Crit Care Med 1992;20:251–262.

71. Slomp J, van der Voort PH, Gerritsen RT, et al. Albumin-adjusted calcium is not suitable for diagnosis of hyper- and hypocalcemia in the critically ill. Crit Care Med 2003;31:1389–1393.

72. Potts JT. Hyperparathyroidism and other hypercalcemic disorders. Adv Intern Med 1996;41:165–212.

73. Zojer N, Keck AV, Pecherstorfer M. Comparative tolerability of drug therapies for hypercalcaemia of malignancy. Drug Saf 1999;21: 389–406.

74. Rude RK. Hyperparathyroidism. Otolaryngol Clin North Am 1996;29: 663–679.

75. Chisholm MA, Mulloy AL, Taylor AT. Acute management of cancer-related hypercalcemia. Ann Pharmacother 1996;30:507–513.

76. Strewler GJ. The physiology of parathyroid hormone-related protein. N Engl J Med 2000;342:177–185.

77. Ralston SH, Coleman R, Fraser WD, et al. Medical management of hypercalcemia. Calcif Tissue Int 2004;74:1–11.

78. Schmidt-Gayk H, Haerdt H. Differential diagnosis of hypercalcemia: Laboratory assessment. Recent Results Cancer Res 1994;137:122–137.

79. Agus ZS, Wasserstein A, Goldfarb S. Disorders of calcium and magnesium homeostasis. Am J Med 1982;72:473–488.

80. Maruani G, Hertig A, Paillard M, Houillier P. Normocalcemic primary hyperparathyroidism: evidence for a generalized target-tissue resistance to parathyroid hormone. J Clin Endocrinol Metab 2003;88:4641–4648.

81. Goodman WG, Goldin J, Kuizon BD, et al. Coronary-artery calcification in young adults with end-stage renal disease who are undergoing dialysis. N Engl J Med 2000;342:1478–1483.

82. Goldsmith DJ, Covic A, Sambrook PA, Ackrill P. Vascular calcification in long-term haemodialysis patients in a single unit: A retrospective analysis. Nephron 1997;77:37–43.

83. Guerin AP, London GM, Marchais SJ, Metivier F. Arterial stiffening and vascular calcifications in end-stage renal disease. Nephrol Dial Transplant 2000;15:1014–1021.

84. Singer FR, Krane SM. Paget's disease of bone. In: Avioli LV, Krane SM, eds. Metabolic Bone Disease and Clinically Related Disorders, 3rd ed. New York, Academic Press, 1998:545–605.

85. Rodman JS, Mahler RJ. Kidney stones as a manifestation of hypercalcemic disorders. Hyperparathyroidism and sarcoidosis. Urol Clin North Am 2000;27:275–285.

86. Yamashita H, Noguchi S, Uchino S, et al. Influence of renal function on clinico-pathological features of primary hyperparathyroidism. Euro J Endocrinol 2003;148:597–602.

87. Dretler SP. The physiologic approach to the medical management of stone disease. Urol Clin North Am 1998;25:613–623.

88. Parks JH, Coe FL. Pathogenesis and treatment of calcium stones. Semin Nephrol 1996;16:398–411.

89. U.S. Renal Data System. 2002 Annual Data Report. Bethesda, MD, The National Institutes of Health, National Institute of Diabetes and Digestive and Kidney Diseases, 2002.

90. Mundy GR, Guise TA. Hypercalcemia of malignancy. Am J Med 1997;103:134–145.

91. Singer FR, Ginger K. Resistance to calcitonin. In: Singer F, Wallach S, eds. Paget's Disease of Bone. Clinical Assessment, Present and Future Therapy. New York, Elsevier, 1991:75–85.

92. Barri YM, Knochel JP. Hypercalcemia and electrolyte disturbances in malignancy. Hematol Oncol Clin North Am 1996;10:775–790.

93. Body JJ. Clinical research update: zoledronate. Cancer 1997;80:1699–1701.

94. Major P, Lortholary A, Hon J, et al. Zoledronic acid is superior to pamidronate in the treatment of hypercalcemia of malignancy: a pooled analysis of two randomized, controlled clinical trials. J Clin Oncol 2001;19:558–567.

95. Body JJ, Lortholary A, Romieu G, et al. A dose-finding study of zoledronate in hypercalcemic cancer patients. J Bone Miner Res 1999;14:1557–1561.

96. Pecherstorfer M, Steinhauer EU, Rizzoli R, et al. Efficacy and safety of ibandronate in the treatment of hypercalcemia of malignancy: a randomized multicenter comparison to pamidronate. Support Care Cancer 2003;11:539–547.

97. Watters J, Gerrard G, Dodwell D. The management of malignant hypercalcemia. Drugs 1996;52:837–848.

98. Rastad J, Benson L, Johansson H, et al. Clodronate treatment in patients with malignancy-associated hypercalcemia. Acta Med Scand 1987;221:489–494.

99. Banerjee D, Asif A, Striker L, et al. Short-term, high-dose pamidronate-induced acute tubular necrosis: the postulated mechanisms of bisphosphonate nephrotoxicity. Am J Kidney Dis 2003;41:E18.

100. Markowitz GS, Fine PL, Stack JI, et al. Toxic acute tubular necrosis following treatment with zoledronate (Zometa). Kidney Int 2003;64:281–289.

101. Leyland-Jones B. Treatment of cancer-related hypercalcemia: the role of gallium nitrate. Semin Oncol 2003;30(2 Suppl 5):13–19.

102. Edelson GW, Kleerekoper M. Hypercalcemic crisis. Med Clin North Am 1995;79:79–92.

103. Manolagas SC, Weinstein RS. New developments in the pathogenesis and treatment of steroid-induced osteoporosis. J Bone Miner Res 1999;14:1061–1066.

104. Block GA, Port FK. Re-evaluation of risks associated with hyperphosphatemia and hyperparathyroidism in dialysis patients: Recommendations for a change in management. Am J Kidney Dis 2000;35:1226–1237.

105. Collins MT, Skarulis MC, Bilezikian JP, et al. Treatment of hypercalcemia secondary to parathyroid carcinoma with a novel calcimimetic agent. J Clin Endocrinol Metab 1998;83:1083–1088.

106. Franceschini N, Joy MS, Kshirsagar A. Cincacet HCl: a calcimimetic agent for the management of primary and secondary hyperparathyroidism. Expert Opin Investig Drugs 2003;12:1413–1421.

107. Guise TA, Mundy GR. Evaluation of hypocalcemia in children and adults. J Clin Endocrinol Metab 1995;80:1473–1478.

108. Jawan B, de Villa V, Luk HN, et al. Ionized calcium changes during living-donor liver transplantation in patients with and without administration of blood-bank products. Transpl Int 2003;16:510–514.

109. Kishimoto M, Ohto H, Shikama Y, et al. Treatment for the decline of ionized calcium levels during peripheral blood progenitor cell harvesting. Transfusion 2002;42:1340–1347.

110. Yarpuzlu AA. A review of clinical and laboratory findings and treatment of tumor lysis syndrome. Clinica Chemica Acta 2003;333:13–18.

111. Alvarez-Hernandez D, Santamaria I, Rodriguez-Garcia M, et al. A novel mutation in the calcium-sensing receptor responsible for autosomal dominant hypocalcemia in a family with two uncommon parathyroid hormone polymorphisms. J Mol Endocrinol 2003;31:255–262.

112. Hu J, Mora S, Colussi G, et al. Autosomal dominant hypocalcemia caused by a novel mutation in the loop 2 region of the human calcium receptor extracellular domain. J Bone Miner Res 2002;17:1461–1469.

113. Singer FR. Medical management of nonparathyroid hypercalcemia and hypocalcemia. Otolaryngol Clin North Am 1996;29:701–710.

114. Juan D. Hypocalcemia: Differential diagnosis and mechanisms. Arch Intern Med 1979;139:1166–1171.

115. Fouser L. Disorders of calcium, phosphorus and magnesium. Pediatr Ann 1995;24:38, 41–46.

116. Choyke PL, Knopp MV. Pseudohypocalcemia with MR imaging contrast agents: a cautionary tale. Radiology 2003;227:639–646.

117. Tohme JF, Bilezikian JP. Hypocalcemic emergencies. Endocrinol Metab Clin North Am 1993;22:363–375.

118. Hruska K, Gupta A. Disorders of phosphate homeostasis. In: Avioli LV, Krane SM, eds. Metabolic Bone Disease and Clinically Related Disorders, 3rd ed. New York, Academic Press, 1998:207–236.

119. Weisinger JR, Bellorin-Font E. Magnesium and phosphorus. Lancet 1998;352:391–396.

120. Fine A, Patterson J. Severe hyperphosphatemia following phosphate administration for bowel preparation in patients with renal failure: Two cases and a review of the literature. Am J Kidney Dis 1997;2: 103–105.

121. Bourke E, Yanagawa N. Assessment of hyperphosphatemia and hypophosphatemia. Clin Lab Med 1993;13:183–207.

122. Kelsler R, McDonald RD, Cadnapaphornchai P. Dynamic changes serum phosphorus levels in diabetic ketoacidosis. Am J Med 1985;7 571–576.

123. Eknoyan G, Levin A, Levin NW. K/DOQI clinical practice guideline for bone metabolism and disease in chronic kidney disease. Am J Kidney Dis 2003;42(Suppl 3):S1–201.

124. Joy MS, Finn WF. Randomized, double-blind, placebo-controlled, dose titration, Phase III study assessing the efficacy and tolerability of lanthanum carbonate: a new phosphate binder for the treatment of hy perphosphatemia. Am J Kidney Dis 2003;42:96–107.

125. D'Haese PC, Spasovski GB, Sikole A, et al. A multicenter study of the effects of lanthanum carbonate (Fosrenol) and calcium carbon ate on renal bone disease in dialysis patients. Kidney Int 2003;8 S73–S78.

126. Perreault MM, Ostrop NJ, Tierney MG. Efficacy and safety of intra venous phosphate replacement in critically ill patients. Ann Pharma cother 1997;31:683–688.

127. Subramanian R, Khardori R. Severe hypophosphatemia. Pathophys iologic implications, clinical presentation, and treatment. Medicin (Baltimore) 2000;79:1–78.

128. Knochel JP. The pathophysiology and clinical characteristics of sever hypophosphatemia. Arch Intern Med 1977;137:203–220.

129. Silvis SE, DiBartolomeo AG, Aaker HM. Hypophosphatemia and neu rological changes secondary to oral caloric intake. Am J Gastroentero 1980;73:215–222.

130. Hoggson SF, Hurley DL. Acquired hypophosphatemia. Endocrine Metab Clin North Am 1993;22:397–409.

131. Michiels JP, Dive A, Donckier J, Installe E. Reversible myocardial dys function in a patient with alcoholic ketoacidosis. Am J Emerg Me 1998;16:371–373.

132. Charron T, Bernard F, Skrobik Y, et al. Intravenous phosphate in th intensive care unit: more aggressive repletion regimens for moder ate and severe hypophosphatemia. Intensive Care Med 2003;29:1273 1278.

133. Lentz RD, Brown DM, Kjellstrand CM. Treatment of severe hypophos phatemia. Ann Intern Med 1978;89:941–944.

134. Clark CL, Sacks GS, Dickerson RN, et al. Treatment of hypophos phatemia in patients receiving specialized nutrition support using a grad uated dosing scheme: Results from a prospective clinical trial. Crit Care Med 1995;23:1504–1511.

135. Prie D, Blanchet FB, Essig M, et al. Dipyridamole decreases renal phos phate leak and augments serum phosphorus in patients with low rena phosphate threshold. J Am Soc Nephrol 1998;9:1264–1269.

50
DISORDERS OF POTASSIUM AND MAGNESIUM HOMEOSTASIS

Donald F. Brophy and Todd W. B. Gehr

Learning Objectives and other resources can be found at *www.pharmacotherapyonline.com.*

KEY CONCEPTS

1. Potassium is the primary intracellular ion in the human body.

2. The normal plasma potassium concentration range is 3.5 to 5 mEq/L (3.5 mmol/L).

3. Potassium regulates many biochemical processes in the body, and is a key ion for electrical action potentials across cellular membranes.

4. Potassium chloride is the preferred potassium supplement for the most common causes of hypokalemia.

5. In patients with concomitant hypokalemia and hypomagnesemia, it is imperative to correct the hypomagnesemia before the hypokalemia.

6. Hyperkalemia commonly results in patients with acute or chronic kidney disease.

7. Magnesium is an important cofactor for many cellular functions.

8. The normal plasma magnesium concentration range is 1.4 to 1.8 mEq/L (0.85 to 1.15 mmol/L).

9. Hypomagnesemia is commonly caused by excessive gastrointestinal or renal magnesium wasting.

10. Hypermagnesemia is commonly observed in patients with acute or chronic kidney disease.

Potassium and magnesium are electrolytes that are responsible for numerous metabolic activities. Disorders of these electrolytes are frequently seen in both the acute care and community ambulatory care settings. Clinicians should have a firm understanding of the etiology, pathophysiology, symptoms, pharmacotherapy, and monitoring of these disorders. This chapter describes the homeostatic mechanisms that are responsible for the maintenance of normal potassium and magnesium serum concentrations. The clinical disorders responsible for the development of hyperkalemia, hypermagnesemia, hypokalemia, and hypomagnesemia are also reviewed.

POTASSIUM

1. Potassium is the most abundant cation in the body, with estimated total body stores of 3,000 to 4,000 mEq.[1] Ninety-eight percent of this amount is contained within the intracellular compartment, and the remaining 2% is distributed within the extracellular compartment. The Na^+-K^+-ATPase pump located in the cell membrane is responsible for the compartmentalization of potassium. This pump is an active transport system that maintains increased intracellular stores of potassium by transporting sodium out of the cell and potassium into the cell at a ratio of 3:2. Consequently the pump maintains a higher concentration of potassium inside the cell.

2. The normal serum concentration range for potassium is 3.5 to 5.0 mEq/L, whereas the intracellular potassium concentration is usually about 140 mEq/L.[2] Approximately 70% of the intracellular potassium is located in skeletal muscle; the remaining 30% is located in the liver and red blood cells. Extracellular potassium is distributed throughout the serum and interstitial space. Potassium is dynamic in that it is constantly moving between the intracellular and extracellular compartments according to the body's needs.[3] Thus the serum potassium concentration alone does not accurately reflect the total body potassium content.

3. Potassium has many physiologic functions within cells, including protein and glycogen synthesis and cellular metabolism and growth. It is also a determinant of the electrical action potential across the cell membrane.[1] The ratio of the intracellular to extracellular potassium concentration is the major determinant of the resting membrane potential across the cell membrane. Thus the resting membrane potential is greatly affected by variations in extracellular potassium concentration. Serum potassium concentrations outside the normal range can have disastrous effects on neuromuscular activity, in particular cardiac conduction. Hypo- and hyperkalemia are both associated with potentially fatal cardiac arrhythmias, along with other neuromuscular disturbances.

CONTROL OF POTASSIUM HOMEOSTASIS

Potassium homeostasis and the maintenance of serum potassium within the normal range are regulated by dietary intake, gastrointestinal and urinary excretion, hormones, acid-base balance, and body fluid tonicity.[4]

The recommended daily allowance for dietary potassium intake is approximately 50 mEq/day.[2] Potassium is found in abundance in fruits, vegetables, and meats. The typical American ingests approximately 50 to 150 mEq of potassium daily.[4] Nearly all of this is absorbed, with only 10 to 20 mEq eliminated in feces. The amount eliminated in the feces increases, however, in patients with diarrhea, and perhaps in those with underlying chronic kidney disease (CKD).[5]

The kidney is the primary route of potassium elimination. Potassium is freely filtered with almost all of it being reabsorbed passively in the proximal tubule and the thick ascending limb of the loop of Henle.[6] Therefore urinary potassium excretion is primarily determined by potassium secretion from the luminal cells of the distal tubule and collecting duct. The normal daily amount of potassium excreted in the urine is generally 40 to 90 mEq/L,[2] but it can vary based on dietary intake, serum potassium concentration, and aldosterone activity.

Hormones such as insulin, catecholamines, and aldosterone dramatically affect potassium homeostasis. Insulin may be the most important hormonal mediator of potassium balance because it stimulates the cellular Na^+-K^+-ATPase pump to increase cellular potassium uptake in the liver, muscle, and adipose tissue.[4] Evidence suggests that a complex negative feedback loop exists in which insulin secretion tightly regulates potassium concentrations.[1] Indeed, serum potassium increases of only a few tenths of a milliequivalent stimulate pancreatic insulin secretion into the portal circulation in an attempt to prevent hyperkalemia from occurring.[1,2] If hyperkalemia occurs, glucagon is released from the liver to protect against insulin-induced hypoglycemia. Conversely, hypokalemia inhibits insulin secretion, which explains why some patients receiving diuretics develop hyperglycemia.[7]

Circulating catecholamines such as epinephrine also result in an intracellular movement of potassium by two mechanisms.[8] They stimulate the β-receptor, which directly activates the Na^+-K^+-ATPase pump. Secondly, they stimulate glycogenolysis, which raises blood glucose levels, thereby increasing insulin secretion. This dual mechanism is often used therapeutically in patients with hyperkalemia to normalize serum potassium concentrations.

Aldosterone is a mineralocorticoid that is secreted from the adrenal glands in response to high serum potassium concentrations. Aldosterone promotes potassium excretion through the kidneys. Aldosterone works at the distal tubule and collecting duct to promote the reabsorption of sodium and water in exchange for potassium. The net result is potassium secretion into the urine. Aldosterone may also have extrarenal activity by stimulating cellular Na^+-K^+-ATPase pump activity.[8]

Changes in acid-base status significantly affect the serum potassium concentration. For example, in an acidotic state, the body compensates for excessive hydrogen ions by moving them from the serum into the cell, in exchange for intracellular potassium, to maintain electroneutrality. However, the process by which this occurs is complex, and a cellular H^+-K^+-ATPase pump has been identified. The efflux of potassium into the serum can result in hyperkalemia. A commonly quoted approximation of the pH effect is that for every 0.1 unit decrease in pH, there is a corresponding increase in serum potassium of 0.6 to 0.8 mEq/L (with a wide range of 0.2 to 1.7).[6] This is often referred to as *false hyperkalemia* because there isn't a true excess of total body potassium. Only metabolic inorganic acids, such as hydrochloric acid, result in an increase in serum potassium. Metabolic acidosis caused by organic acids, such as lactic acidosis and ketoacidosis, do not result in hyperkalemia, because both cation

and anion enter the cell, thus maintaining electroneutrality.[1] Respiratory acidosis does not significantly affect the serum potassium concentration.[8]

Conversely, metabolic alkalosis results in hypokalemia as a result of a net loss of hydrogen ion in the serum. In response, the body releases intracellular hydrogen ion into the serum to increase the acidity of the blood in exchange for extracellular potassium ions. This creates a relative deficiency of serum potassium. Serum potassium falls approximately 0.6 mEq/L for each 0.1 unit rise in blood pH. Similarly this is frequently termed *false hypokalemia* because there isn't a true deficiency in total body potassium.

Finally, hyperosmolality results in enhanced movement of potassium from the cell into the extracellular fluid. This occurs most likely because of the associated cell shrinkage and water loss, which increases the intracellular-to-extracellular potassium gradient.[4] This is seen most commonly in conditions such as diabetic ketoacidosis. Conversely, hypo-osmolality does not seem to affect potassium distribution.

HYPOKALEMIA

EPIDEMIOLOGY

Hypokalemia (defined as a plasma potassium concentration <3.5 mEq/L) is one of the most commonly encountered electrolyte abnormalities in clinical practice.[9,10] However, it is virtually nonexistent in otherwise healthy adults not receiving medication. This is partly explained by the high potassium content in the typical Western diet as well as the effective potassium-sparing mechanisms in the body to autoregulate the plasma potassium concentration. Hypokalemia usually occurs in patients who are receiving diuretic therapy. It has been estimated that as many as 50% of patients who receive diuretics have plasma potassium concentrations less than 3.5 mEq/L.[10] Hypokalemia can be described as mild (serum potassium 3 to 3.5 mEq/L), moderate (serum potassium 2.5 to 3 mEq/L), or severe (<2.5 mEq/L). When hypokalemia is detected, a diagnostic work-up that evaluates the patient's comorbid disease states and concomitant medications should be initiated.

ETIOLOGY AND PATHOPHYSIOLOGY

Hypokalemia results when there is a total body potassium deficit, or when serum potassium is shifted into the intracellular compartment. Total body deficits occur in the setting of poor dietary intake of potassium, or when there are excessive renal and gastrointestinal losses of potassium from the body.

Maintaining a consistent dietary intake of potassium is important because the body has no effective method for storing potassium. At steady state, potassium excretion matches potassium intake; approximately 90% of ingested potassium is renally excreted whereas 10% is excreted in feces.[11] This underscores the importance of eating a well-balanced diet. Elderly patients with chronic diseases, and patients undergoing surgery are at increased risk for developing hypokalemia because of insufficient intake or losses resulting from surgery.

Many drugs may cause hypokalemia by a variety of mechanisms. These mechanisms include intracellular potassium shifting and increased renal or stool losses (Table 50–1). Non–potassium-sparing diuretic administration is the most common cause of drug-induced hypokalemia.[9] Loop and thiazide diuretics inhibit renal sodium reabsorption, which results in increased sodium delivery to the distal tubule. Consequently, hypokalemia develops because the distal

TABLE 50–1. Mechanism of Drug-Induced Hypokalemia

Transcellular Shift	Enhanced Renal Excretion	Enhanced Fecal Elimination
β_2-Receptor agonists	Diuretics	Sodium polystyrene sulfonate
Epinephrine	Acetazolamide	Phenolphthalein
Albuterol	Thiazides	Sorbitol
Terbutaline	Indapamide	
Pirbuterol	Metolazone	
Salmeterol	Furosemide	
Isoproterenol	Torsemide	
Ephedrine	Bumetanide	
Pseudoephedrine	Ethacrynic acid	
Tocolytic agents	High-dose penicillins	
Ritodrine	Nafcillin	
Nylidrin	Ampicillin	
Theophylline	Penicillin	
Caffeine	Mineralocorticoids	
Insulin overdose	Miscellaneous	
	Aminoglycosides	
	Amphotericin B	
	Cisplatin	

Adapted from Gennari.[9]

tubule selectively reabsorbs sodium, and excretes potassium down its concentration gradient. Secondly, because diuretics result in volume contraction, aldosterone is secreted which further promotes the renal excretion of potassium. If concomitant potassium supplements are not provided to patients receiving loop and thiazide diuretics, hypokalemia is inevitable.

The second most common etiology of hypokalemia is loss of potassium-rich GI fluid through diarrhea and vomiting. The typical potassium loss in feces is approximately 10 mEq per day.[9] In diarrheal states, this amount increases proportionally with the volume of stool output. Vomiting also accounts for substantial potassium losses, which have been estimated to be as high as 30 to 50 mEq/L.[2] Metabolic alkalosis can also occur in cases of severe diarrhea and vomiting due to loss of bicarbonate-rich fluids. As discussed above, this causes an intracellular shifting of potassium, which lowers the serum concentration of potassium even further. Prolonged diarrhea and vomiting can significantly affect children and elderly patients because their kidneys are unable to effectively maintain an adequate fluid status.

Hypomagnesemia can also contribute to the development of hypokalemia because it reduces the intracellular potassium concentration and promotes renal potassium wasting.[12] The intracellular potassium concentration falls because hypomagnesemia impairs the function of the Na^+-K^+-ATPase pump. The mechanism of the accelerated renal loss of potassium is unknown.[12] It is unclear whether hypomagnesemia directly causes hypokalemia, because the two are often found together as a result of drugs (diuretic administration) or disease states (diarrhea). When concomitant hypokalemia and hypomagnesemia occur, the magnesium deficiency must be corrected first, otherwise full repletion of the potassium deficit is difficult.[12]

CLINICAL PRESENTATION OF HYPOKALEMIA[9,13–24]

GENERAL
The presence of signs and symptoms with hypokalemia are usually nonspecific and highly variable between patients.

SYMPTOMS
Symptoms are highly dependent on the degree of hypokalemia and its rapidity of onset. Mild hypokalemia is often asymptomatic. Moderate hypokalemia is associated with cramping, weakness, malaise, and myalgias. Severe hypokalemia is associated with cardiac arrhythmias.

SIGNS
Cardiovascular: Essential hypertension and electrocardiographic changes are present (ST-segment depression or flattening, T-wave inversion, and U-wave elevation). Clinical arrhythmias include heart block, atrial flutter, paroxysmal atrial tachycardia, ventricular fibrillation, and digitalis-induced arrhythmias.
Musculoskeletal: Cramping and impaired muscle contraction are seen.

LABORATORY TESTS
Serum potassium concentration less than 3.5 mEq/L is diagnostic. Hypomagnesemia (serum magnesium concentration <1.7 mg/dL) may also be present.

▶ TREATMENT: Hypokalemia

▓ DESIRED OUTCOME

The goals of hypokalemia management are to prevent and to treat serious life-threatening complications, to normalize the serum potassium concentration, to identify and correct the underlying cause of hypokalemia, and to prevent overcorrection of the potassium concentration.

GENERAL APPROACH TO THERAPY

The general approach to therapy depends on the degree and rapidity of hypokalemia, and the presence of symptoms. Serum potassium concentrations between 3.5 and 4 mEq/L are a sign of early potassium depletion. No pharmacologic therapy is recommended at this point; however, these patients should be encouraged to increase their dietary intake of potassium-rich foods. When the serum potassium concentration is between 3 and 3.5 mEq/L, it is still debatable whether pharmacologic therapy should be initiated for all patients. Oral potassium supplementation should be initiated in patients with underlying cardiac conditions that predispose them to cardiac arrhythmias. This includes patients receiving concomitant digoxin therapy.[22] Patients with serum potassium concentrations below 3 mEq/L should always be treated to achieve values >4 mEq/L. In asymptomatic patients, oral therapy is the preferred route of administration. Intravenous potassium may be necessary in symptomatic patients with severe depletion, or in patients who are intolerant to oral supplementation. In patients with concomitant hypomagnesemia, the magnesium deficit should be corrected before potassium supplementation, to prevent refractory hypokalemia.[21]

NONPHARMACOLOGIC THERAPY

Various nonpharmacologic therapies exist to prevent and treat hypokalemia. Probably the best and most abundant source of potassium comes from dietary sources, in particular, fresh fruits and vegetables, fruit juices, and meats.[21] Table 50–2 lists foods that are excellent sources of potassium. Salt substitutes are another effective, inexpensive source of potassium. Increased dietary intake of foods with high potassium content is not recommended long-term because it may add unwanted calories to the patient's diet. Moreover, dietary potassium is almost entirely coupled with phosphate, rather than chloride, so it isn't as effective in correcting potassium loss associated with hypochloremic conditions such as vomiting, nasogastric suctioning, and diuretic therapy.[21]

PHARMACOLOGIC THERAPY

Guidelines for potassium supplementation have been published by the National Council on Potassium in Clinical Practice (Table 50–3).[21] These guidelines provide a comprehensive framework for potassium prophylaxis and replacement in many distinct patient populations. When deciding on appropriate pharmacotherapy to replete potassium, five factors must be considered: (1) the patient's normal baseline potassium concentration; (2) underlying medical conditions that may affect potassium balance; (3) concomitant medications that may affect potassium balance; (4) the patient's dietary and salt intake; and (5) the patient's ability to comply with the therapeutic regimen.[21]

A general rule for potassium replacement is that for every 1-mEq/L fall of potassium below 3.5 mEq/L, there is a corresponding total body potassium deficit of 100 to 400 mEq. Due to the wide variance in projected deficits each patient's therapy must be individualized and adjustments made on the basis of the patients signs, symptoms, and frequent measurements of serum potassium. In patients receiving loop or thiazide diuretics, 40 to 100 mEq of potassium is generally needed to correct mild deficits. Doses up to 120 mEq may be required in more severe deficiencies. The total daily dose should be divided

TABLE 50–2. Foods That Are High in Potassium

Highest content (>1,000 mg/100 g)
  Dried figs
  Molasses
Very high content (>500 mg/100 g)
  Dried fruits (dates, prunes)
  Nuts
  Avocados
  Bran cereals
  Lima beans
High content (>250 mg/100 g)
  Vegetables
    Spinach
    Tomatoes
    Broccoli
    Squash
    Beets
    Cauliflower
    Carrots
    Potatoes
  Fruits
    Bananas
    Cantaloupe
    Kiwi
    Oranges
    Mangos
  Meats
    Ground beef
    Steak
    Pork
    Lamb
    Veal

Adapted from Gennari[9] and Cohn et al.[21]

into three to four doses to prevent GI side effects. Patients receiving diuretics may become chronically hypokalemic and may benefit from combination potassium-sparing diuretic therapy.

CLINICAL CONTROVERSY

The replacement of potassium IV may be accomplished by way of IV piggyback or by buretrol. A pharmacist usually prepares the potassium IV piggyback, double checks the concentration and fluid, then dispenses the final product to the medical unit. However, with buretrol administration, essentially any clinician (e.g., nurse or physician) can prepare the solution on the medical unit, and infuse the potassium solution into the patient.

Whenever possible, potassium supplementation should be administered by mouth. Three salts are available for oral potassium supplementation: chloride, phosphate, and bicarbonate. Potassium phosphate should be used when patients are both hypokalemic and hypophosphatemic; potassium bicarbonate is most commonly used when potassium depletion occurs in the setting of metabolic acidosis. Potassium chloride, however, is the primary salt form used because it is the most effective treatment for the common causes of potassium depletion (i.e., diuretic-induced and diarrhea-induced hypokalemia). Because diarrhea and diuretics such as hydrochlorothiazide and furosemide promote net potassium and chloride losses, supplementation with potassium chloride repletes both electrolytes. Potassium chloride can be administered in either tablet or liquid formulations (Table 50–4). The liquid forms are generally less expensive; however,

TABLE 50–3.   General Consensus Guidelines for Potassium Replacement

Guideline	Comment
Potassium replacement therapy should accompany dietary consumption of potassium-rich foods.	Potassium-rich foods often cannot completely replace potassium associated with chloride losses (vomiting, diuretics, or nasogastric suction) because it is almost entirely coupled to phosphate. Furthermore, increasing dietary intake of these foods may lead to unwanted weight gain.
Potassium replacement is recommended in patients who are sodium sensitive, and in hypertensive patients.	A high-sodium diet often results in excessive urinary potassium excretion.
Potassium replacement is recommended in patients who are subject to vomiting, diarrhea, or diuretic/laxative abuse.	These conditons promote excessive renal and GI potassium loss.
Potassium supplementation is best administered orally in divided doses over several days to achieve full repletion.	
Laboratory measurement of serum potassium is convenient, but not always accurate.	Clinicians should be aware of the factors that result in transcellular potassium shifts. Monitoring 24-hour urinary potassium excretion may be necessary in high-risk patients.
Patient adherence to potassium replacement may be increased with compliance-enhancing regimens.	Microencapsulated products have no bitter smell or aftertaste and have much better GI tolerance. Regimens should be made as simple as possible to follow.
A potassium dosage of 20 mEq/day is usually sufficient to prevent hypokalemia from occurring. Doses of 40–100 mEq are usually sufficient to treat hypokalemia.	

Adapted from Cohn et al.[21]

patient compliance may be low because of their strong, unpleasant taste.[21] Two sustained-release preparations are currently available in the United States: a wax-matrix formulation, and a microencapsulated formulation. The microencapsulated tablet disintegrates better in the stomach as compared to the wax-matrix preparation, and is associated with less GI erosion.[9,21] Regardless of the preparation used, the potassium is generally well absorbed.

Intravenous potassium use should be limited to (1) severe cases of hypokalemia (serum concentration <2.5 mEq/L); (2) patients exhibiting signs and symptoms of hypokalemia such as electrocardiogram (ECG) changes or muscle spasms; or (3) patients unable to tolerate oral therapy. Intravenous supplementation is more dangerous than oral therapy because it is more likely to result in hyperkalemia, thrombophlebitis, and pain at the site of infusion.

The vehicle in which intravenous potassium is administered is important. Whenever possible, potassium should be mixed in saline-containing solutions (e.g., 0.9% or 0.45% NaCl), and not dextrose-containing solutions. Dextrose-containing solutions stimulate insulin secretion, which causes further intracellular shifting of potassium. Indeed, there are reports of enhanced hypokalemia in patients being repleted with potassium in dextrose infusions.[25] Generally, 10 to 20 mEq of potassium is diluted in 100 mL 0.9% NaCl for intravenous administration. These concentrations are generally safe when administered through a peripheral vein over 1 hour. When infusion rates exceed 10 mEq/h, ECG monitoring should be performed to detect cardiac signs of hyperkalemia. The serum potassium concentration should be evaluated following the infusion of each 30 to 40 mEq, to direct further potassium replacement requirements. Multiple doses of potassium can be repeated as needed until the serum potassium concentration normalizes.

In cases of severe potassium depletion, patients may require as much as 300 to 400 mEq/day. In this instance, it is common practice to dilute 40 to 60 mEq in 1,000 mL 0.45% NaCl and infuse at a rate not exceeding 40 mEq/h. If possible, this should be performed in an intensive care unit under continuous ECG monitoring. Because of the high potassium concentration, and the risk for burning pain and peripheral venous sclerosis, the infusion should be through a central intravenous line into a large vein (e.g., superior vena cava). Frequent serum potassium monitoring should be performed to avoid the development of hyperkalemia.

ALTERNATIVE THERAPIES

Potassium-sparing diuretics are an alternative to exogenous potassium supplementation, especially when patients are concomitantly receiving drugs that are known to deplete potassium (e.g., diuretics or amphotericin B). Spironolactone inhibits the effect of aldosterone in the distal convoluted tubule, thereby decreasing potassium elimination in the urine. Spironolactone is especially effective as a potassium-sparing agent in patients with primary or secondary hyperaldosteronism. Amiloride and triamterene act by an aldosterone-independent mechanism; however, the complete mechanism of their potassium sparing is unknown.

Spironolactone is available as 25-mg, 50-mg, and 100-mg tablets. The usual starting dose is 25 to 50 mg daily, and can be titrated to a maximum dose of 400 mg/day. The potassium-retaining effects generally take about 48 hours to occur. Important side effects

TABLE 50–4.   Differentiation of Available Potassium Supplements

Supplement	Comment
Controlled-release microencapsulated tablet	Disintegrates better in GI tract; fewer GI erosions as compared to wax-matrix tablets
Encapsulated controlled-release microencapsulated particles	Fewer erosions as compared to wax-matrix tablets
Potassium chloride elixir	Inexpensive, poor taste, poor compliance, immediate effect
Potassium chloride effervescent tablets for solution	More expensive than elixir, convenient
Wax-matrix extended-release tablets	Easier to swallow; more GI erosions as compared to other therapies

include hyperkalemia, gynecomastia, breast tenderness, and impotence in men.[23]

Triamterene is available as 50-mg and 100-mg capsules. The usual starting dose is 50 mg twice daily, which can be titrated to 100 mg twice daily. Triamterene 50 mg is available as a combination product with hydrochlorothiazide 25 mg and is commonly used for the treatment of stage I and II hypertension. Common side effects include hyperkalemia, sodium depletion, and metabolic acidosis.[22]

Amiloride is available as a 5-mg tablet. The usual starting dose is 5 mg daily; however, 10 mg can be given in those with severe hypokalemia. This is also available as a combination product with hydrochlorothiazide 50 mg. The most common side effects are hyperkalemia and metabolic acidosis.[23]

Generally, concomitant use of potassium supplementation with potassium-sparing diuretics is not necessary. However, conditions that result in excessive urinary potassium wasting, such as congestive heart failure, cirrhosis, or the nephrotic syndrome, may require dual therapy.[23] There is a significant risk of hyperkalemia during combination therapy, especially in patients with underlying renal insufficiency or diabetes mellitus.

PHARMACOECONOMIC CONSIDERATIONS

To date, there have been no pharmacoeconomic evaluations of the different pharmacotherapeutic alternatives to manage hypokalemia. The most economical source of potassium is from the diet. Thus patients receiving diuretic therapy should be instructed to increase their dietary intake of potassium-rich foods. By doing so, they may avert the need for exogenous potassium therapy. Additionally, oral potassium supplementation is much less expensive than intravenous supplementation by virtue of its ease of administration and lack of need

HYPERKALEMIA

Hyperkalemia is defined as a serum potassium concentration greater than 5.5 mEq/L. It can be further classified according to its severity: mild hyperkalemia (serum potassium 5.5 to 6 mEq/L); moderate hyperkalemia (6.1 to 6.9 mEq/L); and severe hyperkalemia (>7 mEq/L).[22]

EPIDEMIOLOGY

Hyperkalemia is much less common than hypokalemia. In fact, if all patients with acute and chronic kidney disease were excluded, the true prevalence of hyperkalemia would be insignificant.[23,26] Indeed, the incidence of hyperkalemia in hospitalized patients has been estimated to be 1.4% to 10%.[27] Most cases of hyperkalemia are the result of overcorrection of hypokalemia with potassium supplements. Severe hyperkalemia occurs more commonly in elderly patients with renal insufficiency who receive potassium supplementation.[27]

ETIOLOGY AND PATHOPHYSIOLOGY

Hyperkalemia develops when potassium intake exceeds excretion (i.e., elevated total body stores), or when the transcellular distribution of potassium is disturbed (i.e., normal total body stores). Generally, there are four primary causes of true hyperkalemia: (1) increased

for ECG monitoring. The pharmacoeconomic difference between the oral products is dependent on several variables, including patient tolerance and compliance.

EVALUATION OF THERAPEUTIC OUTCOMES

Serum potassium concentrations should be monitored regularly while the patient is receiving potassium supplementation. For patients receiving long-term prophylactic potassium supplementation during diuretic therapy, the serum potassium and magnesium concentrations, as well as renal function should be monitored during each clinic visit. In hospitalized patients receiving therapy for mild hypokalemia, the potassium concentration should be monitored every 2 to 3 days. This usually isn't a problem because of the frequent laboratory monitoring performed in hospitalized patients. Generally, the potassium concentration begins to rise within 72 hours. If it doesn't rise appreciably within 96 hours, the clinician should suspect concomitant magnesium depletion.[23] If present, correcting the magnesium deficit generally results in normalization of potassium. Patients receiving IV potassium supplementation require close ECG monitoring if the infusion rate is greater than 10 mEq/h. In addition the patient should be assessed for adverse effects such as burning pain at the infusion site or thrombophlebitis.

potassium intake; (2) decreased potassium excretion; (3) tubular unresponsiveness to aldosterone; and (4) redistribution of potassium into the extracellular space. The four major causes of true hyperkalemia are discussed below.

Hyperkalemia Associated with Increased Potassium Intake

Hyperkalemia in this setting is almost always associated with renal insufficiency. Predialysis and dialysis patients that are noncompliant with dietary potassium restrictions often present with life-threatening hyperkalemia. Many of these patients don't realize that fresh fruits and vegetables contain large amounts of potassium. Anecdotally, in many dialysis centers the incidence of hyperkalemia peaks during the summer months, when fresh garden produce is available. Another common dietary source of hyperkalemia is potassium chloride salt substitutes. Many dialysis patients are instructed to use salt substitutes to avoid excessive sodium intake in an attempt to control volume overload. These patients unwittingly become hyperkalemic because these products contain approximately 10 to 15 mEq potassium per gram, or 200 mEq per tablespoon. Finally, many over-the-counter herbal products may contain unknown concentrations of potassium in their dosage forms. A case of hyperkalemia was recently reported in a patient ingesting noni juice, an herbal product purported to increase energy levels.[28]

It is essential for patients with CKD to receive education regarding dietary sources of potassium as well as information on the potassium content of herbal products, since the ingestion of these may lead to hyperkalemia.

Hyperkalemia Associated with Decreased Renal Potassium Excretion

6 The kidneys excrete 80% of the daily potassium intake. Therefore when the kidney is unable to excrete potassium appropriately, as in acute renal failure and CKD, potassium is retained and often results in hyperkalemia. Moreover, many drugs can inhibit the kidney's ability to excrete potassium by inhibiting aldosterone and thus contribute to an increase in serum potassium levels.

Severe hyperkalemia is more common in acute renal failure (ARF) than in CKD because ARF patients are often hypercatabolic and can have underlying disorders, such as rhabdomyolysis or tumor lysis syndrome, which result in release of potassium from injured or lysed cells.[29] Severe hyperkalemia is rare in stable CKD, perhaps because of enhanced GI and renal potassium excretion.[23,30] A recent study suggests that hyperkalemia actually functions in a homeostatic fashion, directly stimulating renal K+ excretion through an effect that is independent of, and additive to, aldosterone.[30] Renal excretion of potassium is also inhibited by various endocrinologic disorders, including adrenal insufficiency, Addison's disease, and selective hypoaldosteronism. All of these disorders involve a decreased production of aldosterone, which results in the retention of potassium. In addition, several drugs have profound effects on the kidney's ability to secrete potassium. Four drug classes in particular have specific effects at the kidney: angiotensin-converting enzyme inhibitors (ACEIs), angiotensin receptor blockers (ARBs), potassium-sparing diuretics, and prostaglandin inhibitors such as nonsteroidal anti-inflammatory drugs (NSAIDs). Other miscellaneous drugs that cause hyperkalemia are trimethoprim-sulfamethoxazole, heparin, and pentamidine.

Tubular Unresponsiveness to Aldosterone

Certain medical conditions, such as sickle cell anemia, systemic lupus erythematosus, and amyloidosis, can produce a defect in tubular potassium secretion, possibly as the result of an alteration in the aldosterone-binding site. The exact mechanism of the tubular unresponsiveness is unknown.

Redistribution of Potassium into the Extracellular Space

The efflux of potassium into the extracellular fluid is to be expected in the presence of metabolic acidosis, secondary to diabetes mellitus, chronic renal failure, or lactic acidosis. β-Blockers can also result in a transcellular potassium shift.

The serum potassium concentration may also be falsely elevated in some conditions, and not reflect the actual in vivo potassium concentration. This is termed *pseudohyperkalemia*. Pseudohyperkalemia occurs most commonly in the setting of extravascular hemolysis of red blood cells.[26] When a blood specimen is not processed promptly and cellular destruction occurs, intracellular potassium is released into the serum. Pseudohyperkalemia can also occur in conditions of thrombocytosis or leukocytosis. If severe hyperkalemia is found in a patient who is asymptomatic with an otherwise normal laboratory report, the hyperkalemia is most likely pseudohyperkalemia,[23] and a repeat blood sample should be evaluated. Elevated potassium concentrations are normally associated with other laboratory abnormalities,

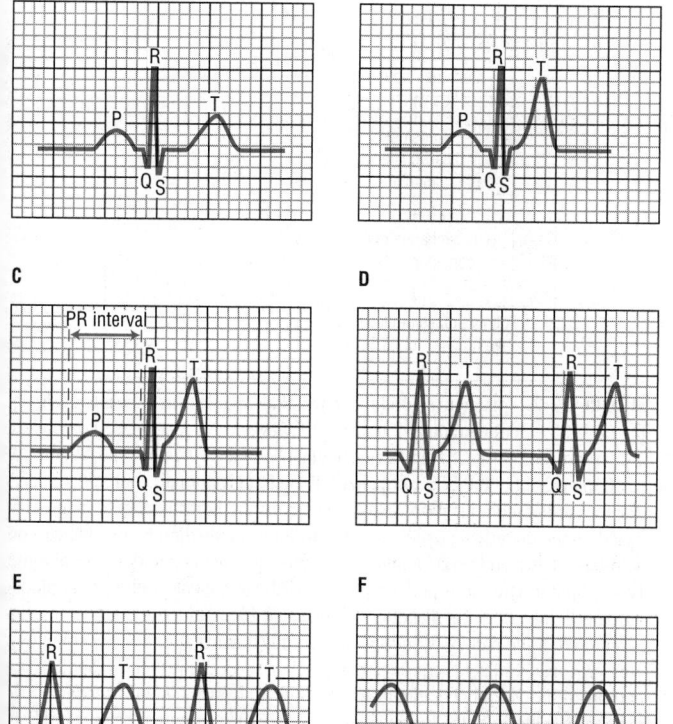

FIGURE 50–1. The earliest electrocardiographic manifestation of hyperkalemia is an increase in the rate of ventricular repolarization, which results in a peaking of the T wave at serum potassium concentrations of ≈5.5 to 6 mEq/L (*B*), relative to the normal ECG presentation (*A*). Further increases in the serum potassium concentration above 6 mEq/L result in conduction delays through the His-Purkinje system, the atrial myocardium, and the ventricular myocardium. The ECG manifestations of these conduction delays and the sequence in which they occur are a widening of the PR interval (*C*), delay through the His-Purkinje system, a loss of the P wave (*D*), delay through the atrial myocardium, a widening of the QRS complex (*E*), and delay through the ventricular myocardium. Finally, there is a merging of the QRS complex with the T wave (*F*), which results in a sine-wave appearance to the tracing.

such as low carbon dioxide (acidosis) or elevated blood urea nitrogen and creatinine concentrations (indicating renal insufficiency).

CLINICAL PRESENTATION OF HYPERKALEMIA

GENERAL
Related to the effects of excessive potassium on neuromuscular, cardiac, and smooth muscle cell function.

SYMPTOMS
Frequently asymptomatic; however, the patient may complain of heart palpitations or skipped heartbeats.

SIGNS
ECG changes (see Fig. 50–1 for description).

LABORATORY TESTS
Serum potassium concentration >5.5 mEq/L.

▶ TREATMENT: Hyperkalemia

▦ DESIRED OUTCOME

The goals of therapy for the treatment of hyperkalemia are to antagonize adverse cardiac effects, reverse any symptoms that may be present, and to return the serum and total body stores of potassium to normal. Severe hyperkalemia (>7 mEq/L) or moderate hyperkalemia (6.1 to 6.9 mEq/L), when associated with clinical symptoms or electrocardiographic changes, requires immediate treatment. Initial treatment of hyperkalemia is focused on antagonism of the membrane actions of hyperkalemia (calcium). Secondarily, one should attempt to decrease extracellular potassium concentration by promoting its intracellular movement (e.g., with glucose, insulin, β_2-receptor agonists, or sodium bicarbonate). Finally, removal of potassium from the body by hemodialysis and/or cation-exchange resins may need to be implemented.[26] The underlying cause of hyperkalemia should be identified and reversed, and exogenous potassium must be withheld.

▦ GENERAL APPROACH TO TREATMENT

The general treatment approach for patients with hyperkalemia is outlined in Fig. 50–2. In patients who are symptomatic, calcium should be administered to prevent or treat any cardiac manifestations of hyperkalemia. Once the patient is hemodynamically stabilized, the serum potassium concentration should be rapidly decreased within minutes by administering drugs that result in an intracellular shift. If the patient is asymptomatic, rapid correction is not necessary. The clinician can administer an ion exchange resin (e.g., sodium polystyrene sulfonate; SPS) that results in removal of potassium from the body over several hours.

▦ NONPHARMACOLOGIC THERAPY

End-stage renal disease (ESRD) patients who present with severe hyperkalemia, or with cardiac manifestations of hyperkalemia, should undergo immediate hemodialysis. Dialysis is the most rapid means of lowering potassium compared to bicarbonate, epinephrine, or insulin plus glucose therapy.[31,32] Other forms of dialysis can be performed (e.g., peritoneal dialysis or continuous renal replacement therapy), although they appear to be less effective means to acutely lower an elevated serum potassium.[31]

▦ PHARMACOLOGIC THERAPY

Various drug therapies exist for lowering the serum potassium concentration. The optimal regimen for a given patient is dependent on the rapidity and degree of lowering that is necessary. Table 50–5

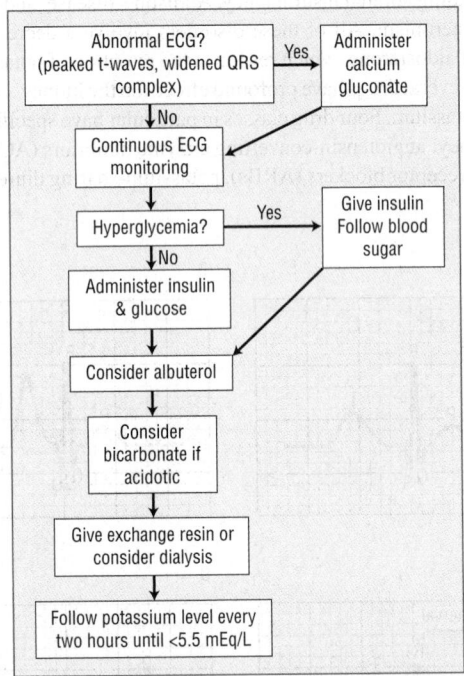

FIGURE 50–2. Treatment algorithm for hyperkalemia. The first step is to evaluate the patient's electrocardiogram. If peaked T waves or widened QRS complexes are present, administer 1 ampule IV calcium gluconate 10% and repeat every 30 to 60 minutes until the ECG normalizes. If the ECG is normal, continue to monitor for cardiac complications. Next, decide on the best therapeutic approach based on the underlying patient symptoms; for example, underlying diabetes or acid-base status, and need for immediate correction. For nonacidotic conditions, IV insulin and glucose is preferred for nondiabetic patients with normal blood glucose. If the patient is diabetic with elevated blood glucose, only IV insulin is required. If the patient is unresponsive to this therapy after 30 to 60 minutes, albuterol via nebulizer is considered adjunctive second-line therapy. Sodium bicarbonate should only be administered when the hyperkalemia is secondary to metabolic acidosis. Potassium exchange resins or dialysis should be used last line for acute situations. If the patient has end-stage renal disease, dialysis may be the preferred first-line therapy. In nonacute situations in which rapid onset is not required, potassium exchange resins are considered a first-line therapy. The patient should be monitored every 2 hours until the serum potassium concentration falls below 5.5 mEq/L.

TABLE 50–5. Therapeutic Alternatives for the Management of Hyperkalemia

Medication	Dose	Route of Administration	Onset/Duration of Action	Acuity	Mechanism of Action	Expected Result
Calcium	1 g (1 ampule)	IV over 5–10 min	1–2 min/10–30 min	Acute	Raises cardiac threshold potential	Reverses electrocardiographic effects
Furosemide	20–40 mg	IV	5–15 min/4–6 hours	Acute	Inhibits renal Na^+ reabsorption	Increased urinary K^+ loss
Regular insulin	5–10 units	IV or SC	30 min/2–6 hours	Acute	Stimulates intracellular K^+ uptake	Intracellular K^+ redistribution
Dextrose 10%	1,000 mL (100 g)	IV over 1–2 hours	30 min/2–6 hours	Acute	Stimulates insulin release	Intracellular K^+ redistribution
Dextrose 50%	50 mL (25 g)	IV over 5 min	30 min/2–6 hours	Acute	Stimulates insulin release	Intracellular K^+ redistribution
Sodium bicarbonate	50–100 mEq	IV over 2–5 min	30 min/2–6 hours	Acute	Raises serum pH	Intracellular K^+ redistribution
Albuterol	10–20 mg	Nebulized over 10 min	30 min/1–2 hours	Acute	Stimulates intracellular K^+ uptake	Intracellular K^+ redistribution
Hemodialysis	4 hours	N/A	Immediate/variable	Acute	Removal from plasma	Increased K^+ elimination
Sodium polystyrene sulfonate	15–60 g	Oral or rectal	1 hour/variable	Nonacute	Resin exchanges Na^+ for K^+	Increased K^+ elimination

provides an overview of the available therapies, and their respective onset and the degree of change one can expect.

In asymptomatic patients with mild to moderate hyperkalemia (serum concentration 5.5 to 6.9 mEq/L), aggressive therapy is usually not indicated. In patients with normal renal function, loop diuretics can be administered in the short term to promote urinary potassium excretion. Furosemide 20 to 40 mg orally is a common starting dose, and this can be titrated to response. Its onset of activity is within minutes, and its duration of activity is approximately 4 to 6 hours. Close monitoring of the patient's volume status and other electrolyte concentrations is required while the patient is receiving loop diuretic therapy. Alternatively, SPS (Kayexalate), a cation-exchange resin, can be administered orally or rectally by enema. SPS is available in powder form or prepackaged as 70% sorbitol suspension. The oral route is more effective than the enema and is better tolerated by the patient. As the resin passes through the intestines, each gram of SPS exchanges 1 mEq of sodium for 1 mEq of potassium ions, which are in a relatively higher concentration in the large intestine. The onset of action of SPS is within 1 hour, and it can be repeated every 4 hours as needed. The sorbitol component of the suspension promotes the excretion of the cationically modified potassium exchange resin by inducing diarrhea.[23] The usual oral dose of SPS is 15 to 60 g in 70% sorbitol suspension. A retention enema prepared by mixing 60 to 100 g SPS in 100 to 200 mL 30% sorbitol or 10% dextrose warmed to body temperature will usually remove 0.5 mEq of potassium per gram of SPS.[23] The enema may be retained in the rectum for several hours as tolerated by the patient.

In symptomatic patients, or in those with severe hyperkalemia (serum potassium >7 mEq/L), emergency care is indicated. Initial therapy in this setting is the administration of intravenous calcium to protect the heart from life-threatening arrhythmias.[11,27,31] Calcium antagonizes the cardiac membrane effect of hyperkalemia and reverses ECG changes within minutes. Its duration of action is 30 to 60 minutes, and it can be repeated as needed based on ECG findings.

Intravenous calcium can be given as either the chloride or gluconate salt; each is available as a 10% solution by weight. Calcium chloride provides approximately three times more calcium than equal volumes of the gluconate salt; however, it can cause tissue necrosis if extravasation occurs. For this reason, calcium gluconate is more commonly administered, with the standard dose being one 10-mL ampule IV bolus over 5 to 10 minutes.

Rapid correction of hyperkalemia may necessitate the administration of drugs that result in an intracellular shift of potassium, such as insulin and dextrose, sodium bicarbonate, and the β_2-receptor agonist albuterol. The treatment of choice depends on the underlying medical disorders accompanying hyperkalemia. For example, in patients with concomitant metabolic acidosis, a sodium bicarbonate bolus or infusion of 50 to 100 mEq is the preferred therapy (see Chap. 51 for additional information). Sodium bicarbonate helps to correct the metabolic acidosis by raising the extracellular pH, in addition to causing a rapid intracellular potassium shift. It should be noted that sodium bicarbonate is much less effective when hyperkalemia is not related to metabolic acidosis.[29] Sodium bicarbonate is also less effective in patients with ESRD, in whom a decrease in serum potassium may not be seen for as long as 4 hours.[32] Sodium bicarbonate can also lead to sodium and volume overload in ESRD patients. Administration of insulin (5 to 10 units IV) and dextrose (dextrose 10% or 50%) is an effective method of reducing potassium. Insulin increases the activity of the Na^+-K^+-ATPase pump, thereby intracellularly shifting potassium. Glucose should be given with insulin unless the serum glucose is greater than 250 mg/dL because hypoglycemia can develop with unopposed insulin therapy. Albuterol is a β_2-adrenergic agonist that has a dual mechanism for lowering serum potassium. First, it stimulates the Na^+-K^+-ATPase pump to promote intracellular potassium uptake. Second, it stimulates pancreatic β receptors to increase insulin secretion. Albuterol can be administered intravenously (0.5 mg given over 15 minutes) or via nebulizer (10 to 20 mg nebulized over 10 minutes); however, it should be noted that injectable albuterol is not available in the United States. The problems with nebulized albuterol therapy are frequent underdosing, and subsequently poor response in as many as 33% of patients.[33] Moreover, cardiac side effects such as tachycardia may be undesirable in patients who already have abnormal ECGs. In summary, albuterol should be reserved as adjunctive therapy in patients already receiving insulin and dextrose therapy, due to its synergistic activity on the Na^+-K^+-ATPase pump.

▓ EVALUATION OF THERAPEUTIC OUTCOMES

In patients who have acute symptomatic hyperkalemia (e.g., ECG changes), frequent potassium concentration and ECG monitoring is warranted. The patient should receive continuous ECG telemetry monitoring until the serum potassium concentration falls below 5 mEq/L, and the ECG abnormalities resolve. Similarly, while the patient is receiving emergent therapy, serial serum potassium concentrations should be obtained every hour until the potassium concentration falls below 5 mEq/L. The patient's medication records should be reviewed to assure the patient is not receiving drug therapy that increases the serum potassium concentration. For patients who receive insulin and dextrose therapy for hyperkalemia, blood glucose monitoring should be performed hourly, or more frequently if patients demonstrate signs and symptoms of hypoglycemia. For patients who receive large doses of sodium bicarbonate therapy for hyperkalemia, an arterial blood gas or serum chemistry profile should be obtained to assess blood acid-base status. Furthermore, the patient should be evaluated for signs of fluid overload secondary to the high sodium load. Patients receiving albuterol therapy should be questioned regularly regarding the development of palpitations and tachycardia. In asymptomatic patients receiving SPS, serum potassium concentrations can be obtained within 4 hours, and the dose repeated as necessary. Furthermore, the patient should be questioned regarding the occurrence of diarrheal stool output.

DISORDERS OF MAGNESIUM HOMEOSTASIS

◀7 Magnesium plays a central role in cellular function and is an important cofactor in more than 300 biochemical reactions in the body, especially those systems that are dependent on adenosine triphosphate.[34,35] Mitochondrial function, protein synthesis, cell membrane function, and parathyroid hormone (PTH) secretion are just a few important functions affected by magnesium. It is the fourth most abundant extracellular cation and second most abundant intracellular cation. Disorders of magnesium homeostasis are commonly encountered in clinical situations and most frequently are manifested as alterations in cardiovascular and neuromuscular function. Life-threatening conditions such as paralysis and cardiac arrhythmias may occur, making the proper recognition and treatment of these problems of paramount importance.

◀8 Magnesium is distributed in three major compartments: extracellular, 1.3%; intracellular, 13%; and bone, 67%.[36,37] Because of its predominantly intracellular distribution, measurement of magnesium in the extracellular compartment may not accurately reflect the total body magnesium content. The majority of magnesium in the extracellular fluid is in the ionized form; only 20% to 30% is protein bound. The normal range for serum magnesium is 1.4 to 1.8 mEq/L, which equals 1.7 to 2.3 mg/dL or 0.85 to 1.15 mmol/L.

The maintenance of magnesium homeostasis depends on the balance between intake and output. Thirty to forty percent of ingested magnesium is absorbed in the small bowel. A small amount is present in intestinal secretions and reabsorbed in the sigmoid colon. The kidneys play a major role in maintaining magnesium balance. Renal magnesium handling is unique in that only 15% to 25% of the filtered magnesium is reabsorbed in the proximal tubule; the majority of reabsorption occurs in the loop of Henle.[36] This explains why loop diuretics often cause profound urinary magnesium wasting. Unlike most other important electrolytes, there is no hormonal regulation of the distribution of magnesium between bone and circulating or intracellular magnesium pools. Because of this, both hypomagnesemia and hypermagnesemia commonly occur.

↓ HYPOMAGNESEMIA

EPIDEMIOLOGY

The prevalence of hypomagnesemia in outpatients and hospitalized patients is approximately 6% to 12%.[38] In patients with concomitant hypokalemia, the incidence rises to nearly 42%.[38] The incidence in critically ill patients may be as high as 65%, principally because of the concomitant use of diuretics and aminoglycosides.[39] Although serum magnesium concentrations are not a reliable index of total body magnesium content, they remain the primary diagnostic tool to evaluate body stores.

ETIOLOGY AND PATHOPHYSIOLOGY

◀9 Hypomagnesemia is usually associated with disorders of the intestinal tract or kidney. Drugs or conditions that interfere with intestinal absorption or increase renal excretion of magnesium can result in hypomagnesemia (Table 50–6). Decreased intestinal absorption as a result of small bowel disease is the most common cause of hypomagnesemia worldwide.[40] These disorders include regional enteritis; radiation enteritis; ulcerative colitis; acute and chronic diarrhea; pancreatic insufficiency and other malabsorptive syndromes; small-bowel bypass surgery; and chronic laxative abuse.[40]

Hypomagnesemia is commonly associated with alcoholism, and occurs in as many as 30% of hospitalized patients.[41] The etiology is often multifactorial, including reduced intake, pancreatic insufficiency, chronic vomiting and diarrhea, and urinary magnesium wasting. In addition, patients who are hospitalized for acute alcohol withdrawal often receive IV glucose and may experience even greater reductions in the serum magnesium concentration.[42] Because hypomagnesemia may contribute to the development of delirium tremens associated with alcohol withdrawal, frequent monitoring and aggressive magnesium replacement is indicated for these patients, especially those with tachyarrhythmias, hypocalcemia, or hypokalemia.

Primary renal magnesium wasting may be due to a defect in renal tubular magnesium reabsorption, or inhibition of sodium reabsorption in those segments in which magnesium transport follows passively. The former condition is associated with hypercalciuria, nephrolithiasis, and progressive renal disease.[40] The latter is associated with Gitelman's and Bartter's syndromes.[40] Much more common than these is renal magnesium wasting secondary to diuretics. Hypomagnesemia occurs with both thiazide and loop diuretics, and may be present in as many as 37% of diuretic users.[43] Other commonly used drugs which may cause renal magnesium wasting include aminoglycosides, amphotericin B, cyclosporine, tacrolimus, cisplatin, pentamidine, and foscarnet.[43]

TABLE 50–6. Causes of Hypomagnesemia

Gastrointestinal	**Renal (continued)**
Reduced intake	Glomerulonephritis
Protein-calorie malnutrition	Pyelonephritis
Total parenteral nutrition without magnesium	Nephrotic syndrome
Prolonged parenteral fluid administration without magnesium	Drug-induced renal losses
Alcoholism	Aminoglycosides
Reduced absorption	Amphotericin B
Primary hypomagnesemia	Cyclosporine
Malabsorption syndromes (e.g., tropical sprue, celiac disease, radiation enteritis or intestinal lymphectasia)	Diuretics
	Digitalis
Short-bowel syndrome (e.g., small-bowel resection or ileal bypass)	Cisplatin
Pancreatic insufficiency	Hormone-induced renal losses
Increased loss	Primary hyperparathyroidism
Excessive vomiting	Hyperthyroidism
Prolonged nasogastric suction	Aldosteronism
Excessive laxative use	"Hungry bone syndrome" after parathyroidectomy
Intestinal and biliary fistulas	**Internal redistribution**
Prolonged diarrhea (ulcerative colitis, Crohn's disease, or cancer of the colon)	Diabetic ketoacidosis
Renal	Glucose, amino acid, or insulin administration
Primary tubular disorders	Massive blood transfusion (citrate)
Primary renal magnesium wasting	Pancreatitis with lipidemia (magnesium soap)
Bartter's syndrome	**Other**
Renal tubular acidosis	Excessive sweating and lactation
Diuretic phase of acute tubular necrosis	Hypercalcemia and hypercalciuria
Postobstructive diuresis	Phosphate depletion
Postrenal transplant diuresis	Chronic alcoholism
	Extracellular fluid volume expansion

CLINICAL PRESENTATION

Because hypomagnesemia is often associated with a variety of other electrolyte abnormalities such as hypokalemia and hypocalcemia, it is difficult to ascribe specific clinical manifestations solely to magnesium deficiency. Hypocalcemia is one of the most prominent symptoms of hypomagnesemia.[40] Hypocalcemia is usually detected first because it is more commonly measured in clinical practice. The etiology of hypocalcemia is not entirely clear, but it is probably caused by decreased secretion of PTH, low 1,25-$(OH)_2$ vitamin D concentrations, and skeletal resistance to PTH.[40] As with hypokalemia, hypocalcemia accompanied by hypomagnesemia is most effectively treated with magnesium administration.

CLINICAL PRESENTATION OF HYPOMAGNESEMIA [40,43,44]

GENERAL
The dominant organ systems involved in hypomagnesemia include the neuromuscular and cardiovascular systems.

SYMPTOMS
The patient may complain of neuromuscular symptoms such as tetany, twitching, and generalized convulsions. Cardiac symptoms include heart palpitations.

SIGNS
Neuromuscular: Presence of Chvostek's sign, Trousseau's sign (see description below), tremor, and tetany.
Cardiovascular: Cardiac arrhythmias (ventricular fibrillation, torsades de pointes, or digoxin-induced arrhythmias), sudden cardiac death, and hypertension may be present. ECG abnormalities include widened QRS complex and peaked T waves with mild hypomagnesemia; and prolonged PR interval, progressive widening of QRS complex, and flattened T waves with moderate to severe hypomagnesemia.

LABORATORY TESTS
Serum magnesium concentration less than 1.4 mEq/L. Serum potassium and calcium concentrations may also be low.

▶ TREATMENT: Hypomagnesemia

▄ DESIRED OUTCOME

The treatment goals in the management of hypomagnesemia are: (1) resolution of the corresponding signs and symptoms; (2) restoration of normal magnesium concentrations; (3) correction of concomitant electrolyte abnormalities; and (4) identifying and correcting the underlying cause of magnesium depletion.

▄ GENERAL APPROACH TO TREATMENT

Magnesium supplementation can be given by the oral, intramuscular (IM), or IV route. Table 50–7 outlines one approach to the hypomagnesemic patient. The severity of the magnesium depletion and the presence of severe signs and symptoms should dictate the route of administration. Because IM administration is painful, it should be

TABLE 50–7. Guidelines for Treatment of Magnesium Deficiency in Adults

1. **Serum magnesium <1 mEq/L (1.2 mg/dL) with life-threatening symptoms (seizure or arrhythmia)**
   Day 1
   2 g MgSO$_4$ (1 g MgSO$_4$ = 8.1 mEq Mg^{2+}) mixed with 6 mL 0.9% NaCl in 10-mL syringe and administer IV push over 1 min
   Follow with 0.5 mEq Mg^{2+}/kg lean body weight IV infusion over 5–6 h, then 0.5 mEq Mg^{2+}/kg lean body weight IV infusion over 17–18 h
   Days 2–5
   0.5 mEq Mg^{2+}/kg lean body weight per day divided in maintenance IV fluids
2. **Serum magnesium <1 mEq/L (1.2 mg/dL) without life-threatening symptoms**
   Day 1
   Total of 1 mEq Mg^{2+}/kg lean body weight per day as continuous IV infusion, or divided and given IM every 4 h for five doses
   Days 2–5
   Total of 0.5 mEq Mg^{2+}/kg lean body weight IV infusion per day as continuous IV infusion or divided and given IM every 6–8 h
3. **Serum magnesium >1 mEq/L (1.2 mg/dL) and <1.5 mEq/L (1.8 mg/dL) without symptoms**
   As in no. 2, above, or
   Milk of magnesia 5 mL four times daily as tolerated, or
   Magnesium-containing antacid 15 mL three times daily as tolerated, or
   Magnesium oxide tablets 300 mg four times daily; increase to two tablets four times daily as tolerated

reserved for those patients with severe hypomagnesemia and limited venous access. IV bolus administration is associated with flushing, sweating, and a sensation of warmth; thus bolus administration should be avoided if possible. Even if severe magnesium depletion is present, approximately 50% of the administered dose is excreted in the urine. Consequently, magnesium replacement should be performed over 3 to 5 days, and continued supplementation should be provided for patients unable to eat and for those patients with continued magnesium wasting.

PHARMACOLOGIC THERAPY

Asymptomatic patients, or those patients with serum magnesium concentrations greater than 1 mEq/L (1.2 mg/dL), can be treated with oral supplements, such as magnesium-containing antacids or laxatives. However, as expected, diarrhea is the most common dose-limiting side effect of oral therapy, which may greatly reduce patient compliance. Moreover, many oral products contain very little magnesium, which necessitates frequent dosing, resulting in the increased risk of side effects.[45]

In cases of severe magnesium depletion (serum levels <1 mEq/L), or if signs and symptoms are present regardless of the

serum level, IV magnesium should be administered. A 50% solution of MgSO$_4$ is available for injection in 2-mL or 10-mL ampules (4 mEq/mL). The 50% solution should be diluted to 20% before injection to prevent venous sclerosis and pain. Therapy should be continued until the signs and symptoms have completely resolved. In patients with renal insufficiency, the dose should be reduced by 50%.

EVALUATION OF THERAPEUTIC ENDPOINTS

Patients being treated for symptomatic severe hypomagnesemia should have their serum magnesium concentration monitored hourly until the serum concentration reaches 1.5 mEq/L and the symptoms resolve. At that point the serum magnesium concentration can be monitored every 6 to 12 hours for the first 24 hours while receiving magnesium supplementation. Once the magnesium concentration is stable in the normal range, a level can be obtained daily. It should be reiterated that it typically takes 3 to 5 days to fully replete total body magnesium stores. Patients receiving oral magnesium-containing antacids or supplements should be asked regularly about the occurrence of diarrhea.

HYPERMAGNESEMIA

EPIDEMIOLOGY

Hypermagnesemia (serum magnesium >2 mEq/L) is a rare occurrence. It is generally seen in the setting of advanced renal failure when magnesium intake exceeds the excretory capacity of the kidneys. The prevalence of hypermagnesemia in hospitalized patients has been estimated to range from approximately 6% to 9%.[46,47] Elderly patients are prone to hypermagnesemia because of their reduced GFR

and because of their consumption of magnesium-containing antacids and vitamins.[37]

ETIOLOGY AND PATHOPHYSIOLOGY

Because absolute magnesium excretion falls as GFR declines, serum magnesium concentrations rise in patients with moderate to severe renal insufficiency. Indeed, magnesium concentrations steadily rise as the GFR falls below 30 mL/min.[48] As long as the patient maintains

TABLE 50–8. Causes of Hypermagnesemia

Decreased renal excretion
Acute renal failure
Chronic renal failure with exogenous intake
Excessive Intake
Treatment of toxemia of pregnancy
Ureteral irrigants (hemiacidrin)
Cathartics
Other
Lithium therapy
Hypothyroidism
Milk-alkali syndrome
Addison's disease
Viral hepatitis
Acute diabetic ketoacidosis

a normal diet, the serum magnesium concentration typically stabilizes at approximately 2.5 mEq/L. If patients with renal insufficiency are taking concomitant magnesium-containing antacids, the serum level can approach 6 mEq/L, a value associated with signs and symptoms of toxicity.[37] Critically ill patients with multiorgan system failure receiving enteral or parenteral nutrition are also prone to develop hypermagnesemia. Finally, the parenteral treatment of eclampsia with magnesium sulfate can lead to hypermagnesemia. Table 50–8 lists other causes of hypermagnesemia.

CLINICAL PRESENTATION

The signs and symptoms of hypermagnesemia reflect magnesium's action on the neuromuscular and cardiovascular systems.[34,48,49] Although there is wide interpatient variability between magnesium concentration and symptoms, they are rare when the serum concentration is less than 4 mEq/L. Figure 50–3 provides a general guide to the clinical findings associated with hypermagnesemia.

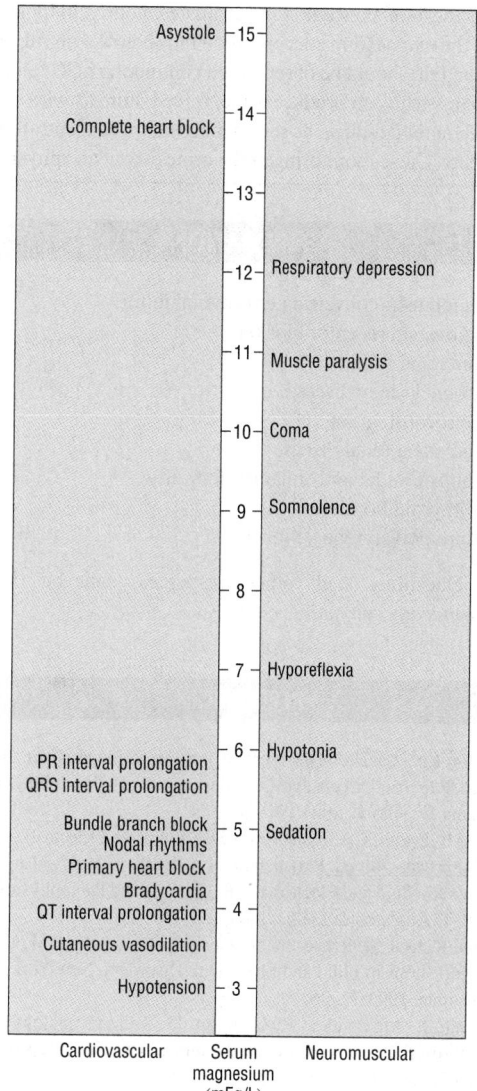

FIGURE 50–3. Clinical findings associated with hypermagnesemia.

▶ TREATMENT: Hypermagnesemia

▨ DESIRED OUTCOME

The goals of therapy are to (1) reverse the neuromuscular and cardiovascular manifestations of hypermagnesemia; (2) decrease the magnesium concentration toward normal values; and (3) diagnose and reverse the underlying cause of hypermagnesemia.

▨ PHARMACOLOGIC THERAPY

The treatment of hypermagnesemia depends on the presence of signs and symptoms, and degree of serum concentration elevation. Intravenous calcium in doses of 100 to 200 mg of elemental calcium directly antagonizes the neuromuscular and cardiovascular effects of hypermagnesemia. The clinical effect of calcium is immediate but the effect is transient; hence repeated intravenous doses of 100 to

200 mg elemental calcium can be administered hourly until the hypermagnesemic symptoms abate and the magnesium concentration is normalized. Supportive care with cardiac pacing, vasopressors, and mechanical ventilation may be necessary in life-threatening situations. In patients with adequate renal function, forced diuresis with saline and loop diuretics can promote magnesium elimination. An initial loop diuretic bolus of furosemide 40 mg intravenously can be used for immediate effects. Subsequent dosing can be determined based on the patient's clinical response. Patients with CKD may require long-term loop diuretic therapy to maintain adequate fluid and electrolyte balance. In patients with ESRD, hemodialysis with a magnesium-free dialysate should be emergently undertaken.

▨ EVALUATION OF THERAPEUTIC ENDPOINTS

Patients who are receiving intravenous calcium salts for the treatment of severe, symptomatic hypermagnesemia should have their serum magnesium concentration evaluated hourly until symptoms abate and the magnesium concentration falls below 4 mg/dL. Furthermore the patient should be observed on continuous ECG telemetry. In CKD patients who can produce urine, forced diuresis with saline and furosemide should reduce the serum magnesium concentration within 6 to 12 hours. Close monitoring of the urine output and physical exam for signs of volume overload are important. For patients who have end-stage renal disease and receive dialysis, emergency hemodialysis will usually correct the hypermagnesemia within 4 hours. To prevent further episodes of hypermagnesemia, the patient should receive dietary education regarding foods and beverages that contain large quantities of magnesium.

ABBREVIATIONS

ACEI: angiotensin-converting enzyme inhibitor
ARB: angiotensin receptor blocker
ARF: acute renal failure
CKD: chronic kidney disease
ECG: electrocardiogram
ESRD: end-stage renal disease
NSAID: nonsteroidal anti-inflammatory drug
PTH: parathyroid hormone
SPS: sodium polystyrene sulfonate

Review Questions and other resources can be found at *www.pharmacotherapyonline.com.*

REFERENCES

1. Peterson LN, Levi M. Disorders of potassium metabolism. In: Schrier RW, ed. Renal and Electrolyte Disorders, 6th Ed. Philadelphia, Lippincott, Williams & Wilkins, 2003:171–215.
2. Lee CAB, Barrett CA, Ignatavicius DD. Fluids and Electrolytes: A Practical Approach, 4th ed. Philadelphia, FA Davis, 1996:57–71.
3. Cogan MG. Fluid and Electrolytes. Physiology and Pathophysiology. Norwalk, CT: Appleton & Lange, 1991:125–163.
4. Sharma K, Cox M. Potassium homeostasis. In: Szerlip HM, Goldfarb S, eds. Workshops in Fluid and Electrolyte Disorders. New York, Churchill Livingstone, 1993:71–96.
5. Agarwal R, Afzalpurkar R, Fordtran JS. Pathophysiology of potassium absorption and secretion by the human intestine. Gastroenterology 1994;107:548–571.
6. Rose BD, Rennke HG. Renal Pathophysiology—The Essentials. Baltimore, Williams & Wilkins, 1994:169–190.
7. Krishna GG. Hypokalemic states: Current clinical issues. Semin Nephrol 1990;10:515–524.
8. Wingo CS, Weiner ID. Disorders of potassium balance. In: Brenner BM, ed. The Kidney, 6th ed. Philadelphia, WB Saunders, 2000:998–1036.
9. Gennari FJ. Hypokalemia. N Engl J Med 1998;339:451–458.
10. Weiner ID, Wingo CS. Hypokalemia—Consequences, causes, and correction. J Am Soc Nephrol 1997;8:1179–1188.
11. Gennari FJ. Disorders of potassium homeostasis: hypokalemia and hyperkalemia. Crit Care Clin 2002;18:273–288.
12. Ryan MP. Interrelationships of magnesium and potassium homeostasis. Miner Electrolyte Metab 1993;19:290–295.
13. Krishna GG, Kapoor SC. Potassium depletion exacerbates essential hypertension. Ann Intern Med 1991;115:77–83.
14. Barri YM, Wingo CS. The effects of potassium depletion and supplementation on blood pressure: A clinical review. Am J Med Sci 1997;314:37–40.
15. Geleijnse JM, Witteman JCM, den Breeijen JH, et al. Dietary electrolyte intake and blood pressure in older subjects: The Rotterdam Study. J Hypertens 1996;14:737–741.
16. INTERSALT Cooperative Research Group. INTERSALT: An international study of electrolyte excretion and blood pressure. Results for 24-hour urinary sodium and potassium excretion. BMJ 1988;297:319–328.
17. Ascherio A, Hennekens C, Willett WC, et al. Prospective study of nutritional factors, blood pressure, and hypertension among US women. Hypertension 1996;27:1065–1072.
18. The Seventh Report of the Joint National Committee on Prevention, Detection, Evaluation, and Treatment of High Blood Pressure. JAMA 2003;289:2560–2572.
19. Whelton PK, He J, Cutler JA, et al. Effects of oral potassium on blood pressure: Meta-analysis of randomized controlled clinical trials. JAMA 1997;277:1624–1632.
20. Langford HG. Dietary potassium and hypertension: Epidemiologic data. Ann Intern Med 1983;98:770–772.
21. Cohn JN, Kowey PR, Whelton PK, Prisant LM. New guidelines for potassium replacement in clinical practice: A contemporary review by the National Council on Potassium in Clinical Practice. Arch Intern Med 2000;160:2429–2436.
22. Siscovick DS, Raghunathan TE, Psaty BM, et al. Diuretic therapy for hypertension and the risk of primary cardiac arrest. N Engl J Med 1994; 330:1852–1857.
23. Mandal AK. Hypokalemia and hyperkalemia. Med Clin North Am 1997; 81:611–639.
24. Sica DA, Struthers AD, Cushman WC, et al. Importance of potassium in cardiovascular disease. J Clin Hypertens 2002;4:198–206.
25. Agarwal A, Wingo CS. Treatment of hypokalemia. N Engl J Med 1999; 340:154–155. Letter.
26. Weiner ID, Wingo CS. Hyperkalemia: A potential silent killer. J Am Soc Nephrol 1998;9:1535–1543.
27. Rastegar A, Soleimani M, Rastergar A. Hypokalaemia and hyperkalaemia. Postgrad Med J 2001;77:759–764.
28. Mueller BA, Scott MK, Sowinski KM, Prag KA. Noni juice (*Morinda citrifolia*): hidden potential for hyperkalemia? Am J Kidney Dis 2000; 35:310–312.
29. Chmielewski CM. Hyperkalemic emergencies: Mechanisms, manifestations and management. Crit Care Nurs Clin North Am 1998;10:449–458.
30. Gennari FJ, Segal AS. Hyperkalemia: An adaptive response in chronic renal insufficiency. Kidney Int 2002;62:1–9.
31. Greenberg A. Hyperkalemia: Treatment options. Semin Nephrol 1998; 18:46–57.
32. Ahmed J, Weisberg LS. Hyperkalemia in dialysis patients. Semin Dial 2001;15:348–356.
33. Wong SL, Maltz HC. Albuterol for the treatment of hyperkalemia. Ann Pharmacother 1999;33:103–106.
34. Toto KH, Yucha CB. Magnesium homeostasis, imbalances, and therapeutic uses. Crit Care Nurs Clin North Am 1994;6:767–783.
35. Wicks TC. AANA Journal course. Update for nurse anesthetists—Magnesium homeostasis and deficiency. AANA J 1999;67:171–179.
36. Quamme GA. Renal magnesium handling: New insights in understanding old problems. Kidney Int 1997;52:1180–1195.
37. Slatopolsky E, Hruska KA. Disorders of phosphorus, calcium and magnesium metabolism. In: Schrier RW, ed. Diseases of the Kidney and Urinary Tract, Vol. 3, 7th ed. Philadelphia, Lippincott, Williams and Wilkins, 2001:2607–2660.
38. Wong ET, Rude RK, Singer FR, Shaw ST Jr. A high prevalence of hypomagnesemia in hospitalized patients. Am J Clin Pathol 1983;79:348–352.
39. Ryzen E. Magnesium homeostasis in critically ill patients. Magnesium 1989;8:201–212.
40. Kelepouris E, Agus ZS. Hypomagnesemia: Renal magnesium handling. Semin Nephrol 1998;18:58–73.
41. Elisaf M, Merkouropolous M, Tsianos EV, et al. Pathogenetic mechanisms of hypomagnesemia in alcoholic patients. J Trace Elem Med Biol 1995;9:210–214.

42. Kobrin SM, Goldfarb S. Magnesium deficiency. Semin Nephrol 1990; 10:525–535.

43. Tso EL, Barish RA. Magnesium: Clinical considerations. J Emerg Med 1992;10:735–745.

44. Whang R, Hampton EM, Whang DD. Magnesium homeostasis and clinical disorders of magnesium deficiency. Ann Pharmacother 1994;28:220–226.

45. Innerarity S. Hypomagnesemia in acute and chronic illness. Crit Care Nurs Q 2000;23:1–19.

46. Whang R, Ryder KW. Frequency of hypomagnesemia and hypermagnesemia requested vs. routine. JAMA 1990:263;3063–3064.

47. Wong ET, Rude RK, Singer FR, et al. A high prevalence of hypomagnesemia and hypermagnesemia in hospitalized patients. Am J Clin Pathol 1983;79:348–352.

48. Van Hook JW. Endocrine crises. Hypermagnesemia. Crit Care Clin 1991; 7:215–223.

49. Clark BA, Brown RS. Unsuspected morbid hypermagnesemia in elderly patients. Am J Nephrol 1992;12:336–343.

51
ACID-BASE DISORDERS

Gary R. Matzke and Paul M. Palevsky

Learning Objectives and other resources can be found at *www.pharmacotherapyonline.com.*

KEY CONCEPTS

1 The kidney plays a central role in the regulation of acid-base homeostasis through the excretion or reabsorption of filtered HCO_3^-, the excretion of metabolic fixed acids and generation of new HCO_3^-.

2 Arterial blood gases, along with serum electrolytes, physical findings, medical and medication history, and the clinical condition of the patient, are the primary tools to determine the cause of an acid-base disorder and to design and monitor a course of therapy.

3 Metabolic acidosis and metabolic alkalosis are generated by a primary change in the serum bicarbonate concentration. In metabolic acidosis, bicarbonate is lost or a nonvolatile acid is gained, whereas metabolic alkalosis is characterized by a gain in bicarbonate or a loss of nonvolatile acid.

4 Renal tubular acidosis refers to a group of disorders characterized by impaired tubular renal acid handling despite normal or near-normal glomerular filtration rates. These patients often present with hyperchloremic metabolic acidosis.

5 Respiratory compensation for a primary metabolic acidosis begins rapidly (within 15 to 30 minutes) but does not reach a steady state for 12 to 24 hours after the onset of metabolic acidosis.

6 Primary therapy of most acid-base disorders must include treatment or elimination of the underlying cause, not just correction of the pH and electrolyte disturbances.

7 Potassium supplementation is always necessary for patients with chronic metabolic acidosis, as the bicarbonaturia resulting from alkali therapy increases the renal potassium wasting.

8 Effective treatment of the underlying cause of some organic acidoses (e.g., ketoacidosis) can result in the regeneration of bicarbonate within hours, thus mitigating the need for alkali therapy.

9 Loss of gastric acid from vomiting or nasogastric suctioning is often responsible for the development of a metabolic alkalosis, characterized by hypochloremia and hyperbicarbonatemia.

10 Aggressive diuretic therapy may produce a metabolic alkalosis, and the accompanying hypokalemia may be serious.

11 The patient's response to volume replacement may be predicted by the urine chloride concentration, and permits the differential diagnosis of metabolic alkalosis.

12 Management of these disorders usually consists of treatment of the underlying cause of mineralocorticoid excess. In patients in whom the mineralocorticoid excess cannot be corrected, chronic pharmacologic therapy may be required.

13 In most cases of acute respiratory acidosis, such as following cardiopulmonary arrest, sodium bicarbonate therapy is not indicated and may be detrimental. Blood gas analysis should guide therapy.

Acid-base disorders are common, and often serious, disturbances that may result in significant morbidity and mortality. This chapter reviews the mechanisms responsible for the maintenance of acid-base balance and the laboratory analyses that aid clinicians in their assessment of acid-base disorders. The pathophysiology of the four primary acid-base disturbances is presented, the therapeutic options are critiqued, and guidelines for the achievement of the desired therapeutic outcomes are presented. Because many drugs affect acid-base homeostasis and many acid-base abnormalities are potentially preventable, clinicians must anticipate drug-related problems in order to avoid or minimize the clinical consequences, and when necessary design appropriate treatment regimens.

ACID-BASE CHEMISTRY

An acid is a substance that can donate protons (hydrogen ions, H^+):

$$(acid)\ HCl \rightarrow H^+ + Cl^-$$

A base is a substance that can accept protons (hydrogen ions):

$$NH_3 + H^+ \rightarrow NH_4^+\quad (base)$$

The acid-base pairs commonly encountered in clinical practice are listed in Table 51–1.

The acidity of body fluids is quantified in terms of the hydrogen ion concentration. By convention, the degree of acidity is expressed

TABLE 51–1. Acid-Base Pairs

Carbonic acid/bicarbonate	H_2CO_3/HCO_3^-
Monobasic/dibasic phosphate	H_2PO_4/HPO_4^-
Ammonium/ammonia	NH_4^+/NH_3
Lactic acid/lactate	$H_6C_3O_2/H_5C_3O_2^-$

as pH, or the negative logarithm (base 10) of the hydrogen ion concentration. Thus hydrogen ion concentration and pH are inversely related. Normally, the pH of blood is maintained at 7.40 ($[H^+]$ of 4×10^{-8} M) with a range of 7.35 to 7.45. A pH of less than 6.7 ($[H^+]$ of 2×10^{-7} M), representing a fivefold increase in hydrogen ion concentration, or greater than 7.7 ($[H^+]$ of 2×10^{-8} M), representing a 50% decrease in hydrogen ion concentration, are considered incompatible with life.

The hydrogen ion concentration in blood may not be indicative of that in other body compartments. For example, the pH within cells, within the cerebrospinal fluid, or on the surface of bone may all be altered without causing an alteration in blood pH.[1] Recognizing this caveat, the acid-base status of the body is usually analyzed based on measurement of blood pH. Alterations in blood pH serve as the basis for the diagnosis of acid-base disorders.

Because the dissociation of acid-base pairs is an equilibrium reaction, the relationship between hydrogen ion concentration or pH and the relative concentrations of the acid and base can be described mathematically in terms of the dissociation constant for the acid-base buffer pair. When expressed as a logarithmic relationship, where pK is the negative logarithm of the dissociation constant K, this is known as the Henderson-Hasselbalch equation:

$$pH = pK + \log([base]/[acid])$$

BUFFERS

The ability of a weak acid and its corresponding anion (base) to resist change in the pH of a solution upon the addition of a strong acid or base is referred to as *buffering*. An acid-base pair is most efficient in functioning as a buffer at a pH close to its pK. The principal extracellular buffer is the carbonic acid/bicarbonate (H_2CO_3/HCO_3^-) system. Other physiologic buffers include plasma proteins, hemoglobin, and phosphates. Because the isohydric principle requires that all buffer systems remain in chemical equilibrium, the complex buffering of biologic fluids can be analyzed based on a single buffer pair.

The carbonic acid/bicarbonate buffer system plays a unique role in acid-base homeostasis. In addition to being the most abundant extracellular buffer, the components of this buffer pair are under dynamic regulation by the body. In the presence of carbonic anhydrase, carbonic acid, $[H_2CO_3]$ is in equilibrium with carbon dioxide (CO_2) gas. Changes in ventilation that alter the partial pressure of CO_2 (P_{CO_2}) in the blood regulates the carbonic acid level in the blood. The bicarbonate concentration is independently regulated by the kidney. Because the pK for the carbonic acid/bicarbonate system is 6.1, the relationship between pH, carbonic acid, and bicarbonate concentrations can be described by the Henderson-Hasselbalch equation. The concentration of carbonic acid is directly proportional to the amount of CO_2 dissolved in blood, which is equal to the product of P_{CO_2} and its solubility in physiologic fluids, ($P_{CO_2} \times 0.03$). This term can therefore be substituted into the equation below in place of $[H_2CO_3]$.

$$pH = 6.1 + \log([HCO_3^-]/[H_2CO_3])$$

$$pH = 6.1 + \log([HCO_3^-]/(P_{CO_2} \times 0.03))$$

Thus, hydrogen ion concentration and pH are determined not by the absolute amounts of bicarbonate and P_{CO_2}, but by their ratio.[1] Under normal physiologic conditions, the kidneys maintain the serum bicarbonate at about 24 mEq/L, while the lungs maintain the P_{CO_2} at approximately 40 mm Hg. The normal physiologic pH is thus 7.4:

$$pH = 6.1 + \log[24/(0.03 \times 40)]$$

$$pH = 6.1 + 1.3 = 7.4$$

If, in response to an acid load, the serum bicarbonate concentration were to fall to 12 mEq/L, the predicted pH would be:

$$[HCO_3^-] = 12 \text{ mEq/L}$$

$$P_{CO_2} = 40 \text{ mm Hg}$$

$$pH = 6.1 + \log[12/(0.03 \times 40)]$$

$$pH = 6.1 + 1.0 = 7.1$$

However, the normal respiratory response to an acid load is hyperventilation. As a result, if the P_{CO_2} fell to approximately 26 mm Hg, the change in pH would be less:

$$[HCO_3^-] = 12 \text{ mEq/L}$$

$$P_{CO_2} = 26 \text{ mm Hg}$$

$$pH = 6.1 + \log[12/(0.03 \times 26)]$$

$$pH = 6.1 + 1.19 = 7.29$$

Thus, the physiologic regulation of both P_{CO_2} and $[HCO_3^-]$ permit the carbonic acid/bicarbonate system to provide more effective buffering of the extracellular fluids than could be achieved on the basis of chemical buffering alone.

REGULATION OF ACID-BASE HOMEOSTASIS

Cellular metabolism results in the production of large quantities of hydrogen that need to be excreted in order to maintain acid-base balance. In addition, small amounts of acid and alkali are also presented to the body through the diet. The bulk of acid production is in the form of CO_2, from the metabolism of carbohydrates, proteins, and lipids. When respiratory function is normal, the amount of CO_2 produced metabolically is equal to the amount lost by respiration, and the blood CO_2 concentration remains constant. The average adult produces approximately 15,000 mmol of CO_2 each day from the catabolism of carbohydrate, protein, and fat.[2]

Digestion of dietary substances and tissue metabolism also results in the production of nonvolatile acids. These acids are derived primarily from the sulfur-containing amino acids cysteine and methionine, as well as from ingested sulfur. In addition, phosphates are generated from the metabolism of proteins and phospholipids. Neutral substances such as glucose may also be incompletely metabolized to intermediates, such as lactic and pyruvic acid, and fatty acids may be incompletely metabolized to acetoacetic acid and β-hydroxybutyric acid. These dietary and metabolic fixed acids are excreted, primarily by the kidney, to maintain acid-base homeostasis. On average, daily fixed acid excretion is approximately 0.8 mEq/kg per day.[3]

Three mechanisms collectively maintain acid-base balance: extracellular buffering, ventilatory regulation of carbon dioxide elimination, and renal regulation of hydrogen ion and bicarbonate excretion. Extracellular buffering is the body's first and fastest defense against a sudden increase in hydrogen ion concentration. Hyperventilation will then result in a decrease in P_{CO_2}, returning blood pH toward normal. Finally, the kidney will excrete the excess hydrogen ion, and return acid-base balance to normal.

EXTRACELLULAR BUFFERING

The body's buffering system can be divided into three components: bicarbonate/carbonic acid, proteins, and phosphates. The bicarbonate buffer is the most important of the body's buffers, because (1) there is more bicarbonate present in the extracellular fluid (ECF) than any other buffer component; (2) the supply of carbon dioxide is unlimited; and (3) the acidity of ECF can be regulated by controlling either the bicarbonate concentration or the P_{CO_2}.

Carbonic acid represents the respiratory component of the buffer pair because its concentration is directly proportional to the P_{CO_2}, which is determined by ventilation. Bicarbonate represents the metabolic component because the kidney may alter its concentration by reabsorption, generating new bicarbonate, or altering elimination.[4] The bicarbonate buffer system easily adapts to changes in acid-base status by alterations in ventilatory elimination of acid (P_{CO_2}) and/or renal elimination of base (HCO_3^-).

The phosphate buffer system consists of serum inorganic phosphate (3.5 to 5 mg/dL), intracellular organic phosphate, and calcium phosphate in bone. Extracellular phosphate is present only in low concentrations, so its usefulness as a buffer is limited; however, as an intracellular buffer, phosphate is more useful. Calcium phosphate in bone is relatively inaccessible as a buffer, but prolonged metabolic acidosis will result in the release of phosphate from bone.

Intracellular and extracellular proteins also act as buffering systems. The charged side chains of amino acids provide the buffering action. Because the concentration of protein is much greater intracellularly than extracellularly, protein is much more important as an intracellular buffer.

RESPIRATORY REGULATION

The second mechanism for maintenance of acid-base homeostasis is control of ventilation. Both the rate and depth of ventilation can be varied to allow for excretion of CO_2 generated by diet and tissue metabolism. Medullary chemoreceptors in the brain stem sense changes in P_{CO_2} and in pH and modulate the control of breathing. Increasing minute ventilation, by increasing either or both respiratory rate or tidal volume, will increase CO_2 excretion and decrease the blood P_{CO_2}. Conversely, decreasing minute ventilation decreases CO_2 excretion and increases blood P_{CO_2}. This system rapidly adjusts, within minutes, to changes in acid-base balance.[2]

RENAL REGULATION

Because bicarbonate is a small ion, it is freely filtered at the glomerulus. The bicarbonate load delivered to the nephron is approximately 4,500 mEq/day. To maintain acid-base balance, this entire filtered load must be reabsorbed. Bicarbonate reabsorption occurs primarily in the proximal tubule (Fig. 51–1). In the tubular lumen, filtered bicarbonate combines with hydrogen ion secreted by the apical Na^+-H^+-exchanger to form carbonic acid. The carbonic acid is rapidly broken down to CO_2 and water by carbonic anhydrase located on the luminal surface of the brush border membrane. The CO_2 then diffuses into the proximal tubular cell, where it reforms carbonic acid in the presence of intracellular carbonic anhydrase. The carbonic acid dissociates to form hydrogen ion, that can again be secreted into the tubular lumen, and bicarbonate that exits the cell across the basolateral membrane and enters the peritubular capillary.

Excretion of metabolic fixed acids and generation of new HCO_3^- is achieved through renal ammoniagenesis and distal tubular hydrogen ion secretion. Ammoniagenesis plays a critical role in acid-base homeostasis, with ammonium ($NH4^+$) excretion comprising approxi-

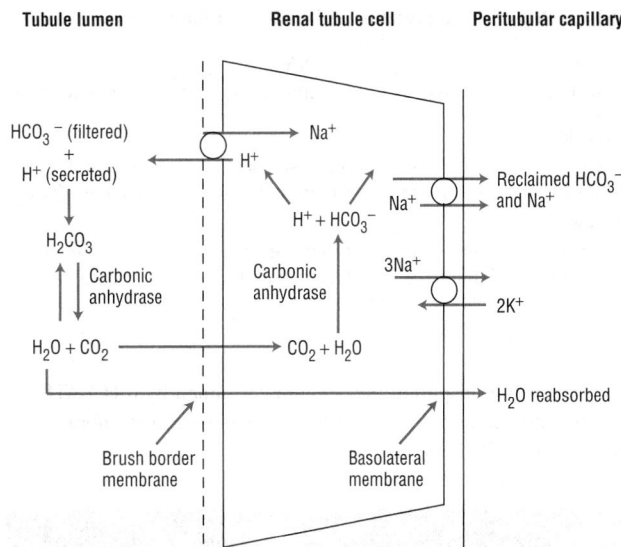

FIGURE 51–1. Proximal tubular bicarbonate reabsorption. In the tubular lumen, filtered bicarbonate combines with hydrogen ion secreted by an apical Na^+-H^+-exchanger to form carbonic acid. The carbonic acid is rapidly broken down to CO_2 and water by carbonic anhydrase located on the luminal surface of the brush border membrane. The CO_2 then diffuses into the proximal tubular cell, where it reforms carbonic acid in the presence of intracellular carbonic anhydrase. The carbonic acid dissociates to form hydrogen ion, that can again be secreted into the tubular lumen, and bicarbonate that exits the cell across the basolateral membrane and enters the peritubular capillary.

mately 50% of renal net acid excretion. Ammonium is generated from the deamination of glutamine in the proximal tubule. For each ammonium ion excreted in the urine, one bicarbonate ion is regenerated and returned to the circulation.[5]

Distal tubular hydrogen ion secretion accounts for the remaining 50% of net acid excretion (Fig. 51–2). In the distal tubular cell, CO_2 combines with water in the presence of intracellular carbonic anhydrase to form carbonic acid, which dissociates to H^+ and HCO_3^-. The

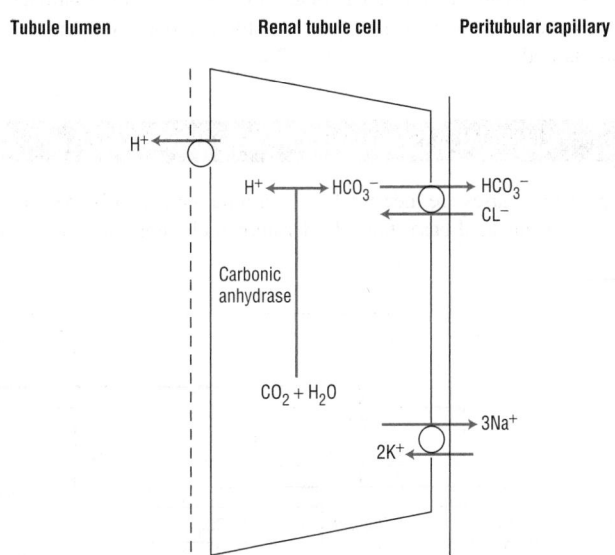

FIGURE 51–2. Collecting duct acid excretion. Hydrogen ion and bicarbonate are generated intracellularly from CO_2 and water, in the presence of intracellular carbonic anhydrase. The hydrogen ion is actively secreted into the tubular lumen by H^+-ATPases located in the apical (luminal) membrane. Bicarbonate exits the cell across the basolateral membrane and enters the peritubular capillary.

TABLE 51–2. Interpretation of Simple Acid-Base Disorders

Acid-Base Disorder	pH	Primary Disturbances	Compensation
Acidosis			
Respiratory	Decrease	Increase Pa_{CO_2}	Increase HCO_3^-
Metabolic	Decrease	Decrease HCO_3^-	Decrease Pa_{CO_2}
Alkalosis			
Respiratory	Increase	Decrease Pa_{CO_2}	Decrease HCO_3^-
Metabolic	Increase	Increase HCO_3^-	Increase Pa_{CO_2}

TABLE 51–3. Normal Blood Gas Values

	Arterial Blood	Mixed Venous Blood
pH	7.40 (7.35–7.45)	7.38 (7.33–7.43)
P_{O_2}	80–100 mm Hg	35–40 mm Hg
Sa_{O_2}	95%	70%–75%
P_{CO_2}	35–45 mm Hg	45–51 mm Hg
HCO_3^-	22–26 mEq/L	24–28 mEq/L

HCO_3^-, bicarbonate; P_{CO_2}: partial pressure of carbon dioxide; P_{O_2}: partial pressure of oxygen; Sa_{O_2}, saturation of arterial oxygen.

H^+ is actively transported into the tubular lumen by a H^+-ATPase. The bicarbonate exits the cell across the basolateral membrane and enters the circulation.[5]

ACID-BASE DISTURBANCES

Alterations in blood pH are designated by the suffix "-emia"; *acidemia* is an arterial blood pH <7.35 and *alkalemia* is an arterial blood pH >7.45. The pathophysiologic processes that result in alterations in blood pH are designated by the suffix "-osis." These disturbances are classified as either metabolic or respiratory in origin. In metabolic acid-base disorders, the primary disturbance is in the plasma bicarbonate concentration. Metabolic acidosis is characterized by a decrease in the plasma bicarbonate concentration while in metabolic alkalosis the plasma bicarbonate concentration is increased. Respiratory acid-base disorders are caused by alterations in alveolar ventilation that produce corresponding changes in the arterial carbon dioxide tension (Pa_{CO_2}). In respiratory acidosis, the Pa_{CO_2} is elevated; in respiratory alkalosis it is decreased. Each disturbance has a compensatory (secondary) response which attempts to correct the $[HCO_3^-]$:Pa_{CO_2} ratio toward normal and mitigate the change in pH (Table 51–2). Although the time course of the respiratory compensatory responses to metabolic disturbances is rapid, the metabolic compensation for respiratory disturbances is slow. As a result, respiratory disturbances are characterized as acute (minutes to hours in duration), indicating that there has not been sufficient time for metabolic compensation, or chronic (days), indicating sufficient time for metabolic compensation has elapsed.

CLINICAL ASSESSMENT OF ACID-BASE STATUS

 Blood gases are measured to determine the patient's oxygenation and acid-base status. Under normal circumstances, there is no clinically significant difference in pH between arterial and mixed venous blood. Arterial samples are designated with the letter "a" (e.g., Pa_{O_2} and Pa_{CO_2}), while mixed venous samples are labeled with the letter "v" or not labeled (e.g., Pv_{O_2} and Pv_{CO_2}). The normal values for arterial and venous blood gases are shown in Table 51–3. Arterial blood provides the added information of how well the lungs are oxygenating the blood (an accurate measurement of partial oxygen pressure $[Pa_{O_2}]$). Arterial blood rather than venous blood should be used whenever possible because venous blood obtained from an extremity may provide misleading information. If metabolism in the extremity is altered by hypoperfusion, exercise, infection, or some other cause, the differences between arterial and venous blood can be dramatic. The venous pH and Pc_{CO_2} during cardiopulmonary resuscitation, may be significantly lower and higher, respectively than the arterial pH and arterial Pc_{CO_2}. This indicates a severe tissue acidosis from CO_2 accumulation due to hypoperfusion.

ANALYSIS OF ARTERIAL BLOOD GAS DATA

Arterial blood gases provide an assessment of the patient's acid-base status. Low pH values (<7.35) indicate an acidemia, whereas high pH values (>7.45) indicate an alkalemia (Fig. 51–3). In a metabolic acidosis, the pH is decreased in association with a decreased serum bicarbonate concentration and a compensatory fall in Pa_{CO_2}. In a respiratory acidosis, the pH is decreased; the Pa_{CO_2}, however, is elevated. The serum bicarbonate concentration is variable, depending on whether it is an acute disturbance (minimal increase in serum bicarbonate) or a chronic respiratory acidosis (substantial increase in serum bicarbonate). In a metabolic alkalosis, the pH is elevated in association with an increased bicarbonate concentration and a compensatory rise in Pa_{CO_2}. In respiratory alkalosis, the pH is also elevated; the Pa_{CO_2}, however, is decreased. As with respiratory acidosis, the metabolic compensation is variable, with a minimal decrease in serum bicarbonate in acute respiratory alkalosis and a larger decrease in $[HCO_3^-]$ in chronic respiratory alkalosis.

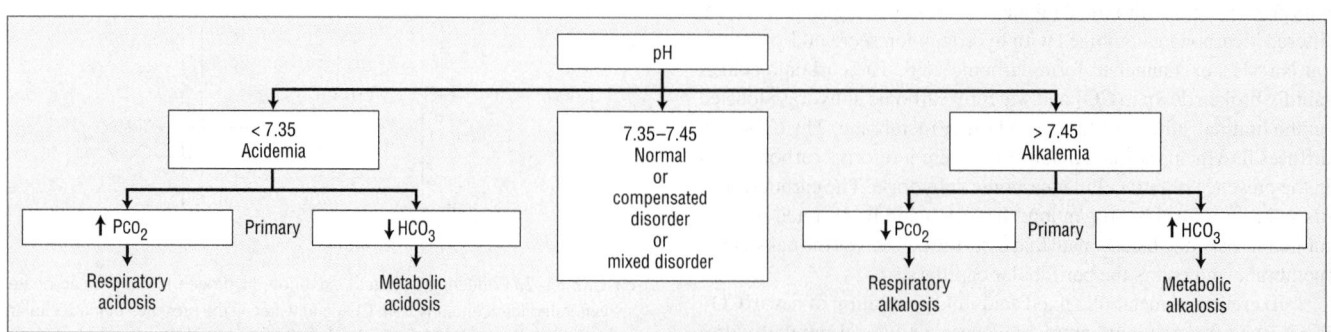

FIGURE 51–3. Analysis of arterial blood gases.

TABLE 51–4. Guidelines for Initial Interpretation of Acid-Base Disorders

Metabolic acidosis	$Paco_2$ (in mm Hg) should fall by 1–1.5 times the fall in plasma $[HCO_3^-]$ (in mEq/L)
Metabolic alkalosis	$Paco_2$ (in mm Hg) should increase by 0.25–1 times the rise in plasma $[HCO_3^-]$ (in mEq/L)
Acute respiratory acidosis	The plasma $[HCO_3^-]$ should rise by 0.1 times the increase in $Paco_2 \pm 3$
Acute respiratory alkalosis	The plasma $[HCO_3^-]$ should fall by 0.1–0.3 times the decrease in $Paco_2$ but usually not to less than 18 mEq/L
Chronic respiratory acidosis	The plasma $[HCO_3^-]$ should rise by 0.4 times the increase in $Paco_2 \pm 4$
Chronic respiratory alkalosis	The plasma $[HCO_3^-]$ should fall by 0.2–0.5 times the decrease in $Paco_2$ but usually not to less than 14 mEq/L

Adapted from Shapiro and Kaehny [4].

The degree of expected compensatory response for each primary disturbance is depicted in Table 51–4. If the observed compensatory response is substantially different than that predicted by these empiric relationships, a mixed acid-base disturbance (i.e., more than one primary disorder) may be present. Nomograms, such as the one shown in Fig. 51–4, may also be used to differentiate between the various acid-base disorders.[4,6] In this nomogram, each pathologic acid-base disorder, together with the appropriate range of in vivo physiologic compensation, is represented as a shaded band. Blood gas values—serum bicarbonate, pH, and carbon dioxide tension—falling within a band usually represent a single disturbance; however, a mixed disturbance may occasionally present in this way. Acid-base values falling outside any band almost certainly represent a mixed acid-base disturbance.[6]

When arterial blood gases differ significantly from those expected on the basis of the patient's clinical condition and previous laboratory determinations, additional venous blood samples should

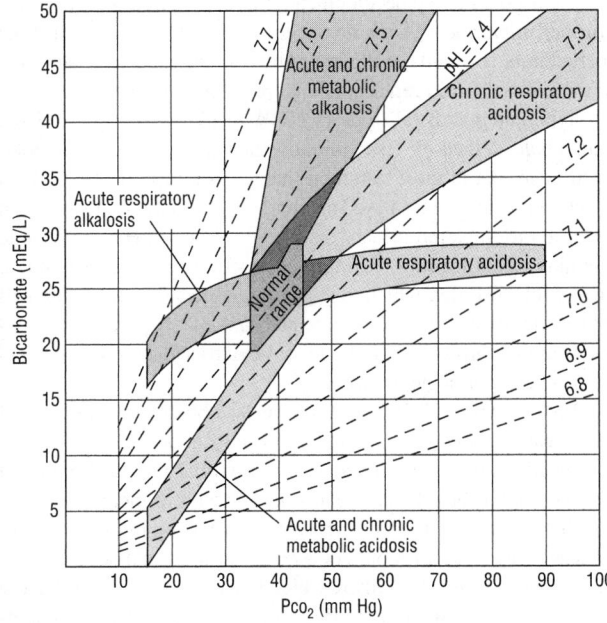

FIGURE 51–4. Acid-base nomogram. (*Reprinted with permission from Arbus.[6]*)

be drawn to assess plasma electrolyte concentrations. The bicarbonate calculated from the patient's $Paco_2$ and pH of the blood gas should be compared with the measured total CO_2 content (the amount of CO_2 gas extractable from plasma, consisting of HCO_3^-, H_2CO_3, and Pco_2). Ordinarily, the blood gas bicarbonate value is approximately 1 to 2 mEq/L less than total CO_2 content.[3] If these values do not correspond, the results should be interpreted with caution because the difference may reflect an error in the blood collection or storage of the sample, or in the calibration of the blood gas analyzer.

METABOLIC ACID-BASE DISORDERS

METABOLIC ACIDOSIS

PATHOPHYSIOLOGY

Metabolic acidosis is characterized by a decrease in pH as the result of a primary decrease in serum bicarbonate concentration. This can result from the buffering (consumption of HCO_3^-) of an exogenous acid, an organic acid accumulating because of a metabolic disturbance (e.g., lactic acid or ketoacids), or the progressive accumulation of endogenous acids secondary to impaired renal function (e.g., phosphates and sulfates).[9] The serum HCO_3^- can also be decreased as the result of a loss of bicarbonate-rich body fluids (e.g., diarrhea, biliary drainage, or pancreatic fistula) or occur secondary to the rapid administration of non–alkali-containing intravenous fluids (dilutional acidosis).

The serum anion gap (SAG), as defined below, may be used to infer whether an organic or mineral acidosis is present.

$$SAG = [Na^+] - [Cl^-] - [HCO_3^-]$$

To maintain electroneutrality, the total concentration of cations in the serum must equal the total concentration of anions.

$$[Na^+] + [UCs] = ([Cl^-] + [HCO_3^-]) + [UAs]$$

The cation concentration is equal to the sodium concentration plus that of "unmeasured" cations (UCs), predominantly magnesium, calcium, and potassium. The anion concentration is equal to the concentrations of chloride, bicarbonate, and "unmeasured" anions (UAs), including proteins, sulfates, phosphates, and organic anions. Therefore, as the result of the combination of the two equations above the SAG can be expressed as:

$$SAG = [UAs] - [UCs]$$

The normal SAG is approximately 9 mEq/L, with a range of 3 to 11 mEq/L. This value is lower than the value of 12 mEq/L cited in the literature in the past because of changes in the instrumentation for measurement of serum electrolytes during the past decade.[8] Increases in the anion gap to values in excess of 17 to 20 mEq/L are indicative of the accumulation of unmeasured anions in ECF.

These unmeasured anions are generated as the result of the consumption of HCO_3^- by endogenous organic acids such as lactic acid, acetoacetic acid, or β-hydroxybutyric acid or from the ingestion of toxins such as methanol or ethylene glycol. The degree of elevation in the SAG is dependent on the clearance of the anion, as well as the multiple factors that influence HCO_3^- concentrations. Thus the SAG is a relative rather than an absolute indication of the cause of metabolic acidosis. The SAG may also be elevated in the metabolic acidosis due to renal failure, as the result of the accumulation of various organic anions, phosphates, and sulfates.

TABLE 51–5. Common Causes of Metabolic Acidosis

Increased Serum Anion Gap	Normal Serum Anion Gap/ Hyperchloremic States
Alcoholic ketoacidosis	Acid ingestion (hydrochloric acid or ammonium chloride)
Diabetic ketoacidosis	Carbonic anhydrase inhibitors
Lactic acidosis	Cholestyramine
Renal failure	Diarrhea
(acute or chronic)	Dilutional acidosis
Methanol ingestion	Gastrointestinal disorders
Ethylene glycol ingestion	Pancreatic fistula
Salicylate overdose	Potassium-sparing diuretic
Starvation	Renal tubular acidosis
	Ureterosigmoidostomy, ileostomy

In hyperchloremic metabolic acidosis, bicarbonate losses from the ECF are replaced by chloride and the SAG remains normal. This decrease in bicarbonate results from losses from the gastrointestinal tract, dilution of bicarbonate in the ECF space by the addition of sodium chloride solutions, or the addition of chloride-containing acids to the ECF. Common causes of metabolic acidosis with an increased or a normal SAG are listed in Table 51–5.

HYPERCHLOREMIC METABOLIC ACIDOSIS

Hyperchloremic metabolic acidosis may result from increased gastrointestinal bicarbonate loss, renal bicarbonate wasting, impaired renal acid excretion, or exogenous acid gain. Gastrointestinal disorders such as diarrhea, biliary drainage, and pancreatic fistula may result in the loss of large volumes of bicarbonate-containing fluids, with diarrhea being the most common cause for hyperchloremic metabolic acidosis. Severe diarrhea can lead to a daily loss of 5 to 10 L of fluid containing 100 to 140 mEq/L of sodium, 20 to 40 mEq/L of potassium, 80 to 100 mEq/L of chloride, and 30 to 50 mEq/L of bicarbonate.[4] Patients who have undergone ureteral diversion into the sigmoid colon or isolated ileal loop may also develop a hyperchloremic metabolic acidosis. In these patients, chloride is reabsorbed and the bicarbonate secreted by the gastrointestinal epithelial cells while urine retained in the colon or bowel loop results in a net loss of bicarbonate. Hyperchloremic metabolic acidosis caused by renal bicarbonate wasting is the defining disturbance in proximal renal tubular acidosis and is a complication of therapy with carbonic anhydrase inhibitors. During the treatment of diabetic ketoacidosis, renal losses of β-hydroxybutyrate and acetoacetate, which would otherwise be metabolized to yield bicarbonate, may contribute to the development of hyperchloremic metabolic acidosis. Impaired renal acid excretion as a result of distal tubular dysfunction characterizes the distal renal tubular acidoses. Impaired renal acid excretion is also characteristic of moderate to severe renal insufficiency. Initially, the metabolic acidosis of renal insufficiency is hyperchloremic, progressing to an anion-gap acidosis as the renal insufficiency worsens and sulfates, phosphates, and other anions accumulate. Hyperchloremic metabolic acidosis may also result from the exogenous administration of acid as hydrochloric acid or ammonium chloride or the unbuffered administration of acid salts of amino acids in parenteral nutrition fluids.

RENAL TUBULAR ACIDOSIS

 Renal tubular disorders may involve the proximal tubule, with a resultant failure to reabsorb filtered bicarbonate, or affect acid excretion in the distal tubule. The distal renal tubular acidoses (RTAs) are the most common and are all characterized by impaired net acid excretion. The distal RTAs are subdivided into those that are associated with hypokalemia (type I) and those associated with hyperkalemia (type IV). Patients with classic distal (type I) RTA have impaired H^+ ion secretion, and are unable to excrete the daily acid load necessary to maintain acid-base balance.[4] These patients are unable to maximally acidify their urine (i.e., attain urine pH of <5.5), even in the face of an acid challenge. Type I RTA may be the result of a primary tubular defect or develop secondary to a wide variety of disorders including hypercalcemia, multiple myeloma, systemic lupus erythematosus, Sjögren's syndrome, sickle-cell disease, and renal transplant rejection, or following the administration of amphotericin B or ingestion of toluene. The primary form of this disorder usually occurs in children and can result in severe acidosis, slowed growth, nephrocalcinosis, and kidney stones.[9,10] In adults, clinical complications include osteomalacia, nephrocalcinosis, and recurrent kidney stones. The hypokalemia associated with classic distal (type I) RTA results from secondary hypoaldosteronism associated with volume depletion. The renal potassium wasting decreases considerably when bicarbonate therapy is begun.

The hyperkalemic distal (type IV) RTAs are a heterogeneous group of disorders characterized by hypoaldosteronism or generalized distal tubule defects. The most common form of type IV RTA is hyporeninemic hypoaldosteronism. This syndrome is most commonly associated with mild renal insufficiency caused by diabetic nephropathy, but may also be seen in a variety of other disorders, including chronic interstitial nephritis, sickle-cell disease, human immunodeficiency virus (HIV) nephropathy, and obstructive uropathy. The clinical presentation of this syndrome is often exacerbated by pharmacologic therapy with agents that can interfere with the renin-angiotensin-aldosterone axis, such as β-adrenergic blockers, angiotensin-converting enzyme inhibitors, angiotensin receptor blockers, and nonsteroidal anti-inflammatory drugs. Heparin may induce the syndrome by inhibiting adrenal aldosterone biosynthesis. Patients with this form of RTA are able to maximally acidify their urine (urine pH <5.5).[9] The primary defect in acid excretion is impaired ammoniagenesis caused by mild renal insufficiency. Hyperaldosteronism predisposes to the development of hyperkalemia, which results in further impairment of ammoniagenesis. Treatment to control the hyperkalemia is usually sufficient to reverse the metabolic acidosis, and mineralocorticoid replacement is frequently unnecessary.

Hyperkalemic distal (type IV) RTA resulting from generalized distal tubule defects is less common than hyporeninemic hypoaldosteronism, but is more common than classic distal (type I) RTA. Patients with this defect have impaired tubular potassium secretion in addition to impaired urinary acidification (urine pH >5.5 despite acidemia or acid loading). Urinary obstruction is the most frequent cause of this disorder, which may also be associated with sickle-cell nephropathy, systemic lupus erythematosus, HIV nephropathy, analgesic abuse nephropathy, amyloidosis, renal transplant rejection, and chronic cyclosporine nephrotoxicity.

Proximal (type II) RTA is characterized by defects in proximal tubular reabsorption of bicarbonate. Normally, more than 85% of filtered bicarbonate is reabsorbed in the proximal tubule. Defects in proximal tubular bicarbonate reabsorption result in increased delivery of bicarbonate to the distal nephron, which has a limited capacity for bicarbonate reabsorption. As a result, at a normal serum bicarbonate concentration, the filtered bicarbonate load is incompletely reabsorbed, and is lost in the urine. As the serum bicarbonate concentration falls, the filtered load of bicarbonate is proportionately decreased. A new equilibrium is established in which the kidney is able to reabsorb the filtered bicarbonate load, albeit at a reduced serum bicarbonate concentration. Thus patients with proximal RTA present with a chronic, nonprogressive hyperchloremic metabolic acidosis. These patients are able to acidify their urine in response to an acid load, but develop bicarbonaturia at a reduced serum bicarbonate concentration following bicarbonate loading. The impaired bicarbonate reabsorption results in salt wasting and secondary hyperaldosteronism. Hypokalemia, which may be severe, develops as a result of the hyperaldosteronism and bicarbonaturia.[4,9] Unlike patients with classic distal (type I) RTA, the hyperkalemia in proximal RTA is exacerbated by alkali replacement. Proximal RTA may develop as an isolated defect or it may be associated with generalized proximal tubular dysfunction (Fanconi's syndrome), with impaired proximal tubular glucose, phosphate, and amino acid reabsorption. Proximal RTA usually presents as an acquired disorder, secondary to a variety of diseases (amyloidosis, multiple myeloma, or nephrotic syndrome) or exposure to toxins (lead, cadmium, mercury, or outdated tetracyclines). Pharmacologic therapy with carbonic anhydrase inhibitors produces an iatrogenic form of proximal RTA.

ELEVATED ANION GAP METABOLIC ACIDOSIS

Metabolic acidosis with an increased SAG commonly results from increased endogenous organic acid production. In lactic acidosis, lactic acid accumulates as a by-product of anaerobic metabolism. Accumulation of the ketoacids β-hydroxybutyric acid and acetoacetic acid defines the ketoacidosis of uncontrolled diabetes mellitus, alcohol intoxication, and starvation (see Table 51–5). In advanced renal failure, ac-cumulation of phosphate, sulfate, and organic anions is responsible for the increased SAG, which is usually less than 24 mEq/L.[11] The severe metabolic acidosis seen in myoglobinuric acute renal failure caused by rhabdomyolysis may be caused by the metabolism of large amounts of sulfur-containing amino acids released from myoglobin.

The presence of mild elevations in the SAG cannot be automatically attributed to the presence of a high SAG metabolic acidosis. Elevations in the SAG are commonly seen in hospitalized patients, especially those who are critically ill.[12] A variety of factors may contribute to this nonspecific elevation in the SAG, including the presence of alkalemia, which increases the anionic charge of albumin and other plasma proteins. The usefulness of the SAG as a marker of acid-base status is dependent on proper interpretation of a patient's clinical status.[8,13] Despite these limitations, when the SAG exceeds 20 to 25 mEq/L a significant organic acidosis is likely to be present.

High anion gap metabolic acidosis may develop in many clinical settings, including uncontrolled diabetes mellitus (see Chap. 72), alcohol intoxication (see Chaps. 37 and 65), and starvation (see Chap. 62). Toxic ingestions of methanol, ethylene glycol, and salicylates are also associated with high anion gap metabolic acidosis (see Chap. 10). The mechanisms responsible for the development of acidosis in these settings are diverse.

Lactic Acidosis

Lactic acidosis is one of the most common causes of high SAG metabolic acidosis. Lactic acid is the end product of anaerobic metabolism of glucose (glycolysis). In normal individuals, lactic acid derived from pyruvate enters the circulation in small amounts and is promptly removed by the liver. In the liver, and to a lesser extent in the kidney, lactic acid is reoxidized to pyruvic acid, which is then metabolized to CO_2 and H_2O. The normal plasma lactate concentration in healthy subjects is approximately 1 mEq/L.[7,14] The diagnosis of lactic acidosis should be considered in all patients with metabolic acidosis

TABLE 51–6. Causes of Lactic Acidosis

Primary decrease in tissue oxygenation
Shock
Severe anemia
Congestive heart failure
Asphyxia
Carbon monoxide poisoning

Deranged oxidative metabolism
Diabetes mellitus
Liver failure
Malignancy
Seizures
Medications (iron, isoniazid, metformin, or salicylates)
Methanol, ethanol, or ethylene glycol
Disorders associated with inborn errors of metabolism

associated with an increased SAG. Lactic acidosis is considered to be present when lactate concentrations exceed 4 to 5 mEq/L in an acidemic patient.

Classically, lactic acidosis has been differentiated into disorders associated with tissue hypoxia (type A lactic acidosis) and disorders associated with deranged oxidative metabolism (type B lactic acidosis), although the distinction between them is blurred (Table 51–6). The etiologies of lactic acidosis can also be categorized on the basis of changes in lactate production and/or utilization.[4,15] Metabolic disturbances can result in increased tissue pyruvate production or impaired utilization, with proportional increases in lactate concentrations. Increased lactate production is more commonly associated with alterations in tissue redox state, resulting in preferential conversion of pyruvate to lactate. During anaerobic metabolism, reduced nicotinamide adenine dinucleotide accumulates, driving the conversion of pyruvate to lactate and increasing the lactate:pyruvate ratio. States of enhanced metabolic activity (e.g., grand mal seizures, strenuous exercise, or hyperthermia), decreased tissue oxygen delivery (e.g., severe anemia, hypoxia, circulatory shock, or carbon monoxide poisoning) or impaired oxygen utilization (e.g., cyanide toxicity) all are associated with lactic acidosis. Impaired hepatic clearance of lactate, as seen in hypoperfusion states, liver failure, and alcohol intoxication, may also result in lactic acidosis.

Cardiovascular and septic shock, with resultant tissue hypoperfusion, are the most common causes of lactic acidosis. Poor tissue perfusion and hypoxia influence enzymatic pyruvate and lactate metabolism to stimulate anaerobic glycolysis and to decrease lactate utilization. This leads to hyperlactatemia and lactic acidosis. The mortality rate of this type of lactic acidosis may be as high as 80% and correlates with the degree of hyperlactatemia.

Lactic acidosis associated with liver disease, drugs (e.g., metformin), toxins, and congenital enzyme deficiency may be due to deranged oxidative metabolism or impaired lactate clearance.[4,15] The exact role of diabetes mellitus in the induction of lactic acidosis is not clear. It may involve a decrease in pyruvate dehydrogenase activity, the enzyme responsible for pyruvate metabolism. Lactic acidosis in neoplastic disease is uncommon and reported mostly in patients with myeloproliferative disorders. Leukocytes and neoplastic cells in general have high rates of glycolysis. In the case of a large tumor or tightly packed bone marrow, oxygenation can be decreased, favoring the accumulation of lactate. Lactic acidosis has been reported in patients with massive liver tumors, and it has been postulated that the liver uptake of lactate is decreased in these patients. Lactic acidosis associated with seizures is usually transient and occurs because of excessive muscle activity.[7]

CLINICAL PRESENTATION

Chronic metabolic acidosis is usually not associated with severe acidemia and is relatively asymptomatic. The major manifestations are in the bones, where chronic acidemia causes bone demineralization with the development of rickets in children and osteomalacia and osteopenia in adults. In infants and children, chronic metabolic acidosis is associated with growth failure and short stature and may be associated with nonspecific symptoms including anorexia, nausea, weight loss, and muscle weakness.

CLINICAL PRESENTATION OF METABOLIC ACIDOSIS

GENERAL
The patient is usually relatively asymptomatic if the acidosis is acute and mild. In those with severe acidemia (pH <7.15 to 7.20) the cardiovascular, respiratory, and central nervous systems may be affected.

SYMPTOMS
The patient may complain of loss of appetite, nausea, and vomiting.

SIGNS
Cardiac: Flushing, a rapid heart rate, wide pulse pressure, and an increase in cardiac output may be seen initially. This may be followed by a reduction in cardiac output, blood pressure, and liver and kidney blood flow.
Cerebral: Obtundation or coma.
Metabolic: Insulin resistance; increased protein degradation; increased metabolic demands.
Gastrointestinal: Nausea, vomiting, loss of appetite.
Respiratory: Dyspnea, hyperventilation with deep, rapid respirations is seen in those with severe acidosis.
Chronic acidemia causes bone demineralization with the development of rickets in children and osteomalacia and osteopenia in adults.

LABORATORY TESTS
Hyperglycemia and hyperkalemia are common. In those with severe acidosis the pH is <7.2

Severe metabolic acidosis is usually associated with acute processes. The manifestations of severe acidemia (pH <7.15 to 7.20) involve the cardiovascular, respiratory, and central nervous systems. Hyperventilation is often the first sign of metabolic acidosis. At a pH of 7.2, pulmonary ventilation increases about fourfold and an eightfold increase has been noted at a pH of 7.[17] Respiratory compensation may occur as Kussmaul's respirations—the deep, rapid respirations seen commonly in patients with diabetic ketoacidosis. In extremely severe acidosis (pH <6.8), central nervous system (CNS) function is disrupted to such a degree that the respiratory center is depressed.

CNS depression correlates more closely with spinal fluid pH than with blood pH. For this reason, neurologic symptoms tend to occur more frequently and to a greater degree in patients with respiratory acidosis, because the CO_2 accumulated in the respiratory form readily crosses the blood-brain barrier to cause acidosis in the CNS.[1] Because of the slow penetration of administered bicarbonate into the CNS, the CNS pH fails to normalize as rapidly as blood pH. Therefore patients continue to hyperventilate because of sustained CNS acidity, and severe respiratory alkalosis may occur. Sustained lowering of the $PaCO_2$ within 12 to 36 hours is to be anticipated during the correction of any metabolic acidosis.[1]

Systemic acidosis can cause peripheral arteriolar dilatation, characterized by flushing, a rapid heart rate, and wide pulse pressure. Initially, cardiac output may be increased, but as acidosis becomes more severe, myocardial contractility becomes impaired and cardiac output falls. The effects of vagal stimulation are also enhanced at pH levels lower than 7.1, probably as a consequence of inhibition of acetylcholinesterase. This increases the danger of vagally mediated bradycardia and heart block during acidosis.

Gastrointestinal symptoms of metabolic acidosis include loss of appetite, nausea, and vomiting. Severe acidosis (pH <7.1) interferes with carbohydrate metabolism and insulin utilization, and results in hyperglycemia. Metabolic acidosis alters potassium homeostasis and contributes to the development of hyperkalemia. The magnitude of the effect on serum potassium depends on the type of acidosis: Acidosis caused by mineral acids (e.g., hydrochloric acid) are associated with a greater change in potassium levels than acidosis caused by organic acids (e.g., lactic acidosis), in which the increase in potassium attributable to the acidosis per se is minimal.

COMPENSATION

5 The patient's primary means to compensate for metabolic acidosis is to increase carbon dioxide excretion by increasing respiratory rate. This results in a decrease in $PaCO_2$. This ventilatory compensation results from stimulation of the respiratory center by changes in cerebral bicarbonate concentration and pH.[1] For every 1-mEq/L decrease in bicarbonate concentration below the average of 24, the $PaCO_2$ decreases by about 1 to 1.5 mm Hg from the normal value of 40 (see Table 51–4).

The anticipated $PaCO_2$ associated with a given bicarbonate concentration for patients with uncomplicated metabolic acidosis can be calculated as:[18]

$$PaCO_2 = (1.5 \times [HCO_3^-]) + 8] \pm 2$$

For example, 95% of patients with a plasma bicarbonate of 16 mEq/L should have an arterial PCO_2 of 30 to 34 mm Hg. An observed arterial PCO_2 within this range is consistent with physiologic respiratory compensation for a metabolic acidosis, and suggests that there is no respiratory disturbance. In contrast, if the PCO_2 is less than 30 mm Hg, a superimposed respiratory alkalosis may be present, whereas if the PCO_2 is greater than 34 mm Hg, a superimposed respiratory acidosis is present.

▶ TREATMENT: Metabolic Acidosis

▨ CHRONIC METABOLIC ACIDOSIS

6 Asymptomatic patients with mild to moderate degrees of acidemia (plasma bicarbonate of 12 to 20 mEq/L; pH of 7.2 to 7.4) do not require emergent therapy. They can usually be managed with gradual correction of the acidemia, over a period of days to weeks, using oral sodium bicarbonate or other alkali preparations (Table 51–7). In all forms of chronic metabolic acidosis, primary therapy should be directed at treating the underlying disease state.

TABLE 51–7. Therapeutic Alternatives for Oral Alkali Replacement

Generic Name	Trade Name(s)	Milliequivalents of Alkali	Dosage Form (s)	Comment
Shohl's solution Sodium citrate/citric acid	Bicitra (Willen)	1 mEq Na/mL; equivalent to 1 mEq bicarbonate	Solution (500 mg Na citrate, 334 mg citric acid/5 mL)	Citrate preparations increase absorption of aluminum
Sodium bicarbonate	Various (e.g., Rugby)	3.9 mEq bicarbonate/tablet (325 mg) 7.8 mEq bicarbonate/ tablet (650 mg)	325 mg tablet 650 mg tablet	Bicarbonate preparations may cause bloating due to CO_2 production
	Baking soda (various)	60 mEq bicarbonate/tsp (5 g/tsp)	Powder	
Potassium citrate	Urocit-K (Mission)	5 mEq citrate/tablet	5 mEq tablet	See above
Potassium bicarbonate/ potassium citrate	K-Lyte (Bristol)	25 mEq bicarbonate/tablet	25 mEq tablet (effervescent)	
	K-Lyte DS (Bristol)	50 mEq bicarbonate/tablet (double strength)	50 mEq tablet (effervescent)	See above
Potassium citrate/citric acid	Polycitra-K (Willen)	2 mEq K/mL; equivalent to 2 mEq bicarbonate 30 mEq bicarbonate/unit dose packet	Solution (1100 mg K citrate, 334 mg citric acid/5 mL) Crystals for reconstitution (3300 mg K citrate, 1002 mg citric acid/unit dose packet)	See above
Sodium citrate/potassium citrate/citric acid	Polycitra (Willen) Polycitra-LC (Willen)	1 mEq K, 1 mEq Na/mL; equivalent to 2 mEq bicarbonate	Syrup (Polycitra) Solution (Polycitra-LC) (Both contain 550 mg K citrate, 500 mg Na citrate, 334 mg citric acid/5 mL)	See above

Gastrointestinal pathology should be treated to reduce ongoing bicarbonate losses, and factors that exacerbate RTA should be treated. If acidemia persists, alkali therapy should be instituted, with the goal of normalization of blood pH. The loading dose (LD) of alkali to initially correct the acidemia can be calculated as follows:[19]

$$LD(mEqs) = (V_D HCO_3^- \times body\ weight\ [BW])$$
$$\times (desired\ [HCO_3^-] - current\ [HCO_3^-])$$

For a 60-kg patient with a serum bicarbonate of 15 mEq/L, the loading dose is calculated thusly:

$$LD(mEqs) = (0.5\ L/kg \times 60\ kg) \times (24\ mEq/L - 15\ mEq/L)$$
$$= 30\ L \times 9\ mEq/L$$
$$= 270\ mEqs$$

The calculated loading dose of alkali should be administered over several days to avoid volume overload from the accompanying sodium load. For this scenario, a regimen of 60 to 70 mEq three times a day for 3 to 5 days should result in an increase in HCO_3^- levels toward normal. In addition to the calculated loading dose, supplemental alkali must also be provided to replace ongoing losses, which can be approximated to be 2 mEq/kg per day or 40 mEq three times a day. In patients with associated volume depletion, bicarbonate replacement can be provided simultaneous with volume resuscitation by substituting bicarbonate for chloride in intravenous crystalloid solutions.

In patients with chronic metabolic acidosis because of gastrointestinal bicarbonate losses, maintenance therapy should provide sufficient alkali to replace ongoing bicarbonate losses. The magnitude of this replacement is variable and may be substantial (>10 mEq/kg per day). In addition, associated losses of other electrolytes, such as potassium and magnesium, may need to be replaced (see Chap. 50).

Proximal (type II) RTA is a bicarbonate-wasting disorder that requires the administration of large maintenance doses of alkali (10 to 15 mEq/kg per day). As alkali replacement raises the serum bicarbon-

ate concentration toward normal, the proximal tubule's capacity to reabsorb bicarbonate is overwhelmed and renal bicarbonate wasting increases. In children, aggressive therapy of proximal RTA is necessary to avoid growth retardation and osteopenia. Because this is generally a mild, nonprogressive acidosis in adults, the benefit of alkali therapy is frequently outweighed by the risks of increased potassium wasting. In patients with classic distal (type I) RTA, maintenance therapy usually requires only enough alkali to buffer the amount of acid generated from dietary intake and metabolism. This usually approximates 1 to 3 mEq/kg per day.

After initial potassium deficits are replaced, ongoing potassium supplementation may not be required, as renal potassium losses decrease following initiation of appropriate alkali therapy. The use of potassium alkali salts may, however, be desirable in patients with associated nephrolithiasis, because sodium salts may increase urinary calcium excretion.

The metabolic acidosis associated with hyperkalemic distal (type IV) RTA with hyporeninemic-hypoaldosteronemia that is often seen in patients with diabetes mellitus may be corrected by the treatment of hyperkalemia alone (see Chap. 50). The use of supplemental alkali (1 to 2 mEq/kg per day) to increase sodium intake and stimulate distal tubular potassium secretion may be beneficial. A minority of patients require the administration of pharmacologic amounts of fludrocortisone.[4] Type IV RTA resulting from a generalized distal tubular disorder often responds to low doses of alkali (1.5 to 2.0 mEq/kg per day).[20] Corrections of the acidosis along with modest dietary potassium restriction (to 1 mEq/kg per day) will often result in the maintenance of serum potassium levels of 5 mEq/L or less.

ACUTE SEVERE METABOLIC ACIDOSIS

The management of patients with life-threatening acute metabolic acidosis (plasma bicarbonate of 8 mEq/L and pH

<7.20) is dependent on the underlying cause and the patient's cardio-vascular status. Patients with hyperchloremic acidosis (e.g., diarrhea-induced) are unable to regenerate bicarbonate, and the generation of new bicarbonate by the kidneys may require several days before one can observe a meaningful change in their status.[14] Thus intravenous alkali therapy is often required for these patients.

CLINICAL CONTROVERSY

The role of alkali therapy in patients with severe lactic acidosis is controversial. Treatment should be directed at the underlying causes since serial bicarbonate administration is often not effective and in some settings may be deleterious.

Although conventional wisdom recommends the use of alkali replacement in patients with severe acidemia caused by the deleterious effects of acidemia on circulatory function,[7,14,15] studies have not demonstrated improved outcome with alkali replacement.[21–24]

There are several therapeutic alternatives available for the acute correction of severe metabolic acidosis. Sodium acetate, sodium citrate, and sodium lactate are unreliable sources of alkali because their alkalinizing effect is dependent on their oxidative conversion to bicarbonate. This process is often impaired in critically ill patients, especially those with liver disease or circulatory failure. Although sodium bicarbonate is the most widely used intravenous alkalitic agent,[14] several studies suggest that it is frequently ineffective and may actually be deleterious, especially in patients with lactic acidosis.[21–24] Two of the three remaining alternatives (carbicarb and dichloroacetate) are investigational and not available in most clinical settings. Tromethamine, or THAM, is a carbon dioxide–consuming, commercially available solution that buffers respiratory as well as metabolic acids.

▒ SODIUM BICARBONATE

In theory, sodium bicarbonate administration provides fluid and electrolyte replacement and increases arterial pH, thereby improving cardiac function, perfusion and oxygenation of peripheral tissues, and intracellular pH, and should therefore decrease lactate production and increase clearance. However, sodium bicarbonate administration can actually have an adverse effect on intracellular pH. When bicarbonate is given by IV infusion, the carbon dioxide generated diffuses more readily than bicarbonate across cell membranes and into cerebrospinal fluid. Therefore the intracellular pH can actually be decreased by administration of bicarbonate.[4]

CLINICAL CONTROVERSY

Although it has been recommended that sodium bicarbonate be administered to raise the arterial pH to about 7.15 to 7.20, there are no controlled clinical trials demonstrating that sodium bicarbonate administration is significantly better than general supportive care in reducing morbidity and mortality in these patients.[4,14,21–24]

Excessive sodium bicarbonate administration may result in (1) a shift of the oxyhemoglobin saturation curve to the left, and thereby impaired oxygen release from hemoglobin to tissues; (2) sodium and water overload, with subsequent pulmonary congestion and hypernatremia; (3) paradoxical acidosis as a result of the production of CO_2 that freely diffuses into myocardial and cerebral cells;[25] and (4) decreased ionized calcium with resultant decreased

myocardial contractility. If there is an endogenous source of bicarbonate, such as can occur in the case of ketoacidosis or lactic acidosis, a bicarbonate "overshoot" may develop because the ketoacids (acetoacetic acid and β-hydroxybutyric acid) or lactic acid are converted in the liver to bicarbonate once the underlying cause of acidosis is corrected.[12,14,26] Alkalosis may also result if too much is given too fast.

If intravenous sodium bicarbonate is used, one must be mindful that the goals are to increase, not normalize, pH (to approximately 7.20) and plasma bicarbonate (to 8 to 10 mEq/L). There is no calculative method that will assure attainment of these goals with a given dose of sodium bicarbonate because of the multiplicity of competing processes that can affect acid-base status (vomiting, potential increases in endogenous acid production, and renal failure) and the marked variability in the volume of distribution of bicarbonate (50% of body weight in patients with mild acidosis to approximately 100% in those with severe acidosis).[19] Adrogue and Madias[14] recommended that the dose of sodium bicarbonate be calculated using a distribution volume of 50% of body weight for all patients to avoid overtreatment. The total dose calculated as described previously in the RTA section should be administered as an infusion over one-half to several hours. Follow-up monitoring of arterial blood gases beginning no sooner than 30 minutes after the end of the infusion should be used to guide further therapeutic decisions.

Bicarbonate therapy is generally not necessary in the routine patient with cardiac arrest, even if the initial arrest was unmonitored. The standards and guidelines from the National Conference on Cardiopulmonary and Emergency Cardiac Care state that sodium bicarbonate is most useful in cardiac life support when combined with ventilation in an attempt to maintain near-normal arterial pH during an arrest.[27] During a cardiac arrest, sodium bicarbonate (initial dose 1 mEq/kg) may be administered by rapid, direct intravenous injection. It should be used only after more proven interventions such as defibrillation, cardiac compression, support of ventilation including intubation, and drug therapies such as epinephrine and antiarrhythmic agents have been employed. Subsequent doses of sodium bicarbonate should be based on measurements of arterial blood pH and Pa_{CO_2}.

▒ TROMETHAMINE

THAM, available as a 0.3 N solution, is a highly alkaline, sodium-free organic amine that acts as a proton acceptor to prevent or correct acidosis.[28] Tromethamine combines with hydrogen ions from carbonic acid to form bicarbonate and a cationic buffer. THAM also acts as an osmotic diuretic to increase urine flow, urine pH, and the excretion of fixed acids, CO_2, and electrolytes. At pH 7.4, 30% of THAM is not ionized and therefore may penetrate into cells and neutralize acidic anions of the intracellular fluid. Intracellular pH increases have been noted within 1 hour after the infusion of THAM. There is, however, no clinical or physiologic evidence that this action is beneficial, or that THAM is more efficacious than sodium bicarbonate.[14,29]

When THAM is used, it must be administered slowly, with careful monitoring to avoid alkalosis. The usual empiric dosage range for tromethamine is 1 to 5 mmol/kg administered intravenously over 1 hour, but doses up to 1.25 mmol/kg may be given over 5 to 15 minutes in acute situations. The dose of THAM can be individualized using the following equation:[28]

$$\text{Dose of THAM (in mLs)} = 1.1 \times \text{BW (in kilograms)}$$

$$\times \text{ base deficit}$$

where base deficit = normal $[HCO_3^-]$ minus current $[HCO_3^-]$.

The need for additional THAM is determined by serial measurements of the serum bicarbonate concentration and calculation of the base deficit. Large doses may cause respiratory depression as a result of an increase in blood pH and a decrease in $PaCO_2$ concentration.[29] Tromethamine solution is highly alkaline and may cause severe inflammation, vascular spasm, or tissue damage (necrosis, sloughing, pain, chemical phlebitis, or thrombosis) if infiltration occurs. Hyperkalemia, hypoglycemia, hypocalcemia, and impaired coagulation have also been reported.[29,30] This agent should only be used with extreme caution in patients with severe liver or kidney failure.

CARBICARB

Carbicarb is an equimolar mixture of sodium carbonate (Na_2CO_3) and sodium bicarbonate ($NaHCO_3$).[31,32] It is no longer commercially available in Canada, and its use in the United States is still investigational. The carbonate ion is a stronger base than bicarbonate, and thus preferentially buffers hydrogen ions. The result of this reaction is the formation of bicarbonate rather than CO_2. Thus carbicarb limits, but does not eliminate, the generation of CO_2. Unlike bicarbonate, which can produce a paradoxical intracellular acidosis and thereby impair cardiac function, carbicarb appears to correct intracellular acidosis if present.[33,34] In a prospective, double-blind, randomized, multicenter trial, Leung and colleagues[31] compared carbicarb to sodium bicarbonate in surgical patients with mild intraoperative metabolic acidosis. Carbicarb proved as effective as sodium bicarbonate in correcting mild metabolic acidosis. Furthermore, cardiac output increased with carbicarb as compared to sodium bicarbonate. Carbicarb also appears to be beneficial in the management of lactic acidosis.

Although the optimal dosage of carbicarb has not been determined, it can be approximated as:[31]

Dose (in milliequivalents of Na)

$$= 0.2 \text{ L/kg} \times \text{BW (in kilograms)} \times \text{(base deficit)}$$

The risk of hypervolemia and hypertonicity after carbicarb administration is similar to that of bicarbonate. The small number of trials reporting the clinical utility of this agent and its continued investigational status in most of the world limits its use and availability for the foreseeable future.

DICHLOROACETATE

Dichloroacetate (DCA), another investigational agent, significantly lowers serum lactate levels and increases blood pH in patients with lactic acidosis.[35,36] DCA facilitates aerobic lactate metabolism by stimulating the activity of lactate dehydrogenase, reverses hyperlactatemia, and decreases morbidity in acquired and congenital forms of lactic acidosis. In a randomized, multicenter, placebo-controlled trial, Stacpoole and associates[35] studied the effects of DCA (50 to 100 mg/kg) in 252 patients with lactic acidosis. Serum lactate was significantly lowered and blood pH increased, but there was no improvement in patient outcome as compared to conventional management. A subsequent study in patients undergoing liver transplantation demonstrated that DCA attenuated lactate acid accumulation and reduced the need for bicarbonate therapy in this high-risk patient population.[37] The drug also improves cardiac output and left ventricular mechanical efficiency under conditions of myocardial ischemia or failure, probably by facilitating myocardial glucose utilization and inhibiting gluconeogenesis. DCA administration has also been reported to reverse the abnormal glucose metabolism, branched chain amino acid utilization, and muscle catabolism in septic patients.[38] DCA can cause a reversible peripheral neuropathy that may be ameliorated or prevented with thiamine supplementation. Mild drowsiness has been reported in approximately half of the adult recipients, but no other drug-related adverse effects have been reported.[36] The future role of DCA in the management of metabolic acidosis, particularly lactic acidosis, remains to be clarified.

METABOLIC ALKALOSIS

PATHOPHYSIOLOGY

Metabolic alkalosis is a simple acid-base disorder that presents as alkalemia (increased arterial pH) with an increase in plasma bicarbonate. It is an extremely common entity in hospitalized patients with acid-base disturbances. Under normal circumstances, the kidney is readily able to excrete an alkali load. Thus evaluation of patients with metabolic alkalosis must consider two separate issues: (1) the initial process that generates the metabolic alkalosis; and (2) alterations in renal function that maintain the alkalemic state.[39,40]

Generation

The generation of metabolic alkalosis can also result from excessive losses of H^+ via the kidneys or from the gain of exogenous bicarbonate-rich fluids. Gastric secretory volume is usually less than 50 mL/h in the basal state, but may increase up to fivefold with stimulation. The gastric juice is rich in chloride and H^+. In the gastric parietal cells, hydrogen ion and bicarbonate are generated from CO_2 and water.[40] The hydrogen ion is secreted into gastric fluid and the bicarbonate is retained in the ECF. Normally, an amount of bicarbonate equal to the bicarbonate generated in the stomach is eliminated in the alkaline pancreatic and small-bowel secretions, maintaining hydrogen ion balance. With vomiting and nasogastric suctioning, hydrogen ion is lost externally and metabolic alkalosis

results. Diarrhea, as seen with secretory villous adenomas and other secretory diarrheas, often results in excessive gastrointestinal losses of chloride-rich, bicarbonate-poor fluid and thus leads to the generation of metabolic alkalosis.

Diuretic agents acting on the thick ascending limb of the loop of Henle (e.g., furosemide, bumetanide, and torsemide) and distal convoluted tubule (thiazides), have most commonly been associated with the generation of metabolic alkalosis.[41] These agents promote the excretion of sodium and potassium almost exclusively in association with chloride, without a proportionate increase in bicarbonate excretion. Collecting duct hydrogen ion secretion is stimulated directly by the increased luminal flow rate and sodium delivery, and indirectly by intravascular volume contraction, which results in secondary hyperaldosteronism. Renal ammoniagenesis may also be stimulated by concomitant hypokalemia, further augmenting net acid excretion.

Increased renal acid excretion may also be the result of excess mineralocorticoid activity. Elevated mineralocorticoid levels directly stimulate collecting duct hydrogen ion secretion and indirectly increase ammoniagenesis by causing hypokalemia.[17] Increased mineralocorticoid activity may result from Cushing's syndrome, primary hyperaldosteronism, or hyperaldosteronism secondary to increased renin activity (e.g., malignant hypertension). In Bartter's and Gitelman's syndromes, defects in sodium transport in the loop of Henle (Bartter's) or distal convoluted tubule (Gitelman's) lead to hypokalemia, secondary hyperaldosteronism, and metabolic alkalosis.[40] In Liddle's syndrome, enhanced sodium reabsorption by the cortical collecting duct epithelial sodium channel results in a syndrome of pseudohyperaldosteronism.[39] Administration of high doses of penicillins (e.g., ticarcillin) may produce metabolic alkalosis because they act as nonreabsorbable anions. High concentrations of poorly reabsorbable anions in the distal renal tubule increase luminal flow rate and luminal electronegativity, which enhances the secretion of potassium and hydrogen ion and results in hypokalemia and metabolic alkalosis.

Metabolic alkalosis may also be generated by the gain of exogenous alkali. This may be seen as a result of bicarbonate administration or from the infusion of organic anions that are metabolized to bicarbonate, such as acetate, lactate, and citrate. The milk-alkali syndrome was historically a common cause of metabolic alkalosis in patients with peptic ulcer disease secondary to the ingestion of large quantities of milk products and antacids. This syndrome has become increasingly uncommon with the advent of alternative effective therapies for dyspeptic syndromes.

Maintenance

No matter which condition initiated the metabolic alkalosis, abnormalities in renal function underlie its maintenance. Normally, the kidneys are capable of excreting all of the excess bicarbonate presented to them, even during periods of increased bicarbonate loads.[4] As the serum bicarbonate concentration increases, the filtered bicarbonate load exceeds the maximal rate for bicarbonate reabsorption, and the excess bicarbonate is excreted in the urine. Under normal circumstances, the excess bicarbonate is rapidly excreted and metabolic alkalosis does not occur, or is corrected in a matter of hours.[40]

Several mechanisms may impair renal bicarbonate excretion, and contribute to the maintenance phase of metabolic alkalosis.[39] In general, these mechanisms can be divided into volume-mediated processes (sodium chloride–responsive) and volume-independent processes (sodium chloride–resistant) that are predominantly associated with excess mineralocorticoid activity and hypokalemia (Table 51–8). Intravascular volume depletion maintains metabolic alkalosis through a number of mechanisms. Decreases in the glomerular filtration rate reduce the filtered load of bicarbonate at any given serum concentration, thereby decreasing the kidney's ability to excrete a bicarbonate load. While this may play a role in patients with chronic kidney disease, it is also an important factor in patients in whom intravascular volume contraction accompanies metabolic alkalosis. Decreased effective arterial blood volume also enhances proximal and distal tubular sodium reabsorption. Sodium reabsorption must be coupled with reabsorption of an anion, such as chloride or bicarbonate, or exchange with a cation, such as potassium or hydrogen, in order to maintain charge neutrality. In the proximal tubule, increased sodium reabsorption stimulates bicarbonate reabsorption. In the distal nephron, enhanced sodium reabsorption, particularly in the setting of hypokalemia, stimulates hydrogen ion secretion.

Mineralocorticoid excess also plays a significant role in the maintenance of metabolic alkalosis. In patients with volume-responsive metabolic alkalosis, intravascular volume depletion stimulates aldosterone secretion. As discussed earlier, excess mineralocorticoid activity may also underlie the generation of metabolic alkalosis. In either situation, the increased mineralocorticoid effect stimulates collecting duct H^+ secretion. Metabolic alkalosis may also be maintained by persistent hypokalemia. Hypokalemia has a multitude of effects on renal acid-base homeostasis, enhancing proximal tubular bicarbonate reabsorption, stimulating ammoniagenesis and increasing distal tubular H^+ secretion.[40]

TABLE 51–8. Courses of Metabolic Alkalosis Differentiated on the Basis of Their Responsiveness to Sodium Chloride

Sodium chloride–responsive (urinary chloride concentration <10 mEq/L)
Gastrointestinal disorders
  Vomiting
  Gastric drainage
  Villous adenoma of the colon
  Chloride diarrhea
Diuretic therapy
Correction of chronic hypercapnia
Cystic fibrosis
Excessive bicarbonate therapy of an organic acidosis
Mild/moderate potassium deficiency

Sodium chloride–resistant (urinary chloride concentration >20 mEq/L)
Excess mineralocorticoid activity
  Hyperaldosteronism
  Cushing's syndrome
  Bartter's syndrome
  Gitelman's syndrome
Excessive black licorice intake
Profound potassium depletion
Magnesium deficiency
Liddle's syndrome

Unclassified
Alkali administration
Milk-alkali syndrome
Massive blood or plasma protein fraction transfusion
Nonparathyroid hypercalcemia
Carbohydrate refeeding after starvation
Large doses of penicillin

CLINICAL PRESENTATION

There are no unique signs or symptoms associated with mild to moderate metabolic alkalosis, but patients may complain of symptoms related to the underlying cause of the disorder (e.g., muscle weakness with hypokalemia or postural dizziness with volume depletion). They may have a history of vomiting, gastric drainage, or diuretic use, all of which contribute to the development of metabolic alkalosis. Severe alkalemia (blood pH >7.60) has been associated with cardiac arrhythmias, particularly in patients with heart disease, and hyperventilation with hypoxemia.[42] Neuromuscular irritability may be present, with signs of tetany or hyperactive reflexes, possibly caused by the decreased ionized calcium concentration that occurs secondary to the increase in pH. This decrease in ionized calcium may be caused by a conformational change in the albumin molecules to which the calcium is bound, resulting in increased binding, or by decreased competition from hydrogen ions for binding sites on the albumin molecule. Mental confusion, muscle cramping, and paresthesias may also occur.

COMPENSATION

The respiratory response to metabolic alkalosis is hypoventilation, which results in an increased $PaCO_2$. Respiratory compensation is initiated within hours when the central and peripheral chemoreceptors sense an increase in pH. The $PaCO_2$ increases 6 to 7 mm Hg for each 10-mEq/L increase in bicarbonate, up to a $PaCO_2$ of about 50 to 60 mm Hg (see Table 51–4) before hypoxia sensors react to prevent further hypoventilation. If the $PaCO_2$ is normal or less than normal, one should consider the presence of a superimposed respiratory alkalosis, which may be secondary to fever, gram-negative sepsis, or pain.

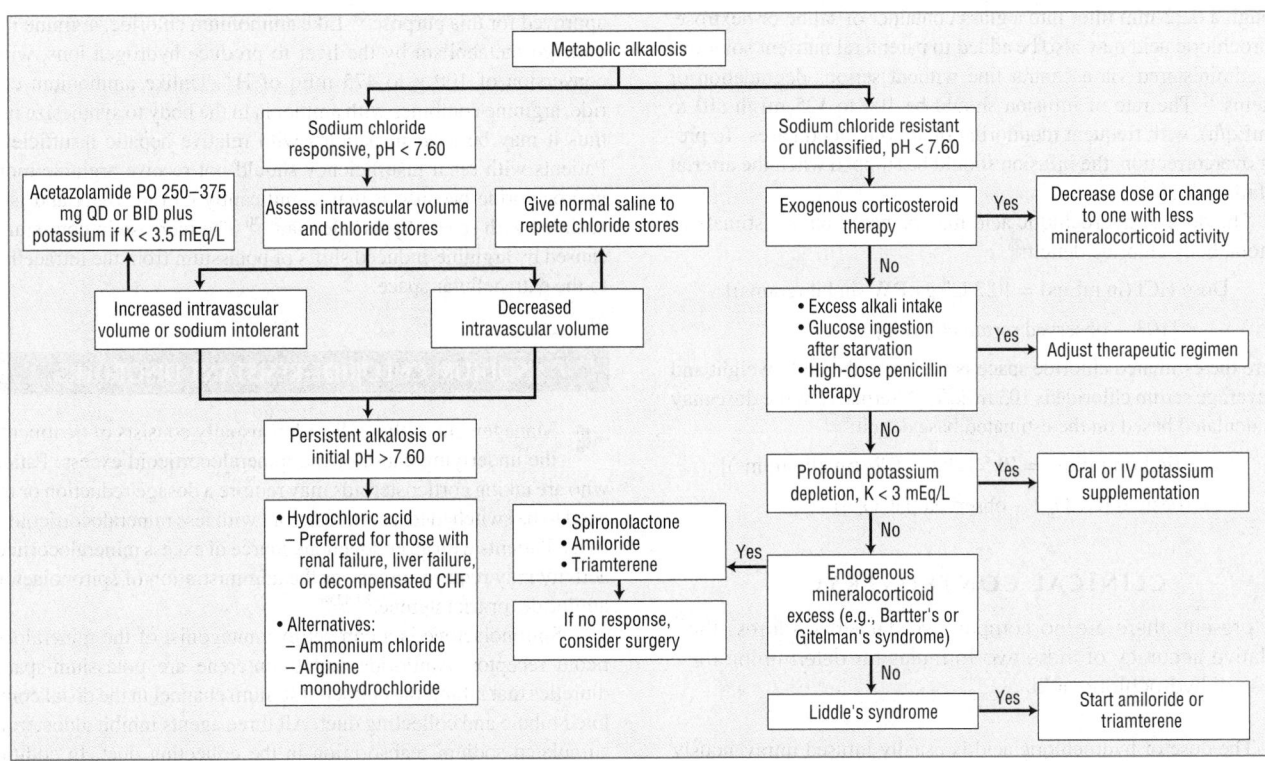

FIGURE 51–5. Treatment algorithm for patients with primary metabolic alkalosis.

▶ TREATMENT: Metabolic Alkalosis

Treatment of metabolic alkalosis should be aimed at correcting the factor(s) responsible for the maintenance of the alkalosis.[39,40,42] For example, vomiting should be treated with antiemetics, gastric losses of H^+ during nasogastric suction may be modulated by giving histamine blockers such as ranitidine or proton pump inhibitors such as omeprazole, and reducing or discontinuing diuretic therapy.[43,44] Metabolic alkalosis will persist until the renal mechanism responsible for maintaining the disorder is corrected, despite the fact that the original cause of the elevated plasma bicarbonate may have resolved. For example, hypovolemia should be treated with sodium chloride (i.e., diuretic abuse or nasogastric suction) to allow excretion of bicarbonate by the kidney. However, patients with severely compromised cardiovascular function may not be able to tolerate this therapeutic approach. In situations such as this and/or the presence of life-threatening alkalosis, some have advocated reduction in pH by control of ventilation.[4] Although controlled hypoventilation, sometimes using inspired CO_2 with supplemental oxygen to prevent hypoxia may be life-saving,[4] this approach is not universally accepted.[40,42] Therapy for metabolic alkalosis can be conceptualized on the basis of the sodium chloride responsiveness of the disorders as shown in Fig. 51–5.

SODIUM CHLORIDE–RESPONSIVE DISORDERS

Sodium chloride–responsive disorders usually result from volume depletion and chloride loss, which may accompany severe vomiting, prolonged nasogastric suction, and diuretic therapy. Initially therapy is directed at expanding intravascular volume and replenishing chloride stores. Sodium and potassium chloride–containing solutions should be administered to patients who can tolerate the volume load.[40,42] Patients with metabolic alkalosis who are volume overloaded or intolerant to volume administration because of congestive heart failure may benefit from the carbonic anhydrase inhibitor acetazolamide. This agent inhibits the action of carbonic anhydrase, thereby inhibiting renal bicarbonate reabsorption. Unfortunately, it also increases the renal losses of potassium and phosphate. Administration of acetazolamide (250 to 375 mg once or twice daily) may promote a sufficient bicarbonate diuresis and return the pH toward normal. However, because the clinical effectiveness of the drug declines as the HCO_3^- concentration falls, only rarely will this approach fully correct the alkalosis.[39]

Acidifying agents including hydrochloric acid, ammonium chloride, and arginine monohydrochloride may be used to treat severe (pH >7.6) symptomatic metabolic alkalosis. In general, this management is reserved for patients who are unresponsive to conventional fluid and electrolyte management or who are unable to tolerate the requisite volume load because of decompensated congestive heart failure or advanced renal failure.[39,42] Alternatively, hemodialysis using a low-bicarbonate dialysate may be used for the rapid correction of metabolic acidosis.

HYDROCHLORIC ACID

Hydrochloric acid is usually infused intravenously via a large central vein as a 0.1 to 0.25 N HCl solution in either 5% dextrose or normal saline, although sterile water has also been used. Extemporaneously prepared solutions can be made by adding 100 to 250 mEq of HCl through a 0.22-mm filter into a glass container of saline or dextrose. Hydrochloric acid may also be added to parenteral nutrient solutions and administered via a central line without serious degradation of proteins.[45] The rate of infusion should be 100 to 125 mL/h (10 to 25 mEq/h), with frequent monitoring of arterial blood gases. To prevent overcorrection, the infusion should be stopped when the arterial pH falls to 7.50.[40]

The dose of hydrochloric acid may be based on an estimate of the total body chloride deficit:[28]

$$\text{Dose HCl (in mEqs)} = [0.2 \text{ L/kg} \times \text{BW (in kilograms)}]$$

$$\times [103 - \text{observed serum chloride}]$$

where the estimated chloride space is 0.2 times the body weight and the average serum chloride is 103 mEq/L. Alternatively, the dose may be calculated based on the estimated base deficit:[42]

$$\text{Dose HCl (in mEqs)} = [0.5 \text{ L/kg} \times \text{BW (in kilograms)}]$$

$$\times (\text{desired } [HCO_3^-] - \text{observed } [HCO_3^-])$$

CLINICAL CONTROVERSY

At present, there are no comparative data that address the relative accuracy of these two formulas for determining the dose of hydrochloric acid.

The dose of hydrochloric acid is usually infused intravenously over 12 to 24 hours.[49] A severe transient respiratory acidosis may occur if the hydrochloric acid is infused too quickly because of the slower reduction of the elevated bicarbonate concentration in the cerebrospinal fluid than in the extracellular fluid. Improvement is usually seen within 24 hours of initiating therapy. Arterial blood gases and serum electrolytes should be drawn every 4 to 8 hours to evaluate and adjust therapy.

AMMONIUM CHLORIDE

Ammonium chloride has a limited role in the treatment of metabolic alkalosis. The liver converts ammonium chloride to urea and free hydrochloric acid:[28]

$$2NH_4Cl + 2HCO_3^- \rightarrow CO(NH_2)_2 + CO_2 + 3H_2O + 2Cl^-$$

The dose of ammonium chloride can be calculated on the basis of the chloride deficit using the same method as for HCl, using the conversion of 20 g ammonium chloride providing 374 mEq of H^+. However, only half of the calculated dose of ammonium chloride should be administered so as to avoid ammonia toxicity. Ammonium chloride is available as a 26.75% solution containing 100 mEq in 20 mL, which should be further diluted prior to administration. A dilute solution may be prepared by adding 100 mEq of ammonium chloride to 500 mL of normal saline and infusing the solution at a rate of no more than 1 mEq/min. Improvement in metabolic status is usually seen within 24 hours. CNS toxicity, marked by confusion, irritability, seizures, and coma, has been associated with more rapid rates of administration. Ammonium chloride must be administered cautiously to patients with renal or hepatic impairment. In patients with hepatic dysfunction, impaired conversion of ammonia to urea may result in increased ammonia levels and worsened encephalopathy. In patients with renal failure, the increased urea synthesis may exacerbate uremic symptoms.[28]

ARGININE MONOHYDROCHLORIDE

Arginine monohydrochloride at a dose of 10 g/h given intravenously has been used to treat metabolic alkalosis, although it was never FDA-

approved for this purpose.[28] Like ammonium chloride, arginine must undergo metabolism by the liver to produce hydrogen ions, with a conversion of 100 g to 475 mEq of H^+. Unlike ammonium chloride, arginine combines with ammonia in the body to synthesize urea; thus it may be used in patients with relative hepatic insufficiency. Patients with renal insufficiency should not receive arginine monohydrochloride because it may significantly elevate BUN and is associated with severe hyperkalemia.[28,30] The increase in potassium is caused by arginine-induced shifts of potassium from the intracellular to the extracellular space.

SODIUM CHLORIDE-RESISTANT DISORDERS

Management of these disorders usually consists of treatment of the underlying cause of the mineralocorticoid excess. Patients who are taking corticosteroids may require a dosage reduction or may need to be switched to a corticosteroid with less mineralocorticoid activity. Patients with an endogenous source of excess mineralocorticoid activity may require surgery or the administration of spironolactone, amiloride, or triamterene.[39,42,46]

Spironolactone is a competitive antagonist of the mineralocorticoid receptor. Amiloride and triamterene are potassium-sparing diuretics that inhibit the epithelial sodium channel in the distal convoluted tubule and collecting duct. All three agents inhibit aldosterone-stimulated sodium reabsorption in the collecting duct. In addition, spironolactone directly inhibits aldosterone-stimulation of the hydrogen ion secretory pump. Thus most patients with mineralocorticoid excess, including Bartter's and Gitelman's syndromes, respond to therapy with these agents.[39,40,46] Liddle's syndrome, which is a form of pseudohyperaldosteronism caused by overactivity of the epithelial sodium channel, is not responsive to spironolactone, but may be treated with either amiloride or triamterene. Although experience is limited, some patients with Bartter's and Gitelman's syndromes may respond to nonsteroidal anti-inflammatory agents or angiotensin-converting enzyme inhibitors.[47,48] Finally, aggressive potassium repletion may correct the alkalosis in those who have not responded to the approaches outlined above.

RESPIRATORY ACID-BASE DISORDERS

As with the metabolic acid-base disturbances, there are two cardinal respiratory acid-base disturbances: respiratory acidosis and respiratory alkalosis. These disorders are generated by a primary alteration in carbon dioxide excretion, which changes the concentration of carbon dioxide, and therefore the carbonic acid concentration in body fluids. A primary reduction in $PaCO_2$ causes a rise in pH (respiratory alkalosis), and a primary increase in $PaCO_2$ causes a decrease in pH (respiratory acidosis). Unlike the metabolic disturbances, for which respiratory compensation is rapid, metabolic compensation for the respiratory disturbances is slow. Hence these disturbances can be further divided into acute disorders, with a duration of minutes to hours that is too short for metabolic compensation to have occurred, and chronic disorders, that have been present long enough for metabolic compensation to be complete.

RESPIRATORY ALKALOSIS

Respiratory alkalosis is characterized by a primary decrease in $PaCO_2$ that leads to an elevation in pH. The $PaCO_2$ falls when the excretion of CO_2 by the lungs exceeds the metabolic production of CO_2. It is the

TABLE 51–9. Causes of Respiratory Alkalosis

Central stimulation of respiration
Anxiety
Pain
Fever
Brain tumors, vascular accidents
Head trauma
Pregnancy
Progesterone
Catecholamines, theophylline, nicotine
Salicylates
Peripheral stimulation of respiration
Pulmonary emboli
Congestive heart failure
Altitude
Asthma
Pulmonary shunts
Hypotension
Pneumonia
"Stiff lungs" without hypoxemia
Multiple mechanisms
Hepatic cirrhosis
Gram-negative sepsis
Mechanical or voluntary hyperventilation

most frequently encountered acid-base disorder, occurring physiologically in normal pregnancy and in persons living at high altitudes.[49] Respiratory alkalosis also occurs frequently among hospitalized patients (Table 51–9).

PATHOPHYSIOLOGY

A decrease in $PaCO_2$ occurs when ventilatory excretion exceeds metabolic production. Because endogenous production of CO_2 is relatively constant, negative CO_2 balance is primarily caused by an increase in ventilatory excretion of CO_2 (hyperventilation). The metabolic production of CO_2, however, may be increased during periods of stress or with excess carbohydrate administration (e.g., parenteral nutrition). Hyperventilation may develop from an increase in neurochemical stimulation via either central or peripheral mechanisms, or be the result of voluntary or mechanical (iatrogenic) hyperventilation.

A decrease in $PaCO_2$ may occur in patients with cardiogenic, hypovolemic, or septic shock because oxygen delivery to the carotid and aortic chemoreceptors is reduced. This relative deficit in PaO_2 stimulates an increase in ventilation. The hyperventilation in sepsis is also mediated via a central mechanism. Hyperventilation-induced respiratory alkalosis with an elevation in cardiac index and hypotension without peripheral vasoconstriction may therefore be an early sign of sepsis.

CLINICAL PRESENTATION

Although most patients are asymptomatic, respiratory alkalosis may cause adverse neuromuscular, cardiovascular, and gastrointestinal effects.[49] During periods of decreased $PaCO_2$, there is a decrease in cerebral blood flow, which may be responsible for symptoms of light-headedness, confusion, decreased intellectual functioning, syncope, and seizures. Nausea and vomiting may occur, probably as a result of cerebral hypoxia. In severe respiratory alkalosis, cardiac arrhythmias may occur, due to sensitization of the myocardium to the

arrhythmogenic effects of circulating catecholamines.[2] Acute respiratory alkalosis has no effect on blood pressure or cardiac output in awake individuals. Anesthetized patients, however, may experience a decrease in both cardiac output and blood pressure, possibly owing to the lack of a tachycardic response.[50]

CLINICAL PRESENTATION OF RESPIRATORY ALKALOSIS

GENERAL
The patient is usually asymptomatic if the condition is chronic and mild.

SYMPTOMS
The patient may complain of light-headedness, confusion, muscle cramps and tetany, and decreased intellectual functioning.
Nausea and vomiting may occur, probably as a result of cerebral hypoxia.

SIGNS
In severe respiratory alkalosis pH >7.60
Syncope and seizures
Cardiac arrhythmias
Hyperventilation

LABORATORY TESTS
Serum chloride concentration is usually slightly increased.
Serum ionized calcium, potassium, and phosphorus concentration may be decreased.

The concentration of serum electrolytes may also be altered secondary to the development of respiratory alkalosis. The serum chloride concentration is usually slightly increased, and serum potassium concentration may be slightly decreased. Clinically significant hypokalemia can be a consequence of extreme respiratory alkalosis, although the effect is usually very small or negligible.[2,50] Serum phosphorus concentration may decrease by as much as 1.5 to 2.0 mg/dL because of the shift of inorganic phosphate into cells. Reductions in the blood ionized calcium concentration may be partially responsible for symptoms such as muscle cramps and tetany. Approximately 50% of calcium is bound to albumin, and an increase in pH results in an increase in binding.[49]

COMPENSATION

The initial response of the body to acute respiratory alkalosis is chemical buffering. Hydrogen ions are released from the body's buffers—intracellular proteins, phosphates, and hemoglobin—and titrates down the serum bicarbonate concentration. This process occurs within minutes. Acutely, the bicarbonate concentration can be decreased by a maximum of 3 mEq/L for each 10–mm Hg decrease in $PaCO_2$[17] (see Table 51–4). When only the physicochemical buffering has occurred, the disturbance is referred to as acute respiratory alkalosis.

Metabolic compensation occurs when respiratory alkalosis persists for more than 6 to 12 hours. In response to the alkalemia, proximal tubular bicarbonate reabsorption is inhibited and the serum bicarbonate concentration falls. Renal compensation is usually complete within 1 to 2 days. The renal bicarbonaturia, as well as decreased NH_4^+ and titratable acid excretion, are direct effects of the reduced $PaCO_2$ and pH on renal reabsorption of chloride and bicarbonate.[2] The acuity of the respiratory alkalosis can be assessed on the basis of the degree of renal compensation (see Table 51–4). In fully compensated respiratory alkalosis, the bicarbonate concentration falls by 4 mEq/L below 24 for each 10–mm Hg drop in $PaCO_2$. For example, a sustained decrease in $PaCO_2$ of 20 mm Hg will lower serum bicarbonate from 24 to 14 mEq/L with a resultant pH of 7.46. Bicarbonate concentrations differing from those anticipated using the preceding guidelines suggest a mixed acid-base disorder (refer to Fig. 51–4).

▶ TREATMENT: Respiratory Alkalosis

Because most patients with respiratory alkalosis, especially chronic cases, have few or no symptoms and pH alterations are usually mild (pH not exceeding 7.50), treatment is often not required.[42] The first consideration in the treatment of acute respiratory alkalosis with pH >7.50 is the identification and correction of the underlying cause. Relief of pain, correction of hypovolemia with intravenous fluids, treatment of fever or infection, treatment of salicylate overdose, and other direct measures may prove effective. A rebreathing device, such as a paper bag, may be useful in controlling hyperventilation in patients with the anxiety/hyperventilation syndrome.[49] Oxygen therapy should be initiated in patients with severe hypoxemia. Patients with life-threatening alkalosis (pH >7.60) and complications such as arrhythmia or seizures may require mechanical ventilation with sedation and/or paralysis to control hyperventilation. Simple respiratory alkalosis rarely requires such aggressive therapy, but it may be necessary for patients with mixed respiratory and metabolic alkalosis.

Respiratory alkalosis in patients receiving mechanical ventilation is usually iatrogenic. It may often be corrected by decreasing the minute ventilation (i.e., the number of mechanical breaths per minute times the volume delivered), although other measures can also be employed. The use of a capnograph and spirometer in the breathing circuit enables a more precise adjustment of the ventilator settings. Another method of treating respiratory alkalosis is to increase the amount of dead space in the ventilator circuit by placing a known length of tubing between the artificial airway and the "Y" piece of the ventilator. This results in "rebreathing" of expired gas, and therefore an increase in the inspired carbon dioxide concentration, which should increase the carbon dioxide tension of the patient, correcting the respiratory alkalosis. In patients breathing more rapidly than the ventilator settings, sedation with or without paralysis may be beneficial.

RESPIRATORY ACIDOSIS

PATHOPHYSIOLOGY

Respiratory acidosis, a primary retention of carbon dioxide that lowers the pH, results from a failure of the lungs to excrete carbon dioxide normally. This may be the result of neuromuscular diseases that inhibit central control of ventilation or neuromuscular function, intrinsic airway or parenchymal pulmonary disease, or interruption in pulmonary perfusion (Table 51–10). Acute respiratory acidosis with hypoxemia, hypercarbia, and acidosis is life-threatening. Those disorders that produce an increase in $PaCO_2$ and hypoxemia to a degree compatible with life (e.g., chronic obstructive pulmonary disease), with or without oxygen therapy, may result in chronic respiratory acidosis (Table 51–11). These patients can function normally without noticeable neurologic defects with $PaCO_2$ concentrations in the range of 90 to 100 mm Hg (normal, 40 mm Hg), provided adequate oxygenation is maintained.[50]

CLINICAL PRESENTATION

Respiratory acidosis may produce neuromuscular symptoms, including altered mental status, abnormal behavior, seizures, stupor, and coma. Hypercapnia may mimic stroke or CNS tumors by producing headache, papilledema, focal paresis, and abnormal reflexes. Carbon dioxide acts as a vasodilator in the brain, thus causing an increase in cerebral blood flow.[2] This increase in cerebral blood flow is thought to be partially responsible for the CNS symptoms. The CNS response to hypercapnia is extremely variable between patients and is also influenced by the acuity of presentation. Chronic hypercapnia blunts the usual respiratory stimulus resulting from increased $PaCO_2$. In patients with severe chronic respiratory acidosis, hypoxemia rather than hypercapnia provides the primary ventilatory stimulus.[50]

The degree to which cardiac contractility and heart rate are altered depends on the severity of the acidosis and the rapidity with which it develops. Modest acute hypercapnia ($PaCO_2$ of 50 to 55 mm Hg) stimulates a stress-like response, with elevated catecholamines and corticosteroid hormone levels, and can result in increased cardiac output and pulmonary artery pressure.[51] As the severity increases, cardiac output declines and vascular resistance decreases. Refractory hypotension may be present in some patients.[2]

TABLE 51–10. Causes of Acute Respiratory Acidosis

Perfusion abnormalities
Massive pulmonary embolism
Cardiac arrest

Airway and pulmonary abnormalities
Severe pulmonary edema
Severe pneumonia
Smoke inhalation
Pneumothorax
Severe bronchospasm
Acute respiratory distress syndrome
Airway obstruction: foreign body, laryngeal edema
Aspiration of vomitus

Neuromuscular abnormalities
Trauma, stroke
Narcotic or sedative overdose
Brain stem or cervical cord injury
Guillain-Barré syndrome
Myasthenia gravis
Status epilepticus

Mechanical ventilator
Ventilator malfunction
Inadequate frequency or tidal volume settings
Large dead space

Total parenteral nutrition (increased CO_2 production)

CLINICAL PRESENTATION OF RESPIRATORY ACIDOSIS

GENERAL
The patient is usually symptomatic.

SYMPTOMS
The patient may complain of confusion or difficulty thinking and headache.

SIGNS
In severe respiratory acidosis:
Cardiac: Increased cardiac output if moderate, that decreases if severe. Refractory hypotension may be present in some patients.
CNS: Abnormal behavior, seizures, stupor, and coma. Papilledema, focal paresis, and abnormal reflexes may also be present.

LABORATORY TESTS
Serum potassium concentration may be modestly increased. Hypercapnia may be moderate ($PaCO_2$ of 50 to 55 mm Hg) to severe ($PaCO_2$ of >80 mm Hg). Hypoxia (PaO_2 is <70 mm Hg) is often present.

In respiratory acidosis, the serum potassium concentration increases modestly secondary to cellular shifts. The increases are less than those seen with inorganic metabolic acidosis and are difficult to predict for individual patients (see Chap. 50).

COMPENSATION

The body responds to acute respiratory acidosis with chemical buffering. The increase in $PaCO_2$ results in increased carbonic acid levels.

TABLE 51–11. Causes of Chronic Respiratory Acidosis

Neuromuscular abnormalities
Brain stem infarct
Obesity-hypoventilation (Pickwickian) syndrome
Tumors
Poliomyelitis
Multiple sclerosis
Diaphragmatic paralysis
Pulmonary abnormalities
Chronic obstructive pulmonary disease
Kyphoscoliosis
Interstitial pulmonary disease
Overzealous parenteral feeding

The carbonic acid dissociates, releasing hydrogen ions, which are buffered by nonbicarbonate buffers (i.e., proteins, phosphate, and hemoglobin) and bicarbonate. Thus on the basis of physicochemical factors, increases in $PaCO_2$ raise the serum bicarbonate concentration. In general, in acute respiratory acidosis, the bicarbonate concentration increases by 1 mEq/L above 24 for each 10–mm Hg increase in $PaCO_2$ above 40 (see Table 51–4).

Metabolic compensation occurs when respiratory acidosis is prolonged beyond 12 to 24 hours. In response to hypercapnia and acidemia, proximal tubular bicarbonate reabsorption, ammoniagenesis, and distal tubular hydrogen secretion are enhanced, resulting in an increase in serum bicarbonate concentration and raising the pH toward normal. Renal compensation for chronic hypercapnia generally results in the plasma bicarbonate concentration increasing by 4 mEq/L above 24 for each 10–mm Hg increase in $PaCO_2$ above 40 (see Table 51–4). The new steady state in acid-base values is generally achieved within 5 days of the onset of hypercapnia in dogs; the time interval necessary for compensation in humans has not been established.

▶ TREATMENT: Respiratory Acidosis

The treatment of respiratory acidosis is dependent on the chronicity of the patient's condition. Respiratory decompensation in patients with chronic elevations in $PaCO_2$ are frequently seen in those with acute infections and those recently started on narcotic analgesics or oxygen therapy.[42] Aggressive treatment of these conditions can offer considerable benefit and should be initiated. Furthermore, tranquilizers and sedatives should be avoided and supplemental oxygen, if used, should be minimized.

ACUTE RESPIRATORY ACIDOSIS

When carbon dioxide excretion is severely impaired ($PaCO_2$ >80 mm Hg) and/or life-threatening hypoxia is present (PaO_2 <40 mm Hg), the immediate therapeutic goal is to provide adequate oxygenation. Under these circumstances, hypoxia, not acidemia, is the principal threat to life. A patent airway needs to be established, which may necessitate intubation. Excessive secretions must be cleared from the airway and oxygen administered to restore adequate oxygenation. Mechanical ventilation is likely to be required.

The underlying cause of the acidosis should be treated aggressively (e.g., bronchodilators for treatment of severe bronchospasm;

narcotic or benzodiazepine antagonists to reverse the effects of these respiratory depressant drugs). Bicarbonate administration is rarely necessary in the treatment of respiratory acidosis. Furthermore, rapid correction of acidosis with bicarbonate may eliminate the patient's respiratory drive or precipitate a metabolic alkalosis. Cautious use of alkali (bicarbonate or THAM) can restore the responsiveness of bronchial muscles to β-adrenergic agonists and thus may be beneficial for those patients with severe bronchospasm.[51] Arterial blood gases should be monitored closely to ensure that the respiratory acidosis is resolving without creating a metabolic alkalosis as the result of compensatory elevation in HCO_3^- and decrease in $PaCO_2$. Arterial blood gases should be obtained every 2 to 4 hours during the acute phase and less frequently (every 12 to 24 hours) as the acidosis improves.

ACUTE RESPIRATORY ACIDOSIS IN A COMPENSATED CHRONIC RESPIRATORY ACIDOTIC PATIENT

Patients with a history of chronic respiratory acidosis (e.g., those with chronic obstructive pulmonary disease) may experience an acute worsening of their respiratory acidosis. This may result in severe life-threatening hypoxemia. As with acute respiratory acidosis, the goals of therapy are maintenance of a patent airway and adequate oxygenation. Individuals with chronic respiratory acidosis are routinely able to tolerate a low PaO_2 and an elevated $PaCO_2$ because of compensation (increased number of red blood cells, hemoglobin content, and 2,3-diphosphoglycerate). The drive to breathe in these patients is dependent on hypoxemia rather than hypercarbia. Administration of oxygen to a patient with chronic respiratory acidosis can eliminate this drive to breathe and result in the syndrome of carbon dioxide narcosis. In this case, if the PaO_2 is 50 mm Hg, no oxygen treatment is necessary. If the PaO_2 is <50 mm Hg, oxygen therapy should be initiated carefully using a controlled flow of oxygen.[2]

Arterial blood gases should be checked periodically to ensure adequate oxygenation. If the $PaCO_2$ increases during oxygen therapy, it may be a sign of impending carbon dioxide narcosis and oxygen therapy may need to be discontinued. The underlying cause of the acute exacerbation should be aggressively managed. Pulmonary infections should be treated with the appropriate antibiotics and bronchodilators administered as necessary. Excess secretions should be cleared from the airway to allow proper gas exchange. This may involve increasing oral fluid intake to decrease the viscosity of secretions, deep breathing, and postural drainage, suction, or bronchoscopy.

MIXED ACID-BASE DISORDERS

DIAGNOSIS

The diagnosis of a mixed disorder depends on an understanding of the appropriate quantitative response of the compensatory mechanisms for each of the simple acid-base disturbances. To diagnose mixed disorders, one must know how each of the four simple disorders alters pH, $PaCO_2$, and $[HCO_3^-]$ (see Table 51–4). If a given set of blood gases does not fall within the range of expected responses for a simple acid-base disturbance (see Fig. 51–4), a mixed disorder should be suspected. In addition to laboratory information, a thorough history and physical examination of the patient will often lead to the diagnosis, even before the laboratory data are available. Examples of common mixed disturbances follow.

MIXED RESPIRATORY ACIDOSIS AND METABOLIC ACIDOSIS

In mixed respiratory and metabolic acidosis, there is a failure of compensation. The respiratory disorder prevents the compensatory decrease in $PaCO_2$ expected in the defense against metabolic acidosis. The metabolic disorder prevents the buffering and renal mechanisms from raising the bicarbonate concentration as expected in the defense against respiratory acidosis. In the absence of compensatory mechanisms, the pH decreases markedly.

Mixed respiratory and metabolic acidosis may develop in patients with cardiorespiratory arrest, in those with chronic lung disease who are in shock, and in metabolic acidosis patients who develop respiratory failure. This mixed disorder should be treated by responding to both the respiratory and metabolic acidosis. Improved oxygen delivery must be initiated to improve hypercarbia and hypoxia. Mechanical ventilation may be needed to reduce $PaCO_2$. During the initial stage of therapy, appropriate amounts of alkali should be given to reverse the metabolic acidosis (see section on treatment of metabolic acidosis earlier in this chapter).

MIXED RESPIRATORY ALKALOSIS AND METABOLIC ALKALOSIS

The combination of respiratory and metabolic alkalosis is the most common mixed acid-base disorder. This mixed disorder occurs frequently in critically ill surgical patients with respiratory alkalosis caused by mechanical ventilation, hypoxia, sepsis, hypotension, neurologic damage, pain, or drugs, and with metabolic alkalosis caused by vomiting or nasogastric suctioning and massive blood transfusions. It may also occur in patients with hepatic cirrhosis who hyperventilate, receive diuretics, or vomit, as well as in patients with chronic respiratory acidosis and an elevated plasma bicarbonate concentration

who are placed on mechanical ventilation and undergo a rapid fall in $PaCO_2$.

The decrease in bicarbonate concentration that usually compensates for respiratory alkalosis is prevented by the complicating metabolic alkalosis. Likewise, the increase in $PaCO_2$ expected to compensate for metabolic alkalosis is prevented by primary respiratory alkalosis. The failure of compensation that occurs with mixed respiratory and metabolic alkalosis may result in a severe alkalemia.

Correction of the metabolic component by administration of sodium chloride and potassium chloride solutions should be undertaken, and readjustment of the ventilator or treatment of an underlying disorder causing hyperventilation may correct or ameliorate the respiratory component of this mixed disorder.

MIXED METABOLIC ACIDOSIS AND RESPIRATORY ALKALOSIS

This mixed disorder is often seen in patients with advanced liver disease, salicylate intoxication, and pulmonary-renal syndromes. The respiratory alkalosis decreases the $PaCO_2$ beyond the appropriate range of the respiratory compensation for metabolic acidosis. The plasma bicarbonate concentration also falls below the level expected in compensation for a simple respiratory alkalosis. In a sense, the defense of pH for either disorder alone is enhanced; thus the pH may be normal or close to normal, with a low $PaCO_2$ and a low $[HCO_3^-]$. Treatment of this disorder should be directed at the underlying cause. Because of the enhanced compensation, the pH is usually closer to normal than in either of the two simple disorders.

MIXED METABOLIC ALKALOSIS AND RESPIRATORY ACIDOSIS

This mixed disorder often occurs in patients with chronic obstructive pulmonary disease and chronic respiratory acidosis who are treated with salt restriction, diuretics, and possibly glucocorticoids. When diuretics are initiated, the plasma bicarbonate may increase because of increased renal bicarbonate generation and reabsorption, providing mechanisms for both generating and maintaining metabolic alkalosis. The elevated pH diminishes respiratory drive and may therefore worsen the respiratory acidosis.

Although the pH may not deviate significantly from normal, treatment may need to be initiated to maintain PaO_2 and $PaCO_2$ at acceptable levels. Because it is often difficult to correctly identify this mixed disorder, it is helpful to observe the patient's response to discontinuation of diuretics and administration of sodium and potassium chloride.[2] If the patient has a simple metabolic alkalosis, the $PaCO_2$ will normalize, but it will only minimally affect the $PaCO_2$ if it is a mixed disorder. Treatment should be aimed at decreasing the plasma bicarbonate with sodium and potassium chloride therapy, thereby allowing the renal excretion of retained bicarbonate from the diuretic-induced metabolic alkalosis. This therapy should be used cautiously to avoid exacerbating any underlying congestive heart failure.

EVALUATION OF THERAPEUTIC OUTCOMES

Because acid-base disorders are such a common and widespread problem, pharmacists may play a key role in identifying, preventing, and properly treating acid-base abnormalities. Acid-base disorders do not occur only in the intensive care unit setting. Patients in ambulatory and extended care settings have many chronic conditions and drug therapies that commonly affect acid-base balance. Thus pharmacists in all practice settings should use their knowledge to identify patients at high risk for developing drug-related problems and to undertake appropriate prevention and treatment measures to improve the quality of life of the patients they care for.

ABBREVIATIONS

BW: body weight
CNS: central nervous system
DCA: dichloroacetate
ECF: extracellular fluid
H_2CO_3: carbonic acid
H^+: hydrogen ion
HCO_3^-: bicarbonate
HIV: human immunodeficiency virus
$NH4^+$: ammonium
$PaCO_2$: partial pressure of carbon dioxide from arterial blood
PaO_2: partial pressure of oxygen from arterial blood
pH: the negative logarithm (base 10) of the hydrogen ion
   concentration
pK: the negative logarithm of the dissociation constant
$PvCO_2$: partial pressure of carbon dioxide from venous blood
PvO_2: partial pressure of oxygen from venous blood
RTA: renal tubular acidosis
SAG: serum anion gap
THAM: tromethamine [tris(hydroxymethyl)aminomethane]
UC: unmeasured cations
UA: unmeasured anions

Review Questions and other resources can be found at *www.pharmacotherapyonline.com.*

REFERENCES

1. Narins RG. Acid-base disorders: Definitions and introductory concepts. In: Narins RG, ed. Maxwell & Kleeman's Clinical Disorders of Fluid and Electrolyte Metabolism, 5th ed. New York, McGraw-Hill, 1994:765–768.
2. Kaehny WD. Pathogenesis and management of respiratory and mixed acid-base disorders. In: Schrier RW, ed. Renal and Electrolyte Disorders, 5th ed. Philadelphia, Lippincott, Williams & Wilkins, 1997:172–191.
3. Adrogue HE, Adrgue HJ. Acid-base physiology. Respir Care 2001;46: 328–341.
4. Shapiro JI, Kaehny WD. Pathogenesis and management of metabolic acidosis and alkalosis. In: Schrier RW, ed. Renal and Electrolyte Disorders, 5th ed. Philadelphia, Lippincott, Williams & Wilkins, 1997:130–171.
5. Halperin ML, Jungas RL, Cheema-Dhadli S, Brosnan JT. Disposal of the daily acid load: An integrated function of the liver, lungs and kidneys. Trends Biochem Sci 1987;12:197–199.
6. Arbus GS. An in-vivo acid-base nomogram for clinical use. Can Med Assoc J 1973;109:291–293.
7. Narins RG, Krishna GG, Yee J, et al. The metabolic acidoses. In: Narins RG, ed. Maxwell & Kleeman's Clinical Disorders of Fluid and Electrolyte Metabolism, 5th ed. New York, McGraw-Hill, 1994:769–826.
8. Kraut JA, Madias NE. Approach to patients with acid-base disorders. Respir Care 2001;46:392–403.
9. Halperin ML, Carlisle EJ, Donnelly S, et al. Renal tubular acidosis. In: Narins RG, ed. Maxwell & Kleeman's Clinical Disorders of Fluid and Electrolyte Metabolism, 5th ed. New York, McGraw-Hill, 1994:875–910.
10. Roth KS, Chan JC. Renal tubular acidosis: a new look at an old problem. Clin Pediatr 2001;40:533–543.
11. Levraut J, Grimaud D. Treatment of metabolic acidosis. Curr Opin Crit Care 2003;9:260–265.
12. Gauthier PM, Szerlip HM. Metabolic acidosis in the intensive care unit. Crit Care Clin 2002;18:289–308.
13. Salem MM, Mujais SK. Gaps in the anion gap. Arch Intern Med 1992; 152:1625–1629.
14. Adrogue HJ, Madias NE. Management of life-threatening acid-base disorders I. N Engl J Med 1998;338:26–34.
15. Kraut JA, Madias NE. Lactic acidosis. In: Adrogue HJ, ed. Contemporary Management in Critical Care, Vol. 1. Baltimore, Williams & Wilkins, 1995:449–457.
16. Saltpeter SR, Greyber E, Pasternak GA, Salpeter EE. Risk of fatal and nonfatal lactic acidosis with metformin use in type 2 diabetes mellitus: systemic review and meta-analysis. Arch Intern Med 2003;163:2594–2602.
17. Narins RG, Emmett M. Simple and mixed acid-base disorders: A practical approach. Medicine (Baltimore) 1980;59:161–187.
18. Albert MS, Dell RB, Winters RW. Quantitative displacement of acid-base equilibrium in metabolic acidosis. Ann Intern Med 1964;66:312–322.
19. Kraut JA. The role of metabolic acidosis in the pathogenesis of renal osteodystrophy. Adv Ren Replace Ther 1995;2:40–51.
20. Morris RC, Ives HE. Inherited disorders of the renal tubule. In: Brenner BM, ed. Brenner and Rector's The Kidney, Vol. II, 5th ed. Philadelphia, WB Saunders, 1996:1764–1827.
21. Sing RF, Branas CA, Sing RF. Bicarbonate therapy in the treatment of lactic acidosis: Medicine or toxin? J Am Ostepath Assoc 1995;95:52–57.
22. Cooper DJ, Walley KR, Wiggs BR, Russell JA. Bicarbonate does not improve hemodynamics in critically ill patients who have lactic acidosis: A prospective controlled clinical study. Ann Intern Med 1990;112:492–498.
23. Mizock BA. Lactic acidosis in critical illness. Crit Care Med 1992; 20:80–89.
24. Forsythe SM, Schmidt GA. Sodium bicarbonate for the treatment of lactic acidosis. Chest 2000;117:260–267.
25. Adrogue HJ, Rashad MN, Gorin AB, et al. Assessing acid-base status in circulatory failure: Differences between arterial and central venous blood. N Engl J Med 1989;320:1312–1316.
26. Faber MD, Kupin WL, Heiling CW, Narins RG. Common fluid-electrolyte and acid-base problems in the intensive care unit: Selected issues. Semin Nephrol 1994;14:8–22.
27. Emergency Cardiac Care Committee and Subcommittees, American Heart Association. Guidelines for cardiopulmonary resuscitation and emergency cardiac care. JAMA 1992;268:2171–2302.
28. McEvoy GK, Litvak K, Welsh OH, et al. American Hospital Formulary Service, Drug Information. Bethesda, MD, American Society of Hospital Pharmacists, 2004.
29. Moon PF, Gabor L, Gleed RD, Erb HN. Acid-base, metabolic, and hemodynamic effects of sodium bicarbonate or tromethamine administration in anesthetized dogs with experimentally induced metabolic acidosis. Am J Vet Res 1997;58:771–776.
30. Marmarou A, Holdaway R, Ward JD, et al. Traumatic brain tissue acidosis: Experimental and clinical studies. Acta Neurochir 1993;57:160–164.
31. Leung JM, Landow L, Franks M, et al. Safety and efficacy of intravenous Carbicarb in patients undergoing surgery: Comparison with sodium bicarbonate in the treatment of mild metabolic acidosis. Crit Care Med 1994; 22:1540–1549.
32. Shapiro JI. Functional and metabolic responses of the isolated heart

during acidosis: Effects of sodium bicarbonate and Carbicarb. Am J Physiol 1990;258:H1835–H1839.

33. Shapiro JI. Pathogenesis of cardiac dysfunction during metabolic acidosis: Therapeutic implications. Kidney Int 1997;51:47–51.

34. Bersin RM, Arieff AI. Improved hemodynamic function during hypoxia with Carbicarb, a new agent for the management of acidosis. Circulation 1988;77:227–233.

35. Stacpoole PW, Wright EC, Baumgartner TG, et al. A controlled clinical trial of dichloroacetate for treatment of lactic acidosis. N Engl J Med 1992;327:1564–1569.

36. Stacpoole PW, Nagaraja NV, Hutson AD. Efficacy of dichloroacetate as a lactate-lowering drug. J Clin Pharmacol 2003;43:683–691.

37. Shangraw RE, Winter R, Hromco J, et al. Amelioration of lactic acidosis with dichloroacetate during liver transplantation in humans. Anesthesiology 1994;81:1127–1138.

38. Vary TC, Siegel JH, Zechnich A, et al. Pharmacologic reversal of abnormal glucose regulation, BCAA utilization, and muscle catabolism in sepsis by dichloroacetate. J Trauma 1988;28:1301–1311.

39. Palmer BF, Alpern RJ. Metabolic alkalosis. J Am Soc Nephrol 1997; 8:1462–1469.

40. Khanna A, Kurtzman NA. Metabolic alkalosis. Respir Care 2001;46:354–365.

41. Miltiadous G, Mikhailidis DP, Elisaf M. Acid-base and electrolyte abnormalities observed in patients receiving cardiovascular drugs. J Cardiovasc Pharmacol Ther 2003;8:267–276.

42. Adrogue HJ, Madias NE. Management of life-threatening acid-base disorders II. N Engl J Med 1998;338:107–111.

43. Rowlands BJ, Tindall SF, Elliot DJ. The use of dilute hydrochloric acid and cimetidine to reverse severe metabolic alkalosis. Postgrad Med J 1978;54:118–123.

44. Barton CH, Vaziri ND, Ness RL, et al. Cimetidine in the management of metabolic alkalosis induced by nasogastric drainage. Arch Surg 1979; 1:70–74.

45. Mirtallo JM, Rogers KR, Johnson JA, et al. Stability of amino acids and the availability of acid in total parenteral nutrition solutions containing hydrochloric acid. Am J Hosp Pharm 1981;38:1729–1731.

46. Colussi G, Rombola G, De Ferrari ME, et al. Correction of hypokalemia with antialdosterone therapy in Gitelman's syndrome. Am J Nephrol 1994; 14:127–135.

47. Hene RJ, Koomans HA, Dorhout Mees EJ, et al. Correction of hypokalemia in Bartter's syndrome by enalapril. Am J Kidney Dis 1987; 9:200–205.

48. Vinci JM, Gill JR Jr, Bowden RE, et al. The kallikrein-kinin system in Bartter's syndrome and its response to prostaglandin synthetase inhibition. J Clin Invest 1987;61:1671–1682.

49. Foster GT, Vaziri ND, Sassoon CS. Respiratory alkalosis. Respir Care 2001;46:384–391.

50. Gennari FJ. Respiratory acidosis and alkalosis. In: Narins RG, ed. Maxwell & Kleeman's Clinical Disorders of Fluid and Electrolyte Metabolism, 5th ed. New York, McGraw-Hill, 1994:957–990.

51. Respiratory pump failure: Primary hypercapnia (respiratory acidosis). In: Adrogue HJ, Tobin MJ, eds. Respiratory Failure. Cambridge, MA, Blackwell Science, 1997:125–134.

52

EVALUATION OF NEUROLOGIC ILLNESS

Susan C. Fagan and Fenwick T. Nichols

Learning Objectives and other resources can be found at *www.pharmacotherapyonline.com.*

KEY CONCEPTS

◀1 The clinical neurologic history and examination are the cornerstones of the neurologic diagnosis and management.

◀2 Through the history, one can determine the main symptoms, the mode of onset (gradual or sudden), progression over time (maximal at onset or steadily gaining intensity), and associated illnesses/risk factors.

◀3 The neurologic examination is directed at localization of the

disease process so that evaluation and management may be planned appropriately.

◀4 The neurologic examination of a specific patient may be adapted to the patient's specific deficit. For example, a patient with double vision may warrant an extensive cranial nerve examination but a less extensive assessment of finger strength.

In order to contribute most effectively to the care of patients with neurologic illness, one must understand the tools used in the diagnosis and management of these patients. In addition, clinicians must be able to gather their own data through a targeted neurologic examination and history taking in order to ensure optimal pharmacotherapy in neurologic patients. Despite technologic advances that have led to the development of sensitive diagnostic tests in neuroscience, the clinical neurologic history and examination are still the cornerstones of the neurologic diagnosis and management.[1]

SIGNS AND SYMPTOMS

◀1 As in all of medicine, obtaining an accurate and complete history is of utmost importance in the evaluation of neurologic diseases. In many instances, the diagnosis can be made on the basis of the history, and the neurologic examination can be tailored to optimally evaluate the patient and confirm the diagnosis. The clinician depends on the patient or family for the details of the illness. Care must be taken to avoid "leading" the patient. Obtaining an accurate history may be difficult because a number of neurologic diseases may affect ◀2 patients' speech and memory. Through the history, one can determine the main symptoms, the mode of onset (gradual or sudden), progression over time (maximal at onset or steadily gaining intensity), and associated illnesses/risk factors (recent head injury from a motor vehicle accident).

The physical examination is important in revealing evidence of systemic disease that may have affected the nervous system secondarily (e.g., a seizure in a patient with elevated temperature and stiff neck may suggest meningitis). The neurologic examination is only one component of a complete general physical examination.

THE NEUROLOGIC EXAMINATION

◀3 An assessment of patient effort is necessary to interpret the results of the neurologic examination. It can identify any abnormalities, particularly asymmetry of function, and help to localize the lesion within the nervous system (central versus peripheral and specific location within the central nervous system or the peripheral nervous system). The neurologic examination consists of six main components: higher cortical function (mental status), cranial nerves, motor function, reflexes, sensory function, and gait. Table 52–1 describes the common approaches to assessing each of the six domains and includes examples of the diseases in which abnormal findings are ◀4 common. A targeted neurologic examination can be performed when a specific deficit is suspected. Table 52–2 describes the cranial nerve examination in more detail. The reader is encouraged to consult other references to better understand the intricacies of the neurologic examination.[2] The clinician must synthesize the results of the history and physical examination to arrive at an anatomic localization of the lesion and create a differential diagnosis.

PROCEDURES USED IN THE DIAGNOSIS

In addition to the neurologic examination, certain imaging techniques and procedures may be essential in the diagnosis of neurologic disorders. Some of the more commonly used procedures are described next.[2]

Lumbar puncture (LP) is used to obtain cerebrospinal fluid (CSF). It is used most often as an evaluation of CNS infections such as meningitis and encephalitis, but it is also useful in subarachnoid hemorrhage, multiple sclerosis, and dementia. Opening pressure, cell count and differential, glucose concentration, total protein

TABLE 52–1. The Neurologic Examination

Domain	Tests Performed	Diseases
Mental status	While obtaining the history: general mental and emotional status, speech, memory, alertness, abstract reasoning, ability to follow commands (motor integration), ability to communicate	Dementias, stroke, metabolic encephalopathies
Cranial nerves	Visual acuity, visual fields, eye movements, jaw strength, corneal reflex, facial symmetry, auditory acuity, gag reflex, shoulder and neck strength	Myasthenia gravis, Parkinson's disease, stroke, amyotrophic lateral sclerosis (ALS)
Motor function	Motor strength with and without resistance, coordination (rapid alternating movements, finger-to-nose), tremors, atrophy, fasiculations	Stroke, myasthenia gravis, Parkinson's disease, ALS
Reflexes	Biceps, triceps, tendon reflexes, plantar response (Babinski sign is an upgoing toe and is abnormal), superficial cutaneous reflexes (abdominal)	Stroke, spinal cord lesions, endocrine diseases (e.g., diabetes, hypothyroidism), peripheral neuropathy
Sensory function	Asymmetry to pin-prick, vibration, temperature	Stroke, peripheral neuropathy, migraine aura, diabetes, spinal cord lesions
Gait	Walking, standing (Romberg test = eyes closed will accentuate disequilibrium)	Stroke, Parkinson's disease, spinal cord lesions

concentration, and culture and sensitivity are obtained routinely. A space-occupying lesion in the brain with mass effect is a relative contraindication to LP because herniation could result. Prior to performing an LP, the patient should be checked for papilledema, which may indicate increased intracranial pressure (ICP). The opening CSF pressure usually is less than 180 mm H$_2$O. Normal CSF is clear and colorless and should not contain any red blood cells (RBCs) or polymorphonuclear cells. The presence of up to five mononuclear cells is considered normal. Total protein in the CSF usually is 45 mg/dL or less. Protein may increase with infection, breakdown of the blood-brain barrier (e.g., tumors, stroke, and trauma), and diabetes.

Electroencephalography (EEG) records the electrical activity of the brain. The record is interpreted by observing the basic rhythms and waveforms, the symmetry of the recording, and abnormal electrical discharges. It also may be used to assess the response to photic stimulation or hyperventilation. It is used primarily in the diagnosis of seizures and may be helpful in the evaluation of patients with altered mental status. EEG also may be used to measure evoked potentials (EPs). The EPs are the EEG response to repetitive stimuli (visual, auditory, or tactile) and provide information about the presence of abnormalities and disturbances (but not the cause) in the specific pathways tested.

Electromyography (EMG) and nerve conduction velocities (NCVs) are used to assess the function of the peripheral nerves, neuromuscular junction, and muscles. NCVs are measured by stimulating the nerve and recording the speed of conduction of the impulse. NCVs can be used to detect the presence of localized peripheral nerve injuries (carpal tunnel, etc.) or diffuse symmetric neuropathies (which may be inherited or acquired). EMG assesses muscle dysfunction due to primary muscle disease or secondary to nerve injury. This test is used to diagnose peripheral neuropathies (inherited and acquired), Guillain-Barré syndrome, myasthenia gravis, amyotrophic lateral sclerosis, radiculopathies, and muscle diseases.

The cerebral circulatory system can be imaged or evaluated in a number of different ways depending on the type and location of the abnormality suspected. Imaging techniques can be used to identify local arterial stenosis, aneurysms, or arteriovenous malformations. Atherosclerosis of the extracranial arteries, a frequent cause of stroke, can be evaluated using ultrasound (referred to as *duplex sonography, carotid Doppler,* or *color-flow Doppler*), magnetic resonance angiography (MRA), spiral computed tomographic angiography (CTA), or intraarterial angiography. The intracranial arterial circulation can be evaluated using transcranial Doppler (TCD), MRA, CTA, or intraarterial angiography. Each technique has its own advantages and disadvantages. Intraarterial angiography provides the best imaging of the

TABLE 52–2. Cranial Nerve Function and Examples of Testing

I. Olfactory nerve. Smell: Identify odors (coffee, cinnamon, lemon; test each nostril separately).

II. Optic nerve. Visual acuity: Eye card; Visual fields: Peripheral vision and blind spot; Funduscopic exam; Pupil size and reaction; Color vision (rarely done).

III. Oculomotor. (Cranial nerves III, IV, and VI have similar functions and are tested as a unit.) Eye movements: Patient is asked to watch a light as it moved up, down, and on both sides, while eye movements are observed.

IV. Trochlear. See III.

V. Trigeminal nerve. Motor: Tests power of jaw opening and sideways deviation against the resistance of a hand placed against the jaw. Sensory: Test corneal reflex by touching cornea (also nasal mucosa) with a wisp of cotton.

VI. Abducens. See III.

VII. Facial nerve. Observe asymmetry of face at rest or on speaking, baring teeth, raising eyebrows, or wrinkling forehead. Reflex eye closure to a threatening movement. Glabellar tap: Repetitive tapping over bridge of nose—initial blinking should cease after the first few taps.

VIII. Auditory nerve. Vestibular division: Observe for nystagmus, positional testing. Auditory division: Test acuity with light sound; watch, whisper, rubbing of fingers close to ear.

IX. Glossopharyngeal nerve. Test for gag reflex by touching back of throat with tongue depressor; test swallowing and coughing and note any drooling or pooling of saliva. Test symmetry of palate movement on vocalizing "ah."

X. Vagus nerve. Test gag reflex as in IX.

XI. Spinal accessory nerve. Trapezius and sternomastoid muscles: Test power of shrugging shoulders and turning the head to one side against resistance.

XII. Hypoglossal nerve. Motor function of tongue. Look for wasting and abnormal movements.

smaller arteries of the cerebral circulation but is more invasive than the other measures.

Computed tomography (CT) uses x-rays to produce images of "slices" of the brain that are 1 to 10 mm in thickness. CT revolutionized the practice of neurology by allowing direct imaging of the brain anatomy. CT is currently available in most communities and is used to evaluate patients with intracranial disease. CT scans are used to identify tumors, hemorrhages, infarctions, hydrocephalus, and atrophy. Intravenous contrast agents (a contrast-enhanced scan) can be administered to enhance the image of blood vessels and areas of blood-brain barrier damage that may be caused by abscesses, other inflammatory conditions, tumors, or stroke.

Magnetic resonance imaging (MRI) uses the magnetic properties of the hydrogen atom nucleus and proton to produce computer-processed scans that provide improved anatomic detail when compared with CT scans. MRI offers the advantages of better differentiating between white and gray matter and delineating lesions close to bone (brain stem and cerebellum) and has no radiation risk; however, it is not as readily available as CT and is more expensive. MRI has a proven advantage over CT in evaluating lesions in the posterior fossa and in detecting lesions in the white matter such as plaques in multiple sclerosis. MRI is also useful in the diagnosis of tumors and very early ischemic stroke (diffusion-weighted imaging, or DWI). Imaging of the spinal canal and its contents can be accomplished either by MRI myelography or CT myelography.

Other imaging techniques such as positron-emission tomography (PET) and single-photon-emission computed tomography (SPECT) are considered tests of brain function. These tests are being studied extensively in epilepsy as well as in cerebrovascular disorders, cerebral tumors, movement disorders, and dementia. PET scans use a positron-emitting isotope to display chemical activity and the rates of biologic processes within the brain. This method can assess regional metabolic changes in the brain. The expense, technical complexity (a cyclotron is needed), and limited availability of this technique limit its clinical utility.

SPECT scans measure radiotracer uptake by tissues and provide cross-sectional images of the brain. This technique has been used extensively to assess cerebral blood flow. Although the resolution of SPECT is not as good as PET, the availability has led to wide clinical use in disorders such as stroke, dementia, and epilepsy.

CONCLUSION

Assessment of the patient with neurologic disease is challenging. The patient by virtue of the neurologic deficit, may or may not be able to provide reliable information regarding medication history or extent of illness. The clinician must develop alternate strategies to obtain a complete data set and develop a pharmacotherapy plan. Ability to interpret and synthesize the results of the neurologic examination and other diagnostic tests will help a great deal in this quest.

ABBREVIATIONS

CSF: cerebrospinal fluid
CT: computed tomography
CTA: computed tomography angiography
DWI: diffusion-weighted imaging
EEG: electroencephalogram
EMG: electromyography
EPs: evoked potentials
LP: lumbar puncture
MRA: magnetic resonance angiography
MRI: magnetic resonance imaging
NCVs: nerve conduction velocities
PET: positron-emission tomography
RBCs: red blood cells
SPECT: single-photon-emission computed tomography
TCD: transcranial Doppler

Review Questions and other resources can be found at *www.pharmacotherapyonline.com.*

REFERENCES

1. Greenberg DA, Aminoff MJ, Simon RP. Clinical Neurology, 5th ed. New York, McGraw-Hill, 2002:355–366.
2. Greenberg DA, Aminoff MJ, Simon RP. Clinical Neurology, 5th ed., New York, McGraw-Hill, 2002:337–354.

53

MULTIPLE SCLEROSIS

Jacquelyn L. Bainbridge and John R. Corboy

Learning Objectives and other resources can be found at *www.pharmacotherapyonline.com.*

KEY CONCEPTS

❶ The etiology of multiple sclerosis (MS) is unknown, and currently there is no cure.

❷ MS appears to be an immunologic disorder that is characterized by central nervous system demyelination and axonal damage.

❸ Diagnosis of MS is made primarily on the basis of clinical examination and magnetic resonance imaging (MRI) findings.

❹ Acute exacerbations or relapses usually are treated with high-dose glucocorticoids, such as methylprednisolone.

❺ In most patients suffering from an acute exacerbation, a clinical response to steroid treatment can be expected within 3 to 5 days.

❻ Treatment with interferon-β or glatiramer acetate (Avonex, Betaseron, Copaxone, and Rebif, or ABC-R, therapy) can reduce annual relapse rate, slow progression of disability, slow cognitive decline, and slow changes seen on the brain MRIs.

❼ Treatment with immunomodulating interferon-β or glatiramer acetate (ABC-R therapy) should begin promptly after the diagnosis of relapsing MS is made and after a single attack if the MRI is suggestive of high risk of further attacks. Therapy after interferon-β or glatiramer acetate (ABC-R therapy) "treatment failure" and in patients with secondary progressive MS and primary progressive MS is not clear.

❽ The only treatments approved for secondary progressive MS are mitoxantrone and interferon-β-1b.

❾ Patients suffering from MS frequently will have symptoms such as spasticity, bladder dysfunction, fatigue, pain, and depression that may require treatment. Patients must be counseled that therapies such as interferon-β and glatiramer acetate will not relieve these symptoms.

❿ Depression is common in MS and may pose the risk of suicide.

Multiple sclerosis (MS) is an inflammatory disease of the central nervous system (CNS) that affects between 250,000 and 350,000 persons in the United States.[1] It is one of the major causes of neurologic disability in young and middle-aged adults. The term *multiple sclerosis* refers to two characteristics of the disease: the numerous affected areas of the brain and spinal cord producing multiple neurologic symptoms that accrue over time and the characteristic plaques or sclerosed areas that are the hallmark of the disease.

❶ Although MS was first described almost 130 years ago, the cause remains a mystery, and a cure is still unavailable. Nevertheless, many advances have been made in treating and managing the complications of the disease and improving the quality of life of individuals affected by MS.

EPIDEMIOLOGY

MS usually is diagnosed in patients between the ages of 20 and 45 years (although cases in children have been reported), with the peak incidence occurring in the fourth decade of life.[2] Reported onset can occur as early as age 10 and as late as the eighth decade, and one of the authors (Corboy) has seen a child with first symptoms at age 4.[3] Women are afflicted more than men by a ratio of approximately 2:1.[3] Men usually develop the first signs of MS at a later

age than women and are also more likely to develop the progressive form of the disease.[3] The most important factors in the determination of individuals at risk for developing the disease are geography, age, environmental influences, and genetics.[2–5]

In general, the greater the distance from the equator, the higher is the prevalence of the disease.[2,6,7] Within the United States, the prevalence of MS is higher in states above the thirty-seventh parallel. MS occurs more frequently in whites of Scandinavian ancestry than in other ethnic groups.[8,9]

It is thought that a crucial environmental agent that may predispose one to developing MS is contacted by susceptible individuals between the ages of 10 and 15 years who usually have lived in a high-risk area for at least 2 years.[9] Interestingly, an individual who migrates from a low- to a high-risk area prior to age of 15 years acquires the same chance of developing MS as those who live in a high-risk area all their lives.[10] If the move is made in the opposite direction, from a high- to a low-risk area, the individual retains the high risk if the move is made after the age of 15 years but acquires the lower risk if the move is made prior to this age.[9,10]

The familial recurrence rate of MS is approximately 5%, with siblings being the most commonly reported relationship.[8] Concordance data show a higher prevalence of MS between monozygotic than between dizygotic twins, and a recent study has confirmed the overall concordance among monozygotic twins at about 25%, with a risk among females of 34% and males just 5%, similar to that seen in dizygotic twins.[11] Genetic studies also have determined an association between MS and the major histocompatibility complex (MHC) and, in particular, with the human leukocyte antigen (HLA) region on the sixth chromosome that is associated with the genetic control of immune mechanisms.[8,12,13] This association between HLA haplotype and MS susceptibility may vary between ethnic groups. In whites, the strongest association appears to be with the MHC class II allele DR2 haplotype. The relative risk of developing MS is approximately four times as great in DR2+ versus DR2− individuals.[12] This association is not specific enough to be used for diagnostic purposes given a 30% to 50% false-negative rate and that the DR2+ haplotype is found in at least 20% of the healthy white population. Although the significance of the association between MS and the HLA region remains unclear, the fact that certain HLA antigens are neither necessary nor sufficient to lead to the development of MS suggests that inheritance is most likely polygenic in nature and that there may only be a genetic susceptibility to developing this disease following an as-yet-unknown etiologic challenge. In addition, a number of genes have been identified that may alter the speed of progression of the illness, such as apolipoprotein E ε4 homozygosity.[14,15]

ETIOLOGY

AUTOIMMUNE THEORY

In the autoimmune theory (Fig. 53–1), MS results from an autoimmune attack against self-myelin or self-oligodendrocyte antigens. The actual mediator of myelin destruction has not been established, but this activity has been attributed to the action of macrophages, killer T cells, lymphokines, antibodies, or a combination of these elements.[16] T-helper cells (CD4+) appear to be key initiators of myelin destruction in MS. These autoreactive CD4+ cells are activated in the periphery, perhaps following a viral infection, and express adhesion molecules on their surfaces that allow them to attach and roll along the endothelial cells that constitute the blood-brain barrier (BBB). These activated T cells also produce matrix metalloproteinases that help to create openings in the BBB, allowing entry of the activated T cells past the BBB and into the CNS. Once inside the CNS, the T cells produce cytokines, which further create openings in the BBB, allowing entry of B cells, complement, macrophages, and antibodies. The T cells also interact within the CNS with the resident microglia, astrocytes, and macrophages, further enhancing production of proinflammatory cytokines and other potential mediators of CNS damage, including reactive oxygen intermediates and nitric oxide. The exact trigger for the activation of the T cells in the periphery remains unclear, but the T cells recognize myelin basic protein (MBP), proteolipid protein, myelin oligodendrocyte glycoprotein, and myelin-associated glycoprotein in the blood of patients with MS. A reduction in T-suppressor cells, or suppressor activity, has been reported during active MS and in patients with progressive disease; however, a relative increase in the T-helper/suppressor ratio is not found consistently and does not always correlate with disease activity.[17–19]

ROLE OF CYTOKINES

Cytokines are molecules whose physiologic functions are numerous and include modulating inflammatory and anti-inflammatory responses in the immune system. Cytokines such as tumor necrosis factor alpha (TNF-α), interleukin-2 (IL-2), and interferon-γ (INF-γ) have been alleged as contributors to the pathogenesis of MS. TNF-α may contribute to demyelination by upregulation of MHC class I expression, direct injury of oligodendrocytes, and/or promotion of BBB breakdown.[20] INF-γ is produced predominantly by CD4+ cells and is involved in antiviral responses. Because of this, INF-γ was at one time evaluated as a potential MS disease-modifying agent. Clinical trials, however, clearly demonstrated that treatment with this compound resulted in disease exacerbation.[21] INF-γ upregulates MHC class II expression on macrophages, microglia, and astrocytes, leading to an inflammatory response. INF-γ also upregulates adhesion molecules, which are crucial in the early stages of inflammation by facilitating the migration of T cells across the endothelial cells of the BBB.[22]

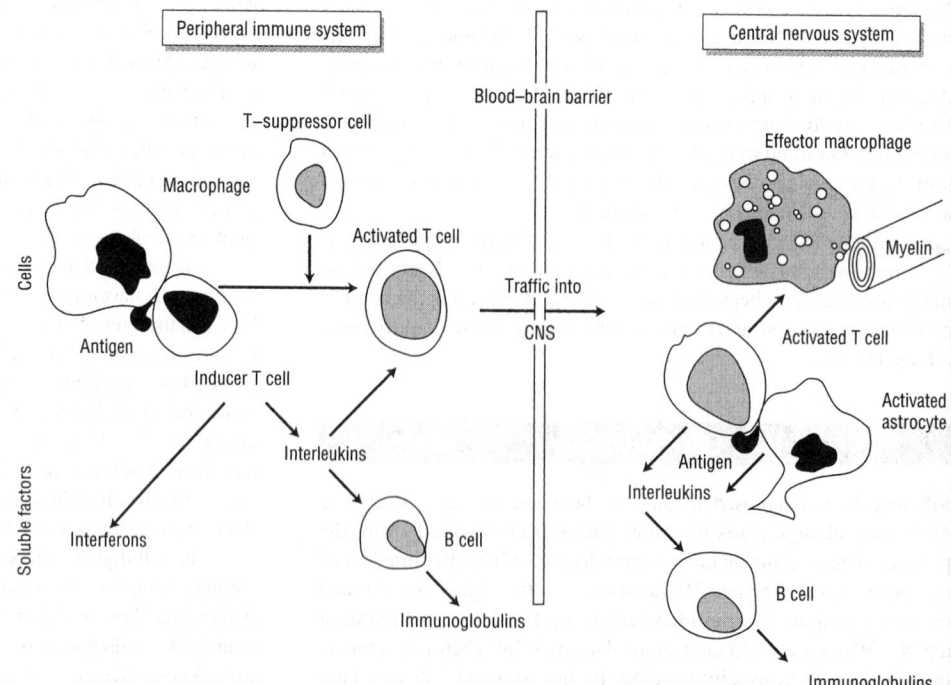

FIGURE 53–1. Autoimmune theory of the pathogenesis of MS. The immune response is initiated in the peripheral immune compartment when antigen is processed and presented to an inducer cell by a macrophage or antigen-presenting cell. The inducer cell becomes activated and releases a number of soluble factors, including interleukins and interferons, that act on both B and T cells to augment the immune response. T-suppressor cells act to dampen the immune response. Activated T cells traffic into the central nervous system, where they again release factors, presumably after having antigen presented to them. In this regard, astrocytes are capable of presenting antigens to T cells. Other cellular elements also enter the CNS (macrophages, B cells), where the potential for a local immune response occurs. B cells are known to produce immunoglobulin locally within the CNS, and macrophages function within the CNS to phagocytose myelin, in addition to their antigen-presenting properties. *(Reprinted with permission from Ann Neurol 1988;23: 214.)*

In contrast, the role of modulating, or downregulating, cytokines also has been described. In patients with stable or mild disease, increased numbers of cells are found that express mRNA for transforming growth factor beta (TGF-β) and IL-10 compared with patients with severe disease.[23,24]

QUESTIONABLE MICROBIAL ETIOLOGY

Although no clear association with any microbial agent has been identified, there are several ways in which a virus or bacteria could play a role in the pathogenesis of MS. These might include either a direct attack on myelin and/or the oligodendrocyte or stimulation of an autoimmune response leading to demyelination.[16,25] Evidence to support a viral etiology includes increased immunoglobulin G (IgG) synthesis in the CNS, increased antibody titers to certain viruses, and epidemiologic studies indicating a childhood exposure factor and suggesting that "viral" infections may precipitate exacerbations. Immunoglobulin patterns in the cerebrospinal fluid (CSF) are similar in subacute sclerosing panencephalitis (SSPE) and MS. SSPE is a chronic measles infection of the CNS known to be associated with the production of oligoclonal bands in the CSF.[26] In addition, viruses have been shown to cause diseases with prolonged incubation periods, myelin destruction, and a relapsing/remitting course in both humans and experimental animal models.[2,27]

The most compelling evidence against a microbial etiology is the fact that no single infectious agent has been identified as the cause of MS. Many possible agents have been implicated, including mycoplasma, spirochetes, rabies virus, herpes simplex, canine distemper virus, coronavirus, human T-cell leukemia virus type I (HTLV-I), MS-associated retrovirus, measles, and most recently, human herpes virus type 6 (HHV-6)[28] and *Chlamydia pneumoniae*.[29] However, to date, no causal relationship has been established.[27,30]

PATHOPHYSIOLOGY

The basic physiologic derangement in MS is the stripping of the myelin sheath surrounding neurons in the CNS. Demyelination, coupled with an inflammatory response, leads to the formation of the characteristic MS lesions, or plaques, that are found primarily in the brain, spinal cord, and optic nerves. Initially, neuronal axons, although stripped bare of their myelin sheath, usually are well preserved.[25] Recent studies, however, have shown that damage to axons can be significant, even early in the course of the illness.[31] Axonal damage may be seen as a hypointense lesion, or T_1 hole, on magnetic resonance imaging (MRI), and these correlate with disability.[32]

Demyelination and axonal transection cause disruption in the transmission of nerve impulses, which leads to neurologic symptoms reflecting the area of the brain or spinal cord that is affected. Demyelinated nerve fibers have prolonged refractory periods that impair conduction of electrical impulse volleys. Maximal electrical impulse frequency may be reduced substantially before impulse conduction is interrupted entirely. A single plaque may extend across several nerve pathways, producing symptoms involving several nervous system functions. Smaller plaques may cause isolated disturbances; however, typically several plaques develop at the same time, causing multiple but unrelated problems such as disturbed vision and decreased sensation.

The pathology of MS lesions is different in early stages of the disease, during chronic MS, and during acute exacerbations.[33] Active and inactive lesions can be found side by side in the brain. Both types of lesions display some degree of perivascular inflammation, but inflammation is much more pronounced and usually associated with BBB damage in active lesions.[33]

Decreased numbers of oligodendrocytes (myelin-producing cells) are observed within the MS plaques, causing speculation as to whether myelin or the oligodendrocyte is the target of an immunologic attack.[18,25,34] Oligodendrocyte destruction appears to occur in a nonspecific manner in early or acute MS, whereas selective destruction of myelin and oligodendrocytes occurs in chronic stages of MS.[33] More recent studies have identified four immunopathologic subtypes of demyelinating lesions, with variable amounts of T cells or immunoglobulins present in the plaques. All type IV patients studied so far have primary progressive multiple sclerosis (PPMS), but otherwise, there is no obvious association of immunopathology and clinical type.[35]

CLINICAL PRESENTATION

The clinical presentation of MS is extremely variable among patients and typically varies over time in a given patient (Table 53–1). The signs and symptoms of MS usually are divided into three categories. Primary symptoms are a direct consequence of conduction disturbances produced by demyelination and axonal damage and reflect the area of the brain or spinal cord that is damaged. Secondary symptoms are complications resulting from primary symptoms. For example, urinary retention, a primary symptom, may lead to frequent urinary tract infections, considered a secondary symptom. Tertiary symptoms relate to the effect of the disease on the patient's everyday life.[36]

The most widely used clinical rating scale in MS is the Expanded Disability Status Scale (EDSS), in which a numerical value ranging from 0 (no disability) to 10 (death from MS) is assigned based on the evaluation of several neurologic functions.[37] The limitations of this scale are the relative insensitivity to clinical changes not involving impairment of gait and ambulation, such as changes in cognition, fatigue, and affect. Other tools, such as the Multiple Sclerosis Functional Composite (MSFC), are being evaluated for possible increased sensitivity and utility in describing changes in MS-related disability over time.[38] Increasingly, MRI is being used as an index of both disease activity and progression.[39,40] Specifically, the appearance of new lesions or changes in lesion number, size, and volume (burden of disease) are being used as outcome measures. It is important to note, however, that the correlation between MRI lesion load and clinical disability is modest at best.[41]

The unpredictable nature of MS makes it impossible to anticipate when an exacerbation will occur. However, certain factors have been reported to aggravate symptoms or even lead to an acute attack (new episode of demyelination). These implicated factors include infections, hyperventilation, heat (including fever), sleep deprivation, stress, malnutrition, anemia, concurrent organ dysfunction, exertion, and childbirth.[2,3,42] Interestingly, many patients experience a significant reduction in acute relapses during the third trimester of pregnancy, followed by a relative increase postpartum.[42] There are no significant epidemiologic data that support an association between physical trauma and the development or worsening of MS, but this may reflect inadequacy of the studies reported to date.[43,44]

The clinical course of MS is classified into four categories[45] (Fig. 53–2). About 85% of patients have attacks—new symptoms lasting at least 24 hours and separated from other new symptoms by at least 30 days—followed by remissions (complete or incomplete) at the outset of the illness. Attacks frequently are referred to as *relapses* or *exacerbations,* and the first attack is called a *clinically isolated*

TABLE 53–1. Presentation of Multiple Sclerosis

General

Most patients with multiple sclerosis will present with nonspecific complaints. Many will have problems with their vision or paresthesias.

Primary Symptoms/Signs	Secondary Symptoms	Tertiary Symptoms
Visual complaints	Recurrent urinary tract infections	Financial problems
Gait problems	Urinary calculi	Personal/social problems
Paresthesias	Decubiti	Vocational problems
Pain	Muscle contractures	Emotional problems
Spasticity	Respiratory infections	
Weakness	Poor nutrition	
Ataxia		
Speech difficulty		
Psychological changes		
Cognitive changes		
Fatigue		
Bowel/bladder dysfunction		
Sexual dysfunction		
Tremor		

Laboratory Tests

Multiple sclerosis is a diagnosis of exclusion. Magnetic resonance imaging, cerebrospinal fluid studies, and sometimes evoked potentials are useful in confirming the diagnosis. Magnetic resonance imaging may be positive for periventricular white matter lesions. Enhancing T_1 gadolinium lesions may show signs of active disease. Cerebrospinal fluid synthesis of immunoglobulin G is increased, presence of two or more oligoclonal bands, and increased protein.

---

syndrome (CIS). This course is called *relapsing-remitting MS* (RRMS). In RRMS patients, attack frequency tends to decrease over time and becomes independent of the development of progressive disabilities.[45,46] Neurologic recovery following an acute exacerbation is usually quite good early in the disease course, but following repeated relapses, recovery tends to be less complete. Given these features, interpretation and evaluation of potential therapeutic interventions must be done quite cautiously, and control groups are essential in the design of clinical studies.

Up to 10% to 20% of RRMS patients have a benign course, characterized by few relapses, often sensory, with minimal disability accruing over time. Most RRMS patients, however, do not have a benign course and eventually enter a progressive phase in which attacks and remissions generally are difficult to identify. This is referred to as *secondary-progressive MS* (SPMS). Disability tends to accumulate more significantly during this phase of the illness. New brain MRI lesions, especially those seen only after the injection of contrast material, are less common, and brain atrophy increases.[47]

About 15% of patients never have acute attacks and remissions but have progressive disease from the outset. These patients with PPMS have symptoms, especially spastic paraparesis, that may worsen rapidly or relatively slowly over time, and they accrue progressively more disability. In general, PPMS patients tend to have a worse prognosis than those who present initially with RRMS. Finally, a small percentage of patients may have a mixture of both progression and relapses, referred to as *progressive-relapsing MS* (PRMS).[45]

MS usually does not directly diminish life expectancy. The development of secondary complications such as pneumonia or septicemia (secondary to aspiration of mouth contents with swallowing difficulties, decubitus ulcers, or urinary tract infections) or rapid progression of primary lesions affecting respiratory function may lead to a shorter than expected life span. Most of this decrease in life span is seen in patients with rapidly progressive disease. Suicide rates as high as seven times that expected in the general population have been reported.[48] Clinical and demographic factors that have been used to predict prognosis of MS are listed in Table 53–2.[49,50] Several MRI

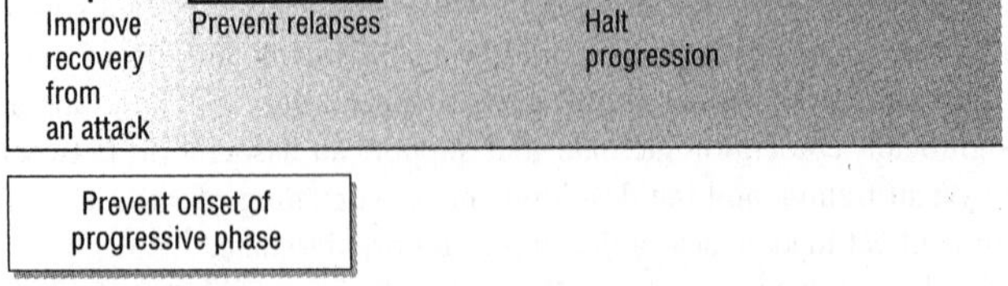

FIGURE 53–2. Clinical course and treatment of multiple sclerosis. The horizontal axis represents time, and the vertical axis represents level of disability. The vertical dotted line represents the onset of the progressive disease phase. The progressive phase may evolve after a number of relapses or, in a subcategory of patients, may be the clinical course of the disease from the onset. *(Reprinted with permission from Ann Neurol 1988;23:212.)*

TABLE 53–2. Prognostic Indicators In Multiple Sclerosis

Indicator	Favorable Prognosis	Unfavorable Prognosis
Age at onset	<40 years	>40 years
Gender	Female	Male
Initial symptoms	Optic neuritis or sensory symptoms	Motor or cerebellar symptoms
Attack frequency in early disease	Low	High
Course of disease	Relapsing/remitting	Progressive

features also have been shown to correlate with progression of disease (see below).[51–53] World Health Organization (WHO) statistics suggest that mortality from MS has decreased up to 25% during the past 30 years, most likely reflecting improvements in overall care.[50]

DIAGNOSIS

MS symptoms frequently can be attributed to other neurologic diseases, just as many syndromes can mimic MS. Some patients may have typical symptoms consistent with classic CIS, whereas many others may have symptoms that are more vague. In the past, the unpredictable nature of MS and the lack of laboratory tests and imaging techniques specific for the disease led to difficulties in making this diagnosis, especially in the early stages of the disease. The diagnosis remains primarily a clinical one that requires the demonstration of "lesions separated in space and time," referring to the occurrence of at least two episodes of neurologic disturbance reflecting distinct sites of damage in the CNS that cannot be explained by another mechanism.[54] Older diagnostic criteria used a complicated system of clinical outcomes and types of laboratory support that might define MS.[55] An international panel of MS experts was convened in 2000 to reevaluate diagnostic criteria and to incorporate MRI knowledge. The result of this panel's work is the McDonald criteria,[56] which allow brain MRI lesions to substitute for clinical lesions in defining "separated in space and time." In the new scheme, diagnostic categories are MS, possible MS (for those individuals at high risk of developing MS), and not MS. In comparison with older criteria, the McDonald criteria allow for earlier diagnosis.[57,58] Indeed, a new consensus panel of the American Association of Neurology endorses the utility of MRI for this purpose,[59] and the Food and Drug Administration (FDA) has now approved one of the immunotherapies to be used after a single attack of demyelination in the context of an appropriately abnormal brain MRI. Thus the definition of MS itself has been altered by the introduction of MRI technology.

LABORATORY STUDIES

To date, there are no tests specific for MS. Tests that are used frequently include MRI of the brain and spine, CSF evaluation, and evoked potentials. Evidence provided by these studies, used in conjunction with the clinical history, aids in establishing the diagnosis of MS.

IMAGING STUDIES

MRI is able to produce images of the brain and spine that reflect damage in the CNS that is characteristic of MS plaques in multiple forms, as well as more generalized abnormalities such as brain atrophy. Images may be referred to as T_1 or T_2 (including proton-density and fluid attenuated inversion recovery [FLAIR] images) and may be visualized before and/or after the injection of contrast material. MRI, especially after the injection of contrast material, is much more sensitive than computed tomographic (CT) scans in the detection of MS lesions[60] and currently is considered the preferred imaging technique. It is extremely helpful for diagnosis but also, in part, useful for prognosis. Patients with a single, typical attack of demyelination (possible MS or CIS, e.g., optic neuritis) and three or more T_2-weighted lesions on the brain MRI have an almost 90% likelihood of developing a second attack (clinically definite MS) over 15 years.[51] In contrast, similar individuals with normal brain MRIs have only a 19% likelihood of

developing MS over 15 years.[51] Total volume of T_2-weighted lesions (called T_2 burden of disease) at the onset of CIS also appears to correlate with the development of disability.[61] Lesions that enhance after injection of the contrast material gadolinium indicate new lesions and disruption of the BBB and are associated with early conversion to MS in CIS/possible MS patients[61] but do not correlate well over time with progression of disability. Brain atrophy, even early in the course of the illness, probably correlates better with progression of disability.[62]

CSF EVALUATION

In MS patients, CNS synthesis of IgG is increased, whereas serum IgG levels are normal. Electrophoretic studies of the CSF show that the IgG separates into a small number of discrete bands, which, when similar bands are not seen in the serum samples taken at the same time, are called *oligoclonal bands* (OCBs).[63] Oligoclonal banding of IgG is present in 90% to 95% of patients with clinically definite, established MS but also may be seen in lower percentages of diseases that mimic MS or are quite different clinically.[63] After CIS (e.g., after initial symptoms), CSF may be positive in only 30% to 50% of patients. Increasingly, with advances in MRI, CSF analysis is reserved only for patients with atypical clinical scenarios or individuals with possible MS[56] in whom a CSF positive for OCBs may help to define a more definite diagnosis of MS. Myelin basic protein is detected in the CSF of 90% of patients shortly after an acute attack but is nonspecific and usually not obtained. Additional nonspecific CSF abnormalities may include increased CSF protein concentrations in approximately 25% of patients and a mild CSF leukocytosis.[64] The presence of greater than 50×10^6 mononuclear cells in the CSF usually indicates a diagnosis other than MS.[64]

EVOKED POTENTIALS

Evoked potentials may be helpful in establishing areas of demyelination that are clinically silent. Slowed conduction of visual, brain stem, and somatosensory potentials can be identified, although the sensitivity and specificity of these tests seem to be somewhat less than that seen with MRI or CSF evaluation.

BLOOD STUDIES

A recent report has documented that in CIS patients with abnormal brain MRIs and abnormal CSF consistent with MS, presence or absence of antimyelin antibodies in serum is very helpful in defining prognosis for further events consistent with clinically definite MS.[65]

DIFFERENTIAL DIAGNOSIS

A number of disorders can mimic MS. Thus most patients are screened with blood tests for rheumatologic, collagen-vascular, infectious, and sometimes inherited metabolic diseases. MRI may rule out tumors and cervical spondylosis. There are many causes of nonspecific T_2 and FLAIR lesions seen in the subcortical white matter on a brain MRI, however, and use of established criteria for distinguishing MS lesions from other etiologies (e.g., migraine, hypertension, age greater than 50 years, and others) enhances diagnostic accuracy. Electromyography may help in diagnosing amyotrophic lateral sclerosis. Magnetic resonance angiography (MRA) and more traditional angiography may be useful in identifying CNS vasculitis and vascular malformations.

▶ TREATMENT: Multiple Sclerosis

Treatment of MS falls into three broad categories: symptomatic therapy, treatment of acute attacks, and disease-modifying therapies to alter the natural course of the disease. Symptomatic management of the disease is of utmost importance to maintain the patient's quality of life. Treatment of acute attacks will shorten the duration and possibly decrease the severity of the attack. Disease-modifying therapies that alter the course of the illness are most important to diminish progressive disability over time. In present usage, both attack therapies and disease-modifying therapies are based on principles of manipulation of the immune system and can be classified as immunotherapies. The basic goals of immunotherapy are to decrease the frequency and severity of exacerbations, diminish the progression of lesions seen on brain and spine MRIs, and slow progression of disability over time. Current therapies are variably successful at achieving these goals, and none is able to restore neurologic function in damaged nervous systems.[66,67]

A number of different treatment modalities have been studied in the last 30 years, but many older trials had flawed designs.[66,67] There are no universally accepted treatment algorithms, and treatments vary among clinicians and centers. Perhaps more important, treatment decisions frequently are based on the wishes and goals of individual patients. One potential algorithm for the immunotherapy of MS is shown in Fig. 53–3.

CLINICAL CONTROVERSY

When patients initially show signs of MS, many practitioners begin treatment with interferon-β or glatiramer acetate (ABC-R medications). However, it is controversial as to which medication to start. Most practitioners assist patients in making the decision of which medication best fits their lifestyle and offers the maximum efficacy. In patients with severe depression, interferon therapy is contraindicated, and patients are encouraged to use glatiramer acetate. None of the therapies should be used during pregnancy, while attempting to get pregnant, or while breastfeeding.

▓ TREATMENT OF ACUTE EXACERBATIONS

◀4 Mild acute exacerbations that do not produce functional decline may not require treatment.[68] When functional ability is affected, although treatment suggestions may vary among clinicians, the standard intervention is intravenous injection of high-dose corticosteroids for 3 to 5 days. Results from a large trial of optic neuritis suggest and the American Academy of Neurology recommends that if treatment with steroids is warranted, it is best to use intravenous methylprednisolone. The mechanism of action for corticosteroids in MS is unknown, but it is speculated that steroids improve recovery by decreasing edema in the area of demyelination.[68]

High-dose methylprednisolone has been shown to shorten the duration of acute exacerbations,[68] and it may delay repeat attacks after optic neuritis, although it has not been shown definitively to affect the progression of disease.[67,69]

Comparative trials of the steroid precursor adrenocorticoid hormone (ACTH) and high-dose intravenous steroids suggest that steroids produce a quicker and more predictable improvement in acute exacerbations. Although the reasons for this are not entirely clear, differences between agents may be due to the variable adrenal secretion

of endogenous glucocorticoids following ACTH stimulation.[65,68,70] The use of ACTH, therefore, largely has been supplanted by methylprednisolone.

◀5 Methylprednisolone doses may range from 500 to 1000 mg/day, given intraveneously. The duration of therapy is variable and may range from 3 to (rarely) 10 days depending on clinical response. A standard time is 3 to 5 days. Some clinicians offer prednisone or other oral tapers to patients after the intravenous injections, but others do not, in an effort to limit lifetime exposure to steroids and resulting side effects. If improvement occurs, it is usually seen in the first 3 to 5 days.

A very small number of patients have very severe attacks, manifested by hemiplegia, paraplegia, or quadriplegia. If these patients fail to improve with aggressive steroid therapy, a recent study suggests that treatment with plasma exchange every other day for seven treatments may be beneficial for about 40% of patients.[71,72]

CLINICAL CONTROVERSY

If a patient taking interferon decompensates and has neutralizing antibodies in the blood, most practitioners will stop the medication. In this situation it is controversial whether to rechallenge the patient at a later date with interferon therapy. Many clinicians will only rechallenge with interferon therapy if the patient does not do well on other therapies.

▓ DISEASE-MODIFYING THERAPY: REDUCTION OF RELAPSES AND PROGRESSION (ABC-R THERAPY WITH AVONEX, BETASERON, COPAXONE, AND REBIF)

▓ INTERFERON-β-1b AND INTERFERON-β-1a

◀6 Interferon-β-1b (Betaseron) was the first agent proven to alter the natural history of the illness.[65] Interferon-β-1b is a nonglycosylated synthetic analog of recombinant interferon-β and is produced synthetically in *Escherichia coli*. Although the exact mechanism of action is unknown, its effect in MS may be due to its immunomodulating properties, including the ability to augment suppressor cell function and reduce interferon-γ secretion by activated lymphocytes, its macrophage-activating effect, and its ability to downregulate the expression of interferon-γ–induced class II MHC gene products on antigen-presenting glial cells.[65] Interferon-β-1b also suppresses T-cell proliferation and may decrease BBB permeability.[65]

Interferon-β-1b is administered every other day subcutaneously at a dose of 8 million IU. Clinical trials have demonstrated that at these doses, interferon-β-1b significantly reduces annual relapse rate and MRI burden of disease compared with placebo. With respect to clinical disability, however, no significant differences were noted between the interferon- and placebo-treated groups.[65] Betaseron is packaged in premixed syringes with a new formulation that does not require refrigeration. Betaseron costs approximately $15,283 per year.

Interferon-β-1a (Avonex and Rebif) is a natural-sequence glycosolated interferon produced in recombinant Chinese hamster ovary cells. Avonex is given as 30 mcg (6 million IU) intramuscularly (IM) once weekly. The prefilled syringes should be refrigerated but may be kept at room temperature for 30 days. Avonex costs approximately $12,915 per year. Rebif is given as 44 mcg subcutaneously three times weekly. It is supplied in a 0.5-mL prefilled syringe with an

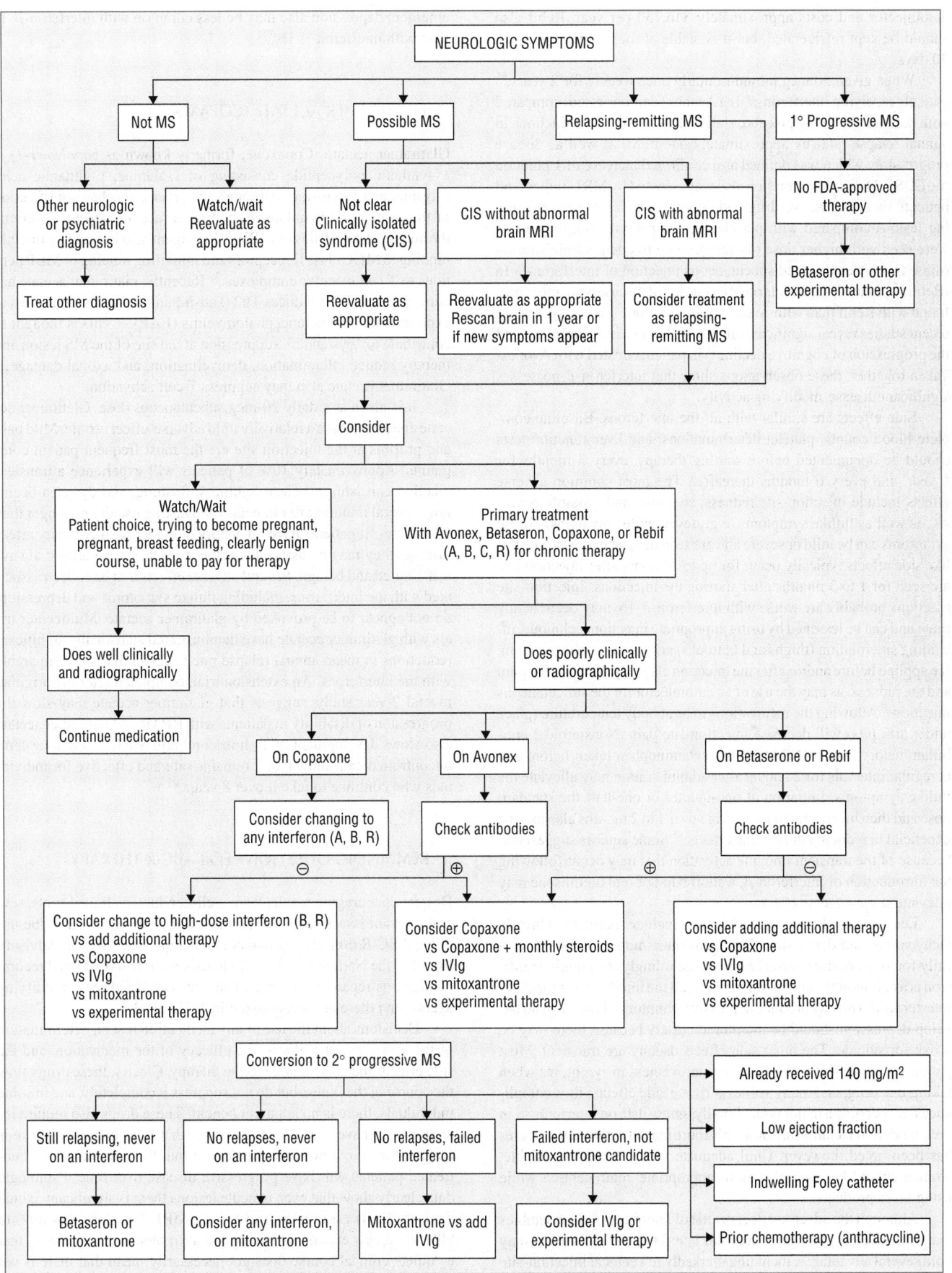

FIGURE 53–3. Algorithm for management of relapsing-remitting multiple sclerosis.

autoinjector and costs approximately $16,730 per year. Rebif also should be kept refrigerated, but it is stable at room temperature for 30 days.

When given 30 mcg intramuscularly once weekly for 2 years,[65] patients receiving interferon-β-1a (Avonex) demonstrated, compared with patients receiving placebo, statistically significant reductions in annual relapse rate (by approximately one-third) as well as disease progression, which was defined as a confirmed increase of 1 point on the EDSS. Disease progression also was assessed by MRI studies, and patients receiving active drug had significantly fewer new enhancing lesions compared with placebo-treated patients. Similar results were seen with higher dose (44 mcg), more frequent administration (three times weekly), and subcutaneous injection of interferon-β-1a (Rebif).[73] Indeed, the effects on MRI burden of disease were more profound with Rebif than with Avonex in studies done separately.[73] More recent studies reveal significant effects on slowing brain atrophy[74] and the progression of cognitive decline[75] in patients treated with Avonex. Taken together, these observations show that interferon-β possesses significant disease-modifying activity.

Side effects are similar with all the interferons. Baseline complete blood counts, platelet determinations, and liver function tests should be documented before starting therapy, every 3 months for 1 year, and every 6 months thereafter. The most common adverse effects include injection-site redness, swelling, and possibly necrosis, as well as flulike symptoms (e.g., fever, chills, myalgias). These symptoms can be mild or severe and are seen in most patients. The flulike side effects typically occur for up to 24 hours after injection and are seen for 1 to 3 months after starting the injections. Injection-site reactions probably are worse with interferon-β-1b, may occur at any time, and can be lessened by using appropriate injection technique, including site rotation (thighs and buttocks) and hydrocortisone cream. Ice applied before and/or after the injection also may decrease the pain and the redness, as may the use of an autoinjector for the subcutaneous injections. Allowing the medications to be at body temperature (place under arm pits) will decrease injection-site pain. Nonsteroidal anti-inflammatory agents (NSAIDs) or acetaminophen taken before and at regular intervals for 24 hours after administration may alleviate the flulike symptoms. Initiation of one-quarter or one-half the standard dose and then increasing to full dosage over 1 to 2 months also may be beneficial in reducing flulike side effects.[76] Some authors suggest that because of the transient immune activation that may occur following the introduction of interferon-β, a short burst of oral prednisone may alleviate some adverse effects.[76]

Less commonly reported side effects include shortness of breath, tachycardia, and depression. Clinicians must monitor patients carefully for signs of depression and treat accordingly. Although depression is a common finding in MS patients, all the interferons, especially interferon-β-1b, may produce depressive symptoms. Patients who develop depression should be monitored closely because there may be a risk for suicide. The other side effects usually are transient. Most patients will not feel better or have improvement in symptoms when taking this drug, and many will experience side effects; thus compliance may become a major issue. Finally, safety data on interferon-β in pregnancy and lactation are lacking. Abortifacient activity in primates has been noted, however. Until adequate safety data are available, women should be counseled as to appropriate contraception while using these products.

Although the adverse-effect profile of interferon-β-1a resembles that of interferon-β-1b, intramuscular interferon-β-1a (Avonex) may hold several advantages, including markedly fewer local injection-site reactions and once-weekly administration versus subcutaneous injection every other day (or three days per week with Rebif). Treatment-

emergent depression also may be less common with interferon-β-1a than with interferon-β-1b.[77]

GLATIRAMER ACETATE (COPAXONE)

Glatiramer acetate (Copaxone, formerly known as *copolymer-1*) is a synthetic polypeptide consisting of L-alanine, L-glutamic acid, L-lysine, and L-tyrosine. Although the precise mechanism of action of this compound is unknown, glatiramer acetate appears to mimic the antigenic properties of MBP.[78] This agent also may act by directly binding to MHC class II receptors and inhibiting binding of MBP peptides to T-cell receptor complexes.[78] Recently, glatiramer acetate has demonstrated that it induces Th2 (anti-inflammatory) lymphocytes in experimental allergic encephalomyelitis (EAE).[78] This is thought to contribute to "bystander" suppression at the site of the MS lesion and thereby reduce inflammation, demyelination, and axonal damage.[79] Glatiramer acetate also may suppress T-cell activation.

It is given as a daily 20-mcg subcutaneous dose. Glatiramer acetate appears to have a relatively mild adverse-effect profile. Mild pain and pruritus at the injection site are the most frequent patient complaints. Approximately 10% of patients will experience a transient reaction consisting of chest tightness, flushing, and dyspnea beginning several minutes after injection and lasting usually no longer than 20 minutes. If patients have no history or evidence of coronary artery disease, they may be assured that these reactions are almost always self-limited and benign. Several adverse effects that have been associated with the interferons, including flulike symptoms and depression, do not appear to be provoked by glatiramer acetate. Multicenter trials with glatiramer acetate have demonstrated statistically significant reductions in mean annual relapse rate ($\sim$25%) that are comparable with the interferons. An extension trial, completed after the original, pivotal 2-year study, suggests that glatiramer acetate may slow the progression of disability in patients with RRMS.[79] Glatiramer acetate also slows development of T_1 holes on brain MRIs,[80] and long-term uncontrolled data show that it remains safe and effective for individuals who continue to take it over 8 years.[81]

REMAINING QUESTIONS FOR ABC-R THERAPY

Despite encouraging results from well-conducted clinical trials, several relevant issues remain. The most important question in the use of the ABC-R drugs is when to begin therapy. The Medical Advisory Board of the National Multiple Sclerosis Society has adopted recommendations regarding the use of the current MS disease-modifying agents, and these are summarized in Table 53–3.[82]

Decisions about the use of any medication rest on determination of the severity of the illness, the efficacy of the medication, and the side effects and costs related to the therapy. Clearly, these drugs slow the course of the illness but do not suppress it completely, and in some individuals, there is no apparent benefit. These drugs also require injections and have side effects and costs that limit their use. There is now, however, overwhelming evidence that the vast majority of untreated patients will have progressive disease over time. Pathologic data clearly show that even in acute lesions there is significant axonal damage that is essentially irreversible. MRI data show that 80% to 90% of all new enhancing lesions are asymptomatic, suggesting that a "quiet" clinical course does not necessarily mean that there is not ongoing disease activity that ultimately will be reflected in cognitive problems and mood disorders.

TABLE 53–3. Disease Management Consensus Statement (Abridged)

- Initiation of therapy is advised as soon as possible following a definite diagnosis of MS and determination of a relapsing course.
- Patients' access to medication should not be limited by the frequency of relapses, age, or level of disability.
- Treatment is not to be stopped during evaluation for continuing treatment.
- Therapy is to be continued indefinitely, unless there is clear lack of benefit, intolerable side effects, new data that reveal other reasons for cessation, or better therapy becomes available.
- All three agents should be included in formularies and covered by third-party payers so that physicians and patients may determine the most appropriate agent on an individual basis.
- Movement from one immunomodulating drug to another should be permitted.
- Most concurrent medical conditions do not contraindicate use of any of these therapies.

Modified from Ref. 82.

Furthermore, it is now known that very early therapy is effective. In patients with CIS and two or more T_2 lesions on brain MRI (i.e., at high risk for developing clinically definite MS), treatment with Avonex produced, compared with patients receiving placebo, a 44% reduction in the likelihood of patients going on to have a second clinical attack over a 2-year period of study. Several MRI measures also were significantly better in treated patients.[61,83] Similar results were seen with low-dose weekly Rebif.[84] Thus not only is very early therapy warranted, but it is also effective and is now approved by the FDA. Indeed, the National MS Society recommends that patients with relapsing disease should be placed on ABC-R therapy immediately after the diagnosis.[82]

A second major issue is which drug to use in which patient. There has not been a single, randomized study comparing all four drugs with one another in a similar patient population at the same time.[85] The pivotal placebo-controlled trials produced results that were more similar than different when comparing across trials, including a nearly identical one-third reduction in relapse rate for all four drugs over 2 years. There has been speculation for some time, however, that higher dose and/or more frequent administration of interferon (Rebif or Betaseron) may be more beneficial than the lower dose once-weekly use of interferon (Avonex). To address this issue, two comparative trials of Avonex versus Betaseron[86] and Avonex versus Rebif[87] have now been completed. In both cases, Avonex was used in the standard 30 mcg per week intramuscular injection, and the other interferons were used at the usual higher dose, more frequent subcutaneous administration, as in a typical clinical practice. In both studies, there were small but statistically significant differences favoring Betaseron or Rebif in a variety of clinical and MRI measures of efficacy, and it was this short-term (6-month) comparative trial[87] that resulted in FDA approval of Rebif in the United States in 2002.

There were many scientific objections to these trials, most important of which was lack of control of dosing versus frequency of administration, absence of blinding of clinical outcomes, and the use of novel primary outcome measures with unclear biologic or clinical significance. In addition, published around the same time was a trial comparing 60 mcg with the standard 30 mcg Avonex in a weekly injection showing no difference over a 2-year study.[88] Thus the significance of these Phase IV marketing-driven studies remains to be determined.

A concern with all three interferon products that further muddies our understanding of the clinical differences between the interferon products is the development of neutralizing antibodies. In clinical trials, 38% of patients receiving interferon-β-1b developed antibodies directed against the drug.[89] In these patients, the exacerbation rate was similar to that in placebo-treated patients. With interferon-β-1a, neutralizing antibodies were found in 22% of early trials of Avonex, but later studies reported that only about 2% to 5% of treated patients developed antibodies.[88] Percentages for Rebif are intermediate, at about 22%.[87] The long-term clinical significance of these findings, however, is still unclear,[65] although most data are similar to the Betaseron data described earlier, i.e., suggesting reduction in clinical efficacy with production of antibodies. Whether these antibodies are truly cross-reactive between products is unknown, as is the duration during which antibodies may be detected. The clinical relevance of neutralizing antibodies must be evaluated prospectively. Significant neutralizing antibodies have not been seen with glatiramer acetate.

Intriguingly, in vitro data suggest a potential synergism between glatiramer acetate and interferon-β. Given the cost of these therapies, as well as the potential for additive adverse effects, this therapeutic combination cannot be recommended until clinical evidence demonstrating benefit is available. A study that will compare glatiramer acetate alone with interferon-β-1a (Avonex) alone versus a combination of the two has just been funded by NIH and is underway, with results expected in several years.

All four of the ABC-R drugs are approved by the FDA for relapsing forms of the disease. Clinical trials of Betaseron, Avonex, and Rebif in SPMS have had mixed results.[90–92] Based primarily on a large European trial of Betaseron,[90] there is a suggestion that patients with SPMS and ongoing attacks or enhancing MRI lesions may benefit from using interferon, whereas those without such findings will not. Indeed, the FDA has now approved interferon-β-1b for use in SPMS when the patient continues to experience superimposed relapses, but neither interferon-β-1a product is approved by the FDA for SPMS. A planned 3-year trial of glatiramer acetate in PPMS was halted after 2 years when it was determined there was little likelihood continuation of the trial would result in a significant difference between the treated and placebo groups. Alternative delivery routes, including nasal and oral, are being studied but have not yet been shown to be effective. Finally, determination of "treatment failure" or inadequacy and treatment options in the event of progression of disease while on ABC-R therapy remains a difficult question.

OTHER THERAPIES

Short-term, intensive pulse doses of corticosteroids, similar to those used in acute exacerbations, initially may decrease disability, but prolonged steroid therapy has no established effects on the progression of disease.[65,69] If progression continues while a patient is on a disease-modifying agent, an immunosuppressive agent may be tried.

Mitoxantrone (Novantrone), a member of the anthracenediene family, has now been approved by the FDA for reducing neurologic disability and/or the frequency of clinical relapses in patients with SPMS (chronic), PRMS, or worsening RRMS.[65] Mitoxantrone is administered as a brief (5- to 15-minute) intravenous infusion dosed at 12 mg/m^2 every 3 months. An evaluation of left ventricular ejection fraction is required prior to administration of the initial dose, before each dose, after an accumulated dosage of 100 mg/m^2 has been reached, and if signs or symptoms of congestive heart failure develop. The maximum allowable lifetime cumulative dose of mitoxantrone is

TABLE 53–4. Treatment of Selected Primary MS Symptoms

Spasticity	Bladder Symptoms	Sensory Symptoms	Fatigue
Baclofen	Propantheline	Carbamazepine	Amantadine
Dantrolene	Oxybutinin	Phenytoin	Pemoline
Diazepam	Dicyclomine	Amitriptyline or other TCAs	Antidepressants
Tizanidine	DDAVP	Gabapentin	Modafinil
Tiagabine	Self-catheterization	Lamotrigine	Methylphenidate
Gabapentin	Imipramine or amitriptyline		Dextroamphetamine
	Prazosin		
	Botulinum toxin type A		

140 mg/m^2.[93] Other potential side effects noted with this agent are nausea, alopecia, menstrual disorder, amenorrhea, upper respiratory tract infection, urinary tract infection, and leukopenia.[93] The role mitoxantrone will play in the treatment of MS remains unclear because potential cardiac toxicity appears to limit its long-term use. Currently, there are no proven therapies for the treatment of PPMS,[94] and a recent trial of Copaxone in PPMS was halted after 2 years of a planned 3-year trial owing to a lack of efficacy.

A number of other agents have been studied over the last 30 years but have either failed to provide definitive benefit, or the data are still evolving. Cyclophosphamide has been studied alone and in combination with other treatment modalities in attempts to slow progression of MS.[95] Maintenance therapy with intermittent (monthly) pulse doses of cyclophosphamide may slow the progression of disease in younger patients with rapidly progressive disease, but further study is required to confirm benefit in these patients. Prolonged therapy with cyclophosphamide usually is intolerable, but it appears that some form of maintenance is necessary.[95] Cyclosporine appears to produce only a modest delay in the progression of disability in chronic progressive MS. A significant number of patients may develop severe side effects, in particular nephrotoxicity and hypertension,[96] which may limit the usefulness of cyclosporine.

Conflicting results have been seen when azathioprine is used alone or in combination with other therapies. Reductions in the exacerbation rate and slowing of disease progression are only modest. It is usually given in doses of 2 to 3 mg/kg until the white blood cell count drops to less than 4000/mm^3. It is then followed with corticosteroid therapy.[67] Although not without serious side effects, azathioprine may be less toxic than cyclophosphamide and may be tolerated for a longer period of time. Methotrexate given as 7.5 mg orally each week also has shown modest benefit in slowing disease progression.[67]

Other experimental modalities include total lymphoid irradiation (TLI), interferon-α, monoclonal antibodies, cladribine, and intraveneous immune globulin (IVIG).[97] IVIG may stimulate remyelination of neurons in established MS lesions. Further studies are required to confirm the observation of reduced exacerbations and improved neurologic function. Two monoclonal antibodies, one[98] directed against a cellular adhesion molecule (natalizumab, Antegren) and the other[99] against the lymphocyte cell marker CD52 (alemtuzumab, Campath), have shown significant activity in preliminary studies, especially with effects on gadolinium-enhancing lesions in relapsing patients, and both are in Phase III studies now. High-dose immunoablation therapy followed by stem cell rescue has been used in a small number of patients around the world with promising preliminary results,[100,101] but this approach has significant potential toxicities that likely will limit its use to those with severe disease. Rituximab directed against CD20 cells may prove to be beneficial in the treatment of MS.

SYMPTOMATIC MANAGEMENT

❾ Many of the symptoms of MS do not require pharmacologic management or do not respond to it. This section covers the primary symptoms in which pharmacologic management may be of benefit (Table 53–4). See the preceding section on the treatment of acute exacerbations for a discussion on optic neuritis.

GAIT DIFFICULTIES AND SPASTICITY

Problems with gait may be due to spasticity, weakness, ataxia, defective proprioception, or a combination of these factors. Spasticity is amenable to pharmacologic intervention, whereas physical therapy may be required in treating gait disturbances owing to any of the other factors. Spasticity is encountered commonly and tends to affect the legs more markedly than the arms. Spasticity may result in falls; however, in the later stages of the disease, the increased muscle tone of a spastic limb often lends strength to patients with underlying weakness. Therefore, when using muscle relaxants, one must be careful not to decrease the tone to an extent where ambulation is actually hindered.[102,103] Baclofen (Lioresal), a γ-aminobutyric acid (GABA) analog, is the preferred agent and usually is started in dosages of 10 mg three times daily and titrated upward to achieve the desired response. Most patients will achieve a satisfactory response with dosages between 40 and 80 mg/day; however, dosages higher than the recommended daily maximum of 80 mg are required by some patients.[102,103] Continuous intrathecal administration of baclofen may be an option for patients unable to tolerate or unresponsive to oral therapy. Baclofen should not be discontinued abruptly to avoid the possibility of seizures.[103] Small doses of diazepam (e.g., 0.5–1 mg) often are added to baclofen in patients in whom optimal response has not been achieved.

A newer agent, tizanidine (Zanaflex), is a short-acting, centrally acting α-adrenergic agonist that can reduce spasticity by increasing presynaptic inhibition of motor neurons. It appears to have efficacy comparable with that of baclofen.[103] Dosage must be titrated slowly over 2 to 4 weeks, starting with 4 mg at bedtime with adjustments based on clinical response. Effective tolerated dosages have ranged from 2–36 mg/day. Sedation, dizziness, and dry mouth are the most commonly reported adverse effects, but hypotension also can occur, as well as a rare but severe hepatotoxicity. Increased aminotransferase activity was noted in 5% of patients during clinical trials. In patients who are unable to tolerate baclofen or tizanidine, diazepam (Valium), clonazepam (Klonopin), or dantrium sodium (Dantrolene) may be considered as alternatives, but they generally are less effective than either baclofen or tizanidine. Mild spasticity also may respond to moderately high doses of gabapentin (Neurontin). Tiagabine (Gabitril) may be useful in some patients with spasticity, but side effects may prohibit its use.

TREMOR

Cerebellar symptoms such as tremor can be troubling and difficult to control. Medications that may be helpful include propranolol, primidone, and isoniazid.

BOWEL AND BLADDER SYMPTOMS

Patients commonly complain of incontinence, urgency, frequency, and nocturia, which are indications of a hyperreflexic bladder (i.e., inability to store urine). A number of anticholinergic agents, including oxybutynin chloride (Ditropan, 10–20 mg/day), tolterodine (Detrol, 2–4 mg/day), propantheline bromide (Probanthine, 45–90 mg/day), and dicyclomine hydrochloride (Bentyl, 30–80 mg/day) are used to treat this problem if symptoms are mild. Ditropan is now also available in an extended-release formulation (5 and 10 mg). In addition, tricyclic antidepressants, such as imipramine (Tofranil) and amitriptyline (Elavil), also have been used for their anticholinergic properties. With all anticholinergic agents, great care must be used to avoid the problem of constipation, which is worsened by the patient's natural instinct to limit fluid intake (owing to the increasing the urge to urinate). As an alternative, the synthetic antidiuretic hormone preparation desmopressin (DDAVP) has been reported to be effective in the treatment of urgency and incontinence.[104] Use of DDAVP probably is best limited to bedtime so as to improve sleep because there may be significant problems with hyponatremia and possible seizures if overused. Patients with significant sphincter activity may benefit from the oral use of α-adrenergic blockers such as prazosin (Minipress) or intramuscular use of botulinum toxin type A (Botox).

Intermittent self-catheterization with or without a concomitant anticholinergic agent is recommended in patients with large postvoid urine residual volumes (>100 mL) or when the urinary problem is hyporeflexic in nature (failure to empty). Patients with large postvoid residual volumes are at risk for developing urinary tract infections and often are prescribed urinary acidifiers such as vitamin C or antiseptics such as methenamine mandelate to prevent infections.

Constipation is the most common bowel complaint. Increases in dietary fiber and hydration may alleviate this problem, but in some instances laxatives or enemas may be necessary.[102]

CLINICAL CONTROVERSY

In a depressed patient with a new diagnosis of MS, it is controversial whether to start interferon therapy because depression is a side effect of the interferon therapies, and the incidence of suicide is higher in this population. Practitioners generally will start patients on an antidepressant along with the interferon and watch them closely. Never should interferon be started in a severely depressed patient.

MAJOR DEPRESSION

Major depression is common in patients with MS, and the risk of suicide may be increased markedly as compared with healthy subjects.[105] Patients should be monitored closely for the development of major depressive symptomatology and treated accordingly (see Chap. 67). Interferon products should be used cautiously in patients with significant depression.

SENSORY SYMPTOMS

Numbness and paresthesias are frequent sensory complaints but usually do not require treatment. Some MS patients may develop acute or chronic pain syndromes,[103] such as trigeminal neuralgia and painful dysasthesias, for which treatment is necessary. Carbamazepine (Tegretol) is the preferred agent for the treatment of trigeminal neuralgia and is used in the same doses that are used for the treatment of seizure disorders. Painful dysasthesias (i.e., burning sensations that occur commonly in the extremities) often respond to treatment with tricyclic antidepressants, carbamazepine, gabapentin, or other anticonvulsant medications such as lamotrigine (Lamictal).

SEXUAL DYSFUNCTION

Sexual dysfunction in both men and women is also common in MS, and counseling should be offered to both partners. Sildenafil citrate (Viagra), tadalafil (Cialis), and vardenafil (Levitra) are very effective for men with MS who have erectile dysfunction. Viagra is currently being studied in the female population with MS and sexual dysfunction.

FATIGUE

Fatigue, one of the most common complaints in MS patients, can be severely disabling. Typically present in the late to middle afternoon, it may increase with heat exposure, exertion, intercurrent infection, spasticity, weakness, and depression. Amantadine hydrocholoride (100 mg twice daily) is used often and may offer significant relief.[103] Pemoline (Cylert) also has been used in doses starting at 18.75 to 37.5 mg/day,[103] but its use is limited by an FDA advisory suggesting very frequent monitoring of liver function tests owing to potential toxicity. Methylphenidate (Ritalin) and dextroamphetamine (Dexedrine) also are used commonly for fatigue in MS. Modafinil (Provigil), at 100 mg twice daily, is also helpful for MS-related fatigue. Antidepressants may be helpful, but only if the patient exhibits symptoms of depression. Otherwise, the sedating effects may worsen fatigue.

The aminopyridines, 4-aminopyridine and 3,4-diaminopyridine,[106] are potassium channel blockers that are currently under investigation in the symptomatic treatment of MS. These agents may improve conduction in demyelinated axons and may improve strength and decrease heat sensitivity.

Each symptom should be assessed individually, and therapy with available agents should be tried and modified when needed. In addition to counseling patients regarding the adverse effects associated with medications, pharmacists also should actively encourage patients to comply with their prescribed regimens.

COMPLEMENTARY AND ALTERNATIVE THERAPIES FOR MS

A large percentage of patients with MS use complementary or alternative medicine (CAM) instead of or in addition to disease-modifying and symptomatic therapies. Common CAM therapies include diet and dietary supplements, such as vitamins, minerals, and herbs. To date, no one diet or dietary supplement has proven to modify the course of MS. Mildly beneficial results have been seen in clinical trials with diets that increase the intake of polyunsaturated fatty acids (PUFAs). Omega-3 fatty acid is an example of polyunsaturated fatty acids and may be obtained through fatty fish, such as salmon or tuna. Suggestive results have been obtained from in vitro and animal studies with vitamin D, ginkgo biloba, cannabinoids, and an herbal medicine known as Padma 28. Antioxidant supplements vitamin A, C, E, α-lipoic acid (ALA), CoQ10, grape seed, and pine bark extracts also have suggestive evidence in benefiting MS patients. However, for patients with MS, there is a theoretical risk involved with taking antioxidant supplements owing to their ability to stimulate the immune system (T cells and macrophages). Stimulating the immune system in a patient with MS could be counterproductive, possibly worsening or exacerbating their disease, and may counteract the effects of immunomodulators. Other immune-stimulating supplements that should be used with caution are garlic, ginseng (Asian and Siberian), echinacea, cat's claw, astragulus, alfalfa, and stinging nettle. A few agents that may pose a problem in MS but also may have benefit are zinc, melatonin (for insomnia), and dehydroepiandrosterone (DHEA).[107]

Even though there is suggestive evidence for some of these CAM therapies, there are insufficient clinical trials supporting their use and safety as disease-modifying therapies for MS. However, for patients with MS who are willing to try new approaches with limited evidence, CAM may be a consideration. Health care providers can be a source of objective information regarding the use of CAM for MS and can assist their patients in making the best decision for them.[107]

PHARMACOECONOMIC CONSIDERATIONS

As with many therapeutic decisions, economic cost both to the individual and to society must be considered. Currently, the annual cost of the new potentially disease-modifying therapies is considerable. The cost to the pharmacist of glatiramer and both currently available interferons is between $10,000 and $17,000 per patient per year. Given this expense, it must be remembered that these therapies are not curative and that individual patients may experience variable results. Future investigations evaluating these therapeutic modalities clearly will need to address not only clinical but also economic and humanistic outcomes.

EVALUATION OF THERAPEUTIC OUTCOMES

Response to treatment of acute exacerbations of MS is seen commonly within days. With respect to disease-modifying treatments, it is important for the clinician to recognize that over the short term (days to weeks), little or no apparent benefit may be noted by either patient or clinician. Evaluation of therapeutic outcomes, such as decreased MS exacerbations and hospitalizations or perhaps slowed disease progression and disability (as measured using scales such as EDSS), must be conducted over a period of months to years. Patients should be provided with realistic goals and expectations of these treatment options and encouraged to participate in the evaluation of therapeutic response. Initially, it may be important to reevaluate patients at relatively short time intervals to monitor for adverse effects.

Safety monitoring of patients on interferon includes regular laboratory monitoring, patient observation and questioning for adverse effects or changing disability, and regular neurologic examinations.

Specific laboratory monitoring should include a complete blood count, platelet count, and liver function tests. These should be completed at baseline, every 3 months for 1 year, and every 6 months yearly thereafter. Copaxone requires no laboratory monitoring.

CONCLUSION

MS is an inflammatory disease of the CNS that appears to strike young, genetically susceptible individuals living in high-risk geographic areas. Although the exact etiology of MS is unknown, it is likely that MS is an autoimmune disease triggered by a viral infection. There is no cure, but quality of life can be improved through symptomatic management. Because of the relapsing-remitting nature of MS, it is often difficult to assess whether improvement is due to treatment or to the natural course of the disease. The paucity of conclusive evidence for many of the described treatments and the lack of specific guidelines make treatment choices difficult.

ACKNOWLEDGMENT

We would like to acknowledge both Jennifer Stone, Pharm.D., and Ruth C. Taggart, MSN, ANP-C, for their contributions to this chapter.

ABBREVIATIONS

ABC-R: Avonex, Betaseron, Copaxone, and Rebif
ACTH: adrenocorticotropic hormone
ALA: α-lipoic acid
BBB: blood-brain barrier
CAM: complementary or alternative medicine
CD4+: T-helper cells
CIS: clinically isolated syndrome
CNS: central nervous system
CSF: cerebrospinal fluid
CT scan: computed tomographic scan
DHEA: dehydroepiandrosterone
EAE: experimental allergic encephalomyelitis
EDSS: expanded disability status scale
GABA: γ-aminobutyric acid
HHV-6: human herpes virus type 6
HLA: human leukocyte antigen
HTLV: human T-cell leukemia virus
IgG: immunoglobulin G
IL-2: interleukin-2
IL-10: interleukin-10
INF-γ: interferon-γ
IVIG: intravenous immunoglobulin
MBP: myelin basic protein
MHC: major histocompatibility complex
MRA: magnetic resonance angiography
MRI: magnetic resonance imaging
MS: multiple sclerosis
MSFC: Multiple Sclerosis Functional Composite
NSAID: nonsteroidal anti-inflammatory drug
OCBs: oligoclonal bands
PPMS: primary-progressive multiple sclerosis
PRMS: primary-relapsing multiple sclerosis
PUFAs: polyunsaturated fatty acids
RRMS: relapsing-emitting multiple sclerosis

PMS: secondary-progressive multiple sclerosis

SPE: subacute sclerosing panencephalitis

GF-β: transforming growth factor β

LI: total lymphoid irradiation

NF-α: tumor necrosis factor alpha

WHO: World Health Organization

Review Questions and other resources can be found at *www.pharmacotherapyonline.com.*

REFERENCES

1. Anderson DW, Ellenberg JH, Leventhal CM, et al. Revised estimate of the prevalence of multiple sclerosis in theUnited States. Ann Neurol 1992; 31:333–336.

2. Wynn DR, Rodriguez M, O'Fallon WM, et al. Update on the epidemiology of multiple sclerosis. Mayo Clin Proc 1989;64:808–817.

3. Sadovnick AD, Ebers GC. Epidemiology of multiple sclerosis: A critical overview. Can J Neurol Sci 1993;20:17–29.

4. Ebers GC, Bulman D. The geography of MS reflects genetic susceptibility. Neurology 1986;36(suppl 1):108.

5. Compston A. Risk factors for multiple sclerosis: Race or place? (Editorial). J Neurol Neurosurg Psychiatry 1990;53:821–823.

6. Kurtzke JF. Epidemiologic contributions to multiple sclerosis: An overview. Neurology 1980;30(suppl 2):61–79.

7. Ebers GC. Genetics and multiple sclerosis: An overview. Ann Neurol 1994;36:S12–S14.

8. Compston A. The epidemiology of multiple sclerosis: Principles, achievements, and recommendations. Ann Neurol 1994;36:S211–S217.

9. Wolfson C, Wolfson EB, Zielinski JM. On the estimation of the distribution of the latent period of multiple sclerosis. Neuroepidemiology 1989;8:239–248.

10. Detels R, Visscher BR, Haile RW, et al. Multiple sclerosis and age at migration. Am J Epidemiol 1978;108:386–393.

11. Willer CJ, Dyment DA, Risch, et al. Twin concordance and sibling recurrence rates in multiple sclerosis. Proc Natl Acad Scs USA 2003; 100:12877–12882.

12. Hillert J. Human leukocyte antigen studies in multiple sclerosis. Ann Neurol 1994;36:S15–S17.

13. Genetics and immunology. In: Kesselring J, ed. Multiple Sclerosis. Cambridge, England, Cambridge, University Press, 1997:30–48.

14. Chapman J, Vinokurov S, Achiron A, et al. APOE genotype is a major predictor of long-term progression of disability in MS. Neurology 2001;56: 2148–2149.

15. Schmidt S, Barcellos LF, DeSombre K, et al. Association of polymorphisms in the apolipoprotein E region with susceptibility to and progression of multiple sclerosis. Am J Hum Genet 2002;70:708–717.

16. Lucchinetti CF, Rodriguez M. The controversy surrounding the pathogenesis of the multiple sclerosis lesion. Mayo Clin Proc 1997;72:665–678.

17. De Keyser J. Autoimmunity in multiple sclerosis. Neurology 1988;38:371–374.

18. McDonald WI. The mystery of the origin of multiple sclerosis. J Neurol Neurosurg Psychiatry 1989;49:113–323.

19. Poser CM. Pathogenesis of multiple sclerosis: A critical reappraisal. Acta Neuropathol 1986;71:1–10.

20. Sharief MK, Thompson EJ. In vivo relationship of tumor necrosis factor alpha to blood-brain barrier damage in patients with active multiple sclerosis. J Neuroimmunol 1992;38:27–33.

21. Panitch HS, Hirsch RL, Schindler J, Johnson KP. Treatment of multiple sclerosis with gamma interferon: Exacerbation associated with activation of the immune system. Neurology 1987;37:1097–1102.

22. Hartung HP, Archelos JJ, Zievasek J, et al. Circulating adhesion molecules and inflammatory mediators in demyelination: A review. Neurology 1995;45(suppl 6):22–32.

23. Link J, Soderstrom M, Olsson T. Increased TGF-β, IL-4, and INF-α in multiple sclerosis. Ann Neurol 1994;36:379–386.

24. Rieckman P, Albrecht M, Kitze B, et al. Cytokine mRNA levels in mononuclear blood cells from patients with multiple sclerosis. Neurology 1994;44:1523–1526.

25. Sobel RA. The pathology of multiple sclerosis. Neurol Clin 1995;13:1–16.

26. Smith-Jensen T, Burgoon M, Anthony J, et al. Comparison of immunoglobulin G heavy-chain sequences in MS and SSPE brains reveals an antigen-driven response. Neurology 2000;54:1227–1232.

27. Johnson RT. The virology of demyelinating diseases. Ann Neurol 1994; 36:S54–S60.

28. Berti R, Soldan SS, Akhyani N, et al. Extended observations on the association of HHV-6 and multiple sclerosis. J Neurovirol 2000;6(suppl 2): S85–S87.

29. Sriram S, Stratton CW, Yao S, et al. *Chlamydia pneumoniae* infection of the central nervous system in multiple sclerosis. Ann Neurol 1999; 46(1):6–14.

30. Swanborg RH, Whittum-Hudson JA, Hudson AP. Infectious agents and multiple sclerosis: Are *Chlamydia* pneumoniae and human herpes virus six involved? J Neuroimmunol 2003;136:1–8.

31. Trapp BD, Peterson J, Ransohoff RM, et al. Axonal transection in the lesions of multiple sclerosis. N Engl J Med 1998;338:278–285.

32. Truyen L, van Wuesberghe JHTM, Barkof F, et al. Accumulation of hypointense lesions ("blackholes") on T_1 spin echo MRI correlates with disease progression in multiple sclerosis. Neurology 1996;47: 1469–1476.

33. Lassman H, Suchanek G, Ozawa K. Histopathology and the blood–cerebrospinal fluid barrier in multiple sclerosis. Ann Neurol 1994;36: S42–S46.

34. Rodriguez M. Multiple sclerosis: Basic concepts and hypothesis. Mayo Clin Proc 1989;64:570–576.

35. Lucchinetti C, Bruck W, Parisi J, et al. Heterogeneity of multiple sclerosis lesions: Implications for the pathogenesis of demyelination. Ann Neurology 2000;47:707–717.

36. Schapiro RT. Symptom management in multiple sclerosis. Ann Neurol 1994;36:S123–S129.

37. Kurtzke JF. Rating neurologic impairment in multiple sclerosis: An expanded disability status scale (EDSS). Neurology 1983;33:1444–1452.

38. Rudick RA, Cutter G, Reingold S. The multiple sclerosis functional composite: A new clinical outcome measure for multiple sclerosis trials. Mult Scler 2002;8:359–365.

39. Noseworthy JH. Clinical scoring methods for multiple sclerosis. Ann Neurol 1994;36:S80–S85.

40. Miller DH. Magnetic resonance imaging in monitoring the treatment of multiple sclerosis. Ann Neurol 1994;36:S91–S94.

41. Filippi M, Paty DW, Kappos L, et al. Correlations between changes in disability and T_2-weighted brain activity in multiple sclerosis: A follow-up study. Neurology 1995;45:255–260.

42. Abramsky O. Pregnancy and multiple sclerosis. Ann Neurol 1994;36: S38–S41.

43. Goodin DS, Ebers GC, Johnson KP, et al. The relationship of MS to physical trauma and psychological stress: Report of the Therapeutics and Technology Assessment Subcommittee of the American Academy of Neurology. Neurology 1999;52:1737–1745.

44. Goodin DS, Ebers GC, Johnson KP, et al. The relationship of MS to physical trauma and psychological stress: Report of the Therapeutics and Technology Assessment Subcommittee of the American Academy of Neurology. Neurology 1999;52:1737–1745.

45. Weinshenker BG. Natural history of multiple sclerosis. Ann Neurol 1994; 36:S6–S11.

46. Confavreux C, Vukusic S, Moreau T, et al. Relapses and progression of disability in multiple sclerosis. N Engl J Med 2000;343:1430–1438.

47. Zivadinov R, Zorzon M. Is gadolinium enhancement predictive of the development of brain atrophy in multiple sclerosis? A review of the literature. J Neuroimag 2002;12:302–309.

48. Sadovnick AD, Eisen K, Ebers GC, Paty DW. Cause of death in patients attending multiple sclerosis clinics. Neurology 1991;41:1193–1196.

49. Swanson JW. Multiple sclerosis: Update in diagnosis and review of prognostic factors. Mayo Clin Proc 1989;64:577–586.

50. Williams ES, Jones DR, McKeran RO. Mortality rates from multiple sclerosis: Geographical and temporal variations revisited. J Neurol Neurosurg Psychiatry 1991;54:104–109.

51. Brex PA, Ciccarelli O, Riordan J, et al. A longitudinal study of abnormalities on MRI and disability from multiple sclerosis. N Engl J Med 2002;346:158–164.

52. Truyen L, van Waesberghe JH, van Walderveen MA, et al. Accumulation of hypointense lesions ("black holes") on T1 spin-echo MRI correlates with disease progression in multiple sclerosis. Neurology 1996;47:1469–1476.

53. Fisher E, Rudick R, Simon J, et al. Eight-year follow-up study of brain atrophy in patients with MS. Neurology 2002;59:1412–1420.

54. McDonald W, Compston A, Edan G, et al. Recommended diagnostic criteria for multiple sclerosis: Guidelines from the international panel on diagnosis of multiple sclerosis. Ann Neurol 2001;50:121–127.

55. Poser C, Paty D, Scheinberg L, et al. New diagnostic criteria for multiple sclerosis: Guidelines for research protocols. Ann Neurol 1983;13:227–231.

56. Tintore M, Rovira A, Rio J, et al. New diagnostic criteria for multiple sclerosis: Application in first demyelinating episode. Neurology 2003;60:27–30.

57. Dalton C, Brex P, Miszkiel K, et al. New T_2 lesions enable an earlier diagnosis of multiple sclerosis in clinically isolated syndromes. Ann Neurol 2003;53:673–676.

58. Frohman EM, Goodin DS, Calabresi PA, et al. The utility of MRI in suspected MS: Report of the Therapeutics and Technology Assessment Subcommittee of the American Academy of Neurology. Neurology 2003;61:1332–1338.

59. McFarland H, Frank JA, Albert PS, et al. Using gadolinium-enhanced magnetic resonance imaging lesions to monitor disease activity in multiple sclerosis. Ann Neurol 1992;32:758–766.

60. O'Riordan JI, Thompson AJ, Kingsley DP, et al. The prognostic value of brain MRI in clinically isolated syndromes of the CNS: A 10-year follow-up. Brain 1998;121:495–503.

61. CHAMPS Study Group. MRI predictors of early conversion to clinically definite MS in the CHAMPS placebo group. Neurology 2002;59:998–1005.

62. Fisher E, Rudick RA, Simon JH, et al. Eight-year follow-up study of brain atrophy in patients with MS. Neurology 2002;59:1412–1420.

63. Olsson T. Cerebrospinal fluid. Ann Neurol 1994;36:S100–S102.

64. Berger T, Rubner P, Schautzer F, et al. Antimyelin antibodies as a predictor of clinically definite multiple sclerosis after a first demyelinating event. N Engl J Med 2003;349:139–145.

65. Goodin DS, Frohman EM, Garmany GP, et al. Disease-modifying therapies in multiple sclerosis: Report of the therapeutics and technology assessment subcommittee of the American Academy of neurology and the MS Council for Clinical Practice Guidelines. Neurology 2002;58:169–178.

66. Myers LW, Ellison GW. The peculiar difficulties of therapeutic trials for multiple sclerosis. Neurol Clin 1990;8:119–141.

67. Hunter SF, Weinshenker BG, Carter JL, Noseworthy JH. Rational clinical immunotherapy for multiple sclerosis. Mayo Clin Proc 1997;72:765–780.

68. Kaufman DI, Trobe JD, Eggenberger ER, Whitaker JN. Practice parameter: The role of corticosteroids in the management of acute monosymptomatic optic neuritis. Report of the quality standards subcommittee of the American Acad Neurol. Neurol 2000;54:2039–2044.

69. Zivadinov R, Rudick RA, De Masi R, et al. Effects of IV methylprednisolone on brain atrophy in relapsing-remitting MS. Neurology 2001;57:1239–1247.

70. Kappos L. Therapy. In: Kesselring J, ed. Multiple Sclerosis. Cambridge, England, Cambridge University Press, 1997:148–167.

71. Weinshenker BG, O'Brian PC, Petterson TM, et al. A randomized trial of plasma exchange in acute central nervous system inflammatory demyelinating disease. Ann Neurol 1999;46:878–886.

72. Weinshenker BG. Therapeutic plasma exchange for acute inflammatory demyelinating syndromes of the central nervous system. J Clin Apheresi 1999;14:144–148.

73. PRISMS Study Group and the University of British Columbia MS/MRI Analysis Group. PRISMS-4: Long-term efficacy of interferon-β-1a in relapsing MS. Neurology 2001;56:1628–1636.

74. Simon JH, Jacobs L, Campion M, et al. A longitudinal study of brain atrophy in relapsing MS. Neurology 1999;58:139–145.

75. Fischer JS, Priore RL, Jacobs LD, et al. Neuropsychological effect of interferon-β-la in relapsing multiple sclerosis. Ann Neurol 2000;48:885–892.

76. Frohman E, Phillips T, Kokel K, et al. Disease-modifying therapy in multiple sclerosis: Strategies for optimizing management. Neurology 2002;8:227–236.

77. Patten SB, Metz LM. Interferon-β-1a and depression in relapsing remitting multiple sclerosis: An analysis of depression data from the PRISMS clinical trial. Mult Scler 2001;7:243–248.

78. Aharoni R, Teitelbaum D, Sela M, et al. Copolymer 1 induces T cells of the T helper type 2 that cross-react with myelin basic protein and suppress experimental autoimmune encephalomyelitis. Proc Natl Acad Sci USA 1997;94:10821–10826.

79. Johnson KP, Brooks BR, Cohen JA, et al. Extended use of glatiramer acetate (Copaxone) is well tolerated and maintains its clinical effect on multiple sclerosis relapse rate and degree of disability. Neurology 1998;50:701–708.

80. Fillippi M, Rovaris M, Rocca MA, et al. Glatiramer acetate reduces the proportion of new MS lesions evolving into "black holes." Neurology 2001;57:731–733.

81. Johnson KP, Brooks BB, Ford CC, et al. Results of the long-term (eight year) prospective, open-label trial of glatiramer acetate for relapsing multiple sclerosis. Neurol Suppl 2002;58:PO6.079.

82. van den Noort S, Eidelman B, Rammohan K, et al. for the National Multiple Sclerosis Society (NMSS). Disease Management Consensus Statement: Clinical Bulletin. New York, National MS Society, 1998:1–8.

83. Jacobs LD, Beck RW, Simon JH, et al. Intramuscular interferon-β-1a therapy initiated during a first demyelinating event in multiple sclerosis. N Engl J Med 2000;343:898–904.

84. Comi G, Filippi M, Barkhof F, et al. Effect of early interferon treatment on conversion to definite multiple sclerosis: A randomised study. Lancet 2001;357:1576–1582.

85. Vartanian T. An examination of the results of the EVIDENCE, INCOMIN, and phase III studies of interferon beta products in the treatment of multiple sclerosis. Clin Ther 2003;1:105–118.

86. Durelli L, Verdun E, Bergui M, et al. Every-other-day interferon-β-1b versus once-weekly interferon-β-1a for multiple sclerosis: Results of a 2-year prospective randomized multicentre study (INCOMIN). Lancet 2002;359:1453–1460.

87. Panitch H, Goodin D, Francis G, et al. Randomized, comparative study of interferon-β-1a treatment regimens in MS: The EVIDENCE Trial. Neurology 2002;59:1496–1506.

88. Clanet M, Radue E, Kappos L, et al. A randomized, double-blind, dose-comparison study of weekly interferon-β-1a in relapsing MS. Neurology 2002;59:1507–1517.

89. Bertolotto A. Neutralizing antibodies to interferon beta: Implications for the management of multiple sclerosis. Curr Opin Neurol 2004;17:241–246.

90. Kappos L, Polman C, Pozzilli C, et al. Final analysis of the European multicenter trial on IFNβ-1b in secondary-progressive MS. Neurology 2001;57:1969–1975.

91. Secondary Progressing Efficacy Clinical Trial of Recombinant Interferon-β-1a in MS (SPECTRIMS) Study Group. Randomized controlled trial of interferon-β-1a in secondary progressive MS: Clinical results. Neurology 2001;56:1496–1504.

92. Cohen J, Cutter G, Fischer J, et al. Benefit of interferon-β-1a on MSFC progression in secondary progressive MS. Neurology 2002;59:679–687.

93. Immunex Corporation. Novantrone (mitoxantrone concentrate for injection) package insert. Seattle, WA, October, 2000.

94. Noseworthy JH, Lucchinetti C, Rodriguez M, Weinshenker BG. Multiple sclerosis. N Engl J Med 2000;343:938–952.

95. La Mantia L, Milanese C, Mascoli N, et al. Cyclophosphamide for multiple sclerosis. Cochrane Database Syst Rev 2002;4:CD002819.

96. The Multiple Sclerosis Study Group. Efficacy and toxicity of cyclosporine in chronic progressive multiple sclerosis: A randomized, double-blinded, placebo-controlled clinical trial. Ann Neurol 1990;27: 591–605.

97. Corboy JR, Goodin DS, Frohman EM. Disease-modifying therapies for multiple sclerosis. Curr Treat Options Neur 2003;5:35–54.

98. Miller DH, Khan OA, Sheremata WA, et al. A controlled trial of natalizumab for relapsing multiple sclerosis. N Engl J Med 2003;348:15–23.

99. Paolillo A, Coles AJ, Molyneux PD, et al. Quantitative MRI in patients with secondary progressive MS treated with monoclonal antibody Campath 1H. Neurology 1999;53:751–757.

100. Nash RA, Bowen JD, McSweeney PA, et al. High-dose immunosuppressive therapy and autologous peripheral blood stem cell transplantation in severe multiple sclerosis. Blood 2003;102:2364–2372.

101. Cohen Y, Polliack A, Nagler A. Treatment of refractory autoimmune diseases with ablative immunotherapy using monoclonal antibodies and/or high dose chemotherapy with hematopoietic stem cell support. Curr Pharm Des 2003;9:279–288.

102. Schapiro RT. Symptom management in multiple sclerosis. Ann Neurol 1994;36:S123–S129.

103. Mitchell G. Update on multiple sclerosis therapy. Med Clin North Am 1993;77:231–249.

104. Kinn AC, Larsson PO. Desmopressin: A new principle for symptomatic treatment of urgency and incontinence in patients with multiple sclerosis. Scand J Urol Nephrol 1990;24:109–112.

105. Stenager EN, Stenager E, Koch Henriksen N, et al. Suicide and multiple sclerosis: An epidemiological investigation. J Neurol Neurosurg Psychiatry 1992;55:542–545.

106. Beaver CT Jr. The current status of studies of aminopyridine in patients with multiple sclerosis. Ann Neurol 1994;36:S118–S121.

107. Bowling AC, Stewart TM. Current complementary and alternative therapies for multiple sclerosis. Curr Treat Options Neurol 2003;5:55–68.

54

EPILEPSY

Barry E. Gidal and William R. Garnett

Learning Objectives and other resources can be found at *www.pharmacotherapyonline.com.*

KEY CONCEPTS

◄1 Accurate diagnosis and classification of seizure/syndrome type is critical to selection of appropriate pharmacotherapy.

◄2 Patient-specific treatment goal(s) should be identified. Treatment goals may change over time. In general, the goal of treatment should be seizure freedom and no adverse effects.

◄3 Patient characteristics such as age, medical condition, ability to comply with prescribed regimen, and insurance coverage also may influence choice of antiepileptic drugs.

◄4 Pharmacotherapy of epilepsy is highly individualized and requires titration of dose to optimize antiepileptic drug therapy (maximal seizure control with minimal or no side effects). About 70% of patients can be maintained on one antiepileptic drug.

◄5 If the therapeutic goal (seizure freedom and no intolerable adverse effects) is not achieved with maximal monotherapy, a second drug may be added or a switch to an alternative single antiepileptic drug can be made. The second antiepileptic drug should have a different mechanism of action from the first.

◄6 Some patients eventually can discontinue antiepileptic drug therapy. Several factors predict successful withdrawal of antiepileptic drugs.

◄7 The appropriate use of antiepileptic drugs requires a thorough understanding of their clinical pharmacology, e.g., mechanism of action, pharmacokinetics, adverse reaction, dosage forms, and drug interactions.

Epilepsy is a disorder that is best viewed as a symptom of disturbed electrical activity in the brain caused by a wide variety of etiologies. It is a collection of many different types of seizures that vary widely in severity, appearance, cause, consequence, and management. Epilepsy implies a periodic recurrence of seizures with or without convulsions.[1] Seizures that are prolonged or repetitive can be life-threatening. The effect epilepsy has on patients' lives can be extremely frustrating. Indeed, studies have shown that patients with epilepsy who do not experience complete seizure control have lower self-reported quality-of-life scores than patients who are seizure-free. It is also important to recognize that seizures may be just one (albeit the most obvious) symptom of an epileptic disorder. Not uncommonly, patients have other comorbid disorders, including depression, anxiety, and potentially neuroendocrine disturbances. Patients with epilepsy also may display neurodevelopmental delay, memory problems, and/or cognitive impairment. While, by convention, the focus of drug treatment is on the abolition of seizures, clinicians also need be attentive to addressing these common comorbidities.

EPIDEMIOLOGY

Each year, 120 per 100,000 people in the United States come to medical attention because of a newly recognized seizure.[2,3] At least 8% of the general population will have at least one seizure in a lifetime. However, it is possible to have a seizure and not have epilepsy. The rate of recurrence of a first unprovoked seizure within 5 years ranges between 23% and 80%. Children with an idiopathic first seizure and a normal electroencephalogram (EEG) have a particularly favorable prognosis. Some seizures may occur as single events resulting from withdrawal

of central nervous system (CNS) depressants (e.g., alcohol, barbiturates, and other drugs) or during acute illnesses (such as meningitis or encephalitis) or toxic conditions (e.g., uremia or eclampsia). Some patients will have seizures only associated with fever. These febrile seizures do not constitute epilepsy.[2]

Epilepsy is a chronic disorder characterized by recurrent seizures.[1] The age-adjusted incidence of epilepsy is 44 per 100,000 person-years. Each year, about 125,000 new epilepsy cases occur; of these, 30% are in people younger than age 18 at the time of diagnosis. There is a bimodal distribution in the occurrence of the first seizure, with one peak occurring in newborn and young children and the second peak occurring in patients older than age 65. The relatively high frequency of epilepsy in the elderly is now being recognized. At least 10% of patients in long-term care facilities are taking at least one antiepileptic drug (AED).

ETIOLOGY

Seizures occur because small numbers of neurons discharge abnormally. Anything that disrupts the normal homeostasis of the neuron and disturbs its stability may trigger abnormal activity and seizures. A genetic predisposition to seizures has been suggested. Patients with mental retardation and cerebral palsy are at increased risk for seizures. The more profound the degree of mental retardation as measured by intelligence quotient (IQ), the greater is the incidence of epilepsy. However, mental retardation is not synonymous with epilepsy. In the elderly, seizures are primarily partial in onset. The causes of seizures in the elderly may be multifactorial and include cerebrovascular disease (both ischemic and hemorrhagic stroke), neurodegenerative disorders, tumor, head trauma, metabolic disorders, and CNS infections. In some cases, if an etiology can be found and corrected, the patient will not require chronic AED treatment. In many cases, patients will present with seizures that do not have an identifiable cause and thus have idiopathic epilepsy. The incidence of idiopathic epilepsy is higher in children.[3]

Many factors have been shown to precipitate seizures in susceptible individuals. Hyperventilation may precipitate absence seizures. Sleep, sleep deprivation, sensory stimuli, and emotional stress may initiate seizures. Hormonal changes occurring around the time of menses, puberty, or pregnancy have been associated with the onset of or an increased frequency of seizures. A careful history should be obtained from patients presenting with seizures because theophylline, alcohol, high-dose phenothiazines, antidepressants (especially maprotiline or buproprion), and street drug use have been associated with provoking seizures. Also, AEDs in toxic concentrations may cause seizures in certain patients. Perinatal factors and subsequent events have been identified as risk factors for the subsequent development of epilepsy. Children who are small for gestational age or with neonatal seizures are also at increased risk for developing epilepsy. The most clearly established risk factors for epilepsy in all age groups are head trauma (especially in patients in whom the dura mater has been breached and in whom there is evidence of loss of conciousness), CNS infections, and stroke. Immunizations have not been associated with an increased risk of epilepsy.

PATHOPHYSIOLOGY

Seizure activity is characterized by paroxysmal discharges occurring synchronously in a large population of cortical neurons.[4] This is characterized on EEG as a sharp wave or *spike*. The basic physiology of a seizure episode is traceable to an unstable cell membrane or its surrounding supportive cells. The seizure originates from the gray matter of any cortical or perhaps subcortical area. Initially, a small number of neurons fire abnormally. Normal membrane conductances and inhibitory synaptic currents break down, and excess excitability spreads, either locally to produce a focal seizure or more widely to produce a generalized seizure. This onset propagates by physiologic pathways to involve adjacent or remote areas. The clinical manifestations depend on the site of the focus, the degree of irritability of the surrounding area of the brain, and the intensity of the impulse.[4]

An abnormality of potassium conductance, a defect in the voltage-sensitive ion channels, or a deficiency in the membrane ATPases linked to ion transport may result in neuronal membrane instability and a seizure. Selected neurotransmitters (e.g., glutamate, aspartate, acetylcholine, norepinephrine, histamine, corticotropin-releasing factor, purines, peptides, cytokines, and steroid hormones) enhance the excitability and propagation of neuronal activity, whereas γ-aminobutyric acid (GABA) and dopamine inhibit neuronal activity and propagation. A relative deficiency of inhibitory neurotransmitters such as GABA or an increase in excitatory neurotransmitters such as glutamate would promote abnormal neuronal activity. Normal neuronal activity also depends on an adequate supply of glucose, oxygen, sodium, potassium, chloride, calcium, and amino acids. Systemic pH is also a factor in precipitating seizures. The different kinds of epilepsies probably arise from different neurophysiologic abnormalities.[4]

Control of abnormal neuronal activity with AEDs is accomplished by elevating the threshold of neurons to electrical or chemical stimuli or by limiting the propagation of the seizure discharge from its origin. Raising the threshold most likely involves stabilization of neuronal membranes, whereas limiting the propagation involves depression of synaptic transmission and reduction of nerve conduction.[4]

During a seizure, there is a large increase in the demand for blood flow to the brain to carry off CO_2 and to bring substrates for neuronal metabolic activity. The more prolonged the seizure, the more likely the brain is to suffer ischemia that may result in neuronal destruction and brain damage. Also, the continued exposure to glutamate, an excitatory neurotransmitter, may contirubte to neuronal damage. Although individual seizures as such do not cause a significant decrease in intelligence, it has been suggested that patients suffering a large number (>100) of generalized tonic-clonic (GTC) seizures who have multiple episodes of status epilepticus may be at risk for eventual cognitive declines.

In addition, there appears to be a positive correlation between the early initiation of appropriate AED therapy and the ability to control seizure activity. The failure to control seizures seems to lead to an increase in seizure activity and also to the occurrence of other seizure types. Therefore, appropriate therapy should be initiated early after the diagnosis of epilepsy.

CLINICAL PRESENTATION

The International League Against Epilepsy (ILAE) has proposed two major schemes for the classification of seizures and epilepsies: the International Classification of Epileptic Seizures and the International Classification of the Epilepsies and Epilepsy Syndromes.[5,6]

The International Classification of Epileptic Seizures (Table 54–1) combines the clinical description with certain electrophysiologic findings in order to classify epileptic seizures. Seizures are divided into two main pathophysiologic groups—partial seizures and generalized seizures—by EEG recordings and clinical symptomatology.

Partial (focal) seizures begin in one hemisphere of the brain and—unless they become secondarily generalized—result in an asymmetric motor manifestation. Partial seizures manifest as alterations in motor functions, sensory or somatosensory symptoms, or automatisms. Partial seizures with no loss of consciousness are classified as *simple partial*. In some cases, patients will describe somatosensory symptoms as a "warning" prior to the development of a GTC seizure.

TABLE 54–1. International Classification of Epileptic Seizures

I. Partial seizures (seizures begin locally)
  A. Simple (without impairment of consciousness)
    1. With motor symptoms
    2. With special sensory or somatosensory symptoms
    3. With psychic symptoms
  B. Complex (with impairment of consciousness)
    1. Simple partial onset followed by impairment of consciousness—with or without automatisms
    2. Impaired consciousness at onset—with or without automatisms
  C. Secondarily generalized (partial onset evolving to generalized tonic-clonic seizures)
II. Generalized seizures (bilaterally symmetrical and without local onset)
  A. Absence
  B. Myoclonic
  C. Clonic
  D. Tonic
  E. Tonic-clonic
  F. Atonic
  G. Infantile spasms
III. Unclassified seizures
IV. Status epilepticus

Ref. 5, 6.

These warnings are in fact simple partial seizures and frequently are termed *auras*.

Partial seizures with an alteration of consciousness are described as *complex partial*. With complex partial seizures, the patient may have automatisms, periods of memory loss, or aberrations of behavior.[1] Some patients with complex partial epilepsy have been mistakenly diagnosed as having psychotic episodes. Complex partial seizures also may progress to GTC seizures. Patients with complex partial seizures typically are amnestic to these events.

Generalized seizures have clinical manifestations that indicate involvement of both hemispheres. Motor manifestations are bilateral, and there is a loss of consciousness. Generalized seizures may be further subdivided by EEG and clinical manifestations. A partial seizure that becomes generalized is referred to as a *secondarily generalized seizure*.

Generalized absence seizures are manifested by a sudden onset, interruption of ongoing activities, a blank stare, and possibly a brief upward rotation of the eyes. They generally occur in young children through adolescence. It is important to differentiate absence seizures from complex partial seizures.

GTC seizures are what many people think of as epilepsy. The seizure results in a sudden sharp tonic contraction of muscles followed by a period of rigidity and clonic movements. During the seizure, the patient may cry or moan, lose sphincter control, bite the tongue, or develop cyanosis. After the seizure, the patient may have altered conciousness, drowsiness, or confusion for a variable period of time (postictal period) and frequently goes into a deep sleep. Tonic and clonic seizures may occur separately.

Brief shocklike muscular contractions of the face, trunk, and extremities are known as *myoclonic jerks*. They may be isolated events or rapidly repetitive. A sudden loss of muscle tone is known as an *atonic seizure*. This may be described as a head drop, the dropping of a limb, or a slumping to the ground. These patients often wear protective headware to prevent trauma.

The International Classification of Epilepsies and Epilepsy Syndromes adds components such as age of onset, intellectual development, findings on neurologic examination, and results of neuroimaging studies to define epilepsy syndromes more fully. Syndromes can include one or many different seizure types (e.g., Lennox Gastaut syndrome). The syndromic approach includes seizure type(s) and possible etiologic classifications (e.g., idiopathic, symptomatic, or unknown). *Idiopathic* describes syndromes that are presumably genetic but also those in which no underlying etiology is documented or suspected. A family history of seizures is commonly present, and neurologic function is essentially normal except for the occurrence of seizures. *Symptomatic* cases involve evidence of brain damage or a known underlying cause. A *cryptogenic* syndrome is assumed to be symptomatic of an underlying condition that cannot be documented. *Unknown* or *undetermined* is used when no cause can be identified. This syndromic classification is more important for prognostic determinations than for a classification based simply on seizure type. The syndrome classification scheme requires more information and,

in return, provides a more powerful tool for comprehensive clinical management. A patient's epilepsy is classified based on seizure type (i.e., generalized versus partial) and syndromic type (i.e., idiopathic, symptomatic, or cryptogenic).

CLINICAL PRESENTATION OF EPILEPSY

GENERAL

In most cases, the health care provider will not be in a position to witness a seizure. Many patients (particularly those with complex partial or generalized tonic-clonic seizures) are amnestic to the actual seizure event. Obtaining an adequate history and description of the ictal event (including time course) from a third party (e.g., significant other, family member, or witness) is critically important.

SYMPTOMS

Symptoms of a specific seizure will depend on seizure type. While seizures can vary between patients, they tend to be stereotyped within an individual.

- Complex partial seizures may include somatosensory or focal motor features.
- Complex partial seizures are associated with altered conciousness.
- Absence seizures may appear relatively bland, with only very brief (seconds) periods of altered conciousness.
- Generalized tonic-clonic seizures are major convulsive episodes and are always associated with a loss of conciousness.

SIGNS

Interictally (between seizure episodes), there are typically no objective, pathognomonic signs of epilepsy.

LABORATORY TESTS

There are currently no diagnostic laboratory tests for epilepsy. In some cases, particularly following generalized tonic-clonic (or perhaps complex partial) seizures, serum prolactin levels may be transiently elevated. Laboratory tests may be done to rule out treatable causes of seizures (e.g., hypoglycemia, altered electrolyted concentrations, infections, etc.) that do not represent epilepsy.

OTHER DIAGNOSTIC TESTS

- EEG is very useful in the diagnosis of various seizure disorders.
- The EEG may be normal in some patients who still have the clinical diagnosis of epilepsy.
- While MRI is very useful (especially imaging of the temporal lobes), CT scan typically is not helpful except in the initial evaluation for a brain tumor or cerebral bleeding.

▶ TREATMENT: Epilepsy

DESIRED OUTCOME

The ultimate goal of treatment for epilepsy is no seizures and no side effects with an optimal quality of life. The best quality of life is associated with a seizure-free state.[7] Often, however, a balance between efficacy and side effects must be reached because with the

older AEDs used as monotherapy, fewer than 50% of patients become seizure-free.

Because therapy is continued for many years (often a lifetime), chronic side effects must be considered. If the patient is overly sedated or develops other significant side effects, some seizure control may have to be sacrificed to improve functioning. The patient should be involved in deciding what balance between frequency of seizures and the occurrence of side effects is most appropriate. The newer AEDs offer alternatives for balancing seizure frequency and drug side effects.

Providing optimal quality of life goes beyond balancing seizures and side effects. It involves assessing all the concerns of a patient with epilepsy. For example, patients with epilepsy are concerned about driving, their future, forming relationships, safety, social isolation, social stigma, and so on. It is also important to recognize that patients with epilepsy may have other neuropsychiatric comorbidities such as depression, anxiety, and sleep disturbances.[8–10] Clinicians should be aware of these potential problems and consider therapy where appropriate.

GENERAL APPROACH TO TREATMENT

◀ The general approach to treatment involves identification of goals, assessment of seizure type and frequency, development of a care plan, and a follow-up evaluation. During the assessment phase, it is critical to establish an accurate diagnosis of the seizure type and classification. This diagnostic step will help to determine the appropriate initial AEDs. Patient-specific treatment goals must be identified, and these may change over time. In all patients, the goal should be "no seizures, no side effects, and an optimal quality of life." It must be recognized that this may not be possible in a significant minority of patients. Despite appropriate AED treatment, approximately 30% to 35% of patients will be refractory to treatment. In this setting, seizure freedom may not be obtained, and more obtainable outcomes should be established (e.g., decrease in the number of seizures and minimized drug adverse effects). Identification of specific goals will help in the development of the short- and long-term treatment plans. Patient characteristics such as age, medical condition, ability to comply with a prescribed regimen, and insurance coverage also should be explored because these may influence AED choices or help to explain a lack of response or unexpected adverse effects.

Once the assessment is complete, the advantages and disadvantages of appropriate AEDs are compared. For patients with new-onset seizures, the choice is whether to use drug therapy and, if so, which one. For a patient with long-standing epilepsy, adequacy of the current medication regimen must be evaluated. An AED should not be considered ineffective unless the patient has experienced unacceptable adverse effects with continued seizures.

◀ If a decision is made to start AED therapy, monotherapy is preferred, and about 50% to 70% of all patients with epilepsy can be maintained on one drug.[11,12] However, many of these patients are not seizure-free. The percentage of patients who are seizure-free on one drug varies by seizure type. The prognosis for 12-month seizure freedom is best for those who have only GTC seizures (48% to 55%), worst for those who have only complex partial seizures (23% to 26%), and intermediate for those with mixed seizure types (25% to 32%).[12] Drugs may be combined in an attempt to help the patient become seizure-free. Combining AEDs with different mechanisms of action may be advantageous, although this approach is as yet unproven.[13] Approximately 65% of patients can be expected to be maintained on one AED and be considered well controlled, although not necessarily seizure-free. Of the 35% of patients with unsatisfactory control, 10% will be well controlled with a two-drug treatment. Of the remaining 25%, 20% will continue to have unsatisfactory control despite multiple drug treatment. It has been suggested recently that there may be a genetic predisposition to epilepsy that is refractory to drug therapy. Some of these patients will become surgical candidates. For some patients, an implantable device such as the vagal nerve stimulator may be an additional nonpharmacologic option.

Once the care plan is established, a prescription is generated for a specific AED. Usually this includes a dose-titration schedule. At this point, patient education and assurance of patient understanding of the plan are essential. Detailed directions regarding titration, what to do in the event of a treatment-emergent side effect, and what to do if a seizure occurs must be provided to patients. Documentation of the assessment, care plan, and educational process is essential. Providing the patient with a seizure and side-effect diary will assist in the follow-up and evaluation phase. At the follow-up stage of treatment (which can be done in the hospital, clinic, or pharmacy or by phone), the treatment goals must be reviewed. If the goal has been achieved, new goals should be identified. For example, if the GTC seizures are now controlled, the goal may be to control partial seizures. If a patient fails to respond to the first AEDs, trials with other AEDs should be attempted. Completion of the evaluation often requires a reassessment of the patient and development of a new care plan. The assessment at this point should evaluate compliance, efficacy, and safety of the initial treatment.

Medication noncompliance may be the single most common reason for treatment failure. It is estimated that up to 60% of patients with epilepsy are noncompliant.[14] The rate of noncompliance is increased by the complexity of the drug regimen and by doses taken three and four times a day. Noncompliance is not influenced by age, sex, psychomotor development, seizure type, or seizure frequency.[14]

CLINICAL CONTROVERSY

Epilepsy is a clinical diagnosis defined by recurrent seizures. Controversy surrounds the most appropriate time to initiate AED therapy. Many clinicians do not initiate treatment until a second unprovoked seizure has occurred. Some clinicians start AED treatment after the first seizure, whereas others may initiate prophylactic treatment following a CNS insult thought likely to cause epilepsy eventually (e.g. stroke or head trauma). Appropriate treatment decisions may vary depending on individual patient clinical characteristics and circumstances.

Drug treatment may not be indicated in patients whose seizures have minimal impact on their lives or those who have had only a single seizure. If a patient presents after a single isolated seizure, one of three treatment decisions can be made: treat, possibly treat, or do not treat. These decisions are based on the probability of the patient having a second seizure (Table 54–2). For patients with no risk factors, the probability of a second seizure is less than 10% in the first year and approximately 24% by the end of 2 years. If risk factors are present, this recurrence rate can increase dramatically and can be as high as 80% after 5 years.[1] Are these rates high enough to warrant AED therapy? This decision often depends on patient-specific factors such as epilepsy syndrome, seizure etiology, presence of an neuroanatomic defect, and the EEG. Clearly, the patient's lifestyle and preference are of paramount importance. Patients who have had two or more seizures generally should be started on AEDs.

WHEN TO STOP ANTIEPILEPTIC DRUGS

◀ The AEDs used initially to control seizures may not need to be given for a lifetime. Polypharmacy may be reduced, and some patients can discontinue AEDs altogether. In reducing polypharmacy

TABLE 54–2. Recurrence Risk for Patients Experiencing One Unprovoked Seizure

Type of Patient	Ist-Yr Risk (%)	5th-Yr Risk (%)
Adults with single unproved seizure		34
No CNS insult	10	29
Influence of family history		
Sibling with seizure	29	46
No sibling with seizures	7	27
EEG patterns		
GSW on EEG	15	58
Normal EEG	9	26
Occurrence of previous seizure	10	39
Due to an illness or childhood febrile seizure		
Remote symptomatic with Todd's	26	48
paresis	41	75
Status epilepticus at onset	37	56
Prior acute seizure	60	80
Idiopathic	10	29

CNS = central nervous system; EEG = electroencephalogram; GSW = generalized spikes and waves.

TABLE 54–3. American Academy of Neurology Guideline for Discontinuing AEDs in Seizure-Free Patients

After assessing the risks and benefits to both patient and society from a recurrent seizure, the discontinuance of antiepileptic drugs may be considered by the physician and informed patient or parent/guardian if the patient meets the following profile:
- Seizure-free 2 to 5 years on AEDs (mean, 3.5 years)
- Single type of partial seizure (simple partial, complex partial, or secondary generalized tonic-clonic seizure) or single type of primary generalized tonic-clonic seizures
- Normal neurologic examination/normal IQ
- EEG normalized with treatment

the drug considered less appropriate for the seizure type (or the agent deemed most responsible for adverse effects) should be discontinued first. In some cases, decreasing the number of AEDs a patient is receiving can decrease side effects and increase cognitive abilities.[15] This improvement in cognition may be small, especially if the patient is on a drug that primarily affects psychomotor speed with less effect on higher-order cognitive functioning.

Factors favoring successful withdrawal of AEDs include a seizure-free period of 2 to 4 years, complete seizure control within 1 year of onset, an onset of seizures after age 2 but before age 35, and a normal neurologic examination and EEG. Factors associated with a poor prognosis in discontinuing AEDs, despite a seizure-free interval, include a history of a high frequency of seizures, repeated episodes of status epilepticus, a combination of seizure types, and development of abnormal mental functioning. Children who have irregular generalized spike and wave activity in EEG recordings prior to discontinuation of treatment may have a higher relapse rate (67%) compared with children without epileptiform activity (33%) or children with other types of epileptiform activity (33%) in their last EEG recordings before discontinuation. A 2-year seizure-free period is suggested for absence and rolandic epilepsy, whereas a 4-year seizure-free period is suggested for simple partial, complex partial, and absence associated with tonic-clonic convulsions. AED withdrawal generally is not suggested for patients with juvenile myoclonic epilepsy, absence with clonic-tonic-clonic seizures, or clonic-tonic-clonic seizures. The American Academy of Neurology has issued guidelines for discontinuing AEDs in seizure-free patients (Table 54–3). When the factors likely to be associated with successful withdrawal are present, the relapse rate is expected to be less than 32% for children and 39% for adults.

If the decision is made to attempt AED withdrawal, this should be done gradually. This may be particularly true for patients with profound developmental disabilities. Some patients will have a recurrence of seizures as the AEDs are withdrawn. Sudden withdrawal is associated with the precipitation of status epilepticus. Withdrawal seizures are of particular concern for agents such as benzodiazepines and barbiturates. Seizure relapse has been reported to be more common if the AEDs are withdrawn over 1 to 3 months than over 6 months.

The risk of seizure relapse has been estimated at 10% to 70%. A meta-analysis determined that the relapse rate was 25% after 1 year and 29% after 2 years. Withdrawal doubles the risk of seizure recurrence for the first 1 to 2 years but does not modify the long-term prognosis of a person's epilepsy. If seizures recur after AED withdrawal, AEDs should be restarted. Ninety percent of patients will regain at least another 2-year remission. In addition to seizure relapse, the withdrawal of AEDs has been associated with the emergence of anxiety and depression.[15]

CLINICAL CONTROVERSY

It is not entirely clear which patients with epilepsy will require lifelong treatment. While many clinicians feel that AED therapy is lifelong, others would argue that certain patients with idiopathic epilepsy and a normal neurologic examination and EEG may be candidates for AED withdrawal following a prolonged period of seizure freedom (e.g., >2 to 3 years). Most of the data supporting discontinuing AEDs have been obtained from children. Some adults will be reticent to discontinue AED therapy even if the clinician is in favor of it because of the fear of having a seizure and the consequences (e.g., loss of driver's license) that it would entail. The patient must be a willing participant in a therapeutic plan to discontinue an AED. The patient should agree to the plan to reduce or withdraw AED therapy.

There may be a significant psychosocial benefit to the patient from AED withdrawal. Withdrawal may need to be scheduled at the convenience of the patient. A follow-up of 5 years is suggested for any patient withdrawn from AED therapy.

NONPHARMACOLOGIC THERAPY

Nonpharmacologic therapy for epilepsy includes diet, surgery, and vagal nerve stimulation (VNS), which is implantation of a vagal nerve stimulator. A vagal nerve stimulator is an implanted medical device approved for use in epilepsy. The NCP system (NeuroCybernetic prosthesis) is indicated for use as an adjunctive therapy in reducing the frequency of seizures in adults and adolescents older than 12 years of age with partial-onset seizures that are refractory to AEDs. The device consists of an implantable, programmable pulse generator connected to a helical lead. The generator is implanted in a subcutaneous infraclavicular pocket and is powered by a lithium battery. The lead is attached to the left vagus nerve and delivers a biphasic current to the

TABLE 54–4. Drugs of Choice for Specific-Seizure Disorders

Seizure Type	First-Line Drugs	Alternative Drugs
Partial seizures	Carbamazepine	Gabapentin
	Phenytoin	Topiramate
	Lamotrigine	Levetiracetam
	Valproic acid	Zonisamide
	Oxcarbazepine	Tiagabine
		Primidone, phenobarbital
		Felbamate
Generalized seizures		
Absence	Valproic acid, ethosuximide	Lamotrigine, levetiracetam
Myoclonic	Valproic acid, clonazepam	Lamotrigine, topiramate, felbamate, zonisamide, levetiracetam
Tonic-clonic	Phenytoin, carbamazepine, valproic acid	Lamotrigine, topiramate, phenobarbital, primidone, oxcarbazepine, levetiracetam

nerve that can be programmed to different parameters by the physician through the skin. In addition, the patient can use a magnet placed over the generator to activate the generator during a seizure or aura.

The mechanisms of antiseizure actions of VNS are unknown, but recent studies have indicated that VNS acutely causes widespread bilateral cortical and subcortical alterations in blood flow, suggesting that it affects synaptic activity in humans.[16]

The VNS device is relatively safe. The most common side effect associated with stimulation is hoarseness, voice alteration, increased cough, pharyngitis, dyspnea, dyspepsia, and nausea. Serious adverse effects reported include infection, nerve paralysis, hyesthesia, facial paresis, left vocal chord paralysis, left facial paralysis, left recurrent laryngeal nerve injury, urinary retention, and low-grade fever. Over all the VNS studies, the percentage of patients who achieved a 50% or greater reduction in their seizure frequency (responders) ranged from 23% to 50%.

Surgery is the most widespread and most useful nonpharmacologic therapy.[17] The use of surgery for intractable epilepsy that significantly interferes with patients' lives and functioning is increasing in both adult and pediatric patients. The success rate is reported to be between 80% and 90% in properly selected patients. A National Institutes of Health Consensus Conference identified three absolute requirements for surgery. They are an absolute diagnosis of epilepsy, failure on an adequate trial of drug therapy, and definition of the electroclinical syndrome. A focus in the temporal lobe has the best chance for a positive outcome; however, extratemporal foci may be excised successfully in more than 75% of patients. The procedure is not without risk. Learning and memory are most susceptible to impairment postoperatively, and general intellectual abilities are also affected in a small number of patients. Surgery may be particularly useful in children with intractable epilepsy. Patients may still need to receive AED therapy for a period of time following successful epilepsy surgery in order to prevent seizure recurrence.[18]

The ketogenic diet was devised in the 1920s.[19] It is high in fat and low in carbohydrates and protein and thus leads to acidosis and ketosis. Protein and calorie intake are set at levels that will meet requirements for growth. Most of the calories are provided in the form of heavy cream and butter. No sugar is allowed. Vitamins and minerals are supplemented. Medium-chain triglycerides may be substituted for the dietary fats. Fluids are also controlled. It requires strict control and parent compliance. Although some centers find this useful for refractory patients, others have found that it is poorly tolerated by patients. Long-term effects are unknown.

▓ PHARMACOLOGIC THERAPY

Optimal management of epilepsy therefore requires that AED treatment be individualized. Specifically, different patient groups (e.g., children, women of child-bearing potential, and the elderly) may be better suited to one AED versus another by virtue not only of seizure type but also of succeptability or relative risk for certain adverse effects. These issues will be highlighted further below.

Selection and optimization of AED therapy require not only an understanding of drug mechanism(s) of action and spectrum of clinical activity but also an appreciation of pharmacokinetic variability as well as patterns of drug-related adverse effects. An AED must demonstrate efficacy for the specific seizure type being treated. The drug treatments of first choice depend on the type of epilepsy, as well as on the interface between drug-specific adverse effects and patient preferences (Table 54–4). Ultimately, AED effectiveness is the result of the interaction of each of these factors. A suggested algorithm for a general approach to the treatment of epilepsy is shown in Fig. 54–1.

The mechanism of action of most AEDs can be categorized as either affecting ion channels, augmenting inhibitory neurotransmission, or modulating excitatory neurotransmission. The ion channels affected include the sodium and calcium channels. Augmentation in inhibitory neurotransmission includes increasing CNS concentrations of GABA, whereas efforts to decrease excitatory neurotransmission are primarily focused on decreasing (or antagonizing) glutatmate and aspartate neurotransmission. AEDs that are effective against GTC and partial seizures probably reduce sustained repetitive firing of action potentials by delaying recovery of sodium channels from activation. Drugs that reduce corticothalmic T-type calcium currents are effective against generalized absence seizures. Myoclonic seizures respond to drugs that enhance $GABA_A$ receptor inhibition.[20] In addition to mechanism of action, awareness of pharmacokinetic properties (Table 54–5), adverse effects (Table 54–6), and drug-drug interactions (Tables 54–7 and 54–8) can aid in the optimization of AED therapy. Pharmacokinetic interactions are a common complicating factor in AED selection. Interactions can occur in any of the pharmacokinetic processes: absorption, distribution, or elimination. Caution should be used when AEDs are added to or withdrawn from a drug regimen.

Adverse effects of AEDs can be divided into acute and chronic (see Table 54–6). Acute effects can be dose/serum concentration–related or idiosyncratic. Concentration-dependent effects are common and troublesome but not usually life-threatening. Neurotoxic

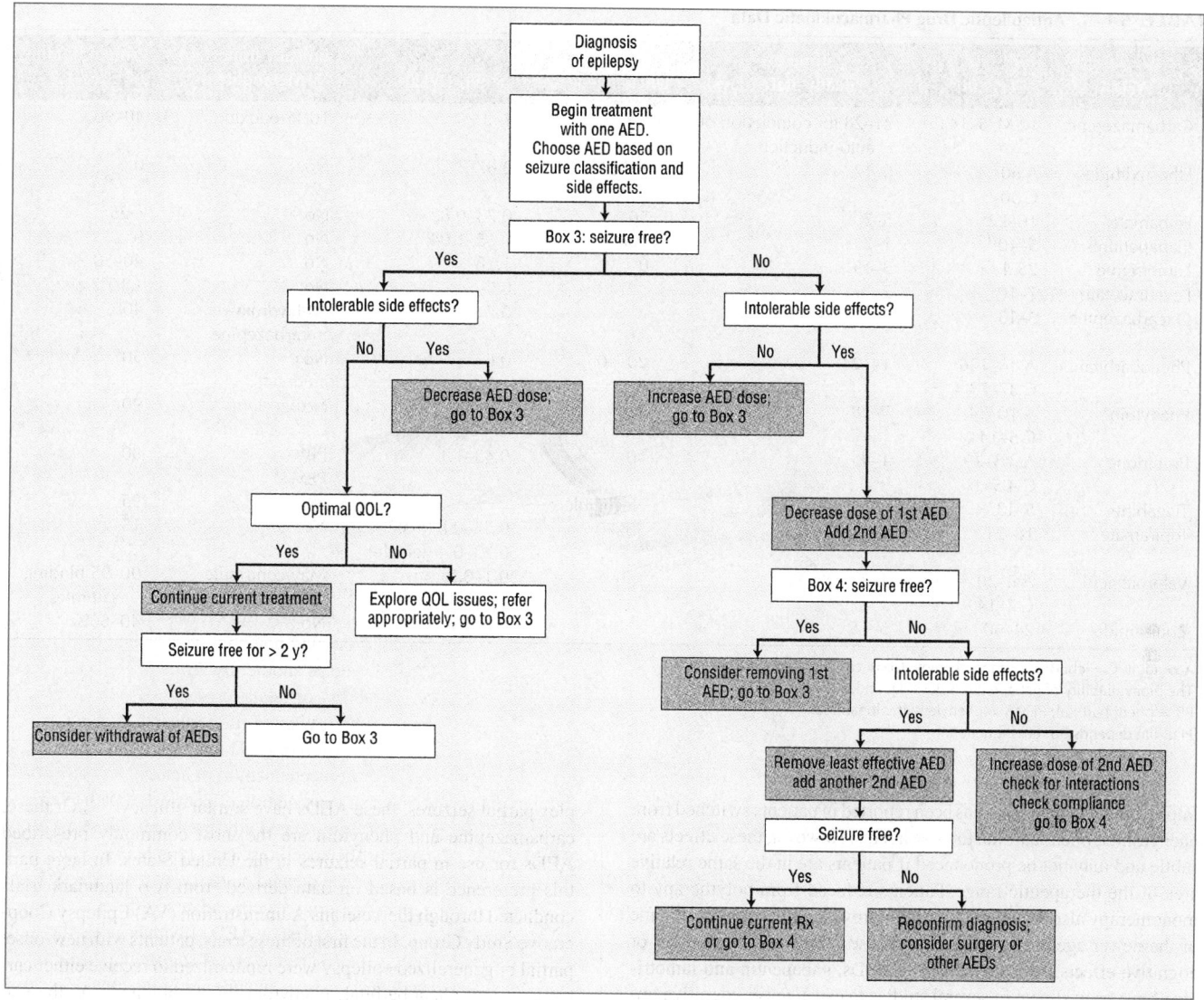

FIGURE 54–1. Algorithm for the treatment of epilepsy.

adverse effects are encountered commonly and can include sedation, dizziness, blurred or double vision, difficulty with concentration, and ataxia. In many cases these effects can be alleviated by decreasing drug dose. Most idiosyncratic reactions owing to an allergic reaction are mild, but they can be more serious if the hypersensitivity involves one or more organ systems. Other idiosyncratic side effects including hepatitis or blood dyscrasias are serious but rare.

Acute organ failure, if it is going to occur, generally occurs within the first 6 months of AED therapy. Unfortunately, screening laboratory evaluations of blood and urine typically are not helpful in predicting or detecting the early stage of severe reactions and generally are not recommended in asymptomatic patients. Laboratory assessment including white blood cell counts and liver function tests may be reasonable if the patient reports an unexplained illness (e.g., lethargy, vomiting, fever, or rash).[21] It is important to recognize that adverse effects can occur despite serum concentrations being within the proposed therapeutic range.[22]

Another potential long-term adverse effect of AED treatment is osteomalacia and osteoporosis.[23] The bone disorders associated with AED use consist of a heterogeneous group of disorders. These include findings ranging from asymptomatic high-turnover disease,

with findings of normal bone mineral density, to markedly decreased bone mineral density sufficient to warrent the diagnosis of osteoporosis. While the etiology of these osteopathies is still uncertain, it has been hypothesized that certain drugs, including phenytoin, phenobarbital, and perhaps carbamazepine and valproic acid, may interfere with vitamin D metabolism. Whether the newer AEDs are associated with these effects is as yet unknown. Common laboratory findings in these patients include elevated bone-specific alkaline phosphatase concentration and decreased serum calcium and 25-OH vitamin D concentrations. Patients receiving these drugs at the least should receive supplemental vitamin D and calcium.

The comparative effects of AEDs on cognition have been difficult to evaluate because of differences or inconsistencies in study design, included seizure types, control for serum drug concentrations, and the neuropsychological tests used. In general, there are not large differences between the older drugs,[24,25] although the barbiturates phenobarbital and primidone appear to cause more cognitive impairment than other commonly used AEDs. Phenytoin, particularly when serum concentrations are above the commonly accepted therapeutic range, may have a greater effect on motor function and speed. Among the older AEDs, valproic acid may cause less impairment of cognition.

TABLE 54–5. Antiepileptic Drug Pharmacokinetic Data

AED	$t_{1/2}$ (h)[a]	Time to Steady State (days)	Unchanged (%)	V_D (1/kg)	Clinically Important Metabolite	Protein Binding (%)
Carbamazepine	12 M; 5–14 Co	21–28 for completion of auto-induction	<1	1–2	10,11-epoxide	40–90
Ethosuximide	A 60 C 30	6–12	10–20	0.67	No	0
Felbamate	16–22	5–7	50	0.73–0.82	No	~25
Gabapentin[b]	5–40[d]	1–2	100	0.65–1.04	No	0
Lamotrigine	25.4 M	3–15	0	1.28	No	40–50
Levetiracetam	7–10	2		0.7	No	<10%
Oxcarbazepine	3–13	2		0.7	10-Hydroxy-carbazepine	40%
Phenobarbital	A 46–136 C 37–73	14–21	20–40	0.6	No	50
Phenytoin	A 10–34 C 5–14	7–28	<5	0.6–8.0	No	90
Primidone	A 3.3–19 C 4.5–11	1–4	40	0.43–1.1	PB[c] PEMA[c]	80
Tiagabine	5–13		Negligible		No	95
Topiramate	18–21	4–5	50–70	0.55–0.8 (male) 0.23–0.4 (female)	No	15
Valproic acid	A 8–20 C 7–14	1–3	<5	0.1–0.5	May contribute to toxicity	90–95 binding saturates
Zonisamide	24–60	5–15		0.8–1.6	No	40–60%

[a]A = adult; C = child; M = monotherapy; Co = combination therapy.
[b]The bioavailability of gabapentin is dose dependent.
[c]PB = phenobarbital; PEMA = phenylethylmalonamide.
[d]Half-life depends on renal function.

Improvement in cognition has been reported in patients switched from phenytoin or phenobarbital to these agents. However, these effects are subtle and may not be pronounced if patients are in the same relative area of the therapeutic range. Patients reduced from polytherapy to monotherapy also may demonstrate improvement in cognition. Some of the newer agents are believed to cause fewer neurobehavioral or cognitive effects. Among the newer AEDs, gabapentin and lamotrigine have been shown in several studies to cause fewer cognitive impairments as compared with older agents such as carbamazepine.[26–28] Conversely, topiramate may cause substantial cognitive impairment, particularly when used at high doses or during rapid dose escalation.[28] Finally, in some cases, AED treatment itself has been suggested to cause worsening of seizures. This may result from either improper selection of an AED for a specific seizure type or syndrome or may represent a paradoxical toxic effect of the drug.[29]

CLINICAL CONTROVERSY

The role and necessity of AED serum concentration monitoring are controversial. Some clinicians feel that therapeutic blood level monitoring is essential for appropriate use of AEDs, whereas other feel that blood level monitoring is overused and, in many cases, unwarranted. AED blood level monitoring should be viewed as a tool to be used as part of overall AED treatment optimization. Acheivement of a specific "therapeutic" level should not be an absolute goal in and of itself.

Because most adult patients have localization-related (partial onset) seizures, the most widely used AEDs traditionally have been carbamazepine, phenobarbital, phenytoin, and valproic acid. For com-plex partial seizures, these AEDs have similar efficacy.[30,31] Of these, carbamazepine and phenytoin are the most commonly prescribed AEDs for use in partial seizures in the United States. In large part, this preference is based on data derived from two landmark trials conducted through the Veterans Administration (VA) Epilepsy Cooperative Study Group. In the first of these trials, patients with new-onset partial or generalized epilepsy were randomized to receive either carbamazepine, phenobarbital, phenytoin, or primidone.[30] At the end of 3 years, patients who received either carbamazepine or phenytoin were equally likely and patients on phenobarbital or primidone were least likely to have remained on their originally assigned treatment. Thus carbamazepine and phenytoin were considered the drugs of first choice in patients with new-onset partial or generalized seizures. Carbamazepine was associated with fewer side effects. A follow-up study using almost identical methods compared carbamazepine and valproic acid.[31] Carbamazepine- and valproic acid–treated groups had equal retention rates for tonic-clonic seizures. Carbamazepine was superior to valproic acid for partial seizures. Valproic acid caused slightly more adverse effects.

Based in large part on the earlier VA cooperative trials, carbamazepine traditionally has been recognized as the AED of first choice for partial seizures. Several of the newer-generation AEDs may prove to be reasonable alternatives. The newer antiepileptic drugs were first approved as adjunctive therapy for patients with refractory partial seizures. Monotherapy trials with several of these newer agents including lamotrigine, gabapentin, topiramate, and oxcarbazepine have been completed.[32–34] Comparisons between lamotrigine and older agents including carbamazepine and phenytoin as initial monotherapy in partial seizures have been conducted in Europe, and the results would suggest comparable effectiveness and perhaps better tolerability, particularly in elderly patients. Preliminary observations

TABLE 54–6. Antiepileptic Drug Side Effects

AED	Acute Side Effects		Chronic Side Effects
	Concentration Dependent	*Idiosyncratic*	
Carbamazepine	Diplopia Dizziness Drowsiness Nausea Unsteadiness Lethargy	Blood dyscrasias Rash	Hyponatremia
Ethosuximide	Ataxia Drowsiness GI distress Unsteadiness Hiccoughs	Blood dyscrasias Rash	Behavior changes Headache
Felbamate	Anorexia Nausea Vomiting Insomnia Headache	Aplastic anemia Acute hepatic failure	Not established
Gabapentin	Dizziness Fatigue Somnolence Ataxia	Pedal edema	Weight gain
Lamotrigine	Diplopia Dizziness Unsteadiness Headache	Rash	Not established
Levetiracetam	Sedation Behavioral disturbance	Not established	Not established
Oxcarbazepine	Sedation Dizziness Ataxia Nausea	Rash	Hyponatremia
Phenobarbital	Ataxia Hyperactivity Headache Unsteadiness Sedation Nausea	Blood dyscrasias Rash	Behavior changes Connective tissue disorders Intellectual blunting Metabolic bone disease Mood change Sedation
Phenytoin	Ataxia Nystagmus Behavior changes Dizziness Headache Incoordination Sedation Lethargy Cognitive impairment Fatigue Visual blurring	Blood dyscrasias Rash Immunologic reaction	Behavior changes Cerebellar syndrome Connective tissue changes Skin thickening Folate deficiency Gingival hyperplasia Hirsutism Coarsening of facial features Acne Cognitive impairment Metabolic bone disease Sedation
Primidone	Behavior changes Headache Nausea Sedation Unsteadiness	Blood dyscrasias Rash	Behavior change Connective tissue disorders Cognitive impairment Sedation
Tiagabine	Dizziness Fatigue Difficulties concentrating Nervousness Tremor Blurred vision Depression Weakness	Spike-wave stupor	Not established
Topiramate	Difficulties concentrating Psychomotor slowing Speech or language problems Somnolence, fatigue Dizziness Headache	Metabolic acidosis Acute angle glaucoma Oligohidrosis	Kidney stones Weight loss

(continued)

TABLE 54–6. (continued)

| AED | Acute Side Effects | | Chronic Side Effects |
	Concentration Dependent	*Idiosyncratic*	
Valproic acid	GI upset Sedation Unsteadiness Tremor Thrombocytopenia	Acute hepatic failure Acute pancreatitis Alopecia	Polycystic ovary-like syndrome(?) Weight gain Hyperammonemia
Zonisamide	Sedation Dizziness Cognitive impairment Nausea	Rash Oligohydrosis	Kidney stones Weight loss

TABLE 54–7. Interactions Between Antiepileptic Drugs

AED	Added Drug	Effect[a]
Carbamazepine (CBZ)	Felbamate	Incr. 10, 11 epoxide
	Felbamate	Decr. CBZ
	Phenobarbital	Decr. CBZ
	Phenytoin	Decr. CBZ
Felbamate (FBM)	Carbamazepine	Decr. FBM
	Phenytoin	Decr. FBM
	Valproic acid	Incr. FBM
Gabapentin	No known interactions	
Lamotrigine (LTG)	Carbamazepine	Decr. LTG
	Phenobarbital	Decr. LTG
	Phenytoin	Decr. LTG
	Primidone	Decr. LTG
	Valproic acid	Incr. LTG
Levetiracetam	No known interactions	
Oxcarbazepine	Carbamazepine	Decrease MHD[b]
	Phenytoin	Decrease MHD[b]
	Phenobarbital	Decrease MHD[b]
Phenobarbital (PB)	Felbamate	Incr. PB
	Phenytoin	Incr. or decr. PB
	Valproic acid	Incr. PB
Phenytoin (PHT)	Carbamazepine	Decr. PHT
	Felbamate	Incr. PHT
	Methsuximide	Incr. PHT
	Phenobarbital	Incr. or decr. PHT
	Valproic acid	Decr. Total PHT
	Vigabatrin	Decr. PHT
Primidone (PRM)	Carbamazepine	Decr. PRM Incr. PB
	Phenytoin	Decr. PRM Incr. PB
	Valproic acid	Incr. PRM Incr. PB
Tiagabine (TGB)	Carbamazepine	Decr. TGB
	Phenytoin	Decr. TGB
Topiramate (TPM)	Carbamazepine	Decr. TPM
	Phenytoin	Decr. TPM
	Valproic acid	Decr. TPM
Valproic acid (VPA)	Carbamazepine	Decr. VPA
	Lamotrigine	Decr. VPA (slight)
	Phenobarbital	Decr. VPA
	Primidone	Decr. VPA
	Phenytoin	Decr. VPA
Zonisamide	Carbamazepine	Decrease zonisamide
	Phenytoin	Decrease zonisamide
	Phenobarbital	Decrease zonisamide

[a]Incr. = increased; Decr. = decreased.
[b]MHD = 10-monohydroxymetabolite.

TABLE 54–8. Interactions With Other Medications

AED	Altered By	Result	Alters	Result
Carbamazepine	Cimetidine	Incr. CBZ	Oral contraceptives (OC)	Decr. efficacy of OC
	Erythromycin	Incr. CBZ	Doxycycline	Decr. doxycycline
	Fluoxetine	Incr. CBZ	Theophylline	Decr. theophylline
	Isoniazid	Incr. CBZ	Warfarin	Decr. warfarin
	Propoxyphene	Incr. CBZ		
Oxcarbazepine			OC	Decr. efficacy of OC
Phenobarbital	Acetazolamide	Incr. PB	OC	Decr. efficacy of OC
Phenytoin	Amiodarone	Incr. PHT		
	Antacids	Decr. absorption of PHT	Oral contraceptives	Decr. efficacy of oral contraceptives
	Cimetidine	Incr. PHT	Bishydroxycoumarin	Decr. anticoagulation
	Chloramphenicol	Incr. PHT	Folic acid	Decr. folic acid
	Disulfiram	Incr. PHT	Quinidine	Decr. quinidine
	Ethanol (acute)	Incr. PHT	Vitamin D	Decr. vitamin D
	Fluconazole	Incr. PHT		
	Fluoxetine	Incr. PHT		
	Isoniazid	Incr. PHT		
	Propoxyphene	Incr. PHT		
	Warfarin	Can both incr./decr. INR		
	Ethanol (chronic)	Decr. PHT		
Primidone	Isoniazid	Decr. metabolism of primidone	Chlorpromazine	Decr. chlorpromazine
	Nicotinamide	Decr. metabolism of primidone	Corticosteroids	Decr. corticosteroids
			Quinidine	Decr. quinidine
			Tricyclics	Decr. tricyclics
			Furosemide	Decr. renal sensitivity to furosemide
Topiramate			OC	Decr. efficacy of OC
Valproic acid	Cimetidine	Incr. VPA		
	Salicylates	Incr. free VPA		

Incr. = increased; Decr. = decreased.

from a recently completed VA cooperative trial designed to compare gabapentin, lamotrigine, and carbamazepine in newly diagnosed elderly patients suggest that gabapentin efficacy is comparable with that of both lamotrigine and carbamazepine and in fact may be better tolerated than carbamazepine in this population (E. R. Ramsay et al., unpublished data, 2003). Clinical data would suggest that in newly diagnosed patients, oxcarbazepine is as effective as phenytoin, valproic acid, and immediate-release carbamazepine, with perhaps fewer adverse effects. Interestingly, close examination of the conversion to monotherapy trials would suggest that oxcarbazepine may demonstrate efficacy even in patients who previously had had an inadequate response to carbamazepine despite their structural similarity.

In addition, several monotherapy trials using an active control or psuedoplacebo design also have been performed. While these particular study designs do provide evidence of efficacy of the newer drugs, because the comparison is between active drug and placebo in patients who continue to have seizures despite current treatment with standard AEDs, it is difficult to compare the efficacy of the newer directly with the older AEDs. A meta-analysis designed to compare some of the newer AEDs[35] indirectly found that because of wide and overlapping confidence intervals for both efficacy and tolerability outcome measures, no statistically significant differences between agents could be found. Generally speaking, the newer AEDs appear to have comparable efficacy to the older agents and are perhaps better tolerated.

To date, among the newer-generation agents, only lamotrigine and oxcarbazepine have received Food and Drug Administration (FDA) approval for use as monotherapy in patients with partial seizures. Phenobarbital and primidone are also useful in partial

seizures, but sedation and cognitive adverse effects limit their utility. Felbamate, which has monotherapy approval, is effective but has been associated with some significant side effects. Interpretation of monotherapy trials with the newer AEDs can be daunting owing to the unique study designs and specific patient populations employed. While a complete discussion of this topic is beyond the scope of this chapter, several reviews and analyses have been published recently.[32]

Primarily generalized seizures such as absence seizures may respond differently pharmacologically than other seizure types. Phenytoin, phenobarbital, and carbamazepine, although effective in GTC and partial seizures, are ineffective in treating absence seizures and in some cases may precipitate an increase in seizure activity. Absence seizures are best treated with ethosuximide, valproic acid, and perhaps lamotrigine. Either levetiracetam, topiramate, or zonisamide also may be effective, although further clinical data are needed to confirm this. Gabapentin and tiagabine do not appear to be effective in treating absence seizures. If the patient has a combination of absence and other generalized or partial seizures, valproic acid is the preferred first choice because it is the only AED effective against absence and other seizure types. If valproic acid is ineffective in treating a mixed seizure disorder that includes absence, ethosuximide should be used in combination with another AED.

The traditional treatment of tonic-clonic seizures is phenytoin or phenobarbital; however, the use of carbamazepine and valproic acid is increasing because these AEDs have a lower incidence of side effects and equal efficacy. Valproic acid generally is considered the drug of first choice for atonic seizures and for juvenile myoclonic epilepsy. Lamotrigine and perhaps topiramate and zonisamide may be alternative agents for these seizure types.

What has become obvious is that individuals may respond differently to each AED and that an understanding of each of these newer agents is needed to optimize therapy for individual patients. In most cases, selection of specific AED will depend on multiple factors, including seizure type, unique patient characteristics, and the expected adverse-effect/pharmacokinetic profile of each AED. An important clinical question remains as to the precise role of the newer-generation drugs. While several studies would suggest that at least some of the newer agents may have comparable efficacy, as well as improved tolerability, to the older drugs, definitive comparative studies with all agents are lacking. In the absence of randomized, double-blind clinical trials with all the AEDs, a recent consensus panel published a set of preferred AED treatment options for a variety of patient scenarios.[36]

Another question that frequently confronts clinicians surrounds the role of therapeutic drug monitoring. Although most of the older AEDs have published therapeutic ranges, the serum concentration should be viewed as a tool with which to optimize therapy for an individual patient, not as a therapeutic end point in and of itself. The serum concentration is a target that should be correlated with clinical outcome. The desired response is the cessation of seizures without side effects. Seizure control may occur before the "minimum" of the published range is achieved, and side effects may appear before the "maximum" of the range is achieved. Some patients may need and tolerate concentrations beyond the maximum. The therapeutic range for AEDs may be different for different seizure types. Serum concentrations may need to be higher to control complex partial seizures than to control tonic-clonic seizures. Clinicians should define a therapeutic range for an individual patient above which there are side effects and below which the patient experiences seizures. The pharmacodynamic response to AEDs may change as the patient ages because elderly patients may be more sensitive to various neurocognitive adverse effects of these drugs. Along with this, elderly patients may demonstrate efficacy (e.g., control of seizures) at relatively lower serum concentrations as well. To date, therapeutic concentration ranges have not been established conclusively for the newer-generation drugs.

▧ THERAPEUTIC CONSIDERATIONS IN WOMEN

Many hormones influence brain electrical excitability, and the steroid hormones estrogen and progesterone may interact in complex ways to alter neuronal excitability and protein synthesis.[37] Estrogen has a seizure-activating effect, whereas progesterone exerts a seizure-protective effect. Estrogen has an inhibitory effect on GABA receptors, potentiates excitatory glutaminergic activity, and may promote the development of kindling. Progesterone has the opposite effect and appears to potentiate GABA receptor activity and reduce neuronal discharge rates. AEDs, especially hepatic metabolizing enzyme inducers, also affect hormones by increasing the metabolism of steroid hormones and inducing the production of sex hormone–binding globulin. This may lead to decreases in the unbound fraction of the hormone. Enzyme-inducing AEDs, including topiramate and oxcarbazepine at higher doses, may cause treatment failures in women taking oral contraceptives owing to induction of both ethinyl estradiol and progestin metabolism. A supplemental form of birth control in addition to oral contraceptives is advised if breakthrough bleeding occurs. Valproic acid, benzodiazepines, and most of the newer AEDs such as lamotrigine, gabapentin, levetiracetam, tiagabine, and zonisamide are not enzyme inducers and have not been associated with this effect.

In some women, vulnerability to seizures is highest just before and during the menstrual flow (catamenial seizures) and at the time of ovulation. The risk of catamenial epilepsy is estimated at 12.5%, but it may occur in as many as 50% of women with epilepsy. This pattern of seizure exacerbation may be related to progesterone withdrawal and changes in the estrogen-to-progesterone ratio. Conventional AEDs should be tried first in these women. Intermittent acetazolamide also has been used, but with variable and limited success. Hormonal therapy with progestational agents, particularly cyclic natural progesterone therapy, also may be effective. Reproductive endocrine disorders are common in women with epilepsy and include menstrual irregularity, infertility, sexual dysfunction, and possibly an increased risk of polycystic ovary syndrome.[38] Potential mechanisms for these disturbances include disruption of the hypothalamic-pituitary-adrenal (HPA) axis via seizure discharges in limbic structures and/or AEDs.[38] AEDs, particularly the enzyme-inducing agents (e.g., carbamazepine, phenytoin, and phenobarbital), also may affect HPA function by altering the metabolism of the neuroactive sex hormones, including testosterone. Although a definitive causal relationship has not yet been established, an apparent increased incidence of polycystic ovary syndrome has been suggested for women with epilepsy who are receiving valproic acid.[38]

Pregnancy raises several concerns, including the possibility of increased maternal seizures, pregnancy complications, and adverse fetal outcome.[39] About 25% to 30% of women have increased seizures during pregnancy, whereas seizures decrease in a similar number. Increased seizure activity may result from either a direct effect on seizure threshold or a reduction in AED concentration. An increase in clearance has been reported for phenytoin, carbamazepine, phenobarbital, ethosuximide, lamotrigine, and clorazepate. Protein binding also may be altered. The altered disposition of AEDs may begin as early as the first 10 weeks of pregnancy and may take up to 4 weeks postpartum to return to normal. The return to the nonpregnant metabolism and binding requires longer for carbamazepine and phenobarbital than it does for phenytoin. There is a higher incidence of adverse pregnancy outcomes in women with epilepsy. Although the risk of congenital malformations is 4% to 6% (twice as high as in nonepileptic women), more than 90% of pregnancies in epileptic mothers have satisfactory outcomes. Barbiturates and phenytoin are associated with congenital heart malformations, orofacial clefts, and other malformations. Valproic acid and carbamazepine are associated predominantly with spina bifida (neural tube defect) and hypospadias. The risk of neural tube defect with valproic acid and carbamazepine has been estimated to be 0.5% to 1%, respectively, and appears to be related to drug exposure during gestational days 0 to 28. Other adverse pregnancy outcomes associated with maternal seizures but not necessarily caused by AEDs are growth, psychomotor, and mental retardation. Women with epilepsy are also more likely to have miscarriages, and 10% to 20% of infants are born with low birth weight. Guidelines have been developed for counseling and managing pregnant women with epilepsy.

Many of these teratogenic effects can be prevented by adequate folate intake; therefore, prenatal vitamins with folic acid ($\sim$ 0.4–5 mg/day) should be given to any woman of child-bearing potential who is taking AEDs.[39] Higher folate doses should be used in women with a history of a previous pregnancy with a neural tube defect. Higher AED doses and serum concentrations, polytherapy, and a family history of birth defects appear to increase the teratogenic risk. Therefore, deciding on the most effective single-drug treatment prior to conception is vitally important. New AEDs are reported to be less teratogenic, and animal reproductive toxicology studies appear to be favorable. At present, clinical data are quite limited, and more experience is needed before the true risk (or lack thereof) can be determined. AEDs also can lead to neonatal hemorrhagic disorder. Vitamin K 10 mg orally given to the mother daily during the last month of pregnancy should prevent this coagulopathy.

Although AEDs pass into the breast milk, the concentrations are very low, and the infant receives a subtherapeutic dose. In general, knowledge of the degree of protein binding of a given AED can allow for prediction of breast milk accumulation, with drugs with less protein binding partitioning more. Treatment with AEDs is not necessarily a reason to discourage breast-feeding. It is advisable that women taking any AED (particularly barbiturates or benzodiazepines) closely observe infants for signs of excess sedation, irritability, or poor feeding.[39]

Little is known regarding the effect of menopause on epilepsy. The perimenopausal period may be associated with worsening of seizures, possibly owing to fluctuations in sex hormones. At menopause, seizures actually may improve, particularly in women who previously presented with a catamenial pattern. The effect of hormone-replacement therapy on seizure control is still unclear, but clinicians should monitor for seizure exacerbation in women receiving supplemental estrogen.

CLINICAL CONSIDERATIONS WITH SPECIFIC DRUGS

Tables 54–5 to 54–9 list specific pharmacokinetic and typical dosing data for each of the commonly used AEDs. Below we summarize the relative properties, advantages and disadvantages, and perspectives as to the place in therapy of each of these agents.

CARBAMAZEPINE

Pharmacology and Mechanism of Action. The exact mechanism by which carbamazepine suppresses seizure spread is obscure, although it is believed to act primarily through inhibition of voltage-gated sodium channels.[40]

Pharmacokinetics. The absorption of carbamazepine from immediate-release tablets is slow and erratic because of its low water solubility. There is also a large variability in the peak-to-trough concentrations of up to 40%. There is no first-pass metabolism. Food may enhance the bioavailability of carbamazepine. The suspension dosage form is absorbed faster than the tablets.[41] Controlled-release (Tegretol-XR) and sustained-release (Carbatrol) preparations are also available. These dosage forms are bioequivalent in twice-daily (every 12 hours) dosing to dosing four times daily (every 6 hours) with immediate-release carbamazepine. Compared with immediate-release carbamazepine, both these formulations have lower peaks and higher troughs, which may decrease side effects and improve seizure control. Patients should be told to take Tegretol-XR with food and that the casing will be excreted in the feces. Tegretol-XR cannot be broken or crushed. Tegrtetol-XR and Carbatrol appear to be bioequivalent; however, there was less variability in the absorption of Carbatrol.[41]

Carbamazepine is a neutral and highly lipophilic drug that results in high body tissue binding. It binds to α_1-acid glycoprotein and to albumin. Most (98% to 99%) of an administered dose of carbamazepine is metabolized by the liver, primarily by CYP3A4.[41] The major metabolite is carbamazepine-10,11-epoxide,[41] which has anticonvulsant activity in animals and humans. The formation of the 10,11-epoxide is influenced by concurrent use of other enzyme-inducing or enzyme-inhibiting drugs; thus the 10,11-epoxide concentration may change with the administration of other drugs (e.g., valproate and felbamate) with no change in parent carbamazepine concentration.[41]

Carbamazepine has the unique ability to induce its own metabolism (autoinduction).[41] The half-life after a single dose is much longer than the half-life after chronic therapy. The presence of enzyme-inducing drugs reduces the half-life even more. The enzyme-induction effect begins within 3 to 5 days of the initiation of therapy and takes 21 to 28 days to complete. Therefore, it is possible to achieve initial concentrations that are within the therapeutic range but have concentrations fall despite continued therapy with good compliance. Some patients who respond well to initial therapy may be labeled refractory or noncompliant if the autoinduction phenomenon is not considered. The autoinduction reverses rapidly if therapy with carbamazepine is discontinued temporarily. This would be very important in epilepsy monitoring units where all drugs are stopped in an attempt to precipitate seizures in patients being evaluated for seizure surgery.[41]

Adverse Effects. Side effects (see Table 54–6) of carbamazepine may fluctuate daily, paralleling the rise and decline of serum concentrations. The side-effect profile also may follow a circadian rhythm. Neurosensory side effects (e.g., diplopia, blurred vision, nystagmus, ataxia, unsteadiness, dizziness, and headache) are the most common, occurring in 35% to 50% of patients. These side effects are more common during initiation of therapy and may dissipate with continued treatment. Patients have variable threshold concentrations for the occurrence of CNS side effects. If the carbamazepine serum concentration is kept below the individual threshold, the CNS side effects can be minimized. Dosage manipulation, including the use of the controlled- or sustained-release preparations, should be tried before the patient is considered to be intolerant of carbamazepine. Carbamazepine may induce a hyponatremic hyposmolar condition that is similar to the syndrome of inappropriate antidiuretic hormone secretion. The incidence may increase with age. Periodic determinations of serum sodium concentration are recommended, especially in the elderly.[41]

Thrombocytopenia and anemia are relatively rare events that usually respond to discontinuation of the offending drug. Leukopenia is the most common hematologic side effect. An incidence as high as 10% has been reported. Leukopenia usually is transient, even when the drug is continued, and may be due to a redistribution of white blood cells (WBCs) rather than a decrease in their production. In about 2% of patients, the leukopenia is persistent, but even patients with WBC counts of 3000/mm^3 or less do not seem to have an increased incidence of infection. A clinical guide is to continue carbamazepine therapy unless the WBC count drops to less than 2500/mm^3 and the absolute neutrophil count drops to less than 1000/mm^3.[41]

Rashes are the most frequent hypersensitivity response. An incidence of approximately 10% has been reported. These usually are mildly eczematous but may progress to Stevens-Johnson syndrome. Other rare side effects reported with carbamazepine include hepatitis, osteomalacia, cardiac conduction defects, and lupus-like reactions.

TABLE 54–9. AED Dosing and Target Serum Concentration Ranges

	Trade Name	Manufacturer	Year Introduced	Usual Initial Dose	Usual Maximum Daily Dose	Target Serum Concentration Range
Barbiturates						
Mephobarbital	Mebaral	Sanofi Winthrop	1935	50–100 mg/day	400–600 mg	Not defined
Phenobarbital	Various	Generic	1912	1–3 mg/kg/day (10–20 mg/kg LD)	180–300 mg	10–40 mcg/mL
Primidone	Mysoline	Wyeth-Ayerst	1954	100–125 mg/day	750–2000 mg	5–10 mcg/mL
Benzodiazepines						
Clonazepam	Klonopin	Roche	1975	1.5 mg/day	20 mg	20–80 ng/mL
Clorazepate	Tranxene	Abbott	1981	7.5–22.5 mg/day	90 mg	Not defined
Diazepam	Valium	Roche/generic	1968	PO: 4–40 mg IV: 5–10 mg	PO: 4–40 mg IV: 5–30 mg	100–1000 ng/mL
Lorazepam	Ativan	Wyeth-Ayerst generic		PO: 2–6 mg IV: 0.05 mg/kg IM: 0.05 mg/kg	PO: 10 mg IV: 0.044 mg/kg	10–30 ng/mL
Hydantoins						
Ethotoin	Peganone	Abbott	1957	<1000 mg/day	2000–4000 mg with food	15–50 mcg/mL
Mephenytoin	Mesantoin	Sandoz	1947	50–100 mg/day	200–800 mg	25–40 mcg/mL
Phenytoin	Dilantin	Pfizer	1938	PO: 3–5 mg/kg (200–400 mg) (15–20 mg/kg LD)	PO: 500–600 mg	Total: 10–20 mcg/mL Unbound: 0.5–3 mcg/mL
Succinimides						
Ethosuximide	Zarontin	Pfizer	1960	500 mg/day	500–2000 mg	40–80 mcg/mL
Methsuximide	Celontin	Pfizer	1957	300 mg/day	300–1200 mg	*N*-desmethyl metabolite 10–40 mcg/mL
Other						
Carbamazepine	Tegretol	Novartis, generic	1974	400 mg/day	400–2400 mg	4–14 mcg/mL
Felbamate	Felbatol	MedPointe	1993	1200 mg/day	3600 mg	40–100 mcg/mL[a]
Gabapentin	Neurontin	Pfizer	1993	900 mg/day	4800 mg	4–16 mcg/mL[a]
Lamotrigine	Lamictal	Glaxo SmithKline	1994	25 mg qod if on VPA; 25–50 mg/day if not on VPA	100–150 mg if on VPA; 300–500 mg if not on VPA	4–20 mcg/mL[a]
Levetiracetam	Keppra	UCB-Pharma	2000	500–1000 mg/day	3000–4000 mg	Not defined
Oxcarbazepine	Trileptal	Novartis	2000	300–600 mg/day	2400–3000 mg	12–30 mcg/mL[a] (MHD)
Tiagabine	Gabitril	Abbott	1997	4–8 mg/day	80 mg	Not defined
Topiramate	Topamax	Ortho McNeil	1997	25–50 mg/day	200–1000 mg	Not defined
Valproic acid	Depakene Depakote Depacon	Abbott	1978	15 mg/kg (500–1000 mg)	60 mg/kg (3000–5000 mg)	50–150 mcg/mL[a]
Zonisamide	Zonegran	Elan	2000	100–200 mg/day	600 mg	10–40 mcg/mL[a]

[a]Based on data from clinical trials—no established therapeutic ranges.

■ *Drug Interactions.* Because of concentration-dependent efficacy and side effects, drug interactions with carbamazepine often are very significant clinically. Valproic acid increases 10,11-epoxide metabolite concentrations without affecting the concentration of carbamazepine via inhibition of epoxide hydrolase. Drugs that inhibit CYP3A4 potentially may increase carbamazepine serum concentrations. Carbamazepine may interact with other drugs by inducing their metabolism.

■ *Dosing and Administration.* The variable contributions of the 10,11-epoxide metabolite and free carbamazepine concentrations have restricted a precise definition of the therapeutic range. Loading doses of carbamazepine are indicated only for critically ill patients. During dosage titration, it should be remembered that carbamazepine clearance increases with time. Doses may be started at one-fourth to one-third the anticipated maintenance dose and increased every 2 to 3 weeks. Because of the auto- and heteroinduction of carbamazepine metabolism, it is necessary to administer the drug two to four times per day. The controlled- and sustained release formulations provide fewer peak-to-trough fluctuations, which may improve adherence, reduce side effects, and improve seizure control. Carbamazepine tablets should not be stored in places where they would be exposed to high heat and high humidity.[41]

■ *Advantages.* Carbamazepine was approved as an AED in 1974 and has been well studied. Oral immediate- and extended-release solid and liquid dosage forms are available. The oral solid dosage form is available as an immediate-release tablet and as a sustained-release capsule and a controlled-release tablet. The sustained- and controlled-release dosage forms allow for twice-daily dosing to reduce the peak-to-trough fluctuations. Compared with other first-generation AEDs, carbamazepine causes minimal cognitive impairment.

Disadvantages. Carbamazepine has an active metabolite that can contribute to efficacy and toxicity. Other drugs can alter the concentration of this metabolite without changing the concentration of the parent carbamazepine. It induces its own metabolism, which requires careful dosage titration. It also induces the metabolism of other medications, and other drugs may interact with it and/or the active metabolite. There is no parenteral formulation. There are clinically meaningful CNS side effects including sedation. There may be fewer side effects with the sustained- or controlled-release formulations, but this has not been evaluated prospectively. Carbamazepine has been associated with a 1% risk of spina bifida. Chronic carbamazepine use also has been associated with alterations in bone mineral density in some studies. The generic formulations of immediate-release tablets have been associated with breakthrough seizures when brands have been switched.

Place in Therapy. Carbamazepine should be considered a first-line therapy for patients with newly diagnosed partial seizures and for patients with primary generalized convulsive seizures who are not in an emergent situation.

ETHOSUXIMIDE

Pharmacology and Mechanism of Action. The exact mechanism of action of ethosuximide remains elusive. Proposed mechanisms include inhibition of NADPH-linked aldehyde reductase, inhibition of the sodium-potassium ATPase system, a decrease in non-inactivating Na^+ currents, blocking of Ca^{2+}-dependent K^+ channels, and inhibition of T-type Ca^{2+} channel currents.[42]

Pharmacokinetics. Metabolism occurs in the liver by hydroxylation, and the metabolites are believed to be inactive. There is some evidence of a nonlinear metabolic process at higher concentrations.

Adverse Effects. The most frequently reported side effects are nausea and vomiting (up to 40%), and these symptoms may be minimized by administration of smaller doses and more frequent dosing. Other common side effects include drowsiness, fatigue, lethargy, dizziness, hiccups, and headaches. Rarely, idiosyncratic reactions such as rashes, lupus, and blood dyscrasias have been reported.[42]

Drug Interactions. Because ethosuximide is not protein bound, displacement interactions cannot occur. The metabolism of ethosuximide may be induced by carbamazepine. A complex interaction between valproic acid and ethosuximide has been reported. Valproic acid may inhibit the metabolism of ethosuximide, but only if the metabolism of ethosuximide is near saturation.[40]

Dosing and Administration. A loading dose of ethosuximide is not required. Titration over 1 to 2 weeks to maintenance doses of 20 mg/kg per day usually results in concentrations of approximately 50 mcg/mL. Data suggest that patients can be managed successfully on once-a-day therapy; however, gastrointestinal distress appears to be dose-related, and the total daily dose is usually divided into two equal doses.[41]

Advantages. This drug is very effective in the treatment of absence seizures. It is generally well tolerated and has few pharmacokinetic interactions.

Disadvantages. Ethosuximide has a very narrow spectrum of activity.

Place in Therapy. Ethosuximide is still a first-line treatment for absence seizures.

FELBAMATE

Pharmacology and Mechanism of Action. Felbamate appears to act as an antagonist of the glycine receptor site on the N-methyl-D-aspartate (NMDA) receptor. This action inhibits the initiation and propagation of seizures.[20] It also may inhibit NMDA/glycine-stimulated increases in intracellular Ca^{2+}.[43]

Pharmacokinetics. Felbamate is rapidly and well absorbed. The absorption is unaffected by food or antacids. About 40% to 50% of a dose of felbamate is metabolized by hydroxylation and conjugation pathways in the liver, with the remainder being excreted unchanged in the urine. Felbamate displays linear pharmacokinetics.[43]

Adverse Effects. The most frequently reported side effects with felbamate prior to marketing were anorexia, weight loss, insomnia, nausea, and headache. Anorexia and weight loss may be especially problematic in children and in patients with diminished caloric intake. In addition, headache occasionally can be severe. After about 1 year of general use and 100,000 patient care exposures, the use of felbamate was found to be associated with aplastic anemia and acute liver failure. The onset was between 68 and 354 days of therapy. The approximate rate of occurrence of aplastic anemia is 1 in 3000 and of hepatitis is 1 in 10,000. Initially, no relationship with dose and no predictors of who is more likely to develop these life-threatening reactions were apparent. Data are now emerging suggesting an increased risk for aplastic anemia in patients, especially women, with a history of cytopenia, AED allergy or significant toxicity, viral infection, and/or immunologic problems.[44–46]

Drug Interactions. Felbamate inhibits the clearance and increases the serum concentration of phenytoin, valproic acid, and phenobarbital. The concentration of carbamazepine decreases in patients on concurrent therapy with felbamate secondary to enzyme induction; however, the concentration of the 10,11-epoxide metabolite increases. It is recommended that the dose of phenytoin, carbamazepine, and valproic acid be decreased by about 30% when felbamate is added. Felbamate does not appear to interact with either gabapentin or lamotrigine. Phenytoin and carbamazepine are enzyme inducers and have been shown to increase the clearance of felbamate. Interactions with warfarin also have been reported.[43]

Dosing and Administration. A therapeutic range for felbamate has not been established. The drug is dosed to clinical response. If felbamate is used as monotherapy, the dose is initiated at 1200 mg/day (15 mg/kg in children) and then is increased by 600 mg every 2 weeks up to a maximum dose of 3600 mg (45 mg/kg in children).

Advantages. Felbamate has a unique mechanism of action. It is approved for treating atonic seizures in patients with the Lennox

Gastaut syndrome and is effective in treating patients with partial seizures.

▨ *Disadvantages.* The use of felbamate is limited by the association with aplastic anemia and hepatotoxicity, as well as multiple drug interactions.

▨ *Place in Therapy.* This agent should be reserved for patients not responding to other AEDs.

▨ GABAPENTIN

▨ *Pharmacology and Mechanism of Action.* Gabapentin was designed to be a GABA agonist but does not react at the GABA receptor, alter GABA uptake, or interfere with GABA transaminase. Gabapentin appears to bind to an amino acid carrier protein and appears to act at a unique receptor. Gabapentin also may modulate specific voltage-sensitive Ca^{2+} channels.[20] It elevates human brain GABA levels, possibly via alterations in GABA synthesis or reversal of the neuronal GABA transporter, resulting in nonvesicular release of GABA.[47]

▨ *Pharmacokinetics.* Gabapentin is a substrate of the L-amino acid carrier protein in the gut (system L), as well as in the CNS.[48] This amino acid carrier protein transports the drug across the gut membrane by an active process. The binding of gabapentin to this system is saturable, and gabapentin therefore displays dose-dependent bioavailability that appears to vary considerably between individuals.[49] Food, including protein-rich meals, does not appear to interfere with gabapentin oral absorption.[50] Concentrations in human CSF are 5% to 35% of plasma levels, and tissue concentrations are approximately 80% of plasma levels.

Because gabapentin is eliminated exclusively by the kidneys, dosage adjustments will be necessary in patients with significantly impaired renal function. In anuric patients, 35% of gabapentin is removed by dialysis.[51]

▨ *Adverse Effects.* Fatigue, somnolence, dizziness, and ataxia are the most frequently reported side effects. Rash is uncommon with this agent. Other side effects reported include nystagmus, tremor, and diplopia. Aggressive behavior has been reported in children.[52] The CNS effects of gabapentin are generally less than those of traditional AEDs. Some clinicians have noted that patients may gain weight while on gabapentin.[44–46]

▨ *Drug Interactions.* Gabapentin does not induce or inhibit liver enzymes; therefore, drug interactions are not likely to occur with gabapentin. There is a 10% reduction in the clearance of gabapentin in patients taking cimetidine and a 20% reduction in the bioavailability if aluminum antacids are taken simultaneously with gabapentin. These interactions are unlikely to be clinically significant.

▨ *Dosing and Administration.* Typical starting doses of gabapentin are 300 mg at bedtime on the first day, increasing to 900 mg/day over 3 days. Faster titration rates (e.g., starting at 300 to 900 mg three times daily) have been well tolerated.[53] The manufacturer recommends maintenance doses of 1800 to 2400 mg/day, but higher doses (5000 to 10,000 mg/day) have been used safely. It is important that clinicians titrate this drug to effect rather that a set preconceived absolute drug dosage. However, it is unclear if higher doses of gabapentin should be given more frequently than three times per day because of

saturable absorption.[54] Gabapentin does not appear to be absorbed rectally. Patients with end-stage renal disease maintained on hemodialysis should receive an initial 300- to 400-mg dose with 200 to 300 mg gabapentin given after every 4 hours of hemodialysis.[51]

▨ *Advantages.* Gabapentin has multiple mechanisms of action and is mechanistically different from first-generation AEDs. It is not metabolized and is excreted unchanged by the kidney. Gabapentin has the additional advantages of a broad therapeutic index with minimal CNS adverse effects and no drug interactions. Doses can be escalated rapidly.

▨ *Disadvantages.* Gabapentin is absorbed by an active process that saturates at higher doses. This may require more frequent daily dosing for patients who need doses greater than 3600 mg/day. Doses exceeding the 3600 mg/day maximum listed in the package insert may be required in some patients to achieve seizure remission. There is no parenteral formulation.

▨ *Place in Therapy.* Gabapentin is a second-line agent for patients with partial seizures who have failed initial treatment. In addition, although monotherapy trials have no proven efficacy in previously diagnosed refractory patients, there may be a role for this drug in patients with less severe seizure disorders, such as new-onset partial epilepsy, particularly in the elderly patient. Gabapentin also has been shown to be useful in the treatment of chronic pain and other nonepilepsy conditions.

▨ LAMOTRIGINE

▨ *Pharmacology and Mechanism of Action.* A primary mechanism of action for lamotrigine appears to be blockade of neuronal sodium channels that is both voltage- and use-dependent. Lamotrigine produces dose-dependent inhibition of high-voltage activation Ca^{2+} currents, possibly through inhibition of presynaptic N-type Ca^{2+} channels, and blocks the release of excitatory amino acid neurotransmitters such as glutamate and aspartate.[20,55]

▨ *Pharmacokinetics.* Lamotrigine is completely and rapidly absorbed, with a bioavailability of 98%. Food does not significantly affect drug absorption. Lamotrigine is also absorbed following rectal administration, although the mean area under the curve (AUC) is approximately 50% of that achieved by oral administration. Lamotrigine is approximately 55% bound to plasma proteins. Lamotrigine is extensively hepatically metabolized by UDP-glucuronosyl tranferase (UGT 1A4), which is inactive. Renal elimination of unchanged drug accounts for a minor fraction of the administered dose (<10%). When given as monotherapy in adults, lamotrigine elimination half-life is approximately 24 to 29 hours. Lamotrigine clearance is higher in children and lower in the elderly compared with young adults. There are only modest differences in the pharmacokinetics of lamotrigine in the elderly versus younger subjects. Hepatic disease, depending on severity, can influence lamotrigine pharmacokinetics. Approximately 17% of a lamotrigine dose may be removed by hemodialysis, with half-life being reduced to about 13 hours. For patients on dialysis, the half-life is much more prolonged between dialyses (57.4 hours) but shorter during dialysis (13 hours).[56]

A well-defined serum concentration–effect range has not been established. The half-life is prolonged in patients with renal failure.

Adverse Effects. The most frequently reported side effects of lamotrigine include diplopia, drowsiness, ataxia, and headache.[55] Adverse effects are more common when lamotrigine is given in combination with other AEDs (e.g., diplopia when given concomitantly with carbamazepine or tremor with valproic acid) as compared with monotherapy and thus may be pharmacodynamic in nature. Lamotrigine may cause rash, which usually appears in the first 3 to 4 weeks of therapy. The rash typically is generalized, erythematous, and morbilliform and generally is mild to moderate in severity. However, Stevens-Johnson reaction also has been reported. Some rashes, especially those which develop early, may necessitate the withdrawal of lamotrigine.[57] Risk factors for the emergence of more serious rashes appear to be concomitant use of valproic acid and situations where high initial doses or rapid dosage escalation is used. Data from several European monotherapy trials suggest that when dosed appropriately, the incidence of rash from lamotrigine is similar to that of older agents such as carbamazepine and phenytoin. The incidence also may be higher in children than in adults. Lamotrigine does not appear to cause significant changes in body weight.[44–46]

Drug Interactions. Lamotrigine does not inhibit or induce liver enzymes and has a low potential for pharmacokinetic interactions with other drugs. Lamotrigine does not interfere with oral contraceptives.

The metabolism of lamotrigine, however, does display substantial interpatient variability, and plasma clearance may be altered by concurrent therapy with other drugs. Lamotrigine elimination half-life is reduced by approximately 50% in the presence of inducing drugs, such as carbamazepine, phenobarbital, primidone, and phenytoin.[55] Concomitant treatment with oral contraceptives may lead to a reduction in the serum concentrations of lamotrigine. While this interaction has not been clearly defined, it may be speculated to result from induction of lamotrigine glucuronidation by the ethinyl estradiol component of the pill.[58] However, lamotrigine does not appear to influence the pharmacokinetics of either the estrogen or progestin component of these preparations.

Valproic acid inhibits the clearance of lamotrigine.[55] Inhibition of lamotrigine metabolism by valproic acid is substantial and appears to occur even at very low serum concentrations. Maximal inhibition of lamotrigine by valproic acid appears to occur at valproic acid doses/serum concentrations of 500 mg/day and 40–50 mcg/mL, respectively. Clinically, this implies that in order to achieve any given plasma concentration, larger maintenance doses of lamotrigine may be required in the presence of an inducer as compared with monotherapy, whereas lower doses may be necessary when given with valproic acid. A pharmacodynamic interaction may occur with concurrent carbamazepine therapy, leading to an increase in CNS side effects.

Dosing and Administration. In patients who are taking enzyme-inducing drugs, lamotrigine can be started more rapidly than in patients receiving valproic acid. The maintenance doses are also different (see Table 54–9). These different doses are critical owing to the relationship between rash, concomitant valproic acid, and the dose escalation rate. Removal of inducers from a lamotrigine regimen may necessitate decreases in lamotrigine doses, whereas removal of valproic acid may necessitate an increase in the lamotrigine dose. A dispersable tablet is available for patients who cannot swallow an oral solid.[44–46]

Advantages. Lamotrigine is potentially a broad-spectrum AED, having efficacy in partial seizures as well as several types of generalized seizures. A pediatric dosage form is available. It does not induce or inhibit the metabolism of other AEDs. Lamotrigine has linear pharmacokinetics and is not highly protein bound. Lamotrigine appears to be generally well tolerated in both children and elderly adult patients and does not cause weight gain.

Disadvantages. Lamotrigine is associated with rash, especially in patients who start at a high dose, have rapid dose escalation, and/or are taking concurrent valproic acid. Therefore, the initial doses must be low (lower if the patient is on valproic acid) and escalated slowly in order to maximize patient safety. There is no parenteral dosage form.

Place in Therapy. Lamotrigine is useful as both adjunctive treatment in patients with partial seizures and as monotherapy. Lamotrigine appears to have comparable effectiveness with more traditional AEDs such as carbamazepine and phenytoin in these patients when used as monotherapy. In addition, lamotrigine may be useful alternative therapy in patients with primary generalized seizure types such as absence.

LEVETIRACETAM

Pharmacology and Mechanism of Action. Levetiracetam, an S-enantiomer pyrolidone derivitive, is chemically unrelated to other available AEDs. While the precise mechanism of action of levetiracetam has yet to be delineated, it is known that this drug is not active in the classic models used to test antiepileptic drugs. This agent may have a unique mechanism of action, including reduction in high-voltage activated Ca^{2+} currents and delayed-rectifer K^+ currents, as well as a unique action on GABA currents. Levetiracetam also appears to bind to a specific presynaptic binding site that may modulate neurotransmitter release. There is some limited evidence that levetiracetam may have *antiepileptogenic effects,* meaning that this compound may be able to prevent the development of epilepsy under certain circumstances.[59] Clinical confirmation of this animal research is still needed, however.

Pharmacokinetics. Levetiracetam is rapidly and completely absorbed following oral administration and displays negligible protein binding (<10%). Renal elimination of unchanged parent drug accounts for the majority of drug clearance (66%), with the remainder being metabolized in blood via nonhepatic enzymatic hydrolysis of an acetamide group to inactive metabolites.[60] This metabolic pathway does not involve either the CYP450 or UGT isozyme systems. The plasma half-life of this drug is approximately 7 hours. Because this drug is eliminated renally, clinicians should anticipate age-related reductions in clearance in elderly patients. Conversely, levetiracetam clearance appears to be approximately 40% higher in children than in adults. Currently, data are sparce regarding serum concentration–effect relationships, so the role of therapeutic drug level monitoring remains unclear.

Adverse Effects. Adverse effects appear to be modest, with sedation, fatigue, and coordination difficulties being the most common CNS effects. Behavioral disturbances, such as agitation, irritability, and occasionally depression, have been reported. The mechanism underlying these effects is unknown. Using a slower rate of dose escalation may be helpful in minimizing these adverse effects. Formal studies evaluating the cognitive effects of this medication have not yet been conducted.[44–46]

Drug Interactions. Levetiracetam neither inhibits nor induces the CYP450, UGT, or epoxide hydrolase enzyme systems, and in vitro data predict a low potential for pharmacokinetic interactions. Levetiracetam does not appear to interact with other AEDs, warfarin, digoxin, or oral contraceptive drugs.[60,61]

Dosing and Administration. Typical initial dosing of this agent is 500 mg orally twice daily, titrating at 1000-mg/day increments every 2 weeks to a maximum recommended dose of 3000 mg/day (1500 mg twice daily). In order to minimize CNS side effects, clinicians may consider initiating the drug at one-half this rate.

Advantages. Levetiracetam has a novel, although unknown, mechanism of action. It has linear pharmacokinetics and is not metabolized by the cytochrome P450 system. No significant drug interactions, including oral contraceptives, have been reported. Initial doses may be effective. The drug appears to be well tolerated, with transient sedation being the most troublesome adverse effect in most individuals.

Disadvantages. Dose adjustments are needed for patients with decreased renal functioning, and slower dose escalation may be needed to avoid CNS adverse effects. Behavioral problems may limit therapy in some patients. Currently, there is no parenteral formulation, but one is in development.

Place in Therapy. Currently, levetiracetam is indicated for patients with partial seizures who have failed initial therapy. Its role as monotherapy for partial seizures and as adjunctive treatment for generalized seizures remains to be clarified.

OXCARBAZEPINE

Pharmacology and Mechanism of Action. Oxcarbazepine, which is structurally related to carbamazepine, is a prodrug that is rapidly converted to a 10-monohydrate derivative (MHD), which is the active component. The mechanism of action of oxcarbazepine is similar to that of carbamazepine and perhaps lamotrigine. Oxcarbazepine and MHD block voltage-sensitive sodium channels, modulate the voltage-activated calcium currents, and increase potassium conductance. Interestingly, however, oxcarbazepine may display differing affinities for both sodium channels and Ca^{2+} channels compared with older drugs such as carbamazepine.[62] Whereas carbamazepine may modulate L-type Ca^{2+} channels, oxcarbazepine appears to modulate N- and P-type Ca^{2+} channels.[63] Whether these receptor differences lead to differing patterns of clinical effectiveness is still uncertain. It has no significant interactions with brain neurotransmitters or modulation of receptor sites.

Pharmacokinetics. Oxcarbazepine is absorbed completely and is metabolized extensively by noninducable cytosolic ketoreductases to MHD.[64] The concentration of MHD peaks 4 to 6 hours after a dose of oxcarbazepine. The MHD is inactivated by glucuronide conjugation and eliminated by the kidneys. The plasma half-life of MHD is 9.3 ± 1.8 hours, and it does not change with repeated dosing because there is no autoinduction. The half-life of MHD is shorter in patients taking enzyme-inducing drugs. The relationship between dose and serum concentration is linear. Oxcarbazepine is 67% protein bound, and MHD is 35% to 40% protein bound. The pharmacokinetics of MHD in children and adolescents are similar to those in adults. Children 2 to 6 years of age need larger doses to achieve the same serum concentration, suggesting a more rapid clearance. The C_{max} and bioavailability of MHD in elderly volunteers were higher than in younger volunteers, and the elimination rate was slower, possibly reflecting decreased renal elimination. Patients with significant renal impairment may require a dosage reduction. The suggested target serum concentration range for MHD is 20–200 mcmol/L.

Adverse Effects. Oxcarbazepine has been in clinical use worldwide since 1990 and was marketed in over 50 countries prior to approval in the United States. In U.S. clinical trials the most frequently reported adverse events were dizziness, nausea, headache, diarrhea, vomiting, upper respiratory tract infections, constipation, dyspepsia, ataxia, and nervousness. In comparative trials, oxcarbazepine generally caused fewer side effects than phenytoin, valproic acid, or carbamazepine. Dizziness may be more common in elderly patients. Overall, CNS adverse effects appear to be far more common at doses greater than 1200 mg/day. Hyponatremia, defined as a plasma sodium concentration of less than 125 mmol/L, has been reported in up to 25% of patients taking oxcarbazepine. As with carbamazepine, hyponatremia appears to occur more often in elderly patients. While the incidence of hyponatremia with oxcarbazepine is higher than that with carbamazepine, data suggest that many patients were asymptomatic, and about 80% were taking sodium-depleting medications. Clinicians should be particularly watchful in patients receiving concomitant sodium-depleting drugs such as diuretics. Hyponatremia appears to occur less frequently in children. Nevertheless, clinicians should consider monitoring serum sodium levels following the initiation of oxcarbazepine and instructing patients regarding the symptoms of hyponatremia. About 25% to 30% of patients who develop a rash with carbamazepine will experience a similar reaction with oxcarbazepine.[44–46] The tolerability of oxcarbazepine has not been compared with that of extended-release formulations of carbamazepine that have lower peaks and potentially fewer side effects than immediate-release carbamazepine formulations.

Drug Interactions. Oxcarbazepine decreases the bioavailability of ethinyl estradiol and levonorgestrel.[65] Women concurrently taking oral contraceptives should be counseled about the potential for contraceptive failure. There are no interactions between cimetidine, erythromycin, or warfarin and oxcarbazepine. The administration of oxcarbazepine in doses greater than 1200 mg with phenytoin has resulted in a 40% increase in the concentration of phenytoin, consistent with inhibition of CYP450 2C19. Oxcarbazepine treatment also may cause modest declines in lamotrigine serum concentrations, suggesting induction of UGT isozymes.[66]

Enzyme-inducing drugs increase the clearance of the active MHD. The replacement of carbamazepine with oxcarbazepine may result in a drug interaction because an enzyme-inducing drug is being removed.

Dosing and Administration. In adults, the starting dose of oxcarbazepine as monotherapy is 300 mg once or twice a day. The dose is titrated upward at a rate of 600 mg/day per week to a maximum dose of 2400 mg/day. Adverse effects frequently are dose-limiting at doses exceeding 1200 mg/day. Most patients require a slower titration rate. For children aged 4 to 16 years, the starting dose is 8 to 10 mg/kg given twice daily, not to exceed 600 mg/day. The dose is titrated to the target dose over 2 weeks. The recommended daily dose according to weight is 20–29 kg, 900 mg/day; 29.1–39 kg, 1200 mg/day; greater than 39 kg, 1800 mg/day. In patients being converted from carbamazepine, the typical maintenance doses of oxcarbazepine are 1.5 times the carbamazepine dose.

Advantages. The efficacy of oxcarbazepine is comparable with that of carbamazepine, phenytoin, and valproic acid. It has been approved in 50 countries, and thus broad international experience has been gained.

Disadvantages. About 30% of patients who have experienced a rash with carbamazepine have a cross-reaction with oxcarbazepine. There are more reports of hyponatremia with oxcarbazepine, especially in patients at risk, including the elderly and patients receiving sodium-depleting drugs such as diuretics. Replacing carbamazepine with oxcarbazepine may result in interactions with the removal of carbamazepine. Enzyme-inducing drugs may increase the clearance of MHD. This drug is not likely to be effective in seizure types where carbamazepine is ineffective, such as absence or myoclonic seizures.

Place in Therapy. Oxcarbazepine is indicated for use as monotherapy or adjunctive therapy in the treatment of partial seizures in adults and as monotherapy and adjunctive therapy in the treatment of partial seizures in patients as young as 4 years of age with epilepsy. It is also a potential first-line drug for patients with primary generalized convulsive seizures. Oxcarbazepine may be effective in patients not demonstrating a response to carbamazepine.

PHENOBARBITAL

Pharmacology and Mechanism of Action. Phenobarbital may elevate seizure threshold by decreasing postsynaptic excitation, possibly by stimulating postsynaptic GABAergic inhibitor responses.[20]

Pharmacokinetics. Phenobarbital is absorbed rapidly and completely regardless of whether it is given orally, intramuscularly, or rectally.[40] Phenobarbital penetrates the brain at a rate comparable with that of phenytoin, and peak concentrations are achieved 3 to 20 minutes after an intravenous dose. Phenobarbital is about 50% bound to plasma proteins, and it has a very long half-life.

Drugs affecting liver enzymes may alter phenobarbital metabolism, but phenobarbital clearance is not affected by liver blood flow. The elimination of phenobarbital is linear. Because tubular reabsorption of phenobarbital is pH dependent, the amount excreted renally can be increased by giving diuretics and urinary alkalinizers.[40]

Adverse Effects. CNS side effects are the primary factors limiting the use of phenobarbital. Tolerance usually develops to initial complaints of fatigue, drowsiness, sedation, and depression. In children, paradoxically, the primary side effect is hyperactivity. Phenobarbital impairs higher cortical function and depresses cognitive performance. Phenobarbital also may cause porphyria and rash, including serious rashes such as Stevens-Johnson[67] (see Table 54–6).

Drug Interactions. Phenobarbital is a potent enzyme inducer and may increase the elimination of any drug metabolized by CYP450- or UGT-mediated metabolism. Valproic acid, phenytoin, felbamate, cimetidine, and chloramphenicol inhibit phenobarbital metabolism, necessitating a decrease in dose. Ethanol increases the metabolism of phenobarbital.[40]

Dosing and Administration. In nonacute situations, phenobarbital should be started in low doses and titrated upward. The dose-concentration relationship is linear. Because the half-life of phenobarbital is long, doses can be given once daily. Bedtime dosing may minimize CNS depression. Because of its long half-life, phenobarbital takes 3 to 4 weeks to reach steady state. Therefore, rapid dosage adjustments should be avoided in a nonacute situation.

Advantages. Phenobarbital has linear and predictable pharmacokinetics. If the dose is doubled, the resulting serum concentrations double. Multiple dosage forms (e.g., oral solid, oral liquid, intramuscular, and intravenous) are available, so the route of administration can be tailored to patient needs, including emergent conditions. It is the most inexpensive AED.

Disadvantages. Phenobarbital is associated with significant side effects. These include delayed intellectual development and hyperactivity in children and significant cognitive impairment in adults. It is an enzyme inducer and interacts with many other drugs metabolized by the cytochrome P450 system. Phenobarbital has a very long half-life, and thus achievement of steady state is delayed. Dosage adjustments should not be made more often than every 2 to 3 weeks.

Place in Therapy. Phenobarbital is the drug of choice for neonatal seizures but in other situations is reserved for patients who have failed other AEDs. It may be useful given intravenously in refractory status epilepticus.

PHENYTOIN

Pharmacology and Mechanism of Action. Proposed mechanisms include alteration of ion fluxes associated with depolarization, repolarization, and membrane stability; alteration of calcium uptake in presynaptic terminals; influence on calcium-dependent synaptic protein phosphorylation and transmitter release; alteration of the sodium-potassium ATP-dependent ionic membrane pump; and prevention of cyclic nucleotide buildup and cerebellar stimulation.[20]

Pharmacokinetics. The pharmacokinetics of phenytoin are complex and fascinating. Space does not permit an in-depth review of phenytoin pharmacokinetics in this chapter. For a more in-depth understanding, the reader is referred to a more extensive review.[68] The oral absorption of phenytoin is almost complete. Dissolution is the rate-limiting step, and absorption may be saturable at higher doses, such as those used for oral loading doses. Absorption following intramuscular administration of phenytoin is erratic and delayed, and intramuscular injections are painful. Intramuscular absorption following fosphenytoin is rapid and well tolerated.

Phenytoin enters the brain rapidly and is redistributed to other body tissues, including breast milk and the placenta. It is highly (>90%) protein bound. Phenytoin competes for albumin sites with other highly protein bound drugs. It is essential to know the patient's serum albumin level in interpreting the serum concentrations of phenytoin.[69] Patients with significant renal dysfunction will have altered phenytoin protein binding. Obesity increases the volume of distribution of phenytoin.

Phenytoin is metabolized in the liver by parahydroxylation. The major isoforms responsible for the metabolism of phenytoin are CYP2C9 and CYP2C19. Phenytoin displays Michaelis-Menton pharmacokinetics, which means that the metabolism of phenytoin saturates at doses used clinically. The clinical importance of this is that a small change in dose can result in a very disproportionally large increase in serum concentrations leading to potential toxicity. The metabolism of phenytoin may saturate even at low serum concentrations within the therapeutic range. The metabolism of phenytoin has been shown to decrease with age.

Adverse Effects.

When phenytoin is initiated, the CNS depressant effects may result in lethargy, fatigue, incoordination, blurred vision, higher cortical dysfunction, and drowsiness (see Table 54–6). These effects usually are transient and may be minimized by slow dosage titration. Nystagmus, ataxia, and altered mental status are associated with higher concentrations. At very high concentrations (>50 mcg/mL), phenytoin may exacerbate seizures.

It is difficult to determine whether the chronic side effects of phenytoin are concentration- or duration-dependent. One of the more common chronic side effects is gingival hyperplasia. Good oral hygeine may minimize ginginval hyperplasia and should be encouraged. Other chronic effects include hirsutism, acne, coarsening of facial features, vitamin D deficiency, osteomalacia, folic acid deficiency, carbohydrate intolerance, immunologic disturbances, hypothyroidism, and peripheral neuropathy. Phenytoin is associated with rare hypersensitivity or idiosyncratic reactions resulting in rashes, Stevens-Johnson syndrome, pseudolymphoma, bone marrow suppression, lupus-like reactions, and hepatitis.[70]

Drug Interactions.

Phenytoin is associated with numerous drug interactions involving altered absorption, metabolism, and protein binding (see Tables 54–7 and 54–8) that can enhance or reduce its effects. Phenytoin is an inducer of both CYP450 and UGT isozymes. The absorption of phenytoin may be increased or decreased with the administration of food depending on the composition of the meal. The bioavailability of phenytoin suspension may be decreased in patients receiving continuous enteral nutrient tube feedings. A single-dose study of simultaneous administration of enteral feeding found no difference in phenytoin bioavailability, suggesting that the mechanism was something other than physical contact.[68]

A complex interaction of phenytoin with folic acid also has been described, making vitamin ingestion an important part of the drug history. Phenytoin reportedly decreases folic acid absorption, but folic acid enhances the clearance of phenytoin. Replacement of folic acid can reduce phenytoin concentrations and result in loss of efficacy.[68]

Dosing and Administration.

Four dosage forms are used for oral administration of phenytoin (Table 54–10). The salt content should be considered when changing from one dosage form to another. Changes between dosage forms may lead to changes in phenytoin concentration. Phenytoin capsules are designated as immediate-release or extended-release. Only the extended-release capsules should be used in once-a-day dosing. Particle size rather than formulation may determine the rate of absorption. Recently, Phenytek has been marketed in the United States as an extended-release dosage form of phenytoin.

If oral administration is not feasible, intravenous administration of phenytoin is preferred over intramuscular administration. Fosphenytoin is a prodrug for phenytoin and is available as a parenteral dosage form. It is very water-soluble and is converted rapidly to phenytoin systemically. Fosphenytoin can be given rapidly intravenously and intramuscularly with reliable absorption and minimal pain. It is significantly better tolerated than phenytoin.

Oral dosing of phenytoin should start at about 5 mg/kg per day for adults. If using oral loading doses, 20 mg/kg is typical, and the total dose should be divided by four and given at 6-hour intervals. Subsequent dosage adjustments should be done cautiously owing to its nonlinear elimination. One author has suggested that if the serum concentration is less than 7 mcg/mL, the dose should be increased by 100 mg/day; if the serum concentration is between 7 and 12 mcg/mL, the dose can be increased by 50 mg/day; and if the serum concentration is greater than 12 mcg/mL, the dose can be increased by 30 mg/day or less. These increases are proposed to result in less than 10% of patients achieving a phenytoin serum concentration greater than 25 mcg/mL.[71]

Advantages.

Phenytoin has been used for over 60 years, and its risk-to-benefit ratio is well developed. It is available in oral solid, oral liquid, extended-release oral solid, and parenteral (phenytoin and fosphenytoin) dosage forms, allowing flexibility in dosing and use in emergent conditions.

Disadvantages.

Phenytoin displays Michales-Menton pharmacokinetics, meaning that the metabolism saturates at doses given clinically. This makes phenytoin a difficult drug to dose. Also, phenytoin is an inducer of cytochrome P450 isozymes, is metabolized by cytochrome P450 enzymes, and is highly protein bound. Therefore, many drug interactions are associated with this agent. Phenytoin also has multiple adverse effects, including gait disorders, cognitive slowing at higher concentrations, gingival hyperplasia, cosmetic alterations, osteomalacia, rash, and teratogenicity.

Place in Therapy.

Phenytoin has long been a first-line AED for primary generalized convulsive and partial seizures. Its use in therapy may be reevaluated as more experience is gained with newer AEDs. Phenytoin or fosphenytoin is a first-line drug for the treatment of status epilepticus.

TIAGABINE

Pharmacology and Mechanism of Action.

Tiagabine is a potent and specific inhibitor of GABA uptake into glial and other neuronal

---

TABLE 54–10. Phenytoin Dosage Forms

Dosage Form	Salt or Acid	Extended or Prompt	Amount of Acid Available
Dilantin capsules	Phenytoin sodium	Extended	
100 mg			92 mg
30 mg			27 mg
Dilantin suspension 125 mg/5 mL	Phenytoin acid	Prompt	125 mg/5 mL
Dilantin Infatabs 50 mg	Phenytoin acid	Prompt	50 mg
Phenytoin injectable 50 mg/mL	Phenytoin sodium	Prompt	46 mg/mL
Fosphenytoin 50 mg PE/mL			50 mg PHT equivalents/mL
Phenytoin capsules (generic)	Phenytoin sodium	Prompt	92 mg

PHT = phenytoin.

elements. Thus tiagabine enhances the action of GABA by decreasing its removal from the synaptic space.[72]

■ *Pharmacokinetics.* Tiagabine is absorbed quickly and nearly completely after oral administration. There is a linear relationship between daily doses and serum concentrations. It is oxidized in the liver by CYP450 3A4 enzymes, and enzyme inducers increase its clearance. Children eliminate tiagabine slightly faster than adults. Subjects with hepatic impairment have higher and more prolonged plasma concentrations of total and unbound drug. Renal dysfunction does not change its pharmacokinetics.[72]

■ *Adverse Effects.* The most frequently reported adverse effects of tiagabine are dizziness, asthenia, nervousness, tremor, diarrhea, and depression. Rash is uncommon with tiagabine. Adverse events usually are mild to moderate in severity and transient, and most were associated with dose titration.[73] CNS side effects may be diminished by taking tiagabine with food, thus slowing the absorption rate. Serious adverse events were uncommon, and no idiosyncratic events, including visual field defects, were reported.[44-46]

■ *Drug Interactions.* Enzyme inducers, such as carbamazepine and phenytoin, increase tiagabine clearance and decrease the half-life. Food decreases the rate but not the extent of absorption. Tiagabine is displaced from protein by naproxen, salicylates, and valproate. However, tiagabine does not displace phenytoin, valproic acid, amitryptyline, tolbutamide, or warfarin.[72]

■ *Dosing and Administration.* A clear dose-response has been demonstrated, and the minimal effective adult dose level is 30 mg/day. The initial dose, 4 mg/day, can be titrated up to 56 mg/day by adding 4 to 8 mg to the daily dose each week. The dosage range typically employed is 32 to 56 mg daily,[72] and the variability can be explained in part by the presence of concomitant enzyme-inducing AEDs. Slow dosage titration is essential to decrease adverse CNS effects.[44-46]

■ *Advantages.* Tiagabine has a specific, known mechanism of action. It is the first drug marketed in the United States that acts only on GABA reuptake. This drug has linear pharmacokinetics and is not reported to interact with other drugs.

■ *Disadvantages.* Initially high and rapid dosage escalation is associated with increased CNS side effects. Therefore, the drug must be started at a low dose and titrated gradually to patient response. Lower doses may be needed in patients with liver disease. Tiagabine is metabolized by CYP450 3A4 enzymes, and other drugs may alter its clearance. There is no parenteral formulation.

■ *Place in Therapy.* Tiagabine is considered a second-line therapy for patients with partial seizures who have failed initial therapy. It does not appear to have a role in primary generalized seizure types.

■ TOPIRAMATE

■ *Pharmacology and Mechanism of Action.* Topiramate is a sulfamate-substituted monosaccharide that has multiple modes of action involving voltage-dependent sodium channels, GABA receptors, and antagonism of α-amino-3-hydroxy-5-methyl-4-isoxazole-4-propionic acid (AMPA) subtype glutamate receptors.[74]

■ *Pharmacokinetics.* While generally considered to have linear absorption and elimination pharmacokinetics, a greater than proportional increase in both maximal peak concentration and area under the concentration-time curve has been observed and probably is explained by saturable binding of the drug to erythrocytes.[75] Topiramate does not display significant protein binding. Approximately 50% of the dose is excreted unchanged renally; however, metabolism is increased by approximately 50% when topiramate is given with enzyme-inducing AEDs. Renal tubular reabsorption may be involved prominently in the renal handling of topiramate.[76]

■ *Adverse Effects.* The main adverse events of topiramate are ataxia, impaired concentration, memory difficulties, attentional deficits, confusion, dizziness, fatigue, paresthesias, somnolence, and "thinking abnormally," which rarely has included psychosis. Word-finding difficulties are a somewhat unique and specific problem with topiramate and may occur in a significant number of patients. Most of these occurred during rapid titration and at higher doses.[77] There may be an increased incidence of cognitive dysfunction in patients receiving concomitant therapy with topiramate and valproic acid. During long-term treatment, weight loss can occur, a phenomenon that may be dose-dependent. Nephrolithiasis has occurred in 1.5% of patients receiving topiramate, which is two to four times the incidence in the general population. Patients should be encouraged to maintain adequate fluid intake in order to minimize this problem. Recently, the use of topiramate was associated with acute narrow-angle glaucoma, oligohydrosis, and metabolic acidosis. Metabolic acidosis in part may explain the anorexia and weight loss seen with this drug.[44]

■ *Drug Interactions.* Topiramate does not change plasma levels of carbamazepine, carbamazepine-epoxide, or lamotrigine. Oral clearance of digoxin is slightly increased when topiramate is added. Topiramate coadministration may result in increased phenytoin serum concentrations in some patients, an effect consistent with in vitro studies showing an inhibitory effect of topiramate on the CYP2C19 isoform. The variable response seen with the interaction of topiramate and phenytoin may be explained by the intersubject variability in the proportion of phenytoin clearance attributed to CYP2C19 metabolism and whether the patient is a homozygous or heterozygous carrier of the mutant allele responsible for the CYP2C9 and/or CYP2C19 "poor metabolilzer" phenotype. Topiramate can increase the oral clearance of valproic acid modestly and increase formation of the 4-ene-VPA metabolite. The clinical significance of this interaction is unclear. Topiramate increases the clearance of ethinyl estradiol in a dose-dependant manner. Topiramate doses of less than 200 mg/day are unlikely to alter oral contraceptive pharmacokinetics. Carbamazepine and phenytoin increase topiramate clearance.[78]

■ *Dosing and Administration.* Topiramate should be titrated slowly in order to avoid adverse events.[74] Starting doses are 12.5 to 50 mg/day, increasing by 12.5 to 50 mg/day every week or every other week. The minimally effective dose of topiramate is approximately 200 mg/day.[79] For patients on other AEDs, doses of greater than 600 mg/day do not appear to lead to improved efficacy and may cause increased adverse effects; however, higher doses may prove beneficial to individual patients who tolerate them.[80] Monotherapy doses as high as 1000 mg/day have been well tolerated and effective in some patients.

■ *Advantages.* Topiramate has multiple mechanisms of action and may be a broad-spectrum AED. The kidney mainly eliminates it, although some liver metabolism occurs. It has liner pharmacokinetics and few drug interactions.

■ *Disadvantages.* With rapid dosage escalation, topiramate may compromise cognitive functioning, including impaired word finding and short-term memory. Therefore, low initial doses should be used, and the dose must be titrated slowly. Renal stones and weight loss also have been associated with topiramate use. The dose should be decreased in patients with renal failure. There is no parenteral formulation.

■ *Place in Therapy.* Topiramate is a second-line AED for patients with partial seizures who have failed initial therapy. Its role as a primary AED and in other seizure types is being evaluated.

■ VALPROIC ACID/DIVALPROEX SODIUM

■ *Pharmacology and Mechanism of Action.* Initially it was believed that valproic acid increased GABA by inhibiting its degradation or by activating its synthesis. Although this may explain in part valproic acid effects, the time course for the increase in GABA compared with the onset of anticonvulsant effects indicates that alterations of the synthesis and degradation of GABA do not fully explain the antiseizure activity of valproic acid. It has been proposed that valproic acid may potentiate postsynaptic GABA responses, may have a direct membrane-stabilizing effect, and may affect potassium channels.[81]

■ *Pharmacokinetics.* Valproic acid appears to be absorbed completely from available oral dosage forms when administered on an empty stomach.[81] However, the rate of absorption differs among preparations. Peak concentrations occur in 0.5 to 1 hour with the syrup, 1 to 3 hours with the capsule, and 2 to 6 hours with the enteric-coated tablet.[81] The extended-release formulation (Depakote-ER) is FDA approved for use in both patients with migraine headache and epilepsy. It should be noted, however, that the bioavailability of this formulation is approximately 15% less than that of enteric-coated divalproex sodium (Depakote).

Valproic acid is extensively bound to albumin, and this binding is saturable. Accordingly, the valproic acid free fraction will increase as the total serum concentration increases. Because of this saturable binding, measurement of unbound serum concentrations may be a better monitoring parameter than the total valproic acid serum concentration, especially at higher concentrations or in patients with hypoalbuminemia.[40]

The primary route of valproic acid metabolism is β-oxidation, although up to 40% of a dose may be excreted as the glucuronide. At least 10 metabolites of valproic acid have been identified. Some of these may have weak anticonvulsant activity, and at least one metabolite may be responsible for the hepatotoxicity reported with valproic acid. One of the lesser oxidative metabolites, 4-en-valproic acid, causes significant hepatotoxicity in rats. The formation of this metabolite is increased when valproic acid is given with enzyme-inducing drugs.[81]

■ *Adverse Effects.* The most frequently reported side effects are gastrointestinal complaints (up to 20%), including nausea, vomiting, anorexia, and weight gain. Pancreatitis is very rare. The gastrointestinal complaints may be minimized but not totally alleviated with the enteric-coated formulation or by giving the drug with food. Other frequently reported side effects (e.g., drowsiness, ataxia, and postural tremor) may respond to a modification of dose (see Table 54–6).

Alopecia and hair changes are temporary, and hair growth returns even with continued dosing. Weight gain can be significant for many patients and may involve stimulation of appetite and/or inhibition of fatty acid β-oxidation leading to reduced metabolic rate.[82] Valproic acid causes minimal cognitive impairment.[81]

The most serious side effect reported with valproic acid is hepatotoxicity. Hyperammonemia is common (50%) but does not necessarily imply liver damage; however, at least 67 fatalities have been attributed to valproic acid hepatotoxicity. Most deaths have occurred in patients who were younger than 2 years of age, mentally retarded, and receiving multiple AEDs. Hepatotoxicity occurred early in the course of therapy. Patients who complain of nausea, vomiting, lethargy, anorexia, and edema in the first 6 to 12 months of therapy should have liver function tests done. Multiple-AED therapy may alter the metabolism of valproic acid, leading to increased formation of the potentially liver-toxic 4-en-valproic acid. Valproic acid has been shown to alter carnitine metabolism, and it has been postulated that a deficiency of carnitine alters fatty acid oxidation that could lead to both liver toxicity and hyperammonemia.[83] However, valproic acid hepatotoxicity has occurred in a patient taking supplemental carnitine, and a prospective study demonstrated no effect on well-being when carnitine was added. While carnitine may ameliorate hyperammonemia in part, it is expensive, and there are only limited data to support routine supplemental use in patients taking valproic acid.[84]

Thrombocytopenia and alterations in platelet aggregation occur in the patients receiving valproic acid, and these phenomena are related to serum concentration. Other hematologic toxicities have been reported, including leukopenia with transient neutropenia, transient erythroblastopenia, and bone marrow changes. Polycystic ovary syndrome and menstrual cycle irregularities also have been associated with valproic acid.[83]

■ *Drug Interactions.* Drugs that affect liver enzymes may alter valproic acid kinetics by increasing or decreasing clearance; for example, phenytoin, phenobarbital, primidone, and carbamazepine all increase valproic acid clearance. Topiramate may reduce valproic acid serum concentrations modestly. Because it is highly protein bound, other highly protein-bound drugs may displace valproic acid. Free fatty acids and aspirin may alter valproic acid binding by displacement. Felbamate may impair valproic clearance via inhibition of β-oxidation.

Valproic acid is an enzyme inhibitor that can inhibit specific cytochrome P450 isozymes, epoxide hydrolase, and UGT isozymes. The addition of valproic acid to phenobarbital results in a 30% to 50% decrease in the clearance of phenobarbital and potential toxicity if the dose of phenobarbital is not reduced. Valproic acid may increase concentrations of 10,11-carbamazepine epoxide without affecting concentrations of the parent drug via inhibition of epoxide hydrolase. Valproic acid is also a potent inhibitor of lamotrigine, via inhibition of UGT enzymes, and can result in a doubling of the half-life of lamotrigine.[85]

■ *Dosing and Administration.* Although some patients may have a half-life sufficiently long to permit once-daily dosing with enteric-coated divalproex, more frequent dosing is the norm. Based on half-life data, twice-daily dosing is feasible with any valproic acid dosage form; however, children and other patients taking enzyme inducers may require dosing three to four times daily.[40] The serum concentration–dose relationship is curvilinear (i.e., the concentration-dose ratio decreases with increasing dose) probably because of increasing free concentrations and a resulting increase in clearance.[40]

Valproic acid is available as a soft gelatin capsule, an enteric-coated tablet, a syrup, a "sprinkle," an extended-release formulation designed for once-daily dosing, and a parenteral (intravenous) formulation for replacement of oral therapy or in situations where rapid loading of valproic acid is deemed necessary.[81] This parenteral formulation must not be given intramuscularly because it may cause tissue necrosis. The sprinkle, designed to be opened and mixed with food, has a slower rate of absorption, which results in fewer fluctuations in the peak-to-trough ratio. The syrup is absorbed more rapidly than any solid dosage form. The enteric-coated tablet is not sustained-release; it consists of sodium divalproex, which must be metabolized in the gut to valproic acid. It is enteric coated to reduce the incidence of gastrointestinal distress. The enteric coating does cause delayed absorption, although once the enteric coating dissolves, sodium divalproex has absorption, metabolism, and elimination rates similar to those of the gelatin capsule. Clinicians may need to monitor serum drug concentrations if converting patients from divalproex (Depakote) to the extended-release formulation (Depakote-ER). If a patient is switched from Depakote to Depakote-ER, the dose should be increased by 14% to 20%. Depakote-ER may be given once daily.

Although 100–120 mcg/mL is widely quoted as the upper end of the therapeutic range, experience indicates that a significant number of patients have improved seizure control when the concentration is above this level. Although some reports have linked tremor, drowsiness, stupor, and decreases in fibrinogen to concentrations greater than 80 to 100 mcg/mL, there are very few clearly defined concentration-dependent side effects of valproic acid. In refractory or partially responding patients, the concentration of valproic acid may be titrated upward cautiously, provided the patient is closely monitored. As the concentration is increased, protein binding may become saturated, and serum concentration monitoring of free drug may be helpful.[40]

▨ *Advantages.* Valproic acid is available in multiple dosage formulations. It has a wide therapeutic index and can be considered a broad-spectrum AED. It also may be useful in other neurologic or psychiatric disorders, including migraine headache and bipolar-affective disorder.

▨ *Disadvantages.* Some patients report significant weight gain with valproic acid, and this may limit compliance. Valproic acid is also associated with other side effects, such as alopecia, tremor, pancreatitis, polycystic ovary disease, and thrombocytopenia. This drug has been associated with hepatic necrosis in young children. Valproic acid is an enzyme inhibitor and is involved in multiple drug-drug interactions.

▨ *Place in Therapy.* Valproic acid is first-line therapy for primary generalized seizures such as myoclonic, atonic, and absence seizures. It can be used as both monotherapy and adjunctive therapy for partial seizures, and it can be very useful in patients with mixed seizure disorders.

▨ ZONISAMIDE

▨ *Pharmacology and Mechanism of Action.* Zonisamide, a synthetic 1,2-benzisoxazole derivative classified as a sulfonamide, is chemically different from other AEDs. In animal testing it was demonstrated to be a broad-spectrum AED. It is believed to exert its antiepileptic effect by reducing repetitive neuronal firing via blockade of voltage-sensitive sodium channels, by reducing voltage-dependent T-type Ca^{2+} channels, by facilitating dopaminergic and serotonergic neurotransmission, by weakly inhibiting carbonic anhydrase, and by blocking K^+ evoked glutamate release. It is also postulated that zonisamide may protect the neurons from free radical damage.[86]

▨ *Pharmacokinetics.* Zonisamide is absorbed completely, reaching a maximum peak concentration in 2 to 6 hours. It is only about 40% protein bound and has a very long half-life of approximately 63 to 69 hours in uninduced subjects. Zonisamide is metabolized by both CYP3A4 (50%) and N-acetylation (20%). Eight inactive metabolites have been identified. About 30% is excreted unchanged. Marked renal impairment ($Cr_{Cl} < 20$ mL/min) was associated with an increase in the AUC of zonisamide by 35%. Zonisamide is distributed to most tissues, but the concentration in red blood cells, liver, kidney, and adrenal gland is twice as high. Zonisamide crosses the placenta. The concentration in breast milk is similar to that in the plasma. Although not firmly established, a target concentration range of 10–40 mcg/mL has been suggested.[87]

▨ *Adverse Effects.* The most common adverse effects of zonisamide include somnolence, dizziness, anorexia, headache, nausea, agitation, and irritability. Adverse effects may be more common during rapid dose escalation. Because zonisamide is structurally related to sulfonamides, hypersensitivity reactions may occur (0.02% of patients), and zonisamide should be used with caution (if at all) in patients with a confirmed history of allergy to sulfonamide compounds. A 2.6% incidence of symptomatic kidney stones has been reported in patients treated in the United States.[88] Because of reports of modest, reversible declines in renal function in some patients, monitoring of renal function may be advisable for certain patients. Oligohydrosis has been reported. In addition, modest weight loss has been reported with this agent.[44–46]

▨ *Drug Interactions.* Zonisamide does not inhibit or induce the cytochrome P450 system. Enzyme inducers and CYP3A4 inhibitors can affect the concentration of zonisamide.[32] Treatment with enzyme inducers can reduce zonisamide half-life to 27 to 36 hours.[89]

▨ *Dosing and Administration.* In adults, the initial recommended dose of zonisamide is 100 mg/day. Doses should be titrated by 100 mg daily every 2 weeks to patient response. The dosage range in adults is 100 to 600 mg/day. In children, zonisamide can be initiated at a dose of 2–4 mg/kg per day and titrated to 4–8 mg/kg per day up to a maximum of 12 mg/kg per day. Zonisamide is stable for 48 hours when mixed with water, apple juice, or pudding for patients who have trouble swallowing oral solid dosage forms.

▨ *Advantages.* Zonisamide has multiple mechanisms of action and may be a broad-spectrum AED. It has been used in other countries, and there is broad international experience with this drug. It has a very long half-life, which is suitable for once- or twice-daily dosing. Once-daily dosing is associated with more fluctuations around the mean concentration and perhaps more side effects. Patients may experience modest weight loss with this drug.

▨ *Disadvantages.* The dose of zonisamide should be titrated slowly to patient response. Renal stones and oligohydrosis also have been associated with zonisamide. In addition, cognitive impairment may occur, especially if dosage is escalated rapidly.

▨ *Place in Therapy.* Zonisamide is currently approved for the adjunctive treatment of partial seizures. Thus far, insufficient data exist to support its use as initial monotherapy. Zonisamide is potentially effective in a variety of partial and primary generalized seizure types.

PHARMACOECONOMIC CONSIDERATIONS

CLINICAL CONTROVERSY

Given the cost differential between the older-generation and newer-generation AEDs, the place in therapy of these newer drugs is controversial. The cost of the newer AEDs generally is much higher that that of the older drugs. Given that, in general, the efficacy of the newer drugs is comparable with that of the older agents, many clinicians (and patients) have been slow to adopt this newer generation of drugs. It is important to recognize that overall effectiveness encompasses both efficacy and tolerability assessments. Generally speaking, the newer generation of AEDs possesses fewer adverse effects and appears to be be better tolerated than older, far less expensive agents such as the barbiturates. Whether these sometimes subjective differences justify the difference in cost needs to be determined on an individual basis.

The direct costs of epilepsy include the cost of the drug, treatment of adverse events, emergency room visits, drug levels, laboratory tests, physician visits, rehabilitation, and transportation. Indirect costs include the costs associated with time lost from work, the inability to get a job, decreased productivity, and mortality.

It is difficult to assess the entire cost of epilepsy to society. Pashko and coworkers,[90] using a cohort of Pennsylvania Medicaid patients, estimated that the total direct cost of epilepsy is in excess of $10 billion annually, with the majority of the per-patient costs incurred for inpatient hospitalization (uncontrolled seizures or treatment-related toxicity). Another study suggested that the direct costs of epilepsy made up about 37% of the total costs, with indirect costs accounting for the remainder.[91] This study also indicated that the costs were much less for a patient who is well controlled than for a patient who is poorly controlled. Drug costs in the Pashko study accounted for about 10% of the total costs of epilepsy. In another study, the cost-effectiveness of some of the newer drugs (lamotrigine, vigabatrin, and gabapentin) was estimated for the first year of drug therapy. There was little difference in initial costs, but gabapentin, with fewer adverse effects, resulted in cost savings.[92] The methodology used in this study has been criticized. There have been no pharmacoeconomic studies comparing the older, less expensive AEDs with the newer, more expensive drugs.

Providing the best quality of life possible is a treatment goal for patients with epilepsy. This concept entails more than a balance between side effects and the number of seizures. Quality of life takes into account all the concerns of patients with epilepsy, including their social and economic concerns. This can best be assessed by the patient. Complete seizure freedom leads to the best quality of life.[13] In one study, driving was listed as the most important concern by 28% of patients, followed by employment (21%), independence (9%), safety (6%), AED side effects (5%), seizure unpredictability (5%), and seizure avoidance (5%).[93] Assessment of quality of life as a therapeutic outcome ultimately may be more meaningful than measuring blood levels of the AEDs. Several quality-of-life instruments have been used, although primarily as research tools.[94] A single seizure can be devastating to a given patient.

It is clear that the cheapest drugs in epilepsy (e.g., phenobarbital) are not the best because of the number of side effects. Further drug therapy that would control seizures, decrease side effects, improve the quality of life, and reduce the use of other health care resources would be cost-effective. Because epilepsy treatment continues to be very patient-specific, the drug or combination of drugs that controls seizures with the least number of side effects will be the drug of choice for that patient no matter how expensive the drug acquisition cost.

Because many patients with epilepsy require minimal variation in blood concentrations to prevent seizures and avoid side effects, generic prescribing for epilepsy remains controversial. One study suggested that the money saved by generic prescribing is outweighed by the negative health gain for the person with epilepsy, increased work in general practice, and increased social costs.[95]

EVALUATION OF THERAPEUTIC OUTCOMES

A therapeutic range should be established for each patient. This range should define concentrations that result in minimal side effects and optimal seizure control. This therapeutic plasma concentration range should be used to identify the appropriate patient-specific dose. Patients should be monitored chronically for seizure control, comorbid conditions, social adjustment (including quality-of-life assessments), drug interactions, compliance, and adverse effects. Periodic screening for comorbid neuropsychiatric disorders such as depression and anxiety is also important. Clinical response is more important than the serum drug concentration.

Outcomes can be assessed by prospective clinical monitoring, drug utilization review, and quality-of-life assessments. Clinical monitoring involves identifying the number and type of seizures. Patients should be given a seizure diary, and the severity as well as the frequency of seizures should be monitored. There should be a decrease in the number and/or severity of seizures. Patients should be questioned regularly to determine whether they are seizure-free. It is important to recall that perhaps as many as 30% of patients will be intractable to current pharmacologic treatments. In these patients, if the clinician has determined that AED dosage has been maximized, one should consider either AED combination therapy or, potentially, evaluation for epilepsy surgery or the vagal nerve stimulator.

The treatment of epilepsy begins with a careful identification of the seizure type and selection of the most appropriate AED. Therapy should be initiated slowly, except in life-threatening situations, to avoid acute toxicity. Although most patients can be managed successfully on monotherapy, some patients' seizures remain uncontrolled despite the use of multiple AEDs. Some patients may be genetically refractory to AED therapy. The newer AEDs, as adjunctive therapy or monotherapy, offer additional opportunity for complete seizure control. There is a continuing need for new AEDs and additional research in this area.

Review Questions and other resources can be found at *www.pharmacotherapy.com.*

REFERENCES

1. Leppik IE. Contemporary Diagnosis and Management of the Patient with Epilepsy, 2d ed. Newtown, PA, Handbooks in Health Care, 1996.
2. Sander JW. The epidemiology of epilepsy revisted. Curr Opin Neurol 2003;16:165–170.
3. Annegers JF. The epidemiology of epilepsy. In: Wylie E, ed. The Treatment of Epilepsy, 3d ed. Philadelphia, Lippincott Williams & Wilkins; 2001:131–138.
4. Najm IM, Janigro D, Babb TL. Mechamisms of epileptogenesis and experimental models of seizures. In: Wylie E, ed. The Treatment of Epilepsy, 3d ed. Philadelphia, Lippincott Williams & Wilkins; 2001:33–44.

5. Commission on Classification and Terminology of the International League Against Epilepsy. Proposal for revised clinical and electroencephalographic classification of epileptic seizures. Epilepsia 1981;22:489–501.

6. Commission on Classification and Terminology of the International League Against Epilepsy. Proposal for revised classification of epilepsies and epileptic syndromes. Epilepsia 1989;30:389–399.

7. Vickrey BG, Hays RD, Rausch R, et al. Quality of life of epilepsy surgery patients as compared with outpatients with hypertension, diabetes,heart disease, and/or depressive symptoms. Epilepsia 1994;35:597–607.

8. Hecimovic H, Goldstein J, Shelie Y, Gilliam FG. Mechanisms of depression in epilepsy from a clinical perspective. Epilepsy Behav 2003;4:S25–30.

9. Plioplys S. Depression in children and adolescents with epilepsy. Epilepsy Behav 2003;4:S39–45.

10. Wiegartz P, Seidenberg M, Woodard A, et al. Co-morbid psychiatric disorder in chronic epilepsy: recognition and etiology of depression. Neurology 1999;53(suppl 2):S3–8.

11. Brodie MJ, French JA. Management of epilepsy in adolescents and adults. Lancet 2000;356:323–328.

12. Mattson RH. Antiepileptic drug monotherapy in adults: selection and use in new-onset epilepsy. In: Levy RH, Mattson RH, Meldrum BS, Perucca E, eds. Antiepileptic Drugs, 5th ed. Philadelphia, Lippincott Williams & Wilkins, 2002:72–95.

13. Perucca E, Levy RH. Combination therapy and drug interactions. In: Levy RH, Mattson RH, Meldrum BS, Perucca E, eds. Antiepileptic Drugs, 5th ed. Philadelphia, Lippincott Williams & Wilkins; 2002:96–102.

14. Garnett WR. Antiepileptic drug treatment: Outcomes and adherence. Pharmacotherapy 2000;20:191S–199S.

15. Shinnar S, Gross-Tsur V. Discontinuing antiepileptic drug therapy. In: Wyllie E, ed. The Treatment of Epilepsy, 3d ed. Philadelphia, Lippincott Williams & Wilkins, 2001:811–819.

16. Wheless J. Vagus nerve stimulation. In: Wyllie E, ed. The Treatment of Epilepsy, 3d ed. Philadelphia, Lippincott Williams & Wilkins, 2001:1007–1015.

17. Benbadis S, Chelune GJ, Stanford LD, et al. Outcome and complications of epilepsy sugery. In: Wyllie E, ed. The Treatment of Epilepsy, 3d ed. Philadelphia, Lippincott Williams & Wilkins, 2001:1197–1211.

18. Schiller Y, Casino GD, So EL, Marsh R. Discontinuation of antiepileptic drugs after successful epilepsy surgery. Neurology 2000;54:346–349.

19. Nordli DRJ, De Vivo DC. The ketogenic diet revisited: Back to the future. Epilepsia 1997;38:743–749.

20. Rho JM, Sankar R. The pharmacological basis of antiepileptic drug action. Epilepsia 1999;40:1471–1483.

21. Harden CL. Therapeutic safety monitoring: What to look for and when to look for it. Epilepsia 2000;41(suppl 8):S37–44.

22. Perucca E. Is there a role of therapeutic drug monitoring of new anticonvulsants. Clin Pharmacokinet 2000;38:191–204.

23. Pack AM, Olarte LS, Morrell MJ, et al. Bone mineral density in an outpatient population receiving enzyme-inducing antiepileptic drugs. Epilepsy Behav 2003;4:169–174.

24. Meador KJ, Gilliam FG, Kanner AM, Pellock JM. Cognitive and behavioral effects of antiepileptic drugs. Epilepsy Behav 2001;2:S1–17.

25. Vermeulen J, Aldenkamp AP. Cognitive side-effects of chronic antiepileptic drug treatment: A review of 25 years of research. Epilepsy Res 1995;22:65–95.

26. Meador KJ, Loring DW, Ray PG, et al. Differential cognitive effects of carbamazepine and gabapentin. Epilepsia 1999;40:1279–1285.

27. Meador KJ, Loring DW, Ray PG. Differential cognitive effects of carbamazepine and lamotrigine (abstact). Neurology 2000;54:A84.

28. Martin R, Kuzniecky R, Ho S, et al. Cognitive effects of topiramate, gabapentin and lamotrigine in healthy young adults. Neurology 1999;52:321–327.

29. Elger CE, Bauer J, Scherrmann J, Widman G. Aggravation of focal epileptic seizures by antiepileptic drugs. Epilepsia 1998;39:S15–18.

30. Mattson RH, Cramer JA, Collins JF, et al. Comparison of carbamazepine, phenobarbital, phenytoin, and primidone in partial and secondarily generalized tonic-clonic seizures. New Engl J Med 1985;313:145–151.

31. Mattson RH, Cramer JA, Collins JF, et al. A comparison of valproate with carbamazepine for the treatment of complex partial seizures and secondarily generalized tonic-clonic seizures in adults. New Engl J Med 1992;327:765–771.

32. Beydoun A, Kutluay E. Conversion to monotherapy: Clinical trials in patients with refractory partial seizures. Neurology 2003;60(suppl 4):S13–25.

33. French JA, Kanner AM, Bautista J, et al. Efficacy and tolerability of the new antiepileptic drugs: I. Treatment of new-onset epilepsy. Epilepsia 2004;45;401–409.

34. French JA, Kanner AM, Bautista J, et al. Efficacy and tolerability of the new antiepileptic drugs: II. Treatment of refractory epilepsy. Epilepsia 2004;45;410–423.

35. Marson AG, Kadir ZA, Chadwick DW. New antiepileptic drugs: A systematic review of their efficacy and tolerability. Br Med J 1996;313:1169–1174.

36. Karceski S, Morrell M, Carpenter D. The expert consensus guideline series: Treatment of epilepsy. Epilepsy Behav 2001;2:A1–A50.

37. Smith S, Wolley CS. Cellular and molecular effects of steroid hormones and CNS excitability. Cleve Clin J Med 2004;71:S5–10.

38. Morrell MJ, Montouris GD. Reproductive disturbances in patients with epilepsy. Cleve Clin J Med 2004;71:S19–24.

39. Yerby MS, Kaplan P, Tran T. Risks and management of pregnancy in women with epilepsy. Cleve Clin J Med 2004;71:S25–37.

40. Garnett WR. Antiepileptics. In: Schumacher GE, ed. Therapeutic Drug Monitoring. Norwalk, CT, Appleton and Lange, 1995:345–395.

41. Garnett WR. Carbamazepine. In: Murphy J, ed. Clinical Pharmacokinetics, 2d ed. Washington, American Society of Health-Systems Pharmacists, 2004.

42. Garnett WR. Ethosuximide. In: Murphy J, ed. Clinical Pharmacokinetics. Washington, American Society of Health-Systems Pharmacists, 2004.

43. Pellock JM, Perhach JL, Sofia RD. Felbamate. In: Levy RH, Mkattson RH, Meldrum BS, et al, eds. Antiepileptic Drugs, 5th ed. Philadelphia, Lippincott Williams & Wilkins, 2002:301–318.

44. LaRoche SM, Helmers SL. The new antiepileptic drugs: Scientific review. JAMA 2004;291:605–614.

45. French JA, Kanner AM, Bautista J, et al. Efficacy and tolerability of the new antiepileptic drugs: I. Treatment of new onset epilepsy. Neurology 2004;62:1252–1260.

46. French JA, Kanner AM, Bautista J, et al. Efficacy and tolerability of the new antiepileptic drugs: II. Treatment of refractory epilepsy. Neurology 2004;62:1261–1273.

47. Taylor CP, Gee NS, Su TZ, et al. A summary of mechanistic hypothesis of gabapentin pharmacology. Epilepsy Res 1998;29:233–249.

48. Luer MS, Hamani C, Dujovny M, et al. Saturable transport of gabapentin at the bloodbrain barrier. Neurol Res 1999;21:559–562.

49. Gidal BE, Radulovic LL, Kruger S, et al. Inter- and intrasubject variability in gabapentin (GBP) absorption and absolute bioavailability. Epilepsy Res 2000;40:123–127.

50. Gidal BE, Maly MM, Kowalski J, et al. Gabapentin absorption: Effect of mixing with foods of varying macronutrient content. Ann Pharmacother 1998;32:405–408.

51. Wong MO, Eldon MA, Keane WF, et al. Disposition of gabapentin in anuric subjects on hemodialysis. J Clin Pharmacol 1995;35:622–626.

52. Lee DO, Steingard RJ, Cesena M, et al. Behavioral side effects of gabapentin in children. Epilepsia 1996;37:87–90.

53. McLean MJ, Gidal BE. Gabapentin in the treatment of epilepsy: A dosing review. Clin Ther 2003;25:1382–1406.

54. Gidal BE, DeCerce J, Bockbrader HR, et al. Gabapentin bioavailability: Effect of dose and frequency of administration in adult patients with epilepsy. Epilepsy Res 1998;31:91–99.

55. Gilman JT. Lamotrigine: An antiepileptic agent for the treatment of partial seizures. Ann Pharmacother 1995;29:144–151.

56. Dickins M, Chen C. Lamotrigine: Chemistry, biotransformation, and pharmacokinetics. In: Levy RH, Mattson RH, Meldrum BS, et al, eds., Antiepiletic Drugs, 5th ed. Philadelphia, Lippincott Williams & Wilkins, 2002:369–379.

57. Messenheimer JA. Rash in adult and pediatric patients treated with lamotrigine. Can J Neurol Sci 1998;25:S14–18.

58. Holdrich T, Whiteman P, Orme M, et al. Effect of lamotrigine on pharmacology of the combined oral contraceptive pill (abstract). Epilepsia 1992;32(suppl 1):96.

59. Loscher W, Honack D, Rundfeldt C. Antiepileptogenic effects of the novel anticonvulsant levetiracetam (ucb LO59) in the kindling model of temporal lobe epilepsy. J Pharm Exp Ther 1998;284:474–479.

60. Welty TE, Gidal BE, Ficker DM, Privitera MD. Levetiracetam: A different approach to the pharmacotherapy of epilepsy. Ann Pharmacother 2002;36:296–304.

61. Perucca E, Gidal BE. Effects of antiepileptic comedication on levetiracetam pharmacokinetics: A pooled analysis of data. from randomized adjunctive therapy trials. Epilepsy Res 2003;53:47–56.

62. Ambrosio AF, Soares-Da-Silva P, Carvalho CM, Carvalho AP. Mechanisms of action of carbamazepine and its derivatives, oxcarbazepine, BIA 2-093 and BIA 2-024. Neurochem Res 2002;27:121–130.

63. Ambrosio AF, Silva AP, Malva JO, et al. Carbamazepine inhibits L-type Ca^{2+} channels in coctrinal RAT hippocampal neurons stimulated with glutamate receptor agonists. Neuropharmacology 1999;38:1349–1359.

64. Lloyd P, Flesch G, Dieterle W. Clinical pharmacology and pharmacokinetics of oxcarbazepine. Epilepsia 1994;35:10–13.

65. Kalis MM, Huff NA. Oxcarbazepine, an antiepileptic agent. Clin Therapeut 2001;23:680–700.

66. May TW, Ramback B, Jurgens U. Influence of oxcarbazepine and methsuximide on lamotrigine concentrations in epileptic patients with and without valproic acid co-medication: results of a retrospective study. Ther Drug Monit 1999;21:175–181.

67. Baulac M, Cramer JA, Mattson RH. Phenobarbital and other barbiturates: Adverse effects. In: Levy RH, Mattson RH, Meldrum BS, et al, eds. Antiepileptic Drugs, 5th ed. Philadelphia, Lippincott Williams & Wilkins, 2002, 528–540.

68. Tozer TN, Winter ME. Phenytoin. In: Evans WE, Schentag JJ, Jusko WJ, eds. Applied Pharmacokinetics, 3d ed. Spokane, WA, Applied Therapeutics 1992:25-1–25.44.

69. Anderson GD, Pak C, Doane KW, et al. Revised Winter-Tozer equation for normalized phenytoin concentrations in trauma and elderly patients with hypoalbuminemia. Ann Pharmacother 1997;31:279–284.

70. Bruni J. Phenytoin and other hydantoins: Adverse effects. In: Levy RH, Mattson RH, Meldrum BS, et al, (eds). Antiepileptic Drugs, 5th ed. Philadelphia, Lippincott Williams & Wilkins, 2002:605–610.

71. Privitera MD. Clinical rules for phenytoin dosing. Ann Pharmacother 1993;27:1169–1173.

72. Schachter SC. Tiagabine: Current status and potential clinical applications. Exp Opin Invest Drugs 1996;5:1377–1387.

73. Leppik IE. Tiagabine: The safety landscape. Epilepsia 1995;36:S10–13.

74. Walker MC, Sander JW. Topiramate: A new antiepileptic drug for refractory epilepsy. Seizure 1996;5:199–203.

75. Gidal BE, Lensmeyer GL. Therapeutic drug monitoring of topiramate: Evaluation of the saturable distribution between erythrocytes and plasma in whole blood using an optimized HPLC Method. Ther Drug Monit 1999;21:567–576.

76. Langtry HD, Gillis JC, Davis R. Topiramate: A review of its pharmacodynamic and pharmacokinetic properties and clinical efficacy in the management of epilepsy. Drugs 1997;54:752–773.

77. Shorvon SD. Safety of topiramate: adverse events and relationship to dosing. Epilepsia 1996;37(suppl 2):S18–22.

78. Gidal BE. Topiramate: Drug interactions. In: Levy RH, Mattson RH, Meldrum BS, et al, eds. Antiepileptic Drugs, 5th ed. Philadelphia, Lippincott Williams & Wilkins, 2002:735–739.

79. Faught E, Wilder BJ, Ramsay RE, et al. Topiramate placebo-controlled dose-ranging trial in refractory partial epilepsy using 200-, 400-, and 600-mg daily dosages. Neurology 1996;46:1684–1690.

80. Privitera M, Fincham R, Penry J, et al. Topiramate placebo-controlled dose-ranging trial in refractory partial epilepsy using 600-, 800-, and 1,000-mg daily dosages. Neurology 1996;46:1678–1683.

81. Davis R, Peters DH, McTavish D. Valproic acid: A reappraisal of its pharmacological properties and clinical efficacy in epilepsy. Drugs 1994;47:332–372.

82. Gidal BE, Anderson GD, Spencer NW, et al. Valproate-associated weight gain in patients with epilepsy: potential relationship to energy expenditure and metabolism. J Epilepsy 1996;9:234–241.

83. Genton P, Gelissse P. Valproic acid: Adverse effects. In: Levy RH, Mattson RH, Meldrum BS, et al, Antiepileptic Drugs, 5th ed. Philadelphia, Lippincott Williams & Wilkins, 2002:837–851.

84. Gidal BE, Inglese CM, Meyer JM, et al. Diet and valproate mediated transient hyperammonemia: Effect of l-carnitine supplementation in children with epilepsy. Pediatr Neurol 1997;16:301–305.

85. Scheyer RD. Valproic acid: Drug interactions. In: Levy RH, Mattson RH, Meldrum BS, et al, eds. Antiepileptic Drugs, 5th ed. Philadelphia, Lippincott Williams & Wilkins, 2002:801–807.

86. Macdonald RL. Zonisamide: Mechanisms of action. In: Levy RH, Mattson RH, Meldrum BS, et al, eds. Antiepileptic Drugs, 5th ed. Philadelphia, Lippincott Williams & Wilkins, 2002:867–872.

87. Shah J, Shellenberger K, Canafax DM. Zonisamide: Chemistry, biotransformation, and pharmacokinetics. In Levy RH, Mattson RH, Meldrum BS, et al, ed. Antiepileptic Drugs, 5th ed. Philadelphia, Lippincott Williams & Wilkins, 2002:873–879.

88. Lee BI. Zonisamide: Adverse effects. In: Levy RH, Mattson RH, Meldrum BS, et al. (ed)., Antiepileptic Drugs. Philadelphia, Lippincott Williams & Wilkins, 2002; 892–898.

89. Mather GG, Shah J. Zonisamide: Drug interactions. In: Levy RH, Mattson RH, Meldrum BS, et al, eds: Antiepileptic Drugs, 5th ed. Philadelphia: Lippincott Williams & Wilkins, 2002:880–884.

90. Pashko S, McCord A, Sena MM. The cost of epilepsy and seizures in a cohort of Pennsylvania Medicaid patients. Med Interface 1993 (November):84.

91. Begley CE, Annegers JF, Lairson DR, et al. Cost of epilepsy in the United States: A model based on incidence and prognosis. Epilepsia 1994; 35:1230–1243.

92. Hughes D, Cockerell OC. A cost minimization study comparing vigabatrin, lamotrigine, and gabapentin for the treatment of intractable partial epilepsy. Seizure 1996;5:89–95.

93. Gilliam F, Kuzniecky R, Faught E, et al. Patient-validated content of epilepsy-specific quality-of-life measurement. Epilepsia 1997;38:233–236.

94. Jacoby A. Assessing quality of life in patients with epilepsy. Pharmaoeconomics 1996;9:399–416.

95. Crawford P, Hall WW, Chappell B, et al. Generic prescribing for epilepsy: Is it safe? Seizure 1996;5:1–5.

55

STATUS EPILEPTICUS

Stephanie J. Phelps, Collin A. Hovinga, and Bradley A. Boucher

Learning Objectives and other resources can be found at *www.pharmacotherapyonline.com.*

KEY CONCEPTS

◀1 Status epilepticus (SE) is a neurologic emergency that may be associated with significant morbidity (i.e., brain damage) and mortality.

◀2 Generalized convulsive status epilepticus (GCSE) is defined as any recurrent or continuous seizure activity lasting longer than 30 minutes in which the patient does not regain baseline mental status. Any tonic-clonic seizure that does not stop automatically within 10 minutes should be treated.

◀3 There are two types of status epilepticus, generalized convulsive status epilepticus (GCSE) and nonconvulsive status epilepticus (NCSE). GCSE is the most common type.

◀4 Most GCSE develops in patients with no history of epilepsy; however, a patient with preexisting epilepsy may experience GCSE as a result of acute anticonvulsant withdrawal, metabolic disorder or concurrent illness, or progression of neurologic disease.

◀5 Although the pathophysiology of GCSE is unknown, experimental models have shown that there is a dramatic decrease in γ-aminobutyric acid (GABA)–mediated inhibitory synaptic transmission and that glutamatergic excitatory synaptic transmission sustains the seizures.

◀6 General treatment includes patient stabilization, adequate oxygenation, preservation of cardiorespiratory function, management of systemic complications, and aggressive assessment of underlying causes.

◀7 The main purpose of treatment is to prevent or decrease cerebral damage by terminating all clinical and electrical seizure activity as soon as possible. The risk of damage is increased after 1 to 2 hours of continuous seizures.

◀8 Lorazepam is the preferred benzodiazepine in treatment of GCSE because of its long duration of action.

◀9 Currently, the hydantoins (phenytoin and fosphenytoin) are the long-acting anticonvulsants used most frequently. Either phenytoin or fosphenytoin should be given concurrently with benzodiazepines.

◀10 The maximum rate of infusion for phenytoin and fosphenytoin in adults is 50 mg/min and 150 mg PE/min, respectively.

◀11 If GCSE is not controlled by a benzodiazepine, hydantoin, or phenobarbital, the GCSE is considered to be refractory, and other therapies should be considered.

◀1 Status epilepticus (SE) is a common neurologic emergency that may be associated with brain damage and death. Although there ◀2 is no consensus on its definition, the International Classification of Epileptic Seizures defines SE as (1) any seizure lasting longer than 30 minutes whether or not consciousness is impaired or (2) recurrent seizures without an intervening period of consciousness between ◀3 seizures.[1] SE can present in several forms (Table 55–1), including nonconvulsive status epilepticus (NCSE) and generalized convulsive status epilepticus (GCSE).[1]

Absence, atypical absence, myoclonic, and complex partial NCSE occurs in about 25% of those with SE. It is characterized by a fluctuating or continuous "twilight" state that produces altered consciousness and/or behavior (e.g., lethargy, decreased mental function). An altered electroencephalogram (EEG) is the most important diagnostic and management tool.[2] In most instances, benzodiazepine and/or valproate remain the drugs of choice for absence and complex partial NCSE.[2] Although intravenous (IV) phenytoin/fosphenytoin or phenobarbital may be tried in patients who are refractory to the preceding therapies, general anesthesia or barbiturate coma is not appropriate.[2] The reader is referred to several reviews

for a more comprehensive discussion of NCSE and its pharmacologic management.[2,3]

◀3 GCSE is the most common and severe form of status epilepticus and is characterized by repeated primary or secondary generalized seizures that involve both hemispheres of the brain and are associated with a persistent postictal state. This chapter will focus on the epidemiology, pathophysiology, presentation, and management of GCSE.

EPIDEMIOLOGY

It is difficult to determine the incidence of GCSE because most studies fail to consider the patient's age, seizure etiology, and type or duration of the seizure. The global incidence of GCSE is thought to range between 1.2 and 5 million cases per year, with an annual incidence of about 100,000 to 152,000 cases each year in the United States.[4] GCSE has no predilection for gender or socioeconomic status but does occur more frequently in nonwhites across all ages.[5] Most episodes of GCSE occur in individuals without a previous history of epilepsy, and

TABLE 55–1. International Classification of Status Epilepticus

Convulsive		Nonconvulsive	
International	*Traditional Terminology*	*International*	*Traditional Terminology*

Primary generalized SE
• Tonic-clonic[a,b]
• Tonic[a,c]
• Clonic[c]
• Myoclonic[b]
• Erratic[d]
Secondary generalized SE[a,b]
• Tonic
• Partial seizures with secondary
  generalization
	Grand mal, epilepticus convulsivus	Absence[c]	Petit mal, spike-and-wave stupor,
			  spike-and-slow-wave or 3/s spike-and-wave,
			  epileptic fugue, epilepsia minora continua,
			  epileptic twilight, minor SE

		Partial SE[a,b]	Focal motor, focal sensory, epilepsia partialis continuans, adversive SE

		Simple partial
		  Somatomotor
		  Dysphasic
		  Other types
			Elementary

		Complex partial	Temporal lobe, psychomotor, epileptic
			  fugue state, prolonged epileptic stupor, prolonged
			  epileptic confusional state, continuous epileptic
			  twilight state

[a]Most common in older children.
[b]Most common in adolescents and adults.
[c]Most common in infants and young children.
[d]Most common in neonates.

about 5% of adults and 10% to 25% of children with known epilepsy will have an episode of GCSE.[3]

ETIOLOGY

Precipitating events for GCSE vary among studies and generally reflect different populations and referral patterns. Most episodes that occur in known epileptics occur because of acute anticonvulsant withdrawal, a metabolic disorder or concurrent illness, or progression of a preexisting neurologic disease. Common etiologies and mortality rates for pediatric and adult populations are shown in Table 55–2.[5,6]

Precipitating events for GCSE are divided into type I and type II etiologies. Type I etiologies are not associated with new structural lesions but do include patients with a history of epilepsy. Elevated serum anticonvulsant concentrations or their acute withdrawal may precipitate GCSE. A number of prescription, over-the-counter (OTC), and recreational medications should be considered in any patient with new-onset GCSE. Type II etiologies are associated with structural lesions and have a poor prognosis.

There are major differences in etiologies for pediatric and adult patients (see Table 55–2). During their first few weeks of life, infants who are born to addicted mothers may develop drug withdrawal seizures. Another subset of the neonatal population may develop GCSE owing to a pyridoxine deficiency. The EEG should normalize within hours following treatment with intravenous pyridoxine (100 mg). Acute encephalopathy and metabolic disorders (inborn errors of metabolism) are the major causes of GCSE in patients younger than 1 year of age. In young children, the cause is frequently idiopathic but may be associated with such symptoms as fever and/or a viral illness. Unless accompanied by an underlying neurologic abnormality, fever-induced GCSE is less likey to be associated with sequelae.

The most frequent precipitating events in adults are cerebrovascular disease, withdrawal of anticonvulsants, and low anticonvulsant serum concentrations. Interestingly, infection is not a major cause of GCSE in adults; however, there have been increasing reports of association with human immunodeficiency virus infection. Cerebrovascular disease is the leading cause of GCSE in those who have their first seizures after age 60.

TABLE 55–2. Etiology and Mortality for Pediatric and Adult Cases of Status Epilepticus

Etiology	Pediatric ($n = 200$) % SE cases (% mortality)	Adult ($n = 512$) % SE cases (% mortality)
Type I (no structural lesion)		
Infection	55 (5)	6 (35)
CNS infection	11 (0)	2 (20)
Metabolic	20 (5)	12 (36)
Low AED levels	16 (0)	24 (7)
Alcohol	0 (0)	13 (8)
Idiopathic	6 (0)	13 (18)
Type II (structural lesion)		
Anoxia/hypoxia	27 (13)	14 (65)
CNS tumor	3 (50)	5 (22)
CVA	5 (0)	26 (27)
Drug overdose	5 (0)	3 (23)
Hemorrhage	5 (11)	4 (35)
Trauma	13 (0)	3 (23)
Remote causes[a]	33 (5)	7 (13)

Percentages do not add up to 100% because some patients had multiple etiologies. (AED = antiepileptic drug; CVA = cerebrovascular accident)
[a]More than half of remote causes were congenital malformations and CVA in pediatric and adult patients, respectively.
Data modified from Refs. 5 and 6.

MORBIDITY

◀ No one would dispute that GCSE is harmful to the brain and is associated with morbidity. However, whether the morbidity occurs from the underlying etiology or as a result of the GCSE itself remains to be determined. Most would contend that it is the GCSE that is responsible for the morbidity. GCSE neuronal damage in animal models is evident following 30 to 60 minutes regardless of the inducing stimulus, and most animals progress to the development of epilepsy following a prolonged seizure. Interestingly, inhibiting the neuronal damage associated with seizures does not prevent the development of epilepsy in these animals, suggesting that the seizures themselves may be harmful. It is difficult to establish a relationship between long-term outcomes in humans with GCSE. This is largely because it is difficult to weigh the effects of seizure type, etiology, duration, concurrent physiologic events, and therapy or lack thereof. However, it has been shown that humans with a history of prolonged febrile seizures who later developed epilepsy share similar histopathologic changes (i.e., hippocampal sclerosis) as those found in animal models of GCSE.[7,8] In these cases the period between the initial prolonged seizure and the first epileptic seizure can take months to decades. This suggests that there may be a link between GCSE and the later development of epilepsy. Importantly, both animal and human studies of GCSE show that the currently available anticonvulsants do not prevent the development of epilepsy following prolonged seizures.[8,9]

Patients who develop epilepsy following prolonged GCSE are less likely to experience remission of their seizures and may have decreased cognitive and memory function, mental retardation, or neurologic deficits.[10] Most studies have found that younger children and those with preexisting epilepsy have a higher propensity for sequelae.

MORTALITY

The estimated mortality rate in the United States following GCSE ranges between 22,000 and 42,000 individuals per year.[6] Recent estimates suggest a mortality rate of up to 10% in children,[11] 20% in adults,[4] and 38% in the elderly.[5] When compared with other populations, neonates with seizures have a higher mortality and more neurologic sequelae (e.g., mental retardation, cerebral palsy, and epilepsy).

Table 55–2 summarizes the etiology for GCSE and their corresponding mortality rates.[5,6] Interestingly, the mortality associated with many etiologies is significantly greater in adults than in children. Unresponsive patients may die from GCSE, but more frequently they die as a result of the acute illness that precipitated the GCSE. For example, patients with serious central nervous system structural changes (e.g., hemorrhage, stroke) have a poor prognosis, whereas the majority (i.e., 80–90%) of patients with no structural lesion generally respond to intravenous phenytoin.

Two variables that affect outcome are the time between onset of GCSE and the initiation of treatment and the duration of the seizure. GCSE lasting longer than 60 minutes has a higher mortality (32%) than seizures lasting less than 60 minutes (2.5%).[6] Although one might expect better outcomes for patients managed in major medical centers, there is no difference in mortality between community hospitals and medical centers.[6] Fortunately, the likelihood of death has decreased over the past decade and probably reflects a change in the definition of GCSE (60 to 30 minutes), recognition of the need to initiate presequenced therapy immediately, and a greater understanding of the pathogenesis of GCSE.

PATHOGENESIS

Brain homeostasis is preserved by a local neuronal network's ability to terminate excessive excitatory impulses before they spread to other networks. Seizures occur when the excitatory neurotransmission overcomes inhibitory impulses in one or more brain regions (i.e., neural networks). Most seizures are brief (≤5 minutes) largely because of the brain's inhibitory mechanisms that restore the balance of normal neurotransmission.[12] Currently, there is little known about why the mechanisms that control normal brain homeostasis fail. However, when repeated seizures occur in close succession or the magnitude of the proconvulsant (i.e., seizure-inducing) stimulus is severe enough, compensatory mechanisms can be overwhelmed and lead to GCSE.

◀ Although the exact cellular mechanisms responsible for the production of abnormal neural impulses are unknown, it appears that seizure *initiation* is caused by an imbalance between excitatory (e.g., glutamate, calcium, sodium, substance P, and neurokinin B) and inhibitory neurotransmission (e.g., γ-aminobutyric acid [GABA], adenosine, potassium, neuropeptide Y [NPY], opioid peptides, and galanin).[12] Seizure *maintenance* associated with GCSE is largely due to the excitatory neurotransmitter glutamate acting on postsynaptic N-methyl-d-aspartate (NMDA) and α-amino-3-hydroxy-5-methyl-4 isoxazolepropionate (AMPA)/kainate receptors. Most of what is known about GCSE has focused on ion channels (receptor-gated or voltage-dependent), with less known about receptor–second messenger systems (e.g., metabotropic glutamate receptors).[12]

◀ During GCSE, glutamate activation of the NMDA and AMPA receptors causes opening of the gated calcium and sodium channels, respectively. Entry of the respective ions causes neuronal depolarization. Sustained depolarization not only may maintain GCSE but also may eventually cause neuronal death through calcium-, free radical–, and kinase-mediated events.[8] Although drugs acting as NMDA and AMPA receptor antagonists seem to be attractive options for the treatment of GCSE, it is likely that glutamate is not the sole mechanism for GCSE and that other mechanisms become increasingly important as the duration of seizures increases.

◀ $GABA_A$ receptors are postsynaptic receptors that control chloride channels to produce hyperpolarization (inhibition) of the postsynaptic cell membrane. These receptors have binding sites for GABA, as well as for select anticonvulsants (e.g., the GABA agonists phenobarbital and benzodiazepines) and enhance $GABA_A$-mediated chloride inhibitory currents. It was once believed that there was a decrease in presynaptic GABA release that led to prolonged seizures during GCSE. Current data, however, suggest that GABA concentrations increase during the early phases of GCSE and continue to be elevated during late GCSE. Prolonged seizures lead to decreased inhibitory $GABA_A$ receptor density because of postsynaptic receptor endocytosis, and $GABA_A$ receptors may be modified during SE such that there is decreased response to both endogenous GABA and GABA agonists.[13] Clinically, this can have a dramatic influence on response to both benzodiazepines and phenobarbital in that their relative potencies can be reduced up to tenfold if seizures persist for 30 minutes or longer.[13] A similar phenomenon occurs with sodium channel antagonists (phenytoin); however, the magnitude of resistance is believed to be less.[12]

PATHOPHYSIOLOGY

As GCSE continues, there are systemic alterations, progression of motor phenomena, and development of specific EEG findings.[14] Two distinct and predictable phases have been identified. Phase I occurs during the first 30 minutes of seizure activity, and phase II begins 60 minutes later. Although the presence of systemic complications affects the prognosis of GCSE, one must remember that prolonged seizures may destroy neurons independent of these systemic events.[8] In fact, the systemic effects of experimentally induced seizures in animals can be blocked, but the damage to the neocortex, cerebellum, and hippocampus persists.

During phase I, each seizure produces marked increases in plasma epinephrine, norepinephrine, and steroid concentrations that may cause hypertension, tachycardia, and cardiac arrhythmias.[14] Within minutes, arterial systolic pressures may rise to values above 200 mm Hg, and heart rate may increase by 83 beats per minute. Although blood pressure returns to normal within 60 minutes, mean arterial pressure does not fall below 60 mm Hg; hence cerebral perfusion pressure is not compromised. In animals, cerebral blood flow is also increased by 200% to 600%, thereby protecting neurons from hypoxic injury.

Seizure-induced increases in sympathetic and parasympathetic stimulation of the heart, in the presence of a hypoxic myocardium, may result in ventricular arrhythmias. Autonomic neuron stimulation also can cause a release of insulin and glucagon. Concurrently, circulating catecholamines cause an elevation of hepatic cyclic adenosine monophosphate, producing glycogenolysis. Although the patient may be hyperglycemic initially, serum glucose concentration begins to fall.

Seizure-induced muscular contractions and hypoxia cause lactic acid release that can produce a severe acidosis that may be accompanied by hypotension and shock. Muscle contractions can be so severe that rhabdomyolysis with secondary hyperkalemia and acute tubular necrosis may occur. The airway may be obstructed, and the patient may become cyanotic or hypoxic at any time. Additionally, an increase in salivation and tracheal and pulmonary secretions may result in aspiration pneumonia. Although transient pleocytosis (i.e., white blood cell counts up to 20,000/mm^3) may develop, it should not be attributed to GCSE until infectious causes have been eliminated.

Between seizures, the EEG slows, and blood pressure normalizes. Although metabolic demands are increased, the brain is able to compensate for these increased demands adequately. If seizure activity exceeds 60 minutes (phase II), the EEG ictal discharge and clonic motor activity become continuous, and the patient begins to decompensate. Despite elevated levels of catecholamines, blood pressure is no longer increased, and the patient may become hypotensive. During the late phase, autoregulation of cerebral blood flow becomes dependent on mean arterial pressure and begins to fail. There continues to be an excessive consumption of oxygen and glucose; however, compensatory mechanisms are no longer able to keep up with demands.

During phase II, the serum glucose concentration may be normal or decreased. Profound hypoglycemia, secondary to hyperinsulinemia, can occur in patients with hepatic dysfunction or in those with reduced glycogen stores (e.g., elderly, neonates). Hyperthermia and respiratory deterioration with hypoxia and ventilatory failure may develop. There also may be metabolic and biochemical complications, including respiratory and metabolic acidosis, hyperkalemia, hyponatremia, and azotemia. There is increased sweating and salivation. Marked elevations in plasma prolactin, glucagon, growth hormone, and adrenocorticotropic hormone concentrations also have been identified. Importantly, during prolonged seizures, motor activity may cease, but electrical seizures may persist. This fact has important clinical ramifications, in that a patient's seizures may appear to have

been terminated without treatment or when an ineffective therapy is given.

CLINICAL PRESENTATION AND DIAGNOSIS

Accurate diagnosis requires observation, physical examination, laboratory assessment, EEG, and neurologic imaging. A careful history of the nature and duration of the seizure should be obtained, and a diagnosis of GCSE should not be made until a clinician has observed at least one seizure in a patient with a history of repeated seizures and impaired consciousness. Most patients have an altered consciousness that ranges from obtunded to marked lethargy and somnolence with pronounced eyes-open unresponsiveness and waxy rigidity. Motor features may include muscle contractions, extensor or flexor posturing, and spasms. Over time, the clinical manifestations become less apparent, and the diagnosis requires careful assessment.

In addition to an assessment of language and cognitive abilities, the physical examination also should assess motor, sensory, and reflex abnormalities and pupillary response, asymmetry, and posturing on neurologic examination. Because generalized seizures may cause physical injury, the patient should be examined for secondary injuries (e.g., tongue lacerations, shoulder dislocations, head trauma, and facial trauma).

Laboratory tests are essential to the diagnosis of various etiologies. Hypoglycemia, hyponatremia, hypernatremia, hypomagnesemia, hypocalcemia, and renal failure all can cause seizures. A urine drug screen may help to rule out the possibility of illicit drug use or drug overdose. Serum drug concentration determination(s) in those on chronic anticonvulsants should be obtained because high concentrations of certain medications can induce seizures, and low or nondetectable concentrations may reflect noncompliance or rapid drug withdrawal. A baseline serum concentration is necessary to determine whether a loading dose of a specific anticonvulsant may or may not be required. Assessment of other laboratory parameters (e.g., albumin, renal function, and hepatic function) that affect anticonvulsant dosing also may be useful. An EEG is a valuable diagnostic tool, but treatment should not be delayed while awaiting testing or results.

A second phase in diagnosis occurs after the seizures have stopped and the patient is stabilized. It is important to determine if the patient is febrile or has a systemic or central nervous system (CNS) infection. Many physiologic consequences of GCSE (e.g., leukocytosis, pleocytosis, and hyperthermia) produce symptoms that may be confused with other conditions. If a CNS infection is suspected, empirical antibiotics should be started, and a spinal tap should be performed. In order to rule out vascular, neoplastic, or infectious etiologies, computed tomography (CT) or magnetic resonance imaging (MRI) should be obtained.

CLINICAL PRESENTATION OF GCSE

GENERAL

Status epilepticus (SE) is a medical emergency that may be associated with significant morbidity and mortality.

SYMPTOMS

- Impaired consciousness (e.g., lethargy to coma)
- Disorientation once GCSE is controlled
- Pain associated with injuries (e.g., tongue lacerations, shoulder dislocations, head trauma, facial trauma)

EARLY SIGNS

- Acute injuries or CNS insults that cause extensor or flexor posturing
- Fever or intercurrent illnesses (signs of sepsis or meningitis)
- Evidence of head or other CNS injury (bradycardia, tachypnea, and hypertension; poor pupillary response; asymmetry on neurologic examination; abnormal posturing
- Generalized convulsions
- Hypothermia or fever suggestive of intercurrent illnesses
- Incontinence
- Muscle contractions, spasms
- Normal blood pressure or hypotension
- Respiratory compromise

LATE SIGNS

- Pulmonary edema with respiratory failure
- Cardiac failure (dysrhythmias, arrest, cardiogenic shock)
- Hyoptension/hypertension
- Disseminated intravascular coagulation, multi-organ failure

- Rhabdomyolysis
- Hyperpyremia

INITIAL LABORATORY TESTS

- Complete blood count (CBC) with differential
- Serum chemistry profile (e.g., electrolytes, calcium, magnesium, glucose, serum creatinine, ALT, AST)
- Urine drug/alcohol screen
- Blood cultures
- Arterial blood gas to assess for metabolic and respiratory acidosis
- Serum drug concentration if previous anticonvulsant suspected or known

OTHER DIAGNOSTIC TESTS

- Lumbar puncture if CNS infection suspected
- EEG—should be obtained on presentation and once clinical seizures are controlled
- CT with and without contrast (to assess for bleeding, infection, arteriovenous malformations, neoplasm)
- MRI later
- X-ray if indicated to diagnose fractures
- ECG, especially if ingestion confirmed

ALT, alanine aminotransferase; AST, aspartate aminotransferase; CBC, complete blood count; CNS, central nervous system; CT, computed tomography; ECG, electrocardiogram; EEG, electroencephalograph; GCSE, generalized convulsive status epilepticus; MRI, magnetic resonance imaging; SE, status epilepticus

▶ TREATMENT: Generalized Convulsive Status Epilepticus

◼ NONPHARMACOLOGIC

Concurrent with initiation of anticonvulsants, vital signs should be assessed, an adequate and protected airway should be established, ventilation should be maintained, and oxygen should be administered. Patients who seize for prolonged periods will require intubation and mechanical ventilation. Arterial blood gas determinations should be done frequently to assess for metabolic and/or respiratory acidosis. Metabolic acidosis resolves quickly following termination of GCSE; however, sodium bicarbonate should be given if the pH is less than 7.2. If the patient has respiratory acidosis, assisted ventilation should correct the imbalance.

Patients who continue to have altered consciousness after clinical control of their seizures should have an EEG performed. Some patients, including those who have been given neuromuscular blockers for airway management, may not have clinical motor manifestations but may continue to have electrical SE. An EEG is essential to detect and diagnose electrical GCSE. Although hypoglycemia is a rare cause of GCSE, all patients should receive glucose. Because Wernicke's encephalopathy can develop in alcoholics, adults should receive thiamine (100 mg) prior to glucose.[11] Initially, adults should be given 50 mL of a 50% dextrose solution, and children should be given 1 mL/kg of a 25% dextrose solution.[11] Serum glucose

concentration should be determined to assess the need for further glucose supplementation.

◼ PHARMACOLOGIC

Although a diagnosis of GCSE technically cannot be made until seizures have persisted for longer than 30 minutes, therapy should not be withheld during this time. When a tonic-clonic seizure does not stop automatically, or when doubt exists regarding the diagnosis, patients should be treated as if they have GCSE. An algorithm of the choice of anticonvulsants, timing, and dosing for the treatment of GCSE in hospitalized patients is provided in the Fig. 55–1.

It is imperative that a clear, presequenced management plan be initiated rapidly. To ensure that this occurs, many institutions have developed and used a seizure protocol. There are four immediate goals in the management of GCSE: (1) patient stabilization, including adequate oxygenation, preservation of cardiorespiratory function, and management of systemic complications, (2) accurate diagnosis of the subtype of GCSE and identification of precipitating factors, (3) termination of clinical and electrical seizures as early as possible, and (4) prevention of seizure recurrence.

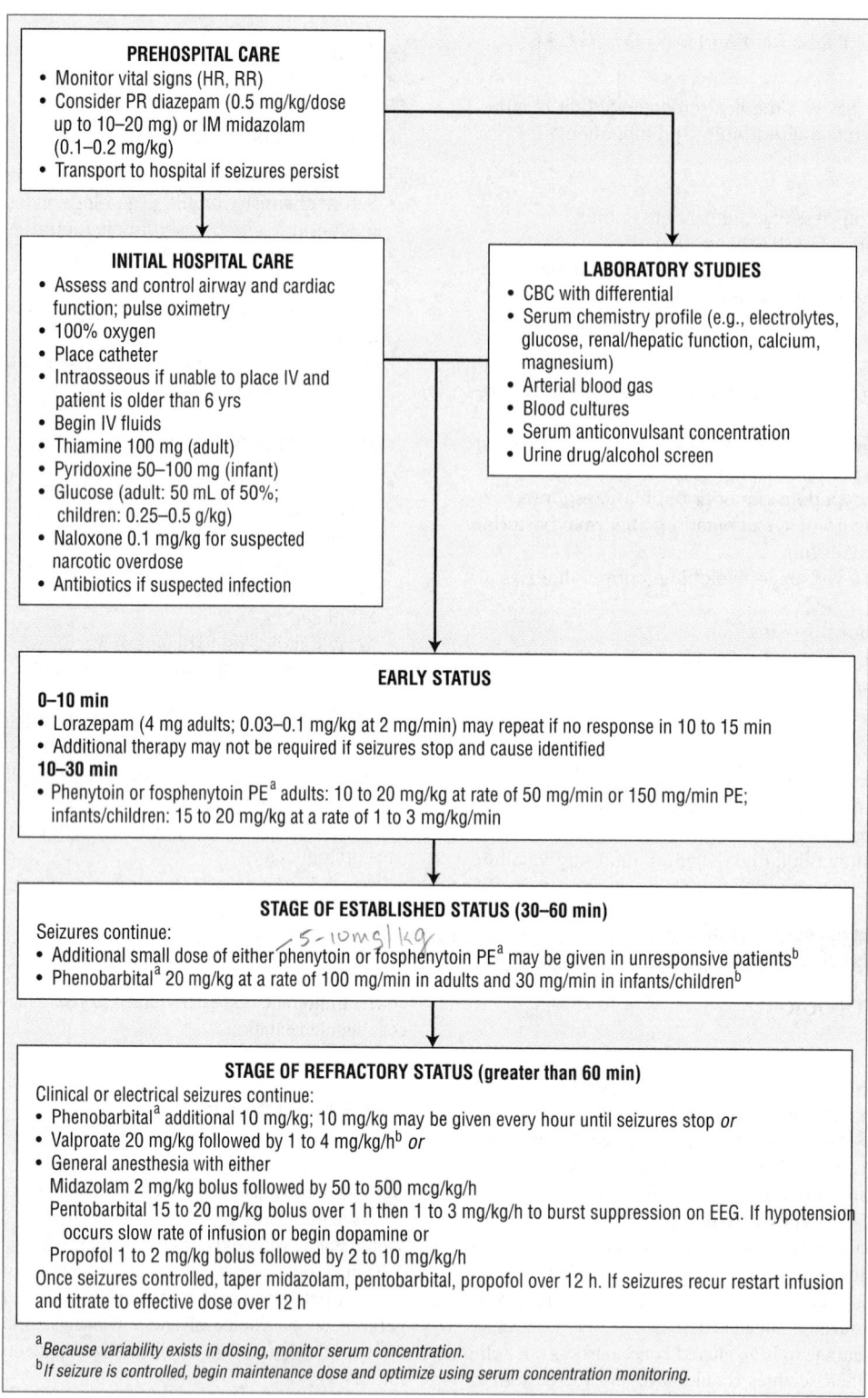

PREHOSPITAL CARE
- Monitor vital signs (HR, RR)
- Consider PR diazepam (0.5 mg/kg/dose up to 10–20 mg) or IM midazolam (0.1–0.2 mg/kg)
- Transport to hospital if seizures persist

INITIAL HOSPITAL CARE
- Assess and control airway and cardiac function; pulse oximetry
- 100% oxygen
- Place catheter
- Intraosseous if unable to place IV and patient is older than 6 yrs
- Begin IV fluids
- Thiamine 100 mg (adult)
- Pyridoxine 50–100 mg (infant)
- Glucose (adult: 50 mL of 50%; children: 0.25–0.5 g/kg)
- Naloxone 0.1 mg/kg for suspected narcotic overdose
- Antibiotics if suspected infection

LABORATORY STUDIES
- CBC with differential
- Serum chemistry profile (e.g., electrolytes, glucose, renal/hepatic function, calcium, magnesium)
- Arterial blood gas
- Blood cultures
- Serum anticonvulsant concentration
- Urine drug/alcohol screen

EARLY STATUS
0–10 min
- Lorazepam (4 mg adults; 0.03–0.1 mg/kg at 2 mg/min) may repeat if no response in 10 to 15 min
- Additional therapy may not be required if seizures stop and cause identified
10–30 min
- Phenytoin or fosphenytoin PE[a] adults: 10 to 20 mg/kg at rate of 50 mg/min or 150 mg/min PE; infants/children: 15 to 20 mg/kg at a rate of 1 to 3 mg/kg/min

STAGE OF ESTABLISHED STATUS (30–60 min)
Seizures continue:
- Additional small dose of either phenytoin or fosphenytoin PE[a] may be given in unresponsive patients[b]   *~5–10 mg/kg*
- Phenobarbital[a] 20 mg/kg at a rate of 100 mg/min in adults and 30 mg/min in infants/children[b]

STAGE OF REFRACTORY STATUS (greater than 60 min)
Clinical or electrical seizures continue:
- Phenobarbital[a] additional 10 mg/kg; 10 mg/kg may be given every hour until seizures stop *or*
- Valproate 20 mg/kg followed by 1 to 4 mg/kg/h[b] *or*
- General anesthesia with either
  Midazolam 2 mg/kg bolus followed by 50 to 500 mcg/kg/h
  Pentobarbital 15 to 20 mg/kg bolus over 1 h then 1 to 3 mg/kg/h to burst suppression on EEG. If hypotension occurs slow rate of infusion or begin dopamine or
  Propofol 1 to 2 mg/kg bolus followed by 2 to 10 mg/kg/h
Once seizures controlled, taper midazolam, pentobarbital, propofol over 12 h. If seizures recur restart infusion and titrate to effective dose over 12 h

[a] *Because variability exists in dosing, monitor serum concentration.*
[b] *If seizure is controlled, begin maintenance dose and optimize using serum concentration monitoring.*

FIGURE 55–1. Algorithm for the treatment of GCSE in hospitalized patients.

The three most commonly used classes of anticonvulsants for the initial treatment of GCSE are the benzodiazepines, hydantoins, and barbiturates. Five prospective, randomized studies have compared these therapies for the treatment of GCSE.[15–19] The first two studies were a blinded comparison of lorazepam versus diazepam in adults[15] and children.[17] The third study was a randomized comparison of phenobarbital with phenytoin plus diazepam.[18] The fourth study compared lorazepam with phenytoin.[17] The fifth study was a multicenter, prospective, randomized, double-blind comparison of phenytoin and diazepam and phenytoin, lorazepam, or phenobarbital.[19] There is no consensus regarding the anticonvulsant of choice, sequencing of therapy, or treatment of refractory GCSE.

BENZODIAZEPINES

The benzodiazepines are effective initial therapy in most patients with GCSE and should be administered as soon as possible. Generally, one or two intravenous doses will stop seizures within 2 to 3 minutes.[4] Diazepam, lorazepam, and midazolam are the only benzodiazepines available in the United States in a parenteral formulation. Because these are equally effective in GCSE, the preferred benzodiazepine is determined by differences in the pharmacokinetic and pharmacoeconomic profiles of the available agents.

Diazepam is an extremely lipophilic moiety with a large volume of distribution (1 to 2 L/kg).[11] Although its initial distribution phase into the brain occurs within seconds, it rapidly redistributes into fat, causing its half-life in the brain to be less than 1 hour and its duration of effect to be less than 30 minutes.[11] If diazepam is the sole anticonvulsant, the rapid fall in brain concentration may cause seizure recurrence; hence a longer-acting anticonvulsant (e.g., phenytoin or phenobarbital) should be given immediately after diazepam. The initial dose of diazepam (Table 55–3) may be repeated if the patient does not respond within 5 minutes.[11] The maximum total dosage is 5 mg in children younger than 5 years of age, 10 mg in children 5 years of age or older, and 40 mg in adults. Although certain serum concentrations have been associated with seizure control, assays for the benzodiazepines are not readily available; hence therapeutic drug monitoring is impractical.

Although lorazepam is not approved by the Food and Drug Administration (FDA) for GCSE, it is currently considered the benzodiazepine of choice.[11] Lorazepam is less lipid soluble than diazepam and takes longer to achieve peak concentrations in the brain; however, it has minimal redistribution that results in a longer duration of action (>12 to 24 hours).[11] It also has a higher-affinity binding to the benzodiazepine receptor than diazepam.[11] For these reasons, significantly fewer patients treated with lorazepam require additional anticonvulsants for seizure termination.

The initial dose of lorazepam can be found in Table 55–3. Data suggest that a single dose produces adequate serum concentrations and provides seizure protection for 24 hours. A second dose may be given after 5 minutes, and if necessary, a third and final dose may be given after another 5 minutes.[11] It is important to remember that patients chronically on a benzodiazepine (e.g., clonazepam) may have developed tolerance and could require large doses before response.

Both diazepam and lorazepam cause vein irritation and should be diluted with an equal volume of compatible diluent before administration. The intravenous forms of both diazepam and lorazepam contain propylene glycol, which may cause dysrhythmia and hypotension if administered too rapidly.[11] Because of slow and erratic absorption, these agents should not be given intramuscularly. If necessary, both medications may be given rectally.

Midazolam is a water-soluble benzodiazepine that diffuses rapidly into the brain. Unfortunately, it has an extremely short half-life that requires it to be given by continuous infusion. Various routes of administration (e.g., buccal, intranasal, and intramuscular) have been used successfully to terminate seizures rapidly when intravenous access cannot be established. Resulting peak serum concentrations occur within minutes and exceed those required for sedation in adults. Unfortunately, heavy breathing and increased nasal discharge may limit or delay intranasal absorption in a seizing patient. Buccal administration is performed easily by drawing up the desired volume of midazolam injection or syrup, parting the patient's lips, and squirting it into the mouth. The volume of fluid is small enough (e.g., 2 to 5 mL) to be placed in the cavity between the cheek and gum without significant concern for aspiration. Because of its increased solubility, intramuscular midazolam has a more reliable absorption than either diazepam or lorazepam. In fact, some practitioners have recommended that intramuscular midazolam be given by emergency medical technicians as first-line treatment in the out-of-hospital setting.[20] Midazolam has been well tolerated with all the aforementioned routes with minimal changes in blood pressure or respiration.

All benzodiazepines can impair consciousness and interfere with neurologic assessment.[11] Although rare, brief (<1 minute) cardiorespiratory depression may occur and can necessitate assisted ventilation or require intubation. This is especially true if a benzodiazepine is used concomitantly with a barbiturate. Hypotension secondary to a reduction in vasomotor tone may occur following large doses of a benzodiazepine.[4]

PHENYTOIN

Phenytoin is a second-line agent in GCSE that is unresponsive to the benzodiazepines or in seizures that recur after successful treatment with a benzodiazepine.[21] While it is effective in terminating seizures in 40% to 91% of patients,[11] one study reported that phenytoin alone was inferior to lorazepam, phenobarbital, or diazepam plus phenytoin at stopping GCSE within 20 minutes of their infusion.[19] Phenytoin has a relatively long half-life (20 to 36 hours) and causes

TABLE 55–3. Medications Used in the Initial Treatment of GCSE

Anticonvulsant (Route)	Loading Dose (Maximum Dose) Adult	Loading Dose (Maximum Dose) Pediatric	Rate of Infusion Adult	Rate of Infusion Pediatric	Maintenance Dose Adult	Maintenance Dose Pediatric
Diazepam (IV bolus)	0.25 mg/kg[a,b,c] (40 mg)	0.25–0.5 mg/kg[a,c] (0.75 mg/kg)	<5 mg/min	<5 mg/min	Not used	Not used
Fosphenytoin IV	15–20 mg PE/kg	15–20 mg PE/kg	150 mg PE/min	3 mg PE/kg/min	4–5 mg PE/kg/day	5–10 mg PE/kg/day
Lorazepam (IV bolus)	4 mg[a,b,c] (8 mg)	0.1 mg/kg[a,c] (4 mg)	2 mg/min	Over 2–5 min	Not used	Not used
Midazolam IV	200 mcg/kg[a,d]	150 mcg/kg[a,d]	0.5–1 mg/min	2–3 min	50–500 mcg/kg/h[e]	60–120 mcg/kg/h[e]
Phenobarbital IV	10–20 mg/kg[e]	15–20 mg/kg[e]	100 mg/min	30 mg/min	1–4 mg/kg/day[e]	3–5 mg/kg/day[e]
Phenytoin IV	15–20 mg/kg[f]	15–20 mg/kg[f]	50 mg/min	1 mg/kg/min	4–5 mg/kg/day[e]	5–10 mg/kg/day[e]

[a]Doses may be repeated every 10 to 15 min until the maximum dosage is given.
[b]Initial doses in the elderly are 2 to 5 mg.
[c]Larger doses may be required if patients chronically on a benzodiazepine (e.g., clonazepam).
[d]May be given by the intramuscular, rectal, or buccal routes.
[e]Titrate dose as needed.
[f]Administer additional loading dose based on serum concentration.

less respiratory depression and sedation than the benzodiazepines or phenobarbital[11]; however, it cannot be delivered rapidly enough to be considered a first-line single agent.

Injectable phenytoin should be diluted to less than or equal to 5 mg/mL in normal saline. Microcrystals will precipitate if it is mixed in a glucose-containing solution. The vehicle (40% propylene glycol) may cause administration-related hypotension and cardiac arrhythmias. These effects are more likely to occur if large loading doses are given to elderly individuals with preexisting cardiac disease or in critically ill patients with marginal blood pressure.[11] Vital signs and an electrocardiogram (ECG) should be obtained during administration. The infusion rate should be slowed if the QT interval widens or if hypotension or arrhythmias develop.[11] The maximum rate of infusion is 50 mg/min in adults and 1 mg/kg per minute in children weighing less than 50 kg.[11] The rate should not exceed 25 mg/min in the elderly or in those with atherosclerotic cardiovascular disease. The rate should be reduced once seizures have stopped.[11]

Suggested intravenous loading doses of phenytoin are provided in Table 55–3.[11] If the patient has been on phenytoin prior to admission and the phenytoin concentration is known, this should be considered in determining a loading dose. A reduction in the loading dose is recommended for elderly patients,[11] and a larger loading dose is required in obese patients.[22] If seizures continue after the initial loading dose, some advocate an additional 5 mg/kg dose. There is no evidence that a total loading dose above 20 mg/kg will be beneficial in unresponsive GCSE. This practice may cause concentrations to exceed the reference range and produce toxicity. Serum concentrations within the reference range generally do not persist more than 24 hours in patients given a loading dose of less than 18 mg/kg. For this reason, maintenance doses (see Table 55–3) should be started within 12 to 24 hours of the loading dose.

Because phenytoin has poor lipid solubility and enters the brain slowly, it may take up to 60 minutes before the pharmacodynamic effect is apparent. This delay in response is important when considering administration of a second mini-loading dose. For a review of the distribution and elimination pharmacokinetics of phenytoin, see Chap. 54.

Phenytoin has an alkaline pH, which is associated with pain and burning during infusion; phlebitis may occur with chronic infusion, and tissue necrosis is likely on infiltration. Intramuscular administration is not recommended because absorption is delayed and erratic, and phenytoin may crystallize in tissue. Although an orally administered loading dose has been used in patients not actively seizing, it may take 4 to 12 hours before adequate serum concentrations are obtained; therefore, this practice is not recommended.

■ FOSPHENYTOIN

Fosphenytoin is a water-soluble phosphate ester that has no known pharmacologic activity.[21] Because it does not contain propylene glycol, it is compatible with most common intravenous fluids. It should be diluted prior to intravenous administration in 5% dextrose or normal saline to a concentration of 1.5 to 25 mg PE/mL.[21] It is converted rapidly (7 to 15 minutes) and completely (100%) to phenytoin by blood and tissue phosphatases after intravenous and intramuscular dosing.[21] This inherent delay in conversion was a concern initially; however, the conversion delay is offset by high protein binding, saturable binding at high concentrations, and the rapid rate of infusion, which results in unbound concentrations exceeding those seen following phenytoin at an infusion rate of 50 mg/min or less.[21]

Nystagmus, dizziness, and ataxia are the most frequent adverse events with fosphenytoin and are attributed to phenytoin. The frequency of ECG or blood pressure changes is less than that reported for phenytoin. Paresthesia and pruritus are related to dose and infusion rate and occur more frequently with fosphenytoin than with phenytoin. These side effects typically have a distribution to the face and groin areas and subside within 5 to 10 minutes after the infusion.[21] They are not allergic reactions and rarely necessitate discontinuation of fosphenytoin.

In order to minimize dosing errors, fosphenytoin should be dosed using phenytoin equivalents (PE), thereby obviating the need for interconversion between phenytoin and fosphenytoin. The loading dose of fosphenytoin can be found in Table 55–3. Because of delays in achieving adequate phenytoin serum concentrations, a loading dose of fosphenytoin should not be given intramuscularly unless intravenous access is impossible. The rate of administration is 100 to 150 mg PE/min and 1 to 3 mg PE/kg per minute in adult and pediatric patients, respectively.[22] Continuous ECG, blood pressure, and respiratory status monitoring is recommended for all loading doses of fosphenytoin.

Tests for fosphenytoin serum concentration are not available commercially and are of no clinical value. Serum phenytoin concentrations are the end point for therapeutic drug monitoring, and the desired serum concentration range is the same as that when phenytoin is administered (10 to 20 mg/L). Because fosphenytoin cross-reacts with several immunoassays for phenytoin to cause a 1.2- to 6-fold overestimation of phenytoin concentration, blood should not be obtained for at least 2 hours after intravenous and 4 hours after intramuscular administration.[21] In order to minimize in vitro conversion to phenytoin, blood should be collected in tubes containing EDTA, and samples should be refrigerated as soon as possible.[21]

CLINICAL CONTROVERSY

The debate continues as to which hydantoin (i.e., phenytoin or fosphenytoin) is the preferred agent in GCSE. Although phenytoin has been used for decades, it is associated with a variety of problems related to its formulation. Conversely, fosphenytoin is associated with less infusion pain and intravenous-site complications and fewer hemodynamic adverse effects than phenytoin. While most practitioners believe that fosphenytoin is clearly a "better" formulation, many practitioners and administrators struggle with the benefit of fosphenytoin when compared with phenytoin given its cost.

■ PHENOBARBITAL

There are three different opinions regarding the use of phenobarbital in GCSE. The most widely held contention is that because barbiturates cause CNS and respiratory depression, as well as hypotension, phenobarbital should be the third-line agent when a benzodiazepine plus phenytoin has failed.[4] The second opinion suggest that the barbiturates are as safe and effective as other anticonvulsants and should be the drug of choice after the benzodiazepines have been administered. This belief is especially evident in pediatric institutions with large emergency departments. The third emerging opinion is that continuous-infusion midazolam should be the third-line anticonvulsant before the barbiturates.[23]

Two studies have compared the efficacy of phenobarbital with other anticonvulsants in GCSE. The first study compared phenobarbital alone with diazepam plus phenytoin in adult patients with GCSE.[18] Phenobarbital acted more rapidly and was as safe and effective as the

TABLE 55–4. Medications Used to Treat Refractory GCSE

Anticonvulsant (Route)	Loading Dose		Rate of Infusion		Maintenance Dose	
	Adult	*Pediatric*	*Adult*	*Pediatric*	*Adult*	*Pediatric*
Lidocaine	50–100 mg	1 mg/kg (maximum dose = 3–5 mg/kg in first hour)		≤2 min	1.5–3.5 mg/kg/h	1.2–3 mg/kg/h
Midazolam IV	200 mcg/kg[a]	150 mcg/kg[a]	0.5–1 mg/min	2–3 min	50–500 mcg/kg/h[b]	60–120 mcg/kg/h[b]
Pentobarbital (IV)	10–20 mg/kg	15–20 mg/kg	1–2 h	1–2 h	1–5 mg/kg/h[b]	1–5 mg/kg/h[b]
Propofol IV	2 mg/kg	3 mg/kg	10 seconds	20–30 seconds	5–10 mg/kg/h	2–18 mg/kg/h[b]
Valproate	15–20 mg/kg	20–25 mg/kg	3 mg/kg/min	3 mg/kg/min	1–4 mg/kg/h[b]	1–4 mg/kg/h[b]

[a]Doses may be repeated twice every 10 to 15 min until the maximum dosage is given.
[b]Titrate dose as needed.

combination of diazepam plus phenytoin.[18] A second multicenter trial reported that phenobarbital was as effective as lorazepam alone or diazepam plus phenytoin in GCSE and was not associated with serious adverse effects.[19] Although there is technically no definitive answer, the Working Group on Status Epilepticus recommends that phenobarbital be given after a benzodiazepine plus phenytoin has failed.[11] Currently, most practitioners agree that phenobarbital is the long-acting anticonvulsant of choice in patients with a hypersensitivity to the hydantoins or in those with cardiac conduction abnormalities.

Following intravenous administration, phenobarbital has two phases of distribution into body organs.[24] During the first phase, the drug distributes into highly vascular organs, but it does not distribute into the brain. With the exception of fat, phenobarbital distributes throughout the body during the second phase[24]; hence body fat should be considered when dosing. In order to avoid overdosing, estimated lean body mass should be used in obese patients.[24] Although phenobarbital penetrates into the brain slowly, the highest brain concentrations occur 12 to 60 minutes after an intravenous dose.[24] On average, seizures are controlled within minutes of the loading dose.[19] Phenobarbital exhibits first-order linear pharmacokinetics, and there is no maximum dose beyond which further doses are likely to be ineffective.[25]

The loading and maintenance dose for phenobarbital are given in Table 55–3. When necessary, larger loading doses (30 mg/kg) have been used in neonates without adverse effects. If the initial loading dose does not stop the seizures within 20 to 30 minutes, an additional 10 to 20 mg/kg dose may be given. If seizures continue, a third 10 mg/kg load may be given.[25] Once GCSE is controlled, the maintenance dose should be started within 12 to 24 hours.

Although injectable phenobarbital contains propylene glycol, it can be given more rapidly than phenytoin (see Table 55–3). Phenobarbital can be given intramuscularly, but its rate of absorption is too slow to be effective in GCSE. Phenobarbital may cause depression of consciousness and respiration. The risk of apnea and hypopnea may be more profound in patients treated initially with benzodiazepines.[4,11] Medical personnel should be ready to provide respiratory support whenever the two agents are used concurrently. If significant hypotension develops, the infusion should be slowed or stopped.[11]

TREATMENT OF REFRACTORY GCSE

When adequate doses of a benzodiazepine, hydantoin, or barbiturate have failed, the condition is termed *refractory*.[23] Approximately 10% to 15% of patients will develop refractory GCSE.[26]

About 30% of patients whose seizures are "clinically" controlled will have persistent electrical manifestations (i.e., still in status) and will remain in GCSE after administration of these anticonvulsants.[23] When a patient develops refractory GCSE, a neurologist with expertise in epilepsy should be consulted, and an intense search should be performed for an acute or progressive cause.[11]

It should be remembered that the longer GCSE lasts, the harder it is to treat and that failure to treat aggressively early in the course of GCSE increases the likelihood of nonresponse.[11] The optimal therapeutic approach for patients with refractory GCSE has not been determined. Approaches used include the continuous infusion of a benzodiazepines, medically induced coma, valproate, propofol, paraldehyde, or lidocaine. Doses for these agents can be found in Table 55–4. Regardless of the therapy selected, the goal is to stop electrical epileptiform activity.

BENZODIAZEPINES

Although refractory GCSE has been treated with a variety of agents, some practitioners have advocated not only that midazolam should be the first-line agent in refractory GCSE but also that it should be the third-line agent in patients unresponsive to lorazepam plus phenytoin.[23,27,28] Table 55–4 contains the loading and maintenance doses for adult and pediatric patients. The continuous-infusion rate should be increased every 15 minutes until seizures are controlled.[29] Most patients respond within 65 minutes.

Because tachyphylaxis can develop, frequent increases in the infusion rate may be necessary, and dosing should be guided by EEG response.[23] Once GCSE is terminated, dosages can be decreased by 1 mcg/kg per minute every 2 hours. Successful discontinuation is enhanced by maintaining the patient's phenytoin serum concentration near 20 mg/L and phenobarbital concentration above 40 mg/L.[23] Because of midazolam's short half-life, patients may return to consciousness more rapidly than those receiving larger doses of more sedating anticonvulsants (e.g., phenytoin, phenobarbital). Generally, continuous-infusion midazolam has been well tolerated, with few cases of hypotension and respiratory depression seen. Hypotension and poikilothermia can occur and may require supportive therapies.

Large-dose continuous-infusion lorazepam and diazepam also have been used successfully in patients unresponsive to phenytoin or phenobarbital.[30,31] Lorazepam contains propylene glycol, which can accumulate in patients receiving continuous infusions. It has been noted to cause a marked osmolar gap, metabolic acidosis, and renal toxicity, which was attributed to the infusion of propylene glycol.[32–34]

MEDICALLY INDUCED COMA

If there is an inadequate response to large doses of midazolam, anesthetizing the patient to suppress the cerebral ictal discharge is recommended.[11,27,28] Although it is likely that the patient is already being mechanically ventilated, intubation and respiratory support are mandatory during barbiturate coma. Because hypotension is a concern, it is essential that vital signs be monitored continuously. A short-acting barbiturate (usually either pentobarbital or thiopental) generally is preferred because it allows a more rapid reversal of coma.

Several sources note that the initial loading dose of pentobarbital is 5 mg/kg.[11] However, this dose is inadequate to produce the serum concentrations (30 to 40 mg/L) necessary to induce an isoelectric EEG. Pentobarbital should be initiated with a loading dose of at least 10 to 20 mg/kg over 40 to 60 minutes[27] (see Table 55–4). If hypotension occurs during the loading dose, the rate of administration should be slowed, or dopamine should be administered. The loading dose should be followed immediately by a continuous infusion.[11] Rates are typically begun at 1 mg/kg/h and titrated as needed up to a dose of 5 mg/kg/h. The maintenance infusion should be increased gradually until there is evidence of burst suppression on EEG (i.e., flat EEG) or prohibitive adverse effects occur. Although the duration of barbiturate coma in most studies has been 2 to 3 days, pentobarbital coma has been used safely for 53 days in an 18-year-old patient.[35] In order to avoid complications (e.g., pneumonia, pulmonary edema), the pentobarbital should be discontinued as soon as possible. Twelve hours after a burst-suppression pattern is obtained, the rate of pentobarbital infusion should be titrated downward every 2 to 4 hours to enable the clinician to determine if the patient's GCSE is in remission.

VALPROATE

Limited human data exist regarding the use of valproate in refractory GCSE. Although an intravenous dosage form has been approved by the FDA, it is not approved for GCSE. A number of loading and continuous-infusion doses (see Table 55–4) have been used to treat GCSE in both adult[36–38] and pediatric patients.[38,39] One study suggested the need to consider the effects of enzyme-inducing anticonvulsants when dosing valproate.[39] This group recommended that the continuous-infusion rate be determined by the presence of concurrent anticonvulsants (no inducers present, 1 mg/kg per hour; one or more inducers [e.g., phenytoin, phenobarbital], 2 mg/kg per hour; and inducers and pentobarbital coma, 4 mg/kg per hour).

Although the manufacturer originally recommended intravenous valproate be given no faster than 20 mg/min, much faster rates have been studied (2 to 6 mg/kg per minute) and are used for administration of the loading dose.[39,40] Currently, the manufacturer recommends that intravenous valproate be administered at a rate of 3 mg/kg per minute. In general, intravenous valproate has been well tolerated, with no cases of respiratory depression. Hemodynamic instability is extremely rare, but patients' vital signs should be monitored closely during the loading dose.

PROPOFOL

Propofol is extremely lipid soluble and has a large volume of distribution. It has a very rapid onset of action and an extremely short half-life (2 to 4 minutes), which promotes rapid awakening on drug discontinuation. Although extensive data are not available, it appears to be effective in GCSE.[27,41] Doses can be found in Table 55–4. It may cause respiratory and cerebral depression and bradycardia. Although metabolic acidosis has been reported, the occurrence of propofol-associated metabolic acidosis is controversial.[42] Finally, a normal adult dose may provide over 1000 calories per day as lipid at a cost to the patient that may exceed $1000 per day.

OTHER AGENTS

Historically, rectal or intravenous paraldehyde has been used for refractory GCSE. Although effective, it is extremely difficult to administer, is associated with serious adverse effects (e.g., hypotension, tachycardia, pulmonary edema, and polyethylene emboli), and is no longer manufactured in the United States. The only available formulation currently licensed is an enteral product that is difficult to obtain in a timely manner. If a rectal dose is given, it should be diluted 1:1 in vegetable oil and given every 20 minutes as needed via a rubber catheter.[11]

Lidocaine has been used in refractory GCSE, but its use is not recommended unless other agents have failed.[43] It is administered intravenously and has a rapid onset of action. Table 55–4 gives the recommended initial loading and continuous-infusion doses. Although the reference serum concentration range for the antiarrhythmic effects of lidocaine is 2 to 6 mg/L, the reference range for GCSE has not been established. Serum lidocaine concentrations should be monitored to avoid drug accumulation and toxicity. CNS toxicity (e.g., fasiculations, visual disturbances, and tinnitus) may occur at concentrations between 6 and 8 mg/L; seizures and obtundation may develop when concentrations exceed 8 mg/L.

Halothane, isoflurane, ketamine, and other inhaled anesthetics have been shown to produce EEG suppression; however, these gases are difficult to deliver outside the operating room and require the presence of an anesthesiologist. No proven advantages have been shown over traditional anticonvulsants (e.g., barbiturate coma or continuous-infusion benzodiazepine), and these gases can increase intracranial pressure. If used, dosing is titrated to obtain EEG burst suppression. It also may be prudent to validate that the patient does not have a low serum magnesium concentration because magnesium deficiency can lower the seizure threshold.

PHARMACOECONOMIC CONSIDERATIONS

Although no prospective pharmacoeconomic studies have been performed in patients with GCSE, a number of economic issues may have an impact on formulary considerations. Clearly, there are intra- and interclass differences in medication costs and in ancillary tests or technologies associated with select therapies. For example, if one assumes five treatment options and hypothetically initiates anticonvulsant therapy in a patient weighing 70 kg, the following differences in average wholesale prices are noted:

- Diazepam (20 mg) plus generic phenytoin (1 g): $15.01
- Lorazepam alone (8 mg): $15.62
- Midazolam alone (0.25 mg/kg load, 0.1 mg/kg/hr): $31.10
- Generic phenytoin (1 g) alone: $13.33
- Diazepam (20 mg) plus fosphenytoin PE (1 g): $181.68
- Phenobarbital (20 mg/kg) alone: $28.22
- Intravenous valproate (15 mg/kg load, 1 mg/kg per hour): $88.20

Although many practitioners have heralded the arrival of fosphenytoin as an important therapeutic advancement, it has created a fiscal and ethical dilemma for many institutions. Fosphenytoin is associated with less infusion pain and fewer intravenous-site complications and hemodynamic adverse effects than phenytoin; however, the cost of this agent ($180/g PE versus $13.33/g phenytoin) has caused many practitioners and administrators to struggle with the practical and ethical importance of the increased safety profile relative to the cost of the product to an institution. When evaluating the difference in cost of these two agents, it is important to remember that phenytoin requires the placement of two intravenous catheters because of its incompatibility with many solutions and medications that are given concurrently. Additionally, some practitioners are giving fosphenytoin intramuscularly in the emergency room for non-SE indications and thereby avoiding the placement of a catheter and use of an infusion device. Many institutions fail to consider the expense associated with a tissue infiltration of phenytoin. Should an infiltration of phenytoin cause tissue necrosis that necessitates plastic surgery or amputation, the expense of a single multimillion-dollar lawsuit likely will offset the difference between phenytoin and fosphenytoin cost to several institutions.

There is little difference in expense if one advocates phenobarbital over midazolam as third-line therapy, but it might be argued that a patient who experiences phenobarbital-induced respiration depression ultimately may be more expensive to the health system. Finally, a 24-hour infusion of propofol to the same patient will cost in excess of $1000.

EVALUATION OF THERAPEUTIC OUTCOMES

Initial success is defined as termination of all clinical and electrical activity, but ultimate success is measured by the patient's quality of life. The morbidity and mortality associated with GCSE are affected by the underlying etiology; however, these can be minimized by the rapid implementation of a rational therapeutic plan. An EEG is an extremely important tool that not only allows practitioners to determine when abnormal electrical activity has been aborted but also may assist in determining which anticonvulsant was effective. Because many of the anticonvulsants affect the cardiorespiratory system, it is imperative that vital signs (e.g., heart rate, respiratory rate, and blood pressure) be monitored during drug infusion. It also may be necessary to monitor the ECG in some patients. Finally, it is imperative that the infusion site be assessed for any evidence of infiltration before and during administration of phenytoin. Information regarding the patient's past medical and drug history and imaging studies (e.g., MRI) also may help to determine if there is a defined etiology for the original episode of GCSE. This information then may be used to guide future medication therapy, as well as help in determining if the patient is at risk for a poor outcome.

CONCLUSION

Our understanding of the cellular basis, physiology, and neuropathology of GCSE continues to evolve. Over the past decade, research into an activated cascade of pathophysiologic changes in neurotransmission, GABAergic inhibition, and NMDA receptor channel–mediated events has enhanced our understanding of this disorder. Although anticonvulsants will continue to be the mainstay of therapy in terminating seizures, specific agents including antagonists of excitatory amino acid neurotransmitters (e.g., glutamate and calcium channel blockers) and agonists of inhibitory neurotransmitters (GABA) may help to block further neuronal damage beyond the epileptogenic focus. Likewise, additional trials investigating the role of newer anticonvulsants in GCSE are warranted.

ABBREVIATIONS

AMPA: α-amino-3-hydroxy-5-methyl-4-isoxazolepropionate
ECG: electrocardiogram
EEG: electroencephalogram, electroencephalography
FDA: Food and Drug Administration
GABA: γ-aminobutyric acid
GCSE: generalized convulsive status epilepticus
MRI: magnetic resonance imaging
NCSE: nonconvulsive status epilepticus
NMDA: N-methyl-D-aspartate
NPY: neuropeptide Y
PE: phenytoin equivalents

Review Questions and other resources can be found at *www.pharmacotherapy.com*.

REFERENCES

1. Commission on Classification of Terminology, International League Against Epilepsy. Proposal for revised clinical and electroencephalographic classification of epileptic seizures. Epilepsia 1981;22:489–501.
2. Walker MC. Diagnosis and treatment of nonconvulsive status epilepticus. CNS Drugs 2001;15:931–939.
3. Shorvon S. The management of status epilepticus. J Neurol Neurosurg Psychiatry. 2001;70(suppl 2):II22–7.
4. Lowenstein DH, Alldredge BK. Status epilepticus. N Engl J Med 1998; 338:970–976.
5. DeLorenzo RJ, Pellock JM, Towne AR, Boggs J. Epidemology of status epilepticus. J Clin Neurophysiol 1995;12:316–325.
6. DeLorenzo RJ, Towne AR, Pellock JM, Ko D. Status epilepticus in children, adults, and the elderly. Epilepsia 1992;33:S15–25.
7. Herman ST, Kapur J, MacDonald RL. Rapid seizure-induced reduction of benzodiazepine and sensitivity of hippocampal dentate granule cells. J Neurosci 1997;17:7532–7540.
8. Pitkanen A. Efficacy of current antiepileptics to prevent neurodegeneration in epilepsy models. Epilepsy Res 2002;50:141–160.
9. Temkin NR. Antiepileptogenesis and seizure prevention trials with antiepileptic drugs: Meta-analysis of controlled trials. Epilepsia 2001;42: 515–524.
10. Treiman DM. Generalized convulsive status epilepticus in the adult. Epilepsia 1993;34(suppl 1):S2–11.
11. Working Group on Status Epilepticus. Treatment of convulsive status epilepticus: Recommendations of the Epilepsy Foundation of America's Working Group on Status Epilepticus. JAMA 1993;270:854–859.
12. Wasterlain CG, Mazarati AM, Naylor D, et al. Short-term plasticity of hippocampal neuropeptides and neuronal circuitry in experimental status epilepticus. Epilepsia 2002;45(suppl 5):20–29.

13. Mazarati AM, Liu H, Wasterlain CG. Opioid peptide pharmacology and immunocytochemistry in an animal model of self-sustaining status epilepticus. Neuroscience 1999;89:167–173.

14. Lothman E. The biochemical basis and pathophysiology of status epilepticus. Neurology 1990;40:13–23.

15. Leppik IE, Derivan AT, Homan RW, et al. Double-blind study of lorazepam and diazepam in status epilepticus. JAMA 1983;249:1452–1454.

16. Treiman DM, De Giorgio CM, Ben-Menachem E, et al. Lorazepam versus phenytoin in the treatment of generalized convulsive status epilepticus: Report of an ongoing study. Neurology 1985;35:284.

17. Appleton R, Sweeney A, Choonara I, et al. Lorazepam versus diazepam in the acute treatment of epileptic seizures and status epilepticus. Dev Med Child Neurol 1995;37:682–688.

18. Shaner DM, McCurdy SA, Herring MO, Gabor AJ. Treatment of status epilepticus: A prospective comparison of diazepam and phenytoin versus phenobarbital and optional phenytoin. Neurology 1988;38:202–207.

19. Treiman DM, Meyers PD, Walton NY, et al. A comparison of four treatments for generalized convulsive status epilepticus. Veterans Affairs Status Epilepticus Cooperative Study Group. N Engl J Med 1998;339:792–798.

20. LeDuc TJ, Goellner WE, Sanadi NE. Out-of-hospital midazolam for status epilepticus. Ann Emerg Med 1996;28:377.

21. Fischer JH, Patel TV, Fischer PA. Fosphenytoin: Clinical pharmacokinetics and comparative advantages in the acute treatment of seizures. Clin Pharmacokinet 2003;42:33–58.

22. Abernethy DR, Greenblatt DJ. Phenytoin disposition in obesity: Determination of loading dose. Arch Neurol 1985;42:468–471.

23. Bleck TP. Advances in the management of refractory status epilepticus. Crit Care Med 1993;21:955–957.

24. Dodson WE, Rust RS. Phenobarbital: Absorption, distribution, and excretions In: Levy R, Mattson R, Meldrum B, eds. Antiepileptic Drugs, 4th ed. New York, Raven Press, 1995:379–387.

25. Crawford TO, Mitchell WG, Fishman LS, Snodgrass SR. Very-high-dose phenobarbital for refractory status epilepticus in children. Neurology 1988;38:1035–1040.

26. Lowenstein DH, Alldredge BK. Status epilepticus at an urban public hospital in the 1980s. Neurology 1993;43:483–488.

27. Claassen J, Hirsch LJ, Emerson RG, Mayer SA. Treatment of refractory status epilepticus with pentobarbital, propofol, or midazolam: A systematic review. Epilepsia 2002;43:146–153.

28. Holmes GL, Riviello JJ. Midazolam and pentobarbital for refractory status epilepticus. Pediatr Neurol 1999;20:259–264.

29. Koul RL, Aithala GR, Chacko A, et al. Continuous midazolam infusion as treatment of status epilepticus. Arch Dis Child 1997;76:445–448.

30. Labar DR, Ali A, Root J. High-dose intravenous lorazepam for the treatment of refractory status epilepticus. Neurology 1994;44:1400–1403.

31. Bell HE, Bertino JS Jr. Constant diazepam infusion in the treatment of continuous seizure activity. Drug Intell Clin Pharm 1984;18:965–970.

32. Chicella M, Jansen P, Parthiban A, et al. Propylene glycol accumulation associated with continuous infusion of lorazepam in pediatric intensive care patients. Crit Care Med 2002;30:2752–2756.

33. Hayman M, Seidl EC, Ali M, Malik K. Acute tubular necrosis associated with propylene glycol from concomitant administration of intravenous lorazepam and trimethoprim-sulfamethoxazole. Pharmacotherapy 2003;23:1190–1194.

34. Yaucher NE, Fish JT, Smith HW, Wells JA. Propylene glycol–associated renal toxicity from lorazepam infusion. Pharmacotherapy 2003;23:1094–1099.

35. Mirski MA, Williams MA, Hanlet DF. Prolonged pentobarbital and phenobarbital coma for refractory generalized status epilepticus. Crit Care Med 1995;23:400–404.

36. Giroud M, Gras D, Escousse A, et al. Use of injectable valproic acid in status epilepticus. Drug Invest 1993;5:154–159.

37. Price DJ. Intravenous valproate: Experience in neurosurgery. In: Fourth International Symposium on Sodium Valproate in Epilepsy. London, Royal Society of Medicine International Congress Symposium Series, 1989:197–203.

38. Chez MG, Hammer MS, Loeffel M, et al. Clinical experience of three pediatric patients and one adult case of spike and wave status epilepticus treated with injectable valproic acid. J Child Neurol 1999;14:239–242.

39. Hovinga CA, Chicella MF, Rose DF, et al. Use of intravenous valproate in three pediatric patients with nonconvulsive or convulsive status epilepticus. Ann Pharmacother 1999;33:579–584.

40. Venkataraman V, Wheless JW. Safety of rapid intravenous infusion of valproate loading doses in epilepsy patients. Epilepsy Res 1999;35:147–153.

41. Brown LA, Levin GM. Role of propofol in refractory status epilepticus. Ann Pharmacother 1998;32:1053–1059.

42. Susla GM. Propofol toxicity in critically ill pediatric patients: Show us the proof. Crit Care Med 1998;26:1959–1960.

43. Aggarwal P, Wali JP. Lidocaine in refractory status epilepticus: A forgotten drug in the emergency department. Am J Emerg Med 1993;2:243–244.

56

ACUTE MANAGEMENT OF
THE BRAIN INJURY PATIENT

Bradley A. Boucher, Stephanie J. Phelps, and Shelly D. Timmons

Learning Objectives and other resources can be found at *www.pharmacotherapyonline.com*.

KEY CONCEPTS

◄1 Cerebral ischemia is the key pathophysiologic event triggering secondary neuronal injury following severe traumatic brain injury (TBI). Intracellular accumulation of calcium is postulated to be a central pathophysiologic process in amplifying and perpetuating secondary neuronal injury via inhibition of cellular respiration and enzyme activation.

◄2 *Guidelines for the Management of Severe Brain Injury,* published by the Brain Trauma Foundation/American Association of Neurological Surgeons, serves as the foundation on which clinical decisions in managing adult neurotrauma patients are based; comparable guidelines for infants, children, and adolescents also have been published recently.

◄3 Correcting and preventing early hypotension (systolic blood pressure < 90 mm Hg) and hypoxemia (PaO_2 < 60 mm Hg) are primary goals during the initial resuscitative and intensive care of severe TBI patients.

◄4 The principal monitoring parameter for severe TBI patients within the intensive care environment is intracranial pressure (ICP). Cerebral perfusion pressure (CPP) is also a critical monitoring parameter and should be maintained at greater than 60 mm Hg (>40 mm Hg in pediatric patients) through

the use of fluids, vasopressors, and/or ICP normalization therapy.

◄5 Nonspecific pharmacologic treatment in the management of intracranial hypertension should include analgesics, sedatives, antipyretics, and paralytics under selected circumstances.

◄6 Specific pharmacologic treatment in the management of intracranial hypertension includes mannitol, furosemide, and high-dose pentobarbital. Neither routine use of corticosteroids nor aggressive hyperventilation (i.e., $PaCO_2$ <25 mm Hg) should be used in the management of intracranial hypertension.

◄7 Use of phenytoin for the prophylaxis of posttraumatic seizures usually should be discontinued after 7 days if no seizures are observed.

◄8 Numerous investigational strategies (e.g., calcium antagonists, glutamate antagonists, antioxidants, and free-radical scavengers) targeted at interrupting the pathophysiologic cascade of events occurring following severe TBI have been employed.

Traumatic brain injury (TBI) has been referred to as America's "invisible epidemic" and is currently the leading cause of death and disability among children and young adults in the industrialized world.[1] Based on an ever-growing understanding of TBI pathophysiology, clinicians and scientists share an optimism that patient outcomes can be improved through the use of evidence-based management guidelines presently and administration of neuroprotective agents in the future. This chapter summarizes TBI epidemiology and pathophysiology and highlights guidelines and systematic reviews of the literature pertaining to the management of severe TBI patients.

EPIDEMIOLOGY

It is estimated that approximately 1.5 million persons sustain a nonfatal brain injury each year in the United States, resulting in 230,000 hospital admissions and 50,000 deaths annually based on data from

1989 to 1998.[2] Importantly, over 5 million Americans currently live with disabilities as a result of their TBI, highlighting the enormous physical and emotional toll of this health care problem in the United States.[1] The economic effects of acute neurotrauma are also enormous, with estimates of spending on TBI patients requiring hospitalization exceeding $56 billion per year in the United States.[3] While the frequency of TBI remains high, the mortality rate following traumatic brain injury has decreased from nearly 25 per 100,000 to 19.4 per 100,000 population per year since 1979.[2] Motor vehicle accidents account for about 50% of all adult cases, whereas falls, assaults, gunshot wounds, sports and recreational accidents, and other miscellaneous causes account for the remaining cases.[4] Motor vehicle–related TBIs were the leading cause of death in individuals aged 0 to 19 years of age.[2] In TBI patients 20 to 74 years of age, gunshot wounds are responsible for the highest number of TBI fatalities, whereas fall-related TBIs caused the greatest number of deaths in patients 75 years of age or older.[2] Furthermore, TBI-related mortality in males exceeds that in females threefold.[2]

PATHOPHYSIOLOGY

PRIMARY BRAIN INJURY

The neurologic sequelae of brain trauma can occur instantaneously as a consequence of the primary injury or can result from secondary injuries that follow within minutes, hours, or days.[5] Primary injury involves the external transfer of kinetic energy to various structural components of the brain (e.g., neurons, nerve synapses, glial cells, axons, and cerebral blood vessels). The biomechanical forces responsible for primary brain injury can be classified broadly as concussive/compressive (e.g., blunt-object blow, penetrating-missile injuries) and acceleration/deceleration (e.g., instantaneous brain movements following motor vehicle accidents). Primary injuries are categorized further as focal (e.g., contusions, hematomas) or diffuse.[6] The latter usually are associated with shearing or stretch forces, which primarily affect axons within the brain (i.e., diffuse axonal injury).[6,7]

SECONDARY BRAIN INJURY

A complex sequence of pathophysiologic events precipitated by primary brain injury may seriously disrupt the normal central nervous system (CNS) balance between oxygen supply and demand.[5] Hypotension during the early posttraumatic period is a major contributor to this imbalance and a primary determinant of outcome.[6,8] The end result of this imbalance may be cerebral ischemia, the key pathophysiologic event triggering secondary injury. Figure 56–1 is a simplified schematic of the processes that constitute secondary brain injury and their various interrelationships. The brain is particularly susceptible to ischemia because of its normally high resting energy requirement and its limited capacity to store oxygen, glucose, and high-energy phosphate compounds (e.g., adenosine triphosphate [ATP]).[5]

Ischemia following brain injury typically occurs in the first 6 to 24 hours following the insult.[9,10] Thereafter, patients can have hyperemia from days 1 to 3.[10] Vasospasm also can occur.[10] These phenomena can result in imbalances in cerebral oxygen delivery (CDo_2) and consumption ($CMRo_2$), processes that are closely autoregulated under normal circumstances.[5] Factors that can diminish cerebral oxygen supply following brain injury include cerebral edema, expanding mass lesions (e.g., epidural, subdural, and intracerebral hematomas), cerebral vasospasm, and loss of vasoregulatory control.[5] Hypoxemia can further exacerbate local decreases in cerebral oxygen supply following acute respiratory failure and systemic hypotension. Metabolic demand also can increase following neurotrauma secondary to seizures, agitation, and temperature elevation.[11] There is evidence that TBI itself can increase metabolic demand as well.

Brain tissue affected by focal ischemia can have a dense core surrounded by a marginally viable region. Cells in this area are electrically silent and unable to perform normal neurologic functions. If adequate cerebral blood flow (CBF) is restored, the affected tissue may recover; however, sustained ischemia can result in further loss of cellular integrity and eventual cell death. The loss of ionic homeostasis is postulated to be a key event in fostering secondary brain injury within this ischemic region. Cellular influx of sodium, chloride, and water (i.e., cytotoxic edema) with a corresponding efflux of potassium and magnesium occurs with Na^+,K^+-ATPase pump dysfunction.[5] An influx of calcium into the presynaptic terminal ends of damaged neurons is mediated by N-type voltage-sensitive calcium channels. This in turn, is postulated to stimulate excessive release of the excitatory amines glutamate and aspartate from the affected neurons.[7] The result is ongoing stimulation of postsynaptic cells, which can result in an extension of neurotoxicity and cell death. Influx of calcium and additional sodium is stimulated by activation of the N-methyl-D-aspartate (NMDA) receptor.[12] Calcium influx and its intracellular

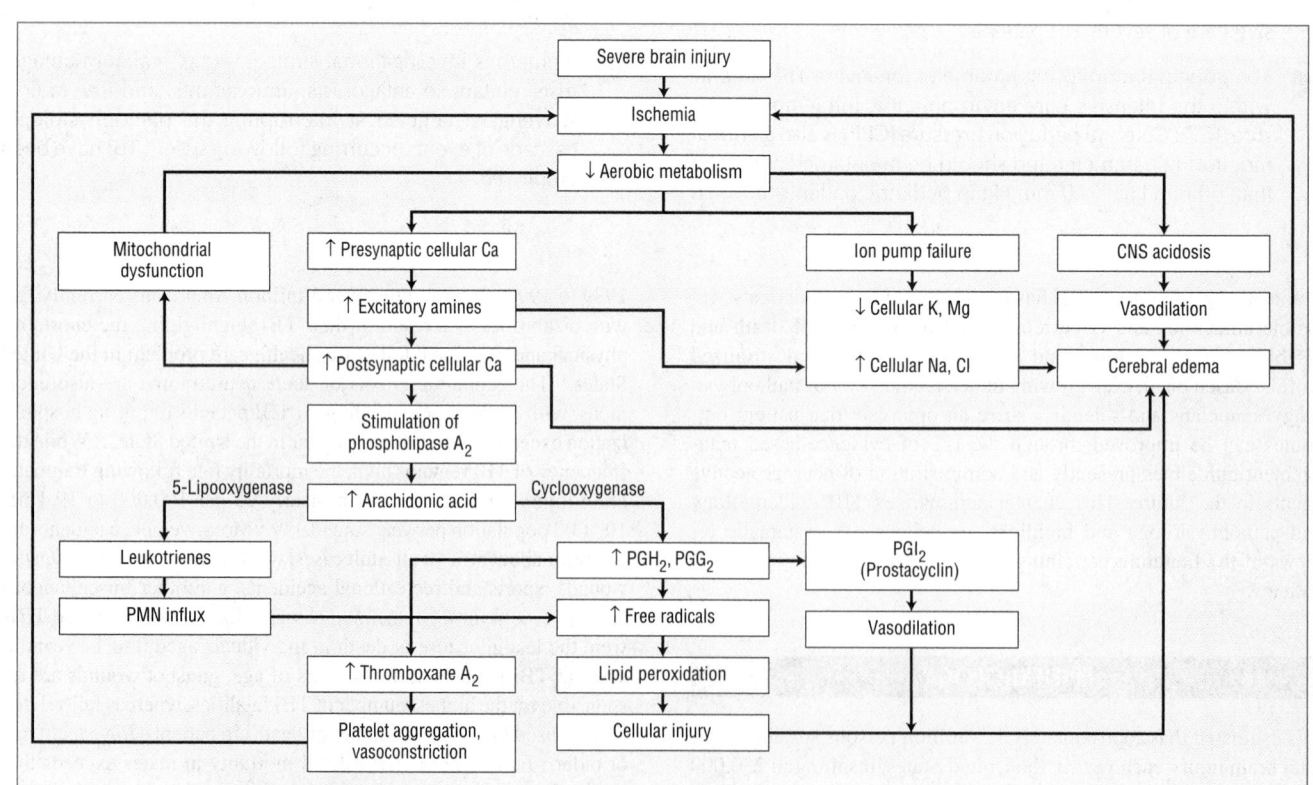

FIGURE 56–1. Schematic illustration of the cascade of biochemical events proposed to occur following severe neurotrauma (secondary brain injury). Ca, calcium; CNS, central nervous system; K, potassium; Mg, magnesium; Na, sodium; Cl, chloride; PMN, polymorphonucleocyte; PG, prostaglandin.

TABLE 56–1. Clinical Presentation of Acute Brain Injury

General	Level of consciousness on admission ranges from awake and alert to completely unresponsive (i.e., GCS 15 to 3, respectively).
Symptoms	Posttraumatic amnesia (e.g., greater than 1 hour), increasing dizziness, a moderate to severe headache, limb weakness, or paresthesia may indicate more severe injury.
Signs	CSF otorrhea or rhinorrhea and seizures may indicate more severe injury.
	A rapid deterioration in mental status strongly suggests the presence of an expanding lesion within the skull.
	Severe TBI may be accompanied by significant alterations or instability in vital signs, including abnormal breathing patterns (e.g., apnea, Cheyne-Stokes respiration, tachypnea), hypotension, or bradycardia.
Laboratory tests	ABGs indicating hypoxia (i.e., decreased PaO_2) or hypercapnia (i.e., increased $PaCO_2$) may indicate compromised ventilation.
	A positive blood ethanol concentration and/or positive urine drug screen indicates that drug intoxication may be affecting the patient's mental status in addition to the TBI.
Other diagnostic tests	CT of the head is an important diagnostic tool for detecting the presence of mass lesions.

GCS, Glasgow Coma Scale; CSF, cerebrospinal fluid; TBI, traumatic brain injury; ABG, arterial blood gas; PaO_2, partial pressure of arterial blood oxygen; $PaCO_2$, partial pressure of arterial blood carbon dioxide; CT, computed tomography.

accumulation initiate a number of events that amplify and perpetuate secondary neuronal injury. High intracellular concentrations of calcium result in mitochondrial dysfunction, which further inhibits cellular respiration, a process already affected by ischemic and/or hypoxic insults.[12] A second major deleterious effect of calcium is to stimulate activation of autodestructive enzymes, including phosphatases, kinases, lipases, and proteases, such as calpain, caspase-1, and caspase-3.[7,13,14] The effect of phospholipase A_2 stimulation includes formation of several arachidonic acid metabolites derived from membrane lipids: thromboxane A_2, prostaglandins, and leukotrienes.[12] The subsequent effects of these metabolites are lipid peroxidation and the formation of oxygen free-radical species.[15] Lipid peroxidation is an especially damaging event because the formation of oxygen free radicals can propagate, resulting in further cellular membrane damage, unless quenched by endogenous antioxidants (e.g., vitamin E, ascorbic acid, superoxide dismutase).[15] Recent data suggest that this event occurs very early after injury (e.g., before hospitalization), which may limit the effectiveness of exogenously administered antioxidants.[16] A common end point with the release of excitatory amines, increases in intracellular calcium, and oxygen free radical generation is apoptosis or programmed cell death and nonprogrammed cellular necrosis.[17]

Cells with a more elaborate dendritic structure (e.g., cortical neurons, hippocampal cells) may be more vulnerable to the effects of apoptosis.[18] Cell-mediated injury involving inflammatory mediators (e.g., cytokines, platelet-activating factor, etc.), nitric oxide, and cell adhesion molecules is yet another possible mechanism involved in secondary neuronal injury.[19] Among the cell lines implicated are polymorphonuclear neutrophils, platelets, endothelial cells, and macrophages. Stimulation of platelet aggregation, vasodilation, and vasoconstriction, intravascularly, also may occur. Vasogenic cerebral edema can develop as a consequence of cerebral capillary endothelial damage.[5] With cytotoxic and vasogenic edema comes expansion of the intracellular and extracellular fluid spaces, respectively. Elevated intracranial pressure (ICP) is the most detrimental consequence of cerebral edema formation and occurs as the brain tissue volume increases within the nondistensible skull. A significant increase in ICP may further compromise cerebral blood flow (CBF) and extend cytotoxic edema. Hence an increase in ICP can be self-perpetuating unless this cycle is reversed.

Lastly, preliminary data suggest that there may be a genetic vulnerability to the effects of TBI.[7] Specifically, a link between the gene that encodes for apolipoprotein E_4 and outcome has been postulated.[20,21] Noteworthy is that this is the same protein that has been associated with the deleterious effects of various types of Alzheimer's disease.[7]

CLINICAL PRESENTATION

The clinical presentation of acute brain injury is summarized in Table 56–1. The Glasgow Coma Scale (GCS) is the most widely used system to grade the arousal and functional capacity of the cerebral cortex.[6] The GCS defines the level of consciousness according to eye opening, motor response, and verbal response (Table 56–2). A GCS score of 15 corresponds to a normal neurologic examination. A GCS score of 3–8, 9–12, and 13–15 is consistent with severe, moderate,

TABLE 56–2. Glasgow Coma Scale

Response	Score
Eyes	
Open spontaneously	4
To verbal command	3
To pain	2
No response	1
Best Motor Response	
To verbal command	
Obeys	6
To painful stimulus (pressure to nailbeds)	
Localizes pain	5
Flexion, withdrawal	4
Flexion, abnormal (decorticate rigidity)	3
Extension (decerebrate rigidity)	2
No response	1
Best Verbal Response (Arouse patient with painful stimulus if necessary)	
Oriented and converses	5
Disoriented and converses	4
Inappropriate words	3
Incomprehensible sounds	2
No response	1
Total	3–15

and mild brain injury, respectively.[6] The possibility of ethanol or drug intoxication, hypotension, hypoxia, postictal state, or hypothermia altering the neurologic examination always should be considered. Because narcotics and muscle relaxants affect the neurologic examination, they should not be administered until the initial examination

is complete if at all possible. Simple, rapidly attainable clinical variables that are predictive of survival include patient age, GCS score (especially the motor score), pupillary reactivity, and presence or absence of a hematoma and ventricular cisterns found on a computed tomographic (CT) scan of the head.[22]

▶ TREATMENT: Traumatic Brain Injury

In July 1995, the Brain Trauma Foundation (BTF) published an extensive document entitled *Guidelines for the Management of Severe Brain Injury* as a joint initiative with the Guidelines Committee of the American Association of Neurological Surgeons (AANS) and the Joint Section on Neurotrauma and Critical Care of the AANS and the Congress of Neurological Surgeons, with subsequent revision in 2000.[23,24] This landmark publication established for the first time a comprehensive series of evidence-based standards, guidelines, and options for the care of severe TBI patients. A recent survey suggested that significant changes consistent with the BTF/AANS guidelines in the acute management of TBI patients have occurred since 1991, providing indirect evidence as to their overall impact on patient care.[25] Since then, the European Brain Injury Consortium has issued guidelines for the management of severe TBI in adults,[26] prehospital TBI management,[27] surgical management, and management of penetrating brain injury. Furthermore, TBI management guidelines for infants, children, and adolescents have been developed.[28] In addition, a series of systematic reviews addressing TBI management emanating from The Cochrane Library has been published.[29–36] These reviews have rigorously evaluated the literature for essentially all the major conventional TBI treatment strategies. The recommendations emanating from the published guidelines on TBI management and published systematic reviews will be highlighted throughout the remaining portion of this chapter. Until further clinical studies become available, recommendations from the published guidelines should serve as the foundation on which all clinical decisions in managing severe TBI are based.[7] Recommendations provided in this chapter pertain to adults and children unless specifically noted to the contrary.

▦ DESIRED OUTCOMES

The overall goal in TBI management is not only reduction in morbidity and mortality but also optimization of long-term functional outcome for these patients. This requires careful attention to the following short-term therapeutic goals: (1) establishment of an adequate airway and maintenance of ventilation and circulation during the initial period of resuscitation and evaluation, (2) maintenance of balance between CDo_2 and $CMRo_2$, (3) prevention or attenuation of secondary neuronal injury, and (4) prevention and/or treatment of associated medical complications.

▦ INITIAL RESUSCITATION

The first priority in the unconscious patient is the establishment of an airway, which ensures adequate oxygenation and prevents aspiration.[6] Thereafter, restoration of circulating blood volume and maintenance of systolic arterial pressure (SBP) greater than 90 mm Hg are of utmost importance.[8] In pediatric patients, the SBP goal should be in

excess of 70 mm Hg + (2 × age in years).[28] Correcting and preventing early hypotension (SBP < 90 mm Hg) and hypoxia ($PaO_2 <$ 60 mm Hg) are essential because these two factors are among the most powerful predictors of outcome.[8,37] Isotonic saline (0.9% normal saline) and lactated Ringer's solution are the most commonly used resuscitation fluids. However, some clinicians believe that hypertonic saline (e.g., 3% or 7.5% saline) should be the fluid of choice in the resuscitation of TBI patients.[8] In children, the recommended infusion rate for 3% saline is 0.1–1 mL/kg per hour.[28] Clinical studies have yielded equivocal results relative to superiority over isotonic solutions.[38–40] Vasopressors and inotropic agents may be needed to maintain an adequate mean arterial pressure (MAP) if hypotension persists after adequate restoration of intravascular volume. Figure 56–2 is an algorithm summarizing treatment priorities in the initial management of acute TBI.

▦ POSTRESUSCITATIVE CARE

Following successful resuscitation, priorities shift toward diagnostic evaluation of intracranial and extracranial injuries and emergent surgical intervention as needed. Evacuation of intracranial hematomas (i.e., epidural, subdural, and intracerebral hematomas) is essential to control ICP and improve outcome. Elevation of depressed skull fractures and débridement of penetrating wound tracts are other important emergent surgical procedures in TBI patients. Continuous ICP monitoring (e.g., intraventricular catheter, intraparenchymal fiberoptic catheter) is indicated in patients with a GCS score of less than or equal to 8 with an abnormal admission CT scan or in high-risk severe TBI patients with a normal CT scan (i.e., age > 40 years, motor posturing, SBP < 90 mm Hg).[23,24] Intraventricular catheters have a therapeutic advantage over the other alternatives but are associated with a higher complication rate and can be difficult to place in the setting of the swollen brain. Specifically, cerebrospinal fluid (CSF) can be drained using this device as a means to lower ICP.[6] Continuous ICP monitoring is the only means to objectively evaluate the success of therapies used to decrease ICP. Once the ICP exceeds 20 to 25 mm Hg, therapy should be initiated to decrease ICP below 20 mm Hg.[23,24,28] Aggressive use of ICP monitors in academic trauma centers across the United States was associated with a reduction in mortality risk as well as a shorter length of stay among survivors.[41] Jugular venous oxygen saturation ($Sjvo_2$) monitoring is strongly advocated by some practitioners for detection of global cerebral hypoxia (i.e., adequacy of CBF relative to $CMRo_2$), although it is not currently addressed within the BTF/AANS guidelines.[42] Hence its role remains unclear at present.[6,43] Cerebral microdialysis techniques have been used successfully as research tools to measure the cerebral extracellular chemistry of TBI patients.[44] While the spread of this methodology to general clinical practice has been deemed unlikely, the use of brain tissue oxygen monitoring in TBI patients is promising.[7] Recently, the roles of several biochemical markers of TBI (e.g., S-100 protein,

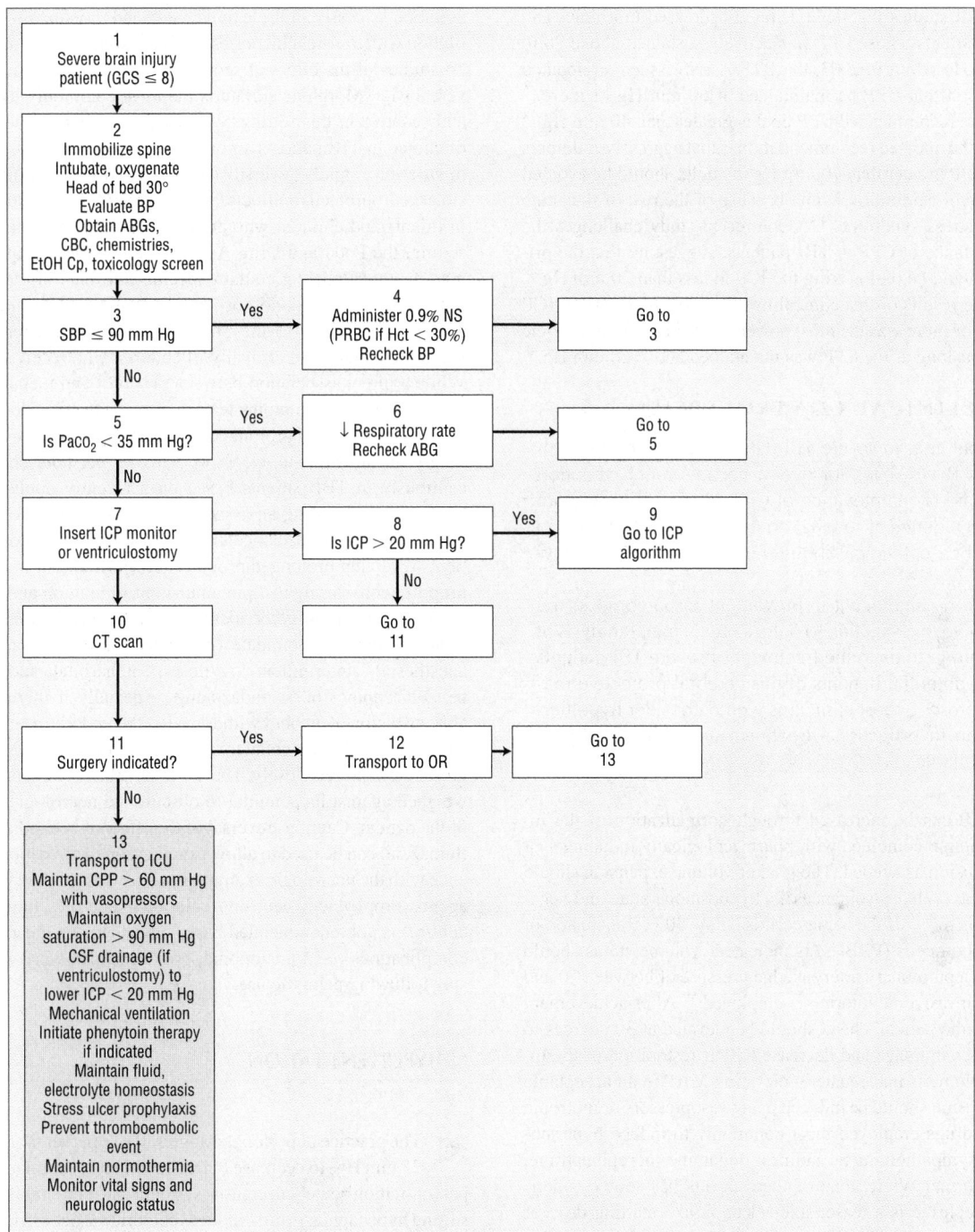

FIGURE 56–2. Algorithm for the acute management of the TBI patient. GCS, Glasgow Coma Scale; BP, blood pressure; ABG, arterial blood gas; CBC, complete blood count; EtOH Cp, ethanol plasma concentration; SBP, systolic blood pressure; NS, normal saline; PRBCs, packed red blood cells; Hct, hematocrit; $Paco_2$, partial pressure of arterial blood carbon dioxide; ICP, intracranial pressure; CT, computed tomography; OR, operating room; ICU, intensive care unit; CPP, cerebral perfusion pressure; CSF, cerebrospinal fluid. *(Adapted with permission from Boucher BA. Neurotrauma: Pharmacotherapy Self Assessment Program, 3d ed., Module 2: Critical Care. New York, American College of Clinical Pharmacy, 1995:215–238.)*

neuron-specific enolase) also were reviewed.[45] The utility of these or other proteins for the detection of secondary injury in TBI and/or as a treatment-monitoring parameter is uncertain at this time.

Another important monitoring parameter for severe TBI patients within the intensive care environment in recent years has been the cerebral perfusion pressure (CPP), which is the difference between MAP and ICP (i.e, CPP = MAP − ICP). The maintenance of an acceptable CPP has been postulated to be critical in reducing cerebral ischemia and secondary injury. The goal CPP can be achieved by increasing MAP through the use of fluids and/or vasopressors or by lowering elevated ICP. The BTF/AANS guidelines originally recommended that CPP be maintained greater than 70 mm Hg based on a number of studies that demonstrated decreased morbidity and mortality in patients whose CPP was actively sustained above 70 to 80 mm Hg.[23] However, in 2003, the BTF/AANS issued an updated recommendation that CPP be maintained at 60 mm Hg or more.[46] In children, the recommended CPP goal is greater than 40 mm Hg.[28] Furthermore, the updated recommendation is that aggressive attempts to maintain CPP greater than 70 mm Hg in adults should be avoided in the absence of cerebral ischemia because of the risk of the acute respiratory distress syndrome.[24,47] One recent study challenges the relative importance of CPP in TBI patients, suggesting that the primary focus should be on lowering the ICP to less than 20 mm Hg.[48] In essence, the results of this clinical investigation were that an ICP of 20 mm Hg or more was the most powerful predictor of neurologic deterioration as long as the CPP was maintained above 60 mm Hg.[48]

CLINICAL CONTROVERSIES

The principal goal in severe TBI patients should be normalization of ICP. However, for over a decade, much attention has been paid to maintenance of CPP (MAP − ICP) without conclusive evidence as to what an ideal goal for CPP should be. In either case, the goal should be to lower the ICP below 20 mm Hg.

Despite no significant improvement in outcome in the most extensive investigation to date, a recent meta-analysis of 12 hypothermia trials in the treatment of severe TBI patients did discern potential benefits of this cerebral-protective maneuver. At present, most clinicians would consider hypothermia to be an investigational treatment until additional data become available.

The MAP can be increased through normalization of the intravascular volume combined with pharmacologically inducing systemic hypertension as needed. The goal of volume expansion should be euvolemia as well as avoidance of a hypoosmolar state and negative fluid balance.[28,49] If the hematocrit is below 30%, transfusion of packed red blood cells (PRBCs) is indicated. Volume status should be targeted to a pulmonary artery wedge pressure of between 10 and 14 mm Hg if invasive monitoring is employed.[50] After achievement of euvolemia, the patient's head should be elevated at 30 degrees to promote venous drainage and decrease ICP. If restoration of the intravascular volume is inadequate in elevating MAP to an acceptable level, hypertension should be induced using vasopressors or inotropic support. The drugs employed most commonly to induce hypertension are the sympathomimetic amines, dopamine, norepinephrine, and phenylephrine. While none of these agents has shown superiority, norepinephrine is a reasonable selection at a starting dose of 0.02 mcg/kg per minute based on its predominant vasoconstrictive properties.[50] Patients should be monitored for renal dysfunction, lactic acidosis, and signs of peripheral ischemia when these agents are used, especially at large doses.

TREATMENT OF INTRACRANIAL HYPERTENSION

GENERAL PHARMACOLOGIC STRATEGIES

◀5 The use of analgesics, sedatives, and paralytics has an important primary role in the management of intracranial hypertension (Fig. 56–3). This is related directly to the association of pain,

agitation, excessive muscle movement, and resisting mechanical ventilation with transient increases in ICP.[51] Nonetheless, there have been no studies of the effect of sedation on outcome in patients with severe TBI.[23] Morphine sulfate is the most commonly used analgesic and sedative in this setting.[6,51,52] Propofol has become the sedative of choice in TBI patients among many clinicians because of its ease of titration, rapidly reversible effects on discontinuation, and possible neuroprotective effects.[6,53,54] Although it is used for sedation in infants and children who are mechanically ventilated in the ICU setting, the Food and Drug Administration (FDA) required that the manufacturer labeling contain specific information that propofol is not approved for sedation of pediatric patients admitted to an ICU. This is due in part to the publication of 10 case reports of fatal metabolic acidosis in critically ill children who received propofol.[55] While a direct association between propofol and metabolic acidosis remains unclear, symptoms tend to occur with large doses (>4.8–30 mg/kg per hour) and prolonged infusions (>48–72 hours). Likewise, long-term infusions in excess of 5 mg/kg per hour should be used cautiously in TBI patients based on a recently published case report series suggesting an association between propofol and cardiac failure.[56] Triglyceride concentrations also should be monitored in patients receiving prolonged propofol infusions and/or high dosages of propofol considering its lipid emulsion formulation and the potential for inducing hypertriglyceridemia under these conditions. Alternative sedatives include etomidate (particularly useful in rapid-induction anesthesia),[6] intermittent low-dose pentobarbital, and short-acting benzodiazepines (e.g., midazolam), especially if there is a reasonable suspicion of alcohol withdrawal as the underlying etiology of the agitation.[51,52] The potential for these agents to decrease MAP and CPP must be monitored closely. The use of any sedative agent also must be weighed against its potential to obscure the neurologic examination of the patient. Cautious reversal of the effect of benzodiazepines with flumazenil can be used to allow examination of the patient.[52] Interference with the neurologic examination is also associated with paralytic agents. Prophylactic neuromuscular blockade (i.e., unrelated to ICP control) is not recommended based on evidence indicating increased complications (e.g., pneumonia, prolonged paralysis) and length of stay following paralytic use.[6]

■ HYPERVENTILATION

◀6 The practice of prolonged aggressive hyperventilation (PaCO$_2$ < 25 mm Hg) to decrease ICP is no longer recommended.[23,24] Hyperventilation acutely decreases systemic and cerebral PaCO$_2$. The resulting hypocapnia, in turn, induces cerebral vasoconstriction, thereby decreasing CBF and cerebral blood volume (CBV).[57,58] For decades, it was a widely held belief that a reduction in CBV and any accompanying decrease in ICP were beneficial. Nonetheless, a systematic review of the literature concluded that data are inadequate to ascertain potential benefit or harm from hyperventilation.[32] Other studies have determined that severe TBI patients with normocapnia versus those receiving aggressive hyperventilation have an improved outcome at 3 and 6 months.[23,24] Furthermore, recent evidence using microdialysis and local CBF techniques suggests that aggressive hyperventilation may increase extracellular glutamate, a mediator of secondary injury, and lactate concentrations.[59] Despite the decrease in CBF during hyperventilation, no detrimental decrease in CMRo$_2$ was observed in a recent study.[58] Nonetheless, the potential for decreased CBF to increase the possibility for cerebral ischemia must be weighed. In consideration of the equivocal data relative to the merits of therapeutic

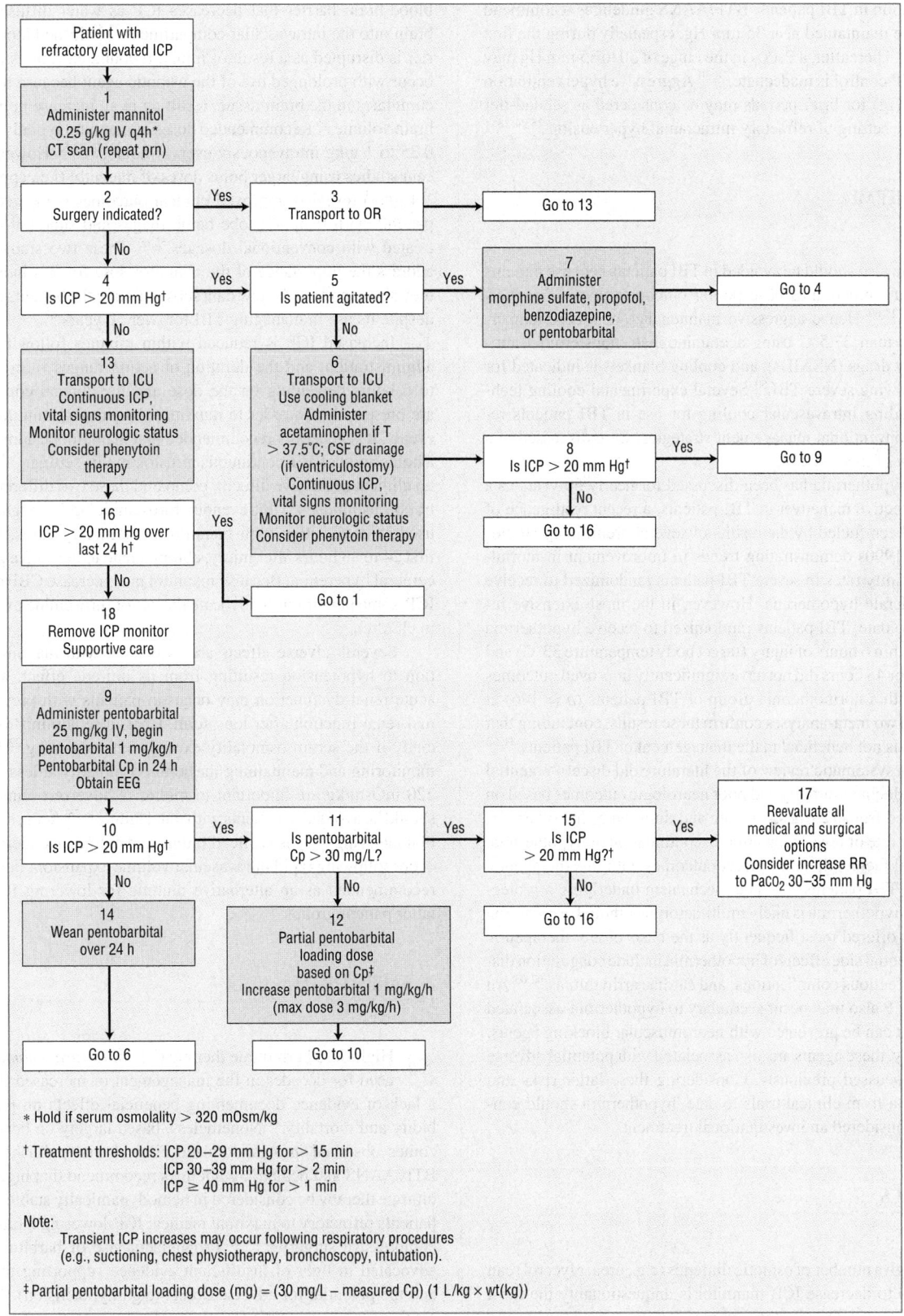

FIGURE 56–3. Algorithm for the management of increased ICP. Cp, plasma concentration; CT, computed tomography; OR, operating room; ICP, intracranial pressure; ICU, intensive care unit; T, temperature; CSF, cerebrospinal fluid; EEG, electroencephalogram; RR, respiratory rate; PaCO₂, partial pressure of arterial blood carbon dioxide. (*Adapted with permission Boucher BA. Neurotrauma: Pharmacotherapy Self Assessment Program, 3d ed., Module 2: Critical Care. Chicago, American College of Clinical Pharmacy, 1999;215–238.*)

hyperventilation in TBI patients, BTF/AANS guidelines recommend that PaCO$_2$ be maintained near 35 mm Hg, especially during the first 24 hours.[23,24] Thereafter, a PaCO$_2$ in the range of 30 to 35 mm Hg may be used if ICP control is inadequate.[28,50] Aggressive hyperventilation (25–30 mm Hg) for brief periods may be considered as second-tier therapy in the setting of refractory intracranial hypertension.[23,24,28]

HYPOTHERMIA

Hyperthermia also should be avoided in TBI patients because patients with elevated temperatures have poorer outcomes than normothermic patients.[28,60] Hence aggressive maintenance of a core temperature of less than 37.5°C using acetaminophen, nonsteroidal anti-inflammatory drugs (NSAIDs), and cooling blankets is indicated for patients following severe TBI.[50] Several experimental cooling techniques, including intravascular cooling for use in TBI patients refractory to conventional management strategies, were discussed in a recent review of this topic.[60]

While hypothermia has been discussed for nearly 50 years as a cerebral protective maneuver in TBI patients, a recent resurgence of interest has been fueled by the results of several preliminary studies in the early 1990s demonstrating trends in improvement in mortality and morbidity rates in severe TBI patients randomized to receive mild to moderate hypothermia. However, in the most extensive investigation to date, TBI patients randomized to receive hypothermia ($n = 199$) within 6 hours of injury (target body temperature 33°C) and maintained for 48 hours did not have significantly improved outcomes compared with a normothermia group of TBI patients ($n = 196$) at 6 months.[61] Two meta-analyses confirm these results, concluding that hypothermia is not beneficial in the management of TBI patients.[31,62] Regardless, a systematic review of the literature did discern potential benefits in reducing mortality and poor neurologic outcomes based on data combined from 12 trials.[63] Depth and duration of hypothermia, as well as the rate of rewarming after discontinuation of hypothermia, are additional factors that may affect outcomes with this therapeutic maneuver in TBI patients.[63,64] The mechanism underlying a protective effect of hypothermia is likely multifactorial, although a reduction in CMR$_{O_2}$ is offered most frequently as the basis of any therapeutic benefits. Potential side effects of hypothermia include coagulation disturbances, infectious complications, and cardiac arrhythmias.[62,63] An increase in ICP also may occur secondary to hypothermia-associated shivering that can be prevented with neuromuscular blocking agents. Unfortunately, these agents are also associated with potential adverse events, as discussed previously. Considering these latter risks and equivocal data from clinical trials to date, hypothermia should continue to be considered an investigational treatment.

DIURETICS

Although a number of osmotic diuretics (e.g., urea, glycerol) can be used to decrease ICP, mannitol is unquestionably the most widely employed.[51] Despite the common practice of administering mannitol to patients with suspected or actual increases in ICP following brain injury, no clinical trial comparing its effects against placebo have been performed.[29] The mechanisms responsible for mannitol's beneficial effects likely relate to (1) an immediate plasma-expanding effect that reduces blood viscosity and increases CBF and (2) establishment of an osmotic concentration gradient across an intact blood-brain barrier that decreases ICP as water diffuses from the brain into the intravascular compartment.[23,51] If the blood-brain barrier is disrupted as a result of injury, rebound elevations of ICP may occur with prolonged use of the osmotic agent because mannitol accumulates in the brain tissue, resulting in an increase in intracellular brain volume.[51] Recommended doses of mannitol typially range from 0.25 to 1 g/kg intravenously every 4 hours.[23,24,52] However, two recent studies using larger bolus doses of mannitol (i.e., approximately 1.4 g/kg) revealed improved clinical outcomes compared with TBI patients with temporal lobe hemorrhages and subdural hematomas treated with conventional dosages.[65,66] These two studies not only address the importance of the mannitol dose for this indication, but they also represent the few data substantiating the benefits of mannitol despite its use in managing TBI for over 50 years.[67]

Increased ICP is reduced within minutes following mannitol administration, and the duration of action ranges from 90 minutes to 6 hours depending on the dose and the clinical conditions that are present.[23,24] In order to maximize benefit and minimize adverse events, it is generally recommended that mannitol be administered as a bolus and not as a continuous infusion in this setting.[23,24] However, no clinical trials have directly compared these two different administration techniques.[29] Intravenous furosemide (0.5–1 mg/kg) may be used in conjunction with mannitol in refractory cases. During the first 24 to 48 hours after injury, children tend to develop a generalized cerebral hyperemia. Because mannitol may increase CBF and worsen ICP, some practitioners advocate the use of furosemide over mannitol in children.

Several adverse effects are associated with mannitol. In addition to hypotension resulting from its diuretic effect, a reversible acute renal dysfunction may occur in patients with previously normal renal function after long-term, large-dose administration, especially if the serum osmolality exceeds 320 mOsm/kg.[23,24,52] Hence monitoring and maintaining the serum osmolality at less than 310 to 320 mOsm/kg are important to minimize adverse events. Mannitol should be avoided in patients with renal failure.[6,28] Acute exacerbation of underlying congestive heart failure and pulmonary edema also may occur following rapid intravascular volume expansion. Furosemide is recommended as an alternative diuretic for lowering ICP in these latter patient groups.

BARBITURATES

High-dose barbiturate therapy (i.e., *barbiturate coma*) has been used for decades in the management of increased ICP despite a lack of evidence documenting beneficial effects on patient morbidity and mortality.[33] Nonetheless, based largely on beneficial outcomes observed in a randomized clinical trial published in 1988, BTF/AANS and pediatric guidelines recommend that high-dose barbiturate therapy be considered in hemodynamically stable severe TBI patients refractory to maximal medical ICP-lowering therapy and decompressive surgery.[23,24,28] Prophylactic use of barbiturates is not advocated in light of insufficient evidence supporting this practice and the potential for adverse events (e.g., hypotension).[24,33] Several mechanisms responsible for the cerebral protective effects of barbiturates have been proposed. These include (1) lowering the regional CMR$_{O_2}$ with a coupled reduction in CBF to these areas, (2) inhibition of lipid peroxidation, and (3) alteration of cerebral vascular tone.[52]

Prior to inducing a barbiturate coma, the severe TBI patient must be mechanically ventilated with continuous monitoring of arterial blood pressure, electrocardiogram (ECG), and ICP. Pentobarbital is the most commonly used barbiturate for this indication, although thiopental also has been used. Pentobarbital should be administered as an intravenous loading infusion totaling 25 mg/kg (i.e., 10 mg/kg over 30 minutes and then 5 mg/kg per hour for 3 hours), followed by an initial maintenance infusion of 1 mg/kg per hour.[41] The maintenance infusion can be titrated upward if needed to a maximum of 2–3 mg/kg per hour.[52] If the systolic blood pressure falls during the loading or maintenance infusions, the rate should be slowed temporarily and blood pressure support initiated. The goal of a barbiturate coma is to maintain ICP and CPP at the previously discussed target thresholds in addition to achieving a pentobarbital steady-state concentration of between 30 and 40 mg/L and EEG burst suppression. Initiation of barbiturate therapy withdrawal can occur when ICP has been controlled satisfactorily for 24 to 48 hours.[24] Barbiturates should be tapered over 24 to 72 hours to prevent ICP spikes.

Side effects associated with high-dose barbiturate therapy involve primarily the cardiovascular system. Hypotension caused by peripheral vasodilation may occur, necessitating decreasing the barbiturate dose or the administration of fluids and vasopressors to maintain blood pressure. A recent systematic review of the literature suggested that one of every four patients receiving barbiturate therapy will develop hypotension.[33] Gastrointestinal (GI) effects of barbiturates include decreased GI muscular tone and decreased amplitude of contraction. On emergence from coma, there may be a period of GI hypermotility. Care should be taken to avoid extravasation of pentobarbital and thiopental solutions because severe tissue damage may occur. Barbiturates should be administered by continuous infusion through a central line dedicated for this purpose. The potential for barbiturates to induce the hepatic drug metabolism of concurrent medications should be also considered. Lastly, the potential for prolonged interference with the proclamation of brain death in TBI patients meeting the locally accepted brain death neurologic criteria must be considered prior to the initiation of high-dose barbiturate therapy.

CORTICOSTEROIDS

Although corticosteroids are effective in preventing or reducing cerebral edema in patients with nontraumatic conditions producing vasogenic edema, most studies in TBI patients have not demonstrated that they lower ICP or improve outcome.[24] In addition, use of corticosteroids following TBI has been associated with increased complications, including GI bleeding, glucose intolerance, electrolyte abnormalities, and infection.[50] Based on several major randomized trials, the BTF/AANS adult and pediatric guidelines recommend that corticosteroids not be used.[24,28] Recent systematic reviews nonetheless have concluded that neither moderate benefits nor moderate harmful effects of corticosteroids in TBI patients can be excluded after review of all clinical trial data collected to date.[34] Noteworthy is that an international investigation known as the CRASH (Corticosteroid Randomization After Significant Head Injury) study was initiated in an attempt to define the merits of corticosteroid therapy in patients with TBI.[68] In this study 10,008 patients with a GCS score ≤ 14 were randomized to receive a 48-hour continuous infusion of methylprednisolone or placebo. Preliminary results of this study indicate a higher risk of death within 2 weeks of enrollment (relative risk 1.18) in those patients receiving corticosteroids compared with patients receiving placebo ($p < 0.001$).[68] Thus, corticosteroids should not be used to treat TBI patients regardless of severity.[68]

TREATMENT AND PROPHYLAXIS OF POSTTRAUMATIC SEIZURES

It is generally agreed that patients who have experienced one or more seizures following a moderate to severe TBI should receive anticonvulsant therapy to avoid increases in CMR_{O_2} that occur with the onset of subsequent seizures. Initial therapy in these persons should consist of incremental intravenous doses of diazepam (5–40 mg adults, 0.1–0.5 mg/kg infants and children) or lorazepam (2–8 mg adults, 0.03–0.1 mg/kg infants and children) to terminate any active seizure activity followed by intravenous phenytoin to prevent seizure recurrence. Phenytoin dosing regimens for adults and pediatric patients include an intravenous loading dose of 15–20 and 10–15 mg/kg, respectively, followed by a maintenance dose of 5 mg/kg per day. Alternatively, fosphenytoin, a water-soluble phosphate ester of phenytoin, can be administered intravenously or intramuscularly using the same doses, specified as phenytoin equivalents (PE). The merits of preventive anticonvulsant therapy in patients who have not had a seizure postinjury historically has been more controversial. Risk factors for early posttraumatic seizures (<7 days after injury) include a GCS score of less than 10, a cortical contusion, a depressed skull fracture, a subdural hematoma, an epidural hematoma, an intracerebral hematoma, a penetrating head wound, or a seizure within the first 24 hours of injury.[24] In a landmark randomized, placebo-controlled study, the incidence of early posttraumatic seizures in patients receiving placebo was 14.2% compared with 3.6% in patients receiving phenytoin ($p < 0.05$) without a significant increase in drug-related side effects.[69,70] A recent systematic review of the literature corroborated these findings, estimating an improved pooled relative risk for early seizure prevention of 0.34 (95% confidence interval: 0.21–0.54) in patients receiving anticonvulsants.[36] Thus it is recommended that phenytoin (or alternatively carbamazepine) should be used to prevent seizures in TBI patients at high risk during the first 7 days after injury.[24,28,71] Valproate therapy is not recommended based on a trend for higher mortality in a study comparing valproate-treated patients with those receiving phenytoin short-term therapy.[72] The benefits of prophylactic anticonvulsants beyond 7 days have not been demonstrated, and thus their use for this indication is not recommended.[24,36,72] Unfortunately, despite reducing the incidence of early seizures following brain injury, no beneficial effects have been documented for anticonvulsants on patient mortality or long-term disability.[36]

SUPPORTIVE CARE

While normalizing ICP and maintaining an adequate CPP are the highest priorities in preventing secondary injury following severe TBI, attention also must be given to preventing and/or treating systemic and extracranial complications. This includes careful ongoing fluid and electrolyte management.[73] Common electrolyte disturbances in TBI patients that should be monitored and treated aggressively include hyponatremia, hypomagnesemia, hypokalemia, and hypophosphatemia. Aggressive nutritional support of the TBI patient is another important therapeutic consideration.[24,28] Evidence suggests that early feeding of TBI patients may be associated with a trend toward better outcomes in terms of survival and disability.[30] Infectious complications commonly encountered in severe TBI patients include nosocomial pneumonia, sepsis, urinary tract infections, and meningitis.[74,75] Treatment of these potentially devastating infections should be aggressive, with careful attention being paid to antibiotic blood-brain barrier penetration for intracranial infections. Adjunctive administration of granulocyte colony-stimulating factor also has received limited attention relative to preventing nosocomial infections in these patients.[76,77] Other important therapeutic interventions include correction of any documented coagulopathy,[78] acute gastritis prophylaxis,[6] prevention of thromboembolic events,[78,79] fever control,[80] and prevention of decubi and contractures.

CLINICAL PATHWAYS/GUIDELINE IMPLEMENTATION

Use of clinical pathways and formal TBI management guidelines has been demonstrated to improve TBI patient outcomes and reduce institutional resource utilization. For example, implementation of a severe TBI clinical pathway resulted in a significant reduction in length of stay, ICU stay, and ventilator days among survivors at one institution.[81] Implementation of published TBI guidelines also has been demonstrated to have significant impact on patient outcomes compared with historical controls in two other institutions.[82,83] Nonetheless, the challenges of using historical controls in evaluating the effects of changes in practice standards was raised as a concern in one of these two investigations.[84] Regardless, few practitioners would dispute the overall importance of integrating current evidence-based management guidelines into clinical practice as a means to optimize care and improve the functional outcome of TBI patients.[84]

INVESTIGATIONAL THERAPY

The steady decrease in morbidity and mortality following severe neurotrauma over the last 30 years can be attributed largely to expeditious and aggressive management of events resulting in secondary injury (i.e., ischemia, hypoxia, increased ICP) using conventional treatment strategies.[7] Numerous neuroprotective agents targeting specific pathophysiologic processes that are theorized to occur following severe TBI have been investigated over the last decade in an attempt to further enhance the prospects for a meaningful recovery. A review of these investigations is presented below. Unfortunately, none of these agents to date has demonstrated a significant reduction in morbidity or mortality following severe TBI in phase III clinical trials with the exception of nimodipine in a subset of patients.

Numerous explanations have been offered as to the variance between benefits observed in animal models of brain injury using a variety of neuroprotective drugs and their lack of effectiveness in patients. These include mechanistic differences in secondary brain injury between animal models and patients,[85–87] patient heterogenicity relative to intracranial and extracranial pathology,[85,86] inadequate sample size,[88] poor drug penetration into the brain,[89,90] insensitive outcome measures,[89,90] patient enrollment imbalances,[89,90] and unrealistic improvement expectations.[86,89] Other issues that require careful attention in future clinical trials to maximize the utility of these agents are the dose, timing, and sequencing of drug administration; duration of therapy relative to the traumatic event; and possibly combination therapy.[85–87] The process of obtaining informed consent in an expeditious manner is also a formidable challenge in this patient subset, as is true of other critically ill patient subsets.[91] Inherent delays in obtaining informed consent prior to investigational drug administration may compromise potential benefits derived from the agent and eliminate the possibility of prehospital treatment of the TBI patient except in the rare instance where waiver of informed consent has

been granted. Despite the investigational study failures to date, the search is likely to continue for neuroprotective agents that eventually may improve the long-term outcome in severe TBI patients by avoiding some of the pitfalls in study design present in previous negative investigations.

MODULATION OF CALCIUM INFLUX

Calcium Antagonists

The calcium antagonists are obvious candidates for potentially attenuating the deleterious effects of calcium influx in acute neurotrauma patients. Nimodipine, a dihydropyridine, has been studied most extensively among the calcium antagonists that block the post-synaptic L-type calcium channel. Unfortunately, two major trials of nimodipine in adult TBI patients did not demonstrate a statistically significant improvement in outcome compared with placebo.[92] A significant benefit was observed in the subgroup of patients with posttraumatic subarachnoid hemorrhage (tSAH) receiving nimodipine that was corroborated in a follow-up investigation.[93] The nimodipine dosage used in the latter investigation was 2 mg/h intravenously for 7 to 10 days, followed by 360 mg daily administered orally until day 21 of treatment.[93] A recent sytematic review of the literature concluded that nimodipine may be beneficial in tSAH patients, although there is insufficient evidence to support the use of calcium antagonists in unselected TBI patients.[35] Systemic hypotension is a relative limitation with the use of other L-type calcium channel antagonists for this indication.

Another target for calcium modulation is the presynaptic N-type voltage-sensitive calcium channels. Omega conotoxin (SNX-111, ziconotide) is one such antagonist that has been evaluated in TBI patients. Unfortunately, a major phase III trial of omega conotoxin was halted prematurely after an interim analysis deemed the likelihood for a favorable outcome to be very small compared with placebo.[85] Profound systemic hypotension requiring vasopressor support was a major concern with use of this agent.

Glutamate Antagonists

A significant amount of experimental evidence has been accumulated confirming the efficacy of NMDA receptor antagonists in attenuating secondary injury events following model brain injury. Based on these results, both competitive and noncompetitive NMDA receptor antagonists have been developed as neuroprotective agents. D-CPP-ene and CGS 19755 (Selfotel) are investigational NMDA antagonists competing with glutamate at the receptor site (i.e., competitive antagonists). Results of two phase III Selfotel clinical trials involving 693 patients did not demonstrate increased efficacy compared with placebo and possible increased mortality and serious brain-related adverse events in the treatment groups during interim analysis of the data.[94] As such, the trials were stopped prematurely.[94] Noncompetitive NMDA antagonists or receptor channel blockers bind to the open NMDA receptor, thereby blocking the ionic current. Compounds within this group include ketamine, phencyclidine, dextromethorphan, dextrorphan, and the investigational agents dizocilpine (MK-801), dexanabinol (which also possesses free-radical scavenging properties),[95] and aptiganel (Cerestat). A phase III trial of aptiganel also was discontinued prematurely based on limited benefit (1.1%) in favor of the treatment over placebo in the first 340 patients studied.[7] Another NMDA receptor antagonist that selectively blocks the NR2B regulatory site on the postsynaptic receptor and has undergone clinical investigation is CP-101,606.[96] A phase III study involving 600 severe TBI patients randomized to receive either CP-101,606 or placebo was completed recently. Results of this investigation are expected in the future. A phase II trial of of dexanabinol in 67 severe TBI patients was completed recently and demonstrates it to be safe and well tolerated; a trend toward faster and superior neurologic outcomes also was observed.[95]

ANTIOXIDANTS/FREE RADICAL SCAVENGERS

The potential role of oxygen free radicals in the pathophysiology of TBI has stimulated interest in the use of antioxidants to interrupt the self-perpetuating cycle of membrane destruction in these patients. Tirilazad (Freedox), a 21-aminosteroid, is one such antioxidant that has undergone phase III testing in TBI, stroke, and subarachnoid hemorrhage (SAH) patients. An attractive feature of this steroid analog is that although it is a potent inhibitor of lipid peroxidation, it is essentially devoid of glucocorticoid activity. Unfortunately, two major trials of tirilazad in TBI patients were unable to demonstrate efficacy compared with placebo.[89,97] An enzymatic free-radical scavenger that has undergone clinical trials in severe TBI patients is superoxide dismutase conjugated to a polyethylene glycol polymer (PEG-SOD; pegorgotein, Dismutec). While results of the preliminary phase II trial were promising, no statistically significant improvement in outcome or mortality was observed in the larger phase III trial in severe TBI patients receiving two doses of pegorgotein compared with placebo.[98]

OTHER TREATMENT STRATEGIES

Formation of inflammatory mediators including the metabolites of arachidonic acid has been implicated in the latter stages of tertiary injury following neurotrauma. As such, both cyclooxygenase inhibitors (e.g., NSAIDs)[99,100] and mixed cyclooxygenase-lipooxygenase inhibitors (e.g., BW7544C) have been studied in experimental neurotrauma models with limited success. Furthermore, the immunosuppressant cyclosporin A has received some attention relative to attenuation of cortical damage in animal models of TBI.[87,101] Inhibitors of inflammatory mediators also are under consideration as neuroprotective agents. These include antagonists to bradykinin,[102] platelet-activating factor, cytokines, leukotriene LT4, and capase-1.[103] Lastly, various growth factors, including brain-derived neurotrophic factor, nerve growth factor, neurotrophin-3, and erythropoietin,[104] and co-factors such as insulin-like growth factor 1[105] and GM1 ganglioside may have a future role in the management of TBI by promoting nerve cell regeneration and differentiation.[37] Such neurorestorative strategies may be classified as structural or functional.[7] Importantly, such strategies may be the most fertile targets for genetic manipulation in the future and may have significant implications for post-TBI rehabilitation.[7]

EVALUATION OF THERAPEUTIC OUTCOMES

The process for evaluation of therapeutic outcomes is summarized in Table 56–3. Patients with severe TBI require ICU monitoring initially with the goals of maintaining or reestablishing neurologic and systemic homeostasis as well as readily detecting any neurologic deterioration.[50] This requires frequent evaluation of the patient's neurologic status (e.g., GCS) and measurement of vital signs, urine output, and arterial oxygen saturation (as well as ICP in patients with an ICP monitor in place). Furthermore, careful attention must be paid to the potential for a variety of electrolyte, mineral, and acid-base disturbances, coagulopathies, and infections by obtaining various laboratory tests on a daily basis initially. The intensity of monitoring will be a function of the relative degree of neurologic and hemodynamic

TABLE 56–3. Evaluation of Therapeutic Outcomes

General	GCS: Record hourly initially, decrease frequency as neurologic status stabilizes
	Vital signs (BP, HR, RR, temperature): Record hourly initially, decrease frequency as neurologic status stabilizes
	Urine output: Record hourly initially, decrease frequency as neurologic status stabilizes
	Arterial oxygen saturation: Continuously while in intensive care unit
Risk of increased ICP	ICP: Record hourly, decrease frequency as ICP stabilizes less than 20 mm Hg
	CPP: Record hourly, decrease frequency as CPP stabilizes in excess of 60 mm Hg[a]
Laboratory tests	Ethanol concentration and urine drug screen: On admission
	ABGs: Daily at a minimum while intubated, repeated as needed based on pulmonary instability requiring ventilator setting changes
	CBC: Daily while in intensive care unit
	Serum electrolytes (Na, K, Cl): Daily while in intensive care unit
	Minerals (Mg, Ca, P): Daily initially until concentrations stable
Radiologic procedures	CT scan: Postresuscitation initially with repeat scan(s) as needed based on degree of neurologic instability (e.g., decrease in GCS)

GCS, Glasgow Coma Scale; BP, blood pressure; HR, heart rate; RR, respiratory rate; CSF, cerebrospinal fluid; TBI, traumatic brain injury; ICP, intracranial pressure; CPP, cerebral perfusion pressure; ABG, arterial blood gas; CBC, complete blood count; Na, sodium; K, potassium; Cl, chloride; Mg, magnesium; Ca, calcium; P, phosphorus; CT, computed tomography.
[a]Continuous monitoring mandated initially if technologically feasible.

stability of the patient in the hours and days following the neurologic insult. Lastly, radiologic tests (e.g., CT scans) are essential not only for the initial diagnostic evaluation of TBI patients but also as means to evaluate the etiology for any subsequent neurologic deterioration as well.

ABBREVIATIONS

AANS: American Association of Neurological Surgeons
ABG: arterial blood gas
ATP: adenosine triphosphate
BTF: Brain Trauma Foundation
CBF: cerebral blood flow
CBV: cerebral blood volume
CDo_2: cerebral oxygen delivery
$CMRo_2$: cerebral oxygen consumption
CNS: central nervous system
CPP: cerebral perfusion pressure
CSF: cerebrospinal fluid
CT: computed tomography
ECG: electrocardiogram
GCS: Glasgow Coma Scale
GI: gastrointestinal
ICP: intracranial pressure
MAP: mean arterial pressure
NMDA: N-methyl-D-aspartate
NSAID: nonsteroidal anti-inflammatory drug
PBRCs: packed red blood cells
SBP: systolic blood pressure
$Sjvo_2$: jugular venous oxygen saturation
TBI: traumatic brain injury
tSAH: traumatic subarachnoid hemorrhage

REFERENCES

1. Centers for Disease Control and Prevention (CDC). Traumatic Brain Injury in the United States: A Report to Congress. Atlanta, CDC, National Center for Injury and Prevention and Control, 1999.
2. Adekoya N, Thurman DJ, White DD, Webb KW. Surveillance for traumatic brain injury deaths—United States, 1989–1998. MMWR Surveill Summ 2002;51:1–14.
3. Centers for Disease Control and Prevention (CDC). Injury Fact Book 2001–2002. Atlanta, CDC, National Center for Injury Prevention and Control, 2001.
4. Kraus JF, McArthur DL, Silverman TA, Jayaraman M. Epidemiology of brain injury. In: Narayan RK, Wilberger JE, Povlishock JT, eds. Neurotrauma. New York, McGraw-Hill, 1996:13–30.
5. Veremakis C, Lindner DH. Central nervous system injury: Essential physiologic and therapeutic concerns. In: Civetta JM, Taylor RW, Kirby RR, eds. Critical Care. Philadelphia, Lippincott-Raven, 1997:273–289.
6. Marik PE, Varon J, Trask T. Management of head trauma. Chest 2002; 122:699–711.
7. Marshall LF. Head injury: Recent past, present, and future. Neurosurgery 2000;47:546–561.
8. Chesnut RM. Avoidance of hypotension: Conditio sine qua non of successful severe head-injury management. J Trauma 1997;42:S4–9.
9. Bouma GJ, Muizelaar JP, Choi SC, et al. Cerebral circulation and metabolism after severe traumatic brain injury: The elusive role of ischemia. J Neurosurg 1991;75:685–693.
10. Martin NA, Patwardhan RV, Alexander MJ, et al. Characterization of cerebral hemodynamic phases following severe head trauma: Hypoperfusion, hyperemia, and vasospasm. J Neurosurg 1997;87:9–19.
11. Woodman T, Robertson CS. Jugular venous oxygen saturation monitoring. In: Narayan RK, Wilberger JE, Povlishock JT, eds. Neurotrauma. New York, McGraw-Hill, 1996.
12. Young W. Death by calcium: A way of life. In: Narayan RK, Wilberger JEJ, Povlishock JT, eds. Neurotrauma. New York, McGraw-Hill, 1996: 1421–1431.
13. Ray SK, Dixon CE, Banik NL. Molecular mechanisms in the pathogenesis of traumatic brain injury. Histol Histopathol 2002;17:1137–1152.
14. Kampfl A, Posmantur RM, Zhao X, et al. Mechanisms of calpain proteolysis following traumatic brain injury: Implications for pathology and therapy—a review and update. J Neurotrauma 1997;14:121–134.
15. Hall ED. Free radicals and lipid peroxidation. In: Narayan RK, Wilberger JE, Povlishock JT, eds. Neurotrauma. New York, McGraw-Hill, 1996: 1405–1419.
16. Cristofori L, Tavazzi B, Gambin R, et al. Early onset of lipid peroxidation after human traumatic brain injury: A fatal limitation for the free radical scavenger pharmacological therapy? J Investig Med 2001;49:450–458.
17. Raghupathi R, Graham DI, McIntosh TK. Apoptosis after traumatic brain injury. J Neurotrauma 2000;17:927–938.
18. Huang PP, Esquenazi S, Le Roux PD. Cerebral cortical neuron apoptosis after mild excitotoxic injury in vitro: Different roles of mesencephalic and cortical astrocytes. Neurosurgery 1999;45:1413–1422.
19. Hsu CY, Hu ZY, Doster SK. Cell-mediated injury. In: Narayan RK, Wilberger JE, Povlishock JT, eds. Neurotrauma. New York, McGraw-Hill, 1996:1433–1444.
20. Teasdale GM, Nicoll JA, Murray G, Fiddes M. Association of apolipoprotein E polymorphism with outcome after head injury. Lancet 1997;350:1069–1071.
21. Graham DI, Horsburgh K, Nicoll JA, Teasdale GM. Apolipoprotein E and the response of the brain to injury. Acta Neurochir Suppl (Wien) 1999; 73:89–92.
22. Signorini DF, Andrews PJ, Jones PA, et al. Predicting survival using simple clinical variables: A case study in traumatic brain injury. J Neurol Neurosurg Psychiatry 1999;66:20–25.
23. Bullock R, Chesnut RM, Clifton GL, et al. Guidelines for the management of severe head injury. Brain Trauma Foundation, American Association of Neurological Surgeons, Joint Section on Neurotrauma and Critical Care. J Neurotrauma 1996;13:641–734.
24. Bullock R, Chesnut RM, Clifton GL, et al. Guidelines for the management of severe head injury. Brain Trauma Foundation, American Association of Neurological Surgeons, Joint Section on Neurotrauma and Critical Care. J Neurotrauma 2000;17:449–627.
25. Marion DW, Spiegel TP. Changes in the management of severe traumatic brain injury: 1991–1997. Crit Care Med 2000;28:16–18.
26. Maas AI, Dearden M, Teasdale GM, et al. EBIC guidelines for management of severe head injury in adults. European Brain Injury Consortium. Acta Neurochir 1997;139:286–294.
27. Gabriel EJ, Ghajar J, Jagoda A, et al. Guidelines for prehospital management of traumatic brain injury. J Neurotrauma 2002;19:111–174.
28. Adelson PD, Bratton SL, Carney NA, et al. Guidelines for the acute medical management of severe traumatic brain injury in infants, children, and adolescents. Crit Care Med 2003;31:S417–491.
29. Roberts I, Schierhout G, Wakai A. Mannitol for acute traumatic brain injury. Cochrane Database Syst Rev 2003.
30. Yanagawa T, Bunn F, Roberts I, et al. Nutritional support for head-injured patients. Cochrane Database Syst Rev 2003.
31. Gadkary CS, Alderson P, Signorini DF. Therapeutic hypothermia for head injury. Cochrane Database Syst Rev 2003.
32. Roberts I, Schierhout G. Hyperventilation therapy for acute traumatic brain injury. Cochrane Database Syst Rev 2003.
33. Roberts I. Barbiturates for acute traumatic brain injury. Cochrane Database Syst Rev 2003.
34. Alderson P, Roberts I. Corticosteroids for acute traumatic brain injury. Cochrane Database Syst Rev 2003.
35. Langham J, Goldfrad C, Teasdale G, et al. Calcium channel blockers for acute traumatic brain injury. Cochrane Database Syst Rev 2003.
36. Schierhout G, Roberts I. Antiepileptic drugs for preventing seizures following acute traumatic brain injury. Cochrane Database Syst Rev 2003.

37. Teasdale GM, Graham DI. Craniocerebral trauma: Protection and retrieval of the neuronal population after injury. Neurosurgery 1998;43: 723–737.

38. Simma B, Burger R, Falk M, et al. A prospective, randomized, and controlled study of fluid management in children with severe head injury: Lactated Ringer's solution versus hypertonic saline. Crit Care Med 1998; 26:1265–1270.

39. Shackford SR, Bourguignon PR, Wald SL, et al. Hypertonic saline resuscitation of patients with head injury: A prospective, randomized clinical trial. J Trauma 1998;44:50–58.

40. Qureshi AI, Suarez JI, Castro A, Bhardwaj A. Use of hypertonic saline/acetate infusion in treatment of cerebral edema in patients with head trauma: Experience at a single center. J Trauma 1999;47:659–665.

41. Bulger EM, Nathens AB, Rivara FP, et al. Management of severe head injury: Institutional variations in care and effect on outcome. Crit Care Med 2002;30:1870–1876.

42. Cruz J. The first decade of continuous monitoring of jugular bulb oxyhemoglobin saturation: Management strategies and clinical outcome. Crit Care Med 1998;26:344–351.

43. Latronico N, Beindorf AE, Rasulo FA, et al. Limits of intermittent jugular bulb oxygen saturation monitoring in the management of severe head trauma patients. Neurosurgery 2000;46:1131–1138.

44. Hutchinson PJ, O'Connell MT, Al-Rawi PG, et al. Clinical cerebral microdialysis: A methodological study. J Neurosurg 2000;93:37–43.

45. Ingebrigtsen T, Romner B. Biochemical serum markers of traumatic brain injury. J Trauma 2002;52:798–808.

46. Brain Trauma Foundation. Guidelines for the Management of Severe Traumatic Brain Injury: Cerebral Perfusion Pressure. January 5, 2003 update, *http://www2.braintrauma.org*.

47. Contant CF, Valadka AB, Gopinath SP, et al. Adult respiratory distress syndrome: A complication of induced hypertension after severe head injury. J Neurosurg 2001;95:560–568.

48. Juul N, Morris GF, Marshall SB, Marshall LF. Intracranial hypertension and cerebral perfusion pressure: Influence on neurological deterioration and outcome in severe head injury. The Executive Committee of the International Selfotel Trial. J Neurosurg 2000;92:1–6.

49. Clifton GL, Miller ER, Choi SC, Levin HS. Fluid thresholds and outcome from severe brain injury. Crit Care Med 2002;30:739–745.

50. Kelly DF, Doberstein C, Becker DP. General principles of head injury management. In: Narayan RK, Wilberger JE, Povlishock JT, eds. Neurotrauma. New York, McGraw-Hill, 1996:71–101.

51. Duhaime AC. Conventional drug therapies for head injury. In: Narayan RK, Wilberger JE, Povlishock JT, eds. Neurotrauma. New York, McGraw-Hill, 1996:365–374.

52. Chesnut RM. Treating raised intracranial pressure in head injury. In: Narayan RK, Wilberger JE, Povlishock JT, eds. Neurotrauma. New York, McGraw-Hill, 1996:445–469.

53. Bao YP, Williamson G, Tew D, et al. Antioxidant effects of propofol in human hepatic microsomes: Concentration effects and clinical relevance. Br J Anaesth 1998;81:584–589.

54. Kelly DF, Goodale DB, Williams J, et al. Propofol in the treatment of moderate and severe head injury: A randomized, prospective double-blinded pilot trial. J Neurosurg 1999;90:1042–1052.

55. Susla G. Propofol toxicity in critically ill pediatric patients. Show us the proof. Crit Care Med 1998;26:1959–1960.

56. Cremer OL, Moons KG, Bouman EA, et al. Long-term propofol infusion and cardiac failure in adult head-injured patients. Lancet 2001;357:117–118.

57. Skippen P, Seear M, Poskitt K, et al. Effect of hyperventilation on regional cerebral blood flow in head-injured children. Crit Care Med 1997; 25:1402–1409.

58. Diringer MN, Yundt K, Videen TO, et al. No reduction in cerebral metabolism as a result of early moderate hyperventilation following severe traumatic brain injury. J Neurosurg 2000;92:7–13.

59. Marion DW, Puccio A, Wisniewski SR, et al. Effect of hyperventilation on extracellular concentrations of glutamate, lactate, pyruvate, and local cerebral blood flow in patients with severe traumatic brain injury. Crit Care Med 2002;30:2619–2625.

60. Thompson HJ, Tkacs NC, Saatman KE, et al. Hyperthermia following traumatic brain injury: A critical evaluation. Neurobiol Dis 2003;12:163–173.

61. Clifton GL, Miller ER, Choi SC, et al. Lack of effect of induction of hypothermia after acute brain injury. N Engl J Med 2001;344:556–563.

62. Harris OA, Colford JM Jr, Good MC, Matz PG. The role of hypothermia in the management of severe brain injury: A meta-analysis. Arch Neurol 2002;59:1077–1083.

63. McIntyre LA, Fergusson DA, Hebert PC, et al. Prolonged therapeutic hypothermia after traumatic brain injury in adults: A systematic review. JAMA 2003;289:2992–2999.

64. Tokutomi T, Morimoto K, Miyagi T, et al. Optimal temperature for the management of severe traumatic brain injury: Effect of hypothermia on intracranial pressure, systemic and intracranial hemodynamics, and metabolism. Neurosurgery 2003;52:102–111.

65. Cruz J, Minoja G, Okuchi K. Improving clinical outcomes from acute subdural hematomas with the emergency preoperative administration of high doses of mannitol: A randomized trial. Neurosurgery 2001;49:864–871.

66. Cruz J, Minoja G, Okuchi K. Major clinical and physiological benefits of early high doses of mannitol for intraparenchymal temporal lobe hemorrhages with abnormal pupillary widening: A randomized trial. Neurosurgery 2002;51:628–637.

67. Schrot RJ, Muizelaar JP. Mannitol in acute traumatic brain injury. Lancet 2002;359:1633–1634.

68. CRASH Trial Collaborators. Effect of intravenous corticosteroids on death within 14 days in 10,008 adults with clinically significant head injury (MRC CRASH trial): Randomised placebo-controlled trial. Lancet 2004;364:1321–1328.

69. Temkin NR, Dikmen SS, Wilensky AJ, et al. A randomized, double-blind study of phenytoin for the prevention of post-traumatic seizures. N Engl J Med 1990;323:497–502.

70. Haltiner AM, Newell DW, Temkin NR, et al. Side effects and mortality associated with use of phenytoin for early posttraumatic seizure prophylaxis. J Neurosurg 1999;91:588–592.

71. Chang BS, Lowenstein DH. Practice parameter: Antiepileptic drug prophylaxis in severe traumatic brain injury: Report of the Quality Standards Subcommittee of the American Academy of Neurology. Neurology 2003;60:10–16.

72. Temkin NR, Dikmen SS, Anderson GD, et al. Valproate therapy for prevention of posttraumatic seizures: A randomized trial. J Neurosurg 1999; 91:593–600.

73. Andrews BT. Fluid and electrolyte management in the head-injured patient. In: Narayan RK, Wilberger JE, Povlishock JT, eds. Neurotrauma. New York, McGraw-Hill, 1996:331–344.

74. Girou E, Stephan F, Novara A, et al. Risk factors and outcome of nosocomial infections: Results of a matched case-control study of ICU patients. Am J Respir Crit Care Med 1998;157:1151–1158.

75. Greenberg SB, Atmar RL. Infectious complications after head injury. In: Narayan RK, Wilberger JE, Povlishock JT, eds. Neurotrauma. New York, McGraw-Hill, 1996:703–722.

76. Heard SO, Fink MP, Gamelli RL, et al. Effect of prophylactic administration of recombinant human granulocyte colony-stimulating factor (filgrastim) on the frequency of nosocomial infections in patients with acute traumatic brain injury or cerebral hemorrhage. The Filgrastim Study Group. Crit Care Med 1998;26:748–754.

77. Ishikawa K, Tanaka H, Takaoka M, et al. Granulocyte colony-stimulating factor ameliorates life-threatening infections after combined therapy with barbiturates and mild hypothermia in patients with severe head injuries. J Trauma 1999;46:999–1007.

78. Lazio BE, Simard JM. Anticoagulation in neurosurgical patients. Neurosurgery 1999;45:838–847.

79. Kim J, Gearhart MM, Zurick A, et al. Preliminary report on the safety of heparin for deep venous thrombosis prophylaxis after severe head injury. J Trauma 2002;53:38–42.

80. Bruder N, Raynal M, Pellissier D, et al. Influence of body temperature, with or without sedation, on energy expenditure in severe head-injured patients. Crit Care Med 1998;26:568–572.

81. Vitaz TW, McIlvoy L, Raque GH, et al. Development and implementation of a clinical pathway for severe traumatic brain injury. J Trauma 2001;51: 369–375.

82. Palmer S, Bader MK, Qureshi A, et al. The impact on outcomes in a community hospital setting of using the AANS traumatic brain injury guidelines. Americans Associations for Neurologic Surgeons. J Trauma 2001; 50:657–664.

83. Elf K, Nilsson P, Enblad P. Outcome after traumatic brain injury improved by an organized secondary insult program and standardized neurointensive care. Crit Care Med 2002;30:2129–2134.

84. Boucher BA, Wood GC. Why not use guidelines for the management of severe traumatic brain injury? Crit Care Med 2002;30:2164–2165.

85. Bullock MR, Lyeth BG, Muizelaar JP. Current status of neuroprotection trials for traumatic brain injury: Lessons from animal models and clinical studies. Neurosurgery 1999;45:207–217; discussion 217–220.

86. Teasdale GM, Maas A, Iannotti F, et al. Challenges in translating the efficacy of neuroprotective agents in experimental models into knowledge of clinical benefits in head injured patients. Acta Neurochir Suppl 1999; 73:111–116.

87. Faden AI. Neuroprotection and traumatic brain injury: Theoretical option or realistic proposition. Curr Opin Neurol 2002;15:707–712.

88. Dickinson K, Bunn F, Wentz R, et al. Size and quality of randomised, controlled trials in head injury: Review of published studies. Br Med J 2000;320:1308–1311.

89. Maas AI, Steyerberg EW, Murray GD, et al. Why have recent trials of neuroprotective agents in head injury failed to show convincing efficacy? A pragmatic analysis and theoretical considerations. Neurosurgery 1999; 44:1286–1298.

90. Doppenberg EM, Choi SC, Bullock R. Clinical trials in traumatic brain injury: What can we learn from previous studies? Ann NY Acad Sci 1997; 825:305–322.

91. Davis N, Pohlman A, Gehlbach B, et al. Improving the process of informed consent in the critically ill. JAMA 2003;289:1963–1968.

92. Murray GD, Teasdale GM, Schmitz H. Nimodipine in traumatic subarachnoid haemorrhage: A reanalysis of the HIT I and HIT II trials. Acta Neurochir 1996;138:1163–1167.

93. Harders A, Kakarieka A, Braakman R. Traumatic subarachnoid hemorrhage and its treatment with nimodipine. German tSAH Study Group. J Neurosurg 1996;85:82–89.

94. Morris GF, Bullock R, Marshall SB, et al. Failure of the competitive N-methyl-D-aspartate antagonist Selfotel (CGS 19755) in the treatment of severe head injury: Results of two phase III clinical trials. The Selfotel Investigators. J Neurosurg 1999;91:737–743.

95. Knoller N, Levi L, Shoshan I, et al. Dexanabinol (HU-211) in the treatment of severe closed head injury: A randomized, placebo-controlled, phase II clinical trial. Crit Care Med 2002;30:548–554.

96. Merchant RE, Bullock MR, Carmack CA, et al. A double-blind, placebo-controlled study of the safety, tolerability and pharmacokinetics of CP-101,606 in patients with a mild or moderate traumatic brain injury. Ann NY Acad Sci 1999;890:42–50.

97. Marshall LF, Maas AI, Marshall SB, et al. A multicenter trial on the efficacy of using tirilazad mesylate in cases of head injury. J Neurosurg 1998; 89:519–525.

98. Young B, Runge JW, Waxman KS, et al. Effects of pegorgotein on neurologic outcome of patients with severe head injury: A multicenter, randomized controlled trial. JAMA 1996;276:538–543.

99. Slavik RS, Rhoney DH. Indomethacin: A review of its cerebral blood flow effects and potential use for controlling intracranial pressure in traumatic brain injury patients. Neurol Res 1999;21:491–499.

100. Hurley SD, Olschowka JA, O'Banion MK. Cyclooxygenase inhibition as a strategy to ameliorate brain injury. J Neurotrauma 2002;19:1–15.

101. Scheff SW, Sullivan PG. Cyclosporin A significantly ameliorates cortical damage following experimental traumatic brain injury in rodents. J Neurotrauma 1999;16:783–792.

102. Marmarou A, Nichols J, Burgess J, et al. Effects of the bradykinin antagonist Bradycor (deltibant, CP-1027) in severe traumatic brain injury: Results of a multi-center, randomized, placebo-controlled trial. American Brain Injury Consortium Study Group. J Neurotrauma 1999;16:431–444.

103. Sanchez Mejia RO, Ona VO, Li M, Friedlander RM. Minocycline reduces traumatic brain injury–mediated caspase-1 activation, tissue damage, and neurological dysfunction. Neurosurgery 2001;48:1393–1399; discussion 1399–1401.

104. Buemi M, Cavallaro E, Floccari F, et al. Erythropoietin and the brain: From neurodevelopment to neuroprotection. Clin Sci (Lond) 2002;103: 275–282.

105. Hatton J, Rapp RP, Kudsk KA, et al. Intravenous insulin-like growth factor-I (IGF-I) in moderate-to-severe head injury: A phase II safety and efficacy trial. J Neurosurg 1997;86:779–786.

57

PARKINSON'S DISEASE

Merlin V. Nelson, Richard C. Berchou, and Peter A. LeWitt

Learning Objectives and other resources can be found at *www.pharmacotherapyonline.com.*

KEY CONCEPTS

◀1 Amantadine and anticholinergic medications are useful for relieving mild features of idiopathic Parkinson's disease (IPD).

◀2 The optimal time to start carbidopa/L-dopa is controversial, but in general, treatment should be started when the disease interferes with the patient's occupation, activities of daily living, or quality of life.

◀3 Anticholinergic medication should be used with caution in the elderly or those with preexisting cognitive difficulties.

◀4 Carbidopa/L-dopa is the most effective medication for symptomatic treatment of IPD.

◀5 L-Dopa response fluctuations may be explained primarily by its pharmacokinetic and pharmacodynamic properties.

◀6 Most carbidopa/L-dopa–treated patients eventually will develop response fluctuations.

◀7 Selegiline, catechol-*O*-methyl-transferase (COMT) inhibitors, and controlled-release carbidopa/L-dopa decrease response fluctuations through pharmacokinetic mechanisms.

◀8 Dopamine agonists are L-dopa–sparing and decrease response fluctuations but are more likely to cause psychiatric symptoms such as hallucinations.

◀9 Close management of medication dosing and administration times is necessary to optimize therapeutic outcomes and avoid adverse effects.

While its clinical manifestations previously had escaped attention, *paralysis agitans* acquired an unmistakable presence following the 1817 publication by an obscure British physician, James Parkinson.[1] Parkinson provided vivid descriptions of such characteristic features as an "involuntary tremulous motion," "the hand failing to answer with exactness to the dictates of the will," and the tendency to "pass from a walking to a running pace." Later observers added a variety of signs and symptoms, among them rigidity and instability of balance, to define idiopathic Parkinson's disease (IPD) as we know it today.

EPIDEMIOLOGY

The annual incidence of IPD increases with age from about 20 per 100,000 persons in the fifth decade of life to about 90 per 100,000 persons in the seventh decade of life, with the usual age of onset at about age 60.[2] Extensive epidemiologic research of IPD suggests that environmental factors such as rural living, drinking well water, and heavy metal and hydrocarbon exposure have small but demonstrable contributions to the risk for IPD. Interestingly, cigarette smoking, caffeine consumption, and nonsteroidal anti-inflammatory drug use are associated with protection against the illness.[3-5]

The onset of IPD in later life implies that cumulative exposures to putative toxins, factors associated with central nervous system (CNS) aging, or other as yet uncharacterized cell death mechanisms may be responsible for the onset and progression of the disease. While IPD is sporadic in most instances, genetic factors may have a role in its etiology, particularly if the disease begins before age 50. Nine genetic linkages and four genes have been identified in parkinsonism.[6]

These include mutations of *α-synuclein* (which transcribes a presynaptic protein) and *parkin* genes. These genes have been associated with autosomal dominant and autosomal recessive early-onset Parkinson's kindreds, respectively. Pathologic findings and some aspects of the phenotype are different from those in IPD; however, *parkin* gene mutations may predispose to both early- and late-onset forms of IPD.[7]

ETIOLOGY

The pathogenesis of IPD is not known. Neurotoxins highly selective for substantia nigra pars compacta (SNc) dopaminergic neurons are instructive because animal models of parkinsonism can be created with 6-hydroxydopamine and with 1-methyl-4-phenyl-1,2,3,6-tetrahydropyridine (MPTP). The latter compound is converted by monoamine oxidase (MAO) type B to the toxic 1-methyl-4-phenylpyridinium ion (MPP^+). MAO-B inhibition by selegiline eliminates the toxicity of MPTP. MPP^+ is toxic to neurons by interfering with mitochondrial metabolism. Another mechanism of toxicity that has received consideration for the pathogenesis of IPD is cellular damage from oxyradicals.[8] Dopamine generates free radicals from autooxidation and from MAO metabolism (Fig. 57–1). Several antioxidative mechanisms are present within and outside neurons to limit any damage that might be produced by free-radical attack, but one possibility is that such protection might be overwhelmed or impaired in IPD. Excitotoxicity, programmed cell death activation, and chronic infection are also under consideration for IPD etiology.[9]

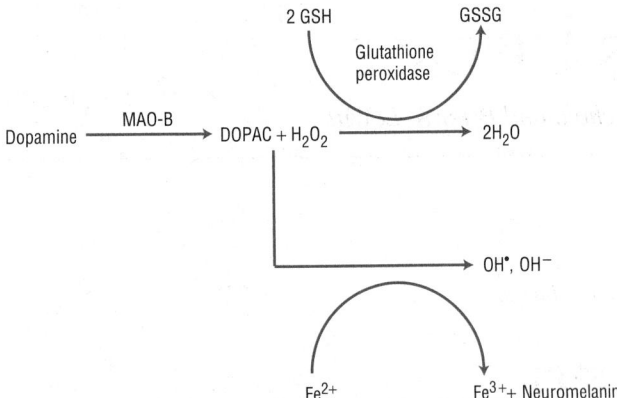

FIGURE 57–1. Dopamine metabolism results in hydrogen peroxide (H_2O_2) formation. If the glutathione system is deficient or excess hydrogen peroxide is present, hydrogen peroxide accepts an electron from ferrous iron (Fe^{2+}), forming ferric iron (Fe^{3+}) and the hydroxyl free radical (OH*). The hydroxyl free radical can cause lipid peroxidation, thereby damaging neuronal cell membranes. MAO-B, monoamine oxidase B; DOPAC, 3,4-dihydroxyphenylacetic acid; H_2O, water; GSH, glutathione; GSSG, glutathione disulfide; OH^-, the hydroxide ion.

PATHOPHYSIOLOGY

Dopaminergic projections from the SNc to the striatum (putamen and caudate) synapse on two populations of efferent neurons (Fig. 57–2). The direct pathway involves activation of striatal D_1 dopamine receptors that stimulate inhibitory γ-aminobutyric acid (GABA)/substance P efferents to the globus pallidus interna (GPi) and substantia nigra pars reticulata (SNr). The indirect pathway involves activation of striatal D_2 dopamine receptors that inhibit inhibitory GABA/enkephalin efferents to the globus pallidus externa (GPe). The GPe projects inhibitory GABA neurons to the subthalamic nucleus (STN). Here, excitatory glutaminergic neurons project to the GPi. GPi output is inhibitory on the ventroanterior and ventrolateral thalamic projections to the frontal cortex. Thus loss of nigrostriatal dopamine neurons in IPD results in reduction of cortical activation (see Fig. 57–2). Virtually all the motor deficits of IPD are attributable to the marked loss in dopaminergic neurons projecting to the putamen.

In actuality, the pathways and interactions involved have a greater complexity than those described in this model.[10] The synaptic organization of the basal ganglia involves a variety of neurotransmitters and neuromodulators, including acetylcholine, dopamine, GABA, glutamate, enkephalins, substance P, adenosine, and serotonin. Each is a target for intervention in IPD. Drugs enhancing dopaminergic or inhibiting acetylcholine or glutamate neurotransmission have been successful in IPD therapeutics. The role for drug modulation of other neurotransmitters active in the basal ganglia has not been explored fully, but recent results with adenosine A_{2A} receptor antagonists are promising.[11,12]

The model of dopaminergic depletion or blockade in producing parkinsonian features provided much of the impetus for development of therapies to augment stimulation of striatal dopamine receptors. Stimulation of D_1 dopamine receptors activates adenylate cyclase. D_2 dopamine receptors are coupled to a guanosine triphosphate (GTP)–binding protein that opens potassium channels to hyperpolarize neurons, thereby reducing the excitability of striatal cells.[13] In IPD, activation of the D_2 receptor appears to be of primary importance for mediating both clinical improvements and some adverse effects (such as hallucinations). Dyskinesias are more likely to occur with L-dopa therapy (D_1 and D_2 agonism) than with dopamine agonist therapy

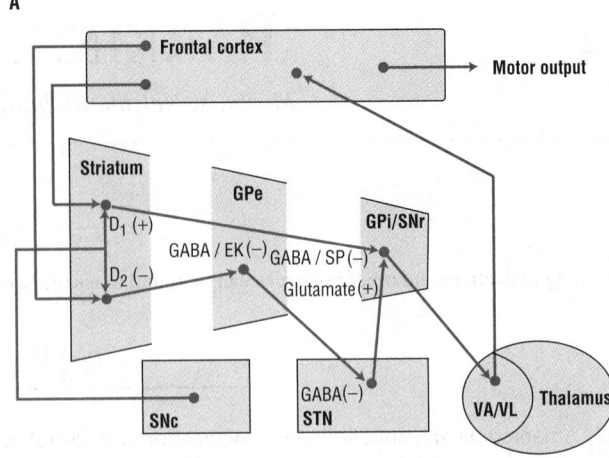

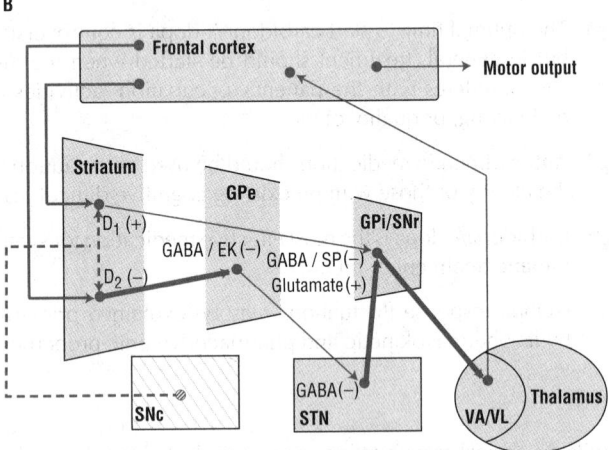

FIGURE 57–2. *A.* The normal balance of the basal ganglia–thalamocortical circuit. GPe, globus pallidus externa; GPi, globus pallidus interna; SNr, substantia nigra pars reticulata; SNc, substantia nigra pars compacta; VA, ventroanterior nuclei of the thalamus; VL, ventrolateral nuclei of the thalamus; STN, subthalamic nucleus. *B.* With nigrostriatal degeneration (*dashed line*), there is loss of inhibition of the GPi by the direct pathway and activation of the GPi via the indirect pathway, resulting in decreased activation of the cortex. See text for details.

(primarily D_2 agonism), suggesting D_1 receptor involvement in producing dyskinesia.

Pathologic findings reveal a markedly decreased number of nigrostriatal neurons and a correlation between the extent of nigrostriatal dopamine loss and the severity of clinical features. The threshold for onset of parkinsonism appears to be the loss of 70% to 80% of these neurons.[14] [^{18}F]Fluorodopa positron-emission tomography (PET) measures aromatic amino acid decarboxylase activity, whereas other PET ligands and [^{123}I]2β-carbomethoxy-3β-(4-iodophenyl)tropane (β-CIT) single-photon-emission computed tomography measure dopamine transporter (DAT) activity. In IPD, these functional imaging studies suggest compensatory responses such as upregulation of dopamine synthesis and downregulation of synaptic dopamine reuptake. These responses may help to explain how such a significant loss of neurons can be relatively asymptomatic.[15,16] Progressive supranuclear palsy (PSP) and other "Parkinson plus" disorders are not responsive to dopamine replacement or dopamine agonist therapies, presumably on the basis of decreased dopamine receptors owing to postsynaptic damage beyond the neuropathologic changes in IPD.

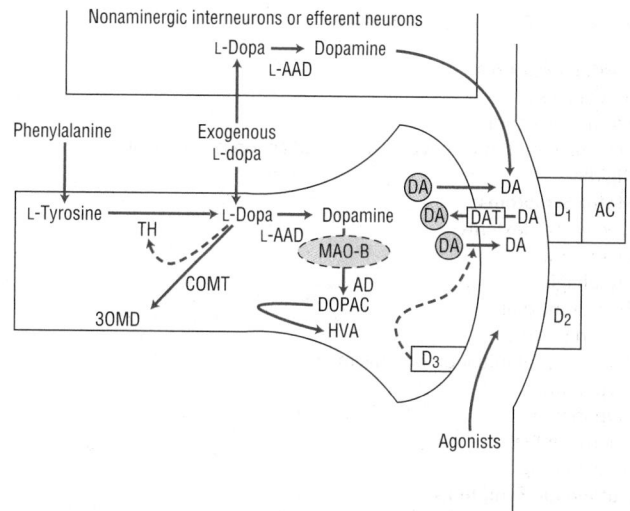

FIGURE 57–3. Dopamine metabolism in presynaptic dopamine neuron (see text for full details). 3OMD, 3-*O*-methyldopa; AC, adenylate cyclase; AD, aldehyde dehydrogenase; COMT, catechol-*O*-methyl transferase; D_1–D_3, dopamine receptors; DA, dopamine; DAT, dopamine transporter; DOPAC, 3,4-dihydroxyphenylacetic acid; HVA, homovanillic acid; L-AAD, L-aromatic amine decarboxylase; MAO-B, monoamine oxidase B; TH, tyrosine hydroxylase.

Dopamine metabolism is shown in Fig. 57–3, and the range of therapeutic interventions for IPD is summarized in Table 57–1. L-Tyrosine, the metabolic precursor of dopamine, is converted by tyrosine hydroxylase (TH) to L-dihydroxyphenylalanine (L-dopa) in a highly regulated synthetic process. L-Dopa is decarboxylated to dopamine by the enzyme L-amino acid decarboxylase (L-AAD). L-AAD is present outside the CNS and in some nonaminergic neurons, whereas TH is found exclusively in aminergic neurons. Peripheral decarboxylation can be blocked by antagonists of L-AAD (carbidopa or benserazide) that do not pass the blood-brain barrier. Use of these drugs with L-dopa increases the CNS penetration of exogenously administered L-dopa and decreases adverse effects from the peripheral metabolism to dopamine. Dopamine is stored in synaptic vesicles until stimulated to be released into the synapse by calcium-dependent mechanisms. Dopamine activity is terminated primarily by reuptake into the presynaptic neuron by means of a specific dopamine transporter. Sequestration into the storage granules of the presynaptic neurons or the actions of catabolic pathways involving MAO or catechol-*O*-methyl-transferase (COMT) leads to inactivation of dopamine.

Since dopamine tonically inhibits acetylcholine neurons in the striatum, the degeneration of nigrostriatal dopamine neurons results in a relative increase of striatal cholinergic interneuron activity. This increased cholinergic activity contributes especially to the tremor of IPD, as evidenced by symptomatic improvement with the use of anticholinergics and worsening with cholinergic agents.

IPD has a characteristic neuropathologic picture that permits differentiation from similar clinical syndromes. In the SNc, loss of neurons and Lewy bodies (a neuronal inclusion body composed of amyloid neurofilaments) is always found. Lewy bodies appear in degenerating neurons in association with adjacent gliosis. The loss of pars compacta neurons is the basis for loss of dopamine projections to the striatum. Small numbers of Lewy bodies can be found in other neurologic disorders and in normal aging. The occurrence of SNc Lewy bodies in patients without parkinsonism indicates that the disease can exist as a pathologic entity with less involvement than necessary for

TABLE 57–1. Mechanisms for Potential IPD Treatments

Increase Endogenous Dopamine
L-Dopa
  Inhibit peripheral metabolism by dopa decarboxylase
    Carbidopa
    Benserazide
  Sustained-release products
  Infusions
    Intravenous
    Duodenal/jejunal
  Inhibit catechol-*O*-methyl-transferase
    Entacapone (peripheral only)
    Tolcapone (peripheral and central)
  Inhibit central and peripheral metabolism by monoamine oxidase B
    Selegiline (deprenyl)
    Rasagiline
Dopamine Agonists
D_2-specific
  Bromocriptine
  Dihydroergocryptine
  Lisuride
  Rotigotine
  Sumanirole
D_2- and D_3-specific
  Pramipexole
  Ropinirole
D_1- and D_2-nonspecific
  Pergolide
  Apomorphine
    Intravenous
    Subcutaneous infusions
    Intranasal
    Sublingual
Partial agonists
  Terguride
Adenosine A_{2a}
Istradefylline (KW-6002)
Anticholinergic
Benztropine
Trihexyphenidyl

causing clinical signs and symptoms (incidental Parkinson's disease). Even patients whose clinical features strongly suggest IPD may lack its characteristic pathology.

CLINICAL PRESENTATION

While the disorder is unmistakable in its advanced form, distinguishing mild IPD from changes seen with normal aging can be challenging. Diagnostic criteria specify that at least two of the following must be present: limb muscle rigidity, resting tremor (at 3–6 Hz and abolished by movement), bradykinesia, or postural instability.[17] For the diagnosis of IPD, other conditions must be excluded (Table 57–2). Medication-induced parkinsonism can mimic the idiopathic disorder, so it is important to establish if such medications have been used (e.g., antipsychotics, antiemetics, or metoclopramide). Several neurodegenerative conditions resemble the clinical picture of IPD, including PSP, striatonigral degeneration, olivopontocerebellar degeneration, and rarely, Huntington's or Wilson's disease. In order to distinguish IPD from secondary parkinsonism, other diagnostic criteria include lack of other neurologic impairments and responsiveness to L-dopa.

TABLE 57–2. Differential Diagnosis of Parkinsonism

Idiopathic parkinsonism (Parkinson's disease, Lewy body parkinsonism)
Secondary parkinsonism
   Drug-induced
      Antipsychotics (phenothiazines, butyrophenones, risperidone,
        others)
      Antiemetics (metoclopramide, prochlorperazine)
      Other drugs (reserpine, alpha-methyldopa)
   Toxic
      Carbon monoxide poisoning
      Hydrogen sulfide
      Manganese
      Methanol
      MPTP (1-methyl-4-phenyl-1-2-5-6-tetrahydropyridine)
      Petrochemicals
   Neoplasms or strokes in the regions of the nigrostriatal pathways
   Traumatic lesions interrupting substantia nigra projections
   Normal-pressure hydrocephalus
Parkinsonism with other neuronal system degenerations
   Wilson's disease (copper deposition in the brain)
   Progressive supranuclear palsy
   Pallidonigral degeneration
   Corticobasalganglionic degeneration
   Alzheimer's disease
   Multiple-system atrophy
      Striatonigral degeneration
      Shy-Drager syndrome
      Olivopontocerebellar atrophy

TABLE 57–3. Clinical Features

Cardinal Features
Bradykinesia
Postural instability
Resting tremor (may have postural and action components)
Rigidity
Motor Symptoms
Decreased dexterity
Dysarthria
Dysphagia
Festinating gait
Flexed posture
"Freezing" at initiation of movement
Hypomimia
Hypophonia
Micrographia
Slow turning
Autonomic Symptoms
Bladder and anal sphincter disturbances
Constipation
Diaphoresis
Orthostatic blood pressure changes
Paroxysmal flushing
Sexual disturbances
Mental Status Changes
Bradyphrenia
Confusional state
Dementia
Psychosis (paranoia, hallucinosis)
Sleep disturbance
Other
Fatigability
Oily skin
Pedal edema
Seborrhea
Weight loss

IPD develops insidiously and progresses slowly in most patients, although progression sometimes arrests. Initial complaints may include sensory symptoms, but as the disease progresses, the patient exhibits one or more classic clinical features: resting tremor, rigidity, bradykinesia, or change in posture. Characteristic problems, even in mildly affected patients, include small handwriting (micrographia), decreased facial animation (hypomimia) and blink rate, diminished arm swing while walking, shuffling gait, soft or indistinct speech (hypophonia), and decreased dexterity in everyday activities. Symptoms can progress to severe functional impairment, at which time patients may require nursing home placement and may be confined to bed or wheelchair. Other clinical characteristics of IPD are listed in Table 57–3.

Bradykinesia refers to slowness of movement. Movement in IPD is often slow throughout an intended action, but initiation of movement may display a hesitation out of proportion to slowness affecting completion of the movement. A progressive slowing and decline in dexterity with repetition may impair tasks such as finger tapping. Intermittent immobility (*freezing*) is another common characteristic. Freezing is especially likely to occur in situations such as when walking in a crowd or when walking through a narrow doorway. Patients also may experience a slow shuffling gait with difficulty halting their steps while in motion.

Tremor occurring at rest is highly typical of IPD and often is the sole presenting complaint; however, only two-thirds of parkinsonian patients have tremor on diagnosis, and some will never develop this sign. Tremor in IPD is present most commonly in the hands, sometimes with a characteristic pill-rolling. It also can involve the jaw or legs. Sometimes the sensory equivalent is perceived as an "internal" sensation of vibration without outward manifestations. Like other symptoms of IPD, resting tremor often begins unilaterally and may persist in this distribution. Stressful situations or use of limbs in other activities may increase tremor amplitude in a limb at rest. Usually, volitional movement abolishes resting tremor, and it is absent during sleep.

Rigidity is the increased muscular resistance to passive range of motion and often has a cog-wheeling quality. Because it can lead to falls, postural instability is one of the most disabling problems of parkinsonism. A disturbance of appropriate responses to the perturbation of balance is common in advanced IPD. Testing for impaired postural responses by means of the pull test (in which a patient is unable to recover balance after sudden backward displacement at the shoulders) can help to identify the risk for falling. Many patients with impaired postural responses also have tendencies for propulsive gait (festination) and a forward flexed posture of their axial structures along with partial flexion of the extremities.

IPD is predominantly a disorder of motor capabilities; however, neuropsychological abnormalities can be detected even in patients with early or mild forms of the disorder and without obvious cognitive impairments. Although intellectual deterioration is not inevitable in IPD, some patients deteriorate in a manner indistinguishable from Alzheimer's disease and other dementing conditions.[18] It is difficult to estimate the number of patients at risk because medications and concomitant illnesses can confound analysis for the extent of cognitive decline owing specifically to IPD. IPD patients are also at increased risk for depression. While the disabilities of IPD may provoke depression in some instances, the biochemical changes in the brain due to IPD also may predispose for endogenous depression.

▶ TREATMENT: Parkinson's Disease

▨ SURGICAL THERAPY

The most effective surgical technique is deep brain stimulation (DBS) of the STN, which decreases outflow from this region (as shown in Fig. 57–2*B*) and thus reduces input to the thalamus.[19] STN DBS is especially useful for tremor, dyskinesias, gait disorder, and start hesitation. Thalamic DBS and thalamotomy (a focal destructive lesion of the thalamus) can reduce disabling tremor. Pallidotomy (a focal destructive lesion of the GPi) and GPi DBS can help with severe dyskinesias and on/off fluctuations but is not as helpful for bradykinesia. Destructive lesions are immediate and permanent, whereas DBS requires lifelong maintenance. Transplantation of autologous adrenal medulla tissue was unsuccessful, as has been more recent experience in most cases of fetal tissue transplantation.

▨ PHARMACOLOGIC THERAPY

Treatment algorithms for early and advanced IPD are shown in Figs. 57–4 and 57–5. More detailed treatment information has been published, as have evidence-based assessments of treatment interventions.[20,21] The only established pharmacologic therapy for IPD is medication that can transiently reverse signs and symptoms.

Patients with mild features of IPD and no disability do not need symptomatic medication. With advancing disability, however, symptomatic therapy is vital for maintaining independence.

The most efficacious treatment for IPD is replacement of the natural neurotransmitter dopamine by the use of its immediate precursor L-dopa. As indicated in the treatment algorithm shown in Fig. 57–4, anticholinergic drugs or amantadine can be used for treating resting tremor as an alternative to L-dopa. While not highly effective against bradykinesia, gait disturbance, or other features of advanced parkinsonism, these medications can be useful for relieving mild disabilities experienced by patients in the first few years after the onset of parkinsonism. The decision to incorporate L-dopa or dopamine agonist therapy comes from advancing disability and ineffectiveness of alternative medications to provide adequate symptomatic control. Depending on profession and lifestyle, the same basic parkinsonian features may result in different degrees of disability, and drug therapy goals may need to be adjusted accordingly. A summary of available antiparkinsonian medications is listed in Table 57-4.

Selegiline and other MAO-B inhibitors (lazabemide and rasagiline) have been studied not only for symptomatic effects but also for possible neuroprotection. Recently, the National Institute of Neurological Disorders and Stroke formed a committee for identifying and implementing studies of potential therapies against the progression of IPD.[22] Twenty-one promising agents were identified from an initial 59

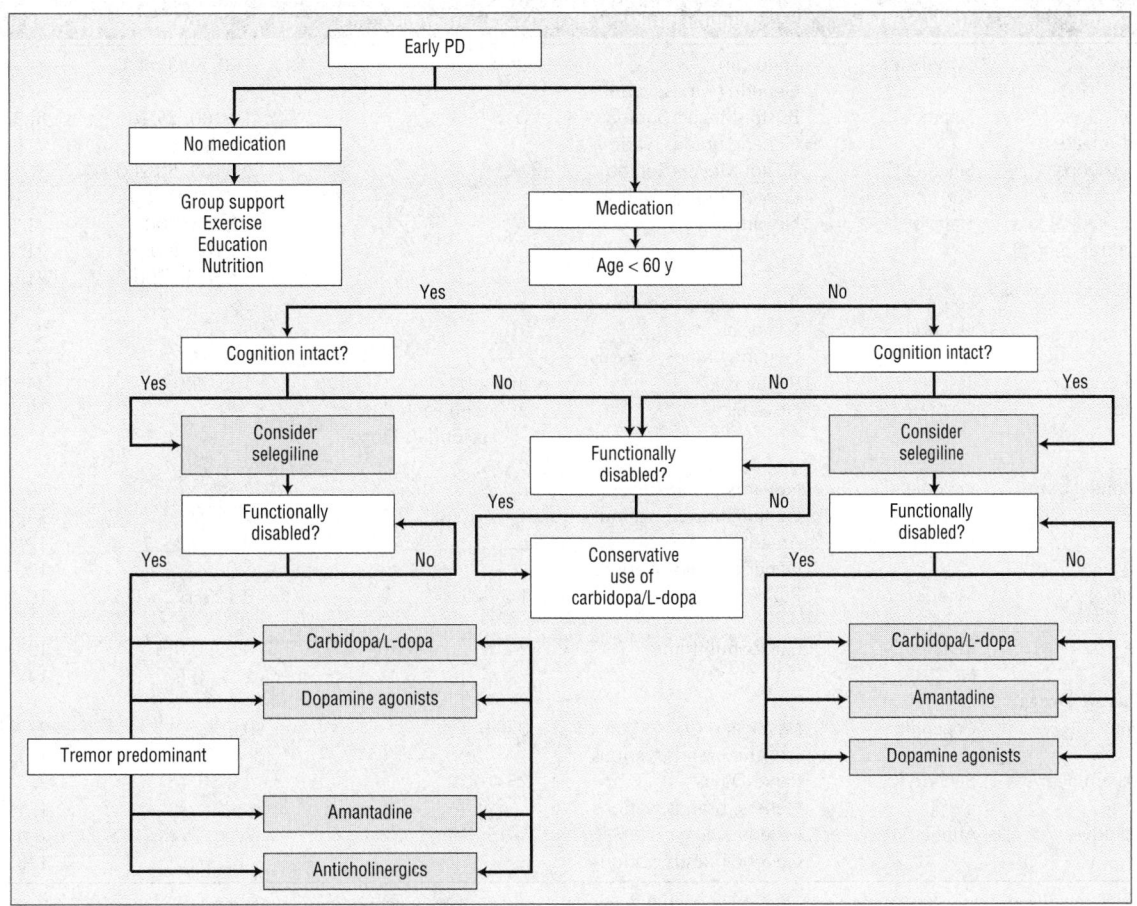

FIGURE 57–4. General algorithm for treating early IPD.

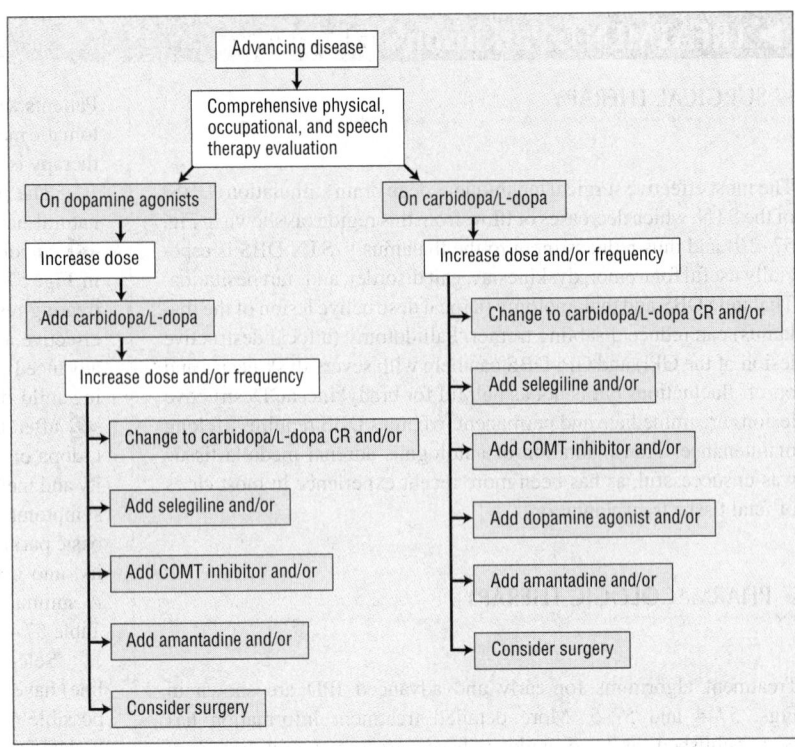

FIGURE 57–5. Algorithm for treating advanced IPD.

TABLE 57–4. Drugs Used in Parkinson's Disease

Generic Name	Trade Name	Manufacturer	Dosage Range (mg/day)	Dosage Forms (mg)	Cost Index[a]
Amantadine	Symmetrel	Endo Labs	200–300	100, 50/5 mL	14, 13
		Generic brands, various			6, 7
Carbidopa/L-Dopa Controlled-release	Sinemet	Bristol-Meyers Squibb	b	10/100, 25/100, 25/250	8, 9, 11
		Generic brands, various			7, 8, 10
Carbidopa/L-Dopa	Sinemet CR	Bristol-Meyers Squibb	b	25/100, 50/200	10, 19,
		Generic brands, various			9, 18
Carbidopa/L-Dopa/ entacapone	Stalevo	Novartis	b	12.5/50/200	21
				25/100/200	21
				37.5/150/200	21
Carbidopa	Lodosyn	Bristol-Meyers Squibb	b	25	6
Selegiline	Eldepryl	Somerset	10	5	27
		Generic brands, various			22
Tolcapone	Tasmar	Roche	300–600	100, 200	24, 26
Entacapone	Comtan	Novartis	200 with each dose of carbidopa/L-Dopa	200	19
Agonists					
Bromocriptine	Parlodel	Novartis	b	2.5, 5	30, 46
		Generic brands, various			23, 27
Pergolide	Permax	Amarin	b	0.05, 0.25, 1	12, 21, 45
		Generic brands, various			12, 19, 40
Pramipexole	Mirapex	Pfizer	1.5–4.5	0.125, 0.25, 0.5 1, 1.5	10, 13, 22 22, 22
Ropinirole	Requip	GlaxoSmithKline	24	0.25, 0.5; 1 2, 3, 4, 5	13, 13, 13 13, 23, 23, 23
Anticholinergic Drugs					
Benztropine	Cogentin	Merck and Co.	0.5–6	0.5, 1, 2	2, 2, 3
		Generic brands, various			1, 1, 1
Diphenhydramine	Benadryl	Parke-Davis	25–100	25, 50	2, 3
		Generic brands, various			1, 1
Trihexyphenidyl	Artane	Lederle	1–15	2, 5, 2/5 mL	2, 4, 4
		Generic brands, various			1, 3

[a]Cost index calculated from February 2004 average wholesale price per 100. Approximate cost per 100 (or per pint for solutions) equivalent to index × $10.00
[b]Dosage must be individualized.

TABLE 57–5. Candidate Medications and Primary Mechanism for Phase II or III Neuroprotection Studies

Caffeine	Adenosine antagonist
Coenzyme Q10	Antioxidant/mitochondrial stabilizer
Creatine	Antioxidant/mitochondrial stabilizer
Estrogen	Undetermined/multiple
GPI 1485	Trophic factor
GM-1 ganglioside	Trophic factor
Minocycline	Anti-inflammatory/antiapoptotic
Pramipexole	Antioxidant/vesicular trafficking
Ropinirole	Antioxidant
Rasagiline	Antioxidant/antiapoptotic
Selegiline	Antioxidant/antiapoptotic

proposed agents. The agents identified as candidates for phase II or III neuroprotection studies are listed in Table 57–5. A recent coenzyme Q10 study in IPD found that 16 months of therapy with 1200 mg/day gave small but statistically beneficial effects at slowing decline in activities of daily living. The investigators concluded that it would be premature to recommend the use of coenzyme Q10 as a neuroprotective treatment of IPD until confirmatory studies are completed.[23] Vitamin E (2000 IU/day) has not proven useful in preventing disease progression. Pramipexole and ropinirole are associated with slower decline in imaging markers of dopaminergic function compared with L-dopa monotherapy, suggesting neuroprotection.[24,25] These results are tempered by alternative explanations for these findings.[26]

L-Dopa and dopaminergic agonists not only act on the nigrostriatal system but also facilitate mesolimbic dopaminergic projections. This may result in psychiatric symptoms, including compulsive behaviors, delirium, agitation, paranoia, delusions, and hallucinations. These effects tend to occur more frequently in older patients and in those with underlying confusion or dementia and are associated with poor outcome.[27] These problems can be managed using the guidelines and antipsychotic medications summarized in Table 57–6.[28,29] Most other antipsychotic medications, including olanzapine and

TABLE 57–6. Stepwise Approach to Drug-Induced Psychosis in Parkinson's Disease

1. General measures such as evaluating for hypoxemia, infection (especially encephalitis, systemic sepsis, or urinary tract infection), or electrolyte disturbance (especially hypercalcemia or hyponatremia).
2. Simplify the antiparkinsonian regimen as much as possible by discontinuing the medications with the highest risk-benefit ratio first.
   a. Discontinue anticholinergics, including other nonparkinsonian medications with anticholinergic activity such as antidepressants, e.g., amitriptyline.
   b. Discontinue selegiline.
   c. Taper and discontinue dopamine agonists.
   d. Taper and discontinue amantadine, being aware that amantadine withdrawal delirium has been reported.
   e. Consider reduction of levodopa (especially at the end of day) and discontinuation of COMT inhibitors.
3. Consider atypical antipsychotic medication if psychosis persists.
   a. Quetiapine 12.5–50 mg at bedtime and gradually increased upward by 12.5–25 mg per week until psychosis controlled, *or*
   b. Clozapine 12.5–50 mg at bedtime and gradually increased upward by 12.5 mg per week until psychosis controlled (requires weekly monitoring for leukopenia).

risperidone, can improve psychotic symptoms but tend frequently to worsen parkinsonian features.

The decision to start L-dopa early (as soon as the diagnosis of IPD is made) or late (only when symptoms compromise social, occupational, or psychological well-being) has generated controversy.[30,31] Proponents for delaying treatment point to evidence suggesting that long-term L-dopa therapy is associated with an increased risk of response fluctuations, an increased risk of dementia, and loss of L-dopa efficacy.[32] L-Dopa therapy hypothetically could increase oxidative stress in dopaminergic neurons and thus increase dopaminergic neuronal loss; however, there is no firm evidence that this mechanism actually affects the course of IPD. The counterargument is that response fluctuations are secondary to disease progression, not L-dopa.[33] A multicenter study found that withholding L-dopa therapy for more than 3 years after diagnosis resulted in a doubling of the excess mortality rate compared with early treatment.[34] A 40-week randomized, double-blind, placebo-controlled clinical trial comparing earlier versus later L-dopa treatment (ELLDOPA) now underway may address this issue.[35] Fortunately, medications other than carbidopa/L-dopa can be initiated in newly diagnosed young and cognitively intact patients (see Fig. 57–4) if symptoms are functionally disabling.

Anticholinergic Medications

The anticholinergic drugs can be effective against tremor but rarely show much benefit for bradykinesia or other disabilities of IPD. Not all patients with tremor respond to these medications. Sometimes dystonic features associated with IPD also will improve. Adverse effects of these drugs include dry mouth, blurred vision, constipation, and urinary retention. More serious reactions include forgetfulness, sedation, depression, and anxiety. An encephalopathic state can evolve gradually in some patients. Increased Alzheimer's disease pathology (amyloid plaques and neurofibrillary tangles) is related to the use of these agents in IPD.[36] Patients with preexisting cognitive deficits and advanced age are at greater risk for central anticholinergic effects. The anticholinergic drugs differ little in their adverse effects and have essentially the same therapeutic potential. Anticholinergic drugs can be used alone or in conjunction with L-dopa and other antiparkinsonian agents.

Amantadine

Amantadine (Symmetrel, Endo; various generic brands) is often effective for relief of most signs and symptoms in patients with mild IPD.[37] More recently, it has been reported to suppress L-dopa–induced dyskinesia (at doses up to 400 mg/day).[38] Therapy with amantadine is also considered an independent predictor of improved survival in IPD.[39] Like anticholinergics, it can be especially effective against tremor. The drug typically is used at 200–300 mg/day. The elderly are particularly prone to confusion at higher doses. Adverse effects that may occur at onset of the drug (e.g., sedation and vivid dreams) may disappear with time. Dry mouth is a common adverse effect reminiscent of anticholinergic drugs, although amantadine does not block cholinergic receptors. Other adverse central effects seen uncommonly include depression, hallucinations, anxiety, dizziness, psychosis, and confusion. A common (and reversible) adverse effect of amantadine is livedo reticularis, a diffuse mottling of the skin.

Amantadine is eliminated renally, and a decreased dose should be administered when renal dysfunction is present (100 mg/day with creatinine clearances of 30–50 mL/min, 100 mg every other day for creatinine clearances of 15–29 mL/min, and 200 mg every 7 days for creatinine clearances of less than 15 mL/min and patients on hemodialysis). Unlike other drugs for IPD, the precise mechanism of action of amantadine is unknown, but it may involve either dopaminergic or nondopaminergic mechanisms such as inhibition of NMDA receptors.

L-Dopa and Carbidopa/L-Dopa

L-Dopa (Larodopa, Roche) was first studied for parkinsonism in the 1960s, and recognition of its unequivocal benefit was reported in 1967.[40] It is still the most effective drug in the management of IPD. L-Dopa is the immediate precursor of dopamine. It crosses the blood-brain barrier, whereas dopamine does not. In the striatum and elsewhere, L-dopa is converted by L-amino acid decarboxylase (L-AAD) to dopamine. Peripherally formed dopamine is responsible for adverse effects such as nausea, vomiting, cardiac arrhythmias, and postural hypotension. By combining L-dopa with the peripherally acting L-AAD inhibitors carbidopa (Sinemet, Bristol-Myers Squibb; various generic brands) or benserazide (Madopar; not available in the United States), peripheral conversion of L-dopa to dopamine is blocked. As a result, increased amounts of L-dopa are transported into the brain, and peripheral adverse effects of dopamine are reduced.[41]

Today, L-dopa is used almost exclusively as a combination product with decarboxylase inhibitors. Starting L-dopa doses of 200–300 mg/day often are adequate for relief of disability. Some patients require larger amounts on a daily basis; however, the usual maximal dose of L-dopa needed by patients even with severe parkinsonism is 800 mg/day. Slow buildup of dose (e.g., increments of 100 mg L-dopa per week) can help to assess the lowest effective dose and minimizes the risk for adverse effects, such as postural hypotension, nausea, vomiting, sedation, and vivid dreams.

Generally, about 75 mg carbidopa is required to prevent peripheral adverse effects, but some patients may benefit from as much as 150 mg/day. Carbidopa/L-dopa is used most widely in a 25-mg/100-mg tablet form, although 25-mg/250-mg and 10-mg/100-mg forms are also available. Controlled-release preparations of carbidopa/L-dopa are available in 50-mg/200-mg and 25-mg/100-mg forms. If peripheral adverse effects are prominent, 25-mg carbidopa (Lodosyn, Bristol-Myers Squibb) tablets are available.

Pharmacokinetics and Pharmacodynamics. The pharmacokinetic and pharmacodynamic properties of L-dopa explain many of its clinical effects, including response fluctuations. There is marked intra- and intersubject variability in the time to peak plasma concentrations after oral L-dopa. Often there may be more than one peak plasma concentration after a single dose, which is attributed to erratic gastric emptying. Meals delay gastric emptying, whereas antacids (which decrease gastric acidity) promote gastric emptying. L-Dopa is absorbed primarily in the proximal duodenum by a saturable large neutral amino acid (LNAA) transport system. Competition for this site by dietary or supplemental LNAAs can reduce L-dopa plasma concentrations. The gut wall also contains a saturable decarboxylase that limits the bioavailability of L-dopa unless it is combined with a peripheral decarboxylase inhibitor such as carbidopa.

L-Dopa is not bound to plasma proteins. It crosses the blood-brain barrier by stereospecific saturable facilitated diffusion and competes with LNAA for transport into the brain. High-dose infusions of phenylalanine and leucine decrease the clinical response to L-dopa without altering L-dopa plasma concentrations. This has led to

recommendations of protein restriction and special diets for improving L-dopa responsiveness, although generally reduction in protein intake is not needed to maintain good L-dopa effect. A metabolite of L-dopa, 3-O-methyldopa (3OMD), also competes for transport, but it is not clear how this affects L-dopa clinical response.

L-Dopa elimination is primarily by decarboxylation to dopamine. Additional pathways are by 3-O-methylation and transamination. With adequate decarboxylase inhibition, increased amounts of L-dopa are metabolized by the other pathways. The elimination half-life of L-dopa is about 1 hour, and this is extended to about $1\frac{1}{2}$ hours with the addition of carbidopa. 3OMD has a half-life of about 15 hours and accumulates with chronic dosing.

Motor Complications of L-Dopa. Between 5% and 10% of IPD patients will develop involuntary movements or motor fluctuations with each year of L-dopa treatment.[42] Movement complications associated with long-term treatment with carbidopa/L-dopa and their suggested treatments are listed in Table 57–7 and have been reviewed recently.[43,44] Initiating therapy with the controlled-release form of carbidopa/L-dopa did not reduce motor complications compared with standard-release carbidopa/L-dopa in a 5-year trial.[45]

> ### CLINICAL CONTROVERSY
>
> Some clinicians are concerned with possible long-term risks (motor fluctuations) of L-dopa and will delay or avoid its use even though it is more effective than other medications currently available. Others believe that motor fluctuations are a consequence of disease severity and progression rather than due to L-dopa itself. Individualized considerations of a patient's disability should guide all interventions for IPD.

Wearing Off. End-of-dose deterioration (the wearing-off effect) has been related to increasing loss of neuronal storage capability for dopamine. Initially, exogenous L-dopa is taken up by the remaining presynaptic neurons, converted to dopamine, and stored in synaptic vesicles. With progressive loss of presynaptic neurons, storage capacity declines, and patients become more dependent on the rate of L-dopa delivery to the brain for the generation of dopamine. Hence the peripheral pharmacokinetic properties of L-dopa increasingly become the determinant of central dopamine synthesis.

With advancement of IPD, a single carbidopa/L-dopa dose may produce benefits for as little as 1.5 to 2 hours. As a result, carbidopa/L-dopa needs to be given more frequently in order to prevent the wearing off of its benefits. Alternatively, a controlled-release product is available (Sinemet CR, Bristol-Myers Squibb; various generic brands) that can extend the duration of L-dopa effect; thus there is a more gradual wearing off of L-dopa effect and a need for fewer daily doses.[46] Some patients will require an increase in L-dopa intake when switched to the sustained-release form because of its decreased bioavailability. Patients maintained on the sustained-release product also may require a conventional carbidopa/L-dopa dose in the morning for its more rapid absorption and response.

Dopamine agonists also can be added to a carbidopa/L-dopa regimen in an attempt to treat wearing off. In addition, either intravenous or duodenal L-dopa infusions will produce constant serum L-dopa concentrations (and presumably striatal dopamine concentrations) and thus reduce response fluctuations.[47,48] Although some patients have been maintained on duodenal and intravenous infusions for long periods of time, these invasive methods of administration require careful planning and generally are not used outside the research setting. Sipping small amounts of carbidopa/L-dopa solution is an easier way to

TABLE 57–7. Motor Fluctuations and Possible Interventions in IPD

Effect	Possible Treatments
End of dose deterioration ("wearing off")	Increase frequency of doses; controlled-release carbidopa/L-dopa; consider dopamine agonists, selegiline, COMT inhibitors, or amantadine; duodenal or intravenous L-dopa infusions; carbidopa/L-dopa oral solution; subcutaneous apomorphine infusions; transdermal dopamine agonists
Delayed onset of response	Give on empty stomach before meals; crush or chew and take with a full glass of water; reduce dietary protein intake; antacids; morning standard-release carbidopa/L-dopa if on sustained-release carbidopa/L-dopa; infusions of L-dopa; dopamine agonists
Drug-resistant "off" periods	Increase carbidopa/L-dopa dose and/or frequency; give on empty stomach before meals; crush or chew and take with a full glass of water; infusions of L-dopa or dopamine agonists; apomorphine subcutaneous injection; consider deep brain stimulation
Random oscillations ("on/off")	Dopamine agonists; controlled-release carbidopa/L-dopa, selegiline; COMT inhibitors; infusions of L-dopa or dopamine agonists; consider drug holiday and deep brain stimulation
Start hesitation ("freezing")	Increase carbidopa/L-dopa dose; dopamine agonists; gait modifications (tapping, rhythmic commands, stepping over objects, rocking)
Peak-dose dyskinesia (I-D-I response[a])	Smaller more frequent doses of carbidopa/L-dopa; controlled-release carbidopa/L-dopa; dopamine agonist; consider amantadine, propranolol, fluoxetine, buspirone, clozapine, deep brain stimulation
Diphasic dyskinesias (D-I-D response[b])	Reduce anticholinergic medication
Dystonia	Baclofen; nighttime carbidopa/L-dopa; morning standard-release carbidopa/L-dopa if on sustained-release carbidopa/L-dopa; dopamine agonists; anticholinergics; selective denervation with botulinum toxin
Myoclonus	Decrease nighttime L-dopa doses; clonazepam
Akathisia	Benzodiazepines; propranolol; dopamine agonists; gabapentin

[a]I-D-I is the improvement-dyskinesia/dystonia-improvement pattern of response.
[b]D-I-D is the dyskinesia-improvement-dyskinesia pattern of response.

noninvasively titrate drug intake to optimal effect.[49] A solution that is stable for 24 hours can be prepared by adding 10 tablets of carbidopa/L-dopa and 2 g crystalline ascorbic acid to 1 L of tap water. Finally, MAO-B inhibitors such as selegiline and the COMT inhibitors tolcapone (Tasmar, Roche) and entacapone (Comtan, Novartis) extend the action of L-dopa. Entacapone is now available in fixed-dose combinations with carbidopa/L-dopa as well (Stalevo, Novartis).

■ *Drug-Resistant Off Periods.* Drug-resistant off periods or delayed response to carbidopa/L-dopa can be due to delayed stomach emptying or decreased absorption in the upper gastrointestinal tract. Chewing a tablet or crushing it and then drinking a full glass of water may decrease disintegration time and facilitate gastric emptying.

■ *Rapid Fluctuations.* Rapid fluctuations from on to off motor states (*yo-yoing*) can develop in patients receiving L-dopa chronically. Rapid transitions from normal or dyskinetic on motor activity to bradykinetic or off states may just be an extension of wearing off. Nonmotor symptoms also may fluctuate. Concentration versus effect data reveal nonlinear (sigmoid E_{max} model) relationships such that small changes in serum L-dopa concentrations may lead to large effect responses, even if the sustained-release product is used.[50] Differences in the pharmacodynamic parameters EC_{50} (concentration at half-maximal effect), K_{e0} (elimination rate constant from the effect compartment), and N (the sigmoidicity constant) have been found between stable and fluctuating IPD patients with no change in pharmacokinetic parameters.[51] These same pharmacodynamic parameters have been found to change significantly in individual patients followed longitudinally over 4 years.[52] With progression of IPD, motor skill performance decreases so that there will be larger differences between baseline capabilities and maximum therapeutic effect; hence there will be an even steeper slope at the EC_{50} and more clinically noticeable dose-by-dose effects. These circumstances contribute to rapid fluctuations in motor responses. Simulations of the number of times a patient could alternately tap two levers 25 cm apart using

mean pharmacodynamic and kinetic values for stable and fluctuating patients are shown in Fig. 57–6 to illustrate further the dramatic differences between these groups. These pharmacodynamic mechanisms have been reviewed in detail by Nutt and Holford.[53]

Infusions of L-dopa or long-acting dopaminergic agonists tend to alleviate these fluctuations. Dopaminergic agonists can be added

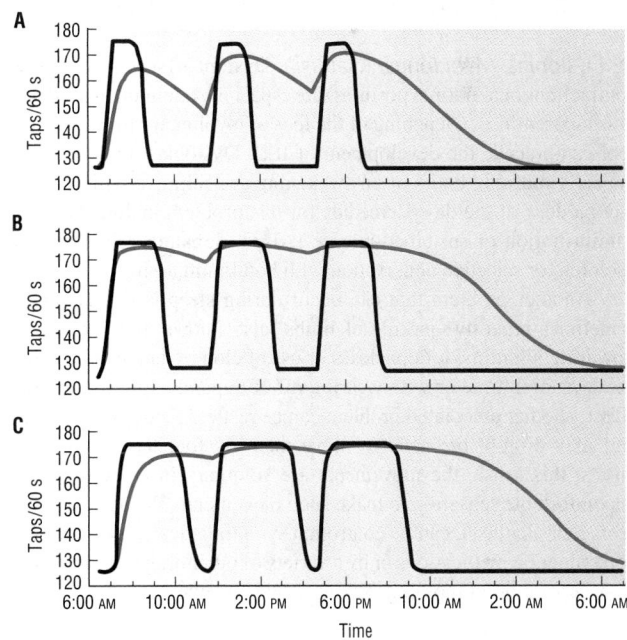

FIGURE 57–6. Effect of change in carbidopa/L-dopa dosage form on tapping effect in stable (*red line*) and fluctuating (*black line*) patients. A. Carbidopa/L-dopa 25 mg/100 mg (K_{e1} of 1.242 h^{-1}, K_a of 3.384 h^{-1}, and V/f of 35.4 L) administered at typical administration times of 7 AM, 12 noon, and 5 PM B. Carbidopa/L-dopa 50 mg/200 mg (same pharmacokinetic parameters as in A) administered at the same times. C. Carbidopa/L-dopa 50 mg/200 mg with a longer half-life of absorption of 1.4 h ($K_a = 0.5$) simulating the controlled-release form.

to L-dopa to treat on/off fluctuations. Other strategies include MAO inhibitors and COMT inhibitors that decrease the clearance of L-dopa. A drug-free period ("drug holiday") has been investigated in an attempt to modify postsynaptic dopamine receptors and thus decrease unpredictable off states. Because of the discomforts and risks, as well as the limited gains for most patients, drug holidays are rarely recommended.

Dyskinesias. Another complication of L-dopa therapy is dyskinesias (choreiform abnormal involuntary movements involving usually the neck, trunk, and upper extremities). These involuntary movements usually are associated with peak antiparkinsonian benefit (peak-effect dyskinesia or improvement-dyskinesia/dystonia-improvement), although they also can develop during the rise and fall of L-dopa effects (the dyskinesia-improvement-dyskinesia or diphasic pattern of response). In the case of peak-effect dyskinesias or dystonias, smaller, more frequent doses of L-dopa, use of the sustained-release preparations, or addition of dopamine agonists sometimes can be beneficial. The optimal treatment for the dyskinesia-improvement-dyskinesia pattern is unknown and actually can worsen with strategies useful for extending L-dopa effect.

Simplistically, dyskinesias can be thought of as too much movement secondary to extension of the pharmacologic effect or too much striatal dopamine receptor stimulation. However, the phenomenology is far more complex, as demonstrated by the occasional patient simultaneously demonstrating parkinsonian features and dyskinesias. An interaction between different classes of dopamine receptors may be involved. A partial dopamine agonist, terguride, has been found to suppress dyskinesias without worsening parkinsonian symptoms, suggesting that some pharmacologic approaches may differentiate the effects of dopaminergic stimulation on different aspects of motor system activation. Propranolol, dextromethorphan, idazoxan (an α_2-antagonist) and sarizotan (a $5HT_{1A}$ agonist) are nondopaminergic agents that have been studied for L-dopa–induced dyskinesia.[54]

Dystonias, Myoclonus, Akathisia. Dystonias (sustained muscle contractions or abnormal postures) are especially common in the distal lower extremities. Clenching of the toes or involuntary turning of the foot can precede the development of IPD. Dystonias often occur in the early morning hours or on awakening and improve with the first L-dopa dose of the day. Remedies for this problem include bedtime administration of sustained-release L-dopa, dopaminergic agonists, baclofen, or selective denervation with botulinum toxin.

Another problem that can occur during sleep is myoclonus, a sometimes repetitive jerking of limbs (also known as *sleep jerks*). Lowering nighttime L-dopa doses or use of clonazepam can be beneficial. At nighttime or with wearing off of dopaminergic medication effect, another associated problem can be restless feelings in the legs that may prompt the need to move them by foot tapping or pacing. In this sense, the movements are voluntary in response to an uncomfortable sensation to make such movements. Restless leg syndrome, or akathisia, can be controlled symptomatically by nighttime dopaminergic medications or by a variety of other drugs, among them clonazepam, propranolol, gabapentin, and codeine.

Monoamine Oxidase B Inhibitors

Selegiline (Eldepryl, Somerset; various generic brands), an irreversible MAO-B inhibitor, also known as deprenyl, is marketed for extending L-dopa effects. By its central action, it modestly extends the duration of action from each dose of L-dopa. This can provide up to 1 hour of extended on time for patients with wearing off of L-dopa actions. Selegiline also increases the peak effects of L-dopa and can worsen preexisting dyskinesias or psychiatric symptoms such as delusions and hallucinations. Often use of selegiline permits reduction of L-dopa intake to as little as one-half its previous optimal dose.

Selegiline has been used widely at a dose of 10 mg/day, although its irreversible inhibition of MAO-B can be achieved at lower doses.[55] In addition, renewal of the enzyme proceeds at a slow rate, so the effect of the drug lingers for weeks. Selegiline is lipophilic and penetrates the blood-brain barrier rapidly. The metabolic pathway of selegiline leads to end products of L-methamphetamine and L-amphetamine. Adverse effects of selegiline are minimal but can include insomnia (especially if administered at bedtime) and jitteriness. The hypertensive "cheese effect," which occurs from ingesting tyramine with the use of MAO-A inhibitors, does not occur with selegiline.[56] Rarely, concomitant selective serotonin reuptake inhibitors can cause the *serotonin syndrome*, characterized by hypertension, diaphoresis, and shivering. A similar reaction has been reported with concomitant selegiline and meperidine.

Selegiline and other MAO-B inhibitors have been investigated for neuroprotective properties. They inhibit the oxidative deamination of dopamine, which generates hydrogen peroxide and ultimately oxyradicals capable of damaging nigrostriatal neurons (see Fig. 57–1). Since MAO-B inhibition diverts dopamine catabolism to an alternate route not generating peroxide, selegiline therapy may spare these neurons from oxidative stress. One study evaluating its neuroprotective properties showed that it delayed the need for L-dopa in newly diagnosed IPD patients by about 9 months. However, the study was inconclusive because of the drug's symptomatic effects and loss of the apparent protective action after approximately 12 months.[57] Rasagiline, an MAO-B inhibitor similar to selegiline but without amphetamine metabolites, has similar effects as selegiline on enhancing L-dopa effects, as well as modest beneficial effects in monotherapy.[58,59]

COMT Inhibitors

Two COMT inhibitors, tolcapone (Tasmar, Roche) and entacapone (Comtan, Novartis), have been developed to extend the effects from each dose of L-dopa. By themselves, they have no effect on IPD symptoms. Both prevent the peripheral conversion of levodopa to 3OMD, thus prolonging the dopaminergic effects of L-dopa. For patients with wearing off, these agents can decrease off time significantly by increasing the L-dopa area under the curve by about 35% without increasing C_{max} or T_{max}.[60] In clinical practice, COMT inhibition is more effective than controlled-release carbidopa/L-dopa in providing consistent extension of effect and avoids the delay in time to maximal effect that affects patients with controlled-release L-dopa preparations. The recently introduced triple-combination product carbidopa/levodopa/entacapone (Stalevo; Novartis) offers variable carbidopa/levodopa content (12.5 mg/50 mg, 25 mg/100 mg, and 37.5 mg/150 mg) with a fixed 200-mg entacapone content. Concomitant use of nonselective MAO inhibitors should be avoided to prevent inhibition of most of the pathways for normal catecholamine metabolism. It remains to be seen whether the use of these adjunctive agents will be more beneficial and cost-effective than maximizing therapy with carbidopa/L-dopa alone.

Tolcapone has effects on both peripheral and central COMT, but it is unclear what role central COMT inhibition has. Its use is limited by reports of three cases of fatal hepatotoxicity such that strict monitoring of hepatic function is required, as outlined in the package nsert. Tolcapone should be discontinued if there is any elevation in iver function tests above the upper limit of normal or if any signs or symptoms develop suggesting hepatic failure (e.g., persistent nausea, fatigue, lethargy, anorexia, jaundice, dark urine, pruritus, or right upper quadrant abdominal tenderness). An informed consent for use s included in the package insert to ensure that patients are informed of the risk of adverse effects. The starting and recommended dose is l00 mg three times per day as an adjunct to carbidopa/L-dopa. Delayed onset of diarrhea (weeks to months later) can occur in up to 5% of patients. Since an alternative similar but safer medication is available, any role for tolcapone is unclear.

Entacapone has a shorter half-life than tolcapone, and 200 mg needs to be given with each dose of carbidopa/L-dopa up to 8 times per day. In clinical trials, both tolcapone and entacapone increased on time by about 1 hour and permitted reduction of L-dopa dose if dyskinesias emerged.[61,62] Dopaminergic adverse effects may occur and generally are manageable by reduction of the carbidopa/L-dopa dosage. Brownish-orange urinary discoloration may occur with entacapone, as with tolcapone, but there are no reports of hepatotoxicity from entacapone.

Dopamine Agonists

The ergot dopamine agonists pergolide (Permax, Amarin; various generic brands) and bromocriptine (Parlodel, Novartis; various generic brands) and the nonergots pramipexole (Mirapex, Pfizer) and ropinirole (Requip, GlaxoSmithKline) are beneficial as adjuncts to L-dopa therapy in patients with deteriorating response to L-dopa, in patients who are experiencing fluctuations in response to L-dopa, and in patients with limited clinical response to L-dopa owing to an inability to tolerate higher doses. The dopamine agonists decrease the frequency of off periods and provide an L-dopa–sparing effect. Crossover studies suggest that pergolide with L-dopa is similar or possibly more efficacious with fewer adverse effects than bromocriptine with L-dopa.[63] Pergolide may improve functional status in patients with deteriorating response to bromocriptine,[64] whereas bromocriptine does not appear to improve function in patients with a deteriorating response to pergolide.[65]

Bromocriptine monotherapy in previously untreated IPD patients is limited by a high incidence of adverse effects and treatment failures necessitating either lowering the dose or the addition of L-dopa.[66] Pergolide, pramipexole, and ropinirole seem to be more effective as monotherapy alternatives to L-dopa, but only pramipexole and ropinirole are approved for monotherapy. Investigations comparing initial therapy with L-dopa with initial therapy with dopamine agonists (to which L-dopa could be added) revealed a decreased risk of developing response fluctuations at a cost of less motor control in the agonist group.[67–69] This has generated controversy as to whether initial treatment of IPD should be with dopamine agonist monotherapy.[70–72] The American Academy of Neurology practice parameter states that either can be used depending on the impact of improving motor function.[73] Younger patients are more likely to develop motor fluctuations, and therefore, dopamine agonists may be preferred. Older patients are more likely to suffer psychosis from the dopamine agonists, and thus carbidopa/L-dopa may be the best starting medication, particularly if cognitive problems or dementia is present. There is no rationale at this time to choose one dopamine agonist over another based on receptor specificity.

A recommended initial dose of bromocriptine is 1.25 mg once or twice daily. The dose of bromocriptine should be escalated slowly by 1.25 to 2.5 mg/day every week and maintained at the minimum amount necessary to accomplish the desired therapeutic effect. Average daily dosages of less than 30 mg may be effective for several years in many patients; however, some patients may require dosages of up to 120 mg/day.

A recommended initial dose of pergolide (which is about 13 times more potent than bromocriptine) is 0.05 mg/day for 2 days, gradually increasing the dose by approximately 0.1–0.15 mg/day every 3 days over a 12-day period. Should more drug be needed, the dose then may be increased by 0.25 mg every 3 days until symptoms are eliminated or adverse effects occur. The mean therapeutic dose in most clinical trials was approximately 3 mg/day.

Pramipexole is initiated at a dose of 0.125 mg three times a day and increased every 5 to 7 days as tolerated. In a fixed-dose study, daily doses of 3, 4.5, and 6 mg were not more effective than 1.5 mg/day, and the higher doses were associated with a higher frequency of adverse effects.[74] When switching from bromocriptine or pergolide to pramipexole, a 10:1 and 1:1 dosage substitution is recommended, respectively.[75] Ropinirole is initiated at 0.25 mg three times a day and increased by 0.25 mg three times a day on a weekly basis to a maximum of 24 mg/day. The dose of dopaminergic agonists is best determined by slow titration to enhance tolerance and to find the least dose that provides optimal benefit.

Adverse effects are often a limiting factor in dopamine agonist therapy. These occur frequently at the start and are more likely at higher doses or with rapid escalation of dose. Nausea is the most common, followed by sedation, light-headedness, and vivid dreams. Asymptomatic postural hypotension is common but does not always require adjustment of medication. Among psychic effects, confusion, hallucinations, and daytime sedation (including sleep attacks) often are dose limiting. Attempts to reduce excessive daytime drowsiness and sleep attacks in patients on agonist therapy should include patient education, eliminating other sedative medications, reducing or changing the drug, and addressing coexisting sleep disorders.[76] The addition of a dopamine agonist to L-dopa therapy can increase the frequency and severity of dyskinesias during periods of good functional status but also can improve motor functioning even with reduction in carbidopa/L-dopa dose. Among other idiosyncratic effects occurring with dopaminergic agonists is pedal edema. In a study of pramipexole, 6% of patients developed this problem, which is dose-related, nonresponsive to diuretics, and resolved with stopping the medication.[77] The ergot dopamine agonists are associated rarely with pleuropulmonary fibrosis, and recently, cases of cardiac valvulopathy have been reported with pergolide.[78,79]

Bromocriptine is fairly rapidly absorbed, exhibits high first-pass metabolism, is highly protein bound, and has multiple metabolites excreted primarily through the bile.[80] The elimination half-life is about 3 hours. A slow-release bromocriptine product has been investigated but is not available. A significant increase in bromocriptine plasma concentrations has been documented with erythromycin. Pergolide has similar properties as bromocriptine except that it has a longer elimination half-life (about 24 hours). Pramipexole is excreted primarily renally with an 8- to 12-hour half-life. The initial dosage must be adjusted in renal insufficiency (0.125 mg twice daily for creatinine clearances of 35–59 mL/min, 0.125 mg once daily for creatinine clearances of 15–34 mL/min). Ropinirole has a 6-hour half-life and is metabolized by cytochrome P450 1A2. A sustained-release form is under development. Potent inhibitors (fluoroquinolones) and inducers (smoking) of this enzyme likely will lead to alterations in ropinirole clearance.

Apomorphine is a dopamine agonist soon to be released in the United States. It will be marketed for subcutaneous injection and already has shown promise for rescue of freezing episodes.[81]

Cabergoline is a selective D_2 ergot agonist with a long half-life (70 hours) that is as effective as bromocriptine but dosed up to 4 mg once a day. It is available in the United States only as a 0.5-mg tablet (Dostinex, Pharmacia) for the treatment of hyperprolactinemia. A transdermal delivery form of the potent dopaminergic agonist rotigotine is being investigated. Specific D_1 receptor agonists do not appear to have much antiparkinsonian effect. Domperidone is a peripheral dopamine receptor blocker (not available in the United States) that can be used to block some of the adverse effects of the dopamine agonists.[82]

PHARMACOECONOMIC CONSIDERATIONS

Few pharmacoeconomic assessments have been reported in IPD treatment. Treatment with anticholinergic medications, amantadine, and carbidopa/L-dopa is inexpensive. For cost-effectiveness, the lowest dose giving adequate results should be used, and optimization of the carbidopa/L-dopa regimen should be attempted before adding more costly medications. In early IPD, a long-duration response can be seen such that a carbidopa/L-dopa dose every 3 days may be all that is required.[83] Initial therapy with the more expensive sustained-release product (Sinemet CR) or combination product (Stalevo) in the absence of response fluctuations is not indicated. As symptoms progress, the addition or continued use of dopamine agonists, selegiline, or COMT inhibitors can add considerable expense, sometimes with minimal or no benefit. A large trial underway in the United Kingdom to determine which class of drugs provides the most effective control with the fewest side effects for both early and later IPD hopefully also will provide information on cost-effectiveness.[84]

EVALUATION OF THERAPEUTIC OUTCOMES

A list of monitoring parameters is given in Table 57–8. It is important to educate patients and caregivers that IPD is a neurodegenerative disease that often progresses with time and that not all symptoms are amenable to treatment. They can participate in treatment by recording medication administration times as well as the duration of on and off times that can be reviewed at each office visit. If a bothersome symptom such as dystonia occurs only infrequently, it can be videotaped by the family to be reviewed with the physician.

TABLE 57–8. Monitoring Parkinson's Disease Therapy

1. Determine medications, medication administration times, relationship to meals, and the time of the last dose. Educate the patient that carbidopa/L-dopa is absorbed best on an empty stomach.
2. Assess patient's general impression of motor functioning, and address any specific concerns the patient may have.
3. Inquire specifically about dose-by-dose effects of medication, wearing off of medication, inadequate response to a single dose of medication, "freezing," abnormal involuntary movements, cramps or spasms, hallucinations (particularly visual hallucinations), and nausea, vomiting, or light-headedness. Offer suggestions to help alleviate these.
4. Inquire about the preceding symptoms from the caregivers, and address any concerns they may have with specific attention to sleep disorders, depression, psychotic features, and dyskinesias that may not be apparent to the patient.
5. Observe the patient and determine if dyskinetic movements are present and if the patient is aware of them. If present, educate the patient about dyskinesias and recommend appropriate interventions.
6. Ensure that the patient and/or caregivers understand the recommended medication regimen.

The history always should include a detailed medication history because patients often may improvise and adjust their own medication schedules. It is important to determine the times of the day that may be most difficult for them to function. Assessment of general level of functioning including activities of daily living will help to determine when L-dopa or dopamine agonists should be added. A history of falls should be investigated further as to the circumstances surrounding them to determine whether falls are secondary to imbalance (such as retropulsion), freezing or stumbling, orthostatic hypotension, or some other etiology. The patient should be questioned about common adverse effects of the antiparkinsonian medications, including nausea, hypotension, pedal edema, sleep disorders, and psychiatric difficulties. The patient also should be observed for dyskinesias and, if present, educated about them. Recommendations always should be made in view of the patient's perception of the severity of symptoms.

CONCLUSIONS

Although the cause of IPD remains unknown, symptomatic therapy has been developed to involve a number of options for early and later stages of the disease. Several directions of neuroprotective therapy are under investigation. Pharmacologic therapy through manipulation of the dopaminergic system can improve a patient's comfort and functional status significantly. Despite problems that can be associated with L-dopa, it remains the standard of therapy for most patients with IPD. The goal of management remains maintaining acceptable functional control with the minimum amount of antiparkinsonian drug necessary.

ABBREVIATIONS

3OMD: 3-O-methyldopa
COMT: catechol-O-methyl-transferase
DAT: dopamine transporter
DBS: deep brain stimulation
GABA: γ-aminobutyric acid
GPe: globus pallidus externa
GPi: globus pallidus interna
GTP: guanosine triphosphate
IPD: idiopathic Parkinson's disease
L-AAD: L-amino acid decarboxylase
LNAA: large neutral amino acid
MAO: monoamine oxidase
MPP+: 1-methyl-4-phenylpyridinium
MPTP: 1-methyl-4-phenyl-1,2,3,6-tetrahydropyridine
PET: positron-emission tomography
PSP: progressive supranuclear palsy
SNc: substania nigra pars compacta
SNr: substantia nigra pars reticulata
STN: subthalamic nucleus
TH: tyrosine hydroxylase

Review Questions and other resources can be found at *www.pharmacotherapyonline.com.*

REFERENCES

1. Factor SA, Weiner WJ. James Parkinson: The man and the essay. In: Factor SA, Weiner WJ, eds. Parkinson's Disease: Diagnosis and Clinical Management. New York, Demos, 2002:1–18.

2. Bower JH, Maraganore DM, McDonnell SK, Rocca WA. Incidence and distribution of parkinsonism in Olmsted County, Minnesota, 1976–1990. Neurology 1999;52:1214–1220.

3. LeWitt PA. Tobacco smoking, nicotine, and neuroprotection. In: Factor SA, Weiner WJ, eds. Parkinson's Disease: Diagnosis and Clinical Management. New York, Demos, 2002:519–529.

4. Di Monte DA. The environment and Parkinson's disease: Is the nigrostriatal system preferentially targeted by neurotoxins? Lancet Neurol 2003;2:531–533.

5. Chen H, Zhang SM, Hernan MA, et al. Nonsteroidal anti-inflammatory drugs and the risk of Parkinson disease. Arch Neurol 2003;60:1059–1064.

6. Hardy J, Cookson MR, Singleton A. Genes and parkinsonism. Lancet Neurol 2003;2:221–228.

7. Oliveira SA, Scott WK, Martin ER, et al. Parkin mutations and susceptibility alleles in late onset Parkinson's disease. Ann Neurol 2003;53:624–629.

8. Alam ZI, Daniel SE, Lees AJ, et al. A generalised increase in protein carbonyls in the brain in Parkinson's but not incidental Lewy body disease. J Neurochem 1997;69;1326–1329.

9. LeWitt PA. Parkinson's disease: Etiologic considerations. In: Ahlskog JE, Adler CA, eds. Parkinson's Disease and Movement Disorders: Diagnosis and Treatment Guidelines for the Practicing Physician. New York, Humana Press, 2000:91–100.

10. Smith Y, Bevan MD, Shink E, Bolam JP. Microcircuitry of the direct and indirect pathways of the basal ganglia. Neuroscience 1998;86:353–387.

11. Bara-Jimenez W, Sherzai A, Dimitrova T, et al. Adenosine A_{2A} receptor antagonist treatment of Parkinson's disease. Neurology 2003;61:293–296.

12. Hauser RA, Hubble JP, Truong DD, and the Istradefylline US-001 Study Group. Randomized trial of the adenosine A_{2A} receptor antagonist Istradefylline in advanced PD. Neurology 2003;61:297–303.

13. Mercuri NB, Calabresi P, Bernardi G. Physiology and pharmacology of dopamine D_2 receptors: Their implications in dopamine-substitute therapy for Parkinson's disease. Neurology 1989;39:1106–1108.

14. Bernheimer H, Birkmayer W, Hornykiewicz O, et al. Brain dopamine and the syndrome of Parkinson's and Huntington: Clinical, morphological, and neurochemical correlations. J Neurol Sci 1973;20:415–455.

15. Tatsch K. Can SPET imaging of dopamine uptake sites replace PET imaging in Parkinson's disease? For. Eur J Nucl Med 2002;5:711–714.

16. Frey KA. Can SPET imaging of dopamine uptake sites replace PET imaging in Parkinson's disease? Against. Eur J Nucl Med 2002;5:715–717.

17. Gelb DJ, Oliver E, Gilman S. Diagnostic criteria for Parkinson disease. Arch Neurol 1999;56:33–39.

18. Emre M. Dementia associated with Parkinson's disease. Lancet Neurol 2003;2:229–237.

19. Hallett M, Litvan I, Task Force on Surgery for Parkinson's Disease. Evaluation of surgery for Parkinson's disease: A report of the therapeutics and technology assessment subcommittee of the American Academy of Neurology. Neurology 1999;53:1910–1921.

20. Olanow CW, Koller WC. An algorithm (decision tree) for the management of Parkinson's disease: Treatment guidelines. Neurology 1998;50 (suppl 3):S1–57.

21. Rascol O, Goetz C, Koller W, et al. Treatment interventions for Parkinson's disease: An evidence-based assessment. Lancet 2002;359:1589–1598.

22. Neuroprotective agents for clinical trials in Parkinson's disease. Neurology 2003;60:1234–1240.

23. Effects of coenzyme Q10 in early Parkinson disease: Evidence of slowing of the functional decline. Arch Neurol 2002;59:1541–1550.

24. Parkinson Study Group. Dopamine transporter brain imaging to assess the effects of pramipexole vs levodopa on Parkinson disease progression. JAMA 2002;287:1653–1661.

25. Whone AL, Watts RL, Stoessl AJ. Slower progression in early Parkinson's disease treated with ropinirole vs levodopa: The REAL-PET study. Ann Neurol 2003;54:93–101.

26. Ahlskog JE. Slowing Parkinson's disease progression: Recent dopamine agonist trials. Neurology 2003;60:381–389.

27. Factor SA, Feustel PJ, Friedman JH, et al. Longitudinal outcome of Parkinson's disease patients with psychosis. Neurology 2003;60:1756–1761.

28. Juncos JL. Management of psychotic aspects of Parkinson's disease. J Clin Psychiatry 1999;60(suppl 8):42–53.

29. Friedman JH, Factor SA. Atypical antipsychotics in the treatment of drug induced psychosis in Parkinson's disease. Mov Disord 2000;15:201–211.

30. Fahn S, Bressman SB. Should levodopa therapy for parkinsonism be started early or late? Evidence against early treatment. Can J Neurol Sci 1984;11:200–206.

31. Muenter MD. Should levodopa therapy be started early or late? Can J Neurol Sci 1984;11:195–199.

32. Rajput AH, Stern W, Laverty WH. Chronic low-dose levodopa therapy in Parkinson's disease: An argument for delaying levodopa therapy. Neurology 1984;34:991–996.

33. Agid Y. Levodopa: Is toxicity a myth? Neurology 1998;50:858–863.

34. Diamond SG, Markham CH, Hoehn MM, et al. Multicenter study of Parkinson mortality with early versus later dopa treatment. Ann Neurol 1987;22:8–12.

35. Fahn S. Parkinson disease, the effect of levodopa, and the ELLDOPA trial. Arch Neurol 1999;56:529–535.

36. Perry EK, Kilford L, Lees AJ, et al. Increased Alzheimer's pathology in Parkinson's disease related to antimuscarinic drugs. Ann Neurol 2003;54:235–238.

37. Fahn S, Isgreen W. Long-term evaluation of amantadine and levodopa combination in parkinsonism by double-blind crossover analysis. Neurology 1975;25:695–700.

38. Metman LV, Del Dotto P, LePoole K, et al. Amantadine for levodopa-induced dyskinesias: A 1-year follow-up study. Arch Neurol 1999;56:1383–1386.

39. Uitti RJ, Rajput AH, Ahlskog JE, et al. Amantadine treatment is an independent predictor of improved survival in Parkinson's disease. Neurology 1996;46:1551–1556.

40. Cotzias CG, Van Woert MH, Schiffer LM. Aromatic amino acids and modification of parkinsonism. N Engl J Med 1967;276:374–379.

41. Papavasilou PS, Cotzias GC, Duby SE, et al. Levodopa in parkinsonism: Potentiation of central effects with a peripheral inhibitor. N Engl J Med 1972;285:8–14.

42. Poewe WH, Wenning GK. The natural history of Parkinson's disease. Neurology 1996;47(suppl 3):S146–152.

43. Ahlskog JE. Medical treatment of later stage motor problems of Parkinson disease. Mayo Clin Proc 1999;74:1239–1254.

44. Van Laar T. Levodopa-induced response fluctuations in patients with Parkinson's disease: Strategies for management. CNS Drugs 2003;17:475–489.

45. Koller WC, Hutton JT, Tolosa E, et al. Immediate-release and controlled release carbidopa/levodopa in PD: A five-year randomized multicenter study. Neurology 1999;53:1012–1019.

46. LeWitt PA, Nelson MV, Berchou RC, et al. Controlled-release carbidopa/levodopa (Sinemet 50/200 CR4): Clinical and pharmacokinetic studies. Neurology 1989;39(suppl 2):45–53.

47. Quinn N, Parkes JD, Marsden CD. Control of on/off phenomenon by continuous intravenous infusion of levodopa. Neurology 1984;34:1131–1136.

48. Nilsson D, Nyholm D, Aquilonius S-M. Duodenal levodopa infusion in Parkinson's disease: Long-term experience. Acta Neurol Scand 2001;104:343–348.

49. Kurth MC, Tetrud JW, Irwin I, et al. Oral levodopa/carbidopa solution versus tablets in Parkinson's patients with severe fluctuations: A pilot study. Neurology 1993;43:1036–1039.

50. Nelson MV, Berchou RC, LeWitt PA, et al. Pharmacodynamic modeling of concentration-effect relationships after controlled release carbidopa/levodopa (Sinemet CR4) in Parkinson's disease. Neurology 1990;40:70–74.

51. Contin M, Riva R, Martinelli P, et al. Pharmacodynamic modeling of oral levodopa: Clinical application in Parkinson's disease. Neurology 1993;43:367–371.

52. Contin M, Riva R, Martinelli P, et al. Longitudinal monitoring of the levodopa concentration-effect relationship in Parkinson's disease. Neurology 1994;44:1287–1292.

53. Nutt JG, Holford NHG. The response to levodopa in Parkinson's disease: Imposing pharmacological law and order. Ann Neurol 1996;39:561–573.

54. LeWitt PA. New and experimental drug treatments for Parkinson's disease. In: Pahwa R, Lyons K, Koller WC, eds. Therapy of Parkinson's Disease. New York, Marcel Dekker, 2004:491–505.

55. Mahmood I. Is 10 milligrams selegiline essential as an adjunct therapy for the symptomatic treatment of Parkinson's disease? Ther Drug Monit 1998;20:717–721.

56. Elsworth JD, Glover V, Reynolds GP, et al. Deprenyl administration in man: A selective MAO-B inhibitor without "cheese-effect." Psychopharmacology 1987;57:33–38.

57. Shoulson I, Parkinson Study Group. DATATOP: A decade of neuroprotective inquiry. Ann Neurol 1998;44(suppl 1):S160–166.

58. Rabey JM, Sagi I, Huberman M, et al. Rasagiline mesylate, a new MAO-B inhibitor for the treatment of Parkinson's disease: A double-blind study as adjunctive therapy to levodopa. Clin Neuropharmacol 2000;23:324–330.

59. Parkinson Study Group. A controlled trial of rasagiline in early Parkinson disease. Arch Neurol 2002;59:1937–1943.

60. Ruottinen HM, Rinne UK. COMT inhibition in the treatment of Parkinson's disease. J Neurol 1998;245(suppl 3):25–34.

61. Rinne UK, Larsen JP, Siden A, Worm-Peterson J. Entacapone enhances the response to levodopa in parkinsonian patients with motor fluctuations. NOMECOMT Study Group. Neurology 1998;51:1309–1314.

62. The Parkinson Study Group. Entacapone improves motor fluctuations in levodopa-treated Parkinson's disease patients. Ann Neurol 1997;42:747–755.

63. Pezzoli G, Martinoni E, Pacchetti C, et al. A crossover, controlled study comparing pergolide with bromocriptine as an adjunct to levodopa for the treatment of Parkinson's disease. Neurology 1995;45(suppl 3):S22–27.

64. Lieberman A, Neophytides A, Liebowitz M, et al. Comparative efficacy of pergolide and bromocriptine in patients with advanced Parkinson's disease. Adv Neurol 1983;37:95–108.

65. Olanow CW. Pergolide, parlodel crossover study. Neurology 1988;38:314–316.

66. Hely MA, Morris JGL, Reid WGJ, et al. The Sidney multicentre study of Parkinson's disease: A randomised, prospective five-year study comparing low-dose bromocriptine with low-dose levodopa-carbidopa. J Neurol Neurosurg Psychiatry 1994;57:903–910.

67. Przuntek H, Welzel D, Gerlach M, et al. Early institution of bromocriptine in Parkinson's disease inhibits the emergence of levodopa-associated motor side effects: Long term results of the PRADO study. J Neurol Transm 1996;103:699–715.

68. Rascol O, Brooks DJ, Korczyn AD, et al. A five-year study of the incidence of dyskinesia in patients with early Parkinson's disease who were treated with ropinirole or levodopa. N Engl J Med 2000;342:1491.

69. Parkinson Study Group. A randomized, controlled trial comparing pramipexole with levodopa in early Parkinson's disease: Design and methods of the CALM-PD study. Clin Neuropharmacol 2000;23:34–43.

70. Weiner WJ. The intial treatment of Parkinson's disease should begin with levodopa. Mov Disord 1999;14:716–724.

71. Montastruc JL, Rascol O, Senard JM. Treatment of Parkinson's disease should begin with a dopamine agonist. Mov Disord 1999;14:725–730.

72. Albin RL, Frey KA. Initial agonist treatment of Parkinson disease: A critique. Neurology 2003;60:390–394.

73. Mijasaki JM, Martin W, Suchowersky O, et al. Practice parameter: Initiation of treatment for Parkinson's disease: An evidence based review. Report of the quality standards subcommittee of the American Academy of Neurology. Neurology 2002:58;11–17.

74. Parkinson Study Group. Safety and efficacy of pramipexole in early Parkinson disease: A randomized dose-ranging study. JAMA 1997;278:125–130.

75. Goetz CG, Blasucci L, Stebbins GT. Switching dopamine agonists in advanced Parkinson's disease: Is rapid titration preferable to slow? Neurology 1999;52:1227–1229.

76. O'Suilleabhain PE, Dewey RB. Contributions of dopaminergic drugs and disease severity to daytime sleepiness in Parkinson's disease. Arch Neurol 2002;59:986–989.

77. Tan E, Ondo W. Clinical characteristics of pramipexole-induced peripheral edema. Arch Neurol 2000;57:729–732.

78. Ling LH, Ahlskog JE, Munger TM, et al. Constrictive pericarditis and pleuropulmonary disease linked to ergot dopamine agonist therapy (cabergoline) for Parkinson's disease. Mayo Clin Proc 1999;74:371–375

79. Pritchett AM, Morrison JF, Edwards WD, et al. Valvular heart disease in patients taking pergolide. Mayo Clin Proc 2002;77:1280–1286.

80. Clinical pharmacokinetic and pharmacodynamic properties of drugs used in the treatment of Parkinson's disease. Clin Pharmacokinet 2002;41:261–309.

81. Dewey RB Jr, Hutton JT, LeWitt PA, Factor SA. A randomized double-blind placebo-controlled trial of subcutaneously injected apomorphine for Parkinsonian "off" states. Arch Neurol 2001;58:1385–1392.

82. Barone JA. Domperidone: A peripherally acting dopamine-2-receptor antagonist. Ann Pharmacother 1999;33:429–440.

83. Quattrone A, Zappia M. Oral pulse levodopa therapy in mild Parkinson's disease. Neurology 1993;43:1161–1166.

84. PD MED: A large randomised assessment of the relative cost-effectiveness of classes of drugs for Parkinson's Disease. Available at the University of Birmingham Web site, *www.pdmed.bham.ac.uk;* accessed October 31, 2003.

58
PAIN MANAGEMENT

Terry J. Baumann

Learning Objectives and other resources can be found at *www.pharmacotherapyonline.com.*

KEY CONCEPTS

◀1 It is important, whenever possible, to ask patients if they have pain, to identify the source of pain, and to assess the characteristics of the pain.

◀2 Patients taking analgesics should be monitored for response and side effects, particularly sedation and constipation associated with the opioids.

◀3 Oral analgesics are preferred whenever feasible, but it is important to adjust the route of administration to the needs of the patient.

◀4 Equianalgesic doses are useful as a guide when converting from one agent to another, but further dose titration usually is required to achieve treatment goals.

◀5 Doses must be individualized for each patient and administered for an adequate duration of time. Around-the-clock regimens should be considered for acute and chronic pain. As-needed regimens should be used for breakthrough pain or when acute pain displays wide variability and/or has subsided greatly.

◀6 Whenever possible, a multidisciplinary approach and nonpharmacologic strategies should be used.

◀7 For neuropathic pain, capsaicins, tricyclic antidepressants, anticonvulsants, and methadone should be considered.

◀8 Placebo therapy should not be used as an attempt to diagnose psychogenic pain.

Although the world is full of suffering, it is also full of the overcoming of it.

Helen Keller[1]

Humans have always known and sought relief from pain.[2] The act of relieving pain is probably as old as the medical profession itself. Today, pain's impact on society is still great, and indeed, pain complaints remain a primary reason patients seek medical advice.[3]

Regrettably, many health care providers do not receive adequate training in this area, and new information is not widely disseminated and/or understood. Clearly, pain management is enhanced when a multidisciplinary approach is applied. Thus, understanding the pathophysiology of pain therapy and maintaining a working knowledge of individual pain regimens are important to clinicians and are key factors in addressing inadequate pain control.

DEFINITION

An acceptable definition of pain remains an enigma. Once thought to be a punishment from the gods, the word is derived from the Latin *peone* and the Greek *poine*, meaning "penalty" or "punishment."[2] Aristotle considered pain a feeling and classified it as a passion of the soul, where the heart was the source or processing center of pain.[2] This Aristotelian concept predominated for the next 2000 years, although Descartes, Galen, and Vesalius postulated that pain was a sensation in which the brain played an important role. In the nineteenth century, Mueller, Van Frey, and Goldscheider hypothesized the concepts of neuroreceptors, nociceptors, and sensory input.[2] These theories developed into the current definition of pain: "an unpleasant sensory and emotional experience associated with actual or potential tissue damage or described in terms of such damage."[4] Pain is often so subjective, however, that many clinicians define pain as whatever the patient says it is. The best care is achieved when (1) the patient comes first and (2) when in doubt remember number 1.[5]

EPIDEMIOLOGY

Fifty million Americans are partially or totally disabled because of pain.[3] The annual cost of pain to American society can be estimated to be in the billions of dollars.[6] These numbers are expected to rise as more and more Americans work beyond 60 years of age and survive into their 80s.[6]

Unfortunately, pain often remains undertreated and continues to be a problem in hospitals, long-term care facilities, and the community. Seriously ill hospitalized patients have reported a 50% incidence of pain; 15% had extremely or moderately severe pain occurring at least 50% of the time, and 15% were dissatisfied with overall pain control.[7] In a follow-up report, the authors state that pain control persists as a major problem in hospitalized patients, and some of these patients were still in pain many months after hospitalization and experienced pain even on their deathbeds.[8] In addition, problems with inadequate use of analgesics have been reported in cancer patients residing in nursing homes.[9] In the Michigan pain study, 70% of chronic pain patients claimed to have pain despite treatment, with 22% believing that treatment worsened pain.[6]

PATHOPHYSIOLOGY

The pathophysiology of pain involves a complex array of neural networks in the brain that are acted on by afferent stimuli to produce

TABLE 58–1. Nociception: Basic Process of Pain Transmission

1. *Stimulation.* Noxious stimulus sensitizes and/or stimulates nociceptors and causes the release of neural chemicals that also sensitize and/or stimulate nociceptors. This activation leads to the production of an action potential.
2. *Transmission.* The action potential continues from the site of noxious stimulus to the dorsal horn of the spinal cord and then ascends to higher centers in the CNS. Transmission takes place in at least five pathways:
   a. Spinothalamic tract
   b. Spinoreticular tract
   c. Spinomesencephalic tract
   d. Dorsal column postsynaptic spinomedullary pathway
   e. Propriospinal multisynaptic ascending systems
3. *Perception.* Conscious experience of pain.
4. *Modulation.* Inhibition of nociceptive impulses. Neurons from the brain stem descend to the spinal cord and release substances such as endogenous opioids, serotonin, and norepinephrine that inhibit transmission of nociceptive impulses.

Compiled from refs. 11, 12, and 13.

the experience we know as pain. These peripheral and central mechanisms are dynamic and are modulated by changes that occur secondary to tissue damage. In acute pain, this modulation is short-lived, but in some situations, the changes may persist, and chronic pain develops.[10] Classification by inferred pathology in terms of nociceptive and neuropathic pathways gives one a better understanding of both acute and chronic pain.[11] Nociceptive pain best outlines the pathophysiology of acute pain, whereas neuropathic pathophysiology is why some chronic pain develops.

NOCICEPTIVE PAIN

Nociceptive pain typically is classified as either somatic (arising from skin, bone, joint, muscle, or connective tissue) or visceral (arising from internal organs such as the large intestine or pancreas). While somatic pain most often presents as throbbing and well localized, visceral pain can manifest as pain feeling as if it is coming from other structures (referred) or as a well-localized phenomenon.[11] We can think of nociception in terms of stimulation, transmission, perception, and modulation[11] (Table 58–1).

STIMULATION

The first step leading to the sensation of pain is stimulation of free nerve endings known as *nociceptors*. These receptors are found in both somatic and visceral structures, distinguish between noxious and innocuous stimuli, and are activated and sensitized by mechanical, thermal, and chemical impulses.[11] The underlying mechanism of these noxious stimuli (which in and of themselves may sensitize/stimulate the receptor) may be the release of bradykinins, K^+, prostaglandins, histamine, leukotrienes, serotonin, and substance P (among others) that sensitize and/or activate the nociceptors.[12,13] Receptor activation leads to action potentials that are transmitted along afferent nerve fibers to the spinal cord[11] (Fig. 58–1).

TRANSMISSION

Nociceptive transmission takes place in Aδ and C-afferent nerve fibers.[11] Stimulation of large-diameter, sparsely myelinated Aδ fibers evokes sharp, well-localized pain, whereas stimulation of unmyelinated, small-diameter C fibers produces dull, aching, and poorly localized pain.[11] These afferent, nociceptive pain fibers synapse in various layers (laminae) of the spinal cord's dorsal horn,[13] releasing a

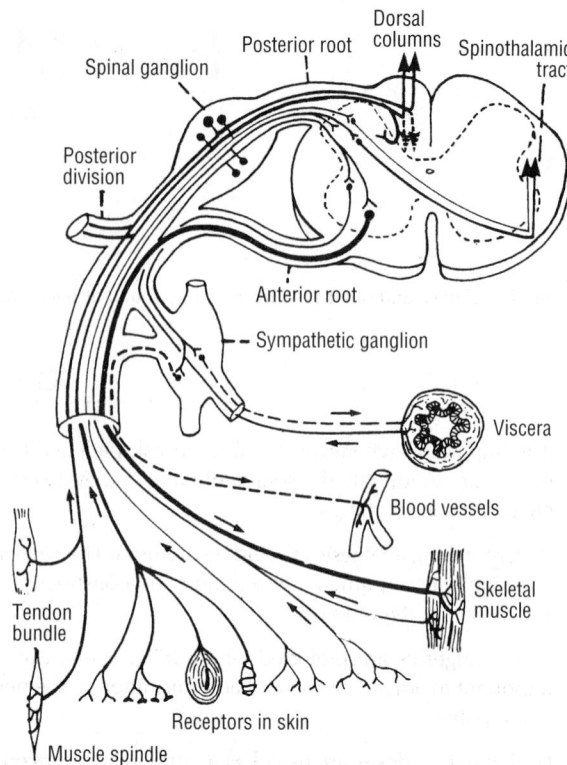

FIGURE 58–1. Schematic representation of dorsal horn nociceptive modulation. *(Adapted from Ref. 13.)*

variety of neurotransmitters, including glutamate, substance P, and calcitonin gene–related peptide.[14] The complex array of events that influence pain can be explained in part by the interactions between neuroreceptors and neurotransmitters that take place in this synapse. For example, by stimulating large sensory myelinated fibers (e.g., Aβ) that mutually connect in the dorsal horn with pain fibers, both noxious and nonnoxious stimuli can have an inhibitory effect on pain transmission[15] (see Fig. 58–1). Functionally, the importance of the interplay between these different fibers and various neurotransmitters and neuroreceptors is evident in the analgesic response produced by topical irritants or transcutaneous electrical nerve stimulation. These pain-initiated processes reach the brain through a complex array of at least five ascending spinal cord pathways, which include the spinothalamic tract[16] (see Table 58–1). Information other than pain is also carried along these pathways. Thus pain is influenced by many factors supplemental to nociception and precludes simple schematic representation. It is postulated that the thalamus acts as a relay station as these pathways ascend and passes the impulses to central structures where pain can be processed further.[11]

PAIN PERCEPTION

At this point in transmission, pain is thought to become a conscious experience that takes place in higher cortical structures. The brain may accommodate only a limited number of pain signals; thus cognitive and behavioral functions can modify pain. Relaxation, distraction, meditation, and guided mental imagery may decrease pain by limiting the number of processed pain signals.[11]

MODULATION

The body modulates pain through a number of complex processes. One, known as the *endogenous opiate system,* consists of neurotransmitters (e.g., enkephalins, dynorphins, and β-endorphins) and receptors (e.g., mu, delta, and kappa) that are found throughout the central nervous system (CNS).[16] Like exogenous opioids, endogenous opioids bind to opioid receptor sites and modulate the transmission of pain impulses.[11] Other receptor types also can influence this system. Activation of *N*-methyl-*D*-aspartate (NMDA) receptors, found in the dorsal horn, can decrease the mu receptors' responsiveness to opiates.[16]

The CNS also contains a highly organized descending system for control of pain transmission. This system can inhibit synaptic pain transmission at the dorsal horn and originates in the brain.[11] Important neurotransmitters here include endogenous opioids, serotonin, norepinephrine, γ-aminobutyric acid (GABA), and neurotensin.[11]

NEUROPATHIC PAIN

Neuropathic pain is distinctly different from nociceptive pain. It is pain sustained by abnormal processing of sensory input by the peripheral or CNS. A large number of neuropathic pain syndromes exist (Fig. 58–2), and they are often difficult to treat.[11] In addition, the pain reported often is not evident by examining physical findings.[11]

The mechanism responsible may be the nervous system's endogenous dynamic nature. Nerve damage or persistent stimulation may cause pain circuits to rewire themselves both anatomically and biochemically.[14] This produces spontaneous nerve stimulation, autonomic neuronal pain stimulation, and a progressive increase in the discharge of dorsal horn neurons.[11,14]

Clinically, patients present with spontaneous pain transmission (often described as burning, tingling, shocklike, or shooting), exaggerated painful response to normally noxious stimuli (hyperalgesia), or painful response to normally nonnoxious stimuli (allodynia).[11,17] This change over time may help to explain why this type pain often manifests long after the actual nerve-related injury.

CLINICAL PRESENTATION

Clinical presentation of pain is best addressed by proper pain assessment. A patient-oriented approach is essential, and evaluation methods should not differ from those used in other medical conditions.[2] Therefore, a comprehensive history and physical examination are imperative to evaluate underlying diseases and possible contributing factors thoroughly.[2] This includes identifying the source of pain when possible.[2] A baseline characterization of pain can be obtained by assessing PQRST characteristics[18] (Table 58–2). Attention also must be given to mental factors that alter the pain threshold. Anxiety, depression, fatigue, anger, and fear in particular are noted to lower this threshold, whereas rest, mood elevation, sympathy, diversion, and understanding raise the pain threshold.[18]

TABLE 58–2. PQRST Characteristics of Pain

P	Palliative factors	What makes the pain better?
	Provocative factors	What makes the pain worse?
Q	Quality	Describe the pain.
R	Radiation	Where is the pain?
S	Severity/intensity	How does this pain compare with other pain you have experienced?
T	Temporal factors	Does the intensity of the pain change with time?

Modified from ref. 18.

CLINICAL PRESENTATION OF PAIN

GENERAL

- Patients may be in obvious acute distress (trauma pain) or appear to have no noticeable suffering (chronic/persistent).

SYMPTOMS

- Pain can be described as sharp, dull, burning, shocklike, tingling, shooting, radiating, fluctuating in intensity, and varying in location.
- Over time, the same pain stimulus may cause symptoms that completely change (e.g., sharp to dull, obvious to vague).
- Nonspecific symptoms include anxiety, depression, fatigue, insomnia, anger, and fear.

SIGNS

- Acute pain can cause hypertension, tachycardia, diaphoresis, mydriasis, and pallor, but these signs are *not diagnostic*.
- In some acute cases and in most chronic/persistent pain, there may be no obvious signs.

LABORATORY TESTS

- Pain is always subjective
- There are *no* laboratory tests that can diagnose pain.
- Thus pain is best diagnosed based on patient description and history.

Source: Compiled from refs. 18 and 22.

Clinicians must evaluate all components of the pain experience, e.g., behavioral (part of our reaction to pain is learned),[19] cognitive (thinking processes alter pain experiences),[20] social (pain expression differs in accordance with social environments),[21] and cultural (cultural background may influence pain tolerance).[21] In addition, separating pain with neuropathic pathophysiology (see Fig. 58–2) from that caused by a known nociceptive pathophysiology (e.g., post-trauma pain) allows for improved treatment regimens. Nociceptive

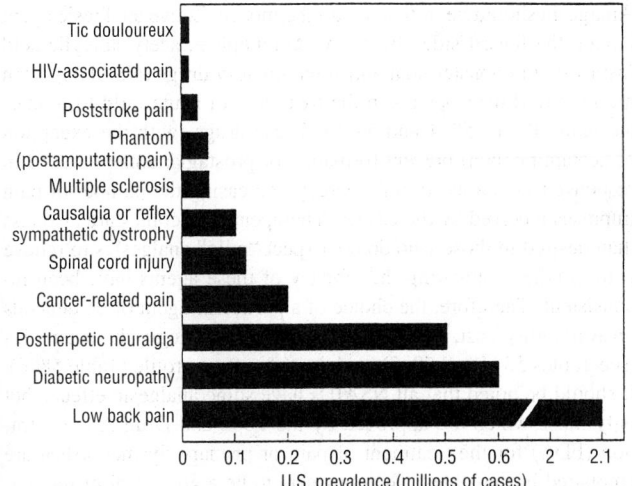

FIGURE 58–2. Estimated prevalence of neuropathic pain. *(Adapted from Ref. 14.)*

pain is often acute, localized, well described, and relieved with conventional analgesic therapy (e.g., opioids, acetaminophen, nonsteroidal anti-inflammatory drugs), whereas neuropathic pain is often chronic, not well recognized, and not easily treated with conventional analgesics. Proper patient assessment also must include an evaluation of pain management. Pain intensity, pain relief, and medication side effects (e.g., opioid-induced sedation or constipation) must be assessed and reassessed on a regular basis. The timing and regularity of this assessment will depend on the type of pain and the medications administered. Postoperative pain and

acute exacerbation of cancer pain may need to be assessed every hour, whereas chronic nonmalignant pain may need only daily assessment. Quality of life also must be assessed on a regular basis in all patients.

The clinician must remember, however, that "pain is always subjective. Objective observations of grimacing, limping, or tachycardia may be helpful in assessing patients, but these signs are often absent in patients with chronic pain caused by structural lesions. No neurophysiological or chemical test can measure pain. The clinician must accept the patient's report of pain"[22]

▶ TREATMENT: Acute and Chronic Pain

Acute pain may be a useful physiologic process warning individuals of disease states and potentially harmful situations. Unfortunately, severe, unremitting, undertreated, acute pain, when it outlives its biologic usefulness, can produce many deleterious effects (e.g., psychological problems). When acute pain is not treated effectively, the stress and concurrent reflex reactions often cause hypoxia, hypercapnia, hypertension, excessive cardiac activity, and emotional difficulties.

Under normal conditions, acute pain subsides quickly as the healing process decreases the pain-producing stimuli; however, in some instances, pain persists for months to years, leading to a chronic pain state with features quite different from those of acute pain (Table 58–3). Chronic pain can be divided into four subtypes: pain that persists beyond the normal healing time for an acute injury, pain related to a chronic disease, pain without identifiable organic cause, and pain that involves both the chronic and acute pain associated with cancer.[23] Patients in chronic pain can develop severe psychological problems caused by fear and memory of past pain. In addition, chronic pain patients may develop dependence on and tolerance to analgesics, have trouble sleeping, and react more readily to environmental changes that can intensify the pain response. Distinguishing between chronic and acute pain states is very important because of differing management techniques.

ACUTE PAIN MANAGEMENT

The obvious way to relieve pain is to eliminate the underlying cause. This is often not possible, however, and symptomatic relief usually

is indicated. Therapeutic interventions include pharmacologic treatment, stimulation therapies, and psychological therapies.

NONPHARMACOLOGIC THERAPY

Stimulation Therapy

Transcutaneous electrical nerve stimulation (TENS) has shown moderate success in managing surgical, traumatic, and oral-facial pain.[15] Although opioid-like side effects certainly are prevented, this technique has not gained wide acceptance in acute pain.

Psychologic Intervention

Even though the cognitive, behavioral, and social aspects of pain are well established, psychologic techniques for the treatment of acute pain are not employed widely. Simple interventions (e.g., introductory information about sensations to expect after certain procedures) reduce patient distress and greatly reduce postprocedure suffering.[24] Other successful psychologic techniques include relaxation training, imagery, and hypnosis.[24]

PHARMACOLOGIC TREATMENT

Nonopioid Agents

Analgesia should be initiated with the most effective analgesic agent having the fewest side effects. Acetaminophen, acetylsalicylic acid (aspirin), and nonsteroidal anti-inflammatory drugs (NSAIDs) often are preferred over opiates in the treatment of acute mild to moderate pain (Tables 58–4 and 58–5). These drugs (with the exception of acetaminophen) prevent formation of prostaglandins produced in response to noxious stimuli, thereby decreasing the number of pain impulses received by the CNS.[22] Therapeutic outcomes are also less than desired in those who do not expect "mild" analgesics to relieve pain. Studies comparing the efficacy of these agents have been inconsistent. Therefore, the choice of a particular agent often depends on availability, cost, pharmacokinetics, pharmacologic characteristics (see Tables 58–4 and 58–5), and the side-effect profile (Table 58–6). It should be noted that all NSAIDs have some analgesic effects, but only those which are approved by the Food and Drug Administration (FDA) for the treatment of pain or primary dysmenorrhea are compared in the tables. There appears to be a great deal of interpatient variability in the therapeutic response to the NSAIDs. After an

TABLE 58–3. Characteristics of Acute and Chronic Pain

Characteristic	Acute Pain	Chronic Pain
Relief of pain	Highly desirable	Highly desirable
Dependence and tolerance to medication	Unusual	Common
Psychological component	Usually not present	Often a major problem
Organic cause	Common	Often not present
Environmental contributions and family involvement	Small	Significant
Insomnia	Unusual	Common component
Treatment goal	Cure	Functionality
Depression	Uncommon	Common

Modified from ref. 2, p. 256

TABLE 58–4. Pharmacokinetic and Pharmacodynamic Profiles of FDA-Approved Nonopioid Analgesics (does not include agents approved only for osteoarthritis or rheumatoid arthritis)

Agent	Time to Peak Concentration (h)	Elimination Half-Life (h)	Analgesic Onset (h)	Analgesic Duration (h)
Aspirin	0.25–2	0.25–0.33	0.5	3–6
Choline salicylate	1.5–2	—[a]	—[a]	4
Magnesium salicylate	1.5–2	—[a]	—[a]	4
Sodium salicylate	0.67	—[a]	—[a]	4
Diflunisal	2–3	8–12	1	8–12
Acetaminophen	0.5–2	1.25–3	0.5–1	3–6
Meclofenamate	0.5–2	0.8–5.3	—[a]	4–6
Mefenamic acid	2–4	2–4	—[a]	6
Etodoloc	1	7	0.5–1	6–8
Diclofenac potassium	1	2	0.5	6–8
Ibuprofen	1–2	1–2.5	0.5	4–6
Fenoprofen	1–2	2–3	0.25–0.5	4–6
Ketoprofen	0.5–2	1.1–4	1	4–8
Naproxen	2–4	12–17	1	Up to 12
Naproxen sodium	1–2	12–13	0.5–1	Up to 12
Ketorolac (parenteral)	0.5–1	4–6	0.17	6
Ketorolac (oral)	0.5–1	4–6	0.5–1	4–6
Celecoxib	3	11	1	12–24
Valdecoxib	3	8–11	1	12–24

[a]Data not available to author.
Complied from refs. 22, 33, 34, 54, 55, 56, 57, 58, 59, and 61.

adequate drug trial of any of these agents, it is considered rational therapy to switch to another member of this drug group for an additional trial period.

Opioid Agents

Most clinicians consider the use of opioids to be the next logical step in the management of acute pain. The classification of these agents, their equianalgesic doses, and dosing guidelines are outlined in Tables 58–7 and 58–8.

The pharmacologic activity of opioids depends on their affinity for opiate receptors.[25] Therapeutic activities and side effects range from those exhibited by the opiate agonists (e.g., morphine) to those seen with the opiate antagonists (e.g., naloxone). Partial agonists and antagonists (e.g., pentazocine) compete with agonists for opiate receptor sites and, depending on the inherent agonist and antagonist properties, exhibit mixed agonist-antagonist activity. Mixed agonist-antagonist agents with analgesic activity appear to exhibit selectivity for analgesic receptor sites.[25] This may result in analgesia with fewer undesirable side effects.

The effects of the opioid analgesics are relatively selective, and at normal therapeutic concentrations, these agents do not affect other sensory modalities,[26] such as sensitivity to touch, sight, or hearing; however, as the dosage increases, so do the undesirable side effects (see Table 58–9). Patients in severe pain may receive very high doses of opioids with no unwanted side effects, but as the pain subsides, they may not tolerate even very low doses.[27] Frequently, when opioids are administered, pain is not eliminated, but its unpleasantness is decreased.[27] Patients report that although their pain is still present, it no longer bothers them.

Opioids share related pharmacologic attributes and exert a profound effect on the CNS and gastrointestinal tract.[27] Mood changes, sedation, respiratory depression, nausea, vomiting, decreased gastrointestinal motility, dependence, and tolerance are evident in varying degrees with all agents. Consideration of efficacy and side-effect profile assists in selection of the most appropriate agent.

The route of administration depends on individual patient needs. With oral analgesics, the onset usually takes about 45 minutes, whereas the peak effect usually occurs 1 to 2 hours after administration.[22] This delay must be a consideration when immediate relief is needed. The opioids differ greatly in equianalgesic dose, as seen in Table 58–7, which should be used only as a guide because the nature of pain makes it necessary to individualize pain regimens. True opioid allergies are rare, but Table 58–7 also can be used when treating a patient who is allergic to opiates. Although caution is always advised, a decrease in potential cross-sensitivity exists when moving from one opioid class to another. The classes are morphine-like agonists, meperidine-like agonists, and methadone-like agonists. When considering cross-sensitivity, the mixed agonist-antagonist class acts much like the morphine-like agonists.[28]

In the initial stages of acute pain, analgesics should be given around the clock. This should commence after administering a typical starting dose and titrating up or down depending on the patient's degree of pain and demonstrated side effects (e.g., sedation).[22] As-needed schedules often produce wide swings in analgesic plasma concentrations that create wide swings in pain and sedation. This may initiate a vicious cycle where increasing amounts of pain medications are needed for relief. As the painful state subsides and the need for medication decreases, however, as-needed schedules can be used. Continuous intravenous and subcutaneous methods of opioid infusion are effective in some postoperative pain, but the probability of unwanted side effects is high.[22] An alternative method that has gained prominence is patient-controlled analgesia (PCA). With this technique, patients can self-administer preset amounts of intravenous opioids via a syringe pump electronically interfaced with a timing device. Using this procedure, patients balance pain control with sedation.

Administration of opiates directly into the CNS (i.e., epidural and intrathecal/subarachnoid routes) has shown considerable promise in

TABLE 58–5. FDA-Approved Nonopioid Analgesics in Adults (does not include agents approved only for osteoarthritis or rheumatoid arthritis)

Class and Generic Name	Usual Dosage Range (mg)	Maximal Dose (mg/day)
Salicylates		
Acetylsalicylic acid[a] (aspirin)	325–650 every 4 h	4000
Choline[a]	870 every 3–4 h	5220
Magnesium[a]	650 every 4 h or 1090 three times daily	4800 in 3–4 divided doses
Sodium[a]	325–650 every 4 h	5400
Diflunisal	500–1000 initial	
	250–500 every 8–12 h	1500
para-Aminophenol		
Acetaminophen[a]	325–1000 every 4–6 h	4000
Fenamates		
Meclofenamate	50–100 every 4–6 h	400
Mefenamic acid	Initial 500	
	250 every 6 h (maximum of 7 days)	1000[b]
Pyranocarboxylic Acid		
Etodoloc	200–400 every 6–8 h (immediate release only)	1000
Acetic Acid		
Diclofenac potassium	In some patients, initial 100,	150[c]
	50 three times a day	
Propionic Acids		
Ibuprofen[a]	200–400 every 4–6 h	3200
		1200[d]
Fenoprofen	200 every 4–6 h	3200
Ketoprofen[a]	25–50 every 6–8 h	300
	12.5–25 every 4–6 h[d]	75[d]
Naproxen	500 initial	
	500 every 12 h or 250 every 6–8 h	1000[b]
Naproxen sodium[a]	In some patients, 440 initial[d]	
	220 every 8–12 h[d]	660[d]
Naproxen delayed-release[e]	500 every 12 h	1000
Naproxen controlled-release[e]	500–1000 every 24 h	1500
Pyrrolizine Carboxylic Acid		
Ketorolac (parenteral)	30–60 (single IM dose only)	30–60
	15–30 every 6 h (maximum of 5 days)	120
Ketorolac (oral) (indicated for continuation	In some patients, initial oral dose 20	40
with parenteral only)	10 every 4–6 h (maximum of 5 days,	
	which includes parenteral doses)	
Cyclooxygenase 2 Inhibitors		
Celecoxib	Initial 400 followed by another 200 on first day	400[f]
	then 200 twice daily[f]	
Valdecoxib	20 twice daily[g]	40[g]

[a]Available both as an over-the-counter preparation and as a precription drug.
[b]Up to 1250 mg on the first day.
[c]Up to 200 mg on the first day.
[d]Over the counter.
[e]Not for the initial treatment of acute pain.
[f]For acute pain primary dysmenorrhea.
[g]For primary dysmenorrhea.
Compiled from refs. 22, 33, and 34.

the control of acute pain[29] (see Table 58–10) and is common in both large and small institutions throughout the United States. Because of reports of marked sedation, respiratory depression, pruritus, nausea, vomiting, urinary retention, and hypotension,[30] these methods of analgesia require careful monitoring and are best employed by experienced practitioners. Respiratory depression is of concern and can occur within the first half hour or manifest as late as 12 hours after a single dose of epidural morphine.[30] Naloxone is used to antagonize this effect, but continual infusion may be required.[30] Analgesia and side effects are evident at lower doses when the opioids are administered intrathecally instead of epidurally. Intrathecally, single morphine doses of 0.1 to 0.3 mg are common, whereas epidurally, doses of 1 to 6 mg are the norm.[29] These intrathecal and epidural opioids often

are administered on a continuous-infusion and/or patient-contolled basis, and when given simultaneously with intrathecal or epidural local anesthetics such as bupivacaine, they have been proven safe and effective.[31] All agents administered directly into the CNS should be preservative-free.

■ *Morphine and Congeners.* Despite the availability of several newer agents, morphine remains the prototype opiate analgesic. As new opioid and nonopioid compounds are developed, their efficacy and side-effect profiles are compared against morphine as the standard. Many clinicians consider morphine the first-line agent when treating moderate to severe pain. Morphine can be given parenterally, orally, or rectally.

TABLE 58–6. Relative Side Effects of FDA-Approved Nonopioid Analgesics (does not include agents approved only for osteoarthritis or rheumatoid arthritis)

Agent	GI Irritation	CNS Effects	Hepatic Toxicity	Renal Toxicity
Aspirin	++++++	+	++	++
Choline salicylate	+++	—[a]	—[a]	—[a]
Magnesium salicylate	+++	—[a]	—[a]	—[a]
Sodium salicylate	+++	—[a]	—[a]	—[a]
Diflunisal	++	+	+	+
Acetaminophen	+	+	++	+
Meclofenamate	++	+	+	++
Mefenamic acid	++	+	+	++
Etodolac	++	+	+	++
Diclofenac potassium	++	+	+	++
Ibuprofen	++	+	+	++
Fenoprofen	++	++	+	++
Ketoprofen	++	+	+	++
Ketorolac[b]	++	+	+	+
Naproxen	++	+	+	++
Celecoxib	+	+	+	++
Valdecoxib	+	+	+	++

[a] No data available to author.
[b] Five-day use only.
Compiled from refs. 33 and 34.

Morphine's CNS effects are numerous. Through direct stimulation of the chemoreceptor trigger zone, morphine causes nausea and vomiting.[27] Opioid-induced nausea is observed most frequently after the initial dose and often subsides with subsequent doses.[32] Although euphoria and dysphoria have been reported, morphine's unpleasant effects are more prominent when administered to those not experiencing pain.[27] As doses of morphine are increased, the respiratory center becomes less responsive to carbon dioxide, resulting in progressive respiratory depression. This effect is less pronounced in those being treated for severe pain. Respiratory depression often manifests as a decrease in respiratory rate (although minute volume and tidal volume are also affected) and is further compounded because the cough reflex is also depressed. Morphine-induced respiratory depression can be reversed by pure opioid antagonists.[27] In patients with underlying pulmonary dysfunction, caution must be employed when using morphine or any related opioid. Although these patients may be functioning normally, they are already using compensatory breathing mechanisms and are at risk for further respiratory compromise.[27] Precaution is also urged when using opiate analgesics with alcohol or other CNS depressants. This combination amplifies CNS depression and is potentially harmful and possibly lethal.

Therapeutic doses of morphine have minimal effects on blood pressure, cardiac rate, or cardiac rhythm when patients are supine; however, morphine does produce venous and arteriolar vessel dilation, and orthostatic hypotension may result. Hypovolemic patients are more susceptible to morphine-induced cardiovascular changes (e.g., decreases in blood pressure).[27] Because morphine prompts a decrease in myocardial oxygen demand in ischemic cardiac patients, it is often considered the drug of choice when using opioids to treat pain associated with myocardial infarction.

Morphine decreases the propulsive contractions of the gastrointestinal tract, and biliary and pancreatic secretions are reduced.[27] The end result, especially when morphine is administered over extended time periods, is constipation. Morphine-induced spasms of the sphincter of Oddi have been observed.[27] However, the clinical significance of such an occurrence should be assessed on an individual basis. Although morphine's effect on the urinary bladder varies, urinary retention can become a problem; tolerance develops to this effect over time.[27] Morphine-induced histamine release often manifests as pruritus, and although not seen often, it may exacerbate bronchospasm in patients with a history of asthma.[27] Therapeutic doses of morphine do not directly affect cerebral circulation, but drug-induced respiratory depression can increase intracranial pressure. Thus caution is advised in head trauma patients who are not ventilated because morphine may exaggerate this pressure[27] while clouding the neurologic examination results.

Hydromorphone is more potent, has better oral absorption characteristics, and is more soluble than morphine, but its overall pharmacologic profile parallels that of morphine. A sustained-release hydromorphone product has recently become available. Oxymorphone can be administered rectally and by injection. Although it is more potent than morphine, it offers no real pharmacologic advantages. Levorphanol has an extended half-life, but its overall therapeutic effects are similar to those of morphine.

Codeine is an analgesic that is effective in the treatment of mild to moderate pain. It is often combined with other analgesic products and enjoys a popularity that makes it the standard for other oral opioids. Unfortunately, codeine has the same propensity to produce tolerance, dependence, and constipation as morphine. Hydrocodone, a derivative of codeine, also is seen most often in combination products and has pharmacologic properties similar to those of morphine. Oxycodone has a similar potency to morphine and is an excellent oral analgesic for moderate to severe pain. This is especially true when the product is used in combination with nonopioids; however, its predilection for causing tolerance and dependence, along with its basic opioid characteristics, likens it to morphine. It should be noted that sustained-release oxycodone is also available.

■ *Meperidine and Congeners (Phenylpiperidines).* The prototype phenylpiperidine, meperidine, has a pharmacologic profile comparable with that of morphine; however, it is not as potent and has a shorter analgesic duration. This necessitates larger doses that often must be administered more frequently for satisfactory pain relief. Although meperidine is effective orally, larger doses must be

TABLE 58–7. Opioid Analgesics

Class and Generic Name	Route	Equianalgesic Dose (mg) (Adults)
Morphine-Like Agonists		
Morphine	IM	10
	PO	30
Hydromorphone	IM	1.5
	PO	7.5
Oxymorphone	IM	1
	R	5[a]
Levorphanol	IM (acute)	2
	PO (acute)	4
	IM (chronic)	1
	PO (chronic)	1
Codeine	IM	15–30[b]
	PO	15–30[b]
Hydrocodone	PO	5–10[b]
Oxycodone	PO	20–30[c]
Meperidine-Like Agonists		
Meperidine	IM	75
	PO	300[c] Not recommended
Fentanyl	IM	0.1–0.2
	Transdermal	25 mcg/h[d]
	Transmucosal for breakthrough pain only	
Methadone-Like Agonists		
Methadone	IM (acute)	Variable[e]
	PO (acute)	Variable[e]
	IM (chronic)	Variable[e]
	PO (chronic)	Variable[e]
Propoxyphene	PO	65[b]
Agonist-Antagonist Derivatives		
Pentazocine	IM	Not recommended
	PO	50[b]
Butorphanol	IM	2
	Intranasal	1[b]
		(one spray)
Nalbuphine	IM	10
Buprenorphine	IM	0.4
Dezocine	IM	10
Antagonists		
Naloxone	IV	0.4–1.2[f]
Central Analgesic		
Tramadol	PO	50–100[b]

[a]Reference 22 considers 5 mg rectal morphine = 5 mg rectal oxymorphone.
[b]Starting dose only (equianalgesia not shown).
[c]Starting doses lower (oxycodone, 5–10 mg).
[d]Equivalent IM morphine dose = 8–22 mg day.
[e]The equianalgesic dose of methadone when compared with other opioids will decrease progressively the higher the previous opioid dose has been.
[f]Starting doses to be used in cases of opioid overdose.
Compiled from refs. 22, 26, 34, and 35.

administered to achieve the same effect as obtained with the parenteral form (Table 58–7). With high doses or in patients with renal failure, the metabolite normeperidine accumulates, causing CNS excitability, manifested as tremor, muscle twitching, and possibly seizures.[33] The combination of monoamine oxidase inhibitors and meperidine should not be used because this mixture can produce severe respiratory depression or excitation, delirium, hyperpyrexia, and convulsions.[27] In most clinical settings, meperidine offers no real advantage over morphine and is largely being replaced by other opioids.

Fentanyl is a synthetic opioid structurally related to meperidine and is used often in anesthesiology as an adjunct to general anesthesia.[33] This agent is more potent and shorter acting than meperidine (see Tables 58–7 and 58–11). Transdermal fentanyl is also available for the treatment of chronic pain in patients requiring opioid analgesics. One patch can provide analgesic support for 72 hours, but it takes 12 to 24 hours to obtain optimal analgesic effect after a patch is applied. In addition, it may take 6 days after increasing a dose before new steady-state levels are achieved. Thus the patch should not be used in patients with acute pain.[34] A fentanyl lozenge on a stick is available for the treatment of breakthrough cancer pain.[34]

■ *Methadone and Congeners.* Methadone has gained considerable popularity because of its oral efficacy, extended duration of action, and ability to suppress withdrawal symptoms in heroin addicts. With

ABLE 58–8. Dosing Guidelines

Agent(s)	Doses (Titrate Up or Down Based on Patient Response)	Notes
NSAIDs/acetaminophen/aspirin	Dose to maximum before switching to another agent (see Table 58–5)	Used in mild to moderate pain May use in conjunction with opioid agents to decrease doses of each Regular alcohol use and high doses of acetaminophen may result in liver toxicity Care must be exercised to avoid overdose when combination products containing these agents are used
Morphine	PO 5–30 mg q 3–4 h[a] IM 5–10 mg q 3–4 h[a] IV 1–2.5 mg q 5 min prn[a] SR 15–30 mg q 12 h (may need to be q 8 h in some patients) Rectal 10–20 mg q 4 h[a]	Drug of choice in severe pain Use immediate-release product with SR product to control "breakthrough" pain in cancer patients Every 24 hour product available
Hydromorphone	PO 2–4 mg q 3–6 h[a] IM 1–4 mg q 3–6 h[a] IV 0.1–0.5 mg q 5 min prn[a] Rectal 3 mg q 6–8 h[a]	Use in severe pain More potent than morphine; otherwise, no advantages Use immediate-release product with sustained-release product to control "breakthrough" pain in cancer patients Use sustained-release product only in those patients who have demonstrated opioid tolerance 12-mg, 16-mg, 24-mg, and 32-mg sustained-release capsules are available and should be dosed every 24 hours
Oxymorphone	IM 1–1.5 mg q 4–6 h[a] IV 0.5 mg initially Rectal 5 mg q 4–6 h[a]	Use in severe pain No advantages over morphine
Levorphanol	PO 2–3 mg q 6–8 h[a] IM 1–2 mg q 6–8 h	Use in severe pain Extended half-life useful in cancer patients In chronic pain, wait 3 days between dosage adjustments
Codeine	PO 15–60 mg q 3–6 h[a] IM 15–60 mg q 3–6 h[a] IV 15–60 mg q 3–6 h[a] (max. 360 mg q day)	Use in moderate pain Weak analgesic; use with NSAIDs or aspirin or acetaminophen
Hydrocodone	PO 5–10 mg q 3–6 h[a]	Use in moderate/severe pain Most effective when used with NSAIDs or aspirin or acetaminophen
Oxycodone	PO 5–10 mg q 3–6 h[a] Controlled release, 10–20 mg q 12 h	Use in moderate/severe pain Most effective when used with NSAIDs or aspirin or acetaminophen Use immediate-release product with controlled-release product to control "breakthrough" pain in cancer patients
Meperidine	IM 50–150 mg q 3–4 h[a] IV 5–10 mg q 5 min prn[a]	Use in severe pain Oral not recommended Do not use in renal failure May precipitate tremors, myoclonus, and seizures Monoamine oxidase inhibitors can induce hyperpyrexia and/or seizures or opioid overdose symptoms
Fentanyl	IV 25–50 mcg/h IM 0.05–0.1 mg q 1–2 h[a] Transdermal 25 mcg/h q 72 h Transmucosal 200 mcg may repeat × 1, 30 minutes after first dose is given then titrate	Used in severe pain Do not use transdermal in acute pain Transmucosal for "breakthrough" cancer pain
Methadone	PO 2.5–10 mg q 3–4 h (acute)[a] IM 2.5–10 mg q 3–4 h (acute)[a] PO 5–20 mg q 6–8 h (chronic)[a]	Effective in severe chronic pain Sedation can be major problem Some chronic pain patients can be dosed every 12 hours The equianalgesic dose of methadone when compared with other opioids will decrease progressively the higher the previous opioid dose has been
Propoxyphene	PO 100 mg q 4 h[a] (napsylate) PO 65 mg q 4 h[a] (HCl) (max. q day 600 mg of napsylate, 390 mg HCl)	Use in moderate pain Weak analgesic; most effective when used with NSAIDs or aspirin or acetaminophen Will cause carbamazepine levels to increase 100 mg of napsylate salt = to 65 mg of HCl salt
Pentazocine	PO 50–100 mg q 3–4 h[b] (max. 600 mg q day)	Third-line agent for moderate to severe pain May precipitate withdrawal in opiate-dependent patients Parenteral doses not recommended

TABLE 58–8. (continued)

Agent(s)	Doses (Titrate Up or Down Based on Patient Response)	Notes
Butorphanol	IM 1–4 mg q 3–4 h[b] IV 0.5–2 mg q 3–4 h[b] Intranasal 1 mg (1 spray) q 3–4 h[b] If inadequate relief after initial spray, may repeat in other nostril × 1 in 30–60 minutes Max 2 sprays (one per nostril) q 3–4 h[b]	Second-line agent for moderate to severe pain May precipitate withdrawal in opiate-dependent patients
Nalbuphine	IM/IV 10 mg q 3–6 h[b] (max 20 mg dose, 160 mg q day)	Second-line agent for moderate to severe pain May precipitate withdrawal in opiate-dependent patients
Buprenorphine	IM 0.3 mg q 6 h[b] Slow IV 0.3 mg q 6 h[b] May repeat x 1, 30–60 min after initial dose	Second-line agent for moderate to severe pain May precipitate withdrawal in opiate-dependent patients Naloxone may not be effective in reversing respiratory depression
Dezocine	IM 5–20 mg q 3–6 h[b] IV 2.5–10 mg q 2–4 h[b]	Second-line agent for moderate to severe pain May precipitate withdrawal in opiate-dependent patients
Naloxone	IV 0.4–1.2 mg	When reversing opiate side effects in patients needing analgesia, dilute and titrate (0.1–0.2 mg q 2–3 min) so as not to reverse analgesia
Tramadol	PO 50–100 mg q 4–6 h[a] If rapid onset not required, start 25 mg/day and titrate over several days	Maximum dose is 400 mg/24 h Decrease dose in renal impairment and in the elderly

SR, sustained release; h, hour; q, every; mg, milligram; mcg, microgram; prn, as needed.

[a]May start with an around-the-clock regimen and switch to prn if/when the painful signal subsides or is episodic.

[b]May reach a ceiling analgesic effect.

Compiled from refs. 22, 24, 25, 26, 33, 34, and 62.

TABLE 58–9. Major Adverse Effects of the Opioid Analgesics

Effect	Manifestation
Mood changes	Dysphoria, euphoria
Somnolence	Lethargy, drowsiness, apathy, inability to concentrate
Stimulation of chemoreceptor trigger zone	Nausea, vomiting
Respiratory depression	Decreased respiratory rate
Decreased gastrointestinal motility	Constipation
Increase in sphincter tone	Biliary spasm, urinary retention (varies among agents)
Histamine release	Urticaria, pruritus, rarely exacerbation of asthma (varies among agents)
Tolerance	Larger doses for same effect
Dependence	Withdrawal symptoms upon abrupt discontinuation

Compiled from 2, 25, and 27.

repeated doses, the analgesic duration of action is prolonged,[34] and excessive sedation also may result. Although methadone is effective in acute pain,[34] it is usually used to treat chronic pain. The pharmacologic profile resembles that of morphine. However, properties unique to methadone when compared with other opioids include the d-isomer's ability to antagonize NMDA receptors and block the reuptake of serotonin and norepinephrine.[35–37] These properties may prove useful in the treatment of neuropathic pain. Contrary to previous thought, the equianalgesic dose of methadone when compared with other opioids will decrease progressively the higher the previous opioid use has been.[35]

CLINICAL CONTROVERSY

Some clinicians believe that methadone should be tried before other opioids in many chronic pain conditions where an opioid is warranted because they believe that neuropathic pain is often present, whereas others believe that sustained-released morphine and oxycodone are better first choices.

TABLE 58–10. Intraspinal Opioids

Agent	Dose (mg) (Single)	Onset of Pain Relief (min)	Duration of Pain Relief (h)	Continual Infusion Dose (mg/h)
Epidural Route				
Morphine	1–6	30	6–24	0.1–1
Hydromorphone	1–2	15	6–16	0.1–0.2
Fentanyl	0.025–0.1	5	1–4	0.025–0.1
Subarachnoid Route				
Morphine	0.1–0.3	15	8–24+	—
Fentanyl	0.005–0.025	5	3–6	—

Modified from ref. 29.

TABLE 58–11. Opioid Analgesic Pharmacokinetics[a]

Agent	Time to Peak (h)	Half-Life (h)	Analgesic Onset (min)	Analgesic Duration (h)
Morphine	0.5–1	2	10–20	3–5
Hydromorphone	0.5–1	2–3	10–20	3–5
Oxymorphone	0.5–1	2–3	10–20	4–6
Levorphanol	0.5–1	12–16	10–20	5–8
Hydrocodone (PO)	1	4	30–60	4–6
Codeine	0.5–1	3	10–20	4–6
Oxycodone (PO)	0.5–1	2–3	30–60	4–6
Meperidine	0.5–1	3–4	10–20	2–5
Fentanyl	0.17–0.33	3–4	7–15	1–2
Methadone	0.5–1	15–30	10–20	4–5 (acute) >8 (chronic)
Propoxyphene (PO)	2–2.5	6–12	30–60	4–6
Pentazocine	0.5–1	4–5	15–20	3–6
Butorphanol	0.5–1	2.5–3.5	10–20	4–6
Nalbuphine	0.5–1	2–5	<15	4–6
Buprenorphine	0.5–1	5	10–20	4–8
Dezocine	0.17–1.5 (IM)	0.6–5 (IV)	15–30 (IV)	2–4 (IV)
Naloxone[c] (IV/IM)	—[b]	1–1.5	1–2 (IV) 2–5 (IM)	0.5–2 (IV) IM may last longer
Tramadol (PO)	2–3	6–7	<60	4–6

[a]Based on intramuscular data unless otherwise indicated.
[b]No data available to author.
[c]Narcotic antagonist.
Compiled from refs. 27, 32, 33, and 34.

Propoxyphene is usually used in combination with acetaminophen in the treatment of moderate pain. The toxicity profile of propoxyphene is similar to that of codeine.

Opioid Agonist-Antagonists Derivatives

Analgesic agents that stimulate the analgesic portion of opioid receptors while blocking or having no effect on the toxicity portion would be considered ideal. The agonist-antagonist derivatives were developed with this in mind. The analgesic class produces analgesia and has a ceiling effect on respiratory depression.[25] These agents also have a lower abuse potential than morphine, but psychotomimetic responses (e.g., hallucinations and dysphoria, as seen with pentazocine), a ceiling analgesic effect, and a propensity to initiate withdrawal in opioid-dependent populations[25] have diminished their widespread clinical use.

Opioid Antagonists

The pure opioid antagonist naloxone binds competitively to opioid receptors but does not produce an analgesic or opioid side-effect response. Therefore, it is used most often to reverse the toxic effects of agonist- and agonist-antagonist–derived opioids.

Central Analgesic

Tramadol has two basic modes of action: mu opiate receptor binding and inhibition of norepinephrine and serotonin reuptake. It is indicated for the relief of moderate to moderately severe pain.[38]

Although associated with less respiratory depression than morphine at recommended doses, tramadol has a side-effect profile that in some ways is similar to that of the previously mentioned opioid analgesics (e.g., dizziness, euphoria, hallucinations, cognitive dysfunction, and constipation).[33] Tramadol alone may enhance the risk of seizures. In addition, concomitant use with serotonin reuptake inhibitors, opioids, tricyclic antidepressants, monoamine oxidase inhibitors, neuroleptics, or other drugs that can reduce the seizure threshold and use in patients with seizure disorders may increase the risk of seizures.[38]

Tramadol may have a place in treating patients with chronic pain, especially that of neuropathic origin.[39] However, this agent has little advantage over the previously mentioned opioid analgesics when treating patients for acute pain.

Combination Therapy

The combination of opioid and nonopioid oral analgesics often results in analgesia superior to that produced by either agent alone.[24] Attacking pain on two fronts, prostaglandins and opiate receptors, enhances pain relief and facilitates the use of lower doses of each agent. This frequently produces a more favorable side-effect profile and is the reason there are so many aspirin- and/or acetaminophen-opioid analgesic combination products on the market. Patients must be cautioned, however, when combination products are used to be aware of the many over-the-counter preparations that contain acetaminophen or aspirin so as not to exceed a safe dose of these agents. The addition of an injectable NSAID (ketorolac) makes this combination possible also in patients who cannot take oral medications. The clinician should not be limited by the availability of commercially established fixed-ratio combinations. For example, the administration of NSAIDs in combination with scheduled opioid regimens is often very effective in the treatment of pain resulting from bone metastases in advanced cancer.[40]

Agents shown to potentiate the analgesic efficacy of parenteral opioids include hydroxyzine and dextroamphetamine.[40] Promethazine and chlorpromazine, once thought to possess this potentiating property, apparently offer no inherent analgesic or potentiating characteristics when combined with narcotics, although unwanted sedation may be increased.[24] Methotrimeprazine, a phenothiazine derivative, does induce analgesia but also produces sedation, orthostatic hypotension, and dizziness.[34]

TABLE 58–12. Local Anesthetics[a]

Agent	Onset (min)	Duration (h)
Esters		
Procaine	2–5	0.25–1
Chloroprocaine	6–12	0.5
Tetracaine	≤15	2–3
Amides		
Mepivacaine	3–5	0.75–1.5
Bupivacaine	5	2–4
Lidocaine	<2	0.5–1
Prilocaine	<2	≥1
Etidocaine	3–5	5–10
Ropivacaine[b]	11–26	1.7–3.2

[a]Unless otherwise indicated, values are for infiltrative anesthesia.
[b]Epidural administration in cesarean section.
Compiled from refs. 34 and 60.

TABLE 58–13. Barriers to Effective Pain Management in Cancer Pain

Problems Related to Health Care Professionals
Inadequate knowledge about pain management
Poor assessment skills
Fear of addiction
Overconcern about opioid side effects
Overconcern about regulation of opioids

Problems Related to Patients
Reluctance to report pain (pain may mean cancer is getting worse)
Fear of addiction
Poor adherence to prescribed regimens

Problems Related to the Health Care System
Inadequate reimbursement
Restrictive regulations on opioids
Opioids unavailable in the pharmacies

Modified from ref. 42.

REGIONAL ANALGESIA

Regional analgesia with properly administered local anesthetics can provide relief of both acute and chronic pain[31] (Table 58–12). These agents can be positioned by injection (i.e., in joints, in the epidural or intrathecal space, along nerve roots, or in a nerve plexus) or topically. Regional anesthetics relieve pain by blocking nociceptive transmission and interrupting sympathetic reflexes.[31] Their lipid solubility, pK_a, percentage of un-ionized drug, drug concentration, vasodilator behavior, and amount of vasoconstrictor (commonly epinephrine) used concomitantly determine the mechanism of action.[31] High plasma concentrations can cause signs of CNS excitation and depression, including dizziness, tinnitus, drowsiness, disorientation, muscle twitching, seizures, and respiratory arrest.[33] Cardiovascular effects include myocardial depression, hypotension, decreased cardiac output, heart block, bradycardia, ventricular arrhythmia, and cardiac arrest.[34] Disadvantages of such methods include the need for skillful technical application, the need for frequent administration, and highly specialized follow-up procedures.

CHRONIC PAIN MANAGEMENT

CANCER PAIN

Managing the pain of malignant diseases encompasses both acute and chronic management techniques. Thus pharmacologic treatment and psychological therapies are best combined with surgical methods, anesthetic procedures, and supportive care measures in a multidisciplinary approach to pain relief.[41] The goal is to provide patients with enough pain amelioration to tolerate diagnostic and therapeutic manipulation and permit them to function at a level that will allow freedom of movement and choice.[40] Unfortunately, a number of patients with cancer suffer significant pain needlessly.[9,42] Barriers to effective pain management in this population are outlined in Table 58–13. A barrier that consistently causes clinicians to misjudge and mistreat pain is the misunderstanding of opioid tolerance, physical dependence, addiction, and pseudoaddiction. "Tolerance is the diminution of drug effect over time as a consequence of exposure to the drug."[43] It develops at different rates and with tremendous patient variation. However, with stable disease, opioid use often stabilizes, and tolerance does not lead to addiction.[43] "Physical dependence is a pharmacological effect of a drug defined by the occurrence of an abstinence syndrome following administration of an antagonist drug

or abrupt dose reduction or discontinuation."[43] Clinicians must understand that physical dependence and tolerance are not equivalent to addiction, and although with chronic opioid use, they are likely to develop, the risk of developing addiction is very small and should not be a concern when treating cancer pain.[22] "Addiction is best defined as a behavioral pattern characterized as loss of control over drug use, compulsive drug use, and continued use of a drug despite harm."[43] When opioids are being used, these behaviors must be evaluated continually, but extreme caution is advised when using the term *addiction* because of its many negative connotations, which can lead to harmful clinician-patient relationship and ineffective pain control.[22,43] In addition, clinicians must be aware that an individual's behaviors may suggest addiction, when in reality the behaviors noted are a reflection of unrelieved pain or pseudoaddiction.[22] Assessment of the factors described in Table 58–2 also apply to cancer patients. Special attention must be given to continual reassessment of the painful state, and individualization of therapy is always required.[40]

Nonpharmacologic Treatment

Psychologic and Supportive Care. Previously mentioned psychologic techniques (e.g., relaxation training, controlled mental imagery) are very helpful in relieving pain experienced in malignant disease[40] and prove especially useful in conjunction with pharmacologic therapy.

Supportive care, in and outside the hospital, using programs such as hospice is one of the cancer patient's greatest allies not only in coping with pain but also in accepting the disease. The positive effect this has on the patient cannot be overstated.

Pharmacologic Treatment

Pharmacologic management is the mainstay of therapy, and a typical progression of analgesic use is outlined in Fig. 58–3. The objective is to prevent the patient from experiencing constant fluctuations between severe pain and pain relief. This is best accomplished by around-the-clock administration schedules that inhibit serum analgesic concentrations from falling below the point at which a patient experiences the suffering of pain. As-needed (prn) schedules are to be employed in conjunction with around-the-clock regimens and are used when patients experience breakthrough pain. Again, nonopioid agents

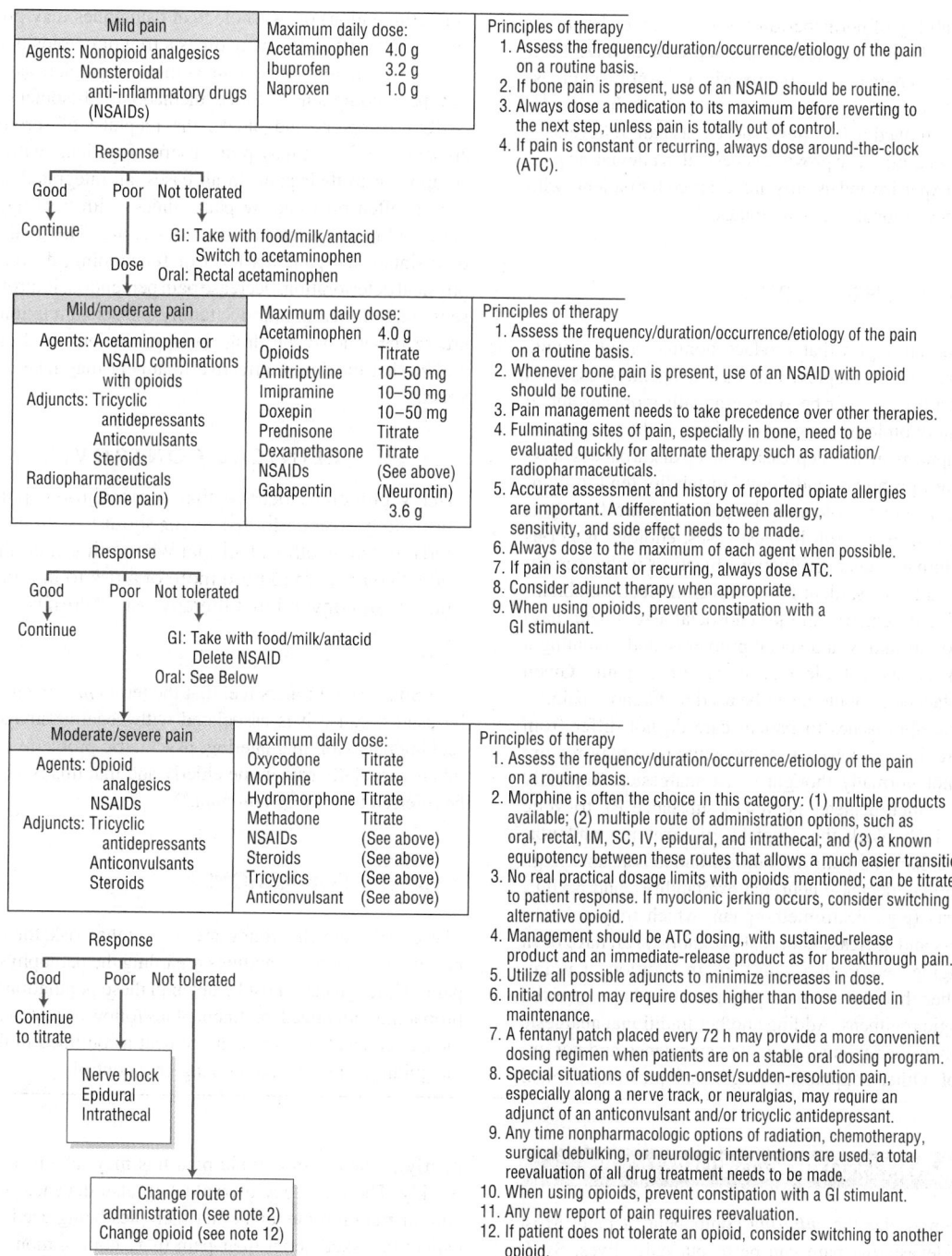

FIGURE 58–3. Algorithm for pain management in oncology patients. *(Adapted from the Kaiser Permanente Algorithm for Pain Management in Patients with Advanced Malignant Disease and Ref. 40.)*

are used as first-line agents, with NSAIDs being especially effective in treating bone pain.[40] Bone pain also can be treated with radiopharmaceuticals. Both strontium-89 and samarium SM 153 lexidronam have been shown to provide pain relief.[34] The choice of opiate should be based on patient acceptance; analgesic effectiveness; and pharmacokinetic, pharmacodynamic, and side-effect profiles. Many clinicians have found morphine both safe and effective when administered by the oral route (sustained-release, liquid, and fast-release), subcutaneous route, rectal route, continual intravenous infusion, patient-controlled intravenous route, and epidural or intrathecal route.[40]

Recently, methadone has regained prominence in treating cancer pain.[42] It has a prolonged mechanism of action, excellent oral

absorption, NMDA receptor antagonist activity (d-isomer),[37] and is inexpensive. However, its unpredictable half-life have make it hard to titrate. In addition, when switching to methadone from another opioid, the dose of the initial opioid used will greatly affect the equianalgesic dose needed. In general, the higher the previous dose of opioid, the lower is the needed dose of methadone.[42] Methadone can be used initially, as an alternative, or in addition to other opioids when managing cancer pain. Epidural clonidine is also effective with epidurally administered opioid analgesics for the treatment of refractory pain.[34] The fentanyl patch may provide a more convenient dosing alternative in patients on stable regimens. Meperidine is not recommended for long-term use because of its relatively short duration of action and the CNS hyperirritability of normeperidine, one of its metabolites.[40] Anticonvulsant drugs and tricyclic antidepressants have been shown to be effective in pain of neuropathic origin.[43] Antihistamines, amphetamines, and steroids are used as adjuvant pain medications[40]; however, they have enjoyed only limited success as pain relievers.

Anesthetic procedures have proven successful in alleviating pain but require special expertise and usually are reserved for patients who are refractory to conventional analgesic routes.[40]

NONMALIGNANT CHRONIC PAIN

The numerous etiologies that produce nonmalignant chronic pain make treatment complex, and its management assumes multidisciplinary aspects. As pain becomes gradually more chronic, it loses many of the autonomic characteristics evident in the acute stage, and additional symptoms such as depression, sleep disturbances, anxiety, irritability, work problems, and family instability tend to dominate. Patients should not be told that the pain they are feeling is "psychosomatic" or in their head. In most cases, etiology is not as important as symptomatic relief. Evaluation objectives include establishing an accurate diagnosis, identifying iatrogenic factors, obtaining a comprehensive psychiatric and psychosocial assessment, paying special attention to family and social problems, and obtaining a description of factors that alleviate or exacerbate pain.[2] Given these objectives, placebo's should never be used to diagnose pain.[2]

Pharmacologic approaches to patient care do not differ from those described previously; however, neuropathic pain may require medications not normally thought of as analgesics. Topically applied capsaicin (which depletes nerves of substance P), tricyclic antidepressants (which block the reuptake of serotonin and norepinephrine, thus enhancing pain inhibition), anticonvulsants (e.g., gabapentin, which may decrease neuronal excitability), and NMDA receptor antagonists (e.g., dextromethorphan, which may enhance opioid effectiveness and decrease neuronal excitability) all have been effective in managing neuropathic pain.[44–46] In addition, it is important to remember that chronic pain patients often have received many pharmacologic regimens. Adding another traditional analgesic (e.g., opioids) to their therapy may promote dependence and not improve pain control. Other nonpharmacologic therapies (e.g., spinal cord stimulation) or psychological techniques may prove more successful. Nevertheless, many times a trial of opioids is warranted, but such a trial should not be done without a complete assessment of the pain complaint.[47] Since methadone (d-isomer)[37] antagonizes NMDA receptors and blocks the reuptake of serotonin and norepinephrine,[35–37] it may prove useful in patients with a neuropathic component to their pain. In all cases, an integrated, systematic approach often provided by pain clinics, with a strong emphasis on patient-clinician relationships, is essential. The goal is to improve or maintain the patient's level of functioning, decrease the rate of physical deterioration, decrease pain perception, improve the patient's sense of well-being, improve family and social relationships, and decrease dependency on drug therapy.[2] Patients and clinicians must realize that maximum effective treatment may take months or even years.

CLINICAL CONTROVERSY

Many clinicians believe that some chronic painful conditions (e.g., osteoarthritis) never should be treated with opioids, whereas others feel that when other modalities are not effective or seem to pose more of a risk to that particular patient than conventional therapy (e.g., NSAIDs), then opioids are necessary.

Some practitioners feel that the term *chronic pain* should never be used because it is associated with negative images (e.g., drug-seeking behavior, malingering, psychiatric problems). They feel that this is especially true in the elderly and that this type of pain should be referred to as *persistent pain*.[48]

SPECIAL POPULATIONS

The elderly and the young are at a higher risk for undertreatment because of misunderstandings regarding the pathophysiology of their pain. Although care must be taken in these populations to ensure that proper individualized treatment plans follow accepted guidelines,[48,49] the key concepts in pain management as outlined in this chapter are the guiding tenets in maximizing pain control.

PHARMACOECONOMIC CONSIDERATIONS

One cannot overemphasize the *suffering* component of pain. Most of us know how devastating pain can be to our daily lives. Swift relief from acute and cancer pain and well-planned treatment regimens in chronic nonmalignant pain will allow patients to concentrate on recovery and regaining control of their lives. Although few well-designed pharmacoeconomic studies have been performed,[50,51] most pain clinicians believe that this approach leads to decreased time in the hospital, decreased time away from work, and an overall increase in the quality of life.

EVALUATION OF THERAPEUTIC OUTCOMES

The key to treating pain effectively is to consistently monitor effectiveness (pain relief) versus side effects (e.g., sedation) and titrate treatment accordingly (see Table 58–8). In acute pain this often needs to be done several times a day (in the early stages, hourly), whereas in chronic pain this may take place daily or even weekly. The frequency of evaluation also depends on the drug, the administration route, and other therapies being used. When patients cannot be asked about their pain (e.g., coma), monitoring agitation and heart rate is appropriate. Given the subjective nature of pain, the most successful therapies will involve not only frequent patient assessment but also a large degree of patient control (as with PCA).

All opioids can cause constipation. The best management of constipation is prevention. Patients should be counseled on the proper intake of fluids and fiber. A laxative may be added, if needed. As noted earlier, CNS depressants (e.g., alcohol, benzodiazepines) amplify CNS depression when used with opioid analgesics and should be monitored closely and discouraged when possible.

CONCLUSIONS

Poor training of health care practitioners in pain assessment and management, improper patient education, and inadequate communication

mong health care professionals are some of the reasons for inadequate pain relief.[52,53] The use of an integrated approach, employ-
ng the expertise of many disciplines, may well be the most overlooked
rinciple of pain pharmacotherapy. Indeed, it is the responsibility of
ll health care professionals who deal with pain to work together to
nsure proper management in an effort to relieve treatable suffering
nd pain.

ABBREVIATIONS

'NS: central nervous system
'DA: Food and Drug Administration
'iABA: γ-aminobutyric acid
M: intramuscular
V: intravenous
'$^{+}$: potassium ion
Max: maximum
'IMDA: N-methyl-D-aspartate
'ISAIDs: nonsteroidal anti-inflammatory drugs
'CA: patient-controlled analgesia
'O : oral
'ENS: transcutaneous electrical nerve stimulation

Review Questions and other resources can be found at
vww.pharmacotheray.com.

REFERENCES

1. www.river.org\dHawk\keller-quotes.html. Selected quotes from Helen
   Keller. David Hawkins Quote Page, 1998; accessed March 6, 2004.
2. Stimmel B. Pain, Analgesia and Addiction: The Pharmacology of Pain.
   New York, Raven Press, 1983:1, 2, 63, 241–245, 259, 266.
3. Joint Commission on Accreditation of Healthcare Organizations
   (JCAHO). Pain Assessment and Management an Organizational Approach. Oakbrook Terrace, IL, JCAHO, 2000:1.
4. Turk DC, Okifuji A. Pain terms and taxonomies of pain. In: Loeser JD,
   Butler SH, Chapman CR, et al, eds. Bonica's Management of Pain.
   Philadelphia, Lippincott Williams & Wilkins, 2000:17–25.
5. Partners Against Pain News, Vol. 4, No. 3. Norwalk, CT, Purdue Pharma
   LP, 2000:1.
6. Gallagher RM. Primary care and pain medicine: A community solution to the public health problem of chronic pain. Med Clin North Am
   1999;83:555–583.
7. Desbiens NA, Wu AW, Broste SK, et al. Pain and satisfaction with pain
   control in seriously ill hospitalized adults: Findings from the SUPPORT
   research investigations. Crit Care Med 1996;24:1953–1961.
8. Desbiens NA, Wu AW. Pain and suffering in seriously ill hospitalized
   patients. J Am Geriatr Soc 2000;48:S183–186.
9. Bernabei R, Gambassi G, Lapane K, et al. Management of pain in elderly
   patients with cancer. JAMA 1998;279:1877–1882.
10. Loeser JD, Melzack R. Pain: An overview. Lancet 1999;353:1607–1609.
11. Pasero C, Paice JA, McCaffery M. Basic mechanisms underlying the
    causes and effects of pain. In: McCaffery M, Pasero C, eds. Pain.
    St. Louis, Mosby, 1999:15–34.
12. Johnson BW. Pain mechanisms: Anatomy, physiology, and neurochem-
    istry. In: Raj PP, Abrams BM, Hahn MB, et al, eds. Practical Management
    of Pain. St. Louis, Mosby, 2000:117–143.
13. Byers MR, Bonica JJ. Peripheral pain mechanisms and nociceptor plastic-
    ity. In: Loeser JD, Butler SH, Chapman CR, et al, eds. Bonica's Manage-
    ment of Pain. Philadelphia, Lippincott Williams & Wilkins, 2000:26–72.
14. Bennett GJ. Neuropathic pain: New insights, new interventions. Hosp
    Pract 1998;October:95–114.
15. Chabal C. Trancutaneous electrical nerve stimulation. In: Loeser JD,
    Butler SH, Chapman CR, et al, eds. Bonica's Management of Pain.
    Philadelphia, Lippincott Williams & Wilkins, 2000:1842–1847.
16. Terman GW, Bonica JJ. Spinal mechanisms and their modulation. In:
    Loeser JD, Butler SH, Chapman CR, et al, eds. Bonica's Management of
    Pain. Philadelphia, Lippincott Williams & Wilkins, 2000:73–152.
17. Elliott, KJ. Taxonomy and mechanisms of neuropathic pain. Semin Neurol
    1994;3:195–205.
18. Twycross RG. Pain and analgesics. Curr Med Res Opin 1978;5:497–505.
19. Kendall NA, Psychosocial approaches to the prevention of chronic
    pain: The low back paradigm. Bailliers Best Pract Res Clin Rheumatol
    1999;September 13:545–54.
20. Feldner MT, Hekmat H. Perceived control over anxiety-related events as
    a predictor of pain behaviors in a cold pressor task. J Behav Ther Exp
    Psychiatry. 2001;32:191–202.
21. Craig KD. Social modelling influences on pain. In: Sternbach RA, ed. The
    Psychology of Pain. New York, Raven Press, 1978:73–109.
22. American Pain Society. Principles of Analgesic Use in the Treatment of
    Acute Pain and Chronic Cancer Pain, 5th ed. 2003:1, 3, 15, 18, 28, 39.
23. Chapman CR, Bonica JJ. Chronic Pain: Current Concepts. Kalamazoo,
    MI, Scope Publications, 1985:4.
24. Clinical Practice Guideline. Acute Pain Management: Operative or Medi-
    cal Procedures and Trauma. Publication No. 92-0032, Rockville, MD, De-
    partment of Health and Human Services, Public Health Service, Agency
    for Health Care Policy and Research (now called Agency for Healthcare
    Research and Quality), 1992.
25. Miyoshi HR, Leckband SG. Systemic opioids and analgesics. In: Loeser
    JD, Butler SH, Chapman CR, et al, eds. Bonica's Management of Pain.
    Philadelphia, Lippincott Williams & Wilkins, 2000:1682–1709.
26. Gutstein HB, Akil H. Opioid analgesics. In: Hardman JG, Limbird G,
    eds. The Pharmacological Basis of Therapeutics. New York, McGraw-
    Hill, 2001:569–619.
27. Reisine T, Pasternak G. Opioid analgesics and antagonists. In: Hardman
    JG, Limbird LE, Molinoff PB, et al, eds. The Pharmacological Basis of
    Therapeutics. New York, McGraw-Hill, 1995:521–555.
28. Baumann TJ. Analgesic selection when the patient is allergic to codeine.
    Clin Pharm 1991;10:658.
29. Ready BL. Regional analgesics with intraspinal opioids. In: Loeser JD,
    Butler SH, Chapman CR, et al, eds. Bonica's Management of Pain.
    Philadelphia, Lippincott Williams & Wilkins, 2000:1953–1966.
30. Littrell RA. Epidural analgesia. Am J Hosp Pharm 1991;48:2460–2474.
31. Buckley PF. Regional anesthesia with local anesthetics. In: Loeser JD,
    Butler SH, Chapman CR, et al, eds. Bonica's Management of Pain.
    Philadelphia, Lippincott Williams & Wilkins, 2000:1893–1952.
32. Pasero C, Portenoy RK, McCaffery M. Opioid analgesics. In: McCaffery
    M, Pasero C, eds. Pain. St. Louis, Mosby, 1999:161–299.
33. Anonymous. American Hospital Formulary Service. In: McVoy GK, ed.
    Drug Information. Bethesda, MD, American Society of Hospital Pharma-
    cists, 1987, 1991, 1994, 1997, 1999, 2001, 2003.
34. Anonymous. Facts and Comparisons. Philadelphia, Lippincott, 1986,
    1991, 1994, 1997, 2000, 2003, 2004.
35. Mancini I, Lossignol DA, Body JJ. Opioid switch to oral methadone in
    cancer pain. Curr Opin Oncol 2000;12:308–313.
36. Codd EE, Shank RP, Schupsky JJ, Raffa RB. Serotonin and nor-
    epinephrine uptake inhibiting activity of centrally acting analgesics: Struc-
    tural determinants and role in antinociception. J Pharmacol Exp Ther
    1995;274:1263–1270.
37. Bennett G, Seratini M, Burchiel K, et al. Evidence-based review of the
    literature on intrathecal delivery of pain medication. J Pain Symptom
    Manage 2000;20:512–536.
38. Package insert. Tramadol. Ortho-McNeil, Raritan, NJ, August 2001.
39. Sindrup SH, Andersen G, Madsen C, et al. Tramadol relieves pain and
    allodynia in polyneuropathy: A randomized, double-blind, controlled trial.
    Pain 1999;83:85–90.
40. Clinical Practice Guideline No. 9. Management of Cancer Pain.
    Publication No. 94-0592, Rockville, MD, Department of Health, Pub-
    lic Health Service, Agency for Health Care Policy and Research (now
    called Agency for Healthcare Research and Quality), 1994.

41. Foley KM. The treatment of cancer pain. N Engl J Med 1985;313: 84–95.
42. Pain. Available at *cancer.gov;* modified 2003:1–54.
43. Portenoy, RK. Pain specialists and addiction medicine specialists unite to address critical issues. American Pain Society Bulletin 1999;March–April:9(2).
44. Sindrup SH, Jensen TS. Efficacy of pharmacologic treatments of neurophathic pain: An update and effect related to mechanism of drug action. Pain 1999;83:389–400.
45. Nelson KA, Park KM, Robinovitz E, et al. High-dose dextromethorphan versus placebo in painful diabetic neuropathy. Neurology 1997;48:1212–1218.
46. Semenchuk M. Adjuvant analgesics for management of neuropathic pain. In: Beizer JL, ed. Clinical Pharmacy Newswatch, Vol. 6. Parke-Davis, 1999:1.
47. The use of opioids for the treatment of chronic pain: A consensus statement from the American Academy of Pain Medicine and American Pain Society. Approved 1996, American Pain Society Web site: *www.ampainsoc.org;* modified September 2003; accessed March 6, 2004.
48. Clinical Practice Guideline, American Geriatrics Society Panel on Persistent Pain in Older Persons. The management of persistent pain in older persons. J Am Geriatr Soc 2002;50:1–20.
49. American Academy of Pediatrics and American Pain Society. The assessment and management of acute pain in infants, children and adolescents. Pediatrics 2001;108:793–797.
50. Thomsen AB, Sorensen J, Sjogren P, Eriksen J. Economic evaluation of multidisciplinary pain management in chronic pain patients: A qualitative systematic review. J Pain Symptom Manage 2001;22:688–698.
51. Varrassi G, Marinageli F, Donatelli F, Beltrutti D. Pharmacoeconomics of pain management. Curr Pain Headache Rep 1998;2:151–156.
52. McCaffery M. Pain management problems and progress. In: McCaffery M, Pasero C, eds. Pain. St. Louis, Mosby, 1999:1–14.
53. Bonica JJ, Loeser JD. History of pain concepts and therapies. In: Loeser JD, Butler SH, Chapman CR, et al, eds. Bonica's Management of Pain. Philadelphia, Lippincott Williams & Wilkins, 2000:3–16.
54. Amadio P. Peripherally acting analgesics. Am J Med 1984;77:17–26.
55. Hopkinson JH, Smith MT, Bare WW, et al. Acetaminophen (500 mg) versus acetaminophen (325 mg) for relief of pain in episiotomy patients. Curr Ther Res 1974;16:194–200.
56. Levy G. Comparative pharmacokinetics of aspirin and acetaminophen. Arch Intern Med 1981;141:279–281.
57. Gaston GW, Mallow RD, Frank JE. Comparison of etodolac, aspirin, and placebo for pain after oral surgery. Pharmacotherapy 1986;6:199–205.
58. Package insert. Diclofenac potassium. Geigy Pharmaceuticals, Ardsley, NJ, February 1996.
59. Package insert. Valecoxib. G. D. Searle LLC, Caguas, PR, October 2002.
60. Package insert. Ropivicaine. Astra, Westborough, MA, January 1999.
61. Package insert. Celecoxib. Pharmacia/Pfizer, New York, October 2001.
62. Package insert. Extended release hydromorphone capsules. Purdue Pharma L. P. Stamford, CT, September 2004.

59

HEADACHE DISORDERS

Deborah S. King and Katherine C. Herndon

Learning Objectives and other resources can be found at *www.pharmacotherapyonline.com.*

KEY CONCEPTS

◀1 Acute migraine therapies should provide consistent, rapid relief and enable the patient to resume his or her normal activities at home, school, or work.

◀2 A stratified care approach, in which the selection of initial treatment is based on headache-related disability and symptom severity, is the preferred treatment strategy for the migraineur.

◀3 Strict adherence to maximum daily and weekly doses of antimigraine medications is essential.

◀4 Preventive therapy should be considered in the setting of recurring migraines that produce significant disability; frequent attacks requiring symptomatic medication more than twice per week; symptomatic therapies that are ineffective, contraindicated, or produce serious side effects; and un-

common migraine variants that cause profound disruption and/or risk of neurologic injury.

◀5 The selection of an agent for migraine prophylaxis should be based on individual patient response, tolerability, convenience of the drug formulation, and comorbid conditions of the patient.

◀6 Each prophylactic medication should be given an adequate therapeutic trial to judge its efficacy, usually 2 to 3 months.

◀7 A general wellness program and avoidance of migraine triggers should be included in the management plan.

◀8 After an effective abortive agent and dose have been identified, subsequent treatments should begin with that same regimen.

Headache is one of the most common complaints encountered by health care practitioners, accounting for over 1% of visits to physicians' offices or emergency departments.[1] As one of the top 10 presenting complaints in ambulatory medical care, headache may be symptomatic of a distinct pathologic process or may occur without an underlying cause.[1,2] In 2004, the International Headache Society (IHS) updated its classification system and diagnostic criteria for headache disorders, cranial neuralgias, and facial pain[3] (Table 59–1). Designed to facilitate headache diagnosis in clinical practice and research, the IHS classification provides more precise definitions and standardized nomenclature for both the primary (tension-type, migraine, and cluster headache) and secondary (symptomatic of organic disease) headache disorders. This chapter focuses on the management of the primary headache disorders.

Most recurrent headaches are the result of a benign chronic primary headache disorder.[1] Less often, headaches are symptomatic of a serious underlying medical condition, such as infection, cerebral hemorrhage, or brain mass lesion. The peak prevalence of tension-type and migraine headache, the most common of the primary headache disorders, occurs during the most productive years of life (20 to 55 years of age).[4] Despite the prevalence of these disorders and their associated disability, studies indicate that most migraine and tension-type headache sufferers do not seek medical care for their headaches.[4,5] An improved understanding of the diagnosis and pathophysiologic mechanisms of the primary headache disorders, particularly migraine, has led to the development of specific medications capable of providing rapid relief from moderate to severe attacks. However, a thorough evaluation of the headache history is essential to establish an accurate

headache diagnosis and identify patients who may benefit from these newer therapeutic options.

MIGRAINE HEADACHE

EPIDEMIOLOGY

Results of the American Migraine Study II indicate that 18.2% of women and 6.5% of men in the United States experience one or more migraine headaches per year.[6] The prevalence of migraine varies considerably by age and gender. Before the age of 12 years, migraine is more common in boys than in girls, but prevalence increases more rapidly in girls after puberty.[4] After age 12, females are two to three times more likely than males to suffer from migraine. Gender differences in migraine prevalence have been linked to menstruation, but these differences persist beyond menopause. Prevalence is highest in both men and women between the ages of 35 and 45 years.[6] The usual age of onset is 10 to 29 years of age, but onset of migraine in early childhood is not uncommon.[7] In the American Migraine Study II, 92% of women and 89% of men with migraine reported some headache-related disability, and 53% were severely disabled or needed bed rest during an attack.[6] A number of neurologic and psychiatric disorders, including stroke, epilepsy, major depression, and anxiety disorder, show increased comorbidity with migraine.[4] Whether this relationship is causal or representative of a common pathophysiologic mechanism is unknown. The economic burden of migraine is substantial; however, the direct medical costs associated with migraine treatment

TABLE 59–1. International Headache Society Classification System: Focus on Migraine Headache

Migraine
  Migraine without aura
  Migraine with aura
    Typical aura with migraine headache (aura lasting less than 1 hour)
    Typical aura with nonmigraine headache
    Typical aura without headache
    Familial hemiplegic migraine
    Sporadic hemiplegic migraine
    Basilar-type migraine
  Childhood periodic syndromes that are commonly precursors of migraine
    Cyclical vomiting (self-limiting episodic condition)
    Abdominal migraine (episodic midline abdominal pain attacks lasting 1 to 72 hours)
    Benign paroxysmal vertigo of childhood (brief episodic vertigo)
  Retinal migraine (repeated attacks of monocular visual disturbance)
  Complications of migraine
    Chronic migraine (occurring on 15 or more days per month for more than 3 months)
    Status migrainosus (debilitating attack lasting for more than 72 hours)
    Persistent aura without infarction (symptoms persisting for more than 1 week)
    Migrainous infarction (aura symptoms associated with an ischemic brain lesion)
    Migraine-triggered seizure
  Probable migraine
    Probable migraine without aura
    Probable migraine with aura
    Probable chronic migraine
Tension-type headache
Cluster headache and other trigeminal autonomic cephalalgias
Other primary headaches
Headache attributed to head and/or neck trauma
Headache attributed to cranial or cervical vascular disorder
Headache attributed to non-vascular intracranial disorder
Headache attributed to a substance or its withdrawal
Headache attributed to infection
Headache attributed to disorder of homeostasis
Headache or facial pain attributed to disorder of cranium, neck, eyes, ears, nose, sinuses, teeth, mouth, or other facial or cranial structures
Headache attributed to psychiatric disorder
Cranial neuralgias and central causes of facial pain
Other headache, cranial neuralgia, central or primary facial pain

Adapted with permission from ref. 3.

are far exceeded by the indirect costs that result from work-related disability.[8]

ETIOLOGY AND PATHOPHYSIOLOGY

The etiologic and pathophysiologic mechanisms of migraine are not completely understood. According to the vascular hypothesis proposed by Harold Wolff in 1938, the migraine aura is caused by intracerebral arterial vasoconstriction that is followed by reactive extracranial vasodilation and associated headache.[4] Although studies of regional blood flow in the brain do not support the vascular hypothesis, the aura phase of migraine is associated with a reduction in cerebral blood flow that begins in the occipital region and moves across the cerebral cortex at a rate of 2 to 3 mm/min.[9] However, most clinicians now believe that the positive and negative symptoms of the migraine aura are caused by neuronal dysfunction, not ischemia.

The neurologic changes of the aura parallel those which occur during spreading depression, a neuronal event characterized by a wave of depressed electrical activity that advances across the brain cortex at a rate that is consistent with the spread of aura symptoms.[9] Migraine without aura is a neurobiologic disorder.[3] Migraine pain is believed to result from activity within the trigeminovascular system, a network of visceral afferent fibers that arises from the trigeminal ganglion and projects peripherally to innervate the pain-sensitive intracranial extracerebral blood vessels, dura mater, and large venous sinuses (see Fig. 59–1). These fibers also project centrally, terminating in the trigeminal nucleus caudalis in the brain stem and upper cervical spinal cord, and thus provide a pathway for nociceptive transmission from meningeal blood vessels into higher centers of the central nervous system (CNS). Activation of trigeminal sensory nerves triggers the release of vasoactive neuropeptides, including calcitonin gene–related peptide (CGRP), neurokinin A, and substance P, from perivascular axons. The released neuropeptides interact with dural blood vessels to promote vasodilation and dural plasma extravasation, resulting in perivascular inflammation.[10] Orthodromic conduction along trigeminovascular fibers transmits pain impulses to the trigeminal nucleus caudalis, where the information is relayed further to higher cortical pain centers. Continued afferent input may result in sensitization of these central sensory neurons, producing a hyperalgesic state that prolongs and intensifies headache pain as the attack progresses.[11]

Despite recent advances in understanding of the pathophysiology of headache pain, there is still a considerable lack of knowledge regarding the mechanisms involved in the initiation of a migraine attack. Although the exact pathophysiology of migraine needs further elucidation, new imaging techniques have provided insight into mechanisms. Previous vascular and neural theories of migraine development have merged into a combined theory of neurovascular mechanisms through evidence provided by neuroimaging. Activity within the trigeminovascular system may be regulated in part by noradrenergic and, most important, serotonergic neurons within the brain stem. Thus the pathogenesis of migraine may be related to an imbalance in the activity of serotonin-containing neurons and/or noradrenergic pathways in brain stem nuclei that modulate cerebral vascular tone and nociception.[10] This imbalance may result in vasodilation of intracranial extracerebral blood vessels and consequent activation of the trigeminovascular system. Future research may further delineate the role of the brain stem as the "migraine generator."

Genetic factors appear to play an important role in an individual's susceptibility to migraine attacks. Studies in monozygotic twins suggest that up to 50% of the contribution to the common migraine variants is genetically based, with a substantial influence from environmental factors.[12] While it may be possible for any individual to experience a migraine attack, it is the recurrence of attacks in the migraineur that is abnormal. Attack occurrence and frequency are governed by the sensitivity of the CNS to migraine-specific triggers. Migraineurs appear to have a lowered threshold of response to specific triggers as a result of genetic factors that govern the balance of excitation and inhibition at various levels in the CNS.[9] Thus trigger factors can be viewed as modulators of the genetic set point that predisposes to migraine headache. The hyperresponsiveness of the migrainous brain may be the result of an inherited abnormality in P/Q-type calcium channels that regulate cortical excitability through the release of serotonin and other neurotransmitters.[4] Low levels of magnesium or dopamine, increased levels of excitatory amino acids, and alterations in levels of endogenous opioids also may affect the migraine threshold.[9]

Serotonin (5-hydroxytryptamine, or 5-HT) has long been implicated as an important mediator of migraine headache. Specific

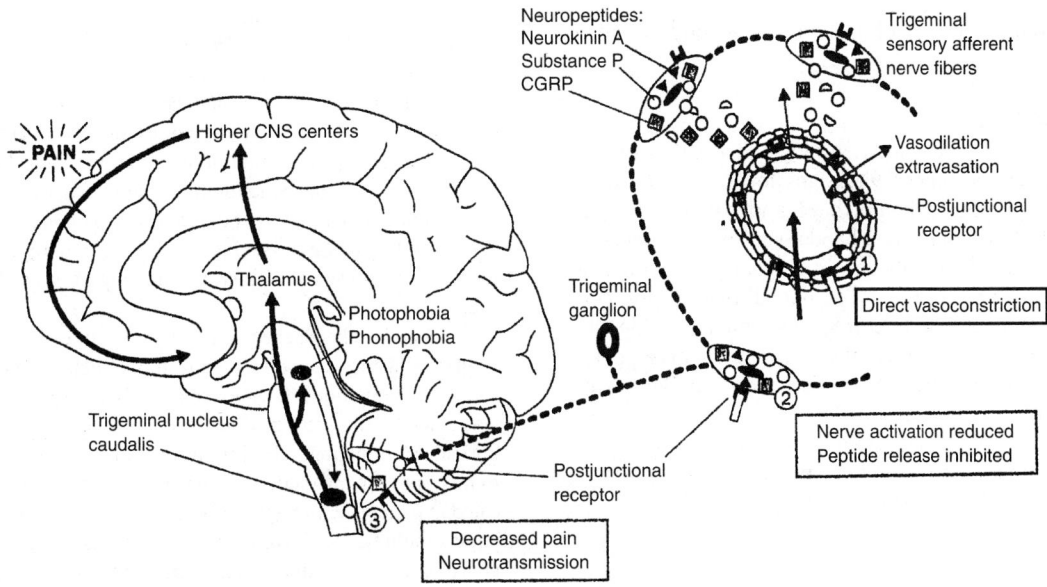

FIGURE 59–1. The pathophysiology of migraine headache. Vasodilation of intracranial extracerebral blood vessels (possibly the result of an imbalance in the brain stem) results in the activation of the perivascular trigeminal nerves that release vasoactive neuropeptides to promote neurogenic inflammation. Central pain transmission may activate other brain stem nuclei, resulting in associated symptoms (nausea, vomiting, photophobia, phonophobia). The antimigraine effects of the 5-HT$_{1B/1D}$ receptor agonists are highlighted at areas 1, 2, and 3. (*Adapted with permission from Ferrari MD. Migraine.* Lancet *1998;351:1043–1051.* © *by The Lancet Ltd.*)

populations of the seven subfamilies of 5-HT receptors (5-HT$_1$ to 5-HT$_7$) appear to be involved in the pathophysiology and treatment of migraine headache.[13] Specific acute antimigraine drugs such as the ergot alkaloids and triptan derivatives are agonists of vascular and neuronal 5-HT$_1$ receptor subtypes, resulting in vasoconstriction of meningeal blood vessels and inhibition of vasoactive neuropeptide release and pain signal transmission.[10] Drugs used for migraine prophylaxis appear to stabilize serotonergic neurotransmission and raise the migraine threshold by antagonizing or downregulating 5-HT$_2$ receptors or by modulating serotonergic neuronal discharge.[13]

CLINICAL PRESENTATION

The migraine attack has been divided into several phases that merit description. *Premonitory symptoms* are experienced by approximately 20% to 60% of migraineurs in the hours or days before the onset of headache.[3,14] The previously popular terms *prodrome* and *warning symptoms* should be avoided because these are often used mistakenly to include aura.[3] Premonitory symptoms vary widely among migraineurs but usually are consistent within an individual. Neurologic symptoms (e.g., phonophobia, photophobia, hyperosmia, and difficulty concentrating) are most common, but psychological (e.g., anxiety, depression, euphoria, irritability, drowsiness, hyperactivity, and restlessness), autonomic (e.g., polyuria, diarrhea, and constipation), and constitutional symptoms (e.g., stiff neck, yawning, thirst, food cravings, and anorexia) also are reported.[4,15]

CLINICAL PRESENTATION OF MIGRAINE HEADACHE

GENERAL

Migraine is a common, recurrent, severe headache that interferes with normal functioning. It is a primary headache disorder divided into two major subtypes, migraine without aura and migraine with aura.

SYMPTOMS

Migraine is characterized by recurring episodes of throbbing head pain, frequently unilateral, that when untreated can last from 4 to 72 hours. Migraine headaches can be severe and associated with nausea, vomiting, and sensitivity to light, sound, and/or movement. Not all symptoms are present at every attack.

In the headache evaluation, diagnostic alarms should be identified. These include: acute onset of the "first" or "worst" headache ever, accelerating pattern of headache following subacute onset, onset of headache after age 50, headache associated with systemic illness (e.g., fever, nausea, vomiting, stiff neck, and rash), headache with focal neurologic symptoms or papilledema, and new-onset headache in a patient with cancer or human immunodeficiency virus (HIV) infection.

SIGNS

A stable pattern, absence of daily headache, positive family history for migraine, normal neurologic examination, presence of food triggers, menstrual association, long-standing history, improvement with sleep, and subacute evolution are all signs of migraine headache. Aura may signal the migraine headache but is not required for diagnosis.

LABORATORY TESTS

In selected circumstances and secondary headache presentation, serum chemistries, urine toxicology profiles, thyroid function tests, lyme studies, and other blood tests such as a complete blood count, antinuclear antibody titer, erythrocyte sedimentation rate, and antiphospholipid antibody titer may be considered.

DIAGNOSTIC TESTS

Perform a general medical and neurologic physical examination. Check for abnormalities: vital signs (fever, hypertension), funduscopy (papilledema, hemorrhage, and exudates), palpation and auscultation of the head and neck (sinus tenderness, hardened or tender temporal arteries, trigger points, temporomandibular joint tenderness, bruits, nuchal rigidity, and cervical spine tenderness), and neurologic examination (identify abnormalities or deficits in mental status, cranial nerves, deep tendon reflexes, motor strength, coordination, gait, and cerebellar function).

Consider neuroimaging studies in patients with abnormal neurologic examination findings of unknown etiology and in those with additional risk factors warranting imaging.

The migraine *aura,* a complex of positive and negative focal neurologic symptoms that precedes or accompanies an attack, is experienced by approximately 31% of migraineurs on some occasions.[16] The aura typically evolves over 5 to 20 minutes and lasts less than 60 minutes. Headache usually occurs within 60 minutes of the end of the aura. Occasionally, aura symptoms begin at the onset of headache or during the attack. The aura is most often visual and frequently affects half the visual field.[3,4] Visual auras vary in their complexity and can include both positive (scintillations, photopsia, teichopsia, or fortification spectrum) and negative (scotoma, hemianopsia) features. Sensory and motor aura symptoms, such as paresthesias or numbness involving the arms and face, dysphasia or aphasia, weakness, and hemiparesis, also are reported.

The average migraineur experiences between one and five attacks per month.[17] Migraine *headache* may occur at any time of the day or night but occurs most often in the early morning hours on awakening. Pain is usually gradual in onset, peaking in intensity over a period of minutes to hours and lasting between 4 and 72 hours in adults. Pain may occur anywhere in the face or head but most often involves the frontotemporal region. The headache is typically unilateral and throbbing or pulsating in nature; however, pain may be bilateral at onset or become generalized during the course of an attack.[9] Gastrointestinal symptoms almost invariably accompany a migraine headache. During an attack, as many as 90% of migraineurs experience nausea, and emesis occurs in approximately one-third of patients.[17] Other systemic symptoms associated with the headache phase include anorexia, food cravings, constipation, diarrhea, abdominal cramps, nasal stuffiness, blurred vision, diaphoresis, facial pallor, and localized facial, scalp, or periorbital edema. Sensory hyperacuity, manifested as photophobia, phonophobia, or osmophobia, is reported frequently. Since headache pain usually is aggravated by physical activity, most migraineurs seek a dark, quiet room for rest and relief. Impaired concentration, depression, irritability, fatigue, or anxiety often accompany the headache. Once headache pain wanes, patients may experience a *resolution phase* characterized by feeling tired, exhausted, irritable, or listless. Impaired concentration may continue, as well as scalp tenderness or mood changes. Some patients many experience depression and malaise, whereas others may feel unusually refreshed or euphoric.[14] The reader is referred to the IHS classification and recent reviews for descriptions of the classic migraine variants and other migraine subtypes[3,4,9,14,18] (see also Table 59–1).

Although headaches have many potential causes, most are caused by the primary headache disorders. A comprehensive headache history is the most important element in establishing the clinical diagnosis of migraine.[9] A thorough headache history always should be obtained from the patient. Information collected should include age at onset, attack frequency and timing, duration of attacks, precipitating or aggravating factors, ameliorating factors, description of neurologic symptoms, characteristics of the headache pain (quality, intensity, location, and radiation), associated signs and symptoms, treatment history, family and social history, and the impact of headaches on daily life.

Secondary headache can be identified or excluded based on the headache history, as well as the results of general medical and neurologic examinations. Diagnostic and laboratory testing also may be warranted in the setting of suspicious headache features or an abnormal examination. The routine use of neuroimaging (computed tomography or magnetic resonance imaging) generally is not indicated in patients with migraine and a normal neurologic examination, but it should be considered in patients with an unexplained abnormal neurologic examination or an atypical headache history.[19] Because migraine headaches usually begin by the second or third decade of life, headaches beginning after age 50 suggest an organic etiology such as a mass lesion, cerebrovascular disease, or temporal arteritis. Table 59–2 lists the IHS diagnostic criteria for migraine with and without aura.[3]

TABLE 59–2. IHS Diagnostic Criteria for Migraine

Migraine without Aura
At least five attacks
Headache attack lasts 4 to 72 hours (untreated or unsuccessfully treated)
Headache has at least two of the following characteristics:
Unilateral location
Pulsating quality
Moderate or severe intensity
Aggravation by or avoidance of routine physical activity (ie, walking or climbing stairs)
During headache at least one of the following:
- Nausea, vomiting, or both
- Photophobia and phonophobia
- Not attributed to another disorder

Migraine with Aura (Classic Migraine)
At least two attacks
Migraine aura fulfills criteria for typical aura, hemiplegic aura, or basilar-type aura
Not attributed to another disorder

Typical Aura
Fully reversible visual, sensory, or speech symptoms (or any combination) but no motor weakness
Homonymous or bilateral visual symptoms including positive features (e.g., flickering lights, spot, lines) or negative features (e.g., loss of vision) or unilateral sensory symptoms including positive features (e.g., visual loss, pins and needles) or negative features (i.e., numbness), or any combination
At least one of the following:
- At least one symptom that develops gradually over a minimum of 5 minutes or different symptoms that occur in succession or both
- Each symptom lasts for at least 5 minutes and for no longer than 60 minutes
- Headache that meets criteria for migraine without aura begins during the aura or follows aura within 60 minutes

Adapted with permission from ref. 3.

▶ TREATMENT: Migraines

▣ DESIRED OUTCOME

Clinicians who care for migraineurs must appreciate the impact of this painful and debilitating disorder on the life of the patient, the patient's family, and the patient's employer. Treatment strategies must ◀ address both immediate and long-term goals. Acute migraine therapies should provide consistent, rapid relief and enable the patient to resume normal activities at home, school, or work. Recurrence of symptoms and treatment-related adverse effects should be minimal. Ideally, patients should be able to manage their own headaches effectively without a visit to a physician's office or emergency room. In addition, migraineurs should take an active role in the creation of a long-term formal management plan. An individualized approach to treatment can result in a reduction in attack frequency and severity, thus minimizing headache-related disability and emotional distress and improving the patient's quality of life. Goals of long-term and acute treatment of migraine are listed in Table 59–3.

▣ GENERAL APPROACH TO TREATMENT

Nonpharmacologic and pharmacologic interventions are available for the management of migraine headache; however, drug therapy remains the mainstay of treatment for most patients. Pharmacotherapeutic management of migraine may be acute (e.g., symptomatic or abortive) or preventive (e.g., prophylactic). When choosing acute or preventive therapies, the clinician should consider the patient's response to specific medications and their tolerability, as well as coexisting illnesses that may limit treatment choices. Abortive or acute therapies can be migraine-specific (e.g., ergots and triptans) or nonspecific (e.g., analgesics, antiemetics, nonsteroidal anti-inflammatory drugs, and corticosteroids) and are most effective at relieving pain and associated symptoms when administered at the onset of migraine[14,20] ◀ (Table 59–4). A stratified care approach in which the selection of

TABLE 59–3. Goals of Therapy in Migraine Management

Goals of Long-Term Migraine Treatment
Reduce migraine frequency, severity, and disability
Reduce reliance on poorly tolerated, ineffective, or unwanted acute pharmacotherapies
Improve quality of life
Prevent headache
Avoid escalation of headache medication use
Educate and enable patients to manage their disease
Reduce headache-related distress and psychological symptoms

Goals for Acute Migraine Treatment
Treat migraine attacks rapidly and consistently without recurrence
Restore the patient's ability to function
Minimize the use of backup and rescue medications[a]
Optimize self-care for overall management
Be cost-effective in overall management
Cause minimal or no adverse effects

[a]Rescue medications are defined as medications used at home when other treatments fail that permit the patient to get relief without a visit to the physician's office or emergency department.
Adapted from refs. 19 and 42.

initial treatment is based on headache-related disability and symptom severity is the preferred treatment strategy for the migraineur.[19,21] Because attack severity varies in individuals, patients may be advised to use nonspecific agents for mild to moderate headache while reserving migraine-specific medications for more severe attacks. The absorption and efficacy of orally administered drugs may be compromised by the gastric stasis or nausea and vomiting that often accompany migraine.[22] Pretreatment with antiemetic agents or the use of nonoral treatment (e.g., suppositories, nasal sprays, or injections) may be advisable when nausea and vomiting are severe. Administration of the prokinetic agent metoclopramide enhances the absorption of oral medications, in addition to its antiemetic effects.[22]

The frequent or excessive use of acute migraine medications can result in a pattern of increasing headache frequency and drug consumption known as *medication-overuse headache* (or *rebound headache*).[21,23,24] The syndrome appears to evolve as a self-sustaining headache-medication cycle in which the headache returns as the medication effect wears off, leading to the consumption of more drug for relief. The headache history often reflects the gradual onset of an atypical daily or near-daily headache with superimposed episodic migraine attacks. Medication overuse is one of the most common causes of chronic daily headache.[4] Agents most commonly implicated in this syndrome include simple and combination analgesics, opiates, ergotamine tartrate, and triptans.[19,23,24] Discontinuation of the offending agent leads to a gradual decrease in headache frequency and severity and a return of the original headache characteristics. While detoxification usually can be accomplished on an outpatient basis, hospitalization may be necessary for the control of refractory rebound headache and other withdrawal symptoms (e.g., nausea, vomiting, asthenia, restlessness, and agitation). Regulation of nociceptive systems and renewed responsiveness to therapy may not occur for 3 to ◀ 12 weeks following medication withdrawal.[4,24] Most experts recommend limiting use of acute migraine therapies to *2 days per week* in order to avoid the development of medication misuse headache.[19,23]

Preventive migraine therapies are administered on a daily basis to reduce the frequency, severity, and duration of attacks and improve responsiveness to symptomatic migraine therapies[19] (Table 59–5). ◀ Preventive therapy should be considered in the setting of recurring migraines that produce significant disability despite acute therapy; frequent attacks requiring symptomatic medication more than twice per week with the risk of developing rebound headache; symptomatic therapies that are ineffective, contraindicated, or produce serious side effects; uncommon migraine variants that cause profound disruption and/or risk of permanent neurologic injury (e.g., hemiplegic migraine, basilar migraine, and migraine with prolonged aura); and patient preference to limit the number of attacks.[19,25] Preventive therapy also may be administered preemptively or intermittently when headaches recur in a predictable pattern (e.g., exercise-induced migraine or menstrual migraine). The efficacy of the various agents used for migraine prophylaxis appears to be similar, but the quality of published data is limited for many commonly used drugs (only propranolol, timolol, and valproic acid are currently approved by the Food and Drug ◀ Administration [FDA] for the indication).[26,27] Thus the selection of an agent typically is based on its side-effect profile and the patient's comorbid conditions.[25] A therapeutic trial of 2 to 3 months is necessary to judge the efficacy of each medication, but some reduction in attack frequency may be evident by the first month of therapy.[19,25] ◀ Drug therapy should be initiated with low doses and advanced slowly until a therapeutic effect is achieved or side effects become

TABLE 59–4. Acute Migraine Therapies[a]

Medication	Dosage	Comments
Analgesics		
Acetaminophen	1000 mg at onset; repeat every 4–6 hours as needed	Maximum daily dose is 4 g
Acetaminophen 250 mg/aspirin 250 mg/caffeine 65 mg	2 tablets at onset and every 6 hours	Available over-the-counter as Excedrin Migraine
Aspirin or acetaminophen with butalbital, caffeine	1–2 tablets every 4–6 hours	Limit dose to 4 tablets/day and usage to 2 days/week
Isometheptene 65 mg/ dichloralphenazone 100 mg/ acetaminophen 325 mg (Midrin)	2 capsules at onset; repeat 1 capsule every hour as needed	Maximum of 6 capsules/day and 20 capsules/month
Nonsteroidal Anti-Inflammatory Drugs		
Aspirin	500–1000 mg every 4–6 hours	Maximum daily dose is 4 g
Ibuprofen	200–800 mg every 6 hours	Avoid doses >2.4 g/day
Naproxen sodium	550–825 mg at onset; may repeat 220 mg in 3–4 hours	Avoid doses >1.375 g/day
Diclofenac potassium	50–100 mg at onset; may repeat 50 mg in 8 hours	Avoid doses >150 mg/day
Ergotamine Tartrate		
Oral tablet (1 mg) with caffeine 100 mg	2 mg at onset; then 1–2 mg every 30 minutes as needed	Maximum dose is 6 mg/day or 10 mg/week; consider pretreatment with an antiemetic
Sublingual tablet (2 mg)		
Rectal suppository (2 mg) with caffeine 100 mg	Insert 1/2 to 1 suppository at onset; repeat after 1 hour as needed	Maximum dose is 4 mg/day or 10 mg/week; consider pretreatment with an antiemetic
Dihydroergotamine		
Injection 1 mg/mL	0.25–1 mg at onset IM or SQ; repeat every hour as needed	Maximum dose is 3 mg/day or 20 mg/week
Nasal spray	One spray (0.5 mg) in each nostril at onset; repeat sequence 15 minutes later (total dose is 2 mg or 4 sprays)	Maximum dose is 3 mg/day; prime sprayer 4 times before using; do not tilt head back or inhale through nose while spraying; discard open ampules after 8 hours
Serotonin Agonists (Triptans)		
Sumatriptan		
Injection	6 mg SC at onset; may repeat after 1 hour if needed	Maximum daily dose is 12 mg
Oral tablets	25, 50, or 100 mg at onset; may repeat after 2 hours if needed	Optimal dose is 50–100 mg; maximum daily dose is 200 mg
Nasal spray	5, 10, or 20 mg at onset; may repeat after 2 hours if needed	Optimal dose is 20 mg; maximum daily dose is 40 mg; single-dose device delivering 5 or 20 mg; administer one spray in one nostril
Zolmitriptan	2.5 or 5 mg at onset as regular or orally disintegrating tablet; may repeat after 2 hours if needed	Optimal dose is 2.5 mg; maximum dose is 10 mg/day Do not divide ODT dosage form
Naratriptan	1 or 2.5 mg at onset; may repeat after 4 hours if needed	Optimal dose is 2.5 mg; maximum daily dose is 5 mg
Rizatriptan	5 or 10 mg at onset as regular or orally disintegrating tablet; may repeat after 2 hours if needed	Optimal dose is 10 mg; maximum daily dose is 30 mg; onset of effect is similar with standard and orally disintegrating tablets; use 5-mg dose (15 mg/day max) in patients receiving propranolol
Almotriptan	6.25 or 12.5 mg at onset; may repeat after 2 hours if needed	Optimal dose is 12.5 mg; maximum daily dose is 25 mg
Frovatriptan	2.5 or 5 mg at onset; may repeat in 2 hours if needed	Optimal dose 2.5–5 mg; maximum daily dose is 7.5 mg (3 tablets)
Eletriptan	20 or 40 mg at onset; may repeat after 2 hours if needed	Maximum single dose is 40 mg; maximum daily dose is 80 mg
Miscellaneous		
Butorphanol nasal spray	1 spray in 1 nostril (1 mg) at onset; repeat in 1 hour if needed	Limit to 4 sprays/day; consider use only when nonopioid therapies are ineffective or not tolerated
Metoclopramide	10 mg IV at onset	Useful for acute relief in the office or emergency department setting
Prochlorperazine	10 mg IV or IM at onset	Useful for acute relief in the office or emergency department setting

[a]Limit use of symptomatic medications to 2 days/week when possible to avoid medication misuse headache.
Compiled from refs. 20, 22, 24, 34, 42, and 47.

TABLE 59–5. Prophylactic Migraine Therapies

Medication	Dose
β-Adrenergic Antagonists	
Atenolol	25–100 mg/day
Metoprolol[a]	50–300 mg/day in divided doses
Nadolol	80–240 mg/day
Propranolol[ab]	80–240 mg/day in divided doses
Timolol[b]	20–60 mg/day in divided doses
Antidepressants	
Amitriptyline	25–150 mg at bedtime
Doxepin	10–200 mg at bedtime
Imipramine	10–200 mg at bedtime
Nortriptyline	10–150 mg at bedtime
Protriptyline	5–30 mg at bedtime
Fluoxetine	10–80 mg/day
Phenelzine[c]	15–60 mg/day in divided doses
Valproic Acid/Divalproex Sodium[b]	500–1500 mg/day in divided doses
Verapamil[a]	240–360 mg/day in divided doses
Methysergide[b,c]	2–8 mg/day in divided doses with food
Nonsteroidal Anti-inflammatory Drugs[c]	
Aspirin	1300 mg/day in divided doses
Ketoprofen[a]	150 mg/day in divided doses
Naproxen sodium[a]	550–1100 mg/day in divided doses
Vitamin B_2	400 mg/day

[a]Sustained-release formulation available.
[b]FDA approved for prevention of migraine.
[c]Daily or prolonged use limited by potential toxicity.
Compiled from refs. 14, 19, 20, and 26.

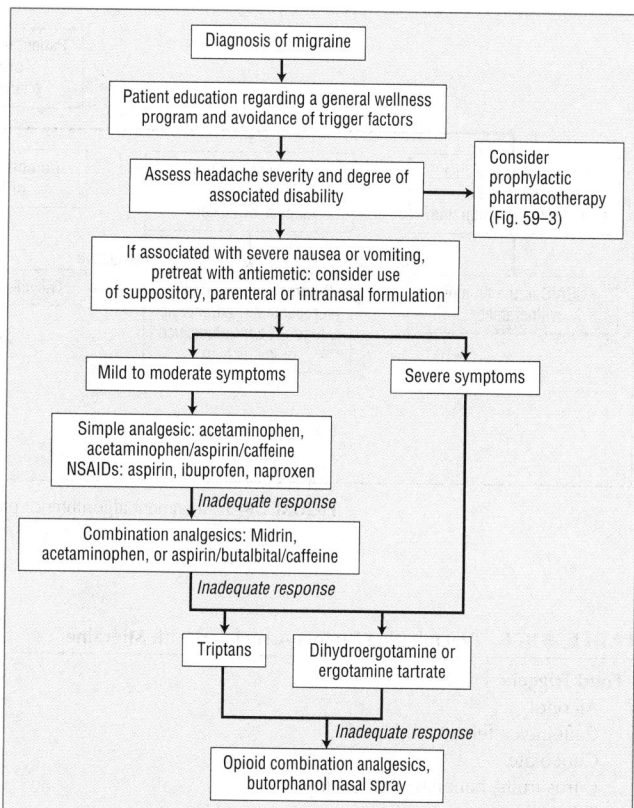

FIGURE 59–2. Treatment algorithm for migraine headaches.

intolerable. Drug doses for migraine prophylaxis are often lower than those necessary for other indications.[4] Overuse of acute headache medications will interfere with the therapeutic effects of preventive treatment.[25] Prophylactic treatment usually is continued for at least 3 to 6 months after the frequency and severity of headaches have diminished and then is tapered gradually and discontinued. Many migraineurs experience fewer and less severe attacks for lengthy periods following discontinuation of prophylactic medications or taper to a lower dose.[25] Figures 59–2 and 59–3 identify treatment and management algorithms for migraine headache.

NONPHARMACOLOGIC THERAPY

Nonpharmacologic therapy of acute migraine headache is limited but may include application of ice to the head and periods of rest or sleep, usually in a dark, quiet environment. Preventive management of migraine should begin with the identification and avoidance of factors that consistently provoke migraine attacks in susceptible individuals[24,28] (Table 59–6). Changes in estrogen levels associated with menarche, menstruation, pregnancy, menopause, oral contraceptive use, and other hormone therapies can trigger, intensify, or alleviate migraine.[29–32] Attacks are linked exclusively to menstruation in approximately 14% of women (i.e., true menstrual migraine).[20,29] A headache diary that records the frequency, severity, and duration of attacks may facilitate identification of migraine triggers. Patients also may benefit from adherence to a wellness program that includes regular sleep, exercise, and eating habits, smoking cessation, and limited caffeine intake. Behavioral interventions, such

as relaxation therapy, biofeedback (often used in combination with relaxation therapy), and cognitive therapy, are preventive treatment options for patients who prefer nondrug therapy or when symptomatic therapies are poorly tolerated, contraindicated, or ineffective.[19]

ACUTE MIGRAINE TREATMENT

CLINICAL CONTROVERSY

The availability of many over-the-counter drugs that were formerly prescription medications enables some migraine patients to self-medicate and delay entry into appropriate medical management. Some clinicians feel that over-the-counter products invite patients to take a less effective step-care approach rather than being treated according to evidence-based guidelines.[33]

Although controversial, some clinicians argue that the efficacy and tolerability of over-the-counter medications for migraine relief are limited because of patient dissatisfaction with the route of administration, the onset of action, the completeness of pain relief, and the length of suffering and prolonged disability.[33]

ANALGESICS AND NONSTEROIDAL ANTI-INFLAMMATORY DRUGS (NSAIDS)

Simple analgesics and NSAIDs are effective medications for the management of many migraine attacks[6,21,34] (see Table 59–4). They offer a reasonable first-line choice for treatment of mild to moderate

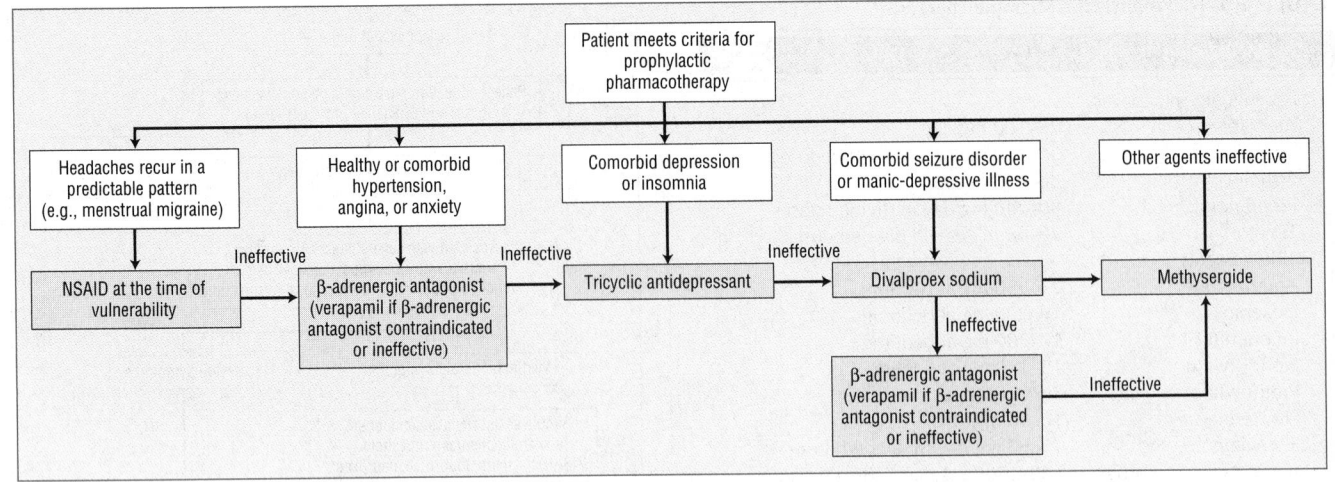

FIGURE 59–3. Treatment algorithm for prophylactic management of migraine headaches.

TABLE 59–6. Precipitating Factors Associated with Migraine

Food Triggers
Alcohol
Caffeine/caffeine withdrawal
Chocolate
Citrus fruits, bananas, figs, raisins
Dairy products
Fermented and pickled foods
Monosodium glutamate (e.g., in Chinese food, seasoned salt, and instant foods)
Nitrate-containing foods (e.g., processed meats)
Saccharin/aspartame (e.g., diet foods or diet sodas)
Sulfites in shrimp
Tyramine-containing foods
Yeast products

Environmental Triggers
Glare or flickering lights
High altitude
Loud noises
Strong smells and fumes
Tobacco smoke
Weather changes

Behavioral-Physiologic Triggers
Excess or insufficient sleep
Fatigue
Menstruation, menopause
Skipped meals
Strenuous physical activity (e.g., prolonged overexertion)
Stress or post-stress

Medications
Analgesic overuse
Benzodiazepine withdrawal
Cimetidine
Decongestant overuse
Ergotamine overuse
Estrogen therapy
Indomethacin
Nifedipine
Nitrates
Oral contraceptives
Reserpine
Theophylline

Compiled from refs. 24 and 28.

migraine attacks or severe attacks that have been responsive in the past to similar NSAIDs or nonopiate analgesics.[19] Of the NSAIDs, aspirin, ibuprofen, naproxen sodium, tolfenamic acid, and the combination of acetaminophen plus aspirin and caffeine have demonstrated the most consistent evidence of efficacy.[28] Although conclusions regarding clinical efficacy are not available, intramuscular ketorolac is an option for physician-supervised settings.[19,34] Evidence for other NSAIDs is either limited (only one study) or inconsistent (some positive and some negative studies).[34] Acetaminophen alone is not generally recommended for migraine because the scientific support is not optimal.[14,19,34] Comparisons with other pharmacotherapeutic classes are limited.

NSAIDs appear to prevent neurogenically mediated inflammation in the trigeminovascular system through the inhibition of prostaglandin synthesis. In general, NSAIDs with a long half-life that preclude their frequent use are preferred.[35] Combination therapy with metoclopramide can speed the absorption of analgesics and NSAIDs and alleviate migraine-related nausea and vomiting.[24] Suppository analgesic preparations and intramuscular ketorolac are also options when nausea and vomiting are severe.[20] Effervescent formulations may offer the advantage of enhanced absorption.[24] Acute NSAID therapy is associated with gastrointestinal (e.g., dyspepsia, nausea, vomiting, and diarrhea) and CNS side effects (e.g., somnolence, dizziness). NSAIDs should be used cautiously in patients with previous ulcer disease, renal disease, or hypersensitivity to aspirin.[34]

The over-the-counter combination of acetaminophen, aspirin, and caffeine was approved for the treatment of migraine in the United States because of its proven efficacy in relieving migraine pain and associated symptoms.[34,36] Aspirin and acetaminophen are also available in prescription combination products containing a short-acting barbiturate (butalbital) or narcotic (codeine, propoxyphene). No randomized, placebo-controlled studies support the efficacy of butalbital-containing products in the treatment of migraine. The use of butalbital-containing analgesics or narcotics should be limited because of concerns about overuse, medication-overuse headache, and withdrawal.[14,19,34] Midrin, a combination of acetaminophen, isometheptene mucate (a sympathomimetic amine), and dichloralphenazone (a chloral hydrate derivative), has demonstrated modest benefits in placebo-controlled studies and generally is viewed as an alternative for patients with mild to moderate migraine attacks.[19,3] Although frequent consumption of aspirin or acetaminophen alone an result in medication overuse headache, combination analgesics appear to pose a greater risk.[23]

OPIATE ANALGESICS

Narcotic analgesic drugs (e.g., meperidine, butorphanol, oxycodone, and hydromorphone) are effective but generally should be reserved for patients with moderate to severe infrequent headaches in whom conventional therapies are contraindicated or as "rescue medication" after patients have failed to respond to conventional therapies.[14] Frequent use of narcotic analgesics may lead to the development of dependency and rebound headache.[34] The intranasal formulation of butorphanol, a synthetically derived opioid agonist-antagonist, is a treatment option and alternative to frequent office or emergency department visits for injectable migraine therapies. Butorphanol is used widely despite the established risk of overuse and dependence. Opioid therapy should be supervised closely.[19,34]

ANTIEMETICS

Adjunctive antiemetic therapy is useful for combating the nausea and vomiting that accompany migraine headaches and the medications used to treat acute attacks (e.g., ergotamine tartrate). A single dose of an antiemetic, such as metoclopramide, chlorpromazine, or prochlorperazine, administered 15 to 30 minutes before ingestion of oral abortive migraine medications is often sufficient. Suppository preparations are available when nausea and vomiting are particularly prominent. Metoclopramide is also useful to reverse gastroparesis and improve absorption from the gastrointestinal tract during severe attacks.[19,34]

In addition to antiemetic effects, dopamine antagonist drugs also have been used successfully as monotherapy for the treatment of intractable headache. Prochlorperazine administered by the intravenous and intramuscular routes and intravenous metoclopramide provided more effective pain relief than placebo. Chlorpromazine also has provided relief of migraine headache comparable to that provided by intravenous metoclopramide and dihydroergotamine when administered parenterally. Domperidone has a possible role for preemptive treatment of migraine. The precise mechanism of action for these agents is unknown. The dopamine antagonists offer an alternative to the narcotic analgesics for the treatment of refractory migraine. Drowsiness and dizziness were reported occasionally with the use of dopamine antagonists in migraineurs. Extrapyramidal side effects were reported infrequently in migraine trials.[34]

MISCELLANEOUS NONSPECIFIC MEDICATIONS

Corticosteroids may be an effective rescue therapy for status migrainosus (a severe, continuous migraine that may last up to 1 week).[19] Open-label studies also suggest that short courses of orally or parenterally administered prednisone, dexamethasone, and hydrocortisone appear to be useful in the management of refractory headache that has persisted for several days.[14]

Limited studies suggest a role for intranasal lidocaine in the treatment of acute migraine headache.[34] Intranasal lidocaine provides rapid pain relief within 15 minutes of administration, but headache recurrence is common. Adverse effects generally are limited to local irritation of the nose or eye, an unpleasant taste, and numbness of the throat.

Preliminary investigations of intramuscular droperidol, nitrous oxide, and intravenous propofol have yielded favorable results in the treatment of acute migraine headache.[37-39] Future studies may establish a more defined role for these agents in migraine management.

ERGOT ALKALOIDS AND DERIVATIVES

Ergotamine tartrate and dihydroergotamine are useful and may be considered for the treatment of moderate to severe migraine attacks.[19] These drugs are nonselective 5-HT$_1$ receptor agonists that constrict intracranial blood vessels and inhibit the development of neurogenic inflammation in the trigeminovascular system.[40] Central inhibition of the trigeminovascular pathway is also reported.[41] These agents also display activity at α-adrenergic, β-adrenergic, and dopaminergic receptors. Venous and arterial constriction occur with therapeutic doses, but ergotamine tartrate exerts more potent arterial effects than dihydroergotamine.[40]

Ergotamine tartrate is available for oral, sublingual, and rectal administration (see Table 59–4). Oral and rectal preparations contain caffeine to enhance absorption and potentiate analgesia. Some patients respond preferentially to rectal dosing.[14] Dosage requirements should be titrated strictly to establish an effective but subnauseating dose for future attacks. Ergotamine is most effective when administered early in the migraine attack.[42] Despite its widespread clinical use since 1925, evidence supporting the efficacy of ergotamine tartrate in migraine is inconsistent.[14,34]

Dihydroergotamine is available for intranasal and parenteral administration by the intramuscular, subcutaneous, and intravenous routes[14,19] (see Table 59–4). Parenteral dihydroergotamine was viewed previously as inpatient or emergency department treatment for moderate to severe migraine, but patients can be trained to self-administer dihydroergotamine intramuscularly or subcutaneously. The bioavailability of dihydroergotamine is approximately 30% following intranasal administration, and maximum plasma concentration is achieved in 30 to 60 minutes.[43]

Nausea and vomiting (resulting from stimulation of the chemoreceptor trigger zone) are among the most common adverse effects of the ergotamine derivatives; however, ergotamine is 12 times more emetic than dihydroergotamine.[40] Pretreatment with an antiemetic agent should be considered with ergotamine and intravenous dihydroergotamine therapy. Other common side effects include abdominal pain, weakness, fatigue, paresthesias, muscle pain, diarrhea, and chest tightness. Occasionally, symptoms of severe peripheral ischemia (ergotism), including cold, numb, painful extremities, continuous paresthesias, diminished peripheral pulses, and claudication, may result from the vasoconstrictor effects of the ergot alkaloids. Gangrenous extremities, myocardial infarction, hepatic necrosis, and bowel and brain ischemia have been reported rarely.[4,40-42] Dihydroergotamine is rarely associated with such side effects.[42,44] Triptans and ergot derivatives should not be used within 24 hours of each other.[42] Recently, reports of severe vasospasm during concomitant therapy with ergotamine and protease inhibitors have appeared in the literature.[45,46] These cases are attributed to protease inhibitor inhibitory effects on the CYP3A4 isoenzyme and a consequent rise in ergotamine blood levels. Ergotamine derivatives are contraindicated in patients with renal or hepatic failure; coronary, cerebral, or peripheral vascular disease; uncontrolled hypertension; and sepsis and in women who are pregnant or nursing.[4,42] Dihydroergotamine does not appear to cause rebound headache, but dosage restrictions for ergotamine tartrate should be observed strictly to prevent this complication.[4]

SEROTONIN RECEPTOR AGONISTS (TRIPTANS)

Introduction of the serotonin receptor agonists, or triptans, represented a significant advance in migraine pharmacotherapy. The first member of this class, sumatriptan, and the second-generation agents zolmitriptan, naratriptan, rizatriptan, almotriptan, frovatriptan, and eletriptan are selective agonists of the 5-HT$_{1B}$ and 5-HT$_{1D}$ receptors. Relief of migraine headache is the result of three key actions: vasoconstriction of pain-producing intracranial blood vessels through stimulation of vascular 5-HT$_{1B}$ receptors, inhibition of vasoactive neuropeptide release from trigeminal perivascular nerves through stimulation of presynaptic 5-HT$_{1D}$ receptors, and interruption of pain signal transmission within the brain stem trigeminal nuclei through stimulation of 5-HT$_{1D}$ receptors (centrally acting agents).[10,22] Individual affinities for 5-HT$_{1B}$ and 5-HT$_{1D}$ receptors vary somewhat but are comparable.[10,47] These agents also display varying affinity for 5-HT$_{1A}$, 5-HT$_{1E}$, and 5-HT$_{1F}$ receptors. The triptans are appropriate first-line therapy for patients with moderate to severe migraine and are used for rescue therapy when nonspecific medications are ineffective.[19,20]

Sumatriptan, the most extensively studied antimigraine therapy, is available for subcutaneous, oral, and intranasal administration.[22] Subcutaneous sumatriptan is consistently superior to placebo in alleviating migraine headache and associated symptoms, with relief reported in 71% of patients at 1 hour (43% pain-free) and 79% at 2 hours (60% pain-free) in a meta-analysis of placebo-controlled studies.[22,47] In addition to enhanced efficacy, subcutaneous sumatriptan has a more rapid onset of action (10 minutes) when compared with the oral formulation (30 minutes).[20,47] The subcutaneous injection is packaged as an autoinjector device for self-administration by patients. Intranasal sumatriptan provides a faster onset of effect (15 minutes) than the oral formulation and produces similar rates of response (relief in 61% of patients at 2 hours) in placebo-controlled studies.[47] Approximately 30% to 40% of patients who respond to sumatriptan experience headache recurrence within 24 hours.[47] This has been attributed to the drug's short half-life, but recurrence is a problem with most acute migraine therapies.[22,47] A second dose given at the time of recurrence usually is effective.

The second-generation triptans appear to offer an improved pharmacokinetic and pharmacodynamic profile compared with oral sumatriptan.[22,47,48] These agents have higher oral bioavailability and longer half-lives than oral sumatriptan, which theoretically could improve within-patient treatment consistency and reduce headache recurrence[16,22,49] (Table 59–7). Despite the fact that oral absorption may be delayed during migraine attacks, most patients prefer oral formulations, and these account for 80% of all triptan prescriptions.[50] Frovatriptan has the longest half-life of the triptans but the slowest onset of action. Penetration of the blood-brain barrier, as a result of increased lipophilicity, allows for a central site of action within the trigeminal nuclei and may hasten the onset of therapeutic effect of the second-generation agents.[10,22] Sumatriptan does not cross the intact blood-brain barrier in experimental systems. However, evidence suggests that the blood-brain barrier may be disrupted during a migraine attack, allowing central access for sumatriptan as well.[10]

Results of placebo-controlled studies with each of the second-generation agents reveal somewhat comparable 2-hour response rates. Direct comparative clinical trials are necessary to determine their relative efficacy, but these are available for only a few of the triptans. A recent meta-analysis summarizes the efficacy and tolerability of the different oral triptans across both published and unpublished studies.[50] At all marketed doses, the oral triptans are effective and well tolerated. Across studies for sumatriptan 100 mg, mean results were a 2-hour headache response of 59%, with 29% pain-free at 2 hours, 20% sustained pain-free, and 67% consistency. Compared with sumatriptan 100 mg, rizatriptan 10 mg showed better efficacy and consistency and similar tolerability; eletriptan 80 mg showed better efficacy, similar consistency, but lower tolerability; almotriptan 12.5 mg showed similar efficacy at 2 hours but better other results; naratriptan 2.5 mg and eletriptan 20 mg showed lower efficacy and better tolerability; and zolmitriptan 2.5 and 5 mg, eletriptan 40 mg, and riaztriptan 5 mg all showed similar results. Available data suggest lower efficacy for frovatriptan.[50]

Clinical response to the triptans can vary considerably among individual patients. Individual responses cannot be predicted, and if one triptan fails, a patient may be switched successfully to another triptan.[14,50] After an effective agent and dose have been identified, subsequent treatments should begin with that same regimen.

Side effects to the triptans are common but usually mild to moderate in nature and of short duration. Adverse effects are consistent among the class and include paresthesias, fatigue, dizziness, flushing,

TABLE 59–7. Pharmacokinetic Characteristics of Triptans

Drug	Half-Life (hours)	Time to Maximal Concentration (t_{max})	Bioavailability	Elimination
Almotriptan	3–4	1.4–3.8 h	70%	MAO-A, CYP450 3A4 and 2D6
Eletriptan	5	1.4–2.8 h	50%	CYP 3A4
Frovatriptan	25	2–4 h	24–30%	CYP 1A2
Naratriptan	5–6	2–3 h	63–74%	CYP450 (various isoenzymes)
Rizatriptan	2–3		40–45%	MAO-A
Oral tablets		1–1.5 h		
Disintegrating		1.6–2.5 h		
Sumatriptan:	2			MAO-A
SC injection		12–15 min	97%	
Oral tablets		2.5 h	14%	
Nasal spray		1–2.5 h	17%	
Zolmitriptan	3		40%	CYP 1A2, MAO-A
Oral		1.5 h		
Disintegrating		3 h		
Nasal		4 h		

Compiled from refs. 16, 35, and 47–49.

arm sensations, and somnolence. Local side effects are reported with the subcutaneous (minor injection-site reactions) and intranasal (taste perversion, nasal discomfort) routes. Doses that provide the best ratio of efficacy and safety are considered optimal. Up to 15% of patients receiving a triptan consistently report "chest symptoms," including tightness, pressure, heaviness, or pain in the chest, neck, or throat.[20,22] The mechanism of these symptoms is unknown, but a cardiac source of pain seems unlikely in most patients.[22] However, all triptans are partial agonists of human 5-HT coronary artery receptors in vitro, resulting in a small but significant vasoconstrictor response.[22,48] Adverse cardiac events are rare because 5-HT$_{2A}$ receptors mediate most of the effects of serotonin on coronary vessels.[20] Isolated cases of myocardial infarction and coronary vasospasm with ischemia have been reported, but myocardial ischemia is unlikely in patients with normal coronary vasculature.[48] The triptans are contraindicated in patients with a history of ischemic heart disease (e.g., angina pectoris, Prinzmetal's angina, or previous myocardial infarction), uncontrolled hypertension, and cerebrovascular disease. Patients at risk for unrecognized coronary artery disease (e.g., postmenopausal women, men over 40 years of age, and patients with multiple risk factors) should receive a cardiovascular assessment prior to triptan use and have their initial dose administered under medical supervision. Triptans are also contraindicated in patients with hemiplegic and basilar migraine. The triptans should not be given within 24 hours of the ergotamine derivatives. Administration of sumatriptan, rizatriptan, and zolmitriptan within 2 weeks of therapy with monoamine oxidase inhibitors is not recommended. Concomitant therapy with the selective serotonin reuptake inhibitors (SSRIs) should be monitored carefully because of isolated reports of serotonin syndrome in sumatriptan-treated patients. Frequent use of the triptans has been associated with the development of medication misuse headache.[16,19,34]

PREVENTIVE THERAPY

β-ADRENERGIC ANTAGONISTS

β-Adrenergic antagonists are the most widely used drugs for migraine prophylaxis.[25] Propranolol, nadolol, timolol, atenolol, and metoprolol have proven efficacy in controlled clinical trials, reducing the frequency of attacks by 50% in 60% to 80% of patients[25,27] (see Table 59–5). Because the relative efficacy of the individual agents has not been established, selection of a β-blocker may be based on β selectivity, convenience of the formulation, and tolerability. β-Blockers with intrinsic sympathomimetic activity are ineffective for migraine prophylaxis.[25] Although their precise mechanism of antimigraine action is unknown, they may raise the migraine threshold by modulating adrenergic or serotonergic neurotransmission in cortical or subcortical pathways. β-Blockers are particularly useful in patients with comorbid anxiety, hypertension, or angina. Side effects can include drowsiness, fatigue, sleep disturbances, vivid dreams, memory disturbance, depression, impotence, bradycardia, and hypotension. β-Blockers should be used with caution in patients with congestive heart failure, peripheral vascular disease, atrioventricular conduction disturbances, asthma, depression, and diabetes. Bronchoconstrictive and hyperglycemic effects may be minimized with β$_1$-selective agents.

ANTIDEPRESSANTS

The beneficial effects of antidepressants in migraine are independent of their antidepressant activity and may be related to downregulation of central 5-HT$_2$ and adrenergic receptors.[25] Amitriptyline, the most widely studied antidepressant for migraine prophylaxis, has demonstrated efficacy in placebo-controlled and comparative studies.[27] Use of other antidepressants is based primarily on clinical and anecdotal experience (see Table 59–5). Other tricyclic antidepressants (TCAs) that have been used successfully for migraine prophylaxis include doxepin, nortriptyline, protriptyline, and imipramine.[19,25] Anticholinergic side effects are common and limit use of these agents in patients with benign prostatic hyperplasia and glaucoma. Evening doses are preferred because of associated sedation. Increased appetite and weight gain may occur. Orthostatic hypotension and cardiac toxicity (slowed atrioventricular conduction) also are reported occasionally. The more favorable side-effect profile of nortriptyline and protriptyline could prove advantageous in patients who are particularly intolerant of the anticholinergic and sedative side effects of amitriptyline.

SSRIs have not been studied extensively for the preventive treatment of migraine headaches, but clinicians have used them nonetheless.[20] Fluoxetine is the most studied SSRI for migraine prevention, but definitive benefit has not been demonstrated in a rigorous clinical study.[25] Prospective data evaluating the other SSRIs (e.g., sertraline, paroxetine, fluvoxamine, and citalopram) are lacking.[19] The SSRIs are considered to be less effective than TCAs for migraine prophylaxis but have gained favor with some clinicians as a result of their more favorable adverse-effect profile.[4] These agents should not be considered as first- or second-line medications for the management of migraine, but they are useful in patients with comorbid depression.[4,25] Preliminary evidence suggests a possible benefit with venlafaxine, an inhibitor of serotonin and norepinephrine reuptake.[51]

Monoamine oxidase inhibitors (MAOIs), such as phenelzine, have been used in the management of refractory headache, but their complex adverse-effect profile limits their use to experienced prescribers.[51] Strict adherence to a tyramine-free diet is necessary to avoid potentially life-threatening hypertensive crisis.

ANTICONVULSANTS

Anticonvulsant medications have emerged as an important therapeutic option for the prevention of migraine headaches. The beneficial effects of these agents are likely due to multiple mechanisms of action, including enhancement of γ-aminobutyric acid (GABA)–mediated inhibition, modulation of the excitatory neurotransmitter glutamate, and inhibition of sodium and calcium ion channel activity.[52] Anticonvulsants, such as divalproex sodium and topiramate, are particularly useful in migraineurs with comorbid seizures, anxiety disorder, or bipolar disorder.[4] The efficacy of valproic acid and divalproex sodium (a 1:1 molar combination of valproate sodium and valproic acid) has been demonstrated in multiple placebo-controlled studies.[25] Nausea and vomiting, the most common early side effects, are self-limited and appear to be less common with divalproex sodium and gradual titration of doses. Alopecia, tremor, asthenia, somnolence, and weight gain are also common complaints.[25,53] The extended-release formulation of divalproex sodium is administered once daily and is better tolerated than the enteric-coated formulation.[53] Hepatotoxicity is the most serious side effect of valproate therapy, but the risk appears to be low in migraineurs (e.g., patients older than 10 years of age who are receiving monotherapy and have no underlying metabolic or neurologic disorder).[25] Baseline liver function tests should be obtained, but routine follow-up studies are not necessary in asymptomatic adults on monotherapy. Patient evaluation is recommended every 1 to 2 months during the first 6 to 9 months of therapy. Valproate is contraindicated in pregnant women (owing to potential teratogenicity) and patients with a history of pancreatitis or chronic liver disease. Although valproate level determinations may be useful for assessing compliance and toxicity, a recent study suggests that serum levels of less than 50 mcg/mL (usual therapeutic level is 50 to 100 mcg/mL) may provide similar benefit to higher levels.[54]

Topiramate is currently undergoing FDA review for a migraine prophylaxis indication based on the results of a randomized, double-blind study that demonstrated significantly greater reductions in mean monthly migraine frequency with 100 and 200 mg topiramate daily compared with placebo.[55] Treatment-emergent adverse events associated with topiramate included paresthesia, fatigue, anorexia, diarrhea, weight loss, difficulty with memory, and nausea. Kidney stones, acute myopia and acute angle-closure glaucoma, and oligohidrosis have been reported infrequently with topiramate use.[56]

A recent study suggests that gabapentin also may be an effective agent for migraine prevention in patients achieving a daily dose of 2400 mg.[25,57] Somnolence, dizziness, and asthenia were the most commonly reported adverse events. Preliminary studies suggest a possible role for other anticonvulsants, including tiagabine, levetiracetam, and zonisamide; however, further clinical studies are needed to confirm their utility in migraine prophylaxis.[56,58]

CALCIUM CHANNEL BLOCKERS

The calcium channel blockers generally are considered second- or third-line options for preventive treatment when other drugs with established clinical benefit are ineffective or contraindicated.[20] Verapamil is the most widely used calcium channel blocker for preventive treatment, but it provided only modest benefit in decreasing the frequency of attacks in two placebo-controlled studies.[4] The therapeutic effect of verapamil may not be noted for up to 8 weeks after initiation of therapy.[51] Side effects of verapamil may include constipation, hypotension, bradycardia, atrioventricular block, and exacerbation of congestive heart failure. Evaluations of nifedipine, nimodipine, diltiazem, and nicardipine have yielded equivocal results.[25]

METHYSERGIDE

The semisynthetic ergot alkaloid methysergide is a potent 5-HT$_2$ receptor antagonist that appears to stabilize serotonergic neurotransmission in the trigeminovascular system to block the development of neurogenic inflammation.[59] Although methysergide is an effective preventive medication, its utility is limited by the rare (1 in 5000 patients) development of retroperitoneal, endocardial, and pulmonary fibrosis during long-term administration.[4] Consequently, a medication-free interval of 4 weeks is recommended following each 6-month treatment period.[59] The dosage should be tapered over a 1-week period to prevent rebound headaches. Monitoring for fibrotic complications should include periodic auscultation of the heart, as well as yearly chest roentgenography, echocardiography, and abdominal magnetic resonance imaging.[25] Methysergide is best tolerated when taken with meals. In addition to gastrointestinal intolerance, muscle aching, leg cramps, claudication, weight gain, and hallucinations are also reported with its use. It is contraindicated in pregnancy, peripheral vascular disorders, coronary artery disease, severe hypertension, thrombophlebitis or cellulitis of the legs, peptic ulcer disease, liver or renal dysfunctions, and valvular heart disease.[59] Peripheral vasospasm and severe claudication have been reported occasionally in patients without a prior history of vascular disease. Methysergide is reserved for patients with refractory headaches that do not respond to other preventive therapies.

NONSTEROIDAL ANTI-INFLAMMATORY DRUGS (NSAIDS)

NSAIDs are modestly effective for reducing the frequency, severity, and duration of migraine attacks, but potential gastrointestinal and renal toxicity may limit the daily or prolonged use of these agents.[25,27] Consequently, NSAIDs have been used intermittently to prevent headaches that recur in a predictable pattern, such as menstrual migraine. Administration of NSAIDs in the perimenstrual period may be beneficial in women with true menstrual migraine.[60] NSAIDs should be initiated 1 to 2 days prior to the expected onset of headache and continued during the period of vulnerability.[4] Prostaglandin production may be enhanced in women with menstrual migraine, and the preventive mechanism of NSAIDs is thought to involve inhibition of prostaglandin synthesis.[4] If long-term NSAID therapy is initiated, monitoring of renal function and occult blood loss is necessary.

MISCELLANEOUS PROPHYLACTIC AGENTS

A double-blind, placebo-controlled study demonstrated the efficacy of riboflavin (vitamin B$_2$) 400 mg daily in migraine prophylaxis. Riboflavin was associated with 50% or greater improvement in attack frequency in 59% of patients.[56] More recently, localized injections of botulinum toxin type A have reduced the frequency, severity, and disability associated with migraine headaches significantly in three small double-blind, placebo-controlled trials.[61] The angiotensin-converting enzyme inhibitor lisinopril and the angiotensin II receptor blocker candesartan provided effective migraine prophylaxis in recent double-blind, placebo-controlled, crossover studies of these agents.[62,63] Further research is needed to establish the safety and efficacy of the herbal medication feverfew (*Tanacetum parthenium*) because studies to date have yielded conflicting results.[4] Authors of a recent double-blind, placebo-controlled study concluded that petasites, an extract from the plant *Petasites hybridus*, may be an effective preventive treatment for migraine.[58] Further study is need to determine the clinical utility and comparative efficacy of these agents for the prophylactic management of migraine.

PHARMACOECONOMIC CONSIDERATIONS

Although migraine is widely recognized as a disease that exacts an enormous toll on the sufferer, the direct and indirect costs associated with migraine headache impose a substantial burden on society as well. The direct costs associated with migraine diagnosis and treatment are substantial. The volume of health care services used by migraineurs is two or more times that of nonmigraineurs, with 2.5 times as many pharmacy claims, more emergency department visits, and more than 6 times the cost of diagnostic procedures.[64] A large portion of the cost of treatment is pharmacotherapy, but this actually represents a small percentage of the total cost of migraine.[64] The indirect costs of the illness related to work absenteeism, decreased productivity, and impairment greatly exceed the direct cost of medical are.[8,65] The estimated indirect cost of migraine-related disability, the most important determinant of the economic impact of migraine, is approximately $13 billion each year.[8,65]

According to the American Migraine Study II, only 48% of those surveyed with clear symptoms of migraine were diagnosed by a physician.[5,6] Although 96% of severe migraine sufferers take some medication for their headaches, only 41% of those with moderate to severe headache-related disability take prescription medication.[5,6] Because many migraineurs who receive inadequate care experience substantial levels of pain and disability, improvement in migraine diagnosis, care, and treatment potentially could result in lower direct and indirect costs of the disease.

Education of headache patients regarding required behavior changes and effective use of acute and prophylactic pharmacotherapy may be time-consuming, but it is also extremely cost-effective. Oversights may lead to decreased efficacy of medications resulting in repeat dosing and polypharmacy, decreased compliance, increased emergency department use, increased "doctor shopping," and, perhaps, increased use of expensive diagnostic procedures and inpatient services. Recent studies demonstrate that effective migraine treatment can reduce productivity loss during a migraine attack.[66] Health care resource use and time lost from workplace productivity and nonworkplace activity also were reduced significantly 3 to 6 months after the initiation of sumatriptan therapy in a managed-care population.[67] Health-related quality of life also improved in these patients. These studies demonstrate that the clinical benefits of effective migraine therapy ultimately may translate into reduced indirect migraine-related costs. Further studies should be conducted to demonstrate the value of effective migraine pharmacotherapies in reducing the overall costs of managing the migraineur.

SUMMARY

Acute and preventive pharmacotherapy for migraine should be individualized based on the individual patient response, tolerability of the available agents, and presence of comorbid conditions. Migraine management should be individualized on the basis of the patient's clinical presentation and medical history. Analgesics and NSAIDs may be considered the drugs of choice for infrequent mild to moderate attacks. The triptans or dihydroergotamine can be used as secondary agents if initial therapies prove ineffective or as first-line therapy in moderate to severe migraine headache. Abortive therapy should be instituted early in the course of the attack to optimize efficacy and minimize migraine-related pain and disability. Preventive therapy should be considered in the setting of recurring migraines that produce significant disability, frequent attacks requiring symptomatic medication more than twice per week, symptomatic therapies that are ineffective, contraindicated, or produce serious side effects, and uncommon migraine variants that cause profound disruption and/or risk of neurologic injury. Efficacy of a prescribed prophylactic regimen should be reassessed periodically. A prolonged headache-free interval could allow for gradual dosage reduction and discontinuation of therapy.

TENSION-TYPE HEADACHE

EPIDEMIOLOGY

Tension-type headache is the most common type of primary headache, with an estimated 1-year prevalence of 63% in men and 86% in women.[2] First onset of tension-type headache typically is early in life (before age 20 in 40% of patients), and prevalence peaks between the ages of 20 and 50 years.[2,4] It is more common among women in adulthood, with a female-to-male ratio of 4:3.[68] The mean frequency of attacks is 2.9 days per month, with most sufferers experiencing fewer than one attack per month.[4] The prevalence of chronic tension-type headache (defined as ≥180 headache days per year) is estimated at 2% to 3%.[4] Although an estimated 60% of tension-type headache sufferers experience some degree of functional impairment during their attacks, only 16% of patients have consulted a general practitioner for their headaches.[4,68]

PATHOPHYSIOLOGY

Although tension-type headache is the most common type of headache, it is the least studied of the primary headache disorders, and there is limited understanding of key pathophysiologic concepts.[68] Some practitioners theorize that migraine and tension-type headaches may represent a continuum of headache severity within the same entity.[69] However, more recently, tension-type headache has been recognized as a distinct disorder. The pain of episodic tension-type headache is thought to originate from the myofascial tissues, although central mechanisms also may be involved.[68] Following activation of supraspinal pain perception structures, a self-limiting headache results in most individuals owing to central modulation of the incoming peripheral stimuli.[68] Chronic tension-type headache may evolve from episodic tension-type headache in predisposed individuals owing to a disturbance of central nociceptive processing and subsequent sensitization of the CNS.[68] It is likely that other pathophysiologic mechanisms also contribute to the development of tension-type headache.

CLINICAL PRESENTATION

Premonitory symptoms and aura are absent with tension-type headache. The pain usually is mild to moderate in intensity and often is described as a dull, nonpulsatile tightness or pressure.[3,4] Bilateral pain is most common, but the location can vary (frontal and temporal pain are most common; occipital and parietal regions also may be affected).[3] The pain is classically described as having a "hatband" pattern. Associated symptoms generally are absent, but mild photophobia or phonophobia may be reported. The disability associated with tension-type headache typically is minor in comparison with migraine headache, and routine physical activity does not affect headache severity.[3,4] Palpation of the pericranial or cervical muscles may reveal tender spots or localized nodules in some patients.[3] Tension-type headache is classified as either episodic (infrequent or frequent) or chronic based on the frequency and duration of the attacks.[4]

▶ TREATMENT: Tension-Type Headaches

GENERAL APPROACH TO TREATMENT

The vast majority of episodic tension-type headache sufferers self-medicate with over-the-counter medications and do not consult a health care professional. While pharmacologic and nonpharmacologic treatments are available, simple analgesics and NSAIDs are the mainstay of acute therapy. Most agents used for tension-type headache have not been studied in controlled clinical trials.[70]

NONPHARMACOLOGIC THERAPY

Psychophysiologic therapy and physical therapy have been used in the management of tension-type headache. Psychophysiologic therapy may consist of reassurance and counseling, stress management, relaxation training, and biofeedback. Relaxation training and biofeedback training (alone or in combination) can result in a 50% reduction in headache activity.[4] Evidence supporting physical therapeutic options, such as heat or cold packs, ultrasound, electrical nerve stimulation, stretching, exercise, massage, acupuncture, manipulations, ergonomic instruction, and trigger point injections or occipital nerve blocks, is somewhat inconsistent.[4] However, patients may benefit from selected modalities (e.g., massage) during an acute episode of tension-type headache.

PHARMACOLOGIC THERAPY

Simple analgesics (alone or in combination with caffeine) and NSAIDs are effective for the acute treatment of mild to moderate tension-type headache. Acetaminophen, aspirin, ibuprofen, naproxen, ketoprofen, indomethacin, and ketorolac have demonstrated efficacy in placebo-controlled and comparative studies.[4] Failure of over-the-counter agents may warrant therapy with prescription drugs. High-dose NSAIDs and the combination of aspirin or acetaminophen with butalbital or, rarely, codeine are effective options. Use of butalbital and codeine combinations should be avoided when possible owing to the high potential for overuse and dependency. As with migraine headache, acute medication should be taken for episodic tension-type headache no more than 2 days per week to prevent the development of chronic tension-type headache.[4,71] There is no evidence to support the efficacy of muscle relaxants (e.g., cyclobenzaprine, baclofen, and methocarbamal) in the management of episodic tension-type headache.[4,70] Preventive treatment should be considered if headache frequency (more than two per week), duration (greater than 3-4 hours), or severity results in medication overuse or substantial disability. The principles of preventive treatment for tension-type headache are similar to those for migraine headache. TCAs are prescribed most often for prophylaxis, but other drugs also can be selected after consideration of comorbid medical conditions and respective side-effect profiles.[4] Injection of botulinum toxin into pericranial muscles has demonstrated efficacy in the prophylaxis of chronic tension-type headache in two recently published placebo-controlled studies.[70]

CLUSTER HEADACHE

EPIDEMIOLOGY

Cluster headache, the most severe of the primary headache disorders, is characterized by attacks of severe, unilateral head pain that occur in series lasting for weeks or months (i.e., cluster periods) separated by remission periods usually lasting months or years.[4,72] Cluster headaches may be episodic or chronic.[3] Cluster headache is relatively uncommon among the primary headache disorders, with an estimated prevalence of approximately 0.4% for men and 0.08% for women.[72] Unlike migraine, men are four to seven times more likely than women to suffer from cluster headache.[4] Onset can occur at any age but is most common in the late twenties. Recent evidence suggests that a genetic predisposition for cluster headache may exist in certain families.[4]

PATHOPHYSIOLOGY

The etiologic and pathophysiologic mechanisms of cluster headache are not completely understood. Similar to migraine headache, the head pain of cluster attacks is thought to involve activation of trigeminovascular neurons with resulting release of vasoactive neuropeptides and the development of sterile, neurogenic inflammation.[72] The characteristic location of head pain appears to implicate the cavernous sinus as the site of the inflammatory process.[9] Triggers of cluster headache attacks may cause periodic discharges of the trigeminovascular system that result in headache pain; however, the mechanisms that activate the trigeminovascular system are not yet understood. The periodicity and regularity of attacks may implicate hypothalamic dysfunction and resulting alterations in circadian rhythms in the pathogenesis of cluster headache.[4,72] Hypothalamus-induced changes in cortisol, prolactin, testosterone, growth hormone, β-endorphin, and melatonin have been demonstrated during periods of cluster headache attack.[72] Neuroimaging studies performed during acute cluster headache attacks have demonstrated activation of the ipsilateral hypothalamic gray area.[9] This region may be the fundamental "driver" of the cluster attack. Because serotonergic systems modulate activity in both the hypothalamus and trigeminovascular neurons, 5-HT may play a significant role in cluster headache pathophysiology. The association of cluster headache with high-altitude hypoxia, rapid-eye-movement sleep, and vasodilator therapy, as well as the efficacy of oxygen inhalation therapy in aborting cluster attacks, suggests that hypoxemia also may play a role in the pathogenesis of cluster headache.[72]

CLINICAL PRESENTATION

Attacks occur in cluster periods lasting 2 weeks to 3 months in most patients, followed by long pain-free intervals.[4,72] Periods of remission average 2 years in length but have been reported to be from 2 months to 20 years in duration. Approximately 10% of patients have chronic symptoms with no remission periods. Cluster headache attacks occur at night in more than 50% of patients and appear to be more common in the spring and fall.[72] Attacks occur suddenly, with pain peaking quickly after onset and generally lasting 15 to 180 minutes.[3] Auras are not present with cluster headaches. The pain is excruciating and penetrating but usually nonthrobbing and is most often unilateral in orbital, supraorbital, and temporal locations.[4,72] The headache is associated with autonomic features consistent with sympathetic system paresis and parasympathetic overdrive. These features are present on the pain side and include conjunctival injection, lacrimation, and nasal stuffiness or rhinorrhea. Ipsilateral scalp and facial tenderness, ptosis, miosis, and periorbital swelling also are described. During the cluster period, attacks occur from once every other day to eight times per day.[4] Whereas migraine patients retreat to a quiet dark room, cluster headache patients generally move about during an attack and may rub or beat their heads against objects in an attempt to alleviate the pain.[72] Male patients often have a history of heavy tobacco and/or alcohol use.[72] Specific diagnostic criteria for cluster headaches are provided within the IHS classification system.[3]

► TREATMENT: Cluster Headaches

As in migraine, therapy for cluster headaches involves both abortive and prophylactic therapy. Abortive therapy is directed at managing the acute attack. Prophylactic therapy is intended to shorten the duration of episodic cluster attacks, in addition to reducing the frequency and severity of attacks in both episodic and chronic cluster headache. Prophylactic therapies are started early in the cluster period and administered daily until the patient is headache-free for at least 2 weeks. The medication is then tapered but may be restarted with the next cluster period. Patients with chronic cluster headache may require prophylactic medications indefinitely.

■ ABORTIVE THERAPY

▌ OXYGEN

The standard acute treatment of cluster headache is inhalation of 100% oxygen by facial mask at a rate of 7–10 L/min for 10 to 15 minutes.[4,72] Repeat administration may be necessary because of recurrence because oxygen appears merely to delay, rather than abort, the attack in some patients.[72] No side effects have been reported with the use of oxygen.

▌ ERGOTAMINE DERIVATIVES

Intravenous or intramuscular dihydroergotamine provides effective relief for acute attacks of cluster headache.[4,72] Onset of effect usually occurs within 10 minutes following intravenous administration.[72] Intramuscular administration is effective within 30 minutes, and patients may be trained to self-administer the intramuscular injection.[72] Repeated intravenous administration of dihydroergotamine for 3 to 7 days can break the cycle of frequent cluster headache attacks with minimal side effects.[72] Ergotamine tartrate also has provided effective relief of cluster headache attacks when administered sublingually or rectally, but the pharmacokinetics of these preparations frequently limit their clinical utility.[4,72] Dosing guidelines are similar to those for migraine headache therapy.

▌ TRIPTANS

Subcutaneous and intranasal sumatriptan is considered safe and effective treatment for acute cluster headaches.[49,73] Adverse events reported in cluster headache patients are similar to those seen in migraineurs. Sumatriptan has been used in the management of cluster headaches for up to 1 year without evidence of tachyphylaxis or increased toxicity.[73] Orally administered sumatriptan has limited use in cluster attacks because of its relatively long onset of action; oral zolmitriptan, however, was efficacious in patients with episodic cluster headache, with 60% of patients experiencing relief (mild or no pain) at 30 minutes.[49,73]

■ PROPHYLACTIC THERAPY

▌ VERAPAMIL

Verapamil, the preferred calcium channel blocker for the prevention of cluster headaches, is effective in approximately 70% of patients.[4] The beneficial effects of verapamil often appear after 1 week of therapy. Effective doses usually range from 240 to 360 mg/day for episodic attacks, but higher doses may be necessary to control chronic cluster headache.

▌ LITHIUM

Lithium carbonate is effective against episodic and chronic cluster headache attacks, with beneficial effects often appearing during the first week of therapy. A positive response is seen in up to 78% of patients with chronic cluster headache and in up to 63% of patients with episodic cluster headache.[4] The usual dose of lithium for cluster headache is 600 to 900 mg/day administered in divided doses. Tachyphylaxis to lithium has been reported occasionally during prolonged therapy.[4,72] Optimal plasma lithium levels for the prevention of cluster headache have not been established, but efficacy has been reported at relatively low serum concentrations (0.3–0.8 mEq/L).[4,72]

Initial side effects are mild and include tremor, lethargy, nausea, diarrhea, and abdominal discomfort. Lithium treatment has been associated with headache symptoms described as episodes of moderately severe, throbbing occipital pain lasting 6 to 12 hours, but these headaches are easily distinguishable from the cluster headache and disappear when lithium is withdrawn. Lithium should be administered with caution to patients with significant renal or cardiovascular disease, dehydration, pregnancy, or concomitant diuretic use.

▌ ERGOTAMINE

Ergotamine can be an efficacious agent for prophylactic as well as abortive therapy of cluster headaches.[4] A 2-mg bedtime dose is often beneficial for the prevention of nocturnal headache attacks. Daily use of 1 to 2 mg ergotamine alone or in combination with verapamil or lithium may provide effective headache prophylaxis in patients refractory to other agents with little risk of ergotism or rebound headache.[4,72]

▌ METHYSERGIDE

In patients unresponsive to other therapies, methysergide 4 to 8 mg/day in divided doses is usually effective in shortening the course of cluster headaches.[72] Response to treatment usually occurs within 1 week of initiation of the drug. Response rates in patients with episodic cluster headache approach 70%, but chronic cluster headache patients receive less benefit.[72] Precautions regarding methysergide use were described earlier in this chapter.

▌ CORTICOSTEROIDS

Corticosteroids are useful for chronic cluster headaches refractory to verapamil, lithium, ergotamine, and methysergide or combinations of these agents.[4,72] Therapy is initiated with 40 to 60 mg/day prednisone and tapered over approximately 3 weeks. Relief appears within 1 to 2 days of initiating therapy. To avoid steroid-induced complications, long-term use is not recommended. Headaches may recur when therapy is tapered or discontinued.

MISCELLANEOUS AGENTS

Other therapies that have been used in the acute management of cluster headache include intranasal lidocaine, intranasal capsaicin, and intramuscular leuprolide.[72] Preliminary evidence also may support the use of divalproex sodium, gabapentin, baclofen, topiramate, and phototherapy treatments, but well-designed, controlled studies are needed.[4,72,75,76] Neurosurgical intervention may be necessary for patients with chronic cluster headache that is resistant to all medical therapies.[4,72]

EVALUATION OF THERAPEUTIC OUTCOMES

Because of the prevalence of headache disorders, clinicians need to be actively involved in patient care issues. Patients should be monitored for frequency, intensity, and duration of headaches, as well as any change in the headache pattern. To this end, migraineurs should be encouraged to keep a headache diary to document the frequency, severity, and duration of migraine attacks, as well as response to medication and potential trigger factors. Careful monitoring is essential to initiate the most appropriate pharmacotherapy, document therapeutic successes and failures, identify medication contraindications, and prevent or minimize adverse events. Patients using acute therapies should be monitored for frequency of use of prescription and over-the-counter medications in order to identify potential medication misuse headache. Patient counseling is necessary to allow for proper medication use (e.g., self-injection with sumatriptan), to encourage early use of medications in the headache cycle, and to enhance patient compliance. Strict adherence to dosing guidelines should be stressed to minimize potential toxicity. Patterns of abortive medication use can be documented to establish the need for prophylactic therapy. Prophylactic therapies also should be monitored closely for adverse reactions, abortive therapy needs, adequate dosing, and compliance. Consultation with other health care practitioners should be encouraged when changes in headache patterns or medication use occur.

CONCLUSIONS

Although headache disorders such as migraine and cluster headaches appear to occur as a result of neuronal dysfunction, the precise etiology and nature of the dysfunction are unknown. Serotonergic neurotransmission and the trigeminovascular system appear to play important roles. A careful patient workup, including patient history, physical examination, and appropriate laboratory tests, should identify most headache patients with major disease. A variety of strategies can be helpful for managing migraine, tension-type and cluster headaches. Management of primary headache disorders is directed at suppressing acute attacks and preventing recurrences. Continuing research will better define pathophysiologic mechanisms and aid the search for less toxic and more efficacious pharmacologic agents.

ABBREVIATIONS

CGRP: calcitonin gene–related peptide
GABA: γ-aminobutyric acid
5-HT: serotonin, 5-hydroxytryptamine
IHS: International Headache Society
MAOIs: monoamine oxidase inhibitors
NSAIDs: nonsteroidal anti-inflammatory drugs
SSRI: selective serotonin reuptake inhibitor
TCA: tricyclic antidepressant

Review Questions and other resources can be found at *www.pharmacotherapyonline.com.*

REFERENCES

1. Silberstein SD, Lipton RB, Dalessio DJ. Overview, diagnosis, and classification of headache. In: Silberstein SD, Lipton RB, Dalessio DJ, eds. Wolff's Headache and Other Head Pain, 7th ed. New York, Oxford University Press, 2001:6–26.
2. Mueller L. Tension-type, the forgotten headache. Postgrad Med 2002;111:25–50.
3. Headache Classification Committee of the International Headache Society. The international classification of headache disorders, 2nd ed. Cephalalgia 2004;24(suppl 1):1–151.
4. Silberstein SD, Lipton RB, Goadsby PJ. Headache in Clinical Practice. London, Martin Dunitz, 2002:21–33, 69–128.
5. Lipton RB, Diamond S, Reed M, et al. Migraine diagnosis and treatment: Results from the American Migraine Study II. Headache 2001;41:638–645.
6. Lipton RB, Stewart WF, Diamond S, et al. Prevalence and burden of migraine in the United States: Data from the American Migraine Study II. Headache 2001;41:646–657.
7. Dahlof CGH. Current concepts of migraine and its treatment. Neurologia 1999;14:67–77.
8. Hu XH, Markson LE, Lipton RB, et al. Burden of migraine in the United States. Arch Intern Med 1999;159:813–818.
9. Lance JW, Goadsby PJ. Mechanism and Management of Headache, 6th ed. Oxford, UK, Butterworth Heinemann, 1998:9–16, 25–157, 176–205, 291–298.
10. Hargreaves RJ, Shepheard SL. Pathophysiology of migraine: New insights. Can J Neurol Sci 1999;26(suppl 3):S12–19.
11. Edvinsson L. On migraine pathophysiology. In: Edvinsson L, ed. Migraine and Headache Pathophysiology. London, Martin Dunitz, 1999:3–15.
12. Gardner K. The genetic basis of migraine: How much do we know? Can J Neurol Sci 1999;26(suppl 3):S37–43.
13. Hamel E. The biology of serotonin receptors: Focus on migraine pathophysiology and treatment. Can J Neurol Sci 1999;26(suppl 3):S2–6.
14. Silberstein SD. Migraine. Lancet 2004;363:381–391.
15. Kaniecki RG. Diagnostic issues in migraine. Curr Pain Headache Rep 2001;5:183–188.
16. Goadsby PJ, Lipton RB, Ferrari MD. Migraine: Current understanding and treatment. N Engl J Med 2002;346:257–270.
17. Dahlof CGH, Solomon GD. The burden of migraine to the individual sufferer: A review. Eur J Neurol 1998;5:525–533.
18. Solomon S. Migraine variants. Curr Pain Headache Rep 2001;5:165–169.
19. Silberstein SD. Practice parameter: Evidence-based guidelines for migraine headache (an evidence-based review). Neurology 2000;55:754–763.
20. Silberstein SD, Goadsby PJ, Lipton RB. Management of migraine: An algorithmic approach. Neurology 2000;55(suppl 2):S46–52.
21. Lipton RB, Stewart WF, Stone AM, et al. Stratified care vs step care strategies for migraine: The disability in strategies of care study. JAMA 2000;284:2599–2605.
22. Ferrari MD. Migraine. Lancet 1998;351:1043–1051.
23. Bartleson JD. Treatment of migraine headaches. Mayo Clin Proc 1999;74:702–708.
24. Moore KL, Noble SL. Drug treatment of migraine: Acute therapy and drug-rebound headache. Am Fam Phys 1997;56:2039–2048.
25. Silberstein SD, Goadsby PJ. Migraine: Preventive treatment. Cephalalgia 2002;22:491–512.
26. Becker WJ. Evidence-based migraine prophylactic drug therapy. Can J Neurol Sci 1999;26(suppl 3):S27–32.
27. Ramadan NM, Silberstein SD, Freitag FG, et al. Evidence-based guidelines for migraine headache in the primary care setting: Pharmacological

management for prevention of migraine. Accessed at *www.aan.com/professionals/practice/guidelines,*2000.

48. Snow V, Weiss K, Wall EM, Mottur-Pilson C. Pharmacologic management of acute attacks of migraine and prevention of migraine headache. Ann Intern Med 2002;137:840–849.

49. Silberstein S, Merriam G. Sex hormones and headache 1999. Neurology 1999;53(suppl 1):S3–13.

50. Becker WJ. Use of oral contraceptives in patients with migraine. Neurology 1999;53(suppl 1):S19–25.

51. Aube M. Migraine in pregnancy. Neurology 1999;53(suppl 1):S26–28.

52. Fettes I. Migraine in menopause. Neurology 1999;53(suppl 1):S29–33.

53. Tonore TB, King DS, Noble SL. Do over-the-counter medications for migraine hinder the physician? Curr Pain Headache Rep 2002;6:162–167.

54. Matchar DB, Young WB, Rosenberg JA, et al. Evidence-based guidelines for migraine headache in the primary care setting: Pharmacological management of acute attacks. The US Headache Consortium, 2000; accessed at *www.aan.com/professionals/practice/guidelines.*

55. del Rio MS, Silberstein SD. How to pick optimal acute treatment for migraine headache. Curr Pain Headache Rep 2001;5:170–178.

56. Lipton RB, Stewart WF, Ryan RE, et al. Efficacy and safety of acetaminophen, aspirin, and caffeine in alleviating migraine headache pain: Three double-blind, randomized, placebo-controlled trials. Arch Neurol 1998;55:210–217.

57. Richman PB, Reischel U, Ostrow A, et al. Droperidol for acute migraine headache. Am J Emerg Med 1999;17:398–400.

58. Krusz JC, Scott V, Belanger J. Intravenous propofol: Unique effectiveness in treating intractable migraine. Headache 2000;40:224–230.

59. Triner WR, Bartfield JM, Birdwell M, Robak N. Nitrous oxide for the treatment of acute migraine headache. Am J Emerg Med 1999;17:278–281.

60. Silberstein SD. The pharmacology of ergotamine and dihydroergotamine. Headache 1997;37(suppl 1):15–25.

61. Tfelt-Hansen P, Saxena PR, Dahlof C, et al. Ergotamine in the acute treatment of migraine: A review and European consensus. Brain 2000;123:9–18.

62. Aukerman G, Knutson D, Miser WF. Management of the acute migraine headache. Am Fam Phys 2002;66:2123–2130, 2140–2141.

63. Logemann CD, Rankin LM. Newer intranasal migraine medications. Am Fam Phys 2000;61:180–186.

64. Lipton R. Ergotamine tartrate and dihydroergotamine mesylate: Safety profiles. Headache 1997;37(suppl 1):S33–41.

65. Rosenthal E, Sala F, Chichmanian RM, et al. Ergotism related to the concurrent administration of ergotamine tartrate and indinavir. JAMA 1999;281:987.

66. Liaudet L, Buclin T, Jaccard C, Eckert P. Severe ergotism associated with interaction between ritonavir and ergotamine. Br Med J 1999;318:771.

67. Tfelt-Hansen P, DeVries P, Saxena PR. Triptans in migraine: A comparative review of pharmacology, pharmacokinetics, and efficacy. Drugs 2000;60:1259–1287.

68. Deleu D, Hanssens Y. Current and emerging second-generation triptans in acute migraine therapy: A comparative review. J Clin Pharmacol 2000;40:687–700.

69. Pringsheim T, Gawel M. Triptans: Are they all the same? Curr Pain Headache Rep 2002;6:140–146.

70. Ferrari MD, Roon KI, Lipton RB, Goadsby PJ. Oral triptans (serotonin 5-HT$_{1B/1D}$ agonists) in acute migraine treatment: A meta-analysis of 53 trials. Lancet 2001;358:1558–1575.

71. Adelman JU, Adelman, RD. Current options for the prevention and treatment of migraine. Clin Ther 2001;23:772–788.

52. Cutrer FM. Antiepileptic drugs: How they work in headache. Headache 2001;41(suppl):S3–10.

53. Freitag FG. Divalproex sodium extended-release for the prophylaxis of migraine headache. Expert Opin Pharmacother 2003;4:1573–1578.

54. Kinze S, Clauss M, Reuter U, et al. Valproic acid is effective in migraine prophylaxis at low serum levels: A prospective open-label study. Headache 2001;41:774–778.

55. Brandes JL, Saper JR, Diamond M, et al. Topiramate for migraine prevention: A randomized controlled trial. JAMA 2004;291:965–973.

56. Krymchantowski AV, Bigal ME, Moreira PF. New and emerging prophylactic agents for migraine. CNS Drugs 2002;16:611–634.

57. Mathew NT, Rapoport A, Saper J, et al. Efficacy of gabapentin in migraine prophylaxis. Headache 2001;41:119–128.

58. Bigal ME, Krymchantowski AV, Rapoport AM. New developments in migraine prophylaxis. Expert Opin Pharmacother 2003;4:433–443.

59. Silberstein SD. Methysergide. Cephalalgia 1998;18:421–435.

60. Boyle C. Management of menstrual migraine. Neurology 1999;53 (suppl 1):S14–18.

61. Dodick DW. Botulinum neurotoxin for the treatment of migraine and other primary headache disorders: From bench to bedside. Headache 2003;43(suppl 1):S25–33.

62. Schrader H, Stovner LJ, Helde G, et al. Prophylactic treatment of migraine with angiotensin converting enzyme inhibitor (lisinopril): Randomized, placebo-controlled, crossover study. Br Med J 2001;322:1–5.

63. Tronvik E, Stovner LJ, Helde G, et al. Prophylactic treatment of migraine with an angiotensin II receptor blocker: A randomized, controlled trial. JAMA 2003;289:65–69.

64. Rapoport AM, Ademlan JU. Cost of migraine management: A pharmacoeconomic overview. Am J Managed Care 998;4:531–545.

65. Johnson K. Migraine therapy: Balancing efficacy and safety with quality of life and cost. Formulary 2002;37:634–644.

66. Cady RC, Ryan R, Jhingram P, et al. Sumatriptan injection reduces productivity loss during a migraine attack: Results of a double-blind, placebo-controlled trial. Arch Intern Med 1998;158:1013–1018.

67. Lofland JH, Johnson NE, Batenhorst AS, Nash DB. Changes in resource use and outcomes for patients with migraine treated with sumatriptan: A managed-care perspective. Arch Intern Med 1999;159:857–863.

68. Jensen R. Pathophysiological mechanisms of tension-type headache: A review of epidemiological and experimental studies. Cephalalgia 1999;19:602–621.

69. Kaniecki RG. Migraine and tension-type headache: An assessment of challenges in diagnosis. Neurology 2002;58(suppl 6):S15–20.

70. Jensen R, Olesen J. Tension-type headache: An update on mechanisms and treatment. Curr Opin Neurol 2000;13:285–289.

71. Solomon S, Newman LC. Episodic tension-type headaches. In: Silberstein SD, Lipton RB, Dalessio DJ, eds. Wolff's Headache and Other Head Pain, 7th ed. New York, Oxford University Press, 2001:238–246.

72. Mendizabal JE, Umana E, Zweifler RM. Cluster headache: Horton's cephalalgia revisited. South Med J 1998;91:606–617.

73. Gobel H, Lindner V, Heinz A, et al. Acute therapy for cluster headache with sumatriptan: Findings of a one-year long-term study. Neurology 1998;51:430–435.

74. Bahra A, Gawel MJ, Hardebo JE, et al. Oral zolmitriptan is effective in the acute treatment of cluster headache. Neurology 2000;54:291–296.

75. Hanit-Hering R, Gadoth N. Baclofen in cluster headache. Headache 2000;40:48–51.

76. Wheeler SD, Carrazana EJ. Topiramate-treated cluster headache. Neurology 1999;53:234–236.

60

EVALUATION OF PSYCHIATRIC ILLNESS

Patricia A. Marken, Mark E. Schneiderhan, and Stuart Munro

Learning Objectives and other resources can be found at *www.pharmacotherapyonline.com.*

KEY CONCEPTS

❶ Patients with psychiatric conditions are treated in all areas of health care. All clinicians need to develop basic skills in psychiatric assessment in order to best care for their patients.

❷ *Diagnostic and Statistical Manual of Mental Disorders*, 4th edition, Text Revision (DSM-IV-TR) is the most widely accepted diagnostic reference. It, along with the American Psychiatric Association (APA) *Practice Guidelines for the Psychiatric Evaluation of Adults*, provides the clinician a standardized approach for the initial assessment and follow-up of patients with mental illness.

❸ At times, it can be challenging to gather needed information from patients suffering from mental illness, as their condition prevents them from fully cooperating with the assessment. A range of strategies can be used to gather the needed

information while increasing the safety and comfort of both patient and clinician.

❹ A thorough medication history that assesses what medications were taken to treat the condition, in what combination, and whether there was an adequate trial (dose and duration) is a cornerstone of effective patient management.

❺ A baseline mental status examination (MSE), along with a specific target symptom list, is a critical tool in monitoring response to treatment.

❻ There is no consensus about what specific physical and laboratory tests are needed in the evaluation of patients with psychiatric conditions. Testing is best individualized based on the patient's age, medical history, current physical health, and current medication use.

❶ Patients with mental illnesses are treated by all disciplines and in all settings of health care and may in fact receive the bulk of their care from nonpsychiatrists. Hence the need for good psychiatric assessment skills is not limited to mental health specialists. Along with traditional assessments used across all medical specialties (laboratory tests, medical history, and physical examination), psychiatrists use additional strategies to manage their patients that are less objective and perhaps less familiar to the nonpsychiatrist. This chapter provides a basic overview of appropriate assessment techniques used by clinicians when working with psychiatric patients to develop an individualized treatment plan. Readers needing greater depth than the materials provided in this chapter are referred to other reference materials.[1-5]

OVERVIEW OF *DIAGNOSTIC AND STATISTICAL MANUAL OF MENTAL DISORDERS*

❷ *Diagnostic and Statistical Manual of Mental Disorders*, 4th edition, Text Revision (DSM-IV-TR) is the most widely accepted and most important diagnostic reference used in the care of the mentally ill. It provides a common language for mental health practitioners to describe and diagnose psychiatric disorders.[6] Common language is essential because there is considerable overlap of symptoms across

many diagnoses. The DSM-I was introduced in 1952 and was the first manual on mental disorders to contain a description of diagnostic categories. The most recent edition, DSM-IV-TR, was released in 2000. The DSM-IV-TR uses essentially the same diagnostic criteria sets as DSM-IV.[6] Its purpose is to correct factual errors in DSM-IV and update the text sections (e.g., associated features, prevalence, and differential diagnosis) with more contemporary data. A more significant rewriting of diagnostic criteria and introduction of new diagnoses will appear in DSM-V, which probably will not be available until 2006.[6] The DSM-IV-TR contains many components that provide a comprehensive understanding of a specific mental illness and assist clinicians in making an accurate diagnosis. For example, the multiaxial patient evaluation ensures that most factors that could contribute to, or complicate, the condition are considered during a patient assessment and treatment planning. Axis I lists the principal psychiatric disorder, developmental disorders, or provisional diagnoses present in the patient. Mental retardation and personality disorders are listed on Axis II. Axis III lists existing physical disorders or conditions. Axis IV lists the severity of psychosocial stressors that may have contributed to a new or recurrent mental disorder or exacerbation of an existing condition. Stressors are rated on a scale of 1 (none) to 6 (catastrophic) and can be acute (lasting less than 6 months) or enduring (lasting longer than 6 months). Examples of stressors include difficulties with interpersonal relationships, parenting, occupation, living circumstances, finances, the legal system, and health. Axis V describes the global assessment of functioning (GAF), rated on a scale from 1 (persistent danger to self or others) to 90 (minimal or absent symptoms). A GAF rating is based on the current level of functioning compared with the highest level of functioning seen in the previous months to a year prior to the current evaluation. By documenting the baseline level of functioning, the GAF helps evaluate progress toward a patient's therapeutic goals.

DSM-IV-TR provides general information on all mental disorders recognized by the American Psychiatric Association (APA) and includes age of onset, clinical course, complications, predisposing factors, prevalence, and differential diagnoses. The specific diagnostic criteria for each mental illness and the number of symptoms required to establish a diagnosis are also listed. The DSM-IV-TR also includes decision trees for differential diagnosis and a glossary of technical terms. *The Clinical Interview Using DSM-IV* is a 2-volume companion publication that provides extensive information on interviewing techniques assisting the clinician in establishing a specific diagnosis using DSM-IV criteria.[7]

Additional information besides the DSM-IV-TR diagnosis is required before a comprehensive treatment plan can be developed. The *American Psychiatric Association Practice Guidelines for Psychiatric Evaluation of Adults* offers a more comprehensive approach to patient assessment. It includes a full discussion of the domains needed for a thorough clinical evaluation, including chief complaint; history of present illness; past psychiatric history; general medical history; social, family, and occupational history; physical and mental status examinations; and diagnostic tests. It further describes issues of privacy, evaluations in the elderly, and techniques for working with multidisciplinary teams.[5]

In summary, by using the DSM-IV-TR and the American Psychiatric Association Practice Guidelines, clinicians can evaluate patients in a systematic manner, thereby creating better treatment plans and a more consistent evaluation of response.

THE CLINICAL INTERVIEW

The interview should be conducted in a quiet, nonstimulating, and comfortable area where the patient and the interviewer feel at ease. The interviewer should introduce himself or herself and explain the procedure in order to facilitate establishment of a trusting relationship. Generally, open-ended questions should come first, followed by questions focused on more specific or personal data. Open-ended questions allow the patient to provide descriptions and other information in his or her own words. Even though more specific questions may then be necessary to fill in the gaps, beginning in this manner minimizes the risk of "leading" the patient. Patients may respond to specific questions and "yes" or "no" questions with answers they think the interviewer wants to hear. The interviewer must be nonjudgmental about the information offered by the patient in order to develop trust and rapport with the patient and to ensure completeness and accuracy of the information. Whether a clinician takes notes during the interview is an individual decision, with the primary considerations being to make an accurate record of the content of the examination and assuring that the patient is comfortable with the note taking. Table 60–1 provides examples of questions that can be used to gather information during the completion of the clinical interview.

THE CHALLENGING PATIENT

 Patient assessment may be challenging when symptoms of the condition prevent effective engagement between the patient

---

TABLE 60–1. Examples of Interview Questions for Assessing Mental Illnesses

Mania
1. Do your thoughts go faster than you can say them?
2. Have you noticed a change in the amount of sleep that you require?
3. Have you spent a lot of money lately and what did you spend it on?
4. Do you have a lot of extra energy?
   (To assess hallucinations and delusions, see schizophrenia section below.)

Depression
1. Do you cry without any reason?
2. Do you still enjoy the same hobbies/activities that you once did?
3. Has your weight changed recently?
4. Have you had changes in your energy level recently?
5. Do you have any guilty feelings?
6. Do you find it difficult to remember phone numbers, names of friends, appointments, etc?
   (To assess sleep and suicidal potential, see sleep and suicide sections below.)

Schizophrenia
Delusions
1. Do you feel that people plot against you?
2. Do you ever feel that you are watched or spied on?
3. Do you have any special abilities?
4. Does anyone ever try to mess with you or bother you?
5. Do others read your thoughts?

Hallucinations
1. Does the TV/radio ever tell you things?
2. Do you hear voices that other people don't hear?
3. What do they say? How many voices?
4. How often do they bother you?

5. Do the voices ever tell you to hurt yourself or someone else?
6. Have you ever heard your name called when there is no one there?
7. Have you ever seen anything strange that you can't explain?
8. Do you ever see things that bother you and no one else?
9. Do you want to act on what the voices say?

Thought broadcasting/insertion
1. If I stood by you could I hear your thoughts?
2. Does your head ever act like a radio?
3. Do you feel that others can put thoughts in your head?

Insight
1. What reasons did your family give you for coming here?
2. What brought you here?
3. Do you consider yourself in need of help?
4. What does your medication do for you?

Sleep
1. Tell me about your sleep.
2. How many hours do you sleep each night at present?
3. How many hours do you usually sleep at night?
4. Do you sleep all through the night?
5. Is there a reason for your waking up?
6. Do you have trouble falling asleep?
7. How do you feel when you wake up?

Suicide potential
1. Do you feel your life is worth living?
2. Do you ever think of hurting yourself?
3. Do you see things improving in the future?
4. Do you think you will try to hurt yourself now?
5. How would you do it?
6. Do you have the means to hurt yourself?

and the clinician. Patients ramble if their speech patterns are circumstantial or tangential in nature, or they ruminate as part of a depression. Patients in the manic phases of bipolar disorder may not pause as they speak, making it difficult for the interviewer to interject. In all cases, the interviewer can regain control of the assessment by politely redirecting the patient back toward the question. Psychotic patients may be paranoid as part of their illness and appear guarded or frightened by the questions. The best approach is to remain calm and respectful with the patient and try using shorter or more close-ended questions to seek the desired information. Patients with mental illnesses can become agitated and occasionally violent. Often the violence is preceded by increasing psychomotor agitation as evidenced by pacing, speaking in a loud voice, or gripping the arms of the chair very firmly. If the interviewer is concerned about safety, he or she should avoid any behavior that could be misconstrued as threatening, such as touching the or staring unnecessarily and should complete the interview in the presence of another health care provider. Both the patient and the interviewer should have equal access to leave the room if either becomes too uncomfortable during the interview. If a patient describes suicidal thoughts, he or she should be further assessed using the questions outlined in Table 60–1, and depending upon the results of further assessment be directed to the appropriate type of care, including hospitalization for patients at immediate risk of harming themselves. A suicidal patient should never be left alone. Asking a patient about suicidal thoughts will not increase the risk, as patients are able to reach these conclusions independently of the interviewer's questioning. Before any conclusions are made about the content of the interview, consideration of the impact of culture on the patient's presentation should be made. Something that sounds delusional in Western culture may be the norm in other cultures. If a clinician is unclear whether culture of origin accounts for some of the patient's symptoms, they should more fully explore these options before any conclusions are drawn.

PSYCHIATRIC HISTORY

Both the patient's and their family's history of mental illness provide important information when formulating a diagnosis and treatment plan. Information should be descriptive and include the current and previous psychiatric diagnoses, presentation of each illness, time frame between episodes, level of functioning between episodes, length of each episode, total duration of illness, and treatment given during each episode. Baseline functioning or the highest level of functioning achieved in the past few years is important information because it provides a target or goal for treatment. Information on the history of the current episode and reasons for coming to the clinician also should be gathered. A family history should include a medication history of the immediate relatives because a family member's response to a given medication may predict an individual patient's response to that same medication.

SOCIAL HISTORY

A social history should include educational and occupational background, religion, marital status, substance use patterns including smoking, and current living situation. By understanding a patient's living environment and social situation, strategies to prevent noncompliance, reduce stress, and increase social support can be developed.

MEDICATION HISTORY

4 A thorough medication history is one of the most important contributions a clinician can make to treatment planning. The history should include medications for both psychiatric and medical conditions. It should list all medications taken by the patient, and report on how each was tolerated and the nature of the response to that drug or combination of drugs. Because most psychiatric medications have a delay in the onset of effect, it is important to determine whether an adequate trial (adequate dose and duration) was provided before the patient was considered nonresponsive to that drug. If a patient has a history of noncompliance, specific causes such as cost, complicated dosing schedules, lack of insight, and adverse effects should be investigated.

MENTAL STATUS EXAMINATION

5 The mental status examination (MSE) is a key patient assessment in psychiatry and is analogous to the physical examination in medicine. The MSE is completed through a direct patient interview, and it results in a description of current patient behavior, thoughts, perceptions, and functioning. The results of an MSE provide an objective evaluation used in diagnosis, assessment of the course of the illness, and response to treatment. The MSE is combined with other components of the patient work-up (history of present illness, physical examination, appropriate labs, and medical and psychiatric history) in order to give a full picture of the presenting problem and factors contributing to the illness. An MSE has several components.[5,7]

APPEARANCE AND ATTITUDE TOWARD EXAMINER

The appearance of the patient throughout the interview should be noted, including age, dress, grooming and hygiene, use of cosmetics, and facial expressions. A description of appearance also should include unusual physical characteristics and the general state of physical health. The interviewer should note whether the patient is cooperative, mute, hostile, paranoid, guarded, or withdrawn.

ACTIVITY

Changes in motor activity include overactivity, underactivity, and catatonia. Overactivity is an increase in purposeful movements or agitation and can include pacing; hand wringing; picking at clothing, skin, or hair; inability to sit still during the interview; and excessive hand gestures. Underactive patients move less than expected. Patients with rigid posture, an absence of movement, and failure to communicate may be catatonic, paranoid, or experiencing medication-induced adverse effects.

SPEECH AND LANGUAGE

The quantity, flow, and speed of speech and the amount of eye contact should be noted. Speech should be assessed as to whether it proceeds logically in a goal-directed manner or whether the content is vague and poorly organized. Abnormal speech characteristics include *blocking*, whereby the person suddenly stops speaking without any obvious reason. *Thought blocking* usually occurs when a hallucination or delusion intrudes into the person's thinking or when upsetting issues are discussed. *Circumstantial speech* lacks a clear direction because of excess unnecessary information, but the circumstantial patient eventually will make his or her point. In *tangential speech,* however, the ultimate point is never made. *Perseveration* is repetition of an original answer to subsequent questions. *Flight of ideas* is overproductive, rapid speech during which the patient jumps rapidly from one idea to the next. *Mutism* is identified when the patient does not respond even though he or she is aware of the discussion.

MOOD AND AFFECT

Affect describes the patient's current emotional tone, as expressed through facial expression and tone of voice, all of which may be objectively observed by the clinician. *Mood* describes more sustained feelings which are subjectively reported by the patient. To properly evaluate a patient's mood and affect, his or her appearance and the content of speech must be considered. Change in facial expression and the presence of tears, flushing, sweating, or tremors should be noted. Affect can be described further by its range, appropriateness, intensity, and stability. For example, in schizophrenia or depression, the affect may be flat, whereby no change in expression occurs throughout the interview. In contrast, during a manic episode, the affect is very intense and often labile. The range of emotional expression is reduced, but not absent, with blunted affect. An example of inappropriate affect is when a patient laughs when he or she is depressed or cries when stating that he or she is happy. A rapidly shifting affect from one extreme to the other is described as labile.

THOUGHT AND PERCEPTUAL DISTURBANCES

A variety of thought disturbances can occur in mental illness. These disturbances generally indicate the presence of psychosis, or impaired reality resting. *Delusions* are fixed, false beliefs that are not based in reality or consistent with the patient's religion or culture. Delusions can be paranoid, somatic, or grandiose in nature. Delusions are often unshakable, and one should not attempt to talk a patient out of a delusion. *Thought broadcasting* is the belief that one's thoughts are audible to others. *Hallucinations* are false sensory impressions or perceptions that occur in the absence of an external stimulus. Hallucinations may be auditory, visual, olfactory, or gustatory, and may be continuous or intermittent. In contrast, *illusions* are visual misperceptions involving a misinterpretation of a real sensory stimulus. For example, a person who initially misperceives a curtain blown by the wind to be an intruder has experienced an illusion. This phenomenon is not indicative of psychiatric illness, and can be seen in normal persons. Other thought disturbances are not considered to be psychotic. For example, the couplet of obsessions and compulsions may be indicative of the presence of obsessive-compulsive disorder, which is not considered to be a psychotic disorder. *Obsessions* are unwanted thoughts or ideas that intrude into a person's thinking. *Compulsions* are actions performed in response to the obsessions or to control anxiety associated with the obsession.

NEUROPSYCHIATRIC EVALUATION

A neuropsychiatric evaluation assesses sensorium, attention, concentration, memory, and higher cognitive functions such as orientation and abstraction. Prior to initiation of the neuropsychiatric evaluation, it should be documented whether the patient has received medications with sedative properties, because the outcome of the examination could be altered if central nervous system depressants have recently been taken.

Sensorium, or level of consciousness, refers to the alertness of the patient, and if he or she is not fully alert, the amount of stimulation needed to awaken the patient. Attention and concentration can be assessed using serial 7s or 3s, whereby the patient subtracts backward from 100 in increments of 7 or 3, respectively. Another concentration test is to have a patient spell a five-letter word backward. Language skills are assessed initially by having a patient read something aloud and silently. General intelligence can be assessed loosely by asking factual information about current news items, recent presidents, or popular television shows or sporting events. Memory is the ability to recall past experiences and is classified as sensory stores, which lasts seconds, short-term memory (the ability to recall information immediately after acquisition), working memory (i.e., immediate application of visual or auditory instructions), and long-term or remote memory (historical facts). Orientation to time, place, person, and situation assesses sensory stores and short-term memory. Asking a patient to recall three objects 5 minutes after they are learned is the definitive test for short-term memory. Patients with depression or anxiety may have deficits in short-term memory. Asking the patient to do a certain task such as pick up a pen with his or her right hand and then fold a piece of paper and pass it to the examiner can assess the patient's working memory. Patients with cognitive deficits such as those seen in dementias and schizophrenia may exhibit deficits in working memory. Remote memory is assessed by asking the patient to recall old facts about their life, such as where they were born or where they went to school. Remote memory usually stays intact the longest in patients with intellectual decline, while the ability to create new memories is generally the first sign of a memory deficit. Abstraction is the ability to interpret information such as a proverb ("People in glass houses shouldn't throw stones") or identify similarities or differences between words (apple and orange). Abstraction is influenced by education and linguistic fluency; thus inability to abstract is not always a sign of a psychiatric disorder.

INSIGHT AND JUDGMENT

Insight refers to patient awareness that they have a mental illness and the consequences of that illness on their life. Patients typically have a lack of insight when they are psychotic. Patients with poor insight are often noncompliant with prescribed medications. *Judgment* is the ability to make decisions appropriate to the situation and may be impaired in a variety of mental illnesses. Often this can be assessed by asking the patient how they would handle either their current or a hypothetical situation. Both insight and judgment can be quite fluid. For example, an intoxicated patient may demonstrate poor insight and judgment which improves over several hours as blood alcohol levels diminish.

PHYSICAL AND LABORATORY ASSESSMENT IN PSYCHIATRY

Patients who present with psychiatric symptoms need a careful medical assessment for many reasons.[1-3]

Both medical illnesses and medications can cause psychiatric symptoms. The rapidity of onset of psychiatric symptoms is an important clue that a medical cause may be present. Most chronic mental illnesses have a prodromal period, whereas medically based psychiatric symptoms often have a more rapid onset of symptoms. Patients over age 40 at first presentation are more likely to have a medical cause for their psychiatric symptoms because major psychiatric illnesses such as schizophrenia and bipolar disorder usually first present in adolescence or early adulthood. A family history of physical illnesses with a psychiatric component, such as Huntington's chorea or systemic lupus erythematosus, may provide an additional clue.

Patients with fluctuating levels of consciousness, disorientation, memory impairment, or visual, tactile, or olfactory hallucinations, substance abuse, and serious medical conditions are more likely to have a medical basis for their illness.

Patients with psychiatric illnesses, especially depression and anxiety disorders, will often present with only physical complaints, leading to inappropriate care for medical problems that are not present or as serious as they may appear, while the root cause is ignored. Psychotropic medications can cause or exacerbate medical conditions, such as diabetes mellitus or cardiac arrhythmias, necessitating an understanding of the patient's other risk factors for these conditions before medication is selected. Finally, patients with chronic psychiatric illnesses often receive inadequate health care and have poorly controlled medical conditions for many reasons, including their appearance or behavior prohibiting a thorough evaluation, inaccurate information from the patient secondary to impaired memory or perception, and incomplete data to make an appropriate diagnosis and treatment recommendation. In a recent retrospective review, it was found that patients with diabetes or hypertension and diagnoses of schizophrenia, bipolar disorder, or posttraumatic stress disorder were statistically less likely to utilize medical services than similar patients without these psychiatric conditions.[8]

There is no consensus about specific laboratory tests needed in the evaluation of a patient with mental illness.[2,5] General laboratory screening is useful for ruling out medical causes of psychiatric illnesses, but extensive testing is usually unnecessary and not cost-effective. Laboratory tests should be individualized to the age, medical history, cooperativeness, and physical health of the patient. For example, a fasting glucose determination is preferred over a random measure when a patient takes medications known to cause significant weight gain and/or induce diabetes mellitus.[9] If available, recent laboratory tests can be used to evaluate medical status, provided that no change in physical status has occurred since they were taken.

A complete physical examination, along with a detailed medical and medication history, vital signs, weight and body mass index, and routine blood chemistry are commonly part of the work-up of persons with mental illness. Clinicians will want diagnostic tests to help evaluate the relative safety of specific medications (e.g., renal status when using lithium or an electrocardiogram when using a tricyclic antidepressant such as amitriptyline or an antipsychotic such as ziprasidone or clozapine) or when baseline information is needed to identify future adverse effects from medications (e.g., lithium-induced hypothyroidism, clozapine-induced leukopenia, antipsychotic-induced diabetes mellitus). Serum concentration monitoring of selected medications is also helpful in increasing probability of response and minimizing the likelihood of adverse effects. Urine drug screens and blood alcohol tests play an important role in identifying the contribution of substances of abuse to the presenting symptoms.

In patients with underlying medical problems, more extensive testing is indicated to rule out possible contributing etiologies or confounding factors which may create similar presenting symptoms. Additional testing can include an electroencephalogram to evaluate for the presence of seizure activity or other neurologic conditions, computed tomography or magnetic resonance imaging to detect structural abnormalities, sedimentation rate and antinuclear antibodies for autoimmune disorders, a test for the human immunodeficiency virus, thyroid function tests, or B_{12} and folate concentrations for anemias.[2]

The identification of biologic markers as diagnostic tools and predictors or indicators of drug response is of great interest but currently of little clinical utility. The most promising was the dexamethasone suppression test, proposed to be a marker for endogenous melancholic depression. However, its lack of sensitivity and specificity has limited its utility as a routine screening tool during a work-up for depression.[2]

In summary, a range of assessments aids the clinician in making an accurate diagnosis and identifying underlying or potential drug-related problems. The MSE is the cornerstone of the psychiatric work-up, although selective medical tests, a good medical, psychiatric and medication history, and a thorough physical exam are also important.

PSYCHIATRIC RATING SCALES

Psychiatric rating scales can be useful tools to provide an objective way of measuring subjective data (i.e., feelings, thoughts, and perceptions), assess certain domains of psychiatric illnesses, and even to diagnose disorders. Unfortunately it may be puzzling to the rater since there are so many types of scales to choose from. The rater needs special training and experience to use and select the most appropriate scale that will assess the specific domain under question. These specific domains may include: cognition, behavior (i.e., aggression), severity of illness including response to treatment and medication side effects, level of functioning, and quality of life. These tools may be used in a variety of settings, including research and patient care and may serve an administrative purpose such as quality control.[4]

Some drawbacks include a substantial time commitment for staff to administer the tests and the inability of some patients to tolerate these interviews, especially patients who are severely paranoid or agitated. In addition, a single psychiatric rating scale score may only provide a limited picture or snapshot of a complex clinical situation. Therefore repeated ratings are usually necessary to objectively describe longitudinal changes over a defined treatment period.

Some rating scales are self-administered and do not require a staff member to interview a patient; thus they require minimal resources to administer. However, there are many cases in which the patient is unable to complete a questionnaire for a variety of reasons, including literacy and severity of symptoms.

In contrast to symptom-based rating scales (i.e., brief psychiatric rating scale [BPRS] or Hamilton Rating Scale for Depression [HAMD]), global rating scales such as the Clinical Global Impression (CGI) scale assess the overall severity of illness based on a rater's clinical experience.[10] The rating scale will not determine the reason for the symptoms. For example, a patient may have a high global severity score; however, the scale will not specifically elucidate whether the severity of illness is due to paranoia or a primary anxiety disorder. Second, when evaluating the results of rating scales either clinically or in the literature, it is important to know the range of clinically significant scores; for example, a patient may have a statistically significant (e.g., p value <0.05) drop in a rating scale score from one week to the next, but remain severely ill.

Psychiatric medication treatment can potentially expose a patient to a myriad of adverse effects. To ensure safe medication use and to decrease clinician liability, rating scales are available to measure adverse side effects. Global and specific assessments of adverse effects are a federal requirement in clinical drug trials. In clinical practice medical professionals should also report significant adverse medication reactions to the U.S. Food and Drug Administration (FDA) using MEDWatch.[11] Often, important adverse effects are realized only after a medication product has been prescribed to a large population in the postmarketing period. Specific adverse side effect measures may be used for specific categories of medications. For example, patients treated with antipsychotic agents may be susceptible to extrapyramidal side effects (EPSs). Tardive dyskinesia is a potentially irreversible

TABLE 60–2. Adverse Effects Measures

Rating Scale	Type	Scoring	Comments
Systematic Assessment for Treatment Emergent Events—General Inquiry (SAFTEE-GI)	Structured interview and global assessment	Summary scores of number of events, average severity, and impairment	5–10 minutes to complete. Baseline and weekly evaluations. Easy to administer. The specific reported information may be more useful than an overall summary score
MED Watch	Global assessment	No scoring involved	Minutes to complete. The one-page form requires a narrative description of the problem or adverse reaction. Online submission: http://www.fda.gov/medwatch/
Abnormal Involuntary Movement Scale (AIMS)	Tardive dyskinesia assessment	12-item, 5-point severity scale. Items 1–4 orofacial movement; 5–7 extremity and truncal movement; 8–10 global severity; 11 and 12 problems with teeth or dentures (yes or no)	5–10 minutes to complete. Commonly used in most clinical settings for dyskinesia assessment. Requires training and clinical experience to make diagnosis. Diagnostic criteria: at least 3 months of antipsychotic treatment. Mild severity score (2) in two discrete areas or moderate severity (3) in one area (i.e., orofacial)
Dyskinesia Identification System: Condensed User Scale (DISCUS)	Tardive dyskinesia assessment	15-item, 5-point severity scale. Items 1, 2 face; 3 eyes; 4, 5 oral; 6–9 lingual; 10, 11 head/neck/trunk; 12, 13 upper limb; 14, 15 lower limb	10–15 minutes to complete. More descriptive criteria for scoring severity than the AIMS. Scoring based on three dimensions: frequency, detectability, and intensity. A flow chart is provided in the user's manual to assign an item score
Rating Scale for Extrapyramidal Side Effects (Simpson-Angus EPS Scale)	Drug-induced Parkinson's and dystonia assessments	10-item, 5-point anchored severity scale. Mean score is obtained by adding all scores and dividing by 10. A mean score of 0.3 is the upper limit for no EPS	10 minutes to complete. Item domains include gait, arm dropping, shoulder shaking, elbow rigidity, wrist rigidity, leg pendulousness, head dropping, glabella tap, tremor, and salivation. Requires training and practice to administer
Barnes Akathisia Rating Scale (BARS)	Drug-induced akathisia	4 items including three 4-point anchored severity scored items and a 5-point global rating score item. Total score of 12 possible	10 minutes to complete. Items 1–3 (objective akathisia, subjective awareness of restlessness, and subjective distress related to restlessness). Diagnostic criteria: requires both objective and subjective ratings of at least 1 in either two subjective items. Pseudoakathisia is suggested with a positive objective rating but no subjective score is noted

EPS, extrapyramidal symptoms.
Adapted from Schooler and Chengappa[11] and Sprague and Kalachnik.[12]

movement disorder (see Chap. 66 on schizophrenia) that requires close monitoring approximately every 3 to 6 months if present during treatment with antipsychotic agents.[12] Table 60–2 provides a summary of the most common rating scales used to assess and quantify the presence and severity of adverse effects.

Sensitivity, specificity, reliability, and validity are important considerations when selecting a rating scale. The sensitivity of a test refers to its ability to detect a symptom or illness, given that the symptom or illness is present. Specificity refers to a test's ability to determine that a symptom or illness is absent given that the person does not have the illness.

Reliability is the extent to which the score on the scale reflects the hypothetical "true" score and how much interference occurs from outside influences.[13] Reliability is reported by the correlation coefficient, which represents a chance correlation (zero) or perfect correlation (one). Rating scales with reliability correlation coefficients of less than 0.7 are usually considered unreliable for clinical studies. Interrater reliability—agreement in rating scores among clinicians—is important to achieve when multiple clinicians rate the same patient or population. Interrater reliability is established by having all raters independently rate individual patients at the same time to determine the correlation of their scores. Other types of reliability include

TABLE 60–3. Schizophrenia Rating Scales

Rating Scale	Type	Scoring	Comments
Brief Psychiatric Rating Scale (BPRS)	Clinician-rated	18 items, 7-point severity scale: score ≥38 indicates moderate severity	The anchored BPRS provides descriptions of each severity rating to increase the interrater reliability. The BPRS has four clusters of symptoms: thinking disturbance, anxious depression, withdrawal-retardation, and hostility-suspiciousness
Scale for Assessment of Negative Symptoms (SANS)	Clinician-rated	30 items, 6-point severity scale: 0 = normal; 5 = severe	Measures degree of: affect, alogia, avolition, anhedonia, and attention
Schedule for Affective Disorders and Schizophrenia—Change (SADS-C)	Clinician-rated	29-item, 6-point scale and global assessment scale. Subsets of items can be combined to score specific affective symptoms	Structured interview to measure change in symptoms and assess anxiety, depression, manic features, and delusions or disorganization
Positive and Negative Syndrome Scale (PANSS)	Clinician-rated	30-item scale, 7-point severity scale	Based on the 18-item brief psychiatric rating scale
Nurses' Observation Scale for Inpatient Evaluation (NOSIE)	Observational	30-item, 5-point severity scale 0 = never; 1 = sometimes; 2 = often; 3 = usually; 4 = always	Patient behavior is rated daily
Clinical Global Impression (CGI) Scale	Observational	Severity of illness 7-point rating scale. Global improvement 7-point rating scale. Efficacy index: 1–4 marked improvement; 5–8 moderate; 9–12 minimal; 13–16 unchanged/worse	Observational rating scale to compare severity of illness compared to other similar patients and measures improvement from baseline. The efficacy index measures therapeutic effect and side effects to determine the score

test-retest reliability (assesses the stability of the scale in producing the same results with repeated use) and internal consistency (the degree to which items in the scale measure different aspects of the same condition without overlap).

Validity, in contrast, is the ability of a scale to measure what it was designed to measure. Content validity measures the extent to which the scale assesses appropriate aspects of the illness. Concurrent validity is a measure of the correlation of the rating scale with an external measure such as diagnosis or clinical change. Construct validity is the extent to which the test appears to measure symptom traits in contrast to measuring a more limited, specific symptom.

Psychiatric rating scales should not be confused with psychological tests such as neuropsychological and intellectual assessments, and are best used as only one part of a comprehensive diagnostic plan. Tables 60–3, 60–4, and 60–5 describe commonly used patient-rated and clinician-rated scales for a variety of disease states.[14-19] In clinical research, a combination of clinician- and self-rated rating scales and diagnostic tests provides the most accurate measurement of drug efficacy and treatment outcome.

TABLE 60–4. Depression Rating Scales

Rating Scale	Type	Scoring	Comments
Hamilton Psychiatric Rating Scale for Depression (HAMD)	Clinician-rated	17-item scale; <6 = normal mood; 17–25 = mild depression; >25 = severe depression	Used to screen patients for drug studies and to determine severity of symptoms, treatment outcome, and is the standard to compare other depression rating scales
Montgomery Asberg Depression Rating Scale (MADRS)	Clinician-rated	10-item, 7-point scale. For each item: 0 = no symptoms; 6 = severe symptoms	Differentiates between all the intermediate grades of depression. Decreases bias in patients with other medical illness and increased somatization
Beck Depression Inventory (BDI)	Patient-rated	21-item scale; 0–9 = normal; 10–15 = mild depression; 16–19 = mild-moderate; 20–29 = moderate-severe; 30–63 = severe depression	The standard for self-rating scales and an objective measure of change in symptoms as a result of treatment
Zung Self-Rating Depression Scale (SDS)	Patient-rated	20-item scale, 4-point severity; <50 normal; 50–59 minimal-mild; 60–69 moderate-marked; ≥70 severe depression	Severity rated by frequency of occurrence of symptoms. May not be as sensitive in measuring changes in severity of symptoms
Raskin's Mood Scales and Modified Mood Scales for Depression (RMS)	Patient-rated	53-item scale	Measures the presence or absence of symptoms. Sensitive in measuring changes resulting from treatment

TABLE 60–5. Anxiety Rating Scales

Rating Scale	Type	Scoring	Comments
Hamilton Anxiety Scale (HAM-A or HAM-AS or HAMRS)	Clinician-rated	14 items, 5-point scales; scores of ≥18–20 for moderate anxiety	Consists of subscales to measure somatic and psychic anxiety
Self-Rating Anxiety Scale (SAS) (Zung)	Patient-rated	20-item scale; 4-point intensity ratings	Correlates to the clinician-rated Anxiety Status Inventory (ASI); however, there is little information on the validity of either test
State Trait Anxiety Inventory (STAI)	Patient-rated	20-item state anxiety (A-state) and 20 items trait anxiety (A- trait); 4-point intensity ratings; total scores range from 20–80	A-Trait scale reflects the patient's general or baseline anxiety. A-State scale reflects the patient's most current anxiety and measures changes in anxiety. The A-State score is sensitive to stress-induced testing
Sheehan Panic and Anticipatory Anxiety Scale (SPAAS)	Patient- and clinician-rated	Three-part scale	Measures panic attacks, anticipatory anxiety, and limited symptom attacks
Yale-Brown Obsessive Compulsive Scale (YBOCS)	Clinician-rated	Semistructured interview	Consists of several clusters of obsessions and compulsions. Used to assess change in treatment studies

SYSTEMATIC MEASUREMENT OF COGNITIVE FUNCTION

Neuropsychiatric rating scales provide specific information such as the rate of change and severity of cognitive decline or improvement. They are useful in situations in which repeated measurements of a patient's mental status are needed because they allow the clinician to determine response to an intervention (e.g., medication) in a more systematic manner. In addition, some cognitive function measures are useful screens for Alzheimer's and other dementias, cerebral infarction, and encephalitis or encephalopathies. A number of cognitive rating scales are available, the most common being the mini-mental status examination (MMSE). The MMSE globally assesses many cognitive domains including orientation, visuospatial organization, memory, and reasoning to determine an overall score of cognitive function. The MMSE takes 5 to 10 minutes to administer and is used routinely in the clinical setting.[20] Other examples of cognitive rating scales include the information-memory-concentration (IMC) test the dementia rating scale (DRS), and the clock drawing and Alzheimer's Disease assessment scale.[20,21] Some scales are useful for identifying deficits in specific cognitive domains such as orientation, speech and language, visuospatial, visuoperceptual and visuomotor skills, memory, arithmetic calculations, and reasoning (Table 60–6).

TABLE 60–6. Selected Neuropsychiatric Measures

Rating Scale	Type	Scoring	Comments
Mini-Mental Status Examination (MMSE)	Structured interview	Maximum score is 30; 23 or less is indicative of cognitive impairment. Level of consciousness also listed	5–10 minutes to administer. Global assessment of orientation, attention, recall and language, memory
Dementia Rating Scale (DRS)	Structured interview	Total scores range from 0–144 (perfect score)	30–40 minutes to administer. Global measure of dementia using 5 subscales: attention, initiation and perseveration, construction, conceptualization, memory
Neurobehavioral Cognitive Status Examination (NCSE, COGNISTAT)	Structured interview	Eight separately scored cognitive domains (11 subsets). The 8 domains are scored and plotted on a graph provided	5–10 minutes to nonimpaired and up to 30 minutes in impaired patients. Distinguishes confusional states from dementias by using separate domain scores such as language, memory, calculations, etc. Requires some practice; however, it is easy to administer.
Clock Drawing	Instructional	Qualitative assessment (template matching). Quantitative scoring. Points awarded for correctness of design	Assessment at bedside which involves either copying a clock, putting hands on a clock, and/or showing a specific time. Cognitive domains: comprehension, conceptualization, visuospatial skills
Alzheimer's Disease Assessment Scale (ADAS)	Structured interview	21 items total; 11 items in the cognitive (COG) subset. 10 items in the noncognitive behavioral subset. Each subset may be scored separately from the total ADAS score	Takes 45 minutes to administer the ADAS and 35 minutes for the ADAS-COG. The ADAS-COG refers to the cognitive assessment subset commonly used to measure cognitive function in clinical drug trials. Requires training for administration and scoring

Adapted from Schneider et al[20] and Salmon.[21]

TABLE 60–7. Common Psychological Tests

Wechsler Adult Intelligence Scale-Revised (WAIS-R) and Wechsler Intelligence Scale for Children-Revised (WISC-R)
Measures abstract thinking, learning from experience, problem solving, adjustment to new situations. Score less than 70 denotes mental retardation
Bender Visual Motor Gestalt Test
Screening test for brain damage, learning problems, emotional difficulties, nonverbal intelligence. Person is asked to reproduce nine geometric designs
Interpretation of Projective Drawings
Patient draws a person, house-tree-person, family, or spontaneously to assess unconscious feeling, conflicts, and strengths
Rorschach
Patient interprets 10 inkblots and explains what they mean. Assesses personality structure
Minnesota Multiphasic Personality Inventory (MMPI-2)
Measures personality traits from 567 true/false questions. Can be affected by intelligence, education, socioeconomic status

Most of the rating scales involve a structured interview that requires clinician training to ensure accurate administration. Noise and distraction can affect the patient's performance ability; therefore the interview should be conducted in a quiet area with adequate lighting. The interviewer should speak slowly and clearly to the patient when providing instructions or asking questions.

PSYCHOLOGICAL TESTING

Although most clinicians do not administer psychological testing, they can use the results to evaluate the role of medication in relationship to the diagnosis. Psychological testing alone cannot establish a firm diagnosis but can be a useful diagnostic tool when coupled with clinical judgment. Types of psychological testing include personality tests, intelligence tests, and neuropsychological tests.[3] Table 60–7 describes common psychological tests.

CONCLUSIONS

Patient assessment is the basis from which a pharmaceutical care plan evolves. Problem identification and therapeutic monitoring cannot occur until a thorough assessment is complete. The initial assessment is also the basis for evaluating response to therapy throughout the course of treatment. Psychiatric assessment requires sensitivity and good listening skills on the part of the clinician because it is based primarily on a subjective interview and not objective tests. With careful data collection, clinicians can make substantial contributions to care that improve patient outcomes.

ABBREVIATIONS

APA: American Psychiatric Association
BRS: brief psychiatric rating scale
CGI: Clinical Global Impression (scale)
DRS: dementia rating scale
DSM-IV-TR: *Diagnostic and Statistical Manual of Mental Disorders*, 4th edition, Text Revision
EPS: extrapyramidal side effect
GAF: global assessment of functioning
HAMD: Hamilton Rating Scale for Depression
IMC: information-memory-concentration (test)
MMSE: mini-mental status examination
MSE: mental status examination

Review Questions and other resources can be found at *www.pharmacotherapyonline.com.*

REFERENCES

1. Manley MRS. The psychiatric interview, history and mental status examination. In: Sadock BJ, Sadock VA, eds. Comprehensive Textbook of Psychiatry, Vol. 1, 7th ed. Philadelphia, Lippincott Williams & Wilkins, 2000: 652–665.
2. Rosse RB, Deutsch LH, Deutsch SI. Medical assessment and laboratory testing and psychiatry. In: Sadock BJ, Sadock VA, eds. Comprehensive Textbook of Psychiatry, Vol. 1, 7th ed. Philadelphia, Lippincott Williams & Wilkins, 2000:732–754.
3. Adams RL, Culbertson JL. Personality assessment of adults and children. In: Sadock BJ, Sadock VA, eds. Comprehensive Textbook of Psychiatry, Vol. 1, 7th ed. Philadelphia, Lippincott Williams & Wilkins, 2000:702–722.
4. Blacker D. Psychiatric rating scales. In: Sadock BJ, Sadock VA, eds. Comprehensive Textbook of Psychiatry, Vol. 1, 7th ed. Philadelphia, Lippincott Williams & Wilkins, 2000:755–783.
5. Fogel BS, Shellow R. Practice guideline for psychiatric evaluation of adults. In: McIntyre JS, Charles SC, Zarin DA, eds. American Psychiatric Association Practice Guidelines for the Treatment of Psychiatric Disorders. Compendium 2000. Washington, American Psychiatric Association, 2000:5–26.
6. American Psychiatric Association. Diagnostic and Statistical Manual of Mental Disorders, 4th ed., Text Revision (DSM-IV-TR). Washington, American Psychiatric Press, 2000.
7. Othemer E, Othmer SC. The Clinical Interview Using DSM-IV, Vol. 1: Fundamentals. Washington, American Psychiatric Press, 1994.
8. Henderson DC, Caliero E, Gray C, et al. Clozapine, diabetes mellitus, weight gain and lipid abnormalities: A five-year naturalistic study. Am J Psychiatry 2000;157:975–981.
9. Cradock-O'Leary J, Young AS, et al. Use of general medical services by VA patients with psychiatric disorders. Psychiatr Serv 2002;53:874–878.
10. Guy W. ECDEU Assessment Manual for Psychopharmacology, rev. ed. DHEW Publication (ADM) 76-338. Washington, U.S. Government Printing Office, 1976:158–169.
11. Schooler NR, Chengappa KNR. Adverse effect measures. In: Rush AJ, Pincus HA, First MB, et al, eds. Handbook of Psychiatric Measures, Vol. 11. Washington, American Psychiatric Association, 2000:151–168.
12. Sprague RL, Kalachnik JE. Reliability, validity, and a total score cutoff for the dyskinesia identification system: Condensed user scale (DISCUS) with mentally ill and mentally retarded populations. Psychopharmacol Bull 1991;27:51–58.
13. Thompson C. Introduction. In: Thompson C, ed. The Instruments of Psychiatric Research. New York, Wiley, 1989:1–16.
14. Fankhauser MP, German ML. Understanding the use of behavioral rating scales in studies evaluating the efficacy of antianxiety and antidepressant drugs. Am J Hosp Pharm 1987;44:2087–2100.

15. Andreasen NC. The scale for assessment of negative symptoms (SANS): Conceptual and theoretical foundations. Br J Psychiatry 1989; 155(Suppl 7):49–58.

16. Kay SR, Opler LA, Lindenmayer JP. The positive and negative syndrome scale (PANSS): Rationale and standardization. Br J Psychiatry 1989;155(Suppl 7):59–65.

17. Montgomery SA, Asberg M. A new depression scale designed to be sensitive to change. Br J Psychiatry 1979;134:382–389.

18. Sheehan DV. The Anxiety Disease. New York, Bantam, 1983: 114–115.

19. Goodman WK, Price LH, Rasmussen SA, et al. The Yale-Brown Obsessive Compulsive Scale (Y-BOCS): II. Validity. Arch Gen Psychiatry 1989;46:1006–1011.

20. Schneider LS, Tariot Pierre N, Olin JT. Brief assessments of cognitive function. In: Manual of Rating Scales for the Assessment of Geriatric Mental Illnesses, Vol. 5. Wilmington, DE, Astra-Zeneca, 2000:19–21.

21. Salmon DP. Neuropsychiatric measures for cognitive disorders. In: Rush AJ, Pincus HA, First MB, et al, eds. Handbook of Psychiatric Measures, Vol. 21. Washington, American Psychiatric Association, 2000: 417–455.

61
CHILDHOOD DISORDERS
Julie A. Dopheide, Karen A. Theesen, and Michael Malkin

Learning Objectives and other resources can be found at *www.pharmacotherapyonline.com*.

KEY CONCEPTS

◄1 Inattention and impulsivity due to attention-deficit/hyperactivity disorder (ADHD) begins before age 7 and can continue into adolescence and adulthood, often requiring ongoing drug treatment.

◄2 Coexisting disorders have an impact on drug selection. A mood stabilizer is appropriate if bipolar disorder coexists, while an antidepressant may be needed if a mood or anxiety disorder coexists.

◄3 Stimulants are first-line treatment for ADHD; atomoxetine, bupropion, and tricyclic antidepressants (TCAs) are second-line agents; clonidine, guanfacine, and other medications are adjunctive treatments.

◄4 Tourette's disorder presents with both motor and vocal tics, which are present during childhood, plateau during adolescence, and may continue during adulthood with a fluctuating course.

◄5 The decision to medicate for Tourette's disorder is based on

the degree of concern perceived by the patient, symptom severity, and comorbid disorders.

◄6 Individuals with Tourette's disorder are particularly sensitive to medication side effects, so medication dosing must be individualized carefully, and close monitoring is essential.

◄7 Nondrug approaches to enuresis management, such as dry-bed training or using moisture-sensitive alarms, are preferred because of higher cure rates and avoidance of drug side effects.

◄8 Desmopressin is effective orally and intranasally for enuresis, but it is expensive and works better in older than in younger children.

◄9 Imipramine and other TCAs are effective for enuresis at wide dosage ranges. TCAs have rapid onset, but side effects may be problematic for some patients.

All neuropsychiatric disorders can first present during childhood.[1] Attention-deficit/hyperactivity disorder (ADHD), Tourette's disorder, and enuresis are the focus of this chapter because the onset of symptoms occurs explicitly during childhood.

Treating children with psychotropic drugs requires a very different approach than treating adults. A child's neurologic, physiologic, and psychosocial status is undergoing constant changes throughout the developmental period. Age-related pharmacodynamic and pharmacokinetic differences can alter drug disposition and response. Well-defined diagnostic criteria guide drug selection;[1] however, frequent comorbid disorders present treatment challenges.[2] In addition, children may not be able to verbalize symptom response or adverse effects of a medication. All factors considered, children generally are given psychotropic drugs to control a group of symptoms or behaviors in order to facilitate the child's learning and development.

The psychiatric assessment of a child requires obtaining information from the child, parents, caregivers, and teachers.

ATTENTION-DEFICIT/HYPERACTIVITY DISORDER

CLINICAL PRESENTATION AND EPIDEMIOLOGY

ADHD evaluation should be considered whenever a child presents with developmentally inappropriate inattention, impulsivity, and or

hyperactivity (Table 61–1). Symptom presence and severity vary with the situation. It is unusual for a child to display signs of the disorder in all settings or even in the same setting at all times.[1] The ◄1 onset of ADHD is typically by the age of 3 years and must occur by age 7, although the disorder may not require professional attention until the child enters school. The National Institutes of Health (NIH) estimate the prevalence in school-age children to be 3% to 5%;[3] however, community sample estimates average 2.9% for girls and 9.2% for boys.[4] Girls display more inattention and less hyperactive and impulsive symptomatology.[3,4] Symptoms may persist lifelong for both sexes, but hyperactivity is much less prominent in adolescence and adulthood.[2,4,5]

It is critical to clarify the diagnosis of ADHD in individuals with these symptoms. Inattention and distractibility can be symptoms of an anxiety disorder, depression, or bipolar disorder.[2,3,6] In other ◄2 cases, these anxiety or mood disorders can coexist with ADHD, just as learning deficiencies and conduct or oppositional disorders are common comorbid conditions.[2,6,7] The presence of multiple comorbid conditions, particularly conduct or oppositional disorder, may increase the likelihood of ADHD chronicity.[2]

ETIOLOGY AND PATHOPHYSIOLOGY

ADHD is a clinical diagnosis with multiple heterogeneous causes.[3,7] Both genetic and nongenetic factors are involved. The child of a

1133

TABLE 61–1. Clinical Presentation of ADHD

Inattention	• Often fails to give close attention to details or makes careless mistakes in schoolwork or other activities
	• Often has difficulty sustaining attention in activities
	• Often has difficulty organizing tasks and activities
	• Avoids tasks that require sustained mental effort
	• Often does not seem to listen when spoken to directly
	• Often does not follow through on instructions and fails to finish schoolwork, chores, or duties in the workplace
	• Is easily distracted by extraneous stimuli
	• Is often forgetful in daily activities
	• Loses things necessary for activities
Hyperactivity and impulsivity	• Often fidgets with hands or feet or squirms in seat
	• Often leaves seat when remaining seated is expected
	• Often runs about or climbs excessively at inappropriate times
	• Often has difficulty playing quietly
	• Is often on the go or acts as if driven by a motor
	• Often talks excessively
	• Often blurts out answers before questions have been completed
	• Often has difficulty waiting to take turns
	• Often interrupts or intrudes on others

Symptoms must be present before age 7; six or more of the symptoms must persist for 6 months; significant impairment must be seen in two or more settings (e.g., home and school); symptoms must be documented by parent, teacher, and clinician.
Adapted from American Psychiatric Association.[1]

parent with ADHD has up to a 50% chance of developing ADHD; monozygotic twins have up to a 92% concordance rate for ADHD.[3,4] In addition, children with fetal alcohol syndrome, lead poisoning, and meningitis have a higher incidence of ADHD symptomatology.[3,4] An association of ADHD with a variety of environmental risks including obstetric adversity, maternal smoking, and adverse parent-child relationships has been noted.[7,8] Dietary causes are unlikely.[3,4]

Although brain studies show no definitive pathophysiologic markers of ADHD, the prefrontal cortex, basal ganglia, and caudate volumes are consistently reported as abnormal, typically smaller.[9–1] In addition, individuals with ADHD are twice as likely to display a defective 7-repeat allele of the dopamine$_4$ receptor gene. This gene has been related to a deficiency in translating the dopaminergic signal to the second messenger system. Norepinephrine and epinephrine are agonists at this receptor as well. Implications of these findings are being studied.[12]

A prevailing pathophysiologic explanation for ADHD symptoms involves deficits in prefrontal cortex–mediated executive brain function also known as *response inhibition*. Children with ADHD are unable to control their behavior, resist distractions, and develop an awareness of space and time.[9,12] In addition, a dysregulation of arousal in frontosubcortical pathways has been proposed. Children with ADHD display insufficient alertness during dull and repetitive tasks, alternating with overarousal.[12]

Effective treatments modulate dopamine (DA) and norepinephrine (NE) to improve executive functioning and regulate arousal for improved performance. The clinical response associated with stimulants is not paradoxical, and is not diagnostic for ADHD because stimulants can increase attention, decrease motor activity, and improve learning tasks in those with subclinical ADHD or in individuals with such problems from other sources (e.g., fatigue).[3,4,13]

▶ TREATMENT: Attention-Deficit/Hyperactivity Disorder

▓ STIMULANTS

Stimulants are considered first-line therapy in most cases of ADHD; however, comorbid conditions have an impact on the drug selection process, calling for a careful, systematic approach. Pharmacotherapy should be considered whenever a thorough diagnostic assessment indicates symptoms of ADHD that cause significant functional impairment. Several studies demonstrate the superiority of stimulants compared with behavioral interventions in alleviating core symptoms of ADHD.[4,14] However, stimulants have not been shown to improve social and academic functioning reliably; therefore multimodal treatment, individualized to the specific needs of the child and family, is crucial for overall positive therapeutic outcome.[3,15] Table 61–2 describes behavioral interventions for ADHD. Multimodal treatment includes parent training, family therapy, classroom interventions, and contingency management (e.g., rewards for good behavior).[3,16] Figure 61–1 provides an algorithm for drug selection in the treatment of ADHD.

Stimulants (e.g., methylphenidate, mixed amphetamine salts, dextroamphetamine, and pemoline) are the most effective drug treatment options, with efficacy ranging from 70% to 96% when a trial of each drug is given using wide dosage ranges.[3,15,16] Mixed amphetamine salts (Adderall), a combination of dextroamphetamine and D, L-amphetamine salts, is a longer-acting alternative to methylphenidate.[17] Pemoline is considered to be a "last-resort" therapy because of the risk of hepatic toxicity.[6,15]

Despite knowledge of the effects of stimulants on neurotransmitter activity, how these drugs affect the primary symptoms of ADHD is unclear. To varying degrees the central nervous system (CNS) stimulants inhibit the reuptake of DA and NE, enhance release of DA and NE from the presynaptic neuron, or inhibit the enzyme monoamine oxidase (MAO). Because stimulants work through slightly different mechanisms, lack of response to one stimulant does not preclude response to another.[6,15]

Dosing of the stimulants should be titrated for maximum individual efficacy and minimum side effects. Table 61–3 provides initial dose and titration recommendations for stimulants based on manufacturer's recommendations and published guidelines developed by experienced clinicians.[6,15,16,18]

Drug response is maximal during the absorption phase, is evident in 15 to 30 minutes, and lasts 2 to 6 hours.[15] With immediate-release stimulants, most patients require a two or three times daily dosing schedule due to the short half-lives of these drugs (2 to 4 hours for methylphenidate and dexmethylphenidate and approximately 6 hours for dextroamphetamine).[15,16,18]

Drug delivery systems of once-daily products (Concerta, Metadate CD, Ritalin LA, Adderall XR) provide 8 to 12 hours of symptom control.[15,19] Concerta uses an oral osmotic (OROS) controlled-release delivery system, while other preparations use combinations of immediate-release or extended-release beads containing drug.[19] Concerta is a nondeformable tablet and it should not be given to children with gastrointestinal narrowing due to the risk of obstruction. Older wax-matrix sustained-release products (e.g., Ritalin SR)

TABLE 61–2. Behavioral Interventions for ADHD

Technique	Description	Example
Positive reinforcement	Providing rewards or privileges contingent on the child's performance	Child completes an assignment and is permitted to play on the computer
Time-out	Removing access to positive reinforcement contingent on performance of unwanted or problem behavior	Child hits sibling impulsively and is required to sit for 5 minutes in the corner of the room
Response cost	Withdrawing rewards or privileges contingent on the performance of unwanted or problem behavior	Child loses free time privileges for not completing homework
Token economy	Combining positive reinforcement and response cost. The child earns rewards and privileges contingent on performing desired behaviors and loses the rewards and privileges based on undesirable behavior	Child earns stars for completing assignments and loses stars for getting out of seat. The child cashes in the sum of stars at the end of the week for a prize

From American Academy of Pediatrics.[16]

are less effective and infrequently used.[15] When choosing between immediate-release or once-daily stimulants, the convenience of once-daily dosing must be weighed against the potential for difficulty falling asleep with once-daily or sustained-release products.[15,16] Adolescents and adults with ADHD are also responsive to stimulants. Methylphenidate is demonstrated effective in adults using doses up to 1 mg/kg per day.[6,15]

ADVERSE EFFECTS

The most common adverse effects of stimulants and their management strategies are listed in Table 61–4. Growth suppression or delay is a possibility. Proposed mechanisms of stimulant effects on growth include alterations in growth hormone secretion and suppression of appetite leading to reduced caloric intake. One study measured the

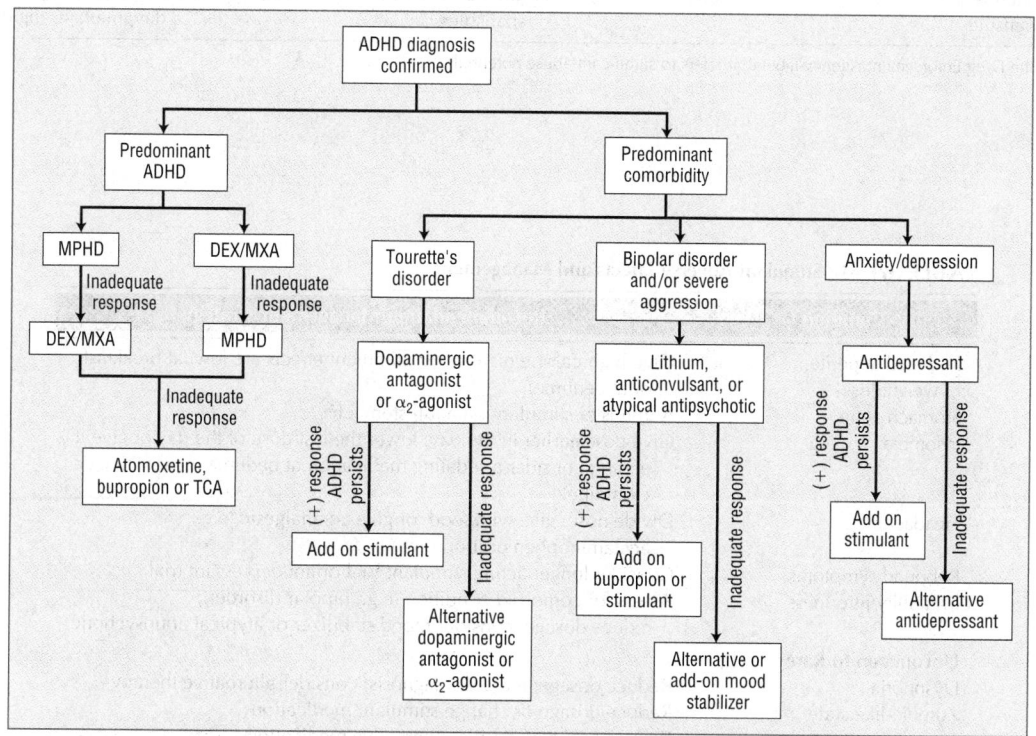

FIGURE 61–1. Algorithm for management of ADHD. Treat predominant disorder first, reassess, and consider alternative or adjunct medications for optimal symptom control. MPHD, methylphenidate; DEX, dextroamphetamine; MXA, mixed amphetamine salts; TCA, tricyclic antidepressant; AD, antidepressant. (Adapted from Pliszka et al,[6] Pliszka et al,[15] MTA Cooperative Group,[16] Caballero,[22] Daviss et al,[24] State et al,[30] Schur et al,[32] Hughes et al,[34] Muller-Vahl,[46] and Jimenez-Jimenez.[47])

TABLE 61–3. **Stimulant Comparison**

Stimulant	Duration of Effect	Initial Dose and Available Strengths	Usual Dosing Range Maximum Dose
Methylphenidate C-II FDA approved for children >6 y old			
Short-acting Immediate release (IR) Ritalin, Methylin, generics	3–5 h	5 mg two or three times a day; increase by 5–10 mg/day at weekly intervals; available as: 5, 10, 20 mg	5–20 mg two or three times a day; max dose: 60 mg/day
Intermediate-acting Ritalin SR (sustained-release) Methylphenidate SR Metadate ER (extended-release) Methylin ER	3–8 h	SR, ER doses; corresponds to the IR dose	20–40 mg every AM or 40 mg every AM and 20 mg in the early afternoon; max dose: 60 mg/day
Long-acting Metadate CD 30% IR beads, 70% ER beads	8–12 h	20 mg every AM; available as: 10, 20, and 30 mg	20–40 mg every AM and 20 mg in early afternoon; max dose: 60 mg/day
Ritalin LA 50% IR, 50% ER beads Concerta (oral osmotic [OROS] controlled-release delivery)		20 mg every AM; available as: 20, 30, and 40 mg	20–60 mg/day, given every AM; max dose: 72 mg/day
ER inner compartments coated with IR methylphenidate		18 mg every AM; available as 18, 27, 36, and 54 mg; 90% bioavailability of IR	
Dexmethylphenidate (Focalin) C-II FDA approved for children ≥6 y old	3–5 h	2.5 mg every AM or twice a day; available as: 2.5, 5, and 10 mg tablets	5–10 mg/day given twice a day; max initial dose: 7.5 mg/day max dose: 20 mg/day
Dextroamphetamine C-II FDA approved for children >3 y old	4–6 h	2.5 mg every AM to two or three times daily dosing	5–15 mg twice a day
Short-acting Dextroamphetamine generics Dexedrine, Dextrostat	3–5 h	5 mg every AM; available as: 5 and 10 mg	10–40 mg/day given twice a day
Intermediate-acting Dexedrine Spansule	5–8 h	Available as: 5-, 10-, and 15-mg spansules	5–30 mg every day or 5–15 mg twice a day; max: 40 mg/day

C-II = schedule II, the Drug Enforcement Agency label that refers to significant abuse potential.

TABLE 61–4. **Stimulant Adverse Effects and Management**

Common	Recommendation/Management Strategy
Reduced appetite, weight loss	Give high-calorie meal when stimulant effects are low (at breakfast or at bedtime)
Stomach ache	Administer stimulant on a full stomach
Insomnia	Give dose earlier in the day; lower the last dose of the day or give it earlier; consider a sedating medication at bedtime (guanfacine or clonidine)
Headache	Divide dose; give with food; or give an analgesic (e.g., acetaminophen or ibuprofen)
Rebound symptoms	Consider longer-acting stimulant trial or antidepressant trial
Irritability/jitteriness	Assess for comorbid condition (e.g., bipolar disorder); reduce dosage; consider mood stabilizer or atypical antipsychotic
Uncommon to Rare	
Dysphoria	Reduce dosage; reassess diagnosis; consider alternative therapy
Zombie-like state	Reduce dosage or change stimulant medication
Tics or abnormal movements	Reduce dosage; consider alternative medication
Hypertension	Reduce dosage; change medication
Hallucinations	Discontinue stimulant; reassess diagnosis; mood stabilizer and/or antipsychotic may be needed

height of 84 children with ADHD treated with methylphenidate and compared their growth to non-ADHD siblings over 2 years. Significant differences in growth were found over a broad range of doses (10 to 80 mg), suggesting that the prevalence of growth-suppressive effects of methylphenidate is greater than previously suggested.[20] Some evidence exists attributing maturational delays to ADHD itself, not stimulant treatment.[21]

A related aspect of stimulant use concerns drug holidays and duration of treatment. Drug holidays are important because they provide time to reassess treatment.[16] All children should be given a drug-free trial every year. Consideration must be given to the risks of negative effects on learning, socialization, and self-image while off stimulant therapy when determining the frequency and duration of drug holidays. Drug dosage often varies from year to year, largely due to age-related pharmacokinetic changes. As a child develops, hepatic metabolism slows and volume of distribution increases.

CLINICAL CONTROVERSY

According to recent studies growth suppression or delay is a possibility with stimulant use in children; however, results are mixed. Some studies indicate that effects are temporary, with normalization in height and weight occurring through mid-adolescence.[3,4,20]

A diagnosis of ADHD confers at least a twofold greater risk of adolescent and adult substance abuse.[42,43] The risk is greater if conduct disorder, antisocial personality, or bipolar disorder coexists.[12,42] Stimulant therapy does not increase the risk of substance abuse, and effective treatment of ADHD may facilitate functioning and participation in substance abuse recovery.[42]

■ NONSTIMULANTS

Atomoxetine, a selective norepinephrine reuptake inhibitor, is the first nonstimulant approved by the Food and Drug Administration (FDA) for the treatment of ADHD. In contrast to the stimulants, it has no apparent abuse potential and is not a controlled substance. Placebo-controlled, short-term trials (6 to 12 weeks) have shown that atomoxetine is effective in reducing ADHD symptoms in children, teens, and adults. It is not clear whether it is as effective as the stimulants, although one preliminary open study suggested comparable efficacy with methylphenidate.[22]

Atomoxetine has a significantly slower onset of therapeutic effect than stimulants (2 to 4 weeks versus 1 hour with an effective stimulant dose). Atomoxetine may be taken once daily or in divided doses in the morning or late afternoon.[22] Table 61–5 provides dosing and titration recommendations for all nonstimulant medications.

TABLE 61–5. Antidepressants and Other Agents for ADHD and Associated Symptoms

Drug	Dosing Range and Titration Schedule	Adverse Effect Monitoring
Atomoxetine (Strattera)	≤70 kg: start at 0.5 mg/kg every AM or twice a day; max: 1.4 mg/kg per day ≥70 kg: start at 40 mg every AM or twice a day; max: 100 mg/day	Nausea, anorexia, ↑ blood pressure, ↑ pulse, insomnia, fatigue, sedation, severe liver injury
Bupropion (Wellbutrin)	50–300 mg/day; 3 mg/kg per day by end of week one; may increase to 6 mg/kg per day or maximum of 300 kg/day as tolerated	Nausea, insomnia, rash, tics; dose-related risk of seizures
Tricyclic antidepressants: desipramine or nortriptyline	50–150 mg/day; start at 0.5–1 mg/kg per day; increase as tolerated to 2–3 mg/kg per day; max: 300 mg/day of desipramine (adults only) or 150 mg/day nortriptyline	Sedation, dizziness, constipation, heart block (check ECG), weight gain, overdose toxicity, rapid heartbeat
Clonidine (Catapres)	0.05 mg two or four times daily; may increase as tolerated to 0.1–0.4 mg/day	Sedation, dizziness, heart block (check ECG), constipation
Guanfacine (Tenex)	0.5 mg once to twice a day; may increase as tolerated to 1–4 mg/day	Same as above with potentially lower risk of sedation
Risperidone[a] (Risperdal)	0.25–0.5 mg twice daily; may titrate every 3–4 days as tolerated to response, (1–4 mg/day)	Extrapyramidal symptoms, dizziness, ↑ prolactin, hepatotoxicity, weight gain
Olanzapine[a] (Zyprexa)	2.5–5 mg every day; may titrate every 3–4 days as tolerated to response (usual range: 7.5–15 mg/day)	Sedation, weight gain, restlessness, diabetes, hyperlipidemia
Ziprasidone[a] (Geodon)	10–20 mg twice daily; may titrate every 3–4 days as tolerated to response (usual range: 40–120 mg/day)	Nausea, restlessness, insomnia, QTc prolongation
Haloperidol[a] (Haldol)	0.5–1 mg twice daily; may titrate every 3–4 days as tolerated to response (usual range: 0.5–5 mg/day)	Extrapyramidal symptoms, dizziness, ↑ prolactin, sedation

[a]Short-term use (1–4 months) only for severe aggression associated with ADHD.

Bupropion, a monocyclic antidepressant, is a DA and NE reuptake inhibitor with no significant direct effect on serotonin or MAO. Its active metabolites augment noradrenergic and dopaminergic function. Investigations with bupropion in children demonstrated efficacy greater than placebo in a controlled trial[6] and efficacy comparable with methylphenidate (n = 15 children) in another controlled trial.[6] Advantages of bupropion include less toxicity on overdose compared with TCAs and less appetite suppression compared with stimulants. Bupropion also may be effective in adults at antidepressant doses.[5]

Imipramine and desipramine are the most systematically studied TCAs in the treatment of ADHD, although nortriptyline is also effective.[6,16] The onset of TCA clinical response occurs within the first 2 to 4 weeks.[6,16] Variability in dosage requirements for TCAs and atomoxetine may be due to interpatient variability in drug plasma concentration achieved at a given dose. Both are metabolized via cytochrome P450 2D6, and bioavailability and half-life may be 4 to 8 times greater in those taking a P450 2D6 inhibitor (e.g., bupropion, fluoxetine, or paroxetine) or in poor metabolizers. For example, atomoxetine's half-life is 5 hours in extensive metabolizers and 19 hours in poor metabolizers.[22,23] If tolerance seems to develop after months of therapy, a dosage adjustment may be necessary to compensate for age-related changes in distribution and metabolism.

◀3 Atomoxetine, bupropion, and TCAs are second-line alternatives to the stimulants for treatment of ADHD in children, teens, and adults. The potential benefits of these agents in comparison with stimulants include reduced risk of abuse and somewhat lower potential for sleep disturbance. TCAs are the most dangerous in overdose and pose the greatest risk for cardiovascular side effects.[5,6,16,22] The monoamine oxidase inhibitor tranylcypromine is effective but used infrequently due to the potential for dangerous drug and dietary interactions.[5] Selective serotonin reuptake inhibitors (SSRIs) are not effective for ADHD.[6,16]

▨ ADVERSE EFFECTS

Possible adverse effects and management for atomoxetine are listed in Table 61–5 and are strikingly similar to those of stimulants. Atomoxetine has a greater risk of fatigue and sedation compared to stimulants. The relative risk of all potential adverse events compared to stimulants (decreased appetite, growth delay, sleep disturbance, gastrointestinal side effects, and tics) and bupropion require further study.[22,23] Atomoxetine labeling has recently been updated to include a bolded warning of potential for severe liver injury following reports in two patients.

Bupropion's adverse effects and their management are listed in Table 61–5 and include nausea, which may resolve over time or with slower dosage titration, and rash, which may require discontinuation of therapy if severe. Bupropion can cause or exacerbate tics and therefore should be used with caution in individuals with tics or a family history of tics.[24]

TCAs are effective for control of impulsivity and hyperactivity, but they are not as effective as stimulants in increasing attention.[5,6,16] TCAs should be taken throughout the week and not just during school days. TCA withdrawal effects are common in children and include nausea, vomiting, and diarrhea.[25]

Possible CNS adverse effects of TCAs include dizziness, aggressiveness, excitement, nightmares, insomnia, forgetfulness, and irritability. Signs of CNS toxicity are confusion, impaired concentration, hallucinations, and delusions.

◀3 Clonidine and guanfacine are less effective alternatives to stimulant monotherapy. They are prescribed more frequently as adjuncts to reduce disruptive behavior, control aggression, or to improve sleep.[6,16,26] Clonidine and guanfacine, central α_2-adrenergic agonists, inhibit noradrenergic activity by decreasing the release of NE from the presynaptic neuron. Both reduce the firing rate within the locus ceruleus, decrease excessive arousal, and are thought to "prime" the posterior attention system to external stimuli.[13,26] Guanfacine has a longer elimination half-life (12 to 18 hours) compared with clonidine (2.5 to 4 hours).[27]

The most common side effect of clonidine is dose-dependent sedation that usually subsides after 2 to 3 weeks of therapy.[6,26] Of concern are reports of bradycardia, rebound hypertension, heart block, and sudden death.[6,26] Four children have died on the combination of methylphenidate and clonidine; however, complicating factors make it impossible to link the drug combination directly with the cause of death.[6] Of 10,060 children exposed to clonidine and assessed by a poison control center over a 7-year period, moderate (19%) to major (2%) toxic effects (bradycardia, hypotension, and respiratory depression) including one death were reported. Overdoses, concurrent clonidine and stimulant administration, as well as missed doses of clonidine all add to the risk of adverse cardiovascular events.[28,29] Similar adverse-effect concerns apply to treatment with guanfacine, although its α_{2a} selectivity may result in less sedation and hypotension than clonidine.[27]

◀2 Lithium and anticonvulsants are used increasingly to control aggression and explosive behavior in patients with a diagnosis of ADHD. Some patients actually may have childhood-onset bipolar disorder or combined ADHD-intermittent explosive disorder.[6,30] Lithium, valproate, and carbamazepine are effective for explosive behavior, aggression, and impulsivity, but they are not beneficial treatments for a child with the inattentive subtype of ADHD. Dosing starts in low divided doses with titration over 1 to 2 weeks to therapeutic response.[2,6,31]

Conventional antipsychotics improve symptoms of hyperactivity and impulsivity, but may have negative effects on learning and cognitive functioning as well as extrapyramidal side effects (e.g., dystonia and tardive dyskinesia) that limit their usefulness.[6] The atypical antipsychotics risperidone, olanzapine, quetiapine, and ziprasidone have been used to control severe aggression in refractory cases of ADHD, particularly if conduct disorder or bipolar disorder coexists. More studies are needed to clarify their place in therapy.[6,32,33]

If multiple drugs are started simultaneously, it is impossible to determine the impact of each drug. The predominance and urgency of symptoms guide the drug-selection process (see Fig. 61–1). For example, if a child presents as severely anxious or depressed with associated attentional problems, then an antidepressant should be initiated first with monitoring to determine if attentional symptoms improve.[34] When a child presents with severe ADHD and associated anxiety or depression, a stimulant should be initiated to treat the more severe ADHD. If ADHD symptoms improve significantly but anxiety or depression persists, then an antidepressant can be added. Careful monitoring is needed to detect drug interactions that lead to higher drug plasma levels and increased adverse effects.[6] Studies show that stimulants do not routinely make anxiety disorders worse, but they may not improve symptoms either.[6,16] In children with epilepsy, methylphenidate is effective; however, the child must be stabilized and seizure-free on an anticonvulsant prior to initiation of the stimulant.[35] Patients with seizure disorders should not receive bupropion.

PHARMACOECONOMIC CONSIDERATIONS

A study comparing medical care use and costs between persons with and without ADHD over 9 years found that the median cost for a person with ADHD was more than double ($4306 vs. $1944; p <0.001) that of someone without ADHD. Increased costs are attributed to accidental injuries, diagnostic assessments, hospital visits, and outpatient visits.[36] The cost-effectiveness of drug treatment has not been assessed. Immediate-release generic methylphenidate, dextroamphetamine, and mixed amphetamine salts appear to provide the most effective and economic therapy due to relatively low drug cost. The cost of once-daily Concerta, Ritalin LA, Metadate CD, Adderall XR, and Strattera is approximately 2 to 4 times that of an immediate-release generic stimulant. Generic bupropion is the least expensive nonstimulant treatment. Imipramine, desipramine, clonidine, and mood stabilizers are relatively inexpensive, but ongoing electrocardiographic and blood-level monitoring can increase costs significantly.[6,29]

EVALUATION OF THERAPEUTIC OUTCOMES

Careful documentation of baseline symptoms and complaints over a 1-month predrug period is essential to the evaluation of therapeutic and adverse outcomes. Baseline symptoms can be measured using videotapes, clinician rating scales (e.g., Child Behavioral Checklist or ADHD Rating Scale-IV), or both. In addition, height, weight, and eating and sleeping patterns should be recorded at baseline and every 3 months.[6,37]

After the initiation and titration of any drug treatment, it is necessary that parents, teachers, and clinicians assess the overall functioning of the child using standardized rating scales to determine if significant therapeutic benefit justifies continuing medication.[6,15,37,38] Therapeutic effects of the stimulants include decreased motor activity and impulsivity and increased attention span. Improved cognitive performance may result from an overall improvement in attention and concentration and may not be a direct drug effect on cognition.[9,15] This suggests that stimulants are indicated for ADHD symptoms and not for primary learning disorders. The benefits of drug therapy must outweigh the adverse effects.[39–41]

Atomoxetine and bupropion require monitoring to detect changes in appetite, weight, and sleep patterns, or if pulse or blood pressure changes occur. A therapeutic trial of atomoxetine or bupropion consists of 1 month of maximum tolerated doses.[5,22,24]

When clonidine or guanfacine are given, careful clinical monitoring for fatigue, dizziness, and autonomic changes (e.g., blood pressure and pulse) is recommended.[6] The American Heart Association has stated that electrocardiographic monitoring is not required for clonidine treatment in children, although many clinicians continue to assess for electrocardiogram changes. When discontinuing treatment, clonidine and guanfacine should be withdrawn slowly (0.05 mg clonidine/0.5 mg guanfacine reductions every 3 days) to prevent rebound hypertension or behavioral dyscontrol.[28] A therapeutic trial takes 1 to 2 months, although increased sleep can be seen immediately.

The effects of TCAs on the electrocardiogram should be monitored carefully. Of more concern are reports of sudden death in children taking desipramine or imipramine.[38] Children and adolescents given TCAs should have pretreatment and follow-up electrocardiograms to assess the effects of TCA therapy on cardiac rate and rhythm.[6,16,38]

CONCLUSION

At this time, the preferred first-line drug therapy for ADHD is either methylphenidate, dexmethylphenidate, mixed amphetamine salts, or dextroamphetamine. Atomoxetine, bupropion, or TCAs are good options for those unresponsive to or unable to tolerate stimulants. Clonidine and guanfacine are third-line options or adjuncts that require careful cardiovascular monitoring. Mood stabilizers (e.g., lithium, divalproex, and carbamazepine) and atypical antipsychotics are adjuncts for control of aggression or comorbid bipolar disorder. Other agents require further investigation before their status in the treatment of ADHD can be fully determined.

TOURETTE'S DISORDER

EPIDEMIOLOGY AND CLINICAL PRESENTATION

Once considered rare, Tourette's disorder is present in 0.7% to 1.1% of boys and 0.4% of girls.[44,45] The essential features of this CNS disorder are multiple motor tics and one or more vocalizations. A tic is a sudden, rapid, recurrent, nonrhythmic, stereotyped motor movement or vocalization. See Table 61–6 and the accompanying references for examples of motor and vocal tics.[45,46] The clinical presentation may vary from barely noticeable to debilitating, and the type of tic expressed may change over time.[1,45,46]

Presence of both motor and vocal tics is necessary for more than 1 year before the diagnosis of Tourette's disorder is made. The median age of onset of motor tics is 6 years, with an average delay in diagnosis of 6.8 years.[1,45,46]

Transient tic disorder is diagnosed if motor or vocal tics occur for less than 1 year, with chronic tic disorder diagnosed if motor or vocal tics are present for longer than 1 year.[1,45] Tics are most prominent during childhood and may plateau or attenuate during adolescence. The early 20s frequently bring stabilization of symptoms, although exacerbations occur during adulthood with characteristic fluctuating symptom severity.[1,45,46]

Over 90% of children with Tourette's disorder have coexisting conditions such as ADHD (75%), mood disorders (60%), obsessive-compulsive disorder (40%), other anxiety disorders, or a combination of comorbidities.[45–47] Tourette's disorder itself does not cause diminished intellectual functioning; however, the severity of tics and associated illnesses can result in significant impairment in school functioning, sometimes necessitating special education classes.[45–47]

TABLE 61–6. Clinical Presentation of Tourette's Disorder

- Onset before age 18 years
- Multiple motor or one or more vocal tics present
- Motor and vocal tics do not need to occur concurrently

Motor Tics	Vocal Tics
Eye blinking, lip licking	Clicks, grunts
Facial twitching	Barking, yelping
Shoulder shrugging	Throat clearing, echolalia
Squatting, twirling	Coprolalia, palilalia

The tics occur many times a day (usually in bouts) nearly every day or intermittently throughout a period of more than 1 year, and during this period there was never a tic-free period of more than 3 consecutive months.
Data from American Psychiatric Association.[1]

ETIOLOGY AND PATHOPHYSIOLOGY

Tourette's disorder is transmitted in a complex polygenic pattern, whereas symptoms and severity of the disorder vary from one generation to another.[45-47] The neurochemical pathophysiology involves an imbalance in the interaction of dopaminergic, serotonergic, γ-aminobutyric acid (GABA)-ergic, glutamatergic, cholinergic, noradrenergic, and opioid systems in multiple brain regions, most notably the basal ganglia and caudate nucleus. The imbalance may cause a lack of regulation of the brain's inhibitory mechanisms, resulting in tics and associated behavior disorders. This multisystem etiology best explains the success of a variety of treatment options.[46,47]

▶ TREATMENT: Tourette's Disorder

5 Whenever symptoms are severe enough to impair the child's ability to function, drug therapy should be initiated. Haloperidol and pimozide (dopamine [D_2] receptor antagonists) are approved by the FDA and are highly effective with a relatively rapid onset. Clonidine is significantly less effective but has no risk of extrapyramidal side effects. Psychotherapy and behavioral treatment are useful adjuncts.[45-47]

Therapy with haloperidol or pimozide should be initiated at very low doses of 0.25 to 0.5 mg/day given at bedtime and then increased gradually. Gradual titration over 2 to 3 weeks helps minimize extrapyramidal and sedative effects while permitting careful assessment of response. Symptoms may regress within 48 to 72 hours after an effective dose is reached. Doses less than 5 mg/day are effective in controlling tics for most patients, but occasionally up to 10 mg/day or even 20 mg/day are required.[46,47] Pimozide is considered comparable or possibly superior to haloperidol in efficacy when equivalent doses are used.[45,46]

Risperidone, a serotonin (5-HT$_2$)/D_2 receptor antagonist, was significantly more effective than placebo in decreasing motor and vocal tic severity according to two controlled trials.[48,49] The mean daily dose was 2.5 mg/day (range 1 to 6 mg/day). In addition, in parallel comparison trials risperidone was found to be as effective as pimozide or clonidine. The mean risperidone dose in the pimozide trial was 3.8 mg/day, while the dose of risperidone ranged from 0.6 to 2.4 mg/day in the clonidine trial.[50,51] Ziprasidone, another 5HT$_2$/D_2 antagonist, showed significant efficacy versus placebo in a controlled study at an average dose of 30 mg/day titrated from a starting dose of 5 mg/day.[52,53] An open trial with olanzapine at a mean dose of 10.9 mg/day showed a 50% reduction in global tic severity.[54] Clozapine, a 5-HT$_2$ antagonist with minimal D$_1$-blocking and no significant D$_2$-blocking effects, was found to be ineffective with worsening of symptoms in some Tourette's patients.[46,47]

Clonidine is the most widely prescribed treatment for Tourette's disorder, according to an international database of 3500 cases, but its efficacy is not robust, and it is not more effective than DA antagonists.[46,47] In some patients, the response is limited to improvement in attention and behavior with no changes in the frequency of tics. A clonidine trial should be initiated carefully, usually 0.025 to 0.05 mg given in the morning or divided two to three times daily with gradual titration every 4 to 7 days to the usual therapeutic trial dose of 0.15 to 0.25 mg/day (maximum 0.6 mg/day).[45-47] Doses usually are divided during maintenance therapy for more continuous symptom control and to minimize adverse effects. Case reports describe a positive response from the clonidine patch as well. The onset of therapeutic effects for both tablet and patch is slow, ranging from 2 weeks to a few months.[46,47]

CLINICAL CONTROVERSY

The decision to treat Tourette's disorder with a D$_2$ receptor antagonist vs. an α_2-agonist can be controversial and challenging. The choice is usually based on whether high efficacy (D$_2$ antagonist) or milder adverse effect burden (α_2-agonist) is more desirable in an individual patient.[45-47]

COMORBIDITY

Pharmacotherapy of Tourette's disorder is challenging due to multiple coexisting disorders typically requiring medication combinations. Often the behavioral problems precede and are more disturbing than the involuntary movements, making them a treatment priority.

TOURETTE'S AND ADHD

Pharmacotherapy with stimulants increases dopaminergic and noradrenergic activity, which has the potential to aggravate or precipitate tics. One study examined the comparative effects of methylphenidate and dextroamphetamine on tics in children and found the majority experienced improvement in ADHD symptoms with acceptable effects on tics.[46,55] Methylphenidate was better tolerated than dextroamphetamine. Another double-blind placebo-controlled trial compared methylphenidate or clonidine monotherapy to combination methylphenidate and clonidine in patients with ADHD and Tourette's disorder. Combination therapy demonstrated the greatest benefit in reducing symptoms of ADHD and tics ($p < 0.0001$).[56] Clonidine appeared most helpful for impulsivity and hyperactivity, while methylphenidate was most helpful for inattention. All treatments were well tolerated.

Patients and caregivers should be aware of the risks of using stimulants in children with Tourette's disorder (see ADHD section); careful monitoring is essential.[46,47,55]

Controlled trials of TCA therapy for comorbid ADHD and chronic tics or Tourette's disorder show significant improvement in inattentive and hyperactive/impulsive symptoms without worsening of tics.[57] In one study, both tics and symptoms of ADHD improved.[57] TCAs offer an alternative to clonidine or combined clonidine/methylphenidate therapy that may be more effective for some patients.

Clonidine or guanfacine monotherapy is a less effective alternative to stimulants in the treatment of children with Tourette's disorder and ADHD. Guanfacine, a central α_{2a}-selective noradrenergic receptor agonist, was administered to 34 children (mean age 10.4 years), with ADHD and tic disorder during an 8-week placebo-controlled trial at a dose of 1.5 to 3 mg/day. Tic severity decreased by 31% in the guanfacine group compared to 0% in the placebo group.[27,46] There was a mean improvement of 37% on the teacher-rated ADHD scale compared to 8% improvement with placebo. Due to its similarity to clonidine, guanfacine's cardiovascular effects warrant careful clinical monitoring.[6,28,46,47]

Nicotine administration by gum or patch may potentiate the effects of dopamine-blocking agents in relieving tics, according to small controlled trials.[45,46,58] ADHD symptoms may improve as well.[46,58] The long-term adverse effects of nicotine on overall health may limit usefulness.

TOURETTE'S AND ANXIETY OR MOOD DISORDERS

Therapeutic trials (6 to 8 weeks) of an SSRI or clomipramine should be tried when obsessive-compulsive, anxiety, or depressive symptoms cause functional impairment in patients with Tourette's disorder.[46,47] Careful monitoring for behavioral activation, disinhibition, and motor restlessness is essential during SSRI or clomipramine therapy, because these symptoms occur in 20% to 40% of children and may require drug discontinuation.[45,46,59]

ADJUNCTIVE OR ALTERNATIVE TREATMENTS

For those who are unresponsive, partially responsive, or unable to tolerate DA antagonists or α_2-agonists, there are several adjuncts or alternative treatments available. Clonazepam, selegiline, or baclofen appear to offer the most promise in relieving tics and associated symptoms. Opioid agonists or antagonists are not effective. Botulinum toxin requires further study.[45-47] Nonpharmacologic interventions include support groups, "habit-reversal therapy," and even neurosurgery.[45,46,60]

ADVERSE EFFECTS

Adverse effects have been reported with haloperidol doses of 2 mg/day or greater. In one review of 24 patients treated with haloperidol for Tourette's disorder, 66.7% discontinued treatment due to intolerable side effects (e.g., dysphoria, akathisia, nervousness, sedation,

dystonia, and cognitive dulling or feeling drugged).[61] Lowering the dose may alleviate side effects. An antiparkinsonian agent such as benztropine (at a starting dose of 0.5 mg orally twice daily) generally will reverse extrapyramidal side effects. Whether a patient with Tourette's disorder is developing a new symptom or is developing tardive dyskinesia can be difficult to determine. Dosage titration of the medication and careful monitoring will assist in this clinical decision-making process.[46,47]

Pimozide is less likely to cause extrapyramidal side effects compared to haloperidol. Anticholinergic side effects may occur in addition to drowsiness, and occasionally, anxiety will occur. Electrocardiographic changes, including T- and U-wave abnormalities and prolongation of the QTc interval, are found rarely with recommended therapeutic doses for Tourette's disorder; however, drugs that inhibit cytochrome P450 isoenzyme 3A4 (e.g., clarithromycin or fluoxetine) should not be combined with pimozide due to the risk of excessively elevating pimozide blood levels and lethal QTc prolongation.[6,46,47]

Adverse effects reported during clinical studies in children taking risperidone and olanzapine include light-headedness, sedation, akathisia or agitation, weakness, insomnia, depressed mood, aggressive behavior, tachycardia, weight gain, hepatotoxicity, and extrapyramidal side effects including tardive dyskinesia.[32,46,47] Risperidone is more likely to be associated with hyperprolactinemia and extrapyramidal effects compared to olanzapine. However, olanzapine has been associated with greater weight gain and more cases of new-onset diabetes compared to risperidone. Ziprasidone carries a risk of QTc prolongation, hyperprolactinemia, extrapyramidal effects, restlessness, nausea, and mild sedation, but minimal to no weight gain.[32,53]

For clonidine and guanfacine the most common adverse effect is sedation. Fortunately, tolerance usually develops to this effect over days to weeks. The most potentially serious side effects are cardiovascular (see the ADHD section).[28] Other α_2-agonist side effects include dry mouth, constipation, headache, mood changes, and even a temporary worsening of tics in 10% of patients.

PHARMACOECONOMIC CONSIDERATIONS

No pharmacoeconomic studies have been published on Tourette's disorder. Haloperidol provides the most economic therapy due to high efficacy and low drug cost. Pimozide is more expensive than generic haloperidol. Although generic clonidine is inexpensive, delayed onset of effect and significantly lower efficacy substantially increase total costs of treatment. 5-HT$_2$/D$_2$ antagonists such as risperidone are expensive alternatives due to high medication costs.

EVALUATION OF THERAPEUTIC OUTCOMES

Evaluating therapeutic interventions is challenging, as most patients can suppress their tics voluntarily for minutes to hours.[45,46] Also numerous factors such as stress, concentration, and relaxation can impact tic frequency and severity. The use of regular videotaped assessments in conjunction with standardized rating scales (Yale Global Tic Severity Scale) is helpful in objectively evaluating symptoms, side effects, and overall drug response.[45-47]

Individuals with Tourette's disorder are particularly sensitive to medication side effects, so medication dosing must be

individualized with low starting doses and careful weekly titration to response, realizing that it may take 1 to 2 months for an adequate therapeutic trial. Children taking any dopamine-blocking medication should receive monitoring every 3 to 6 months for extrapyramidal effects with a standardized rating scale (e.g., abnormal involuntary movement scale [AIMS]).[32,33] Patients given pimozide should receive baseline and follow-up electrocardiograms.[6,46,47] Adult patients with Tourette's disorder still may be responsive to drug treatments that were effective during childhood, although the dose and schedule may require adjustment.[45-47]

CONCLUSION

Haloperidol, pimozide and potentially risperidone have the advantage of greatest efficacy and rapid onset in the treatment of Tourette's disorder. Ziprasidone shows promise; however, comparison studies with haloperidol, pimozide, or risperidone are needed to determine its relative safety and efficacy. Clonidine and guanfacine have the advantage of no extrapyramidal side effects, but they are significantly less effective and require ongoing cardiovascular monitoring. Drug treatment must be highly individualized, considering comorbid disorders, side-effect sensitivity, and drug interactions.

ENURESIS

ETIOLOGY, PATHOPHYSIOLOGY, AND CLINICAL PRESENTATION

The essential feature of enuresis is repeated involuntary or intentional voiding of urine by day or night that is not caused by a general medical condition (Table 61–7).[1] Medical causes of inappropriate voiding (e.g., diabetes mellitus, diabetes insipidus, seizure disorders, or urinary tract infections) should be ruled out. Enuresis may be primary or secondary. Primary enuresis, the most common type, is diagnosed if the child has never established urinary continence. Secondary enuresis follows an established period (3 to 6 months) of urinary continence.

At age 5, prevalence is 15% to 20%; at age 10 it is 5%; for adolescents it is 1%, and 0.5% of adults wet the bed at least once a month. There is a 15% annual rate of spontaneous remission. The ratio of males to females with enuresis is 3:2.[62–64] Factors that predispose a child to either type of enuresis include a positive family history,

TABLE 61–7. Clinical Presentation of Enuresis

- Age 5 years or older
- Child repeatedly voids urine into bed or clothes
- May be involuntary or intentional
- Clinically significant problem for child
- Either a frequency of twice a week for at least 3 consecutive months or presence of distress or impairment in social, academic, or occupational functioning.

Modified from American Psychiatric Association.[1]

reduced functional bladder capacity, delayed or lax toilet training, constipation, psychological factors, and developmental delay. Some children with nocturnal enuresis lack the normal circadian variation in urine excretion rate, urine osmolality, and antidiuretic hormone (ADH) secretion. Nocturnal enuresis is not associated with a particular sleep stage, although children with enuresis are more difficult to arouse.[63–65]

▶ TREATMENT: Enuresis

The first step in treating the child with enuresis is to educate the family about the high frequency of the problem, dispel any misconceptions, provide emotional support, and strongly discourage punishment. For younger children who have not been toilet trained properly, the conditioning technique of dry-bed training should be tried first. This technique encourages extra fluids during the day and restricts fluids close to bedtime. Children are encouraged to use the toilet before bedtime. If this method is unsuccessful, then a bed-wetting alarm can be used. After 3 to 4 months of using a bed-wetting alarm, enuresis is cured in more than 70% of children.[66,67]

Teaching continence skills and various behavioral and conditioning methods remain the primary treatments for enuresis, and drug treatment remains a secondary approach.[63,64,68,69] Combined treatment with an enuresis alarm and desmopressin may be successful for severe enuresis.[70]

DESMOPRESSIN

Desmopressin acetate, a synthetic analog of the natural human ADH arginine vasopressin, is currently available in a nasal spray and oral tablet for the treatment of nocturnal enuresis. Desmopressin raises overnight urinary osmotic concentration by increasing water reabsorption and reducing the volume of urine entering the bladder.[71,72] Desmopressin is effective in reducing the number of wet nights in 70% of children.[73] In a short-term (2-week) controlled study, 24.5% of adolescents/adults became completely dry,[67] whereas in a naturalistic 6-week trial, 22% of children became completely dry.[74] Patients with colds or allergies that affect the nasal mucosa may have a less-than-optimal response to desmopressin nasal spray.

Predictors of best response to desmopressin include older age (>9 years), fewer initial wet nights, and larger bladder capacity.[75,76] For children 6 years of age and older, the initial recommended nasal dose is 20 mcg at bedtime, increasing to 40 mcg at bedtime after 3 days if there is no response. Some patients may respond to as little as 10 mcg. One-half of each dose is administered in each nostril. About 10% of the dose of desmopressin is absorbed from the nasal mucosa,

and plasma concentrations reach a maximum about 45 minutes after administration. Less than 1% of oral desmopressin is absorbed, with effective dosages ranging from 200 to 600 mcg/day.[71] Biologic half-life is 4 to 6 hours, and the duration of action varies from 6 to 24 hours.[71]

TRICYCLIC ANTIDEPRESSANTS

Imipramine significantly increases the number of dry nights for 70% to 80% of children with enuresis.[77] Imipramine is the most studied TCA, although desipramine, amitriptyline, and nortriptyline are also effective. The exact mechanism of action of TCAs in treating enuresis is unknown; proposed mechanisms include an anticholinergic effect, an α-adrenergic agonist effect, and an increase in ADH.[63,71] An initially effective dose often becomes ineffective in 2 to 6 weeks, but increasing the dose usually re-establishes control. For children 6 years of age and older, the initial dose of imipramine should be 25 mg at bedtime, with weekly increases of 25 mg if necessary. A nightly dose greater than 75 mg is rarely necessary, although doses up to 150 mg have been required in teenagers.[25,78]

ADVERSE EFFECTS

Infrequent adverse effects of desmopressin spray include nasal irritation, epistaxis, rhinitis, and nasal congestion, whereas desmopressin tablets or spray may cause transient headache, chills, dizziness, nausea, and abdominal pain. Rarely, water intoxication, hyponatremia, and subsequent tonic-clonic seizures have been reported,[74] particularly in children with concurrent physical disorders, intentional overdoses, or excessive fluid intake. When desmopressin is administered, evening fluids should be limited to 8 ounces to prevent hyponatremia or water intoxication.[79,80]

TCA adverse effects are dose related and include sedation, dizziness, dry mouth, constipation, weight gain, and the risk of electrocardiographic changes, heart block, and lowering of the seizure threshold.[25]

PHARMACOECONOMIC CONSIDERATIONS

No pharmacoeconomic studies on enuresis are available. The use of a bed-wetting alarm provides the highest overall cure rate, and drugs are a secondary approach. However, insurance companies commonly reimburse drug therapy, whereas they do not reimburse for alarms. The most inexpensive drug therapy is low-dose TCA; however, electrocardiographic and TCA blood level monitoring increases overall costs. Therapy with desmopressin is substantially more expensive than with TCAs due to higher drug cost.

EVALUATION OF THERAPEUTIC OUTCOMES

Before treatment begins, an accurate baseline of bed-wetting frequency must be established. A 50% or greater increase in dry nights is considered a therapeutic response. For example, if baseline dry nights are 2 out of 7 days per week, and drug treatment results in 4 or more dry nights per week, the drug is considered effective. If only one more dry night per week occurs and the drug is at the low end of the dosing range, a dosage increase is needed.[66,67,71,72]

At least 1 week is needed to evaluate the efficacy of TCAs, and 2 weeks may be needed for evaluation of desmopressin. If drug treatment is ongoing for several months, particularly if enuresis has resolved, attempts to discontinue the drug every 3 to 6 months are recommended to assess for spontaneous remission. Slow tapering of the medication may decrease the frequency of relapse. Unfortunately, therapeutic drug efficacy does not extend beyond drug discontinuation.[73,77,81,82] Drug plasma level monitoring is not established for desmopressin; however, plasma concentrations of imipramine plus desipramine of greater than 116 ng/mL have been correlated with increased clinical response.[77]

CONCLUSION

Overall, both desmopressin and TCAs are effective in the treatment of nocturnal enuresis as long as the drug is maintained. Drug selection is based on adverse-effect profiles, ease of administration, and cost. Imipramine has a higher adverse effect burden compared to desmopressin, and the risk of accidental overdose is of concern, especially in very disorganized families. In contrast, desmopressin is markedly more expensive than imipramine.

ABBREVIATIONS

ADH: antidiuretic hormone
ADHD: attention-deficit/hyperactivity disorder
AIMS: abnormal involuntary movement scale
DA: dopamine
D_2, D_4: dopamine receptors
GABA-γ-aminobutyric acid
5-HT$_2$: serotonin
MAO: monoamine oxidase
NE: norepinephrine
SSRI: selective serotonin reuptake inhibitor
TCA: tricyclic antidepressant

Review Questions and other resources can be found at *www.pharmacotherapyonline.com*.

REFERENCES

1. American Psychiatric Association. Diagnostic and Statistical Manual of Mental Disorders, 4th ed., Text Revision. Washington, American Psychiatric Press, 2000:39–134.
2. Barkley RA. Major life activity and health outcomes associated with attention-deficit/hyperactivity disorder. J Clin Psychiatry 2002;63(Suppl 12):10–15.
3. NIH Consensus Development Conference Statement on the Diagnosis and Treatment of ADHD. J Am Acad Child Adolesc Psychiatry 2000;39:182–193.
4. American Academy of Pediatrics. Clinical practice guideline: Diagnosis and evaluation of the child with attention-deficit/hyperactivity disorder. Pediatrics 2000;105:1158–1170.
5. Wilens TE, Biederman J, Spencer TJ. Attention deficit/hyperactivity disorder across the lifespan. Ann Rev Med 2002;53:113–131.
6. Pliszka SR, Greenhill LL, Crismon ML, et al. The Texas medication algorithm project: Report of the Texas consensus conference panel on medication treatment of childhood attention-deficit/hyperactivity disorder, parts 1 and 2. J Am Acad Child Adolesc Psychiatry 2000;39:908–927.
7. Buitelaar JK, Montgomery SA, van Zwieten-Boot. Attention deficit hyperactivity disorder: Guidelines for investigating efficacy of pharmacological intervention. Eur Neuropsychopharmacology 2003;13:297–304.
8. Mick E, Biederman J, Faraone SV, et al. Case-control study of attention-deficit hyperactivity disorder and maternal smoking, alcohol use, and drug use during pregnancy. J Am Acad Child Adolesc Psychiatry 2002;41:378–385.
9. Barkley RA. Attention-deficit hyperactivity disorder. Sci Am 1998;279:66–71.
10. Castellanos FX, Lee PP, Sharp W, et al. Developmental trajectories of brain volume abnormalities in children and adolescents with attention-deficit/hyperactivity disorder. JAMA 2002;288:1740–1748.
11. Castellanos FX, Sharp WS, Gottesman RF, et al. Anatomic brain abnormalities in monozygotic twins discordant for attention deficit hyperactivity disorder. Am J Psychol 2003;160:1693–1696.
12. Spencer TJ, Biederman J, Wilens TJ, et al. Overview of neurobiology of attention-deficit/hyperactivity disorder. J Clin Psychiatry 2002;63(Suppl 12):3–9.
13. Pliszka SR, McCracken JT, Maas JW. Catecholamines in attention-deficit hyperactivity disorder: Current perspectives. J Am Acad Child Adolesc Psychiatry 1996;35:264–272.
14. MTA Cooperative Group. A 14-month randomized clinical trial of strategies for attention-deficit/hyperactivity disorder. Arch Gen Psychiatry 1999; 56:1073–1086.
15. Greenhill LL, Pliszka S, Dulcan MK, et al. Practice parameter for the use of stimulant medications in the treatment of children, adolescents and adults. J Am Acad Child Adolesc Psychiatry 2002;41(Suppl 2):26S–49S.
16. American Academy of Pediatrics. Clinical practice guideline: Treatment of the school-aged child with ADHD. Pediatrics 2001;108:1033–1044.
17. Pliszka SR, Browne RG, Olvera RL, et al. A double-blind, placebo-controlled study of Adderall and methylphenidate in the treatment of ADHD. J Am Acad Child Adolesc Psychiatry 2000;39:619–626.
18. Keating GM, Figgitt DP. Dexmethylphenidate. Drugs 2002;62:1899–1904.
19. Swanson J, Gupta S, Lam A, et al. Development of a new once-a-day formulation of methylphenidate for the treatment of attention-deficit/hyperactivity disorder: Proof-of-concept and proof-of-product studies. Arch Gen Psychiatry 2003;60:204–211.
20. Lisska MC, Rivkees SA. Daily methylphenidate use slows the growth of children: A community based study. J Pediatr Endocrinol 2003;16:711–718.
21. Kramer JR, Loney J, Ponto LB, et al. Predictors of adult height and weight in boys treated with methylphenidate for childhood behavior problems. J Am Acad Child Adolesc Psychiatry 2000;39:517–524.
22. Caballerro J, Nahata MC. Atomoxetine hydrochloride for the treatment of ADHD. Clin Ther 2003;25:3065–3083.

23. Wernicke JF, Kratochvil CJ. Safety profile of atomoxetine in the treatment of children and adolescents with ADHD. J Clin Psychiatry 2002;63(Suppl 12):50–55.

24. Daviss WB, Bentivoglio P, Racusn R, et al. Bupropion sustained release in adolescents with comorbid attention-deficit/hyperactivity disorder and depression. J Am Acad Child Adolesc Psychiatry 2001;40:307–314.

25. Daly JM, Wilens T. The use of tricyclic antidepressants in children and adolescents. Pediatr Clin North Am 1998;45:1123–1135.

26. Hazell PL, Stuart JE. A randomized controlled trial of clonidine added to psychostimulant medication for hyperactive and aggressive children. J Am Acad Child Adolesc Psychiatry 2003;42:886–894.

27. Scahill L, Chappell PB, Kim Young S, et al. A placebo-controlled study of guanfacine in the treatment of children with tic disorders and attention deficit hyperactivity disorder. Am J Psychol 2001;158:1067–1074.

28. Cantwell DP, Swanson J, Connor DF. Case study: Adverse response to clonidine. J Am Acad Child Adolesc Psychiatry 1997;36:539–544.

29. Klein-Schwartz W. Trends and toxic effects from pediatric clonidine exposures. Arch Pediatr Adolesc Med 2002;156:392–396.

30. State RC, Altshuler LI, Frye MA. Mania and attention deficit hyperactivity disorder in a prepubertal child: Diagnostic and treatment challenges. Am J Psychiatry 2002;159:918–925.

31. Silva R, Munoz D, Alpert M. Carbamazepine use in children and adolescents with features of attention-deficit hyperactivity disorder: A meta-analysis. J Am Acad Child Adolesc Psychiatry 1996;35:352–358.

32. Schur SB, Sikich L, Fingling RL, et al. Treatment recommendations for the use of antipsychotics for aggressive youth (TRAAY) Part 1: A review. J Am Acad Child Adolesc Psychiatry 2003;42:132–144.

33. Pappadopulos E, Macintyre J, Crismon ML, et al. Treatment recommendations for the use of antipsychotics for aggressive youth (TRAAY) Part 2. J Am Acad Child Adolesc Psychiatry 2003;42:145–161.

34. Hughes CW, Emslie GJ, Crismon ML, et al. The Texas children's medication algorithm project: Report of the Texas consensus conference panel on medication treatment of childhood major depressive disorder. J Am Acad Child Adolesc Psychiatry 1999;38:1442–1454.

35. Gross-Tsur V, Manor O, van der Meere J, et al. Epilepsy and attention deficit hyperactivity disorder: Is methylphenidate safe and effective? J Pediatr 1997;130:40–44.

36. Leibson CL, Katusic SK, Barbaresi WJ, et al. Use and costs of medical care for children and adolescents with and without attention-deficit/hyperactivity disorder. JAMA 2001;285:60–66.

37. Collett BR, Ohan JL, Myers KM. Ten-year review of rating scales: Scales assessing attention-deficit/hyperactivity disorder. J Am Acad Child Adolesc Psychiatry 2003;42:1015–1037.

38. Dopheide JA. Management of depression in children and adolescents. J Pharm Pract 2001;14:488–497.

39. LeFever GB, Dawson KV, Morrow AL. The extent of drug therapy for attention deficit-hyperactivity disorder among children in public schools. Am J Public Health 1999;89:1359–1364.

40. Angold A, Alaattin E, Egger HL, et al. Stimulant treatment for children: A community perspective. J Am Acad Child Adolesc Psychiatry 2000;39:975–984.

41. Hoagwood K, Kelleher KJ, Feil M, et al. Treatment services for children with ADHD: A national perspective. J Am Acad Child Adolesc Psychiatry 2000;39:198–206.

42. Wilens TE, Faraone SV, Biederman J, et al. Does stimulant therapy of attention-deficit/hyperactivity disorder beget later substance abuse? A meta-analytic review of the literature. Pediatrics 2003;111:179–185.

43. Tapert SF, Baratta MV, Abrantes AM, et al. Attention dysfunction predicts substance involvement in community youths. J Am Acad Child Adolesc Psychiatry 2002;41:680–686.

44. Kadesjo B, Gillberg C. Tourette's disorder: Epidemiology and comorbidity in primary school children. J Am Acad Child Adolesc Psychiatry 2000;39:548–555.

45. Jankovic J. Medical progress: Tourette's syndrome. N Engl J Med 2001;345:1184–1192.

46. Muller-Vahl JT. The treatment of Tourette's syndrome: Current opinions. Expert Opin Pharmacother 2002;3:899–914.

47. Jimenez-Jimenez FJ. Pharmacological options for the treatment of Tourette's disorder. Drugs 2001;61:2207–2200.

48. Dion Y, Annable L, Sandor P, et al. Risperidone in the treatment of Tourette syndrome: A double-blind, placebo-controlled trial. J Clin Psychopharmacol 2002;22:31–39.

49. Scahill L, Leckman JF, Schultz RT, et al. A placebo-controlled trial of risperidone in Tourette's syndrome. Neurology 2003;60:1130–1135.

50. Gaffney GR, Perry P, Lund BC, et al. Risperidone versus clonidine in the treatment of children and adolescents with Tourette's syndrome. J Am Acad Child Adolesc Psychiatry 2002;41:330–336.

51. Bruggeman R, van der Linden, Buitelaar JK, et al. Risperidone versus pimozide in Tourette's disorder: A comparative double-blind parallel-group study. J Clin Psychiatry 2001;62:50–56.

52. Sallee FR, Kurlan R, Goetz CG, et al. Ziprasidone treatment of children and adolescents with Tourette's syndrome: A pilot study. J Am Acad Child Adolesc Psychiatry 2000;39:292–299.

53. Sallee FR, Gilbert DL, Vinks AA, et al. Pharmacodynamics of ziprasidone in children and adolescents: Impact on dopamine transmission. J Am Acad Child Adolesc Psychiatry 2003;42:902–907.

54. Budman CL, Gayer A, Lesser M, et al. An open label study of the treatment of Tourette's disorder. J Clin Psychiatry 2001;62:290–294.

55. Castellanos FX, Giedd JN, Elia J, et al. Controlled stimulant treatment of ADHD and comorbid Tourette's syndrome: Effects of stimulant and dose. J Am Acad Child Adolesc Psychiatry 1997;36:589–596.

56. Tourette's Syndrome Study Group. Treatment of ADHD in children with tics: A randomized controlled trial. Neurology 2002;58:527–536.

57. Spencer T, Biederman J, Coffey B, et al. A double-blind comparison of desipramine and placebo in children and adolescents with chronic tic disorder and comorbid attention-deficit/hyperactivity disorder. Arch Gen Psychiatry 2002;59:649–656.

58. Silver AA, Shytle D, Philipp MK. Transdermal nicotine and haloperidol in Tourette's disorder: A double-blind placebo-controlled study. J Clin Psychiatry 2001;62:707–714.

59. Leonard HL, March J, Rickler KC, et al. Pharmacology of the selective serotonin reuptake inhibitors in children and adolescents. J Am Acad Child Adolesc Psychiatry 1997;36:725–736.

60. Wilhelm S, Deckersbach T, Coffey BJ, et al. Habit reversal versus supportive psychotherapy for Tourette's disorder: A randomized controlled trial. Am J Psychiatry 2003;160:1175–1177.

61. Silva RR, Munoz DM, Daniel W, et al. Causes of haloperidol discontinuation in patients with Tourette's disorder: Management and alternatives. J Clin Psychiatry 1996;57:129–135.

62. Hjalmas K. Nocturnal enuresis: Basic facts and new horizons. Eur Urol 1998;33:53–57.

63. Jalkut MW, Lerman SE, Churchill BM. Enuresis. Pediatr Clin North Am 2001;48:1461–1488.

64. Mikkelsen EJ. Enuresis and encopresis: Ten years of progress. J Am Acad Child Adolesc Psychiatry 2001;40:1146–1158.

65. Issenman RM, Filmer RB, Gorski PA. A review of bowel and bladder control development in children: How gastrointestinal and urologic conditions relate to problems in toilet training. Pediatrics 1999;103:1346–1352.

66. Rushton HG. Nocturnal enuresis: Epidemiology, evaluation and currently available treatment options. J Pediatr 1998;114:691–696.

67. Monda JM, Husmann DA. Primary nocturnal enuresis: A comparison among observation, imipramine, desmopressin acetate and bedwetting alarm systems. J Urol 1995;154:745–748.

68. Moffatt MEK. Nocturnal enuresis: A review of the efficacy of treatments and practical advice for clinicians. Dev Behav Pediatr 1997;18:49–56.

69. Lackgren G, Hjalmas K, van Gool J, et al. Nocturnal enuresis: A suggestion for a European treatment strategy. Acta Paediatr 1999;88:679–690.

70. Bradbury MG, Meadow SR. Combined treatment with enuresis alarm and desmopressin for nocturnal enuresis. Acta Paediatr 1995;84:1014–1018.

71. Gimpel GA, Warzak WJ, Kuhn BR, Walburn JN. Clinical perspectives in primary nocturnal enuresis. Clin Pediatr 1998;37:23–30.

72. Janknegt RA, Zweers HM, Delaere KP, et al. Oral desmopressin as a new treatment modality for primary nocturnal enuresis in adolescents and

adults: A double-blind, randomized, multicenter study. Dutch Enuresis Study Group. J Urol 1997;157:513–517.

3. Glazener CM, Evans JH. Desmopressin for nocturnal enuresis in children. Cochrane Database Syst Rev 2002;3:CD002112.

74. Hjalmas K, Hanson E, Hellstrom AL, et al. Long-term treatment with desmopressin in children with primary monosymptomatic nocturnal enuresis: An open multicentre study. Swedish Enuresis Trial (SWEET) Group. Br J Urol 1998;82:704–709.

75. Rushton HG, Belman AB, Skoog S, et al. Predictors of response to desmopressin in children and adolescents with monosymptomatic nocturnal enuresis. Scand J Urol Nephrol 1995;173:109–111.

76. Eller DA, Austin PF, Tanguay S, Homsy YL. Daytime functional bladder capacity as a predictor of response to desmopressin in monosymptomatic nocturnal enuresis. Eur Urol 1998;S33:25–29.

77. Fritz GK, Rockney RM, Yeung AS. Plasma levels and efficacy of

imipramine treatment for enuresis. J Am Acad Child Adolesc Psychiatry 1994;33:60–64.

78. Donoghue MB, Latimer E, Pillsbury HL, Hertzog JH. Hyponatremic seizure in a child using desmopressin for nocturnal enuresis. Arch Pediatr Adolesc Med 1998;152:290–292.

79. Robson WL, Norgaard JP, Leung AK. Hyponatremia in patients with nocturnal enuresis treated with DDAVP. Eur J Pediatr 1996;155:959–962.

80. Owens RG, Karram MM. Comparative tolerability of drug therapies used to treat incontinence and enuresis. Drug Saf 1998;19:123–139.

81. Glazener CM, Evans JH. Tricyclic and related drugs for nocturnal enuresis in children. Cochrane Database Syst Rev 2000;3:CD002117.

82. Riccabona M, Oswald J, Glauninger P. Long-term use and tapered dose reduction of intranasal desmopressin in the treatment of enuretic children. Br J Urol 1998;81(Suppl 3):S24–S25.

62
EATING DISORDERS

Patricia A. Marken and Roger W. Sommi

Learning Objectives and other resources can be found at *www.pharmacotherapyonline.com.*

KEY CONCEPTS

◀1 The causes of eating disorders are complex, so ongoing multidisciplinary treatment is needed to ensure a positive outcome. Outpatient treatment is appropriate for the majority of patients.

◀2 Careful medical and psychiatric assessments are needed at baseline to determine severity of illness and comorbid conditions.

◀3 Nonpharmacologic measures such as cognitive behavioral therapy (CBT), nutritional counseling, family therapy, and interpersonal psychotherapy are the cornerstone of management of anorexia nervosa (AN).

◀4 In patients with AN, one goal is to achieve and maintain a body weight within 85% of the normal weight for age and height. If the patient is malnourished, oral refeeding with the daily caloric intake slowly titrated upward to 2,000 to 3,000 kcal/day is preferred. Parenteral refeeding is a treatment of last resort.

◀5 Antidepressants in AN are reserved for patients with mood, anxiety, and obsessional symptoms that persist after weight has improved.

◀6 Antidepressants can improve both mood and specific target symptoms in bulimia nervosa (BN), but they remain adjunctive to nonpharmacologic treatments.

◀7 Selective serotonin reuptake inhibitors (SSRIs) are first-line agents when medications are indicated for BN, because of improved tolerability and safety, but they do not have superior efficacy compared with other antidepressant classes. The dose of fluoxetine in BN is higher (60 mg/day) than the dose usually used in depression.

◀8 An adequate drug therapy trial is 4 to 8 weeks. If drug treatment fails, consider a lack of absorption as a cause, since the patient may be vomiting up the drug.

◀9 The optimal duration of antidepressant treatment is unknown, but most clinicians will continue them for 6 to 12 months in patients who respond and then re-evaluate the need for ongoing medication management. The long-term course is variable, but there is the potential for a fatal outcome from cardiac arrest or suicide.

◀10 Monitoring in BN should include frequency and severity of binge/purge episodes, exercise patterns, use of laxatives or ipecac, mood and anxiety symptoms, eating habits, daily caloric intake, weight, and changes in laboratory abnormalities.

The eating disorders encompass several complex diseases that share a central pathologic feature of overevaluation of shape and weight. Eating disorders arise from the interaction between environmental, societal, developmental, psychosocial, genetic, and biologic factors. It is estimated that 5 to 10 million women and 1 million men in the United States have an eating disorder. The urbanization of society and an increasing obsession with perfection have led to an increasing prevalence of eating disorders, most alarmingly in an increasingly younger population.[1-3] Anorexia nervosa (AN) was described over a century ago; bulimia nervosa (BN) emerged as a distinct disorder in 1979, and other eating disorders and subtypes continue to be defined.[4-6] Extensive research has improved our understanding of these severely disabling and potentially fatal disorders. Management, however, remains difficult, and pharmacologic management is only a small part of a comprehensive plan that emphasizes cognitive behavioral therapy and psychotherapy.

EPIDEMIOLOGY

ANOREXIA NERVOSA

AN occurs predominantly in females (90%) and usually presents in late adolescence. The median age of onset is 17, with new cases rarely occurring after age 40. Its reported prevalence in the United States ranges from 1 in 100 to 1 in 800 for females between the ages of 12 and 18 years.[7] AN is reportedly on the rise, with the prevalence increasing sixfold in the 1970s versus the 1960s, and a rise in the number of prepubertal teens and males with the disease.[3]

BULIMIA NERVOSA

BN also occurs predominantly in females (90%) and usually presents in adolescence or early adult life.[4] Between 1% and 4.6% of adolescent and young adult females meet diagnostic criteria for BN, with the prevalence being 10 times higher than in males.[3,7,8]

EATING DISORDER NOT OTHERWISE SPECIFIED

Eating disorder not otherwise specified is also described in the American Psychiatric Association's *Diagnostic and Statistical Manual of Mental Disorders,* 4th Edition, Text Revision (DSM-IV-TR).[3,7] Its prevalence is 4.7% of the population and up to 50% of eating disorder patients admitted to tertiary care settings have this condition.[9] Individuals present with symptoms characteristic of eating disorders, but they do not meet the diagnostic criteria for a specific eating disorder.

BINGE EATING DISORDER

Binge eating disorder (BED) is currently a research diagnosis, although there is significant interest in treatment. The diagnostic criteria for BED describe recurrent episodes of binge eating without compensatory behavior (purging, excessive exercise, or fasting). BED typically presents later in life (40s), and approximately one-fourth of BED patients are male.[9,10]

ETIOLOGY AND PATHOPHYSIOLOGY

1 The potential etiologic or exacerbating factors for eating disorders represent an array of physiologic, biochemical, developmental, genetic, psychological, psychosocial, and psychiatric phenomena. The biologic basis for eating disorders is difficult to delineate because it is unclear whether the observed biologic changes are caused by or are a result of the aberrant eating behavior.

Abnormalities of the hypothalamic-pituitary-gonadal, hypothalamic-pituitary-adrenal, and hypothalamic-pituitary-thyroid axes are described as potential causes of AN. An extensive review of the psychoendocrinology of AN is provided by the Work Group on Eating Disorders.[9] Although many endocrine abnormalities occur in other forms of starvation, a primary difference with AN is that the dysfunction may not correct despite weight normalization, suggesting a primary biologic abnormality.[10] Amenorrhea is found in the majority of females with AN, supporting the role of the hypothalamic-pituitary-gonadal axis, and in particular, the function of the gonadotropins luteinizing hormone, follicle-stimulating hormone, and gonadotropin-releasing hormone.[8] Up to 25% of females have amenorrhea before the onset of AN, and the return of menses lags behind weight normalization.

The roles of serotonin, norepinephrine, and dopamine have been studied extensively, as these neurotransmitters have important functions in controlling eating behaviors. Dysfunctions in these systems have been found, although many are thought to be secondary to associated weight loss. Some aspects of serotonin function do remain abnormal after weight restoration, leading investigators to propose that other mechanisms are involved.[11,12]

Reasonably strong genetic influences are present in AN, and genetics may play a role in the occurrence of BN as well. In twin studies, concordance of approximately 55% and 35% in monozygotic twins and 5% and 30% in dizygotic twins for AN and BN, respectively, has been reported. Genetic mutation studies have focused on polymorphisms of the serotonin 2A receptor, with mixed preliminary results.[10]

A great deal of emphasis is placed on psychological and developmental issues in the pathogenesis of eating disorders, especially regarding the role of the family. Family separations, losses, and dysfunction (sexual or physical abuse, neglect, and substance dependence) may trigger abnormal eating behavior.[3,8,9,13] Whether family-related issues are truly etiologic for eating disorders remains controversial, although the prognosis is better when a relatively healthy family environment is present. Finally, athletes are at special risk for eating disorders, especially female gymnasts, figure skaters, distance runners, swimmers, and male wrestlers and body builders.[14]

Eating disorders are complex and cannot be explained by a simple physiologic, biochemical, developmental, psychological, or psychiatric model. Instead a multifaceted perspective will best serve the clinician in making decisions about treatment alternatives.

DIAGNOSTIC CRITERIA AND CLINICAL PRESENTATION

2 AN and BN occur together in about 30% to 64% of patients with eating disorders, and may not be distinct diagnostic entities, but rather occur along a continuum of symptoms.[15–17] Many patients initially present with either AN or BN and alternate from one eating disorder to the other or with an atypical eating disorder. Figure 62–1 presents symptoms that are specific to AN or BN and those symptoms that are shared between the disorders.

The medical consequences of eating disorders are many and are related primarily to self-induced starvation and purging. Patients commonly present with vague complaints of lethargy and pain. Metabolic and electrolyte disturbances along with dehydration are common

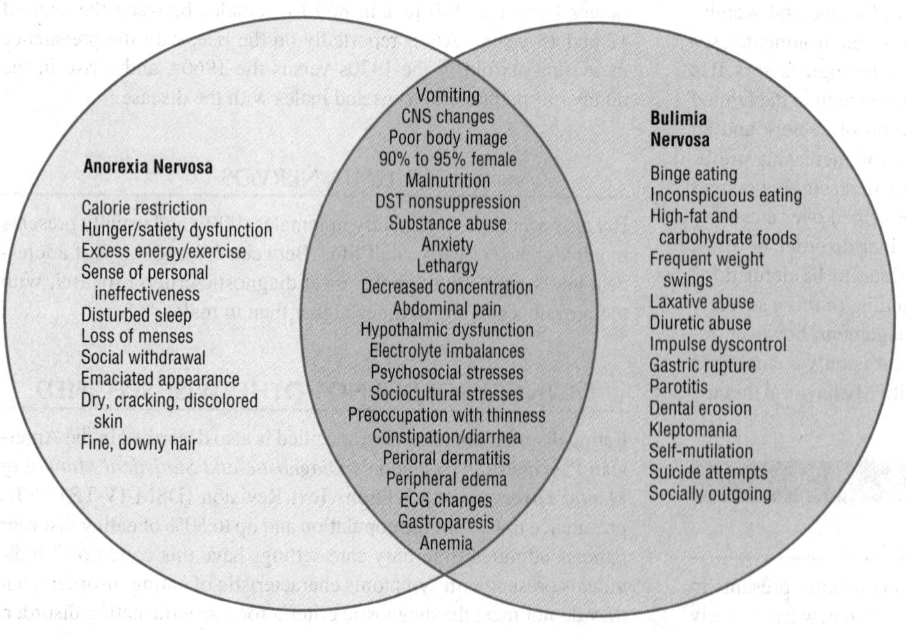

Anorexia Nervosa

Calorie restriction
Hunger/satiety dysfunction
Excess energy/exercise
Sense of personal
  ineffectiveness
Disturbed sleep
Loss of menses
Social withdrawal
Emaciated appearance
Dry, cracking, discolored
  skin
Fine, downy hair

Vomiting
CNS changes
Poor body image
90% to 95% female
Malnutrition
DST nonsuppression
Substance abuse
Anxiety
Lethargy
Decreased concentration
Abdominal pain
Hypothalmic dysfunction
Electrolyte imbalances
Psychosocial stresses
Sociocultural stresses
Preoccupation with thinness
Constipation/diarrhea
Perioral dermatitis
Peripheral edema
ECG changes
Gastroparesis
Anemia

Bulimia Nervosa

Binge eating
Inconspicuous eating
High-fat and
  carbohydrate foods
Frequent weight
  swings
Laxative abuse
Diuretic abuse
Impulse dyscontrol
Gastric rupture
Parotitis
Dental erosion
Kleptomania
Self-mutilation
Suicide attempts
Socially outgoing

FIGURE 62–1. Signs and symptoms of anorexia nervosa and bulimia nervosa.

nd occur because of poor dietary intake, self-induced vomiting, or hronic laxative and diuretic abuse. Severe electrolyte disturbances an cause cardiac disturbances and even sudden death. Abnormali- ies of the hypothalamic-pituitary-gonadal axis are likely the result of tarvation. These abnormalities include effects on estradiol, the go- nadotropins (e.g., luteinizing hormone, follicle-stimulating hormone, nd gonadotropin-releasing hormone), thyroid function, adrenal func- ion, and growth hormone.[8] Osteoporosis and infertility are potential ong-term complications of endocrine changes. Vomiting can cause ental problems, including decalcification, erosion of the enamel and entin layers, and staining of the surfaces of the teeth.[7] Chronic starva- ion can cause brain atrophy visible on computed tomographic scan s an increase in ventricular:brain ratio. Decreases in white matter nd cerebrospinal fluid volumes return to normal after a healthy veight is achieved, but gray matter loss may continue to persist. Gray matter loss can be demonstrated during neuropsychological esting.[9,18,19] A thorough physical and laboratory evaluation, as de- cribed in Table 62–1, is needed to determine the severity of medical omplications.[7,13,20] The presence of a particular medical complica- ion depends on whether the patient engages in starvation or purging vomiting or laxative abuse) and the frequency and severity of the ehavior.

Depression, schizophrenia, obsessive-compulsive disorder, and onversion disorders should be included in the differential diagno- is of AN and BN because eating abnormalities can be a compo- ent of these illnesses. The salient difference between these psy- hiatric disorders and eating disorders is the overriding drive for hinness, a disturbed body image, increased energy directed toward osing weight, and binge eating episodes that are relatively specific for the eating disorders. Additionally, many patients will experi- nce relief of the psychiatric symptoms on refeeding and not require psychotropics.[9]

TABLE 62–1. Physical and Laboratory Assessment of Eating Disorders

Evaluation	Target Symptoms
Pulse	Bradycardia
Blood pressure	Hypotension, orthostasis
Respiratory rate	Rapid if heart failure occurs during refeeding
Temperature	Hypothermia, cold intolerance
Electrocardiogram	ST depression, flat T waves, U waves, increased QT interval, atrioventricular block
Gastrointestinal	Hypoactive bowel sounds, gastritis, abdominal distention
Skin	Dry, scaling, lanugo, hair loss, calluses on fingers and hands
Menses	Amenorrhea
Complete blood count	Leukopenia, anemias, thrombocytopenia
Electrolytes	Hypokalemia, hypomagnesemia, hypo- or hyperphosphatemia
pH	Metabolic alkalosis (acidosis if laxative abuse)
Amylase	Elevated, pancreatitis rare
Liver	Hypoalbuminemia, γ-glutamyl transferase if alcohol abuse
Thyroid	Low to low normal, but not true disease
Cortisol	Elevated with lack of suppression on dexamethasone suppression test
Bone density	Osteoporosis

Modified from American Psychiatric Association[7] and Halmi.[13]

ANOREXIA NERVOSA

The core features of AN include refusal to maintain a minimal nor- mal body weight (e.g., >85% normal body weight or body mass index >17.5 kg/m^2) or failure to make expected weight gains, intense fear and obsession about weight gain or being "fat," a distorted body im- age, and amenorrhea for at least three consecutive cycles. Patients typically lack an appreciation for the degree of weight loss experi- enced, or are preoccupied with the idea that a part of their body is too large, despite evidence to the contrary. DSM-IV-TR further clas- sifies AN into restricting type (the person does not regularly engage in binge eating or purging behavior), or binge eating/purging type, in which they regularly participate in such behavior.[7] The AN patient has difficulty sensing when he or she is full (satiety) and commonly complains of feeling bloated soon after they start eating. Patients also describe not feeling in control of various aspects of their life, and in particular, of caloric intake. When patients with AN are underweight, they often present with features of major depression, but these symp- toms should initially be considered to be secondary to starvation and not indicative of a true mood disorder.

CLINICAL PRESENTATION OF ANOREXIA NERVOSA

GENERAL
Patients refuse to maintain body weight and have distorted perceptions about their body.

SYMPTOMS
- Patients have obsessions and fears about eating and gaining weight.
- They complain about feeling full even when they have eaten very little food.
- Denial of symptoms and low self-esteem is the norm. They often feel ineffective and have a lack of self-control.

SIGNS
Weakness, lethargy, cachexia, amenorrhea, vomiting, re- stricted food intake, inappropriate exercise, delayed sexual development, edema, delayed gastric emptying, constipation, bradycardia, hypotension, osteoporosis, dry cracking skin, lanugo, callus on dorsum of hand, perioral dermatitis, ero- sion of dental enamel

LABORATORY TESTS
Hypokalemia, hypokalemic alkalosis, hypomagnesemia, leukopenia, QT interval prolongation, ST-segment depres- sion, U Waves, hypercholesterolemia, anemia

OTHER DIAGNOSTIC TESTS
Nonspecific EEG changes

Psychiatric comorbidity is common, as up to 75% of patients have a primary mood disorder.[21] A link between AN and anxiety disorders, especially social phobia (fear of eating in public) and obsessive-compulsive disorder, has been noted. The lifetime preva- lence of obsessive-compulsive disorder in patients with AN is re- ported to be as high as 25%, much higher than the lifetime prevalence in the general population (2.5%).[21,22] Personality disorders are also more common among people with AN, especially the avoidant and obsessive-compulsive types, than in the general population.[23,24]

CLINICAL PRESENTATION OF BULIMIA NERVOSA

GENERAL

- Patients binge eat and stop when they have abdominal pain or self-induced vomiting or are interrupted by another individual.
- They have a pattern of severe dieting followed by binge-eating episodes.
- They are concerned about their body image but do not have the drive to thinness as do patients with AN.

SYMPTOMS

- Patients do not eat regular meals and do not feel satiety at the end of a meal.
- May use laxatives for weight control.
- They have guilt, depression, and self-disparagement after binges.
- Social isolation can result from frequent bingeing.
- Chaotic and troubled personal relationships and substance abuse are common.

SIGNS

Bingeing, vomiting, salivary gland inflammation, erosion of dental enamel, callus on dorsum of hand, perioral dermatitis, caries, parotid gland enlargement, abdominal pain. Upper end of normal weight or slightly overweight. Frequent weight fluctuations. Diminished masticatory ability.

LABORATORY TESTS

Hypokalemia, hypochloremic metabolic acidosis, elevated serum amylase

OTHER DIAGNOSTIC TESTS

None

BULIMIA NERVOSA

The core feature of BN is recurrent episodes of binge eating (an excessive intake of calorie-laden food over a short period of time). Persons with BN are overly sensitive about their weight and have a distorted body image. Most have normal weight, although they may fluctuate between being slightly underweight to slightly overweight for body size and age. Patients lack control over their eating and participate in recurrent compensatory behavior to prevent weight gain. This can include self-induced vomiting; misuse of laxatives, diuretics, enemas, or other medications; strict dieting or fasting; or excessive exercise. To meet DSM-IV-TR criteria, the binges and compensatory behaviors must occur on average at least twice weekly for 3 months. DSM-IV-TR further differentiates an episode of BN into purging type (the person regularly engages in self-induced vomiting or the misuse of laxatives, diuretics, or enemas) or nonpurging type (the person uses other inappropriate compensatory behaviors, such as fasting or excessive exercise, but doesn't engage in purging activities).[7]

Patients typically binge one or more times daily and vomit at least once daily. Patients can consume between 5,000 and 20,000 calories during a single binge, although caloric intake can be smaller. Patients tend to consume foods that are easy to ingest, do not require much chewing or preparation, and are high in carbohydrates or fat (e.g., ice cream, bread, candy, or doughnuts). Binge eating typically is secretive, and episodes are often precipitated by a stressful event. Because patients lose control over their eating behavior, they are often remorseful after a binge. Binges typically last less than 2 hours, but can last for more than 8 hours. To compensate for the excessive caloric intake, many patients fast for prolonged periods, exercise compulsively, purge, or abuse laxatives.

Psychiatric comorbidity includes depression (up to 80%), impulse-control problems, and substance abuse. Approximately 30% to 37% of bulimic patients have a personal history of substance abuse.[25] Kleptomania is reported more commonly in patients with BN than in the general public. Patients commonly steal comfort items such as laxatives, candies, and clothes.[8] Personality disorders, especially borderline and avoidant types, are more common in these patients than in the general population.[23,24]

BINGE EATING DISORDER

Binge eating disorder presents with recurrent episodes of binge eating without the compensatory behaviors associated with bulimia or anorexia. It is estimated that 5% to 10% of patients seeking treatment for obesity have the disorder. BED patients are likely to have comorbid depressive disorder, although the self-deprecating focus on body image is less severe than in AN or BN.[10,24]

▶ TREATMENT: Eating Disorders

▪ PROGNOSIS

▪ ANOREXIA NERVOSA

The long-term prognosis of AN patients is not clear, as studies focus on people who receive treatment and not all who experience the condition. The course of AN most commonly consists of a single episode with subsequent return to normal weight. These patients may still experience issues with disturbed body image, disordered eating, and other psychiatric problems.[9] Some patients experience an unremitting course leading to death, while others suffer episodically. One study found that 50% of AN patients had a "good" outcome, 30% had a "medium" outcome, and 20% a "poor" outcome.[26] More recent data showed that only 10% of patients met full criteria for AN a decade after initial treatment, although chronic symptoms including lower body weight and perfectionism continued. Many later developed BN, but in most cases it remitted. Finally, their rates of anxiety disorders, major depression, and alcohol dependence were higher than in the general population.[27] A poorer prognosis is associated with a longer duration of illness, presenting with a lower initial weight, having a premorbid history of poor family relationships, and the presence of BN or purging behavior.[10,28,29] The actual mortality rates in AN are unclear, but they are among the highest of all psychiatric disorders. Long-term follow-up shows that over 10% of AN patients eventually die, primarily from cardiac arrest or suicide.[7]

▪ BULIMIA NERVOSA

The prognosis of BN has not been well studied. Overall, BN patients appear to have a better prognosis than AN patients. Patients with milder presenting symptoms who are treated as outpatients tend to do better, whereas patients with electrolyte imbalances, esophagitis, dental caries, and salivary gland enlargement have a more complicated course.[8] A 6-year follow-up of patients who received intensive treatment found that 60% were "good," 29% had "intermediate" response, 10% were doing "poorly," and 1% had died.[30] It is important to note that even in cases in which patients respond, they continue to exhibit symptoms, the severity of which waxes and wanes over time in response to their external environment. Total absence of symptoms is a less common outcome. The actual definition of recovery varies, since once-a-month binge/purge episodes are considered by some to be recovery if their episodes were previously more frequent, whereas others consider a patient recovered only when complete absence of these behaviors occurs.[28] Of concern is that ongoing symptoms may predispose patients to relapse.[31]

GENERAL APPROACH TO TREATMENT

The overall goals for patients with AN, BN, and BED are to reduce distorted body image, restore and maintain healthy body weight, reestablish normal eating patterns, improve associated psychological and physical problems, resolve contributory family problems, and prevent relapse. An individualized treatment plan is based on the specific core features of the eating disorder and comorbid medical and psychiatric conditions present in the patient, along with the severity of those symptoms. Psychiatrists, nutrition specialists, psychologists, nurses, and pharmacists all play a role in the care of these complex patients. The patient and their close friends and relatives must all be engaged in treatment planning, as denial is a common problem, and without their active participation, treatment will not be a success. Even with a comprehensive treatment approach, complete recovery can be difficult to attain. A critical first step is to determine the illness severity, as that drives both the intensity and the setting for delivery of care. For example, a patient with severe medical complications from starving and purging will require hospitalization, as opposed to the patient who binges and purges daily, but is medically stable and can be managed as an outpatient. Hospitalization is based on the criteria outlined in Table 62–2 and is limited to only the most severely ill patients.[10,13,14] Patients with BN are usually managed in the outpatient setting, as they are usually medically stable. Medications are rarely indicated as a sole treatment for eating disorders, but are part of a comprehensive treatment strategy.[32–34]

TABLE 62–2. Criteria for Hospitalization of Patients with Eating Disorders

- Significant weight loss of 20% or more of normal weight, particularly if weight loss has been recent and rapid, severe starvation symptoms are present, or the patient has been ill for more than 2 years
- Medical complications (e.g., edema) and metabolic abnormalities (e.g., hypoproteinemia) from bingeing, purging, and starvation (e.g., heart rate <40 bpm, blood pressure <90/60 mm Hg, glucose <60 mg/dL, potassium <3 mEq/L, temperature <97°F)
- Suicidal ideation or psychotic depression
- Nonresponsive to outpatient treatment (after 3–4 months) and poor motivation to recover
- Demoralization or nonfunctional family
- Continuous supervision required to prevent purging (vomiting or laxative abuse)

Modified from Fairburn and Harrison,[10] Halmi,[13] and Powers.[14]

ANOREXIA NERVOSA

Nonpharmacologic Treatments

Evidence supports that nonpharmacologic treatments have the greatest likelihood of causing a response in AN patients.[9,32] Behavioral management, cognitive behavioral therapy (CBT), interpersonal psychotherapy (IP), nutritional counseling, and family therapy, especially for adolescent patients, are all options available to the clinician.[9,13] CBT helps the patient overcome distorted thinking, self-worth that is measured by body image, feelings of being fat despite evidence to the contrary, and denial of the seriousness of the condition. CBT also teaches patients how to use strategies besides food to cope. IP focuses on interpersonal relationships and functioning, whereas behavioral therapy provides positive reinforcement for weight gain.[21] The benefit of treatment based on an addiction model (12-step program) is not supported by the literature.[9,10] It is critical to note that many psychiatric symptoms in an acutely ill patient, such as depression and anxiety, will diminish or disappear entirely after normal weight is restored. Hence, initial treatment is directed toward restoring a healthy weight (>90% of normal weight for age-matched controls) and treating food phobias.[35] After the patient is medically stable and at their appropriate weight, therapy can be redirected toward addressing ongoing interpersonal problems, weight maintenance, cognitive restructuring, and finally, skill development for relapse prevention.[36] Oral refeeding, initially with liquid formulas if necessary, is the most common approach to weight restoration.

Total parenteral nutrition is reserved for the initial management of severely malnourished patients, or when oral refeeding fails. The decision to administer total parenteral nutrition must be made carefully because of the potentially devastating psychological effect on patients who do not wish to gain weight. A controlled weight gain of no more than two to three pounds each week is recommended. Patients usually start by consuming 1000 to 1600 calories per day and slowly titrate upwards until they demonstrate sustained weight gain. Some patients may need as many as 70 to 100 kcal/day during the weight gain phase. Patients may also need 200 to 400 extra calories a day to maintain their weight gain.[10,37] Slow refeeding is important in order to minimize medical and psychological consequences that can occur with a more rapid weight gain.[10] Complications can include circulatory overload and severe anxiety.

Pharmacologic Therapy

Antidepressants. Antidepressants currently play no role in treating acute AN. Antidepressants, and in particular selective serotonin reuptake inhibitors (SSRIs), theoretically work because of their impact on serotonin, a neurotransmitter which is involved with many of the behaviors that are disturbed in AN.[13] This recommendation is based on recent analyses of the literature and the most recent practice guidelines from the American Psychiatric Association.[9,10,32]

Data suggest that medication is ineffective if a patient weighs less than 85% of their expected weight.[35,38] Antidepressants should be initiated only if depression, anxiety, obsessions, or compulsions persist after the target weight is achieved.[10] The duration of treatment when antidepressants are used in this manner is unclear, but the trial that found a benefit treated patients for 1 year.[3] Antidepressants, along with psychotherapy, have been used to help maintain weight and prevent relapse, although the data are limited.[39] If antidepressants are indicated, most clinicians prefer the SSRIs because they are better tolerated and have greater cardiovascular safety than tricyclic antidepressants (TCAs), especially in low-weight patients.[40] Patients are sensitive to anticholinergic and cardiovascular effects, and if TCAs are used at all, low starting doses and a slow titration toward an effective dose are needed. The risk of cardiotoxicity in a malnourished population must not be underestimated, especially in chronic purgers, who may have hypokalemia. A baseline electrocardiogram (ECG) must be obtained before beginning an antidepressant. Open trials used fluoxetine, 20 to 60 mg/day.[37,41] The one long-term trial that found a benefit used 20 mg/day.[39] Since dosing information is limited, most clinicians will initiate patients at lower doses, for example 20 mg/day, and increase to a maximum of 60 mg/day if there is an inadequate response or relapse and the drug is tolerated.

Antipsychotics. Typical antipsychotics were the first medications used to treat AN because of their potential to reduce obsessive thoughts, paranoid ideation about weight gain and anxiety, and promote weight gain.[42] Clinical experience found little specific improvement secondary to typical antipsychotic administration in AN patients and that the risks outweighed the benefits. However, interest in antipsychotics for acutely ill AN patients has re-emerged because of the introduction of atypical agents whose safety profile is improved over older agents. Most of the data are from case reports or small trials using risperidone 0.5 to 1.5 mg daily or olanzapine 5 to 10 mg daily.[43-45] Improvement has been shown in some, but not all trials, hence these agents require further study before they become a routine part of care. Caution is important as revealed by a case report of increased QTc interval in an AN patient taking rispiridone.[46] Any change in QTc interval must be taken seriously in a population at risk for hypokalemia. Optimal treatment duration is unknown, as most of the larger studies were ≤3 months in length. In some case studies symptoms remained in remission even after the medication was discontinued.[47]

Miscellaneous Agents. Metoclopramide may be helpful in reducing the bloating, early satiety, and abdominal pain commonly found in AN, but it does not impact weight gain.[9] Low-dose short-acting benzodiazepines (0.25 mg alprazolam or 0.5 mg lorazepam) given before meals are useful when severe anxiety limits eating.[9] Estrogen replacement has been used, but restoring menses through refeeding is a better approach to minimizing bone density loss. Estrogen use to restore menses may reinforce the patient's denial of their illness.[35]

Overall, the treatment goals in AN are for the patient to recognize their need for treatment, restore and maintain their weight at a healthy level, normalize eating habits, and improve psychosocial functioning (body image and peer interactions). The value of family therapy for treating adolescents has been demonstrated in the literature and should be provided to AN patients. Overall, CBT is the most commonly applied strategy in eating disorder programs. Currently antidepressants have no role in acutely ill patients, while the data in weight maintenance are limited but suggestive of some value.[9,10] Atypical antipsychotics may be used in acutely ill patients, but further data are needed to determine their precise role.

CLINICAL CONTROVERSY

Clinicians continue to look for medications that are beneficial during the acute phase of AN. Atypical antipsychotics are being used by some clinicians in acutely ill patients with severe obsessions and paranoia about eating, although the data supporting this are limited.

BULIMIA NERVOSA

Nonpharmacologic Therapy

The nondrug strategies used in BN are similar to those used with AN and are equally critical to success. CBT has the strongest evidence supporting its benefit in managing BN.[9,10] IP also plays a role and has a moderate degree of evidence to support its use.[9,10] Behavioral approaches such as planned meals and self-monitoring can help interrupt the binge-purge cycle. Nutritional counseling and family therapy are also important components of treatment. Family therapy in BN patients is less critical than with AN, as these patients tend to be older. Programs using guided self-manuals based on CBT as a nonpharmacologic approach are also showing promise, although further study is indicated.[13,48] Twelve-step programs for BN play an adjunctive role at best, as the data supporting their efficacy are lacking.[9,1] Supportive counseling encouraging medication compliance may be needed early in treatment while the patient becomes tolerant to adverse effects.

Pharmacologic Therapy

Antidepressants. Antidepressants are used in the acute and maintenance phase of BN management, although they are adjunctive to nonpharmacologic approaches. Theoretically, the benefit is derived from an increase in central serotonin concentrations.[8] A wide array of antidepressants, including TCAs, monoamine oxidase inhibitors, trazodone, and SSRIs, have been studied in numerous clinical trials since the 1980s, and many of these studies were placebo controlled.[49-5] Additionally, several recent reviews analyzing this body of literature have been published, although there is limited new literature since the mid-1990s.[10,32] Antidepressants are reported to reduce depression, anxiety, obsessions, impulsive behaviors such as binge eating and purging, and improve eating habits, although their impact on body dissatisfaction remains unclear. The presence of comorbid mood disorders is not necessary for an antidepressant response, as patients with and without depression responded equally well to the medication.[10,59,60]

The benefit appears to be more robust in the acute phase of the illness, as relapse despite continued antidepressant use is common in patients who are in or near remission.[10,13,34] Short-term (6 to 8 weeks) antidepressant response varies across trials, and reduction in frequency of binge/purge behavior has been as high as 73% and as low as zero.[32] Abstinence rates with short-term use range from none to 68%. More data are needed to determine the long-term benefits of antidepressants for preventing relapse of BN symptoms. One recent trial evaluating the impact of fluoxetine versus placebo in the maintenance of response was promising, as it found a better outcome in patients receiving fluoxetine 60 mg/day. It should be noted that dropout rates were high in both groups, somewhat blurring the overall benefit of active medication.[61]

SSRIs are the preferred agents because of their tolerability and because they may have been studied in the largest number of patients. Fluoxetine is the only agent to have Food and Drug Administration approval for BN. Tolerability is the primary criterion for selecting an antidepressant in BN because of patients' heightened sensitivity to adverse effects and lack of a clear difference in efficacy between the classes. Even though there is a suggestion that monoamine oxidase inhibitors produce the most robust effect, the complications of using these medications in impulsive patients and the fact that the data are more than 10 years old limits their use.[34] Bupropion is not used in patients with BN because of an unacceptably high risk of seizures.

A careful baseline physical examination, ECG, and laboratory work-up are essential. Underlying ECG changes (U waves, prolonged QT interval, or flattened T waves) secondary to hypokalemia or bradycardia and atrioventricular block from starvation may be present. All antidepressants can cause seizures; thus a careful risk-benefit assessment is warranted if the patient has predisposing factors such as a personal or family history of seizures, cerebrovascular disease, or alcohol or sedative-hypnotic withdrawal.

Doses in BN are in the same range as for patients with depression. Readers are referred to Chap. 67 on depressive disorders for a discussion of dosing ranges for antidepressants. For fluoxetine, the higher end of the dosing range, 60 mg/day, may be necessary for response.[56] With other agents, most clinicians will initially target the bottom to the middle of the dosing range and increase the dose if there is an inadequate response and the patient is known to be compliant. Slow titration is needed to allow time to develop tolerance to adverse effects. TCA serum concentration monitoring is recommended to ensure that absorption is not compromised by purging. The same TCA serum concentration ranges are used in depression and BN.

The time for antidepressant onset of effect in BN is unclear. In the absence of data, the definition of a therapeutic trial from the depression literature (4 to 8 weeks at a therapeutic dose) should be used. Since the majority of subjects will not experience a complete remission, and there are few data on predictors of response or whether switching to another class will improve response, a clear and specific target should be stated initially.[9] For example, will the medication be continued if the patient has a 50% reduction in binge-purge episodes, or if abstinence from such behavior is the ultimate therapeutic goal.

Optimal duration of treatment after response is also poorly defined. Most clinicians will treat for 6 months to 1 year and then re-evaluate the need for ongoing treatment. The evidence is mixed as to whether any early benefit is sustained, hence the decision to continue treatment should be made based on both initial response and the maintenance of that benefit. If the symptoms return within a few months after the antidepressant is discontinued, then the treatment may need to be reinitiated.

Table 62–3 describes potential guidelines for medication use in BN, but it must be noted that no evidence-based consensus for treatment has been endorsed, even with the recent meta-analyses and reviews of the literature.[3,10,32,34,40] The selection of an effective treatment approach is especially challenging when patients fail CBT.[10]

Mood Stabilizers (Lithium and Anticonvulsants). Due to the lack of evidence demonstrating their benefit, lithium and anticonvulsants are reserved for BN patients with a comorbid bipolar affective disorder.[9,62–66] Target serum concentrations and doses are similar to those used for patients with seizure or mood disorders. Lithium must be used cautiously, because purging and laxative abuse increases the risk of toxicity. The adverse effect of weight gain often makes mood stabilizers and anticonvulsants unacceptable to patients in the long term.

Miscellaneous Agents. Low-dose benzodiazepines, such as 0.25 mg alprazolam three times a day administered before meals, may help reduce anxiety associated with refeeding, although long-term use is not warranted for many patients because of the risk of dependence. One double-blind trial with ondansetron has shown benefit, but the data remain too limited to recommend a specific role for the agent.[67]

TABLE 62–3. Guidelines for Medication Use in Bulimia Nervosa

1. Determine baseline frequency of binge and vomiting episodes, laxative abuse, obsessive thoughts, and compulsive behavior. Document weight and patient's subjective feelings of self-image. Describe a baseline level of functioning.
2. Identify comorbid psychiatric conditions (e.g., depression, anxiety disorder, substance abuse, or bipolar disorder).
3. Determine baseline physical status (especially nutritional status, electrocardiogram, and fluid status [dehydration and electrolytes]).
4. Consider whether an antidepressant is part of a comprehensive treatment plan that includes nonpharmacologic measures, especially cognitive behavioral therapy.
5. If antidepressant is indicated, start at a low dose, and use a selective serotonin reuptake inhibitor unless there is a medical reason not to do so.
6. Monitor carefully for response, adverse effects, and compliance. Response usually is seen after 6–12 weeks. Response is determined by change from baseline frequency and severity of target symptoms.
7. If patient responds and response is sustained, continue treatment for 6–12 months, then reassess.
8. If response is poor, evaluate compliance and whether patient is vomiting medication. Ensure that the patient is receiving nonpharmacologic therapy.
9. There is no good evidence as to what treatment to try if medication is not effective.

Antipsychotics and appetite suppressants do not play a role in managing this condition.[10]

Nonpharmacologic versus Pharmacologic Approaches

Antidepressants have been compared directly to CBT and other forms of psychotherapy. The results were mixed, and some studies had very high dropout rates, making interpretation difficult. Overall, nonpharmacologic methods were superior to medication alone, and in many cases were better accepted by the patient.[32,68] There are limited data to suggest that some patients who fail psychotherapy (CBT or IP) respond to antidepressants.[69,70] Antidepressants without some form of psychotherapy have also been proposed as a first step in the primary care setting before referral to specialty care occurs. Primary care settings are generally ill-prepared to provide the type of specialty psychotherapy required in BN patients, but can manage antidepressant issues.[10]

The most common scenario, and one recommended by most clinicians, is a combination of drug and nondrug approaches.[9] The literature is somewhat mixed as to whether the addition of antidepressants offers significant benefit, but there is enough positive literature to recommend this course of treatment.[49,71–74] A serious challenge in the care of these and other eating disorder patients is that quality CBT and other nonpharmacologic approaches are often unavailable.

In summary, the combination of pharmacologic and nonpharmacologic measures appears to produce the best chance for a positive outcome for patients with BN.[32] Antidepressants are the class of choice in patients with BN, while other medications such as mood stabilizers are reserved for patients with comorbid psychiatric conditions. Only in unusual circumstances should patients be treated with antidepressants alone, as the chances for success are not high. SSRIs are the antidepressant class of choice for managing BN patients. Evidence suggests the greatest benefit in the acute phase of treatment, whereas data are more mixed for their role in the prevention of relapse.

CLINICAL CONTROVERSY

The optimal time to continue antidepressant therapy in BN patients after a response is unclear. Some patients will maintain their response, while others will deteriorate and become symptomatic while continuing on medication. Most clinicians advise the patient to continue the antidepressant for 6 to 12 months if they respond, then re-evaluate whether further treatment is needed.

BINGE EATING DISORDER

The treatment goals for BED are different from those of the other eating disorders because patients are often obese and in need of significant weight loss along with control of their binge eating behavior. Many patients also experience depression. As with the other eating disorders, CBT and IP appear to be the most effective interventions.[10] Antidepressants, anticonvulsants, and appetite suppressants are the pharmacologic agents with the greatest promise in BED, but data are limited, trials are short in duration (16 weeks or less), and

the issue of sustained benefit is unclear.[75] Antidepressants have demonstrated efficacy during the acute phases of the illness compared to placebo.[10,76–78] The majority of the data are with SSRIs given at antidepressant doses.[75] Topiramate 50 to 600 mg daily (a median dose is approximately 200 mg daily) is receiving attention in treating BED because anticonvulsants have been used with some benefit in patients with impulse control disorder and because it promotes weight loss. Short-term data demonstrating superiority over placebo have been published, but long-term data are lacking.[79] Sibutramine 15 mg/day has also demonstrated benefit in reducing weight and binge frequency in obese patients with BED compared to placebo.[80]

In summary, the question of where BED fits on the diagnostic spectrum continues to be explored. An increasing body of literature suggests that three different types of pharmacologic agents (SSRIs, topiramate, and sibutramine) hold promise in the short term, but long-term data are lacking. As with other eating disorders, nonpharmacologic treatments are key to a successful outcome. Control of both weight and binge eating is important, as these patients are at risk for developing cardiovascular and endocrine complications as well as the negative consequences from the psychiatric sequelae.

PHARMACOECONOMIC CONSIDERATIONS

There are no formal evaluations of the economic impact of eating disorders on individual patients, on global health care costs, or on indirect costs such as unemployment, premature death, or disability payments. Certainly the chronic course, the disability found in severe cases, and the lack of improvement in up to a third of patients suggest a significant cost impact. Clinicians should contribute to the appropriate use of resources by ensuring that medications are used in situations in which there is evidence demonstrating their benefit and that they are never used as the sole treatment modality. For example, antidepressants are started after normal weight is restored in AN patients and not to treat depressive symptoms in significantly malnourished patients. One study evaluating the relative costs of CBT alone, medication alone, or combination treatment of BN concluded that if overall effectiveness was the prime consideration, then CBT, with medication added if the response was inadequate, was the best approach. If cost-effectiveness was the basis for making treatment decisions, then antidepressants alone as a first step, followed by the addition of CBT when response was inadequate, was the preferred direction to take.[81] These data were published in 1994, and clearly more study is needed to make evidence-based decisions about the best order and combination of treatment.

EVALUATION OF THERAPEUTIC OUTCOMES

ANOREXIA NERVOSA

A combination of subjective and objective measures is used to assess patient response. A reduction in the frequency and severity of abnormal eating habits, normalized exercise patterns and laboratory tests, and a sustained weight close to age-matched normals are key indicators of response. A diary recording exercise frequency, menses, food intake, patterns of eating, and associated feelings while eating is a useful tool to track progress, especially in the outpatient setting. Weekly weigh-ins on the same scale, preferably at a clinician's office, help monitor progress early in treatment and reduce the focus on weight and anxiety due to the variability found among different

scales.[36] Follow-up laboratory tests and ECGs are not part of routine monitoring unless the patient is restricting food intake, is purging, or continues to lose weight despite treatment. Inpatients require daily assessment of weight and caloric intake, vital signs, and urine output because of the more severe nature of their illness. They also may need monitoring of bathroom privileges early in their care. A healthy weight gain of no more than two to three pounds per week toward a goal of 90% to 95% of normal weight or a body mass index >18.5 kg/m^2 is a critical sign of treatment success. A patient's use of coping skills and contingencies for dealing with stress other than manipulating food consumption also should be assessed. Antidepressants may assist in alleviation of persistent depression, anxiety, and obsessions, after weight restoration. Improvement in mood is expected to occur within 8 weeks. Patients receiving TCAs should be evaluated for anticholinergic effects, especially dry mouth and constipation, hypotension, and sedation. Patients receiving SSRIs should be monitored for agitation, drug-induced anorexia, nausea, weight loss, and insomnia. The decision to use long-term medication must be based on specific and sustained improvement in the target symptoms already mentioned, balanced against tolerance of adverse effects.

BULIMIA NERVOSA

An individualized treatment and monitoring plan begins with a thorough assessment describing the baseline frequency and severity of treatment-responsive target symptoms and other associated findings. The assessment must be comprehensive, as a patient may hide their illness by shifting from one type of behavior to another. For example, they may switch from compulsive exercise to purging after meals as a way to compensate for bingeing.

A comprehensive assessment includes a description of psychiatric symptoms, physical findings, frequency and severity of binge/purge episodes, laxative and ipecac use, exercise patterns, and laboratory and ECG abnormalities.[6] Interpersonal and relationship problems should also be evaluated. Some findings indicating a more chronic course of illness, such as salivary gland inflammation or erosion of dental enamel, may take months to reverse or may never normalize, hence these are not sensitive indicators of early treatment sponse. Data describing a patient's baseline level of functioning nd previous response to treatment should be used to set goals in the urrent treatment plan.

Antidepressant response usually occurs within 4 to 8 weeks after the onset of treatment. If response does not occur, binge/purge ehavior should be considered as a contributing factor. If this behavior is not present, then every attempt should be made to maximize ie dose. Serum concentration monitoring, when appropriate as with CAs, should be done periodically (every 3 to 6 months if a patient is esponding and tolerating the medication, or more frequently if clincally indicated). Evaluation of previously described adverse effects lso should be part of the monitoring plan. If the patient responds, iey should be followed for 6 to 12 months, then the need for onoing medication should be reassessed. If the patient relapses upon iedication discontinuation, then the medication should be restarted.

Ambulatory eating disorder patients present a particular chalenge to clinicians. Impulsivity associated with BN may increase the isk for suicide. Prescriptions should be limited to small supplies. In ddition, pharmacists should be alert to persons who make large or requent purchases of laxatives or ipecac syrup, as this is an indicator f possible bulimic behaviors.

CONCLUSIONS

)ur understanding of the pathophysiology and symptomatology of ating disorders has improved significantly over the past several years. Medication serves an adjunctive role to a variety of psychosocial herapies in AN, whereas it plays a more central role in BN and 3ED treatment. By gaining a greater understanding of the underlying >hysiologic changes and the psychosocial complications associated vith eating disorders, treatment plans can be specifically designed for n individual patient with the goal of improving their quality of life.

ABBREVIATIONS

AN: anorexia nervosa
3ED: binge eating disorder
3N: bulimia nervosa
CBT: cognitive behavioral therapy
P: interpersonal psychotherapy
SSRI: selective serotonin reuptake inhibitor
TCA: tricyclic antidepressant

Review Questions and other resources can be found at www.pharmacotherapyonline.com.

REFERENCES

1. Bulik CM, Tozzi FC, Anderson C, et al. The relationship between eating disorders and components of perfectionism. Am J Psychiatry 2003; 160:366–368.
2. McKnight Investigators. Risk factors for the onset of eating disorders in adolescent girls: Results of the McKnight longitudinal risk factor study. Am J Psychiatry 2003;160:248–254.
3. Favaro A, Ferrara S, Santonastaso P. The spectrum of eating disorders in young women: A prevalence study in a general population sample. Psychosom Med 2003;65:701–708.
4. Gull WW. Anorexia nervosa. Trans Clin Soc (Lond) 1874. In: Kaufman RM, Heifman M, eds. Evolution of Psychosomatic Concepts. Anorexia Nervosa: A Paradigm. New York, International Universities Press, 1964: 22–28.
5. Lesegue C. De l'anorexic hysterique. Arch Gen Med 1873. In: Kaufman RM, Heifman M, eds. Evolution of Psychosomatic Concepts. Anorexia Nervosa: A Paradigm. New York, International Universities Press, 1964: 385–395.
6. Russel G. Bulimia nervosa: An ominous variant of anorexia nervosa. Psychol Med 1979;9:429–448.
7. American Psychiatric Association. Diagnostic and Statistical Manual of Mental Disorders, 4th ed., Text Revision. Washington, American Psychiatric Press, 2000:583–596.
8. Sadock BJ, Sadock VA, eds. Kaplan and Sadock's Synopsis of Psychiatry. Behavioral Sciences/Clinical Psychiatry, 9th ed. Philadelphia, Lippincott Williams & Wilkins, 2003:739–750.
9. Work Group on Eating Disorders. American Psychiatric Association Practice Guidelines. Practice guidelines for eating disorders. Am J Psychiatry 2000;157(Suppl):1–39.
10. Fairburn CG, Harrison PJ. Eating disorders. Lancet 2003;361:407–416.
11. Kaye WH, Frank GK, Meltzer CC, et al. Altered 5-HT2A receptor activity in women who have recovered from bulimia nervosa. Am J Psychiatry 2001;158:1152–1155.
12. Frank GK, Kaye WH, Meltzer CC, et al. Reduced 5-HT2A receptor binding after recovery from anorexia nervosa. Biol Psychiatry 2002;52:896–906.
13. Halmi K. Eating disorders. In: Sadock BJ, Sadock VA, eds. Comprehensive Textbook of Psychiatry, 7th ed. Philadelphia, Lippincott Williams & Wilkins, 2000:1663–1676.
14. Powers PS. Initial assessment and early treatment options for anorexia nervosa and bulimia nervosa. Psychiatr Clin North Am 1996;19: 639–655.
15. Casper RC, Hedeker D, McClough JF. Personality dimensions in eating disorders and their relevance for subtyping. J Am Acad Child Adolesc Psychiatry 1992;31:830–840.
16. Eckert ED, Halmi KA, Marchi P, et al. Ten-year follow-up of anorexia nervosa: Clinical course and outcome. Psychol Med 1995;25:143–156.
17. Garner DM, Garfinkel PE, O'Shaughnessy M. Validity of the distinction between bulimia with and without anorexia nervosa. Am J Psychiatry 1985;142:581–587.
18. Kingston K, Szmukler G, Andrews D, et al. Neuropsychological and structural brain changes in anorexia nervosa before and after refeeding. Psychol Med 1996;26:15–28.
19. Lambe EK, Katzman DK, Mikulis DJ, et al. Cerebral gray matter volume deficits after weight recovery from anorexia nervosa. Arch Gen Psychiatry 1997;54:537–542.
20. Carney CP, Anderson AE. Eating disorders: Guide to medical evaluation and complications. Psychiatr Clin North Am 1996;19:657–679.
21. Halmi KA. Eating disorders: Anorexia nervosa, bulimia nervosa, and obesity. In: Hales RE, Yudofsky SC, eds. Essentials of Clinical Psychiatry, 3d ed. Washington, American Psychiatric Press, 1999:667–685.
22. Braun DL, Sunday SR, Halmi KA. Psychiatric comorbidity in patients with eating disorders. Psychol Med 1994;24:859–867.
23. Skodol AE, Oldham JM, Hyler SE, et al. Comorbidity of DSM-III-R eating disorders and personality disorders. Int J Eat Disord 1993;14:403–416.
24. O'Brien KM, Vincent NK. Psychiatric comorbidity in anorexia and bulimia nervosa: Nature, prevalence, and causal relationships. Clin Psychol Rev 2003;23:53–74.
25. Herzog DB, Keller MB, Sacks NR, et al. Psychiatric comorbidity in treatment seeking anorexics and bulimics. J Am Acad Child Adolesc Psychiatry 1992;31:810–818.
26. Steinhaus HC, Rauss-Mason C, Seidel R. Follow-up studies of anorexia nervosa: A review of four decades of research. Psychol Med 1991;21:447–454.
27. Sullivan PF, Bulik CM, Fear JL, Pickering A. Outcome of anorexia nervosa: A case-controlled study. Am J Psychiatry 1998;155:939–946.
28. Herzog DB, Nussbaum KM, Marmor AK. Comorbidity and outcome in eating disorders. Psychiatr Clin North Am 1996;19:843–859.
29. Ward A. Anorexia nervosa subtypes: Differences in recovery. J Nerv Ment Dis 2003;191:197–200.
30. Fichter MM, Quadfleig N. Six year course of bulimia nervosa. Int J Eat Disord 1997;22:361–384.

31. Crow SJ, Mitchell JE. Integrating cognitive therapy and medications in bulimia nervosa. Psychiatr Clin North Am 1996;19:755–760.

32. Mitchell JE, deZwaan M, Roerig JL. Drug therapy for patients with eating disorders. Curr Drug Targets CNS Neurol Disord 2003;2:17–29.

33. Bacaltchuk J, Hay P. Review: Antidepressants increase remission and clinical improvement in bulimia nervosa. Cochrane Database Syst Rev 2001;4:CD003391.

34. Nakash-Eisikovits O, Dierberger A, Westen D. A multidimensional meta-analysis of pharmacotherapy for bulimia nervosa: Summarizing the range of outcomes in controlled clinical trials. Harv Rev Psychiatry 2002;10:190–211.

35. Zerbe KJ. Multimodal treatment of severe eating disorders. Essent Psychopharmacol 2000;3:1–17.

36. Kleifield EI, Wagner S, Halmi KA. Cognitive-behavioral treatment of anorexia nervosa. Psychiatr Clin North Am 1996;19:715–737.

37. Kaye WH, Weltzin TE, Hsu G, Bulik CM. An open trial of fluoxetine in patients with anorexia nervosa. J Clin Psychiatry 1991;52:464–471.

38. Berg C, Eriksson M, Lindberg G, Sodersten P. Selective serotonin reuptake inhibitors in anorexia. Lancet 1996;348:1459–1450.

39. Kaye WH, Nagata T, Weltzin TE, et al. Double-blind placebo-controlled administration of fluoxetine in restricting- and restricting-purging-type anorexia nervosa. Biol Psychiatry 2001;4:644–652.

40. Jimerson DC, Wolfe BE, Brotman AW, Metzger ED. Medication in the treatment of eating disorders. Psychiatr Clin North Am 1996;19:739–754.

41. Gwirtsman HE, Guze BH, Yager J, Gainsley B. Fluoxetine treatment of anorexia nervosa. An open clinical trial. J Clin Psychiatry 1990;51:378–382.

42. Dally PJ, Sargant W. A new treatment for anorexia nervosa. Br Med J 1960;1:1770–1773.

43. Carver AE, Miller S, Hagman J, Sigel E. Academy of Eating Disorders Annual Meeting, Boston, April 2002.

44. Powers PS, Santana CA, Bannon YS. Olanzapine in the treatment of anorexia nervosa: An open label trial. Int J Eat Disord 2002;32:146–154.

45. Jensen VS, Mejlhede A. Anorexia nervosa: Treatment with olanzapine. Br J Psychiatry 2000;177:87.

46. Newman-Toker JJ. Risperidone in anorexia nervosa. Am Acad Child Adolesc Psychiatry 2000;39:941–942.

47. Mehler C, Wewetzer C, Schulze U, et al. Olanzapine in children and adolescents with chronic anorexia nervosa. A study of five cases. Eur Child Adolesc Psychiatry 2000;10:151–157.

48. Mitchell JE, Fletcher L, Hanson K, et al. The relative efficacy of fluoxetine and manual-based self-help in the treatment of outpatients with bulimia nervosa. J Clin Psychiatry 2001;21:298–304.

49. Pope HG, Hudson JI, Jonas JM, Yurgelun-Todd D. Bulimia treated with imipramine: A placebo-controlled, double-blind study. Am J Psychiatry 1983;140:554–558.

50. Pope HG, Hudson JI, Jonas JM, Yurgelun-Todd D. Antidepressant treatment of bulimia: A two-year follow-up study. J Clin Psychopharmacol 1985;5:320–327.

51. Mitchell JE, Pyle RL, Eckert ED, Hatsakami D, et al. Response to alternative antidepressants in imipramine nonresponders. J Clin Psychopharmacol 1989;9:291–293.

52. Barlow J, Blouin J, Blouin A, Perez E. Treatment of bulimia with desipramine: A double-blind crossover study. Can J Psychiatry 1988;33:129–133.

53. McCann UD, Angras WS. Successful treatment of nonpurging bulimia nervosa with desipramine: A double-blind, placebo-controlled study. Am J Psychiatry 1990;147:1509–1513.

54. Walsh BT, Gladis M, Roose SP, et al. Phenelzine vs placebo in 50 patients with bulimia. Arch Gen Psychiatry 1988;45:471–475.

55. Pope HG, Keck PE, McElroy SL, Hudson JI. A placebo-controlled study of trazodone in bulimia nervosa. J Clin Psychopharmacol 1989;9:254–259.

56. Fluoxetine Bulimia Nervosa Collaborative Study Group. Fluoxetine in the treatment of bulimia nervosa: A multicenter, placebo-controlled, double-blind trial. Arch Gen Psychiatry 1992;49:139–147.

57. Goldstein DJ, Wilson MG, Thompson VL, et al. Long-term fluoxetine treatment of bulimia nervosa. Br J Psychiatry 1995;166:660–666.

58. Fitcher MM, Kruger R, Rief W, et al. Fluvoxamine in prevention of relapse in bulimia nervosa: Effects on eating-specific psychopathology. J Clin Psychopharmacol 1996;16:9–18.

59. Mitchell JE, Groat R. A placebo-controlled, double-blind trial of amitriptyline in bulimia. J Clin Psychopharmacol 1984;4:186–193.

60. Hughes PL, Wells LA, Cunningham CJ, Ilstrup DM. Treating bulimia with desipramine: A double-blind, placebo controlled trial. Arch Gen Psychiatry 1986;43:182–186.

61. Romano SJ, Halmi KA, Sarkar NP, et al. A placebo-controlled study of fluoxetine in continued treatment of bulimia nervosa after successful fluoxetine treatment. Am J Psychiatry 2002;159:96–102.

62. Green RS, Rau JH. Treatment of compulsive eating disorders with anticonvulsant medication. Am J Psychiatry 1974;131:428–432.

63. Wermuth BM, Davis KL, Hollister LE, Stunkard AJ. Phenytoin treatment of binge eating syndrome. Am J Psychiatry 1977;136:1249–1253.

64. Kaplan AS, Garfinkel PE, Darby PL, Garner DM. Carbamazepine in the treatment of bulimia. Am J Psychiatry 1983;140:1225–1226.

65. Herridge PL, Pope HG. Treatment of bulimia and rapid cycling bipolar disorder with sodium valproate: A case report. J Clin Psychopharmacol 1985;5:229–230.

66. Hsu LKG, Clement L, Santhouse R. Treatment of bulimia with lithium. A preliminary study. Psychopharmacol Bull 1987;2:45–48.

67. Faris PL, Kim SW, Meller WH, et al. Effect of decreasing afferent vagal activity with ondansetron on the symptoms of bulimia nervosa: A randomized double-blind trial. Lancet 2000;355:792–797.

68. Bacaltchuk J, Trefiglio RP, de Oliveira R, et al. Antidepressants versus psychotherapy for bulimia nervosa: A systematic review. J Clin Pharm Ther 1999;24:23–31.

69. Mitchell JE, Halmi K, Wilson GT, et al. A randomized secondary treatment study of women with bulimia nervosa who fail to respond to CBT. Int J Eat Disord 2002;32:271–281.

70. Walsh BT, Wilson GT, Loeb KL, et al. Medication and psychotherapy in the treatment of bulimia nervosa. Am J Psychiatry 1997;154:523–531.

71. Angras WS, Walsh BT, Fairburn CG, et al. A multicenter comparison of cognitive-behavioral therapy and interpersonal psychotherapy for bulimia nervosa. Arch Gen Psychiatry 2000;57:459–466.

72. Mitchell JE, Pyle RL, Eckert ED, et al. A comparison study of antidepressants, structured interview and group psychotherapy in the treatment of bulimia nervosa. Arch Gen Psychiatry 1990;47:149–157.

73. Angras WS, Rossiter EM, Arnow B, et al. Pharmacological and cognitive-behavioral treatment for bulimia nervosa: A controlled comparison. Am J Psychiatry 1992;149:82–87.

74. Walsh BT, Wilson GT, Loeb KL, et al. Medication and psychotherapy in the treatment of bulimia nervosa. Am J Psychiatry 1997;154:523–531.

75. Carter WP, Hudson JI, Lalonde JK, et al. Pharmacologic treatment of binge eating disorder. Int J Eat Disord 2003;34:S74–S88.

76. Kaplan AS. Academy for Eating Disorders International Conference on Eating Disorders. Expert Opin Investig Drugs 2003;12:1441–1443.

77. McElroy SL, Casuto LS, Nelson EB, et al. Placebo-controlled trial of sertraline in the treatment of binge eating disorder. Am J Psychiatry 2000;157:1004–1006.

78. Hudson J, McElroy SL, Raymond NC, et al. Fluvoxamine in the treatment of binge eating disorder: A multicenter, placebo-controlled, double-blind trial. Am J Psychiatry 1998;155:1756–1762.

79. McElroy SL, Arnold LM, Shapira NA, et al. Topiramate in the treatment of binge eating disorder associated with obesity: A randomized, placebo-controlled trial. Am J Psychiatry 2003;160:255–261.

80. Appolinario JC, Gody-Matos A, Fontanelle LF, et al. An open trial of sinbutramine in obese patients with BED. J Clin Psychiatry 2002;63:28–30.

81. Angras WS, Rossiter EM, Arnow B, et al. One year follow up of psychosocial and pharmacologic treatments for bulimia nervosa. J Clin Psychiatry 1994;55:179–183.

63

ALZHEIMER'S DISEASE

Jennifer D. Faulkner, Jody Bartlett, and Paul Hicks

Learning Objectives and other resources can be found at *www.pharmacotherapyonline.com*.

KEY CONCEPTS

1 The prevalence of Alzheimer's disease (AD) increases with each decade of life and is more common in females.

2 The etiology of AD is unknown, and pharmacotherapy neither cures nor arrests the pathophysiology.

3 Neuritic plaques and neurofibrillary tangles are the pathologic hallmarks of AD; however, the definitive cause of this disease is yet to be determined.

4 AD affects multiple areas of cognition and is characterized by a gradual onset with a slow progressive decline.

5 A thorough physical and neurologic exam, as well as laboratory and imaging studies, are required to rule out other disorders and diagnose AD before considering drug therapy.

6 Early initiation and continued, uninterrupted treatment provide the optimal cognitive benefit.

7 Pharmacotherapy for AD focuses on impacting three domains: cognition, psychiatric symptoms, and activities of daily living.

8 Nondrug therapy and social support for the patient and family are the primary treatment interventions for AD.

9 Cholinesterase inhibitors and memantine are used to treat cognitive symptoms of AD; other medications have been suggested to be beneficial because of their potential preventive or cognitive effects.

10 Slow medication dosage titration with careful monitoring should be done to minimize the incidence of troubling adverse drug reactions.

11 A thorough behavioral assessment and plan with careful examination of environmental factors should be conducted before initiating drug therapy for behavioral symptoms.

12 Pharmacotherapy may reduce the total cost of treating AD by delaying cognitive decline and time to nursing home placement.

> *I now begin the journey that will lead me into the sunset of my life.*
>
> Ronald Reagan

Alzheimer's disease (AD), first characterized by Alois Alzheimer in 1907, is a gradually progressive dementia affecting both cognition and behavior. The exact pathophysiologic mechanisms underlying AD are not entirely known, and no cure exists.[1] Although drugs may reduce AD symptoms for a time, the disease is eventually fatal.

AD profoundly affects the family as well as the patient. The need for supervision and assistance increases until the late stages of the disease, when AD patients become totally dependent on a family member, spouse, or other caregiver for all of their basic needs. These are the all-too-common experiences of the millions of people in the United States who have AD.

EPIDEMIOLOGY

AD is the most common cause of dementia, accounting for over 60% of cases of late-life cognitive dysfunction.[1] Table 63–1 lists etiology-based subclasses of dementia. This chapter focuses exclusively on dementia of the Alzheimer's type. However, the reader is encouraged to use the nonpharmacologic approaches and management of behavioral problems outlined in this chapter to assist in the general treatment approach to other types of dementia that may share similar features with AD.

Approximately 4.5 million Americans have AD.[2] By the year 2050, one of five people will be over age 65 years, and the number of AD patients is projected to be 13.2 million (Fig. 63–1). AD is generally associated with the elderly because most cases present in persons older than age 65, but in about 5% of cases onset can be as early as age 40, resulting in the arbitrary age classifications of early-onset (ages 40 to 64 years) and late-onset (age 65 years and older).[3,4]

1 The prevalence of AD increases exponentially with age, affecting approximately 7% of individuals aged 65 to 74 years, 53% aged 75 to 84, and 40% of persons aged 85 years and older.[2] AD affects two times as many women as men, and family history of AD may increase the risk of inheriting the disease by up to fourfold.[3] Although genetic inheritance is a significant factor in its transmission, other factors may contribute. Factors determining age of onset and rate of progression remain largely undefined.

Survival following AD onset is estimated to be 3 to 20 years, with an average of 8 years after the onset of symptoms.[3] Approximately 100,000 individuals with AD die every year. AD is the eighth leading cause of death in United States.[5] This is somewhat of a misrepresentation, as AD does not cause death directly, but indirectly by

TABLE 63–1. Classification of Dementia

Dementia of the Alzheimer's type
Vascular dementia
Dementia due to human immunodeficiency viral disease
Dementia due to head trauma
Dementia due to Parkinson's disease
Dementia due to Huntington's disease
Dementia due to Pick's disease
Dementia due to Creutzfeldt-Jakob disease
Dementia due to other general medical condition (e.g, normal-pressure
    hydrocephalus, hypothyroidism, brain tumor, vitamin B_{12} deficiency,
    intracranial radiation)
Substance-induced persisting dementia (e.g., alcohol, inhalant,
    sedative, hypnotic, anxiolytic, or other substance)
Dementia due to multiple etiologies
Dementia not otherwise specified

Adapted from American Psychiatric Association.[27]

predisposing patients to sepsis, pneumonia, choking and aspiration, nutritional deficiencies, and trauma.[6]

ETIOLOGY

The exact etiology of AD is unknown; however, several genetic and environmental causes have been explored as potential causes of AD.

GENETICS

Genetic factors have been investigated in both early- and late-onset AD. Almost all early-onset cases of AD can be attributed to alterations on chromosomes 1, 14, or 21. The majority and most aggressive early-onset cases are attributed to mutations of an Alzheimer's gene located on chromosome 14, which produces a protein called presenilin 1.[7] Similar in structure to presenilin 1 is a protein produced by a gene on chromosome 1 called presenilin 2. Presenilin 2 is responsible for early-onset AD in a family of Germans living in Russia's Volga Valley.[8] Both presenilin 1 and presenilin 2 encode

for membrane proteins that may be involved in amyloid precursor protein (APP) processing. It has been suggested, but not proven, that presenilins are either γ-secretase or that presenilins affect γ-secretase activity.[7] APP is encoded on chromosome 21. Only a small number of early-onset familial AD cases have been associated with mutations in the APP gene, resulting in overproduction of beta-amyloid protein (βAP).[7,8]

Genetic susceptibility to late-onset AD is thought to be primarily influenced by the apolipoprotein E (apo E) genotype. The gene responsible for the production of apo E is located on chromosome 19 in a region previously associated with late-onset AD. Three major subtypes or alleles of apo E occur, and are termed apo E2, apo E3, and apo E4.[7,8] Humans inherit one copy of the apo E gene from each parent. Apo E3 is the most common type, occurring in 40% to 90% of the population, with apo E2 and apo E4 occurring less frequently.[7] However, rather than being causative, the apo E4 allele is a risk factor for development of AD.

Inheritance of the apo E4 isoform increases risk for late-onset AD; however, the degree of risk depends on such factors as the number of apo E4 copies, age, ethnicity, and gender.[4,7] Overall, about 40% of patients with late-onset AD have at least one copy of apo E4. Individuals homozygous for apo E4 are at increased risk, and as many as 90% of persons inheriting two copies of apo E4 will develop AD by age 80 years. Moreover, onset of symptoms occurs at a relatively younger age as compared to patients having zero or only one copy of apo E4 in their genotype.[4,7] In Caucasians, inheriting a single copy of apo E4 increases AD risk, whereas inheriting the apo E2 allele may protect against AD.[7,9] Differences also exist with regard to gender; inheriting one copy of apo E4 increases risk in females more than in males.[3]

Although inheritance of the apo E4 allele increases the risk of AD, it is not diagnostic or even essential for disease presence. AD occurs in persons with no copies of apo E4 and not all persons with two alleles of apo E4 develop AD. If a person homozygous for apo E4 does not develop AD by age 80 years, it is unlikely to occur.

Genetic factors have been linked to both early- and late-onset AD. Alterations to chromosomes 1, 14, and 21 have been associated with early-onset AD, whereas the presence of apo E4 alleles increase a person's risk of developing late-onset AD. However, genetic causes of AD have been associated with only a small percentage of Alzheimer's patients, and the exact cause of AD remains unknown.

ENVIRONMENTAL AND OTHER FACTORS

A number of environmental factors have been associated with an increased risk of AD, including stroke, alcohol abuse, small head circumference, repeated or severe head trauma, Down syndrome, and lower levels of education.[10–12] In particular, traumatic head injury in combination with the apo E4 genotype has been associated with an increased risk of AD.[13]

PATHOPHYSIOLOGY

STRUCTURAL CHANGES

AD is defined by both neuropathologic and clinical criteria. Neuropathologically, AD destroys neurons in the cortex and limbic structures of the brain, particularly the basal forebrain, amygdala, hippocampus, and cerebral cortex. These areas are responsible for higher learning, memory, reasoning, behavior, and emotional control. Anatomically, four major alterations in brain structure are seen:

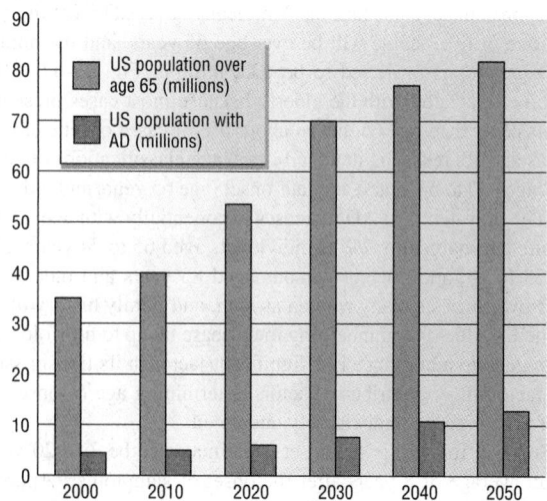

FIGURE 63–1. Our aging population. The percentage of U.S. population over age 65 years and the percentage with AD projected from years 2000 to 2050. (Estimates based on data from Crismon and Eggert[1] and U.S. Census Bureau.[106])

ortical atrophy, degeneration of cholinergic and other neurons, presence of neurofibrillary tangles (NFTs), and the accumulation of neuritic plaques.[1,7,14] NFTs and neuritic plaques are considered the signature lesions of AD; without them AD does not occur. Plaques and tangles may also be present in other diseases, even in normal aging, but there is a much higher concentration of plaques and tangles in patients with AD. To understand the causes of AD, researchers must discern the circumstances in which these lesions lead to the clinical picture of AD.[13]

NFTs are comprised of paired helical filaments that aggregate in dense bundles. Paired helical filaments are formed from tau protein. Tau protein provides structural support to microtubules, the cell's transportation and skeletal support system.[7,13] When tau filaments undergo abnormal phosphorylation at a specific site, they cannot bind effectively to microtubules, and the microtubules collapse. Without an intact system of microtubules, the cell cannot function properly and eventually dies.[13] Overactivity of kinases such as microtubule affinity-regulating kinase, or underactivity of phosphatases could theoretically produce or prevent breakdown of abnormally phosphorylated tau protein.[7,13] NFTs are found in other dementing illnesses besides AD, and may represent a common method by which various inciting factors culminate in cell death.[7]

Neuritic plaques (also termed amyloid or senile plaques) are extracellular lesions found in the brain and cerebral vasculature (amyloid angiopathy). Plaques are comprised of βAP, and an entwined mass of broken neurites (axon and dendrite projections of neurons).[1,7,13] Many of these broken neurites contain neuropil filaments made up of the abnormally phosphorylated tau protein found in NFTs.[7,13] Two types of glial cells, astrocytes and microglia, are also found in plaques.[1,7,13] Among other functions, glial cells secrete inflammatory mediators and serve as scavenger cells, which may be important in causing the inflammatory processes that occur in the development of AD. While the number of NFTs is strongly correlated with the severity of dementia, the number of neuritic plaques is not.[7] Clinical development of AD may inversely correlate with the number of normal neurons and synapses remaining despite plaque presence,[7,13,14] thus introducing the concept of neurologic reserve.

Forming the center of the neuritic plaque are aggregates of a 39- to 43-amino acid protein segment called βAP.[7] The βAP accumulating in the brain and cerebral blood vessels in AD is different from other disease-producing amyloid proteins.[7] βAP is cleaved from the APP, a transmembrane protein.[1,7,13] Proteases cleave APP in several different ways (Fig. 63–2). In the normal secretory pathway APP is cleaved through the βAP region, first using an enzyme called

α-secretase, and then by an enzyme termed γ-secretase. The resulting product, p3, is soluble and harmless.[7] In the potentially pathologic process, the endosomal pathway cleaves on both sides of βAP, first with β-secretase and then with γ-secretase, resulting in the formation of a βAP fragment which is released into the extracellular space.[7,13] Most of these βAP strings contain 40 amino acids, but it was recently determined that a version of βAP containing 42 amino acids damages nerve cells. Although it is not known how βAP causes neuronal damage, it does cause dysregulation in calcium and damage to mitochondria.[7] This in turn may trigger inflammatory mediators. Taken as a whole, these data suggest that βAP deposition occurs early in the disease process, rather than being simply an end-product of neuronal death, and likely initiates the process of plaque formation and nerve cell destruction.

AD is a neuronal degenerative process that is characterized by the presence of NFTs, neuritic plaques, and cellular atrophy in the cortex and limbic structures of the brain. Though the presence of these structural changes are the hallmark of definitive AD diagnosis, the initial precipitating event remains uncertain.

INFLAMMATORY MEDIATORS

Inflammatory mediators and other immune system constituents are present near areas of plaque formation, suggesting that the immune system plays an active role in the pathogenesis of AD. Although perhaps not the disease-initiating event, an immune response generated against some brain insult could facilitate neuronal destruction. Evidence supporting significant involvement of the immune system includes the increased presence of acute-phase proteins, such as α_1-antichromotrypsin and α_2-macroglobulin, both in the serum and within amyloid plaques of patients with AD.[15] Glial cells (microglial cells and astrocytes), cytokines (e.g., interleukin-1 and interleukin-6), and components of the classic complement cascade are also markedly increased in plaque-infested areas.[15] These inflammatory mediators increase βAP toxicity and aggregation. Chronic production of cytotoxic agents and free radicals by activated microglia can result in accelerated neurodegeneration.

Microglial cells located around and within amyloid plaques are thought to release inflammatory mediators, which locally destroy neuronal tissue. Glial cells also function as phagocytes, similar to macrophages and monocytes in the periphery. Another component of the complement cascade, the membrane attack complex, is found associated with broken neurites and areas containing NFTs, implicating the membrane attack complex as a promoter of the vast neuronal destruction characterizing AD.[15] As stated earlier, the acute-phase proteins α_1-antichromotrypsin and α_2-macroglobulin also act as protease inhibitors, and could influence proteolytic breakdown of APP into βAP.[7,15] As is the case in many chronic inflammatory illnesses, specific factors responsible for initiating the immune response are not known. One theory is that breaks in the blood-brain barrier caused by trauma, leaky endothelial cells, or other conditions trigger an immune response to brain proteins previously unexposed to the periphery.[15,16] Another possibility is that the immune system is activated by plaque precursors or by-products of damaged cells, resulting in further destruction of adjacent neurons.[16]

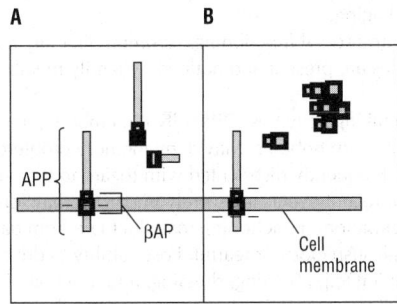

FIGURE 63–2. Representation of two physiologic cleavage sites of APP. APP is pictured as a transmembrane protein, with the βAP subunit anchored within the membrane. In part A, α-secretase and then γ-secretase cut APP through the βAP region. In part B, β-secretase and then γ-secretase cut βAP on either side of the βAP subunit. βAP is then released intact into the extracellular fluid, where it can aggregate, forming insoluble preamyloid plaques. (Adapted from St George-Hyslop[7] and Mortimer.[13])

THE CHOLINERGIC SYSTEM

Multiple neuronal pathways are destroyed in AD. Damage occurs in any nerve cell population located in or traveling through plaque-laden areas.[7] Widespread cell destruction results in a variety of neurotransmitter deficits. Most profoundly damaged are the cholinergic pathways, particularly a large system of neurons located at the base of the forebrain in the nucleus basalis of Meynert, a brain area believed to be involved in thought integration.[1,7] Axons of these cholinergic neurons project to the frontal cortex and hippocampus, areas strongly associated with memory and cognition.

The discovery of vast cholinergic cell loss led to the development of a cholinergic hypothesis linked to the pathophysiology of AD. The cholinergic hypothesis targeted cholinergic cell loss as the source of memory and cognitive impairment in AD. Therefore it was presumed that increasing cholinergic function would improve symptoms of memory loss. This approach is flawed for two reasons. First, cholinergic cell loss appears to be a secondary consequence of Alzheimer's pathology, not the disease-producing event; second, cholinergic neurons are only one of many neuronal pathways destroyed in AD. It is increasingly clear that simple addition of acetylcholine cannot compensate for the loss of neurons, receptors, and other neurotransmitters lost during the course of the illness. The goal then is to minimize or improve symptoms through augmentation of neurotransmission at remaining synapses.

OTHER NEUROTRANSMITTER ABNORMALITIES

Although the cholinergic system has received the lion's share of attention in AD pharmaceutical research, deficits also exist in other neuronal pathways. For example, serotonergic neurons of the raphe nuclei and noradrenergic cells of the locus ceruleus are lost, while monoamine oxidase type B activity is increased. Monoamine oxidase type B is found predominantly in the brain and in platelets, and is responsible for metabolizing dopamine. In addition, abnormalities appear in glutamate pathways of the cortex and limbic structures, where a loss of neurons leads to a focus on excitotoxicity models as possible contributing factors to AD pathology.

Glutamate is the major excitatory neurotransmitter in the cortex and hippocampus. Many neuronal pathways essential to learning and memory use glutamate as a neurotransmitter, including the pyramidal neurons (a layer of neurons with long axons carrying information out of the cortex), hippocampus, and entorhinal cortex. Glutamate and other excitatory amino acid neurotransmitters have been implicated as

potential neurotoxins in AD.[16] If glutamate is allowed to remain in the synapse for extended periods of time, it can destroy nerve cells. Toxic effects are thought to be mediated through increased intracellular calcium and accumulation of intracellular free radicals.[1,16] The presence of βAP renders cells more susceptible to glutamate-mediated excitotoxicity in vitro. Dysregulated glutamate activity is thought to be one of the primary mediators of neuronal injury after stroke or acute brain injury. Although intimately involved in cell injury, the role of excitatory amino acids in AD is as yet unclear; however, blockade of N-methyl-D-aspartate (NMDA) receptors decreases activity of glutamate in the synapse and may lessen the degree of cellular injury in AD.

CHOLESTEROL

Research has found multiple links between cholesterol and the occurrence of AD. Some evidence suggests that cellular membranes contain lipid rafts rich in cholesterol. These rafts are small conglomerates of protein and cholesterol that float within the cellular membrane of the lipid bilayer. The APP in the lipid rafts is cleaved by β- and γ-secretases to produce β-amyloid fragments that could eventually form amyloid plaques.[17,18] It is theorized that cholesterol depletion can inhibit the amyloidogenic pathway and prevent or slow down the plaque formation process. In addition, the APP in the lipid rafts may alter the shape of the membrane, which could promote further amyloid formation via a seeding-type mechanism.[17,18] Depleting cellular cholesterol appears to decrease this process. Another potential theory linking cholesterol to AD involves the apo E4 allele. The apo E4 allele is thought to be involved in cholesterol metabolism, and neuronal cholesterol levels have been theorized to be increased in the presence of this allele.[17] The elevated cholesterol levels in brain neurons may alter membrane functioning and result in the cascade leading to plaque formation and AD.

ESTROGEN

Estrogen is thought to be involved in promoting neuronal growth, and in preventing oxidative damage, which would benefit cells exposed to βAP.[19] Estrogen receptors are present in the brain, and are

TABLE 63–2. Stages of Cognitive Decline: The Global Deterioration Scale (GDS)

Stage 1	Normal	No subjective or objective change in intellectual functioning.
Stage 2	Forgetfulness	Complaints of losing things or forgetting names of acquaintances. Does not interfere with job or social functioning. Generally a component of normal aging.
Stage 3	Early confusion	Cognitive decline causes interference with work and social functioning. Anomia, difficulty remembering right word in conversation, and recall difficulties are present and noticed by family members. Memory loss may cause anxiety for patient.
Stage 4	Late confusion (early AD)	Patient can no longer manage finances or homemaking activities. Difficulty remembering recent events. Begins to withdraw from difficult tasks and to give up hobbies. May deny memory problems.
Stage 5	Early dementia (moderate AD)	Patient can no longer survive without assistance. Frequently disoriented with regard to time (date, year, season). Difficulty selecting clothing. Recall for recent events is severely impaired; may forget some details of past life (e.g., school attended or occupation). Functioning may fluctuate from day to day. Patient generally denies problems. May become suspicious or tearful. Loses ability to drive safely.
Stage 6	Middle dementia (moderately severe AD)	Patients need assistance with activities of daily living (e.g., bathing, dressing, and toileting). Patients experience difficulty interpreting their surroundings; may forget names of family and caregivers; forget most details of past life; have difficulty counting backward from 10. Agitation, paranoia, and delusions are common.
Stage 7	Late dementia	Patient loses ability to speak (may only grunt or scream), walk, and feed self. Incontinent of urine and feces. Consciousness reduced to stupor or coma.

Adapted from Reisberg et al.[103]

istributed in a pattern consistent with areas destroyed in AD.[19,20] In he hippocampus, cerebral cortex, and basal forebrain, estrogen receptors colocalize with receptors for nerve growth factor on cholinergic erve terminals.[20,21] The presence of estrogen increases the number f nerve growth factor receptors. The ability of estrogen to interact with nerve growth factor may explain estrogen's ability to promote ynaptic growth, stimulating axons and dendrites to sprout new terminals. Estrogen supplementation also prevents decrements in choline ptake and choline acetyltransferase concentrations, which occurs in ats following ovariectomy. This suggests that estrogen is important in naintaining normal cholinergic neurotransmission.[20] Estrogen may lso increase NMDA receptor numbers in brain areas involved in ecording new memories. In addition to promoting growth, estrogen revents cell damage by acting as an antioxidant.[19] In culture, estrogen rotects hippocampal neurons exposed to glutamate and β-amyloid rom cytotoxic and free radical damage.

A single common mechanism for producing AD does not exist. Regardless of the source, however, the features remain the same: legeneration of neurons in higher brain areas; accumulation of NFTs nd neuritic plaques; profound destruction of cholinergic pathways; nd an insidious dementia, slowly progressive until death.

CLINICAL PRESENTATION

The onset of AD is almost imperceptible, without abrupt changes in cognition or function. Deficits occur progressively over time, ffecting multiple areas of cognition.[1,22] For treatment and assessnent purposes, it is helpful to divide Alzheimer's symptoms into two asic categories: cognitive symptoms and noncognitive (behavioral) ymptoms.[22] Cognitive symptoms are present throughout the illness, whereas behavioral symptoms are less predictable.[22] Table 63–2 sumnarizes the stages of AD.

GENERAL

The patient may have vague memory complaints initially, or the paient's significant other may report that the patient is "forgetful." Cognitive decline is gradual over the course of illness. Behavioral listurbances may be present in moderate stages. Loss of daily funcion is common in advanced stages.

SYMPTOMS

Cognitive: Memory loss (poor recall and losing items); aphasia (circumlocution and anomia); apraxia; agnosia; disorientation (impaired perception of time and unable to recognize familiar people); impaired executive function

Noncognitive: Depression, psychotic symptoms (hallucinations and delusions), behavioral disturbances (physical and verbal aggression, motor hyperactivity, uncooperativeness, wandering, repetitive mannerisms and activities, and combativeness)

Functional: Inability to care for self (dressing, bathing, toileting, and eating)

LABORATORY TESTS

• Rule out vitamin B_{12} and folate deficiency
• Rule out hypothyroidism with thyroid function tests

OTHER DIAGNOSTIC TESTS

• CT or MRI scans may aid diagnosis

DIAGNOSIS

A family member rather than the patient often first brings memory complaints to the attention of a primary care clinician. Up to 50% of patients who meet criteria for dementia are not given a diagnosis in the primary care setting, leading some to believe that an appropriate screening tool may be helpful in aiding diagnosis and leading to earlier treatment.[23] Despite the phenomenon of underdiagnosis, the United States Preventative Services Task Force recently concluded that there are insufficient data to recommend for or against cognitive screening for AD because it could not be determined if the benefits outweigh the risks.[24] Similarly, the Quality Standards Subcommittee of the American Academy of Neurology (AAN) recommended against screening in asymptomatic patients; however, screening and monitoring were useful in patients who were classified as having mild cognitive impairment (patients do not meet criteria for dementia, but do have some impairment of memory), because they are at increased risk for developing dementia.[25]

At present the only way to definitively diagnose AD is through direct examination of brain tissue at autopsy or biopsy. In 1984 the National Institute of Neurological and Communicative Disorders and Stroke (NINCDS) and the Alzheimer's Disease and Related Disorders Association (ADRDA) developed criteria for diagnosing patients with probable AD, reducing the percentage of erroneously diagnosed AD cases to less than 10%. The NINCDS-ADRDA criteria (Table 63–3) remain the standard.[26] *Diagnostic and Statistical Manual of Mental Disorders*, 4th ed., Text Revision (DSM-IV-TR) criteria are also considered appropriate for making the diagnosis.[27,28] Other recommendations from the AAN include noncontrast computed

---

TABLE 63–3. NINCDS-ADRDA Criteria and Diagnostic Work-Up for Probable Alzheimer's Disease

I. History of progressive cognitive decline of insidious onset
 • In-depth interview of patient and caregivers
II. Deficits in at least two or more areas of functioning
III. No disturbance of consciousness
 • Confirmation with use of dementia rating scale (e.g., Mini-Mental Status Exam [MMSE] or Blessed Dementia Scale)
IV. Age between 40 and 90 years (usually >65 years)
V. No other explainable cause of symptoms
 • Normal laboratory tests including hematology, full chemistries, B_{12} and folate, thyroid function tests, Venereal Disease Research Lab test (to rule out venereal disease or syphilis)
 • Normal electrocardiogram and electroencephalogram
 • Normal physical exam, including thorough neurologic exam
 • Neuroimaging: CT or MRI scanning: No focal lesions signifying other possible causes of dementia are present. Abnormalities which are common, but not diagnostic for AD include general cerebral wasting, widening of sulci, widening of the ventricles, and lesions of white matter surrounding the ventricle deep in the brain

The Mini-Mental Status Exam is a commonly used scale that measures orientation, recall, short-term memory, concentration, constructional praxis, and language. The MMSE is scored from 0 to 30, with a score of 10–26 typical of mild to moderate Alzheimer's disease.
Adapted from McKhann et al.[26]

tomography (CT) or magnetic resonance imaging (MRI) scanning, which can be useful neuroimaging tests for initial evaluation; screening and treatment of depression, B_{12} deficiency, and hypothyroidism are also recommended.[28] Other tests such as linear or volumetric MRI or CT, positron emission tomography, single photon emission computed tomography, apo E genotyping, cerebrospinal fluid or other biomarkers, or syphilis serology are not recommended at this time.[28] Following diagnosis, functional assessment can be obtained from the patient and caregiver using the functional activities questionnaire (FAQ).[29]

▶ TREATMENT: Alzheimer's Disease

■ DESIRED OUTCOMES

2 None of the current treatments for AD are curative or are known to directly reverse or halt the pathophysiologic processes of the disorder. Therefore the primary goal of treatment in AD is to symptomatically treat cognitive difficulties and preserve patient function as long as possible. Secondary goals include treating the psychiatric and behavioral sequelae that occur as a result of the disease.

■ GENERAL TREATMENT APPROACH

6 Clinical trials have consistently shown the need for early and continuous treatment with cholinesterase inhibitors.[30-32] **7** Following this approach allows for maximum gain and maintenance of cognition and activities of daily living. A symptomatic approach is used to treat psychiatric symptoms as they arise.

Also essential to treatment is the provision of education to the patient and family at the time of diagnosis. Discussion of the course of illness, treatment options, as well as legal and financial decisions allows the family to plan for these more effectively. Good communication skills are important to maintain a therapeutic environment and minimize stress.

■ NONPHARMACOLOGIC THERAPY

Treatment of AD must include both nonpharmacologic and pharmacologic approaches because AD has a profound effect on both the **8** patient and family. It is emphasized that nonmedication interventions are the current primary interventions for management of AD, and medications should be used in the context of multimodal interventions. Upon initial diagnosis, the patient and caregiver should be educated on the course of illness, prognosis, available treatments, legal decisions, and quality-of-life issues. Education, including short- and long-term programs, has been demonstrated to improve caregiver knowledge and confidence and in some cases delay time to nursing home placement.[33] Table 63–4 lists basic principles of care for the AD patient. Communication between the patient and family members is essential in order to minimize stress on everyone.

While encouraging as much function and self-reliance as possible, life for the AD patient must become progressively more simple and structured in order to compensate for the deficits in cognition and to ensure safety. Education and guidance need to be provided regarding the patient's independence in conducting activities of daily living, including use of power tools, household repairs, cooking, and especially driving. Latches may need to be installed on doors and cabinets to prevent wandering or rummaging through household items. The patient will need frequent reminders in the beginning, but increasing assistance later with personal hygiene and other personal activities of daily living. A night light and a bedside commode may help prevent confusion and wandering when the patient awakens in the middle of the night for toileting.

Caregiver communication is essential at all stages of AD. For example, overly technical or detailed directions may confuse and upset patients. Family members may not realize at first the degree of impairment of the Alzheimer's patient's memory and ability to reason. Simple instructions or a demonstration of the desired activity improves patient understanding. Caregivers with good intentions may try to push patients to continue doing familiar tasks in the hope that this will preserve existing function as long as possible. As the patient becomes increasingly unable to accomplish a task because of disease progression, the patient may easily become frustrated and upset. A simple change to a less demanding lifestyle may decrease agitated behaviors substantially. For example, the patient may accuse a family member of stealing an item that has been misplaced. The family member becomes upset at this accusation and attempts to rationalize or argue with the patient. This frequently causes agitated behavior to escalate. Although difficult, the caregiver may find that by ignoring accusations or changing the subject, the patient will calm down.

The caregiver must be prepared to face the changes in life that will occur, and acceptance of this does not come easily. Denial on the part of the patient and rationalization on the part of the family are common. The clinician should encourage the family to address legal and financial matters and designate a durable power of attorney for execution of financial and medical decisions once the patient is incompetent. The caregiver will need to address issues such as respite services to provide time for rest, relaxation, and conduct of personal business. Eventually the caregiver will need to face critical questions with respect to institutionalization. The two primary reasons for institutionalization of patient with AD are behavioral disturbances and incontinence, problems that most caregivers find difficult to manage in the home. This is probably the most difficult decision for the caregiver.

TABLE 63–4. Basic Principles of Care for the Alzheimer's Patient

- Keep requests and demands of the patient simple, and avoid complex tasks that might lead to frustration.
- Avoid confrontation, and defer requests that lead to frustration.
- Remain calm, firm, and supportive if the patient becomes upset.
- Maintain a consistent environment and avoid unnecessary changes.
- Provide frequent reminders, explanations, and orientation cues.
- Recognize declines in capacity and adjust expectations for patient performance.
- Bring sudden declines in function and the emergence of new symptoms to professional attention.

Adapted from Rabins.[34]

TABLE 63–5. Resources for Caregivers of Persons with Alzheimer's Disease

The following organizations provide educational literature and information on diagnosis, treatment, social support, and ongoing research in Alzheimer's disease:

U.S. Administration on Aging
1 Massachusetts Avenue
Suites 4100 and 5100
Washington, DC 20201
Phone: 202-619-0724
E-Mail: AoAInfo@aoa.gov
Web: http://www.aoa.dhhs.gov/

Alzheimer's Disease Education and Referral Center (ADEAR)
P.O. Box 8250
Silver Springs, MD 20907-8250
Phone: (800) 438-4380
Web: http://www.alzheimers.org

The Alzheimer's Association
225 North Michigan Avenue, Suite 1700
Chicago, IL 60611
Phone: (800) 272-3900
Web: http://www.alz.org

The Eldercare Locator
Phone: (800) 667-1116
Web: http://www.eldercare.gov

Suggested reading
Davies HD, Jensen MP. Alzheimer: The Answers You Need. Forest Knolls, CA, Elder Books, 1998.
Gruetzner H. Alzheimer's: The Complete Guide for Families and Loved Ones. New York, Wiley, 1997.
Mace NL, Robins PV. The 36-Hour Day: A Family Guide to Caring for Persons with Alzheimer's Disease, Related Dementing Illnesses, and Memory Loss in Later Life. Baltimore, Johns Hopkins University Press, 1991.
McGowin DF. Living in the Labyrinth: A Personal Journal Through the Maze of Alzheimer's Disease. New York, Dell, 1994.

Clinician support and referral to social services is vitally important in assisting the caregiver at that moment. The family should also be referred to local resources, such as the Alzheimer's Association, that can provide detailed information regarding support services. Table 63–5 lists some referral sources and references for caregivers.

Education, communication, and planning are the key nonpharmacologic components of caring for an AD patient. Preparation in the early stages of illness will lessen some of the caregiver stress as the illness progresses.

PHARMACOLOGIC THERAPY

PHARMACOTHERAPY FOR COGNITIVE SYMPTOMS

The cholinesterase inhibitors are indicated for treatment of mild to moderate AD. None of the agents in this class have been compared in head-to-head clinical trials; therefore no conclusions on the effectiveness of one agent versus another can be made. The latest treatment guidelines, which were written prior to memantine becoming available, recommend the use of cholinesterase inhibitors as beneficial treatment for AD, and no preference has been suggested for a specific agent.[33–35]

CLINICAL CONTROVERSIES

Several cholinesterase inhibitors are now available, raising the question of whether it is appropriate to switch a patient from one to another if the first is not considered effective. Theoretical differences exist in their mechanisms of action, but some clinicians feel that these differences will not be clinically meaningful; therefore switching is not helpful. Switching is recommended if a patient is not tolerating the initial treatment. Most clinicians probably switch to another agent, and initial data seem to indicate that some patients do respond to an alternative cholinesterase inhibitor.

Disagreement exists about how to determine effectiveness of cholinesterase inhibitors. Selection of qualitative versus quantitative assessment may bias a clinician's impression of response. Subtle changes are often detected only by psychometric testing rather than with routine questioning. No standard has been suggested to define the effectiveness of these medications; therefore great variation exists between clinicians, and the duration of treatment ranges from months to years.

Additionally, two of these guidelines recommend consideration for concomitant treatment with vitamin E.[33,34] The AAN guidelines consider selegiline as an option for treatment, recommend against estrogen, and feel evidence is insufficient to support anti-inflammatory agents.[33] In practice, with the exception of tacrine, any of the cholinesterase inhibitors are appropriate as initial treatment. Some clinicians prefer donepezil because more data are available on long-term use, and it can be given once daily.

Cholinesterase inhibitors should be used throughout the course of illness because of the cognitive benefits, possible treatment of behavioral symptoms, and economic factors. Additionally, vitamin E should be used adjunctively with the cholinesterase inhibitors throughout treatment. Vitamin E is recommended solely based on the results of one study that showed no cognitive benefit, but a delayed requirement for nursing home placement with vitamin E. Figure 63–3 shows pharmacotherapeutic treatment algorithms for AD. These recommendations are made based on available efficacy, safety, and tolerability data.

Unfortunately, clinical trials have failed to provide answers to key questions in treating AD patients. Information from clinical trials is insufficient to know if a cholinesterase inhibitor dose-response relationship exists, or if additional cognitive improvement may be gained by increasing to the maximum tolerated dose, rather than continuing with the usual recommended daily dosage. Guidance in extrapolating data related to changes in cognition is needed so that a reasonable duration of clinical treatment with cholinesterase inhibitors can be determined.

In natural disease progression studies, scores on the Alzheimer's Disease Assessment Scale—Cognition (ADAS-COG) have been shown to worsen (increase) by an average of four points over 6 months and seven points over 1 year. Based on these findings, the general consensus is that a four-point change in the ADAS-COG represents a clinically significant change. Therefore if a pharmacotherapeutic agent decreases the ADAS-COG by four points, one could think of this as having reversed progression of disease symptoms by 6 months. The utility of the ADAS-COG in clinical practice is limited due to the time required for administration; it is much more practical to assess changes in disease severity using the mini-mental

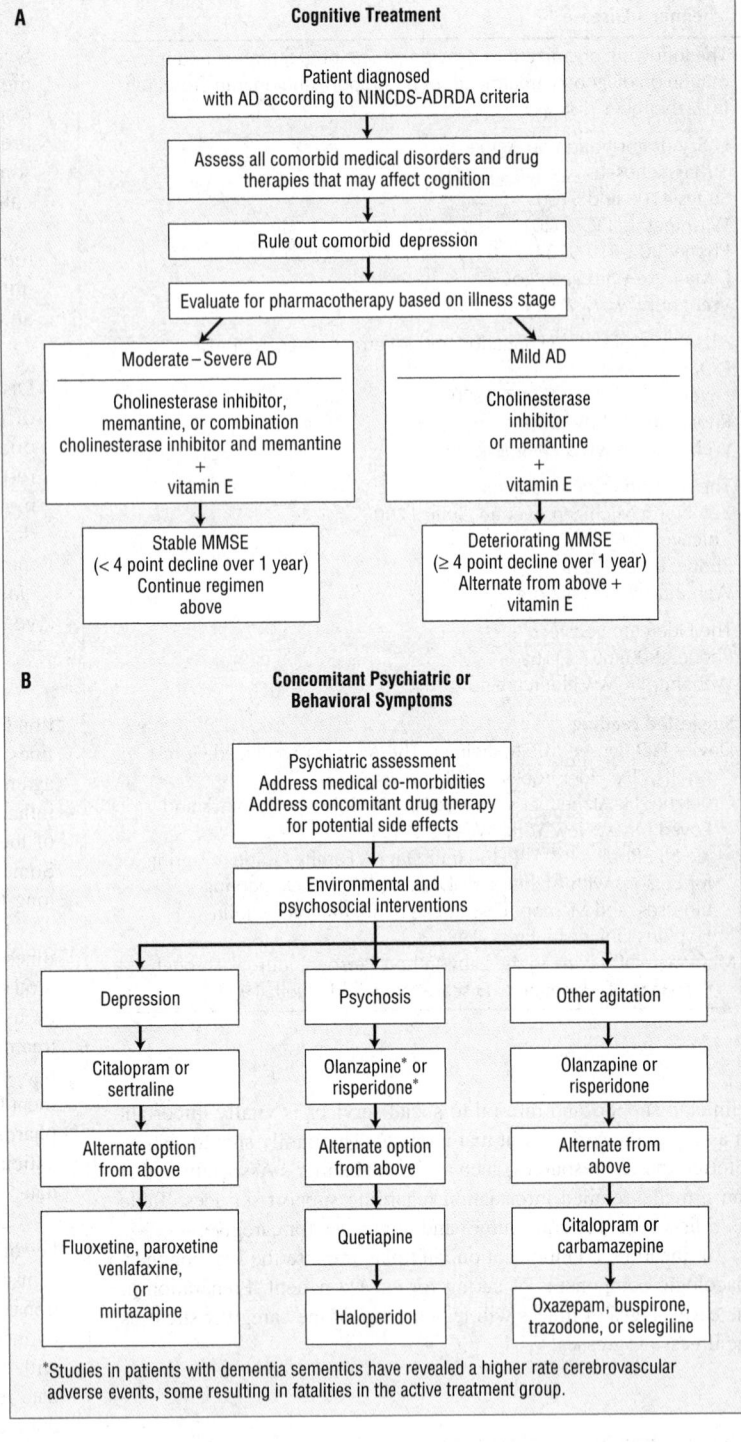

FIGURE 63–3. Proposed treatment algorithms for Alzheimer's disease. *A.* Cognitive treatment. *B.* Concomitant psychiatric or behavioral symptoms.

status exam (MMSE). An untreated patient has an average decline of 2 to 4 points in MMSE score per year. Successful treatment would therefore reflect a decline of less than 2 points a year. It is reasonable to change to a different cholinesterase inhibitor if the decline in MMSE score is greater than 2 to 4 points after 1 year with the initial agent.

The AAN has also provided guidelines for treatment of noncognitive symptoms of AD. For agitation and psychosis, atypical and traditional antipsychotics are effective; however, the atypicals are better tolerated. Selective serotonin reuptake inhibitors (SSRIs), monoamine oxidase type B inhibitors, and selected tricyclic antidepressants are recommended for treatment of depression.[33]

CLINICAL CONTROVERSY

Disagreement exists about the utility of cholinesterase inhibitors in advanced stages of AD. Some clinicians feel that patients should be taken off cholinesterase inhibitors once they have reached severe stages of AD, while others believe that these medications may continue to be helpful with managing psychiatric symptoms and maintaining function. Most clinicians probably discontinue cholinesterase inhibitors once the AD patient is bedridden and unable to perform activities of daily living.

TABLE 63–6. Recommended Dosing Strategies for Cholinesterase Inhibitors

	Tacrine	Donepezil	Rivastigmine	Galantamine
Starting dose	10 mg four times a day	5 mg daily	1.5 mg twice a day	4 mg twice a day
Maintenance dose	20–40 mg four times a day	5–10 mg daily	3–6 mg twice a day	8–12 mg twice a day
Time between dose adjustment	4–6 weeks	4–6 weeks	2 weeks	4 weeks

Cholinesterase Inhibitors

Just as levodopa was developed as replacement therapy for dopaminergic deficiency in Parkinson's disease, in the early 1980s researchers began to examine means to enhance cholinergic activity in patients with AD. Tacrine was the first such drug to be examined in a systematic fashion. However, tacrine is fraught with significant side effects, including hepatotoxicity, that severely limit the ability of patients to adhere to treatment. For all practical purposes the use of tacrine has been replaced by the use of safer, more tolerable cholinesterase inhibitors.

Donepezil. Donepezil[36] is a piperidine cholinesterase inhibitor with specificity for inhibition of acetylcholinesterase as compared to butyrylcholinesterase. This specificity is claimed to result in fewer peripheral side effects (such as nausea, vomiting, and diarrhea) than with nonspecific cholinesterase inhibitors such as tacrine.[37]

Donepezil is approved for treatment of cognitive impairment in mild to moderately severe AD (MMSE score 10 to 26) at doses of 5 mg and 10 mg daily. Preliminary evidence suggests that it may also be beneficial in patients with moderate to severe AD.[38] Cognitive improvement is generally modest with a sustained cognitive benefit of 6 to 9 months, followed by a gradual decline thereafter.[39]

Donepezil should be initiated at a 5-mg/day dose in the morning and titrated to 10 mg/day after 4 to 6 weeks if it is well tolerated. Table 63–6 summarizes cholinesterase inhibitor dosing recommendations. The most common donepezil side effects are nausea, vomiting,

and diarrhea—typical cholinergic side effects; however, the medication is well tolerated in most patients.[37] Table 63–7 compares the side effects of various AD medications.

Few drug interactions have been reported with donepezil. Pharmacokinetic studies in healthy male patients revealed increased donepezil concentrations when administered with either ketoconazole or cimetidine, inhibitors of the cytochrome P450 (CYP450) 3A4 system.[40] Four case reports in AD patients have cited potential interactions with paroxetine, risperidone, or tiapride.[40] The effects of enzyme inducers on donepezil kinetics have not been studied. Though highly protein bound (96%), donepezil has no effect on the kinetics of theophylline, warfarin, or digoxin.[40] Clinically significant interactions are unlikely with donepezil; however, monitoring for possible increased peripheral cholinergic side effects such as nausea, vomiting, or diarrhea is advisable when adding a CYP450 2D6 or 3A3/4 inhibitor to a donepezil regimen.

Rivastigmine. Butyrylcholinesterase is thought to play an important role in acetylcholine degradation following the depletion of acetylcholinesterase. Additionally, acetylcholinesterase is found in two forms: globular G4 and globular G1. The highest concentrations of globular G1 can be found in the hippocampus and cortex, two regions known to be affected in AD. Interestingly, although the globular G4 form is significantly depleted in postmortem studies, globular G1 remains abundant. By blocking this particular form of the acetylcholinesterase enzyme, higher concentrations of acetylcholine may be obtained.[41]

TABLE 63–7. Comparative Common Adverse Effects of AD Medications from Clinical Trials Data

Adverse Event	Tacrine (n = 634)	Donepezil (n = 747)	Rivastigmine (n = 1189)	Galantamine (n = 1040)	Memantine (n = 940)
Elevated liver function tests	29%	NR	NR	NR	NR
Nausea or vomiting	28%	NR	NR	NR	NR
Nausea	NR	11%	47%	24%	NR[a]
Vomiting	NR	5%	31%	13%	3%
Diarrhea	16%	10%	19%	9%	NR[a]
Headache	11%	10%	17%	8%	6%
Dizziness	12%	8%	21%	9%	7%
Muscle cramps	9%	6%	NR	NR	NR
Insomnia	6%	9%	9%	5%	NR[a]
Fatigue	4%	5%	9%	5%	NR
Anorexia	9%	4%	17%	9%	NR[a]
Depression	4%	3%	6%	7%	NR[a]
Abnormal dreams	NR	3%	NR	NR	NR
Weight decrease	3%	3%	3%	7%	NR
Somnolence	4%	2%	5%	4%	3%
Abdominal pain	8%	NR	13%	5%	NR
Tremor	2%	NR	4%	3%	NR
Agitation	7%	NR	NR	NR	NR[a]
Rhinitis	8%	NR	NR	NR	NR

[a]Reported in at least 2% of patients but exact percentage is unknown.
NR, not reported.
Compiled from package inserts for Aricept (donepizil),[36] Reminyl (galantamine),[45] Namenda (memantine),[47] Excelon (rivastigmine),[104] and Cognex (tacrine).[105]

Rivastigmine has central activity at acetylcholinesterase and butyrylcholinesterase, but low activity at these sites in the periphery. At least theoretically, this should result in a lower incidence of peripheral side effects.[37] Rivastigmine activity at the acetylcholinesterase globular G1 site is higher than at G4, and this may be theoretically advantageous because it may prevent degradation of acetylcholine via this enzyme over the course of the disease as compared to other cholinesterase inhibitors without this activity. It is difficult to say what this means clinically, and long-term head-to-head trials with other cholinesterase inhibitors are needed.

Rivastigmine is efficacious at doses of 6 to 12 mg/day.[31,42,43] Cognitive improvement was modest and sustained for 6 to 12 months in the treatment groups. Improvement in activities of daily living have also been demonstrated in this dosing range.[43] Rivastigmine has not been evaluated in patients with severe dementia or for treatment of behavioral symptoms.

Rivastigmine should be initiated at a dose of 1.5 mg twice daily and titrated upward at a minimum of 2-week intervals to a maximum daily dose of 12 mg. In addition to capsules, rivastigmine is also available as a 2-mg/mL oral solution (Table 63–6 provides dosing guidelines). Tolerability and absorption are improved when rivastigmine is given with food. The potential for drug interactions is low because of low protein binding, and it is not metabolized through the CYP450 enzyme system.[40] Cholinergic side effects are the most common adverse effects with rivastigmine, but they were well tolerated in clinical studies.[31,42,43]

Galantamine.
Galantamine is the fourth approved cholinesterase inhibitor, and it also has activity as an allosteric nicotinic receptor agonist. Though galantamine has been shown to be efficacious at dosages of 16 mg/day, 24 mg/day, and 32 mg/day, the maximum dosage recommended by the manufacturer at this time is 24 mg/day.[32,44,45] Cognitive improvement was similar to that of other cholinesterase inhibitors, producing modest and sustained improvement for approximately 9 months. It is recommended that a patient be continued on the maximum tolerated dosage, as accelerated cognitive deterioration has been seen with dosage reductions.[32] Improvement in activities of daily living has also been demonstrated with galantamine.[32] Psychiatric and behavioral symptoms have been shown to remain stable, but not improved.[44]

Galantamine should be initiated at 8 mg/day with dosage titration of 8 mg/day occurring at 4-week intervals. This slower titration rate resulted in better patient tolerance and fewer reported adverse drug reactions; therefore adjustment at 4-week intervals is recommended in clinical practice. Galantamine is also available as a 4-mg/mL oral solution.

Galantamine is metabolized through the CYP450 2D6 and CYP450 3A4 pathways, and pharmacokinetic studies with inhibitors of these systems have resulted in increased galantamine concentrations or reductions in clearance.[40] Studies with CYP450 3A4 inducers have not been conducted. As with donepezil, monitoring for increased cholinergic side effects is recommended if inhibitors of these enzyme systems are added to galantamine.

Cholinesterase inhibitors are the primary treatment for patients with AD. Early and continued use seem to offer patients the optimal benefit. While no differences in effectiveness have been demonstrated to date, tolerability, dosing frequency, and ease of titration may be used for selection of the initial agent. The MMSE may be helpful as a monitoring tool for changes in severity of illness. Unless patients are not tolerating the initial medication, it is recommended to continue for at least a year before considering an alternative agent.

Other Agents

Memantine.
Memantine, an NMDA-antagonist, is a novel agent for treating AD. By blocking NMDA receptors, excitotoxic reactions, which ultimately lead to cell death, may be prevented.[46]

Memantine has been studied in patients with vascular dementia, and in patients with moderate and severe AD as monotherapy and in combination with donepezil with favorable results.[46] It is currently indicated for use in AD patients with moderate to severe illness.

Memantine has 100% bioavailability regardless of administration with or without food. Protein binding is low. Metabolism is minimal, and memantine is excreted renally unchanged. The half-life ranges from 60 to 100 hours. Based on its pharmacologic profile, memantine should be associated with few drug interactions. Preliminary in vitro tests did not reveal any CYP450 inhibition or any effect on acetylcholinesterase inhibitors.[46]

Overall, memantine has been well tolerated in clinical trials. The most frequent adverse events associated with memantine include constipation, confusion, dizziness, headache, coughing, and hypertension.[47] As some of these side effects are also reported with cholinesterase inhibitors, caution should be used when administering memantine with this class of medications.[46]

Memantine is likely to be used as monotherapy and also in combination with cholinesterase inhibitors, particularly in patients with moderate to severe AD. Memantine should be initiated at 5 mg once a day and increased weekly by 5 mg a day to the effective dose of 10 mg twice daily.[47] It may be given with or without food. Dosing of 10 mg daily is recommended in patients with creatinine clearance of 40 to 60 mL/min and patients with severe renal impairment (creatinine clearance <40 mL/min) should not receive memantine.[46]

CLINICAL CONTROVERSY

Because of its potential effectiveness, tolerability, and low cost, some clinicians recommend the addition of vitamin E. However, some feel that there is insufficient evidence to broadly recommend this as an additive treatment.

Vitamin E and Selegiline.
Based on pathophysiologic theories involving free radicals, significant interest has evolved regarding the use of antioxidants in the treatment of AD. Vitamin E is often recommended as adjunctive treatment for AD patients. This recommendation is based on data from the only published clinical trial to date, which evaluated the time to critical endpoints (i.e., death, institutionalization, loss of ability to perform activities of daily living, or severe dementia) in patients treated with vitamin E, selegiline, the combination, or placebo.[48] Although vitamin E and selegiline were superior to placebo, this study has been criticized because of differences in baseline cognitive severity, calling the validity of the results into question. Nonetheless, vitamin E's potential effectiveness, favorable side effect profile, and low cost have perpetuated its use as adjunctive therapy. Although potential benefits of vitamin E combined with a cholinesterase inhibitor have not been evaluated, there are no known complications from their combined use. Vitamin E should be titrated to a maintenance dose of 1000 international units twice a day.[48]

Additional clinical data are lacking in support of selegiline, and it is not recommended as adjunctive therapy in AD.[49]

Estrogen.
Interest in estrogen use has increased over the last decade. Most, but not all, epidemiologic studies show a lower incidence of AD in women who took estrogen replacement therapy

postmenopausally. Results from these epidemiologic trials prompted researchers to look at the use of estrogen preventively and as a treatment for cognitive decline.

Recent clinical trials have not supported the use of estrogen as a treatment for cognitive decline. Two studies evaluating the potential benefit of conjugated estrogens as a treatment for cognitive decline did not show any benefit[50,51]; behavioral and functional outcomes were not improved either.

The Women's Health Initiative Memory Study, the largest trial to date, enrolled over 4500 healthy women 65 and older to evaluate the incidence of dementia and mild cognitive impairment in patients taking estrogen plus progestin versus placebo.[52] The mean time from entry until final cognitive assessment was 4 years, with the number of probable dementia cases in the estrogen plus progestin group almost double that of the placebo group (45 versus 22, respectively). Overall, the incidence of probable dementia was low (67 total cases), but suggests 23 more cases of dementia for every 10,000 women per year if they are treated with combination estrogen and progestin. The risk of developing mild cognitive impairment was no different between the treatment and placebo groups. These studies do not support a role for estrogen in treating symptoms of AD. Ongoing clinical trials are being conducted to determine the potential role of estrogen as a preventive treatment for AD.

Other health risks of estrogen use have also been raised recently. The estrogen plus progestin arm of the Women's Health Initiative was terminated early because this treatment group exceeded the threshold for breast cancer risk.[53,54] Average follow-up was 5.2 years and showed increased risk in coronary heart disease, breast cancer, stroke, and pulmonary embolism. Benefits included reduced risk of colorectal cancer and hip fracture. The effect of estrogen in AD as a treatment of cognition has not been established, and other health risks are also of concern; therefore estrogen should only be used in those patients who have another medical reason for estrogen replacement therapy.

Anti-Inflammatory Agents. Epidemiologic studies have also suggested a protective effect against AD in patients who have taken nonsteroidal anti-inflammatory drugs (NSAIDs).[55-57] Treatment for less than 2 years has been associated with a lower relative risk of AD; however, longer treatment duration lowered this risk further.[56,57]

The benefits of anti-inflammatory agents on cognition have been less compelling in clinical studies. Indomethacin, prednisone, and diclofenac/misoprostol administration have had no cognitive benefit in AD patients.[58-60] Tolerability was also problematic.[58,59] Additionally, prednisone treatment was associated with worsening behavioral symptoms,[59] and data from other patient populations suggest that prednisone may be associated with cognitive impairment.[61] Because there is a lack of compelling data and also a significant incidence of adverse effects, particularly gastritis and the possibility of gastrointestinal bleeds, NSAIDs and prednisone are not recommended for general use in the treatment or prevention of AD at the present time.

Recent attention has shifted to the potential benefit of the cyclooxygenase-2 inhibitors in light of their anti-inflammatory properties. Rofecoxib has been compared to naproxen and placebo with no demonstrated cognitive benefit after 1 year.[62] Perhaps the duration of treatment has been inadequate in clinical trials studying anti-inflammatory agents and longer-term exposure as seen in epidemiologic trials is necessary. Until clinical trials establish clinical benefit of the cyclooxygenase-2 inhibitors, their general use as preventive treatment for AD cannot be recommended. Market withdrawal of rofecoxib and other safety concerns within this class may limit further study in AD.

Lipid-Lowering Agents. Interest in the potential protective effects in AD patients of lipid-lowering agents, particularly the 3-hydroxy-3-methylglutaryl-CoA (HMG-CoA)-reductase inhibitors, is growing based on animal and recent epidemiologic studies. Longitudinal population-based studies have suggested an association between elevated midlife total cholesterol levels and AD.[63,64] Other studies suggested that the incidence of AD is lower in patients who have taken either a statin[65,66] or another lipid-lowering agent,[67] but not in patients who were taking other cardiovascular medications.[66] Interestingly, pravastatin and lovastatin, but not simvastatin, were associated with a lower prevalence of AD,[66] suggesting that individual agents rather than a class effect impact AD prevalence. Although these studies have linked cholesterol levels to increased risk of AD, others have yielded conflicting results.[68]

Prospective clinical trials will need to address the cognitive benefit, duration of treatment, class effect versus effectiveness of individual agents, and optimal dosing. Simvastatin has been studied in one clinical trial showing a reduction in β-amyloid in patients with milder AD, but not in those with severe illness.[69] Mixed results were also seen in cognitive outcomes.[69] Atorvastatin is currently being studied in clinical trials. Further studies, including randomized prospective statin trials, are needed to determine cholesterol's role, if any, in the pathogenesis of AD. For now these agents should be reserved for patients who have other indications for their use.

Ginkgo Biloba. Egb 761, an extract of ginkgo biloba, is claimed to improve memory. Although it is thought to be an antioxidant and to affect inflammation and neuromodulation, the mechanisms of the multiple compounds in Egb 761 have not been elucidated. A recent meta-analysis determined that only 4 of 57 ginkgo biloba studies that were identified met minimal scientific standards for clinical trials; however, cognitive benefit, though modest, has been demonstrated.[70] Standardized doses of gingko ranged from 120 to 240 mg/day. No significant adverse events were reported; however, some case reports have shown an association with hemorrhaging.

Even if the herbal extract is effective, significant problems exist with its use. The content of herbal products is poorly standardized, and significant variation in supposed active ingredient content for some herbals exists from lot to lot and between manufacturers. Until these products are better standardized and their manufacturing and stability better assured, it is recommended that they be used with caution. Furthermore, little is known about potential adverse reactions, drug interactions, or long-term toxicity with their use.

Because the effects of cholinesterase inhibitors are modest, there is great interest in developing alternative or additional treatments for AD. Most of these alternatives have shown promise in epidemiologic studies; however, benefit in prospective clinical trials has been limited or insufficiently studied. Memantine is the first non–cholinesterase inhibitor approved for AD treatment. Its role in treatment will become more clearly defined in the next several years.

PHARMACOTHERAPY OF NONCOGNITIVE SYMPTOMS

The majority of patients with AD manifest noncognitive symptoms at some point in the illness.[22] These symptoms can be roughly divided into three categories: psychotic symptoms, inappropriate or disruptive behavior, and depression. Effective management of these problems is important because behavioral symptoms are distressing to both the patient and the caregiver, necessitate increased caregiver supervision and patience, and are a leading reason for nursing home placement.

TABLE 63–8. Medications Used in Treating Noncognitive Symptoms of Dementia

Drugs	Suggested Dosage in Dementia (mg/day)	Indications
Antipsychotics		Psychosis: hallucinations, delusions, suspiciousness
Haloperidol	0.5–4 mg	Disruptive behaviors: agitation, aggression
Olanzapine	2.5–10 mg	
Quetiapine	12.5–200 mg	
Risperidone	0.25–2 mg	
Antidepressants		Depression: poor appetite, insomnia, hopelessness,
Citalopram	10–20 mg	anhedonia, withdrawal, suicidal thoughts, agitation
Fluoxetine	5–20 mg	
Mirtazapine	15–45 mg	
Paroxetine	10–40 mg	
Sertraline	50–200 mg	
Trazodone	75–400 mg[a]	
Venlafaxine	37.5–150 mg	
Anticonvulsants		Agitation or aggression
Carbamazepine	100–1,000 mg[ab]	
Others		
Buspirone	10–45 mg	Disruptive behaviors
Oxazepam	10–60 mg[a]	Disruptive behaviors
Selegiline	10 mg	Disruptive behaviors, agitation, anxiety, depression

[a]Administer in divided doses.
[b]Dosage adjustment should be guided by drug serum concentrations.
Adapted from Borson and Raskind,[71] Defilippi and Crismon,[79] and Rabins et al.[87]

In fact, presence of neuropsychiatric symptoms increases caregiver burden more than loss of cognition or self-care.

Strategies for treatment of psychotic or behavioral symptoms should include both environmental and pharmacologic interventions (e.g., antipsychotics, antidepressants, mood stabilizers, and anxiolytics). The potential harm to the patient or caregiver should be used as a guide for selecting the appropriate intervention. For example, hallucinations or delusions that are of a nonstressful, nonthreatening nature can generally be ignored or redirected by family members. Nonaggressive behaviors can generally be managed with environmental interventions, such as distracting the patient from the behavior, creating a structured environment, providing reassurance to calm the patient, and attending support groups for the caregiver. Patients with aggressive behaviors should be approached similarly; however, pharmacologic treatment is often an additional necessity.

Despite the widespread nature of noncognitive symptoms in AD, until recently little research has been conducted in these patients. Data from clinical trials of antidepressants and antipsychotics are now emerging, although more research is needed. Because of limited clinical data, side-effect profiles have been used as a guide in selecting the appropriate treatment. Psychotropic medications with anticholinergic effects should be avoided because they may actually worsen cognition. Other side effects in the elderly include sedation, medication-induced postural instability, and extrapyramidal side effects, which can decrease the clinical utility of traditional psychotropic agents.

General guidelines governing therapy can be summarized as follows: Use reduced doses, monitor closely, titrate dosage slowly, and document carefully. Caregivers often have erroneous expectations regarding the effects of psychotropic medications, and the anticipated benefits and risks of therapy should be clearly explained. Disruptive behaviors and delusions wax and wane with disease progression. Attempts to slowly taper and discontinue antipsychotic medication should be undertaken in minimally symptomatic patients at least every 3 months, because many patients who initially respond to these medications show no change in symptoms and occasionally improve on medication withdrawal.[71] Table 63–8 outlines suggested doses of medications.

Antipsychotics

Antipsychotic medications have traditionally been used to treat disruptive behaviors and psychosis in AD patients. Symptoms responding to antipsychotics include assaultiveness, extreme agitation, hyperexcitability, hallucinations, delusions, suspiciousness, hostility, and uncooperativeness; whereas withdrawal, apathy, cognitive deficits, wandering, and incontinence are not responsive.[72]

Until the advent of the atypical antipsychotics, conventional agents were widely used, although available placebo-controlled studies suggested that they were moderately effective at best.[72,73] More recently, risperidone has been shown to have modest effects in patients with psychotic symptoms or behavioral disturbances associated with dementia.[74–76] It is recommended to begin with 0.25 mg daily and to titrate in 0.25- to 0.5-mg increments to 1 mg daily, which is usually considered the optimal dose. If response is inadequate, further titrating to a maximum of 2 mg daily may be necessary if the patient is tolerating the medication; however, side effects, particularly extrapyramidal effects, somnolence, and orthostasis, increase with increased dose.

Olanzapine has been studied in AD patients with modest results on psychiatric symptoms at doses of 5 and 10 mg/day. It should be noted that 15 mg/day has also been studied and was no more effective than placebo.[77] Because the pharmacologic profile of olanzapine includes cholinergic blockade, some concern has been raised as to the utility of this agent in the AD population. Clinical studies have not shown any deleterious cognitive effects in the short-term; however, these results cannot be extrapolated over the long-term.

No placebo-controlled trials are currently available evaluating quetiapine, ziprasidone, or aripiprazole in psychosis of dementia. An open-label study suggests possible effect and good tolerability with quetiapine.[78] For patients who respond inadequately, have elevated cardiovascular risk, or who have unacceptable side effects with risperidone or olanzapine, quetiapine is a reasonable alternative. Ziprasidone and aripiprazole require formal study in this population prior to recommending their use.

Patients with AD are more sensitive to antipsychotic side effects than other patient groups. Increased sensitivity to antipsychotic side effects in the elderly appears to be the result of altered pharmacodynamics rather than altered pharmacokinetics.[79] Particularly problematic side effects are extrapyramidal side effects, postural hypotension caused by α-adrenergic blockade, and anticholinergic effects, including increased confusion, urinary retention, constipation, and dry mouth.[79] For a more detailed description of antipsychotic side effects see Chap. 66 on schizophrenia. Overall, fewer side effects are seen with the newer atypical antipsychotics, making them a preferred choice for treatment of psychosis or aggression in the AD patient.[79] Effective doses of antipsychotic medications are much lower than those typically used to treat schizophrenia (see Table 63–8). The rule of thumb is to "start low and go slow."

Antidepressants

Prevalence estimates of depression in AD differ widely, ranging from less than 10% to 80%. Actual prevalence rates of major depression in AD are probably 5% to 15% in community-based patients and 15% to 20% among institutionalized patients.[71] The inconsistency in these figures is largely attributed to symptom overlap, diagnostic differences, and the patient population sampled. Early in the course of AD, depression presents much the same as in other elderly persons, but later in the disease course, diagnosis can be difficult. Apathy, decreased initiative and socialization, decreased concentration, psychomotor retardation, agitation, and changes in appetite and sleep patterns are all symptoms intrinsic to both dementia and depression.[71] Because of the inherent difficulty and variation in diagnosing depression in AD, criteria have recently been suggested to facilitate uniformity in diagnosis.[80] These criteria were based on DSM-IV-TR criteria for major depression with the following differences: presence of only three or more symptoms, symptoms need not be present nearly every day, irritability and social isolation or withdrawal were added as symptoms, and finally loss of interest or pleasure were revised to a decreased positive affect or pleasure. In determining whether or not a patient with these symptoms is depressed, it is particularly important to assess the patient's affect and ability to experience pleasure. Affective signs of depression might include crying spells, staying in bed, decreased food intake, asking to be killed, moaning, or sorrowful facial expression. An interview with the patient's caregiver can be helpful in obtaining a more accurate record of symptoms. Depression may be more common in the early stages of AD as the patient attempts to adjust to limitations associated with cognitive loss.

The bulk of literature examining antidepressant use in AD is made up of case reports and uncontrolled studies. Most of these report a favorable response to antidepressants,[72] but several placebo-controlled trials have demonstrated mixed results. Of the antidepressants studied, citalopram, sertraline, clomipramine, and moclobemide (a monoamine oxidase inhibitor not marketed in the U.S.) were considered efficacious in at least one study[81]; but fluoxetine and imipramine were no better than placebo. It should be noted that citalopram and sertraline have both been studied in other placebo-controlled trials in this population with no difference over placebo.[81]

A controlled comparator trial of fluoxetine 10 mg/day and amitriptyline 25 mg/day found that both were equally effective; however, the fluoxetine group tolerated the medication much better and had significantly lower dropout rates.[81,82] Similarly, a study comparing paroxetine 40 mg/day and imipramine 100 mg/day showed equal effectiveness.[81] The available literature also suggests that antidepressant response, as measured by reductions in Hamilton Depression Rating scores, is not as dramatic as in depressed nondemented patients. Because depressive target symptoms are difficult to distinguish from dementia, it is unclear whether this modest decrease in Hamilton Depression Rating scores is a result of poor drug response or of difficulty in assessing symptoms in this population.[80,81] Some clinicians have noted that a longer duration of treatment (e.g., up to 12 weeks) is required before elderly patients experience an antidepressant effect.

It is desirable to document symptoms of depression for several weeks prior to initiating antidepressant therapy in a patient with AD. A significant nonspecific treatment response occurs in this population, and it is possible that simply visiting with a clinician or increasing the patient's activity level may be sufficient to improve symptoms. Should this approach fail, a trial of an antidepressant may be initiated. Pharmacotherapy should be initiated with an antidepressant possessing a favorable side-effect profile. Citalopram and sertraline have been recommended as first-line agents because of demonstrated efficacy in placebo-controlled trials.[81] Other SSRIs such as fluoxetine, paroxetine, or serotonin/norepinephrine reuptake inhibitors such as venlafaxine or mirtazapine may be alternatives.[81] While tricyclics have antidepressant efficacy in the dementia population, their very significant anticholinergic effects, which could exacerbate confusion and memory disturbances, should preclude their use unless other alternatives have been exhausted.

In addition to their demonstrated effectiveness, SSRIs also have a low propensity to cause anticholinergic effects, orthostatic hypotension, and sedation, and can usually be dosed once daily. These medications are not risk free, however. Gastrointestinal adverse effects, confusion, agitation, dizziness, and insomnia have been reported in patients with AD taking fluoxetine, especially at higher doses (>20 mg of fluoxetine daily).[83] Paroxetine reportedly causes more anticholinergic effects than other SSRIs. For a more complete discussion of treatment of depression refer to Chap. 67 on depressive disorders.

Miscellaneous Therapies

Because antipsychotic therapy has shown only modest efficacy and poses a substantial risk of undesirable side effects, medications traditionally used to treat disruptive behaviors and aggression in other psychiatric and neurologic disorders have been suggested as potential alternatives. These alternatives include benzodiazepines, buspirone, carbamazepine, selegiline, and SSRIs.

In addition to antipsychotics, citalopram (10 to 20 mg/day) and carbamazepine (mean dose of 300 mg/day) have been shown to decrease psychosis and behavioral disturbances of dementia.[84,85] Carbamazepine was well tolerated in AD patients.[86]

Benzodiazepines, particularly oxazepam, have been used to treat anxiety, agitation, and aggression, but they generally show inferior efficacy when compared to antipsychotics. Because benzodiazepines impair cognition, can result in disinhibition, and may increase the risk of falls in AD patients, their routine use is not advised.[87] Conversely, the 5-HT$_{1A}$ partial agonist buspirone has shown benefit in treating agitation and aggression in a limited number of patients with minimal adverse effects.[88,89] Selegiline decreases anxiety, depression, and agitation in open-label and controlled studies.[90,91] Trazodone reportedly decreases insomnia, agitation, and dysphoria in AD patients, and is often used to treat sundowning.

Should antipsychotics fail to manage noncognitive behaviors, available evidence suggests that a trial of citalopram or carbamazepine may be appropriate second-line alternatives. Only minimal evidence exists to support the use of valproate in this population. Lithium has shown no benefit and frequent toxicity.[87] Clearly, more rigorous placebo-controlled studies are needed to determine the relative efficacy and place in therapy for these medication alternatives.

Interest has grown regarding the potential use of cholinesterase inhibitors for treatment of psychiatric symptoms in AD. Studies assessing noncognitive symptoms in clinical trials with tacrine, donepezil, and galantamine suggest that these agents have positive effects on psychiatric and behavioral symptoms.[92] Unfortunately, these have been post-hoc analyses or small open-label trials, making it difficult to draw conclusions. Significant differences were seen in hallucination and apathy scores. Additional research is needed in this area before specific treatment recommendations can be made with confidence.

Noncognitive symptoms are often the most difficult aspect of AD for the caregiver. Without effective treatment, nursing home placement is often needed. Selected antipsychotics and antidepressants have been useful for effective management of behavioral, psychotic, and depressive symptoms; this helps to ease caregiver burden and allow the patient to spend additional time at home. Alternative treatments are also available in case initial choices are not successful. Improved tolerability with newer medications should also make treatment easier for these patients.

PHARMACOECONOMIC CONSIDERATIONS

The economic and social costs of AD are staggering. It is the third most expensive illness in the United States after heart disease and cancer, and the majority of medical and caregiving expenses are left to the patients' families. The total national cost of Alzheimer's disease is estimated at approximately $100 billion annually.[93,94] Annual Medicare costs in 2000 were estimated at $31.9 billion and Medicaid costs for institutionalized AD patients were estimated at $18.2 billion.[95] With life expectancy and the number of AD cases increasing, the cost of AD is projected to quadruple over the next 50 years.[93] The potential financial burden of this disease on the health care system could reach crisis proportions in the near future unless more effective avenues are developed to provide care for these individuals, to prevent the disease from occurring, or to slow its progression.

Seventy-five percent of care for AD patients is provided by family and friends.[3] Lifetime cost of care for AD is estimated at $174,000.[3] Higher levels of home care have been associated with poorer health and higher rates of emotional stress in caregivers, increasing the likelihood of placing patients in institutionalized care, which is considered the greatest financial cost in treating patients with AD.[3] On average, the cost of yearly nursing home care is $42,000.[3] Clearly, the economic burden for the home-living AD patient is the time spent in caring for the patient, whereas in the nursing home burden is the cost for others to provide care.

Economic data in AD are increasing, and several studies have evaluated the cost benefits of medications. The Assessment of Health Economics in Alzheimer's Disease trial projected health and economic outcomes of AD patients treated with galantamine in the Netherlands over a 10-year period.[96] Full-time patient care was predicted to be delayed by 10% in AD patients treated with galantamine. Studies with donepezil and rivastigmine have also predicted decreases in total costs of therapy and delayed nursing home placement.[84,97,98]

Studies with agents other than cholinesterase inhibitors are rare but should increase in number as the understanding of AD and its potential treatments improve. A 28-week placebo-controlled trial with memantine reported cost savings and a lower incidence of institutionalization than in the placebo group.[99] Caregiver costs decreased by $824/month and societal costs by $1090/month with memantine therapy. However, direct medical costs to the patient treated with memantine were higher than placebo due to cost of the medication.

Other trials have suggested that patients may require longer treatment with medication therapy before cost savings become apparent. In a study of Medicare-managed patients, 204 AD patients receiving donepezil were compared with 204 AD patients receiving no medication therapy.[84] Health care costs were $3891 lower in patients receiving donepezil than those with no medications, and greater savings were reported with longer therapy (>270 days). A study with rivastigmine estimated cost savings to be $1595 per patient after projecting 3 years of continuous medication therapy.[100] Cost reductions were reported as higher when treatment was begun earlier in the course of the illness.

Caregiver time has been difficult to quantify into actual dollar amounts, but several studies have shown a decrease in caregiver time associated with medication treatment. A 1-year prospective double-blind trial of 286 patients receiving donepezil or placebo reported a decrease of 66 minutes per day of assisting with activities of daily living.[101] This resulted in $1033 of cost savings per patient in the donepezil group. A study with memantine reported a 103-minute-per-day reduction in caregiver time over 28 weeks of therapy.[99] Depending on the severity of illness, caregivers may spend up to 8 hours or more per day providing care to AD patients. Medication therapy that can reduce caregiver time or improve patient functioning may help with caregiver burden and delay time to nursing home placement.

Other pharmacoeconomic studies have evaluated cholinesterase inhibitor effects on cognitive functioning. Ernst and associates modeled potential cost savings of cholinesterase inhibitor treatment, and found potential cost savings for most mild or severely ill patients to be small. However, for home-dwelling patients with a baseline MMSE score of 7, potential cost savings from treatment were significant, with prevention of a 2-point decline saving $3700 annually.[102] The extent to which these types of studies predict economic outcomes in real practice is unclear.

Data from current pharmacoeconomic studies in AD suggest that medication therapy may reduce costs of treating this illness; however, the true cost effectiveness of these therapies has yet to be established. If AD treatments delay cognitive decline and time to nursing home placement, then they not only have potential economic benefit, but significant effects on the quality of life of patients and caregivers. Future studies, including prospective pharmacoeconomic trials of longer duration and more detailed cost evaluation modeling, are needed to determine the role and benefits of pharmacotherapy on AD.

EVALUATION OF THERAPEUTIC OUTCOMES

An evaluation of therapeutic outcomes in the patient with AD begins with a thorough assessment at baseline and a clear definition of therapeutic goals. Cognitive status, physical status, functional performance, mood, thought processes, and behavior all need to be evaluated before initiation of drug therapy. The clinician should interview both the patient and the caregiver to assess response to drug therapy. Because caregivers often have difficulty giving honest and frank information about their loved one's condition in his or her presence, it is often necessary to interview family caregivers separately. In evaluating response to cognitive agents, the clinician should ask questions about the patient's ability to perform daily functional tasks and about mood and behavior, as well as questions about memory and orientation. Objective assessments such as the MMSE for cognition and the FAQ for activities of daily living, should be used to quantify changes in symptoms and function.[85]

Because target symptoms of psychiatric disorders may respond differently in demented patients, a detailed list of symptoms to be treated should be documented in the pharmacotherapy plan to aid in monitoring. These could include, for example, "striking at spouse because patient believes spouse is an impostor," "verbal threats and refusal to allow clothes to be changed," and so on, as opposed to documenting vague symptoms such as "aggression" or "delusions." To make an accurate assessment of depression, multiple symptoms (e.g., sleep, appetite, and activity and interest levels) need to be assessed in addition to the patient's stated mood.

The patient should be observed carefully for potential side effects of drug therapy. Depending on the therapeutic agent being employed, patients should be assessed for potential side effects such as diarrhea, gastrointestinal distress, dizziness, sedation, extrapyramidal side effects, or worsening of behavior. The specific side effects to be monitored and the method and frequency of monitoring should be documented. Periodic assessments for drug effectiveness, side effects, compliance, need for dosage adjustment, or change in treatment should occur at least monthly. However, patients need to be treated for an adequate duration to see a therapeutic effect from a given intervention. Because the effects of cognition-enhancing medications are not great, a treatment period of several months to a year may be necessary before it can be determined whether therapy is beneficial. Cognitive effects of the drug are often noticed only as a plateauing during treatment or as deterioration following drug discontinuation. In general, cognitive agents should be continued if the patient is demonstrating no change in clinical status. However, if there is doubt, the medication can be slowly tapered and discontinued, and the patient monitored off the drug for 4 to 6 weeks to determine the need for continued therapy.

ABBREVIATIONS

AAN: American Academy of Neurology
AD: Alzheimer's disease
ADAS-COG: Alzheimer's Disease Assessment Scale—Cognition
ADRDA: Alzheimer's Disease and Related Disorders Association
apo E: apolipoprotein E
APP: amyloid precursor protein
βAP: beta-amyloid protein
CYP450: cytochrome P450 enzyme system
DSM-IV-TR: *Diagnostic and Statistical Manual of Mental Disorders*, 4th ed., Text Revision
FAQ: functional activities questionnaire
MMSE: mini-mental status exam
NFT: neurofibrillary tangle
NINCDS: National Institute of Neurological and Communicative Disorders and Stroke
NMDA: N-methyl-D-aspartate
NSAID: nonsteroidal anti-inflammatory drug
SSRI: Selective serotonin reuptake inhibitor

Review Questions and other resources can be found at *www. pharmacotherapyonline.com.*

REFERENCES

1. Crismon ML, Eggert AE. Pharmacist care of patients with Alzheimer's disease. In: Pharmacist Care: Mental Health. Alexandria, VA, National Institute for Pharmacist Care Outcomes, 2000:ALZ 1–29.
2. Hebert LE, Scherr PA, Bienias JL, et al. Alzheimer's disease in the U.S. population: Prevalence estimates using the 2000 census. Arch Neurol 2003;60:1119–1122.
3. Alzheimer's Association. Available at: http://www.alz.org/. Accessed May 1, 2003.
4. Nussbaum RL, Ellis CE. Alzheimer's disease and Parkinson's disease. N Engl J Med 2003;348:1356–1364.
5. Arias E, Smith BL. Deaths: Preliminary data for 2001. National Vital Statistics Reports, Vol. 51 No. 5. Hyattsville, MD, National Center for Health Statistics, 2003:1–48.
6. Chandra V, Bharucha NE, Schoenberg BS. Conditions associated with Alzheimer's disease at death: Case-control study. Neurology 1986;36:209–211.
7. St George-Hyslop PH. Piecing together Alzheimer's. Sci Am 2000; 283:76–83.
8. Blacker D. New insights into genetic aspects of Alzheimer's disease. Postgrad Med 2000;108:119–122, 125, 126, 129.
9. Corder EH, Saunders AM, Risch NJ, et al. Protective effect of apolipoprotein E type 2 allele for late-onset Alzheimer's disease. Nat Genet 1994;7:180–184.
10. Tsuang D, Larson E, Bowen J, et al. The utility of apolipoprotein E genotyping in the diagnosis of Alzheimer's disease in a community-based case series. Arch Neurol 1999;56:1489–1495.
11. American Federation for Aging Research. Available at: http://www. infoaging.org. Accessed September 10, 2003.
12. Alzheimer's Disease.com. Available at: http://www.alzheimersdisease. com. Accessed September 10, 2003.
13. Mortimer JA. Is Alzheimer's disease a lifelong illness? Risk factors for pathological and clinical disease. In: Heston LL, ed. Progress in Alzheimer's Disease and Similar Conditions. Washington, American Psychiatric Press, 1997:9–20.
14. Mirra SS. Alzheimer's disease and other dementias: Neuropathological considerations. In: Heston LL, ed. Progress in Alzheimer's Disease and Similar Conditions. Washington, American Psychiatric Press, 1997: 21–34.
15. McGeer EG, McGeer PL. Innate immunity in Alzheimer's disease: A model for local inflammatory reactions. Mol Interventions 2001;1: 22–29.
16. Wenk GL. Neuropathologic changes in Alzheimer's disease. J Clin Psychiatry 2003;64(Suppl 9):7–10.
17. Simons M, Keller P, Dichgans J, et al. Cholesterol and Alzheimer's disease. Is there a link? Neurology 2001;57:1089–1093.
18. Simons K, Ehehalt R. Cholesterol, lipid rafts, and disease. J Clin Invest 2002;110:597–603.
19. Czlonkowska A, Ciesielska A, Joniec I. Influence of estrogens on neurodegenerative processes. Med Sci Monit 2003;9:RA247–RA256.
20. Simpkins JW, Singh M, Bishop J. The potential role for estrogen replacement therapy in the treatment of the cognitive decline and neurodegeneration associated with Alzheimer's disease. Neurobiol Aging 1994;15:S195–S197.
21. Wickelgren I. Estrogen stakes claim to cognition. Science 1997;276: 675–678.
22. Mohs RC, Haroutunian V. Alzheimer disease: From earliest symptoms to end stage. In: Davis KL, Charney D, Coyle JT, Nemeroff C, eds. Neuropsychopharmacology: The Fifth Generation of Progress. New York, Lippincott Williams & Wilkins, 2002:1189–1198.
23. Boustani M, Peterson B, Hanson L, et al. Screening for dementia in primary care: A summary of the evidence for the U.S. Preventive Services Task Force. Ann Intern Med 2003;138:927–937.
24. U.S. Preventative Services Task Force. Screening for dementia: Recommendation and rationale. Ann Intern Med 2003;138:925–926.

25. Petersen RC, Stevens JC, Ganguli M, et al. Practice parameter: Early detection of dementia: Mild cognitive impairment (an evidence-based review). Neurology 2001;56:1133–1142.

26. McKhann G, Drachman D, Folstein M, et al. Clinical diagnosis of Alzheimer's disease: Report of the NINCDS-ADRDA work group under the auspices of the department of health and human services task force on Alzheimer's disease. Neurology 1984;34:939–944.

27. American Psychiatric Association. Diagnostic and Statistical Manual of Mental Disorders, 4th ed., Text Revision. Washington, American Psychiatric Association, 2000:154–158.

28. Knopman DS, DeKosky ST, Cummings JL, et al. Practice parameter: Diagnosis of dementia (an evidence-based review). Neurology 2001;56:1143–1153.

29. Pfeffer RI, Kurosaki TT, Harrah CH, et al. Measurement of functional activities of older adults in the community. J Gerontol 1982;37:323–329.

30. Rogers SL, Friedhoff LT, Donepezil Study Group. The efficacy and safety of donepezil in patients with Alzheimer's disease: Results of a U.S. multicentre, randomized, double-blind, placebo-controlled trial. Dementia 1996;7:293–303.

31. Corey-Bloom J, Anand R, Veach J. A randomized trial evaluating the efficacy and safety of ENA 713 (rivastigmine tartrate), a new acetylcholinesterase inhibitor, in patients with mild to moderately severe Alzheimer's disease. Int J Geriatr Psychopharmacol 1998;1:55–65.

32. Raskind MA, Peskind ER, Wessel T, et al. Galantamine in AD: A 6-month randomized, placebo-controlled trial with a 6-month extension. Neurology 2000;54:2261–2268.

33. Doody RS, Stevens JC, Beck C, et al. Practice parameter: Management of dementia (an evidence-based review). Neurology 2001;56:1154–1166.

34. Rabins P. Practice guideline for the treatment of patients with Alzheimer's disease and other dementias of late life. Am J Psychiatr 1997;154(Suppl 5):1–39.

35. Small GW, Rabins PV, Barry PP, et al. Diagnosis and treatment of Alzheimer disease and related disorders: Consensus statement of the American Association for Geriatric Psychiatry, the Alzheimer's Association, and the American Geriatrics Society. JAMA 1997;278:1363–1371.

36. Eisai. Aricept (donepezil hydrochloride) package insert. Teaneck, NJ, 2002.

37. Nordberg A, Svensson A. Cholinesterase inhibitors in the treatment of Alzheimer's disease: A comparison of tolerability and pharmacology. Drug Saf 1998;19:465–480.

38. Feldman H, Gauthier S, Hecker J, et al. A 24-week, randomized, double-blind study of donepezil in moderate to severe Alzheimer's disease. Neurology 2001;57:613–620.

39. Rogers SL, Doody RS, Pratt RD, Ieni JR. Long-term efficacy and safety of donepezil in the treatment of Alzheimer's disease: Final analysis of a U.S. multicentre open-label study. Eur Neuropsychopharmacol 2000;10:195–203.

40. Defilippi JL, Crismon M. Drug interactions with cholinesterase inhibitors. Drugs Aging 2003;20:437–444.

41. Jann MW. Rivastigmine, a new-generation cholinesterase inhibitor for the treatment of Alzheimer's disease. Pharmacotherapy 2000;20:1–12.

42. Agid Y, Dubois B, Anand R, et al. Efficacy and tolerability of rivastigmine in patients with dementia of the Alzheimer type. Current Therapeutic Research 1998;59:837–845.

43. Rosler M, Anand R, Cicin-Sain A, et al. Efficacy and safety of rivastigmine in patients with Alzheimer's disease: International randomized controlled trial. BMJ 1999;318:633–640.

44. The Galantamine USA-10 Study Group. A 5-month, randomized, placebo-controlled trial of galantamine in AD. Neurology 2000;54:2269–2276.

45. Janssen Pharmaceutica. Reminyl (galantamine hydrobromide) package insert. Titusville, NJ, 2001.

46. Jarvis B, Figgitt DP. Memantine. Drugs Aging 2003;20:465–476.

47. Forest Laboratories, Inc. Namenda (memantine hydrochloride) package insert. New York, 2004.

48. Sano M, Ernesto C, Thomas RG, et al. A controlled trial of selegiline, alpha-tocopherol, or both as treatment for Alzheimer's disease. N Engl J Med 1997;336:1216–1222.

49. Birks J, Flicker L. Selegiline for Alzheimer's disease (Cochrane Review). In: The Cochrane Library, Issue 4, 2003. Chichester, UK, John Wiley & Sons, Ltd.

50. Henderson VW, Paganini-Hill A, Miller BL, et al. Estrogen for Alzheimer's disease in women: Randomized, double-blind, placebo-controlled trial. Neurology 2000;54:295–301.

51. Mulnard RA, Cotman CW, Kawas C, et al. Estrogen replacement therapy for treatment of mild to moderate Alzheimer disease: A randomized controlled trial. JAMA 2000;283:1007–1015.

52. Shumaker SA, Legault C, Thal SL, et al. Estrogen plus progestin and the incidence of dementia and mild cognitive impairment in postmenopausal women. JAMA 2003;289:2651–2662.

53. Writing Group for the Women's Health Initiative Investigators. Risks and benefits of estrogen plus progestin in healthy postmenopausal women. JAMA 2002;288:321–333.

54. Hays J, Ockene JK, Brunner RL, et al. Effects of estrogen plus progestin on health-related quality of life. N Engl J Med 2003;348:1839–1854.

55. McGeer PL, Schulzer M, McGeer EG. Arthritis and anti-inflammatory agents as possible protective factors for Alzheimer's disease: A review of 17 epidemiologic studies. Neurology 1996;47:425–432.

56. Stewart WF, Kawas C, Corrada M. Risk of Alzheimer's disease and duration of NSAID use. Neurology 1997;48:626–632.

57. Etminan M, Gill S, Samii A. Effect of non-steroidal anti-inflammatory drugs on risk of Alzheimer's disease: Systematic review and meta-analysis of observational studies. BMJ 2003;327:128–132.

58. Rogers J, Kirby LC, Hempelman SR, et al. Clinical trial of indomethacin in Alzheimer's disease. Neurology 1993;43:1609–1611.

59. Aisen PS, Davis KL, Berg JD, et al. A randomized controlled trial of prednisone in Alzheimer's disease. Neurology 2000;54:588–593.

60. Scharf S, Mander A, Ugoni A, et al. A double-blind, placebo-controlled trial of diclofenac/misoprostol in Alzheimer's disease. Neurology 1999;53:197–201.

61. Schmidt LA, Fox NA, Goldberg MC. Effects of acute prednisone administration on memory, attention and emotion in healthy human adults. Psychoneuroendocrinology 1999;24:461–483.

62. Aisen PS, Schafer KA, Grundman M, et al. Effects of rofecoxib or naproxen vs placebo on Alzheimer disease progression. JAMA 2003;289:2819–2826.

63. Notkola IL, Sulkava R, Pekkanen J, et al. Serum total cholesterol, apolipoprotein E4 allele, and Alzheimer's disease. Neuroepidemiology 1998;17:14–20.

64. Kivipelto M, Helkala EL, Laasko MP, et al. Midlife vascular risk factors and Alzheimer's disease in later life: Longitudinal population based study. BMJ 2001;322:1447–1451.

65. Jick H, Zornberg GL, Jick SS, et al. Statins and the risk of dementia. Lancet 2000;356:1627–1631.

66. Wolozin B, Kellman W, Rousseau P, et al. Decreased prevalence of Alzheimer disease associated with 3-hydroxy-3-methylglutaryl coenzyme A reductase inhibitors. Arch Neurol 2000;57:1439–1443.

67. Rockwood K, Kirkland S, Hogan D, et al. Use of lipid-lowering agents, indication bias, and the risk of dementia in community-dwelling elderly people. Arch Neurol 2002;59:223–227.

68. Tan ZS, Seshadri S, Beiser A, et al. Plasma total cholesterol levels as a risk factor for Alzheimer's disease: The Framingham study. Arch Intern Med 2003;163:1053–1057.

69. Cooper JL. Dietary lipids in the aetiology of Alzheimer's disease. Drugs Aging 2003;20:399–418.

70. Oken BS, Storzbach DM, Kaye JA. The efficacy of ginkgo biloba on cognitive function in Alzheimer disease. Arch Neurol 1998;55:1409–1415.

71. Borson S, Raskind MA. Clinical features and pharmacologic treatment of behavioral symptoms of Alzheimer's disease. Neurology 1997;48:S17–S24.

72. Raskind MA, Barnes RF. Alzheimer's disease: Treatment of noncognitive behavioral abnormalities. In: Davis KL, Charney D, Coyle JT, Nemeroff C, eds. Neuropsychopharmacology: The Fifth Generation of Progress. New York, Lippincott Williams & Wilkins, 2002:1253–1265.

73. Lanctot KL, Best TS, Mittman N, et al. Efficacy and safety of neuroleptics in behavioral disorders associated with dementia. J Clin Psychiatry 1998;59:550–561.

74. Katz IR, Jeste DV, Mintzer JE, et al. Comparison of risperidone and placebo for psychosis and behavioral disturbances associated with dementia: A randomized, double-blind trial. J Clin Psychiatry 1999;60:107–115.

75. Brodaty H, Ames D, Snowdon J, et al. A randomized placebo-controlled trial of risperidone for the treatment of aggression, agitation, and psychosis of dementia. J Clin Psychiatry 2003;64:134–143.

76. De Deyn PP, Rabheru K, Rasmussen A, et al. A randomized trial of risperidone, placebo, and haloperidol for behavioral symptoms of dementia. Neurology 1999;53:946–955.

77. Street JS, Clark WS, Gannon KS, et al. Olanzapine treatment of psychotic and behavioral symptoms in patients with Alzheimer disease in nursing care facilities. Arch Gen Psychiatry 2000;57:968–976.

78. Scharre DW, Chang SI. Cognitive and behavioral effects of quetiapine in Alzheimer disease patients. Alzheimer Dis Assoc Disord 2002;16:128–130.

79. Defilippi JL, Crismon ML. The use of antipsychotic agents in patients with dementia. Pharmacotherapy 2000;20:23–33.

80. Olin JT, Schneider LS, Katz IR, et al. Provisional diagnostic criteria for depression of Alzheimer disease. Am J Geriatr Psychiatry 2002;10:125–128.

81. Lyketsos CG, Olin J. Depression in Alzheimer's disease: Overview and treatment. Biol Psychiatry 2002;52:243–252.

82. Taragano FE, Lyketsos CG, Mangone CA, et al. A double-blind, randomized, fixed-dose trial of fluoxetine vs. amitriptyline in the treatment of major depression complicating Alzheimer's disease. Psychosomatics 1997;38:246–252.

83. Geldmacher DS, Waldman AJ, Doty L, Heilman KM. Fluoxetine in dementia of the Alzheimer's type: Prominent adverse effects and failure to improve cognition. J Clin Psychiatry 1994;55:161.

84. Hill JW, Futterman R, Mastey V, et al. The effect of donepezil therapy on health costs in a Medicare managed care plan. Manag Care Interface 2002;15:63–70.

85. Costa PT Jr., Williams TF, Somerfield M, et al. Recognition and Initial Assessment of Alzheimer's Disease and Related Dementias. Clinical Practice Guideline No. 19. Rockville, MD, U.S. Department of Health and Human Services, Public Health Service, Agency for Health Care Policy and Research, 1996. AHCPR No. 97–0702.

86. Schneider LS, Pollock VE, Lyness SA. A meta-analysis of controlled trials of neuroleptic treatment in dementia. J Am Geriatr Soc 1990;38:553–563.

87. Rabins P, Blacker D, Bland W, and the Workgroup on Alzheimer's Disease and Related Dementias. Practice guideline for the treatment of patients with Alzheimer's disease and other dementias of late life. Am J Psychiatry 1997;154(Suppl 5):1–39.

88. Sakuye KM, Camp CJ, Ford PA. Effects of buspirone on agitation associated with dementia. Am J Geriatr Psychiatry 1993;1:82–84.

89. Hermann N, Eryavec G. Buspirone in the management of agitation and aggression associated with dementia. Am J Geriatr Psychiatry 1993;1:249–253.

90. Tariot PN, Cohen RM, Sunderland T, et al. L-Deprenyl in Alzheimer's disease. Arch Gen Psychiatry 1987;44:427–433.

91. Schneider LS, Pollock VE, Zemansky MF, et al. A pilot study of low-dose L-deprenyl in Alzheimer's disease. J Geriatr Psychiatry Neurol 1991;4:143–148.

92. Cummings JL. Cholinesterase inhibitors: A new class of psychotropic compounds. Am J Psychiatry 2000;157:4–15.

93. Koppel R. Alzheimer's disease: The costs to U.S. businesses in 2002. Social Research Corporation, Wyncote, PA. Prepared for the Alzheimer's Association.

94. Johnson N, Davis T, Bosanquet N. The epidemic of Alzheimer's disease: How can we manage the costs? Pharmacoeconomics 2000;18:215–223.

95. Medicare and Medicaid costs for people with Alzheimer's disease. Washington, April 2001, The Lewin Group, pg. 1.

96. Garfield FB, Getsios D, Caro JJ, et al. Assessment of Health Economics in Alzheimer's Disease (AHEAD); treatment with galantamine in Sweden. Pharmacoeconomics 2002;20:629–637.

97. Lamb HM, Goa KL. Rivastigmine. A pharmacoeconomic review of its use in Alzheimer's disease. Pharmacoeconomics 2001;19:303–318.

98. Wolfson C, Oremus M, Shukla V, et al. Donepezil and rivastigmine in the treatment of Alzheimer's disease. A best evidence synthesis of the published data on their efficacy and cost effectiveness. Clin Ther 2002;24:862–886.

99. Wimo A, Winblad B, Stoffler A, et al. Resource utilization and cost analysis of memantine in patients with moderate to severe Alzheimer's disease. Pharmacoeconomics 2003;21:327–340.

100. Fenn P, Gray A. Estimating long term cost savings from treatment of Alzheimer's disease: A modeling approach. Pharmacoeconomics 1999;16:165–174.

101. Wimo A, Winblad B, Engedal K, et al. An economic evaluation of donepezil in mild to moderate Alzheimer's disease: results of a 1 year double blind randomized trial. Dement Geriatr Cogn Disord 2003;15:44–54.

102. Ernst RL, Hay JW, Fenn C, et al. Cognitive function and the costs of Alzheimer disease: An exploratory study. Arch Neurol 1997;54:687–693.

103. Reisberg B, Ferris SH, DeLeon MJ, Crook T. The global deterioration scale for assessment of primary degenerative dementia. Am J Psychiatry 1982;139:1136–1139.

104. Novartis Pharmaceuticals. Exelon (rivastigmine tartrate) package insert. East Hanover, NJ, 2001.

105. First Horizon Pharmaceutical Corporation. Cognex (tacrine hydrochloride) package insert. Roswell, GA, 2000.

106. U.S. Census Bureau. Available at: http://www.census.gov/population/www/projections/natsum-T3.html. Accessed January 23, 2003.

64

SUBSTANCE-RELATED DISORDERS: OVERVIEW AND DEPRESSANTS, STIMULANTS, AND HALLUCINOGENS

Paul L. Doering

Learning Objectives and other resources can be found at *www.pharmacotherapyonline.com.*

KEY CONCEPTS

❶ Problems related to abuse of chemical substances can occur acutely (e.g., respiratory arrest from using heroin) or after some length of time (e.g., dependence or withdrawal from continued use of an opiate). The treatment approach is distinctly different depending on the type of problem.

❷ Pharmacotherapy of substance-related disorders is most often adjunctive to other modes of therapy such as counseling and intense psychotherapy.

❸ Withdrawal from certain classes of drugs (e.g., benzodiazepines or barbiturates) can be life-threatening, and steps must be taken to ensure that withdrawal is gradual and that it takes place in closely supervised settings.

❹ While there is much research focusing on drugs to treat the underlying addictive processes, to date the successes have been few. Whereas methadone, levo-alpha-acetylmethadol (LAAM), and now buprenorphine are used for narcotic maintenance, the logical approach at present should center on prevention. Because of their knowledge of pharmacology and the actions of drugs on the body, health professionals can play a key role in education of young people on the dangers of recreational drug use.

Abuse of alcohol, tobacco, and other drugs (ATOD) is the nation's number one health problem, according to a Robert Wood Johnson health care report prepared by the Institute for Health Policy, Brandeis University.[1] There are more deaths, illnesses, and disabilities from substance abuse than from any other preventable health condition. The economic cost of substance abuse to the U.S. economy each year is staggering, and it is estimated at over $414 billion.[1] A heavy smoker will stay 25% longer when hospitalized than a nonsmoker, and a problem drinker will stay four times as long as a nondrinker.[1] According to the Robert Wood Johnson health report, "Without a reduction in ATOD abuse, health care costs cannot be curtailed effectively." Of the more than 2 million deaths each year in the United States, approximately one in four is attributable to alcohol, illicit drug, or tobacco use: 100,000 people die as a result of alcohol, 16,000 die from illicit drug use and deaths related to the acquired immune deficiency syndrome, and 430,700 from tobacco-related illnesses.

In addition, one-half to two-thirds of homicides and serious crimes involve alcohol. Nearly one-half of men arrested for homicide and assault actually test positive for an illegal drug.[1] ATOD abuse contributes to family problems, with one in four Americans reporting that alcohol has been a cause of trouble in the family, and alcohol abuse plays a part in one of three failed marriages.[1]

Since publication of the last edition of this textbook, a disturbing new trend in drug abuse has emerged: increase in the use of medicinal drugs for nonmedicinal purposes. Between 1995 and 2002 there was a 163% increase in the number of emergency room visits tied to the abuse of prescription drugs, according to the Substance Abuse & Mental Health Services Administration (SAMHSA).[2] SAMHSA estimates that 9 million people now abuse prescription drugs, meaning that they use them for nonmedical, and often recreational, purposes. Three million abusers are children between the ages of 12 and 17 years old. The abuse of such drugs can be deadly. Prescription drugs now are a factor in a quarter of all overdose deaths reported in the United States.

This chapter and the next focus on the problems associated with the abuse of chemical substances and the things clinicians can do to help deal with these problems.

TERMINOLOGY

The lack of a common vocabulary in substance abuse treatment and prevention leads to several problems. There is a wide array of terms in common use, many without precise meaning. A number of professional disciplines are involved in research, treatment, and education regarding alcohol and other drug-related problems, and each discipline tends to use its own terminology. This lack of universal agreement on language hampers effective communication among professionals and leads to difficulties in formulating public policy and administering third-party reimbursement programs. The Liaison Committee on Pain and Addiction, a collaborative effort of the American Academy of Pain Medicine, the American Pain Society, and the

American Society of Addiction Medicine has developed definitions related to the use of medications for the treatment of pain that purport to be consistent with current understanding of relevant neurobiology, pharmacology, and appropriate clinical practice. The ultimate goal of their project was to achieve acceptance and use of uniform definitions by clinicians, regulators, and the public, both nationally and internationally, in order to promote appropriate treatment of pain throughout the world. The definitions have been approved by each of the three collaborating organizations. The following definitions resulted from this particular consensus development committee:[3]

- *Addiction* is a primary, chronic, neurobiologic disease, with genetic, psychosocial, and environmental factors influencing its development and manifestations. It is characterized by behaviors that include one or more of the following 5Cs: *c*hronicity, impaired *c*ontrol over drug use, *c*ompulsive use, *c*ontinued use despite harm, and *c*raving.
- *Physical dependence* is a state of adaptation that is manifested by a drug class–specific withdrawal syndrome that can be produced by abrupt cessation, rapid dose reduction, decreasing blood level of the drug, and/or administration of an antagonist.
- *Tolerance* is a state of adaptation in which exposure to a drug induces changes that result in a diminution of one or more of the drug's effects over time.

EPIDEMIOLOGY

NATIONAL SURVEY ON DRUG USE & HEALTH

The National Survey on Drug Use & Health (NSDUH) (formerly called the National Household Survey on Drug Abuse)[4] is the primary source of statistical information on the use of illegal drugs by the U.S. population. Conducted by the federal government since 1971, the survey collects data from a representative sample of the population at their place of residence.

In 2002, there were 19.5 million Americans (8.3% of the population ages 12 or older) who currently used illicit drugs. An estimated 22 million Americans suffered from substance dependence or abuse due to drugs, alcohol, or both. The 2002 survey found that marijuana is the most commonly used illicit drug, used by 14.6 million Americans. The second most popular category of drug use after marijuana is the nonmedical use of prescription drugs. An estimated 6.2 million people, 2.6% of the population ages 12 or older, were current users of prescription drugs taken nonmedically. Of these, an estimated 4.4 million used narcotic pain relievers, 1.8 million used antianxiety medications, 1.2 million used stimulants, and 0.4 million used sedatives.[4]

THE MONITORING THE FUTURE STUDY

Every year the Institute for Social Research of the University of Michigan conducts its Monitoring the Future Study (MTFS), supported under a series of research grants from the National Institute on Drug Abuse.[5] The project has many purposes. Among them is to study changes in the beliefs, attitudes, and behavior of young people in the United States. This study focuses on youth because of their significant involvement in today's social changes, and most importantly because youth in a very literal sense will constitute our future society.[5]

In 2002, 43,700 eighth, tenth, and twelfth grade students in 394 public and private secondary schools were surveyed. Use of a number of illicit drugs showed broad declines (most notably in the use of ecstasy) for the first time, cigarette smoking dropped sharply in all grades, and drinking alcohol and getting drunk were also down in all grades. For eighth graders the annual prevalence of marijuana use in 2002 of 14.6% is down from the recent peak of 18.3% in 1996. At 30.3% in 2002, the annual prevalence of use of marijuana in tenth graders is now somewhat below the recent 1997 peak of 34.8%; but twelfth graders are down only modestly, from the recent 1997 peak of 38.5% to 36.2% in 2002. The rates of daily use in 2002 are approximately where they stood in 2000 in all five populations. Among twelfth graders 6% are now current daily marijuana users, as are 4.1% of college students and 4.5% of all young adults. Daily use among eighth graders is considerably lower, at 1.2%. Other interesting trends have emerged for the following drugs:

- *Ecstasy.* Use of this so-called club drug showed a decline over previous years. The rates of annual prevalence in 2002 for ecstasy were: 2.9%, 4.9%, and 7.4% among eighth, tenth, and twelfth graders, respectively, 6.8% among college students, and 6.2% among all young adults.
- *Inhalants.* Inhalants, the only class of drug that tends to be more popular among younger teens than older ones, include a wide variety of common household products that youngsters inhale or "huff" in order to get high, such as glues, solvents, butane, gasoline, and aerosols. Some 7.7% of the 2002 eighth graders and 5.8% of the tenth graders indicated inhalant use in the prior 12 months, making inhalants the second most widely used class of illicitly used drugs for eighth graders (after marijuana), and the third most widely used (after marijuana and amphetamines) for tenth graders. The annual prevalence rate among twelfth-grade students was 6.5% in 1979, but only 1.1% in 2002.
- *Amphetamine and methamphetamine.* For eighth graders, inhalant use is followed closely in the rankings by amphetamines, with a lifetime prevalence of use rate of 8.7%. But amphetamine use comes ahead of inhalant use in the rankings for tenth and twelfth graders, with 15% of tenth graders and 17% of twelfth graders reporting some use in their lifetime.
- *Prescription drugs.* In 2002 data were gathered for the first time on two prescription drugs in the narcotic class: Vicodin (hydrocodone with acetaminophen) and OxyContin (oxycodone controlled-release). MTFS results found that Vicodin had attained surprisingly high prevalence rates in the five populations under study—an annual prevalence of 2.5% in eighth graders, 6.9% in tenth graders, 9.6% in twelfth graders, 6.9% among college students, and 8.2% among young adults. Considerably lower rates were found for OxyContin, but considering that it is a highly addictive narcotic drug when used inappropriately, the rates are not inconsequential—1.3%, 3%, 4%, 1.5%, and 1.9% in the same five populations, respectively.

TRENDS IN SUBSTANCE ABUSE EMERGENCIES: THE DAWN PROGRAM

Since the early 1970s, the Drug Abuse Warning Network (DAWN),[2] an ongoing national survey of hospital emergency departments (EDs), has collected information on patients seeking hospital ED treatment related to their use of an illegal drug or the nonmedical use of a legal drug. DAWN serves as an early warning system to the ever-changing patterns of use of illegal drugs. These data allow health care professionals to be better prepared to react to medical emergencies arising from illegal drug use and to target prevention and education programs to specific drug-using groups or populations.

DAWN defines a *drug-related episode* as an ED visit that was induced by or related to the use of an illegal drug(s) or the nonmedical use of a legal drug for patients aged 6 to 97 years. A *drug mention* refers to a substance that was mentioned during a drug-related ED episode.

In 2002, there were 670,307 drug abuse–related ED episodes in the coterminous United States, with 1,209,938 drug mentions (on average, 1.8 drug mentions per episode). Cocaine-related episodes constituted 30% of all ED drug-related episodes in 2002, more than any other illicit substance measured by DAWN. About one-fifth of the cocaine mentions in 2002 (21%, 42,146 mentions) were attributed to crack cocaine. No significant changes from 2001 to 2002 were evident for the club drugs ecstasy (MDMA) (4,026 mentions in 2002), γ-hydroxybutyrate (GHB) (3,330 mentions), or ketamine (260 mentions). Heroin accounted for 14% (93,519 mentions) in 2002, and amphetamines and methamphetamine were each mentioned in 3% of drug abuse–related ED episodes (21,644 mentions of amphetamines; 17,696 mentions of methamphetamine). When considered together, narcotic analgesics and combinations comprised 119,185 mentions or 10% of ED mentions estimated for the coterminous United States in 2002. From 2001 to 2002, ED mentions of narcotic analgesics and combinations rose 20% (from 99,317 to 119,185 mentions). From 2000 to 2002, the increase was 45% (from 82,373), and over the 8-year period from 1995 to 2002, mentions of narcotic analgesics and combinations rose 163% (from 45,254).

ECONOMIC IMPACT OF SUBSTANCE ABUSE

Substance abuse and addiction have an enormous impact on the economy. Over the years, the Center on Addiction and Substance Abuse (CASA) at Columbia University has conducted numerous studies aimed at quantifying the costs to local, state, and federal governments and agencies. CASA recently reported the results[6] of an intensive 3-year analysis of the impact of substance abuse on state budgets. They discovered that in 1998 states spent $620 billion of their own funds to operate state government and provide public services such as education, Medicaid, child welfare, mental health, and highway safety. Of this amount, a full 13.1%—$81.3 billion—went to dealing with the aftermath of substance abuse and addiction.[6] This figure does not include the financial toll such abuse extracts from federal or local spending or the private costs such as lost productivity or premature death. Each American paid $277 per year in state taxes to deal with the burden of substance abuse and addiction in their social programs and only $10 a year for prevention and treatment. Of every dollar states spend on substance abuse, 95.8 cents goes to pay for the burden of this problem on public programs. For example, untreated substance abuse increases the cost of every state's criminal justice system; elementary and secondary schools; Medicaid; child welfare, juvenile justice and mental heath systems, highways, and state payrolls. These costs totaled $77.9 billion in 1998.[6]

The majority of the substance abuse–related diseases in the Medicaid population are linked to tobacco and illicit drugs, many related to birth complications resulting from cocaine use. More than 60 Medicare ailments are attributable to ATOD abuse. The majority of the substance abuse–related diseases in the Medicare population are associated with tobacco, which accounts for 80% of these diseases. If substance abuse and addiction do not decrease, it will cost the Medicare program alone more than $1 trillion over the next 20 years.[9] Needless to say, reducing the problem of substance abuse and dependence would result in tremendous savings for local, state, and federal governments and would have a net positive impact on the quality of life of our citizens.

ACUTE VERSUS CHRONIC PROBLEMS

Misuse of chemical substances causes problems of two types: those that occur acutely and those that arise after continued use of a drug. Acute problems are usually predictable, given the pharmacology of the drug. Acute drug intoxications usually occur at doses in excess of that normally taken. Chronic abuse of chemical substances can cause a wide array of physical, psychological, and psychiatric ailments. The substance-induced disorders to be discussed here mainly include intoxication and withdrawal. Psychiatric problems associated with substance abuse, including dementia, psychosis, mood disorders, and anxiety, are discussed elsewhere. Physical illnesses associated with chronic use of chemicals (e.g., alcoholic liver disease) are likewise covered in other chapters.

The essential feature of substance dependence is the continued use of the substance despite adverse substance-related problems. The criteria for substance dependence are the same for each of the drugs or drug classes, varying only to fit the unique pharmacologic properties of each drug. Patients who take prescribed drugs for appropriate medical indications and in correct doses may still show tolerance, physical dependence, and withdrawal symptoms if the drug is stopped abruptly rather than being tapered. Tolerance and physical dependence are inevitable consequences of chronic treatment with opioids and certain other drugs, but by themselves, tolerance and physical dependence do not imply "addiction." To meet *Diagnostic and Statistical Manual of Mental Disorders*, 4th ed., Text Revision (DSM-IV-TR) criteria[7] for the diagnosis of substance dependence, at least three of the following must be present at any time in a 12-month period:

1. Tolerance
2. Withdrawal, indicated by the appearance of the characteristic withdrawal syndrome or the use of the same or related drug to relieve or avoid withdrawal symptoms
3. Substance taken in larger amounts or over a longer period of time than was intended
4. Persistent desire or unsuccessful efforts to cut down or control substance use
5. Time spent in activities necessary to obtain the substance, use the substance, or recover from its effects
6. Social, occupational, or recreational activities given up or reduced because of substance use
7. Substance use continued despite knowledge of having a persistent or recurrent physical or psychological problem caused or exacerbated by the substance

The characteristic feature of *substance abuse* is a maladaptive pattern of substance use indicated by repeated adverse consequences related to the repeated use of the substance. Examples include failure to fulfill important obligations at work, school, or home; repeated use in situations in which it is physically dangerous, such as driving under the influence; legal problems; and social or interpersonal problems such as arguments and fights.[7] *Intoxication* refers to the development of a substance-specific syndrome after recent ingestion and presence in the body of a substance, and it is associated with maladaptive behavior during the waking state caused by the effect of the substance on the central nervous system (CNS). Examples include belligerence, mood lability, impaired judgment, and impaired social or occupational functioning. Evidence for recent intake of the substance can be obtained from the history, physical examination, or laboratory examination. The most common changes involve disturbances in perception, wakefulness, attention, thinking, judgment, motor behavior, and interpersonal behavior.

In addition to the previous definition, *withdrawal* can be further described as the development of a substance-specific syndrome after cessation of or reduction in intake of a substance that was used regularly by the individual to induce a state of intoxication. Withdrawal causes significant distress to the individual and is associated with impairment in social, occupational, or other areas of functioning. Withdrawal is usually associated with substance dependence. Withdrawal generally is also associated with a craving to readminister the drug to relieve the symptoms.

As with most illnesses, the course and prognosis of the disorders of substance use and dependence are variable. Untreated physical withdrawal from the CNS depressants is potentially life-threatening, but withdrawal almost always can be managed successfully with proper medical care. Getting patients who are drug dependent to stop using drugs is very difficult, and many patients return to drug use even after treatment. As many as 75% of treated substance-dependent patients relapse at least once. Many patients, however, are able to obtain recovery with treatment and continued care in programs such as Alcoholics Anonymous (AA) or Narcotics Anonymous (NA). Substance dependence or addiction can be viewed as a chronic illness that can be controlled successfully with treatment, but cannot be cured and is associated with a high relapse rate. Without treatment, the course can progress to life-threatening severity, resulting from the effects of the drug, drug contaminants, or medical complications of use.[7] Although an in-depth discussion of the mechanism of drug addiction is beyond the scope of this chapter, the interested reader is directed to a recent concise review article that presents the current understanding of the biology of drug addiction.[8]

CNS DEPRESSANTS

BENZODIAZEPINES AND OTHER SEDATIVE-HYPNOTICS

The past several years have witnessed a sharp rise in the abuse of prescription drugs. In 2002, an estimated 6.2 million persons were current users of prescription-type drugs nonmedically.[4] Benzodiazepines are among the most popular "party drugs" both on college campuses and in the population at large. DAWN estimates show that from 1995 to 2002, increases were evident for the most frequently mentioned benzodiazepines, alprazolam (62%, from 17,082 to 27,659), clonazepam (33%, from 12,802 to 17,042), and unnamed benzodiazepines (199%, from 11,587 to 34,697).[2]

In clinical practice, the benzodiazepines largely have replaced the short-acting barbiturates and other nonbarbiturate sedative-hypnotics. Benzodiazepines with faster onset (e.g., diazepam) tend to be preferred by the recreational drug user because they are reinforcing. Flunitrazepam emerged in the mid-1990s as an illegal drug in the United States that was predominantly abused recreationally and associated with sexual assaults.[9] Medically, this benzodiazepine is used in the short-term treatment of insomnia and as a preanesthetic

medication. As with other benzodiazepines, flunitrazepam is most commonly ingested orally, frequently in conjunction with alcohol or other drugs. The drug's effects begin within 30 minutes, peak within 2 hours, and may persist for up to 8 hours or more depending on the dosage.[9]

Adverse effects associated with the use of benzodiazepines include decreased blood pressure, memory impairment, drowsiness, visual disturbances, dizziness, confusion, gastrointestinal disturbances, and urinary retention.

Even when used alone, benzodiazepines can cause users to appear extremely intoxicated, with slurred speech, poor coordination, swaying, and bloodshot eyes, with no odor of alcohol. When surreptitiously slipped into a drink, young women have reported waking up in strange surroundings having been sexually assaulted while under the influence of the drug.[10] For this reason, flunitrazepam has come to be called the "date rape drug."

A dramatic drop in cases of flunitrazepam abuse followed the legal reclassification of the drug as a schedule I substance in Florida in February 1997. A recent rise in alprazolam and clonazepam cases coincides with the decreased use of flunitrazepam and represents a new trend in abuse of the benzodiazepines. Alprazolam (Xanax) has become particularly popular and is known on the street by its slang names, Z-Bars, Zandy bars, footballs, and Zannies, among others. Young people will often take alprazolam or other benzodiazepines before going to the bar or dance club, ostensibly to lower the amount of alcoholic beverage needed to attain the desired level of intoxication. Unfortunately, this "pre-partying" is especially popular among women who do not like the taste of beer or find the caloric burden of drinking to be limiting. Sadly, whether taking it intentionally or being given the drug without their knowledge or consent, these women become targets for sexual predators who know that the victim will have diminished recall of the events that take place. When a victim is unable to give precise details of what happened and when it happened, and is unable to identify the perpetrator, the chances of successful prosecution are greatly diminished.

Because all benzodiazepines have abuse and dependence liability, patients cannot be switched from one benzodiazepine to another in hopes of decreasing a pattern of drug abuse or dependence behavior. Zolpidem, a nonbenzodiazepine nonbarbiturate sedative, has been suggested to have little liability for physical dependence, but tolerance and withdrawal have been reported in association with its use as well.[11]

Benzodiazepines generally do not cause life-threatening respiratory depression, as do the barbiturate-like drugs.[12] Long-term use of even therapeutic doses of benzodiazepines may cause physical dependence and withdrawal symptoms after abrupt discontinuation.[13] Signs and symptoms of withdrawal are similar in many respects to those of alcohol withdrawal, but the time courses may be quite different. While withdrawal from shorter-acting agents (e.g., lorazepam and alprazolam) has an onset within 12 to 24 hours of the last dose, others (e.g., diazepam, chlordiazepoxide, clorazepate, phenobarbital, and amobarbital) have elimination half-lives or active metabolites with elimination half-lives of 24 to over 100 hours. As a result, the onset of withdrawal symptoms may be delayed for several days after discontinuation of the drug.[13] The likelihood and severity of withdrawal are a function of both dose and duration of exposure. Gradual tapering of dosage is also associated with less withdrawal and rebound anxiety than abrupt discontinuation. Dependence on sedative-hypnotics and benzodiazepines is summarized in Table 64–1.

Occurrence of hallucinations or seizures would indicate severe physical withdrawal. For additional information on benzodiazepine withdrawal, refer to Chap. 69.

TABLE 64–1. Dependence on Sedative-Hypnotics

Generic Name	Common Trade Names (Manufacturer)	Oral Sedating Dose (mg)	Physical Dependence Dose and Time Needed to Produce Dependence	Time Before Onset of Withdrawal (h)	Peak Withdrawal Symptoms (d)
Benzodiazepines					
Diazepam	Valium (Roche)	5–10	40–100 mg × 42–120 days	12–24	5–8
Chlordiazepoxide	Librium, Libritabs (Roche)	10–25	75–600 mg × 42–120 days	12–24	5–8
Clorazepate	Tranxene (Abbott)	7.5–15	45–180 mg × 42–120 days (est.)	12–24	5–8
Alprazolam	Xanax (Upjohn)	0.25–8	8–16 mg × 42 days (est.)	8–24	2–3
Flunitrazepam	Rohypnol (Roche)	1–2	8–10 mg × 42 days (est.)	24–36	2–3
Barbiturates					
Secobarbital	Seconal, Seco-8 (Lilly)	100	800–2200 mg × 35–37 days	6–12	2–3
Pentobarbital	Nembutal (Abbott)	100	Same	6–12	2–3
Equal parts of secobarbital and amobarbital	Tuinal (Lilly)	100	Same	6–12	2–3
Amobarbital	Amytal (Lilly)	65–100	Same	8–12	2–5
Nonbarbiturate sedative-hypnotics					
Ethchlorvynol	Placidyl (Abbott)	200	1–1.5 g × 30 days	6–12	2–3
Chloral hydrate	Noctec (various)	250	Exact dose unknown; 12 g/day chronically has led to delirium upon sudden withdrawal	6–12	2–3
Meprobamate	Equanil, Miltown, Meprotabs (various)	400	1.6–3.2 g × 270 days	8–12	3–8

Withdrawal symptoms are tremor, tachycardia, diaphoresis, nausea, vomiting, elevated blood pressure, delirium, seizures, and hallucinations.

γ-HYDROXYBUTYRATE

γ-Hydroxybutyrate (GHB) is a chemical compound structurally similar to the inhibitory brain neurotransmitter γ-aminobutyric acid. Powdered forms of GHB were marketed in health food stores as a nutritional supplement before being removed from the retail market by the Food and Drug Administration (FDA) in 1991. At that time it was used primarily by body builders for its purported ability to increase growth hormone, but it proved to cause serious illness and death when taken in excess doses or in combination with alcohol or other drugs. Primary groups using GHB include party and nightclub attendees. Like flunitrazepam, GHB is also characterized as a date rape drug.[10] Manifestations of acute GHB toxicity include coma, seizures, respiratory depression, and vomiting. Other documented effects of GHB include amnesia and hypotonia (associated with doses of 10 mg/kg of body weight), abnormal sequence of rapid eye movement (REM) and non-REM sleep (doses of 20 to 30 mg/kg), and anesthesia (doses of approximately 50 mg/kg). Doses greater than 50 mg/kg can decrease cardiac output and produce severe respiratory depression, seizure-like activity, and coma[14,15]; coma and respiratory depression may be potentiated by concomitant use of alcohol.[15] There is no antidote for GHB overdose, and treatment is restricted to nonspecific supportive care. Figure 64–1 shows a protocol recommended for treating suspected GHB overdose.

In the United States, GHB has been produced clandestinely in widely varying degrees of purity. Today GHB is sold mostly as a liquid under such names as "grievous bodily harm," "Georgia home boy," "liquid ecstasy," "scoop," "easy lay," "salty water," and "organic quaalude."

In March 2000, GHB was placed into schedule I of the Controlled Substances Act. Until recently, the majority of GHB sold on the streets was manufactured using inexpensive kits obtained over the Internet. It is mixed largely by nonchemists from recipes that can be flawed or incomplete, and finished products are often of questionable purity, and more important, unknown potency. Improper preparation of GHB can result in a mixture of GHB and sodium hydroxide that can be severely toxic because of the combined effects of the GHB and the direct caustic effects of sodium hydroxide. Since there is no way to tell the strength of homemade GHB, what might be a safe dose today (e.g., "one capful") could produce a toxic dose tomorrow if a different batch is used. Fortunately, crackdowns in 1997 by the FDA, the Department of Justice, and other enforcement groups has led to decreased availability of ready-made kits on the Internet. Despite the FDA's action, GHB remains available to consumers.

The decreased Internet availability of kits to make GHB has been accompanied by an increased availability of chemical precursors to GHB as well as GHB analogs. Also available in gyms and health food stores, these substances include γ-butyrolactone (GBL) and 1,4-butanediol.[16] GBL is converted in the body to GHB. Labels of marketed products may use unfamiliar synonyms to disguise the actual content. GBL is also known by the chemical names 2(3H)-furanone dihydro, butyrolactone, 4-butyrolactone, dihydro-2(3H)-furanone, 4-butanolide, 2(3H)-furanone, dihydro, tetrahydro-2-furanone, and butyrolactone-γ.

Withdrawal resulting in severe agitation, mental status changes, elevated blood pressure, and tachycardia has been reported hours after stopping chronic use of GHB. In one case the patient admitted to substantial GHB abuse on a daily basis for 2.5 years. Previous attempts at cessation reportedly resulted in diaphoresis, tremors, and agitation. The patient required 507 mg lorazepam and 120 mg diazepam over 90 hours to control agitation.[17]

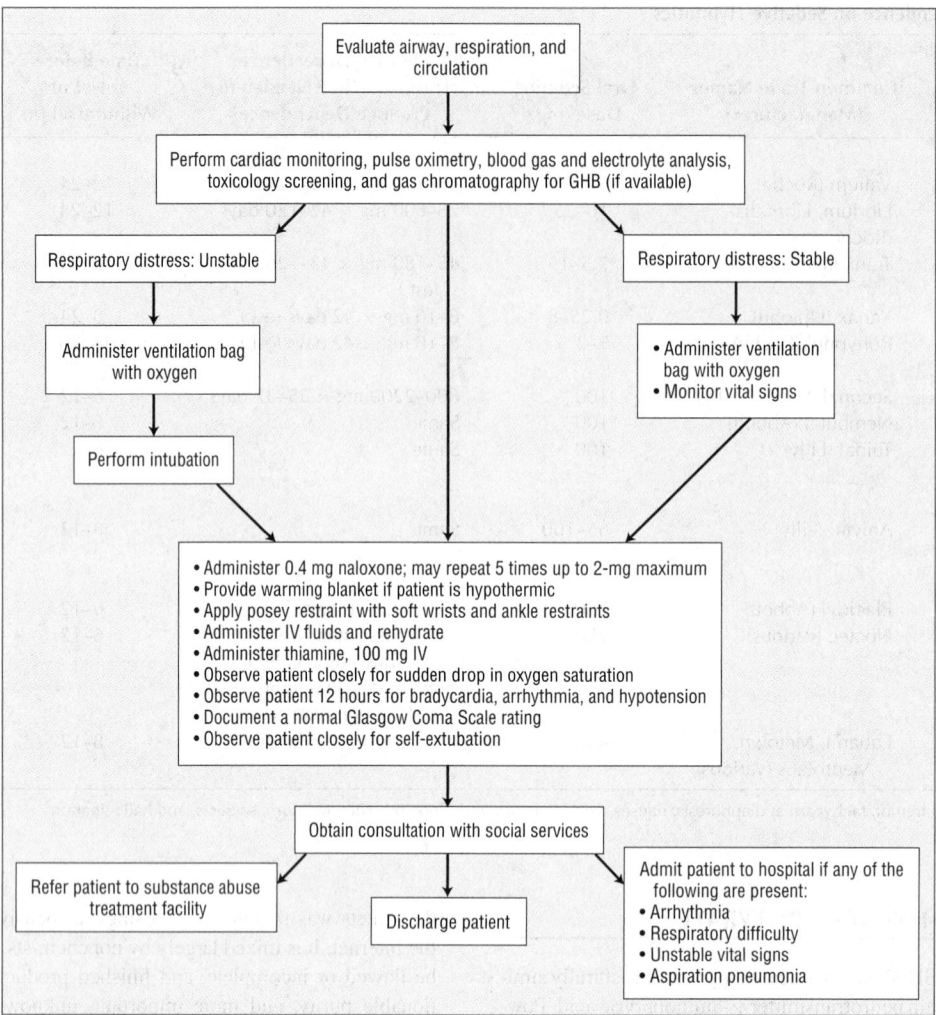

FIGURE 64–1. Protocol for treatment of suspected GHB overdose.

OPIATES

Incidence and prevalence of opiate use are widely variable depending on the drug. In 2002, there were 166,000 current heroin users. Collectively, use of opiates other than heroin is far more common. An estimated 4.4 million people used narcotic pain relievers and 1.9 million persons ages 12 or older used what SAMHSA classified as "OxyContin" nonmedically at least once in their lifetime.[4]

Signs and symptoms of opioid intoxication and withdrawal are summarized in Table 64–2. Onset of the acute phase of withdrawal varies with the drug consumed, but ranges from a few hours after stopping heroin to 3 to 5 days after stopping methadone. The duration of withdrawal ranges from 3 to 14 days. Opioid withdrawal is significantly different from withdrawal from alcohol or other sedative-hypnotics. The biggest difference is that opioid withdrawal is not fatal unless there is a concurrent medical problem of major concern. This has significant treatment implications. Although patients in opioid withdrawal may be in great discomfort and incapacitated, they are not delirious. The presence of delirium should raise the question of concurrent withdrawal from another drug, such as alcohol, or another cause of delirium possibly secondary to drug use.

Many of the complications of opiate use, especially intravenous use, are related not only to the drug itself, but also to varying purity, contaminants, and techniques of administration such as dirty equipment and use of shared needles. Overdoses, anaphylactic reactions

to impurities, nephrotic syndrome, septicemia, endocarditis, and acquired immune deficiency syndrome are examples.

Increased recreational use of pharmaceutical dosage forms of opiates has sparked nationwide debate on both the illegal and legal use of these drugs. OxyContin has been a target of much of this criticism. Introduced in 1995, OxyContin is a controlled-release dosage form of oxycodone that gradually releases steady amounts of narcotics for 12 hours. By crushing the OxyContin tablets, drug abusers can get the full 12-hour narcotic effect almost immediately. Snorting or injecting

TABLE 64–2. Signs and Symptoms of Opioid Intoxication and Withdrawal

Intoxication	Withdrawal
Euphoria	Lacrimation
Dysphoria	Rhinorrhea
Apathy	Mydriasis
Motor retardation	Piloerection
Sedation	Diaphoresis
Slurred speech	Diarrhea
Attention impairment	Yawning
Miosis	Fever
	Insomnia
	Muscle aching

the crushed tablet can lead to overdose and death. Abuse of this drug has caused a nationwide discussion on whether drugs of this nature should be more closely regulated. In September 2003 a federal drug advisory panel rejected requests from members of Congress and drug enforcement officials that sales of OxyContin be severely restricted. According to testimony at the hearings, OxyContin is responsible for 500 to 1000 deaths a year.[18] But these data are refuted in a careful examination of data from an oxycodone postmortem database.[19] Created from 1243 solicited cases from medical examiner and coroner offices in 23 states in the United States, the database included information collected from August 27, 1999 through January 17, 2002. Researchers examined records of the 919 deaths related to oxycodone and discovered that in only 12 of the cases was OxyContin the only agent found at autopsy. The remaining victims had taken either an overdose of other oxycodone-containing drugs (for example, Percocet) or a combination of drugs. In fact, 97% had at least three other drugs in their systems, mostly alcohol, benzodiazepines, cocaine, antidepressants, or other narcotics like heroin. From these data, the authors concluded that oxycodone-related deaths overwhelmingly occur in drug-abusing individuals, and rarely is OxyContin an exclusive cause of death.

Various groups have weighed in on the pros and cons of prescribing opiates for chronic pain and the debate at times is emotional. Various position statements and points of view have been expressed, but the limited space here precludes an exhaustive review of the issues. An excellent review of the appropriate use of opioid therapy for chronic pain has recently been published, and the interested reader is directed there for more information.[20]

CLINICAL CONTROVERSY

There is considerable debate about the appropriate use of prescribed opiates and how this might contribute to the overuse or abuse of these same drugs for nonmedicinal purposes. Some clinicians believe that use of opiates in patients with chronic pain is inappropriate because it leads to physical dependence and addiction. Practitioners should strive to balance the therapeutic imperative that says "Always use analgesics when they are appropriate for a patient" against the regulatory imperative that says "Never use analgesics when they are inappropriate for a patient."

CNS STIMULANTS

COCAINE

Cocaine is perhaps the most behaviorally reinforcing of all drugs of abuse. Clinicians estimate that approximately 10% of people who begin to use the drug recreationally will go on to serious, heavy use. Once having tried cocaine, an individual cannot predict or control the extent to which he or she will continue to use the drug.

The most characteristic systemic effect of cocaine is stimulation of the CNS.[21] In the CNS, cocaine appears to mediate its effects primarily by blocking reuptake of catecholamine neurotransmitters such as norepinephrine and dopamine. The most common clinical manifestations of cocaine stimulation of the CNS are intense euphoria, decreased fatigue, and increased alertness.

In 2002, an estimated 2 million persons (0.9% of the U.S. population) were current cocaine users, 567,000 of whom used crack during the same time period (0.2%).[4] About half of these meet the criteria for dependence on cocaine.

Cocaine is absorbed rapidly from virtually all sites of application. For many years, cocaine has been administered as the hydrochloride salt form, usually by inhalation, but also by injection. In the last 15 to 18 years, as the purity of cocaine hydrochloride obtained on the street declined, many users converted the cocaine hydrochloride to cocaine base, also known as "crack" or "rock." Smoking the drug leads to almost instant absorption and intense euphoria. Peak plasma concentrations of more than 900 ng/mL have been achieved following inhalation of cocaine base vapors, compared with concentrations of only 150 to 200 ng/mL achieved after inhalation of similar amounts of pure cocaine hydrochloride powder.[21]

The high from snorting may last 15 to 30 minutes, whereas that from smoking may last 5 to 10 minutes. Increased use can reduce the period of stimulation. Some users of cocaine report feelings of restlessness, irritability, and anxiety. An appreciable tolerance to the high may be developed, and many addicts report that they seek but fail to achieve as much pleasure as they did from their first exposure. Scientific evidence suggests that the powerful neuropsychological reinforcing property of cocaine is responsible for an individual's continued use despite harmful physical and social consequences. In rare instances, sudden death can occur on the first use of cocaine or unexpectedly thereafter. However, there is no way to determine who is prone to sudden death.

High doses of cocaine and/or prolonged use can trigger paranoia. Smoking crack cocaine can produce a particularly aggressive paranoid behavior in users. When addicted individuals stop using cocaine they often become depressed. This may lead to further cocaine use to alleviate depression. Prolonged cocaine snorting can result in ulceration of the mucous membranes of the nose and can damage the nasal septum enough to cause it to collapse. Cocaine-related deaths are often a result of cardiac arrest or seizures followed by respiratory arrest.

Recent research has helped clarify certain patterns of cocaine use such as combining cocaine and alcohol. Such drug use would seem counterintuitive because cocaine is a CNS stimulant and alcohol a CNS depressant. In the presence of alcohol, cocaine is metabolized to cocaethylene, a longer-acting but potent psychoactive compound as compared with the parent drug.[22] The risk of death from cocaethylene is greater than from cocaine.[23] The cocaine-alcohol combination is one of the most commonly identified among individuals who come to hospital emergency departments with acute substance abuse problems.

Cocaine is metabolized and eliminated rapidly. The elimination half-life of cocaine is approximately 1 hour, and the duration of effect is very short.[21] The short duration of effect provides a powerful incentive for repeated use of the drug. Many users experience intense drug use cycling, sometimes lasting days, characterized by rapidly repeating doses of cocaine until their supply is exhausted. Laboratory monkeys, given a choice between food and cocaine around the clock for 8 days, consistently choose cocaine.[24]

Complications of cocaine use frequently involve cardiovascular events.[25] At higher doses it increases heart rate because of an overall systemic increase in sympathetic tone. At toxic doses, cocaine causes cardiac failure due to a direct effect on myocardial contractility. Cocaine is also pyrogenic, and hyperthermia is observed frequently in cocaine poisoning. Death is usually related to arrhythmias, shock, or convulsions.

Cocaine is a psychotomimetic drug, sometimes even at systemically nontoxic doses. A kindling phenomenon has been described with cocaine in which neuronal function becomes altered with each dose of the drug. This causes a type of reverse tolerance with increased receptor sensitivity to cocaine, and psychosis may be caused by doses that formerly did not cause psychosis. The toxic psychosis is characterized by auditory, visual, and frequently tactile hallucinations, paranoid thinking, and looseness of associations. The psychosis is qualitatively very similar to a paranoid schizophrenic psychosis.[26]

TABLE 64–3. Signs and Symptoms of Cocaine Intoxication and Withdrawal

Intoxication	Withdrawal
Motor agitation	Fatigue
Elation/euphoria	Sleep disturbance
Grandiosity	Nightmares
Loquacity	Depression
Hypervigilance	Increased appetite
Tachycardia	
Mydriasis	
Elevated or lowered blood pressure	
Sweating or chills	
Nausea and vomiting	

Signs and symptoms of cocaine intoxication are summarized in Table 64–3. Although there is some controversy as to whether cocaine is associated with physical withdrawal on abrupt discontinuation, most clinicians feel that there is a characteristic syndrome of withdrawal effects, although they are not life-threatening.[13,27] Cocaine withdrawal consists primarily of fatigue, sleep disturbance, nightmares, and depression; it begins within hours of discontinuing the drug and lasts up to several days.

AMPHETAMINE, METHAMPHETAMINE, AND OTHER STIMULANTS

During the 1940s the Japanese government distributed amphetamines to soldiers, sailors, and pilots, as well as to arms factory workers, to mobilize all their reserves for the war effort. Pilots routinely used the drug to remain awake and alert for long periods on long-distance bombing missions. After 1945 large quantities of the drug from looted military supplies flooded the market. In the United States in the 1950s and 1960s, legally manufactured tablets of methamphetamine were used nonmedically by college students, truck drivers, and athletes, who usually did not become severely addicted. This pattern changed drastically in the later 1960s with the increased availability of injectable methamphetamine.

There were an estimated 378,000 new methamphetamine users in 1998, up from 149,000 in 1990.[4] Street methamphetamine is referred to by many names, such as "speed," "meth," and "crank." Methamphetamine hydrochloride, clear chunky crystals resembling ice which can be inhaled by smoking, is referred to as "ice," "crystal," and "glass."

The physiologic and psychological effects of amphetamines and other stimulants are qualitatively similar to those of cocaine—they diminish fatigue, increase alertness, and suppress appetite. Pharmacologically, amphetamines increase the activity of catecholamine neurotransmitters (e.g., norepinephrine and dopamine) by blocking reuptake, increasing release of neurotransmitters, and inhibiting the degradative enzyme monoamine oxidase.[28] The longer duration of effect of methamphetamine has led to a shift away from cocaine and toward the longer-acting drug.

Methamphetamine is taken orally or intranasally, by intravenous injection, and by smoking. Immediately after inhalation or intravenous injection, the methamphetamine user experiences an intense sensation, called a "rush" or "flash," that lasts only a few minutes and is described as extremely pleasurable.

Because methamphetamine elevates mood, people who experiment with it tend to use it with increasing frequency and in increasing doses, although this was not their original intent. The CNS actions that result from taking even small amounts of methamphetamine include increased wakefulness, increased physical activity, decreased appetite, increased respiration, hyperthermia, and euphoria. Other CNS effects include irritability, insomnia, confusion, tremors, convulsions, anxiety, paranoia, and aggressiveness. Hyperthermia and convulsions can result in death.

Cardiovascular side effects, which include chest pain and hypertension, also can result in cardiovascular collapse and death. In addition, methamphetamine causes increased heart rate and blood pressure and can cause irreversible damage to blood vessels in the brain, producing strokes. Other effects of methamphetamine include respiratory problems, irregular heartbeat, and extreme anorexia.

Methamphetamine can be injected, smoked, snorted, or ingested orally or anally. The timing and intensity of the "rush" that accompanies the use of methamphetamine, which is a result of the release of high levels of dopamine into the brain, depends in part on the method of administration. Specifically, the effect is almost instantaneous when smoked or injected, while it takes approximately 5 minutes after snorting or 20 minutes after oral ingestion. Immediate physiologic changes associated with the use of methamphetamine are similar to those produced by the fight-or-flight response and include increased blood pressure, body temperature, heart rate, and respiratory rate. Negative side effects include high body temperature, stroke, cardiac arrhythmias, stomach cramps, and shaking, as well as increased anxiety, insomnia, aggressive tendencies, paranoia, and hallucinations.

Prolonged use of methamphetamine may result in a tolerance for the drug and increased use at higher dosage levels, creating dependence. Such continual use of the drug with little or no sleep leads to an extremely irritable and paranoid state. Discontinuing use of methamphetamine often results in a state of depression, as well as fatigue, anergia, and some types of cognitive impairment that last anywhere from 2 days to several months.[29]

Both short- and long-term health effects have also been documented. Negative consequences of methamphetamine abuse range from anxiety and insomnia to convulsions, paranoia, and brain damage, but in addition to the many direct effects on methamphetamine users are the indirect impacts on individuals and society. Children of methamphetamine abusers are at high risk of neglect and abuse, and pregnant women's use of methamphetamine can cause growth retardation, premature birth, and developmental disorders in neonates. Extensive evidence indicates that in many Western U.S. cities, methamphetamine is used extensively by gay males and is frequently associated with high-risk sexual behavior, a major factor in the transmission of the human immunodeficiency virus (HIV). Within this particular group, effective treatment for methamphetamine dependence may be one of the most important strategies in reducing the spread of HIV and other associated communicable diseases.[30] Treatment for methamphetamine dependence is very difficult, with a low success rate.[31]

The expanding global market is fed by an increase in clandestine manufacture of methamphetamine. Not only are there more laboratories in more countries, but their size and sophistication is also increasing. The number of clandestine methamphetamine laboratories seized nationwide by the U.S. Drug Enforcement Administration (DEA) increased from 263 in 1994 to 1815 in 2000, a 590% increase. In addition, state and local police agencies seized almost 4,600 clandestine laboratories in the United States during 2000. So-called "kitchen" laboratories are still detected, but today clandestine laboratories with 100-kilogram capacities per week are also found. Initially the clandestine manufacture of methamphetamine was based primarily in the West and Southwest. Today methamphetamine can be found in cities across the United States. Methamphetamine is manufactured using the ephedrine or pseudoephedrine reduction method. In this process, ephedrine or pseudoephedrine is extracted from over-the-counter cold and allergy tablets. Pharmacists should be wary of persons wishing to purchase large quantities of products containing nonprescription sympathomimetic products.

Prices for methamphetamine vary throughout different regions of the United States, ranging from $3500 per pound in parts of California and Texas to $21,000 per pound in southeastern and northeastern regions of the country. Retail prices range from $400 to $3000 per ounce.[32] This corresponds to a cost of $10 to $60 per dosage unit.[33]

ECSTASY AND OTHER METHAMPHETAMINE ANALOGS

Several dozen analogs of amphetamine and methamphetamine are hallucinogenic. Two methamphetamine analogs of most concern are 3,4-methylenedioxyamphetamine (MDA) and especially 3,4-methylenedioxymethamphetamine (MDMA or ecstasy). Use of this latter drug has skyrocketed in recent years. The drug is particularly popular among young people at all-night dance parties referred to as "raves," and the drug is classified among the "club drugs." As stated earlier, among high school seniors annual use rates have actually declined from 9.2% to 7.4%.[5]

Decreased usage of a drug is usually tied to increases in the perceived risk of using that drug. Disapproval of ecstasy use rose sharply in all three grades in 2002, indicating that peer norms against the use of this drug are strengthening. In 2000, only 38% of twelfth graders said there was a great risk of harm associated with trying ecstasy. That figure jumped to 46% in 2001 and again in 2002 to 52%.[5]

The vast majority of ecstasy consumed domestically is produced in Europe. It costs as little as 25 to 50 cents to manufacture an ecstasy tablet in Europe, but the street value of that same ecstasy tablet can be as high as $40, with a tablet typically selling for between $20 and $30.[34] A limited number of ecstasy laboratories operate in the United States. Law enforcement seized 17 clandestine ecstasy laboratories in the United States in 2001 compared to 7 seized in 2000.[34] United States Customs Service statistics show a dramatic increase in seizures of MDMA tablets. In fiscal year 1997, approximately 400,000 MDMA tablets were seized, compared to approximately 7.2 million tablets seized in fiscal year 2001. On July 22, 2000, approximately 2.1 million tablets worth an estimated $40 million were seized in Los Angeles. To date this is the largest seizure of MDMA tablets in the United States.[35]

MDMA is structurally similar to methamphetamine and mescaline and stimulates the CNS, producing a mild hallucinogenic effect. Known most commonly on the street as ecstasy, it is also called "Adam," "X," "X-TC," "Stacy," "beans," "e," or simply "pills." Users under the influence of MDMA are said to be "rolling." Those taking both MDMA and lysergic acid diethylamide (LSD) are referred to as "trolling," a combination of the slang terms "tripping" and "rolling." MDMA is usually taken by mouth in tablet, capsule, or powder form, but it also may be smoked, snorted, or injected.

The effects of MDMA usually last approximately 4 to 6 hours. Users of the drug say that it produces profoundly positive feelings, empathy for others, elimination of anxiety, and extreme relaxation. MDMA is also said to suppress the need to eat, drink, or sleep, enabling users to endure 2- to 3-day parties. Consequently MDMA use sometimes results in severe dehydration or exhaustion. MDMA generally reduces inhibitions and creates a sense of euphoria, but it also can evoke anxiety and paranoia. Heavier doses generate depression, irrationality, and psychosis. Users claim they experience feelings of closeness with others and a desire to touch them.

MDMA use can result in a variety of acute psychiatric disturbances, including panic, anxiety, depression, and paranoid thinking.[36] Physical symptoms include muscle tension, nausea, blurred vision, faintness, chills, and sweating. MDMA also increases the heart rate and blood pressure. Other effects include hyperthermia, dehydration, vomiting, tremors, loss of control over body movements, insomnia, convulsions, rapid eye movements, and teeth and jaw clenching.

MDMA is perceived to be a harmless drug by many of its users, based in part on the fact that the risk of death is low compared with other drugs like heroin and cocaine. However, mounting evidence points to neurotoxic effects of MDMA, involving a complex and incompletely understood mechanism. MDMA has been clearly shown to destroy serotonin-producing neurons in animals.[37] Doses of MDMA that produce neurotoxicity are only two or three times more than the minimum dose needed to produce a psychotropic response. This suggests that individuals who are self-administering the drug may be getting a neurotoxic dose.[38]

Researchers have found that heavy MDMA users have memory problems that persist for at least 2 weeks after they have stopped using the drug.[39] The authors compared 24 abstinent MDMA users and 24 control subjects on several standardized tests of memory, after matching subjects for age, gender, educational level, and vocabulary score (a surrogate of verbal intelligence). The authors also explored correlations between changes in memory function and decrements in cerebrospinal fluid (CSF) 5-hydroxyindoleacetic acid (5-HIAA), which serves as a marker of central serotonin neural function. These researchers were able to show that greater use of MDMA (total milligrams per month) was associated with greater impairment in immediate verbal memory and delayed visual memory. Furthermore, lower vocabulary scores were associated with stronger dose-related effects, with men having greater dose-related deficits than women. Lastly, lower concentrations of CSF 5-HIAA were associated with poorer memory performance. The authors concluded that abstinent MDMA users have impairment in verbal and visual memory, and that the extent of memory impairment correlates with the degree of MDMA exposure and the reduction in brain serotonin, as indexed by CSF 5-HIAA.

McCann and colleagues[40] conducted a study to determine the effects of MDMA use on cognitive performance. Twenty-two MDMA users who had not used MDMA for at least 3 weeks and 23 control subjects were tested repeatedly with a computerized cognitive performance assessment battery while participating in a 5-day controlled inpatient study. CSF measures of monoamine metabolites also were collected as an index of brain monoaminergic function. MDMA users and controls were found to perform similarly on several cognitive tasks. However, MDMA subjects had significant performance deficits on a sustained-attention task requiring arithmetic calculations, a task requiring complex attention and incidental learning, a task requiring short-term memory, and a task of semantic recognition and verbal reasoning. MDMA users also had significant selective decreases in CSF 5-HIAA. The authors believe that their data provide further evidence that MDMA is neurotoxic to brain serotonin neurons in humans, and the behavioral data suggest that brain serotonin injury is associated with subtle but significant cognitive deficits. Additional evidence has been accruing.[41]

Manufacturers of illicit drugs sometimes substitute other, potentially more dangerous substances for the one the buyer is expecting. Other suppliers produce products adulterated with chemical byproducts of the incomplete synthesis of active ingredients. One such chemical, *para*-methoxyamphetamine, is a drastically more potent hyperthermic agent than MDMA.[42] Deaths from the drug likely will rise as a result of these poor-quality tablets.

PHENCYCLIDINE AND KETAMINE

Phencyclidine (PCP), commonly referred to as "angel dust" and "crystal," was popular in the 1970s, but as its adverse effects became better known, use declined. PCP is most often a substitute for or contaminant of other drugs, and its most common pattern of use may now

TABLE 64–4. Signs and Symptoms of Phencyclidine Intoxication

Nystagmus	Euphoria
Increased blood pressure	Motor agitation
Tachycardia	Anxiety and emotional lability
Paresthesias	Hostility
Ataxia	Delusions
Slurred speech	Hallucinations
Muscle rigidity	

be unintentional. The actual extent of its use is unclear. It is often misrepresented as LSD or Δ^9-tetrahydrocannabinol (THC). With the exception of the pharmaceutical dosage form of dronabinol, THC is virtually unavailable on the street because it is highly unstable when isolated from the marijuana plant. When used intentionally, PCP is commonly smoked with marijuana and referred to as a "crystal joint," but it also may be taken orally or intravenously.

PCP has widely varied actions including CNS stimulation, depression, and hallucinogenic properties. Pharmacologically, it is known to block reuptake of serotonin, dopamine, and norepinephrine, but neurotransmitter antagonists do not effectively block its effects. In low doses, PCP causes sedation, ataxia, nystagmus, slurred speech, and paresthesias. At higher doses, users experience an increase in heart rate, blood pressure, temperature, diaphoresis, and muscle rigidity. At acutely toxic doses, coma and seizures may occur.[43]

Behavioral effects of PCP range from sleep to catatonic detachment to paranoid psychosis to violent hostility. Users are sometimes amnestic for events that occur under the influence of the drug. Psychoses sometimes last for weeks. Users with a previous history of schizophrenia are especially susceptible to the psychotomimetic effects of the drug. The only truly characteristic behavioral effect of PCP use is its high unpredictability. The signs and symptoms of PCP intoxication are summarized in Table 64–4.

Ketamine, a compound chemically related to PCP, is used primarily as a veterinary anesthetic but has gained popularity recently as a recreational drug.[44] Once used extensively in human medicine, it has fallen out of favor because of "emergence delirium," characterized by hallucinations, delirium, vivid dreams, and other psychiatric effects. This untoward effect as a medicinal agent is precisely the effect that recreational users are seeking.

Known as "special K," "jet," "green," and other names on the street, ketamine is sometimes injected, but can be evaporated to solid crystals, powdered, and smoked, snorted, or swallowed. Marijuana cigarettes are sometimes soaked in the ketamine solution, allowed to dry, and then smoked. Ketamine has become popular as a "rave" club drug. Side effects include significant transient increases in blood pressure and heart rate, respiratory depression, airway obstruction, apnea, muscular hypertonia, psychomotor and psychotomimetic effects, and acute dystonic reactions. Following overdose, seizures, polyneuropathy, increased intracranial pressure, respiratory arrest, and cardiac arrest may occur.[45,46]

The effects of a ketamine "high" usually last an hour, but they can last for 4 to 6 hours, and 24 to 48 hours are generally required before the user will feel completely normal again. Effects of chronic use of ketamine may take from several months to 2 years to disappear completely. Low doses (25 to 100 mg) produce psychedelic effects quickly. Large doses can produce vomiting and convulsions and may lead to hypoxia of the brain and muscles; 1 g can cause death. Flashbacks may even occur 1 year after use. Long-term effects include tolerance and possible physical and/or psychological dependence.

Since its emergence as a drug of abuse in the late 1960s, PCP has been described as one of the most dangerous of all synthetic hallucinogens. Its niche in the drug world is usually one characterized by

abusers exhibiting hostile behavior that manifests itself in extremely violent episodes.[45,46]

Despite the negative effects associated with PCP, there remains an illicit market for the drug. Illicit organizations producing and distributing PCP are still active in the United States.[47] These organizations, operating mainly in Los Angeles and to a lesser extent in Houston, supply most of the PCP available in the nation. The recent emergence of large PCP laboratories in other locations, such as Indiana and Maryland, are cause for concern because this may be an indication that the demand for PCP is on the rise. Lending support to this claim is a DAWN survey indicating that the number of PCP-related ED visits increased 78% from 1998 to 2001; mentions of PCP increased 25% (from 6,102 to 7,648) from 2001 to 2002.[2]

HALLUCINOGENS

The drugs commonly classified as hallucinogens are LSD, psilocybin, dimethyltryptamine (DMT), mescaline, and other related compounds. LSD is one of the most potent mood-changing chemicals. It is manufactured from lysergic acid, which is found in ergot, a fungus that grows on rye and other grains.

Pharmacologically, LSD and related drugs stimulate both presynaptic (5-HT$_{1A}$ and 5-HT$_{1B}$) and postsynaptic (5-HT$_2$) serotonin recognition sites in the brain, which functionally may cause either agonist or antagonist effects on serotonin activity.[48] Precisely how the hallucinogens exert their effects remains unclear. LSD, often referred to as "acid," is an extraordinarily potent compound, producing observable CNS effects at doses as low as 25 mcg.[48]

LSD is sold on the street in tablets, capsules, and occasionally in liquid form. It is odorless, colorless, and tasteless and usually is taken by mouth. Often LSD is added to absorbent paper, such as blotter paper, and divided into small decorated squares, with each square representing one dose.

The DEA reports that the strength of LSD samples obtained recently from illicit sources ranges from 20 to 80 mcg of LSD per dose. This is considerably less than the levels reported during the 1960s and early 1970s, when the dosage ranged from 100 to 200 mcg or higher per unit.

The effects of LSD are unpredictable. They depend on the amount taken; the user's personality, mood, and expectations; and the surroundings in which the drug is used. Usually the user feels the first effects of the drug 30 to 90 minutes after taking it. The physical effects include dilated pupils, higher body temperature, increased heart rate and blood pressure, sweating, loss of appetite, sleeplessness, dry mouth, and tremors.

Sensations and feelings change much more dramatically than the physical signs. The user may feel several different emotions at once or swing rapidly from one emotion to another. If taken in a large enough dose, the drug produces delusions and visual hallucinations. The user's sense of time and self changes. Sensations may seem to "cross over," giving the user the feeling of hearing colors and seeing sounds. These changes can be frightening and can cause panic.

Many LSD users experience flashbacks, or recurrence of certain aspects of a person's experience, without the user having taken the drug again. A flashback occurs suddenly, often without warning, and may occur within a few days or more than a year after LSD use. Flashbacks usually occur in people who use hallucinogens chronically or have an underlying personality problem; however, otherwise healthy people who use LSD occasionally also may have flashbacks.

Most users of LSD voluntarily decrease or stop its use over time. LSD is not considered an addictive drug because it does not

TABLE 64–5. Signs and Symptoms of Hallucinogen Intoxication

Psychologic	Physical
Perceptual intensification	Mydriasis
Depersonalization	Tachycardia
Derealization	Diaphoresis
Illusions	Palpitations
Hallucinations	Blurred vision
Synesthesias	Tremor
	Incoordination
	Dizziness
	Weakness
	Drowsiness
	Paresthesias

produce compulsive drug-seeking behavior. However, as with many of the addictive drugs, LSD use produces tolerance, so some users who take the drug repeatedly must take progressively higher doses to achieve the state of intoxication that they had achieved previously.

Signs and symptoms of hallucinogen intoxication are summarized in Table 64–5. Psychological symptoms of intoxication include a subjective intensification of perceptions, depersonalization, illusions, hallucinations, and synesthesias, the overflow of one sensory modality to another (colors are heard, sounds are seen). Among the hallucinogenic drugs, LSD is the most potent and long acting; it is hundreds of times more potent than both psilocybin and mescaline. DMT is inactive when ingested orally but can be smoked, inhaled, or injected. There is cross-tolerance among LSD, psilocybin, and mescaline. There is no observable physical withdrawal syndrome after abrupt discontinuation of hallucinogenic drugs.[49]

Complications from hallucinogen use are primarily psychological. Users sometimes experience prolonged episodes of panic—the so-called "bad trip." The flashbacks noted above are common, occurring in approximately 15% of users and occurring episodically up to several years after the last exposure to the drug. Flashbacks may occur spontaneously but are also triggered by other drugs, including marijuana, and by anxiety-provoking stimuli. Physical effects of hallucinogen use are relatively nontoxic. Contrary to a widely held notion in the 1960s and early 1970s, there is no reliable evidence that hallucinogen use causes chromosome damage or genetic defects.[48]

Few LSD laboratories have ever been seized in the United States because of infrequent and irregular production cycles. In 2000, the DEA seized one LSD laboratory that was located in a converted missile silo in Kansas. This was the largest LSD lab seizure ever made by the DEA, and agents seized approximately 41.3 kilograms (90.86 pounds) of LSD and approximately 23.6 kilograms (51.92 pounds) of iso-LSD, a by-product of the manufacture of LSD.[50]

MARIJUANA

Marijuana, referred to as "reefer," "pot," "grass," or "weed," remains the most commonly used illicit drug. In 2002, it was used by 75% of current illicit drug users. Approximately 55% of current illicit drug users used only marijuana, 20% used marijuana and another illicit drug, and the remaining 25% used an illicit drug but not marijuana in the past month. Ninety-five million people 12 years and older (40.4%) have tried marijuana at least once.[4] There were an estimated 2.6 million new marijuana users in 2001. In 2001, about two-thirds (67%) of new marijuana users were under age 18. This proportion has generally increased since the 1960s, when less than half of initiates were under

18. The average age of marijuana initiates was around 19 in the late 1960s and 17.1 in 2001.

Most users smoke marijuana in hand-rolled cigarettes called joints, among other names; some use pipes or water pipes called bongs. Marijuana cigars called blunts have also become popular. To make blunts, users slice open cigars and replace the tobacco with marijuana, often combined with another drug, such as crack cocaine. Marijuana also is used to brew tea and is sometimes mixed into foods.[51]

Marijuana's effects begin immediately after the drug enters the brain and last from 1 to 3 hours. If marijuana is consumed in food or drink, the short-term effects begin more slowly, usually in $^1/_2$ to 1 hour, and last longer, for as long as 4 hours. Smoking marijuana deposits several times more THC into the blood than does eating or drinking the drug.[51]

Within minutes of inhaling marijuana smoke, the heart rate increases, the bronchial passages relax and become enlarged, and blood vessels in the eyes dilate, causing the eyes to appear bloodshot. As THC enters the brain, it causes a user to feel euphoric, activating the reward system by stimulating brain cells to release dopamine. A marijuana user may experience pleasant sensations, colors and sounds may seem more intense, and time appears to pass very slowly. The user's mouth feels dry, and he may suddenly become very hungry and thirsty. The hands may tremble and grow cold. The euphoria passes after awhile, and then the user may feel sleepy or depressed. Occasionally, marijuana use produces anxiety, fear, distrust, or panic.[51]

Marijuana use impairs a person's ability to form memories, recall events, and shift attention from one thing to another.[52] THC also disrupts coordination and balance by binding to receptors in the cerebellum and basal ganglia. Through its effects on the brain and body, marijuana intoxication can cause accidents. Studies show that approximately 6% to 11% of fatal accident victims test positive for THC. In many of these cases alcohol is detected as well.

In a study conducted by the National Highway Traffic Safety Administration, a moderate dose of marijuana alone was shown to impair driving performance; however, the effects of even a low dose of marijuana combined with alcohol were markedly greater than for either drug alone. Driving indices measured included reaction time, visual search frequency (driver checking of side streets), and the ability to perceive and/or respond to changes in the relative velocity of other vehicles.[53]

Marijuana users who have taken high doses of the drug may experience acute toxic psychosis, which includes hallucinations, delusions, and depersonalization—the persistent or recurrent feelings of being detached from one's body or mental processes and usually a feeling of being an outside observer of one's own life. Although the specific causes of these symptoms remain unknown, they appear to occur more frequently when a high dose of cannabis is consumed in food or drink rather than smoked.[51]

The principal psychoactive component of marijuana is THC. Hashish, the dried resin of the top of the plant, is much more potent than the plant itself. Increasingly sophisticated growing techniques have resulted in plants of greater potency. In a recent study, the amount of Δ^9-THC found in the samples ranged from 1.41% to 12.62% by dry weight. The average Δ^9-THC content was 6.20%, which is almost identical to the 2002 value reported by The University of Mississippi's Potency Monitoring Project.[52]

Marijuana has been used widely and is believed by many to be a relatively harmless, nonaddictive intoxicant. Chronic low doses of marijuana usually are not associated with significant physical withdrawal on abrupt discontinuation, but many chronic users exhibit compulsive drug-seeking and drug-use behaviors characteristic of addiction or dependence. Acutely, marijuana has many of the effects of

TABLE 64–6. Signs and Symptoms of Marijuana Intoxication

Tachycardia	Euphoria
Conjunctival congestion	Sensory intensification
Increased appetite	Apathy
Dry mouth	Hallucinations

alcohol—sedation, a decrease in reactivity and ability to perform complex tasks, and disinhibition. Marijuana also causes hallucinations with high enough doses. Chronic use is associated with all the risks of tobacco smoking, although marijuana smokers are commonly also tobacco smokers, and thus differentiation of effects is often difficult. Endocrine effects including amenorrhea, decreased testosterone production, and inhibition of spermatogenesis have been demonstrated. Marijuana is associated with an amotivational syndrome characterized by a behavioral pattern of apathy, dullness, impaired judgment, decreased concentration and memory, loss of interest in personal hygiene, and a general reduction of goal-directed behavior.[54]

The signs and symptoms of marijuana intoxication are summarized in Table 64–6. Although the duration of effect of marijuana may be only several hours, THC is detectable on toxicologic screening for up to 4 to 5 weeks, especially in chronic users.

Marijuana smoke is irritating to the lungs. Researchers have found that the daily use of one to three marijuana joints appears to produce approximately the same lung damage and potential cancer risk as smoking five times as many cigarettes.[55] The study results suggest that the way smokers inhale marijuana, in addition to its chemical composition, increases the adverse physical effects. The study findings refute the argument that marijuana is safer than tobacco because users smoke only a few joints a day.

Clearly, there is much more work to be done before the precise health and psychological effects of marijuana use are well understood. In fact, many of these health issues remain the subject of much debate. Undoubtedly, opinions on its risks are polarized along the lines of proponents' views on what its legal status should be. This polarization of opinion has prevented the development of any consensus on what health information the medical profession should give to patients who are users or potential users of marijuana. There is conflicting evidence about many of the effects of marijuana use. Readers are referred to an excellent article that attempts to summarize in a dispassionate way the evidence on the most probable adverse health and psychological consequences of acute and chronic use of marijuana.[56]

INHALANTS

Inhalants are a diverse group of substances that include volatile solvents, gases, and nitrites that are sniffed, snorted, huffed, or bagged to produce intoxicating effects similar to those of alcohol. These substances are found in common household products like glues, lighter fluid, cleaning fluids, paint products, nail polish remover, gasoline, rubber glue, waxes, and varnishes. Chemicals found in these products include toluene, benzene, methanol, methylene chloride, acetone, methylethyl ketone, methylbutyl ketone, trichloroethylene, and trichlorethane. The gas used as a propellant in canned whipped cream and in small metallic containers called "whippets" (used to make whipped cream) is nitrous oxide or "laughing gas." Tiny cloth-covered ampules called "poppers" or "snappers" by abusers contain amyl nitrite, a medication used to dilate blood vessels. Butyl nitrite, sold as tape head cleaner and referred to as "rush," "locker room," or "climax," is often sniffed or huffed to get high.

The easy accessibility, low cost, legal status, and ease of transport and concealment make inhalants one of the first substances abused by children. Survey data indicate that about 15% to 20% of junior and senior high school students have tried inhalants, with about 2% to 6% reporting current use. The highest incidence of use is among 10- to 12-year-old children, with rates of use declining with age.[5] Parents worry about alcohol, tobacco, and drug use, but may be unaware of the hazards associated with products found throughout their homes.

Inhalants may be sniffed directly from an open container or huffed from a rag soaked in the substance and held to the face. Alternatively, the open container or soaked rag can be placed in a bag where the vapors can concentrate before being inhaled. Although inhalant abusers may prefer one particular substance because of taste or odor, a variety of substances may be used because of similar effects, availability, and cost. Once inhaled, the extensive capillary surface area of the lungs allows rapid absorption of the substance and blood levels peak rapidly. Entry into the brain is fast, and the intoxicating effects are intense but short-lived. Intoxication is often accompanied by headache and nausea, and users may experience hallucinations and delusions. The most serious physical risk of acute use is sudden death, usually from cardiac arrhythmias. Some users die from suffocation by plastic bags that contain the solvent. With chronic use, the drugs are toxic to virtually all organ systems. Psychological impairment; impaired pulmonary, renal, and hepatic function; neuropathies; encephalopathy; and brain damage have all been observed.[57]

Inhalants depress the CNS, producing decreased respiration and blood pressure. Users report distortion in perceptions of time and space. Many users experience headaches, nausea, slurred speech, and loss of motor coordination. Mental effects may include fear, anxiety, or depression. A rash around the nose and mouth may be seen, and the abuser may start wheezing. An odor of paint or organic solvents on clothes, skin, and breath is sometimes a sign of inhalant abuse. Other indicators of inhalant abuse include slurred speech or staggering gait; red, glassy, watery eyes; and excitability or unpredictable behavior.

▶ TREATMENT: Substance-Related Disorders

▓ ACUTE DRUG INTOXICATIONS

Treatment of drug intoxication, summarized in Table 64–7, is primarily supportive. Vital functions are maintained while waiting for the drug to be eliminated. When absolutely necessary, physical restraint may be required temporarily while a diagnostic evaluation is initiated to rule out other causes for the behavior (e.g., metabolic or fluid and electrolyte disturbances). Whenever possible, drug therapy should be avoided because psychotropic drug therapy has the potential for worsening a toxic reaction to another psychoactive agent; however, when patients are agitated, combative, assaultive, hallucinatory, or delusional, drug therapy may be required. Drug therapy also may be indicated in the treatment of an acute, potentially fatal drug overdose. Toxicology screens are useful in the evaluation and treatment process, but knowledge of the metabolism of the suspected drug and its excretion patterns is important for proper interpretation of test results. When toxicology screens are desired, blood or urine should be collected immediately upon the patient's arrival.

TABLE 64–7. Treatment of Substance Intoxication

Drug Class	Pharmacologic Therapy	Nonpharmacologic Therapy
Benzodiazepines	Flumazenil 0.2 mg/min IV initially, repeat up to 3 mg maximum	Support vital functions
Alcohol, barbiturates, and sedative-hypnotics (nonbenzodiazepines)	None	Support vital functions
Opiates	Naloxone 0.4–2 mg IV every 3 min	Support vital functions
Cocaine and other CNS stimulants	Lorazepam 2–4 mg IM every 30 min to 6 h as needed for agitation	Monitor cardiac function
	Haloperidol 2–5 mg (or other antipsychotic agent) every 30 min to 6 h as needed for psychotic behavior	
Hallucinogens, marijuana, and inhalants	Lorazepam and/or haloperidol as above	Reassurance; "talk-down therapy"; support vital functions
Phencyclidine	Lorazepam and/or haloperidol as above	Minimize sensory input

For alcohol and barbiturate intoxication, supportive treatment is the rule. For benzodiazepine intoxication, the benzodiazepine antagonist flumazenil can be used to reverse toxic effects. However, it is not indicated in all cases of suspected drug overdose, and is specifically contraindicated in cases in which cyclic antidepressant involvement is known or suspected because of the risk of seizures. In addition, it should be used with caution in patients when benzodiazepine physical dependence is suspected because of the risks of induction of benzodiazepine withdrawal. In the case of opiate intoxication, if the patient is unconscious and respiration is depressed, the opiate antagonist naloxone can be used to revive the patient. The usual dosage for naloxone in acute opiate toxicity is 0.4 to 2 mg intravenously, given approximately every 3 minutes as necessary.[58] Although naloxone is effective in reversing opiate overdose, it also may precipitate physical withdrawal in physically dependent patients. Patients who fail to respond to a total dosage of 10 mg naloxone probably have a cause of acute intoxication other than an opiate.

Intoxication with stimulants, including cocaine, is treated pharmacologically only if the patient is overtly psychotic and agitated. Injectable benzodiazepines, usually lorazepam 2 to 4 mg intramuscularly every 30 minutes to 6 hours as necessary, can be used for agitation. As a back-up to lorazepam, antipsychotic drugs can be used on a short-term basis, primarily in patients with psychotic symptoms, and usually at relatively low doses, such as haloperidol 2 to 5 mg intramuscularly every 30 minutes to 6 hours as necessary, followed by 5 to 15 mg orally per day in single or divided doses if the patient is still psychotic after initial treatment.[27] Cardiovascular complications are treated symptomatically with antiarrhythmic agents or other interventions as necessary. Seizures generally are treated supportively. Intravenous lorazepam or diazepam can be used if seizures progress to status epilepticus.

Hallucinogen intoxication is treated in a manner similar to stimulant intoxication. Drug therapy often can be avoided because patients may respond to careful reassurance, or so-called talk-down therapy. When necessary, short-term antianxiety and/or antipsychotic drug therapy can be used, as described previously. The same approach applies to marijuana and inhalant intoxication.

PCP intoxication is more unpredictable and more difficult to treat than other psychosis-producing drugs. Most clinicians suggest that sensory input be minimized to the extent possible; thus talk-down therapy is not recommended and may in fact make the patient worse. If PCP intoxication is suspected, patients should be left alone in a quiet, dimly lit room. If behavior is uncontrollable, antianxiety and/or antipsychotic drug therapy may be necessary.

WITHDRAWAL

Treatment of drug withdrawal is the primary indication for drug therapy in substance-related disorders. Goals of drug therapy include prevention of progression of withdrawal to life-threatening severity, enabling the patient to be sufficiently comfortable and functional in order to participate in a behavioral treatment program, and supportive drug therapy. The clinician should remember that withdrawal is usually part of a substance dependence disorder. Patients with drug dependence generally cope with almost any stress through the use of a drug. In drug therapy for withdrawal, it is important to avoid reinforcing the patient's drug-seeking and drug-use behavior to the extent possible. Drug withdrawal in the best of circumstances is uncomfortable. Patients must be educated to deal with the stress of withdrawal without seeking drugs. The use of drugs as needed for anxiety or insomnia should be avoided. A recent review on the management of drug and alcohol withdrawal has been published.[13] Treatment of drug withdrawal is summarized in Table 64–8.

CNS DEPRESSANT WITHDRAWAL

Benzodiazepines

Treatment of benzodiazepine withdrawal is very similar to the treatment of alcohol withdrawal, and the same drugs and dosages may be used.[59] The major difference in management is the length of treatment. The onset of withdrawal symptoms in patients physically dependent on the long-acting benzodiazepines may be delayed up to 7 days after discontinuation of the drug.[13] A common approach in detoxification of such patients is to initiate treatment at usual dosages (chlordiazepoxide 50 mg three times a day; lorazepam 2 mg three times a day) and to maintain the initial dosage for 5 days, with gradual tapering over an additional 5 days. Detoxification in patients physically dependent on shorter-acting benzodiazepines is similar to treatment of alcohol withdrawal. Among the benzodiazepines, alprazolam has been suggested to be more difficult to taper and discontinue than the other benzodiazepines. Whether the difficulty is related to a different patient population commonly treated with alprazolam (e.g., panic disorder) or to intrinsic differences between alprazolam and other benzodiazepines is not clear. A longer, more gradual taper of the benzodiazepine used for detoxification may be needed. With all benzodiazepines, protracted minor abstinence symptoms—such as

TABLE 64–8. Treatment of Withdrawal from Some Common Drugs of Abuse

Drug or Drug Class	Pharmacologic Therapy
Benzodiazepines	
Short- to intermediate-acting	Chlordiazepoxide 50 mg three to four times a day or lorazepam 2 mg three to four times a day; taper over 5–7 days
Long-acting	Chlordiazepoxide 50 mg three to four times a day or lorazepam 2 mg three to four times a day; taper over additional 5–7 days
Barbiturates	Pentobarbital tolerance test; initial detoxification at upper limit of tolerance test; decrease dosage by 100 mg every 2–3 days
Opiates	Methadone 20–80 mg orally daily; taper by 5–10 mg daily or clonidine 2 mcg/kg three times a day × 7 days; taper over additional 3 days
Mixed-substance withdrawal	
Drugs are cross-tolerant	Detoxify according to treatment for longer-acting drug used
Drugs are not cross-tolerant	Detoxify from one drug while maintaining second drug (cross-tolerant drugs), then detoxify from second drug
CNS stimulants	Supportive treatment only; pharmacotherapy often not used; bromocriptine 2.5 mg three times a day or higher may be used for severe craving associated with cocaine withdrawal

anxiety, insomnia, irritability, sensitivity to light and sound, and muscle spasms—may remain for several weeks in patients with a history of long exposure, even after the acute phase of benzodiazepine withdrawal is complete.

Barbiturates and Other Sedative-Hypnotic Drugs

While once used extensively, barbiturates and other nonbenzodiazepine sedating medications have been largely replaced by safer and more effective medications. Abuse problems with barbiturates resemble those seen with benzodiazepines in many ways. Withdrawal from barbiturates should be handled similarly to interventions for the abuse of alcohol and benzodiazepines.[11]

Opiates

Opiate withdrawal syndrome is similar to a severe case of influenza.[13] Opiate withdrawal is not life-threatening unless there is a concurrent life-threatening medical condition. Although most patients complain of symptoms of withdrawal such as cramping or insomnia, these symptoms are tolerable, and initiation of drug therapy may be avoided in many cases. Because opiate withdrawal is not life-threatening, observable signs of withdrawal, such as mydriasis, pilomotor erection, diaphoresis, or diarrhea should be noted before initiation of drug therapy. Characteristic signs and symptoms of opiate withdrawal include pupillary dilatation, lacrimation, rhinorrhea, piloerection ("gooseflesh"), yawning, sneezing, anorexia, nausea, vomiting, and diarrhea. Seizures do not occur. Onset and duration of withdrawal symptoms and the time of peak occurrence depends on the half-life of the drug involved. Typically heroin withdrawal reaches a peak within 36 to 72 hours of discontinuation and can last for 7 to 10 days. For methadone, symptoms peak at 72 hours but can last for 2 weeks or more.[13]

The conventional drug therapy for opioid withdrawal has been methadone, a synthetic opiate. Recently, buprenorphine has been approved for opioid withdrawal and will be discussed in detail below. In detoxification treatment, methadone is administered in decreasing doses over a period not exceeding 30 days (short-term detoxification) or 180 days (long-term detoxification). There are many tapering schedules recommended in the literature. Most patients in withdrawal

continue to complain of mild symptoms after detoxification is completed. Some patients who are unable to discontinue methadone completely or habitually return to drug use when methadone is discontinued are placed in methadone-maintenance treatment programs and receive methadone chronically.[60]

Levo-alpha-acetylmethadol (LAAM) was approved by the FDA in 1993 as a potential alternative to methadone maintenance. LAAM forms two long-acting metabolites which allow three-times-a-week dosing.[58]

Typically, opioid dependency is treated initially with detoxification, usually as an inpatient. Except in a few individuals who remain drug free, detoxification is followed by long-term maintenance therapy. In the past, opioid-dependent patients relied on methadone or levomethadyl acetate, but federal restrictions limited distribution of these drugs to a small number of methadone clinics, which are not only inconvenient, but also expose patients to other drug users, and can stigmatize patients if friends, family, or coworkers are aware of their trips to the clinic. There were limited provisions for take-at-home dosing of methadone or levomethadyl because of concern about the diversion of these drugs to illicit use.

In October 2003, the FDA approved two new products for treatment of opiate dependence. These products represent two new formulations of buprenorphine. The first of these formulations, Subutex, contains only buprenorphine and is intended for use at the beginning of treatment for opiate abuse. The other, Suboxone, contains both buprenorphine and the opiate antagonist naloxone, and is intended to be the formulation used in maintenance treatment of opiate addiction. Naloxone has been added to Suboxone to guard against intravenous abuse of buprenorphine by individuals physically dependent on opiates.

These drugs represent the first therapy for in-office prescribing for opioid dependence under the federal Drug Addiction Treatment Act (DATA) of 2000.[61] Prior to the passage of the DATA, office-based management of opioid therapy was illegal because existing federal laws prohibited physicians from prescribing narcotics for the sole purpose of maintaining a patient in a narcotic-addicted state. However, not every physician is permitted to prescribe these new drugs.

To qualify, physicians must be board certified in addiction medicine/psychiatry or hold other special credentials, and physicians are required to obtain 8 hours of authorized training before they can prescribe medications for office-based treatment of opioid dependence. They also must agree to treat no more than 30 opioid-dependent patients at any one time, and they must obtain special DEA numbers indicating that they are authorized to prescribe under the provisions of the DATA.

The two formulations of the drug have been placed into schedule III by the DEA. Each product is available in two dosage strengths, 2 mg and 8 mg. Once-daily doses are titrated to a target of 16 mg/day of buprenorphine, but the dosing range extends from 4 mg/day to 24 mg/day.

Office-based maintenance therapy is well studied for patients who are already receiving treatment.[62–65]

In a multicenter, randomized, placebo-controlled trial,[62] 326 opiate-addicted persons were assigned to office-based treatment with sublingual tablets consisting of buprenorphine (16 mg) in combination with naloxone (4 mg), buprenorphine alone (16 mg), or placebo given daily for 4 weeks. The primary outcome measures were the percentage of urine samples negative for opiates and the subjects' self-reported craving for opiates. Safety data were obtained on 461 opiate-addicted persons who participated in an open-label study of buprenorphine and naloxone (at daily doses of up to 24 mg and 6 mg, respectively), and another 11 persons who received this combination only during the trial. The double-blind trial was terminated early because buprenorphine and naloxone in combination and buprenorphine alone were found to have greater efficacy than placebo. The proportion of urine samples that were negative for opiates was greater in the combined-treatment and buprenorphine groups (17.8% and 20.7%, respectively) than in the placebo group (5.8%; p <0.001 for both comparisons); the active-treatment groups also reported less opiate craving (p <0.001 for both comparisons with placebo). Rates of adverse events were similar in the active-treatment and placebo groups. During the open-label phase, the percentage of urine samples negative for opiates ranged from 35.2% to 67.4%. Results from the open-label follow-up study indicated that the combined treatment was safe and well tolerated. The authors concluded that buprenorphine and naloxone in combination and buprenorphine alone are safe and reduce the use of opiates and the craving for opiates among opiate-addicted persons who receive these medications in an office-based setting.

To check to see if the prescriber is authorized to treat patients under the DATA, pharmacists can call 1-866-BUP-CSAT or send an e-mail message to info@buprenorphine.samhsa.gov. Physicians generally use Subutex during induction and give a small supply of the product directly to the patient (clinical studies used buprenorphine-only tablets for the first 2 days). If patients present prescriptions for either agent from more than one prescriber for the same time period, a pharmacist should assume that diversion or abuse is occurring, refuse to fill the prescriptions, and notify both prescribers. Likewise, prescriptions for Subutex should be verified with prescribers, as the Suboxone formulation is preferred for long-term therapy.[65]

A rapid detoxification (RD) technique has been developed that is designed to shorten detoxification by precipitating withdrawal through the administration of opioid antagonists such as naloxone hydrochloride or naltrexone.[66] This approach is thought to have the advantage of getting patients though detoxification rapidly, minimizing the risk of relapse, and initiating treatment more quickly with naltrexone maintenance combined with suitable psychosocial interventions. Ultrarapid detoxification (URD) represents a variant of this technique in which patients undergo opioid antagonist–precipitated withdrawal while under general anesthesia or heavy sedation. Although it is difficult to estimate the extent of their clinical use, these techniques are becoming increasingly available in response to rising demand for opioid-dependence treatment services. In the United States there has been a rapid proliferation of programs offering URD, with some programs charging up to $7500 per treatment.[66]

A recent meta-analysis was performed to assess the evidence for the efficacy of both RD and URD to determine their role among the available treatment options for opioid dependence. Analysis was performed on 12 studies of RD and 9 studies of URD. The authors concluded that more research is needed using more rigorous research methods, longer-term outcomes, and comparisons with other methods of treatment for opioid dependence before these techniques can gain widespread acceptance.[66]

CLINICAL CONTROVERSY

Ultrarapid detoxification from opiates remains somewhat controversial in terms of its efficacy, safety, and cost. Before consenting to such treatment, patients should inquire of the practitioner regarding previous experience with this technique, including success rates of patients remaining drug-free, and also rates of complications that have occurred.

▨ WITHDRAWAL FROM OTHER SUBSTANCES

Withdrawal from other drugs, including cocaine and other stimulants, is primarily supportive. However, pharmacotherapy recently has assumed a greater role in treating cocaine withdrawal and dependence. Bromocriptine, a dopamine antagonist at low dosages and an agonist at high dosages, is usually used in the treatment of parkinsonism and hyperprolactinemia and has been used to treat cocaine withdrawal symptoms and to reduce the craving for cocaine. Use of bromocriptine is based on the hypothesis that chronic use of cocaine causes dopamine depletion; therefore higher dosages should be used (i.e., 2.5 mg three times daily or higher). Despite initially promising pilot studies, recent evidence does not support the efficacy of bromocriptine to reduce cocaine use or craving.[67]

▨ SUBSTANCE DEPENDENCE

The treatment of drug dependence is primarily behavioral. The patient generally is taught that complete abstinence is the only realistic alternative to a life of uncontrollable drug use and despair that ultimately will end in death, and that there is no intermediate, controllable level of drinking or use of another drug. However, complete and permanent abstinence as the sole route to recovery is controversial. There may be an extremely few individuals who can return to controllable levels of drinking alcohol, but it is impossible to predict who these individuals are; most treatment programs continue to advocate complete abstinence. The prospect of life without alcohol or other drugs is incomprehensible to many patients. Entry into treatment often is facilitated by some type of leverage that the drug-dependent person associates with negative consequences, such as potential loss of job, divorce, legal problems, or deteriorating physical health. Early treatment is directed at penetrating the denial of a problem that is always present. The patient must be educated as to the disease of addiction, the effects of drugs, and the permanence of the condition.

As evidenced by the approval of the two buprenorphine products, there has been a trend toward outpatient treatment for drug dependence, due in part to cost-containment efforts. Inpatient treatment programs can cost as much as $20,000 for a 4-week stay. When withdrawal symptoms are mild to moderate and there are no other medical indications for hospitalization, outpatient treatment may be an attractive alternative to inpatient treatment. One critical criterion for outpatient treatment is the patient's compliance with complete abstinence from the dependence-producing drug during the treatment experience.

Families must be involved in treatment. The course of the patient's illness often has a devastating effect on other family members. Severely depleted self-esteem, denial of the family member's addiction, feelings of responsibility for the family member's drug use, and other behaviors that parallel the addiction process are often present. Treatment must be a lifelong process. Aftercare, or what is now being called *continued care,* should include regular and frequent treatment in some form. Most drug-dependence treatment programs embrace a treatment approach based on the twelve steps to recovery. Alcoholics Anonymous (AA) is one of the most successful of all self-help groups. Associated groups include Alanon (a group for family members of alcoholics), Narcotics Anonymous (self-help groups based on the AA concept for users of other drugs), Overeaters Anonymous (a group for individuals with eating disorders), Gamblers Anonymous, and several other similar programs. Among chemically dependent health care professionals, treatment that incorporates both AA and peer-led self-help groups may be most effective.[68]

CONCLUSIONS

Substance use disorders remain one of the great public health issues of contemporary society. Dependence on drugs is a powerful emotional and political issue. Because we live in a chemically oriented society, everyone is affected in some way by drug abuse and drug dependence. Health care professionals must be particularly vigilant for problems associated with drug use, not only for our patients, but also for ourselves.

ABBREVIATIONS

AA: Alcoholics Anonymous
ATOD: alcohol, tobacco, and other drugs
CASA: Center on Addiction and Substance Abuse
CSF: cerebrospinal fluid
DATA: Drug Addiction Treatment Act
DAWN: Drug Abuse Warning Network
DEA: U.S. Drug Enforcement Administration
DMT: dimethyltryptamine
GBL: γ-butyrolactone
GHB: γ-hydroxybutyrate
5-HIAA: 5-hydroxyindoleacetic acid
LAAM: levo-alpha-acetylmethadol
LSD: lysergic acid diethylamide
MDA: 3,4-methylenedioxyamphetamine
MDMA: 3,4-methylenedioxymethamphetamine
MTFS: Monitoring the Future Study
NA: Narcotics Anonymous
NSDUH: National Survey on Drug Use & Health
PCP: Phencyclidine
RD: rapid detoxification
REM: rapid eye movement
SAMHSA: Substance Abuse & Mental Health Services Administration
THC: Δ^9-tetrahydrocannabinol
URD: ultrarapid detoxification

Review Questions and other resources can be found at *www.pharmacotherapyonline.com.*

REFERENCES

1. Schneider Institute for Health Policy, Brandeis University. Substance Abuse: The Nation's Number One Health Problem. Key Indicators for Policy—Update. Princeton, NJ, Robert Wood Johnson Foundation, 2001:1–128.
2. Substance Abuse & Mental Health Services Administration, Office of Applied Studies. Emergency Department Trends from the Drug Abuse Warning Network (DAWN), Final Estimates 1995–2002. DAWN Series: D-24, DHHS Publication No. (SMA) 03-3780, Rockville, MD, 2003:1–148.
3. Savage SR, Joranson DE, Covington EC, et al. Definitions related to the medical use of opioids: Evolution towards universal agreement. J Pain Symptom Manage 2003;26:655–667.
4. Substance Abuse & Mental Health Services Administration. Results from the 2002 National Survey on Drug Use and Health: National Findings. Office of Applied Studies, NHSDA Series H-22, DHHS Publication No. SMA 03–3836. Rockville, MD. Last accessed February 2004. Available from: http://www.samhsa.gov/oas/nhsda/2k2nsduh/Results/2k2Results.htm#fig3.3.
5. Johnston LD, O'Malley PM, Bachman JG. Monitoring the Future national results on adolescent drug use: Overview of key findings, 2002. NIH Publication No. 03-5374. Bethesda, MD, National Institute on Drug Abuse. Last accessed February 27, 2004. Available from: www.monitoringthefuture.org.
6. The National Center on Addiction and Substance Abuse at Columbia University. Shoveling Up: The Impact of Substance Abuse on State Budgets. January 2001:2–3.
7. Diagnostic and Statistical Manual of Mental Disorders, 4th ed., Text Revision. Washington, American Psychiatric Press, 2000:191–198.
8. Cami J, Farre M. Drug addiction. N Engl J Med 2003;349:975–986.
9. Woods JH, Winger G. Abuse liability of flunitrazepam. J Clin Psychopharmacol 1997;17(Suppl 2):1S–57S.
10. Schwartz RH, Milteer R, LeBeau MA. Drug-facilitated sexual assault ("date rape"). South Med J 2000;93:558–561.
11. Hajak G, Muller WE, Wittchen HU, et al. Abuse and dependence potential for the non-benzodiazepine hypnotics zolpidem and zopiclone: A review of case reports and epidemiological data. Addiction 2003;98:1371–1378.
12. Hobbs WR, Rall TW, Verdoorn TA. Hypnotics and sedatives: Ethanol. In: Hardman JG, Limbird LE, eds. Goodman and Gilman's The Pharmacological Basis of Therapeutics, 9th ed. New York, McGraw-Hill, 1996:361–396.
13. Kosten TR, O'Connor PG. Management of drug and alcohol withdrawal. N Engl J Med 2003;348:1786–1795.
14. Centers for Disease Control and Prevention. Gamma-hydroxy butyrate use—New York and Texas, 1995–1996. MMWR Morb Mortal Wkly Rep 1997;46:281–283.
15. Kam PC, Yoong FF. Gamma-hydroxybutyric acid: An emerging recreational drug. Anaesthesia 1998;53:1195–1198.
16. Zvosec DL, Smith SW, McCutcheon JR, et al. Adverse events, including death, associated with the use of 1,4-butanediol. N Engl J Med 2001;344:87–94.
17. Craig K, Gomez HF, McManus JL, Bania TC. Severe gamma-hydroxybutyrate withdrawal: A case report and literature review. J Emerg Med 2000;18:65–70.
18. Anonymous. Department of Health and Human Services, Food and Drug Administration, Center for Drug Evaluation and Research, Anesthetic and Life Support Drugs Advisory Committee, September 9, 2003, Bethesda, MD. Last accessed February 27, 2004. Available from: http://www.fda.gov/ohrms/dockets/ac/03/transcripts/3978T1.pdf.
19. Cone EJ, Fant RV, Rohay JM, et al. Oxycodone involvement in drug abuse deaths: A DAWN-based classification scheme applied to an oxycodone postmortem database containing over 1000 cases. J Anal Toxicol 2003;27:57–67.

20. Ballantyne JC, Mao J. Opioid therapy for chronic pain. N Engl J Med 2003;349:1943–1953.

21. Gold MS, Miller NS. Cocaine (and crack): Neurobiology. In: Lowinson JH, Ruiz P, Millman RB, Langrod JG, eds. Substance Abuse: A Comprehensive Textbook, 3rd ed. Baltimore, Williams & Wilkins, 1997:166–181.

22. Hart CL, Jatlow P, Sevarino KA, McCance-Katz EF. Comparison of intravenous cocaethylene and cocaine in humans. Psychopharmacology (Berl) 2000;149:153–162.

23. McCance-Katz EF, Kosten TR, Jatlow P. Concurrent use of cocaine and alcohol is more potent and potentially more toxic than use of either alone: A multiple-dose study. Biol Psychiatry 1998;44:250–259.

24. Aigner TG, Balster RL. Choice behavior in rhesus monkeys: Cocaine versus food. Science 1978;201:534–535.

25. Stein MD. Medical consequences of substance abuse. Psychiatr Clin North Am 1999;22:351–370.

26. Harris D, Batki SL. Stimulant psychosis: Symptom profile and acute clinical course. Am J Addict 2000;9:28–37.

27. Mendelson JH, Mello NK. Management of cocaine abuse and dependence. N Engl J Med 1996;334:965–972.

28. King GR, Ellinwood EH. Amphetamines and other stimulants. In: Lowinson JH, Ruiz P, Millman RB, Langrod JG, eds. Substance Abuse: A Comprehensive Textbook, 3rd ed. Baltimore, Williams & Wilkins, 1997:207–223.

29. Simon SL, Domier C, Carnell J, et al. Cognitive impairment in individuals currently using methamphetamine. Am J Addict 2000;9:222–231.

30. Frosch D, Shoptaw S, Huber A, et al. Sexual HIV risk among gay and bisexual male methamphetamine abusers. J Subst Abuse Treat 1996;13:483–486.

31. Rawson RA, Gonzales R, Brethen P. Treatment of methamphetamine use disorders: An update. J Subst Abuse Treat 2002;23:145–150.

32. Anonymous. Drug Trafficking in the United States, Drug Enforcement Administration, Washington. Last accessed February 27, 2004. Available from: http://www.dea.gov/pubs/intel/01020/index.html.

33. Anonymous. Illegal Drug Price and Purity Report, Drug Enforcement Administration, Washington. Last accessed February 27, 2004. Available from: http://www.dea.gov/pubs/intel/02058/02058.html#9

34. Anonymous. MDMA (Ecstasy), Drug Enforcement Administration, Washington. Last accessed February 27, 2004. Available from: http://www.dea.gov/concern/mdma/mdma_factsheet.html.

35. Anonymous. Drug Trafficking in the United States, Drug Enforcement Administration, Washington. Last accessed February 27, 2004. Available from: http://www.dea.gov/concern/drug_trafficking.html.

36. Miller NS, Gold MS. LSD and ecstasy: Pharmacology, phenomenology, and treatment. Psychiatr Ann 1994;24:131–133.

37. McCann UD, Eligulashvili V, Ricaurte GA. (+/−) 3,4-Methylenedioxymethamphetamine ("Ecstasy")-induced serotonin neurotoxicity: Clinical studies. Neuropsychobiology 2000;42:11–16.

38. Seiden LS, Sabol KE. Methamphetamine and methylenedioxymethamphetamine neurotoxicity: Possible mechanisms of cell destruction. NIDA Res Monogr 1996;163:251–276.

39. Bolla KI, McCann UD, Ricaurte GA. Memory impairment in abstinent MDMA ("ecstasy") users. Neurology 1998;51:1532–1537.

40. McCann UD, Mertl M, Eligulashvili V, Ricaurte GA. Cognitive performance in (+/−) 3,4-methylenedioxymethamphetamine (MDMA, "ecstasy") users: A controlled study. Psychopharmacology (Berl) 1999;143:417–425.

41. Ricaurte GA, McCann UD, Szabo Z, Scheffel U. Toxicodynamics and long-term toxicity of the recreational drug, 3,4-methylenedioxymethamphetamine (MDMA, "Ecstasy"). Toxicol Lett 2000;112–113, 143–146.

42. James RA, Dinan A. Hyperpyrexia associated with fatal paramethoxyamphetamine (PMA) abuse. Med Sci Law 1998;38:83–85.

43. Zukin SR, Sloboda Z, Javitt DC. Phencyclidine (PCP). In: Lowinson JH, Ruiz P, Millman RB, Langrod JG, eds. Substance Abuse: A Comprehensive Textbook, 3rd ed. Baltimore, Williams & Wilkins, 1997:238–246.

44. Freese TE, Miotto K, Reback CJ. The effects and consequences of selected club drugs. J Subst Abuse Treat 2002;23:151–156.

45. Jansen KL. A review of the nonmedical use of ketamine: Use, users and consequences. J Psychoactive Drugs 2000;32:419–433.

46. Jansen KL, Darracot-Cankovic R. The nonmedical use of ketamine, part two: A review of problem use and dependence. J Psychoactive Drugs 2001;33:151–158.

47. Anonymous. Drug Intelligence Brief, PCP: The Threat Remains. Drug Enforcement Administration, May 2003, Washington. Last accessed February 27, 2004. Available from: http://www.dea.gov/pubs/intel/03013/index.html.

48. Glennon RA. Classical hallucinogens: An introductory overview. NIDA Res Monogr 1994;146:4–32.

49. Pechnick RN, Ungerleider JT. Hallucinogens. In: Lowinson JH, Ruiz P, Millman RB, Langrod JG, eds. Substance Abuse: A Comprehensive Textbook, 3rd ed. Baltimore, Williams & Wilkins, 1997:230–238.

50. News Release from the Drug Enforcement Administration. Pickard and Apperson Convicted of LSD Charges, Largest LSD Lab Seizure in DEA History, March 31, 2003, Washington. Last accessed February 27, 2004. Available from: http://www.dea.gov/pubs/states/newsrel/sanfran033103.html.

51. National Institute on Drug Abuse (NIDA) Research Report—Marijuana Abuse. Washington, NIH Publication No. 02-3859, October 2002:1–8.

52. ElSohly MA, Ross SA, Mehmedic Z, et al. Potency trends of delta 9-THC and other cannabinoids in confiscated marijuana from 1980–1997. J Forensic Sci 2000;45:24–30.

53. National Highway Traffic Safety Administration (NHSTA) Notes. Marijuana and alcohol combined severely impede driving performance. Ann Emerg Med 2000;35:398–399.

54. Grinspoon L, Bakalar JB. Marihuana. In: Lowinson JH, Ruiz P, Millman RB, eds. Substance Abuse: A Comprehensive Textbook, 3rd ed. Baltimore, Williams & Wilkins, 1997:199–206.

55. Sarafian TA, Magallanes JA, Shau H, et al. Oxidative stress produced by marijuana smoke: An adverse effect enhanced by cannabinoids. Am J Respir Cell Mol Biol 1999;20:1286–1293.

56. Hall W, Solowij N. Adverse effects of cannabis. Lancet 1998;352:1611–1616.

57. Sharp CW, Rosenberg NL. Inhalants. In: Lowinson JH, Ruiz P, Millman RB, Langrod JG, eds. Substance Abuse: A Comprehensive Textbook, 3rd ed. Baltimore, Williams & Wilkins, 1997:246–264.

58. Greenstein RA, Fudala PJ, O'Brien CP. Alternative pharmacotherapies for opiate addiction. In: Lowinson JH, Ruiz P, Millman RB, Langrod JG, eds. Substance Abuse: A Comprehensive Textbook, 3rd ed. Baltimore, Williams & Wilkins, 1997:415–425.

59. Smith DE, Wesson DR. Benzodiazepines and other sedative-hypnotics. In: Galanter M, Kleber HD, eds. Textbook of Substance Abuse Treatment. Washington, American Psychiatric Press, 1994:179–186.

60. Jaffe JJ, Clifford CM, Ciraulo DA. Opiates: Clinical aspects. In: Lowinson JH, Ruiz P, Millman RB, Langrod JG, eds. Substance Abuse: A Comprehensive Textbook, 3rd ed. Baltimore, Williams & Wilkins, 1997:158–166.

61. Drug Addiction Treatment Act of 2000 (DATA), title XXXV of the Children's Health Act of 2000 (Pub. L. 106-310; 116 Stat. 1222).

62. Fudala PJ, Bridge TP, Herbert S, et al. Buprenorphine/Naloxone Collaborative Study Group. Office-based treatment of opiate addiction with a sublingual-tablet formulation of buprenorphine and naloxone. N Engl J Med 2003;349:949–958.

63. Fiellin DA, O'Connor PG. Office-based treatment of opioid-dependent patients. N Engl J Med 2002;347:817–823.

64. Boatwright DE. Buprenorphine and addiction: Challenges for the pharmacist. J Am Pharm Assoc 2002;42:432–438.

65. Anonymous. Food and Drug Administration. Information for pharmacists—Suboxone and Subutex. October 8, 2002, Bethesda, MD. Last accessed February 27, 2004. Available from: http://www.fda.gov/cder/drug/infopage/subutex_suboxone/default.htm.

66. O'Connor PG, Kosten TR. Rapid and ultrarapid opioid detoxification techniques. JAMA 1998;279:229–234.

67. Handelsman L, Rosenblum A, Palij M, et al. Bromocriptine for cocaine dependence: A controlled clinical trial. Am J Addict 1997;6:54–64.

68. Beeder AB, Millman RB. Patients with psychopathology. In: Lowinson JH, Ruiz P, Millman RB, Langrod JG, eds. Substance Abuse: A Comprehensive Textbook, 3rd ed. Baltimore, Williams & Wilkins, 1997:551–563.

65

SUBSTANCE-RELATED DISORDERS: ALCOHOL, NICOTINE, AND CAFFEINE

Paul L. Doering

Learning Objectives and other resources can be found at *www.pharmacotherapyonline.com.*

KEY CONCEPTS

◀1 Tobacco is the number one preventable cause of death in the United States.

◀2 Between 12 and 16 million Americans report current heavy alcohol use or alcohol abuse.

◀3 Pharmacogenomics studies have identified genotypic and functional phenotypic variants that either serve to protect patients or predispose them toward alcohol dependence.

◀4 Alcohol is a central nervous system depressant that shares many pharmacologic properties with the nonbenzodiazepine sedative hypnotics.

◀5 The metabolism of alcohol is considered to follow zero-order pharmacokinetics, and this has important implications for the time course in which alcohol can exert its effects.

◀6 Benzodiazepines are the treatment of choice for alcohol withdrawal.

◀7 Disulfiram and naltrexone are the only two drugs FDA approved for the treatment of alcohol dependence, although the clinical utility of these agents remains controversial.

◀8 More than three-quarters of smokers are nicotine dependent. Tobacco dependence is a chronic condition that requires repeated interventions.

◀9 Use of nicotine replacement therapy along with behavioral counseling doubles cessation rates.

◀10 Bupropion is efficacious alone and in combination with nicotine replacement therapy for smoking cessation.

◀11 Caffeine's pharmacologic actions are similar to those of other stimulant drugs. As such, abstinence from caffeine induces a distinct withdrawal syndrome that includes headache, drowsiness, and fatigue.

◀1 Alcohol, nicotine, and caffeine are considered by most to be socially acceptable drugs, yet they impose an enormous social and economic cost on our society. More than 440,000 deaths each year are attributable to tobacco use, making tobacco the number one preventable cause of death and disease in this country.[1] Smoking is responsible for 85% of all lung cancer deaths, approximately 80% of all chronic obstructive pulmonary disease deaths, and 30% of overall health disease deaths.[2]

◀2 Approximately 12.9 million persons in the United States report current heavy use of alcohol or alcohol abuse.[3] Almost one-half of these persons meet *Diagnostic and Statistical Manual of Mental Disorders,* 4th ed., Text Revision (DSM-IV-TR) criteria for alcohol dependence,[4] and more than 700,000 persons are in treatment for alcoholism at any one time.[5] Population-based surveys of current drinkers have found rates of 7% to 16% for alcohol abuse or dependence.[6] In 1995, 2.7% of the annual emergency department visits were related to alcohol abuse. These alcohol-related visits were 1.6 times as likely to be associated with injuries and with a chief complaint of pain. Alcohol dependence was diagnosed in 20% of these cases.[7] According to the Drug Abuse Warning Network 2002 survey, ED visits related to drug abuse most frequently involved alcohol, and included 31% of the observed cases.[8]

An estimated 100,000 U.S. citizens die each year because of alcohol-related causes, including traffic collisions and cirrhosis of the liver.[9] Direct and indirect health and social costs of alcoholism to the nation are estimated to be $180 billion annually.[10]

Caffeine is currently the most widely used psychoactive substance in the world.[11] In the United States, 80% to 90% of adults regularly consume behaviorally active doses of caffeine.[11] Although research has shown that caffeine can cause a compulsive pattern of use, the prevalence of caffeine dependence and its clinical significance are difficult to determine.

The subjects of alcohol, tobacco, and caffeine abuse deserve much more attention than space permits in this chapter. Therefore the information here should serve as a brief overview of these topics, and the reader desiring more details is urged to consult one or more of the many textbooks and articles devoted to these subjects.

ALCOHOL

EPIDEMIOLOGY OF ALCOHOL USE

Roughly half (51%) of Americans ages 12 and older reported being current drinkers of alcohol according to the National Survey on

TABLE 65–1. Genotypic, Phenotypic, and Environmental Factors that Affect Alcohol Dependence Risk

Susceptibility Genes	Phenotype	Environment
Regions on chromosomes 1 and 4 that code for the following receptors:	Personality traits that include:	Religious background
GABA$_A$	Novelty seeking	Urban residence vs. rura
Serotonin 1b	Impulsivity	History of sexual abuse
DRD4 (dopamine 2)	Aggression	Being single
Tryptophan hydroxylase	Depression	Having deceased parent
Neuropeptide Y	Maximum number of alcoholic drinks consumed per day	
Gene that codes for:		
ALDH2 (alcohol dehydrogenase, type 2; on chromosome 12)		
5HTTLPR (serotonin transporter promoter)		

Drug Use & Health (formerly called the National Household Survey on Drug Abuse).[3] This translates to an estimated 120 million people. Approximately one-fifth of persons 12 years of age and older (54 million people) participated in binge drinking, defined as having five or more drinks on the same occasion, at least once in the 30 days prior to the survey. In 2002 there were 15.9 million heavy drinkers, meaning that they drank five or more drinks on the same occasion on at least five different days in the past month.[3]

Among youths aged 12 to 17 years, an estimated 22.9% used alcohol in the month prior to the survey interview. The prevalence of current alcohol drinking increases with increasing age, from 2% among youths aged 12 to a peak of 70.9% for persons 21 years of age. In 2002, 57.4% of males (age 12 and older) were current drinkers compared with 44.9% of females. In contrast to the pattern for illicit drugs, the higher the level of educational attainment, the more likely was the current use of alcohol. In 2002, 67.4% of adults with college degrees were current drinkers compared with only 37.8% of those having less than a high school education.[3]

THE DISEASE MODEL OF ADDICTION AS APPLIED TO ALCOHOLISM

Individuals who are drug dependent frequently are regarded as constitutionally weak people who have brought their problems on themselves and deserve the consequences of their behavior. Even when the lay public and health care professionals acknowledge addiction as a disease process, it is often felt to be self-induced. The disease concept of addiction, using alcoholism as a model, states that addiction is a disease and that individuals who suffer from the disease do not choose to contract the disease any more than someone who suffers from heart disease or diabetes mellitus chooses to contract that illness. A *disease* is defined as "any deviation from or interruption of the normal structure or function of any part, organ, or system (or combination thereof) of the body that is manifested by a characteristic set of symptoms and signs and whose etiology, pathology, and prognosis may be known or unknown."[4] Alcoholism, which is discussed as a prototype, meets all the definitional criteria. Diagnostic criteria for alcoholism do not specify frequency of drinking or amount of alcohol consumed. The key determinant is whether drinking is compulsive, out of control, and consequential when one drinks.

It has long been recognized that alcoholism is heritable, since 50% to 60% of first-degree relatives of alcoholics become alcohol dependent themselves.[12] Past discussions have focused on whether this heritable risk is due to genetics, environment, or both. Recent research has identified several traits (or phenotypes), that attenuate one's risk of alcohol dependence. Initially based on data from pre clinical studies, pharmacogenomics studies have identified genotypic and functional phenotypic variants that either serve to protect patients or predispose them toward alcohol dependence.[13] Large-scale pharmacoepidemiologic studies have further elucidated the environmental risk factors that are associated with either protective effects or predisposition toward alcoholism.[14] This is referred to as the "genome x environment interaction effect. The known susceptibility genes, phenotypic characteristics, and environmental risk factors are summarized in Table 65–1. Interplay between the nonmodifiable interpatient variability due to functional polymorphisms that directly influence alcohol metabolism, as well as those functional genetic variants of proteins involved in the physiologic response to alcohol has increased our understanding of alcohol pharmacokinetics and pharmacodynamics. Yet, further elucidation of the gene-environment interactions are needed before these data are used to (1) create alcohol abuse prevention programs that target high-risk populations, and (2) to develop targeted treatments to prevent and treat alcohol dependence.[15]

Based on this and other information, the belief that addiction is a self-induced disease or a constitutional weakness has been dismissed by clinicians in the addiction treatment field. Willpower and self-discipline cannot control genetics or environment. Since most patients will consume alcohol at some point in their lives, and over half drink alcohol regularly, the determination of who becomes alcoholic must be multifactorial.

PHARMACOLOGY AND PHARMACOKINETICS OF ALCOHOL

ALCOHOL AS A DRUG

Alcohol is a central nervous system (CNS) depressant that shares many pharmacologic properties with the nonbenzodiazepine sedative-hypnotic drugs. It affects the CNS in a dose-dependent fashion, producing sedation that progresses to sleep, unconsciousness, coma, surgical anesthesia, and finally fatal respiratory depression and cardiovascular collapse. Alcohol affects endogenous opiates and several neurotransmitter systems in the brain, including γ-aminobutyric acid (GABA), glutamine, and dopamine. Alcohol intake results in an increase in endogenous opioids,[16] and this may be responsible for the euphoria experienced with alcohol consumption. Currently there are no clinically useful antagonists that can reverse all the pharmacologic effects of alcohol.

Alcohol is available in a variety of concentrations in various alcoholic beverages. There are approximately 14 g of alcohol in a 12-oz can of beer (approximately 5%), 4 oz of nonfortified wine (approximately 10% to 14%), or one shot (1.5 oz) of 80-proof whiskey (40%). This amount will cause an increase in blood alcohol level of about 20 to 25 mg/dL in a healthy 70-kg male, although this varies with the time frame over which the alcohol is consumed, the type of alcoholic beverage, whether food is consumed along with it, and many patient variables. The lethal dose of alcohol in humans is variable, but deaths generally occur when blood alcohol levels are greater than 400 to 500 mg/dL.[17]

PHARMACOKINETICS

Absorption of alcohol begins in the stomach within 5 to 10 minutes of oral ingestion. The onset of clinical effects follows fairly rapidly. It is absorbed primarily from the duodenum, but in smaller amounts from the stomach, esophagus, and mucous membranes. Peak serum concentrations of alcohol usually are achieved 30 to 90 minutes after finishing the last drink, although it is quite variable depending on the type of alcoholic beverage consumed, what and when the person last ate, and other factors.[18]

Over 90% of alcohol in the plasma is metabolized in the liver by three enzyme systems that operate within the hepatocyte. The remainder is excreted by the lungs and in urine and sweat. Alcohol is metabolized to acetaldehyde by alcohol dehydrogenase in the cell. In turn, acetaldehyde is metabolized to carbon dioxide and water by the enzyme aldehyde dehydrogenase. A second pathway for oxidation of alcohol uses catalase, an enzyme located in the peroxisomes and microsomes. The third enzyme system, the microsomal alcohol oxidase system, has a role in the oxidation of alcohol to acetaldehyde. These last two mechanisms are of lesser importance than the alcohol dehydrogenase-aldehyde dehydrogenase system.

The metabolism of alcohol generally is said to follow zero-order pharmacokinetics.[18] This may in fact be an oversimplification because at very high or very low concentrations of alcohol the metabolism may follow first-order pharmacokinetics.[19] On average, the blood alcohol concentration is lowered from 15 to 22.2 mg/dL per hour in the nontolerant individual, assuming that the individual is in the postabsorptive state. Alcohol has a volume of distribution of 0.6 to 0.8 L/kg, representing the total body water.[18]

ACUTE EFFECTS OF ALCOHOL

At lower serum concentrations, euphoria and disinhibition may be noted. Slurred speech, altered perception of the environment, impaired judgment, ataxia, incoordination, nystagmus, and hyperreflexia may occur. As plasma levels increase or in different individuals, combative and destructive behavior may occur. With higher levels still, somnolence and respiratory depression may ensue. The typical effects of various blood alcohol concentrations (BACs) are shown in Table 65–2, although effects vary from individual to individual.

ALCOHOL POISONING

If the BAC gets high enough, death becomes a very real possibility, especially if there is coadministration of other sedative-hypnotics. Acute alcohol poisoning usually occurs with rapid consumption of large quantities of alcoholic beverages, because this type of drinking

TABLE 65–2. Specific Effects of Alcohol Related to the Blood Alcohol Concentration (BAC)

BAC (%)	Effect
0.02–0.03	No loss of coordination, slight euphoria and loss of shyness. Depressant effects are not apparent.
0.04–0.06	Feeling of well-being, relaxation, lower inhibitions, sensation of warmth. Euphoria. Some minor impairment of reasoning and memory, lowering of caution.
0.07–0.09	Slight impairment of balance, speech, vision, reaction time, and hearing. Euphoria. Judgment and self-control are reduced, and caution, reason, and memory are impaired. It is illegal to operate a motor vehicle in some states at this level of intoxication.
0.10–0.125	Significant impairment of motor coordination and loss of good judgment. Speech may be slurred; balance, vision, reaction time, and hearing will be impaired. Euphoria. It is illegal to operate a motor vehicle at this level of intoxication.
0.13–0.15	Gross motor impairment and lack of physical control. Blurred vision and major loss of balance. Euphoria is reduced and dysphoria is beginning to appear.
0.16–0.20	Dysphoria (anxiety, restlessness) predominates, nausea may appear. The drinker has the appearance of a "sloppy drunk."
0.25	Needs assistance in walking; total mental confusion. Dysphoria with nausea and some vomiting.
0.30	Loss of consciousness.
≥0.40	Onset of coma, possible death due to respiratory arrest.

Grams of ethyl alcohol per 100 mL of whole blood.

delivers a large bolus of alcohol to the gastrointestinal (GI) tract. Normally, one passes out before a toxic dose of alcohol can be ingested, and/or the person vomits to rid the stomach of its toxic reservoir. With rapid drinking as described, the person may fall asleep or pass out without vomiting, allowing continued absorption from the GI tract until fatal BACs are achieved.

In the clinical setting, it is important to differentiate acute alcohol intoxication from certain other medical or surgical illnesses. Mental status changes may result from head trauma, and if the diagnosis is missed, the consequences could be disastrous. Appropriate diagnostic measures such as computed tomography (CT) should be performed on any patient with deteriorating mental status, focal neurologic findings, failure to improve over time, new-onset seizures, or mental status out of proportion to the degree of intoxication.

LABORATORY STUDIES

In the emergency room, a BAC should be ordered in any patient in whom alcohol ingestion is suspected, regardless of the presenting complaint. For clinical purposes, most laboratories report BAC in units of milligrams per deciliter. In legal cases, results are reported in percent (grams of ethyl alcohol per 100 mL of whole blood). For example, a whole blood alcohol level of 150 mg/dL reported in the hospital corresponds to 0.15% BAC obtained by law enforcement.

If the diagnosis is unclear, if the intoxication seems atypical, or when there is suspicion of multiple drug ingestions, a complete toxicologic screen to rule out the presence of other substances may be useful.

▶ TREATMENT: Alcohol-Related Disorders

▦ ALCOHOL WITHDRAWAL

The DSM-IV-TR definition of alcohol withdrawal includes two main components.[4] The first component is a history of cessation or reduction in heavy and prolonged alcohol use. The second includes the presence of two or more of the symptoms of alcohol withdrawal. Signs and symptoms of alcohol withdrawal as well as acute alcohol intoxication are shown in Table 65–3.

Goals for alcohol-dependent persons trying to decrease or discontinue alcohol intake include (1) the prevention and treatment of withdrawal symptoms (including seizures and delirium tremens) and medical or psychiatric complications, (2) long-term abstinence after detoxification, and (3) entry into ongoing medical and alcohol-dependence treatment.

CLINICAL CONTROVERSY

The use of phenobarbital for acute alcohol withdrawal remains controversial. Despite its time-honored place in therapy, there is a lack of published evidence-based support for its efficacy and safety for acute alcohol withdrawal.

▦ PHARMACOLOGIC THERAPY

◀6   A meta-analysis was performed to provide evidence-based recommendations on the pharmacologic management of alcohol withdrawal.[20] Trials comparing different benzodiazepines demonstrated that all appear similarly efficacious in reducing signs and symptoms of withdrawal. However, there is some evidence that longer-acting agents may be more effective in preventing seizures. Evidence shows, however, that longer-acting agents contribute to an overall smoother withdrawal course with fewer breakthrough or rebound symptoms.

Another consideration in the choice of benzodiazepine is their potential for abuse. Individuals with addictive disorders prefer certain agents to others. Agents with rapid onset of action, such as diazepam or alprazolam, demonstrate higher abuse potential because of their reinforcing effects. Those with slower onset of action, such as chlordiazepoxide, oxazepam, and halazepam, are less likely to be abused. This consideration may be relevant in an outpatient setting or for patients with a history of benzodiazepine or other substance abuse.[20]

TABLE 65–3. Signs and Symptoms of Alcohol Intoxication and Withdrawal

Intoxication	Withdrawal
Slurred speech	Tremor
Ataxia	Tachycardia
Nystagmus	Diaphoresis
Sedation	Labile blood pressure
Flushed face	Anxiety
Mood change	Nausea and vomiting
Irritability	Hallucinations
Euphoria	Seizures
Loquacity	Hyperthermia
Impaired attention	Delirium

Although barbiturates are used by approximately 10% of detoxification programs in the United States, there is less evidence-based support for their use versus the benzodiazepines.[21] Their use is, however, supported by uncontrolled studies, including a recent randomized open-label pilot study that compared phenobarbital with valproic acid. Both were found to have similar efficacy for decreasing withdrawal symptoms.[22] Unlike other barbiturates, phenobarbital has low abuse potential. It is long acting; it can be administered reliably by oral, intramuscular, and intravenous routes; it has well-documented anticonvulsant activity; and it is inexpensive. However, the barbiturates (including phenobarbital) pose a greater risk of respiratory depression, particularly when combined with alcohol, and an overall lower safety profile than benzodiazepines when used in high doses.

Although phenothiazines, clonidine, carbamazepine, γ-hydroxybutyric acid, and valproic acid may reduce symptoms of alcohol withdrawal, their ability to prevent seizures or delirium tremens has yet to be proven,[23] and in fact, the phenothiazines may lower the seizure threshold. Other drugs used to treat symptoms of alcohol withdrawal include other barbiturates, alcohol itself, sympatholytics such as atenolol, thiamine, magnesium, and other neuroleptics such as haloperidol. At the time of this writing, gabapentin is being compared to lorazepam for acute alcohol withdrawal in a phase II clinical trial.

▦ Treatment Regimens

▦ *Fixed-Schedule Therapy.* Over the years, benzodiazepines given regularly at a fixed dosing interval have been considered the gold standard therapy for alcohol withdrawal. Chlordiazepoxide 50 to 100 mg orally every 6 hours for 1 day followed by 2 days at 25 to 50 mg every 6 hours is known to prevent delirium tremens and seizures.

The treatment guideline,[20] however, takes exception with this rigid approach, urging clinicians to allow for some degree of individualization within fixed-schedule therapy. Patients should be monitored and given additional medication when indicated by symptoms. This type of regimen is useful in patients with a history of seizures, patients with acute medical or surgical illness, or patients with a history of delirium tremens. It also may be preferable for pregnant women.[20]

▦ *Front Loading.* *Front loading* refers to regimens in which frequent, high doses of medication are given to treat the early signs and symptoms of withdrawal. Diazepam is given in 20-mg doses every 2 hours until resolution of withdrawal symptoms. A total of 60 mg typically is required. Because of the long half-life of diazepam and its active metabolites, further doses are not required. This regimen also has been shown to decrease the incidence of seizures. Advantages of front loading are that medication administration and intensive monitoring are limited to the early symptomatic period of withdrawal.[20]

▦ *Symptom-Triggered Therapy.* With symptom-triggered therapy, medication is given only when the patient has symptoms. This approach results in treatment that is shorter, potentially avoiding oversedation and allowing the physician to focus on specific therapy for alcohol dependence.[20] A typical regimen would include diazepam 10 to 20 mg administered every hour when a structured assessment scale such as the Clinical Institute Withdrawal Assessment-Alcohol—Revised indicates that symptoms are moderate to severe.[24]

Treatment of Alcohol Withdrawal Seizures

Alcohol withdrawal seizures do not require treatment with an anticonvulsant drug unless they progress to status epilepticus because seizures usually end before diazepam or another drug can be administered.[20,23] Phenytoin, which is not cross-tolerant to alcohol, does not prevent or treat withdrawal seizures, and without an intravenous loading dose, therapeutic blood levels of phenytoin are not reached until acute withdrawal is complete. Patients experiencing seizures should be treated supportively. An increase in the dosage and slowing of the tapering schedule of the benzodiazepine used in detoxification or a single injection of a benzodiazepine may be necessary to prevent further seizure activity. Patients with a history of withdrawal seizures can be predicted to experience an especially severe withdrawal syndrome. In such patients, a higher initial dosage of a benzodiazepine and a slower tapering period of 7 to 10 days are advisable.

Treatment Settings

Alcohol withdrawal treatment can take place in hospitals, inpatient detoxification units, or outpatient settings. Inpatient treatment may be necessary when there are coexisting acute or chronic medical (including pregnancy), surgical, or psychiatric conditions that would complicate alcohol withdrawal. Only patients with mild to moderate symptoms should be considered for outpatient treatment, and it is a good idea to have a responsible, sober person available to help the patient monitor symptoms and administer medications. Patients with a strong craving for alcohol, those concurrently using other drugs, and those with a history of seizures or delirium tremens are not good candidates for outpatient treatment.

ALCOHOL DEPENDENCE

PHARMACOLOGIC MANAGEMENT

◁   In the United States, disulfiram and naltrexone are the only two drugs specifically indicated for the treatment of alcohol dependence. Disulfiram acts as a deterrent to the resumption of drinking, and naltrexone is a competitive opioid antagonist that has been shown to reduce cravings for alcohol. Other drugs, including nalmefene,[25] acamprosate,[26] bupropion, various serotonergic agents (including selective serotonin reuptake inhibitors and serotonin₃ receptor antagonists), and lithium also have been used either abroad or in the United States for off-label indications.[27] Recently, an evidence-based review of the pharmacologic treatment of alcohol dependence was published.[27] Recommendations from this report will be incorporated into the discussion that follows.

CLINICAL CONTROVERSY

The theory behind deterrent therapy with disulfiram is intuitively simple, and thus it would seem to be an attractive treatment option for chronic alcoholism. However, many clinicians question its overall role in achieving long-term abstinence. Studies have failed to prove it effective, and it is poorly tolerated. For this reason, most clinicians rarely recommend the use of disulfiram.

Disulfiram

Disulfiram deters a patient from drinking by producing an aversive reaction if the patient drinks. Note that although disulfiram appeared to be effective in a series of small-scale studies, these were largely uncontrolled.[27] In the absence of alcohol, disulfiram has minimal effects. It inhibits the liver enzyme aldehyde dehydrogenase in the biochemical pathway for alcohol metabolism, allowing acetaldehyde to accumulate. The resulting increase in acetaldehyde causes severe facial flushing, throbbing headache, nausea and vomiting, chest pain, palpitations, tachycardia, weakness, dizziness, blurred vision, confusion, and hypotension. Severe reactions including myocardial infarction, congestive heart failure, cardiac arrhythmia, respiratory depression, convulsions, and death can occur, particularly in vulnerable individuals.

The disulfiram-alcohol interaction sometimes can be intense, causing serious problems for patients with cerebrovascular, cardiovascular, or severe pulmonary disease or chronic renal failure. The use of disulfiram in patients who may have occult vascular disease, such as those over 60 years of age and patients with diabetes, also should be avoided.[27] Vomiting during a disulfiram reaction can cause severe bleeding in a patient with esophageal varices, and for this reason disulfiram is contraindicated in patients with cirrhosis with portal hypertension. Disulfiram can lower the seizure threshold and cause peripheral neuropathy and should be avoided in patients with these conditions. It has been linked to birth defects and therefore should not be used during pregnancy. Because disulfiram can cause drowsiness, it should be taken first on the weekend at bedtime and discontinued if the patient continues to be drowsy on awakening after 2 to 3 days of medication.

A rare but potentially fatal idiosyncratic hepatotoxicity can occur with disulfiram. As a result, baseline liver function tests should be obtained and the patient monitored for hepatotoxicity by monitoring for symptoms and by repeating the liver function tests at 2 weeks, 3 months, 6 months, and then twice yearly thereafter.

The prescriber should wait at least 24 hours after the last drink before starting disulfiram, usually at a dose of 250 mg/day. At this dose there are fewer side effects than at 500 mg, although some research suggests that higher doses are needed to reliably produce an aversive reaction if the patient drinks.[27]

Naltrexone

Naltrexone, an opiate antagonist that has been available in the United States since 1984 for the treatment of opioid dependence, blocks the effects of exogenous opioids. In 1994 the Food and Drug Administration (FDA) approved its use in the treatment of alcohol dependence. Naltrexone is thought to attenuate the reinforcing effects of alcohol,[28] and those who consume alcohol while taking naltrexone report feeling less intoxicated and having less craving for alcohol.[28]

The efficacy of naltrexone for use in alcohol dependence has been investigated in three placebo-controlled clinical trials, and is currently being evaluated in several phase IV clinical trials. Patients randomized to receive 50 mg naltrexone daily for 12 weeks were more likely to remain abstinent and to avoid relapse to heavy drinking; 31% of placebo-treated patients remained abstinent compared with 54% of patients on naltrexone; 48% of placebo-treated patients avoided heavy drinking, whereas 75% of naltrexone-treated patients avoided drinking to excess successfully. Craving for alcohol also was significantly lower for patients on naltrexone.

Naltrexone should not be given to patients currently dependent on opiates because it can precipitate a severe withdrawal syndrome. Naltrexone is associated with dose-related hepatotoxicity, but this generally occurs at doses higher than those recommended for treatment of alcohol dependence. Nevertheless, it is considered contraindicated in patients with hepatitis or liver failure, and liver function tests should be monitored monthly for the first 3 months and every 3 months thereafter.

Nausea is the most common side effect of naltrexone, occurring in about 10% of patients. Other side effects are headache, dizziness, nervousness, fatigue, insomnia, vomiting, anxiety, and somnolence.

Naltrexone should be given in a dose of 50 mg/day, which effectively blocks μ opioid receptors. Documentation is lacking to support routine use of higher doses.[29]

Other Drugs

Nalmefene is a newer opioid antagonist that is structurally similar to naltrexone, but with a number of potential pharmacologic advantages for the treatment of alcohol dependence, including no dose-dependent association with liver toxicity, greater oral bioavailability, longer duration of antagonist action, and more competitive binding with opioid receptor subtypes that are thought to reinforce drinking.[29] A meta-analysis of controlled clinical trials that include naltrexone, nalmefene, and other opioid antagonists evaluated efficacy in alcoholic abstinence maintenance versus placebo. Naltrexone decreased the number of patients that returned to drinking significantly, yet short-term dropout rates were high for both naltrexone and placebo groups. The other opioid antagonists did not differ from placebo.

Acamprosate is a drug that has been studied extensively in Europe, but is also not commercially available in the United States. Clinical trial results with this drug have been consistently positive for reducing drinking frequency, with some evidence of enhancing abstinence. Its future impact on U.S. practice is not yet clear.[26,27] At the time of this writing, acamprosate was in phase III clinical trials alone and in combination with naltrexone to enhance abstinence.

Using the limited data on serotonergic agents in the evidence-based analysis,[27] these drugs were deemed not very promising, although most studies were confounded by high rates of comorbid mood disorders. Topiramate, a fructopyranose derivative that is FDA approved for seizure prevention, looks promising as a treatment for alcohol dependence. A recent randomized, double-blind, 12-week trial demonstrated topiramate efficacy for preventing alcoholic relapse in patients who have already been detoxified from alcohol. Pharmacologically, this therapy is quite rational since topiramate binds to a nonbenzodiazepine site on the $GABA_A$ receptor.[30]

NICOTINE

Cigarette smoking is an enormous national health problem, and as health care professionals, we are not doing enough to help people quit smoking. A telephone survey of adult cigarette smokers was conducted to determine the types of smoking cessation counseling interventions they received during their physician office visits in the past year. Only about one-half of the current smokers surveyed reported that their doctors talked with them about their smoking, less than half were advised to stop smoking, 15% were offered smoking cessation assistance in the form of education and support groups, and only 9% were prescribed drug therapies to assist smoking cessation efforts.[31] A second observational study was conducted to determine the effects of community-based academic detailing interventions on the quit rates of a sample of smokers (n = 4295). Detailed interventions were delivered to physicians that encouraged smoking cessation efforts with patients to comply with the National Cancer Institute and the Agency for Healthcare Quality and Research smoking intervention standards.[31,32] A small, significant effect was observed in a subgroup of patients residing in the intervention area.[32] Other health care professionals did an even poorer job, with only 22% of dentists, 24% of nurses, and 4% of pharmacists helping their patients to quit smoking.[33]

EPIDEMIOLOGY OF TOBACCO USE

An estimated 71.5 million Americans reported current use (past month use) of a tobacco product in 2002, a prevalence rate of 30.4% for the population aged 12 or older.[34] Among that same population, 61.1 million (26% of the total population aged 12 or older) smoked cigarettes, 12.8 million (5.4%) smoked cigars, 7.8 million (3.3%) used smokeless tobacco, and 1.8 million (0.8%) smoked tobacco in pipes.

The rate of lifetime cigarette use among youths aged 12 to 17 has remained between 29% and 39% for every year since 1965. Although the rate increased during the 1990s from 30.3% in 1990 to 37.8% in 1999, there was a significant decline from 2001 to 2002 (from 37.3% to 33.3%). One of the national health objectives for 2010 is to reduce the prevalence of cigarette smoking among adults to less than 12%.[34]

ECONOMIC IMPACT OF SMOKING

The direct medical costs associated with smoking total more than $75 billion per year, and the costs associated with lost productivity are estimated to be $80 billion. About 14% of all Medicaid expenditures are for smoking-related illnesses. This estimate does not include the costs of smoking-related neonatal disorders.

HEALTH RISKS OF SMOKING

Each year more than 440,000 deaths, or 20% of the total deaths in the United States, are caused by smoking.[35] Cigarette smoking substantially increases the risk of (1) cardiovascular diseases such as stroke, sudden death, and heart attack, (2) nonmalignant respiratory diseases including emphysema, asthma, chronic bronchitis, and chronic obstructive pulmonary disease, (3) lung cancer, and (4) other cancers (e.g., mouth, pharynx, larynx, esophagus, stomach, pancreas, uterus, cervix, kidney, ureter, and bladder).

Exposure to environmental tobacco smoke (*passive exposure*) has been cited as the cause of 3,000 lung cancer deaths and 35,000 to 40,000 heart disease deaths in the United States every year.[35] When children are exposed to environmental smoke, they have a higher risk of respiratory infection, asthma, and middle ear infections than those who are not exposed. Sudden infant death syndrome occurs more often in infants whose mothers smoked during pregnancy than in offspring of nonsmoking mothers.[35] The harmful effects of smoking on reproduction and pregnancy include reduced fertility and fetal

owth, as well as increased risk of ectopic pregnancy and sponta-
eous abortion.[35]

PHARMACOLOGY OF NICOTINE

icotine is a ganglionic cholinergic receptor agonist whose pharmacologic effects are highly dependent on dose. These effects
include central and peripheral nervous system stimulation and
epression, respiratory stimulation, skeletal muscle relaxation, cat-
cholamine release by the adrenal medulla, peripheral vasoconstric-
ion, and increased blood pressure, heart rate, cardiac output, and
xygen consumption.[36] Cigarette smoking or low doses of nicotine
roduce an increased alertness and increased cognitive functioning by
imulating the cerebral cortex. At higher doses, nicotine stimulates
e "reward" center in the limbic system of the brain.[36]

Chronic nicotine ingestion may lead to physical and psycho-
gic dependence and tolerance to some of its pharmacologic effects.
brupt smoking cessation in physically dependent smokers results in

TABLE 65–4. Withdrawal Symptoms of Nicotine

Anxiety	Gastrointestinal disturbances
Craving for tobacco	Headache
Decreased blood pressure and heart rate	Hostility
	Increased appetite and weight gain
Depression	Increased skin temperature
Difficulty concentrating	Insomnia
Drowsiness	Restlessness
Frustration, irritability, impatience	

withdrawal symptoms (Table 65–4). Onset of these symptoms usually
occurs within 24 hours and may last for days, weeks, or longer. The
craving for tobacco may last for years.

8 Although some smokers do not develop physical or psychologic
dependence, most people who smoke 10 to 15 cigarettes daily
for several weeks or longer do. Between 77% and 92% of smokers
are addicted to nicotine in cigarettes.[37]

▶ TREATMENT: Nicotine Dependence

AGENCY FOR HEALTHCARE RESEARCH AND QUALITY CLINICAL PRACTICE GUIDELINE: TREATING TOBACCO USE AND DEPENDENCE

he Agency for Healthcare Research and Quality (AHRQ) periodi-
ally convenes expert panels to develop clinical guidelines for health
are practitioners when the need dictates. Because of the widespread
revalence of smoking-related illnesses, its related morbidity and
nortality, and the economic burden imposed, the agency convened
panel of experts in 1994 to develop guidelines on the treatment of
obacco addiction. The resultant guideline for smoking cessation was
eleased in 1996. In June 2000, an updated version of the 1996 Smok-
ng Cessation Clinical Practice Guideline was issued by AHRQ.[38]

The revised guideline suggests strategies for providing appro-
riate treatments for every patient. The panel reminds us that ef-
ective treatments for tobacco dependence now exist and that every

patient should receive at least minimal treatment every time he or
she visits a clinician. The first step in this process, identification and
assessment of tobacco use status, separates patients into three treatment categories:

1. Patients who use tobacco and are willing to quit should
   be treated using the 5 A's (*a*sk, *a*dvise, *a*ssess, *a*ssist,
   and *a*rrange).
2. Patients who use tobacco but are unwilling to quit at
   this time should be treated with the 5 R's of
   motivational intervention (*r*elevance, *r*isks, *r*ewards,
   *r*oadblocks, and *r*epetition).
3. Patients who have quit using tobacco recently should
   be provided relapse-prevention treatment.

Figure 65–1 shows an overall approach to evaluating patients'
needs and desires to quit smoking. Figure 65–2 is an algorithm for
treating tobacco use.

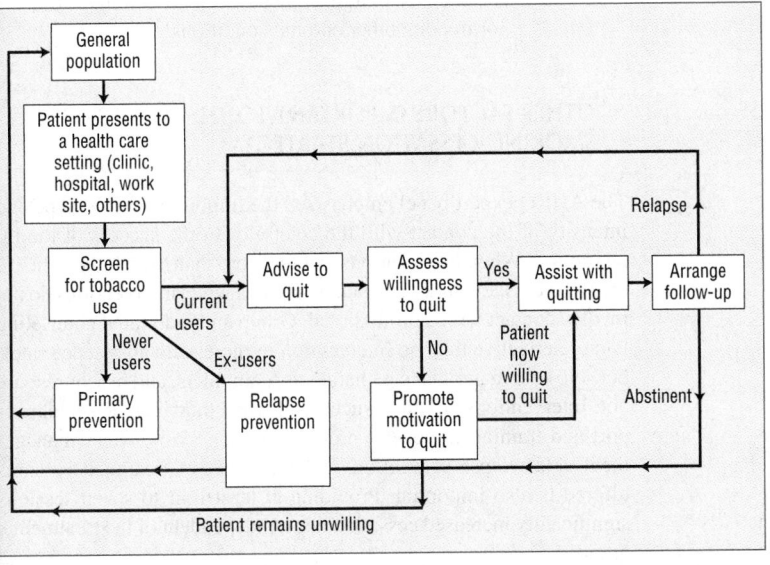

FIGURE 65–1. Model for treatment of tobacco use and dependence.

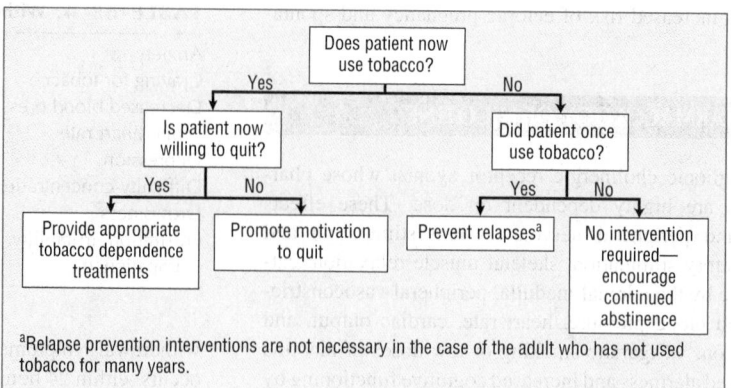

FIGURE 65–2. Algorithm for treating tobacco use.

KEY FINDINGS

The guideline identified a number of key findings that clinicians should use:

1. Tobacco dependence is a chronic condition that often requires repeated intervention. However, effective treatments exist that can produce long-term or even permanent abstinence.

2. Because effective tobacco dependence treatments are available, every patient who uses tobacco should be offered at least one of these treatments:
    - Patients willing to try to quit tobacco use should be provided with treatments that are identified as effective in the guideline.
    - Patients unwilling to try to quit tobacco use should be provided with a brief intervention that is designed to increase their motivation to quit.

3. It is essential that clinicians and health care delivery systems (including administrators, insurers, and purchasers) institutionalize the consistent identification, documentation, and treatment of every tobacco user who is seen in a health care setting.

4. Brief tobacco dependence treatment is effective, and every patient who uses tobacco should be offered at least brief treatment.

5. There is a strong dose-response relationship between the intensity of tobacco dependence counseling and its effectiveness. Treatments involving person-to-person contact (via individual, group, or proactive telephone counseling) are consistently effective, and their effectiveness increases with treatment intensity (e.g., minutes of contact).

6. Three types of counseling and behavioral therapies were found to be especially effective and should be used with all patients who are attempting tobacco cessation:
    - Provision of practical counseling (problem-solving/skills training).
    - Provision of social support as part of treatment (intratreatment social support).
    - Help in securing social support outside treatment (extratreatment social support).

7. Numerous effective pharmacotherapies for smoking cessation now exist. Except in the presence of contraindications, these should be used with all patients who are attempting to quit smoking. Five first-line pharmacotherapies were identified that reliably increase long-term smoking abstinence rates:
    - Bupropion sustained-release (SR)
    - Nicotine gum
    - Nicotine inhaler
    - Nicotine nasal spray
    - Nicotine patch

    Two second-line pharmacotherapies were identified as efficacious and may be considered by clinicians if first-line pharmacotherapies are not effective:
    - Clonidine
    - Nortriptyline

8. Tobacco dependence treatments are both clinically effective and cost-effective relative to other medical and disease-prevention interventions. As such, insurers and purchasers should ensure that
    - All insurance plans include as a reimbursed benefit the counseling and pharmacotherapeutic treatments that are identified as effective in this guideline.
    - Clinicians are reimbursed for providing tobacco dependence treatment just as they are reimbursed for treating other chronic conditions.

OTHER FACTORS IMPORTANT TO THE SUCCESS OF A SMOKING-CESSATION STRATEGY

The AHRQ expert panel emphasized the importance of the type and intensity of the contact with the counselor to the success of the intervention. When interventions last for more than 10 minutes, the increase in cessation rates is much better than when interventions do not involve contact with a professional. Group and individual counseling is more effective than no intervention in increasing abstinence rates, but self-help materials (e.g., handouts, pamphlets, and brochures) are not. Interventions are more successful when they include social support and training in general problem-solving skills, stress management, and relapse prevention.[38] The number of treatment sessions offered is also important. Providing at least four to seven sessions significantly increased cessation rates, independent of the treatment's intensity.[38]

Comprehensive behavioral interventions are more effective in helping people quit smoking and remain abstinent, but less intensive treatments are beneficial as well. Even minimal contacts lasting less than 3 minutes and simple advice to quit are more successful in increasing cessation rates than intervention involving no contact.[38]

Counseling efficacy is further augmented by the addition of nicotine-replacement products. The cessation rates of nicotine patch users are approximately double the cessation rates of smokers who receive placebos, according to a meta-analysis.[39] Although absolute quit rates have varied greatly, abstinence rates for the nicotine patch are estimated at 27% (ranging from 14% to 69%) at the end of treatment and 22% (ranging from 13% to 34%) at 6 months posttreatment.[39]

Although comprehensive programs are most effective, few smokers (10% to 15%) seek formal assistance in quitting.[39] A health care professional who merely advises his or her patient to quit smoking is providing at least minimal assistance in the efforts.

PHARMACOLOGIC THERAPY FOR SMOKING CESSATION

All patients attempting to quit should be encouraged to use effective pharmacotherapies for smoking cessation except in the presence of special circumstances. Long-term smoking-cessation pharmacotherapy should be considered as a strategy to reduce the likelihood of relapse. As with other chronic diseases, the most effective treatment of tobacco dependence encompasses multiple modalities. Pharmacotherapy is a vital element of a multicomponent approach. The clinician should encourage all patients initiating a quit attempt to use one or a combination of efficacious pharmacotherapies, although pharmacotherapy use requires special consideration with some patient groups (e.g., those with medical contraindications, those smoking fewer than 10 cigarettes a day, pregnant or breast-feeding women, and adolescent smokers). The role of pharmacotherapy is summarized in Table 65–5.

TABLE 65–5. Summary of Clinical Guidelines for Prescribing Pharmacotherapy for Smoking Cessation

Who should receive pharmacotherapy for smoking cessation?	All smokers trying to quit, except in the presence of special circumstances. Special consideration should be given before using pharmacotherapy with selected populations: those with medical contraindications, those smoking fewer than 10 cigarettes/day, pregnant/breast-feeding women, and adolescent smokers.
What are the first-line pharmacotherapies recommended in this guideline?	All five of the FDA-approved pharmacotherapies for smoking cessation are recommended, including bupropion SR, nicotine gum, nicotine inhaler, nicotine nasal spray, and the nicotine patch.
What factors should a clinician consider when choosing among the five first-line pharmacotherapies?	Because of the lack of sufficient data to rank order these five medications, choice of a specific first-line pharmacotherapy must be guided by factors such as clinician familiarity with the medications, contraindications for selected patients, patient preference, previous patient experience with a specific pharmacotherapy (positive or negative), and patient characteristics (e.g., history of depression, concerns about weight gain).
Are pharmacotherapeutic treatments appropriate for lighter smokers (e.g., 10–15 cigarettes/day)?	If pharmacotherapy is used with lighter smokers, clinicians should consider reducing the dose of first-line nicotine replacement pharmacotherapies. No adjustments are necessary when using bupropion SR.
What second-line pharmacotherapies are recommended in this guideline?	Clonidine and nortriptyline.
When should second-line agents be used for treating tobacco dependence?	Consider prescribing second-line agents for patients unable to use first-line medications because of contraindications or for patients for whom first-line medications are not helpful. Monitor patients for the known side effects of second-line agents.
Which pharmacotherapies should be considered with patients particularly concerned about weight gain?	Bupropion SR and nicotine replacement therapies, in particular nicotine gum, have been shown to delay, but not prevent, weight gain.
Are there pharmacotherapies that should be especially considered in patients with a history of depression?	Bupropion SR and nortriptyline appear to be effective with this population.
Should nicotine replacement therapies be avoided in patients with a history of cardiovascular disease?	No. The nicotine patch in particular is safe and has been shown not to cause adverse cardiovascular effects.
May tobacco-dependence pharmacotherapies be used long term (e.g., 6 months or more)?	Yes. This approach may be helpful with smokers who report persistent withdrawal symptoms during the course of pharmacotherapy or who desire long-term therapy. A minority of individuals who successfully quit smoking use ad libitum nicotine replacement medications (gum, nasal spray, inhaler) long term. The use of these medications long term does not present a known health risk. Additionally, the FDA has approved the use of bupropion SR for long-term maintenance.
May pharmacotherapies ever be combined?	Yes. There is evidence that combining the nicotine patch with either nicotine gum or nicotine nasal spray increases long-term abstinence rates over those produced by a single form of nicotine replacement therapy.

*Reprinted from Hurt et al.[48]

NICOTINE-REPLACEMENT THERAPY

A Systematic Review of Nicotine Replacement Therapy

In 2002 a systematic review[39] of published studies was performed to determine the effectiveness of the different forms of nicotine replacement therapy (NRT; e.g., chewing gum, transdermal patches, nasal spray, inhalers, and tablets) in achieving abstinence from cigarettes or a sustained reduction in the amount smoked. The review was also designed to determine whether the effect is influenced by the clinical setting in which the smoker is recruited and treated, the dosage and form of the NRT used, or the intensity of additional advice and support offered to the smoker; to determine whether combinations of NRT are more effective than one type alone; and to determine its effectiveness compared to other pharmacotherapies.

The review was limited to randomized trials in which NRT was compared to placebo or no treatment, or where different doses of NRT were compared. The main outcome measure was abstinence from smoking after at least 6 months of follow-up. For each trial, researchers used the most rigorous definition of abstinence, and confirmation with biochemical markers where available. The review includes 110 studies, 96 of which included a placebo or non–nicotine control arm. These studies were used in the primary analysis. In this group there were 51 trials of nicotine gum, 34 of transdermal nicotine patch, 4 of intranasal nicotine spray, 4 of inhaled nicotine, and 3 of an oral tablet. Five trials compared combinations of two forms of nicotine therapy with only one form (patch with gum to patch alone; patch with gum to gum alone; patch with nasal spray to patch alone; patch with inhaler to inhaler alone; and patch with inhaler to either one alone).[39]

The odds ratio (OR) for abstinence with NRT compared to control was 1.74 (95% confidence interval [CI] 1.64 to 1.86). The ORs for the different forms of NRT were 1.66 for gum, 1.74 for patches, 2.27 for nasal spray, 2.08 for inhaled nicotine, and 2.08 for nicotine sublingual tablet/lozenge. These odds were not a function of the duration of therapy, the intensity of additional support provided, or the setting in which the NRT was provided. The 4-mg gum provided a significant benefit over 2-mg gum (OR 2.67; 95% CI 1.69 to 4.22) in highly dependent smokers. Higher doses of nicotine patch may produce additional small increases in quit rates compared to lower doses. Only one study directly compared NRT to another pharmacotherapy, in which bupropion was significantly more effective than nicotine patch or placebo.[39]

The authors of this review concluded that all of the commercially available forms of NRT (nicotine gum, transdermal patch, the nicotine nasal spray, nicotine inhaler, and nicotine sublingual tablets/lozenges) are effective as part of a strategy to promote smoking cessation. They increase quit rates approximately 1.5- to twofold regardless of setting.[39]

The percentage of smokers who were abstinent after 12 months (excluding trials with shorter follow-up; data not shown) was 18% (95% CI 17% to 19%) among smokers who had been allocated to receive nicotine gum, and 14% (95% CI 13% to 15%) among those who had used transdermal patches. For intranasal spray, nicotine inhaler, and sublingual tablet, the corresponding figures were 24% (95% CI 20% to 28%), 17% (95% CI 14% to 21%), and 20% (95% CI 15% to 25%), respectively.

The AHRQ guidelines recommend use of NRT in the forms of transdermal nicotine patches, nicotine gum, nicotine sprays, and nicotine inhalers.[38] The use of NRT is relatively safe, but it is not recommended for all smokers. Although cardiovascular disease is not an independent risk factor for acute myocardial events, NRT should be used with caution among particular cardiovascular patient group those in the immediate (within 2 weeks) post–myocardial infarctio period, those with serious arrhythmias, and those with serious or wor ening angina pectoris.[38]

In a recent study of survey data from California,[40] use of NR increased short-term cessation success in moderate to heavy smoke in each survey year. However, a long-term cessation advantage wa only observed before NRT became widely available over the counte (August 1996). In 1999, no advantage for pharmaceutical aid use was observed in either the short or long term for the nearly 60% c California smokers classified as light smokers (<15 cigarettes/day Authors contend that since becoming available over the counter, NR appears no longer effective in increasing long-term successful cessa tion in California smokers.

Nicotine Gum

Clinicians should offer 4-mg rather than 2-mg nicotine gum to highl dependent smokers. The 2-mg nicotine gum improves long-term absti nence rates by approximately 30% to 80% as compared with placebc The 2-mg gum is recommended for patients smoking less than 2 cigarettes per day, whereas the 4-mg gum is recommended for pa tients smoking 25 or more cigarettes per day. Generally, the gur should be used for up to 12 weeks, no more than 24 pieces chewe per day. The dosage and duration of therapy should be tailored to mee the needs of each patient.

Nicotine gum currently is available exclusively as an over-the counter medication and is packaged with important instructions o correct use, including chewing instructions. There is currently littl evidence to suggest that combined use of the patch and gum increase abstinence beyond 24 weeks.

Gum should be chewed slowly until a peppery or minty tast emerges and then "parked" between cheek and gums to facilitat nicotine absorption through the oral mucosa. It should be chewe slowly and intermittently and parked for about 30 minutes or until th taste dissipates. Acidic beverages (e.g., coffee, juices, or soft drinks interfere with the buccal absorption of nicotine, so eating and drinkin; anything except water should be avoided for 15 minutes before an during chewing. Patients often do not use enough gum to get th maximum benefit: They chew too few pieces per day, and they do nc use the gum for a sufficient number of weeks. Instructions to chev the gum on a fixed schedule (at least one piece every 1 to 2 hours) fo at least 1 to 3 months may be more beneficial than ad libitum use.

Nicotine Patch

The nicotine patch approximately doubles long-term abstinenc rates over those produced by placebo interventions. The nico tine patch is available both as an over-the-counter medication anc as a prescription medication. Treatment of 8 weeks or less has beer shown to be as efficacious as longer treatment periods. The 16- anc 24-hour patches are of comparable efficacy.[38] Clinicians should con sider individualizing treatment based on specific patient characteris tics, such as previous experience with the patch, amount smoked, anc degree of addiction, among others. Finally, clinicians should conside starting treatment on a lower patch dose in patients smoking 10 o fewer cigarettes per day.[38]

At the start of each day, the patient should place a new patch or a relatively hairless location, typically between the neck and waist There are no restrictions on activity while using the patch. Patches

...ould be applied as soon as the patient wakes on the quit day. Patients ...ho experience sleep disruption should remove the 24-hour patch ...ior to bedtime or use the 16-hour patch.

Nicotine Nasal Spray

...icotine nasal spray more than doubles long-term abstinence rates ...hen compared with a placebo spray. Nicotine nasal spray is available ...xclusively as a prescription medication. A dose of nicotine nasal ...pray consists of one 0.5-mg delivery to each nostril (1 mg total). ...itial dosing should be one to two doses per hour, increasing as ...eeded for symptom relief. The minimum recommended treatment is ...doses per day, with a maximum limit of 40 doses per day (5 doses per ...our). Each bottle contains approximately 100 doses. Recommended ...uration of therapy is 3 to 6 months. Patients should not sniff, swallow, ...r inhale through the nose while administering doses because this ...creases irritating effects. The spray is best delivered with the head ...ted slightly back.[38]

Instructing Patients in the Use of NRT

...ompliance with NRT improves when the patient is presented a clear ...ationale for its use and a realistic expectation about the response.[41] ...: should be explained to the patient that nicotine is responsible for ...ddiction and that discontinuation of the nicotine causes craving for ...igarettes, tension, irritability, sadness, problems with sleep, and dif-...culty concentrating. These are partly due to nicotine withdrawal. ...he patient should be told that using the patch results in less desire to ...moke and provides an opportunity for a new nonsmoker to practice ...ll the new nonsmoking skills without being burdened by craving. ...he patient should understand that with smoking, there are natu-...ally peaks and valleys in the amount of nicotine in the bloodstream. ...Vith the patch there is a steady gradual rise in the blood nicotine ...oncentration that levels off and remains constant for much of the day ...nd then gradually decreases while the person is asleep. Maintaining ...n adequate blood level of nicotine lessens withdrawal symptoms.[42]

A similar rationale can be used if patients are using gum. It ...hould be emphasized that NRT is not a "magic bullet" and that the ...se of coping skills is essential for abstinence. The patch or the gum ...nly buys time by reducing withdrawal symptoms and giving indi-...iduals a chance to figure out alternatives that they can use in place ...f smoking.[43]

CLINICAL CONTROVERSY

Some clinicians are hesitant to prescribe nicotine replacement therapy for smoking cessation during pregnancy because the safety and efficacy of nicotine replacement therapy has not been established in controlled clinical trials in this population.

Side Effects

...icotine replacement products have relatively few side effects. Nau-...ea and light-headedness are possible signs of nicotine overdose that ...varrant a reduction of the nicotine dose.

The most frequent side effect with the nicotine patch is skin irri-...ation related to the adhesive or the medium containing nicotine and ...ot to the nicotine itself. About 50% of patients report skin irritation ...uring the course of treatment with the patch. The patch site can be

rotated to diminish this problem. The use of over-the-counter hydro-cortisone cream (1%) or triamcinolone cream (0.5%) is recommended as a local treatment for patch-related skin irritations. Switching to a different brand of patch also may alleviate the problem because different products use different adhesives or media. The gum can be used instead of the patch when the skin irritation is severe. Less than 5% of patients were forced to discontinue therapy because of skin reactions.

About 23% of patients using the patch report sleep disturbances, but the insomnia is hard to differentiate from the sleeplessness that often accompanies withdrawal itself, especially during the first few weeks of quitting.

More research regarding the safety and efficacy of pharmacother-apy during pregnancy is needed to define the risk/benefit profile of smoking cessation medications in this population.[44] Clearly, expo-sure of the fetus to nicotine delivered by smoking is known to be detrimental to the fetus. Because total nicotine levels are lower with NRT than smoking, if the alternative is active smoking, NRT is almost certainly safer if cessation can be achieved. Nicotine does cross the placenta, whether delivered by cigarette smoking or through nicotine replacement. Nicotine transdermal systems and inhalers are classified as FDA pregnancy risk category D, and nicotine gum is classified as FDA pregnancy category C, but there are conflicting data regarding pregnancy safety ratings of nicotine replacement products, and the pregnancy categories cannot be used in isolation from other informa-tion sources. Nicotine replacement is not contraindicated and could be appropriately used in well-selected pregnant patients.

A recent study[45] of women using various doses of transdermal nicotine while breast-feeding confirms that nicotine is transferred via milk to the infant. The absolute infant dose of nicotine and its metabo-lite cotinine decreases by about 70% while using the 7-mg patch com-pared to when they were smoking or using the 21-mg patch. The use of the nicotine patch had no significant influence on milk intake by the breast-fed infant. The authors conclude that undertaking maternal smoking cessation with the nicotine patch is therefore a safer option than continued smoking. Ultimately, the choice of whether to use pharmacotherapy for smoking cessation should be made jointly by the pregnant or breast-feeding smoker and her health care provider.

Duration

Those who commit to quitting smoking using the nicotine patch should be told to expect a minimum of 6 to 8 weeks of treatment. Us-ing the therapy beyond 8 weeks is not associated with better success rates.[38] However, some patients will experience severe withdrawal even beyond 8 weeks, and these people may need to use the patch longer.

The duration of therapy with the gum should be at least 1 to 3 months on a fixed schedule rather than when one has the urge to smoke.[39] Studies have found, however, that 15% to 20% of abstainers continue to use the gum for longer than 12 months. Patients should be encouraged to stick with the patch and/or gum for the minimally acceptable duration of treatment.

Economic and Pharmacoeconomic Considerations

Most health insurers provide coverage for the chronic illnesses caused by smoking (e.g., chronic obstructive pulmonary disease, cancer, and myocardial infarction), yet few provide coverage for treating the nico-tine addiction that caused those ailments.[38] For each of the approx-imately 22 billion packs of cigarettes sold in the United States in

1999, $3.45 was spent on medical care attributable to smoking, and $3.73 in productivity losses were incurred, for a total cost of $7.18 per pack.[1] Even after adding the cost of the nicotine patch to physician counseling, costs from the standpoint of a third-party payer range from $1441 to $3445 per quality-adjusted life year saved for NRT (based on 15 minutes of physician counseling and 1 to 2 months of NRT).[46] Treating tobacco dependence is particularly important economically in that it can prevent a variety of costly chronic diseases, including heart disease, cancer, and pulmonary disease. A recent meta-analysis conducted by the Cochrane Collaboration determined that a 36% reduction in risk of death from coronary heart disease was obtained by quitting smoking. This decrease in risk is comparable, if not greater, than that obtained from lowering LDL cholesterol or blood pressure lowering.[47] This is but one reason why smoking cessation treatment is referred to as the gold standard of preventive interventions.

It is important to note that smoking cessation is also cost effective in special populations such as hospitalized patients and pregnant women. For hospitalized patients, successful tobacco abstinence not only reduces general medical costs in the short term, but also reduces the number of future hospitalizations.[38] Smoking cessation interventions for pregnant women are especially cost effective because they result in fewer low-birth-weight babies and perinatal deaths; result in fewer physical, cognitive, and behavioral problems during infancy and childhood; and also yield important health benefits for the mother.[38]

The failure of a health plan to cover tobacco dependence treatment could reduce the number of people seeking and receiving these services.

BUPROPION

In 1997, the antidepressant drug bupropion, available since 1989 under the brand name Wellbutrin, was approved by the FDA in a sustained-release formulation (Zyban) for use as an aid in smoking cessation. Bupropion inhibits neuronal reuptake and potentiates the effects of norepinephrine and dopamine. Although its precise mechanism in smoking cessation is not well understood, dopamine has been associated with the rewarding effects of addictive substances. Withdrawal symptoms may be decreased by virtue of bupropion inhibition of norepinephrine uptake. The AHRQ panel concluded that sustained-release (SR) bupropion is an efficacious smoking cessation treatment that patients should be encouraged to use.[38] Two large multicenter studies met selection criteria and were included in the meta-analysis comparing bupropion SR with placebo. The use of bupropion SR approximately doubles long-term abstinence rates when compared with placebo.

Bupropion requires a prescription and is contraindicated in patients with a seizure disorder, a current or prior diagnosis of bulimia or anorexia nervosa, use of a monoamine oxidase inhibitor within the previous 14 days, or in patients on another medication that contains bupropion. Bupropion SR can be used in combination with NRT.

One study compared the effects of 100, 150, or 300 mg/day of bupropion SR or placebo for 7 weeks in 615 patients who visited the clinic each week for evaluation and counseling.[48] When the study was concluded, smoking cessation rates were 19% with placebo and 28.8%, 38.6%, and 44.2% with the respective doses of the drug. The differences between the 150- and 300-mg doses and placebo were statistically significant. After 1 year, the respective rates were 12.4%, 19.6%, 22.9%, and 23.1%, indicating a fairly high rate of relapse in all groups.

Bupropion at a dose of 150 mg twice daily of sustained-release tablets was compared with the 21-mg nicotine patch separately and as combined therapy and with placebo in nearly 900 patients studied for 9 weeks. At the 10-week mark, smoking cessation had been accomplished in 20% of the placebo group, 32% of the group using the patch alone, 46% of the group using bupropion alone, and 51% of the group using combined therapy. All three active treatments were significantly better than placebo.[49] Unlike its use as an antidepressant, no seizures occurred with bupropion in smoking cessation trials. Insomnia and dry mouth were the most frequent adverse effects. Other side effects noted in the trials were tremor, rash, and a few anaphylactoid reactions characterized by pruritus, urticaria, angioedema, and dyspnea. Insomnia also was reported.[49]

For smoking cessation, the manufacturer recommends a dosage of 150 mg once daily for 3 days and then twice daily for 7 to 12 weeks or longer, with or without nicotine replacement. Patients are instructed to stop smoking during the second week of treatment and are encouraged to use counseling and support services along with the medication. For maintenance therapy, consider bupropion SR 150 mg twice daily for up to 6 months.[38] In addition, bupropion SR appears to be effective for smokeless tobacco cessation.[50]

Cost per quality-adjusted life year saved after smoking cessation ranged from $920 to $2150 for bupropion alone, and $1282 to $2836 for NRT plus bupropion.[46]

SECOND-LINE MEDICATIONS

Second-line medications are pharmacotherapies for which there is evidence of efficacy for treating tobacco dependence, but they have a more limited role than first-line medications because (1) the FDA has not approved them for a tobacco-dependence treatment indication and (2) there are more concerns about potential side effects than exist with first-line medications.[38] Second-line treatments should be considered for use on a case-by-case basis after first-line treatments have been used or considered.

Clonidine

Clonidine, a prescription drug, is an efficacious smoking cessation treatment. It may be used under a clinician's supervision as a second-line agent to treat tobacco dependence. A recent meta-analysis of six trials showed that clonidine increased smoking cessation rates by 11% (OR 1.89; CI 1.30 to 2.14). There was a high incidence of dose-dependent side effects, particularly dry mouth and sedation.[51] It should be noted that abrupt discontinuation of clonidine can result in symptoms such as nervousness, agitation, headache, and tremor, accompanied or followed by a rapid rise in blood pressure and elevated catecholamine levels.

Because clonidine is used primarily as an antihypertensive medication and has not been approved by the FDA as a smoking cessation medication, clinicians need to be aware of the specific warnings regarding this medication as well as its side-effect profile. Additionally, a specific dosing regimen for the use of clonidine in smoking cessation has not been established. Because of the warnings associated with clonidine discontinuation, the variability in dosages used to test this medication, and a lack of FDA approval, the guideline panel chose to recommend clonidine as a second-line agent. Doses used in various clinical cessation trials have varied significantly, from 0.15 to 0.75 mg/day orally to 0.10 to 0.20 mg/day transdermally, without a clear dose-response relation to cessation. Initial dosing typically is

1 mg orally twice daily or 0.1 mg/day transdermally, increasing y 0.1 mg/day each week if needed. The dose duration also varied cross the clinical trials, ranging from 3 to 10 weeks. Most commonly eported side effects include dry mouth, drowsiness, dizziness, sedaion, and constipation. As an antihypertensive medication, clonidine an be expected to lower blood pressure in most patients. Thereore clinicians may need to monitor blood pressure when using this aedication.[38]

Nortriptyline

ortriptyline is also considered to be efficacious as a second-line agent o treat tobacco dependence. Based on very limited data, the use of ortriptyline appears to increase abstinence rates when compared with lacebo.

Nortriptyline should be considered for smoking cessation under a clinician's direction in patients unable to use first-line medications because of contraindications or in patients who failed using first-line medications. Therapy is initiated 10 to 28 days before the quit date to allow nortriptyline to reach steady state at the target dose. Smoking cessation trials have initiated treatment at a dose of 25 mg/day, increasing gradually to a target dose of 75 to 100 mg/day. Duration of treatment used in smoking cessation trials has been approximately 12 weeks. Most commonly reported side effects include sedation, dry mouth, blurred vision, urinary retention, light-headedness, and shaky hands.

Trials have investigated the use of other antidepressants for smoking cessation, including other tricyclics and selective serotonin reuptake inhibitors. Because of a paucity of data, the AHRQ panel drew no conclusions about the use of other antidepressants for smoking cessation.[38]

CAFFEINE

affeine is the most widely consumed behaviorally active substance in ne world.[52] *Caffeinism* is the term coined to describe the clinical synrome produced by acute or chronic overuse of caffeine.[53] The synrome usually is characterized by CNS and peripheral manifestations, lost notably anxiety, psychomotor alterations, sleep disturbances, nood changes, and psychophysiologic complaints. Table 65–6 ummarizes typical manifestations of caffeine overuse syndrome.

As many as one in five adults consumes doses of caffeine generally considered large enough to cause clinical symptoms.[54–55] Conrolled double-blind studies demonstrate that caffeine has reinforcenent properties in most people with a history of heavy prior use[56] and hat this reinforcement is a function of dose and prior exposure.

Pharmacologically, the risk of developing some meaningful clincal manifestations becomes high when intake exceeds 500 mg/day. 'his places 20% to 30% of North Americans at risk.[54] Recognizng that there are individual variations and accepting a conservative pproach, these data suggest that perhaps 10% to 20% of the North .merican adult population probably has meaningful clinical sympoms consistent with a diagnosis of caffeinism, a prevalence rate exeeding that of most other substances of abuse.

Caffeine has been proposed as a "model of drug abuse" despite he facts that its sale is largely unrestricted and that heavy consumption f caffeine-containing beverages is not considered to be drug abuse. . recent exhaustive review of caffeine dependence focused on the poential for abuse of caffeine and the nature of tolerance and withdrawal nd presents a symposium of current knowledge as to the site(s) and nechanism of action of caffeine.[55] A second comprehensive review f human and animal data on coffee and caffeine consumption and affeine dependence, withdrawal, and reinforcement also has been ublished.[54] The information below represents a broad overview of hese topics, and the reader interested in more detail is urged to consult hese two reviews.[54,55]

EPIDEMIOLOGY OF CAFFEINE USE AND ABUSE

Caffeine is used by 80% of the population of the United States,[57] and its use can be problematic for some people. In 1999 there were 108,000,000 coffee consumers in the United States spending approximately $9.2 billion in the retail sector and $8.7 billion in the food service sector every year.[58] It can be inferred, therefore, that a coffee drinker spends on average $164.71 per year on coffee. The National Coffee Association found in 2001 that 52% of the adult population of the United States drinks coffee daily.[59] More than 107 million Americans drink an average of 3.3 cups of coffee per day.

Average caffeine consumption in humans can range in different cultures and nations from 80 to 400 mg per person per day. In the United States caffeine consumption exceeds several billion kilograms annually. Per capita intake for the entire world's population approximates 70 mg/day. In the United States this figure is considerably larger, at 210 to 238 mg. The majority of caffeine users progress to a pattern of frequent or daily consumption. Approximately one-fourth eventually begin consuming large quantities, exceeding 500 mg/day, and conservatively, 10% of all adults then progress to develop the syndrome of caffeinism. Mean daily consumption of caffeine in American children is surprisingly high. The Framingham Children's Study[60] looked at the amounts of caffeine consumed each day by children between the ages of 6 and 10 years (mean 8.4 years for boys and 8.1 years for girls). Mean intake of caffeine was 16.0 ± 9.6 mg/day. Caffeinated soft drinks and chocolate furnished almost all of the caffeine.

Caffeine is an added ingredient in approximately 70% of soft drinks consumed in the United States.[57] Soft drink manufacturers' justification to regulatory agencies and the public for adding caffeine to soft drinks is that caffeine is a flavoring agent. In a recent study, only 8% of a group of regular cola soft drink consumers could detect the taste effect of the caffeine concentration found in most cola soft drinks. Thus soft drinks serve as a major source of caffeine intake without any apparent purpose beyond its stimulant effects.[57]

DIFFERENTIAL DIAGNOSIS

Caffeine intoxication is the only official diagnosis associated with caffeinism in the DSM-IV-TR. Caffeine-induced anxiety may manifest as restlessness, nervousness, excitement, insomnia, diuresis, flushing, gastrointestinal disturbance, muscle twitching, irritability, and jitteriness. If caffeine-induced insomnia requires specific treatment, caffeine-induced sleep disorder (DSM-IV-TR) is an appropriate diagnosis.[4,53]

TABLE 65–6. Signs and Symptoms of Excessive Caffeine Intake

Restlessness	Gastrointestinal disturbances
Nervousness	Muscle twitching
Excitement	Rambling flow of thought or speech
Insomnia	Tachycardia or cardiac arrhythmia
Flushed face	Periods of inexhaustibility
Diuresis	Psychomotor agitation

Because excessive caffeine consumption is so widespread, a thorough history of caffeine use should be included in the routine assessment of all new patients in primary care medical settings. In this manner, the practitioner can use the information gathered to uncover high levels of caffeine intake and then use the information to pinpoint the cause of clinical signs and symptoms typical of caffeinism. Clinical manifestations of caffeinism almost always will lessen in intensity or disappear completely within 1 to 2 weeks after removing the drug.[4]

PHARMACOLOGY OF CAFFEINE

Caffeine is rapidly and completely absorbed from the gastrointestinal tract, reaching a peak blood level within 30 to 45 minutes of oral ingestion. It easily crosses the blood-brain barrier, and levels achieved in the brain are proportional to the dose administered.

The half-life of caffeine in humans is approximately 3.5 to 5 hours. It is metabolized extensively according to a complex metabolic pathway occurring primarily in the liver. Serious problems rarely result from overdoses of caffeine. In fact, the amount of caffeine needed to cause death in an average adult male is 5 to 10 g, the equivalent of 50 to 100 cups of regular brewed coffee. Thus the risk of overdose from dietary sources of caffeine is virtually nonexistent.

Caffeine increases the heart rate and force of contraction. It also has a strong diuretic effect. The key factor promoting caffeine use and dosage increases may be the drug's reinforcing effect on pleasure and reward centers of the brain. Caffeine's pharmacologic actions appear comparable (although less potent) in some aspects with those of other stimulants, such as amphetamines and cocaine. After years of uncertainty, it is apparent from both preclinical research and human studies that regular caffeine use does induce tolerance.

CAFFEINE DEPENDENCE

Research has shown that abstinence from caffeine induces a distinct withdrawal syndrome. Evidence for the existence of a caffeine dependence syndrome was presented by Strain and associates.[52] In a structured psychiatric interview, subjects self-identified as having problems with caffeine use were evaluated for features of a DSM-IV-TR diagnosis of drug dependence. Those judged as caffeine dependent manifested at least three of four criteria (i.e., tolerance, withdrawal, persistent desire, or an unsuccessful attempt to reduce consumption and persistent use despite adverse psychological or physical consequences). Of 99 people screened, 27 were evaluated by means of a structured psychiatric interview modified for the diagnosis of caffeine dependence; 16 of those subjects (59%) met the criteria. In a second phase of the study, 11 of the 16 caffeine-dependent individuals participated in a 2-day double-blind crossover study of caffeine deprivation. Nine showed evidence of caffeine withdrawal during the placebo phase, a finding that validated one of the criteria for the diagnosis of dependence.

CAFFEINE WITHDRAWAL

The frequency of the caffeine withdrawal syndrome is not well known, but it may be common. Withdrawal can occur when individuals who previously have been consuming caffeine on a regular basis suddenly discontinue its intake.[4] The syndrome can be characterized by the occurrence of headache, drowsiness, fatigue, and sometimes impaired psychomotor performance, difficulty concentrating, nausea, excessive yawning, and craving. These symptoms usually appear within 18 to 24 hours of discontinuation of intake, corresponding to the time required for the drug to leave the body.

TABLE 65–7. Signs and Symptoms of Caffeine Withdrawal

Headache	Difficulty concentrating
Drowsiness	Nausea
Fatigue	Excessive yawning
Impaired psychomotor performance	Craving

The caffeine withdrawal headache is somewhat unique, starting with a sense of fullness in the head and progressing to throbbing and diffuse pain that is made worse by movement. The maximum intensity of the pain occurs 3 to 6 hours after beginning. Symptoms of caffeine withdrawal are summarized in Table 65–7.

In an effort to understand the relationship between caffeine dosing conditions and the emergence of withdrawal, Evans and Griffiths[61] performed a series of double-blind experiments in independent groups of healthy participants to assess the conditions under which withdrawal symptoms occur on cessation of low to moderate doses of caffeine. Their results show that significant caffeine withdrawal symptoms can occur reliably when individuals are maintained on as little as 100 mg caffeine each day, and the severity of caffeine withdrawal is an increasing function of the caffeine maintenance dose. Administration of caffeine as a single daily dose produces physical dependence similar to that produced by three divided doses over the day, suggesting that the daily dose of caffeine consumed is more relevant to the development of caffeine dependence than the pattern of caffeine intake within the day. They showed that caffeine withdrawal occurs after as little as 3 consecutive days of caffeine exposure, with a somewhat increased severity of withdrawal observed after a week of caffeine exposure. Finally, when individuals were maintained on 300 mg caffeine per day, a substantial reduction in caffeine consumption or complete elimination is necessary for the manifestation of the full, classic withdrawal symptoms.

When caffeine is reintroduced, relief of withdrawal symptoms tends to occur within 30 to 60 minutes. At present, this appears to be the most effective "treatment" for the caffeine-withdrawal syndrome.

EFFECT ON SLEEP

Caffeine interferes with sleep in most nontolerant individuals.[4,53] Once tolerance has developed, people are much less likely to self-report sleep abnormalities, or they may sense that the insomnia has disappeared altogether. To illustrate, 53% of those consuming less than 250 mg/day agreed that caffeine before bedtime would prevent sleep, compared with 43% of those consuming 250 to 749 mg/day, and only 22% of those taking 750 mg/day or more. Even though the higher-level consumers denied that caffeine interferes with their sleep, studies done in the sleep laboratory confirm that caffeine consumers do have greater sleep latency, more frequent awakenings, and altered sleep architecture, and that these effects are dose related.

CAFFEINE-RELATED SOMATIC MANIFESTATIONS

Caffeine can cause other problems in addition to anxiety and nervousness. Users of high doses of caffeine often experience one or more of the following problems: urinary frequency and diuresis, headache, tachycardia, arrhythmias, tremulousness, diarrhea, gastrointestinal pain or discomfort, and light-headedness. Less frequent symptoms include seeing "spots" in front of the eyes, ringing in the ears, a feeling of being unable to breathe, tingling in fingers and toes, and excessive perspiration. Caffeine also may precipitate a true panic attack.

COMORBID SUBSTANCE-RELATED DISORDERS

It is not uncommon for heavy users of caffeine to also be taking a variety of other psychoactive medications, mostly of the CNS depressant variety. Sedative-hypnotics and antianxiety agents are used significantly more often in those consuming high doses of caffeine than in those consuming low or moderate amounts. Approximately two-thirds of heaviest caffeine users reported using an antianxiety agent within the past month. Similar effects on the brain reward pathways may help explain why excessive caffeine, alcohol, and tobacco use tend to occur in the same individuals.

▶ TREATMENT: Caffeinism

Caffeinism is treated by reducing or discontinuing the drug. It may be necessary to wean the patient off the drug because going "cold turkey" may produce such serious symptoms that the drug must be restarted. Decaffeinated beverages may be substituted slowly for the caffeinated type. However, relapses are less likely to occur when the drug is discontinued all at once, probably due to the considerable self-discipline required to continue weaning the drug when one knows that an increase in dose will cause the symptoms to abate.

It may be possible for some individuals simply to reduce their dosage of caffeine rather than discontinue it altogether. Others may be particularly sensitive to the drug, and they may not be able to handle even reduced intake of caffeine. Patients with cardiovascular disease, especially arrhythmias, should refrain totally, as should people with prior stroke or transient ischemic attacks. Peptic ulcer patients and those with bipolar mood disorder and schizophrenia should be encouraged to avoid caffeine altogether.

CONCLUSIONS

Use of alcohol, tobacco, and caffeine is so commonly accepted in our society that people take notice only when their use causes serious problems. When these problems do occur, the human and economic costs are enormous. Health professionals must be committed to helping people free themselves of the addictions that can occur with these common drugs.

ABBREVIATIONS

AHRQ: Agency for Healthcare Research and Quality
BAC: blood alcohol concentration
DSM-IV-TR: *Diagnostic and Statistical Manual of Mental Disorders,* 4th ed., Text Revision
GABA: γ-aminobutyric acid
NRT: nicotine replacement therapy

Review Questions and other resources can be found at *www.pharmacotherapyonline.com.*

REFERENCES

1. Annual smoking attributable mortality, years of potential life lost, and economic costs—United States, 1995–1999. MMWR Morb Mortal Wkly Rep 2002;51:300–303.
2. Smoking and Health: A National Status Report, 2nd ed. DHHS Publication No. (CDC) 87-8396. Rockville, MD, U.S. Department of Health and Human Services, 1990.
3. Substance Abuse and Mental Health Services Administration. Results from the 2002 National Survey on Drug Use and Health: National Findings. Office of Applied Studies, NHSDA Series H-22, DHHS Publication No. SMA 03–3836. Rockville, MD. Last accessed February 23, 2004. Available from: http://www.samhsa.gov/oas/nhsda/2k2nsduh/Results/2k2Results.htm#fig3.3.
4. Diagnostic and Statistical Manual of Mental Disorders, 4th ed., Text Revision. Washington, American Psychiatric Association, 2000:212–214.
5. National Institute on Alcohol Abuse and Alcoholism. Chapter 8: Treatment Research. Tenth Special Report to the U.S. Congress on Alcohol and Health, 2000. Washington, U.S. Department of Health and Human Services, 2000. Last accessed February 23, 2004. Available from: http://www.niaaa.nih.gov/publications/10report/chap08.pdf.
6. Fiellin DA, Reid MC, O'Connor PG. Outpatient management of patients with alcohol problems. Ann Intern Med 2000;133:815–827.
7. Li G, Keyl PM, Rothman R, et al. Epidemiology of alcohol-related emergency department visits. Acad Emerg Med 1998;5:788–795.
8. Substance Abuse and Mental Health Services Administration, Office of Applied Studies. Emergency Department Trends from the Drug Abuse Warning Network, Final Estimates 1995–2002. DAWN Series: D-24, DHHS Publication No. (SMA) 03-3780. Rockville, MD, 2003. Available at: http://dawninfo.samhsa.gov/pubs_94_02/.
9. Alcohol, injuries, and the emergency department. Last accessed February 23, 2004. Available at: http://www.cdc.gov/ncipc/fact_book/09_Alcohol_%20Injuries_%20ED.htm.
10. Price D. Alcohol-related injury and violence project staff. Economic costs of substance abuse, 1995. Proc Assoc Am Physicians 1999;111:119–125.
11. Griffiths RR, Juliano LM, Chausmer AL. Caffeine pharmacology and clinical effects. In: Graham AW, Schultz TK, Mayo-Smith MF, et al, eds. Principles of Addiction Medicine, 3rd ed., pp. 193–224. Chevy Chase, MD, American Society of Addiction, 2003. Available at: http://www.caffeinedependence.org/caffeine_dependence.html.
12. Enoch MA. Pharmacogenomics of alcohol response and addiction. Am J Pharmacogenomics 2003;3:217–232.
13. Bierut LJ, Saccone NL, Rice JP, et al. Defining alcohol-related phenotypes in humans. The Collaborative Study on the Genetics of Alcoholism. Alcohol Res Health 2002;26:208–213.
14. Heath AC, Nelson EC. Effects of the interaction between genotype and environment. Research into the genetic epidemiology of alcohol dependence. Alcohol Res Health 2002;26:193–201. Last accessed February 23, 2004. Available at: http://www.niaaa.nih.gov/publications/arh26-3/193-201.htm.
15. Radel M, Goldman D. Pharmacogenetics of alcohol response and alcoholism: The interplay of genes and environmental factors in thresholds for alcoholism. Drug Metab Dispos 2001;29:489–494.
16. Hutchison KE, Wooden A, Swift RM, et al. Olanzapine reduces craving for alcohol: A DRD4 VNTR polymorphism by pharmacotherapy interaction. Neuropsychopharmacology 2003;28:1882–1888.
17. Jones AW, Holmgren P. Urine/blood ratios of ethanol in deaths attributed to acute alcohol poisoning and chronic alcoholism. Forensic Sci Int 2003;135:206–212.
18. Ramchandani VA, Kwo PY, Li TK. Effect of food and food consumption on alcohol elimination rates in healthy men and women. J Clin Pharmacol 2001;41:1345–1350.
19. Norberg A, Jones AW, Hahn RG, Gabrielsson JL. Role of variability in explaining ethanol pharmacokinetics: Research and forensic applications. Clin Pharmacokinet 2003;42:1–31.
20. Mayo-Smith MF. Pharmacological management of alcohol withdrawal. A meta-analysis and evidence-based practice guideline. American Society

of Addiction Medicine Working Group on Pharmacological Management of Alcohol Withdrawal. JAMA 1997;278:144–151.

21. Kosten TR, O'Connor PG. Management of drug and alcohol withdrawal. N Engl J Med 2003;348:1786–1795.

22. Rosenthal RN, Perkel C, Singh P, et al. A pilot open randomized trial of valproate and phenobarbital in the treatment of acute alcohol withdrawal. Am J Addict 1998;7:189–197.

23. Hillbom M, Pieninkeroinen L, Leone M. Seizures in alcohol-dependent patients. CNS Drugs 2003;17:1013–1030.

24. Reoux JP, Miller K. Routine hospital alcohol detoxification practice compared to symptom triggered management with an objective withdrawal scale (CIWA-Ar). Am J Addict 2000;9:135–144.

25. Mason BJ, Salvato FR, Williams LD, et al. A double-blind, placebo-controlled study of oral nalmefene for alcohol dependence. Arch Gen Psychiatry 1999;56:719–724.

26. Zornoza T, Cano MJ, Polache A, Granero L. Pharmacology of acamprosate: An overview. CNS Drug Rev 2003;9:359–374.

27. Garbutt JC, West SL, Carey TS, et al. Pharmacological treatment of alcohol dependence: A review of the evidence. JAMA 1999;281:1318–1325.

28. Morris PL, Hopwood M, Whelan G, et al. Naltrexone for alcohol dependence: a randomized controlled trial. Addiction 2001;96:1565–1573.

29. Srisurapanont M, Jarusuraisin N. Opioid antagonists for alcohol dependence. Cochrane Database Syst Rev 2002;2:CD001867.

30. Johnson BA, Ait-Daoud N, Bowden CL, et al. Oral topiramate for treatment of alcohol dependence: A randomized controlled trial. Lancet 2003;361:1677–1685.

31. Goldstein MG, Niaura R, Willey-Lessne C, et al. Physicians counseling smokers. A population-based survey of patients' perceptions of health care provider-delivered smoking cessation interventions. Arch Intern Med 1997;157:1313–1319.

32. Goldstein MG, Niaura R, Willey C, et al. An academic detailing intervention to disseminate physician-delivered smoking cessation counseling: Smoking cessation outcomes of the Physicians Counseling Smokers Project. Prev Med 2003;36:185–196.

33. McClure JB, Skaar K, Tsoh J, et al. Smoking cessation treatment 3: Needed health care policy changes. Behav Med 1997;23:29–34.

34. U.S. Department of Health and Human Services. Healthy People 2010, 2nd ed. Understanding and Improving Health and Objectives for Improving Health (2 vols). Washington, U.S. Department of Health and Human Services, 2000.

35. American Cancer Society. Cancer Facts and Figures 2004. Atlanta, American Cancer Society, 2004. Available at: http://www.cancer.org/ docroot/PED/ped_10.asp?sitearea=WHO&level=1.

36. Balfour DJ. Neuroplasticity within the mesoaccumbens dopamine system and its role in tobacco dependence. Curr Drug Targets CNS Neurol Disord 2002;1:413–421.

37. Anonymous. Industry watch: Blowing smoke: How cigarette manufacturers argued that nicotine is not addictive. Tob Control 1999;8:210–213.

38. U.S. Department of Health and Human Services. Treating tobacco use and dependence: Clinical Practice Guideline. Available at: http://www.surgeongeneral.gov/tobacco/treating_tobacco_use.pdf.

39. Silagy C, Lancaster T, Stead L, et al. Nicotine replacement therapy for smoking cessation. Cochrane Database Syst Rev 2002;4:CD000146.

40. Pierce JP, Gilpin EA. Impact of over-the-counter sales on effectiveness of pharmaceutical aids for smoking cessation. JAMA 2002;288:1260–1264.

41. Tsoh JY, McClure JB, Skaar KL, et al. Smoking cessation: 2. Components of effective intervention. Behav Med 1997;23:15–27.

42. Benowitz NL, Zevin S, Jacob P 3rd. Sources of variability in nicotine and cotinine levels with use of nicotine nasal spray, transdermal nicotine, and cigarette smoking. Br J Clin Pharmacol 1997;43:259–267.

43. Sorensen G, Barbeau E, Hunt MK, Emmons K. Reducing social disparities in tobacco use: a social-contextual model for reducing tobacco use among blue-collar workers. Am J Public Health 2004;94:230–239.

44. Wisborg K, Henriksen TB, Jespersen LB, et al. Nicotine patches for pregnant smokers: A randomized controlled trial. Obstet Gynecol 2000;96:967–971.

45. Ilett KF, Hale TW, Page-Sharp M, et al. Use of nicotine patches in breast feeding mothers: Transfer of nicotine and cotinine into human milk. Clin Pharmacol Ther 2003;74:516–524.

46. Song F, Raftery J, Aveyard P, et al. Cost-effectiveness of pharmacological interventions for smoking cessation: A literature review and a decision analytic analysis. Med Decis Making 2002;22:s26–s37.

47. Critchley J, Capewell S. Smoking cessation for the secondary prevention of coronary heart disease (Cochrane Review). In: The Cochrane Library, Issue 4, 2003.

48. Hurt RD, Sachs DP, Glover ED, et al. A comparison of sustained release bupropion and placebo for smoking cessation. N Engl J Med 1997;337:1195–1202.

49. Jorenby DE, Leischow SJ, Nides MA, et al. A controlled trial of sustained release bupropion, a nicotine patch, or both for smoking cessation. N Engl J Med 1999;340:685–691.

50. Glover ED, Glover PN, Sullivan CR, et al. A comparison of sustained release bupropion and placebo for smokeless tobacco cessation. Am Health Behav 2002;26:386–393.

51. Gourlay SG, Stead LF, Benowitz NL. Clonidine for smoking cessation. Cochrane Database Syst Rev 2000;2:CD000058.

52. Strain EC, Mumford GK, Silverman K, et al. Caffeine dependence syndrome: Evidence from case histories and experimental evaluations. JAMA 1994;272:1043–1048.

53. Hughes JR, Oliveto AH, Liguori A, et al. Endorsement of DSM-IV dependence criteria among caffeine users. Drug Alcohol Depend 1998;52:99–107.

54. Nehlig A. Are we dependent upon coffee and caffeine? A review of human and animal data. Neurosci Biobehav Rev 1999;23:563–576.

55. Daly JW, Fredholm BB. Caffeine: An atypical drug of dependence. Drug Alcohol Depend 1998;52:99–107.

56. Garrett BE, Griffiths RR. Physical dependence increases the relative reinforcing effects of caffeine versus placebo. Psychopharmacology 1998;139:195–202.

57. Griffiths RR, Singer MR. Is caffeine a flavoring agent in cola soft drinks? Arch Fam Med 2000;9:727–734.

58. Gorman L. 2001 Specialty Coffee Market Research Report. The Gourmet Retailer 2001;98–106. Available at: http://www.gourmetretailer.com. gourmetretailer/images/pdf/coffee.pdf.

59. The Coffee Science Source. Coffee Facts and Figures. National Coffee Association Annual Survey 2001. Last accessed February 25, 2004. Available at: http://www.coffeescience.org/factrend.html.

60. Ellison RC, Singer MR, Moore LL, et al. Current caffeine intake of young children: Amount and sources. J Am Diet Assoc 1995;95:802–804.

61. Evans SM, Griffiths RR. Caffeine withdrawal: A parametric analysis of caffeine dosing conditions. J Pharmacol Exp Ther 1999;289:285–294.

66

SCHIZOPHRENIA

M. Lynn Crismon and Peter F. Buckley

Learning Objectives and other resources can be found at *www.pharmacotherapyonline.com.*

KEY CONCEPTS

1. The pathophysiology of schizophrenia may occur in one or more different neurotransmitter systems.

2. The clinical presentation of schizophrenia is characterized by positive symptoms, negative symptoms, and impairment in cognitive functioning.

3. Comprehensive care for individuals with schizophrenia must occur in the context of a multidisciplinary mental health care environment that offers psychotropic medication management and comprehensive psychosocial services.

4. A thorough patient evaluation (e.g., history, mental status exam, physical exam, and laboratory analysis) should occur to establish a diagnosis of schizophrenia and to identify potential co-occurring disorders, including substance abuse and general medical disorders.

5. Given that one cannot distinguish among the newer second-generation antipsychotics based upon efficacy, side-effect profiles become important in choosing an antipsychotic for an individual patient.

6. Pharmacotherapy algorithms should emphasize monotherapies with antipsychotics of optimal efficacy:side-effect ratios and progress to medications with greater side-effect risks and to combination regimens in treatment-resistant patients.

7. Adequate time on a given medication at a therapeutic dose is the most important variable in predicting medication response.

8. Long-term maintenance antipsychotic treatment is necessary for the vast majority of patients with schizophrenia in order to prevent relapse.

9. Thorough patient and family psychoeducation should occur, including education about the illness, symptoms, prognosis, medication, psychosocial treatments, and methods to improve adaptive functioning.

10. Pharmacotherapy decisions should be guided by systematic monitoring of patient symptoms, preferably with the use of brief symptom rating scales.

Schizophrenia is one of the most complex and challenging of psychiatric disorders. It represents a heterogeneous syndrome of disorganized and bizarre thoughts, delusions, hallucinations, inappropriate affect, and impaired psychosocial functioning. From the time that Kraepelin first described dementia praecox in 1896 until publication of the *Diagnostic and Statistical Manual of Mental Disorders,* 4th edition, Text Revision (DSM-IV-TR) in 2000, the description of this illness has continuously evolved.[1] Scientific advances that increase our knowledge of central nervous system (CNS) physiology, pathophysiology, and genetics will likely improve our understanding of schizophrenia in the future.

EPIDEMIOLOGY

According to the Epidemiologic Catchment Area Study, the U.S. lifetime prevalence of schizophrenia ranges from 0.6% to 1.9%, with an average of approximately 1%.[2] With only a few possible exceptions, the worldwide prevalence of schizophrenia is remarkably similar among all cultures. Schizophrenia most commonly has its onset in late adolescence or early adulthood and rarely occurs before adolescence or after the age of 40 years. Although the prevalence of schizophrenia is equal in males and females, the onset of illness tends

to be earlier in males. Males most frequently have their first episode during their early twenties, whereas with females it is usually during their late twenties to early thirties.[1,2]

ETIOLOGY

Although the etiology of schizophrenia is unknown, research has demonstrated various abnormalities in brain structure and function.[3] However, these changes are not consistent among all individuals with a diagnosis of schizophrenia, and much has yet to be learned about its pathogenesis. The cause of schizophrenia is likely multifactorial; that is, multiple pathophysiologic abnormalities may play a role in producing the similar but varying clinical phenotypes we refer to as schizophrenia.

A neurodevelopmental model has been evoked as one possible explanation for the etiology of schizophrenia.[4] This model proposes that schizophrenia has its origins in some as yet unknown in utero disturbance, possibly occurring during the second trimester of pregnancy. Evidence for this is provided by the abnormal neuronal migration demonstrated in most studies of schizophrenic brains. This "schizophrenic lesion" may result in abnormalities in cell shape, position, symmetry, and connectivity, and functionally to the development of abnormal brain circuits.[3,4] Changes are consistent with a cell migration abnormality during the second trimester of pregnancy, and some studies associate upper respiratory infections during the second trimester of pregnancy with a higher incidence of schizophrenia.[5] Other studies show a relationship between obstetric complications or neonatal hypoxia and schizophrenia. Some studies also associate low birth-weight (<2,500 g) with schizophrenia.[2] The resulting secondary "synaptic disorganization" associated with such insults is thought not to produce overt clinical manifestations of psychosis until adolescence or early adulthood because this is the corresponding time period of neuronal maturation.

Additional support for a developmental model is provided by the fact that although studies have shown decreased cortical thickness and increased ventricular size in the brains of many patients with schizophrenia, this occurs in the absence of widespread gliosis.[3] Gliosis, or the proliferation of glial cells, is thought to occur as a compensatory change in degenerative diseases of the brain. One hypothesis is that obstetric complications and hypoxia, in combination with a genetic predisposition, could activate a glutamatergic cascade that results in increased neuronal pruning. It is hypothesized that this genetic predisposition may be related to genes controlling N-methyl-D-aspartate (NMDA) receptor activity. As a part of the normal neurodevelopmental process, pruning of dendrites occurs. In the normal individual, about 35% of the peak number of dendrites at 2 years of age are pruned by midadolescence. Some studies have shown a higher percentage of pruning in individuals with schizophrenia. Furthermore, synaptic pruning predominantly involves glutamatergic dendrites. Hypoxia or other prenatal insult may result in a decreased number of basal neurons from which to start, and glutamatergic activation may exaggerate the pruning process. This is consistent with studies showing perinatal hypoxia being associated with earlier age of onset of schizophrenia. Others have suggested that altered membrane phospholipid metabolism may result in a cascade of effects leading to the expression of schizophrenia.[6]

Numerous studies have shown neuropsychological abnormalities as early as 4 years of age in individuals who later develop schizophrenia.[1,2] Impairment in reaching normal motor milestones, and abnormal movements in children as young as 8 months of age, have been associated with the development of schizophrenia.[2] These findings indicate abnormalities in brain function long before the onset of psychotic symptomatology and provide empiric evidence for schizophrenia being a neurodevelopmental disorder.[7] However, the progressive clinical deterioration in some patients suggests that this illness may also have a neurodegenerative component. This is consistent with recent brain imaging studies that show deteriorative brain changes in patients whose illness course is of frequent relapses.[8,9] This had led our field not so much to consider schizophrenia as *either* neurodevelopmental *or* neurodegenerative in origin, but rather to reconceptualize the illness as exhibiting neurodegenerative propensity based upon a vulnerable neurodevelopmental substrate.[10] This notion has substantial implications for early detection and treatment of this debilitating condition.[11]

GENETICS

Although a specific abnormality has not been discovered, increasing evidence suggests a genetic basis for schizophrenia. Although the risk of developing schizophrenia is 0.6% to 1.9% in the general population, this increases to approximately 10% if a first-degree relative has the illness and to 3% if a second-degree relative has the illness.[12] If both parents have schizophrenia, the risk of producing a

schizophrenic offspring increases to approximately 40%. Twin studies in dizygotic twins report that the risk of the second twin developing schizophrenia if one twin has the illness is between 12% and 14%. However, in monozygotic twins the risk increases to 48%.[12] Numerous adoption studies indicate that the risk for schizophrenia lies with the biologic parents, and change in the environment during the child's developmental stages does not alter this. If schizophrenia occurs in siblings, the onset of illness tends to occur at the same age in each, thus lessening the possibility of an environmental precipitant. A search for a genetic linkage in schizophrenia has been difficult, and any genetic etiologies in schizophrenia are likely heterogeneous, but present with similar phenotypes. Potential loci have been identified on chromosomes 6, 8, 13, and 22.[12] Beyond traditional familial and twin association studies, the study of the genetics of schizophrenia has become increasingly molecular in focus.[3,12] Recent work has shown that polymorphism in the VAL/MET alleles of the catecholamine-o methyl transferase gene may explain some of the frontal lobe functional deficits in patients with schizophrenia.[12] Other recent studies have shown abnormalities in several genes that code for neurodevelopment and for trophic factors.[12–14]

PATHOPHYSIOLOGY

Computed axial tomography (CAT) scans and magnetic resonance imaging (MRI) studies show increased ventricular size, particularly in the third and lateral ventricles, in subtypes of schizophrenics. Recent studies also show a small but definite decrease in brain size as compared to matched controls. These changes appear to be consistent with brain asymmetry, the ventricular enlargement being most pronounced in the left temporal horn, and the decreased cortical size being most obvious in the left temporal lobe.[3,8] Not only does premorbid lower hippocampal volume predict onset of symptoms in high-risk individuals, these changes may progress throughout the course of the illness.[15] Changes in hippocampal volume may correspond with impairment in neuropsychological testing, and these patients may have poorer response to first-generation antipsychotics (FGAs).[8] Rather than a decrease in the number of neurons in affected brain areas, a decrease in axonal and dendritic communications between cells may result in a loss of connectivity that may be important with respect to neuronal adaptivity and CNS homeostasis.[3] These changes are likely consistent with the evidence for abnormal neuronal pruning.[4]

NEUROTRANSMITTER CHANGES

Since the discovery of the role of dopamine (DA) as a neurotransmitter in 1958, and the observations that antipsychotic drugs are postsynaptic DA-receptor antagonists, interest in a dopaminergic hypothesis for the pathophysiology of schizophrenia has existed. However, these theories may be more appropriately oriented toward the treatment of psychosis with antipsychotics.

Four dopaminergic tracts are of primary interest. Table 66–1 outlines the origin, innervation, and primary functional activity of each tract, as well as the effects of dopamine antagonists.[7]

Increasing evidence supports the presence of a DA-receptor defect in schizophrenia. Numerous positron emission tomography (PET) studies have shown regional brain abnormalities, including increased glucose metabolism in the caudate nucleus, and decreased blood flow and glucose metabolism in the frontal lobe and left temporal lobe.[2,3]

TABLE 66–1. Dopaminergic Tracts and Effects of Dopamine Antagonists

Dopamine Tract	Origin	Innervation	Function	Dopamine Antagonist Effect
Nigrostriatal	Substantia nigra (A9 area)	Caudate nucleus Putamen	Extrapyramidal system, movement	Movement disorders
Mesolimbic	Midbrain ventral tegmentum (A10 area)	Limbic areas (e.g., amygdala, olfactory tubercle, septal nuclei), cingulate gyrus	Arousal, memory, stimulus processing, motivational behavior	Relief of psychosis
Mesocortical	Midbrain ventral tegmentum (A10 area)	Frontal and prefrontal lobe cortex	Cognition, communication, social function, response to stress	Relief of psychosis Akathisia?
Tuberoinfundibular	Hypothalamus	Pituitary gland	Regulates prolactin release	Increased prolactin concentrations

this may indicate dopaminergic hyperactivity in the head of the caudate nucleus and dopaminergic hypofunction in the frontotemporal regions. PET studies using D_2-specific ligands provide data suggesting increased densities of D_2 receptors in the head of the caudate nucleus with decreased densities in the prefrontal cortex.[2,3] PET studies assessing D_1 function suggest that subpopulations of schizophrenics may have decreased densities of D_1 receptors in the caudate nucleus and the prefrontal cortex. Hypofrontality may be associated with lack of volition, one of the core negative symptoms seen in schizophrenia. It is important to emphasize that it is unknown whether these changes represent a primary event or whether they are secondary processes related to other pathophysiologic abnormalities in schizophrenia. Because of the heterogeneity in the clinical presentation of schizophrenia, it has also been suggested that the DA hypothesis may be more applicable to "neuroleptic-responsive psychosis," with multiple different etiologies possibly being responsible for causing schizophrenia.[16] Attempts have been made to develop relationships between these abnormal findings and behavioral symptoms present in schizophrenic patients. The positive symptoms are possibly more closely associated with DA-receptor hyperactivity in the mesocaudate, whereas negative symptoms are most closely related to DA-receptor hypofunction in the prefrontal cortex. Presynaptic D_1 receptors in the prefrontal cortex are thought to be involved in modulating glutamatergic activity, and this may be important with regard to working memory in individuals with schizophrenia.[15]

Glutamatergic dysfunction has been suggested as being etiologic in schizophrenia. The glutamatergic system is one of the most widespread excitatory neurotransmitter systems in the brain. Alterations in its function, either hypo- or hyperactivity, can result in toxic neuronal reactions.[2,3,15] Dopaminergic innervation from the ventral striatum decreases the limbic system's inhibitory activity (perhaps through γ-aminobutyric acid [GABA] interneurons); thus, dopaminergic stimulation increases arousal. The corticostriatal glutamate pathways have the opposite effect, inhibiting dopaminergic function from the ventral striatum, therefore allowing the limbic system to have increased inhibitory activity. Descending glutamatergic tracts interact with dopaminergic tracts directly as well as through GABA interneurons. Glutamatergic deficiency produces symptoms similar to those of dopaminergic hyperactivity and possibly those seen in schizophrenia. Clinical support for this hypothesis comes from the fact that phencyclidine, a potent psychotomimetic, is a noncompetitive antagonist at the NMDA receptor, a major glutamate receptor. It is proposed that schizophrenia may involve some currently unknown in utero assault that leads to a developmental defect in NMDA receptor function—so-called NMDA hypofunction. This defect is proposed

to have latent clinical expression with neuropsychological pathology from NMDA hypofunction not being seen until late adolescence or early adulthood. It has been shown that excess D_2 stimulation can impair NMDA transmission via GABAergic neurons. Thus the use of antipsychotic drugs could potentially enhance glutamatergic transmission.[15]

Serotoninergic receptors are present on dopaminergic axons, and it is known that stimulation of these receptors will decrease DA release, at least in the striatum.[7] Although somewhat more diffuse, the distribution of serotonergic neurons is similar to that of dopaminergic neurons, thus allowing these two neurotransmitter systems to innervate the same areas. In fact, 5-hydroxytryptamine$_2$ (serotonin$_2$; 5-HT$_2$) receptors and D_4 receptors have been found to be colocalized in the cortex.[3,7,15] Patients with schizophrenia with abnormal brain scans have higher whole-blood 5-HT concentrations, and these concentrations are correlated with increased ventricular size.[17] Atypical antipsychotics with potent 5-HT$_2$ receptor antagonist effects reverse worsening of symptomatology induced by 5-HT agonists in patients with schizophrenia.[17]

The primary pathophysiologic abnormality in schizophrenia may occur in one of a number of different neurotransmitters (e.g., dopaminergic, glutamatergic, or serotonergic systems), with changes in other neurotransmitters occurring secondarily. For example, a primary defect resulting in abnormal presynaptic release of DA from the neuron and ineffective feedback mechanisms could lead to postsynaptic DA receptor hypersensitivity. The NMDA hypofunction model is another approach that could lead to dysregulation among neurotransmitter systems.

Schizophrenia is a complex disorder, and multiple etiologies likely exist for the clinical syndrome we refer to as schizophrenia. Based on current knowledge, it is naive to think that any currently proposed etiology can adequately explain the genesis of this complex disease. Molecular research involving genetically determined subtle changes in G proteins, protein metabolism, and other subcellular processes may well identify the biologic disturbances associated with schizophrenia.[3,7,15]

CLINICAL PRESENTATION

Schizophrenia is the most common functional psychosis, and there are as many clinical presentations of schizophrenia as there are individuals with the disorder. Despite numerous attempts to portray a stereotype in movies and on television, the stereotypic schizophrenic essentially does not exist. Moreover, schizophrenia does not mean "split personality." Schizophrenia is a chronic disorder of thought and affect with the individual having a significant disturbance in interpersonal relationships and ability to function in society on a daily basis.

The first psychotic episode may be sudden in onset with few premorbid symptoms, or commonly may be preceded by withdrawn, suspicious, peculiar behavior (schizoid). During the acute psychotic episodes, the patient loses touch with reality, and in a sense, the brain creates a false reality to replace it. The patient experiences a variety of acute psychotic symptoms, such as hallucinations (especially hearing voices), delusions (fixed false beliefs), and ideas of influence (beliefs that one's actions are controlled by external influences). Thought processes are disconnected (loose associations), the patient may not be able to carry on logical conversation (alogia), and may have simultaneous contradictory thoughts (ambivalence). The patient's affect may be flat (no emotional expression), or it may be inappropriate and labile. The patient is often withdrawn and inwardly directed (autism). Uncooperativeness, hostility, and verbal or physical aggression may be seen because of the patient's misperception of reality. Self-care skills are impaired, and the patient is frequently dirty, unkempt, and in general has poor hygiene. Sleep and appetite are often disturbed. When the acute psychotic episode remits, the patient typically has residual features. This is an important point in differentiating schizophrenia from other psychotic disorders. Although residual symptoms and their severity vary, patients may have difficulty with anxiety management, suspiciousness, and lack of volition, motivation, insight, and judgment. Therefore they often have difficulty living independently in the community. Because of poor anxiety management and suspiciousness, they are frequently withdrawn socially, and have difficulty forming close relationships with others. In addition, impaired volition and motivation contribute to poor self-care skills and make it difficult for the patient with schizophrenia to maintain employment.

Patients with schizophrenia frequently experience a lack of historicity, or difficulty in learning from their experiences. They may repeatedly make the same mistakes in social conduct and situations requiring judgment. They have difficulty understanding the importance of treatment, including medications, in maintaining their ability to function in society. Therefore they tend to discontinue medications and other treatments, and this increases the risk of relapse and rehospitalization.

Although the course of the illness is variable, the long-term prognosis for many schizophrenic patients is poor. The disease is marked by intermittent acute psychotic episodes and impaired psychosocial functioning between acute episodes, with most of the deterioration in psychosocial functioning occurring within 5 years after the first psychotic episode.[18] By late life, the patient may appear "burned out," that is, the patient ceases to have acute psychotic episodes, but residual symptoms, as previously described, persist. However, functional skills may actually improve compared with earlier in the patient's life. In a subpopulation of patients, probably 5% to 15%, psychotic symptoms are nearly continuous, and response to typical antipsychotics is poor.[19]

The DSM-IV-TR places a greater emphasis on the chronicity of schizophrenia and negative symptoms than do previous editions. Schizophrenia is a chronic disorder, and the patient's history must be carefully assessed for dysfunction that has persisted for longer than 6 months. After their first episode, patients with schizophrenia rarely have a level of adaptive functioning as high as before the onset of the disorder. Table 66–2 summarizes the DSM-IV-TR criteria, and this reference should be consulted for a more detailed discussion of the differential diagnosis.[1]

TABLE 66–2. DSM-IV-TR Diagnostic Criteria for Schizophrenia

A. Characteristic symptoms: Two or more of the following, each persisting for a significant portion of at least a 1-month period:
   (1) delusions
   (2) hallucinations
   (3) disorganized speech
   (4) grossly disorganized or catatonic behavior
   (5) negative symptoms
   Note: Only one criterion A symptom is required if delusions are bizarre or if hallucinations consist of a voice keeping a running commentary on the person's behavior or two or more voices conversing with each other.
B. Social/occupational dysfunction: For a significant portion of the time since onset of the disorder, one or more major areas of functioning such as work, interpersonal relations, or self-care are significantly below the level prior to onset.
C. Duration: Continuous signs of the disorder for at least 6 months. This must include at least 1 month of symptoms fulfilling criterion A (unless successfully treated). This 6 months may include prodromal or residual symptoms.
D. Schizoaffective or mood disorder has been excluded.
E. Disorder is not due to a medical disorder or substance use.
F. If a history of a pervasive developmental disorder is present, there must be symptoms of hallucinations or delusions present for at least 1 month.

Adapted from American Psychiatric Association.[1]

❷ The DSM-IV-TR classifies the symptoms of schizophrenia into two categories: positive and negative. Recently greater emphasis has been placed on a third symptom category, cognitive dysfunction (Table 66–3).[19] The areas of cognition found to be abnormal in schizophrenia include attention, working memory, and executive function. Positive symptoms have traditionally attracted the most attention and are the ones most affected by traditional antipsychotic drugs. However, negative symptoms and impairment in cognition are more closely associated with poor psychosocial function. This fact merits attention when one is examining pharmacologic options for treatment.

Numerous authors have attempted to construct subtypes of schizophrenia, and it has been suggested that symptom complexes may correlate with prognosis, cognitive functioning, structural abnormalities in the brain, and response to antipsychotic drugs. Negative symptoms and cognitive impairment may be more closely associated with prefrontal lobe dysfunction and positive symptoms with temporolimbic abnormalities. Many patients demonstrate both positive and negative symptoms. Patients with negative symptoms frequently have more antecedent cognitive dysfunction, poor premorbid adjustment, low level of educational achievement, and a poorer overall prognosis.[19]

TABLE 66–3. Schizophrenia Symptom Clusters

Positive	Negative	Cognitive
Suspiciousness	Affective flattening	Impaired attention
Unusual thought content (delusions)	Alogia	Impaired working memory
Hallucinations	Anhedonia	Impaired executive function
Conceptual disorganization	Avolition	

From American Psychiatric Association,[1] Lehman et al,[19] and Velligan et al.[119]

▶ TREATMENT: Schizophrenia

DESIRED OUTCOME

Pharmacotherapy is the mainstay of treatment in schizophrenia, and it is essentially impossible in most patients to implement effective psychosocial rehabilitation programs in the absence of antipsychotic treatment.[19] Elements of the comprehensive care of patients with schizophrenia are listed in Table 66–4. A pharmacotherapeutic treatment plan should be developed that delineates drug-related aspects of therapy. Because most deterioration in psychosocial functioning occurs within the first 5 years of the initial psychotic episode, treatment interventions should be particularly assertive during this period.[18] Explicit endpoints should be defined, including realistic goals of the target symptoms most likely to respond, and the relative time course for response.[2,19] Other goals include avoiding unwanted side effects, using the minimum effective dose, emphasizing adequate time as a primary variable in determining response, and limiting augmentation medications to nonresponsive patients.

NONPHARMACOLOGIC THERAPY

Psychosocial rehabilitation programs oriented toward improving patients' adaptive functioning are the mainstay of nondrug treatment for schizophrenia. These programs may include basic living skills, social skills training, basic education, work programs, and supported housing. In particular, programs aimed at employment and housing have been the more effective interventions and are considered "best practices" for persons with serious and persistent mental disorders. Programs that involve families in the care and life of the patient have also been shown to decrease rehospitalization and to improve functioning in the community. For particularly low-functioning patients, assertive intervention programs referred to as active community treatment (ACT) are effective in improving patients' functional outcomes. ACT teams are available on a 24-hour basis and work in the patient's home and place of employment to provide comprehensive treatment, including medication, crisis intervention, daily living skills, and supported employment and housing.[2,19] A listing of psychotherapeutic approaches to the treatment of schizophrenia is given in Table 66–5.

PHARMACOLOGIC THERAPY

ASSESSMENT PRIOR TO TREATMENT

The importance of initial assessment for accurate diagnosis cannot be overemphasized in a patient presenting with acute psychosis. A thorough mental status examination, physical and neurologic examination, complete family and social history, and laboratory work-up must be performed to confirm the diagnosis and exclude general medical or substance-induced causes of psychosis, such as acute or chronic drug ingestion. Laboratory tests, biologic markers, and commonly available brain imaging techniques do not assist in diagnosis or selection of medication. A pretreatment patient work-up is not only important in excluding other pathology, but in serving as a baseline for monitoring potential medication-related side effects, and should include: vital signs, complete blood count, electrolytes, hepatic function, renal function, electrocardiogram, fasting serum glucose, serum lipids, thyroid function, and urine drug screen.

ANTIPSYCHOTIC MEDICATION CHOICES

Second-Generation Antipsychotics

Second-generation antipsychotics (SGAs) (with the exception of clozapine) have become the agents of first choice in the treatment of schizophrenia, and most practice guidelines and consensus statements support this recommendation.[19–21] The nomenclature for these drugs is at present confusing. No absolute criterion distinguishes atypical (second-generation) from typical (traditional or conventional first-generation) antipsychotics, and no universally accepted definition exists for an atypical antipsychotic.[17] Thus in many respects, "second-generation antipsychotic" is a more appropriate term. Common to all definitions is the ability of the drug to produce antipsychotic response with few or no acutely occurring extrapyramidal side effects (EPS). Other attributes that have been ascribed to SGAs include enhanced efficacy, particularly for negative symptoms and cognition; absence or near absence of tardive dyskinesia; and lack of effect on serum prolactin.[19] To date, the only approved SGA that fulfills all of these criteria is clozapine, the prototypical agent.[17] Growing, but still controversial, evidence suggests that SGAs have superior efficacy for the treatment of negative symptoms, cognition, mood, and general psychopathology.[19–21] Whether these differences are a result of differences in core efficacy or differences in side-effect profile is unknown. The major advantage of atypical antipsychotics may be in their side-effect profiles with respect to motor effects, as they generally have better overall tolerability than the FGAs. While information from maintenance studies is beginning to accrue, there is still a relative lack of information to adequately define the long-term clinical outcomes resulting from their widespread use. However, some experts believe that their use during the first 5 years of onset of the

TABLE 66–4. Comprehensive Care Elements in the Treatment of Schizophrenia

- Medication treatment
- Individual supportive therapy
- Cognitive and psychosocial therapies
- Family psychoeducation and support
- Social support
- Case management
- Housing
- Financial support
- Vocational support

TABLE 66–5. Psychotherapeutic Approaches to the Treatment of Schizophrenia

Individual	Group	Cognitive Behavioral
Supportive/counseling Personal therapy Social skills therapies Vocational sheltered employment rehabilitation therapies	Interactive/social	Cognitive behavioral therapy Compliance therapy

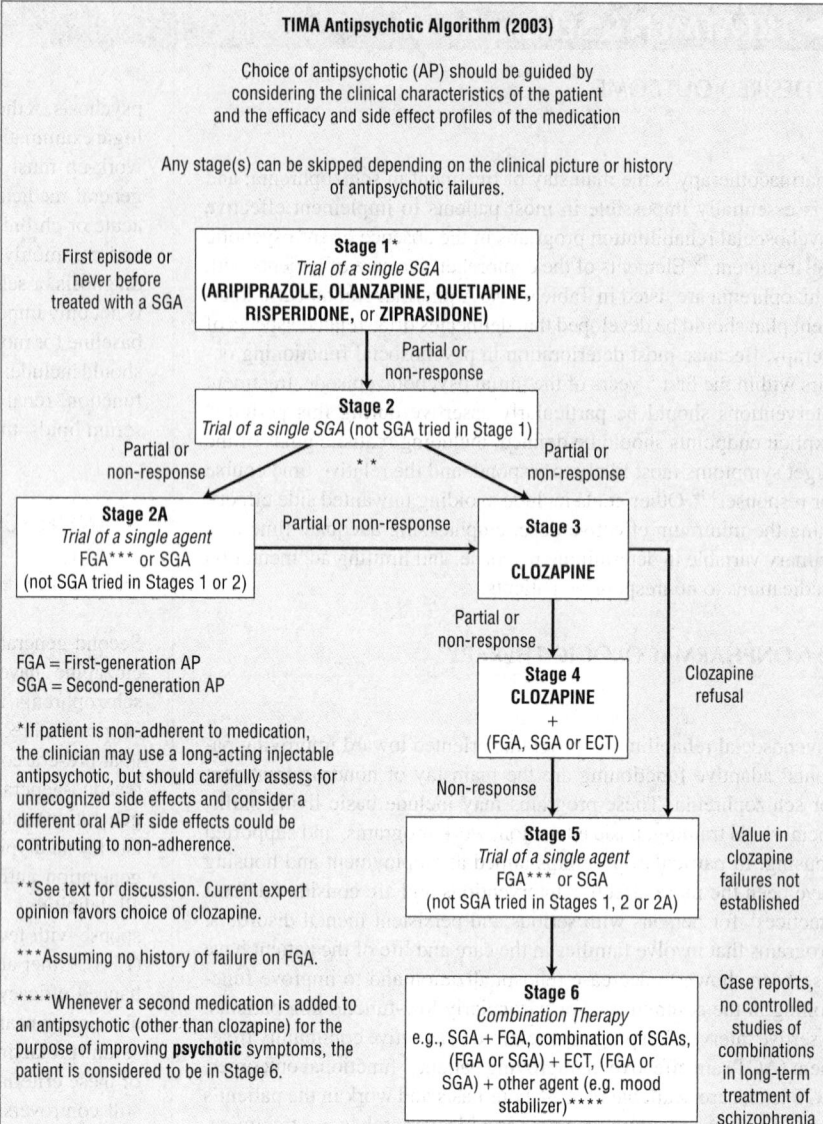

FIGURE 66–1. Patient entry into the algorithm is determined by individual patient history and clinical presentation. Algorithm stages can be skipped if clinically appropriate, and one may go back stages if indicated. In general, inadequately responding patients should not remain in stages 1 or 2 longer than 12 weeks at therapeutic doses. Stage 3 may be up to 6 months. TIMA = Texas Implementation of Medication Algorithms. (From Miller et al[20] and Miller et al.[22] This figure is in the public domain and may be reproduced with appropriate citation of the authors and source. Algorithm updates may be obtained at *http://www.mhmr.state.tx.us/centraloffice/medicaldirector/timasczman.pdf.*)

illness could help prevent some of the deterioration associated with the disease.[18,22] However, adequate psychosocial rehabilitation programs must be used in conjunction with atypical antipsychotics if patients are to achieve their maximum functional capacity.

Risperidone fulfills the atypical criterion of having a low incidence of EPS at low to moderate doses. The mean optimal dose in parallel, fixed-dose studies was 4 to 6 mg daily. At doses greater than 6 mg daily, risperidone's profile is more similar to that of an FGA.[22,23] Because risperidone appears to lose its atypical profile at higher doses, the lowest possible dose should be used in treatment. This may include gradual dose titration downward if patients do not respond initially, rather than upward titration as has been the traditional approach to dosing antipsychotics.[19,22]

Olanzapine has a very low incidence of EPS when used within the approved dose range of 10 to 20 mg daily.[2,19,22] However, many patients are being treated at doses above the currently recommended limit in the approved product labeling of 20 mg/day. Quetiapine is an efficacious antipsychotic with an excellent EPS profile.[22,24] Although contrary to efficacy studies, doses above 500 mg are often used to achieve optimal effects, with dose titration to 800 mg/day being a common occurrence. From a clinical perspective, the optimal daily quetiapine dose appears unclear.

Ziprasidone 40 to 160 mg/day appears to have efficacy similar to other SGAs, with response rates increasing at doses greater than 80 mg daily.[2,22,25] Aripiprazole has established efficacy at 15 to 30 mg/day.[19,20,26] Both aripiprazole and ziprasidone have significantly less potential to produce weight gain than other SGAs.

The side-effect profiles of individual atypical antipsychotics and individual patient characteristics should be used in deciding which drug to use in an individual patient. Information from the algorithm (Fig. 66–1) and the adverse effects sections should be utilized in arriving at this decision.

First-Generation or Typical Antipsychotics

Because of the risk of EPS, particularly tardive dyskinesia, FGAs are not usually considered first-line treatments.[19,20,21] All FGAs are equal in efficacy when used in equipotent doses. Selection of medication should be based on the need to avoid certain side effects and

ABLE 66–6. Available Antipsychotics: Doses and Dosage Forms

Generic Name	Trade Name	Traditional Equivalent Dose (mg)[a]	Usual Dosage Range (mg/day)	Manufacturer's Maximum Dose (mg/day)	Dosage Forms[b]
Traditional antipsychotics (first-generation antipsychotics)					
Chlorpromazine	Thorazine	100	100–800	2,000	T, L, LC, I, C-ER, SR
Fluphenazine	Prolixin	2	2–20	40	T, L, LC, I, LAI
Haloperidol	Haldol	2	2–20	100	T, LC, I, LAI
Loxapine	Loxitane	10	10–80	250	C, LC
Molindone	Moban	10	10–100	225	T, LC
Mesoridazine	Serentil	50	50–400	500	T, LC, I
Perphenazine	Trilafon	10	10–64	64	T, LC, I
Thioridazine	Mellaril	100	100–800	800	T, LC
Thiothixene	Navane	4	4–40	60	C, LC
Trifluoperazine	Stelazine	5	5–40	80	T, LC, I
Atypical antipsychotics (second-generation antipsychotics)					
Aripiprazole	Abilify	NA	15–30	30	T
Clozapine	Clozaril	NA	50–500	900	T
Olanzapine	Zyprexa	NA	10–20	20	T, I, O
Quetiapine	Seroquel	NA	250–500	800	T
Risperidone	Risperdal	NA	2–8	16	T, O, L
Risperidone	Risperdal	NA	25–50	50	LAI
	Consta		Every 2 weeks	Every 2 weeks	
Ziprasidone	Geodon	NA	40–160	200	C, I

NA. This parameter does not apply to atypical antipsychotics.

T, tablet; C, capsule; ER or SR, extended- or sustained-release; I, injection; L, liquid solution, elixir, or suspension; LC, liquid concentrate; O, orally disintegrating tablets; AI, long-acting injectable.

oncurrent medical or psychiatric disorders. No differences exist in ef-cacy between low- and high-potency FGAs, and high-potency drugs e.g., haloperidol) are as effective in treating acute agitation as otency, highly sedating FGAs (e.g., chlorpromazine).

Previous patient or family history of response to an antipsychotic s helpful in the selection of an agent. Traditional dosage equivalents expressed in "chlorpromazine equivalent dosages"—the equipotent osage of any traditional FGA compared with 100 mg of chlorpro-nazine) may assist in determining the effective dosage range if the eed arises to treat a patient with a different FGA. However, because GAs differ in mechanism of action, the dose equivalents have little elevance when comparing dosages of SGAs. Table 66–6 lists an-ipsychotics and their usual dosage ranges.

Pharmacotherapeutic Algorithm

Figure 66–1 outlines a suggested pharmacotherapeutic algo-rithm for schizophrenia.[20,22] Newer SGAs are recommended s first-line treatment (i.e., stages 1, 2, and 2A) because of a lower ncidence of acutely occurring EPS and tardive dyskinesia, and some vidence for a superior effect on negative symptoms and cognition. Although it is unclear how many newer SGAs to try before proceed-ng to clozapine, because of safety concerns and the need for white lood cell (WBC) monitoring, it is generally recommended that pa-ients be tried on two newer SGAs as monotherapy before proceeding o a trial of clozapine (stage 3).[20,22] Clozapine has been shown to have uperior efficacy in decreasing suicidal behavior, and it should also be onsidered as a higher treatment option in the suicidal patient.[27] If a atient will not consent to taking clozapine, then a trial of a different GA or an FGA is recommended (stage 2A).

Treatment algorithm recommendations after clozapine (stages 4, , and 6) are based more on anecdotal experiences and clinical opin-ons than on empirical research.[20,22] These combination strategies are imed at a small percentage of patients who have responded poorly to

stages 1 through 3. These interventions should be implemented with careful evaluation of a patient's symptom response and discontinua-tion of the combination if improvement does not occur. See the later section on the treatment-resistant patient for a discussion of these strategy options.

If partial or poor adherence contributes to inadequate clinical im-provement, then long-acting or depot injectable antipsychotics should be considered.[19] Risperidone long-acting injection is currently the only long-acting SGA available. Because of a lower risk of EPS com-pared to fluphenazine or haloperidol depot injection, it is a preferred agent. In addition to individuals who are identified as partially ad-herent, some other patients may elect a once-every-2-week injection instead of taking daily oral medications. Long-acting injectable an-tipsychotics can be substituted for an oral antipsychotic at any point in the algorithm where they are thought to be indicated.

CLINICAL CONTROVERSY

Some effectiveness studies and meta-analyses of SGA effi-cacy studies have shown minimal superiority of these medi-cations in improving psychotic symptoms (especially positive symptoms), particularly when compared with lower doses of haloperidol. However, other studies have reported that SGAs are superior to FGAs in improving negative symptoms. Nearly all studies have demonstrated a lower incidence of EPS with SGAs than FGAs. Tension exists between policy decision mak-ers who are responsible for managing finite resources and clinicians who see clinical benefits of the SGAs in the pa-tients they treat.

The use of antipsychotic combinations is controver-sial, as no research evidence supports increased efficacy for combination antipsychotic treatment. Combination antipsy-chotics are frequently used by clinicians, and testimonies at-test to clinical benefits when a second SGA is added.

PREDICTORS OF RESPONSE

Obtaining a thorough medication history is important, and previous antipsychotic treatment should help guide the selection of current drug therapy, in that either a good prior response favors the use of the same agent or a negative prior response suggests the selection of a dissimilar drug. Nonprescription and illicit drug use may influence psychiatric presentation and thus diagnosis or antipsychotic response. Amphetamine and other CNS stimulants, cocaine, corticosteroids, digitalis glycosides, indomethacin, marijuana, pentazocine, phencyclidine, and other drugs can induce psychosis in susceptible individuals or exacerbate psychosis in patients with preexisting psychiatric illness.[28] Schizophrenic patients who continue to abuse alcohol or drugs usually have a poor response to medications and a poor prognosis. Alcohol, caffeine, and nicotine use potentially results in drug interactions.

Individual differences in patient response have been either proposed or identified, which may be clinically useful predictors of response.[29] Acute onset and short duration of illness, presence of acute stressors or precipitating factors, later age of onset, family history of affective illness, and good premorbid adjustment as reflected in stable interpersonal relationships or employment are all predictors of good response.[29]

Negative schizophrenic symptoms are generally less responsive to antipsychotic therapy. Although controversial, affective symptoms may correlate with an overall good response. However, other than these caveats, few data support a relationship between drug response and schizophrenic subtypes. Neuropsychological deficits related to cognition and neurologic soft signs may correlate with poor antipsychotic response.[29] A patient's subjective response within the first 48 hours after being administered an FGA may be associated with drug responsiveness.[30] An initial dysphoric response, demonstrated by stating a dislike of the medication, or feeling worse or zombie-like, combined with anxiety or akathisia-like symptoms, is associated with poor drug response, and likely adverse effects. If continued on the same medication, the patient will likely be nonadherent.

The importance of developing a therapeutic alliance between the patient and the clinician cannot be underestimated. Patients who form positive therapeutic alliances are more likely to be adherent with all aspects of therapy, experience a better outcome at 2 years, and generally require smaller antipsychotic doses.

A certain minority of patients fail to benefit from antipsychotic therapy, and their psychosocial functioning may actually worsen. Unfortunately, no accepted method is available to identify these people before treatment.[29]

INITIAL TREATMENT IN AN ACUTE PSYCHOTIC EPISODE

Initial dosing should follow the goals described in the individualized pharmacotherapeutic treatment plan. The goals during the first 7 days should be decreased agitation, hostility, combativeness, anxiety, tension, and aggression, and normalization of sleep and eating patterns. The usual recommendation is to initiate therapy and to titrate over the first few days to an average effective dose, unless the patient's physiologic status or history indicates that this dose may result in unacceptable adverse effects. Table 66–6 lists the usual dosage range, and an average dose is typically midrange. If "cheeking" of medication is suspected, liquid formulations and orally disintegrating tablets of different antipsychotics are available (see Table 66–6). If a patient has shown absolutely no improvement after 3 to 4 weeks at therapeutic doses, then an alternative antipsychotic should be considered (i.e., moving to the next treatment stage in the algorithm; see Fig. 66–1).[20,22]

Although some clinicians believe that larger daily doses are necessary in more severely symptomatic patients, data are not available to support this practice. Some symptoms, such as agitation, tension, aggression, and increased motor activity, may respond more quickly, but side effects may be more common with higher doses. However, interindividual differences in dosage and patient response do occur. In partial but inadequate responders who are tolerating the chosen antipsychotic well, it may be reasonable to titrate above usual dose ranges. However, this tactic should be time-limited (i.e., 2 to 4 weeks), and if the patient does not achieve further improvement, the dose should either be decreased, or an alternative treatment strategy tried.[19,22] In general, rapid titration of antipsychotic dosage is not indicated.[19,22] However, intramuscular antipsychotic administration (e.g., ziprasidone 10 to 20 mg IM, olanzapine 2.5 to 10 mg IM, or haloperidol 2 to 5 mg IM) can be used to assist in calming a severely agitated patient. Agitation can be manifested by loud, physically or verbally threatening behavior, motor hyperactivity, or physical aggression. Although this technique may assist in calming an acutely agitated psychotic patient, it does not improve the extent of or time to remission, or the length of hospitalization. If IM haloperidol is used, the occurrence of EPS may eliminate some of the advantages of using an SGA. If the patient is receiving an antipsychotic within the usual therapeutic range, the use of lorazepam 2 mg IM as needed in combination with the maintenance antipsychotic is a rational alternative to an injectable antipsychotic.

CLINICAL CONTROVERSY

Minimal research evidence supports the use of antipsychotic doses beyond the dose range in the Food and Drug Administration (FDA) approved product labeling. Clinicians frequently titrate doses above the approved range, and often attest to symptom improvement when this is done.

STABILIZATION THERAPY

Improvement is usually a slow but steady process over 6 to 12 weeks or longer. During the first 2 to 3 weeks, goals should include increased socialization and improvement in self-care habits and mood. Improvement in formal thought disorder should follow and may take an additional 6 to 8 weeks to respond. Patients who are early in the course of their illness may experience a more rapid resolution of symptoms than individuals who are more chronically ill. In general, if a patient has not received a robust decrease in positive and negative symptoms within 8 to 12 weeks at adequate doses, then an alternate monotherapy antipsychotic in the algorithm should be considered. In a more chronically ill patient, symptoms may continue to improve for 3 to 6 months. During acute stabilization, usual labeled doses of SGAs are recommended (see Table 66–6); with FGAs, a range of 300 to 1,000 mg of chlorpromazine equivalents daily is recommended.[19,22] An optimum dose of the chosen drug should be estimated in the initial treatment plan. If the patient begins to show adequate response before or at this dosage, then the patient should remain at this dosage as long as symptoms continue to improve. In general, adequate time on a therapeutic antipsychotic dose is the most important factor in predicting medication response. However, if necessary, dose titration may continue within the therapeutic range every week or two as long as the patient has no side effects.

Before changing medications in a poorly responding patient, the following should be considered: Were the initial target symptoms indicative of schizophrenia or did they represent manifestations of a different diagnosis, a long-standing behavioral problem, a substance

buse disorder, or a general medical condition? Is the patient ad-
erent with pharmacotherapy? Are the persistent symptoms poorly
esponsive to antipsychotics (e.g., impaired insight or judgment, or
xed delusions)? How does the patient's current status compare with
esponse during previous exacerbations? Would this patient poten-
ally benefit from a change to a different treatment stage (see Fig.
6–1)? Does this patient have a treatment-refractory schizophrenic
lness?

The conclusion that a partially responding patient has achieved
s much symptomatic improvement as possible is one that must be
ade with great care and after considering all possible treatment
lternatives. However, treatment goals must be realistic. Medications
re effective at decreasing many of the symptoms of schizophrenia
and are thus referred to as *palliative*), but they are not curative, and
ll symptoms may not abate. This being said, the treatment approach
hould be assertive. While one should expect none to minimal residual
ositive symptoms with effective treatment, it is still unclear what a
ealistic goal is with regard to maximum improvement in negative
ymptoms.

It is important to screen patients for co-occurring mental disor-
ers, and their presence may become more apparent during the stabi-
ization or maintenance phases of schizophrenia treatment. Examples
nclude substance abuse disorders, depression, obsessive-compulsive
isorder, and panic disorder. As co-occurring disorders will limit
ymptom and functional improvement and increase the risk of re-
apse, it is critical that they be appropriately treated. Pharmacological
nd nonpharmacological interventions specific for the co-occurring
isorder should be implemented in combination with evidence-based
reatment for schizophrenia.

MAINTENANCE TREATMENT

Maintenance drug therapy prevents relapse, as shown in numerous
ouble-blind studies. The average relapse rate after 1 year is 18% to
2% with active drug (including some nonadherent patients) versus
0% to 80% for placebo.[19,23,31]

Available evidence suggests that the 1-year relapse rate may be
ower with SGAs, with an average 1-year relapse rate of 15%.[23,31]
After treatment of the first psychotic episode in a schizophrenic paient, medication should be continued for at least 12 months after
emission.[19,22] Although maintenance treatment in patients with mul-
iple acute episodes is more difficult to define, good medication re-
ponders should be treated for at least 5 years. It is still unknown
hereafter whether low-dose strategies or complete drug tapering and
vithdrawal should be considered in an effort to determine the need for
continued treatment. Continuous or lifetime pharmacotherapy is
ecessary in the majority of patients to prevent relapse. This should
e approached with the lowest effective dose of the antipsychotic that
s likely to be tolerated by the patient.[32] Targeted medication adminis-
ration based on prodromal symptoms was historically recommended
s an alternative to continuous antipsychotic treatment in stabilized
atients. However, studies show continuous medication to be more
ffective than targeted medication in preventing decompensation, in
ecreasing need for hospitalization, and in improving the extent and
uality of employment.[2,19] Therefore the approach of intermittent or
argeted therapy has now been abandoned.

Antipsychotics should be tapered slowly before discontinuation.
Abrupt discontinuation of antipsychotics, especially low-potency
'GAs and clozapine, can result in withdrawal symptoms, felt to be a
nanifestation of rebound cholinergic outflow. Insomnia, nightmares,
eadaches, gastrointestinal symptoms (e.g., abdominal cramps, stom-
ch pain, nausea, vomiting, and diarrhea), restlessness, increased

salivation, and sweating are reported. In general, when switching from
one antipsychotic to another, the first antipsychotic should be tapered
and discontinued over at least 1 to 2 weeks after the second antipsychotic is initiated.[19,20,33] Tapering often needs to occur more slowly,
especially with clozapine.[19,20]

LONG-ACTING OR DEPOT INJECTABLE ANTIPSYCHOTICS

Depot or long-acting antipsychotics are recommended for patients
who are unreliable in taking oral medication on a daily basis, and
thus are not usually used as first-line therapy. Before a long-acting
antipsychotic is initiated, it should be determined whether the patient's medication nonadherence is because of side effects. If so, an
alternative medication with a more favorable side-effect profile should
be considered before a long-acting injectable antipsychotic.

The patient's motivation for treatment is a major factor influencing outcome. Conversion from oral therapy to a long-acting injectable
is most successful in patients who have been stabilized on oral therapy. The ideal patient for a long-acting injectable is the individual
who does not like the daily reminder of oral medication or is unreliable in taking medications. Risperidone recently became available as
the first long-acting injectable formulation of an SGA.[34] Long-acting
risperidone has demonstrated efficacy, with an optimum dose range
likely between 25 and 50 mg given IM every 2 weeks. Doses above
50 mg every 2 weeks are not recommended, as results from one study
showed no greater efficacy but more EPS.[35] The pattern of adverse
effects, especially low propensity to induce EPS and tardive dyskinesia, is similar to that of oral risperidone, and it appears to be well
tolerated by patients.[34,35]

Conversion from an oral antipsychotic to a long-acting medication should start with stabilization on an oral dosage form of the same
agent, or at least a short trial (3 to 7 days), to determine whether the
patient tolerates the medication without significant side effects. Long-
acting risperidone is a suspension of drug in glycolic acid-lactate
copolymer microspheres that must be reconstituted before administration. The microspheres are degraded via hydrolysis with significant
risperidone serum concentrations being measurable approximately
3 weeks after single-dose administration. Thus it is important that the
oral antipsychotic be administered for at least 3 weeks after beginning the injections. Dose adjustments are recommended to be made
no more often than once every 4 weeks.[35]

For fluphenazine decanoate, the simplest dosing conversion
method recommends 1.2 times the oral fluphenazine daily dose for
stabilized patients, rounding up to the nearest 12.5-mg interval, administered in weekly doses for the first 4 to 6 weeks; or 1.6 times
the oral daily dose for more acutely ill patients.[36] Subsequently,
fluphenazine decanoate may be administered once every 2 to 3 weeks.
Oral fluphenazine may be overlapped for 1 week. For haloperidol decanoate, a factor of 10 to 15 times the oral haloperidol daily dose is
commonly recommended, rounding up to the nearest 50-mg interval,
administered in a once-monthly dose with an oral haloperidol overlap
for the first month. A more assertive conversion method recommends
20 times the oral daily dose, but dividing the injection into consecutive doses of 100 to 200 mg every 3 to 7 days until the entire amount is
given.[37] With this method, oral medication overlap was unnecessary.
The haloperidol decanoate dose is decreased by 25% at the second
and third months.

Injection site reactions have been reported with the haloperidol decanoate 100 mg/mL preparation, consisting of painful pruritic swelling at the injection site.[38] Acute EPS can be seen following injections of either fluphenazine or haloperidol decanoate. These

effects are minimized with the use of risperidone microspheres. Both haloperidol and fluphenazine decanoate should be administered by a deep, "Z-tract" intramuscular method. Long-acting risperidone is injected by deep IM injection in the gluteus maximus, but Z-tracting is not necessary. For patients not exposed to the oral drug, an oral test dose of the medication is recommended before administering the first IM dose of the long-acting antipsychotic.

METHODS TO ENHANCE PATIENT ADHERENCE

It is often a challenge for individuals with chronic illnesses to maintain high levels of medication adherence, and partial compliance is thus a reality in the treatment of all chronic illnesses.[39] Individuals with serious mental disorders have somewhat higher nonadherence rates than those with general medical disorders, with the following explanations provided: denial of illness, lack of insight, grandiosity or paranoia, no perceived need for medication, perceived lack of input into choice of medication or dosage, side effects, misperceived "allergies," or the number of medications prescribed or doses received daily. In fact, clinicians should expect partial compliance to be the norm with regard to medication-taking behavior. This should be approached in a nonjudgmental manner, with the clinician actively engaging the patient in care as a mechanism to enhance therapeutic alliance and patient adherence.

Education geared toward patients becoming more informed about their illness and the effectiveness and risks of treatment may help to increase adherence.[40] These programs should be staged so that patients initially receive basic information about their disorder and its symptoms and basic information about their medication and self-monitoring techniques. As the patient is capable of dealing with more complex information, more detailed information regarding schizophrenia, psychosocial treatments, and prognosis should be discussed. Patients and families should be taught self-monitoring techniques and when to report symptom exacerbation or medication side effects to the clinician.[40] Psychoeducation strategies should involve individual counseling as well as group activities.

Recent evidence suggests that the use of cognitive behavioral therapy that focuses on medication adherence can improve patient outcome.[41] This approach is called *compliance therapy*. Groups facilitated by trained individuals who have the illness may be more effective in enhancing awareness and acceptance of schizophrenia and necessary treatment than groups led only by professionals. Active involvement of family members further increases the likelihood of patient adherence with treatment. In addition to programs provided by community mental health centers, support groups operated by consumer groups such as the National Alliance for the Mentally Ill (NAMI) are available in most urban areas. Contact information for local NAMI chapters can be accessed at *http://www.nami.org/Template.cfm?Section=Your_Local_NAMI*. In the hospital, self-medication administration often reinforces the patient's perception of their active role in their own treatment. When patients miss outpatient appointments, active outreach interventions must be implemented to enhance patient engagement in treatment. These include both phone calls and home visits.[19,40,42]

MANAGEMENT OF TREATMENT-RESISTANT SCHIZOPHRENIA

An official definition of "treatment resistance" does not exist.[19] In general, it reflects a patient who has had inadequate symptom response

from multiple antipsychotic trials. Traditionally, treatment resistance has been defined as lack of improvement in positive symptoms, but it can be defined by poor improvement in negative symptoms, or even by medication intolerance. Between 10% and 30% of patients receive minimal symptomatic improvement after multiple FGA monotherapy trials.[19] An additional group of patients (30% to 60%) has partial but inadequate improvement in symptoms or unacceptable side effects associated with antipsychotic use.[19,20]

Atypical Antipsychotics

Only clozapine has shown superiority over other antipsychotics in randomized clinical trials for the management of treatment-resistant schizophrenia. Most other SGAs have either not been studied in treatment-refractory patients or evaluated in small open trials. In a seminal study, clozapine was effective in approximately 30% of patients with treatment-resistant schizophrenia, compared with only 4% treated with a combination of chlorpromazine and benztropine.[43] The results of this study not only demonstrated the efficacy of clozapine in this population, but provided a definition for treatment-resistant schizophrenia. This definition includes treatment failures on three different FGAs from at least two different chemical classes and a history of poor social functioning for the past 5 years.[43] It is significant that when using these criteria for treatment resistance, almost no patients improved with trials of haloperidol and chlorpromazine. These criteria have been subsequently modified to require only two treatment failures, and includes both FGAs and SGAs. Other treatment candidates for clozapine include those patients who cannot tolerate even conservative doses of other antipsychotics.

Symptomatic improvement with clozapine in the treatment-resistant patient often occurs slowly, and as many as 60% of patients may improve if clozapine is used for up to 6 months.[44] This, in combination with clozapine's adverse effects profile, provides sufficient information to conclude that clozapine is not a panacea for schizophrenia. However, as an SGA with proven efficacy in the treatment-resistant population, a therapeutic trial of clozapine is recommended at algorithm stage 3 for those patients who consent to its use and are willing to have the weekly to biweekly blood draws for WBCs. Polydipsia and hyponatremia (psychogenic water drinking) is a frequent problem among treatment-resistant patients, and clozapine reportedly decreases water drinking and increases serum sodium in such patients.[45]

Because of the risk of orthostatic hypotension, clozapine is usually titrated more slowly than other antipsychotics, particularly on an outpatient basis. If a 12.5-mg test dose does not produce hypotension, then clozapine 25 mg at bedtime is recommended, increased to 25 mg twice a day after 3 days, and then increased in 25- to 50-mg/day increments every 3 days until a dose of at least 300 mg/day is reached. Because high doses are associated with significantly increased side effects, including seizures, a clozapine serum concentration is recommended before exceeding 600 mg/day. Although some clinicians add valproate when exceeding this dose to prevent the occurrence of seizures, no evidence supports this intervention, and it is more prudent to start valproate if a seizure occurs.

Augmentation and Combination Strategies

Little empirical evidence exists to guide treatment decisions for patients who do not respond to clozapine.[19,46] Numerous suggestions have been made regarding augmentation of clozapine or other SGAs and using combinations of antipsychotics (see Fig. 66–1).[20,47] Augmentation therapy involves the addition of a nonantipsychotic drug to an antipsychotic drug in a poorly or partially responsive patient, whereas combination treatment involves using two antipsychotics simultaneously. Several guidelines should be followed regarding augmentation: (a) augmentation should be used only in inadequately responding patients; (b) augmentation agents are rarely effective for schizophrenic symptoms when used alone; (c) augmentation responders usually improve rapidly; and (d) if augmentation does not improve symptomatology, the augmenting agent should be discontinued.[22,47]

Mood stabilizers are frequently used as an augmentation strategy. Lithium does not enhance antipsychotic effect, but may improve labile affect and agitated behavior in selected patients. However, a recent meta-analysis showed its effects as an augmenting agent to be inconclusive.[48] Valproic acid and carbamazepine have also been used. A large placebo-controlled trial supports faster symptom improvement when divalproex was used in combination with either olanzapine or risperidone.[49] Enzyme induction with carbamazepine may cause a decrease in antipsychotic serum concentrations and potentially worsen psychotic symptoms in some patients. Dosing of mood stabilizers in treatment-resistant schizophrenia is similar to dosing in bipolar disorder[19] (see Chap. 68).

Selective serotonin (5-HT) reuptake inhibitors (SSRIs), particularly fluoxetine and fluvoxamine, have reasonable evidence for improving negative symptoms when used as augmentation of FGAs. Potential benefits of combining SSRIs with SGAs require more study.[50] Consistently positive results have been reported when using SSRIs to treat obsessive-compulsive symptoms that worsen or arise during clozapine treatment.

β-Blockers such as propranolol, pindolol, and nadolol have been reported to have an antiaggression effect when used in a variety of psychiatric disorders, but particularly in the organic aggressive syndrome.[19] Doses are typically higher than those required for cardiovascular β-blockade, but patients should be monitored carefully for β-blocker–related side effects. Patients may need to be treated with adequate doses for 6 to 8 weeks in order to evaluate an antiaggression response.

Combining an FGA with an SGA and combining different SGAs have been suggested as intervention strategies for treatment-resistant patients. These treatments are based on the hypothesis that using antipsychotics with different mechanisms of action will result in greater efficacy than using any medication individually. Critics argue that combining an FGA with an SGA will negate the advantages of the SGA (e.g., fewer EPS). Pharmacodynamically, no clear rationale exists for explaining how combinations of antipsychotics would produce enhanced efficacy, and increased side effects is a possible result. Increased EPS, elevated prolactin levels, and increased D_2 binding were demonstrated in one small study after the addition of haloperidol 4 mg/day to stable doses of clozapine.[51] In general, a series of antipsychotic monotherapies, including clozapine, are preferred over antipsychotic combinations.[20] However, when this fails to produce desired outcomes, a time-limited combination trial may be attempted (see Fig. 66–1, stages 4 or 6).[19,20,22] As is evidenced in Figure 66–1, this is usually indicated only after inadequate response to clozapine, or in a patient who refuses to give consent for clozapine treatment. Such antipsychotic combination treatment trials should be time limited (6 to 12 weeks) and the patient carefully evaluated with rating scales for changes in symptomatology. If no apparent improvement is observed, then one of the medications should be tapered and discontinued.

ANTIPSYCHOTIC DRUG MECHANISMS OF ACTION

The exact mechanism of action of antipsychotic medications is unknown. Research has centered on antipsychotics' relative affinities to block various neurotransmitter receptors, with recent work focusing on the relative affinity to block D_2 versus 5-HT_{2A} receptors. It has been suggested that current antipsychotics be classified into three different categories: (a) typical or traditional (high D_2 antagonism and low 5-HT_{2A} antagonism); (b) atypical (moderate to high D_2 antagonism and high 5-HT_{2A} antagonism); and (c) atypical clozapine-like (low D_2 antagonism and high 5-HT_{2A} antagonism).[52,53] With the exception of aripiprazole, all current SGAs have a greater affinity for 5-HT_{2A} receptors than D_2 receptors. Aripiprazole is a potent 5-HT_{1A} agonist, and it has been suggested that 5-HT_{1A} agonism may produce a clinical effect similar to 5-HT_{2A} blockade, resulting in an atypical clinical profile.[26,53]

Studies of antipsychotic receptor binding in humans have utilized PET scans to examine neurotransmitter receptor binding at 12 hours postdose in small numbers of individuals who have been dosed to steady state. Using this methodology, at least 60% to 65% occupation of D_2 receptors has been thought necessary to decrease positive psychotic symptoms, whereas blockade of approximately 77% or more of D_2 receptors is associated with EPS.[52,54] FGAs are dopaminergic antagonists with high affinity for D_2 receptors. During chronic treatment with these agents, between 70% and 90% of D_2 receptors in the striatum are usually occupied. Thus treatment with FGAs frequently exceeds the threshold for production of EPS. In contrast, during clozapine treatment only 38% to 47% of D_2 receptors are occupied. Even with doses as high as 900 mg daily, less than 50% of D_2 receptors are occupied.[52,55] Newer SGAs have variable D_2 binding. With low-dose risperidone (2 to 5 mg/day), D_2 binding ranges from 60% to 79%, but with doses greater than 6 mg daily, binding commonly exceeds the 77% threshold associated with the development of EPS. Risperidone 2 mg/day produces 5-HT_{2A} binding greater than 70%, and with 4 mg/day it is nearly 100%.[52,55]

Olanzapine 10 to 20 mg/day produces D_2 binding ranging from 71% to 80%, while at 30 to 40 mg/day, it ranges from 83% to 88%. At 5 mg/day, 5-HT_{2A} receptors are near saturation of binding.[52] Thus risperidone 6 mg and olanzapine 20 mg/day have similar D_2 binding, while both drugs have high 5-HT_{2A} occupancy even at the lower end of the usual therapeutic dose range.[55]

Ziprasidone has the highest 5-HT_{2A}:D_2 affinity ratio of any of the currently available antipsychotics. It is also a potent 5-HT_{1A} agonist.[56]

Quetiapine has the lowest D_2 binding. At doses of 300 to 600 mg/day, D_2 binding ranges from 0% to 27%. Even at quetiapine 800 mg/day, only 30% of D_2 receptors are occupied. At these same daily doses, 45% to 90% of 5-HT_{2A} receptors are occupied. However, when quetiapine D_2 binding is examined 2 to 3 hours postdose, 58% and 64% of receptors were occupied with 400 mg and 450 mg, respectively. This led to the conclusion that transient blockade of dopamine receptors may be adequate to produce antipsychotic effect (and transient rise in serum prolactin concentrations), but long-term D_2 blockade is required for production of EPS and sustained hyperprolactinemia. It was further concluded that low D_2 binding, and thus atypicality, may be directly associated with how rapidly the antipsychotic disassociates from the D_2 receptor.[52,55]

The recent availability of aripiprazole, a partial agonist at D_2 receptors, represents a further elaboration of the dopamine hypothesis of antipsychotic action.[26,53] Based on extensive preclinical studies, it is proposed that aripiprazole works as a functional partial agonist in the hypodopaminergic state, and as a functional but weak dopamine antagonist in the hyperdopaminergic state. Aripiprazole is a rather weak 5-HT$_{2A}$ antagonist, but a potent 5-HT$_{1A}$ agonist, which is also thought to contribute to its atypicality.[26,53] Thus it is clear that the SGAs differ in their mechanisms of action and most likely in the manner in which they produce an atypical clinical profile.

The primary therapeutic effects of FGAs are thought to occur in the limbic system, including the ventral striatum, whereas EPS are thought to be related to DA blockade in the dorsal striatum. Tolerance often develops to the acutely occurring EPS within a few weeks, but tolerance to the antipsychotic effects appears to be less common, if not rare. 5-HT$_{2A}$ antagonism in combination with modest D$_2$ blockade leads to release of dopamine in the prefrontal cortex, and this is one explanation for the decrease in negative symptoms and improvement in cognition reported with atypical antipsychotics. It has also been suggested that polymorphism in the 5-HT$_{2A}$ receptor gene may explain some of the variance in response to clozapine.[53]

Antipsychotics vary in their effects on other neurotransmitter receptor systems, including the antagonism of D$_1$, D$_4$, 5-HT$_{2C}$, 5-HT$_6$, 5-HT$_7$, muscarinic, α_1-adrenergic, and histaminic receptors.[52,53,55] Additionally, clozapine is a partial agonist at D$_1$ receptors, and ziprasidone is a modest inhibitor of the presynaptic reuptake of NE and 5-HT.[53] Although any potential effects of these different mechanisms on differential efficacy is unclear, they do explain some potential differences in the side-effect profiles among antipsychotics. For example, this offers an explanation for side effects such as dry mouth, constipation, sinus tachycardia, and orthostatic hypotension with some antipsychotics. These differences in pharmacodynamic profiles also point out that the SGAs are not all alike, and that patients obtaining an inadequate clinical response (either efficacy or side effects) with one antipsychotic may have a superior response on an alternate drug. Thus serial SGA monotherapy trials should be tried in patients receiving a suboptimal clinical response (see Fig. 66–1).

PHARMACOKINETICS

As a class, antipsychotics are highly lipophilic and highly bound to membranes and plasma proteins. They distribute readily into most tissues with a high blood supply and may accumulate in tissues;

therefore they have large volumes of distribution.[57] Most antipsychotics are largely metabolized, primarily through the cytochrome P450 pathways in the liver, except for ziprasidone, which is largely metabolized by aldehyde oxidase. Risperidone and its active metabolite 6-OH-risperidone are both metabolized through CYP 2D6, and thus are susceptible to polymorphic metabolism. This should be considered in individuals who experience side effects at low doses. In particular, 30% to 35% of Africans and Asians are slow to intermediate metabolizers, in addition to about 7% and 2%, respectively, who are poor metabolizers.[58] Thus approximately 40% of patients in these racial/ethnic groups may have increased sensitivity to side effects with drugs such as risperidone that are primarily metabolized through CYP 2D6. Table 66–7 outlines the prominent metabolic pathways of selected antipsychotics.

Most antipsychotics have fairly long elimination half-lives, in the range of 20 to 40 hours, with the exception of quetiapine and ziprasidone, which have short half-lives.[26,57,59] Thus after dosage stabilization most antipsychotics can be dosed once daily. Although not systematically studied, brain receptor kinetics are different than peripheral kinetics, and it may be possible to dose these SGAs less often than their plasma kinetics would suggest. Efforts to develop relationships between antipsychotic plasma concentrations and clinical response have been hampered by several factors, including the variable lag time between beginning antipsychotic treatment and symptom change, the subjective and relatively imprecise methods of measuring drug effect or symptom change in schizophrenia, the presence of multiple metabolites, and perhaps differences between receptor kinetics and peripheral pharmacokinetics. Among the SGAs, only clozapine has an established therapeutic range, with efficacy being associated with a clozapine plasma concentration greater than 250 to 350 ng/mL. A 12-hour postdose clozapine serum concentration of at least 250 ng/mL is recommended if the patient is receiving divided clozapine doses, or 350 ng/mL if the patient is being dosed once daily. Whether increased symptom improvement occurs with continued dosage increases above these serum concentrations, and a potential maximum therapeutic clozapine serum concentration exists, are poorly defined. However, side effects do increase with increased clozapine serum concentrations. It is likely not cost effective to

TABLE 66–7. Pharmacokinetic Parameters of Selected Antipsychotics

Drug	Bioavailability (%)	Half-life (h)	Major Metabolic Pathways	Active Metabolites
Selected first-generation antipsychotics				
Chlorpromazine	10–30	8–35	FMO3, CYP 3A4	7-hydroxy, others
Fluphenazine	20–50	14–24	CYP 2D6	?
Fluphenazine decanoate		14.2 ± 2.2[a] days		
Haloperidol	40–70	12–36	CYP 1A2, 2D6, 3A4	Reduced haloperidol
Haloperidol decanoate		21 days		
Second-generation antipsychotics				
Aripiprazole	87	48–68	CYP 3A4, 2D6	Dehydroaripiprazole
Clozapine	12–81	11–105	CYP 1A2, 3A4, 2C19	Desmethylclozapine
Olanzapine	80	20–70	CYP 1A2, 3A4, FMO3	N-glucuronide; 2-OH-methyl; 4-N-oxide
Quetiapine	9 ± 4	6.88	CYP 3A4	7-OH-quetiapine
Risperidone	68	3–24	CYP 2D6	9-OH-risperidone
Risperidone Consta		3–6 days	CYP 2D6	9-OH-risperidone
Ziprasidone	59	4–10	Aldehyde oxidase, CYP 3A4	None

[a]Based on multiple-dose data. Single-dose data indicate a β half-life of 6–10 days.
Adapted from De Leon et al,[26] Harrison and Goa,[35] Ereshefsky et al,[36] Ereshefsky et al,[37] Ereshefsky,[57] and ziprasidone package insert.[59]

outinely monitor clozapine serum concentrations in all patients. However, they should be monitored before exceeding 600 mg daily; in patients who develop unusual or severe adverse side effects; in patients who are taking concomitant medications that may cause drug interactions; in patients who have age or pathophysiologic changes suggesting a change in pharmacokinetics; or for assessment of patient adherence.[31]

Long-acting risperidone is a suspension of drug in glycolic acid-lactate copolymer microspheres.[35] After IM injection the polymer is slowly hydrolyzed, and significant risperidone begins being released after about 3 weeks, with therapeutic concentrations achieved in weeks 3 and 4. The apparent β-phase half-life is 3 to 6 days.[35] With dosing every 2 weeks, steady-state risperidone concentrations are achieved after approximately 2 months. Steady-state risperidone concentrations have been reported to be similar in elderly and younger individuals.[35]

The depot FGAs fluphenazine decanoate (also available in an enanthate salt) and haloperidol decanoate are esterified drugs formulated in sesame seed oil for deep intramuscular injection. Their absorption from the muscle and metabolism to the free base is sufficiently slow to cause absorption to be the rate-limiting step in determining their respective apparent half-lives.[36]

ADVERSE EFFECTS

Table 66–8 presents the relative incidence of common categories of antipsychotic side effects. The precise incidence of many of these side effects has not been systematically evaluated. Side effects are discussed below with respect to organ system affected. A general approach to monitoring and assessing side effects requires prospective monitoring by clinicians, preferably using a thorough review of systems approach. Patient-oriented self-rated side-effect scales may also be helpful, because many patients with schizophrenia do not readily complain of side effects, because of a lack of volition, a lack of perception of having input into their treatment, poor understanding, or because of the actual interference of side effects themselves (e.g., sedation).

With the variety of antipsychotics currently available, using an alternative drug should be considered in patients who complain of poorly tolerated side effects. Because medication side effects are one of the primary predictors of patient nonadherence, the clinician should take advantage of the treatment options currently available in an attempt to improve patient outcomes. As new antipsychotics become available, side effects and risks associated with different drugs should be re-evaluated. As we learn more about relative side-effect risks (e.g., weight gain, glucose intolerance, QTc prolongation, acute extrapyramidal side effects, and tardive dyskinesia), it will be necessary to regularly reconsider which antipsychotics should be considered first-line treatment alternatives.

Endocrine System

DA blockade in the tuberoinfundibular tract results in increased prolactin levels, because DA is the major prolactin-inhibiting factor. Galactorrhea may occur in up to 57% of women, and menstrual irregularities or amenorrhea in up to 97%. These effects may be dose related and are more common with the use of FGAs and risperidone. Gynecomastia and galactorrhea are reported in men as well. Tolerance does not appear to develop to these effects.[60] Switching to the SGAs olanzapine, quetiapine, ziprasidone, or aripiprazole, which have no appreciable sustained effect on prolactin, is the most reasonable treatment option. Bromocriptine in doses up to 15 mg daily, or amantadine in doses up to 300 mg daily, has been used to treat prolactin-related symptoms.

The potential risk of osteoporosis is of concern with the long-term use of medications that cause osteoporosis. Inadequate evidence is currently available regarding the potential effects on bone density of long-term antipsychotic-related hyperprolactinemia.

Weight gain is frequently reported in both adults and children receiving antipsychotics.[61,62] Although the exact mechanism is uncertain, weight gain has been associated with antihistaminic effects, antimuscarinic effects, and blockade of 5-HT$_{2C}$ receptors. However, dietary factors and activity levels may play a significant role in this population, as does renourishment after a period of poor self-care. Weight gain may be seen with most atypical antipsychotics. In particular, significant weight gain, as defined by $\geq$7% of the baseline body weight, is associated with clozapine and olanzapine therapy in 40% or more of patients.[61,63] Risperidone and quetiapine may cause weight gain, but much less than that caused by clozapine or olanzapine. Ziprasidone and aripiprazole both have been associated with minimal weight gain.

The clinical significance of weight gain during antipsychotic therapy is substantial. The risk of cardiovascular-related mortality is higher in individuals with schizophrenia,[64,65] and this is further

TABLE 66–8. Relative Side Effect Incidence of Commonly Used Antipsychotics

	Sedation	EPS	Anticholinergic	Orthostasis	Weight Gain	Prolactin
Aripiprazole	+	+	±	±	±	±
Chlorpromazine	++++	+++	+++	++++	++	+++
Clozapine	++++	±	++++	++++	++++	±
Fluphenazine	+	++++	+	+	+	++++
Haloperidol	+	++++	+	+	+	++++
Olanzapine	++	++	++	++	++++	+
Perphenazine	++	++++	++	+	+	++++
Quetiapine	++	±	+	++	++	±
Risperidone	+	++	+	++	++	++++
Thioridazine	++++	+++	++++	++++	+	+++
Thiothixene	+	++++	+	+	+	++++
Ziprasidone	++	++	±	+	±	+

Side effects shown are relative risk based on doses within the recommended therapeutic range.
Individual patient risk varies depending on patient-specific factors.
EPS, extrapyramidal side effects; Relative side-effect risk: ±, negligible; +, low; ++, moderate; +++, moderately high; ++++, high.

aggravated by drug-related weight gain. Additionally, obesity is a risk factor for diabetes mellitus.[66] Weight gain during treatment is a major reason for poor patient medication adherence, and patients commonly report weight gain as being a concern.[67]

As in all patient populations, interventions for weight reduction in persons with schizophrenia are far from perfect. A number of pharmacological interventions have been attempted for antipsychotic-related weight gain, but in general these should be discouraged. Switching patients to an SGA less likely to cause weight gain, dietary restriction, exercise, and behavior modification programs are reported to be successful in small short-term studies.[68] An American Diabetes Association consensus task force recommends consideration of a change in antipsychotic if a patient gains more than 5% of baseline body weight after starting the drug.[69]

Schizophrenic patients have a higher prevalence of type II diabetes than the nonschizophrenic population. Beyond this, antipsychotics may adversely affect glucose levels in diabetic patients. The extent to which these effects are related to drug-induced weight increase is unclear.[63,70,71] A single-dose study suggests that SGAs impair glucose tolerance and increase insulin secretion, which supports a potential effect on glucose regulation independent of weight increase. A naturalistic study of patients taking clozapine found a 5-year rate of new-onset diabetes totaling 52%.[71] New-onset diabetes has been reported during treatment with risperidone, olanzapine, quetiapine, and ziprasidone; aripiprazole is too new in clinical practice to draw conclusions regarding any association with diabetes. Although there are more reports of diabetes during treatment with clozapine or olanzapine, epidemiologic studies provide conflicting data regarding the relative risk of different SGAs to produce diabetes mellitus.[70] At present, the overall incidence, relative occurrence across agents, and treatment-patient related risk factors for diabetes during antipsychotic therapy are unknown. In March 2004 the FDA issued a safety alert requiring revisions in the labeling of all SGAs, that describes the increased risk of diabetes mellitus in patients taking atypical antipsychotics.[72] Given the public health significance of diabetes, clarifying the diabetogenic effect of SGAs is a major focus of current research. Moreover, designing care models and standards for managing diabetes in patients with schizophrenia is another major consideration. Clozapine and olanzapine should be used with caution in patients with preexisting diabetes.

CLINICAL CONTROVERSY

The relative role of individual SGAs in precipitating diabetes mellitus is unclear. Clinicians are increasingly concerned about the escalating number of new cases of diabetes mellitus being reported in patients taking SGAs. It is clear, however, that obesity is associated with an increased risk of type II diabetes mellitus; olanzapine and clozapine have been shown to cause more weight gain than other SGAs.

Cardiovascular System

Orthostatic Hypotension. Postural or orthostatic hypotension, defined as a greater than 20-mm Hg drop in systolic pressure, is caused by α-adrenergic blockade, which inhibits reflex vasoconstriction when rising to a sitting or standing position; this appears to be a combination of local vasodilatory effects and central inhibition of the vasomotor center, as well as sympatholysis leading to an unopposed β-adrenergic effect.[73] Patients may experience light-headedness or syncope. Associated with lower potency FGAs and SGAs (especially

on intramuscular or intravenous administration), orthostatic hypotension can occur in any patient, but diabetic patients with preexisting cardiovascular disease and the elderly seem particularly predisposed. For mild cases, patient education should address slow changes in posture to allow for adaptation and/or the use of support hose. For most patients, tolerance to this effect occurs within 2 to 3 months. If tolerance does not occur, lower doses or a change to an antipsychotic with less α-blockade can be attempted.

Electrocardiographic Changes. Among the antipsychotics, thioridazine, mesoridazine, clozapine, and ziprasidone are most likely to cause electrocardiogram (ECG) changes. ECG changes include increased heart rate (through sinus tachycardia from anticholinergic effects, or reflex tachycardia from α-adrenergic blockade), flattened T waves, ST segment depression, and prolongation of QT and PR intervals. The most clinically important of these potential changes is prolongation of the QTc interval, which has been associated with ventricular arrhythmias, including torsades de pointes syndrome. Thioridazine has been shown to prolong the QTc interval on average about 20 milliseconds (ms) longer than haloperidol, risperidone, olanzapine, or quetiapine.[63,74] Thioridazine's effects on QTc prolongation appear to be dose related. For this reason, thioridazine and mesoridazine (an active metabolite of thioridazine) have a black box warning in the FDA-approved product labeling with regard to this effect. Torsades de pointes has been reported with thioridazine, which may cause cardiac sudden death. Given the number of antipsychotic options currently available, few reasons exist to use either thioridazine or mesoridazine. In the same study, ziprasidone prolonged the QTc interval about 10 ms longer than did haloperidol, risperidone, olanzapine, or quetiapine—about one-half of the effect of thioridazine.[63] Ziprasidone effects were not dose related. Widespread clinical use suggests that ziprasidone's effects on the ECG are not associated with clinical sequelae, unless the patient has baseline risk factors.[20] Although the precise point at which QTc prolongation becomes clinically dangerous is unclear, it has been recommended to discontinue a medication associated with QTc prolongation if the interval consistently exceeds 500 ms.

Greater caution regarding antipsychotic choice and use is necessary in the elderly, in patients with preexisting cardiac disease, and in patients taking diuretics or medications that may prolong the QTc interval.[20,59,63] In patients older than 50 years of age, a pretreatment ECG is recommended, as are baseline serum potassium and magnesium levels. These factors should be considered in antipsychotic selection.[59]

Lipid Changes

Treatment with at least some SGAs and phenothiazines appears associated with elevations in serum triglycerides and cholesterol. As with diabetes, the extent to which this adverse event differs among agents is unclear, although less risk for change in serum lipid or cholesterol levels may occur with risperidone, ziprasidone, or aripiprazole.[65]

The occurrence of weight gain, diabetes, and lipid abnormalities during antipsychotic therapy is consistent with the development of metabolic syndrome (i.e., syndrome X). The metabolic syndrome consists of raised triglycerides (≥150 mg/dL), low HDL cholesterol (≤40 mg/dL for males, ≤50 mg/dL for females), elevated fasting glucose (≥100 mg/dL), blood pressure elevation (≥130/85 mm Hg), and weight gain (abdominal circumference >102 cm for males, >88 cm in females).[65] These abnormalities, either alone or in combination, dictate an important role for general health screening and monitoring n patients with schizophrenia, and prompt intervention when such abnormalities occur. The propensity of individual antipsychotics to produce metabolic disturbances should be considered in the context of individual patient risk factors at the time of drug selection, and in patient monitoring during treatment.

Autonomic Nervous System

Patients receiving antipsychotics, or antipsychotics in combination with anticholinergics, may experience anticholinergic side effects (e.g., dry mouth, constipation, tachycardia, blurred vision, inhibition or impairment of ejaculation, urinary retention, or impaired memory). This is particularly so with low-potency FGAs, and the elderly are especially sensitive to these effects. Of the SGAs, clozapine and olanzapine have moderately high rates of anticholinergic effects. System-specific effects are discussed under the appropriate heading. Dry mouth can be managed with increased intake of fluids, oral lubricants (Xerolube), ice chips, or use of sugarless chewing gum or hard candy. Constipation, caused by slowed peristaltic movement and decreased intestinal fluid content, should be closely monitored and treated, especially in the elderly. Paralytic ileus and necrotizing enterocolitis may also occur. Constipation can be treated with increases in fluid and dietary fiber intake, and exercise.

Central Nervous System

Extrapyramidal System

DYSTONIA

Dystonia is defined as a state of abnormal tonicity, sometimes described simplistically as a severe "muscle spasm."[75] Dystonias may be dramatic, frightening, and painful. More accurately, they are prolonged tonic contractions, with a rapid onset, usually within 24 to 96 hours of dosage initiation or dosage increase. They may be life-threatening, as in the case of pharyngeal-laryngeal dystonias, and can contribute to patient nonadherence. Types of dystonic reactions include trismus, glossospasm, tongue protrusion, pharyngeal-laryngeal dystonia, blepharospasm, oculogyric crisis, torticollis, and retrocollis. Dystonic reactions occur primarily with FGAs. Risk factors include younger patients (especially males), the use of high-potency agents, and high dosage. The overall incidence from the 1960s through the mid-1970s ranged from 2.3% to 10%, but as higher-potency traditional antipsychotics became more widely used, the rate increased to as high as 64%.

Intramuscular or intravenous anticholinergics (Table 66–9) or benzodiazepines are the treatments of choice for dystonia. Benztropine mesylate 2 mg or diphenhydramine 50 mg may be given intramuscularly or intravenously. Diazepam 5 to 10 mg by slow IV push or lorazepam 1 to 2 mg intramuscularly are treatment alternatives. Relief is typically seen within 15 to 20 minutes of an intramuscular injection and within 5 minutes of intravenous administration. If no response is seen within 15 minutes of intravenous injection or within 30 minutes of intramuscular injection, the dose can be repeated. The antipsychotic may be continued, with concomitant short-term use of oral anticholinergic agents. In general, prophylactic anticholinergic medications are not recommended routinely with all FGAs. However, prophylaxis is reasonable when using high-potency FGAs (e.g., haloperidol or fluphenazine) in young men, and in patients with a history of dystonia.[75] Dystonias may also be minimized by the use

TABLE 66–9. Agents Used to Treat Extrapyramidal Side Effects

Generic Name	Equivalent Dose (mg)	Daily Dosage Range (mg)
Antimuscarinics		
Benztropine[a]	1	1–8[b]
Biperiden[a]	2	2–8
Trihexyphenidyl	2	2–15
Anithistaminic		
Diphenhydramine[a]	50	50–400
Dopamine agonist		
Amantadine	N/A	100–400
Benzodiazepines		
Lorazepam[a]	N/A	1–8
Diazepam	N/A	2–20
Clonazepam	N/A	2–8
β-Blockers		
Propranolol	N/A	20–160

[a]Injectable dosage form can be given intramuscularly for relief of acute dystonia.
[b]Dosage may be titrated to 12 mg/day with care; nonlinear pharmacokinetics have been demonstrated.

of lower initial FGA doses. Anticholinergics are good choices for prophylaxis, whereas amantadine has not been proved effective for this purpose. The risk of dystonia is greatly reduced with SGAs. The availability of olanzapine and ziprasidone injectables introduces a rapid-acting injection with a low risk of dystonia.

AKATHISIA

Akathisia is defined as the inability to sit still and as being functionally motor restless. The most accurate diagnosis is made by combining subjective complaints with objective symptoms (pacing, shifting, shuffling, or tapping feet). Subjectively, patients may describe a feeling of inner restlessness or disquiet or a compulsion to move or remain in constant motion. Akathisia occurs in 20% to 40% of patients treated with high-potency FGAs.[75] The majority of patients receiving FGAs may actually experience akathisia, but the reported incidence reflects only patients who can verbalize their feelings or recognize akathisia as being different from psychosis. Akathisia is frequently accompanied by dysphoria. Detection of akathisia requires a high degree of interviewer sensitivity, and symptoms can be quantified by use of the Barnes Akathisia Scale.

Many treatments for akathisia, although accepted to be effective, are based on anecdotal data. Treatment with anticholinergic agents, usually considered the standard treatment for all acute extrapyramidal side effects, is disappointing for akathisia, but may be helpful in patients with concomitant pseudoparkinsonism.[75] Traditionally, reduction in antipsychotic dosage has been considered the best intervention; however, this may not be a realistic goal in an acutely psychotic patient. A logical alternative is to switch to an SGA, an SGA with a lower risk of akathisia, or an antipsychotic previously used in the patient without adverse effect. Akathisia may occasionally occur with SGAs, and this seems to be the most common EPS-like symptom reported with SGAs. Although head-to-head comparisons are not widely available, quetiapine and clozapine appear to have the lowest risk of producing akathisia.[22,59]

Benzodiazepines have been used for treatment of akathisia, but the high prevalence of co-occurring substance abuse in schizophrenia discourages their prescribing.[75] The β-blockers propranolol in doses up to 160 mg daily, nadolol in doses up to 80 mg daily, and metoprolol in β_2-selective doses of 100 mg daily or less are reported as effective.[75]

Clonidine has also been investigated, and hypotension and sedation were the only observed side effects. Preventive measures for akathisia include using the lowest possible FGA dose, or preferably, the use of SGAs.

PSEUDOPARKINSONISM

Pseudoparkinsonism, produced by D_2 blockade in the nigrostriatum, resembles idiopathic Parkinson's disease. A patient with pseudoparkinsonism may present with any of four cardinal symptoms: (1) akinesia, bradykinesia, or decreased motor activity including difficulty initiating movement, as well as extreme slowness, mask-like facial expression, micrographia, slowed speech, and decreased arm swing; (2) tremor, known as pill-rolling type, that is predominant at rest and decreases with movement, usually involving the fingers and hands, although tremors may also be seen in the arms, legs, neck, head, and chin (it may often be activated in resting body parts by having the patient perform mechanical movements with one extremity); (3) cogwheel rigidity, seen as the patient's limbs yielding in jerky, ratchet-like fashion when passively moved by the examiner (a mild form may present as stiffness); and (4) postural abnormalities and instability manifested as stooped posture, difficulty in maintaining stability when changing body position, and a gait that ranges from slow and shuffling to festinating (a result of autonomic dysfunction combined with a shift in the center of gravity due to the stooped posture). Accessory symptoms include the autonomic manifestations seborrhea, sialorrhea, and hyperhidrosis.[75] Fatigue and weakness may be noted, as well as oral abnormalities including dysphagia and dysarthria, and abnormal palmomental and glabellar reflexes. A variant of pseudoparkinsonism is rabbit syndrome, a perioral tremor. The overall incidence of pseudoparkinsonism from FGAs ranges from 15.4% to 36%, depending on the drug and dose. Akinesia alone can be seen in 59% of patients on high-potency FGAs. Other risk factors include increasing age and possibly female gender. The onset of symptoms is typically 1 to 2 weeks after initiation of antipsychotic therapy or a dose increase.

The efficacy of anticholinergic medications in alleviating or attenuating symptoms of pseudoparkinsonism is well established.[75] Benztropine is advantageous in that its longer half-life allows once- to twice-daily dosing. Typical dosing is 1 to 2 mg twice a day up to a usual maximum dosage of 8 mg daily, although some patients will continue to respond to doses up to 12 mg. Dosage titration should be slow, as benztropine displays nonlinear pharmacokinetics, and side effects may become unacceptable. Trihexyphenidyl (2 to 5 mg three times a day), diphenhydramine (25 to 50 mg three times a day), and biperiden (2 mg three times a day) usually require thrice-daily administration. Diphenhydramine produces more sedation than the other agents. Although it has been suggested that trihexyphenidyl is more likely to be abused, all of the anticholinergics have been abused for their euphoriant effects.[76] With all of these agents, symptoms typically begin to resolve within 3 to 4 days after initiation of treatment, but a minimum of at least 2 weeks of treatment is normally required for full response. Amantadine is generally as efficacious for pseudoparkinsonism as anticholinergics, with significantly less effect on memory function.[75] Its mechanism of action involves enhancement of dopaminergic tone in the striatum. Excessive doses may produce anxiety, agitation, restlessness, or uncommonly exacerbation of psychosis. Dosage adjustment is necessary with renal insufficiency. The need for prophylactic use of these agents against pseudoparkinsonism is less convincing than with dystonias, and is unnecessary when using SGAs.[75] The long-term treatment of pseudoparkinsonism with antiparkinsonism medication

is somewhat controversial, and an attempt should be made to taper and discontinue these agents 6 weeks to 3 months after symptom resolution. If symptoms reappear, then switching to an SGA should be considered. The risk of pseudoparkinsonism with SGAs is extremely low. When risperidone is used in doses greater than 6 mg/day, the risk of pseudoparkinsonism symptoms approaches that with FGAs. However, in doses lower than 6 mg/day, the risk of pseudoparkinsonism appears similar to that of olanzapine or ziprasidone.[20] Quetiapine, aripiprazole, or clozapine are reasonable alternatives in a patient experiencing extrapyramidal side effects with other SGAs.[20,22,26,75]

TARDIVE DYSKINESIA

Tardive dyskinesia is a syndrome characterized by abnormal involuntary movements occurring late in onset in relation to initiation of antipsychotic therapy. Tardive dyskinesia is sometimes irreversible and continues to be a controversial issue, clinically, legally, and ethically.

The classic description of tardive dyskinesia is the buccolingualmasticatory (BLM) syndrome, or orofacial movements. The onset of BLM movements is usually insidious. Typically, they are the first detectable signs of tardive dyskinesia, and begin with mild forward, backward, or lateral movements of the tongue. As the disorder progresses, more obvious or frank BLM movements appear, including tongue thrusting, rolling, or fly-catching movements, and chewing or lateral jaw movements. Tardive dyskinesia symptoms may interfere with the patient's ability to chew, speak, or swallow. Further complications include oral ulcerations, inability to wear dentures, and inflammation and loosening of mandibular joints. Eating difficulties and malnutrition may be primary physical complications of tardive dyskinesia. Weight loss may be seen in patients with esophageal or respiratory manifestations but not in those with truncal movements. Facial movements include frequent blinking, brow arching, grimacing, upward deviation of the eyes, and lip smacking. Involvement of the extremities sometimes occurs, with the appearance of restless choreiform (irregular spasmodic) and distal athetosis (slow, writhing movement) of limbs including twisting, spreading, flexion (bending) and extension of fingers, toe tapping, and toe dorsiflexion (upward turning). Unusual posture, hyperextension, pelvic thrusting, axial hyperkinesia (excessive muscular activity of head and trunk), ballismus (jerking or shaking), exaggerated lordosis (bending backward), rocking, and swaying are occasionally observed. Among the more common differential diagnoses are withdrawal dyskinesias occurring after short-term use of antipsychotics, spontaneous orofacial dyskinesias in the elderly, orofacial dyskinesias in the edentulous, stereotypic movements in schizophrenics, Huntington's disease, and congenital torsion dystonia. Orofacial movements are reported more commonly in older patients, whereas the truncal axial movements are classically reported in young adults. Movements may worsen with stress, decrease with sedation, and disappear during sleep. Concentration on motor tasks or attempts to suppress the movements voluntarily may actually increase them.

Early signs of tardive dyskinesia may be reversible, but if allowed to persist or if not detected in the early stages, they may become irreversible, even with drug discontinuation. When the antipsychotic dose is decreased or tapered and discontinued, there is often a worsening of abnormal movements and then possibly a slow improvement after months or years if the patient remains on lower doses or discontinues treatment. No standardized diagnostic criteria for tardive dyskinesia are available. Abnormal involuntary movements can be detected early through physical assessment and the use of rating scales. Available

ating scales include the abnormal involuntary movement scale (AIMS) and the Dyskinesia Identification System: Condensed User Scale.[75,77] Neither scale is diagnostic in itself.

Risk factors include increasing age, the occurrence of acute extrapyramidal side effects, poor antipsychotic drug response, diagnosis of organic mental disorder, diabetes mellitus, mood disorders, and possibly female gender.[78,79] Duration of antipsychotic therapy, daily dosage, and possibly total cumulative dosage are probably the most significant risk factors. However, persistent dyskinesias may occur with as little as 6 months of therapy. Overall morbidity and mortality are greater in tardive dyskinesia patients, and patients with tardive dyskinesia show a greater incidence of respiratory tract infections and cardiovascular illness.

With FGAs, the reported incidence of tardive dyskinesia ranges from 0.5% to 62%.[78] In a first episode of schizophrenia, the incidence is estimated at about 5% per year, with the overall prevalence ranging from 20% to 25% with long-term treatment. Among the elderly, the overall risk of tardive dyskinesia is higher, with the 3-year FGA treatment prevalence estimated at 53%.[79] Tardive dyskinesia is not always permanent, with remission of symptoms observed in 25% of patients after 5 years of continued treatment.[75,78,79]

The risk of tardive dyskinesia with SGAs is significantly lower. A systematic review of 11 studies with SGAs lasting 1 year or more found an overall risk of tardive dyskinesia to be about 0.8% per year in nonelderly adults and 5.3% per year in the elderly. For individual agents, the annual incidence rates ranged from zero to 0.5% for olanzapine to 0.6% to 0.7% for risperidone or quetiapine. Given that most of the patients in these studies had been previously treated with FGAs, the true risk of tardive dyskinesia with SGAs could potentially be lower.[80] To date, there are no reports of tardive dyskinesia with clozapine monotherapy. Although introduced in the United States in 1990, it has been used in some European countries since the early 1970s.

Prevention of tardive dyskinesia is important, as treatment of the movements once they occur is difficult. Because of data suggesting a lower risk of tardive dyskinesia with SGAs, these agents are considered treatments of first choice[19,20,22,80] (see Fig. 66–1). Regular neurologic examinations (AIMS or other scales) should be performed at baseline and at least quarterly to assess for early signs of tardive dyskinesia. At the first signs of tardive dyskinesia, the need for continuing antipsychotic treatment should be reassessed. In such situations, if the patient is taking an FGA and continuing treatment is indicated, the medication should be switched to an SGA.

Numerous drugs have been used in an attempt to treat tardive dyskinesia, representing various strategies affecting CNS neurotransmission. In two controlled trials lasting 22 to 52 weeks, clozapine decreased abnormal involuntary movements.[79,81] Switching antipsychotic therapy to clozapine is a favored first-line pharmacotherapeutic strategy, particularly in patients with moderate to severe dyskinesias.[78,79,81] Limited evidence suggests that olanzapine may decrease symptoms, and no data are available with other SGAs.[81] A systematic review of studies with vitamin E suggest that it may help prevent deterioration in tardive dyskinesia symptoms, but have no effect on symptom improvement.[82]

Sedation and Cognition. Sedation must be recognized as an antipsychotic side effect and not as an indication of therapeutic effect. It occurs more frequently with antipsychotics with antihistaminic properties. Chlorpromazine, thioridazine, mesoridazine, clozapine, olanzapine, and quetiapine are most frequently implicated. Administration of most or all of the daily dosage at bedtime (depending on the drug half-life) can decrease daytime sedation and in some patients eliminate the need for hypnotic agents. Sedation occurs early in treatment

and may decrease over time.[73] Oversedation may play a large role in cognitive, perceptual, and motor dysfunction. With acute dosing, tasks requiring vigilance, attention, or motor behavior may be impaired. However, the positive effects of medication are seen with chronic administration, evidenced by improvements in tasks involving visual-motor skills, attention to task, and working memory. Compared with FGAs, several studies have shown cognitive benefits of SGAs. Comparative effects of different SGAs on cognition are as yet unclear, but available studies suggest that different SGAs may have effects on varying cognitive domains.[83] An algorithm-driven disease management program utilizing SGAs as first-line treatment was shown to improve cognition over a 9-month period.[84] Since SGAs appear to have beneficial effects on cognition, ongoing research is evaluating the clinical significance of this effect, and the relative effects of different SGAs.

Seizures. Antipsychotics lower the seizure threshold through GABA depletion, changes in CNS permeability leading to enhanced conduction of a discharge, disruption of DA-acetylcholine balance, or the activation of a latent seizure focus. There is an increased risk of drug-induced seizures in all patients treated with antipsychotics. However, this risk is greater if the following predisposing factors are present: preexisting seizure disorder, history of drug-induced seizure, abnormal electroencephalogram (EEG), and preexisting CNS pathology or head trauma. Seizures are more closely associated with the use of higher doses, rapid dosage increases, and upon initiation of treatment. When an isolated seizure occurs, a dosage decrease is first recommended; anticonvulsant therapy is not recommended. Although spontaneously occurring seizures have been reported with most antipsychotics, the highest potential risk for an antipsychotic-related seizure is with clozapine or chlorpromazine. Based on EEG findings, olanzapine may also be associated with greater risk. If a change in antipsychotic therapy is required because of a drug-induced seizure, risperidone, molindone, thioridazine, haloperidol, pimozide, trifluoperazine, and fluphenazine are associated with the lowest potential.[85]

Thermoregulation. Poikilothermia, the body temperature adjusting to the ambient temperature, can be a serious side effect of antipsychotic therapy in temperature extremes.[86] Hyperpyrexia can be a danger in hot weather or during exercise. Inhibition of sweating, a result of anticholinergic properties impairing the peripheral mechanisms of heat dissipation, can also contribute to this problem, which in its severest form can lead to heat stroke. Hypothermia is also a risk, particularly in the elderly and in cold climates. All patients receiving antipsychotics should be educated about these potential problems. Thermoregulatory problems are reportedly more common with the use of low-potency FGAs and may occur with the more anticholinergic SGAs.

Neuroleptic Malignant Syndrome. Neuroleptic malignant syndrome (NMS) occurs in 0.5% to 1% of patients receiving FGAs. The rate of NMS has diminished since the introduction of SGAs, and reliable current estimates are not available. NMS may occur more frequently in patients receiving high-potency FGAs, injectable or depot FGAs, and in patients who are dehydrated, with physical exhaustion, or organic mental disorders. Although less common than with FGAs, NMS has been reported with SGAs, including clozapine. The onset of symptoms varies from early in treatment to months later. It develops rapidly, over the course of 24 to 72 hours. NMS may occur after antipsychotic discontinuation, especially when depot agents are used. Possible mechanisms of NMS include disruption of the central thermoregulatory process or excess production of heat secondary to skeletal muscle contractions. The differential diagnosis includes heat stroke, lethal catatonia, anesthetic-associated malignant hyperthermia, anticholinergic toxicity, and monoamine oxidase inhibitor drug interactions. Cardinal signs and symptoms of NMS are body temperature exceeding 38°C (100.4°F), altered level of consciousness, autonomic dysfunction (tachycardia, labile blood pressure, diaphoresis, tachypnea, or urinary or fecal incontinence), and rigidity. Laboratory evaluation, although considered nonspecific, frequently shows leukocytosis with or without a left shift, increases in creatine kinase (CK), aspartate aminotransferase, alanine aminotransferase, lactate dehydrogenase, and myoglobinuria.[87,88]

Treatment should always begin with antipsychotic discontinuation and supportive care. In many cases that alone is effective. The role of adjunctive agents is unclear, yet they are often practical in clinical settings. The DA agonist bromocriptine, used in theory to reverse DA blockade, reduces rigidity, fever, or CK in up to 94% of patients, whereas the use of another DA agonist, amantadine, has been successfully used in up to 63% of patients. Dantrolene has been used as a skeletal muscle relaxant, with effects on temperature, heart rate, respiratory rate, and CK in up to 81% of patients.[87,88] Wide recognition and rapid antipsychotic discontinuation has drastically reduced mortality from 20% 15 years ago to 4% in the mid-1990s.

Many patients with schizophrenia, despite having had NMS, will require future antipsychotic pharmacotherapy. Patient selection for rechallenge is important, as only those patients in need of reinstitution of antipsychotics should receive future trials. A review of antipsychotic rechallenges suggests that the risk of rechallenge is acceptable in most patients, provided that the patient is observed for an extended period of time (2 weeks or more is suggested) without antipsychotics, that there is careful monitoring and slow dose titration, and that the patient is maintained on the lowest possible dose.[87] Only SGAs should be used for rechallenge following an episode of NMS. Neither patient-specific demographic variables nor antipsychotic agent used assist in predicting recurrence.

Psychiatric Side Effects. Antipsychotic-induced akathisia, akinesia, and dysphoria may have unfortunate sequelae, resulting in what has been termed "behavioral toxicity."[30] Akathisia has resulted in impulsivity and in extreme cases, violence and suicide. Akinesia, characterized by "diminished spontaneity," results in symptoms of apathy and withdrawal, often mistaken for the negative symptoms of schizophrenia; these patients may actually appear depressed on formal evaluation.

Delirium and psychosis are reported with larger doses of FGAs or combinations of anticholinergics with FGAs. Chronic confusion and disorientation can occur in the elderly as a result of antipsychotic treatment.[89] Unfortunately, the link is not always made between initiation of antipsychotic therapy, and the patient may be misdiagnosed with an organic mental disorder. This clinical presentation, called a "pseudodementia," is easily reversible on discontinuation of the antipsychotic.

Exacerbation and new onset of obsessive-compulsive symptoms have been reported with clozapine, and has anecdotally been reported to improve with addition of an SSRI.[90]

Ophthalmologic Effects. Anticholinergic effects of antipsychotics or concomitant antiparkinson medications can exacerbate narrow-angle (angle closure) glaucoma. Antipsychotics with low anticholinergic effects should be used in such individuals, and they should be appropriately monitored.[91]

Opaque deposits in the cornea and lens occur with chronic phenothiazine treatment, most frequently with chlorpromazine. Although visual acuity is not usually affected, periodic slit-lamp ophthalmologic examinations are frequently recommended in patients receiving long-term treatment with phenothiazines.

Because of cataract development and lenticular changes in animals, baseline and periodic eye exams are recommended in the product labeling for patients receiving quetiapine.[92] However, clinical experience with quetiapine since marketing has not supported a significant risk of cataracts.[22,92] Retinitis pigmentosa can result from use of thioridazine doses greater than 800 mg daily. It is caused by melanin deposits, and can result in permanent visual impairment or blindness. There is no evidence that it is a function of cumulative dose.[91]

Hepatic System

Cholestatic hepatocanalicular jaundice has been reported in up to 2% of patients receiving phenothiazines. Additionally, liver function test (LFT) abnormalities (elevated aminotransferases and alkaline phosphatase), often asymptomatic, were reported in up to 50% of patients.[93] If aminotransferases are greater than three times the upper limit of normal, antipsychotic therapy should be changed to a chemically unrelated antipsychotic.

Overall, LFT abnormalities are uncommon with SGAs. However, cholestatic hepatitis has been reported with risperidone,[94] and LFT abnormalities, mostly transient, have been reported to be more frequent with clozapine than haloperidol.[95]

Genitourinary System

Urinary hesitancy and retention is reported with low-potency FGAs and with clozapine. Anticholinergic effects cause smooth muscle slowing and paralyze the detrusor muscle of the bladder, requiring greater urine volume to evoke muscle contraction. Men with benign prostatic hypertrophy are especially prone to this effect.[89]

Urinary incontinence is thought to be caused by α-blockade, and among the SGAs, it appears to be particularly problematic with clozapine. The incidence has been reported to be as high as 44%, and it may be persistent in 25% of patients.[96]

Numerous different mechanisms have been suggested to cause sexual dysfunction, including dopaminergic blockade, hyperprolactinemia, histaminergic blockade (sedation), anticholinergic effects, and α-adrenergic blockade. This area is inadequately studied, and multiple mechanisms are likely responsible for producing sexual dysfunction. Unmedicated individuals with schizophrenia report decreased libido. However, to varying degrees antipsychotics produce decreased libido and sexual dysfunction. Most but not all studies have shown a relationship between hyperprolactinemia and sexual dysfunction, including decreased libido, erectile dysfunction, difficulty achieving orgasm, and ejaculatory abnormalities. While risperidone produces at least as much sexual dysfunction as FGAs, other SGAs, which have weak effects on prolactin or are "prolactin-sparing," produce less sexual dysfunction. It is unclear whether hyperprolactinemia directly impairs sexual functioning, reflects high dopaminergic blockade from risperidone and FGAs, or is associated with other mechanisms of producing sexual dysfunction. Some evidence suggests that hyperprolactinemia may be associated with low testosterone concentrations, which could be associated with altered sexual functioning. Patients experiencing sexual dysfunction with FGAs or risperidone should be switched to an SGA with less effect on prolactin.[97]

Hematologic System

Transient leukopenia may occur during initial treatment with antipsychotics; however, it typically does not progress to clinically significant parameters.[98] If the WBC count is less than 3,000/mm^3, or if the absolute neutrophil count (ANC) is less than 1,000/mm^3, the antipsychotic should be discontinued, and the WBC monitored closely until it returns to normal. Agranulocytosis reportedly occurs in 0.01% of patients receiving FGAs, and more frequently with chlorpromazine and thioridazine. The onset is usually within the first 8 weeks of therapy. Agranulocytosis may initially manifest clinically as a local infection, with sore throat, leukoplakia, erythema, and ulcerations of the pharynx. These symptoms in any patient receiving antipsychotics should signal the immediate need for a WBC count. If either the WBC or ANC falls below these parameters, the drug should be discontinued immediately and the patient monitored closely for the development of secondary infections. Isolated rare cases of thrombocytopenia and eosinophilia have been reported.

Agranulocytosis with clozapine significantly limits the clinical utility of this agent. Data on the incidence since the release of clozapine in February 1990 following stringent monitoring guidelines reveal that the 1-year treatment risk of developing agranulocytosis with clozapine is approximately 0.8%, and the 18-month risk is 0.91%.[99] Increasing age and female gender are associated with greater risk. Based on available data, the time period for greatest risk appears to be between months 1 and 6 of treatment, and weekly WBC monitoring for the first 6 months of therapy is mandated in the FDA-approved product labeling.[100] After the first 6 months, the labeling allows the frequency of WBC monitoring to be decreased to every 2 weeks. If the total WBC count drops to less than 2,000/mm^3, or the ANC is less than 1,000/mm^3, clozapine should be discontinued and the patient monitored closely. Some clinicians have used the granulocyte colony-stimulating factor filgrastim with hopes of improving the outcome by hastening resolution or decreasing morbidity. One case series that used filgrastim (starting dose of 300 mcg/day SC, increased by 300 mcg/day until 900 mcg/day is reached, and then continued until the agranulocytosis is resolved) demonstrated a decrease in time to resolution and decreased intensive care bed costs when compared to historical controls.[101] In cases of mild to moderate neutropenia (granulocytes between 2,000/mm^3 and 3,000/mm^3, or ANC between 1,000/mm^3 and 500/mm^3), which occurs in up to 2% of patients, clozapine should be discontinued with daily monitoring of complete blood counts until values return to normal.

Dermatologic System

Allergic reactions are rare and usually occur within 8 weeks of initiating therapy, manifesting as maculopapular, erythematous, pruritic rashes that are evident on the face, neck, trunk, or extremities. Drug discontinuation and topical steroids are recommended. Contact dermatitis, including the oral mucosa, may occur in patients or medical personnel. For patients, mixing the antipsychotic concentrate in a sufficient quantity of a nonacidic liquid and swallowing it quickly decreases problems in susceptible patients. Care should be taken in the handling and preparation of liquid FGAs.

Phenothiazine structures can absorb ultraviolet light and energy, resulting in the formation of free radicals, which can have damaging effects on the skin. Both SGAs and FGAs cause photosensitivity. Erythema and severe sunburns can occur. Exposure to sunlight should be limited, and patients should be educated about the use of a maximally blocking sunscreen, hats, protective clothing, and sunglasses.[102]

Blue-gray or purplish skin coloration in areas exposed to sunlight occurs in patients receiving higher doses of low-potency phenothiazines during long-term administration, especially with chlorpromazine. It commonly occurs with concurrent corneal or lens pigmentation.

Miscellaneous Adverse Effects

A particularly curious and sometimes troubling side effect with clozapine is sialorrhea, which may occur in up to 54% of patients taking clozapine. The mechanism of clozapine-induced drooling is unclear, although α-adrenergic blockade and muscarinic$_4$ receptor agonism have been suggested as potential etiologies. α-Agonists such as clonidine and antimuscarinics such as benztropine have been suggested as potential treatments.[103]

TOXICITY WITH OVERDOSE

Acute overdose with antipsychotics rarely results in serious symptomatology. Mild intoxication manifests as sedation, hypotension, and miosis, whereas with severe intoxication, agitation and delirium may typically progress to motor retardation, seizures, cardiac arrhythmias, respiratory arrest, and coma. Dystonias and pseudoparkinsonism symptoms also occur. Supportive measures, gastric lavage, and activated charcoal are recommended. Induction of emesis may be difficult because of effects on the chemoreceptor trigger zone, and dialysis is ineffective because of the degree of drug-protein binding. Phenytoin or sodium bicarbonate are useful in the treatment of quinidine-like cardiac conduction effects on the QRS or QTc intervals. Physostigmine is not generally recommended to reverse anticholinergic toxicity because of deleterious effects on arrhythmias and seizure threshold.[104]

USE IN PREGNANCY AND LACTATION

Minimal data exist regarding the effects of pregnancy on schizophrenia. However, the disorganized thought processes, impaired cognition, and negative symptoms can have a detrimental effect on the functioning and self-care of the mother, and therefore adversely affect the fetus.[105] Currently available data assessing the risk of teratogenesis with antipsychotic agents are insufficient. Epidemiologic studies show a slightly increased risk of birth defects with low-potency FGAs. Haloperidol is the best studied of all antipsychotics, and no relationship between its use and teratogenicity has been found. SGAs have been inadequately studied. However, concern has been expressed regarding the use of clozapine in pregnancy.[106] The weight gain associated with olanzapine and clozapine and potential risk of gestational diabetes should be considered in drug selection.

The risk of antipsychotic use must be weighed against the benefits of pharmacotherapy in pregnant women who may be experiencing disorganized thoughts, delusions about change in body image or pregnancy, or who are unable to provide adequate prenatal care.[105] Other potential but largely unknown risks of antipsychotics throughout pregnancy are the possibility of behavioral teratogenicity on the neonate, receptor changes, perinatal effects (e.g., tonicity, strength, and sucking), extrapyramidal side effects, jaundice, respiratory depression, and intestinal obstruction.

Antipsychotics appear in breast milk with milk:plasma ratios of 0.5 to 1. However, 1 week after delivery, clozapine milk concentrations have been found to be as much as 279% of serum concentrations. Its use during breast-feeding is not recommended.[106] Overall, little is known about breast-feeding and the potential effects of antipsychotics on the neonate. Although not contraindicated, the lowest dosage should be used in the mother, and the infant should be carefully monitored.

DRUG INTERACTIONS

Although drug interactions may occur through a variety of mechanisms, most occur because of pharmacodynamic or pharmacokinetic interactions. Common examples of pharmacodynamic interactions resulting in enhanced effect include the excess sedation that can occur when antipsychotics are used concomitantly with other medications that have sedative side effects (e.g., mood stabilizers, hypnotics, alcohol, antidepressants, anxiolytics, or antihistamines).

Additive antimuscarinic effects of antipsychotics used with other medications with antimuscarinic effects (e.g., antihistamines, antidepressants, or antiparkinsonism agents) may result in urinary retention, constipation, blurred vision, or other anticholinergic side effects.[30] Both combined sedative and anticholinergic effects from multiple medications may result in impaired cognition, particularly in the elderly and other patients predisposed to such problems.[63] Patients may be more likely to experience symptomatic orthostatic hypotension when an antipsychotic is used with other medications that cause orthostasis (e.g., antidepressants with α-blockade, antihypertensive agents, or diuretics). Although metoclopramide is a commonly prescribed medication for treating esophageal reflux, it is a DA antagonist, and patients are more likely to experience akathisia and other extrapyramidal side effects if it is used concomitantly with antipsychotics.[63] Although some SSRIs may interact with antipsychotics through enzyme inhibition, they may also interact through pharmacodynamic mechanisms. 5-HT$_2$ receptors are present on the presynaptic dopaminergic neuron, and their activation leads to decreased dopamine release from the presynaptic terminal. Increased availability of serotonin through SSRI effect may activate these receptors, decrease dopamine release, and add to the dopaminolytic effects of antipsychotic agents.[63] Thus in the absence of enzyme inhibition, SSRIs may still precipitate akathisia or extrapyramidal side effects when added to a patient stabilized on an antipsychotic medication. A potentially more dangerous interaction may occur when medications that slow myocardial conduction (e.g., quinidine, procainamide, or tricyclic antidepressants), and thus prolong the QTc interval, are used in combination with antipsychotics that significantly prolong the QTc interval, such as ziprasidone, thioridazine, or mesoridazine.[63,74,107] Medications that prolong the QTc interval should also be monitored carefully in patients taking concomitant diuretics.[59] These effects may all increase the risk of clinically significant side effects.

Although atypical antipsychotics may be affected to varying degrees by enzyme inhibitors and inducers, none of the available atypical antipsychotics have been shown to significantly affect the pharmacokinetics of other medications. Table 66–7 lists the major pathways thought to be involved in the metabolism of SGAs. Risperidone is metabolized primarily by CYP 2D6 to its active metabolite, 9-OH-risperidone, which is metabolized by the same pathway.[57] 9-OH-risperidone is thought to have a pharmacodynamic profile similar to risperidone. Paroxetine has been reported to increase the total risperidone plus active metabolite concentrations by 76% over the baseline. This was also associated with EPS in some individuals.[108] As indicated, SSRIs may also interact with antipsychotics through pharmacodynamic mechanisms. Carbamazepine has been reported to decrease risperidone plasma concentrations.[108]

After single-dose administration, the mean bioavailability of quetiapine is 9% with significant interindividual variation.[57] If a CYP 3A4 inhibitor (e.g., cimetidine, ketoconazole, nefazodone, grapefruit juice, or erythromycin) is added to quetiapine, increased side effect (e.g., sedation or orthostasis) may occur. Fluoxetine may also decrease clearance of a medication such as quetiapine metabolized through CYP 3A4. However, with fluoxetine, it is the long-acting metabolite norfluoxetine, and not fluoxetine, that is the primary inhibitor of 3A4 metabolism. If an enzyme inducer such as carbamazepine or St. John's wort is added to quetiapine, then decreased antipsychotic effects may occur.[108,109]

Based on current information, inhibitors of CYP 1A2 have the greatest potential for causing interactions with olanzapine.[109] Examples include cimetidine, fluvoxamine, and fluoroquinolone antibiotics (e.g., ciprofloxacin) to varying degrees. To date, however, no serious inhibition interactions have been reported with olanzapine, which may be a result of olanzapine's wide therapeutic index. Carbamazepine has been reported to increase olanzapine elimination by as much as 50%.[110] Cigarette smoking is a potent inducer of CYP 1A2, and one would expect lower mean olanzapine serum concentrations in smokers compared to nonsmokers.

Because of the risk of seizures with higher clozapine tissue concentrations, inhibition interactions with clozapine are potentially significant. In particular, fluvoxamine has been reported to increase clozapine serum concentrations by an average of two- to threefold and up to fivefold.[111,112] Fluoxetine and erythromycin may increase clozapine serum concentrations in some patients, but to a lesser degree.[111] Mean clozapine serum concentrations are reported to be 32% lower in smokers compared with nonsmokers.[110] Carbamazepine may also induce clozapine metabolism and lead to lower serum concentrations.[110]

A study with the potent CYP 3A4 inhibitor ketoconazole showed minimal effects on ziprasidone single-dose pharmacokinetics, with only a 33% mean increase in the ziprasidone area under the time-versus-concentration curve.[59,74] These results are consistent with data suggesting that aldehyde oxidase is the major metabolic pathway for ziprasidone, with only 30% to 35% being metabolized by CYP 3A4.[59,113]

Modest elevations of aripiprazole serum concentration occur in the presence of ketoconazole or quinidine, which inhibit CYP 2D6 and 3A4, respectively. Carbamazepine has been reported to decrease aripiprazole serum concentrations.[26]

Antidepressants are commonly used in combination with antipsychotics to treat depressive symptoms in individuals with schizophrenia. Different antidepressants have been reported to inhibit metabolism of different P450 pathways.[110] Table 66–10 summarizes the potential metabolic drug interactions between antidepressants and SGAs. Potential enzyme inhibitor interactions with clozapine are the most clinically significant. Increased clozapine serum concentrations with a CYP 1A2 inhibitor such as fluvoxamine may precipitate seizures.[110] With the newer atypical antipsychotics, enzyme inhibitors are more likely to cause side effects such as increased sedation, orthostatic hypotension, or increased risk of akathisia and other extrapyramidal side effects.

PHARMACOECONOMIC CONSIDERATIONS

It is estimated that approximately 80% of individuals suffering their first schizophrenic break will have recurrent episodes and significant lifetime psychosocial dysfunction. In 1994, the direct cost of treating schizophrenia in the United States was estimated to be $45 billion.[114] The public mental health care sector provides the majority of services for individuals with schizophrenia. Mental health care costs

TABLE 66–10. Antidepressant/Antipsychotic P450 Inhibitor Drug Interactions

Inhibitor (Inhibits Substrate)	Substrate (Drug Metabolized By Pathway)		
	1A2	2D6	3A3/4
Bupropion (Wellbutrin)		**Phenothiazines (some)**	
Citalopram (Celexa)		Phenothiazines	
Fluoxetine (Prozac)		**PHENOTHIAZINES** **Risperidone**, Aripiprazole	**Clozapine, Quetiapine,** Ziprasidone[a]
Fluvoxamine (Luvox)	**CLOZAPINE, THIORIDAZINE, HALOPERIDOL, OLANZAPINE, THIOTHIXENE**		**Clozapine, Quetiapine,** Ziprasidone[a]
Nefazodone (Serzone)			**QUETIAPINE, Clozapine,** Ziprasidone[a]
Paroxetine (Paxil)		**PHENOTHIAZINES, Risperidone,** Aripiprazole	
Sertraline (Zoloft)		Phenothiazines	Clozapine, Quetiapine, Ziprasidone[a]

The inhibitor drug inhibits the metabolism of the substrate drug; therefore increasing the amount of substrate drug in the body, and the potential for side effects from the substrate drug. Bold type and capital letters reflect the relative potential for the interaction to be clinically significant (i.e., **HIGH**, **Moderate**, Low).
[a]Indicates that this is a minor pathway for this substrate, and therefore the possibility of a clinically significant interaction through this pathway is decreased.

for schizophrenia represent disproportionate expenditures for crisis intervention and hospitalization as compared to comprehensive outpatient services oriented toward maintaining remission and improving psychosocial functioning. The suboptimal or inadequate funding provided for efficient ambulatory mental health services further increases the demand for hospitalization, which diverts additional revenues that might be available for outpatient services. This created a vicious revolving door cycle and is a major challenge facing public mental health care.

The advent of more expensive SGAs, accompanied by limited resources, has forced mental health care organizations to examine the outcomes and related economics of treating patients with the SGAs compared with the traditional, largely generic FGAs. Although medication costs are higher with SGAs than with FGAs, studies with various SGAs have fairly consistently shown total mental health costs to be no higher or even lower with SGAs.[114] Similarly, some studies have shown clozapine to result in lower overall mental health care costs, while others have shown no difference in costs compared to FGAs. Additionally, clozapine decreases suicidality more than comparator antipsychotics, and it is more effective in treatment-resistant schizophrenia.[115,116]

Of greater debate is whether differences in cost-effectiveness exist among the SGAs. Significant differences in acquisition costs among the SGAs have produced controversy regarding formulary decisions in organized health care settings.[114] For example, although olanzapine has a higher acquisition cost, some studies have found no difference in total mental health care direct costs (i.e., medications plus services) when comparing olanzapine and risperidone.[114,117] However, these findings are inconsistent, and the comparative pharmacoeconomics of SGAs remain controversial.[114]

EVALUATION OF THERAPEUTIC OUTCOMES

Assessment of response has traditionally been done subjectively or empirically (a relative sense of how the clinician feels the patient is doing). A formal mental status examination (MSE) is used to structure the patient interview and focus on items related to appearance, mood, sensorium, intellectual functioning, and thought processes. However, the MSE is not specific for the measurement of drug response. Clinicians should be trained to use simple, standardized psychiatric rating scales to assist in objectively rating patient drug responses.[20,22,118] The brief psychiatric rating scale (BPRS) and the Positive and Negative Symptom Scale (PANSS) were developed for use in clinical trials as research tools to quantify symptoms and improvement seen with antipsychotic treatment.[118] Objectively, the use of a numeric indicator (e.g., 20%, 30%, or 40% reduction in BPRS score) has been used to quantify overall symptom reduction and classify patients according to different degrees of response. However, these types of rating scales are too long and unwieldy to be routinely used within the time constraints of most clinical practices. Symptom scales used in clinical practice must be sufficiently brief to be used during an ordinary clinic visit (e.g., 15 to 30 minutes) while measuring both positive and negative symptoms, and being sufficiently representative of overall symptomatology. The four-item Positive Symptom Rating Scale and the Brief Negative Symptom Assessment are brief scales that meet such criteria (Fig. 66–2).[22,118] It is increasingly recognized that clinicians should be examining cognition as an outcome in treatment of schizophrenia. Although multiple lengthy research batteries are available, brief, simple assessments have not been readily available. However, a brief cognition battery has recently been developed and validated, and it can be completed in 15 to 20 minutes.[119]

Similarly, the pharmacotherapeutic plan should include specific monitoring parameters for potential side effects. The plan should include the side effects to be monitored (e.g., EPS and weight increase), how the potential side effect will be evaluated, and the frequency of assessment (e.g., daily or weekly). Given the risk of weight gain, diabetes, and lipid abnormalities associated with many of the SGAs, a consensus task force led by the American Diabetes Association recommends the following baseline parameters before beginning antipsychotics: family history, weight, height, body mass index, waist circumference, blood pressure, fasting plasma glucose, and fasting lipid profile.[69] They also recommend follow-up monitoring of these parameters after beginning or changing SGAs. Weight should be monitored monthly for the first 3 months, and quarterly thereafter. The

BRIEF CLINICAL ASSESSMENTS FOR MONITORING ANTIPSYCHOTIC RESPONSE IN SCHIZOPHRENIA

4-Item Positive Symptom Rating Scale (PSRS)

Use each item's anchor points to rate the patient.

1	Suspiciousness	NA	1	2	3	4	5	6	7
2	Unusual thought content	NA	1	2	3	4	5	6	7
3	Hallucinations	NA	1	2	3	4	5	6	7
4	Conceptual disorganization	NA	1	2	3	4	5	6	7

SCORE ________

Each item is scored from 1 (not present) to 7 (extremely severe); NA = not able to be assessed

Brief Negative Symptom Assessment (BNSA)

Use each item's anchor points to rate the patient.

1	Prolonged time to respond	1	2	3	4	5	6
2	Emotion: unchanging facial expression, blank, expressionless face	1	2	3	4	5	6
3	Reduced social drive	1	2	3	4	5	6
4	Poor grooming and hygiene	1	2	3	4	5	6

SCORE ________

Each item is scored from 1 (normal) to 6 (severe)

FIGURE 66–2. Brief clinical assessments for monitoring antipsychotic response in schizophrenia. To enhance consistency in ratings, the structured probes in the administration manual should be used each time the scales are used. (Data from Miller et al[22] and Miller et al.[118] The complete administration manual for the Positive Symptom Rating Scale and the Brief Negative Symptom Assessment can be accessed from the appendices in the TIMA Procedure Manual: Schizophrenia Module at *http://www.dshs.state.tx.us/mhprograms/timasczman.pdf.* This rating scale is in the public domain and may be reproduced with appropriate citation of the authors and source.)

other parameters should be assessed at the end of 3 months and then annually. If normal, serum lipids can be monitored less often.

Self-assessments can be a useful adjunct in treating the patient. Although the patient with schizophrenia may not always be accurate in evaluating symptom severity (in fact, just the opposite may occur), the use of patient self-assessments increases patient engagement in care, enhances therapeutic alliance, and gives the clinician an opportunity to identify misconceptions the patient may have regarding symptoms associated with the illness, medication side effects, and the like.[40,42,118] Traditionally, clinicians have often accepted partial symptom response in schizophrenia as success, and have not been aggressive in attempting to achieve greater symptomatic remission. In many respects the side-effect profile of FGAs encouraged the acceptance of partial response and a tendency to not "rock the boat" in a patient with partial improvement. However, the advent of multiple different SGAs with varying, but overall favorable, side-effect profiles should encourage clinicians to be more assertive in attempting to achieve symptom remission.

CONCLUSIONS

Schizophrenia is a complex disease with multiple ramifications for patients and their families. Treatment issues remain clouded by the fact that the etiology of the illness is unknown. It is clear, however, that no single treatment modality is adequate to properly manage a patient with schizophrenia. Antipsychotics are the bedrock of treatment. SGAs have substantially advanced the care of people with schizophrenia. However, notwithstanding such advances, the SGAs are not a panacea and have multiple adverse effects in addition to the limitations of their efficacy. However, when used within the context of multidisciplinary treatment, SGAs improve positive and negative symptoms and cognition so that patients can appropriately participate in psychosocial rehabilitation programs. Scientific advances continue to expand our understanding of CNS physiology and the abnormalities present in schizophrenia. Advances in our understanding of the pathophysiology of schizophrenia should, in turn, result in the development of treatments that are more specific and more effective. In practice, it is mandatory that clinicians appropriately use their expanding armamentarium. It is important that clinicians appreciate the pharmacodynamic basis for treatment interventions so that they can effectively design and implement rational pharmacotherapeutic regimens. Finally, it is critical that clinicians more objectively evaluate individual patient response to medication so that treatment can be optimized. With these strategies, the gap between practice and science can be narrowed and patients' lives benefited.

ABBREVIATIONS

ACT: active community treatment
AIMS: abnormal involuntary movement scale
ANC: absolute neutrophil count
BLM: buccolingual-masticatory (syndrome)
BPRS: brief psychiatric rating scale
CK: creatine kinase
DA: dopamine
DSM-IV-TR: *Diagnostic and Statistical Manual of Mental Disorders,* 4th edition, Text Revision
EPS: extrapyramidal side effects
FGA: first-generation antipsychotic
GABA: γ-aminobutyric acid
5-HT_2: 5-hydroxytryptamine$_2$
LFT: liver function test
MSE: mental status examination
NAMI: National Alliance for the Mentally Ill
NMDA: N-methyl-D-aspartate
NMS: neuroleptic malignant syndrome
PANSS: Positive and Negative Symptom Scale
PET: positron emission tomography

SGA: second-generation antipsychotic
SSRI: selective serotonin reuptake inhibitor

Review Questions and other resources can be found at *www.pharmacotherapyonline.com.*

REFERENCES

1. American Psychiatric Association. Schizophrenia and other psychotic disorders. In: Diagnostic and Statistical Manual of Mental Disorders, 4th ed., Text Revision. Washington, American Psychiatric Association, 2000:297–319.

2. Jones P, Buckley P. Schizophrenia. London, Mosby, 2003:168.

3. Harrison P. The neuropathology of schizophrenia. A critical review of the data and their interpretation. Brain 1999;122:593–624.

4. Lewis DA, Levitt P. Schizophrenia as a disorder of neurodevelopment. Ann Rev Neurosci 2002;25:409–432.

5. Brown AS, Susser ES. In utero infection and adult schizophrenia. Ment Retard Dev Disabil Res Rev 2002;8:51–57.

6. Mahadik, SP, Evans DR. Is schizophrenia a metabolic brain disorder? Membrane phospholipid dysregulation and its therapeutic implications. Psychiatr Clin North Am 2003;26:41–46.

7. Weinberger D. Schizophrenia as a neurodevelopmental disorder. In: Weinberger DR, Hirsch SR, eds. Schizophrenia. Oxford, Blackwell Science, 2003:326–348.

8. Mathalon DH, Sullivan EV, Lim KO, Pfefferbaum A. Progressive brain volume changes and the clinical course of schizophrenia in men: A longitudinal magnetic resonance imaging study. Arch Gen Psychiatry 2001;58:148–157.

9. Ho BC, Andreasen NC, Nopoulos P, et al. Progressive structural brain abnormalities and their relationships to clinical outcome: A longitudinal magnetic resonance imaging study early in schizophrenia. Arch Gen Psychiatry 2003;60:585–594.

10. McClure RK, Lieverman JA. Neurodevelopmental and neurodegenerative hypothesis of schizophrenia: A review and critique. Curr Opin Psychiatry 2003;16(Suppl 2):S15–S28.

11. Buckley PF, Mahadik S, Evans D, Stirewalt E. Causes, course, and neurodevelopment of schizophrenia. Current Psychosis and Therapeutic Reports 2003;1:41–49.

12. McDonald C, Murphy KC. The new genetics of schizophrenia. Psychiatr Clin North Am 2003;26:41–63.

13. Wei J, Jemmings GP. The NOTCH4 locus is associated with susceptibility to schizophrenia. Nat Genet 2002;25:376–377.

14. Novak G, Kim D, Seeman P, Tallerico T. Schizophrenia and Nogo: Elevated mRNA in cortex, and high prevalence of a homozygous CAA insert. Brain Res Mol Brain Res 2002;107:183–189.

15. Frankle WG, Lerma J, Laruelle M. The synaptic hypothesis of schizophrenia. Nature 2003;39:205–216

16. Lieberman JA, Sheitman BB, Kinon BJ. Neurochemical sensitisation in the pathophysiology of schizophrenia: Deficits and dysfunction in neuronal regulation and plasticity. Neuropsychopharmacology 1997;17:205–229.

17. Meltzer HY. What's atypical about atypical antipsychotic drugs? Curr Opin Pharmacol 2004;4:53–57.

18. Lieberman JA. Atypical antipsychotic drugs as a first-line treatment of schizophrenia: A rationale and hypothesis. J Clin Psychiatry 1996;57 (Suppl 11):68–71.

19. Lehman AF, Lieberman JA, Dixon LB, et al. American Psychiatric Association Practice Guidelines; Work Group on Schizophrenia. Practice guideline for the treatment of patients with schizophrenia, second edition. Am J Psychiatry 2004;161(2 Suppl):1–56.

20. Miller AL, Hall CS, Buchanan RW, et al. The Texas Medication Algorithm Project antipsychotic algorithm for schizophrenia: 2003 Update. J Clin Psychiatry 2004;65:500–508.

21. Marder SR, Essock SM, Miller AL, et al. The Mount Sinai conference on schizophrenia. Schizophrenia Bull 2002;28:5–16.

22. Miller AL, Hall CS, Crismon ML, Chiles J. TIMA procedural manual: schizophrenia algorithm. Austin, TX, Texas Department of Mental Health and Mental Retardation, 2003. Available at *http://www.dshs.state.tx.us/mhprograms/timasczman.pdf.*

23. Csernansky JG, Mahmoud R, Brenner R. Risperidone-USA-7 Group: A comparison of risperidone and haloperidol for the prevention of relapse in patients with schizophrenia. N Engl J Med 2002;346:16–22.

24. Small JG, Hirsch SR, Arvanitis LA, et al. Quetiapine in patients with schizophrenia. A high-and low-dose double-blind comparison with placebo. Arch Gen Psychiatry 1997;54:549–557.

25. Daniel DG, Zimbroff DL, Potkin SG, et al. Ziprasidone 80 mg/day and 160 mg/day in the acute exacerbation of schizophrenia and schizoaffective disorder: A 6-week placebo-controlled trial. Neuropsychopharmacology 1999;20:491–505.

26. De Leon A, Patel NC, Crismon ML. Aripiprazole: A comprehensive review of its pharmacology, clinical efficacy, and tolerability. Clin Therapeutics 2004;26:649–666.

27. Meltzer HY, Alphs L, Green AI, et al. Clozapine treatment for suicidality in schizophrenia: International Suicide Prevention Trial (InterSePT). Arch Gen Psychiatry 2003;60:82–91.

28. Green AL, Canuso CM, Brenner MJ, Wojcik JD. Detection and management of comorbidity in patients with schizophrenia. Psychiatr Clin North Am 2003;26:115–139.

29. Awad AG. Drug therapy in schizophrenia: Variability of outcome and prediction of response. Can J Psychiatry 1989;34:711–720.

30. Van Putten T, Marder SR. Behavioral toxicity of antipsychotic drugs. J Clin Psychiatry 1987;48(Suppl 9):13–19.

31. Leucht S, Barnes TR, Kissling W, et al. Relapse prevention in schizophrenia with new-generation antipsychotics: A systematic review and exploratory meta-analysis of randomized, controlled trials. Am J Psychiatry 2003;160:1209–1222.

32. Marder SR, Glynn SM, Wirshing WC, et al. Maintenance treatment of schizophrenia with risperidone or haloperidol: 2-year outcomes. Am J Psychiatry 2003;160:1405–1412.

33. Kinon BJ, Burson BR, Gilmore J, et al. Strategies for switching from conventional antipsychotic drugs to risperidone or olanzapine. J Clin Psychiatry 2000;61:833–840.

34. Kane JM, Eerdekens M, Lindenmayer JP, et al. Long-acting injectable risperidone: Efficacy and safety of the first long-acting atypical antipsychotic. Am J Psychiatry 2003;160:1125–1132.

35. Harrison TS, Goa KL. Long-acting risperidone: A review of its use in schizophrenia. CNS Drugs 2004;18:113–132.

36. Ereshefsky L, Saklad SR, Jann MW, et al. Future of depot neuroleptic therapy: Pharmacokinetics and pharmacodynamic approaches. J Clin Psychiatry 1984;45(5 pt 2):50–59.

37. Ereshefsky L, Toney G, Saklad SR, Seidel DR. A loading dose strategy for converting from oral to depot haloperidol. Hosp Comm Psychiatry 1993;44:1155–1161.

38. Hamann GL, Egan TM, Wells BG, et al. Injection site reactions after intramuscular administration of haloperidol decanoate 100 mg/mL. J Clin Psychiatry 1990;51:502–504.

39. Cramer JA, Rosenheck R. Compliance with medication regimens for mental and physical disorders. Psychiatr Serv 1998;49:196–201.

40. Toprac MG, Rush AJ, Conner TM, et al. The Texas Medication Algorithm Project patient and family education program: A consumer-guided initiative. J Clin Psychiatry 2000;61:477–486.

41. O'Donnell C, Donohoe G, Sharkey L, et al. Compliance therapy: A randomised controlled trial in schizophrenia. BMJ 2003;327:834.

42. Rush AJ, Crismon ML, Toprac MG, et al. Implementing guidelines and systems of care: Experiences with the Texas Medication Algorithm Project (TMAP). J Pract Psychiatry Behav Health 1999;5:75–86.

43. Kane J, Honigfeld G, Singer J, et al. Clozapine for the treatment-resistant schizophrenic: A double-blind comparison with chlorpromazine. Arch Gen Psychiatry 1988;45:789–796.

44. Kane JM. Treatment-resistant schizophrenic patients. J Clin Psychiatry 1996;57(Suppl 9):35–40.

45. Spears NM, Leadbetter RA, Shutty MS. Clozapine treatment in polydipsia and intermittent hyponatremia. J Clin Psychiatry 1996;57:123–128.

46. Buckley PF, Miller AL, Olsen J, et al. When symptoms persist: Clozapine augmentation strategies. Schiozphr Bull 2001;27:615–628.

47. Canales PL, Olsen J, Miller AL, Crismon ML. The role of antipsychotic polypharmacotherapy in the treatment of schizophrenia. CNS Drugs 1999;12:179–188.

48. Leucht S, Kissling W, McGrath J. Lithium for schizophrenia revisited: A systematic review and meta-analysis of randomized controlled trials. J Clin Psychiatry 2004;65:177–186.

49. Casey DE, Daniel DG, Wassef AA, et al. Effect of divalproex combined with olanzapine or risperidone in patients with an acute exacerbation of schizophrenia. Neuropsychopharmacology 2003;28:182–192.

50. Silver H. Selective serotonin reuptake inhibitor augmentation in the treatment of negative symptoms of schizophrenia. Int Clin Psychopharmacol 2003;18:305–313.

51. Kapur S, Roy P, Daskalakis J, Remington G. Increased dopamine D_2 receptor occupancy and elevated prolactin level associated with addition of haloperidol to clozapine. Am J Psychiatry 2001;158:311–314.

52. Kapur S, Mamo D. Half a century of antipsychotics and still a central role for dopamine D_2 receptors. Prog Neuropsychopharmacol Biol Psychiatry 2003;27:1081–1090.

53. Meltzer L, Li Z, Kaneda Y, Ichikawa J. Serotonin receptors: Their key role in drugs to treat schizophrenia. Prog Neuropsychopharmacol Biol Psychiatry 2003;27:1159–1172.

54. Nyberg S, Eriksson B, Oxenstierna G, et al. Suggested minimal effective dose of risperidone based on PET measured D_2 and $5-HT_{2A}$ receptor occupancy in schizophrenic patients. Am J Psychiatry 1999;156:869–875.

55. Kapur S, Zipursky RB, Remington G. Clinical and theoretical implications of $5-HT_2$ and D_2 receptor occupancy of clozapine, risperidone, and olanzapine in schizophrenia. Am J Psychiatry 1999;156:286–293.

56. Stahl SM, Shayegan DK. The psychopharmacology of ziprasidone: Receptor-binding properties and real-world psychiatric practice. J Clin Psychiatry 2003;64(Suppl 19):6–12.

57. Ereshefsky L. Pharmacokinetics and drug interactions: Update for new antipsychotics. J Clin Psychiatry 1996;57(Suppl 11):12–25.

58. Bradford LD. CYP2D6 allele frequency in European Caucasians, Asians, Africans, and their descendants. Pharmacogenetics 2002;3:229–243.

59. Pfizer Inc. Ziprasidone (Geodon) package insert. New York, revised December 2003.

60. Zito JM, Sofair JB, Jaeger J. Self-reported neuroendocrine effects of APs in women: A pilot study. DICP 1990;24:176–180.

61. Allison DB, Mentore JL, Heo M, et al. Antipsychotic induced weight gain: A comprehensive research synthesis. Am J Psychiatry 1999;156:1686–1696.

62. Patel NC, Kistler JL, James EB, Crismon ML. A retrospective analysis of olanzapine and quetiapine on weight and body mass index in children and adolescents. Pharmacotherapy 2004;24:824–830.

63. Miller AL, Dassori A, Ereshefsky L, Crismon ML. Recent issues and developments in antipsychotic use. In Dunner DL, Rosenbaum JF, eds. Psychiatric Clinics of North America Annual Review of Drug Therapy 2001. Philadelphia, WB Saunders, 2001;8:209–235.

64. Harris EC, Barraclough B. Excess mortality of mental disorder. Br J Psychiatry 1998;173:11–53.

65. Meyer JM. Cardiovascular illness and hyperlipidemia in patients with schizophrenia. In: Meyer JM, Nasarallah HA, eds. Medical Illness and Schizophrenia. Washington, American Psychiatric Press, 2003:53–80.

66. Wirshing D, Boyd J, Meng LR, et al. The effects of novel antipsychotics on glucose and lipid levels. J Clin Psychiatry 2002;63:856–865.

67. Weiden PJ, Ross R. Why do patients stop their antipsychotic medications? A guide for family and friends. J Psychiatr Pract 2002;8:413–416.

68. Vreeland B, Minsky S, Menza M, et al. A program for managing weight gain associated with atypical antipsychotics. Psychiatr Serv 2003;54:1155–1157.

69. American Diabetes Association. Consensus development conference on antipsychotic drugs and obesity and diabetes. Diabetes Care 2004;27:596–601.

70. Citrome LL, Jaffe AB. Relationship of atypical antipsychotics with development of diabetes. Ann Pharmacother 2003;37:1849–1857.

71. Henderson DC, Cagliero E, Gray C, et al. Clozapine, diabetes mellitus, weight gain and lipid abnormalities: A five-year naturalistic study. Am J Psychiatry 2000;157:975–981.

72. Zyprexa (olanzapine). MedWatch, U.S. Food and Drug Administration. Available at: *http://www.fda.gov/medwatch/SAFETY/2004/safety04.htm#zyprexa*. Accessed March 28, 2004.

73. Tandon R. Safety and tolerability: how do newer generation "atypical" antipsychotics compare? Psychiatr Q 2002;73:297–311.

74. Briefing document for Zeldox capsules (ziprasidone HCl). FDA Psychopharmacological Drugs Advisory Committee. New York, Pfizer Pharmaceuticals, July 19, 2000.

75. Holloman LC, Marder SR. Management of acute extrapyramidal effects induced by antipsychotic drugs. Am J Health Syst Pharm 1997;54:2461–2477.

76. Wells BG, Marken PA, Rickman LA, et al. Characterizing anticholinergic abuse in community mental health. J Clin Psychopharmacol 1989;9:431–435.

77. Sprague RL, Kalachnik JE. Reliability, validity, and a total score cut-off for the Dyskinesia Identification System Condensed User Scale (DISCUS) with mentally ill and mentally retarded populations. Psychopharmacol Bull 1991;27:51–58.

78. Egan MF, Apud J, Wyatt RJ. Treatment of tardive dyskinesia. Schizophr Bull 1997;23:583–609.

79. Tandon R, Kasper S, Kane J, Juncos J. The scourge of extrapyramidal side effects: Have atypical antipsychotics solved the problem? J Clin Psychiatry 2000;61:955–962.

80. Correll CU, Leucht S, Kane JM. Lower risk for tardive dyskinesia associated with second-generation antipsychotics: A systematic review of 1-year studies. Am J Psychiatry 2004;161:414–425.

81. Tamminga CA, Woerner MG. Clinical course and cellular pathology of tardive dyskinesia. In Davis KL, Charney D, Coyle JT, Nemeroff C, eds. Neuropsychopharmacology: The Fifth Generation of Progress. Philadelphia, Lippincott Williams & Wilkins, 2002:1831–1841.

82. Soares KV, McGrath JJ. Vitamin E for neuroleptic-induced tardive dyskinesia. Cochrane Database Syst Rev 2001;4:CD000209.

83. Bilder RM, Goldman RS, Volavka J, et al. Neurocognitive effects of clozapine, risperidone, and haloperidol in patients with chronic schizophrenia or schizoaffective disorder. Am J Psychiatry 2002;159:1018–1028.

84. Miller AL, Crismon ML, Rush AJ, et al. The Texas Medication Algorithm Project: clinical results for schizophrenia. Schizophr Bull (in press).

85. Pisani F, Oteri G, Costa C, et al. Effects of psychotropic drugs on seizure threshold. Drug Saf 2002;25:91–110.

86. Simpson GM, Pi EH, Sramek JJ. Adverse effects of antipsychotic agents. Drugs 1981;21:138–151.

87. Chandron GJ, Mikler JR, Keegan DL. Neuroleptic malignant syndrome: Case report and discussion. CMAJ 2003;169:439–442.

88. Buckley PF, Adityanjee, Sajatovic M: Neuroleptic malignant syndrome. In Bashier Y, et al eds. Textbook of Neuromuscular Disorders. Philadelphia, Butterworth-Heinemann, 2001:1264–1278.

89. Crismon ML. Psychotropic drugs in the elderly: Principles of use. Am Pharm 1990;NS30:57–63.

90. Levin Z, Hwang MY, Rotrosen J. The relationship between clozapine and obsessive-compulsive disorder. Compr Psychiatry 1996;37:74.

91. Oshika T. Ocular adverse effects of neuropsychiatric agents: Incidence and management. Drug Saf 1995;12:256–263.

92. Shahzad S, Suleman MI, Shahab H, et al. Cataract occurrence with antipsychotic drugs. Psychosomatics 2002;43:354–359.

93. Regal RE, Billi JE, Glazer HM. Phenothiazine-induced cholestatic jaundice. Clin Pharm 1987;6:787–794.

94. Krebs S, Dormann H, Muth-Selbach U, et al. Risperidone-induced cholestatic hepatitis. Eur J Gastroenterol Hepatol 2001;13:67–69.

95. Hummer M, Kurz M, Kurzthaler I, et al. Heptatotoxicity of clozapine. J Clin Psychopharmacol 1997;17:314–317.

96. Lin CC, Bai YM, Chen JY, et al. A retrospective study of clozapine and urinary incontinence in Chinese in-patients. Acta Psychiatr Scand 1999;100:158–161.

97. Knegtering H, van der Moolen AEGM, Castelein S, et al. What are the effects of antipsychotics on sexual dysfunctions and endocrine functioning? Psychoneuroendocrinology 2003;28(Suppl 2):109–123.

98. Hall RL, Smith AG, Ewards JG. Haematological safety of antipsychotic drugs. Expert Opin Drug Saf 2003;2:395–399.

99. Alvir JMJ, Lieberman JA, Safferman AZ, et al. Clozapine induced agranulocytosis: Incidence and risk factors in the United States. N Engl J Med 1993;329:162–167.

00. Zhang M, Owen RR, Pope SK, Smith GR. Cost-effectiveness of clozapine monitoring after the first 6 months. Arch Gen Psychiatry 1996;53:954–958.

01. Gullion G, Yeh HS. Treatment of clozapine-induced agranulocytosis with recombinant granulocyte colony stimulating factor. J Clin Psychiatry 1994;55:401–405.

02. Meltzer HY, Fatemi SH. Treatment of schizophrenia. In Schatzberg AF, Nemeroff CB, eds. Textbook of Psychopharmacology, 2nd ed. Washington, American Psychiatric Press, 1998:747–774.

03. Davydov L, Botts SR. Clozapine-induced hypersalivation. Ann Pharmacother 2000;34:662–665.

04. Perry PJ, Alexander B, Liskow B. Psychotropic Drug Handbook, 7th ed. Washington, American Psychiatric Press, 1997:1–129.

05. American Academy of Pediatrics Committee on Drugs. Use of psychoactive medication during pregnancy and possible effects on the fetus and newborn. Pediatrics 2000;105:880–887.

06. Ernst CL, Goldberg JF. The reproductive safety profile of mood stabilizers, atypical antipsychotics, and broad-spectrum psychotropics. J Clin Psychiatry 2002;63(Suppl 4):42–55.

07. Hartigan-Go K, Bateman DN, Nyberg G, et al. Concentration-related pharmacodynamic effects of thioridazine and its metabolites in humans. Clin Pharmacol Ther 1996;60:543–553.

08. Spina E, Scordo MG, D'Arrigo C. Metabolic drug interactions with new psychotropic agents. Fund Clin Pharmacol 2003;17:517–538.

09. DeVane CL, Nemeroff CB. Psychotropic drug interactions 2000. TEN 2000;2:55–75.

110. DeVane CL, Markowitz JS. Antipsychotics. In Levy RH, Thummel KE, Trager WF, et al. Metabolic Drug Interactions. Philadelphia, Lippincott Williams & Wilkins, 2000:245–258.

111. Chang WH, Augustin B, Lane HY, et al. In vitro and in vivo evaluation of drug-drug interaction between fluvoxamine and clozapine. Psychopharmacology 1999;145:91–98.

112. Wetzel H, Anghelescu I, Szegedi A, et al. Pharmacokinetic interactions of clozapine with selective serotonin reuptake inhibitors: Differential effects of fluvoxamine and paroxetine in a prospective study. J Clin Psychopharmacol 1998;18:2–9.

113. Prakash C, Kamel A, Cui D, et al. Identification of the major human liver cytochrome P450 isoform(s) responsible for the formation of the primary metabolites of ziprasidone and prediction of possible drug interactions. Br J Clin Pharmacol 2000;49(Suppl 1):35S–42S.

114. Liu GG, Sun SX, Christensen DB, Luo X. Cost comparisons of olanzapine and risperidone in treating schizophrenia. Ann Pharmacother 2004;38:134–141.

115. Hayhurst KP, Brown P, Lewis SW. The cost-effectiveness of clozapine: A controlled, population-based mirror-image study. J Psychopharmacol 2002;16:169–175.

116. Duggan A, Warner J, Knapp M, Kerwin R. Modeling the impact of clozapine on suicide in patients with treatment-resistant schizophrenia. Br J Psychiatry 2003;182:505–508.

117. Rascati KL, Johnsrud MT, Crismon ML, et al. Olanzapine versus risperidone in the treatment of schizophrenia: A comparison of costs among Texas Medicaid patients. Pharmacoeconomics 2003;21;683–697.

118. Miller AL, Chiles JA, Chiles JK, et al. The TMAP schizophrenia algorithms. J Clin Psychiatry 1999;60:649–657.

119. Velligan DI, DiCocco M, Bow-Thomas C, et al. A brief cognitive assessment (BCA) for use with schizophrenia patients in a community clinic. Schizophr Res 2004;71:273–283.

67

DEPRESSIVE DISORDERS

Judith C. Kando, Barbara G. Wells, and Peggy E. Hayes

Learning Objectives and other resources can be found at *www.pharmacotherapyonline.com.*

KEY CONCEPTS

◀ **1** When counseling patients with depression who are receiving pharmacotherapeutic interventions, the patient should be informed that adverse effects might occur immediately, while resolution of symptoms may take 2 to 4 weeks.

◀ **2** When evaluating a patient for the presence of depression, it is essential to rule out medical causes of depression and drug-induced depression.

◀ **3** The goal of pharmacological treatment of depression is the resolution of current symptoms and the prevention of further episodes of depression.

◀ **4** When determining if a patient has been nonresponsive to a particular pharmacotherapeutic intervention, it must be determined whether the patient has received an adequate dose for an adequate duration. If tricyclic antidepressants are being used, a serum level may be useful, especially in special populations such as the elderly, and those with concurrent medications that may alter the pharmacokinetic profile of the TCAs.

◀ **5** Childhood depression occurs commonly and can present with nonspecific symptoms. The dosage range, titration, and adverse effects of fluoxetine, imipramine, and sertraline are similar in children and adults.

◀ **6** An assessment of compliance should be made with every patient interaction. Remember that accurate capsule or tablet counts do not mean the patient has consumed the medication or consumed it in the manner prescribed.

◀ **7** If a patient exhibits a partial response to a pharmacotherapeutic agent, augmentation therapy should be considered before the trial is abandoned and the patient is treated with an alternative therapeutic agent.

◀ **8** When evaluating response to an antidepressant agent, in addition to target signs and symptoms, consider quality-of-life issues such as role, social functioning, and occupational function. In addition, the tolerability of the agent should be assessed because the occurrence of side effects may lead to nonadherence to the regimen.

Major depressive disorder is a disorder of mood in which the individual experiences one or more major depressive episodes without a history of manic, mixed, or hypomanic episodes. A major depressive episode is defined by the criteria listed in the *Diagnostic and Statistical Manual of Mental Disorders,* 4th ed., Text Revision (DSM-IV-TR), published by the American Psychiatric Association.[1] Depression is associated with significant functional disability, morbidity, and mortality.

Newer generations of antidepressants have provided pharmacological interventions that are effective and better tolerated than older agents like the tricyclic antidepressants (TCAs) and the monoamine oxidase inhibitors (MAOIs). In addition, substantial efforts have been undertaken to improve the ability of clinicians to recognize the signs and symptoms of depression and to treat. This chapter focuses exclusively on the diagnosis and treatment of major depressive disorder.

EPIDEMIOLOGY

The true prevalence of depressive disorders in the United States is unknown. The National Comorbidity Survey Replication recently found that 16.2% of the population studied had a history of major depressive disorder in their lifetime, and more than 6.6% had an episode within the past 12 months.[2] Women are at increased risk of depression from early adolescence until their mid-50s, with a lifetime rate of depression that is 1.7 to 2.7 times greater than for men.[3] Although depression can occur at any age, adults 25 to 44 years of age experience the highest rates of major depression.[4] The estimated lifetime prevalence of major depression in individuals aged 65 to 80 recently was reported to be 20.4% in women and 9.6% in men.[5] Depressive disorders are common during adolescence, with comorbid substance abuse, suicide attempts, and deaths occurring frequently in these young patients.[6,7] Depressive disorders and suicide tend to occur within families, and first-degree relatives of patients with depression are 1.5 to 3 times more likely to develop depression than normal controls.[1,8,9] Approximately 8% to 18% of patients with major depression have at least one first-degree relative (father, mother, brother, or sister) with a history of depression, compared with 5.6% of the first-degree relatives of a normal control group.[8] A twin study found that the heritability of liability for major depression was 39% and was the same in men and women, whereas the remaining 61% of the variance in liability was due to individual-specific environment.[10] Therefore major depressive disorder is relatively common, occurs more frequently in women than men, and prevalence is influenced by both genetic and environmental factors.

ETIOLOGY

The etiology of depressive disorders is too complex to be totally explained by a single social, developmental, or biologic theory. Several factors appear to work together to cause or precipitate depressive disorders. The symptoms reported by patients with major depression consistently reflect changes in brain monoamine neurotransmitters, specifically norepinephrine (NE), serotonin (5-HT), and dopamine (DA).[11-13]

PATHOPHYSIOLOGY

BIOGENIC AMINE HYPOTHESIS

The biogenic amine hypothesis evolved as a result of several observations made in the early 1950s. It was noted that the antihypertensive drug reserpine depleted neuronal storage granules of NE, 5-HT, and DA and produced clinically significant depression in 15% or more of patients.[14] In addition, it was discovered that the hallucinogen lysergic acid diethylamide blocked peripheral serotonin receptors, and it was proposed that the mind-altering effects of lysergic acid diethylamide were secondary to similar effects on central nervous system (CNS) serotonin receptors.[13]

◄ Therefore, several years before the introduction of antidepressants, the cause of depression was linked to decreased brain levels of the neurotransmitters NE, 5-HT, and DA, although the actual cause remains unknown. Although the reuptake blockade of monoamines (e.g., NE and 5-HT) occurs immediately upon administration of an antidepressant, the clinical antidepressant effects generally are not observed until after 4 weeks of dosing.[15] The reason for this delay in onset of action has caused researchers to focus on the adaptive changes induced by antidepressants, as discussed below.[12]

THEORIES OF POSTSYNAPTIC CHANGES IN RECEPTOR SENSITIVITY

A more perplexing aspect of the observed effects of antidepressants is the discrepancy between monoamine reuptake blockade (immediate) and any measurable improvement in depressive symptoms (delayed therapeutic response). Accordingly, theories that focus on adaptive (or chronic) changes in amine receptor systems compared with acute changes have emerged over the past decade.

In the mid-1970s it was recognized that chronic, but not acute, administration of antidepressants to animals caused desensitization of NE-stimulated cyclic adenosine monophosphate synthesis. In fact, for most antidepressants, downregulation of β-adrenergic receptors accompanies this desensitization.[16]

Studies of many antidepressants have demonstrated that either desensitization or downregulation of NE receptors corresponds to a clinically relevant time course for antidepressant effects.[11] Other studies have revealed downregulation of 5-HT$_2$ receptors following chronic administration of antidepressants.[17,18] Thus a theory based on postsynaptic changes in receptor sensitivity provides a cogent explanation of the delayed onset of activity of antidepressant drugs.[11]

DYSREGULATION HYPOTHESIS

The dysregulation hypothesis incorporates the diversity of antidepressant activity with the adaptive changes occurring in receptor sensitization over several weeks.[19] In this theory, emphasis is placed on a failure of homeostatic regulation of neurotransmitter systems rather than on absolute increases or decreases in their activities.[15] According to this hypothesis, effective antidepressant agents restore efficient regulation to the dysregulated neurotransmitter system.[19,20]

5-HT/NE LINK HYPOTHESIS

It is apparent that no single neurotransmitter theory of depression is adequate. The 5-HT/NE link hypothesis maintains that both the serotonergic and noradrenergic systems need to be functional for an antidepressant effect to be exerted.[12,17] The 5-HT/NE hypothesis is also consistent with the rationale of the postsynaptic alteration theory of depression, which emphasizes the importance of β-adrenergic receptor downregulation for achieving an antidepressant effect.[16] Again, it has been proposed that both NE and 5-HT are necessary for homologous desensitization of central β-adrenergic receptors by antidepressants.[17]

ROLE OF DA IN DEPRESSION

Traditional explanations of the biologic basis of depressive disorders have focused largely on NE and 5-HT; however, most of the evidence that coalesced into the biogenic amine hypothesis of depression does not clearly distinguish between NE and DA.[21]

Several reviews suggest that increased DA neurotransmission in the nucleus accumbens may represent a final common pathway for at least part of the mechanism of action of antidepressant medications.[22] The mechanisms by which antidepressant drugs sensitize DA transmission remain unclear, but may be mediated indirectly by primary actions at NE or 5-HT terminals.

The evidence supporting a dopaminergic mechanism of antidepressant action is entirely preclinical, and clinical studies evaluating the role of DA mechanisms in the action of classical antidepressants have not been conducted.[21]

The complexity of the interaction between 5-HT, NE, and possibly DA is gaining greater appreciation, but a more in-depth understanding of the precise mechanism is needed.

BIOLOGIC MARKERS

Investigators continue to search for biologic or pharmacodynamic markers to assist in the diagnosis and treatment of depressed patients. Although no biologic marker has been discovered, several biologic abnormalities are present in many depressed patients. Approximately 45% to 60% of patients with major depression have a neuroendocrine abnormality, including hypersecretion of cortisol, lack of cortisol suppression after dexamethasone administration (i.e., a positive dexamethasone suppression test), or an abnormal or diminished thyroid-stimulating hormone response to the administration of thyrotropin-releasing hormone. The dexamethasone suppression test is the most specific measure of hypothalamic-pituitary-adrenal axis overactivity. Dexamethasone administration suppresses adrenal corticosteroid production in normal subjects for 24 hours. Failure of dexamethasone to suppress plasma cortisol concentrations indicates overactivity or dysregulation of the hypothalamic-pituitary-adrenal axis. Unfortunately, the high rate of false-positive and false-negative results limits the usefulness of testing for these markers, and has led to their relative lack of use in clinical practice.

Sleep studies in patients with major depression have identified several abnormalities that become more pronounced with advancing age. In depressed patients, the onset of rapid eye movement (REM) sleep occurs earlier during sleep (decreased REM latency) and there is a shift of REM sleep to the first half of the night. There also may be a decrease in slow-wave sleep (stages 3 and 4), increased awakenings during sleep, and early morning awakening.[23] Sleep abnormalities occur in other psychiatric disorders and are not diagnostic for major depression.

CLINICAL PRESENTATION

When a patient has depressive symptoms, it is necessary to investigate the possibility of a medical, psychiatric, and/or drug-induced cause (Table 67–1).[24] Up to 25% of patients with chronic medical conditions (e.g., diabetes, myocardial infarction, carcinoma, or stroke) develop major depression during the course of their medical condition, and the depression often is not accurately diagnosed, especially in the elderly.[25]

All depressed patients should have a complete physical examination, mental status examination, and basic laboratory work-up, including a complete blood count with differential, thyroid function tests, and electrolyte determinations to identify any potential medical problems. A complete medication review should be performed because many drugs may precipitate or worsen a depressive episode (see Table 67–1).

A patient diagnosed with major depressive disorder can expect to have one or more episodes of major depression during their lifetime. According to the DSM-IV-TR a single major depressive episode is characterized by five or more of the symptoms described in Table 67–2. At least one of the symptoms is depressed mood (often an irritable mood in children or adolescents) or loss of interest or pleasure in nearly all activities.[1] These symptoms must have been present nearly every day for at least 2 weeks and must represent a change from the patient's previous level of functioning. The clinician must consider presenting symptoms, their duration, and the patient's current level of social, occupational, or other important areas of functioning. Significant stressors or life events may trigger depression in some individuals but not others; and there may be an important precipitant at the beginning of the disorder.[1,13]

EMOTIONAL SYMPTOMS

A major depressive episode is characterized by a persistent, diminished ability to experience pleasure. A loss of interest and pleasure in usual activities, hobbies, or work is common. Patients appear sad or depressed, and they are often pessimistic and believe that nothing will help them feel better. The presence of intense hopelessness and complete or near-total loss of interest and pleasure in usual activities may identify patients at risk for suicide.[26] Anxiety symptoms are present in almost 90% of depressed outpatients.

Patients often have guilt feelings that are unrealistic, and these may reach delusional proportions. Patients may feel that they deserve punishment and may view their present illness as a punishment. A patient suffering from major depression with psychotic features may hear voices (auditory hallucinations) saying that he or she is a bad person and that he or she should commit suicide. Depression with psychotic features may require hospitalization, especially if the patient becomes a danger to self or others.

PHYSICAL SYMPTOMS

Physical symptoms often motivate patients, especially the elderly, to seek medical attention. Chronic fatigue is a common complaint, with a decreased ability to perform normal daily tasks. Fatigue often appears worse in the morning and does not improve with rest. Complaints of pain, especially headache, often accompany fatigue.

Sleep disturbances generally present as frequent early morning awakening (terminal insomnia), with difficulty returning to sleep. This may coexist with difficulty falling asleep (initial insomnia) and frequent nighttime awakening. Less frequently, depressed patients complain of increased sleep (hypersomnia), although they experience daytime exhaustion or fatigue.

Appetite disturbances, including complaints of decreased appetite, often result in substantial weight loss, especially in the elderly.[25] Some patients lose 2 pounds or more per week without dieting. Other patients, especially in the ambulatory setting, may overeat and gain weight, although they actually may not enjoy eating. They may crave specific foods.

Some patients exhibit gastrointestinal complaints, others cardiovascular complaints, especially palpitations. Patients frequently present with a loss of sexual interest or libido.

TABLE 67–1. Common Medical Disorders, Psychiatric Disorders, and Drug Therapy Associated With Depression

Medical disorders	Metabolic disorders	**Psychiatric disorders**
Endocrine diseases	Electrolyte imbalance	Alcoholism
Hypothyroidism	Hypokalemia	Anxiety disorders
Addison's disease	Hyponatremia	Eating disorders
Cushing's disease	Hepatic encephalopathy	Schizophrenia
Deficiency states	Cardiovascular disease	**Drug therapy**
Pernicious anemia	Coronary artery disease	Antihypertensives
Wernicke's encephalopathy	Congestive heart failure	Clonidine
Severe anemia	Myocardial infarction	Diuretics
Infections	Neurologic disorders	Guanethidine sulfate
AIDS	Alzheimer's disease	Hydralazine hydrochloride
Encephalitis	Epilepsy	Methyldopa
Influenza	Huntington's disease	Propranolol
Mononucleosis	Multiple sclerosis	Reserpine
Sexually transmitted diseases	Pain	**Hormonal therapy**
Tuberculosis	Parkinson's disease	Oral contraceptives
Collagen disorder	Poststroke	Steroids/adrenocorticotropic
Systemic lupus erythematosus	Malignant disease	hormone
		Acne therapy
		Isotretinoin
		Other
		Interferon-beta-1a

Compiled from Katon and Sullivan.[24]

TABLE 67–2. DSM-IV-TR Criteria for Major Depressive Episode

A. Five (or more) of the following symptoms have been present during the same 2-week period and represent a change from previous functioning; at least one of the symptoms is either (1) depressed mood or (2) loss of interest or pleasure.

Note: Do not include symptoms that are clearly due to a general medical condition or mood-incongruent delusions or hallucinations.

1. Depressed mood most of the day nearly every day
2. Markedly diminished interest or pleasure in all, or almost all, activities most of the day nearly every day
3. Significant weight loss when not dieting or weight gain (e.g., a change of more than 5% of body weight in a month), or decrease or increase in appetite nearly every day
4. Insomnia or hypersomnia nearly every day
5. Psychomotor agitation or retardation nearly every day (observable by others, not merely subjective feelings of restlessness or being slowed down)
6. Fatigue or loss of energy nearly every day
7. Feelings of worthlessness or excessive or inappropriate guilt (which may be delusional) nearly every day
8. Diminished ability to think or concentrate, or indecisiveness, nearly every day
9. Recurrent thoughts of death (not just fear of dying), recurrent suicidal ideation without a specific plan, or a suicide attempt or a specific plan for committing suicide

B. The symptoms cause clinically significant distress or impairment in social, occupational, or other important areas of functioning.
C. The symptoms are not due to the direct physiological effects of a substance (e.g., a drug of abuse, a medication) or a general medical condition (e.g., hypothyroidism).
D. The symptoms are not better accounted for by bereavement (i.e., after the loss of a loved one), the symptoms persist for longer than 2 months or are characterized by marked functional impairment, morbid preoccupation with worthlessness, suicidal ideation, psychotic symptoms, or psychomotor retardation.

Modified and reprinted with permission from the Diagnostic and Statistical Manual of Mental Disorders, 4th ed., Text Revision. Washington, American Psychiatric Association, 2000.

INTELLECTUAL OR COGNITIVE SYMPTOMS

Intellectual or cognitive symptoms include a decreased ability to concentrate, slowed thinking, and a poor memory for recent events. Patients may appear confused and indecisive. Depression should be considered when cognitive symptoms are present in the elderly.[25]

PSYCHOMOTOR DISTURBANCES

Patients may appear noticeably slowed or retarded in physical movements, thought processes, and speech (psychomotor retardation). Conversely, depression may be accompanied by psychomotor agitation, manifesting as purposeless, restless motion (e.g., pacing, wringing of hands, or outbursts of shouting).

SUICIDE RISK EVALUATION AND MANAGEMENT

Suicide is the eighth leading cause of death in the United States, and most patients who committed suicide were suffering from depression around the time of their death.[27] All patients suffering from major depression should be assessed for suicidal thoughts. Widely held myths regarding suicide include the belief that people are more likely to commit suicide if they are asked about it, that people who attempt or talk about suicide are just looking for attention and are not serious, that suicidal people are crazy, and that most suicides are caused by a sudden traumatic event.

Factors that increase the risk for suicide include increasing age, being widowed, being unmarried, being unemployed, living alone, a history of a previous psychiatric admission, substance abuse, depression, feelings of hopelessness, prior attempts, family history of suicide, anniversary of a loss, presence of a serious medical problem, lack of a social support system, and refusal to seek help.[26] The presence of a very detailed plan with the intention and ability to carry it out indicates a high risk of suicide. Although women attempt suicide two to three times more often than men, men succeed about three times more frequently. Suicide is almost twice as common in the elderly as in the general population.[28] This appears to be a result of more determination, carefully planned acts, and fewer warning signs.[28] To assess the severity of suicidal thoughts, the clinician must be sensitive to hints of suicidal ideation, including a change in personality, a sudden decision to make a will or give away possessions, and any recent purchase of a gun or obtaining (or hoarding) a large supply of medications or other potentially toxic substances. It is important to remember that the risk of suicide in those recovering from major depression may increase as they develop the energy and capacity to act on a plan made earlier in a course of illness. It is not always possible to predict whether or when a depressed person will attempt suicide.

When suicidal intent is suspected, it is important to ask, "Are you thinking about harming or killing yourself?" If the risk is significant, the patient must be referred immediately to an appropriate health care professional.

▶ TREATMENT: Depressive Disorders

DESIRED OUTCOME

The goals of treatment are to reduce the symptoms of acute depression, facilitate the patient's return to a premorbid level (before the onset of the illness) of functioning, and prevent further episodes of depression. Whether or not to hospitalize the patient is often the first decision that is made in consideration of the patient's risk of suicide, physical state of health, social support system, and presence of a psychotic and/or catatonic depression.

GENERAL APPROACH TO TREATMENT

Studies have found that antidepressants are of equivalent efficacy when administered in comparable doses. Because one cannot predict which antidepressant will be the most effective in an individual patient, the initial choice is made empirically. Factors that often influence the choice of an antidepressant include the patient's history of response, pharmacogenetics (history of familial antidepressant response), subtype of depression, patient's concurrent medical history, potential for drug-drug interactions, adverse events profile, and drug cost.

Although the pathophysiology of major depression remains elusive, the clinician can now select from multiple drug therapies with different mechanisms of action.[29] Failure to respond to one antidepressant class or one antidepressant drug within a class does not predict a failed response to another drug class or another drug within the class.

Approximately 65% to 70% of patients with varying types of depression improve with drug therapy, compared with 30% to 40% who improve with placebo. A preferential response to MAOIs has been reported in patients with atypical depression.[30] In atypical depression, two or more of the following are present: (1) weight gain or increase in appetite, (2) hypersomnia, (3) heavy feelings in arms or legs, and (4) interpersonal rejection sensitivity. Depressed individuals with psychotic symptoms should be treated with an antidepressant plus an antipsychotic agent or electroconvulsive therapy (ECT).[31]

NONPHARMACOLOGIC THERAPY

In addition to pharmacologic interventions, psychotherapy should be employed whenever the patient is able and willing to participate. Psychotherapy alone is not recommended for the acute treatment of patients with severe and/or psychotic major depressive disorder. However, if the depressive episode is mild to moderate in severity, psychotherapy may be the first-line therapy.[32] The effects of psychotherapy and antidepressant medications are considered to be additive. Combined treatment may be advantageous for patients with partial responses to either treatment alone and for those with a chronic course of illness. However, for uncomplicated, nonchronic major depressive disorder, combined treatment may provide no unique advantage.[32] Although not extensively evaluated, cognitive therapy, behavioral therapy, and interpersonal psychotherapy appear equally effective.[32] Maintenance psychotherapy as the sole treatment to prevent recurrence generally is not recommended. Often, medication alone may prevent a depressive recurrence during the maintenance phase.[32]

ECT is a safe and effective treatment for certain severe mental illnesses, including all subtypes of major depressive disorder as well as other selected psychiatric illnesses.

Patients are candidates for ECT when a rapid response is needed, risks of other treatments outweigh potential benefits, there is a history of poor response to drugs and a good response to ECT, and the patient expresses a preference for ECT.[33]

A course of ECT generally consists of 6 to 12 treatments administered either unilaterally or bilaterally two to three times weekly. A rapid therapeutic response (10 to 14 days) has been reported. Although there are no absolute contraindications to the use of ECT, several conditions are associated with increased risk. These include increased intracranial pressure, cerebral lesions, recent myocardial infarction, recent intracerebral hemorrhage, bleeding, or otherwise unstable vascular condition. The use of an anesthetic as well as a nondepolarizing neuromuscular blocking agent decreases the morbidity associated with ECT.[33]

Adverse effects of ECT include cognitive dysfunction, cardiovascular dysfunction, prolonged apnea, treatment-emergent mania, headache, nausea, and muscle aches. Cognitive changes associated with ECT include confusion immediately after the seizure and retrograde and anterograde memory disturbance. Most cognitive disturbances are transient, but some patients may report permanent loss of memory for events occurring over the months before, after, or during treatment.[33]

Relapse rates during the year immediately following ECT are high unless maintenance antidepressant medication is prescribed. Guidelines developed by the American Psychiatric Association include indications and contraindications for the appropriate use of ECT, procedures for obtaining informed consent, and issues in administering ECT.[33]

Some individuals experience depressive episodes during a particular season of the year. This condition is referred to as *seasonal affective disorder* (SAD) and occurs most commonly in the winter, with remission in spring or summer.[34] Reduced environmental light may be the main precipitating factor of winter depression,[34] and may result from a disturbance of the circadian rhythm caused by desynchronization between the solar clock and the human biologic clock during short photoperiods.[34] Bright-light therapy is used to resynchronize the disturbed rhythm,[35–37] and requires the patient to gaze into a light box in the morning or evening for approximately 2 hours.[36] Some individuals will require antidepressant therapy in addition to light therapy or antidepressants for nonseasonal episodes of major depression.

Light therapy is well tolerated, with minor visual complaints being the most frequently reported event.[36] Consequently, anyone undergoing light therapy should receive baseline and periodic eye examinations.

PHARMACOLOGIC THERAPY

Antidepressants can be classified in several ways, including by chemical structure and the presumed mechanism of antidepressant activity. Although the link between the presumed mechanism of drug action and antidepressant response is tenuous, this classification has the advantage of being based on established pharmacology and clearly explains some of the common, but expected, adverse effects. The knowledgeable clinician can use these facts to tailor treatment to individual patient needs and thereby optimize treatment outcome. Currently available antidepressants and initial dosages are shown in Table 67–3.

MIXED SEROTONIN AND NOREPINEPHRINE REUPTAKE INHIBITORS

Although TCAs are effective in treating all depressive subtypes, especially the severe melancholic subtype of major depressive disorder, their use has diminished greatly due to the availability of equally effective therapies that are much safer and better tolerated. All TCAs potentiate the activity of NE and 5-HT by blocking their reuptake. However, the potency and selectivity of TCAs for the inhibition of reuptake of NE and 5-HT vary greatly among these agents (Table 67–4). Because TCAs affect other receptor systems including the anticholinergic, neurologic, and cardiovascular systems, adverse events are reported frequently during TCA therapy.[38]

Venlafaxine, a structurally novel antidepressant, is a potent inhibitor of 5-HT and NE reuptake and a weak inhibitor of dopamine reuptake. Unlike the TCAs, it has virtually no affinity for muscarinic, histaminergic, and α_1-adrenergic receptors.[39]

Maprotiline and amoxapine are both inhibitors of NE reuptake, with less effect on 5-HT reuptake. Maprotiline is associated with

TABLE 67–3. Adult Dosages for Currently Available Antidepressant Medications[a]

Generic Name	Trade Name	Suggested Therapeutic Plasma Concentration (ng/mL)	Initial Dose (mg/day)	Usual Dosage Range (mg/day)
Selective serotonin reuptake inhibitors				
Citalopram	Celexa		20	20–60
Escitalopram	Lexapro		10	10–20
Fluoxetine	Prozac		10–20	10–80
Fluvoxamine	Luvox		50	50–300
Paroxetine	Paxil		20	20–50
Sertraline	Zoloft		50	100–200
Serotonin/norepinephrine reuptake inhibitor				
Venlafaxine	Effexor		75	75–375
Aminoketone				
Bupropion	Wellbutrin		200	300–450
Triazolopyridines				
Nefazodone	Serzone		200	300–600
Trazodone	Desyrel		50–150	150–400
Tetracyclines				
Maprotiline	Ludiomil	200–300[b]	50–75	100–225
Mirtazapine	Remeron		15	15–45
Tricyclic antidepressants				
Tertiary amines				
Amitriptyline	Elavil	120–250[b]	50–75	100–300
Clomipramine	Anafranil		25	100–250
Doxepin	Sinequan	110–250[b]	50–75	100–300
Imipramine	Tofranil	200–300[b]	50–75	100–300
Trimipramine	Surmontil		50–75	100–300
Secondary amines				
Desipramine	Norpramin	125–300	50–75	100–300
Nortriptyline	Pamelor	50–150	25–50	50–150
Protriptyline	Vivactil	70–240	10–20	15–60
Dibenzoxazepine				
Amoxapine	Asendin	200–400[c]	50–150	100–400
Monoamine oxidase inhibitors				
Phenelzine	Nardil		15	15–90
Tranylcypromine	Parnate		20	20–60

[a]Doses listed are total daily doses; elderly patients are usually treated with approximately one-half of the dose listed.
[b]Parent drug plus demethylated metabolite.
[c]Parent drug plus hydroxymetabolite.
Compiled from Baldessarini,[15] Horst and Preskorn,[41] Andrews et al,[53] Wells,[68] Task Force on the Use of Laboratory Tests in Psychiatry,[75] and Waugh and Goa.[81]

a higher incidence of seizures than imipramine or amitriptyline.[19] Amoxapine, while less sedating than some antidepressants, blocks cholinergic receptors, causing clinically significant anticholinergic effects.

SELECTIVE SEROTONIN REUPTAKE INHIBITORS

The efficacy of SSRIs is superior to placebo and equal to the TCAs in treating patients with major depression, and the SSRIs cause minimal anticholinergic effects.[29]

TRIAZOLOPYRIDINES

Trazodone and nefazodone have dual actions on serotonergic neurons, acting as both 5-HT$_2$ antagonists and 5-HT reuptake inhibitors,[40] and they may enhance 5-HT$_{1A}$-mediated neurotransmission. These drugs have negligible affinity for cholinergic and histaminergic receptors. Trazodone's use as an antidepressant agent has diminished secondary to side effects (e.g., dizziness and sedation) and increased availability of alternative better-tolerated agents. Nefazodone also has low affinity for α_1-adrenergic receptors. The triazolopyridines are effective agents in treating major depression with no substantial evidence to support a unique spectrum of therapeutic activity.

AMINOKETONE

Bupropion, the only marketed aminoketone antidepressant, appears to have a unique mechanism of drug action.[41] It has no appreciable effect on the reuptake of NE or 5-HT, and its most potent neurochemical action is blockade of DA reuptake.

MIXED SEROTONIN-NOREPINEPHRINE EFFECTS

Mirtazapine, a TCA, enhances central noradrenergic and serotonergic activity through the antagonism of central presynaptic α_2-adrenergic autoreceptors and heteroreceptors.[42]

TABLE 67–4. Relative Potencies of Norepinephrine and Serotonin Reuptake Blockade and Side-Effect Profile of Antidepressant Drugs

	Reuptake Antagonism		Anticholinergic Effects	Sedation	Orthostatic Hypotension	Seizures	Conduction Abnormalities
	Norepinephreine	*Serotonin*					
Selective serotonin reuptake inhibitors							
Citalopram	0	++++	0	+	0	++	0
Escitalopram	0	++++	0	0	0	0	0
Fluoxetine	0	+++	0	0	0	++	0
Fluvoxamine	0	++++	0	0	0	++	0
Paroxetine	0	++++	+	+	0	++	0
Sertraline	0	++++	0	0	0	++	0
Serotonin/norepinephrine reuptake inhibitor							
Venlafaxine	++++	++++	+	+	0	++	+
Aminoketone							
Bupropion	+	+	+	0	0	++++	+
Triazolopyridines							
Nefazodone	0	++	0	+++	+++	++	+
Trazodone	0	++	0	++++	+++	++	+
Tetracyclines							
Maprotiline	+++	+	+++	+++	++	++++	++
Mirtazapine	0	0	+	++	++		+
Tricyclic antidepressants							
Tertiary amines							
Amitriptyline	++	++++	++++	++++	+++	+++	+++
Clomipramine	++	+++	++++	++++	++	++++	+++
Doxepin	++	++	+++	++++	++	+++	++
Imipramine	+++	+++	+++	+++	++++	+++	+++
Trimipramine	++	++	++++	++++	+++	+++	+++
Secondary amines							
Desipramine	++++	+	++	++	++	++	++
Nortriptyline	+++	++	++	++	+	++	++
Protriptyline	+++	++	++	+	++	++	+++
Dibenzoxazepine							
Amoxapine[a]	+++	++	+++	++	++	+++	++
Monoamine oxidase inhibitors							
Phenelzine	++	++	+	++	++	+	
Tranylcypromine	++	+	+	+	++	+	+

++++, high; +++, moderate; ++, low; +, very low; 0, absent.
[a]Also blocks dopamine receptors.
Compiled from Baldessarini,[15] Bryant and Brown,[19] Horst and Preskorn,[41] Andrews et al,[53] Wells,[68] Task Force on the Use of Laboratory Tests in Psychiatry,[75] DeVane,[78] and Waugh and Goa.[81]

MONOAMINE OXIDASE INHIBITORS

MAOIs increase the concentrations of NE, 5-HT, and DA within the neuronal synapse through inhibition of the MAO enzyme. Studies have demonstrated that similarly to TCAs, chronic therapy causes changes in receptor sensitivity (i.e., downregulation of β-adrenergic, α-adrenergic, and serotonergic receptors).[43,44] The MAOIs currently marketed in the U.S., phenelzine and tranylcypromine, are nonselective inhibitors of MAO A and MAO B.

ST. JOHN'S WORT

Increasingly, consumers are choosing alternative forms of therapy, such as herbal medications including St. John's wort.[45,46] Some evaluations have found that the active ingredient in St. John's wort, hypericum, is a safe and effective treatment for mild to moderate depression[45,46] when compared with placebo, TCAs, and fluoxetine.[47,48] In most cases, side effects appear to be mild. St. John's wort is available as an over-the-counter medication. Although this

may allow certain advantages such as reduced cost of therapy and self-treatment, it also has the potential to result in circumvention of the health care system. St. John's wort has been found to have several significant drug interactions with medications used to treat human immunodeficiency virus (e.g., indinavir) and digoxin.[49] Perhaps most disconcerting is the fact that herbal medications are not regulated by the Food and Drug Administration (FDA), and manufacturers are not required to adhere to good manufacturing practices. St. John's wort should be administered under the guidance of a clinician trained in the treatment of depression, and a single-source product should be used continuously from a reputable and trusted manufacturer.

CLINICAL CONTROVERSY

The treatment of depression with herbal agents or nutriceuticals remains controversial. Studies evaluating the efficacy of therapies such as St. John's wort have been conflicting. In addition, concerns regarding the safety and integrity of the products have been raised.

ADVERSE EFFECTS

TCAs and Other Heterocyclics

The most commonly reported adverse effects of antidepressant therapy are summarized in Table 67–4. The TCAs affect several neurotransmitters and produce a wide range of pharmacologic actions, including many unwanted, but expected, adverse effects. The side effects most frequently associated with the TCAs (e.g., dry mouth, constipation, blurred vision, urinary retention, dizziness, tachycardia, memory impairment, and at higher doses, delirium) may result from blockade of cholinergic receptors.[43] These adverse effects often have an impact on patient compliance, particularly in the elderly and those receiving long-term maintenance therapy. A common and potentially problematic effect, orthostatic hypotension, has been attributed to the affinity of the TCAs for adrenergic receptors.[50] TCAs also cause cardiac conduction delays and may even induce heart block in patients with a preexisting conduction disorder. TCA overdose can produce severe arrhythmias.[50] Therefore caution should be exercised when prescribing these agents to patients with clinically significant cardiac disease. Other adverse effects that lead to patient noncompliance include weight gain, excessive perspiration, and sexual dysfunction.[50]

Abrupt withdrawal of TCAs is often associated with symptoms suggestive of cholinergic rebound (e.g., dizziness, nausea, diarrhea, insomnia, and restlessness), especially if the daily dose exceeds 300 mg.[51,52] Therefore the dose should be tapered over several days.

Amoxapine, the demethylated metabolite of loxapine, has intermediate sedative and anticholinergic potency.[51] Because of its postsynaptic receptor DA-blocking effects, extrapyramidal side effects, including pseudoparkinsonism, dystonia, akathisia, and tardive dyskinesia have been reported.[19] Amoxapine offers no advantage over standard TCAs or other antidepressants.

Maprotiline, a tetracyclic drug, blocks reuptake of NE with minimal effect on 5-HT. It has intermediate sedative and anticholinergic effects and may cause less orthostatic hypotension than imipramine; however, an exanthematous rash occurs in approximately 4% of patients.[19] Maprotiline is also associated with a higher incidence of seizures than standard TCAs and is contraindicated in patients with a history of a seizure disorder.

Venlafaxine

The most commonly reported adverse effects with venlafaxine include nausea, constipation, somnolence, dry mouth, dizziness, nervousness, sweating, asthenia, abnormal ejaculation/orgasm, and anorexia.[44,53] These side effects may be dose related. Venlafaxine may cause a dose-related increase in diastolic blood pressure, and baseline blood pressure is not a useful predictor of the occurrence of this phenomenon. Blood pressure should be monitored regularly during venlafaxine therapy, and dosage reduction or discontinuation may be necessary if sustained hypertension occurs.[53,54]

Selective Serotonin Reuptake Inhibitors

The SSRIs include fluoxetine, citalopram, sertraline, paroxetine, escitalopram, and fluvoxamine. The SSRIs have a low affinity for histaminic, α_1-adrenergic, and muscarinic receptors, and therefore produce fewer anticholinergic and cardiovascular adverse effects than the TCAs, and are not associated with weight gain.[55,56] The most common adverse effects, which generally are mild and short lived, are gastrointestinal symptoms (i.e., nausea, vomiting, and diarrhea), sexual dysfunction in both males and females, headache, insomnia, and fatigue.[56]

Although the SSRIs are known to improve the anxiety symptoms associated with depression, a few patients experience an increase in anxiety symptoms or agitation early in treatment.

Triazolopyridines

Trazodone and nefazodone have minimal anticholinergic effects and 5-HT agonist side effects, but they can cause orthostatic hypotension. Sedation, cognitive slowing, and dizziness are the most frequent dose-limiting side effects associated with trazodone.[43] Prescribing information for nefazodone was recently updated to include a black box warning related to cases of life-threatening hepatic failure. Treatment with nefazodone should not be initiated in individuals with active liver disease or with elevated baseline serum transaminases.[57] Common adverse effects associated with nefazodone include light-headedness, dizziness, orthostatic hypotension, somnolence, dry mouth, nausea, and asthenia.[45]

A rare but potentially serious adverse effect of trazodone is priapism, which is reported to occur in approximately 1 in 6000 male patients. Some cases have required surgical intervention (1 in 23,000) and permanent impotence may result.[58] There have been no reports of priapism associated with nefazodone use in men, but there is a published case report of nefazodone-induced clitoral priapism.[59]

Aminoketone

Adverse effects associated with bupropion include nausea, dizziness, tremor, insomnia, vomiting, constipation, dry mouth, and skin reactions. The occurrence of seizures in patients taking bupropion appears to be strongly associated with dose, and may be increased by predisposing factors such as history of head trauma and CNS tumor. At daily doses of 450 mg (the FDA-approved ceiling dose) or less the incidence of seizures is 0.4%.[60,61]

Mixed Serotonin-Norepinephrine Effects

The most common adverse effects of mirtazapine are somnolence, weight gain, dry mouth, and constipation. In premarketing clinical trials, both agranulocytosis and liver function test (LFT) elevations were noted. However, the incidence appears to be rare, and therefore routine laboratory monitoring is not recommended.[47] Additionally, LFT elevations were observed 1.4 times more frequently than with other antidepressants and 1.6 times more frequently than with placebo. Prescribers should consider obtaining baseline LFTs and monitoring these periodically throughout the course of therapy.[47]

Monoamine Oxidase Inhibitors

The most common adverse effect of MAOIs is postural hypotension; this is more likely to occur with phenelzine than with tranylcypromine.[48] Hypotensive reactions may be minimized through divided dosage scheduling. Anticholinergic side effects, especially dry mouth and constipation, are common but are milder in severity compared with those associated with the TCAs.

TABLE 67–5. Dietary Restrictions for Patients Taking Monoamine Oxidase Inhibitors

Aged cheeses[a]
Sour cream[b]
Yogurt[b]
Cottage cheese[b]
American cheese[b]
Mild Swiss cheese[b]
Wine[c] (especially Chianti and sherry)
Beer
Herring[a] (pickled, salted, dry)
Sardines
Snails
Anchovies
Canned, aged, or processed meats
Monosodium glutamate
Liver (chicken or beef, more than 2 days old)
Fermented foods
Canned figs
Raisins
Pods of broad beans[a] (fava beans)
Yeast extract[a] and other yeast products
Meat extract (marmite)
Soy sauce
Chocolate[d]
Coffee[d]
Ripe avocado
Sauerkraut
Licorice

[a] Clearly warrants absolute prohibition (e.g., English Stilton, blue, Camembert, cheddar).
[b] Up to 2 oz daily is acceptable.
[c] 3 oz white wine or a single cocktail is acceptable.
[d] Up to 2 oz daily is acceptable: larger amounts of decaffeinated coffee are acceptable.

TABLE 67–6. Medication Restrictions for Patients Taking Monoamine Oxidase Inhibitors

Amphetamines	Levodopa
Appetite suppressants	Local anesthetics containing
Asthma inhalants	sympathomimetic vasoconstrictors
Buspirone	Meperidine
Carbamazepine	Methyldopa
Cocaine	Methylphenidate
Cyclobenzaprine	Other antidepressants[a]
Decongestants (topical	Other MAOIs
and systemic)	Reserpine
Dextromethorphan	Rizatriptan
Dopamine	Stimulants
Ephedrine	Sumatriptan
Epinephrine	Sympathomimetics
Guanethidine	Tryptophan

[a] Tricyclic antidepressants may be used with caution by experienced clinicians in treatment-resistant populations.

be taught to recognize the symptoms of hypertensive crisis and to seek treatment should those symptoms occur.

Phenelzine, the most frequently prescribed MAOI, has mild to moderate sedating effects. Tranylcypromine may exert a stimulating effect, and insomnia may occur, so the last dose of the day should be administered in the early afternoon. Dose-related impotence and anorgasmia in males and orgasmic inhibition in females have been reported.[62,63] In addition, fever, myoclonic jerking, and brisk deep tendon reflexes may occur.[48,64]

Hypertensive crisis, a potentially fatal but rare adverse reaction, may occur when MAOIs are taken concurrently with certain foods, especially those high in tyramine (Table 67–5) or drugs (Table 67–6). Ten milligrams of tyramine can cause a marked pressor effect, and 25 mg can result in serious hypertensive crisis,[65] and these incidents may culminate in cerebrovascular accident and death.[48] Symptoms of hypertensive crisis include occipital headache, stiff neck, nausea, vomiting, sweating, and sharply elevated blood pressure. Hypertensive crises were previously treated with sublingual nifedipine, but recent reports of adverse events secondary to an uncontrollable fall in blood pressure and resulting rebound catecholamine release have led to concerns.[66] Alternative agents, such as captopril, should be considered.[67]

Education of patients taking MAOIs regarding dietary and medication restrictions is extremely important. Printed and verbal patient instructions should be provided. Patients unable to read and those with difficulty understanding or remembering medication instructions should not be prescribed MAOIs unless they have competent caregivers. Patients should be instructed to consult a health care professional before taking over-the-counter medications. Patients should

PHARMACOKINETICS

The pharmacokinetics of the antidepressants are summarized in Table 67–7. In general, the TCAs are absorbed rapidly after oral administration. Bioavailability is low (30% to 70% for most TCAs) as a result of the first-pass effect, which shows great interindividual variation.[68]

The TCAs have a large volume of distribution and concentrate in brain and cardiac tissue in laboratory animals. They are bound extensively and strongly to plasma albumin, erythrocytes, α_1-acid glycoprotein, and lipoprotein.[68]

The major metabolic pathways are demethylation, aromatic and aliphatic hydroxylation, and glucuronide conjugation. Enterohepatic cycling has been described.[68,69] Metabolism of TCAs appears to be linear within the usual dosage range. The elimination half-lives of the TCAs vary greatly among individual patients, and this may be determined genetically.[68]

The diversity of the SSRIs is evident not only in their chemical structures, but also in their pharmacokinetic profiles.[70] Fluoxetine has an elimination half-life of 2 to 3 days (4 to 5 days with multiple dosing). The single-dose half-life of norfluoxetine, the active metabolite, is 7 to 9 days. Paroxetine and sertraline have half-lives of approximately 24 hours. Unlike paroxetine, sertraline has an active metabolite, but the metabolite contributes minimally to the pharmacologic effects. Escitalopram has a half-life of approximately 30 hours. Peak plasma concentrations of citalopram are observed within 2 to 4 hours after dosing, and the elimination half-life is about 30 hours. The SSRIs, with the exception of fluvoxamine, escitalopram, and citalopram, are extensively bound to plasma proteins (94% to 99%). The SSRIs are extensively distributed to the tissues, and all, with the possible exception of citalopram, may have a nonlinear pattern of drug accumulation with long-term administration.[70]

Mirtazapine undergoes biotransformation via demethylation and hydroxylation followed by glucuronide conjugation.[47] The 1A2 and the 2D6 isoenzymes of the cytochrome P450 system may be responsible for the formation of the hydroxymetabolite, whereas the 3A4 isoenzyme may be responsible for the formation of the N-desmethyl and the N-oxide metabolite.[47] Although these metabolites are

TABLE 67–7. Pharmacokinetic Properties of Antidepressants

Generic Name	Elimination Half-Life (h)[a]	Time of Peak Plasma Concentration (h)	Plasma Protein Binding (%)	Percentage Bioavailable	Clinically Important Metabolites
Selective serotonin reuptake inhibitors					
Citalopram	33	2–4	80	≥80	Desmethyl- and didemethylcitalopram
Escitalopram	27–32	5	56	80	None
Fluoxetine	4–6 days[b]	4–8	94	95	Norfluoxetine
Fluvoxamine	15–26	2–8	77	53	None
Paroxetine	24–31	5–7	95		None
Sertraline	27	6–8	99	36[c]	N-Desmethylsertraline
Serotonin/norepinephrine reuptake inhibitor					
Venlafaxine	5	2	27–30		O-Desmethylvenlafaxine
Aminoketone					
Bupropion	10–21	3	82–88	[d]	Bupropion threoamino alcohol; bupropion morpholinol
Triazolopyridines					
Nefazodone	2–4	1	99	20	Meta-chlorophenylpiperazine hydroxynefazodone; triazoledione
Trazodone	6–11	1–2	92	[d]	Meta-chlorophenyl piperazine
Tetracyclines					
Maprotiline	28–105	4–24	88	79–87	Desmethylmaprotiline
Mirtazapine	20–40	2	85	50	None known
Tricyclic antidepressants					
Tertiary amines					
Amitriptyline	9–46	1–5	90–97	30–60	Nortriptyline; 10-hydroxynortriptyline
Clomipramine	20–24	2–6	97	36–62	
Doxepin	8–36	1–4	68–82	13–45	Desmethyldoxepin
Imipramine	6–34	1.5–3	63–96	22–77	2-Hydroxyimipramine; desipramine 2-hydroxydesipramine
Trimipramine	7–40	3	94–96	18–63	None
Secondary amines					
Desipramine	11–46	3–6	73–92	33–51	2-Hydroxydesipramine
Nortriptyline	16–88	3–12	87–95	46–70	10-Hydroxynortriptyline
Protriptyline	54–198	6–12	90–94	75–90	None
Dibezoxazepine					
Amoxapine	8–30[e]	1–2	90	[d]	8-Hydroxyamoxapine
Monoamine oxidase inhibitors					
Phenelzine	1.5–4	[d]	[d]	[d]	
Tranylcypromine	1.5–3	[d]	[d]	[d]	

[a]Biologic half-life in slowest phase of elimination.
[b]4–6 days with chronic dosing; norfluoxetine, 4–16 days.
[c]Increases 30–40% when taken with food.
[d]No data available.
[e]Amoxapine, 8 hours; 8-hydroxyamoxapine, 30 hours.

theoretically active, they are present at such low plasma concentrations as to contribute little to the overall pharmacologic profile of mitazapine.

Altered Pharmacokinetics

Factors reported to influence TCA plasma concentrations include disease states, genetics, age, cigarette smoking, and concurrent drug administration. Hepatic disease may reduce metabolic clearance of TCAs.[77] Renal failure does not alter nortriptyline metabolism, but the 10-hydroxy metabolite may accumulate, and protein binding may be diminished, with resulting enhanced sensitivity to the drug.[68] Clinicians should be alert to the possibility of higher-than-expected plasma concentrations of some TCAs in the elderly. Because dose-related

kinetics cannot be ruled out in the elderly, dosage adjustments based on plasma concentration monitoring may be difficult.

In cirrhotics, the half-lives of fluoxetine and norfluoxetine increased to 7.6 and 12 days, respectively.[70] Patients with hepatic impairment had a twofold increase in plasma concentrations of paroxetine.[71] Similarly, in patients with mild stable cirrhosis, the half-life of sertraline was 2.5 times greater than in patients without liver disease.[72] Patients with renal impairment had a two- to fourfold increase in paroxetine plasma concentrations compared with normal volunteers.[71] Plasma concentrations of SSRIs in the elderly are reported to be greater than in younger patients.[70]

The area under the curve of nefazodone and hydroxynefazodone is 25% greater in cirrhotics than in normal volunteers.[73] Patients with cirrhosis accumulate metabolites of bupropion to concentrations two to three times those seen in normal individuals.

Plasma Concentration and Clinical Response

tudies in acutely depressed patients have demonstrated a correlation between antidepressant effect and plasma concentrations for ome TCAs. The patient's clinical response, not plasma concentraon, dictates dosage adjustments. Some patients with plasma concenrations outside the suggested therapeutic plasma concentration range espond, whereas others are nonresponsive regardless of their plasma oncentration. See Table 67–3 for a listing of suggested therapeutic lasma concentration ranges.

For four TCAs (nortriptyline, desipramine, imipramine, and mitriptyline) there is more consistent evidence to support a mininal plasma concentration for clinical response. The best established herapeutic range is for nortriptyline.[74] Studies suggest a curvilinear lasma concentration-response relationship for nortriptyline, with a uggested therapeutic range of 50 to 150 ng/mL. Using logistic regresion analysis of data from multiple published studies, it was found that vithin this range, 70% of patients with major depression responded ersus only 29% of patients with plasma concentrations outside this ange. Interestingly, the response rate generally was higher at the ower end of this range than at the upper limit.[74]

For the newer antidepressants, a correlation has not been established between plasma concentration and clinical response or adverse effects.

Plasma Concentration Monitoring

Because of interindividual variations in plasma concentrations ichieved by a given dose, approximately 40% of patients receiving standard doses of TCAs may not obtain plasma concentrations vithin the desired therapeutic range.[75] Although plasma level monitoring is not performed routinely, some indications include inadequate response, relapse, serious or persistent adverse effects, use of nigher-than-standard doses, suspected toxicity, elderly patients, pregnant patients, patients of African or Asian descent (because of slower netabolism), cardiac disease, suspected noncompliance, suspected pharmacokinetic drug interactions, and when the manufacturer of the product changes. Plasma concentration monitoring of TCAs, when used appropriately, can improve efficacy and minimize drug-related problems. Plasma concentrations should be obtained at steady state, usually after a minimum of 1 week at constant dosage. Sampling should be performed during the drug elimination phase, usually in the morning, 12 hours after the last dose. Samples collected in this manner are comparable for patients on once-, twice-, or thrice-daily regimens.[68]

DRUG INTERACTIONS

TCAs

Because the TCAs are metabolized in the liver through the cytochrome P450 system, they may interact with other drugs that modify hepatic enzyme activity or hepatic blood flow. TCAs are also extensively protein bound, which can cause drug interactions through displacement from protein-binding sites. Many commonly used medications can interact when given concurrently with TCAs. Pharmacokinetic and pharmacodynamic drug interactions involving TCAs are shown in Tables 67–8 and 67–9, respectively.

TCAs may reverse the hypotensive effects of certain sympatholytic antihypertensives (e.g., guanethidine, methyldopa, and clonidine) because of inhibition of presynaptic uptake of the

TABLE 67–8. Pharmacokinetic Drug Interactions Involving Tricyclic Antidepressants

Elevates plasma concentrations of TCAs
Cimetidine
Diltiazem
Ethanol, acute ingestion
SSRIs
Haloperidol
Labetalol
Methylphenidate
Oral contraceptives
Phenothiazines
Propoxyphene
Quinidine
Verapamil
Lowers plasma concentrations of TCAs
Barbiturates
Carbamazepine
Ethanol, chronic ingestion
Phenytoin
Elevates plasma concentrations of interacting drug
Hydantoins
Oral anticoagulants
Lowers plasma concentrations of interacting drug
Levodopa

Compiled from Wells.[68]

TABLE 67–9. Pharmacodynamic Drug Interactions Involving Tricyclic Antidepressants

Interacting Drug	Effect
Alcohol	Increased CNS depressant effects
Amphetamines	Increased effect of amphetamines
Androgens	Delusions, hostility
Anticholinergic agents	Excessive anticholinergic effects
Bepredil	Increased antiarrhythmic effect
Clonidine	Decreased antihypertensive efficacy
Disulfiram	Acute organic brain syndrome
Estrogens	Increased or decreased antidepressant response; increased toxicity
Guanadrel	Decreased antihypertensive efficacy
Guanethidine	Decreased antihypertensive efficacy
Insulin	Increased hypoglycemic effects
Lithium	Possible additive lowering of seizure threshold
Methyldopa	Decreased antihypertensive efficacy; tachycardia; CNS stimulation
Monoamine oxidase inhibitors	Increased therapeutic and possibly toxic effects of both drugs; hypertensive crisis; delirium; seizures; hyperpyrexia; serotonin syndrome
Oral hypoglycemics	Increased hypoglycemic effects
Phenytoin	Possible lowering of seizure threshold and reduced antidepressant response
Sedatives	Increased CNS depressant effects
Sympathomimetics	Increased pharmacologic effects of direct-acting sympathomimetics; decreased effects of indirect-acting sympathomimetics
Thyroid hormones	Increased therapeutic and possibly toxic effects of both drugs; CNS stimulation; tachycardia

Compiled from Wells.[68]

antihypertensive or desensitization of the α_2-adrenergic receptor.[76] Similarly, because of inhibition of presynaptic uptake, TCAs may increase the vasopressor response to direct-acting sympathomimetics such as phenylephrine, epinephrine, and NE. The vasopressor response to indirect-acting sympathomimetics such as ephedrine is decreased.[76] Adverse effects of any TCA would be additive with those of other drugs with similar pharmacologic effects (e.g., anticholinergic, sedative, or hypotensive drugs).[76]

Although MAOIs and TCAs may be coadministered safely in refractory patients with apparent increased efficacy compared with monotherapy, severe reactions and fatalities have occurred. These reactions include hypertensive crises, hyperpyrexia, excitation, and convulsions, and they usually occur when TCAs are added to established MAOI therapy.[76]

SSRIs

Table 67–10 summarizes the drug interactions of non-TCA antidepressants. Drug-drug interactions may occur when an SSRI is coadministered with another drug metabolized through the cytochrome P450 system.[76] Two of the isoenzymes of the cytochrome P450 system, 2D6 and 3A4, are responsible for the metabolism of over 80% of currently marketed drugs.[77] The ability of an SSRI, or any antidepressant, to inhibit or induce the activity of these enzymes will be a significant contributory factor in determining its capability to cause a pharmacokinetic drug interaction when administered concomitantly.[77,78] Table 67–11 shows the cytochrome P450 enzyme inhibitory, potential of the second- and third-generation antidepressant agents.[77]

The long half-lives of fluoxetine (2 to 5 days in young healthy subjects) and of its active metabolite, norfluoxetine (7 to 9 days), ensure that following discontinuation of the drug, active compounds persist in the body for weeks. The very slow elimination of fluoxetine makes it critical to ensure a 5-week washout after fluoxetine discontinuation before starting an MAOI.[77] For all other SSRIs, a 2-week washout is recommended. Serious and potentially fatal reactions may occur when any SSRI is coadministered with an MAOI, and coadministration is contraindicated.[76]

Patients prescribed concomitant phenytoin or carbamazepine with fluoxetine may have increased anticonvulsant plasma concentrations and symptoms of toxicity.[76] Markedly increased plasma concentrations of TCAs with resulting symptoms of toxicity have been reported in patients taking fluoxetine.

Although no significant pharmacokinetic changes were present with the coadministration of warfarin and fluoxetine, altered anticoagulation effects, including bleeding, have been documented.[79] Similar findings have been noted with paroxetine and sertraline, and consequently careful monitoring of prothrombin time is recommended when warfarin and an SSRI are administered concomitantly. The risk of using SSRIs in combination with other CNS-active medications has not been evaluated systematically. Although coadministration appears relatively safe, caution should be used when prescribing an SSRI and other CNS-active drugs such as benzodiazepines.[55] There are case reports of elevated levels of TCAs when administered concomitantly with fluoxetine, sertraline, and paroxetine. In a patient on a stable dose of a TCA in whom therapy with an SSRI is being initiated, it is recommended that a blood level of the TCA be obtained. Therapy with the SSRI should be initiated carefully and conservatively. Consideration of a dose reduction of the TCA is appropriate for susceptible populations such as the elderly or those with cardiovascular disease.

Data to date suggest that citalopram may cause only moderate or no pharmacokinetic interactions when coadministered with TCAs.

Coadministration of cimetidine reduced citalopram oral clearance by 29%, whereas the addition of fluvoxamine caused a significant increase in plasma concentrations of citalopram.[80] At this time, escitalopram is considered unlikely to be involved in clinically important pharmacokinetic interactions, although coadministration of escitalopram and desipramine resulted in a doubling of the area under the curve for desipramine.[81]

Other Agents

Venlafaxine and its active metabolite, O-desmethylvenlafaxine, are only 30% protein bound, permitting coadministration with other highly protein-bound drugs.[53] Venlafaxine did not cause any significant change in the pharmacokinetics of ethanol, diazepam, or lithium.[53] Venlafaxine is metabolized to its active metabolite by the cytochrome P450 2D6 isoenzyme, which is the source of the genetic polymorphism present in the metabolism of many antidepressants. Venlafaxine does not have an inhibitory effect on isoenzymes 1A2, 2C9, 2D6, or 3A4.[82] Although nefazodone is highly protein bound in vitro, nefazodone does not alter the in vitro protein binding of chlorpromazine, desipramine, diazepam, phenytoin, lidocaine, prazosin, propranolol, verapamil, or warfarin. However, it is unknown whether or not displacement of either nefazodone or other drugs occurs in vivo.[73] Triazolobenzodiazepines, such as triazolam and alprazolam, interacted significantly with nefazodone. When triazolam is coadministered with nefazodone, a 75% reduction in the dose of triazolam is recommended. If alprazolam is coadministered with nefazodone, a 50% reduction in the dose of alprazolam is recommended.[73] Astemizole is metabolized by the cytochrome P450 3A4 isoenzyme. Ketoconazole, erythromycin, and other inhibitors of 3A4 can block the metabolism of terfenadine and astemizole, resulting in an increased plasma concentration of parent drug. Increased plasma concentrations of terfenadine and astemizole are associated with QT prolongation and with rare cases of serious cardiovascular adverse events, including death. Nefazodone is an in vitro inhibitor of 3A4. The concurrent use of mirtazapine and the MAOIs should be avoided. In addition, 14 days should elapse between the discontinuation of an MAOI and the initiation of mirtazapine, and vice versa. Mirtazapine is metabolized by cytochrome P450 isoenzymes 1A2, 2D6, and 3A4.

SPECIAL POPULATIONS

Elderly Patients

Depression in the elderly is a major public health problem. Many elderly depressed patients are often inadequately treated, or depression is missed or mistaken for another disorder, such as dementia. In the elderly, depressed mood, the typical signature symptom of depression, may be less prominent than other depressive symptoms such as loss of appetite, cognitive impairment, sleeplessness, anergia, and loss of interest in and enjoyment of the normal pursuits of life.[83] Somatic (physical) complaints are quite frequently the presenting symptoms in elderly depressed patients. The increased suicidal attempts present in the depressed elderly may be due to access to firearms, diminished cognitive functions, sleep disruptions, poor social interactions, and inattention among primary caregivers.[84] Approximately every 95 minutes an elderly person commits suicide.[84]

Before initiating antidepressant treatment, a complete physical examination should be performed. In prescribing antidepressants, elderly patients may be either over- or undertreated. Overtreatment

ABLE 67–10. Drug Interactions of Non-TCA Antidepressants

Non-TCA	Interacting Drug/Drug Class	Effect
Dibenzoxazepine		
Amoxapine	Many of the drugs that interact with the TCAs	Similar response to that seen with TCA interaction
Tetracyclines		
Maprotiline	Many of the drugs that interact with the TCAs	Similar response to that seen with TCA interaction
Mirtazapine	MAOIs	Theoretically central serotonin syndrome could occur
Triazolopyridines		
Nefazodone	Alprazolam	Increased plasma concentrations of alprazolam
	Astemizole	Theoretically increased plasma concentrations of astemizole with potentially serious cardiovascular adverse effects
	Digoxin	Increased C_{max}, C_{min}, and AUC of digoxin by 29%, 27%, and 15%, respectively
	Haloperidol	Decreased clearance of haloperidol by 35%
	MAOIs	Hypertensive crisis; serotonin syndrome; delirium; coma; seizures; hyperpyrexia
	Propranolol	Decreased C_{max} and AUC of propranolol; increased C_{max}, C_{min}, and AUC of m-CCP metabolite of nefazodone
	Ritonavir	Increased AUC of ritonavir with potential for increased adverse events: headaches, dry mouth, nausea, somnolence, dizziness
	Terfenadine	Theoretically increased plasma concentrations of terfenadine with potentially serious cardiovascular adverse effects
	Triazolam	Increased plasma concentrations of triazolam; increased psychomotor impairment
Trazodone	CNS depressants	Increased CNS depression
	Digoxin	Increased serum concentrations of digoxin
	Ethanol	Additive impairment in motor skills
	Fluoxetine	Increased plasma concentrations of trazodone
	MAOIs	Theoretically central serotonin syndrome could occur
	Neuroleptics	Increased hypotension
	Phenytoin	Increased serum concentrations of phenytoin
	Tryptophan	Agitation, restlessness, poor concentration, nausea
	Warfarin	Decreased hypoprothrombinemic response
Aminoketone		
Bupropion	MAOIs	Increased toxicity of bupropion
	Medications that lower seizure threshold	Increased incidence of seizures
	Levodopa	Increased incidence of adverse experiences
	Ritonavir	Increased blood level of bupropion with increased risk of seizures
Selective serotonin reuptake inhibitors		
Citalopram	Cimetidine	Reduced oral clearance of citalopram
	Fluvoxamine	Increased plasma concentrations of citalopram
	TCAs	Possible increased AUC of TCA
Fluoxetine	Alprazolam	Increased plasma concentrations and half-life of alprazolam; increased psychomotor impairment
	Anticoagulants	Possible increased risk of bleeding
	β-Adrenergic blockers	Increased metoprolol serum concentrations and bradycardia; possible heart block
	Buspirone	Decreased therapeutic response to buspirone
	Carbamazepine	Increased plasma concentrations of carbamazepine with symptoms of carbamazepine toxicity
	Dextromethorphan	Visual hallucinations (one patient only)
	Haloperidol	Increased haloperidol concentrations and increased extrapyramidal side effects
	Lithium	Neurotoxicity—confusion, ataxia, dizziness, tremor, absence, seizures
	MAOIs	Severe or fatal reactions—confusion, nausea, double vision, hypomania, hypertension, tremor, serotonin syndrome
	Phenytoin	Increased plasma concentrations of phenytoin and symptoms of phenytoin toxicity
	TCAs	Markedly increased TCA plasma concentration with symptoms of TCA toxicity
	Terfenadine	Arrhythmias, shortness of breath, and orthostasis
	Trazodone	Headaches, dizziness, sedation
	Tryptophan	Agitation, restlessness, poor concentration, nausea
	Valproate	Increased valproate serum concentrations

TABLE 67–10. (Continued)

Non-TCA	Interacting Drug/Drug Class	Effect
Fluvoxamine	Alprazolam	Increased AUC of alprazolam by 96%, increased alprazolam half-life by 71%, and increased psychomotor impairment
	Astemizole	Theoretically increased plasma concentrations of astemizole with potentially serious cardiovascular effects
	β-Adrenergic blockers	Fivefold increase in propranolol serum concentration; bradycardia and hypotension with combined fluvoxamine and metoprolol
	Carbamazepine	Possible carbamazepine toxicity, although a controlled study did not support this
	Clozapine	Increased clozapine serum concentrations and increased risk for seizures and orthostatic hypotension
	Diazepam	Decreased clearance of diazepam and its active metabolite
	Diltiazem	Bradycardia
	Haloperidol	Increased haloperidol plasma concentrations
	Lithium	Increased serotonergic effects; seizures, nausea, tremor
	MAOIs	Potential for hypertensive crisis, serotonin syndrome, seizures, delirium
	Methadone	Increased methadone plasma concentrations with symptoms of methadone toxicity
	TCAs	Increased TCA plasma concentration
	Terfenadine	Theoretically increased plasma concentrations of terfenadine with potentially serious cardiovascular effects
	Theophylline	Increased serum concentrations of theophylline with symptoms of theophylline toxicity
	Tryptophan	Increased serotonergic effects and severe vomiting
	Warfarin	Increased hypoprothrombinemic response to warfarin
Paroxetine	Cimetidine	Increased paroxetine serum concentrations
	Desipramine	Increased plasma concentrations and half-life of desipramine
	MAOIs	Potential for hypertensive crisis, serotonin syndrome, seizures, delirium
	Warfarin	Possible increased risk for bleeding
Sertraline	Carbamazepine	Increased plasma concentrations of carbamazepine
	Diazepam	Small decrease in clearance of diazepam
	MAOIs	Serotonin syndrome, myoclonus, violent shaking
	TCAs	Increased plasma concentrations of secondary amine TCAs (desipramine, nortriptyline)
	Tolbutamide	Decreased clearance of tolbutamide (16%)
	Warfarin	Increased prothrombin time
Serotonin/norepinephrine reuptake inhibitor		
Venlafaxine	Cimetidine	Reduced clearance of venlafaxine by 43%
		AUC and peak serum concentration of venlafaxine increased by 60%
	MAOIs	Potential for hypertensive crisis, serotonin syndrome, seizures, delirium

AUC, area under the curve, C_{max}, maximum concentration; C_{min}, minimum concentration; MAOI, monoamine oxidase inhibitor.
Compiled from Wells,[68] Hansten and Hon,[76] and Mitchell.[77]

occurs when age-related pharmacokinetic and pharmacodynamic factors are overlooked. Undertreatment results from an overly conservative approach as a result of the patient's advanced age or concurrent medical problems. The SSRIs are usually selected as first-choice antidepressants in the elderly, and may enable the clinician to avoid some of the problematic adverse effects commonly associated with the TCAs (e.g., sedative, anticholinergic, and cardiovascular side effects). Nefazodone, bupropion, and venlafaxine are also chosen because of milder anticholinergic and less frequent cardiovascular side effects.[83] If a TCA is prescribed, a secondary amine (e.g., desipramine or nortriptyline) should be selected because of the defined therapeutic plasma concentration ranges and lower incidence of side effects compared to the tertiary amines. Plasma concentration monitoring can be a useful tool for managing drug therapy in this patient population.[83]

Although the MAOI phenelzine may be used in carefully selected patients, in general, MAOIs are usually reserved for treatment-resistant patients because of the hypotensive side effects of the MAOIs

and the availability of newer, better tolerated drugs. Dietary and medication restrictions are also a concern.[83]

Pediatric Patients

5   Accumulating evidence indicates that childhood depression occurs quite commonly. Symptoms of depression in the young may vary from accepted diagnostic criteria and include several nonspecific symptoms such as boredom, anxiety, failing adjustment, and sleep disturbance.[85]

Data collected under controlled conditions that support the efficacy of antidepressants in children and adolescents are sparse, and no antidepressant, except fluoxetine, is FDA-approved for the treatment of depression in patients less than 18 years of age. In fact, the FDA now requires all antidepressants to carry a black box warning linking the antidepressants to increased suicidal thoughts and behavior

TABLE 67–11. Second- and Third-Generation Antidepressants and Cytochrome (CYP) P450 Enzyme Inhibitory Potential

Drug	CYP Enzyme			
	1A2	2C	2D6	3A4
Buproprion	0	0	0	0
Citalopram	0	0	0	+++
Escitalopram	0	0	0	0
Fluoxetine	0	++	++++	++
Fluvoxamine	++++	++	0	++
Mirtazapine	0	0	0	0
Nefazodone	0	0	0	++++
Paroxetine	0	0	++++	0
Sertraline	0	+++	++	+
Venlafaxine	0	0	0	0

++++, high; +++, moderate; ++, low; +, very low; 0, absent.
Compiled from Task Force on the Use of Laboratory Tests in Psychiatry,[75] DeVane,[78] and Waugh and Goa.[81]

children and adolescents. The FDA also recommends specific monitoring parameters when antidepressants are used in children and adolescents. Detailed information is available from the FDA or from the FDA-approved labeling of these agents. Conversely, a recent report of two double-blind placebo-controlled trials of sertraline in the treatment of children and adolescents with major depressive disorder found that sertraline-treated patients did better than patients on placebo.[86] In addition, sertraline was well-tolerated with the major side effects being diarrhea, vomiting, anorexia and agitation.[86] In a double-blind study by Preskorn and associates, imipramine was superior in efficacy to placebo only through the first 3 weeks of treatment.[87] Demonstration of efficacy in this population is confounded by a high placebo response rate. However, the TCAs and several of the SSRIs remain viable treatment options. Toxicity in overdose is important in the adolescent population, where suicide is a major concern and must be considered when prescribing TCAs.[88]

Antidepressants are used to treat depressed children and adolescents because no other definitive effective therapies are currently available. Plasma concentration monitoring of TCAs is important to ensure safety. As in the adult population, plasma concentrations above 450 ng/mL are associated with increased risk of serious adverse effects including delirium, seizures, delayed cardiac conduction, and sudden death.[89]

Several cases of sudden death have been reported in children and adolescents taking desipramine. A baseline electrocardiogram (ECG) is recommended before initiating treatment with a TCA in children and adolescents, and many clinicians recommend an additional ECG when steady-state plasma concentrations are achieved.[89]

Although several antidepressants are FDA-approved for use in children, only one, fluoxetine, is currently approved for childhood depression. Imipramine is approved for the treatment of enuresis, clomipramine for obsessive-compulsive disorder in children 12 years and older, and fluvoxamine along with fluoxetine is approved for obsessive-compulsive disorder in children.[90] The treatment of depression in children remains challenging, as depression can be difficult to diagnose and treat once identified. The studies involving imipramine, sertraline, and fluoxetine found that the dose range and titration as well as adverse effects were similar to those in adults.[86,90–92]

Pregnant and Lactating Patients

Approximately 10% of pregnant women develop a serious depression during pregnancy. No major teratogenic effects are currently associated with the SSRIs or TCAs.[93–94] Studies have been conducted evaluating birth anomalies, growth impairment, and behavioral teratogenicity. A meta-analysis of first-trimester exposure to TCAs found no significant association between exposure to TCAs and congenital malformations.[93] An additional evaluation compared birth defects in neonates born to women who were exposed to fluoxetine, TCAs, and agents felt not to increase baseline teratogenetic risk (such as penicillin or dental x-rays). Comparable rates of malformations were found across all three groups. However, a higher rate of miscarriages was present in the fluoxetine- and TCA-treated groups (13.5% and 12.2%, respectively) compared with the control group (6.8%). This raised questions about the effect of both depression and antidepressant treatment on the rate of miscarriage.[94] Some studies, but not all, have reported higher rates of perinatal complications associated with third-trimester use of fluoxetine.[95]

Studies evaluating the development of children exposed prenatally to TCAs, fluoxetine, or nonteratogens found no important differences in the rates of prenatal complications, incidence of major malformations, and mean global IQ scores.[95]

Concern regarding the use of fluoxetine arose as a result of an evaluation of neonates exposed to fluoxetine before 25 weeks of gestation only (early exposure) versus exposure during the third trimester (late exposure) versus exposure to nonteratogens. Premature birth occurred in 14.3% of late-exposure neonates versus 4.1% of early-exposure neonates, and 5.9% in the control group.[93] Additionally, birth weight, birth length, and maternal weight gain were less in the late-exposure group compared with the early-exposure and control groups. Evaluations to date do not support any teratogenic effects of fluoxetine, but do raise questions regarding premature birth and fetal growth rate.[94]

If a TCA is withdrawn during pregnancy, it should be tapered gradually to avoid maternal or fetal withdrawal symptoms. If possible, drug tapering is usually begun 5 to 10 days before the estimated day of confinement.[94] Although MAOIs have demonstrated teratogenicity in animals, there are insufficient data in humans to permit firm conclusions. Similarly, there are inadequate data on the use of other antidepressants during pregnancy.

In summary, the risks and benefits of drug therapy during pregnancy must always be weighed, and concerns about the risks of untreated depression during pregnancy should be considered. These include the possibility of low birth weight secondary to poor maternal weight gain, suicidality, potential for hospitalization, potential for marital discord, inability to engage in appropriate obstetric care, and difficulty caring for other children.[95] Several different approaches exist for dealing with pregnancy and antidepressant use.[95] First, discontinuation of an antidepressant before conceptions is an option for women who are stable and appear likely to remain well while not taking antidepressant medication. Secondly, continuation of the antidepressant until conception may be reasonable. For those who have a history of depressive relapse after medication discontinuation, the antidepressant should be continued throughout pregnancy. Further evaluations of the newer antidepressant agents are needed to fully understand the risks associated with their use at various stages of the gestational period. Additionally, the risks of not treating depression in a pregnant woman should not be underestimated or minimized.

Refractory Patients

⟨6⟩ The majority of "treatment resistant" depressed patients are likely the result of inadequate therapy (relative resistance).[29] Issues to be addressed in assessing the patient who has not responded to treatment include the following:

1. Is the diagnosis correct?
2. Does the patient have a psychotic depression?
3. Has the patient received an adequate dose and adequate duration of treatment?
4. Do adverse effects preclude adequate dosing?
5. Has the patient adhered to the prescribed regimen?
6. Was a stepwise approach to treatment used?
7. Was treatment outcome adequately measured?
8. Is there a coexisting or preexisting medical or psychiatric disorder?
9. Are there other factors that interfere with treatment?

⟨7⟩ When a patient has failed to respond, nondrug modalities including environmental manipulation, family counseling, cognitive therapy, or interpersonal psychotherapy are often beneficial.[29]

Three primary pharmacologic approaches are used when dealing with treatment nonresponse. The current antidepressant may be stopped and a trial with an unrelated agent initiated. For example, the patient may be switched from a TCA to an SSRI or an MAOI. Second, the current antidepressant can be augmented (potentiated) by the addition of lithium, liothyronine, or an anticonvulsant such as carbamazepine or valproic acid. A recently published study evaluated the efficacy of high-dose fluoxetine (40 to 60 mg/day), fluoxetine plus lithium, and fluoxetine plus desipramine in a group of patients who had failed to respond to 8 weeks of treatment with fluoxetine 20 mg per day.[96] There was no significant difference in response rates or drop rates across the three treatment groups, although the high-dose fluoxetine group was associated with a numerically greater response (42.4% vs. 29.4% vs. 23.5%, respectively). More recent evaluations have explored the addition of a novel antipsychotic agent (e.g., olanzapine or risperidone) to an antidepressant agent.[97] A third approach to the treatment-resistant patient is to use two different classes of antidepressants concurrently (e.g., a TCA plus an MAOI).[29] As discussed previously, the combination of an SSRI and an MAOI should never be used.

There are accumulating data to support that 50% to 60% of previously treatment-resistant depressed patients respond to adequate doses of SSRIs. MAOIs can be considered in the truly treatment-resistant population, especially for the patient with atypical features.[29]

Augmenting strategies, such as the addition of lithium to a TCA regimen, have been found to benefit some previously unresponsive patients. Several older trials support that addition of liothyronine to a TCA regimen may induce antidepressant response.[29]

Only a prescriber experienced in the use of such combination should undertake concurrent use of a TCA and an MAOI. When th is undertaken, the MAOI is slowly added to the TCA. Desipramine not recommended to be used in combination with an MAOI. When th combination is discontinued, the MAO inhibitor should be stoppe first. Patients with psychotic depression usually require the combination of an antidepressant and an antipsychotic.[29]

The American Psychiatric Association practice guideline for th treatment of patients with major depressive disorder offers guideline for managing patients who fail to respond. This publication advise that if patients fail to respond to medication after 6 to 8 weeks, a reap praisal of the treatment regimen should be considered.[29] For thos with no response, options include changing to a second antidepressar or the addition of psychotherapy or ECT. Partial responders shoul consider changing the dose, augmenting the antidepressant, or addin psychotherapy or ECT. Comorbid medical or psychiatric condition should be identified and treated because they may complicate trea ment. Before changing a patient's treatment, the clinician is advise to evaluate the adequacy of the medication dosage and complianc with the prescribed regimen. A combination of two drugs should n be used when one drug will suffice.

CLINICAL CONTROVERSY

There are no universally agreed upon algorithms or guidelines for individuals experiencing treatment-resistant depression. Approaches include discontinuing the current antidepressant and initiating treatment with a different agent, augmenting the current treatment, or beginning a trial of combination antidepressant therapy (see Fig. 67–1).

CLINICAL APPLICATION

A suggested algorithm for the management of depression is shown i Figure 67–1.

Dosing

Recommended initial doses and dosage ranges are shown in Tabl 67–3. The usual initial adult dose of most TCAs is 50 mg at bedtime and the dose may be increased by 25 to 50 mg every third day. Th recommended initial dose for the SSRIs is fluoxetine, 10 to 20 mg paroxetine, 20 mg; sertraline, 50 mg; citalopram, 20 mg; and esci talopram 10 mg.

Bupropion is usually initiated at 100 mg twice daily, and this dos may be increased to 100 mg three times daily after 3 days. Most pa tients will respond at 300 mg/day; however, an increase to 450 mg/day given as 150 mg three times daily, may be considered in patients wit no clinical response after several weeks of treatment at 300 mg/day Additionally, a sustained-release formulation of bupropion is cur rently available and may be given as 200 mg twice a day in those individuals requiring higher dosages.

Typically, phenelzine is initiated at 15 mg in the morning and then increased by 15 mg every third day up to 60 mg/day. The dos should be given three times daily to minimize postural hypotension with the last dose given in the early afternoon to lessen the likelihoo of insomnia. Maintenance doses may be as low as 15 mg/day.

The usual starting dose of venlafaxine is 75 mg/day given i two or three divided doses and taken with food. Depending on toler ability, the dose is then increased to 150 mg/day. If needed, the dos

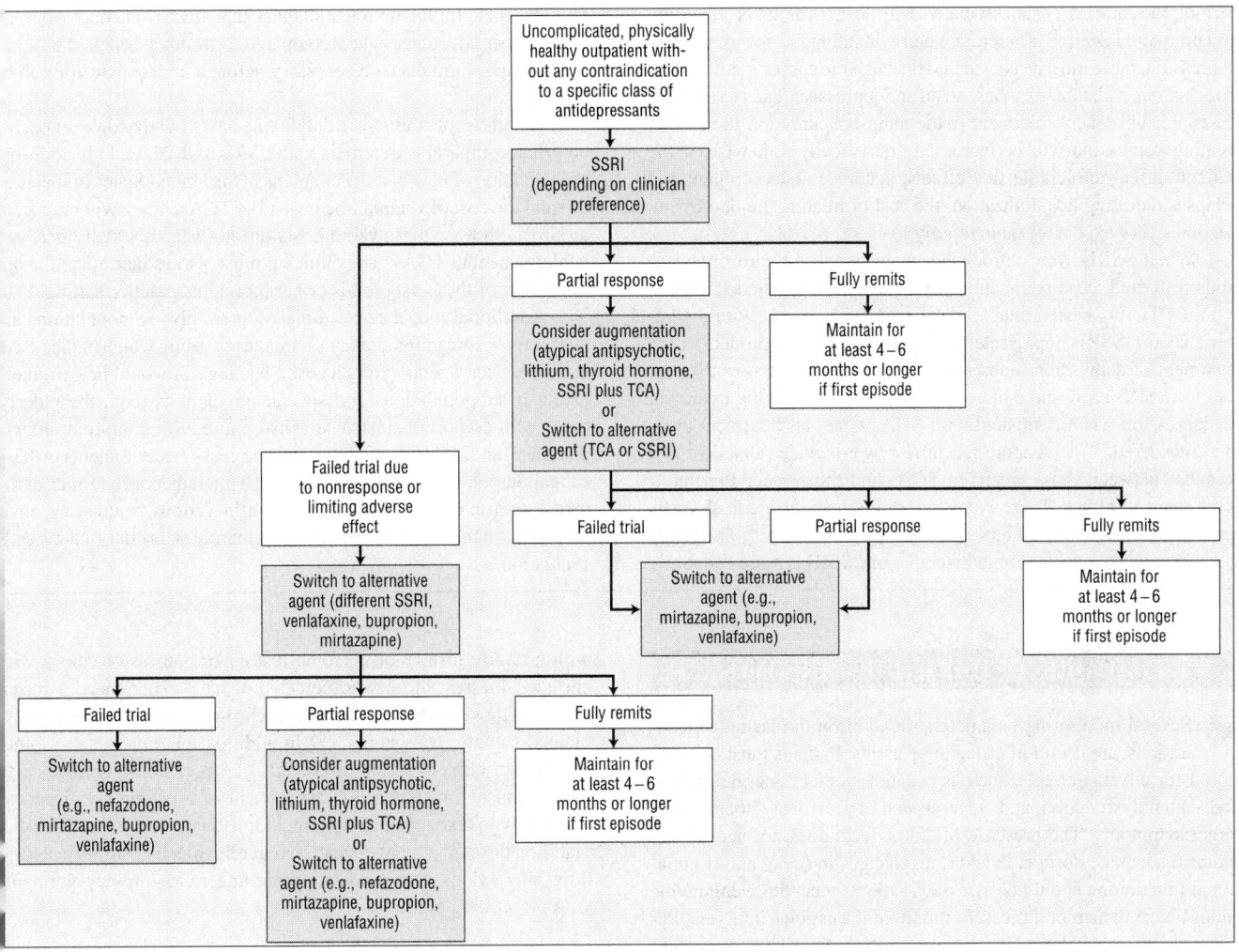

FIGURE 67–1. Algorithm for treatment of uncomplicated major depression.

may be further increased to 225 mg/day. Certain patients, including severely depressed patients, may need a dose up to 375 mg/day. A sustained-release formulation of venlafaxine is also available. The recommended starting dose is 75 mg/day administered with food. Dosage increases should occur in 75-mg/day increments with a maximum daily dose of 225 mg.

The starting dose of nefazodone is 100 mg given twice daily. Dose increases should occur in increments of 100 mg/day, on a twice-daily schedule, at intervals of no less than 1 week, with the usual effective dose range between 300 and 600 mg/day.

The recommended starting dose of mirtazapine is 15 mg/day administered in a single dose at bedtime. The maximum dose recommended is 45 mg/day. Dosage increases should occur every 1 to 2 weeks as indicated.

Caution is urged when switching from one antidepressant to another. It is important to remember that 3 to 4 weeks is usually required before a mood-elevating response is seen. A 6-week trial at a maximum dosage is considered an adequate trial.[29] It is crucial to explain to the patient about the expected lag time before the onset of clinical response. Patients uneducated in this regard often fail to comply with their prescribed regimens.

In elderly patients, as a general rule dosing is initiated at half the initial dose administered to younger adults, and the dose is increased at a slower rate. Thus desipramine or nortriptyline may be initiated at

10 to 25 mg/day, or fluoxetine at 10 to 20 mg/day, or alternatively 20 mg every second or third day. Six to twelve weeks of treatment may be required to achieve the desired antidepressant response in elderly patients. A remission is achieved when symptoms of depression are no longer present. A relapse is a return of symptoms within 6 months after remission. To prevent relapse, antidepressants should be continued at full therapeutic doses for 4 to 9 months after remission.[29] This period of treatment is termed *continuation therapy*. A recurrence is a separate episode of depression, which may occur after years of normal functioning. Five years after the first episode of depression, only 25% of patients had recovered and remained well.[98] The risk of recurrence increases as the number of past episodes and age at onset of the first episode increase. The duration of antidepressant therapy depends on the risk of recurrence. Some investigators recommend lifelong maintenance therapy for persons at greatest risk for recurrence (persons below 40 years of age with two or more prior episodes and persons of any age with three or more prior episodes).[29]

PHARMACOECONOMIC CONSIDERATIONS

Drug costs account for only about 1% to 2% of total costs of the treatment of depression and about 10% to 12% of direct costs of depression.[99] Other costs associated with depression primarily include the indirect costs associated with lost earnings/productivity and premature death.[99] Therefore when evaluating the cost of treating depression, more must be considered than just the cost of medications. For example, if lack of response to an antidepressant leads to an overdose and subsequent treatment in the intensive care unit, the cost of treating depression will be increased dramatically. Likewise, if the patient suffers intolerable side effects, becomes noncompliant, and relapses requiring hospitalization, the cost of treating the depression becomes very expensive quite rapidly.

When SSRIs were introduced, many managed care organizations restricted these medications to those who had failed treatment with the TCAs or been unable to tolerate these agents, with the belief that the SSRIs represented a more expensive approach to the treatment of depression. Subsequent evaluations have shown that in fact the SSRIs represent a more economic approach to the treatment of depression when compared with TCAs when all treatment costs are considered.[100,101] A more recent review concluded that cost differences between those receiving TCAs and those receiving fluoxetine were minimal. There were few differences in medical costs, depression outcomes, and health-related quality of life.[102] The larger question seems to center around whether one SSRI is more economic

than another. Initial findings suggest that fluoxetine may offer an overall cost advantage when compared with other SSRIs, but additional longer-term data are necessary before a final conclusion can be reached.[103]

A number of studies of venlafaxine have found a lower expected cost than comparable treatment with SSRIs and TCAs.[104] In addition, an evaluation of nine health care plans in the United States of resource use and the cost of venlafaxine instead of TCAs, after switching from an SSRI, showed that overall costs did not vary markedly between venlafaxine and TCAs. The clinician must always determine the applicability of these data to his or her individual practice setting.[104]

Additional longer-term studies in more diverse populations are necessary before judgments can be made regarding which of the newer antidepressant agents offers a cost advantage. It would be extremely useful if subpopulations and special populations (e.g., the elderly, those with comorbid substance abuse, those with comorbid anxiety disorders, and children) were studied and cost-effective agents in these subpopulations were identified. Also, the pharamacoeconomics of the medication management of depression in various health care environments such as public, private psychiatry, or primary care needs evaluation.

EVALUATION OF THERAPEUTIC OUTCOMES

8 Several monitoring parameters, in addition to plasma concentrations, are useful in managing patients. Patients must be monitored for adverse effects, such as sedation, anticholinergic effects, and sexual dysfunction, and for remission of previously documented target symptoms. The presence of side effects does not necessarily indicate adequate dosage. In addition, changes in social and occupational functioning should be assessed. Patients receiving venlafaxine should have their blood pressure monitored at regular intervals. Patients older than 40 should receive a pretreatment ECG before starting TCA therapy, and follow-up ECGs should be performed periodically. Patients should be monitored for the emergence of suicidal ideation after initiation of any antidepressant.

In addition to the clinical interview, psychometric rating instruments (e.g., patient-rated and clinician-rated scales) allow for rapid and reliable measurement of the nature and severity of depressive and associated symptoms (see Chap. 60). It is helpful to administer the rating scales prior to treatment, 6 to 8 weeks after initiation of therapy, and periodically thereafter. Interviewing a family member or friend (with the patient's permission) regarding symptoms and daily functioning also can assist in assessment of progress. Patients should be monitored at more frequent intervals early in treatment. Monitoring is then continued at regular intervals throughout the continuation and maintenance phases of treatment. Regular monitoring for re-emergence of side effects should be continued for several months after antidepressant therapy is discontinued.

COLLABORATIVE PRACTICE

Significant evidence exists to show that depression is common, chronic, and causes significant morbidity and mortality.[105] Pharmacists in conjunction with other health care providers can play a crucial role in the screening, recognition, and treatment of this disorder. In fact, the United States Preventive Services Task Force has recommended that clinicians "maintain an especially high index of suspicion for depressive symptoms in adolescents and young adults, persons

with a family history or personal history of depression, those with chronic illnesses, those who perceive or have experienced a recent loss, and those with sleep disorders, chronic pain or multiple unexplained somatic complaints."[106] In addition, pharmacists and other health care clinicians play a crucial role in ensuring adherence to medication regimens through assessment of a patient's willingness and ability to take a medication, including an assessment of financial viability, through patient education regarding dosing, side effects and drug interactions, and guidance regarding follow-up appointments with prescribing clinicians.[107]

CONCLUSIONS

Major depressive disorder remains one of the most commonly occurring mental illnesses in adults, and it is often undiagnosed and untreated. Pharmacologic intervention is the cornerstone of antidepressant treatment. Antidepressant medications have a broad spectrum of neurochemical effects and influence a variety of receptors peripherally and centrally. Safe and effective use of antidepressants requires a thorough understanding of the pharmacology of these drugs and of the principles of monitoring efficacy and adverse effects. In addition, clinicians must have a thorough understanding of antidepressant drug interactions and other factors that may influence the pharmacokinetics of antidepressant drugs. Plasma concentration monitoring is unnecessary for most patients, but can improve the outcome in some situations. The search for more effective antidepressants with more favorable adverse-effect profiles must continue.

ABBREVIATIONS

DA: dopamine
DSM-IV-TR: *Diagnostic and Statistical Manual of Mental Disorders,* 4th ed., Text Revision
ECT: electroconvulsive therapy
5-HT: serotonin
LFT: liver function test

MAOI: monoamine oxidase inhibitor
NE: norepinephrine
REM: rapid eye movement
SAD: seasonal affective disorder
TCA: tricyclic antidepressant

Review Questions and other resources can be found at *www.pharmacotherapyonline.com.*

REFERENCES

1. American Psychiatric Association. Diagnostic and Statistical Manual of Mental Disorders, 4th ed., Text Revision. Washington, American Psychiatric Association, 2000:356.

2. Kessler RC, Berglund P, Demler O. The epidemiology of major depressive disorders: Results from the National Comorbidity Survey Replication (NCS-R). JAMA 2003;289:3095–3105.

3. Burt VK, Stein K. Epidemiology of depression throughout the female life cycle. J Clin Psychol 2002;63(Suppl 7):9–15.

4. Kessler RC, McGonagle KA, Zhao S, et al. Lifetime and 12-month prevalence of DSM-III-R psychiatric disorders in the United States: Results from the National Comorbidity Survey. Arch Gen Psychiatry 1994;51:8–19.

5. Steffens DC, Skoog I, Norton MC, et al. Prevalence of depression and its treatment in an elderly population. The Cache County study. Arch Gen Psychiatry 2000;57:601–607.

6. Kessler RC, Walters EE. Epidemiology of DSM-III-R major depression and minor depression among adolescents and young adults in the National Comorbidity Survey. Depress Anxiety 1998;7:3–14.

7. Larsson B, Ivarsson T. Clinical characteristics of adolescent psychiatric inpatients who have attempted suicide. Eur Child Adolesc Psychiatry 1998;7:201–208.

8. Weissman MM, Gershon ES, Kidd KK, et al. Psychiatric disorders in the relatives of probands with affective disorder. Arch Gen Psychiatry 1984;41:13–21.

9. Warner V, Weissman MM, Mufson L, Wickramaratne PJ. Grandparents, parents, and grandchildren at high risk for depression: A three-generation study. J Am Acad Child Adolesc Psychiatry 1999;38:289–296.

10. Kendler KS, Prescott CA. A population based twin study of lifetime major depression in men and women. Arch Gen Psychiatry 1999;56:39–44.

11. Stahl SM. Blue genes and the mechanism of action of antidepressants. J Clin Psychiatry 2000;61:164–165.

12. Delgado PL. Depression: The case for a monoamine deficiency. J Clin Psychiatry 2000;61(Suppl 6):7–11.

13. Hirschfield RM. History and the evolution of the monoamine hypothesis of depression. J Clin Psychiatry 2000;61(Suppl 6):4–6.

14. Delgado PL, Moreno FA, Potter R, et al. Norepinephrine and serotonin in antidepressant action: Evidence from neurotransmitter depletion studies. In: Briley M, Montgomery SA, eds. Antidepressant Therapy at the Dawn of the Third Millennium. London, Marin Dunitz, 1997:141–163.

15. Baldessarini RJ. Drugs and the treatment of psychiatric disorders: Depression and anxiety disorders. In: Hardman JG, Limbrid LE, Goodman A, et al, eds. Goodman and Gilman's The Pharmacological Basis of Therapeutics, 10th ed. New York, McGraw-Hill, 2000:447–484.

16. Feighner JP. Mechanism of action of antidepressant medications. J Clin Psychiatry 1999;60(Suppl 4):4–11.

17. Frazer A. Pharmacology of antidepressants. J Clin Psychopharmacol 1997;17:2S–18S.

18. Stahl S. Basic psychopharmacology of antidepressants, part 1: Antidepressants have seven distinct mechanisms of action. J Clin Psychiatry 1998;59(Suppl 4):5–14.

19. Bryant SG, Brown CS. Current concepts in clinical therapeutics: Major affective disorders, part 1. Clin Pharmacol 1986;5:304–318.

20. Siever LJ, Davis KL. Overview: Toward a dysregulation hypothesis of depression. Am J Psychiatry 1985;142:1017–1031.

21. Willner P. Dopaminergic mechanisms in depression and mania. In: Bloom FE, Kupfer DJ, eds. Psychopharmacology: The Fourth Generation of Progress. New York, Raven, 1995:921–931.

22. Reddy PL, Khanna S, Subhash MN, et al. CSF amine metabolites in depression. Biol Psychiatry 1992;31:112–118.

23. Thase ME, Fasiczka AL, Berman SR, et al. Electroencephalographic sleep profiles before and after cognitive behavior therapy of depression. Arch Gen Psychiatry 1998;55:138–144.

24. Katon W, Sullivan MD. Depression and chronic medical illness. J Clin Psychiatry 1990;51(Suppl):3–11.

25. Lebowitz BD, Pearson JL, Schneider LS, et al. Diagnosis and treatment of depression in late life: Consensus statement update. JAMA 1997;278:1186–1190.

26. Malone KM, Oquendo MA, Haas GL, et al. Protective factors against suicidal acts in major depression: Reasons for living. Am J Psychiatry 2000;157:1084–1088.

27. Oquendo MA, Ellis SP, Greenwald S, et al. Ethnic and sex differences in suicide rates relative to major depression in the United States. Am J Psychiatry 2001;158:1652–1658.

28. Alexopoulois GS, Bruce HL, Hull J, et al. Clinical determinant of suicidal ideation and behavior in geriatric depression. Arch Gen Psychiatry 1999;56:1048–1053.

29. American Psychiatric Association. Practice guideline for the treatment of patients with major depressive disorder (revision). Am J Psychiatry 2000;157(Suppl):1–45.

30. Nierenberg AA, Alpert JE, Pava J, et al. Course and treatment of atypical depression. J Clin Psychiatry 1998;59(Suppl 18):5–9.

31. Rothschild AJ. Management of psychotic treatment-resistant depression. Psychiatr Clin North Am 1996;19:237–252.

32. Blackbum IM, Moore RG. Controlled acute and follow-up trial of cognitive therapy and pharmacotherapy in outpatients with recurrent depression. Br J Psychiatry 1997;171:328–334.

33. Klapheke MM. Electroconvulsive therapy consultation: An update. Convuls Ther 1997;13:227–241.

34. Partonen T, Partinen M. Light treatment for seasonal affective disorder: Theoretical considerations and clinical implications. Acta Psychiatr Scand 1994;377:41S–45S.

35. Partonen T, Lonnavist J. Seasonal affective disorder. Lancet 1998;352:1369–1374.

36. Lafer B, Sachs GS, Labbate LA, et al. Side effects induced by bright light therapy. Am J Psychiatry 1994;151:1081–1083.

37. Labbate LA, Lafter B, Thibault A, Sachs GS. Phototherapy for seasonal affective disorder: A blind comparison of three different schedules. J Clin Psychiatry 1994;55:189–191.

38. Burke MJ, Preskorn SH. Short term treatment of mood disorders with standard antidepressants. In: Bloom FE, Kupfer DJ, eds. Psychopharmacology: The Fourth Generation of Progress. New York, Raven, 1995:1053–1065.

39. Ballenger JC. Clinical evaluation of venlafaxine. J Clin Psychopharmacol 1996;16(Suppl 2):29S–35S.

40. Davis R, Whittington R, Bryson HM. Nefazodone: A review of its pharmacology and clinical efficacy in the management of major depression. Drugs 1997;53:608–636.

41. Horst WD, Preskorn SH. Mechanism of action and clinical characteristics of three atypical antidepressants: Venlafaxine, nefazodone, bupropion. J Affect Disord 1998;51:237–254.

42. Gorman JM. Mirtazapine: Clinical overview. J Clin Psychiatry 1999;60(Suppl 17):9–13.

43. Bryant SG, Brown CS. Current concepts in clinical therapeutics: Major affective disorders, part 2. Clin Pharmacol 1986;5:385–395.

44. Peroutka SJ, Snyder SH. Long term antidepressant treatment decreases spiroperidol-labeled serotonin receptor binding. Science 1980;210:88–90.

45. Josey ES, Hackett RL. St. John's wort: A new alternative for depression? Int J Clin Pharmacol Ther 1999;37:111–119.

46. Gastor B, Holroyd J. St. John's wort for depression: A systematic review. Arch Intern Med 2000;160:152–156.

47. Shelton RC, Keller MB, Gelenberg A, et al. Effectiveness of St. John's wort in major depression: A randomized controlled trial. JAMA 2001; 285:1978–1986.

48. Schrader E. Equivalence of St. John's wort extract (Ze 117) and fluoxetine: A randomized, controlled study in mild-moderate depression. Int Clin Psychopharmacol 2000;15:61–68.

49. McIntyre M. A review of the benefits, adverse events, drug interactions, and safety of St. John's wort (Hypericum perforatum): The implications with regard to the regulation of herbal medicines. J Altern Complement Med 2000;6:115–124.

50. Settle ED Jr. Antidepressant drugs: disturbing and potentially dangerous adverse effects. J Clin Psychiatry 1998;59(Suppl 16):25–30.

51. Haddad P. Antidepressant discontinuation reactions. In: Thompson C, chairperson. Discontinuation of antidepressant therapy: Emerging complications and their relevance [Academic Highlights]. J Clin Psychiatry 1998;59:541–548.

52. Moller HJ, Volz HP. Drug treatment of depression in the 1990s: An overview of achievements and future possibilities. Drugs 1996;52: 625–638.

53. Andrews JM, Ninan PT, Nemeroff CB. Venlafaxine: A novel antidepressant that has a dual mechanism of action. Depression 1996;4:48–56.

54. Feighner JP. Cardiovascular safety in depressed patients: Focus on venlafaxine. J Clin Psychiatry 1995;56:574–579.

55. Preskorn SH. Clinically relevant pharmacology of selective serotonin reuptake inhibitors: An overview with emphasis on pharmacokinetics and effects on oxidative drug metabolism. Clin Pharmacokinet 1997; 32(Suppl 1):1–21.

56. Goldstein BJ, Goodnick PJ. Selective serotonin reuptake inhibitors in the treatment of affective disorders: III. Tolerability, safety and pharmacoeconomics. J Psychopharmacol 1998;12(3 Suppl B):S55–S87.

57. Bristol-Myers Squibb Company. Nefazadone (Serzone) package insert. Princeton, NJ, 2002.

58. Aranoff GM. Trazodone associated with priapism. Lancet 1984;1:856.

59. Brodie-Meijer CC, Diemont WL, Buijs PJ. Nefazodone-induced clitoral priapism. Int Clin Psychopharmacol 1999;14:257–258.

60. Johnston JA, Lineberry CG, Ascher JA. A 102 center prospective study of seizures in association with bupropion. J Clin Psychiatry 1991;52: 450–456.

61. Nierenberg AA, Cole JO. Antidepressant adverse drug reactions. J Clin Psychiatry 1991;52(Suppl):40–47.

62. Rapp MS. Two cases of ejaculatory impairment related to phenelzine. Am J Psychiatry 1979;136:1200–1201.

63. Barton JL. Orgasmic inhibition by phenelzine. Am J Psychiatry 1979; 136:1616–1617.

64. Rabkin JG, Quitkin FM, McGrath P, et al. Adverse reactions to monoamine oxidase inhibitors: II. Treatment correlates and clinical management. J Clin Psychopharmacol 1985;5:2–9.

65. Neil JF, Licata SM, May SJ, Himmelhoch JM. Dietary noncompliance during treatment with tranylcypromine. J Clin Psychiatry 1979;40: 33–37.

66. Grossman E, Messerli FH, Grodzicki T, Kowey P. Should a moratorium be placed on sublingual nifedipine capsules given for hypertensive emergencies and pseudoemergencies? JAMA 1996;276:1328–1331.

67. Varon J, Marik PE. The diagnosis and management of hypertensive crises. Chest 2000;118:214–227.

68. Wells BG. Tricyclic antidepressants. In: Taylor WJ, Caviness MHD, eds. A Textbook for the Clinical Application of Therapeutic Drug Monitoring. Irving, TX, Abbott Laboratories, 1986:449–465.

69. Rudorfer MV, Polter WZ. Metabolism of tricyclic antidepressants. Cell Mol Neurobiol 1999;19:373–409.

70. DeVane CL. Metabolism and pharmacokinetics of the selective serotonin reuptake inhibitors. Cell Mol Neurobiol 1999;19:443–466.

71. Krastev Z, Terzivoanov D, Vlahov V, et al. The pharmacokinetics of paroxetine in patients with liver cirrhosis. Acta Psychiatry Scand 1989; 350(Suppl):91–92.

72. Demolis JL, Angebaud P, Grange JD, et al. Influence of liver cirrhosis on sertraline pharmacokinetics. Br J Clin Pharmacol 1996;42: 394–397.

73. Green DS, Barvhaiya RH. Clinical pharmacokinetics of nefazodone. Clin Pharmacokinet 1997;33:260–275.

74. Perry PJ, Pfohl BM, Holstad SC. The relationship between antidepressant response and tricyclic antidepressant plasma concentrations. Clin Pharmacokinet 1987;13:381–392.

75. Task Force on the Use of Laboratory Tests in Psychiatry. Tricyclic antidepressants—Blood level measurements and clinical outcomes: An APA task force report. Am J Psychiatry 1985;142:155–162.

76. Hansten PD, Horn JR. Drug Interactions and Updates. Vancouver, WA, Applied Therapeutics, 1997:127–842.

77. Mitchell PB. Drug interactions of clinical significance with serotonin reuptake inhibitors. Drug Saf 1997;17:390–406.

78. DeVane CL. Differential pharmacology of newer antidepressants. J Clin Psychiatry 1998;59(Suppl 20):85–93.

79. Rosenbaum JR, Managing SSRI-drug interactions in clinical practice. Clin Pharmacokinet 1995;29(Suppl 1):53–59.

80. Bezchlibnyk-Butler K, Alexksic I, Kennedy SH. Citalopram and drug interactions. J Psychiatry Neurosci 2000;25:241–254.

81. Waugh J, Goa KL. Escitalopram: A review of its use in the management of depressive and anxiety disorders. CNS Drugs 2003;17:343–362.

82. Ereshefsky L. Drug-drug interactions involving antidepressants: focus on venlafaxine. J Clin Psychopharmacol 1996;(3 Suppl 2):37S–50S.

83. Zisook S, Downs NS. Diagnosis and treatment of depression in late life. J Clin Psychiatry 1998;59(Suppl 4):80–91.

84. Turvey CL, Conwell Y, Jones MP, et al. Risk factors for late-life suicide. Am J Psychiatry 2002;10:398–406.

85. Cosgrave E, McGorry P, Allen N, Jackson H. Depression in young people: A growing challenge for primary care. Aust Fam Physician 2000; 29:123–127.

86. Wagner KD, Ambrosini P, Rynn M, et al. Efficacy of sertraline in the treatment of children and adolescents with major depressive disorder. JAMA 2003;290:1033–1041.

87. Preskorn S, Weller E, Hughes C, et al. Depression in prepubertal children: DST nonsuppression predicts differential response to imipramine versus placebo. Psychopharmacol Bull 1987;23:128–133.

88. Larsson B, Ivarsson T. Clinical characteristics of adolescent psychiatric inpatients who have attempted suicide. Eur Child Adolesc Psychiatry 1998;7:201–208.

89. Leonard HL, Meyer HC, Swedo SE, et al. Electrocardiographic changes during desipramine and clomipramine treatment in children and adolescents. J Am Acad Child Adolesc Psychiatry 1995;34:1460–1468.

90. Emslie GJ, Heiligenstein JH, Wagner KD, et al. Fluoxetine for acute treatment of depression in children and adolescents: A placebo controlled randomized trial. J Am Acad Child Adolesc Psych 2002;10. 1205–1215.

91. Hamilton JD, Bridge J. Outcome at 6 months for 50 adolescents with major depression treated in a health maintenance organization. J Am Acad Child Adolesc Psychiatry 1999;38:1340–1346.

92. Alderman J, Wolkow R, Chung M, Johnston HF. Sertraline treatment of children and adolescents with obsessive compulsive disorder or depression: Pharmacokinetics, tolerability, and efficacy. J Am Acad Child Adolesc Psychiatry 1998;37:386–394.

93. Wisner KL, Gelenberg AJ, Leonard H, et al. Pharmacologic treatment of depression during pregnancy. JAMA 1999;282:1264–1269.

94. Baum AL, Misri S. Selective serotonin-reuptake inhibitors in pregnancy and lactation. Harvard Rev Psychiatry 1996;4:117–125.

95. Hendrick V, Altshuler L. Management of major depression during pregnancy. Am J Psychiatry 2002;159:1667–1673.

96. Fava M, Jonathan A, Nierenberg A, et al. Double-blind study of high dose fluoxetine versus lithium or desipramine augmentation of fluoxetine in partial responders and nonresponders to fluoxetine. J Clin Psychopharmacol 2002;22:279–387.

97. Thase ME. What role do atypical antipsychotic drugs have in treatment resistant depression? J Clin Psychiatry 2002;63:95–103.

98. Keller MB, Lavori PW, Mueller TI. Time to recovery, chronicity, and levels of psychopathology in major depression: A five year prospective follow up of 431 subjects. Arch Gen Psychiatry 1992;49:809–816.

99. Smith W, Sherill A. A pharmacoeconomic study of the management of major depression: Patients in a TennCare HMO. Med Interface 1996; 9:88–92.

100. Greenberg PE, Stiglin LE, Finkelstein LM, et al. The economic burden of depression in 1990. J Clin Psychiatry 1993;54:405–418.

101. LePen C, Levy E, Ravily V, et al. The cost of treatment dropout in depression: A cost-benefit analysis of fluoxetine versus tricyclics. J Affective Disord 1994;31:1–18.

102. Frank L, Revicki DA, Sorenssen SV, et al. The economics of selective serotonin reuptake inhibitors in depression: A critical review. CNS Drugs 2001;15:59–83.

103. Sclar DA, Robinson LM, Skaer TL, et al. Antidepressant pharma-cotherapy: Economic evaluation of fluoxetine, paroxetine, and sertraline in a health maintenance organization. J Int Med Res 1995;23: 395–412.

104. Morrow TJ. The pharmacoeconomics of venlafaxine in depression. Am J Managed Care 2001;7:S386–S392.

105. American College of Physicians-American Society of Internal Medicine. Pharmacist Scope of Practice. Ann Intern Med 2002;136:79–85.

106. U.S. Preventive Services Task Force. Guide to Clinical Preventive Services, 2nd ed. Baltimore, Williams & Wilkins, 1996:541–546.

107. Finely P, Rens HR, Pont JT, et al. Impact of a collaborative pharmacy practice model on the treatment of depression in primary care. Am J Health-Sys Pharm 2002;59:1518–1526.

68

BIPOLAR DISORDER

Martha P. Fankhauser and Marlene P. Freeman

Learning Objectives and other resources can be found at *www.pharmacotherapyonline.com.*

KEY CONCEPTS

❶ Bipolar disorder is a cyclic mental illness with recurrent mood episodes that occur over a person's lifetime. The symptoms, course, severity, and response to treatment differ among individuals.

❷ Bipolar disorder is likely caused by genetic factors, environmental triggers, and the dysregulation of neurotransmitters, neurohormones, and secondary messenger systems in the brain.

❸ The goal of therapy for bipolar disorder should be to eliminate mood episodes, maximize adherence to therapy, improve the functioning of the patient, and limit adverse effects.

❹ Patients and family members should be educated about bipolar disorder and treatments. Long-term monitoring and adherence to treatment are major factors in obtaining stabilization of the disorder.

❺ Lithium and valproate are the mainstays of treatment for both acute mania and prophylaxis for recurrent manic and depressive episodes. Anticonvulsants such as lamotrigine, carbamazepine, and oxcarbazepine and atypical antipsychotics such as aripizrazole, olanzapine, risperidone, queti-

apine, and ziprasidone are alternatives or adjunctive agents for acute mania. Anticonvulsants may be more effective than lithium in several mood subtypes (e.g., mixed states and rapid cycling). Lamotrigine and lithium may be more effective for recurrent bipolar depression.

❻ Practice guidelines have been developed for bipolar disorder and are generally based on available efficacy and safety data and on opinions from a consensus panel of experts. Algorithms help the clinician select treatment options based on the type of mood episode, response to treatment, and patient-specific characteristics.

❼ Some patients can be stabilized on one mood stabilizer, but others may require combination therapies or adjunctive agents for the acute treatment of mood episodes and for the continuation phase. If possible, adjunctive agents should be tapered and discontinued when the acute mood episode remits and the patient is stabilized.

❽ Baseline and follow-up laboratory tests are required for some medications to monitor for adverse effects. Serum drug concentrations (applicable for lithium, carbamazepine, and valproate) help to adjust the dose and are used for both the acute and maintenance phase of treatment.

❶ Bipolar disorder (manic-depressive illness) is one of the most common of the severe chronic psychiatric disorders. The cyclic mood disorder is characterized by recurrent fluctuations in mood, energy, and behavior encompassing the extremes of human experiences.[1-4] Bipolar disorder differs from recurrent major depression (or unipolar depression) in that a manic, hypomanic, or mixed episode occurs during the course of the illness.[2] Bipolar disorder is a lifelong illness with a variable course and requires both nonpharmacologic and pharmacologic treatments for mood stabilization.[2,3]

EPIDEMIOLOGY

Approximately 1% to 3% of the adult population has either bipolar I or II disorder, but broader definitions suggest prevalence rates up to 5% if the full spectrum of recurrent mood disorders are included.[2-4,6] A national comorbidity survey reported that the lifetime prevalence rate of a manic episode is $1.6\% \pm 0.3\%$ for men and $1.7\% \pm 0.3\%$ for women in the United States (approximately 4 million people).[7] The

lifetime prevalence of bipolar I disorder (one or more manic or mixed episodes) is 0.4% to 1.6%; that for bipolar II disorder (recurrent major depressive episodes with hypomanic episodes) is approximately 0.5%.[2,3] Bipolar I disorder occurs equally in men and women, whereas bipolar II disorder is more common in women.[2,3] Of the 1.9 million Americans who have either bipolar I or II disorder, it is estimated that only 50% of these individuals are receiving any type of treatment for their illness.[1]

ETIOLOGY

❷ The exact etiology of bipolar disorder is unknown. Bipolar disorder is thought to be genetically based, environmentally influenced, and caused by a wide range of biological abnormalities. Stressful life events, alcohol or substance use, and changes in the sleep-wake cycle may elicit the expression of genetic or biological vulnerabilities that cause dysregulation of neurotransmitters, neuroendocrine pathways, and secondary messenger systems.[4] Table 68–1 summarizes the etiologic theories of bipolar disorder.[1,4,8-12]

TABLE 68–1. Etiologic Theories of Bipolar Disorder

Genetic factors

80–90% of patients with bipolar disorder have a biologic relative with a mood disorder (e.g., bipolar disorder, major depression, cyclothymia, or dysthymia).

    First-degree relatives of bipolar patients have a 15–35% lifetime risk of developing any mood disorder and a 5–10% lifetime risk for developing bipolar disorder.

    The concordance rate of mood disorders is 60–80% for monozygotic twins and 14–20% for dizygotic twins.

Linkage studies suggest that certain loci on genes and the X chromosome may contribute to genetic susceptibility of bipolar disorder.

Nongenetic factors

Perinatal insult

Head trauma

Environmental factors

    Desynchronization of circadian or seasonal rhythms cause diurnal variations in mood and sleep patterns and may result in seasonal recurrences of mood episodes.

    Changes in the sleep-wake cycle or light-dark cycle may precipitate episodes of mania or depression.

    Bright light therapy may be used for the treatment of winter depression, and may precipitate hypomania, mania, or mixed episodes.

Psychosocial or physical stressors

    Stressful life events often precede mood episodes and may increase recurrence rates and prolong time to recovery from mood episodes.

Nutritional factors

    Deficiency of essential amino acid precursors in the diet may cause a dysregulation of neurotransmitter activity (e.g., L-tryptophan deficiency causes a decrease in 5-HT and melatonin synthesis and activity).

    Deficiency in essential fatty acids (e.g., omega-3 fatty acids) may cause a dysregulation of neurotransmitter activity.

Neurotransmitter/neuroendocrine/hormonal theories

    Dysregulation between excitatory and inhibitory neurotransmitter systems; excitatory: NE, DA, glutamate, and aspartate; inhibitory: 5-HT and GABA.

Monoamine hypothesis

    An excess of catecholamines (primarily NE and DA) cause mania.

    Agents that decrease catecholamines are used for the treatment of mania (e.g., DA antagonists and α_2-adrenergic agonists).

    Deficit of neurotransmitters (primarily NE, DA, and/or 5-HT) cause depression.

    Agents that increase neurotransmitter activity are used for the treatment of depression (e.g., 5-HT and NE/DA reuptake inhibitors and MAOIs).

Dysregulation of amino acid neurotransmitters

    Deficiency of GABA or excessive glutamate activity causes dysregulation of neurotransmitters (e.g., increased DA and NE activity).

    Agents that increase GABA activity or decrease glutamate activity are used for the treatment of mania and for mood stabilization (e.g., benzodiazepines, lamotrigine, lithium, or valproic acid).

Cholinergic hypothesis

    Deficiency of acetylcholine causes an imbalance in cholinergic-adrenergic activity and may increase the risk of manic episodes.

    Agents that increase acetylcholine activity may decrease manic symptoms (e.g., use of cholinesterase inhibitors or augmentation of muscarinic cholinergic activity).

    Increased central acetylcholine levels may increase the risk of depressive episodes.

    Agents that decrease acetylcholine activity may alleviate depressive symptoms (i.e., anticholinergic agents).

Secondary messenger system dysregulation

    Abnormal G protein functioning dysregulates adenylate cyclase activity, phosphoinositide responses, sodium/potassium/calcium channel exchange, and activity of phospholipases. Abnormal cyclic adenosine monophosphate and phosphoinositide secondary messenger system activity.

    Abnormal protein kinase C activity and signaling pathways.

Hypothalamic-pituitary-thyroid axis dysregulation

    Hyperthyroidism may precipitate a mania.

    Hypothyroidism may precipitate a depression and be a risk factor for rapid cycling; thyroid supplementation used for refractory rapid cycling and augmentation of antidepressants in unipolar depression.

    Positive antithyroid antibody titers reported in patients with bipolar disorder.

    Hormonal changes during the female life cycle may cause dysregulation of neurotransmitters (e.g., premenstrual, postpartum, and perimenopause).

Membrane and cation theories

    Abnormal neuronal calcium and sodium activity and homeostasis causes neurotransmitter dysregulation.

    Hypocalcemia associated with causing anxiety, mood irritability, mania, psychosis, and delirium.

    Hypercalcemia associated with causing depression, stupor, and coma.

    Extracellular and intracellular calcium concentrations may affect the synthesis and release of NE, DA, and 5-HT, as well as the excitability of neuronal firing.

Sensitization and kindling theories

    Recurrences of mood episodes causes behavioral sensitivity and electrophysiologic kindling (similar to the amygdala-kindling models for seizures in animals) and may result in rapid or continuous mood cycling.

    Anticonvulsants with antikindling properties are effective for stabilizing mood (e.g., carbamazepine, valproic acid).

DA, dopamine; GABA, γ-aminobutyric acid; 5-HT, serotonin; MAOI, monoamine oxidase inhibitor; NE, norepinephrine.

Compiled from Torrey and Knable,[1] Goldberg and Harrow,[4] Kelso,[8] Manji et al,[9] Lenox et al,[10] Baron,[11] Bezchlibnyk and Young,[12] Goodnick,[18] Soares,[19] Manji et al,[20] Gould and Manji,[21] Sobczak et al,[22] Freeman et al,[23] Ketter and Wang,[24] White,[25] Rasgon et al,[26] and Mahmood and Silverstone.[27]

ABLE 68–2. Secondary Causes of Mania

edical conditions that induce mania
CNS disorders (brain tumor, strokes, head injuries, subdural hematoma, multiple sclerosis, systemic lupus erythematosus, temporal lobe seizures, Huntington's disease)
Infections (encephalitis, neurosyphilis, sepsis, human immunodeficiency virus)
Electrolyte or metabolic abnormalities (calcium or sodium fluctuations, hyper- or hypoglycemia)
Endocrine or hormonal dysregulation (Addison's disease, Cushing's disease, hyper- or hypothyroidism, menstrual-related or pregnancy-related or perimenopausal mood disorders)
Vitamin and nutritional deficiencies (essential amino acids, essential fatty acids, vitamin B_{12})
edications or drugs that induce mania
Alcohol intoxication
Drug withdrawal states (alcohol, α_2-adrenergic agonists, antidepressants, barbiturates, benzodiazepines, opiates)
Antidepressants (MAOIs, TCAs, 5-HT and/or NE and/or DA reuptake inhibitors, 5-HT antagonists)
DA-augmenting agents (CNS stimulants: amphetamines, cocaine, sympathomimetics; DA agonists, releasers, and reuptake inhibitors)
Hallucinogens (LSD, PCP)
Marijuana intoxication precipitates psychosis, paranoid thoughts, anxiety, and restlessness
NE-augmenting agents (α_2-adrenergic antagonists, β-agonists, NE reuptake inhibitors)
Steroids (anabolic, adrenocorticotropic hormone, corticosteroids)
Thyroid preparations
Xanthines (caffeine, theophylline)
Over-the-counter weight loss agents and decongestants (ephedra, pseudoephedrine)
Herbal products (St. John's wort)
matic therapies that induce mania
Bright light therapy
Sleep deprivation

NS, central nervous system; DA, dopamine; 5-HT, serotonin; LSD, lysergic acid diethylamide; MAOI, monoamine oxidase inhibitor; NE, norepinephrine; PCP, phencyclidine; A, tricyclic antidepressant.
mpiled from Torrey and Knable,[1] American Psychiatric Association,[2] American Psychiatric Association,[3] and Goodnick.[18]

SECONDARY CAUSES

everal medical, medication-induced, or substance-related causes of ania and depression have been identified (see Table 68–2 for causes mania and Table 67–1 in Chap. 67 on depressive disorders for uses of depression).[1–3] A complete medical, psychiatric, and med- ation history; physical examination; and laboratory testing are nec- sary to rule out any organic causes of mania or depression.[3] An ccurate diagnosis is important because some psychiatric and neu- logic disorders present with manic-like symptoms.[3,4] For exam- e, attention-deficit/hyperactivity disorder and a manic episode have milar characteristics; thus individuals with bipolar disorder may be isdiagnosed and prescribed central nervous system stimulants.[13,14] se of any substance that affects the central nervous system (e.g., cohol, antidepressants, caffeine, central nervous system stimulants, llucinogens, or marijuana) can worsen symptoms and decrease the sponse to treatment.[3,15–18]

PATHOPHYSIOLOGY

Many theories have been proposed regarding the pathophysi- ology of mood disorders.[4] Family, twin, and adoption studies port an increased lifetime prevalence risk of having mood disor- ers among first-degree relatives of patients with bipolar disorder.[3,5] enetic linkage studies suggest multiple gene loci may be in- olved in the heredity of mood disorders.[8–11,18] Neuroimaging stud- s have found neurochemical, anatomic, and functional abnormali- es in bipolar patients.[18,19] Environmental or psychosocial stressors, utritional deficiencies, infections, immunologic reactions, sleep eprivation, and disruption of circadian rhythms may cause dysregu- tion in neurotransmitters, hormones, endocrine function, neuropep-

tides, cations, intracellular second messengers, and signal transduc- tion pathways.[3,4,9,18–24]

NEUROCHEMICAL THEORIES

The kindling and behavioral sensitization model postulates that psy- chosocial stressors can result in manic or depressive episodes because various brain networks are sensitized for exaggerated and spontaneous reactions secondary to neurotransmitter imbalances or dysregulation and voltage-gated ion channel abnormalities.[4,25] Dysregulation be- tween neurotransmitters, neuropeptides, hormones, and secondary messenger systems may produce a cyclic rhythm disturbance in the central nervous system.[1,4,9,18,25] Abnormal calcium, potassium, and sodium homeostasis may alter neurotransmitter release and the sec- ondary messenger system.[9,25] Hormonal changes during the menstrual cycle, postpartum period, and perimenopausal phase may contribute to mood dysregulation.[23,26]

The "permissive serotonin hypothesis" proposes that serotonin (5-hydroxytryptamine or 5-HT) plays a critical role in modulating brain activity (e.g., stabilization of the catecholamine system and inhibition of dopamine [DA] release), and is low in both mania and depression.[18,27] L-tryptophan or 5-HT deficiency and changes in the light-dark cycle may result in reduced melatonin secretion from the pineal gland that disrupts the sleep-wake cycle, alters circadian rhythms, and causes seasonal affective changes.[1,18,27]

The catecholamine hypothesis of mood disorders suggests that increased DA and norepinephrine (NE) activity contribute to hyperac- tivity and psychosis associated with the severe stages of mania, and re- duced activity causes depression.[4,18] A γ-aminobutyric acid (GABA) deficiency theory has been proposed for mania since it inhibits NE and DA activity.[4,9,18] Glutamate and aspartate, excitatory amino acid neurotransmitters, may be overactive and involved in causing manic episodes.[9] Cholinergic underactivity has been proposed to cause mania and overactivity of acetylcholine to cause depression.[9,18] Acetylcholine is an antagonist of the catecholamine system and contributes to the interaction between phosphatidylinositol and phosphatidylcholine secondary messenger systems.[9]

CLINICAL PRESENTATION

◀ The essential feature of bipolar disorder is a history of mania or hypomania that is not caused by any other medical condition, substance, or psychiatric disorder (see Table 68–2 for secondary causes of mania).[2,3] The *Diagnostic and Statistical Manual of Mental Disorders,* 4th ed., Text Revision (DSM-IV-TR) of the American Psychiatric Association (APA) details the present understanding of mood disorders.[2] Bipolar disorder is divided into four subtypes based on the identification of specific mood episodes: bipolar I, bipolar II, cyclothymic disorder, and bipolar disorder not otherwise specified. See Table 68–3 for a definition of mood disorders by type of episode. The mood states are further separated into four subcategories to differentiate the current or most recent mood episode: major depressive, manic, hypomanic, or mixed. See Table 68–4 for the evaluation and diagnostic criteria of mood episodes. A new concept of "bipolar spectrum disorder" has been suggested that broadens the diagnosis to include dysthymia, cyclothymia, drug-induced hypomania, and recurrent unipolar depression.[4,28] Comorbid psychiatric disorders associated with bipolar disorder include alcohol and substance abuse, personality disorders, and anxiety disorders such as panic disorder, social anxiety, and obsessive-compulsive disorder.[2–4,15,17,18,29,30]

MAJOR DEPRESSIVE EPISODE

Bipolar depression is often underdiagnosed and is frequently misdiagnosed as major depressive disorder.[3,31] Compared to manic episodes, depressive episodes are more frequent, longer lasting, and occur more often in bipolar II than in bipolar I disorder.[4,32] Over a person's lifetime, depressive episodes may account for up to 80% of all mood episodes. Compared to men, women have twice the lifetime risk for major depression and a higher prevalence of seasonal affective disorder.[2,23] In bipolar depression, patients have an increased suicide risk and often have mood lability, hypersomnia, low energy, psychomotor retardation, cognitive impairment, anhedonia, decreased sexual activity, slowed speech, carbohydrate craving, and weight gain (also called atypical depressive features).[4,32,33] Delusions, hallucinations, and suicide attempts are more common in bipolar depression than in unipolar depression.[4]

MANIC EPISODE

For a diagnosis of mania, the symptoms must last at least 1 week, the mood must be elevated (expansive or irritable), and there must be a impairment in functioning.[2] Acute mania usually begins abruptly and symptoms escalate over several days. Common symptoms of mania include grandiosity, decreased need for sleep or food, pressured speech, flight of ideas (racing thoughts), distractibility, increased activity, poor judgment, and involvement in pleasurable activities with potentially negative consequences.[2] The severe stages of a manic episode resemble paranoid schizophrenia with bizarre behavior, hallucinations, and paranoid or grandiose delusions. Seasonal changes, stressors, sleep deprivation, antidepressants, central nervous system stimulants, or bright light can precipitate a manic episode. Bipolar patients may use cocaine or other stimulants during a manic phase to intensify and prolong mania.[4]

HYPOMANIC EPISODE

Hypomania is a less severe form of mania, and by definition does not cause a marked impairment in social or occupational functioning, and no delusions or hallucinations are present.[2,4] Patients with hypomania often do not seek treatment until they have a depressive episode, thus hypomania may not be recognized or reported.[3] Symptoms found in hypomanic episodes are similar to those of cocaine- or antidepressant-induced mood disorders; thus the differential diagnosis should rule out any substance-induced or medical conditions that present with elevated mood.[17] Hypomanic states should be closely monitored, because 5% to 15% of patients may rapidly switch to a manic episode.[4]

TABLE 68–3. Mood Disorders Defined by Episodes

Disorder Subtype	Episode(s)[a]
Major depressive disorder, single episode	Major depressive episode
Major depressive disorder, recurrent	Two or more major depressive episodes
Bipolar disorder, type I[b]	Major depressive episode + manic or mixed episode
Bipolar disorder, type II[c]	Major depressive episode + hypomanic episode
Dysthymic disorder	Chronic subsyndromal depressive episodes
Cyclothymic disorder[d]	Chronic fluctuations between subsyndromal depressive and hypomanic episodes (2 years for adults and 1 year for children and adolescents)
Mood disorder due to a general medical condition	Disturbance in mood that is secondary to a general medical condition (see Table 68–2)
Substance-induced mood disorder	Disturbance in mood that is secondary to the effects of a substance (e.g., medication, toxin, drug abuse, somatic treatments; see Table 68–2)
Bipolar disorder not otherwise specified	Mood states do not meet criteria for any specific bipolar disorder

[a]The length and severity of a mood episode and the interval between episodes varies from patient to patient. Manic episodes are usually briefer and end more abruptly than major depressive episodes. The average length of untreated manic episodes ranges from 4 to 13 months. Episodes may occur regularly (at the same time or season of the year) and often cluster at 12-month intervals. Women have more depressive episodes than manic episodes, whereas men have a more even distribution of episodes.
[b]For bipolar I disorder, 90% of individuals who experience a manic episode later have multiple recurrent major depressive, manic, hypomanic, or mixed episodes alternating with a normal mood state.
[c]Approximately 5–15% of patients with bipolar II disorder will develop a manic episode over a 5-year period. If a manic or mixed episode develops in a patient with bipolar II disorder, the diagnosis is changed to bipolar I disorder.
[d]Patients with cyclothymic disorder have a 15–50% risk of later developing a bipolar I or II disorder.
Compiled from American Psychiatric Association,[2] Goldberg and Harrow,[4] and Goodnick.[18]

TABLE 68–4. Evaluation and Diagnostic Criteria of Mood Episodes

Diagnostic work-up depends on clinical presentation and findings	• Mental status examination • Psychiatric, medical, and medication history • Physical and neurological examination • Basic laboratory tests: complete blood count, blood chemistry screen, thyroid function, urinalysis, urine drug screen • Psychological testing • Brain imaging: magnetic resonance imaging and functional scan; alternative: computed tomography scan, positron emission tomography scan • Lumbar puncture • Electroencephalogram

Diagnosis

Episode	Impairment of Functioning or Need for Hospitalization[a]	DSM-IV-TR Criteria[b]
Major depressive	Yes	>2-Week period of either depressed mood or loss of interest or pleasure in normal activities, associated with at least five of the following symptoms: • Depressed, sad mood (adults); may be irritable mood in children • Decreased interest and pleasure in normal activities • Decreased appetite, weight loss • Insomnia or hypersomnia • Psychomotor retardation or agitation • Decreased energy or fatigue • Feelings of guilt or worthlessness • Impaired concentration and decision making • Suicidal thoughts or attempts
Manic	Yes	>1-Week period of abnormal and persistent elevated mood (expansive or irritable), associated with at least three of the following symptoms (four if the mood is only irritable): • Inflated self-esteem (grandiosity) • Decreased need for sleep • Increased talking (pressure of speech) • Racing thoughts (flight of ideas) • Distractible (poor attention) • Increased activity (either socially, at work, or sexually) or increased motor activity or agitation • Excessive involvement in activities that are pleasurable but have a high risk for serious consequences (buying sprees, sexual indiscretions, poor judgment in business ventures)
Hypomanic	No	At least 4 days of abnormal and persistent elevated mood (expansive or irritable); associated with at least three of the following symptoms (four if the mood is only irritable): • Inflated self-esteem (grandiosity) • Decreased need for sleep • Increased talking (pressure of speech) • Racing thoughts (flight of ideas) • Increased activity (either socially, at work, or sexually) or increased motor activity or agitation • Excessive involvement in activities that are pleasurable but have a high risk for serious consequences (buying sprees, sexual indiscretions, poor judgment in business ventures)
Mixed	Yes	Criteria for both a major depressive episode and manic episode (except for duration) occur nearly every day for at least a 1-week period
Rapid cycling	Yes	>4 Major depressive or manic episodes (manic, mixed, or hypomanic) in 12 months

Impairment in social or occupational functioning; need for hospitalization due to potential self-harm, harm to others, or psychotic symptoms.
The disorder is not due to a medical condition (e.g., hypothyroidism) or substance-induced disorder (e.g., antidepressant treatment, medications, electroconvulsive therapy).
Compiled from Torrey and Knable,[1] American Psychiatric Association,[2] American Psychiatric Association.[3]

MIXED EPISODE

Bipolar "mixed episode" (previously known as mixed state, dysphoric mania, or depressive mania) is defined as the simultaneous occurrence of manic and depressive symptoms.[2,4] Mixed mood states occur in up to 40% of all episodes, and are more common in younger and older patients and in females.[4] Mixed episodes are often difficult to diagnose and treat because of the fluctuating clinical presentation. Patients with mixed states often have comorbid alcohol and substance abuse, severe anxiety symptoms, a higher suicide rate, and a poorer prognosis.[4,17]

COURSE OF ILLNESS

Bipolar disorder is frequently not recognized and treated for many years because of its fluctuating course and episodic mood states.[3,4,18] The onset of bipolar disorder is rare before puberty, but its incidence increases during late adolescence and into early adulthood (usually between the ages of 15 and 30).[2] The average age of onset of a first manic episode is 21 for both men and women.[3] The first episode in females is more likely to be a major depressive episode, whereas males are more likely to first experience a manic episode.[2,3]

Women are more likely to have mixed states, depressive episodes, and rapid cycling compared to men.[2,3] Onset of manic episodes after the age of 60 is rare and is likely caused by a medical or neurological condition (e.g., stroke, tumor, or dementia), medications, or substance use.[3]

Approximately 95% of patients with bipolar disorder experience episodes of depression during their lifetime.[2,4] Recurrent depressive episodes are more common in women compared to men.[4] Unipolar mania (i.e., with no depressive episodes) occurs in less than 5% to 9% of patients. More than 80% of patients have more than four mood episodes during their lifetime; untreated patients may have ten or more episodes during their lifetime.[3] There may be a longer duration of episodes and more frequent episodes with aging.[3] Usually there is a period of normal functioning between episodes, but approximately 20% to 30% of patients with bipolar I type and 15% with bipolar II type have no period of euthymia because of mood lability, residual mood symptoms, or a direct switch to the opposite polarity.[2]

Rapid cycling (more than four mood episodes per year) occurs in approximately 10% to 20% of bipolar I and II disorder patients, and 70% to 90% of rapid-cycling patients are women.[1–4,16,23] Frequent and severe episodes of depression appear to be the most common hallmark of rapid cycling. Use of alcohol, stimulants such as cocaine and antidepressants, sleep deprivation, hypothyroidism, and seasonal changes may play a role in rapid cycling.[4,16,34] Seasonal patterns of mania in the summer and depression during the winter have been observed.[1] A rare form of bipolar disorder is characterized by "ultrarapid" cycles (e.g., every 24 to 48 hours) or "continuous" cycles with no free interval between episodes.[4] Rapid-cycling patients have a poorer long-term prognosis and often require combination therapies.[4]

Bipolar disorder affects an estimated 1% of children and adolescents and is often harder to recognize, diagnose, and treat than in a typical adult patient.[2,3,16,18,35] Late adolescence (ages 15 to 19) is a period with increased vulnerability for the onset of bipolar disorder.[18] Approximately 10% to 15% of adolescents with recurrent major depressive episodes have a subsequent episode of mania or hypomania.[2] Stimulants, hallucinogens, and excessive caffeine can precipitate a mania or mixed state.[18] Early stressful experiences in childhood (e.g., physical or sexual abuse) may precipitate an earlier onset and result in faster cycling, increased suicide risk, and alcohol or substance abuse.[4,18] Before the onset of mania, adolescents may exhibit irritability, hyperactivity, impulsivity, emotional lability, poor judgment, marked anxiety, insomnia, depression, and psychosis.[2,14,18] Acute mania often has psychotic symptoms, thus adolescents may be misdiagnosed as having schizophrenia.[18]

Early-onset bipolar disorder (before age 7 years) often presents similarly to attention-deficit/hyperactivity disorder with extreme irritability or rages.[36] The misdiagnosis of attention-deficit/hyperactivity disorder and use of central nervous system stimulants may be a factor in causing treatment-refractory mixed states or rapid cycling. Child-onset bipolar disorder is associated with a higher genetic loading for affective illness, a high comorbidity of disruptive behavior and attention disorders, an increased risk of anxiety and psychotic features, more frequent mood recurrences (mixed states and rapid cycling), a more chronic course, and a less favorable response to treatment.[3,4,13,18,35,36]

Fluctuations in hormones and neurotransmitters during the luteal phase of the menstrual cycle, postpartum period, and during perimenopause (starting approximately 10 years before menopause) may precipitate mood changes and increase cycling that resembles bipolar II disorder.[2,23,26] Women with bipolar I disorder are at greater risk for relapse into mania, depression, or psychosis during the postpartum period.[3] If a severe mood episode occurs postpartum, there is an increased risk for recurrences during subsequent postpartum periods.[3] Prophylactic medications such as lithium or valproate may prevent postpartum episodes in women with bipolar disorder.[3]

Alcohol and substance abuse is common among patients with bipolar disorder and may have a significant impact on the age of onset, course of the illness, and response to treatment.[4,15,18,30] Alcohol and drug abuse or dependence has been reported in 46% and 41% of bipolar patients, respectively.[3,18] Patients with substance use disorders are more likely to have an earlier onset of their illness, mixed states, higher rates of relapse, a poorer response to treatment, comorbid personality disorders, increased suicide risk, and more psychiatric hospitalizations.[4] Bipolar patients may self-medicate during episodes (e.g., cocaine during mania and alcohol during depression), resulting in further impairment of judgment, poor impulse control, treatment nonadherence, and a worsening of the clinical course.[3,4,17]

More than one-half (55% to 65%) of bipolar I patients have some degree of functional disability after the onset of their illness, and approximately 10% to 20% of bipolar patients have severe impairment in their psychosocial and occupational functioning.[1–4,37] In a 1-year longitudinal study in 258 bipolar patients, two-thirds had four or more mood episodes a year despite comprehensive pharmacologic treatment, and approximately 33.2% of the year was spent being depressed compared to 10.8% of the time in a manic phase.[37]

Compared with the general population, individuals with bipolar disorder have a 2.3-times higher mortality rate.[1] Suicide attempts occur in up to 50% of patients with bipolar disorder, and approximately 10% to 19% of individuals with bipolar I disorder commit suicide.[2–4,38] Recent studies suggest patients with bipolar II disorder have more suicide attempts than bipolar I patients.[33] Suicidal ideation and attempts are most likely to occur in a depressive or mixed state and in patients with personality disorders, psychotic features, and/or a comorbid alcohol and substance use disorder.[3,4,39] Accidental deaths are more frequent during manic episodes when the person has grandiosity, hallucinations, or delusions that result in risk-taking behaviors.[1,3] In addition, bipolar patients have a higher mortality from endocrine, respiratory, and cardiovascular disease that may be related to higher rates of obesity, smoking, alcohol and substance abuse, infections, and lack of medical care.[1,3]

Acutely manic or depressed patients may need protection (or hospitalization) because they are suicidal, have violent or aggressive behavior, or lack appropriate judgment and insight.[3] Nonadherence with pharmacologic treatment and alcohol or substance abuse are major factors in relapse and hospitalizations.[3,4] Medication discontinuation occurs in up to 50% of patients secondary to intolerance of drug-induced side effects.[40] The best predictor for level of functioning during a person's lifetime is adherence with medication treatment. Because of failure to recognize the disorder, reluctance to acknowledge it, or poor adherence with treatment, an estimated two-thirds of patients with bipolar disorder do not receive appropriate treatment.[1]

Severe psychiatric illnesses such as bipolar disorder often manifest themselves during adolescence and young adulthood, and result in disruption of educational, occupational, marital, and other pursuits. Residual symptoms are often common between mood episodes, and more than one-half of bipolar patients manifest some degree of functional disability after the onset of the illness. Poorer outcome is associated with rapid cycling, mixed states, concurrent alcohol and substance abuse, nonadherence to treatment, and poor psychosocial support.

▶ TREATMENT: Bipolar Disorder

■ DESIRED OUTCOME

The desired outcome for bipolar disorder is to alleviate or shorten the duration of an acute manic, hypomanic, or depressive episode, to maintain good functioning, and to prevent further cycles of mania or depression.[1,3,4] The general principles and goals for the management of bipolar disorder are found in Table 68–5.

■ GENERAL APPROACH TO TREATMENT

Treatment of bipolar disorder must be individualized because the clinical presentation, severity, and frequency of episodes vary widely among patients. Treatment approaches should include both nonpharmacologic and pharmacologic strategies (Table 68–6).[4] Patients and family members should be educated about bipolar disorder (e.g., symptoms, causes, and course) and treatment options. Long-term adherence to treatment is the most important factor in achieving stabilization of the disorder.

■ NONPHARMACOLOGIC THERAPY

The basics of nonpharmacologic approaches should address issues of adequate nutrition, sleep, exercise, and stress reduction.[1,4] Sleep deprivation, high stress, and deficiencies in dietary essential amino acids, fatty acids, vitamins, and minerals may exacerbate mood episodes and result in poorer outcomes.[4] Another effective treatment is to combine medications with adjunctive psychoeducational programs, supportive counseling, insight-oriented psychotherapy (individual or group), couples or family therapy, cognitive behavioral therapy, and communication enhancement training.[1,3,4,18,41]

Most communities have self-help, support groups, and mental health organizations that provide information, educational materials, and support. For public information, individuals may contact the Depression and Bipolar Support Alliance at 800-826-3632 and *www.dbsalliance.org*; the National Alliance for the Mentally Ill (NAMI) at 800-950-6264 (helpline) and *www.nami.org*; the National Foundation for Depressive Illness at 800-248-4344 or 800-239-1265 and *www.depression.org*; National Mental Health Association at 800-433-5959 or 800-969-6642 (resource center) and *www.nmha.org*; and National Institute of Mental Health at 866-615-6464 or *www.nimh.nih.gov*.[1,3] A recently published book for patients, families, and providers called *Surviving Manic Depression* is an excellent educational resource about the disorder.[1]

Several nonpharmacologic treatment strategies (e.g., electroconvulsive therapy [ECT], high-intensity bright light therapy, phase-advanced sleep schedule, and partial or complete sleep deprivation) have been used for bipolar disorder.[1,3,4] Bilateral ECT is an effective treatment for severe mania, psychotic depression, rapid cycling, and mixed states with high suicidal risk (approximately an 80% response rate).[3] Repetitive transcranial magnetic stimulation has been reported to be effective in depression, but the effectiveness in bipolar disorder is unknown.[3,4,42]

■ PHARMACOLOGIC THERAPY

Pharmacotherapy is crucial for the acute and maintenance treatment of bipolar disorder and includes lithium, valproate, carbamazepine, oxcarbazepine, lamotrigine, atypical antipsychotics, and adjunctive agents such as antidepressants and benzodiazepines.

TABLE 68–5. General Principles for the Management of Bipolar Disorder

Goals of treatment
- Eliminate mood episode with complete remission of symptoms (i.e., acute treatment)
- Prevent recurrences or relapses of mood episodes (i.e., continuation phase treatment)
- Return to complete psychosocial functioning
- Maximize adherence with therapy
- Minimize adverse effects
- Use medications with the best tolerability and fewest drug interactions
- Treat comorbid substance use and abuse
  Eliminate alcohol, marijuana, cocaine, amphetamines, and hallucinogens
  Minimize nicotine use and stop caffeine intake at least 8 hours prior to bedtime
- Avoidance of stressors or substances that precipitate an acute episode

Monitor for:
- Mood episodes: document symptoms on a daily mood chart (document life stressors, type of episode, length of episode, and treatment outcome); monthly and yearly life charts are valuable for documenting patterns of mood cycles
- Medication adherence (missing doses of medications is a primary reason for nonresponse and recurrence of episodes)
- Adverse effects, especially sedation and weight gain (manage rapidly and vigorously to avoid noncompliance)
- Suicidal ideation or attempts (suicide completion rates with bipolar I disorder are 10–15%; suicide attempts are primarily associated with depressive episodes, mixed episodes with severe depression or presence of psychosis)

Frequency of visits:
- Severely ill patients should be seen more often (i.e., weekly) compared with less ill patients who are symptomatic (i.e., every 2 weeks)
- When starting new medications or switching therapies, frequent monitoring is recommended (e.g., every 2 weeks) to assess adherence, efficacy, dosing, and adverse effects
- When a patient is stabilized on medication, less frequent monitoring is possible during the continuation phase (e.g., every month for the first 3 months, then every 2–3 months)
- Patients should be encouraged to call their clinician if any problems or adverse events occur or if mood episodes occur between scheduled appointments; rapidly identifying and correcting potential problems or making dosage adjustments is essential in achieving mood stabilization

Compiled from Torrey and Knable,[1] American Psychiatric Association,[3] Goodnick,[18] and Suppes et al.[45]

TABLE 68–6. General Guidelines for Nonpharmacologic and Pharmacologic Treatments for Bipolar Disorder

Nonpharmacologic therapies
- Psychoeducation about bipolar disorder, treatment, and monitoring for the patient and family
  - Early signs and symptoms of mania and depression and charting mood changes
  - Importance of compliance with therapy
  - Psychosocial or physical stressors that may precipitate an episode
  - Limiting substances and drugs that can trigger mood episodes
  - Strategies for coping with stressful life events
  - Development of a crisis intervention plan
- Psychotherapy (e.g., individual, group, and family), interpersonal therapy, and/or cognitive behavioral therapy
- Stress reduction techniques, relaxation therapy, massage, yoga, etc.
- Sleep (regular bedtime and awake schedule; avoid alcohol or caffeine intake prior to bedtime)
- Nutrition (regular intake of protein-rich foods or drinks and essential fatty acids; supplemental vitamins and minerals)
- Exercise (regular aerobic and weight training at least three times a week)

Pharmacologic treatments
- Use an established mood stabilizer for the treatment of an acute mood episode and for continuation therapy (see Table 68–7 for efficacy ratings and recommendations based on clinical trials, guidelines, and algorithms)
  - If a patient responded well to a specific pharmacologic agent in the past and it was well tolerated, then use the same treatment again
  - If a patient had intolerance or adverse reactions to a specific pharmacologic agent in the past or has a strong preference against an agent, then do not use it
  - It is preferable to slowly taper off a medication than to abruptly discontinue it
- There are no specific guidelines for when to switch therapies or when combination approaches should be started
  - In general, if a patient with mania or mixed states has not responded within 2 to 4 weeks with an established mood stabilizer (e.g., lithium, lamotrigine, or valproate), a second first-line agent can be added to the regimen for augmentation; alternative treatment options include adding carbamazepine, oxcarbazepine, or an atypical antipsychotic in lieu of a first-line agent
  - Patients who are nonresponsive or intolerant to adverse effects of first-line pharmacologic approaches should be switched to another agent; when necessary, electroconvulsive therapy may be used to rapidly reduce manic or depressive symptoms and may be used for maintenance treatment
  - Changes in medication therapies and doses should be based on treatment response (or change in symptoms), tolerability of side effects, serum drug levels when applicable, and avoidance of drug interactions
- For patients with rapid cycling(>4 mood episodes per year):
  - Evaluate and treat underlying hypothyroidism, hormonal imbalance, or drug or alcohol abuse
  - For antidepressant-induced rapid cycling, taper off antidepressant and other agents that increase norepinephrine or dopamine activity (e.g., central nervous system stimulants, sympathomimetics, and caffeine)
- Use combination therapies for patients who are partially responsive or unresponsive to monotherapy with an established mood stabilizer
  - Combination therapies may be needed for the treatment of acute mania or mixed episodes, breakthrough depression, and rapid cycling
  - Reassessment of combination and adjunctive therapies should be done routinely and unnecessary medications should be tapered off gradually and discontinued
  - Use antidepressants or stimulants cautiously in patients with rapid cycling or with a history of antidepressant-induced mania; patients with recurrent depressive episodes may need long-term antidepressant therapy to minimize relapses
- Some mood stabilizers have an increased teratogenic risk during the first trimester (e.g., carbamazepine, lithium, oxcarbazepine, and valproate); this risk is greater if the patient is on multiple agents
  - Prenatal monitoring suggested: maternal serum α-fetoprotein screening for neural tube defects before the twentieth week of gestation and high-resolution ultrasound at 16–18 weeks' gestation to detect cardiac abnormalities; fetal echocardiography is recommended if lithium is used during the first trimester
  - Routine serum level monitoring of medications (when applicable) is recommended during pregnancy, with dosage adjustments if indicated
- Electroconvulsive therapy may be considered for patients with severe or treatment-resistant mania or depression and in pregnant women; maintenance drug therapy may be considered for patients whose acute episodes responded to electroconvulsive therapy
- After the resolution of the mood episodes, maintenance treatment is generally recommended for both bipolar I and II disorder: lithium or valproate (first choices) and carbamazepine, lamotrigine, and oxcarbazepine (alternative choices)
  - Patients should be maintained on a 6-month continuation phase of the mood stabilizer while the adjunctive treatment(s) are tapered and discontinued if possible
  - Patients who have had only one manic episode and who have responded to treatment should be continued on a mood stabilizer for 12 months, then gradually tapered off over several months (usually after 6 months of complete remission)
- Lifetime prophylaxis with a mood stabilizer is recommended for:
  - Bipolar I: after two manic episodes, after one severe manic episode, in the presence of a strong family history of bipolar disorder or major depressive disorder, with frequent episodes (more than one per year), or with rapid onset of manic episodes
  - Bipolar II: after three hypomanic episodes or if the patient becomes hypomanic with antidepressant therapy

Compiled from American Psychiatric Association,[3] Goldberg and Harrow,[4] Goodnick,[18] and Suppes et al.[45]

▪ Drug Treatments of First Choice

▪ *Published Guidelines and Treatment Protocols.* Currently there are no published evidence-based studies that compare different agents and combination therapies for the treatment of acute mania, mixed

states, and depression, and for the maintenance phase.[3,43–49] An example of efficacy ratings for various medications used in bipolar disorder is found in Table 68–7.[47]

The term "mood stabilizer" is often used to describe the class of medications used in the treatment of bipolar disorder, bu

TABLE 68–7. Efficacy Ratings of Pharmacological Treatments Used in Bipolar I Disorder

Drug	Acute Mania or Mixed States	Acute Bipolar Depression	Continuation or Maintenance Therapy
Lithium			
Lithium carbonate	A+: monotherapy	A	A+
Anticonvulsants			
Carbamazepine	A: monotherapy	B	B
Divalproex	A+: monotherapy	C	A
Gabapentin	X: monotherapy and adjunctive	D	D
Lamotrigine	C: monotherapy B: rapid cycling	A	A+
Levetiracetam	D	D	D
Oxcarbazepine	B: monotherapy	D	B
Tiagabine	X: monotherapy D: adjunctive	D	D
Topiramate	C: monotherapy or adjunctive	C: adjunctive	C: adjunctive
Zonisamide	C: monotherapy	D	D
Antipsychotics			
Aripiprazole	A+: monotherapy	D	D
Clozapine	A: monotherapy for treatment-resistant patients	D	D
Haloperidol	A: monotherapy or adjunctive	D	D
Olanzapine	A+: monotherapy or adjunctive	B: adjunctive with fluoxetine	D
Risperidone	A+: monotherapy or adjunctive	B: adjunctive	D
Quetiapine	A+: monotherapy or adjunctive	D	D
Ziprasidone	A+: monotherapy	D	D

Definition of Ratings:

A = Efficacy established by two or more randomized, double-blind, placebo-controlled or comparator trials and/or recommended as a first-line agent by APA Practice Guidelines for the Treatment of Patients with Bipolar Disorder (Revision) or Texas Consensus Panel on Medication Treatment of Bipolar Disorder; + = approved by the FDA.

B = Efficacy suggested by one randomized, double-blind, placebo-controlled or comparator trial; recommended as a second-line (alternative) agent by APA Practice Guidelines for the Treatment of Patients with Bipolar Disorder (Revision) or Texas Consensus Panel on Medication Treatment of Bipolar Disorder; not approved by the FDA.

C = Efficacy suggested by two or more open-label and/or non–placebo-controlled trials; not approved by the FDA.

D = No controlled clinical trials and/or efficacy not established for monotherapy in bipolar disorder.

X = Not recommended due to negative results or no significant difference from placebo on a randomized, placebo-controlled or comparator trial.

APA, American Psychiatric Association, FDA, Food and Drug Administration.

Compiled from American Psychiatric Association,[3] Suppes et al,[45] Sachs,[47] Keck and McElroy,[50] and Kusmakar.[64]

this may not be accurate since some medications are more effective for acute mania, some for the depressive episode, and others for the maintenance phase.[3,50,51] Lithium, divalproex sodium (or valproate), and olanzapine are currently approved by the Food and Drug Administration (FDA) for the treatment of acute mania in bipolar I disorder, and only lithium and lamotrigine are approved for the maintenance treatment of bipolar I disorder. Lithium is the drug of choice for classic bipolar disorder, whereas valproate has better efficacy for mixed states and rapid cycling compared to lithium.[3] Carbamazepine and oxcarbazepine are not approved for bipolar disorder, but are often alternative treatments (or adjunctive agents) for acute mania and maintenance therapy.[3,52]

Several atypical antipsychotics (e.g., aripiprazole, quetiapine, risperidone, and ziprasidone) have been approved by the FDA for acute mania (e.g., monotherapy and adjunctive with lithium or valproate) and are under investigation for maintenance treatment of bipolar I disorder. Combination therapies (e.g., lithium plus valproate or carbamazepine; lithium or valproate plus an atypical antipsychotic) may provide better acute response and long-term prevention of relapse and recurrence than monotherapy in some bipolar patients with mixed states or rapid cycling.[3,4,52] Controlled efficacy and safety studies addressing the combination of specific antidepressants with mood-stabilizing agents for acute versus long-term therapy are lacking.[3,4,49]

Several guidelines and algorithms have been published regarding the treatment of bipolar disorder, and these are generally based on the best available data and the clinical consensus of experts.

One excellent reference is the Practice Guideline for the Treatment of Patients with Bipolar Disorder (Revision) that was published in 2002 by the APA.[3] The APA guidelines address the diagnosis, clinical course, epidemiology, and treatment strategies for adults, but are not intended to be used as a standard of psychiatric care. Texas has developed and implemented algorithms in the public mental health system to improve treatment outcomes with bipolar I disorder.[45,53] In addition, an international task force of the World Federation of Societies of Biological Psychiatry has published guidelines for the treatment of bipolar depression and mania.[46,54]

There are few controlled studies in children and adolescents with bipolar disorder, thus little is known about the long-term efficacy and safety of specific agents or for combination therapies in this population.[3,4,13,35,55] The only published guidelines for children and adolescents are the Practice Parameters for the Assessment and Treatment of Children and Adolescents with Bipolar Disorder by the American Academy of Child and Adolescent Psychiatry,[13] and a proposed treatment algorithm for pediatric bipolar disorder.[35] A more complete review of using mood stabilizers and antipsychotics in children and adolescents can be found elsewhere.[56]

Based on the APA guidelines,[3] the Texas algorithms for bipolar disorder,[45] available research, and current marketing of medications, an example of treatment algorithms and guidelines for acute mood episodes in adult patients with bipolar I disorder are listed in Table 68–8.[47] Because newer anticonvulsants, atypical antipsychotics, and combination therapies are under investigation for bipolar disorder, published guidelines, algorithms, and decision trees may be

TABLE 68–8. Algorithm and Guidelines for the Acute Treatment of Mood Episodes in Patients with Bipolar I Disorder

Acute Manic or Mixed Episode		Acute Depressive Episode	
General guidelines • Assess for secondary causes of mania or mixed states (e.g., alcohol or drug use) • Taper off antidepressants, stimulants, and caffeine if possible • Treat substance abuse • Encourage good nutrition (with regular protein and essential fatty acid intake), exercise, adequate sleep, stress reduction, and psychosocial therapy • Optimize the dose of mood stabilizing medication(s) before adding on benzodiazepines; if psychotic features are present, add on antipsychotic; ECT used for severe or treatment-resistant manic/mixed episodes or psychotic features		**General guidelines** • Assess for secondary causes of depression (e.g., alcohol or drug use) • Taper off antipsychotics, benzodiazepines or sedative-hypnotic agents if possible • Treat substance abuse • Encourage good nutrition (with regular protein and essential fatty acid intake), exercise, adequate sleep, stress reduction, and psychosocial therapy • Optimize the dose of mood stabilizing medication(s) before adding on lithium, lamotrigine or antidepressant (e.g., bupropion or an SSRI); if psychotic features are present, add on an antipsychotic; ECT used for severe or treatment-resistant depressive episodes or for psychosis or catatonia	
Mild to moderate symptoms of mania or mixed episode	**Moderate to severe symptoms of mania or mixed episode**	**Mild to moderate symptoms of depressive episode**	**Moderate to severe symptoms of depressive episode**
First, initiate and/or optimize mood-stabilizing medication: lithium[a] or valproate[a] or atypical antipsychotic (e.g., olanzapine, quetiapine, risperidone) Alternative anticonvulsants: carbamazepine, lamotrigine,[b] or oxcarbazepine	First, two-drug combinations: lithium[a] or valproate[a] **plus** an atypical antipsychotic (e.g., olanzapine, quetiapine, risperidone) for short-term adjunctive treatment of psychotic features (e.g., delusions or hallucinations) Alternative anticonvulsants: carbamazepine, lamotrigine,[b] or oxcarbazepine	First, initiate and/or optimize mood-stabilizing medication: lithium[a] or lamotrigine.[b] Alternative anticonvulsants: carbamazepine, oxcarbazepine, or valproate	First, two-drug combinations: lithium[a] or lamotrigine[b] **plus** an antidepressant[c]; lithium **plus** lamotrigine Alternative anticonvulsants: carbamazepine, oxcarbazepine, or valproate
Second, if response is inadequate, consider adding a benzodiazepine (lorazepam or clonazepam) for short-term adjunctive treatment of agitation or insomnia if needed	Second, if response is inadequate, consider adding a benzodiazepine (lorazepam or clonazepam) for short-term adjunctive treatment of agitation or insomnia if needed; lorazepam is recommended for catatonia		Second, if response is inadequate, consider adding an atypical antipsychotic for short-term adjunctive treatment of psychotic features (e.g., delusions or hallucinations) if needed
Third, if response is inadequate, consider a two-drug combination: • Lithium **plus** an anticonvulsant or an atypical antipsychotic • Anticonvulsant **plus** an anticonvulsant or atypical antipsychotic	Third, if response is inadequate, consider a three-drug combination: • Lithium **plus** an anticonvulsant **plus** an atypical antipsychotic • Anticonvulsant **plus** an anticonvulsant **plus** an atypical antipsychotic Fourth, if response is inadequate, consider ECT for mania with psychosis or catatonia;[d] or add clozapine for treatment-refractory illness Fifth, if response is inadequate, consider adding adjunctive therapies[e]		Third, if response is inadequate, consider a three-drug combination: • Lithium **plus** an anticonvulsant **plus** an antidepressant • Lamotrigine[b] **plus** an anticonvulsant **plus** an antidepressant Fourth, if response is inadequate, consider ECT for treatment-refractory illness and depression with psychosis or catatonia[d] Fifth, if response is inadequate, consider adding adjunctive therapies[e]

[a]Utilize standard therapeutic serum concentration ranges; if partial response or breakthrough episode, adjust dose to achieve higher serum concentrations without causing intolerable adverse effects; valproate is preferred over lithium for mixed episodes and rapid cycling; lithium and/or lamotrigine is preferred over valproate for bipolar depression

[b]Lamotrigine is not approved for the acute treatment of depression, and the dose must be started low and slowly titrated up to decrease adverse effects if used for maintenance therapy of bipolar I disorder. A drug interaction and a severe dermatologic rash may occur when lamotrigine is combined with valproate (i.e., lamotrigine doses must be halved from standard dosing titration).

[c]Antidepressant monotherapy is not recommended for bipolar depression. Bupropion, selective serotonin reuptake inhibitors (SSRIs; e.g., citalopram, escitalopram, or sertraline), and serotonin-norepinephrine reuptake inhibitors (SNRIs; e.g., venlafaxine) have shown good efficacy and fewer adverse effects in the treatment of unipolar depression; monoamine oxidase inhibitors (MAOIs) and tricyclic antidepressants (TCAs) have more adverse effects (e.g., weight gain) and may have a higher risk of causing antidepressant-induced mania; fluoxetine, fluvoxamine, nefazodone, and paroxetine inhibit liver metabolism and should be used with caution in patients on concomitant medications that require cytochrome P450 clearance; paroxetine and venlafaxine have a higher risk for causing a discontinuation syndrome.

[d]Electroconvulsive therapy (ECT) is used for severe mania or depression during pregnancy and for mixed episodes; prior to treatment, anticonvulsants, lithium, and benzodiazepines should be tapered off to maximize therapy and minimize adverse effects.

[e]There are minimal or no efficacy data for some adjunctive (add-on) therapies: α_2-adrenergic agonists, calcium channel blockers, gabapentin, tiagabine, topiramate, and zonisamide; topiramate may have efficacy as an adjunctive agent with standard agents for maintenance therapy, based on initial trials.

Compiled from American Psychiatric Association,[3] Suppes et al,[45] Sachs,[47] Keck and McElroy,[50] and Kusmakar.[64]

out of date as new scientific knowledge evolves. Selection of treatments for acute mood episodes (e.g., manic or mixed, depressive, or rapid cycling) and for maintenance strategies to prevent relapses of mood episodes should be individualized. Treatment plans should be based on patient-specific characteristics, comorbid psychiatric and medical conditions, and avoidance of drug interactions and adverse effects.[3]

General Information Regarding Efficacy and Safety. Lithium was first utilized in 1949 as a treatment for mania and was approved in 1972 in the United States for the treatment of acute mania and for maintenance therapy. Lithium was the first established mood stabilizer, and is still considered a first-line agent for acute mania and continuation treatment of bipolar I and II disorder.[50,57,58] Lithium is the only bipolar medication approved for children and adults aged 12 and older. Long-term lithium treatment has been shown to reduce suicide risk in several studies.[3,59] Patients with rapid cycling or mixed states may not respond as well to lithium monotherapy compared to some anticonvulsants.[34,57] Lithium requires regular assessment of renal and thyroid functioning and lithium blood level monitoring to minimize adverse effects.[3]

In the 1980s, anticonvulsants were investigated for manic-depressive illness since the disorder had similar characteristics to episodic neurological disorders like epilepsy and migraines. Divalproex sodium (known as sodium valproate) was marketed in 1995 for the acute treatment of mania in adults and is now the most prescribed mood stabilizer in the United States. Although carbamazepine has been used for both acute and maintenance therapy, it is not approved in the United States for bipolar disorder and may cause more adverse effects and drug interactions compared to oxcarbazepine, a 10-keto analogue of carbamazepine that is used extensively in Europe.[3,4] Valproate, carbamazepine, and oxcarbazepine each have a wide range of neurological, gastrointestinal, electrolyte, and hematologic adverse effects that requires regular assessment as well as routine blood level monitoring (for valproic acid and carbamazepine).

Lamotrigine, a newer anticonvulsant, was approved in 2003 in the United States for the maintenance treatment of bipolar I disorder.[60,61] Lamotrigine add-on or monotherapy has been used for treatment-refractory bipolar depression without increasing cycling or inducing a switch to mania.[3,60] Lamotrigine is associated with causing hypersensitivity reactions and rare life-threatening skin rashes and requires slow dosage titration.[3]

Atypical antipsychotics such as aripiprazole, olanzapine, quetiapine, risperidone, and ziprasidone are effective as monotherapy or adjunctive therapy with lithium and valproate in the treatment of acute mania.[62] Some antipsychotics have the potential to cause adverse effects such as extrapyramidal reactions, sedation, depression, emotional blunting, sexual dysfunction, weight gain, and orthostatic hypotension.[18,63] Prophylactic use of antipsychotics may be needed for some patients with recurrent mania or mixed states, but the risks versus benefits must be weighed because of long-term adverse effects (e.g., obesity, type 2 diabetes, hyperlipidemia, hyperprolactinemia, cardiac disease, and tardive dyskinesia).[64,65]

Few randomized controlled trials have been done to evaluate different approaches for the treatment of acute and recurrent bipolar depression.[3,51,66,67] Nonpharmacologic treatment that may have augmenting effects include phototherapy for seasonal-pattern depression and sleep deprivation for rapid cycling.[4,68] The use of ECT for severe episodes of mania/mixed episodes, depression, psychotic features (e.g., hallucinations or delusions), or rapid cycling is still considered the best acute treatment approach for those patients who do not respond to first-line mood stabilizers such as lithium and valproate.[3,4]

Alternative Drug Treatments

Although monotherapy with an established mood stabilizer is preferred for long-term maintenance, combinations of different types of medications may be necessary for patients with acute depressive, manic, or mixed episodes who have partial or nonresponse to monotherapy, and for those who experience rapid cycling.[3,64,69]

Benzodiazepines. High potency benzodiazepines such as clonazepam and lorazepam are common alternatives to antipsychotics when patients are experiencing acute mania, agitation, anxiety, panic, and insomnia, or cannot take mood stabilizers (e.g., during the first trimester of pregnancy).[3,4,29,70,71] Lorazepam is available for intramuscular injection and is useful in the acute management of agitation. Benzodiazepines cause minimal adverse effects compared to antipsychotics, and at higher doses, rapidly sedate agitated patients.[4] Benzodiazepines may cause central nervous system depression, sedation, cognitive and motor impairment, dependence, and withdrawal reactions. Relative contraindications for long-term therapy with benzodiazepines are drug or alcohol abuse or dependency. When no longer required, benzodiazepines should be gradually tapered over several weeks and discontinued to avoid withdrawal symptoms.

Antidepressants. Antidepressants are routinely added for the treatment of acute depression, but some studies have reported that specific classes such as the tricyclic antidepressants may cause an increased risk of inducing mania in bipolar I disorder and possibly cause rapid cycling.[3,4] Some guidelines recommend avoiding antidepressants in the treatment of bipolar depression or limiting their use to brief intervals, but recent evidence suggests that the coadministration of mood stabilizers can reduce the risk of antidepressant-induced switching.[51] Before the addition of an antidepressant, the patient should be on a therapeutic dosage or blood level of a primary mood stabilizer.[3] Patients who have a history of mania after a depressive episode or who have frequent cycling should be treated cautiously with antidepressants.[3,4] In general, the antidepressant should be gradually withdrawn 2 to 6 months after remission, and the patient maintained on a mood-stabilizing agent.[32,44] For patients with recurrent depressive episodes, the use of long-term adjunctive treatment with antidepressants may be required to avoid relapses, particularly in bipolar II disorder.[3,64,72] Treatment-resistant depression is often associated with using inadequate dosages and duration of treatment for mood-stabilizing agents and antidepressants, alcohol and substance abuse, poor compliance, and rapid cycling. For more information, see Chapter 67 for comparisons between antidepressants.

Alternative augmenting or adjunctive treatments for depression include: atypical antipsychotics such as olanzapine for mixed states, psychotic features, or rapid cycling; estradiol replacement therapy for perimenopausal women with rapid cycling; thyroid hormones for rapid cycling or augmentation of antidepressants; calcium channel blockers (e.g., nimodipine) for rapid cycling; and DA agonists (e.g., pramipexole) for augmentation of DA.[3,4]

Calcium Channel Antagonists. Calcium channel antagonists inactivate voltage-sensitive calcium channels, thus inhibiting neurotransmitter synthesis and release and neuronal signal transmission.[9,18] Verapamil, a nondihydropyridine, has demonstrated mood stabilizing properties in some studies but negative results were found in other trials.[3,4,18,75] Nimodipine, a dihydropyridine, may be more effective than verapamil for rapid-cycling bipolar disorder because of its anticonvulsant properties, high lipid solubility, and good penetration into the brain.[3,4,9,18,34,75] Calcium channel blockers are generally well tolerated, and the most common adverse effects are bradycardia and hypotension. The low teratogenic effects of these agents may make them a preferable choice over lithium or anticonvulsants during pregnancy and breastfeeding.[18]

Newer Anticonvulsants.

Third-generation anticonvulsants have been investigated for treating bipolar disorder with the hope that a different mechanism of action would be beneficial for mood stabilization.[1,76,77] Despite early reports of efficacy based on open-label trials, agents such as gabapentin and topiramate were not effective for acute mania in double-blind comparator trials.[78–80] Both gabapentin and topiramate require slow dosing titration to avoid initial adverse effects, thus they may have a delayed onset of efficacy until therapeutic doses can be attained.[81,82] Gabapentin has virtually no drug interactions but requires three-times-daily dosing because of a short half-life.[4] Gabapentin causes sedation, dizziness, and weight gain with high-dose therapy.[65,74] Topiramate may cause drug interactions and has dose-related adverse effects (e.g., sedation, fatigue, psychomotor slowing, dizziness, speech and language disorders, difficulty with memory and concentration, paresthesia, nystagmus, tremor, nausea, anorexia, and weight loss).[3,82] Although topiramate has been used as an add-on weight-reduction medication, there are no randomized controlled trials supporting its use in bipolar disorder.[65,74] The effectiveness of gabapentin and topiramate as adjunctive agents for bipolar depression, comorbid anxiety and insomnia, refractory patients, or for the maintenance phase still needs to be evaluated in controlled studies.[4,77–79]

Newer anticonvulsants such as levetiracetam and zonisamide have several published case reports or open trials showing efficacy in mania and treatment-refractory rapid cycling, but it is too early to predict whether they have a place in either acute or maintenance therapy.[49,77,79] Tiagabine has caused seizures in patients with bipolar disorder and has two negative open-label trials, thus there is little support for its safety and efficacy as a mood stabilizer.

Novel Agents and Dietary Intake.

Disturbances in 5-HT neurotransmission secondary to inadequate dietary L-tryptophan or abnormalities in tryptophan hydroxylase, 5-HT transporters, and 5-HT receptors was implicated in the pathophysiology of manic-depressive illness as early as 1958.[18] Low 5-HT activity may be a trait marker for bipolar disorder.[27] If available 5-HT is low, the synthesis and secretion of melatonin may be disrupted, thus causing circadian rhythm changes.[18] Acute tryptophan depletion has been shown to reverse the antidepressant effects of 5-HT reuptake inhibitors in depressed patients in remission, but may not negatively affect mood changes in lithium-stabilized bipolar patients.[83] Randomized controlled studies of L-tryptophan or 5-hydroxytryptophan have shown positive results in the acute treatment and prophylaxis of bipolar disorder.[18] Because 5-HT synthesis in the brain is dependent on dietary L-tryptophan intake, the importance of adequate and regular ingestion of animal-derived protein should be discussed with patients.[18]

A dietary deficiency in essential fatty acids (found in certain fish oils and flaxseed oil that contains α-linolenic acid) has been proposed as a potential cause of mood disorders.[84,85] Omega-3 fatty acids have been shown to suppress neuronal pathways and inhibit kindling processes by several mechanisms (e.g., inhibition of phosphatidylinositol and G-protein secondary messengers and blocking L-type calcium channels). Seafood and fish are rich dietary sources of omega-3 essential fatty acids, specifically docosahexaenoic acid and eicosapentaenoic acid. A relationship between greater seafood consumption and lower prevalence rates of bipolar disorders has been reported.[84] A double-blind, placebo-controlled study with high doses of omega-

3 fatty acids reported some positive benefits in patients with bipolar disorder.[85]

Several novel agents have been tried in bipolar disorder, but randomized controlled trials are needed to determine their efficacy and safety.[3] High doses of levothyroxine sodium (0.15 to 0.4 mcg/day) have been reported to have mood-stabilizing properties in rapid cycling bipolar patients when combined with traditional mood stabilizing agents.[3]

SPECIAL POPULATIONS

Approaches for treating bipolar disorder in special populations (e.g., comorbid medical or psychiatric disorders, pregnancy, or breast feeding) are found in Table 68–9. Patients with comorbid medical conditions or concomitant substance abuse, those over 65 years of age, and pregnant patients may require different treatment approaches. Approximately 20% to 50% of women with bipolar disorder relapse postpartum; therefore prophylaxis with mood stabilizers is recommended immediately postpartum to decrease the risk of relapse.[86]

DRUG CLASS INFORMATION

Product information, dosing and administration, clinical use and proposed mechanism of action for agents used in the treatment of bipolar disorder are found in Table 68–10. Pharmacokinetic and therapeutic serum concentrations of lithium and selected anticonvulsants are listed in Table 68–11. Table 68–12 includes recommendations for baseline and routine laboratory testing for patients receiving carbamazepine, lamotrigine, lithium, olanzapine, oxcarbazepine, and valproate.

Antipsychotics

Pharmacology and Mechanism of Action.

Typical (conventional) antipsychotic agents that block DA_2 receptors and newer atypical antipsychotics that block both DA_2 and 5-HT_{2A} receptors are used to decrease DA activity in the treatment of mania and mixed states.

Pharmacokinetics.

A summary of pharmacokinetic parameters and metabolism pathways for antipsychotics is found in Chapter 66.

Efficacy.

Typical antipsychotic agents are effective in up to 70% of patients with acute mania, particularly those with psychosis and psychomotor agitation. Atypical antipsychotics such as olanzapine, quetiapine, and risperidone have demonstrated similar efficacy and fewer side effects than typical antipsychotics (e.g., chlorpromazine and haloperidol) for the treatment of acute mania associated with agitation, aggression, and psychosis.[3,62,63,87,88] Currently aripiprazole, olanzapine, quetiapine, risperidone, and ziprasidone are FDA approved for the treatment of acute manic episodes in bipolar I disorder. Depot antipsychotics (e.g., haloperidol decanoate, fluphenazine decanoate, and risperidone long-acting injection) may have a place in the maintenance of patients with noncompliance or treatment-resistant bipolar disorder.[3] Controlled studies in acute mania with lithium or valproate plus an antipsychotic suggest greater efficacy with combination therapies compared with any of these agents alone.[3,62] Adjunctive atypical antipsychotics may be beneficial in the treatment of breakthrough manic episodes or if there is incomplete response to monotherapy with lithium or valproate.

Olanzapine has shown efficacy in the treatment of acute manic, mixed, and depressive phases with or without psychotic features in

TABLE 68–9. Approaches to Treating Bipolar Disorder in Special Populations and with Comorbidities

Population Type or Comorbid Condition	First-Line Therapies	Second-Line Therapies
Aggression/violence/homicidal	Hospitalization: optimize dose and/or serum concentrations of lithium or valproate, then lithium or valproate ± atypical antipsychotic[a] Alternative: carbamazepine or oxcarbazepine ± atypical antipsychotic[a]	Lithium ± valproate ± atypical antipsychotic[a] ± benzodiazepines Alternative: carbamazepine or oxcarbazepine ± atypical antipsychotic[a] ± benzodiazepines
Anxiety disorders (panic or obsessive-compulsive disorder)	Valproate or add antidepressant (e.g., 5-HT reuptake inhibitor)	Adjunctive: benzodiazepine (short-term)
Attention deficit hyperactivity disorder	Add bupropion or atomoxetine; DA or NE augmenting agents may exacerbate mood changes and make it difficult to monitor bipolar disorder	CNS stimulants (use cautiously): amphetamine, dextroamphetamine, methylphenidate
Breast-feeding	All medications used in the treatment of bipolar disorder are secreted in breast milk, thus the risks versus benefits must be weighed.	There are no recommendations or treatment guidelines at this time. Valproate or carbamazepine are compatible with breast-feeding, but potential risks should be considered.
Cardiac disease/heart failure	Valproate: monitor for hypertension, tachycardia, peripheral edema	Calcium channel blocker: monitor for bradycardia, hypotension, peripheral edema
Catatonia (mutism, motor excitement, and stereotypic movements)	Benzodiazepines (lorazepam) for acute treatment	ECT for acute treatment
Children and adolescents	Lithium or valproate: maintenance treatment should continue for a minimum of 18 months after stabilization to decrease risk of relapse	Carbamazepine or oxcabazepine. Alternative: atypical antipsychotics (for psychosis) or combination therapies
Geriatric patients (over 65 years of age and in good health)	Rule out general medical conditions, medications, or substance use that may cause a manic syndrome; valproate and lithium require lower doses, regular laboratory and serum concentration monitoring; concomitant medications and medical conditions may alter the metabolism and excretion of medications	Carbamazepine or oxcarbazepine induce liver enzymes and may affect the metabolism and blood levels of concomitant medications; lithium, antipsychotics, and benzodiazepines increase the risk of adverse effects and cognitive impairment
Liver disease	Lithium: not metabolized by the liver Alternative: gabapentin (no efficacy data)	All anticonvulsants (except gabapentin), atypical antipsychotics, benzodiazepines, and calcium channel blockers require liver metabolism, and dosage adjustments may be needed (e.g., 25–50% reduction of normal doses)
Neurologic disorders (migraine, seizures)	Valproate	Carbamazepine or oxcarbazepine Alternative: lamotrigine
Pregnancy[b]	Pregnancy should be planned in consultation with a psychiatrist and obstetrician to weigh risks versus benefits of treatment options (e.g., discontinuing medications before conception or at the beginning of pregnancy, discontinuing medications only for the first trimester, or continuing medications throughout pregnancy). Medications should be tapered off slowly to avoid recurrent mood episodes. Prophylactic medications such as lithium or valproate may prevent postpartum mood episodes. Alternative: ECT used for patients with severe mania, mixed states, depression, or psychosis.	Acute mania or mixed episode: first choice: lithium After first trimester: carbamazepine, lamotrigine, oxcarbazepine, or valproate Second choice: benzodiazepine (lorazepam) Third choice: calcium channel blocker With psychosis: first choice: adjunctive high-potency typical antipsychotic (haloperidol, perphenazine, thiothixene, or trifluoperazine) Second choice: adjunctive atypical antipsychotic[b] Acute depression: First choice: adjunctive 5-HT or 5-HT/NE reuptake inhibitors Second choice: adjunctive bupropion
Psychosis (delusions, hallucinations)	Optimize dose and/or serum concentrations of lithium or anticonvulsant Alternative: add atypical or typical antipsychotic for short-term adjunctive therapy	ECT
Renal disease or impairment	Carbamazepine and valproate: if creatinine clearance is <10 mL/min, administer 75% of standard dose; combining medications in patients with renal impairment should be done cautiously; use agents that have a therapeutic serum concentration range for blood level monitoring	Oxcarbazepine: initiate dosing at one-half the usually starting dose (300 mg/day) and increase slowly

TABLE 68–9. (Continued)

Population Type or Comorbid Condition	First-Line Therapies	Second-Line Therapies
Substance use disorders (e.g., alcohol, cocaine, methamphetamine)	Dual-diagnosis treatment program: substance abuse plus standard pharmacologic/ nonpharmacologic treatments for bipolar disorder; hepatic dysfunction from chronic alcohol abuse or from hepatitis may alter the metabolism of some agents	Lithium or valproate Alternative: carbamazepine or oxcarbazepine or topiramate (alcohol dependence)
Suicidal behavior or attempts	Lithium: long-term treatment associated with reduction of suicide risk and mortality	

[a]Olanzapine, quetiapine, and risperidone are preferred; alternative atypicals: aripiprazole and ziprasidone are newer agents and may initially cause akathisia-like reactions; clozapine is usually reserved for treatment-resistant mania or mixed states.
[b]Teratogenic ratings: gabapentin, lamotrigine, olanzapine, oxcarbazepine, quetiapine, risperidone, topiramate, and verapamil are category C; carbamazepine, clonazepam, lithium, lorazepam, and valproate are category D. Lithium may have fewer teratogenic effects than previously thought and may be considered during the first trimester. Carbamazepine, oxcarbazepine, and topiramate increase the metabolism of oral contraceptives and may make them ineffective.
DA, dopamine; ECT, electroconvulsive therapy; 5-HT, serotonin; NE, norepinephrine.
Compiled from American Psychiatric Association,[3] Goldberg and Harrow,[4] Goodnick,[18] and Suppes et al.[45]

double-blind trials (compared with placebo, lithium, valproate, and haloperidol).[62,87] Patients with a younger onset of illness, no prior substance abuse, and those who are antipsychotic naïve may respond better to olanzapine.[89] Olanzapine is under investigation for the long-term maintenance treatment of bipolar disorder.[51]

Clozapine monotherapy has acute and long-term mood-stabilizing effects in refractory bipolar disorder, including conditions with mixed mania and rapid cycling, but requires regular white blood cell monitoring for agranulocytosis.[3,18,62,86] Risperidone, in combination with other mood-stabilizing agents (lithium or valproate), and as monotherapy (versus haloperidol, lithium, and placebo) has demonstrated efficacy in several double-blind acute mania trials.[3,18,62,90] Quetiapine at higher doses (e.g., 400 to 800 mg/day) has been reported to be effective for monotherapy and as an adjunctive agent with standard mood stabilizers in acute mania in a double-blind, placebo-controlled trial.[62] Ziprasidone was more effective than placebo in a double-blind, placebo-controlled study in acute mania, but has been associated with inducing mania or hypomania.[3,62] Aripiprazole, a partial agonist at the DA_2 receptor, has been evaluated in two randomized, placebo-controlled studies in bipolar I disorder patients with an acute manic or mixed episode and in one comparative trial with haloperidol in acute mania.[62] Aripiprazole was significantly better than placebo in one 3-week study at doses of 30 mg/day (but was no different from placebo in the second study), and was significantly better than haloperidol by week 12.[62]

The long-term safety and efficacy of antipsychotics for monotherapy or as an adjunctive treatment for bipolar depression and as a prophylactic agent in bipolar disorder still needs to be evaluated.[3,51,87,88]

■ *Adverse effects.* Low-potency typical antipsychotics (chlorpromazine and thioridazine) are more sedating and cause more orthostatic hypotension and weight gain, but have the advantage of causing fewer extrapyramidal side effects.[3] The high-potency typical agents (haloperidol and fluphenazine) and moderate-potency agents (perphenazine and thiothixene) cause less sedation and fewer blood pressure changes, but are more likely to cause extrapyramidal side effects such as akathisia and pseudoparkinsonism.[3] Patients with bipolar disorder may be at increased risk of developing extrapyramidal side effects, tardive dyskinesia, and depression from antipsychotic agents.[4,18]

Atypical antipsychotics cause fewer extrapyramidal side effects and may have a lower risk of causing tardive dyskinesia than typ-

ical agents.[3,87] At dosages under 6 mg/day, risperidone has few extrapyramidal side effects; however, the incidence increases with higher dosages, and several cases of tardive dyskinesia have occurred. Although olanzapine and clozapine have a lower incidence of extrapyramidal side effects than risperidone, they may cause sedation, dry mouth, constipation, orthostatic hypotension, increased appetite, weight gain, and hepatic transaminase elevations.[3,18] Weight gain may lead to obesity, impaired glucose tolerance, hyperglycemia, an increased risk of type 2 diabetes, elevation of cholesterol and triglyceride levels, hypertension, and mortality.[74] Elevated plasma prolactin concentrations have been reported with risperidone and olanzapine, and may result in sexual dysfunction, galactorrhea, menstrual disorders, impaired fertility, and decreased bone density.[3]

Quetiapine has sedative effects and may cause weight gain, but it causes minimal extrapyramidal side effects or prolactin elevations. Ziprasidone causes few extrapyramidal side effects, does not significantly increase prolactin levels, and has a lower risk of causing weight gain. Aripiprazole has low extrapyramidal side effects (except for initial akathisia), minimal effect on prolactin levels, and is considered to be weight neutral.

■ *Drug-Drug Interactions.* Combining antipsychotics with other agents with antimuscarinic, antihistaminic, α_1-adrenergic blockade, and DA blockade may result in additive adverse effects.[1] DA-augmenting agents may reverse the effect of DA receptor blockade, and 5-HT–augmenting agents may work against the 5-HT_{2A} receptor blockade, thus decreasing DA release and worsening extrapyramidal side effects. Several atypical antipsychotic agents may be affected by enzyme inhibitors or inducers. Cigarette smoking is a potent inducer of cytochrome P450 1A2 and can significantly lower clozapine and olanzapine serum concentrations. Agents that inhibit the cytochrome P450 1A2 or 3A3/4 pathways may significantly increase clozapine serum concentrations and result in toxicity and an increased risk of seizures. A summary of drug interactions with antipsychotics can be found in Chapter 66.

■ *Dosing and Administration.* For acute mania, higher initial doses of antipsychotics may be required (e.g., olanzapine 15 mg/day was more effective than 10 mg/day in hospitalized patients).[3] Once acute mania is controlled (usually within 7 to 28 days), the antipsychotic can be gradually tapered and discontinued, and the patient maintained on the mood stabilizer alone.

TABLE 68–10. Product Formulations, Dosage and Administration, Clinical Use, and Proposed Mechanism of Action of Agents Used in the Treatment of Bipolar Disorder

Generic Name	Trade Name	Formulations	Dosage and Administration	Clinical Use	Proposed Mechanism of Action
Lithium salts: FDA-approved for bipolar disorder					
Lithium carbonate	Eskalith	Capsule: 300 mg	900–2400 mg/day in 2–4 divided doses, preferably with meals. There is wide variation in the dosage needed to achieve therapeutic response and trough serum lithium concentration (i.e., 0.6–1.2 mEq/L for maintenance therapy and 1.0–1.2 mEq/L for acute mood episodes taken 8–12 hours after the last dose).	Use alone or in combination with other drugs (e.g., valproate, carbamazepine, antipsychotics) for the acute treatment of mania and for maintenance treatment.	• Normalizes or inhibits secondary messenger systems (e.g., inhibits phosphoinositide and adenylate cyclase signaling; normalizes guanine nucleotide-binding protein [G protein] signal transduction system)
	Eskalith CR	Extended-release tablet: 450 mg			
	Lithobid	Extended-release tablet: 300 mg			
	Generic	Tablet: 300 mg (scored) Capsule: 150, 300, 600 mg			• Decreases 5-HT reuptake and increases postsynaptic 5-HT receptor sensitivity
Lithium citrate	Cibalith-S	8 mEq/5 mL			• Inhibits the synthesis of DA, decreases the number of β-adrenergic receptors and inhibits DA_2 and β-adrenergic receptor supersensitivity
					• Enhances GABAergic activity and normalizes GABA levels
					• Reduces glutaminergic activity (e.g., increases glutamate uptake) with chronic therapy
					• Decreases Ca^+ transport into cells, interferes with Ca^+-Na^+ active transport system, increases renal tubular reabsorption of Ca^+ and increases serum Ca^+ and parathyroid concentrations
					• Increases choline in red blood cells and potentiates the cholinergic secondary messenger system
Anticonvulsants: FDA-approved for bipolar disorder					
Divalproex sodium	Depakote	Enteric-coated, delayed-release tablet: 125, 250, 500 mg Sprinkle capsule: 125 mg	750–3000 mg/day (20–60 mg/kg per day) in 2–3 divided doses for delayed-release divalproex or valproic acid.	Use alone or in combination with other drugs (e.g., lithium, carbamazepine, antipsychotics) for the acute treatment of mania and for maintenance treatment.	• Increases GABA levels in plasma and CNS; inhibits GABA catabolism, increases synthesis, and release; may prevent GABA reuptake; enhances the action of GABA at the $GABA_A$ receptor
	Depakote ER	Enteric-coated extended release tablet: 250, 500 mg	Extended-release divalproex may be given once daily at bedtime after stabilization.		• Normalizes Na^+ and Ca^+ channels
Valproic acid	Depakene	Capsule: 250 mg	A loading dose of divalproex (20–30 mg/kg per day) can be given, then 20 mg/kg per day and titrated to a serum concentration of 50–125 mcg/mL.	Use caution when combining with lamotrigine due to potential drug interaction.	• Reduces intracellular inositol and protein kinase C isozymes
Valproate sodium	Depakene	Syrup: 250 mg/5 mL			• May modulate gene expression
					• Antikindling properties may decrease rapid cycling and mixed states

TABLE 68–10. (Continued)

Generic Name	Trade Name	Formulations	Dosage and Administration	Clinical Use	Proposed Mechanism of Action
Lamotrigine	Lamictal	Tablet: 25, 100, 150, 200 mg Chewable tablet: 2, 5, 25 mg	50–400 mg/day in divided doses. Dosage should be slowly increased (e.g., 25 mg/day for 2 weeks, then 50 mg/day for weeks 3 and 4, then 50-mg/day increments at weekly intervals up to 200 mg/day). When combined with valproate, initial and titration dosing should be decreased by 50% to minimize the risk of a serious rash.	Use alone or in combination with other drugs (e.g., lithium, carbamazepine) for long-term maintenance treatment for bipolar I disorder. Lamotrigine may have efficacy for prevention of bipolar depression.	• Blocks voltage-sensitive Na^+ and Ca^+ channels • Modulates or decreases presynaptic aspartate and glutamate release • Antikindling properties may decrease rapid cycling and mixed states

Anticonvulsants: Not FDA-approved for bipolar disorder

Generic Name	Trade Name	Formulations	Dosage and Administration	Clinical Use	Proposed Mechanism of Action
Carbamazepine	Tegretol, Epitol Tegretol Tegretol-XR Carbatrol	Tablet: 200 mg Chewable tablet: 100 mg Suspension: 100 mg/5 mL Extended-release tablet: 100, 200, 400 mg Extended-release capsule: 200, 300 mg	200–1800 mg/day in 2–4 divided doses. Dosage should be slowly increased according to response and adverse effects (e.g., 100–200 mg twice daily and increase by 200 mg/day at weekly intervals). Administer conventional tablets and suspension with meals. Extended-release tablets should be swallowed whole and not be broken or chewed. Carbatrol capsules may be opened and contents sprinkled over food.	Use alone or in combination with other drugs (e.g., lithium, valproate, antipsychotics) for the acute and long-term maintenance treatment of mania or mixed episodes for bipolar I disorder. APA guidelines recommend reserving it for patients unable to tolerate or who have inadequate response to lithium or valproate.	• Blocks voltage-sensitive Na^+ channels • Stimulates the release of antidiuretic hormone and decreases Na^+ serum concentrations • Blocks Ca^+ influx through the NMDA glutamate receptor and decreases Ca^+ serum concentrations • Modulates presynaptic asparate and glutamate release • Antikindling properties may decrease rapid cycling and mixed states
Oxcarbazepine	Trileptal	Tablet: 150, 300, 600 mg Suspension: 300 mg/5 mL	300–1200 mg/day in two divided doses. Dosage should be slowly adjusted up and down according to response and adverse effects (e.g., 150–300 mg twice daily and increase by 300–600 mg/day at weekly intervals).	May have fewer adverse effects and be better tolerated than carbamazepine	• Oxcarbazepine and its monohydroxy metabolite increase K^+ conductance; modulates the activity of hight-voltage activated Ca^+ channels; and blocks Na^+ channels
Clonazepam	Klonopin	Tablet: 0.5, 1, 2 mg	0.5–20 mg/day in divided doses or one dose at bedtime. Dosage should be slowly adjusted up and down according to response and adverse effects.	Use in combination with other drugs (e.g., antipsychotics, lithium, valproate) for the acute treatment of mania or mixed episodes. Use as a short-term adjunctive sedative-hypnotic agent.	• Binds to the benzodiazepine site and augments the action of $GABA_A$ by increasing the frequency of Cl^- channel opening, which causes hyperpolarization (a less excitable state) and inhibits neuronal firing
Lorazepam	Ativan	Tablet: 0.5, 1, 2 mg Oral solution: 2 mg/mL Injection: 2, 4 mg/mL	2–40 mg/day in divided doses or one dose at bedtime. Dosage should be slowly adjusted up and down according to response and adverse effects.		

ABLE 68–10. (Continued)

Generic Name	Trade Name	Formulations	Dosage and Administration	Clinical Use	Proposed Mechanism of Action
Gabapentin	Neurontin	Capsule: 100, 300, 400 Solution: 250 mg/5 mL Tablets: 600, 800 mg	900–3600 mg/day in 3–4 divided doses. Dosage should be slowly increased to minimize adverse effects (e.g., 300 mg three times daily, and increase by 300 mg/day every 3–7 days up to 1800 mg/day).	Not recommended for the acute treatment of mania or mixed episodes for bipolar I disorder due to lack of efficacy. Used as an adjunctive agent for comorbid anxiety states and insomnia.	• Exact mechanism is unknown; although gabapentin is structurally related to GABA, it does not interact with GABA receptors • May modulate the action of the GABA synthetic enzyme (glutamic acid decarboxylase) and the glutamate synthetic enzyme; alters the synthesis and release of GABA; increases GABA levels
Topiramate	Topamax	Tablet: 25, 100, 200 mg Sprinkle capsule: 15, 25 mg	50–200 mg/day in divided doses. Dosage should be slowly increased to minimize adverse effects (e.g., 25 mg at bedtime for 1 week, then 25–50 mg/day increments at weekly intervals).	Not recommended for the acute treatment of mania or mixed episodes due to lack of efficacy; used as an adjunctive agent with established mood stabilizers	• Modulates voltage-sensitive Na^+ channels • Inhibits Ca^+ channels • Blocks glutamate activity • Potentiates GABAergic activity and levels • Inhibits protein kinases A and C • Weak carbonic anhydrase inhibitor
Atypical antipsychotics: FDA-approved for bipolar disorder					
Aripiprazole	Abilify	Tablet: 5, 10, 15, 20, 30 mg	10–30 mg/day once daily	Use in combination with lithium or valproate for the acute treatment of mania or mixed states (primarily with psychotic features) for bipolar I disorder. Only olanzapine is FDA-approved at this time.	• Antagonist of postsynaptic DA_2 receptors; atypical agents also block $5\text{-}HT_{2A}$ receptors that increase the presynaptic release of DA, thus lowering the risk of extrapyramidal symptoms and prolactin release • Receptor blockade varies by agent: DA_{1-4}, $5\text{-}HT_{2A-2C}$, α_{1-2}-adrenergic, muscarinic, and histamine$_1$
Olanzapine	Zyprexa	Tablet: 2.5, 5, 7.5, 10, 15, 20 mg	5–20 mg/day in 1 or 2 doses		
	Zyprexa Zydis	Tablet, orally disintegrating: 5, 10, 15, 20 mg			
Quetiapine	Seroquel	Tablet: 25, 100, 200, 300 mg	50–800 mg/day in divided doses or once daily when stabilized		
Risperidone	Risperdal	Tablet: 0.25, 0.5, 1, 2, 3, 4 mg Oral solution: 1 mg/mL	0.5–6 mg/day in 1 or 2 doses		
Ziprasidone	Geodon	Capsule: 20, 40, 60, 80 mg	40–160 mg/day in divided doses		
Calcium channel blockers: Not FDA-approved for bipolar disorder					
Nimodipine	Nimotop	Capsule: 30 mg	30–120 mg/day	Use as third-line agent for combination with other drugs (e.g., carbamazepine, valproate, antipsychotics).	• Blocks Ca^+ influx through L-type Ca^+ channels • Alters Ca^+-Na^+ exchange • Decreases 5-HT, DA, and endorphin activity
Verapamil	Verelan	Capsule: 120, 180, 240, 360 mg	80–480 mg/day		
	Calan, Isoptin	Film-coated tablet: 40, 80, 120 mg Extended-release tablet: 120, 180, 240 mg			

APA, American Psychiatric Association; Ca^+, calcium; Cl^-, chloride; DA, dopamine; FDA, Food and Drug Administration; GABA, γ-aminobutyric acid; 5-HT, serotonin; K^+, potassium; Na^+, sodium; NMDA, N-methyl-D-aspartate; NE, norepinephrine.

Compiled from Torrey and Knable,[1] American Psychiatric Association,[3] Goldberg and Harrow,[4] Manji et al,[9] Goodnick,[18] and White.[25]

Carbamazepine

Pharmacology and Mechanism of Action. Carbamazepine, a dibenzazepine derivative, is structurally related to tricyclic antidepressants.[18,91] The precise mechanism of action of carbamazepine in affective disorders remains to be elucidated.[9] Proposed mechanisms of action for carbamazepine are listed in Table 68–10.

Pharmacokinetics. A summary of the absorption, distribution, metabolism, and elimination data for carbamazepine is found in Table 68–11.

Efficacy. Carbamazepine is not a first-line agent for bipolar disorder, and is generally reserved for lithium-refractory patients, rapid cyclers, or for mixed states.[1,3,18] Carbamazepine has acute antimanic

TABLE 68–11. Pharmacokinetics and Therapeutic Serum Concentrations of Lithium and Anticonvulsants Used in the Treatment of Bipolar Disorder

	Lithium	Carbamazepine	Oxcarbazepine	Divalproex (DVPX) Sodium/ Valproic Acid (VPA)	Lamotrigine
Gastrointestinal absorption					
Regular release	Rapid: 95–100% within 1–6 hours	Slow and erratic: 85–90%	Slow and complete: 100%	Rapid and complete (VPA)	Rapid: 98%
Syrup/suspension/ solution	Faster rate of absorption: 100%	Faster rate of absorption	Unknown	Faster rate of absorption than tablets	NA
Extended-release/ enteric-coated tablets	Delayed absorption: 60–90%	Delayed absorption: 89% of the suspension; and less than regular-release tablets	NA	Extended release: 90% of intravenous dose Delayed release: 81–90% of intravenous dose Delayed absorption with delayed-release tablets; valproate is rapidly converted to VPA in the stomach, then is rapidly and almost completely absorbed from the GI tract	NA
Delay in absorption by food	Yes	No; reports of increased rate of absorption with fatty meals (extended-release capsule)	Unknown	Yes; food slows the rate of absorption but not the extent for DVPX	Bioavailability not affected by food
Time to reach peak serum concentrations	0.5–3 hours (regular-release) 4–12 hours (extended-release) 0.25–1 hours (oral solution)	4.5 hours (regular-release); 1.5 hours (suspension); 3–12 hours (extended-release tablets); 4.1–7.7 hours (extended-release capsules); higher peak concentrations with chewable tablets	4.5 hours (range of 3–13 hours)	1–4 hours (VPA) 3–5 hours (DVPX single dose) 7–14 hours (DVPX extended-release multiple dosing)	1–4 hours
Distribution					
Volume of distribution	Initial: 0.3–0.4 L/kg Steady-state: 0.7–1 L/kg	0.6–2 L/kg (adults)	10-monohydroxy carbazepine (metabolite): 49 L/kg	11 L/1.73 m^2 (total valproate); 92 L/1.73 m^2 (free valproate)	0.9–1.3 L/kg
Crosses the placenta	Yes; pregnancy risk category: D Risk of cardiac defects: 0.1–0.5%	Yes; pregnancy risk category: D	Yes; pregnancy risk category: C	Yes; pregnancy risk category: D Risk of neural tube defects: 1–5%	Yes; pregnancy risk category: C
Crosses into breast milk	Yes: 35–50% of mother's serum concentration; breast-feeding not recommended	Yes: ratio of concentration in breast milk to plasma is 0.4 for drug and 0.5 for epoxide metabolite; considered compatible with breast-feeding	Yes: both drug and active metabolite; breast-feeding not recommended	Yes: considered compatible with breast-feeding	Yes: breast-feeding not recommended
Protein binding	No	75–90%	40% of active metabolite	80–90% (dose dependent)	55%

TABLE 68–11. (Continued)

	Lithium	Carbamazepine	Oxcarbazepine	Divalproex (DVPX) Sodium/ Valproic Acid (VPA)	Lamotrigine
Renal clearance	Yes: 10–40 mL/min with 90–98% of dose excreted in urine; 80% of lithium that is filtered by the renal glomeruli is reabsorbed	Yes: 1–3% excreted unchanged in urine	Yes: 95% excreted in the urine; less than 1% excreted unchanged	Yes: 30–50% excreted as glucuronide conjugate; less than 3% excreted unchanged	Yes: 94% excreted as glucuronide conjugate
Metabolism					
Hepatic metabolism	No	Yes: oxidation and hydroxylation Induces liver enzymes to increase its metabolism and other drugs	Yes: oxidation and conjugation	Yes: oxidation and glucuronide conjugation	Yes: glucuronic acid conjugation Induces its own metabolism in normal volunteers
Metabolites	No	Yes: 10, 11-epoxide (active)	Yes: 10-monohydroxy carbazepine (active)	Yes (not active)	No
Kinetics	First-order	First-order after initial enzyme induction phase	First-order	First-order	First-order
Half-life (t$_{1/2}$)	18–27 hours (adult); greater than 36 hours (elderly or patients with renal impairment)	t$_{1/2}$ decreases over time due to autoinduction: 25–65 hours (initial) 12–17 hours (adult multiple dosing) 8–14 hours (children multiple dosing)	2 hours (parent) 9 hours (metabolite)	5–20 hours (adult)	25 hours; increases to 59 hours with concomitant valproic acid therapy
Cytochrome P450 (CYP450) isoenzyme					
CYP450 substrate	No	2C8 and 3A3/4	Unknown	2C19	Unknown
CYP450 inhibitor	No	No	2C19	2C9, 2D6, and 3A3/4	Unknown
CYP450 inducer	No	1A2, 2C9/10, and 3A3/4	3A3/4	No	Unknown
Therapeutic serum/plasma concentrations					
Obtain blood level 10–12 hours postdose	1–1.5 mEq/L: for adult, acute mania 0.4–0.6 mEq/L: for elderly or medically ill 0.6–1.2 mEq/L: for adult, maintenance	4–12 mcg/mL: for adult, acute mania and maintenance 4–8 mcg/mL: for elderly or medically ill	No established therapeutic range; 12–30 mcg/mL for 10-hydroxy carbazepine based on epilepsy trials	50–125 mcg/mL: adult, acute mania and maintenance 40–75 mcg/mL: elderly or medically ill	No established therapeutic range; 4–20 mcg/mL based on epilepsy trials

NA, not applicable.

Compiled from American Psychiatric Association,[3] Goodnick,[18] Yatham et al,[90] McEvoy et al,[94] McEvoy et al,[96] McEvoy et al,[98] and McEvoy et al.[99]

effects comparable to lithium and chlorpromazine, but its long-term effectiveness is unclear.[3,18] One comparison trial in hospitalized manic patients indicated that carbamazepine was less effective and needed more rescue adjunctive medications than valproate.[3] Other comparison studies with lithium have reported carbamazepine to be less effective than lithium for maintenance therapy.[3] In a double-blind, placebo-controlled crossover study and in an open study, carbamazepine showed efficacy in the treatment of bipolar depression.[3,18] Studies with treatment-refractory patients have reported that carbamazepine has both acute and long-term prophylactic effects.[4,18] A gradual loss of efficacy over time (similar to lithium and valproate) has been reported in some patients.[4,18]

The combination of carbamazepine with lithium, valproate, and antipsychotics is often utilized for treatment-resistant manic patients.[18] Carbamazepine increases the hepatic metabolism of antide-

pressants, anticonvulsants, and antipsychotics; thus dosage increases may be necessary (see drug-drug interactions).[18,91] Calcium channel blockers (i.e., verapamil and diltiazem) increase carbamazepine blood levels; thus combination therapy should be closely monitored.[91] The combination of carbamazepine with nimodipine for treatment-refractory bipolar illness may have potential benefit.

Adverse Effects. The most common adverse effects of carbamazepine involve central nervous system toxicity, which occurs in up to 60% of patients.[3,91] Neurologic side effects include drowsiness, dizziness, fatigue, clumsiness, ataxia, vertigo, blurred vision, diplopia, nystagmus, dysarthria, confusion, and headache.[3,18,91] These side effects usually occur during the first few weeks of therapy, so initiating therapy with low doses, gradually increasing the dose, changing to a slow-release product, or giving a larger bedtime dose may

TABLE 68–12. Guidelines for Baseline and Routine Laboratory Tests and Monitoring for Agents Used in the Treatment of Bipolar Disorder

	Baseline: Physical Exam & General Chemistry[a]	Hematologic Tests[b]		Metabolic Tests[c]		Liver Function Tests[d]		Renal Function Tests[e]		Thyroid Function Tests[f]		Serum Electrolytes[g]		Dermatologic[h]	
	Baseline	Baseline	6–12 mo	Baseline	6–12 mo	Baseline	6–12 mo	Baseline	6–12 mo	Baseline	6–12 mo	Baseline	6–12 mo	Baseline	3–6 mo
Atypical antispychotics[i]	X			X	X										
Carbamazepine[j]	X	X	X			X	X	X				X	X	X	X
Lamotrigine[k]	X													X	X
Lithium[l]	X	X	X	X	X			X	X	X	X	X	X	X	X
Oxcarbazepine[m]	X											X	X		
Valproate[n]	X	X	X	X	X	X	X							X	X

[a]Screen for drug abuse and serum pregnancy.

[b]Complete blood cell count (CBC) with differential and platelets.

[c]Fasting glucose, serum lipids, weight.

[d]Lactate dehydrogenase, aspartate aminotransferase, alanine aminotransferase, total bilirubin, alkaline phosphatase.

[e]Serum creatinine, blood urea nitrogen, urinalysis, urine osmolality, specific gravity.

[f]Triiodothyronine, total thyroxine, thyroxine uptake, and thyroid-stimulating hormone.

[g]Serum sodium.

[h]Rashes, hair thinning, alopecia.

[i]Atypical antipsychotics: Monitor for increased appetite with weight gain (primarily in patients with initial low or normal body mass index); monitor closely if rapid or significant weight gain occurs during early therapy; cases of hyperlipidemia and diabetes reported.

[j]Carbamazepine: Manufacturer recommends CBC and platelets (and possibly reticulocyte counts and serum iron) at baseline, and that subsequent monitoring be individualized by the clinician (e.g., CBC, platelet counts, and liver function tests every 2 weeks during the first 2 months of treatment, then every 3 months if normal). Monitor more closely if patient exhibits hematologic or hepatic abnormalities or if the patient is receiving a myelotoxic drug; discontinue if platelets are <100,000/mm³, if white blood cell (WBC) count is <3,000/mm³ or if there is evidence of bone marrow suppression or liver dysfunction. Serum electrolyte levels should be monitored in the elderly or those at risk for hyponatremia. Carbamazepine interferes with some pregnancy tests.

[k]Lamotrigine: If renal or hepatic impairment, monitor closely and adjust dosage according to manufacturer's guidelines. Serious dermatologic reactions have occurred within 2–8 weeks of initiating treatment and are more likely to occur in patients receiving concomitant valproate, with rapid dosage escalation, or using doses exceeding the recommended titration schedule.

[l]Lithium: Obtain baseline electrocardiogram for patients over age 40 or if preexisting cardiac disease (benign, reversible T-wave depression may occur). Renal function tests should be obtained every 2–3 months during the first 6 months, then every 6–12 months; if impaired renal function, monitor 24-hour urine volume and creatinine every 3 months; if urine volume >3L/d, monitor urinalysis, osmolality, and specific gravity every 3 months. Thyroid function tests should be obtained once or twice during the first 6 months, then every 6–12 months; monitor for signs and symptoms of hypothyroidism; if supplemental thyroid therapy is required, monitor thyroid function tests and adjust thyroid dose every 1–2 months until thyroid function indices are within normal range, then monitor every 3–6 months.

[m]Oxcarbazepine: Hyponatremia (serum sodium concentrations <125 mEq/L) has been reported and occurs more frequently during the first 3 months of therapy; serum sodium concentrations should be monitored in patients receiving drugs that lower serum sodium concentrations (e.g., diuretics or drugs that cause inappropriate antidiuretic hormone secretion) or in patients with symptoms of hyponatremia (e.g., confusion, headache, lethargy, and malaise). Hypersensitivity reactions have occurred in approximately 25–30% of patients with a history of carbamazepine hypersensitivity and requires immediate discontinuation.

[n]Valproate: Weight gain reported in patients with low or normal body mass index. Monitor platelets and liver function during first 3–6 months if evidence of increased bruising or bleeding. Monitor closely if patients exhibit hematologic or hepatic abnormalities or in patients receiving drugs that affect coagulation, such as aspirin or warfarin; discontinue if platelets are <100,000/mm³/L or if prolonged bleeding time. Pancreatitis, hyperammonemic encephalopathy, polycystic ovary syndrome, increased testosterone, and menstrual irregularities have been reported; not recommended during first trimester of pregnancy due to risk of neural tube defects.

Compiled from American Psychiatric Association,[3] Goodnick,[18] McEvoy et al,[91] McEvoy et al,[94] McEvoy et al,[96] McEvoy et al,[98] and McEvoy et al.[99]

minimize these effects.[91] Gastrointestinal side effects (nausea, vomiting, abdominal pain, diarrhea, constipation, and anorexia) occur early in therapy in up to 15% of patients.[3,18] Hyponatremia occurs in 6% to 31% of patients and may be related to fluid retention secondary to carbamazepine's antidiuretic effect.[3,91] Carbamazepine has been noted to produce weight gain, although it occurs less frequently than with valproate.[3,66,74]

Mild asymptomatic leukopenia may occur in 25% of patients and return to normal with dosage reduction or with discontinuation.[3] Patients with low- or below-normal pretreatment white blood cell and neutrophil counts should be monitored more closely because of their increased risks of developing leukopenia. Mild thrombocytopenia has been reported and may respond to dosage reduction.[3,18] Serious hematologic dyscrasias such as agranulocytosis and aplastic anemia are rare. Patients should be educated about the signs and symptoms of leukopenia and thrombocytopenia (oral ulcers, sore throat, easy bruising, bleeding, and fever).[1,18]

Other side effects of carbamazepine include hypersensitivity and dermatologic reactions (e.g., pruritic and erythematous rashes, urticaria, photosensitivity reactions, and a systemic lupus erythematosus–like syndrome).[18,91] Patients should be instructed to seek medical attention if they develop a rash. A mild transient elevation of liver enzyme levels occurs in 5% to 15% of patients; hepatitis and a significant increase in liver enzyme levels can occur.[3,91] Carbamazepine may decrease total and free thyroxine levels and increase free cortisol levels.[3]

Acute overdoses of carbamazepine are potentially lethal, and serum levels above 15 mcg/mL are associated with ataxia, choreiform movements, diplopia, nystagmus, cardiac conduction changes, seizures, and coma.[3] Gastric lavage, hemoperfusion, and symptomatic treatment are recommended for the management of carbamazepine toxicity.

Because the safe use of carbamazepine during pregnancy has not been established, caution should be used in prescribing carbamazepine during the first trimester of pregnancy or in women of reproductive age.[92] Carbamazepine may cause craniofacial deformities, spina bifida (0.5% to 1%), and low birth weight.[18,91] Carbamazepine is excreted in breast milk (the milk-to-maternal plasma ratio of carbamazepine is about 0.4).[4] There are two case reports of transient cholestatic hepatitis and jaundice in nursing infants.

■ *Drug-Drug Interactions.* Carbamazepine induces the hepatic cytochrome P450 isoenzymes (1A2, 3A4, 2C9/10, and 2D6), which increases the metabolism of many medications, such as anticonvulsants (i.e., lamotrigine, topiramate, and valproate), antidepressants (i.e., tricyclics and bupropion), antipsychotics (i.e., clozapine, haloperidol, fluphenazine, olanzapine, and thiothixene), benzodiazepines, oral contraceptives, and protease inhibitors.[3,4,91] Women who receive carbamazepine require higher dosages of oral contraceptives or alternative contraceptive methods.[4]

Carbamazepine is metabolized to an active 10,11-epoxide metabolite, thus medications that inhibit 3A4 isoenzymes may result in carbamazepine toxicity (e.g., cimetidine, diltiazem, erythromycin, fluoxetine, fluvoxamine, isoniazid, itraconazole, ketoconazole, nefazodone, propoxyphene, and verapamil).[3,4,18,91] When carbamazepine is combined with valproate, the carbamazepine dose should be reduced because valproate displaces carbamazepine from protein binding sites, thus increasing free levels.[4,18] Combining clozapine and carbamazepine is not recommended because of the possibility of bone marrow suppression with both agents.[18]

■ *Dosing and Administration.* Carbamazepine must be titrated up gradually to avoid adverse effects. During an acute manic episode, carbamazepine can be started at 200 to 400 mg/day in divided doses with meals and increased by 200 mg/day every 2 to 4 days up to 10 to 15 mg/kg per day.[91] If there is no response after 2 weeks, then the dosage can be gradually increased to obtain serum concentrations between 6 and 10 mcg/mL. During the first month of therapy, serum concentrations of carbamazepine may decrease due to its autoinduction of cytochrome P450 3A4 enzymes, and the dose may need to be increased to maintain serum concentrations.[91] Carbamazepine should be withdrawn slowly to avoid precipitating the recurrence of bipolar symptoms.

Carbamazepine serum levels are usually obtained every 1 to 2 weeks during the first 2 months, and then every 3 to 6 months during maintenance therapy. Serum levels should be drawn 10 to 12 hours after the dose (trough levels) and at least 5 to 7 days after a dosage change. Although there is no correlation between carbamazepine serum concentration and degree of antimanic or antidepressant response, most clinicians attempt to maintain levels between 6 and 10 mcg/mL (although some treatment-resistant patients may require serum concentrations of 12 to 14 mcg/mL).[1] Recommended baseline and routine laboratory tests for carbamazepine are listed in Table 68–12.

■ **Lamotrigine**

■ *Pharmacology and Mechanism of Action.* Lamotrigine blocks voltage-sensitive sodium channels, modulates or decreases glutamate and aspartate release, and has antikindling properties (see Table 68–10).[4,9,61,93,94]

■ *Pharmacokinetics.* Lamotrigine is rapidly and completed absorbed (with little first-pass metabolism), has 55% protein binding, is metabolized predominantly by hepatic glucuronic acid conjugation, and is renally excreted.[93,94] The normal half-life is approximately 25 hours; with concomitant valproic acid it increases to 59 hours, and with carbamazepine it decreases to 15 hours (see Table 68–11).[18,61]

■ *Efficacy.* The effectiveness of lamotrigine for the maintenance treatment of bipolar I disorder in adult patients was established in two multicenter double-blind, placebo-controlled studies.[3] Doses of 200 mg/day were more effective than lower doses and there were no advantages to using 400 mg/day. Lamotrigine has both antidepressant and mood-stabilizing effects, it may have augmenting properties when combined with lithium or valproate, and has low rates of switching patients to mania.[73,93] Although lamotrigine is less effective for acute mania compared to standard mood stabilizers, it may be beneficial in the maintenance therapy of treatment-resistant bipolar I and II disorders, in rapid-cycling dysphoric mania, and in mixed states.[3,4,80,93]

■ *Adverse Effects.* Lamotrigine has fewer side effects with slow titration during the initiation of therapy.[93,94] Common adverse effects include headache, nausea, dizziness, ataxia, diplopia, drowsiness, tremor, rash, and pruritus.[93,94] Lamotrigine is considered to be weight-neutral compared to lithium and valproate.[74] Approximately 10% of patients in premarketing clinical trials developed a maculopapular rash and required discontinuation of therapy.[93,94] Although most rashes are self-limiting and resolve with continued treatment, some cases progressed to life-threatening conditions such as Stevens-Johnson syndrome. The incidence of rash appears to be greatest with coadministration of valproate, with higher than recommended initial doses, and with rapid dose escalation.[94] If a slow titration schedule is used, the incidence of a serious rash is 0.01% in adults. Patients should be warned about the rash, and the need for discontinuing lamotrigine if the rash is diffuse, involves mucosal membranes, and is accompanied by a fever or sore throat.

■ *Drug-Drug Interactions.* Valproate decreases the clearance of lamotrigine (i.e., more than doubles the half-life) and lamotrigine must be administered at a reduced dosage (approximately half the standard dose).[94] Carbamazepine, phenytoin, and phenobarbital increase the clearance of lamotrigine. Lamotrigine has no effect on the pharmacokinetics of lithium and does not inhibit the cytochrome P450 isoenzymes.

■ *Dosing and Administration.* For the maintenance treatment of bipolar disorder, the usual dosage range of lamotrigine is 50 to 300 mg/day. The target dose is generally 200 mg/day (100 mg/day in combination with valproate and 400 mg/day in combination with carbamazepine).[93,94] For patients not taking medications that affect lamotrigine's clearance, the dose is 25 mg/day for the first 2 weeks of therapy, 50 mg/day for weeks 3 and 4, 100 mg/day for week 5, and 200 mg/day for week 6 and beyond.[3,93,94] Lamotrigine should not be abruptly discontinued, and doses should be reduced by approximately 50% per week over 2 weeks when discontinued. Patients who stop lamotrigine therapy for more than a few days should be restarted on the recommended dosage escalation titration schedule.

■ **Lithium**

■ *Pharmacology and Mechanism of Action.* Despite numerous investigations into the biologic and clinical properties of lithium, there is no unified theory for its mechanism of action (see Table 68–10).[9,18,20,95] Chronic lithium administration may modulate gene expression and have neuroprotective effects.

■ *Pharmacokinetics.* Lithium has unique pharmacokinetics because it is a monovalent cation. Lithium is rapidly absorbed, is widely distributed with no protein binding, is not metabolized, and is excreted unchanged in the urine and in other body fluids (see Table 68–11).[96]

■ *Efficacy.* Early placebo-controlled studies with lithium reported up to a 78% response rate in aborting an acute manic or hypomanic episode, but more recent studies suggest a slower onset of action and a more moderate effectiveness when compared to other agents.[3,4,58] Lithium has displayed efficacy in acute mania trials similar to that of valproate, carbamazepine, risperidone, olanzapine, chlorpromazine, and other typical antipsychotics.[3] In placebo-controlled studies in bipolar depression, lithium has been found to have efficacy, but there may be a 6- to 8-week delay for its antidepressant effects.[3] Lithium is more effective for pure or elated (classic) mania, and may be less effective for severe mania with psychotic features, mixed episodes, rapid or continuous cycling, alcohol and drug abuse, and in organic-induced mood states.[3,4,57]

Long-term lithium therapy is more effective in patients with fewer prior episodes, with a history of euthymia or good functioning between episodes, and with a family history of bipolar illness with a positive response to lithium.[4,18] Lithium produces a prophylactic response in up to two-thirds of patients and reduces suicide risk by 8- to 10-fold.[3,57–59]

Patients maintained on standard serum concentrations of lithium (between 0.8 and 1 mEq/L) may have fewer relapses than patients maintained on lower serum concentrations (0.4 to 0.6 mEq/L).[3,4] Abrupt discontinuation or noncompliance with lithium therapy may increase the risk of relapse.[3,4] Discontinuation-induced refractoriness has been reported in approximately one-fifth of patients who previously were stabilized on lithium.[3,4]

Lithium augmentation of antidepressants, carbamazepine, lamotrigine, and valproate may improve treatment response in bipolar I disorder.[3,97] Concomitant use of lithium with valproate or carbamazepine appears to be well tolerated, but may increase the risk of sedation, weight gain, gastrointestinal complaints, and tremor. Initial reports of combining lithium and lamotrigine suggest that the combinations are safe and effective, but further studies are necessary.

Lithium is frequently combined with both traditional and atypical antipsychotics in euphoric acute mania with psychotic features. Case reports of neurotoxicity (e.g., delirium, cerebellar dysfunction, extrapyramidal symptoms, and severe tremors) have been reported in elderly patients receiving lithium and traditional antipsychotics.[96] Combining lithium with calcium channel blockers is not recommended because of reports of neurotoxicity and severe bradycardia with verapamil and diltiazem.[96] Acute neurotoxicity and delirium have been reported in patients receiving ECT with lithium (even at reduced dosages); therefore lithium should be withdrawn and discontinued at least 2 days before ECT and should not be resumed until 2 to 3 days after the last treatment.

Adverse Effects. Approximately 35% to 93% of patients treated with lithium will experience adverse effects. These are divided into those that occur early in therapy but are generally innocuous and transient, those that occur with long-term therapy and are usually not dose-related, and toxic effects that occur with high serum concentrations.[1,3,96]

Initial side effects are often dose-related and are worse at peak serum concentrations (1 to 2 hours postdose).[3] Standard approaches for minimizing adverse effects include lowering the dose, taking smaller doses with food, using extended-release products, and trying once-daily dosing at bedtime.[3] Gastrointestinal distress (e.g., nausea, vomiting, dyspepsia, and diarrhea) can be minimized by the standard approaches or by adding antacids or antidiarrheal agents.[3] Muscle weakness and lethargy develop in about 30% of patients, but these symptoms are usually transient. Polydipsia with polyuria and nocturia occurs in up to 70% of patients and can be managed by changing to once-daily bedtime dosing.

As many as 40% of patients complain of headache, memory impairment, confusion, poor concentration, and impaired motor performance.[18] A fine hand tremor may be evident in up to 50% of patients. Stress, concomitant use of antidepressants or antipsychotics, caffeine, sympathomimetics, and impending toxicity may exacerbate the tremor. Strategies to reduce the tremor include standard approaches or adding a β-adrenergic antagonist (e.g., propranolol 20 to 120 mg/day, atenolol 50 mg/day, or metoprolol 20 to 80 mg/day).

Lithium reduces the kidney's ability to concentrate urine and may cause a nephrogenic diabetes insipidus characterized by low urine specific gravity and a low osmolality polyuria (urine volumes >3 L/day).[3,96] Lithium-induced nephrogenic diabetes insipidus is treated with loop diuretics, thiazide diuretics, or triamterene. If a thiazide diuretic is used (e.g., hydrochlorothiazide 50 mg/day), lithium doses should be decreased by 50%, and potassium levels need to be monitored.[3] Amiloride, a potassium-sparing diuretic, has weaker natriuretic effects than thiazides and appears to be relatively safe with minimal effect on lithium clearance. Potassium supplements have been suggested as another treatment for lithium-induced polyuria.[18] Fluid restriction is not recommended because dehydration increases the risk of lithium toxicity. If edema occurs, treatment approaches include lowering sodium intake or using a diuretic (e.g., spironolactone); close monitoring for lithium toxicity is necessary because these treatments often increase lithium concentrations.

Patients on long-term lithium therapy have a 10% to 20% risk of developing morphological renal changes (e.g., glomerular sclerosis, tubular atrophy, and interstitial nephritis) that is associated with impairment of water resorption and increased serum creatinine concentrations.[3] Lithium rarely causes nephrotoxicity if patients are maintained on the lowest effective dose, if once-daily dosing is used, if adequate hydration is maintained, and if toxicity is avoided.[18] Lithium should be avoided in patients with preexisting renal disease unless there is frequent monitoring.

Lithium is concentrated in the thyroid gland, interferes with thyroid hormone synthesis, and may induce the formation of thyroid antibodies.[96] Up to 30% of patients on maintenance lithium therapy develop transiently elevated thyroid-stimulating hormone concentrations, and 5% to 35% of patients develop a goiter and/or hypothyroidism.[3] Lithium-induced hypothyroidism is not dose-related, is observed 10 times more frequently in women (particularly in those with rapid cycling), and usually occurs after 6 to 18 months of therapy.[3] Hypothyroidism does not require discontinuation of lithium, because exogenous thyroid hormone (i.e., levothyroxine) can be added to the regimen. When lithium is discontinued, the need for exogenous thyroid hormone should be reassessed, because hypothyroidism is almost always reversible.

Lithium may cause a variety of benign and reversible cardiac effects, particularly T-wave flattening or inversion (in up to 30% of patients), atrioventricular block, and bradycardia.[3,18,96] Lithium rarely causes myocarditis, sinus node dysfunction, or sinoatrial block, but may aggravate ventricular arrhythmias and atrial premature contractions. If a patient has significant preexisting cardiac disease, consultation with a cardiologist and an electrocardiogram is recommended at baseline and during lithium therapy.

Other late-appearing lithium side effects include benign reversible leukocytosis and a variety of dermatologic effects (e.g., acne and acneiform eruptions, alopecia, exacerbation of psoriasis, pruritic dermatitis, maculopapular rashes, and folliculitis).[3,18] Weight gain is common (approximately 20% of patients gain more than 10 kg) and may be related to fluid retention, the consumption of high-calorie beverages as a result of polydipsia, or to a decreased metabolic rate due to hypothyroidism.[18,66,74] Decreased libido, sexual dysfunction, dry mouth, alterations in taste, changes in glucose tolerance, hypercalcemia, and hyperparathyroidism have been reported.[3,18,96] Severe neurologic disturbances such as coarse hand tremors, ataxia, slurred speech, myasthenia gravis, extrapyramidal syndrome, pseudotumor cerebri, and papilledema are occasionally observed.

Lithium is an extremely toxic drug if accidentally or intentionally taken in overdose. Lithium toxicity can occur with blood levels greater than 1.5 mEq/L, but elderly patients may have symptoms at therapeutic levels.[3] Severe lithium intoxication occurs when concentrations are higher than 2 mEq/L, and there is a worsening in several key symptoms: *gastrointestinal* (e.g., vomiting, diarrhea, or incontinence); *coordination* (e.g., severe fine to coarse hand tremor, unstable gait, slurred speech, and muscle twitching); and *cognition* (e.g., poor concentration, drowsiness, disorientation, apathy, and coma).[3] Several reports of seizures, cardiac dysrhythmia, permanent neurologic impairments with ataxia and deficits in memory, and kidney damage with reduced glomerular filtration rate have been reported after lithium intoxication.[3]

Situations that predispose patients to lithium toxicity include: sodium restriction, dehydration, vomiting, diarrhea, and drug interactions that decrease lithium clearance. Heavy exercise, sauna baths, hot weather, and fever may promote sodium loss. Patients should be cautioned to maintain adequate sodium and fluid intake (2.5 to 3 quarts per day of fluids) and to avoid the excessive use of coffee, tea, cola, and other caffeine-containing beverages and alcohol.

If lithium toxicity is suspected, the person should go to an emergency room to be monitored, and lithium should be discontinued.[3] Gastric lavage and intravenous fluids may be needed, and the patient should be monitored for fluid balance, renal and electrolyte status, and neurologic changes. In cases of overdose with sustained-release lithium products, the development and duration of toxicity can be prolonged.[3] When lithium concentrations are above 3.5 to 4 mEq/L, intermittent hemodialysis (12 hours on and 12 hours off) can be started and continued until the lithium concentration is below 1 mEq/L when taken 12 hours after the last dialysis. Hemodialysis is generally required when serum lithium levels are above 4 mEq/L for patients on long-term treatment, and greater than 6 to 8 mEq/L after acute poisoning.[3] Rebound increases in serum lithium concentrations may occur 5 to 8 hours after dialysis, thus repeat dialysis may be needed.[3]

Infants whose mothers took lithium during the first trimester of pregnancy may have a lower incidence of cardiovascular defects (particularly Epstein's anomaly) than was previously thought.[3,18] Lithium freely crosses the placenta and is found in equal concentrations in maternal and fetal blood.[96] When lithium is used during pregnancy, it should be tapered down to the lowest effective dose necessary to decrease the risk of relapse. Lithium may cause a "floppy" infant syndrome (e.g., low Apgar scores, lethargy, hypotonia, bradycardia, cyanosis, shallow respiration, and poor sucking), hypothyroidism, and nontoxic goiters. Milk concentrations of lithium range from 30% to 50% of the mother's serum concentration, and serum concentrations in the nursing infant are 10% to 50% of the mother's; thus breastfeeding is usually discouraged.[3,18,92]

Drug-Drug Interactions. Neurotoxicity may occur when lithium is combined with carbamazepine, diltiazem, losartan, methyldopa, metronidazole, phenytoin, and verapamil.[3,96] Thiazide diuretics, nonsteroidal anti-inflammatory drugs, cyclooxygenase-2 inhibitors, angiotensin-converting enzyme inhibitors, fluoxetine, and salt-restricted diets can elevate lithium levels.[1,3] Analgesics such as acetaminophen or aspirin and loop diuretics are less likely to interfere with lithium clearance. Caffeine and theophylline may enhance the renal elimination of lithium. Because lithium has no effect on the hepatic metabolizing enzymes, it has fewer drug-drug interactions compared with carbamazepine, oxcarbazepine, and valproate.

Dosing and Administration. Lithium dosing depends on the patient's age and weight, tolerance to adverse effects, and the acuity of the illness. Dosing is generally titrated up to achieve steady-state serum lithium concentrations of 0.6 to 1.2 mEq/L.[3] Lithium therapy is usually initiated with low to moderate doses (600 mg/day) for prophylaxis and higher doses (900 to 1,200 mg/day) for acute mania, using a two- to three-times-a-day dosing regimen.[3,96] Immediate-release lithium preparation should be given in two or three divided daily doses, whereas extended-release products may be given once or twice daily. If lithium is discontinued, a gradual tapering down of the dose by 300 mg/day each month has been recommended to reduce the risk of relapse.

When lithium is first started, a non–steady-state serum concentration is recommended every 2 to 3 days in patients prone to toxicity.[96] Once a desired serum concentration has been achieved, levels should be drawn every 1 to 2 weeks for 2 months or until lithium concentrations are stabilized.

Maintenance lithium serum concentrations are usually measured every 3 months, but can be adjusted to every 6 months for stabilized patients, and every 1 to 2 months for patients with frequent mood episodes.[3] Lithium clearance rates increase by 50% to 100% during pregnancy and return to normal postpartum; thus lithium levels should be determined monthly during pregnancy and weekly the month before delivery. At delivery, rapid fluid changes may significantly increase lithium levels, thus a reduction to prepregnancy lithium doses and adequate hydration are recommended.[3]

The recommended guidelines for baseline and routine laboratory testing for lithium are listed in Table 68–12. The 12-hour postdose lithium serum concentration may be 12% to 33% higher with extended-release preparations and lower with regular-release tablets with divided dosage schedules. The dose should be adjusted based on the steady-state serum concentration drawn 12 hours (±30 minutes) after the last dose.[96] A therapeutic trial (lithium serum concentrations of 0.6 to 1.2 mEq/L) should last a minimum of 4 to 6 weeks. Acutely manic patients may require serum concentrations of 1 to 1.2 mEq/L, and some need up to 1.5 mEq/L to achieve a therapeutic response. Although serum concentrations less than 0.6 mEq/L are associated with higher rates of relapse, some patients may do well at 0.4 to 0.7 mEq/L.[3] For bipolar prophylaxis in elderly patients, serum concentrations of 0.4 to 0.6 mEq/L are recommended because of increased sensitivity to adverse effects.[3]

Oxcarbazepine

Pharmacology and Mechanism of Action. Oxcarbazepine, a 10-keto analog of carbamazepine, blocks voltage-sensitive sodium channels, modulates voltage-activated calcium currents, and increases potassium conductance.[98]

Pharmacokinetics. A summary of the absorption, distribution, metabolism, and elimination data for oxcarbazepine is found in Table 68–11.[98]

Efficacy. Initial trials suggest oxcarbazepine has mood-stabilizing effects similar to those of carbamazepine, as well as the advantages of milder adverse effects, no autoinduction of liver enzymes, and fewer drug interactions.[3]

■ *Adverse Effects.* Oxcarbazepine has dose-related adverse effects of dizziness, sedation, headache, ataxia, fatigue, vertigo, abnormal vision, diplopia, nausea, vomiting, and abdominal pain.[98] Hyponatremia has been reported in up to 3% of patients.

■ *Drug-Drug Interactions.* Oxcarbazepine, a cytochrome P450 2C19 enzyme inhibitor and a 3A3/4 enzyme inducer, has the potential for causing drug interactions.[98] Oxcarbazepine induces the metabolism of oral contraceptives, thus alternative contraceptive measures are required.[3]

■ *Dosing and Administration.* Initial dosing is usually 150 to 300 mg twice daily and doses may be increased by 300 to 600 mg/day every 3 to 6 days up to 1,200 mg/day in divided doses (with or without food).[98]

▒ Valproate Sodium and Valproic Acid

■ *Pharmacology and Mechanism of Action.* The exact mechanism of action of valproic acid is not known (see Table 68–10).[9,18,20,99]

■ *Pharmacokinetics.* Valproate sodium is rapidly converted to valproic acid in the stomach, whereas divalproex sodium delayed-release and extended-release tablets must pass into the small intestine to be converted to valproic acid.[99] Valproic acid is highly bound to albumin and other plasma proteins, and it is extensively metabolized in the liver.[18] A summary of the absorption, distribution, metabolism, and elimination data for valproate is found in Table 68–11.[99]

■ *Efficacy.* Valproic acid is a branched chain fatty acid and was originally utilized as an organic solvent before it was discovered in the 1960s to have anticonvulsant properties. Valproate has antimigraine, mood-stabilizing, antianxiety, antipanic, and antiaggressive effects.[99] In 1995 the enteric-coated formulation divalproex sodium (valproate) was approved for the acute treatment of mania. Several controlled studies have shown valproate to be as effective as lithium and olanzapine in patients with pure mania, and it may be more effective than lithium in certain subtypes of bipolar disorder (e.g., rapid cycling, mixed states, secondary bipolar disorder, and comorbid substance abuse).[3,4,16,18,100] Placebo- and lithium-controlled and open studies report that valproate reduces or prevents recurrent manic, depressive, and mixed episodes.[3,4,18] Although valproate is not approved for bipolar disorder in children and adolescents, studies suggest that it is effective and well tolerated.[18,35]

Predictors of a positive response with valproate include rapid cycling, mixed episodes, comorbid panic disorder, organic mental disorders (e.g., head trauma), and mental retardation.[1,4,18] Low-dose valproate (125 to 500 mg/day) has been reported to be effective in reducing mood cycling in bipolar II disorder and cyclothymia. Oral loading with divalproex sodium, 20 mg/kg per day, may produce a rapid reduction in manic and psychotic symptoms within 4 days without causing major side effects, although there may be a lag time to obtain full antimanic efficacy. Development of tolerance and loss of efficacy with valproate occurs in some patients after several years of treatment.[4]

Giving lithium, carbamazepine, antipsychotics, or benzodiazepines with valproate may augment its antimanic effects. The addition of valproate to lithium may have synergistic effects in treatment-refractory rapid cycling and mixed states, and the combination has demonstrated efficacy in maintenance therapy for bipolar I disorder.[16]

Combinations of valproate and carbamazepine may have synergistic effects, but the potential drug interactions make blood level monitoring of both agents essential.[18] Valproate has been combined with traditional and atypical antipsychotics (e.g., olanzapine and risperidone) for patients with mixed state, depression, rapid cycling, or psychotic features.[51] Adding adjunctive atypical antipsychotics to valproate may be effective for breakthrough mania or if there is incomplete or partial response to monotherapy. Clozapine and olanzapine may increase the risk of sedation and weight gain when combined with valproate. The combination of valproate and lamotrigine may be effective, but there is an increased risk of rashes, ataxia, tremor, sedation, and fatigue.[93,99]

■ *Adverse Effects.* The most frequent dose-related adverse effects with valproate are gastrointestinal complaints (anorexia, nausea, indigestion, vomiting, mild diarrhea, and flatulence), fine hand tremors and sedation.[3,18,99] The gastrointestinal complaints are usually transient, but giving the drug with food, using lower initial doses with gradual increases in doses, switching to divalproex sodium extended-release tablets, or adding a histamine$_2$ antagonist such as famotidine or ranitidine can minimize them.[3,18] Reduction of the dose or the addition of a β-blocker may alleviate tremors, and giving the total daily dose at bedtime may minimize daytime sedation.[3,18]

Other adverse effects of valproate include ataxia, lethargy, alopecia, changes in the texture or color of hair, pruritus, prolonged bleeding due to inhibition of platelet aggregation, transient increases in liver enzymes, and hyperammonemia.[18,99] Increased appetite and weight gain occurs in approximately 50% of patients on long-term valproate therapy. Weight gain may be related to changes in metabolic rates and not to excessive food intake; excessive weight gain may result in obesity-induced hyperinsulinemia and insulin resistance.[66,74] Valproate may chelate trace metals such as selenium or zinc, which contributes to hair loss; therefore supplementation of selenium and zinc may help to manage hair thinning.[18]

Mild cases of asymptomatic leukopenia and rare cases of agranulocytosis and hepatitis have been reported with valproate.[3,18,99] Thrombocytopenia may occur at higher doses, and patients should be monitored for bleeding and bruising. Lowering the valproate dose may restore platelet counts to normal levels.[3] Fatal necrotizing hepatitis is a rare idiosyncratic, non–dose-related adverse effect that has occurred in children with epilepsy receiving multiple anticonvulsants.[18,99] Children receiving valproate should be monitored for the signs and symptoms of hepatitis (nausea, vomiting, abdominal pain, malaise, lethargy, fever, and jaundice).[18] A life-threatening hemorrhagic pancreatitis has been reported in both children and adults.[3,18,99] Patients should be warned that nausea, vomiting, abdominal pain, and anorexia can be symptoms of pancreatitis, which requires prompt medical attention. Polycystic ovarian syndrome, menstrual irregularities, hyperandrogenemia, and peripheral insulin resistance (possibly associated with significant weight gain) have been reported in women taking valproate.[3,74,99,100]

Valproate has a wide therapeutic range, so toxicity from overdoses is uncommon.[3] Signs of overdose include coma, visual hallucinations, deep sleep, and heart block. Hemodialysis can be used to remove unbound valproic acid in overdose situations.[3,99]

Valproate is usually not recommended during the first trimester of pregnancy due to a 1% to 5% risk of neural tube birth defects, primarily spina bifida.[92,99] Administration of folate may reduce the risk of neural tube defects; therefore the risks versus benefits of using valproate during pregnancy must be discussed with the patient.[18] Valproic acid is excreted into human breast milk in low concentrations (less than 1% to 10% of the mother's serum level), so is considered to be compatible with breast-feeding.[4] One case report of thrombocytopenia and anemia from valproate exposure has been reported in a nursing infant. If the mother receives valproate during breast-feeding, the infant should have routine blood level and laboratory monitoring like the mother.

■ *Drug-Drug Interactions.* There are several complex interactions between valproate and other medications.[99] Valproic acid is a weak inhibitor of liver enzymes, it may displace other drugs that are highly protein-bound (e.g., warfarin), and it may be displaced from protein binding sites by aspirin.[3,4,18,99] The antiplatelet effects of valproic acid may potentiate the anticoagulant effects of warfarin and aspirin. Valproate tends to increase serum concentrations of other anticonvulsants and tricyclic antidepressants.[18] Valproic acid may displace carbamazepine from serum protein binding sites and inhibit the metabolism of carbamazepine 10,11-epoxide, thereby causing carbamazepine toxicity.[4] Hepatic metabolism induced by carbamazepine may decrease valproic acid serum concentrations. Chlorpromazine, cimetidine, erythromycin, felbamate, and fluoxetine may inhibit liver metabolism of valproic acid and result in toxicity.[18] Valproic acid inhibits the metabolism of lamotrigine by competing with the glucuronidation enzyme site in the liver, thus lamotrigine should be initiated at half the starting dose and titrated up more slowly to 50% of the standard dose.[3,93]

■ *Dosing and Administration.* For acute mania, the initial starting dosage of valproate is 500 to 1,000 mg/day (5 to 10 mg/kg per day) in divided doses, and the dose is adjusted up by 250 to 500 mg/day every 1 to 3 days (based on clinical response and tolerability) to 1,000 to 3,000 mg/day (i.e., 15 to 20 mg/kg per day up to 60 mg/kg per day) (see Table 68–10).[3,18,99] For outpatients who are hypomanic, euthymic, or for elderly patients, the initial starting dose can be lower and gradually titrated to avoid adverse effects.[3] Once an optimal dosage has been achieved, the total daily dose may be given twice daily or at bedtime if tolerated.[3,18,99] Extended-release divalproex can be administered once daily, but bioavailability may be 15% lower than immediate-release products, thus requiring slightly higher doses.[3] Higher initial loading doses of divalproex sodium (20 to 30 mg/kg per day in divided doses) have been used in acutely agitated manic inpatients, resulting in therapeutic serum levels within 5 days.[3,4]

Recommended baseline and routine laboratory tests for valproate are listed in Table 68–12. Data from clinical trials in acutely manic patients indicated that there was an earlier response when trough serum levels were greater than 45 mcg/mL during the first week of treatment.[4] Although therapeutic serum concentrations of valproic acid have not been established in bipolar disorder, most clinicians use the anticonvulsant therapeutic range of 50 to 125 mcg/mL taken 12 hours after the last dose.[3,18] Patients with cyclothymia or mild bipolar II disorder may have a therapeutic response to lower doses and blood levels, whereas some patients with a more severe form of bipolar disorder may require up to 150 mcg/mL. Serum valproic acid levels are usually determined every 1 to 2 weeks during the first 2 months, and then every 3 to 6 months during maintenance therapy.[99]

■ PHARMACOECONOMIC CONSIDERATIONS

Bipolar disorder is one of the leading causes of chronic disability worldwide and shares characteristics of both major depressive disorder and schizophrenia.[4,101] Bipolar disorder is primarily treated in the public mental health sector, and a majority of patients receive lifelong disability coverage because of compromised functioning.[4] The total cost to society for bipolar disorder is enormous and is exceeded only by the costs for treating individuals with schizophrenia.[18] It is estimated that the total economic impact of bipolar disorder in the United States is approximately $45 billion.[1]

Despite the prevalence, morbidity, mortality, and costs associated with the illness, there are few pharmacoeconomic or evidence-based outcome studies.[4,102,103] To address some of these issues, The Stanley Foundation Bipolar Network was created to obtain longitudinal data (among five core sites and a number of affiliated sites) from double-blind, randomized controlled trials using consistent methodology and reliable and validated instruments.[104] A Systematic Treatment Enhancement Program for Bipolar Disorder (STEP-BD) is a 5-year outpatient study funded by the National Institute of Mental Health (*www.stepbd.org*) to determine which treatments or combination of treatments are most effective for bipolar disorder. The results from these controlled studies will help to provide the data for evidence-based outcomes and pharmacoeconomic considerations. Recently published data from a 12-month outpatient bipolar study (the Texas Algorithm Project) suggested that an algorithm-driven treatment had better initial and long-term improvement on outcome measures compared to a treat-as-usual group.[53]

CLINICAL CONTROVERSIES

The place in therapy of the newer anticonvulsants, such as gabapentin, levetiracetam, tiagabine, topiramate, and zonisamide, is controversial. Many clinicians consider these agents to be less effective than established mood stabilizers based on initial studies and avoid them for monotherapy in bipolar disorder.

No published algorithms and guidelines have addressed the long-term use of combination therapies; thus the concurrent use of psychotropic agents from different classes remains controversial. At present the best approach is to maximize the dose and/or blood levels of the established mood stabilizer, and if possible, to taper off any adjunctive agent once the mood episode has resolved.

The issue of medication-induced weight gain in psychiatric patients has received considerable attention in the literature because of the medical complications of obesity. The management of weight gain and its consequences on physical and mental health remains controversial. Clinicians must strive to reduce weight gain because it decreases adherence to treatment and results in increased morbidity and mortality.

EVALUATION OF THERAPEUTIC OUTCOMES

The establishment and maintenance of a therapeutic alliance with a clinician is essential in monitoring a patient's psychiatric status and safety; enhancing treatment adherence; promoting good nutrition, sleep, and exercise; identifying stressors; recognizing new mood episodes; and minimizing adverse reactions and drug interactions.[1,3] Patients who have a partial response or nonresponse to established bipolar therapies should be reassessed for an accurate diagnosis, concomitant medical or psychiatric conditions, and medications or substances that exacerbate mood symptoms. Nonadherence to medication treatment, delusional symptoms, alcohol or substance abuse, rapid cycling, or mixed states are often associated with poorer treatment outcomes.

The evaluation of therapeutic outcomes for bipolar disorder requires regular monitoring by a clinician. More frequent office visits, telephone calls, and intensive outpatient programs are first-line strategies to prevent hospitalization during the acute treatment phase of a manic or depressive episode.[3] Patients (and family members if needed) should be actively involved with their treatment and help to monitor target symptoms, efficacy of treatment, and adverse effects.[1,3]

Standardized rating scales for mania and depression are used to measure severity and changes in symptoms in clinical trials (e.g., Young Mania Rating Scale, brief bipolar disorder symptoms scale, Hamilton Rating Scale for Depression, and Montgomery-Asberg Depression Rating Scale). Patient-rated life mood charts, a timeline of stressful life events, and a graphic display of sleep patterns are helpful in recognizing early symptoms of mood episodes and in documenting patterns and lengths of episodes.[3] A mood disorder questionnaire, a 13-item self-reported screening tool, was recently developed to differentiate bipolar disorder from other mood disorders (*www.dbsalliance.org/questionnaire/screening_intro.asp*).[3,28] Health-related quality of life scales such as the Short Form (SF)-36 and the Psychological General Well Being Scale have been recommended to assess the quality of life in individuals with bipolar disorder.[105]

ABBREVIATIONS

DA: dopamine
ECT: electroconvulsive therapy
GABA: γ-aminobutyric acid
5-HT: serotonin
NE: norepinephrine
SSRI: selective serotonin reuptake inhibitor

Review Questions and other resources can be found at *www.pharmacotherapyonline.com*.

REFERENCES

1. Torrey EF, Knable MB. Surviving Manic Depression: A Manual on Bipolar Disorder for Patients, Families, and Providers. New York, Basic Books, 2002.
2. American Psychiatric Association. Diagnostic and Statistical Manual of Mental Disorders, Fourth Edition, Text Revision. Washington, American Psychiatric Association, 2000:382–401.
3. American Psychiatric Association. Practice Guideline for the Treatment of Patients with Bipolar Disorder (Revision). Am J Psychiatry 2002; 159:1–50.
4. Goldberg JF, Harrow M, eds. Bipolar Disorders: Clinical Course and Outcome. Washington, American Psychiatric Press, 1999.
5. Taylor L, Farone SV, Tsuang MT. Family, twin, and adoption studies of bipolar disease. Curr Psychiatry Rep 2002;4:130–133.
6. Judd LL, Akiskal HS. The prevalence and disability of bipolar spectrum disorders in the U.S. population: Re-analysis of the ECA database taking into account subthreshold cases. J Affect Disord 2003;73:123–131.
7. Kessler RC, McGonagle KA, Zhao S, et al. Lifetime and 12-month prevalence of DSM-III-R psychiatric disorders in the United States: Results from the national comorbidity survey. Arch Gen Psychiatry 1994;51: 8–19.
8. Kelso JR. Arguments for the genetic basis of the bipolar spectrum. J Affect Disord 2003;73:183–197.
9. Manji HK, Bowden CL, Belmaker RH, eds. Bipolar Medications: Mechanisms of Action. Washington, American Psychiatric Press, 2000.
10. Lenox RH, Gould TD, Manji HK. Endophenotypes in bipolar disorder. Am J Med Genet 2002;114:391–406.
11. Baron M. Manic-depressive genes and the new millennium: Poised fo discovery. Mol Psychiatry 2002;7:342–358.
12. Bezchlibnyk Y, Young LT. The neurobiology of bipolar disorder: Focu on signal transduction pathways and the regulation of gene expression Can J Psychiatry 2002;47:135–148.
13. Practice Parameters for the Assessment and Treatment of Children an Adolescents with Bipolar Disorder. J Am Acad Child Adolesc Psychiatr 1997;36:138–157.
14. Kim EY, Miklowitz DJ. Childhood mania, attention deficit hyperactivit disorder and conduct disorder: A critical review of diagnostic dilemmas Bipolar Disord 2002;4:215–225.
15. Salloum IM, Thase ME. Impact of substance abuse on the course an treatment of bipolar disorder. Bipolar Disord 2000;2:269–280.
16. Calabrese JR, Shelton MD, Rapport DJ, et al. Current research on rapi cycling bipolar disorder and its treatment. J Affect Disord 2001;67 241–255.
17. Sherwood Brown E, Suppes T, Adinoff B, Rajan Thomas N. Drug abus and bipolar disorder: Comorbidity or misdiagnosis? J Affect Disor 2001;65:105–115.
18. Goodnick PJ, ed. Mania: Clinical and Research Perspectives Washington, American Psychiatric Press, 1998.
19. Soares JC. Can brain imaging studies provide a "mood stabilizer signa ture?" Mol Psychiatry 2002;7(Suppl 1):S64–S70.
20. Manji HK, Moore GJ, Chen G. Bipolar disorder: leads from the molecula and cellular mechanisms of action of mood stabilizers. Br J Psychiatr Suppl 2001;41:S107–S119.
21. Gould TD, Manji HK. Signaling networks in the pathophysiology an treatment of mood disorders. J Psychosom Res 2002;53:687–697.
22. Sobczak S, Honig A, van Duinen MA, Riedel WJ. Serotonergic dysfunc tion in bipolar disorders: A literature review of serotonergic challeng studies. Bipolar Disord 2002;4:347–356.
23. Freeman MP, Wosnitzer Smith K, Freeman SA, et al. The impact o reproductive events on the course of bipolar disorder in women. J Cli Psychiatry 2002;63:284–287.
24. Ketter TA, Wang PW. The emerging differential roles of GABAergic an antiglutamatergic agents in bipolar disorders. J Clin Psychiatry 2003 64(Suppl 3):15–20.
25. White HS. Mechanism of action of newer anticonvulsants. J Cli Psychiatry 2003;64(Suppl 8):5–8.
26. Rasgon N, Bauer M, Glenn T, et al. Menstrual cycle related mood change in women with bipolar disorder. Bipolar Disord 2003;5:48–52.
27. Mahmood T, Silverstone T. Serotonin and bipolar disorder. J Affec Disord 2001;66:1–11.
28. Hirschfeld RM. Bipolar spectrum disorder: improving its recognitio and diagnosis. J Clin Psychiatry 2001;62(Suppl 14):5–9.
29. Freeman MP, Freeman SA, McElroy SL. The comorbidity of bipola and anxiety disorders: Prevalence, psychobiology, and treatment issues J Affect Disord 2002;68:1–23.
30. Cassidy F, Ahearn EP, Carroll BJ. Substance abuse in bipolar disorder Bipolar Disord 2001;3:181–188.
31. Bowden CL. Strategies to reduce misdiagnosis of bipolar depression Psychiatr Serv 2001;52:51–55.
32. Sachs GS, Koslow CL, Ghaemi SN. The treatment of bipolar depression Bipolar Disord 2000;2:256–260.
33. Rihmer Z, Kiss K. Bipolar disorders and suicidal behavior. Bipola Disord 2002;4(Supp 1):21–25.
34. Barrios C, Chaudhry TA, Goodnick PJ. Rapid cycling bipolar disorder Expert Opin Pharmacother 2001;2:1963–1973.
35. Chang KD, Ketter TA. Special issues in the treatment of paediatric bipola disorder. Expert Opin Pharmacother 2001;2:613–622.
36. Wozniak J, Biederman J, Richards JA. Diagnostic and therapeutic dilem mas in the management of pediatric-onset bipolar disorder. J Clin Psychiatry 2001;62(Suppl 14):10–15.
37. Post RM, Denicoff KD, Leverich GS, et al. Morbidity in 258 bipolar outpatients followed for 1 year with daily prospective ratings on the NIMH life chart method. J Clin Psychiatry 2003;64:680–690.
38. Jamison KR. Suicide and bipolar disorder. J Clin Psychiatry 2000; 61(Suppl 9):47–51.

39. Dalton EJ, Cate-Carter TD, Mundo E, et al. Suicide risk in bipolar patients: the role of co-morbid substance use disorders. Bipolar Disord 2003;5:58–61.

40. Lingam R, Scott J. Treatment non-adherence in affective disorders. Acta Psychiatr Scand 2002;105:164–172.

41. Otto MW, Reilly-Harrington N, Sachs GS. Psychoeducational and cognitive-behavioral strategies in the management of bipolar disorder. J Affect Disord 2003;73:171–181.

42. Hasey G. Transcranial magnetic stimulation in the treatment of mood disorder: A review and comparison with electroconvulsive therapy. Can J Psychiatry 2001;46:720–727.

43. Goldberg JF. Treatment guidelines: current and future management of bipolar disorder. J Clin Psychiatry 2000;61(Suppl 13):12–18.

44. Sachs GS, Printz DJ, Kahn DA, et al. The Expert Consensus Guideline Series: Medication Treatment of Bipolar Disorder 2000. Postgrad Med 2000;Spec No:1–104.

45. Suppes T, Dennehy EB, Swann AC, et al. Report of the Texas Consensus Conference Panel on medication treatment of bipolar disorder 2000. J Clin Psychiatry 2002;63:288–299.

46. Grunze H, Kasper S, Goodwin G, et al. World Federation of Societies of Biological Psychiatry (WFSBP) guidelines for biological treatment of bipolar disorders. Part I: Treatment of bipolar depression. World J Biol Psychiatry 2002;3:115–124.

47. Sachs GS. Decision tree for the treatment of bipolar disorder. J Clin Psychiatry 2003;64(Suppl 80):35–40.

48. Möller JH, Nasrallah HA. Treatment of bipolar disorder. J Clin Psychiatry 2003;64(Suppl 6):9–17.

49. Mondimore FM, Fuller GA, DePaulo JR Jr. Drug combinations for mania. J Clin Psychiatry 2003;64(Suppl 5):25–31.

50. Keck PE Jr., McElroy SL. Redefining mood stabilization. J Affect Disord 2003;73:163–169.

51. Keck PE Jr., Nelson EB, McElroy SL. Advances in the pharmacologic treatment of bipolar depression. Biol Psychiatry 2003;53:671–679.

52. Keck PE Jr., McElroy SL. Carbamazepine and valproate in the maintenance treatment of bipolar disorder. J Clin Psychiatry 2002;63(Suppl 10):13–17.

53. Suppes T, Rush AJ, Dennehy EB, et al. Texas Medication Algorithm Project, phase 3 (TMAP-3): Clinical results for patients with a history of mania. J Clin Psychiatry 2003;64:370–382.

54. Grunze H, Kasper S, Goodwin G, et al. The World Federation of Societies of Biological Psychiatry (WFSBP) Guidelines for the Biological Treatment of Bipolar Disorders, Part II: Treatment of Mania. World J Biol Psychiatry 2003;4:5–13.

55. Weller EB, Danielyan AK, Weller RA. Somatic treatment of bipolar disorder in children and adolescents. Child Adolesc Psychiatric Clin North Am 2002;11:595–617.

56. Kowatch RA, DelBello MP. The use of mood stabilizers and atypical antipsychotics in children and adolescents with bipolar disorders. CNS Spectr 2003;8:273–280.

57. Goodwin FK. Rationale for long-term treatment of bipolar disorder and evidence for long-term lithium treatment. J Clin Psychiatry 2002;63(Suppl 10):5–12.

58. Baldessarini RJ, Tondo L, Hennen J, Viguera AC. Is lithium still worth using? An update of selected recent research. Harv Rev Psychiatry 2002;10:59–75.

59. Baldessarini RJ, Tondo L, Hennen J. Lithium treatment and suicide risk in major affective disorders: Update and new findings. J Clin Psychiatry 2003;64(Suppl 5):44–52.

60. Calabrese JR, Shelton MD, Rapport DJ, et al. Long-term treatment of bipolar disorder with lamotrigine. J Clin Psychiatry 2002;63(Suppl 10):18–22.

61. Hurley SC. Lamotrigine update and its use in mood disorders. Ann Pharmacother 2002;36:860–873.

62. Hirschfeld RMA. The efficacy of atypical antipsychotics in bipolar disorders. J Clin Psychiatry 2003;64(Suppl 8):15–21.

63. Yatham LN. The role of novel antipsychotics in bipolar disorders. J Clin Psychiatry 2002;63(Suppl 3):10–14.

64. Kusmakar V. Antidepressants and antipsychotics in the long-term treatment of bipolar disorder. J Clin Psychiatry 2002;63(Suppl 10):23–28.

65. Nemeroff CB. Safety of available agents used to treat bipolar disorder: focus on weight gain. J Clin Psychiatry 2003;64:532–539.

66. Altshuler LL, Frye MA, Gitlin MJ. Acceleration and augmentation strategies for treating bipolar depression. Biol Psychiatry 2003;53:691–700.

67. Keck PE Jr., Nelson EB, McElroy SL. Advances in the pharmacologic treatment of bipolar depression. Biol Psychiatry 2003;53:671–679.

68. Riemann D, Voderholzer U, Berger M. Sleep and sleep-wake manipulations in bipolar depression. Neuropsychobiology 2002;45(Suppl 1):7–12.

69. Goodwin FK. Rationale for using lithium in combination with other mood stabilizers in the management of bipolar disorder. J Clin Psychiatry 2003;64(Suppl 5):18–24.

70. McEvoy GK, Miller J, Snow EK, et al. Benzodiazepines. AHFS Drug Information 2004. Bethesda, MD, American Society of Health-System Pharmacists, 2004:2372–2380.

71. Alderfer BS, Allen MH. Treatment of agitation in bipolar disorder across the life cycle. J Clin Psychiatry 2003;64(Suppl 4):3–9.

72. Keck PE Jr., McElroy SL. New approaches in managing bipolar depression. J Clin Psychiatry 2003;64(Suppl 1):13–18.

73. Malhi GS, Mitchell PB, Salim S. Bipolar depression: Management options. CNS Drugs 2003;17:9–25.

74. Aronne LJ, Segal KR. Weight gain in the treatment of mood disorders. J Clin Psychiatry 2003;64(Suppl 8):22–29.

75. Levy NA, Janicak PG. Calcium channel antagonists for the treatment of bipolar disorder. Bipolar Disord 2000;2:108–119.

76. White HS. Mechanism of action of newer anticonvulsants. J Clin Psychiatry 2003;64(Suppl 8):5–8.

77. Evins AE. Efficacy of newer anticonvulsant medications in bipolar spectrum mood disorders. J Clin Psychiatry 2003;64(Suppl 8):9–14.

78. Macdonald KJ, Young LT. Newer antiepileptic drugs in bipolar disorder: Rationale for use and role in therapy. CNS Drugs 2002;16:549–562.

79. Yatham LN, Kusumakar V, Calabrese JR, et al. Third generation anticonvulsants in bipolar disorder: a review of efficacy and summary of clinical recommendations. J Clin Psychiatry 2002;63:275–283.

80. Calabrese JR, Shelton MD, Rapport DJ, Kimmel SE. Bipolar disorders and the effectiveness of novel anticonvulsants. J Clin Psychiatry 2002;63(Suppl 3):5–9.

81. McEvoy GK, Miller J, Snow EK, et al. Gabapentin. AHFS Drug Information 2004. Bethesda, MD, American Society of Health-System Pharmacists, 2004:2130–2134.

82. McEvoy GK, Miller J, Snow EK, et al. Topiramate. AHFS Drug Information 2004. Bethesda, MD, American Society of Health-System Pharmacists, 2004:2148–2152.

83. Johnson L, El-Khoury A, Aberg-Wistedt A, et al. Tryptophan depletion in lithium-stabilized patients with affective disorder. Int J Neuropsychopharmacol 2001;4:329–336.

84. Noaghiul S, Hibbelm JR. Cross-national comparisons of seafood consumption and rates of bipolar disorders. Am J Psychiatry 2003;160:2222–2227.

85. Stoll AL, Severus WE, Freeman MP, et al. Omega-3 fatty acids in bipolar disorder: A preliminary double-blind, placebo-controlled trial. Arch Gen Psychiatry 1999;56:407–412.

86. Viguera AC, Cohen LS, Baldessarini RJ, Nonacs R. Managing bipolar disorder during pregnancy: Weighing the risks and benefits. Can J Psychiatry 2002;47:426–436.

87. Brambilla P, Barale F, Soares JC. Atypical antipsychotics and mood stabilization in bipolar disorder. Psychopharmacology 2003;166:315–332.

88. Strakowski SM, Del Bello MP, Adler CM, Keck PE Jr. Atypical antipsychotics in the treatment of bipolar disorder. Expert Opin Pharmacother 2003;4:751–760.

89. Baldessarini RJ, Hennen J, Wilson M, et al. Olanzapine versus placebo in acute mania treatment responses in subgroups. J Clin Psychopharmacol 2003;23:370–376.

90. Yatham LN, Grossman F, Augustyns I, et al. Mood stabilizers plus risperidone or placebo in the treatment of acute mania. Br J Psychiatry 2003;182:141–147.

91. McEvoy GK, Miller J, Snow EK, et al. Carbamazepine. AHFS Drug Information 2004. Bethesda, MD, American Society of Health-System Pharmacists, 2004:2122–2127.

92. Ernst CL, Goldberg JF. The reproductive safety profile of mood stabilizers, atypical antipsychotics, and broad-spectrum psychotropics. J Clin Psychiatry 2002;63(Suppl 4):42–55.

93. Bowden CL, Karren NU. Lamotrigine in the treatment of bipolar disorder. Expert Opin Pharmacother 2002;3:1513–1519.

94. McEvoy GK, Miller J, Snow EK, et al. Lamotrigine. AHFS Drug Information 2004. Bethesda, MD, American Society of Health-System Pharmacists, 2004:2134–2140.

95. Shaldubina A, Agam G, Belmaker RH. The mechanism of lithium action: state of the art, ten years later. Prog Neuropsychopharmacol Biol Psychiatry 2001;25:855–866.

96. McEvoy GK, Miller J, Snow EK, et al. Lithium salts. AHFS Drug Information 2004. Bethesda, MD, American Society of Health-System Pharmacists, 2004:2425–2434.

97. Goodwin FK. Rationale for using lithium in combination with other mood stabilizers in the management of bipolar disorder. J Clin Psychiatry 2003;64(Suppl 5):18–24.

98. McEvoy GK, Miller J, Snow EK, et al. Oxcarbazepine. AHFS Drug Information 2004. Bethesda, MD, American Society of Health-System Pharmacists, 2004:2146–2147.

99. McEvoy GK, Miller J, Snow EK, et al. Valproate sodium, valproic acid, divalproex sodium. AHFS Drug Information 2004. Bethesda, MD, American Society of Health-System Pharmacists, 2004:2152–2158.

100. Macritchie K, Geddes JR, Scott J, et al. Valproate for acute mood episodes in bipolar disorder. Cochrane Database Syst Rev 2003;1:CD004052.

101. Bauer M, Unutzer J, Pincus HA, Lawson WB, NIMH Affective Disorders Workgroup. Bipolar disorder. Ment Health Serv Res 2002;4:225–229.

102. Baldessarini RJ. Treatment research in bipolar disorder: Issues and recommendations. CNS Drugs 2002;16:721–729.

103. Kusumakar V. Antidepressants and antipsychotics in the long-term treatment of bipolar disorder. J Clin Psychiatry 2002;63(Suppl 10):23–28.

104. Post RM, Nolen WA, Kupka RW, et al. The Stanley Foundation Bipolar Network. I. Rationale and methods. Br J Psychiatry Suppl 2001;41:S69–S76.

105. Namjoshi MA, Buesching DP. A review of the health-related quality of life literature in bipolar disorder. Qual Life Res 2001;10:105–115.

69

ANXIETY DISORDERS I: GENERALIZED ANXIETY, PANIC, AND SOCIAL ANXIETY DISORDERS

Cynthia K. Kirkwood and Sarah T. Melton

Learning Objectives and other resources can be found at *www.pharmacotherapyonline.com.*

KEY CONCEPTS

◀1 The long-term goal in generalized anxiety disorder is remission with minimal or no anxiety symptoms and no functional impairment.

◀2 Antidepressants are the agents of choice for long-term management of generalized anxiety disorder.

◀3 Antidepressants have a lag time of 2 to 4 weeks or longer before antianxiety effects occur in generalized anxiety disorder.

◀4 When monitoring the effectiveness of antidepressants in panic disorder, it is important to allow an adequate amount of time (8 to 12 weeks) to achieve full therapeutic response.

◀5 Clonazepam and alprazolam extended-release are alternatives to alprazolam immediate-release for patients with panic disorder having breakthrough panic symptoms at the end of a dosing interval.

◀6 The optimal duration of panic therapy is unknown; 12 to 24 months of pharmacotherapy is recommended before

gradual drug discontinuation over 4 to 6 months is attempted.

◀7 Social anxiety disorder is a chronic long-term illness requiring extended therapy. After improvement, at least a 1-year maintenance period is recommended to maintain response and decrease the rate of relapse.

◀8 The selective serotonin reuptake inhibitors or venlafaxine are considered first-line pharmacotherapy for social anxiety disorder, especially in patients with comorbid depression, other anxiety disorders, or substance abuse.

◀9 An adequate trial of antidepressants in generalized social anxiety disorder lasts at least 8 weeks, and maximal benefit may not be seen until 12 weeks.

◀10 The three principal domains in which improvement should be observed in generalized social anxiety disorder include symptoms, functionality, and well being or overall improvement.

Anxiety is an emotional state commonly caused by the perception of real or perceived danger that threatens the security of an individual. It allows a person to prepare for or react to environmental changes. Everyone experiences a certain amount of nervousness and apprehension when faced with a stressful situation. This is an adaptive response, and is transient in nature.

Anxiety can produce uncomfortable and potentially debilitating psychological (e.g., worry or feeling of threat) and physiological arousal (e.g., tachycardia or shortness of breath) if it becomes excessive. Some individuals experience persistent, severe anxiety symptoms and possess irrational fears that significantly impair normal daily functioning. These persons often suffer from an anxiety disorder.[1]

Anxiety disorders are among the most frequent mental disorders encountered in clinical practice. Health care professionals often mistake anxiety disorders for physical illnesses, and only 23% of patients receive appropriate treatment.[2] Failure to diagnose and manage anxiety disorders results in negative outcomes including overuse of health care resources, increased morbidity, and mortality.[3] Individuals with anxiety disorders develop cardiovascular, cerebrovascular, gastroin-

testinal, and respiratory disorders at a significantly higher rate than the general population.[4]

To treat anxiety appropriately, the clinician must make a reliable diagnosis. It is essential that the distinction between short-term symptoms of anxiety and anxiety disorders be understood. Common or situational anxiety is a normal response to a stressful circumstance. Although symptoms can be severe, they are temporary and usually last no more than 2 or 3 weeks. While short-term, "as needed" treatment with an anxiolytic agent such as a benzodiazepine is common and may provide some symptomatic relief, prolonged drug therapy is unnecessary.[5]

EPIDEMIOLOGY

The prevalence rates of anxiety disorders was recently adjusted to reflect clinically significant disorders in the community.[6] According to the revised prevalence estimates of mental disorders in the

United States, the 1-year prevalence rate for anxiety disorders was 13.3% in persons aged 18 to 54 years and 10.6% in those over age 55 years.[6] Specific phobias were the most common anxiety disorder, with a 12-month prevalence of 8%; however, patients were not seriously impaired in terms of daily functioning, and few persons sought treatment.[1,6] The 1-year prevalence of generalized anxiety disorder (GAD) was 2.8%, that of panic disorder was 1.7%, and that of social anxiety disorder (SAD) was 3.7%.[6]

In general, anxiety disorders are a group of heterogeneous illnesses that develop before age 30 and are more common in women, individuals with social issues, and those with a family history of anxiety and depression. Patients often develop another anxiety disorder, major depression, or substance abuse.[1–3] The clinical picture of mixed anxiety and depression is much more common than an isolated anxiety disorder.[7,8]

ETIOLOGY

The differential diagnosis of anxiety disorders includes medical and psychiatric illnesses and certain drugs.[8] Family studies show that SAD can be inherited, with a threefold increase in the rate of SAD in relatives of patients.[9] Behavioral inhibition, characterized by wariness, decreased social interaction, and withdrawal, is a genetic trait that may contribute to SAD.[10] Patients with SAD commonly report having overprotective parents. Parental dysfunction and abuse are potential risk factors for developing SAD.[10]

MEDICAL DISEASES ASSOCIATED WITH ANXIETY

Anxiety symptoms are an inherent part of the initial clinical presentation of several diseases, thus complicating the distinction between anxiety disorders and medical disorders.[7] If the anxiety symptoms are secondary to a medical illness, they usually will subside as the medical situation stabilizes. However, the knowledge that one has a physical illness (e.g., cancer and diabetes) can trigger anxious feelings and further complicate therapy. Persistent anxiety subsequent to a physical illness requires further assessment for an anxiety disorder.[7] Symptoms of anxiety frequently present in medical disorders include palpitations, tachycardia, chest pain or tightness, shortness of breath, and hyperventilation. Medical disorders most closely associated with anxiety are listed in Table 69–1.[7,8,11] About 50% of patients with GAD have irritable bowel syndrome.[12]

TABLE 69–1. Common Medical Illnesses Associated with Anxiety Symptoms

Cardiovascular
Angina, arrhythmias, congestive heart failure, ischemic heart disease, myocardial infarction

Endocrine and metabolic
Cushing's disease, hyperparathyroidism, hyperthyroidism, hypothyroidism, hypoglycemia, hyponatremia, hyperkalemia, pheochromocytoma, vitamin B_{12} or folate deficiencies

Neurologic
Dementia, migraine, Parkinson's disease, seizures, stroke, neoplasms, poor pain control

Respiratory system
Asthma, chronic obstructive pulmonary disease, pulmonary embolus, pneumonia

Others
Anemias, systemic lupus erythematosus, vestibular dysfunction

Compiled from House and Stark,[7] Gliatto,[8] and Chen et al.[11]

TABLE 69–2. Drugs Associated with Anxiety Symptoms

Anticonvulsants: carbamazepine
Antidepressants: selective serotonin reuptake inhibitors, tricyclic antidepressants
Antihypertensives: felodipine
Antibiotics: quinolones, isoniazid
Bronchodilators: albuterol, theophylline
Corticosteroids: prednisone
Dopa agonists: levodopa
Herbals: ma huang, ginseng, ephedra
Nonsteroidal anti-inflammatory drugs: ibuprofen
Stimulants: amphetamines, methylphenidate, caffeine, cocaine
Sympathomimetics: pseudoephedrine
Thyroid hormones: levothyroxine
Toxicity: anticholinergics, antihistamines, digoxin
Withdrawal: alcohol, sedatives

Compiled from American Psychiatric Association,[1] House and Stark,[7] and Chen et al.[11]

PSYCHIATRIC DISEASES ASSOCIATED WITH ANXIETY

Anxiety can be a presenting feature of several major psychiatric illnesses. Anxiety symptoms are extremely common in patients with mood disorders, schizophrenia, delirium, dementia, and substance-use disorders. Most psychiatric patients will have two or more concurrent psychiatric disorders (comorbidity) within their lifetime.[6] It is important to diagnose and treat all comorbid psychiatric conditions in patients with anxiety disorders.

DRUG-INDUCED ANXIETY

Drugs are a common cause of anxiety symptoms (Table 69–2). Anxiety occurs during the use of central nervous system (CNS) stimulating drugs in a dose-dependent manner, but ingestion of minimal amounts can result in marked anxiety, including panic attacks, in some individuals. The onset of drug-induced anxiety is usually rapid after the initiation of therapy; look for a recent drug or dosage change to rule out drug etiologies for anxiety.

Anxiety occurs occasionally during the use of CNS depressants, especially in children and the elderly; however, anxiety complaints are more common as complications of drug withdrawal after the abrupt discontinuation of these agents.[7,11]

PATHOPHYSIOLOGY

Data from biochemical and neuroimaging studies indicate that the modulation of normal and pathologic anxiety states is associated with multiple regions of the brain and abnormal function in several neurotransmitter systems, including norepinephrine (NE), γ-aminobutyric acid (GABA), and serotonin (5-HT). Current neuroanatomic models of fear (i.e., the response to danger) and anxiety (i.e., the feeling of fear that is disproportionate to the actual threat) include some key brain areas. The amygdala, a temporal lobe structure, plays a critical role in the assessment of fear stimuli and learned response to fear.[13] The locus ceruleus (LC), located in the brain stem, is the primary NE-containing site in the brain, with widespread projections to areas responsible for implementing fear responses (e.g., vagus, lateral and paraventricular hypothalamus). The hippocampus is integral in the consolidation of traumatic memory, and along with the entorhinal cortex, contextual fear conditioning that is involved in overgeneralization f the fear response. The hypothalamus is the principal area for inte-rating neuroendocrine and autonomic responses to a threat.[13]

NEUROCHEMICAL THEORIES

NORADRENERGIC MODEL

The basic premise of the noradrenergic theory is that the autonomic nervous system of anxious patients is hypersensitive and overreacts to various stimuli. Many anxious patients clearly display symptoms of peripheral autonomic hyperactivity. In response to threat or fear-ful situations, the LC serves as an alarm center, activating NE re-lease and stimulating the sympathetic and parasympathetic nervous systems. Chronic central noradrenergic overactivity downregulates α_2-adrenoreceptors in patients with GAD. This receptor is hypersen-sitive in some patients with panic disorder.[13] Patients with SAD appear to have a hyperresponsive adrenocortical response to psychological stress.[14]

By administering drugs that have a relatively specific effect on the LC, researchers have further explored the NE theory of anxiety and panic disorder. Drugs with anxiogenic effects (e.g., yohimbine [an α_2-adrenergic receptor antagonist]) stimulate LC firing and in-crease noradrenergic activity. NE in turn increases glutamate release (an excitatory neurotransmitter).[13] This produces subjective feelings of anxiety and can precipitate a panic attack in those with panic dis-order, but not in normal volunteers or those with other psychiatric illnesses.[15] Drugs with anxiolytic or antipanic effects (e.g., benzodi-azepines, antidepressants, and clonidine) inhibit LC firing, decrease noradrenergic activity, and block the effects of anxiogenic drugs.[13]

GABA RECEPTOR MODEL

There are two superfamilies of GABA protein receptors: $GABA_A$ and $GABA_B$. Drugs to reduce anxiety and produce sedation target the $GABA_A$ receptor. The $GABA_B$ receptor is a G-protein coupled recep-tor postulated to be involved in the presynaptic inhibition of GABA release.[13] $GABA_A$ receptors are ligand-gated ion channels. The open-ing of the channel is composed of five peptide subunits (i.e., α, β, γ, δ, or ρ subunits) that surround a central pore that crosses the neu-ronal cell membrane and is permeable to chloride. Benzodiazepine ligands either enhance or diminish the inhibitory effects of GABA.[13] GABA, the major inhibitory neurotransmitter in the CNS, has a strong regulatory or inhibitory effect on the 5-HT, NE, and dopamine (DA) systems. When GABA binds to the $GABA_A$ receptor, the chloride ion channel opens and permits the influx of negatively charged chlo-ride ions; this results in hyperpolarization of the cell membrane and decreases nerve cell excitability.

The specific role of the GABA receptors in anxiety disorders has not been established. The number of $GABA_A$ receptors can change with alterations in the environment (e.g., chronic stress) and the sub-unit expression can be altered by hormonal changes.[16] In patients with GAD, benzodiazepine binding in the left temporal lobe is reduced.[16] Abnormal sensitivity to antagonism of the benzodiazepine binding site and decreased binding was demonstrated in panic disorder.[13,16] This is consistent with the suggestion that panic disorder is secondary to a lack of central inhibition that results in uncontrolled elevations in anxiety during panic attacks.[16] Growth hormone response to ba-clofen in patients with generalized SAD suggests an abnormality of central $GABA_B$ receptor function.[17] Antidepressant potentiation of the $GABA_A$ modulatory effects of neurosteroids may contribute to their mechanism of action in anxiety disorders.[16]

SEROTONIN MODEL

Although there are data suggesting that the 5-HT system is dysregu-lated in patients with anxiety disorders, definitive evidence that shows a clear abnormality in 5-HT function is lacking. 5-HT is primarily an inhibitory neurotransmitter that is used by neurons originating in the raphe nuclei of the brain stem and projecting diffusely throughout the brain (e.g., cortex, amygdala, hippocampus, and limbic system). The diverse actions of 5-HT are regulated by at least 14 different postsynaptic receptor subtypes.[13] Abnormalities in serotonergic func-tioning through release and uptake at the presynaptic autoreceptors ($5-HT_{1A/1D}$), the serotonin reuptake transporter site (SERT), or ef-fect of 5-HT at the postsynaptic receptors (e.g., $5-HT_{1A}$, $5-HT_{2A}$, and $5-HT_{2C}$) may play a role in anxiety disorders.[13] Preclinical models sug-gest that greater 5-HT function facilitates avoidance behavior; how-ever, primate studies show that reducing 5-HT increases aggression.[13] It is postulated that greater 5-HT activity reduces NE activity in the LC, inhibits defense/escape response via the periaqueductal gray re-gion, and reduces hypothalamic release of corticotropin-releasing factor. The selective serotonin reuptake inhibitors (SSRIs) acutely increase 5-HT levels by blocking the SERT to increase the amount of 5-HT available postsynaptically, and are efficacious in blocking the manifestations of panic and anxiety.[13] The precise role of 5-HT in panic disorder is unclear; however, 5-HT may play a role in the development of anticipatory anxiety.[15]

Low 5-HT activity may lead to a dysregulation of other neuro-transmitters. NE and 5-HT systems are closely linked, and interactions between the two are reciprocal and vary. NE may act at presynaptic 5-HT terminals to decrease 5-HT release, and its activity at postsy-naptic receptors can cause increased 5-HT release. Stimulation of the postsynaptic $5-HT_{2A}$ receptors in the limbic system results in anxiety and avoidance behavior.

Buspirone is a selective $5-HT_{1A}$ partial agonist that is effective for GAD but not for panic disorder. Because the selective $5-HT_{1A}$ partial agonists reduce serotonergic activity, GAD symptoms may reflect excessive 5-HT transmission or overactivity of the stimulatory 5-HT pathways. Patients with SAD have greater prolactin response to buspirone challenge compared with healthy controls, indicating an enhancement of central serotonergic response.[18]

NEUROIMAGING STUDIES

Functional neuroimaging studies suggest that frontal and occipital brain areas are integral to the anxiety response. There is some evi-dence that patients with panic disorder have abnormal activation of the parahippocampal region and prefrontal cortex at rest. Panic anxiety is associated with activation of brain stem and basal ganglia areas.[15] In GAD patients there is an abnormal increase in cortical activity and a decrease in basal ganglia activity. After benzodiazepine treatment, basal ganglia activity increases, and cortical activity is reduced.[15] Neuroimaging studies implicate abnormalities in the amygdala, hip-pocampus, and varied cortical regions in patients with SAD.[19]

CLINICAL PRESENTATION

The *Diagnostic and Statistical Manual of Mental Disorders,* Fourth Edition, Text Revision classifies anxiety disorders into several categories: GAD, panic disorder (with or without agoraphobia), agoraphobia, SAD, specific phobia, obsessive-compulsive disorder, posttraumatic stress disorder, and acute stress disorder.[1] The charac-teristic features of these illnesses are anxiety and avoidance behavior.

TABLE 69–3. Presentation of Generalized Anxiety Disorder

Psychological and cognitive symptoms
- Excessive anxiety
- Worries that are difficult to control
- Feeling keyed up or on edge
- Poor concentration or mind going blank

Physical symptoms
- Restlessness
- Fatigue
- Muscle tension
- Sleep disturbance
- Irritability

Impairment
- Social, occupational, or other important functional areas
- Poor coping abilities

Screening questions
- What is going on in your life?
- How do you feel about it?
- What troubles you the most?
- How are you handling that?

Compiled from American Psychiatric Association[1] and Hildago and Davidson.[20]

Obsessive-compulsive disorder and posttraumatic stress disorder are discussed in Chap. 70.

GENERALIZED ANXIETY DISORDER

The diagnostic criteria for GAD require persistent symptoms for most days for at least 6 months.[1] The essential feature of GAD is unrealistic or excessive anxiety and worry about a number of events or activities.[1] The clinical presentation of GAD appears in Table 69–3. The anxiety or apprehensive expectation is accompanied by at least three psychological or physiological symptoms. Anxiety and worry are not confined to features of another psychiatric illness (e.g., having a panic attack, being embarrassed in public). The persistent worry must cause significant distress, and impairment in social, occupational, or other important areas of functioning. Anxiety and worry should not be secondary to a drug or illicit substance or a general medical disorder, and not occur solely as part of another psychiatric disorder (e.g., mood disorder).[1]

The onset, course of illness, and comorbid conditions of GAD are important considerations. GAD has a gradual onset with an average age of 21 years; however, there is a bimodal distribution. If GAD is the primary disorder, the patient can present in their teens. If it develops secondary to another anxiety disorder, the onset can be as late as age 30 years and even extend into the mid-50s. Most patients report onset of symptoms in childhood or adolescence. The median duration of illness at the time of diagnosis is 15.6 years.[20] GAD can be exacerbated or precipitated in later life by severe psychological stressors. Tense life events also can play a role in the persistence of symptoms. The course of the illness is chronic (i.e., episodes can last for a decade or longer); there is a high percentage of relapse and low rates of recovery. The likelihood of remission at 2 years is 25%.[1,20] Patients report substantial interference with their lives and have a high probability of seeking treatment.[3] The majority of patients with GAD eventually will develop another mental disorder. GAD is usually the primary disorder in patients with comorbid anxious depression.

PANIC DISORDER

Panic disorder begins as a series of unexpected (spontaneous) panic attacks involving an intense, terrifying fear similar to that caused by life-threatening danger. The unexpected panic attacks are followed

TABLE 69–4. Symptoms of a Panic Attack

Psychological symptoms
- Depersonalization
- Derealization
- Fear of losing control
- Fear of going crazy
- Fear of dying

Physical symptoms
- Abdominal distress
- Chest pain or discomfort
- Chills
- Dizziness or light-headedness
- Feeling of choking
- Hot flushes
- Palpitations
- Nausea
- Paresthesias
- Shortness of breath
- Sweating
- Tachycardia
- Trembling or shaking

From American Psychiatric Association.[1]

by at least 1 month of persistent concern about having another panic attack, worry about the possible consequences of the panic attack, or a significant behavioral change related to the attacks.[1] During an attack, patients often describe an overwhelming sense of doom, a fear of dying or losing control, and at least four physical symptoms (Table 69–4).[1] Panic attacks usually last no more than 20 to 30 minutes, with the peak intensity of symptoms within the first 10 minutes. Often patients seek help at a physician's office or emergency department, only to have their symptoms resolve before or on arrival. Because panic symptoms mimic those present in several medical conditions, patients often are misdiagnosed, and multiple referrals are common.[1]

Secondary to the panic attacks, many patients eventually develop agoraphobia. Agoraphobia is anxiety about being in places or situations in which escape might be difficult or where help might not be available in the event of a panic attack.[1] As a result, patients often avoid specific situations (e.g., flying or elevators) in which they fear a panic attack might occur.[1]

Panic disorder has an adverse impact on the patient's quality of life (QOL), including a significant degree of social and work impairment. Complications include depression (10% to 65% have major depressive disorder), alcohol abuse, and high use of health services and emergency rooms.[1] Patients with panic disorder have a high lifetime risk for suicide attempts compared with the general population.[21] The usual course is chronic but waxing and waning.

SOCIAL ANXIETY DISORDER

SAD is characterized by an intense, irrational, and persistent fear of being negatively evaluated or scrutinized in at least one social or performance situation. Exposure to the feared circumstance usually provokes an immediate situation-related panic attack. Symptoms of SAD are found in Table 69–5. Blushing is the principal physical indicator and distinguishes SAD from other anxiety disorders. Adults with SAD usually recognize their fear is excessive and unreasonable; however, they are unable to overcome it without treatment. If necessary, the feared situation is avoided or endured with significant distress.[1] The avoidance, anxious anticipation, or distress in the feared social or performance situation must interfere significantly with the person's normal routine, occupational or academic functioning, or social activities or relationships, or cause significant distress about having

TABLE 69–5. Presentation of Social Anxiety Disorder

Fears
  Being scrutinized by others
  Being embarrassed
  Being humiliated
Some feared situations
  Addressing a group of people
  Eating or writing in front of others
  Interacting with authority figures
  Speaking in public
  Talking with strangers
  Use of public toilets
Physical symptoms
  Blushing
  "Butterflies in the stomach"
  Diarrhea
  Sweating
  Tachycardia
  Trembling
Types
  Generalized type: fear and avoidance extend to a wide range of
  social situations
  Nongeneralized type: fear is limited to one or two situations
Screening questions
  Are you uncomfortable or embarrassed at being the center of
  attention?
  Do you find it hard to interact with people?

Compiled from American Psychiatric Association[1] and Ballenger et al.[22]

the phobia. In individuals under 18 years of age, the duration of symptoms is at least 6 months. The fear or avoidance is not caused by a drug or other substance (e.g., cocaine), or a general medical or psychiatric disorder.[1]

The mean age of onset of SAD is during the mid-teens. Rates of SAD are slightly higher among women than men and more frequent in younger cohorts. It is a chronic disorder with a mean duration of 20 years.[1]

Differentiating SAD from other anxiety disorders can be difficult. Panic attacks occur in both SAD and panic disorder, but the distinction between the two is the rationale behind fear; fear of anxiety symptoms is characteristic of panic disorder, while fear of embarrassment from social interaction typifies SAD.[1] GAD is likely the diagnosis if anxiety regarding social situations are part of a pattern of worries about multiple life areas or numerous potential negative outcomes. A majority of SAD patients have a comorbid mood, anxiety, or substance abuse disorder.[22] The SAD typically precedes the development of comorbid disorders, which is associated with increased suicidal ideation.[22]

SPECIFIC PHOBIA

Specific phobia is marked and persistent fear of a circumscribed object or situation (e.g., insects, heights, blood, or public transportation). Apart from contact with the feared object or situation, the patient is usually free of symptoms. Most persons simply avoid the feared object and adjust to certain restrictions on their activities.[1]

▶ TREATMENT: Generalized Anxiety Disorder

■ DESIRED OUTCOME

The short-term goals of therapy in the acute management of GAD are to reduce the severity and duration of the anxiety symptoms and to improve overall functioning. The long-term goal in GAD is remission with minimal or no anxiety symptoms and no functional impairment.[23] Patients with comorbid depression should have minimal depressive symptoms.[23]

■ GENERAL APPROACH TO TREATMENT

Once GAD is diagnosed, a patient-oriented treatment plan, which usually consists of both psychotherapy and drug therapy, is devel-

oped. The plan depends on the patient's degree of emotional distress, age, drug history, medical status, and the potential outcomes of pharmacologic treatment. Psychotherapy is the least invasive and safest treatment modality.[8] Antianxiety medication is indicated for patients experiencing anxiety symptoms severe enough to produce functional disability. Table 69–6 lists drug choices for GAD, panic disorder, and SAD. Many questions remain unanswered regarding how to manage treatment-resistant GAD.

■ NONPHARMACOLOGIC THERAPY

Nonpharmacologic treatment modalities in GAD include psychoeducation, short-term counseling, stress management, psychotherapy, meditation, or exercise. Psychoeducation includes information on the

TABLE 69–6. Drug Choices for Anxiety Disorders

Anxiety Disorder	First-Line Drugs	Second-Line Drugs	Alternatives
Generalized anxiety	Venlafaxine XR Paroxetine Escitalopram	Benzodiazepines Imipramine Buspirone	Hydroxyzine
Panic disorder	SSRIs	Imipramine Clomipramine Alprazolam Clonazepam	Phenelzine
Social anxiety disorder	Paroxetine Sertraline Venlafaxine XR	Citalopram Escitalopram Fluvoxamine Clonazepam	Buspirone Gabapentin Phenelzine

SSRI, selective serotonin reuptake inhibitor; XR, extended-release.
Compiled from Ballenger et al,[12] Ballenger et al,[22] Bandelow et al,[24] and Work Group on Panic Disorder.[25]

etiology and management of GAD. Anxious patients should be instructed to avoid caffeine, nonprescription stimulants, diet pills, and excessive use of alcohol. Most patients with GAD require psychological therapy, alone or in combination with antianxiety drugs, to overcome fears and to learn to manage their anxiety and worry.[5] Cognitive behavioral therapy (CBT) is the most effective psychological therapy in GAD patients. Controlled trials comparing the efficacy of combining CBT with medication or using it alone are lacking.[24] The current literature is not clear regarding when to use CBT. Certified therapists can be identified through the Web sites of the Academy of Cognitive Therapy (*www.academyofct.org*) or the American Board of Professional Psychology (*www.abpp.org*).[12]

■ PHARMACOLOGIC THERAPY

The benzodiazepines are the most effective, safe, and commonly prescribed drugs for the rapid relief of acute anxiety symptoms. They are also used intermittently or adjunctively for acute GAD exacerbations and for sleep disturbances at the outset of antidepressant therapy.[12]

All benzodiazepines are equally effective anxiolytics, and consideration of pharmacokinetic properties and the patient's clinical situation will assist in the selection of the most appropriate agent. Pharmacokinetic differences vary, and the clinician must monitor response to the initial treatment regimen after 2 to 4 weeks.[5]

Because of the lack of dependency and tolerable adverse effect profile, antidepressants have emerged as the treatment of choice for the long-term management of chronic anxiety, especially in the presence of comorbid depressive symptoms. Buspirone is an additional anxiolytic option (Table 69–7) in patients without comorbid depression or other anxiety disorders (e.g., panic disorder and SAD). Because of the high risk of adverse effects and toxicity, barbiturates, antipsychotics, antipsychotic-antidepressant combinations, and antihistamines generally are not indicated in the treatment of GAD.[12,24] The benzodiazepines are more effective in treating the somatic and autonomic symptoms of GAD as opposed to the psychic symptoms (e.g., apprehension and worry), which are reduced by antidepressants.[5]

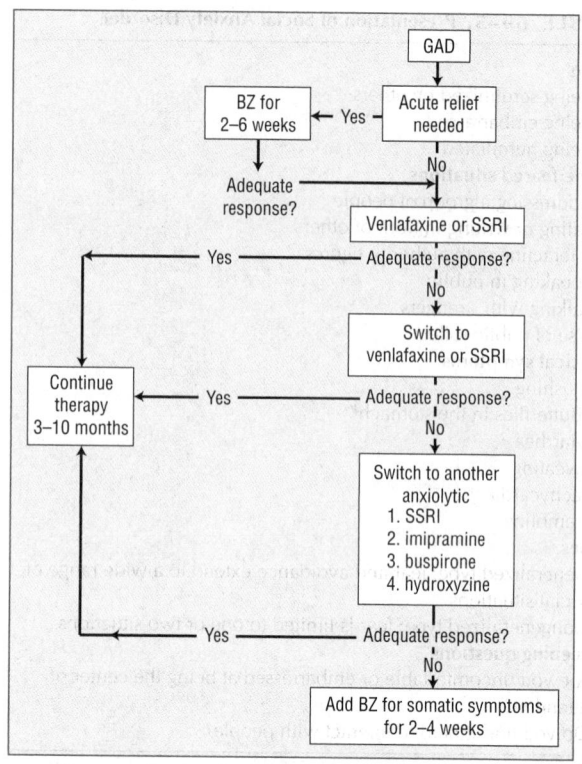

FIGURE 69–1. Algorithm for the pharmacotherapy of GAD. SSRI = selective serotonin reuptake inhibitor, BZ = benzodiazepine. (Compiled from Rickels and Rynn,[5] Ballenger et al,[12] and Bandelow et al.[24])

Two published algorithms outline the pharmacotherapy of GAD[5] and management of anxiety disorders in patients with chemical dependency.[30] A consensus report on the management of anxiety in primary care[12] and guidelines on the pharmacological treatment of GAD from the World Federation on Societies of Biological Psychiatry were published.[24] An algorithm for the pharmacologic management of GAD is shown in Figure 69–1, but the current literature is not conclusive on the optimal sequence of pharmacologic therapies.

TABLE 69–7. Nonbenzodiazepine Antianxiety Agents for Generalized Anxiety Disorder

Generic Name	Trade Name	Starting Dose	Dosage Range (mg/day)[a]
Antidepressants			
Escitalopram[b]	Lexapro	10 mg per day	10–20
Imipramine[c]	Tofranil	50 mg per day	75–200
Paroxetine[b,c]	Paxil	20 mg per day	20–50
Venlafaxine[b]	Effexor XR	37.5 or 75 per day	75–225[d]
Azapirones			
Buspirone[b,c]	BuSpar	7.5 mg twice per day	15–60[d]
Diphenylmethane			
Hydroxyzine[b,c,e]	Vistaril, Atarax	25 or 50 mg four times daily	200–400

[a]Elderly patients are usually treated with approximately one-half of the dose listed.
[b]FDA-approved for generalized anxiety disorder.
[c]Available generically.
[d]No dosage adjustment is required in elderly patients.
[e]FDA-approved for anxiety and tension in children in divided daily doses of 50–100 mg.
Compiled from Bandelow et al,[24] Lexapro package insert,[26] Paxil package insert,[27] Effexor XR package insert,[28] and Vistaril package insert.[29]

ALTERNATIVE DRUG TREATMENTS

Hydroxyzine and kava kava are two alternatives. Patients with GAD demonstrated continued efficacy for 3 months with hydroxyzine or bromazepam (not marketed in the United States), but not with placebo.[31] Efficacy was maintained in 86% of the hydroxyzine group and 88% of the bromazepam group.[31] A meta-analysis of randomized trials comparing the herbal preparation kava kava found it was more effective than placebo for anxiety during trial durations of 1 to 24 weeks. Many patients experienced CNS effects (e.g., tremors, drowsiness, restlessness, and headaches) and abdominal discomfort during short-term treatment.[32] Because of recent reports of hepatotoxicity, kava kava is not recommended as an anxiolytic.[33]

SPECIAL POPULATIONS

The management of anxiety in pregnancy, children, elderly patients, and those with hepatic impairment requires special consideration in the choice of anxiolytic. The literature is unclear if the potential risks of anxiolytic therapy outweigh the benefits of treating anxiety during pregnancy. Clinical practice guidelines for anxiety disorders indicate that the use of SSRIs or tricyclic antidepressants (TCAs) in pregnancy does not pose increased risk; however, neonatal complications and prematurity were reported.[24] Cleft lip, cleft palate, and other teratogenic effects are associated with benzodiazepine use, but a causal relationship is inconclusive.[24] Diazepam and chlordiazepoxide are the two benzodiazepines with the longest safety records. Diazepam should not be used if the mother is nursing because infants can experience sedation, lethargy, and weight loss.[34] Clinicians should avoid benzodiazepine use during the first trimester, use the lowest dosage for the shortest period of time, divide the total daily dosage into two or three doses to prevent high peak plasma levels, and use the agent as monotherapy.[34]

In the elderly, secondary to a decreased capacity for oxidation and alterations in the volume of distribution, drug accumulation can result. Patients with hepatic disease also are at risk for drug accumulation and subsequent complications. Therefore, intermediate- or short-acting benzodiazepines without active metabolites are preferred for chronic use in the elderly and those with liver disorders. Elderly patients are also sensitive to the CNS adverse effects of benzodiazepines (regardless of half-life) and their use is associated with a high frequency of falls and hip fractures.[35]

There are few controlled clinical trials of drugs in children and adolescents with GAD. CBT alone or in conjunction with antidepressants can have long-term benefits.[36] Randomized controlled trials of sertraline and fluvoxamine, and open trials of alprazolam, clonazepam, and fluoxetine indicate short-term efficacy;[36–38] however, behavioral activation was reported with clonazepam.[36,37] To date, fluoxetine is FDA-indicated for treatment of both depression and OCD, and fluvoxamine and sertraline are FDA-indicated for OCD in children and adolescents. Other SSRIs and venlafaxine have not been proved safe and effective in children and adolescents.[39] There are reports of hostility, suicidal ideation, and self-harm with paroxetine in children with major depression, and venlafaxine in children with major depression or GAD.[40,41] Increased monitoring for behavioral activation with benzodiazepines and suicide-related adverse effects with SSRIs is necessary if these agents are prescribed for anxiety in children and adolescents. The FDA recently placed a black box warning on the use of all antidepressants in children and adolescents, and specific monitoring parameters were defined. The reader is referred to the official approved labeling for each antidepressant and to the FDA for additional information.

ANTIDEPRESSANT THERAPY

Antidepressants are considered first-line agents in the long-term management of GAD. Venlafaxine extended-release, paroxetine, and escitalopram are FDA-approved antidepressants for GAD. Imipramine is considered when patients fail to respond to SSRIs or venlafaxine (see Table 69–7). The antianxiety response of antidepressants is delayed by 2 to 4 weeks or longer.[24] The pharmacokinetics and drug interactions of the antidepressants are reviewed in the chapter on depressive disorders (Chap. 67).

Efficacy

Venlafaxine extended-release, a serotonin-norepinephrine reuptake inhibitor (SNRI), alleviates anxiety in patients with and without co-morbid depression. The reduction in psychic symptoms of anxiety and tension is not accompanied by significant reductions in somatic symptoms. Venlafaxine (dosed once daily) was effective at doses of 150 and 225 mg for 2 months in patients with GAD, and efficacy was maintained for an additional 6 months of therapy.[42] Paroxetine was significantly more effective than placebo at achieving response in 62% and 68% of patients at 20 and 40 mg daily, respectively, after 2 months. Remission occurred in 30% and 36% of patients taking 20 and 40 mg of paroxetine, respectively.[43] Escitalopram was more efficacious than placebo in three 8-week trials in patients with GAD.[26] In a four parallel-group comparison, diazepam and trazodone were found to be equivalent in anxiolytic activity (remission rates of 66% and 69%, respectively) compared with placebo (47% remission rate), but imipramine's rate of remission (73%) exceeded that of the other three treatments.[37]

Mechanism of Action

The mechanism of action of antidepressants in anxiety disorders is not fully understood. Research indicates that antidepressants modulate receptor activation of neuronal signal transduction pathways connected to the neurotransmitters 5-HT, DA, and NE. As a result these cascades modify the expression of certain genes and the proteins that are produced (e.g., increase messenger RNA for glucocorticoid receptors and brain-derived neurotropic factor for trkB receptors, and reduce mRNA expression for corticotropin-releasing hormone).[44] It is theorized that by activating stress-adapting pathways, SSRIs and SNRIs reduce the somatic anxiety symptoms and the general distress experienced by patients.[44]

Adverse Effects

The most common adverse events of venlafaxine in patients with GAD were nausea, somnolence, and dry mouth.[42] Paroxetine was associated with a high rate of somnolence, nausea, abnormal ejaculation, dry mouth, decreased libido, and asthenia compared with placebo.[43] Escitalopram caused nausea, insomnia, fatigue, decreased libido, ejaculation disorders, and decreased libido at a higher rate than placebo in patients with GAD.[26] The use of TCAs may be limited by troublesome adverse events (e.g., sedation, orthostatic hypotension,

TABLE 69–8. Benzodiazepine Antianxiety Agents

Generic Name	Brand Name	Approved Dosage Range (mg/day)[a]	Approximate Equivalent Dose (mg)
Alprazolam[b]	Xanax	0.75–4	0.5
	Xanax XR	1–10[c]	
Chlordiazepoxide[b]	Librium	25–100	25
Clonazepam[b]	Klonopin	1–4[c]	0.25
Clorazepate[b]	Tranxene	7.5–60	7.5
Diazepam[b]	Valium	2–40	5
Lorazepam[b]	Ativan	0.5–10	0.75–1
Oxazepam[b]	Serax	30–120	15

[a]Elderly patients are usually treated with approximately one-half of the dose listed.
[b]Available generically.
[c]Panic disorder dose.
Equivalent doses from Shader and Greenblatt.[45]

anticholinergic effects, and weight gain) in some patients and the risk of toxicity in overdose.[5] However in a meta-analysis of antidepressant trials there was no difference in dropout rates between antidepressants (i.e., paroxetine, venlafaxine, and imipramine) compared with placebo, suggesting equivalent tolerability between antidepressants.[37]

Dosing and Administration

The antidepressants can be dosed once a day (see Table 69–7). The initial dose of venlafaxine extended-release is 75 mg once a day; 37.5 mg can be used in some patients. The dose can be increased every 4 days up to a maximum of 225 mg once daily, although a dose-response relationship has not been established.[28] Paroxetine is administered in a single daily dose (with or without food) of 20 mg. Doses greater than 20 mg/day have not been found to be more effective, but it can be increased by 10 mg/day every week.[27] Escitalopram dosing begins with 10 mg daily.[26]

BENZODIAZEPINE THERAPY

The benzodiazepines are the most frequently prescribed drugs for treating anxiety.[8] Although all benzodiazepines possess anxiolytic properties, only 7 of the 13 currently marketed agents have Food and Drug Administration (FDA) approval for the treatment of GAD (Table 69–8). Estazolam, flurazepam, temazepam, quazepam, and triazolam are marketed as sedative-hypnotic agents. Clonazepam is marketed as an antipanic agent and anticonvulsant,[46] and midazolam is labeled for preoperative sedation. Alprazolam is indicated for the treatment of panic disorder with or without agoraphobia, as well as GAD, and is also available in once-daily dosed extended-release tablets.[47]

Pharmacology and Mechanism of Action

The GABA receptor model of anxiety (described in the pathophysiology section) theorizes that benzodiazepines ameliorate anxiety through potentiation of the inhibitory activity of GABA.[13] The GABA receptor is composed of protein subunits arranged in a pentamer with a chloride ion channel in the center. Benzodiazepines bind on the $GABA_A$ receptor at the α_1, α_2, α_3, and α_5 sites; the anxiolytic effects of benzodiazepines are mediated at the α_2 site.[13] When benzodiazepines bind to the $GABA_A$ receptor, the frequency of the chloride ion channels opening and the influx of chloride ions into the neuronal cell are increased. The resulting negatively charged hyperpolarized membrane prevents further depolarization by excitatory neurotransmitters. Other neurotransmitters (e.g., 5-HT, NE, and DA) may be involved in benzodiazepine activity.

Pharmacokinetics

A wide difference in milligram potency exists between the benzodiazepine compounds; however, when dosage adjustments are made, all agents share similar anxiolytic and sedative-hypnotic activity. The variations in lipid solubility between compounds influence the pharmacokinetic properties of benzodiazepines. Different pharmacokinetic and pharmacodynamic properties can assist the clinician in choosing an appropriate anxiolytic (Table 69–9). After a single dose, the onset, intensity, and duration of pharmacological effects are important factors to consider when using benzodiazepines for the short-term, intermittent, or as-needed treatment of anxiety.

The primary determinant of a drug's onset of effect after a single oral dose is the rate of drug absorption. Because of high lipophilicity, diazepam and clorazepate are absorbed rapidly and distributed quickly into the CNS. Therefore the onset of anxiolytic effect occurs within 30 to 60 minutes, which results in a rapid and intense relief of anxiety. High lipophilicity increases the extent of drug redistribution into the periphery, particularly adipose tissue, resulting in a shorter duration of effect after a single dose than indicated by single-dose elimination half-life studies.[48] Clinically, patients perceive a rapid onset of action, but some experience an unpleasant feeling of drowsiness or loss of control. This "rush" can be euphoric and contribute to abuse. Chlordiazepoxide's onset of action is much slower because of decreased lipophilicity, slower absorption, and delayed passage into the CNS.

Compared with diazepam, lorazepam and oxazepam are relatively less lipophilic and have a slower onset of effect. These benzodiazepines have smaller volumes of distribution and a resulting longer duration of action.[48] Oxazepam absorption is slow, and peak levels are not obtained until 2 to 4 hours after a single dose; however, like lorazepam, oxazepam's anxiolytic effects are long lasting because extensive distribution does not occur.

Parenteral administration via the intramuscular route should be avoided with diazepam and chlordiazepoxide secondary to variability in the rate and extent of drug absorption. Intramuscular lorazepam provides rapid, reliable, and complete absorption; however, the preparation requires refrigeration.

After multiple dosing, the rate and extent of drug accumulation are functions of the drug's elimination half-life in relation to dosing intervals, clearance, and formation of active metabolites. Differences

TABLE 69–9. Pharmacokinetics of Benzodiazepine Antianxiety Agents

Generic Name	Time to Peak Plasma Level (h)	Elimination Half-Life, Parent (h)	Metabolic Pathway	Clinically Significant Metabolites	Protein Binding (%)
Alprazolam	1–2	12–15	Oxidation	—	80
Chlordiazepoxide	1–4	5–30	N-Dealkylation Oxidation	Desmethylchlordiazepoxide Demoxepam DMDZ[a]	96
Clonazepam	1–4	30–40	Nitroreduction	—	85
Clorazepate	1–2	Prodrug	Oxidation	DMDZ	97
Diazepam	0.5–2	20–80	Oxidation	DMDZ Oxazepam	98
Lorazepam	2–4	10–20	Conjugation	—	85
Oxazepam	2–4	5–20	Conjugation	—	97

Desmethyldiazepam (DMDZ) half-life 50–100 h.
Compiled from Bailey et al.[48]

The clinical effects that occur during and after repeated dosages with the benzodiazepines are related in part to variability in metabolism and metabolite accumulation.[48]

The benzodiazepines undergo two primary metabolic processes, hepatic oxidation (catalyzed by cytochrome P450 3A4) and glucuronide conjugation. With the exception of lorazepam and oxazepam (which are conjugated only) and clonazepam (which undergoes nitroreduction), all benzodiazepines are oxidized first and then conjugated and excreted renally.[48,49] Diazepam's metabolism is also catalyzed by cytochrome P450 2C19.[49] Oxidation can be impaired in patients with liver disease, in the elderly, and in those who simultaneously use drugs that inhibit oxidation. Impaired oxidation results in higher levels of the parent drug and/or an active metabolite.

Many benzodiazepines are converted to desmethyldiazepam (DMDZ), an active metabolite with a long elimination half-life of about 100 hours[48] (see Table 69–9). DMDZ is further oxidized to oxazepam and then conjugated and excreted. After multiple dosing, accumulation of DMDZ is slow and extensive, providing a long-lasting antianxiety effect. If oxidation of DMDZ is impaired, the half-life is prolonged, and drug accumulation can result with repeated dosing.

Clorazepate is a prodrug and possesses no anxiolytic effects until metabolism to DMDZ. Before absorption, clorazepate is metabolized rapidly in the stomach through a pH-dependent process under acidic conditions.

Benzodiazepines with shorter half-lives (e.g., alprazolam, lorazepam, and oxazepam) reach steady-state plasma concentrations rapidly, and drug accumulation after repeated dosing is minimal. Oxazepam and lorazepam are not converted into active metabolites.

Benzodiazepine protein binding is extensive, especially for the drugs with a long elimination half-life. After a single dose of a benzodiazepine with a long elimination half-life, the expected duration of clinical activity may not parallel the drug's pharmacokinetic half-life because of drug redistribution.[48] After multiple dosing, drugs with long elimination half-lives and active metabolites require 1 to 2 weeks to reach steady state.

Efficacy

Clinical trials of benzodiazepines show that 65% to 75% of patients with GAD have a marked to moderate response, with most of the improvement occurring in the first 2 weeks of therapy.[50] Benzodiazepines are more effective on the somatic symptoms of anxiety and fail to obviate the cognitive or psychic symptoms (e.g., worry).

Adverse Effects

The most common adverse events associated with benzodiazepine therapy involve CNS depression. This is manifested clinically as drowsiness, sedation, psychomotor impairment, and ataxia.[51] A transient mild drowsiness is experienced commonly by patients during the first few days of treatment; however, tolerance often develops. Disorientation, depression, confusion, irritability, aggression, and excitement are reported.[52]

Impairment of memory and recall also may occur during benzodiazepine treatment. The memory loss induced by the benzodiazepines typically is limited to events occurring after drug ingestion (anterograde amnesia).[52] Anterograde amnesia is secondary to disordered consolidation processes that store information and is not impairment in the perception or retrieval of information.[7] Benzodiazepines with high affinity for binding to the benzodiazepine receptor (e.g., lorazepam) appear to possess a higher potential for amnesia.

Abuse, Dependence, Withdrawal, and Tolerance

Two serious complications of benzodiazepine therapy are the potential for abuse and development of physical dependence. Benzodiazepine abuse is rare in the general population of users; however, individuals with a history of multiple drug abuse (e.g., alcohol or sedatives) are at the greatest risk for becoming benzodiazepine abusers.[26]

Because of the chronicity of illness, persons with GAD and panic disorder are at high risk of developing benzodiazepine dependence.[50] Benzodiazepine dependence is a physiologic phenomenon demonstrated by the appearance of a predictable abstinence syndrome (withdrawal symptoms) on abrupt discontinuation of therapy. Withdrawal symptoms may result because of the sudden dissociation of a benzodiazepine from its receptor site. After abrupt discontinuation, an acute decrease in GABA neurotransmission results, producing a less inhibited CNS.

Benzodiazepine Discontinuation

After benzodiazepine therapy is discontinued suddenly, several events can occur. Rebound anxiety represents an immediate but transient return of original symptoms having an increased intensity compared with baseline. Recurrence or relapse is the return of original symptoms with similar intensity as before treatment. About half of the patients using benzodiazepines relapse within 6 weeks of discontinuation, so some patients will be able to taper the benzodiazepine at this point in therapy.[50]

Withdrawal symptoms are the emergence of new symptoms and a worsening of pre-existing symptoms after benzodiazepine discontinuation. Symptoms may persist for days to weeks and resolve gradually over months.

Common symptoms of benzodiazepine withdrawal include anxiety, insomnia, restlessness, muscle tension, and irritability. Less frequently occurring symptoms are nausea, malaise, coryza, blurred vision, diaphoresis, nightmares, depression, hyperreflexia, and ataxia. Tinnitus, confusion, paranoid delusions, hallucinations, seizures, and psychosis occur rarely. Seizures may occur with both therapeutic and high doses of benzodiazepines with a short elimination half-life, usually within 3 days of drug discontinuation. They may occur approximately 1 week after discontinuation of agents with a long elimination half-life. High benzodiazepine doses, a long duration of therapy, and concurrent ingestion of drugs that lower the seizure threshold are risk factors for withdrawal seizures.

The onset of withdrawal symptoms in patients ingesting benzodiazepines with short elimination half-lives occurs much earlier (within 24 to 48 hours) than in those taking benzodiazepines with long elimination half-lives (within 3 to 8 days). Other factors associated with an increased incidence and severity of benzodiazepine withdrawal include high doses and long-term benzodiazepine therapy.

Several strategies to minimize the severity of benzodiazepine withdrawal include a 25% per week reduction in dosage until 50% of the dose is reached, and then dosage reduction by one-eighth every 4 to 7 days. If therapy exceeds 8 weeks, a slow dosage taper over 2 to 3 weeks is recommended; however, if the duration of treatment is 6 months, a taper over 4 to 8 weeks should ensue.[5] Long-term use of benzodiazepines (i.e., 1 year or longer) requires a 2 to 4 month slow taper.[5] Tapering will not eliminate the emergence of withdrawal symptoms entirely, but will prevent severe withdrawal. Slow drug taper is extremely important for the drugs with a short elimination half-life because some individuals have greater difficulty with discontinuation. Adjunctive use of certain drugs (e.g., imipramine, valproic acid, or buspirone) or CBT can help to reduce withdrawal symptoms during the benzodiazepine taper.[5] If patients experience difficulties, especially with the agents with a short elimination half-life, then substitution of an agent with a long elimination half-life should be considered. Using this approach, diazepam can be initiated as a loading dose (40% of daily consumption), followed by daily tapering of 10%. Clonazepam is an alternative agent.

Although tolerance develops to the sedative, muscle relaxant, and anticonvulsant activities, the benzodiazepines do not appear to lose anxiolytic or antipanic efficacy.[24] The anxiolytic efficacy of benzodiazepines in long-term clinical trials (>6 to 8 months of chronic use) has not been reported.[5]

Drug Interactions

Drug interactions with the benzodiazepines generally fall into two categories: pharmacodynamic and pharmacokinetic (Table 69–10).[49] Simultaneous use of alcohol and a benzodiazepine results in additive CNS depressant effects and lowers the therapeutic index of the benzodiazepine. In addition, concurrent use of a benzodiazepine and drugs with CNS depressant properties (e.g., narcotic agonists, antipsychotics, and antihistamines) can potentiate the adverse sedative effects. When ingested alone in an overdose attempt, benzodiazepines are rarely life-threatening; however, the combination of

TABLE 69–10. Pharmacokinetic Drug Interactions with the Benzodiazepines

Drug	Effect
Alcohol (chronic)	Increased Cl of BZs
Carbamazepine	Decreased Cl of alprazolam
Cimetidine	Decreased Cl of alprazolam, diazepam, chlordiazepoxide, and clorazepate and increased $t_{1/2}$
Disulfiram	Decreased Cl of alprazolam and diazepam
Erythromycin	Decreased Cl of alprazolam
Fluoxetine	Decreased Cl of alprazolam and diazepam
Fluvoxamine	Decreased Cl of alprazolam and prolonged $t_{1/2}$
Itraconazole	Potentially decreased Cl of alprazolam and diazepam
Ketaconazole	Potentially decreased Cl of alprazolam
Nefazodone	Decreased Cl of alprazolam, AUC doubled, and $t_{1/2}$ prolonged
Omeprazole	Decreased Cl of diazepam
Oral contraceptives	Increased free concentration of chlordiazepoxide and slightly decreased Cl; decreased Cl and increased $t_{1/2}$ of diazepam and alprazolam
Paroxetine	Decreased Cl of alprazolam
Phenobarbital	Increased Cl of clonazepam and reduced $t_{1/2}$
Phenytoin	Increased Cl of clonazepam and reduced $t_{1/2}$
Probenecid	Decreased Cl of lorazepam and prolonged $t_{1/2}$
Propranolol	Decreased Cl of diazepam and prolonged $t_{1/2}$
Ranitidine	Decreased absorption of diazepam
Rifampin	Increased metabolism of diazepam
Theophylline	Decreased alprazolam concentrations
Valproate	Decreased Cl of lorazepam

AUC, area under the plasma concentration curve; BZ, benzodiazepine; Cl, clearance; $t_{1/2}$, elimination half-life.
Compiled from Tanaka.[49]

benzodiazepines with alcohol or other CNS depressant agents is potentially fatal. SSRIs can affect benzodiazepine metabolism by inhibition of cytochrome P450 3A4 and 1A2 enzymes.[49] Nefazodone and fluvoxamine increase alprazolam concentrations; thus the alprazolam dose should be reduced by 50% when these agents are added.[49]

Dosing and Administration

Benzodiazepine dosage requirements vary widely among patients and must be individualized. Therapy should be initiated using low doses (e.g., diazepam 2 mg three times daily, alprazolam 0.25 mg three times a day or equivalent doses of other benzodiazepines) and titrated upward to relieve anxiety symptoms and avoid adverse events. After an initial treatment response is achieved, agents with long elimination half-lives can be dosed at bedtime. Dosage adjustments should be made weekly. Three to four weeks of a daily dose at the maximum dose constitutes an adequate clinical trial.[5]

The duration of benzodiazepine therapy for the acute management of anxiety generally should not exceed 2 to 4 weeks. Benzodiazepines can be prescribed on an as-needed basis, and if several acute courses are necessary a benzodiazepine-free period of 2 to 4 weeks should be implemented between courses.[5] Individuals with persistent symptoms should be managed with antidepressants or buspirone because of the risk of dependence with continued benzodiazepine therapy.[12]

Patient education should include the anticipated length of drug therapy, potential side effects, and consequences of the ingestion of alcohol and other CNS depressants. Patients should understand that benzodiazepines provide symptomatic relief but do not solve underlying psychological problems. Patients should be instructed not to decrease or discontinue benzodiazepine usage without contacting their prescriber.

BUSPIRONE THERAPY

Buspirone is a nonbenzodiazepine anxiolytic that lacks anticonvulsant, muscle relaxant, hypnotic, motor impairment, and dependence properties. It is considered to be a second-line agent for GAD because of inconsistent reports of efficacy, delayed onset of effect (i.e., 2 weeks or longer), and lack of efficacy for other potential comorbid depressive and anxiety disorders (e.g., panic disorder or SAD).[12,24]

Pharmacology and Mechanism of Action

Buspirone's anxiolytic mechanism of action is unknown. It is thought to exert its anxiolytic effect through $5-HT_{1A}$ partial agonist activity at the presynaptic 5-HT receptors by reducing the firing of 5-HT neurons.[51] Unlike benzodiazepines, buspirone is effective for the cognitive symptoms of anxiety.[51]

Pharmacokinetics

After an oral dose, buspirone is absorbed rapidly and completely and undergoes extensive first-pass metabolism. The mean elimination half-life is 2.5 hours and it must be dosed 2 to 3 times daily, which adversely affects adherence to the drug regimen.[51]

Adverse Effects

A major advantage of buspirone is its lack of sedative properties. Adverse events include dizziness, nausea, and headaches.[51]

Drug Interactions

Drugs that inhibit cytochrome P450 3A4 (e.g., verapamil, diltiazem, itraconazole, fluvoxamine, nefazodone, and erythromycin) can increase buspirone levels. Rifampin caused a 10-fold reduction in buspirone levels. Buspirone reportedly increases haloperidol levels and elevates blood pressure in patients taking a monoamine oxidase inhibitor (MAOI).

Dosing and Administration

The recommended initial dose of buspirone is 7.5 mg two times daily with dosage increments of 5 mg/day every 2 to 3 days as needed.[50] The usual therapeutic dose of buspirone is 30 to 60 mg/day.[24,50] The onset of improvement in cognitive symptoms (2 weeks or longer) precedes the relief of somatic symptoms; maximum therapeutic benefit may not be evident for 4 to 6 weeks.

Buspirone is an agent of choice in the management of uncomplicated GAD, in patients who fail other anxiolytic therapies, or in patients with a history of substance abuse. It is not useful in clinical situations requiring immediate anxiolysis or for situations requiring as-needed anxiolytic therapy. The use of benzodiazepines within the previous month of initiation of buspirone therapy was associated with reduced efficacy because of its delayed onset in the reduction of somatic symptoms.[50] Patients who responded to benzodiazepines in the past often perceive that buspirone is ineffective because they do not experience the same effect on their somatic symptoms of anxiety.[50]

PHARMACOECONOMIC CONSIDERATIONS

The annual economic burden of anxiety disorders in the United States was estimated to be $42.3 billion in 1990 ($63.1 billion in 1998 dollars).[3] Nonpsychiatric medical treatment costs represented more than half of this figure ($23 billion), with expenses of $13.3 billion for psychiatric treatment, $4.1 billion for indirect workplace costs, and $1.2 billion in mortality costs.

GAD is associated with high rates of health care use and disability. The number of days missed increases when GAD is comorbid with one or more other psychiatric disorders. Patients with GAD tend to use family practitioners and gastroenterologists more frequently than healthy controls.[12] GAD ranks third among anxiety disorders in the rate of use of primary care physician time and it is the leading cause of disability in the workplace in the United States.[12] Pharmacoeconomic analyses in the management of GAD have not been conducted.

CLINICAL CONTROVERSIES

The optimal duration of treatment with antidepressants in patients with GAD is controversial. The longest study duration (6 months) occurred with venlafaxine extended-release. Many clinicians recommend treating patients for up to 1 year.

The role of combined benzodiazepines and antidepressants in the first few weeks of GAD therapy has not been resolved. In practice, despite a lack of evidence of clinical benefits, many clinicians combine a benzodiazepine and an antidepressant for the first few weeks of therapy until the antidepressant begins to work.

EVALUATION OF THERAPEUTIC OUTCOMES

The goals of treatment and expected duration of therapy should be discussed with the patient at the beginning of therapy. Initially, anxious patients should be monitored twice weekly for a reduction in the frequency, duration, and severity of anxiety symptoms and improvement in occupational, social, and interpersonal functioning. The clinician should assess the patient for response to treatment by asking about specific target symptoms of anxiety and emergence of adverse events. Ideally, the patient should have no or minimal anxiety or depressive symptoms and no functional impairment. After achieving an optimal drug dosage, the patient can be evaluated monthly until drug discontinuation. Use of an objective measurement of remission of GAD (e.g., Hamilton Rating Scale for Anxiety score <7 to 10 and a Sheehan Disability Scale Score ≤1 on each item) can assist in the evaluation of drug response.[23] If a patient has only a partial response, the dose should be increased after 4 to 6 weeks of antidepressant therapy (or 2 weeks for acute therapy with benzodiazepines). The length of therapy should be individualized, with some patients requiring up to 1 year of antidepressant therapy.[5]

▶ TREATMENT: Panic Disorder

▧ DESIRED OUTCOME

The goal of therapy in panic disorder is remission. Patients should be free of panic attacks, have no or minimal anticipatory anxiety and agoraphobic avoidance, and no functional impairment.[23] Naturalistic studies indicate that after pharmacotherapy, over 50% of patients have occasional panic attacks, 40% experience agoraphobic avoidance, and most continue to take medications.[53]

▧ GENERAL APPROACH TO TREATMENT

Therapeutic options include single or combined pharmacologic agents, concurrent psychotherapy, or psychotherapy followed by pharmacotherapy. Most patients without agoraphobic avoidance will improve with pharmacotherapy alone; however, if avoidance is present, CBT typically is initiated concurrently. With all effective drug therapies, resolution of agoraphobic avoidance tends to occur slowly.

In the most comprehensive study to date, efficacy of imipramine alone and CBT alone were equivalent in acute therapy for 3 months and during 6 months of maintenance therapy. Combined imipramine and CBT therapy was not significantly better than CBT or imipramine alone for acute therapy, but was significantly better during maintenance. At 6 months after discontinuation, only CBT maintained improvement (4% relapse) compared with a 25% relapse rate in patients treated with imipramine.[54] Patients who failed to respond to CBT and had paroxetine added to therapy had a significant improvement in agoraphobic behavior and anxiety symptoms.[55]

▧ NONPHARMACOLOGIC THERAPY

Patients should be educated to avoid substances that can precipitat panic attacks, including caffeine, drugs of abuse, and nonprescriptio stimulants.[1,56] CBT focuses on the correction of a patient's maladap tive thoughts and behaviors that initiate, perpetuate, or exacerbat panic symptoms.[56] Through CBT, the patient learns to decrease th fear and avoidance of internal and external signals associated wit panic attacks. The cognitive restructuring and in vivo exposure (t feared stimuli) components of CBT target panic attacks and phobic avoidance behavior.[56] For patients who cannot or will not take med ications, CBT alone is certainly indicated. CBT is associated wit short-term improvement in 80% to 90% of patients and 6-month im provement in 75% of patients.[56]

▧ PHARMACOLOGIC THERAPY

Panic disorder is treated effectively with several drugs including th SSRIs, the TCA imipramine, the benzodiazepines alprazolam an clonazepam, and the MAOI phenelzine[8] (Table 69–11). Alprazolam clonazepam, sertraline, and paroxetine are approved for this indica tion. SSRIs are the first-line agents because of their tolerability;[24,25,5] however, the benzodiazepines are the most commonly used drug fo panic disorder.[59] In a meta-analysis of the pharmacotherapy of pani disorder, the effect size of SSRIs and TCAs did not differ; however, th number of dropouts in the TCA group (31%) was significantly highe than in the SSRI group (18%).[60] Three practice guidelines[24,25,53] an one consensus statement for the treatment of panic disorder wer

TABLE 69–11. Drugs Used in the Treatment of Panic Disorder

Class/Generic Name	Brand Name	Starting Dose	Antipanic Dosage[a] Range (mg)
Selective serotonin reuptake inhibitors			
Citalopram	Celexa	10 mg per day	20–60
Escitalopram	Lexapro	5 mg per day	10–20
Fluoxetine[b]	Prozac	5 mg per day	10–20
Fluvoxamine[b]	Luvox	25 mg per day	100–300
Paroxetine[b]	Paxil	10 mg per day	20–60[c]
Sertraline	Zoloft	25 mg per day	50–200[c]
Benzodiazepines			
Alprazolam[b]	Xanax	0.25 mg three times a day	4–10[c]
	Xanax XR	0.5–1 mg per day	1–10[c]
Clonazepam[b]	Klonopin	0.25 mg once or twice per day	1–4[c]
Diazepam[b]	Valium	2–5 mg three times a day	5–20
Lorazepam[b]	Ativan	0.5–1 mg three times a day	2–8
Tricyclic antidepressants			
Clomipramine[b]	Anafranil	25 mg twice a day	75–250
Imipramine[b]	Tofranil	10–25 mg per day	75–250
Monoamine oxidase inhibitor			
Phenelzine	Nardil	15 mg per day	45–90

[a]Dosage used in clinical trials but not FDA-approved.
[b]Available generically.
[c]Dosage is FDA-approved.
Compiled from Bandelow et al,[24] Work Group on Panic Disorder,[25] Zamorski and Albucher,[57] and Stahl et al.[58]

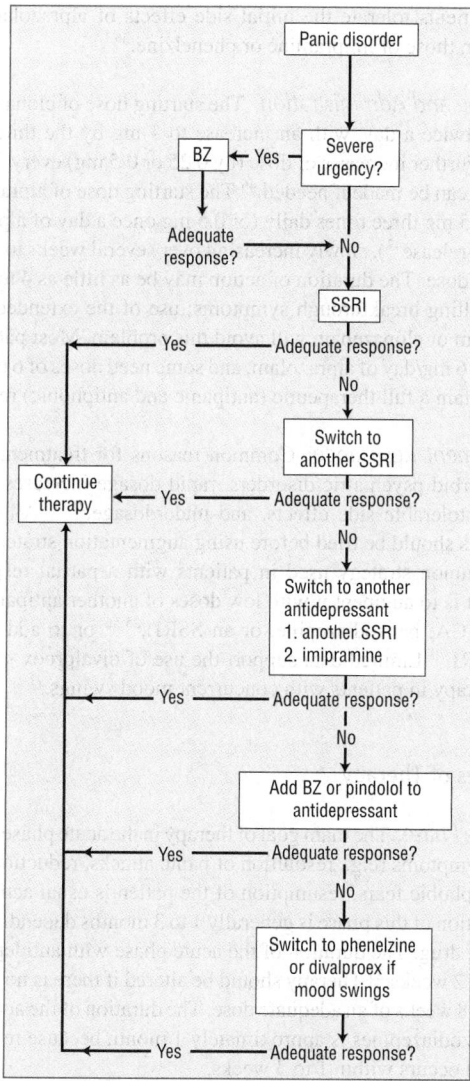

FIGURE 69–2. Algorithm for the pharmacotherapy of panic disorder. SSRI = selective serotonin reuptake inhibitor, BZ = benzodiazepine. (Compiled from Bandelow et al,[24] Work Group on Panic Disorder,[25] Ballenger et al,[61] and Sheehan.[69])

published.[61] An algorithm for the pharmacologic therapy of panic disorder appears in Figure 69–2.

Except in instances in which rapid response is required (i.e., loss of a job), benzodiazepines are considered second-line agents. Because of the risk of dependency, benzodiazepines should be used only after several trials of antidepressants have failed.[24,25] Because of potential emergence of depressive symptoms during treatment, benzodiazepines should not be used as monotherapy in a patient who is clinically depressed or has a history of depression. In patients whose illness is complicated by a history of alcohol or drug abuse, benzodiazepine use should be avoided.[8,26] Data support the combined use of SSRIs and benzodiazepines in the first weeks of treatment to offset the delay in the SSRI effect.[62,63]

ALTERNATIVE DRUG TREATMENTS

Buspirone, trazodone, bupropion, and β-blockers are ineffective in panic disorder.[24,53,55] Venlafaxine was effective in a small trial.[24]

SPECIAL POPULATIONS

Elderly patients with panic disorder have fewer, less intense symptoms and avoidant behavior than younger patients.[64] Youth often present with fear that they are dying or being smothered, and agoraphobia can be manifested as a fear of leaving home.[39] Antidepressants, especially the SSRIs, are preferred for management of panic disorder in elderly patients and youth.[39,64] Benzodiazepines are second-line agents because of potential problems with disinhibition in these two populations.

ANTIDEPRESSANT THERAPY

Tricyclic Antidepressants

Efficacy. Imipramine is the most studied TCA, alleviating panic attacks in 75% of patients with panic disorder. Imipramine effectively blocks panic attacks within at least 4 weeks; however, maximal improvement (including antiphobic response) does not occur until 8 to 12 weeks.[25] The sequence of patient response is an initial decrease in the number of panic attacks, then diminution of anticipatory anxiety, followed by a reduction in agoraphobic avoidance.[25]

Adverse Effects. Up to 40% of patients experience stimulant-like side effects, including anxiety, insomnia, jitteriness, and irritability.[25,63] These side effects often affect patient compliance significantly, prevent medication dosage increases, and interfere with the overall treatment outcome.

Problems with TCA use in panic disorder are well documented and include stimulatory side effects, anticholinergic effects, orthostatic hypotension, delayed onset of antipanic effects, and toxicity in overdose.[25] Approximately 25% of patients reportedly discontinue treatment because of side effects.[63] Weight gain is a problematic side effect associated with long-term therapy.[25]

Dosing and Administration. When using imipramine, treatment should be conservatively initiated with 10 mg/day at bedtime and slowly increased by 10 mg every 2 to 4 days as tolerated to 75 to 100 mg/day, and then increased by 25 mg every 2 to 4 days over a 2- to 4-week period.[56,57] Most patients require at least 150 mg/day of imipramine (or a combined imipramine-desipramine plasma concentration of 100 to 150 ng/mL).[63] If this dose is not effective, a higher dose (up to 300 mg/day) can be used.

Selective Serotonin Reuptake Inhibitors

Efficacy. Clinical studies indicate that all SSRIs are effective in panic disorder.[53,65–68] The percentage of patients who become panic-free ranges between 60% and 80%.[25] The antipanic effect of SSRIs is delayed for at least 4 weeks, and some patients do not respond for 8 to 12 weeks.[25]

Adverse Effects. Typical antidepressant doses of SSRIs can cause side effects of insomnia, jitteriness, restlessness, and agitation, and lead to drug discontinuation in patients with panic disorder. Transient gastrointestinal disturbances occur more frequently with SSRIs than with TCAs. Thus low initial SSRI doses should be prescribed.[24,57] Sleep disturbances, headaches, and sexual dysfunction often are problematic.[24]

▓ *Dosing and Administration.* Low initial doses of SSRIs are recommended (see Table 69–11) to avoid stimulatory side effects (e.g., insomnia or nervousness). The initial doses are much smaller than those used in depression and should be maintained for the first week of therapy. Paroxetine can be increased by 10 mg weekly; the target dose is 40 mg.[66] The starting dose of fluoxetine is 5 mg/day, with dosage increases every 2 or 3 days to a dosage range of 10 to 20 mg/day by the end of 2 weeks.[57] Fluvoxamine can be increased to 150 mg/day in divided doses over 2 weeks.[67]

Monoamine Oxidase Inhibitors

▓ *Efficacy.* The majority of studies assessing the efficacy of MAOIs in treating panic disorder were open-labeled. These trials lacked sufficient dosage and duration of treatment, adequate sample size, and valid ratings of panic attacks. No maintenance trials of MAOIs are published. The course of response mimics that of TCAs.[25] MAOIs are reserved for the most refractory or difficult patients.[24,57]

▓ *Adverse Effects.* Side effects and dietary restrictions adversely affect patient acceptance.[25] Anticholinergic side effects are less severe with phenelzine than with TCAs, but orthostatic hypotension and insomnia are often more of a problem. After 3 weeks, most unpleasant side effects subside.

Hypertensive crisis following the ingestion of tyramine-containing foods or sympathomimetic drugs is the most serious, potentially life-threatening event encountered with phenelzine[57] (see Chapter 67 for food and drug restrictions and side effects). Patients should observe the food, beverage, and drug restrictions for at least 24 hours before starting the first dose of phenelzine and for 2 weeks after stopping therapy.

▓ *Dosing and Administration.* The starting dose of phenelzine is 15 mg/day after the evening meal, increasing by 15 mg/day every 3 to 4 days until a minimum dose of 45 mg/day (in two or three divided doses) is reached. Dosages can be increased (up to 90 mg/day) if improvement is not achieved after 8 to 12 weeks. If a patient was on an antidepressant previously, it should be discontinued 2 weeks before phenelzine is started to prevent a potential drug interaction. Fluoxetine must be stopped 5 weeks before phenelzine (or another MAOI) can be started.

Benzodiazepines

▓ *Efficacy.* Although benzodizaepines are effective antipanic agents, concerns over their use are prevalent. The development of dependency, risk of withdrawal, lack of efficacy for comorbid depression, and the need for multiple daily dosing (i.e., alprazolam immediate-release) with possible interdose rebound anxiety can limit their usefulness. The high-potency benzodiazepines clonazepam and alprazolam are used frequently.[56] Diazepam and lorazepam are possibly effective in treating panic disorder when taken in sufficiently high doses.[25] Therapeutic response to benzodiazepines occurs in 1 to 2 weeks. It is estimated that 60% to 80% of panic disorder patients respond to benzodiazepines.[69] Alprazolam is an ideal agent for patients who need rapid relief. Relapse rates of 50% or higher are common despite slow drug tapering.[25]

▓ *Adverse Effects.* Patient acceptance of benzodiazepines usually is not a problem, and except for sedation, side effects are reported rarely. Patients tolerate the initial side effects of alprazolam much better than those of imipramine or phenelzine.[56]

▓ *Dosing and Administration.* The starting dose of clonazepam is 0.25 mg twice a day, with an increase to 1 mg by the third day of therapy. Further increases of dose (by 0.25 or 0.5 mg) every 3 days to 4 mg/day can be made if needed.[46] The starting dose of alprazolam is 0.25 to 0.5 mg three times daily (or 0.5 mg once a day of alprazolam extended-release[47]), slowly increasing over several weeks to reach an ◀**5** ideal dose. The duration of action may be as little as 4 to 6 hours with resulting breakthrough symptoms; use of the extended-release alprazolam or clonazepam will avoid this problem. Most patients require 3 to 6 mg/day of alprazolam, and some need doses of 6 to 10 mg/day to obtain a full therapeutic (antipanic and antiphobic) response.

▓ *Treatment Resistance.* Common reasons for treatment failures are comorbid psychiatric disorders, rapid dosage increases with resulting intolerable side effects, and underdosage.[25,56] All standard treatments should be tried before using augmentation strategies. The most common strategy used in patients with a partial response to one agent is to augment it with low doses of another antipanic agent (e.g., a TCA, benzodiazepine, or an SSRI),[25,56] or to add pindolol to an SSRI.[70] Limited data support the use of divalproex sodium as monotherapy in patients with concurrent mood swings.[71]

Phases of Therapy

▓ *Acute Phase.* The main goal of therapy in the acute phase is reduction of symptoms (e.g., resolution of panic attacks, reduction in anxiety and phobic fears, resumption of the patient's usual activities).[25] The duration of this phase is generally 1 to 3 months depending on the choice of drug. The duration of the acute phase with antidepressants is about 12 weeks.[25] Therapy should be altered if there is no response after 6 to 8 weeks of an adequate dose. The duration of the acute phase with benzodiazepines is approximately 1 month because response is rapid and occurs within 1 to 3 weeks.

The guiding principle for using drugs in panic disorder is to start low, use an adequate dose, and treat for an appropriate period of time.[57] Side effects with the antidepressants, often from too high an initial dose, may prevent achievement of an optimal dosage, compromise treatment response, and contribute to patient noncompliance.

▓ *Maintenance Phase and Discontinuation.* The optimal ◀**6** length of therapy is unknown; however, the total duration of therapy appears to be 12 to 24 months before drug discontinuation over 4 to 6 months is attempted.[24,25] The dose used in the acute phase is continued into the maintenance phase.[24] Successful maintenance with single weekly doses of fluoxetine was described.[72] Citalopram, clomipramine, fluoxetine, and imipramine maintained clinical effects for up to 1 year of treatment.[24] When drugs are discontinued too early, a high rate of relapse occurs; thus longer periods of treatment are associated with more sustained response. Reinstitution of drug usually results in renewed clinical response.[25] Patients successfully treated with imipramine for 6 months had the same rate of relapse after discontinuation as those treated for 12 to 30 months.[73] Pharmacotherapy, even at long duration, may not prevent relapse, and many patients require long-term therapy.

Patients taking alprazolam, clonazepam, or imipramine for up to 8 months maintained antipanic efficacy without dosage increases, suggesting that tolerance does not develop to the antipanic effects of these agents.[5,74] The most important determinant of compliance with maintenance therapy is the tolerability of adverse events.[25] Some adverse events which are experienced short term become unbearable during long-term management (e.g., sexual dysfunction and weight gain). The primary risk of long-term benzodiazepine use is the development of dependency and withdrawal reactions on discontinuation. Abuse of benzodiazepines usually is confined to patients with a personal or family history of substance or alcohol use.[5] Both TCAs and SSRIs can be associated with discontinuation symptoms.

Some patients receiving high-dose alprazolam (>4 mg/day) can have an extremely difficult time with drug taper, and the withdrawal schedule for all patients should be individualized. The taper phase is most successful when it is accomplished over a 4- to 6-month period. Approximately 30% of the patients receiving high doses, even with slow taper, may experience transient, mild to moderate withdrawal symptoms (as discussed in the earlier section on benzodiazepines) and relapse of panic attacks. Adjunctive CBT reportedly facilitates benzodiazepine discontinuation.[5] If a TCA is discontinued abruptly a substantial number of patients develop severe cholinergic rebound with upset stomach, nausea, vomiting, and abdominal cramping; thus TCAs should be reduced by 25 mg every 2 to 4 weeks.[56] The dose of phenelzine should be reduced by 15 mg every 2 to 4 weeks.

Patient education is essential. Patients should be informed regarding the lag time before a therapeutic response will occur and any problematic side effects. Many patients are reluctant to take drugs for fear that their illness will worsen or that they will become addicted. Adverse events are often perceived as a worsening of the illness and can contribute to nonadherence or prevent necessary dosage increases. Patients receiving benzodiazepines should be told not to decrease or discontinue therapy unless authorized by their clinician.

PHARMACOECONOMIC CONSIDERATIONS

Patients with panic disorder have high rates of unemployment, receiving welfare, disability benefits, and health care services.[3] They also have impaired emotional and physical health status and experience poor marital and social functioning.[21] After 6 weeks of clonazepam, work productivity improved (from 71% to 88%), and personal happiness also increased.[21] Measures of quality of life (QOL) improved with imipramine, clonazepam, and sertraline. Treatment with clomipramine, paroxetine, or fluoxetine improved work, social, and family responsibilities. Improvements in anxiety and phobic avoidance were significantly associated with QOL improvements but not reduction in the frequency of panic attacks, which is used most often as the measure of success in drug efficacy trials.[21] In a cost comparison, group CBT was more cost-beneficial than pharmacotherapy for the initial 4 months of therapy.[75]

CLINICAL CONTROVERSY

The role of benzodiazepines in the management of panic disorder is controversial. The treatment guidelines for panic disorder recommend SSRIs as first-line agents, especially when long-term therapy is being considered. In clinical practice benzodiazepines are the most commonly prescribed pharmacotherapeutic agents for panic disorder, despite the risk of dependence with long-term therapy.

EVALUATION OF THERAPEUTIC OUTCOMES

During the first few weeks of the acute phase of therapy, patients with panic disorder should be seen at least weekly to adjust drug dosages based on improvement in panic symptoms and to monitor for adverse events. Subsequently, monthly visits should suffice. The patient should be counseled to maintain a diary to record the date, time, frequency, and duration of panic episodes and the severity of panic symptoms, anticipatory anxiety, and agoraphobic avoidance. Treatment outcomes can be assessed objectively by use of the Hamilton Rating Scale for Anxiety (score ≤ 7 to 10) for anxiety.[23] At scheduled visits, the clinician can inquire about the level of disability experienced by the patient and have the patient complete the Sheehan Disability Scale (with a goal of ≤ 1 on each item).[23] During drug discontinuation, the frequency of appointments should be increased to evaluate for emergence of withdrawal symptoms and monitor for relapse.

▶ TREATMENT: Social Anxiety Disorder

DESIRED OUTCOME

The goals of therapy in the acute phase of treatment are to reduce physiological symptoms of anxiety (e.g., tachycardia, flushing, and sweating), social anxiety, and phobic avoidance. The duration of this phase is 4 to 12 weeks, depending on the drug therapy.

The goals of therapy in the continuation phase are to extend the therapeutic benefits of the acute phase, especially the patient's ability to participate in social activities, and improve QOL. This phase usually lasts 3 to 6 months.

SAD is a chronic, long-term illness requiring extended therapy. After improvement, at least a 1-year maintenance period is recommended to maintain improvement and decrease the rate of relapse.[22] Situations suggesting a possible need for long-term treatment include the presence of unresolved symptoms or comorbidity, an early onset of disease, and a prior history of relapse.[22] The long-term goal in the treatment of SAD is remission with the disappearance of the core symptoms of social anxiety, little or no anxiety, and no functional impairment or comorbid depressive symptoms.[23]

GENERAL APPROACH TO TREATMENT

Generalized SAD is associated with significant morbidity, and patients should be treated aggressively. Obstacles to effective treatment include patient avoidance of therapy secondary to fear and shame, treatment directed toward somatic symptoms or comorbid conditions, and financial barriers.[76] Patients with SAD often respond to treatment more slowly and less completely than patients with other anxiety disorders. Therefore it is important to set reasonable expectations for response to therapy. The patient's symptoms, prior treatments, comorbid conditions, and history of substance abuse direct treatment selections.

CBT and pharmacotherapy are effective in the treatment of SAD.[77–79] Pharmacotherapy is often the most practical choice because CBT may not be available outside of large urban areas secondary to the lack of trained therapists and high treatment costs. Studies suggest the acute treatment outcomes for CBT and pharmacotherapy are equal; however, they may differ in long-term effects.[78,79] Drug therapy tends to be superior on some measures in acute treatment (e.g., independent assessment, self-report, and behavior test measures), while CBT can lead to a greater likelihood of maintaining response after treatment termination.[79] It is not possible to predict which patients will respond best to pharmacotherapy, CBT, or a combination.[79]

There are no data to predict which patients will maintain gains after discontinuing pharmacotherapy. Some patients elect lifelong therapy. Many patients are reluctant to attempt drug discontinuation because of fear of relapse. The relapse rate 12 to 24 weeks after discontinuation of acute paroxetine therapy ranged from 39% to 63%.[77] Data show that relapse rates after discontinuation of CBT are significantly less than those after discontinuation of effective pharmacotherapy.[79] Sertraline is the only medication approved for the long-term treatment of SAD, although paroxetine, escitalopram, and venlafaxine are also effective in preventing relapse over an extended time period.[80–82]

NONPHARMACOLOGIC THERAPY

Patients should be educated about SAD, the symptoms they experience, and effective therapeutic options. Support groups are helpful for some patients. Self-help group programs that focus on effective communication can benefit people with public-speaking phobia.

CBT for SAD consists of exposure therapy, cognitive restructuring, relaxation training techniques, and social skills training.[9] Through CBT, patients learn to overcome anxiety in social situations and change the beliefs and responses that maintain this behavior. Therapy usually lasts several months and often is conducted in a group setting.

PHARMACOLOGIC THERAPY

SPECIAL POPULATIONS

SAD can present in children of preschool to elementary school age. If the disorder is not treated, it can persist into adulthood and increase the risk of depression and substance abuse. CBT and social skills training are effective nonpharmacological therapies in children.[10] Pharmacological evidence is limited to case studies or open-label trials. SSRIs are considered first-line therapy because of tolerability and effectiveness. Fluoxetine, fluvoxamine, sertraline, and paroxetine were effective in children with SAD.[10,38] Headache, nausea, drowsiness, insomnia, jitteriness, and stomach aches were reported in children receiving SSRIs.

Benzodiazepines are prescribed in children with SAD after all other types of drugs fail to show improvement.[10] If prescribed, they should be used for the shortest time period possible. The adverse effects of benzodiazepines in children include drowsiness, oppositional behavior, disinhibition, fatigue, and nausea.

Approximately one-fifth of patients with SAD also suffer from an alcohol use disorder (AUD). Many people with SAD report that they use alcohol to cope with their anxiety. Most clinical trials evaluating pharmacotherapy for SAD excluded patients with AUD. Paroxetine significantly reduced social anxiety and decreased the frequency and severity of alcohol use in patients with SAD and an AUD.[77] MAOIs and benzodiazepines are not appropriate therapy for these patients. The tyramine present in many alcoholic beverages can precipitate hypertensive crisis in patients on an MAOI. People who abuse alcohol are at risk for abusing or becoming dependent on benzodiazepines. SSRI therapy is the treatment of choice in this patient population.

ANTIDEPRESSANT THERAPY

The SSRIs and venlafaxine have the benefits of antidepressant activity for comorbid depression and safety when used in patients with substance abuse. Paroxetine, sertraline, and venlafaxine extended-release are approved for the treatment of generalized SAD and are considered first-line agents because of their efficacy and tolerability (Table 69–12). Venlafaxine and paroxetine were equivalent in efficacy for SAD over a 12-week acute period.[83] The International Consensus Group on Depression and Anxiety published a consensus statement on SAD.[22] An algorithm on the pharmacotherapy of SAD appears in Figure 69–3.

Selective Serotonin Reuptake Inhibitors

Efficacy. The efficacy and safety of paroxetine and sertraline were established in large placebo-controlled trials.[84,85] Response rates to SSRIs in SAD ranged from at least 50% in controlled trials to up to 80% in open trials.[77]

Patients treated with paroxetine or sertraline showed improvement in anxiety and avoidance symptoms and a decrease in disability.[84,85] Daily doses up to 60 mg of paroxetine and 200 mg of sertraline were well tolerated, and emergent adverse effects were similar to those of depression trials (e.g., nausea, sexual dysfunction, sweating, and somnolence). The onset of effect was delayed 4 to 8 weeks, and maximum benefit was often not observed until 12 weeks or longer. Sertraline is also effective in disabled patients suffering from the marked to severe form of generalized SAD.[85] Limited data suggest that citalopram, escitalopram, and fluvoxamine are also effective in treating SAD.[86–88] Fluoxetine was not effective in SAD.[89]

Dosing and Administration. SSRIs should be initiated at doses similar to those used for the treatment of depression and administered as a single daily dose with or without food (except for fluvoxamine). If the patient suffers from comorbid panic disorder, the SSRI dose should be started at one-fourth or one-half of the normal antidepressant dose. Patients should receive the starting dose for 2 to 4 weeks before it is increased slowly (i.e., paroxetine 10 mg/day and sertraline 50 mg/day) in weekly intervals as necessary to obtain a response. Safety for paroxetine in SAD was demonstrated in doses up to 60 mg/day, but additional therapeutic benefits above 20 mg/day were not shown.[90] The maximum dosage of sertraline used in patients with SAD was 200 mg/day.[85]

The starting dose for fluvoxamine is 50 mg/day, which is then increased as tolerated and needed up to 300 mg/day divided into twice-daily doses.[88] If citalopram is used, the initial dose is 20 mg/day, and it may be increased to 40 mg/day after 2 weeks.[86] The starting dose for escitalopram is 10 mg/day, and it can be increased to a maximum of 20 mg/day.[81] The dosage should be tapered slowly (i.e., decreasing sertraline by 50 mg/month or paroxetine by 10 mg/month) to decrease

TABLE 69–12. Drugs Used in the Treatment of Social Anxiety Disorder

Class/Generic Name	Brand Name	Starting Dose	Dosage Range[a] (mg/day)
Selective serotonin reuptake inhibitors			
Citalopram[b]	Celexa	20 mg per day	20–40
Escitalopram	Lexapro	10 mg per day	10–20
Fluvoxamine[b]	Luvox	50 mg per day	150–300
Paroxetine[b]	Paxil	10–20 mg per day	20–60[c]
Sertraline	Zoloft	25–50 mg per day	50–200[c]
Serotonin-norepinephrine reuptake inhibitor			
Venlafaxine	Effexor XR	75 mg per day	75–225[c]
Benzodiazepine			
Clonazepam[b]	Klonopin	0.25 mg per day	1–3
Monoamine oxidase inhibitor			
Phenelzine[b]	Nardil	15 mg q pm	60–90
Alternate agents			
Buspirone[b,d]	Buspar	10 mg twice per day	45–60
Gabapentin[b]	Neurontin	100 mg three times a day	900–3600

[a]Dosage used in clinical trials but not FDA-approved.
[b]Available generically.
[c]Dosage is FDA-approved.
[d]Used as augmenting agent.
Compiled from Ballenger et al,[22] Paxil package insert,[27] Effexor XR package insert,[28] Blanco et al,[93] and Pollack.[96]

the risk of relapse during discontinuation. Patients should be observed for signs of relapse for several months.[77]

Venlafaxine

Efficacy. Venlafaxine extended-release was significantly better than placebo in improving social interaction, performance, avoidance factors, and some fear factors (e.g., public speaking).[91] Beneficial effects were seen by week 3. Venlafaxine was effective in patients who failed to respond to therapy with SSRIs.[92]

Adverse Effects. Adverse effects included anorexia, dry mouth, nausea, insomnia, and sexual dysfunction.

Dosing and Administration. The starting dose of venlafaxine extended-release is 75 mg/day administered in a single dose. The dose may be increased in increments of 75 mg/day at an interval of not less

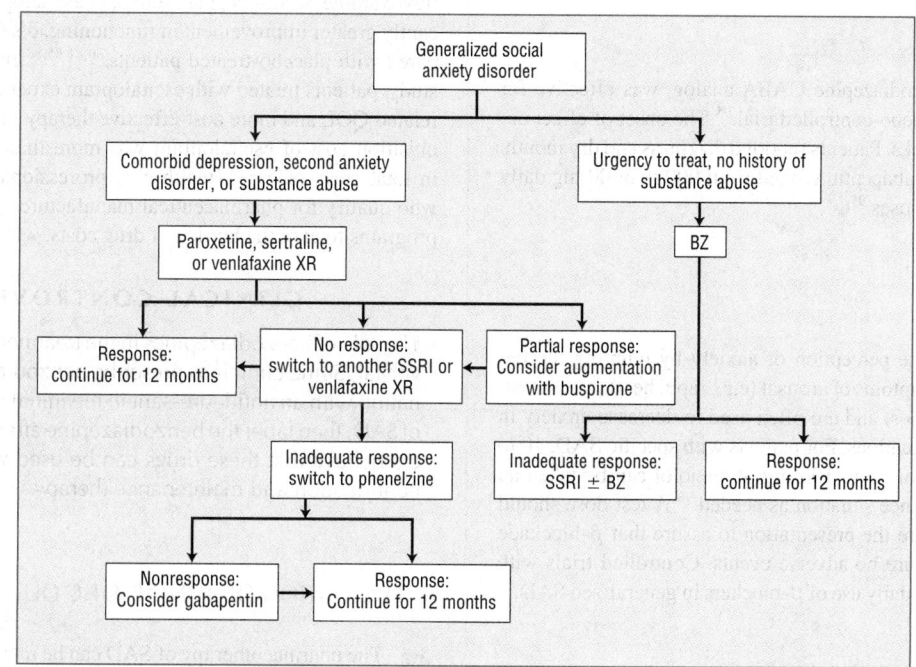

FIGURE 69–3. Algorithm for the pharmacotherapy of social anxiety disorder. SSRI = selective serotonin reuptake inhibitor, BZ = benzodiazepine. (Compiled from Ballenger et al,[22] Van Amerigen and Mancini,[77] and Blanco et al.[93])

than 4 days to a maximum of 225 mg/day.[77,91,93] Venlafaxine should be tapered slowly (i.e., decreasing by 37.5 mg/month) over several months to decrease the risk of relapse during discontinuation.[77]

ALTERNATE AGENTS

Benzodiazepines

Benzodiazepines are prescribed commonly for SAD. Clonazepam is the most extensively studied benzodiazepine for the treatment of generalized SAD.[94] Clonazepam improved fear and phobic avoidance, interpersonal sensitivity, fears of negative evaluation, and disability measures.[78,94] Adverse effects included sexual dysfunction, unsteadiness, dizziness, and poor concentration.[94] Clonazepam is often prescribed in conjunction with an antidepressant, psychotherapy, or both for initial symptom relief.[22] Comorbid alcohol or substance abuse are contraindications to the use of benzodiazepines. Other limitations of clonazepam therapy include lack of efficacy in depression and difficulty with discontinuation. Because of the risk of dependency, benzodiazepines should be reserved for patients at a low risk of substance abuse, those who require rapid relief of symptoms, or those who have not responded to other therapies.

For patients requiring a rapid onset of effect, clonazepam is effective within 1 to 2 weeks. The acute phase of benzodiazepine therapy is about 1 month. The initial dose of 0.25 mg/day can then be increased as tolerated over several weeks up to 3 mg/day. The average daily dose in clinical trials was 2.5 mg.[77,93] Patients should be instructed not to decrease or discontinue clonazepam without consulting their clinician.

Benzodiazepines must be slowly tapered on discontinuation. Patients on clonazepam for 6 months who were slowly tapered over 5 months maintained their treatment response.[94]

Gabapentin

Gabapentin, a nonbenzodiazepine GABA analog, was effective for SAD in a 14-week placebo-controlled trial.[95] The onset of effect occurred within 2 to 4 weeks. Patients reported dizziness and dry mouth. The effective dose of gabapentin ranged from 900 to 3600 mg daily given in three divided doses.[95]

Beta-Blockers

β-Blockers decrease the perception of anxiety by blunting the peripheral autonomic symptoms of arousal (e.g., rapid heart rate, sweating, blushing, and tremor) and are often used to decrease anxiety in performance-related situations. For patients with specific SAD, 10 to 80 mg of propranolol or 25 to 100 mg of atenolol can be taken an hour before a performance situation as needed.[96] A test dose should be taken at home before the presentation to assure that β-blockade is sufficient and there are no adverse events. Controlled trials with atenolol do not support daily use of β-blockers in generalized SAD.[77]

Treatment Resistance

There are no data to guide clinicians in the choice of treatments if there is a lack of response to antidepressants. Patients who have an incomplete response to a first-line agent may benefit from augmentation with buspirone at an initial dose of 10 mg twice daily. The dose of buspirone can be increased as needed to 45 to 60 mg/day.[93]

An adequate trial usually consists of 8 to 12 weeks (at maximum dosages) to confirm efficacy. Subsequent options include a trial of a second SSRI or venlafaxine extended-release. Some patients experience clinical benefit during the first 4 weeks of therapy. If nonresponsiveness continues, a trial of an alternative agent is warranted.

Phenelzine

The MAOIs are reserved for treatment-resistant patients. Although phenelzine is effective in 77% of patients with SAD,[22,77,93] dietary restrictions, potential drug interactions and adverse effects (e.g., postural hypotension, insomnia, weight gain, sedation, and hypertensive crisis) have limited its use.

The starting dose of phenelzine is 15 mg/day. It can be increased weekly by 15 mg/day to a maximum of dose of 90 mg (in divided doses).[93] Patients must avoid tyramine-containing foods and sympathomimetic drugs to prevent hypertensive crisis. If a patient is switched from another antidepressant to phenelzine, an appropriate washout period should be followed.

PHARMACOECONOMIC CONSIDERATIONS

Generalized SAD is associated with lower health-related QOL, higher rate of lifetime suicide attempts, diminished educational and occupational attainment, and increased use of health care resources.[2] Patients with SAD have a low employment status.

Early intervention is important in the treatment of SAD. Pharmacotherapy can dramatically improve QOL. Patients treated with fluvoxamine, sertraline, paroxetine, or escitalopram showed a significantly greater improvement in functioning, disability, and QOL compared with placebo-treated patients.[80,81,85,88] In a relapse prevention study, patients treated with escitalopram experienced a better health-related QOL and more cost-effective therapy than placebo.[81] The acquisition cost of escitalopram was more than offset by a decrease in total costs of care. Health care professionals can assist patients who qualify for pharmaceutical manufacturer patient access-to-care programs to ease the burden of drug costs.

CLINICAL CONTROVERSY

The role of benzodiazepines in the treatment of SAD is controversial. Some clinicians prescribe benzodiazepines in combination with an antidepressant in the initial acute management of SAD, then taper the benzodiazepine after 3 to 4 weeks. Others believe that these drugs can be used without risk during continuation and maintenance therapy.

EVALUATION OF THERAPEUTIC OUTCOMES

The pharmacotherapy of SAD can be monitored in three principal domains. The domains include SAD symptoms (e.g., fear and physical symptoms), functionality, and well being or overall improvement.[22] Response to pharmacotherapy in SAD is defined as a stable, clinically meaningful improvement; patients no longer have the full range of symptoms but typically continue to experience more than minimal symptoms.[22]

During the acute phase of treatment, patients should be seen weekly while the drug dosage is titrated. Once the patient responds and the dosage is stabilized, the patient can be seen monthly. At each visit, the patient should be asked about adverse effects and improvement in symptoms. The patient should be instructed to keep a diary to record fear levels, physical symptoms, cognitions, and anxious behaviors in actual exposures to social situations. The Liebowitz Social Anxiety Scale is a clinician-rated scale that rates clinical severity and change in SAD that can be used to monitor response.[22] Patients can use the Social Phobia Inventory for self-assessment of SAD symptoms.[22] Full remission is a complete resolution of symptoms across the three SAD domains that is maintained for 3 months[22] or a Liebowitz Social Anxiety Scale score of ≤ 30.[23]

Patient counseling is important. The patient should be instructed about the gradual onset of effect and that the full therapeutic effect may not be achieved for up to 12 weeks. Patients should be told that long-term therapy is required. When drug therapy is discontinued, the dosage will need to be gradually decreased over several months, and the patient should be seen more frequently to monitor for signs and symptoms of relapse or withdrawal.

It is important to remember that while pharmacotherapy usually leads to improvement in social and occupational functioning, most patients do not achieve a full remission. Many patients require additional treatment, often in the form of CBT.

▶ TREATMENT: Specific Phobia

Specific phobia is considered unresponsive to drug therapy, although highly responsive to behavioral therapy. The use of antidepressant drugs can be detrimental in patients with specific phobias.

CONCLUSIONS

Anxiety disorders are common in the population and are commonly comorbid with other psychiatric disorders. The proper management of anxiety disorders begins with the correct diagnosis; not all patients should receive antianxiety agents. Nonpharmacologic interventions often are effective alone or when combined with drug therapy.

There are several subtypes of anxiety disorders, and the diagnosis determines the type of drug and nonpharmacologic intervention selected. Although benzodiazepines remain the drugs of choice for situational anxiety, antidepressants have emerged as first-line therapy for GAD, panic disorder, and SAD. The antidepressants are the drugs of choice for patients who need chronic therapy for GAD. Benzodiazepines are reserved for use in situations requiring immediate anxiety relief or for use on an as-needed basis. Antidepressants, including the SSRIs and the benzodiazepines clonazepam and alprazolam, are used extensively in patients with panic disorder. Research in the area of SAD has resulted in new pharmacologic treatment strategies with antidepressants.

The long-term goal of therapy for GAD, panic disorder, and SAD is remission of core anxiety symptoms with no impairment in functionality, minimal anxiety, and no depressive symptoms. Clinicians can use the pharmacological armamentarium effectively to achieve this goal for patients.

ABBREVIATIONS

AUD: alcohol use disorder
CBT: cognitive behavioral therapy
DA: dopamine
DMDZ: desmethyldiazepam
GABA: γ-aminobutyric acid
GAD: generalized anxiety disorder
5-HT: serotonin
LC: locus ceruleus
MAOI: monoamine oxidase inhibitor
NE: norepinephrine

QOL: quality of life
SAD: social anxiety disorder
SERT: serotonin reuptake transporter site
SNRI: serotonin-norepinephrine reuptake inhibitor
SSRI: selective serotonin reuptake inhibitor
TCA: tricyclic antidepressant

Review Questions and other resources can be found at *www.pharmacotherapyonline.com*.

REFERENCES

1. American Psychiatric Association. Diagnostic and Statistical Manual of Mental Disorders, Fourth Edition, Text Revision. Washington, American Psychiatric Association, 2000:429–484.
2. Young AS, Klap R, Sherbourne CD, Wells KB. The quality of care for depressive and anxiety disorders in the United States. Arch Gen Psychiatry 2001;58:55–61.
3. Lépine J. The epidemiology of anxiety disorders: Prevalence and societal costs. J Clin Psychiatry 2002;63(Suppl 14):4–8.
4. Bowen RC, Senthilselvan A, Barale A. Physical illness as an outcome of chronic anxiety disorders. Can J Psychiatry 2000;45:459–464.
5. Rickels K, Rynn M. Pharmacotherapy of generalized anxiety disorder. J Clin Psychiatry 2002;63(Suppl 14):9–16.
6. Narrow WE, Rae DS, Robins LN, Reigier DA. Revised prevalence estimates of mental disorders in the United States: Using a clinical significance criterion to reconcile 2 surveys' estimates. Arch Gen Psychiatry 2002; 59:115–123.
7. House A, Stark D. Anxiety in medical patients. Br Med J 2002;325: 207–209.
8. Gliatto MF. Generalized anxiety disorder. Am Fam Physician 2000;62: 1591–1600, 1602.
9. den Boer JA. Social anxiety disorder/social phobia: Epidemiology, diagnosis, neurobiology, and treatment. Compr Psychiatry 2000;41:405–415.
10. Beidel DC, Ferrell C, Alfano CA, Yeganeh R. The treatment of childhood social anxiety disorder. Psychiatr Clin North Am 2001;24:831–846.
11. Chen J, Reich L, Chung H. Anxiety disorders. West Med J 2002;176: 249–253.
12. Ballenger JC, Davidson JRT, Lecrubier Y, et al. Consensus statement on generalized anxiety disorder from the International Consensus Group on Depression and Anxiety. J Clin Psychiatry 2001;62(Suppl 11):53–58.

13. Kent JM, Mathew SJ, Gorman JM. Molecular targets in the treatment of anxiety. Biol Psychiatry 2002;52:1008–1030.

14. Condren RM, O'Neill A, Ryan MC, et al. HPA axis response to a psychological stressor in generalised social phobia. Psychoneuroendocrinology 2002;27:693–703.

15. Gorman JM, Kent JM, Sullivan GM, Coplan JD. Neuroanatomical hypothesis of panic disorder, revised. Am J Psychiatry 2000;157:493–505.

16. Malizia AL. Receptor binding and drug modulation in anxiety. Eur Neuropsychopharmacol 2002;12:567–574.

17. Condren RM, Lucey TV, Thakore JH. A preliminary study of baclofen-induced growth hormone release in generalised social phobia. Hum Psychopharmacol 2003;18:135–130.

18. Condren RM, Dinan TG, Thakore JH. A preliminary study of buspirone stimulated prolactin release in generalised social phobia: Evidence for enhanced serotonergic responsivity? Eur Neuropsychopharmacol 2002;12:349–354.

19. Furmark TF, Tillfors M, Marteinsdottir I, et al. Common changes in cerebral blood flow in patients with social phobia treated with citalopram or cognitive-behavioral therapy. Arch Gen Psychiatry 2002;59:425–433.

20. Hildago RB, Davidson JRT. Generalized anxiety disorder: An important clinical concern. Med Clin North Am 2001;85:691–710.

21. Mendlowicz MV, Stein MB. Quality of life in individuals with anxiety disorders. Am J Psychiatry 2000;157:669–682.

22. Ballenger JC, Davidson JRT, Lecrubier Y, et al. Consensus statement on social anxiety disorder from the International Consensus Group on Depression and Anxiety. J Clin Psychiatry 1998;59(Suppl 17):54–60.

23. Doyle AC, Pollack MH. Establishment of remission criteria for anxiety disorders. J Clin Psychiatry 2003;64(Suppl 15):40–45.

24. Bandelow B, Zohar J, Hollander E, et al. Guidelines for the pharmacological treatment of anxiety, obsessive-compulsive and posttraumatic stress disorders. World J Biol Psychiatry 2002;3:171–199.

25. Work Group on Panic Disorder. Practice guideline for the treatment of patients with panic disorder. Am J Psychiatry 1998;155(Suppl 5):1–34.

26. Lexapro package insert. Forest Pharmaceuticals, Inc., St. Louis, MO, December 2003.

27. Paxil package insert. GlaxoSmithKline, Research Triangle Park, NC, August 2003.

28. Effexor XR package insert. Wyeth Pharmaceuticals, Inc., Philadelphia, December 2003.

29. Vistaril package insert. Pfizer Labs, New York, October 2001.

30. Osser DN, Renner JA, Bayog R. Algorithms for the pharmacotherapy of anxiety disorders in patients with chemical abuse and dependence. Psychiatr Ann 1999;29:285–299.

31. Llorca P, Spadone C, Sol O, et al. Efficacy and safety of hydroxyzine in the treatment of generalized anxiety disorder: A 3-month double-blind study. J Clin Psychiatry 2002;63:1020–1027.

32. Pitler MH, Ernst E. Kava extract for treating anxiety (Cochrane Review). In: The Cochrane Library, Issue 3, 2003. Oxford, Update Software.

33. Humberston CL, Akhtar J, Krenzelok ED. Acute hepatitis induced by kava kava. J Toxicol Clin Toxicol 2003;41:109–113.

34. Ibqual MM, Sobhan T, Ryals T. Effects of commonly used benzodiazepines on the fetus, the neonate, and the nursing infant. Psychiatr Serv 2002;53:39–49.

35. Wang PS, Bohn RL, Glynn RJ, et al. Hazardous benzodiazepine regimens in the elderly: Effects of half-life, dosage, and duration on risk of hip fracture. Am J Psychiatry 2001;158:892–898.

36. Wagner CD. Generalized anxiety disorder in children and adolescents. Psychiatric Clin North Am 2001;24:139–153.

37. Kapczinski F, Lima MS, Souza JS, Schmitt R. Antidepressants for generalized anxiety disorder (Cochrane Review). In: The Cochrane Library, Issue 3, 2003. Oxford, Update Software.

38. The Research Unit on Pediatric Psychopharmacology Anxiety Study Group. Fluvoxamine for the treatment of anxiety disorders in children and adolescents. N Engl J Med 2001;344:1279–1285.

39. Varley C, Smith CJ. Anxiety disorders in the child and teen. Pediatric Clin North Am 2003;50:1107–1138.

40. Wyeth Pharmaceuticals. Important update to prescribing information. August 22, 2003, *http://www.effexorxr.com/pdf/Wyeth_HCP.pdf*. Accessed January 15, 2004.

41. U.S. Food and Drug Administration. Reports of suicidality in pediatric patients being treated with antidepressant medications for major depressive disorder. FDA Public Health Advisory, October 27, 2003. *http://fda.gov/cder/drug/advisory/mdd.html*. Accessed January 15, 2004.

42. Gelenberg AJ, Lydiard RB, Rudolph RL, et al. Efficacy of venlafaxine extended-release capsules in nondepressed outpatients with generalized anxiety disorder: A 6-month randomized controlled trial. JAMA 2000; 283:3082–3088.

43. Rickels K, Zaninelli R, McCafferty J, et al. Paroxetine treatment of generalized anxiety disorder: A double-blind, placebo-controlled study. Am J Psychiatry 2003;160:749–756.

44. Shelton RC, Brown LL. Mechanisms of action in the treatment of anxiety. J Clin Psychiatry 2001;62(Suppl 12):10–15.

45. Shader RI, Greenblatt DJ. Can you provide a table of equivalences for benzodiazepines and other marketed benzodiazepine agonists? J Clin Psychopharmacol 1997;17:331.

46. Klonopin package insert. Roche Laboratories, Nutley, NJ, July 2001.

47. Xanax XR package insert. Pharmacia & Upjohn Company, Kalamazoo, MI, January 2003.

48. Bailey L, Ward M, Musa M. Clinical pharmacokinetics of benzodiazepines. J Clin Pharmacol 1994;34:804–811.

49. Tanaka E. Clinically significant pharmacokinetic drug interactions with benzodiazepines. J Clin Pharmacol Ther 1999;24:347–355.

50. Sramek JJ, Zarotsky V, Cutler NR. Generalised anxiety disorder. Drugs 2002;62:1635–1648.

51. Gorman JM. Treating generalized anxiety disorder. J Clin Psychiatry 2003; 64(Suppl 2):24–29.

52. Longo LP, Johnson B. Benzodiazepines: Side effects, abuse risk and alternatives (Addiction Part 1). Am Fam Physician 2000;61:2121–2128.

53. Royal Australian and New Zealand College of Psychiatrists Clinical Practice Guidelines Team for Panic Disorder and Agoraphobia. Australian and New Zealand clinical practice guidelines for the treatment of panic disorder and agoraphobia. Aust N Z J Psychiatry 2003;37:641–656.

54. Barlow DH, Gorman JM, Shear MK, Woods SW. Cognitive-behavioral therapy, imipramine, or their combination for panic disorder. JAMA 2000; 283:2529–2536.

55. Kampman M, Keijsers GPJ, Hoogduin CAL, Hendriks G. A randomized, double-blind, placebo-controlled study of the effects of adjunctive paroxetine in panic disorder patients unsuccessfully treated with cognitive-behavioral therapy alone. J Clin Psychiatry 2002;63:772–777.

56. Saeed SA, Bruce TJ. Panic disorder: Effective treatment options. Am Fam Physician 1998;57:2405–2412.

57. Zamorski MA, Albucher RC. What to do when SSRIs fail: Eight strategies for optimizing treatment of panic disorder. Am Fam Physician 2002; 66:1471–1484.

58. Stahl SM, Gergel I, Li D. Escitalopram in the treatment of panic disorder: A randomized, double-blind, placebo-controlled trial. J Clin Psychiatry 2003;64:1322–1327.

59. Bruce SE, Vasile RG, Goisman RM, et al. Are benzodiazepines still the medication of choice for patients with panic disorder with or without agoraphobia? Am J Psychiatry 2003;160:1432–1438.

60. Bakker A, van Balkom AJ, Spinhoven P. SSRIs vs. TCAs in the treatment of panic disorder: A meta-analysis. Acta Psychiatr Scand 2002;106:163–167.

61. Ballenger JC, Davidson JRT, Lecrubier Y, et al. Consensus statement on panic disorder from the International Consensus Group on Depression and Anxiety. J Clin Psychiatry 1998;59(Suppl 8):47–54.

62. Goddard AW, Brouette T, Almai A, et al. Early coadministration of clonazepam with sertraline for panic disorder. Arch Gen Psychiatry 2001; 58:681–686.

63. Pollack MH, Simon M, Worthington JJ, et al. Combined paroxetine and clonazepam treatment strategies compared to paroxetine monotherapy for panic disorder. J Psychopharmacol 2003;17:275–281.

64. Flint AJ, Gagnon N. Diagnosis and management of panic disorder in older adults. Drugs Aging 2003;20:881–891.

65. Pollack MH, Otto MW, Worthington JJ, et al. Sertraline in the treatment of panic disorder: A flexible-dose multicenter trial. Arch Gen Psychiatry 1998;55:1010–1016.

66. Ballenger JC, Wheadon DE, Steiner M, et al. Double-blind, fixed-dose, placebo-controlled study of paroxetine in the treatment of panic disorder. Am J Psychiatry 1998;155:36–42.

67. Sandman J, Lörch B, Bandelow B, et al. Fluvoxamine or placebo in the treatment of panic disorder and relationship to blood concentration of fluvoxamine. Pharmacopsychiatry 1998;31:117–121.

68. Lepola UM, Wade AG, Leinonen EV, et al. A controlled, prospective, 1-year trial of citalopram in the treatment of panic disorder. J Clin Psychiatry 1998;59:528–534.

69. Sheehan DV. The management of panic disorder. J Clin Psychiatry 2002; 63(Suppl 14):17–21.

70. Hirshman S, Dannon PN, Iancu I, et al. Pindolol augmentation in patients with treatment-resistant panic disorder: A double-blind, placebo-controlled trial. J Clin Psychopharmacol 2000;20:556–559.

71. Baetz M, Bowen RC. Efficacy of divalproex sodium in patients with panic disorder and mood instability who have not responded to conventional therapy. Can J Psychiatry 1998;43:73–77.

72. Emmanuel NP, Ware MR, Brawn-Mintzer O, et al. Once-weekly dosing of fluoxetine in the maintenance of remission in panic disorder. J Clin Psychiatry 1999;60:299–301.

73. Mavissakalian MR, Perel JM. Duration of imipramine therapy and relapse in panic disorder with agoraphobia. J Clin Psychopharmacol 2002; 22:294–299.

74. Moroz G, Rosenbaun JF. Efficacy, safety, and gradual discontinuation of clonazepam in panic disorder: A placebo-controlled, multicenter study using optimized dosages. J Clin Psychiatry 1999;60:604–612.

75. Otto MW, Pollack MH, Maki KM. Empirically supported treatments for panic disorder: Costs, benefits, and stepped care. J Consult Clin Psychol 2000;68:556–563.

76. Olfson M, Guardino M, Struening E, et al. Barriers to the treatment of social anxiety. Am J Psychiatry 2000;157:521–527.

77. Van Amerigen M, Mancini C. Pharmacotherapy of social anxiety disorder at the turn of the millennium. Psychiatr Clin North Am 2001;24:783–803.

78. Otto MW, Pollack MH, Gould RA, et al. A comparison of the efficacy of clonazepam and cognitive-behavioral group therapy for the treatment of social phobia. J Anxiety Disord 2000;14:345–358.

79. Liebowitz MR, Heimberg RG, Schneir FR, et al. Cognitive-behavioral group therapy versus phenelzine in social phobia: Long term outcome. Depress Anxiety 1999;10:89–98.

80. Stein DJ, Versiani M, Hair T, Kumar R. Efficacy of paroxetine for relapse prevention in social anxiety disorder: A 24-week study. Arch Gen Psychiatry 2002;59:1111–1118.

81. Montgomery SA. Escitalopram-treatment shows better cost-effectiveness and improved quality of life versus placebo in social anxiety disorder [poster]. 23rd Annual Congress of the Anxiety Disorder Association of America, Toronto, May 2003.

82. Stein MB. Long-term treatment of generalized social anxiety disorder with venlafaxine XR [poster]. 23rd Annual Congress of the Anxiety Disorder Association of America, Toronto, May 2003.

83. Liebowitz MR. Comparison of venlafaxine XR and paroxetine in the short-term treatment of SAD [poster]. 23rd Annual Congress of the Anxiety Disorder Association of America, Toronto, May 2003.

84. Stein DJ, Stein MB, Pitts CD, et al. Predictors of response to pharmacotherapy in social anxiety disorder: An analysis of 3 placebo-controlled paroxetine trials. J Clin Psychiatry 2002;63:152–155.

85. Liebowitz MR, DeMartinis NA, Weihs K, et al. Efficacy of sertraline in severe generalized social anxiety disorder: Results of a double-blind, placebo-controlled study. J Clin Psychiatry 2003;64:785–792.

86. Schneier FR, Blanco C, Campeas R, et al. Citalopram treatment of social anxiety disorder with comorbid major depression. Depress Anxiety 2003;17:191–196.

87. Montgomery SA. Escitalopram prevents relapse in patients suffering from social anxiety disorder (SAD) [poster]. 23rd Annual Congress of the Anxiety Disorder Association of America, Toronto, May 2003.

88. Stein MB, Fyer AJ, Davidson JR, et al. Fluvoxamine treatment of social phobia (social anxiety disorder): A double-blind, placebo-controlled study. Am J Psychiatry 1999;156:756–760.

89. Kobak KA, Greist JH, Jefferson JW, Katzelnick DJ. Fluoxetine in social phobia: A double-blind, placebo-controlled pilot study. J Clin Psychopharmacol 2002;22:257–262.

90. Liebowtiz MR, Stein MB, Tancer M, et al. A randomized, double-blind, fixed-dose comparison of paroxetine and placebo in the treatment of generalized social anxiety disorder. J Clin Psychiatry 2002;63:66–74.

91. Davidson JRT, Manguano RM. Venlafaxine XR in social anxiety disorder [poster]. XII World Congress of Psychiatry, Yokohama, Japan, August 2002.

92. Altamura AC, Pioli R, Vitto M, et al. Venlafaxine in social phobia: A study in selective serotonin reuptake non-responders. Int Clin Psychopharmacol 1999;14:239–245.

93. Blanco C, Antia SX, Liebowitz MR. Pharmacotherapy of social anxiety disorder. Biol Psychiatry 2002;51:109–120.

94. Jefferson JW. Benzodiazepines and anticonvulsants for social phobia (social anxiety disorder). J Clin Psychiatry 2001;62:50–53.

95. Pande AC, Davidson JR, Jefferson JW, et al. Treatment of social phobia with gabapentin: A placebo-controlled study. J Clin Psychopharmacol 1999;19:341–348.

96. Pollack MH. Social anxiety disorder: Designing a pharmacologic treatment strategy. J Clin Psychiatry 1999;60(Suppl 9):20–26.

70

ANXIETY DISORDERS II: POSTTRAUMATIC STRESS DISORDER AND OBSESSIVE-COMPULSIVE DISORDER

Cynthia K. Kirkwood, Eugene H. Makela, and Barbara G. Wells

Learning Objectives and other resources can be found at *www.pharmacotherapyonline.com.*

KEY CONCEPTS

① The short-term goal in posttraumatic stress disorder is reduction in core symptoms, while the long-term goal is remission.

② Cognitive and behavioral approaches are the most effective nonpharmacologic methods to reduce symptoms of posttraumatic stress disorder.

③ The selective serotonin reuptake inhibitors (SSRIs) are considered first-line treatment for posttraumatic stress disorder.

④ An adequate trial for an antidepressant in posttraumatic stress disorder is 8 to 12 weeks.

⑤ The duration of pharmacotherapy for posttraumatic stress disorder is at least 12 months.

⑥ The SSRIs are the drugs of choice for the treatment of obsessive-compulsive disorder.

⑦ Clomipramine should be considered after 2 or 3 failed SSRI trials for obsessive-compulsive disorder.

⑧ Antidepressant taper can be considered after 1 to 2 years of treatment for obsessive-compulsive disorder.

⑨ Long-term or lifetime prophylactic maintenance medication is recommended for obsessive-compulsive disorder after 2 to 4 severe relapses or 3 to 4 mild to moderate relapses.

Recent world events (e.g., wars, terrorist attacks, and earthquakes) have placed a renewed focus on posttraumatic stress disorder (PTSD). Initially diagnosed in veterans of war, PTSD is now acknowledged as a significant psychiatric illness in the civilian population.[1] PTSD continues to be poorly recognized and diagnosed in clinical practice.[2] Because of its co-occurrence with other anxiety disorders, depression, and substance abuse, the overlapping symptoms can lead to diagnostic uncertainty. Advances in the science and treatment of PTSD can assist clinicians in all fields of health care to screen patients for a history of trauma and effectively manage PTSD if it is present.

Obsessive-compulsive disorder (OCD) is one of the ten leading causes of disability.[3] Patients with OCD experience significant impairment in their quality of life (QOL), with reductions in social, family, and occupational functioning.[4] OCD affects far more individuals than was thought in the past. Because of the nature and potential severity of signs and symptoms and the resultant negative effects on QOL, OCD is considered a major medical condition. Clinicians should be able to identify OCD and understand the current treatment options.

EPIDEMIOLOGY

The prevalence rates of anxiety disorders were recently revised to encompass clinically significant cases in the community.[5] According to the modified prevalence estimates of mental disorders in the United States, the 1-year prevalence rate of PTSD was 3.6%.[5] The

1-year prevalence rate for obsessive-compulsive disorder was 2.4% in persons aged 18 to 54 years and 1.5% in those over age 55 years.[5]

The epidemiology of PTSD is associated with the incidence of trauma. It is estimated that about 50% of men and 60% of women are exposed to a life-threatening traumatic event. Of these individuals 8.2% of men and 20% of women will develop PTSD.[6] Previous exposure to a trauma and the intensity of response to the event increase the risk of PTSD.[6] Individuals with a history of childhood sexual abuse are at higher risk of developing PTSD as adults.[7] Men tend to be assaulted more frequently, but women have a higher rate of PTSD after assault. The incidence of PTSD is equal between men and women after rape (i.e., 50%) and natural disasters (i.e., <5%).[6] Genetic factors can increase vulnerability to PTSD if an individual is exposed to a traumatic event. Offspring of Holocaust survivors had a higher lifetime prevalence rate of PTSD compared with a control group.[6]

OCD usually begins early in life, with 20% of cases occurring in childhood, 29% in adolescence, and 49% of cases occurring by age 20. The onset of illness is earlier in men than women. OCD tends to be a chronic disorder.[1] Twin studies revealed significantly higher concordance rates in monozygotic versus dizygotic twins, but OCD probably has nongenetic as well as genetic influences over expression of the illness, because the concordance rate for monozygotic twins is less than 100%. Individuals have an 11% to 12% risk of developing the illness if a first-degree relative has OCD; however, this familial relationship may be age-sensitive. In one epidemiological study, no cases of OCD were found in relatives of patients developing the illness after 18 years of age.[8]

ETIOLOGY

The exact etiologies of PTSD and OCD are not known. It is likely that abnormalities in several areas of brain functioning interact to cause these chronic anxiety disorders. Genetics may play a role in expression of PTSD and OCD, but environmental factors likely are also involved. A neurodevelopmental model of OCD has been proposed.[9]

OCD has been characterized as a pediatric autoimmune neuropsychiatric disorder associated with streptococcal infections. In response to streptococcal infection, antibodies are produced in some individuals that temporally precipitate sudden onset or exacerbation of symptoms of OCD. Neuroimaging studies suggest that in these patients the antibodies produce inflammation of the basal ganglia. This leads to increased volumes of the caudate, putamen, and the globus pallidus, and subsequently to smaller caudate volumes potentially reflective of scarring or atrophy related to streptococcal infection. Although most patients with OCD do not have a streptococcal etiology, an accurate medical history regarding onset of illness is imperative because specific treatment strategies are indicated.[10]

PATHOPHYSIOLOGY

Research findings in the areas of neuroendocrinology, neurobiology, and neuroimaging have advanced a number of theories on the pathophysiology of anxiety disorders. Neuroendocrine changes in the hypothalamic-pituitary-adrenal (HPA) axis are implicated in the pathophysiology of PTSD.[6] As reviewed in the previous chapter (Chap. 69), data from neurochemical and neuroimaging studies indicate that the modulation of normal and pathologic anxiety states is associated with multiple regions of the brain (e.g., amygdala, hippocampus, thalamus, and prefrontal cortex). Abnormal function in several neurotransmitter systems, including norepinephrine (NE), γ-aminobutyric acid (GABA), glutamate, dopamine (DA), and serotonin (5-HT) may affect the manifestations of anxiety disorders.[11,12]

NEUROENDOCRINE THEORIES

Neuroendocrine studies provide data that abnormalities occurring pretrauma, during trauma, and posttrauma contribute to PTSD.[6] Normally the immediate reaction to stress occurs as an automatic response from the amygdala to the sympathetic and parasympathetic systems and the HPA axis. The release of corticotropin-releasing factor stimulates cortisol release from the adrenal gland. Both catecholamines and cortisol levels rise in tandem. Cortisol reduces the stress response by tempering the sympathetic reaction through negative feedback on the pituitary and hypothalamus.[6] These systems return to normal after a few hours.

Patients with PTSD have a hypersecretion of corticotropin-releasing factor but demonstrate subnormal levels of cortisol at the time of trauma and chronically.[6] Dysregulation of the HPA axis is postulated to be a risk factor for eventual development of PTSD.[6]

NEUROCHEMICAL THEORIES

Several neurotransmitters may be involved in the pathophysiology of PTSD. 5-HT and NE are associated with the processing of

emotional and somatic contents of memories in the amygdala. The cortex and hippocampus are involved in storing the facts and related cues of memory.[13] The noradrenergic theory posits that the autonomic nervous system of anxious patients is hypersensitive and overreacts to stimuli. The alarm center, the locus ceruleus, releases NE to stimulate the sympathetic and parasympathetic nervous systems. Patients with PTSD tend to experience sustained elevated heart rates during trauma and enhanced startle effects starting a month after trauma exposure. Patients with chronic central noradrenergic overactivity have downregulated α_2-adrenoreceptors.[14] Dysregulation of the processing of sensory input and memories may contribute to the dissociative and hypervigilant symptoms in PTSD. Preliminary data indicate that the 5-HT and 5-HT$_2$ antagonist *meta*-chlorophenylpiperazine (*m*-CPP) causes increased anxiety symptoms in patients with PTSD.[13] Abnormalities of GABA inhibition may lead to increased awareness or response to stress, as seen in PTSD.[13]

Both 5-HT and DA are implicated in the pathogenesis of OCD. Pharmacologic trials involving selective and potent serotonergic reuptake inhibitors have consistently shown these agents to be effective for symptoms of the illness. Results of challenge studies using 5-HT agonists support a role for this neurotransmitter as well. However, to date there is no specific identified abnormality in the 5-HT system with OCD.[12] DA dysregulation may contribute to some forms of OCD. Neurologic symptoms (e.g., tics) are part of the clinical presentation in some patients with OCD. Tourette's disorder, a disorder of DA dysfunction, is often comorbid with OCD.[1] Patients with OCD and tics benefit from the addition of an antipsychotic drug to their treatment regimen.[12]

NEUROIMAGING STUDIES

Neuroimaging studies suggest that certain areas of the brain are altered by psychological trauma. The most consistent finding is decreased hippocampal volumes in patients with PTSD.[15] In twin studies, the unaffected twin of patients with PTSD also demonstrated smaller hippocampi compared with twins without PTSD.[15] These findings suggest that lower hippocampal volumes in patients with PTSD are likely a precursor associated with vulnerability for subsequent development of PTSD.[11]

Findings of increased activation of the amygdala after symptom provocation (e.g., via personal trauma script, visual imagery, or audiotape of combat sounds) indicate that this structure plays a role in the formation of emotional memory. Concurrent reductions in the activity in Broca's area (functioning here is required to attach meaning to experiences that can be translated into words) may explain why patients with PTSD have problems in labeling and understanding their extreme emotions.[16,17] Neuroimaging data suggest that the biological changes after trauma can also involve alterations in brain structure and function.[16]

Progress has been made in elucidating the pathophysiologic mechanisms that are the underpinnings of OCD. Functional neuroimaging studies indicate that individuals with OCD show hyperactivity in the ventral prefrontal cortex (VPFC) of the brain. In adult patients with OCD there is a correlation between symptom severity and VPFC and striatal activity. Lesions of the VPFC in patients with OCD result in decreased obsessive-compulsive symptoms. The VPFC dysfunction may be related to a loss of inhibitory processes that results in increased metabolic rates in this region and difficulty in inhibiting thoughts and rituals that otherwise would seem senseless.[9]

CLINICAL PRESENTATION

The *Diagnostic and Statistical Manual of Mental Disorders,* Fourth Edition, Text Revision classifies anxiety disorders into several categories: generalized anxiety disorder, panic disorder (with or without agoraphobia), social anxiety disorder, specific phobia, OCD, PTSD, and acute stress disorder (ASD).[1] The characteristic features of these illnesses are anxiety and avoidance behavior. Generalized anxiety disorder, panic disorder, and social anxiety disorder are discussed in Chap. 69.

POSTTRAUMATIC STRESS DISORDER

Exposure to a traumatic event is required for a diagnosis of PTSD.[1] The person must have witnessed, experienced, or have been confronted with a situation that involved definite or threatened death or serious injury, or possible harm to themselves or others. The patient's response to the trauma must include intense fear, helplessness, or horror.[1] Some examples of traumatic events include motor vehicle accidents, natural disasters, rape, being held hostage, child sexual abuse, and witnessing a murder or injury of another.

The resulting PTSD symptoms include persistent re-experiencing of the traumatic event, avoidance of stimuli associated with the trauma, numbing of general responsiveness, and persistent symptoms of hyperarousal (Table 70–1). Patients must have at least one re-experiencing symptom that can include recurrent images, thoughts, perceptions, or dreams of the event; dissociative flashbacks,

TABLE 70–1. Presentation of Posttraumatic Stress Disorder

Re-experiencing symptoms
  Recurrent, intrusive distressing memories of the trauma
  Recurrent, disturbing dreams of the event
  Feeling that the traumatic event is recurring (e.g., dissociative flashbacks)
  Physiologic reaction to reminders of the trauma
Avoidance symptoms
  Avoidance of conversations about the trauma
  Avoidance of thoughts or feelings about the trauma
  Avoidance of activities that are reminders of the event
  Avoidance of people or places that arouse recollections of the trauma
  Inability to recall an important aspect of the trauma
  Anhedonia
  Estrangement from others
  Restricted affect
  Sense of a foreshortened future (e.g., does not expect to have a career, marriage)
Hyperarousal symptoms
  Decreased concentration
  Easily startled
  Hypervigilance
  Insomnia
  Irritability or angry outbursts
Subtypes
  Acute: duration of symptoms is less than 3 months
  Chronic: symptoms last for longer than 3 months
  With delayed onset: onset of symptoms is at least 6 months posttrauma
Screening questions
  Have you ever experienced a significant trauma in your life?
  Did this experience have a lasting negative impact or change your life?

Adapted from American Psychiatric Association[1] and Ballenger et al.[11]

illusions, hallucinations, or a sense of reliving the event; physiologic reactivity (e.g., increased heart rate) on exposure to internal or external cues that symbolize a feature of the trauma.[1] At least three signs or symptoms of persistent avoidance of stimuli associated with the trauma or numbing are required and can include the following: efforts to avoid feelings, conversations, and thoughts about the trauma; avoidance of places, activities, or individuals that stimulate recollections of the event; restricted range of affect; feelings of estrangement from others; anhedonia; dissociative amnesia; and sense that they lack a future.[1] At least two symptoms of increased arousal are present, including insomnia, exaggerated startle response, difficulty concentrating, hypervigilance, and irritability.[1] Symptoms from each category need to be present for longer than 1 month and cause significant distress or impairment in functioning. Most persons diagnosed with PTSD also meet criteria for another mental disorder.[1]

Anxiety and dissociative symptoms (e.g., sense of numbing or absence of emotional responsiveness, derealization, depersonalization, inability to recall important features of the event) emerging within 1 month after exposure to a traumatic stressor are classified as ASD. Symptoms of ASD are experienced during or immediately after the trauma, last for at least 2 days, and resolve within 4 weeks.[1]

The age of onset and course of PTSD are variable. PTSD can occur at any age. The presentation is not predictable because symptoms are related to the duration and intensity of the trauma, the presence of other psychiatric disorders, and how the patient deals with the trauma. The average duration of symptoms in patients in treatment is about 36 months. In those not receiving treatment, symptoms can last for a mean of 5 years. About one-third of patients with PTSD have a poor prognosis for recovery.[7] About 80% of patients with PTSD have a concurrent depression or anxiety disorder.[7] Over half of men with PTSD suffer from comorbid alcohol abuse or dependence.[7] About 20% of patients with PTSD attempt suicide.[7]

OBSESSIVE-COMPULSIVE DISORDER

Patients with OCD exhibit a great variety of symptoms upon presentation to clinicians (Table 70–2). The diversity and oddity of symptoms that manifest can obscure accurate diagnosis and delay appropriate treatment of the disorder. Patients may be secretive about symptoms and purposefully refuse to report or deny symptoms.[18] Patients can present in a seemingly incongruous manner to nonpsychiatrists for

TABLE 70–2. Presentation of Obsessive-Compulsive Disorder

Obsessions
- Repetitive thoughts (e.g., feeling contaminated after touching an object, doubting whether the stove was turned off)
- Repetitive images (e.g., recurrent sexually explicit pictures)
- Repetitive impulses (e.g., need for symmetry or putting things in specific order, impulse to shout out obscenities in a church)

Compulsions
- Repetitive activities (e.g., hand washing, checking, ordering, need to ask, need to confess)
- Repetitive mental acts (e.g., counting, repeating words silently, praying)

Screening questions
- Do you have repetitive thoughts that make you anxious and that you cannot get rid of?
- Do you check things excessively?
- Do you feel the need to wash your hands frequently?
- Do you keep things exceptionally clean?

Adapted from American Psychiatric Association[1] and Jenike.[18]

other complaints—dermatologists for eczema or chapped skin, pediatricians for parental concerns over a child's compulsive hand washing, neurologists for tics, or dentists for gum lesions from compulsive teeth brushing.

The diagnostic criteria for OCD requires the presence of either obsessions and/or compulsions (although most patients have both) that are severe enough to cause marked distress, to be time-consuming (occupy more than 1 hour per day), or to cause significant impairment in social or occupational functioning.[1] An obsession is a recurrent, persistent idea, thought, impulse, or image that is experienced as intrusive and inappropriate and produces marked anxiety. Common obsessions involve thoughts about contamination (e.g., concern with germs, dirt, or toxic chemicals), repeated doubts, and needing to have things in a particular order.[1]

Individuals must recognize that their obsessions or compulsions are excessive or unreasonable. Obsessions must be acknowledged as products of the individual's own mind and attempts must be made to ignore or suppress them. The obsessions produce marked feelings of anxiety and are not simply excessive worry about a real life situation.[1]

A compulsion is defined as a repetitive behavior or mental act generally performed in response to an obsession. The most common compulsions involve washing and cleaning, counting, checking, and requesting or demanding assurances. Diagnostically, compulsive behavior is not pleasurable and is designed to prevent discomfort or the occurrence of a dreaded event that is often unknown. For example, many patients are obsessed with feelings of doubt (e.g., whether a door was left unlocked), causing them marked distress, and leading to repetitive checking (or compulsive behaviors). These behaviors are usually performed according to certain rules or in a stereotyped fashion. The individual recognizes compulsions as senseless. Because patients recognize their behavior as silly, they become extremely adept at denying symptoms, disguising their rituals, and concealing their illness from friends and family.[1]

Patients with OCD often have comorbid depression, anxiety disorders, and alcohol abuse or dependence.[18] It is a chronic illness in most patients, with severity of symptoms varying in intensity over time. Many patients with OCD have significantly impaired QOL and ability to function.[18]

▶ TREATMENT: Posttraumatic Stress Disorder

▦ DESIRED OUTCOME

1 The short-term goal of therapy in the management of PTSD is reduction in core symptoms (i.e., intrusive re-experiencing, avoidance, and hyperarousal). Patients should also have improvements in disability, comorbid conditions, and QOL. The long-term goal in PTSD is remission.[19]

▦ GENERAL APPROACH TO TREATMENT

In general, patients who seek treatment acutely after a trauma and are in intense distress should receive therapy based on their presenting symptoms (e.g., a nonbenzodiazepine hypnotic for difficulty sleeping). Short courses of cognitive behavioral therapy (CBT) can be helpful. If symptoms (e.g., hyperarousal, avoidance, dissociation, sleep difficulties, or depressed mood) persist for 3 to 4 weeks and the patient experiences marked social, occupational, and/or interpersonal impairment, they should be treated with pharmacotherapy, psychotherapy, or both. Many patients with PTSD will improve substantially with pharmacotherapy but retain some symptoms. Treatment regimens usually combine psychoeducation, psychosocial support and/or treatment, and pharmacotherapy.[11]

▦ NONPHARMACOLOGIC THERAPY

Psychotherapy can be used when a patient suffers from mild symptoms, in patients who prefer not to use medications, or in conjunction with drugs in patients with severe symptoms to improve response.[11] Patients who have experienced trauma should be educated that they can experience anxiety, depression, nightmares, and even flashbacks as a normal reaction to the event.[11] Brief courses of CBT in close proximity to the traumatic event resulted in lower rates of PTSD

3 and 6 months later.[11] Single-session critical incident stress debriefing was not shown to be effective in preventing development of PTSD and actually may cause harm.[11]

2 Psychotherapies for treating PTSD include anxiety management (e.g., stress-inoculation training, relaxation training, biofeedback, distraction techniques), CBT (e.g., exposure therapy, cognitive processing therapy, and eye movement desensitization reprocessing), insight-oriented therapies (e.g., psychodynamic therapy, and hypnosis), and psychoeducation.[20,21] Short-term reductions in symptoms can be achieved with anxiety management, group therapy, hypnosis, or psychodynamic therapy.[20] Cognitive and behavioral approaches are the most effective nonpharmacologic methods to reduce symptoms of PTSD. Follow-up studies after a 3-month course of CBT demonstrated continued benefit for 3 to 12 months.[22] Psychoeducation includes information about the disease state, treatment options, and avoidance of excessive use of alcohol, nicotine, and other substances of abuse.

▦ PHARMACOLOGIC THERAPY

3 Antidepressants are the major pharmacotherapeutic treatment for PTSD. In addition to their efficacy in PTSD, these agents are also effective for comorbid depression and anxiety disorders. The selective serotonin reuptake inhibitors (SSRIs) are the first-line pharmacotherapy of PTSD. Other antidepressants (e.g., tricyclic antidepressants [TCAs] and monoamine oxidase inhibitors [MAOIs]) may also be effective, but they have less favorable side-effect profiles (Table 70–3). Sertraline and paroxetine are both approved for the acute treatment of PTSD,[24,25] and sertraline is approved for the long-term (i.e., 52 weeks) management of PTSD.[25] A number of drugs can be used as augmentation agents (e.g., anticonvulsants, antiadrenergic drugs, and antipsychotics).[21] Benzodiazepines are not effective in the management of PTSD.[23] Two practice guidelines[20,21] and two consensus statements for the treatment of PTSD are published.[11,21] An algorithm for the treatment of PTSD appears in Fig. 70–1.

TABLE 70–3. Antidepressants Used in the Treatment of Posttraumatic Stress Disorder

Class/Generic Name	Brand Name	Starting Dose	Dosage Range[a] (mg/day)
Selective serotonin reuptake inhibitors			
Citalopram[c]	Celexa	20 mg per day	20–40
Escitalopram	Lexapro	10 mg per day	10–20
Fluoxetine[c]	Prozac	10–20 mg per day	10–60
Fluvoxamine[c]	Luvox	50 mg per day	100–250
Paroxetine[c]	Paxil	10–20 mg per day	20–60[b]
Sertraline	Zoloft	25–50 mg per day	50–200[b]
Other agents			
Amitriptyline	Elavil	25–50 mg per day	75–200
Imipramine	Tofranil	25–50 mg per day	75–200
Lamotrigine	Lamictal	25 mg per day	50–500
Phenelzine	Nardil	15 mg every night	45–75

[a]Dosage used in clinical trials but not FDA-approved.
[b]Dosage is FDA-approved.
[c]Available generically.
Compiled from Ballenger et al,[11] The Expert Consensus Guideline Series,[21] Bandelow et al,[23] Paxil package insert,[24] and Zoloft package insert.[25]

SPECIAL POPULATIONS

Children who experience stress and trauma (e.g., sexual or physical abuse or loss of a parent) are predisposed to develop mood and anxiety disorders. The SSRIs are the initial pharmacologic agents of choice in this patient population. Psychotherapy is also a treatment option (e.g., play therapy).[21,26]

ANTIDEPRESSANT THERAPY

Selective Serotonin Reuptake Inhibitors

The SSRIs act pharmacologically to enhance serotonergic functioning. Large prospective studies documented the efficacy of sertraline and paroxetine in the acute management of PTSD. In a 12-week trial sertraline (mean dose 146 mg/day) was effective across the spectrum of PTSD-specific, global, and functional outcome measures. About 60% of the patients improved on symptom clusters of arousal and avoidance/numbing but not on re-experiencing.[27] Sixty percent of patients with PTSD receiving a paroxetine dose of 20 mg/day and 54% of patients receiving 40 mg/day responded; response was not related to dose.[28] In a flexible-dose trial, paroxetine significantly improved all three PTSD symptom clusters and disability compared with placebo at 12 weeks.[29] Fluoxetine showed efficacy in a placebo-controlled trial,[30] and fluvoxamine was efficacious in an open trial in acute PTSD.[31] In a comparison between sertraline and citalopram, PTSD symptoms improved significantly in both groups, but sertraline was significantly better in reducing avoidance/numbing than citalopram.[32] In general, the SSRIs reduced the numbing symptoms of PTSD, whereas other drugs have not. Adverse reactions reported in patients with PTSD treated with SSRIs include gastrointestinal symptoms, sexual dysfunction, insomnia, and agitation.

The results of two long-term trials indicate that sertraline (12 months) and fluoxetine (9 months) were effective in preventing relapse.[30,33] Sertraline also improved QOL compared with placebo.[33]

Other Antidepressants

The TCAs amitriptyline and imipramine and the MAOI phenelzine can be considered second- or third-line antidepressants if therapeutic

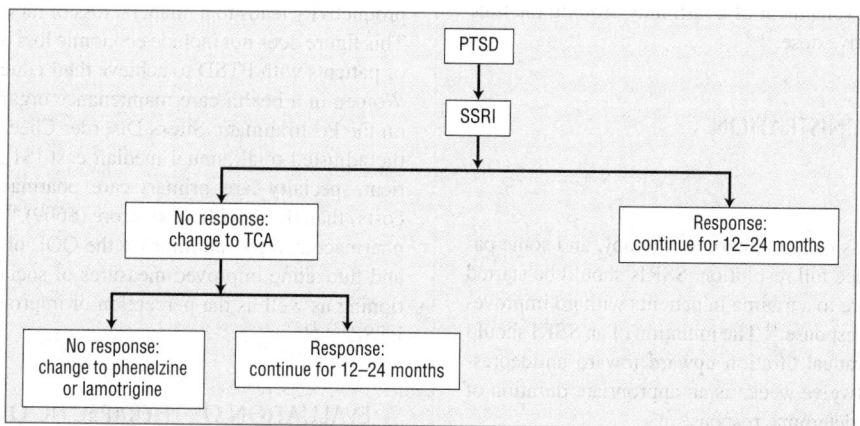

FIGURE 70–1. Algorithm for the pharmacotherapy of posttraumatic stress disorder. (Adapted from Ballenger et al[11] and Bandelow et al.[23])

trials of SSRIs have failed. Phenelzine decreased insomnia, nightmares, and flashbacks, and may be an alternative for patients who do not respond to SSRIs. TCAs are associated with a higher burden of adverse effects compared with SSRIs (e.g., daytime drowsiness, toxicity in overdose, and poor compliance).[21,23]

Other antidepressants have been studied in open-label trials. Trazodone and mirtazapine decreased some symptoms of PTSD.[34,35] Patients with PTSD who used trazodone in the past reported that it helped to relieve nightmares.[34] The sedating effect of trazodone is used frequently to treat insomnia induced by SSRIs. Mirtazepine was effective on global ratings of symptoms in 64% of patients with PTSD in doses up to 45 mg/day.[35] Venlafaxine improved PTSD symptom severity and global assessment of functioning in five refugees.[36] Although bupropion decreased symptoms of depression and hyperarousal, most PTSD symptoms were unchanged.[37] Patients who have failed therapy with other drugs may respond to a trial of nefazodone,[38] but the risk of hepatotoxicity must be considered.

ALTERNATIVE DRUG TREATMENTS

Mood stabilizers can be used as augmentation therapy in cases of partial response to antidepressant therapy, especially those with prominent irritability or anger.[21] Anticonvulsants (thought to exert their mechanism in part through antikindling effects) have been effective in treating PTSD. In a retrospective review topiramate reduced nightmares and flashbacks.[39] Divalproex sodium was effective in an open trial.[40]

Prazosin, an α_1-adrenergic antagonist, decreased nightmares and sleep disturbances, and improved the core PTSD symptoms in daily doses of 1 to 4 mg. Its presumed mechanism of action is reduction of noradrenergic transmission.[41]

Initial case reports of risperidone's improvement in aggressive behavior, hyperarousal, and flashbacks has led to further investigation into the adjunctive use of atypical antipsychotics in refractory PTSD.[42] Quetiapine (mean dose 100 mg/day; range, 25 to 300 mg/day) reduced core PTSD symptoms over a 6-week period when added to current therapy.[43] Olanzapine (mean dose 15 mg/day) added adjunctively to SSRIs decreased PTSD symptoms and significantly improved sleep compared with placebo. Patients gained an average of 13.2 pounds over the course of the 8-week trial.[44]

Anticonvulsants can be useful in some patients with PTSD. The response rate for patients receiving lamotrigine was twice that of patients receiving placebo (50% and 25%, respectively) over an 8-week period.[45] However, the slow dosage escalation of lamotrigine needed to avoid the development of a rash may prolong the time required to reach an effective dose.[23]

DOSAGE AND ADMINISTRATION

Acute Phase

PTSD symptoms respond slowly to pharmacotherapy, and some patients may never experience full resolution. SSRIs should be started 3 to 4 weeks after exposure to a trauma in patients with no improvement in their acute stress response.[11] The initiation of an SSRI should be at a low dose with gradual titration upward toward antidepressant doses. Eight to twelve weeks is an appropriate duration of antidepressant therapy to determine response.[21]

The initial dose of sertraline is 25 mg given once daily, with an increase to 50 mg/day after 1 week. The dose can be increased in weekly intervals by 50 mg/day up to a maximum dosage of 200 mg/day. Paroxetine can be initiated at 20 mg/day and increased by 10 mg/day in weekly intervals to a target dose of 40 mg/day and a maximum dosage of 60 mg/day. The initial dose of phenelzine is 15 mg given in the evening, and the dose is titrated to 45 to 60 mg/day. Dietary precautions must be followed and drug interactions carefully avoided to prevent hypertensive crisis. The dosing of other antidepressants is shown in Table 70–3.

Continuation Phase

Many patients may be undergoing psychotherapy during the continuation phase of therapy, and dosages can vary as patients deal with past traumatic experiences. During this phase symptoms continue to improve, and the maximal drug benefit (i.e., improvement of disability) accrues. Patients who responded to fluoxetine after 3 months of treatment continued to improve at 15 months.[46] Clinical response at 3 months was identified as a predictor of long-term outcome.[46]

Maintenance and Discontinuation

Patients with PTSD who respond to pharmacotherapy should continue treatment for at least 12 months.[21,23] If residual symptoms persist, drug therapy should be continued for at least 24 months.[21] The decision about when to discontinue therapy is based on response to therapy, presence of ongoing stresses, and adverse effects.[21] The patient must be confident in the discontinuation plan and requires extra support throughout the process. Drug therapy should be withdrawn and tapered slowly over a period of at least 1 month to reduce the potential for relapse.[21]

> ### CLINICAL CONTROVERSY
>
> The sequence of antidepressant use in PTSD after the first trial of SSRIs fails is controversial. It is not known if a second trial of a different SSRI should be undertaken or if an antidepressant of a different class should be used.

PHARMACOECONOMIC CONSIDERATIONS

PTSD compares with depression in the level of disability it imposes on patients with the disorder.[47] Individuals fail to realize their potentials for career development, marriage, and education. Decreased productivity leads to a financial loss of more than $3 billion per year. This figure does not include economic loss associated with the failure of patients with PTSD to achieve their educational or career goals.[47] Women in a health care maintenance organization with high scores on the Posttraumatic Stress Disorder Checklist had more than twice the adjusted total annual median cost ($1,283) of care (i.e., outpatient, specialty care, primary care, pharmacy and mental health care costs) than those with a low score ($609).[48] Treatment with effective pharmacotherapy can improve the QOL of these patients. Sertraline and fluoxetine improved measures of social and occupational functioning as well as the perception of improved QOL in patients with PTSD.[34,49]

EVALUATION OF THERAPEUTIC OUTCOMES

During the acute phase of therapy, patients should be seen weekly for a month and then every other week.[21] During months 3 to 6 of therapy, the patient can be seen monthly. In months 6 to 12 of therapy, visits can be extended to every 1 to 2 months. After a year of pharmacotherapy patients can be seen every 3 months. The patient should be asked about target symptoms of PTSD as well as other symptoms including sleep, anger outbursts, irritability, and disability.[21] The patient should maintain a diary to record the date and presence of symptoms of re-experiencing, avoidance behavior, and hyperarousal, as well as comorbid conditions (e.g., panic attacks, obsessions and compulsions, or suicidal ideation). A remission or good response in patients with PTSD is defined as a greater than 75% reduction in symptoms and response maintained for at least 3 months. Patients who have a 25% to 75% reduction in symptoms are considered partial responders.

Patients who are nonresponsive to therapy have less than 25% reduction in symptoms.[21] Before deciding that a patient is not responsive to pharmacotherapy, the clinician should ensure that the medication trial has been adequate in both dose and duration.[21] Use of an objective measurement of remission of PTSD (e.g., a Treatment Outcome PTSD Scale [TOPS-8] score ≤ 5 and a Sheehan Disability Scale ≤ 1 on each item) can assist in the evaluation of drug response.[19]

Many patients with PTSD are sensitive to the adverse effects of drugs. They should be monitored carefully for adverse reactions that may delay the escalation of drug dosages or cause the patient distress. When pharmacotherapy is discontinued, patients should be seen more frequently and monitored carefully for signs of relapse or withdrawal.

► TREATMENT: Obsessive-Compulsive Disorder

▓ DESIRED OUTCOMES

Goals of therapy for OCD include reduction in the frequency of obsessive thoughts and in the time spent performing compulsive acts and reduction in the degree of anxiety. Treatment for OCD may not completely eliminate obsessions or compulsions, but patients may feel remarkably improved with partial resolution of their symptoms. Treatment should provide the patient with an optimal level of psychosocial and occupational functioning and an overall improved QOL. Efforts should be made to minimize adverse drug events and prevent drug interactions.

▓ GENERAL APPROACH TO TREATMENT

It is important at the outset of therapy to identify and document the specific target symptoms for pharmacotherapy. Rating scales may be used to measure symptom severity, and a baseline determination is indicated if these tools are used (e.g., Leyton Obsessional Inventory, Symptom Check List 90-OC, and the National Institutes of Mental Health Global Scale). The most widely used scale is the Yale-Brown Obsessive Compulsive Scale (YBOCS).[50,51]

The Food and Drug Administration (FDA) has approved five antidepressants for the management of OCD: clomipramine, fluoxetine, fluvoxamine, paroxetine, and sertraline. In adolescents with OCD, CBT is generally selected first for mild OCD, but CBT plus an SSRI (e.g., fluoxetine, fluvoxamine, sertraline, or paroxetine) are used for more severe OCD. In adults, CBT is the initial choice for mild OCD, and CBT plus an SSRI or an SSRI alone is selected for more severe OCD. Figure 70–2 is an algorithm for the treatment of OCD.

▓ NONPHARMACOLOGIC TREATMENTS

CBT is the treatment of choice for mild OCD in both adolescents and adults. In the management of OCD, CBT involves exposure plus response prevention combined with cognitive therapy. When available, CBT should be offered to every OCD patient.[52] Exposure involves having the patient perform actions that were formerly avoided. For instance, if a patient avoided touching the flush handle on a bathroom toilet, exposure would involve holding onto the handle. Response

prevention involves having the patient resist the compulsive rituals that are performed. The ritualistic washing behavior often associated with a contamination obsession might be the focus: the patient would be asked to delay the washing behavior as long as possible. At the beginning of CBT treatment patients are often unable to perform these activities, and imaginal exposure is used as the first step in the treatment process. Over time in a gradual manner the patient is exposed to feared objects/activities and is trained to resist rituals for longer periods of time.

Two-thirds to three-fourths of patients who continue in CBT therapy generally respond.[54] CBT should be added to the regimen when a patient is a nonresponder or a partial responder to SSRI or clomipramine monotherapy. CBT should be used alone if the patient is intolerant to adverse drug effects, is pregnant, or has a medical condition that contraindicates medication.[52] Behavioral therapy appears to have stronger effects on compulsive rituals than for the associated obsessions.

Exposure and response prevention therapies have longer-lasting effects after discontinuation and produce greater improvement compared with drug therapy.[55] Techniques such as teaching patients to prevent relapse through self-exposure and self-imposed ritual prevention are suggested to foster optimal nonpharmacologic therapy.[55] Exposure with response prevention is particularly helpful for contamination or other fears, symmetry rituals, counting/repeating, hoarding, and aggressive urges. Cognitive therapy is beneficial for scrupulosity, moral guilt, and pathologic doubt. Thirteen to twenty sessions are typically required to treat uncomplicated OCD.[52]

A major barrier to the application of nonpharmacologic therapy is availability of treatment. CBT requires specific training. Many psychiatrists are not adequately trained and/or do not have the time or desire necessary to apply this therapy. Psychologists and social workers may have skills in this discipline; however, the availability of their services is often restricted in certain areas.

▓ PHARMACOLOGIC THERAPY

The Expert Consensus Panel report reflects the most recent comprehensive opinions of a large number of leading authorities in the field of OCD treatment.[52] The SSRIs are considered to be the drugs of choice in the treatment of OCD. Drug therapy is reserved for patients with moderate to severe symptoms. Antidepressants may be combined with CBT or used alone in adults with moderate to severe symptoms. An SSRI should be added when there has been no response or partial response to CBT alone. Generally, an SSRI is selected

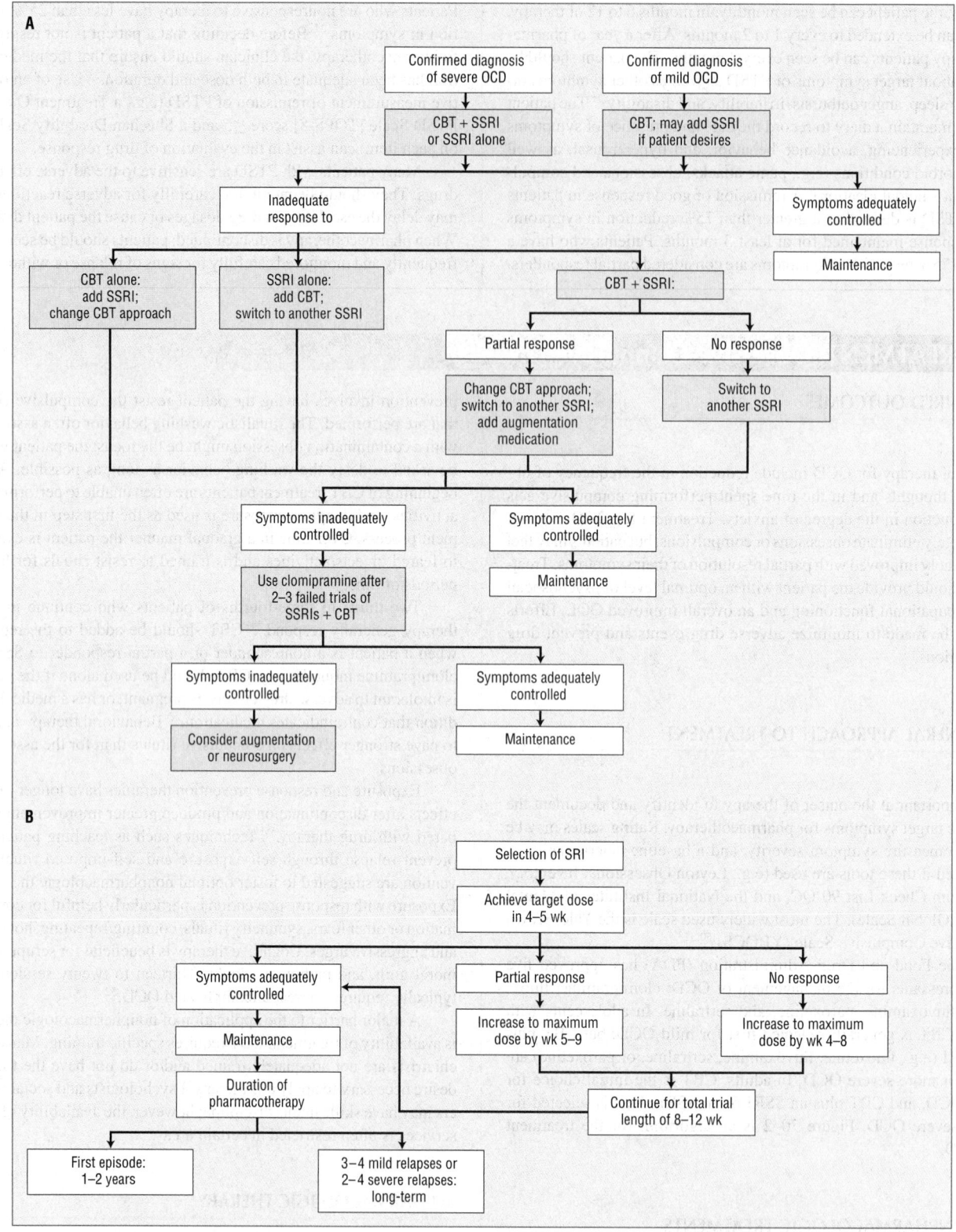

FIGURE 70–2. Algorithm for management of obsessive-compulsive disorder in adults. *A.* Overall approach to treatment. *B.* Pharmacotherapeutic approach to treatment. CBT, cognitive behavioral therapy; SSRI, selective serotonin reuptake inhibitor. (Derived from Expert Consensus Panel for Obsessive-Compulsive Disorder[52] and American Pharmaceutical Association.[53])

before clomipramine, and whenever anticholinergic, cardiovascular, sexual, sedative, or weight gain adverse effects are a major concern. If one SSRI is ineffective, then another SSRI should be tried. Treatment resistance can be defined as failure to achieve at least a 25% reduction in baseline scores on the YBOCS.[18,52] Clomipramine may be selected after two to three failed SSRI trials. Clomipramine can be used to augment an SSRI in partially responsive or nonresponsive patients.[52]

SPECIAL POPULATIONS

Children and Adolescents

Clomipramine, fluvoxamine, sertraline, and fluoxetine are approved by the FDA for treatment of OCD in children and adolescents.[56] Childhood and adult OCD appear to respond similarly to drug therapy. The SSRIs appear to be effective and well tolerated in treatment of OCD in children and are generally considered first-line agents.[57] Treatment with an SSRI produces a favorable response in 75% of children and adolescents with OCD. A combination of SSRIs and CBT is preferred in most cases.[58] In children, the most commonly described side effects of SSRI therapy include nausea, headache, tremor, gastrointestinal complaints, drowsiness, akathisia, insomnia, disinhibition, and agitation.[58] Clomipramine was significantly better than placebo in the treatment of OCD in children and adolescents, with 75% of patients having a moderate to marked improvement.[59] Clomipramine was also more effective than desipramine in children and adolescents.[60]

Hepatic and Renal Disease

Clomipramine, fluoxetine, sertraline, paroxetine, fluvoxamine, and citalopram are extensively metabolized in the liver, and patients with significant liver disease should be prescribed these drugs cautiously and in lower doses than those used in healthy subjects. The pharmacokinetics of fluoxetine and fluvoxamine were similar in patients with renal failure and in healthy subjects; however, the manufacturer recommends starting with a lower dose in patients with renal impairment. The pharmacokinetics of sertraline are not altered in patients with significant renal dysfunction, and dosage adjustment is not necessary in these patients.[25] Increased plasma concentrations of paroxetine occur in subjects with renal impairment.[26] The initial dose of paroxetine should be reduced in patients with severe renal impairment, and upward titration should occur more slowly.[26] No dosage adjustment is necessary for patients with mild to moderate renal impairment receiving citalopram.

Elderly

Little information is available on treating OCD in the elderly. Case reports and anecdotal information suggest that the antiobsessional drugs are likely to be equally effective in the elderly and in younger adults.[61] Selection of medication for an elderly person with OCD, however, should be based on history of response and adverse side-effect profile. Treatment should be initiated with low doses in elderly patients, and doses should be increased slowly, with vigilance for emergence of side effects. Some elderly patients may ultimately require doses similar to those used in younger adults, but doses must be individualized according to response and tolerance of side effects.

In elderly patients refractory to SSRIs, an augmentation strategy with minimal risk is to add buspirone to SSRI therapy. The use of clonazepam should be avoided because of the potential for excess sedation, particularly in frail elderly patients and those with gait disturbances.[62] Because of clomipramine's sedative and anticholinergic side effects, it is not usually chosen as first-line therapy for elderly OCD patients.[62]

The multiple-dose elimination half-life of fluvoxamine was 17.4 and 25.9 hours in the elderly as compared to 13.6 and 15.6 hours in younger subjects at steady state for 50- and 100-mg doses, respectively.[63] The safety of fluvoxamine has not been adequately studied in the elderly and patients with cardiovascular disease. Dosage should be titrated slowly during initiation of fluvoxamine therapy in elderly patients.

Sertraline plasma clearance in elderly patients was approximately 40% lower than in a group of younger individuals. Clearance of desmethylsertraline was also decreased in elderly men but not in elderly women.[25]

In a multiple-dose study in the elderly, the minimal concentrations of paroxetine were 70% to 80% greater than in nonelderly subjects. The manufacturer recommends that the initial dose be reduced in the elderly (10 mg/day), and total daily doses should not exceed 40 mg.[24]

Pregnancy

In general, CBT alone should be used for pregnant patients except in cases in which the risks of untreated OCD outweigh the risks of drug use (e.g., a pregnant woman who will not eat because of contamination fears).[52] Women with a history of OCD should be informed that OCD may worsen during pregnancy and during the postpartum period. OCD symptoms may exacerbate during the first trimester, especially if pharmacotherapy is discontinued just before conception or early in pregnancy. Symptoms often improve during the second trimester and worsen during the third trimester. The use of SSRIs in pregnancy and lactation is discussed in the chapter on depression (Chap. 67).

If drug therapy during pregnancy is required, fluoxetine appears to be the safest choice. However, the neurobehavioral effects of prenatal exposure on the neonate and the child have not been fully elucidated. Clomipramine should be avoided during pregnancy.[64] Clonazepam can be considered for OCD symptoms in pregnant women with disabling anxiety, but with higher doses (2 to 5 mg/day), hypotonia, apnea, and failure to feed have been observed in newborns.[64]

ANTIDEPRESSANT THERAPY

Serotonergic Antidepressants

The only medications consistently demonstrating efficacy in controlled trials are the TCA clomipramine and the SSRIs fluoxetine, fluvoxamine, paroxetine, and sertraline. Sixty-five to seventy percent of patients with OCD respond to their first SSRI treatment, and up to 90% ultimately respond with additional drug trials. Improvement in symptoms is incomplete, and ranges from 25% to 60%. Most patients continue to have symptoms that limit their functioning.[56] Obsessive-compulsive symptoms improve over a 4- to 10-week treatment period.[65]

Current evidence indicates that 5-HT is important for the antiobsessional effects of medication. The SSRIs and clomipramine inhibit

5-HT reuptake into the presynaptic neuron. Inhibiting reuptake of 5-HT makes more 5-HT available to postsynaptic receptors and reduces formation of the 5-HT metabolite 5-hydroxyindoleacetic acid. Although other antidepressants, such as imipramine and amitriptyline, inhibit 5-HT reuptake, they are less potent and selective than the SSRIs and clomipramine. Prolonged exposure to increased amounts of 5-HT after chronic antidepressant treatment (2 to 3 weeks) leads to altered responsiveness of postsynaptic 5-HT receptors or presynaptic autoregulatory receptors that govern 5-HT release in specific brain regions.[65]

The most impressive and consistent evidence supporting a role for 5-HT in treating OCD is that only potent 5-HT reuptake inhibitors appear to be effective. Furthermore, an improvement in obsessional symptoms may correlate with plasma concentrations of clomipramine but not desmethylclomipramine, the metabolite of clomipramine with less selectivity for 5-HT reuptake inhibition. With clomipramine treatment, the decrease in obsessional symptoms correlates with a decrease in the concentration of 5-hydroxyindoleacetic acid in cerebrospinal fluid, and a decrease in platelet 5-HT content. The effectiveness of serotonergic agents in treating OCD lends support to the role of 5-HT in the etiology of OCD. However, because many patients fail to respond to these agents, the role of other neurotransmitter systems in the pathophysiology of OCD must continue to be explored.

PHARMACOKINETICS

Clomipramine is rapidly absorbed following oral administration. Maximum plasma concentrations occur within 2 hours. It is highly protein-bound (>90%) in the blood and has a half-life of 19 to 37 hours.[63] The drug is metabolized to desmethylclomipramine, which is pharmacologically active.[63] The pharmacokinetics of the SSRIs are discussed in Chapter 67.

EFFICACY

In a 10-week randomized study of 31 patients treated with fluvoxamine, paroxetine, or citalopram, there was no significant difference between treatments in antiobsessional effects.[66] Clomipramine was equivalent in efficacy when compared with fluoxetine or fluvoxamine.[59] A meta-analysis supported the superiority of clomipramine over fluoxetine, fluvoxamine, and sertraline.[67] Six of seven head-to-head comparisons of either fluoxetine, fluvoxamine, or paroxetine versus clomipramine found similar efficacy, but with a lower incidence of side effects with the SSRI.[73]

Most experts agree that the SSRIs are better tolerated than clomipramine.[52] The SSRIs are less likely to cause cardiovascular, sedative, anticholinergic, and weight gain side effects. Clomipramine is less likely than the SSRIs to cause insomnia, akathisia, nausea, and diarrhea. Side effects may be more severe when larger doses are used and with faster dose escalation. Tolerance to adverse effects often develops over 6 to 8 weeks of treatment, and tolerance is more likely to develop to nausea, diarrhea, sedation, diminished libido and/or orgasm, anxiety, restlessness, insomnia, and anticholinergic side effects than to akathisia.[52]

Other Antidepressants

Venlafaxine, which acts as a serotonin and norepinephrine reuptake inhibitor, may be effective for OCD. In an open-label naturalistic trial, venlafaxine was studied in 39 patients with OCD (with 29 of the group being treatment resistant). Sixty-nine percent responded as rated by the Clinical Global Impressions-Improvement scale.[69] In a double-blind switch study of paroxetine and venlafaxine using the YBOCS as a measurement of severity, 37 of 75 patients receiving venlafaxine were initial responders. However, in the switch phase open to nonresponders, only 3 patients out of 16 responded. In this study phase paroxetine was found to be more efficacious than venlafaxine.[70]

ALTERNATIVE DRUG TREATMENTS

If there is no response or partial response to combined CBT and three antidepressant trials (one of which is clomipramine), augmentation with another drug and more intensive CBT can be tried. 5-HT enhancers and agents involving other neurotransmitter systems can be initiated, but controlled augmentation trials have been disappointing. Because of this disparity in results, it is suggested that attempts at augmentation be conducted with the use of rating scales or careful symptom severity assessment so that the benefit of the added drug therapy is clearly evident. Controlled studies of lithium or buspirone augmentation of clomipramine or fluvoxamine failed to demonstrate improvement in OCD symptoms.[71] When buspirone is used as augmentation therapy, the initial dose is 5 mg three times daily, and the target dose should be 60 to 90 mg/day.[52] In a randomized open-label trial, citalopram (40 mg/day) plus clomipramine (150 mg/day) was more effective in refractory patients than was citalopram alone.[7] These are preliminary findings that await confirmation in a larger double-blind trial.[72]

DA receptor antagonists alone are not effective in the treatment of the core symptoms of OCD. In an open-case series of 17 fluvoxamine nonresponders, 88% of patients with comorbid tic disorder diagnose responded after pimozide was added and 22% of patients without these comorbid diagnoses responded.[73] The recommended initial dose of pimozide is 0.5 mg, and the target dose is 1 to 6 mg/day. Pimozide can cause cardiovascular problems, and it should not be used concurrently with clomipramine.[52] Haloperidol was significantly more effective than placebo in reducing obsessive-compulsive symptoms. Furthermore, those with a concurrent chronic tic disorder demonstrated a preferential response to the fluvoxamine-haloperidol combination.[7] The recommended initial dose of haloperidol is 0.5 mg, and the target dose is 0.25 to 6 mg/day.[52] Patients should be nonresponsive to at least two antidepressant trials (including clomipramine) before haloperidol is tried because of the risk of tardive dyskinesia and other movement disorders with long-term use.[71]

Results of low-dose risperidone (0.5 to 2 mg/day) added to antidepressant therapy in refractory patients are encouraging. Treatment response over 6 weeks was rapid and consistent.[71] An additional 8-week, open-label study reported that 50% of patients previously unresponsive to clomipramine responded after risperidone 3 mg/day was added. The recommended initial dose of risperidone is 0.25 mg, and the target dose is 0.5 to 5 mg/day.[52] Thirty-six patients unresponsive to antidepressants were given risperidone, up to 6 mg/day, or placebo in a double-blind trial. Risperidone treatment resulted in a significant reduction in YBOCS scores.[74] In an open-label trial of olanzapine augmentation of SSRIs for 8 weeks, most patients experienced complete or partial remission in doses of 1.25 to 20 mg/day.[75]

Dosage and Administration

Table 70–4 summarizes dosing guidelines for the SSRIs and clomipramine. If there is inadequate response to an average dose, then

TABLE 70–4. Dosing of Selective Serotonin Reuptake Inhibitors in Treatment of OCD

Generic Name	Usual Initial Daily Dose (mg)	Usual Daily Dosage Range (mg)	Average Target Daily Dose (mg)
Citalopram[a]	20	20–60	40
Clomipramine	10	100–250	150–200
Fluoxetine	20	20–80	40–60
Fluvoxamine	50	100–300	200
Paroxetine	20	20–60	40
Sertraline	50	75–200	150

[a]Not FDA-approved for treatment of OCD. Optimal dosing guidelines are not well established.
Modified from Expert Consensus Panel for Obsessive-Compulsive Disorder.[52]

it should be incrementally increased to the maximum dose within 4 to 9 weeks from the start of treatment. If there is an inadequate response after 4 to 6 weeks at the maximum dose, then another SSRI should be tried. Eight to thirteen weeks is considered an adequate trial before changing to another drug or augmenting with another agent.

After patients have responded to the acute phase of treatment, treatment gains are maintained with maintenance-phase ◀❽ strategies. Monthly follow-up visits are recommended for at least 3 to 6 months, and a medication taper can be considered after 1 to 2 years of treatment. Medication should not be rapidly discontinued, and booster CBT sessions may reduce the risk of relapse when medication is withdrawn. The drug dosage can be decreased by 25%, and then 2 months should lapse before again decreasing the dose, ◀❾ depending on response. Long-term or lifelong prophylaxis with pharmacotherapy is recommended after two to three severe relapses or three to four mild relapses.[52] Although the appropriate maintenance dose of SSRIs is unknown, it is notable that one investigator was successful in reducing the dose of clomipramine from a mean of 270 mg/day to 165 mg/day in the maintenance phase. Mundo and colleagues studied patients successfully treated with clomipramine or fluvoxamine and reduced their doses by 33 to 66% for maintenance therapy. They found that the maintenance therapy was successful with reduced dosages of the antiobsessional drug, with clear advantages for tolerability and compliance. However, study duration was only 102 days.[76]

CLINICAL CONTROVERSY

The role of atypical antipsychotics as adjunctive agents in managing treatment-resistant OCD is controversial, especially in view of the documentation that the addition of an atypical agent may also precipitate or worsen OCD symptoms. Most clinicians use the atypical antipsychotics cautiously as an add-on to antidepressant therapy in nonresponding or partially responding patients, especially those with concurrent tic disorder.

▓ PHARMACOECONOMIC CONSIDERATIONS

The annual outpatient direct costs for patients seeking treatment for OCD in the United States in 1995 were $5.1 billion. Aggregate inappropriate treatment costs were up to $2.4 billion.[75] In 1990, the total cost to the economy was $8 billion, which includes expenditures for direct ($2.1 billion) and indirect costs. Direct costs include costs of hospitalization, outpatient professional services, and drugs. Indirect costs include costs associated with lost productivity, work loss, early retirement, and absenteeism. As OCD frequently has its onset in childhood or adolescence, loss of income over a lifetime is substantial.[77]

▓ EVALUATION OF THERAPEUTIC OUTCOMES

Target symptoms of OCD should be monitored closely. The degree of response may indicate a need to modify dosage, change drug, or augment therapy. Rating scales can be used to monitor symptom response to therapy for OCD. The clinician should inquire about and address problematic adverse effects (including the emergence of suicidal ideation) reported by the patient. Drug interactions should be monitored. Changes in social and occupational functioning should be assessed.

Patients older than 40 years of age should receive a pretreatment electrocardiogram before starting clomipramine. In patients with liver disease, baseline and periodic liver function tests are recommended when clomipramine is used. If clomipramine is given concurrently with sympatholytic antihypertensive agents, blood pressure should be regularly monitored. Patients receiving clomipramine who develop fever and sore throat should have leukocyte and differential white blood cell counts assessed to evaluate for agranulocytosis.

CONCLUSIONS

The past five years have brought a renewed interest in the recognition and management of PTSD. Health care workers are sensitized to the devastating effects that PTSD can have on patients' functioning, QOL, and use of health care resources. Adequately detecting and appropriately managing PTSD is important to improving the lives of patients who suffer from this chronic illness. Data on the efficacy of the SSRIs supports their use for both acute and long-term management of the symptoms of PTSD. The SSRIs are the first-line pharmacotherapy of PTSD and OCD. Research in OCD has resulted in new pharmacologic treatment strategies, especially with augmentation therapies.

ABBREVIATIONS

ASD: acute stress disorder
CBT: cognitive behavioral therapy
DA: dopamine
5-HT: serotonin
GABA: γ-aminobutyric acid
HPA: hypothalamic-pituitary-adrenal axis
MAOI: monoamine oxidase inhibitor
NE: norepinephrine
OCD: obsessive-compulsive disorder
PTSD: posttraumatic stress disorder
QOL: quality of life
SSRI: selective serotonin reuptake inhibitor
TCA: tricyclic antidepressant
VPFC: ventral prefrontal cortex
YBOCS: Yale-Brown Obsessive Compulsive Scale

Review Questions and other resources can be found at *www.pharmacotherapyonline.com.*

REFERENCES

1. American Psychiatric Association. Diagnostic and Statistical Manual of Mental Disorders, Fourth Edition, Text Revision. Washington, American Psychiatric Association, 2000:429–484.
2. Lecrubier Y. Posttraumatic stress disorder in primary care: A hidden diagnosis. J Clin Psychiatry 2004;65(Suppl 1):49–54.
3. Murray CJL, Lopez AD, eds. Global Burden of Disease: A Comprehensive Assessment of Mortality and Disability for Diseases, Injuries, and Risk Factors in 1990 and Projected to 2020, Vol. 1. Cambridge, MA: Harvard University Press, World Health Organization, 1996:1–43.
4. Stein DJ. Neurobiology of the obsessive-compulsive spectrum disorders. Biol Psychiatry 2000;47:296–304.
5. Narrow WE, Rae DS, Robins LN, Reigier DA. Revised prevalence estimates of mental disorders in the United States: Using a clinical significance criterion to reconcile 2 surveys' estimates. Arch Gen Psychiatry 2002;59: 115–123.
6. Yehuda R. Risk and resilience in posttraumatic stress disorder. J Clin Psychiatry 2004;65(Suppl 1):29–36.
7. Grinage BD. Diagnosis and management of post-traumatic stress disorder. Am Fam Physician 2003;68:2401–2408.
8. Pato MT, Schindler KM, Pato CN. The genetics of obsessive-compulsive disorder. Curr Psychiatry Rep 2001;3:163–168.
9. Rosenberg DR, Keshavan MS. Toward a neurodevelopmental model of obsessive-compulsive disorder. Biol Psychiatry 1998;43:623–640.
10. Leonard HL, Topol D, Bukstein O, et al. Clonazepam as an augmenting agent in the treatment of childhood-onset obsessive-compulsive disorder. J Am Acad Child Adolesc Psychiatry 1994;33:792–794.
11. Ballenger JC, Davidson JRT, Lecrubier Y, et al. Consensus statement update on posttraumatic stress disorder from the International Consensus Group on Depression and Anxiety. J Clin Psychiatry 2004;65(Suppl 1): 55–62.
12. Stein DJ, Allen A, Bobes J, Eisen JL, et al. Quality of life in obsessive-compulsive disorder. CNS Spectr 2000;5(Suppl 4):37–39.
13. Nutt DJ. The psychobiology of posttraumatic stress disorder. J Clin Psychiatry 2000;61(Suppl 5):24–29.
14. Kent JM, Mathew SJ, Gorman JM. Molecular targets in the treatment of anxiety. Biol Psychiatry 2002;52:1008–1030.
15. Nutt DJ, Malizia AL. Structural and functional brain changes in posttraumatic stress disorder. J Clin Psychiatry 2004;65(Suppl 1):11–17.
16. Hull AM. Neuroimaging findings in posttraumatic stress disorder: Systematic review. Br J Psychiatry 2002;181:102–110.
17. Taber KH, Rauch SL, Lanius RA, Hurley RA. Functional magnetic resonance imaging: Applications to posttraumatic stress disorder. J Neuropsychiatry Clin Neurosci 2003;15:125–129.
18. Jenike MA. Obsessive-compulsive disorder. N Engl J Med 2004;350: 259–265.
19. Doyle AC, Pollack MH. Establishment of remission criteria for anxiety disorders. J Clin Psychiatry 2003;64(Suppl 15):40–45.
20. Work Group on ASD and PTSD. Practice guideline for the treatment of patients with acute stress disorder and posttraumatic stress disorder. Am J Psychiatry 2004;161(11 [suppl]):1–61.
21. The Expert Consensus Guideline Series. Treatment of posttraumatic stress disorder. The Expert Consensus Panel for Posttraumatic Stress Disorder. J Clin Psychiatry 1999;60(Suppl 16):3–76.
22. Davidson JRT. Long-term treatment and prevention of posttraumatic stress disorder. J Clin Psychiatry 2004;65(Suppl 1):44–48.
23. Bandelow B, Zohar J, Hollander E, et al. Guidelines for the pharmacological treatment of anxiety, obsessive-compulsive and posttraumatic stress disorders. World J Biol Psychiatry 2002;3:171–199.
24. Paxil package insert. GlaxoSmithKline, Research Triangle Park, NC. August 2003.
25. Zoloft package insert. Pfizer, New York. September 2003.
26. Donnelly CL. Pharmacologic treatment approaches for children and adolescents with posttraumatic stress disorder 2003;12:251–269.
27. Brady K, Pearlstein T, Asnis GM, et al. Efficacy and safety of sertraline treatment of posttraumatic stress disorder: A randomized controlled trial. JAMA 2000;283:1837–1844.
28. Marshall RD, Beebe KL, Oldham M, Zaninelli R. Efficacy and safety of paroxetine treatment for chronic PTSD: A fixed-dose, placebo-controlled study. Am J Psychiatry 2001;158:1982–1988.
29. Tucker P, Zaninelli R, Yehuda R, et al. Paroxetine in the treatment of chronic posttraumatic stress disorder: Results of a placebo-controlled flexible-dosage trial. J Clin Psychiatry 2001;62:860–868.
30. Martenyi F, Brown EB, Zhang H, et al. Fluoxetine versus placebo in posttraumatic stress disorder. J Clin Psychiatry 2002;63:199–206.
31. Tucker P, Smith KL, Marx B, et al. Fluvoxamine reduces physiologic reactivity to trauma scripts in posttraumatic stress disorder. J Clin Psychiatry 2000;20:367–372.
32. Tucker P, Potter-Kimball R, Wyatt DB, et al. Can physiologic assessment and side effects tease out differences in PTSD trials? A double-blind comparison of citalopram, sertraline, and placebo. Psychopharmacol Bull 2003;37:135–149.
33. Davidson JRT, Pearlstein T, Londborg P, et al. Efficacy of sertraline in preventing relapse of posttraumatic stress disorder: Results of a 28-week double-blind, placebo-controlled study. Am J Psychiatry 2001;158:1974–1981.
34. Warner MD, Dorn MR, Peabody CA. Survey on the usefulness of trazodone in patients with PTSD with insomnia or nightmares. Pharmacopsychiatry 2001;34:128–131.
35. Davidson JRT, Weisler RH, Butterfield MI, et al. Mirtazapine vs. placebo in posttraumatic stress disorder: A pilot study. Biol Psychiatry 2003;53: 188–191.
36. Smajkic A, Weine S, Djueric-Bijedic Z, et al. Sertraline, paroxetine, and venlafaxine in refugee posttraumatic stress disorder with depression symptoms. J Traumatic Stress 2001;14:445–452.
37. Canive JM, Clark RD, Calais LA, et al. Bupropion treatment in veterans with posttraumatic stress disorder: An open study. J Clin Psychopharmacol 1998;18:379–383.
38. Zisook S, Chentsova-Dutton YE, Smith-Vaniz A, et al. Nefazodone in patients with treatment-refractory posttraumatic stress disorder. J Clin Psychiatry 2000;61:203–208.
39. Berlant J, van Kammen DP. Open-label topiramate as primary or adjunctive therapy in chronic civilian posttraumatic stress disorder: A preliminary report. J Clin Psychiatry 2002;63:15–20.
40. Clark RD, Canive JM, Calais LA, et al. Divalproex in posttraumatic stress disorder: An open-label clinical trial. J Trauma Stress 1999;12:395–401.
41. Raskind MA, Preskind ER, Kanter ED, et al. Reduction of nightmares and other PTSD symptoms in combat veterans by prazosin: A placebo-controlled study. Am J Psychiatry 2003;160:371–373.
42. Krashin D, Oates EW. Risperidone as an adjunct therapy for post-traumatic stress disorder. Mil Med 1999;164:605–606.
43. Hamner MB, Deitsch SE, Brodrick PS, et al. Quetiapine treatment in patients with posttraumatic stress disorder: An open trial of adjunctive therapy. J Clin Psychopharmacol 2003;23:15–20.
44. Stein MB, Kline NA, Matloff JL. Adjunctive olanzapine for SSRI-resistant combat-related PTSD: A double-blind, placebo-controlled study. Am J Psychiatry 2002;159:1777–1779.
45. Hertzberg MA, Butterfield MI, Feldman ME, et al. A preliminary study of lamotrigine for the treatment of posttraumatic stress disorder. Biol Psychiatry 1999;45:1226–1229.
46. Davidson JRT. Pharmacotherapy of posttraumatic stress disorder: Treatment options, long-term follow-up, and predictors of outcome. J Clin Psychiatry 2000;61(Suppl 5):52–56.
47. Friedman MJ, Davidson JRT, Mellman TA, Southwick SM. Pharmacotherapy. In: Foa EB, Keane TM, Friedman MJ, eds. Effective Treatments of Posttraumatic Stress Disorder. New York, Guilford Press, 2000:84–105.
48. Walker EA, Katon W, Russo J, et al. Health care costs associated with posttraumatic stress disorder symptoms in women. Arch Gen Psychiatry 2003; 60:369–374.
49. Malik ML, Connor KM, Sutherland SM, et al. Quality of life and PTSD: A pilot study assessing changes in SF-36 scores before and after treatment in a placebo-controlled trial of fluoxetine. J Trauma Stress 1999;12:387–393.
50. Kim SW, Dysken MW, Katz R. Rating scales for obsessive compulsive disorder. Psychiatr Ann 1989;192:74–79.
51. Goodman WK, Price LH, Rasmussen SA, et al. The Yale-Brown obsessive compulsive scale. Arch Gen Psychiatry 1989;46:1006–1011.

52. Expert Consensus Panel for Obsessive-Compulsive Disorder. Obsessive-compulsive disorder executive summary: Recommendations for first-line treatments by clinical situation. J Clin Psychiatry 1997;58(Suppl 4):2–72.

53. American Pharmaceutical Association. Management of obsessive-compulsive disorder. In: APhA Guide to Drug Treatment Protocols: A Resource for Creating and Using Disease-Specific Pathways. Washington, American Pharmaceutical Association, 1997:OCDi–OCDii.

54. Baer L. Behavior therapy for obsessive-compulsive disorder in the office-based practice. J Clin Psychiatry 1993;54(Suppl 6):10–15.

55. Marks I. Behavior therapy for obsessive-compulsive disorder: A decade of progress. Can J Psychiatry 1997;42:1021–1027.

56. Hollander E, Pallanti S. Current and experimental therapeutics of OCD. In: Davis KL, Charney D, Coyle JT, Nemeroff C, eds. Neuropsychopharmacology: The Fifth Generation of Progress. Philadelphia, Lippincott Williams & Wilkins, 2002:1647–1664.

57. King RA, Leonard H, March J, et al. Practice parameters for the assessment of children and adolescents with obsessive-compulsive disorder. J Am Acad Child Adolesc Psychiatry 1998;37(Suppl 10):27S–45S.

58. Thomsen PH. Obsessive-compulsive disorder: Pharmacologic treatment. Eur Child Adolesc Psychiatry 2000;9(Suppl 1):176–184.

59. Flament MF, Bisserbe JC. Pharmacologic treatment of obsessive-compulsive disorder: Comparative studies. J Clin Psychiatry 1997;58(Suppl 12):18–22.

60. Leonard HL, Swedo SE, Rapoport JL, et al. Treatment of obsessive compulsive disorder with clomipramine and despiramine in children and adolescents. Arch Gen Psychiatry 1989;46:1088–1092.

61. Sheikh JL, Salzman C. Anxiety in the elderly, Psychiatr Clin North Am 1995;18:871–883.

62. Pollard CA, Carmin CN, Ownby R. Obsessive-compulsive disorder in later life. In: Dickstein LJ, Riba MB, et al, eds. OCD across the life cycle. Section III of Review of Psychiatry, Vol. 16. Washington, American Psychiatric Press, 1997:57–72.

63. Luvox package insert. Solvay Pharmaceuticals, Marietta, GA, 2002.

64. Diaz SF, Grush LR, Sichel DA, Cohen LS. Obsessive-compulsive disorder in pregnancy and the puerperium. In: Dickstein LJ, Riba MB, et al, eds. OCD across the life cycle. Section III of Review of Psychiatry, Vol. 16. Washington, American Psychiatric Press, 1997:97–112.

65. Ellingrod VL. Pharmacotherapy of primary obsessive-compulsive disorder: Review of the literature. Pharmacotherapy 1998;18:936–960.

66. Mundo E, Bianchi L, Bellodi L. Efficacy of fluvoxamine, paroxetine, and citalopram in the treatment of obsessive-compulsive disorder. J Clin Psychopharmacol 1997;17:267–271.

67. Greist JH, Jefferson JW, Kobah KA, et al. Efficacy and tolerability of serotonin transport inhibitors in obsessive-compulsive disorder. Arch Gen Psychiatry 1995;52:53–60.

68. Pigott TA, Seay SM. A review of the efficacy of selective serotonin reuptake inhibitors in obsessive-compulsive disorder. J Clin Psychiatry 1999;60:101–106.

69. Hollander E, Friedberg J, Wasserman AA, et al. Venlafaxine in treatment-resistant obsessive-compulsive disorder. J Clin Psychiatry 2003;64:546–550.

70. Denys D, vanMegen HJGM, van der Wee N, Westenberg HGM. A double-blind switch study of paroxetine and venlafaxine in obsessive-compulsive disorder. J Clin Psychiatry 2004;65:37–43.

71. McDougle CJ. Update on the pharmacologic management of OCD: Agents and augmentation. J Clin Psychiatry 1997;58(Suppl 12):11–17.

72. Pallanti S, Quercioli L, Paiva RS, Koran LM. Citalopram for treatment-resistant obsessive-compulsive disorder. Eur Psychiatry 1999;14:101–106.

73. Goodman WK, McDougle CJ, Price LH, et al. Dopamine antagonists in tic-related and psychotic spectrum obsessive compulsive disorder. J Clin Psychiatry 1994;55(Suppl 3):24–31.

74. McDougle CJ, Epperson CN, Pelton GH, et al. A double-blind placebo-controlled study of risperidone addition in serotonin reuptake inhibitor-refractory obsessive-compulsive disorder. Arch Gen Psychiatry 2000;57:794–801.

75. Weiss EL, Potenza MN, McDougle CJ, et al. Olanzapine addition in obsessive-compulsive disorder refractory to selective serotonin reuptake inhibitors: An open-label case series. J Clin Psychiatry 1999;60:524–527.

76. Mundo E, Bareggi SR, Pirola R, et al. Long-term therapy of obsessive-compulsive disorder: A double-blind controlled study. J Clin Psychiatry 1997;17:4–10.

77. Hollander E, Stein DJ, Kwon JH, et al. Psychosocial function and economic costs of obsessive-compulsive disorder. CNS Spectr 1997;2:16–25.

71

SLEEP DISORDERS

Cherry W. Jackson and Judy L. Curtis

Learning Objectives and other resources can be found at *www.pharmacotherapyonline.com.*

KEY CONCEPTS

1. Common causes of insomnia include jet lag, significant psychosocial stressors, excessive alcohol use, caffeine intake, and nicotine use.

2. Patients experiencing insomnia lasting longer than 3 weeks should be evaluated for symptoms of a medical or psychiatric disorder.

3. Monitoring mood symptoms of a patient experiencing a sleep disturbance after a significant loss or during a difficult time is important to prevent a long-term problem with insomnia and to provide appropriate therapy if a mood disorder occurs.

4. Sleep hygiene principles, such as relaxing before bedtime, exercising regularly, establishing a regular bedtime and wake-up time, and discontinuing alcohol, caffeine, and nicotine should be taught to individuals with insomnia.

5. Bedtime doses of antidepressants such as trazodone may

be considered an alternative for patients experiencing insomnia.

6. Long-acting benzodiazepines should be avoided in the elderly.

7. Benzodiazepine tolerance and dependence are avoided by using low-dose therapy for the shortest possible duration.

8. Nonpharmacologic interventions such as weight loss, removing an obstruction in the airway, and or nasal continuous positive airway pressure are considered first-line therapies for obstructive sleep apnea.

9. Obstructive sleep apnea and central sleep apnea patients should avoid central nervous system depressants such as alcohol, benzodiazepines, and zolpidem.

10. Modafinil is the standard of treatment for daytime sleepiness associated with narcolepsy.

Approximately 70 million Americans suffer with a sleep-related problem, with as many as 60% experiencing a chronic disorder.[1] In a study by the National Institute of Aging, of 9000 patients age 65 and older, over 80% report a sleep-related disturbance.[1]

SLEEP PHYSIOLOGY

SLEEP CYCLES

Sleep is divided into two phases: non–rapid eye movement (NREM) sleep and rapid eye movement (REM) sleep. Humans typically experience four to six cycles of NREM and REM sleep, with each cycle lasting between 70 and 120 minutes.[2]

There are four stages of NREM sleep. Healthy sleep will typically progress through the four stages of NREM sleep prior to the first REM period. From wakefulness, sleep typically progresses quickly through stages 1 and 2. During stages 3 and 4 NREM, both metabolic activity and brain waves slow. This slow-wave sleep occurs most frequently early in the sleep cycle. After stage 4, the first REM cycle occurs and typically lasts between 5 and 7 minutes. REM cycles tend to lengthen in the later stages of the sleep cycle.[2]

REM sleep involves a dramatic physiological change from stage 4 NREM slow-wave sleep, to a state in which the brain becomes electrically and metabolically activated.[2] REM occurs in bursts, and is accompanied by a 62% to 173% increase in cerebral blood flow,

generalized muscle atonia, poikilothermia, vivid dreaming, and fluctuations in respiratory and cardiac rate.[2]

CIRCADIAN RHYTHM

At birth human infants spend up to 20 hours a day sleeping, and it is not until between 3 and 6 months of age that differentiation between REM and NREM sleep occurs.[2] By age 3, the ultradian sleep-wake rhythm changes to a circadian pattern, with most sleep occurring at night. The suprachiasmic nucleus of the brain serves as the biological clock and paces the circadian rhythm. Although the length of a day is 24 hours, in environments devoid of light cues, the sleep-wake cycle lasts 24.2 hours.[3] Without environmental cues (*zeitgebers*) such as alarm clocks and lights, it would be difficult to set our internal clocks.[3,4] In midlife, there is a gradual decline in sleep efficiency and sleep time.[2] In the elderly, sleep is lighter in depth and more fragmented, with intermittent arousals, shifts in the sleep stages, and a gradual disappearance of slow wave sleep.[4]

NEUROCHEMISTRY

The neurochemistry of sleep is complex since sleep cannot be localized to either a specific area of the brain or a specific neurotransmitter. NREM sleep appears to be controlled by the basal forebrain, the area surrounding the solitary tract in the medulla and the dorsal raphe nucleus, which is primarily serotonergic.[3] Sleep is reduced when there are decreases in serotonin or destruction of the dorsal raphe nucleus in the brain stem, which contains most of the brain's serotonergic bodies. REM sleep appears to be turned on by cholinergic cells in the mesencephalic, medullary, and pontine gigantocellular regions. REM sleep appears to be turned off by the dorsal raphe nucleus, the locus ceruleus, and the nucleus peribrachialis lateris, the latter two of which are primarily noradrenergic. The ascending reticular activating system and the posterior hypothalamus facilitate arousal and wakefulness.[5] Dopamine has an alerting effect. Drugs that increase dopamine in the brain cause increased wakefulness, and those that decrease dopamine cause sleepiness.[4] Neurochemicals involved in wakefulness include norepinephrine and acetylcholine in the cortex and histamine and neuropeptides such as substance P and corticotropin-releasing factor in the hypothalamus.[4,6]

ELECTROPHYSIOLOGY

Sleep is typically measured and observed in sleep laboratories by electroencephalograms (EEGs), electro-oculograms (EOGs) of each eye, and electromyograms (EMGs) of the mentalis and submentalis muscles. This information in total is used to evaluate the character of sleep.

The EEG is characterized during wakefulness by low-voltage, rapid-frequency alpha (8 to 13 Hz) and beta rhythms (>13 Hz). Stage 1 of NREM sleep is the stage between wakefulness and sleep during which alpha waves evolve into slower theta waves (4 to 7 Hz). Individuals describe this experience as being awake, being drowsy, or as being asleep. Stage 2 is characterized by theta rhythms with sleep spindles (brief bursts of electrical activity at 12 to 14 Hz) and K complexes (an electronegative wave followed by an electropositive wave). Stage 3 and stage 4 sleep is called *delta sleep* since more than 20% to 50% of the sleep is characterized by high-amplitude slow activity known as delta waves (0.5 to 3 Hz). In this stage eye movements are absent and muscle tone is atonic.[3]

REM sleep is characterized by a low-amplitude, mixed-frequency EEG, absence of muscle tone, and bursts of bilateral rapid eye movements. Dreaming occurs during REM sleep, and if an individual is awakened during or at the end of one of these periods, 80% to 90% can report the content of their dream.[5,6]

CLASSIFICATION OF SLEEP DISORDERS

The *Diagnostic and Statistical Manual of Mental Disorders,* Fourth Edition, Text Revision classifies sleep disorders into four categories based on etiology (Table 71–1) and requires a minimum of 1 month before a sleep disorder can be diagnosed.[7,8] Primary sleep disorders are those disorders in which there is no other etiology (mental disorder, substance-related disorder, or medical condition) responsible for the disorder. Primary sleep disorders appear to be based on an endogenous abnormality of the sleep-wake cycle, or circadian rhythm, and they are divided into dyssomnias or parasomnias. A *dyssomnia* is defined as an abnormality in the amount, quality, or timing of sleep, while a *parasomnia* is defined as abnormal behavioral or physiological events associated with sleep.

INSOMNIA

Insomnia is defined as a complaint of difficulty falling asleep, difficulty maintaining sleep, or experiencing nonrestorative sleep

TABLE 71–1. DSM-IV-TR Classification of Sleep Disorders

Primary sleep disorders
Dyssomnias
  Primary insomnia
  Primary hypersomnia
  Narcolepsy
  Breathing-related sleep disorder
  Circadian rhythm sleep disorder
    Delayed sleep phase type
    Jet lag type
    Shift work type
    Unspecified type
  Dyssomnia not otherwise specified
Parasomnias
  Nightmare disorder
  Sleep terror disorder
  Sleepwalking disorder
  Parasomnia not otherwise specified
Sleep disorders related to another mental disorder
  Insomnia related to another mental disorder
  Hypersomnia related to another mental disorder
Other sleep disorders
  Sleep disorder due to a general medical condition
  Substance-induced sleep disorder

(sleeping but not feeling rested) that lasts at least 1 month.[8] This sleep disorder causes distress, frequently due to fear that they may not be able to fall asleep at bedtime, or impaired occupational functioning due to daytime fatigue or drowsiness. While young adults are more likely to complain that they have difficulty falling asleep, middle-aged and elderly adults are more likely to complain that they have middle-of-the-night awakening or early morning awakening.

It is important to evaluate insomnia based on its duration. A sleep complaint lasting two or three nights is considered to be transient insomnia. Short-term insomnia usually resolves in less than 3 weeks, and is typically due to illness, jet lag, or stress. According to the *Diagnostic and Statistical Manual,* insomnia lasting longer than 1 month is considered chronic.

EPIDEMIOLOGY

Insomnia is the most common complaint in general medical practice settings.[9] Primary insomnia usually begins in young adulthood or middle age, and is rare in childhood or adolescence. More than 50% of the population complains of insomnia in their lifetime.[1] A 1-year prevalence study of insomnia in the United States reports that one-third of the individuals surveyed complained of insomnia, and 17% reported that the symptoms were serious.[1] Conservative estimates of chronic insomnia range from 9% to 12% in adulthood and up to 20% in the elderly.[1,10] Women complain of insomnia twice as frequently as men. Individuals who are elderly, unemployed, separated or widowed, or those with a lower socioeconomic status reported a significantly higher incidence of insomnia. Forty percent with insomnia also had a concurrent psychiatric disorder (anxiety, depression, or substance abuse).[9]

Despite the prevalence of insomnia, only 5% of individuals seek medical attention for management of their insomnia. Approximately 10% to 20% use nonprescription drugs or alcohol to self-treat. Of he 3% of the population who are prescribed sedative-hypnotics for nsomnia, 11% report usage exceeding 1 year.[11]

DIFFERENTIAL DIAGNOSIS

Primary insomnia is considered to be an endogenous disorder due to either a neurochemical or structural disorder affecting the sleep-wake cycle. Individuals with primary insomnia may be light sleepers who are easily aroused by noise, temperature, or anxiety. Some studies have suggested that primary insomnia is a "hyperarousal state," in that insomnia patients have an increased metabolic rate compared with controls, and have longer-than-average sleep latencies in sleep studies.[2]

◀1 Evaluation of patients with a complaint of short-term or transient insomnia should focus on recent stressors, such as a separation, a death in the family, a job change, or college exams. Another common cause is jet lag. These individuals often develop situational anxiety based on fear of not being able to fall asleep. Environmental cues such as alarm clocks may also cause situational anxiety.[2]

◀2 Chronic insomnia is frequently associated with a psychiatric or medical condition, and individuals with such a complaint should receive a complete diagnostic examination. This evaluation should include routine laboratory tests and physical and mental status examinations, as well as ruling out any medication- or substance-related causes.[12] Common causes of insomnia are listed in Table 71–2.

TABLE 71–2. Common Etiologies of Insomnia

Situational
Work or financial stress
Interpersonal conflicts
Major life events
Jet lag or shift work
Medical
Cardiovascular (angina, arrhythmias, heart failure)
Respiratory (asthma, sleep apnea)
Chronic pain
Endocrine disorders (diabetes, hyperthyroidism)
Gastrointestinal (gastroesophageal reflux disease, ulcers)
Neurologic (delirium, epilepsy, Parkinson's disease)
Pregnancy
Psychiatric
Mood disorders (depression, mania)
Anxiety disorders (generalized anxiety disorder,
    obsessive-compulsive disorder, or panic disorder)
Substance abuse (alcohol or sedative-hypnotic withdrawal)
Pharmacologically induced
Anticonvulsants
Central adrenergic blockers
Diuretics
Selective serotonin reuptake inhibitors
Steroids
Stimulants

▶ TREATMENT: Insomnia

The therapeutic management of insomnia is initially based on whether the individual has experienced a short-term, transient, or chronic sleep disturbance. Clinicians should assess the symptoms based on a description of the symptoms, onset, duration, frequency, effect on daytime function, sleep hygiene habits, and history of previous symptoms or treatment.[13]

◀3 General therapeutic management should be used for all patients with insomnia. Management includes identifying the cause of the insomnia, patient education on sleep hygiene, and stress management. Monitoring mood symptoms of a patient experiencing a sleep disturbance after a significant loss or during a difficult time is important to prevent a long-term problem with insomnia and to provide appropriate therapy if a mood disorder occurs. Any unnecessary pharmacotherapy should be eliminated.[10] Transient insomnia, which occurs as a result of an acute stressor, is expected to resolve quickly, and should be treated with good sleep hygiene and careful use of sedative-hypnotics.[14] Short-term insomnia, which lasts up to 3 weeks, is associated with situational, personal, or medical stress. Nonpharmacologic treatment is important in this type of insomnia, and if sedative-hypnotics are used, prevention of tolerance or dependence is an important consideration.[13] Chronic insomnia requires careful assessment for the medical reason for the insomnia, as well as nonpharmacologic techniques and careful and less frequent use of sedative-hypnotics to prevent tolerance and dependence.[12]

NONPHARMACOLOGIC THERAPY

◀4 In many cases insomnia can be treated without sedative-hypnotics. Education about normal sleep and habits for good sleep hygiene are often sufficient interventions.[2] Nonpharmacologic interventions for insomnia frequently consist of short-term cognitive behavioral therapies. The ones most studied include: stimulus control therapy, sleep restriction, relaxation therapy, cognitive therapy, paradoxical intention, and sleep hygiene (Table 71–3).[10,15,16]

TABLE 71–3. Nonpharmacologic Recommendations for Insomnia

Stimulus control procedures
1. Establish regular times to wake up and to go to sleep (including weekends).
2. Sleep only as much as necessary to feel rested.
3. Go to bed only when sleepy. Avoid long periods of wakefulness in bed. Use the bed only for sleep or intimacy; do not read or watch television in bed.
4. Avoid trying to force sleep; if you do not fall asleep within 20–30 minutes, leave the bed and perform a relaxing activity (e.g., read, listen to music, or watch television) until drowsy. Repeat this as often as necessary.
5. Avoid daytime naps.
6. Schedule worry time during the day. Do not take your troubles to bed.

Sleep hygiene recommendations
1. Exercise routinely (three to four times weekly), but not close to bedtime because this may cause arousal.
2. Create a comfortable sleep environment by avoiding temperature extremes, loud noises, and illuminated clocks in the bedroom.
3. Discontinue or reduce the use of alcohol, caffeine, and nicotine.
4. Avoid drinking large quantities of liquids in the evening to prevent nighttime trips to the restroom.
5. Do something relaxing and enjoyable before bedtime.

CLINICAL CONTROVERSY

Some clinicians believe that sleep restriction is an effective form of treatment for chronic insomnia. Evidence from studies varies, and use of sleep restriction in many studies was part of combination therapy, and the specific contribution of sleep restriction toward sleep improvement was unclear.

▧ PHARMACOLOGIC THERAPY

▧ NONBENZODIAZEPINE HYPNOTIC AGENTS

Antihistamines exhibit sedating properties and are included in many over-the-counter sleep agents. They are effective in the treatment of mild insomnia and are generally safe.[13] Diphenhydramine and doxylamine are more sedating than pyrilamine, and in addition, pyrilamine causes more gastrointestinal discomfort. In one study, patients reported that diphenhydramine causes sedation equivalent to that of pentobarbital 60 mg.[13] Increasing the dose of antihistamines will not produce a linear increase in response. The safety and efficacy of antihistamines over placebo have been documented in several studies. In all studies, side effects were considered to be minimal.[18] Antihistamines are considered to be less effective than benzodiazepines, and have the disadvantages of anticholinergic side effects, which are especially troublesome in the elderly.[13,18]

The amino-acid L-tryptophan, a precursor of serotonin, was once popular as a natural sedative. Cases of eosinophilia-myalgia syndrome, which were most likely due to contamination of excipients, caused this product to be removed from the market.[11]

Antidepressants are alternatives for patients with nonrestorative sleep who should not receive benzodiazepines, especially those who have depression, pain, or a risk of substance abuse. Using antidepressants for insomnia without depression is common but not well studied.[18] Sedating antidepressants such as amitriptyline, doxepin, and nortriptyline are effective for inducing sleep continuity, although daytime sedation can be significant.[18] Disadvantages include anticholinergic activity, adrenergic blockage, and cardiac conduction prolongations which are problematic in the elderly and in overdose situations.[18]

Trazodone is very sedating and improves sleep continuity.[11] Trazodone is popular for the treatment of insomnia in patients prone to substance abuse, since addiction and tolerance are not a problem. Trazodone is frequently used in patients with selective serotonin reuptake inhibitor (SSRI) and bupropion-induced insomnia in doses of 25 to 75 mg.[11] Adverse effects of trazodone include serotonin syndrome when used in combination with other antidepressants. Other side effects include oversedation and α-adrenergic blockade. Orthostasis may occur at any age, but it is more dangerous in the elderly. Priapism is a rare but serious side effect reported to occur in one in 6000 men. One in 23,000 will require surgical intervention, which can lead to permanent impotence.[19]

Some SSRIs are sleep promoting, while others may cause insomnia. Some of the new generation of antidepressants such as mirtazapine and nefazodone are also sedating. Sedating antidepressants may be effective in nondepressed patients, especially those who have insomnia and a dependency problem. Since many of these medications affect the cytochrome P450 system, it is important to evaluate for the potential of drug interactions with these agents.[19]

Melatonin is a hormone released by the pineal gland during the night. It is available as an over-the-counter agent and is promoted as a sleep aid. Although the dosage varies, the typical starting dose is 3 mg. Most studies with melatonin have been in children with neurological impairment and in individuals with jet lag.[11] Since it is marketed as a dietary supplement, there may be inconsistencies in potency. This must be taken into consideration when recommending this agent.

Valerian is an herbal sleep remedy that has been studied for its sedative-hypnotic properties in patients with insomnia. The mechanism of action of this herb is still unknown, but it may involve inhibition of the enzyme that breaks down γ-aminobutyric acid (GABA). The recommended dose for insomnia ranges from 300 to 600 mg. An equivalent dose of dried herbal valerian root is 2 to 3 grams soaked in 1 cup of hot water for 20 to 25 minutes.[20] As with melatonin, and other herbal products not regulated by the Food and Drug Administration (FDA), valerian is not regulated for quality or consistency.

Zolpidem, an imidazopyridine chemically unrelated to benzodiazepines or barbiturates, has a short half-life of 6 to 8 hours.[21] It acts selectively at the GABA benzodiazepine-1 receptor and has minimal anxiolytic and no muscle relaxant or anticonvulsant properties. It is comparable in efficacy to benzodiazepine hypnotics, reducing latency to sleep and increasing total sleep time and efficiency. Zolpidem is effective for reducing sleep latency and nocturnal awakenings and increasing total sleep time and does not appear to have significant effects on next-day psychomotor performance. Rebound effects on withdrawal and tolerance with prolonged use are minimal; however, theoretical concerns about abuse exist.[21]

The safety and efficacy of zolpidem for insomnia is similar to that of the benzodiazepines. As with other sedative medications, treatment optimally should not exceed 4 weeks to minimize tolerance and dependence. Zolpidem is less disruptive of sleep stages than benzodiazepines. The most common adverse effects include drowsiness, amnesia, dizziness, headache, and gastrointestinal complaints.[21] Several cases of brief psychotic reactions have been reported in women.[21]

The recommended daily dose of zolpidem is 10 mg, but 5 mg is used in elderly patients and those with hepatic impairment. The dosage may be increased to 20 mg per night, but the incidence of adverse effects is dose related.[21]

Zaleplon is a pyrazolopyrimidine, and like zolpidem it binds selectively to the benzodiazepine-1 receptor. Zaleplon has a rapid onset of action, a half-life of 1 hour, and is metabolized to inactive metabolites.[22] It is effective for decreasing time to sleep onset, but not for reducing nighttime awakening or for increasing the total sleep time. Zaleplon may be best used as a sleep aid for middle-of-the-night awakenings.

Zaleplon does not appear to cause rebound insomnia and has no effect on next-day psychomotor performance.[23] At doses of 5 to 20 mg, it has been shown to reduce sleep latency, and at 20 mg to increase sleep duration when compared with placebo. The recommended dose is 10 mg in adults and 5 mg in the elderly.[24]

The most common adverse effects with zaleplon are dizziness, headache, and somnolence. There is some concern about the possible occurrence of dependence, but insufficient data exist to determine whether this will be an issue with this agent. Development of tolerance does not appear to be significant.[21] There are two drug interactions of note: zaleplon plasma levels are increased when combined with cimetidine and decreased with rifampin.[21]

▧ BENZODIAZEPINE HYPNOTICS

The most commonly used treatment for insomnia has been the benzodiazepines. All benzodiazepines are effective as sedative-hypnotics, although only five have been marketed for that purpose (Table 71–4).

TABLE 71–4. Pharmacokinetics of Benzodiazepine Hypnotic Agents

Generic Name	t_{max} (h)[a]	Parent $t_{1/2}$ (h)	Daily Dose Range (mg)	Metabolic Pathway	Clinically Significant Metabolites
Estazolam	2	12–15	1–2	Oxidation	—
Flurazepam	1	8	15–30	Oxidation	Hydroxyethylflurazepam Flurazepam aldehyde
				N-dealkylation	N-DAF[b]
Quazepam	2	39	7.5–15	Oxidation	2-Oxo-quazepam
				N-dealkylation	N-DAF[b]
Temazepam	1.5	10–15	15–30	Conjugation	—
Triazolam	1	2	0.125–0.25	Oxidation	—

[a] Time to peak plasma concentration.
[b] N-desalkylflurazepam, mean half-life 47 to 100 hours.

Benzodiazepines bind to GABA receptors in the brain resulting in stimulatory effects on GABAergic transmission and hyperpolarization of neuronal membranes. They have sedative, anxiolytic, muscle relaxant, and anticonvulsant properties. Benzodiazepines relieve insomnia by reducing sleep latency and increasing total sleep time. Benzodiazepines increase stage 2 sleep while decreasing REM, stage 3, and stage 4 sleep.[11] Benzodiazepines are very safe, and fatal overdoses are rare unless they are taken in combination with CNS depressants or alcohol.[11]

Pharmacokinetics

The choice of a particular benzodiazepine is based on its pharmacokinetic profile. When used as a single dose, the extent of distribution and elimination half-life is important in predicting the duration of action. However, after multiple dosing, the elimination half-life and formation of active metabolites determine the extent of drug accumulation and resultant clinical effects.[11] The benzodiazepine pharmacokinetic profiles are summarized in Table 71–4. The onset of action depends on the rate of absorption. Flurazepam and triazolam are absorbed rapidly. Temazepam is less lipophilic and has a slower onset of effect. Sedation after flurazepam, estazolam, and quazepam occurs within 1 to 2 hours after ingestion.[11] Triazolam is redistributed quickly because of its high lipophilicity and thus has a short duration of effect.[11] Estazolam and temazepam are intermediate in their duration of action. The therapeutic effects of flurazepam and quazepam are long in comparison because of the active metabolites.

With the exception of temazepam, which is eliminated by conjugation, all benzodiazepine hypnotics are metabolized by hepatic microsomal oxidation and then undergo glucuronide conjugation. Oxidation may be inhibited in patients with impaired liver function, advanced age, or concurrent use of drugs that inhibit oxidation. Drugs that inhibit the cytochrome P450 3A4 enzyme (e.g., erythromycin, nefazodone, fluvoxamine, and ketoconazole) reduce the clearance of triazolam and increase its plasma concentrations.[11]

Triazolam, which has a short elimination half-life, and estazolam and temazepam, which have intermediate elimination half-lives, lack clinically significant metabolites. Flurazepam and quazepam have long elimination half-lives. Flurazepam is metabolized rapidly to two short-acting metabolites, hydroxyethylflurazepam and flurazepam aldehyde. These metabolites contribute to sleep induction on the first night of therapy, but are eliminated within 13 hours.[11] N-desalkylflurazepam (N-DAF) is an active metabolite that has a very long half-life and accumulates extensively during multiple dosing.

N-DAF accounts for most flurazepam pharmacologic effects. Quazepam and one of its metabolites, 2-oxo-quazepam, have elimination half-lives of 39 hours.[11] Quazepam's oxo-quazepam metabolite is metabolized to N-DAF. If oxidation of N-DAF is impaired its half-life becomes prolonged, and complications of drug accumulation may result with repeated dosing; however, tolerance may develop to these effects. N-DAF may be useful when daytime anxiety or early morning awakening are complaints, but daytime sedation and impaired psychomotor performance may complicate therapy.[11]

Adverse Effects

Side effects are dose dependent and vary according to the pharmacokinetics of the individual benzodiazepine. High doses with long or intermediate elimination half-lives have a greater potential for producing daytime sedation and performance impairment. These effects include excessive drowsiness, psychomotor incoordination, decreased concentration, and cognitive deficits. Tolerance may develop with time. Rapidly eliminated benzodiazepines have less potential for daytime sedation.[11]

Tolerance to benzodiazepine hypnotic effects develops sooner with triazolam (after 2 weeks of continuous use) than with other benzodiazepine hypnotics.[11] The hypnotic efficacy of flurazepam, quazepam, and temazepam is maintained for 1 month of continuous nightly use.[11] Estazolam reportedly maintains the duration and quality of sleep at the maximum dosage (2 mg nightly) for up to 12 weeks.[11] Long-term use (greater than 6 months) of benzodiazepines was associated with a low risk of abuse, side effects, and tolerance in patients with severe, chronic sleep disorders; however, efficacy has not been established.[11]

Anterograde amnesia, an impairment of memory and recall, occurs more frequently with triazolam than with temazepam; however, it has been reported with most benzodiazepines.[11] The lowest effective dosage should be used to avoid adverse effects on memory. When compared with temazepam, triazolam use was associated with a higher reported rate of confusion, bizarre behavior, agitation, and hallucination. These CNS effects occurred with higher doses and in older patients.[11] Because of the high incidence of CNS adverse effects, the United Kingdom suspended sales of triazolam in 1991.[11] Controversy surrounding triazolam led the FDA to review the agent in 1990 and 1992. Triazolam was considered safe and effective, but caution was noted regarding possible memory problems.

Rebound insomnia is characterized by increased wakefulness beyond baseline amounts that last for one to two nights after abrupt discontinuation of benzodiazepine hypnotics with short or intermediate elimination half-lives. Rebound insomnia occurs more frequently after high doses of triazolam, even when ingested intermittently.[11] The occurrence of rebound insomnia can be minimized by using the lowest effective dose and tapering the dose on discontinuation.[11]

The incidence of CNS side effects increases with age secondary to prolonged benzodiazepine half-lives, which may increase the potential for drug accumulation. Prolonged sedation and cognitive and psychomotor impairment are concerns in the elderly. Drugs with short and intermediate elimination half-lives are associated with fewer performance deficits; however, they may be associated with more daytime anxiety in elderly patients. There is an association between falls and hip fractures and the use of benzodiazepines with long elimination half-lives; thus flurazepam and quazepam should be avoided in elderly patients.[25]

EVALUATION OF THERAPEUTIC OUTCOMES

Hypnotic therapy is indicated in individuals with transient or short-term insomnia.[15] Patients should be counseled that sleep will return to normal when the precipitating stressor is eliminated, and they should also be educated on strategies for stimulus control and good sleep hygiene (see Table 71–3). If the stressor is expected to last more than 1 week, intermittent hypnotic use (three or four nights per week) should be prescribed for no more than 3 weeks.

For patients with chronic insomnia, medical, psychiatric, and pharmacologic causes should be identified and managed.[11] If treatment of an underlying disorder fails to result in improvement, intermittent pharmacotherapy may be indicated. If the insomnia is psychophysiologic, several months of supervised hypnotic therapy may help alleviate anxiety and re-establish a regular sleep pattern on drug discontinuation; however, these patients require nonpharmacologic therapy as well.[17]

Tolerance and dependence can be avoided by using hypnotics at the lowest possible dose, intermittently, and for the shortest duration possible. From the outset of therapy, patients should receive instruction on frequency of drug use and the expected duration of therapy, to prevent development of dependence.

Withdrawal symptoms can be diminished by tapering the dosage gradually. Patients should be counseled on rebound insomnia when benzodiazepine therapy is terminated. Patients with difficulty initiating sleep and those who require daytime alertness should receive the short-acting benzodiazepine hypnotics or zaleplon. Those with difficulty maintaining sleep or those with early morning awakening may benefit from an agent with an intermediate elimination half-life if daytime performance is required. Benzodiazepines with long elimination half-lives should be considered if management of daytime anxiety is required. There is no rationale for the concurrent use of two benzodiazepines to treat anxiety and insomnia.

Benzodiazepine hypnotics should not be prescribed for individuals with sleep apnea, a history of substance abuse, or during pregnancy. Patients should be instructed to avoid alcohol; even taking alcohol on the day after ingestion of a benzodiazepine with a long elimination half-life can result in additive CNS impairment. Prescriptions for benzodiazepine hypnotics should be accompanied by printed information and verbal counseling on precautions.

SLEEP APNEA

Sleep apnea is defined as the cessation of airflow at the nose and mouth lasting at least 10 seconds. Sleep apnea is quantified using polysomnography (PSG) and is classified into two major categories: obstructive and central. Central sleep apnea involves impairment of the respiratory drive, while obstructive sleep apnea is caused by intermittent upper airway obstruction. Some patients will experience both central and obstructive sleep apnea. Patients with this sleep disorder have a high risk of morbidity and mortality.[26]

Sleep apnea is very common. Approximately 9% of females and 24% of males experience sleep apnea. Sleep apnea is two to three times more common in men, and it is more common in middle-aged men than in younger men.[26] As many as 80% of middle-aged men snore, and 25% of heavy snorers have sleep apnea. Sleep apnea may be less prevalent in elderly patients, and it is theorized that this may be evidenced by sleep apnea's effect on mortality.[26]

OBSTRUCTIVE SLEEP APNEA

Obstructive sleep apnea (OSA) is a potentially life-threatening condition characterized by snoring. At one end of the spectrum are those individuals who snore intermittently with little sleep disruption, and at the other end are patients who snore heavily and have severe gas exchange disturbances and respiratory failure, causing them to gasp for air. These episodes are repeated as often as 600 times per night.[26] As a result of these frequent arousals, hypoxia and sleep fragmentation occur. Hypoxia may lead to daytime sleepiness, impaired attention and memory, and personality changes. Individuals with sleep apnea are usually not aware of the snoring or respiratory pauses, and symptoms are most frequently reported by their bed partner.[26]

OSA is caused by occlusion of the upper airway due to factors such as obesity, and fixed upper airway lesions such as polyps, as well as enlarged tonsils or adenoids or the tongue. It can also be caused by acromegaly, amyloidosis, and hypothyroidism, as well as neurological conditions that impair upper airway muscle tone.[26] Medical complications include arrhythmias, hypertension, cor pulmonale, and sudden death.[26]

Treatment of OSA must be individualized and depends on the severity of the disordered breathing and the amount of sleep disruption. Patients with severe apnea (>20 episodes per hour on PSG and excessive daytime somnolence) and those with moderate apneas (5 to 20 episodes per hour on PSG and excessive daytime somnolence or other daytime symptoms) have shown significant improvement and reduction in mortality with treatment.[27] Nonpharmacologic measures are the treatments of choice.

Weight loss may eliminate the apnea and reduce daytime hypersomnia; however, improvement is only limited. Treatment of underlying causes of obstruction (e.g., tonsillectomy, nasal septal repair, and nonsedating antihistamines for allergic rhinitis) may eliminate apneas during sleep. In patients with mild apnea and snoring with no daytime symptomatology, management may include avoidance of a supine sleep position.[27]

Continuous positive airway pressure (CPAP) during sleep is the standard treatment for most patients with OSA. CPAP acts as a splint to maintain the patency of the oropharynx during respiration. Compliance is variable, ranging from 25% to 70%, and is the major limitation of this treatment.[26] One night of noncompliance results in a complete reversal of the gains made in daytime alertness.[27]

The most important pharmacologic intervention is the avoidance of all CNS depressants (e.g., alcohol, anxiolytics, hypnotics, narcotics, and zolpidem). Preliminary studies suggest that zaleplon does not interfere with respiratory function. CNS depressant use is potentially lethal since it inhibits the brain's reflex ability to cause a mini-arousal and resume breathing. Medication therapy should be reserved for patients with mild OSA and those who are treatment resistant. Protriptyline in doses of 10 to 30 mg daily reduces the frequency of apneas and increases oxygen saturation.[26,28] The mechanism of action may be related to a decrease in REM sleep, the sleep stage in which most apneas occur. Imipramine was found to exert similar effects to protriptyline in two uncontrolled studies.[28] Fluoxetine and paroxetine have shown results similar to those of protriptyline, with fewer adverse effects. The SSRIs may be preferable to tricyclic antidepressants due to their similar efficacy but fewer adverse effects.[28] Medroxyprogesterone (MPG) has proved disappointing in OSA, showing no results in curing nighttime apnea. In contrast, MPG does appear to have a beneficial effect in daytime hypercapnia. At present the only role for MPG is in OSA patients with awake respiratory failure or noncompliance with CPAP. Theophylline is a respiratory stimulant that has been frequently used in patients with OSA. Studies with theophylline have shown questionable efficacy. Some studies have shown a reduction in obstructive events, but an increase in the number of arousals, increasing daytime sleepiness.[26] Mixed reviews have also been found for antihypertensive agents. Studies have evaluated the effects of angiotensin-converting enzyme inhibitors, calcium channel blockers, metoprolol, and clonidine, showing reduction in the frequency of apnea. Studies have also shown that antihypertensives can increase OSA.[26] Thus the efficacy of these agents is unclear.

CENTRAL SLEEP APNEA

Central sleep apnea (CSA) is a form of apnea in which breathing effort is not detected, in contrast to obstructive apnea, in which attempts at breathing are vigorous. CSA makes up only 10% of all apneas. Hypercapnic patients usually present with a morning headache and daytime somnolence, while nonhypercapnic patients complain of insomnia and nocturnal awakenings with shortness of breath or gasping. Although the majority of cases are idiopathic, identifiable causes are nasal obstruction, autonomic nervous system lesions (e.g., cervical cordotomy), neurological diseases (e.g., poliomyelitis, encephalitis, and myasthenia gravis), and congestive heart failure.[26]

The primary treatment approach for CSA is supplemental oxygen and CPAP.[29] Pharmacologic treatments include acetazolamide, theophylline, and MPG. Acetazolamide induces a metabolic acidosis that stimulates respiratory drive. Long-term studies have shown a 70% reduction in CSA with acetazolamide, and no effect on obstructed breathing events. It has been suggested that acetazolamide induces a resetting of the CO_2 response threshold. Clinical use is limited because of adverse effects such as electrolyte changes, paresthesias, and precipitation of calcium phosphate salts in alkaline urine.[26,29] Theophylline may have some efficacy in CSA related to congestive heart failure. In one trial there was a 60% reduction in central apneas per hour of sleep compared with 20% with placebo,[29] but further study is needed. In nonhypercapnic CSA patients, treatment may consist of benzodiazepines (triazolam or temazepam) to reduce arousals, and acetazolamide, CPAP, and oxygen to stabilize breathing patterns.[26]

NARCOLEPSY

Narcolepsy is a severely debilitating neurologic disease that affects an estimated 140,000 Americans.[30] Despite the debilitating nature of the symptoms, the disease may go undiagnosed or misdiagnosed for many years. Prevalence estimates differ between studies, but narcolepsy is estimated to occur in 0.03% to 0.06% of the adult population.[30] The diagnosis appears to be equal in men and women, although there may be a higher diagnostic rate in men. Narcolepsy has been noted in children and adolescents, but it is typically recognized in the second decade of life and increases in severity through the third or fourth decade.[30]

Four characteristic symptoms differentiate narcolepsy from other sleep disorders, and are known as the *narcolepsy tetrad*: sleep attacks, cataplexy, hypnagogic hallucinations, and sleep paralysis. Individuals with narcolepsy complain of excessive daytime sleepiness, with sleep attacks that last up to 30 minutes. Individuals complain of hypersomnia, fatigue, impaired performance, and disturbed nighttime sleep.

Cataplexy is an episode of sudden bilateral loss of muscle tone resulting in the individual collapsing and is often precipitated by situations characterized by high emotion (e.g., laughter, anger, or excitement). The individual remains conscious, and the episode is brief, lasting seconds to several minutes. Cataplexy occurs in 70% to 80% of people with narcolepsy.[30] Sleep paralysis occurs when the individual is falling asleep or when waking. It is an episodic loss of voluntary muscle tone. The individual is awake, but is unable to move or speak. Hypnagogic (meaning at the threshold of sleep) and hypnopompic (meaning upon awakening) hallucinations are brief, dream-like experiences that intrude into wakefulness. Nearly 70% of narcoleptics experience these hallucinations, and unfortunately these symptoms sometimes lead to an incorrect diagnosis of mental illness.[30] Disturbed nighttime sleep has been recognized as an essential feature in almost all patients with narcolepsy.

Narcolepsy may have multiple causes, including a genetic predisposition, since 3% of patients have a first-degree relative with the disorder.[31] Molecular studies including human leukocyte antigen (HLA) typing have found a high incidence of HLA-DR2 haplotypes among narcoleptics, although this does not appear to be the only determinant. In spite of the high incidence of HLA-DR2 haplotypes in narcoleptics, there is also a high incidence in the non-narcoleptic population that could lead to misdiagnosis.[31]

It is now generally accepted that narcolepsy results from one or more defects in the functioning of the hypocretin-orexin neurotransmitter system. Neurons containing hypocretin-orexin are found in the lateral hypothalamus and project to various parts of the brain that are thought to regulate sleep. In 75% of narcoleptic patients, hypocretin-orexin is undetectable in cerebrospinal fluid.[34] On postmortem examination, individuals with narcolepsy have deficiencies in hypocretin-orexin–producing neurons.[35] Despite the strong association between hypocretin-orexin deficiency and narcolepsy, the primary cause is unknown. Available data do suggest that the destruction of hypocretin-orexin–producing cells is part of an autoimmune process.[36,37]

In the sleep laboratory, individuals with narcolepsy have impairment of both the onset and offset of REM and NREM sleep. Narcoleptics are unable to maintain either REM or NREM sleep, which results in multiple arousals during the night. It is thought that the REM sleep disturbance during the night causes the symptoms of cataplexy, sleep paralysis, and hypnagogic hallucinations.[31]

▶ TREATMENT: Narcolepsy

Nonpharmacologic management of narcolepsy includes counseling the patient and family concerning the illness to alleviate misconceptions around the individual's behavior. Good sleep hygiene should be encouraged as well as two or more brief daytime naps. Daytime naps lasting 15 minutes each may help the individual with narcolepsy stay refreshed for several hours.

Doses of medications used to treat narcolepsy are summarized in Table 71–5. Pharmacologic management of narcolepsy is focused on two primary areas: treatment of excessive daytime sleepiness (EDS) and treatment of cataplexy.

Modafanil, a racemic compound unrelated to psychostimulants, is the current standard for the treatment of EDS.[38] Modafinil selectively targets neuronal pathways in the hypothalamus that regulate the normal sleep-wake cycle. The precise mechanism by which modafinil promotes wakefulness is unknown. Modafinil is readily absorbed, reaches peak plasma concentrations in 2 to 4 hours, and has a half-life of 15 hours. The dose is between 200 and 400 mg/day.[39] The efficacy of modafinil in treating EDS has been demonstrated in several randomized studies. EDS may also be treated with stimulants to improve alertness and to increase daytime performance. Cataplexy is not significantly treated with modafinil and must be treated with anticataplectic agents.[40]

Modafinil is well tolerated, with the most commonly reported adverse effects being headache, nausea, nervousness, anxiety, and insomnia. Adverse effects are usually mild in severity. Preliminary evidence for modafinil suggests no signs of tolerance, withdrawal after abrupt discontinuation, or risk of abuse.[41]

Dextroamphetamine and methylphenidate also have FDA approval for the treatment of narcolepsy. Methamphetamine has also been used on an off-label basis. Methylphenidate and amphetamines have a fast onset of effect and durations of 6 to 10 and 3 to 4 hours, respectively. The dose may range from 5 to 60 mg daily and divided doses are recommended, although more expensive sustained-release forms are available.

The stimulants improve alertness and increase daytime performance. In addition to increasing alertness, they may elevate mood and prevent sleep. Side effects may include insomnia, hypertension, palpitations, and irritability. Tolerance to long-term stimulant therapy may occur, necessitating dosage increases. Amphetamine use is associated with more likelihood of abuse and tolerance, especially when prescribed in high doses. Compliance with stimulants is generally poor, especially when high doses are required.[40]

Pemoline, a mild CNS stimulant, has been used for the treatment of narcolepsy. It has a delayed onset of effect, but it has a duration of 8 to 10 hours. Pemoline's dosage range is 18.75 to 112.5 mg/day. Although less potent than the amphetamines, adherence tends to be better. Unfortunately, rare but potentially lethal liver toxicity and the need for frequent liver function testing limit the acceptance of this agent for the treatment of narcolepsy.[38]

Stimulants do not treat cataplexy effectively. The most effective treatment for cataplexy is tricyclic antidepressants or fluoxetine. The mechanism of antidepressants in relieving cataplexy, hypnagogic hallucinations, and sleep paralysis is unknown. Imipramine, protriptyline, clomipramine, fluoxetine, and nortriptyline are effective in approximately 80% of patients. Selegiline improves hypersomnolence and cataplexy through REM suppression and an increase in REM latency. The cost of the medication is high, and experience with the high doses needed for narcolepsy is limited.

Sodium oxybate (γ-hydroxybutyrate) shows the most promise of new agents for the treatment of narcolepsy. Early investigations demonstrated that the nightly administration of sodium oxybate changed sleep architecture to close to that of normal sleep. Sodium oxybate has been shown to increase slow-wave sleep, decrease nighttime awakenings, and increase REM efficiency. Not only does it

TABLE 71–5. Drugs Used to Treat Narcolepsy

Generic Name	Trade Name (Manufacturer)	Daily Dosage Range (mg)
Excessive daytime somnolence		
Dextroamphetamine	Dexadrine (GlaxoSmithKline) generics (various)	5–60
Dextroamphetamine/amphetamine salts[a]	Adderall (Shire US)	5–60
Methamphetamine[b]	Desoxyn (Abbott)	5–15
Methylphenidate	Ritalin (Novartis), generics (various)	30–80
Modafinil	Provigil (Cephalon)	200–400
Pemoline	Cylert (Abbott)	37.5–112.5
Adjunct agents for cataplexy		
Fluoxetine	Prozac (Lilly), generics (various)	20–80
Gamma-hydroxybutyrate	Xyrem (Orphan Medical)	60 mg/kg per night
Imipramine	Tofranil (Novartis), generics (various)	50–250
Nortriptyline	Aventyl (Lilly), Pamelor (Sandoz), generics (various)	50–200
Protriptyline	Vivactil (Merck), generics (various)	5–30
Selegiline	Eldepryl (Somerset)	20–40

[a] Dextroamphetamine sulfate, dextroamphetamine saccharate, amphetamine aspartate, and amphetamine sulfate.
[b] Not available in some states.
Compiled from U.S. Modafinil in Narcolepsy Multicenter Study Group[41] and Standard of Practice Committee of the American Sleep Disorders Association. Practice parameters for the use of stimulants in the treatment of narcolepsy. Sleep 1994;17:348–351.

improve the symptoms of EDS, it also decreases episodes of sleep paralysis, cataplexy, and hypnagogic hallucinations. The FDA approved sodium oxybate (Xyrem) in 2002.[42]

EVALUATION OF THERAPEUTIC OUTCOMES

The primary objective of pharmacologic treatment of narcolepsy is to reduce symptoms that adversely impact the quality of life. This includes alleviating daytime sleepiness with modafinil or stimulants. The goal is to produce the fullest possible return of normal function for patients at work, school, home, and socially. Cataplexy, hypnagogic hallucinations, and sleep paralysis should be treated when they are present and troublesome. The health care provider should consider

the benefit:risk ratio for the individual patient, the cost of medication, the convenience of administration, and cost of laboratory tests when selecting a medicine for the treatment of narcolepsy.[38]

CLINICAL CONTROVERSY

Some clinicians believe that combinations of long- and short-acting stimulants are effective for the treatment of narcolepsy. Some stimulants have a short effective period, while others have a longer duration of activity and slower onset of action. By combining stimulants with different activities it may be possible to achieve alertness more rapidly and for a longer period. In addition, although published evidence is limited, combinations of stimulants and antidepressants may be of benefit for treatment of sleepiness and cataplexy.

CIRCADIAN RHYTHM DISORDERS

The sleep-wake cycle is under the circadian control of oscillators and can be disrupted by misalignment between an individual's biological clock and external demands on the sleep cycle. Circadian rhythm sleep disorders usually present with either insomnia or hypersomnia, depending on the individual's performance requirements. Two commonly occurring circadian rhythm sleep disorders are jet lag and shift work sleep problems.

JET LAG

Jet lag occurs when individuals travel through multiple time zones and have dramatic changes in zeitgebers. Sleep disturbances typically last for 2 to 3 days, but may last as long as 7 to 10 days if the time zone changes are greater than 8 hours. Compared to westward travel, eastward travel is associated with a longer duration of jet lag. Jet lag also leads to decreased alertness, decreased performance, and an increased incidence of gastrointestinal disturbances.

Treatment of jet lag includes nonpharmacologic and pharmacologic management. Jet lag can be avoided in coast-to-coast travel in the U.S. if the duration is less than 7 days and the normal sleep-wake cycle is observed. For travel lasting longer than 7 days, adjustment to a westbound time zone can be made by staying up and arising one to two hours later several days prior to the trip. If traveling east, an earlier bedtime and wake time for several days prior to the trip will help. Pharmacologic treatment of jet lag includes the use of short-acting benzodiazepines. Melatonin has also been used to restore the circadian rhythm.

SHIFT WORK SLEEP PROBLEMS

Shift workers comprise approximately 20% of the work force.[43] Night shift work causes a misalignment in the sleep-wake cycle and circadian rhythm that is associated with a decrease in alertness, performance, and quality of daytime sleep. More than 65% of workers on rotating shifts complain of insomnia compared with only 20% who work one shift.[43] Shift workers have a higher injury rate, rate of divorce, occurrence of on-the-job sleepiness, and incidence of substance use. Night shift workers are usually in a state of permanent circadian misalignment due to the tendency to revert to conventional sleep schedules on their days off.[43] The treatment approach for shift work sleep problems is to promote good sleep hygiene, recommending a day shift job, extending daytime sleep by sleeping in the afternoon, or

scheduling a 2- to 3-hour nap on days off from work. Hypnotics may be useful. Scheduled exposure to bright lights at night and darkness in the daytime improves adaptation to night work and daytime sleep.[43] Melatonin has also been used successfully.

DYSSOMNIA NOT OTHERWISE SPECIFIED

A sleep disorder that is not endogenous or due to a medical condition or substance-related condition is categorized as "not otherwise specified." Restless leg syndrome and periodic limb movements are two sleep disturbances that do not meet criteria for any of the other sleep disorders.

RESTLESS LEG SYNDROME

Restless leg syndrome (RLS), or Ekbom's syndrome, is characterized by paresthesias that are felt deep in the calf muscles and cause the urge to keep the legs in motion. Sometimes it is verbalized as feeling like pins and needles or a crawling or cramping sensation. Although it usually occurs in the calves, it may also occur in the thighs or arms. RLS can be very distressing, and in some cases it has led to suicide.[44] RLS occurs in both males and females, and occurs more frequently in the elderly. It has been associated with uremia, anemia, and pregnancy; caffeine, stress, and fatigue all tend to worsen symptoms. The diagnosis is made on the clinical presentation. The sensation is bilateral and occurs only during rest and inactivity and is relieved by either walking or moving the legs. The discomfort returns when the person tries to sleep, resulting in insomnia.[44]

Pharmacologic treatment of RLS includes dopaminergic agents, benzodiazepines, opioids, or anticonvulsants. In mild cases of RLS, benzodiazepines may be first-line agents. Clonazepam, lorazepam, triazolam, and temazepam have been effective. Clonazepam 0.5 to 2 mg is most frequently studied. Opiates such as methadone 5 to 20 mg, codeine 30 to 120 mg, and oxycodone 2.5 mg are very effective, but the development of tolerance is a concern. Abuse potential with opiates is also a concern due to the chronic nature of the condition.[2] Other agents that have been used include apomorphine, amantadine, tramadol, magnesium, oxycodone, propoxyphene, gabapentin, bromocriptine, clonidine, and carbamazepine.[45–50] Tolerance may develop with any agent used. Patients should take the agent early enough to allow for drug absorption prior to bedtime. In severe cases, levodopa and the dopamine agonists cabergoline, pergolide, pramipexole, and ropinirole may be useful. The initial dose of levodopa is 50 mg 30 minutes before bedtime. This dose may be titrated, with most patients achieving benefit from levodopa 200 mg/carbidopa 50 mg.[44] Rebound symptoms may occur; however, dosing during the day or using sustained-release products may alleviate rebound.

NOCTURNAL MYOCLONUS (PERIODIC LEG MOVEMENTS)

Most patients with RLS also have periodic leg movements (PLMs), and approximately one-third of patients with PLMs have RLS.[48] Unlike RLS, PLMs are diagnosed in the sleep laboratory. A burst of muscle activity lasting 0.5 to 5 seconds is noted in the anterior tibialis EMG recording. Confirmation of diagnosis is at least 40 bursts within 8 hours of sleep.[48]

PLMs are stereotypic, repetitive, periodic movements of the legs that occur during sleep every 20 to 40 seconds and last 10 minutes to several hours.[48] The movements usually involve the big toe, but the ankle, knee, and hip may also flex. They may be terminated by a violent kick or other body movement. The person does not recognize the problem and only notes the daytime consequence of insufficient sleep and morning leg cramps. Often the bed partner describes the person as a restless sleeper and notes that the bedcovers are in disarray. Renal failure may predispose to PLMs.[51] Benzodiazepine withdrawal and TCAs may precipitate the condition. The treatment approach for PLMs is similar to that of RLS. While mild cases may not require treatment, more severe cases may require clonazepam, baclofen, or opiates. TCAs usually worsen the problem, although in one case series, imipramine 25 mg improved symptoms in five patients. Lamotrigine 100 mg has improved symptoms.[52] The most severe cases are treated with levodopa or dopamine agonists. Patients should take their medications early enough prior to bedtime to allow for drug absorption.

PARASOMNIAS

Parasomnias are adverse events that either occur during sleep or are exaggerated by sleep. Many of these disorders are considered to be disorders of partial arousal from various sleep stages. Examples of parasomnias are sleepwalking disorder, sleep terror disorder, and nightmare disorder.

Sleepwalking and sleep terrors are found normally in children between the ages of 4 and 12 and usually resolve in adolescence. These disorders are associated with psychopathology only if they persist into adulthood.[53] Sleep terrors may begin in adults between the ages of 20 and 30. Onset of sleepwalking in adults without a history of sleepwalking as children should prompt a search for a neurological or substance use condition.[53] Sleepwalking and sleep terror disorder involve intrusions of wakefulness into NREM sleep during the first third of the night. In sleepwalking, individuals become ambulatory, are difficult to awaken, and are amnestic for the event. Sleep terrors involve intense fear and autonomic arousal. Individuals are difficult to awaken, inconsolable, and amnestic for the event.[53]

Treatment of sleepwalking involves protecting the individual from harm by putting safety latches on doors and windows, removing hazardous objects from bedrooms, and covering glass doors with heavy curtains. Benzodiazepines, SSRIs, or TCAs may be beneficial in adults. Benzodiazepines may also be helpful in curtailing sleep terrors in adults.[53]

Nightmares are anxiety-provoking dreams characterized by vivid recall. Treatment is directed at reducing stress, anxiety, and sleep deprivation. In extreme cases, low-dose benzodiazepines may be indicated. Cyproheptadine may be useful for adults with frequent, extremely disturbing nightmares.[53]

PHARMACOECONOMIC CONSIDERATIONS

Despite the prevalence of sleep disorders, most cases go undiagnosed and untreated. The direct cost of insomnia alone adds an estimated $13.9 billion to the national health care bill each year.[1,54] The direct and indirect costs of sleep disorders including medications, treatment, absenteeism, decreased productivity, accidents, hospitalizations, and increased morbidity and mortality is estimated to be between $92.5 and $107.5 billion annually. Improvements in recognition and treatment may decrease the economic burden and prevent progression to both medical and psychiatric disorders.[54]

Quality of life may be improved by appropriate treatment. For example, treatment of OSA with nasal CPAP improved the number of years of good health by 5.5 quality-adjusted life years. Hypnotic therapy has also been found to markedly improve both the disorder and quality of life in shift workers.[54]

EVALUATION OF THERAPEUTIC OUTCOMES

A decision analysis for dyssomnias is shown in Figure 71–1. Patients with short-term or chronic insomnia should be evaluated after 1 week of therapy to assess for drug efficacy, adverse effects, and adherence to nonpharmacologic recommendations. Patients should be instructed to keep a sleep diary. The diary requires daily recording of bedtime, wake time, latency of sleep onset, number and duration of awakenings, medication ingestion, naps, and an index of sleep quality.

Individuals with sleep apnea treated with weight reduction and CPAP or drug therapy should be evaluated after 2 to 4 weeks of treatment for improvement in alertness and daytime symptoms (reduction in headache frequency and severity, improvement in memory, and decreased irritability) and weight reduction. The bed partner can be consulted regarding reduced snoring and gasping episodes. A repeat PSG is indicated if the patient has not shown clinical improvement. Overall, the goals of therapy are to reduce the number of apneic episodes and improve oxygen saturation.

In individuals with narcolepsy, reduction in daytime sleepiness, cataplexy, hypnagogic and hypnopompic hallucinations, and sleep paralysis are monitored. Patients should be evaluated monthly until an optimal dose is achieved, and then every 6 to 12 months to assess for the development of adverse drug effects (e.g., mood changes, sleep disturbances, and cardiovascular abnormalities). If symptoms increase during therapy, PSG should be performed.

Patients with RLS or PLMs should be evaluated monthly to monitor for excessive daytime somnolence, tolerance, efficacy, and adverse effects of the medication. Because the conditions are chronic, assessment should occur every 6 to 12 months and should include monitoring for depression because it is a frequent complication that should be treated.

CONCLUSION

Disturbances of sleep affect approximately one-third of the population. Effective management of sleep disturbances requires an accurate diagnosis. Treatment of sleep disorders involves both nonpharmacologic and pharmacologic management. Identifiable causes of insomnia should be managed if possible before instituting pharmacologic

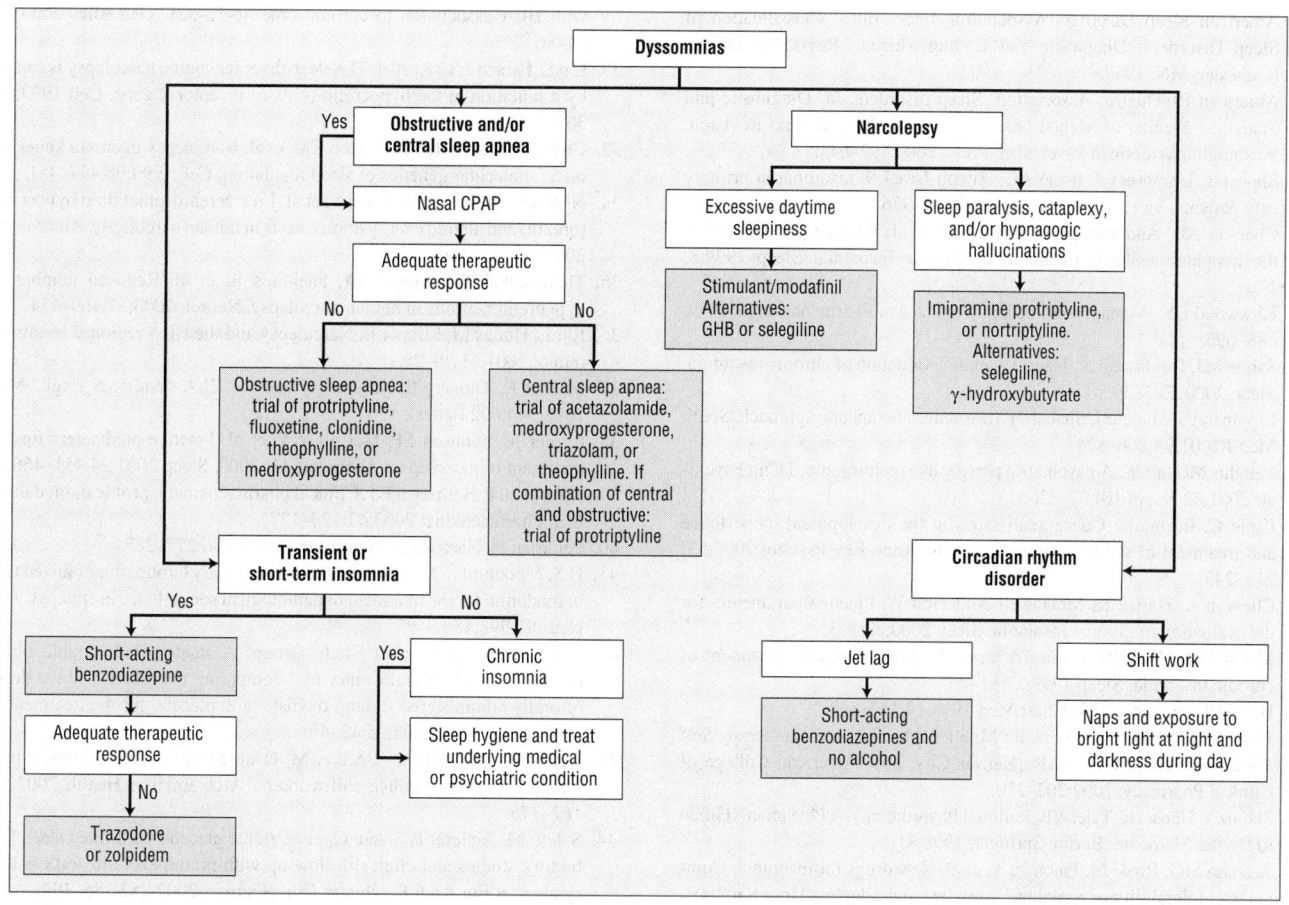

FIGURE 71–1. Algorithm for treatment of dyssomnias. (Adapted and reprinted with permission from Jermain DM. Sleep disorders. In: Jann M (ed): Pharmacotherapy Self-Assessment Program, 2nd ed. Kansas City, MO, American College of Clinical Pharmacy, 1995:139–154.)

therapy. Benzodiazepines are preferable for the treatment of short-term insomnia; however, their use is contraindicated in sleep apnea. Antidepressants are an alternative treatment for insomnia, and they effectively treat sleep apnea and some of the symptoms of narcolepsy. Modafinil, psychostimulants, TCAs, and fluoxetine are effective treatments for narcolepsy. Parasomnias and circadian rhythm disorders are usually managed nonpharmacologically. Mild cases of RLS and PLMs may be managed nonpharmacologically; more severe cases are treated with clonazepam, levodopa-carbidopa, or opiates.

ABBREVIATIONS

CPAP: continuous positive airway pressure
CSA: central sleep apnea
EDS: excessive daytime sleepiness
EEG: electroencephalogram
EMG: electromyogram
EOG: electro-oculogram
GABA: γ-aminobutyric acid
HLA: human leukocyte antigen
MPG: medroxyprogesterone
N-DAF: N-desalkylflurazepam
NREM: non–rapid eye movement (sleep)
OSA: obstructive sleep apnea

PLM: periodic leg movement
PSG: polysomnography
REM: rapid eye movement (sleep)
SSRI: selective serotonin reuptake inhibitor

Review Questions and other resources can be found at *www.pharmacotherapyonline.com.*

REFERENCES

1. Walsh JK, Engelhardt CL. The direct economic costs of insomnia in the United States for 1995. Sleep 1999;22:S386–S393.
2. Neylan TC, Reynolds CF, Kupfer DJ. Sleep disorders. In: Yudofsky SC, Hales RE, eds. American Psychiatric Press Textbook of Neuropsychiatry, 3rd ed. Washington, American Psychiatric Press, 2000:583–606.
3. Gillin CJ, Seifritz E, Zoltoski RK, et al. Basic science of sleep. In: Sadock BJ, Sadock VA, eds. Kaplan and Sadock's Comprehensive Textbook of Psychiatry, 7th ed. Philadelphia, Lippincott Williams & Wilkins, 2000: 199–209.
4. Dagan Y, Abadi J. Sleep-wake disorder disability: A lifelong untreatable pathology of the circadian time structure. Chronobiol Int 2001;18:1019–1027.
5. Franken P. Long-term vs. short-term processes regulating REM sleep. J Sleep Res 2002;11:17–28.
6. Stickgold R, Hobson JA, Fosse R, Fosse M. Sleep, learning and dreams: Off-line memory reprocessing. Science 2001;294:1052–1058.

7. American Sleep Disorders Association. International Classification of Sleep Disorders: Diagnostic and Coding Manual: Revised Addition. Rochester, MN, 1997.

8. American Psychiatric Association. Sleep disorders. In: Diagnostic and Statistical Manual of Mental Disorders, Fourth Edition, Text Revision. Washington, American Psychiatric Press, 2000:597–644.

9. Shocat T, Umphress J, Isreal AG, Ancoli-Israel S. Insomnia in primary care patients. Sleep 1999;22(Suppl 2):S359–S365.

10. Chesson AL, Anderson WM, Littner M, et al. Practice parameters for the nonpharmacologic treatment of chronic insomnia. Sleep 1999;8: 1–6.

11. Kirkwood CK. Management of insomnia. J Am Pharm Assoc 1999;39: 688–696.

12. Sateia MJ, Doghramji K, Hauri PJ, et al. Evaluation of chronic insomnia. Sleep 2000;23:1–39.

13. Lippmann S, Mazour I, Shabab H. Insomnia: Therapeutic approach. South Med J 2001;94:866–874.

14. Vaughn-McCall W. A psychiatric perspective on insomnia. J Clin Psychiatr 2001;62(Suppl 10):27–32.

15. Espie C. Insomnia: Conceptual issues in the development, persistence and treatment of sleep disorders in adults. Annu Rev Psychol 2002;53: 215–243.

16. Chesson A, Hartse K, McDowell-Anderson W. Practice parameters for the evaluation of chronic insomnia. Sleep 2000;23:1–5.

17. Morin CM, Hauri PJ, Espie CA, et al. Nonpharmacologic treatment of chronic insomnia. Sleep 1999;22:81–23.

18. Hauri PJ. Insomnia. Clin Chest Med 1998;19:157–168.

19. Jackson CW. Mood disorders. In: Mueller BA, ed. Pharmacotherapy Self Assessment Program (PSAP). Kansas City, MO, American College of Clinical Pharmacy, 2002:203–250.

20. Schulz V, Hansel R, Tyler VE. Rational Phytotherapy. A Physician's Guide to Herbal Medicine. Berlin, Springer, 1998:81.

21. Terzano MG, Rossi M, Palomba V, et al. New drugs for insomnia: Comparative tolerability of zopiclone, zolpidem and zaleplon. Drug Saf 2003; 26:261–282.

22. Elie R, Ruteher E, Farr IK, et al. Sleep latency is shortened during 4 weeks of treatment with zaleplon, a novel nonbenzodiazepine hypnotic. J Clin Psychiatry 1999;60:536–544.

23. Walsh JK, Fry J, Erwin CS, et al. Efficacy and tolerability of 14-day administration of zaleplon 5 mg and 10 mg for the treatment of primary insomnia. Clin Drug Invest 1998;16:347–354.

24. Walsh JK, Pollack CP, Shark MMB, et al. Lack of residual sedation following middle-of-the-night zaleplon administration in sleep maintenance insomnia. Clin Neuropharmacol 2000;23:17–21.

25. Ancoli-Isreal S. Insomnia in the elderly: A review for the primary care practitioner. Sleep 2000;23:S23–S30.

26. Grunstein RR, Hedner J, Grote L. Treatment options for sleep apnoea. Drugs 2001;61:2:237–251.

27. Kribbs NB, Pack AJ, Kline LR, et al. Effects of one night without nasal CPAP treatment on sleep and sleepiness in patients with obstructive sleep apnea. Am Rev Respir Dis 2003;147:1162–1168.

28. Kraiczi H, Hedner J, Dahlof P, et al. Effect of serotonin uptake inhibition on breathing during sleep and daytime symptoms in obstructive sleep apnoea. Sleep 1999;22:61–67.

29. Naughton MT, Bradley TD. Sleep apnoea in congestive heart failure. Clin Chest Med 1998;19:99–113.

30. Mitler M, Hayduk R. Benefits and risks of pharmacotherapy for narcolepsy. Drug Saf 2002;25(11):791–809.

31. Nakayama J, Miura M, Honda M, et al. Linkage of human narcolepsy with HLA association to chromosome 4p-13-q21. Genomics 2000;65: 84–86.

32. Lin L, Faraco J, Li R, et al. The sleep disorder canine narcolepsy is caused by a mutation in the hypocretin (orexin) receptor 2 gene. Cell 1999;98: 365–376.

33. Chemelli RM, Willie JT, Sinton CM, et al. Narcolepsy in orexin knockout mice: molecular genetics of sleep regulation. Cell 1999;98:437–451.

34. Nishin S, Ripley B, Overeem S, et al. Low cerebrospinal fluid hypocretin (orexin) and altered energy homeostasis in human narcolepsy. Ann Neurol 2001;50:381–388.

35. Thannicakal TC, Moore RY, Nienhuis R, et al. Reduced number of hypocretin neurons in human narcolepsy. Neuron 2000;27:469–474.

36. Lin L, Hungs M, Mignot E. Narcolepsy and the HLA region. J Neuroimmunol 2001;117:9–20.

37. Mignot E, Thorsby E. Narcolepsy and the HLA system. N Engl J Med 2001;344:692 (letter).

38. Littner M, Johnson SF, McCall WV, et al. Practice parameters for the treatment of narcolepsy: An update for 2000. Sleep 2001;24:451–466.

39. Robertson P, Hellriegel ET. Clinical pharmacokinetic profile of modafinil. Clin Pharmacokinet 2003;42:123–127.

40. Feldman N. Narcolepsy. South Med J 2003;96:277–287.

41. U.S. Modafinil in Narcolepsy Multicenter Study Group. Randomized trial of modafinil for the treatment of pathological somnolence in epilepsy. Ann Neurol 1998;43:88–97.

42. U.S. Xyrem Multicenter Study Group. A randomized, double blind, placebo-controlled multicenter trial comparing the effect of three doses of orally administered sodium oxybate with placebo for the treatment of narcolepsy. Sleep 2002;25:42–49.

43. Garbarino S, Nobili L, Beelke, M, et al. Sleep disorders and daytime sleepiness in state police shiftworkers. Arch Environ Health 2002;57: 167–175.

44. Saletu M, Anderer P, Saletu G, et al. Acute placebo-controlled sleep laboratory studies and clinical follow-up with pramipexole in restless legs syndrome. Eur Arch Psychiatry Clin Neurosci 2002;252:185–194.

45. Reuter I, Ellis CM, Ray-Chaudhuri K. Nocturnal subcutaneous apomorphine infusion: I. Parkinson's disease and restless legs syndrome. Acta Neurol Scand 1999;100:163–167.

46. Evidente VG, Adler CH, Caviness JN, et al. Amantadine is beneficial in restless legs syndrome. Mov Disord 2000;15:324–337.

47. Lauerma H, Markkula J. Treatment of restless legs syndrome with tramadol: An open study. J Clin Psychiatry 1999;60:241–244.

48. Chesson AL, Wise M, Davila D, et al. Practice parameters for the treatment of restless legs syndrome and periodic limb movements. Sleep 1999;22: 961–968.

49. Stiasny K, Robbecke J, Schuler P, Oertel WH. Treatment of idiopathic restless legs syndrome (RLS) with the D2-agonist cabergoline: An open clinical trial. Sleep 2000;23:349–354.

50. Wetter TC, Stiasny K, Winkelmann J, et al. A randomized controlled study of pergolide in patients with restless legs syndrome. Neurology 1999;52: 944–950.

51. Montplaisir J, Nicolas A, Denesle R, Gomez-Mancilla B. Restless legs syndrome improved by pramipexole: A double-blind randomized trial. Neurology 1999;52:938–943.

52. Ondo W. Ropinirole for restless legs syndrome. Mov Disord 1999;14: 18–40.

53. Schenck CH, Mahowald MW. Parasomnias managing bizarre sleep-related behavior disorders. Postgrad Med 2000;107:145–156.

54. Leger D. Public health and insomnia: Economic impact. Sleep 2000; 23(Suppl 3):S69–S76.

72

DIABETES MELLITUS

Curtis L. Triplitt, Charles A. Reasner, and William L. Isley

Learning Objectives and other resources can be found at *www.pharmacotherapyonline.com.*

KEY CONCEPTS

◀1 Diabetes mellitus is a group of metabolic disorders of fat, carbohydrate, and protein metabolism that results from defects in insulin secretion, insulin action (sensitivity), or both.

◀2 The incidence of type 2 diabetes mellitus (DM) is increasing. This has been attributed in part to increasing obesity, sedentary lifestyle, and an increasing minority population.

◀3 The two major classifications of diabetes mellitus are type 1 (insulin deficient) and type 2 (combined insulin resistance and relative deficiency in insulin secretion). They differ in clinical presentation, onset, etiology, and progression of disease. Both are associated with microvascular and macrovascular disease complications.

◀4 Diagnosis of diabetes is made by three criteria: fasting plasma glucose ≥126 mg/dL, a 2-hour value from a 75-g oral glucose tolerance test ≥200 mg/dL, or a casual plasma glucose level of ≥200 mg/dL with symptoms of diabetes; with results confirmed by any of the three criteria on a separate day.

◀5 Goals of therapy in diabetes mellitus are directed at reducing symptoms of hyperglycemia, reducing the onset and progression of retinopathy, nephropathy, and neuropathy complications, intensive therapy for associated cardiovascular risk factors, and improving quality and quantity of life.

◀6 Metformin should be included in the therapy for all type 2 DM patients, if tolerated and not contraindicated, as it is the only oral antihyperglycemic medication proven to reduce the risk of total mortality and cardiovascular death, according to the United Kingdom Prospective Diabetes Study.

◀7 Intensive glycemic control is paramount for reduction of microvascular complications (neuropathy, retinopathy, and nephropathy) as evidenced by the Diabetes Control and Complications Trial in type 1 DM and the United Kingdom Prospective Diabetes Study (UKPDS) in type 2 DM. The UKPDS also reported that control of hypertension in patients with diabetes will not only reduce the risk of retinopathy and nephropathy, but also reduce cardiovascular risk.

◀8 Knowledge of the patient's quantitative and qualitative meal patterns, activity levels, pharmacokinetics of insulin preparations, and pharmacology of oral antihyperglycemic agents are essential to individualize the treatment plan and optimize blood glucose control while minimizing risks for hypoglycemia and other adverse effects of pharmacologic therapies.

◀9 Type 1 treatment necessitates insulin therapy. Currently, the basal-bolus insulin therapy or pump therapy in motivated individuals often leads to successful glycemic outcomes. Basal-bolus therapy often includes a basal insulin for fasting and postabsorptive control, and rapid acting bolus insulin for mealtime coverage. Therapeutically, use of basal-bolus therapy in type 2 DM is increasing.

◀10 Treatment of type 2 DM often necessitates use of multiple therapeutic agents (combination therapy), including oral antihyperglycemics and insulin to obtain glycemic goals.

◀11 Aggressive management of cardiovascular disease risk factors in type 2 DM is necessary to reduce the risk for adverse cardiovascular events or death. Smoking cessation, use of antiplatelet therapy as a primary prevention strategy, aggressive management of dyslipidemia minimally to goal low-density lipoprotein-cholesterol (LDL-C) (<100 mg/dL) and secondarily to raise high-density lipoprotein-cholesterol (HDL-C) to ≥40 mg/dL, and treatment of hypertension (again often requiring multiple drugs) minimally to <130/80 mm Hg are vital.

◀12 Prevention strategies for type 1 DM have been unsuccessful. Prevention strategies for type 2 DM are established. Lifestyle changes, dietary restriction of fat, aerobic exercise for 30 minutes 5 times a week, and weight loss, form the backbone of successful prevention. To date, medications have been less effective than lifestyle changes to prevent progression to type 2 DM.

◀13 Patient education and ability to demonstrate self-care and adherence to therapeutic lifestyle and pharmacologic interventions are crucial to successful outcomes. Multidisciplinary teams of health care professionals including physicians (primary care, endocrinologists, ophthalmologists, and vascular surgeons), podiatrists, dietitians, nurses, pharmacists, social workers, behavioral health specialists, and certified diabetes educators are needed to optimize these outcomes in persons with diabetes mellitus.

Diabetes mellitus (DM) is a group of metabolic disorders characterized by hyperglycemia; is associated with abnormalities in carbohydrate, fat and protein metabolism; and results in chronic complications including microvascular, macrovascular, and neuropathic disorders. Nearly 18.2 million Americans have DM, yet only about two-thirds of them have been diagnosed.[1] The economic burden of DM approximated 132 billion dollars in 2002, including direct medical and treatment costs as well as indirect costs attributed to disability and mortality.[1] DM is the leading cause of blindness in adults aged 20 to 74 years, and the leading contributor to development of end-stage renal disease. It also accounts for approximately 82,000 lower extremity amputations annually.[1] Finally, a cardiovascular event is responsible for 75% of deaths in individuals with type 2 DM.[1]

Although efforts to control hyperglycemia and associated symptoms are important, the major challenges in optimally managing the patient with DM are targeted at reducing or preventing complications, and improving life expectancy and quality of life. Research and drug development efforts over the past several decades have provided valuable information that applies directly to improving outcomes in patients with DM and have expanded the therapeutic armamentarium. Additionally, interventions in an attempt to prevent disease in high-risk populations have been reported for type 1 and 2 DM.

EPIDEMIOLOGY

Typical type 1 DM is an autoimmune disorder developing in childhood or early adulthood, although some latent forms do occur. Type 1 DM accounts for up to 10% of all cases of DM and is likely initiated by the exposure of a genetically susceptible individual to an environmental agent.[2] Candidate genes and environmental factors are reportedly prevalent in the general population, but development of β-cell autoimmunity occurs in less than 10% of the population and progresses to diabetes mellitus in less than 1% of the population.[3]

The prevalence of β-cell autoimmunity appears proportional to the incidence of type 1 DM in various populations. For instance, the countries of Sweden, Sardinia, and Finland have the highest prevalence of islet cell antibody (3% to 4.5%) and are associated with the highest incidence of type 1 DM, 22 to 35 per 100,000.[4]

Markers of autoimmunity have been detected in 14% to 33% of persons with type 2 DM in some populations and manifest with early failure of oral agents and insulin dependence. This type of DM has also been referred to as latent autoimmune diabetes in adults (LADA).[4]

Type 1 DM idiopathic is a nonimmune form of diabetes frequently seen in minorities with intermittent insulin requirements.[5] The prevalence of type 1 DM has been increasing over the last one hundred years.[6] Maturity onset diabetes of youth (MODY), which has an identifiable genetic defect in the glucokinase gene, and endocrine disorders such as acromegaly and Cushing's syndrome, can be secondary causes of DM.[7] These unusual etiologies, however, only account for 1% to 2% of the total cases of type 2 DM. See the section on other forms of diabetes mellitus later in this chapter for further discussion.

The prevalence of type 2 DM is increasing. Type 2 DM accounts for as much as 90% of all cases of DM, and overall the prevalence of type 2 DM in the United States is about 8.7% in persons age 20 or older. However, there is likely one person undiagnosed for every two persons currently diagnosed with the disease.[1] Multiple

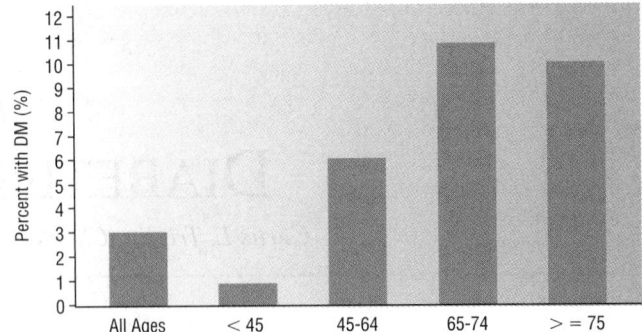

FIGURE 72–1. Percentage of the population with diagnosed diabetes by age for the period 1991–1993. (Adapted from National Institutes of Health. Diabetes in America, 2nd ed. 1995.)

risk factors for the development of type 2 DM have been identified, including family history (i.e., parents or siblings with diabetes); obesity (i.e., ≥20% over ideal body weight, or body mass index [BMI] ≥25 kg/m²); habitual physical inactivity; race or ethnicity (see list below); previously identified impaired glucose tolerance or impaired fasting glucose; hypertension (≥140/90 mm Hg in adults); high-density lipoprotein (HDL) cholesterol ≤35 mg/dL and/or a triglyceride level ≥250 mg/dL; history of gestational diabetes mellitus or delivery of a baby weighing >9 pounds; history of vascular disease; and polycystic ovary disease.[8] The prevalence of type 2 DM increases with age, it is more common in women than in men in the United States, and varies widely among various racial and ethnic populations, being especially increased in some groups of Native Americans, Hispanic-American, Asian-American, African-American, and Pacific Island people[4] (Figs. 72–1 and 72–2). While the prevalence of type 2 DM increases with age, the disorder is increasingly being recognized in adolescence. Much of the rise in adolescent type 2 DM is related to an increase in adiposity and sedentary lifestyle, in addition to an inheritable predisposition.[9] Most cases of type 2 DM do not have a well-known cause; therefore it is uncertain whether it represents a few or many independent disorders manifesting as hyperglycemia.[10] With increasing worldwide obesity, the prevalence of type 2 DM is increasing, though this has been recently disputed, suggesting that we are primarily just finding more cases through more aggressive screening.[11]

Gestational diabetes mellitus (GDM) complicates roughly 7% of all pregnancies in the United States.[12] Most women will return to normoglycemia postpartum, but 30% to 50% will develop type 2 DM or glucose intolerance later in life.

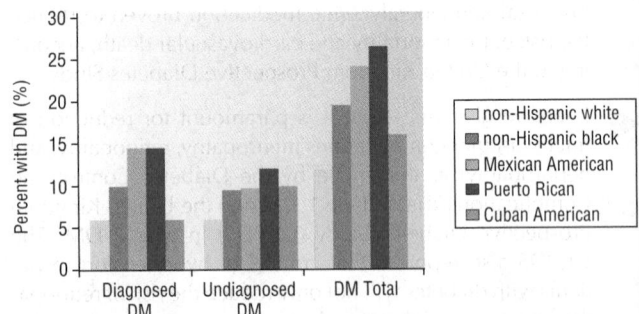

FIGURE 72–2. Prevalence of diabetes mellitus (ages 45–74 years) in U.S. whites, blacks (1976–1980), and Latinos (1982–1984). (Adapted from National Institutes of Health. Diabetes in America, 2nd ed. 1995.)

PATHOGENESIS, DIAGNOSIS, AND CLASSIFICATION

CLASSIFICATION OF DIABETES

Diabetes is a metabolic disorder characterized by resistance to the action of insulin, insufficient insulin secretion, or both.[13] The clinical manifestation of these disorders is hyperglycemia. The vast majority of diabetic patients are classified into one of two broad categories: type 1 diabetes caused by an absolute deficiency of insulin, or type 2 diabetes defined by the presence of insulin resistance with an inadequate compensatory increase in insulin secretion. Women who develop diabetes due to the stress of pregnancy are classified as having gestational diabetes. Finally, uncommon types of diabetes caused by infections, drugs, endocrinopathies, pancreatic destruction, and known genetic defects are classified separately (Table 72–1).

TYPE 1 DIABETES

This form of diabetes results from autoimmune destruction of the β cells of the pancreas. Markers of immune destruction of the β cell are present at the time of diagnosis in 90% of individuals and include islet cell antibodies, antibodies to glutamic acid decarboxylase, and antibodies to insulin. While this form of diabetes usually occurs in children and adolescents, it can occur at any age. Younger individuals typically have a rapid rate of β-cell destruction and present with ketoacidosis, while adults often maintain sufficient insulin secretion to prevent ketoacidosis for many years, which is often referred to as latent autoimmune diabetes in adults (LADA).[4]

TYPE 2 DIABETES

This form of diabetes is characterized by insulin resistance and at least initially, a relative lack of insulin secretion. Most individuals with type 2 diabetes exhibit abdominal obesity which itself causes insulin resistance. In addition, hypertension, dyslipidemia (high triglyceride levels and low HDL-cholesterol levels), and elevated inhibitor plasminogen activator-1 (PAI-1) levels are often present in these individuals. This clustering of abnormalities is referred to as the "insulin resistance syndrome" or the "metabolic syndrome." Because of these abnormalities, patients with type 2 diabetes are at increased risk of developing macrovascular complications. Type 2 diabetes has a strong genetic predisposition and is more common in all ethnic groups other than those of European ancestry. At this point the genetic cause of most cases of type 2 diabetes is not well defined.[14]

GESTATIONAL DIABETES MELLITUS

Gestational diabetes mellitus (GDM) is defined as glucose intolerance which is first recognized during pregnancy. Gestational diabetes complicates about 7% of all pregnancies. Clinical detection is important, as therapy will reduce perinatal morbidity and mortality.

OTHER SPECIFIC TYPES OF DIABETES

Genetic Defects

Maturity onset diabetes of youth (MODY) is characterized by impaired insulin secretion with minimal or no insulin resistance. Patients typically exhibit mild hyperglycemia at an early age. The disease is inherited in an autosomal dominant pattern with at least three different loci identified to date. Genetic inability to convert proinsulin to insulin results in mild hyperglycemia and is inherited in an autosomal dominant pattern. Similarly, the production of mutant insulin molecules has been identified in a few families and results in mild glucose intolerance.

Several genetic mutations have been described in the insulin receptor and are associated with insulin resistance. Type A insulin resistance refers to the clinical syndrome of acanthosis nigricans, virilization in women, polycystic ovaries, and hyperinsulinemia. Leprechaunism is a pediatric syndrome with specific facial features and severe insulin resistance due to a defect in the insulin receptor gene. Lipoatrophic diabetes probably results from postreceptor defects in insulin signaling.

SCREENING

TYPE 1 DIABETES MELLITUS

There is still a low prevalence of type 1 DM in the general population and due to the acuteness of symptoms, screening for type 1 DM is not recommended.[15]

TYPE 2 DIABETES MELLITUS

Based on expert opinion, the American Diabetes Association (ADA) recommends screening for type 2 DM every 3 years in all adults beginning at age 45 years.[16] Testing should be considered at an earlier age and more frequently in individuals with risk factors. The recommended screening test is the fasting plasma glucose. An oral glucose tolerance test (OGTT) (more costly, less convenient) can be performed alternatively or in addition to fasting plasma glucose when a high index of suspicion for the disease is present.[5]

CHILDREN AND ADOLESCENTS

Despite a lack of clinical evidence to support widespread testing of children for type 2 DM, it is clear that more children and adolescents are developing type 2 DM. The ADA recommends that overweight (defined as BMI >85th percentile for age and sex, weight for height >85th percentile, or weight >120% of ideal [50th percentile] for height) youths with at least two of the following risk factors: a family history of type 2 diabetes in first- and second-degree relatives; Native Americans, African-Americans, Hispanic-Americans, and Asians/South Pacific Islanders; and those with signs of insulin resistance or conditions associated with insulin resistance (acanthosis nigricans, hypertension, dyslipidemia, or polycystic ovary syndrome) be screened. Testing should be done every 2 years starting at 10 years of age or at the onset of puberty if it occurs at a younger age.[16]

GESTATIONAL DIABETES

Risk assessment for GDM should occur at the first prenatal visit. Women at high risk (positive family history, history of GDM, marked obesity, or member of a high-risk ethnic group) should be screened as soon as feasible. If the initial screening is negative they should undergo retesting at 24 to 28 weeks' gestation. Evaluation for GDM can be done in one of two ways. The one-step approach involves an OGTT only and may be cost-effective in high-risk patient populations. The two-step approach uses a screening test to measure plasma or serum glucose concentration 1-hour after a 50-g oral glucose load

TABLE 72–1. Etiologic Classification of Diabetes Mellitus

1. **Type 1 diabetes**[a] (β-cell destruction, usually leading to absolute insulin deficiency)
   Immune mediated
   Idiopathic
2. **Type 2 diabetes**[a] (may range from predominantly insulin resistance with relative insulin deficiency to a predominantly insulin secretory defect with insulin resistance)
3. **Other specific types**
   Genetic defects of β-cell function (42)
      Chromosome 20q, HNF-4α (MODY1)
      Chromosome 7p, glucokinase (MODY2)
      Chromosome 12q, HNF-1β (MODY3)
      Chromosome 13q, insulin promoter factor (MODY4)
      Chromosome 17q, HNF-1β (MODY5)
      Chromosome 2q, neurogenic differentiation 1/b-cell e-box transactivator 2 (MODY 6)
      Mitochondrial DNA
      Others
   Genetic defects in insulin action
      Type 1 insulin resistance
      Leprechaunism
      Rabson-Mendenhall syndrome
      Lipoatrophic diabetes
      Others
   Diseases of the exocrine pancreas
      Pancreatitis
      Trauma/pancreatectomy
      Neoplasia
      Cystic fibrosis
      Hemochromatosis
      Fibrocalculous pancreatopathy
      Others
   Endocrinopathies
      Acromegaly
      Cushing's syndrome
      Glucagonoma
      Pheochromocytoma
      Hyperthyroidism
      Somatostatinoma
      Aldosteronoma
      Others
   Drug- or chemical-induced
      Vacor (pyriminil)
      Pentamidine
      Nicotinic acid
      Glucocorticoids
      Thyroid hormone
      Diazoxide
      β-Adrenergic agonists
      Thiazides
      Phenytoin
      α-Interferon
      Others
   Infections
      Congenital rubella
      Cytomegalovirus
      Others
   Uncommon forms of immune-mediated diabetes
      "Stiff-man" syndrome
      Anti-insulin receptor antibodies
      Others
   Other genetic syndromes sometimes associated with diabetes
      Down's syndrome
      Klinefelter's syndrome
      Turner's syndrome
      Wolfram's syndrome
      Friedreich's ataxia
      Huntington's chorea
      Laurence-Moon-Bieldel syndrome
      Myotonic dystrophy
      Porphyria
      Prader-Willi syndrome
      Others
4. **Gestational diabetes mellitus (GDM)**

[a] Patients with any form of diabetes may require insulin treatment at some stage of their disease. Such use of insulin does not in itself classify the patient.
Adapted with permission from Report of the Expert Committee.[13]

TABLE 72–2. Diagnosis of Gestational Diabetes Mellitus with a 100-g or 75-g Glucose Load

100-g Glucose load

Time	Plasma Glucose
Fasting	≥95 mg/dL (5.3 mmol/L)
1 hour	≥180 mg/dL (10.0 mmol/L)
2 hours	≥155 mg/dL (8.6 mmol/L)
3 hours	≥140 mg/dL (7.8 mmol/L)

75-g Glucose load

Fasting	≥95 mg/dL (5.3 mmol/L)
1 hour	≥180 mg/dL (10.0 mmol/L)
2 hours	≥155 mg/dL (8.6 mmol/L)

Two or more values must be met or exceeded for a diagnosis of diabetes to be made. The test should be done in the morning after an 8- to 14-hour fast.

(glucose challenge test [GCT]), followed by a diagnostic OGTT on the subset of women exceeding a glucose threshold of either >140 mg/dL (80% sensitive) or >130 mg/dL (90% sensitive). The diagnosis of GDM is based on a 75-g (not as well validated) or 100-g OGTT. Criteria for diagnosis of GDM based on the OGTT are summarized in Table 72–2.

DIAGNOSIS OF DIABETES

The diagnosis of diabetes requires the identification of a glycemic cut point, which discriminates normals from diabetics (Table 72–3). The present cut points reflect the level of glucose above which microvascular complications have been shown to increase. Cross-sectional studies from Egypt, in Pima Indians, and in a representative sample from the United States have shown a consistent increase in the risk of developing retinopathy at a fasting glucose level above 99 to 116 mg/dL (5.5 to 6.4 mmol/L), at a 2-hour postprandial level above 125 to 185 mg/dL (6.9 to 10.3 mmol/L), and a hemoglobin A₁c (HbA₁c) above 5.9 to 6.0% (Fig. 72–3).[13,17,18]

The ADA recommends using the fasting glucose as the principal tool for the diagnosis of diabetes mellitus in nonpregnant adults. In addition, as shown in Table 72–4, they defined a new category of glycemia, impaired fasting glucose (IFG). IFG is a plasma glucose of at least 100 mg/dL (5.6 mmol/L) but less than 126 mg/dL (7.0 mmol/L). This category corresponds to the category of impaired glucose tolerance (IGT), defined as a 2-hour glucose value ≥140 mg/dL (7.8 mmol/L), but less than 200 mg/dL (11.0 mmol/L) during an OGTT. Patients with either IFG or IGT are now commonly referred to as having "prediabetes" due to a higher risk of developing diabetes in the future.

TABLE 72–4. Categorization of Glucose Status

Fasting plasma glucose (FPG)
Normal
• FPG <100 mg/dL (5.6 mmol/L)
Impaired fasting glucose (IFG)
• 100–125 mg/dL (5.6–6.9 mmol/L)
Diabetes mellitus[a]
• FPG ≥126 mg/dL (7.0 mmol/L)

2-Hour postload plasma glucose (oral glucose tolerance test)
Normal
• Postload glucose <140 mg/dL (7.8 mmol/L)
Impaired glucose tolerance (IGT)
• 2-hour postload glucose 140–199 mg/dL (7.8–11.1 mmol/L)
Diabetes mellitus[a]
• 2-hour postload glucose ≥200 mg/dL (11.1 mmol/L)

[a]Provisional diagnosis of diabetes (diagnosis to be confirmed; see Table 72–3).

The fasting and postprandial glucose levels do not measure the same physiologic processes and do not identify the same individuals as having diabetes. The fasting glucose reflects hepatic glucose production, which depends on insulin secretory capacity of the pancreas. The postprandial glucose reflects uptake of glucose in peripheral tissues (muscle and fat) and depends on insulin sensitivity of these tissues.

The ADA recommends use of hemoglobin A₁c (HbA₁c) determinations to monitor glycemic control in known diabetic patients. Because there is no gold standard assay and several countries do not have ready access to the test, an HbA₁c determination is not recommended to diagnose diabetes at the present time.

PATHOGENESIS

TYPE 1 DIABETES MELLITUS

Type 1 DM is characterized by an absolute deficiency of insulin. Most often this is the result of an immune-mediated destruction of pancreatic β cells, but rare unknown or idiopathic processes may contribute. What is evident are four main features: (1) a long preclinical period marked by the presence of immune markers when β-cell destruction is thought to occur; (2) hyperglycemia when 80% to 90% of β cells are destroyed; (3) transient remission (the so-called, "honeymoon" phase); and (4) established disease with associated risks for complications and death. Unknown is whether there is one or more inciting factors (e.g., cow's milk, or viral, dietary, or other environmental exposure) that initiate the autoimmune process[2] (Fig. 72–4).

The autoimmune process is mediated by macrophages and T lymphocytes with circulating autoantibodies to various β-cell

TABLE 72–3. Criteria for the Diagnosis of Diabetes Mellitus[a]

Symptoms of diabetes plus casual[b] plasma glucose concentration ≥200 mg/dL (11.1 mmol/L)

or

Fasting[c] plasma glucose ≥126 mg/dL (7.0 mmol/L)

or

2-hour postload glucose ≥200 mg/dL (11.1 mmol/L) during an OGTT[d]

[a]In the absence of unequivocal hyperglycemia, these criteria should be confirmed by repeat testing on a different day. The third measure (oral glucose tolerance test; OGTT) is not recommended for routine clinical use.
[b]Casual is defined as any time of day without regard to time since last meal. The classic symptoms of diabetes include polyuria, polydipsia, and unexplained weight loss.
[c]Fasting is defined as no caloric intake for at least 8 hours.
[d]The test should be performed as described by the World Health Organization, using a glucose load containing the equivalent of 75 g anhydrous glucose dissolved in water.

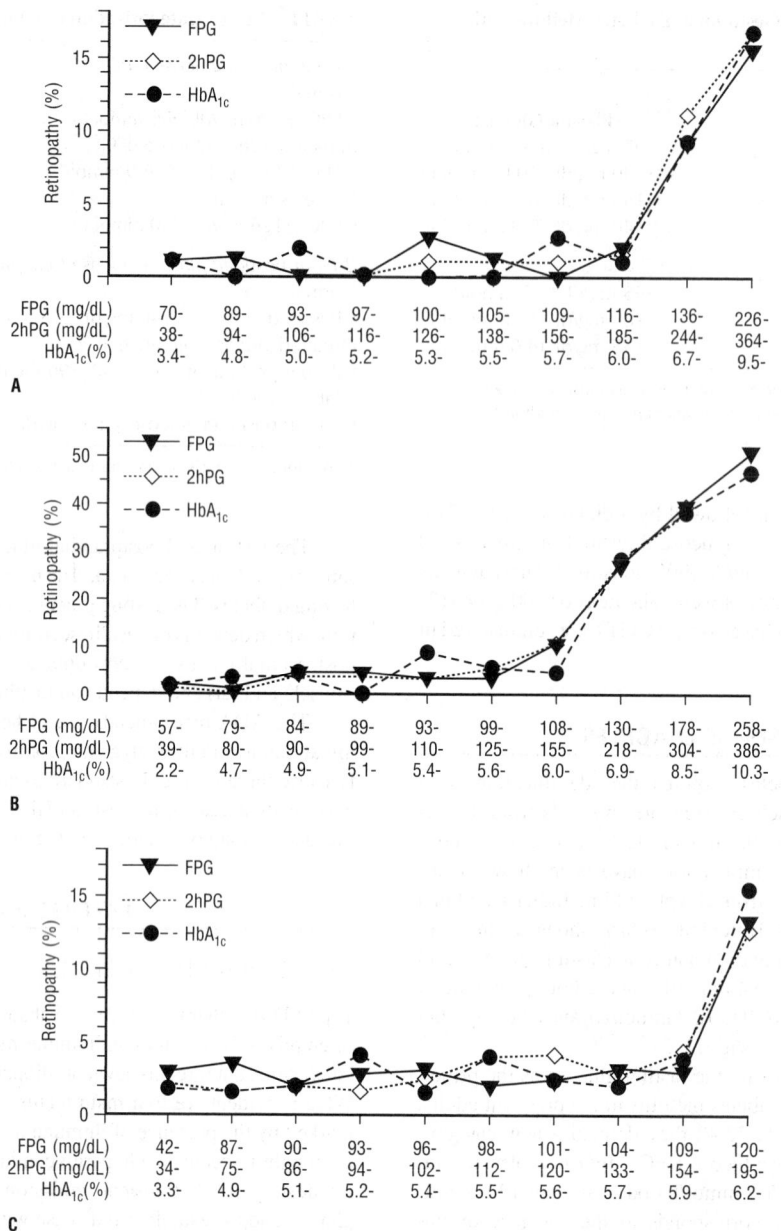

FIGURE 72–3. Prevalence of retinopathy by deciles of the distribution of fasting plasma glucose (FPG), 2-hour postprandial glucose (2-h PG), and hemoglobin A_{1c} (HbA_{1c}) in (A) Pima Indians,[12] (B) Egyptians,[11] and (C) in 40- to 74-year old participants in National Health and Nutrition Examination Survey (NHANES) III.[13] The x-axis labels indicate the lower limit of each decile group. Note that these deciles and the prevalence rates of retinopathy differ considerably among the studies, especially the Egyptian study, in which diabetic subjects were oversampled. Retinopathy was ascertained by different methods in each study; therefore the absolute prevalence rates are not comparable between studies, but their relationships with FPG, 2-h PG, and HbA_{1c} are very similar within each population.

antigens. The most commonly detected antibody associated with type 1 DM is the islet cell antibody. The test for islet cell antibody, however, is difficult to standardize across laboratories. Other more readily measured circulating antibodies include insulin autoantibodies, antibodies directed against glutamic acid decarboxylase, insulin antibodies against islet tyrosine phosphatase, and several others. More than 90% of newly diagnosed persons with type 1 DM have one or another of these antibodies, as will 3.5% to 4% of unaffected first-degree relatives. Preclinical β-cell autoimmunity precedes the diagnosis of type 1 DM by up to 9 to 13 years. Autoimmunity may remit in some perhaps less-susceptible persons, or can progress to β-cell failure in

others. These antibodies are generally considered markers of disease rather than mediators of β-cell destruction. They have been used to identify individuals at risk for type 1 diabetes mellitus in evaluating disease prevention strategies. Other nonpancreatic autoimmune disorders are associated with type 1 DM, most commonly Hashimoto's thyroiditis, but the extent of organ involvement can range from no other organs to polyglandular failure.[19]

There are strong genetic linkages to the DQA and B genes and certain human leukocyte antigens (HLAs) may be predisposing (DR3 and DR4) or protective (DRB1*04008-DQB1*0302 and DRB1*0411-DQB1*0302) on chromosome 6.[19] Other candidate genes

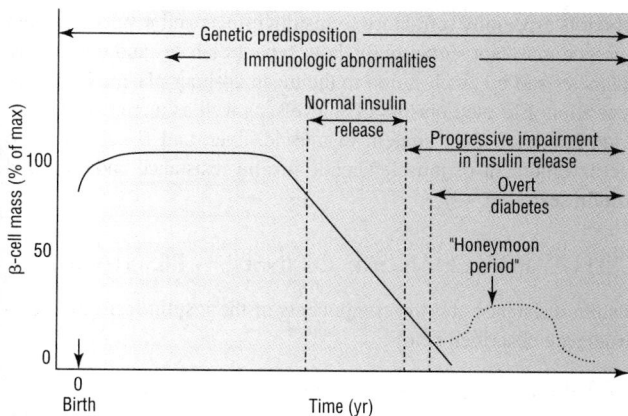

FIGURE 72–4. Scheme of the natural history of the β-cell defect in type 1 diabetes mellitus. (From ADA Medical Management of Type of 1 Diabetes, 3rd ed. 1998.)

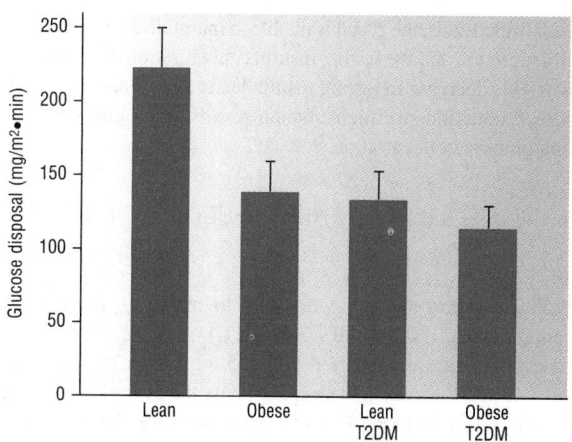

FIGURE 72–5. Whole body glucose disposal, a measure of insulin resistance, is reduced 40% to 50% in obese nondiabetic and lean type 2 diabetic individuals. Obese diabetic individuals are slightly more resistant than lean diabetic patients. (From DeFronzo RA. Diabetes Reviews 1977;5:177–269.)

regions have been identified on several other chromosomes as well. Because twin studies do not show 100% concordance, environmental factors such as infectious agents, chemical agents, and dietary agents are likely contributing factors in the expression of the disease.

TYPE 2 DIABETES MELLITUS

Normal Insulin Action

In the fasting state 75% of total body glucose disposal takes place in non–insulin dependent tissues: the brain and splanchnic tissues (liver and gastrointestinal tissues).[20] In fact, brain glucose uptake occurs at the same rate during fed and fasting periods and is not altered in type 2 diabetes.

The remaining 25% of glucose metabolism takes place in muscle, which is dependent on insulin.[21] In the fasting state approximately 85% of glucose production is derived from the liver, and the remaining amount is produced by the kidney.[20–22] In the fed state, carbohydrate ingestion increases the plasma glucose concentration and stimulates insulin release from the pancreatic β cells. The resultant hyperinsulinemia (1) suppresses hepatic glucose production and (2) stimulates glucose uptake by peripheral tissues.[20,23] The majority (~80% to 85%) of glucose that is taken up by peripheral tissues is disposed of in muscle,[20,23] with only a small amount (~4% to 5%) being metabolized by adipocytes.

Although fat tissue is responsible for only a small amount of total body glucose disposal, it plays a very important role in the maintenance of total body glucose homeostasis. Small increments in the plasma insulin concentration exert a potent antilipolytic effect, leading to a marked reduction in the plasma free fatty acid (FFA) level. The decline in plasma FFA concentration results in increased glucose uptake in muscle[24] and reduces hepatic glucose production.[25] Thus a decrease in the plasma FFA concentration lowers plasma glucose by both decreasing its production and enhancing the uptake in muscle.[26,27]

Type 2 diabetic individuals are characterized by: (1) defects in insulin secretion; and (2) insulin resistance involving muscle, liver, and the adipocyte. Insulin resistance is present even in *lean* type 2 diabetic individuals (Fig. 72–5).

Impaired Insulin Secretion

The pancreas in people with a normal-functioning β cell is able to adjust its secretion of insulin to maintain normal glucose tolerance.

Thus in nondiabetic individuals, insulin is increased in proportion to the severity of the insulin resistance and glucose tolerance remains normal. Impaired insulin secretion is a uniform finding in type 2 diabetic patients and the evolution of β-cell dysfunction has been well characterized in diverse ethnic populations.

DeFronzo and colleagues[28] measured the fasting plasma insulin concentration and performed oral glucose tolerance tests in 77 normal-weight type 2 diabetic patients and over 100 lean subjects with normal or impaired glucose tolerance (Fig. 72–6). The relationship between the fasting plasma glucose concentration and the fasting plasma insulin concentration resembles an inverted U or horseshoe. As the fasting plasma glucose concentration rises from 80 to 140 mg/dL, the fasting plasma insulin concentration increases progressively, peaking at a value that is 2- to 2.5-fold greater than in normal weight nondiabetic controls. When the fasting plasma glucose concentration

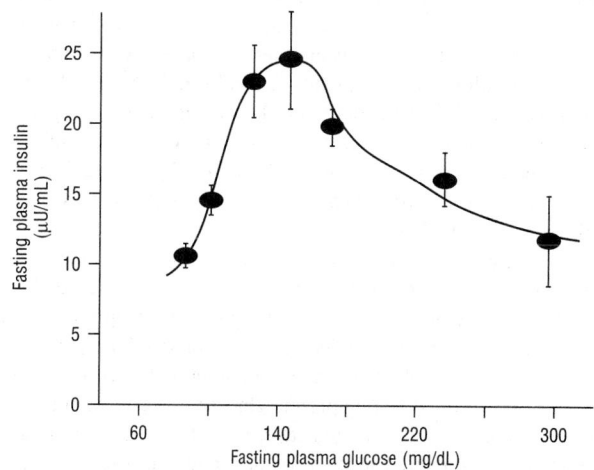

FIGURE 72–6. The relationship between fasting plasma insulin and fasting plasma glucose in 177 normal weight individuals. Plasma insulin and glucose increase together up to a fasting glucose of 140 mg/dL. When the fasting glucose exceeds 140 mg/dL, the β cell makes progressively less insulin, which leads to an overproduction of glucose by the liver and results in a progressive increase in fasting glucose. (Adapted from DeFronzo,[28] with permission.)

exceeds 140 mg/dL, the β cell is unable to maintain its elevated rate of insulin secretion and the fasting insulin concentration declines precipitously. This decrease in fasting insulin leads to an increase in hepatic glucose production overnight, which results in an elevated fasting plasma glucose concentration.[28]

SITE OF INSULIN RESISTANCE IN TYPE 2 DIABETES

Liver

In type 2 diabetic subjects with mild to moderate fasting hyperglycemia (140 to 200 mg/dL, 7.8 to 11.1 mmol/L), basal hepatic glucose production is increased by ~0.5 mg/kg per minute. Consequently, during the overnight sleeping hours the liver of an 80-kg diabetic individual with modest fasting hyperglycemia adds an additional 35 g of glucose to the systemic circulation. This increase in fasting hepatic glucose production is the cause of fasting hyperglycemia.[20]

Following glucose ingestion, insulin is secreted into the portal vein and carried to the liver, where it suppresses hepatic glucose output. If the liver is resistant to insulin and continues to produce glucose, there will be two inputs of glucose into the body, one from the liver and another from the gastrointestinal tract, and marked hyperglycemia will ensue.

Peripheral (Muscle)

Muscle is the major site of glucose disposal in man, and approximately 80% of total body glucose uptake occurs in skeletal muscle.[20] In response to a physiologic increase in plasma insulin concentration, muscle glucose uptake increases linearly, reaching a plateau value of 10 mg/kg per minute. In contrast, in lean type 2 diabetic subjects, the onset of insulin action is delayed for ~40 minutes, and the ability of insulin to stimulate leg glucose uptake is reduced by 50%. Therefore the primary site of insulin resistance in type 2 diabetic subjects resides in muscle tissue.

Peripheral (Adipocyte)

In obese nondiabetic and diabetic humans, basal plasma FFA levels are increased and fail to suppress normally after glucose ingestion. FFAs are stored as triglycerides in adipocytes and serve as an important energy source during conditions of fasting. Insulin is a potent inhibitor of lipolysis, and restrains the release of FFAs from the adipocyte by inhibiting the hormone-sensitive lipase enzyme. It is now recognized that chronically elevated plasma FFA concentrations can lead to insulin resistance in muscle and liver,[20,24,27,29] and impair insulin secretion.[26,30,31] In addition to FFAs that circulate in plasma in increased amounts, type 2 diabetic and obese nondiabetic individuals have increased stores of triglycerides in muscle[32,33] and liver,[34,35] and the increased fat content correlates closely with the presence of insulin resistance in these tissues.

In summary, insulin resistance involving both muscle and liver are characteristic features of the glucose intolerance in type 2 diabetic individuals. In the basal state, the liver represents a major site of insulin resistance, and this is reflected by overproduction of glucose. This accelerated rate of hepatic glucose output is the primary determinant of the elevated fasting plasma glucose concentration in type 2 diabetic individuals. In the fed state, both decreased muscle glucose uptake and impaired suppression of hepatic glucose production contribute to the insulin resistance. In obese individuals and in the majority (>80%) of type 2 diabetic subjects, there is an expanded fat cell mass and the adipocytes are resistant to the antilipolytic effects of insulin. Most obese and diabetic individuals are characterized by expanded visceral adiposity, discussed in detail later in the chapter,

which is especially refractory to insulin effects and results in a high lipolytic rate. Not surprisingly, both type 2 diabetes and obesity are characterized by an elevation in the mean 24-hour plasma FFA concentration. Elevated plasma FFA levels, as well as increased triglyceride/fatty acyl CoA content in muscle, liver, and β cells, lead to the development of muscle/hepatic insulin resistance and impaired insulin secretion.

CELLULAR MECHANISMS OF INSULIN RESISTANCE

Insulin resistance and the components of the insulin resistance syndrome are described below.

Obesity and Insulin Resistance

Weight gain leads to insulin resistance, and obese nondiabetic individuals have the same degree of insulin resistance as lean type 2 diabetic patients.[36] In 1,146 nondiabetic, normotensive individuals, Ferrannini and associates showed a progressive loss of insulin sensitivity when the BMI increased from 18 kg/m^2 to 38 kg/m^2.[37] The increase in insulin resistance with weight gain is directly related to the amount of visceral adipose tissue.[38,39]

The term *visceral adipose tissue* (VAT) refers to fat cells located within the abdominal cavity and includes omental, mesenteric, retroperitoneal, and perinephric adipose tissue. VAT has been shown to correlate with insulin resistance and explain much of the variation in insulin resistance seen in a population of African-Americans.[4] Visceral adipose tissue represents 20% of fat in men and 6% of fat in women. This fat tissue has been shown to have a higher rate of lipolysis than subcutaneous fat, resulting in an increase in free fatty acid production. These fatty acids are released into the portal circulation and drain into the liver, where they stimulate the production of very-low-density lipoproteins and decrease insulin sensitivity in peripheral tissues.[38] VAT also produces a number of cytokines which cause insulin resistance. These factors drain into the portal circulation and reduce insulin sensitivity in peripheral tissues.[41]

The fat cell also has the capability of producing at least one hormone that improves insulin sensitivity: adiponectin. This factor is made in decreasing amounts as an individual becomes more obese.[42,43] In animal models, adiponectin decreases hepatic glucose production and increases fatty acid oxidation in muscle.[44,45]

The Metabolic Syndrome

The association of insulin resistance with a clustering of cardiovascular risk factors including hyperinsulinemia, hypertension, abdominal obesity, dyslipidemia, and coagulation abnormalities has been referred to by a variety of names including "the insulin resistance syndrome," "the metabolic syndrome," "the dysmetabolic syndrome," and "the deadly quartet," to name a few. Since the description of the "insulin resistance syndrome" by Reaven in 1988,[46] the number of associated factors has continued to grow.

The most widely used criteria to define this syndrome were published as part of The National Cholesterol Education Program Adult Treatment Panel (NCEP-ATP) III Guidelines for the treatment of hypercholesterolemia.[47] The NCEP components of the metabolic syndrome are outlined in Table 72–5. The ATP guidelines establish a diagnosis of the metabolic syndrome when at least three of the five criteria are present. The metabolic syndrome has been assigned the diagnostic code 277.7 by the International Classification of Diseases, Ninth Revision,[48] which enables reimbursement for treating patients with this condition. The standard for the individual risk factors vary between NCEP-ATP and other expert panels including the World Health Organization and The American College of Endocrinology.

TABLE 72–5. Five Components of the Metabolic Syndrome (Individuals Having at Least Three Components Meet the Criteria for Diagnosis)

Risk Factor	Defining Level
Abdominal obesity	Waist circumference
Men	>102 cm (>40 in)
Women	>88 cm (>35 in)
Triglycerides	≥150 mg/dL
High-density-lipoprotein C	
Men	<40 mg/dL
Women	<50 mg/dL
Blood pressure	≥130/≥85 mm Hg
Fasting glucose	≥110 mg/dL

Reproduced from Expert Panel on Detection.[47]

For example, NCEP-ATP uses waist circumference to define obesity, while other expert committees use the body mass index (BMI). The ATP guidelines base glucose intolerance on a fasting glucose while others prefer the results of an oral glucose tolerance test (OGTT). As we are better able to quantify the relationship between these factors and the development of cardiovascular disease, the definition of the syndromes and the individual component values will no doubt continue to be refined.

Prevalence. The insulin resistance syndrome (IRS) is common in the United States. Ford and colleagues analyzed the data from the Third National Health and Nutrition Evaluation Survey (NHANES III) carried out in 1988–1994.[49] The sample included 20,050 persons age 17 years and over, with glucose tolerance testing performed in 8,302 persons aged 40 to 74 years. Twenty six percent of this population had three or more of the metabolic abnormalities defined by the NCEP-ATP. The prevalence of the IRS increases with age, with 33% affected at age 40, 40% at age 50, and 50% by 60 years of age. The prevalence of the IRS also differs in various ethnic groups, with 32% of Mexican-Americans affected, compared to 36% of African-Americans and 40% of Caucasians.

The impact of treating the clinical components of the metabolic syndrome was demonstrated in the Steno-2 Study.[50] In this prospective study, 63 patients with diabetes and microalbuminuria were randomized to the usual therapy group and 67 patients were treated intensively. Intensive therapy consisted of diet and exercise and pharmacologic intervention aimed at hyperglycemia, hypertension, dyslipidemia, microalbuminuria, and increased coagulopathy (aspirin therapy). Treatment goals for intensive therapy included a blood pressure <130/80 mm Hg, HbA$_{1c}$ <6.5%, total cholesterol <175 mg/dL, and triglycerides <150 mg/dL. All patients in the intensive treatment group were given an aspirin and treated with an angiotensin-converting enzyme (ACE) inhibitor. Patients in the intensively treated group showed a 53% reduction in cardiovascular disease and a 61% reduction in nephropathy. The magnitude of this reduction is greater than has been demonstrated with individual interventions, stressing the importance of targeting all the components of the metabolic syndrome. The study design did not allow conclusions regarding which interventions had the most impact.

CLINICAL PRESENTATION

The clinical presentations of type 1 DM and type 2 DM are very different (Table 72–6). Autoimmune type 1 DM can occur at any age. Approximately 75% will develop the disorder before age 20 years, but the remaining 25%, including relatives of index patients, develop the disease as adults. Individuals with type 1 diabetes mellitus are often thin and are prone to develop diabetic ketoacidosis if insulin is withheld, or under conditions of severe stress with an excess of insulin counterregulatory hormones.[2] Twenty to forty percent of patients with type 1 DM present with diabetic ketoacidosis after several days of polyuria, polydipsia, polyphagia, and weight loss. Occasionally, patients are diagnosed as short of "metabolic bankruptcy" when they have blood tests drawn for other reasons or for early symptoms. Because newly diagnosed patients with type 1 DM often have a small amount of residual pancreatic β-cell function, they may enter a "honeymoon" phase, when their blood glucose concentrations are relatively easy to control and small amounts of insulin are needed.

TABLE 72–6. Clinical Presentation of Diabetes Mellitus[a]

Characteristic	Type 1 DM	Type 2 DM
Age	<30 years[b]	>30 years[b]
Onset	Abrupt	Gradual
Body habitus	Lean	Obese or history of obesity
Insulin resistance	Absent	Present
Autoantibodies	Often present	Rarely present
Symptoms	Symptomatic[c]	Often asymptomatic
Ketones at diagnosis	Present	Absent[d]
Need for insulin therapy	Immediate	Years after diagnosis
Acute complications	Diabetic ketoacidosis	Hyperosmolar hyperglycemic state
Microvascular complications at diagnosis	No	Common
Macrovascular complications at or before diagnosis	Rare	Common

[a]Clinical presentation can vary widely.
[b]Age of onset for type 1 DM is generally <20 years of age, but can present at any age. The prevalence of type 2 DM in children, adolescents, and young adults is increasing. This is especially true in ethnic and minority children.
[c]Type 1 may present acutely with symptoms of polyuria, nocturia, polydipsia, polyphagia, and weight loss.
[d]Type 2 children and adolescents are more likely to present with ketones, but after the acute phase may be treated with oral agents. Prolonged fasting can also produce ketones in individuals.

Once this residual insulin secretion wanes, the patients are completely insulin deficient and have more labile glycemia.

Patients with type 2 DM often present without symptoms, even though complications tell us that they may have had type 2 DM for several years.[10] Often these patients are diagnosed secondary to unrelated blood testing. Lethargy, polyuria, nocturia, and polydipsia can be seen at diagnosis in type 2 diabetes, but significant weight loss at diagnosis is less common.

► TREATMENT: Diabetes Mellitus

▓ DESIRED OUTCOME

⑤　The primary goals of DM management are to reduce the risk for microvascular and macrovascular disease complications, to ameliorate symptoms, to reduce mortality, and to improve quality of life.[51] Near-normal glycemia will reduce the risk for development of microvascular disease complications, but current evidence targets aggressive management of traditional cardiovascular risk factors (i.e., smoking cessation, treatment of dyslipidemia, intensive blood pressure control, and antiplatelet therapy) to reduce the likelihood of development of macrovascular disease.

Hyperglycemia not only increases the risk for microvascular disease, but contributes to poor wound healing, compromises white blood cell function, and leads to classic symptoms of DM. Diabetic ketoacidosis and hyperosmolar hyperglycemic state are severe manifestations of poor diabetes control, invariably requiring hospitalization. Reducing the potential for microvascular complications is targeted at adherence to therapeutic lifestyle intervention (i.e., diet and exercise programs) and drug-therapy regimens, as well as at maintaining blood pressure as near normal as possible.

▓ GENERAL APPROACH TO TREATMENT

Appropriate care requires goal setting for glycemia, blood pressure, and lipid levels, regular monitoring for complications, dietary and exercise modifications, medications, appropriate self-monitoring of blood glucose (SMBG), and laboratory assessment of the aforementioned parameters.[51] Glucose control alone does not sufficiently reduce the risk of complications in persons with DM.

▓ GLYCEMIC GOAL SETTING AND THE HEMOGLOBIN A_{1c}

Controlled clinical trials provide ample evidence that glycemic control is paramount in reducing microvascular complications in both type 1 DM[52] and type 2 DM.[53] HbA_{1c} measurements are the gold standard for following long-term glycemic control for the previous 3 months.[54] Hemoglobinopathies, anemia, and red cell membrane defects can affect HbA_{1c} measurements. Other strategies (e.g., measurement of fructosamine) may be necessary to assess diabetes control in these patients. Unless the risk outweighs the benefit (as in elderly patients, patients with advanced complications, and patients with other advanced disease), an HbA_{1c} target of <7% is appropriate (Table 72–7), and lower values may be targeted if significant hypoglycemia and/or weight gain can be avoided.[51]

▓ MONITORING COMPLICATIONS

The ADA recommends initiation of complications monitoring at the time of diagnosis of diabetes mellitus.[8] Current recommendations continue to advocate yearly dilated eye examinations in type 2 DM, and an initial eye exam in the first 3 to 5 years in type 1 DM, then yearly thereafter. Less frequent testing (every 2 to 3 years) can be implemented upon the advice of an eye care specialist. The feet should be examined and the blood pressure should be assessed at each visit. A urine test for microalbumin once yearly is appropriate. Yearly testing for lipid abnormalities, and more frequently if needed to achieve lipid goals, is recommended.

▓ SELF-MONITORING OF BLOOD GLUCOSE

The advent of SMBG in the early 1980s revolutionized the treatment of DM, enabling patients to know their blood glucose concentration at any moment easily and relatively inexpensively. Frequent SMBG is necessary to achieve near-normal blood glucose concentrations and to assess for hypoglycemia, particularly in patients with type 1 DM.[54] The more intense the insulin regimen is, the more intense the SMBG needs to be (four or more times daily in patients on multiple insulin injections or pump therapy). The utility and optimal frequency of SMBG for patients with type 2 DM is unresolved. Frequency of monitoring in type 2 DM should be sufficient to facilitate reaching glucose

TABLE 72–7. Glycemic Goals of Therapy

Biochemical Index	ADA	ACE and AACE
Hemoglobin A_{1c}	<7%[a]	≤6.5%
Preprandial plasma glucose	90–130 mg/dL (5.0–7.2 mmol/L)	<110 mg/dL
Postprandial plasma glucose	<180 mg/dL[b] (<10 mmol/L)	<140 mg/dL

[a]Referenced to a nondiabetic range of 4.0–6.0% using a DCCT-based assay. More stringent glycemic goals (i.e., a normal HbA_{1c}, <6%) may further reduce complications at the cost of increased risk of hypoglycemia (particularly in those with type 1 diabetes).
[b]Postprandial glucose measurements should be made 1–2 hours after the beginning of the meal, generally the time of peak levels in patients with diabetes.
ADA, American Diabetes Association; ACE, American College of Endocrinology; AACE, American Association of Clinical Endocrinologists; DCCT, Diabetes Control and Complications Trial.

als. The role of SMBG in improving glycemic control in type 2 DM atients is unproven.[55] Patients must be empowered to change their erapeutic regimen (lifestyle and medications) in response to test sults, or no meaningful change is likely to be effected.

NONPHARMACOLOGIC THERAPY

DIET

Medical nutrition therapy is recommended for all persons with DM.[56] aramount for all medical nutrition therapy is the attainment of opmal metabolic outcomes and the prevention and treatment of comications. For individuals with type 1 DM, the focus is on regulating isulin administration with a balanced diet to achieve and maintain healthy body weight. Although still debated, most people with diaetes require a meal plan that is moderate in carbohydrates and low in aturated fat, with a focus on balanced meals. It is imperative that paents understand the connection between carbohydrates and glucose ontrol. In addition, patients with type 2 DM often require caloric estriction to promote weight loss. Rather than a set diabetic diet, dvocate a diet using foods that are within the financial reach and ultural milieu of the patient. Bedtime and between-meal snacks are ot usually needed if pharmacologic management is appropriate.

ACTIVITY

n general, most patients with DM can benefit from increased ctivity.[57] Aerobic exercise improves insulin resistance and glycemic ontrol in the majority of individuals, and reduces cardiovascular risk actors, contributes to weight loss or maintenance, and improves welleing. The patient should choose an activity that she or he is likely

to continue. Start exercise slowly in previously sedentary patients. Older patients, patients with long-standing disease (age >35 years, or >25 years with DM ≥10 years), patients with multiple cardiovascular risk factors, presence of microvascular disease, and patients with previous evidence of atherosclerotic disease should have a cardiovascular evaluation, probably including a graded exercise test with imaging, prior to beginning a moderate to intense exercise regimen. In addition, several complications (autonomic neuropathy, insensate feet, and retinopathy) may require restrictions on the activities recommended.

PHARMACOLOGIC THERAPY

Until 1995, only two options for pharmacologic treatment were available for patients with diabetes; sulfonylureas (for type 2 DM only) and insulin (for type 1 or 2). After 1995, a number of new oral agents and insulins have been introduced in the United States.

Currently, five classes of oral agents are approved for the treatment of type 2 diabetes: α-glucosidase inhibitors, biguanides, meglitinides, peroxisome proliferator activated receptor γ agonists (which are also commonly identified as thiazolidinediones or glitazones), and sulfonylureas. Oral agents are indicated for use in type 2 DM patients who are unable to achieve glycemic control goals despite diet and exercise. Oral antidiabetic agents are often grouped according to their glucose-lowering mechanism of action. Biguanides and thiazolidinediones are often categorized as insulin sensitizers due to their ability to reduce insulin resistance. Sulfonylureas and meglitinides are often categorized as insulin secretagogues because they enhance endogenous insulin release.

New options for implementation of insulin therapy are now available. Rapid-acting insulins (lispro and aspart) are available in insulin mixtures (Humalog Mix 75/25 and NovoLog Mix 70/30), and the long-acting basal insulin glargine has increased the ease of implementation of intensive insulin therapy for many patients. Glulisine, another rapid-acting insulin analog, has received Food and Drug Administration (FDA) approval for treatment of type 1 and 2 DM, and is expected to be marketed in 2005. Research on alternative delivery of insulin through inhalation or oral routes is continuing, though the latest information targets 2005 or 2006 as a likely time frame for the earliest FDA approval of a product.

The subsequent sections describe the current antidiabetic medications that are available to treat type 1 and type 2 diabetes mellitus.

DRUG CLASS INFORMATION

Insulin

Pharmacology. Insulin is an anabolic and anticatabolic hormone. It plays major roles in protein, carbohydrate, and fat metabolism. For a complete review of insulin action, the reader is referred to a diabetes physiology text.[58] Endogenously produced insulin is cleaved from the larger proinsulin peptide in the β cell to the active peptide of insulin and C-peptide, which can be used as a marker for endogenous insulin production. All commercially available insulin preparations contain only the active insulin peptide.

Characteristics. Characteristics that are commonly used to categorize insulins include source, strength, onset, and duration of action.

TABLE 72–8. Available Insulin Preparations

Generic Name	Manufacturer	Analog[a]	Administration Options	Room Temperature[b] Expiration
Rapid-acting insulins				
Humalog (insulin lispro)	Lilly	Yes	Insulin pen, vial, or 1.5-mL and 3-mL pen cartridge	28 days
NovoLog (insulin aspart)	Novo-Nordisk	Yes	Insulin pen, vial, or 3-mL pen cartridge	28 days
Apidra (insulin glulisine)[c]	Aventis	Yes	Vial	28 days
Short-acting insulins				
Humulin R (regular)	Lilly	No	U-100, 10-mL vial	28 days
Available in: U-100 and U-500			U-500, 20-mL vial	
Novolin R (regular)	Novo-Nordisk	No	Insulin pen, vial, or 3-mL pen cartridge, and InnoLet[d]	Vial: 30 days; others: 28 days
Intermediate-acting insulins				
NPH				
Humulin N	Lilly	No	Vial, prefilled pen	Vial: 28 days; pen: 14 days
Novolin N	Novo-Nordisk	No	Vial, prefilled pen, and InnoLet[d]	Vial: 30 days; others: 14 days
Lente				
Humulin L	Lilly	No	Vial	28 days
Long-acting insulins				
Humulin U (ultralente)	Lilly	No	Vial	28 days
Lantus (insulin glargine)	Aventis	Yes	Vial	28 days
Pre-mixed insulins				
Pre-mixed insulin analogs				
Humalog Mix 75/25 (75% neutral protamine lispro, 25% lispro)	Lilly	Yes	Vial, prefilled pen	Vial: 28 days; pen: 10 days
Novolog Mix 70/30 (70% aspart protamine suspension, 30% aspart)	Novo-Nordisk	Yes	Vial, prefilled pen, 3-mL pen cartridge	Vial: 28 days; others: 14 days
NPH-regular combinations				
Humulin 70/30	Lilly	No	Vial, prefilled pen	Vial: 28 days; pen: 10 days
Novolin 70/30	Novo-Nordisk	No	Vial, pen cartridge, InnoLet[d]	Vial: 30 days; others: 10 days
Humulin 50/50	Lilly	No	Vial	28 days

[a]All insulins available in the U.S. are now made by human recombinant DNA technology. An insulin analog is a modified human insulin molecule that imparts particular pharmacokinetic advantages.
[b]Room temperature defined as 59–86°F.
[c]FDA approved, possible launch in 2005.
[d]InnoLet: A prefilled insulin pen with a "kitchen timer" type of dial for determining the number of insulin units. May be useful in patients with impaired eyesight or dexterity.

Additionally, insulins may be characterized as analogs, defined as insulins that have had amino acids within the insulin molecule modified to impart particular physiochemical and pharmacokinetic advantages. Table 72–8 summarizes available insulin preparations.

U-100 and U-500, 100 units/mL and 500 units/mL, respectively, are the strengths of insulin currently available in the United States. U-500 regular insulin is available for individuals that may require large doses of insulin to control their diabetes. In the United States, all other insulins are available only in U-100 strength. For some type 1 diabetes patients who require extremely low doses of insulin, dilution of U-100 insulin to obtain accurate insulin doses may be necessary. Diluents and empty bottles can be obtained from the manufacturers for dilution.

Historically, insulin came from either beef or pork sources. Beef insulin differs by three amino acids and pork by one amino acid when compared to human insulin. Manufacturers in the United States have discontinued production of beef and pork source insulins as of December 2003, and now exclusively use recombinant DNA technology to manufacture insulin. Eli Lilly and Aventis currently use

a non–disease producing strain of *Escherichia coli* for synthesis of human insulin, whereas Novo Nordisk uses *Saccharomyces cerevisiae*, or bakers' yeast, for synthesis.

Purity of insulin refers to the amount of proinsulin and other impurities present in a given insulin product. Prior to 1980, most insulin contained enough impurities (300 to 10,000 ppm) to cause local reactions upon injection, as well as systemic adverse effects from antibody production. Modern technology has provided less expensive techniques to purify insulin. As a result, all insulin products contain ≤10 ppm of proinsulin, with purified preparations (all recombinant DNA human insulin and insulin analogs) containing <1 ppm of proinsulin.

Regular crystalline insulin naturally self-associates into a hexameric (six insulin molecules) structure when injected subcutaneously. Before absorption through a blood capillary can occur, the hexamer must dissociate first to dimers, and then to monomers. This principle is the premise for additives such as protamine and zinc described below and modification of amino acids for insulin analogs. Lispro, aspart, and glulisine insulins dissociate rapidly to monomers, thus absorption is rapid. Lispro (B-28 lysine and B-29 proline human insulin; monomeric) insulin with two amino acids transposed, aspart (B-28 aspartic acid human insulin; mono- and dimeric) insulin with replacement of one amino acid, and glulisine (B-3 lysine and B-29 glutamic acid) are rapidly absorbed, peak faster, and have shorter durations of action when compared to regular insulin. In comparison to human insulin, with an isoelectric point of 5.4, the analog glargine insulin (A-21 glycine, B-30a-arginine, B-30a L-arginine, and B-30b L-arginine human insulin) has an isoelectric point of 6.8. In the bottle, glargine is buffered to a pH of 4, a level at which it is completely soluble, resulting in a clear colorless solution. When injected into the neutral pH of the body, it rapidly forms microprecipitates that slowly dissolve into monomers and dimers which are then subsequently absorbed. The result is a long-acting, peakless, 24-hour duration insulin analog.

Insulin analogs are modified human insulin molecules, and safety is paramount for FDA approval. Key factors that should be considered in the approval process include local injection reactions, antigenicity, efficacy compared to human insulin, insulin receptor binding affinity, and insulin-like growth factor 1–receptor affinity (which is compared to that of human insulin to determine mitogenic potential).

Pharmacokinetics. Subcutaneous injection kinetics are dependent on onset, peak, and duration of action, and are summarized in Table 72–9. Absorption of insulin from a subcutaneous depot is dependent on several factors, including: source of insulin, concentration of insulin, additives to the insulin preparations (e.g., zinc, protamine, etc), blood flow to the area (rubbing of injection area, increased skin temperature, and exercise in muscles near the injection site may enhance absorption), and injection site. Insulin is commonly injected in (from most rapid to slowest absorption): abdominal fat, posterior upper arms, lateral thigh area, and superior buttocks area. Insulin analogs, unlike other preparations of insulin, appear to retain their kinetic profile at all sites of injection. U-500 regular insulin has a delayed onset and requires a lower dose when compared to U-100 insulin. Addition of protamine (NPH, NPL, and aspart protamine suspension) or excess zinc (lente or ultralente insulin) will delay onset, peak, and duration of the insulin's effect. Variability in absorption, inconsistent suspension of the insulin by the patient or health care provider when drawing up a dose, and inherent insulin action based on the pharmacokinetics of the products may all contribute to a labile glucose response. All insulin suspensions should be inverted or rolled gently at least 10 times to fully resuspend the insulin.

The half-life of an intravenous (IV) injection of regular insulin is about 9 minutes. Thus the effective duration of action of a single IV injection is short, and changes in IV insulin rates will reach steady state in approximately 45 minutes. Intravenous pharmacokinetics of other soluble insulins (lispro, aspart, glulisine, and even glargine) appear similar to IV regular insulin, but they have no advantages over IV regular insulin and are more expensive.

Insulin is degraded in the liver, muscle, and kidney. Liver deactivation is 20% to 50% in a single passage. Approximately 15% to 20% of insulin metabolism occurs in the kidney. This may partially explain the lower insulin dosage requirements in patients with end-stage renal disease.

The pharmacokinetics of the inhaled insulin products under development appear to be similar to those of rapid-acting insulin preparations, but inhaled insulin has not been released as of this writing.[59]

Efficacy. The efficacy of traditional insulins (e.g., regular, NPH, and lente insulins) is unequivocal. Insulin analog efficacy is measured via the same ways as traditional insulins. Insulin analogs in most studies have not shown superior HbA$_{1c}$ levels when compared to traditional insulins, but are often preferred by patients and practitioners. Lispro, aspart, and glulisine are advantageous due to the ability to inject within 10 minutes of a meal, as compared to the recommendation to inject regular insulin approximately 30 minutes prior. Rapid-acting analogs have shown superior postprandial lowering of glucose when compared to regular insulin. Glargine insulin injected at bedtime has shown significantly less nocturnal hypoglycemia when compared to NPH injected at bedtime.

An educated patient in conjunction with a skilled practitioner can achieve excellent glycemic control with insulin therapy. Efficacy with insulin therapy is related to achieving glycemic control while minimizing the risk of potential side effects, specifically hypoglycemia and weight gain. Insulin is recommended in patients with: extremely high fasting plasma glucose levels (>280 to 300 mg/dL), patients with ketonuria or ketonemia, symptomatic patients (weight loss with polyuria, polydipsia, and/or nocturia), gestational diabetes mellitus, and if deemed appropriate by the clinician and patient.[60–63]

Microvascular Complications. Insulin has been shown to be as efficacious as any oral agent for treating DM. The United Kingdom Prospective Diabetes Study, which used sulfonylureas or insulin, showed equal efficacy in lowering the risk of microvascular events in newly diagnosed type 2 DM.[53] Similarly, in type 1 DM the Diabetes Control and Complications Trial (DCCT) showed efficacy in reducing microvascular complications.[52]

TABLE 72–9. Pharmacokinetics of Various Insulins Administered Subcutaneously

Type of Insulin	Onset (Hours)	Peak (Hours)	Duration (Hours)	Maximum Duration (Hours)	Appearance
Rapid-acting					
Aspart	15–30 min	1–2	3–5	5–6	Clear
Lispro	15–30 min	1–2	3–4	4–6	Clear
Glulisine[a]	15–30 min	1–2	3–4	5–6	Clear
Short-acting					
Regular	0.5–1.0	2–3	3–6	6–8	Clear
Intermediate-acting					
NPH	2–4	4–6	8–12	14–18	Cloudy
Lente	3–4	6–12	12–18	20	Cloudy
Long-acting					
Ultralente	6–10	10–16	18–20	24	Cloudy
Glargine	4–5	—	22–24	24	Clear

[a]FDA approved, possible launch in 2005.

Macrovascular Complications. The connection between high insulin levels (hyperinsulinemia), insulin resistance, and cardiovascular events incorrectly leads some clinicians to believe that insulin therapy may cause macrovascular complications. The UKPDS and DCCT found no differences in macrovascular outcomes with intensive insulin therapy. One study, the Diabetes Mellitus, Insulin Glucose Infusion in Acute Myocardial Infarction study[64] reported reductions in mortality with insulin therapy. This group assessed the effect of an insulin-glucose infusion in type 2 DM patients who had experienced an acute myocardial infarction. Those randomized to insulin infusion followed by intensive insulin therapy lowered their absolute mortality risk by 11% over a mean follow-up period of approximately 3 years. This was most evident in subjects who were insulin-naïve or had a low cardiovascular risk prior to the acute myocardial infarction.[64]

Adverse Effects. The most common adverse effects reported with insulin are hypoglycemia and weight gain. Hypoglycemia is more common in patients on intensive insulin therapy regimens versus those on less-intensive regimens. Also, patients with type 1 DM tend to have more hypoglycemic events compared to type 2 DM patients. In the UKPDS study, performed over 10 years, the percentage of diabetic patients that needed assistance (third-party or hospitalization) due to a hypoglycemic reaction was 2.3%. The UKPDS reported a rate of 36.5% for risk of any hypoglycemic event, including mild, self-treated events. In the DCCT, tighter control produced a risk three times higher for severe hypoglycemia compared to conventional therapy. Glycemic goals should incorporate hypoglycemic risk vs. the benefit of lowering the glucose, when HbA$_{1c}$ levels are near normal, especially in type 1 DM.

Minimization of risk for patients on insulin should include education about the signs and symptoms of hypoglycemia, proper treatment of hypoglycemia, and blood glucose monitoring. Blood glucose monitoring is essential for those on insulin, and is particularly of value in patients with hypoglycemia unawareness. Patients with hypoglycemia unawareness do not experience the normal sympathetic symptoms of hypoglycemia (tachycardia, tremulousness, and sweating). Initial symptoms are often neuroglycopenic in nature (confusion, agitation, loss of consciousness, and/or progression to coma). Patients with hypoglycemia unawareness should check their blood glucose level prior to any activities that may be dangerous with a low blood sugar (e.g., driving and certain sports, among others). Proper treatment of hypoglycemia dictates ingestion of carbohydrates, with glucose being preferred. Unconsciousness is an indication for either IV glucose, or glucagon injection, which increases glycogenolysis in the liver. Glucagon use would be appropriate in any situation in which the patient does not have or cannot have ready IV access for glucose administration. Education for reconstitution and injection of glucagon is recommended for close friends and family of a patient who has recurrent neuroglycopenic events. The patient and close contacts should be informed that it can take 10 to 15 minutes for the injection to start raising glucose levels, and patients often vomit during this time. Proper positioning to avoid aspiration should be emphasized.

Weight gain is predominantly from increased truncal fat, and tends to be related to daily dose and plasma insulin levels present. Weight gain is undesirable in most type 2 DM, but may be seen as beneficial in underweight type 1 DM. Weight gain appears to be related to intensive insulin therapy, and can be somewhat minimized by physiologic replacement of insulin.

The two forms of lipodystrophy, though less common today in people with diabetes, still occur. Lipohypertrophy is caused by many injections into the same injection site. Due to insulin's anabolic actions, a raised fat mass is present at the injection site with resultant variable insulin absorption. Lipoatrophy, in contrast, is thought to be due to insulin antibodies, with destruction of fat at the site of injection. Injection away from the site with more purified insulin is recommended, though several reports of lipoatrophy with lispro have been reported.

Drug-Drug Interactions. There are no significant drug-drug interactions with insulin, though other medications that may affect glucose control can be considered. Table 72–10 lists common medications known to affect blood glucose levels.

TABLE 72–10. Medications That May Affect Glycemic Control[a]

Drug	Effect on Glucose	Mechanism/Comment
Angiotensin-converting enzyme inhibitors	Slight reduction	Improves insulin sensitivity
Alcohol	Reduction	Reduces hepatic glucose production
α-Interferon	Increase	Unclear
Diazoxide	Increase	Decreases insulin secretion, decreases peripheral glucose use
Diuretics	Increase	May increase insulin resistance
Glucocorticoids	Increase	Impairs insulin action
Nicotinic acid	Increase	Impairs insulin action, increases insulin resistance
Oral contraceptives	Increase	Unclear
Pentamidine	Decrease, then increase	Toxic to β cells; initial release of stored insulin, then depletion
Phenytoin	Increase	Decreases insulin secretion
β-Blockers	May increase	Decreases insulin secretion
Salicylates	Decrease	Inhibition of I-kappa-B kinase-beta (IKK-beta) (only high doses, e.g., 4–6 g/day)
Sympathomimetics	Slight increase	Increased glycogenolysis and gluconeogenesis
Clozapine and olanzapine	Increase	Unclear; weight gain

[a]This list is not inclusive of all medications reported to cause glucose changes.

Dosing and Administration. The dose of insulin for any person with altered glucose metabolism must be individualized. In type 1 DM, the average daily requirement for insulin is 0.5 to 0.6 units/kg, with approximately 50% being delivered as basal insulin, and the remaining 50% dedicated to meal coverage. During the honeymoon phase it may fall to 0.1 to 0.4 units/kg. During acute illness or with ketosis or states of relative insulin resistance, higher dosages are warranted. In type 2 DM a higher dosage is required for those patients with significant insulin resistance. Dosages vary widely depending on underlying insulin resistance and concomitant oral insulin sensitizer use. Strategies on how to initiate and monitor insulin therapy will be described later in the therapeutics section.

Storage. It is recommended that unopened insulins be refrigerated (36° to 46°F) prior to use. The manufacturer's expiration date printed on the insulin is used for unopened, refrigerated insulin. Once the insulin is in use, the manufacturer-recommended expiration dates will vary based on the insulin and delivery device. Table 72–8 outlines manufacturer-recommended expiration dates for room temperature (59° to 86°F) insulin. For financial reasons, patients may attempt to use insulins longer than their expiration dates, but careful attention must be paid to monitoring glycemic control and signs of insulin decay (clumping, precipitates, discoloration, etc) if this is attempted.

Sulfonylureas

Pharmacology. The primary mechanism of action of sulfonylureas is enhancement of insulin secretion. Sulfonylureas bind to a specific sulfonylurea receptor (SUR) on pancreatic β cells. Binding closes an adenosine triphosphate–dependent K^+ channel, leading to decreased potassium influx and subsequent depolarization of the membrane. Voltage-dependent Ca^{+2} channels open and allow an inward flux of Ca^{+2}. Increases in intracellular Ca^{+2} cause translocation of secretory granules of insulin to the cell surface and resultant exocytosis of the granule of insulin. Elevated secretion of insulin from the pancreas travels via the portal vein and subsequently suppresses hepatic glucose production.

Classification. Sulfonylureas are classified as first-generation and second-generation agents. The classification scheme is largely derived from differences in relative potency, relative potential for selective side effects, and differences in binding to serum proteins (i.e., risk for protein-binding displacement drug interactions). First-generation agents consist of acetohexamide, chlorpropamide, tolazamide, and tolbutamide. Each of these agents is lower in potency relative to the second-generation drugs: glimepiride, glipizide, and glyburide (Table 72–11). It is important to recognize that all sulfonylureas are equally effective at lowering blood glucose when administered in equipotent doses.

Pharmacokinetics. All sulfonylureas are metabolized in the liver; some to active, others to inactive metabolites (see Table 72–11). Cytochrome P450 (CYP450) 2C9 is involved with the hepatic metabolism of the majority of sulfonylureas. Agents with active metabolites or parent drug that are renally excreted require dosage adjustment or use with caution in patients with compromised renal function. The half-life of the sulfonylurea also relates directly to the risk for hypoglycemia. The hypoglycemic potential is therefore higher with chlorpropamide and glyburide. The long duration of effect of chlorpropamide may be particularly problematic in elderly individuals,

whose renal function declines with age, and therefore it has great potential for accumulation, resulting in severe and protracted hypoglycemia. Individuals at high risk for hypoglycemia (e.g., elderly individuals and those with renal insufficiency or advanced liver disease) should be started at a very low dose of a sulfonylurea with a short half-life. Hypoglycemia on low-dose sulfonylureas may dictate a short-acting insulin secretagogue (nateglinide or repaglinide) in lieu of a sulfonylurea.

Efficacy. As mentioned earlier, when given in equipotent doses, all sulfonylureas are equally effective at lowering blood glucose. On average, HbA_{1c} will fall 1.5% to 2%, with fasting plasma glucose reductions of 60 to 70 mg/dL. A majority of patients will not reach glycemic goals with sulfonylurea monotherapy. Patients who fail sulfonylurea usually fall into two groups: Those with low C-peptide levels and high (>250 mg/dL) fasting plasma glucose (FPG) levels. These patients are often primary failures on sulfonylureas (<30 mg/dL drop of FPG) and have significant glucose toxicity or slow-developing type 1 DM. The other group is those with a good initial response (>30 mg/dL drop of FPG), but which is insufficient to reach their glycemic goals. Over 75% of patients fall into the second group. Factors that portend a positive response include newly diagnosed patients with no indicators of type 1 DM, high fasting C-peptide levels, and moderate fasting hyperglycemia (<250 mg/dL). If glycemic goals are met, a secondary failure rate of approximately 5% to 7% per year can be expected.

Microvascular Complications. Sulfonylureas showed a reduction of microvascular complications in type 2 DM patients in the UKPDS.[53] A more in-depth discussion follows later in the chapter.

Macrovascular Complications. In the largest study to date, the UKPDS, no significant benefit or harm was seen in newly diagnosed type 2 DM patients given sulfonylureas over 10 years. The University Group Diabetes Program study documented higher rates of coronary artery disease in type 2 patients given tolbutamide, when compared to patients given insulin or placebo, though this study has been widely criticized.[65,66] Some sulfonylureas bind to the SUR-2A receptor that is found in cardiac tissue. Binding to the SUR-2A receptor has been implicated in blocking ischemic preconditioning via K^+ channel closure in the heart. Ischemic preconditioning is the premise that prior ischemia in cardiac tissue can provide greater tolerance of subsequent ischemia. Thus patients with heart disease potentially have one compensatory mechanism to protect the heart from ischemia blocked. Conclusions are controversial and readers are referred to the pertinent articles for further discussion.[67–69]

Adverse Effects. The most common side effect of sulfonylureas is hypoglycemia. The pretreatment fasting plasma glucose is a strong predictor of hypoglycemic potential. The lower the FPG is upon initiation, the higher the potential for hypoglycemia. Also, in addition to the high-risk individuals outlined in the pharmacokinetics section, those who skip meals, exercise vigorously, or lose substantial amounts of weight are also more likely to experience hypoglycemia.

Hyponatremia (serum sodium <129 mEq/L) is reportedly associated with tolbutamide, but it is most common with chlorpropamide and occurs in as many as 5% of individuals treated. An increase in antidiuretic hormone secretion is the mechanism for hyponatremia. Risk factors include age >60 years, female gender, and concomitant use of thiazide diuretics.

Weight gain is common with sulfonylureas. In essence, patients who are no longer glycosuric and who do not reduce caloric intake

TABLE 72–11. Oral Agents for the Treatment of Type 2 Diabetes Mellitus

Generic Name (generic version available? Y = yes, N = no)	Brand	Dose (mg)	Recommended Starting Dosage (mg/day) Nonelderly	Elderly	Equivalent Therapeutic Dose (mg)	Maximum Dose (mg/day)	Duration of Action	Metabolism or Therapeutic Notes
Sulfonylureas								
Acetohexamide (Y)	Dymelor	250, 500	250	125–250	500	1500	Up to 16 hours	Metabolized in liver; metabolite potency equal to parent compound; renally eliminated
Chlorpropamide (Y)	Diabinese	100, 250	250	100	250	500	Up to 72 hours	Metabolized in liver; also excreted unchanged renally
Tolazamide (Y)	Tolinase	100, 250, 500	100–250	100	250	1000	Up to 24 hours	Metabolized in liver; metabolite less active than parent compound; renally eliminated
Tolbutamide (Y)	Orinase	250, 500	1000–2000	500–1000	1000	3000	Up to 12 hours	Metabolized in liver to inactive metabolites that are renally excreted
Glipizide (Y)	Glucotrol	5, 10	5	2.5–5	5	40	Up to 20 hours	Metabolized in liver to inactive metabolites
Glipizide (N)	Glucotrol XL	2.5, 5, 10, 20	5	2.5–5	5	20	24 hours	Slow-release form; do not cut tablet
Glyburide (Y)	Diaβeta Micronase	1.25, 2.5, 5	5	1.25–2.5	5	20	Up to 24 hours	Metabolized in liver; elimination 1/2 renal, 1/2 feces
Glyburide, micronized (Y)	Glynase	1.5, 3, 6	3	1.5–3	3	12	Up to 24 hours	Equal control, but better absorption from micronized preparation
Glimepiride (N)	Amaryl	1, 2, 4	1–2	0.5–1	2	8	24 hours	Metabolized in liver to inactive metabolites
Short-acting insulin secretagogues								
Nateglinide (N)	Starlix	60, 120	120 with meals	120 with meals	NA	120 mg three times a day	Up to 4 hours	Metabolized by cytochrome P450 (CYP450) 2C9 and 3A4 to weakly active metabolites; renally eliminated
Repaglinide (N)	Prandin	0.5, 1, 2	0.5–1 with meals	0.5–1 with meals	NA	16	Up to 4 hours	Metabolized by CYP 3A4 to inactive metabolites; excreted in bile
Biguanides								
Metformin (Y)	Glucophage	500, 850, 1000	500 mg twice a day	Assess renal function	NA	2550	Up to 24 hours	No metabolism; Renally secreted and excreted
Metformin extended-release (N)	Glucophage XR	500, 750 (generic available for 500 mg)	500–1000 mg with evening meal	Assess renal function	NA	2550	Up to 24 hours	Take with evening meal or may split dose; may consider trial if intolerant to immediate-release
Thiazolidinediones								
Pioglitazone (N)	Actos	15, 30, 45	15	15	NA	45	24 hours	Metabolized by CYP 2C8 and 3A4; two metabolites have longer half-lives than parent compound
Rosiglitazone (N)	Avandia	2, 4, 8	2–4	2	NA	8 mg/day or 4 mg twice a day	24 hours	Metabolized by CYP2C8 and 2C9 to inactive metabolites that are renally excreted
α-Glucosidase inhibitors								
Acarbose (N)	Precose	25, 50, 100	25 mg one to three times a day	25 mg one to three times a day	NA	25–100 mg three times a day	1–3 hours	Eliminated in bile
Miglitol (N)	Glyset	25, 50, 100	25 mg one to three times a day	25 mg one to three times a day	NA	25–100 mg three times a day	1–3 hours	Eliminated renally

(continued

ABLE 72–11. (*Continued*)

Generic Name (generic version available? Y = yes, N = no)	Brand	Dose (mg)	Recommended Starting Dosage (mg/day)		Equivalent Therapeutic Dose (mg)	Maximum Dose (mg/day)	Duration of Action	Metabolism or Therapeutic Notes
			Nonelderly	*Elderly*				
Combination products								
Glyburide/metformin (Y)	Glucovance	1.25/250 2.5/500 5/500	2.5–5/500 twice a day	1.25/250 twice a day; assess renal function	NA	20 of glyburide, 2000 of metformin	Combination medication	Use as initial therapy: 1.25/250 mg twice a day
Glipizide/metformin (N)	Metaglip	2.5/250 2.5/500 5/500	2.5–5/500 twice a day	2.5/250; assess renal function	NA	20 of glipizide, 2000 of metformin	Combination medication	Use as initial therapy: 2.5/250 mg twice a day
Rosiglitazone/ metformin (N)	Avandamet	1/500 2/500 4/500 2/1000 4/1000	1–2/500 twice a day	1/500 twice a day	NA	8 of rosiglitazone; 2000 of metformin	Combination medication	FDA-approved for secondline therapy, but could be used as initial therapy

ith improvement of blood glucose will store excess calories. Other otable, although much less common, adverse effects of sulfonylureas re skin rash, hemolytic anemia, gastrointestinal upset, and cholesta-is. Disulfiram-type reactions and flushing have been reported with olbutamide and chlorpropamide when alcohol is consumed.

Drug Interactions. Several drugs are thought to interact with sulonylureas, and Table 72–12 summarizes them by proposed mechnisms of action.[70] Drug interactions from protein-binding changes hould occur shortly after the interacting medication is given, as the oncentration of free (thus active) sulfonylurea will acutely increase. irst-generation sulfonylureas, which bind to proteins ionically, are nore likely to cause drug-drug interactions than second-generation ulfonylureas, which bind nonionically.[71] Of note, the clinical importance of protein-binding interactions has been questioned, as the najority of these drug interactions have been found to truly be due to epatic metabolism. Drugs that are inducers or inhibitors of CYP450 C9 should be monitored carefully when used with a sulfonylurea. Additionally, other drugs known to alter blood glucose should be onsidered (see Table 72–10).

Dosing and Administration. The usual starting dose and maxinum dose of sulfonylureas are summarized in Table 72–11. Lower osages are recommended for most agents in elderly patients and those vith compromised renal or hepatic function. The dosage should be trated every 1 to 2 weeks (use a longer interval with chlorpropamide) o achieve glycemic goals. This is possible due to the rapid increase of nsulin secretion in response to the sulfonylurea. Of note, immediate-elease glipizide's maximal dose is 40 mg/day, but its maximal effec-

tive dose is about 10 to 15 mg/day. The maximal effective dose of sulfonylureas tends to be about 60% to 75% of their stated maximum dose.

Short-Acting Insulin Secretagogues

Pharmacology. Though the binding site is adjacent to the binding site of sulfonylureas, nateglinide and repaglinide stimulate insulin secretion from the β cells of the pancreas, similarly to sulfonylureas. Repaglinide, a benzoic acid derivative, and nateglinide, a phenylalanine amino acid derivative, both require the presence of glucose to stimulate insulin secretion. As glucose levels diminish to normal, stimulated insulin secretion diminishes.

Pharmacokinetics. Both nateglinide and repaglinide are rapid-acting insulin secretagogues that are rapidly absorbed ($\sim$0.5 to 1 hour) and have a short half-life (1 to 1.5 hours). Nateglinide is highly protein-bound, primarily to albumin, but also to a_1-acid glycoprotein. Nateglinide is predominantly metabolized by CYP2C9 (70%) and CYP3A4 (30%) to less active metabolites. Glucuronide conjugation then allows rapid renal elimination. Repaglinide is mainly metabolized by the CYP3A4 system to inactive metabolites that are excreted in the bile.

Efficacy. In monotherapy, both significantly reduce postprandial glucose excursions and reduce HbA$_{1c}$ levels. Repaglinide, dosed 4 mg three times a day, when compared to glyburide in diet-treated drug-naïve patients reduced HbA$_{1c}$ levels less (1% vs. 2.4%, from baseline, respectively).[72] Nateglinide, dosed 120 mg three times a day in a similar population reduced HbA$_{1c}$ values by 0.8%.[73] The lower efficacy of these agents vs. sulfonylureas should be considered when patients are >1% above their HbA$_{1c}$ goal. These agents can be used to provide increased insulin secretion during meals, when it is needed, in patients close to glycemic goals. Also, it should be noted that addition of either agent to a sulfonylurea will not result in any improvement in glycemic parameters.

Adverse Effects. Hypoglycemia is the main side effect noted with both agents. Hypoglycemic risk appears to be less vs. sulfonylureas. In part, this is due to the glucose-sensitive release of insulin. If the glucose concentration is normal, less glucose-stimulated release of

ABLE 72–12. **Drug Interactions with Sulfonylureas**

Interaction	Drugs
Displacement from protein binding sites[a]	Warfarin, salicylates, phenylbutazone, sulfonamides
Alters hepatic metabolism (cytochrome P450)	Chloramphenicol, monoamine oxidase inhibitors, cimetidine, rifampin[b]
Altered renal excretion	Allopurinol, probenecid

Many of these drug interactions may be metabolism-based.
Inducer.
eproduced from Gerich.[70]

insulin will occur. In two separate studies, nateglinide rates of hypoglycemia were 3% and repaglinide 15% vs. glyburide and glipizide rates of 15% and 19%, respectively. Weight gain of 2 to 3 kg has been noted with repaglinide, whereas weight gain with nateglinide appears to be <1 kg.

Drug Interactions. Glycemic control and hypoglycemia should be closely monitored when inducers or inhibitors of CYP3A4 are given with repaglinide. Gemfibrozil, a common medication used to treat hypertriglyceridemia in DM, more than doubles the half-life of repaglinide and has resulted in prolonged hypoglycemic reactions. Nateglinide appears to be a weak inhibitor of CYP2C9 based on tolbutamide metabolism, though no significant drug-drug interactions have been reported.

Dosing and Administration. Nateglinide and repaglinide should be dosed prior to each meal (up to 30 minutes prior). The recommended starting dose for repaglinide is 0.5 mg in subjects with HbA$_{1c}$ <8% or treatment-naïve patients, increased weekly to a total daily dose of 16 mg (see Table 72–11). The maximal effective dose of repaglinide is likely 2 mg with each meal, as a dose of 1 mg prior to each meal provides approximately 90% of the maximal glucose-lowering effect. Nateglinide should be dosed at 120 mg prior to meals, and does not require titration. A 60-mg dose is available, but the HbA$_{1c}$ decrement is small (0.3% to 0.5%). If a meal is skipped, the medication can be skipped, and meals extremely low in carbohydrate content may not need a dose. Both agents may be used in patients with renal insufficiency, and offer an excellent alternative in patients experiencing hypoglycemia with low-dose sulfonylurea. Caution is advised for patients with moderate to severe hepatic impairment, as nateglinide has not been studied and the half-life is prolonged with use of repaglinide.

Biguanides

Pharmacology. Metformin is the only biguanide available in the United States. Metformin has been used clinically for 45 years, and has been approved in the U.S. since 1995. Metformin enhances insulin sensitivity of both hepatic and peripheral (muscle) tissues. This allows for an increased uptake of glucose into these insulin-sensitive tissues. The exact mechanisms of how metformin accomplishes insulin sensitization are still being investigated, though adenosine 5'-monophosphate–activated protein kinase activity, tyrosine kinase activity enhancement, and glucose transporter 4 all play a part. Metformin has no direct effect on the β cells, though insulin levels are reduced, reflecting increases in insulin sensitivity.

Pharmacokinetics. Metformin has approximately 50% to 60% oral bioavailability, low lipid solubility, and a volume of distribution that approximates body water. Metformin is not metabolized and does not bind to plasma proteins. Metformin is eliminated by renal tubular secretion and glomerular filtration. The average half-life of metformin is 6 hours, though pharmacodynamically, metformin's antihyperglycemic effects last >24 hours.

Efficacy. Metformin consistently reduces HbA$_{1c}$ levels by 1.5% to 2.0%, fasting plasma glucose levels by 60 to 80 mg/dL, and retains the ability to reduce fasting plasma glucose levels when they are extremely high (>300 mg/dL). The sulfonylureas' ability to stimulate insulin release from β cells at extremely high glucose levels

is often impaired, a concept commonly referred to as *glucose toxicity*. Metformin also has positive effects on several components of the insulin resistance syndrome. Metformin decreases plasma triglycerides and LDL-C by approximately 8% to 15%, as well as increasing HDL-C very modestly (2%). Metformin reduces levels of plasminogen activator inhibitor-1 and causes a modest reduction in weight (2 to 3 kg).

Microvascular Complications. Metformin (n = 342) was compared to intensive glucose control with insulin or sulfonylureas in the UKPDS. No significant differences were seen between therapies with regard to reducing microvascular complications.

6 *Macrovascular Complications.* Metformin reduced macrovascular complications in obese subjects in the UKPDS.[74] Metformin significantly reduced all-cause mortality and risk of stroke vs. intensive treatment with sulfonylureas or insulin. Metformin also reduced diabetes-related death and myocardial infarctions vs. the conventional treatment arm of the UKPDS. Metformin should be included in the therapy for all type 2 DM patients, if tolerated and not contraindicated, as it is the only oral antihyperglycemic medication proven to reduce the risk of total mortality and cardiovascular death.

Adverse Effects. Metformin causes gastrointestinal side effects including abdominal discomfort, stomach upset, and/or diarrhea in approximately 30% of patients. Anorexia and stomach fullness is likely part of the reason loss of weight is noted with metformin. These side effects are usually mild and can be minimized by slow titration. Gastrointestinal side effects also tend to be transient, lessening in severity over several weeks. If encountered, make sure patients are taking metformin with or right after meals, and reduce the dose to a point at which no gastrointestinal side effects are encountered. Increases in the dose may be tried again in several weeks. Anecdotally, extended release metformin (Glucophage-XR) may lessen some of the GI side effects. Metallic taste, interference with vitamin B$_{12}$ absorption, and hypoglycemia during intense exercise has been documented, but are clinically uncommon.

Metformin therapy rarely (3 cases per 100,000 patient-years) causes lactic acidosis. Any disease state that may increase lactic acid production or decrease lactic acid removal may predispose to lactic acidosis. Tissue hypoperfusion, such as that due to congestive heart failure, hypoxic states, shock, or septicemia, via increased production of lactic acid; and severe liver disease or alcohol, via reduced removal of lactic acid in the liver, all increase the risk of lactic acidosis. The clinical presentation of lactic acidosis is often nonspecific flu-like symptoms, thus the diagnosis is usually made by laboratory confirmation. Metformin use in renal insufficiency, defined as a serum creatinine of 1.4 mg/dL in women and 1.5 mg/dL in men or greater is contraindicated, as it is renally eliminated. Elderly patients, who often have reduced muscle mass, should have their glomerular filtration rate estimated by a 24 hour urine creatinine collection. If the calculated glomerular filtration rate is less than 70 to 80 mL/min, metformin should not be given. Due to the risk of acute renal failure during intravenous dye procedures, metformin therapy should be withheld starting the day of the procedure and resumed in 2 to 3 days when normal renal function has been documented.

Drug Interactions. Cimetidine competes for renal tubular secretion of metformin and concomitant administration leads to higher metformin serum concentrations. At least one case report of lactic acidosis with metformin therapy implicates cimetidine. Other cationic ugs may interact similarly such as procainamide, digoxin, quinine, trimethoprim, and vancomycin.[75]

Dosing and Administration. Metformin immediate-release usually dosed 500 mg twice a day with the largest meals to minimize astrointestinal side effects. Metformin may be increased by 500 mg eekly until glycemic goals or 2000 mg/day is achieved (see Table 2–11). Metformin 850 mg may be dosed daily, and then increased ery 1 to 2 weeks to the maximum dose of 850 mg three times a day 550 mg/day). Approximately 80% of the glycemic-lowering effect ay be seen at 1500 mg, and 2000 mg/day is the maximal effective ose.

Extended-release metformin can be initiated at 500 mg a day ith the evening meal and titrated weekly by 500 mg as tolerated to single evening dose of 2000 mg/day. Twice daily to three times a ay dosing of extended-release metformin may help to minimize gasointestinal side effects and improve glycemic control. Metformin xtended-release 750 mg tablets may be titrated weekly to the maxmum dose of 2250 mg/day, though as stated above, 1500 mg/day ovides the majority of the glycemic-lowering effect.

Thiazolidinediones

Pharmacology. Thiazolidinediones are also referred to as TZDs glitazones. Pioglitazone and rosiglitazone are the two currently aproved thiazolidinediones for the treatment of type 2 DM (see Table 2–11). Thiazolidinediones work by binding to the peroxisome proferator activator receptor-γ (PPAR-γ), which are primarily located fat cells and vascular cells. The concentration of these receptors in e muscle is very low; thus this is unlikely to be the main site of acon. Thiazolidinediones enhance insulin sensitivity at muscle, liver, d fat tissues indirectly. Thiazolidinediones cause preadipocytes to fferentiate into mature fat cells in subcutaneous fat stores. Small fat lls are more sensitive to insulin and more able to store free fatty ids. The result is a flux of free fatty acids out of the plasma, visceral t, and liver into subcutaneous fat, a less insulin-resistant storage ssue. Muscle intracellular fat products, which contribute to insulin sistance, also decline.

Pharmacokinetics. Pioglitazone and rosiglitazone are well absorbed with or without food. Both are highly (>99%) protein bound albumin. Pioglitazone is primarily metabolized by CYP2C8, and to lesser extent by CYP3A4 (17%), with the majority being eliminated the feces. Rosiglitazone is metabolized by CYP2C8, and to a lesser xtent by CYP2C9, then conjugated with two-thirds found in urine d one-third in feces. The half-life of pioglitazone and rosiglitazone 3 to 7 hours and 3 to 4 hours, respectively. Two active metabolites of ioglitazone with longer half-lives deliver the majority of activity at eady state. Both medications have a duration of antihyperglycemic ction of over 24 hours.

Efficacy. Pioglitazone and rosiglitazone, given for about 6 months, educe HbA$_{1c}$ values ~1.5% and reduce FPG levels by approximately 0 to 70 mg/dL at maximal doses. Glycemic-lowering onset is slow, nd maximal glycemic-lowering effects may not be seen until 3 to months of therapy. It is important to inform patients of this fact and at they should not stop therapy even if minimal glucose lowering initially encountered. The efficacy of both drugs is dependent on ufficient insulinemia. If there is insufficient endogenous insulin prouction (β-cell function) or exogenous insulin delivery via injections, either will lower glucose concentrations efficiently. Interestingly,

patients who are more obese, or who gain weight on either medication tend to have a larger reduction in HbA$_{1c}$ values. Pioglitazone consistently decreases plasma triglyceride levels by 10% to 20%, whereas rosiglitazone tends to have a neutral effect. LDL-C concentrations tend to increase with rosiglitazone 5% to 15%, but do not significantly increase with pioglitazone. Both appear to convert small, dense LDL particles, which have been shown to be highly atherogenic, to large, fluffy LDL particles, that are less dense. Large, fluffy LDL particles may be less atherogenic, but any increase in LDL must be of concern. Both drugs increase HDL similarly, up to 3 to 9 mg/dL. Thiazolidinediones also affect several components of the insulin resistance syndrome. Plasminogen-activator inhibitor-1 (PAI-1) levels are decreased, and many other adipocytokines are affected, endothelial function improves, and blood pressure may decrease slightly.

Microvascular Complications. Thiazolidinediones reduce HbA$_{1c}$ levels, which have been shown to be related to the risk of microvascular complications.

Macrovascular Complications. Macrovascular outcome studies are in progress. Thiazolidinediones improve endothelial function, raise HDL levels, slightly lower blood pressure, and have been shown to reduce restenosis after percutaneous transluminal coronary artery stenting.

Adverse Effects. Troglitazone, the first thiazolidinedione approved, caused idiosyncratic hepatotoxicity and had 28 deaths from liver failure, which prompted removal from the U.S. market in March 2000. Approximately 1.9% of patients placed on troglitazone had alanine aminotransferase (ALT) levels more than three times the upper limit of normal. The incidence, using these criteria for elevated liver enzymes, with pioglitazone (0.25%) and rosiglitazone (0.2%) has been low. No evidence of hepatotoxicity was reported in an analysis of more than 5,000 patients given rosiglitazone or pioglitazone.[76,77] Several case reports of hepatotoxicity with rosiglitazone or pioglitazone have been reported, but improvement in ALT was consistently noted when the drug was discontinued. Prior to therapy, it is recommended that an ALT be checked. ALT monitoring vigilance has been lowered, and it is now recommended that the ALT be checked periodically at the practitioner's discretion. Prior guidelines recommended every 2 months for the first year of therapy, then periodically. Patients with ALT levels >2.5 times the upper limit of normal should not start either medication, and if the ALT is >3 times the upper limit of normal the medication should be discontinued.

Retention of fluid leads to many different possible side effects with rosiglitazone and pioglitazone. The etiology of the fluid retention has not been fully elucidated, but appears to include peripheral vasodilation and/or improved insulin sensitization with a resultant increase in renal sodium and water retention. A reduction in plasma hemoglobin (2% to 4%), attributed to a 10% increase in plasma volume, may result in a dilutional anemia which does not require treatment. Edema is also commonly (4% to 5% in mono- or combination therapy) reported. When a thiazolidinedione is used in combination with insulin, the incidence of edema (~15%) is increased. Thiazolidinediones are contraindicated in patients with New York Heart Association Class III and IV heart failure, and great caution should be exercised when given to patients with Class I and II heart failure or other underlying cardiac disease, as pulmonary edema and heart failure have been reported. Edema tends to be dose related and if not severe, a reduction in the dose as well as use of diuretics will allow the continuation of therapy in the majority of patients.[78]

Weight gain, which is also dose related, can be seen with both rosiglitazone and pioglitazone. Mechanistically, both fluid retention and fat accumulation play a part in explaining the weight gain. Thiazolidinediones, besides stimulating fat cell differentiation, also reduce leptin levels, which stimulate appetite and food intake. Average weight gain varies, but a 1.5- to 4-kg weight gain is not uncommon. Rarely, a patient will gain large amounts of weight in a short period of time, and this may necessitate discontinuation of therapy. Weight gain positively predicts a larger HbA_{1c} reduction, but must be balanced with the well documented effects of long term weight gain.

As a caution, anovulatory patients may resume ovulation on thiazolidinediones. Adequate pregnancy and contraception precautions should be explained to all women capable of becoming pregnant, as both agents are pregnancy category C.

■ *Drug Interactions.* No significant drug interactions have been noted with either medication. Neither pioglitazone nor rosiglitazone appear to be inhibitors or inducers of CYP3A4/2C8 or CYP2C8/CYP2C9, respectively, though drugs that are strong inhibitors or inducers of these pathways necessitate close monitoring.

■ *Dosing and Administration.* The recommended starting dosages of pioglitazone and of rosiglitazone are 15 mg once daily and 2 to 4 mg once daily, respectively. Dosages may be increased slowly based on therapeutic goals and side effects. The maximum dose and maximum effective dose of pioglitazone is 45 mg, and rosiglitazone is 8 mg once daily, though 4 mg twice a day may reduce HbA_{1c} by 0.2% to 0.3% more vs. 8 mg once daily.

■ α-Glucosidase Inhibitors

■ *Pharmacology.* Currently, there are two α-glucosidase inhibitors available in the United States (acarbose and miglitol). α-Glucosidase inhibitors competitively inhibit enzymes (maltase, isomaltase, sucrase, and glucoamylase) in the small intestine, delaying the breakdown of sucrose and complex carbohydrates.[79,80] They do not cause any malabsorption of these nutrients. The net effect from this action is to reduce the postprandial blood glucose rise.

■ *Pharmacokinetics.* The mechanism of action of α-glucosidase inhibitors is limited to the luminal side of the intestine. Some metabolites of acarbose are systemically absorbed and renally excreted, whereas the majority of miglitol is absorbed and renally excreted unchanged.

■ *Efficacy.* Postprandial glucose concentrations are reduced (40 to 50 mg/dL), while fasting glucose levels are relatively unchanged (~10% reduction). Efficacy on glycemic control is modest (average reductions in HbA_{1c} of 0.3% to 1%), affecting primarily postprandial glycemic excursions. Thus patients near target HbA_{1c} levels with near normal fasting plasma glucose levels, but high postprandial levels, may be candidates for therapy.

■ *Microvascular Complications.* α-Glucosidase inhibitors modestly reduce HbA_{1c} levels, which have been shown to be related to the risk of microvascular complications.

■ *Macrovascular Complications.* The STOP-NIDDM study demonstrated that acarbose can decrease the conversion rate of impaired glucose tolerance to diabetes, as well as reduce the risk of

cardiovascular events.[81,82] Currently, no medication is FDA approved for the prevention of type 2 DM.

■ *Adverse Effects.* The gastrointestinal side effects, such as flatulence, bloating, abdominal discomfort, and diarrhea, are very common and greatly limit the use of α-glucosidase inhibitors. Mechanistically, these side effects are caused by distal intestinal degradation of undigested carbohydrate by the microflora, which results in gas (CO_2 and methane) production. α-Glucosidase inhibitors should be initiated at a low dose and titrated slowly to reduce gastrointestinal intolerance. Beano, an α-glucosidase enzyme, may help to decrease gastrointestinal side effects, but may decrease efficacy slightly.[83]

If a patient develops hypoglycemia within several hours of ingesting an α-glucosidase inhibitor, oral glucose is advised because the drug will inhibit the breakdown of more complex sugar molecules. Milk, with lactose sugar, may be used as an alternative when no glucose is available, as acarbose only slightly (10%) inhibits lactase.

Rarely, elevated serum aminotransferase levels have been reported with the highest doses of acarbose. It appeared to be dose and weight related, and is the premise for the weight-based maximum doses.

■ *Dosing and Administration.* Dosing for both miglitol and acarbose are similar. Initiate with a very low dose (25 mg with one meal a day); increase very gradually (over several months) to a maximum of 50 mg three times a day for patients ≤60 kg or 100 mg three times a day for patients >60 kg (see Table 72–11). Both α-glucosidase inhibitors should be taken with the first bite of the meal so that drug may be present to inhibit enzyme activity. Only patients consuming a diet high in complex carbohydrates will have significant reductions in glucose levels. α-Glucosidase inhibitors are contraindicated in patients with short-bowel syndrome or inflammatory bowel disease, and neither should be administered in patients with serum creatinine >2 mg/dL, as this population has not been studied.

■ PIVOTAL TRIALS

■ DIABETES CONTROL AND COMPLICATIONS TRIAL

◀ Much of the last century in diabetes care was dominated by the debate over whether glycemic control actually was causative in complications of DM. Animal studies and some human studies suggested that the worse the glycemia the greater the risk of complications. But "the glucose hypothesis" was not ultimately accepted and proven until the publication of the DCCT in 1993.[52] One thousand four hundred forty-one patients with type 1 DM were divided into two groups: those without complications (726 subjects, primary prevention), and those with early microvascular complications (715 subjects, secondary prevention). These two groups were then again divided into two groups, one randomized to receive conventional therapy (one or two shots of insulin daily and infrequent SMBG with no attempt to change therapy based on home blood glucose readings), and the other to receive intensive therapy (3+ injections of insulin daily or insulin pump, with frequent SMBG and alteration of insulin therapy based on SMBG results, plus frequent contact with a health professional). After 6.5 years mean follow-up with a difference in HbA_{1c} between the two groups being ≈2% (≈9% vs. ≈7%), retinopathy was decreased by 76% in the primary prevention cohort, with retinopathy progression reduced 54% in the secondary prevention group. Neuropathy was decreased by 60% in both groups combined. Microalbuminuria as decreased 39%, while macroproteinuria was reduced 54% with tensive therapy. Hypoglycemia was more common and weight gain eater with intensive therapy. A non–statistically significant reduc- on in coronary events was seen in the intensively treated group as mpared to the conventional group. Follow-up studies 8 years after e DCCT ended continued to show an advantage of good glycemic ntrol over what was previously considered conventional therapy.[84] ie DCCT revolutionized therapy of DM, demanding that stricter ycemic control be the goal.

IMPLICATIONS OF THE UNITED KINGDOM PROSPECTIVE DIABETES STUDY

ie UKPDS was a landmark study for the care of patients with type DM, confirming the importance of glycemic control for reducing the sk of microvascular complications.[53] More than 5000 patients with wly diagnosed type 2 DM were entered into the study. Patients were llowed for an average of 10 years. The major portion of the study ssessed "conventional therapy" (no drug therapy unless the patient as symptomatic or had fasting plasma glucose >270 mg/dL), versus tensive therapy starting with either sulfonylureas or insulin, aimed keeping the fasting plasma glucose <108 mg/dL. A subset of obese itients was studied using metformin as the primary therapeutic agent.

CLINICAL CONTROVERSY

Preservation of β-cell function, and thus arresting the progression of type 2 diabetes, appears to be the future goal of treatment. The UKPDS clearly showed that sulfonylureas, metformin, and insulin are ineffective in stopping the progressive β-cell failure. In animal models thiazolidinediones (TZDs) have been able to arrest β-cell failure, and in humans short-term indirect β-cell function measures have shown improvements. This could mean that TZDs arrest the progressive β-cell decline in type 2 DM. Based on these data and the large amount of indirect evidence showing that TZDs may be cardioprotective, some clinicians have started using TZDs as first-line therapy. Glucagon-like peptide-1 derived therapies have also shown promise in this area, though no agents are FDA approved at the face of this writing. Long-term studies are underway.

Significant findings from the study include:

Microvascular complications (predominantly the need for laser photocoagulation on retinal lesions) are reduced by 25% when median HbA$_{1c}$ is 7% as compared to 7.9%.[53]

A continuous relationship exists between glycemia and microvascular complications, with a 35% reduction in risk for each 1% decrement in HbA$_{1c}$. No glycemic threshold for microvascular disease exists.[85]

Glycemic control has minimal effect on macrovascular disease risk.[53] Excess macrovascular risk appears to be related to conventional risk factors such as dyslipidemia and hypertension.[86]

Sulfonylureas and insulin therapy do not increase macrovascular disease risk.[53]

Metformin reduces macrovascular risk in obese patients.[74]

Vigorous blood pressure control reduces microvascular and macrovascular events.[86] There was no evidence for a threshold systolic blood pressure above 130 mm Hg for protection

against complications. β-Blockers and angiotensin-converting enzyme (ACE) inhibitors appear to be equally efficacious.[87]

THERAPEUTICS

⏴8 Knowledge of the patient's quantitative and qualitative meal patterns, activity levels, pharmacokinetics of insulin preparations, and pharmacology of oral antidiabetic agents for type 2 DM are essential to individualize the treatment plan and optimize blood glucose control while minimizing risks for hypoglycemia and other adverse effects of pharmacologic therapies.

TYPE 1 DIABETES MELLITUS

The choice of therapy for type 1 DM is simple: all patients need insulin. However, how that insulin is delivered to the patient is a matter of considerable practice difference among patients and clinicians. Historically, after the discovery of insulin by Banting and Best in 1921, frequent injections of regular insulin (initially the only insulin available) were given. Modifications of insulin led to longer-acting insulin suspensions and the use by many patients of one or two shots of longer-acting insulin each day. Because SMBG and HbA$_{1c}$ testing were not available at that time, patients and practitioners had no idea how well their patients' blood glucose concentrations were controlled, other than a vague sense from an indirect method, measurement of glucose in the urine. While the renal threshold for glucose is relatively predictable in young healthy subjects, it is highly variable in older patients and patients with renal disease. The advent of SMBG and HbA$_{1c}$ testing in the 1980s revolutionized the care of diabetes, enabling patients and practitioners to directly access blood glucose for assessment, and enabling the patient to make instantaneous changes in the insulin regimen if need be. Modern diabetes management would be impossible without these two tools.

Contemporary management of type 1 DM attempts to match carbohydrate intake with glucose-lowering processes, most commonly insulin, as well as with exercise. Diet is still the cornerstone of diabetes therapy, but unlike in previous years, attempts are made to allow the patient to live as normal a life as possible. Understanding the principles of glucose input and glucose egress from the blood will allow the practitioner and the patient great latitude in the management of patients with type 1 DM.

Simplistically speaking, one can break down normal insulin secretion into a relatively constant background level of insulin ("basal") for the fasting and postabsorptive period, and prandial spikes of insulin after eating ("bolus") (Fig. 72–7).[88] Insulin sensitivity and insulin secretion are not constant throughout the day, rendering the basal concept inaccurate. However, in most clinical situations, this approach provides a useful paradigm for understanding and applying insulin treatment for type 1 DM. The other basic principle to consider is that the timing of insulin onset, peak, and duration of effect must match meal patterns and exercise schedules to achieve near-normal blood glucose values throughout the day.

Historically, complexity of insulin regimens has usually been related to the number of injections of insulin administered per day. This is a reasonable classification. Clearly one injection of any insulin preparation daily will in no way mimic normal physiology, and therefore is unacceptable. Similarly, two injections of any insulin daily will fail to replicate normal insulin release patterns. Injection regimens that begin to approximate physiologic insulin release start with

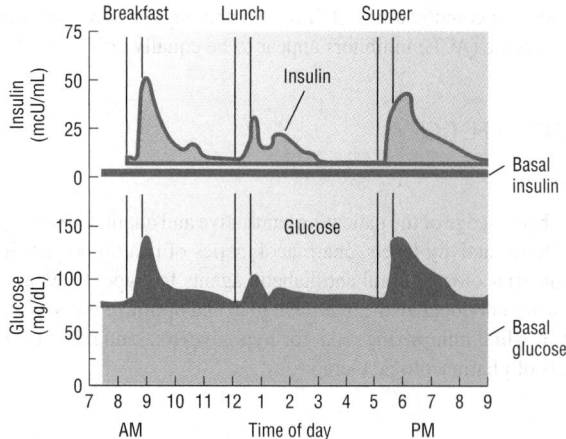

Intensive insulin therapy regimens

	7AM	11AM	5PM	HS
1. 2 doses, R + N or L	R + N or L		R + N or L	
2. 3 doses, R or rapid + N or L	R, Lis or A + N or L	R, Lis or A	R, Lis or A + N or L	
3. 4 doses, R or rapid acting + intermediate or ultralente	R, Lis or A + N, L or UL	R, Lis or A	R, Lis or A	N, L or UL
4. 4 doses, R or rapid acting + long acting	R, Lis or A	R, Lis or A	R, Lis or A	G
5. CS-II pump	Bolus	←——— Adjusted Basal ———→ Bolus	Bolus	

FIGURE 72–7. Relationship between insulin and glucose over the course of a day and how various insulin regimens could be given. A, aspart; CS-II, continuous subcutaneous insulin infusion; G, glargine; L, lente; Lis, lispro; N, NPH; R, regular; UL, ultralente.

"split-mixed" injections of a morning dose of neutral protamine Hagedorn (NPH) and regular insulin before breakfast, and again before the evening meal. The presumption is made that the morning NPH insulin gives basal insulin for the day and covers the midday meal, the morning regular insulin covers breakfast, the evening NPH insulin gives basal insulin for the rest of the day, and the evening regular covers the evening meal. If patients are very compulsive about consistency of timing of their injections and meals and intake of carbohydrate, such a strategy may be successful. However, most patients are not sufficiently predictable in their schedule and food intake to allow "tight" glucose control with such an approach.

The first modification that is frequently made to such a regimen is the movement of the evening NPH to bedtime (now three total injections per day) because the fasting glucose in the morning is too high. This approach improves glycemic control and reduces hypoglycemia, sufficiently intensifying the insulin therapy for some patients.[89] However, many patients need a more intense approach that also allows greater flexibility in their lifestyle.

The basal-bolus concept is an attempt to replicate normal insulin physiology with a combination of intermediate- or long-acting insulin to give the basal component, and short-acting insulin to give the bolus component. Various strategies have been used for the former, including once- or twice-daily NPH, lente, or ultralente insulin, or once-daily insulin glargine. Most patients require two shots of all of the above insulins except insulin glargine. Also, all of the above

insulins, with the exception of insulin glargine, have some degree of peak effect that must be considered in planning meals and activity. Insulin glargine is a feasible basal insulin supplement for most patients with type 1 DM. The bolus insulin component is given before meals with regular insulin, lispro insulin, or insulin aspart. The rapid onset of action and short time course of lispro insulin and insulin aspart more closely replicate normal physiology. This approach allows the patient to vary the amount of insulin injected, depending on the preprandial SMBG level, the anticipated activity (upcoming exercise may reduce insulin requirement), and anticipated carbohydrate intake. Most patients will have a prescribed dose of insulin preprandially that they vary by use of a "sliding scale." This type of adjusted scale insulin is intended to optimize the insulin regimen. In light of the negative connotation of the term "sliding scale" (usually referring to giving insulin only after the blood glucose increases, rather than treating the underlying disorder), a better descriptor for the adjusted-dose insulin is *variable-dose prandial insulin* or insulin algorithm. Carbohydrate counting is a very effective tool for determining the amount of insulin to be injected preprandially. Although general algorithms give rough guidelines, each patient will have to adjust the prescribed preprandial insulin dosage to achieve optimal glucose control.

As a rough estimate, patients may be begun on ≈0.6 units/kg per day with basal insulin 50% of total dose and prandial insulin 20% of total dose prebreakfast, 15% prelunch, and 15% presupper. Type 1 DM patients generally require between 0.5 and 1 unit/kg per day. The need for significantly higher amounts of insulin suggests the presence of insulin antibodies or insulin resistance (coexistent endocrinopathy or type 2 DM).

Obviously, insulin pump therapy (continuous subcutaneous insulin infusion [CSII], generally using lispro or aspart insulin to diminish aggregation) is the most sophisticated form of basal bolus insulin delivery system. CSII may be slightly more efficacious in achieving good glycemic control than multiple-dose insulin injections.[90,91] Extensive discussion of this mode of therapy is beyond the scope of this text.[92] Nevertheless, the basic principles for implementation are the same. The one advantage of pump therapy is that the basal insulin dose may be varied, consistent with changes in insulin requirements throughout the day. In selected patients, this feature will allow greater glycemic control with CSII. However, insulin pumps require even greater attention to detail and frequency of SMBG than four injections daily.[93] In appropriately selected patients willing to pay sufficient attention to detail of SMBG and insulin administration, CSII can be a very useful form of therapy.

Intensive therapy (basal bolus) to all adult patients with type 1 DM at the time of diagnosis is recommended to reinforce the importance of glycemic control from the outset rather than change strategies over time after lack of control. Occasional patients with an extended honeymoon period may need less intense therapy initially, but should be converted to basal bolus therapy at the onset of glycemic lability. For patients insisting on two injections daily, NPH and regular insulin (starting at 0.6 units/kg with two-thirds in the morning, two-thirds of morning dose as NPH, and one-half of evening dose as NPH) may be sufficient. Regardless of the regimen chosen, gross adjustments in the total insulin dose can be made based on HbA$_{1c}$ measurements and symptoms such as polyuria, polydipsia, and weight gain or loss. Fine insulin adjustments can be determined on the basis of the results of frequent SMBG.

All patients receiving insulin should have extensive education in the recognition and treatment of hypoglycemia. Yearly (or more often) questioning about the recognition of hypoglycemia is warranted. Documentation of frequency of hypoglycemia, particularly that requiring assistance of another person, visit to an emergent of urgent care facility, or hospitalization, should be recorded. In type 1 DM, the development of hypoglycemia unawareness is common. It may result from progression of disease with autonomic neuropathy. Loss of adrenergic warning signs in such a situation is a relative contraindication to intensive insulin therapy. More commonly, type 1 DM patients have loss of warning signs because of a presumed lower set-point for release of counterregulatory hormones as a result of frequent episodes of hypoglycemia ("hypoglycemia begets hypoglycemia").[94] In such situations, more normal hypoglycemia awareness may be restored by reduction or redistribution of the insulin dose to eliminate significant hypoglycemic episodes. A recent publication has found that short-term treatment with theophylline will improve hypoglycemia awareness.[95] Whether this therapy should routinely be employed is still unknown.

Children and pubescent adolescents are relatively protected from microvascular complications and must be managed with consideration of what is practical. Therefore it is not unreasonable to use less-intense management (two shots per day, premixed insulins) until the patient is postpubertal.[96]

Occasional patients have antibodies to injected insulin, but the significance of the antibodies is minimal.[97] Human insulin therapy has not totally eliminated insulin allergies, although most patients have a local reaction that will dissipate over time. If the allergic reaction does not improve or is systemic, insulin desensitization can be carried out.[98] Protocols for desensitization are available from major insulin manufacturers. While more common in the animal insulin era, lipohypertrophy is still seen in some patients with long-standing type 1 DM. Such patients give their insulin injections in the same site to minimize discomfort. Because insulin absorption from an area of lipohypertrophy is unpredictable, avoidance of injections into these areas is mandatory.

Several common errors can occur in the therapy of patients with type 1 DM, causing erratic glucose fluctuations:

- Failure to take into account peaks of insulin action when using a peaking insulin and planning meals and/or activity. Eating should be planned around the peaks of the insulin.
- Random rotation of insulin injection sites. There is sufficient variability of insulin absorption from site to site that this practice alone may cause wide glucose swings. The most consistent absorption of insulin is from the abdominal wall. We try to get our patients to take all their injections in the abdomen. If the patient is unable or unwilling to follow this advice, then systematic site rotation is the next preferable option. The patient always gives the insulin injection in the same region of the body the same time of the day each day. For instance, the arms are always used every morning. Needless to say, the patient would not inject in a limb and then go out and exercise that limb, increasing blood flow and insulin absorption. Overinsulinization is a very common problem. The answer to all high blood glucose is not necessarily more insulin, as the patient may be insulinopenic, or may be "rebounding" from a previous low glucose and treating it with excessive amounts of carbohydrate. Fastidious SMBG, particularly during the night (or selected use of continuous glucose monitoring) will help sort this out. Also, practitioners sometimes do not adequately differentiate type 1 DM from type 2 DM when using insulin. Patients with type 1 DM are insulinopenic but have normal insulin sensitivity. Patients with type 2 DM have varying degrees of insulin resistance. Therefore one unit change in the dose of insulin for a patient with type 1 DM may have a dramatic effect on glucose concentrations, whereas in some

patients with type 2 DM 10 to 20 times that amount of insulin may have little effect on glucose. Large changes in insulin dose in patients with type 1 DM are not usually indicated unless the patient's blood glucose control is very poor. Widely erratic SMBG results and/or weight gain often suggest overinsulinization.

- When in doubt, always double check the patient's technique for insulin dosing, insulin injection, and SMBG. Sometimes the simplest of errors results in miserable glycemic control.

Islet cell and whole pancreas transplantation are occasionally used in patients, usually renal transplants, who require immunosuppressive therapy for other reasons.[99] There has been considerable interest in islet cell transplantation since investigators in Edmonton reported success without using glucocorticoids as immunosuppressive agents.[100] Some of these patients are able to come off insulin altogether.

TYPE 2 DIABETES MELLITUS

Pharmacotherapy for type 2 DM has changed dramatically in the last few years with the addition of several new drug classes and recommendations to achieve more stringent glycemic control. Symptomatic patients may initially require treatment with insulin or combination oral therapy to reduce glucose toxicity (which may reduce β-cell insulin secretion and worsen insulin resistance). Patients with HbA_{1c} $\approx$7% or less are usually treated with therapeutic lifestyle measures with or without an insulin sensitizer. Those with HbA_{1c} >7% but <8% are initially treated with single oral agents. Patients with higher initial HbA_{1c} may benefit from initial therapy with two oral agents.

Depending on patient motivation and adherence to therapeutic lifestyle changes, most patients with HbA_{1c} greater than 9% to 10% will likely require therapy with two or more agents to reach glycemic goals. Treatment of type 2 DM often necessitates use of multiple therapeutic agents (combination therapy), including oral antihyperglycemics and insulin to obtain glycemic goals.

The best initial oral therapy for patients with type 2 DM is widely debated. Based on the results of the UKPDS and safety record, obese patients (>120% ideal body weight) without contraindications should be started on metformin titrated to $\approx$2,000 mg/d.[101] Near-normal weight patients may be treated with insulin secretagogues. Failure of initial therapy should result in addition rather than substitution (reserve substitution for intolerance to a drug due to side effects) of another class of drug. For cost and efficacy reasons, metformin and an insulin secretagogue are often first- and second-line therapy. Initial oral combination therapy for patients with HbA_{1c} >9% to 10% should be considered, and several oral combination products (Glucovance and Metaglip) have been approved as a first-line treatment. Figure 72–8 is an algorithm developed by the Texas Diabetes Council for glycemic control. Thiazolidinediones may be substituted in situations in which a patient is intolerant of, or has a contraindication to, metformin as an insulin sensitizer. In the UKPDS, insulin, metformin, or sulfonylureas did not halt β-cell failure. Thiazolidinediones, in a Zucker diabetic fatty rat model, preserved β-cell function.[102] Short-term human studies have reinforced these results through indirect measures of β-cell function, and if similar results are found long-term, thiazolidinediones could become first-line therapy. For dual therapy, HbA_{1c} reductions vary according to the medication added to the current therapy (Table 72–13). After a patient has inadequate control on two drugs, adding a third class of oral agents (usually a thiazolidinedione) can be considered, though triple therapy is not presently FDA approved. (Triple

TABLE 72–13. Add-On Dual Therapy: Average HbA₁c Reductions[a]

Drug Combination	Change in HbA$_{1c}$ (%)	Number of Studies	Number of Subjects
Sulfonylurea + metformin	−2.2	8	458
Sulfonylurea + insulin	−1.9	17	88
Meglitinide + thiazolidinedione	−1.7	1	434
Metformin + insulin	−1.7	8	138
Sulfonylurea + α-glucosidase inhibitor	−1.6	3	177
Metformin + meglitinide	−1.4	3	226
Insulin + α-glucosidase inhibitor	−1.2	1	20
Insulin + thiazolidinedione	−1.2	7	850
Sulfonylurea + thiazolidinedione	−1.1	12	1315
Metformin + thiazolidinedione	−0.9	3	284
Metformin + α-glucosidase inhibitor	−0.4	3	173

[a]Reductions are averages and do not imply superiority or inferiority of a combination.
Unpublished data compiled by Tina Lopez, PharmD and Curtis Triplitt, PharmD.

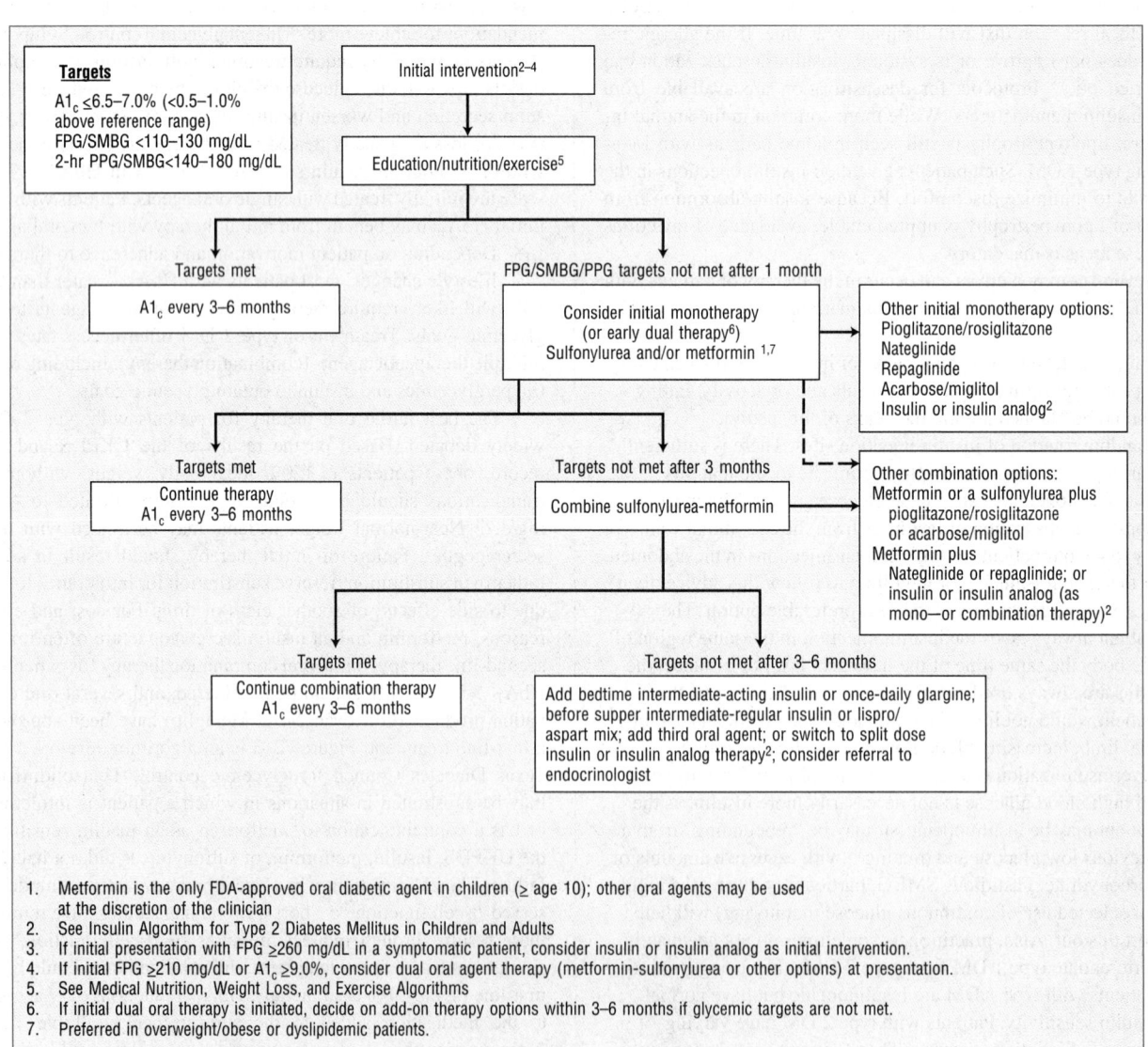

1. Metformin is the only FDA-approved oral diabetic agent in children (≥ age 10); other oral agents may be used at the discretion of the clinician
2. See Insulin Algorithm for Type 2 Diabetes Mellitus in Children and Adults
3. If initial presentation with FPG ≥260 mg/dL in a symptomatic patient, consider insulin or insulin analog as initial intervention.
4. If initial FPG ≥210 mg/dL or A1c ≥9.0%, consider dual oral agent therapy (metformin-sulfonylurea or other options) at presentation.
5. See Medical Nutrition, Weight Loss, and Exercise Algorithms
6. If initial dual oral therapy is initiated, decide on add-on therapy options within 3–6 months if glycemic targets are not met.
7. Preferred in overweight/obese or dyslipidemic patients.

FIGURE 72–8. Glycemic control algorithm for type 2 DM in children and adults. See *www.texasdiabetescouncil.org* for current algorithms. (*Reprinted with permission from the Texas Diabetes Council.*)

combination therapy with a sulfonylurea, metformin, and troglitazone as approved,[103] but troglitazone is no longer available for use.) An alternative is to add an intermediate-acting or long-acting insulin at bedtime, to the initial oral agent used or two-drug combination. Sulfonylureas are often stopped when insulin is added, but continuing the sulfonylurea is permissible until multiple daily injections are started, at which time it should definitely be discontinued.

Virtually all patients with type 2 DM ultimately become relatively insulinopenic and will require insulin therapy. Insulin therapy for type 2 DM has changed dramatically in the last few years. Specifically, patients are often "transitioned" to insulin by using a bedtime injection of an intermediate- or long-acting insulin, using oral agents primarily for control during the day.[104,105] This strategy leads to less hyperinsulinemia during the day and is associated with less weight gain than the more traditional insulin strategies. Because most patients are insulin resistant, insulin sensitizers are commonly used with insulin therapy. Patients with type 2 DM are usually well buffered against hypoglycemia. Patients should be monitored for hypoglycemia by asking about nocturnal sweating, nightmares (both indicative of nocturnal hypoglycemia), palpitations, tremulousness, and neuroglycopenic symptoms, as well as SMBG. When bedtime insulin plus daytime oral medications fails, a conventional multiple daily dose insulin regimen while continuing the insulin sensitizers should be tried. Concerns and problems with insulin administration is addressed in the section on type 1 DM generally relate to the therapy of type 2 DM. However, patients with type 2 DM rarely have hypoglycemia unawareness. Also, the variability of insulin resistance means that insulin doses may range from 0.7 to 2.5 units/kg or more. Figure 72–9 is an algorithm for insulin therapy options in type 2 diabetes developed by the Texas Diabetes Council.

The availability of short-acting insulin secretagogues, very short-acting insulin, and α-glucosidase inhibitors, all of which target postprandial glycemia, has reminded practitioners that glycemic control is a function of fasting and preprandial glycemia and postprandial glycemic excursions.[106] Therefore postprandial glucose measurements may need more emphasis if the HbA_{1c} is near the glycemic goal. Currently, it remains to be seen whether targeting after-meal glucose excursions will have more of an effect on complications risk than more conventional strategies. Importantly, postprandial excursions proportionally contribute more than the fasting plasma glucose to the HbA_{1c} percentage obtained as the HbA_{1c} nears goals, and thus will need to be targeted for optimal glycemic control in many patients. In epidemiologic studies post–glucose challenge glucose measurements are a better predictor of macrovascular disease risk and form the basis for American College of Endocrinology/American Association of Clinical Endocrinologists postprandial glycemic goals (see Table 72–7).[107]

SPECIAL POPULATIONS

CHILDREN AND ADOLESCENTS WITH TYPE 2 DM

Type 2 DM is increasing in adolescence.[10] Obesity and physical inactivity seem to be particular culprits in the pathogenesis of this disease. Given the many years that the patient will have to live with diabetes, and recent evidence that the timeline for complications may mimic that of older adults, extraordinary efforts should be expended on lifestyle modification measures in an attempt to normalize glucose levels. Failing that strategy, the only labeled oral agent for use in children (10 to 16 years) is metformin, though sulfonylureas are also commonly used in therapy. Thiazolidinediones have not been studied

in children, but studies to ascertain safety and efficacy are currently underway. In adolescent females, the possibility of future pregnancy should be considered in the prescription of any drug regimen.

ELDERLY PATIENTS WITH DM

Elderly patients with newly diagnosed DM (almost always type 2 DM) present a different therapeutic challenge. Consideration of the risks of hypoglycemia in this population and the probable life span should help determine if less-stringent glycemic goals should be set. Thinner, older patients may primarily be treated with shorter-acting insulin secretagogues, low-dose sulfonylureas (preferably not long-acting ones), or α-glucosidase inhibitors. Risk for lactic acidosis, which increases with older age and the age-related decline in renal function, makes metformin therapy more problematic. Thiazolidinediones may offer another alternative in patients in whom some weight gain is not unwelcome. Simple insulin regimens may be another easy approach to glycemic control in elderly patients with newly diagnosed DM.

GESTATIONAL DM

Gestational DM is diagnosed as previously described. Dietary therapy to minimize wide fluctuations in blood glucose is of paramount importance.[5] Intensive educational efforts are usually necessary. Pregnant women without DM maintain plasma glucose concentrations between 50 and 130 mg/dL. Frequent SMBG is needed to tell whether dietary interventions are successful. If fasting plasma glucose is >105 mg/dL, or 1-hour postprandial plasma glucose levels are >155 mg/dL, or if 2-hour postprandial plasma glucose levels are >130 mg/dL, insulin therapy is usually begun. One shot of NPH or a mixture of NPH and regular insulin in a 2:1 ratio given before breakfast may be adequate to reach glucose targets. Titration of insulin and switching to more complicated regimens is guided by SMBG results. In spite of the long-standing labeling of sulfonylureas as contraindicated in pregnancy, one randomized, open-label, controlled trial evaluated the efficacy of glyburide as compared to insulin initiated after 11 weeks' gestation.[108] Adequate control of blood glucose was achieved as compared to traditional insulin therapy, with less hypoglycemia in the glyburide group. No evidence of any difference in complications, specifically cord-serum insulin concentrations, incidence of macrosomia, cesarean delivery, or neonatal hypoglycemia between regimens were noted. Glyburide was not detected in the cord serum of any infant. As the study limited enrollment beyond 11 weeks' gestation, no conclusions regarding teratogenicity can be made from this study. The ADA cites this study in a position paper and mentions its utility, but also warns that it is not a labeled use of the drug and suggests further studies are needed to establish its safety.[12] Patients with gestational DM should be evaluated 6 weeks after delivery to ensure that normal glucose tolerance has returned. Because these patients' long-term risk for the development of DM is considerable, periodic assessment after that is warranted.

SPECIAL SITUATIONS

SICK DAYS

Acute self-limited illness rarely presents a major problem for patients with type 2 DM, but can be a significant challenge for insulinopenic type 1 DM patients.[109] While caloric intake generally declines, insulin

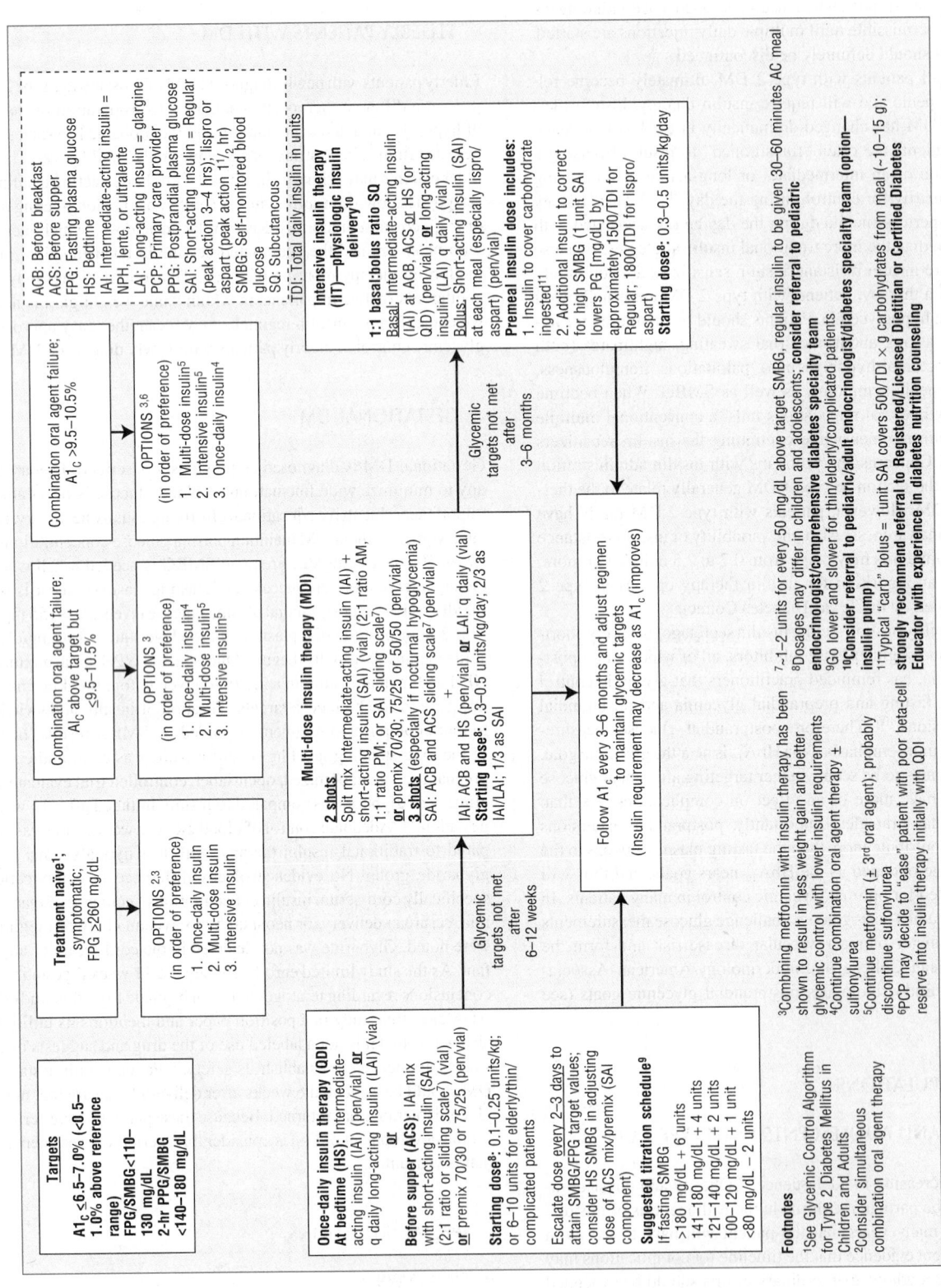

FIGURE 72–9. Insulin algorithm for type 2 DM in children and adults. See www.texasdiabetescouncil.org for current algorithms. (*Reprinted with permission from the Texas Diabetes Council.*)

sensitivity also decreases, meaning that it may take greater amounts of insulin to control blood glucose concentrations. Patients need to be adept at frequent SMBG, checking urine ketones, use of short-acting insulin, and understanding that sugar intake in this situation is not "bad" but may be necessary to "cover" the insulin therapy given to keep the patient out of diabetic ketoacidosis. We encourage patients to continue their usual insulin regimen and to use supplemental rapid-acting insulin based on SMBG results, with further additional insulin given if ketonuria develops. Sugar and electrolyte solutions, such as sports drinks, can be used to maintain hydration, to provide needed electrolytes if there are significant gastrointestinal or urinary losses, and to provide sugar to keep the patient from developing hypoglycemia because of the extra insulin that is usually needed. In contrast, type 2 patients may need to switch to sugar-free drinks if blood glucose levels are continually elevated. Most patients can be taught how to sufficiently manage sick days and avoid hospitalization.

DIABETIC KETOACIDOSIS AND HYPEROSMOLAR HYPERGLYCEMIC STATE

Diabetic ketoacidosis and hyperosmolar hyperglycemic state are true diabetic emergencies.[110,111] A comprehensive discussion of their treatment is beyond the scope of this book. In patients with known diabetes, diabetic ketoacidosis is usually precipitated by insulin omission in type 1 DM, and intercurrent illness, particularly infection, in both type 1 and type 2 DM. However, patients with type 1 or type 2 DM (the latter being usually non-whites or Hispanics) may present at initial presentation.[112] It is possible that some of the patients deemed to have type 2 DM actually have type 1 idiopathic DM. Patients with diabetic ketoacidosis may be alert, stuporous, or comatose at presentation. The hallmark diagnostic laboratory values include hyperglycemia, anion gap acidosis, and large ketonuria. Afflicted patients have fluid deficits of several liters and sodium and potassium deficits of several hundred milliequivalents. Restoration of intravascular volume acutely with normal saline, followed by hypotonic saline to replace free water, potassium supplements, and constant infusion insulin restore the patient's metabolic status relatively quickly. A flow sheet is often helpful in tracking the fluid and insulin therapies and laboratory parameters in these patients. Bicarbonate administration is generally not needed and may be harmful, especially in children.[113] Treatment of the inciting medical condition is also vital. Hourly bedside monitoring of glucose and frequent monitoring (every 2 to 4 hours) of potassium is essential. Metabolic improvement is manifested by an increase in the serum bicarbonate or pH. Serum phosphorus usually starts high and plummets to lower-than-normal levels, though replacing phosphorus, while not unreasonable, is of questionable benefit in most patients. Fluid administration alone will reduce the glucose concentration, so a decrement in glucose values does not necessarily mean that the patient's metabolic status is improving. Rare patients will require larger amounts of insulin than those usually given (5 to 10 units/h). We double the patient's insulin dose if the serum bicarbonate has not improved after the first 4 hours of insulin therapy. Constant infusion of a fixed dose of insulin and the administration of intravenous glucose when the blood glucose level decreases to <250 mg/dL is preferable to titration of the insulin infusion based on the glucose level. The latter strategy may delay clearance of the ketosis and prolong treatment. The insulin infusion should be continued until the urine ketones clear and the anion gap closes. Long-acting insulin should be given 1 to 2 hours prior to discontinuing the insulin infusion. Intramuscular regular insulin or subcutaneous insulin lispro or aspart given every 1 to 2 hours can be utilized rather than an insulin infusion in patients without hypoperfusion. Patients may develop hyperchloremic metabolic acidosis with treatment if they have been given large volumes of normal saline in the course of their treatment. Such a situation does not require any specific treatment.

Hyperosmolar hyperglycemic state usually occurs in older patients with type 2 DM, at times undiagnosed, or in younger patients with prolonged hyperglycemia and dehydration or significant renal insufficiency. A large ketonemia is usually not seen, as residual insulin secretion suppresses the production of ketones. Infection or another medical illness is the usual precipitant. Fluid deficits are usually greater and blood glucose concentrations higher (at times >1000 mg/dL) in these patients than in patients with diabetic ketoacidosis. Blood glucose levels should be lowered very gradually with hypotonic fluids and low-dose insulin infusions (1 to 2 units/h). Rapid correction of the glucose levels, a drop greater than 75 to 100 mg/dL per hour, is not recommended, as it can result in cerebral edema. This is especially true for children with diabetic ketoacidosis. Mortality is high with the hyperosmolar hyperglycemic state.

HOSPITALIZATION FOR INTERCURRENT MEDICAL ILLNESS

Patients on oral agents may need transient therapy with insulin to achieve adequate glycemic control. In patients requiring insulin, patients should receive scheduled doses of insulin with additional short-acting insulin. "Sliding-scale" insulin is to be discouraged, as it is notorious for not controlling glucose and for sometimes resulting in therapeutic misadventures, with wide swings in the blood glucose as the patient "bounces" from hypoglycemia to hyperglycemia.[114] In-hospital mortality is increased in many hyperglycemic conditions. Recent work documented a reduction in mortality in type 2 diabetes patients with acute myocardial infarctions[115] who receive constant intravenous insulin during the acute phase of the event to maintain near-normal glucose concentrations. In the case of cardiac ischemia, the beneficial effects may be a result of reducing free fatty acids or inflammation with insulin therapy. Similar mortality results have been documented in several intensive care unit settings using intravenous insulin and tight glucose control.[116,117] Recently, the American College of Endocrinology released a position statement on inpatient glycemic control which recommended preprandial levels <110 mg/dL, and postprandial levels <180 mg/dL.[118] It is prudent to stop metformin in all patients who arrive in acute care settings until full elucidation of the reason for presentation can be ascertained, as contraindications to metformin are prevalent in hospitalized patients.[119]

PERIOPERATIVE MANAGEMENT

Surgical patients may experience worsening of glycemia for reasons similar to those listed above for intercurrent medical illness.[120] Patients on oral agents may need transient therapy with insulin to control blood glucose. In patients requiring insulin, scheduled doses of insulin or continuous insulin infusions are preferred. For patients who can eat soon after surgery, the time-honored approach of giving one-half of the usual morning NPH insulin dose with dextrose 5% in water intravenously is acceptable, with resumption of scheduled insulin, perhaps at reduced doses, within the first day. For patients requiring more prolonged periods without oral nutrition and for major surgery, such as coronary artery bypass grafting and major abdominal surgery, constant infusion intravenous insulin is preferred. Metformin should be discontinued temporarily after any major surgery until it is clear that the patient is hemodynamically stable and normal renal function is documented.

REPRODUCTIVE-AGE WOMEN AND PRECONCEPTION CARE FOR WOMEN

An increasing prevalence of DM has been noted in reproductive-age women.[121,122] Prepregnancy planning is absolutely mandatory, as organogenesis is largely completed within 8 weeks, so good glycemic control should be obtained prior to conception. Unfortunately, major congenital malformations due to poor glucose control remain the leading cause of mortality and serious morbidity in infants of mothers with type 1 or type 2 diabetes. For women with diabetes mellitus controlled by lifestyle measures alone, conversion to insulin as soon as the pregnancy is confirmed is appropriate. For women with polycystic ovary disease who ovulate and become pregnant with insulin sensitizer therapy, conversion to insulin is mandatory as soon as pregnancy is confirmed. Insulin is the only acceptable pharmacologic therapy during pregnancy for women with diabetes mellitus in the United States. In Europe, metformin is sometimes used in pregnancy for type 2 DM, but its use is eschewed in the United States. Patients previously treated with insulin may need intensification of their regimen to achieve therapeutic goals. Normal pregnancy is associated with a decrease in the blood glucose concentration as fuel is diverted to the fetus. Pregnant patients will be ingesting both meals and snacks daily. SMBG is generally intensified to try to reach glycemic targets and reduce fetal and maternal morbidity. Whether preprandial or postprandial glucose concentrations should be the target of therapy is hotly debated. Ketosis should be avoided, requiring urine monitoring for ketones in the morning and if the blood sugar is >200 mg/dL.

There has been some concern about the safety of insulin analogs in pregnancy, both for fetal development and advancement of microvascular complications. One study has shown no increase in retinopathy or progression of same with the use of insulin lispro in pregnancy.[123]

SPECIAL TOPICS

PREVENTION OF DIABETES MELLITUS

Efforts to prevent type 1 DM with immunosuppressives[124] or injected[125] or oral insulin therapy[126] have been unsuccessful. The Diabetes Prevention Program[127] confirmed that modest weight loss in association with exercise can have a dramatic impact on insulin sensitivity and the conversion from impaired glucose tolerance to type 2 diabetes. In this study approximately 2,000 individuals with impaired glucose tolerance were randomized to lifestyle changes (diet, exercise, and weight loss) vs. usual care. The study, which was originally planned to be ongoing for 5 years, was stopped after 2.8 years because the results were so conclusive. The usual care group developed diabetes at the rate of 11% each year. The lifestyle arm developed diabetes at a rate of 5% per year, a 58% reduction in the risk of developing diabetes.[127] Surprisingly, a modest amount of diet and exercise yielded impressive results. The exercise program in the lifestyle group was walking 30 minutes 5 days each week. The mean weight loss over the 2.8 year study period was only 8 pounds. Similar results were seen in the Finnish Diabetes Study.[128] In the Diabetes Prevention Program[127] discussed above, approximately 1,000 of the study patients were randomized to metformin therapy. The metformin-treated patients showed a 4-pound weight loss on average, and a reduction in the risk of developing diabetes of 31% compared to placebo.[12] Interestingly, young and overweight individuals on metformin had a greater reduction in the risk of developing diabetes than normal weight and older study patients.[127]

The TRIPOD study[129] evaluated the ability of troglitazone to prevent the development of diabetes in women with a history of gestational diabetes. The rate of development of diabetes in the placebo arm of the study was approximately 12% per year, compared to about 5% in the treatment group. Total preservation of β-cell function was demonstrated over a 5-year period in women who had near normal β-cell function at baseline and who initially responded to the drug.[129] The preservation of β-cell function was observed 8 months after the drug had been discontinued. It should be noted that no pharmacologic agents are currently FDA approved or recommended for prevention of type 2 diabetes, though prevention studies are underway using rosiglitazone, pioglitazone, nateglinide, ramipril, and valsartan.[130]

CLINICAL CONTROVERSY

Diabetes mellitus is associated with a substantially higher risk of morbidity and mortality. Pharmacologic prevention or delay of type 2 DM has been widely discussed since the release of the Diabetes Prevention Program results. Though lifestyle changes were more effective, with a 58% lower relative risk of progression to diabetes, metformin 850 mg twice a day reduced the risk by 31%. Acarbose, troglitazone, and orlistat all have been able to prevent or delay the onset of type 2 DM. Despite these data, there are no FDA-approved or ADA-recommended medications for the delay or prevention of type 2 DM. Medications require monitoring, can have serious side effects, and have been documented to be less effective than lifestyle changes. Despite this, many clinicians are giving high-risk patients medication for the delay or prevention of diabetes, in combination with lifestyle changes.

PATIENT EDUCATION

It is not satisfactory to give patients with DM brief instruction with a few pamphlets and expect them to manage their disease adequately. Thinking that diabetes education is limited to one or two encounters is misguided; education is a lifetime exercise. Successful treatment of DM involves lifestyle changes for the patient (e.g., medical nutrition therapy, physical activity, self-monitoring of blood glucose and possibly of urine for ketones, and taking prescribed medications). The patient must be involved in the decision-making process and must learn as much about the disease and associated complications as possible. Emphasis should be placed on the evidence that indicates that complications can be prevented or minimized with glycemic control and management of risk factors for cardiovascular disease. Recognition of the need for proper patient education to empower them into self-care has generated programs for certification in diabetes education. Certified diabetes educators (CDEs) must document their patient education hours and sit for a certification examination that assesses the knowledge, tasks, and skills of an educator in order to become certified. An increasing number of nurses, pharmacists, dietitians, and

ysicians are becoming CDEs to document to the public that they
eet a minimum standard for diabetes education, and to fulfill quality
itiatives in meeting guidelines for education recognition.[131]

TREATMENT OF CONCOMITANT CONDITIONS AND COMPLICATIONS

RETINOPATHY

atients with established retinopathy should see an ophthalmologist
optometrist trained in diabetic eye disease.[132] A dilated eye exam
required to fully evaluate diabetic eye disease. Early background
tinopathy may reverse with improved glycemic control. More ad-
nced retinopathy will not regress with improved glycemia, and may
tually worsen with short-term improvements in glycemia. Studies
e underway to determine whether medical therapy independent of
ucose control will prevent the development of advanced retinopathy.
aser photocoagulation has markedly improved sight preservation in
abetic patients.

NEUROPATHY

eripheral neuropathy is the most common complication seen in type
DM patients in outpatient clinics.[133] Paresthesias, numbness, or
ain may be the predominant symptom. The feet are involved far
ore often than the hands. Improved glycemic control may alleviate
me of the symptoms. If neuropathy is painful, symptomatic therapy
empiric, including low-dose tricyclic antidepressants, anticonvul-
nts (gabapentin, carbamazepine, and maybe phenytoin), duloxetine,
nlafaxine, topical capsaicin, and various pain medications, includ-
g tramadol and nonsteroidal anti-inflammatory drugs. Recently, an-
her anticonvulsant, topiramate, has shown promise in the reduction
f symptoms, with the positive side effect of weight loss in type
diabetes patients. The numb variant of peripheral neuropathy is
t treated with medication. Clinical manifestations of diabetic auto-
mic neuropathy include resting tachycardia, exercise intolerance,
thostatic hypotension, constipation, gastroparesis, erectile dysfunc-
on, sudomotor dysfunction (anhidrosis, heat intolerance, gustatory
eating, and/or dry skin), impaired neurovascular function, and hy-
glycemic autonomic failure. Gastroparesis can be a severe and
ebilitating complication of DM. Improved glycemic control, discon-
nuation of medications that slow gastric motility, and the use of meto-
opramide (preferably for only a few days at a time) or erythromycin
ay be helpful. Gastric pacemakers as therapeutic hardware are rarely
sed, though available. Orthostatic hypotension may require pharma-
ologic management with mineralocorticoids or adrenergic agonist
gents. In severe cases, supine hypertension is extreme, mandating
at the patient sleep in a sitting or semirecumbent position. Patients
ith cardiac autonomic neuropathy are at a higher risk for silent my-
cardial infarction and mortality. The hallmark of diabetic diarrhea is
s nocturnal occurrence. Diabetic diarrhea frequently responds to a
)- to 14-day course of an antibiotic such as doxycycline or metron-
azole. In more unresponsive cases, octreotide may be useful. Erec-
le dysfunction is common in diabetes, and initial treatment should
clude a trial of one of the oral medications currently available to treat
ectile dysfunction. People with diabetes often require the highest
ses of these medications to have an adequate response. Sudomotor
sfunction, as earlier defined, results in loss of sweating and resultant
y, cracked skin. Use of hydrating creams and ointments is needed.

MICROALBUMINURIA AND NEPHROPATHY

Diabetes mellitus, and particularly type 2 DM, is the biggest contributor statistically to the development of end-stage renal disease in the
United States.[134] The American Diabetes Association recommends a
screening urinary analysis for albumin at diagnosis in persons with
type 2 DM. Precise onset of type 2 DM can rarely be ascertained,
and patients will often present at diagnosis with microvascular complications. In type 1 DM, microalbuminuria rarely occurs with short
duration of disease or before puberty. Screening individuals with type
1 DM should begin with puberty and after 5 years' disease duration.
There are three methods for assessing microalbuminuria: (1) measurement of the urine albumin:creatinine ratio in a random spot collection
(preferably the first morning void); (2) 24-hour timed collection; and
(3) timed (e.g., 4-hour or 10-hour overnight) collection. Microalbuminuria on a spot urine specimen is defined as a ratio of 30 to 300
mg/g albumin:creatinine. On timed collections, microalbuminuria is
defined as 30 to 300 mg/24 hours or an albumin excretion rate of 20
to 200 mcg/min. Because of day-to-day variability, microalbuminuria should be confirmed on at least two of three samples over 3 to
6 months. Additionally, when assessing urine protein or albumin,
conditions that may cause transient elevations in urinary albumin excretion should be excluded. These conditions include: intense exercise, recent urinary tract infections, hypertension, short-term hyperglycemia, heart failure, and acute febrile illness.[134]

In type 2 DM, the presence of microalbuminuria is a strong risk
factor for macrovascular disease and is frequently present at the time
of diagnosis. Microalbuminuria may be a weaker predictor for future
kidney disease in type 2 vs. type 1 DM.

Glucose and blood pressure control are most important for the
prevention of nephropathy, and blood pressure control is the most
important for retarding the progression of established nephropathy.
Angiotensin-converting enzyme (ACE) inhibitors and angiotensin receptor blockers, considered first-line recommended treatment modalities, have shown efficacy in preventing the clinical progression of
renal disease in patients with type 2 diabetes mellitus.[135–137] Diuretics frequently are necessary due to the volume-expanded state of the
patient and are recommended second-line therapy. The American Diabetes Association and the National Kidney Foundation blood pressure
goal of <130/80 mm Hg can be difficult to achieve. Three or more
antihypertensives are often needed to treat to goal blood pressures.

PERIPHERAL VASCULAR DISEASE AND FOOT ULCERS

Claudication and nonhealing foot ulcers are common in type 2 DM
patients.[138] Smoking cessation, correction of lipid abnormalities, and
antiplatelet therapy are important strategies in treating claudicants.
Pentoxifylline or cilostazol may be useful in selected patients. Revascularization is successful in selected patients. Local débridement and
appropriate footwear and foot care are vitally important in the early
treatment of foot lesions. In more advanced lesions, topical treatments
may be of benefit. Diabetic foot care is an excellent example of the
adage, "an ounce of prevention is worth a pound of cure."

CORONARY HEART DISEASE

The risk for coronary heart disease (CHD) is two to four times
greater in diabetic patients than in nondiabetic individuals. CHD

TABLE 72–14. Classification of Lipid and Lipoprotein Levels in Adults

Parameter	Goal		Treatment (In Order of Preference)
LDL cholesterol	<100 mg/dL		Lifestyle; HMG-CoA reductase inhibitors; cholesterol absorption inhibitor; niacin or fenofibrate
HDL cholesterol	Men >40 mg/dL	Women >50 mg/dL	Lifestyle; nicotinic acid; fibric acid derivatives
Triglycerides	<150 mg/dL		Lifestyle; glycemic control; fibric acid derivatives; high-dose statins (in those with high LDL)

HDL, high-density lipoprotein; HMG-CoA, 3-hydroxy-3-methylglutaryl coenzyme A; LDL, low-density lipoprotein.

is the major source of mortality in patients with DM. Recent studies suggest that multiple risk-factor intervention (lipids, hypertension, smoking cessation,[139] and antiplatelet therapy)[140] will reduce the burden of excess macrovascular events. Epidemiologic data suggest that CHD prevention guidelines for type 2 DM apply equally to patients with type 1 DM.[141] β-Blocker therapy supplies an even greater protection from recurrent CHD events in diabetic patients than in nondiabetic subjects. Masking of hypoglycemic symptoms is a greater problem in type 1 DM patients than in patients with type 2 DM.

Lipids

The Scandinavian Simvastatin Survival Study showed 42% reduction in CHD events in diabetic patients with known CHD and very high LDL-C levels with simvastatin therapy (mean dose, 27 mg/day with LDL-C reduction of approximately 35%).[142] Lesser degrees of risk reduction have been shown in other secondary prevention studies in patients treated with pravastatin with mild-to-moderate LDL-C elevation at baseline.[143] The Heart Protection Study randomized 5,963 patients age >40 years with diabetes and total cholesterol >135 mg/dL. A significant 22% reduction (95% confidence interval [CI] 13 to 30) in the event rate for major cardiovascular events was seen with simvastatin 40 mg per day. This was evident even at lower LDL levels (<116 mg/dL), and suggests that ~30% reduction in LDL levels regardless of starting LDL levels may be appropriate.[144] The diabetic subgroup in the Veterans Administration HDL Intervention Trial of CHD patients with low HDL-C and low LDL-C showed approximately 22% reduction in CHD events in diabetic patients with known CHD when HDL-C was increased by approximately 6% by gemfibrozil.[145]

The new National Cholesterol Education Program Adult Treatment Panel III (NCEP-ATP)[47] guidelines classify the presence of DM as a CHD risk equivalent, and therefore recommend that LDL-C be lowered to <100 mg/dL. Unlike previous guidelines, more consideration is now given to HDL-C and triglycerides. The primary target is the treatment of LDL-C. After the LDL-C goal is reached (usually with a statin), triglycerides are considered for pharmacologic management, assuming unresponsiveness to glycemic control efforts, weight management, and exercise. In such situations, a non-HDL-C goal is established (a surrogate for all apolipoprotein B–containing particles). The non-HDL-C goal for patients with DM is <130 mg/dL. Niacin or a fibrate can be added to reach that goal if triglycerides are 201 to 499 mg/dL. Niacin or a fibrate can also be added if the LDL-C goal is reached, but the patient has low HDL-C (<40 mg/dL). Patients with marked hypertriglyceridemia (≥500 mg/dL) are at risk for pancreatitis. Efforts to reduce triglycerides with glycemic control, elimination

of other secondary causes (including medications), and drug therapy (fibrate and/or niacin) are effective treatment strategies. The American Diabetes Association also recommends similar LDL goals, but places raising HDL as the second priority (Table 72–14).

HYPERTENSION

The role of hypertension in increasing microvascular and macrovascular risk in patients with DM has been confirmed in the UKPDS[86] and Hypertension Optimization Treatment[146] trials. The American Diabetes Association recommends aggressive goals for blood pressure (<130/80 mm Hg) in patients with DM.[51] ACE inhibitors and angiotensin receptor blockers are generally recommended for initial therapy. The National Kidney Foundation also suggests that the blood pressure goal be less than 130/80 mm Hg, as well as recommending diuretics as second-line therapy in patients with diabetic kidney disease.[147] Many patients require multiple agents, on average three agents, to obtain goals, so diuretics, calcium channel blockers, and β-blockers frequently are useful as second and third agents. Blood pressure goals are generally more difficult to achieve than glycemic goals or lipid goals in most diabetic patients.[148]

CLINICAL CONTROVERSY

Initial therapy choices for hypertension in diabetes mellitus usually include angiotensin-converting enzyme inhibitors or an angiotensin receptor blocker due to their well documented renoprotective effects. Currently, angiotensin receptor blockers have less robust data to support cardiovascular reduction compared to other therapeutic choices, yet the data that exists appears to be positive in patients with type 2 DM. Also, diuretics have shown superior results to an ACE inhibitor in the ALLHAT trial. The ADA currently recommends the use of any class (ACE inhibitors, angiotensin receptor blockers, β-blockers, diuretics, or calcium channel blockers) of antihypertensive medication that has shown benefit in prevention of poor cardiovascular outcomes. Choice of monotherapy may not be important, as an average of two to three antihypertensive medications are needed to reach blood pressure goals.

TRANSPLANTATION

Whole pancreas and islet cell transplantation are still relatively experimental procedures in patients with type 1 DM; those with end-stage renal disease also receive kidney transplantation.[149]

PHARMACOECONOMIC CONSIDERATIONS

As described in the introduction, the direct and indirect costs of DM are substantial. Much of the indirect costs are related to loss of productivity due to the significant morbidity (hospitalizations, loss of vision, lower extremity amputations, kidney failure, and cardiovascular events) associated with the disease. For a disease that affects only 5% to 6% of the population, it is responsible for 11% to 12% of health expenditures. With evidence from the DCCT and UKPDS to support intensive blood glucose control to reduce the risk of complications, the question of cost effectiveness comes into play.

An economic model based on the DCCT approximates that 120,000 persons in the U.S. would meet criteria for intensive intervention. The cost of implementing intensive therapy over the lifetime of the population is estimated at $4 billion dollars. The benefits of this strategy are net gains of 920,000 years of sight, 691,000 years free from end-stage renal disease, and 678,000 years free from lower extremity amputations. The incremental cost per year of life gained is $28,661. This is well within the limits of a cost-effective strategy and compares favorably to treatment of high blood pressure or hypercholesterolemia.

Economic analysis of intensive therapy for type 2 DM is more complex. Outcomes must also factor in the burden of cardiovascular disease as the major cause of mortality. One model analyzed the health benefits and economics of treating type 2 DM with the goal of achieving normoglycemia, but using outcomes based on the DCCT trial results. Accounting for the prevalence of cardiovascular disease in type 2 DM, an estimate of $16,002 incremental cost per quality-adjusted life year gained was obtained. The limitation of this analysis is that while the UKDPS did demonstrate an improvement in diabetes-related outcomes, the overall efficacy on microvascular disease complications was not mirrored by the DCCT.

Two economic analyses were performed on data generated from the UKPDS, one assessing cost effectiveness of an intensive blood glucose control policy in type 2 DM, and the other assessing improved blood pressure control in hypertensive patients with type 2 DM. In the first analysis, outcome was measured as the incremental cost per event-free year gained within the trial. Based on trial outcomes and assumptions, the incremental cost in the intensive treatment group per event-free year gained is $1,366. While intensive treatment costs were higher, the cost per event-free year gained appears cost-effective. The second analysis showed the incremental cost per extra year free from microvascular and macrovascular end points from intensive blood pressure control in a standard clinical practice model to be $1498. The incremental cost per life year gained was estimated at $619, again demonstrating the cost-effectiveness of intensive intervention.[151,152]

EVALUATION OF THERAPEUTIC OUTCOMES

MONITORING OF THE PHARMACEUTICAL CARE PLAN

A comprehensive pharmaceutical care plan for the patient with DM will integrate considerations of goals to optimize blood glucose control and protocols to screen for, prevent, or manage microvascular and macrovascular complications. In terms of standards of care for persons with DM, one can review the document published by the American Diabetes Association that outlines initial and ongoing assessments for patients with DM.[51] For quality-of-care measures, one can refer to the National Diabetes Quality Improvement Alliance web site at

www.nationaldiabetesalliance.org, whose members include many of the governmental and physician organizations concerned with diabetes quality-of-care measures.

The major performance measures should assess the ability to meet current standards of care and recognize the minimal treatment goals for glycemia, lipids, and hypertension, and provide targets for monitoring and adjusting pharmacotherapy as discussed in various sections above. Unfortunately, current publicly-reported quality measures often fall short of current guidelines. Glycemic control (percentage of patients with <9%) lipid (percentage of patients with LDL <130 mg/dL), and hypertension (percentage of patients with blood pressure <140/90 mm Hg) quality measures are not congruent with the current goals recommended by the American Diabetes Association or American College of Endocrinology/American Association of Clinical Endocrinologists. Glycemic control is paramount in managing type 1 or type 2 DM, but as readily identified from the above discussion, it requires frequent assessment and adjustment in diet, exercise, and pharmacologic therapies. Minimally, HbA$_{1c}$ should be measured twice a year in patients meeting treatment goals on a stable therapeutic regimen. Quarterly assessments are recommended for those whose therapy has changed or who are not meeting glycemic goals. Fasting lipid profiles should be obtained as part of an initial assessment and thereafter at each follow-up visit if not at goal, annually if stable and at goal, or every 2 years if the lipid profile suggests low risk. Documenting regular frequency of foot exams (each visit), urine albumin assessment (annually), dilated ophthalmologic exams (yearly or more frequently with identified abnormalities), and office visits for follow-up are also important. Assessment for pneumococcal vaccine administration, annual administration of influenza vaccine, and routine assessment for and management of other cardiovascular risks (i.e., smoking and antiplatelet therapy) are components of preventive medicine strategies. The multiplicity of assessments for each patient visit are likely to be better facilitated utilizing an integrative computer program, standardized progress note forms, or flow sheets, which assist the clinician in identifying whether the patient has met standards of care in the frequency of monitoring and achievement of defined targets of therapy.

ABBREVIATIONS

ACE: angiotensin-converting enzyme
ADA: American Diabetes Association
ALT: alanine aminotransferase
BMI: body mass index
CDE: certified diabetes educator
CHD: coronary heart disease
CSII: continuous subcutaneous insulin infusion
CYP450: cytochrome P450
DCCT: Diabetes Control and Complications Trial
DM: diabetes mellitus
FFA: free fatty acid
GCT: glucose challenge test
GDM: gestational diabetes mellitus
HbA$_{1c}$: hemoglobin A$_{1c}$
HDL-C: high-density lipoprotein cholesterol
IFG: impaired fasting glucose
IGT: impaired glucose tolerance
IRS: insulin resistance syndrome
LADA: latent autoimmune diabetes in adults
LDL-C: low-density lipoprotein cholesterol

MODY: maturity onset diabetes of youth

NCEP-ATP: National Cholesterol Education Program Adult Treatment Panel

NHANES III: The Third National Health and Nutrition Evaluation Survey

NPH: neutral protamine Hagedorn

OGTT: oral glucose tolerance test

PAI-1: activator-1 plasminogen-inhibitor

PPAR-γ: peroxisome proliferator activator receptor-γ

SUR: sulfonylurea receptor

SMBG: self-monitoring of blood glucose

TZD: thiazolidinedione

UKPDS: United Kingdom Prospective Diabetes Study

VAT: visceral adipose tissue

Review Questions and other resources can be found at *www.pharmacotherapyonline.com*.

REFERENCES

1. American Diabetes Association. Diabetes facts and figures. Available at: http://diabetes.org/diabetes-statistics.jsp. Accessed January 27, 2004.
2. Atkinson MA, Eisenbarth GS. Type 1 diabetes: New perspectives on disease pathogenesis and treatment. Lancet 2001;358:221–229.
3. Raffel LJ, Scheuner MT, Rotter JI. Genetics of diabetes. In: Porte D Jr, Sherwin RS, eds. Ellenberg & Rifkin's Diabetes Mellitus, 5th ed. Stamford, CT, Appleton & Lange, 1997:401–454.
4. Bennett P, Rewers M, Knowler W. Epidemiology of diabetes mellitus. In: Porte D Jr, Sherwin RS, eds. Ellenberg & Rifkin's Diabetes Mellitus, 5th ed. Stamford, CT, Appleton & Lange, 1997:373–400.
5. American Diabetes Association. Diagnosis and classification of diabetes mellitus. Diabetes Care 2004;27(Suppl 1):S5–S10.
6. Gale EA. The rise of childhood type 1 diabetes in the 20th century. Diabetes 2002;51:3353–3361.
7. Froguel P, Zouali H, Vionnet N, et al. Familial hyperglycemia due to mutations in glucokinase. Definition of a subtype of diabetes mellitus. N Engl J Med 1993;328:697–702.
8. American Diabetes Association. Standards for medical care: Screening for diabetes. Diabetes Care 2004;27(Suppl 1):S15–S17.
9. American Diabetes Association. Type 2 diabetes in children and adolescents. Diabetes Care 2000;23:381–389.
10. Kahn SE, Porte D Jr. The pathophysiology of type II (non-insulin dependent) diabetes mellitus: Implications for treatment. In: Porte D Jr, Sherwin RS, eds. Ellenberg & Rifkin's Diabetes Mellitus, 5th ed. Stamford, CT, Appleton & Lange, 1997:487–512.
11. Gale EA. Is there really an epidemic of type 2 diabetes? Lancet 2003; 362:503–504.
12. American Diabetes Association. Gestational diabetes mellitus. Diabetes Care 2004;27(Suppl)1:S88–S90.
13. Report of the expert committee on the diagnosis and classification of diabetes mellitus. Diabetes Care 1997;20:1183–1197.
14. van Tilburg J, van Haeften TW, Pearson P, Wijimenga C. Defining the genetic contribution of type 2 diabetes mellitus. J Med Genet 2001;38: 569–578.
15. American Diabetes Association. Prevention of type 1 diabetes mellitus. Diabetes Care 2004;27(suppl 1):S133.
16. American Diabetes Association. Screening for type 2 diabetes. Diabetes Care 2004;27(Suppl 1):S11–S14.
17. Engelgau MM, Thompson TJ, Herman WH, et al. Comparison of fasting and 2-hour glucose and HbA$_{1c}$ levels for diagnosing diabetes: Diagnostic criteria and performance revisited. Diabetes Care 1997;20:785–791.
18. McCance DR, Hanson RL, Charles MA, et al. Comparison of tests for glycated haemoglobin and fasting and two hour plasma glucose concentrations as diagnostic methods for diabetes. BMJ 1994;308:1323–1328.
19. Janeway CA Jr. Immunology relevant to diabetes. In: Porte D Jr, Sherwin RS, eds. Ellenberg & Rifkin's Diabetes Mellitus, 5th ed. Stamford, CT Appleton & Lange, 1997:287–300.
20. DeFronzo RA. Pathogenesis of type 2 diabetes mellitus: Metabolic an molecular implications for identifying diabetes genes. Diabetes 1997 5:117–269.
21. Gerich JE, Meyer C, Woerle HJ, Stumvoll M. Renal gluconeogenesis Its importance in human glucose homeostasis. Diabetes Care 2001;24 382–391.
22. Ekberg K, Landau BR, Wajngot A, et al. Contributions by kidney an liver to glucose production in the postabsorptive state and after 60 h c fasting. Diabetes 1999;48:292–298.
23. Mandarino L, Bonadonna R, McGuinness O, Wasserman D. Regulatio of muscle glucose uptake in vivo. In: Jefferson LS, Cherrington AL eds. Handbook of Physiology, Section 7, The Endocrine System, Vol. I The Endocrine Pancreas and Regulation of Metabolism. Oxford, Oxfor University Press, 2001:803–848.
24. Santomauro A, Boden G, Silva M, et al. Overnight lowering of free fatt acids with acipimox improves insulin resistance and glucose tolerance i obese diabetic and non-diabetic subjects. Diabetes 1999;48:1836–184
25. Bergman RN. Non-esterified fatty acids and the liver: Why is insuli secreted into the portal vein? Diabetologia 2000;43:946–952.
26. Boden G. Role of fatty acids in the pathogenesis of insulin resistanc and NIDDM. Diabetes 1997;46:3–10.
27. McGarry JD. Banting lecture 2001: Dysregulation of fatty aci metabolism in the etiology of type 2 diabetes. Diabetes 2002;51:7–18.
28. DeFronzo RA, Ferrannini E, Simonson DC. Fasting hyperglycemia i non-insulin-dependent diabetes mellitus: Contributions of excessive hep atic glucose production and impaired tissue glucose uptake. Metabolisr 1989;38:387–395.
29. Kelley De, Mandarino LJ. Fuel selection in human skeletal muscle i insulin resistance. A reexamination. Diabetes 2000;49:677–683.
30. Kashyap S, Belfort R, Pratipanawatr T, et al. Chronic elevation in plasm free fatty acids impairs insulin secretion in non-diabetic offspring wit a strong family history of T2DM. Diabetes 2002;51(Suppl 2):A12.
31. Carpentier A, Mittelman SD, Bergman RN, et al. Prolonged elevatio of plasma free fatty acids impairs pancreatic beta-cell function in obes nondiabetic humans but not in individuals with type 2 diabetes. Diabete 2000;49:399–408.
32. Goodpaster BH, Thaete FL, Kelley BE. Thigh adipose tissue distributio is associated with insulin resistance in obesity and in type 2 diabete mellitus. Am J Clin Nutr 2000;71:885–892.
33. Greco AV, Mingrone G, Giancaterini A, et al. Insulin resistance i morbid obesity. Reversal with intramyocellular fat depletion. Diabete 2002;51:144–151.
34. Ryysy L, Hakkinen AM, Goto T, et al. Hepatic fat content and insuli action on free fatty acids and glucose metabolism rather than insulin ab sorption are associated with insulin requirements during insulin therap in type 2 diabetic patients. Diabetes 2000;49:749–758.
35. Miyazaki Y, Mahankali A, Matsuda M, et al. Effect of pioglitazone on ab dominal fat distribution and insulin sensitivity in type 2 diabetic patients J Clin Endocrinol Metab 2002;87:2784–2791.
36. DeFronzo RA. Pathogenesis of type 2 diabetes: Metabolic and molec ular implications for identifying diabetes genes. Diabetes Rev 1997;4 177–269.
37. Ferrannini E, Natali A, Bell P, et al. On behalf of the European Grou for the Study of Insulin Resistance (EGIR). Insulin resistance and hy persecretion in obesity. J Clin Invest 1997;100:1166–1173.
38. Montague CT, O'Rahilly S. The perils of portliness: Causes and conse quences of visceral adiposity. Diabetes 2000;49:883–888.
39. Kelley DE, Williams KV, Price JC, et al. Plasma fatty acids, adiposity an variance of skeletal muscle insulin resistance in type 2 diabetes mellitus J Clin Endocrinol Metab 2001;86:5412–5419.
40. Banerji MA, Lebowitz J, Chaiken RL. Relationship of visceral adipos tissue and glucose disposal is independent of sex in black NIDDM sub jects. Am J Physiol 1997;273:E425–E432.
41. Kelley DE. The impact of obesity, regional adiposity and ectopic fat o the pathophysiology of type 2 diabetes. Council on Obesity Diabete Education 2003;12–20.

42. Weyer C, Funahashi T, Tanaka S, et al. Hypoadiponectinemia in obesity and type 2 diabetes: close association with insulin resistance and hyperinsulinemia. J Clin Endocrinol Metab 2000;86:1930–1935.

43. Arita Y, Kihara S, Ouchi N, et al. Paradoxical decrease of an adipose-specific protein, adiponectin, in obesity. Biochem Biophys Res Commun 1999;257:79–83.

44. Berg AH, Combs TP, Du X, et al. The adipocyte-secreted protein Acrp30 enhances hepatic insulin action. Nat Med 2001;7:947–953.

45. Yamauchi T, Kamon J, Waki H, et al. The fat-derived hormone adiponectin reverses insulin resistance associated with both lipoatrophy and obesity. Nat Med 2001;7:941–946.

46. Reaven GM. Role of insulin resistance in human disease. Diabetes 1988; 37:1595–1607.

47. Expert Panel on Detection, Evaluation, and Treatment of High Blood Cholesterol in Adults. Executive Summary of the Third Report of the National Cholesterol Education Program (NCEP) Expert Panel on Detection, Evaluation, and Treatment of High Blood Cholesterol in Adults (Adult Treatment Panel III). JAMA 2001;285:2486–2496.

48. Park Y-W, Zhu S, Palaniappan L, et al. The metabolic syndrome: prevalence and associated risk factor findings in the US population from the Third National Health and Nutrition Examination Survey, 1988–1994. Arch Intern Med 2003;163:427–436.

49. Ford ES, Giles WH, Dietz WH. Prevalence of the metabolic syndrome among US adults: findings from the third National Health and Nutrition Examination Survey. JAMA 2002;287:356359.

50. Gaede P, Vedel P, Larsen N, et al. Multifactorial intervention and cardiovascular disease in patients with type 2 diabetes. N Engl J Med 2003; 348:383–393.

51. American Diabetes Association. Standards of medical care for patients with diabetes mellitus. Diabetes Care 2004;27(Suppl 1):S15–S35.

52. Diabetes Control and Complications Trial Research Group. The effect of intensive treatment of diabetes on the development and progression of long-term complications in insulin-dependent diabetes mellitus. N Engl J Med 1993;329:977–986.

53. UK Prospective Diabetes Study Group. Intensive blood-glucose control with sulphonylureas or insulin compared with conventional treatment and risk of complications in patients with type 2 diabetes (UKPDS 33). Lancet 1998;352:837–853.

54. American Diabetes Association. Self-monitoring of blood glucose. Diabetes Care 1994;17:81–86.

55. Kennedy L. Self-monitoring of blood glucose in type 2 diabetes: Time for evidence of efficacy. Diabetes Care 2001;24:977–978.

56. American Diabetes Association. Nutrition principles and recommendations in diabetes. Diabetes Care 2004;27(Suppl 1):S36–S46.

57. American Diabetes Association. Diabetes mellitus and exercise. Diabetes Care 2004;27(Suppl 1):S58–S62.

58. Alberti KGMM, Zimmet P, DeFronzo RA, Keen H, eds. International Textbook of Diabetes Mellitus, 2nd ed., Vol. 1. New York, John Wiley & Sons, 1997:469–610.

59. Skyler JS, Cefalu WT, Kourides IA, et al. Efficacy of inhaled human insulin in type 1 diabetes mellitus: a randomised proof-of-concept study. Lancet 2001;357:331–335.

60. Dewitt DE, Dugdale DC. Using new insulin strategies in the outpatient treatment of diabetes: clinical applications. JAMA 2003;289:2265–2269.

61. DeWitt DE, Hirsch IB. Outpatient insulin therapy in type 1 and type 2 diabetes mellitus: scientific review. JAMA 2003;289:2254–2264.

62. Gerich JE. Novel insulins: Expanding options in diabetes management. Am J Med 2002;113:308–316.

63. Lepore M, Pampanelli S, Fanelli C, et al. Pharmacokinetics and pharmacodynamics of subcutaneous injection of long-acting human insulin analog glargine, NPH insulin, and ultralente human insulin and continuous subcutaneous infusion of insulin lispro. Diabetes 2000;49:2142–2148.

64. Malmberg K, for the DIGAMI Study Group. Prospective randomised study of intensive insulin treatment on long term survival after acute myocardial infarction in patients with diabetes mellitus. BMJ 1997;314: 1512–1515.

65. Schor S. The University Group Diabetes Program. A statistician looks at the mortality results. JAMA 1971;217:1673–1675.

66. Kilo C, Miller L, Williamson J. The crux of the UGDP. Spurious results and biologically inappropriate data analysis. Diabetologia 1980;18: 179–185.

67. Brady PA, Jovanovic A. The sulfonylurea controversy: Much ado about nothing or cause for concern? J Am Coll Cardiol 2003;42:1022–1025.

68. Klamann A, Sarfert P, Lanhardt V, et al. Myocardial infarction in diabetic vs. non-diabetic subjects: survival and infarct size following therapy with sulfonylureas (glibenclamide). Eur Heart J 2000;21:220–229.

69. Riddle MC. Sulfonylureas differ in effects on ischemic preconditioning—is it time to retire glyburide? J Clin Endocrinol Metab 2003;88:528–530.

70. Gerich JE. Oral hypoglycemic agents. N Engl J Med 1989;321: 1231–1245.

71. White JR, Campbell RK. Dangerous and common drug interactions in patients with diabetes mellitus. Endocrinol Metab Clin North Am 2000; 29:789–802.

72. Wolffenbuttel BH, Landgraf R, for the Dutch and German repaglinide study group. A 1-year multicenter randomized double-blind comparison of repaglinide and glyburide for the treatment of type 2 diabetes. Diabetes Care 1999;22:463–467.

73. Horton ES, Clinkingbeard C, Gatlin M, et al. Nateglinide alone and in combination with metformin improves glycemic control by reducing mealtime glucose levels in type 2 diabetes. Diabetes Care 2000;23: 1660–1665.

74. UK Prospective Diabetes Study (UKPDS) Group. Effect of intensive blood-glucose control with metformin on complications in overweight patients with type 2 diabetes (UKPDS 34). Lancet 1998;352:854–865.

75. Dawson D, Conlon C. Case study: Metformin associated lactic acidosis: could orlistat be relevant? Diabetes Care 2003;26:2471–2472.

76. Lebovitz HE, Kreider M, Freed MI. Evaluation of liver function in type 2 diabetic patients during clinical trials: evidence that rosiglitazone does not cause hepatic dysfunction. Diabetes Care 2002;25:815–821.

77. Baba S. Pioglitazone: A review of Japanese clinical studies. Curr Med Res Opin 2001;17;166–189.

78. Nesto RW, Bell D, Bonow RO, et al. Thiazolidinedione use, fluid retention, and congestive heart failure. A consensus statement from the American Heart Association and the American Diabetes Association. Diabetes Care 2004;27:256–263.

79. Mooradian AD, Thurman JE. Drug therapy of postprandial hyperglycemia. Drugs 1999;57:19–29.

80. Campbell LK, Baker DE, Campbell RK. Miglitol: Assessment of its role in the treatment of patients with diabetes mellitus. Ann Pharmacother 2000;34:1291–1301.

81. Chiasson JL, Josse RG, Gomis R, et al. Acarbose for prevention of type 2 diabetes mellitus: The STOP-NIDDM randomized trial. Lancet 2002; 359:2072–2077.

82. Chiasson JL, Josse RG, Gomis R, et al. Acarbose treatment and the risk of cardiovascular disease and hypertension in patients with impaired glucose tolerance: the STOP-NIDDM trial. JAMA 2003;290:486–494.

83. Lettieri JT, Dain B. Effects of beano on the tolerability and pharmacodynamics of acarbose. Clin Ther 1998;20:497–504.

84. EDIC writing group. Sustained effect of intensive treatment of type 1 diabetes mellitus on development and progression of diabetic nephropathy: The Epidemiology of Diabetes Interventions and Complications of Study. JAMA 2003;290:2159–2167.

85. Stratton IM, Adler AI, Neil HA. Association of glycaemia with macrovascular and microvascular complications of type 2 diabetes (UKPDS 35): Prospective observational study. BMJ 2000;321:405–412.

86. Adler AI, Stratton IM, Neil HA: Association of systolic blood pressure with macrovascular and microvascular complications of type 2 diabetes (UKPDS 36): Prospective observational study. BMJ 2000;321: 412–419.

87. UK Prospective Diabetes Study Group. Efficacy of atenolol and captopril in reducing risk of macrovascular and microvascular complications in type 2 diabetes: UKPDS 39. BMJ 1998;317:713–720.

88. Strowig S, Raskin P. Intensive management of insulin-dependent diabetes mellitus. In: Porte D Jr, Sherwin RS, eds. Ellenberg & Rifkin's Diabetes Mellitus, 5th ed. Stamford, CT, Appleton & Lange, 1997:709–733.

89. Fanelli CG, Pampanelli S, Porcellati F, et al. Administration of neutral protamine Hagedorn insulin at bedtime versus with dinner in type 1 diabetes mellitus to avoid nocturnal hypoglycemia and improve control. A randomized, controlled trial. Ann Intern Med 2002;136:504–514.

90. DeVries JH, Snoek FJ, Kostense PJ, et al, on behalf of the Dutch Insulin Pump Study Group. A randomized trial of continuous subcutaneous insulin infusion and intensive injection therapy in type 1 diabetes for patients with long-standing poor glycemic control. Diabetes Care 2002;25:2074–2080.

91. Pickup J, Mattock M, Kerry S. Glycaemic control with continuous subcutaneous insulin infusion compared with intensive insulin injections in patients with type 1 diabetes: Meta-analysis of randomised controlled trials. BMJ 2002;324:705.

92. Lenhard MJ, Reeves GD. Continuous subcutaneous insulin infusion: A comprehensive review of insulin pump therapy. Arch Intern Med 2001; 161:2293–2300.

93. Schade DS, Valentine V. To pump or not to pump. Diabetes Care 2002; 25:2100–2102.

94. Cryer PE. Hypoglycemia is the limiting factor in the management of diabetes. Diabetes Metab Res Rev 1999;15:42–46.

95. de Galan BE, Tack CJ, Lenders JW, et al. Theophylline improves hypoglycemia unawareness in type 1 diabetes. Diabetes 2002;51:790–796.

96. Rosenbloom AL, Schatz DA, Krischer JP, et al. Therapeutic controversy: Prevention and treatment of diabetes in children. J Clin Endocrinol Metab 2000;85:494–522.

97. Binder C, Brange J. Insulin chemistry and pharmacokinetics. In: Porte D Jr, Sherwin RS, eds. Ellenberg & Rifkin's Diabetes Mellitus, 5th ed. Stamford, CT, Appleton & Lange, 1997:689–708.

98. Kelly DB, ed. Management of Type 1 Diabetes Mellitus, 3rd ed. Alexandria, VA, American Diabetes Association, 1998:211–222.

99. Halvorsen T, Levine F. Diabetes mellitus-cell transplantation and gene therapy approaches. Curr Mol Med 2001;1:273–286.

100. Shapiro AM, Lakey JR, Ryan EA, et al. Islet transplantation in seven patients with type 1 diabetes mellitus using a glucocorticoid-free immunosuppressive regimen. N Engl J Med 2000;343:230–238.

101. DeFronzo RA. Pharmacologic therapy for type 2 diabetes mellitus. Ann Intern Med 1999;131:281–303.

102. Higa M, Zhou YT, Ravazzola M, et al. Troglitazone prevents mitochondrial alterations, beta cell destruction, and diabetes in obese prediabetic rats. Proc Natl Acad Sci USA 1999;96:11513–11518.

103. Yale JF, Valiquett TR, Ghazzi MN, et al. The effect of a thiazolidinedione drug, troglitazone, on glycemia in patients with type 2 diabetes mellitus poorly controlled with sulfonylurea and metformin. A multicenter, randomized, double-blind, placebo-controlled trial. Ann Intern Med 2001;134:737–745.

104. Shank ML, Del Prato S, DeFronzo RA. Bedtime insulin/daytime glipizide. Effective therapy for sulfonylurea failures in NIDDM. Diabetes 1995;44:165–172.

105. Yki-Jarvinen H, Ryysy L, Nikkila K. Comparison of bedtime insulin regimens in patients with type 2 diabetes mellitus. A randomized, controlled trial. Ann Intern Med 1999;130:389–396.

106. Bastyr EJ 3rd, Stuart CA, Brodows RG. Therapy focused on lowering postprandial glucose, not fasting glucose, may be superior for lowering HbA1C. IOEZ Study Group. Diabetes Care 2000;23:1236–1241.

107. European Diabetes Epidemiology Group. Glucose tolerance and mortality. Comparison of WHO and American Diabetes Association diagnostic criteria. The DECODE study group. Diabetes Epidemiology: Collaborative analysis of diagnostic criteria in Europe. Lancet 1999;354:617–621.

108. Langer O, Conway DL, Berkus MD, et al. A comparison of glyburide and insulin in women with gestational diabetes mellitus. N Engl J Med 2000;343:1134–1138.

109. Laffel L. Sick-day management in type 1 diabetes. Endocrinol Metab Clin North Am 2000;29:707–723.

110. American Diabetes Association. Hyperglycemic crises in patients with diabetes mellitus. Diabetes Care 2001;24(Suppl 1):S83–S90.

111. Kitabchi AE, Umpierrez GE, Murphy MB, et al. Management of hyperglycemic crises in patients with diabetes. Diabetes Care 2001;24: 131–153.

112. Balasubramanyam A, Zern JW, Hyman DJ, Pavlik V. New profiles of diabetic ketoacidosis: Type 1 vs type 2 diabetes and the effect of ethnicity. Arch Intern Med 1999;159:2317–2322.

113. Glaser N, Barnett P, McCaslin I, et al. Pediatric Emergency Medicine Collaborative Research Committee of the American Academy of Pediatrics. N Engl J Med 2001;344:264–269.

114. Sawin CT. Action without benefit. The sliding scale of insulin use. Arch Intern Med 1997;157:489.

115. Malmberg K, Norhammar A, Wedel H. Glycometabolic state at admission: Important risk marker of mortality in conventionally treated patients with diabetes mellitus and acute myocardial infarction: Long-term results from the Diabetes and Insulin-Glucose Infusion in Acute Myocardial Infarction. Circulation 1999;99:2626–2632.

116. van den Berghe G, Wouters P, Weekers F, et al. Intensive insulin therapy in the critically ill patients. N Engl J Med 2001;345:1359–1367.

117. Montori VM, Bistrian BR, McMahon MM. Hyperglycemia in acutely ill patients. JAMA 2002;288:2167–2169.

118. http://www.aace.com/clin/guidelines/InpatientDiabetesPosition-Statement.pdf. Accessed January 27, 2004.

119. Dumo P, Knapp E, Wesley G. Inappropriate metformin use in hospitalized patients. Abstract 503-P, ADA 63rd Annual Scientific Sessions, New Orleans, LA, 2002.

120. Jacober SJ, Sowers JR. An update on perioperative management of diabetes. Arch Intern Med 1999;159:2405–2411.

121. American Diabetes Association. Preconception care of women with diabetes. Diabetes Care 2004;27(Suppl 1):S76–S78.

122. Ryan EA. Pregnancy in diabetes. Med Clin North Am 1998;82:823–845.

123. Buchbinder A, Miodovnik M, McElvy S, et al. Is insulin lispro associated with the development or progression of diabetic retinopathy during pregnancy? Am J Obstet Gynecol 2000;183:1162–1165.

124. Schernthaner G. Progress in the immunointervention of type 1 diabetes mellitus. Horm Metab Res 1995;27:547–554.

125. Diabetes Prevention Trial-type 1 diabetes study group. Effects of insulin in relatives of patients with type 1 diabetes mellitus. N Engl J Med 2002; 346:1685–1691.

126. Kakka R, Koda-Kimble MA. Can insulin therapy delay or prevent insulin-dependent diabetes mellitus? Pharmacotherapy 1997;17: 38–44.

127. Diabetes Prevention Program Research Group. Reduction in the incidence of type 2 diabetes with lifestyle intervention or metformin. N Engl J Med 2002;346:393–403.

128. Tuomilehto J, Lindstrom J, Eriksson JG, et al, for the Finnish Diabetes Prevention Study Group. Prevention of type 2 diabetes mellitus by changes in lifestyle among subjects with impaired glucose tolerance. N Engl J Med 2001;344:1343–1350.

129. Buchanan TA, Xiang AH, Peters RK, et al. Preservation of pancreatic β-cell function and prevention of type 2 diabetes by pharmacologic treatment of insulin resistance in high-risk Hispanic women. Diabetes 2002;51:2796–2803.

130. American Diabetes Association. Prevention or delay of type 2 diabetes. Diabetes Care 2004;27(Suppl 1):S47–S54.

131. Mensing C, Boucher J, Cypress M, et al. National standards for diabetes self-management education. Diabetes Care 2000;23:682–689.

132. American Diabetes Association. Retinopathy in diabetes. Diabetes Care 2004;27(Suppl 1):S84–S87.

133. Vinik AI. Diabetic neuropathy: Pathogenesis and therapy. Am J Med 1999;107:17S–26S.

134. American Diabetes Association. Diabetic nephropathy. Diabetes Care 2004;27(Suppl 1):S79–S83.

135. Lewis EJ, Hunsicker LG, Clarke WR, et al. Renoprotective effect of the angiotensin-receptor antagonist irbesartan in patients with nephropathy due to type 2 diabetes. N Engl J Med 2001;345:851–860.

136. Brenner BM, Cooper ME, deZeeuw D, et al. Effects of losartan on renal and cardiovascular outcomes in patients with type 2 diabetes and nephropathy. N Engl J Med 2001;345:861–869.

137. Parving HH, Lehnert H, Brochner-Mortensen J, et al. The effect of irbesartan on the development of diabetic nephropathy in patients with type 2 diabetes. N Engl J Med 2001;345:870–878.

138. American Diabetes Association. Consensus development conference on diabetic foot wound care, 7–8 April 1999, Boston, MA. Diabetes Care 1999;22:1354–1360.

139. Haire-Joshu D, Glasgow RE, Tibbs TL. Smoking and diabetes (technical review). Diabetes Care 1999;22:1887–1898.

140. American Diabetes Association. Aspirin therapy. Diabetes Care 2004; 27(Suppl 1):S72–S73.

141. Orchard TJ, Forrest KY, Kuller LH, Becker DJ. Lipid and blood pressure treatment goals for type 1 diabetes: 10-year incidence data from the Pittsburgh Epidemiology of Diabetes Complications Study. Diabetes Care 2001;24:1053–1059.

142. Haffner SM, Alexander CM, Cook TJ. Reduced coronary events in simvastatin-treated patients with coronary heart disease and diabetes or impaired fasting glucose levels: Subgroup analyses in the Scandinavian Simvastatin Survival Study. Arch Intern Med 1999;159:2661–2667.

143. Goldberg RB, Mellies MJ, Sacks FM, et al. Cardiovascular events and their reduction with pravastatin in diabetic and glucose-intolerant myocardial infarction survivors with average cholesterol levels: Subgroup analyses in the cholesterol and recurrent events (CARE) trial. The Care Investigators. Circulation 1998;98:2513–2519.

144. Heart Protection Study Collaborative Group. MRC/BHF Heart Protection Study of cholesterol-lowering with simvastatin in 5963 people with diabetes: A randomised placebo-controlled trial. Lancet 2003;361: 2005–2016.

145. Rubins HB, Robins SJ, Collins D, et al. Gemfibrozil for the secondary prevention of coronary heart disease in men with low levels of high-density lipoprotein cholesterol. Veterans Affairs High-Density Lipoprotein Cholesterol Intervention Trial Study Group. N Engl J Med 1999;341:410–418.

146. Hansson L, Zanchetti A, Carruthers SG. Effects of intensive blood-pressure lowering and low-dose aspirin in patients with hypertension: principal results of the Hypertension Optimal Treatment (HOT) randomised trial. HOT Study Group. Lancet 1998;351:1755–1762.

147. Bakris GL, Williams M, Dworkin L, et al. Preserving renal function in adults with hypertension and diabetes: A consensus approach. National Kidney Foundation Hypertension and Diabetes Executive Committees Working Group. Am J Kidney Dis 2000;36:646–661.

148. Deedwania PC. Hypertension and diabetes: new therapeutic options. Arch Intern Med 2000;160:1585–1594.

149. Robertson RP, Davis C, Larsen J, et al. Pancreas and islet transplantation for patients with diabetes mellitus (technical review). Diabetes Care 2000;23:112–116.

150. American Diabetes Association. Dyslipidemia management in adults with diabetes. Diabetes Care 2004;27:S68–S71.

151. Gray A. Raikou M, McGuire A, et al. Cost effectiveness of an intensive blood glucose control policy in patient with type 2 diabetes: Economic analysis alongside randomized controlled trial (UKPDS 41). BMJ 2000;320:1373–1378.

152. Anonymous. Cost effectiveness analysis of improved blood pressure control in hypertensive patients with type 2 diabetes: UKPDS 40. BMJ 1998;317:720–726.

73

THYROID DISORDERS

Robert L. Talbert

Learning Objectives and other resources can be found at *www.pharmacotherapyonline.com.*

KEY CONCEPTS

1 The molecular biology of the thyroid hormones and their receptors has provided an in-depth understanding of the various mutations that give rise to hyper- and hypothyroidism.

2 Thyrotoxicosis is most commonly caused by Graves' disease, which is an autoimmune disorder in which thyroid-stimulating antibody (TSAb) directed against the thyrotropin receptor elicits the same biologic response as thyroid-stimulating hormone (TSH).

3 Hyperthyroidism may be treated with antithyroid drugs such as propylthiouracil (PTU) or methimazole (MMI), radioactive iodine (RAI; e.g., ^{131}I), or surgical removal of the thyroid gland; selection of the initial treatment approach is based on patient characteristics such as age, concurrent physiology (e.g., pregnancy), comorbidities (e.g., chronic obstructive lung disease), and convenience.

4 PTU and MMI reduce the synthesis of thyroid hormones and are similar in efficacy and adverse effects, but their dosing ranges differ by 10-fold.

5 Response to PTU and MMI is seen in 4 to 6 weeks with a maximal response in 4 to 6 months; treatment usually continues for 1 to 2 years and therapy is monitored by clinical signs and symptoms and by measuring the serum concentrations of TSH and free thyroxine (T_4).

6 Many patients choose to have ablative therapy with ^{131}I rather than undergo repeated courses of PTU or MMI; most receiving RAI eventually become hypothyroid and require thyroid hormone supplementation.

7 Adjunctive therapy with β-blockers controls the adrenergic symptoms of thyrotoxicosis, but does not correct the underlying disorder; iodine may also be used adjunctively in preparation for surgery and acutely for thyroid storm.

8 Hypothyroidism is most often due to an autoimmune disorder known as Hashimoto's thyroiditis, and the drug of choice for replacement therapy is T_4.

9 Monitoring of thyroxine replacement therapy is done by clinical signs and symptoms and by measuring the TSH (elevated for underreplacement) and free T_4 (below normal for underreplacement).

Thyroid hormones affect the function of virtually every organ system. In the child, thyroid hormone is critical for normal growth and development. In the adult, the major role of thyroid hormone is to maintain metabolic stability. Substantial reservoirs of thyroid hormone in the thyroid gland and blood provide constant thyroid hormone availability. In addition, the hypothalamic-pituitary-thyroid axis is exquisitely sensitive to small changes in circulating thyroid hormone concentrations, and alterations in thyroid hormone secretion maintain peripheral free thyroid hormone levels within a narrow range. Patients seek medical attention for evaluation of symptoms owing to abnormal thyroid hormone levels or because of diffuse or nodular thyroid enlargement.

THYROID HORMONE PHYSIOLOGY

THYROID HORMONE SYNTHESIS

The thyroid hormones thyroxine (T_4) and triiodothyronine (T_3) are formed on thyroglobulin, a large glycoprotein synthesized within the thyroid cell (Fig. 73–1). Because of the unique tertiary structure of this glycoprotein, iodinated tyrosine residues present in thyroglobulin are able to bind together to form active thyroid hormones.[1,2]

Iodide is actively transported via a Na^+/I^- symporter from the extracellular space into the thyroid follicular cell against both electrical and biochemical gradients.[3] Structurally related anions such as SCN^- (thiocyanate), ClO_4^- (perchlorate), and TcO_4^- (pertechnetate) are competitive inhibitors of iodine transport.[4] In addition, bromine, fluorine, and lithium block iodide transport into the thyroid (Table 73–1). Inorganic iodide that enters the thyroid follicular cell is oxidized by thyroid peroxidase and is covalently bound (organified) to tyrosine residues of thyroglobulin (Fig. 73–2). It is interesting that although salivary glands and the gastric mucosa are able to actively transport iodide, they are unable to effectively incorporate iodide into proteins. Similarly, when tyrosine molecules are iodinated on proteins other than thyroglobulin, they lack the proper tertiary structure needed to allow the formation of active thyroid hormones.

The iodinated tyrosine residues monoiodotyrosine (MIT) and diiodotyrosine (DIT) combine to form iodothyronines (Fig. 73–3). Thus, two molecules of DIT combine to form T_4, whereas MIT and DIT constitute T_3. In addition to its role in iodine organification,

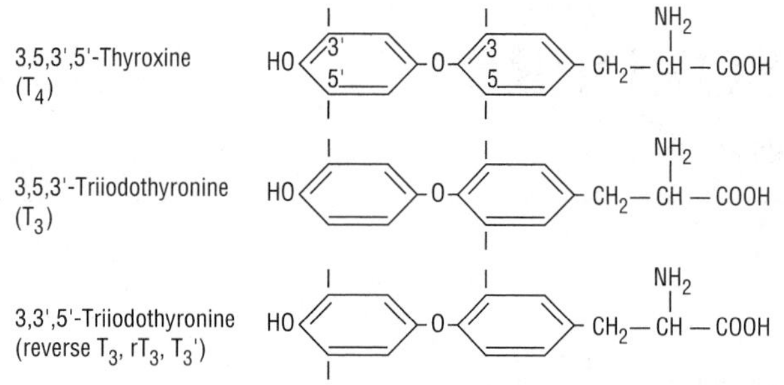

3,5,3',5'-Thyroxine (T$_4$)

3,5,3'-Triiodothyronine (T$_3$)

3,3',5'-Triiodothyronine (reverse T$_3$, rT$_3$, T$_3$')

FIGURE 73–1. Structure of thyroid hormones.

the hemoprotein thyroid peroxidase also catalyzes the formation of iodothyronines (coupling).

Iodine deficiency causes an increase in the ratio of MIT to DIT in thyroglobulin and leads to a relative increase in the production of T$_3$. Because T$_3$ is more potent than T$_4$, the increase in T$_3$ production in iodine-depleted areas may be beneficial. The thionamide drugs used to treat hyperthyroidism inhibit thyroid peroxidase and thus block thyroid hormone synthesis.

Thyroglobulin is stored in the follicular lumen and must re-enter the cell, where the process of proteolysis liberates thyroid hormone into the bloodstream. Thyroid follicles active in hormone synthesis are identified histologically by columnar epithelial cells lining follicular lumens, which are depleted of colloid. Inactive follicles are lined by cuboidal epithelial cells and are replete with colloid. Both iodide and lithium block the release of preformed thyroid hormone, through poorly understood mechanisms.

T$_4$ and T$_3$ are transported in the bloodstream by three proteins: thyroid-binding globulin (TBG), thyroid-binding prealbumin (TBPA), and albumin.[5] It is estimated that 99.96% of T$_4$ and 99.5% of T$_3$ are bound to these proteins. Only the unbound (free) thyroid hormone is able to diffuse into the cell, elicit a biologic effect, and regulate thyroid-stimulating hormone (TSH; also known as thyrotropin) secretion from the pituitary.

Whereas T$_4$ is secreted solely from the thyroid gland, less than 20% of T$_3$ is produced in the thyroid. The majority of T$_3$ is formed from the breakdown of T$_4$ catalyzed by the enzyme 5'-monodeiodinase found in peripheral tissues. Because T$_3$ may be five times more active than T$_4$, the deiodinase enzymes play a pivotal role in determining overall metabolic activity. Three different 5'-monodeiodinase enzymes are present in the body.[6] Type I enzymes are present in peripheral tissues, whereas type II enzymes are found in the central nervous system, pituitary, and thyroid. Type III en-

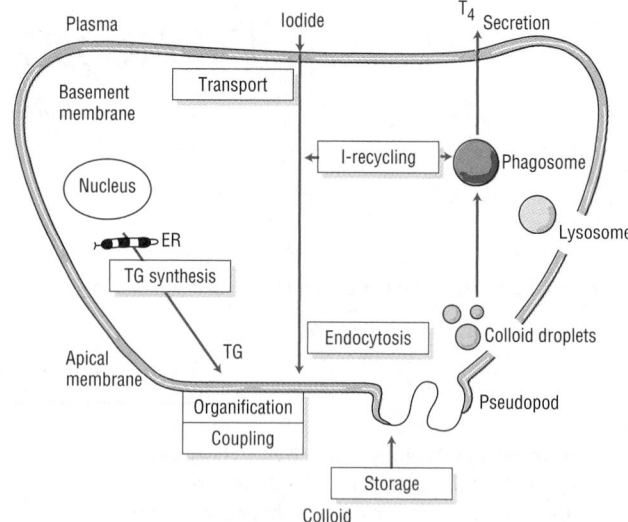

FIGURE 73–2. Thyroid hormone synthesis. Iodide is transported from the plasma, through the cell, to the apical membrane where it is organified and coupled to the thyroglobulin (TG) synthesized within the thyroid cell. Hormone stored as colloid re-enters the cell through endocytosis and moves back toward the basal membrane, where T$_4$ is secreted.

zymes, found in the placenta, skin, and developing brain, inactivate T$_4$ and T$_3$.[5,7] The principal characteristics of these enzymes are listed in Table 73–2. T$_4$ may also be acted on by the enzyme 5'-monodeiodinase to form reverse T$_3$. Reverse T$_3$ has no known significant biologic activity. T$_3$ is removed from the body by deiodinative degradation and through the action of sulfotransferase enzyme systems to T$_3$ sulfate and 3,3-diiodothyronine sulfates.

The growth and function of the thyroid are stimulated by activation of the thyrotropin receptor by thyroid-stimulating hormone. This receptor belongs to the family of G-protein–coupled receptors. The thyrotropin receptor is coupled to the α subunit of the stimulatory guanine-nucleotide–binding protein (G$_s\alpha$), activating adenylate cyclase and increasing the accumulation of cyclic adenosine

TABLE 73–1. Thyroid Hormone Synthesis and Secretion Inhibitors

Mechanism of Action	Substance
Blocks iodide transport into the thyroid	Bromine
	Fluorine
	Lithium
Impairs organification and coupling of thyroid hormones	Thionamides
	Sulfonylureas
	Sulfonamide(?)
	Salicylamide(?)
	Antipyrine(?)
Inhibits thyroid hormone secretion	Iodide (large doses)
	Lithium

Tyrosine

Monoiodotyrosine (MIT)

Diiodotyrosine (DIT)

Triiodothyronine (T$_3$)

Thyroxine (tetraiodothyronine, T$_4$)

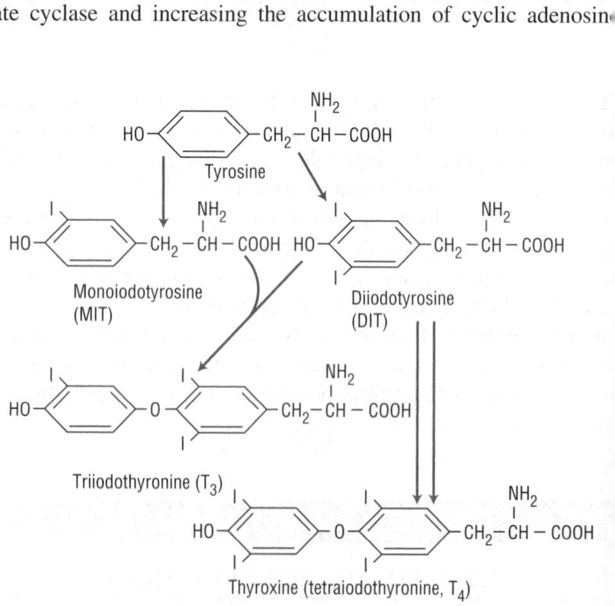

FIGURE 73–3. Scheme of coupling reactions. After tyrosine is iodinated to form MIT or DIT (organification of the iodine), MIT and DIT combine to form triiodothyronine (T$_3$), or two molecules of DIT form T$_4$.

TABLE 73–2. Properties of Iodothyronine 5'-Deiodinase Isoforms

Property	Type I	Type II	Type III
Effect of propylthiouracil	Increase	Decrease	Increase
Tissue localization	Thyroid, liver, kidney	Pituitary, thyroid, CNS, brown adipose tissue	Placenta, developing brain, skin
Preferred substrate	$rT_3 > T_4 > T_3$	$T_4 > T_3$	T_3 (sulfate) $> T_4$
Physiologic role	Extracellular T_3 production for peripheral tissue	Intracellular T_3 production, especially for brain in hypothyroidism or iodine deficiency	Inactivation of T_4 and T_3
Developmental expression	Expressed latest in development; predominant deiodinase in adult	Expressed second; especially high in brain and brown adipose tissue	Expressed first; high in developing brain; may be important for fetal thyroid hormone metabolism

rT_3, reverse T_3; T_3, triiodothyronine; T_4, thyroxine.

monophosphate. This regulates the expression of thyroglobulin and thyroid peroxidase genes. A mutation in the receptor that results in chronic stimulation causes diffuse thyroid enlargement and hyperthyroidism (germline mutations) or autonomously functioning thyroid nodules (somatic mutation in an epithelial cell).[9] Conversely, thyrotropin resistance would result from point mutations, leading to abnormalities in the thyrotropin receptor–adenylate cyclase system.[8] Individuals with this abnormality have high levels of TSH, but decreased thyroglobulin levels and a normal or small gland.

Thyroid hormone receptors[10,11] regulate the transcription of target genes in the presence of physiologic concentrations of T_3. Thyroid receptors translocate from the cytoplasm to the nucleus and interact in the nucleus with T_3, and target genes and other proteins required for basal and T_3-dependent gene transcription. Thyroid receptors exist in multiple isoforms such as TRβ2, TRβ1, TRα1, and others in man and animals. There is some evidence that the genes that encore for these receptors, THRA and THRB, may be linked to some human cancers.[12]

The production of thyroid hormone is regulated in two main ways. First, thyroid hormone is regulated by TSH secreted by the anterior pituitary. The secretion of TSH is itself under negative feedback control by the circulating level of free thyroid hormone and the positive influence of hypothalamic thyrotropin-releasing hormone (TRH). Second, extrathyroidal deiodination of T_4 to T_3 is regulated by a variety of factors including nutrition, nonthyroidal hormones, drugs, and illness.

THYROTOXICOSIS

Thyrotoxicosis results when tissues are exposed to excessive levels of T_4, T_3, or both.[13] In the National Health and Nutrition Examination Survey III, 0.2% of those surveyed who were not taking thyroid medications and had no history of thyroid disease had subclinical hyperthyroidism (TSH <0.1 milli-international units/L; and T_4 normal), and 0.2% had "clinically significant" hyperthyroidism (TSH <0.1 milli-international units/L; and T_4 >13.2 mcg/dL).[14] The prevalence of suppressed TSH peaked in people aged 20 to 39, declined in those 40 to 79, and increased again in those 80 or older. Elevated and suppressed TSH levels were more common among women than among men.

CLINICAL PRESENTATION OF THYROTOXICOSIS

GENERAL
Patients may have symptoms for an extended time period before the diagnosis of hyperthyroidism is made.

SYMPTOMS
The clinical manifestations of thyrotoxicosis include nervousness, anxiety, palpitations, emotional lability, easy fatigability, and heat intolerance. A cardinal sign is loss of weight concurrent with an increased appetite.

SIGNS
A variety of physical signs may be elicited including warm, smooth, moist skin, exophthalmos, pretibial myxedema, and unusually fine hair. Separation of the end of the fingernails from the nail beds (onycholysis) may be noted. Ocular signs that result from thyrotoxicosis include retraction of the eyelids and lagging of the upper lid behind the globe when the patient looks downward (lid lag). Physical signs of a hyperdynamic circulatory state are common and include tachycardia at rest, a widened pulse pressure, and a systolic ejection murmur. Gynecomastia is sometimes noted in men. Neuromuscular examination often reveals a fine tremor of the protruded tongue and outstretched hands. Deep tendon reflexes are generally hyperactive. Thyromegaly is usually present.

DIAGNOSIS
- Elevated free and total T_3 and T_4 serum concentrations. Low thyroid-stimulating hormone (TSH) serum concentration[15]
- Elevated radioactive iodine uptake (RAIU) by the thyroid gland

OTHER TESTS
- Thyroid stimulating antibodies (TSAb)
- Thyroglobulin
- Thyrotropin receptor antibodies
- Thyroid biopsy

TABLE 73–3. Differential Diagnosis of Thyrotoxicosis

Increased RAIU	Decreased RAIU
TSH-induced hyperthyroidism	Inflammatory thyroid disease
TSH-secreting tumors	Subacute thyroiditis
Selective pituitary resistance to T$_4$	Painless thyroid
Thyroid stimulators other than TSH[a]	Ectopic thyroid tissue
TSAb (Graves' disease)	Struma ovarii
hCG (trophoblastic diseases)	Metastatic follicular carcinoma
Thyroid autonomy	Exogenous sources of thyroid hormone
Toxic adenoma	Medication
Multinodular goiter	Food

hCG, human chorionic gonadotropin; RAIU, radioactive iodine uptake; TSAb, thyroid-stimulating antibodies; TSH, thyroid-stimulating hormone.
[a]The RAIU may be decreased if the patient has been recently exposed to excess iodine.
Adapted from Ingbar SH, Braverman LE, Werner S. The Thyroid, 5th ed. Philadelphia, JB Lippincott, 1986, with permission.

In the elderly patient and in the patient with very severe disease, anorexia may be present as well. Elderly patients are also more likely to develop atrial fibrillation with thyrotoxicosis than younger patients. The frequency of bowel movements may increase but frank diarrhea is unusual. Palpitations are a prominent and distressing symptom, particularly in the patient with pre-existing heart disease. Proximal muscle weakness is common and is noted on climbing stairs or in getting up from a sitting position. Women may note their menses are becoming scanty and irregular. Extremely thyrotoxic (thyrotoxic storm) patients may have tachycardia, heart failure, psychosis, hyperpyrexia, and coma.[13]

DIFFERENTIAL DIAGNOSIS

Measurement of the radioactive iodine uptake (RAIU) is critical in the evaluation of the clinically thyrotoxic patient (Table 73–3). The normal 24-hour RAIU ranges from 10% to 30% with some regional variation owing to differences in iodine intake. An elevated RAIU indicates true hyperthyroidism, that is, the patient's thyroid gland is actively overproducing T$_4$, T$_3$, or both. Conversely, a low RAIU indicates the excess thyroid hormone is not a consequence of thyroid gland hyperfunction. The importance of differentiating true hyperthyroidism from other causes of thyrotoxicosis lies in the widely different prognosis and treatment of the diseases in these two categories. Therapy of thyrotoxicosis associated with thyroid hyperfunction is mainly directed at decreasing the rate of thyroid hormone synthesis, secretion, or both. Such measures are ineffective in treating thyrotoxicosis that is not the result of true hyperthyroidism, because hormone synthesis and regulated hormone secretion are already at a minimum.

CAUSES OF THYROTOXICOSIS ASSOCIATED WITH ELEVATED RAIU

TSH-INDUCED HYPERTHYROIDISM

To better understand these syndromes we must first review TSH biosynthesis and secretion. TSH is synthesized in the anterior pituitary as separate α- and β-subunit precursors. The α subunits from luteinizing hormone (LH), follicle-stimulating hormone (FSH), human chorionic gonadotropin (hCG), and TSH are similar, whereas the β subunits are unique and confer immunologic and biologic speci-

ficity. Free β subunits are devoid of receptor binding and biologic activity and require combination with an α subunit to express their activity. Criteria for the diagnosis of TSH-induced hyperthyroidism include (1) evidence of peripheral hypermetabolism, (2) diffuse thyroid gland enlargement, (3) elevated free thyroid hormone levels, and (4) elevated serum immunoreactive TSH concentrations. Because the pituitary gland is extremely sensitive to even minimal elevations of free T$_4$, a detectable TSH level in any thyrotoxic patient indicates the inappropriate production of TSH.

TSH-SECRETING PITUITARY ADENOMAS

TSH-secreting pituitary tumors[16,17] occur sporadically and release biologically active hormone that is unresponsive to normal feedback control. The mean age at diagnosis is around 40 years, with women being diagnosed more commonly than men (8:7). These tumors may co-secrete prolactin or growth hormone; therefore the patients may present with amenorrhea/galactorrhea or signs of acromegaly. Most patients present with classic symptoms and signs of thyrotoxicosis. Visual-field defects may be present owing to impingement of the optic chiasm by the tumor. Tumor growth and worsening visual-field defects have been reported following treatment of thyrotoxicosis.

Diagnosis of a TSH-secreting adenoma should be made by demonstrating lack of TSH response to TRH stimulation, elevated α-subunit levels, and radiologic imaging. Note that some small tumors are not identified by MRI. Moreover, 10% of "normal" individuals may have pituitary tumors noted on pituitary imaging.[18]

Transsphenoidal pituitary surgery is the treatment of choice for TSH-secreting adenomas. Pituitary gland irradiation is often given following surgery to prevent tumor recurrence. Bromocriptine has been used to treat tumors that co-secrete prolactin.

PITUITARY RESISTANCE TO THYROID HORMONE

Pituitary resistance to thyroid hormone (PRTH) refers to selective resistance of the pituitary thyrotrophs to thyroid hormone.[8,19] About twice as many women as men have been reported with this rare, probably familial syndrome. Multiple abnormalities have been reported in the initial 50 reported cases including schizophrenia (three patients), mental retardation (two patients), short fourth metacarpals (one patient), and Marfanoid habitus (one patient). About 90% of patients studied have an appropriate increase in TSH in response to TRH; conversely, the TSH will be suppressed by T$_3$ administration.

Patients with PRTH require treatment to reduce their elevated thyroid hormone levels. Determining the appropriate serum T$_4$ level is difficult because TSH cannot be used to evaluate adequacy of therapy. Any reduction in thyroid hormone carries the risk of inducing thyrotroph hyperplasia. Ideally, agents that suppress TSH secretion could be used to treat these individuals. Glucocorticoid, dopaminergic drugs, somatostatin and its analog, and thyroid hormone analogs with reduced metabolic activity have all been tried. None is ideal.

THYROID STIMULATORS OTHER THAN TSH

GRAVES' DISEASE

Graves' disease[22–24] is an autoimmune syndrome that may include hyperthyroidism, diffuse thyroid enlargement, exophthalmos, pretibial myxedema, and thyroid acropachy (Figs. 73–4 and 73–5).[21,22] Graves' disease is the most common cause of hyperthyroidism. The prevalence of Graves' disease is estimated to be 3 per

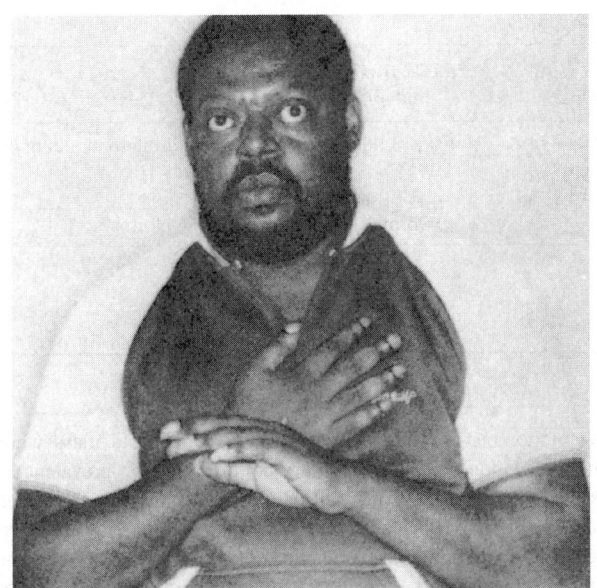

FIGURE 73–4. A 33-year-old male with Graves' disease manifested by bilateral exophthalmos, acropachy (clubbing), and extensive pretibial myxedema. When this photograph was taken, he already had been treated with radioactive ^{131}I, had become hypothyroid, and was receiving replacement therapy with exogenous l-thyroxine. *(Reproduced with permission from Becker KL, ed. Principles and Practice of Endocrinology and Metabolism. Philadelphia, Lippincott, 1990.)*

1000 population in the United States. Hyperthyroidism results from the action of thyroid-stimulating antibodies (TSAb), which are directed against the thyrotropin receptor on the surface of the thyroid cell. When these immunoglobulin G antibodies bind to the receptor, they activate the enzyme adenylate cyclase in the same manner as TSH. Autoantibodies that react with orbital muscle and fibroblast tissue in the skin are responsible for the extrathyroidal manifestations of Graves' disease, and these autoantibodies are encoded by the same germline genes that encode for other autoantibodies for striated muscle and thyroid peroxidase. The defect leading to abnormal antibody production may be a genomic point mutation in the extracellular domain of the thyrotropin receptor.[8] Clinically, the extrathyroidal disorders may not appear at the same time that hyperthyroidism develops.

There is now compelling evidence that heredity and gender both play a role in the development of clinically overt thyroid disease. Several lines of evidence support a role for heredity. First, there is a well-recognized clustering of Graves' disease within some families. Twin studies in Graves' disease have revealed that a monozygotic twin has a 50% likelihood of ultimately developing the disease compared to a 9% likelihood for a dizygotic twin. Second, the occurrence of other autoimmune diseases, including Hashimoto's thyroiditis, is also increased in families of patients with Graves' disease. Third, several studies have demonstrated an increased frequency of certain human leukocyte antigens (HLAs) in patients with Graves' disease. In Whites, HLA-D3 is present in at least one-half of patients, and the presence in an individual of both HLA-B8 and -D3 confers a fourfold greater risk for developing Graves' disease. A role for gender in the emergence of Graves' disease is suggested by the fact that hyperthyroidism is approximately eight times more common in women than men.

The thyroid gland is diffusely enlarged in the majority of patients and is commonly 40 to 60 g (two to three times the normal size). The surface of the gland is smooth and the consistency varies from soft to firm. In patients with severe disease, a thrill may be felt and a systolic bruit may be heard over the gland. The presence of any of the extrathyroidal manifestations of this syndrome including exophthalmos, thyroid acropachy, or pretibial myxedema in a thyrotoxic patient is pathognomonic of Graves' disease (see Fig. 73–4).

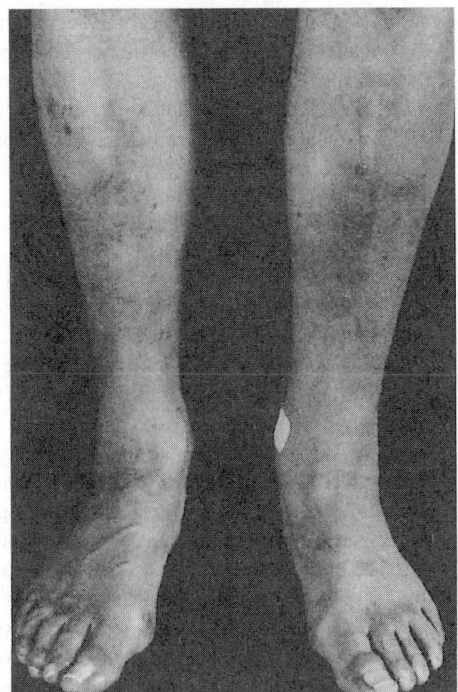
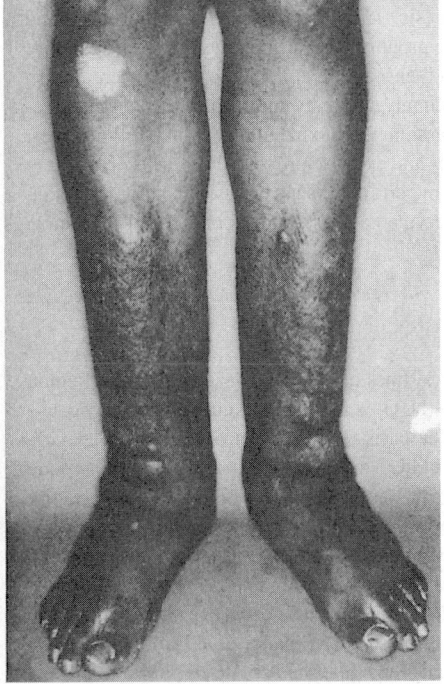

A   B

FIGURE 73–5. *A* and *B*. Different degrees of involvement of tissues with pretibial myxedema. *(Reproduced with permission from Becker KL, ed. Principles and Practice of Endocrinology and Metabolism. Philadelphia, Lippincott, 1990.)*

TABLE 73–4. Thyroid Function Test Results in Different Thyroid Conditions

	Total T$_4$	Free T$_4$	Total T$_3$	T$_3$ Resin Uptake	Free Thyroxine Index	TSH
Normal	4.5–12.5 mcg/dL	0.8–1.5 ng/dL	80–220 ng/dL	22% to 34%	1.0–4.3 units	0.25–6.7 milli-international units/
Hyperthyroid	↑↑	↑↑	↑↑↑	↑	↑↑↑	↓↓
Hypothyroid	↓↓	↓↓	↓	↓↓	↓↓↓	↑↑
Increased TBG	↑	Normal	↑	↓	Normal	Normal

TBG, thyroid-binding globulin; TSH, thyroid-stimulating hormone.

An important clinical feature of Graves' disease is the occurrence of spontaneous remissions. The abnormalities in TSAb production may decrease or disappear over time in many patients.

The results of laboratory tests in thyrotoxic Graves' disease include an increase in the overall hormone production rate with a disproportionate increase in T$_3$ relative to T$_4$ (Table 73–4). In an occasional patient, the disproportionate overproduction of T$_3$ is exaggerated, with the result that only the serum T$_3$ concentration is increased (T$_3$ toxicosis). The saturation of thyroid-binding globulin (TBG) is increased owing to the elevated levels of serum T$_4$ and T$_3$. This is reflected in elevated values for the T$_3$ resin uptake. As a result, the concentration of free T$_4$, free T$_3$, and the free T$_4$ and T$_3$ indices are increased to an even greater extent than are the measured serum total T$_4$ and T$_3$ concentrations. The TSH level will be undetectable owing to negative feedback by elevated levels of thyroid hormone at the pituitary.

In the patient with manifest disease, measurement of the serum T$_4$ concentration, T$_3$ resin uptake (or free T$_4$), and the TSH value will confirm the diagnosis of thyrotoxicosis. If the patient is not pregnant, a 24-hour RAIU should be obtained. An increased RAIU documents that the thyroid gland is inappropriately utilizing the iodine to produce more thyroid hormone at a time when the patient is thyrotoxic.

Hypokalemic periodic paralysis is a rare complication of hyperthyroidism commonly observed in Asian and Hispanic populations. It presents as recurrent proximal muscle flaccidity ranging from mild weakness to total paralysis. The paralysis may be asymmetric and usually involves muscle groups that are strenuously exercised before the attack. Cognition and sensory perception are spared, whereas deep tendon reflexes are commonly markedly diminished. Hypokalemia results from a shift of potassium from extracellular to intracellular sites. High carbohydrate loads and exercise provoke the attacks. Treatment includes correcting the hyperthyroid state, potassium administration, spironolactone to conserve potassium, and propranolol to minimize intracellular shifts.[25]

TROPHOBLASTIC DISEASES

In the past decade several lines of evidence have shown that human chorionic gonadotropin (hCG) is a thyroid stimulator and may cause hyperthyroidism.[20,26] The basis for the thyrotropic effect of hCG is the structural similarity of hCG to TSH (similar α subunits and unique β subunits). In hyperthyroid patients with very high hCG levels, serum TSH may be inappropriately detectable owing to the weak cross-reactivity of hCG in the radioimmunoassay for TSH. In patients with hyperthyroidism caused by trophoblastic tumors, serum hCG levels usually exceed 300 units/mL and always exceed 100 units/mL. The mean peak hCG level in normal pregnancy is 50 units/mL. On a molar basis, hCG has only 1/10,000 the activity of pituitary TSH in mouse bioassays. Nevertheless, this thyrotropic activity may be very substantial in patients with trophoblastic tumors, whose serum hCG concentrations may reach 2000 units/mL.

THYROID AUTONOMY

TOXIC ADENOMA

An autonomous thyroid nodule is a discrete thyroid mass whose function is independent of pituitary control.[27,28] The prevalence of toxic adenoma ranges from about 2% to 9% of thyrotoxic patients and depends on iodine availability and geographic location. Toxic adenomas arise from gain-of-function somatic or germline mutation of the G$_s\alpha$ protein or the TSH receptor; more than a dozen TSH receptor mutations have been described.[27] These nodules may be referred to as a toxic adenoma or a "hot" nodule because of their appearance on a radioiodine thyroid scan (Fig. 73–6). The amount of thyroid hormone produced by an autonomous nodule is mass related. Therefore hyperthyroidism usually occurs with larger nodules (i.e., those >4 cm in diameter). Older patients (>60 years) are more likely (up to 60%) to be thyrotoxic from autonomous nodules than are younger patients (12%). There are many reports of isolated elevation of serum T$_3$ in patients with autonomously functioning nodules. Therefore if the T$_4$ level is normal, a T$_3$ level must be measured to rule out T$_3$ toxicosis. Once a radioiodine scan has demonstrated that the toxic thyroid adenoma would collect more radioiodine than the surrounding tissue, independent function may be documented by a failure of the autonomous nodule to decrease its iodine uptake during exogenous T$_3$ administration. RAI ablation, subtotal thyroidectomy, thionamides, and percutaneous ethanol injection are treatment options, but since thionamides do not halt the proliferative process in the nodule, definitive therapies are recommended. Because thyroid carcinoma is not a major consideration in an autonomously functioning thyroid nodule, observation is usually recommended for patients with autonomously functioning nodules who are euthyroid.

MULTINODULAR GOITERS

In multinodular goiters (MNGs; Plummer's disease),[27] follicles with a very high degree of autonomous function coexist with normal or even nonfunctioning follicles. Thyrotoxicosis in a multinodular goiter occurs when the follicles with a high degree of autonomy generate enough thyroid hormone to exceed the needs of the patient. The pathogenesis of multinodular goiter is thought to be similar to that of toxic adenoma.[29] It is not surprising that this type of hyperthyroidism develops insidiously over a period of several years and predominantly affects older individuals with long-standing goiters. Often, elderly women present with subtle signs of hyperthyroidism that are superimposed on underlying heart disease. The patient's complaints of weight loss, depression, anxiety, and insomnia may be attributed to old age. Any unexplained chronic illness in an elderly patient presenting with a multinodular goiter calls for the exclusion of hidden thyrotoxicosis. Third-generation TSH assays and T$_3$ suppression testing may be useful in detecting subclinical hyperthyroidism.[30]

A thyroid scan will show patchy areas of autonomously functioning thyroid tissue. The preferred treatment for toxic MNG is RAI or

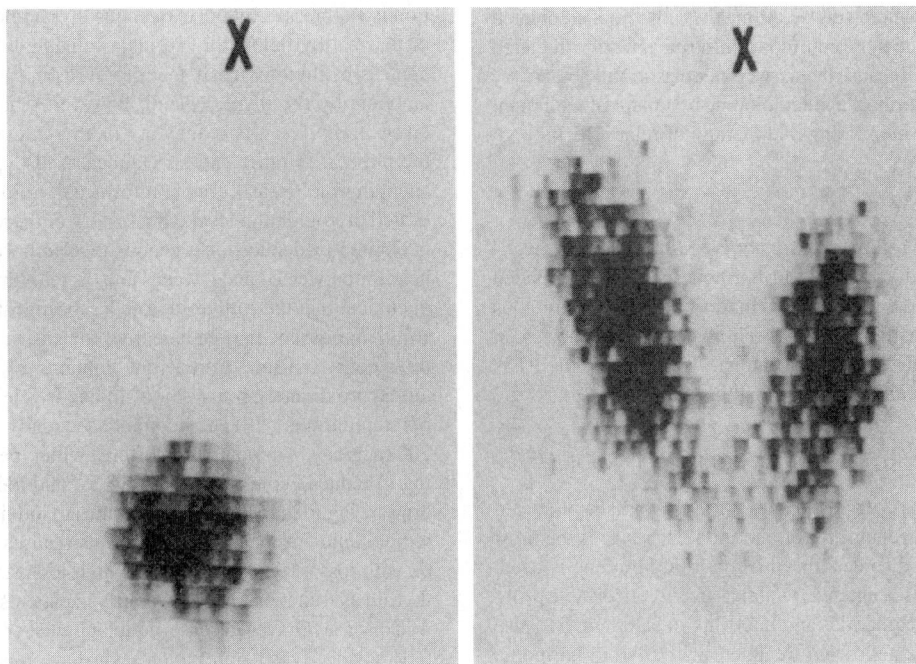

FIGURE 73–6. *Left.* Autonomously functioning nodule is suppressing the remainder of the thyroid gland. *Right.* Previously suppressed lobes of thyroid gland are visualized 3 months after radioiodine treatment of hyperfunctioning nodule. The "X" is a marker for thyroid cartilage. *(Reproduced with permission from Becker KL, ed. Principles and Practice of Endocrinology and Metabolism. Philadelphia, Lippincott, 1990.)*

surgery. Surgery is usually selected for younger patients and patients in whom large goiters impinge on vital organs. Alternatively, percutaneous injection of 95% ethanol has also been used to destroy single or multinodular adenomas with a 5-year success rate approaching 80%.

CAUSES OF THYROTOXICOSIS ASSOCIATED WITH SUPPRESSED RAIU

INFLAMMATORY THYROID DISEASE

Subacute Thyroiditis

Painful subacute (viral or deQuervain's) thyroiditis may be caused by viral invasion of thyroid parenchyma. Typically, patients complain of severe pain in the thyroid region, which often extends to the ear on the affected side. With time, the pain may migrate from one side of the gland to the other. Low-grade fever is common. Systemic symptoms owing to thyrotoxicosis are present. On physical examination, the thyroid gland is firm and exquisitely tender. Signs of thyrotoxicosis are present.

Thyroid function tests typically run a triphasic course. Initially, serum thyroxine levels are elevated owing to release of preformed thyroid hormone from disrupted follicles. The 24-hour RAIU during this time is less than 2% owing to thyroid inflammation and TSH suppression by the elevated thyroxine level. As the disease progresses, intrathyroidal hormone stores are depleted and the patient may become mildly hypothyroid with an appropriately elevated TSH level. During the recovery phase thyroid hormone stores are replenished and serum TSH elevation gradually returns to normal. Recovery is generally complete within 2 to 6 months. Most patients remain euthyroid and recurrences of painful thyroiditis are extremely rare. The patient with painful thyroiditis should be reassured that the disease is self-limited and is unlikely to recur. Thyrotoxic symptoms may be relieved with β-blockers. Aspirin (650 mg orally every 6 hours)

will usually relieve the pain. Occasionally, prednisone (20 mg orally three times a day) must be used to suppress the inflammatory process. Antithyroid drugs are not indicated because they do not decrease the release of preformed thyroid hormone.

Painless Thyroiditis

Since its description in 1975, painless (silent, lymphocytic, postpartum) thyroiditis has been recognized as a common cause of thyrotoxicosis and may represent up to 15% of cases of thyrotoxicosis in North America. The etiology is not fully understood and may be heterogeneous. The triphasic course of this illness mimics that of painful thyroiditis. Most patients present with mild thyrotoxic symptoms. Lid retraction and lid lag are present but exophthalmos is absent. The thyroid gland may be diffusely enlarged but thyroid tenderness is absent.

The 24-hour RAIU will be suppressed to less than 2% during the thyrotoxic phase of painless thyroiditis.[31,32] Antithyroglobulin and antimicrosomal antibody levels are elevated in more than 50% of patients. Painless thyroiditis frequently occurs during the immediate postpartum period, and individual patients may experience recurrence of the disease with subsequent pregnancies. Patients with mild hyperthyroidism and painless thyroiditis should be reassured that they have a self-limited disease. Adrenergic symptoms may be ameliorated with propranolol. Antithyroid drugs are not indicated because they do not decrease the release of preformed thyroid hormone.

ECTOPIC THYROID TISSUE

Struma Ovarii

Struma ovarii is a teratoid tumor of the ovary that is capable of making thyroid hormone. This extremely rare cause of thyrotoxicosis is suggested by the absence of thyroid enlargement in a thyrotoxic patient with a suppressed RAIU. The diagnosis is established by localizing functioning thyroid tissue in the ovary with whole-body radioactive iodine (^{131}I) scanning. Interestingly, struma ovarii without associated hyperthyroidism is much more common than struma ovarii associated with hyperthyroidism. Because the tissue is neoplastic and potentially malignant, combined surgical and radioiodine treatment of malignant struma ovarii for both monitoring and therapy of relapse is the recommended treatment.[33]

Follicular Cancer

In widely metastatic follicular carcinomas with relatively well-preserved function, sufficient thyroid hormone can be synthesized and secreted to produce thyrotoxicosis. In most instances, a previous diagnosis of thyroid malignancy has been made. The diagnosis can be confirmed by whole-body ^{131}I scanning. Treatment with ^{131}I is generally effective at ablating functioning thyroid metastases.

EXOGENOUS SOURCES OF THYROID HORMONE

The term *thyrotoxicosis factitia* denotes hyperthyroidism produced by the ingestion of exogenous thyroid hormone. Obesity is the most common nonthyroidal disorder for which thyroid hormone is used, but thyroid hormone has been used for almost every conceivable problem from menstrual irregularities and infertility to baldness. Because these patients do not benefit from treatment with thyroid hormone, the physician or patient may gradually increase the dose of hormone employed in an attempt to gain the desired effect. Obviously, thyrotoxicosis factitia can also occur when too large a dose of thyroid hormone is employed for conditions in which it is likely to be beneficial, such as hypothyroidism or nontoxic goiter. Rarely, thyrotoxicosis factitia is caused by the purposeful and secretive ingestion of thyroid hormone by disturbed patients (usually with a medical background) who wish to obtain attention or lose weight.

Thyrotoxicosis factitia should be suspected in a thyrotoxic patient without infiltrative ophthalmopathy or thyroid enlargement. The RAIU uptake is at low levels because the patient's thyroid gland function is suppressed by the exogenous thyroid hormone. Measurement of plasma thyroglobulin (TG) is a valuable laboratory aid in the diagnosis of thyrotoxicosis factitia. TG is normally secreted in small amounts by the thyroid gland; however, when thyroid hormone is taken orally, very low amounts of thyroglobulin are detectable in the plasma. In other entities characterized by a low RAIU, such as silent thyroiditis, leakage of preformed thyroid hormone results in elevated thyroglobulin levels. If a history of thyroid hormone ingestion is elicited or deduced, exogenous thyroid hormone should be withheld for between 4 and 6 weeks and thyroid function tests repeated to document that the euthyroid state has been restored.[34]

Amiodarone may induce thyrotoxicosis (2% to 3% of patients) or hypothyroidism. Amiodarone contains 37.2% iodine by weight and approximately 6 mg/day of iodine is released for each 200 mg of amiodarone.[4,35] The recommended daily amount of iodine is 200 mcg/day. Amiodarone interferes with type I 5′-deiodinase, leading to reduced conversion of T_4 to T_3, and iodide released from the drug owing to deiodination contributes to iodine excess, especially in iodine-deficient areas. Amiodarone also causes a destructive thyroiditis with loss of thyroglobulin and thyroid hormones. Iodine-induced thyroid dysfunction occurs primarily in patients with pre-existing thyroid disease (Graves' disease, nodular goiter, or Hashimoto's thyroiditis) known as type I, or in patients who have apparently normal thyroid glands (type II). The two types may be differentiated using color flow Doppler ultrasonography.[36] Type I amiodarone-induced hyperthyroidism responds well to thionamides, whereas type II may require glucocorticoids or iopanoic acid.[37] An inflammatory process induced by amiodarone or iodine, which also leads to follicular cell damage and subacute thyroiditis with leakage of thyroid hormones into the circulation, is associated with elevated interleukin-6 levels. The manifestations may be atypical symptoms such as ventricular tachycardia and exacerbation of underlying chronic obstructive pulmonary disease. Prednisone has been reported to normalize interleukin-6 and thyroid hormone values.[38]

▶ TREATMENT: Hyperthyroidism

▦ DESIRED OUTCOMES

◀3 Three common treatment modalities are used in the management of hyperthyroidism: surgery, antithyroid medications, and radioactive iodine (RAI) (Table 73–5). The overall therapeutic objectives are to eliminate the excess thyroid hormone and minimize the symptoms and long-term consequences of hyperthyroidism. Therapy must be individualized based on the type and severity of hyperthyroidism, patient age and gender, existence of nonthyroidal conditions, and response to previous therapy.[20,39,40] Clinical guidelines for the treatment of hyperthyroidism have been published by various groups.[41–44]

▦ NONPHARMACOLOGIC THERAPY

Surgical removal of the hypersecreting thyroid gland became feasible in 1923 when Plummer discovered that iodine reduced the gland's vascularity, making this definitive procedure possible. Surgery should be considered in patients with a large thyroid gland (>80 g), severe ophthalmopathy, and a lack of remission on antithyroid drug treatment. In case of cosmetic or pressure symptoms, the choice in multinodular goiter stands between surgery, which is still the first choice, and radioiodine if uptake is adequate (hot). In addition to surgery, the solitary nodule, whether hot or cold, can be treated with percutaneous ethanol injection therapy. If hot, radioiodine is the therapy of choice.[45] Traditional preparation of the patient for thyroidectomy includes propylthiouracil (PTU) or methimazole (MMI) until the patient is biochemically euthyroid (usually 6 to 8 weeks), followed by the addition of iodides (500 mg/day) for 10 to 14 days before surgery to decrease the vascularity of the gland. Levothyroxine may be added to maintain the euthyroid state while the thionamides are continued. Iodine supplementation in iodine-deficient areas of the country may lead to a greater reduction in remnant volume in nontoxic goiter.[46] Propranolol for several weeks preoperatively and 7 to 10 days after surgery has also been used to maintain a pulse rate of less than 90 beats/min. Combined pretreatment with propranolol and 10 to 14 days of potassium iodide also has been advocated.

The overall morbidity rate with surgery is 2.7%. Hyperthyroidism persists or recurs in 0.6% to 17.9% of patients after thyroidectomy for Graves' disease and is more common in children. The most common complications of surgery include hypothyroidism (up to about 49%), hypoparathyroidism (up to 3.9%), and vocal cord abnormalities (up to 5.4%). The frequent occurrence of hypothyroidism following surgery requires periodic follow-up for identification and treatment of these patients.[47–49]

TABLE 73–5. Treatments for Hyperthyroidism Caused by Graves' Disease

Treatment	Advantages	Disadvantages	Comment
Antithyroid drugs	Noninvasive Lower initial cost Low risk of permanent hypothyroidism Possible remissions due to immune effects	Low cure rate (30%–80%; average 40%–50%) Adverse drug reactions Drug compliance	First-line treatment in children, adolescents, and in pregnancy Initial treatment in severe cases or preoperative preparation
Radioactive iodine (^{131}I)	Cure of hyperthyroidism Most cost effective	Permanent hypothyroidism almost inevitable Might worsen ophthalmopathy Pregnancy must be deferred for 6–12 months; no breast-feeding Small potential risk of exacerbation of hyperthyroidism	Best treatment for toxic nodules and toxic multinodular goiter
Surgery	Rapid, effective treatment, especially in patients with large goiters	Most invasive Potential complications (recurrent laryngeal nerve damage, hypoparathyroidism) Most costly Permanent hypothyroidism Pain, scar	Potential in pregnancy if major side-effect from antithyroid Useful when coexisting suspicious nodule present Option for patients who refuse radioiodine

PHARMACOLOGIC THERAPY

ANTITHYROID MEDICATIONS

Thiourea Drugs

Two drugs within this category, PTU and MMI, are approved for the treatment of hyperthyroidism in the United States.[50,51] They are classified as thioureylenes (thionamides), which incorporate a N—C—S = N group into their ring structures.

❹ *Mechanism of Action.* PTU and MMI share several mechanisms to inhibit the biosynthesis of thyroid hormone.[13] These drugs serve as preferential substrates for the iodinating intermediate of thyroid peroxidase and divert iodine away from potential iodination sites in thyroglobulin. This prevents subsequent incorporation of iodine into iodotyrosines and ultimately iodothyronine ("organification"). Second, they inhibit coupling of monoiodotyrosine and diiodotyrosine to form T_4 and T_3. The coupling reaction may be more sensitive to these drugs than the iodination reaction. Experimentally, these drugs exhibit immunosuppressive effects, although the clinical relevance of this finding is unclear. In patients with Graves' disease, antithyroid drug treatment has been associated with lower TSAb titers and restoration of normal suppressor T-cell function. However, perchlorate, which has a different mechanism of action, also decreases TSAbs, suggesting that normalization of the thyroid hormone level may itself improve the abnormal immune function. PTU inhibits the peripheral conversion of T_4 to T_3. This effect is acutely dose-related and occurs within hours of PTU administration. MMI does not have this effect. Over time, depletion of stored hormone and lack of continuing synthesis of thyroid hormone results in the clinical effects of these drugs.

Pharmacokinetics. Both antithyroid drugs are well absorbed (80% to 95%) from the gastrointestinal tract, with peak serum concentrations about 1 hour after ingestion. The plasma half-life ranges of PTU and MMI are 1 to 2.5 hours and 6 to 9 hours, respectively, and are not appreciably affected by thyroid status. Urinary excretion is about 35% for PTU and less than 10% for MMI. These drugs are actively concentrated in the thyroid gland, which may account for the disparity between their relatively short plasma half-lives and the effectiveness of once-daily dosing regimens even with PTU. Approximately 60% to 80% of PTU is bound to plasma albumin, whereas MMI is not protein-bound. Methimazole readily crosses the placenta and appears in breast milk. Older studies suggested that PTU crosses the placental membranes only one-tenth as well as MMI; however, these studies were done in the course of therapeutic abortion early in pregnancy. Newer studies show little difference between fetal concentrations of PTU and MMI, and both are associated with elevated TSH in about 20% and low T_4 in about 7% of the fetuses.[52]

❺ *Dosing and Monitoring.* PTU is available as 50-mg tablets and MMI as 5- and 10-mg tablets. MMI is approximately 10 times more potent than PTU. Initial therapy with PTU ranges from 300 to 600 mg daily, usually in three or four divided doses. MMI is given in three divided doses totaling 30 to 60 mg/day. Although the traditional recommendation is for divided doses, evidence exists that both drugs can be given as single daily doses. Patients with severe hyperthyroidism may require larger initial doses, and some may respond better at these larger doses if the dose is divided. The maximal blocking doses of PTU and MMI are 1200 and 120 mg daily, respectively. Once the intrathyroidal pool of thyroid hormone is reduced and new hormone synthesis is sufficiently blocked, clinical improvement should ensue. Usually within 4 to 8 weeks of initiating therapy, symptoms are diminished and circulating thyroid hormone levels are returning to normal. At this time the tapering regimen can be started. Changes in dose for each drug should be made on a monthly basis, because the endogenously produced T_4 will reach a new steady-state concentration in this interval. Typical ranges of daily maintenance doses for PTU and MMI are 50 to 300 mg and 5 to 30 mg, respectively.

If the objective of therapy is to induce a long-term remission, the patient should remain on continuous antithyroid drug therapy for 12 to 24 months. Antithyroid drug therapy induces permanent remission rates of 10% to 98%, with an overall average of about 40% to 50%.[53] This is much higher than the remission rate seen with propranolol alone, which is reported to range from 22% to 36%. Patient characteristics for a favorable outcome include older patients (>40 years), low ratio of T_4 to T_3 (<20), a small goiter (<50 g), short duration of disease (<6 months), no previous history of relapse with antithyroid drugs, duration of therapy 1 to 2 years or longer, and low TSAb titers at baseline or a reduction with treatment.[13] It is important that patients be followed every 6 to 12 months after remission occurs. If a relapse occurs, alternate therapy with RAI is preferred to a second course of antithyroid drugs. Relapses seem to plateau after about 5 years and eventually 5% to 20% of patients will develop spontaneous hypothyroidism.

Concurrent administration of thyroxine with thionamide therapy for thyrotoxicosis and subclinical hyperthyroidism may reduce autoantibodies directed toward the thyroid gland and improve the remission rate; however, these effects have not been consistently observed in all studies.[53,54] In a Japanese study, adjunctive treatment with thyroxine was associated with a 20-fold reduction in the recurrence rate of Graves' disease compared with the recurrence rate seen in patients treated with antithyroid drugs alone. Attempts to reproduce these results in American and European patients with Graves' disease have failed to show any delay or reduction in the recurrence of Graves' disease with thyroxine administration.[55]

Adverse Effects. Minor adverse reactions to PTU and MMI have an overall incidence of 5% to 25% depending on the dose and the drug, whereas major adverse effects occur in 1.5% to 4.6% of patients receiving these drugs.[13,56,57] Pruritic maculopapular rashes (sometimes associated with vasculitis based on skin biopsy), arthralgias, and fevers occur in up to 5% of patients and may occur at greater frequency with higher doses and in children. Rashes often disappear spontaneously, but if persistent, may be managed with antihistamines.

Perhaps one of the most common side effects is a benign transient leukopenia characterized by a white blood cell (WBC) count of less than 4000/mm^3. This condition occurs in up to 12% of adults and 25% of children, and sometimes can be confused with mild leukopenia seen in Graves' disease. This mild leukopenia is not a harbinger of the more serious adverse effect of agranulocytosis, so therapy can usually be continued. If a minor adverse reaction occurs with one antithyroid drug, the alternate thiourea may be tried, but cross-sensitivity occurs in about 50% of patients.[50]

Agranulocytosis is the most serious adverse effect of thiourea drug therapy and is characterized by fever, malaise, gingivitis, oropharyngeal infection, and a granulocyte count less than 250/mm^3.[50] These drugs are concentrated in granulocytes and this reaction may represent a direct toxic effect rather than hypersensitivity. This toxic reaction has occurred with both thioureas, and the incidence varies from 0.5% to 6%. It is higher in patients over age 40 receiving a methimazole dose greater than 40 mg/day or the equivalent dose of PTU, and is linked to HLA class II genes containing the DRB1*08032 allele.[58] Agranulocytosis almost always develops in the first 3 months of therapy. Because the onset is sudden, routine monitoring is not recommended. Colony-stimulating factors have been used with some success to restore cell counts to normal, but it is unclear how effective this form of therapy is to routine supportive care.[59,60] Peripheral lymphocytes obtained from patients with PTU-induced agranulocytosis undergo transformation in the presence of other thioamides, suggesting that these severe reactions are immunologically mediated and patients should not receive other thionamides. Aplastic anemia has been reported with MMI and may be associated with an inhibitor to colony-forming units. Once antithyroid drugs are discontinued, clinical improvement is seen over several days to weeks. Patients should be counseled to discontinue therapy and contact their physician when flu-like symptoms such as fever, malaise, or sore throat develop.

Arthralgias and a lupus-like syndrome (sometimes in the absence of antinuclear antibodies) have been reported in 4% to 5% of patients. This generally occurs after 6 months of therapy. Uncommonly, polymyositis, presenting as proximal muscle weakness and elevated creatine phosphokinase, has been reported with PTU administration. Gastrointestinal intolerance is also reported to occur in 4% to 5% of patients. Hepatotoxicity, which usually occurs within the first 3 months of therapy, may be seen with both methimazole and PTU with a prevalence of about 1.3%.[61] In mice, MMI undergoes epoxidation of the C-4,5 double bond by cytochrome P450 enzymes, and after being hydrolyzed, the resulting epoxide is decomposed to form N-methylthiourea, a proximate toxicant.[62] At moderate doses, some authors have found that initial enzyme elevations eventually normalize in most patients with continued therapy.[63] High doses of PTU are more likely to produce severe hepatitis and even death. Discontinuation of therapy usually results in complete resolution of hepatitis. Patients receiving interferon products for hepatitis C or other disorders may develop hyper- or hypothyroidism along with liver enzyme abnormalities.[64] Although older reports suggested that congenital skin defects (aplasia cutis) may be caused by methimazole and carbimazole, a registry review from the Netherlands could not find an association between maternal use of these drugs and skin defects.[65] Hypoprothrombinemia is a rare complication of thionamide therapy. Patients who have experienced a major adverse reaction to one thiourea drug should not be converted to the alternate drug because of cross-sensitivity.

Iodides

Iodide was the first form of drug therapy for Graves' disease. Its mechanism of action is to acutely block thyroid hormone release, inhibit thyroid hormone biosynthesis by interfering with intrathyroidal iodide utilization (the Wolff-Chaikoff effect), and decrease the size and vascularity of the gland. This early inhibitory effect provides symptom improvement within 2 to 7 days of initiating therapy, and serum T_4 and T_3 concentrations may be reduced for a few weeks. Despite the reduced release of T_4 and T_3, thyroid hormone synthesis continues at an accelerated rate, resulting in a gland rich in stored hormones. The normal and hyperfunctioning thyroid soon escapes from this inhibitory effect within 1 to 2 weeks by decreasing the active transfer of iodide into the gland. Iodides are often used as adjunctive therapy to prepare a patient with Graves' disease for surgery, to acutely inhibit thyroid hormone release and quickly attain the euthyroid state in severely thyrotoxic patients with cardiac decompensation, or to inhibit thyroid hormone release following radioactive iodine therapy. However, large doses of iodine may exacerbate hyperthyroidism or indeed precipitate hyperthyroidism in some previously euthyroid individuals (Jod-Basedow disease).[66] This Jod-Basedow phenomenon is most common in iodine-deficient areas, particularly in patients with pre-existing nontoxic goiter. Iodide is contraindicated in toxic multinodular goiter.

Potassium iodide is available either as a saturated solution (SSKI), which contains 38 mg of iodide per drop, or as Lugol's solution, which contains 6.3 mg of iodide per drop. The typical starting dose of SSKI is 3 to 10 drops daily (120 to 400 mg) in water or juice. There is no documented advantage to using doses in excess of 6 to 8 mg/day. When used to prepare a patient for surgery, it should be administered 7 to 14 days preoperatively. As an adjunct to RAI, SSKI should not be used before, but rather 3 to 7 days after RAI treatment, so that the radioactive iodide can concentrate in the thyroid. The most frequent toxic effect with iodide therapy is hypersensitivity reactions (skin rashes, drug fever, rhinitis, and conjunctivitis); salivary gland swelling; "iodism" (metallic taste, burning mouth and throat, sore eeth and gums, symptoms of a head cold, and sometimes stomach pset and diarrhea); and gynecomastia.

Other compounds containing organic iodide have also been used herapeutically for hyperthyroidism. These include various radiologic ontrast media that share a triiodo- and monoaminobenzene ring with propionic acid chain (e.g., iopanoic acid and sodium ipodate). The ffect of these compounds is a result of the iodine content inhibit-ng thyroid hormone release as well as competitive inhibition of 5'-nonodeiodinase conversion related to their structures, which resem-le thyroid analogs.[4]

Adrenergic Blockers

Because many of the manifestations of hyperthyroidism are me-diated by β-adrenergic receptors, β-blockers (especially pro-ranolol) have been used widely to ameliorate thyrotoxic symptoms uch as palpitations, anxiety, tremor, and heat intolerance. Although -blockers are quite effective for symptom control, they have no ef-ect on the urinary excretion of calcium, phosphorus, hydroxypro-ine, creatinine, or various amino acids, suggesting a lack of effect n peripheral thyrotoxicosis and protein metabolism. Furthermore, -blockers do not reduce TSAb nor prevent thyroid storm. Propra-olol and nadolol partially block the conversion of T_4 to T_3, but this ontribution to the overall therapeutic effect is small in magnitude. nhibition of conversion of T_4 to T_3 is mediated by d-propranolol, vhich is devoid of β-blocking activity, and l-propranolol, which is esponsible for the antiadrenergic effects and has little effect on the onversion.

β-Blockers are usually used as adjunctive therapy with antithy-oid drugs, RAI, or iodides when treating Graves' disease or toxic odules; in preparation for surgery; or in thyroid storm. The only onditions for which β-blockers are primary therapy for thyrotoxico-is are thyroiditis and iodine-induced hyperthyroidism. The dose of ropranolol required to relieve adrenergic symptoms is variable, but n initial dose of 20 to 40 mg four times daily is effective (heart rate <90 beats/min) for most patients. Younger or more severely toxic pa-ients may require as much as 240 to 480 mg/day because there seems o be an increased clearance rate in these patients. β-Blockers are ontraindicated in patients with decompensated heart failure unless t is caused solely by tachycardia (high output). Nonselective agents nd those lacking intrinsic sympathomimetic activity should be used vith caution in patients with asthma and bronchospastic chronic ob-tructive lung disease. β-Blockers that are cardioselective and have ntrinsic sympathomimetic activity may have a slight margin of safety n these situations. Other patients in whom contraindications exist re those with sinus bradycardia, those receiving monoamine oxi-lase inhibitors or tricyclic antidepressants, and those with sponta-eous hypoglycemia. β-Blockers may also prolong gestation and la-oor during pregnancy. Other side effects include nausea, vomiting, nxiety, insomnia, light-headedness, bradycardia, and hematologic listurbances.

Antiadrenergic agents such as centrally acting sympatholytics nd calcium channel antagonists may have some role in the symp-omatic treatment of hyperthyroidism. These drugs might be use-ul when contraindications to β-blockade exist. When compared to adolol 40 mg twice daily, clonidine 150 mcg twice daily reduced lasma catecholamines, whereas nadolol increased both epinephrine nd norepinephrine after 1 week of treatment. Diltiazem 120 mg given very 8 hours reduced heart rate by 17%; fewer ventricular extrasys-oles were noted after 10 days of therapy, and diltiazem has been hown to be comparable to propranolol in lowering heart rate and lood pressure.

Radioactive Iodine

Although other radioisotopes have been used to ablate thyroid tissue, sodium iodide 131 (^{131}I) is considered to be the agent of choice for Graves' disease, toxic autonomous nodules, and toxic multinodular goiters.[22,67] RAI is administered as a colorless and tasteless liquid that is well absorbed and concentrates in the thyroid. Sodium iodide 131 is a β-emitter with a tissue penetration of 2 mm and a half-life of 8 days. Other organs take up ^{131}I, but the thyroid gland is the only organ in which organification of the absorbed iodine takes place. Initially, RAI disrupts hormone synthesis by incorporating into thyroid hormones and thyroglobulin. Over a period of weeks, follicles that have taken up RAI and surrounding follicles develop evidence of cellular necrosis, breakdown of follicles, development of bizarre cell forms, nuclear pyknosis, and destruction of small vessels within the gland, leading to edema and fibrosis of the interstitial tissue. Pregnancy is an absolute contraindication to the use of RAI.

β-Blockers may be given any time without compromising RAI therapy, accounting for their role as a mainstay of adjunctive ther-apy to RAI treatment. If iodides are administered, they should be given 3 to 7 days after RAI to prevent interference with the uptake of RAI in the thyroid gland. Because thyroid hormone levels will transiently increase following RAI treatment owing to release of pre-formed thyroid hormone, patients with cardiac disease and elderly patients are often treated with thionamides prior to RAI ablation. Oc-casionally, in patients with underlying cardiac disease, it may be nec-essary to reinstitute antithyroid drug therapy following radioactive io-dine ablation. The standard practice is to withdraw the thionamide 4 to 6 days prior to RAI treatment and to reinstitute it 4 days after therapy is concluded. Administering antithyroid drug therapy following RAI treatment may result in a higher rate of posttreatment recurrence or persistent hyperthyroidism.[67]

Corticosteroid administration will blunt and delay the rise in antibodies to the TSH receptor, thyroglobulin, and thyroid per-oxidase while reducing T_3 and T_4 concentrations following RAI. Bartalena and associates found no progression in ophthalmopathy in patients receiving prednisone after RAI compared with methima-zole (2% to 3% worsened), or no other treatment (5% with persistent worsening).[68] Theoretically, if shared thyroidal and orbital antigen is involved in the pathogenesis of Graves' ophthalmopathy, antigen released with RAI treatment could aggravate pre-existing eye dis-ease. Note also that thyroid ablation may decrease eye disease in the long term by removing the source of antigen, but it is unclear if RAI differs from surgery or thionamide for the risk of worsening eye disease.[69]

Destruction of the gland attenuates the hyperthyroid state, and hypothyroidism commonly occurs months to years following RAI.[70] The goal of therapy is to destroy overactive thyroid cells, and a sin-gle dose of 4000 to 8000 rads results in a euthyroid state in 60% of patients at 6 months or less. The remaining 40% become euthyroid within 1 year, requiring two or more doses. It is advisable that a sec-ond dose of RAI be given 6 months after the first RAI treatment if the patient remains hyperthyroid. Variables that influence the outcome of RAI include gender (men are less likely to develop hypothyroidism), race (blacks are more resistant to ^{131}I), the size of the thyroid, sever-ity of disease, and perhaps the level of TSAb. The acute, short-term side effects of ^{131}I therapy are minimal and include mild thyroidal tenderness and dysphagia. Concern over the development of thyroid carcinoma and leukemia and increased risk of mutations and congeni-tal defects now appears to be unfounded because long-term follow-up studies have not revealed increased risk for these complications.[50,71] Although RAI is very effective in the treatment of hyperthyroidism, long-term follow-up from Great Britain suggests that among patients with hyperthyroidism treated with RAI, mortality from all causes and mortality resulting from cardiovascular and cerebrovascular disease and fracture are increased.[72]

A common approach to Graves' hyperthyroidism is to administer a single dose of 5 to 15 mCi(80 to 120 mcCi/g of tissue).[50,67] The optimal method for determining ^{131}I treatment doses for Graves' hyperthyroidism is unknown, and techniques have varied from a fixed dose to more elaborate calculations based on gland size, iodine uptake, and iodine turnover. In a trial of 88 patients with Graves' disease, no difference in outcome was seen among high or low, fixed or adjusted doses.[73] Thyroid glands estimated to weigh >80 g may require larger doses of RAI. Larger doses are likely to induce hypothyroidism and are seldom given outside the United States owing to the imposition of stringent safety restrictions. For example, in the United Kingdom, a nursery school teacher is advised to stay out of school for 3 weeks following a 15-mCi dose of ^{131}I.[74]

EVALUATION OF THERAPEUTIC OUTCOMES: HYPERTHYROIDISM

After therapy (surgery, thionamides, or RAI) for hyperthyroidism has been initiated, patients should be evaluated on a monthly basis until they reach a euthyroid condition. Clinical signs of continuing thyrotoxicosis (tachycardia, weight loss, and heat intolerance, among others) or the development of hypothyroidism (bradycardia, weight gain, and lethargy, among others) should be noted. β-Blockers may be used to control symptoms of thyrotoxicosis until the definitive treatment has returned the patient to a euthyroid state. Once thyroxine replacement is initiated, the goal is to maintain both the free thyroxine level and the TSH concentration in the normal range. Once a stable dose of thyroxine is identified, the patient may be followed-up every 6 to 12 months.

Finally, a common, potentially confusing clinical situation should be mentioned. Why are the TSH concentrations suppressed in some patients who are clinically hypothyroid and who have a low free T_4 level? In patients with long-standing hyperthyroidism, the pituitary thyrotrophs responsible for making TSH become atrophic. The average amount of time required for these cells to resume normal functioning is 6 to 8 weeks.[75] Therefore if a thyrotoxic patient has his or her free T_4 concentration lowered rapidly, before the thyrotrophs resume normal function, a period of "transient central hypothyroidism" will be observed.

SPECIAL CONDITIONS

GRAVES' DISEASE AND PREGNANCY

Inappropriate production of human chorionic gonadotropin (hCG) is a cause of abnormal thyroid function tests during the first half of pregnancy, and hCG can cause either subclinical (normal T_4, suppressed TSH) or overt hyperthyroidism.[76-78] This is owing to the homology of hCG and TSH as well as their receptors. Hyperthyroidism during pregnancy is almost solely caused by Graves' disease, with approximately 0.1% to 0.4% of pregnancies affected. Although the increased metabolic rate is usually well tolerated in pregnant women, two symptoms suggestive of hyperthyroidism during pregnancy are failure to gain weight despite good appetite, and persistent tachycardia. There is no increase in maternal mortality or morbidity in well-controlled patients; however, postpartum thyroid storm has been reported in about 20% of untreated individuals. Fetal loss is also more common, owing to the facts that spontaneous abortion and premature delivery are more common in untreated pregnant women, as are low-birth-weight infants and eclampsia. Transplacental passage of thyroid-stimulating antibodies may occur, causing fetal as well as neonatal hyperthyroidism.[79] An uncommon cause of hyperthyroidism is molar pregnancy; women present with a large-for-dates uterus and evacuation of the uterus is the preferred management approach.[80-84]

Because RAI is contraindicated in pregnancy and surgery is usually not recommended (especially during the first trimester), antithyroid drug therapy is usually the treatment of choice. Methimazole readily crosses the placenta and appears in breast milk.

PTU is considered to be the drug of choice in pregnancy, with the lowest possible doses used to maintain the maternal T_4 level in the high-normal range, but as described previously, there appears to be little difference between PTU and methimazole.[52] To prevent fetal goiter and suppression of fetal thyroid function, PTU is usually prescribed in daily doses of 300 mg or less and tapered to 50 to 150 mg daily after 4 to 6 weeks. PTU doses of less than 200 mg daily are unlikely to produce fetal goiter.[85] During the last trimester, TSAbs fall spontaneously, and some patients will go into remission so that antithyroid drug doses may be reduced. A rebound in maternal hyperthyroidism occurs in about 10% of women and may require more intensive treatment postpartum than in the last trimester of pregnancy.[79]

NEONATAL AND PEDIATRIC HYPERTHYROIDISM

Following delivery, some babies will be hyperthyroid owing to placental transfer of TSAbs, which stimulates thyroid hormone production in utero and postpartum.[86,87] This is likely if the maternal TSAb titers were quite high. The disease is usually expressed 7 to 10 days postpartum and treatment with antithyroid drugs (PTU 5 to 10 mg/kg per day or methimazole 0.5 to 1 mg/kg per day) may be needed for as long as 8 to 12 weeks until the antibody is cleared (immunoglobulin G half-life is about 2 weeks). Iodide (potassium iodide 1 drop/day or Lugol's solution 1 to 3 drops/day) and sodium ipodate may be used for the first few days to acutely inhibit hormone release.

Childhood hyperthyroidism is usually managed with either PTU or methimazole. Long-term follow-up studies suggest that this form of therapy is quite acceptable, with 25% of a cohort experiencing remission every 2 years.[88]

THYROID STORM

Thyroid storm is a life-threatening medical emergency characterized by severe thyrotoxicosis, high fever (often >103°F), tachycardia, tachypnea, dehydration, delirium, coma, nausea, vomiting, and diarrhea.[89,90] Precipitating factors for thyroid storm include infection, trauma, surgery, RAI treatment, and withdrawal from antithyroid drugs. It may occur at any age and has an average duration of 72 hours, although symptoms may persist up to 8 days if treatment is not aggressive. With aggressive treatment, the mortality rate has been lowered to 20%. The following therapeutic measures should be instituted promptly: (1) suppression of thyroid hormone formation and secretion, (2) antiadrenergic therapy, (3) administration of corticosteroids, and (4) treatment of associated complications or coexisting factors that may have precipitated the storm. Specific agents used in thyroid storm are outlined in Table 73–6. PTU in large doses is the preferred thionamide because it interferes with the production of thyroid hormones and blocks the peripheral conversion of T_4 to T_3. If patients are unable to take medications orally, the tablets can be crushed into suspension and instilled by gastric tube. Iodides, which

TABLE 73–6. Drug Dosages Used in the Management of Thyroid Storm

Drug	Regimen
Propylthiouracil	900–1200 mg/day orally in four or six divided doses
Methimazole	90–120 mg/day orally in four or six divided doses
Sodium iodide	Up to 2 g/day IV in single or divided doses
Lugol's solution	5–10 drops three times a day in water or juice
Saturated solution of potassium iodide	1–2 drops three times a day in water or juice
Propranolol	40–80 mg every 6 h
Dexamethasone	5–20 mg/day orally or IV in divided doses
Prednisone	25–100 mg/day orally in divided doses
Methylprednisolone	20–80 mg/day IV in divided doses
Hydrocortisone	100–400 mg/day IV in divided doses

rapidly block the release of preformed thyroid hormone, should be administered after PTU is initiated to inhibit iodide utilization by the overactive gland. If iodide is administered first, it could theoretically provide the substrate, permitting the synthesis and storage of a large amount of thyroid hormone in the thyroid gland, which would prolong the duration of hyperthyroidism thereafter.

Antiadrenergic therapy with the short-acting agent esmolol may be used in the patient with pulmonary disease or at risk for cardiac failure because its effects may be rapidly reversed.[91] Corticosteroids are generally recommended, although there is no convincing evidence of adrenocortical insufficiency in thyroid storm, and the benefits derived from steroids may be owing to their antipyretic action and their effect of stabilizing blood pressure.[92] General supportive measures, including acetaminophen as an antipyretic (do not use aspirin or other nonsteroidal anti-inflammatory agents because they may displace bound thyroid hormone), fluid and electrolyte replacement, sedatives, digitalis, antiarrhythmics, insulin, and antibiotics should be given as indicated. Plasmapheresis and peritoneal dialysis have been used to remove excess hormone when the patient has not responded to more conservative measures, although these measures do not always work.[93]

HYPOTHYROIDISM

Hypothyroidism is defined as the clinical and biochemical syndrome resulting from decreased thyroid hormone production.[94] Overt hypothyroidism occurs in 1.5% to 2% of women and 0.2% of men, and its incidence increases with age.[95–97] In the Third National Health and Nutrition Examination Survey, levels of serum thyroid-stimulating hormone (TSH) and total thyroxine (T4) were measured in a representative sample of adolescents and adults (age 12 or older). Among 16,533 people who neither were taking thyroid medication nor reported histories of thyroid disease, 3.9% had subclinical hypothyroidism (TSH >4.5 milli-international units/L; and T4 normal), and 0.2% had "clinically significant" hypothyroidism (TSH >4.5 milli-international units/L; and T4 <4.5 mcg/dL).[14] The vast majority of hypothyroid patients have thyroid gland failure (primary hypothyroidism). Special populations with higher risk of developing hypothyroidism include postpartum women, individuals with a family history of autoimmune thyroid disorders and patients with previous head and neck or thyroid irradiation or surgery, other autoimmune endocrine conditions (e.g., type 1 diabetes mellitus, adrenal insufficiency, and ovarian failure), some other nonendocrine autoimmune disorders (e.g., celiac disease, vitiligo, pernicious anemia, Sjögren's syndrome, and multiple sclerosis), primary pulmonary hypertension,

and Down's and Turner's syndromes.[94] Pituitary failure is an uncommon cause of hypothyroidism, but should be suspected in a patient with decreased levels of thyroxine and inappropriately normal or low TSH levels. Most patients with secondary hypothyroidism will have clinical signs of more generalized pituitary insufficiency, such as abnormal menses and decreased libido, or evidence of a pituitary adenoma, such as visual field defects, galactorrhea, or acromegaloid features. Generalized (peripheral and central) resistance to thyroid hormone is extremely rare.

Thyroid hormone is essential for normal growth and development during embryonic life. Thyroid hormone deficiency during fetal and neonatal development results in mental retardation. There is slowing of physical and mental activity, as well as of cardiovascular, gastrointestinal, and neuromuscular function. Depression may result from untreated hypothyroidism.[98]

CLINICAL PRESENTATION OF HYPOTHYROIDISM

GENERAL
Hypothyroidism can lead to a variety of end-organ effects and a wide range of disease severity, from entirely asymptomatic individuals to patients in coma with multisystem failure. In the adult, manifestations of hypothyroidism are varied and nonspecific. In the child, thyroid hormone deficiency may manifest as growth retardation.

SYMPTOMS
Common symptoms of hypothyroidism include dry skin, cold intolerance, weight gain, constipation, and weakness. Complaints of lethargy and fatigue or loss of ambition and energy are also common but are less specific. Muscle cramps, myalgia, and stiffness are frequent complaints of hypothyroid patients.

SIGNS
Objective weakness is common, with proximal muscles being affected more than distal muscles. Slow relaxation of deep tendon reflexes is common. The most common signs of decreased levels of thyroid hormone include coarse skin and hair, cold or dry skin, periorbital puffiness, and bradycardia. Speech is often slow as well as hoarse. Reversible neurologic syndromes such as carpal tunnel syndrome, polyneuropathy, and cerebellar dysfunction may also occur.

DIAGNOSIS
TSH serum concentration should be elevated.
Free and/or total T4 and T3 serum concentrations should be low.

OTHER TESTS
Antithyroid perioxidase antibodies and antithyroglobulin antibodies are likely to be elevated.

A rise in the TSH level is the first evidence of primary hypothyroidism. Many patients will have a T4 level within the normal range (compensated hypothyroidism) and few, if any, symptoms of hypothyroidism. As the disease progresses the T4 concentration will drop below the normal level. Interestingly, the T3 concentration will often be maintained in the normal range in spite of a low T4. The RAIU is not a useful test in the evaluation of a hypothyroid patient.

CAUSES OF HYPOTHYROIDISM

Table 73–7 outlines the causes of hypothyroidism.

TABLE 73–7. Causes of Hypothyroidism

Primary hypothyroidism
Hashimoto's disease
Iatrogenic hypothyroidism
Others
   Iodine deficiency
   Enzyme defects
   Thyroid hypoplasia
   Goitrogens
Secondary hypothyroidism
Pituitary disease
Hypothalamic disease

CHRONIC AUTOIMMUNE THYROIDITIS

Autoimmune thyroiditis (Hashimoto's disease) is the most common cause of spontaneous hypothyroidism in the adult. Patients may present with either goitrous thyroid gland enlargement and mild hypothyroidism, or thyroid gland atrophy and more severe thyroid hormone deficiency. Both forms of autoimmune thyroiditis probably result from cell- and antibody-mediated thyroid injury. The bulk of evidence suggests that the presence of specific defects in suppressor T-lymphocyte function leads to the survival of a randomly mutating clone of helper T lymphocytes, which are directed against normally occurring antigens on the thyroid membrane. Once these T lymphocytes interact with thyroid membrane antigen, B lymphocytes are stimulated to produce thyroid antibodies.[99,100]

Antimicrosomal antibodies are present in virtually all patients with Hashimoto's thyroiditis and appear to be directed against the enzyme thyroid peroxidase, thyroglobulin, and other thyroid cell-membrane antigens. These antibodies are capable of fixing complement and inducing cytotoxic changes in thyroid cells. Antibodies that are capable of stimulating thyroid growth are also present in the goitrous variety of Hashimoto's disease; conversely, antibodies that inhibit the trophic effects of TSH are present in the atrophic type.[101]

IATROGENIC HYPOTHYROIDISM

Iatrogenic hypothyroidism follows exposure to radiation (radioiodine or external radiation) or surgery. Hypothyroidism occurs within 3 months to a year after ^{131}I therapy in most patients treated for Graves' disease. Thereafter it occurs at a rate of approximately 2.5% each year. External radiation therapy to the region of the thyroid using doses of greater than 2500 rads for therapy of neck carcinoma also causes hypothyroidism. This effect is dose-dependent, and more than 50% of patients who receive more than 4000 rads to the thyroid bed develop hypothyroidism. Total thyroidectomy causes hypothyroidism within 1 month.

OTHER CAUSES OF PRIMARY HYPOTHYROIDISM

Iodine deficiency, enzymatic defects within the thyroid gland, thyroid hypoplasia, and maternal ingestion of goitrogens during fetal development may cause cretinism. Early recognition and treatment of the resultant thyroid hormone deficiency is essential for optimal mental development. Large-scale screening programs in North America, Europe, Japan, and Australia are now in place.[102,103] The frequency of congenital hypothyroidism in North America and Europe is 1 per 3500 to 4000 live births. In the United States, there are racial differences in the incidence of congenital hypothyroidism, with whites being affected seven times as frequently as blacks.[104–107]

In the adult, hypothyroidism may rarely be caused by iodine deficiency and goitrogens. Rarely, iodine ingestion in the form of expectorants can lead to hypothyroidism. In sensitive persons, the iodide blocks the synthesis of thyroid hormone, leading to an increased secretion of TSH, which causes thyroid enlargement.[4] Thus both iodine excess and iodine deficiency can cause decreased secretion of thyroid hormone.

CAUSES OF SECONDARY HYPOTHYROIDISM

Pituitary Disease

TSH is required for normal thyroid secretion. Thyroid atrophy and decreased thyroid secretion follow pituitary failure. Pituitary insufficiency may be caused by destruction of thyrotrophs by either functioning or nonfunctioning pituitary tumors, surgical therapy, external pituitary radiation, postpartum pituitary necrosis (Sheehan's syndrome), infiltrative processes of the pituitary such as metastatic tumors, tuberculosis, histiocytosis, and autoimmune mechanisms. In all these situations, TSH deficiency most often occurs in association with other pituitary hormone deficiencies.

In most hypothyroid patients with pituitary disease, serum TSH concentrations are low or normal. A serum TSH concentration in the normal range is clearly inappropriate if the patient's T_4 is low.

Note that pituitary enlargement in hypothyroidism does not invariably indicate the presence of a primary pituitary tumor. Pituitary enlargement is seen in patients with severe primary hypothyroidism owing to compensatory hyperplasia and hypertrophy of the thyrotrophs. Serum TSH concentrations and pituitary enlargement decline during thyroid hormone replacement therapy, indicating that the TSH secretion is not autonomous. These patients are easily separated from patients with primary pituitary failure by measuring a TSH level.

Hypothalamic Hypothyroidism

TRH deficiency also causes hypothyroidism. In both adults and children it may occur as a result of cranial irradiation, trauma, infiltrative diseases, or neoplastic diseases. Hypothalamic hypothyroidism is rare.

▶ TREATMENT: Hypothyroidism

▌ PHARMACOLOGIC THERAPY

▌ DESIRED OUTCOMES

The goals of therapy are to restore normal thyroid hormone concentrations in tissue, provide symptomatic relief, prevent neurologic deficits in newborns and children, and reverse the biochemical abnormalities of hypothyroidism.

▌ GENERAL APPROACH

Any of the commercially available thyroid preparations accomplish this goal (Table 73–8); however, levothyroxine (l-thyroxine) is considered to be drug of choice. The thyroid preparations are either natural (i.e., desiccated thyroid and thyroglobulin) or synthetic (levothyroxine, liothyronine, and liotrix) in origin. The availability of sensitive and specific assays for total and free hormone levels as well as TSH

TABLE 73–8. Thyroid Preparations Used in the Treatment of Hypothyroidism

Drug/Dosage Form	Content	Relative Dose	Comments/Equivalency
Thyroid USP Armour Thyroid (T_4:T_3 ratio) 9.5 mcg:2.25 mcg, 19 mcg:4.5 mcg, 38 mcg:9 mcg, 57 mcg:13.5 mcg, 76 mcg:18 mcg, 114 mcg:27 mcg, 152 mcg:36 mcg, 190 mcg:45 mcg tablets	Desiccated beef or pork thyroid gland	1 grain (equivalent to 60 mcg of T_4)	Unpredictable hormonal stability, inexpensive generic brands may not be bioequivalent
Thyroglobulin Proloid 32-mg, 65-mg, 100-mg, 130-mg, 200-mg tablets	Partially purified pork thyroglobulin	1 grain	Standardized biologically to give T_4:T_3 ratio of 2.5:1; more expensive than thyroid extract; no clinical advantage
Levothyroxine Synthroid, Levothroid, and other generics 25-, 50-, 75-, 88-, 100-, 112-, 125-, 137-, 150-, 175-, 200-, 300-mcg tablets; 200- and 500-mcg/vial injection Levoxyl, Thyro-Tabs, Unithroid	Synthetic T_4	50–60 mcg	Stable; predictable potency; generics are bioequivalent; when switching from natural thyroid to L-thyroxine, lower dose by 1/2 grain; variable absorption between products; half-life = 7 days, so daily dosing; considered to be drug of choice
Liothyronine Cytomel 5-, 25-, and 50-mcg tablets	Synthetic T_3	15–37.5 mcg	Uniform absorption, rapid onset; half-life = 1.5 days, monitor TSH assays
Liotrix Thyrolar 1/4-, 1/2-, 1-, 2-, and 3-strength tablets	Synthetic T_4:T_3 in 4:1 ratio	50–60 mcg T_4 and 12.5–15 mcg T_3	Stable; predictable; expensive; lacks therapeutic rationale because T_4 is converted to T_3 peripherally

TSH, thyroid-stimulating hormone.

now allow more definitive dose titration to allow adequate replacement without inadvertent overdose. The response of TSH to TRH had been advocated for use by some for "fine-tuning" thyroid replacement, but this is not necessary if the sensitive immunoradiometric assays for TSH are used. Minimum clinical guidelines for the treatment of hypothyroidism have been published by the American Thyroid Association.[42]

NATURAL THYROID HORMONES

Desiccated thyroid is derived from hog, beef, or sheep thyroid gland. The United States Pharmacopeia, 23th ed., requires Thyroid USP to contain 38 mcg (±15%) of levothyroxine and 9 mcg (±10%) of liothyronine for each 65 mg (1 grain) of the labeled content of thyroglobulin. Thyroglobulin USP should contain 36 mcg (±15%) of levothyroxine and 12 mcg (±10%) of liothyronine for each 65 mg (1 grain) of the labeled content of thyroglobulin. Not all generic brands may be bioequivalent, and switching among brands in patients stabilized on one product should be discouraged. Thyroid USP, as an animal protein–derived product, may be antigenic in allergic or sensitive patients. Even though desiccated thyroid is inexpensive, its limitations preclude it from being considered as a drug of choice for hypothyroid patients. Thyroglobulin is a purified hog-gland extract, but it has no clinical advantages and is not widely used.

SYNTHETIC THYROID HORMONES

Levothyroxine (T_4; l-thyroxine) is the drug of choice for thyroid replacement and suppressive therapy because it is chemically stable, relatively inexpensive, and free of antigenicity, and has uniform potency. Whereas T_3 and not T_4 is the biologically more active form of thyroid hormone, levothyroxine administration results in a pool of thyroid hormone that is readily and consistently converted to T_3; in this regard levothyroxine may be thought of as a prohormone. The half-life of levothyroxine is approximately 7 days. This long half-life is responsible for a stable pool of prohormone and the need for only once-daily dosing with levothyroxine. Older studies with levothyroxine suggested that bioavailability was low and erratic; however, this product has been reformulated and the average bioavailability is now approximately 80%.[108–110] The bioavailability of Synthroid, Levoxine, and generic levothyroxine preparations were compared in a blinded, randomized, four-way cross-over trial.[111] The study was sponsored by the manufacturers of Synthroid, who have challenged the authors' conclusions that the levothyroxine preparations are bioequivalent and should be interchangeable for the majority of patients. However, because the relationship between T_4 concentration and TSH is not linear, very small changes in T_4 concentration can lead to substantial changes in TSH, which is a more accurate reflection of hormone replacement status. To avoid over- and undertreatment, once a product is selected, therapeutic interchange should be discouraged. Currently, no products are AB rated for Synthroid. The time to maximal absorption is 2 hours, and this should be considered when T_4 and TSH concentrations are determined. Mucosal diseases such as sprue, diabetic diarrhea, and ileal bypass surgery may also reduce absorption. Cholestyramine, calcium carbonate, sucralfate, aluminum hydroxide,[112] ferrous sulfate,[113] soybean formula,[114] and dietary fiber supplements[115] may also impair the absorption of levothyroxine from the gastrointestinal tract. Drugs that increase nondeiodinative T_4 clearance include rifampin, carbamazepine, and possibly phenytoin. Selenium deficiency and amiodarone may block the conversion of T_4 to T_3.

Liothyronine (T_3) is chemically pure with known potency and has a shorter half-life of 1.5 days. Although it is widely used diagnostically in the T_3-suppression test, T_3 has some clinical disadvantages, including a higher incidence of cardiac adverse effects, higher cost, and difficulty in monitoring with conventional laboratory tests. Liotrix is a combination of synthetic T_4 and T_3 in a 4:1 ratio that attempts to mimic natural hormonal secretion. It is chemically stable and pure and has a predictable potency. The major limitations to this product are high cost and lack of therapeutic rationale, because about 35% of T_4 is peripherally converted T_3.

Recently a trial comparing levothyroxine alone to a combination of levothyroxine plus partial replacement with liothyronine (triiodothyronine) has been published.[116] Patients received a regimen in which 50 mcg of the usual dose of thyroxine was replaced by 12.5 mcg of triiodothyronine. The order in which each patient received the two treatments was randomized. Biochemical, physiologic, and psychological tests were performed at the end of each treatment period. Although lower serum free and total thyroxine concentrations and higher serum total triiodothyronine concentrations after treatment with thyroxine plus triiodothyronine were noted, the TSH concentrations were not significantly different. Cognitive function was higher on some rating scales, but neurophysiologic test scores were similar. In another recent trial of combination therapy, when compared with levothyroxine alone, treatment of primary hypothyroidism with combination levothyroxine plus liothyronine demonstrated no beneficial changes in body weight, serum lipid levels, hypothyroid symptoms as measured by a health-related quality of life questionnaire, and standard measures of cognitive performance.[117]

Dosing and Monitoring

During the mid-1980s the average dose of levothyroxine was about 160 mcg/day. With the advent of more sensitive assay methods for TSH and the reformulation of levothyroxine, it is now apparent that many patients have been treated with excessive amounts of levothyroxine. More recent studies suggest that the average maintenance dose for most adults should be closer to about 125 mcg per day.[94] Indeed, as many as one-third of patients receiving levothyroxine 150 mcg daily will be overreplaced. There is, however, a wide range of replacement doses, necessitating individualized therapy and appropriate monitoring to determine an adequate but not excessive dose.

The initial dose of levothyroxine is dependent on the patient's age, and the presence of associated disorders, as well as the severity and duration of hypothyroidism.[118] In young patients with long-standing disease and patients over age 45 without known cardiac disease, therapy should be initiated with 50 mcg daily of levothyroxine and increased to 100 mcg daily after 1 month. The recommended initial daily dose for older patients or those with known cardiac disease is 25 mcg per day titrated upward in increments of 25 mcg at monthly intervals to prevent stress on the cardiovascular system. Some patients may experience an exacerbation of angina with higher doses of thyroid hormone. Although the TSH is very sensitive for under- or overreplacement, clinicians often fail to alter the dose of T_4 based on TSH clearly outside of the normal range.[119]

Patients with subclinical hypothyroidism (seen more commonly in the elderly and particularly in women) have no or few signs or symptoms, normal serum T_3 and T_4 concentrations, and an elevated basal TSH concentration.[97] The prevalence of this disorder is thought to be about 8%, but the reported range is quite wide.[120,121] Although the treatment of subclinical hypothyroidism is controversial, patients presenting with marked elevations in TSH (>10 milli-international

units/L) and high titers of TSAb or prior treatment with ^{131}I may be most likely to benefit from treatment.[122] Other patients who may improve with replacement include those with mild symptoms of hypothyroidism and depression. It should be noted that some studies find that only one of four treated patients experienced improvement.[121] Conservative treatment goals in this situation would be to maintain serum T_4 and T_3 levels in the normal range and reduce TSH to a value of 1 milli-international unit/L.

❾ Once euthyroidism is attained, the daily maintenance dose of levothyroxine does not fluctuate greatly. As patients age, the dosing requirement may need to be reduced.[123] The ability to measure serum TSH concentrations has improved the accuracy with which thyroid hormone replacement can be monitored. Many clinicians now consider serum TSH concentration to be the most sensitive and specific monitoring parameter for adjustment of levothyroxine dose. Plasma TSH concentrations begin to fall within hours and are usually normalized within 2 weeks, but may take up to 6 weeks in some patients, depending on the baseline value. TSH and T_4 concentrations are both used to monitor therapy, and they should be checked every 6 weeks until a euthyroid state is achieved. Serum T_4 concentrations can be useful in detecting noncompliance, malabsorption, or changes in levothyroxine product bioequivalence. An elevated TSH concentration indicates insufficient replacement. The appropriate dose maintains the TSH concentration in the normal range. Thyroxine disposal is accelerated by nephritic syndrome, other severe systemic illnesses, and several antiseizure medications (phenobarbital, phenytoin, and carbamazepine) and rifampin. Pregnancy increases the thyroxine dose requirement in 75% of women, probably because of increased degradation by the placental deiodinase. Initiating postmenopausal hormone replacement therapy increases the dose needed in 35% of women, perhaps due to an increased circulating thyroxine-binding globulin level. Patient noncompliance with prescribed thyroxine, the most common cause of inadequate treatment, might be suspected in patients with a dose that is higher than expected, variable thyroid function test results that do not correlate well with prescribed doses, and an elevated serum thyrotropin concentration with serum free thyroxine at the upper end of the normal range, which can suggest improved compliance immediately before testing due to a lag in the thyrotropin response. The metabolism of other pharmacologic agents can be altered in patients with hypothyroidism. The mechanism might be decreased expression of hepatic enzymes involved in drug metabolism, as seen in hypothyroid rats. As a result, increased sensitivity to anesthetic and sedative agents, and higher serum levels of phenytoin have been reported. Hypothyroidism can also cause higher serum digoxin values, an effect attributed to a decreased volume of drug distribution. Conversely, hypothyroidism might decrease sensitivity to warfarin due to slowed metabolism of the vitamin K–dependent clotting factors, and restoration of euthyroidism can then increase the warfarin dose requirement.

In patients with hypothyroidism caused by hypothalamic or pituitary failure, alleviation of the clinical syndrome and restoration of serum T_4 to the normal range are the only criteria available for estimating the appropriate replacement dose of levothyroxine. Concurrent use of dopamine, dopaminergic agents (bromocriptine), somatostatin or somatostatin analogs (octreotide), and corticosteroids suppresses TSH concentrations and may confound the interpretation of this monitoring parameter.[124]

TSH-suppressive levothyroxine therapy may also be given to patients with nodular thyroid disease and diffuse goiter, to patients with a history of thyroid irradiation, and to patients with thyroid cancer. The rationale for suppression therapy is to reduce TSH secretion, which promotes growth and function in abnormal thyroid tissue. In patients with solitary nodules who have not received radiation, TSH should be suppressed to 0.05 to 0.1 milli-international unit/L in premenopausal women and in men <60 years old. A dose of levothyroxine of 100 to 150 mcg per day is usually sufficient. In men over 60 years of age and postmenopausal women, TSH levels should be reduced to 0.1 to 0.3 milli-international unit/L, owing to the risk of more serious adverse effects in this population and reduced clearance of levothyroxine with advanced age. Levothyroxine may be given in nontoxic multinodular goiter to suppress the TSH to low-normal levels of 0.5 to 1 milli-international unit/L if the baseline TSH is >1 milli-international unit/L. Goiter size and thyroid volume may be reduced with suppression therapy. Diffuse goiter associated with autoimmune thyroiditis may also be treated with levothyroxine to reduce goiter size and thyroid volume. In patients with follicular or papillary thyroid cancer, current recommendations are to suppress the TSH to <0.02 milli-international unit/L. Doses of levothyroxine of up to 2.2 to 2.5 mcg/kg may be needed to provide TSH levels of <0.02 milli-international unit/L in this population, and free T_3 and T_4 levels are useful in detecting hyperthyroidism.[125]

Adverse Effects

Serious untoward effects are unusual if dosing is appropriate and the patient is carefully monitored during initial treatment. Levothyroxine replacement in athyrotic hypothyroid patients restores systolic and diastolic left ventricular performance within 2 weeks, and the use of levothyroxine may increase the frequency of atrial premature beats, but not necessarily ventricular premature beats. Excessive doses of thyroid hormone may lead to heart failure, angina pectoris, and myocardial infarction; rarely, the latter may be caused by coronary artery spasm. Allergic or idiosyncratic reactions can occur with the natural animal-derived products such as desiccated thyroid and thyroglobulin, but these are extremely rare with the synthetic products used today. The 0.05-mg Synthroid tablet is the least allergenic (owing to a lack of dye and few excipients) and should be tried in the patient suspected to be allergic to thyroid hormone.

Hyperremodeling of cortical and trabecular bone due to hyperthyroidism leads to reduced bone density and may increase the risk of fracture. Compared with normal controls, excess exogenous thyroid hormone results in histomorphometric and biochemical changes similar to those observed in osteoporosis and untreated hyperthyroidism; however, at routinely used replacement doses, bone mineral density loss is less than that seen with untreated hyperthyroidism and only slightly greater than in controls.[126] The risk for this complication of therapy seems to be related to the dose of levothyroxine, patient age, and gender. Markers for bone turnover include urinary cross-linked N-telopeptides, pyridinoline of type I collagen, osteocalcin, and bone-specific alkaline phosphatase. When doses of levothyroxine are used to suppress TSH concentrations to below-normal values (less than 0.3 milli-international unit/L) in postmenopausal women, this adverse effect is more likely to be seen. Cortical bone is affected to a greater degree than trabecular bone at suppressive doses of l-thyroxine. In contrast, it appears to be much less likely in men and in premenopausal women. Maintaining the TSH between 0.7 and 1.5 milli-international units/L with approximately 150 mcg/day of levothyroxine does not alter bone mineral density in premenopausal women.

SPECIAL CONDITIONS

MYXEDEMA COMA

Myxedema coma is the end stage of long-standing, uncorrected hypothyroidism.[127] Clinical features include hypothermia, advanced stages of hypothyroid symptoms, and altered sensorium ranging from delirium to coma. Mortality rates of 60% to 70% necessitate immediate and aggressive therapy with intravenous bolus thyroxine 300 to 500 mcg. Glucocorticoid therapy with intravenous hydrocortisone 100 mg every 8 hours should be given until coexisting adrenal suppression is ruled out. Consciousness, lowered TSH concentrations, and normal vital signs are expected within 24 hours. Maintenance doses are typically 75 to 100 mcg given intravenously until the patient stabilizes and oral therapy is begun. Supportive therapy must be instituted to maintain adequate ventilation, euglycemia, blood pressure, and body temperature. Any underlying disorder, such as sepsis, myocardial infarction, and the like obviously must be diagnosed and treated.

CONGENITAL HYPOTHYROIDISM

In congenital hypothyroidism, full maintenance therapy should be instituted early to improve the prognosis for mental and physical development.[128] The average maintenance dose in infants and children depends on the age and weight of the child. Several studies demonstrate that aggressive therapy with levothyroxine is important for normal development and current recommendations are for initiation of therapy within 45 days of birth at a dose of 10 to 15 mcg/kg per day.[129] This dose is used to keep T_4 concentrations at about 10 mcg/dL within 30 days of starting therapy and is associated with improved IQs in treated infants. The dose is progressively decreased to a typical adult dose as the child ages, the adult dose being given in the age range of 11 to 20 years. In utero treatment of fetal goiter and hypothyroidism has been accomplished with the injection of thyroxine into the amniotic fluid.[130]

HYPOTHYROIDISM IN PREGNANCY

Hypothyroidism during pregnancy leads to an increased rate of stillbirths and possibly lower psychological scores in infants born of women who received inadequate replacement during pregnancy.[131,132] Thyroid hormone is necessary for fetal growth and must come from the maternal side during the first 2 months of gestation. Although liothyronine may cross the placental membrane slightly better than levothyroxine, the latter is considered to be the drug of choice. The objective of treatment is to decrease TSH to 1 unit/mL and maintain free T_4 concentrations in the normal range. Based on elevated TSH levels during pregnancy, it was found that the mean dose of levothyroxine had to be increased by 36 mcg/day to suppress TSH into the normal range. Increased production of binding proteins, a marginal decrease in free hormone concentration, modification of peripheral thyroid hormone metabolism, and increased thyroxine metabolism by the fetal-placental unit also contributes to increased thyroid hormone demand and the need for increased doses decreases after delivery.[77] Only about 20% of women need to have levothyroxine dose adjustment during pregnancy. After delivery the levothyroxine may need to be reduced based on T_3 concentrations and measurement of TSH.[133]

EFFECTS OF HYPOTHYROIDISM ON SELECTED MEDICATIONS

Hypothyroidism may affect the metabolism and clinical efficacy of several medications. Digitalis preparations have a decreased volume of distribution in the hypothyroid state, resulting in increased sensitivity to the digitalis effect. Therefore, many hypothyroid patients achieve a therapeutic effect at lower digitalis doses. Insulin degradation may be delayed in hypothyroidism, thereby requiring a lower insulin dose. Hypothyroidism delays the catabolism of clotting factors, and if a patient stabilized on warfarin is made euthyroid with levothyroxine, the patient may become excessively anticoagulated. Respiratory depressants such as barbiturates, phenothiazines, and opioid analgesics should be avoided, because increased sensitivity may increase carbon dioxide retention and precipitate myxedema coma.

RECOMBINANT TSH IN THYROID CANCER

Patients with previously treated thyroid carcinoma require lifelong monitoring for recurrent disease.[134,135] Two diagnostic tests that play a central role in follow-up of these patients—radioiodine whole body scanning and serum thyroglobulin measurement—are most accurate during thyroid-stimulating hormone (TSH) stimulation. Temporary discontinuation of thyroid hormone therapy was previously the sole effective approach for TSH-stimulated testing. However, hormone withdrawal was associated with the morbidity of hypothyroidism and occasional tumor progression. The introduction of recombinant TSH (rTSH)-stimulated testing offers an alternative therapy. Recent clinical trials have shown that the sensitivity of combined rTSH-stimulated radioiodine scanning and serum thyroglobulin measurement has equivalent sensitivity to testing after thyroid hormone withdrawal. Furthermore, measurement of the rTSH-stimulated thyroglobulin concentration is a more sensitive way to detect residual thyroid cancer or normal tissue than thyroglobulin measurement or thyroid hormone therapy alone.

NONTHYROIDAL ILLNESS

A wide variety of abnormalities of pituitary-thyroid function, serum thyroid hormone binding, and extrathyroidal thyroid hormone metabolism occur in patients with nonthyroidal illness. These abnormalities frequently result in decreased serum T_3 concentrations and less often lead to a decreased serum T_4 concentration. Serum TSH concentrations are usually within the normal range. The presence of coexisting primary hypothyroidism can be recognized in patients who have other illnesses by an elevation in the TSH concentration.

The degree and extent of the abnormality in thyroid function generally correlates with the severity of the nonthyroidal illness. These conditions are frequently referred to as the "euthyroid sick syndrome." It is likely that these changes represent adaptive forms of hypothyroidism that serve to reduce the availability of thyroid hormones to lessen the impact of the nonthyroidal illness.[136]

Decreased serum T_3 concentrations occur in patients with both acute and chronic illnesses. The fundamental cause of decreased serum T_3 concentrations in these situations is decreased extrathyroidal conversion of T_4 to T_3. This reaction is normally mediated by T_4-5'-deiodinase. A circulating inhibitor of this enzyme, perhaps interleukin-6, is present in patients with nonthyroidal illness.[137] Serum total and free T_4 concentrations are usually normal. The serum reverse T_3 concentration is characteristically high because the same enzyme, 5'-deiodinase, that is necessary to convert T_4 to T_3, is necessary to convert reverse T_3 to its breakdown products. Acute respiratory infections and surgery acutely elevate interleukin-6, and T_3 concentration is inversely correlated.[138]

Low serum T_4 is seen in most critically ill patients. This change is caused by diminished serum T_4 binding, resulting either from decreased serum concentrations of thyroid-binding globulin, thyroid-binding prealbumin, or albumin, or from inhibitors of T_4 binding. The free T_4 concentration is generally normal. This more severe degree of hypothyroidism, which occurs in severely ill patients, produces a greater reduction in thyroid hormone availability. The low serum T_4 concentrations in patients with nonthyroidal illness indicates a grave prognosis. In two studies, more than 60% of hospitalized patients with a low serum free T_4 index died. T_4 or T_3 supplementation has been of no benefit in this situation and in fact has increased morbidity.

To confuse matters, some patients with nonthyroidal illness have elevation of their serum T_4 concentration. Most commonly, this is seen in patients with psychiatric disorders during acute psychotic breaks. Thyroid hormone levels return to normal within 2 weeks after successful treatment of the underlying psychiatric disease. The occurrence of these abnormalities requires that care be taken in diagnosing hypothyroidism or hyperthyroidism in patients who have nonthyroidal illnesses.

GOITROUS THYROID DISEASE

Endemic goiter is the major thyroid disease throughout the world, affecting more than 200 million people. Many goitrous glands contain one or more nodules. The introduction of iodide supplementation has eliminated goiter as a major medical problem in developed countries, though it continues to be a problem in developing countries whose geographic position makes them more susceptible to iodide deficiency. In 1924, Marine postulated that periods of iodide deficiency resulted in cyclic hyperplasia and involution of thyroid follicular cells with eventual development of nodular hyperplasia.[102] This hypothesis is still used to explain goiter formation today. Whatever the specific cause, the final common pathway appears to result from an inadequate thyroid hormone secretion with compensatory TSH secretion and eventual thyroid gland enlargement. The essential factor for the conversion of a hyperplastic iodine-deficiency goiter into a colloid goiter appears to be an acute reduction of TSH stimulation; therefore, any situation that would result in a cyclical increase and decrease in TSH secretion might eventually result in the production of a nodular goiter.

There has been an interest in the possibility that growth factors other than TSH play a role in the development of a goiter. Immunoglobulin fractions capable of stimulating thyroid growth have been found in patients with nontoxic goiter and Graves' disease. In these patients, thyroid growth–promoting immunoglobulin titers correlates with goiter size rather than with the thyroid hormone concentration.

Sporadic goiter is defined as a goiter occurring in a nonendemic goiter region. Although a number of known goitrogens and errors in thyroid hormone biosynthesis may cause goiter, the majority of cases of sporadic goiter have no known etiology.

Treatment of all goiters is a trial of thyroid hormone suppression in an effort to eliminate TSH as a possible stimulus for continued thyroid growth. Large, long-standing goiters seldom undergo significant reduction in size. If the patient is symptomatic (with dysphagia dyspnea) or there is a question of malignant thyroid involvement, urgery is recommended.

PHARMACOECONOMIC CONSIDERATIONS

lthough the initial expense of surgery would seem to make it the nost expensive treatment option, the relapse rates for thionamides nd RAI are higher and in longer-term follow-up, there is not much ifference between treatment options nor patients' opinions concern- ng treatment preferences.[139] The cost proportion between the medical nd surgical treatment in younger patients is 1:2.5 (1 = $1126 U.S.) efore and 1:1.3 (1 = $2284 U.S.) after inclusion of the relapse costs. he proportion between the medical, surgical, and ^{131}I treatment in lder patients is 1:2.5:1.6 (1 = $1164 U.S.) before and 1:1.6:1.4 1 = $1972 U.S.) after inclusion of the relapse costs.

CLINICAL CONTROVERSIES

Although the current FDA standards of bioavailability for thy- roxine products suggest that several products are bioequiv- alent, the relationship between T_4 serum concentration and TSH response suggests that the products are not truly bio- equivalent. New standards of bioequivalency may need to be developed for drug products like thyroxine.

Combination therapy of $T_4 + T_3$ for hypothyroidism seems to improve cognitive function over monotherapy with T_4; however, there are not corresponding improvements in biochemical markers of thyroid hormone nor differences in TSH response.

Multiple studies have addressed the role of thyroid supplemen- ation in critically ill patients with cardiac disease, sepsis, pulmonary isease (e.g., acute respiratory distress syndrome), or severe infection, r with burn and trauma patients. In spite of a very large number of ublished studies, it is very difficult to form clear recommendations or treatment with thyroid hormone in the intensive care unit.

EVALUATION OF THERAPEUTIC OUTCOMES

Patients on optimal thyroid hormone replacement therapy should have SH and free T_4 serum concentrations in the normal range with id- opathic hypothyroidism and Hashimoto's thyroiditis. Those who are eing treated for thyroid cancer should have TSH suppressed to very ow levels and thyroglobin should be undetectable. Given the half-life f 7 days of T_4, the appropriate monitoring interval is no more of- en than 4 weeks. The signs and symptoms of hypothyoidism should e improved or absent (see clinical presentation of hypothyroidism, bove), although this may take several months for most to improve.

ABBREVIATIONS

ClO$_4$$^-$: perchlorate
DIT: diiodotyrosine
FSH: follicle-stimulating hormone
G$_s$α: the α subunit of the stimulatory guanine-nucleotide-binding protein
hCG: human chorionic gonadotropin
HLA: human leukocyte antigen
[131]I: sodium iodide 131
L-thyroxine: levothyroxine

LH: luteinizing hormone
MIT: monoiodotyrosine
MMI: methimazole
MNG: multinodular goiter
PRTH: pituitary resistance to thyroid hormone
PTU: propylthiouracil
RAI: radioactive iodine
RAIU: radioactive iodine uptake
rTSH: recombinant thyroid-stimulating hormone
SCN$^-$: thiocyanate
SSKI: saturated solution of potassium iodide
T_3: triiodothyronine
T_4: thyroxine
TBG: thyroid-binding globulin
TBPA: thyroid-binding prealbumin
TcO$_4$$^-$: pertechnetate
TG: thyroglobulin
TRβ2, TRβ1, TRα1: thyroid hormone receptors
TRH: thyrotropin-releasing hormone
TSAb: thyroid-stimulating antibody
TSH: thyroid-stimulating hormone

Review Questions and other resources can be found at *www.pharmacotherapyonline.com.*

REFERENCES

1. Cavalieri RR. Iodine metabolism and thyroid physiology: Current con- cepts. Thyroid 1997;7:177–181.
2. Arvan P, Kim PS, Kuliawat R, et al. Intracellular protein transport to the thyrocyte plasma membrane: Potential implications for thyroid physiol- ogy. Thyroid 1997;7:89–105.
3. De La Vieja A, Dohan O, Levy O, Carrasco N. Molecular analysis of the sodium/iodide symporter: Impact on thyroid and extrathyroid patho- physiology. Physiol Rev 2000;80:1083–1105.
4. Wolf J. Perchlorate and the thyroid gland. Pharmacol Rev 1998;50: 89–105.
5. Motomura K, Brent GA. Mechanisms of thyroid hormone action. Im- plications for the clinical manifestation of thyrotoxicosis. Endocrinol Metab Clin North Am 1998;27:1–23.
6. Salvatore D, Tu H, Harney JW, Larsen PR. Type 2 iodothyronine deio- dinase is highly expressed in human thyroid. J Clin Invest 1996;98: 962–968.
7. Salvatore D, Low SC, Berry M, et al. Type 3 Iodothyronine deiodinase: Cloning, in vitro expression, and functional analysis of the placental selenoenzyme. J Clin Invest 1995;96:2421–2430.
8. Paschke R, Ludgate M. The thyrotropin receptor in thyroid diseases. N Engl J Med 1997;337:1675–1681.
9. Leclere J, Bene MC, Aubert V, et al. Clinical consequences of activating germline mutations of TSH receptor, the concept of toxic hyperplasia. Horm Res 1997;47:158–162.
10. Brent GA. Thyroid hormone action: Down novel paths. Focus on "thy- roid hormone induces activation of mitogen-activated protein kinase in cultured cells." Am J Physiol 1999;276:C1012–C1013.
11. Apriletti JW, Ribeiro RC, Wagner RL, et al. Molecular and structural biology of thyroid hormone receptors. Clin Exp Pharmacol Physiol Suppl 1998;25:S2–S11.
12. Gonzalez-Sancho JM, Garcia V, Bonilla F, Munoz A. Thyroid hormone receptors/THR genes in human cancer. Cancer Lett 2003;192:121–132.
13. Cooper DS. Hyperthyroidism. Lancet 2003;362:459–468.
14. Hollowell JGJ. Serum TSH, T_4, and thyroid antibodies in the United States population (1988 to 1994): National Health and Nutrition Ex- amination Survey (NHANES III). J Clin Endocrinol Metab 2002;87: 489–499.

15. Ladenson PW, Singer PA, Ain KB, et al. American Thyroid Association guidelines for detection of thyroid dysfunction. Arch Intern Med 2000;160:1573–1575.

16. Russo D, Arturi F, Chiefari E, Filetti S. Molecular insights into TSH receptor abnormality and thyroid disease. J Endocrinol Invest 1997;20: 36–47.

17. Beck-Peccoz P, Brucker-Davis F, Persani L, et al. Thyrotropin-secreting pituitary tumors. Endocr Rev 1996;17:610–638.

18. Beck-Peccoz P, Persani L, Mantovani S, et al. Thyrotropin-secreting pituitary adenomas. Metab Clin Exp 1996;45:75–79.

19. Refetoff S. Resistance to thyroid hormone. Curr Ther Endocrinol Metab 1997;6:132–134.

20. Kannan CR, Seshadri KG. Thyrotoxicosis. Dis Mon 1997;43:601–677.

21. Weetman AP. Graves' disease. N Engl J Med 2000;343:1236–1248.

22. Wartofsky L. Radioiodine therapy for Graves' disease: Case selection and restrictions recommended to patients in North America. Thyroid 1997;7:213–216.

23. Prummel MF, Wiersinga WM. Medical management of Graves' ophthalmopathy. Thyroid 1995;5:231–234.

24. Ginsberg J. Diagnosis and management of Graves' disease [see comment]. Can Med Assoc J 2003;168:575–585.

25. Kodali VR, Jeffcote B, Clague RB. Thyrotoxic periodic paralysis: A case report and review of the literature. J Emerg Med 1999;17:43–45.

26. Fantz CR, Dagogo-Jack S, Ladenson JH, Gronowski AM. Thyroid function during pregnancy. Clin Chem 1999;45:2250–2258.

27. Siegel RD, Lee SL. Toxic nodular goiter. Toxic adenoma and toxic multinodular goiter. Endocrinol Metab Clin North Am 1998;27: 151–168.

28. Mazzaferri EL. Evaluation and management of common thyroid disorders in women. Am J Obstet Gynecol 1997;176:507–514.

29. Tonacchera M, Pinchera A. Thyrotropin receptor polymorphisms and thyroid diseases. J Clin Endocrinol Metab 2000;85:2637–2639.

30. Koutras DA. Subclinical hyperthyroidism. Thyroid 1999;9:311–315.

31. Slatosky J, Shipton B, Wahba H. Thyroiditis: Differential diagnosis and management. Am Fam Physician 2000;61:1047–1052, 1054.

32. Kennedy JW, Caro JF. The ABCs of managing hyperthyroidism in the older patient. Geriatrics 1996;51:22–24, 27, 31–32.

33. Dardik RB, Dardik M, Westra W, Montz FJ. Malignant struma ovarii: Two case reports and a review of the literature. Gynecol Oncol 1999;73: 447–451.

34. Braverman LE. Evaluation of thyroid status in patients with thyrotoxicosis. Clin Chem 1996;42:174–178.

35. Ross DS. Syndromes of thyrotoxicosis with low radioactive iodine uptake. Endocrino Metab Clin North Am 1998;27:169–185.

36. Loh KC. Amiodarone-induced thyroid disorders: A clinical review. Postgrad Med J 2000;76:133–140.

37. Bogazzi F, Bartalena L, Cosci C, et al. Treatment of type II amiodarone-induced thyrotoxicosis by either iopanoic acid or glucocorticoids: A prospective, randomized study. J Clin Endocrinol Metab 2003;88: 1999–2002.

38. Ajjan RA, Watson PF, Weetman AP. Cytokines and thyroid function. Adv Neuroimmunol 1996;6:359–386.

39. Lazarus JH, Obuobie K. Thyroid disorders—an update. Postgrad Med J 2000;76:529–536.

40. Woeber KA. Update on the management of hyperthyroidism and hypothyroidism. Arch Family Med 2000;9:743–747.

41. Franklyn JA. Management guidelines for hyperthyroidism. Baillieres Clin Endocrinol Metab 1997;11:561–571.

42. Singer PA, Cooper DS, Levy EG, et al. Treatment guidelines for patients with hyperthyroidism and hypothyroidism. Standards of Care Committee, American Thyroid Association. JAMA 1995;273:808–812.

43. Surks MI, Ortiz E, Daniels GH, et al. Subclinical thyroid disease: Scientific review and guidelines for diagnosis and management [see comment]. JAMA 2004;291:228–238.

44. Gittoes NJ, Franklyn JA. Hyperthyroidism. Current treatment guidelines. Drugs 1998;55:543–553.

45. Hegedus L, Bonnema SJ, Bennedbaek FN. Management of simple nodular goiter: Current status and future perspectives. Endocr Rev 2003;24: 102–132.

46. Carella C, Mazziotti G, Rotondi M, et al. Iodized salt improves the effectiveness of L-thyroxine therapy after surgery for nontoxic goitre: A prospective and randomized study. Clin Endocrinol 2002;57:507–513.

47. Alsanea O, Clark OH. Treatment of Graves' disease: The advantages of surgery. Endocrinol Metab Clin North Am 2000;29:321–337.

48. Gough IR, Wilkinson D. Total thyroidectomy for management of thyroid disease. World J Surg 2000;24:962–965.

49. Witte J, Goretzki PE, Dotzenrath C, et al. Surgery for Graves' disease: Total versus subtotal thyroidectomy—results of a prospective randomized trial. World J Surg 2000;24:1303–1311.

50. Cooper DS. Antithyroid drugs for the treatment of hyperthyroidism caused by Graves' disease. Endocrinol Metab Clin North Am 1998;27: 225–247.

51. Woeber KA. The year in review: The thyroid. Ann Intern Med 1999; 131:959–962.

52. Momotani N, Noh JY, Ishikawa N, Ito K. Effects of propylthiouracil and methimazole on fetal thyroid status in mothers with Graves' hyperthyroidism. J Endocrinol Metab 1997;82:3633–3636.

53. Raber W, Kmen E, Waldhausl W, Vierhapper H. Medical therapy of Graves' disease: Effect on remission rates of methimazole alone and in combination with triiodothyronine. Eur J Endocrinol 2000;142:117–124.

54. Rittmaster RS, Abbott EC, Douglas R, et al. Effect of methimazole, with or without L-thyroxine, on remission rates in Graves' disease. J Clin Endocrinol Metab 1998;83:814–818.

55. McIver B, Rae P, Beckett G, et al. Lack of effect of thyroxine in patients with Graves' hyperthyroidism who are treated with an antithyroid drug. N Engl J Med 1996;334:220–224.

56. Werner MC, Romaldini JH, Bromberg N, et al. Adverse effects related to thionamide drugs and their dose regimen. Am J Med Sci 1989;297: 216–219.

57. Bartalena L, Bogazzi F, Martino E. Adverse effects of thyroid hormone preparations and antithyroid drugs. Drug Saf 1996;15:53–63.

58. Tamai H, Sudo T, Kimura A, et al. Association between the DRB1*08032 histocompatibility antigen and methimazole-induced agranulocytosis in Japanese patients with Graves disease. Ann Intern Med 1996;124: 490–494.

59. Fukata S, Kuma K, Sugawara M. Granulocyte colony-stimulating factor (G-CSF) does not improve recovery from antithyroid drug-induced agranulocytosis: A prospective study. Thyroid 1999;9:29–31.

60. Tamai H, Mukuta T, Matsubayashi S, et al. Treatment of methimazole-induced agranulocytosis using recombinant human granulocyte colony-stimulating factor (rhG-CSF). J Clin Endocrinol Metab 1993;77: 1356–1360.

61. Woeber KA. Methimazole-induced hepatotoxicity. Endocr Pract 2002;8:222–224.

62. Mizutani T, Yoshida K, Murakami M, et al. Evidence for the involvement of N-methylthiourea, a ring cleavage metabolite, in the hepatotoxicity of methimazole in glutathione-depleted mice: Structure-toxicity and metabolic studies. Chem Res Toxicol 2000;13:170–176.

63. Gurlek A, Cobankara V, Bayraktar M. Liver tests in hyperthyroidism: Effect of antithyroid therapy. J Clin Gastroenterol 1997;24:180–183.

64. Benelhadj S, Marcellin P, Castelnau C, et al. Incidence of dysthyroidism during interferon therapy in chronic hepatitis C. Horm Res 1997;48: 209–214.

65. Van Dijke CP, Heydendael RJ, De Kleine MJ. Methimazole, carbimazole, and congenital skin defects. Ann Intern Med 1987;106:60–61.

66. Stanbury JB, Ermans AE, Bourdoux P, et al. Iodine-induced hyperthyroidism: Occurrence and epidemiology. Thyroid 1998;8:83–100.

67. Kaplan MM, Meier DA, Dworkin HJ. Treatment of hyperthyroidism with radioactive iodine. Endocrinol Metab Clin North Am 1998;27:205–223.

68. Bartalena L, Marcocci C, Bogazzi F, et al. Relation between therapy for hyperthyroidism and the course of Graves' ophthalmopathy. N Engl J Med 1998;338:73–78.

69. Tallstedt L, Lundell G. Radioiodine treatment, ablation, and ophthalmopathy: A balanced perspective. Thyroid 1997;7:241–245.

70. Lazarus JH, Clarke S. Use of radioiodine in the management of hyperthyroidism in the UK: development of guidelines. Thyroid 1997;7:229–231.

71. Franklyn JA, Maisonneuve P, Sheppard M, et al. Cancer incidence and mortality after radioiodine treatment for hyperthyroidism: A population-based cohort study. Lancet 1999;353:2111–2115.

72. Franklyn JA, Maisonneuve P, Sheppard MC, et al. Mortality after the treatment of hyperthyroidism with radioactive iodine. N Engl J Med 1998;338:712–718.

73. Leslie WD, Ward L, Salamon EA, et al. A randomized comparison of radioiodine doses in Graves' hyperthyroidism [see comment]. J Clin Endocrinol Metab 2003;88:978–983.

74. Franklyn JA. The management of hyperthyroidism. N Engl J Med 1994;330:1731–1738.

75. Uy HL, Reasner CA, Samuels MH. Pattern of recovery of the hypothalamic-pituitary-thyroid axis following radioactive iodine therapy in patients with Graves' disease. Am J Med 1995;99:173–179.

76. Mestman JH. Hyperthyroidism in pregnancy. Endocrinol Metab Clin North Am 1998;27:127–149.

77. Glinoer D. What happens to the normal thyroid during pregnancy? Thyroid 1999;9:631–635.

78. Lazarus JH, Kokandi A. Thyroid disease in relation to pregnancy: A decade of change. Clin Endocrinol 2000;53:265–278.

79. Momotani N, Noh J, Ishikawa N, Ito K. Relationship between silent thyroiditis and recurrent Graves' disease in the postpartum period. J Clin Endocrinol Metab 1994;79:285–289.

80. Coukos G, Makrigiannakis A, Chung J, et al. Complete hydatidiform mole. A disease with a changing profile. J Reprod Med 1999;44:698–704.

81. Ngowngarmratana S, Sunthornthepvarakul T, Kanchanawat S. Thyroid function and human chorionic gonadotropin in patients with hydatidiform mole. J Med Assoc Thailand 1997;80:693–699.

82. Ayhan A, Tuncer ZS, Halilzade H, Kucukali T. Predictors of persistent disease in women with complete hydatidiform mole. J Reprod Med 1996;41:591–594.

83. Soto-Wright V, Bernstein M, Goldstein DP, Berkowitz RS. The changing clinical presentation of complete molar pregnancy. Obstet Gynecol 1995;86:775–779.

84. Goldstein DP, Berkowitz RS. Current management of complete and partial molar pregnancy. J Reprod Med 1994;39:139–146.

85. Momotani N, Yamashita R, Makino F, et al. Thyroid function in wholly breast-feeding infants whose mothers take high doses of propylthiouracil. Clin Endocrinol 2000;53:177–181.

86. Zimmerman D, Lteif AN. Thyrotoxicosis in children. Endocrinol Metab Clin North Am 1998;27:109–126.

87. Zimmerman D. Fetal and neonatal hyperthyroidism. Thyroid 1999;9:727–733.

88. Segni M, Leonardi E, Mazzoncini B, et al. Special features of Graves' disease in early childhood. Thyroid 1999;9:871–877.

89. Dillmann WH. Thyroid storm. Curr Ther Endocrinol Metab 1997;6:81–85.

90. Ringel MD. Management of hypothyroidism and hyperthyroidism in the intensive care unit. Crit Care Clin 2001;17:59–74.

91. Knighton JD, Crosse MM. Anaesthetic management of childhood thyrotoxicosis and the use of esmolol. Anaesthesia 1997;52:67–70.

92. Burch HB, Wartofsky L. Life-threatening thyrotoxicosis. Thyroid storm. Endocrinol Metab Clin North Am 1993;22:263–277.

93. Samaras K, Marel GM. Failure of plasmapheresis, corticosteroids and thionamides to ameliorate a case of protracted amiodarone-induced thyroiditis. Clin Endocrinol 1996;45:365–368.

94. Roberts CG, Ladenson PW. Hypothyroidism [see comment]. Lancet 2004;363:793–803.

95. Wang C, Crapo LM. The epidemiology of thyroid disease and implications for screening. Endocrinol Metab Clin North Am 1997;26:189–218.

96. Arem R, Escalante D. Subclinical hypothyroidism: Epidemiology, diagnosis, and significance. Adv Intern Med 1996;41:213–250.

97. Adlin V. Subclinical hypothyroidism: Deciding when to treat. Am Fam Physician 1998;57:776–780.

98. Stagnaro-Green A. Recognizing, understanding, and treating postpartum thyroiditis. Endocrinol Metab Clin North Am 2000;29:417–430, ix.

99. Mukuta T, Yoshikawa N, Arreaza G, et al. Activation of T lymphocyte subsets by synthetic TSH receptor peptides and recombinant glutamate decarboxylase in autoimmune thyroid disease and insulin-dependent diabetes. J Clin Endocrinol Metab 1995;80:1264–1272.

100. Roura-Mir C, Catalfamo M, Sospedra M, et al. Single-cell analysis of intrathyroidal lymphocytes shows differential cytokine expression in Hashimoto's and Graves' disease. Eur J Immunol 1997;27:3290–3302.

101. Kasagi K, Kousaka T, Higuchi K, et al. Clinical significance of measurements of antithyroid antibodies in the diagnosis of Hashimoto's thyroiditis: comparison with histological findings. Thyroid 1996;6:445–450.

102. Delange F. Iodine deficiency in Europe and its consequences: An update. Eur J Nucl Med Mol Imaging 2002;29:S404–S416.

103. But B, Chan CW, Chan F, et al. Consensus statement on iodine deficiency disorders in Hong Kong. Hong Kong Med J 2003;9:446–453.

104. Grant DB. Congenital hypothyroidism: Optimal management in the light of 15 years' experience of screening. Arch Dis Child 1995;72:85–89.

105. Glinoer D, Delange F. The potential repercussions of maternal, fetal, and neonatal hypothyroxinemia on the progeny. Thyroid 2000;10:871–887.

106. Mestman JH. Diagnosis and management of maternal and fetal thyroid disorders. Curr Opin Obstet Gynecol 1999;11:167–175.

107. Gruters A, Krude H, Biebermann H, et al. Alterations of neonatal thyroid function. Acta Paediatr Suppl 1999;88:17–22.

108. Blouin RA, Clifton GD, Adams MA, et al. Biopharmaceutical comparison of two levothyroxine sodium products. Clin Pharm 1989;8:588–592.

109. Berg JA, Mayor GH. A study in normal human volunteers to compare the rate and extent of levothyroxine absorption from Synthroid and Levoxine. J Clin Pharmacol 1992;32:1135–1140.

110. Gottwald R, Lorkowski G, Petersen G, et al. Bioequivalence of two commercially available levothyroxine-Na preparations in athyreotic patients. Methods Find Exp Clin Pharmacol 1994;16:645–650.

111. Dong BJ, Hauck WW, Gambertoglio JG, et al. Bioequivalence of generic and brand-name levothyroxine products in the treatment of hypothyroidism. JAMA 1997;277:1205–1213.

112. Liel Y, Sperber AD, Shany S. Nonspecific intestinal adsorption of levothyroxine by aluminum hydroxide. Am J Med 1994;97:363–365.

113. Shakir KM, Chute JP, Aprill BS, Lazarus AA. Ferrous sulfate-induced increase in requirement for thyroxine in a patient with primary hypothyroidism. South Med J 1997;90:637–639.

114. Jabbar MA, Larrea J, Shaw RA. Abnormal thyroid function tests in infants with congenital hypothyroidism: The influence of soy-based formula. J Am Coll Nutr 1997;16:280–282.

115. Liel Y, Harman-Boehm I, Shany S. Evidence for a clinically important adverse effect of fiber-enriched diet on the bioavailability of levothyroxine in adult hypothyroid patients. J Clin Endocrinol Metab 1996;81:857–859.

116. Bunevicius R, Kazanavicius G, Zalinkevicius R, Prange AJ Jr. Effects of thyroxine as compared with thyroxine plus triiodothyronine in patients with hypothyroidism. N Engl J Med 1999;340:424–429.

117. Clyde PW, Harari AE, Getka EJ, Shakir KM. Combined levothyroxine plus liothyronine compared with levothyroxine alone in primary hypothyroidism: A randomized controlled trial [see comment]. JAMA 2003;290:2952–2958.

118. Kabadi UM. Influence of age on optimal daily levothyroxine dosage in patients with primary hypothyroidism grouped according to etiology. South Med J 1997;90:920–924.

119. De Whalley P. Do abnormal thyroid stimulating hormone level values result in treatment changes? A study of patients on thyroxine in one general practice. Br J Gen Pract 1995;45:93–95.

120. Kabadi UM, Cech R. Normal thyroxine and elevated tyrotropin concentrations: Evolving hypothyroidism or persistent euthyroidism with reset thyrostat. J Endocrinol Invest 1997;20:319–326.

121. Jaeschke R, Guyatt G, Gerstein H, et al. Does treatment with L-thyroxine influence health status in middle-aged and older adults with subclinical hypothyroidism? J Gen Intern Med 1996;11:744–749.

122. Zulewski H, Muller B, Exer P, et al. Estimation of tissue hypothyroidism by a new clinical score: Evaluation of patients with various grades of hypothyroidism and controls. J Clin Endocrinol Metab 1997;82: 771–776.

123. Lindsay RS, Toft AD. Hypothyroidism. Lancet 1997;349:413–417.

124. Behnia M, Gharib H. Primary care diagnosis of thyroid disease. Hosp Pract (Office Ed) 1996;31:121–126, 131–134.

125. Taimela E, Koskinen P, Nuutila P, et al. Free thyroid hormones and a third-generation TSH assay in the detection of hyperthyroidism during long-term thyroxine treatment in thyroid carcinoma patients. Scand J Clin Lab Invest 1995;55:181–186.

126. Rosen CJ. Endocrine disorders and osteoporosis. Curr Opin Rheumatol 1997;9:355–361.

127. Fliers E, Wiersinga WM. Myxedema coma. Rev Endocr Metab Disord 2003;4:137–141.

128. Rovet J, Daneman D. Congenital hypothyroidism: A review of current diagnostic and treatment practices in relation to neuropsychologic outcome. Paediatr Drugs 2003;5:141–149.

129. Anonymous. American Academy of Pediatrics AAP Section on Endocrinology and Committee on Genetics, and American Thyroid Association Committee on Public Health: Newborn screening for congenital hypothyroidism: Recommended guidelines. Pediatrics 1993;91: 1203–1209.

130. Bruner JP, Dellinger EH. Antenatal diagnosis and treatment of fetal hypothyroidism. A report of two cases. Fetal Diagn Ther 1997;12:200–204.

131. Atkins P, Cohen SB, Phillips BJ. Drug therapy for hyperthyroidism in pregnancy: Safety issues for mother and fetus. Drug Saf 2000;2: 229–244.

132. Montoro MN. Management of hypothyroidism during pregnancy. Cli Obstet Gynecol 1997;40:65–80.

133. Girling JC. Thyroid disease in pregnancy. Hosp Med (Lond) 200 61:834–840.

134. Ladenson PW. Strategies for thyrotropin use to monitor patients wi treated thyroid carcinoma. Thyroid 1999;9:429–433.

135. Ladenson PW. Recombinant thyrotropin versus thyroid hormone wit drawal in evaluating patients with thyroid carcinoma. Semin Nucl M 2000;30:98–106.

136. Chopra IJ. Clinical review 86: Is it a misnome J Clin Endocrinol Metab 1997;82:329–334.

137. Yamazaki K, Yamada E, Kanaji Y, et al. Interleukin-6 (IL-6) inhibi thyroid function in the presence of soluble IL-6 receptor in culture human thyroid follicles. Endocrinology 1996;137:4857–4863.

138. Murai H, Murakami S, Ishida K, Sugawara M. Elevated seru interleukin-6 and decreased thyroid hormone levels in postoperativ patients and effects of IL-6 on thyroid cell function in vitro. Thyro 1996;6:601–606.

139. Ljunggren JG, Torring O, Wallin G, et al. Quality of life aspects and cos in treatment of Graves' hyperthyroidism with antithyroid drugs, surger or radioiodine: Results from a prospective, randomized study. Thyro 1998;8:653–659.

74

ADRENAL GLAND DISORDERS

John G. Gums and John M. Tovar

Learning Objectives and other resources can be found at *www.pharmacotherapyonline.com.*

KEY CONCEPTS

◀1 Glucocorticoid secretion from the adrenal cortex is stimulated by corticotropin or adrenocorticotropic hormone (ACTH) that is released from the anterior pituitary in response to hypothalamic-mediated release of corticotropin-releasing hormone (CRH).

◀2 To ensure the proper treatment of Cushing's syndrome, diagnostic procedures should (1) establish the presence of hypercortisolism and (2) discover the underlying etiology of the disease.

◀3 The rationale for treating Cushing's syndrome is to reduce the morbidity and mortality resulting from disorders such as diabetes mellitus, cardiovascular disease, and electrolyte abnormalities.

◀4 The treatment of choice for both ACTH-dependent and ACTH-independent Cushing's syndrome is surgery, whereas pharmacologic agents are reserved for adjunctive therapy, refractory cases, or inoperable disease.

◀5 Pharmacologic agents that may be used to manage the patient with Cushing's syndrome include: steroidogenic inhibitors, adrenolytic agents, neuromodulators of ACTH release, and glucocorticoid-receptor blocking agents.

◀6 Spironolactone, a competitive inhibitor of aldosterone, is the drug of choice in bilateral adrenal hyperplasia (BAH)-dependent hyperaldosteronism.

◀7 Addison's disease (primary adrenal insufficiency) is a deficiency in cortisol, aldosterone, and various androgens resulting from the loss of function of all regions of the adrenal cortex.

◀8 Secondary adrenal insufficiency usually results from exogenous steroid use, leading to hypothalamic-pituitary-adrenal (HPA)-axis suppression followed by a decrease in ACTH release, and low levels of androgens and cortisol.

◀9 Virilism results from the excessive secretion of androgens from the adrenal gland and is usually seen as hirsutism in females.

The adrenal glands were first characterized by Eustachius in 1563. After Addison identified a case of adrenal insufficiency in man, adrenal anatomy and physiology flourished. Most of the work done in the early and mid-1900s centered on the glucocorticoid cortisol. With the discovery of aldosterone by Simpson and Tait in 1952, adrenal pharmacology turned toward the mineralocorticoid. Conn[1] followed with his classical description of primary aldosteronism in 1955, and numerous clinicians and investigators have continued the discovery of the variety of disease processes promoted through the adrenal gland.

PHYSIOLOGY, ANATOMY, AND BIOCHEMISTRY

There are two adrenal glands located extraperitoneally to the upper poles of each kidney (Fig. 74–1). On average, each adrenal gland weighs 4 g and is 2 to 3 cm in width and 4 to 6 cm in length. The gland is fed by small arteries from the abdominal aorta and renal and phrenic arteries. Drainage of the adrenal gland occurs via the renal vein on the left and the inferior vena cava on the right.

The adrenal medulla occupies 10% of the total gland and is responsible for the secretion of catecholamines. The adrenal cortex accounts for the remaining 90% and is responsible for the secretion of three types of hormones (Fig. 74–2) from three separate zones.[2]

The zona glomerulosa, 15% of the total adrenal cortex, is responsible for mineralocorticoid production, of which aldosterone is the principal end product. Aldosterone maintains electrolyte and volume homeostasis by altering potassium and magnesium secretion and renal tubular sodium reabsorption. The zona fasciculata, the middle zone, makes up 60% of the cortex, is high in cholesterol, and is responsible for basal and stimulated glucocorticoid production. Glucocorticoids, mainly cortisol, are responsible for the regulation of fat, carbohydrate, and protein metabolism. The zona reticularis occupies 25% of the adrenal cortex, and is responsible for all adrenal androgen production. The androgens, testosterone and estradiol, are the major end products and have influence within the reproductive system as well as affecting primary and secondary sex characteristics.

HORMONE PRODUCTION AND METABOLISM

Cortisol production is accomplished via two successive hydroxylations: the first at the 21-position by 21-hydroxylase (yielding 11-deoxycortisol) and the second at the 11-position by 11-hydroxylase, yielding cortisol or hydrocortisone.

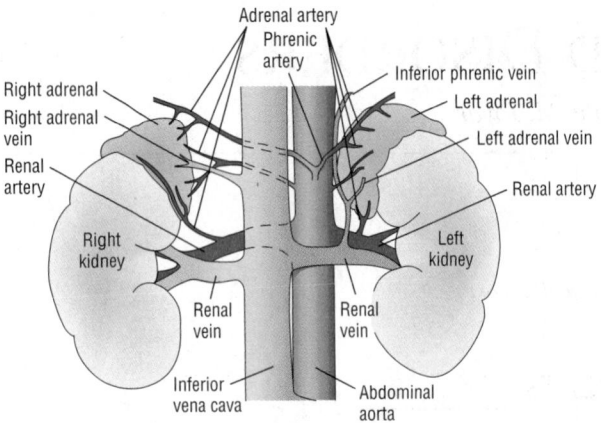

FIGURE 74–1. Anatomy of the adrenal gland.

Aldosterone is a by-product of the 21-hydroxylation of pregnenolone to form deoxycorticosterone. The oxidation of 18-hydroxycorticosterone to aldosterone is a unique feature of the zona glomerulosa, explaining why aldosterone is not affected during disease processes limited to the fasciculata and/or reticularis.

Androgens have a 19-carbon nucleus and serve as precursors to more potent analogs produced in the periphery. The adrenal gland can synthesize estradiol and estrone from testosterone and androstenedione, respectively; however, the quantities are extremely small. The rates of production for the various steroids produced by the adrenal gland are listed in Table 74–1.

Metabolism of glucocorticoids occurs in the liver, and is responsible for converting inactive steroids to active metabolites, as well as deactivating the active steroids to less active or inactive metabolites. Most pharmaceutical steroid products are active; however, in the case of prednisone and cortisone, metabolism is necessary for the conversion to the active prednisolone and cortisol, respectively. Following metabolic conversion, glucocorticoids are excreted renally as less active or inactive metabolites.

After metabolism, glomerular filtration is primarily responsible for the elimination of endogenously produced glucocorticoids. The

TABLE 74–1. Rates of Adrenal Production and Plasma Concentrations of Various Steroids

Steroid	24-Hour Secretion (mg)	Plasma Concentration (ng/mL)
Aldosterone	0.15	0.15–0.17
Androstenedione	2.50 (female)	1.80 ± 0.21 (female)
	2.20 (male)	1.14 ± 0.21 (male)
Corticosterone	1–4	2.4 ± 1.5 (female)
		4.2 ± 2.2 (male)
Cortisol	8–25	20–140 (female)
		40–180 (male)
11-Deoxycorticosterone	0.60	0.15–0.17
11-Deoxycortisol	0.40	0.95–2.50
Progesterone	0.0	0.20 ± 0.09 (female)[a]
		11.8 ± 7.0 (female)[b]
		0.18 ± 0.10 (male)
Testosterone	0.23 (female)	0.48 ± 0.14 (female)
		5.59 ± 1.51 (male)

[a]Follicular phase of menstrual cycle
[b]Luteal phase of menstrual cycle

half-life of cortisol is 70 to 120 minutes; with aldosterone, the half-life is only 15 minutes because of an extremely high intrinsic clearance.

Metabolism and conversion of the various steroids can be altered by a variety of disease states and medicinal compounds. Drugs and diseases known to result in enhanced clearance of steroids include phenytoin, phenobarbital, rifampin, mitotane, aminoglutethimide, hyperthyroidism, and renal disease (dexamethasone only). Drugs and diseases known to result in reduced clearance of steroids include estrogens and estrogen-containing oral contraceptives, liver disease, age, pregnancy, hypothyroidism, anorexia nervosa, protein-calorie malnutrition, and renal disease (prednisolone only). Plasma glucocorticoids are bound to one of three plasma proteins in varying degrees. Corticosteroid-binding globulin (CBG), albumin, and α_1-glycoprotein are capable of binding glucocorticoids, with CBG being the principal binding protein.

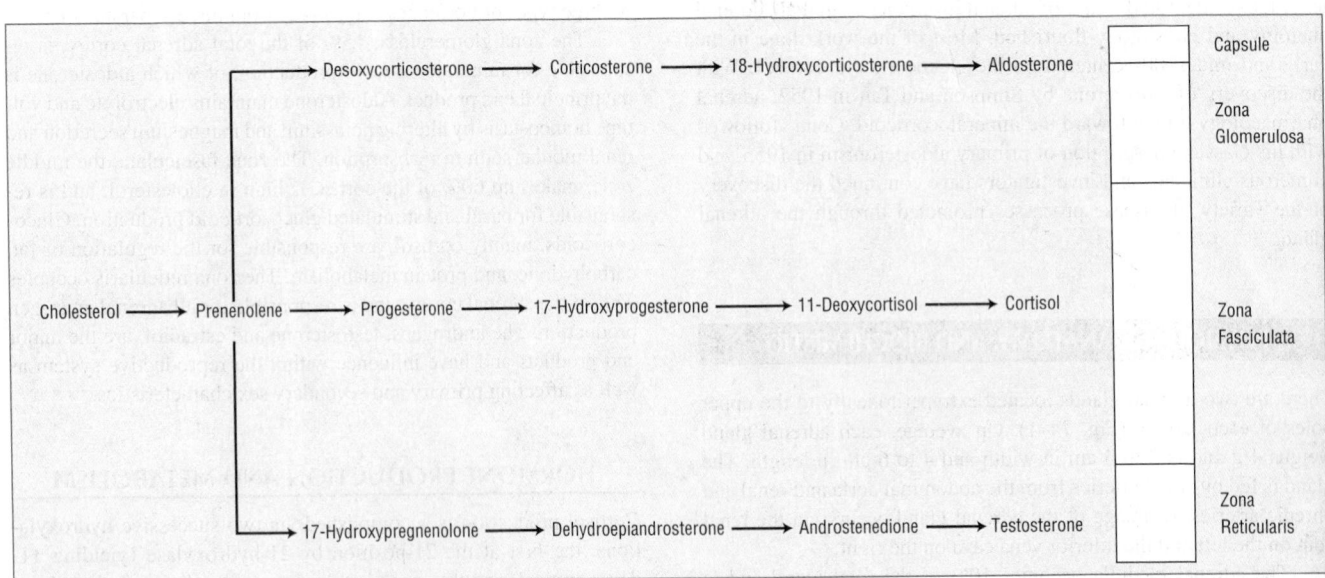

FIGURE 74–2. Hormone synthetic pathways in relation to the zones of the adrenal gland.

The function of steroid binding is to serve as a reservoir of steroids in their inactive state. This binding may change the availability of glucocorticoids to receptor-activating sites. Therefore, a final but important variable in altered plasma concentration of free (active) steroids is concentration of plasma proteins.

REGULATION OF HORMONE SECRETION

The regulation of glucocorticoid secretion is accomplished by the pituitary hormone, adrenocorticotropic hormone (ACTH). Under normal conditions, ACTH is released from the anterior pituitary in response to corticotropin-releasing hormone (CRH), which is secreted by the median eminence of the hypothalamus (Fig. 74–3).

Additionally, histochemical studies have demonstrated that certain neurotransmitters have the unique ability to stimulate production of CRH or ACTH directly. 5-Hydroxytryptamine and norepinephrine have both been shown to increase levels of ACTH. 5-Hydroxytryptamine causes a release of CRH through excitation of a cholinergic intervention. Norepinephrine can cause direct stimulation of ACTH release, although this effect is still controversial. After release, ACTH stimulates the adrenal gland to release cortisol and to a lesser extent aldosterone and androgens. The rising cortisol concentration inhibits the secretion of CRH and ACTH through a negative-feedback mechanism.

Regulation of adrenal androgens is accomplished in a manner similar to cortisol regulation. When plasma androgen reaches sufficient concentrations, production is terminated via a negative-feedback loop. Androgen release is increased during puberty and in women with hirsutism. Adrenal androgen release is decreased in fasting, anorexia nervosa, and aging.

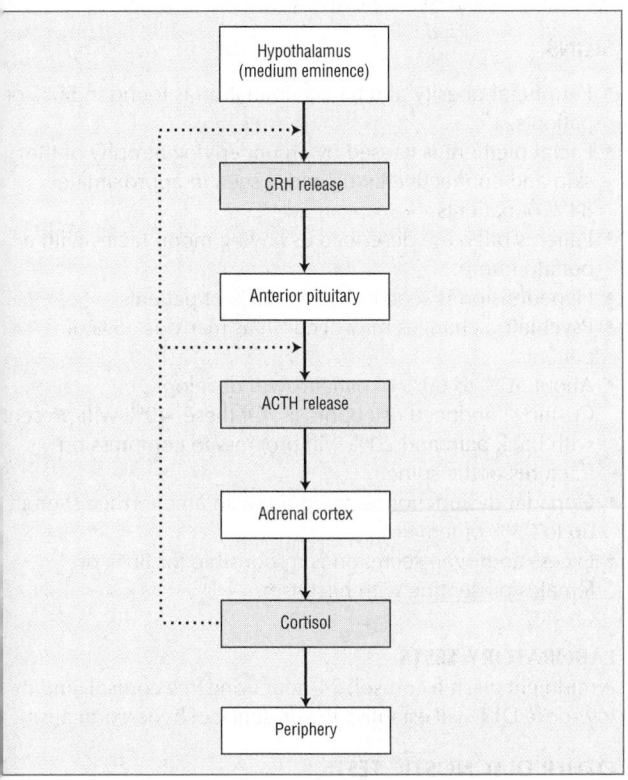

FIGURE 74–3. Negative feedback system involved in the regulation of cortisol secretion under normal conditions. CRH, corticotropin-releasing hormone; ACTH, adrenocorticotropic hormone.

Regulation of aldosterone secretion is considerably more complex. The renin-angiotensin system has the ability to respond to electrolyte and volume changes to increase or decrease aldosterone secretion. Renin production and subsequent aldosterone secretion is stimulated by blood pressure lowering, erect posture, salt depletion, β-adrenergic stimulation, and central nervous system excitation. Renin production is inhibited by salt loading, angiotensin II, vasopressin, potassium, calcium, blood pressure increases, and a variety of drugs. The conversion of renin substrate angiotensinogen to angiotensin I and subsequently to angiotensin II is the initial stimulus for aldosterone synthesis. Angiotensin II is acted on by aminopeptidase and converted to angiotensin III. Angiotensin II and III are both capable of stimulating the zona glomerulosa to secrete aldosterone. Following aldosterone secretion, increases in renal sodium and water retention as well as blood pressure are seen, thereby turning off the stimulus for renin release.

HYPERFUNCTION OF THE ADRENAL GLAND

CUSHING'S SYNDROME

In 1932, Cushing first described a syndrome of pituitary basophilism that attracted national attention. It was not until this time that patients with unexplained central obesity, cutaneous striae, osteoporosis, weakness, hypertension, diabetes mellitus, and congestion had a definite diagnosis. Cushing emphasized that the disease was of pituitary origin. Ten years later, Albright[3] focused his attention on the sugar hormone, which he believed originated from the adrenal cortex.

After the development of the method for measuring urinary steroids, Daughaday discovered elevated steroids in the urine of patients with Cushing's disease. Finally, the end product was identified and Cushing's syndrome was correctly explained as an excess of cortisol in the plasma (hypercortisolism).

ETIOLOGY

Cushing's syndrome results from the effects of supraphysiologic levels of glucocorticoids originating either from exogenous administration or from endogenous overproduction by the adrenal glands (ACTH-dependent) or by abnormal adrenocortical tissues (ACTH-independent). ACTH-dependent Cushing's syndrome is usually (~70% of Cushing's cases) caused by overproduction of ACTH by the pituitary gland, causing adrenal hyperplasia (Cushing's disease). Pituitary adenomas account for approximately 85% of these cases. Ectopic ACTH-secreting tumors and nonneoplastic corticotropin hypersecretion, possibly secondary to excess CRH production, are felt to be responsible for the remaining 12% of ACTH-dependent causes. Ectopic ACTH syndrome refers to excessive ACTH production resulting from an endocrine or nonendocrine tumor, usually of the pancreas, thyroid, or lung. Small-cell carcinoma of the lung will lead to ectopic ACTH secretion in 0.5% to 2% of cases. To distinguish between the various etiologies, a careful history and some pertinent laboratory work are required (Table 74–2).

The remaining 18% of Cushing's syndrome cases are ACTH-independent and are almost equally divided between adrenal adenomas and adrenal carcinomas, with rare cases caused by micronodular or macronodular hyperplasia.[4–5] The majority of adrenal cortex tumors are benign adenomas. Adrenal carcinoma is found more often in children than in adults with Cushing's syndrome.

TABLE 74–2. Various Etiologies of Cushing's Syndrome and Their Respective Differences

	Pituitary Dependent	Ectopic ACTH Syndrome	Adrenal Adenoma	Adrenal Carcinoma
Course	Slow	Rapid	Slow	Rapid
Symptoms	Mild to moderate	Atypical	Mild to moderate	Severe
Dominant sex/age	Female/male	Male	None noted	Children
Virilization	+	+	+	+++
Abdominal mass	0	0	0	++
Plasma ACTH concentration	Slightly elevated	High	0	0
Dexamethasone suppression test	≥50% Suppression	No suppression	No suppression	No suppression
Iodocholesterol scan	Bilateral uptake	Bilateral uptake	Unilateral	None

ACTH, adrenocorticotropic hormone.

CLINICAL PRESENTATION

The most common findings in patients with Cushing's syndrome, which are present in 90% of patients, are central obesity and facial rounding. In addition, about 50% of patients will exhibit some peripheral obesity and fat accumulation. Fat accumulation in the dorsocervical area (buffalo hump) can be associated with any major weight gain, whereas increased supraclavicular fat pads are more specific for Cushing's syndrome.[5] Striae are usually present along the lower abdomen and take on a red to purple color. Hypertensive complications have traditionally been major contributors to the morbidity and mortality of Cushing's syndrome. Hypertension is seen in 75% to 85% of patients, with diastolic blood pressures greater than 119 mm Hg noted in over 20% of patients.[6]

DIAGNOSIS

The diagnosis of Cushing's syndrome involves two steps: (1) establishing the presence of hypercortisolism, which is relatively easy, and (2) differentiating between etiologies, which can be quite a challenge (Fig. 74–4).[4,5,7] The presence of hypercortisolism can be established via the following tests: 24-hour urine free cortisol, midnight plasma cortisol, and/or the low-dose dexamethasone suppression test (DST) (using 1 mg for the overnight test or 0.5 mg/ 6 h for the classic 2-day study). However, because these tests cannot determine the etiology of Cushing's syndrome, other tests and procedures subsequently will be employed. They may include any of the following: high-dose DST; plasma ACTH via immunoradiometric assay (IRMA) or radioimmunoassay (RIA); adrenal vein catheterization; metyrapone stimulation test; adrenal, chest, or abdominal computed tomography (CT); CRH stimulation test; inferior petrosal sinus sampling; and pituitary magnetic resonance imaging (MRI). Other possible tests and procedures include insulin-induced hypoglycemia; somatostatin receptor scintigraphy; the desmopressin stimulation test; naloxone CRH stimulation test; loperamide test; the hexarelin stimulation test; and radionuclide imaging.[4–17] Table 74–3 summarizes some of the tests used to diagnose Cushing's syndrome.

Elevated urinary free cortisol concentrations are highly suggestive of Cushing's syndrome. Normal reference values for urinary free cortisol are 20 to 90 mcg per 24-hour period. It is not unusual to detect a twofold or threefold increase in urine cortisol in the patient with hyperfunction of the adrenal gland. Starvation, topical steroid application, hydration from water loading, and acute stress all are capable of elevating the urine cortisol concentrations. Because other pathologic conditions can increase the amount of free cortisol, additional tests should be performed to confirm the diagnosis, or the diagnostic evaluation should be repeated when the acute stress has resolved. Of all urinary measures, urinary free cortisol is the most useful for assessment of any patient with suspected Cushing's syndrome.[7]

CLINICAL PRESENTATION: CUSHING'S SYNDROME

GENERAL

The most common findings, which are present in 90% of patients, are central obesity and facial rounding.

SYMPTOMS

About 65% and 58% of patients complain of myopathies and muscular weakness, respectively.

SIGNS

- Peripheral obesity and fat accumulation is found in 50% of patients.
- Facial plethora is caused by an underlying atrophy of the skin and connective tissue and is seen in approximately 84% of patients.
- Patients often are described as having moon facies with a buffalo hump.
- Hypertension is seen in 75% to 85% of patients.
- Psychiatric changes may occur in as many as 55% of patients.
- About 50% to 60% of patients will develop Cushing's-induced osteoporosis. Of these, 40% will present with back pain and 20% will progress to compression fractures of the spine.
- Gonadal dysfunction is common, with amenorrhea seen in up to 75% of females.
- Excess androgen secretion is responsible for 80% of females presenting with hirsutism.

LABORATORY TESTS

A midnight plasma cortisol, 24-hour urine free cortisol, and/or low-dose DST will establish the presence of hypercorticalism.

OTHER DIAGNOSTIC TESTS

The high-dose DST, plasma ACTH test, metyrapone stimulation test, and CRH stimulation test will help determine the etiology.

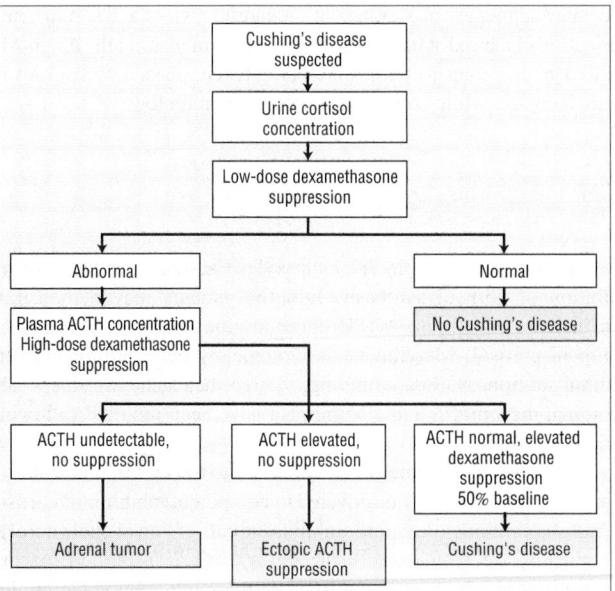

GURE 74-4. Algorithm for diagnosing Cushing's syndrome. ACTH, adrenocorticotropic hormone.

in metabolism from these drug interactions, individual variability, or patient noncompliance.

The first test used to determine the etiology of Cushing's syndrome is the plasma ACTH test. Plasma ACTH concentrations can be measured via RIA or IRMA.[7,16] In the ACTH-dependent Cushing's syndromes, ACTH may be normal or elevated. Very high levels of ACTH favor ectopic production. ACTH values are low in ACTH-independent (adrenal) Cushing's syndrome. ACTH levels may appear artificially low in some ectopic ACTH-producing tumors because ACTH can be secreted as an active prohormone that is not detected by the assay.

The high-dose DST operates under the same principle as the low-dose test.[5,7] The high-dose test has its main application in differentiating the Cushing's disease patient from the patient with another form of hypercortisolism. The Cushing's disease patient will generally demonstrate a 50% reduction in urinary steroids over baseline, whereas the others will generally not suppress. The high-dose test is based on the principle that patients with Cushing's syndrome not caused by adrenal tumors or ectopic ACTH production will suppress their hypothalamic-pituitary axis in the presence of glucocorticoids, but it takes much higher-than-normal doses. An overnight high-dose DST has been developed, whereby the patient has a baseline serum cortisol drawn at 8:00 A.M. and dexamethasone 8 mg is taken at 11:00 P.M. The next morning, at 8:00 A.M., another serum cortisol is drawn.[7,16] The high-dose test is most useful when the low-dose test and other diagnostic studies have confirmed the diagnosis of Cushing's syndrome. The high-dose DST has been studied in combination with ACTH and metapyrone testing, and results in better specificity than either test alone.

Abnormal adrenal anatomy is effectively identified using high-resolution CT scanning and perhaps MRI. Nodules as small as 1 to 1.5 cm on the adrenal cortex are easily identified by CT. With the use of thin-section scanning, nodules as small as 3 to 5 mm can be visualized.[7,19,20]

The normal circadian rhythm of cortisol will demonstrate a 60% to 80% decline between 8:00 A.M. and 11:00 P.M. This rhythm is lost in the Cushing's syndrome patient. Thus while many patients with Cushing's syndrome will have serum cortisol values in the high normal range if the serum is assayed in the morning, only 3.4% will have normal values if measured late at night.[7] Thus a midnight serum cortisol greater than 7.5 mcg/dL is a highly sensitive assay for Cushing's. However, this test requires that patients be admitted for more than 48 hours to avoid false-positive responses secondary to the stress of hospitalization. Also if a patient is sleeping, a lower serum cortisol value (>1.8 mcg/dL) should be used. An alternative assay that may prove useful in the future is measurement of salivary cortisol.

In the overnight DST, 1 mg of dexamethasone is administered at 11:00 P.M. The following morning at 8:00 A.M. plasma cortisol is obtained for analysis. The Cushing's syndrome patient will not exhibit a suppressed cortisol concentration via the negative-feedback loop, and the morning cortisol concentration will be elevated above 5 mcg/dL, or as low as 1.8 mcg/dL.[5,18] The overnight DST is useful only as a screening tool for Cushing's syndrome, because of a high sensitivity, but a rather low specificity. Phenytoin, rifampin, phenobarbital, and other drugs that induce liver enzymes may cause an increase in the clearance rate of the dexamethasone, causing decreased levels leading to a false-positive suppression test.[7] Plasma dexamethasone measured at the conclusion of this test can clarify results clouded by differences

DIFFERENTIAL DIAGNOSIS

Although the diagnosis of Cushing's disease is not a difficult one, at times the clinician will need to differentiate it from syndromes that mimic Cushing's. Pseudo-Cushing's syndrome refers to a group of diseases that can mimic Cushing's disease. Patients with obesity, chronic alcoholism, depression, and acute illness of any type can cloud the diagnosis of Cushing's disease. Depressed patients, though mimicking the urinary steroid abnormalities of Cushing's disease, will not resemble a cushingoid patient in appearance. The chronic alcoholic will have his laboratory panel returned to baseline after he or she stops drinking. The obese patient often will have normal cortisol concentrations on both serum and urinary screening.

TABLE 74–3. Summary of Tests Used to Diagnose Cushing's Syndrome

Test	Normal	Hyperplasia	Adenoma	Carcinoma
Plasma				
Cortisol (mcg/dL, A.M./P.M.)	170/80	↑/↑↑	↑↑/↑↑	↑↑↑/↑↑↑
After low-dose DST	↓	↔	↔	↔
After high-dose DST	↓	↓/↔	↔	↔
ACTH (pg/mL)	10–80	↑↑	↓	↓
Urine				
Cortisol (mcg/24 h)	20–90	↑↑	↑↑	↑↑↑

ACTH, adrenocorticotropic hormone; DST, dexamethasone suppression test.

Iatrogenic Cushing's syndrome, induced by pharmacologic agents, often is indistinguishable from Cushing's disease. This syndrome can occur from administration of oral, inhaled, intranasal, and topical glucocorticoids, as well as progestins such as medroxyprogesterone acetate and megestrol acetate.[21-24] A careful history and serum determination in a basal state can aid the clinician in making the diagnosis. If exogenous glucocorticoids are being taken, plasma cortisol levels may increase, while corticosterone levels remain low.[7,25]

▶ TREATMENT: Cushing's Syndrome

③ If left untreated, Cushing's syndrome is associated with a high percentage of morbidity and mortality owing to associated disorders such as diabetes mellitus, cardiovascular disease, and electrolyte abnormalities. These disorders limit the survival of the Cushing's disease patient to 4 to 5 years following initial diagnosis. The desired outcomes of treatment are to limit the morbidity and mortality and return the patient to a normal functional state by removing the source of hypercortisolism without causing any pituitary or adrenal deficiencies.

④ Once the etiology of the disease is identified, the treatment of choice for both ACTH-dependent and ACTH-independent Cushing's syndrome is surgical resection of any offending tumors.[22] However, several pharmacologic secondary treatment plans are available, depending on the etiology of the disease (Table 74–4).[4,5,26]

■ PHARMACOLOGIC THERAPY

⑤ Pharmacotherapy of Cushing's syndrome (dosing can be found in Table 74–4)[27,28] can be divided into four categories based on the anatomic site of action of the agent: (1) steroidogenic inhibitors; (2) adrenolytic agents; (3) neuromodulators of ACTH release; and (4) glucocorticoid-receptor blocking agents.[26,29,30]

Steroidogenic inhibition may be accomplished with the following agents: metyrapone, aminoglutethimide, and ketoconazole. Either metyrapone or aminoglutethimide used alone has limited efficacy, with relapse occurring after discontinuation of therapy. Neither agent should be used after successful surgery. Their use should be restricted to the refractory patient who is not a surgical candidate. Combination therapy with these agents appears more effective than single-agent therapy and may cause fewer side effects.

Metyrapone inhibits 11-hydroxylase activity, resulting in inhibition of cortisol synthesis. Initially, patients may demonstrate an increase in plasma ACTH concentrations because of a sudden drop in cortisol. Metyrapone is biologically active following oral administration. Nausea, vomiting, vertigo, headache, dizziness, abdominal discomfort, and allergic rash have been reported following administration.[26-30]

Initially, aminoglutethimide was used to treat refractory forms of epilepsy, but it was later discovered to be a potent inhibitor of cortisol synthesis. Aminoglutethimide inhibits the conversion of cholesterol to pregnenolone early in the cortisol pathway.[26,30,31] Plasma cortisol concentrations are reduced by up to 50% following aminoglutethimide therapy. Side effects include severe sedation, nausea, ataxia, and skin rashes.[26,31] Most of these reactions are dose-dependent and limit the use of aminoglutethimide in most patients. Aminoglutethimide may decrease the anticoagulant effect of warfarin. As aminoglutethimide can induce the metabolism of exogenous glucocorticoids, careful titration is required with steroid replacement.

Alone, aminoglutethimide is indicated for short-term use in inoperable Cushing's disease with ectopic ACTH syndrome as the suspected underlying etiology. Aminoglutethimide may be used in combination with metyrapone. Smaller doses of both drugs can be used, thereby minimizing the toxicity associated with either agent. The combination therapy appears effective for various etiologies of Cushing's disease and is useful in the inoperable patient.

The imidazole derivative antifungal ketoconazole[26,29,30] is highly effective in lowering cortisol in Cushing's disease, resulting in normal corticosteroid values in 84% of patients, with an additional 11% of patients reporting improvement. Patients can be maintained successfully for months to years on ketoconazole therapy. In addition to lowering serum cortisol levels, ketoconazole can cause gynecomastia

TABLE 74–4. Possible Treatment Plans in Cushing's Syndrome Based on Etiology

Etiology	Nondrug	Generic (Brand) Drug Name	Treatment Dosing Initial	Usual	Max
Ectopic ACTH syndrome	Surgery, chemotherapy, irradiation	Metyrapone (Metopirone) 250-mg tabs	1–1.5 g/day, divided every 4–6 h	1–6 g/day, divided every 4–6 h	6 g/day
		Aminoglutethimide (Cytadren) 250-mg tabs	0.5–1 g/day, divided two to four times a day for 2 weeks	1 g/day, divided every 6 h	2 g/day
Pituitary-dependent	Surgery, irradiation	Cyproheptadine 2 mg/5 mL syrup or 4-mg tabs	4 mg twice a day	24–32 mg/day, divided four times a day	32 mg/day
		Mitotane (Lysodren) 500-mg tabs	1–6 g/day, increased by 1–2 g/day every 3–7 days	9–10 g/day, divided three to four times a day	16 g/day
		Metyrapone	See above	See above	See above
Adrenal adenoma	Surgery, postoperative replacement	Ketoconazole (Nizoral) 200-mg tabs	200 mg once or twice a day	600–800 mg/day, divided twice a day	1200 mg/day
Adrenal carcinoma	Surgery	Mitotane	See above	See above	See above

ACTH, adrenocorticotropic hormone.

nd lower plasma testosterone values. All of these effects are attributed its inhibition of a variety of cytochrome P450 enzymes, including 1-hydroxylase and 17-hydroxylase.[27] The most common adverse effects are reversible elevation of hepatic transaminases, gynecomastia, nd gastrointestinal upset.[27]

The adrenolytic agent mitotane is a cytotoxic drug that structurally resembles the insecticide dichlorodiphenyltrichloroethane DDT). Mitotane inhibits the 11-hydroxylation of 11-desoxycortisol nd 11-desoxycorticosterone in the cortex. The net result is a reduced synthesis of cortisol and corticosterone. It decreases the cortisol secretion rate, plasma cortisol concentrations, urinary free cortisol, and plasma concentrations of the 17-substituted steroids.[27] This drug appears to selectively inhibit adrenocortical function without causing cellular destruction. Degeneration of cells within the zona fasciculata and reticularis occurs with resultant atrophy of the adrenal cortex. The zona glomerulosa is minimally affected during acute therapy, but can become damaged following long-term treatment.[26,27,30]

Because mitotane can severely reduce cortisol production, the patient should be hospitalized before initiating therapy. Mitotane should be continued as long as clinical benefits occur. Cortisol secretion rate, plasma cortisol concentration, urinary free cortisol, and urinary steroid production should be monitored to assess response to mitotane. If necessary, steroid replacement therapy can be given. Nausea and diarrhea are common adverse effects that occur at doses greater than 2 g/day and may be avoided by gradually increasing the dose and/or administering the agent with food. Approximately 80% of mitotane-treated patients develop lethargy and somnolence, and other central nervous system adverse drug reactions occur in approximately 40% of patients. Furthermore, significant but reversible hypercholesterolemia can result from mitotane use.

Neuromodulatory agents include cyproheptadine, bromocriptine, valproic acid, ritanserin, and octreotide. None of the neuromodulatory agents has demonstrated consistent clinical efficacy in the treatment of Cushing's disease. The existence of a bromocriptine-responsive subset of patients remains controversial.[26,30]

Cyproheptadine can decrease ACTH secretion in the Cushing's disease patient. Morning plasma cortisol concentrations, as well as 24-hour urinary cortisol (free) concentrations should be monitored. Side effects are minor and include sedation and hyperphagia. Cyproheptadine should be reserved for nonsurgical candidates who fail more conventional therapy. Because the response rate is no more than 30%, patients should be followed closely for relapses.

Glucocorticoid receptor antagonism may be accomplished via RU-486 (mifepristone). RU-486 is a progesterone- and glucocorticoid-receptor antagonist that inhibits dexamethasone suppression and raises endogenous cortisol and ACTH values in normal subjects.[26,32] Limited clinical experience in Cushing's suggests that RU-486 is highly effective in reversing the manifestation of hypercortisolism. Because of its novel site of action as a receptor antagonist leading to higher cortisol and ACTH levels, the diagnosis of treatment-induced glucocorticoid insufficiency must rest on clinical signs only. The efficacy and long-term effects of RU-486 remain to be determined.

Spironolactone has been used for its competitive antagonism of aldosterone in the treatment of Cushing's syndrome. Spironolactone can provide symptomatic relief of the hypertension and hypokalemia often seen in Cushing's syndrome.

Close monitoring of 24-hour urinary free cortisol levels and serum cortisol levels are essential to monitor for adrenal insufficiency. Steroid secretion should be monitored with all of these drugs and steroid replacement given as needed. Whatever the choice, pharmacologic therapy in pituitary-dependent disease is mainly centered around patient stabilization prior to surgery or in patients waiting for potential response to other therapies.

NONPHARMACOLOGIC THERAPY

SURGERY

During the last decade, the treatment of choice for Cushing's disease has been transsphenoidal resection of the pituitary microadenoma.[4,5,33] The advantages to this procedure include preservation of pituitary function, low complication rate, and high clinical improvement rate. The overall cure rate of histologically proven tumors approaches 90%.

Bilateral adrenalectomy surgery had been the mainstay of therapy for years. It is used now only in patients for whom transsphenoidal surgery and pituitary irradiation have failed or cannot be used.[5] Bilateral adrenalectomy rapidly reverses hypercortisolism. However, patients may develop Nelson's syndrome, which involves sella turcica enlargement and hyperpigmentation, caused by postoperative hypothalamic stimulation. Therefore if bilateral adrenalectomy is used it should be accompanied by some form of hypothalamic inhibition, such as cyproheptadine.

Irradiation (4000 to 5000 rads) of the pituitary has provided clinical improvement in approximately 50% of patients. Improvement is usually not seen until 6 to 12 months after therapy and can create pituitary-dependent hormone deficiencies. Most clinicians will reserve pituitary irradiation for the patient with a mild case of Cushing's disease or as an adjunct to another therapy.[34]

Adrenal Adenoma

Surgical resection of benign adrenal adenoma is associated with relatively few side effects and a high cure rate (95%). The contralateral gland in the patient with adrenal adenoma is usually atrophic, therefore steroid replacement is needed both perioperatively and postoperatively. Table 74–5 outlines an approach to steroid replacement for three separate routes of hydrocortisone. Therapy should be continued for 6 to 12 months following surgery. Before replacement therapy is discontinued, recovery of the adrenal axis may be assessed by administering ACTH and measuring cortisol response at 30 and 60 minutes. Cortisol levels should exceed 18 mcg/dL before discontinuance of the exogenous steroids.[4]

Adrenal Carcinoma

Unlike the benign adenoma patient, patients with adrenal carcinoma have an unpredictable and unfavorable outcome with surgical resection.[5] Often the complete tumor cannot be excised, leaving the patients with some degree of symptomatology and extra-adrenal involvement. Irradiation can be used if metastases are discovered. In the patient with adrenal carcinoma who is not a surgical candidate, the focus of treatment is on palliative pharmacologic intervention (e.g., mitotane).

Mitotane appears to be the drug of choice in inoperable functional and nonfunctional adrenal carcinoma. Tumor regression is seen in approximately 35% to 50% of patients, with most regression occurring between the second and fourth month of therapy. Seventy-five percent of patients will exhibit a 30% fall in urinary steroids, with 50% of patients showing an improved clinical response after 5 months of

TABLE 74–5. Alternative Steroid Replacement Regimens in the Adrenal Adenoma Patient

| | Hydrocortisone Dose (mg) | | |
Time	IV	IM	PO
Operation day	300	50 before surgery and 50 after surgery	
Postoperative day 1	200	50 every 12 h	
Postoperative day 2	150	50 every 12 h	
Postoperative day 3	100	50 every 12 h	
Postoperative day 4		50 every 12 h	25 every 6 h
Postoperative day 5		25 every 12 h	25 every 6 h[a]
Postoperative day 7			25 every 6 h
Postoperative days 8–10			25 every 8 h
Postoperative days 11–20			25 every 12 h
Postoperative days 21+			20 at 8 A.M.
			10 at 4 P.M.

[a]Add fludrocortisone 0.05–2 mg orally once daily starting on postoperative day 5. Adjust dose based on blood pressure, body weight, and serum electrolytes.

treatment. Patient survival appears prolonged, although no adequate clinical trials are available to support this assumption.

Metyrapone, aminoglutethimide, and ketoconazole may be given to attempt control of steroid hypersecretion. 5-Fluorouracil has also been used in combination therapy.

Ectopic ACTH Syndrome

In the ectopic ACTH syndrome multiple sites of tumors exist, and locating the ectopic site is essential but often difficult.

Therefore only approximately 10% of patients are cured following surgery, and the remaining 90% receive postoperative medication.

Pharmacologic management with metyrapone is effective and remains the agent of choice in the ectopic ACTH syndrome.[35] Aminoglutethimide and ketoconazole are alternative agents.[4,35,36] Mitotane has been tried in patients with ectopic ACTH syndrome; however, its side-effect profile generally limits its use. RU-486 and the somatostatin analog octreotide have been reported to reduce the clinical signs of the ectopic ACTH syndrome.[30,35] Further evaluation of these agents is needed.

HYPERALDOSTERONISM

Excess aldosterone is categorized as either primary or secondary hyperaldosteronism.[37–48]

PRIMARY ALDOSTERONISM

Etiology

Primary aldosteronism implies that the physiologic abnormality is within the adrenal cortex. The most common causes include a solitary adrenal adenoma (60%) or idiopathic adrenocortical hyperplasia (35% bilateral and 5% unilateral). Other rare causes include adrenal cortex carcinoma, primary adrenocortical hyperplasia, renin-responsive adrenocortical adenoma, and genetic mutations, such as in glucocorticoid-suppressible hyperaldosteronism.[39,40,42]

Clinical Presentation

The incidence of primary aldosteronism is disputed, with estimates ranging from approximately 0.5% to 9.5% of all hypertensive patients.[39,49] The disease is more common in women aged 30 to 50 years. Signs and symptoms may include arterial hypertension, muscle weakness, fatigue, and headache, though many patients are asymptomatic.

Diagnosis

The absolute diagnosis is relatively easy based on clinical findings and pertinent laboratory findings. However, as in Cushing's disease, the discovery of the underlying etiology is mandatory to ensure proper treatment. Table 74–6 lists the various abnormalities that must be ruled out when suspicion of hyperaldosteronism is high.

CLINICAL PRESENTATION: PRIMARY HYPERALDOSTERONISM

SYMPTOMS
Patients may complain of muscle weakness, fatigue, paresthesias, and headache.

SIGNS
- Hypertension
- Reduced glucose tolerance is seen in 25% of patients.
- Metabolic alkalosis
- Tetany/paralysis
- Polydipsia/nocturnal polyuria

LABORATORY TESTS
A serum potassium concentration of less than 3.5 mEq/L with a concurrent urinary potassium content greater than 30 mEq per 24 hours is suggestive of primary aldosteronism.

Common laboratory findings include hypokalemia (80% to 90%), suppressed renin activity, elevated plasma aldosterone concentrations, hypernatremia (>142 mEq/L), hypomagnesemia, and elevated bicarbonate concentration (>31 mEq/L).

OTHER DIAGNOSTIC TESTS
A plasma-aldosterone-to-plasma-renin-activity ratio (PA:PRA) greater than 25 is indicative of primary hyperaldosteronism.

A serum potassium concentration of less than 3.5 mEq/L with a concurrent urinary potassium content greater than 30 mEq pe

TABLE 74–6. Differential Diagnosis of Primary Aldosteronism

Disease	Plasma Renin Concentration	Plasma Aldosterone Concentration	Blood Pressure
Primary aldosteronism	Low	High	High
Edematous disorders	High	High	Normal
Malignant hypertension	High	High	High
Congenital adrenal hyperplasia	Low	Low	High
Cushing's syndrome	Low to normal	Low to normal	High
Liddle's syndrome	Low	Low	High
Bartter's syndrome	High	High	Low to normal
Licorice ingestion	Low	Low	High
Low-renin essential hypertension	Low	Low to normal	High

4 hours is suggestive of primary aldosteronism.[36] Normokalemia does not exclude the diagnosis of primary aldosteronism. Between _% and 38% of patients with primary aldosteronism will have serum otassium concentrations greater than 3.6 mEq/L. The diagnosis _f primary aldosteronism can be made with a plasma-aldosterone-_-plasma-renin-activity ratio (PA:PRA). Hirohara and colleagues[44] _ound a PA:PRA greater than 32% to be 100% sensitive and 61% _pecific in patients with aldosterone-producing adenomas. However, _ower cutoffs of 20 and 25 ng/dL per ng/mL have been proposed to _earch for primary hyperaldosteronism.[44–46]

Differentiating between an aldosterone-producing adenoma _APA) and bilateral adrenal hyperplasia (BAH) is imperative to for-_ulate a proper treatment plan. A majority of the adenomas are sin-_ular and small, less than 1 cm. The left adrenal gland is affected at _ higher rate than the right. Patients with APA generally have more _evere hypertension, more profound hypokalemia, and higher plasma _nd urinary aldosterone levels compared to patients with BAH. CT _canning can usually detect most adenomas, though nonfunctional _denomas may occasionally cause confusion.

The underlying abnormality in BAH remains a mystery, but _ome investigators believe that a hormone factor stimulates the zona _lomerulosa, resulting in increased sensitivity to angiotensin II.[34] In _ontrast to APA patients, patients with BAH are able to maintain con-_rol of the renin-angiotensin system, with little effect following doses _f ACTH.

Therapeutic Management

_6_ *BAH-Dependent Hyperaldosteronism.* Spironolactone, _he drug of choice in BAH-dependent hyperaldosteronism, competi-_ively inhibits aldosterone biosynthesis within the adrenal gland, mak-_ng it extremely useful in overstimulated BAH patients.[40,41] It is avail-_ble in oral form, with most patients responding to doses of 25 to _00 mg/day. The clinician should wait 4 to 8 weeks before reassess-_ng the patient for urinary electrolytes and blood pressure control. _dverse effects of spironolactone include gastrointestinal discomfort, _mpotence, gynecomastia, and menstrual irregularities. Additionally, _ecause salicylates increase the renal secretion of canrenone, the _ctive metabolite, patients should be advised to avoid concomi-_ant therapy with salicylates. Because spironolactone blocks testo-_terone biosynthesis, it often is not used in men. The drug of choice _n men and patients intolerant of spironolactone is amiloride.[37,39] The _sual dose is 5 mg twice a day up to 30 mg/day if necessary. More _ecently, eplerenone, a new aldosterone antagonist with high affin-_ty for the aldosterone receptor and low affinity for androgen and _rogesterone receptors, was approved for the treatment of hyper-_ension. It appears to be more beneficial than spironolactone due

to its limited progestational and antiandrogenic side effects. How-ever, its role in the management of hyperaldosteronism has not been established.[37,41]

Second-line therapy is often required to control the blood pres-sure of patients with BAH. Agents useful as second-line choices in-clude the calcium channel blockers, angiotensin-converting enzyme inhibitors, and low-dose diuretics such as hydrochlorothiazide.[38,40,41]

Therapeutic Management

APA-Dependent Hyperaldosteronism. The treatment of choice for APA-dependent aldosteronism remains laparoscopic re-section of the adenoma.[50] If no primary lesion is found, resection of one and a half of the adrenal glands may be attempted, followed by supplemental spironolactone therapy. However, a recent retrospective analysis of patients with aldosterone-producing adenomas who chose medical management instead of surgical resection, revealed medical management to be efficacious in this population and should be consid-ered as an alternative in patients in whom surgery is contraindicated.[51]

Summary

The diagnosis of primary aldosteronism is made through the obser-vation of elevated blood pressure, low serum potassium, high urinary potassium, elevated serum and urinary aldosterone, and an elevated PA:PRA (Fig. 74–5). Differentiating between the various etiologies is mandatory. Patients with adrenal adenomas can be distinguished from patients with hyperplasia by CT scan. Treatment depends on the etiology with surgical resection, well accepted as the treatment of choice in adenomas, and spironolactone or amiloride plus second-line agents in patients with hyperplasia.

SECONDARY ALDOSTERONISM

Secondary hyperaldosteronism results from stimulation of the zona glomerulosa by an extra-adrenal factor, usually the renin-angiotensin system. Excessive potassium intake can create a physiologic increase in aldosterone, as can oral contraceptive use, pregnancy (10 times normal by the third trimester), and menses. Congestive heart failure, cirrhosis, renal artery stenosis, and Bartter's syndrome also can lead to elevated aldosterone concentrations.

Treatment of secondary aldosteronism is dictated by etiology. Control or correction of the extra-adrenal stimulation of aldosterone secretion should resolve the disorder. Medical therapy with spirono-lactone is the mainstay of treatment until an exact etiology can be located.

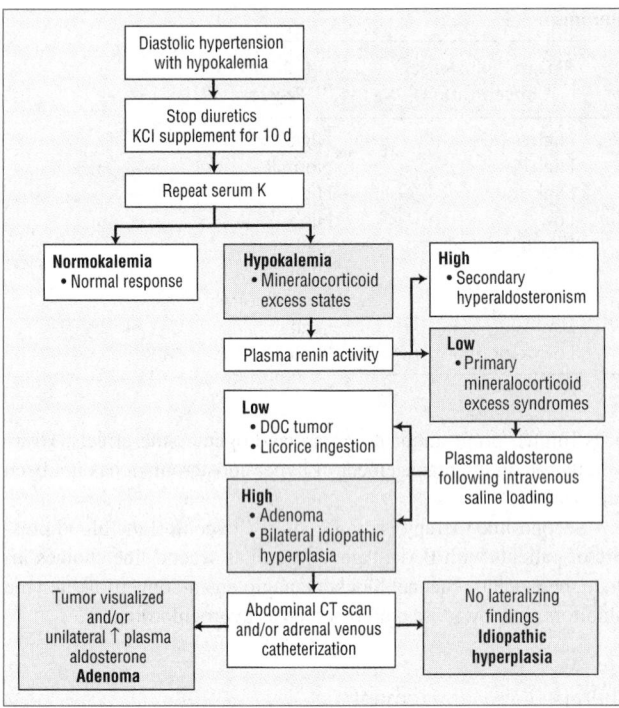

FIGURE 74–5. Algorithm for the diagnosis of primary aldosteronism.

TABLE 74–7. Etiologies of Primary and Secondary Adrenal Insufficiency

Primary Insufficiency	Secondary Insufficiency
Slow onset	
Acquired immunodeficiency syndrome	Craniopharyngioma
Adrenomyeloneuropathy	Cure of Cushing's syndrome
Amyloidosis	Empty sella syndrome
Autoimmune adrenalitis[a]	Tumors of the third ventricle
Bilateral adrenalectomy	Histiocytosis
Congenital adrenal hypoplasia	Hypothalamic tumors
Hemochromatosis	Hypopituitarism
Isolated glucocorticoid deficiency	Long-term corticosteroid administration
Metastatic neoplasia	Lymphocytic hypophysitis
Systemic fungal infection	Pituitary surgery, radiation, or tumor
Tuberculosis[b]	Sarcoidosis
Fast onset	
Adrenal thrombosis, hemorrhage, or necrosis	Postpartum pituitary necrosis
	Necrotic or bleeding pituitary macroadenoma
	Head trauma, lesions of the pituitary stalk
	Pituitary or adrenal surgery for Cushing's syndrome

[a]Accounts for approximately 70% of cases.
[b]Accounts for approximately 20% of cases.

HYPOFUNCTION OF THE ADRENAL GLAND

Primary adrenal insufficiency, or Addison's disease, involves the destruction of all regions of the adrenal cortex. Deficiencies arise in cortisol, aldosterone, and the various androgens. Approximately 40% to 53% of patients with idiopathic primary adrenal insufficiency present with one or more clinical disorders involving multiple endocrine organs. The organs involved can include ovary, thyroid, pancreas, and parathyroid gland. This polyglandular failure syndrome is associated with the idiopathic etiology only and has not been seen with adrenal insufficiency associated with tuberculosis or other invasive diseases.

Secondary insufficiency most commonly results from exogenous steroid use, leading to suppression of the hypothalamic-pituitary-adrenal (HPA)-axis and decreased release of ACTH, resulting in impaired androgen and cortisol production. This has been reported from oral, inhaled, intranasal, and topical glucocorticoid administration.[52–54] Other drugs reported to induce secondary adrenal insufficiency include rifampin, ketoconazole, phenytoin, phenobarbital, mirtazapine, and progestins such as medroxyprogesterone acetate and megestrol acetate.[55–57] Chronic suppression also can result in atrophy of the anterior pituitary and hypothalamus, impairing recovery of function if the exogenous steroid is reduced. Secondary disease classically presents with normal concentrations of mineralocorticoids.

Approximately 90% of the adrenal cortex must be destroyed before adrenal insufficiency symptoms will occur.[58] Specific etiologies for both primary and secondary insufficiency are listed in Table 74–7. Adrenal hemorrhage can result from multiple etiologies including traumatic shock, coagulopathies, ischemic disorders, and other situations of severe stress, but septicemia is the most common. Symptoms include truncal pain, fever, shaking, chills, hypotension preceding shock, anorexia, headache, vertigo, vomiting, rash, psychiatric symptoms, abdominal rigidity or rebound, and death in 6 to 48 hours if not treated. The most common organisms found on autopsy are

Streptococcus pneumoniae, Staphylococcus spp., and *Haemophilus influenzae.*[53]

ADDISON'S DISEASE

Distinguishing Addison's disease from secondary insufficiency is difficult; however, the following guidelines may be helpful:

1. Hyperpigmentation usually is not seen in secondary adrenal insufficiency because of low amounts of melanocyte-stimulating hormone. Low amounts of melanocyte-stimulating hormone are present owing to a deficient pituitary secretion of ACTH and β-lipotropin, all of which are synthesized together in a common precursor peptide, pro-opiomelanocortin (POMC).
2. Aldosterone secretion usually is preserved in secondary insufficiency.
3. Weight loss, dehydration, hyponatremia, hyperkalemia, and elevated blood urea nitrogen are common in Addison's disease.
4. Addison's disease will have an abnormal response to the rapid ACTH-stimulation test. Plasma ACTH levels are usually 400 to 2000 pg/mL in primary insufficiency, versus normal to low (0 to 50 pg/mL; see Table 74–3) in secondary insufficiency. A normal cosyntropin-stimulation test does not rule out secondary adrenal insufficiency.

The short cosyntropin-stimulation test can be used to assess patients suspected of hypocortisolism. Patients are given 250 mcg of synthetic ACTH intravenously or intramuscularly, with serum cortisol levels drawn at baseline and 30 to 60 minutes after the injection. An increase to a cortisol level ≥18 mcg/dL (500 mmol/L) rules out renal insufficiency.[59] While this test remains the most commonly ed method, in some patients with secondary adrenal insufficiency or ild primary adrenal insufficiency, this test will be normal. This result ay be owing to the high dose of corticotropin given. Thus some sug-st that higher cutoff values (≥ 22 to 25 mcg/dL) should be used.[60] lternatively, studies have demonstrated that equivalent results can be en using 1 mcg of cosyntropin. The normal response is an increase a cortisol level ≥ 18 mcg/dL 30 minutes after the injection. Other sts include the insulin hypoglycemia test, the metyrapone test, and e corticotropin-releasing hormone stimulation test.[59,61,62]

Cortisol levels greater than 18 to 20 mcg/dL 30 minutes after a osyntropin-stimulation test are not useful in patients who are acutely l.[63] Severe infection, trauma, burns, illnesses, or surgery can increase rtisol production by as much as a factor of six, making the recog-tion of adrenal insufficiency in this population extremely difficult. the critically ill, a random cortisol level below 15 mcg/dL is in-cative of adrenal insufficiency, while a level greater than 34 mcg/dL ggests that adrenal insufficiency is unlikely.[63] For patients who fall etween these two values, a poor response to corticotropin (less than mcg/dL increase in plasma cortisol from baseline at 30 or 60 min-es) indicates the possibility of adrenal insufficiency and a need for rticosteroid supplementation.[63]

Treatment of Addison's disease must include adequate patient lucation, so that the patient is aware of treatment complications, xpected outcome, missed doses, and drug side effects. The agents of noice are prednisone, hydrocortisone, and cortisone, administered vice daily with the treatment objective being the establishment of e lowest effective dose while mimicking the normal diurnal adrenal ythm.[59] Usually a twice-daily dosing schedule is adequate with the ose depending on the agent used.

Recent studies[64,65] indicate that the daily cortisol production aries between 5 and 10 mg/m^2. Hence, the 12- to 15-mg/m^2 per ay rule for cortisol supplementation, which is roughly equivalent to 5 to 25 mg of hydrocortisone or 25 to 37.5 mg of cortisone acetate aily. A morning dose of cortisone (20 mg), hydrocortisone (15 mg), r prednisone (2.5 mg) followed by an evening dose of the same agent 33% to 50% of the morning dose is usually sufficient to duplicate e normal circadian rhythm of cortisol production. To replace the ineralocorticoid loss, fludrocortisone acetate can be used. A dose of 05 to 0.2 mg by mouth once a day is adequate. If parenteral therapy needed, 2 to 5 mg of deoxycorticosterone trimethylacetate in oil tramuscularly every 3 to 4 weeks can be used. The main reason or adding the mineralocorticoid is to minimize the development of yperkalemia. Adverse effects must be monitored closely. Symptoms clude gastric upset, edema, hypertension, hypokalemia, insomnia, xcitability, and diabetes mellitus. In addition, patient weight, blood ressure, and electrocardiogram should be monitored regularly.[61]

Most adrenal crises occur secondary to glucocorticoid dose re-uction or lack of stress-related dose adjustments. It is recommended at patients receiving corticosteroid-replacement therapy add 5 to 0 mg hydrocortisone to their normal daily regimen shortly before renuous activities such as hiking.[61] Likewise, during times of se-ere physical stress such as febrile illnesses or after accidents, patients nould be instructed to double their daily dose until recovery.[66]

The end point of therapy is difficult to assess in most patients, ut a reduction in excess pigmentation is a good clinical marker. The evelopment of features of Cushing's syndrome indicates excessive placement. Treatment of secondary adrenal insufficiency is identical primary disease treatment with the exception that mineralocorticoid eplacement usually is not necessary. Patient education still should e stressed with emphasis placed on establishing an alternate-day egimen.

ACUTE ADRENAL INSUFFICIENCY

Adrenal crisis, or Addisonian crisis, is characterized by an acute adrenocortical insufficiency. Adrenal crisis represents a true endocrine emergency. Anything that increases adrenal requirements dramati-cally can precipitate an adrenal crisis. Stressful situations, surgery, infection, and trauma all are potential triggering events, especially in the patient with some underlying adrenal or pituitary insufficiency. The most common cause of adrenal crisis is hypothalamic-pituitary-adrenal (HPA)-axis suppression brought on by chronic use of exoge-nous glucocorticoids and abrupt withdrawal.

Treatment of adrenal crisis involves the administration of par-enteral glucocorticoids. Hydrocortisone is the agent of choice owing to its combined mineralocorticoid and glucocorticoid activity. Hydro-cortisone is started at 100 mg intravenously through rapid infusion, and followed by a continuous infusion or intermittent bolus of 100 to 200 mg every 24 hours. Intravenous administration is continued for 24 to 48 hours, at which time if the patient is stable, oral hydrocor-tisone may be started at a dose of 50 mg every 8 hours for another 48 hours. Following oral maintenance therapy, a hydrocortisone taper is initiated until the dosage is 30 to 50 mg/day in divided doses. Fluid replacement often is required and may be accomplished with 5% dex-trose and isotonic saline (D_5NS) at a rate to support blood pressure. If hyperkalemia is present after the hydrocortisone maintenance phase, additional mineralocorticoid usually is required. Fludrocortisone ac-etate in a dose of 0.1 mg by mouth daily is the agent of choice.

Patients with adrenal insufficiency should be instructed to carry a card or wear a bracelet or necklace, such as MedicAlert, that con-tains information about their condition. Patients should also have easy access to injectable hydrocortisone or glucocorticoid suppositories in case of an emergency or during times of physical stress, such as febrile illness or injury.[61]

CLINICAL PRESENTATION: ADRENAL INSUFFICIENCY

SYMPTOMS

- Patients commonly complain of weakness, weight loss, gastrointestinal symptoms, craving for salt, headaches, memory impairment, depression, and postural dizziness.
- Early symptoms of acute adrenal insufficiency also include myalgias, malaise, and anorexia. As the situation progresses, vomiting, fever, hypotension, and shock will develop.

SIGNS

- Increased pigmentation
- Hypotension (postural)
- Fever
- Decreased body hair
- Vitiligo
- Features of hypopituitarism (amenorrhea and cold intolerance)

LABORATORY TESTS

The short cosyntropin stimulation test can be used to assess patients suspected of hypercortisolism.

OTHER DIAGNOSTIC TESTS

Other tests include the insulin hypoglycemia test, the me-tyrapone test, and the corticotropin-releasing hormone stim-ulation test.

HYPOALDOSTERONISM

Hypoaldosteronism is rare and usually is associated with low renin status, diabetes, complete heart block, or severe postural hypotension, or it may occur postoperatively following tumor removal.[2] Hypoaldosteronism may be part of a larger adrenal insufficiency or be the only defect the patient has. In nonselective hypoaldosteronism, the etiology of the low aldosterone is most likely generalized adrenocortical insufficiency (see Addison's disease). In selective hypoaldosteronism, the etiology is usually a specific defect in the stimulation of adrenal aldosterone secretion (21-hydroxylase deficiency being most common) or a defect in peripheral aldosterone action (decreased aldosterone receptors).

Laboratory analysis reveals low serum sodium and high serum potassium concentrations. Patients often will present with hyperchloremic metabolic acidosis. Because the deficiency is in the mineralocorticoid, replacement with fludrocortisone in a dose of 0.1 to 0.3 mg is usually effective. Patients should be followed for blood pressure response as well as electrolyte status.

CONGENITAL ADRENAL HYPERPLASIA

Because many enzyme systems are needed to complete the complex cholesterol-to-cortisol pathway, enzyme deficiencies may lead to disruptions of the normal cascade of events (see Fig. 74–2). This group of enzyme disorders is known as congenital adrenal hyperplasia, mainly because of the resultant chronic adrenal gland stimulation that occurs following enzyme deficiency.[67,68] The most frequent is steroid 21-hydroxylase deficiency, accounting for more than 90% of cases. Any enzyme deficiency is capable of affecting any one or all three of the steroid pathways. Therefore treatment should be focused on replacement of the deficient hormone, as well as cessation of the chronic stimulation causing the hyperplasia. In Table 74–8, six of the most common enzyme deficiencies are briefly outlined.

ADRENAL VIRILISM

Virilism, excessive secretion of androgens from the adrenal gland, is more commonly seen in females, with hirsutism being the dominant feature. Women who present with hirsutism also may have voice deepening, increased muscle mass, menstrual abnormalities, clitoral enlargement, redistribution of body fat and loss of female body contour, breast atrophy, and hair recession and crown balding.[69] Though virilism may be easy to diagnose based on clinical symptoms, making the diagnosis on a biochemical basis is difficult. The most common etiology of virilism involves one of many possible congenital enzyme defects. Depending on the enzyme deficiency, accumulation of a variety of androgens, notably testosterone, can develop.

Treatment of virilism centers around suppression of the pituitary-adrenal axis with exogenous glucocorticoids. Choice of steroids is variable. In adults, the usual steroids used are dexamethasone (0.25 to 0.5 mg), prednisone (2.5 to 5 mg), or hydrocortisone (10 to 20 mg).[69] Antiandrogen use may allow lower steroid doses to be used.

HIRSUTISM

Hirsutism (hypertrichosis) is defined as more hair than is cosmetically acceptable. The majority of cases occur in women with some degree of excess androgen production, though certain drugs also may induce hirsutism. Examples of such drugs include minoxidil, phenytoin, cyclosporine, methyldopa, danazol, metoclopramide, phenothiazines, reserpine, and diazoxide. Androgen excess can be derived from either the ovaries or the adrenal glands, with a small fraction coming from pituitary disorders. Ovarian excess is typically associated with obesity and menstrual abnormalities. In the patient with hirsutism, congenital adrenal hyperplasia, adrenal tumors, and ovarian tumors should be ruled out.[69,70]

TABLE 74–8. Congenital Adrenal Hyperplasia (CAH)

Enzyme Deficiency (Disorder)	Symptoms	Lab Tests	Comments
20-Hydroxylase (nonvirilizing CAH)	Enlarged female genitalia and adrenal gland (due to cholesterol)	All steroids are low in blood and urine	Poor prognosis for infants
17-Hydroxylase (nonvirilizing CAH)	Hypertension usually present	Low concentrations of cortisol and estrogens	Mineralocorticoid replacement not necessary
21-Hydroxylase (virilizing CAH)	Pubertal irregularities (acne, early pubic hair, voice lowering, and increased muscularity); mature normally with replacement	High progesterone, renin, 17-hydroxyprogesterone and ACTH; low cortisol, sodium, and aldosterone	Most common form of CAH (90% of total), incidence of 1/10,000; monitor growth velocity, bone age, renin, and 17-hydroxyprogesterone
11-Hydroxylase (virilizing CAH)	Hypertension secondary to high deoxycortisol and virilism from androgen excess; mistaken for Cushing's, but no glucose intolerance	Low plasma cortisone and aldosterone; high ACTH and MSH concentrations	Second most common form of CAH (9% of total), incidence of 1/100,000; final step in biosynthesis of corticosterone and cortisol; found only in adrenal cortex
3-Hydroxysteroid dehydrogenase (mixed CAH)	Both cortisol and aldosterone deficiencies	Decreased aldosterone, cortisol, estrogens, and androgens; increased pregnenolone and cholesterol	Defect affects both adrenals and gonads
18-Hydroxysteroid dehydrogenase (corticosterone methyloxidase deficiency)	Hypotension	Restricted to zona glomerulosa; sole aldosterone defect; hyponatremia, hyperkalemia, increased renin	Mineralocorticoid replacement without glucocorticoid replacement

TABLE 74–9. Relative Potencies of Glucocorticoids

Glucocorticoid	Anti-Inflammatory Potency	Equivalent Potency (mg)	Approximate Half-Life (min)	Sodium-Retaining Potency
Cortisone	0.8	25	30	2
Hydrocortisone	1	20	90	2
Prednisone	3.5	5	60	1
Prednisolone	4	5	200	1
Triamcinolone	5	4	300	0
Methylprednisolone	5	4	180	0
Betamethasone	25	0.6	100–300	0
Dexamethasone	30	0.75	100–300	0

Cosmetic approaches are generally tried first, with laser photothermodestruction offering the greatest long-term success. Only when cosmetic surgery is ineffective should suppressive therapy be used. Glucocorticoids, such as dexamethasone, can be used if the androgen source is adrenal, but may induce cushingoid symptoms even at doses of 0.5 mg/day. Oral contraceptives can be used in patients who require contraception concurrently. If oral contraceptives are used, a progestin with low androgen activity (norethynodrel or ethynodiol diacetate) should be employed. Gonadotropin-releasing hormone may be an effective adjunct to oral contraceptives if the source of androgen is ovarian. Antiandrogens are often added to the more specific therapies. The most common include spironolactone, flutamide, and finasteride, although none of these is approved by the Food and Drug Administration for the treatment of hirsutism. It can take 4 months for the antiandrogens to alleviate the hirsutism, and duration of therapy is unclear.[69,70]

CLINICAL CONTROVERSY

Some clinicians believe that the usual starting doses for glucocorticoid supplementation are high and unnecessarily increase a patient's risk for adverse outcomes such as osteoporosis.

PRINCIPLES OF GLUCOCORTICOID ADMINISTRATION

Originally, the term *glucocorticoid* was given to these agents to describe their glucose-regulating properties. However, carbohydrate metabolism is only one of a multitude of effects that steroids can exhibit. The activity produced is a function of the receptor activated (glucocorticoid versus mineralocorticoid) as well as the agent and dose prescribed.

The mechanism of glucocorticoids is complex and not fully known. The glucocorticoid enters the cell through passive diffusion and binds to its specific receptor. There are between 5000 and 100,000 receptors per cell. Steroids exhibit various binding affinities to the vast number of receptors in almost every tissue and therefore elicit a wide variety of biologic effects.

After binding to the receptor, there is a structural change that occurs in the receptor, known as *activation*. After activation, the receptor-steroid complex binds to deoxyribonucleic acid sites in the cell called *glucocorticoid regulatory elements* (GREs). This binding to the GREs stimulates or inhibits transcription of nearby genes.

The pharmacokinetics of the glucocorticoids varies with the agent given and the route of administration. In general, most steroids given by the oral route are well absorbed. Water-soluble agents are more rapidly absorbed following intramuscular injection than are lipid-soluble agents. Intravenous administration is recommended when a quick onset of action is needed. A summary of the steroids is provided in Table 74–9.

In addition to systemic steroids causing iatrogenic Cushing's syndrome, they also can lead to increased susceptibility to infection, osteoporosis, sodium retention with resultant edema, hypokalemia, hypomagnesemia, cataracts, peptic ulcer disease, seizures, and generalized suppression of the HPA-axis. Long-term complications tend to be insidious and less likely to respond to steroid withdrawal.

Suppression of the HPA-axis is a major concern whenever systemic steroids are tapered or withdrawn. Single doses of glucocorticoids can prevent the axis from responding to major stressors for several hours. In general, the longer the steroid is administered and the higher the dose used, the more suppression of the axis occurs. However, the possibility of suppression occurs any time the patient is exposed to supraphysiologic doses of a steroid.[62,71] Symptoms of steroid withdrawal resemble those seen in a patient with adrenocortical deficiency.

A variety of recommendations for steroid tapering are available.[62,72,73] In general, patients who have been on long-term steroid therapy will need to be gradually withdrawn toward physiologic doses over months. On average, the normal adult produces approximately 20 to 30 mg of cortisol per day with the peak concentration occurring around 8:00 A.M. As the steroid or steroid-equivalent dose approaches the 20- to 30-mg level, the taper should be slowed and the patient checked for axis function. The primary mode to test HPA integrity is the ACTH test, either high- or low-dose. A normal ACTH test would indicate that daily steroid maintenance therapy is not needed. More recently, the use of exogenous human CRH was found to be nearly as useful in the assessment of pituitary-adrenal function.[74] Caution should be used to prevent disease exacerbation during the steroid taper to prevent the need for rebolusing the patient with another course of high-dose steroids. The dilemma of prolonged steroid administration is sometimes lessened by the use of an alternate-day therapy (ADT) regimen.[72,73] ADT theoretically minimizes the hypothalamic-pituitary suppression as well as some of the adverse effects seen with once-daily therapy. This can be especially important in the treatment of the child and young adult, in whom growth suppression is a major concern. ADT is not recommended for initial management, but rather in the management of the stabilized patient who needs long-term therapy. The patient will be exposed to "on" and "off" days, with the "on" day dose gradually increased with concurrent reduction in the "off" day dose over a period of 14 days. By the fourteenth day, the patient will be consuming medication only on the "on" day. It should be noted that not all patients will have

TABLE 74–10. Factors in Successful Glucocorticoid Therapy

Monitoring	Glucose concentrations (serum and urine)
	Electrolytes (serum and urine)
	Ophthalmologic exams
	Stool tests for occult blood loss
	Growth and development (children and adolescents)
Counseling	Take with food to minimize gastrointestinal discomfort
	Never discontinue medication on your own; check with your physician; gradual dose reduction is usually necessary
	Carry or wear medical identification indicating that you are on long-term glucocorticoid therapy
	Dosage increases may be necessary at times of increased stress (surgery or emergency treatments)
	Be aware of potential side effects (i.e., visual disturbances, bruising, and delayed wound healing)
	What to do if you miss a dose: If your dosing schedule is
	Every other day: Take as soon as possible if remembered that morning. If not remembered until later, skip that day. Take the next morning, then skip the following day.
	Every day: Take as soon as possible, but skip if almost time for the next dose. Never double doses.
Recognizing complications	Early in therapy and essentially unavoidable: insomnia, enhanced appetite, weight gain
	Common in patients with underlying risk factors: hypertension, diabetes mellitus, peptic ulcer disease
	Long-term intense treatment: cushingoid habitus, hypothalamic-pituitary-adrenal suppression, impaired wound healing
	Delayed and insidious: cataracts, atherosclerosis
	Rare and unpredictable: psychosis, glaucoma, pancreatitis

From United States Pharmacopeial Convention[75] and Barlow.[76]

equivalent disease control on ADT, and it should be avoided in certain indications.[73]

EVALUATION OF THERAPEUTIC OUTCOMES

Successful glucocorticoid therapy involves counseling the patient, monitoring the patient, and recognizing complications of therapy (Table 74–10). The risk:benefit ratio of glucocorticoid administration should always be considered, especially with concurrent disease states such as hypertension, diabetes mellitus, peptic ulcer disease, and uncontrolled systemic infections.

CLINICAL CONTROVERSY

Some clinicians believe that twice-daily administration of glucocorticoids in patients with adrenal insufficiency is not as effective as three-times daily. If a twice-daily regimen is used, the second dose should be administered 6 to 8 hours after the first.

ABBREVIATIONS

ACTH: adrenocorticotropic hormone
ADT: alternate-day therapy
APA: aldosterone-producing adenoma
BAH: bilateraladrenalhyperplasia
CBG: corticosteroid-binding globulin
CRH: corticotropin-releasing hormone
CT: computed tomography

D₅NS: 5% dextrose and isotonic saline
DDT: dichlorodiphenyltrichloroethane
DST: dexamethasone suppression test
GRE: glucocorticoid regulatory element
HPA: hypothalamic-pituitary-adrenal
IRMA: immunoradiometric assay
MRI: magnetic resonance imaging
PA:PRA: plasma-aldosterone-to-plasma-renin-activity ratio
RIA: radioimmunoassay
RU-486: mifepristone

Review Questions and other resources can be found at *www.pharmacotherapyonline.com.*

REFERENCES

1. Conn JW. Primary aldosteronism, a new clinical syndrome. J Lab Clin Med 1955;45:6–17.
2. Orth DN, Kovacs WJ. The adrenal cortex. In: Wilson JD, Foster DW, Kronenberg HM, Larsen PR eds. Williams' Textbook of Endocrinology. Philadelphia, Saunders, 1998:517–664.
3. Albright F. Cushing syndrome. Harvey Lect 1942–1943;38:123–186.
4. Boscaro M, Barzon L, Sonino N. The diagnosis of Cushing's syndrome: atypical presentations and laboratory shortcomings. Arch Intern Med 2000;160:3045–3053.
5. Orth DN. Cushing's syndrome. N Engl J Med 1995;332:791–803.
6. Williams GH, Duly RG. Diseases of the adrenal cortex. In: Isselbacher KJ, Braunwald E, Wilson JD et al, eds. Harrison's Principles of Internal Medicine, 13th ed. New York, McGraw-Hill, 1994:1953–1976.
7. Newell-Price J, Trainer P, Besser M, Grossman A. The diagnosis and differential diagnosis of Cushing's syndrome and Pseudo-Cushing's states. Endocr Rev 1998;19:647–672.

Pharmacotherapy

A Pathophysiologic Approach, 6/e

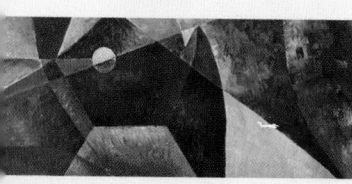

ONLINE LEARNING CENTER (OLC)

www.pharmacotherapyonline.com

- The online resource to accompany Pharmacotherapy: A Pathophysiologic Approach, Sixth Edition.
- Self-testing program and Learning Objectives for each chapter.
- Access to daily updates on important drug-related news through PNN Pharmacotherapy Line.

E-BOOK VERSION OF PHARMACOTHERAPY: A PATHOPHYSIOLOGIC APPROACH, 6/e

- ONE free download to ONE computer for purchasers of the book available from www.pharmacotherapyonline.com.
- Fast access to the complete content of PHARMACOTHERAPY: A PATHOPHYSIOLOGIC APPROACH, SIXTH EDITION from your laptop or desktop computer. It is completely searchable and it can be annotated with your comments.
- Technical support information available at **http://books.mcgraw-hill.com/techsupport/**

FOLLOW THESE DIRECTIONS TO OBTAIN THESE VALUABLE RESOURCES:

1) Use your Web browser to go to **http://www.pharmacotherapyonline.com.**

2) Register Now.

3) Fill in the required fields.

4) Enter your registration code.

5) Set up your User ID and Password.

Important Note: You must be logged in to the Online Learning Center in order to download the e-book version of PHARMACOTHERAPY, 6e.

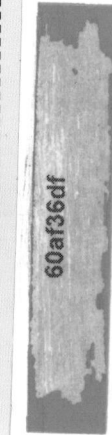

60af36df

E-BOOK DOWNLOAD CODE

Scratch off coating above to reveal a code for obtaining one download of an e-book of Pharmacotherapy: A Pathophysiologic Approach, Sixth Edition. See details above.

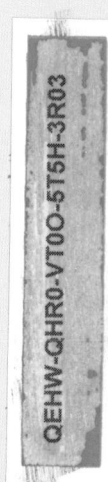

QEHW-QHR0-VT0O-5T5H-3R03

ONLINE LEARNING CENTER CODE

Scratch off the coating above to reveal a code for obtaining access to www.pharmacotherapyonline.com. See details above.

p/n 146393-3

28. Avgerinos PC, Nieman LK, Oldfield EH, Cutler GB Jr. A comparison of the overnight and the standard metyrapone test for the differential diagnosis of adrenocorticotrophin-dependent Cushing's syndrome. Clin Endocrinol 1996;45:483–491.

29. Cremonini N, Furno A, Sforza A, et al. 111In-octreotide scintigraphy in endocrine tumors. Preliminary data. Q J Nucl Med 1995;39(4 Suppl 1): 116–120.

30. Sakai Y, Horiba N, Tozawa F, et al. Desmopressin stimulation test for diagnosis of ACTH-dependent Cushing's syndrome. Endocr J 1997;44: 687–695.

31. Jackson RV, Hockings GI, Torpy DJ, et al. New diagnostic tests for Cushing's syndrome: Uses of naloxone, vasopressin and alprazolam. Clin Exp Pharmacol Physiol 1996;23:579–581.

32. Ambrosi B, Bochicchio D, Colombo P, et al. Loperamide to diagnose Cushing's syndrome. JAMA 1993;270:2301–2302.

33. Wiggam MI, Heaney AP, McIlrath EM, et al. Bilateral inferior petrosal sinus sampling in the differential diagnosis of adrenocorticotropin-dependent Cushing's syndrome: a comparison with other diagnostic tests. J Clin Endocrinol Metab 2000;85:1525–1532.

34. Yanovski JA, Cutler GB Jr, Chrousos GP, Nieman LK. The dexamethasone-suppressed corticotropin-releasing hormone stimulation test differentiates mild Cushing's disease from normal physiology. J Clin Endocrinol Metab 1998;83:348–352.

35. al-Saadi N, Diederich S, Oelkers W. A very high dose dexamethasone suppression test for differential diagnosis of Cushing's syndrome. Clin Endocrinol 1998;48:45–51.

36. Findling JW, Raff H. Newer diagnostic techniques and problems in Cushing's disease. Endocrinol Metab Clin North Am 1999;28: 191–210.

37. Arvat E, Giordano R, Ramunni J, et al. Adrenocorticotropin and cortisol hyperresponsiveness to hexarelin in patients with Cushing's disease bearing a pituitary microadenoma, but not in those with macroadenoma. J Clin Endocrinol Metab 1998;83:4207–4211.

38. Findling JW, Raff H, Aron DC. The low-dose dexamethasone suppression test: a reevaluation in patients with Cushing's syndrome. J Clin Endocrinol Metab 2004;89:1222–1226.

39. Peppercorn PD, Reznek RH. State-of-the-art CT and MRI of the adrenal gland. Eur Radiol 1997;7:822–836.

40. Sosa JA, Udelsman R. Imaging of the adrenal gland. Surg Oncol Clin North Am 1999;8:109–127.

41. Harte C, Henry MT, Murphy KD, Mitchell TH. Progestogens and Cushing's syndrome. Ir J Med Sci 1995;164:274–275.

42. Priftis K, Everard ML, Milner AD. Unexpected side-effects of inhaled steroids: a case report. Eur J Pediatr 1991;150:448–449.

43. Wilson AM, Blumsohn A, Jung RT, Lipworth BJ. Asthma and Cushing's syndrome. Chest 2000;117:593–594.

44. Teelucksingh S, Bahall M, Coomansingh D, et al. Cushing's syndrome from topical glucocorticoids. West Indian Med J 1993;42:77–78.

45. Cizza G, Chrousos GP. Adrenocorticotrophic hormone-dependent Cushing's syndrome. Cancer Treat Res 1997;89:25–40.

46. Sonino N, Boscaro M. Medical therapy for Cushing's disease. Endocrinol Metab Clin North Am 1999;28:211–222.

47. McEvoy GK, ed. American Hospital Formulary Service (AHFS) Drug Information. American Society of Hospital Pharmacists 2004;15–17, 507–513, 1092–1094.

48. United States Pharmacopeial Convention Inc. USPDI: Drug information for the health care professional, Vol. I, 19th ed. Taunton, MA, Rand-McNally, 1999:67–69.

49. Engelhardt D. Steroid biosynthesis inhibitors in Cushing's syndrome. Clin Invest 1994;72:481–488.

50. Morris D, Grossman A. The medical management of Cushing's syndrome. Ann N Y Acad Sci 2002;970:119–133.

51. Cocconi G. First generation aromatase inhibitors-aminoglutethimide and testololactone. Breast Cancer Res Treat 1994;30:57–80.

52. Baulieu EE. RU 486 (mifepristone). A short overview of its mechanisms of action and clinical uses at the end of 1996. Ann N Y Acad Sci 1997;828:47–58.

33. Semple PL, Vance ML, Findling J, Laws ER. Transsphenoidal surgery for Cushing's disease: outcome in patients with a normal magnetic resonance imaging scan. Neurosurgery 2000;46:553–558.

34. Estrada J, Boronat M, Mielgo M, et al. The long-term outcome of pituitary irradiation after unsuccessful transsphenoidal surgery in Cushing's disease. N Engl J Med 1997;336:172–177.

35. Comi RJ, Gorden P. Long-term medical treatment of ectopic ACTH syndrome. South Med J 1998;91:1014–1018.

36. Berwaerts JJ, Verhelst JA, Verhaert GC, et al. Corticotropin-dependent Cushing's syndrome in older people: Presentation of five cases and therapeutical use of ketoconazole. J Am Geriatr Soc 1998;46:880–884.

37. Young WF Jr. Primary aldosteronism: management issues. Ann N Y Acad Sci 2002;970:61–76.

38. Corry DB, Tuck ML. Secondary aldosteronism. Endocrinol Metab Clin North Am 1995;24:511–529.

39. Stewart PM. Mineralocorticoid hypertension. Lancet 1999;353: 1341–1347.

40. Ganguly A. Primary aldosteronism. N Engl J Med 1998;339:1828–1834.

41. Blumenfeld JD, Vaughan ED Jr. Diagnosis and treatment of primary aldosteronism. World J Urol 1999;17:15–21.

42. Fardella CE, Mosso L. Primary aldosteronism. Clin Lab 2002;48: 181–190.

43. Wheeler MH, Harris DA. Diagnosis and management of primary aldosteronism. World J Surg 2003;27:627–631.

44. Hirohara D, Nomura K, Okamoto T, et al. Performance of the basal aldosterone to renin ratio and of the renin stimulation test by furosemide and upright posture in screening for aldosterone-producing adenoma in low renin hypertensives. J Clin Endocrinol Metab 2001;86:4292–4298.

45. Loh KC, Koay ES, Khaw MC, et al. Prevalence of primary aldosteronism among Asian hypertensive patients in Singapore. J Clin Endocrinol Metab 2000;85:2854–2859.

46. Fardella CE, Mosso L, Gomez-Sanchez C, et al. Primary hyperaldosteronism in essential hypertensives: Prevalence, biochemical profile, and molecular biology. J Clin Endocrinol Metab 2000;85:1863–1867.

47. Torpy DJ, Stratakis CA, Chrousos GP. Hyper- and hypoaldosteronism. Vitam Horm 1999;57:177–216.

48. Young WF. Primary aldosteronism: A common and curable form of hypertension. Cardiol Rev 1999;7:207–214.

49. Fardella CE, Mosso L, Gomez-Sanchez C, et al. Primary hyperaldosteronism in essential hypertensives: Prevalence, biochemical profile, and molecular biology. J Clin Endocrinol Metab 2000;85:1863–1867.

50. Gagner M, Pomp A, Heniford BT, et al. Laparoscopic adrenalectomy: lessons learned from 100 consecutive procedures. Ann Surg 1997; 226:238–246.

51. Ghose RP, Hall PM, Bravo EL. Medical management of aldosterone-producing adenomas. Ann Intern Med 1999;131:105–108.

52. Levin C, Maibach HI. Topical corticosteroid-induced adrenocortical insufficiency: Clinical implications. Am J Clin Dermatol 2002;3:141–147.

53. Bello CE, Garrett SD. Therapeutic issues in oral glucocorticoid use. Lippincotts Prim Care Pract 1999;3:333–341.

54. Sizonenko PC. Effects of inhaled or nasal glucocorticosteroids on adrenal function and growth. J Pediatr Endocrinol Metab 2002;15:5–26.

55. Goodman A, Cagliero E. Megestrol-induced clinical adrenal insufficiency. Eur J Gynaecol Oncol 2000;21:117–118.

56. Schule C, Baghai T, Bidlingmaier M, et al. Endocrinological effects of mirtazapine in healthy volunteers. Prog Neuropsychopharmacol Biol Psychiatry 2002;26:1253–1261.

57. Werbel SS, Ober KP. Acute adrenal insufficiency. Endocrinol Metab Clin North Am 1993;22:303–328.

58. Carey RM. The changing clinical spectrum of adrenal insufficiency. Ann Intern Med 1997;127:1103–1105.

59. Dorin RI, Qualls CR, Crapo LM. Diagnosis of adrenal insufficiency. Ann Intern Med 2003;139:194–204.

60. Oelkers W. The role of high- and low-dose corticotropin tests in the diagnosis of secondary adrenal insufficiency. Eur J Endocrinol 1998;139:567–570.

61. Arlt W, Allolio B. Adrenal insufficiency. Lancet 2003;361:1881–1893.

62. Krasner AS. Glucocorticoid-induced adrenal insufficiency. JAMA 1999; 282:671–676.

63. Cooper MS, Stewart PM. Corticosteroid insufficiency in acutely ill patients. N Engl J Med 2003;348:727–734.

64. Brandon DD, Isabelle LM, Samuels MH, et al. Cortisol production rate measurement by stable isotope dilution using gas chromatography-negative ion chemical ionization mass spectrometry. Steroids 1999;64: 372–378.

65. Kraan GP, Dullaart RP, Pratt JJ, et al. The daily cortisol production reinvestigated in healthy men. The serum and urinary cortisol production rates are not significantly different. J Clin Endocrinol Metab 1998;83:1247–1252.

66. Coursin DB, Wood KE. Corticosteroid supplementation for adrenal insufficiency. JAMA 2002;287:236–240.

67. Speiser PW, White PC. Congenital adrenal hyperplasia. N Engl J Med 2003;349:776–788.

68. Deaton MA, Glorioso JE, McLean DB. Congenital adrenal hyperplasia: Not really a zebra. Am Fam Phys 1999;59:1190–1196.

69. Rittmaster RS. Hirsutism. Lancet 1997;349:191–195.

70. Bergfeld WF. Hirsutism in women: Effective therapy that is safe for long term use. Postgrad Med 2000;107:93–104.

71. Henzen C, Suter A, Lerch E, et al. Suppression and recovery of adrenal response after short-term, high-dose glucocorticoid treatment. Lancet 2000; 355:542–545.

72. Kountz DS, Clark CL. Safely withdrawing patients from chronic glucocorticoid therapy. Am Fam Physician 1997;55:521–552.

73. Baxter JD. Advances in glucocorticoid therapy. Adv Intern Med 2000; 45:317–349.

74. Choi CH, Tiu SC, Shek CC, et al. Use of the low-dose corticotropin stimulation test for the diagnosis of secondary adrenocortical insufficiency. Hong Kong Med J 2002;8:427–434.

75. United States Pharmacopeial Convention Inc. USPDI: Advice for the patient: Drug Information in Lay Language, Vol. II, 19th ed. Taunton, MA: Rand-McNally 1999:612–616.

76. Barlow JE. Complications of therapy. In: Boumpas DT, moderator. Glucocorticoid therapy for immune mediated diseases: Basic and clinical correlates. Ann Intern Med 1993;119:1198–1208.

75

PITUITARY GLAND DISORDERS

Amy Heck Sheehan, Jack A. Yanovski, and Karim Anton Calis

Learning Objectives and other resources can be found at *www.pharmacotherapyonline.com.*

KEY CONCEPTS

◀1 Pharmacologic therapy for acromegaly should be considered when surgery and irradiation are contraindicated, when rapid control of symptoms is needed, or when other treatments have failed to normalize growth hormone (GH) and insulin-like growth factor-I (IGF-I) concentrations.

◀2 Dopamine agonists provide advantages of oral dosing and reduced cost when compared to somatostatin analogs and pegvisomant. However, dopamine agonists effectively normalize IGF-I concentrations in only 10% of patients.

◀3 Octreotide therapy should be initiated using the short-acting subcutaneous formulation. Patients who have been maintained on subcutaneous octreotide for at least 2 weeks, and have shown response to therapy, may be converted to the long-acting depot form of octreotide.

◀4 Blood glucose concentrations should be monitored frequently in the early stages of octreotide therapy in all acromegalic patients.

◀5 Pegvisomant appears to be the most effective agent for normalizing IGF-I concentrations. However, further study is needed to determine the long-term safety and efficacy of this agent for the treatment of acromegaly.

◀6 Recombinant GH is currently considered the mainstay of therapy for the treatment of children with growth-hormone-deficient (GHD) short stature. Prompt diagnosis of GHD and initiation of replacement therapy with recombinant GH is crucial for optimizing final adult heights.

◀7 All GH products are generally considered to be equally efficacious. The recommended dose for treatment of GHD short stature in children is 0.3 mg/kg per week.

◀8 Pharmacologic agents that antagonize dopamine or increase the release of prolactin can induce hyperprolactinemia. Discontinuation of the offending medication and initiation of an appropriate therapeutic alternative usually normalizes serum prolactin concentrations.

◀9 Cabergoline appears to be more effective than bromocriptine for the medical management of prolactinomas and offers the advantage of less-frequent dosing and decreased adverse events.

◀10 Patients receiving cabergoline who plan to become pregnant should discontinue the medication at least 1 month before planned conception.

◀11 Pharmacologic treatment of panhypopituitarism consists of glucocorticoids, thyroid-hormone preparations, sex steroids, and recombinant growth hormone, where appropriate, as lifelong replacement therapy.

In the 1950s Geoffrey Harris and his colleagues uncovered the physiologic importance of pituitary hormones and proposed the theory of neurohormonal regulation of the pituitary by the hypothalamus.[1] Today the pituitary gland is recognized for its essential role in body homeostasis, and for this reason it is often referred to as the "master gland." The hypothalamus and the pituitary gland are closely connected, and together they provide a means of communication between the brain and many of the body's endocrine organs. The hypothalamus uses nervous input and metabolic signals from the body to control the secretion of pituitary hormones that regulate growth, thyroid function, adrenal activity, reproduction, lactation, and fluid balance.

ANATOMY AND PHYSIOLOGY

The hypothalamus (Fig. 75–1) is a small region at the base of the brain that receives autonomic nervous input from different areas of the body to regulate limbic functions, food and water intake, body temperature, cardiovascular function, respiratory function, and diurnal rhythms. In addition, the hypothalamus controls the release of hormones from the anterior and posterior regions of the pituitary gland. Neurons in the hypothalamus produce vasopressin and oxytocin and make many hormone-releasing factors that stimulate or inhibit the release of trophic hormones. At the base of the hypothalamus, a projection known as the *median eminence* is rich with nerve axons and blood vessels and provides both chemical and physical connections between the hypothalamus and the pituitary gland.

The pituitary gland, also referred to as the hypophysis, is located at the base of the brain in a cavity of the sphenoid bone known as the *sella turcica.* The pituitary is separated from the brain by an extension of the dura mater known as the *diaphragma sella.* The pituitary is a very small gland, weighing between 0.4 and 1 g in adults. It is divided into two distinct regions, the anterior lobe, or adenohypophysis, and the posterior lobe, or the neurohypophysis (see Fig. 75–1).

The posterior pituitary gland secretes two major hormones, oxytocin and vasopressin (antidiuretic hormone) (Table 75–1). Oxytocin

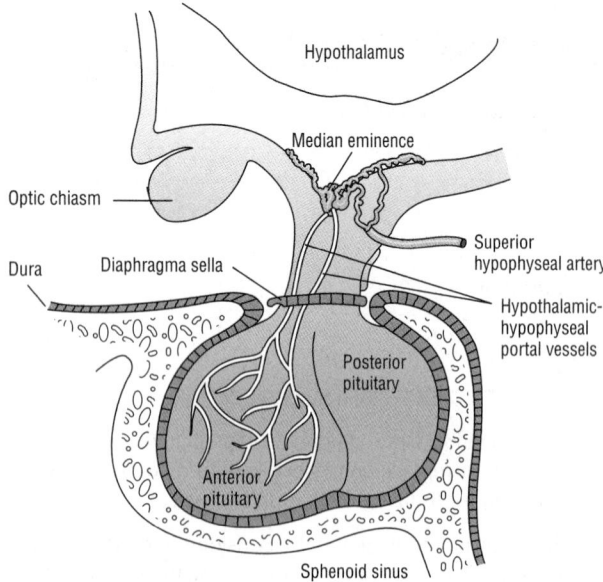

FIGURE 75–1. Pituitary gland.

release from the posterior pituitary causes contraction of the smooth muscles in the breast during lactation and also plays a role in uterine contraction during parturition. Vasopressin is essential for proper fluid balance and acts on the renal collecting ducts to conserve water. Oxytocin and vasopressin are synthesized in the paraventricular and supraoptic nuclei of the hypothalamus. The posterior pituitary gland contains the terminal nerve endings of these two nuclei as well as specialized secretory granules that release hormones in response to appropriate signals. Loss of anterior pituitary function does not necessarily affect the release of vasopressin or oxytocin, because these hormones are actually synthesized in the hypothalamus.

Unlike the posterior pituitary, the release of anterior pituitary hormones is not regulated by direct nervous stimulation, but rather is controlled by specific hypothalamic releasing and inhibitory hormones. The median eminence of the hypothalamus contains a large number of capillaries that converge to form a network of veins known as the hypothalamic-hypophysial portal circulation. Inhibiting and releasing hormones synthesized in the neurons of the hypothalamus reach the anterior pituitary via the hypothalamic-hypophysial portal vessels to control release of anterior pituitary hormones. Although there is a direct arterial blood supply to the anterior pituitary lobe, the hypothalamic-hypophysial portal vessels provide the primary blood supply (see Fig. 75–1). In contrast to the posterior pituitary, the anterior pituitary lobe is extremely vascular and has the highest rate of blood flow of all body organs.

The specialized secretory cells of the anterior pituitary lobe secrete six major polypeptide hormones (see Table 75–1). These include growth hormone (GH) or somatotropin, adrenocorticotropic hormone (ACTH) or corticotropin, thyroid-stimulating hormone (TSH) or thyrotropin, prolactin, follicle-stimulating hormone (FSH), and luteinizing hormone (LH). The release of these hormones is regulated primarily by hypothalamic releasing and inhibiting hormones. Thyrotropin-releasing hormone (TRH) stimulates anterior pituitary release of TSH and prolactin, corticotropin-releasing hormone (CRH) stimulates anterior pituitary release of ACTH, growth hormone-releasing hormone (GHRH) stimulates anterior pituitary release of GH, and gonadotropin-releasing hormone (GnRH) stimulates anterior pituitary release of LH and FSH. Hypothalamic release of somatostatin inhibits release of growth hormone, and hypothalamic release

of dopamine (prolactin-inhibitory hormone) inhibits the secretion of prolactin. Prolactin differs from the other anterior lobe hormones in that an inhibiting factor, rather than a stimulating factor, is primarily responsible for controlling its secretion. In the absence of hypothalamic input, an excess of prolactin is produced, whereas a deficiency state of other anterior pituitary hormones results. Physiologic regulation and action of anterior and posterior pituitary hormones are summarized in Table 75–1.[2–4]

Destruction of the pituitary gland may result in secondary hypothyroidism, hypogonadism, adrenal insufficiency, growth hormone deficiency, and hypoprolactinemia. The formation of certain types of pituitary tumors may result in pituitary hormone excess. Pituitary tumors may also physically compress the pituitary and prevent the release of the trophic hypothalamic factors that regulate pituitary hormones. In this chapter, the pathophysiology and role of pharmacotherapy in the treatment of acromegaly, short stature, hyperprolactinemia, and panhypopituitarism will be discussed.

GROWTH HORMONE

Growth hormone has direct anti-insulin effects on lipid and carbohydrate metabolism. GH decreases utilization of glucose by peripheral tissues, increases lipolysis, and increases muscle mass. GH also stimulates gluconeogenesis in hepatocytes, impairs tissue glucose uptake, decreases insulin-receptor sensitivity, and impairs postreceptor insulin action. The growth-promoting effects of GH are largely mediated by insulin-like growth factors (IGFs) also known as somatomedins. GH stimulates the formation of IGF-I in the liver, as well as in other peripheral tissues. This anabolic peptide acts as a direct stimulator of cell proliferation and growth. There are two types of insulin-like growth factors, IGF-I and IGF-II. IGF-I regulates growth to some extent before, and largely after, birth. In contrast, IGF-II is thought to primarily regulate growth in utero.[5] Growth hormone is secreted by the anterior pituitary in a pulsatile fashion with several short bursts that occur mostly at night. Because of the short half-life of growth hormone in the plasma (approximately 30 minutes), measurements of circulating GH concentrations throughout the waking hours are usually very low or undetectable. Daytime GH pulses are most likely to occur after meals, following exercise, or during periods of stress. The greatest amount of GH secretion occurs during the night within the first 1 to 2 hours of slow-wave sleep (stages III or IV). Secretion of growth hormone is lowest during infancy, increases slightly during childhood, reaches its peak during adolescence, and then begins to gradually decline during the middle-age years.[3]

GROWTH HORMONE EXCESS

Acromegaly is a pathologic condition characterized by excessive production of growth hormone. This is a rare disorder that affects approximately 50 to 70 adults per million.[6] Gigantism, which is even more rare than acromegaly, is the excess secretion of growth hormone prior to epiphyseal closure in children.[7] Patients diagnosed with acromegaly are reported to have a two- to threefold increase in mortality, usually related to cardiovascular, respiratory, or neoplastic disease.[8–10] Most patients are middle-aged at the time of diagnosis, and this disorder does not appear to affect one gender to a greater extent than the other. The most common cause of excess GH secretion in acromegaly, accounting for approximately 98% of all cases, is a growth hormone-secreting pituitary adenoma.[8] Rarely, acromegaly may be caused by ectopic GH-secreting adenomas, GH cell hyperplasia, excess growth hormone-releasing hormone secretion, or as one of the manifestations of the multiple endocrine neoplasia

TABLE 75–1. Pituitary Hormones

Hormone	Stimulation	Inhibition	Physiologic Effects
Anterior pituitary hormones			
Growth hormone (GH)	*Physiologic* GH-releasing hormone Ghrelin ADH GABA Norepinephrine Dopamine Serotonin Estrogen Sleep Stress Exercise *Pharmacologic* α-Adrenergic agonists (e.g., clonidine) β-Adrenergic antagonists (e.g., propranolol) Dopamine agonists (e.g., bromocriptine) GABA agonists (e.g., muscimol)	*Physiologic* Somatostatin Elevated IGF-I Growth hormone Progesterone Glucocorticoids Postprandial hyperglycemia Elevated free fatty acids *Pharmacologic* Dopamine antagonists (e.g., phenothiazines) α-Adrenergic antagonists (e.g., phentolamine) β-Adrenergic agonists (e.g., isoproterenol) Serotonin antagonists (e.g., methysergide)	Stimulates IGF-I production IGF-I and GH promote growth in all body tissues
Prolactin	*Physiologic* TRH VIP Estrogen Serotonin Histamine Endogenous opioids Pregnancy and nursing *Pharmacologic* Dopamine antagonists (e.g., phenothiazines, haloperidol, methyldopa) Opiates Estrogens H$_2$-antagonists (e.g., cimetidine) MAO inhibitors	*Physiologic* Dopamine GABA *Pharmacologic* Dopamine agonists (e.g., levodopa, bromocriptine, pergolide, cabergoline)	Lactation
Adrenocorticotropic hormone (ACTH)	CRH	Elevated cortisol	Glucocorticoid effects Pigmentation
Thyroid-stimulating hormone (TSH)	TRH Estrogens Norepinephrine Serotonin	Thyroxine Triiodothyronine Somatostatin Glucocorticoids Dopamine	Iodine uptake and thyroid hormone synthesis
Luteinizing hormone (LH)	*Physiologic* GnRH *Pharmacologic* Clomiphene	Estradiol Testosterone Fasting	Ovulation Maintains corpus luteum
Follicle-stimulating hormone (FSH)	*Physiologic* GnRH Menopause Ovarian disorders *Pharmacologic* Clomiphene	Estradiol Inhibin Fasting	Ovarian follicle development Stimulates estradiol and progesterone
Posterior pituitary hormones			
Vasopressin (antidiuretic hormone; ADH)	Hyperosmolality Volume depletion	Hypervolemia Hypoosmolality	Acts on renal collecting ducts to prevent diuresis
Oxytocin	Parturition Suckling		Uterine contraction Milk ejection

CRH, corticotropin-releasing hormone; GABA, γ-aminobutyric acid; GnRH, gonadotropin-releasing hormone; IGF-I, insulin-like growth factor; MAO, monoamine oxidase; TRH, thyrotropin-releasing hormone; VIP, vasoactive intestinal peptide.
From Amar et al,[2] Cuttler,[3] and Molitch.[4]

TABLE 75–2. Clinical Presentation of Acromegaly

General

The patient will experience slow development of soft-tissue overgrowth affecting many body systems. Signs and symptoms may gradually progress over 10 to 15 years.

Symptoms

The patient may complain of symptoms related to local effects of the growth hormone (GH)-secreting tumor such as headache and visual disturbances. Other symptoms related to elevated GH and insulin-like growth factor-I (IGF-I) concentrations include excessive sweating, neuropathies, joint pain, and paresthesias.

Signs

The patient may exhibit coarsening of facial features, increased hand volume, increased ring size, increased shoe size, an enlarged tongue, and various dermatologic conditions.

Laboratory tests

The patient's GH concentration will be greater than 1 mcg/L following an oral glucose tolerance test (OGTT) and IGF-I serum concentrations will be elevated. Glucose intolerance may be present in up to 50% of patients.

Additional clinical sequelae

- Cardiovascular diseases such as hypertension, coronary heart disease, cardiomyopathy, and left ventricular hypertrophy are common in patients with acromegaly.
- Osteoarthritis and joint damage develops in up to 90% of acromegalic patients.
- Respiratory disorders and sleep apnea occur in up to 60% of acromegalic patients.
- Type 2 diabetes develops in approximately 25% of acromegalic patients.
- Patients with acromegaly may also have an increased risk for the development of esophageal, colon, and stomach cancer.

From Ben-Shlomo et al,[8] Molitch,[9] Melmed,[10] Fatti et al,[11] Vitale et al,[12] and Webb et al.[13]

syndrome type 1, the McCune-Albright syndrome, or the Carney complex, all very rare hypersecretory endocrinopathies.[8]

The clinical signs and symptoms of acromegaly develop gradually over an extended period of time. In fact, because of the subtle and slowly developing changes in physical appearance that GH excess causes, most patients are not definitively diagnosed with acromegaly until 10 to 15 years after the presumed onset of excessive growth-hormone secretion.[9] Excessive secretion of GH and IGF-I adversely affects several organ systems. Almost all acromegalic patients will present with physical signs and symptoms of soft-tissue overgrowth. Table 75–2 summarizes the classic clinical presentation of patients with acromegaly.[8–13] Some patients with acromegaly may present with few of these classic signs and symptoms, making recognition of this disease extremely difficult.

The diagnosis of acromegaly is based on a combination of diagnostic tests and clinical signs and symptoms. Random measures of plasma GH levels are not usually dependable because of the pulsatile pattern of release. The oral glucose tolerance test (OGTT) is commonly used as an important diagnostic tool. Postprandial hyperglycemia inhibits the secretion of growth hormone for at least 1 to 2 hours. Therefore an oral glucose load would be expected to suppress growth-hormone concentrations.

However, patients with acromegaly continue to secrete growth hormone during the OGTT, and GH concentrations remain elevated after oral glucose loads of 50 to 100 g in 80% of acromegalics.[14] Since GH stimulates the production of IGF-I, serum IGF-I concentrations can also be measured to aid in the diagnosis of acromegaly. Circulating IGF-I is cleared from the body at a much slower rate than GH, and measurements can be collected at any time of the day to identify patients with GH excess.[14] Current criteria for the diagnosis of acromegaly include failure of GH suppression below 1 mcg/L following an OGTT in the presence of elevated IGF-I serum concentrations.[14] With the development of more sensitive GH and IGF-I assays, the cut-off value for diagnosis of acromegaly will likely decrease in the future. Insulin-like growth factor-I-binding-protein-3 (IGFBP-3) can also be measured because it is positively regulated by GH and binds to circulating IGF-I with high affinity. This test may be useful in monitoring response to therapy.[8] Computed tomography and magnetic resonance imaging of the pituitary are important diagnostic tests to confirm the presence of a pituitary adenoma.[9,14]

▶ TREATMENT: Acromegaly

The primary treatment goals for patients diagnosed with acromegaly are to reduce GH and IGF-I concentrations, improve the clinical signs and symptoms of the disease, and decrease mortality.[15–17] Many clinicians define cure of acromegaly as suppression of GH concentrations to lower than 1 mcg/L after a standard OGTT in the presence of normal IGF-I serum concentrations.[15–18] The treatment of choice for acromegaly is transsphenoidal surgical resection of the growth-hormone secreting adenoma.[15,17,18] Postsurgical cure rates have been reported to range from 50% to 90%, depending on the type of adenoma and the expertise of the neurosurgeon.[8,17,18] Complications of transsphenoidal surgery are relatively infrequent and include cerebrospinal fluid leak, meningitis, arachnoiditis, diabetes insipidus, and pituitary failure.[8] For patients who are poor surgical candidates, those who have failed surgical interventions, or others who refuse surgical treatment, radiation therapy may be considered. Radiation, however, may take several years to relieve the symptoms of acromegaly.

Because neither radiation therapy nor surgery will cure all patients with acromegaly, adjuvant drug therapy is often needed to control symptoms.[15,17,18]

PHARMACOLOGIC THERAPY

Drug therapy should be considered for acromegalic patients in whom surgery and irradiation are contraindicated, when rapid control of symptoms is indicated, or when other treatments have failed to normalize GH and IGF-I concentrations. Pharmacologic treatment options include dopamine agonists, somatostatin analogs, and the GH receptor antagonist, pegvisomant. Dopamine agonists such as bromocriptine, pergolide, or cabergoline are effective in a small subset of patients and provide the advantages of oral dosing and reduced cost. Somatostatin analogs are more effective than dopamine agonists, reducing GH concentrations and normalizing IGF-I in approximately 50% to 60% of patients. Pegvisomant is a newly approved GH receptor antagonist that is highly effective, normalizing IGF-I concentrations in up to 97% of patients. However, additional long-term data are needed to establish safety and efficacy of pegvisomant in the management of acromegaly.

DOPAMINE AGONISTS

In normal healthy adults, dopamine agonists cause an increase in growth hormone production. However, when these agents are given to patients with acromegaly, there is a paradoxical decrease in GH production. Most clinical experience with the use of dopamine agonists in acromegaly is with bromocriptine. Other agents such as pergolide, cabergoline, and lisuride have also been used. Bromocriptine is a semisynthetic ergot alkaloid that acts as a dopamine-receptor agonist. Most trials assessing the efficacy of bromocriptine in the treatment of acromegaly were conducted in the 1970s and early 1980s. It was determined from these studies that certain subsets of acromegalic patients have a favorable response to drug therapy with bromocriptine. These patients include individuals with high circulating concentrations of prolactin and patients who experience GH suppression following a single dose of 2.5 mg of bromocriptine, known as a bromocriptine challenge.[19] A review evaluating 34 studies concluded that therapy with bromocriptine was effective in suppressing mean serum GH levels to less than 5 mcg/L in approximately 20% of patients.[20] Only 10% of patients experience normalization of IGF-I concentrations with bromocriptine therapy, but over 50% of patients treated with bromocriptine experience improvement in acromegalic symptoms.[15,21]

Bromocriptine is commercially available in the United States as 2.5-mg oral tablets and 5-mg oral capsules. In acromegalic patients, significant reductions in growth hormone concentrations are observed within 1 to 2 hours of oral dosing. This effect persists for at least 4 to 5 hours. An overall clinical response in acromegalic patients typically occurs following 4 to 8 weeks of continuous bromocriptine therapy. For the treatment of acromegaly, bromocriptine is initiated at a dose of 1.25 mg at bedtime and is increased by 1.25-mg increments every 3 to 4 days as needed.[14,19,20] Doses as high as 80 mg per day have been used for the treatment of acromegaly, but clinical studies have shown that dosages greater than 20 or 30 mg daily do not offer additional benefits in the suppression of GH.[18,20,21] When used for the treatment of acromegaly, the duration of action of bromocriptine is shorter than for the treatment of hyperprolactinemia. Therefore the total daily dose of bromocriptine should be divided into three or four doses.[18,19,21]

The most common adverse effects of bromocriptine therapy include central nervous system symptoms such as headache, lightheadedness, dizziness, nervousness, and fatigue. Gastrointestinal effects such as nausea, abdominal pain, or diarrhea also are very common. Some patients may need to take bromocriptine with food to decrease the incidence of adverse gastrointestinal effects. Most adverse effects are seen early in the course of therapy and tend to decrease with continued treatment.[18,21] Bromocriptine may cause thickening of bronchial secretions and nasal congestion. There have been rare cases of psychiatric disturbances, pleural diseases, and an erythromelalgic syndrome

(painful paroxysmal dilation of the blood vessels in the skin of the feet and lower extremities) reported with the use of bromocriptine. These conditions appear to be associated with higher doses and prolonged duration of therapy.[20,21]

Bromocriptine generally should be discontinued if a woman becomes pregnant while taking the drug. Surveillance of women who took bromocriptine throughout pregnancy do not suggest that bromocriptine is associated with an increased risk of birth defects.[21] If a woman becomes pregnant while taking bromocriptine, the risks and benefits of therapy should be fully considered. In most cases, the benefits of successful therapy outweigh the risks, and bromocriptine therapy should be continued if it is effective in improving symptoms and reducing the elevated GH concentrations.

Other dopamine agonists that have been used to treat acromegaly include pergolide, cabergoline, lisuride, and quinagolide. Cabergoline may be especially useful in patients with pituitary tumors that secrete both prolactin and growth hormone.[21,22] Quinagolide, a dopamine agonist available in Europe, has been shown to be more effective than both bromocriptine and cabergoline in normalizing GH and IGF-I values in acromegalic patients.[19] Because of the potential cost advantages and convenience of oral administration, dopamine agonists are often considered for the treatment of acromegaly prior to initiation of somatostatin analogs. However, the recent development of long-acting somatostatin analogs has made these agents more attractive for first-line treatment of acromegaly.

SOMATOSTATIN ANALOGS

Octreotide is a long-acting somatostatin analog that is approximately 40 times more potent in inhibiting GH secretion than endogenous somatostatin.[23,24] It also suppresses the LH response to GnRH; decreases splanchnic blood flow; and inhibits the secretion of insulin, vasoactive intestinal peptide (VIP), gastrin, secretin, motilin, serotonin, and pancreatic polypeptide. Lanreotide is another somatostatin analog, currently not available in the United States, which is a slow-release depot formulation administered twice monthly.[23]

Octreotide (Sandostatin) injection is commercially available in the United States for subcutaneous or intravenous administration. A long-acting intramuscular formulation of octreotide (Sandostatin LAR) is also available for monthly administration. In addition to the treatment of acromegaly, octreotide has many other therapeutic uses, including the treatment of carcinoid tumors, vasoactive intestinal peptide tumors (VIPomas), gastrointestinal fistulas, variceal bleeding, diarrheal states, and irritable bowel syndrome.

The efficacy of octreotide for the treatment of acromegaly has been determined by two major multicenter trials.[25,26] These studies determined that drug therapy with octreotide suppresses mean serum GH concentrations to less than 5 mcg/L and normalizes serum IGF-I concentrations in 50% to 60% of acromegalic patients. Octreotide is also beneficial in reducing the clinical signs and symptoms of acromegaly. In a 6-month multicenter trial, 70% of patients experienced significant relief of headaches.[26] In some patients, relief of headache symptoms occurred within minutes of octreotide administration. In addition, middle-finger circumference was reduced significantly, and 50% to 75% of the patients experienced improvement in symptoms of excessive perspiration, fatigue, joint pain, and cystic acne. A 2-year follow-up of 103 patients treated with octreotide showed that octreotide therapy is safe and effective for long-term use in acromegalic patients.[27] Several small studies have shown that octreotide improves the cardiovascular manifestations of acromegaly; it decreased left-ventricular mass, decreased heart rate, and increased exercise capacity.[28-30] Octreotide also improves oxygen desaturation, sleep quality, and subjective symptoms of sleepiness in acromegalic patients suffering from sleep apnea.[31] Data from two major multicenter trials indicate that pituitary tumor growth is halted during octreotide treatment, and a small number of patients experience tumor regression.[25,26] A more recent study determined that the growth of pituitary tumors during octreotide therapy is suppressed by approximately 83%.[32]

The pharmacodynamic effects of long-acting octreotide are similar to those of subcutaneously administered octreotide. Single monthly doses of long-acting octreotide have been shown to be at least as effective as daily doses of 300 or 600 mcg of subcutaneous octreotide administered in divided doses three times daily in normalizing IGF-I levels and maintaining suppression of mean serum GH concentrations.[33] A large multicenter trial evaluating the efficacy of long-acting octreotide in acromegalic patients who had previously responded to subcutaneously administered octreotide reported suppression of GH concentrations to below 5 mcg/L in 94% of patients and normalization of IGF-I in 66% of patients following 1 year of therapy.[34]

Response to long-term therapy with octreotide is related to the presence and increased quantity of functioning somatostatin receptors located in the pituitary adenoma.[26,27] Identification of patients who will most likely respond to octreotide, prior to the initiation of therapy, is important when considering the high cost of this medication and the inconvenience of subcutaneous or intramuscular drug administration. Suppression of serum GH concentrations after a single 50-mcg dose of octreotide has been used to predict a favorable long-term response (GH concentrations <1 mcg/L after a standard OGTT in the presence of normal IGF-I serum concentrations) to octreotide therapy. Somatostatin-receptor imaging and serum GH concentrations after short-term (1 month) administration of octreotide appear to be even more accurate in predicting which patients will respond to long-term octreotide therapy than acute suppression of GH by a single dose of octreotide.[35]

❸ The initial dose of octreotide for the treatment of acromegaly is 100 mcg administered every 8 hours.[17,20,24] Some clinicians recommend a starting dose of 50 mcg every 8 hours, then increasing the dose to 100 mcg every 8 hours after 1 week, to improve the patient's tolerance of the adverse gastrointestinal effects.[14,18] The dose may be increased by increments of 50 mcg every 1 to 2 weeks based on mean serum GH and IGF-I concentrations. Patients who experience a significant rise in GH prior to the end of the 8-hour dosing interval may benefit from decreasing the dosing interval to every 4 to 6 hours. Although doses as high as 1500 mcg per day have been used, doses above 600 mcg daily generally do not offer additional benefits, and most patients are adequately managed with 100 to 200 mcg three times daily.[18,25-27] Patients who have been maintained on subcutaneous octreotide for at least 2 weeks and have shown response to therapy, may be converted to the long-acting depot form of octreotide. The initial dose of long-acting octreotide is 20 mg administered intramuscularly in the gluteal region every 28 days. Steady-state serum concentrations are not obtained until after 3 months of therapy. Therefore dosage adjustments for long-acting octreotide should not be considered until after this time. Some patients may require additional subcutaneous injections during the initial dose-titration phase in order to control symptoms. Long-acting octreotide doses higher than 30 mg every 4 weeks have not been studied.

The most common adverse effects of octreotide therapy are gastrointestinal disturbances such as diarrhea, nausea, abdominal cramps, malabsorption of fat, and flatulence.[17,18,23] These effects are dose dependent and can be seen within a few hours of the first octreotide injection. Gastrointestinal adverse effects occur in approx-

imately 75% of patients, but usually subside within 10 to 14 days of continued treatment.[17,18,23] Octreotide has also been reported to cause injection-site pain (4% to 31%), conduction abnormalities and arrhythmias (9%), biochemical hypothyroidism (2% to 12%), biliary tract disorders (4% to 50%), and abnormalities in glucose metabolism (2% to 18%).[20,23]

Octreotide also inhibits cholecystokinin release and gall bladder motility, predisposing patients to the development of cholelithiasis.[17,18,23] The development of gallstones is a long-term adverse effect of octreotide use and is largely dependent on geographic factors, dietary habits, and length of therapy.[14,20,24] The incidence of gallstones in acromegalic patients receiving octreotide increases with length of therapy and has been reported to range from 20% to 50%.[14,24-27] Most patients, however, are asymptomatic, and the diagnosis of cholelithiasis is usually made following an ultrasonographic study that is not prompted by patient symptoms. It has been estimated that only 1% of patients will develop symptomatic gallstones during 1 year of octreotide treatment.[14,24] Because octreotide-induced gallstones are usually present without clinical symptoms, the latest U.S. Acromegaly Therapy Consensus Development Panel recommended that treatment of octreotide-induced gallstones be the same as that for gallstones in the general population.[15] Prophylactic cholecystectomy or medical therapy with ursodeoxycholic acid for acromegalic patients with asymptomatic gallstones are usually not recommended. However, limited data suggest that concomitant therapy with ursodeoxycholic acid may reverse the formation of sludge and gallstones in acromegalic patients receiving octreotide.[36] A small number of studies have suggested that the incidence of gallstone development may be lower with long-acting ocreotide as compared to subcutaneous octreotide.[33,34] However, further studies are needed to confirm this observation.

❹ The effect of octreotide on glucose metabolism in patients with acromegaly is multifactorial. Decreases in serum GH concentrations induced by octreotide should result in decreased hepatic gluconeogenesis and increased insulin-receptor sensitivity. However, octreotide also decreases insulin secretion and increases IGFBP-1 which is known to inhibit the insulin-like effects of IGF-I. In addition, octreotide delays the gastrointestinal absorption of glucose, which may further alter glucose metabolism in acromegalic patients. Small studies conducted in acromegalic patients with glucose intolerance have reported improvement in insulin sensitivity associated with octreotide therapy.[37,38] However, one study of 90 acromegalics reported that 11 (12%) patients developed impaired glucose tolerance and 16 (18%) patients developed frank diabetes mellitus while receiving octreotide.[39] In the same study, 27% of subjects who were diabetic at the beginning of the trial experienced an improvement in their glycemic control by the end of the 6-month study period. Risk factors associated with worsening glucose tolerance included female gender and elevated baseline insulin values. Although octreotide appears to have a beneficial effect on glucose tolerance in most patients, glucose determinations should be obtained frequently in the early stages of octreotide therapy in all acromegalic patients.

■ DOPAMINE AGONIST AND SOMATOSTATIN ANALOG COMBINATION THERAPY

Somatostatin analogs are more effective than dopamine agonists in reducing mean serum GH concentrations and normalizing IGF-I in patients with acromeagaly.[14,15,17,18,20] However, several small studies have suggested that combination therapy with octreotide and bromocriptine or cabergoline may be more beneficial than either drug alone.[20,23,40] Because of the potential for additive adverse effects, combination therapy should be considered as a therapeutic option only for refractory patients who have not fully responded to either therapy alone.

GH RECEPTOR ANTAGONIST

Pegvisomant (Somavert) is a new genetically engineered GH derivative that binds to GH receptors in the liver and inhibits IGF-I. This agent is different from other medications used in the management of acromegaly because it does not inhibit GH production, but rather blocks the physiologic effects of GH on target tissues. Therefore GH concentrations remain elevated during therapy, and response to treatment is evidenced by a reduction in IGF-I concentrations. Unlike somatostatin analogs, the pharmacologic activity of pegvisomant does not depend on the presence and quantity of somatostatin receptors in the pituitary tumor.[41]

Studies evaluating the clinical efficacy of pegvisomant in acromegalic patients have reported a dose-dependent normalization of IGF-I concentrations in 54% to 89% of patients after 12 weeks of therapy, and in 97% of patients after 1 year of therapy.[42,43] Significant improvements in the clinical signs and symptoms of acromegaly were also reported and persisted throughout the 1-year treatment period.[43] Adverse effects appeared to be minimal and included injection-site pain, gastrointestinal complaints such as nausea and diarrhea, and flu-like symptoms. Significant elevations in hepatic aminotransferase concentrations, which were reversible upon discontinuation of the drug, were reported in two patients.[42] As a result, hepatic function tests should be monitored very closely during therapy as outlined in the product labeling, and the drug should be used with caution in patients with baseline elevations in hepatic aminotransferase con-

centrations. Growth hormone concentrations increased significantly during the first 6 months of therapy. Although tumor size did not change significantly during clinical trials, there are theoretical concerns that persistently elevated GH concentrations may stimulate tumor growth or result in other unfavorable long-term effects.

Pegvisomant is commercially available in the United States for daily subcutaneous use. The first dose should be administered under the supervision of a physician as a 40-mg loading dose. Subsequent doses are self-administered by the patient starting at a dose of 10 mg daily. The dose can be adjusted in 5-mg increments based on serum IGF-I concentrations every 4 to 6 weeks, up to a maximum daily dose of 30 mg.[44]

Based on the available data, pegvisomant appears to be among the most effective agents for normalizing IGF-I serum concentrations. However, given the limited clinical data, further study is needed to determine the long-term safety and efficacy of pegvisomant in the treatment of acromegaly.

PHARMACOECONOMIC CONSIDERATIONS

Cost-effectiveness comparisons of the various treatment options for patients with acromegaly have not been performed. Considering that approximately 40% of patients are not completely cured after transsphenoidal surgery, pharmacologic treatment often becomes necessary. Bromocriptine and cabergoline are considerably less expensive than octreotide and pegvisomant. However, these agents are not effective in the majority of patients. Long-acting octreotide offers a convenient method of octreotide administration for acromegalic patients. Although this formulation is approximately two times the cost of subcutaneous octreotide, it may result in improved patient

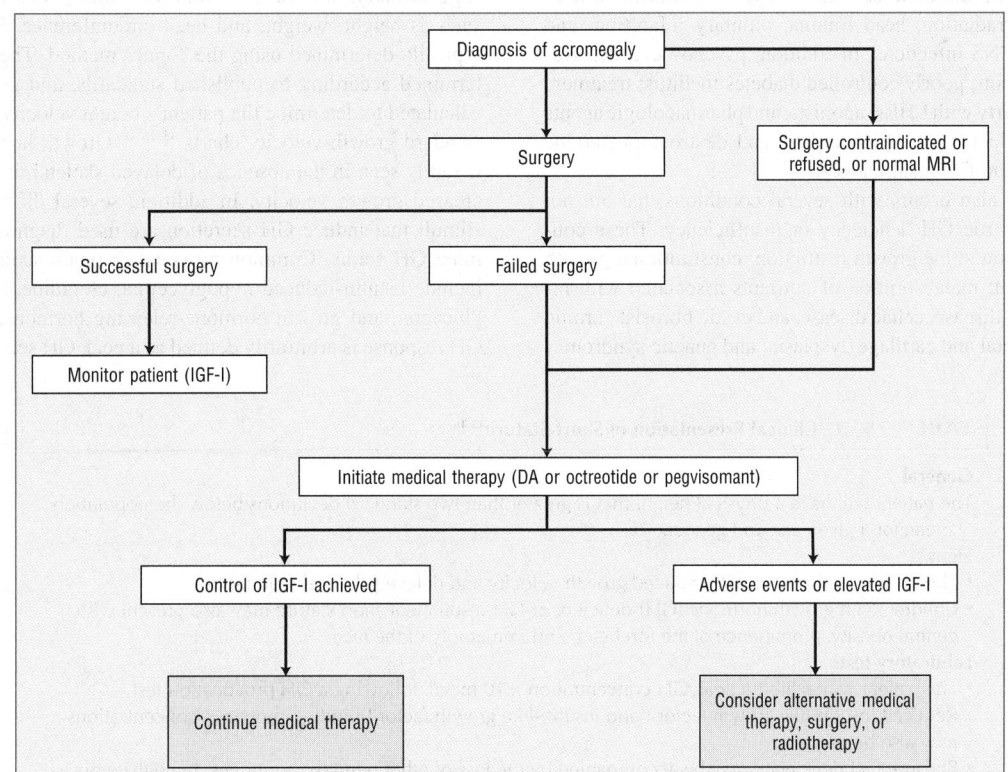

FIGURE 75–2. Treatment algorithm for acromegaly. DA, dopamine agonist; MRI, magnetic resonance imaging; IGF-I, insulin-like growth factor type I. (*Reprinted with permission from Clemmons et al.*[41])

compliance, quality of life, and overall disease management. Pegvisomant appears to the most effective agent for normalizing IGF-I concentrations, and may be useful in patients who are intolerant to or have failed therapy with dopamine agonists or somatostatin analogues. However, pegvisomant is significantly more expensive than long-acting octreotide and requires daily subcutaneous injections. Long-term studies evaluating the safety of pegvisomant are needed to clearly define its role in the management of acromegaly. The drug therapy of choice for an acromegalic patient should be determined by careful consideration of several patient-specific factors including clinical response, compliance, tolerability, and cost of therapy.

CLINICAL CONTROVERSY

Some clinicians advocate the use of somatostatin analogues for primary therapy of acromegaly in place of surgery. However, others believe that sufficient long-term safety and efficacy data are lacking.

CONCLUSIONS

Acromegaly is a chronic debilitating disease characterized by excess growth hormone secretion most commonly caused by a GH-secreting pituitary adenoma. Transsphenoidal surgical resection of the adenoma is the current treatment of choice for patients with acromegaly. Patients who are poor surgical candidates may receive radiation therapy or long-term pharmacologic therapy. Drug therapy options within the U.S. for acromegaly include dopamine agonists, the somatostatin analog octreotide, and pegvisomant. Figure 75–2 illustrates a treatment algorithm for the management of acromegaly.[41]

GROWTH HORMONE DEFICIENCY

Short stature is a condition that is commonly defined by a physical height that is more than two standard deviations below the population mean and lower than the third percentile for height in a specific age group.[45–47] It has been estimated that more than 1.8 million children in the United States can be characterized as having short stature.[47] Short stature is a very broad term describing a condition that may be the result of many different causes. A true lack of GH is among the least common causes and is known as growth-hormone-deficient (GHD) short stature. Absolute GH deficiency is a congenital disorder that can result from various genetic abnormalities such as GHRH deficiency, GH gene deletion, or developmental disorders including pituitary aplasia or hypoplasia.[45,46] GH insufficiency is an acquired condition that can result secondary to hypothalamic or pituitary tumors, cranial irradiation, head trauma, pituitary infarction, and various types of CNS infections. In addition, psychosocial deprivation; hypothyroidism; poorly controlled diabetes mellitus; treatment of precocious puberty with LHRH agonists; and pharmacologic agents such as glucocorticoids, methylphenidate, and dextroamphetamine may induce transient GH insufficiency.[45,48]

Short stature also occurs with several conditions that are not associated with a true GH deficiency or insufficiency. These conditions include intrauterine growth restriction; constitutional growth delay; malnutrition; malabsorption of nutrients associated with inflammatory bowel disease, celiac disease, and cystic fibrosis; chronic renal failure; skeletal and cartilage dysplasia; and genetic syndromes such as Turner's syndrome.[45,46,48] In addition, many children are diagnosed with idiopathic or normal variant short stature. These patients have heights that are significantly lower than the third percentile, but present with normal GH serum concentrations and no specific underlying explanation for short stature.[47]

Children with GHD short stature are usually born with an average birth weight. Decreases in growth velocity generally become evident between the age of 6 months and 3 years.[45,48] In contrast, GH insufficiency may arise at any age during growth and development. The clinical characteristics of GH-deficient or GH-insufficient children are presented in Table 75–3.[45,46]

Several factors must be considered in the diagnosis of GH deficiency or insufficiency. Standard epidemiologic growth charts developed by the National Center for Health Statistics are typically used to determine the percentile of anthropometric measurements such as height, weight, and head circumference. Pubertal stage is typically determined using the Tanner method. The bone age is determined according to published standards, and growth velocity is calculated to determine the patient's height velocity percentile using standard growth-velocity charts.[45,46,48] Growth hormone deficiency is rarely seen in the absence of delayed skeletal maturation and decreased growth velocity. In addition, several different provocative stimuli that induce GH secretion are used diagnostically to determine GH status. Common provocative pharmacologic GH stimuli include insulin-induced hypoglycemia, clonidine, L-dopa, arginine, glucagon, and growth hormone-releasing hormone.[46] A subnormal GH response is arbitrarily defined as a peak GH serum concentration

---

TABLE 75–3. Clinical Presentation of Short Stature[45,46]

General
The patient will have a physical height that is greater than two standard deviations below the population mean for a given age and gender.

Signs
- The patient will present with reduced growth velocity and delayed skeletal maturation.
- Children with growth hormone (GH)-deficient or GH-insufficient short stature may also present with central obesity, prominence of the forehead, and immaturity of the face.

Laboratory tests
- The patient will exhibit a peak GH concentration <10 mcg/L following a GH provocation test. Reduced insulin-like growth factor-I and insulin-like growth factor-I-binding-protein-3 concentrations may also be present.
- Because GH deficiency may be accompanied by the loss of other pituitary hormones, hypoglycemia and hypothyroidism may also be noted.

From Hindmarsh et al[45] and American Association of Endocrinologists.[46]

of <10 mcg/L during a 2-hour period after administration of one of these agents.[46] However, this maximum may be lower, depending on the specific assay and GH reference product used. Assessment of IGF-I and IGFBP-3 serum concentrations should also be made, with measurements exceeding two standard deviations below the standard reference range strongly suggestive of GH deficiency.[46] The three generally accepted criteria for the definitive diagnosis of GH deficiency are a subnormal growth velocity, a delayed bone age, and a subnormal GH response to at least two provocative stimuli.[49] For prepubertal and early-pubertal patients (Tanner stage less than III), priming with sex hormones to improve the specificity of GH provocation tests is often considered. Some patients may exhibit clinical signs of GH deficiency, subnormal growth velocity, and delayed bone age, despite GH levels that are within normal limits after provocative testing. This makes diagnosis in this group of patients very difficult. Diagnosis based on GH stimulation tests becomes further complicated because of the paucity of data reporting the normal range of GH concentrations after provocative testing in healthy children and the fact that commercial GH assays currently available may not be equivalent. One study comparing several different GH assays found a significant variation between measured GH serum concentrations.[49] Because of these limitations, careful consideration of multiple factors by a pediatric endocrinology specialist is required to diagnose growth hormone deficiency correctly.

▶ TREATMENT: Growth Hormone Deficiency

■ PHARMACOLOGIC THERAPY

The treatment of growth hormone deficiency with pituitary-derived human growth hormone was first reported in the late 1950s. The National Hormone and Pituitary Program was founded by the National Institutes of Health in 1963 to coordinate the collection of human pituitary glands and purification of GH for administration to children with GH deficiency. In 1985, three deaths linked to Creutzfeldt-Jakob disease (CJD) were identified in young individuals who were previously treated with human pituitary growth hormone. An evaluation of National Hormone and Pituitary Program data identified 26 cases of fatal CJD in a cohort of 6,107 patients who received treatment with human pituitary–derived growth hormone in the United States between 1963 and 1985.[50] Human pituitary growth hormone was withdrawn from the U.S. market because of the strong likelihood that the CJD was transmitted through contaminated human pituitary–derived growth hormone. Shortly after the withdrawal of human pituitary growth hormone, the U.S. Food and Drug Administration approved the first recombinant DNA–derived growth hormone for the treatment of GH insufficiency. Prior to the introduction of recombinant growth hormone, the number of individuals who received treatment for GH insufficiency was relatively small owing to the limited availability of human pituitary tissue for GH extraction. Currently, with the widespread availability of recombinant growth hormone products, a large number of children can receive growth hormone replacement therapy at higher doses. Unfortunately, human pituitary–derived growth hormone continues to be used today in some underdeveloped countries.

Recombinant GH is currently considered the mainstay of therapy for the treatment of GHD short stature. GH replacement therapy in children with documented GHD short stature produces a significant improvement in growth velocity within the first year of therapy and significantly improves final adult height.[51–54] The initial increase in growth velocity is often referred to as catch-up growth. Most of the initial studies evaluating the efficacy of GH therapy in GHD children were conducted for short periods of time in small numbers of patients, and until recently, information about the long-term outcome of GH therapy was limited. Initial data suggested that final adult height is not substantially improved, with an average final adult height reported to be two standard deviations below the population mean.[55–58] Although these results were disappointing, it is important to note that a substantial percentage of patients included in these studies had initially received human pituitary growth hormone in relatively low doses because of its limited availability. In addition, current growth hormone dosing regimens have changed with regard to frequency of administration, making these data difficult to interpret and apply to patients who are receiving GH replacement therapy today. Recent studies evaluating the adult height of children who received only recombinant GH therapy with currently recommended dosing regimens suggest that current recombinant GH therapy has a greater impact on final adult height than was previously reported.[51–54] These studies have reported average final adult heights ranging from 0.5 to 1.7 standard deviations below the population mean. Initiation of therapy at an early chronologic age, prior to the onset of puberty, is associated with a more favorable increase in final height.[46,52,53] Therefore prompt diagnosis of growth hormone deficiency and early initiation of replacement therapy with recombinant GH are crucial factors in optimizing the final adult height of children with GH deficiency.

Recombinant growth hormone has also been shown to increase the short-term growth rate in patients with chronic renal insufficiency, intrauterine growth restriction, Turner's syndrome, idiopathic short stature, and Prader-Willi syndrome, and is approved by the FDA for treatment of growth failure associated with these conditions.[46] GH is also FDA approved for the treatment of adult growth hormone deficiency and the acquired immunodeficiency syndrome wasting syndrome. Long-term GH therapy in growth-hormone-deficient adults significantly decreases body fat, increases muscle mass, and improves exercise capacity.[46] GH therapy in adults has been shown to improve the cardiac risk profile, bone mineral density, and psychological well being.[59–61] In addition, GH is currently being investigated for a variety of disorders, including infertility, chronic fatigue, obesity, and natural aging.[46] Use of GH as an anabolic agent for management of acute catabolism is not recommended.[46]

The majority of short children in the United States do not have an identifiable medical cause for their condition, but with widespread availability of several recombinant growth hormone formulations, many children have received GH therapy regardless of the underlying etiology of their short stature.[62] The use of recombinant growth hormone therapy in children with non–growth-hormone-deficient short stature, also referred to as idiopathic short stature, has been studied by several investigators. Of note, a recent meta-analysis of 38 clinical studies evaluating the efficacy of GH treatment in non–growth-hormone-deficient children reported average increases in final adult height of 4 to 5 cm (1.6 to 2 inches) following a mean duration of therapy of 4.7 years.[63] This corresponded to an increase above the predicted final adult height of 0.56 to 0.63 standard deviations of the population mean. Given the significant cost of growth hormone therapy, the authors estimated a cost of $35,000 per inch of height gained.[62] Humatrope was recently approved by the FDA for management of idiopathic short stature. However, the use of GH therapy in this patient population remains controversial.

CLINICAL CONTROVERSY

Most pediatric endocrinologists in the U.S. believe that GH therapy is an appropriate treatment in certain patients with non-GHD short stature. However, given the high cost of therapy and small increases in height, use of GH in this patient population remains controversial.

Nine different recombinant growth hormone products are currently available for use in the United States. Somatrem (Protropin) was the first recombinant GH product developed and used for the treatment of GH deficiency. This formulation contains the same 191-amino-acid sequence as human pituitary growth hormone, with the exception of the terminal addition of a methionine amino acid group.

The remaining GH formulations (Genotropin, Norditropin, Nutropin, Nutropin AQ, Nutropin Depot, Humatrope, Serostim, and Saizen) contain somatropin. Somatropin is composed of the same amino-acid sequence as human pituitary GH. Recombinant GH formulations must be administered by intramuscular or subcutaneous injection. Nutropin AQ is the only GH product that is available as a liquid formulation. The remaining products are formulated as lyophilized powders for injection, and patients must be instructed regarding proper reconstitution, storage, and administration. A newly formulated long-acting depot form of growth hormone, Nutropin Depot, is also available for once- or twice-monthly subcutaneous injection. This product may be particularly useful for patients who are noncompliant or experience significant adverse effects from frequent injections. The potency of GH products is expressed as international units per milligram (international units/mg) with 1 mg containing approximately 2.6 international units of growth hormone. Direct comparisons between the different recombinant growth hormone products have not been published. However, all GH products are generally considered to be equally efficacious. The recommended dose for treatment of GHD short stature in children is 0.3 mg/kg per week.[46] Recombinant GH may be administered daily or in equal doses six times per week, depending on the specific GH product used.[46] Dosing regimens with greater frequency of administration have been shown to provide more favorable short-term growth responses.[46] Growth hormone replacement therapy should be initiated as early as possible after diagnosis of GH insufficiency and continued until a desirable height is reached or growth velocity has decreased to less than 2.5 cm per year after the pubertal growth spurt. However, the suitable time point for discontinuation of therapy with growth-promoting doses remains controversial. Glucocorticoids may inhibit the growth-promoting effects of recombinant GH, and concomitant administration of androgens, estrogens, thyroid hormones, or anabolic steroids may accelerate epiphyseal closure and compromise final height.

Three large databases, the National Cooperative Growth Study, the Kabi International Growth Study, and the Australian and New Zealand growth database (OZGROW), have been developed to collect postmarketing adverse effect data or reports associated with recombinant growth hormone. Development of these databases was prompted by the unexpected and tragic cases of CJD reported in patients treated with human pituitary growth hormone. These databases are maintained by pharmaceutical companies that manufacture GH products.[64] Recombinant GH is generally well tolerated in children, and adverse effects are relatively uncommon.[64,65] A small number of patients may complain of injection-site pain or arthralgias. Idiopathic intracranial hypertension, also known as pseudotumor cerebri, has been reported in a very small number of children receiving GH therapy. This condition usually develops within the first 8 to 12 of weeks of treatment and presents with symptoms such as headache, blurred vision, diplopia, nausea, and vomiting.[64] The symptoms of idiopathic intracranial hypertension usually resolve after discontinuation of GH therapy, and long-term complications are rare. Cases of slipped capital femoral epiphysis have been reported in children with growth-hormone deficiency who are receiving GH therapy.[64] This condition is thought to occur as a result of the increased width of the femoral plate during GH treatment, but it has also been reported in GH-deficient children who are not receiving GH replacement. Patients with this condition typically complain of hip or knee pain. Slipped capital femoral epiphysis can be managed by an orthopedic surgeon, and GH therapy does not need to be withdrawn. Because growth hormone is known to cause decreased insulin sensitivity, hyperglycemia and diabetes mellitus may develop.[66] Patients who have specific predisposing risk factors for diabetes mellitus are at greatest risk for this adverse effect.[64–66] Glycosylated hemoglobin concentrations should be monitored in all patients receiving GH products.[46] GH may promote the growth of various types of neoplasms and increase tumor recurrence rates in patients with a history of malignancy.[46,64,65] For this reason, GH should not be administered to patients with an active malignant tumor or a history of recurrent tumor growth. In 1988, a Japanese report indicated that children receiving GH therapy were twice as likely to develop leukemia as children who were not receiving the hormone.[67] A more recent analysis of all collected reports of leukemia associated with GH therapy determined that these children had other leukemia risk factors (Fanconi anemia, Bloom's syndrome, or a prior history of cancer).[68] GH therapy in children without these risk factors does not appear to predispose children to develop leukemia.[64,65,68] Some patients may develop antibodies to recombinant GH. The development of antibodies during replacement therapy with recombinant-GH products has been reported to be relatively low, affecting approximately 15% to 20% of patients.[69,70] More importantly, the presence of GH antibodies has not been shown to adversely affect growth response and appears to be clinically insignificant except in patients with GH gene deletions. Finally, recent postmarketing reports suggest an increased risk of death associated with long-term GH treatment in children with Prader-Willi syndrome who are severely obese or have severe respiratory impairment. GH treatment is contraindicated in patients with Prader-Willi syndrome who have any of these risk factors.

GROWTH HORMONE-RELEASING HORMONE

A synthetic growth hormone-releasing hormone (GHRH) product known as sermorelin (Geref) is currently FDA approved for the treatment of idiopathic growth hormone deficiency in children. Sermorelin [GH-RH (1-29)-NH₂] is composed of 29 amino acid residues that are identical to the amino-terminal segment of human GHRH. Although not as effective as recombinant GH therapy, sermorelin has been shown to increase short-term growth velocity in children with idiopathic growth hormone deficiency.[71] This product has also been shown to increase growth velocity in children who have GH deficiency secondary to hypothalamic damage rather than pituitary abnormalities, as is observed with radiation-induced GH deficiency.[72] In most cases of radiation-induced GH deficiency, pituitary somatotropes are capable of secreting endogenous GH, and stimulation of these cells by exogenously administered GHRH may restore the natural pulsatile secretion of GH and result in increased growth rate.

The recommended dose of sermorelin is 0.03 mg/kg administered daily by subcutaneous injection. No serious adverse events have been identified. The most common adverse effect reported by patients receiving sermorelin therapy is pain at the site of injection. Because normal pituitary function is needed for sermorelin to stimulate GH secretion, children should not receive GHRH therapy with sermorelin unless adequate capacity to secrete GH is documented by provocative GH-stimulation testing. Sermorelin may prove to be a beneficial therapeutic option in the treatment of various types of non-GHD short stature. However, owing to its mechanism of action, sermorelin does not have a role in the treatment of true GHD short stature.

EVALUATION OF THERAPEUTIC OUTCOMES

Appropriate monitoring of therapy for GHD and non-GHD short stature includes regular assessments of height, weight, growth velocity, serum alkaline phosphatase, and bone age every 6 to 12 months. Additional laboratory tests to monitor for potential adverse effects include serum glucose and thyroid function. The dose of GH will periodically need to be increased as weight increases in growing children.

PHARMACOECONOMIC CONSIDERATIONS

The treatment of short stature with recombinant GH is very expensive. Despite the prohibitive cost, recombinant GH remains the mainstay of therapy for children with GHD short stature. However, treatment of non-GHD short stature with recombinant GH is not widely accepted. The benefits in final adult height and increases in growth velocity, particularly in children with true GH deficiency, are associated with significant psychosocial benefits. Many clinicians believe that GH therapy can improve quality of life and should be made available to all children with short stature, regardless of whether or not they are GH deficient.[73] Until studies using recombinant GH more definitively demonstrate improvements in both final adult height and quality of life, the cost-effectiveness of GH, particularly for non-GHD short stature, remains uncertain.

CONCLUSIONS

Growth hormone deficiency during childhood results in short stature. Replacement with recombinant GH is considered the mainstay of therapy for patients with GHD short stature, but its use for the treatment of non-GHD short stature remains controversial, albeit such treatment is FDA approved. Recombinant GH has proven to be safe for use in children and is associated with very few adverse effects. New therapeutic agents such as the synthetic growth hormone-releasing hormone sermorelin, and other growth hormone-releasing peptides may provide benefit for patients with non-GHD short stature. Growth hormone regimens can be particularly demanding and inconvenient for pediatric patients because they must be administered by subcutaneous injection. Knowledge of the long-term benefits and risks is critical to the development of rational, cost-effective treatments for patients with short stature.

PROLACTIN

PHYSIOLOGIC EFFECTS

Prolactin is secreted in a pulsatile fashion by the lactotroph cells of the anterior pituitary, with the highest peak concentrations observed during sleep.[4] The secretion of prolactin is regulated primarily by tonic hypothalamic inhibitory effects of dopamine. As described earlier in this chapter and listed in Table 75–1, many factors can affect prolactin secretion. During pregnancy, prolactin serum concentrations rise substantially above normal. All other conditions characterized by excess prolactin serum concentrations, known as hyperprolactinemia, are considered pathologic.

HYPERPROLACTINEMIA

Hyperprolactinemia is a state of persistent serum prolactin elevation. Prolactin concentrations greater than 20 mcg/L observed on multiple occasions are generally considered indicative of hyperprolactinemia.[74,75] Hyperprolactinemia usually affects women of reproductive age.[74] The incidence of hyperprolactinemia in the general population is reported to be less than 1%.[75]

Hyperprolactinemia has several etiologies. The most common causes are benign prolactin-secreting pituitary tumors, known as prolactinomas, and various medications. Prolactinomas are classified according to size. Prolactin-secreting microadenomas are less than 10 mm in diameter and often do not increase in size.[4,75,76] In contrast, macroadenomas are tumors with a diameter greater than 10 mm that continue to grow and can cause invasion of surrounding tissues.[4,75,76] In the presence of a prolactinoma, prolactin serum concentrations

may remain normal or may be markedly elevated to thousands of micrograms per liter.

8 ◀ Any pharmacologic agent that antagonizes dopamine or increases the release of prolactin can induce hyperprolactinemia (Table 75–4). Serotonin is a strong stimulator of prolactin secretion, and selective serotonin reuptake inhibitors (SSRIs) such as

TABLE 75–4. Drug-Induced Hyperprolactinemia

Dopamine antagonists
  Antipsychotics
  Phenothiazines
  Metoclopramide
  Domperidone
Prolactin stimulators
  Methyldopa
  Reserpine
  Selective serotonin reuptake inhibitors (SSRIs)
  Dexfenfluramine
  Estrogens
  Progestins
  Protease inhibitors
  Gonadotropin-releasing hormone analogs
  Benzodiazepines
  Tricyclic antidepressants
  Monoamine oxidase inhibitors
  H_2-Receptor antagonists
  Opioids
Other
  Verapamil

From Molitch,[4] Mah et al,[75] Molitch,[76] and Davies.[77]

TABLE 75–5. Clinical Presentation of Hyperprolactinemia

General
Hyperprolactinemia most commonly affects women and is very rare in men.

Signs and symptoms
- The patient may complain of symptoms related to local effects of the prolactin-secreting tumor, such as headache and visual disturbances, that result from tumor compression of the optic chiasm.
- Female patients experience oligomenorrhea, amenorrhea, galactorrhea, infertility, decreased libido, hirsutism, and acne.
- Male patients experience decreased libido, erectile dysfunction, infertility, reduced muscle mass, galactorrhea, and gynecomastia.

Laboratory tests
Prolactin serum concentrations at rest will be >20 mcg/L on multiple occasions.

Additional clinical sequelae
- The prolonged suppression of estrogen in premenopausal women with hyperprolactinemia leads to decreases in bone mineral density and significant risk for the development of osteoporosis.
- Risk for ischemic heart disease may be increased with untreated hyperprolactinemia.

From Molitch,[4] Schlechte,[74] Mah et al,[75] and Molitch.[76]

fluoxetine, paroxetine, sertraline, and fluvoxamine are the medications most frequently associated with hyperprolactinemia.[77] Prior to the increased use of SSRIs, antipsychotic medications with potent dopamine-receptor blockade, such as the phenothiazine derivatives and haloperidol, were most often identified as the cause of drug-induced hyperprolactinemia.[78] Metoclopramide and domperidone, an antiemetic available in Europe, are potent dopamine-receptor antagonists reported to induce hyperprolactinemia.[77] Hormones such as estrogen and progesterone, commonly prescribed as oral contraceptives, can stimulate lactotroph growth to promote prolactin secretion and have been implicated in drug-induced hyperprolactinemia. Although the exact mechanism of action remains to be determined, the calcium-channel-blocking agent verapamil has been associated with cases of hyperprolactinemia.[4,77] Methyldopa and reserpine, although not used frequently in clinical practice today, are antihypertensive agents that can stimulate prolactin secretion.[77] Prolactin concentrations may increase with the administration of gonadotropin-releasing hormone analogs like leuprolide or goserelin.[77] Other medications rarely reported to cause hyperprolactinemia include H_2-receptor blocking agents, benzodiazepines, tricyclic antidepressants, dexfenfluramine, opioids, protease inhibitors, and monoamine oxidase inhibitors.[4,75–77] Prolactin levels do not typically rise to greater than 150 mcg/L in cases of drug-induced hyperprolactinemia. Measurement of serum prolactin concentrations prior to the initiation of therapy with medications known to cause prolactin elevation may obviate the need for extensive examination of pituitary function and aid with the appropriate diagnosis of drug-induced hyperprolactinemia.

Less common etiologies include central nervous system lesions that physically compress the pituitary stalk and interrupt tonic hypothalamic dopamine secretion, resulting in hyperprolactinemia.[75,76] Increased thyroid-releasing hormone (TRH) concentrations in hypothyroidism can stimulate prolactin secretion and cause hyperprolactinemia. During conditions of renal or liver compromise, the

clearance of prolactin is decreased, resulting in elevated prolactin concentrations.[4] Despite vigorous diagnostic effort, the cause of hyperprolactinemia cannot always be determined. This is known as idiopathic hyperprolactinemia and is most likely a result of the presence of very small tumors that are not detected by standard imaging techniques.[74] It should be noted that many physiologic factors, such as stress (including the stress of phlebotomy), sleep, exercise, coitus, and eating can also induce transiently elevated prolactin levels.[4,74] This emphasizes the importance of obtaining multiple prolactin measurements to confirm the diagnosis. Ideally, after an intravenous line is placed in the patient's arm, the patient should rest in a supine position or in a chair for 2 hours before prolactin samples are collected.

Elevated prolactin serum concentrations inhibit gonadotropin secretion and sex-steroid synthesis.[74] Because prolactin concentrations higher than 60 mcg/L are associated with anovulation, women with hyperprolactinemia typically present with menstrual irregularities such as oligomenorrhea or amenorrhea and infertility.[7,74,75] In addition, approximately 40% to 80% of women with hyperprolactinemia will have galactorrhea.[74,75] The clinical presentation of patients with hyperprolactinemia is summarized in Table 75–5.[4,74–76]

The diagnosis of hyperprolactinemia, as defined by multiple prolactin serum concentrations above 20 mcg/L, is relatively simple. However, identifying the underlying cause of this abnormality may be more challenging. Patients with modest prolactin elevations should have multiple prolactin serum determinations to minimize the potential for detecting only transient increases in prolactin. A careful medication history is essential, and the presence of hypothyroidism, renal failure, or hepatic dysfunction should be evaluated. If the cause of hyperprolactinemia remains ambiguous, a computed tomography scan or magnetic resonance imaging study should be performed to determine the presence of a pituitary tumor.[74,75] If an underlying cause of elevated prolactin serum concentration is not determined, the hyperprolactinemia is considered to be idiopathic.

▶ TREATMENT: Hyperprolactinemia

The treatment of hyperprolactinemia depends on the underlying cause of the abnormality. In cases of drug-induced hyperprolactinemia, discontinuation of the offending medication and initiation of an appropriate therapeutic alternative usually normalizes serum prolactin concentrations.[77] In cases for which an appropriate therapeutic alternative does not exist, medical therapy with dopamine agonists is

warranted. Sex-steroid replacement should also be considered.[75] Treatment options for the management of prolactinomas include clinical observation, medical therapy with dopamine agonists, radiation therapy, and transsphenoidal surgical removal of the tumor.[4,74–76] Because prolactin-secreting microadenomas are very small and typically do not increase in size, treatment of these tumors is primarily directed toward alleviating symptoms.[74−76] The goal of therapy is to normalize prolactin serum concentrations and re-establish gonadotropin secretion to restore fertility and reduce the risk of osteoporosis. In patients with asymptomatic elevations in serum prolactin, observation and close follow-up are appropriate.[74−76] Treatment goals are more aggressive in patients with prolactin-secreting macroadenomas because these tumors are larger and can cause invasion of local tissues with significant visual defects.[76] Therefore in addition to normalizing prolactin concentrations, tumor shrinkage and correction of visual defects are primary goals of treatment.

Medical therapy with dopamine agonists is usually more effective than transsphenoidal surgery for both types of pituitary prolactinomas.[4,74−76] Postsurgical cure rates differ depending on tumor type and expertise of the neurosurgeon. Long-term cure rates are reported to be approximately 60% for microprolactinomas and only 25% for macroprolactinomas.[4] Transsphenoidal surgery for the removal of prolactinomas is usually reserved for patients who are refractory to or cannot tolerate therapy with dopamine agonists, and for patients with very large tumors that cause severe compression of adjacent tissues.[4,74−76] Radiation therapy may require several years for effective tumor shrinkage and reduction in serum prolactin concentrations, and is usually used only in conjunction with surgery.[4]

PHARMACOLOGIC THERAPY

Medical therapy with dopamine agonists has proven to be very effective in normalizing prolactin serum concentrations, restoring menstruation, and reducing tumor size in approximately 80% to 90% of patients within 3 to 6 months of therapy.[4,75] Bromocriptine has been the mainstay of therapy since the 1970s, and pergolide has been used as an effective alternative in patients who are intolerant of the adverse effects associated with bromocriptine. Cabergoline is a new long-acting dopamine agonist that offers the advantage of less-frequent dosing. In recent years cabergoline has replaced bromocriptine as the agent of choice for the medical management of prolactinomas.

BROMOCRIPTINE

Bromocriptine was the first D_2-receptor agonist to be used in the treatment of hyperprolactinemia and has been the mainstay of therapy for over 20 years. It inhibits the release of prolactin by directly stimulating postsynaptic dopamine receptors in the hypothalamus. Hypothalamic release of dopamine (prolactin-inhibitory hormone) inhibits the release of prolactin. Decreases in serum prolactin concentrations occur within 2 hours of oral administration with maximal suppression occurring after 8 hours, and suppressive effects persisting for up to 24 hours. Medical therapy with bromocriptine normalizes prolactin serum concentrations, restores gonadotropin production, and shrinks tumor size in approximately 90% of patients with prolactinomas.[76]

For the management of hyperprolactinemia, bromocriptine therapy is typically initiated at a dose of 1.25 to 2.5 mg once daily at bedtime to minimize adverse effects.[74,75] The dose can be gradually increased by 1.25-mg increments every week to obtain desirable serum prolactin concentrations. Usual therapeutic doses of bromocriptine range from 2.5 to 15 mg per day, although some patients may require doses as high as 40 mg per day.[75] Bromocriptine is usually administered in two or three divided doses, but once-daily dosing has also been shown to be effective.[79]

The most common adverse effects associated with bromocriptine therapy include central nervous system symptoms such as headache, lightheadedness, dizziness, nervousness, and fatigue. Gastrointestinal effects such as nausea, abdominal pain, and diarrhea are also common. Bromocriptine should be administered with food to decrease the incidence of adverse gastrointestinal effects. Although most of these adverse effects diminish with continued treatment, about 12% of patients will not tolerate the adverse effects associated with bromocriptine therapy.[79] Vaginal preparations of bromocriptine have been studied in an effort to decrease the incidence of adverse effects associated with oral dosage forms.[4,75,80]

Because most patients with hyperprolactinemia are women with a principal complaint of infertility, the safety of bromocriptine in pregnancy must be considered. One report of over 2000 pregnancies in women who received bromocriptine during part or all of their gestation did not detect an increase in the risk for spontaneous abortion or incidence of congenital anomalies.[79] Although bromocriptine does not appear to be teratogenic, most clinicians discontinue therapy as soon as pregnancy is detected because the effects of in utero exposure to bromocriptine on gonadal function and fertility of the offspring remain unknown.[4,74−76] In patients with macroprolactinomas undergoing rapid tumor expansion, bromocriptine therapy may need to be continued throughout pregnancy.

PERGOLIDE

Pergolide is a dopamine-receptor agonist with affinity for both D_1- and D_2-receptors. This agent is 10 to 1000 times more potent than bromocriptine on a per milligram basis. In the United States, pergolide is not FDA-approved for the treatment of hyperprolactinemia and is most commonly prescribed for the treatment of parkinsonism. However, pergolide has been used for many years as a safe and effective alternative to bromocriptine in the management of patients with hyperprolactinemia and offers the advantage of once-daily dosing.[4,76]

For the treatment of hyperprolactinemia, pergolide therapy is initiated at a dose of 25 mcg given once daily at bedtime. The average dose that achieves optimal suppression of prolactin serum concentrations is 50 mcg/day given as a single dose.[76] Adverse effects of pergolide are similar to those of bromocriptine and include nausea, headache, vomiting, and dizziness in about 30% of patients. A few cases of cardiac valvulopathy have been reported during pergolide therapy. Pathologic assessment suggests that the valvulopathy associated with pergolide appears to be similar to that reported with other ergot alkaloids. In addition, a small number of patients receiving pergolide have recently reported abruptly falling asleep while performing activities of daily living. This adverse effect has been reported up to 1 year after initiation of therapy. Therefore patients should be made aware of this potentially dangerous adverse effect. The use of pergolide during pregnancy has not been as extensively evaluated as bromocriptine, and should be avoided until additional data become available.

CABERGOLINE

Cabergoline is a long-acting dopamine agonist with high selectivity and affinity for dopamine D_2-receptors. This agent is approved for the treatment of hyperprolactinemia and has been shown to effectively reduce serum prolactin concentrations in 80% to 90% of hyperprolactinemic patients.[81−83] Cabergoline also effectively reduces tumor size in patients with both micro- and macroprolactinomas.[81,84] In a multicenter randomized trial comparing the efficacy of cabergoline and bromocriptine, serum prolactin levels were normalized in 83% of patients receiving cabergoline and 58% of patients receiving bromocriptine after 6 months of therapy.[85] Cabergoline has also proved effective in patients who are intolerant of or resistant to bromocriptine, and recent data suggest that cabergoline is as effective in men as it is in women with micro- and macroprolactinomas.[86–88]

Cabergoline is commercially available as 0.5-mg oral tablets. The initial dose of cabergoline for the treatment of hyperprolactinemia is 0.5 mg once weekly or in divided doses twice weekly. This dose may be increased by increments of 0.5 mg at 4-week intervals based on serum prolactin concentrations. The usual dose is 1 to 2 mg weekly; however, doses as high as 4.5 mg weekly have been used.[89] Recent studies have also evaluated the efficacy of a vaginal dosage form of cabergoline to reduce the adverse effects associated with oral therapy.[90]

Following oral administration, peak serum concentrations are obtained within 2 hours, and food does not affect absorption. Data from animal studies indicate that cabergoline is widely distributed to well-perfused organs, including the pituitary gland.[89] The elimination of cabergoline from the pituitary appears to be very slow; this rate may explain the long duration of action. Cabergoline is extensively metabolized in the liver by hydrolysis, and the dose should be reduced in patients with severe hepatic failure. This drug is eliminated primarily in the feces, and the elimination half-life ranges from 79 to 155 hours in hyperprolactinemic patients.[89]

The most common adverse effects reported with the use of cabergoline are nausea, vomiting, headache, and dizziness.[81,84,89] These are similar to the adverse effects reported with bromocriptine and pergolide. However, in a large comparative study evaluating bromocriptine and cabergoline, fewer patients receiving cabergoline reported adverse effects than patients receiving bromocriptine, and only 3% of the patients in the cabergoline group withdrew from the study because of adverse effects, versus 12% of patients taking bromocriptine.[85] Other adverse events associated with the use of cabergoline include gastrointestinal complaints, drowsiness, fatigue, paresthesias, dyspnea, suffocation sensation, and epistaxis.[85,89] As with other dopamine agonists, adverse events usually occur early in therapy and subside with continued treatment. However, in one study 15% to 20% of patients receiving cabergoline experienced a recurrence of early symptoms or an onset of new symptoms after several weeks of treatment.[85] Mild to moderate decreases in blood pressure have been observed in up to 50% of patients taking cabergoline; however, the incidence of symptomatic orthostatic hypotension has not been significant.[81,82,85] Transient increases in serum alkaline phosphatase, bilirubin, and aminotransferases have been reported in small numbers of patients receiving cabergoline.[85] Pleuropulmonary disease has been reported with cabergoline, but only with larger doses used in the treatment of Parkinson's disease.[87]

The use of cabergoline in pregnancy has not been extensively studied. However, several case reports of women who received cabergoline therapy during the first and second trimesters of pregnancy have not documented an increased risk of spontaneous abortion, congenital abnormalities, or tubal pregnancy.[89] However, prospective data in large numbers of pregnancies is lacking. Owing to the long half-life and limited data on cabergoline use in pregnancy, most clinicians recommend that women receiving cabergoline therapy who plan to become pregnant should discontinue the medication 1 month before planned conception.[91]

Other dopamine agonists that have been used in the treatment of hyperprolactinemia but are not commercially available in the United States include lisuride, terguride, metergoline, dihydroergocristine, and quinagolide.[79] Quinagolide is a D_2-receptor agonist used frequently in Europe which is dosed once daily. Quinagolide has been shown to be as effective as bromocriptine for the management of hyperprolactinemia and may also be effective in the treatment of patients who are resistant to or intolerant of bromocriptine.[79]

EVALUATION OF THERAPEUTIC OUTCOMES

Prolactin serum concentrations should be monitored every 3 to 4 weeks after the initiation of any dopamine-agonist therapy to assess efficacy and appropriately titrate medication dosage.[74] In addition, symptoms such as headache, visual disturbances, menstrual cycles in women, and sexual function in men should be evaluated to assess clinical response to therapy. Once prolactin concentrations have normalized and clinical symptoms of hyperprolactinemia have resolved with dopamine-agonist therapy, prolactin serum concentrations should be monitored every 6 to 12 months. In patients receiving long-term treatment, the dose of the dopamine agonist can be gradually reduced or discontinued in some patients. For patients with microprolactinomas who have normal serum prolactin concentrations and at least a 50% reduction in tumor size, medical therapy may be withdrawn every 2 to 5 years to assess if remission has been achieved. In the case of macroprolactinomas, the dose of the dopamine agonist can be gradually reduced in some cases, but complete drug discontinuation should be attempted only if careful monitoring for renewed tumor growth can be ensured.[74,75,92]

PHARMACOECONOMIC CONSIDERATIONS

Medical therapy with dopamine agonists is more effective than transsphenoidal surgery or radiation for the management of hyperprolactinemia. Because most patients receive therapy for long periods of time, the medical management of hyperprolactinemia may result in considerable cost. Although bromocriptine has been frequently used to manage hyperprolactinemia, therapy with pergolide, which has been shown to be equally effective, costs considerably less and offers the advantage of once-daily dosing. Cabergoline has been shown to be more effective than bromocriptine and offers additional advantages such as a decreased incidence of adverse effects and improved patient compliance. Most clinicians agree that cabergoline is the most efficacious dopamine agonist currently available. However, the cost of cabergoline therapy is approximately two times greater than that of bromocriptine. Pharmacoeconomic studies are needed to assess whether the higher cost of cabergoline therapy is balanced by the potential added benefits.

CONCLUSIONS

Hyperprolactinemia is a common disorder that can have a significant impact on fertility. Hyperprolactinemia is most commonly caused by the presence of prolactin-secreting pituitary tumors and various medications that antagonize dopamine or increase the secretion of prolactin. Available treatment options for this disorder include medical therapy with dopamine agonists, radiation therapy, and transsphenoidal surgery. In most cases, medical therapy with dopamine agonists is considered the most effective treatment. Cabergoline has replaced bromocriptine as the mainstay of medical therapy, as it appears to be better tolerated and more effective. However, due to limited data regarding the safety of cabergoline during pregnancy, bromocriptine remains the preferred agent when fertility is the primary purpose for treatment.

PANHYPOPITUITARISM

⏴**11** Panhypopituitarism is a condition of complete or partial loss of anterior and posterior pituitary function resulting in a complex disorder characterized by multiple pituitary-hormone deficiencies. Patients with panhypopituitarism may have ACTH deficiency, gonadotropin deficiency, growth hormone deficiency, hypothyroidism, and hyperprolactinemia. Panhypopituitarism can be classified as either primary or secondary depending on the etiology. Primary panhypopituitarism involves an abnormality within the secretory cells of the pituitary, whereas secondary panhypopituitarism is caused by a lack of proper external stimulation needed for normal release of pituitary hormones. Some of the most common causes of panhypopituitarism include primary pituitary tumors, ischemic necrosis of the pituitary, surgical trauma, irradiation, and various types of central nervous system infections. Pharmacologic treatment of panhypopituitarism is essential and consists of replacement of specific pituitary hormones after careful assessment of individual deficiencies. Replacement most often consists of glucocorticoids, thyroid-hormone preparations, and sex steroids. The administration of recombinant growth hormone also may be necessary. Patients with panhypopituitarism will need lifelong replacement therapy and constant monitoring of multiple homeostatic functions.

ABBREVIATIONS

ACTH: adrenocorticotropic hormone
CJD: Creutzfeldt-Jakob disease
CRH: corticotropin-releasing hormone
FSH: follicle-stimulating hormone
GH: growth hormone
GHD: growth-hormone-deficient
GnRH: gonadotropin-releasing hormone
GHRH: growth hormone-releasing hormone
IGFBP-3: Insulin-like growth factor-I-binding-protein-3
IGF: insulin-like growth factor
IIH: idiopathic intracranial hypertension
LH: luteinizing hormone
OGTT: oral glucose tolerance test
SSRI: selective serotonin reuptake inhibitor
TRH: thyrotropin-releasing hormone
TSH: thyroid-stimulating hormone
VIP: vasoactive intestinal peptide

Review Questions and other resources can be found at *www.pharmacotherapyonline.com.*

REFERENCES

1. Raisman G. An urge to explain the incomprehensible: Geoffrey Harris and the discovery of the neural control of the pituitary gland. Ann Rev Neurosci 1997;20:533–566.
2. Amar AP, Weiss MH. Pituitary anatomy and physiology. Neurosurg Clin North Am 2003;14:11–23.
3. Cuttler L. The regulation of growth hormone secretion. Endocrinol Metab Clin North Am 1996;25:541–571.
4. Molitch ME. Disorders of prolactin secretion. Endocrinol Metab Clin North Am 2001;30:585–610.
5. Le Roith D. Insulin-like growth factors. N Engl J Med 1997;336:633–640.
6. Holdaway M, Rajasoorya C. Epidemiology of acromegaly. Pituitary 1999; 2:29–41.
7. Eugster EA, Pescovitz OH. Gigantism. J Clin Endocrinol Metab 1999;84:4379–4384.
8. Ben-Shlomo A, Melmed S. Acromegaly. Endocrinol Metab Clin North Am 2001;30:565–583.
9. Molitch ME. Clinical manifestations of acromegaly. Endocrinol Metab Clin North Am 1992;21:597–614.
10. Melmed S. Unwanted effects of growth hormone excess in the adult. J Pediatr Endocrinol Metab 1996;9(Suppl 3):369–374.
11. Fatti LM, Scacchi M, Pincelli AI, et al. Prevalence and pathogenesis of sleep apnea and lung disease in acromegaly. Pituitary 2001;4:259–262.
12. Vitale G, Pivonello R, Galderisi M, et al. Cardiovascular complications in acromegaly: methods of assessment. Pituitary 2001;4:251–257.
13. Webb SM, Casanueva F, Wass JA. Oncological complications of excess GH in acromegaly. Pituitary 2002;5:21–25.
14. Patel YC, Ezzat S, Chik CL, et al. Guidelines for the diagnosis and treatment of acromegaly: A Canadian perspective. Clin Invest Med 2000;23: 172–187.
15. Acromegaly Treatment Consensus Workshop Participants. Consensus guidelines for acromegaly management. J Clin Endocrinol Metab 2002; 87:4054–4058.
16. Giustina A, Barkan AL, Casanueva FF, et al. Criteria for cure of acromegaly: A consensus statement. J Clin Endocrinol Metab 2000;85:526–529.
17. Sheppard MC. Primary medical therapy for acromegaly. Clin Endocrinol 2003;58:387–399.
18. Melmed S, Vance ML, Barkan AL, et al. Current status and future opportunities for controlling acromegaly. Pituitary 2002;5:185–196.
19. Colao A, Ferone D, Marzullo P, et al. Effect of different dopaminergic agents in the treatment of acromegaly. J Clin Endocrinol Metab 1997;82:518–523.
20. Jaffe CA, Barkan AL. Acromegaly recognition and treatment. Drugs 1994; 47:425–445.
21. Orrego JJ, Barkan AL. Pituitary disorders. Drugs 2000;59:93–106.
22. Abs R, Verhelst J, Maiter D, et al. Cabergoline in the treatment of acromegaly: A study of 64 patients. J Clin Endocrinol Metab 1998;83: 374–378.
23. Freda PU. Somatostatin analogs in acromegaly. J Clin Endocrinol Metab 2002;87:3013–3018.
24. Lamberts SE, Van der Lely A, de Herder WW, Hofland LJ. Drug therapy: Octreotide. N Engl J Med 1996;334:246–254.
25. Vance ML, Harris AG. Long-term treatment of 189 acromegalic patients with the somatostatin analog octreotide. Results of the international multicenter acromegaly study group. Arch Intern Med 1991;151:1573–1578.
26. Ezzat S, Snyder PJ, Young WF, et al. Octreotide treatment of acromegaly: A randomized, multicenter study. Ann Intern Med 1992;117:211–218.
27. Newman CB, Melmed S, Snyder PJ, et al. Safety and efficacy of long term octreotide therapy of acromegaly: Results of a multicenter trial in 103 patients—A clinical research center study. J Clin Endocrinol Metab 1995;80:2768–2775.
28. Merola B, Cittadini A, Colao A, et al. Chronic treatment with the somatostatin analog octreotide improves cardiac abnormalities in acromegaly. J Clin Endocrinol Metab 1993;77:790–793.
29. Padayatty SJ, Perrins EJ, Belchetz PE. Octreotide treatment increases exercise capacity in patients with acromegaly. Eur J Endocrinol 1996;134: 554–559.

30. Giustina A, Boni E, Romanelli G. Cardiopulmonary performance during exercise in acromegaly, and the effects of acute suppression of growth hormone hypersecretion with octreotide. Am J Cardiol 1995;75:1042–1047.

31. Grunstein RR, Ho KKY, Sullivan CE. Effect of octreotide, a somatostatin analog, on sleep apnea in patients with acromegaly. Ann Intern Med 1994;121:478–483.

32. Thapar K, Kovacs KT, Stefaneanu L, et al. Antiproliferative effect of the somatostatin analogue octreotide on growth hormone-producing pituitary tumors: Results of a multicenter randomized trial. Mayo Clin Proc 1997;72:893–900.

33. McKeage K, Cheer S, Wagstaff AJ. Octreotide long-acting release (LAR): A review of its use in the management of acromegaly. Drugs 2003;63:2473–2499.

34. Lancranjan L, Brew Atkinson A, and the Sandostatin LAR Group. Results of European multicentre study with sandostatin LAR in acromegaly patients. Pituitary 1999;1:105–114.

35. Coloa A, Ferone D, Lastoria S, et al. Prediction of efficacy of octreotide therapy in patients with acromegaly. J Clin Endocrinol Metab 1996;81:2356–2362.

36. Avila NA, Shawker TH Roach P, et al. Sonography of gallbladder abnormalities in acromegaly patients following octreotide and ursodiol therapy: incidence and time course. J Clin Ultrasound 1998;26:289–294.

37. Ho KK, Jenkins AB, Furier SM, et al. Impact of octreotide, a long-acting somatostatin analogue, on glucose tolerance and insulin sensitivity in acromegaly. Clin Endocrinol 1992;36:271–279.

38. Sato K, Takamatsu K, Hashimoto K. Short-term effects of octreotide on glucose tolerance in patients with acromegaly. Endocr J 1995;42:739–745.

39. Koop BL, Harris AG, Ezzat S. Effect of octreotide on glucose tolerance in acromegaly. Eur J Endocrinol 1994;130:581–586.

40. Flogstad AK, Halse J, Grass P, et al. A comparison of octreotide, bromocriptine, or a combination of both drugs in acromegaly. J Clin Endocrinol Metab 1994;79:461–465.

41. Clemmons DR, Chihara K, Freda PU, et al. Optimizing control of acromegaly: Integrating a growth hormone receptor antagonist into the treatment algorithm. J Clin Endocrinol Metab 2003;88:4759–4767.

42. Trainer PJ, Drake WM, Katznelson L, et al. Treatment of acromegaly with the growth hormone-receptor antagonist Pegvisomant. N Engl J Med 2000;342:1171–1177.

43. Van Der Lely AJ, Hutson R, Trainer PJ, et al. Long-term treatment of acromegaly with pegvisomant, a growth hormone receptor antagonist. Lancet 2001;358:1754–1759.

44. Anonymous. Pegvisomant (Somavert) for acromegaly. Med Lett Drugs Ther 2003;45:55–56.

45. Hindmarsh PC, Brook CGD. Short stature and growth hormone deficiency. Clin Endocrinol 1995;43:133–142.

46. American Association of Clinical Endocrinologists. Medical guidelines for clinical practice for growth hormone use in adults and children—2003 Update. Endocr Pract 2003;9:64–76.

47. Pasquino AM, Albanese A, Bozzola M, et al. Idiopathic short stature. J Pediatr Endocrinol Metab 2001;(Suppl 2):967–974.

48. Schwartz ID, Grunt JA. Growth, short stature, and the use of growth hormone: Considerations for the practicing pediatrician—an update. Curr Prob Pediatr 1997;27:14–40.

49. Lawson Wilkins Pediatric Endocrine Society Executive Committee. Guidelines for the use of growth hormone in children with short stature. A report by the drug and therapeutics committee of the Lawson Wilkins Pediatric Endocrine Society. J Pediatr 1995;127:857–867.

50. Mills JL, Schonberger LB, Wysowski DK, et al. Long-term mortality in the United States cohort of pituitary-derived growth hormone recipients. J Pediatr 2004;144:430–436.

51. Blethen SL, Bapitista J, Kuntze J, et al. Adult height in growth hormone (GH)-deficient children treated with biosynthetic GH. J Clin Endocrinol Metab 1997;82:418–420.

52. August GP, Julius JR, Blethen SL. Adult height in children with growth hormone deficiency who are treated with biosynthetic growth hormone: The national cooperative growth study experience. Pediatrics 1998;102:512–516.

53. Frinkik JP, Baptista J. Adult height in growth hormone deficiency: Historical perspective and examples from the nation cooperative growth study. Pediatrics 1999;104:1000–1004.

54. Thomas M, Massa G, Bourguignon JP, et al. Final height in children with idiopathic growth hormone deficiency treated with recombinant human growth hormone: The Belgian experience. Horm Res 2001;55:88–94.

55. Rikken B, Massa GG, Wit JM, and the Dutch Growth Hormone Working Group. Final height in a large cohort of Dutch patients with growth hormone deficiency treated with growth hormone. Horm Res 1995;43:136–137.

56. Chipman JJ, Hicks JR, Holcombe JH, Draper MW. Approaching final height in children treated for growth hormone deficiency. Horm Res 1995;43:129–131.

57. Serveri F. Final height in children with growth hormone deficiency. Horm Res 1995;43:138–140.

58. Coste J, Letrait M, Carel JC, et al. Long term results of growth hormone treatment in France in children of short stature: Population, register based study. BMJ 1997;315:708–713.

59. Cuneo RC, Judd S, Wallace JD, et al. The Australian multicenter trial of growth hormone (GH) treatment in GH-deficient adults. J Clin Endocrinol Metab 1998;83:107–116.

60. Kann P, Piepkorn B, Schehler B, et al. Effect of long-term treatment with GH on bone metabolism, bone mineral density and bone elasticity in GH-deficient adults. Clin Endocrinol 1998;48:561–568.

61. Wiren L, Bengtsson BA, Johannsson G. Beneficial effects of long-term GH replacement therapy on quality of life in adults with GH deficiency. Clin Endocrinol 1998;48:613–620.

62. Cuttler L, Silvers JB, Singh J, et al. Short stature and growth hormone therapy: A national study of physician recommendation patterns. JAMA 1996;276:531–537.

63. Finkelstein BS, Imperiale TF, Speroff T, et al. Effect of growth hormone therapy on height in children with idiopathic short stature. Arch Pediatr Adolesc Med 2002;156:230–240.

64. Blethen SL, MacGillivray MH. A risk-benefit assessment of growth hormone use in children. Drug Saf 1997;17:303–316.

65. Thorner MO and the Growth Hormone Research Society. Critical evaluation of the safety of recombinant human growth hormone administration. J Clin Endocrinol Metab 2001;86:1868–1870.

66. Jeffcoate W. Growth hormone therapy and its relationship to insulin resistance, glucose intolerance and diabetes mellitus. Drug Saf 2002;25:199–212.

67. Wantanabe S, Tsunematsu Y, Fujimoto J, et al. Leukaemia in patients treated with growth hormone. Lancet 1988;1:1159–1160.

68. Ogilvy-Stuart A, Gleeson H. Cancer risk following growth hormone use in childhood: Implications for current practice. Drug Saf 2004;24:369–382.

69. Rougeot C, Marchand P, Dray F, et al. Comparative study of biosynthetic human growth hormone immunogenicity in growth hormone deficient children. Horm Res 1991;35:76–81.

70. Pirazzoli P, Cacciari E, Mandini M, et al. Follow-up of antibodies to growth hormone in 210 growth hormone-deficient children treated with different commercial preparations. Acta Paediatr 1995;84:1233–1236.

71. Thorner M, Rochiccioli P, Colle M, et al. Once daily subcutaneous growth hormone-releasing hormone accelerates growth in growth-hormone deficient children during the first year of therapy. J Clin Endocrinol Metab 1996;81:1189–1196.

72. Ogilvy-Stuart AL, Stirling HF, Kelnart CJH, et al. Treatment of radiation-induced growth hormone deficiency with growth hormone-releasing hormone. Clin Endocrinol 1997;46:571–578.

73. American Academy of Pediatrics Committee on Drugs and Committee on Bioethics. Considerations related to the use of recombinant human growth hormone in children. Pediatrics 1997;99:122–129.

74. Schlechte JA. Prolactinoma. N Engl J Med 2003;349:2035–2041.

75. Mah PM, Webster J. Hyperprolactinemia: etiology, diagnosis and management. Semin Reprod Med 2002;20:365–373.

76. Molitch ME. Medical treatment of prolactinomas. Endocrinol Metab Clin North Am 1999;28:143–169.

77. Davies PH. Drug-related hyperprolactinaemia. Adverse Drug React Toxicol Rev 1997;16:83–94.

78. Marken PA, Haykal RF, Fisher JN. Management of psychotropic-induced hyperprolactinemia. Clin Pharm 1992;11:851–856.

79. Webster J. A comparative review of the tolerability profiles of dopamine agonists in the treatment of hyperprolactinaemia and inhibition of lactation. Drug Saf 1996;14:228–238.

80. Carranza-Lira S, Gonzalez-Sanchez JL, Martinez-Chequer JC. Vaginal bromocriptine administration in patients with hyperprolactinemia. Int J Gynaecol Obstet 1999;65:77–78.

81. Verhelst J, Abs R, Maiter D, et al. Cabergoline in the treatment of hyperprolactinemia: A study in 455 patients. J Clin Endocrinol Metab 1999;84:2518–2522.

82. Cannavo S, Curto L, Squadrito S, et al. Cabergoline: A first-choice treatment in patients with previously untreated prolactin-secreting pituitary adenoma. J Endocrinol Invest 1999;22:354–359.

83. Colao A, DiSarno A, Landi ML, et al. Macroprolactinoma shrinkage during cabergoline treatment is greater in naïve patients than in patients pretreated with other dopamine agonists: A prospective study in 110 patients. J Clin Endocrinol Metab 2000;85:2247–2252.

84. Ferrari CI, Abs R, Bevan JS, et al. Treatment of macroprolactinoma with cabergoline: A study of 85 patients. Clin Endocrinol 1997;46:409–413.

85. Webster J, Piscitelli G, Polli A, et al. A comparison of cabergoline and bromocriptine in the treatment of hyperprolactinemic amenorrhea. N Engl J Med 1994;331:904–909.

86. DiSarno A, Landi ML, Cappabianca P, et al. Resistance to cabergoline as compared with bromocriptine in hyperprolactinemia: prevalence, clinical definition, and therapeutic strategy. J Clin Endocrinol Metab 2001; 86:5256–5261.

87. Colao A, Di Sarno A, Landi ML, et al. Macroprolactinoma shrinkage during cabergoline treatment is greater in naïve patients than in patients pretreated with other dopamine agonists: A prospective study in 110 patients. J Clin Endocrinol Metab 2000;85:2247–2252.

88. Colao A, Vitale G, Cappabianca P, et al. Outcome of cabergoline treatment in men with prolactinoma: Effects of a 24-month treatment on prolactin levels, tumor mass, recovery of pituitary function, and semen analysis. J Clin Endocrinol Metab 2004;89:1704–1711.

89. Rains CP, Bryson HM, Fitton A. Cabergoline: A review of its pharmacological properties and therapeutic potential in the treatment of hyperprolactinaemia and inhibition of lactation. Drugs 1995;49:255–279.

90. Motta T, Colombo N, DeVincentiis S, et al. Vaginal cabergoline in the treatment of hyperprolactinemic patients intolerant to oral dopaminergics. Fertil Steril 1996;65:440–442.

91. Colao A, di Sarno A, Pivonello R, et al. Dopamine receptor agonists for treating prolactinomas. Expert Opin Investig Drugs 2002;11:787–800.

92. Colao A, DiSarno A, Cappabianca P, et al. Withdrawal of long-term cabergoline therapy for tumoral and nontumoral hyperprolactinemia. N Engl J Med 2003;349:2023–2033.

76

PREGNANCY AND LACTATION: THERAPEUTIC CONSIDERATIONS

Denise L. Walbrandt Pigarelli, Connie K. Kraus, and Beth E. Potter

Learning Objectives and other resources can be found at *www.pharmacotherapyonline.com.*

KEY CONCEPTS

1 Altered drug pharmacokinetics during pregnancy can influence drug selection and dosing. Physiologic changes during pregnancy typically result in changes in absorption, protein binding, distribution, and elimination.

2 Although drug-induced teratogenicity is a serious concern during pregnancy, most drugs required by pregnant women can be used safely. Informed selection of drug therapy is essential.

3 Health care practitioners must know where to find and how to evaluate evidence related to the safety of drugs used during pregnancy.

4 Pregnancy-influenced health issues such as constipation, gastroesophageal reflux disease, and nausea/vomiting of pregnancy (and others) for many years have been treated safely and effectively with carefully selected drug therapy. Some acute and chronic illnesses may pose special risks during pregnancy, and they should be treated with appropriately selected and monitored drug therapies to avoid harm to both the woman and the fetus.

5 Understanding the physiology of lactation and pharmacokinetic factors affecting drug distribution, metabolism, and elimination can assist the clinician with more appropriate and safe use of medications during lactation.

Drug use in pregnancy and lactation is a critically important topic that is underemphasized in the education of health professions. Interestingly, the subject encompasses a dichotomous discussion of the benefits of drug therapy for the mother and the potential risks for the embryo/fetus. Drug use in pregnancy and lactation is a controversial and emotionally charged area because of medicolegal and ethical implications.

It is the clinician's responsibility to ensure safe and effective therapy before conception, during pregnancy, and after delivery, and the patient's active participation is essential. Both acute and chronic illnesses must be managed during pregnancy, and optimal treatments sometimes are different from those in the nonpregnant patient. Pharmacotherapeutic issues also apply to selection of drugs during parturition and the postpartum period. Principles of drug use during lactation, although similar, are not the same as those applicable during pregnancy.

In many instances, medication dosing recommendations for acute or chronic illness treatment in pregnant women are the same as for the general population. On the other hand, there are some instances where dosing or selection of medications in pregnancy is quite different from that in the general population. We have sought to highlight unique dosing and drug selection considerations in this chapter.

NATURAL COURSE OF PREGNANCY

PHYSIOLOGY

Because of the complexity of fertilization and subsequent pregnancy events, approximately 50% of embroyos do not survive.[1] Most of these losses occur in the first 2 weeks after fertilization, and many women may not realize that they were pregnant. About 15% of the pregnancies that survive the first 2 weeks of gestation will be lost spontaneously later in the course of the pregnancy.[1]

Fertilization occurs when a sperm joins to an egg by attaching to a receptor on the outer protein layer of the egg, the zona pellucida.[1] Immediately, the egg becomes unresponsive to other sperm. The attached sperm releases enzymes that cause the egg's chromosomes to mature and also allow the sperm to fully penetrate the zona pellucida and contact the egg's cell membrane. The membranes of the sperm and egg are then fused to create a new, single cell. Male and female chromosomes join in the new cell, fuse to create a single nucleus, and organize to set the stage for cell division.[1]

Fertilization usually occurs in the fallopian tube.[1] Cell division continues for the first 2 days while the fertilized egg travels down the fallopian tube, reaching the uterine cavity on the third day. Cell division continues for 2 to 3 more days in the uterine cavity before implantation begins.[1] Approximately 6 days after fertilization, the cell mass is termed a *blastocyst*.[1] Human chorionic gonadotropin is now produced in amounts that may be detected in commercial laboratories. The blastocyst sloughs the zona pellucida and rests directly on the endometrium, which now responds to the denuded blastocyst by allowing it to begin to grow into the endometrial wall. After 6 days of this growth, the blastocyst lies implanted under the endometrium's surface and begins to receive nutrition from maternal blood.[1] It is now called an *embryo*.[2]

The embryonic period lasts from approximately 2 weeks after fertilization until 8 weeks after fertilization, when the conceptus is renamed a *fetus*.[2] Most body structures are formed during the embryonic period, and they continue to grow and mature during the fetal period. The fetal period continues until the pregnancy reaches term, approximately 40 weeks after the last menstrual period.[2]

Gravidity refers to the number of times that a woman experiences pregnancy.[2] A multiple birth is counted as a single pregnancy. *Parity* refers to the number of a woman's pregnancies that exceeded 20 weeks of gestation and also relates information regarding the outcome of each pregnancy. In sequence, the numbers reflect (1) term deliveries, (2) premature deliveries, (3) aborted and/or ectopic pregnancies, and (4) number of living children. A woman who has been pregnant four times; has experienced two term deliveries, one premature delivery, and one ectopic pregnancy; and has three living children would be designated by G_4P_{2113}.[2]

PREGNANCY DATING

Approximately 280 days (about 40 weeks or 9 months) constitute the duration of a pregnancy; this time period extends from the first day of the last menstrual period to birth.[2] *Gestational age* or *menstrual age* refers to the age of the embryo or fetus beginning with the first day of the last menstrual period, which is about 2 weeks prior to fertilization. To calculate an approximate pregnancy due date, the clinician adds 7 days to the first day of the last menstrual period and subtracts 3 months.[2]

For simple description purposes, pregnancy is divided into three periods of 3 calendar months, and each period of 3 months is called a *trimester*.

PREGNANCY SIGNS AND SYMPTOMS

The early symptoms of pregnancy include fatigue and increased frequency of urination.[3] At approximately 6 weeks' gestation, the pregnant woman may experience nausea and vomiting; this is commonly known as *morning sickness* but may occur at any time of the day. Nausea and vomiting usually resolve at 12 to 18 weeks' gestation. Fetal movement is detected in the woman's lower abdomen at 16 to 20 weeks of gestation.[3]

Signs of pregnancy may include sudden cessation of menses, changes in consistency of the cervical mucus, a bluish discoloration of the vaginal mucosa, increased skin pigmentation, and anatomic breast changes.[3]

MATERNAL PHARMACOKINETIC CHANGES IN PREGNANCY

During pregnancy, a woman's reduced gastrointestinal motility, increased gastric pH, and increased pulmonary alveolar drug uptake affect drug absorption.[4] Drug distribution in pregnancy may change because maternal plasma volume increases by 50%. Of the approximately 8-L increase in total-body water during pregnancy,

40% is distributed to maternal compartments, and 60% is distributed to the amniotic fluid, placenta, and fetus. Serum albumin binding capacity is decreased during pregnancy, which results in increased unbound drug. However, decreased amounts of ingested drug per kilogram of body weight and increased hepatic and renal elimination of drugs result in a net impact on drug distribution of unaltered free drug serum concentration for many (but not all) drugs.[4]

Pregnancy also affects drug elimination. The maternal hormones progesterone and estradiol affect hepatic drug metabolism in various ways; they enhance the hepatic metabolism of some drugs (e.g., phenytoin) but inhibit the metabolism of others (e.g., theophylline).[4] In addition, the clearance of drugs excreted into the biliary system may slow because estrogen can cause cholestasis. Renal drug clearance may be affected by an increased renal blood flow of 25% to 50% and an increased glomerular filtration rate of 50%. Fortunately, these changes usually do not result in a need for altered drug dosing.[4]

TRANSPLACENTAL DRUG TRANSFER

Although once thought to be a barrier to drug transfer, the placenta is fundamentally the organ of exchange for a number of substances, including drugs, between the mother and fetus.[5] The placenta functions fully for such transport by the fifth week after conception. Most drugs move across the membranes by passive diffusion, both to the fetus from the mother and from the fetus to the mother, as maternal serum levels decline. Such considerations as maternal dose, route of administration, maternal pharmacokinetic handling of the ingested substance, and maternal plasma protein binding may influence the actual amount of drug that reaches the fetus. Characteristics of the ingested substance also influence the degree of transfer. High lipophilicity, low ionization, low maternal protein binding, and low molecular weight all enhance the degree of transfer.[5]

The degree to which exposure to a drug influences the embryo/fetus also may be a function of the timing of the exposure. It is generally thought that drug exposure during the embryonic period has the greatest potential influence on organ development.[5,6] Indeed, the most obvious teratogenic effects occur during this period.[5] Teratogenic effects may include loss of pregnancy, structural abnormalities, growth impairment, and functional loss.[6] However, more subtle changes in function or behavior may be associated with drug exposure at other times during pregnancy.[5]

DRUG SELECTION DURING PREGNANCY

The greatest concern regarding the use of medications in pregnant women is the potential risk of abnormal development in the child. Although some drugs have the potential to cause teratogenic effects, most medications required by pregnant women can be used safely. There are many misconceptions related to the role medications play in causing birth defects.

The vast majority of children are born healthy. The overall incidence of congenital malformations is approximately 3% to 5%.[7,8] Although many people assume that medications play a large role in causing birth defects, it is estimated that medication exposure accounts for less than 1% of all birth defects.[8] Genetic causes are responsible for 15% to 25%, other environmental issues (e.g., maternal conditions, infection, and mechanical deformations) account for 10%, and the remaining 65% to 75% of congenital malformations result from unknown causes.[8]

Despite the greater potential of harm with certain drugs, not every exposure will result in a birth defect. Factors such as the stage of pregnancy when the exposure occurred, the route of administration, and dose all can influence outcomes.[7] In the first 2 weeks after conception, exposure to a teratogen may result in an "all or nothing" effect, which could either destroy the embryo or cause no problems. The period from 18 to 60 days postconception (organogenesis) is the time when organ systems are developing, and teratogenic exposures may result in structural anomalies. In the remainder of the pregnancy, exposure to teratogenic agents may result in retardation of growth, central nervous system (CNS) abnormalities, or death. Examples of medications associated with teratogenic effects in the period of organogenesis include chemotherapy drugs (e.g., methotrexate, cyclophosphamide), sex hormones (e.g., diethylstilbesterol), lithium, retinoids, thalidomide, certain antiepileptic drugs, and coumarin derivatives. Medications such as angiotensin-converting enzyme inhibitors, nonsteroidal anti-inflammatory agents, and tetracycline derivatives are more likely to exhibit effects in the second or third trimesters.[7]

Finally, there is a growing interest in discovering the role that genetic susceptibility plays in whether an exposure to a medication will result in a birth defect. Maternal and fetal genotypes may influence the effect a drug might have on the fetus by influencing the absorption, metabolism, distribution, and binding of a drug.[7] There is some evidence that certain unique anomalies associated with maternal smoking may be more likely in people with specific genetic variants.[9]

In summary, a small number of medications are associated with the potential to cause congenital malformations. Many of these agents can be avoided easily during pregnancy. In situations where a drug may be harmful to the developing child but is necessary for maternal care, considerations related to route of administration and dosing may lessen the risk of congenital malformations.

METHODS OF DETERMINING SAFETY OF DRUGS IN PREGNANCY

Even though most medications are likely to be safe during pregnancy, clinicians will struggle to make decisions about choosing therapy. Information about medication safety in pregnancy comes from a variety of sources. One of the most important questions for the clinician is how to evaluate the quality of the evidence related to the safety of medications used in pregnancy.

Although randomized, controlled trials form the basis for some of the most reliable assessments of drug safety, pregnant women usually are not eligible for participation in clinical trials. Other types of data often are used to estimate the risk associated with medication use during pregnancy, such as animal studies, case reports, case-control studies, prospective cohort studies, historical cohort studies, and voluntary reporting systems.

Although animal studies are a required component of drug testing, extrapolation of the results of such testing to humans is not always accurate. One example is thalidomide, which was found to be safe in some animal models but proved to have teratogenic effects in human offspring.[10]

Case reports may be of limited value because an isolated occurrence of a birth defect in the infant of a woman who used a medication during her pregnancy may have occurred by chance.[10] Because most pregnant women use drugs infrequently, and the overall risk of drug-related teratogenic effects is low, it would take a very large number of exposures to appreciate an increased risk. The few instances in which case reports have been helpful in establishing teratogenic risk were situations in which a drug was used infrequently but was associated with a high rate of birth defects (isotretinoin); or it was used widely and caused reproducible malformations (thalidomide).[11]

Case-control studies identify an outcome (congenital anomaly), match subjects with and without that outcome, and report how often there was exposure to a suspected agent.[10] The concern with this type of study is recall bias, because a woman with an affected pregnancy may be more likely to recall drugs used during the course of pregnancy than would a woman who had a normal pregnancy outcome.[10]

Cohort studies look at the intervention (use of a particular drug) in a group of persons and compare outcomes in a similar group of subjects without the intervention.[10] The fact that the study is prospective eliminates some of the problems with recall bias. This approach has several potential disadvantages, however, such as the need for large numbers of participants, time involved, and potential loss to follow-up. Despite these disadvantages, cohort studies are used often for evaluating the effects of a drug exposure on pregnancy outcomes.[10]

An example of a cohort study is the Michigan Medicaid study, which consisted of data collected from 229,101 pregnancies over 7 years.[10] Teratology information services provide pregnant women with information about potential exposures during pregnancy and, in turn, follow these women throughout the pregnancy to assess the outcomes of the pregnancy. These services may report pooled data to facilitate information sharing about medications used in pregnancy. In addition, some pharmaceutical companies have organized voluntary reporting systems for drugs used in pregnancy. One such example is the Acyclovir in Pregnancy Registry.[10]

RESOURCES

Unfortunately, there is no one place for the clinician to collect information regarding the safety of a medication for pregnant patients. Computerized databases (e.g., the Canadian database, *www.motherisk.org*) and textbooks with information from large cohorts of treated women offer valuable assistance. New information regarding drug use in pregnancy also may be obtained from searches of the primary literature for cohort and case studies.

One commonly used source of information about drug safety is the category system of the Food and Drug Administration (FDA). The FDA created drug categories to provide guidance regarding the risk versus benefit for drug use during pregnancy.[11] The reliability of this resource has been of concern for several reasons.[11,12] When compared with two other risk classification systems from other countries, only 61 of 236 drugs (26%) in common to all three systems were ranked in the same risk category.[12] The FDA ranks very few drugs as considered safe during pregnancy (category A) because it has a requirement for a controlled trial to establish safety. Therefore, the impression from this source would be that few drugs are safe. Another concern about use of the FDA categories involves the difficulty of changing a drug's classification when new information becomes available.[11] An example of this issue is that oral contraceptives are classified by the FDA as category X drugs (studies in animals or pregnant women demonstrated evidence of fetal abnormality), but there is little current evidence that such exposure results in congenital abnormalities.[11,12] In contrast, the Swedish and Australian classification systems do not categorize oral contraceptives as teratogenic agents.[12]

GENERAL RECOMMENDATIONS FOR SELECTION OF MEDICATIONS IN PREGNANCY

Several principles may be helpful in selecting medications for use during pregnancy. The first is to consider selecting drugs that have been used for the longest periods of time with safety.[11] Whenever possible, the amount of drug administered should be at the lower end of the dosing range to minimize fetal exposure. Finally, patients should be discouraged from self-medicating during pregnancy and encouraged to consult their clinician for advice.[11]

PRECONCEPTION PLANNING

There are approximately 4 million births in the United States each year,[13] and almost 50% of these are unplanned.[14] In addition, many women may not seek health care for pregnancy until after the first trimester.[13] Given the dynamic changes that occur during the first trimester, there is growing effort to encourage preconception planning. Not only would such planning assist the prospective mother in identifying areas of risk for pregnancy, but it also would provide education and interventions to improve birth outcomes.[13] Several preconception interventions have been shown to improve pregnancy outcomes significantly. One of the interventions with strong scientific evidence for benefit is the ingestion of folic acid to reduce the risk for neural tube defects,[13] which affect approximately 4000 pregnancies in the United States each year.[14,15] Of these pregnancies, one-third are aborted spontaneously or electively.[15] Controlled clinical trials have shown that folic acid supplementation prior to and during the early stages of pregnancy can reduce the incidence of neural tube defects by 50%. Because the neural tube closes within the first 4 weeks of pregnancy, and because so many pregnancies are unplanned and unrecognized until after this time, it is necessary to encourage women of childbearing potential either to consume folate-enriched foods or to use supplements prior to pregnancy.[15]

The American Academy of Pediatrics Committee on Genetics endorses the recommendation from the U.S. Public Health Service that all women of childbearing age ingest 400 mcg of folic acid daily to reduce the risk of neural tube defects in their potential offspring.[15] Because the consumption of food naturally containing folic acid is variable from day to day, and because folate from these sources is less well absorbed, it is suggested that women fulfill the daily requirement for folic acid through either folate-enriched foods or supplements.[14] Women who have had a pregnancy affected by a neural tube defect or who use certain seizure medications should receive 4000 mcg (4 mg) of folic acid daily beginning 1 to 3 months prior to conception and continuing throughout the first trimester.[15] These higher doses of folic acid require the use of supplements. Although folic acid supplementation potentially may mask the hematologic effects of vitamin B_{12} deficiency, the risk of this occurring in women of childbearing potential is rare. In contrast, the level of evidence of reduction in birth defects with supplementation of other vitamins and nutrients prior to pregnancy is weaker than that for supplementation of folic acid.[13]

Other preconception interventions with evidence of improving pregnancy outcomes include screening and immunization for rubella and varicella.[13] Influenza vaccine is also recommended for women who will be in the second or third trimester during the influenza season.[16] Pregnant women who contract influenza may have greater morbidity and mortality owing to the risk of pneumonia.[16]

Another important component of preconception and early pregnancy care involves the assessment and reduction of risks associated with the use of tobacco.[13] Cigarette smoking is said to be the most significant modifiable cause of adverse events in pregnancy.[17] It is estimated that up to 20% of women smoke during pregnancy.[18] Smoking during pregnancy commonly results in fetal growth retardation.[17] Preterm delivery, perinatal mortality, and sudden infant death syndrome are also associated with the use of tobacco during pregnancy.[17,18] One strategy to reduce the number of women who

smoke during pregnancy is to encourage young women not to begin smoking.[17] This is important because even though women are more likely to quit smoking when they become pregnant than at any other time, many will restart smoking before delivery or soon thereafter.[1]

Behavioral therapy is considered the intervention of first choice to assist pregnant women with smoking cessation.[18] As little as a single 5- to 15-minute counseling session by a provider has resulted in a doubling of the rate of pregnant women who stop smoking versus no counseling (20% versus 5% to 10%). Some pregnant women may be unable to quit smoking with behavioral interventions alone,[19] especially those who use a greater number of cigarettes per day.[17] Use of nicotine replacement in pregnant women who are unable to quit may be helpful.[17] Nicotine has been shown to cause CNS toxicity in fetal animal studies.[19] Cigarette smoking, however, delivers over 300 chemicals in addition to nicotine. One of these chemicals, carbon monoxide, is a factor in reducing fetal growth. Thus, although there are potential risks with nicotine replacement in the pregnant patient, these risks may be more than offset by the benefits if the patient can stop smoking. Some authors recommend intermittently used products (such as gum) to decrease the total daily dose of nicotine or suggest removal of patches at bedtime to allow a drug-free interval. The dose of nicotine initially should be selected to be comparable with that obtained from smoking.[19]

Health care providers can use many different types of encounters with young women of reproductive age to share information about improving their personal health, as well as the future health of their children. Pharmacotherapeutic interventions may include recommendations about folic acid supplementation, appropriate immunizations, and strategies to stop smoking.

PREGNANCY-INFLUENCED ISSUES

Pregnant women commonly experience health issues that are either caused by or exacerbated by the pregnant state. Constipation, gastroesophageal reflux, hemorrhoids, and nausea and vomiting may affect many women during pregnancy. Gestational diabetes, gestational hypertension, and venous thromboembolism have the potential to cause adverse pregnancy consequences. Gestational thyrotoxicosis is usually a self-limiting condition.

GASTROINTESTINAL TRACT

Constipation occurs commonly in pregnancy. Contributing factors may include changes in dietary habits, fluid intake, and physical activity; delayed intestinal transit (most likely because of hormonal changes during pregnancy); and possibly obstruction.[20] Therapy for the constipation of pregnancy should be instituted first with nondrug modalities, such as education, physical exercise, biofeedback, and increased intake of dietary fiber and fluid. If additional therapy is warranted, the use of supplemental fiber and/or a stool softener such as docusate is appropriate. Lactulose, sorbitol, and bisacodyl are acceptable treatments for constipation in pregnancy but should be reserved for occasional rather than routine use. Senna also may be used occasionally. Castor oil should be avoided in pregnancy because it can cause uterine contractions; mineral oil can reduce the absorption of fat-soluble vitamins, such as vitamin K, and the decreased serum levels can lead to neonatal hemorrhage.[20]

Gastroesophageal reflux disease occurs in approximately 50% to 80% of pregnant women, and decreased lower esophageal sphincter pressure (due to estrogen and progesterone causing smooth muscle relaxation) and increased intragastric pressure (due to the gravid uterus are the most likely etiologic factors.[21] Therapy for gastroesophageal reflux disease in pregnancy includes lifestyle and dietary modifications (e.g., small, frequent meals, caffeine avoidance, food avoidance 3 hours before bedtime, elevation of the head of the bed) just as for nonpregnant patients and pharmacologic therapy for pregnant patients who do not receive adequate relief from nondrug therapies.[21] Drug therapy for gastrointestinal reflux disease in pregnancy may be initiated with aluminum, calcium, or magnesium antacid preparations, although the use of sodium bicarbonate should be avoided because of the potential for causing electrolyte and fluid abnormalities in the mother and fetus. Magnesium trisilicate probably should be avoided as well because fetal renal, respiratory, cardiovascular, and muscular problems may occur with long-term, high-dose exposure. Sucralfate is another option for gastroesophageal reflux disease in pregnancy. Evidence also supports the use of ranitidine and cimetidine, but little literature is available regarding the use of famotidine and nizatidine in pregnancy.[21] Combination antacids and nonprescription ranitidine have been shown in one small trial to be effective in patients unresponsive to antacids alone.[22] If a patient does not respond to histamine-2 receptor blockers, lansoprazole and metoclopramide are also viable options for pregnant patients.[21]

The exact prevalence of hemorrhoids during pregnancy is unkown. Pathophysiologic causes of hemorrhoids during pregnancy may include constipation, venous dilation and engorgement due to pregnancy, and laxity of pelvic connective tissue.[20] Therapy of hemorrhoids during pregnancy is generally conservative; high intake of dietary fiber, adequate oral fluid intake, and use of sitz baths are helpful. Topical anesthetics, skin protectants, and astringents also may be used. Other options for refractory hemorrhoids include rubber band ligation, sclerotherapy, and surgery.[20]

Nausea and vomiting affect up to 80% of pregnant women; however, hyperemesis gravidarum (i.e., severe nausea and vomiting requiring hospitalization for hydration and nutrition) occurs in only about 0.5% of pregnant women.[23] Possible causes of nausea and vomiting in pregnancy include elevated serum concentrations of human chorionic gonadotropin, estrogens and progesterone, prostaglandin E_2, *Helicobacter pylori* seropositivity, abnormal autonomic nervous system function and resulting abnormal peristalsis, elevated serum concentrations of thyroid hormones, and psychosocial factors. Dietary modifications such as eating frequent, small meals and avoiding fatty and fibrous foods may be helpful; acupressure and acustimulation also may be beneficial.[23]

A number of pharmacotherapeutic approaches have been tried for the treatment of nausea and vomiting in pregnancy.[23,24] Pyridoxine (vitamin B_6) and cyanocobalamin (vitamin B_{12}) also have shown efficacy.[25] Antihistamines (including doxylamine) have not been proved to be toxic during pregnancy and have shown efficacy in treating this disorder.[24] The anticholinergic agents dicyclomine and scopolamine have not been shown to increase fetal malformation rates above those expected in the general population; however, dicyclomine has no proven efficacy, and no trials exist that evaluate the effects of scopolamine for this disorder.[24] Phenothiazines, with the exception of one study, have not been shown to increase the risk of fetal malformation, and this drug class has demonstrated efficacy in treating nausea and vomiting in pregnancy. Metoclopramide has been used widely for nausea and vomiting in pregnancy, although no randomized clinical trials support its use; the drug has not been linked to an increased risk of malformations.[24] Limited efficacy and safety information is available regarding ondansetron use in pregnancy.[24] Ginger has shown efficacy for hyperemesis in a small trial and probably is safe to use for nausea and vomiting in pregnancy.[23] Corticosteroids (dexamethasone and prednisolone) have shown efficacy for hyperemesis gravidarum, but a small increase in the risk of oral clefts may be associated with first-trimester use.[24]

GESTATIONAL DIABETES

About 7% of pregnant women develop gestational diabetes, although the prevalence may range from 1% to 14% depending on the study population and tests used for diagnosis.[26] Whether or not to screen for gestational diabetes is an issue of significant controversy. The U.S. Preventative Services Task Force Independent Expert Panel has concluded that there is a lack of evidence to prove that screening for gestational diabetes decreases adverse maternal and fetal outcomes.[27] The American Diabetes Association, however, favors screening a woman who has risk factors for developing gestational diabetes mellitus (e.g., obesity, history of the condition, glycosuria, or a strong family history of diabetes) at her first prenatal visit.[26] If this screen is normal, testing should be repeated between weeks 24 and 28 of gestation. Pregnant women without these risk factors should undergo screening for gestational diabetes mellitus between weeks 24 and 28 of gestation unless they are considered low risk. To be low risk, a woman must fulfill *all* the following criteria: (1) age younger than 25 years, (2) normal prepregnancy weight, (3) no known diabetes in first-degree relatives, (4) not a member of an ethnic group with a high prevalence of gestational diabetes mellitus, (5) no history of abnormal glucose tolerance, and (6) no history of abnormal obstetric outcome.[26]

Screening for gestational diabetes mellitus uses the oral glucose challenge test.[26] Initial screening involves measuring plasma glucose concentrations 1 hour after a 50-g oral glucose load; if the results are abnormal, a diagnostic 100-g oral glucose tolerance test should be completed. Of women with gestational diabetes mellitus, 80% will be identified if the glucose threshold value is more than 140 mg/dL; 90% will be identified if the glucose threshold value is more than 130 mg/dL.[26]

According to the American Diabetes Association, first-line therapy for gestational diabetes mellitus includes nutritional and exercise interventions for all women and caloric restriction for obese women.[26] Daily self-monitoring of blood glucose levels is necessary for all women with this condition. If nutritional and exercise interventions fail to result in a fasting whole-blood glucose concentration equal to or less than 95 mg/dL and a 2-hour postprandial whole-blood glucose level equal to or less than 120 mg/dL, insulin therapy with recombinant human insulin should be instituted[26]; glyburide may be considered after 11 weeks of gestation.[28] Women who require insulin therapy also should continue to monitor their glucose levels postprandially. Goals for self-monitored blood glucose levels while on insulin therapy are as follows: preprandial plasma glucose level, 80–110 mg/dL; 2-hour postprandial plasma glucose level, <155 mg/dL.[29]

In contrast to the American Diabetes Association dietary recommendations, a Cochrane Review revealed that there is insufficient evidence to recommend dietary interventions for women with abnormal glucose tolerance in pregnancy.[30] Neither large-birth-weight deliveries nor need for cesarean delivery was influenced by adherence to dietary interventions for gestational diabetes.[30]

CLINICAL CONTROVERSY

Despite a lack of evidence for benefit of screening for gestational diabetes or for implementation of dietary interventions as a therapy for gestational diabetes, many clinicians offer screening and dietary guidelines for women with impaired glucose tolerance results.

HYPERTENSION

In pregnancy, the spectrum of hypertension includes chronic hypertension, gestational hypertension, preeclampsia-eclampsia, and preeclampsia superimposed on chronic hypertension.[31] Chronic hypertension is hypertension present either before pregnancy or before 20 weeks' gestation; gestational hypertension is blood pressure more than 140 mm Hg systolic or more than 90 mm Hg diastolic after 20 weeks' gestation. Preeclampsia-eclampsia is a syndrome consisting of gestational blood pressure elevation with proteinuria (i.e., ≥300 mg in a 24-hour urine collection). The syndrome is also suspected if proteinuria is absent, but the woman has gestational blood pressure elevation with symptoms of blurred vision, abdominal pain, headache, thrombocytopenia (platelet count <100,000 cells/mm³), or elevated liver enzymes (alanine aminotransferase or aspartate aminotransferase or both). Edema is no longer part of the definition for preeclampsia. Eclampsia is defined as preeclampsia with seizures.[31]

A recent meta-analysis including 12,416 women at high-risk for preeclampsia (i.e., history of preeclampsia, chronic hypertension, diabetes, or kidney disease) revealed that 50 to 150 mg aspirin daily significantly reduced rates of perinatal death and preeclampsia.[32] Rates of spontaneous preterm birth were decreased and mean birth weight increased by 215 g with aspirin therapy.[32] No evidence exists for aspirin benefit for women at low risk for preeclampsia. Similar findings exist for calcium supplementation during pregnancy. An evidence-based review suggests that calcium may be beneficial in women at high risk of developing preeclampsia and in those who have low dietary calcium intake.[33]

Nondrug therapeutic approaches for hypertension in pregnancy traditionally have focused on activity restriction, psychosocial therapy, and biofeedback. There is currently no evidence that any of these approaches improves pregnancy outcome, and prolonged bed rest may increase a pregnant woman's risk of venous thromboembolic disease.

Antihypertensive drug therapy for women with gestational hypertension or preeclampsia has not been shown to improve fetal outcomes.[31] If antihypertensive drug therapy is required during pregnancy, methyldopa is preferred because of its established efficacy and safety for mother and fetus.[31] Other alternatives include labetolol, β-blockers (except atenolol), prazosin, nifedipine, isradipine, hydralazine, clonidine, and diuretics.[31,34] The cure for preeclampsia is delivery of the fetus if the pregnancy is at term. Preeclampsia may progress rapidly to eclampsia, a medical emergency, so weight, edema, and blood pressure must be monitored studiously in patients with preeclampsia. For acute severe hypertension in preeclampsia, parenteral hydralazine and labetolol in addition to oral nifedipine for hypertension control and magnesium sulfate for seizure prevention are standard therapy.[31]

THYROID ABNORMALITIES

Human chorionic gonadotropin may stimulate the thyroid gland because the structure of human chorionic gonadotropin is similar to that of thyrotropin.[35] Pregnant patients with excessive thyroid gland stimulation by this mechanism have gestational thyrotoxicosis. Thyrotoxic patients usually present with vomiting, which can be severe; an increased serum level of free thyroxine; and a depressed thyrotropin level. The degree of the thyroxine and thyrotropin abnormalities correlates with the severity of the vomiting, and no other findings are present to support the diagnosis of true thyrotoxicosis. Gestational thyrotoxicosis resolves with declining human chorionic gonadotropin concentrations at the completion of the first trimester.[35] Nausea and vomiting may be treated as for patients without this pseudohyperthyroid state.

Within 3 to 6 months postpartum, women may experience either hypothyroidism or hyperthyroidism owing to thyroiditis secondary to autoimmune factors.[35,36] The thyroiditis is usually self-limiting. This disorder is thought to occur in about 5% of postpartum women without a prior history of thyroid abnormalities. If women are asymptomatic, treatment is not indicated. Women who have hyperthyroid symptoms should undergo further testing to determine the cause of the disorder. If thyroiditis is suspected, only symptomatic treatment of hyperthyroid symptoms is indicated, although the patient should be monitored carefully because transient hypothyroidism may follow. Women who have both symptoms and laboratory evidence of hypothyroidism may be treated with thyroxine therapy, although the decision to initiate therapy depends on the degree of abnormality and symptoms. Again, careful monitoring is required because the condition usually resolves, and thyroxine therapy may be discontinued.[35,36]

THROMBOEMBOLISM

The incidence of venous thromboembolism during pregnancy varies with age. In women younger than 35 years of age, the rate of thromboembolism is 6.15 events per 10,000 pregnancies; in women older than age 35, the rate is 12.16 events per 10,000 pregnancies.[37] Other major risk factors for thromboembolism during pregnancy include history of thromboembolism, hypercoaguable conditions, operative vaginal delivery or cesarean section, obesity, and a family history of thrombosis that suggests an inheritable hypercoagulable condition.[37]

Therapy to prevent or treat venous thromboembolism during pregnancy must not include warfarin after the first 6 weeks of gestation because this drug may cause fetal bleeding, malformations of the nose, stippled epiphyses, or CNS anomalies.[37,38] Low-molecular-weight heparins are the preferred agents for prophylaxis or treatment of venous thromboembolism during pregnancy. Unfractionated heparin also may be used but is associated with a higher incidence of heparin-induced thrombocytopenia and a lower lumbar spine bone mineral density than are the low-molecular-weight heparins.[37,38] Dextran and hirudin should not be used in pregnancy.[37] Aspirin may offer some benefit in prevention of thromboembolism, but it is likely to be less effective than heparin. Compression stockings are recommended for prevention and treatment of venous thromboembolism.[37]

CONCLUSIONS

Many women with pregnancy-influenced gastrointestinal issues can be treated safely with lifestyle modification or medications, many of them nonprescription. Gestational diabetes, hypertension, and thyrotoxicosis may or may not require drug therapy; venous thromboembolism usually will require therapy with a low-molecular-weight heparin and compression stockings.

ACUTE CARE ISSUES IN PREGNANCY

Acute illnesses that occur in pregnant women may present challenges for providers. In some cases, the risks associated with the illness may be magnified during pregnancy, and early screening and treatment become critical. Such is the case for asymptomatic bacteriuria, where the risk of progression to pyelonephritis may have profound effects on the health of both the mother and the infant. In other cases, such as in the treatment of certain sexually transmitted diseases, the urgency regarding treatment comes from an increased likelihood of infection leading to preterm labor. Ocassionally, common acute care issues, such as migraine headache, actually may improve during pregnancy. In all cases, it is important to select therapies that are effective and safe for the pregnant patient.

URINARY TRACT INFECTION

◀ With an estimated incidence of 8%, urinary tract infections are common in pregnancy.[39] The American College of Obstetrics and Gynecology recommends a urine culture both at the initial prenatal visit and during the third trimester to screen pregnant women for such infections.[40] In contrast, the U.S. Preventive Task Force recommends a urine culture between 12 and 16 weeks' gestation. A urine culture is the preferred method for screening because other methods, such as dipsticks that measure leukocytes and esterase, may fail to identify as many as 50% of patients with asymptomatic bacteriuria.[40]

As with the general population, *Escherichia coli* is the principal infecting organism, present in 80% to 90% of infections.[40] Other gram-negative rods, such as *Proteus mirabilis* and *Klebsiella pneumoniae,* also account for some infections. Group B *Streptococcus* bacteriuria is sometimes discovered in pregnant women and is associated with preterm delivery.[41] The presence of group B *Streptococcus* in the urine also may correspond to heavy colonization of the genitourinary tract, increasing the risk for group B *Streptococcus* infection in the newborn. Treatment of group B *Streptococcus* bacteriuria at the time of discovery reduces the rate of preterm delivery from this infection. Additionally, women with group B *Streptococcus* bacteriuria also should receive antibiotics at the time of delivery to prevent infection in the newborn.[41] (Please refer to group B *Streptococcus* under "Labor and Delivery" below.)

In general, urinary tract infections during pregnancy may occur as asymptomatic bacteriuria, acute cystitis, or pyelonephritis. Asymptomatic bacteriuria may be present in 2% to 7% of pregnant women.[43] The most worrisome aspect of asymptomatic bacteriuria is that approximately 25% of untreated pregnant women will develop a pyelonephritis, compared with only 3% to 4% of women who receive treatment. Other adverse effects of asymptomatic bacteriuria include increased risk for preterm labor and low birth weight. These adverse effects in both mothers and infants underscore the need for screening and treatment in the pregnant population.[43]

Even though ampicillin and amoxicillin are considered safe medications for the treatment of asymptomatic bacteriuria, the incidence of *E. coli* resistance to these drugs may be 20% to 30%.[39,40] Nitrofurantoin is considered safe and effective for use in pregnancy; cephalexin is also considered a good alternative. Sulfa-containing drugs may increase the risk for kernicterus in the newborn, and they should be avoided during the third trimester. Folate antagonists, such as trimethoprim, are relatively contraindicated during the first trimester of pregnancy. Fluoroquinolones and tetracyclines are contraindicated in pregnancy. The optimal duration of therapy for urinary tract infection in pregnancy has not been determined. Courses of 7 to 10 days are common, but some studies have demonstrated that shorter courses may be sufficient. A repeat culture to confirm cure is recommended.[39,40]

Acute cystitis occurs in 0.3% to 1.3% of pregnancies.[39] In addition to having significant amounts of bacteria in the urine, women with acute cystitis complain of urinary frequency and pain.[40] The risks of low birth weight and preterm labor associated with acute cystitis have not been defined. Treatment for acute cystitis is the same as described for asymptomatic bacteriuria.[40]

Acute pyelonephritis complicates 1% to 2% of pregnancies,[39] sometimes leading to maternal sepsis and preterm labor and delivery.[40] Patients usually present with bacteriuria and systemic symptoms of fever, flank pain, nausea, and vomiting. Hospitalization often is necessary for pregnant women with pyelonephritis.[40] Inpatient therapy for pyelonephritis has included intravenous administration of cephalosporins (e.g., cefazolin) and ampicillin with gentamicin or the intramuscular administration of ceftriaxone. Outpatient antibiotic therapy for pyelonephritis may be considered if the woman is able to take medications orally and is not exhibiting symptoms of sepsis or preterm labor; cephalexin has been used for this purpose. The total duration of antibiotic therapy for acute pyelonephritis is 10 to 14 days.[39] This course may be followed by bedtime prophylaxis with nitrofurantoin for the duration of the pregnancy.[39]

In summary, the early recognition of asymptomatic bacteriuria in pregnant women is an important primary prevention strategy in reducing morbidity and mortality from severe renal infections. Treatment of pregnant women requires careful consideration of medications with good efficacy and also low likelihood of risks to the infant. The aminopenicillins, cephalosporins, and nitrofurantoin often are viewed as first-line agents for most indications.

SEXUALLY TRANSMITTED DISEASES

◀ Sexually transmitted diseases in pregnant women range from infections that may be transmitted across the placenta and infect the infant prenatally (e.g., syphilis) to organisms that may be transmitted during birth and cause neonatal infection (e.g., *Chlamydia trachomatis, Neisseria gonorrhoeae,* or herpes simplex virus) to infections that pose a threat for preterm labor (e.g., bacterial vaginosis). In the case of bacterial infections, treatment will cure the infection. For viral infections, such as herpes, the goal is not cure but control of outbreaks at the time of delivery. Screening is essential for early detection of most sexually transmitted diseases but may not be beneficial in other instances (bacterial vaginosis in low-risk patients). Medications used to treat sexually transmitted diseases in pregnant women should be chosen to decrease risks to the fetus. In women with certain infections (e.g., syphilis, *N. gonorrhoeae, C. trachomatis*), sexual partners also will require treatment to prevent recurrence of infection.

SYPHILIS

It is recommended that all pregnant women be screened for syphilis at the first prenatal visit.[44] Additional testing may be warranted in areas where the prevalence of syphilis is high. Penicillin is the drug of choice for the treatment of syphilis during pregnancy and is effective in preventing transmission to the fetus as well as treating the fetus, if already infected. The dose and route of administration are determined by the stage of syphilis and are the same for pregnant women as for other patients. One special consideration is the issue that no alternatives for penicillin are acceptable for pregnant women allergic to penicillin. Erythromycin does not cross the placenta well enough to treat an infected fetus adequately. Penicillin skin testing and penicillin desensitization are required for the penicillin-allergic pregnant woman requiring treatment for syphilis.[44]

N. GONORRHOEAE

N. gonorrhoeae cervicitis is a risk factor for preterm delivery, and treatment has been associated with a reduction of risk.[41] Coinfection with *C. trachomatis* is common, and treatment of most *N. gonorrhoeae* infections also includes treatment for *C. trachomatis.* The treatment of choice for *N. gonorrhoeae* cervical infection during pregnancy is ceftriaxone 125 mg intramuscularly as a single dose.[44] For women unable to use a cephalosporin, spectinomycin 2 g intramuscularly as a single dose is appropriate. The quinolones should be avoided in pregnant women.[44] (Please note that although the guidelines include cefixime as a treatment option, the drug is no longer manufactured.)

C. TRACHOMATIS

C. trachomatis is thought to be the most common sexually transmitted organism.[41] The prevalence of infection with this organism in pregnant patients ranges from 5% to 26%. Transmission of *Chlamydia* at the time of delivery represents a risk of 10% to 20% for neonatal pneumonitis and 20% to 50% for conjunctivitis.[45] There is conflicting evidence for the association of *C. trachomatis* with an increased risk for preterm labor. The recommended treatment for *C. trachomatis* cervicitis is erythromycin base 500 mg four times daily for 7 days.[44] Erythromycin estolate should be avoided in pregnant women owing to an increased risk of hepatitis. Amoxicillin also may be used as an alternative treatment at a dose of 500 mg three times daily for 7 days. Azithromycin 1 g as a single dose also appears to be a safe and effective alternative treatment[44] (Table 76-1).

GENITAL HERPES

◀ It is estimated that approximately one of every four women in the United States over the age of 12 is infected with genital herpes simplex virus 2.[46] A smaller number of people have infections caused by herpes simplex virus 1, which is more commonly associated with orolabial infections.[46]

Primary infection in the mother occurs approximately 2 to 14 days after exposure.[46] Patients with a primary infection may be asymptomatic or may have vaginal discharge, pain, malaise, and other systemic symptoms. Recurrence of symptoms is common with people infected with herpes simplex virus 2, although subsequent outbreaks may be milder.[46]

Infants born of infected women may come in contact with the virus as they move down the birth canal, and this may result in a severe or even life-threatening neonatal infection.[46] It is estimated that 1 in 350 infants is delivered vaginally during viral shedding, but the incidence of severe herpetic infection in the newborn is approximately 1 in 20,000.[46]

Several factors may affect transmission from mother to infant.[46] The risk of transmission for an infant born to a mother with a primary infection is 30% to 50%. Conversely, the risk of transmission is less than 1% in women with a history of recurrent herpes at the time of delivery or in women who became infected during the first half of pregnancy.[44]

TABLE 76–1. Recommended Regimens for Treatment of Cervical Infections Due to *Chlamydia* in Pregnancy

First-Line Treatment
Erythromycin base 500 mg orally four times a day for 7 days *or*
Amoxicillin 500 mg orally three times daily for 7 days.

Alternative Regimens
Erythromycin base 250 mg orally four times a day for 14 days *or*
Erythromycin ethylsuccinate 800 mg orally four times a day for 7 days *or*
Erythromycin ethylsuccinate 400 mg orally four times a day for 14 days *or*
Azithromycin 1 g orally, single dose

Ref. 44.

The goal for treating women with a history of genital herpes during pregnancy is to avoid exposure of the infant to infected lesions during the process of birth.[44]

Women who have no signs or symptoms of an outbreak may deliver vaginally. Many physicians will recommend cesarean section for women with outbreaks at the time of delivery. For women who newly acquire herpes near the end of their pregnancy, some specialist clinicians will recommend antiviral therapy, some will recommend cesarean section, and some will recommend both.[44]

Of the agents available for treatment, acyclovir has had the longest period of use and has not demonstrated an increased risk of birth defects with first-trimester use.[44] More data will need to be collected to strengthen the safety data. Both valacyclovir and famciclovir are newer, and data on safety are more limited. Most women will receive oral acyclovir therapy for first episodes of genital herpes or with recurrence. Intravenous acyclovir can be used for severe infections.

CLINICAL CONTROVERSY

Some practitioners provide prophylaxis late in pregnancy with acyclovir for patients with a history of recurrent herpes. At the present time, it is unknown if this practice reduces the need for cesarean section.

BACTERIAL VAGINOSIS

Although not a sexually transmitted disease, bacterial vaginosis during pregnancy is a risk factor for premature rupture of membranes, preterm labor, preterm birth, and spontaneous abortion.[47] It is found in 9% to 23% of pregnant women.[47]

Pregnant women with a history of preterm delivery should undergo screening for bacterial vaginosis at the first prenatal visit.[44] If the infection is present, the recommended regimen is metronidazole 250 mg three times a day for 7 days or clindamycin 300 mg twice a day for 7 days.[44]

Conflicting data exist with regard to treating pregnant women at low risk for preterm labor.[44] Symptomatic women should be treated using the preceding metronidazole or clindamycin regimen. Vaginal creams have not been found to be effective in reducing the risk of adverse pregnancy outcomes associated with bacterial vaginosis.[44]

CONCLUSIONS

One of the unifying themes in this section is the importance of treating genital infections in the pregnant mother not only for her care but also to reduce risks to the developing infant. Genital infections may infect the developing child in utero, may infect the developing child during birth, or may lead to preterm labor and its consequences. Drugs selected for use in pregnant women with genital infections are chosen to lessen risks to the developing child. Ironically, erythromycin may not be used to treat syphilis because it does not cross the placenta well, but it is the drug of choice for *Chlamydia* and is safe because it does not pass to the fetus. Tetracyclines are not used for pregnant women with *Chlamydia*, but other choices are available, including amoxicillin, which generally is not used in the general population as treatment for this condition.

HEADACHE

◀ Headaches are common, acute care conditions reported by more than 80% of women of childbearing age.[48] Headaches in pregnant women can be classified into three different types: tension migraine, or secondary to an underlying disorder. Migraine and tension headaches are the most common types.[48]

In more than 70% of pregnant women with a history of migraine headaches, symptoms will either improve or go into remission during pregnancy.[48] One explanation for this observation is that hormone levels stay consistently elevated during pregnancy. (The improvement in symptoms is more likely to occur in women whose migraine headaches are associated with hormone fluctuations during the menstrual cycle.) Migraines often have a tendency to worsen at the time of delivery and in the early postpartum period. New onset of migraines during pregnancy is rare.[48]

Tension headaches have been less studied during pregnancy.[48] Some women have increases in tension headaches during pregnancy, whereas 25% report improvement. Since psychological and musculoskeletal stresses play a key role in tension headaches, nonpharmacological interventions serve as the treatment mainstay.[48]

Acetaminophen is the drug of first choice for pain relief from migraine and tension headaches.[48] Nonsteroidal anti-inflammatory agents may be used during early pregnancy but generally are contraindicated after 37 weeks' gestation. Narcotics may be used for refractory migraine headaches. The use of sumatriptan in pregnant women is controversial, but some clinicians choose to continue use in women who have tried other agents for migraine headaches without success. Patients with nausea associated with migraine headaches may be treated with metoclopramide. Both ergotamine and dihydroergotamine should be avoided during pregnancy.[48]

CHRONIC ILLNESSES IN PREGNANCY

❹ Pharmacotherapeutic considerations in pregnant women with chronic conditions pose unique challenges. For the majority of women and their health care providers, pregnancy will be a new consideration for a previously diagnosed health condition. Medications used to treat the chronic illness potentially may be used throughout the pregnancy and during breast-feeding.

ALLERGIC RHINITIS, ASTHMA

❹ Asthma and rhinitis represent two of the most common chronic illnesses in pregnant women. Although rhinitis itself is unlikely to cause harm to the mother or fetus, untreated rhinitis may be associated with a diminished quality of life. Asthma control may change during pregnancy, and worsening asthma may have significant health consequences to both the mother and the developing fetus. Use of medications is an integral part of providing care to pregnant women with these conditions.

It is estimated that asthma affects up to 4% of pregnant women.[49] Asthma severity can change during pregnancy, with an almost equal proportion of patients having their symptoms worsen, improve, or remain unchanged. Typically, asthma symptoms may exacerbate during the early part of the third trimester (weeks 24–36), but it is less common to see worsening of symptoms closer to the time of delivery.[49]

Appropriate treatment of asthma is critical to the health of mother and infant.[49] Undertreated asthma in the mother is associated with preterm labor, gestational hypertension, preeclampsia, and uterine hemorrhage.[50] In the infant, intrauterine growth retardation, low birth weight, and congenital malformations may result from poor asthma control.

The goals for care of the pregnant woman with asthma are (1) birth of a healthy baby, (2) achievement of normal or near-normal pulmonary function, (3) lack of adverse effects of treatment, (4) control of symptoms without nighttime awakenings, (5) ability to continue normal activities, (6) ability to exercise, and (7) avoidance of acute exacerbations.[51] It is critical that the pregnant woman avoid things that may exacerbate asthma. Reducing exposure to allergens and irritants, such as cigarette smoke, are important nonpharmacologic interventions.[51]

The American College of Allergy, Asthma, and Immunology and the American College of Obstetrics and Gynecology published guidelines for the medical management of asthma during pregnancy in 2000.[51] Anti-inflammatory therapy is the cornerstone of chronic asthma care. For pregnant women who need to add anti-inflammatory therapy to their regimen, inhaled cromolyn is recommended because of low toxicity and extensive clinical experience. For asthma unresponsive to cromolyn, inhaled budesonide or beclomethasone is recommended, again because of the clinical experience using these agents in pregnancy. For women using other inhaled corticosteroids effectively at the time they become pregnant, the guidelines suggest that continuation of current therapy is reasonable. Rescue medications, the inhaled β-agonists (e.g., terbutaline, metaproterenol, and albuterol), are considered safe in pregnancy. Oral theophylline has a long history of use and may be considered as add-on therapy to inhaled corticosteroids for moderate or severe persistent asthma, or alternatively, the inhaled long-acting β-agonist salmeterol may be used.[51] Leukotriene antagonists may be continued if required prior to pregnancy to control asthma, but these agents are not considered drugs of choice in patients who have not used them prior to pregnancy. Oral corticosteroids are essential therapy for the treatment of severe, acute asthma and appear to be safe.[51]

The various forms of rhinitis—allergic, vasomotor, drug-induced, and bacterial sinusitis—are seen in more than 20% of pregnant women.[49] Vasomotor rhinitis of pregnancy is a unique condition caused by increased blood flow to the nasal turbinates. This condition peaks in the second trimester and generally resolves shortly after delivery. As with asthma, the first approach to treatment of rhinitis is avoidance of exacerbating factors, such as allergens, cigarette smoke, or strong odors. Irrigation of the nose with nasal saline also may be helpful. Occasional use of nasal decongestants, such as oxymetazoline, may be warranted, but frequent use may lead to rebound congestion.

Cromolyn nasal spray is considered a drug of first choice for treatment of chronic allergic rhinitis. Antihistamines also may be used during pregnancy. Chlorpheniramine and tripelenamine have a long history of safety in pregnancy, but the nonsedating antihistamines loratadine or cetirizine also could be considered if the older drugs are not tolerated. Pseudoephedrine may be used as a decongestant, although a very rare gastrointestinal birth defect has been linked to its use. Nasal corticosteroids may be considered for pregnant women who do not respond to other therapies. As with asthma care, budesonide and beclomethasone nasal sprays are recommended as first-line choices because of longer clinical experience in the treatment of pregnant women. If the pregnant woman is receiving immunotherapy before pregnancy, it may be continued. Escalation of therapy or initiation of new therapy is not recommended during pregnancy.[49]

CLINICAL CONTROVERSY

Selection of first-line therapy for allergic rhinitis and asthma and pregnancy is controversial. Topical corticosteroids are a well-established treatment in the general population as drugs of first choice for both conditions; corticosteroids also appear safe to use in pregnancy. However, guidelines still provide advice about use of less effective treatments that have a longer history of use in pregnancy for these conditions.

DERMATOLOGIC CONDITIONS

◁ The treatment of dermatologic conditions during pregnancy often may be delayed until after the delivery. Sometimes, however, it is necessary to implement treatment during pregnancy. The major categories of medications used in dermatology are antiacne agents, antibiotics, antiviral agents, antihistamines, and antifungal agents.[52] Of all the dermatologic agents used commonly during pregnancy, only topical nystatin has been shown to have no fetal risk in controlled studies. Recommended topical agents with minimal pregnancy risk include bacitracin, benzoyl peroxide, ciclopirox, clindamycin, erythromycin, metronidazole, mupirocin, permethrin, and terbinafine, among others. Topical corticosteroids are also thought to be safe for use in pregnancy. Systemic agents that may be used safely in pregnancy for dermatologic conditions include acyclovir, amoxicillin, azithromycin, cephalosporins, chlorpheniramine, cyproheptadine hydrochloride, dicloxacillin, diphenhydramine, erythromycin (except estolates), nystatin, and penicillin. Lidocaine and lidocaine with epinephrine may be used safely topically during pregnancy.[52]

DIABETES

◁ The American Diabetes Association recommends that women with diabetes defer pregnancy until the condition is under control with medication and lifestyle interventions.[29] This recommendation is based on knowledge of increased fetal loss and malformations resulting from suboptimally controlled diabetes. In addition, it is known that diabetic retinopathy may worsen, hypertension may develop, and renal function may deteriorate during pregnancy in diabetic patients. Enhanced monitoring for these target-organ problems is essential during pregnancy.[29]

Insulin is the drug treatment of choice for patients with both type 1 and type 2 diabetes during pregnancy.[29] However, it may be acceptable to use glyburide after the eleventh week of gestation in patients with type 2 diabetes.[28] Medical nutrition therapy and supervised physical activity programs should be continued throughout pregnancy as well.[29] Goals for self-monitored blood glucose are as follows: preprandial plasma glucose level, 80 to 110 mg/dL; 2-hour postprandial plasma glucose level, <155 mg/dL.[29] These goals are the same as for gestational diabetes.

EPILEPSY

◁ Maternal epilepsy is present in about 1% of all pregnancies.[53]
About 35% of women with epilepsy experience an increase in seizure frequency during pregnancy, and approximately 65% of women experience no change or a decrease in seizure frequency. Seizures may become more frequent because of hormonal changes in pregnancy, sleep deprivation, and medication adherence problems[53] because of a perceived teratogenic risk of antiepileptic drug therapy. In addition, free serum concentrations of the antiepileptic drug may change during pregnancy as a result of maternal increased volume of distribution, decreased protein binding because of hypoalbuminemia, increased hepatic drug metabolism, and increased renal drug clearance.[53] A woman's clinical condition rather than solely the free serum concentrations of antiepileptic drug should be the basis for any adjustments in dosage. Postpartum concentrations also must be monitored because drug requirements probably will decrease as pregnancy-induced pharmacokinetic changes resolve. If a woman chooses to breast-feed, her antiepileptic drug requirements will not change until breast-feeding stops.[53]

Major malformations occur in 4% to 6% of the offspring of epileptic women taking benzodiazepines, carbamazepine, phenobarbital, phenytoin, and valproic acid.[53] Minor malformations occur in 6% to 20% of pregnancies affected by epilepsy, which is twice the rate in the general population.[53] The malformations are considered a result of fetal exposure to antiepileptic drug therapy rather than a result of maternal epilepsy.[54] Combination regimens of antiepileptic drugs are associated with higher malformation rates.[54]

For the management of pregnant women with epilepsy, the American Academy of Neurology has recommended the use of antiepileptic drug monotherapy, if possible, and optimization of any drug therapy prior to conception.[55] Medication change exclusively to minimize teratogenic risk, such as the prior recommendation to switch to phenobarbital from other antiepileptic drugs, is *no longer* recommended. If drug withdrawal is planned, it should be attempted at least 6 months before conception is attempted. In addition, all women with epilepsy should take folic acid supplementation of 0.4 to 5 mg daily.[53,55] To correct vitamin K deficiency in newborns, 10 mg oral vitamin K should be supplemented daily in the mother during the last month of gestation.[55]

For women who remain on carbamazepine, divalproex sodium, or valproic acid, an α-fetoprotein check at 14 to 16 weeks' gestation and a level II ultrasound at 16 to 20 weeks' gestation are recommended to screen for neural tube defects.[55]

HUMAN IMMUNODEFICIENCY VIRUS (HIV) INFECTION

◁ Zidovudine is the mainstay of antiretroviral therapy and is recommended for use during pregnancy, labor, and delivery, as well as the postpartum period.[56] During pregnancy, the continuation of any other therapies that the woman may be taking, except for efavirenz and hydroxyurea, should be strongly considered. Additionally, inclusion of zidovudine is recommended after 14 weeks' gestation, whether it is added to the other agents or replaces another nucleoside analog. The current zidovudine dosing recommendation during pregnancy is 100 mg five times daily, 200 mg three times daily, or 300 mg two times daily; zidovudine should be initiated at 14 to 34 weeks' gestation and continued for the duration of the pregnancy. Intravenous zidovudine is recommended during labor, and the infant should receive the drug beginning 8 to 12 hours after birth and continued for the first 6 weeks of life.[56]

A single dose of oral nevirapine administered to women at the beginning of labor and to newborns at 72 hours after birth may be an alternative to zidovudine, especially in developing countries.[57]

HYPERTENSION

◁ For women with stage 1 or 2 chronic hypertension (blood pressure 140 to 179 mm Hg systolic or 90 to 109 mm Hg diastolic), the decision of whether to continue or stop antihypertensive therapy during pregnancy is controversial because most of the increase in adverse fetal and maternal outcomes is due to preeclampsia superimposed on chronic hypertension.[31] If medication is discontinued and women are monitored closely, therapy should be restarted if blood pressure exceeds 150 to 160 mm Hg systolic or 100 to 110 mm Hg diastolic or if target-organ damage is present. Alternatively, antihypertensive drugs may be continued during pregnancy (except for angiotensin-converting enzyme inhibitors and angiotensin II receptor blockers) at the lowest effective dose. Use of diuretics is controversial, but the Working Group on High Blood Pressure in Pregnancy has determined that diuretic use is acceptable in women with chronic hypertension. When considering drug therapy in the treatment of chronic hypertension during pregnancy, the clinician and patient must jointly assess the risks and benefits of any therapy. For women with severe hypertension (diastolic blood pressure ≥ 100 mm Hg), the benefit of drug therapy may outweigh the risks.[31]

No evidence exists for superior efficacy of one agent versus another for blood pressure reduction during pregnancy.[34] Occasionally, it may be necessary to consider changing from one agent to another prior to or during pregnancy, such as switching from an angiotensin-converting enzyme inhibitor before beginning the second trimester of pregnancy in order to reduce teratogenic risk.[34] However, some women may not tolerate medications other than those found to be efficacious prior to pregnancy, or the other drugs may not be as effective. In such cases, the risks and benefits of changing to a different agent solely for the purpose of avoiding teratogenicity must be considered carefully.

MENTAL HEALTH CONDITIONS

Nonpharmacologic and pharmacologic treatments for chronic mental health conditions during pregnancy are important for the health of mother and baby. Misunderstandings regarding the safety of certain psychotropic medications may result in undertreatment of pregnant women, resulting in potential harm to both mother and developing infant.

This point is clearly illustrated by a review of pregnant women who consulted the Motherisk Program, a counseling service for pregnant women and health providers, between 1996 and 1997.[58] All these women had decided to stop taking benzodiazepines or antidepressants when they learned they were pregnant. They were followed throughout the course of their pregnancies. Of the 44 women who agreed to be followed, 4 were lost to follow-up, and 3 others did not become pregnant during the study period. Thirty-four women stopped medications abruptly, and 3 used tapering methods. Nearly one-third of the women reported thinking about suicide for unbearable symptoms, and 4 needed to be hospitalized. One woman had a therapeutic abortion because of how she felt, and one woman used alcohol to deal with benzodiazepine withdrawal symptoms. Most women who discontinued medication did so with the advice of their health care provider. After consultation with Motherisk, approximately 60% of patients resumed medication. Two of these women experienced spontaneous abortions, one had a therapeutic abortion, and there were 35 live births (two sets of twins). All babies were reported to be healthy and normal. Two babies appeared to have mild medication (paroxetine and amitriptyline) withdrawal symptoms that did not require intervention.[58]

DEPRESSION

The prevalence of depression in pregnant women is estimated to be approximately 10%.[59] Of these, one-third represent a new onset of the illness. Concerns about the safety of medications used to treat depression are common among health practitioners. However, untreated depression may, by itself, have adverse effects on the developing fetus, including preterm birth, low birth weight, small head circumference, and low Apgar scores. Nonpharmacologic approaches are an important component of care. Psychotherapy may be helpful alone or in conjunction with pharmacotherapy. Electroconvulsant therapy may be considered as an alternative to long-term use of medications or for women who fail to respond to pharmacotherapy. Safety of electroconvulsant therapy has been established in pregnancy.

Pharmacotherapy is required frequently by pregnant women for optimal treatment of depression. Potential fetal risks from medications used during pregnancy include (1) teratogenic effects from use early in pregnancy, (2) withdrawal symptoms after birth, and

(3) long-term neurologic consequences.[59] Tricyclic antidepressants have a long history of use in pregnant women. Both prospective and retrospective studies have found these agents to be safe for use in pregnancy. Desipramine and nortriptyline are recommended frequently for use because of fewer anticholinergic side effects (constipation) and less likelihood of orthostasis. Although less information is available with respect to the use of selective serotonin reuptake inhibitors (SSRIs), they are emerging as first-line agents in treating depression during pregnancy.[60] The largest body of information exists for fluoxetine and does not suggest an increased rate of major malformations.[59] Less information is available about other SSRIs, but a small prospective study of mostly users of citalopram and a retrospective review of a small group of users of paroxetine did not demonstrate an increase in risk for birth defects.

Decisions about the use of antidepressants during pregnancy need to be made jointly among the patient, her partner, and her health care practitioners.[59] For pregnant women with mild depression, it may be possible to discontinue drug therapy and continue psychotherapy. For women who relapse or have more severe forms of depression, it is reasonable to continue medications in conjunction with psychotherapy. Consideration may be given to switching medications to those with a better-understood safety profile. In a situation where a woman has tried several agents to find the optimal selection, it may be of value to continue that agent. Finally, although it is generally recommended that medications be used at the lowest dosage possible during pregnancy, it is very likely that doses of antidepressants actually may need to be increased during pregnancy to maintain therapeutic effect owing to changes in plasma volume, liver metabolism, and renal clearance.

Many of the selective serotonin reuptake inhibitors are well tolerated by breast-fed infants.[60] Fluoxetine has resulted in some reports of gastrointestinal problems, irritability, and insomnia.[60]

MOOD DISORDERS

It is commonplace for women diagnosed with bipolar disorder to receive mixed messages from health care providers about the advisability of becoming pregnant or maintaining a pregnancy while under treatment for their psychiatric condition.[61] Most of the medications used to treat mood disorders have known potential toxicities for the developing fetus. Patients require well-researched information from their providers to make informed decisions about the care they will need to optimize their own health and the health of their infants during pregnancy.

Bipolar disorder has a lifetime prevalence of approximately 1%.[61] During pregnancy, untreated bipolar disorder may result in hospitalization, suicidal ideation, violence, loss of employment, malnutrition, and an increased risk of postpartum psychosis.[62] It does not appear that pregnancy provides protection for the risk of recurrence of symptoms.[61] Women who discontinue the use of mood stabilizing drugs abruptly before conception or who have had four or more episodes of recurrence of symptoms have a substantial risk for recurrence during pregnancy. Risk for recurrence in the first 3 to 6 months postpartum has been estimated at 20% up to 80%. Postpartum psychosis may occur in 10% to 20% of women with bipolar disorder.

A number of strategies have been used to optimize the use of medications in treating bipolar disorder in pregnancy.[61] Patients who have had a single episode of mania with good recovery may be able to taper medication before conception. Those with multiple and frequent recurrences of symptoms (depression or mania) could attempt to discontinue medications before conception or wait until the pregnancy is diagnosed and then taper medications. Medications could be resumed if symptoms occur or after the first trimester to decrease the risk of recurrence. For women who opt to discontinue medications and stay symptom-free throughout the pregnancy, postpartum prophylaxis with a drug such as lithium should be considered. Women with more severe forms of bipolar disorder may benefit most from continuing medications throughout the pregnancy.

The most commonly used mood-stabilizing medications used for the treatment of bipolar disorder include lithium, valproic acid, and carbamazepine. Each of these agents has unique therapeutic profiles to consider in the context of treatment of pregnant and lactating women.

Lithium

Lithium is currently considered the first-line medication for the treatment of bipolar disorder during pregnancy.[61] Lithium's place in therapy has been controversial because of past concerns about cardiovascular anomalies, especially Epstein's anomaly, in exposed infants. With more recent reviews of epidemiologic data, the risk of Epstein's anomaly is estimated to be 0.05% to 0.1% in infants exposed during the first trimester. Other reported side effects in the newborn include cases of muscular hypotonia with impaired breathing and cyanosis ("floppy baby syndrome"), neonatal hypothyroidism, nephrogenic diabetes insipidus, atrial flutter, tricuspid regurgitation, and congestive heart failure.[61,62] Long-term (5-year) behavioral follow-up in 60 children exposed to lithium during pregnancy did not reveal significant behavioral problems.[61] Lithium concentrations in breast milk may be up to 40% of the serum concentration in the mother.[62] Several case reports describe adverse effects in infants thought to be due to lithium use by lactating mothers. It is recommended that breast-feeding be partially or totally discontinued in mothers using lithium.[62] The American Academy of Pediatrics considers lithium incompatible with breast-feeding.[61]

Valproic Acid

Valproic acid is associated with a 2- to 3-fold increase in the frequency of congenital anomalies.[62] A 10- to 20-fold increase in the risk of spina bifida in infants born to women treated with valproic acid compared with the general population has been reported. The absolute risk of spina bifida in exposed infants appears to be 1% to 2%. Other problems associated with use in pregnancy include intrauterine growth retardation, hypoglycemia, and coagulopathy. Some investigators have reported developmental delays in up to 90% of children with prenatal exposure to valproic acid.[62]

Strategies to reduce the risk of adverse reactions to valproic acid include using divided doses to minimize peak concentrations, recommending folic acid 4 mg to be started before conception and continuing until the twelfth week of pregnancy, prescribing 10 to 20 mg daily of vitamin K to the mother during the last month of pregnancy, and ensuring that the infant receives 1 mg vitamin K intramuscularly at birth to prevent hemorrhage. Valproic acid is excreted into the breast milk in concentrations ranging 2% to 8% of the serum levels of the mother. Several case reports of side effects in nursing infants have been reported, including anemia, thrombocytopenia, and hepatotoxicity. These reports are rare, and valproic acid is considered compatible with breast-feeding.

Carbamazepine

As with valproic acid, a 2- to 3-fold increase in the frequency of congenital malformations has been attributed to the use of carbamazepine.[62] A 10-fold increase in the risk of spina bifida compared with the general population or an absolute risk of 1% has been described. Other birth defects reported from either monotherapy or combination therapy with other agents include facial roundness, nasal bridge defects, nail defects, and other head anomalies. Developmental delay has been reported in up to 20% of children in prospective studies. Carbamazepine has been associated with vitamin K deficiency. Vitamin K and folate supplementation should be provided at doses similar to that with valproic acid. Carbamazepine use appears to be compatible with breast-feeding because it is found in breast milk in only very small quantity.

THYROID DISORDERS

Untreated hypothyroidism during pregnancy may result in significant cognitive and other neurologic deficits in the fetus. It also increases the risk of preeclampsia, premature birth, and low birth weight.[35,36] The causes of hypothyroidism during pregnancy include autoimmune diseases such as Hashimoto's thyroiditis, iodine deficiency (uncommon in the United States), and thyroid dysfunction following surgery or ablative therapy for Graves' disease. Thyroid replacement therapy should be instituted if hypothyroidism is diagnosed during pregnancy; the goal is to attain normal thyrotropin concentrations. Women who receive thyroid replacement therapy prior to pregnancy can expect an increased dosage requirement of 25% to 50% during pregnancy. After delivery, maternal thyroid supplementation requirements decrease.[35,36]

Hyperthyroidism during pregnancy may precipitate outcomes of fetal death, low birth weight, malformations, and maternal heart failure.[35,36] Graves' disease is the most common cause of hyperthyroidism in pregnancy. Therapy for hyperthyroidism in pregnancy includes thioamides (e.g., propylthiouracil, methimazole) and surgery.[35,36] Propylthiouracil historically was the preferred agent because it was thought to cross the placenta less readily and was less likely to cause fetal malformations; recent evidence does not support these tenets.[36] Iodine-131 is contraindicated in pregnancy owing to the risk of thyroid damage in the fetus.[36] The goal of therapy for hyperthyroidism in pregnancy is to attain free thyroxine index concentrations or free thyroxine concentrations in the upper end of the normal range; this allows for minimization of the thioamide dose.[35,36] An additional factor that allows a reduction in the propylthiouracil dose is partial disease resolution as a result of the natural course of Graves' disease during pregnancy.[35]

LABOR AND DELIVERY

The mechanism of labor onset has been elucidated in mammalian and nonhuman primate systems, but the sequence in humans is still unclear.[63] The transition from phase 0 (quiescence) to phase 1 (activation) may be explained by the loss of inhibition of uterine activity mediators, such as progesterone, prostacyclin, and others. Once activation occurs, oxytocin, prostaglandin E_2, and prostaglandin $F_{2\alpha}$ increase and stimulate contractions of the uterus.[63]

PRETERM LABOR

Preterm labor is defined as cervical changes and uterine contractions that occur before 37 weeks' gestation.[63,64] In the United States, the incidence of preterm births is 11% despite a strong national effort to decrease the incidence of preterm labor.[65] Accounting for 35% of health care spending on infants, preterm labor is the leading cause of infant morbidity and mortality.[63,65] Risk factors for preterm delivery include previous preterm delivery, infections (e.g., bacterial vaginosis, upper and lower urinary tract infections, and sexually transmitted infections), multiple gestation, poverty, nonwhite race, maternal complication factors (e.g., smoking and use of illicit drugs or cohol), uterine functional causes (e.g., incompetent cervix and uterine septum), and fetal causes (e.g., congenital anomalies and growth retardation).[63]

Despite knowledge of the risk factors for preterm labor, there have not been good tests to monitor and prevent preterm labor. No evidence supports the use of routine cervical assessments or home monitoring of uterine activity to improve outcomes.[63,64] The presence of fetal fibronectin, an extracellular protein in cervical and vaginal secretions, in the cervix or vagina after 20 weeks is associated with a threefold risk of preterm delivery.[64] Also, a cervical length of <30 mm is associated with increased risk of preterm delivery. However, fetal fibronectin determinations and cervical ultrasonography have not helped to prevent preterm labor but have been more useful for their negative predictive value.[66]

TOCOLYTIC THERAPY

The management of preterm labor has centered on the use of tocolytic drugs. The goal of tocolytic therapy is to postpone delivery long enough to reduce the incidence of problems associated with prematurity. Tocolytics have not been shown to reduce the number of premature deliveries, but they may allow sufficient time for the administration of antenatal corticosteroids to improve pulmonary maturity and for transportation of the mother to a facility equipped to deal with high-risk deliveries.[63,64]

Tocolytic therapy should not be used in cases of intrauterine infection, fetal distress, severe preeclampsia, vaginal bleeding, and maternal hemodynamic instability.[64] The criteria for starting tocolysis are regular uterine contractions with cervical change. In women with cervical dilatation >3 cm, tocolytic therapy is less effective.[64]

There are five classes of tocolytic therapy: β-adrenergic agents, calcium channel blockers, magnesium, nonsteroidal anti-inflammatory agents, and ethanol.[65] The first four therapies are similar in effectiveness for prolonging pregnancy from 48 hours to 1 week. Ethanol has not been shown to be effective in prolonging pregnancy.[65]

The β-adrenergic agents terbutaline and ritodrine have been the first-line in tocolytic therapy.[64,65] (Of the two, only ritodrine has FDA approval for this use, but it was withdrawn from the market in 1997 and 1998 because the manufacturers were no longer interested in producing the drug.[65]) These drugs reduce intracellular calcium levels and reduce the sensitivity of the contractile unit to calcium.[64] Relative to other agents, β-agonists have a higher incidence of maternal side effects, including hyperkalemia, arrhythmias, hyperglycemia, hypotension, and pulmonary edema. Recommended terbutaline doses range from 250 to 500 mcg subcutaneously every 3 to 4 hours.[64]

Magnesium sulfate may be used in an intravenous infusion as a tocolytic agent. Its mechanism of action is to suppress nerve impulses to the uterine smooth muscles by antagonizing intracellular calcium.[64] Maternal side effects are rare but can include pulmonary edema. At toxic levels, hypotension, muscle paralysis, tetany, cardiac arrest, and respiratory depression may occur.[64]

Nifedipine is associated with fewer side effects than magnesium or β-agonist therapy.[64,65] A few studies have suggested that calcium channel blockers are better at prolonging labor than β-agonists.[65] One of the concerns regarding the use of nifedipine is the potential negative effect on blood flow between the placenta and the uterus. However, a meta-analysis has not shown increased harm to infants in the calcium channel blocker group.[65] With the initial diagnosis of preterm labor, 5 to 10 mg nifedipine may be administered sublingually every 15 to 20 minutes for three doses. Once the patient is stabilized and there is no evidence of continuing cervical dilatation, 10 to 20 mg

nifedipine may be administered by mouth every 4 to 6 hours for preterm contractions.[64]

Nonsteroidal anti-inflammatory agents such as indomethacin also have been used for tocolysis. The mechanism of action is to inhibit cervical prostaglandin activity.[64] The drug is first given orally or rectally in a dose of 50 to 100 mg, followed by an oral dose of 25 to 50 mg every 6 hours.[64] An increased rate of premature constriction of the ductus arteriosus has been noted in infants.[65]

Because infection has been thought to play a role in the etiology of preterm labor, antibiotics have been used, in addition to tocolytics and corticosteroids, to improve the outcome of preterm labor.[67] Most studies of antibiotic use in preterm labor do not demonstrate a reduction in the incidence of preterm delivery, and a meta-analysis shows a trend toward neonatal mortality in those who receive antibiotics.[67] Routine use of antibiotics therefore is not recommended.

CLINICAL CONTROVERSY

After acute tocolysis has been achieved, continuation of tocolytic therapy is controversial. Maintenance therapy with tocolytics has not been shown to be of value.[65] However, some clinicians will use maintenance tocolytics such as β-agonists or nifedipine to treat patients who experience frequent contractions without cervical change.[65]

ANTENATAL CORTICOSTEROIDS

A number of clinical trials have demonstrated the benefit of administering antenatal corticosteroids for the prevention of respiratory distress syndrome, intraventricular hemorrhage, and death in infants delivered prematurely.[68] The current clinical recommendation is to administer betamethasone 12 mg intramuscularly every 24 hours for two doses or dexamethasone 6 mg intramuscularly every 12 hours for four doses to pregnant women between 24 and 34 weeks' gestation who are at risk for preterm delivery within the next 7 days.[68] Benefits from antenatal corticosteroids are believed to begin within 24 hours. It has been found that repeat corticosteroid administration does not produce any improvement in outcomes for infants and may trend toward harm.[69]

GROUP B *STREPTOCOCCUS* INFECTION

Maternal infection with group B *Streptococcus* is associated with invasive disease in the newborn.[70] Women colonized with group B *Streptococcus* during pregnancy have an increased risk of premature delivery and transmission of the bacteria to the infant during delivery. Between 10% and 30% of pregnant women are colonized with group B *Streptococcus*.[70]

With active prevention efforts in the 1990s, the incidence of early-onset disease is now 0.5 cases per 1000 births, decreased from 1.8 cases per 1000 births.[70] There has not been any change in the incidence of late-onset group B *Streptococcus* disease, which remains consistent at 0.35 cases per 1000 births.[70] The consequences of neonatal infections include bacteremia, pneumonia, and meningitis in the newborn. The case-fatality rate is approximately 4%.[70]

In 2002, the Centers for Disease Control and Prevention revised the recommendations for the prevention of group B *Streptococcus* infection.[70] Instead of the risked-based screening strategy that was developed in 1996, the Centers for Disease Control and Prevention now recommends universal prenatal screening for group B *Streptococcus* colonization of all pregnant women at 35 to 37 weeks' gestation. Vaginal and rectal cultures should be obtained at 35 to 37 weeks' gestation. If the cultures are positive, if the woman had a previous infant with invasive group B *Streptococcus* disease, or if the woman had group B *Streptococcus* bacteriuria, antibiotics are given. If negative, no antibiotics are given. If a woman presents for delivery and no screening information is available, antibiotics are given for fever of 100.4°F or greater, for membrane rupture of 18 or more hours, or if less than 37 weeks' gestation.[70]

The currently recommended regimen for group B *Streptococcus* disease is penicillin G 5 million units given intravenously, followed by 2.5 million units given every 4 hours until delivery.[70] Alternatively, ampicillin 2 g may be given intravenously, followed by 1 g every 4 hours. If the patient is penicillin-allergic and not at risk for anaphylaxis, cefazolin 2 g intravenously, followed by 1 g every 8 hours, should be used. In patients at high risk for anaphylaxis, clindamycin 900 mg intravenously every 8 hours or erythromycin 500 mg intravenously every 6 hours should be used. In the case of penicillin-allergic women, the group B *Streptococcus* cultures should be sent for sensitivities. If the group B *Streptococcus* is resistant to clindamycin or erythromycin, the woman should receive vancomycin 1 g intravenously every 12 hours until delivery.[70]

CERVICAL RIPENING AND LABOR INDUCTION

Throughout most of pregnancy, the cervix is closed and firm.[71] During the last few weeks of pregnancy, the cervix becomes softer and thinner to facilitate labor. This process is mediated by hormonal changes, including final mediation by prostaglandins E_2 and $F_{2\alpha}$, which cause an increase in the collagenase activity in the cervix leading to thinning and dilatation.[71]

The rate of pregnancy induction ranges from 9.5% to 33.5%.[71] The most common reason for induction is postdatism (>42 weeks), which occurs in 10% of all pregnancies.[72] Other reasons for induction include suspected fetal growth retardation, maternal hypertension, premature rupture of membranes with no active onset of labor, or social factors. Contraindications for induction include placenta previa, oblique or transverse lie, pelvic structure abnormality, prolapsed umbilical cord, and active herpes. The concerns associated with induction of labor are that the labor may be ineffective or that side effects such as uterine hyperstimulation may adversely affect the infant, increasing the likelihood of cesarean section.

A scoring system has been used to determine the likelihood of successful labor induction. The most commonly used system is the Bishop scoring system, which was based originally on the labor patterns of multiparous women. The score is based on five parameters: cervical dilatation, cervical effacement (thinning), station of the baby's head, consistency of the cervix, and position of the cervix. A Bishop score of less than 6 means that a patient requires cervical ripening, and a score of greater than 8 means that the patient most likely will have a successful vaginal delivery.[71]

There are a number of nonpharmacologic methods for cervical ripening. Castor oil, hot baths, sexual intercourse, and nipple stimulation all have been recommended for labor induction. However, there is minimal evidence to support the efficacy of these methods.[71] The use of a Foley catheter placed in an unfavorable cervix for ripening has been found as effective as prostaglandin E_2. A safe and inexpensive method, membrane stripping, is particularly of value.[71]

Herbal supplements also have been used to induce labor. The most commonly mentioned agents are evening primrose oil, black haw, black and blue cohosh, and red raspberry leaves.[71] Midwives have been the most common group of clinicians using these agents. Currently, there is no evidence to support the safety and efficacy of herbal agents.[71]

Prostaglandin E_2 analogs (e.g., dinoprostone, Prepidil, and Cervidil) are commonly used pharmacologic agents for cervical ripening. Prepidil gel is administered intracervically in a dose of 500 mcg. This may be repeated after 6 hours with up to three doses in 24 hours. After administration, the patient remains supine for 30 minutes. Cervidil, a vaginal insert, contains 10 mg dinoprostone with a slower, more constant release of medication than the gel. The insert may be removed when labor begins or after a maximum of 24 hours. Patient must be on a fetal heart rate monitor for the duration of the use of Cervidil and for 15 minutes after its removal.[71]

Misoprostol, a prostaglandin E_1 analog, is an effective and inexpensive method for cervical ripening and labor induction.[73] Misoprostol is not approved by the FDA for cervical ripening, and the manufacturer has no interest in pursing this indication. Because labor induction is not an indicated use of this agent, and because of its association with uterine rupture, some hospitals have discontinued its use as an induction agent. Intravaginal administration of 25 mcg misoprostol every 4 hours for up to six doses is more effective than other prostaglandin agents and results in a shorter time to delivery. The most commonly encountered side effects are uterine hyperstimulation and meconium-stained amniotic fluid. The use of misoprostol is contraindicated in women with a previous uterine scar because of its association with uterine rupture, a catastrophic medical event.[73]

Mifepristone is an antiprogesterone agent that is currently being studied as an induction agent.[71] Preliminary studies show that mifepristone compared with placebo results in a shorter time to delivery and fewer cesarean sections.[74] There is little information on fetal and maternal outcomes because of the small sample sizes.[74]

Oxytocin is the most commonly used agent for labor induction after cervical ripening. At the end of pregnancy, the number of oxytocin receptors has increased by 300-fold.[71] A solution of 10 milliunits/mL is used for infusion. Oxytocin has been shown to be effective in both low-dose (physiologic) and high-dose (pharmacologic) regimens.[71]

LABOR ANALGESIA

During the first phase of labor, women perceive a visceral pain associated with uterine contractions; during the second phase, the pain is associated with perineal stretching.[75,76] Pain perception is variable from woman to woman as a result of physiologic, psychosocial, cultural, and environmental influences.[75]

NONPHARMACOLOGIC APPROACHES TO ANALGESIA

A number of nonpharmacologic strategies have been used to reduce the pain of childbirth. Women who receive continuous support from a doula, a laywoman trained in labor support, have a decrease in operative vaginal deliveries, cesarean deliveries, and requests for pain medication.[75] Intermittent support from a caregiver and continuous support from nursing staff have not been shown to affect birth outcomes.[75] Warm water baths provide temporary pain relief but have not been shown to decrease the use of pharmacologic pain treatments.[75] Intradermal injections of sterile water in the sacral area have been shown to decrease back pain during labor for 45 to 90 minutes. However, there was no decrease in requests for pain medication.[75]

PHARMACOLOGIC APPROACHES TO LABOR PAIN

In 2000, the American College of Obstetrics and Gynecology, along with the American Society of Anesthesiologists, published a joint position statement on pain in labor. They stated that labor results in severe pain and that if a women requests pain medications, it is a medical indication to receive pain relief.[77] Two main types of pharmacologic methods exist in the United States: parenteral opioids and epidural analgesia.

Between 39% and 56% of women in the United States receive parenteral narcotics to alleviate labor pain.[77] Meperidine, morphine, and fentanyl are the most commonly used agents. In comparison with epidural analgesia, parenteral opioids have lower rates of oxytocin augmentation, result in shorter stages of labor, and require fewer instrumental deliveries.[77] However, women are less satisfied with their pain relief with parenteral opioids than with epidural analgesia.[77]

Approximately 60% of women choose an epidural for pain relief during labor.[76] Epidural analgesia involves introducing a catheter into the epidural space and administering a drug (e.g., bupivacaine or fentanyl) to provide pain relief during labor. Another method is the combined spinal-epidural, in which a single bolus of an opioid is injected into the subarachnoid space, providing instant pain relief, and placement of an epidural catheter with a local anesthetic. Women who receive epidural anesthesia report better pain relief than those with other modalities.[76,77] Epidural analgesia is associated with prolongation of the first and second stages of labor, higher numbers of instrumental deliveries, and maternal fever.[76,77] A rare complication of epidural anesthesia is a puncture of the subarachnoid space leading to a severe headache. This occurs in approximately 2% of women.[76] Other complications include hypotension, nausea, vomiting, itching, and urinary retention. Low back pain has not been shown to be associated with the use of epidural analgesia.[76]

Paracervical blocks using local anesthesia may decrease pain associated with the first phase of labor.[77] However, these types of blocks have been associated with fetal bradycardia and are used rarely in clinical practice.

Finally, nitrous oxide is not used in the United States but is a common analgesic in many developed countries.[77] A 50-50 blend of nitrous oxide and oxygen is the most commonly used mixture. Women can self-administer the medication or receive it continuously under medical supervision. Women report significant pain relief.[77] The side effects include nausea, vomiting, and poor recall of labor.[77]

CLINICAL CONTROVERSY

Many clinicians believe that epidural analgesia is associated with a higher number of cesarean deliveries. However, two systematic reviews have not substantiated an increased rate of cesarean delivery with epidural analgesia compared with parenteral opioids. One of the reviews, however, cautioned that there may not be sufficient data to rule out such an association.[77]

POSTPARTUM ISSUES

DRUG USE DURING LACTATION

5 Although most drugs will diffuse into breast milk, there are very few instances where breast-feeding has to be discontinued. Health care providers should encourage breast-feeding women who need to use medications to continue breast-feeding whenever possible. Medications that require the mother to pump and discard milk are few.

There is strong evidence for the benefits associated with breast-feeding. Breast milk has the perfect composition of nutrients, growth factors, enzymes, immune factors, and hormones for infants.[78]

Breast-fed infants have fewer respiratory illnesses, allergies, otitis media, lymphoma, and gastroenteritis than do bottle-fed infants. There also may be improved neurologic development in breast-fed infants.[78]

There are also benefits for the nursing mother.[78] Women who breast-feed infants lose the weight gained during pregnancy more quickly, postpone resumption of their menstrual periods, and have a decreased risk of ovarian cancer, premenopausal breast cancer, and osteoporosis.[78]

Nursing mothers typically produce 600 to 1000 mL per day of milk for their infants.[79] The transfer of medication ingested by the mother into the breast milk occurs by passive diffusion of nonionized and non–protein-bound medication.[80] The higher the concentration of drug in the mother's serum, the higher the concentration will be in the breast milk. Drugs with higher molecular weights, lower lipid solubility, or higher protein binding are less likely to cross into the breast milk. As mother's serum concentration drops from metabolism and excretion of drug, the concentration of drug in the breast milk may redistribute back into the mother's bloodstream.[80]

Several factors influence the amount of drug an infant will receive through breast-feeding.[78] The amount of milk produced, the composition of the milk (mature milk versus colostrum), the concentration of the medication, and the extent to which the breast was emptied during a previous feeding session will influence the amount of drug the infant ingests.[78]

Infants also may vary in their ability to absorb, metabolize, and excrete ingested medication.[78] Premature and full-term infants may not have optimal liver function for the first 2 weeks of life.[79] Kidney function in full-term infants does not reach maturity until 2 to 4 months of age. Older infants may receive calories from other sources besides breast milk and actually ingest less total drug.[78]

Safety of a drug in pregnancy does not always ensure safety for breast-feeding, but the converse also may be true.[80] Fortunately, most of the medications listed in the position statement from the American Academy of Pediatrics are compatible with breast-feeding.[80]

Strategies to reduce the amount of drug transferred to the infant may include selection of medicines that also would be considered safe to use in the infant and use of topical medications, if possible.[80] Medications that have shorter half-lives tend to accumulate less, and those which are more protein bound do not cross into breast milk as well. Drugs with lower oral bioavailability and lower lipid solubility are also good choices. If the mother is using a once-daily medication, administration at bedtime may be advised to increase the interval to the next feeding. For medications taken multiple times per day, administration of medication immediately after a breast-feeding session also will give the longest interval to allow backdiffusion of drug from the breast milk as the mother's serum concentration decreases.[80]

MASTITIS

Women who experience mastitis often will feel fatigued initially, note breast tenderness, and complain of flulike symptoms.[81] Often the breast tenderness affects one breast only and generally is localized to the upper outer quadrant. The highest incidence of mastitis occurs within 1 to 2 weeks of beginning breast-feeding.[82] The risk of developing mastitis may be higher in situations where the feeding pattern has been altered, the number of feedings per day has decreased, the first breast is not emptied before switching to the other side, the infant is latching on poorly, the mother is overproducing milk, or the child or mother is ill.

Staphylococcus aureus is the most common organism associated with mastitis.[82] Antibiotics that are used for treatment of mastitis include penicillinase-resistant penicillins (e.g., cloxacillin, dicloxacillin, and oxacillin) and cephalosporins (e.g., cephalexin). Antibiotics are often given for 10 to 14 days. Anti-inflammatory agents, such as ibuprofen, also may be considered for pain. Prevention of recurrence includes strategies to transfer milk such as frequent feedings or pumping and reduction of breast inflammation.[82]

POSTPARTUM DEPRESSION

Postpartum major depression has been reported to affect 12 % to 16% of women; the incidence may be up to 26% in adolescent women.[83] The actual incidence of postpartum major depression varies in reports and may depend on the time after delivery that depression screening is conducted.

Both nondrug and drug options exist for the treatment of postpartum depression. Nondrug therapies include emotional support from family and friends, education about the condition, and psychotherapy. Bright-light therapy (effective for seasonal affective disorder and nonseasonal depression) also may provide benefit.[84] Pharmacologic therapy may need to be initiated because untreated depression may have negative effects on the mother's care of and relationship with the infant.[83] Guidelines for postpartum antidepressant use include (1) careful drug selection taking into account patient factors and available literature related to potential adverse effects in breast-feeding infants, (2) continual monitoring of drug dosage needs as related to efficacy and potential toxicity of the drug, (3) use of an agent that is known to result in limited infant exposure, (4) use of a single agent whenever possible, (5) continual assessment of possible infant toxicity from a drug, and (6) attention to pharmacokinetics of an agent as related to administration of the agent in relation to breast-feeding as well as selection of an agent with few or no active metabolites.[83] The most common medications used to treat postpartum major depression include selective serotonin reuptake inhibitors and tricyclic antidepressants. The small number of case reports and studies published to date suggest the relative safety of these agents for breast-feeding infants.[83]

RELACTATION

Declining serum prolactin concentrations cause a decrease in or cessation of lactation, and this can be problematic, as well as distressing, for mothers who desire to breast-feed their infants. Relactation is the process of increasing the breast milk supply for such women.[85] Lactation also can be induced in women who have not recently delivered a baby, such as adoptive mothers. The mainstay of therapy for this condition involves nipple stimulation either by the infant's nursing or by pumping of the breast with a mechanical pump or the hand.[85] One small study showed that a substance in beer and nonalcoholic beer can stimulate prolactin secretion and thus increase milk production.[86]

Recommended pharmacologic therapy in the United States for relactation is metoclopramide, which should be used only if nondrug therapy is ineffective.[85] The most commonly used dose is 10 mg taken orally three times daily for 7 to 14 days. Breast milk production can be increased up to 100% or more in women who are 1 month postpartum or less; in mothers who are 8 to 12 weeks postpartum, milk production may be increased up to 40%. Breast milk production may decrease after metoclopramide therapy is discontinued, but if lactation has been established successfully, it will continue.[85]

CONCLUSIONS

Providing pharmacologic care to women during pregnancy can be rewarding and, at times, difficult. Many women perceive a high inherent risk of birth defects with drug exposure during pregnancy. This perception, linked with a high rate of unplanned pregnancies, may create anxiety because of drug exposure prior to the discovery of pregnancy.

Some medications are considered to be safe for use in pregnancy because of frequent use with no apparent increase in the rate of congenital problems. Women using these medications should be reassured that these choices are unlikely to increase the risk of birth defects. In some cases, medications that have been associated with a higher risk of adverse effects to the fetus will need to be selected or continued to ensure the health of the mother and, in some instances, the fetus. In these instances, realistic information about types and likelihood of adverse effects will aid the patient and her family in making decisions.

Health care providers who care for pregnant women need to work in collaboration to seek, evaluate, and present the most contemporary information to their patients. Use of technology to access evidence-based resources, databases related to drug use in pregnancy, and primary literature may assist health care practitioners in accessing relevant medication information to manage drug therapy needs during pregnancy and lactation.

ABBREVIATIONS

CNS: central nervous system
FDA: Food and Drug Administration

Review Questions and other resources can be found at *www.pharmacotherapyonline.com.*

REFERENCES

1. Namnoun AB, Hatcher RA. The menstrual cycle. In: Hatcher RA, Trussell J, Stewart F, et al, eds. Contraceptive Technology, 17th ed. New York, Ardent Media, 1998:69–76.
2. Fetal growth and development. In: Cunningham FG, Gant NF, Leveno KJ, et al, eds. Williams' Obstetrics, 21st ed. New York, McGraw-Hill, 2001: 129–166.
3. Bovone S, Pernoll ML. Normal pregnancy and prenatal care. In: DeCherney AH, Nathan L, eds. Current Obstetric Gynecologic Diagnosis and Treatment, 9th ed. New York, McGraw-Hill, 2003:193–212.
4. Loebstein R, Koren G. Clinical relevance of therapeutic drug monitoring during pregnancy. Ther Drug Monit 2002;24:15–22.
5. Wagner CL, Katikaneni LD, Cox TH, Ryan RM. The impact of prenatal drug exposure on the neonate. Obstet Gyencol Clin North Am 1998; 25:169–194.
6. Larimore WL, Petrie KA. Drug use during pregnancy and lactation. Prim Care 2000;27:35–53.
7. Polifka JE, Friedman JM. Medical genetics: 1. Clinical teratology in the age of genomics. Can Med Assoc J 2002;167:265–273.
8. Brent RL. Immunization of pregnant women: Reproductive, medical and societal risks. Vaccine 2003;21:3414–3421.
9. Shepard TH, Brent RL, Friedman JM, et al. Update on new developments in the study of human teratogens. Teratology 2002;65:153–161.
10. Irl C, Hasford J. Assessing the safety of drugs in pregnancy. Drug Saf 2000;22:169–177.
11. Koren G, Pastuszak A, Ito S. Drug therapy: Drugs in pregnancy. N Engl J Med 1998;338:1128–1137.
12. Addis A, Sharabi S, Bonati M. Risk classifications systems for drug use during pregnancy: Are they a reliable source of information? Drug Saf 2000;23:245–253.
13. Morrison EH. Preconception care. Prim Care 2000;27:1–12.
14. Botto LD, Moore CA, Khoury MJ, Erickson JD. Neural-tube defects. N Engl J Med 1999;341:1509–1519.

15. Committee on Genetics, American Academy of Pediatrics. Folic acid for the prevention of neural tube defects. Pediatrics 1999;104:325–327.

16. Englund JA. Maternal immunization with inactivated influenza vaccine: Rationale and experience. Vaccine 2003;21:3460–3464.

17. Klesges LM, Johnson KC, Ward KD, Barnard M. Smoking cessation in pregnant women. Obstet Gynecol Clin 2001;28:269–282.

18. Benowitz NL, Dempsey DA, Goldenburg RL, et al. The use of pharmacotherapies for smoking cessation during pregnancy. Tobacco Control 2000;9(suppl 3):S91–94.

19. Dempsey DA, Benowitz NL. Risks and benefits of nicotine to aid smoking cessation in pregnancy. Drug Saf 2001;24:277–322.

20. Wald A. Constipation, diarrhea, and symptomatic hemorrhoids during pregnancy. Gastroenterol Clin 2003;32:309–322.

21. Richter JE. Gastroesophageal reflux disease during pregnancy. Gastroenterol Clin 2003;32:235–261.

22. Rayburn W, Liles E, Christensen H, Robinson M. Antacids vs antacids plus non-prescription ranitidine for heartburn during pregnancy. Int J Gynaecol Obstet 1999;66:35–37.

23. Koch KL, Frissora CL. Nausea and vomiting during pregnancy. Gastroenterol Clin 2003;32:201–234.

24. Magee LA, Mazzotta P, Koren G. Evidence-based view of safety and effectiveness of pharmacologic therapy for nausea and vomiting of pregnancy (NVP). Am J Obstet Gynecol 2002;186:S256–261.

25. Mazzotta P, Magee LA. A risk-benefit assessment of pharmacological and nonpharmacological treatments for nausea and vomiting of pregnancy. Drugs 2000;59:781–800.

26. American Diabetes Association. Gestational diabetes mellitus. Diabetes Care 2003;26(suppl 1):S103–105.

27. U.S. Preventive Services Task Force (USPSTF). Screening for gestational diabetes mellitus: Recommendations and rationale. Obstet Gynecol 2003;101:393–395.

28. Langer O, Conway DL, Berkus MD, et al. A comparison of glyburide and insulin in women with gestational diabetes mellitus. N Engl J Med 2000;343:1134–1138.

29. American Diabetes Association. Preconception care of women with diabetes. Diabetes Care 2003;26(suppl 1):S91–93.

30. Walkinshaw SA. Dietary regulation for "gestational diabetes." Cochrane Review 2003;3.

31. National High Blood Pressure Eduction Program Working Group on High Blood Pressure in Pregnancy. Report of the National High Blood Pressure Education Program Working Group on high blood pressure in pregnancy. Am J Obstet Gynecol 2000;183:S1–22.

32. Coomarasamy A, Honest H, Spyros Papaiannou S, et al. Aspirin for prevention of preeclampsia in women with historical risk factors: A systemic review. Obstet Gynecol 2003;101:1319–1332.

33. Hofmeyr GJ, Atallah AN, Duley L. Calcium supplementation during pregnancy for preventing hypertensive disorders and related problems. Cochrane Review 2003;3.

34. Magee LA. Treating hypertension in women of child-bearing age and during pregnancy. Drug Saf 2001;24:457–474.

35. Mulder JE. Thyroid disease in women. Med Clin North Am 1998;82:103–125.

36. American College of Obstetrics and Gynecology, Committee on Practice Bulletin. Clinical management guidelines for obstetricians-gynecologists, Number 32, November 2001 (replaces Technical Bulletin Number 181, June 1993, and Committee Opinion Number 241, September 2000). Thyroid disease in pregnancy. Obstet Gynecol 2001;98:879–888.

37. Greer IA. Prevention and management of venous thromboembolism in pregnancy. Clin Chest Med 2003;24:123–137.

38. Ginsberg JS, Greer I, Hirsch J. Use of antithrombotic agents during pregnancy. Chest 2001;119:122S–131.

39. Connolly A, Thorp JM. Urinary tract infections in pregnancy. Urol Clin North Am 1999;26:779–787.

40. Delzell JE, Lefevre ML. Urinary tract infections during pregnancy. Am Fam Phys 2000;61:713–721.

41. Cram LF. Genitourinary infections and their association with preterm labor. Am Fam Phys 2002;65:241–248.

43. Gilstrap LC, Ramin SM. Urinary tract infections during pregnancy. Obstet Gynecol Clin North Am 2001;28:581–591.

44. Centers for Disease Control and Prevention. Sexually transmitted diseases treatment guidelines, 2002. MMWR 2002;51:1–78.

45. Brocklehurst P. Update on the treatment of sexually transmitted infections in pregnancy-1. Int J STD AIDS 1999;10:571–580.

46. Baker DA. Issues and management of herpes in pregnancy. Int J Fertil 2002;47:129–135.

47. Guise JM, Mahon SM, Aickin M, et al. Screening for bacterial vaginosis in pregnancy. Am J Prevent Med 2001;20:67–72.

48. Von Wald T, Walling AD. Headache during pregnancy. Obstet Gynecol Surv 2002;57:179–185.

49. Blaiss MS. Management of rhinitis and asthma in pregnancy. Ann Allergy Asthma Immunol 2003;90(suppl 3):16–22.

50. Tan KS, Thomson NC. Asthma in pregnancy. Am J Med 2000;109:727–733.

51. Luskin AT, Lipkowitz MA. The diagnosis and management of asthma during pregnancy. Immunol Allergy Clin North Am 2000;20:745–761.

52. Reed BR. Dermatologic drugs, pregnancy, and lactation: A conservative guide. Arch Dermatol 1997;133:894–898.

53. Morrell MJ. Reproductive and metabolic disorders in women with epilepsy. Epilepsia 2003 44(suppl.4):11–20.

54. Holmes LB, Harvey EA, Coull BA, et al. The teratogenicity of anticonvulsant drugs. N Engl J Med 2001;344:1132–1138.

55. Practice parameter: Management issues for women with epilepsy (summary statement). Report of the Quality Standards Subcommittee of the American Academy of Neurology. Neurology 1998;51:944–948.

56. Public Health Service Task Force. Recommendations for the use of antiretroviral drugs in pregnant HIV-1-infected women for maternal health and interventions to reduce prenatal HIV-1 transmission in the United States. Available at *http://www.aidsinfo.nih.gov;* accessed September 18, 2003.

57. Jackson JB, Musoke P, Fleming T, et al. Intrapartum and neonatal single-dose nevirapine compared with zidovudine for prevention of mother-to-child transmission of HIV-1 in Kampala, Uganda: 19-month follow-up of the HIVNET 012 randomized trial. Lancet 2003;362:859–868.

58. Einarson A, Selby P, Koren G. Abrupt discontinuation of psychotropic drugs during pregnancy: Fear of teratogenic risk and impact of counseling. J Psychiatry Neurosci 2001;26:44–48.

59. Nonacs R, Cohen LS. Depression during pregnancy: Diagnosis and treatment options. J Clin Psychiatry 2002;63(suppl 7):24–30.

60. Brown CS. Depression and anxiety disorders. Obstet Gynecol Clin North Am 2001;28:241–268.

61. Viguera AC, Cohen LS, Baldessarini RJ, Nonacs R. Managing bipolar disorder during pregnancy: Weighing the risks and benefits. Can J Psychiatry 2002;47:426–436.

62. Iqbal MM, Gundlapalli SP, Ryan WG, et al. Effects of antimania mood-stabilizing drugs on fetuses, neonates, and nursing infants. South Med J 2001;94:304–322.

63. Slattery MM, Morrison JJ. Preterm delivery. Lancet 2002;360:1489–1497.

64. Weismiller DG. Preterm labor. Am Fam Phys 1999;59:593–602.

65. Berkman ND, Thorp JM, Lohr KN, et al. Tocolytic treatment for the management of preterm labor: A review of the evidence. Am J Obstet Gynecol 2003;188:1648–1659.

66. Iams JD. Prediction and early detection of preterm labor. Obstet Gynecol 2003;101:402–412.

67. King J, Flenady V. Prophylactic antibiotics for inhibiting preterm labor with intact membranes. Cochrane Review 2003;2.

68. Antenatal corticosteroids revisited: Repeat courses. Washington, NIH Consensus Statement Online, August 17–18, 2000; http://consensus.nih.gov/cons/112/112_intro.htm; accessed September 16, 2003.

69. Guinn DA, Atkinson MW, Sullivan L, et al. Single vs weekly courses of antenatal corticosteroids for women at risk of preterm delivery: A randomized, controlled trial. JAMA 2001;286:1581–1587.

70. Centers for Disease Control and Prevention. Prevention of perinatal Group B streptococcal disease. Available at: http://www.cdc.gov/mmwr/preview/mmwrhtml/rr5111al.htm; accessed November 24, 2004.

71. Tenore JL. Methods for cervical ripening and induction of labor. Am Fam Phys 2003;67:2213–2218.

72. Rand L, Robinson JN, Economy KE, Norwitz ER. Post-term induction of labor revisited. Obstet Gynecol 2000;96:779–783.

73. Hofmeyr GJ, Gulmezoglu AM. Vaginal misoprostol for cervical ripening and induction of labor. Cochrane Database Syst Rev 2003;1:CD000941.

74. Neilson JP. Mifepristone for induction of labour. Cochrane Database Syst Rev 2000;4:CD002865.

75. Leeman L, Fontaine P, King V, et al. The nature and management of labor pain: I. Nonpharmacologic pain relief. Am Fam Phys 2003;68: 1109–1112.

76. Eltzschig HK, Lieberman ES, Camann W. Regional anesthesia and analgesia for labor and delivery. N Engl J Med 2003;348:319–322.

77. Leeman L, Fontaine P, King V, et al. The nature and management of labor pain: II. Pharmacologic pain relief. Am Fam Phys 2003;68:1115–1120.

78. Chaudron LH, Jefferson JW. Mood stabilizers during breastfeeding: A review. J Clin Psychiatry 2000;61:79–90.

79. Burt VK, Suri R, Altshuler L, et al. The use of psychotropic medications during breast-feeding. Am J Psychiatry 2001;158:1001–1009.

80. Spencer JP, Gonzalez LS, Barnhart DJ. Medications in the breast-feeding mother. Am Fam Phys 2001;64:119–126.

81. Prachniak GK. Common breastfeeding problems. Obstet Gynecol Clin North Am 2002;29:77–88.

82. Marchant DJ. Inflammation of the breast. Obstet Gynecol Clin North Am 2002;29:89–102.

83. Misri S, Kostaras X. Benefits and risks to mother and infant of drug treatment for postnatal depression. Drug Saf 2002;25:903–911.

84. Corral M, Kuan A, Kostaras D. Bright light therapy's effect on postpartum depression. Am J Psychiatry 2000;157:303–304.

85. Anderson PO, Valdes V. Therapy consultation: Increasing breast milk supply. Clin Pharmacol Ther 1993;12:479–480.

86. Carlson HE, Wasser HL, Feidelberger RD. Beer-induced prolactin secretion: A clinical and laboratory study of the role of salsolinol. J Clin Endocrinol Metab 1985;60:673–677.

77
CONTRACEPTION

Lori M. Dickerson and Kathryn K. Bucci

earning Objectives and other resources can be found at *www.pharmacotherapyonline.com.*

KEY CONCEPTS

1. The attitude of both the patient and the sexual partner toward various contraceptive methods, the reliability of the patient in using it correctly (which may affect the effectiveness of the method), and the patient's ability to pay must be considered carefully when selecting a contraceptive method.

2. Patient-specific factors (e.g., frequency of intercourse, age, smoking status, and concomitant diseases, conditions, or medications) that may prove to be a consideration or precaution for use of a specific method must be evaluated when selecting a contraceptive method.

3. Side effects or difficulties using the chosen method should be monitored carefully and managed in consideration of patient-specific factors.

4. The utility and satisfaction of the patient and partner(s) with a contraceptive method must be reevaluated periodically.

5. Many practitioners recommend progestin-only contraceptives for breast-feeding women because progestins provide effective contraception without diminishing the amount of breast milk produced.

6. Accurate and timely counseling on the optimal use of the contraceptive method and strategies to minimize sexually transmitted diseases must be provided to all patients when contraceptive pharmacotherapy is initiated and on an ongoing basis.

7. Certain oral contraceptives in high doses can be used as emergency contraception to prevent pregnancy after unprotected intercourse. Administration must occur within 72 hours of unprotected intercourse with a follow-up dose 12 hours after the first.

Unintended pregnancy is a significant public health problem with economic, health, personal, and social consequences. The most recent data reveal that 49% of pregnancies are unintended and that 54% of unintended pregnancies end in abortion. Between 1987 and 1994, the unintended pregnancy rate dropped by 16%, from 54 to 45 per 1000 women of reproductive age.[1] Slightly more than half these unintended pregnancies occurred in the 94% of sexually active couples who claimed to use some method of contraception.[2] If the goal of contraception is that pregnancies are planned and desired, education about the use and efficacy of contraceptive methods must be improved.

ETIOLOGY AND PATHOPHYSIOLOGY

Comprehension of the hormonal regulation of the normal menstrual cycle is essential to understanding contraception in women. The cycle of menstruation begins with menarche, usually around age 12, and continues to occur in nonpregnant women until menopause; usually around age 50.[3,4] The cycle includes the vaginal discharge of sloughed endometrium called *menses* or *menstrual flow.* Three phases comprise the menstrual cycle: the follicular (or preovulatory), the ovulatory, and the luteal (or postovulatory).[3,4]

THE MENSTRUAL CYCLE

The first day of menses is referred to as *day 1 of the menstrual cycle* and marks the beginning of the follicular phase.[3,4] This continues until ovulation, which typically occurs on day 14. The time after ovulation is referred to as the *luteal phase,* which lasts until the beginning of the next menstrual cycle. The median menstrual cycle length is 28 days, but it can range from 21 to 40 days. Generally, variation is greatest and follicular and luteal phases are longest in the years immediately after menarche and before menopause, when anovulatory cycles are more common.[5]

The menstrual cycle is influenced by the hormonal relationships between the hypothalamus, anterior pituitary, and ovaries[3] (Fig. 77–1). In response to epinephrine and norepinephrine stimulation, the hypothalamus secretes gonadotropin-releasing hormone (GnRH) in a pulsatile fashion every 60 to 90 minutes.[3,4] These GnRH bursts stimulate the anterior pituitary to secrete bursts of gonadotropins, follicle-stimulating hormone (FSH), and luteinizing hormone (LH). These gonadotropins, FSH, and LH direct events in the ovarian follicles that result in the production of a fertile ovum.

FOLLICULAR PHASE

In the first 4 days of the menstrual cycle, FSH levels rise and allow the recruitment of a small group of follicles for continued growth and development[3,4] (Fig. 77–2). Between days 5 and 7, one becomes the dominant follicle, which will later rupture and release the oocyte. The dominant follicle develops increasing amounts of estradiol and inhibin, which cause a negative feedback on the hypothalamic secretion of GnRH and pituitary secretion of FSH, causing atresia of the remaining follicles recruited during the cycle.

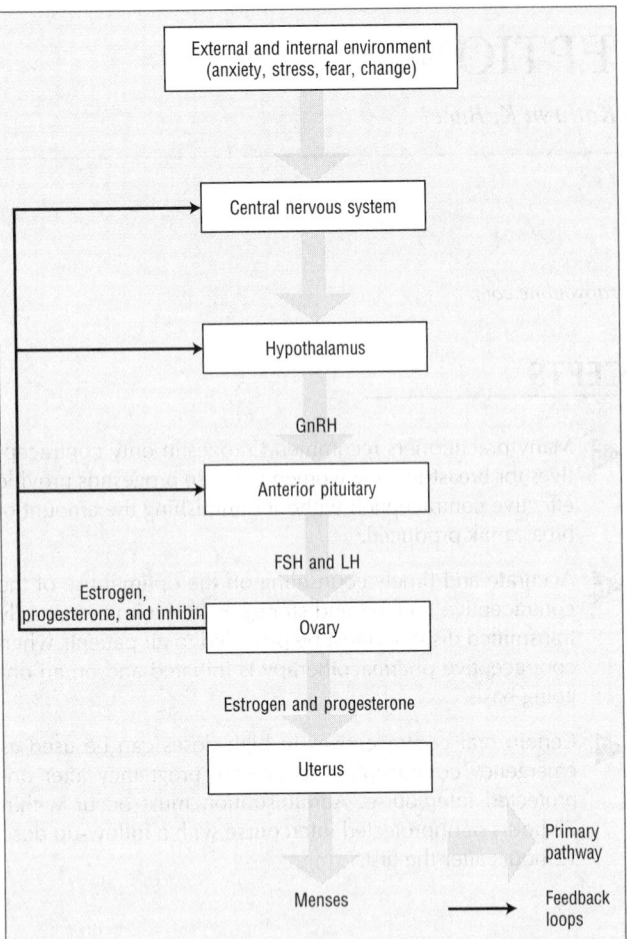

FIGURE 77–1. Regulation of the menstrual cycle. Primary hormone pathways in the reproductive system are modulated by both negative and positive feedback loops. Prostaglandins, secreted by the ovary and by uterine endometrial cells, also play a role in ovulation and may modulate hypothalamic function as well. *(Reproduced courtesy of Hatcher RA, Nelson AL, Zieman M, et al. A Pocket Guide to Managing Contraception. Tiger, GA, Bridging the Gap Foundation, 2003:1–146. This figure may be reproduced at no cost to the reader.)*

Once the follicle has received FSH stimulation, it must have continued FSH stimulation or it will die.[3,4] Gonadotropin-dependent growth allows the follicle to enlarge, produce other layers of receptors for FSH and LH, and synthesize estradiol, progesterone, and androgen. Estradiol serves to stop the menstrual flow from the previous cycle, thickening the endometrial lining of the uterus to prepare it for embryonic implantation. Estrogen is also responsible for the increased production of thin, watery cervical mucus, which will enhance sperm transport during fertilization. FSH also regulates the aromatase enzymes that convert androgens to estrogens in the follicle. If a follicle has insufficient aromatase, androgen will accumulate, and the follicle will not survive. Therefore, follicles with the most FSH stimulation have the lowest androgen-estrogen ratios.

OVULATION

When estradiol levels remain elevated for a sustained period of time (200 pg for at least 50 hours), the pituitary releases a midcycle LH surge[3,4] (see Fig. 77–2). This LH surge stimulates the final stages of follicular maturation and ovulation (follicular rupture and release of the oocyte). On average, ovulation occurs 24 to 36 hours after estradiol peak and 10 to 16 hours after the LH peak. The LH surge, occurring 28 to 32 hours before a follicle ruptures, is the most clinically useful predictor of approaching ovulation. After ovulation, the oocyte is released and travels to the fallopian tube, where it can be fertilized and transported to the uterus for embryonic implantation. Conception is most successful when intercourse takes place from 2 days before ovulation to the day of ovulation.

LUTEAL PHASE

After rupture of the follicle and release of the ovum, the remaining luteinized follicles become the corpus luteum, which synthesizes androgen, estrogen, and progesterone[3,4] (see Fig. 77–2). Progesterone helps to maintain the endometrial lining, which sustains the implanted embryo and maintains the pregnancy. It also inhibits GnRH and gonadotropin release, preventing the development of new follicles. If pregnancy occurs, human chorionic gonadotropin (hCG) prevents regression of the corpus luteum and stimulates continued production of estrogen and progesterone secretion to maintain the pregnancy until the placenta is able to fulfill this role (usually 6 to 8 weeks' gestation).

If fertilization or implantation does not occur, the corpus luteum degenerates, and progesterone production declines.[3,4] The life span of the corpus luteum depends on the continuous presence of small amounts of LH, and its average duration of function is 9 to 11 days. As the progesterone levels decline, endometrial shedding (menstruation) occurs, and a new menstrual cycle begins. At the end of the luteal phase, with low estrogen and progesterone levels, FSH levels start to rise, and follicular recruitment for the next cycle begins.

EPIDEMIOLOGY

Contraception generally implies the prevention of pregnancy following sexual intercourse by inhibiting viable sperm from coming into contact with a mature ovum (i.e., methods that act as barriers or prevent ovulation) or by preventing a fertilized ovum from implanting successfully in the endometrium (i.e., mechanisms that create an unfavorable uterine environment).

Commonly used methods of reversible contraception include oral and transdermal contraceptives, long-acting injectable estrogen and progestins, implantable progestins, condoms, spermicides, withdrawal, the diaphragm, periodic abstinence, and the intrauterine device. These methods differ in their relative effectiveness, safety, and patient acceptability.[4,6]

The actual effectiveness of any contraceptive method is difficult to determine because many factors affect contraceptive failure. A failure inherent to the proper use of the contraceptive alone is considered a method failure or perfect-use failure. User failure or typical-use failure takes into account the user's ability to follow directions correctly and consistently[4,6] (Table 77–1). In a survey of women having abortions in 2000–2001, 46% had not used a contraceptive method in the month they conceived owing to a perceived low risk of pregnancy (33%) and concerns about the use of contraceptives (32%). The male condom was the most commonly used method (28%), from which inconsistent use was the cited cause of pregnancy in 49% of cases. Oral

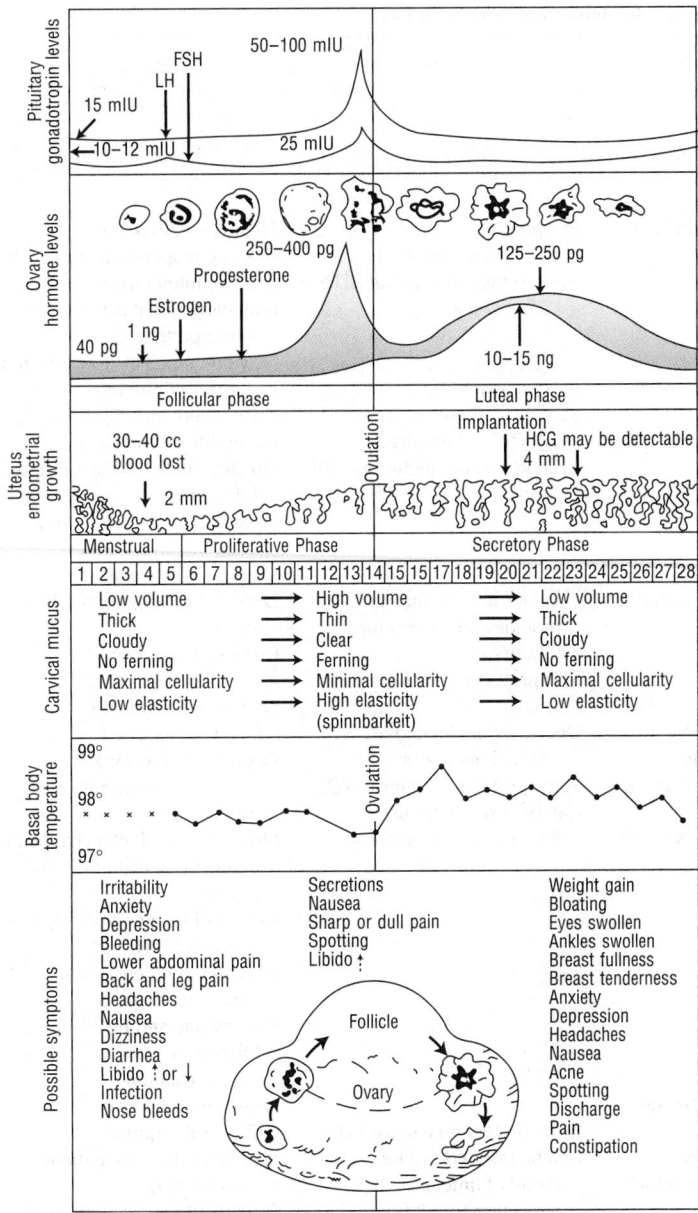

FIGURE 77–2. Menstrual cycle events—idealized 28-day cycle. FSH = follicle-stimulating hormone, HCG = human chorionic gonadotropin, LH = luteining hormone. *(Reproduced courtesy of Hatcher RA, Nelson AL, Zieman M, et al. A Pocket Guide to Managing Contraception. Tiger, GA, Bridging the Gap Foundation, 2003:1–146. This figure may be reproduced at no cost to the reader.)*

contraceptives (OCs) were used by 14% of women, 76% of whom reported inconsistent use resulting in pregnancy.[7]

CLINICAL PRESENTATION

For many young women, a major reason for visiting a clinician is to seek contraception. Clinicians may use this opportunity to provide health maintenance/disease prevention by counseling about reproductive health and sexually transmitted diseases. It always has been tradition that hormonal contraception is provided with clinical breast and pelvic examinations. However, the need for the physical examination may delay access to contraception, resulting in unintended pregnancies and other health risks. In addition, requiring the breast and pelvic examination prior to the prescription of hormonal contraception reinforces the incorrect perception that these methods of pregnancy prevention are harmful or dangerous. Therefore, recent recommendations from the American College of Obstetrics and Gynecology (ACOG) and other national organizations have changed to allow provision of hormonal contraception after a simple medical history and blood pressure measurement.[8] Other preventive measures, such as pelvic and breast examinations, screening for cervical neoplasia, and counseling for prevention of sexually transmitted diseases, can be done during routine annual office visits.

TABLE 77–1. Comparison of Reversible Methods of Contraception

Method	Absolute Contraindications	Advantages	Disadvantages	Percent of Women With Pregnancy[a] Lowest Expected	Typical Use
Episodic Contraceptive Methods					
Spermicides alone	Allergy to spermicide	Inexpensive No office visit required Some protection against STDs	High user failure rate Must be reapplied before each act of intercourse May cause local irritation in either partner May enhance HIV transmission	3	21
Condoms, male	Allergy to latex or rubber	Inexpensive Readily available No office visit required STD protection, including HIV (latex only)	High user failure rate Poor acceptance Possibility of breakage Efficacy decreased by oil-based lubricants Possible-allergic reactions to latex in either partner	2	12
Condoms, female (Reality)	Allergy to polyurethane History of toxic shock syndrome	Can be inserted just before intercourse or ahead of time; provides protection for 8 hours STD protection, including HIV	High user failure rate Dislike ring hanging outside vagina Cumbersome	5.0	21.0
Diaphragm with spermicide	Allergy to latex, rubber, or spermicide Recurrent UTIs History of toxic shock syndrome Abnormal gynecologic anatomy	Low cost Decreased incidence of cervical neoplasia Some protection against STDs Can be inserted for up to 6 hours before intercourse	High user failure rate Office visit required Decreased efficacy with increased frequency of intercourse Must be refitted after significant change in weight (+/−10 pounds) Increased incidence of vaginal yeast and UTIs Increased incidence of toxic shock syndrome Efficacy affected by oil-based lubricants Cervical irritation	6	18
Cervical cap (Prentif)	Allergy to rubber or spermicide Recurrent UTIs History of toxic shock syndrome Abnormal gynecologic anatomy Abnormal Papanicolaou smear	Low cost Some protection against STDs Can be inserted just before or ahead of time; provides protection for 48 hours	High user failure rate Office visit required May be difficult for patient to use correctly Decreased efficacy with parity Cannot be used during menses	6	18
Sponge (Today)	Allergy to spermicide Recurrent UTIs History of toxic shock syndrome Abnormal gynecologic anatomy	Inexpensive No office visit required Some protection against STDs Can be inserted just before or ahead of time; provides protection for 24 hours	High user failure rate Problems removing the sponge due to vaginal dryness Cannot be used during menses Not yet available in U.S.	Parous 9 Nulliparous 6	Parous 28 Nulliparous 18
Hormonal Methods					
Oral contraceptives	Hepatic adenomas Thromboembolic disorders or history thereof Cerebrovascular or coronary artery disease	Decreased risk of PID, ovarian and endometrial cancer Improvement in endometriosis (probably) Fewer functional ovarian cysts (possibly)	Office visit required Increased risk of benign hepatocellular adenomas Mild increased risk of thromboembolism and stroke May elevate blood pressure	0.1	3

TABLE 77–1. (*Continued*)

Method	Absolute Contraindications	Advantages	Disadvantages	Percent of Women With Pregnancy[a]	
				Lowest Expected	Typical Use
	Known or suspected breast cancer Undiagnosed abnormal gynecologic bleeding Jaundice with pregnancy or previous pill use	Less salpingitis and ectopic pregnancy Prevention of benign breast disease (fibroadenoma and fibrocystic changes) Less rheumatoid arthritis (possibly) Increased bone density (possibly) Improvement in acne/hirsutism Significant improvement in menstruation-related problems: fewer cramps, less flow for fewer days, less iron deficiency anemia, more predictable menses, elimination of mittelschmerz, less dysmenorrhea and premenstrual syndrome	No protection against most STDs Estrogenic side effects (nausea, breast tenderness, fluid retention) Progestin side effects (acne, increased appetite, depression) Increased risk of myocardial infarction in older women, smokers		
Progestin-only oral contraceptives	Undiagnosed abnormal gynecologic bleeding	May be used by lactating women and women with cardiovascular risk Allows avoidance of estrogen-related side effects Protection against PID, iron deficiency anemia, and dysmenorrhea	Frequent spotting and amenorrhea Increased risk of ectopic pregnancy Must take every day at the same time	0.5	3
Transdermal contraceptives (Ortho-Evra)	Same as above for oral contraceptives	Same as above for oral contraceptives Convenience of weekly application	Same as above for oral contraceptives	1	Up to 9 in women >90 kg
Contraceptive rings (NuvaRing)	Same as above for oral contraceptives	Same as above for oral contraceptives Convenience of monthly insertion	Same as above for oral contraceptives	1	?
Progestin implants: levonorgestrel (Norplant and Norplant II,[b] Jadelle,[b] Capronor[b]), 3 ketodesogestrel (Implanon[b]), nomegestrol acetate (uniplant[b])	Pregnancy Undiagnosed abnormal gynecologic bleeding Acute liver disease Benign or malignant liver tumors Known or suspected breast cancers Active thrombophlebitis or thromboembolic disease	Passive contraception Duration of efficacy varies; effective up to 5 years with Norplant in women <154 pounds Effects are quickly reversible Less menstrual cramping and mittelschmerz pain No suppression of lactation No metabolic disturbances Can be considered for use in women who have diabetes, hypertension, gall bladder disease, history of cardiovascular or thromboembolic disease and in women who are smokers or lactating	Requires outpatient surgical procedure Irregular menstrual bleeding, headaches, weight gain, acne Progestin side effects Local infection or bruising on insertion; removal may be difficult Expensive initially High discontinuation rate Unacceptable in patients using some anticonvulsants	0.3	0.3

(*continued*)

TABLE 77–1. (*Continued*)

Method	Absolute Contraindications	Advantages	Disadvantages	Percent of Women With Pregnancy[a]	
				Lowest Expected	Typical Use
Depo-Provera	Pregnancy Undiagnosed abnormal gynecologic bleeding Known or suspected breast cancers Liver disease (relative contraindication) Severe depression (relative contraindication) Severe cardiovascular disease (relative contraindication)	Passive contraception No suppression of lactation No increased risk of thromboembolism May decrease seizure frequency Effective for 3 months Can be considered for use in women who have seizure disorders, diabetes, hypertension, gall bladder disease, history of cardiovascular or thromboembolic disease and in women who are smokers or lactating	Office visit required every 3 months Irregular menstrual bleeding, headache, weight gain, acne Delayed return of fertility Possible increased risk of breast cancer in younger users Decreased HDL Progestin side effects Decreased bone density in long-term users	0.3	0.3
Lunelle	Pregnancy Undiagnosed abnormal gynecologic bleeding Known or suspected breast cancers Thromboembolic disorders or history thereof Cerebrovascular or coronary artery disease Jaundice of pregnancy or with prior pill use	Effects quickly reversible Less menstrual cramping and mittelschmerz pain Less menstrual irregularity than other injectable or implantable methods	Office visit required monthly Progestin side effects Estrogen side effects	0.1	0.1
Intrauterine Devices (Hormonal and Nonhormonal)					
Copper-T 380A (ParaGard)	Multiple sexual partners or partner with multiple partners (high risk for STDs) History of PID or ectopic pregnancy, acute pelvic infection Abnormal uterine cavity/pelvic surgery/undiagnosed gynecologic bleeding Uterine or cervical cancer Wilson's disease Allergy to copper	Passive contraception Long-term contraception (can remain in place for up to 10 years) Less expensive per year and easier for some patients No delay in return of fertility after removal	Increased heavy bleeding Spotting between periods Increased cramping and dysmenorrhea Increased risk of ectopic pregnancy Office visit required Rarely, uterine perforation	0.8	3
Progesterone T (Progestasert)	Postpartum endometritis or infected abortion in previous 3 months Acute cervicitis or vaginitis (including BV) until infection controlled	Remains in place for 1 year Decreased cramping and dysmenorrhea Decrease in menstrual blood loss No delay in return of fertility after removal	Office visit required Must be changed each year Increased risk of ectopic pregnancy Rarely, uterine perforation	1.5	2

TABLE 77–1. (*Continued*)

Method	Absolute Contraindications	Advantages	Disadvantages	Percent of Women With Pregnancy[a]	
				Lowest Expected	Typical Use
Levonorgestrel IUD (Mirena)	Conditions associated with increased susceptibility to infections, including leukemia, AIDS, IV drug abuse, and corticosteroid use Valvular heart disease (relative contraindication) Nulliparity (relative contraindication) Genital actinomyces Wilson's disease Allergy to copper	Constant rate of hormone release for 5 years Possibly the single most effective reversible contraceptive method over 5-year period Decreased cramping, dysmenorrhea, menorrhagia Combines benefits of Norplant and Copper-T	Office visit required Irregular menstrual bleeding Rarely, uterine perforation	0.1	0.1

STD, sexually transmitted disease; HIV, human immunodeficiency virus; UTI, urinary tract infection; PID, pelvic inflammatory disease; HDL, high-density lipoprotein cholesterol; BV, bacterial vaginosis; AIDS, acquired immunodeficiency syndrome; IV, intravenous.
[a] Failure rates during first year of use, United States.
[b] Products in development.
Compiled from refs. 3, 4, 6, 12, 13, and 18.

▶ TREATMENT: Contraception

DESIRED OUTCOME

The obvious goal of treatment with all methods of contraception is to avoid pregnancy. However, there are many health benefits associated with contraceptive methods, including prevention of sexually transmitted diseases (condoms), improvements in menstrual cycle regularity (hormonal contraceptives), prevention of malignancies and other health conditions (OCs), and management of perimenopause.[9]

NONPHARMACOLOGIC THERAPY

PERIODIC ABSTINENCE

❶ ❷ Highly motivated couples may use the abstinence (rhythm) method of contraception, avoiding sexual intercourse during the days of the menstrual cycle when conception is likely to occur. These women rely on physiologic changes, such as the basal body temperature and cervical mucus, during each cycle to determine the fertile period. The major reasons for the lack of acceptance are the relatively high pregnancy rates among users and the need to avoid intercourse for several days during each menstrual cycle. To overcome these drawbacks, many women use barrier methods or spermicides during the fertile period.[4,6]

BARRIER TECHNIQUES

The effectiveness of barrier methods and spermicides depends almost exclusively on a couple's motivation to use them consistently and correctly. These methods include the diaphragm, cervical cap, sponge, condom, and spermicides. Besides contraception, an advantage to using these methods is that they can reduce the rate of sexually transmitted disease (STD) transmission.[4,6]

The diaphragm, a reusable dome-shaped rubber cap with a flexible rim that is inserted vaginally, fits over the cervix in order to decrease access of sperm to the ovum. The diaphragm is available in 11 sizes and requires a prescription from a physician who has fitted the patient for the correct size.[4,6] The effectiveness of the diaphragm depends on its function as a barrier and on the spermicidal cream or jelly placed in the diaphragm before insertion. The diaphragm may be inserted as long as 6 hours before intercourse and must be left in place for at least 6 hours after intercourse. If intercourse occurs more than once within 6 hours, the patient must not remove the diaphragm but rather should insert more spermicide and wear the diaphragm for 6 hours after subsequent acts of intercourse or use a condom. Contraindications to the diaphragm are listed in Table 77–1. Users of diaphragms appear to have a lower incidence of cervical neoplasia, which may be attributed to the adjunctive spermicide and the diaphragm's barrier effect against the human papilloma virus. Diaphragm use also has been associated with an increased incidence of urinary tract and yeast infections.

The Prentif cervical cap is a soft, deep, rubber cup with a firm round rim that is smaller than a diaphragm and fits over the cervix like a thimble.[4,6] Spermicide is used to fill the cap one-third full prior to insertion and is held in place against the cervix until the cap is removed. The cap remains effective for more than one episode (up to 48 hours) of intercourse without adding more spermicide; thus it is less messy to use than a diaphragm. However, because of the limited number of sizes, it may not be possible to fit some women with this device. It is recommended that women not wear the cap for longer than 48 hours to reduce the risk of toxic shock syndrome. A recent review by the Cochrane Library found that the Prentif cap was as effective as the diaphragm in preventing pregnancy and was less often associated with vaginal ulcerations or lacerations.[10]

Condoms are devices that create a mechanical barrier, preventing direct contact of the vagina with semen, genital lesions and discharges, and infectious secretions.[4,6] Most condoms made in the United States are made of latex rubber, which is impermeable to viruses; the small proportion (5%) made from young lamb intestine is not, however. Condoms are used worldwide as protection from STDs. When used in conjunction with any other barrier methods, their effectiveness theoretically approaches 95%. Spillage of semen or perforation and tearing of the condom can occur, but proper use minimizes these problems.[4] Mineral oil–based vaginal drug formulations (e.g., Cleocin vaginal cream, Premarin vaginal cream, Vagistat 1, Femstat, and Monistat Vaginal suppositories), lotions, or lubricants can decrease the barrier strength of latex by 90% in just 60 seconds, thus making water-soluble lubricants preferable if they are to come in contact with latex condoms.[4]

The female condom (Reality) appears to be as effective as the diaphragm in preventing pregnancy.[3] The female condom is a prelubricated, soft, loose-fitting polyurethane sheath, closed at one end, with flexible rings at both ends. Properly positioned, the ring at the closed end covers the cervix, and the sheath lines the walls of the vagina. The outer ring remains outside the vagina, covering the labia; this may make it more effective than the male condom in preventing transmission of diseases such as herpes because it protects the labia from contact with the base of the penis. The pregnancy rate is reported to be 26% per year, based on a 6-month follow-up study of 200 women.[3]

PHARMACOLOGIC THERAPY

SPERMICIDES

Spermicides, most of which contain nonoxynol-9, are chemical surfactants that destroy sperm cell walls and offer some protection against STDs and cervical cancer.[4] They are available as foams, creams, suppositories, jellies, and film.[4] Spermicidal tablets or suppositories require 10 to 30 minutes to dissolve. Spermicides can cause local irritation in both men and women. Additional spermicide must be used each time intercourse is repeated.

SPERMICIDE-IMPLANTED BARRIER TECHNIQUES

The vaginal contraceptive sponge (Today) is pillow shaped and contains 1 g of the spermicide nonoxynol-9.[4,11] It has a concave dimple on one side (to fit over the cervix and decrease the risk of dislodgement during intercourse) and a loop on the other side (to facilitate removal). After being moistened with tap water, the sponge is inserted into the vagina up to 6 hours before intercourse. The sponge provides protection for 24 hours, regardless of the frequency of intercourse during this time. After intercourse, the sponge must be left in place for at least 6 hours before removal. Sponges should not be left in place for more than 24 to 30 hours in order to reduce the risk of toxic shock syndrome. After use, sponges should be discarded (they are not effective for reuse). The sponge comes in one size and will soon be available over the counter. Production of the sponge was discontinued temporarily in 1995, and it is now being reviewed by the Food and Drug Administration (FDA) for rerelease in the United States.[4,11] The sponge is currently available in Canada, Europe, and the United Kingdom.

ORAL CONTRACEPTIVES

OCs are highly effective[4,6,12] (see Table 77–1). When used correctly, their effectiveness approaches that of surgical sterilization.

Composition and Formulations

The currently available OCs contain either a combination of a synthetic estrogen and synthetic progestin or a progestin alone. Estrogens suppress FSH and thus prevent the development of a dominant follicle. Estrogens also potentiate the action of the progestin component, which suppresses the LH surge. As a result, even if the estrogen component does not blunt follicular growth adequately, the action of the progestin blocks ovulation. Estrogen also serves to stabilize the endometrial lining (bleeding cycle control), whereas the progestin contributes to other contraceptive effects on cervical mucus (thickened/impermeable) and the endometrium (involution/atrophy).[4,6,12]

The low-dose combination OCs that are currently available are modifications of the original products introduced in 1960; these modified products contain approximately one-third to one-fourth the estrogen and one-tenth the progestin dose found in the earlier pills.[3] Over the past decade, combination multiphasic (biphasic and triphasic) formulations have further lowered the total monthly hormonal dose without clearly demonstrating a significant clinical advantage.[3,4,6] Also introduced in 1960, the progestin-only "minipills" (28 days of active hormone per cycle) are still available. Containing even lower doses of progestin than found in combination OCs and lacking the contribution of estrogen, minipills tend to be less effective than combination OCs with typical use and generally are reserved for women who must avoid estrogen.[3,4,6]

Components

Two synthetic estrogens commonly used in OCs in the United States, ethinyl estradiol (EE) and mestranol, differ only by the presence of a methyl group attached to mestranol at the C-3 site. Mestranol, which must be converted by the liver to ethinyl estradiol before it is pharmacologically active, is estimated to be 50% less potent than EE.[4,6,13]

Progestins currently used in OCs include drospirenone, ethynodiol diacetate, desogestrel, gestodene (not available in the United States), norgestimate, norethindrone, norethindrone acetate, norethynodrel, norgestrel, and norgestrel's active isomer levonorgestrel. Progestins vary in their progestational activity and differ with respect to inherent estrogenic, antiestrogenic, and androgenic effects.[4,6,13–15] Estrogenic and antiestrogenic properties are secondary to the extent of progestins' metabolism to estrogenic substances, whereas androgenic activity results from the structural similarity of the progestin to testosterone (receptor binding and activity) and the ability to affect free testosterone concentrations through impact on sex hormone–binding globulin, a major carrier protein for testosterone.[13,14]

Third-generation OCs contain newer progestins (e.g., desogestrel, drospirenone, gestodene, and norgestimate). These progestins are potent progestational agents that appear to have no estrogenic effects and are less androgenic when compared with levonorgestrel on a weight basis. Therefore, these agents are thought to be more effective in improving mild to moderate acne.[16] Drospirenone also has antimineralocorticoid or antialdosterone activities, which may result in less weight gain when compared with OCs containing levonorgestrel.

TABLE 77–2. Composition of Commonly Prescribed Oral Contraceptives

Product	Estrogen	mcg	Progestin	mg	Spotting and BTB
50 mcg Estrogen					
Necon 1/50M, Nelova 1/50M, Norinyl 1/50, Norethin 1/50M, Ortho-Novum 1/50	Mestranol	50	Norethindrone	1	10.6
Norlestrin 1/50	E. estradiol	50	Nor. acetate	1	103.6
Ovcon 50	E. estradiol	50	Norethindrone	1	11.9
Ovral, Ogestrel	E. estradiol	50	Norgestrel	0.5	4.5
Demulen 1/50, Zovia 1/50	E. estradiol	50	Ethy. diacetate	1	13.9
Sub-50 mcg Estrogen Monophasic					
Alesse, Levlite	E. estradiol	20	Levonorgestrel	0.1	26.5
Brevicon, Modicon, Necon 0.5/30	E. estradiol	35	Norethindrone	0.5	25.2
Demulen 1/35, Zovia 1/35	E. estradiol	35	Ethy. diacetate	1	37.4
Desogen, Ortho-Cept	E. estradiol	30	Desogestrel	0.15	13.1
Levlen, Levora 0.15/30, Nordette	E. estradiol	30	Levonorgestrel	0.15	14.0
Loestrin 1/20,[a] Microgestin 1/20	E. estradiol	20	Nor. acetate	1	29.7
Loestrin 1.5/30,[a] Microgestin 1.5/30	E. estradiol	30	Nor. acetate	1.5	25.2
Lo-Ovral, Low-Ogestrel	E. estradiol	30	Norgestrel	0.3	9.6
Necon 1/35, Norinyl 1/35, Norethin 1/35, Ortho-Novum 1/35	E. estradiol	35	Norethindrone	1	14.7
Ortho-Cyclen	E. estradiol	35	Norgestimate	0.25	14.3
Ovcon-35	E. estradiol	35	Norethindrone	0.4	11
Seasonale[b]	E. estradiol	30	Levonorgestrel	0.15	?
Yasmin	E. estradiol	30	Drospirenone	3	14.5
Sub-50 mcg Estrogen Multiphasic					
Cyclessa	E. estradiol	25 (7)	Desogestrel	0.1 (7)	11.1
		25 (7)		0.125 (7)	
		25 (7)		0.150 (7)	
Estrostep[a]	E. estradiol	20 (5)	Norethindrone	1 (5)	26.2
	E. estradiol	30 (7)	Norethindrone	1 (7)	
	E. estradiol	35 (9)	Norethindrone	1 (9)	
Mircette	E. estradiol	20 (21)	Desogestrel	0.15 (21)	19.7
	E. estradiol	10 (5)	Desogestrel		
Necon 10/11	E. estradiol	35 (10)	Norethindrone	0.5 (10)	17.6
Nelova 10/11	E. estradiol	35 (11)	Norethindrone	1 (11)	
Ortho-Novum 10/11					
Ortho-Novum 7/7/7	E. estradiol	35 (7)	Norethindrone	0.5 (7)	14.5
	E. estradiol	35 (7)	Norethindrone	0.175 (7)	
	E. estradiol	35 (7)	Norethindrone	1 (7)	
Ortho Tri-Cyclen	E. estradiol	35 (7)	Norgestimate	0.18 (7)	17.7
	E. estradiol	35 (7)	Norgestimate	0.215 (7)	
	E. estradiol	35 (7)	Norgestimate	0.25 (7)	
Tri-Levlen, Triphasil	E. estradiol	30 (6)	Levonorgestrel	0.05 (6)	15.1
Trivora	E. estradiol	40 (5)	Levonorgestrel	0.075 (5)	
	E. estradiol	30 (10)	Levonorgestrel	0.125 (10)	
Tri-Norinyl	E. estradiol	35 (7)	Norethindrone	0.5 (7)	25.5
Progestin Only					
Micronor/Nor-Q.D.	E. estradiol	—	Norethindrone	0.35	42.3
Ovrette	E. estradiol	—	Norgestrel	0.075	34.9

OK; products approved but not yet available.
91-day regimen.
Compiled from refs.13 and 14.

Unfortunately, clinical trials comparing the differences between OCs are few, and sample size is small, so the actual relevance of these purported improvements in progestational selectivity and lower androgenic activity remains unknown.[12,14] For example, a recent review by the Cochrane Library concluded that there was no evidence supporting a causal association between combination OCs or combination skin patches and weight gain.[17] Table 77–2 lists available OCs products by brand name and specifies hormonal composition.

Considerations with Oral Contraceptive Use

Oral contraceptives, when used properly, are extremely safe.[9] Numerous noncontraceptive benefits, including relief from menstruation-related problems (e.g., decreased menstrual cramps, decreased ovulatory pain [mittelschmerz], and decreased menstrual blood loss) and prevention of several diseases (e.g., ovarian and endometrial cancer, ovarian cysts, ectopic pregnancy, pelvic inflammatory disease [PID], and benign breast disease) have been attributed to the use of OCs (see Table 77–1). A complete medical history and blood pressure measurement should be obtained before a patient begins using OCs, and the risks and precautions associated with OC use warrant careful consideration.[4,6,7,12,13] The World Health Organization (WHO) has developed a graded list of precautions for clinicians to consider when they are providing OCs, and these precautions have replaced the traditional absolute and relative contraindications to the use of OCs. Many patient-specific characteristics and concomitant disease states increase the patient's risk for adverse effects relating to OC use[4,6,18] (Table 77–3).

Women Over 35 Years of Age. Generally, OCs are an acceptable form of birth control for nonsmoking women up to the time of menopause, with women over 35 using the lowest-dose estrogen products.[4,6,13,18] An ex-smoker for at least 1 year can be regarded as a nonsmoker.[6] A recent case-controlled study of healthy, nonsmoking women over age 35 years indicated that the use of OCs increased the risk of myocardial infarction (MI) and stroke.[19,20] As women approach the perimenopausal stage, OCs confer a benefit with respect to bone mineral density and vasomotor symptoms.[21] If women choose to use hormone therapy, they should switch from OCs in the perimenopausal period.[18,22]

Smoking. Women who smoke more than 20 cigarettes per day and are over age 35 should not use OCs containing estrogen. Those who smoke fewer than 20 cigarettes per day and are over age 35 should use them only with caution.[4,10,18,23] If smoking women use OCs, the 20-mcg estrogen formulation should be used.[23,24] This extremely low dose of OC does not appear to have an impact on clotting factors and platelet activation, even in smokers.[25] Progestin-only pills generally are acceptable for women in whom an estrogen is contraindicated.[26] In smoking women older than age 35, the risk of using OCs is likely to exceed the risk of pregnancy.[18]

Hypertension. Combination OCs, even those containing less than 35 mcg estrogen, can cause small increases in blood pressure, although clinically significant increases are rare with low-dose agents.[4,6,26] If an OC-related increase in blood pressure occurs, discontinuing the OC usually restores blood pressure to pretreatment values within 3 to 6 months.[4,6] The use of low-dose OCs is acceptable in women with well-controlled and well-monitored hypertension.[18] However, hypertensive women who have end-organ vascular disease (e.g., coronary artery disease, congestive heart failure, or cerebrovascular disease) or who smoke should not use combination OCs.[18] Women with hypertension taking potassium-sparing diuretics, angiotensin-converting enzyme inhibitors, angiotensin-receptor blockers, or aldosterone antagonists may see an increase in serum potassium concentration if they are also using an OC containing drospirenone (e.g., Yasmin), which has antialdosterone properties.[15]

Diabetes. Oral contraceptives appear to affect carbohydrate and lipid metabolism, possibly through the progestin component.[4,26,27] With the exception of some levonorgestrel-containing products, formulations containing low doses of progestins do not significantly alter insulin, glucose, or glucagon release after a glucose load in healthy women or in those with a history of gestational diabetes.[4,27] The new progestins are believed to have little, if any, effect on carbohydrate metabolism.[4,27] Studies of women with type 1 diabetes did not find any association between blood glucose control and the use of OCs.[28] In the Nurses' Health Study, women using OCs did not demonstrate any increased risk of developing type 2 diabetes.[29] Nonsmoking women

with diabetes but no associated vascular disease can use OCs safely.[18] However, diabetic women with vascular disease (e.g., hypertension, nephropathy, retinopathy, or neuropathy) should not use OCs.[18]

Dyslipidemia. Generally, synthetic progestins adversely affect lipid metabolism by decreasing the level of high-density lipoprotein (HDL) and increasing the level of low-density lipoprotein (LDL). Estrogens tend to have more beneficial effects by increasing the removal of LDL from the circulation and increasing the level of HDL through increases in ApoA$_1$. Estrogens also may alter the composition of very low density lipoprotein (VLDL) and increase the level of triglycerides.[27] Most low-dose combination OCs, with the possible exception of monophasic levonorgestrel (0.15 mg) pills, have no significant impact on HDL, LDL, triglycerides, or total cholesterol.[6,14,26,27]

Although the lipid effects of OCs theoretically can influence cardiovascular risk, the mechanism of the increased incidence of cardiovascular disease in OC users is believed to be secondary to thromboembolic and thrombotic changes, not atherosclerosis. Numerous epidemiologic studies have failed to find an association between OC use and cardiovascular disease.[18,30] Women with controlled dyslipidemia can use low-dose OCs, although they need frequent monitoring by means of a fasting lipid panel after they begin using these agents.[18] Women with uncontrolled dyslipidemia (LDL > 160 mg/dL, HDL < 35 mg/dL, triglycerides > 250 mg/dL) and additional risk factors (e.g., coronary artery disease, diabetes, hypertension, smoking, or a positive family history) should use an alternative method of contraception.[18]

Thromboembolism. Estrogens play a dose-related role in the development of venous thromboembolism (VTE) and consequent pulmonary embolism, especially in women who smoke or have other underlying inherited conditions (e.g., deficiencies in antithrombin III, protein C, and protein S levels or factor V Leiden mutation) or acquired conditions (e.g., immobility, trauma, surgery, and certain malignancies) that predispose them to coagulation abnormalities.[4,6,31] Early observational studies reported the incidence of VTE to be much higher in OC users than in nonusers, but a recent reevaluation of these data suggest that the risk of VTE is much less with non-third-generation OCs (less than a threefold increase in relative risk) than originally thought.[15,32,33] In addition, the absolute risk is low (15 cases per 100,000 woman-years). The increased risk of VTE and pulmonary embolism appears to be limited to current users, with disappearance of the risk within 3 months after the use of the OC ceases.[6,15,34] The 20-mcg EE formulations do not appear to have an effect on clotting parameters, even in smokers, but whether these products lower the risk of thrombotic events has not been studied.[26,35]

European studies of third-generation OCs reported a possible relationship between these agents and the procoagulant effects of OCs. In early studies, researchers found that users of third-generation agents containing gestodene or desogestrel had a twofold greater risk of nonfatal VTE than women using the older low-dose combination OCs.[3,4,6] More recent data have shown a small increase in the risk of VTE but do not establish a cause-and-effect relationship.[35,36] There also have been reports of VTE in patients receiving OCs containing drospirenone.[15] Some clinicians argue that this difference reflects preferential prescribing of the newer, and perceived safer, progestin products for women at greater risk for VTE.[13,24,37–39] The FDA has concluded that this evidence is not persuasive enough to support any changes in current prescribing patterns or to recommend discontinuation of third-generation OCs.[12,24]

Currently, OCs are contraindicated in any woman with a history of VTE or pulmonary embolism (see Table 77–3). Women who

TABLE 77–3. Precautions in the Provision of Combined Oral Contraceptives (OCs)

Precautions	Rationale/Discussion
World Health Organization Category #4: Refrain from providing combined oral contraceptives for women with the following diagnoses.	
• Deep vein thrombosis or pulmonary embolism, or a history thereof	• Estrogens promote blood clotting. Thromboembolic events related to known trauma or an intravenous needle are not necessarily a reason to avoid use of pills.
• Cerebrovascular accident (stroke), coronary artery or ischemic heart disease, or a history thereof	• Estrogens promote blood clotting.
• Structural heart disease, complicated by pulmonary hypertension, atrial fibrillation, or history of subacute bacterial endocarditis	• Estrogens promote blood clotting.
• Diabetes with nephropathy, retinopathy, neuropathy, or other vascular disease; diabetes of more than 20 years' duration	• Estrogens promote blood clotting.
• Breast cancer	• Breast cancer is a hormonally sensitive tumor. In theory, the hormones in OCs might cause some masses to grow.
• Pregnancy	• Current data do not show that hormonal contraceptives taken during pregnancy cause any significant risk of birth defects. However, hormonal contraceptives should not be given to pregnant women.
• Lactation (<6 weeks postpartum)	• There is some theoretical concern that the neonate may be at risk owing to exposure to steroid hormones during the first 6 weeks postpartum. OCs can diminish the volume of breast milk.
• Liver problems: benign hepatic adenoma or liver cancer, or a history thereof; active viral hepatitis; severe cirrhosis	• OCs are metabolized by the liver, and their use may adversely affect prognosis of existing disease.
• Headaches, including migraine (with aural), with focal neurologic symptoms	• Focal neurologic symptoms such as blurred vision, seeing flashing lights or zigzag lines, or trouble speaking or moving may be an indication of an increased risk of stroke.
• Major surgery with prolonged immobilization or any surgery on the legs	• Risk for deep vein thrombosis and pulmonary embolism is increased.
• Over 35 years old and currently a heavy smoker (20 or more cigarettes a day)	• Smoking increases the risk for cardiovascular disease.
• Hypertension, 160+ mmHg/100+ mmHg or with vascular disease	• Hypertension is an important risk factor for cardiovascular disease.
World Health Organization Category #3: Exercise caution if combined oral contraceptives are used or considered in the following situations and carefully monitor for adverse effects.	
• Postpartum <21 days	• There is some theoretical concern regarding the association between OC use up to 3 weeks postpartum and risk of thrombosis.
• Lactation (6 weeks to 6 months)	• In the first 6 months postpartum, use of OCs during breastfeeding diminishes the quantity of breast milk and may adversely affect the health of the infant.
• Undiagnosed abnormal vaginal/uterine bleeding	• Although OCs are often used to manage heavy bleeding, clinicians should be sure that the cause of the bleeding is known before prescribing OCs.
• Over 35 years of age and light smoker (fewer than 20 cigarettes/day)	• Smoking increases the risk for cardiovascular disease. All smokers should be warned of this risk and should be encouraged and advised to stop smoking.
• Past history of breast cancer, but no evidence of recurrence for 5 years	• Breast cancer is a hormonally sensitive tumor.
• Use of drugs that affect liver enzymes (rifampicin, rifabutin and griseofulvin); use of drugs that affect liver enzymes (phenytoin, carbamazepine, barbiturates, topiramate, and primidone)	• OCs are metabolized by the liver. Drugs that affect liver enzymes could reduce the contraceptive effectiveness of OCs.
• Gallbladder disease: medically treated and current biliary tract disease and history of OC-related cholestasis	• Recent reports show that OCs may be weakly associated with the development of gallbladder disease. There is also concern that OCs may worsen existing gallbladder disease.
World Health Organization Category #2: Advantages generally outweigh theoretical or proven disadvantages and generally can be provided without restrictions in these conditions.	
• Severe headaches that definitely start after initiation of OCs; migraine headaches without focal neurologic symptoms (without aura)	• Migraine headaches with focal neurologic symptoms have been associated with an increased risk of stroke; any headaches clearly starting after initiation of pills may be related to pill use.
• Diabetes mellitus: gestational diabetes or diabetes without vascular disease	• Women with diabetes are at increased risk of heart disease and stroke, particularly if the woman smokes. Estrogens and progestins may slightly decrease glucose tolerance, but this is unlikely to happen with low-dose OCs.
• Major surgery without prolonged immobilization	• With the current low-dose pills, the problems associated with pill use and elective surgery have decreased.
• Sickle cell disease or sickle C disease	• Women with sickle cell disease are predisposed to occlusion of the microvasculature (because of abnormal, inflexible red blood cells). Studies of women with sickle cell disease have shown no significant differences between OC users and non-users with regard to coagulation studies, blood viscosity measurements, or incidence or severity of painful sickle cell crisis.

(continued)

TABLE 77–3. (*Continued*)

Precautions	Rationale/Discussion
• Moderate blood pressure (140–159 mmHg/100–109 mmHg)	• Monitor blood pressure periodically. Hypertension is an important risk factor for cardiovascular disease.
• Undiagnosed breast mass	• Some clinicians and clinical protocols suggest that women found to have a breast mass should not be provided combined OCs until cancer of the breast has been ruled out. Other clinicians are comfortable prescribing pills while the cause of the breast mass is being evaluated.
• Cervical cancer awaiting treatment and cervical intraepithelial neoplasia	• The risk of cervical cancer appears to be increased slightly in OC users. OC users may get Papanicolaou smears more regularly so that early dysplasia is more likely to be recognized. They also tend to have more sexual partners. Pill use may also alter susceptibility to infection with human papilloma virus a known risk factor for cancer of the cervix.
• Over 50 years of age	• Women over 50 are at increased risk for heart and cerebrovascular disease.
• Conditions likely to make it very difficult for a woman to take OCs consistently and correctly	• Mental retardation, major psychiatric illness, alcoholism, or other chemical abuse, and/or a history of repeatedly taking OCs or other medications incorrectly, make compliance with OC regimens difficult.
• Family history of hyperlipidemia	• Some types of hyperlipidemia increase a woman's risk for heart disease. Routine screening is not recommended by WHO because of the rarity of the conditions and the high cost of screening.
• Family history of death of a parent or sibling due to myocardial infarction before age 50	• Myocardial infarction in a mother or sister is especially significant and suggests a need for lipid evaluation.

World Health Organization Category #1: Do not restrict use of combined oral contraceptives for the following conditions.

- Postpartum ≥21 days
- Postabortion after first or second trimester or immediately after postseptic abortion
- History of gestational diabetes
- Varicose veins
- Mild headaches
- Irregular vaginal bleeding patterns, without or with heavy or prolonged bleeding and not anemia
- Past history of pelvic inflammatory disease (PID)
- Current or recent history of (within last 3 months) PID
- Current or recent history of (within last 3 months) sexually transmitted infection (STI)
- Vaginitis without purulent cervicitis
- Increased risk of STI (i.e., multiple partners or partner who has multiple partners)
- Infection with human immunodeficiency virus (HIV), high risk or HIV or acquired immunodeficiency syndrome (AIDS)
- Benign breast disease
- Family history of breast cancer
- Cervical ectropion
- Endometrial or ovarian cancer
- Viral hepatitis carrier
- Uterine fibroids
- Past ectopic pregnancy
- Obesity
- Thyroid conditions: simple goiter, hyperthyroidism, hypothyroidism
- Benign or malignant gestational trophoblastic disease
- Iron deficiency anemia
- Epilepsy
- Schistosomiasis (uncomplicated or with fibrosis of the liver)
- Malaria
- Current use of antibiotics
- Nulliparity or parity
- Severe dysmenorrhea
- Tuberculosis, including pelvic
- Endometriosis
- Benign ovarian tumors
- Prior pelvic surgery

Compiled from refs. 4 and 18.

evelop thrombotic complications while taking a low-dose OCs
ould have an examination for an underlying coagulation
isorder.[4,6,13,18] Some experts support the use of OCs in women with
oagulation disorders *who have been properly anticoagulated,* citing
e potential advantages of lowering the risk of fetal exposure to war-
arin, bleeding corpus luteum cysts, and excessive blood loss during
enses.[4,6,18]

Cerebrovascular Disease. Both thrombotic and hemorrhagic
troke have been associated with the use of OCs. However, early
udies used higher-dose products and did not take into account in-
ependent risk factors for vascular disease (e.g., smoking, hyperten-
on, and advancing age). Recent studies evaluating low-dose OCs
und the risk for stroke to be extremely low in healthy young
omen.[19,20,40,41] These results suggest that the effect of smoking in
omen younger than 35 years of age is minimal in the absence of
ypertension and that hypertension may be the major risk factor for
troke.[13,42,43] Cerebrovascular accidents often are preceded by persis-
ent headaches (for weeks or months) and/or by temporary hemipare-
is. Patients should be screened carefully and counseled to recognize
arning signs of cerebrovascular accidents in order to decrease risk.

Migraine Headaches. Women in their reproductive years fre-
uently experience headaches, ranging in variety from tension
eadache to simple (without aura) and classic migraine (with aura).[18]
)Cs usually decrease the frequency of migraine headaches, but they
xacerbate symptoms in some women; headaches may even occur
uring the hormone-free interval (during menses). There is some ev-
dence that migraine headaches are a risk factor for stroke and that
lassic migraine (with aura) may increase the risk of stroke more than
imple migraine (without aura) does.[18,44] The absolute risk of stroke
n women using OCs who experience simple migraines is relatively
ow, but the risk of stroke among those with classic migraines is still
ndetermined. Combination OCs may be used in young (less than
5 years of age), healthy, nonsmoking women with migraine
eadaches if they do not have focal neurologic signs.[18]

Myocardial Infarction. Generally, myocardial infarction (MI) in
)C users occurs primarily in those older than 35 years of age who
ave additional risk factors for cardiovascular disease (e.g., smoking,
iabetes, hypertension, and obesity).[4,6,13] These risk factors, in par-
icular smoking, appear to act synergistically with OCs to increase the
isk of cardiovascular disease.[13] A large British study found a 21-fold
ncrease in MI among women taking OCs who smoke more than 15
igarettes daily but no apparent increased risk in healthy, nonsmoking
vomen regardless of age.[45] Since the FDA lifted its restrictions on OC
ise in healthy, nonsmoking women over 40 years of age in 1989, OCs
ontaining 30 mcg estrogen or less are being used more frequently
n these women up to the age of menopause without evidence of sig-
ificantly increased risk of cardiovascular events.[4,6,13,43] Recent data
uggest that the use of low-dose OCs containing third-generation pro-
estins may reduce the incidence of MI to a rate that is similar to that
f MI in nonusers.[43,46] Therefore, healthy, nonsmoking women can
ise OCs safely without an increased risk of MI. Women with a history
f coronary artery disease and those who smoke and have other risk
actors for MI should not use combined OCs but rather should use
rogestin-only or nonhormonal methods of contraception.[18]

Cancer. The risk for ovarian and endometrial cancer decreases by
0% to 50% with OC use, and the beneficial effect is believed to persist
or at least 15 years after the use ceases.[4,6,9,23,24] The relationship
etween OCs and other cancers is controversial. OCs increase cervical
ctopy, but the association with cervical cancer is unclear.

Worldwide epidemiologic data from 54 studies in 25 countries
(many of which studied high-dose OCs) were reanalyzed recently
to assess the relationship between the use of OCs and the risk of
breast cancer.[47,48] Researchers concluded that women who began to
use these agents before age 20 had a higher relative risk compared
with users who began at later ages. They also found that women
currently taking OCs and those within 10 years of ceasing to take them
have a small increase in the risk of breast cancer, but these cancers
were less clinically advanced than in women who had never used
OCs.[21,47,48] Prospective data from the Nurses' Health Study cohort
showed no overall relationship between the duration of OC use and
breast cancer, even in long-term users (>10 years), and researchers
concluded that long-term past use, either overall or prior to a full-term
pregnancy, did not increase the risk of breast cancer in women over
40 years of age.[49] This was confirmed by a recent case-control study
that demonstrated that former or current OC use was not associated
with an increased risk of breast cancer in women 35 to 64 years of
age.[50] It will take many years to discover what, if any, impact the low-
dose OCs will have on breast cancer risk. The current recommendation
is that a positive family history of breast cancer in a mother or sister,
or both, or a history of benign breast disease should not be regarded
as a contraindication to OC use.[18]

Systemic Lupus Erythematosus. The use of hormonal contraception is important in women with systemic lupus erythematosus (SLE)
because the risk associated with pregnancy is high in this population.
It has been thought that hormonal contraception may exacerbate the
symptoms of SLE.[18,51] Retrospective studies have not found an association between combined OCs and disease flare-ups in these patients,
but there does appear to be an association between VTE and OC use
in women with SLE and antiphospholipid antibodies.[18,51] Progestin-
only contraceptives should be used in women with SLE and in women
with a history of vascular disease or antiphospholipid antibodies, and
combination OCs should be avoided.[18,51]

Choice of an Oral Contraceptive

◁ ◁ Before prescribing an OC, the clinician must ask and answer
several questions. Are there any precautions to consider in
the use of OCs (see Table 77–3)? Does this form of contraception fit
the patient's lifestyle, and will the patient be compliant? The clinician should discuss the advantages and disadvantages of all available
forms of contraception with the patient to ensure that she can make
an informed choice (see Table 77–1).

Progestin-only pills (minipills) tend to be less effective than combination OCs with typical use and are associated with irregular and
unpredictable menstrual bleeding, as well as an increased frequency
of functional ovarian cysts.[4,6,13] Irregular menstrual cycles indicate
that ovulation has been inhibited; however, this is one of the most
frequent reasons for the discontinuation of the minipill. Unlike combination OCs, minipills are always begun on the first day of menses
and must be taken every day at approximately the same time to maintain contraceptive efficacy. Since minipills may not block ovulation
(nearly 40% of women continue to ovulate normally), the risk of ectopic pregnancy is higher with their use than with the use of other
hormonal contraceptives.

All combined OCs (monophasic and multiphasic) are similarly
effective in preventing pregnancy (see Table 77–1). Although multiphasic pills have a lower total hormone dose per cycle, there is no
convincing evidence that they provide any advantage or cause fewer
side effects than monophasic pills. In addition, some women find
monophasic pills to be simpler to take. A reasonable first choice of an

TABLE 77-4. Symptoms of a Serious or Potentially Serious Nature Associated With Oral Contraceptives (OCs)

Symptom	Possible Cause
Serious: OCs Should Be Stopped Immediately	
Loss of vision, proptosis, diplopia, papilledema	Retinal artery thrombosis
Unilateral numbness, weakness, or tingling	Hemorrhagic or thrombotic stroke
Severe pains in chest, left arm, or neck	Myocardial infarction
Hemoptysis	Pulmonary embolism
Severe pains, tenderness or swelling, warmth, or palpable cord in legs	Thrombophlebitis
Slurring of speech	Hemorrhagic or thrombotic stroke
Hepatic mass or tenderness	Liver neoplasm
Potentially Serious: OCs May Be Continued With Caution While Patient Is Being Evaluated	
Absence of menses	Pregnancy
Spotting or breakthrough bleeding	Cervical, endometrial, or vaginal cancer
Breast mass, pain, or swelling	Breast cancer
Right upper-quadrant pain	Cholecystitis, cholelithiasis, or liver neoplasm
Midepigastric pain	Thrombosis of abdominal artery or vein, myocardial infarction, or pulmonary embolism
Migraine (vascular or throbbing) headache	Vascular spasm which may precede thrombosis
Severe nonvascular headache	Hypertension, vascular spasm
Galactorrhea	Pituitary adenoma
Jaundice, pruritus	Cholestatic jaundice
Depression	Vitamin B_6 deficiency
Uterine size increase	Leiomyomata, adenomyosis, pregnancy

From ref. 13, with permission.

OC is a monophasic pill containing 30 to 35 mcg EE[3,4,6,24] (see Table 77-2). This strategy is based on evidence that the most serious side effects of combination OCs (i.e., thromboembolic events, stroke, or MI) result from excessive estrogen content.[4,6,13,24]

Products containing 20 mcg EE may cause less bloating and breast tenderness, and women over 40 years of age may prefer them. However, these low-estrogen OCs lead to more breakthrough bleeding and an increased risk of contraceptive failure if doses are missed.[3,4,6,13] Because all combined OCs raise sex hormone–binding globulin and decrease free testosterone levels, women may experience an improvement in acne symptoms.[52] Norgestimate-containing OCs also have been shown to improve acne symptoms, and Ortho Tri-Cyclen and Estrostep are specifically approved by the FDA for this indication[53-55] (see Table 77-2).

3 Many symptoms occurring in the first cycle of OC use (e.g., breakthrough bleeding and side effects related to estrogen excess) improve spontaneously by the second or third cycle of use as the body adjusts to the altered hormone level.[6,13] Therefore, initial OC use should be reevaluated during the first 3 to 6 months of therapy to determine if the patient is experiencing any adverse effects and if th patient wishes to continue medication.

If the patient complains of symptoms related to the use of th OC, it is necessary to determine if the symptom indicates the pres ence or potential development of a serious illness[4,13] (Tables 77– and 77–5). Nearly all OC-induced side effects parallel the symptom and physiologic changes of pregnancy (hormone excess) or the peri menopausal period (hormone deficiency). In some cases, symptom relating to the hormonal imbalance may improve with adjustments i the specific combination of estrogen and progestin because progestin can contribute to estrogenic and antiestrogenic activity. However, th clinically significant differences between the low-dose OCs used to day are difficult to distinguish. Several useful handbooks and article are available to the practitioner in managing side effects associate with OCs.[3,4,6,12,13]

For example, women who continue to experience nausea afte 3 months of OC use may benefit from a change to a pill with lowe estrogenic activity. In addition, taking the OC with food or at bedtim also has been recommended.

TABLE 77-5. Symptoms That May Be Warnings of Serious Trouble[a]

Five Signals	Possible Problem
Abdominal pain (severe)	Gallbladder disease, hepatic adenoma, blood clot, pancreatitis
Chest pain (severe), shortness of breath, or coughing up blood	Blood clot in lungs or myocardial infarction (heart attack)
Headaches (severe)	Stroke, hypertension, or migraine headache
Eye problems: blurred vision, flashing lights, or blindness	Stroke, hypertension, or temporary vascular problem of many possible sites
Severe leg pain (calf or thigh)	Blood clot in legs

[a] See your clinician if you have any of these problems, or if you develop depression, yellow jaundice, or a breast lump.
From ref. 4, with permission.

CLINICAL CONTROVERSY

There is a widely held belief that antibiotics reduce the efficacy of OCs, increasing the risk of pregnancy. However, there are little data to support this drug interaction with most antibiotics, with the exception of rifampin. Because of this potential risk, and considering the fact that OCs are not 100% effective, many practitioners still counsel patients about this issue. The Council on Scientific Affairs at the American Medical Association recommends that women be informed about the small risk of interactions with antibiotics and, if desired, provided with additional nonhormonal contraceptive agents.

Drug Interactions

The effectiveness of an OC is sometimes limited by drug interactions that interfere with gastrointestinal absorption, increase intestinal motility by altering gut bacteriologic flora, and alter the metabolism, excretion, or binding of the OC[4,12,13,18,24,57] (Table 77–6).

TABLE 77–6. Interactions of Oral Contraceptives (OCs) With Other Drugs

Interacting Drugs	Adverse Effects (Probable Mechanism)	Comments and Recommendation
Acetaminophen (Tylenol and others)	Possible decreased pain-relieving effect (increased metabolism)	Monitor pain-relieving response
Alcohol	Possible increased effect of alcohol	Use with caution
Ampicillin	Decreased contraceptive effect	Low but unpredictable incidence; use backup method of contraception
Anticoagulants (oral)	Decreased anticoagulant effect	Use with caution, monitor INR
Anticonvulsants (barbiturates, including phenobarbital and primidone; carbamazepine; felbamate; phenytoin; topiramate; vigabatrin)	Possible decreased contraceptive effect	Avoid simultaneous use; use alternative contraceptive (DMPA) for patients with seizure disorder
Antidepressants (Elavil, Norpramin, Tofranil, and others)	Possible increased antidepressant pharmacologic effect	Monitor for adverse effects
Benzodiazepine tranquilizers (Ativan, Librium, Serax, Tranxene, Valium, Xanax, and others)	Possible increased or decreased tranquilizer effects including psychomotor impairment	Use with caution; greatest impairment during drug-free week in oral contraceptive dosage
β-Blockers (Corgard, Inderal, Lopressor, Tenormin)	Possible increased β-blocker pharmacologic effect	Monitor cardiovascular status
Corticosteroids (cortisone)	Possible increased corticosteroid toxicity	Clinical significance not established
Griseofulvin (Fulvicin, Grifulvin V, and others)	Decreased contraceptive effect	Use backup method of contraception
Hypoglycemics (Tolbutamide, Diabinese, Orinase, Tolinase)	Possible decreased hypoglycemic effect	Monitor blood glucose
Methyldopa (Aldoclor, Aldomet, and others)	Possible decreased antihypertensive effect, especially with high-dose OCs	Monitor blood pressure
Non-nucleoside reverse transcriptase inhibitors (Sustiva, Viramune)	Decreased contraceptive effect (Viramune), possible decreased contraceptive effect (Sustiva)	Use alternative method of contraception
Phenytoin (Dilantin)	Decreased contraceptive effect, possible increased phenytoin effect	Use alternative contraceptive (DMPA); monitor phenytoin concentration
Pioglitazone (Actos)	Decreased contraceptive effect documented with previous thiazolidinedione, troglitazone (Rezulin); no documented interaction with rosiglitazone (Avandia); interaction with pioglitazone (Actos) not studied	Use alternative method of contraception
Protease inhibitors (Agenerase, Crixivan, Norvir, Viracept)	Decreased contraceptive effect (Agenerase, Norvir, Viracept), possible decreased contraceptive effect (Crixivan)	Use alternative method of contraception
Rifampin	Decreased contraceptive effect	Use backup method of contraception; use alternate method if planned concomitant use is long term
Sulfonamides	Decreased contraceptive effect	Use backup method of contraception
Tetracycline	Decreased contraceptive effect	Use backup method of contraception
Theophylline (Bronkotabs, Marax, Primatene, Quibron, Tedral, TheoDur, and others)	Decreased contraceptive effect, increased theophylline effect	Monitor theophylline concentration
Troleandomycin (TAO)	Jaundice (additive)	Avoid simultaneous use
Vitamin C	Increased serum concentration and possible increased adverse effects of estrogens with 1 g or more per day of vitamin C	Avoid high dose of vitamin C

INR, International Normalized Ratio; DMPA, depomedroxyprogesterone acetate.
Compiled from refs. 4, 12, 13, 18, 24, and 56.

The lower the dose of hormone in the OC, the greater is the risk that a drug interaction will compromise its efficacy. Women should be instructed to use a an alternative method of contraception (e.g., condoms) if there is a possibility of a drug interacting altering the efficacy of the OC.[4] Several recent reviews of the interaction between antibiotics and OCs have documented a true pharmacokinetic interaction with rifampin in which the efficacy of OCs is impaired. Pharmacokinetic studies of other antibiotics have not shown any consistent interaction, but case reports of individual patients have shown a reduction in EE levels when taken with tetracyclines and penicillin derivatives.[57,58] The Council on Scientific Affairs at the American Medical Association recommends that women taking rifampin should be counseled about the risk of OC failure and advised to use an additional nonhormonal contraceptive agent during the course of rifampin therapy. The council also recommends that women should be informed about the small risk of interactions with other antibiotics, and if desired, appropriate additional nonhormonal contraceptive agents should be considered. In addition, women who develop breakthrough bleeding during concomitant use of antibiotics and OCs should be advised to use an alternate method of contraception during the period of concomitant use.[57]

Women receiving anticonvulsants for a seizure disorder require special attention with regard to hormonal contraception. Giving a hormonal contraceptive concomitantly with phenobarbital, carbamazepine, or phenytoin reduces the contraceptive's efficacy, and many anticonvulsants (e.g., phenytoin) are known teratogens. The use of condoms in conjunction with high-estrogen OCs, injectable progestin-only contraceptives, or intrauterine devices may be considered for these women.[18]

Patient Instructions

◀1 ◀4 ◀6 Many women who take OCs are poorly informed about the proper use of these medications. The patient first should be given the package insert that accompanies all estrogen products and instructed to read it carefully. The written information in the package insert should be supplemented with verbal information describing the way in which the medication works (primarily by stopping release of the egg from the ovary), both common and serious side effects, and the management of those side effects. Although there often are several transient self-limiting side effects (e.g., breast tenderness, bloating, breakthrough bleeding, spotting, and nausea), the patient should be aware of the danger signals (see Table 77–5) that require immediate medical attention[3,4,6] (see Table 77–4). Also, the benefits and risks should be discussed in terms that the patient can understand, including the fact that OCs provide no physical barrier to the transmission of STDs, including the human immunodeficiency virus (HIV). Detailed instructions for when to start taking the medication should be provided. Patients can either start taking the OC on the first Sunday after menses (which provides for period-free weekends) or on the first day of the next menses—either option is appropriate. Patients should be told the importance of routine daily administration to ensure consistent plasma concentrations and improve compliance, and specific instructions should be given regarding what to do if a pill is not taken. Important drug interactions should be discussed.

The patient taking combination OCs should expect her menses to start within 1 to 3 days after taking the last active pill. She should start another pack of pills immediately after finishing a 28-day pack (no days between) or 1 week after finishing the previous 21-day pack, even if her menses is not completed.[4,6,13] The use of an additional contraceptive method is advisable while the patient is taking the first pack of pills (especially if she began 5 days or more after the start of her menses), if she misses more than one pill per cycle, or if she experiences severe diarrhea or vomiting for several days. Patients taking progestin-only pills should be advised to use a backup method for 48 hours if they are 3 or more hours late in taking their daily progestin dose.

There is increasing interest in the use of continuous OCs to eliminate monthly withdrawal bleeding. Several prospective studies have assessed the efficacy of continuous OCs in preventing withdrawal bleeding and have found monophasic OCs to be most useful for this purpose. Although patients may experience increased breakthrough bleeding and spotting, there may be a decrease in headache and other menstruation-associated symptoms. With continued use for 1 year, there have not been any significant changes in blood pressure, weight, or hemoglobin when compared with cyclic users. However, long-term studies have not been done to assess the risk of cancer, VTE, or changes in fertility.[59,60] As an alternative to continuous OCs, a product has been approved recently by the FDA that will produce four menstrual periods per year.[61] This OC pill will provide 12 weeks (84 days) of active EE and levonorgestrel and then 1 week of inactive pills. Therefore, it will allow for one menstrual period per season and is marketed as Seasonale. However, reports from clinical trials demonstrated more breakthrough bleeding and spotting, particularly in the first few cycles, than in women taking a conventional 28-day-cycle OC.

Discontinuation of the Oral Contraceptive, Return of Fertility, and Breast-Feeding

Women who have used OCs may take longer to return to their baseline fertility than women who have used barrier contraception methods. Eventually, the percentage of women who conceive after discontinuing the use of OCs becomes the same as for barrier method users.[4,6,13]

Traditionally, women are counseled to allow two to three normal menstrual periods before becoming pregnant to permit the reestablishment of menses and ovulation.[4,6,13] However, in several large cohort and case-controlled studies, the infants conceived in the first month after an oral contraceptive was discontinued had no greater chance of miscarriage or being born with a birth defect than those born in the general population.[13]

CLINICAL CONTROVERSY

Existing randomized, controlled trials are insufficient to establish an effect of hormonal contraception, if any, on milk quality and quantity. Current recommendations are to avoid combined OCs in the first 6 weeks postpartum and to use them with caution during the 6-month postpartum period.

It is acceptable to begin any method of hormonal contraception immediately after first- or second-trimester termination of pregnancy (spontaneous or induced). Following third-trimester childbirth, ovulation usually does not begin again for 3 weeks (even in a non-breast-feeding woman), and the risk of maternal thromboembolic disease is increased for approximately the same time period.[4,6,62,63] Ideally, therefore, estrogen-containing contraceptives are withheld until the third week after delivery, but progestin-only formulations can be initiated immediately.[4,6,24]

◀5 Because the hormones in OCs are excreted into breast milk, breast-feeding generally is regarded as a relative contraindication to OC use. This contraindication was based on earlier formulations containing higher doses of hormones and probably does not apply to current formulations.[63] Another concern is that estrogens inhibit the action of prolactin at breast tissue receptors, resulting in decreased milk production and protein content.[3,4,6,13] Although this is not a particular problem in well-nourished lactating women, many practitioners recommend progestin-only contraceptives because progestins do not diminish the amount of breast milk and provide highly effective contraception in breast-feeding women.[4,6,13,18,64]

A recent review by the Cochrane Library indicated that existing randomized, controlled trials are insufficient to establish an effect of hormonal contraception, if any, on milk quality and quantity.[64] Furthermore, the review stated that current recommendations are for breast-feeding women to avoid combined OCs in the first 6 weeks postpartum and to use them with caution in the 6-month postpartum period.[64]

CLINICAL CONTROVERSY

Emergency contraception is likely to be available over the counter because prescription use is thought to limit access, leading to unintended pregnancies. Prior to this change, some states allowed pharmacists to dispense emergency contraception without a prescription, and others were considering collaborative practice agreements to increase pharmacists' ability to provide emergency contraception and counsel women receiving this regimen. Regardless of prescription status, the pharmacist can play an important role in assisting women to use this method correctly.

EMERGENCY CONTRACEPTION

High doses of estrogens can inhibit ovulation, in addition to causing a rapid shedding of the endometrium and preventing implantation of the fertilized ovum.[3,4,12,65] OCs in one-time high doses are safe and effective as emergency contraception (EC) to prevent pregnancy after unprotected intercourse (e.g., condom breakage, diaphragm dislodging, or sexual assault). The FDA has approved two hormonal contraceptive products (Preven and Plan B) specifically packaged for this use. In most states, EC is available by prescription only. This is viewed as a public health problem, leading to more unintended pregnancies by limiting access to the regimen. Some states allow pharmacists to dispense EC without a physician's prescription, and many others are considering this legislation.[66,67] Several organizations (AMA, ACOG) support over-the-counter availability of EC and are lobbying the FDA to change this policy.[66-68]

The Preven Emergency Contraceptive Kit contains four blue tablets, each containing 50 mcg EE and 0.25 mg levonorgestrel (similar to four tablets of Ovral, also known as the Yuzpe regimen). The kit also contains a patient education booklet and a urine pregnancy test to determine if the woman is already pregnant. Plan B contains two white tablets, each containing 0.75 mg levonorgestrel (similar to two 10-tablet doses of Ovrette). The first dose of each of these regimens is to be taken within 72 hours of unprotected intercourse (although the sooner, the more effective); the second dose, 12 hours later.[3,4,12,65] One study found single-dose Plan B (1.5 mg levonorgestrel) to be as effective as two-dose Plan B or mifepristone, but this regimen is not yet approved by the FDA.[69]

Despite the availability of the new products, it is still permissible to use regular contraceptives for EC. Specifically, the FDA has declared the following regimens safe and effective methods of EC: Ovral (2 tablets/dose); Nordette, Levlen, Levora, Lo/Ovral, Triphasil, Tri-Levlen, or Trivora (4 tablets/dose); and Alesse or Levlite (5 tablets/dose).[3,4,13] In addition, progestin-only pills can be used as EC, but a large number of tablets must be taken: Ovrette (20 tablets/dose).[3,4,13] When these regular contraceptives are used, the first dose should be taken within 72 hours of unprotected intercourse, with a follow-up dose 12 hours after the first.[3,4,13]

The efficacy of any of the regimens for EC declines if they begin more than 72 hours after intercourse.[3,4,13] Treatment is totally ineffective by 7 days, when implantation usually occurs. Patients may experience nausea, vomiting, and breast tenderness with this regimen. Although some clinicians prescribe antiemetics prophylactically, others recommend simply repeating the dose if the patient vomits within an hour of taking the pills.

TRANSDERMAL CONTRACEPTIVES

[handwritten: Q wk then 3rd wk off]

A new combination contraceptive is available as a transdermal patch (Ortho Evra), which includes 0.75 mg EE and 6 mg norelgestromin, the active metabolite of norgestimate.[70,71] In comparative trials, it has been shown to be as effective as combined OCs. Of the 15 pregnancies reported with the patch, 5 were among women with a baseline weight of greater than 90 kg, so efficacy may be compromised as weight increases. Some patients experience application-site reactions, but other side effects are similar to OCs (i.e., breast discomfort, headache, nausea, and menstrual cramps).

The patch should be applied to the abdomen, buttocks, upper torso, or upper outer arm at the beginning of the menstrual cycle and replaced every week for 3 weeks (the fourth week is patch-free).[70,71] About 5% of patches will need to be replaced because they become partly detached or fall off all together, so single replacements are also available. Two trials have demonstrated greater compliance with the patch than with an OC, but it remains to be seen if this results in reduced pregnancy rates or safety advantages.

CONTRACEPTIVE RINGS

[handwritten: Q 3 wks then 1 wk off]

Hormonal contraception also can be delivered through a vaginal ring. In 2002, the first vaginal ring (NuvaRing) was approved for contraception by the FDA, containing EE and etonogestrel, a progestin.[72] The ring releases approximately 15 mcg/day EE and 120 mcg/day etonogestrel over a 3 week period of time, thus preventing pregnancy. On first use, the ring should be inserted on or prior to the fifth day of the menstrual cycle, remain in place for 3 weeks, then be removed for 1 week to allow for withdrawal bleeding. The new ring should be inserted on the same day of the week as it was during the last cycle, similar to starting a new OC pack on the same day of the week. A second form of contraception should be used for the first 7 days of ring use or if the ring has been expelled accidentally for more than 3 hours.[72]

Side effects, precautions, and contraindications for the hormonal ring are similar to those for combined OCs. The most common reported reasons for discontinuation of use were device-related issues, such as foreign-body sensation, device expulsion, and vaginal symptoms. Cycle control with the vaginal ring appears to be as good as or better than with combined OCs, with a low incidence of breakthrough bleeding and spotting after the second cycle of use.[72,73]

LONG-ACTING INJECTABLE AND IMPLANTABLE CONTRACEPTIVES

Steroid hormones provide long-term contraception when injected or implanted into the skin. The most commonly used steroids for injectable or implantable contraception are progestins, either alone or in combination with estrogen.[4,6] Sustained progestin exposure blocks the LH surge, thus preventing ovulation; should ovulation occur, progestins reduce ovum motility in the fallopian tubes; and even if fertilization occurs, progestins thin the endometrium, reducing the chance of implantation. Progestins also thicken the cervical mucus, producing a barrier to sperm penetration. However, FSH is not intensely suppressed by progestin-only contraception; therefore, follicular growth and estrogen concentrations, although lower than normal at times, are maintained.

Women who particularly benefit from progestin-only methods, including minipills, are those who are breast-feeding, those who are intolerant to estrogens (i.e., have a history of estrogen-related headache, breast tenderness, or nausea), those with concomitant medical conditions in which estrogen is not preferred (i.e., have a history of uncontrolled hypertension or dyslipidemia, history of VTE, or history of SLE); and those who smoke and are older than 35 years of age.[4,6] Pregnancy failure rates with long-acting progestin contraception are comparable with that of female sterilization. Previous reports stated an increased risk of ectopic pregnancy in pregnancies occurring while using one of the progestin-only methods, but a recent study did not find an increase in ectopic pregnancies or fetal anomalies in the 0.42 pregnancies per 1000 women using injectable progestin-only contraception each year. These long-acting methods of contraception do not offer protection from STDs, but the thickened cervical mucus may help to prohibit the entry of bacteria into the upper pelvic region, thus preventing pelvic inflammatory disease.

▣ INJECTABLE PROGESTINS

Medroxyprogesterone acetate is similar in structure to naturally occurring progesterone. Depomedroxyprogesterone acetate 150 mg administered by deep intramuscular injection in the gluteal or deltoid muscle within 5 days of the onset of menstrual bleeding inhibits ovulation for more than 3 months.[4,74] Although this injection may inhibit ovulation for up to 14 weeks, the dose should be repeated every 3 months (12 weeks) to ensure continuous contraception. The manufacturer recommends excluding pregnancy in women more than 1 week late for repeat injection. Depo-Provera is available as a 150 mg/mL injection.[56]

Depomedroxyprogesterone acetate can be used in lactating women, and it may increase the length of time that a woman can breast-feed.[6] Although depomedroxyprogesterone acetate is safe postpartum and no adverse effects have occurred in infants exposed to depomedroxyprogesterone acetate through breast milk, the manufacturer recommends initiating depomedroxyprogesterone acetate at 6 weeks postpartum in women who are breast-feeding. Depomedroxyprogesterone acetate does not alter blood pressure or increase the risk of VTE. It may be used in women with seizure disorders; not only do anticonvulsant drugs have less effect on depomedroxyprogesterone acetate's efficacy, but also it may decrease the frequency of seizures independently.[4,75] Noncontraceptive benefits observed in women using depomedroxyprogesterone acetate include reducing the risk of anemia because less menstrual blood is lost and decreasing the incidence of menstrual cramps and pain at ovulation. The incidence of *Candida* vulvovaginitis, ectopic pregnancy, and pelvic inflammatory disease, as well as endometrial and ovarian cancer, is decreased in women using depomedroxyprogesterone acetate for contraception compared with women using no contraception.

Return of fertility may be delayed after discontinuation of depomedroxyprogesterone acetate. The median time to conception from the first omitted dose is 10 months. Sixty-eight percent of women will be able to conceive within 12 months, 83% within 15 months, and 93% within 18 months of the last injection.[56]

Menstrual irregularities, including irregular, unpredictable spotting or, more rarely, continuous heavy bleeding, are the most frequent adverse effects of depomedroxyprogesterone acetate. In some cases, bleeding may be severe enough to cause a significant drop in hemoglobin. Women who cannot tolerate prolonged bleeding may benefit from a short course of estrogen (e.g., 7 days of 2 mg estradiol or 1.25 mg conjugated estrogen given orally).[74] The incidence of irregular bleeding decreases from 30% in the first year to 10% thereafter (such that most women are amenorrheic after the first year). After 12 months of therapy, 57% of women report amenorrhea, with the incidence increasing to 68% after 2 years.[56]

Because estrogen concentrations may be lower than normal in women using depomedroxyprogesterone acetate, women can lose bone density. The clinical significance of this bone loss is unknown; it has not resulted in an increase in fracture rates.[74,76] Breast tenderness, weight gain, and depression occur less commonly (<5%). Weight gain averages 1 kg annually and may not resolve until 6 to 8 months after the last injection. Whether weight gain can be attributed directly to depomedroxyprogesterone acetate is debatable.[74,76] Minor alterations in total, LDL, and HDL cholesterol have been noted after depomedroxyprogesterone acetate exposure. A decrease in glucose tolerance has been observed in some patients. Clotting factors VII, VIII, IX, and X may be increased. The clinical significance of these minor alterations in metabolism is unknown.[56,74]

Although used in developing countries for decades, depomedroxyprogesterone acetate was not approved as a contraceptive in the U.S. market until 1992 because of a concern about a possible increased incidence of breast cancer. Overall, the risk of breast cancer in women who have used depomedroxyprogesterone acetate is not increased.[4,74] However, two studies suggest that the risk may be increased in some groups. One study from the WHO found a very slight increased risk in the first 4 years of use, but the risk did not increase with a longer duration of use.[77,78] Another study found a possible increased risk in women initiating use at an early age.[79] These studies suggest that if any effect exists at all, medroxyprogesterone may enhance the growth of already existing tumors. Depomedroxyprogesterone acetate was approved for use in the United States as a contraceptive because worldwide data in millions of women showed benefit on maternal mortality and demonstrated other noncontraceptive benefits, outweighing any possible increased risk of breast cancer.

▣ INJECTABLE ESTROGEN/PROGESTINS

◀1 ◀2 Lunelle is a new once-a-month injectable contraceptive agent containing 5 mg estradiol cypionate and 25 mg medroxyprogesterone acetate.[80] Like Depo-Provera, it acts by suppressing ovulation. The addition of estrogen has minimal impact on contraceptive efficacy but promotes regular bleeding patterns.[81] Lunelle is administered by an intramuscular injection given every 23 to 32 days. Its efficacy is similar to that of other injectable/implantable contraceptives, and body weight does not appear to affect it.[81,82] It is a reversible form of contraception, and fertility returns as early as 1 month after discontinuation.[83]

Most women using Lunelle have regular monthly menstrual cycles, similar to women using nonhormonal contraceptive methods. Menstrual irregularities, such as breakthrough bleeding and spotting, are more common in the first three cycles of use, and less than 1% of women experience amenorrhea.[81] Other adverse events associated with Lunelle include headache, breast tenderness, weight gain, and acne. Precautions and drug interactions associated with Lunelle are similar to those for other estrogen- and progestin-containing contraceptive methods.

SUBDERMAL PROGESTIN IMPLANTS

◀1 ◀2 Norplant, developed by the Population Council, became the first subdermal progestin implant approved for use in the United States in 1990.[4] The Norplant contraceptive system is currently a set of six implantable, nonbiodegradable, soft silicone rubber capsules, each filled with 36 mg crystalline levonorgestrel. Capsules are inserted just under the skin to provide continuous contraception for up to 5 years. Early clinical trials included implants with a hard capsule, but they resulted in higher contraceptive failure rates.[4] Because the cumulative pregnancy rate in all groups of women using Norplant increases significantly during the sixth year, Norplant should be replaced after 5 years. Even with the softer capsules currently available in the United States, failure rates may be unacceptable during the fourth and fifth years of use in women weighing more than 154 pounds. Replacement after 3 years in heavier women helps to ensure effectiveness.[4,84]

A new system can be inserted immediately after removal of the old system. Removal of a Norplant system often becomes complicated as a result of poor insertion technique, broken capsules, or impedance by fibrous tissue. A U technique of Norplant removal using a 4-mm incision located parallel to the third and fourth implant appears to be an improvement over the manufacturer-recommended technique, especially for personnel who are not highly experienced in this procedure.[84,85] Norplant II or Jadelle, a levonorgestrel two-rod, 150-mg implant system that provides 3 years of contraception, may prove to be easier to insert and remove than the older system.[86–88] Implanon is the newest contraceptive implant system, a single rod containing 68 mg 3-keto-desogestrel, that lasts for 3 years. However, none of these products is available currently in the United States.[89] Other progestin implants, some of which are biodegradable, are under development.[86]

As with other progestin-only methods, the most common side effect of subdermal progestin implants is irregular menstrual bleeding. Approximately 60% to 70% of women using Norplant experience irregular bleeding during the first year of insertion. Prolonged bleeding can be treated with a short course of estrogen (e.g., 2 mg estradiol or 1.25 mg conjugated estrogen daily for 7 to 10 days).[4,6] Spotting and bleeding decrease in amount and duration with time, but adding several cycles of a low-dose combined OC can resolve repeated monthly menstrual bleeding.[4] However, by the fifth year of use, regular bleeding cycles may resume in more than 60% of users. Regular cyclic bleeding in a woman who is using Norplant indicates return of ovulation and a higher risk of method failure.[84]

Fertility returns quickly after the removal of Norplant. Most women return to baseline ovulatory patterns within the first month after removal of the system. Other progesterone-related adverse effects that usually occur in the first year include headache (common), dizziness, breast tenderness, nervousness, nausea, acne, breast discharge, and weight gain. Because of the extremely low concentrations of levonorgestrel released from the Norplant system, drugs that significantly increase hepatic enzymes, including most antiepileptic medications (e.g., phenobarbital, carbamazepine, and phenytoin) and rifampin, lower the efficacy of the contraceptive. Ovarian cysts may occur but usually regress spontaneously within 1 month of detection.[4,6]

The noncontraceptive benefits of Norplant are similar to those of Depo-Provera, and no clinically significant adverse effects have been observed on carbohydrate metabolism in nondiabetic women, on bone density, on blood coagulation, or on lipid metabolism.[4,56,90,91]

INTRAUTERINE DEVICES

◀1 ◀2 The low-grade intrauterine inflammation and increased prostaglandin formation caused by intrauterine devices (IUDs) appear to be primarily spermicidal, although interference with implantation is a backup mechanism. The IUD has several contraindications (see Table 77–1). The risk of pelvic inflammatory disease among IUD users ranges from 1% to 2.5%. Because the increase in the risk of infection appears to be related to the introduction of bacteria into the genital tract during IUD insertion, the risk is highest during the first 20 days after the procedure.[92] Ideal patients for IUD use include parous, monogamous women who are not at risk for STDs or pelvic inflammatory disease. Three IUDs are currently marketed in the United States; all are shaped like a T and are medicated, one with copper (ParaGard), one with progesterone (Progestasert), and the newest one with levonorgestrel (Mirena). ParaGard provides better contraceptive effectiveness than previous copper devices and can be left in place for 10 years. A disadvantage of Progestasert is that it must be replaced annually, but it has been associated with less blood loss during menstruation and less dysmenorrhea. Mirena releases levonorgestrel over a period of 5 years and appears to lead to less systemic levonorgestrel absorption than the levonorgestrel implants (Norplant).[93]

PHARMACOECONOMIC CONSIDERATIONS

More than half of all pregnancies in the United States are unintended.[4,6] Not all unintended pregnancies are unwanted; many are just "mis-timed." Nevertheless, the United States has a higher rate of induced abortions than most other industrialized Western nations. Whatever method is used, preventing unintended pregnancy is highly cost-effective. With regard to the acquisition cost of reversible contraception, spermicides alone are the least expensive method, followed by use with condoms. Depo-Provera is slightly less expensive than Norplant and IUDs. Implantable and injectable methods carry a higher initial cost that can be prohibitive for some women, and the annual cost is greater if they are removed prior to their expiration. The diaphragm and cervical cap (with spermicide) are midrange in cost, with the female condom being slightly more expensive than the other female barrier methods. OCs, the contraceptive patch, and the vaginal ring are the most expensive forms of reversible contraception. These cost estimates are based on the assumption of 100 acts of intercourse annually. However, with regard to direct medical costs (i.e., method use, side effects, and unintended pregnancies) over 5 years, the copper IUD, vasectomy, Norplant, and Depo-Provera are the most cost-effective. Oral contraceptives are more cost-effective than methods with high failure rates (i.e., barrier methods, spermicides, withdrawal, and periodic abstinence), but even these methods are more cost-effective than no method.[94]

EVALUATION OF THERAPEUTIC OUTCOMES

◀4 Patients should receive both verbal and written instructions concerning the chosen method of contraception. Follow-up appointments can increase compliance, allow time for the patient to ask questions, and provide opportunities to address other health maintenance issues (e.g., self-breast examination, Papanicolaou smears, STD risk).[4]

At least annual blood pressure monitoring is recommended in all users of OCs. When a patient with a history of glucose intolerance or overt diabetes mellitus begins or discontinues the use of an OC, it is necessary to monitor the glucose level closely for deterioration of the condition. OC users should receive at least annual (more frequent if they are at risk for STDs) cytologic screening. Finally, OC users should undergo examination for clinical problems possibly relating to the OC (e.g., breakthrough bleeding, amenorrhea, weight gain, and acne).

Women using Norplant should be monitored for menstrual cycle disturbances, weight gain, local inflammation or infection at the implant site, acne, breast tenderness, headaches, and hair loss. Women using depomedroxyprogesterone acetate should be asked at 3-month follow-up visits about weight gain, any problems or concerns they may have, menstrual cycle disturbances, and STD risks. Patients on depomedroxyprogesterone acetate also should be weighed and have their blood pressure checked and receive annual examinations (e.g., complete physical examination, Papanicolaou smear, and mammogram) as indicated based on the patient's age.

Choosing a contraceptive method most suited to the patient's needs will reduce the chance of unintended pregnancy significantly. Typical failure rates for some of the commonly used methods of reversible contraception are listed in Table 77–1. A medical and sexual history and a thorough physical examination are essential when evaluating the various methods available. Understanding the risks and precautions associated with the methods available is essential for both the patient and the prescriber (see Tables 77–1 and 77–3).

ABBREVIATIONS

ACOG: American College of Obstetrics and Gynecology
AMA: American Medical Association
BTB: breakthrough bleeding
EC: emergency contraception
FDA: Food and Drug Administration
FSH: follicle-stimulating hormone
GnRH: gonadotropin-releasing hormone
hCG: human chorionic gonadotropin
HDL: high-density lipoprotein
HIV: human immunodeficiency virus
IUD: intrauterine devices
LDL: low-density lipoprotein
LH: luteinizing hormone
MI: myocardial infarction
OC: oral contraceptive
PAP: Papanicolaou smear
SLE: systemic lupus erythematosus
STD: sexually transmitted diseases
VLDL: very low density lipoprotein
VTE: venous thromboembolism
WHO: World Health Organization

Review Questions and other resources can be found at *www.pharmacotherapyonline.com*.

REFERENCES

1. Henshaw SK. Unintended pregnancy in the United States. Family Planning Perspectives 1998;30:24–29, 46.
2. Abma JC, Chandra A, Mosher WD, et al. Fertility, family planning, and women's health: New data from the 1995 National Survey of Family Growth. Vital Health Stat 1997;23:1–114.
3. Hatcher RA, Nelson AL, Zieman M, et al. A Pocket Guide to Managing Contraception. Tiger, GA, Bridging the Gap Foundation, 2003:1–146.
4. Hatcher RA, Trussel J, Stewart F, et al. Contraceptive Technology, 17th ed. New York, Ardent Media, 1998:211–544.
5. Rebar RW, Erickson GF. Menstrual cycle and fertility. In Goldman L, Bennett JC, eds. Cecil Textbook of Medicine, 21st ed. Philadelphia, Saunders, 2000:1327–1332.
6. Speroff L, Darnet P. A Clinical Guide for Contraception, 2d ed. Baltimore, Williams & Wilkins, 1996:25–262.
7. Jones RK, Darroch JE, Henshaw SK. Contraceptive use among US women having abortions in 2000–2001. Perspect Sex Reprod Health 2002;34:294–303.
8. Stewart FH, Harper CC, Ellertson CE, et al. Clinical breast and pelvic examination requirements for hormonal contraception: Current practice versus evidence. JAMA 1991;285:2232–2239.
9. Jensen JT, Speroff L. Health benefits of oral contraceptives. Obstet Gynecol Clin North Am 2000;27:705–721.
10. Gallo MF, Grimes DA, Schulz KF. Cervical cap versus diaphragm for contraception. Cochrane Review 2003;3.
11. The Today Sponge. Available at *http://www.todayssponge.us/*; accessed December 30, 2003.
12. Cerel-Suhl SL, Yeager BF. Update on oral contraceptive pills. Am Fam Phys 1999;60:2073–2084.
13. Anonymous. Oral contraceptives. Med Lett Drugs Ther 2000;42:42–44.
14. Dickey RP. Managing Contraceptive Pill Patients, 11th ed. Dallas, Essential Medical Information Systems, 2002:12–113.
15. Anonymous. Yasmin: An oral contraceptive with a new progestin. Med Let Drug Ther 2002;44:55–57.
16. Worret I, Arp W, Zahradnik HP, et al. Acne resolution rates: Results of a single-blind, randomized, controlled, parallel phase III trial with EE/CMA (Belara) and EE/LNG (Microgynon). Dermatology 2001;203:38–44.
17. Gallo MF, Grimes DA, Schulz KF, Helmerhorst FM. Combination contraceptives: Effects on weight. Cochrane Review 2003;3.
18. ACOG Committee on Practice Bulletins—Gynecology. The use of hormonal contraception in women with coexisting medical conditions. ACOG Practice Bulletin 2000;18.
19. Sidney S, Siscovick DS, Petitti DB, et al. Myocardial infarction and use of low-dose oral contraceptives: A pooled analysis of two US studies. Circulation 1998;98:1058–1063.
20. Schwartz SM, Petitti DB, Siscovick DS, et al. Stroke and use of low-dose oral contraceptives in young women: A pooled analysis of two US studies. Stroke 1998;29:2277–2284.
21. Williams JK. Contraceptive needs of the perimenopausal woman. Obstet Gynecol Clin North Am 2002;29:575–588.
22. Mosca L, Grundy SM, Judelson D, et al. Guide to preventive cardiology for women. AHA/ACC Scientific Statement Consensus Panel statement. Circulation 1999;99:2480–2484
23. Kaunitz AM. Oral contraceptive estrogen dose considerations. Contraception 1998;58:15S–21S.
24. Burkman RT, Shulman LP. Oral contraceptive practice guidelines. Contraception 1998;58:35S–43S.
25. Fruzzetti F, Ricci C, Fioretti P. Haemostasis profile in smoking and non-smoking women taking low-dose oral contraceptives. Contraception 1994;49:579–592.
26. Neinstein L. Contraception in women with special medical needs. Compr Ther 1998;24:229–250.
27. Godsland IF, Crook D. Update on the metabolic effects of steroidal contraceptives and their relationship to cardiovascular disease. Am J Obstet Gynecol 1994;170:1528–1536.
28. Garg SK, Chase HP, Marshall G, et al. Oral contraceptives and renal and

retinal complications in young women with insulin-dependent diabetes mellitus. JAMA 1994;271:1099–1102.

29. Chasan-Taber L, Willett WC, Stampfer MJ, et al. A prospective study of oral contraceptives and NIDDM among US women. Diabetes Care 1997; 20:330–335.

30. Chasan-Taber L, Stampfer MJ. Epidemiology of oral contraceptives and cardiovascular disease. Ann Intern Med 1998;128:467–477.

31. Bloemenkamp KWM, Rosendall FR, Helmerhorst FM, Vandenbroucke JP. Higher risk of venous thrombosis during early use of oral contraceptives in women with inherited clotting defects. Arch Intern Med 2000;160: 49–52.

32. Douketis JD, Ginsberg JS, Holbrook A, et al. A reevaluation of risk for venous thromboembolism with use of oral contraception and hormone replacement. Arch Intern Med 1997;157:1522–1530.

33. Grodstein F, Stampfer MJ, Goldhaber SZ, et al. Prospective study of exogenous hormone and risk of pulmonary embolism in women. Lancet 1996; 348:983–987.

34. Basdevant A, Conrad J, Pelissier C, et al. Hemostatic and metabolic effects of lowering the ethinyl estradiol dose from 30 mcg to 20 mcg in oral contraceptives containing desogestrel. Contraception 1993;48:193–204.

35. Herings RMC, Urquhart J, Leufkens HGM. Venous thromboembolism among new users of different oral contraceptives. Lancet 1999;354: 127–128.

36. Jick H, Vandenbroucke JP, Bloemenkamp KWM, et al. Incidence of venous thromboembolism in users of combined oral contraceptives. Br Med J 2000;320:57.

37. Vandenbroucke JP, Helmerhorst FM, Rosendall FR. Competing interests and controversy about third generation oral contraceptives. Br Med J 2000; 320:381–382.

38. Speroff L. Third-generation oral contraceptives and venous thrombosis. OB/GYN Clin Alert 1997;June:11–12.

39. Lewis MA, Heinemann LAJ, MacRae KD, et al (Transnational Research Group on Oral Contraceptives and the Health of Young Women). The increased risk of venous thromboembolism and the use of third generation progestogens: Role of bias in observational research. Contraception 1996; 54:5–13.

40. Petitti DB, Sidney S, Bernstein A, et al. Stroke in users of low-dose oral contraceptives. New Engl J Med 1996;335:8–15.

41. Poulter NR, Chang CL, Farley TMM, et al. Haemorrhagic stroke, overall stroke risk, and combined oral contraceptives: Results of an international, multicentre, case-control study. Lancet 1996;348:498–510.

42. Speroff L. Low-dose oral contraceptives and stroke. OB/GYN Clin Alert 1996;13:49–51.

43. Consensus conference on combination oral contraceptives and cardiovascular disease. Fertil Steril 1999;71(suppl 3):1S–6S.

44. Chang CL, Donaghy M, Poulter N. Migraine and stroke in young women: a case-control study. The World Health Organisation Collaborative Study of Cardiovascular Disease and Steroid Hormone Contraception. Br Med J 1999;318:13–18.

45. Croft P, Hannaford PC. Risk factors for acute myocardial infarction in women: Evidence from the Royal College of General Practitioners' Oral Contraception Study. Br Med J 1989;298:165–168.

46. Dunn N, Thorogood M, Faragher B, et al. Oral contraceptives and myocardial infarction: Results of the MICA case-control study. Br Med J 1999; 12:1579–1583.

47. Collaborative Group on Hormonal Factors in Breast Cancer. Breast cancer and hormonal contraceptives: Collaborative reanalysis of individual data on 53,297 women with breast cancer and 100,239 women without breast cancer from 54 epidemiological studies. Lancet 1996;347:1713–1727.

48. Collaborative Group on Hormonal Factors in Breast Cancer. Breast cancer and hormonal contraceptives: Further results. Contraception 1996; 54(suppl 3):1S–106S.

49. Hankinson SE, Colditz GA, Manson JE, et al. A prospective study of oral contraceptive use and risk of breast cancer (Nurses' Health Study, United States). Cancer Causes Control 1997;8:65–72.

50. Marchbanks PA, McDonald JA, Wilson HG, et al. Oral contraceptives and the risk of breast cancer. New Engl J Med 2002;346:2025–2032.

51. Petri M, Robinson C. Oral contraceptives and systemic lupus erythematosus. Arthritis Rheum 1997;40:797–803.

52. Thorneycroft IH. Update on androgenicity. Am J Obstet Gynecol 1999; 180:S28–94.

53. Thiboutot D. New treatments and therapeutic strategies for acne. Arch Fam Med 2000;9:179–187.

54. Redmond GP, Olson WH, Lippman JS, et al. Norgestimate and ethinyl estradiol in the treatment of acne vulgaris: A randomized, placebo-controlled trial. Obstet Gynecol 1997;89:615–622.

55. Lucky AW, Henderson TA, Olson WH, et al. Effectiveness of norgestimate and ethinyl estradiol in treating moderate acne vulgaris. J Am Acad Dermatol 1997;37:746–754.

56. Facts and Comparisons. St. Louis, Facts and Comparisons, 1999:234–245.

57. Dickinson BD, Altman RD, Neilsen NH, Sterling ML. Drug interactions between oral contraceptives and antibiotics. Obstet Gynecol 2001;98: 853–860.

58. Archer JS, Archer DF. Oral contraceptive efficacy and antibiotic interaction: A myth debunked. J Am Acad Dermatol 2002;46:917–923.

59. Clarke AK, Miller SJ. The debate regarding continuous use of oral contraceptives. Ann Pharmacother 2001;35:1480–1484.

60. Miller L, Hughes JP. Continuous combination oral contraceptive pills to eliminate withdrawal bleeding: A randomized trial. Obstet Gynecol 2003; 101:653–661.

61. FDA Talk Paper. FDA Approves Seasonale Oral Contraceptive. Available at *http://www.fda.gov/bbs/topics/ANSWERS/2003/ANS01251.html;* accessed December 30, 2003.

62. Gray RH, Campbell OM, Zacur HA, et al. Postpartum return of ovarian activity in nonbreastfeeding women monitored by urinary assays. J Clin Endocrinol Metab 1987;64:645–651.

63. American Academy of Pediatrics Committee on Drugs. The transfer of drugs and other chemicals into human milk. Pediatrics 1994;93:137–150.

64. Truitt ST, Fraser AB, Grimes DA, et al. Combined hormonal versus non-hormonal versus protestin-only contraception in lactation. Cochrane Review 2003;3.

65. Wanner MS, Couchenour RL. Hormonal emergency contraception. Pharmacotherapy 2002;22:43–53.

66. APhA Special Report. Emergency Contraception: The Pharmacist's Role. Washington, DC, American Pharmaceutical Association, 2000.

67. Grimes DA. Switching emergency contraception to over-the-counter status. New Engl J Med 2002;347:846–849.

68. FDA Advisory Committee. Plan B emergency contraceptive OTC switch will get committee review Dec. 16. Available at *http://www.fdaadvisorycommittee.com/FDC/AdvisoryCommittee/Committees/Nonprescription+Drugs/121603_PlanB/121603_PlanbA.htm;* accessed on December 30, 2003.

69. VonHertzen H, Piaggio G. Low dose mifeprostone and two regimens of levonorgestrel for emergency contraception: A WHO multicenter randomized trial. Lancet 2002;360:1803–1810.

70. Anonymous. Ortho evra: A contraceptive patch. Med Lett Drugs Ther 2002;44:8.

71. Sicat BL. Ortho evra, a new contraceptive patch. Pharmacotherapy 2003; 23:472–480.

72. NuvaRing product information. West Orange, NJ, Organon Inc., May 2001.

73. Bjarnadottir RI, Tuppurainen M, Killick SR. Comparison of cycle control with a combined contraceptive vaginal ring and oral levonorgestrel/ethinyl estradiol. Am J Obstet Gynecol 2002;186:389–395.

74. Kaunitz AM. Injectable depot medroxyprogesterone acetate contraception: An update for US clinicians. Int J Fertil Women's Med 1998;43: 73–83.

75. American Academy of Neurology. Practice parameter: Management issues for women with epilepsy (summary statement). Neurology 1998;51: 944–948.

76. Kaunitz AM. Long-acting hormonal contraception: Assessing impact on bone density, weight, and mood. Int J Fertil Women's Med 1999;44: 110–117.

77. World Health Organization Collaborative Study of Neoplasia and Steroid Contraceptives. Breast cancer and depo-medroxyprogesterone acetate: A multinational study. Lancet 1991;44:419–430.

78. Bonhomme MG, Potts DM, Fortney JA, Allen MY. Safety of depot medroxyprogesterone acetate. Lancet 1991;338:942.

79. Paul C, Skett DCG, Spears GFS. Depo-medroxyprogesterone (Depo-Provera) and risk of breast cancer. Br Med J 1989;299:759–762.

80. Kaunitz AM, Mishell DR. Lunelle monthly contraceptive injection (medroxyprogesterone acetate and estradiol cypionate injectable suspension): A contraceptive method for women in the US and worldwide. Contraception 1999;60:177–178.

81. Garceau RJ, Wajszczuk CJ, Kaunitz AM, and the Lunelle Study Group. Bleeding patterns of women using Lunelle monthly contraceptive injections (medroxyprogesterone acetate and estradiol cypionate injectable suspension) compared with those of women using Ortho-Novum 7/7/7 (norethindrone/ethinyl estradiol triphasic) or other oral contraceptives. Contraception 2000;62:289–295.

82. Rahimy MH, Cromie MA, Hopkins NK, Tong DM. Lunelle monthly contraceptive injection (medroxyprogesterone acetate and estradiol cypionate injectable suspension): Effects on body weight and injection sites on pharmacokinetics. Contraception 1999;60:201–208.

83. Rahimy MH, Ryan KK. Lunelle monthly contraceptive injection (medroxyprogesterone acetate and estradiol cypionate injectable suspension): Assessment of return of ovulation after three monthly injections in surgically sterile women. Contraception 1999;60:189–200.

84. Harrison PF, Rosenfield A. Research, introduction, and use: advancing from Norplant. Contraception 1998;58:323–334.

85. Rosenberg MJ, Alvarez F, Barone MA, et al. A comparison of U and standard techniques for Norplant removal. Obstet Gynecol 1997;89: 168–173.

86. Newton JR. New hormonal methods of contraception. Ballieres Clin Obstet Gynaecol 1996;10:87–101.

87. Reproductive Health Online. Levonorgestrel rod implants (formerly known as Norplant II Implants). Available at *http://www.reproline.jhu.edu/english/6read/6multi/tgwg/pdf/tgn2_e.pdf;* accessed December 30, 2003.

88. Population Council. Jadelle implants. Available at *www.popcouncil.org/faqs/jadellefaq.html;* accessed on December 30, 2003.

89. Le J, Tsourounis C. Implanon: a critical review. Ann Pharmacother 2001; 35:329–336.

90. Diaz S, Reyes MV, Zepeda A, et al. Norplant implants and progesterone vaginal rings do not affect maternal bone turnover and density during lactation and after weaning. Hum Reprod 1999;11:2499–2505.

91. Suherman SK, Affandi B, Korver T. The effects of Implanon on lipid metabolism in comparison with Norplant. Contraception 1999;60: 281–287.

92. Grimes DA. Intrauterine device and upper-genital-tract infection. Lancet 2000;356:1013–1019.

93. Anonymous. A progestin-releasing intrauterine device for long-term contraception. Med Lett 2001;43:7–8.

94. Chiou CF, Trussell J, Reyes E, et al. Economic analysis of contraceptives for women. Contraception 2003;68:3–10.

78

MENSTRUATION-RELATED DISORDERS

Martha P. Fankhauser and Marlene P. Freeman

Learning Objectives and other resources can be found at *www.pharmacotherapyonline.com.*

KEY CONCEPTS

1 Menstruation-related disorders occur commonly during the reproductive years and are characterized by cyclic, somatic, and/or psychological symptoms during the late luteal phase of the menstrual cycle, and often symptoms become more episodic and severe prior to menopause.

2 Approximately 90% of women experience symptoms of premenstrual syndrome (PMS), and more than 80% of women report that psychological and physical symptoms worsen during the perimenopause phase. Up to 3% to 5% of menstruating women experience severe mood and anxiety symptoms and meet criteria for the diagnosis of premenstrual dysphoric disorder (PMDD).

3 Menstruation-related disorders are the result of a complex interaction between genetic predisposition and cyclic changes in ovarian steroids, neurotransmitters, neurohormones, and neuropeptides.

4 A correct diagnosis of dysmenorrhea, PMS, PMDD, and perimenopause is essential. An evaluation and careful work-up should rule out other possible causes of the symptoms.

5 Premenstrual and perimenopausal syndromes can manifest with a wide variety of symptoms, including depression, mood lability, irritability, anxiety, insomnia, fatigue, abdominal pain, breast tenderness, muscle aches, headaches, hot flashes, decreased libido, and concentration difficulties. Although some degree of these symptoms may be a normal phenomenon, up to 10% of women have significant impairment in social and/or occupational functioning and require treatment.

6 The goals of treatment are to ameliorate or eliminate symptoms, to improve or restore social and occupational functioning, and to minimize adverse effects.

7 There are no specific laboratory tests that are diagnostic for PMS or PMDD. A prospective self-rated symptom diary with severity ratings is most helpful in diagnosing and monitoring menstruation-related disorders.

8 A stepwise approach is recommended, starting with lifestyle changes and nonpharmacologic treatments, then first-line pharmacologic agents, and finally, second-line agents that may have more adverse effects. After a 3-month trial, nonpharmacologic and/or pharmacologic treatments should be

evaluated for efficacy and adverse effects. Combination therapies may be needed for refractory or severe symptoms, if monotherapy is ineffective, and if multiple symptoms persist.

9 Perimenopausal women should be evaluated for hormone-replacement therapy (HRT) because deficiency states may cause physical, psychological, and cognitive symptoms. Although hormone concentrations (e.g., 17β-estradiol, inhibin, testosterone, and follicle-stimulating hormone) are diagnostic for menopause, these tests may not be accurate during the perimenopause phase because of erratic and fluctuating hormone levels secondary to changes in ovarian function. Estradiol-replacement therapy has been identified as a successful treatment for perimenopausal women with vasomotor and depressive symptoms. Testosterone-replacement therapy has been reported to improve mood, well-being, and sexual functioning in perimenopausal women. Assessment of the risks versus benefits of HRT should be done regularly during treatment.

10 Education, psychotherapy, well-balanced meals and snacks, regular exercise, dietary changes (e.g., limiting caffeine, alcohol, and salt), relaxation therapy, stress reduction, and sleep hygiene are first-line nonpharmacologic approaches for menstruation-related disorders.

11 Serotonin (5-hydroxytryptamine, 5-HT)–augmenting antidepressants are effective for treating premenstrual and perimenopausal mood and anxiety symptoms. Serotonin reuptake inhibitors (SRIs) may be given continuously or intermittently during the luteal phase of the menstrual cycle for PMDD.

12 Nonsteroidal anti-inflammatory agents (NSAIDs) are the treatment of choice for dysmenorrhea, muscle aches, and headaches. Diuretics such as spironolactone may provide some relief for bloating and fluid retention if sodium restriction is not effective. Vitamin E supplementation may reduce fibrocystic breast changes if caffeine restriction is not helpful.

13 Ovulation suppression (e.g., oral contraceptives, danazol, gonadotropin-releasing hormone agonists) should be used before resorting to surgical therapy in women with severe PMDD.

During their reproductive years, women are vulnerable to mood and physical changes secondary to hormonal triggers associated with the menstrual cycle.[1-3] *Dysmenorrhea* is the most common menstrual problem in adolescents. *Premenstrual molimina* describes the mild physical symptoms of breast tenderness and bloating that occur premenstrually. *Premenstrual headache* or *migraine* occurs during the late luteal phase of the menstrual cycle and subsides after the onset of menses.[4] *Mastalgia* or *mastodynia* is breast pain that is associated with premenstrual syndrome and fibrocystic breast disease. *Premenstrual tension* or *premenstrual syndrome* (PMS) is the cyclic recurrence of a combination of psychological, behavioral, and physical symptoms that occur during the luteal phase of ovulatory menstrual cycles and resolve with menopause.[3] A more severe subtype of premenstrual syndrome, previously called *late luteal phase dysphoric disorder* and later renamed *premenstrual dysphoric disorder* (PMDD), is associated with significant mood and anxiety symptoms and an impairment in functioning.[3,5,6]

Premenopause describes years preceding menopause when women still have regular menstrual cycles but can experience a worsening of mood, sleep, and cognition.[7,8] The *perimenopausal phase* reflects the transition to menopause and includes the 3 to 5 years before and 1 year after the cessation of menstrual flow. Perimenopause is associated with irregular menstrual cycles, reduced fertility, decreased 17β-estradiol production, a worsening of premenstrual symptoms (e.g., sleep disturbances, irritability, anxiety, depression, fatigue, mood swings, and cognitive changes), and vasomotor complaints (e.g., hot flashes and night sweats).[7,8]

Depression is often associated with declining levels of ovarian hormones (i.e., depression is worse prior to menses, immediately after pregnancy, and prior to menopause).[8,9] Women also have more sleep problems compared with men, and sleep disruption (and deprivation) has a negative impact on mood, energy level, and cognition.[10] Menstruation-associated sleep complaints are secondary to cyclic changes in the levels of reproductive hormones, vasomotor symptoms, and an increase in sleep disorders (e.g., sleep apnea and periodic leg movements) in peri- and postmenopausal women.[11]

EPIDEMIOLOGY

Up to 90% of women experience one or more mood or somatic symptoms just before or during menses in ovulatory cycles.[1,3,5,12] Common symptoms include dysphoric mood, irritability, anxiety, sleep disturbances, changes in appetite, poor concentration, fluid retention, breast tenderness, and various types of pain syndromes.[1,13] After menarche, the type and severity of symptoms may change during the reproductive age span.[6]

The prevalence of *dysmenorrhea* increases from early to late adolescence and decreases after age 30 to 35 years. Approximately 40% to 50% of women have painful menstrual cramps, and up to 10% have impaired functioning for 1 to 3 days per month, such as missing work or school, because of pain.[14] Up to 75% of women younger than age 55 experience premenstrual breast pain, and 11% to 30% have moderate to severe *mastalgia* for at least 5 days or more each month that interferes with their daily functioning.[15,16] Menstruation-related *migraine* affects approximately a third of women at menarche, and peak incidence occurs during adolescence.[4] Approximately 60% of women complain of menstrual migraine attacks, and 8% to 14% experience only premenstrual migraines.[4] Migraines often are associated with other somatic compliants (e.g., backache, cramps, nausea, and breast tenderness). Although migraine prevalence decreases with advancing age, migraines can recur and worsen during menopause, with hormone-replacement therapy, and with oral contraceptive (OC) use.[4] *Fibromyalgia* (a syndrome of chronic musculoskeletal pain, tenderness over trigger points, fatigue, and sleep disturbances) is more common in women, the incidence increases with age, and the syndrome can cause significant disability.[17]

Premenstrual syndrome (variably defined with over 100 possible symptoms) typically begins between the ages of 25 and 35 years.[18] Point-prevalence studies report that up to 50% of menstruating women have PMS (defined as a luteal phase onset of symptoms that resolve midmenses). Approximately 5% to 10% of women have symptoms severe enough to impair their daily functioning during the week prior to and during menses.[1,4-6,12,18] An estimated 3% to 5% of women have severe affective symptoms and meet criteria for PMDD[6] (Table 78–1).

Approximately 50% of women with premenstrual complaints have an exacerbation of an underlying psychiatric or medical disorder.[1,3,6,19] Women with a history of anxiety disorders, dysthymia, major depressive disorder, bipolar disorder, postpartum depression, and mood changes induced by OCs and a family history of mood disorders or premenstrual depression have an increased risk for developing PMDD.[6,19] Compared with controls, women with PMDD are at higher risk for developing other affective disorders, have lower parity rates, and have higher rates of alcohol and drug use.[2] Women with PMDD have an increased risk of experiencing depression during pregnancy and the postpartum period (e.g., 10% to 16% develop a major depression during pregnancy, and up to 70% experience depressive symptoms postpartum).[20] For more information regarding mood disorders occurring during pregnancy and postpartum, see Chap. 76.

More than 80% of women report that psychological and physical symptoms worsen during the perimenopausal phase.[6,21] The menopausal transition (when hot flashes begin and there are changes in bleeding patterns) usually begins in the middle to late 40s, and the last menses occurs in the early 50s.[2] Hot flashes or flushes are one of the most common complaints associated with perimenopause, along with sleep disruption, mood disturbance, and cognitive difficulties.[22] Up to 85% of women have vasomotor symptoms during the year preceding and following menopause. Approximately 25% of women report that hot flashes and night sweats are severe enough to impair their sleep and social functioning and will seek treatment from health care providers.[22-24] Perimenopausal women with vasomotor symptoms are reported to be 4.4 times more likely to be depressed than those without vasomotor symptoms.[22,25] It is estimated that as many as 80% of perimenopausal women develop mood symptoms, and these individuals have higher prevalence rates of major depression (16% to 20%) during the climacteric.[2] Perimenopausal women with a previous history of depression, PMDD, or postpartum depression are at increased risk of a recurrent major depressive episode during the climacteric.[2]

ETIOLOGY

Several biologic, cognitive, genetic, psychological, environmental, and social theories have been proposed for menstruation-related disorders, but there are no definite conclusions regarding the etiology.[2,10,26] The menstrual cycle is a rapidly changing biologic process that involves the hypothalamic-pituitary-gonadal (HPG) axis with input from gonadotropin-releasing hormones (GnRHs), gonadotropins, ovarian hormones, endogenous opioids, neurotransmitters, and neuropeptides.[8,27-29] The hormonal feedback

TABLE 78–1. Assessment and Diagnosis of Premenstrual Dysphoric Disorder

Assessment

Interview
- Retrospective history of premenstrual syndrome
- Psychiatric and medical evaluation (past and current history)
- Medication and over-the-counter drug use (including alternative/complementary therapies)
- Exercise, sleep, and nutritional evaluation

Medical review
- Complete physical examination
- Laboratory testing (e.g., thyroid function, anemia, gonadal hormones)

Daily charting
- Prospective daily self-rating of symptoms for two menstrual cycles (e.g., Prospective Record of the Impact and Severity of Menstruation [PRISM], the Calendar of Premenstrual Experiences [COPE], Menstrual Distress Questionnaire [MDQ], Visual Analogue Scale [VAS])

Diagnostic Criteria for Premenstrual Dysphoric Disorder

A 1-year duration of symptoms that are present for the majority of cycles (occurs during the luteal phase and remits during the follicular phase)

Five of the following symptoms (with at least one of the symptoms marked with an asterisk) must occur during the week before menses and remit within days of menses:
- Irritability*
- Affective lability* (sudden mood swings)
- Depressed mood or hopelessness*
- Tension or anxiety*
- Decreased interest in activities
- Difficulty concentrating
- Lack of energy
- Change in appetite, e.g., food cravings
- Change in sleep
- Feeling out of control or overwhelmed
- Other physical symptoms, e.g., breast tenderness, bloating, headaches

Seriously interferes with work, social activities, relationships

Not an exacerbation of another psychiatric disorder

Confirmed by prospective daily charting/ratings during a minimum of two consecutive symptomatic menstrual cycles

Compiled from refs. 6 and 19.

system that controls neuroendocrine functioning is extremely complex and vulnerable to familial factors, psychosocial and environmental stresses, circadian rhythms, and the normal aging process.[2,5] A circadian rhythm dysregulation theory has been suggested as a possible link between mood disorders and the reproductive cycle.[2,30]

PATHOPHYSIOLOGY

Because medical conditions, emotional/behavioral symptoms, and physiologic indices change during the premenstrual and perimenopause phases, it is important to rule out other disorders that may contribute to mood fluctuations or pain syndromes[1,13] (Table 78–2). For example, dysmenorrhea may be "primary," which occurs during ovulatory cycles, or "secondary," which relates to pelvic pathology e.g., infection caused by the placement of intrauterine devices, endometriosis, pelvic inflammatory disease, ovarian cyst, endometrial cancer, adhesions, and benign uterine tumors).

PREMENSTRUAL PAIN SYNDROMES

Primary dysmenorrhea is a prostaglandin-mediated hypertonicity of the uterine smooth muscle that constricts uterine blood vessels and leads to ischemia and menstrual pain.[14] At menstruation, the shedding of the uterine lining releases arachidonate and stimulates

prostaglandin synthesis that cause uterine and gastrointestinal smooth muscle contraction and ischemia. Women with PMDD have lower β-endorphin levels in the luteal phase and report greater premenstrual pain, suggesting that endogenous opioids may be involved in the pathophysiology of pain sensitivity.[31]

Mastalgia frequently coexists with fibrocystic breast disease and is commonly a benign condition that occurs during ovulatory cycles.[16] The association between caffeine consumption and mastalgia is unclear, but the reduction or elimination of methylxanthines appears to reduce fibrocystic changes.[15] The cause of premenstrual mastalgia is unknown, but theories include estrogen dominance, an augmented response to prolactin during the luteal phase, high dietary fat intake, and abnormalities in fatty acid metabolism.[15,16]

PREMENSTRUAL SYNDROME (PMS)

The HPG axis is responsible for the cyclic hormone secretion that regulates and controls ovulation and plays a major role in menstruation-related disorders.[7,12,27] The menstrual cycle is characterized by cyclic alterations in the production of gonadal hormones (estradiol and progesterone), pituitary hormones (gonadatropins, prolactin, growth hormone), melatonin, and cortisol and in temperature rhythms. Menstruation-related disorders are likely the result of a complex interaction between ovarian steroids and central neurotransmitters, neurohormones, and neuropeptides.[5,8,12] The occurrence of physical

TABLE 78–2. Conditions and Symptoms that Change or Worsen Premenstrually

Medical Conditions	Physical Symptoms
Acute porphyria	Abdominal bloating
Adrenal disorders	Acne
Allergies	Breast swelling/tenderness
Anemia	Cold sores
Arthritis	Constipation
Asthma	Dizziness
Chronic fatigue syndrome	Fatigue
Chronic pelvic pain	Fluid retention/edema
Diabetes	Headaches
Dysmenorrhea	Hot flashes
Endometriosis	Muscle aches/pains
Fibrocystic breast disease	Nausea/vomiting
Fibromyalgia	Palpitations
Genital herpes	Weight gain
Hyperprolactinemia	**Physiologic Symptoms**
Hypoglycemia	Arteriolar responses to hormones and catecholamines
Irritable bowel syndrome	Body temperature
Migraine headaches	Blood pressure and pulse
Multiple sclerosis	Gastrointestinal absorption and transit time
Polycystic ovarian disease	Hepatic metabolism
Seizures	Mucous cytology
Systemic lupus erythematosus	Renal clearance/elimination
Thyroid disorders	Sodium retention
Urticaria	Urinary excretion
Emotional/Behavioral Symptoms	Weight
Aggression/anger/irritability/hostility	
Altered libido/sex drive	
Amotivation	
Anxiety/nervousness	
Depression/feeling blue/crying	
Food cravings (sugar, carbohydrates, chocolate, salty food)	
Impulse control problems	
Obsessive-compulsive behaviors	
Panic attacks	
Poor concentration/memory impairment	
Psychosis/paranoia/hallucinations	
Sleep changes (insomnia, hypersomnia)	
Suicidal ideation/attempts	

Compiled from refs. 1, 13, and 53.

and psychological symptoms is closely linked to the rise and fall of gonadotropins, ovarian hormones, 5-hydroxytryptamine (5-HT), endorphins, and prostaglandins.[2,7,12,26] The hypothesis that ovarian hormones are important for the pathophysiology of reproductive-related physical and mood disorders is supported by the fact that the onset and disappearance of symptoms are linked to ovulatory menstrual cycles and with the administration of progesterone and estrogen products.[12] Symptoms decline during pregnancy, after drug-induced inhibition of ovulation, with surgical ovariectomy, and after menopause.

Ovarian hormones are potent modulators of neurotransmitters in the brain. Although no differences in plasma levels of 17β-estradiol and progesterone have been found between women with PMS and controls, these ovarian steroids have an important role in the development and severity of symptoms.[12,32] Gonadal hormones such as 17β-estradiol, inhibin, progesterone, and testosterone are the most potent peripherally generated chemical signals in the central nervous system (CNS) that affect neurotransmitter synthesis, release, reuptake, and enzymatic inactivation.[12,27] 17β-Estradiol has been shown to affect 5-HT synthesis, levels, and receptors (e.g., promotes tryptophan hydroxylase, the rate-limiting enzyme in the synthesis of 5-HT; reduces 5-HT reuptake transporter activity; and increases the

density of the $5\text{-}HT_{2A}$ receptor in the brain regions associated with mood).[8,26]

PREMENSTRUAL DYSPHORIC DISORDER (PMDD)

Central serotonergic system dysfunction has been one of the leading theories for the pathogenesis of premenstrual and perimenopausal anxiety and mood changes.[5,12,28] Women with premenstrual dysphoria have been found to have reduced platelet [³H]paroxetine binding sites compared with controls, which may reflect abnormalities with brain serotonergic transmission at the presynaptic reuptake pumps.[33] Further evaluation of 5-HT transporter gene polymorphism was not associated with the decreased platelet 5-HT transporter density in women with PMDD.[33] A premenstrual reduction in protein intake has been reported in overweight women with PMS that could decrease the availability of L-tryptophan and its conversion to 5-HT.[34]

5-HT is converted to melatonin in the pineal gland under the influence of darkness, and its production is controlled by a circadian temperature rhythm and synchronized by the light-dark cycle. Several studies have reported reduced and earlier secretion of nocturnal melatonin in women with PMDD.[35] The pineal gland secretes melatonin under the influence of darkness, and the suprachiasmatic nuclei of the hypothalamus controls its release through β-adrenergic receptors. β-Adrenergic blockers such as propranolol suppress melatonin production and may cause insomnia, whereas tryptophan- and 5-HT-augmenting agents increase melatonin levels.

The GABAergic system appears to be involved in the pathophysiology of PMDD.[36] γ-Aminobutyric acid (GABA) neuronal function is modulated by gonadal steroids, and brain levels have been found to fluctuate across the menstrual cycle.[36] Plasma GABA levels have been reported to be lower across the menstrual cycle in women with PMDD compared with controls.[37] Cortical levels of GABA were found to decrease across the menstrual cycle in healthy women, whereas there was an increase in levels from the follicular phase to the midluteal and late luteal phase in women with PMDD compared with the controls.[36] Plasma allopregnanolone levels, a metabolite of progesterone that binds to the $GABA_A$ receptor, were reported to be higher in untreated women with PMDD[38] and lower in women with PMDD who responded to antidepressant treatment compared with controls.[32]

A genetic factor has been proposed for PMDD because several twin studies have found higher concordance rates in monozygotic twins than in dizygotic twins. Premenstrual mood symptoms and postpartum depression also may be linked genetically. During the postpartum period, hormonal changes are more extreme and sustained than they are in the normal menstrual cycle; thus women are particularly vulnerable to the development or exacerbation of anxiety and mood disorders during these times.[26] PMDD and seasonal affective disorder (SAD) may share a genetic vulnerability based on a study of polymorphism in the 5-HT transporter-promoter gene (i.e., women with PMDD and SAD were heterozygous for the 5-HTTLPR *l* and *s* alleles).[39] Women with severe PMDD have been found to have a higher prevalence of SAD compared with controls.[40]

PERIMENOPAUSE

Perimenopause is associated with erratic ovarian function that causes variation in the amount or duration of menstrual flow, change in the length of the menstrual cycle, and skipped menstrual periods.[7,21] The number of ovarian follicles diminishes gradually during a woman's reproductive life, but by the fortieth year, the decline becomes more rapid; by menopause, only a few follicles remain. Menopause generally occurs between the ages of 47 and 53 years, and 90% of women experience menopause by age 55.[7] In natural menopause, the ovaries continue to secrete the precursor to testosterone, androstenedione, which can be converted to estrone and estriol, both weak estrogens. The deficiency of testosterone and its conversion to 17β-estradiol, the primary active estrogen, is associated with causing physical and cognitive changes. Surgical menopause occurs when the ovaries are removed and results in an abrupt and complete loss of the ovarian secretion of testosterone, 17β-estradiol, and progesterone. After menopause, there is an absence of ovarian steroids as well as decreased serotonergic functioning.[8,41]

Compared with controls, perimenopausal women with depression have lower follicular phase plasma 17β-estradiol levels and higher luteinizing hormone (LH) levels.[42] Women with a lifetime history of major depression may have an earlier decline in ovarian function and onset of perimenopause (e.g., higher follicle-stimulating hormone [FSH] and LH levels and lower 17β-estradiol levels).[43] The perimenopausal transition is a time of increased vulnerability for depressive episodes, particularly in women with a history of mood disorders.[43]

CLINICAL PRESENTATION

PREMENSTRUAL SYNDROME (PMS)

5 Premenstrual symptoms begin at menarche and are absent during anovulatory cycles, pregnancy, and after menopause. Sequential hormone replacement with estrogen and progestogen products can produce the same symptoms associated with hormone fluctuations.[29] Although some women experience positive premenstrual changes, such as increased energy and productivity, most women experience negative changes in mood, appetite, sleep, and energy.[1] Women with PMS usually rank anxiety, irritability, mood lability, and fatigue as the most distressing symptoms.[44] Common emotional and behavioral symptoms include sadness, anhedonia, feelings of insecurity, low self-esteem, anger attacks, oversensitivity, crying episodes, decreased concentration, and food cravings. Physical changes (e.g., back pain, breast tenderness, headaches, water retention, and bloating sensations) may be better tolerated and cause less dysfunction than mood or behavioral changes do.[44] Cystic mastalgia is a common problem with PMS and is usually bilateral and nonlocalized (with no sign of pathology on mammographic testing).[14,16] Breast pain can be severe and often interferes with social and occupational functioning and sexual activity; thus women often seek medical care for the problem.[14]

PREMENSTRUAL DYSPHORIC DISORDER (PMDD)

PMDD is listed as an example of a category called *depressive disorder not otherwise specified* in the *Diagnostic and Statistical Manual of Mental Disorders,* Fourth Edition, *Text Revision* (see Table 78–1 for diagnostic criteria).[6] In order to confirm a diagnosis of PMDD, women must chart symptoms for at least two cycles using standardized prospective instruments.[45] The onset of PMDD typically occurs during the late teens to twenties (average age of onset is about 26 years), and the symptoms usually peak in the third or fourth decade.[2] During the perimenopause phase (up to 10 years prior to menopause), PMDD may become more severe and refractory to standard 5-HT-augmenting treatments secondary to the decline in the ovarian production of estradiol.[43] Common negative outcomes of PMDD include marital discord, physical and verbal abuse of others, difficulties in parenting, criminal behavior, poor work or school performance, work absenteeism, social isolation, accidents, hospitalizations, and suicide ideation.[1,2,19,46]

PERIMENOPAUSE

In the climacteric phase preceding menopause, women report trouble sleeping, hot flashes, anxiety attacks, nervous tension, depression, irritability, mood swings, short-term memory loss, and decreased libido.[7,21] Hot flashes and night sweats may disrupt sleep, which can cause irritability, fatigue, and poor concentration.[2] Irregular menstrual periods, vaginal dryness, urogenital atrophy, and urinary incontinence are caused by declining 17β-estradiol levels. A self-reported symptom checklist can be used to determine menopause-related symptoms over three dimensions—psychological, somatic, and vasomotor symptoms.[47] Women with a past history of mood disorders, premenstrual and postpartum depression, and a lengthy and symptomatic menopause transition may be at risk for major depressive episodes.[2,7,21,43] Predictors of an earlier age of perimenopause and menopause include an early age at menarche, cigarette smoking, a hysterectomy, a family history of early menopause, and a lifetime history of depression.[21,42,43]

▶ TREATMENT: Menstruation-Related Disorders

▦ DESIRED OUTCOME

6 The goals of treating menstruation-related disorders are to minimize symptoms and to improve functioning and well-being without causing adverse effects.

▦ GENERAL APPROACH TO TREATMENT

7 Before a diagnosis of a menstruation-related disorder is made, other medical or psychiatric conditions should be excluded (see Table 78–2). Mood and anxiety disorders often first occur during childbearing years and may require standard pharmacologic approaches. Effective treatment depends on an accurate diagnosis, identification and avoidance of triggers, and the development of a treatment plan that reduces the impact of the most disturbing symptoms.[19] A self-rated daily diary or calendar helps to establish a relationship between symptoms and the menstrual cycle and to monitor changes with different treatment approaches. Women should prospectively rate themselves daily for at least two menstrual cycles to determine baseline severity ratings so that treatments can be tailored to the most bothersome symptoms.[2,19] Women with severe PMDD may require immediate pharmacologic interventions because of the disruption in their lives.

8 It is recommended that the clinician follow a stepwise approach beginning with lifestyle modifications and nondrug therapies before resorting to pharmacologic treatments.[3] The weighing of risk versus benefit of pharmacologic interventions is important because some medications cause significant adverse effects and may have teratogenic properties.

In general, five different treatment strategies are used for menstruation-related disorders: (1) lifestyle changes to minimize precipitants, (2) physical and behavioral symptom relief, (3) modification of neurotransmitter/hormonal imbalances, (4) suppression of ovulation, and (5) removal of ovaries.

CLINICAL CONTROVERSY

Laboratory tests such as FSH and 17β-estradiol determinations are used frequently to diagnose perimenopause. The value and accuracy of these levels are controversial because levels fluctuate considerably each month depending on whether ovulation has occurred. No one symptom or laboratory test is accurate by itself to diagnosis perimenopause or PDD.

9 Perimenopausal women have varying degrees of severity of their symptoms (i.e., psychological, somatic, and vasomotor) that fluctuate based on hormonal changes in the late reproductive phase. Longitudinal monitoring of perimenopausal symptoms using a standardized rating scale is helpful to assess the severity and fluctuations during this period.[3,47,48] The use of serum hormone concentrations for diagnosing perimenopause may not be accurate because hormone levels vary widely from woman to woman, and levels change during the day and month based on ovarian functioning. In early perimenopause, there are reduced inhibin B levels (owing to fewer follicles) and a rise in FSH levels, with no significant change in 17β-estradiol or inhibin A levels.[21] FSH levels fluctuate considerably depending on whether ovulation has occurred, and 17β-estradiol levels may be normal or elevated depending on the activity of the ovaries. Thus laboratory tests may not be reflective of perimenopause.[21] An elevated serum FSH level (>25 IU/L), in conjunction with a low free 17β-estradiol level (<40 pg/mL) measured on day 2 or 3 after the onset of menses and a low inhibin B level (<30 ng/L), is suggestive of perimenopause.[21] At menopause, FSH levels are usually higher than 40 IU/L, 17β-estradiol levels are under 25 pg/mL, and both inhibin A and inhibin B levels are reduced.

Middle-aged women with somatic and mood symptoms should undergo evaluation for perimenopausal depression. Transdermal 17β-estradiol replacement can reduce vasomotor symptoms significantly; improve mood, sleep, and cognition; and decrease the risk of osteoporosis.[49–51] Transdermal testosterone therapy has been shown to improve mood, well-being, and sexual functioning in perimenopausal women.[52]

Hormonal fluctuations during the menstrual cycle, postpartum period, and peri- and postmenopause phases may cause differences in the pharmacokinetics and pharmacodynamics of drugs (e.g., changes in drug absorption, distribution, metabolism, and excretion). Thus clinicians must be aware of gender differences when prescribing medications.[53–55]

▦ NONPHARMACOLOGIC THERAPY

10 A great number of lifestyle changes and nonpharmacologic treatments are promoted for menstruation-related disorders without evidence-based studies.[1,3,5,14,19,24,56–61] Examples of lifestyle modifications and nondrug remedies recommended for menstruation-related disorders are listed in Table 78–3.

▦ PHARMACOLOGIC THERAPY

After women have tried lifestyle changes, nutritional supplements, and nonpharmacologic treatment approaches, some may require pharmacologic therapies if there is limited response. Women with less severe PMS generally self-treat headaches and cramps with aspirin, acetaminophen, and nonsteroidal anti-inflammatory drugs (NSAIDs). NSAIDs, such as naproxen and ibuprofen, are the treatments of choice for dysmenorrhea, menstrual headaches or migraines, and mastalgia.

For PMDD, the first-line strategy is to augment serotonergic neurotransmission, and the second-line strategy is to induce an anovulatory state using different types of hormonal treatments. For the perimenopause syndrome, augmentation of 5-HT neurotransmission and hormone-replacement therapy are the most common treatment strategies. Clinical studies have reported that 17β-estradiol replacement improves mood in perimenopausal and postmenopausal women with no or mild depression.[8] In postmenopausal women, 17β-estradiol therapy alone or in combination with antidepressants may be used to treat a major depressive episode.

▦ DRUG TREATMENTS OF FIRST CHOICE

▦ Published Guidelines or Treatment Protocols

There are no published consensus guidelines for the treatment of menstruation-related disorders.[3,19] Information about pharmacologic

TABLE 78–3. Nonpharmacologic Treatments for Menstruation-Related Disorders

- Education about the symptoms, treatment approaches, and strategies to reduce target behaviors
- Daily charting for two menstrual cycles to identify target symptoms
- Reduction or discontinuation of alcohol, caffeine, nicotine, and drugs of abuse
- Regular conditioning or aerobic exercise at least three times a week (with an increase in the daily workout routine by 30 minutes during the premenstrual week) and weight-bearing exercises to prevent osteoporosis
- Bright, white morning light (and possibly evening light) for 1 week premenstrually for seasonal worsening of premenstrual syndrome
- Regular, well-balanced, scheduled meals with adequate fiber, protein, essential fatty acids, complex carbohydrates, vitamins, calcium, and minerals
- Reduced intake of salt, fat, and simple sugars
- Increased intake of phytoestrogen-rich foods (soybean products) and tryptophan-containing foods (fish, poultry, and dairy products)
- Reduce weight to obtain a normal body mass index
- Adequate rest and a regular sleep cycle in a cool, dark room
- Dress in layers, consume cool foods and drinks, and use a fan for hot flashes
- Stress management, relaxation training, yoga, massage, biofeedback, and self-hypnosis
- Acupuncture, electroacupuncture, or acupressure treatment for dysmenorrhea, headaches, and pain symptoms
- Low-level topical heat for dysmenorrhea
- Individual, group, or family therapy, cognitive behavioral therapy, support groups, anger management, and assertiveness training

Compiled from refs. 1, 3, 5, 14, 19, 24, 56–61, and 96.

treatments and nonprescription remedies used for specific symptoms appears in Table 78–4. Examples of treatment approaches for different menstruation-related disorders are found in Table 78–5. An example of an algorithm for the diagnosis and management of PMDD is given in Fig. 78–1.

General Information Regarding Efficacy and Safety

PMDD should first be treated with 5-HT-augmenting antidepressants.[5,28,58,62–64] Fluoxetine, sertraline, and paroxetine are the only agents currently approved by the Food and Drug Administration (FDA) to treat PMDD, but other serotonin reuptake inhibitors (SRIs) are also effective.[65] These agents work by blocking presynaptic 5-HT transporter pumps, and their efficacy depends on 5-HT synthesis and release from the neuron. Patients should be reminded that adequate and regular intake of L-tryptophan (e.g., animal-derived protein such as dairy products, eggs, poultry, fish, and other meat sources) is important for the synthesis and storage of 5-HT in the brain and for the efficacy of SRIs.[28,34] Although benzodiazepines may be useful in the treatment of acute anxiety and intermittent insomnia, these agents should be used only as adjuncts to 5-HT-augmenting antidepressants because they do not alleviate the core symptoms of depression.

For women with premenstrual exacerbation of an underlying depression, severe PMDD, or climacteric depression, a 6- to 12-month course of an antidepressant is recommended. Some women benefit from continuous antidepressant dosing with an intermittent increase in dose prior to the onset of symptoms and a reduction in dose at the onset of menses. Varying the antidepressant dosage and adding supplemental medications based on menstruation-related symptoms have been shown empirically to be helpful. It may be necessary to try several different treatments to find an acceptable therapy.

Perimenopausal symptoms often respond to transdermal 17β-estradiol replacement therapy, along with a 5-HT-augmenting antidepressant if severe mood or anxiety symptoms are present.[26,41,49–51,66] Equine conjugated estrogens may not be effective because of the low content of 17β-estradiol in the product and the high content of other estrogen components that are not bioidentical to human estradiol metabolites.[67] Perimenopausal depression should be treated with standard antidepressant therapy such as 5-HT and norepinephrine (NE) reuptake inhibitors. Synthetic progestogens (e.g., medroxyprogesterone) may increase depressive symptoms and reduce the beneficial effects of estradiol.[2,26]

CLINICAL CONTROVERSY

Women often seek relief for premenstrual and perimenopausal symptoms from alternative or nontraditional treatments without consulting their health care providers. Herbal therapies, phytoestrogens, progesterone creams, megavitamins, folk remedies, and homeopathy are marketed to women without scientific evidence of efficacy or safety. Clinicians should ask women if they use alternative/complementary therapies and become familiar with the products (e.g., mechanism of action, efficacy, dosing, side effects, monitoring, and drug-herb and herb-herb interactions).

ALTERNATIVE DRUG TREATMENTS

Vitamin, Mineral, Herbal, Nutritional, and Hormonal Therapies

Complementary (or alternative) medical approaches are used widely by women to treat menstruation-related disorders.[23,24,56–61,67,68] Daily supplementation of vitamins, minerals, and calcium, along with a well-balanced diet, is the first-line therapy for all menstruation-related disorders and helps to reduce deficiency states, particularly in peri- and postmenopausal women.[68] Vitamin E supplementation in doses of 300 and 400 IU/day may be effective in relieving some premenstrual symptoms based on a few controlled studies.[14] Over-the-counter products that contain megadoses of vitamins, as well as minerals and trace elements, have been marketed for PMS without clinical trials to document their effectiveness or safety. There are several brands of products for PMS (e.g., a combination preparation of a mild diuretic,

TABLE 78-4. Pharmacologic Treatments and Nonprescription Remedies for Menstruation-Related Disorders

Vitamins and Minerals

Supplementation

Pyridoxine	50–100 mg/day (>200 mg/day associated with risk of peripheral neuropathy)
Calcium	1200–1600 mg/day in divided doses 2–4 times/day (minimum of 1000 mg/day for ages 19–50 and 1200 mg/day for ages >51 years) plus adequate vitamin D intake (e.g., 200–600 IU/day)
Magnesium	100–360 mg/day in divided doses during the luteal phase

Over-the-Counter/Herbal Products

Hot flashes

Black cohosh	Various products (e.g., tablets, drops) and dosages used; 27-deoxyactein content 1 mg per 20-mg tablet for Remifemin product
Dietary isoflavones	Soy-derived isoflavones (40–80 mg/day); red clover-derived isoflavones (40–80 mg/day)
Vitamin E	400–800 IU/day

Mastalgia

Evening primrose oil	500 mg/day to 1000 mg three times daily on days 16–28 of menstrual cycle
Chaste tree or chasteberry	30–40 mg/day on days 16–28 of menstrual cycle
Vitamin E	400–800 IU/day

Insomnia

Melatonin	0.1–1 mg at bedtime
Valerian	400–900 mg at bedtime

Depressive/anxiety symptoms (mild)

St. John's wort	300 mg (standardized to 0.3% hypericum) three times daily

Diuretics

Fluid retention/swelling

Spironolactone	50–100 mg/day in divided doses starting on days 12–16 until onset of menses

Nonsteroidal Anti-Inflammatory Drugs

Headache, backache, dysmenorrhea, and mastalgia

Ibuprofen	200–400 mg every 4–6 hours or 600 mg twice daily starting 1 week before menses and during first few days of bleeding
Mefenamic acid	250–500 mg three times daily starting as early as day 16 of cycle or at start of symptoms
Naproxen sodium	550 mg and then 275–550 mg twice daily starting 1 week before menses and during first few days of bleeding

Anxiolytics

Anxiety symptoms: Treat only during the luteal phase and only if serotonin reuptake inhibitors are ineffective.

Alprazolam	0.25–1.5 mg/day in divided doses during the luteal phase to reduce the risk of dependence
Buspirone	16–60 mg/day in divided doses continuously or on days 16–28 of menstrual cycle

Antidepressants

Affective symptoms: Use serotonin reuptake inhibitors only during the luteal phase (e.g., 7–14 days premenstrual) for a 2-month trial. Switch to continuous daily administration if response is inadequate and increase dose 7–14 days premenstrually if needed. A discontinuation syndrome may occur if using higher doses without tapering dose down gradually over several days.

Citalopram	10–40 mg/day
Escitalopram	5–20 mg/day
Fluoxetine	10–40 mg/day
Fluvoxamine	50–200 mg/day (may require tapering off)
Paroxetine	10–30 mg/day (may require tapering off)
Sertraline	50–150 mg/day
Venlafaxine	75–375 mg/day in divided doses (may require tapering on and off)

Dopamine Agonist

Mastalgia

Bromocriptine	2.5 mg twice daily on days 10–28 of menstrual cycle

Hormonal Therapies

Perimenopausal symptoms (vasomotor symptoms, atrophic vaginitis, emotional symptoms, sexual dysfunction)

17β-Estradiol	25–200 mcg transdermal patch (once-weekly patch or twice-weekly patch replacement); vaginal cream, ring, and tablets used primarily for vaginal atrophy and urogenital symptoms
Micronized progesterone	100–200 mg/day orally on days 17–28 or continuous (with intact uterus); progesterone topical products may not provide adequate serum progesterone levels to prevent estrogen-induced endometrial hyperplasia
Testosterone	150 mcg/day transdermal patch twice weekly (for low libido)

Suppression of ovulation (severe premenstrual syndrome or premenstrual dysphoric disorder)

Oral contraceptives	Estradiol + progesterone/progestogen (monophasic products on a continuous basis; biphasic products may cause more mood changes)
Estradiol	100–200 mcg transdermal patch every 3–7 days with add-back progesterone
Danazol	200–400 mg/day in divided doses at onset of breast pain until first day of menses (for mastalgia or premenstrual migraines)
Leuprolide	3.75–7.5 mg intramuscular injection monthly plus add-back estradiol and progesterone
Buserelin	400–900 mcg/day intranasal plus add-back estradiol and progesterone
Goserelin	3.6 mg subcutaneous injection monthly plus add-back estradiol and progesterone

Compiled from refs. 12, 13, 18, 19, 68, 77, and 96.

TABLE 78–5. Treatment Approaches for Menstruation-Related Disorders

First-Line Treatment Approaches

Lifestyle changes
  Regular, frequent, and small balanced meals with complete proteins, essential fatty acids, and complex carbohydrates
  Low dietary intake of fat and sodium
  Caffeine restriction
  Regular exercise
  Smoking cessation
  Alcohol restriction
  Regular sleep

Nonpharmacologic treatments
  Patient education about the cause, diagnosis, and treatment
  Stress reduction and management
  Anger management
  Self-help support group
  Individual and couples therapy
  Cognitive-behavioral therapy
  Light therapy with 10,000-lx cool-white florescent light (morning or evening)
  Acupuncture

Nutritional supplements
  Multiple vitamin with minerals once daily
  Essential fatty acids (omega-3 fatty acids), various products and dosages
  Pyridoxine up to 100 mg/day
  Vitamin E up to 800 IU/day
  Calcium carbonate up to 2000 mg/day
  Magnesium up to 400 mg/day

Second- and Third-Line Treatment Approaches

Dysmenorrhea
  Nonsteroidal anti-inflammatory drugs: ibuprofen, ketoprofen, naproxen sodium
  Alternative: mefenamic acid, acupuncture

Bloating/fluid retention
  Sodium reduction/restriction
  Spironolactone
  Alternative: amiloride, metalozone, hydrochlorthiazide, triamterene

Mastalgia
  Caffeine restriction (for fibrocystic breast disease)
  Evening primrose oil
  Chasteberry (minimal evidence for efficacy)
  Vitamin E (for fibrocystic breast disease)
  Nonsteroidal anti-inflammatory drugs: ibuprofen, ketoprofen, naproxen sodium
  Alternative: bromocriptine, danazol, oral contraceptives, gonadotropin releasing hormone agonist ± estradiol/progesterone add-back therapy

Migraines
  Caffeine restriction
  Nonsteroidal anti-inflammatory drugs: ibuprofen, ketoprofen, naproxen sodium
  Alternative: mefenamic acid, cyclooxygenase-2 inhibitors, acupuncture, oral contraceptives, triptans, intermittent 17β-estradiol, gonadotropin-releasing hormone agonist ± estradiol/progesterone add-back therapy

Insomnia
  Caffeine restriction
  Melatonin or valerian
  Alternative: trazodone, short-acting benzodiazepine, zaleplon, zolpidem (short-term use only)

Anxiety
  Caffeine restriction
  Serotonin reuptake inhibitor (intermittent during luteal phase)
  Alternative: buspirone (intermittent during luteal phase), alprazolam (short-term use only)

Depression
  Serotonin reuptake inhibitor (intermittent luteal phase therapy or continuous)
  Alternative: St. John's wort (mild symptoms only)

Severe premenstrual dysphoric disorder (multiple severe symptoms)
  Serotonin reuptake inhibitor (intermittent or continuous with increase in dose during luteal phase)
  Alternative: danazol or gonadotropin-releasing hormone agonist for 2–3 cycles (if longer treatment, estradiol ± progesterone add-back therapy may be required)

Perimenopausal symptoms (hot flushes, sleep disturbances, mood and congnitive changes)
  17β-transdermal estradiol (with progesterone if intact uterus)
  Alternative: serotonin reuptake inhibitors; gabapentin for hot flushes only

Compiled from refs. 1, 2, 7, 18, 20, 68, 77, and 96.

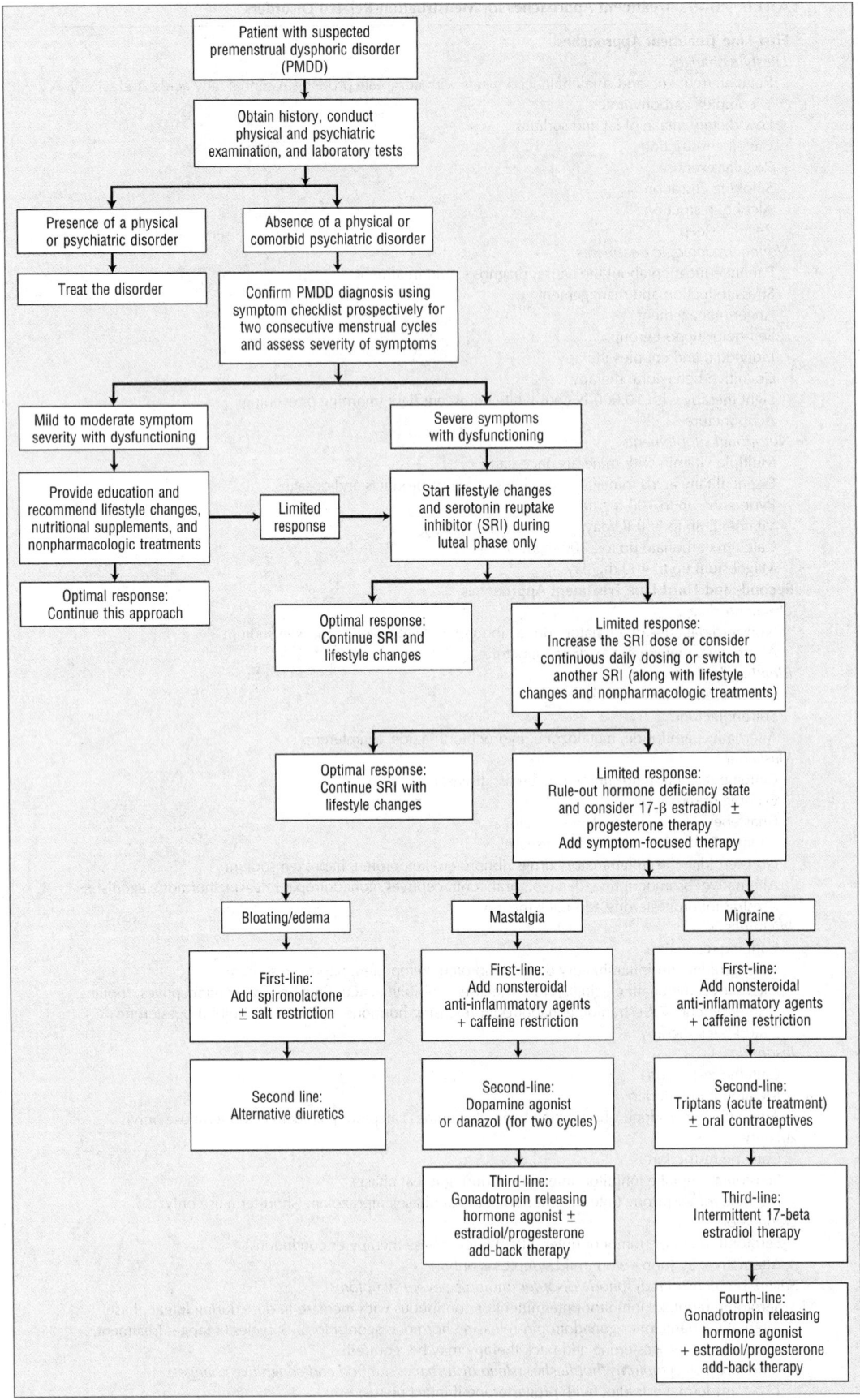

FIGURE 78–1. Algorithm for the treatment of premenstrual dysphoric disorder (PMDD).

an analgesic, and an antihistamine), but no efficacy data are available for these products.

Although pyridoxine (vitamin B_6) is used commonly as a treatment for PMS in doses of 50–100 mg/day, there is no evidence that women have a premenstrual pyridoxine deficiency. Pyridoxine has been reported to reduce the severity of premenstrual depression, fatigue, irritability, headache, and edema, but controlled studies have provided little support for its efficacy in PMS.[14,68] After a meta-analysis of nine published studies with pyridoxine, the authors suggested that doses of 50–100 mg/day pyridoxine may be beneficial in relieving premenstrual symptoms despite the lack of randomized, controlled studies.[69] Pyridoxine has been reported to cause peripheral neuropathy in excessive doses (e.g., 2000–6000 mg/day), and a reversible peripheral neuropathy has occurred with daily dosages of 200 mg.[14,69]

Magnesium is involved with many neuromuscular activities and cellular pathways that may affect PMS.[68] Low intracellular magnesium levels have been reported in women with PMS compared with controls.[70] It has been suggested that PMS may be related to an increased serum calcium-to-magnesium ratio.[71] Daily or luteal magnesium supplementation of 200–360 mg/day was reported to be minimally helpful in reducing premenstrual fluid retention in women with PMS.[18,72] A daily supplementation of 200 mg magnesium and 50 mg pyridoxine was found to reduce anxiety-related premenstrual symptoms in women with PMS compared with placebo.[73]

Abnormalities in calcium or parathyroid hormone homeostasis may be a factor in depression.[61] Significant fluctuations in calcitonin, a calcium-regulating hormone, and low plasma calcium levels during the menstrual cycle may play a part in the etiology of PMS.[74,75] Calcium influx into brain cells is involved with the release of many neurotransmitters. Calcium supplementation (e.g., 1200–1600 mg/day of calcium carbonate in two divided doses) has been shown to reduce premenstrual symptoms such as anxiety, depression, irritability, mood swings, headache, fluid retention, and cramps.[14,68,74–76] Calcium supplementation may help to prevent osteoporosis later in life, and it is a relatively safe and inexpensive treatment.[76]

Although herbal products and nutritional supplements are promoted for PMS and menopause, little is known about their dosing, efficacy, or safety.[23,24,57,60,61,77,78] Up to 80% of peri- and postmenopausal women have reported using botanical dietary supplements (e.g., soy, green tea, chamomile, ginkgo, ginseng, echinacea, St. John's wort, black cohosh, garlic, red clover, kava, valerian, evening primrose, and ephedra).[23,24] Because the FDA does not regulate herbal preparations and dietary supplements, active ingredients may vary from brand to brand.

St. John's wort (*Hypericum perforatum*), the most popular herbal remedy for mild depression, was reported to have efficacy in randomized, controlled trials and in one open-label PMS trial.[14,57,79] For the treatment of menopausal symptoms, only one observational study has reported that women had substantial improvement in physical and psychological symptoms.[14,80] The usual dose recommended for mild depression is 300 mg three times daily of a standardized product (hypericum 0.3%).[57] Several in vitro and human studies suggest that St. John's wort induces the hepatic cytochrome P450 3A4 enzymes and may decrease the efficacy of OCs and should not be combined with SRIs because of the potential risk of a 5-HT syndrome.[77,78,81]

Ginkgo biloba is marketed for improving memory and is often added to combination products to help relieve depression, anxiety, and memory impairment in menopausal women despite the lack of scientific evidence.[14,24] For PMS, *Ginkgo biloba* has been shown to improve mood and reduce breast tenderness and fluid retention when taken at 80 mg twice daily during the luteal phase.[57] Ginkgo inhibits platelet-activating factors and may increase bleeding in some people. Ginkgo also interacts at the cytochrome 450 enzymes in the liver and may cause drug interactions when combined with multiple medications.[57]

Dong quai (*Angelica sinensis*) is used widely in China for menstrual cramps and irregular menses and often is mixed with other herbs.[24] Chaste tree or chasteberry (*Vitex agnus castus*) has been used for PMS, mastodynia, and menstrual irregularities.[14,57,77,82] Three double-blind, placebo-controlled trials suggest that chasteberry may be effective in relieving premenstrual symptoms.[58] Black cohosh (*Actaea racemosa*) has been used for the treatment of dysmenorrhea and menopausal hot flashes, and blue cohosh has been used for menstrual cramps and stimulation of menstrual flow.[14,77,83] A review of clinical studies and drug surveillance reports of black cohosh products suggests that its side effects are mild and reversible.[83] Other herbal products that women often take are valerian, an herbal sleep aid; chamomile, a sedative, antispasmodic, antipyretic, and anti-inflammatory agent; and kava (*Piper methysticum*), an agent used to relieve pain and treat mild anxiety and insomnia.[14,24,57,77,78] Because of recent medical reports of kava causing hepatotoxicity, clinicians should monitor liver function tests if patients use kava.[57]

Products promoted for perimenopausal symptoms without scientific testing include dehydroepiandrosterone, a steroid hormone produced by the adrenal glands and ovaries that is a precursor in the steroid hormone synthesis pathway for testosterone; passion flower for insomnia, pain, and climacteric complaints; wild yam root, which contains diosgenin, a precursor to progesterone; and phytoestrogens, plant-based hormones found in soybean products such as tofu that promote estrogenic effects.[14,77,84] Phytoestrogens have a similar structure to 17β-estradiol but are 100 to 1000 times weaker at estrogen receptors.[14] The results of using soy isoflavones for vasomotor symptoms in peri- and postmenopausal women have been mixed (e.g., no differences in the number and severity of hot flushes compared with placebo treatment).[14,24,85] Controlled studies suggest that standard doses of soy isoflavone extracts (e.g., genistein and daidzein) may not be an effective treatment for vasomotor symptoms.[24,85] Women treated with soy protein also have a high discontinuation rate because the products cause a bad taste, gastrointestinal upset, gas, cramps, and stomach pains.[24] Consumption of soy protein instead of animal protein may decrease the serum concentrations of triglycerides, total cholesterol, and low-density lipoproteins, which may help to decrease cardiovascular risks.[14]

Various progesterone-like skin creams derived from extracts of the Mexican wild yam are available from health food stores. There is controversy as to whether diosgenin, the plant steroid, can be absorbed through the human skin and be converted to a biologically active progestogen.[86] When natural progesterone is added to creams or gels and applied topically, the circulating progesterone levels are low and may not induce a biologic change in the endometrium compared with orally administered micronized progesterone.[24,86,87]

SYMPTOM-BASED APPROACHES: SPECIAL POPULATIONS AND DRUG CLASS INFORMATION

Dysmenorrhea and Cramps

Dietary supplements such as thiamine, calcium, magnesium, omega-3 fatty acids, and herbal products have been reported to be effective in the treatment of both premenstrual and menstrual pain syndromes, but few have been evaluated for the treatment of dysmenorrhea.[14] Other modes of therapy for menstrual pain include biofeedback, transcutaneous electrical nerve stimulation, spinal manipulation, and application of local heat.[14] Acupuncture has been used for over 2500 years for pain syndromes and may be efficacious in the management of menstrual pain based on initial randomized studies.[14,88]

Prostaglandin inhibitors are effective in treating dysmenorrhea, headaches, and other pain syndromes.[58] NSAIDs inhibit prostaglandin synthesis and exhibit anti-inflammatory, analgesic, and antipyretic activity. Mefenamic acid has been reported to be effective in reducing menstrual pain, as well as breast tenderness, bloating, irritability, and depression. Agents such as ibuprofen, ketoprofen, and naproxen are also effective for dysmenorrhea and menstrual migraine. A comparison of nonprescription doses of naproxen (400 mg) and naproxen/naproxen sodium (200/220 mg) indicated that these agents were more effective than acetaminophen (1000 mg), ibuprofen (200 mg), or placebo in the treatment of dysmenorrhea.[89]

NSAIDs may cause gastrointestinal side effects and are contraindicated in patients with aspirin sensitivity, peptic ulcer disease, gastritis, bleeding disorders, and renal insufficiency. NSAIDs should be prescribed for short-term use only and in the lowest effective dosages (e.g., 1 week before the onset of menses and continued through the first few days of bleeding).[58] If primary dysmenorrhea does not respond to first-line agents, OCs (e.g., low-dose ethinyl estradiol combined with desogestrel) may be tried as an alternative approach for menstrual pain.[90]

Headaches and Migraines

The first-line acute treatment approach for menstrual migraines is NSAIDs.[4] If migraines do not respond to these agents, 5-HT$_{1D}$ agonists (triptans) can be used for abortive migraine therapy; however, these agonists should not be combined with 5-HT-augmenting antidepressants such as SRIs or monoamine oxidase inhibitors (MAOIs).[4] For more information on the treatment of acute migraines, see Chap. 59.

Low-dose intermittent estradiol therapy (oral or transdermal patch) started on days 24 to 26 and continued for 7 days through menstruation may help an "estradiol withdrawal" migraine.[4] If a women experiences a worsening of migraines with cyclic estradiol therapy, the dose can be lowered or changed to continuous transdermal therapy.[4] Estradiol-replacement therapy (alone or in combination with progestogens) is used frequently to treat menopausal migraines.[4] Selective estrogen receptor modulators such as raloxifene may be an option for menopausal women who cannot tolerate or take standard estrogen therapies.[4]

Other preventative treatments for menstrual migraine include the use of β-adrenergic blockers, calcium channel blockers, tricyclic antidepressants, and valproate. Agents that suppress ovulation, such as OCs, estrogen implants, danazol, and gonadotropin-releasing hormone agonists (GnRH-As), have been used for menstrual migraines that are refractory to standard migraine therapies.[4]

Bloating and Fluid Retention

Women with premenstrual syndrome commonly complain of bloating, swelling, and weight gain despite little evidence that they actually retain fluid. Dietary salt restriction should be the first-line treatment. If sodium restriction is not effective and there is a documented weight gain of 5 lb or more, diuretic therapy may be indicated. Spironolactone, an aldosterone receptor antagonist with potassium-sparing properties, is the only diuretic recommended for premenstrual weight gain and bloating.[18] Spironolactone has antian-

drogenic effects, and women should not use it during pregnancy and lactation. Other diuretics (e.g., hydrochlorothiazide, metolazone, and triamterene) have been used in treating premenstrual fluid retention, but there is no conclusive evidence that these agents are beneficial for women with PMS.[18] Magnesium supplements have been reported to reduce premenstrual fluid retention after 2 months of treatment.[72]

Mastalgia

Mastalgia, or mastodynia, is a common premenstrual problem and frequently coexists with fibrocystic breast disease.[14–16] Vitamin E (α-tocopherol) has been reported to decrease breast tenderness and swelling and is recommended often for fibrocystic breast disease despite a lack of randomized, controlled studies.[14] Caffeine restriction may not reduce breast pain, but it may be helpful for reducing fibrocystic breast changes.[15] Analgesics, evening primrose oil, chaste tree, and flaxseed have been advocated as therapies for breast pain based on a few open-label and randomized, controlled trials.[14] Diuretics, pyridoxine, and vitamin E have not been shown to be more effective than placebo for mastalgia.[16] A low-fat diet may be helpful because a high intake of saturated fatty acids has been implicated in causing breast pain.[15,16] Acupuncture and physical support (a well-fitted bra) are alternative modes of therapy for mastodynia.[14]

A deficiency of prostaglandin E$_1$ has been proposed to cause breast pain on the rationale that low levels may increase prolactin's effect on breast tissue and cause mastodynia.[18] cis-Linolenic acid, an essential fatty acid contained in vegetable oils, is converted to γ-linolenic acid, the precursor to prostaglandin E$_1$. cis-Linolenic acid, magnesium, pyridoxine, zinc, and vitamin C are all involved in the synthesis of prostaglandin E$_1$. Products that promote the synthesis of prostaglandin E$_1$ (e.g., evening primrose oil, which contains γ-linolenic acid) have been used for breast pain, but a meta-analysis of placebo-controlled studies concluded that evening primrose oil was not effective.[14,91] Although the oil may have little value in treating the other symptoms of PMS, it is used widely as a nutritional supplement for breast tenderness at doses of 500 mg three times daily during the luteal phase.[13,24,57,58]

Dopamine agonists bromocriptine and lisuride have been used to inhibit prolactin secretion and to significantly reduce breast swelling, engorgement, and tenderness in premenstrual women with mastalgia.[16,92] OCs also have demonstrated a reduction in premenstrual breast pain.[12] Antiestrogenic agents that inhibit ovulation (such as danazol and tamoxifen) have been used to treat endometriosis and cystic mastitis.[16] Danazol in doses of 100 mg twice daily was reported to be highly effective for the relief of premenstrual mastalgia when given during the luteal phase only but was less effective in treating the general symptoms of PMS.[93] Danazol has androgenic adverse effects at higher doses (e.g., increased lipids, acne, vocal changes, and negative mood) and should be reserved for the short-term treatment of breast pain or for co-occurring endometriosis and cystic mastitis.[12]

Insomnia

Histamine-1 receptor antagonists (e.g., diphenhydramine) and antidepressants with high histamine-1 blockade (e.g., doxepin and amitriptyline) have been used for acute sleep disturbances but may cause anticholinergic side effects, daytime sedation, and weight gain. Trazodone, a serotonin-2A and α_1-adrenergic antagonist, has sedative properties at lower doses and may be useful to promote sleep. The chronic use of benzodiazepines is not recommended for insomnia ecause such use may lead to tolerance and physical dependence. If enzodiazepines are used for the acute treatment of insomnia, agents vith shorter half-lives should be used (e.g., lorazepam or temazepam). Jltra-short-acting hypnotic benzodiazepines (e.g., triazolam) are less ikely to cause daytime sedation but have an increased risk of causing nterograde amnesia, early-morning insomnia, delirium, and with-lrawal reactions. Zolpidem and zaleplon, nonbenzodiazepines that ind to the benzodiazepine omega-1 receptor subtype, are alternative igents for the treatment of premenstrual insomnia but should be used only for short-term or intermittent therapy.

Melatonin has been used to regulate the sleep-wake cycle and is ised often to treat insomnia. It is not recommended during pregnancy and breast-feeding because of a lack of information about its safety.[94] Lower doses of melatonin (e.g., 0.1–1 mg at bedtime) are effective in nitiating sleep; higher doses may not improve the hypnotic effect.[94] The reduction in daytime sunlight, which increases melatonin secre-ion, may exacerbate PMS in the winter; this type of seasonal mood disorder may respond to phototherapy.[59] Early sleep deprivation also may help to correct circadian rhythm disturbances in PMDD.[95]

Hot Flashes, Vasomotor Symptoms, and Night Sweats

17β-Estradiol therapy (preferably transdermal patches) is an ef-fective treatment for moderate to severe vasomotor symptoms. Although venlafaxine, paroxetine, and fluoxetine have been used for hot flashes in postmenopausal women with a contraindication or intol-erance to estrogen therapy, the role of 5-HT- and NE-augmenting an-tidepressants has not been established in perimenopausal women with hot flashes.[22,96] Gabapentin, an anticonvulsant used in several pain syndromes, was found to reduce hot flushes in doses of up to 1200 mg/day in uncontrolled studies with women who were unwilling to take or who had a contraindication to estrogen exposure.[97] Gabapentin at 900 mg/day was reported to be more effective than placebo treatment in reducing hot flushes in postmenopausal women.[98]

The North American Menopause Society position statement for treatment of mild menopause-associated vasomotor symptoms rec-ommends first trying lifestyle changes, either alone or in combination with nonprescription remedies such as dietary isoflavones, black co-hosh, or vitamin E.[14,23,24,96] Studies suggest that there is a modest reduction in vasomotor symptoms with soy supplementation and that higher doses of soy isoflavones may be needed.[85,99] Black cohosh does not have phytoestrogenic effects, and the evidence of its efficacy for menopausal symptoms is weak.[14,22,57,83,100] Dong quai, a traditional Chinese medicine used for a wide range of gynecologic problems, was reported to have some estrogen-like properties (i.e., it stimu-lates cell proliferation of a human breast cancer cell line).[24,100] To date, there are no controlled efficacy or safety studies with dong quai for perimenopausal women.[24,100] Vitamin E has been promoted as being effective for vasomotor symptoms and vaginal dryness, but placebo-controlled studies have shown no effect on hot flashes.[14] Although chaste tree (*Vitex agnum-castus*), licorice (*Glycyrrhiza glabra*), and wild yam (*Dioscorea villosa*) have been promoted to help with hot flashes and vaginal dryness, no controlled studies have supported their efficacy.[14]

Anxiety

Before the advent of 5-HT-augmenting antidepressants, the treat-ment of premenstrual anxiety symptoms commonly included benzo-diazepines. Although benzodiazepines have the advantage of acting quickly to reduce anxiety symptoms and promote sleep, they have the disadvantage of causing sedation, cognitive and motor impair-ment, tolerance, dependence, and withdrawal reactions. Alprazolam, a triazolobenzodiazepine marketed for the treatment of generalized anxiety and panic disorder, has been evaluated for the treatment of PMDD in six double-blind, placebo-controlled studies. Four of these studies reported that alprazolam was more effective than placebo.[68] Intermittent dosing (e.g., 0.75–4 mg/day in divided doses 8 to 12 days before menses and gradually tapered down at menses by no more than 25% per day) and continuous dosing of alprazolam (e.g., 0.25 mg three times per day) reduced anxiety, irritability, tension, and feelings of being out of control in comparison with placebo. Because of the potential for dependency and worsening of mood, benzodiazepines should be used only for short-term treatment of menstruation-related mood disorders and should be avoided in dependency-prone patients.

Buspirone, a partial 5-HT$_{1A}$ agonist, has anxiolytic properties without causing sedation, cognitive impairment, or muscle relaxation. Buspirone is administered chronically for the treatment of general-ized anxiety disorder, but some studies used intermittent dosing (for 12 days before menstruation). Buspirone has minimal side effects and has the advantage over benzodiazepines of not causing dependence or a withdrawal syndrome after abrupt discontinuation. Comparative efficacy studies of buspirone and SRIs for PMDD are lacking.

Depression

5-HT deficiency or dysregulation (secondary to low levels of estradiol, high levels of MAO, or tryptophan depletion) dur-ing the premenstrual and perimenopausal phases may be a cause of anxiety, depression, and irritability.[5,28,50,62] Controlled studies using 5-HT-augmenting antidepressants (either continuous or intermittent dosing) have reported positive benefits in reducing dysphoria, irri-tability, and tension.[5,28,35,63–65,101] In addition, SRI antidepressants increase the bioavailability of 5-HT in the synapse and have been ef-fective in reducing a premenstrual exacerbation of major depression.

Nortriptyline and clomipramine, TCAs that inhibit the reuptake of 5-HT and NE, have been effective in the treatment of PMDD.[64] Nefazodone, a 5-HT$_{2A}$ antagonist with weak 5-HT reuptake inhibi-tion, was reported to improve symptoms significantly in a preliminary study, but a recent comparison study with buspirone reported that nefa-zodone was not superior to placebo treatment.[102] Venlafaxine, a 5-HT and NE reuptake inhibitor, was reported to be superior to placebo treatment in the treatment of PMDD[64,103,104] and may have efficacy in alleviating pain associated with fibromyalgia.[105] L-Tryptophan (the essential amino acid precursor for 5-HT) is currently not available as a dietary supplement, but it has been reported to be beneficial in PMDD.[105] NE-augmenting antidepressants such as bupropion, de-sipramine, and maprotiline are less effective than serotonergic agents in the treatment of PMDD.[5,28,62]

Compared with other classes of antidepressants, SRIs have a more favorable side-effect profile and better efficacy data.[62] A re-view of randomized, controlled trials with SRIs for the treatment of PMDD reported that the agents were well tolerated and effective in treating physical as well as behavioral symptoms with either intermit-tent or continuous dosing.[63,64,101] Citalopram, fluoxetine, paroxetine, sertraline, and venlafaxine all have been effective in PMDD placebo-controlled trials (60% to 90% efficacy rates with almost complete relief of symptoms).[63,64] For fluvoxamine, there are mixed results because one controlled study reported that it had similar efficacy to placebo treatment in PMDD.[64] Although antidepressants usually take

3 weeks or more to relieve the symptoms of major depression, the 5-HT-augmenting agents work more quickly in PMDD to relieve premenstrual anxiety, depression, irritability, food cravings, overeating, and weight gain. Side effects usually are dose-related and are worse during the first few weeks of therapy (e.g., tiredness, sedation, upset stomach, nausea, decreased appetite, headache, dizziness, sweating, nervousness, insomnia, and difficulty concentrating). A common long-term adverse effect is sexual dysfunction (e.g., decreased libido and delayed orgasm). SRIs have the advantage of not causing the significant weight gain, drowsiness, cardiovascular changes, and anticholinergic side effects compared with TCAs. Further, SRIs appear to have minimal teratogenic risk when used in recommended doses during pregnancy.[106,107]

SRIs may be effective in the treatment of PMDD at lower daily dosages than those required in major depression (e.g., fluoxetine 10 mg/day, sertraline 50 mg/day).[65] Doses should be increased gradually if the agent's effectiveness erodes after several months of treatment.[35] If one SRI is not effective or not tolerated, others should be tried until one is found to be effective.[108] The use of intermittent dosing during the luteal phase is gaining popularity because the SRIs work rapidly to attenuate depressive symptoms. The issue of a 5-HT discontinuation syndrome (e.g., sensory disturbances, flulike symptoms, sleep disturbances, or irritability) needs to be monitored when the agents are used intermittently.[65,109]

Intermittent dosing with fluoxetine 20 mg/day (during the 2 weeks before the onset of menses) has been approved for the treatment of PMDD.[110] Recent studies suggest that fluoxetine is also effective at 10 mg/day during the luteal phase or at 90 mg/day administered weekly at 2 and 1 weeks prior to menses.[65,111] The intermittent administration of citalopram (10–30 mg/day) during the luteal phase was reported to be more effective than continuous or semi-intermittent administration.[112] Controlled studies with intermittent luteal phase administration of clomipramine (25–75 mg/day) and sertraline (50–100 mg/day) reported a 1- to 2-day onset of effects with an improvement in the quality of life and functioning outcomes. A study comparing full- or half-cycle sertraline treatment (50–150 mg/day) reported that both regimens were effective and that side effects were similar for both groups.[113] With luteal phase administration, SRIs may improve mood symptoms more than the physical discomforts. Intermittent therapy with 5-HT-augmenting agents should be recommended before continuous daily dosing in the treatment of PMDD.[63]

For perimenopausal depression, antidepressants usually are dosed daily at standard dosages for major depression, although some women may respond to lower doses. Estradiol deficiency may decrease the activity of 5-HT and decrease the efficacy of antidepressants.[55] Two open-label studies have reported that citalopram in doses of 20–60 mg/day was effective in treating depression in peri- and postmenopausal women and had augmenting effects in depressed subjects who were still symptomatic after treatment with transdermal estradiol (i.e., improved symptoms of anxiety and somatic complaints).[114]

■ HORMONAL THERAPIES

By inducing anovulation with various hormonal therapies, the cyclicity of PMS disappears. Anovulation can be induced by estradiol implants, high doses of progesterones, OCs, GnRH-As, and danazol.[12] For the perimenopausal syndrome, the replacement of hormones such as 17β-estradiol, progesterone (if the uterus is intact), and testosterone is used to stabilize the deficiency and fluctuations in hormone levels.

■ Estradiol

17β-Estradiol, the active estrogen produced by the ovaries, is effective for menstrual migraines and to control perimenopausal symptomatology (i.e., vasomotor symptoms, vaginal dryness, and cognitive function). Given sublingually or transdermally, 17β-estradiol may be helpful for postpartum depression and psychosis.[20,26] Estradiol implants (subcutaneous pellets) and transdermal estradiol patches (two × 100 mcg) have been used to suppress ovulation in controlled studies in women with PMS.[12] Both routes of administration of estradiol were beneficial in reducing premenstrual mental and physical symptoms.

Transdermal administration of 17β-estradiol (combined with the cyclic or continuous administration of progestogens if the uterus is present) is recommended in perimenopausal women with significant mood and physical symptoms. Estradiol-replacement therapy has been beneficial in treating perimenopausal depression as well as in reducing hot flashes and sleep disturbances.[115,116] Preliminary studies suggest that transdermal 17β-estradiol can enhance the efficacy of serotonergic antidepressants in perimenopausal women.[117] Soy-based isoflavone extracts (genistein and daidzein) have been tried as an alternative therapy to estrogen replacement, but they are not a functional equivalent to 17β-estradiol, and long-term safety and efficacy studies are needed in peri- and postmenopausal women.[14]

Available estradiol products include a micronized and an ethinyl estradiol tablet, a cypionate and a valerate estradiol parenteral oil injection, a transdermal 17β-estradiol topical system, topical estradiol gel and emulsion, a vaginal estradiol cream and ring, and several oral and transdermal combination products with progestins (e.g., norgestimate and norethindrone).[110] The transdermal 17β-estradiol patches may cause skin irritation and should be replaced at a new application site every 3 to 7 days depending on the product formulation. With oral administration, 17β-estradiol is rapidly metabolized to estrone, which is not as active biologically and is less likely to help with mood and cognitive symptoms. Oral equine conjugated estrogens should not be used because of the very low content of 17β-estradiol (i.e., approximately 0.005 mg per 0.625-mg tablet), and the product is not bioidentical to human hormone.[67]

Unopposed estrogen therapy increases the risk for endometrial hyperplasia and adenocarcinoma; thus the use of cyclic, intermittent, or continuous progestogen therapy is recommended in women with an intact uterus.[118] Progestins decrease cellular proliferation and synthesis of estradiol receptors in the endometrium and increase the conversion of estradiol to estrone, which has a lower affinity for estrogen receptors. Estradiol with intermittent progestogen therapy (e.g., norethisterone 5 mg/day for 7 days each month to induce regular menses) may cause premenstrual-like side effects.[12] Chronic estrogen-only therapy has certain risks (e.g., increasing risk of endometrial, ovarian, and breast cancer and gallbladder disease).[66] Contraindications to the use of estrogens include breast cancer (relative contraindication), estrogen-dependent cancer, thrombophlebitis or thromboembolic disorders, undiagnosed abnormal uterine bleeding, and pregnancy.[66]

CLINICAL CONTROVERSY

Progesterone therapy has long been advocated for the treatment of PMS, but it is the most controversial treatment. Placebo-controlled trials do not support the use of progesterone or progestogen products in the management of premenstrual or perimenopausal syndrome.

Progesterone

A progesterone-deficiency theory had been proposed as causing PMS; thus for many years the administration of progesterone products during the luteal phase was a common hormonal treatment.[12] A meta-analysis of double-blind, placebo-controlled studies of different progesterone therapies in the management of PMS reported that these products are no better than placebo and that progestogens can induce negative mood changes.[119] Because of its questionable efficacy and risk of adverse effects, progesterone or progestin-only therapy is not recommended as a treatment in premenstrual syndromes.

During the perimenopausal phase, progesterone therapy is indicated if a woman has an intact uterus and is placed on estrogen-replacement therapy. An oral micronized form of natural progesterone is better absorbed but is metabolized rapidly by enzymes in the gut and liver to 5α and 5β reduced metabolites that have anxiolytic and hypnotic effects.[118] Oral administration of progesterone is associated with irregular and variable plasma levels, and transdermal progesterone creams do not achieve adequate plasma levels of progesterone; thus synthetic progestogens usually are added to hormonal regimens for OCs and for menopausal therapy.[87] Progesterone metabolites (especially allopregnanolone) are neuroactive and have benzodiazepine-like effects.[12,32,38] Very high doses of progesterone have been shown to cause confusion, memory impairment, and fatigue.[118] Vaginal administration and possibly topical administration decrease progesterone's conversion to allopregnanolone and may reduce CNS side effects.[118] Progestogens should be used with caution in certain medical conditions (e.g., migraine, seizure disorders, asthma, and cardiac or renal disease). Progestogens are contraindicated in patients with thrombophlebitis and thromboembolic disorders.

Estrogen-Progestin Combinations

OCs cause anovulation and may reduce dysmenorrhea, depression, and irritability in approximately 30% of women with PMS. Most women with PMS taking OCs continue to have cyclic mood changes, although the physical symptoms such as breast tenderness and menstrual pain may improve.[12] Differences in OC products (e.g., monophasic, biphasic, or triphasic and the type of estrogen and progestin) may result in variations in efficacy and adverse effects. Monophasic OCs appear to cause fewer mood changes than triphasic products, whereas monophasic products may result in more fluid retention.[12]

Placebo-controlled studies with drospirenone (a spironolactone-like progestin with antiandrogenic and antimineralocorticoid activity) along with ethinyl estradiol have been disappointing in reducing mood-associated symptoms in women with PMDD, although the product did decrease acne, appetite, and food cravings.[12,120,121] OCs high in progestin or progestin-only contraceptive agents may produce breakthrough bleeding and/or spotting, amenorrhea, acne, hirsutism, increased appetite and food cravings, fatigue, and depression. Pyridoxine-replacement therapy at 50 mg/day is recommended for women who become depressed while taking OCs. Because of the progestogen effects, estrogen-progestin combinations have an increased risk of causing thrombophlebitis, pulmonary embolism, and cerebral thrombosis.

Testosterone

Testosterone-replacement therapy, combined with 17β-estradiol-replacement therapy, has been used in peri- and postmenopausal women and after surgically induced menopause to increase libido, decrease fatigue, and improve well-being.[52,122] Testosterone products have been marketed primarily for male andropause, impotence, hypogonadism, delayed puberty, and palliative treatment of metastatic breast cancer in women. Testosterone is available as a transdermal patch, topical gel, buccal product, an intramuscular injection, and a subcutaneous pellet for implantation for men. A testosterone patch for female sexual dysfunction is under investigation for women with decreased libido after their ovaries have been removed. Methyltestosterone, a synthetic androgenic anabolic steroid, is available as an oral product and as a combination oral product with esterified estrogens for women.

Special testosterone formulations for women (e.g., troches, creams, and gels) with lower doses and in combination with estradiol are compounded frequently by pharmacists. When using testosterone products in perimenopausal women for decreased libido, the lowest effective dose should be used, serum testosterone levels should be monitored, and adverse effects should be assessed regularly.[122] Adverse effects of testosterone include acne, edema, hirsutism, hoarseness, clitoral enlargement, menstrual irregularities, abnormal liver function tests, irritability, anxiety, mental depression, and insomnia. Absolute contraindications include pregnancy and lactation.

Gonadotropin-Releasing Hormone Agonists (GnRH-As)

Because of their downregulation of pituitary gonadotropin secretion, GnRH-As (e.g., buserelin, goserelin, leuprolide, nafarelin, and triptorelin) cause a "medical ovariectomy" or pseudomenopausal state.[12,123] These agents are used for the management of endometriosis, dysfunctional uterine bleeding, uterine leiomyomata (fibroids), and severe PMDD.[123] GnRH-As can be administered subcutaneously, intranasally, by implants, or by intramuscular depot injections. The initial administration stimulates the release of FSH and LH from the pituitary, and then a downregulation of the pituitary decreases ovarian stimulation to release 17β-estradiol and progesterone.[123] Initially, some women report a "flare" in symptoms during the first few weeks of treatment, which is followed by a reduction in the physical and behavioral symptoms.

GnRH-As may improve cyclic mood changes and migraines during short-term therapy, but the chronic effects of suppressing ovarian hormone secretion could result in significant antiestrogen effects (osteoporosis and cardiovascular disease) and worsening of mood without hormone-replacement therapy.[12] GnRH-As therapy alone should not continue for longer than 6 to 9 months because of the risk of osteoporosis.[12] The use of a combination of a GnRH-As plus an "add back" of 17β-estradiol/progesterone may help to reverse antiestrogen and antiprogesterone effects but may decrease the effectiveness of GnRH-As. Low and ultralow dosages of GnRH-As (e.g., buserelin 400- and 100-mcg nasal spray once daily) have reduced cyclic mood changes in women with severe PMDD.[12] Until the long-term safety is established, GnRH-As should be used only for the most severe cases of PMS.

CLINICAL CONTROVERSY

Surgical treatment such as bilateral ovariectomy is controversial because it is irreversible and is associated with severe hormonal deficiency states unless there is add-back therapy. In addition, a tubal ligation or a partial hysterectomy is not effective for menstrual-related disorders. Clinicians usually reserve a complete hysterectomy as a last-resort treatment in severely affected patients who do not respond to standard therapies.

■ SURGICAL THERAPY

◄13 Surgical ablation of the ovaries (oophorectomy or bilateral ovariectomy) should be reserved as the last resort for the treatment of severe PMDD.[12] Before radical surgery, a 3- to 6-month trial of a GnRH-As or danazol is recommended to determine if anovulation is effective because the ovariectomy is not reversible. A hysterectomy without an ovariectomy is not effective for PMS.[12] A woman who has an ovariectomy without a hysterectomy needs both estradiol and progesterone-replacement therapy. Women who have both the ovariectomy and hysterectomy can receive continuous estradiol without intermittent progesterone therapy because there is no risk for endometrial cancer.

PHARMACOECONOMIC CONSIDERATIONS

Few studies have prospectively documented the degree of functional impairment before or after specific treatments or have evaluated the pharmacoeconomic differences in treatments for premenstrual and perimenopausal disorders. Data on the economic burden (i.e., health care utilization, related costs, and the loss of productivity) from different menstrual-related disorders are still lacking.[124] Several PMDD studies have reported greater improvement in psychosocial functioning and work capacity with SRIs compared with placebo.[125,126] In all studies, the degree of functional impairment was substantial at baseline and similar to that seen in studies of major depression. The functional improvement correlated with the improvement in premenstrual symptoms and was evident by the second cycle of treatment.

The peri- and postmenopausal periods are associated with significant physical and psychosocial changes in women's lives that can affect quality of life (e.g., occupational, health, emotional, and sexual).[47,48] Untreated depression may contribute to the development of a chronic and refractory mood disorder that significantly impairs psychosocial functioning. More studies are needed because severe menstruation-related disorders are disabling; prompt diagnosis and efficacious treatments are essential to improve functioning, to reduce morbidity and mortality, and to decrease the negative impact on women and their families.

EVALUATION OF THERAPEUTIC OUTCOMES

A trial of at least three menstrual cycles is needed to determine the treatment efficacy of one therapy and to adjust dosing before resorting to another therapy. Self-rating of prominent symptoms using a severity rating scale helps to monitor the efficacy of different treatment approaches.[1,45] A reduction of baseline premenstrual ratings (the average score for 5 to 7 days prior to menses) by 50% should be the minimum goal of therapy. Ideally, relief would be complete when premenstrual ratings are similar to postmenstrual ratings 5 to 7 days after the cessation of menses for several menstrual cycles.

MONITORING OF THE PHARMACOTHERAPEUTIC CARE PLAN

Patients who are undergoing therapy for menstruation-related disorders should have a monthly examination by a clinician to assess efficacy and adverse effects and adjust dosing, if needed. If first-line treatment approaches are not effective after several months, then alternative or combination therapies should be considered. Perimenopausal women should be monitored every 1 to 2 months to determine the effectiveness of treatment. Once a patient is stable and responding to the treatment plan, monitoring may be extended to every 3 to 6 months. Peri- and postmenopausal women should be monitored regularly because of the increased risk of osteoporosis, cardiovascular disease, and dementia. Throughout therapy, patients should be encouraged to eat well-balanced meals, to engage in regular exercise, to limit caffeine, to avoid drinking excessive alcohol or using drugs of abuse, to practice good sleep hygiene, and to take medications as prescribed to maximize treatment outcomes.

Menstruation-related disorders are common and cause significant disability and impairment in functioning if not treated properly. Therapeutic strategies should be individualized and targeted to the most distressing symptoms. If possible, medications should not be prescribed unless nonpharmacologic approaches have failed or unless symptoms disrupt the patient's functioning. The regular assessment and monitoring of menstruation-related disorders are necessary throughout a woman's reproductive years.

ABBREVIATIONS

DA: dopamine
FDA: Food and Drug Administration
FSH: follicle-stimulating hormone
GABA: γ-aminobutyric acid
GnRH: gonadotropin-releasing hormone
GnRH-A: gonadotropin-releasing hormone agonist
HPG axis: hypothalamic-pituitary-gonadal axis
5-HT: 5-hydroxytryptamine, serotonin
LH: luteinizing hormone
MAOI: monoamine oxidase inhibitor
NE: norepinephrine
NSAID: nonsteroidal anti-inflammatory drug
OC: oral contraceptive
OTC: over the counter
PMDD: premenstrual dysphoric disorder
PMS: premenstrual syndrome
SAD: seasonal affective disorder
SRI: serotonin reuptake inhibitor
TCA: tricyclic antidepressant

Review Questions and other resources can be found at *www.pharmacotherapyonline.com.*

REFERENCES

1. Pearlstein T, Stone AB. Premenstrual syndrome. Psychiatr Clin North Am 1998;21:577–590.
2. Haynes P, Parry BL. Mood disorders and the reproductive cycle: Affective disorders during the menopause and premenstrual dysphoric disorder. Psychopharmacol Bull 1998;34:313–318.
3. Moline ML, Zendell SM. Evaluating and managing premenstrual syndrome. Medscape Womens Health 2000;5:1.
4. Silberstein SD. Hormone-related headache. Med Clin North Am 2001; 85:1017–1035.
5. Steiner M, Pearlstein T. Premenstrual dysphoria and the serotonin system: Pathophysiology and treatment. J Clin Psychiatry 2000; 61(suppl 12):17–21.

6. American Psychiatric Association. Diagnostic and Statistical Manual of Mental Disorders, 4th ed., text revision. Washington, American Psychiatric Press, 2000:771–774.

7. Burt VK, Altshuler LL, Rasgon N. Depressive symptoms in the perimenopause: Prevalence, assessment, and guidelines for treatment. Harvard Rev Psychiatry 1998;6:121–132.

8. Shors TJ, Leuner B. Estrogen-mediated effects on depression and memory formation in females. J Affect Disord 2003;74:85–96.

9. Kessler RC. Epidemology of women and depression. J Affect Disord 2003;74:5–13.

10. Kravitz HM, Ganz PA, Bromberger J, et al. Sleep difficulty in women at midlife: A community survey of sleep and menopausal transition. Menopause 2003:10:19–28.

11. Moline ML, Broch L, Zak R, Gross V. Sleep in women across the life cycle from adulthood through menopause. Sleep Med Rev 2003;2:155–177.

12. Bäckström T, Andreen L, Birzniece V, et al. The role of hormones and hormonal treatments in premenstrual syndrome. CNS Drugs 2003;17:325–342.

13. Frye GM, Silverman SD. Is it premenstrual syndrome? Keys to focused diagnosis, therapies for multiple symptoms. Postgrad Med 2000;107:151–159.

14. Sidani M, Campbell J. Gynecology: Select topics. Prim Care Clin Office Pract 2002;29:297–321.

15. Ader DN, South-Paul J, Adera R, Deuster PA. Cyclic mastalgia: Prevalence and associated health and behavioral factors. J Psychosom Obstet Gynecol 2001;22:71–76.

16. Norlock FE. Benign breast pain in women: A practical approach to evaluation and treatment. JAMA 2002;57:85–90.

17. Goldenberg DL. Fibromyalgia syndrome a decade later: What have we learned? Arch Intern Med 1999;159:777–785.

18. Dickerson LM, Mazyck PJ, Hunter MH. Premenstrual syndrome. Am Fam Phy 2003;67:1743–1753.

19. Steiner M, Born L. Diagnosis and treatment of premenstrual disorder: An update. Int Clin Psychopharmacol 2000;15(suppl 3):S5–17.

20. Nonacs R, Cohen LS. Postpartum mood disorders: Diagnosis and treatment guidelines. J Clin Psychiatry 1998;59(suppl 2):34–40.

21. Bastian LA, Smith CM, Nanda KI. Is this woman perimenopausal? JAMA 2003;289:895–902.

22. Joffe J, Soares CN, Cohen LS. Assessment and treatment of hot flushes and menopausal mood disorders. Psychiatr Clin North Am 2003;26:563–580.

23. Mahady GB, Parrot J, Lee C, et al. Botanical dietary supplement use in peri- and postmenopausal women. Menopause 2003;10:65–72.

24. Taylor M. Alternative medicine and the perimenopause: An evidence-based review. Obstet Gynecol Clin 2002;29:555–573.

25. Joffe H, Hall J, Soares CN, et al. Vasomotor symptoms are associated with depression in perimenopausal women seeking primary care. Menopause 2002;9:392–398.

26. Joffe H, Cohen LS. Estrogen, serotonin, and mood disturbance: Where is the therapeutic bridge? Biol Psychiatry 1998;44:798–811.

27. Sundstrom I, Backstrom T, Wang M, et al. Premenstrual syndrome, neuroactive steroids and the brain. Gynecol Endocrinol 1999;13:206–220.

28. Parry BL. The role of central serotonergic dysfunction in the aetiology of premenstrual dysphoric disorder: Therapeutic implications. CNS Drugs 2001;15:277–285

29. Halbreich U. The pathophysiological background for current treatments of premenstrual syndromes. Curr Psychiatry Rep 2002;4:429–434.

30. Parry BL, Newton RP. Chronobiological basis of female-specific mood disorders. Neuropsychopharmacology 2001;25:S102–108.

31. Straneva PA, Maixner W, Light KC, et al. Menstrual cycle, β-endorphins, and pain sensitivity in premenstrual dysphoric disorder. Health Psychol 2002;21:358–367.

32. Freeman E, Frye CA, Kickels K, et al. Allopregnanolone levels and symptom improvement in severe premenstrual syndrome. J Clin Psychopharmacol 2002;22:516–520.

33. Melke J, Westberg L, Landén M, et al. Serotonin transporter gene polymorphisms and platelet [^{3}H]paroxetine binding in premenstrual dysphoria. Psychoneuroendocrinology 2003;28:446–458.

34. Cross BG, Marley J, Miles H, Wilson K. Changes in nutrient intake during the menstrual cycle of overweight women with premenstrual syndrome. Br J Nutr 2001;85:475–482.

35. Gold JH. Premenstrual dysphoric disorder: An update. J Pract Psychiatr Behav Health 1999;5:209–215.

36. Epperson CN, Haga K, Mason GF, et al. Cortical γ-aminobutyric acid levels across the menstrual cycle in healthy women and those with premenstrual dysphoric disorder: A proton magnetic resonance spectroscopy study. Arch Gen Psychiatry 2002;59:851–858.

37. Halbreich U, Petty F, Yonkers K, et al. Low plasma γ-aminobutyric acid levels during the late luteal phase of women with premenstrual dysphoric disorder. Am J Psychiatry 1996;153:718–720.

38. Girdler SS, Straneva PA, Light KC, et al. Allopregnanolone levels and reactivity to mental stress in premenstrual dysphoric disorder. Biol Psychiatry 2001;49:788–797.

39. Praschak-Rieder N, Willeit M, Winkler D, et al. Role of family history and 5-HTTLPR polymorphism in female seasonal affective disorder patients with or without premenstrual dysphoric disorder. Eur Neuropsychopharmacol 2002;12:129–134.

40. Praschak-Rieder N, Willeit M, Neumeister A, et al. Prevalence of premenstrual dysphoric disorder in female patients with seasonal affective disorder. J Affect Disord 2001;63:239–242.

41. Halbreich U, Rojansky N, Palter S, et al. Estrogen augments serotonergic activity in postmenopausal women. Biol Psychiatry 1995;37:434–441.

42. Young EA, Midgley AR, Carlson NE, Brown MB. Alteration in the hypothalamic-pituitary-ovarian axis in depressed women. Arch Gen Psychiatry 2000;57:1157–1162.

43. Harlow BL, Wise LA, Otto MW, et al. Depression and its influence on reproductive endocrine and menstrual cycle markers associated with perimenopause: The Harvard Study of Moods and Cycles. Arch Gen Psychiatry 2003;60:29–36.

44. Bloch M, Schmidt PJ, Rubinow DR. Premenstrual syndrome: Evidence for symptom stability across cycles. Am J Psychiatry 1997;154:1741–1746.

45. Haywood A, Slade P, King H. Assessing the assessment measures for menstrual cycle symptoms: A guide for researchers and clinicians. J Psychosom Res 2002;52:223–237.

46. Roca CA, Schmidt PJ, Rubinow DR. A follow-up study of premenstrual syndrome. J Clin Psychiatry 1999;60:763–766.

47. Freeman EW, Sammel MD, Liu L, Martin P. Psychometric properties of a menopausal symptom list. Menopause 2003;10:258–265.

48. Utian W, Janata J, Kingsberg SA, et al. The Utian Quality of Life (UQOL) Scale: Development and validation of an instrument to quantify quality of life through and beyond menopause. Menopause 2002;9:402–410.

49. Archer JSM. Relationship between estrogen, serotonin, and depression. Menopause 1999;6:71–78.

50. Rubinow DR, Schmidt PJ, Roca CA. Estrogen-serotonin interactions: Implications for affective regulation. Biol Psychiatry 1998;44:839–850.

51. Rodriguez MM, Grossberg GT. Estrogen as a psychotherapeutic agent. Clin Geriatr Med 1998;14:177–189.

52. Goldstat R, Briganti E, Tran J, et al. Transdermal testosterone therapy improves well-being, mood, and sexual function in premenopausal women. Menopause 2003;10:390–398.

53. Kashuba ADM, Nafziger AN. Physiological changes during the menstrual cycle and their effects on the pharmacokinetics and pharmacodynamics of drugs. Clin Pharmacokinet 1998;34:203–218.

54. Frackiewicz EJ, Sramek JJ, Cutler NR. Gender differences in depression and antidepressant pharmacokinetics and adverse events. Ann Pharmacother 2000;34:80–88.

55. Yonkers KA, Brawman-Mintzer O. The pharmacologic treatment of depression: Is gender a critical factor? J Clin Psychiatry 2002;63:610–615.

56. Manber R, Allen JJB, Morris MM. Alternative treatments for depression: Empirical support and relevance to women. J Clin Psychiatry 2002;63:628–640.

57. Girman A, Lee R, Kligler B. An integrative medicine approach to premenstrual syndrome. Am J Obstet Gynecol 2003;188:S56–65.

58. Mitwally MF, Kahn LS, Halbreich U. Pharmacotherapy of premenstrual syndromes and premenstrual dysphoric disorder: Current practices. Expert Opin Pharmacother 2002;3:1577–1590.

59. Lam RW, Carter D, Misri S, et al. A controlled study of light therapy in women with late luteal phase dysphoric disorder. Psychiatry Res 1999; 86:185–192.

60. Stevinson C, Ernst E. Complementary/alternative therapies for premenstrual syndrome: A systematic review of randomized, controlled trials. Am J Obstet Gynecol 2001;185:227–235.

61. Singh BB, Berman BM, Simpson RL, et al. Incidence of premenstrual syndrome and remedy usage: A national probability sample study. Altern Ther Health Med 1998;4:75–79.

62. Eriksson E. Serotonin reuptake inhibitors for the treatment of premenstrual dysphoria. Int Clin Psychopharmacol 1999;14(suppl 2): S27–33.

63. Luisi AF, Pawasauskas JE. Treatment of premenstrual dysphoric disorder with selective serotonin reuptake inhibitors. Pharmacotherapy 2003; 23:1131–1140.

64. Pearlstein T. Selective serotonin reuptake inhibitors for premenstrual dysphoric disorder: The emerging gold standard? Drugs 2002;62: 1869–1885.

65. Pearlstein T, Yonkers KA. Review of fluoxetine and its clinical applications in premenstrual dysphoric disorder. Expert Opin Pharmacother 2002;3:979–991.

66. Stahl SM. Basic psychopharmacology of antidepressants: 2. Estrogen as an adjunct to antidepressant therapy. J Clin Psychiatry 1998;59(suppl 4): 15–42.

67. Dey M, Lyttle CR, Pickar JH. Recent insights into the varying activity of estrogens. Maturitas 2000;34:S25–33.

68. Pearlstein T, Steiner M. Non-antidepressant treatment of premenstrual syndrome. J Clin Psychiatry 2000;61(suppl 12):22–27.

69. Wyatt KM, Dimmock PW, Jones PW, O'Brien PSM. Efficacy of vitamin B_6 in the treatment of premenstrual syndrome: A systematic review. Br Med J. 1999;318:1375–1381.

70. Chuong CJ, Dawson EB. Critical evaluation of nutritional factors in the pathophysiology and treatment of premenstrual syndrome. Clin Obstet Gynecol 1992;35:679–692.

71. Muneyvirci-Delale O, Nacharaju VL, Altura BM, et al. Sex steroid hormones modulate serum ionized magnesium and calcium levels throughout the menstrual cycle in women. Fertil Steril 1998;69:958–962.

72. Walker AF, DeSouza MC, Vickers MF, et al. Magnesium supplementation alleviates premenstrual symptoms of fluid retention. J Womens Health 1998;7:1157–1165.

73. De Souza MC, Walker AF, Robinson PA, et al. A synergistic effect of a daily supplement for 1 month of 200 mg magnesium plus 50 mg vitamin B_6 for the relief of anxiety-related premenstrual symptoms: A randomized, double-blind, crossover study. J Womens Health Gend Based Med. 2000;9:131–139.

74. Thys-Jacobs S, Starkey P, Bernstein D, et al. Calcium carbonate and the premenstrual syndrome: Effects on premenstrual and menstrual symptoms. Am J Obstet Gynecol 1998;179:444–452.

75. Thys-Jacobs S. Micronutrients and the premenstrual syndrome: The case for calcium. J Am Coll Nutr 2000;19:220–227.

76. Ward MW, Holimon TD. Calcium treatment for premenstrual syndrome. Ann Pharmacother 1999;33:1356–1358.

77. Wong AHC, Smith M, Boon HS. Herbal remedies in psychiatric practice. Arch Gen Psychiatry 1998;55:1033–1044.

78. Klepser TB, Klepser ME. Unsafe and potentially safe herbal therapies. Am J Health Syst Pharm 1999;56:125–138.

79. Stevinson C, Ernest E. A pilot study of *Hypericum perforatum* for the treatment of premenstrual syndrome. Br J Obstet Gynaecol 2000; 107:870–876.

80. Grube B, Walper A, Wheatley D. St John's wort extract: Efficacy for menopausal symptoms of psychological origin. Adv Ther 1999;16: 177–186.

81. Markowitz JS, Donovan JL, Devane CL, et al. Effect of St John's wort on metabolism by induction of cytochrome P450 3A4 enzymes. JAMA 2003;290:1500–1504.

82. Loch E-G, Selle H, Boblitz N. Treatment of premenstrual syndrome with a phytopharmaceutical formulation containing *Vitex agnus castus*. J Womens Health Gend Based Med 2000;9:315–320.

83. Huntley A, Ernst E. A systematic review of the safety of black cohosh. Menopause 2003;10:58–64.

84. Brzezinski A, Adlercreutz H, Shaoul R, et al. Short-term effects of phytoestrogen-rich diet on postmenopausal women. Menopause 1997; 4:89–94.

85. Burke GL, Legault C, Anthony M, et al. Soy protein and isoflavone effects on vasomotor symptoms in peri- and postmenopausal women: The Soy Estrogen Alternative Study. Menopause 2003;10:147–153.

86. Gambrell RD. Progesterone skin cream and measurements of absorption. Menopause 2003;10:1–3.

87. Wren BG, Champion SM, Manga RZ, Eden JA. Transdermal progesterone and its effect on vasomotor symptoms, blood lipid levels, bone metabolic markers, moods, and quality of life for postmenopausal women. Menopause 2003;10:13–18.

88. Wilson M, Farquhar C, Kennedy S, et al. Transcutaneous electrical nerve stimulation and acupuncture for primary dysmenorrhea. Cochrane Review 2001;2.

89. Milsom I, Minic M, Dawood MY, et al. Comparison of the efficacy and safety of nonprescription doses of naproxen and naproxen sodium with ibuprofen, acetaminophen, and placebo in the treatment of primary dysmenorrhea: A pooled analysis of five studies. Clin Ther 2002;24: 1384–1400.

90. Hendrix SL, Alexander NJ. Primary dysmenorrhea treatment with a desogestrel-containing low-dose oral contraceptive. Contraception 2002; 66:393–399.

91. Budeiri D, Li Wan Po A, Dornan JC. Is evening primrose oil of value in the treatment of premenstrual syndrome? Control Clin Trials 1996;17: 60–68.

92. Kaleli S, Aydin Y, Erel CT, Colgar U. Symptomatic treatment of premenstrual mastalgia in premenstrual women with lisuride maleate: A double-blind, placebo-controlled, randomized study. Fertil Steril 2001;75: 718–723.

93. O'Brien PMS, Abukhlil IEH. Randomized, controlled trial of the management of premenstrual syndrome and premenstrual mastalgia using luteal phase-only danazol. Am J Obstet Gynecol 1999;180:18–23.

94. Avery D, Lenz M, Landis C. Guidelines for prescribing melatonin. Ann Med 1998;30:122–130.

95. Parry BL, Mostofi N, LeVeau B, et al. Sleep EEG studies during early and late partial sleep deprivation in premenstrual dysphoric disorder and normal control subjects. Psychiatr Res 1999;85:127–143.

96. Treatment of menopause-associated vasomotor symptoms: Position statement of The North American Menopause Society. Menopause 2004; 11:11–33.

97. Albertazzi P, Bottazzi M, Purdie DW. Gabapentin for the management of hot flushes: A case series. Menopause 2003;10:214–217.

98. Guttuso T Jr, Kurlan R, McDermott MP, Kieburtz K. Gabapentin's effects on hot flashes in postmenopausal women: A randomized controlled trial. Obstet Gynecol 2003;101:337–345.

99. Faure ED, Chantre P, Mares P. Effects of a standardized soy extract on hot flushes: A multicenter, double-blind, randomized, placebo-controlled study. Menopause 2002:9:329–334.

100. Amato P, Christophe S, Mellon PL. Estrogenic activity of herbs commonly used as remedies for menopausal symptoms. Menopause 2002; 9:145–150.

101. Wyatt KM, O'Brien PMS. Selective serotonin reuptake inhibitors for premenstrual syndrome. Cochrane Review 2003;3.

102. Landén M, Eriksson O, Sundblad C, et al. Compounds with affinity for serotonergic receptors in the treatment of premenstrual dysphoria: A comparison of buspirone, nefazodone and placebo. Psychopharmacology (Berl) 2001;155:292–298.

103. Freeman EW, Rickels K, Yonkers KA, et al. Venlafaxine in the treatment of premenstrual dysphoric disorder. Obstet Gynecol 2001;98:737–744.

104. Sayer K, Aksu G, Ak I, Tosun M. Venlafaxine treatment of fibromyalgia. Ann Pharmacother 2003;37:1561–1565.

105. Steinberg S, Annable L, Young SN, et al. A placebo-controlled clinical

trial of L-tryptophan in premenstrual dysphoria. Biol Psychiatry 1999; 45:313–320.

106. Kulin NA, Pastuszak A, Sage SR, et al. Pregnancy outcome following material use of the new selective serotonin reuptake inhibitors: A prospective controlled multicenter study. JAMA 1998;279:609–610.

107. Wisner KL, Gelenberg AJ, Leonard H, et al. Pharmacologic treatment of depression during pregnancy. JAMA 1999;282:1264–1269.

108. Freeman EW, Jabara S, Sondheimer SJ, Auletto R. Citalopram in PMS patients with prior SSRI treatment failure: A preliminary study. J Womens Health Gend Based Med 2002;11:459–464.

109. Zajecka J, Tracy KA, Mitchell S. Discontinuation symptoms after treatment with serotonin reuptake inhibitors: A literature review. J Clin Psychiatry 1997;58:291–297.

110. Cohen LS, Miner C, Brown EW, et al. Premenstrual daily fluoxetine for premenstrual dysphoric disorder: A placebo-controlled, clinical trial using computerized diaries. Obstet Gynecol 2002;100:435–444.

111. Miner C, Brown E, McCray S, et al. Weekly luteal-phase dosing with enteric-coated fluoxetine 90 mg in premenstrual dysphoric disorder: A randomized, double-blind, placebo-controlled clinical trial. Clin Ther 2002;24:417–433.

112. Wikander I, Sundblad C, Andersch B, et al. Citalopram in premenstrual dysphoria: Is intermittent treatment during luteal phases more effective than continuous medication throughout the menstrual cycle? J Clin Psychopharmacol 1998;18:390–398.

113. Freeman EW, Rickels K, Arredondo F, et al. Full- or half-cycle treatment of severe premenstrual syndrome with a serotonergic antidepressant. J Clin Psychopharmacol 1999;19:3–8.

114. Soares CN, Poitras JR, Prouty J, et al. Efficacy of citalopram as a monotherapy or as an adjunctive treatment to estrogen therapy for perimenopausal and postmenopausal women with depression and vasomotor symptoms. J Clin Psychiatry 2003;64:473–479.

115. Schmidt PJ, Nieman L, Danaceau MA, et al. Estrogen replacement in perimenopause-related depression: A preliminary report. Am J Obstet Gynecol 2000;183:414–420.

116. Soares CN, Almeida OP, Joffe H, et al. Efficacy of estradiol for the treatment of depressive disorders in perimenopausal women: A double-blind, randomized, placebo-controlled trial. Arch Gen Psychiatry 2001; 58:529–534.

117. Tam LW, Parry BL. Does estrogen enhance the antidepressant effects of fluoxetine? J Affect Disord 2003;77:87–92.

118. Role of progestogen in hormone therapy for postmenopausal women: Position statement of The North American Menopause Society. Menopause 2003;10:113–132.

119. Wyatt K, Dimmock P, Jones P, et al. Efficacy of progesterone and progestogens in management of premenstrual syndrome: Systematic review. Br Med J 2001;323:1–8.

120. Dickerson V. Quality of life issues: Potential role for an oral contraceptive containing ethinyl estradiol and drospirone. J Reprod Med 2002;47: 985–993.

121. Freeman EW, Kroll R, Rapkin A, et al. Evaluation of a unique oral contraceptive in the treatment of premenstrual dysphoric disorder. J Womens Health Gend Based Med 2001;10:561–569.

122. Davis SR. Androgen treatment in women. Med J Aust 1999;170: 545–549.

123. Moghissi KS. A clinician's guide to the use of gonadotropin-releasing hormone analogues in women. Medscape Womens Health 2000;5:5.

124. Chawla A, Swindle R, Long S, et al. Premenstrual dysphoric disorder: Is there an economic burden of illness? Med Care 2002;40:1101–1112.

125. Pearlstein TB, Halbreich U, Batzar ED, et al. Psychosocial functioning in women with premenstrual dysphoric disorder before and after treatment with sertraline and placebo. J Clin Psychiatry 2000;61:101–109.

126. Steiner M, Brown E, Trzepacz P, et al. Fluoxetine improves functional work capacity in women with premenstrual dysphoric disorder. Arch Womens Ment Health 2003;6:71–77.

79

ENDOMETRIOSIS

Deborah A. Sturpe and Alkesh D. Patel

Learning Objectives and other resources can be found at *www.pharmacotherapyonline.com.*

KEY CONCEPTS

1. The etiology of endometriosis is likely multifactorial, with no single theory satisfactory to explain all cases. Retrograde menstruation is the most widely accepted proposed mechanism.

2. Endometriosis should be suspected in any woman of reproductive age, including adolescents, with recurring cyclic or acyclic pelvic pain and/or subfertility.

3. There are no physical examination findings or laboratory tests that are considered diagnostic for endometriosis. A definitive diagnosis can be made only via surgical visualization of lesions. Confirmation of diagnosis is not necessary in all cases.

4. Treatment goals of endometriosis include improvement of painful symptoms and maintenance or improvement of fertility. Therapy is considered successful based on resolution of the patient's symptoms or achievement of pregnancy.

5. All medical therapies (nonsteroidal anti-inflammatory drugs, oral contraceptives, progestins, danazol, or gonadotropin-releasing hormone agonists) are equally efficacious in treating endometriosis-related pain based on available evidence. Choice among agents is determined primarily by side-effect profile, cost, and individual patient response.

6. Endometriosis-related pain may be treated by medical or surgical therapy. Empirical medical therapy is likely more cost-effective and is recommended based on consensus guidelines.

7. Recurrence rates of endometriosis-related pain are high after both medical and surgical therapies. Extended use of medical therapy or postoperative use of medical therapy may be needed to maintain efficacy.

8. Endometriosis-related infertility is unresponsive to medical therapy. Conservative surgical therapy is the preferred treatment.

Endometriosis is a common cause of chronic pelvic pain in women and is also associated with infertility. Characterized by the presence of endometrial tissue outside the uterus, endometriosis is a chronic, recurring disease. Therapy is targeted at relieving symptoms and improving fertility.

EPIDEMIOLOGY

Endometriosis is the cause of pelvic pain (dysmenorrhea, dyspareunia) and infertility in more than 35% of women of reproductive age, but the exact prevalence of the disease is unknown because surgical visualization is necessary to make a definitive diagnosis. In the general population, prevalence is estimated at approximately 10% of women.[1] An estimated 71% to 87% of women presenting with chronic pelvic pain have endometriosis, and approximately 38% of women with infertility have the disorder.[1] The disease typically presents during the reproductive years but has been documented over a wide age range of 8 to 76 years, with some cases occurring prior to menarche.[2,3] In the adolescent population, 45% to 70% of chronic pelvic pain and dysmenorrhea cases are thought to be secondary to endometriosis, and symptoms are often more severe than in the adult population.[3,4] Endometriosis progression generally is slow, and the disease may remain stable or regress in 50% of women.[5]

ETIOLOGY

1. The etiology of endometriosis is unknown. The mechanism for development of these lesions is likely to be multifactoral and includes theories of retrograde menstrual flow, coelomic metaplasia, lymphatic and vascular spread, and immunologic abnormalities.[1,3,6–8] Retrograde menstruation is the most popular theory of endometriosis development. It proposes that endometrial tissue flows back through the fallopian tubes with subsequent implantation into the peritoneal cavity. However, a low percentage of women with retrograde menstrual flow develop endometriosis, thus supporting other mechanisms of pathogenesis. One of the mechanisms gaining increasing recognition is the involvement of immune system factors in the development and progression of endometriosis. This theory is supported by abnormal B- and T-cell function, decreased apoptosis, and altered levels of prostanoids, cytokines, growth factors, and interleukins found in endometrial lesions and peritoneal fluid of affected women.[8,9] Based on these findings, it has been hypothesized that an underlying immunologic disorder is responsible for endometriosis development in most women.[8]

Several causal associations have been identified in the development of endometriosis despite the uncertainty regarding etiology. Factors associated with endometriosis include obstruction of menstrual flow, frequent or heavy menstruation, genital tract abnormalities, high estrogen levels, and elevated peripheral body fat.[1,7,10,11] Genetic predisposition also has been identified as a contributing factor, with the disease being linked between first-degree female relatives and monozygotic twins.[3,8] The decreased estrogen levels associated with oral contraceptive use, menopause, exercise, and smoking appear to protect against the development of endometriosis.[1,11]

PATHOPHYSIOLOGY

PELVIC PAIN

Endometriosis-associated pain is secondary to structural and/or inflammatory causes. The lesions may cause pain by compression of nerve fibers.[8,12] Increased pressure within endometriomas (cysts within the ovary) has been linked to dyspareunia.[12] Endometrial lesions also generate local inflammation with prostaglandin release and increase the risk of developing adhesions.[8,12] Endometrial lesions contain estrogen and progesterone receptors, and symptoms may correlate with the cyclic release of hormones during the menstrual cycle.

INFERTILITY

In severe endometriosis, infertility likely results from distortion of the pelvic structure secondary to endometrial lesions, inflammation, and adhesions.[8,12,13] In milder disease, the cause-effect relationship is more controversial. Decreased oocyte viability and/or production resulting from the altered uterine environment may be a contributing factor.[12]

CLINICAL PRESENTATION

❷ ❸ Endometriosis should be suspected in women with subfertility, dysmenorrhea, dyspareunia, or chronic pelvic pain. A definitive diagnosis can be made only by direct surgical visualization of endometrial lesions. Lesions typically are found in the pelvis

TABLE 79–1. Clinical Presentation of Endometriosis

Symptoms
Asymptomatic
Dysmenorrhea
Dyspareunia
Chronic pelvic pain (cyclic or acyclic)
Premenstrual spotting
Gastrointestinal disturbances
Urinary disturbances (dysuria, hematuria)
Low back pain
Painful defecation (dyschezia)
Signs
Cul de sac or uterosacral ligament tenderness
Adneal enlargement or tenderness
Pelvic mass
Subfertility
Laboratory Tests
None
Other Diagnostic Modalities
Red "flame" lesions (early disease)
Blue/brown/gray "powder burn" lesions
"White lesions" (healed or inactive disease)
"Chocolate cysts" (endometriomas containing blood)

Compiled from refs. 1, 3, 8, and 12.

but also have been described in the bowel, lung, bladder, and ureter.[8] The American Association of Reproductive Medicine has developed a staging system for endometriosis ranging from stage I (mild) to stage IV (severe) disease. In stage I endometriosis, lesions are scattered and superficial, and adhesions or scarring typically has not yet developed. Conversely, in stage IV endometriosis, large ovarian endometriomas, adhesions, obstruction, and lesions in nonpelvic areas develop. Unfortunately, this staging system is not useful in clinical practice because the size, location, and number of lesions do not correlate with painful symptoms, nor does the staging system predict pregnancy rates.[1,8] Characteristics of the clinical presentation are shown in Table 79–1.

▶ TREATMENT: Endometriosis

■ DESIRED OUTCOME

❹ Treatment goals for endometriosis depend on patient presentation. Women with endometriosis may be asymptomatic, or they may present with pain, infertility, or a combination of both. Depending on the primary complaint, goals of endometriosis treatment include (1) minimization or removal of endometrial deposits, (2) prevention of disease progression, (3) minimization of associated pain, and (4) prevention or correction of associated infertility.

■ GENERAL APPROACH TO TREATMENT

❺ The treatment for an asymptomatic patient with endometriosis consists of expectant management (watchful waiting) only because therapy is not indicated unless symptoms develop. For symptomatic patients, the foundation of therapy includes medical treatment, surgical treatment, or both. To date, no studies have compared medical and surgical treatment directly as first-line therapy. Furthermore,

determining the optimal medical or surgical approach is difficult secondary to a paucity of well designed, randomized, controlled trials. Medical therapy relieves endometriosis-related pain by regressing lesions via induction of a pseudopregnancy or pseudomenopausal state but does not eradicate lesions or improve fertility. Choice of initial therapy therefore depends on multiple factors such as the patient's primary complaint, location and extent of the disease, desire for future fertility, cost of therapy, contraindications to therapy, and potential side effects or complications of therapy.

❻ Consensus recommendations for the treatment of chronic pelvic pain suspected to be secondary to endometriosis advocate empirical medical therapy with nonsteroidal anti-inflammatory drugs (NSAIDs), oral contraceptives (OCs), progestins, danazol, or gonadotropin-releasing hormone agonists (GnRH-a).[5] Conservative surgical therapy is also recommended to treat painful symptoms in women who fail or have contraindications to medical therapy or in instances in which other compelling reasons exist for surgery. Of note, ❼ 30% to 70% of women will experience recurrence of pain within 6 to 18 months after initial treatment with either medical or surgical means, and extended use of medical therapy or postoperative adjunctive medical therapy may be necessary.[8,14] Definitive treatment for

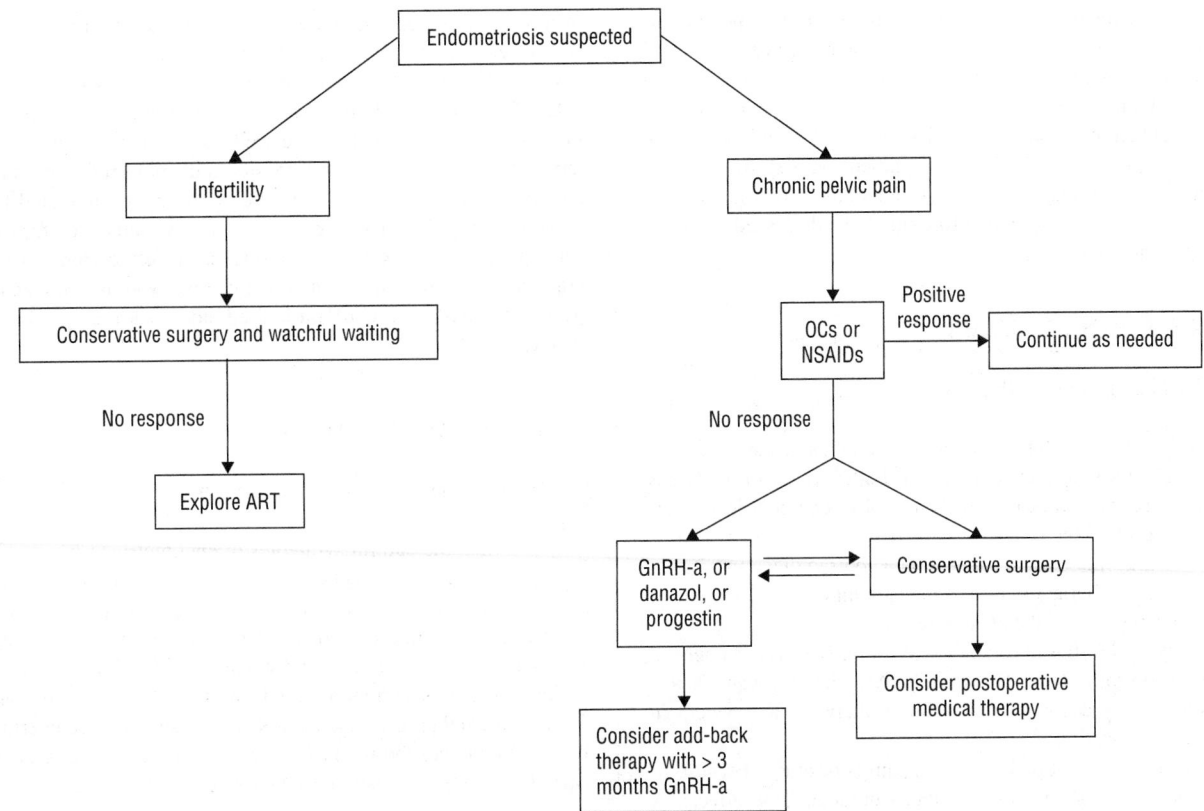

FIGURE 79–1. General treatment algorithm for endometriosis-related problems.

endometriosis involves nonconservative surgical therapy via bilateral salpingo-oophorectomy, with or without hysterectomy. This therapy should be reserved for women not desiring future fertility who accept the potential complications of surgically induced menopause.

For women presenting with infertility as a primary complaint, first-line therapy involves surgical resection of the lesions to restore normal anatomy followed by watchful waiting.[15] Medical therapy is ineffective for endometriosis-related infertility and should be avoided.[12,15–18] For women in whom surgical intervention does not result in pregnancy within 6 months, controlled ovarian stimulation with intrauterine insemination or in vitro fertilization is commonly employed.[19] Pretreatment with GnRH-a prior to in vitro fertilization cycles may increase success rates.[19,20] No clear guidelines or recommendations exist to guide the choice of one therapy or technique over another. A general treatment algorithm for endometriosis-related pain and infertility is shown in Fig. 79–1.

NONPHARMACOLOGIC THERAPY

SURGERY

Surgical intervention in endometriosis may be used as both a diagnostic and a therapeutic tool. Goals of conservative surgical therapy include destruction of endometrial implants, removal of lesions, and restoration of normal pelvic structure to treat associated pain and infertility.[12] Although considered the only "definitive" therapy for endometriosis, radical surgery to remove the uterus and ovaries should be considered only in women not desiring future fertility.

Laparoscopic procedures (versus laparotomy) have become the primary standard of care for endometriosis surgery because of lower complication rates, a lower incidence of postoperative adhesions, and more rapid patient recovery.[1,8] One form of laparoscopic procedure cannot be recommended over another because no studies exist that compare these types of interventions directly. Ultimately, the choice of surgical intervention should be guided by the patient's desire for future fertility, the extent and location of disease, and the expertise and experience of the surgeon.[5]

A systematic review concluded that conservative laparoscopic procedures are superior to watchful waiting in treating the pain of minimal, mild, and moderate endometriosis.[22] Approximately 60% to 100% of affected women will obtain relief of pain from surgery, but up to 44% of women will experience recurrence of symptoms at 1 year.[1,8,14] This recurrence is due to failure to visualize and remove all endometrial lesions and to regrowth of endometrial tissue. Use of adjunctive medical therapy postoperatively may extend the pain-free interval, but routine use of such therapy remains controversial because the small amount of available data show conflicting efficacy results.[1,20] Regimens studied for adjunctive medical therapy include 6 months of treatment with danazol (with or without OCs), medroxyprogesterone, and GnRH-a.[1,5,14,20] Choice of agent depends primarily on patient preference and prior response to medical therapy.[5]

Conservative surgical therapy is a primary treatment for endometriosis-associated infertility. Data support efficacy of surgery at all stages of disease but are limited by lack of well-designed, randomized trials. Patients with advanced disease causing distortion of the pelvic structure may benefit most from surgical intervention. Pregnancy rates in this population are nearly 0 percent, and uncontrolled studies consistently support efficacy of surgery to improve pregnancy rates.[20] For women with mild to moderate disease, spontaneous conception occurs at a rate of approximately 20%; this makes evaluation of surgical efficacy more difficult.[13] A systematic review highlights the inconsistent treatment efficacy from surgery in this population with milder disease. Results suggest that the number needed to treat to achieve one pregnancy ranges from 3 to 100 women with mild to moderate endometriosis.[13]

Surgical therapy is not without risk. Potential complications include uterine prolapse, adhesion development with subsequent reduced fertility, and damage to or denervation of the pelvic structure.[16] Risks and benefits of surgery therefore should be discussed on an individual patient basis.

PHARMACOLOGIC THERAPY

DRUG TREATMENTS OF FIRST CHOICE

5 First-line therapy for endometriosis-associated pain includes NSAIDs, OCs, or a combination of both.[5] These drug classes are considered effective and less costly than other endometriosis treatments. Choice of agent depends on patient characteristics such as desire for contraception, pain patterns, and contraindications. Long-term maintenance therapy with these agents may be considered for women achieving a good therapeutic response.

Efficacy of NSAIDs in patients with endometriosis has not been evaluated in controlled trials. However, NSAIDs have proven efficacy in treating primary dysmenorrhea and are likely to have benefit in endometriosis as well.[5]

Use of OCs to treat endometriosis pain is desirable because of the potential for long-term use without significant side effects. A low-dose OC administered cyclically was compared with a GnRH-a in a randomized trial.[23] Both groups showed overall improvement in dyspareunia, nonmenstrual pain, and dysmenorrhea at 6 months. The rate of recurrent symptoms 6 months after cessation of therapy was equal between groups.

ALTERNATIVE DRUG TREATMENTS

6 Chronic pelvic pain not responding to NSAIDs or OCs should be treated with either advanced medical therapy or conservative surgery according to consensus recommendations.[5] Choice of medical versus surgical therapy should include consideration of patient preference, potential for adverse reactions, cost, and impact on future fertility.

Agents that may be used as advanced medical therapy include progestins, danazol, or GnRH-a.[5] Systematic reviews have concluded that all three classes of agents are effective choices, and no one agent has been proven superior to another.[20,24-26] The primary difference between treatments is the side-effect profile and available dosage forms; choice of agent, therefore, depends on patient preference and tolerance of side effects. A 2-month trial of the agent should be employed, and treatment should be continued for a minimum of 6 months if relief is obtained.[5] For women treated with GnRH-a, add-back therapy with estrogens or progestins should be considered to minimize vasomotor side effects and bone mineral density loss.[5] Surgical therapy should be considered in women failing to respond to advanced medical therapy, in women with contraindications to medical therapy, or in women unable to tolerate side effects caused by medical therapy.[5]

SPECIAL POPULATIONS: ADOLESCENTS

4 Treatment goals for endometriosis in the adolescent patient are focused on management of pain.[27] Medical therapy is preferred over surgical therapy in this population in order to minimize adhesion development from repeated surgeries.[27] Most experts recommend first-line therapy with OCs in adolescents secondary to the minimal side-effect profile and ability to continue treatment indefinitely.[2,27] Progestins are also likely to be well tolerated, although the long-term effects on bone mineral density and lipid profile are still not clearly defined.[27] Danazol is not likely to be well tolerated by the adolescent population and generally is not recommended for use.[2,27] Therapy with a GnRH-a is efficacious, but effects on bone mineral density are of concern in young women who have not achieved peak bone mass. If a GnRH-a is used, add-back therapy should be included.[2,27]

DRUG CLASS INFORMATION

Nonsteroidal Anti-Inflammatory Drugs

NSAIDs treat the painful symptoms of endometriosis by interfering with prostaglandin production but do not affect the structure of the endometrial lesions directly.[8] Long-term use of these agents may be limited by gastrointestinal or renal toxicity. They also may aggravate reactive airways disease and should be used with caution in such patients. The most commonly used NSAIDs in treatment of gynecologic pain are ibuprofen and naproxen.[14] Dosing may be intermittent or continuous depending on whether the pain is cyclic or acyclic.[5] Specific dosing information can be found in Table 79–2.

Oral Contraceptives

OCs treat the pain of endometriosis by decreasing menstrual flow and regressing endometrial implants.[28] The OCs are likely equal in efficacy to GnRH-a and medroxyprogesterone for relieving endometrial pain.[29] OCs are also effective in preventing recurrence of pain after surgical intervention for endometriosis.[30] There is no evidence to suggest that one OC is superior to another.

Side effects of these agents are typically mild and may include nausea, bloating, headache, and breakthrough bleeding. Because of this favorable side-effect profile, OCs are the drug of choice in adolescents with endometriosis. OCs do carry a risk of thromboembolism and should not be used in women with a history of thromboembolism or in smokers over the age of 35.

Administration of OCs may be cyclic or continuous. Although no studies have compared the two methods directly, continuous administration is more likely to induce amenorrhea and therefore may be more beneficial in treating dysmenorrhea.[14,20]

Progestins

Multiple progestins have been studied in the treatment of endometriosis. Agents available in the United States include oral and depot medroxyprogesterone, megestrol, norethindrone, and the levonorgestrel-releasing intrauterine device. The progestins treat endometriosis via atrophy and decidualization of endometrial tissue. They tend to be less expensive and better tolerated than other endometriosis treatments. Most studies have examined use of medroxyprogesterone. A systematic review concluded that continuous medroxyprogesterone (oral or depot) is no more or less effective than other therapies.[26] Overall, 80% to 90% of women report improvement of endometriosis-related pain when using medroxyprogesterone.[14]

TABLE 79–2. Medical Therapy for Endometriosis-Associated Pain

Drug	Dose	Comments
OCs (various)	1 orally daily	Continuous administration may lessen dysmenorrhea
		Contraindicated in women with history of thromboembolism and in women greater than age 35 years old who smoke
NSAIDs		
Ibuprofen	400 mg orally every 4–6 hours	Use with caution in women with reactive airways disease, renal disease, or history of gastrointestinal ulcer
Naproxen	250 mg orally every 6–8 hours	
Progestins		
MPA	30–100 mg orally daily	Generally well-tolerated and less costly than GnRH-as or danazol
	150 mg IM every 3 months	
NE	15 mg orally daily (5 mg daily × 2 weeks, then titrate by 2.5 mg daily every 2 weeks)	May delay return of fertility
Megestrol	40 mg orally daily	
	3.75 mg IM monthly	
GnRH-a		
Leuprolide	11.25 mg IM every 3 months	Vasomotor symptoms and bone loss may limit use
Goserelin	3.6 mg SQ monthly	Add-back therapy improves side effects and reduces bone loss
Nafarelin	200 mcg (one spray) intranasally twice daily	Not preferred in adolescent patients secondary to bone loss
Other		
Danazol	600–800 mg orally daily in divided doses	Androgenic side effects limit use; not preferred in adolescent patients secondary to side-effect profile

Abbreviations: OCs = oral contraceptives; MPA = medroxyprogesterone acetate; IM = intramuscular; NE = norethindrone; GnRH-a = gonadotropin-releasing hormone agonists; SQ = subcutaneous; mcg = micrograms; NSAIDs = nonsteroidal anti-inflammatory drugs.

Common side effects of progestins include breakthrough bleeding, weight gain, fluid retention, and mood swings. Also of concern are the unknown long-term effects on bone mineral density and lipid profile. For women desiring immediate future fertility, progestins may not be optimal secondary to prolonged amenorrhea and anovulation after cessation of therapy. This effect has been noted specifically with the depot form of medroxyprogesterone. Specific progestin dosing information can be found in Table 79–2.

Gonadotropin-Releasing Hormone Agonists

The GnRH-a create a functional oophorectomy via inhibition of follicle-stimulating hormone (FSH) and luteinizing hormone (LH) secretion. This, in turn, diminishes endometrial implants. When first initiated, the GnRH-a create an initial gonadotropin flare prior to receptor downregulation that may cause a temporary increase in pain. Initiating therapy during the midluteal phase may minimize such effects.

Therapy with GnRH-a is superior to placebo and comparable with danazol for relief of endometriosis-associated pain.[25] Response rates are approximately 85% to 100% after 6 months of therapy, but recurrence rates at 5 years are 53%.[1,20,25,29] Although typically taken for 6 months' duration, one comparative study has shown equivalent efficacy and recurrence rates between 3 and 6 months of GnRH-a therapy.[31] Therapy also may need to be extended beyond 6 months to maintain efficacy, although data are limited regarding such extended usage.

Three GnRH-a are currently available in the United States: goserelin, leuprolide, and nafarelin. These agents differ primarily by route of administration. Choice of therapy, therefore, depends on patient preference. Specific dosing information for the GnRH-a can be found in Table 79–2.

Side effects are the primary limitation of GnRH-a use. The pharmacologically induced hypoestrogenic environment results in bone loss and vasomotor symptoms such as hot flashes, vaginal dryness, and insomnia. Loss of bone mineral density is estimated at 4% to 6% over 6 months of GnRH-a therapy, but this loss is recoverable on cessation of the drug.[32] Bone loss is progressive as use of the drugs is extended beyond 6 months, and it is unknown if reversibility is maintained after such longer treatment periods.[33] Add-back therapy with estrogens, progestins, or bisphosphonates has been studied as a way to treat vasomotor symptoms and prevent bone loss while maintaining efficacy of the drug.

The theory behind use of add-back therapy centers on the idea that the level of estrogen needed to prevent GnRH-a side effects is less than the estrogen level that allows growth of endometrial implants.[14] Multiple add-back regimens have been studied, but only three have consistently prevented bone mineral density loss, treated vasomotor symptoms, and maintained efficacy of the GnRH-a. These include norethindrone plus etidronate, norethindrone alone, and low-dose conjugated equine estrogens plus norethindrone.[32] Specific dosing information for add-back therapy regimens can be found in Table 79–3.

The optimal time to initiate add-back therapy remains controversial. The cost of the regimen must be balanced against the potential benefit. Add-back therapy is not recommended for GnRH-a regimens of less than 3 months' duration.[1,32] Use of add-back therapy for GnRH-a regimens of 3 to 6 months' duration is for the primary purpose of relief of vasomotor symptoms and improved adherence

TABLE 79–3. Add-Back Therapy for GnRH Agonists

Drug(s)	Dose	Comments
NE	5 mg orally daily	
NE + CEE	5 mg orally daily (NE) + 0.625 mg orally daily (CEE)	Recommend supplemental calcium
NE + etidronate	2.5 mg orally daily (NE) + 400 mg orally daily × 14 days cycled every 8 weeks (etidronate)	

NE = norethindrone; CEE = conjugated equine estrogens.

because the bone loss sustained at 6 months is recoverable.[32] For GnRH-a therapy lasting longer than 6 months, add-back therapy should be used for the purpose of preventing bone loss along with preventing vasomotor symptoms.[32] In all instances, supplemental calcium should be recommended.

Danazol

Danazol is a synthetic steroid analogue of 17α-ethinyl testosterone. It induces anovulation, amenorrhea, and endometrial atrophy through pituitary suppression of the midcycle LH and FSH surge and induction of a high-androgen, low-estrogen environment. The drug also has immunosuppressive activity that may contribute to its efficacy. Formerly the "gold standard" of endometriosis treatment, danazol's popularity has decreased as agents with more favorable side-effect profiles have been developed.

Danazol has been proven effective as empirical therapy as well as postoperative therapy. Symptomatic improvement has been reported in up to 80% to 90% of women using the drug, with the best results seen in women achieving amenorrhea.[14] A systematic review concluded that 6 months of danazol therapy is superior to placebo in relieving painful symptoms.[24] Therapy for only 3 months has not been as successful, especially when used postoperatively.[1,5,14]

The primary limitation of danazol therapy is the high occurrence of androgenic side effects, including weight gain, acne, hot flashes, decreased breast size, hirsutism, and increased low-density lipoprotein cholesterol. Lowering the dose of danazol may alleviate some of these side effects, but drug efficacy is also compromised.[14] Danazol should not be initiated in women with hyperlipidemia or liver disease. Danazol is also teratogenic, and barrier forms of contraception must be used. The dose of danazol ranges from 200–800 mg/day, but most studies used doses of 600–800 mg. Specific dosing information can be found in Table 79–2.

PHARMACOECONOMIC CONSIDERATIONS

Several cost considerations must be made when choosing endometriosis therapy. Costs of medical therapy must be weighed against the cost of surgical therapy, and the costs of each type of medical therapy must be weighed against another.

❹ Two studies have determined that empirical pain therapy with GnRH-a is less expensive than empirical surgical therapy by laparotomy. Cost savings estimates from these studies range from $1000 to $2500 per treated patient, although the results of these studies are limited by the lack of consideration of the cost of add-back therapy and/or postoperative medical therapy.[34–36] Because the rate of recurrence of symptoms is high for both conservative surgical therapy and medical therapy, empirical medical therapy appears to be the most reasonable option. Generally speaking, the GnRH-a are the most expensive agents, and OCs and progestins are the least expensive. For add-back therapy, norethindrone monotherapy is likely to be most cost-effective.

CLINICAL CONTROVERSIES

Treating endometriosis-related pain by medical therapy versus surgical therapy is controversial. In the past, surgical diagnosis was deemed necessary prior to starting therapy, and surgical intervention, therefore, seemed logical. More recently, evidence supports empirically starting medical therapy and awaiting symptomatic improvement.

Add-back therapy alleviates the vasomotor symptoms and bone density loss associated with GnRH-a. Controversy exists as to when to initiate such therapy. Some practitioners believe that add-back therapy should be prescribed only after 6 months of GnRH-a treatment because bone loss until this point is reversible. Other clinicians recommend immediate use of add-back therapy to minimize side effects and improve adherence.

Recurrence of endometriosis-related pain is frequent after conservative surgery. Some experts therefore recommend routine use of postoperative medical therapy to delay return to symptoms. Data supporting the efficacy of this practice is conflicting, and the cost of such therapy may not be warranted.

EVALUATION OF THERAPEUTIC OUTCOMES

❹ Monitoring of endometriosis therapy is focused on subjective relief of symptoms.[5,14] Although objective confirmation of lesion regression by laparotomy is feasible, the results typically are misleading because the number and size of lesions do not correlate well with patient symptoms.[14]

Endometriosis-related pain should be relieved within 2 months of initiating medical therapy. If symptoms persist, consideration should be given to different medical and/or surgical therapy. For endometriosis-related infertility, most experts recommend 6 months of watchful waiting after surgical intervention. If pregnancy is not achieved within that time, assisted reproductive techniques can be considered.

ABBREVIATIONS

ART: assisted reproductive technology
FSH: follicle-stimulating hormone
GnRH: gonadotropin-releasing hormone
GnRH-a: gonadotropin-releasing hormone agonist
LH: leuteinizing hormone
NSAIDs: nonsteroidal anti-inflammatory drugs
OC: oral contraceptive

Review Questions and other resources can be found at *www.pharmacotherapyonline.com.*

REFERENCES

1. Bulletins—Gynecology ACoP. ACOG practice bulletin: Medical management of endometriosis. Int J Gynaecol Obstet 2000;71:183–196.
2. Laufer MR, Sanfilippo J, Rose G. Adolescent endometriosis: Diagnosis and treatment approaches. J Pediatr Adolesc Gynecol 2003;16.
3. Propst AM, Laufer MR. Endometriosis in adolescents: Incidence, diagnosis and treatment. J Reprod Med 1999;44:751–758.
4. Ballweg ML. Big picture of endometriosis helps provide guidance on approach to teens: Comparative historical data show endo starting younger, is more severe. J Pediatr Adolesc Gynecol 2003;16:S21–26.
5. Gambone JC, Mittman BS, Munro MG, et al. Consensus statement for the management of chronic pelvic pain and endometriosis: Proceedings of an expert-panel consensus process. Fertil Steril 2002;78:961–972.
6. Lessey BA. Medical management of endometriosis and infertility. Fertil Steril 2000;73:1089–1096.
7. Witz CA. Current concepts in the pathogenesis of endometriosis. Clin Obstet Gynecol 1999;42:566–585.
8. Valle RF. Endometriosis: Current concepts and therapy. Int J Gynaecol Obstet 2002;78:107–119.
9. Kim JG, Suh CS, Kim SH, et al. Insulin-like growth factors (IGFs), IGF-binding proteins (IGFBPs), and IGFBP-3 protease activity in the peritoneal fluid of patients with and without endometriosis. Fertil Steril 2000;73:996–1000.
10. Duleba AJ. Diagnosis of endometriosis. Obstet Gynecol Clin North Am 1997;24:331–346.
11. Eskenazi B, Warner ML. Epidemiology of endometriosis. Obstet Gynecol Clin North Am 1997;24:235–258.
12. Child TJ, Tan SL. Endometriosis: Aetiology, pathogenesis and treatment. Drugs 2001;61:1735–1750.
13. Jacobson TZ, Barlow DH, Koninckx PR, et al. Laparoscopic surgery for subfertility associated with endometriosis. Cochrane Review 2003;1.
14. Mahutte NG, Arici A. Medical management of endometriosis-associated pain. Obstet Gynecol Clin North Am 2003;30:133–150.
15. Olive DL, Pritts EA. Treatment of endometriosis. N Engl J Med 2001;345:266–275.
16. Farquhar CM. Extracts from the "clinical evidence": Endometriosis. Br Med J 2000;320:1449–1452.
17. Hughes E, Fedorkow D, Collins J, Vandekerckhove P. Ovulation suppression for endometriosis. Cochrane Review 2003;1.
18. Adamson GD, Pasta DJ. Surgical treatment of endometriosis-associated infertility: Meta-analysis compared with survival analysis. Am J Obstet Gynecol 1994;171:1488–1504.
19. Surrey ES, Schoolcraft WB. Management of endometriosis-associated infertility. Obstet Gynecol Clin North Am 2003;30:193–208.
20. Olive DL, Pritts EA. The treatment of endometriosis: A review of the evidence. Ann NY Acad Sci 2002;955:360–372; discussion 389–93, 396–406.
21. Martin DC, O'Conner DT. Surgical management of endometriosis-associated pain. Obstet Gynecol Clin North Am 2003;30:151–162.
22. Jacobson TZ, Barlow DH, Garry R, Koninckx P. Laparoscopic surgery for pelvic pain associated with endometriosis. Cochrane Review 2003;1.
23. Vercellini P, Trespidi L, Colombo A, et al. A gonadotropin-releasing hormone agonist versus a low-dose oral contraceptive for pelvic pain associated with endometriosis. Fertil Steril 1993;60:75–79.
24. Selak V, Farquhar C, Prentice A, Singla A. Danazol for pelvic pain associated with endometriosis. Cochrane Review 2003;1.
25. Prentice A, Deary AJ, Goldbeck-Wood S, et al. Gonadotrophin-releasing hormone analogues for pain associated with endometriosis. Cochrane Review 2003;1.
26. Prentice A, Deary AJ, Bland E. Progestagens and anti-progestagens for pain associated with endometriosis. Cochrane Review 2003;1.
27. Attaran M, Gidwani GP. Adolescent endometriosis. Obstet Gynecol Clin North Am 2003;30:379–390.
28. Rice VM. Conventional medical therapies for endometriosis. Ann NY Acad Sci 2002;955:343–352.
29. Winkel CA, Scialli AR. Medical and surgical therapies for pain associated with endometriosis. J Womens Health Gend Based Med 2001;10:137–162.
30. Muzii L, Marana R, Caruana P, et al. Postoperative administration of monophasic combined oral contraceptives after laparoscopic treatment of ovarian endometriomas: A prospective, randomized trial. Am J Obstet Gynecol 2000;183:588–592.
31. Hornstein MD, Yuzpe AA, Burry KA, et al. Prospective randomized double-blind trial of 3 versus 6 months of nafarelin therapy for endometriosis associated pelvic pain. Fertil Steril 1995;63:955–962.
32. Surrey ES. Add-back therapy and gonadotropin-releasing hormone agonists in the treatment of patients with endometriosis: Can a consensus be reached? Add-Back Consensus Working Group. Fertil Steril 1999;71:420–424.
33. Hornstein MD, Surrey ES, Weisberg GW, Casino LA. Leuprolide acetate depot and hormonal add-back in endometriosis: A 12-month study. Lupron Add-Back Study Group. Obstet Gynecol 1998;91:16–24.
34. Winkel CA. A cost-effective approach to the management of endometriosis. Curr Opin Obstet Gynecol 2000;12:317–320.
35. Winkel CA. Modeling of medical and surgical treatment costs of chronic pelvic pain: New paradigms for making clinical decisions. Am J Manag Care 1999;5:S276–290.
36. Kephart W. Evaluation of Lovelace Health Systems chronic pelvic pain protocol. Am J Manag Care 1999;5:S309–315.

80

HORMONE THERAPY IN WOMEN

Sophia N. Kalantaridou, Susan R. Davis, and Karim Anton Calis

Learning Objectives and other resources can be found at *www.pharmacotherapyonline.com.*

KEY CONCEPTS

◀1 Estrogen-based postmenopausal hormone therapy should be used for the treatment of menopausal symptoms (i.e., vasomotor and urogenital symptoms) and, when specifically indicated, for osteoporosis prevention.

◀2 A progestogen should be added for endometrial protection when estrogen therapy is prescribed. Thus women with an intact uterus should not receive unopposed estrogen, whereas women who have undergone hysterectomy always should receive estrogen alone.

◀3 Lower doses of hormone therapy than previously used should be considered as standard initial therapy. Clinicians should prescribe hormone therapy at the lowest effective dose for the shortest duration, carefully and individually weighing treatment goals and risks for each woman.

◀4 The major indication for estrogen-containing hormone therapy is the relief of menopausal symptoms, and the benefits of short-term perimenopausal and postmenopausal hormone therapy for the relief of severe menopausal symptoms outweigh the risks in many women.

◀5 Osteoporosis prevention remains an approved indication for estrogen-based hormone therapy, but alternative strategies are available and should be considered as first-line agents for asymptomatic women. Vitamin D deficiency should be excluded before any other treatment is prescribed

for the prevention or treatment of bone loss, and adequate calcium intake should be ensured.

◀6 Postmenopausal hormone treatment with oral combined estrogen plus progestogen has no benefit for cardiovascular disease prevention and increases the risk of breast cancer, coronary heart disease events, stroke, and venous thromboembolic events. However, it reduced the rates of hip fracture and colorectal cancer.

◀7 Hormone therapy improves mood and well-being primarily in women with hot flushes, night sweats, and sleep disturbance, but it does not improve gross quality-of-life measures in postmenopausal women who do not experience vasomotor symptoms.

◀8 Evaluation of each individual woman is essential in determining the appropriateness of perimenopausal and postmenopausal hormone therapy, and collaboration between a woman and her primary care provider in the decision-making process is essential. The benefits and risks of hormone therapy should be reassessed annually.

◀9 Results from randomized trials of hormone therapy in postmenopausal women cannot be extrapolated to premenopausal women with ovarian dysfunction. Women with premature ovarian failure (i.e., those younger than 40 years of age) need exogenous sex steroids to compensate for the decreased production by their ovaries.

Menopause is the permanent cessation of menses following the loss of ovarian follicular activity.[1] By definition, it is a physiologic event that occurs after 12 consecutive months of amenorrhea—so the time of the final menses is determined retrospectively. Women who have undergone hysterectomy must rely on their symptoms to estimate the actual time of menopause.

Many women seek therapy for alleviation of symptoms that arise from loss of ovarian function at the time of menopause. However, the use of hormone therapy (estrogen ± progestogen) for the prevention of diseases of aging has attracted considerable public attention since the premature termination of the estrogen-progestogen arm of the Women's Health Initiative (WHI) in 2002.[2] The estrogen-alone arm of the trial also was discontinued recently after 7 years of follow-up because it was found that estrogen alone did not affect (either increase or decrease) heart disease.[3] Breast cancer risk was not increased during the study period.[3]

The median age at the onset of menopause in the United States is 51 years, whereas the average life expectancy for women is 81 years. Thus American women can expect to be postmenopausal for more than one-third of their lives.

Although the age at menarche has declined steadily throughout the centuries, probably a result of improved nutrition, the age at menopause onset appears to be relatively stable. However, on average, cigarette smokers experience menopause 2 years earlier than nonsmokers. Women who have undergone hysterectomy also are more likely to have an earlier menopause despite preservation of their ovaries. Approximately 1% of women develop ovarian failure before the age of 40 years (premature menopause or premature ovarian failure).[4]

Prior to publication of the WHI results, about 38% of postmenopausal women in the United States took hormone therapy.[5] Approved indications of postmenopausal hormone therapy include treatment of menopausal symptoms (i.e., hot flushes, night sweats, and urogenital atrophy) and osteoporosis prevention.[6]

Results from recent randomized clinical trials evaluating the effects of hormone therapy have differed substantially from previous observational studies. These trials showed that the risks of hormone therapy exceed the potential benefits for chronic disease prevention in postmenopausal women.[2,3,6a] Weighing the risks and benefits, the Food and Drug Administration (FDA) recently mandated the addition of new safety warnings to the labels of all systemic estrogens (regardless of route or dosage form), including estrogen-only and combined estrogen-progestogen products. The labels now caution that use of estrogen-containing hormone therapy regimens by postmenopausal women may be associated with an increased risk of myocardial infarction, stroke, breast cancer, and thromboembolism. Nonetheless, hormone therapy remains the most effective therapy for the management of hot flushes and vaginal atrophy in the postmenopausal woman.[6a]

MENOPAUSE AND PERI- AND POSTMENOPAUSAL HORMONE THERAPY

PHYSIOLOGY

Characteristics of the human menstrual cycle throughout reproductive life have been well described.[7] A woman is born with approximately two million primordial follicles in her ovaries. During a normal reproductive life span, she ovulates less than 500 times. The vast majority of follicles undergo atresia.

The hypothalamic-pituitary-ovarian axis dynamically controls reproductive physiology throughout the reproductive years. The pituitary is regulated by pulsatile secretion of gonadotropin-releasing hormone (GnRH) from the hypothalamus. Follicle-stimulating hormone (FSH) and luteinizing hormone (LH), produced by the pituitary in response to GnRH, regulate ovarian function. These gonadotropins also are influenced by negative feedback from estradiol and progesterone. Ovarian follicular activity is reflected by the circulating concentrations of sex steroids and by peptide hormones (such as inhibin and activin). The sex steroids include estradiol, produced by the dominant follicle; progesterone, produced by the corpus luteum after maturation of the dominant ovarian follicle; and androgens, primarily testosterone and androstenedione, secreted by the ovarian stroma. Sex steroids are important for the healthy functioning of many organs, including the bones, brain, skin, and reproductive and urogenital tracts. They act primarily by regulating gene expression.

Pathophysiologic changes associated with menopause are caused by the loss of ovarian follicular activity.[1] Ovarian primordial follicle numbers decrease with advancing age, and at the time of the menopause, few follicles remain in the ovary. Hence the postmenopausal ovary is no longer the primary site of estradiol or progesterone synthesis. The postmenopausal ovary secretes primarily androstenedione and testosterone. In contrast to the acute fall in circulating estrogen at the time of menopause, the decline in circulating androgens commences in the decade leading up to the average age of natural menopause and closely parallels increasing age.[8] Androgens are secreted by both the ovaries and the adrenal glands. Following menopause, direct ovarian androgen secretion appears to account for as much as 50% of testosterone production, with the adrenal gland being a less important source. Hypertrophy of the ovarian stroma may develop after menopause, probably secondary to high LH concentrations, thereby resulting in increased ovarian testosterone production.

Alternatively, the ovaries may become fibrotic and a poor source of sex steroids.

No endocrine event clearly signals the time just prior to final menses.[9] Nonetheless, as women age, a progressive rise in circulating FSH[10] and a concomitant decline in ovarian inhibin[9] are observed. In women who continue to experience menstrual bleeding, FSH determinations on day 2 or 3 of the menstrual cycle are considered elevated when concentrations exceed 10–12 IU/L, an indication of diminished ovarian reserve. Clear elevations in serum FSH are seen in women around the age of 40.[9] When ovarian function has ceased, serum FSH concentrations are greater than 40 IU/L.

The perimenopause is the period immediately prior to the menopause and the first year after menopause. The menopausal transition is the period of time when the endocrinologic, biologic, and clinical features of the approaching menopause commence.[9] The menopausal transition usually begins approximately 4 years prior to menopause and is characterized by menstrual cycle irregularity caused by increased frequency of anovulatory cycles. Vasomotor symptoms (hot flushes and night sweats), psychological symptoms (anxiety, mood swings, and depression), and disturbances of sexuality are increased markedly in the perimenopause. Menopause is characterized by a 10- to 15-fold increase in circulating FSH concentrations as compared with concentrations of FSH in the follicular phase of the cycle, a four- to fivefold increase in LH, and a more than 90% decrease in circulating estradiol concentrations.[9] During the perimenopause, FSH concentrations may rise to the postmenopausal range during some cycles but return to premenopausal levels during subsequent cycles. Thus high concentrations of FSH should not be used to diagnose menopause in perimenopausal women. However, vasomotor symptoms in perimenopausal women may require treatment despite the presence of menstrual bleeding. Abnormal thyroid function and other conditions that may cause similar symptomatology should be excluded first. Dysfunctional uterine bleeding may occur during the perimenopausal years because of anovulatory cycles, but other gynecologic causes also should be considered. Treatment options for dysfunctional uterine bleeding include progestins or low-dose oral contraceptives.

An observational study of more than 9000 postmenopausal women examined the relationship between endogenous estrogens and bone mineral density, bone loss, fractures, and breast cancer.[11–14] Women with detectable serum estradiol concentrations (5–25 pg/mL) had a 6% to 7% higher bone mineral density at the total hip and spine as compared with women with undetectable levels (less than 5 pg/mL).[11] They also had significantly less bone loss at the hip than women with undetectable levels.[12] Women with undetectable serum estradiol concentrations had a relative risk of 2.5 for subsequent hip and vertebral fractures.[13] However, women with the highest estradiol serum concentrations had the greatest risk of developing breast cancer.[14]

CLINICAL PRESENTATION OF PERIMENOPAUSE AND MENOPAUSE

SYMPTOMS

- Vasomotor symptoms (hot flushes and night sweats)
- Sleep disturbances
- Mood changes
- Sexual dysfunction
- Problems with concentration and memory
- Vaginal dryness and dyspareunia

SIGNS

- *Perimenopause:* Dysfunctional uterine bleeding owing to anovulatory cycles (other gynecologic disorders should be excluded)
- *Menopause:* Signs of urogenital atrophy

LABORATORY TESTS

- *Perimenopause:* FSH on day 2 or 3 of the menstrual cycle greater than 10–12 IU/L
- *Menopause:* FSH greater than 40 IU/L

OTHER RELEVANT DIAGNOSTIC TESTS

- Thyroid function tests
- Iron stores

CLINICAL PRESENTATION OF MENOPAUSE

Vasomotor symptoms, hot flushes, and night sweats are common symptoms of estrogen withdrawal. Hot flushes are the classic sign of menopause and the major clinical complaint of American women during the perimenopausal and early menopausal years. Hot flushes are a sensation of warmth, frequently accompanied by skin flushing and perspiration. A chill may follow as the core body temperature drops. Hot flushes may occur in women of any age who experience acute estrogen withdrawal. They can be occasional or frequent, last from seconds to an hour, and are characterized by symptoms ranging from mild warmth to profuse sweating. For some women, hot flushes are a minor nuisance, but for others, they can be a disturbing symptom that disrupts their sense of well-being and causes problems in their social and professional lives. They usually occur spontaneously but often are increased in frequency or severity in hot or humid weather or after ingestion of caffeine, alcohol, or spicy foods. The prevalence of hot flushes is higher in the first two postmenopausal years. Women who have undergone surgical menopause tend to have more intense menopausal symptoms than those who experience a natural menopause.

Vaginal dryness is also directly related to estrogen insufficiency, but some women can find adequate relief from nonestrogenic vaginal creams. Most women with significant vaginal dryness, however, require local or systemic estrogen therapy to replenish moisture.

Although some would accept a range of other symptoms to be typical of estrogen deficiency (e.g., mood swings, tiredness, poor concentration, depression, insomnia, migraines, formication, arthralgia, myalgia, and urinary frequency), the relationship between these symptoms and the absolute decline in estrogen is more controversial. Many women, nonetheless, experience relief of such symptoms with estrogen therapy.

▶ TREATMENT: Menopause

Postmenopausal hormone therapy is a subject of major interest in the field of women's health. Treatment of menopausal symptoms can be managed effectively in some women with lifestyle modifications, including exercise, weight control, smoking cessation, and a healthful diet. More recently, however, dietary supplements and nonpharmacologic therapies have been promoted as "complementary medicine" alternatives to hormone therapy. To date, there is little to support the use of such nonprescription products, which include various herbal remedies and soy-based supplements.

PHYTOESTROGENS

Phytoestrogens have physiologic effects in humans[15]; they are plant compounds with estrogen-like biologic activity and relatively weak estrogen-receptor-binding properties. Epidemiologic studies suggest that consumption of a phytoestrogen-rich diet, as seen in traditional Asiatic societies, is associated with a lower risk of breast cancer.[16]

The biologic potencies of phytoestrogens vary, and most of these compounds are nonsteroidal in structure and less potent than the synthetic estrogens. There are three main classes of phytoestrogens: isoflavones, lignans, and coumestans, all of which are found in plants or their seeds.[15] The most commonly studied phytoestrogen is the isoflavone class. Genistein and daidzein are the most abundant active components of isoflavones. Of note, the concentration of isoflavones per gram of soy protein varies considerably among preparations. Also, a single plant often contains more than one class of phytoestrogen. Common food sources of phytoestrogens include soybeans (isoflavones), cereals, oilseeds such as flaxseed (lignans), and alfalfa sprouts (coumestans).

Mild estrogenic effects have been seen in postmenopausal women,[15] but current data suggest that phytoestrogen supplementation is no more effective than placebo in relieving hot flushes or other symptoms of menopause in postmenopausal women.[17]

Phytoestrogens decrease low-density lipoprotein (LDL) cholesterol and triglyceride concentrations with no significant change in high-density lipoprotein (HDL) cholesterol concentrations.[18] Furthermore, phytoestrogens have the ability to inhibit LDL oxidation and normalize vascular reactivity in estrogen-deprived primates.[18] In addition, bone density may be improved by phytoestrogens.[15] Common adverse effects include constipation, bloating, and nausea.[19]

Larger, long-term studies are needed to document the effects of phytoestrogens on the breast, bone, and endometrium. Furthermore, differences among classes of phytoestrogens must be identified clearly, including dosing and biologic activity, before phytoestrogens can be considered an alternative to conventional hormone therapy in postmenopausal women.

Black cohosh (*Cimicifuga racemosa*) is used widely and has been shown to be an effective alternative for the relief of vasomotor symptoms in some randomized, controlled trials.[20] It does not appear to have strong intrinsic estrogenic properties but rather may act through the serotonergic system.

HORMONAL REGIMENS

Approved indications of hormone therapy include treatment of menopausal symptoms and osteoporosis prevention. Therapy directed at menopausal symptoms, such as hot flushes, is often short term. However, therapy directed at prevention of osteoporosis should be long term. For osteoporosis prevention, the advantages of hormone therapy must be weighed against risks, including thrombosis and the increased incidence of cardiovascular disease and breast cancer,[2] and consideration should be given to approved nonestrogen alternatives.

In women with an intact uterus, hormone therapy consists of an estrogen plus a progestogen. In women who have undergone hysterectomy, estrogen therapy is given unopposed by a progestogen.

The continuous combined oral estrogen-progestogen arm of the randomized Women's Health Initiative (WHI) study was terminated prematurely. This arm included 16,608 relatively healthy postmenopausal women aged 50 to 79 years at enrollment (mean age 63.2 years). The primary outcome was coronary heart disease events, defined as nonfatal myocardial infarction and coronary artery disease death, with invasive breast cancer as the primary adverse outcome.[2] The study also examined secondary outcomes, including stroke, thromboembolic disease, fractures, colon cancer, and endometrial cancer.[2] After a mean of 5.2 years of follow-up (planned duration was 8.5 years), the Data and Safety Monitoring Board recommended stopping this arm of the trial because of the occurrence of a prespecified level of invasive breast cancer. That is, women receiving the active drug had an increased risk of invasive breast cancer (hazard ratio [HR] 1.26, 95% confidence interval [CI] 1–1.59), and the overall risks exceeded benefits.[2] The study also found increased coronary disease events (HR 1.29, 95% CI 1.02–1.63), stroke (HR 1.41, 95% CI 1.07–1.85), and pulmonary embolism (HR 2.13, 95% CI 1.39–3.25). Beneficial effects included decreases in hip fracture (HR 0.66, 95% CI 0.45–0.98) and colorectal cancer (HR 0.63, 95% CI 0.43–0.92).[2] Results from this study indicated that short-term use (less than 1 year) has risks for coronary heart disease and thromboembolic disease events. The number of deaths was similar among the groups.

After a mean of 7 years of follow-up, the Data and Safety Monitoring Board also recommended stopping the oral estrogen-alone arm of the study. This arm consisted of 10,739 women who had undergone hysterectomy. Estrogen-only therapy had no effect on coronary heart disease risk and no increased breast cancer risk.[3]

Among women in the estrogen-progestogen arm, there was one serious adverse event for every 100 women treated for 5 years. Specifically, it suggested that for every 10,000 women taking combined hormone therapy, there would be 8 more cases of breast cancer, 7 more cases of myocardial infarctions, 8 more cases of stroke, and 8 more cases of pulmonary embolism. However, 6 fewer colorectal cancers and 5 fewer hip fractures would be expected.[2] For the majority of women who had never used hormone therapy before enrolling in the study (6280 treated with estrogen-progestogen and 6024 treated with placebo), the hazard ratio for breast cancer was 1.06 (95% CI 0.81–1.38), indicating that the burden of risk for breast cancer was from hormone therapy use beyond 5 years. Subsequently, a large epidemiologic study reported a greater risk estimate for combined estrogen-progestogen use, as well as increased risk for estrogen-only therapy and tibolone.[21] However, interpretation of these findings is limited by selection bias because the women who used hormone therapy were significantly different from nonusers in their risk profiles.[21] It is unclear if the type of estrogen compound or the dose, route, or administration method could at least in part be responsible for the risks observed in the WHI trial.

ESTROGEN AND PROGESTOGEN TREATMENT

Estrogens

The primary accepted indication for estrogen-based hormone therapy is the relief of vasomotor symptoms, and the initial dose should be the lowest effective dose for symptom control. Estrogens are naturally occurring hormones or synthetic steroidal or nonsteroidal compounds with estrogenic activity. Various systemically administered estrogens (typically oral and transdermal) are suitable for replacement therapy (Table 80–1). Estrogens can be administered orally, transdermally (patches and other topical products), intravaginally (creams, tablets, or rings), intranasally, intramuscularly, and even in the form of subcutaneously implanted pellets. The choice of estrogen delivery (product, route, and method) should be determined in consultation with the patient to ensure acceptability and enhance compliance. In general, the oral and transdermal routes are used most frequently, with oral conjugated equine estrogens (CEEs) being particularly popular in the United States. There is no evidence that one estrogen compound is more effective than another in relieving menopausal symptoms or preventing osteoporosis.

TABLE 80–1. Systemic Estrogen Products[a,b]

Estrogen	Dosage Strength	Comments
Oral estrogens		
Conjugated equine estrogens	0.3, 0.45, 0.625, 0.9, 1.25 mg	Orally administered estrogens stimulate the synthesis of hepatic proteins and increase the circulating concentrations of sex hormone-binding globulin, which, in turn, may compromise the bioavailability of androgens and estrogens.
Synthetic conjugated estrogens	0.3, 0.45, 0.625, 0.9, 1.25 mg	
Esterified estrogens	0.3, 0.625, 1.25, 2.5 mg	
Estropipate (piperazine estrone sulfate)	0.625, 1.5, 2.5 mg	
Micronized estradiol	0.5, 1, 1.5, 2 mg	
Parenteral estrogens		
Transdermal 17β-estradiol (patch)	14, 25, 37.5, 50, 75, 100 mcg per 24 h	Women with elevated triglyceride concentrations or significant liver function abnormalities may benefit from parenteral therapy
Estradiol vaginal ring	0.05, 0.1 mg per 24 h (replaced every 3 months)	
Estradiol topical emulsion	4.35 mg of estradiol hemihydrate	
Estradiol topical gel	0.75 mg of estradiol	
Intranasal estradiol[c]	One spray per nostril delivers 150 mcg	

[a]Systemic oral and transdermal estrogen and progestogen combination products are available in the United States.
[b]Systemic oral estrogen and androgen combination products are available in the United States.
[c]Not available in the United States.

Oral Estrogen. Oral CEE has been available for more than 50 years. CEE is prepared from the urine of pregnant mares and is composed of estrone sulfate (50% to 60%) and multiple other equine estrogens such as equilin and 17α-dihydroequilin.[22]

Estradiol is the predominant and most active form of endogenous estrogens. A micronized form of estradiol (produced by a technique that yields extremely small particles of the pure hormone) is readily absorbed from the small intestines.[22] When given orally, estradiol is metabolized by the intestinal mucosa and the liver during the first hepatic passage, and only 10% reaches the circulation as free estradiol. Metabolism of estrogen is partly mediated by the cytochrome P-450 3A4 isoenzyme. Gut and liver metabolism converts a large proportion of estradiol to the less potent estrone. Thus measurement of serum estradiol is not useful for monitoring oral estrogen replacement. The principal metabolites of micronized estradiol are estrone and estrone sulfate. Administration of estradiol via the oral route results in estrone concentrations that are three to six times those of estradiol. Ethinyl estradiol is a highly potent semisynthetic estrogen that has similar activity following administration by the oral or parenteral routes.

Orally administered estrogens stimulate the synthesis of hepatic proteins and increase the circulating concentrations of sex hormone–binding globulin, which, in turn, may compromise the bioavailability of androgens and estrogens.

Other Routes. Parenteral estrogens (including transdermal, intranasal, and vaginal) bypass the gastrointestinal tract and thereby avoid first-pass liver metabolism. Parenteral routes of estrogen delivery result in a more physiologic estradiol-to-estrone ratio (estradiol concentrations greater than estrone concentrations), as seen in the normal premenopausal state. Parenteral estrogen therapy also is less likely to affect sex hormone–binding globulin as compared with oral therapy. Parenteral regimens produce little or no change in circulating lipids, coagulation parameters, or C-reactive protein levels.[23]

Transdermal estrogens share the advantages of other parenteral estrogen routes. Transdermal systems have the added advantage of delivering estradiol to the general venous circulation at a continuous rate. Reactions at the application site occur in about 10% of women who use reservoir (alcohol-based) patches. The newer matrix systems (estrogen in adhesive) generally are better tolerated, and fewer than 5% of women experience skin reactions.[24] The incidence of skin irritation diminishes when the application site is rotated. Topical anti-inflammatory products can be applied for managing the rashes, and switching to another transdermal patch is often a viable option.

Percutaneous preparations (gels, creams, and emulsions) are convenient, but variability in drug absorption is common. This form of estrogen is used for systemic therapy. Topical emulsion and gel formulations were approved for use recently in the United States.

Estradiol pellets (implants) containing pure crystalline 17β-estradiol have been available for more than 50 years. They are inserted subcutaneously into the anterior abdominal wall or buttock. Pellets are difficult to remove and may continue to release estradiol for a long time after insertion. Implantation should not be repeated until serum estradiol concentrations have fallen to values similar to those at the midfollicular phase of the menstrual cycle. Estradiol pellets have not gained popularity in the United States.

Intranasal 17β-estradiol spray, which enables single-daily or twice-daily dosing, has been shown to have clinical therapeutic equivalence to oral and transdermal estradiol and is associated with significantly lower reporting of mastalgia.[25]

Vaginal creams, tablets, and rings are used for the treatment of urogenital (vulval and vaginal) atrophy. However, this route of administration can have more than just a local effect. Systemic estrogen absorption is lower with the vaginal tablets and rings (specifically Estring) when compared with the vaginal creams. Nonetheless, local application of the cream at low doses can reverse atrophic vaginal changes and avoid significant systemic exposure. Nonestrogen vaginal moisturizers and lubricants also may provide local symptom relief. These products can be used alone or in combination with locally acting vaginal estrogens. Vaginal rings are a sustained-release delivery system composed of a biologically inert liquid polymer matrix with pure crystalline estradiol that can maintain adequate estradiol concentrations. One such vaginal ring product (Femring) is designed to achieve systemic concentrations of estrogen and is indicated for the treatment of moderate to severe vasomotor symptoms.

The standard dose of estrogen previously believed to be effective in alleviating vasomotor symptoms is equivalent to 0.625 mg CEE,[26] but new evidence indicates that lower doses of estrogen are also effective in controlling postmenopausal symptoms and reducing bone loss[27–30] (Table 80-2). Surprisingly, even ultralow doses of 17β-estradiol delivered by a vaginal ring (Estring) improved the serum lipid profiles and prevented bone loss in elderly women.[31] In general, if adverse effects such as breast tenderness occur with initial

TABLE 80–2. Estrogen for the Treatment of Menopausal Symptoms and Osteoporosis Prevention

Regimen	Standard Dose	Low Dose	Route	Frequency
Conjugated equine estrogens	0.625 mg	0.3 or 0.45 mg	Oral	Once daily
Synthetic conjugated estrogens	0.625 mg	0.3 mg	Oral	Once daily
Esterified estrogens	0.625 mg	0.3 mg	Oral	Once daily
Estropipate (piperazine estrone sulfate)	1.5 mg	0.625 mg	Oral	Once daily
Ethinyl estradiol	5 mcg	2.5 mcg	Oral	Once daily
Micronized 17β-estradiol	1–2 mg	0.25–0.5 mg	Oral	Once daily
Transdermal 17β-estradiol	50 mcg	25 mcg	Transdermal (patch)	Once or twice weekly
Intranasal 17β-estradiol[a]	150 mcg, per nostril	—	Intranasally	Once daily
Implanted 17β-estradiol	50–100 mg pellets	25-mg pellets	Pellets implanted subcutaneously	Every 6 months
Percutaneous 17β-estradiol	0.04 mg (gel) 0.05 mg (emulsion)		Transdermal (emulsion, gel)	Once daily

[a]Not available in the United States.

doses, lowering the dose may resolve the problem and improve patient compliance. Alternatively, if vasomotor symptoms are not controlled adequately with a lower-dose regimen, increasing the estrogen dose may be a reasonable option.

Adverse Effects. Common adverse effects of estrogen include nausea, headache, breast tenderness, and heavy bleeding. More serious adverse effects include increased risk for coronary heart disease, stroke, venous thromboembolism, breast cancer, and gallbladder disease.

Initiating therapy with low doses of estrogen often will minimize breast tenderness, unscheduled bleeding, and potentially other adverse effects. Transdermal estrogen is less likely than oral estrogen to cause nausea and headache. Also, transdermal estrogen is associated with a lower incidence of breast tenderness and deep vein thrombosis than oral estrogen.[32,33] Changing from one estrogen regimen to another in many cases can alleviate certain adverse effects.

Progestogens

Because of the increased risk of endometrial hyperplasia and endometrial cancer with estrogen monotherapy (unopposed estrogen), women who have not undergone hysterectomy should be treated concurrently with a progestogen in addition to the estrogen.[34] Progestogens reduce nuclear estradiol receptor concentrations, suppress DNA synthesis, and decrease estrogen bioavailability by increasing the activity of endometrial 17-hydroxysteroid dehydrogenase, an enzyme responsible for the conversion of estradiol to estrone.[35]

Several progestogen regimens designed to prevent endometrial hyperplasia are available (Table 80–3). Progestogens must be taken for a sufficient period of time during each cycle. A minimum of 12 to 14 days of progestin therapy each month is required for complete protection against estrogen-induced endometrial hyperplasia.[36] It should be noted that even use of low-dose estrogen, including some vaginal preparations, requires progestogen coadministration for endometrial protection in women with an intact uterus.[37] However, rarely is there a need for progestogen administration in women who have undergone hysterectomy.

Four combination estrogen and progestogen regimens are currently in use: continuous-cyclic (sequential), continuous-combined, continuous long-cycle (or cyclic withdrawal), and intermittent-combined (or continuous-pulsed) hormone therapy.[38] The latter two have been introduced recently. Sequential hormone therapy results in

TABLE 80–3. Progestogen Doses for Endometrial Protection (Oral Cyclic Administration)

Progestogen	Dose
Dydrogesterone[a]	10–20 mg for 12 to 14 days per calender month
Medroxyprogesterone acetate	5–10 mg for 12 to 14 days per calender month
Micronized progesterone	200 mg for 12 to 14 days per calender month
Norethisterone[a]	0.7–1 mg for 12 to 14 days per calender month
Norethindrone acetate	5 mg for 12 to 14 days per calender month
Norgestrel	0.15 mg for 12 to 14 days per calender month
Levonorgestrel[a]	150 mcg for 12 to 14 days per calender month

[a]Not available in the United States in a progestogen-only oral dosage form.

scheduled vaginal withdrawal bleeding, although in older women this is often scant or completely absent. For many women, the scheduled withdrawal bleeding is one of the main reasons for avoiding or discontinuing hormone therapy. Because there is no physiologic need for bleeding, new hormone therapy regimens that reduce monthly bleeding (such as continuous long-cycle regimens) or prevent monthly bleeding (such as continuous-combined and intermittent-combined regimens) have been developed. Various hormone therapy regimens that combine an estrogen and a progestogen are available (Table 80–4).

The first generation of progestogens included the C-19 androgenic progestogens norethisterone, norgestrel, and levonorgestrel. More recent preparations have included the C-21 progestogens dydrogesterone and medroxyprogesterone acetate, which are less androgenic. Micronized progesterone also has become available for use in postmenopausal women. The most commonly used oral progestogens are medroxyprogesterone acetate, micronized progesterone, and norethisterone acetate. The latter also can now be administered transdermally in the form of a combined estrogen-progestogen patch.

Adverse Effects. Common adverse effects of progestogens include irritability, depression, and headache. Changing from a cyclic to a continuous-combined regimen or changing from one progestogen to another may decrease the incidence or severity of these

TABLE 80–4. Common Combination Postmenopausal Hormone Therapy Regimens

Regimen	Doses
Oral Continuous-Cyclic Regimens	
CEE + MPA[a]	0.625 mg + 5 mg; 0.625 mg + 10 mg
Oral Continuous-Combined Regimens	
CEE + MPA	0.625 mg + 2.5 mg; 0.625 mg + 5 mg; 0.45 mg + 2.5 mg; 0.3 mg + 1.5 mg/day
17β-Estradiol + NETA	1 mg + 0.1 mg; 1 mg + 0.25 mg; 1 mg + 0.5 mg/day
Ethinyl estradiol + NETA	1 mcg + 0.2 mg; 2.5 mcg + 0.5 mg; 5 mcg + 1 mg; 10 mcg + 1.0 mg/day
Transdermal Continuous-Cyclic Regimens	
17β-Estradiol + NETA[a]	50 mcg + 0.14 mg; 50 mcg + 0.25 mg
Transdermal Continuous-Combined Regimens	
17β-Estradiol + NETA	50 mcg + 0.14 mg; 50 mcg + 0.25 mg; 25 mcg + 0.125 mg

[a]Estrogen alone for days 1–14, followed by estrogen-progestogen on days 15–28. CEE, conjugated equine estrogens; MPA, medroxyprogesterone acetate; NETA, norethindrone acetate.

untoward effects. Adverse effects of progestogens are difficult to evaluate and can vary with the agent administered. Some women experience "premenstrual-like" symptoms, such as mood swings, bloating, fluid retention, and sleep disturbance. New methods and routes of progestogen delivery (e.g., parenterally by an intranasal spray or locally by an intrauterine device that releases levonorgestrel or a progesterone-containing bioadhesive vaginal gel) may be associated with fewer adverse effects. Women who are unable to tolerate a progestogen may be given unopposed estrogen if they are informed of the significant increased risk for endometrial cancer and have endometrial biopsy annually or whenever breakthrough vaginal bleeding occurs.

Methods of Estrogen and Progestogen Administration

Continuous Cyclic Estrogen/Progestogen Treatment. Estrogen typically is administered continuously (daily). A progestogen is coadministered with the estrogen for at least 12 to 14 days of a 28-day cycle.[36] The progestogen causes scheduled withdrawal bleeding in approximately 90% of women. With this regimen, bleeding usually begins 1 to 2 days after the last progestin dose. Occasionally, however, bleeding can begin during the latter phase of progestogen administration.

Continuous-Combined Estrogen/Progestogen Treatment. Continuous-combined estrogen-progestogen administration results in endometrial atrophy and the absence of vaginal bleeding. However, initially it causes unpredictable spotting or bleeding, which usually resolves within 6 to 12 months. Decreasing the estrogen dose or increasing the progestin dose usually decreases or stops the spotting. Occasionally, a drug-free period of 1 or 2 weeks may be useful to stop the bleeding.

Women who have undergone menopause recently have a higher risk for excessive, unpredictable bleeding while receiving continuous therapy; thus this regimen is best reserved for women who are at least 2 years postmenopause. Continuous-combined hormone therapy is more acceptable than traditional cyclic therapy.

Continuous Long-Cycle Estrogen/Progestogen Treatment. To decrease the incidence of uterine bleeding, a modified sequential regimen has been developed.[38] In the continuous long-cycle (or cyclic-withdrawal) estrogen-progestogen regimen, estrogen is given daily, and progestogen is given six times a year, every other month for 12 to 14 days, resulting in six periods a year. Bleeding episodes may be heavier and last for more days than withdrawal bleeding with continuous-cyclic regimens. The effect of continuous long-cycle estrogen-progestogen treatment on endometrial protection is unclear.

Intermittent-Combined Estrogen/Progestogen Treatment. The intermittent combined estrogen-progestogen regimen, also called continuous-pulsed estrogen-progestogen or pulsed-progestogen, consists of 3 days of estrogen therapy alone, followed by 3 days of combined estrogen and progestogen, which is then repeated without interruption.[38] This regimen is designed to lower the incidence of uterine bleeding. It is based on the assumption that pulsed progestogen administration will prevent downregulation of progesterone receptors that continuous-combined regimens can produce. The lower progestogen dose induces fewer side effects and can be better tolerated. The long-term effect of intermittent-combined regimens in endometrial protection is undetermined.

CLINICAL CONTROVERSY

Although some clinicians believe that estrogen can be used safely at lower doses to treat postmenopausal women with severe and protracted vasomotor symptoms, others caution that such long-term therapy even with lower doses of estrogen may be associated with unacceptable risks.

Low-Dose Hormone Therapy

Increasingly, it has become recognized that use of hormone therapy at doses lower than prescribed historically is effective in the management of menopausal symptoms (see Table 80–2). The Women's Health, Osteoporosis, Progestin/Estrogen (HOPE) trial demonstrated equivalent symptom relief and bone density preservation without an increase in endometrial hyperplasia using lower doses of hormone therapy (CEE 0.45 mg and medroxyprogesterone acetate 1.5 mg/day).[27–31] Whether lower doses of estrogen will be safer (lower incidence of venous thromboembolism and breast cancer) remains to be proven. Nonetheless, recent evidence of harm associated with a standard dose of hormone therapy has prompted many patients to either discontinue such therapy or taper to lower doses.

ANDROGENS

The therapeutic use of testosterone in women, although controversial, is becoming more widespread.[39] Data to support this practice are limited; however, several randomized trials of transdermal testosterone therapy have been conducted and provide evidence for benefits in selected women. There is a cluster of symptoms that appears to characterize androgen insufficiency in women: loss of sexual desire, diminished well-being, loss of energy, and over time, decreased bone mass and reduced muscle strength.[39] There is evidence that androgen therapy, usually in the form of testosterone, is effective in alleviating these physical and psychological symptoms of androgen insufficiency. Symptoms are more pronounced in women who have undergone surgical menopause because of the abrupt cessation of testosterone production by the ovaries. Following oophorectomy, testosterone and androstenedione serum concentrations decrease by about 50%. Testosterone therapy generally is accepted for women who have undergone surgical menopause but also should be considered for naturally menopausal women and those who have experienced premature ovarian failure.

In women, androgens may act directly via the androgen receptor or indirectly after conversion to estrogen. Androgens are the precursor hormones for estrogen production in the ovaries, as well as in extragonadal sites, including bone, adipose tissue, and the brain.

Although estrogen therapy improves vaginal dryness, vasomotor symptoms, and general well-being, it has minimal effect on libido. Estrogen combined with androgen significantly improves sexual activity, satisfaction, and pleasure more than that reported with estrogen monotherapy. In addition, estrogen combined with androgen increases bone density sooner and to a greater degree than estrogen therapy,[40,41] but data confirming a reduction in fracture rate are lacking.

Testosterone therapy appears to be effective and safe when given in doses that achieve circulating serum free testosterone concentrations within the physiologic range for young reproductive women. The goal is to produce beneficial effects on well-being and quality of life without incurring undesirable virilizing adverse effects.[39]

TABLE 80–5. Androgen Regimens Used for Women

Regimen	Dose	Frequency	Route
Methyltestosterone in combination with esterified estrogen	1.25–2.5 mg	Daily	Oral
Mixed testosterone esters	50–100 mg	Every 4 to 6 weeks	Intramuscular
Testosterone pellets	50 mg	Every 6 months	Subcutaneous (implanted)
Transdermal testosterone system[a]	150–300 mcg/day	Every 3 to 4 days	Transdermal patch
Nandrolone decanoate	50 mg	Every 8 to 12 weeks	Intramuscular

[a]Undergoing clinical trials in the United States.

Nonetheless, oral testosterone therapy can decrease HDL cholesterol and apolipoprotein A₁ and also can lower triglycerides.[40] However, exogenous testosterone therapy increases brachial artery flow-mediated vasodilation and the vasodilation induced by glyceryl trinitrate in postmenopausal women stabilized on hormone therapy.[41]

There are no data regarding the effects of exogenous androgen therapy on the incidence of breast cancer. However, androgen receptors are found in approximately 50% of mammary tumors, and their presence is associated with longer survival in women with operable breast cancer.[39]

Testosterone is available as oral methyltestosterone in the United States and as testosterone implants in the United Kingdom. Of the available oral preparations, methyltestosterone in combination with esterified estrogen (either 0.625 mg esterified estrogen plus 1.25 mg methyltestosterone or 1.25 mg esterified estrogen plus 2.5 mg methyltestosterone) is the most widely studied.

Relative contraindications to testosterone therapy include moderate to severe acne, clinical hirsutism, and androgenic alopecia. Absolute contraindications to androgen replacement include pregnancy or lactation and known or suspected androgen-dependent neoplasia.

Adverse effects from excessive dosage include virilization, fluid retention, and potentially adverse lipoprotein lipid effects, which are more likely with oral administration.

Testosterone replacement for women is now available in a variety of formulations[39] (Table 80–5). The recent development of a transdermal testosterone matrix patch specifically for use in women may provide a new option for women requiring testosterone replacement.[43,44] Testosterone treatment should not be administered to postmenopausal women who are not receiving concurrent estrogen therapy.

SELECTIVE ESTROGEN-RECEPTOR MODULATORS

Selective estrogen-receptor modulators (SERMs), such as raloxifene, prevent bone loss and spinal fractures. Raloxifene does not alleviate vasomotor symptoms, and it may even exacerbate them. The effects of SERMs on the cardiovascular system are currently being evaluated.

SERMs, a new type of nonhormonal therapy, bind to estrogen receptors and function as tissue-specific estrogen antagonists or agonists. The ideal SERM would protect against osteoporosis and decrease the incidence of breast, endometrial, and colorectal cancer and coronary heart disease without exacerbating menopausal symptoms or increasing the risk of venous thromboembolism or gallbladder disease. To date, no SERM meets these ideals. Tamoxifen, the first-generation SERM, has estrogen antagonist activity on the breast and estrogen-like agonist activity on bone and endometrium.[45] The second generation of SERMs, most notably raloxifene (a non-

steroidal benzothiophene derivative), recently became available for the prevention of osteoporosis. Raloxifene decreases bone loss in recently menopausal women without affecting the endometrium and has estrogen-like actions on lipid metabolism.[46,47] The Multiple Outcomes of Raloxifene Evaluation (MORE) study, a multicenter randomized, blinded, placebo-controlled trial, showed that raloxifene increases bone mineral density in the spine and femoral neck and reduces the risk of vertebral fractures.[46] More important, the same study[48] and the Continuing Outcomes Relevant to Evista (CORE) trial[48a] suggest that raloxifene use is associated with a lower incidence of breast cancer compared with placebo. Nonetheless, raloxifene use increases the risk of venous thromboembolism to a degree similar to that of oral estrogen.[46] The Study of Tamoxifen and Raloxifene (STAR) is currently evaluating the ability of these SERMs to reduce breast cancer incidence in high-risk postmenopausal women.

Raloxifene generally is well tolerated. Its adverse effects include leg cramps and hot flushes. Raloxifene is used specifically to reduce the risk of osteoporosis in postmenopausal women.

TIBOLONE

Tibolone is a gonadomimetic synthetic steroid in the norpregnane family with combined estrogenic, progestogenic, and androgenic activity.[49] Tibolone has been used for almost two decades in Europe for the treatment of menopausal symptoms and prevention of osteoporosis. Approval of Organon's new drug application for tibolone (Xyvion) in the United States is expected in 2004. The hormonal effects of this synthetic steroid depend on its metabolism and activation in peripheral tissues. The parent compound has been described as a prodrug that is metabolized quickly in the gastrointestinal tract. It has several active metabolites, including a Δ4-isomer and 3α-OH and 3β-OH compounds.[49] The Δ4-isomer metabolite confers significant progestogenic and androgenic properties. Tibolone has beneficial effects on mood and libido and improves menopausal symptoms and vaginal atrophy. Tibolone protects against bone loss, and its effect on fracture rates is currently being evaluated.[50] In addition, it causes endometrial atrophy and, therefore, does not usually cause withdrawal bleeding when used in women who have had amenorrhea for at least 1 year. Tibolone is not recommended during perimenopause because it may cause irregular bleeding. Its use is associated with a low rate of bleeding, ranging from 10% to 15%, during the initial months of treatment to about 4% after 6 months of treatment.[22]

Tibolone reduces concentrations of total cholesterol, triglycerides, and lipoprotein(a) but significantly decreases HDL cholesterol and thus may increase overall cardiovascular risk.[22] Tibolone increases fibrinolysis parameters without significantly altering coagulation parameters.[51] Long-term safety data are lacking. The Million Women Study, a cohort study, showed that current users of tibolone may be at increased risk for breast cancer (adjusted relative risk 1.45, 95% CI 1.25–1.68).[21] The major adverse effects of tibolone include weight gain and bloating. Further studies are necessary to identify the true risk-benefit ratio of tibolone with respect to its overall effect on coronary artery disease and breast cancer.

TREATMENT CONSIDERATIONS

Hormone therapy is contraindicated in women with endometrial cancer, breast cancer, undiagnosed vaginal bleeding, thromboembolism (including a recent spontaneous thrombosis or in the presence of a thrombophilia), or active liver disease.[52] Relative contraindications include uterine leiomyoma, migraine headaches, and seizure disorder.[53] In addition, oral estrogen should be avoided in women with hypertriglyceridemia, liver disease, and gallbladder disease. For these women, transdermal administration is a safer approach. The main reasons for discontinuing hormone therapy are side effects such as bleeding, breast tenderness, bloating, and "premenstrual-like symptoms." Reducing the dose or changing the regimen or the route of administration can minimize these effects.

Pretreatment Assessment

The initial visit of a perimenopausal or postmenopausal woman is the most appropriate time to obtain a complete medical history, perform a physical examination, and educate the patient.[53] Medical history should include determination of a personal or family history of thrombotic problems. The physical examination should include a complete cardiovascular examination, clinical assessment of thyroid status, and breast and pelvic examinations. Papanicolaou cervical cytologic examination and screening mammography negative for malignancy are required before initiating hormone therapy. Thyroid function tests and lipoprotein lipid profile also should be performed at the discretion of the clinician.

Each patient should be evaluated for the presence of indications (i.e., menopausal symptoms such as hot flushes or vaginal dryness) and possible contraindications. The risks and benefits of hormone therapy should be discussed with the patient so that she can weigh the risks and benefits versus alternatives and make a rational decision about whether to use hormone therapy.

BENEFITS OF HORMONE THERAPY

Relief of Menopausal Symptoms

Vasomotor Symptoms. The major indication for postmenopausal hormone therapy is the management of vasomotor symptoms. Most women with vasomotor symptoms require hormone treatment for less than 5 years, and thus the risk appears to be small.

Fewer than 25% of women experience a menopausal transition without symptoms, whereas over 25% suffer severe menopausal symptoms, most commonly hot flushes and night sweats.[54]

Without treatment, hot flushes in most women typically disappear within 1 to 2 years, but in some untreated women they continue for more than 20 years.[32] Women with mild vasomotor symptoms often experience relief by lifestyle modification (e.g., wear layered clothing that can be removed or added as necessary); reduction in intake of hot spicy foods, caffeine, and hot beverages; exercise; and other good general health practices. At least 25% of women in clinical trials report significant improvement in their vasomotor symptoms when taking placebo. However, no therapy has been shown to be as effective as estrogen therapy in alleviating significant vasomotor symptoms. Estrogens diminish hot flushes in most women, and all types and routes of administration of estrogen are equally effective.[55] A dose-dependent relationship between estrogen administration and suppression of hot flushes is well established. Some women, especially younger women, may require a higher than average dose of estrogen to suppress symptoms. On the other hand, many women with hot flushes at the time of menopause require lower dose of estrogen. Hormone therapy for menopausal symptoms can be stopped about 2 or 3 years after starting. If treatment can be tapered and stopped within 5 years, there is no evidence of increased risk of breast cancer.[2]

Alternatives to estrogen for the treatment of hot flushes include tibolone, selective serotonin reuptake inhibitors (e.g., paroxetine, fluoxetine), venlafaxine, medroxyprogesterone acetate, megestrol acetate, clonidine, and gabapentin[56] (Table 80–6). Progestogens alone may be an option for some women (e.g., those with a history of breast cancer or venous thrombosis), but weight gain, vaginal bleeding, and other adverse effects often limit their use. Selective serotonin reuptake inhibitors and venlafaxine are considered by some to be a first-line therapy for the treatment of hot flushes in women for whom hormone therapy is contraindicated.[56–59] Clonidine often is effective for symptom control, but it is not always well tolerated by women.

To date, randomized, placebo-controlled trials of non-hormonal therapies have been equivocal and have not established the safety and

---

TABLE 80–6. Alternatives to Estrogen for Treatment of Hot Flushes

Drug	Dose (Oral)	Interval	Comments
Tibolone	2.5–5 mg	Once daily	Tibolone is not recommended during the perimenopause because it may cause irregular bleeding
Venlafaxine	37.5–150 mg	Once daily	Side effects include dry mouth, decreased appetite, nausea, and constipation
Paroxetine	12.5–25 mg	Once daily	12.5 mg is an adequate and well-tolerated starting dose for most women; adverse effects include headache, nausea, and insomnia
Fluoxetine	20 mg	Once daily	Modest improvement seen in hot flushes
Megestrol acetate	20–40 mg	Once daily	Progesterone may be linked to breast cancer etiology; also, there is concern regarding the safety of progestational agents in women with preexisting breast cancer
Clonidine	0.1 mg	Once daily	Can be administered orally or transdermally; drowsiness and dry mouth can occur, especially with higher doses
Gabapentin	900 mg	Divided in three daily doses	Adverse effects include somnolence and dizziness; these symptoms often can be obviated with a gradual increase in dosing

efficacy of herbal remedies, homeopathic treatments, or acupuncture for the prevention or treatment of hot flushes.

Vaginal Atrophy. Estrogen receptors have been demonstrated in the lower genitourinary tract, and at least 50% of postmenopausal women suffer symptoms of urogenital atrophy caused by estrogen deficiency.[60] Atrophy of the vaginal mucosa results in vaginal dryness and dyspareunia. Lower urinary tract symptoms include urethritis, recurrent urinary tract infection, urinary urgency, and frequency. Most women with significant vaginal dryness because of vaginal atrophy require the use of local or systemic estrogen therapy for symptom relief. Such treatment also reduces the risk of recurrent urinary tract infections, possibly by modifying the vaginal flora.[61] Vaginal dryness and dyspareunia can be treated with a topical estrogen cream, tablet, or vaginal ring. In clinical trials, topical estrogen appears to be better than systemic estrogen for relieving these symptoms and avoids high levels of circulating estrogen. Concomitant progestogen therapy generally is unnecessary if women are using low-dose micronized 17β-estradiol. However, the regular use of CEE vaginal creams and other products that potentially promote endometrial proliferation in women with an intact uterus requires intermittent progestogen challenges (i.e., for 10 days every 12 weeks). This is an important caveat because vaginal atrophy requires long-term estrogen treatment.[61]

Urinary incontinence, which becomes more prevalent with increasing age, usually is not improved by estrogen therapy, and in one large clinical trial, estrogen-progestogen therapy actually increased incontinence.[62]

Osteoporosis Prevention

Postmenopausal osteoporosis is a serious age-related disease that affects millions of women throughout the world. The WHI randomized trial was the first study to demonstrate that hormone therapy reduces the risk of fractures at the hip, spine, and wrist.[2,63] Hip and clinical vertebral fractures are reduced by 34%, and total osteoporotic fractures are reduced by 24%.[63] These findings are in agreement with observational data and several meta-analyses regarding the efficacy of hormone therapy in reduction of fractures in postmenopausal women.[64]

Menopause is accompanied by accelerated bone loss, and the central role of estrogen deficiency in postmenopausal osteoporosis is well established. Osteoporosis is characterized by reduced bone mass associated with architectural deterioration of the skeleton and increased risk for fracture.[65] Estrogen deficiency results in bone loss through its actions in accelerating bone turnover and uncoupling bone formation from resorption. In fact, annual decrements in bone mass of 3% to 5% are common in the years soon after the menopause, and 0.5% to 1% decrements are seen after 65 years of age.[66] Estrogen therapy reduces bone turnover and increases bone density in postmenopausal women of all ages. Nonetheless, the protective effect persists as long as the treatment is maintained. With cessation of therapy, postmenopausal bone loss resumes at the same rate as that in untreated women. The standard bone-sparing daily estrogen dose is equivalent to 0.625 mg CEE[26] (see Table 80–2). Even low doses of estrogen may increase bone mass when they are supplemented with adequate calcium intake.[26]

Osteoporosis prevention remains an indicated use of estrogen products; however, nonestrogen products, such as raloxifene and bisphosphonates, are as effective as hormone therapy for preventing osteoporosis (Table 80–7). The FDA has withdrawn the "osteoporosis treatment" indication from estrogen products.

Raloxifene decreases the risk of vertebral fracture by 30% to 50%, although it has not been shown to decrease the risk of hip fracture.[46] The bisphosphonates reduce the risk of both hip and vertebral fractures by 30% to 50%.[65] Bisphosphonates are analogues of pyrophosphate that inhibit bone resorption. Drugs in this class include alendronate, etidronate, pamidronate, risedronate, tiludronate, and zoledronate. Bisphoshonates have no known impact on the incidence of cardiovascular disease or breast or endometrial cancer. Adverse effects include upper gastrointestinal side effects, especially if not taken properly. A few trials have shown improved bone density over single therapy when a bisphosphonate is combined with estrogen or raloxifene, but there are no fracture data.[67]

Tibolone can prevent bone loss in early postmenopausal women.[50] A placebo-controlled study investigating the effects of tibolone on fractures is currently ongoing.

TABLE 80–7. Alternatives to Hormone Therapy for Osteoporosis Prevention

Drug	Dose	Comments
Raloxifene	60 mg/day	Raloxifene reduces the risk of vertebral fractures. Adverse effects include hot flushes and leg cramps. Slowly increasing the dose of raloxifene may help reduce the incidence and severity of hot flushes.
Tibolone	1.25 mg or 2.5 mg/day	Tibolone prevents bone loss. No data are yet available regarding fracture rates.
Alendronate	5 mg/day or 35 mg/week	A 50% reduction in the risk of fractures is observed in women with osteoporosis. In younger postmenopausal women without osteoporosis, therapy with alendronate protected all women from bone loss for up to 4 years. Side effects include upper gastrointestinal symptoms, especially if the drug is not taken as directed.
Risedronate	5 mg/day or 35 mg/week	A 40% reduction in vertebral and nonvertebral fractures is observed in women with osteoporosis. In postmenopausal women without osteoporosis, risedronate increases bone mineral density over 2 years. Significant side effects were not observed.
Etidronate	Intermittent administration of 400 mg/day (in 2-week cycles); dose repeated every 3 months	Calcium is taken between the cycles of etidronate. Continuous daily use may cause abnormalities in bone mineralization. A 37% reduction is observed in the risk of vertebral fractures (but not nonvertebral fractures) in women with osteoporosis. Therapy in women without osteoporosis prevents bone loss over 2 years. Side effects include diarrhea and nausea.
Zoledronic acid	4 mg as a single intravenous infusion once yearly	Effects on bone turnover and bone density were similar to those with daily oral bisphosphonates. Efficacy against fractures has not yet been established. Adverse effects include myalgia and pyrexia.

General protective measures, such as adequate calcium intake (1200 mg/day),[68] regular weight-bearing exercise, and the avoidance of detrimental lifestyle habits such as smoking and alcohol abuse, are appropriate for all women. Most women require calcium supplementation to their dietary intake. Also, adequate exposure to sunlight is believed to protect against vitamin D deficiency, but many Western women are deficient in this vitamin. The current recommended dietary intake for vitamin D is 400 IU/day for women aged 51 to 70 years and 600 IU/day for women older than age 70.[68]

Low bone density is the most important risk factor for osteoporosis. According to the World Health Organization, a woman with a bone mineral density greater than 2.5 standard deviations below the mean peak density has osteoporosis.[65] The rates of osteoporosis vary with ethnicity; it is more common in whites and those of Asian descent and less common in blacks.[65] In the United States, approximately 20% of white women aged 50 years or older have osteoporosis.[65]

Bone mass measurement accurately determines the bone density in the spine and hip. The current "gold standard" method of bone density testing is dual-energy x-ray absorptiometry (DEXA).[65] Bone density testing is recommended in the United States for all women with medical causes of bone loss and for all women aged 65 years or older. Bone density testing should be assessed in conjunction with clinical risk profile evaluation. For women at high fracture risk (i.e., T-score <2, previous nonspine fracture, family history of hip or spine fracture, and low body weight), bisphosphonates are the treatment of choice because of the demonstrated fracture protection.[65] There are no clear indications for treating women at low risk for fracture (T-score >2), but raloxifene, tibolone, and bisphosphonates may be used. Long-term hormone therapy is no longer an appropriate first-choice option for osteoporosis prevention because of the risks associated with its long-term use. Therefore, hormone therapy should be considered for osteoporosis prevention only in women at significant risk for osteoporosis who cannot take nonestrogen regimens.

Colon Cancer Risk Reduction

Colorectal cancer is the fourth most common cancer and the second leading cause of cancer death in the United States (see Chap. 127). The WHI was the first randomized, controlled trial to confirm that hormone therapy reduces colon cancer risk. Compared with placebo, 6 fewer colorectal cancers are reported per year in every 10,000 women taking hormone therapy.[2]

Other

Diabetes. In healthy postmenopausal women, hormone therapy appears to have a beneficial effect on fasting glucose level among women with elevated fasting insulin concentrations.[69] Also, in women with coronary artery disease, hormone therapy reduces the incidence of diabetes by 35%.[70] These findings provide important insights into the metabolic effects of hormone therapy but are insufficient to recommend the long-term use of hormone therapy in women with diabetes.

Body Weight. A meta-analysis of randomized, controlled trials showed that unopposed estrogen or estrogen combined with a progestin has no effect on body weight, suggesting that hormone therapy does not cause weight gain in excess of that normally observed at the time of menopause.[71]

RISKS OF HORMONE THERAPY

Cardiovascular Disease

Cardiovascular disease, including coronary artery disease, stroke, and peripheral vascular disease, is the leading cause of death among women. The American Heart Association recommends that postmenopausal hormone therapy should not be used for reducing the risk of coronary heart disease.[72]

In the last decade, an expectation of coronary benefit had been a major reason for postmenopausal hormone use because observational studies indicated that women who use hormone therapy have a 35% to 50% lower risk of coronary heart disease than nonusers.[73] In addition, previous studies have shown that estrogen exerts protective effects on the cardiovascular system, including lipid-lowering,[74] antioxidant,[75] and vasodilating effects.[76] Nevertheless, recent randomized clinical trials have provided no evidence of cardiovascular disease protection and even some evidence of harm with hormone therapy[2,77-82] (Table 80–8).

The primary findings of the WHI trial showed an overall increase in the risk of coronary heart disease (HR 1.24, 95% CI 1–1.54) among healthy postmenopausal women 50 to 79 years of age receiving combined estrogen-progestogen hormone therapy compared with those receiving placebo.[2,82] New findings from the Women's Health Initiative, in women taking estrogen alone, showed no effect (either increase or decrease) in the risk of coronary heart disease.[3]

In the estrogen-progestogen arm of the WHI trial, the elevation in coronary heart disease risk was most apparent at 1 year (HR 1.81, 95% CI 1.09–3.01). The increased risk for stroke and venous thromboembolism continued throughout the 5 years of therapy.[2] Increased risk was observed only for ischemic stroke and not for hemorrhagic stroke.[83] In the estrogen-alone arm of the study, a similar increased risk for stroke was observed. The lack of cardiac protection observed in the WHI trial is consistent with recent findings from randomized trials of postmenopausal hormone therapy in women with coronary heart disease. In the Heart Estrogen/Progestin Replacement Study (HERS), combined hormone therapy had no overall effect on the risk of recurrent coronary events after 4.1[77] and 6.8 years[84] of follow-up. Similar to the WHI, the elevated risk of coronary heart disease was largely limited to the first year of therapy. The Estrogen Replacement in Atherosclerosis (ERA) trial found that neither unopposed estrogen nor estrogen plus progestin slowed the progression of atherosclerosis, measured by quantitative angiography, among women with preexisting coronary heart disease.[78] The Papworth trial,[81] which tested transdermal 17β-estradiol with or without norethindrone, and the ESPRIT trial,[80] which tested estradiol valerate without progestin in women with a history of myocardial infarction, also demonstrated no cardiac protection with hormone therapy. Finally, the Women's Estrogen for Stroke Trial (WEST), which tested oral 17β-estradiol (without progestin), found no overall effect in the risk of coronary events and stroke and an increased risk of stroke in the first 6 months of treatment.[79]

Raloxifene therapy for 4 years in osteoporotic postmenopausal women did not significantly affect the risk of cardiovascular events (myocardial infarction, unstable angina, coronary ischemia, stroke, or transient ischemic attack).[85] Among women at high risk of coronary heart disease, those receiving raloxifene had statistically significant reductions in the risk of cardiovascular events.[85] These findings must be evaluated by a randomized trial designed specifically to assess cardiovascular events.

Hormone therapy should not be initiated or continued for the prevention of cardiovascular disease. Adherence to a healthful lifestyle

TABLE 80–8. Randomized Clinical Trials of Cardiovascular Disease and Postmenopausal Hormone Therapy

Trial	Population	Medication	Results	Comments
WHI (estrogen/ progestogen arm)[2]	16,608 apparently healthy postmenopausal women	Conjugated estrogen 0.625 mg plus medroxyprogesterone acetate 2.5 mg daily or placebo	29% increased risk of coronary heart disease among women taking hormone therapy	The trial was planned to last for 8.5 years but was stopped after 5.2 years owing to increased risk of breast cancer after 5 years of treatment.
WHI (estrogen-alone arm)[3]	10,739 apparently healthy postmenopausal women with prior hysterectomy	Conjugated estrogen 0.625 mg daily or placebo	No effect on cardiovascular disease risk among women taking estrogen therapy	The trial was stopped after 6.8 years because of an increased risk of stroke (hazard ratio 1.39, 95% CI 1.10–1.77)
HERS[77]	2,763 postmenopausal women with coronary heart disease	Conjugated estrogen 0.625 mg plus medroxyprogesterone acetate 2.5 mg daily or placebo	No difference in risk of coronary heart disease events (myocardial infarction or coronary heart disease death) among women in the two groups	A 50% increased risk of coronary heart disease events was observed among women in the hormone therapy group in the first year of treatment.
ERA[78]	309 postmenopausal women with coronary heart disease	Conjugated estrogen 0.625 mg plus medroxyprogesterone acetate 2.5 mg daily or placebo	No difference in changes in coronary diameter in either group after 3 years of treatment	Atherosclersis progression was measured by quantitative angiography.
PAPWORTH[81]	255 postmenopausal women with coronary heart disease	Transdermal 17β-estradiol 80 mcg/day alone for women with hysterectomy; transdermal 17β-estradiol, 80 mcg/day plus cyclic transdermal norethisterone 120 mcg/day for 14 days or placebo	No reduction in the incidence of acute coronary events (coronary disease death, myocardial infarction, unstable angina) among women in the hormone therapy group	During the first 2 years of follow-up, the hormone-therapy group had a higher acute coronary event rate than the control group.
WEST[79]	664 postmenopausal women with recent stroke or transient ischemic attack	Oral 17β-estradiol, 1 mg/day or placebo	No reduction in risk of stroke, death, or coronary events among women in the hormone therapy group during 2.8 years of treatment	In the first 6 months of treatment, a 2.3-fold increase in the risk of stroke was observed among women in the hormone therapy group.
ESPRIT[80]	1017 postmenopausal women with previous myocardial infarction	Oral estradiol valerate 2 mg or placebo	No reduction in the incidence of acute coronary events (coronary disease death, myocardial infarction) among women in the estrogen group	In the estradiol group, there were slightly more nonfatal myocardial infarctions but fewer cardiac deaths.

WHI, Women's Health Initiative; HERS, Heart and Estrogen/Progestin Replacement Study; ERA, Estrogen Replacement in Atherosclerosis; WEST, Women's Estrogen for Stroke Trial; ESPRIT, Estrogen in the Prevention of Reinfarction.

(cessation of smoking, regular exercise, healthy diet, and body mass index less than 25) may prevent the onset of cardiovascular disease in postmenopausal women.[86,87]

Breast Cancer

The WHI trial found that combined estrogen-progestin therapy has an increased risk of invasive breast cancer (HR 1.26, 95% CI 1.0–1.59) and a trend toward increasing risk with increasing duration of therapy.[2] The estrogen-only arm of the WHI found no increased risk for breast cancer during the 7-year follow-up period.[3] In the estrogen-progestogen arm, the increased breast cancer risk did not appear until after 3 years of study participation[2] (Table 80–9). The breast cancers diagnosed in women in the hormone therapy group had similar histology and grade but were more likely to have advanced stage compared with women in the placebo

group.[88] In an unselected postmenopausal population, the Million Women Study found that current use of hormone therapy increased breast cancer risk and breast cancer mortality (relative risk 1.66 and 1.22, respectively). Increased incidence was observed for estrogen-only use (relative risk 1.30), for estrogen-progestin (relative risk 2), and for tibolone (relative risk 1.45).[21]

The lifetime risk of developing breast cancer in the United States is approximately one in eight women,[89] and the greatest incidence occurs in women over the age of 60 years (see Chap. 125). In a collaborative reanalysis of data from 51 studies evaluating over 52,000 women with breast cancer and 108,000 controls, less than 5 years of therapy with estrogen combined with progestogen was associated with a 15% increase in the risk of breast cancer, and the increase was greater with longer duration (relative risk of 1.53 after 5 or more years of use).[90] However, 5 years after discontinuing hormone-replacement therapy, the risk of breast cancer was no longer increased.[90]

ABLE 80–9. Randomized Clinical Trials of Postmenopausal Hormone Therapy and Breast Cancer

Trial	Population	Medication	Results	Comments
WHI (estrogen/ progestogen arm)[2]	16,608 healthy postmenopausal women	Conjugated estrogen 0.625 mg plus medroxyprogesterone acetate 2.5 mg daily or placebo	26% increased risk of breast cancer	The increased risk did not appear until 5 years of study. There was a trend toward increasing risk over time.
WHI (estrogen-alone arm)[3]	10,739 apparently healthy postmenopausal women with prior hysterectomy	Conjugated estrogen 0.625 mg daily or placebo	No increased risk for breast cancer	The possible reduction in breast cancer risk requires further investigation (hazard ratio 0.77, 95% CI 0.59–1.01)
MORE[48]	7705 postmenopausal women with osteoporosis	Raloxifene 60 or 120 mg/ day or placebo	76% lower risk of estrogen receptor-positive breast cancer after 4 years of raloxifene therapy	Raloxifene can cause or exacerbate hot flushes. Also, it increases the risk of venous thromboembolism by about 2-fold.
CORE[48a]	5213 postmenopausal women with osteoporosis	Raloxifene 60 mg daily or placebo	76% lower risk of estrogen receptor-positive breast cancer after 8 years of raloxifene therapy	No new safety concerns were identified during the CORE study. The risk of venous thromboembolism remained increased by about 2-fold.

WHI, Women's Health Initiative; MORE, Multiple Outcomes of Raloxifene Evaluation; CORE, Continuing Outcomes Relevent to Evista.

Addition of progestogens to estrogen may increase breast cancer risk beyond that observed with estrogen alone.[91] The Iowa Women's Health Study showed that exposure to hormone therapy is associated with an increased risk of breast cancer that has a favorable prognosis.[92] These findings have been attributed to an increased use of breast cancer screening in women taking hormone therapy. A study of the effects of hormone therapy in women with a family history of breast cancer found that those who were current users had approximately the same increased relative risk compared with those who did not have a family history.[93] The overall mortality for women with a family history of breast cancer from all causes was reduced significantly among hormone therapy users.[93] These data suggest that hormone therapy use in women with a family history of breast cancer is not associated with a significantly increased incidence of the disease.

Sex steroid deficiency during menopause results in lipomatous involution of the breast that is reflected by decreased mammographic breast density and markedly improved radiotransparency of breast tissue. Thus mammographic changes indicating breast cancer can be recognized more easily and earlier after the menopause. Conversely, combination hormone therapy results in increased mammographic breast density,[94] and increased density on mammography has been associated with higher breast cancer risk.[95] Of note, increased mammographic density is not observed with estrogen-only therapy.[94]

Although raloxifene is not approved for prevention or treatment of breast cancer, a 4-year trial of raloxifene in women with osteoporosis (not at increased risk for breast cancer) showed a 76% risk reduction for estrogen-receptor-positive breast cancer[48] (relative risk 0.24, 95% CI 0.13–0.44). Furthermore, the CORE trial, a study evaluating the efficacy of an additional 4 years of raloxifene therapy in women with osteoporosis, showed that the reduction in estrogen-receptor positive breast cancer incidence continues for up to 8 years[48a] (hazard ratio 0.24, 95% CI 0.15–0.40) (see Table 80–9). Raloxifene does not increase breast density.[96] A trial comparing raloxifene with tamoxifen is underway.

Endometrial Cancer

The WHI trial suggests that combined hormone therapy does not increase endometrial cancer risk compared with placebo (HR 0.81, 95%

CI 0.48–1.36).[97] Estrogen given alone to women with an intact uterus significantly increases uterine cancer risk.[35] With unopposed estrogen therapy, the risk of endometrial cancer increases within 2 years.[35] The excess risk increases with dose and duration of estrogen (10 years of unopposed estrogen increases the risk 10-fold), is apparent within 2 years of the start of treatment, and persists for many years after estrogen replacement is discontinued. Estrogen-induced endometrial cancer is usually of a low stage and grade at the time of diagnosis,[32] and it can be prevented almost entirely by progestogen coadministration. The sequential addition of progestin to estrogen for at least 10 days of the treatment cycle or continuous combined estrogen-progestogen does not increase the risk of endometrial cancer.[98]

Also, lower doses of estrogen may be associated with a lower risk of endometrial hyperplasia.[99] Raloxifene does not result in endometrial hyperplasia, has no effect on endometrial thickness, is not associated with polyp formation, and has virtually no proliferative effect on the endometrium.[100] A 4-year trial of raloxifene in women with osteoporosis showed no increased risk of endometrial cancer.[48]

Ovarian Cancer

Lifetime risk of ovarian cancer is low (1.7%). The WHI trial suggests that combined hormone therapy may increase the risk of ovarian cancer (HR 1.58, 95% CI 0.77–3.24).[97] However, a recent study reported an increased risk of ovarian cancer in women taking postmenopausal estrogen therapy for more than 10 years (relative risk 1.8, 95% CI 1.1–3.0) but no increased risk of ovarian cancer among women receiving combination estrogen-progestin therapy.[101] Additional large, controlled studies are needed to confirm these findings.

Venous Thromboembolism

Venous thromboembolism, including thrombosis of the deep veins of the legs and embolism to the pulmonary arteries, is uncommon in the general population. The absolute risk of venous thromboembolism in non-hormone therapy users is approximately 1 in 10,000 women.[102] Women taking hormone therapy have a twofold increase in risk for thromboembolic events, with the highest risk occurring in the first year of use.[103] The absolute increase in risk is small, with 1.5 venous thromboembolic events per 10,000 women in 1 year.[103] Lower doses of estrogen are associated with a decreased risk for thromboembolism as compared with higher doses.[102]

Currently, there is no indication for thrombophilia screening before initiating hormone therapy. However, hormone therapy should be avoided in women at high risk for thromboembolic events.

Gallbladder Disease

Gallbladder disease is a commonly cited complication of oral estrogen use.[104] The Nurses' Health Study showed that the age-adjusted relative risk of cholecystectomy is 2.2 for women currently taking 0.625 mg CEE.[104] In this study, the risk of cholecystectomy increased with duration of hormone therapy use and did not resolve after discontinuation.[104] Transdermal estrogen is an alternative to oral therapy for women at high risk for cholelithiasis.

CLINICAL CONTROVERSY

Some clinicians believe that hormone therapy may improve well-being and quality of life of postmenopausal women, whereas others believe that hormone therapy, at best, has no effect. Hormone therapy improves mood and well-being mainly in women with vasomotor symptoms and sleep disturbance.

OTHER EFFECTS OF HORMONE THERAPY

Quality of Life, Mood, Cognition, and Dementia

Hormone therapy improves depressive symptoms in symptomatic menopausal women most probably by relieving flushing and improving sleep.[105,106] Women with vasomotor symptoms receiving hormone therapy have improved mental health and fewer depressive symptoms compared with those receiving placebo; however, hormone therapy may worsen quality of life in women without flushes.[107]

There is no evidence that hormone therapy improves quality of life or cognition in older, asymptomatic women.[107–110] Postmenopausal hormone therapy should not be used for treatment of major depression.[111]

More than 33% of women aged 65 years or older will develop dementia during their lifetime.[112] Several observational studies have suggested that estrogen therapy may be protective against Alzheimer disease (see Chap. 63). The WHI Memory Study, an ancillary study of WHI including 4532 women aged 65 years or older, evaluated the effect of combined hormone therapy on dementia and cognition.[1C] The study found that postmenopausal women aged 65 years or older taking estrogen plus progestogen therapy had twice the rate of dementia, including Alzheimer disease, of women taking placebo[1C] (HR 2.05, 95% CI 1.21–3.48). In addition, in these women, estrogen plus progestogen therapy did not prevent mild cognitive impairment, a cognitive and functional state between normal aging and dementia

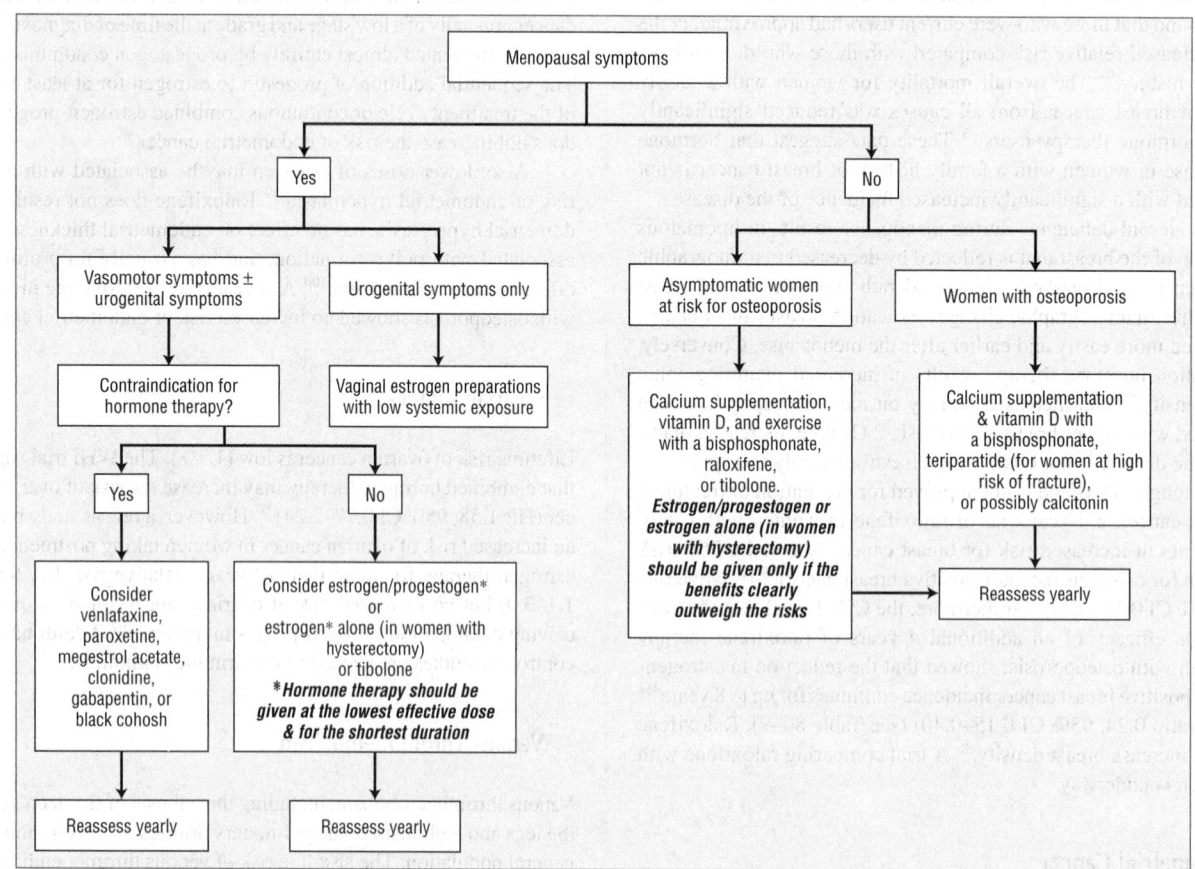

FIGURE 80–1. Treatment algorithm for postmenopausal women. Tibolone is currently not yet approved for use in the United States.

that frequently progresses to dementia.[109] The estrogen-alone arm of the WHI study showed similar findings.[110a,110b]

Raloxifene does not have a significant effect on cognitive function; however, there is a trend toward a smaller decline in verbal memory and attention scores among women receiving raloxifene.[113]

Hormone therapy improves mood and well-being mainly in postmenopausal women with vasomotor symptoms and sleep disturbance, whereas it does not improve quality of life in postmenopausal women without vasomotor symptoms. Hormone therapy does not improve cognitive function when compared with placebo, and more important, a small increased risk of clinically meaningful cognitive decline occurs among women aged 65 years or older taking hormone therapy.[110,110a,110b]

INDIVIDUALIZING HORMONE THERAPY

8 Menopause is a natural life event, not a disease. The decision to take hormone therapy must be individualized and based on several parameters, including menopausal symptoms, osteoporosis risk, coronary artery disease risk, breast cancer risk, and thromboem-

bolism risk. Recommendations should be specific to each woman and her background. Thus the menopausal treatment should be based on each woman's clinical profile and concerns. Approved indications of hormone therapy include treatment of vasomotor symptoms and urogenital atrophy and prevention of osteoporosis. Weighing risks and benefits, the FDA determined that the indication for vasomotor symptoms (hot flushes and night sweats) should remain unchanged, but the other two indications for hormone therapy should be revised. For the treatment of vasomotor symptoms, systemic hormone therapy remains the most effective pharmacologic intervention (Fig. 80–1). For symptoms of urogenital atrophy, such as vaginal dryness, topical products should be considered. In addition, although prevention of postmenopausal osteoporosis remains an indicated use of hormone therapy, consideration should be given to approved nonestrogen products, such as raloxifene and bisphosphonates (see Fig. 80–1). Clinicians should prescribe the lowest effective dose of hormone therapy for the shortest duration, weighing the potential benefits and risks for the individual woman. Furthermore, measures to reduce the risks of cardiovascular disease (such as treating hypertension and avoid smoking) and osteoporosis (such as taking calcium supplements and vitamin D, changing diet, and performing weight-bearing exercise) should be addressed.

EVALUATION OF THERAPEUTIC OUTCOMES

After the menopausal woman begins hormone therapy, a brief follow-up visit 6 weeks later may be useful to discuss patient concerns about hormone therapy and to evaluate the patient for symptom relief, adverse effects, and patterns of withdrawal bleeding. The FDA recommends that women who choose estrogen-based therapy should have yearly breast examinations, perform monthly breast self-examinations, and receive periodic mammograms (to be scheduled based on their age and risk factors). Also, women receiving hormone therapy should undergo annual monitoring, including a medical history and physical examination, pelvic examination, blood pressure measurement, and routine endometrial cancer surveillance, as indicated. Additional follow-up should be determined based on the patient's initial response to therapy and the need for any modification of the regimen. Endometrial biopsy should be considered in women taking cyclic hormone therapy if vaginal bleeding occurs at any time other than the expected time of withdrawal bleeding or when heavier or more prolonged withdrawal bleeding occurs. In women taking continuous combined hormone therapy, endometrial evaluation should be considered when irregular bleeding persists for more than 6 months after initiating therapy. Endovaginal ultrasonography also has been used in the evaluation of abnormal uterine bleeding in women receiving hormone therapy. However, there is no universal agreement that endovaginal ultrasonography is adequate to exclude endometrial pathology.

The main indication for hormone therapy is the relief of menopausal symptoms, and hormone therapy should be used only as long as symptom control is necessary (typically for about 2 to 3 years). When used under such conditions, the absolute risk of harm to an individual woman is very small.[2]

Many women have no difficulty stopping hormone therapy abruptly; others develop vasomotor symptoms after discontinuation. Although these symptoms are usually mild and resolve over a few months, in some women they may be severe and intolerable. Slowly tapering the hormone therapy over several months—reducing the

frequency of administration, the dose, or both—may ameliorate the symptoms.[114]

Women older than 65 years of age or younger with risk factors for osteoporosis should have their bone mineral density measured. Although bone densitometry has been shown to predict fractures, at present there are no guidelines for follow-up bone mineral density testing. However, in women with significant bone loss, repeat testing should be performed as clinically indicated.

PHARMACOECONOMIC CONSIDERATIONS

Estrogens and progestogens used for postmenopausal hormone therapy still are prescribed commonly in the United States, especially for the management of menopausal vasomotor symptoms. Even before publication of the WHI findings, only a fraction of women filled their hormone therapy prescriptions, and only 25% to 40% continued to take postmenopausal hormone therapy for more than 1 year.[115] This may be due to women's attitudes toward hormone therapy or a result of fear about adverse effects and associated risks. Hormone therapy use in the United States declined substantially after dissemination of the WHI study results.[115a]

Use of hormone therapy for the management of vasomotor symptoms is cost-effective, and data to support the use of nonhormonal alternatives are limited. The cost of hormone therapy can vary depending on the route and method of delivery. Transdermal preparations are about twice as expensive as their equivalent oral preparations.[116] Women who have undergone hysterectomy use hormone therapy more frequently than do women with an intact uterus (58.7% versus 19.6%).[5]

Raloxifene adversely affects hot flushes, but it is likely to be used for osteoporosis prevention. For women with a history of breast cancer or thromboembolic disease, alternative means of reducing the risk of osteoporosis, such as bisphosphonates, should be considered.

The results of randomized trials suggest that hormone therapy should not be used for cardiovascular disease prevention. Women with coronary disease risk factors (e.g., hypertension, lipid abnormalities) can benefit from reduction of these risk factors through interventions such as weight loss, lipid lowering, use of aspirin, use of antioxidants, and physical activity.

CONCLUSIONS

During the past decade, postmenopausal hormone therapy became one of the most frequently prescribed therapies in the United States. Menopause is a natural life event, not a disease. Therefore, the decision to use hormone therapy must be individualized based on the severity of menopausal symptoms, risk of osteoporosis, and consideration of such factors as coronary artery disease, breast cancer, and thromboembolism.

Recent large prospective, randomized trials have shown that postmenopausal hormone therapy prescribed for disease prevention may cause more harm than good.[2,77] The WHI study reported increased risk of cardiovascular disease, breast cancer, stroke, and thromboembolic disease among women using continuous-combined therapy with CEE plus medroxyprogesterone acetate compared with placebo.[2] In the estrogen-alone arm of the study, CEE had no effect on cardiovascular disease or breast cancer risk compared to placebo, but an increased risk of stroke and thromboembolic disease was noted in those who received estrogen.[3] The WHI study also demonstrated that quality of life[108] and cognition[109,110,110a,110b] are no better in the group receiving hormone therapy than in the placebo group.

Postmenopausal symptoms, such as hot flushes and vaginal dryness, remain a valid indication for hormone therapy in the absence of contraindications. For short-term use of hormone therapy for the relief of menopausal symptoms, the benefits for many women generally outweigh the risks. For symptoms of genital atrophy alone, local estrogen and/or nonhormonal lubricants should be considered.

Long-term use of hormone therapy cannot be recommended routinely for osteoporosis prevention given the availability of alternative therapies, such as raloxifene and the bisphosponates. For long-term hormone therapy use, the potential harm (cardiovascular disease, breast cancer, and thromboembolism) outweighs the potential benefits.

PREMATURE OVARIAN FAILURE AND PREMENOPAUSAL HORMONE REPLACEMENT

PATHOPHYSIOLOGY

Premature ovarian failure is a condition characterized by sex-steroid deficiency, amenorrhea, and infertility in women younger than 40 years of age. At one time, premature ovarian failure was considered irreversible and was described as "premature menopause." Premature ovarian failure is not an early natural menopause. Normal menopause results from ovarian follicle depletion, whereas premature ovarian failure is characterized by intermittent ovarian function in one-half of affected women.[117] These women produce estrogen intermittently and may ovulate despite the presence of high gonadotropin concentrations. Pregnancies have occurred in 5% to 10% of women after the diagnosis of premature ovarian failure—even in women with no follicles observed on ovarian biopsy.

Premature ovarian failure may occur on the basis of ovarian follicle dysfunction or ovarian follicle depletion and may present as either primary amenorrhea (absence of menses in a girl who has reached the age of 16) or secondary amenorrhea (cessation of menses in a woman previously menstruating for 6 months or more).

TABLE 80–10. Etiology of Premature Ovarian Failure

Idiopathic: *karyotypically normal spontaneous premature ovarian failure*

Autoimmunity: (a) isolated autoimmune premature ovarian failure or (b) as a component of an autoimmune polyglandular syndrome in association with Addison's disease, hypothyroidism, hypoparathyroidism, or mucocutaneous candidiasis

Iatrogenic: *(chemotherapy, radiation, extensive ovarian surgery)*

X-chromosome abnormalities

Gonadotropin and gonadotropin-receptor abnormalities: signal defects

Enzyme deficiencies: *cholesterol desmolase, 17α-hydroxylase, 17, 20-desmolase*

Galactosemia

Blepharophimosis, ptosis, and epicantus inversus syndrome type 1: rare autosomal dominant syndrome in which premature ovarian failure is the predominant syndrome

Perrault's syndrome: familial autosomal recessive premature ovarian failure in association with deafness

In most cases, the etiology cannot be identified (Table 80–10). In the majority of patients, ovarian failure develops after the establishment of regular menses. Young women with premature ovarian failure who develop ovarian dysfunction before they achieve peak adult bone mass sustain sex steroid deficiency for more years than do naturally menopausal women. This deficiency can result in a significantly higher risk for osteoporosis[118] and cardiovascular disease.[119,119a] Importantly, a survey of more than 19,000 women between the ages of 25 and 100 years suggests that ovarian failure occurring before 40 years of age is associated with significantly increased mortality, with the age-adjusted odds ratio for all-cause mortality being 2.14 (95% CI 1.15–3.99).[120]

CLINICAL PRESENTATION OF PREMATURE OVARIAN FAILURE

SYMPTOMS

- *Primary amenorrhea*: No symptoms of estrogen deficiency
- *Secondary amenorrhea*: Vasomotor symptoms (hot flushes and night sweats), sleep disturbances, mood changes, sexual dysfunction, problems with concentration and memory, vaginal dryness, and dyspareunia

SIGNS

- *Primary amenorrhea*: Incomplete development of secondary sex characteristics
- *Secondary amenorrhea*: Normal development of secondary sex characteristics, signs of urogenital atrophy

LABORATORY TESTS

- FSH greater than 40 IU/L
- Other relevant diagnostic tests
- Thyroid function tests and fasting glucose

CLINICAL PRESENTATION

There is no characteristic menstrual pattern or history that precedes premature ovarian failure. Approximately 50% of patients with this condition have a history of oligomenorrhea or dysfunctional uterine bleeding (prodromal premature ovarian failure), and about 25% develop amenorrhea acutely. Some patients develop amenorrhea postpartum, whereas others experience it after discontinuing oral contraceptives. Primary amenorrhea is not associated with symptoms of estrogen deficiency. In cases of secondary amenorrhea, symptoms may include hot flushes, night sweats, fatigue, and mood changes. Prodromal premature ovarian failure may present with hot flushes even in women who menstruate regularly. Incomplete development of secondary sex characteristics may occur in women with primary amenorrhea, whereas these characteristics are typically normal in women with secondary amenorrhea. In general, women with premature ovarian failure have normal fertility before the disorder develops.

Approximately 50% of women with premature ovarian failure have been found to have documented ovarian follicle function.[117]

Premature ovarian failure is defined by the presence of at least 4 months of amenorrhea and at least two serum FSH concentrations measuring greater than 40 IU/L (obtained at least 1 month apart) in women younger than 40 years of age. A complete history should be taken regarding other factors that can affect ovarian function such as prior ovarian surgery, chemotherapy, radiation, and autoimmune disorders. In patients with primary amenorrhea, particular attention should be paid to breast and pubic hair development according to Tanner stages. Short stature, stigmata of Turner's syndrome, and other dysmorphic features of gonadal dysgenesis should be considered. Ideally, a pelvic examination should be performed, but this is not always clinically appropriate. Alternatively, transabdominal ultrasonography can be performed in primary amenorrhea to confirm the presence of normal anatomic structures. In the majority of cases, physical examination is completely normal. A karyotype should be performed in all patients experiencing premature ovarian failure. Women with ovarian failure and a karyotype containing a Y chromosome should undergo bilateral gonadectomy because there is a substantial risk for gonadal germ cell neoplasia.[121] Ovarian biopsy and antiovarian antibody testing are investigational procedures with no proven clinical benefit in premature ovarian failure. As clinically indicated, the workup should include tests for the diagnosis of other possible associated autoimmune disorders such as hypothyroidism, diabetes mellitus, and Addison's disease.

Young women find the diagnosis of premature ovarian failure particularly traumatic and frequently need extensive emotional and psychological support. While most of these women will, in fact, be infertile, it is important to emphasize that premature ovarian failure can be transient and that spontaneous pregnancies have occurred even years after diagnosis.

▶ TREATMENT: Premature Ovarian Failure

Postmenopausal women who take hormone therapy prolong their exposure to estrogen beyond the average age of completion of their reproductive phase. In contrast, women with premature ovarian failure need exogenous sex steroids to compensate for the decreased production by their ovaries. Importantly, 47% of young women with premature ovarian failure have significantly reduced bone mineral density within 1.5 years of their diagnosis despite taking standard hormone therapy.[118]

The goal of therapy in young women with premature ovarian failure is to provide a hormone-replacement regimen that maintains sex steroid status as effectively as the normal, functioning ovary. This usually requires the administration of estrogen at a dose greater than the standard dose given to older women experiencing natural menopause.

PHARMACOLOGIC THERAPY: HORMONAL REGIMENS

Optimal hormone therapy depends on whether the patient has primary or secondary amenorrhea. Young women with primary amenorrhea in whom secondary sex characteristics have failed to develop should be exposed initially to very low doses of estrogen in an attempt to mimic the gradual pubertal maturation process. A typical regimen is as follows: 0.3 mg CEE unopposed (i.e., no progestogen) daily for 6 months with incremental dose increases at 6-month intervals until the required maintenance dose is achieved. Gradual dose escalation often results in optimal breast development and allows time for the young woman to adjust psychologically to her physical maturation. Cyclic progestogen therapy, given 12 to 14 days per month, should be instituted toward the end of the second year of treatment.

Women with secondary amenorrhea who have been estrogen deficient for 12 months or longer also should be given low-dose estrogen replacement initially to avoid adverse effects such as mastalgia and nausea. However, the dose can be titrated up to maintenance levels over a 6-month period, and progestin therapy can be instituted with the initiation of estrogen therapy. Women with a brief history of secondary amenorrhea are less likely to experience undesired effects from hormone therapy if they are given a reduced dose for the first month of therapy followed by a full dose from the second month onward.

An estrogen dose equivalent to at least 1.25 mg CEE (or 100 mcg transdermal estradiol) is needed to achieve adequate estrogen replacement in young women. A progestin should be given for 12 to 14 days per calendar month to prevent endometrial hyperplasia (Table 80–11). Estrogens given in usual replacement doses do not suppress spontaneous follicular activity or ovulation. Because women with premature ovarian failure can have spontaneous pregnancies, hormone therapy should produce regular, predictable menstrual flow patterns (i.e., only cyclic regimens should be used). If these patients miss an expected menses, they should be tested for pregnancy and should discontinue hormone therapy. Because most young women negatively associate hormone therapy with menopause in older women, some clinicians prefer to prescribe oral contraceptives for hormone replacement in premenopausal women with hypogonadism. Oral contraceptives, however, may not inhibit ovulation or effectively prevent pregnancy in young women with elevated gonadotropins.

Androgen replacement also should be considered for women with premature ovarian failure experiencing persistent fatigue, poor well-being, and low libido despite adequate estrogen replacement. In these young women, testosterone replacement may be important for the development and maintenance of normal muscle mass and preservation of bone mineral content. An ongoing study at the National Institutes of Health is evaluating the effectiveness of long-term testosterone supplementation, in addition to standard hormone replacement, in protecting women with premature ovarian failure from bone loss. This study employs a transdermal system that delivers the equivalent of the normal daily ovarian testosterone production (150 mcg/day).

Importantly, all women with premature ovarian failure should understand that hormone therapy must be continued at least until the average age of natural menopause and that long-term follow-up is necessary.

TABLE 80–11. Premenopausal Hormone-Replacement Therapy for Young Women with Premature Ovarian Failure

Regimen	Dose	Frequency	Route
Estrogen Therapy			
Conjugated equine estrogen	1.25 mg	Daily	Oral
Piperazine estrone sulphate	2.5 mg	Daily	Oral
Micronized 17β-estradiol	4.0 mg	Daily	Oral
Transdermal estrogen system	100 mcg/24 h	Once or twice weekly	Transdermal
Progestogen Therapy			
Medroxyprogesterone acetate	10 mg	12–14 days[a]	Oral
Dydrogesterone[b]	20 mg	12–14 days[a]	Oral
Norethindrone acetate	10 mg	12–14 days[a]	Oral
Norethisterone[b]	1 mg	12–14 days[a]	Oral
Micronized progestrerone	200 mg	12–14 days[a]	Oral
Transdermal norethindrone[c]	250 mcg/24 h	Twice weekly for 14 days per calendar month	Transdermal

[a]Per calendar month.
[b]Not available in the United States in a progestogen-only oral dosage form.
[c]Available only in combination with estradiol.

EVALUATION OF THERAPEUTIC OUTCOMES

Young women with premature ovarian failure should be monitored annually for their response to treatment, and their compliance with hormone therapy should be assessed regularly. These patients also should be evaluated continuously for the presence of signs and symptoms of associated autoimmune endocrine disorders, such as hypothyroidism, adrenal insufficiency, and diabetes mellitus. Baseline bone mineral density testing should be performed in all women with premature ovarian failure. Mammography should be performed annually after the age of 40 years in accordance with accepted guidelines. Additional mammography screening in premenopausal women younger than age 40 years who are receiving physiologic hormone therapy is not warranted. Other tests should be performed as clinically indicated.

CONCLUSIONS

Approximately 1% of women spontaneously develop ovarian failure before the age of 40 years.[5] Premature ovarian failure is not an early natural menopause. Most affected women produce estrogen intermittently and may ovulate despite the presence of high gonadotropin concentrations. However, these women sustain sex steroid deficiency for more years than do naturally menopausal women, resulting in a significantly higher risk for osteoporosis[118] and cardiovascular disease.[119]

Women with premature ovarian failure need exogenous sex steroids to compensate for the decreased production by their ovaries. Thus premenopausal hormone therapy is required at least until these women reach the age of "natural menopause."

The goal of therapy is to provide a hormone-replacement regimen that maintains sex steroid status as effectively as the normal, functioning ovary. This usually requires the administration of estrogen at a dose greater than the standard dose given to older women experiencing natural menopause.

Because women with premature ovarian failure can have spontaneous pregnancies, the hormone therapy should produce regular, predictable menstrual flow patterns. If these patients miss an expected menses, they should be tested for pregnancy and promptly discontinue the hormone treatment.

Annual follow-up should include assessment of hormone therapy compliance and evaluation for signs and symptoms of associated endocrine disorders.[117]

ABBREVIATIONS

CEE: conjugated equine estrogens
CORE: Continuing Outcomes Relevant to Evista
ERA: Estrogen Replacement in Atherosclerosis Trial
ESPRIT: Estrogen in the Prevention of Re-infarction Trial
FSH: follicle-stimulating hormone
GnRH: gonadotropin-releasing hormone
HERS: Heart and Estrogen/Progestin Replacement Study
LH: luteinizing hormone
MORE: Multiple Outcomes of Raloxifene Evaluation
NETA: norethindrone acetate
POF: premature ovarian failure
SERM: selective estrogen-receptor modulator
WEST: Women's Estrogen for Stroke Trial
WHI: Women's Health Initiative

Review Questions and other resources can be found at *www.pharmacotherapyonline.com.*

REFERENCES

1. Richardson SJ, Senikas JF, Nelson JF. Follicular depletion during the menopausal transition: Evidence for accelerated loss and ultimate exhaustion. J Clin Endocrinol Metab 1987;65:1231–1237.
2. Writing Group for the Women's Health Initiative Investigators. Risks and benefits of estrogen plus progestin in healthy postmenopausal women: Principal results from the Women's Health Initiative randomized controlled trial. JAMA 2002;288:321–333.
3. Anderson GL, Limacher M, Assaf AR, et al. Effects of conjugated equine estrogen in postmenopausal women with hysterectomy: The Women's Health Initiative randomized controlled trial. JAMA. 2004; 291:1701–1712.
4. Coulam CB, Adamson SC, Annegers JF. Incidence of premature ovarian failure. Obstet Gynecol 1986;67:604–606.
5. Keating NL, Cleary PD, Rossi AS, et al. Use of hormone replacement therapy by postmenopausal women in the United States. Ann Intern Med 1999;130:545–553.
6. Stephenson J. FDA orders estrogen safety warnings: Agency offers guidance for HRT use. JAMA 2003;289:537–538.
6a. American College of Obstetricians and Gynecologists Women's Health

Care Physicians. Executive Summary. Hormone Therapy. Obstet Gynecol 2004;104 (4 Suppl):1–4.

7. Treloar AE, Boynton RE, Behn BG, Brown BW. Variation of the human menstrual cycle through reproductive life. Int J Fertil 1967;12:77–126.

8. Zumoff B, Strain GW, Miller LK, Rosner W. Twenty-four-hour mean plasma testosterone concentration declines with age in normal premenopausal women. J Clin Endocrinol Metab 1995;80:1429–1430.

9. Burger HG. The endocrinology of the menopause. J Steroid Biochem Mol Biol 1999;69:31–35.

10. Lee SJ, Lenton EA, Sexton L, Cooke ID. The effect of age on the cyclical patterns of plasma LH, FSH, oestradiol and progesterone in women with regular menstrual cycles. Hum Reprod 1988;3:851–855.

11. Ettinger B, Pressman A, Sklarin P, et al. Associations between low concentrations of serum estradiol, bone density, and fractures among elderly women: The study of osteoporotic fractures. J Clin Endocrinol Metab 1998;83:2239–2243.

12. Stone K, Bauer DC, Black DM, et al. Hormonal predictors of bone loss in elderly women: A prospective study. J Bone Miner Res 1998;13:1167–1174.

13. Cummings SR, Browner WS, Bauer D. Endogenous hormones and the risk of hip and vertebral fractures among older women. N Engl J Med 1998;339:733–738.

14. Cauley JA, Lucas FL, Kuller LH, et al. Elevated serum estradiol and testosterone concentrations are associated with a high risk for breast cancer. Ann Intern Med 1999;130:270–277.

15. Murkies AL, Wilcox G, Davis SR. Phytoestrogens: Clinical review. J Clin Endocrinol Metab 1998;83:297–303.

16. Yamamoto S, Sobue T, Kobayashi M, et al. for the Japan Public Health Center–Based Prospective Study on Cancer and Cardiovascular Diseases (JPHC) Study Group. Soy, isoflavones, and breast cancer risk in Japan. J Natl Cancer Inst 2003;95:906–913.

17. Tice JA, Ettinger B, Ensrud K, et al. Phytoestrogen supplements for the treatment of hot flashes: The isoflavone clover extract (ICE) study. A randomized, controlled trial. JAMA 2003;290:207–214.

18. Wroblewski-Lissin L, Cooke JP. Phytoestrogens and cardiovascular health. J Am Coll Cardiol 2000;35:1403–1410.

19. Albertazzi P, Pansini F, Bonaccorsi G, et al. The effect of dietary soy supplementation on hot flushes. Obstet Gynecol 1998;91:6–11.

20. Kronenberg F, Fugh-Berman A. Complementary and alternative medicine for menopausal symptoms: A review of randomized, controlled trials. Ann Intern Med 2002;137:805–813.

21. Beral V, Million Women Study Collaborators. Breast cancer and hormone-replacement therapy in the Million Women Study. Lancet 2003;362:419–427.

22. Sturdee DW. Newer HRT regimens. Br J Obstet Gynaecol 1997;104:1109–1115.

23. Lowe G, Upton M, Rumley A, et al. Different effects of oral and transdermal hormone replacement regimens on factor IX, APC-resistance, t-PA, PAI and C-reactive protein: A cross-sectional population survey. Thromb Haemost 2001;86:550–556.

24. Greendale GA, Lee NP, Arriola ER. The menopause. Lancet 1999;353:571–580.

25. Mattsson LA, Christiansen C, Colau J, et al. Clinical equivalence of intranasal and oral 17β-estradiol for postmenopausal symptoms. Am J Obstet Gynecol 2000;182:545–552.

26. Lindsay R, Hart DM, Clark DM. The minimum effective dose of estrogen for postmenopausal bone loss. Obstet Gynecol 1984;63:759–763.

27. Archer DF, Dorin M, Lewis V, et al. Effects of lower doses of conjugated equine estrogens and medroxyprogesterone acetate on endometrial bleeding. Fertil Steril 2001;75:1080–1087.

28. Lindsay R, Gallagher JC, Kleerekoper M, Pickar JH. Effect of lower doses of conjugated equine estrogens with and without medroxyprogesterone acetate on bone in early postmenopausal women. JAMA 2002;287:2668–2676.

29. Pickar JH, Wheeler JE, Cunnane MF, Speroff L. Endometrial effects of lower doses of conjugated equine estrogens and medroxyprogesterone acetate. Fertil Steril 2001;76:25–31.

30. Utian WH, Shoupe D, Bachmann G, et al. Relief of vasomotor symptoms and vaginal atrophy with lower doses of conjugated equine estrogens and medroxyprogesterone acetate. Fertil Steril 2001;75:1065–1079.

31. Naessen T, Rodriguez-Macias K, Lithell H. Serum lipid profile improved by unltra-low doses of 17β-estradiol in elderly women. J Clin Endocrinol Metab 2001;86:2757–2762.

32. Barrett-Connor E. Hormone-replacement therapy. Br Med J 1998;317:457–461.

33. Scarabin PY, Oger E, Genevieve PB, on behalf of the Estrogen and Thromboembolism Risk (ESTHER) Study Group. Differential association of oral and transdermal oestrogen-replacement therapy and venous thromboembolism risk. Lancet 2003;362:428–432.

34. Lethaby A, Farquhar C, Sarkis A, et al. Hormone-replacement therapy in postmenopausal women: Endometrial hyperplasia and irregular bleeding. Cochrane Database Syst Rev 2000;2:CD000402

35. Casper RF. Estrogen with interrupted progestin HRT: A review of experimental and clinical studies. Maturitas 2000;34:97–108.

36. The Writing Group for the Postmenopausal Estrogen/Progestin Interventions (PEPI) Trial. Effects of hormone-replacement therapy on endometrial histology in postmenopausal women. JAMA 1996;275:370–375.

37. Cushing KL, Weiss NS, Voight LF, et al. Risk of endometrial cancer in relation to use of low-dose, unopposed estrogens. Obstet Gynecol 1998;91:35–39.

38. North American Menopause Society. Role of progestogen in hormone therapy for postmenopausal women: Position statement of the North American Menopause Society. Menopause 2003;10:113–132.

39. Davis S. Androgen replacement in women: A commentary. J Clin Endocrinol Metab 1999;84:1886–1891.

40. Davis SR, McCloud P, Strauss BJG, Burger H. Testosterone enhances estradiol's effects on postmenopausal bone density and sexuality. Maturitas 1995;21:227–236.

41. Watts NB, Notelovitz T, Timmons MC, et al. Comparison of oral estrogens and estrogens plus androgens on bone mineral density, menopausal symptoms, and lipid-lipoprotein profiles in surgical menopause. Obstet Gynecol 1995;85:529–537.

42. Worboys S, Kotsopoulos D, Teede H, et al. Evidence that parenteral testosterone therapy may improve endothelium-dependent and -independent vasodilation in postmenopausal women already receiving estrogen. J Clin Endocrinol Metab 2001;86:158–161.

43. Shifren JL, Braunstein GD, Simon JA, et al. Transdermal testosterone treatment in women with impaired sexual function after oophorectomy. N Engl J Med 2000;343:682–688.

44. Kalantaridou SN, Calis KA, Godoy H, et al. Transdermal testosterone replacement for young women with spontaneous premature ovarian failure: A pilot study. Abstract No. 2322 from the Endocrine Society 82nd Annual Meeting, Toronto, Canada, June 21–24, 2000.

45. Burger HG. Selective oestrogen receptor modulators. Horm Res 2000;53(suppl 3):25–29.

46. Ettinger B, Black DM, Mitlak BH, et al. Reduction of vertebral fracture risk in postmenopausal women with osteoporosis treated with raloxifene: Results from a 3-year randomized clinical trial. Multiple Outcomes of Raloxifene Evaluation (MORE) investigators. JAMA 1999;282:637–645.

47. Walsh BW, Kuller LH, Wild RA, et al. Effects of raloxifene on serum lipids and coagulation factors in healthy postmenopausal women. JAMA 1998;279:1445–1451.

48. Cummings SR, Eckert S, Krueger KA, et al. The effect of raloxifene on risk of breast cancer in postmenopausal women: Results from the MORE randomized trial. JAMA 1999;281:2189–2197.

48a. Martino S, Cauley JA, Barrett-Connor E, et al. for the CORE Investigators. Continuing outcomes relevant to Evista: Breast cancer incidence in postmenopausal osteoporotic women in a randomized trial of raloxifene. J Natl Cancer Inst 2004;96:1751–1761.

49. Moore RA. Livial: A review of clinical studies. Br J Obstet Gynaecol 1999;106(suppl):1–21.

50. Gallagher JC, Baylink DJ, Freeman R, McClung M. Prevention of bone loss with tibolone in postmenopausal women: Results of two randomized, double-blind, placebo-controlled, doses finding studies. J Clin Endocrinol Metab 2001;869:4717–4726.

51. Winkler U, Altkemper R, Kwee B, et al. Effects of tibolone and continuous combined hormone-replacement therapy on parameters in the clotting cascades: A multicenter, double blind randomized study. Fertil Steril 2000;74:10–19.

52. American College of Obstetrics and Gynecology. Hormone-Replacement Therapy Technical Bulletin. No. 166. Washington, American College of Obstetrics and Gynecology, 1992.

53. McNagny SE. Prescribing hormone-replacement therapy for menopausal symptoms. Ann Intern Med 1999;131:605–616.

54. Porter M, Penney GC, Russell D, et al. A population based survey of women's experience of the menopause. Br J Obstet Gynaecol 2002;103:1025–1028.

55. MacLennan A, Lester S, Moore V. Oral estrogen replacement therapy versus placebo for hot flushes: A systematic review. Climacteric 2001;4:58–74

56. Loprinzi CL, Barton DL, Rhodes D. Management of hot flashes in breast-cancer survivors. Lancet Oncol 2001;2:199–204.

57. Stearns V, Beebe KL, Iyengar M, Dube E. Paroxetine controlled release in the treatment of menopausal hot flashes: A randomized, controlled trial. JAMA 2003;289:2827–2834.

58. Loprinzi CL, Sloan JA, Perez EA, et al. Phase III evaluation of fluoxetine for treatment of hot flashes. J Clin Oncol 2002;20:1578–1583.

59. Loprinzi CL, Kugler JW, Sloan JA, et al. Venlafaxine in management of hot flashes in survivors of breast cancer: A randomized, controlled trial. Lancet 2000;356:2059–2063.

60. Bachmann GA. A new option for managing urogenital atrophy in postmenopausal women. Cont Obstet Gynecol 1997;42:13–28.

61. Davis SR. Hormone-replacement therapy: Indications, benefits and risks. Aust Fam Phys 1999;28:437–445.

62. Grady D, Brown JS, Vittinghoff E, et al. Postmenopausal hormones and incontinence: The Heart and Estrogen/Progestin Replacement Study. Obstet Gynecol 2001;97:116–120.

63. Cauley JA, Robbins J, Chen Z, et al. Effects of estrogen plus progestin on risk of fracture and bone mineral density: The Women's Health Initiative Randomized Trial. JAMA 2003;290:1729–1738.

64. Wells G, Tugwell P, Shea B, et al. Meta-analysis of the efficacy of hormone replacement therapy in treating and preventing osteoporosis in postmenopausal women. Endocr Rev 2002;23:529–539.

65. North American Menopause Society. Management of postmenopausal osteoporosis: Position statement of the North American Menopause Society. Menopause 2002;9:84–101.

66. Greenspan SL, Maitland LA, Myers ER, et al. Femoral bone loss progresses with age: A longitudinal study in women over age 65. J Bone Miner Res 1994;9:1959–1965.

67. Lindsay R, Cosman F, Lobo RA, et al. Addition of alendronate to ongoing hormone replacement therapy in the treatment of osteoporosis: A randomized controlled clinical trial. J Clin Endocrinol Metab 1999;84:3076–3081.

68. North American Menopause Society. The role of calcium in peri- and postmenopausal women: Consensus opinion of the North American Menopause Society. Menopause 2001;8:84–95.

69. Espeland MA, Hogan PE, Fineberg SE, et al. for the PEPI investigators. Effect of postmenopausal hormone therapy on glucose and insulin concentrations. Diabetes Care 1998;21:1589–1595.

70. Kanaya AM, Herrington D, Vittinghoff E, et al. Glycemic effects of postmenopausal hormone therapy: The Heart and Estrogen/Progestin Replacement Study. A randomized, double-blind, placebo-controlled trial. Ann Intern Med 2003;138:1–9.

71. Norman RJ, Flight IH, Rees MC. Oestrogen and progestogen hormone replacement therapy for perimenopausal and post-menopausal women: Weight and body fat distribution. Cochrane Database Syst Rev 2000;CD001018.

72. Mosca L, Collins P, Herrington DM, et al. Hormone replacement therapy and cardiovascular disease: A statement for healthcare professionals from the American Heart Association. Circulation 2001;104:499–503.

73. Grodstein F, Manson JE, Colditz GA, et al. A prospective observational study of postmenopausal hormone therapy and primary prevention of cardiovascular disease. Ann Intern Med 2000;133:933–941.

74. The Writing Group for the Postmenopausal Estrogen/Progestin Interventions (PEPI) Trial. Effects of estrogen or estrogen/progestin regimens on heart disease risk factors in postmenopausal women. JAMA 1995;273:199–208.

75. Sack MN, Rader JR, Cannon RO. Oestrogen and inhibition of oxidation of low-density lipoproteins in postmenopausal women. Lancet 1994;343:269–270.

76. Koh KK, Jin DK, Yang SH, et al. Vascular effects of synthetic or natural progestogen combined with conjugated equine estrogen in healthy postmenopausal women. Circulation 2001;103:1961–1966.

77. Hulley S, Grady D, Bush T, et al. Randomized trial of estrogen plus progestin for secondary prevention of coronary heart disease in postmenopausal women. JAMA 1998;280:605–613.

78. Herrington DM, Reboussin DM, Brosnihan KB, et al. Effects of estrogen replacement on the progression of coronary artery atherosclerosis. N Engl J Med 2000;343:522–529.

79. Viscoli CM, Brass LM, Kernan WN, et al. A clinical trial of estrogen replacement therapy after ischemic stroke. N Engl J Med 2001;345:1243–1249.

80. Cherry N, Gilmour K, Hannaford P, et al. Oestrogen therapy for prevention of reinfarction in postmenopausal women: A randomized, placebo controlled trial. Lancet 2002;360:2001–2008.

81. Clarke SC, Kelleher J, Lloyd-Jones H, et al. A study of hormone replacement therapy in postmenopausal women with ischaemic heart disease: The Papworth HRT Atherosclerosis Study. Br J Obstet Gynaecol 2002;109:1056–1062.

82. Manson JE, Hsia J, Johnson KC, et al. Estrogen plus progestin and the risk of coronary heart disease. N Engl J Med 2003;349:523–534.

83. Wassertheil-Smoller S, Hendrix S, Limacher M, et al. Effect of estrogen plus progestin on stroke in postmenopausal women: The Women's Health Initiative. JAMA 2003;289:2673–2684.

84. Grady D, Herrington D, Bittner V, et al. Cardiovascular disease outcomes during 6.8 years of hormone therapy: Heart and Estrogen/Progestin Replacement Study follow-up (HERS II). JAMA 2002;288:49–57.

85. Barrett-Connor E, Grady D, Sashegyi A, et al. Raloxifene and cardiovascular events in osteoporotic postmenopausal women: Four-year results from the MORE (Multiple Outcomes of Raloxifene Evaluation) randomized trial. JAMA 2002;287:847–857.

86. Hu FB, Stampfer MJ, Manson JE, et al. Trends in the incidence of coronary heart disease and changes in diet and lifestyle in women. N Engl J Med 2000;343:530–537.

87. Stampfer MJ, Hu FB, Manson JE, et al. Primary prevention of coronary heart disease in women through diet and lifestyle. N Engl J Med 2000;343:16–22.

88. Chlebowski RT, Hendrix SL, Langer RD, et al. Influence of estrogen plus progestin on breast cancer and mammography in healthy postmenopausal women. The Women's Health Initiative Randomized Trial. JAMA 2003;289:3243–3253.

89. Swanson GM. Breast cancer risk estimation: A translational statistic for communication to the public. J Natl Cancer Inst 1993;85:848–849.

90. Collaborative Group on Hormonal Factors in Breast Cancer. Breast cancer and hormone replacement therapy: Collaborative reanalysis of data from epidemiological studies of 52,705 women with breast cancer and 108,411 women without breast cancer. Lancet 1997;350:1047–1059.

91. Schairer C, Lubin J, Troisi R, et al. Menopausal estrogen and estrogen-progestin replacement therapy and breast cancer risk. JAMA 2000;283:485–491.

92. Gapstur SM, Morrow M, Sellers TA. Hormone replacement therapy and risk of breast cancer with a favorable histology. JAMA 1999;281:2091–2097.

93. Sellers TA, Mink PJ, Cerhan JR, et al. The role of hormone replacement therapy in the risk of breast cancer and total mortality in women with a family history of breast cancer. Ann Intern Med 1997;127:973–980.

94. Greendale GA, Reboussin BA, Slone S, et al. Postmenopausal hormone therapy and change in mammographic density. J Natl Cancer Inst 2003;95:30–37.

95. Boyd NF, Byng JW, Jong RA, et al. Quantitative classification of mammographic densities and breast cancer risk: Results from the Canadian National Breast Cancer Screening Study. J Natl Cancer Inst 1995;87:670–675.

96. Freedman M, Martin JS, O'Gorman J, et al. Digitized mammography: A clinical trial of postmenopausal women randomly assigned to receive raloxifene, estrogen, or placebo. J Natl Cancer Inst 2001;93:51–56.

97. Anderson GL, Judd HL, Kaunitz AM, et al. Effects of estrogen plus progestin on gynecologic cancers and associated diagnostic procedures. The Women's Health Initiative randomized trial. JAMA 2003;290:1739–1748.

98. Pike MC, Peters RK, Cozen W, et al. Estrogen-progestin replacement therapy and endometrial cancer. J Natl Cancer Inst 1997;89:1110–1116.

99. Genant HK, Lucas J, Weiss S, et al. Low-dose esterified estrogen therapy: Effects on bone, plasma estradiol concentrations, endometrium, and lipid concentrations. Estratab/Osteoporosis Study Group. Arch Intern Med 1997;157:2609–2615.

100. Goldstein SR, Scheele WH, Rajagopalan SK, et al. A 12-month comparative study of raloxifene, estrogen, and placebo on the postmenopausal endometrium. Obstet Gynecol 2000;95:95–103.

101. Lacey JV, Mink PJ, Lubin JH, et al. Menopausal hormone replacement therapy and risk of ovarian cancer. JAMA 2002;288:3343–3341.

102. Jick H, Derby LE, Myers MW, et al. Risk of hospital admission for idiopathic venous thromboembolism among users of postmenopausal oestrogens. Lancet 1996;348:981–983.

103. Nelson HD, Humphrey LL, Nygren P, et al. Postmenopausal hormone replacement therapy: Scientific review. JAMA 2002;288:872–881.

104. Grodstein F, Colditz GA, Stampfer MJ. Postmenopausal hormone use and cholecystectomy in a large prospective study. Obstet Gynecol 1994;83:5–11.

105. Schmidt PJ, Nieman L, Danaceau MA, et al. Estrogen replacement in perimenopause-related depression: A preliminary report. Am J Obstet Gynecol 2000;183:414–420.

106. LeBlanc ES, Janowsky J, Chan BKS, Nelson HD. Hormone replacement therapy and cognition: Systematic review and meta-analysis. JAMA 2001;285:1489–1499.

107. Hlatky MA, Boothroyd D, Vittnghoff E, et al. for the HERS research group. Quality of life and depressive symptoms in postmenopausal women after receiving hormone therapy: Results from the Heart and Estrogen/Progestin Replacement Study (HERS) Trial. JAMA 2002;287:591–597.

108. Hays J, Ockene JK, Brunner RL, et al. Effects of estrogen plus progestin on health-related quality of life. N Engl J Med 2003;348:1839–1854.

109. Shumaker SA, Legault C, Rapp SR, et al. Estrogen plus progestin and the incidence of dementia and mild cognitive impairment in postmenopausal women. The Women's Health Initiative Memory Study: A randomized, controlled trial. JAMA 2003;289:2651–2662.

110. Rapp SR, Espeland MA, Shumaker SA, et al. Effect of estrogen plus progestin on global cognitive function in postmenopausal women. The Women's Health Initiative Memory Study: A randomized, controlled trial. JAMA 2003;289:2663–2672.

110a. Espeland MA, Rapp SR, Shumaker SA, et al. Conjugated equine estrogens and global cognitive function in postmenopausal women: Women's Health Initiative Memory Study. JAMA 2004;291:2959–2968.

110b. Shumaker SA, Legault C, Kuller L, et al. Conjugated equine estrogens and incidence of probable dementia and mild cognitive impairment in postmenopausal women: Women's Health Initiative Memory Study. JAMA 2004;291:2947–2958.

111. Saletu B, Brandstatter N, Metka M, et al. Double-blind, placebo-controlled, hormonal, syndromal and EEG mapping studies with transdermal estradiol therapy in menopausal depression. Psychopharmacology 1995;122:321–329.

112. Ott A, Breteler MM, Van Harskamp F, et al. Incidence and risk of dementia: The Rotterdam Study. Am J Epidemiol 1998;147:574–580.

113. Yaffe K, Krueger K, Sarkar S, et al. Cognitive function in postmenopausal women treated with raloxifene. N Engl J Med 2001;344:1207–1213.

114. Grady D. A 60-year-old woman trying to discontinue hormone replacement therapy. JAMA 2002;287:2130–2137.

115. Ettinger B, Pressman A. Continuation of postmenopausal hormone replacement therapy in a large health maintenance organization: Transdermal matrix versus oral estrogen therapy. Am J Manag Care 1999;7:779–785.

115a. Majumdar SR, Almasi EA, Stafford RS. Promotion and prescribing of hormone therapy after report of harm by the Women's Health Initiative. JAMA 2004;292:1983–1988.

116. Torgerson DJ, Reid DM. The pharmacoeconomics of hormone replacement therapy. Pharmacoeconomics 1999;16:9–16.

117. Kalantaridou SN, Davis SR, Nelson LM. Premature ovarian failure. Endocrinol Metab Clin North Am 1998;27:989–1006.

118. Anasti JN, Kalantaridou SN, Kimzey LM, et al. Bone loss in young women with karyotypically normal spontaneous premature ovarian failure. Obstet Gynecol 1998;91:12–15.

119. Van Der Schouw YT, Van Der Graaf Y, Steyerberg EW, et al. Age at menopause as a risk for cardiovascular mortality. Lancet 1996;347:714–717.

119a. Kalantaridou SN, Naka KK, Papanikolaou E, et al. Impaired endothelial function in young women with premature ovarian failure: Normalization with hormone therapy. J Clin Endocrinol Metab 2004;89:3907–3913.

120. Snowdon DA, Kane RL, Beeson WL, et al. Is early natural menopause a biologic marker of health and aging? Am J Public Health 1989;79:709–714.

121. Davis SR. Premature ovarian failure. Maturitas 1996;28:1–8.

81

ERECTILE DYSFUNCTION

Mary Lee

Learning Objectives and other resources can be found at *www.pharmacotherapyonline.com*.

KEY CONCEPTS

◀1 The incidence of erectile dysfunction is low in men less than 40 years of age. It increases as men age, likely as a result of concurrent medical conditions that impair the vascular, neurologic, psychogenic, and hormonal systems necessary for a normal penile erection.

◀2 Many commonly used drugs have sympatholytic, anticholinergic, sedative, or antiandrogenic effects that may exacerbate or contribute to the development of erectile dysfunction. Clinicians should be familiar with these agents and be prepared to make adjustments in drug regimens to minimize adverse effects of these drugs on a patient's erectile function.

◀3 Specific treatments for erectile dysfunction include medical devices, pharmacologic treatments, psychotherapy, and surgery.

◀4 The ideal treatment for erectile dysfunction should have a fast onset, be effective, be convenient to administer, be cost-effective, have a low incidence of serious adverse effects, and be free of serious drug interactions. Currently, no ideal treatment for erectile dysfunction exists.

◀5 Specific treatment is first initiated with least invasive forms of treatment, including vacuum erection devices and oral phosphodiesterase inhibitors, followed by intracavernosal injections or intraurethral inserts, and finally by surgical insertion of a penile prosthesis.

◀6 Vacuum erection devices have a slow onset of action (30 minutes) and therefore are most effective in elderly couples in a stable relationship.

◀7 Although phosphodiesterase inhibitors are convenient and effective regardless of the etiology of erectile dysfunction, they fail in 30% to 40% of patients. Also, phosphodiesterase inhibitors are contraindicated in patients taking any form of nitrate, including topical nitrates.

◀8 Testosterone supplementation can improve erectile function in patients who have decreased libido secondary to primary or secondary hypogonadism. Testosterone supplementation should not be used in patients with erectile dysfunction who have normal serum testosterone levels.

◀9 Although intracavernosal alprostadil injections are effective independent of the etiology for erectile dysfunction, these fail in one-third of patients. Also, they should be used cautiously in patients at risk of priapism, which includes those with sickle cell disease or lymphoproliferative disorders.

The National Institutes of Health Consensus Development Panel on Impotence defines erectile dysfunction as the failure to achieve a penile erection suitable for sexual intercourse.[1] Patients may refer to it as impotence.

Erectile dysfunction must be distinguished from disorders of libido, ejaculatory disorders, or infertility, which are caused by different pathophysiologic mechanisms and are treated with alternative agents (Table 81–1). A patient may suffer from one or more disorders of sexual dysfunction. For example, an elderly man with primary hypogonadism may suffer from decreased libido and erectile dysfunction. Diagnosis of the type of sexual disorder that a patient has is a key to initiating the most appropriate treatment.

EPIDEMIOLOGY

◀1 The incidence of erectile dysfunction is low in men younger than 40 years of age, but it increases as men age.[2-4] The Massachusetts Male Aging Study, a cross-sectional survey of a random sample of 1290 men in the Boston area, was conducted during the period from 1987 to 1989. It reported an overall prevalence of 52% for any degree of erectile dysfunction in men aged 40 to 70 years, with a 40% prevalence in men aged 40 years, and a 67% prevalence in men aged 70 years.[1,2] In the most recent Health Professional Follow-Up Study of more than 31,000 male health professionals aged 53 to 90 years, the prevalence of erectile dysfunction was 33%.[3]

TABLE 81–1. Types of Sexual Dysfunction in Men

Type of Dysfunction	Definition
Decreased libido	Decreased sexual drive or desire
Increased libido	Precocious puberty. Inappropriate and excessive sexual drive or desire
Erectile dysfunction (impotence)	Failure to achieve a penile erection suitable for sexual intercourse
Delayed ejaculation	Commonly referred to as "dry sex"; ejaculation is delayed or absent
Retrograde ejaculation	Ejaculate passes retrograde into the bladder, instead of toward the anterior urethra (antegrade) and out of the penis
Infertility	Sperm are insufficient in number or have inadequate motility and fail to fertilize the ovum

Although erectile dysfunction is sometimes assumed to be a symptom of the aging process in men, it is unclear if the incidence is directly related to increasing patient age. Erectile dysfunction more likely results from concurrent medical conditions of the patient (e.g., hypertension, arteriosclerosis, hyperlipidemia, diabetes mellitus, or psychiatric disorders) or from medications that patients may be taking for these diseases.[2–5] For example, up to 50% of patients with diabetes mellitus develop erectile dysfunction, and medications such as β-blockers are associated with a high incidence of erectile dysfunction.

PHYSIOLOGY OF A NORMAL PENILE ERECTION

A normal penile erection requires the full functioning of several physiologic systems: vascular, nervous, and hormonal. The patient must also be psychologically receptive to sexual stimuli.

VASCULAR SYSTEM

The penis comprises two corpora cavernosa on the dorsal side and one corpus spongiosum on the ventral side. The corpus spongiosum surrounds the urethra and forms the glans penis. The corpora are composed of multiple interconnected sinuses, which can fill with blood to produce an erection. The corpora are encased by the tunica albuginea, a fibrous tissue membrane, which has limited distensibility. In the flaccid state, arterial flow into and venous outflow from the corpora are balanced. During the erectile phase, arterial blood flow increases and blood fills the sinusoids within the corpora, which causes penile swelling and elongation. The erection is prolonged by a decrease in venous outflow from the corpora, which is caused by compression of subtunical venules by the swollen corpora (Fig. 81–1).

Arterial flow into the corpora is enhanced by acetylcholine mediated vasodilation. Acetylcholine does not directly enhance arterial flow to the corpora or increase sinusoidal filling of the corpora tissue. Rather, acetylcholine is a co-neurotransmitter, which works along with other nonpeptidinergic intracellular neurotransmitters—including cyclic guanosine monophosphate (cGMP), cyclic adenosine monophosphate (cAMP), or vasoactive intestinal polypeptide—to produce vasodilation.

Acetylcholine probably works through two different pathways to produce an erection. In the presence of sexual stimulation to genital tissue, acetylcholine through one pathway enhances the production

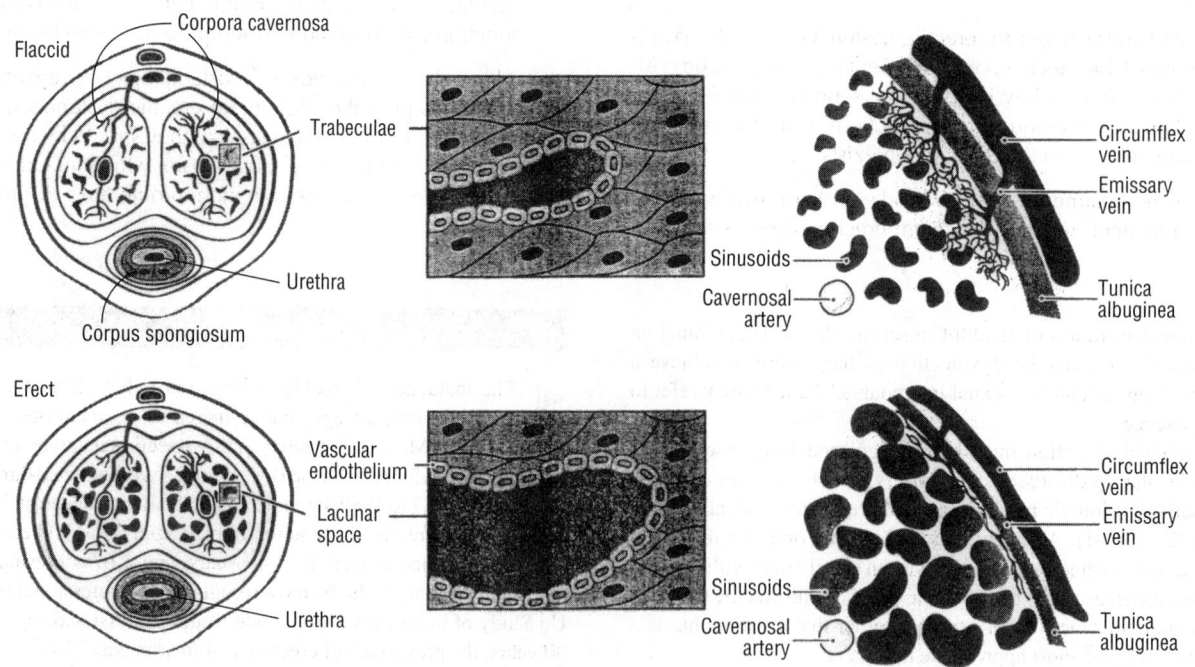

FIGURE 81–1. Microanatomy of and vascular changes in the penis in flaccid and erect states. In the flaccid state, arterial flow into and venous outflow from the corpora are balanced. During the erectile phase, arterial blood flow increases and blood fills the sinusoids within the corpora, which causes penile swelling and elongation. The erection is prolonged by a decrease in venous outflow from the corpora, which is caused by compression of subtunical venules by the swollen corpora. (*Adapted from Korenman.*[22])

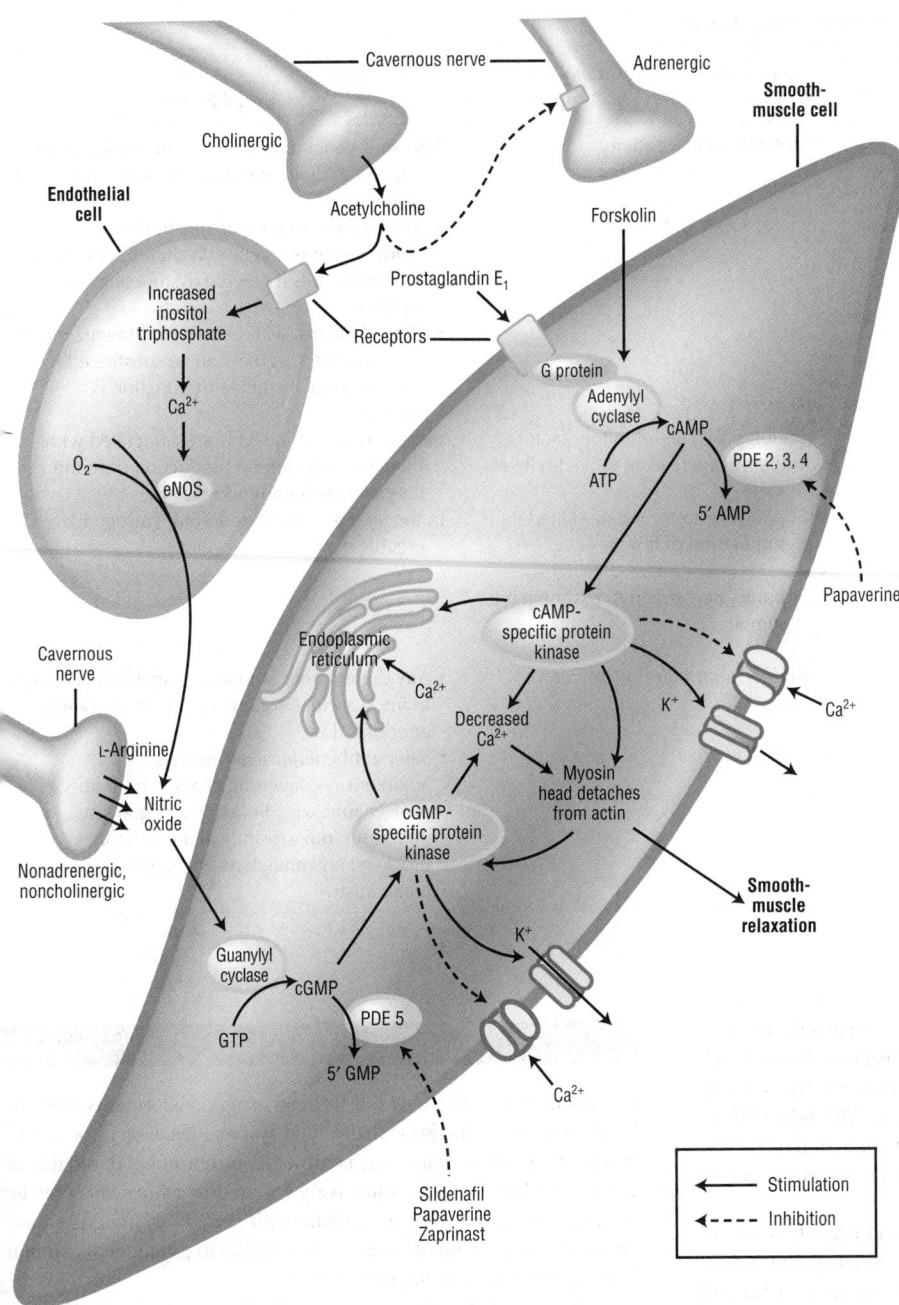

FIGURE 81–2. Molecular mechanism of penile smooth muscle relaxation. cAMP and cGMP, the intracellular second messengers mediating smooth-muscle relaxation, activate their specific protein kinases, which phosphorylate certain proteins to cause opening of potassium channels, closing of calcium channels, and sequestration of intracellular calcium by the endoplasmic reticulum. The resultant fall in intracellular calcium leads to smooth muscle relaxation. Sildenafil inhibits the action of phosphodiesterase (PDE) type 5, thus increasing the intracellular concentration of cGMP. Papaverine is a nonspecific inhibitor. GTP, guanosine triphosphate; eNOS, endothelial nitric oxide synthetase. (*Adapted with permission from Lue.*[6])

of nitric oxide by endothelial cells and nonadrenergic-noncholinergic neurons. Nitric oxide enhances the activity of guanylate cyclase, which increases the conversion of cyclic guanosine triphosphate to cGMP. cGMP decreases intracellular calcium concentrations in smooth-muscle cells of penile arteries and cavernosal sinuses. As a result, smooth-muscle relaxation occurs, which enhances arterial blood flow to and blood filling of the corpora.[5] An erection results (Fig. 81–2).

In an alternative pathway, acetylcholine stimulates a smooth-muscle cell-membrane receptor to enhance the activity of adenyl cyclase. Adenyl cyclase increases the conversion of cyclic adenosine triphosphate to cAMP, a potent muscle relaxant. Similarly to cGMP, cAMP decreases intracellular calcium concentrations to produce smooth-muscle relaxation in cells of the arteries and cavernosal sinuses. Arterial blood flow to and blood filling of the corpora are enhanced, and a penile erection results (see Fig. 81–2).[6]

NERVOUS SYSTEM AND PSYCHOGENIC STIMULI

Some erections are mediated by a sacral nerve reflex arc (e.g., erections can occur while the patient is sleeping). However, in the conscious patient, sensory sexual stimulation mediates erections via the central nervous system. That is, when a patient sees an attractive partner, hears sweet words, smells a particular scent, or tastes or touches a pleasant object, this can result in an erection. In this case, the patient's brain processes this information and the nervous impulse is carried down the spinal cord to peripheral cholinergic nerves that innervate the vascular supply to the corpora, resulting in an erection.

The medial preoptic area of the hypothalamus is thought to be that portion of the brain responsible for integrating external stimuli. Here dopamine exerts a proerectogenic effect, whereas, α_2-adrenergic stimulation causes the penis to become and/or remain flaccid. After moving down the spinal cord, nerve impulses travel to the penis by efferent peripheral nerves, including inhibitory sympathetic

TABLE 81–2. Medication Classes That Can Cause Erectile Dysfunction[7]

Drug Class	Proposed Mechanism by Which Drug Causes Erectile Dysfunction	Special Notes
Anticholinergic agents: antihistamines, antiparkinsonian agents, tricyclic antidepressants, phenothiazines	Anticholinergic activity	• Second-generation nonsedating antihistamines (e.g., loratadine) are not associated with erectile dysfunction. • Selective serotonin reuptake inhibitor antidepressants can be substituted for tricyclic antidepressants if erectile dysfunction is a problem. • Phenothiazines with less anticholinergic effect (e.g., chlorpromazine) can be substituted in some patients if erectile dysfunction is a problem.
Dopamine agonists (e.g., metoclopramide, phenothiazines)	Inhibit prolactin inhibitory factor, thereby increasing prolactin levels	Increased prolactin levels are associated with blocking testosterone production from the testes. Depressed libido results.
Estrogens, antiandrogens (e.g., luteinizing hormone–releasing hormone superagonists, digoxin, spironolactone, ketoconazole, cimetidine)	Suppress testosterone-mediated stimulation of libido	In the face of a decreased libido, a secondary erectile dysfunction develops.
Central nervous system depressants (e.g., barbiturates, narcotics, benzodiazepines, short-term use of large doses of alcohol)	Suppress perception of psychogenic stimuli	
Agents that decrease penile blood flow (e.g., diuretics, peripheral β-adrenergic antagonists, or central sympatholytics (methyldopa, clonidine, guanethidine)	Reduce arteriolar flow to corpora	• Any diuretic that produces a significant decrease in intravascular volume can decrease penile arteriolar flow. • Safer antihypertensives include angiotensin-converting enzyme inhibitors, postsynaptic α_1-adrenergic antagonists (terazosin, doxazosin), calcium-channel blockers, and angiotensin II receptor antagonists.

neurons (T_{11} through L_2), proerectogenic parasympathetic neurons (S_2 through S_4), and proerectogenic somatic neurons (S_2 through S_4).

In summary, acetylcholine produces an erection by working along with other co-neurotransmitters, including cGMP and cAMP, as described earlier. Thus an erection is initiated by the action of nerves, maintained by arterial blood filling of the corpora, and sustained by occlusion of venous outflow from the corpora.

Detumescence, or the progression of an erect penis to a flaccid state, results from the actions of norepinephrine, which contracts vascular smooth muscle to decrease arterial inflow to the corpora and contracts sinusoidal tissue in the corpora. As a result, venous outflow from the corpora increases.

HORMONAL SYSTEM

Testosterone stimulates libido or sexual drive in males. Within the normal physiologic serum concentration range (normal, 300 to 1100 ng/dL), sexual drive is normal. Approximately one-third of men older than 50 years of age have hypogonadism, which is characterized by subphysiologic serum testosterone levels. Such patients complain of loss of energy, loss of muscle strength, depressive mood, and decreased libido.

When libido is decreased, a patient may not develop erections. The relationship between erectile dysfunction and serum testosterone levels is a complicated one. Patients with normal serum testosterone levels may have erectile dysfunction, and patients with subnormal serum testosterone levels may have normal sexual function.[7]

PATHOPHYSIOLOGY

Erectile dysfunction can result from any single abnormality or combination of abnormalities of the four systems necessary for a normal penile erection. Vascular, neurologic, or hormonal etiologies of erectile dysfunction are collectively referred to as *organic erectile dysfunction*. About 80% of patients with erectile dysfunction have the organic type. Patients who fail to respond to psychogenic stimuli have *psychogenic erectile dysfunction*.

Diseases that compromise vascular flow to the corpora cavernosum (e.g., peripheral vascular disease, arteriosclerosis, and essential hypertension) are associated with an increased incidence of erectile dysfunction. Diseases that impair nerve conduction to the brain (e.g., spinal cord injury or stroke) or conditions that impair peripheral nerve conduction to the penile vasculature (e.g., diabetes mellitus) can result in erectile dysfunction.

Diseases associated with hypogonadism, primary or secondary, result in subphysiologic levels of testosterone, which cause diminished sexual drive (decreased libido) and secondary erectile dysfunction. Primary hypogonadism can be associated with the normal aging process in men or surgical removal of the testes for the treatment of prostate or testicular cancer. Secondary hypogonadism may result from hypothalamic or pituitary disorders of luteinizing hormone–releasing hormone or luteinizing hormone, respectively; or elevated prolactin levels, which can result from pituitary tumors or can occur in patients with chronic renal failure.

Questions	Response options
1. How often were you able to get an erection during sexual activity? 2. When you had erections with sexual stimulation, how often were your erections hard enough for penetration?	0 = No sexual activity 1 = Almost never/never 2 = A few times (much less than half the time) 3 = Sometimes (about half the time) 4 = Most times (much more than half the time) 5 = Almost always/always
3. When you attempted sexual intercourse, how often were you able to penetrate (enter) your partner? 4. During sexual intercourse, how often were you able to maintain your erection after you had penetrated (entered) your partner?	0 = Did not attempt intercourse 1 = Almost never/never 2 = A few times (much less than half the time) 3 = Sometimes (about half the time) 4 = Most times (much more than half the time) 5 = Almost always/always
5. During sexual intercourse, how difficult was it to maintain your erection to completion of intercourse?	0 = Did not attempt intercourse 1 = Extremely difficult 2 = Very difficult 3 = Difficult 4 = Slightly difficult 5 = Not difficult
6. How many times have you attempted sexual intercourse?	0 = No attempts 1 = One to two attempts 2 = Three to four attempts 3 = Five to six attempts 4 = Seven to ten attempts 5 = Eleven plus attempts
7. When you attempted sexual intercourse, how often was it satisfactory for you?	0 = Did not attempt intercourse 1 = Almost never/never 2 = A few times (much less than half the time) 3 = Sometimes (about half the time) 4 = Most times (much more than half the time) 5 = Almost always/always
8. How much have you enjoyed sexual intercourse?	0 = No intercourse 1 = No enjoyment 2 = Not very enjoyable 3 = Fairly enjoyable 4 = Highly enjoyable 5 = Very highly enjoyable
9. When you had sexual stimulation or intercourse, how often did you ejaculate? 10. When you had sexual stimulation or intercourse, how often did you have the feeling of orgasm or climax?	0 = No sexual stimulation/intercourse 1 = Almost never/never 2 = A few times (much less than half the time) 3 = Sometimes (about half the time) 4 = Most times (much more than half the time) 5 = Almost always/always
11. How often have you felt sexual desire?	1 = Almost never/ never 2 = A few times (much less than half the time) 3 = Sometimes (about half the time) 4 = Most times (much more than half the time) 5 = Almost always/always
12. How would you rate your level of sexual desire?	1 = Very low/none at all 2 = Low 3 = Moderate 4 = High 5 = Very high
13. How satisfied have you been with your overall sex life? 14. How satisfied have you been with your sexual relationship with your partner?	1 = Very dissatisfied 2 = Moderately dissatisfied 3 = About equally satisfied and dissatisfied 4 = Moderately satisfied 5 = Very satisfied
15. How do you rate your confidence that you can get and keep an erection?	1 = Very low 2 = Low 3 = Moderate 4 = High 5 = Very high

FIGURE 81–3. International Index of Erectile Function Questionnaire. All questions are preceded by the phrase, "Over the past 4 weeks." (*Reprinted with permission from Kirby R, Carson C, Goldstein I. Erectile Dysfunction, A Clinical Guide. Oxford, England, ISIS Medical Media, 1999:30–31.*)

Finally, patients must be in the proper mental frame of mind to be receptive to sexual stimuli. Patients who suffer from malaise, have reactive depression or performance anxiety, are sedated, have Alzheimer's disease, have hypothyroidism, or have mental disorders, commonly complain of erectile dysfunction. In most studies, patients with psychogenic erectile dysfunction generally exhibit a higher response rate to various interventions than do patients with organic erectile dysfunction, as their disease is often less severe.

Social habits of patients have also been linked to erectile dysfunction. The vasoconstrictor effect of cigarette smoking may compromise blood flow to the corpora and decrease cavernosal filling. Excessive ethanol intake may lead to androgen deficiency, peripheral neuropathy, or chronic liver disease, all of which can contribute to erectile dysfunction.

❷ Medications may cause erectile dysfunction through similar pathophysiologic mechanisms (Table 81–2).[8–13] Medications are estimated to be responsible for approximately 10% to 25% of cases of erectile dysfunction. An excellent review of medication-induced erectile dysfunction is available.[8]

CLINICAL PRESENTATION: ERECTILE DYSFUNCTION

Affects men emotionally in many different ways (e.g., depression, performance anxiety, or embarrassment).

Marital difficulties and avoidance of sexual intimacy; patients are often brought to a physician by their mates.

Nonadherence to medications patient believes are causing erectile dysfunction may be a problem.

DIAGNOSIS

With the availability in the late 1990s of effective medications for erectile dysfunction independent of the etiology, diagnostic evaluation of erectile dysfunction became streamlined.[14,15] Key assessments include a description of the severity of the erectile dysfunction, a medical history, a review of concurrent medications, a physical examination, and selected clinical laboratory tests.[16]

To assess the severity of the erectile dysfunction, the patient should be asked about onset and frequency. A standardized questionnaire, such as the International Index of Erectile Dysfunction, is often used. It includes 15 questions about the quality of erectile function and sexual intercourse (Fig. 81–3).[17] The physician should carefully assess the patient's expectations and motivations for erectile function to ensure that they are reasonable.

A medical history should be obtained to identify concurrent medical illnesses that are risk factors for organic or psychogenic erectile dysfunction. If these underlying diseases are not optimally responding to treatment, this should be addressed before specific treatment for erectile dysfunction is initiated. Also, if the patient smokes cigarettes, drinks excessive amounts of ethanol, or uses recreational drugs, these social habits should be discontinued before specific treatment for erectile dysfunction is started.

A complete listing of the patient's prescription and over-the-counter medications should be reviewed by the clinician, who should identify drugs that may be contributing to erectile dysfunction. If possible, causative agents should be discontinued or the dose should be reduced.

A physical examination of the patient should include a check for hypogonadism (i.e., signs of gynecomastia, small testicles, and decreased body hair). The penis should also be evaluated for diseases associated with penile curvature (e.g., Peyronie's disease), which are also associated with erectile dysfunction. Femoral and lower extremity pulses should be assessed to provide an indication of vascular supply to the genitals. Anal sphincter tone and other genital reflexes should be checked to provide an indication of the integrity of the nerve supply to the penis.

Selected laboratory tests should be obtained to identify the presence of underlying diseases that could cause erectile dysfunction. These include a serum blood glucose, lipid profile, and thyroxine level. Serum testosterone levels should be checked in patients older than 50 years of age and in younger patients who complain of decreased sexual drive. Serum testosterone levels follow a circadian pattern of secretion, with the highest levels occurring during the morning hours. To interpret serum testosterone levels properly, serum samples should be obtained in the mornings. At least two serial serum testosterone levels are needed to confirm the presence of hypogonadism.[18]

▶ TREATMENT: Erectile Dysfunction

▦ MANAGEMENT OPTIONS

❸ The goal of treatment is an improvement in the quantity and quality of penile erections suitable for intercourse. Simple as this may sound, health care providers need to ensure that patients have reasonable expectations for any therapies that are initiated. Furthermore, only patients with erectile dysfunction should be treated. Patients who have normal sexual function should not seek—or be encouraged to seek—treatment in an effort to enhance sexual function or enable increased activity.

▦ GENERAL APPROACH TO TREATMENT

The first step in clinical management of erectile dysfunction is to identify, and if possible to reverse, underlying causes. Risk factors for erectile dysfunction, including hypertension, diabetes mellitus, smoking, or chronic ethanol abuse, should be addressed and mini-

mized. Patients should have heart-healthy lifestyles, which includes physical fitness, weight loss to achieve a normal body mass index, low-cholesterol diets, and no smoking. In some cases, these types of interventions are sufficient to restore erectile function. However, if erectile dysfunction fails to respond to these measures, specific treatment is indicated.

For patients with psychogenic erectile dysfunction, psychotherapy may be used as monotherapy, or as an adjunct to specific treatments for the disorder. To enhance the relevance of psychotherapy, both the patient and his partner should be included in the counseling sessions. Also, treatment should be individualized and should address those immediate factors that may be causing performance anxiety or depression, rather than the remote, deep-seated reasons for psychological disorders.[19] The effectiveness of psychotherapy is generally low, and long-term psychotherapy is often necessary.

❹❺ Specific treatments for erectile dysfunction include medical devices, pharmacologic treatments, and surgery. The ideal treatment for this disorder should have a fast onset, be effective, be convenient to administer, be cost-effective, have a low incidence of serious adverse effects, and be free of serious drug interactions

TABLE 81–3. Dosing Regimens for Selected Drug Treatments for Erectile Dysfunction

Route of Administration	Generic Name (Brand Name)	Dosage Form	Common Dosing Regimen
Oral	Yohimbine (Aphrodyne, Yocon, Yohimex)	5.4-mg tablet or capsule	5.4 mg three times a day
	Sildenafil (Viagra)	25-mg, 50-mg, 100-mg tablets	25–100 mg 1 hour before intercourse
	Apomorphine (Uprima)[a]	Sublingual tablets	
	Methyltestosterone (Oreton, Android)	10-mg, 25-mg tablets and capsules	10–40 mg daily
	Fluoxymesterone (Halotestin)	2-mg, 5-mg, 10-mg tablets	5–20 mg daily
	Trazodone (Desyrel)[b]	50-mg, 100-mg, 150-mg, 300-mg tablet	50–150 mg daily
	Phentolamine (Spontane, Vasomax)[a]	Oral or buccal tablets	
	Vardenafil (Levitra)	2.5-mg, 5-mg, 10-mg, 20-mg tablets	5–10 mg 1 hour before intercourse
	Tadalafil (Cialis)	5-mg, 10-mg, 20-mg tablets	5–20 mg prior to intercourse
Topical	Testosterone patch (Testoderm)	4 mg/patch, 6 mg/patch	4–6 mg/day; apply to scrotum
	Testosterone patch (Testoderm TTS)	4 mg/patch, 6 mg/patch	4–6 mg/day; apply to arm, buttock, back
	Testosterone patch (Androderm)	2.5 mg/patch	2.5–5 mg/day; apply to arm, back, abdomen, thigh
	Testosterone gel (AndroGel 1%)	5 g/pkt, 10 g/pkt	5–10 g/day; apply to shoulders, upper arms, abdomen
Intramuscular	Testosterone cypionate (Depo-Testosterone)	100 mg/mL, 200 mg/mL	200–400 mg every 2 to 4 weeks
	Testosterone enanthate (Delatestryl)	100 mg/mL, 200 mg/mL	200–400 mg every 2 to 4 weeks
	Testosterone propionate	100 mg/mL	25–50 mg two to three times a week
Intraurethral	Alprostadil (MUSE)	125-mcg, 250-mcg, 500-mcg, 1000-mcg pellets	125–1000 mcg 5 to 10 minutes before intercourse
Intracavernosal	Alprostadil (Caverject)	5 mcg, 10 mcg, 20 mcg injection	2.5–60 mcg 5 to 10 minutes before intercourse
	Alprostadil (Edex)	5 mcg, 20 mcg, 20 mcg, 40 mcg injection	2.5–60 mcg 5 to 10 minutes before intercourse
	Papaverine[b]	30 mg/mL injection	Variable, usually used in combination
	Phentolamine[b]	2.5 mg/mL injection	Variable, usually used in combination

[a]Not yet commercially available in the United States at the time this chapter was written.
[b]Not FDA-approved for this use.

Currently no treatment for erectile dysfunction is ideal (Table 81–3). Generally, when choosing among treatment approaches, those that are least invasive are chosen first, while more invasive therapies are reserved for patients who fail to respond to first-line agents. A sample algorithm that guides selection of treatment is shown in Fig. 81–4.

■ VACUUM ERECTION DEVICES

A vacuum erection device (VED) has three parts: a pump to generate a negative vacuum pressure; a cylinder, which is closed at one end and into which the penis is inserted; and tubing to connect the pump to the cylinder. The patient inserts his penis into the cylinder, which is then pushed up flush against his lower abdomen to create a vacuum chamber. Then the patient activates the pump to produce vacuum pressure, which draws arteriolar blood into the corpora cavernosa. To prolong the erection, the patient may also use constriction bands or tension rings, which are placed at the base of the penis, to keep the arteriolar blood in and to reduce venous outflow from the penis. With the assistance of loading cones to protect the glans, these bands or rings can be rolled over the glans penis and up the shaft. Alternatively, they can be first threaded onto the plastic cylinder before the penis is inserted. Once the penis is erect, the band or ring can be rolled off the cylinder onto the base of the penis (Fig. 81–5).

The VED's onset of action is comparatively slow (30 minutes), which requires patience from both the patient and his sexual partner. For this reason, VEDs appear to work best in older patients who are married or have stable sexual relationships. In this group, VEDs are considered first-line therapy, and the overall satisfaction rate is 60% to 80%.[20–22] However, 6% to 11% of patients' partners complain that the penis is cool to the touch or is discolored (bluish) in appearance.

VEDs may also be used as second-line therapy in patients who fail oral or injectable drug treatments for erectile dysfunction. The combination of VED with intracavernosal[23] or intraurethral[24] alprostadil is associated with a higher rate of efficacy than use of the VED alone. As a result, combination therapy may sometimes be attempted before surgery is considered in the patient who fails VED monotherapy.

VEDs are available with manual or battery-operated pumps. The latter offer greater convenience, particularly in patients with arthritis of the hands, who find the pumps to be too difficult and tiring to operate. The American Urological Association recommends the use of commercially available VEDs by prescription only.[25]

Pain or injury from VEDs most often is caused by the rubber rings or tension bands used to sustain an erection. Because these rings trap blood in the corpora and reduce arteriolar flow into the penis, the penile shaft may feel cold and numb. If the rings or bands are applied for longer than 30 to 60 minutes, the penile shaft may turn bluish and hurt. Patients may complain that a hinge-like erection is produced in

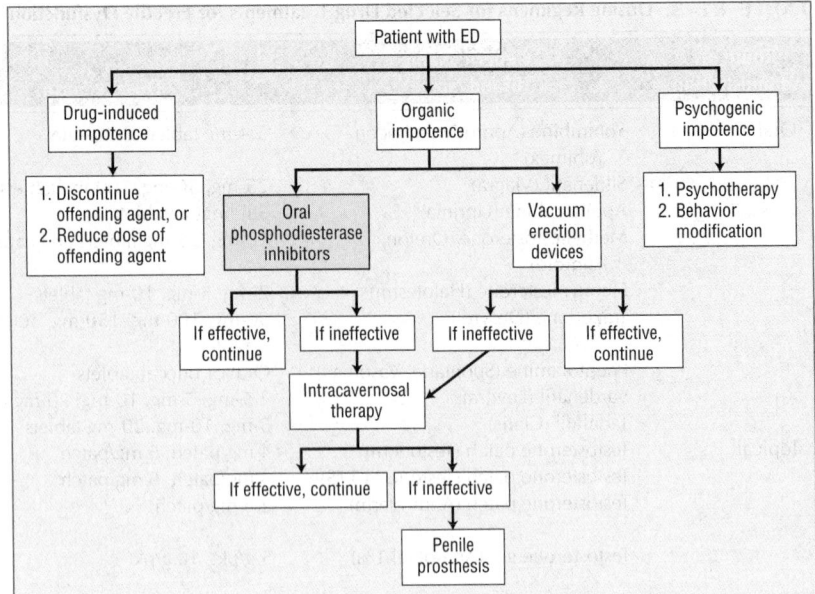

FIGURE 81–4. Algorithm for selecting treatment for erectile dysfunction.

that the penis pivots on the rubber ring or tension band. Patients may also sometimes fail to ejaculate.

VEDs are contraindicated in patients with sickle cell disease. These patients are prone to priapism, which can be exacerbated by the use of rubber rings or tension bands with VEDs. The devices should also be used cautiously in patients on oral anticoagulants. This is also because warfarin, through a poorly understood and idiosyncratic mechanism, can cause priapism.

PHOSPHODIESTERASE INHIBITORS

MECHANISM

In the presence of sexual stimulation, nitric oxide is released by neurons or endothelial cells in penile tissue, thereby enhancing the activity of guanylate cyclase, the enzyme responsible for the conversion of guanylate triphosphate to cGMP (Fig. 81–6).[26] cGMP is a vasodilatory neurotransmitter in corporal tissue. Catabolism of cGMP is mediated by phosphodiesterase.

Three highly selective inhibitors of the phosphodiesterase isoenzyme type 5 found in genital tissue have been marketed in the United States (Table 84–4). These decrease catabolism of cGMP. However, phosphodiesterase isoenzyme type-5 is also found in peripheral vascular tissue, tracheal smooth muscle, and platelets. Inhibition of phosphodiesterase in these nongenital tissues can produce adverse effects.

The three marketed phosphodiesterase inhibitors differ in their pharmacokinetic profiles, drug-food interactions, and adverse effects, and precautions are necessary in patients with cardiovascular disease (Table 81–5). Because sildenafil has been marketed longer and is better studied, it is emphasized in this section, with important differences among the three drugs highlighted as appropriate.

EFFICACY

Because of their apparent effectiveness, convenient route of administration, and comparatively low incidence of serious adverse effects, phosphodiesterase inhibitors are considered first-line therapy for erectile dysfunction, particularly in younger patients.

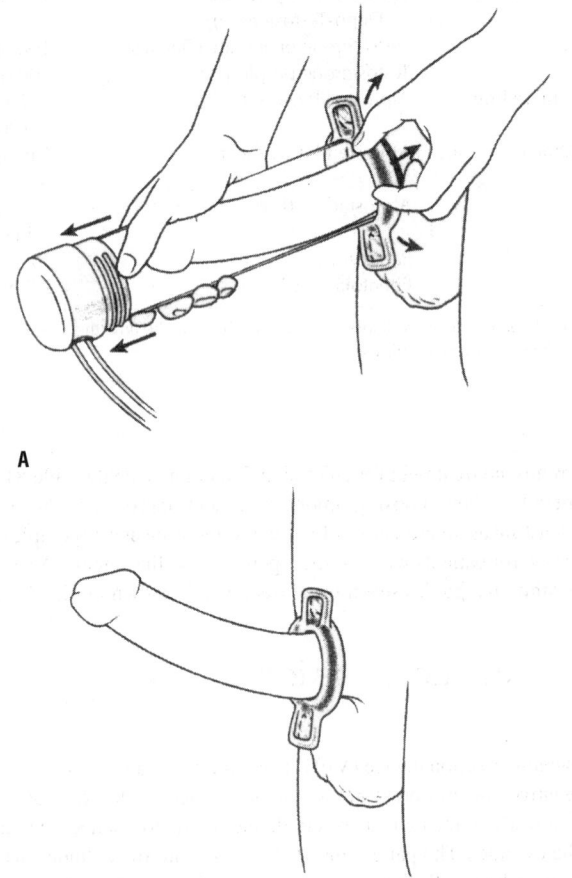

A

B

FIGURE 81–5. Technique for using a vacuum erection device with tension band or rubber constriction ring. *A.* The patient inserts his penis into the cylinder, which is then pushed up flush against his lower abdomen to create a vacuum chamber. Then the patient activates the pump to produce a vacuum pressure, which draws arteriolar blood into the corpora cavernosa. *B.* To prolong the erection, the patient may also use constriction bands or tension rings, which are placed at the base of the penis, to keep the arteriolar blood in and reduce venous outflow from the penis. (*Reprinted with permission from Kirby R, Carson C, Goldstein I. Erectile Dysfunction, A Clinical Guide. Oxford, England, ISIS Medical Media, 1999:52.*)

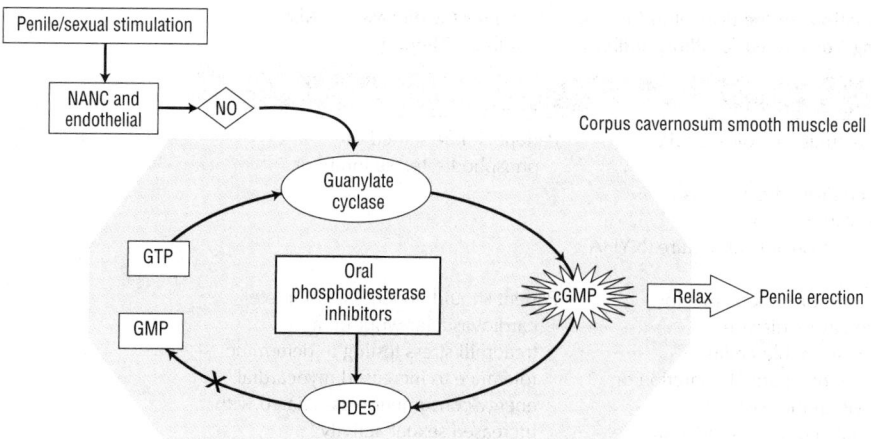

FIGURE 81–6. Nitric oxide (NO)-cyclic guanosine monophosphate (cGMP) mechanism of penile erection and the NO-enhancing effect of the phosphodiesterase type 5 (PDE5) inhibitor sildenafil. GTP, guanosine triphosphate; NANC, nonadrenergic-noncholinergic neurons. (*Adapted with permission from Zusman RM. Cardiovascular data on sildenafil citrate: Introduction. Am J Cardiol 1999;83(5A):2C.*)

In the presence of sexual stimulation and in doses of 25 to 100 mg, sildenafil produces satisfactory erections in 56% to 82% of patients, independent of the etiology of erectile dysfunction. Similar values are documented in the product labeling for the other two agents in this class (65% to 80% for vardenafil and 62% to 77% for tadalafil). Response rates for sildenafil in the lower range have been documented in patients following radical prostatectomy, probably due to postoperative nerve damage.[27] The drugs' effectiveness appears to be dose related.[28–30]

Approximately 30% to 40% of patients fail to respond to the phosphodiesterase inhibitors. For sildenafil, approximately 55% of nonresponders can be salvaged with education on proper use of the drugs, and this will likely prove true for the other agents. Education of patients should include these points: (1) patients must engage in sexual stimulation (foreplay) for the best response; (2) sildenafil should be taken on an empty stomach, at least 2 hours before meals, for the fastest response, but the other two agents may be taken without regard to meals; (3) taking sildenafil or vardenafil with a fatty meal can decrease absorption, but tadalafil's absorption is not affected by this; (4) a patient who does not respond to the first dose should continue with the phosphodiesterase inhibitor for at least five to eight doses before failure is declared; and (5) some patients may require dosage

TABLE 81–4. Pharmacodynamics and Pharmacokinetics of Phosphodiesterase Inhibitors

	Sildenafil[a]	Vardenafil[a]	Tadalafil[a]
Trade name	Viagra	Levitra	Cialis
Inhibits PDE-5	Yes	Yes	Yes
Inhibits PDE-6	Yes	Minimally	No
Inhibits PDE-11	No	No	Yes
Time to peak plasma level (h)	0.5–1	0.7–0.9	2
Fatty meal decreases rate of oral absorption?	Yes	Yes	No
Mean plasma half-life (h)	3.7	4.4–4.8	18
Percentage of dose excreted in feces	80	91–95	61
Percentage of dose excreted in urine	13	2–6	36
Duration (h)	4	4	24–36
Usual daily dose (mg)	25–100	5–20	5–20
Daily dose in elderly patients (mg)	25	5	5–20
Daily dose in moderate renal impairment (mg)	25–100	5–20	5
Daily dose in severe renal impairment (mg)	25	5–20	5
Daily dose in mild hepatic impairment (mg)	25–100	5–20	10
Daily dose in moderate hepatic impairment (mg)	25–100	5–10	10
Daily dose in severe hepatic impairment (mg)	25	Not evaluated	Not recommended
Dose in patients taking cytochrome P450 3A4 inhibitors[a]	25 mg daily	2.5–5 mg every 24–72 hours	10 mg every 72 hours

[a]Sildenafil doses should be decreased when any potent cytochrome P450 3A4 inhibitor is used (e.g., cimetidine, erythromycin, clarithromycin, ketoconazole, itraconazole, ritonavir, and saquinavir). Vardenafil doses vary according to which agent is used (2.5 mg every 72 hours for ritonavir, 2.5 mg every 24 hours for indinavir, ketoconazole 400 mg daily, and itraconazole 400 mg daily; and 5 mg every 24 hours for ketoconazole 200 mg daily, itraconazole 200 mg daily, and erythromycin). Tadalafil doses are reduced only when it is used with the most potent cytochrome P450 3A4 inhibitors (e.g., ketoconazole or ritonavir).
PDE, phosphodiesterase.
From Gresser et al,[34] Porst et al,[35] Ormrod et al,[36] and Young.[37]

TABLE 81–5. Recommendations of the Princeton Consensus Panel for Cardiovascular Risk Stratification of Patients Being Considered for Phosphodiesterase Inhibitor Therapy

Risk Category	Description of Patients' Conditions	Management Approach
Low risk	Has asymptomatic cardiovascular disease Has well-controlled hypertension Has mild, stable angina Has mild congestive heart failure (NYHA Class 1)	Patient can be started on phosphodiesterase inhibitor
Moderate risk	Has three or more risk factors for coronary artery disease Has moderate, stable angina Had a recent myocardial infarction or stroke within the past 6 weeks Has moderate congestive heart failure (NYHA Class 2)	Patient should undergo a complete cardiovascular work-up and treadmill stress testing to determine tolerance to increased myocardial energy consumption associated with increased sexual activity
High risk	Has unstable or symptomatic angina, despite treatment Has poorly controlled hypertension Has severe congestive heart failure (NYHA Class III or IV) Had a recent myocardial infarction or stroke within past 2 weeks Has moderate or severe valvular heart disease	Phosphodiesterase inhibitor is contraindicated

NYHA, New York Heart Association.
From Jarow et al,[29] Rendell et al,[30] McCullough et al,[31] Guay,[33] and Padma-Nathan et al.[33]

titration up to 100 mg of sildenafil, 20 mg of vardenafil, or 20 mg of tadalafil for a response.[31,32]

The phosphodiesterase inhibitors should not be used in patients with normal erectile function. Also, according to FDA-approved labeling, the drugs should not be used in combination with other forms of therapy for erectile dysfunction, as prolonged erections may result.[33]

■ PHARMACOKINETICS

Pharmacokinetic parameters of the phosphodiesterase inhibitors are presented in Table 84–4.

Vardenafil and sildenafil are similar in their pharmacokinetic profiles. Both drugs share a similar 1-hour onset of action, short duration of action, and oral absorption that is significantly delayed when the drug is taken within 2 hours of a fatty meal. In contrast, tadalafil has a delayed onset of action of 2 hours, a prolonged duration of action up to 36 hours, and food does not affect its rate of absorption. Thus tadalafil offers greater spontaneity for patients, as one dose can last through an entire weekend.[34–37]

All three phosphodiesterase inhibitors are hepatically catabolized by the cytochrome P450 3A4 microsomal isoenzyme as well as by other P450 isoenzymes (minor routes) and/or other hepatic enzymes. The drugs and their metabolites (some of which are active) are excreted primarily in the feces, but also in the urine to varying degrees (see Table 84–4).

■ DOSING

The usual oral doses of the phosphodiesterase inhibitors are listed in Table 84–4. The agents vary as to whether doses must be adjusted for elderly patients (over age 65) and compromised hepatic or renal func-

tion. Patients should be advised to take no more than what is prescribed and to use only one dose per day (or less often in the case of some patients taking tadalafil). Doses greater than those recommended have not consistently produced improved erectile responses.[26]

■ ADVERSE EFFECTS

Most adverse effects of the phosphodiesterase inhibitors are mild or moderate and self-limited, rarely requiring treatment discontinuation. In usual doses the most common adverse effects are headache, facial flushing, dyspepsia, nasal congestion, and dizziness, all of which result from inhibition of phosphodiesterase isoenzyme type 5 in extragenital tissues.[26]

Sildenafil produces an 8- to 10-mm decrease in systolic and a 5- to 6-mm decrease in diastolic blood pressure starting about 1 hour after a dose and lasting for 4 hours, and vardenafil has similar vasodilatory actions. Although most patients are asymptomatic as a result of these blood pressure changes, some patients, particularly those taking multiple antihypertensives or nitrates, or those with baseline hypotension, may develop adverse effects as a consequence of these peripheral vascular effects.[26,38] Tadalafil does not produce decreases in blood pressure, but it too must be used with caution in patients with cardiovascular disease, given the cardiac risk inherent in sexual activity. A management approach for such patients, developed based on an analysis of deaths in men who were using sildenafil, and commonly referred to as the recommendations of the Princeton Consensus Panel, can be applied to all the phosphodiesterase inhibitors (see Table 81–5).[39–42]

Sildenafil causes increased sensitivity to light, blurred vision, or loss of blue-green color discrimination in 3% to 10% of patients. This results from the agent's inhibition of phosphodiesterase type 6 in the photoreceptor cells in the retina, particularly at doses larger than

100 mg.[43,44] Although this adverse effect is mild and reversible, caution is recommended in airplane pilots, who rely on green and blue lights for landing planes. Sildenafil is contraindicated in patients at risk of ophthalmologic problems (e.g., retinitis pigmentosa, a genetic disease associated with phosphodiesterase deficiency).[33]

Visual adverse effects occur less frequently with vardenafil when compared with sildenafil (less than 0.1% versus 10%, respectively). Tadalafil has minimal to no inhibitory activity against type 6 phosphodiesterase, and no visual adverse effects have been reported.

Unlike the other two marketed phosphodiesterase inhibitors, tadalafil does inhibit type 11 phosphodiesterase, which is found in skeletal muscle. It is believed that this is linked to back and muscle pain, which occurs in a dose-related fashion in 7% to 30% of patients treated with doses of 10 to 100 mg.[34]

Sildenafil inhibits phosphodiesterase isoenzyme type 5 in platelets, which theoretically could inhibit platelet aggregation. Although sildenafil has not caused bleeding in healthy subjects, it should be used cautiously in patients taking aspirin or other antiplatelet agents and in patients with bleeding tendencies.

Priapism is a rare adverse effect of phosphodiesterase inhibitors, particularly sildenafil and vardenafil, which have shorter plasma half-lives than tadalafil. When priapism has occurred, this has been associated with excessive doses of the phosphodiesterase inhibitor or concomitant therapy involving other erectogenic drugs.

DRUG INTERACTIONS

Patients taking organic nitrates may develop severe hypotension if used with phosphodiesterase inhibitors. This is a result of two major factors: (1) organic nitrates on their own produce hypotension and (2) organic nitrates supply extra nitric oxide, which can stimulate the activity of guanylate cyclase and increase tissue levels of cGMP. For this reason, use of any of the three phosphodiesterase inhibitors is contraindicated in patients taking nitrates given by any route at scheduled times or intermittently.[38,39]

If severe hypotension occurs after exposure to nitrates and a phosphodiesterase inhibitor, the patient should be placed in a Trendelenburg position and aggressive fluid administration should be initiated. If severe hypotension continues, parenteral α-adrenergic agonists (e.g., dopamine, levarterenol, or epinephrine) should be cautiously administered.

Interestingly, dietary sources of nitrates, nitrites, or L-arginine (a precursor for nitrates) do not interact with the phosphodiesterase inhibitors. This is because these dietary sources do not increase circulating levels of nitric oxide in humans.[38]

Sildenafil does not appear to interact with antihypertensive medications. In one retrospective analysis of patients taking sildenafil in combination with α-adrenergic blocking agents, β-adrenergic blocking agents, diuretics, angiotensin-converting enzyme inhibitors, or calcium channel blockers, the incidence of hypotension was similar to that reported in patients taking sildenafil alone.[45] This has been confirmed by a retrospective analysis of pooled data on more than 4800 patients in 35 clinical trials.[33]

However, largely because of postmarketing data showing small decreases in blood pressure with symptomatic hypotension in patients taking sildenafil and α-adrenergic blocking agents, manufacturers of phosphodiesterase inhibitors include a caution to allow a 4-hour interval between doses of these drugs when concomitantly prescribed in the same patient.

The hepatic metabolism of all three phosphodiesterase inhibitors can be inhibited by cytochrome P450 hepatic microsomal enzyme inhibitors of CYP 3A4, including cimetidine, erythromycin, clarithromycin, ketoconazole, itraconazole, ritonavir, and saquinavir.[46,47] In these patients, lower starting doses should be used (see Table 84–4).[26,42]

CLINICAL CONTROVERSY

Some clinicians believe that tachyphylaxis may develop with continuous use of sildenafil, but others believe that a lack of responsiveness may be due to worsening of underlying diseases that may be contributing to the development of erectile dysfunction.

TESTOSTERONE REPLACEMENT REGIMENS

MECHANISM

Testosterone replacement regimens supply exogenous testosterone and restore serum testosterone levels to the normal range (300 to 1100 ng/dL). In so doing, testosterone replacement regimens correct symptoms of hypogonadism, which include malaise, loss of muscle strength, depressed mood, and decreased libido. Testosterone can directly stimulate androgen receptors in the central nervous system and is thought to be responsible for maintaining normal sexual drive.

INDICATIONS

Testosterone replacement regimens are indicated in symptomatic patients with primary or secondary hypogonadism, as confirmed by the presence of a decreased libido and low serum concentrations of testosterone.[48] Simultaneous serum luteinizing hormone levels help to distinguish patients with primary hypogonadism, who have elevated luteinizing hormone levels, from those with secondary hypogonadism, who have decreased luteinizing hormone levels.

Testosterone replacement regimens should never be administered to men with normal serum testosterone levels.

EFFICACY

Testosterone replacement regimens restore muscle strength and sexual drive and improve mood in patients with hypogonadism. Improvements are generally observed within days or weeks of the start of testosterone replacement. Administration of testosterone will correct the serum testosterone level to the normal range. No additional benefit has been demonstrated for large doses of testosterone, which increase the serum testosterone level from the low end to the upper end of the normal range, or to the above-normal range.[7] Testosterone replacement regimens do not directly correct erectile dysfunction; instead, they improve libido, thereby correcting secondary erectile dysfunction.

Testosterone replacement regimens can be administered orally, parenterally, and topically (see Table 81–3). Injectable testosterone replacement regimens are preferred for treatment of symptomatic patients with primary or secondary hypogonadism because they are effective, inexpensive, and not associated with the bioavailability problems or hepatotoxic adverse effects of oral androgens.[6,48] Although convenient for the patient, testosterone patches and gels are much more expensive than other forms of androgen replacement; therefore they should be reserved for those patients who refuse injectable testosterone.[49]

PHARMACOKINETICS

Natural testosterone has poor oral bioavailability because of extensive first-pass hepatic metabolism, and large doses must therefore be taken. To improve oral bioavailability, alkylated derivatives were formulated. Of these, methyltestosterone and fluoxymesterone are more resistant to hepatic catabolism, and can be taken in smaller daily doses, which are potentially safer. However, oral alkylated derivatives of testosterone are associated with a higher incidence of serious hepatotoxicity, and therefore are not preferred for management of sexual dysfunction.

Several testosterone esters have been formulated for intramuscular injection, with different durations of action (see Table 81–3). The shorter-acting testosterone propionate, which requires dosing three times a week, has largely been replaced with testosterone cypionate or enanthate, as they can be dosed every 2, 4, or 6 weeks in most patients. However, these testosterone salts produce suprapharmacologic patterns of serum testosterone during the dosing interval, which have been linked to mood swings in some patients.

Topical testosterone replacement regimens can be delivered as once-daily patches or gel. Testosterone patches increase serum testosterone levels into the normal range in 2 to 6 hours. Serum testosterone levels return to baseline 24 hours after patch administration. However, unlike oral or injectable supplements, topical testosterone products, usually applied each morning, produce physiologic patterns of serum testosterone levels throughout the day. The clinical importance of this biochemical effect is unknown.[50]

The original Testoderm brand patch was formulated for scrotal application. Scrotal skin is thinner and has a richer vascular supply than does the skin on the arms or thighs. Therefore application of Testoderm patches produced excellent absorption of the hormone. However, the patch could fall off when the scrotum became damp or moist, when the patient exercised, or if the scrotum was excessively hairy.

For improved convenience, Androderm and Testoderm TTS patches were formulated for application to the arms, buttocks, or back; Androderm can also be applied to the thighs. The addition of absorption enhancers and different adhesives has been linked to a higher incidence of contact dermatitis with Androderm patches, as compared with the original Testoderm scrotal patch.[51]

Testosterone gel 1% formulation (Androgel) is applied in much larger doses—5 or 10 g each day—to the skin of the shoulders, upper arms, or abdomen. The hormone is absorbed quickly, within 30 minutes, but it may take several hours for complete absorption of the dose. For this reason, the patient should be reminded to wait at least 5 to 6 hours after application before showering. To prevent inadvertent transfer of testosterone gel to others, the patient should thoroughly wash his hands with soap and water after administration of a dose.

DOSING

Table 81–3 lists the usual doses for testosterone replacement regimens. An adequate treatment trial with a particular dose is considered to be 2 to 3 months. Thus a dose should not be increased until the patient has used one particular dose for at least this time period.[52]

Before initiating any testosterone replacement regimen in patients 40 years of age or older, the patient should be screened for the presence of benign prostatic hyperplasia and prostate cancer. Both of these diseases are testosterone-dependent conditions and theoretically could be worsened by the exogenous administration of testosterone. Prostate cancer is a contraindication to androgen supplementation.

ADVERSE EFFECTS

Testosterone replacement regimens can cause sodium retention, which can cause weight gain, or exacerbate hypertension, congestive heart failure, and edema. Gynecomastia can also occur as a result of conversion of testosterone to estrogen in peripheral tissues. This has most often been reported in patients with liver cirrhosis.

Deleterious serum lipoprotein changes have also been reported, including decreasing high-density lipoprotein cholesterol levels. However, no cases of cardiovascular disease have been reported with testosterone replacement regimens.

Large doses of testosterone can stimulate erythropoiesis, and polycythemia may result.[53] Thus patients on long-term testosterone replacement regimens must undergo clinical laboratory testing for serum testosterone, a lipid profile, and a hematocrit every 6 to 12 months.[53] Repeated serum testosterone levels that exceed the normal range require a dosage reduction or increased interval between drug doses. An abnormal lipid profile may require lifestyle and dietary modification, and if necessary, antihyperlipidemic drug therapy. If the hematocrit exceeds 55%, the testosterone replacement regimen should be withheld temporarily.

Oral testosterone replacement regimens have caused hepatotoxicity, which has ranged from mild elevations of hepatic transaminases to serious liver diseases, including peliosis hepatis (hemorrhagic liver cysts), hepatocellular and intrahepatic cholestasis, and benign or malignant tumors. For this reason, parenteral testosterone replacement regimens are preferred.

Topical testosterone patches may cause contact dermatitis, which responds well to topical corticosteroids.

ALPROSTADIL

MECHANISM

Alprostadil, also known as prostaglandin E_1, stimulates adenyl cyclase, resulting in increased production of cAMP, a neurotransmitter that causes smooth-muscle relaxation of the arterial blood vessels to and sinusoidal tissues in the corpora. This results in enhanced blood flow to and blood filling of the corpora (see Fig. 81–1).

Alprostadil is commercially available as an intracavernosal injection (Caverject and Edex) and as an intraurethral insert (medicated urethral system for erection; MUSE).

INDICATIONS

Both commercially available formulations of alprostadil are FDA-approved as monotherapy for the management of erectile dysfunction. Alprostadil is more effective by the intracavernosal than by the intraurethral route.[54,55]

The enhanced efficacy of the intracavernosal injection may be related to the excellent bioavailability of the drug when injected directly into the corpora cavernosum. In contrast, intraurethral alprostadil doses generally are several hundred times larger than intracavernosal doses. Intraurethral alprostadil must be absorbed from the urethra, through the corpus spongiosum, and into the corpus cavernosum, where it exerts its full proerectogenic effect.

Although many other agents, including papaverine and phentolamine, have been used off-label for intracavernosal therapy, alprostadil is preferentially prescribed. This is because the FDA has approved intracavernosal alprostadil for erectile dysfunction, and because it has a low potential for causing prolonged erections and priapism.

Both formulations of alprostadil are considered more invasive than VEDs or phosphodiesterase inhibitors. For this reason, intracavernosal alprostadil is generally prescribed after patients fail to respond to or cannot use the less invasive interventions. Intracavernosal alprostadil is preferred over intraurethral alprostadil because the former is more effective than the latter. Also, intracavernosal alprostadil may be preferred in patients with diabetes mellitus, who are accustomed to injectable drug therapy and may suffer from peripheral neuropathies, which decreases the patient's perception of pain upon injection. Intraurethral alprostadil is generally reserved as a treatment of last resort for patients who fail other less invasive and more effective forms of therapy and also refuse surgery.

INTRACAVERNOSAL ALPROSTADIL

Efficacy

In various controlled and uncontrolled studies, the overall efficacy of intracavernosal alprostadil is 70% to 90%.[6,56,57] In a large parallel design, double-blind, multicenter study, Linet and associates[56] documented three relevant characteristics of intracavernosal alprostadil:

1. The effectiveness of alprostadil is dose related over the range of 2.5 to 20 mcg. The mean duration of erection is directly related to the dose of alprostadil administered and ranges from 12 to 44 minutes.
2. The median effective dose ranged from 3 mcg to 5 mcg. A higher percentage of patients with psychogenic and neurogenic erectile dysfunction responded to alprostadil and at a lower dose when compared to patients with vasculogenic erectile dysfunction.

3. Tolerance does not appear to develop with continued use of intracavernosal alprostadil at home.

Although 70% to 75% of patients respond to intracavernosal alprostadil, a high proportion of patients elect to discontinue its use over time. Depending on the study and the length of observation, 30% to 50% of patients voluntarily discontinue therapy, usually during the first 6 to 12 months. Common reasons for this include lack of perceived effectiveness; inconvenience of administration; an unnatural, nonspontaneous erection; needle phobia; loss of interest; and cost of therapy.[6,58]

Approximately one-third of patients will not respond to usual doses of intracavernosal alprostadil. In these patients, intracavernosal alprostadil has been used successfully along with VEDs. Such combination therapy may be tried in patients before transitioning to more invasive surgical procedures.[23] Alternatively, intracavernosal injections of synergistic combinations of vasoactive agents that act by different mechanisms have been used.[59] Table 81–6 lists examples of such mixtures. Intracavernosal drug combinations typically produce an erection that lasts longer than an erection produced by any one of the agents in the mixture. In addition, because of the low dosage of each agent in the combination, fewer systemic and local fibrotic adverse effects develop compared with high-dose monotherapy. For example, when used in low-dose combination regimens, papaverine is less likely to induce hypotension and liver dysfunction, and phentolamine is less likely to induce tachycardia and hypotension.[65]

Pharmacokinetics

Intracavernosal injection should be made into one corpus cavernosum only. From this injection site, the drug will reach the other corpus cavernosum through vascular communications between the two corpora. Alprostadil acts rapidly, with an onset in 5 to 15 minutes. The duration is directly related to the dose, and within the usual dosage range of 2.5 to 20 mcg, the duration of the erection lasts no more than 1 hour. Local enzymes in the corpora cavernosum quickly metabolize alprostadil. Any alprostadil that escapes into the systemic circulation is deactivated on first passage through the lungs.[6,56,57] Hence the plasma half-life of alprostadil is approximately 1 minute. Also, dose modification is not necessary in patients with renal or hepatic diseases.

TABLE 81–6. Combination Intracavernosal Injection Regimens

Reference	Papaverine Concentration (mg/mL)[a]	Phentolamine Concentration (mg/mL)[a]	Alprostadil Concentration (mcg/mL)[a]	Atropine Concentration (mg/mL)[a]
De la Taile et al.[b]	20	0.67	67	
Zaher[60]	5		5	
Gasser et al.[61]	30	0.5		
Floth et al.[62]	7.5		5	
Floth et al.[62]	7.5	0.005		
Shenfeld et al.[63]	9	0.5		
Shenfeld et al.[63]	4.5	0.25	5	
Montorsi et al.[64]	12.1	1.01	10.1	0.15
Garcia-Reboll et al.[c]	30	1.5	10	
Garcia-Reboll et al.[c]	30	1.0		
Garcia-Reboll et al.[c]	30	2.0	20	

[a]Concentration of each drug is expressed as the amount of medication per milliliter of the final formulation.
[b]From De la Taile A, Delmas V, Amar E, Boccon-Gibod L. Reasons of dropout from short- and long-term self-injection therapy for impotence. Eur Urol 1999;35:312–317.
[c]From Garcia-Reboll L, Mulhall JP, Goldstein I. Drugs for the treatment of impotence. Drugs Aging 1997;11:140–151.

Dosing

The usual dose of intracavernosal alprostadil is 10 to 20 mcg, with a maximum recommended dose of 60 mcg. Doses greater than 60 mcg have not produced any greater improvement in penile erection, but they may cause prolonged erections lasting more than 1 hour or systemic hypotension.[6,56,57] The dose should be administered 5 to 10 minutes before intercourse. The manufacturer recommends that patients be slowly titrated up to the minimally effective dosage. Under a physician's supervision, patients should be started with a 1.25-mcg dose, and this can be increased in increments of 1.25 to 2.50 mcg at 30-minute intervals up to the lowest dose that produces a firm erection for 1 hour and does not produce adverse effects. In clinical practice, this is rarely done because it is time-consuming. Thus many physicians start the patient on 10 mcg and move quickly up the dosage range to identify the best dose for the patient. To avoid adverse effects patients should receive no more than one injection per day and not more than three injections per week.[57]

Intracavernosal injections should be performed using a 0.5-inch, 27- or 30-gauge needle. Also, a tuberculin syringe or a syringe prefilled with diluent as supplied by the manufacturer should be used to ensure precise measurement of doses. Patients with needle phobia, poor vision, or poor manual dexterity can use commercially available autoinjectors (e.g., PenInject) to facilitate the administration of intracavernosal alprostadil.

Intracavernosal injections require that the patient or his sexual partner practice good aseptic technique (to avoid infection), have good manual skills and visual ability, and be comfortable with injection techniques. When practicing self-injection, the patient should use one hand to firmly hold the glans penis against his thigh to expose the lateral surface of the shaft. The injection should be made at right angles into one of the lateral surfaces of the proximal third of the penis. The injection should never be made into the dorsal or ventral surface of the penis. This will prevent inadvertent injection of the drug into arteries on the dorsal surface or the urethra on the ventral surface, respectively. After the injection, the penis should be massaged to help distribute the drug into the opposite corpus cavernosum. Injection sites should be rotated with each dose. Finally, manual pressure should be applied to the injection site for 5 minutes to reduce the likelihood of hematoma formation (Fig. 81–7).[57]

Once the optimal dosage of intracavernosal alprostadil is established, the patient should return for routine medical follow-up every 3 to 6 months. Some patients may subsequently require dosage adjustment, and this is largely attributed to worsening of the underlying disease that is contributing to the erectile dysfunction.

Adverse Effects

Intracavernosal alprostadil is most commonly associated with local adverse effects, which occur most often during the first year of therapy. However, improved administration technique with continued use is believed to account for the lower frequency of adverse effects during subsequent treatment periods.

Intracavernosal injections are associated with several local adverse effects. Cavernosal plaques or areas of fibrosis at injection sites form in approximately 2% to 12% of patients. When these occur, the patient should suspend further injections until the plaques resolve.[66] These plaques may cause penile curvature, similar to Peyronie's disease, which make sexual intercourse difficult or impossible. The cause for corporal fibrosis and plaque formation is unknown. This adverse effect may be caused by poor injection technique[67,68] or by

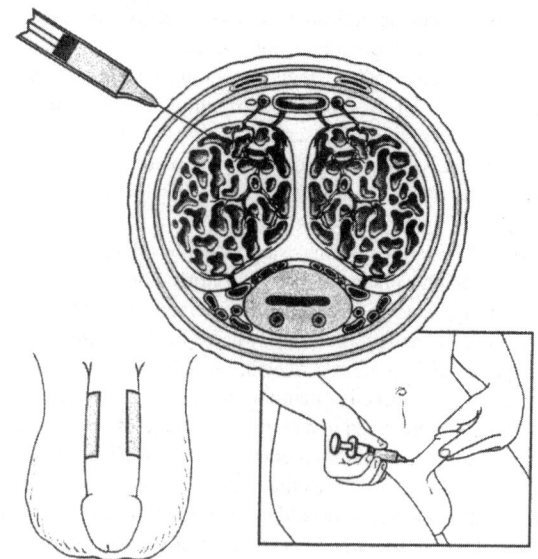

FIGURE 81–7. Technique for administration of intracavernosal injections. (*Reprinted with permission from Kirby R, Carson C, Goldstein I. Erectile Dysfunction, A Clinical Guide. Oxford, England, ISIS Medical Media, 1999:58.*)

alprostadil itself. Although patients have developed corporal fibrosis, alprostadil may be less likely to cause this adverse effect as compared to other intracavernosal drug combinations, such as phentolamine or papaverine.[69] Unlike cavernosal fibrosis associated with large dose and repeated administration of papaverine, penile scarring secondary to alprostadil appears to be unpredictable.

Alprostadil causes penile pain in approximately 10% to 44% of patients.[57,70–72] This has been described as a burning discomfort or dull pain near the injection site or during the erection, which generally does not persist after the penis becomes flaccid. The pain is usually mild, generally does not require discontinuation of therapy, and often abates even with continued treatment. However, 2% to 5% of patients require discontinuation of alprostadil because of severe pain. The pain may be managed by oral analgesics (e.g., acetaminophen) if necessary. One investigator has recommended adding procaine to intracavernosal alprostadil, but this may mask the signs of more serious adverse effects of the drug or of penile injury during intercourse, and it is not recommended.[70] The mechanism of this adverse reaction is poorly understood. Alprostadil may intrinsically produce pain.[72] Also, this may be a result of the pH of the parenteral solution. Alprostadil is acidic and the commercially available Caverject formulation is buffered with sodium citrate, a weak base, to reduce pain on injection.[71]

Priapism, a prolonged, painful erection lasting more than 1 hour, occurs in 1% to 15% of treated patients.[57] It most often occurs during the dose titration period and is rare thereafter. Blood sludging in the corpora can lead to tissue hypoxia and cavernosal fibrosis and scarring, particularly if priapism develops. The risk for this is greatest for erections that persist beyond 4 hours. Patients are advised to seek medical attention immediately when drug-induced erections last more than 1 hour, as this is considered a urologic emergency. Its management includes supportive care, including analgesics for pain and sedatives for anxiety. In addition, needle aspiration of sludged blood in the corpora or intracavernosal injection of α-adrenergic agonists (e.g., phenylephrine) has been used.[72] These procedures facilitate venous drainage of the corpora, allowing the venous outflow to "catch up" with arterial inflow.

The likelihood of prolonged erections with intracavernosal alprostadil is dose-related. Therefore to prevent this adverse effect, the lowest effective dose should be used, and the dose should be titrated to ensure that the duration of the erection is no more than 1 hour.

Other local adverse effects include injection site hematomas and bruising. These are largely the result of unskillful injection techniques. To minimize the risk of injection site hematomas, patients should be advised to apply pressure to the injection site for 5 minutes following each dose. Similarly, infection at the injection site has been reported. Meticulous aseptic technique is recommended to avoid this complication.

Intracavernosal alprostadil rarely causes systemic adverse effects, owing to the agent's localized injection and rapid catabolism. However, large doses greater than 20 mcg are associated with dizziness and hypotension in some patients. This is one reason why such large doses are not commonly used.

Intracavernosal injection therapy should be used cautiously in patients at risk of priapism, which includes patients with sickle cell disease or lymphoproliferative disorders. It should also be used cautiously in patients who may develop bleeding complications secondary to injections, including patients with thrombocytopenia or those on anticoagulants. It should also be used cautiously in patients who may use poor-quality injection technique, including patients with psychiatric disorders, obese patients (who may not be able to reach or see the penile injection site), patients who are blind, and patients with severe arthritis.

INTRAURETHRAL ALPROSTADIL

Efficacy

Intraurethral alprostadil inserts are marketed as MUSE, which contains a pellet inside a prefilled urethral applicator. Multiple studies show this product to have an overall effectiveness rate of 43% to 60%,[54–55] as compared with 70% to 90% for intracavernosal alprostadil. Its decreased effectiveness and inconvenient administration method have resulted in this product being considered a second-line treatment option for patients with erectile dysfunction. However, some patients respond to intraurethral alprostadil even when intracavernosal alprostadil did not work for them.[73]

To improve treatment response to intraurethral alprostadil, it has been combined with an adjustable penile constriction band.[74]

Pharmacokinetics

Following intraurethral instillation, alprostadil is absorbed quickly through the urethra, into the corpus spongiosum, and into the corpora cavernosum. As much as 90% of each dose is absorbed by the urethra and corpus spongiosum in less than 10 minutes, with peak absorption occurring in 20 to 25 minutes. An estimated 20% of each dose is delivered to the corpora cavernosum. As with intracavernosal injections of alprostadil, any drug absorbed into the systemic circulation is rapidly metabolized on first pass through the lungs.

The onset after intraurethral insertion is similar to that of intracavernosal injection, 5 to 10 minutes.

Dosing

The usual dose for intraurethral alprostadil is 125 to 1000 mcg. The dose should be administered 5 to 10 minutes before sexual intercourse.

No more than one dose per day is recommended. Before administration, the patient should be advised to empty his bladder, voiding completely.

Similarly to intracavernosal injection treatments, intraurethral insertion of alprostadil requires good manual and visual skills to minimize the risk of urethral injuries. Intraurethral alprostadil is supplied in a prefilled intraurethral applicator. With one hand the patient holds the glans penis, and with the other hand the patient inserts the intraurethral applicator 0.5-inch into the urethra. The drug pellet is then pushed into the urethra. The penis should then be massaged to enhance drug absorption (Fig. 81–8).

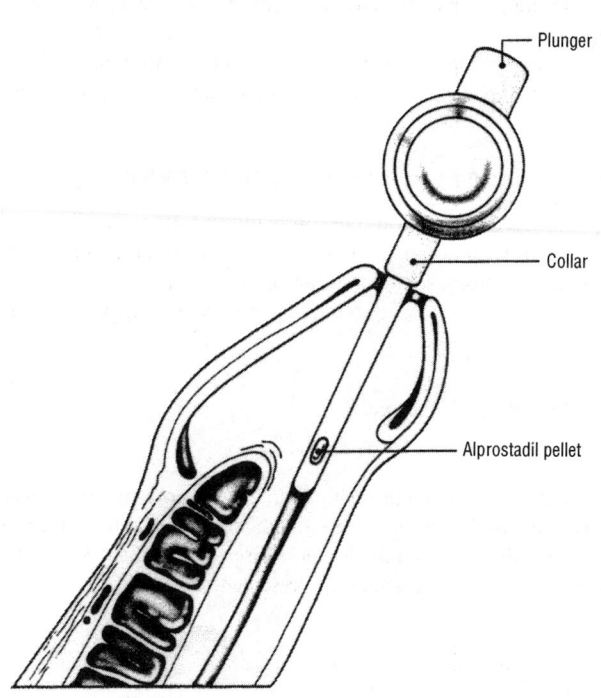

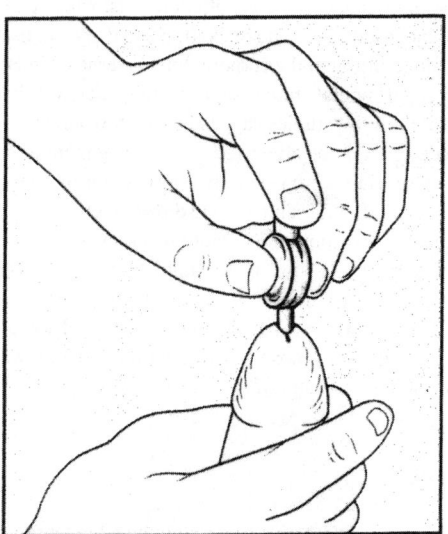

FIGURE 81–8. Technique for administration of intraurethral alprostadil with a MUSE applicator. (*Reprinted with permission from Kirby R, Carson C, Goldstein I. Erectile Dysfunction, A Clinical Guide. Oxford, England, ISIS Medical Media, 1999:62.*)

Adverse Effects

The urethra can be injured because of improper administration technique. Injuries can lead to urethral stricture and difficulty in voiding. Patients should receive complete education about optimal administration procedures before the start of treatment.

Urethral pain has been reported in 24% to 32% of patients. Usually it is mild and does not require discontinuation of treatment. Female sexual partners may experience vaginal burning, itching, or pain, which is probably related to transfer of alprostadil from the man's urethra to the woman's vagina during intercourse. However, the resumption of sexual intercourse could also produce such symptoms.

Prolonged painful erections (priapisms) have been rarely reported.[6,57]

Also, syncope and dizziness have been reported rarely, in only 2% to 3% of patients, and these are likely related to excessively large doses.

CLINICAL CONTROVERSY

Although combinations of proerectogenic drugs may be used in some patients (e.g., sildenafil plus alprostadil intracavernosal injection), such combinations are not recommended by the FDA and may lead to prolonged erections and priapism.

UNAPPROVED AGENTS

A variety of other commercially available and investigational agents have been used for management of erectile dysfunction. Although it is beyond the scope of this chapter to discuss all of them, some of the more commonly used agents are presented.

TRAZODONE

The mechanism by which trazodone produces an erection is not clear. It likely acts peripherally to antagonize α-adrenergic receptors. As a result, a predominant cholinergic effect results, which causes peripheral arteriolar vasodilation and relaxation of cavernosal tissues, which enhances blood filling of the corpora. Intracavernosal injection of trazodone in experimental studies supports this likely mechanism.[75]

Although initial studies suggested that trazodone 50 to 200 mg by mouth daily might be effective in the management of erectile dysfunction, these trials were generally poorly controlled, were nonrandomized, included small samples, and did not include validated objective parameters of response.[76,77] More recent well-controlled studies show that trazodone 50 mg[78] or 150 mg[79] by mouth daily is no more effective than placebo in most patients with erectile dysfunction.

The adverse effects of trazodone, when used for erectile dysfunction, are similar to those reported with trazodone when used to treat depression (see Chap. 67).

YOHIMBINE

Yohimbine, a tree-bark derivative also known as yohimbe, is widely used as an aphrodisiac. This can be explained by yohimbine's central α_2-adrenergic antagonistic effects, which increase catecholamines and improves mood. However, some investigators believe that yohimbine has peripheral proerectogenic effects. It has been postulated that yohimbine may reduce peripheral α-adrenergic tone, thereby permitting a predominant cholinergic tone. This could result in a vasodilatory response.[6]

The usual oral dose is 5.4 mg three times a day.

A controlled clinical trial has shown high-dose yohimbine (100 mg daily) to be no more effective than placebo.[80] Based on a meta-analysis of published studies that came to the same conclusion, the American Urological Association has cautioned against the use of yohimbine.[25] In addition, yohimbine can cause many systemic adverse effects, including anxiety, insomnia, tachycardia, and hypertension.

PAPAVERINE

Papaverine inhibits cavernosal phosphodiesterase, thereby decreasing metabolic catabolism of cAMP in cavernosal tissue. As a result of the enhanced tissue levels of cAMP, smooth-muscle relaxation occurs. Cavernosal sinusoids fill with blood and a penile erection results.[6,81]

Papaverine is not FDA approved for erectile dysfunction. Intracavernosal papaverine alone is not commonly used for management of erectile dysfunction because large doses are required, and these produce dose-related adverse effects: priapism, corporal fibrosis, hypotension, and hepatotoxicity.[82,83] Papaverine is more often administered in lower doses combined with phentolamine and/or alprostadil. A variety of formulae have been used, but no one mixture has been proven better than other mixtures (see Table 81–6). Combination formulations are considered to be safer and associated with the potential for fewer serious adverse effects than high doses of any one of these agents.[82,83]

A portion of each papaverine dose is systemically absorbed, and its prolonged plasma half-life of 1 hour contributes to adverse effects. The usual dose of papaverine is 7.5 to 60 mg when used as a single agent for intracavernosal injection. When used in combination, the dose decreases to 0.5 to 20 mg (see Table 81–6).

If treated with papaverine, patients with a history of underlying liver disease or alcohol abuse should have liver function tests routinely checked at baseline and every 6 to 12 months during continued treatment.[82]

PHENTOLAMINE

Phentolamine is a competitive nonselective α-adrenergic blocking agent. It reduces peripheral adrenergic tone and enhances cholinergic tone. As a result, it improves cavernosal filling and is proerectogenic.

Phentolamine has most often been administered as an intracavernosal injection. Monotherapy is avoided, as large doses are required for an erection, and at these doses systemic hypotensive adverse effects would be prevalent. Most often, phentolamine has been used in combination with other vasoactive agents for intracavernosal administration. A ratio of 30 mg papaverine to 0.5 to 1 mg phentolamine is typical, and the usual dose ranges from 0.1 mL to 1 mL of the mixture. Such a mixture promotes local effects of phentolamine and minimizes systemic hypotensive adverse effects (see Table 81–6).[6]

Hypotension is the most common adverse effect of intracavernosal phentolamine. It is more common and more severe with large doses or in patients with poor injection technique who have injected into a vein (rather than the cavernosa). Prolonged erections have also been reported in patients who used excessive doses of combination intracavernosal therapy.

PENILE PROSTHESES

...urgical insertion of a penile prosthesis is the most invasive treatment ...r erectile dysfunction. It is reserved for those patients who fail to ...spond to or who are not candidates for less invasive oral or injectable ...eatments.

Prosthesis insertion requires anesthesia and skilled urologists. ...wo prostheses are widely used: malleable and inflatable. Malleable ...rostheses consist of two bendable rods that are inserted into the ...orpora cavernosa. The patient appears to have a permanent erection ...ter the procedure; the patient is able to bend the penis into position ... the time of intercourse.

The inflatable prosthesis has several parts, including two inflat-...ble rods and a pump-reservoir mechanism. When activated, the de-...ice pumps saline solution from the reservoir into the rods, causing ...flation. The inflatable prosthesis produces a more natural erection, ... that the patient only develops an erection when the device is acti-...ated. Some newer advances in inflatable prosthesis technology have ...sulted in devices with the pump, reservoir, and rods all in one unit, ...nd these can be placed during shorter surgical procedures and are ...ss likely to malfunction (Fig. 81–9).

Penile prostheses provide penile rigidity suitable for vaginal ...tercourse and are associated with a greater than 90% patient sat-...faction rate. The surgical success rate after insertion is 82% to ...8%.[6]

Adverse effects of prosthesis insertion can occur early or late ...ter the surgical procedure. The most common early complication ... infection. Late complications include mechanical failure of the ...rosthesis, particularly when inflatable prostheses have been inserted. ...Vith improved technology, the mechanical failure rate has decreased ...o 5%.[6] Other late complications include erosion of the rods through

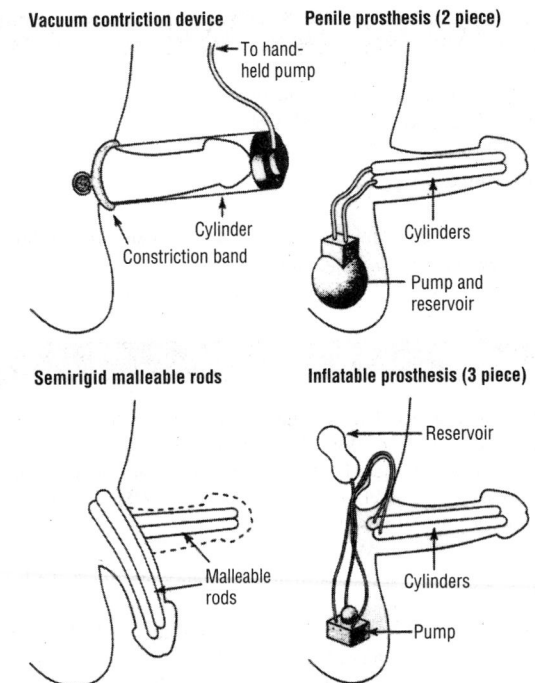

FIGURE 81–9. Devices and prostheses for surgical implantation in patients with erectile dysfunction. (*Adapted with permission from Wagner G, de Tegada IS. Update on male erectile dysfunction. BMJ 1998;316:681.*)

the penis or late-onset infection. Although some salvage procedures have been devised, in many cases the prosthesis may require removal.

EVALUATION OF THERAPEUTIC OUTCOMES

...he primary therapeutic outcomes of specific treatments for erectile ...ysfunction include (1) improvement in the quantity and quality of ...enile erections suitable for intercourse and (2) avoidance of adverse ...rug reactions and drug interactions.

At baseline and after the patient has completed a clinical trial ...eriod of 1 to 3 weeks with a specific treatment for erectile dysfunc-...ion, the physician should conduct assessments to determine whether ...he quality and quantity of penile erections has improved. It should ...e noted that a patient's level of satisfaction is highly individualized ...epending on his lifestyle and expectations. Therefore a patient who ...as successful intercourse once a week might be completely satis-...ied; another patient might judge this to be unsatisfactory. Patients ...vith unrealistic expectations in this regard need to be identified and ...ounseled by their physicians to avoid adverse effects of excessive ...se of proerectogenic agents.

Failure to improve the quality and quantity of penile erections ...uitable for intercourse after an appropriate clinical trial period with a ...pecific treatment for erectile dysfunction occurs in a significant per-...entage of patients, as previously described. In this case, physicians ...enerally take these steps in this order:

1. Ensure that the patient has been prescribed a maximum tolerated dose and has an adequate clinical trial of a specific treatment before discarding it as ineffective.
2. Switch to another drug, usually one with a greater potential for adverse effects and complications than the first drug initiated (see Fig. 81–4).
3. Reserve surgical treatment for patients who fail to respond to drug treatment.

CONCLUSIONS

Erectile dysfunction is a common disorder of aging men. Its inci-dence is higher in patients with underlying medical disorders that compromise the vascular, neurologic, hormonal, or psychogenic sys-tems necessary for a normal penile erection. Medications are common causes of erectile dysfunction. By correcting the underlying etiology, erectile dysfunction can often be reversed without the use of specific treatments.

When treatments for erectile dysfunction are needed, the least in-vasive forms of treatment should be used first, as they produce the low-est incidence of serious adverse effects. VEDs or phosphodiesterase inhibitors are therefore considered first-line treatments. If these fail, intracavernosal alprostadil injection therapy can be initiated. If this fails, the patient can be tried on a combination of intracavernosal alprostadil plus VED, combination intracavernosal therapy, or intra-urethral alprostadil. If this fails, the patient may require insertion of a penile prosthesis.

Some insurance companies do not reimburse for drug treatments for erectile dysfunction; therefore cost is an important issue for some patients.

Clinicians should provide clear and simple advice. Patient con-fidentiality and privacy, which are extremely important to men with erectile dysfunction, should be maintained at all times.

Review Questions and other resources can be found at *www.pharmacotherapyonline.com.*

REFERENCES

1. NIH Consensus Conference. NIH Consensus Development Panel on Impotence. Impotence. JAMA 1993;270:83–90.
2. Feldman HA, Goldstein I, Hatzichristou DG, et al. Impotence and its medical and psychosocial correlates: Results of the Massachusetts Male Aging Study. J Urol 1994;151:54–61.
3. Bacon CG, Mittleman MA, Kawach I, et al. Sexual function in men older than 50 years of age: Results from the Health Professionals Follow-UP Study. Ann Intern Med 2003;139:161–168.
4. Laumann EO, Paik A, Rosen RC. Sexual dysfunction in the United States prevalence and predictors. JAMA 1999;281:537–544.
5. Melman A, Gingell JC. The epidemiology and pathophysiology of erectile dysfunction. J Urol 1999;161:5–11.
6. Lue TF. Erectile dysfunction. N Engl J Med 2000;342:1802–1813.
7. Buena F, Swerdloff RS, Steiner BS, et al. Sexual function does not change when serum testosterone levels are pharmacologically varied within the normal male range. Fertil Steril 1993;59:1118–1123.
8. Keene LC, Davies P. Drug-related erectile dysfunction. Adverse Drug React Toxicol Rev 1999;18:5–24.
9. Hollander E, McCarley A. Yohimbine treatment of sexual side effects induced by serotonin reuptake blockers. J Clin Psychol 1992;53:207–209.
10. Weiss RJ. Effects of antihypertensive agents on sexual function. Am Fam Physician 1991;44:2075–2082.
11. Barksdale JD, Gardner SF. The impact of first-line antihypertensive drugs on erectile dysfunction. Pharmacotherapy 1999;19:573–581.
12. TOMHS Study Group. Long-term effects on sexual function of five antihypertensive drugs and nutritional hygienic treatment in hypertensive men and women. Treatment of mild hypertension study (TOMHS). Hypertension 1997;29:8–14.
13. Morley JE, Kaiser FE. Impotence in elderly men. Drugs Aging 1992;2:330–334.
14. Jarow JP, Burnett AL, Geringer AM. Clinical efficacy of sildenafil citrate based on etiology and response to prior treatment. J Urol 1999;162:722–725.
15. Carson CC, Burnett AL, Levine LA, et al. The efficacy of sildenafil citrate (Viagra) in clinical populations: An update. J Urol 2002;60(Suppl 2B):12–27.
16. Lue TF. Erectile dysfunction: Problems and challenges. J Urol 1993;149:1256–1257.
17. Rosen RC, Riley A, Wagner G, et al. The International Index of Erectile Function (IIEF): A multidimensional scale for assessment of erectile dysfunction. Urology 1997;49:822–830.
18. Buvat J, Lemaire A. Endocrine screening in 1,022 men with erectile dysfunction: Clinical significance and cost-effective strategy. J Urol 1997;158:1764–1767.
19. Masters WH, Johnson VE. Human Sexual Inadequacy. Boston, Little, Brown, 1970.
20. Witherington R. Vacuum constriction device for management of erectile impotence. J Urol 1989;141:320–324.
21. Soderdahl DW, Thrasher JB, Hansberry KL. Intracavernosal drug-induced erection therapy versus external vacuum devices in the treatment of erectile dysfunction. Br J Urol 1997;79:952–957.
22. Korenman SG. New insights into erectile dysfunction: A practical approach. Am J Med 1998;105:135–144.
23. Chen J, Godschalk MF, Katz PG, Mulligan T. Combining intracavernous injection and external vacuum as treatment for erectile dysfunction. J Urol 1995;153:1476–1477.
24. John H, Lehmann K, Hauri D. Intraurethral prostaglandin improves quality of vacuum erection therapy. Eur Urol 1996;29:224–226.
25. Montague DK, Barada JH, Belker AM, et al. Clinical guidelines panel on erectile dysfunction: Summary report on the treatment of organic erectile dysfunction. J Urol 1996;156:2007–2011.
26. Langtry HD, Markham A. Sildenafil: A review of its use in erectile dysfunction. Drugs 1999;57:967–989.
27. Fink HA, Mac Donald R, Rutks IR, et al. Sildenafil for male erectile dysfunction: A systematic review and meta-analysis. Arch Intern Med 2002;162;1349–1360.
28. Goldstein I, Lue TF, Padma-Nathan H, et al. Oral sildenafil in the treatment of erectile dysfunction. N Engl J Med 1998;338:1397–1404.
29. Jarow JP, Burnett AL, Geringer AM. Clinical efficacy of sildenafil citrate based on etiology and response to prior treatment. J Urol 1999;162:722–725.
30. Rendell MS, Rajfer J, Wicker PA, Smith MD for the Sildenafil Diabetes Study Group. Sildenafil for the treatment of erectile dysfunction in men with diabetes. JAMA 1999;281:421–426.
31. McCullough AR, Barada JH, Fawzy A, et al. Achieving treatment optimization with sildenafil citrate (Viagra) in patients with erectile dysfunction. Urology 2002;60(Suppl 2B):28–38.
32. Guay AT. Optimizing response to phosphodiesterase therapy: Impact of risk-factor management. J Androl 2003;24(Suppl):S59–S62.
33. Padma-Nathan H, Eardley I, Kloner RA, et al. A 4-year update on the safety of sildenafil citrate (Viagra). Urology 2002;60(Suppl 2B):67–90.
34. Gresser U, Gleiter CH. Erectile dysfunction: comparison of efficacy and side effects of the PDE-5 inhibitors sildenafil, vardenafil, and tadalafil—review of the literature. Eur J Med Res 2002;7:435–446.
35. Porst H, Padma-Nathan H, Giuliano F, et al. Efficacy of tadalafil for the treatment of erectile dysfunction at 24 and 36 hours after dosing: A randomized controlled trial. Urology 2003;62:121–126.
36. Ormrod D, Easthope SE, Figgett DP. Vardenafil. Drugs Aging 2002;19:217–227.
37. Young JM. Vardenafil. Expert Opin Invest Drugs 2002;11:1487–1496.
38. Cheitlin MD, Hutter AM, Brindis RG, et al. Use of sildenafil (Viagra) in patients with cardiovascular disease. Circulation 1999;99:168–177.
39. Arruda-Olson AM, Mahoney DW, Nehra A, et al. Cardiovascular effects of sildenafil during exercise in men with known or probable CAD. JAMA 2002;287:719–725.
40. DeBusk R, Drory Y, Goldstein I, et al. Management of sexual dysfunction in patients with cardiovascular disease. Recommendations of the Princeton Consensus Panel. Am J Cardiol 2000;86:175–181.
41. Kloner RA, Jarow JP. Erectile dysfunction and sildenafil citrate and cardiologists. Am J Cardiol 1999;83:576–582.
42. Carson CC (program chair). Experience and Progress in the Management of Erectile Dysfunction (symposium). April 28, 2000, University of North Carolina, Chapel Hill, North Carolina.
43. Marmor MF, Kessler R. Sildenafil (Viagra) and ophthalmology. Surv Ophthalmol 1999;44:153–162.
44. Vobig MAM, Klotz T, Staak M, et al. Retinal side effects of sildenafil. Lancet 1999;353:375–376.
45. Zusman RM, Morales A, Glasser DB, et al. Overall cardiovascular profile of sildenafil citrate. Am J Cardiol 1999;83:35C–44C.
46. Hall MCS, Ahmad S. Interaction with sildenafil and HIV-1 combination therapy. Lancet 1999;353:2071–2072.
47. Muirhead GJ, Wulff MB, Fielding H, et al. Pharmacokinetic interactions between sildenafil and saquinavir/ritonavir. Br J Clin Pharmacol 2000;59:99–197.
48. Tenover JL. Male hormone replacement therapy including "andropause." Endocrin Metab Clin North Am 1998;27:969–987.
49. Anonymous. Testosterone patches for hypogonadism. Med Lett Drugs Ther 1996;38:49–50.
50. Cunningham GR, Cordero E, Thomby JI. Testosterone replacement with transdermal therapeutic systems. JAMA 1989;261:2525–2530.
51. Jordan WP. Allergy and topical irritation associated with transdermal

testosterone administration: A comparison of scrotal and nonscrotal transdermal systems. Am J Contact Dermatol 1997;8:108–113.

52. Morales A, Tenover JL. Androgen deficiency in the aging male: When, who, and how to investigate and treat. Urol Clin North Am 2002;29: 975–982.

53. Hajjar RR, Kaiser FE, Morley JE. Outcomes of long-term testosterone replacement in older hypogonadal males: A retrospective analysis. J Clin Endocrinol Metab 1997;82:3793–3796.

54. Porst H. Transurethral alprostadil with MUSE (medicated urethral system for erection) vs intracavernous alprostadil—A comparative study in 103 patients with erectile dysfunction. Int J Impot Res 1997;9:187–192.

55. Fulgham PF, Cochran JS, Denman JL, et al. Disappointing initial results with transurethral alprostadil for erectile dysfunction in a urology practice setting. J Urol 1998;160:2041–2046.

56. Linet OI, Ogring FG for the Alprostadil Study Group. Efficacy and safety of intracavernosal alprostadil in men with erectile dysfunction. N Engl J Med 1996;334:873–877.

57. Meinhardt W, Kropman RF, Vermeij P. Comparative tolerability and efficacy of treatments for impotence. Drug Saf 1999;20:133–146.

58. Mulhall JP, Jahoda AE, Cairney M, et al. The causes of patient dropout from penile self-injection therapy for impotence. J Urol 1999;162: 1291–1294.

59. Israilov S, Niv E, Livine PM, et al. Intracavernosal injections for erectile dysfunction in patients with cardiovascular diseases and failure or contraindications for sildenafil citrate. Int J Impot Res 2002;14:38–43.

60. Zaher TF. Papaverine plus prostaglandin E1 versus prostaglandin E1 alone for intracorporal injection therapy. Int Urol Nephrol 1998;30:193–196.

61. Gasser TC, Roach RM, Larsen EH, et al. Intracavernous self-injection with phentolamine and papaverine for the treatment of impotence. J Urol 1987; 137:678–680.

62. Floth A, Schramek P. Intracavernous injection of prostaglandin E1 in combination with papaverine: Enhanced effectiveness in comparison with papaverine plus phentolamine and prostaglandin E1 alone. J Urol 1999; 145:56–59.

63. Shenfeld O, Hanani J, Shalhav A, et al. Papaverine-phentolamine and prostaglandin E1 versus papaverine-phentolamine alone for intracorporeal injection therapy: A clinical double-blind study. J Urol 1995;154: 1017–1019.

64. Montorsi F, Guazzoni G, Bergamaschi F, et al. Four-drug intracavernous therapy for impotence due to corporal veno-occlusive dysfunction. J Urol 1993;140:1291–1295.

65. Leungwattanakij S, Flynn V, Hellstrom WJG. Intracavernosal injection and intraurethral therapy for erectile dysfunction. Urol Clin North Am 2001;28:343–353.

66. Chew KK, Stuckey BGA, Earle CM, et al. Penile fibrosis in intracavernosal prostaglandin E1 injection therapy for erectile dysfunction. Int J Impot Res 1997;9:225–229.

67. Chen RN, Laken MM, Montague DK, et al. Penile scarring with intracavernosal injection therapy using prostaglandin E1: A risk factor analysis. J Urol 1996;155:138–140.

68. The European Alprostadil Study Group. The long-term safety of alprostadil (prostaglandin-E1) in patients with erectile dysfunction. Br J Urol 1998;82:538–543.

69. Saenz de Tejada I, Moreland RB. Physiology of erection, pathophysiology of impotence and implications of PGE1 in the control of collagen synthesis in the corpus cavernosum. In: Goldstein I, Lue TF, eds. The Role of Alprostadil in the Diagnosis and Treatment of Erectile Dysfunction. Princeton, Excerpta Medica, 1993:3–16.

70. Schramek P, Plas EG, Hubner WA, Pfluger H. Intracavernous injection of prostaglandin E1 plus procaine in the treatment of erectile dysfunction. J Urol 1994;152:1108–1110.

71. Moriel EZ, Rajfer J. Sodium bicarbonate alleviates penile pain induced by intracavernous injections for erectile dysfunction. J Urol 1993;149: 1299–1300.

72. Chen J, Godschalk MF, Katz PG, Mulligan T. Incidence of penile pain after injection of a new formulation of prostaglandin E1. J Urol 1995;154: 77–79.

73. Engel JD, McVary KT. Transurethral alprostadil as therapy for patients who withdrew from or failed prior intracavernous injection therapy. Urology 1998;51:687–692.

74. Lewis RW. Combined use of transurethral alprostadil and an adjustable penile constriction band in men with erectile dysfunction: Results from a multicenter clinical trial. J Urol 1998;159(Suppl):237 (Abstract).

75. Azadzoi KM, Payton T, Krane RJ, et al. Effects of intracavernosal trazodone hydrochloride: Animal and human studies. J Urol 1990;144: 1277–1282.

76. Montorsi F, Strambi LF, Guazzoni G, et al. Effect of yohimbine-trazodone on psychogenic impotence: A randomized double-blind, placebo-controlled study. Urology 1995;44:732–736.

77. Lance R, Albo M, Costabile RA, et al. Oral trazodone as empirical therapy for erectile dysfunction: A retrospective review. Urology 1995;46: 117–120.

78. Costabile RA, Spevak M. Oral trazodone is not effective therapy for erectile dysfunction: A double-blind, placebo controlled trial. J Urol 1999; 161:1819–1822.

79. Meinhardt W, Schmitz PIM, Kropman RF, et al. Trazodone, a double-blind trial for treatment of erectile dysfunction. Int J Impot Res 1997;9:163–165.

80. Teloken C, Rhoden EL, Sogari P, et al. Therapeutic effects of high-dose yohimbine hydrochloride on organic erectile dysfunction. J Urol 1998; 159:122–124.

81. Fallon B. Intracavernous injection therapy for male erectile dysfunction. Urol Clin North Am 1995;22:833–845.

82. Brown SL, Haas CA, Koehler M, et al. Hepatotoxicity related to intracavernous pharmacotherapy with papaverine. Urology 1998;52:844–847.

83. Nehra A, Barrett DM, Moreland RB. Pharmacotherapeutic advances in the treatment of erectile dysfunction. Mayo Clin Proc 1999;74:709–721.

82

MANAGEMENT OF BENIGN PROSTATIC HYPERPLASIA

Mary Lee

Learning Objectives and other resources can be found at *www.pharmacotherapyonline.com*.

KEY CONCEPTS

◀1 Although benign prostatic hyperplasia (BPH) is rare in men younger than 50 years of age, it is very common in men 60 years of age and older as a result of androgen-driven growth in the size of the prostate. Symptoms commonly result from both static factors and dynamic factors.

◀2 While most elderly men have hyperplasia of the prostate, only about 50% of men have symptoms.

◀3 BPH symptoms may be caused by medications, including antihistamines, phenothiazines, tricyclic antidepressants, or anticholinergic agents. In this case discontinuing the causative agent can ameliorate symptoms.

◀4 Specific treatments for BPH include watchful waiting, drug therapy, and surgery.

◀5 No therapy is needed for men with no or few symptoms. They should be managed with watchful waiting, which includes return visits to the physician at 6- to 12-month intervals for reassessment.

◀6 If symptoms progress to moderate severity, drug therapy or surgery is indicated, as waiting longer will not avoid the need for prostatectomy. Drug therapy is an interim measure which delays symptom progression.

◀7 By interfering with testosterone's stimulatory effect on prostate gland enlargement, 5α-reductase inhibitors reduce the static factor. By relaxing prostatic smooth muscle, the α_1-adrenergic antagonists reduce the dynamic factor.

◀8 The drugs of choice are α-adrenergic antagonists. These are all equally effective in relieving BPH symptoms. Older second-generation α-adrenergic antagonists (i.e., terazosin or doxazosin) can cause adverse cardiovascular effects, chiefly hypotension and dizziness. In patients who cannot tolerate hypotensive effects of α-adrenergic agents, the third-generation, pharmacologically uroselective agent tamsulosin is a good alternative. An extended-release formulation of alfuzosin, a second-generation functionally uroselective agent, has fewer cardiovascular adverse effects than terazosin or doxazosin; however, it is unclear if alfuzosin has the same cardiovascular safety profile as tamsulosin.

◀9 5α-Reductase inhibitors are useful primarily in patients with large prostates who wish to avoid surgery and cannot tolerate the side effects of α-adrenergic antagonists.

◀10 Surgery is the gold standard of treatment, as it is the only intervention that relieves symptoms in the greatest number of men with BPH. However, the two most widely used techniques are associated with the highest rates of complications, including retrograde ejaculation and erectile dysfunction.

◀11 Although widely used in Europe for BPH, phytotherapy should be avoided. Studies of these herbal medicines are inconclusive, and the purity of available products is questionable.

Benign prostatic hyperplasia (BPH) is the most common benign neoplasm of American men. A nearly ubiquitous condition among elderly men, BPH is of major societal concern, given the large number of men affected, the long-term nature of the condition, and the health care costs associated with it.

This chapter discusses BPH and its available treatments: "watchful waiting," 5α-reductase inhibitors, α-adrenergic antagonists, and surgery.

EPIDEMIOLOGY

◀1 About 80% of elderly men develop microscopic evidence of BPH, according to the results of autopsy studies. About one-half of the patients with microscopic changes develop an enlarged prostate gland, and as a result have difficulty emptying the contents of the urinary bladder. About one-half of symptomatic patients eventually require treatment.

The peak incidence of clinical BPH occurs at 63 to 65 years of age. Symptomatic disease is uncommon in men younger than 50 years of age, but some urinary voiding symptoms are present by the time men turn 60 years of age. The Boston Area Normative Aging Study estimated that the cumulative incidence of clinical BPH was 78% in patients at age 80 years.[1] Similarly, the Baltimore Longitudinal Study of Aging projected that approximately 60% of men of at least 60 years of age develop clinical BPH.[2]

NORMAL PROSTATE PHYSIOLOGY

Located anterior to the rectum, the prostate is a small heart-shaped, chestnut-sized gland located below the urinary bladder. It surrounds the proximal urethra like a doughnut.

Round, soft, symmetric, and mobile on palpation, a normal prostate gland in an adult man weighs 4 to 20 g. Physical examination of the prostate must be done by digital rectal examination (i.e., the prostate is manually palpated by inserting a finger into the rectum). Thus the prostate is examined through the rectal mucosa.

The prostate has two major functions: (1) to secrete fluids that make up a portion (20% to 40%) of the ejaculate volume; and (2) to provide secretions with possible antibacterial effect related to a high concentration of zinc.[3]

At birth, the prostate is pea-sized and weighs approximately 1 g. The prostate stays that size until the boy reaches puberty. At that time, the prostate undergoes its first growth spurt, growing to its normal adult size of 15 to 20 g by the time the young man is 25 to 30 years of age. The prostate remains this size until the patient reaches age 40, when a second growth spurt begins and continues until the man is 70 to 80. During this period, the prostate can double or triple in size. At surgery, patients with severely symptomatic BPH can have prostates that can exceed 100 g.

The prostate gland comprises three types of tissue: epithelial tissue, stromal tissue, and the capsule. Epithelial tissue, also known as glandular tissue, produces prostatic secretions. These secretions are delivered into the urethra during ejaculation and contribute to the ultimate ejaculate volume. Epithelial tissue is under androgen control (i.e., androgens stimulate epithelial tissue growth). Stromal tissue, also known as smooth muscle tissue, is embedded with α_1-adrenergic receptors. Stimulation of these receptors by norepinephrine causes smooth-muscle contraction, which results in an extrinsic compression of the urethra, reduction of the urethral lumen, and decreased urinary bladder emptying. The normal prostate is composed of a higher amount of stromal tissue than epithelial tissue, as reflected by a stromal-to-epithelial tissue ratio of 2:1. This ratio is further exaggerated to 5:1 in patients with BPH, which explains why α_1-adrenergic antagonists are quickly effective in symptomatic management, and why 5α-reductase inhibitors only reduce an enlarged prostate gland by 25%.[3,4] The capsule, or outer shell of the prostate, is composed of fibrous connective tissue and smooth muscle, which is also embedded with α_1-adrenergic receptors. When stimulated with norepinephrine, the capsule also contracts around the urethra (Fig. 82–1).

Testosterone is the principal testicular androgen in males, whereas androstenedione is the principal adrenal androgen. These two hormones are responsible for penile and scrotal enlargement, increased muscle mass, and maintenance of the normal male libido. These androgens are converted by 5α-reductase in target cells to dihydrotestosterone (DHT), an active metabolite. Two types of 5α-reductase exist. Type I enzyme is localized to hair follicles, sebaceous glands in the frontal scalp, liver, and skin. DHT produced at these target tissues causes acne, increased body and facial hair, and

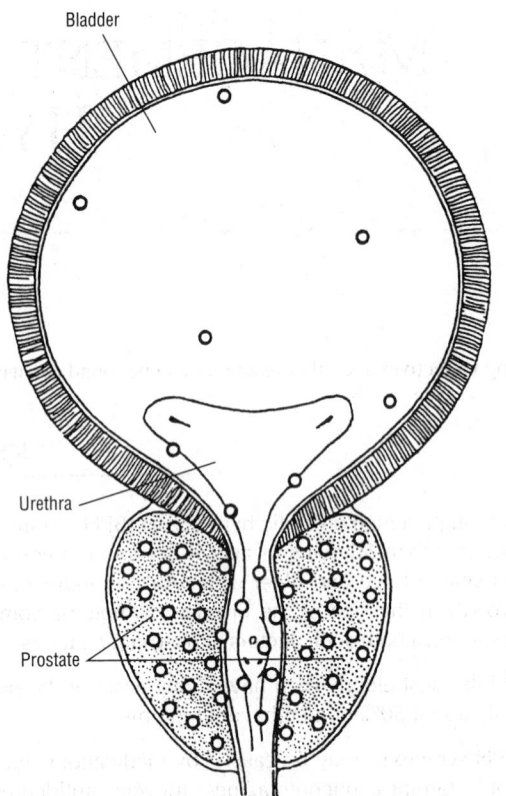

FIGURE 82–1. Representation of the anatomy of and α-adrenergic receptor distribution in the prostate, urethra, and bladder. (*Reproduced with permission from the Western Journal of Medicine 1994;161:501.*)

male pattern baldness. Type II enzyme is localized to the prostate, genital tissue, and scalp. In these target tissues, DHT causes prostate enlargement and prostate growth (Table 82–1).[3]

In prostate cells, DHT has greater affinity for intraprostatic androgen receptors than testosterone, and DHT forms a more stable complex with the androgen receptor. Thus DHT is considered a more potent androgen than testosterone. It is largely responsible for the normal growth of the prostate during the first growth spurt, as well as the development of BPH during the second growth spurt. It should also be noted that despite the decrease in testicular androgen production in the aging male, intracellular DHT levels in the prostate remain normal. This is probably due to increased activity of intraprostatic 5α-reductase.

Estrogen, a product of peripheral metabolism of androgens, is believed to stimulate the growth of the stromal portion of the prostate gland. Estrogens are produced when testosterone and androstenedione are converted by aromatase enzymes in adipose tissues. In addition, estrogens may induce the androgen receptor.[5] As men age, the ratio of serum levels of testosterone to estrogen decreases as a result of a decline in testosterone production by the testes and also increased adipose tissue conversion of androgen to estrogen.

PATHOPHYSIOLOGY

While the precise pathophysiologic mechanisms that cause BPH remain unclear, the role of intraprostatic DHT and type II 5α-reductase in the development of BPH is evidenced by several observations:

- BPH does not develop in men who are castrated before puberty.
- Castration causes an enlarged prostate to shrink.

TABLE 82–1. Characteristics of 5α-Reductase Isoenzymes in Various Target Tissues

Characteristics	Type I	Type II
Localized sites	Scalp, skin (all over the body), sebaceous glands, and liver	Prostate, scalp, liver, genital skin
Clinical manifestations of the presence of the hormone	Acne; increased body and facial hair	Male pattern baldness; BPH; virilization of the fetus
Clinical manifestations of the absence of the hormone	Unknown at this time	Involution of the prostate, ambiguous genitalia in newborns even though the patient is genetically a male (also referred to as pseudohermaphroditism)
Inhibited by finasteride	+	+++

Patients with type II 5α-reductase enzyme deficiency do not develop BPH.

Administration of testosterone to orchiectomized dogs of advanced age produces BPH.

The pathogenesis of BPH is often described as resulting from both static and dynamic factors. Static factors relate to anatomic enlargement of the prostate gland, which produces a physical block at the bladder neck and thereby obstructs urinary outflow. Enlargement of the gland depends on androgen stimulation of epithelial tissue and estrogen stimulation of stromal tissue in the prostate. Dynamic factors relate to excessive α-adrenergic tone of the stromal component of the prostate gland, bladder neck, and posterior urethra, which results in contraction of the prostate gland around the urethra and narrowing of the urethral lumen.

Symptoms of BPH disease may result from static and/or dynamic factors, and this must be recognized when drug therapy is considered. For instance, some patients may present with obstructive voiding symptoms but have prostates of normal size. In these patients, dynamic factors are likely responsible for the symptoms. But in patients with enlarged prostate glands, static and dynamic factors are likely working in concert to produce the observed symptoms.

Static factors may be accentuated by environmental factors. Patients who are stressed or in pain may experience an exacerbation of voiding difficulty. In these situations, increased α-adrenergic tone may precipitate excessive contraction of prostatic stromal tissue. When the stressful event resolves, voiding symptoms often disappear.[6]

MEDICATION-RELATED SYMPTOMS

Medications in several pharmacologic categories should be avoided in patients with BPH, as they may exacerbate symptoms. Testosterone replacement regimens, used to treat primary or secondary hypogonadism, deliver additional substrate that can be metabolized to DHT by the prostate. Although no cases of BPH have been reported as a result of exogenous testosterone administration, cautious use is advised in patients with prostatic enlargement. α-Adrenergic agonists, used as oral or intranasal decongestants (e.g., pseudoephedrine, ephedrine, or phenylephrine), can stimulate α-adrenergic receptors in the prostate, resulting in muscle contraction. By decreasing the caliber of the urethral lumen, bladder emptying may be compromised. Also, drugs with significant anticholinergic adverse effects (e.g., antihistamines, phenothiazines, tricyclic antidepressants, or anticholinergic drugs used as antispasmodics or to treat Parkinson's disease) may

decrease (urinary bladder) detrusor muscle contractility. For patients with BPH, who have a narrowed urethral lumen, the loss of effective detrusor contraction could result in acute urinary retention. Diuretics, particularly large doses, can produce polyuria, which may present as urinary frequency, similar to that experienced in patients with BPH.

CLINICAL PRESENTATION

Patients with BPH can present with a variety of symptoms and signs of disease. All symptoms of BPH can be divided into two categories: obstructive and irritative.

CLINICAL PRESENTATION OF BENIGN PROSTATIC HYPERPLASIA

GENERAL
Patient is in no acute distress unless he has severe complications of the BPH.

SYMPTOMS
Urinary frequency, urgency, intermittency, nocturia, decreased force of stream, hesitancy, and straining

SIGNS
Digital rectal examination reveals an enlarged prostate (>20 g)

LABORATORY TESTS
Increased BUN and serum creatinine, elevated PSA

OTHER DIAGNOSTIC TESTS
Increased AUA Symptom Score and decreased urinary flow rate (<10 mL/s), and increased postvoid residual urine volume

Obstructive symptoms, also known as prostatism or bladder outlet obstruction, result when dynamic and/or static factors reduce bladder emptying. The force of the urinary stream becomes diminished, urinary flow rate decreases, and bladder emptying is incomplete or takes a longer time. Patients report urinary hesitancy and straining and a weak urine stream. Urine dribbles out of their penis, and their bladder always feels full, even after they have voided. Some patients state that they need to press on their bladder to force urine out. In severe cases, patients may go into urinary retention when bladder emptying is not possible. In these cases, suprapubic pain can result from bladder overdistension.

About 50% to 80% of patients have irritative voiding symptoms, which typically occur late in the disease course. Irritative voiding symptoms result from long-standing obstruction at the bladder neck. To compensate, the bladder muscle undergoes hypertrophy so that it can generate a greater contractile force to empty urine past the anatomic obstruction at the bladder neck. Although initially helpful, decompensation eventually occurs, and the hypertrophied bladder muscle is no longer able to generate adequate contractile force, as it becomes hypersensitive and ineffective in storing urine. As a result, small amounts of urine irritate the bladder and initiate a bladder emptying response. Patients complain of urinary frequency and urgency. Bedwetting or clothes wetting occurs. Patients report waking up every 1 to 2 hours at night to void (nocturia), which significantly reduces quality of life.

Symptoms of BPH vary over time. Symptoms may improve, remain stable, or worsen spontaneously. Thus BPH is not necessarily a progressive disease; in fact, some patients experience symptom regression. Between one-third and two-thirds of men with mild disease stabilize or improve without treatment over 2.5 to 5 years.[6,7] However, other patients experience a slow progression of disease.

Obstructive and irritative voiding symptoms are collectively referred to as lower urinary tract symptoms (LUTS). However, LUTS are not pathognomonic for BPH and LUTS may be caused by other diseases.[8]

Another characteristic of BPH is that some men suffer from silent prostatism. While they have obstructive or irritative voiding symptoms, they adapt to them and do not voluntarily complain about them. Such patients do not present for medical treatment until complications of BPH disease arise.

Complications of untreated BPH include:

- Chronic renal failure from long-standing bladder outlet obstruction
- Gross hematuria when tissue growth exceeds its blood supply
- Overflow urinary incontinence or unstable bladder
- Recurrent urinary tract infection that results from urinary stasis
- Bladder diverticula
- Bladder stones

All of these complications can be potentially serious and life-threatening. Approximately 20% of patients with symptomatic BPH require treatment because of disease complications.[5] Symptoms, signs, and complications of BPH (both obstructive and irritative voiding symptoms, decreasing peak urinary flow rate, and acute urinary retention) generally worsen in severity over time, with symptom severity greatest in older men. Prostate size also increases with age, at a rate approximating 0.6 g/y. Older men with prostates greater than 40 g were three times as likely to have severe symptoms or suffer from acute urinary retention, and require prostatectomy.[9–11]

DIAGNOSTIC EVALUATION

Because the common obstructive and irritative voiding symptoms associated with BPH are not unique to the disease and can be presenting symptoms of other genitourinary tract disorders, including prostate or bladder cancer, neurogenic bladder, prostatic calculi, or urinary tract infection, the patient presenting with signs and symptoms of BPH must be thoroughly evaluated.

A careful medical history should be taken to ensure that a complete listing of symptoms is collected, as well as to identify concomitant disorders that may be contributing to voiding symptoms. The medical history should be followed by a thorough medication history, including all prescription and nonprescription medications and dietary supplements that the patient is taking. Any drugs that could be causing the patient's symptoms should be identified. If possible, the suspected drugs should be discontinued or the dosing regimen modified to ameliorate the voiding symptoms.

The patient should also undergo a physical examination, including a digital rectal examination, although the size of the prostate gland does not always correspond to symptoms. BPH usually presents as an enlarged, soft, smooth, symmetric gland, greater than 20 g in size. Some patients have only a slightly enlarged gland and yet have bothersome or even serious voiding difficulties, usually the result of dynamic factors. Other patients have an intravesical enlargement of the prostate gland (i.e., the gland grows into the urinary bladder and produces a ball-valve blockage of the bladder neck). This type of prostate enlargement is not palpable on manual examination.

The patient's perception of the severity of BPH symptoms guides development of a therapeutic plan. To evaluate perceptions objectively, validated instruments, such as the American Urological Association (AUA) Symptom Index, are commonly used. Using the AUA index, the patient rates the "bothersomeness" of seven obstructive and irritative voiding symptoms.[2,9,12] Each item is rated for severity on a scale of 1 to 5 such that 35 is the maximum score and is consistent with the most severe symptoms.

Objective measures of bladder emptying include peak and average urinary flow rate (normal is at least 10 to 15 mL/s). This is determined using a uroflowmeter, which literally checks the rate of urine flow out of the bladder. This is a quick noninvasive outpatient procedure in which the patient's urinary flow is clocked during voiding. A low urinary flow rate implies failure of bladder emptying, but the degree of bladder outlet obstruction correlates poorly with peak urinary flow rate.

Another objective measure is postvoid residual (PVR) urine volume (normal is 0 mL). This is a simple outpatient procedure and is determined after the patient has attempted to empty his bladder. A straight catheter is inserted to drain any urine remaining in the bladder. A high PVR urine volume (more than 25 to 30 mL) implies failure of bladder emptying and a predisposition for urinary tract infections. Because there is a weak correlation among voiding symptoms, prostate size, and urinary flow rate, most physicians use a combination of measures, including the patient's assessment of symptoms along with objective evaluation of urinary outflow and presence of complications of BPH, to determine the need for treatment.

Clinical laboratory tests can also be helpful in evaluating the patient with possible BPH. Elevated serum blood urea nitrogen (BUN) and creatinine values can indicate development of renal insufficiency caused by long-standing bladder outlet obstruction. Abnormal urinalysis results may be caused by hematuria or urinary tract infection, which can cause voiding symptoms. Prostate-specific antigen (PSA) is used in combination with digital rectal examination of the prostate to screen for prostate cancer, which can also cause voiding difficulty.

Many other tests can be performed if additional information is needed to assess the severity of BPH disease and its complications, or assist in the preoperative assessment of the patient, including a voiding cystometrogram, transrectal ultrasound of the prostate, intravenous pyelogram, renal ultrasound, and prostate biopsy.

▶ TREATMENT: Benign Prostatic Hyperplasia

As a disease of symptoms, BPH is treated by relieving manifestations that are bothering the patient. Patients are usually stratified into three severity groups for assessing the need for treatment (Table 82–2). However, recent literature about the natural history of BPH and the significant risk of disease complications suggests that physicians should also consider prevention of serious complications of BPH as a goal of treatment in selected patients. This is a controversial topic, which is complicated by many issues, including the variable costs of treatment options, the inability to clearly distinguish patients who experience spontaneous regression or disease stabilization from those in whom symptoms progress, and the potential benefit that may occur in a comparatively small number of treated patients.

Management options include watchful waiting, drug treatment, or surgical intervention. The most definitive recommendation for BPH treatment is the 2003 American Urological Association Guideline on Management of BPH (Fig. 82–2).[13] This guideline supersedes the older 1994 Guideline on BPH: Diagnosis and Treatment published by the Agency for Health Care Policy and Research.[12] The primary change in the 2003 Guideline is that treatment selection should be based on the patient's perception of the bothersomeness of symptoms, which may not correlate with the AUA Symptom Index Score, but may be more related to the patient's perception of the impact of LUTS on their quality of life.[13,14]

▨ NONPHARMACOLOGIC THERAPY

4 ◀ 5 Patients with mild disease are asymptomatic or have mildly bothersome symptoms and have no complications of BPH disease. In these patients, no specific treatment is indicated. These patients can be managed with "watchful waiting," which entails having the patient return for reassessment at regular 6- to 12-month intervals.

At each return visit, the patient should complete a standardized, validated survey tool to assess severity of symptoms. A digital rectal examination, urinary flow rate, postvoid residual urine volume, and routine laboratory tests (BUN and serum creatinine)

TABLE 82–2. Categories of BPH Disease Severity Based on Symptoms and Signs

Disease Severity	AUA Symptom Score	Typical Symptoms and Signs
Mild	≤7	Asymptomatic Peak urinary flow rate <10 mL/s Postvoid residual urine volume >25–50 mL Increased BUN and serum creatinine
Moderate	8–19	All of the above signs plus obstructive voiding symptoms and irritative voiding symptoms (signs of detrusor instability)
Severe	≥20	All of the above plus one or more complications of BPH

AUA, American Urological Association; BUN, blood urea nitrogen.

should be obtained. Watchful waiting also includes thorough patient education about the disease and behavior modification to avoid practices that exacerbate voiding symptoms. Behavior modification includes fluid restriction close to bedtime, avoiding caffeine and alcohol intake, frequent emptying of the bladder during waking hours (to avoid overflow incontinence and urgency), and avoiding drugs that could exacerbate voiding symptoms.

If symptoms progress to moderate or severe severity or the patient perceives his symptoms to be bothersome, the patient should be offered specific treatment. In these patients, watchful waiting delays—but does not decrease—the need for prostatectomy. In symptomatic patients, watchful waiting can lead to intractable urinary retention, increased PVR urine volumes, and significant voiding symptoms. Therefore watchful waiting is not recommended for symptomatic patients.[15] For patients with BPH of moderate or severe severity, treatment options include drug therapy and surgery.

6 Patients with serious complications of BPH should be offered surgical correction (i.e., prostatectomy). Drug therapy is considered an interim measure in such patients, as it likely only delays worsening of complications and the need for surgical intervention.[15]

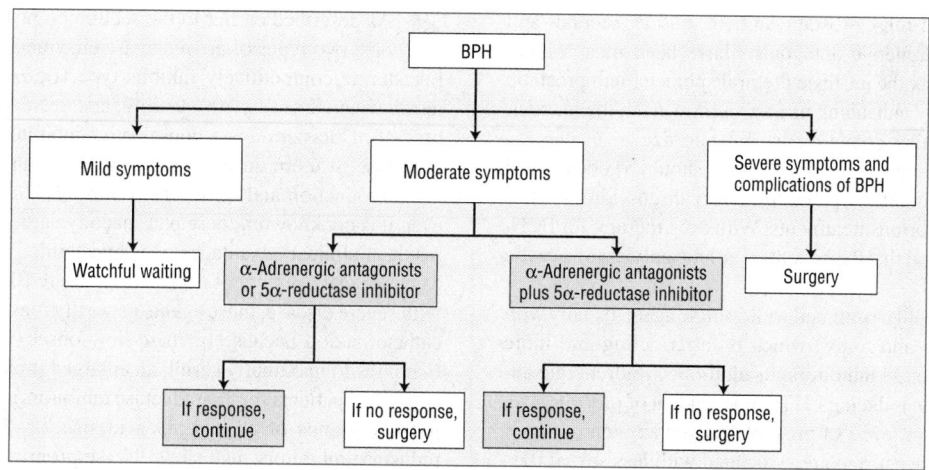

FIGURE 82–2. Management algorithm for benign prostatic hyperplasia.

TABLE 82–3. Summary of Medical Treatment Options for BPH

Category	Mechanism	Drug (Brand Name)	Daily Dose
Reduces static factor	Blocks 5α-reductase enzyme	Finasteride (Proscar)	5 mg by mouth daily
		Dutasteride (Avodart)	0.5 mg by mouth daily
	Blocks dihydrotestosterone at its intracellular receptor	Bicalutamide (Casodex)	50 mg by mouth daily
		Flutamide (Eulexin)	100–250 mg by mouth three times daily
	Blocks pituitary release of luteinizing hormone	Leuprolide (Lupron)	7.5 mg intramuscularly monthly **or** 22.5 mg intramuscularly every 3 months
		Nafarelin	400 mcg subcutaneously daily
	Blocks pituitary release of luteinizing hormone and blocks androgen receptor	Megestrol acetate	40–250 mg by mouth three times daily
Reduces dynamic factor	Blocks α₁-adrenergic receptors in prostatic stromal tissue	Prazosin (Minipress)	2 mg by mouth two to three times daily
		Alfuzosin (UroXatral)	10 mg by mouth daily
		Terazosin (Hytrin)	1–10 mg by mouth daily
		Doxazosin (Cardura)	1–8 mg by mouth daily
	Blocks α₁A receptors in the prostate	Tamsulosin (Flomax)	0.4–0.8 mg by mouth daily

■ PHARMACOLOGIC THERAPY

◀7 Drug therapy for BPH can be categorized into three types: agents that interfere with testosterone's stimulatory effect on prostate gland enlargement (reducing the static factor), agents that relax prostatic smooth muscle (reducing the dynamic factor; Table 82–3), and combination therapy with a 5α-reductase inhibitor plus an α₁-adrenergic antagonist. Of the agents that interfere with testosterone's stimulatory effect on prostate gland size, the only agents approved by the U.S. Food and Drug Administration (FDA) are 5α-reductase inhibitors (e.g., finasteride or dutasteride). Other agents that interfere with androgen stimulation of the prostate have not been popular in the United States because of the many adverse effects associated with their use. The luteinizing hormone-releasing hormone superagonists leuprolide and goserelin produce decreased libido, erectile dysfunction, gynecomastia, and hot flashes. Antiandrogens (e.g., bicalutamide and flutamide) produce nausea, diarrhea, and hepatotoxicity.[16]

Of the agents that relax prostatic smooth muscle, second- and third-generation α₁-adrenergic antagonists have been most widely used. These agents relax the intrinsic urethral sphincter and prostatic smooth muscle, thereby enhancing urinary outflow from the bladder. α₁-Adrenergic antagonists do not reduce prostate size.

Selection of a particular agent for a patient should be determined on a case-by-case basis after a patient-provider discussion of risks, benefits, and costs of various treatments. With drug therapy for BPH, patients must understand that the benefits continue only as long as the medication is taken.[16]

◀8 Drug therapy should be initiated with a single agent, usually with an α₁-adrenergic antagonist, which is faster acting and more effective than 5α-reductase inhibitors. In addition, α₁-adrenergic antagonists are effective in reducing LUTS independent of prostate size, have no effect on serum levels of prostate-specific antigen (a tumor marker for prostate cancer), and are associated with less sexual dysfunction than 5α-reductase inhibitors. A 5α-reductase inhibitor is a good first choice agent in patients with a significantly enlarged prostate, greater than 40 g, who cannot tolerate the cardiovascular adverse effects of α₁-adrenergic antagonists. If a therapeutic dose regimen of a single drug fails, combination drug therapy with a 5α-reductase inhibitor and an α-adrenergic antagonist could be attempted in patients with an enlarged prostate gland that is greater than 40 g,[17,18] and an elevated serum prostate-specific antigen level (>1.3 ng/mL).[19] The rationale for such a combination is that using two drugs with different mechanisms of action can be pharmacologically beneficial. Combination regimens that have been clinically evaluated include terazosin plus finasteride,[20] and doxazosin plus finasteride.[18] It should be noted that combination therapy is more expensive and has more adverse effects than monotherapy regimens. Alternatively, surgery is a choice. Finally, any severely symptomatic patient with BPH disease complications should undergo surgical correction.[13]

■ 5α-REDUCTASE INHIBITORS

◀9 As described earlier in the section on normal prostate physiology, two types of 5α-reductase enzyme exist (see Table 82–1). Finasteride competitively inhibits type II 5α-reductase, suppresses intraprostatic DHT by 80% to 90%, and decreases serum DHT levels by 70%. Dutasteride is a nonselective inhibitor of type I and II 5α-reductase. It more quickly and completely suppresses intraprostatic DHT production and decreases serum DHT levels by 90%.[21] However, it is not known if these pharmacodynamic actions of dutasteride result in clinical advantages over finasteride. These agents are indicated for management of moderate to severe BPH disease. In patients with severe disease, these agents generally must be used with urethral catheterization because of their slow onset (i.e., these agents take 6 months to maximally shrink an enlarged prostate gland).

Ideal patients for 5α-reductase inhibitors are those with enlarged prostate glands of at least 50 g in size.[21,22] In such patients, 5α-reductase inhibitors may slow disease progression and decrease the risk of disease complications, thereby decreasing the ultimate need for surgical intervention.[23] When taken continuously for 4 years

asteride has been shown to decrease the risk of acute urinary re-
ntion and prostatectomy.[23] 5α-Reductase inhibitors may also be
eferred in patients with BPH who have uncontrolled arrhythmias,
oorly controlled angina, patients taking multiple antihypertensive
gents, or those unable to tolerate hypotensive adverse effects of
cond-generation α_1-adrenergic antagonists.

5α-Reductase inhibitors reduce prostate size by 25%, increase
eak urinary flow rate by 1.6 to 2.0 mL/s, improve voiding symp-
ms in approximately 30% of treated patients, and produce very few
rious adverse effects. Compared to α_1-antagonists, 5α-reductase in-
ibitors have several disadvantages. 5α-Reductase inhibitors have a
elayed onset of action, which is undesirable in patients with bother-
ome symptoms, and an adequate clinical trial is 6 to 12 months. In ad-
tion, the percentage of patients who experience objective improve-
ent is less with 5α-reductase inhibitors than with α_1-adrenergic
ntagonists. Finally, 5α-reductase inhibitors cause more sexual
ysfunction than α-adrenergic antagonists. Therefore physicians con-
der 5α-reductase inhibitors to be second-line agents for treatment
BPH.[23–26]

CLINICAL CONTROVERSY

Dutasteride is a nonselective 5α-reductase inhibitor that more
quickly and effectively lowers intraprostatic DHT production
and lowers plasma DHT levels than finasteride. Whether these
hormonal changes result in clinical advantages remains to be
determined.[37]

Finasteride is well absorbed from the gastrointestinal tract
5%), and its absorption is unaffected by food. Peak serum con-
ntrations are reached 1 to 2 hours after the dose. Finasteride is
ghly protein bound. The liver extensively metabolizes finasteride to
active metabolites, which are largely excreted in stool. The plasma
lf-life is 4.7 to 7.1 hours, but its biologic half-life is probably longer,
cause decreased serum DHT levels persist for up to 2 weeks after
asteride dosing is stopped.[27]

For BPH, finasteride is given in doses of 5 mg by mouth daily
r at least 6 to 12 months. The dose can be taken with meals or on an
npty stomach, and no dosage adjustment is needed in patients with
nal dysfunction. Although no dosage reduction is recommended
patients with hepatic insufficiency, patients should be monitored
refully. Maximal reductions in prostate volume or symptom im-
rovement may not be evident for 12 months, but noticeable changes
om baseline should occur after 6 months of continuous treatment.
o clinically relevant drug interactions have been reported with 5α-
ductase inhibitors.

Patients must continue to take 5α-reductase inhibitors as long
; they respond. Upon discontinuation of the drug, prostate size and
oiding symptoms generally return to baseline.

5α-Reductase inhibitors have few adverse effects. Ejaculation
sorders (dry sex or delayed ejaculation) have been reported in 3%
15% of treated patients. A possible result of decreased prostatic
cretion, these disorders are reversible with drug discontinuation.

Erectile dysfunction has been reported in 3% to 5% of patients.[16]
may be secondary to ejaculation disorders, or may be due to drug-
duced inhibition of nitric oxide synthase (which is needed for pro-
icing nitric oxide, a vasodilatory substance) in cavernosal tissue.[28]
he role of 5α-reductase inhibitors in causing erectile dysfunction
not clear, as elderly men with BPH commonly develop erectile
ysfunction as they age, or have concurrent medical illnesses or con-
omitant drug therapies that may predispose to the development of
exual dysfunction.[29]

Other minor adverse effects include nausea, abdominal pain,
asthenia, dizziness, flatulence, headache, rash, muscle weakness, and
gynecomastia.

5α-Reductase inhibitors are in FDA pregnancy category X,
which means that they are contraindicated in pregnant females. Exposure of the fetus to finasteride may produce pseudohermaphroditic
offspring with ambiguous genitalia, similar to those of patients with
a rare genetic deficiency of type II 5α-reductase. Because of this teratogenic effect, women who are pregnant or seeking to become pregnant should not handle 5α-reductase inhibitor tablets and should not
have contact with semen from men being treated with 5α-reductase
inhibitors. Women pharmacists of childbearing age should handle
this product with rubber gloves if there is any chance that they are
pregnant.

Normal doses of 5α-reductase inhibitors reduce serum PSA levels by 50%. For this reason, PSA levels must be measured before
treatment begins, and the patient should have a digital rectal examination. After 6 months of therapy, the patient should have a repeat
PSA. If the level does not decline by 50% and the patient has been
adherent to the 5α-reductase inhibitor regimen, he should be evaluated for prostate cancer. Annually thereafter, the patient should have
a PSA assay and digital rectal examination, and patients with any rise
in PSA levels should be evaluated for prostate cancer.[30] To interpret
a PSA level in a patient being treated with a 5α-reductase inhibitor, it
is generally recommended that the actual measured level be doubled
to get an estimate of the true level.

CLINICAL CONTROVERSY

5α-Reductase inhibitors have been shown to delay disease
progression, which is linked to shrinkage of an enlarged
prostate gland. This benefit of treatment remains to be demonstrated for α-adrenergic antagonists.[37]

α-ADRENERGIC ANTAGONISTS

Three generations of α-adrenergic antagonists have been used to
treat BPH through their relaxation of smooth muscle in the prostate
and bladder neck. Because of their dose-limiting adverse effects on
the heart (tachycardia and arrhythmias), first-generation agents such
as phenoxybenzamine have been replaced by the second-generation
postsynaptic α_1-adrenergic antagonists and third-generation uroselective postsynaptic α_{1A}-adrenergic antagonists.[31]

The second- and third-generation α_1-adrenergic antagonists are
considered to be equally effective for BPH. These agents generally
increase urinary flow rates by 2 to 3 mL/s in 60% to 70% of treated
patients, and reduce postvoid residual urine volume. They have no effect on decreasing prostate volume. Terazosin and tamsulosin produce
durable responses for 3 to 4 years, provided that the patient continues
to take the drug.[32,33] A preliminary study of alfuzosin has showed
that α-adrenergic antagonists may lower the incidence of acute urinary retention.[34] Finally, α-adrenergic antagonists do not reduce PSA
levels, preserving the utility of this prostate cancer marker in this
high-risk population.[35]

Second-generation agents include prazosin, terazosin, doxazosin, and alfuzosin. These differ in terms of duration of action
and dosing schedule. Whereas prazosin requires dosing two to three
times a day, terazosin, doxazosin, and alfuzosin offer more convenient once-daily dosing. Prazosin, terazosin, and doxazosin antagonize peripheral vascular α_1-adrenergic receptors, in addition to
those in the prostate, at the usual doses used to treat BPH. As a result, first-dose syncope, orthostatic hypotension, and dizziness are

TABLE 82–4. Dosing Schedule of α-Adrenergic Antagonists in Patients with BPH

Drug	Half-Life (h)	Usual Daily Dosage	Time to Peak Effect on BPH Symptoms[a]
Prazosin (Minipress)	2–3	2–10 mg in two to three divided doses	2–4 weeks
Terazosin (Hytrin)	12	1–10 mg as a single dose; max 20 mg	2–4 weeks
Doxazosin (Cardura)	19–22	1–4 mg as a single dose; max 8 mg	2–4 weeks
Alfuzosin (UroXatral)		10 mg as a single dose	
Tamsulosin (Flomax)	14–15	0.4–0.8 mg as a single dose	1 day

[a]Time to peak effect on BPH symptoms is dependent on the titration period to full therapeutic doses.
This table is adapted with permission from Lee M, Sharifi R. Benign prostatic hyperplasia: Diagnosis and treatment guideline. Ann Pharmacother 1997;31:481–486.

characteristic adverse effects. To improve tolerance to these adverse effects, it is recommended that patients be started with a low dose of 1 mg daily, and slowly titrated up to a full therapeutic dose over several weeks. Additive blood pressure lowering effects commonly occur when these agents are used along with antihypertensive agents, which limits use of these agents in some patients. Because prazosin requires twice- to thrice-daily dosing and has significant cardiovascular adverse effects, it is not recommended in the current American Urological Association Guidelines for treatment of BPH.[13] Finally, it should be noted that an α-adrenergic antagonist is not preferred as single-drug therapy in patients with BPH and hypertension. In one study of men with hypertension, doxazosin produced more congestive heart failure than other antihypertensives.[36,37] Thus it is recommended that in patients with BPH and hypertension that appropriate and separate drug treatment be initiated for each medical condition.

Alfuzosin is considered to be functionally and clinically uroselective in that usual doses used to treat BPH are less likely than other second-generation agents to cause cardiovascular adverse effects in animal or human models.[36] This clinical observation has more often been seen with the once-daily, extended-release formulation of alfuzosin, which is the only commercially available formulation in the United States, as compared to the immediate-release formulation that is dosed three times a day that is available in Europe.[37,38] It has been postulated that this may be due to higher concentrations of alfuzosin achieved in the prostate versus serum after usual doses,[39] decreased blood-brain barrier penetration of alfuzosin,[16] and the absence of high peak serum levels with the extended-release formulation.[40] Extended-release alfuzosin dosing is FDA-approved for 10 mg daily, with no titration increase.[41–43] This is convenient for physician prescribers and patients who are started on the medication.

Tamsulosin is the only third-generation α_{1A}-adrenergic antagonist available in the United States It represents an advance over second-generation agents in that it is selective for prostatic α_{1A}-receptors, which comprise approximately 70% of the adrenergic receptors in the prostate gland.[44,45] Blockade of these receptors results in smooth-muscle relaxation of the prostate and bladder neck without causing peripheral vascular smooth-muscle relaxation. Tamsulosin has low affinity for vascular α_{1B}-receptors, which explains why hypotension is not a common adverse effect and why the agent has not been studied as a therapy for hypertension.

Tamsulosin's selectivity for α_{1A}-receptors has multiple implications. Dose titration is minimal; therefore patients can begin therapy with the lowest effective maintenance dose, 0.4 mg orally once a day. Patients can be instructed to take the dose anytime during the day, unlike terazosin and doxazosin, which should be taken at bedtime. For best effect, tamsulosin should be taken on an empty stomach, as food decreases its bioavailability. The onset of peak action is quicker, in the range of 2 weeks, because only a minority of patients will require a higher daily dose. No decreases in blood pressure or increases in heart rate have been reported in normotensive patients, subgroups of patients with well-controlled hypertension, or those with uncontrolled hypertension.[46,47] Thus tamsulosin allows initiation of treatment with a therapeutic dose that is not limited by cardiovascular adverse effects, unlike terazosin and doxazosin.[48–52] Finally, the addition of tamsulosin to selected antihypertensive regimens of patients does not result in potentiation of the hypotensive effect of furosemide, enalapril, nifedipine, and atenolol.[53] Therefore tamsulosin represents a good choice, particularly when patients cannot tolerate hypotension; have severe coronary artery disease, volume depletion, cardiac arrhythmias, severe orthostasis, or liver failure; are taking multiple antihypertensives; or when the titration would be too complicated for the patient or produce an unacceptable delay in onset for a particular patient.

A summary of the usual doses of α-adrenergic antagonists is included in Table 82–4.

When using the second-generation α_1-adrenergic antagonists terazosin or doxazosin, slow titration up to a therapeutic maintenance dose is necessary to minimize orthostatic hypotension and first-dose syncope. Conservatively, dosage increases should be done in an orderly stepwise process, with dosage increases occurring at 2- to 7-day intervals, depending on the patient's response to the medication. A faster titration schedule can be used as long as the patient does not develop orthostatic hypotension or dizziness. Two sample titration schedules for terazosin are described here:

- Schedule 1: Slow titration

    Days 1 to 3: 1 mg at bedtime
    Days 4 to 14: 2 mg at bedtime
    Weeks 2 to 6: 5 mg at bedtime
    Weeks 7 and on: 10 mg at bedtime

- Schedule 2: Quicker titration

    Days 1 to 3: 1 mg at bedtime
    Days 4 to 14: 2 mg at bedtime
    Weeks 2 to 3: 5 mg at bedtime
    Weeks 4 and on: 10 mg at bedtime

Patients should continue taking the drug as long as they continue to respond to it. If BPH symptoms worsen, the patient should see his physician for a dosage increase or discuss an alternative form of treatment.

No dosage adjustments are recommended for α_1-adrenergic antagonists in patients with renal failure. Because these drugs are hepatically catabolized, the lowest effective dose should be used in patients with hepatic dysfunction, and patients should be monitored carefully for adverse effects. No specific dosing guidelines are yet available in this patient population.[51]

Approximately 10% to 12% of patients discontinue second-generation α_1-adrenergic antagonists because of adverse effects, especially those affecting the cardiovascular system (e.g., syncope, dizziness, and hypotension).[54]

Patients who tolerate hypotension poorly should avoid second-generation α_1-adrenergic antagonists. This includes patients with poorly controlled angina, serious cardiac arrhythmias, patients with reduced circulating volume, and patients on multiple antihypertensives.[52] These patients are candidates for tamsulosin or finasteride, if drug therapy is deemed necessary. Whether extended-release alfuzosin is also a good choice remains to be elucidated in controlled comparison trials with tamsulosin.

Tiredness and asthenia, ejaculatory dysfunction, flu-like symptoms, and nasal congestion are the most common adverse effects of tamsulosin. These adverse effects are unavoidable, but by properly educating the patient, they should not lead to discontinuation of treatment.

Caution is needed when cimetidine or diltiazem is used with tamsulosin or other α-adrenergic antagonists, as a drug-drug interaction leads to decreased metabolism of the latter agents. In contrast, carbamazepine and phenytoin may increase hepatic catabolism of α-adrenergic antagonists.

Sildenafil, vardenafil, and tadalafil may produce systemic hypotension if used in large doses. Therefore package labeling for these drugs includes a warning to avoid α-adrenergic antagonists for 4 hours after taking a dose of one of these phosphodiesterase inhibitors.

CLINICAL CONTROVERSY

Among the α-adrenergic antagonists, tamsulosin and extended-release alfuzosin have been associated with the highest and lowest incidences of ejaculatory dysfunction, respectively. Although some clinicians claim that this difference should be considered when selecting one agent over another, this adverse effect is of variable clinical significance. Some patients may complain of decreased sexual satisfaction because of ejaculatory dysfunction, whereas other patients will not.

COMBINATION THERAPY

Combination therapy with a 5α-reductase inhibitor and an α_1-adrenergic antagonist is ideal in patients with severe symptoms, who also have an enlarged prostate gland of at least 40 to 50 g and an increased PSA level.[13] A regimen of finasteride and doxazosin for 5 years was shown to prevent symptom progression and decrease the risk of developing acute urinary retention, urinary tract infection, and the need for prostate surgery.[55] Although not proven by direct comparison trials, it is probable that any combination of 5α-reductase inhibitor and α_1-adrenergic antagonist is similarly effective.[13] The disadvantages of a combination regimen include increased cost to the patient and increased incidence of adverse drug effects.

SURGICAL INTERVENTION

The gold standard for treatment of patients with complications of BPH is prostatectomy performed either transurethrally or suprapubically.[15,56] Surgical intervention is also used in patients who are not responsive to drug therapy, those who are noncompliant with

drug therapy, or those who prefer surgical intervention. Surgical removal of the prostate offers the highest rate of symptom improvement, but it also has the highest complication rate.

With transurethral resection of the prostate (TURP), an endoscopic resectoscope inserted through the urethra is used to remove the inside core of the prostate. This enlarges the urethral opening at the bladder neck. TURP is performed only in men with enlarged prostates that are less than 50 g so that the resection can be completed in less than 1 hour. Often performed as outpatient surgery, this procedure produces on average a peak urinary flow increase of 125% and improvement of voiding symptoms by almost 90% in approximately 90% of patients.[6] A common complication of TURP is retrograde ejaculation, occurring in up to 75% of patients. Significant bleeding, urinary incontinence, and erectile dysfunction occur in smaller but significant numbers of patients (2% to 15%).[57,58] Approximately 12% to 15% of patients require second surgeries within 8 years.[56]

Men with larger prostates (>50 g) require an open surgical procedure (open prostatectomy), which can be performed retro- or suprapubically. This necessitates hospitalization for at least a few days, anesthesia, and a longer recuperation time. Adverse effects of open prostatectomy include bleeding, urinary and soft tissue infection, retrograde ejaculation in 77% of patients, erectile dysfunction in 16% to 33% of patients, and urinary incontinence in 2% of patients. The reoperation rate is 3% to 5% at 10 years.[56]

Prostatectomy is ineffective for relieving irritative voiding symptoms of BPH because prostatectomy does not affect the detrusor muscle of the bladder.[59] These patients may respond to oral anticholinergic agents (e.g., oxybutynin or L-hyoscyamine), which improve bladder compliance and decrease detrusor muscle irritability, as discussed in Chap. 83.

A new trend in surgical treatment is use of less invasive or minimally invasive outpatient surgical procedures to remove excessive prostate tissue.[6] These procedures use an energy source, (e.g., heat, cold, or laser) to eliminate excessive prostate tissue, characteristically are short (lasting minutes), have a lower potential to produce adverse effects, are less expensive than continuous drug therapy lasting years, and may be particularly useful in debilitated patients. One significant disadvantage of all minimally invasive surgical procedures is that many patients may require retreatment after an initial improvement in symptoms.[60] Of the procedures available, only transurethral incision of the prostate (TUIP) has been thoroughly evaluated. This procedure is ideal for patients with moderate or severe BPH symptoms who have an enlarged prostate gland less than 30 g in size. TUIP is as effective as TURP, but requires less operation time, causes less blood loss, and produces fewer adverse effects.[61,62] TUIP involves making two to three incisions at the bladder neck to widen the opening. These incisions are made using an endoscopic resectoscope.

Other minimally invasive surgical procedures include visual laser ablation of the prostate (VLAP), transurethral electrovaporization of the prostate (TUVP), transurethral needle ablation of the prostate (TUNA), and transurethral microwave thermotherapy of the prostate (TUMT).[8,63]

PHYTOTHERAPY

Although phytotherapy is widely used in Europe for the management of BPH, the published data on herbal agents are largely inconclusive and conflicting. Studies often lack placebo controls, which are essential in assessing treatments for BPH because spontaneous regression of symptoms can occur. Furthermore, as these agents are marketed under the Dietary Supplements Health and Education Act, their efficacy, safety, and quality are not regulated by the FDA. For these reasons, herbal products—including saw palmetto berry (*Serenoa repens*),[64-67] stinging nettle (*Urtica dioica*),[68] and African plum (*Pygeum africanum*)[69]—are not recommended for BPH.[13] An excellent review on phytotherapy for BPH has been published.[70]

EVALUATION OF THERAPEUTIC OUTCOMES

The primary therapeutic outcome of BPH therapy is restoration of adequate urinary flow without adverse effects. As a disease in which therapy is directed at those symptoms the patient finds most bothersome, assessment of outcomes likewise depends on how the patient perceives the effectiveness and acceptability of therapy. Use of a validated, standardized instrument, such as the AUA Symptom Index, for assessing patient quality of life is important in this process.[2,9,12,13]

In patients being treated with pharmacotherapy, objective measures of bladder emptying are also useful at an appropriate time after drug therapy begins (6 to 12 months for 5α-reductase inhibitors, 3 to 4 weeks after the start of α1-adrenergic antagonists). These include the uroflowmeter and PVR urine volume, as described in the section on diagnostic evaluation section in this chapter.

Key laboratory tests to monitor on an ongoing basis are serum BUN and creatinine and urinalysis. Because this patient population is at high risk for prostate cancer, PSA should be measured and a digital rectal examination performed annually. For patients taking 5α-reductase inhibitors, PSA must be compared with baseline and 6-month responses, as described in the section on 5α-reductase inhibitor.

SUMMARY

A ubiquitous disease of aging men, symptomatic BPH requires medical attention to preserve patient quality of life and avoid complications, many of which can be life-threatening in this patient population. In men who have no or minor symptoms, watchful waiting is the therapeutic option of choice, as BPH remains stable or even regresses in about one-half of these men.

For those with moderate to severe symptoms but no complications, pharmacotherapy is indicated. An α1-adrenergic antagonist is the agent of first choice. Second-generation agents including terazosin, doxazosin, or alfuzosin are also useful. Terazosin and doxazosin cause more cardiovascular adverse effects than extended-release alfuzosin and tamsulosin. Whether extended-release alfuzosin is as well tolerated as tamsulosin in patients at risk of hypotension or hypotension-related morbidity remains to be elucidated. 5α-Reductase inhibitors are preferred drug treatment in patients with enlarged prostates, who are likely to poorly tolerate the hypotensive adverse effects of α1 adrenergic antagonists (Table 82-5). However, 5α-reductase inhibitors have a slow onset of action. For patients who fail monotherapy, combination drug therapy could be attempted and such regimens have been found to be most effective in patients with enlarged prostates greater than 40 g. Alternatively, surgery is an option.

In patients who have complications of BPH, surgery is required. Although it has more adverse complications than does pharmacotherapy or watchful waiting, transurethral resection of the prostate is considered the gold standard.

ACKNOWLEDGMENT

Some portions of this chapter were adapted with permission from Lee M. Health issues in the elderly male. In: Pharmacotherapy Self-Assessment Program Module 6, Respiratory and Endocrinology, 3rd ed. Kansas City, MO, American College of Clinical Pharmacy, 1999:181–207.

ABBREVIATIONS

AUA: American Urological Association
BPH: benign prostatic hyperplasia
BUN: blood urea nitrogen
DHT: dihydrotestosterone
LUTS: lower urinary tract symptoms
PSA: prostate-specific antigen
PVR: postvoid residual
TUIP: transurethral incision of the prostate
TUMT: transurethral microwave thermotherapy of the prostate
TUNA: transurethral needle ablation of the prostate
TURP: transurethral resection of the prostate
TUVP: transurethral electrovaporization of the prostate
VLAP: visual laser ablation of the prostate

Review Questions and other resources can be found at *www.pharmacotherapyonline.com*.

TABLE 82–5. Comparison of 5α-Reductase Inhibitors and α-Adrenergic Antagonists

	5α-Reductase Inhibitors	α-Adrenergic Antagonists
Decreases prostate size	Yes	No
Peak onset	3–6 months	1–6 weeks
Efficacy	++ (in patients with enlarged prostates)	++
Frequency of dosing	Once a day	1–2 times a day, depending on the agent
Decreases prostate-specific antigen	Yes	No
Sexual dysfunction	++	+
Cardiovascular adverse effects	No	Yes

REFERENCES

1. Glynn RJ, Campion EW, Bouchard GR, Silbert JE. The development of benign prostatic hyperplasia among volunteers in the normative aging study. Am J Epidemiol 1985;131:79–90.
2. Roehrborn CG. The Agency for Health Care Policy and Research Clinical guidelines for the diagnosis and treatment of BPH. Urol Clin North Am 1995;22:445–453.
3. Uzzo RG, Herzlinger D, Vaughan D. Prostate development: hormonal and cellular considerations. American Urological Association Update Series 1996;15:1.

. Steers WD. 5α reductase activity in the prostate. Urology 2001;58(Suppl 1):17–24.

. Walsh PC. The role of estrogen/androgen synergism in the pathogenesis of benign prostatic hyperplasia. J Urol 1988;139:826.

. Tammela T. Benign prostatic hyperplasia: Practical treatment guidelines. Drugs Aging 1997;10:349–366.

. Barry MJ. Epidemiology and natural history of benign prostatic hyperplasia. Urol Clin North Am 1990;17:495–507.

. Thorpe A, Neal D. Benign prostatic hyperplasia. Lancet 2003;361: 1359–1367.

. Girman C, Panser L, Chute C, et al. Natural history of prostatism: Urinary flow rates in a community-based study. J Urol 1993;150:887–892.

. Marberger MJ, Andersen JT, Nickel JC, et al. Prostate volume and serum prostate specific antigen as predictors of acute urinary retention. Combined experience from three large multicenter national placebo-controlled trials. Eur Urol 2000;38:563–568.

. Jacobsen SJ, Jacobson DJ, Girman CJ, et al. Treatment for benign prostatic hyperplasia among community dwelling men: The Olmsted County Study of urinary symptoms and health status. J Urol 1999;162:1301–1306.

. U.S. Department of Health and Human Services Public Health Service Agency for Health Care Policy and Research. Clinical practice guideline number 8. Benign prostatic hyperplasia: Diagnosis and treatment. Rockville, MD, U.S. Department of Health and Human Services, 1994: 1–215.

. American Urological Association Practice Guidelines Committee. AUA guidelines on management of benign prostatic hyperplasia (2003). Chapter 1: Diagnosis and treatment recommendations. J Urol 2003;170:530–547.

. Desgrandchamps F. Importance of individual response in symptom score evaluation. Eur Urol 2001;40(Suppl 3):2–7.

. Wasson JH, Reda DJ, Bruskewitz RC, et al, for the Veterans Affairs Cooperative Study Group on Transurethral Resection of the Prostate. A comparison of transurethral surgery with watchful waiting for moderate symptoms of benign prostatic hyperplasia. N Engl J Med 1995;332:75–79.

. Dutkiewics S. Efficacy and tolerability of drugs for treatment of benign prostatic hyperplasia. Int Urol Nephrol 2001;32:423–432.

. Lepor H, Williford WO, Barry MJ, et al. The impact of medical therapy on bother due to symptoms, quality of life and global outcome, and factors predicting response. Veterans Affairs Cooperative Studies Benign Prostatic Hyperplasia Study Group. J Urol 1998;160:1358–1367.

. Kirby RS, Roehrborn C, Boyle P, et al. Efficacy and tolerability of doxazosin and finasteride alone or in combination in treatment of symptomatic benign prostatic hyperplasia—the Prospective European Doxazosin Combination Therapy (PREDICT) Trial. Urology 2003;61:119–126.

. Roehrborn CG, McConnell J, Bonilla J, et al. Serum prostate specific antigen is a strong predictor of future prostate growth in men with benign prostatic hyperplasia—Proscar long term efficacy and safety study. J Urol 2000;163:13–20.

. Lepor H, Williford WO, Barry MJ, et al, for the Veterans Affairs Cooperative Studies Benign Prostatic Hyperplasia Study Group. The efficacy of terazosin, finasteride, or both in benign prostatic hyperplasia. N Engl J Med 1996;335:533–539.

. Anonymous. Dutasteride (Avodart) for benign prostatic hyperplasia. Med Lett Drugs Ther 2002;44:109–110.

. Boyle P, Gould AL, Roehrborn CG. Prostate volume predicts outcome of treatment of benign prostatic hyperplasia with finasteride: Meta-analysis of randomized clinical trials. Urology 1996;48:398–405.

. McConnell JD, Bruskewitz R, Walsh P, et al, for the Finasteride Long-Term Efficacy and Safety Study Group. The effect of finasteride on the risk of acute urinary retention and the need for surgical treatment among men with benign prostatic hyperplasia. N Engl J Med 1998;338:557–563.

. Wasson JH. Finasteride to prevent morbidity from benign prostatic hyperplasia. N Engl J Med 1998;338:612–613.

. Andersen JT, Nickel JC, Marshall VR, et al. Finasteride significantly reduces acute urinary retention and need for surgery in patients with symptomatic benign prostatic hyperplasia. Urology 1997;49:839–845.

. Marberger MJ on behalf of the Prowess Study Group. Long-term effects of finasteride in patients with benign prostatic hyperplasia: A double-blind, placebo-controlled, multicenter study. Urology 1998;51:677–686.

27. Rittmaster RS. Finasteride. N Engl J Med 1994;330:120–125.

28. Park KH, Kim SW, Kim KD, et al. Effects of androgens on the expression of nitric oxide synthase mRNA in rat corpus cavernosum. BJU Int 1999;83:327–333.

29. Rosen R, O'Leary M, Altwein J, et al. Ejaculatory disorders are frequent and bothersome in aging males with LUTS: A worldwide survey (MSAM-7). J Urol 2003;169(Suppl 1):365 (abstract).

30. Pannek J, Marks LS, Pearson JD, et al. Influence of finasteride on free and total serum prostate specific antigen levels in men with benign prostatic hyperplasia. J Urol 1998;159:449–453.

31. Caine P, Perlberg S, Shapiro A. Phenoxybenzamine for benign prostatic obstruction. Urology 1981;17:542–546.

32. Lepor H for the Terazosin Research Group. Long-term efficacy and safety of terazosin in patients with benign prostatic hyperplasia. Urology 1995;45:406–413.

33. Schulman CC, Lock TMTW, Buzelin JM, and the European Tamsulosin Study Group. Tamsulosin: 3-Year follow-up of efficacy and safety in 516 patients with LUTS suggestive of BPO. J Urology 1998;159:256 (Abstract #983).

34. Lukacs B, Grange JC, Comet D, et al, for the BPH Group in General Practice. Three year prospective study of 3,228 clinical BPH patients treated with alfuzosin in general practice. Prostate Cancer Prostatic Dis 1998;5:276–283.

35. Roehrborn CG, Oesterling JE, Olson PJ, Padley RJ, for the HYCAT Investigator Group. Serial prostate-specific antigen measurements in men with clinically benign prostatic hyperplasia during a 12-month placebo-controlled study with terazosin. Urology 1997;50:556–561.

36. Djavan B, Marberger M. A meta analysis on the efficacy and tolerability of α₁ adrenoceptor antagonists in patients with lower urinary tract symptoms suggestive of benign prostatic obstruction. Eur Urol 1999;36: 1–13.

37. ALLHAT Officers and Coordinators for the ALLHAT Collaborative Research Group. Major cardiovascular events in hypertensive patients randomized to doxazosin vs chlorthalidone: The antihypertensive and lipid-lowering treatment to prevent heart attack trial (ALLHAT). JAMA 2000;288:2981–2997.

38. vanKerrebroeck P, Jardin A, Laval KU, et al. Efficacy and safety of a new prolonged release formulation of alfuzosin 10 mg once daily versus alfuzosin 2.5 mg thrice daily and placebo in patients with symptoms of benign prostatic hyperplasia. Eur Urol 2000;37:306–313.

39. Mottet N, Bressolle F, Delmas V, et al. Prostatic tissue distribution of alfuzosin in patients with benign prostatic hyperplasia following repeated oral administration. Eur Urol 2003;44:101–105.

40. Roehrborn CG. Efficacy and safety of once daily alfuzosin in the treatment of lower urinary tract symptoms and clinical benign prostatic hyperplasia: A randomized, placebo-controlled trial. Urology 2001;58:953–959.

41. McKeage K, Plosker GL. Alfuzosin. Drugs 2002;62:633–653.

42. Roehrborn CG. Are all α-blockers created equal? An update. Urology 2002;59(Suppl 2A):3–6.

43. Roehrborn CG for the ALFUS Study Group. Efficacy and safety of once daily alfuzosin in the treatment of lower urinary tract symptoms and clinical benign prostatic hyperplasia: A randomized placebo-controlled trial. Urology 2001;58:953–959.

44. Chapple CR, Burt RP, Andersson PO, et al. α-1-Adrenoreceptor subtypes in the human prostate. Br J Urol 1994;74:585–589.

45. Chapple CR. Pharmacotherapy for benign prostatic hyperplasia—The potential for α1-adrenoceptor subtype-specific blockade. Br J Urol 1998;81(Suppl):34–47.

46. Chapple CR, Wyndaele JJ, Nordling J, et al, on behalf of the European Tamsulosin Study Group. Tamsulosin, the first prostate selective alpha-1A-adrenoreceptor antagonist. Eur Urol 1996;29:155–167.

47. Lowe FC. Coadministration of tamsulosin and three antihypertensive agents in patients with benign prostatic hyperplasia: Pharmacodynamic effect. Clin Ther 1997;19:730–742.

48. Lee E, Lee C. Clinical comparison of selective and non-selective α1-adrenoreceptor antagonists in benign prostatic hyperplasia: Studies on tamsulosin in a fixed dose and terazosin in increasing doses. Br J Urol 1997;80:606–611.

49. Djavan B, Marberger M. A meta-analysis on the efficacy and tolerability of $\alpha 1$ adrenoceptor antagonists in patients with lower urinary tract symptoms suggestive of benign prostatic obstruction. Eur Urol 1999;36:1–13.

50. Fulton B, Wagstaff AJ, Sorkin EM. Doxazosin. Drugs 1995;49:295–320.

51. Wilde MI, McTavish D. Tamsulosin. Drugs 1996;52:883–898.

52. DeMey C, Michel MC, McEwen J, Moreland T. A double-blind comparison of terazosin and tamsulosin on their differential effects on ambulatory blood pressure and nocturnal orthostatic stress testing. Eur Urol 1998;33:481–488.

53. DeMey C. Cardiovascular effects of alpha-blockers used for the treatment of symptomatic BPH: Impact on safety and well being. Eur Urol 1998;34(Suppl 2):18–28.

54. Kaplan SA, D'Alisera PM. Tolerability of α-blockade with doxazosin as a therapeutic option for symptomatic benign prostatic hyperplasia in the elderly patient: A pooled analysis of seven double-blind, placebo-controlled studies. J Gerontol 1998;53A:M201–M206.

55. McConnell JD for the MTOPS Steering Committee. The long term effects of medical therapy on the progression of BPH: Results from the MTOPS trial. J Urol 2002;167:1042.

56. Roos NP, Ramsey EW. A population based study of prostatectomy: Outcomes associated with different surgical procedures. J Urol 1987;37:1184–1187.

57. Mebust WK, Holtgrewe HL, Cockett AT, et al. Transurethral prostatectomy: Immediate and postoperative complications. A cooperative study of 13 participating institutions evaluating 3,885 patients. J Urol 1989;141:243–247.

58. Kassabian VS. Sexual function in patients treated for benign prostatic hyperplasia. Lancet 2003;361:60–62.

59. Kuo HC, Chang SC, Hsu T. Predictive factors for successful surgical outcome of benign prostatic hypertrophy. Eur Urol 1993;24:12–16.

60. Tanuguntla HS, Evans CP. Minimally invasive therapies for benign prostatic hyperplasia. World J Urol 2002;20:197–206.

61. Hellstrom P, Lukkarinen O, Kontturi M. Bladder neck incision or transurethral electroresection for the treatment of urinary obstruction caused by small prostate? A randomized urodynamic study. Scand J Urol Nephrol 1986;20:187–192.

62. Christensen MM, Aagaard J, Madsen PO. Transurethral resection versus transurethral incision of the prostate: A prospective randomized study. Urol Clin North Am 1990;17:621–630.

63. Blute ML, Larson T. Minimally invasive therapies for benign prostatic hyperplasia. Urology 2001;58(Suppl 6a):33–41.

64. Debruyne F, Koch G, Boyle P, et al. Comparison of phytotherapeutic agent (Permixon) with an α-blocker (tamsulosin) in the treatment of benign prostatic hyperplasia: A 1-year randomized international study. Eur Urol 2002;41:497–507.

65. Gerber GS, Kuznetsov D, Johnson BC, et al. Randomized double blind controlled trial of saw palmetto in men with lower urinary tract symptoms. Urology 2001;58:960–964.

66. Marks LS, Tyler VE. Saw palmetto extract: Newest (and oldest) treatment alternative for men with symptomatic benign prostatic hyperplasia. Urology 1999;53:457–461.

67. Wilt TJ, Ishani A, Stark G, et al. Saw palmetto extracts for treatment of benign prostatic hyperplasia. JAMA 1998;280:1604–1609.

68. Wagner H, Flachsbarth H, Vogel G. A new antiprostatic principal of stinging nettle (*Urtica dioica*) roots. Phytomedicine 1994;1:213–224.

69. Andro MC, Riffaud JP. *Pygeum africanum* extract for the treatment of patients with benign prostatic hyperplasia: A review of 25 years of published experience. Curr Ther Res 1995;56:796–817.

70. Lowe FC, Fagelman E. Phytotherapy in the treatment of benign prostatic hyperplasia: An update. Urology 1999;53:671–678.

83

URINARY INCONTINENCE

Eric S. Rovner, Jean Wyman, Thomas Lackner, and David Guay

Learning Objectives and other resources can be found at *www.pharmacotherapyonline.com.*

KEY CONCEPTS

1 In evaluating urinary incontinence, drug-induced or drug-aggravated etiologies must be ruled out.

2 Accurate diagnosis and classification of urinary incontinence type is critical to the selection of appropriate pharmacotherapy.

3 Nonpharmacologic therapy is the cornerstone of management of urinary incontinence, should be the first therapy initiated, and should be continued even if drug therapy must be initiated.

4 Anticholinergic/antispasmodic agents are the therapies of choice for bladder overactivity (urge incontinence).

5 Duloxetine (when approved for treatment of urinary incontinence), α-adrenergic receptor agonists, and topical (vaginal) estrogens (alone or together) are the therapies of choice in urethral underactivity (stress incontinence).

6 Patient-specific treatment goals should be identified. They are not static and may change over time. Choice of therapy may also be influenced by characteristics such as patient age, comorbidities, concurrent medications, and ability to adhere to the prescribed regimen. If therapeutic goals are not achieved with a given agent at optimal dosage, consider adding a second agent or switching to an alternative single agent.

Urinary incontinence (UI) is defined as the complaint of involuntary leakage of urine.[1] It is frequently accompanied by other bothersome lower urinary tract symptoms such as urgency, increased daytime frequency, and nocturia. It is a common yet underdetected and underreported health problem that can significantly affect quality of life. Patients with UI may have depression as a result of the perceived lack of self-control, loss of independence, and lack of self-esteem, and they often curtail their activities for fear of an "accident." It may also have serious medical and economic ramifications for untreated or undertreated patients, including perineal dermatitis, worsening of pressure ulcers, urinary tract infections, and falls.

This chapter highlights the epidemiology, etiology, pathophysiology, and treatment of stress, urge, mixed, and overflow UI in men and women.

EPIDEMIOLOGY

Determining the true prevalence of UI is difficult because of problems with definition, reporting bias, and other methodologic issues.[2] Epidemiologic studies have not historically used a standard definition of the condition or a standard methodology for data recording, with some studies including "postvoid dribbling," while other studies specify "urinary leakage causing a social or hygienic problem." The number of people suffering with UI is certainly great, and the impact of this condition is substantial, crossing all racial, ethnic, and geographic boundaries. Compared with continent controls, patients with UI have an overall poorer quality of life.[3] Several studies have objectively shown that UI is associated with reduced levels of social and personal activities, increased psychological distress, and overall decreased quality of life as measured by numerous indices.[4,5] The condition can affect people of all age groups but the peak incidence of UI, at least in women, appears to occur around the age of menopause, with a slight decrease in the age group 55 to 60 years, and then a steadily increasing prevalence after age 65.

One of the earliest comprehensive epidemiologic studies on UI was conducted by Diokno and colleagues using a standardized survey questionnaire.[6] The Medical, Epidemiologic, and Social Aspects of Aging survey found that the prevalence of UI in noninstitutionalized women 60 years of age and older was approximately 38%. Almost one-third of those surveyed noted urine loss at least once weekly and 16% noted UI daily. A recent publication from a National Institutes of Health working group conference estimated the median level of UI prevalence to be approximately 20% to 30% during young adult life, with a broad peak around middle age (30% to 40% prevalence) which increases in the elderly (30% to 50% prevalence).[7]

In the United States, chronic UI is one of the most common reasons cited for institutionalization of the elderly, and the condition is frequently encountered in the nursing home setting.[8] Little is known about the basic differences in clinical and epidemiologic characteristics of incontinence across racial or ethnic groups.

Some studies report a higher incidence of UI overall in white populations[9,10] as compared to African-Americans, but differences in access to health care as well as cultural attitudes and mores may contribute to these differences.

Consistent across all studies in unselected, noninstitutionalized populations, is the fact that UI is at least half as common in men as in women.[11,12] Overall, the prevalence of UI in men has been recently estimated to be about 9%.[13] Unlike in women, the prevalence of UI in men increases with age across most studies, with the highest prevalence recorded in the oldest patient cohorts.[13]

ETIOLOGY AND PATHOPHYSIOLOGY

ANATOMY

The lower urinary tract consists of the bladder, urethra, urinary or urethral sphincter, and the surrounding musculofascial structures including connective tissue, nerves, and blood vessels. The urinary bladder is a hollow organ composed of smooth muscle and connective tissue located deep in the bony pelvis in men and women. The urethra is a hollow tube that acts as a conduit for urine flow out of the bladder. The interior surface of both the bladder and urethra is lined by an epithelial cell layer termed *transitional epithelium,* which is in constant contact with urine. Previously considered inert and inactive, transitional epithelium may actually play an active role in the pathophysiology of many lower urinary tract disorders, including interstitial cystitis and UI. The urinary or urethral sphincter is a combination of smooth and striated muscle within and surrounding the most proximal portion of the urethra adjacent to the bladder in both men and women. This is a functional but not anatomic sphincter that includes a portion of the bladder neck or outlet as well as the proximal urethra.

URINARY CONTINENCE

To prevent incontinence during the bladder filling and storage phase of the micturition cycle, the urethra, or more accurately the urethral sphincter, must maintain adequate resistance to the flow of urine from the bladder at all times until voluntary voiding is initiated. Urethral resistance or closure is maintained to a large degree by the proximal (under involuntary control) and distal (under both voluntary and involuntary control) urinary sphincters, a combination of smooth and striated muscles within and external to the urethra. Variable contributions to urethral resistance may also come from the urethral mucosa, submucosal spongy tissue, and the overall length of the urethra. During bladder filling and storage, the bladder accommodates increasing volumes of urine flowing in from the upper urinary tract without a significant increase in bladder (intravesical) pressure. In addition, bladder or detrusor smooth muscle activity is normally suppressed during the filling phase by centrally mediated neural reflexes. Normal bladder emptying occurs with a decrease in urethral resistance concomitant with a volitional bladder contraction. The bladder contraction occurs in a coordinated fashion, resulting in a rise in intravesical pressure. The rise in intravesical pressure is ideally of adequate magnitude and duration to empty the bladder to completion. A concomitant decrease in urethral resistance and funneling of the bladder outlet results in opening of the functional urinary sphincters and urine flow into the urethra until the bladder is emptied completely.

The primary motor input to the detrusor muscle of the bladder is along the pelvic nerves emanating from spinal cord segments S_2 to S_4. Parasympathetic impulses travel to the bladder along the efferent fibers of the pelvic nerves. The impulses pass through ganglia situated in the bladder wall before reaching their target. Acetylcholine appears to be the primary neurotransmitter at the neuromuscular junction in the human lower urinary tract. Both volitional and involuntary contractions of the detrusor muscle are mediated by activation of postsynaptic muscarinic receptors by acetylcholine. Of the five known subtypes of muscarinic receptors, bladder smooth-muscle cholinergic receptors are mainly of the M_2 variety. However, M_3 receptors are responsible for both the emptying contraction of normal micturition, as well as involuntary bladder contractions that may result in UI.[14] Thus most pharmacologic antimuscarinic therapy is primarily anti-M_3–based (see discussion below).

The bladder and urethra normally operate in unison during the bladder filling and storage phase, as well as the bladder emptying phase of the micturition cycle. The smooth and striated muscles of the bladder and urethra are organized during the micturition cycle by a number of reflexes coordinated at the pontine micturition center in the midbrain. Disturbances in the neural regulation of micturition at any level (brain, spinal cord, or pelvic nerves) often lead to characteristic changes in lower urinary tract function that may result in UI.

MECHANISMS OF URINARY INCONTINENCE

Simply stated, UI may occur only as a result of abnormalities of the urethra (including the bladder outlet and urinary sphincter) or the bladder, or from a combination of abnormalities of both structures. Abnormalities may result in either overfunction or underfunction of the bladder and/or urethra with the resulting development of UI. While this simple classification scheme excludes extremely rare causes of UI such as congenital ectopic ureters and urinary fistulas, it is useful in gaining a working understanding of the condition.

Urethral Underactivity (Stress Urinary Incontinence)

Some patients characteristically note UI during exertional activities such as exercise, running, lifting, coughing, and sneezing. This implies that the compromised urethral sphincter is no longer able to resist the flow of urine from the bladder during periods of physical activity. In essence, increases in intra-abdominal pressure during physical activity are transmitted to the bladder (an intra-abdominal organ), compressing it and forcing urine through the weakened sphincter.

This type of UI is known as *stress urinary incontinence* (SUI). Although the exact etiology of urethral underactivity and SUI in the woman is incompletely understood, clearly identifiable risk factors include pregnancy, childbirth, menopause, cognitive impairment, obesity, and age.[16,17] The prevalence of SUI in women appears to peak during or after the onset of menopause. This implies that hormonal factors are important in maintaining continence.

In men, SUI is most commonly the result of prior lower urinary tract surgery or injury, with resulting compromise of the sphincter mechanism within and external to the urethra. Radical prostatectomy for treatment of adenocarcinoma of the prostate is probably the most common setting in which surgical manipulation leads to UI. Overall SUI in the male is uncommon, and in the absence of prior prostate surgery, severe trauma, or neurologic illness, is extraordinarily rare. Transurethral resection of the prostate for benign prostatic hyperplasia (see Chap. 82) may also lead to SUI in men.

Bladder Overactivity (Urge Urinary Incontinence)

Bladder overactivity—including bladder filling and urinary storage characterized by involuntary bladder contractions—is termed *urge urinary incontinence* (UUI). Symptoms of bladder overactivity occur because the detrusor muscle is overactive and contracts inappropriately during the filling phase.

The symptoms caused by the overactive bladder are typically urinary frequency, urgency, and urge incontinence. Frequency is defined as emptying the bladder more often than eight times per day. Urgency is described as a sudden, strong desire to urinate. People suffering from bladder overactivity typically have to empty their bladders frequently, and when they experience a sensation of urgency, they may leak urine if they are unable to reach the toilet quickly or if the sensation of urgency is very strong. Many patients may also have associated nocturia (>2 micturitions per night) and/or nocturnal incontinence (enuresis).

The amount of urine lost may be large, as the bladder may empty completely. Sleep may be disturbed, as the need to void may be experienced during the night. Nocturia and enuresis are often particularly disruptive.

Most patients with overactive bladder and UUI have no identifiable underlying etiology. In fact, the most common cause of bladder overactivity and UUI is "idiopathic." Clearly identifiable risk factors for UUI include normal aging, neurologic disease (including stroke, Parkinson's disease, multiple sclerosis, and spinal cord injury), and bladder outlet obstruction (e.g., due to benign prostatic hyperplasia [BPH] or prostate cancer).

The mechanism for bladder overactivity must be either neurogenic or myogenic. The neurogenic hypothesis ascribes the overactive bladder and UUI to disease-related changes within the central or peripheral nervous system.[18] The myogenic hypothesis states that overactive bladder and UUI result from changes within the smooth muscle of the bladder wall itself.[19] Precipitating factors such as bladder outlet obstruction can cause a partial denervation of smooth muscle, leading to a state of decreased responsiveness to activation of intrinsic nerves, but supersensitivity to contractile agonists and direct electrical activation.[20] However, in practice, UUI is difficult to categorize as either neurogenic or myogenic in origin, as these etiologies often seem to be interconnected and complementary.

Urethral Overactivity and/or Bladder Underactivity (Overflow Incontinence)

Overflow incontinence, the result of urethral overactivity and bladder underactivity, is an important but uncommon type of UI in both men and women. Overflow incontinence results when the bladder is filled to capacity at all times but is unable to empty, causing urine to leak from a distended bladder past a normal outlet and sphincter.

In the setting of urethral overactivity, the resistance to the flow of urine during volitional voiding is increased, resulting in functional or anatomic obstruction and incomplete bladder emptying. Common causes of urethral overactivity in men include BPH and prostate cancer. In women, urethral overactivity is rare, but may result from cystocele formation, or surgical overcorrection (iatrogenic obstruction) following anti-SUI surgery. In both sexes, overflow UI may be associated with systemic neurologic dysfunction or diseases, such as spinal cord injury or multiple sclerosis.

Bladder underactivity may also result in overflow incontinence. Under certain circumstances, the detrusor muscle of the bladder may become progressively weakened and eventually lose the ability to voluntarily contract. In the absence of adequate contractility, the bladder is unable to empty completely, and large volumes of residual urine are left after micturition. Both myogenic and neurogenic factors have been implicated in producing the impaired contractility seen in this condition. Clinically, overflow incontinence is most commonly seen in the setting of long-term chronic bladder outlet obstruction in the male such as that due to BPH or prostate cancer.

Mixed Incontinence and Other Types of Urinary Incontinence

Various types of UI may coexist in the same patient. The combination of bladder overactivity and urethral underactivity is termed *mixed incontinence*. This is often a difficult diagnosis to make because of the often-confusing array of presenting symptoms. Bladder overactivity may also coexist with impaired bladder contractility. This is most common in the elderly and is termed *detrusor hyperactivity with impaired contractility*.[21]

Functional incontinence is not caused by bladder- or urethra-specific factors. Rather, in patients with conditions such as dementia or cognitive or mobility deficits, the UI is linked to the primary disease process more than any extrinsic or intrinsic deficit of the lower urinary tract. An example of functional incontinence occurs in the postoperative orthopedic surgery patient. Following extensive orthopedic reconstructions such as total hip arthroplasty, patients are often immobile secondary to pain or traction. Therefore the patient may be unable to access toileting facilities in a reasonable period of time and may become incontinent as a result. The treatment of this type of UI may involve only placing a urinal or commode at the bedside that allows for simplified access to toileting.

Finally, many localized or systemic illnesses may also result in UI because of their effects on the lower urinary tract or the surrounding structures, including:

- Dementia/delirium
- Depression
- Urinary tract infection (cystitis)
- Postmenopausal atrophic urethritis or vaginitis
- Diabetes mellitus
- Neurologic disease (e.g., stroke, Parkinson's disease, multiple sclerosis, or spinal cord injury)
- Pelvic malignancy
- Constipation
- Congenital malformations

 Many commonly used medications may also precipitate or aggravate existing voiding dysfunction and UI (Table 83–1).

TABLE 83–1. Medications Influencing Lower Urinary Tract Function

Medication	Effect
Diuretics	Polyuria, frequency, urgency
α-Receptor antagonists	Urethral relaxation and stress urinary incontinence in women
α-Receptor agonists	Urethral constriction and urinary retention in men
Calcium channel blockers	Urinary retention
Narcotic analgesics	Urinary retention from impaired contractility
Sedative hypnotics	Functional incontinence caused by delirium, immobility
Antipsychotics	Anticholinergic effects and urinary retention
Anticholinergics	Urinary retention
Antidepressants, tricyclic	Anticholinergic effects, α-antagonist effects
Alcohol	Polyuria, frequency, urgency, sedation, delirium
Angiotensin-converting enzyme inhibitors (ACEIs)	Cough as a result of ACEIs may aggravate stress urinary incontinence by increasing intra-abdominal pressure

CLINICAL PRESENTATION OF URINARY INCONTINENCE RELATED TO URETHRAL UNDERACTIVITY

GENERAL

The patient usually notes UI during activities like exercise, running, lifting, coughing, or sneezing. Much more common in females (seen only in males with lower urinary tract surgery or injury compromising the sphincter).

SYMPTOMS

Urine leakage with physical activity (volume is proportional to activity level). No UI with physical inactivity, especially when supine (no nocturia). May develop urgency and frequency as a compensatory mechanism (or as a separate component of bladder overactivity).

DIAGNOSTIC TESTS

Observation of urethral meatus while patient coughs or strains.

CLINICAL PRESENTATION OF URINARY INCONTINENCE RELATED TO BLADDER OVERACTIVITY

GENERAL

Can have bladder overactivity and UI without urgency if sensory input from the lower urinary tract is absent.

SYMPTOMS

Urinary frequency (>8 micturitions/day), urgency with or without urge incontinence; nocturia (≥2 micturitions/night) and enuresis may be present as well.

DIAGNOSTIC TESTS

Urodynamic studies are the gold standard for diagnosis. Also urinalysis and urine culture should be negative (rule out urinary tract infection as cause of frequency).

CLINICAL PRESENTATION OF URINARY INCONTINENCE RELATED TO URETHRAL OVERACTIVITY AND/OR BLADDER UNDERACTIVITY

GENERAL

Important but rare type of UI in both sexes. Urethral overactivity usually due to prostatic enlargement (males) or cystocele formation or surgical overcorrection following antiurethral underactivity (stress incontinence) surgery (females).

SYMPTOMS

Lower abdominal fullness, hesitancy, straining to void, decreased force of stream, interrupted stream, sense of incomplete bladder emptying. May have urinary frequency and urgency, too. Abdominal pain if acute urinary retention is also present.

SIGNS

Increased postvoid residual urine volume.

DIAGNOSTIC TESTS

Digital rectal exam or transrectal ultrasound to rule out prostatic enlargement. Renal function tests to rule out renal failure due to acute urinary retention.

UI may present in a number of ways, depending on the underlying pathophysiology. Generally, SUI is considered the most common type of UI and probably accounts for at least a portion of UI in more than half of all incontinent females. Some studies have found that mixed UI (SUI + UUI) represents the most common type of UI.[6] However, the proportions of SUI versus UUI versus mixed UI vary considerably with age group and sex of patients studied, study methodology, and a variety of other factors. A complete medical history, including an assessment of symptoms and a physical examination, is essential in correctly classifying the type of incontinence and thereby assuring appropriate therapy.

URINE LEAKAGE

UI represents a spectrum of severity in terms of both volume of leakage and degree of bother to the patient. To carefully consider the level of patient discomfort when discussing urine leakage, the clinician must probe during the patient interview to accurately determine the precise nature of the problem.

The use of absorbent products such as panty liners, pads, or briefs is an obvious point to discuss, but the clinician must keep in mind that their use varies among patients. The number and type of pads may not relate to the amount or type of incontinence, as their use is a function of personal preference and hygiene. A high number of absorbent pads may be used every day by a patient with severe, high-volume UI, or alternatively, by a fastidiously hygienic patient with low-volume leakage who simply changes pads often to avoid a sense of wetness or odor. Nevertheless, a large number of pads that are described by the patient as "soaked" is indicative of high-volume urine loss.

Regardless of the volume of urine loss, the desire to seek evaluation and therapy for UI in all patients is almost always elective and contingent on the degree of bother to the individual patient. As with use of absorbent products, patients differ in the amount of urine loss they will tolerate before considering the condition bothersome enough to seek assistance.

SYMPTOMS

Under the best of circumstances, UI is difficult to categorize based on symptoms alone (Table 83–2).[22] In a study of patients who appeared to have SUI based on symptoms and patient history, urodynamics showed that only 72% of patients had SUI as the sole cause of incontinence.[23]

Patients with urethral underactivity or SUI characteristically complain of urinary leakage with physical activity. Volume of leakage is proportional to the level of activity. They will often leak urine during periods of exercise, coughing, sneezing, lifting, or even when rising from a seated to a standing position. Patients with pure SUI will not have leakage when physically inactive, especially when they are supine. Often they will have little or no UI at night, will not awaken to void during the night (nocturia), will not wet the bed, and often do not even wear absorbent products at bedtime. Urinary urgency and frequency may be associated with SUI, either as a separate component caused by bladder overactivity (mixed incontinence), or as a

TABLE 83–2. Differentiating Bladder Overactivity from Urethral Underactivity

Symptoms	Bladder Overactivity	Urethral Underactivity
Urgency (strong, sudden desire to void)	Yes	Sometimes
Frequency with urgency	Yes	Rarely
Leaking during physical activity (e.g., coughing, sneezing, lifting)	No	Yes
Amount of urinary leakage with *each episode* of incontinence	Large if present	Usually small
Ability to reach the toilet in time following an urge to void	No or just barely	Yes
Nocturnal incontinence (presence of wet pads or undergarments in bed)	Yes	Rare
Nocturia (waking to pass urine at night)	Usually	Seldom

Adapted from Rovner et al.[22]

compensatory mechanism wherein the patient with SUI learns to toilet frequently to avoid large-volume urine loss during physical activity.

Typical symptoms of bladder overactivity include frequency, urgency, and urge incontinence. Nocturia and nocturnal incontinence are often present. Urine leakage is unpredictable and the volume loss may be large. Patients will often wear protection both day and night. Urinary frequency can be affected by a number of factors unrelated to bladder overactivity, including excessive fluid intake (polydipsia) and bladder hypersensitivity states such as interstitial cystitis and urinary tract infection, and these should be ruled out. In some patients, bladder overactivity may manifest as UI without awareness in the absence of a sense of urinary urgency or frequency. Urinary urgency, a sensation of impending micturition, requires intact sensory input from the lower urinary tract. In patients with spinal cord injury, sensory neuropathies, and other neurologic diseases, a diminished ability to perceive or process sensory input from the lower urinary tract may result in bladder overactivity and UI without urgency or urinary frequency. When the bladder contraction occurs without warning and sensation is absent, the condition is referred to as reflex incontinence.

Patients with overflow incontinence may present with lower abdominal fullness as well as considerable obstructive urinary symptoms, including hesitancy, straining to void, decreased force of urinary stream, interrupted stream, and a vague sense of incomplete bladder emptying. These patients may also have a significant component of urinary frequency and urgency. In patients with acute urinary retention and overflow incontinence, lower abdominal pain may also be present. Although these symptoms are not specific for overflow incontinence, they may warrant further investigation including an assessment of postvoid residual urine volume.

SIGNS

A presenting complaint of UI mandates a directed physical examination and a brief neurologic assessment. This should ideally include an abdominal examination to exclude a distended bladder, a neurologic assessment of the perineum and lower extremities, a pelvic exam in women (looking especially for evidence of prolapse or hormonal deficiency), and a genital and prostate examination in men.

SUI can usually be objectively demonstrated by having the patient cough or strain during the examination and observing the urethral meatus for a sudden spurt of urine. In women, SUI may be associated with varying degrees of vaginal prolapse including cystourethrocele (bladder and urethral prolapse), enterocele (small bowel prolapse),

rectocele (rectal prolapse), and uterine prolapse. These conditions may have important implications for therapy.

Perineal skin maceration, erythema, breakdown, and ulceration may be indicative of chronic, severe UI. Patients with chronic incontinence may also manifest fungal infections of the skin of the perineum and upper thighs.

In both sexes, digital rectal examination provides an opportunity to check ambient rectal tone, the integrity of the sacral reflex arc (e.g., anal wink), as well as assess the patient's ability to perform a voluntary pelvic floor muscle contraction (i.e., Kegel exercise), which may be an important factor in deciding on appropriate therapy. In men, a digital examination of the prostate assesses for the presence of prostate cancer, inflammation, and BPH.

A targeted neurologic examination includes an assessment of reflexes, rectal tone, and sensory or motor deficits in the lower extremities, which might be indicative of systemic or localized neurologic disease. As noted previously, neurologic diseases have the potential to affect bladder and sphincter function and thus may have significant implications in the incontinent patient.

PRIOR MEDICAL OR SURGICAL ILLNESS

UI may present in the setting of concurrent, seemingly unrelated illnesses. New-onset UI may be the initial manifestation of certain systemic illnesses such as diabetes mellitus, metastatic malignancies, multiple sclerosis, and other neurologic illnesses. Central nervous system disease, or injury above the level of the pons, generally results in symptoms of bladder overactivity and UUI. Spinal cord injury or disease may manifest as bladder overactivity and UUI or as overflow incontinence, depending on the spinal level and completeness of the injury or disease.

Medications may have wide-ranging effects on lower urinary tract function (see Table 83–1). A thorough inquiry into the use of new medications in the setting of recent-onset UI may show a relationship.

Acute UI manifest in the immediate postoperative setting may be secondary to a number of factors, including surgical manipulation and immobility, and to a number of medications, including analgesics. In the postoperative setting, acute urinary retention and overflow incontinence is commonly related to the administration of anesthetic agents and/or opioid analgesics in the perioperative period. These agents may have profound effects on bladder contractility that are completely reversible once the agents are metabolized and excreted.

Prior surgery may have effects on lower urinary tract function. UI following prostate surgery in men is very suggestive of injury to the sphincter and resultant SUI. Pelvic surgery for benign and malignant conditions may result in denervation or injury to the lower urinary tract. This includes bowel surgery and gynecologic procedures. For example, new-onset total UI following gynecologic surgery for uterine fibroids suggests the possibility of intraoperative bladder injury and subsequent development of a postoperative vesicovaginal fistula. Radiation therapy to the pelvis for malignant disease (e.g., prostate cancer or cervical cancer) may result in injury to the bladder or urethra and subsequent UI.

In women, UI may be related to several gynecologic factors, including childbirth, hormonal status, and prior gynecologic surgery. Pregnancy and childbirth, particularly vaginal delivery, are associated with SUI and pelvic prolapse. Significant SUI in the nulliparous woman is rather uncommon. UI that becomes progressive at or around menopause suggests a hormonal component that may potentially be responsive to estrogen or hormone replacement therapy.

Finally, UI may present in the setting of other significant pelvic floor disorders, signs, and symptoms. Constipation, diarrhea, fecal incontinence, dyspareunia, sexual dysfunction, and pelvic pain may be related to UI. A history of gross hematuria in the setting of UI mandates further urologic investigation, including radiologic imaging of the upper urinary tract and cystoscopy. Acute dysuria with or without hematuria in the setting of UI suggests cystitis. A urinalysis and urine culture should be performed in these patients.

▶ TREATMENT: Urinary Incontinence

NONPHARMACOLOGIC TREATMENT

❸ Nonpharmacologic treatment of UI constitutes the chief form of incontinence management at a primary care level. For patients in whom pharmacologic or surgical management is inappropriate or undesired, nondrug treatment is the only option. Examples of patients fulfilling these criteria include patients who are not medically fit for surgery or those who plan future pregnancies (as these may adversely affect long-term surgical outcomes); those with overflow incontinence whose condition is not amenable to surgery or drug therapy; those with comorbid conditions that place them at high risk for adverse effects from drug therapy; those who are delaying surgery or do not want to undergo surgery; and those with mild to moderate symptoms who do not want to take medication.

For additional information on nonpharmacologic interventions for UI, readers are referred to comprehensive literature reviews and consensus opinions of treatment guidelines on nonpharmacologic interventions by multidisciplinary experts.[24] Table 83–3 summarizes the basic nondrug approaches.

Behavioral interventions are the first line of treatment for SUI, UUI, and mixed UI. These include lifestyle modifications, scheduling regimens, and pelvic floor muscle rehabilitation. Because the key to the success with any type of behavioral intervention is the motivation of the patient or caregiver, these individuals must be active participants in developing a treatment plan. Regular follow-up is needed to help motivate patients and caregivers, provide reassurance and support, and to monitor treatment outcomes.

PHARMACOLOGIC TREATMENT

URGE URINARY INCONTINENCE

Pharmacotherapy is useful when UUI symptoms are not adequately controlled with nonpharmacologic therapies, particularly in patients with a low functional bladder capacity. In many cases, the combined use of pharmacotherapy with nonpharmacologic therapy produces a better response than either intervention alone.

❹ Proven to be the most effective agents in suppressing premature detrusor contractions, enhancing bladder storage, and relieving UUI symptoms and complications, anticholinergic/antispasmodic drugs constitute the pharmacotherapy of first choice for UUI (Tables 83–4 and 83–5).[25–44] Drugs with anticholinergic activity act by antagonizing muscarinic cholinergic receptors, through which efferent parasympathetic nerve impulses evoke detrusor contraction. In addition, women with mixed UI or UUI plus urethritis or vaginitis may benefit from a topical or systemic estrogen (alone or in combination with an anticholinergic drug).

Immediate-Release Oxybutynin

Even though a substantial proportion of patients may discontinue oxybutynin immediate-release (IR) therapy because of its nonurinary antimuscarinic effects, oxybutynin IR remains the drug of first choice for UUI and the gold standard against which other drugs are compared. In addition to these antimuscarinic effects (e.g., dry mouth, constipation, vision impairment, confusion, cognitive dysfunction, and tachycardia), oxybutynin IR is associated with orthostatic hypotension secondary to α-adrenergic receptor blockade, as well as sedation and weight gain from histamine H_1-receptor blockade.[26,31,45–49] Furthermore, adverse effects jeopardize medication adherence and can prevent dose escalation to that needed for optimal benefit.

Emerging evidence suggests that the high incidence of adverse effects, especially dry mouth, of oxybutynin IR, and to a lesser extent oxybutynin extended-release (XL) and oxybutynin transdermal system (TDS), may be largely due to the active metabolite, N-desethyloxybutynin (DEO). This metabolite is generated by extensive first-pass metabolism in the liver and upper gastrointestinal tract.[50] Since many of the adverse effects seen with oxybutynin are felt to be related to the primary hepatic metabolite DEO, the lower DEO plasma concentrations seen with oxybutynin TDS and oxybutynin XL (which are due to reduced first-pass metabolism) compared to those of oxybutynin IR may explain their lesser propensity to cause dry mouth and other anticholinergic adverse effects.

Another factor associated with the adverse effects of oxybutynin IR, especially in older patients, is the transient high peak serum oxybutynin plasma concentration and area under the plasma concentration-versus-time curve (AUC), which is twofold higher in elderly patients than in younger adults, after both single and multiple doses.[51] Oxybutynin IR is best tolerated when the dose is gradually escalated from no more than 2.5 mg twice daily to start, to 2.5 mg three times daily after 1 month, then further increased in increments of 2.5 mg/day every 1 to 2 months until the desired response or the maximum recommended or tolerated dose is attained. The optimal response usually requires no more than 5 mg three times daily (see Table 83–4).[26,52]

Adverse effects of oxybutynin IR can sometimes be managed by a dose reduction if this does not significantly compromise drug efficacy. Dry mouth can be relieved by the use of sugarless hard

ABLE 83–3. Nonpharmacologic Management of Urinary Incontinence

Intervention	Description	Patient Characteristics
Lifestyle modifications	Self-management strategies targeted toward reducing or eliminating risk factors that cause or exacerbate urinary incontinence	Smoking cessation for patients with cough-induced stress incontinence; weight reduction for obese patients with stress incontinence; good bowel hygiene for patients with constipation; caffeine reduction, selected dietary and fluid modifications for patients with urge incontinence (e.g., eliminate aspartame, spicy foods, citrus fruits, carbonated beverages)
Scheduling regimens		
Timed voiding	Toileting on a fixed schedule whose interval does not change, typically every 2 hours during waking hours	Used for stress, urge, and mixed incontinence in patients with cognitive or physical impairments; also used in patients without impairments who have infrequent voiding patterns
Habit retraining	Scheduled toiletings with adjustments of voiding intervals (longer or shorter) based on patient's voiding pattern	Used for stress, urge, and mixed incontinence in institutionalized or homebound patients with cognitive or physical impairments; may also be used in patients who have diuretic-induced incontinence
Patterned urge response toileting (PURT)	A specialized type of habit training that involves the use of an electronic monitoring device to identify the timing of incontinent episodes	Used for stress, urge, and mixed incontinence in institutionalized and homebound elderly populations
Prompted voiding	Scheduled toiletings that require prompts to void from a caregiver, typically every 2 hours; patient assisted in toileting only if response is positive; used in conjunction with operant conditioning techniques for rewarding patients for maintaining continence and appropriate toileting	Used for stress, urge, and mixed incontinence in patients who are functionally able to use toilet or toilet substitute, able to feel urge sensation, and able to request toileting assistance appropriately; primarily used in institutional settings or in homebound patients with an available caregiver
Bladder training	Scheduled toiletings with progressive voiding intervals; includes teaching of urge control strategies using relaxation and distraction techniques, self-monitoring, and use of reinforcement techniques; sometimes combined with drug therapy	Used for stress, urge, and mixed incontinence in patients who are cognitively intact, able to toilet, and motivated to comply with training program
Pelvic floor muscle rehabilitation		
Pelvic floor muscle exercises (e.g., Kegel exercises)	Regular practice of pelvic floor muscle contractions; may involve use of pelvic floor muscle contraction for urge inhibition	Used for stress, urge, and mixed incontinence in patients who can correctly contract their pelvic floor muscles without use of accessory muscles; requires a cognitively intact and highly motivated patient
Vaginal weight training	Active retention of increasing vaginal weights; typically used in combination with pelvic floor muscle exercises at least twice a day	Women with stress incontinence who are cognitively intact, can correctly contract pelvic floor muscles, able to stand, and who have sufficient vaginal vault and introitus to retain cone and are highly motivated; contraindicated in patients with moderate to severe pelvic organ prolapse
Biofeedback	Use of electronic or mechanical instruments to display visual or auditory information about neuromuscular or bladder activity; used to teach correct pelvic floor muscle contraction and/or urge inhibition	Used for stress, urge, and mixed incontinence in patients who are able to understand analog or digital signals, who are motivated, and who have the capability to learn voluntary control through observation
Nonimplantable electrical stimulation	Application of electrical current to sacral and pudendal afferent fibers through vaginal, anal, or surface electrodes; used to inhibit bladder overactivity and to improve awareness, contractility, and efficiency of pelvic muscle contraction	Used for stress, urge, and mixed incontinence in patients who are highly motivated; contraindicated in patients with diminished sensory perception, moderate or severe pelvic organ prolapse, urinary retention, history of cardiac arrhythmia, or demand cardiac pacemaker
Extracorporeal magnetic innervation	Pulsed magnetic stimulation to pelvic floor musculature causing depolarization of motor neurons, thus inducing pelvic floor muscle contraction; stimulation is provided through a specially designed chair that contains a device for producing a pulsing magnetic field (e.g., Neotonus, Inc., Marietta, GA)	Initially tested in women with stress incontinence; contraindicated in patients with demand cardiac pacemakers, or with metallic joint replacements; may be useful treatment option when other approaches fail or are not feasible
Anti-incontinence devices		
Intravaginal support device (pessaries and bladder neck support prostheses)	Pessaries and other intravaginal devices designed to support the bladder neck, relieve minor pelvic organ prolapse, and change pressure transmission to the urethra (e.g., Coloplast AS, Humelbaek, Denmark)	Used for female stress incontinence; in postmenopausal women, estrogen replacement is typically prescribed to prevent ulceration and breakdown of vaginal tissue; requires good manual dexterity to manipulate device

(continued)

TABLE 83–3. (*Continued*)

Intervention	Description	Patient Characteristics
External occlusive device	Small, single-use device that covers the urethral meatus which is removed for voiding in women (e.g., FemAssist, Apple Medical, Marlboro, MA; CapSure, Bard Urological, Covington, GA); a penile clamp (e.g., Cunningham clamp) is available for men	Used for female and male stress incontinence; used in cognitively intact patients with good manual dexterity
Intraurethral occlusive device (urethral plug)	Small, single-use device that is worn in the urethra to provide mechanical obstruction to prevent urine leakage; removed for voiding (e.g., FemSoft Insert, Rochester Med. Corp., Stewartville, MN)	Used for female stress incontinence patients who are cognitively intact with good manual dexterity; contraindicated with primary urge incontinence, urinary tract infection, urethral stricture, and any anatomic or pathologic condition making catheter passage difficult
Complex valved catheter (investigational)	Intraurethral occlusive device that has a unidirectional valve that can be opened to permit voiding and resealed; may be left indwelling over a longer period of time than intraurethral occlusive devices, but requires a clinician to insert and remove; several devices are currently undergoing testing	Female stress incontinence and overflow incontinence
Supportive interventions		
Toileting substitutes and other environmental modifications	Urinals, bedside commodes, elevated toilet seats	Used for patients with mobility impairments that make it difficult to reach a toilet in a timely fashion
Physical therapy	Gait and/or strength training	Used for frail elderly patients with mobility impairments that make it difficult to reach a toilet in a timely fashion
Absorbent products	Variety of reusable and disposable pads and pant systems; some products contain a polymer that absorbs urine and wicks it away from the body	Used for all types of incontinence
External collection devices (men only)	Condom catheter with leg bag	Used in men with urge, stress, and overflow incontinence and in those with functional impairments
Catheters	Disposable, intermittent catheters and indwelling urethral and suprapubic catheters	Used for overflow incontinence; also used in patients who are bed-bound or with significant mobility impairments and severe incontinence, those with terminal illness, and those with sacral pressure ulcers until healing occurs

candy, gum, or a saliva substitute. Constipation can be minimized by increasing the intake of water, dietary fiber, physical activity such as walking, or laxative therapy. The need for multiple daily dosing of oxybutynin IR can further jeopardize adherence, especially in people who take multiple medications or those who are cognitively impaired.

Extended-Release Oral Oxybutynin

Because of problems noted with oxybutynin IR, oxybutynin extended-release (XL) was developed. It can be considered an alternative for the first-line therapy of UUI (see Table 83–5).

Oxybutynin XL (Ditropan XL) is an extended-release formulation of oxybutynin.[53] Its extended-release system consists of an osmotically active bilayer core (comprising a drug layer and a push layer containing osmotically active components) surrounded by a semipermeable membrane. Throughout the gastrointestinal tract, water permeates through the rate-controlling membrane into the tablet core, causing the drug to go into suspension and the push layer to expand, pushing the suspended drug out through an orifice.[31] Following oral administration, oxybutynin XL is completely absorbed, and neither the rate nor extent of absorption are significantly affected by administration with food.

Unlike oxybutynin IR, oxybutynin XL delivers a controlled amount of oxybutynin chloride continuously throughout the gastrointestinal tract over a 24-hour time period, reducing first-pass metabolism by cytochrome P450 (CYP450) isoenzyme 3A4, which is

present in higher concentrations in the upper portion of the small intestine than the lower gastrointestinal tract.[53,54] This results in relative bioavailabilities of oxybutynin and its active *N*-desethyloxybutynin metabolite of 153% and 69%, respectively, for oxybutynin XL compared with oxybutynin IR.[55] The greater ratio of parent drug to active metabolite after oxybutynin XL administration, and probably less importantly a lower peak plasma drug concentration, are believed to be the reasons for fewer dose- and concentration-dependent adverse effects and better patient tolerance with the XL preparation as compared to oxybutynin IR.[56] The elimination of oxybutynin XL is not known to be altered in patients with renal or hepatic impairment or in geriatric patients (up to 78 years of age).[53] The absence of an effect of advanced age on oxybutynin XL pharmacokinetics is unexpected since the clearance of oxybutynin IR is significantly lower in elderly individuals.

Controlled studies have demonstrated that oxybutynin XL is significantly more effective than placebo and equally effective as oxybutynin IR in terms of reducing the mean number of UUI episodes, restoring continence, decreasing the number of micturitions per day, and increasing urine volume voided per micturition (see Table 83–5).[30,31,45–47,57–59]

In short-term studies of up to 12 weeks' duration, oxybutynin XL was better tolerated than oxybutynin IR, with approximately 7% of patients discontinuing treatment because of adverse effects (as compared to approximately 27% in those taking oxybutynin IR).[26,31,45,46,52,5?] The rate and severity of adverse effects did not differ significantly between elderly persons (65 years of age and older) and younger adults

TABLE 83–4. Pharmacotherapeutic Options in Patients with Urinary Incontinence

Type	Drug Class	Drug Therapy (Usual Dose)	Comments
Overactive bladder	Anticholinergic agents/antispasmodics	Oxybutynin IR (2.5–5 mg two, three or four times a day), oxybutynin XL (5–30 mg daily), oxybutynin TDS (3.9 mg/day) (apply 1 patch twice weekly), tolterodine IR (1–2 mg twice a day), tolterodine LA (2–4 mg daily), trospium chloride 20 mg twice a day, solifenacin 5–10 mg daily, darifenacin 7.5–15 mg daily	Anticholinergics are the first-line drug therapy (oxybutynin or tolterodine are preferred).
	Tricyclic antidepressants (TCAs)	Imipramine, doxepin, nortriptyline, or desipramine (25–100 mg at bedtime)	TCAs are generally reserved for patients with an additional indication (e.g., depression, neuralgia)
	Topical estrogen (only in women with urethritis or vaginitis)	Conjugated estrogen 0.5 g vaginal cream three times per week for up to 8 months. Repeat course if symptom recurrence. Or use estradiol vaginal insert/ring [2 mg (1 ring)] and replace after 90 days if needed.	Marginally effective. Few adverse effects with cream and vaginal insert
Dual serotonin-norepinephrine reuptake inhibitors	Duloxetine[a]	40–80 mg/day (1 or 2 doses)	Once approved, will become first-line therapy. Most adverse events diminish with time so support patient during initial period of use
Stress	α-Adrenergic agonists	Pseudoephedrine (15–60 mg three times a day) with food, water, or milk	Pseudoephedrine is first-line therapy for women with no contraindication (notably hypertension) (second-line once duloxetine is approved) Phenylpropanolamine was the preferred agent until its removal from the U.S. market in 2000.
	Estrogen	See estrogens (above). Works best if urethritis or vaginitis are present.	Considered a somewhat less-effective alternative to pseudoephedrine. Combined pseudoephedrine and estrogen is somewhat more effective than pseudoephedrine alone in postmenopausal women.
	Imipramine	25–100 mg at bedtime	Imipramine is an optional therapy when first-line therapy is inadequate.
Overflow (atonic bladder)	Cholinomimetics	Bethanechol (25–50 mg three or four times a day) on an empty stomach	Avoid use if patient has asthma or heart disease. Short-term use only. Never give IV or IM because of life-threatening cardiovascular and severe gastrointestinal reactions.

R, immediate-release; LA, long-acting; XL, extended-release, TDS, transdermal system.
[a]Investigational. Doses provided are those best supported by clinical trials to date.

with the XL preparation. A 12-week study demonstrated the superiority of oxybutynin XL over tolterodine IR in reducing the mean number of weekly incontinent episodes and micturitions.[39]

In the OPERA trial, oxybutynin XL was comparable to tolterodine long-acting (LA) in decreasing the mean number of incontinence episodes, but was superior in reducing weekly micturition frequency and achieving total dryness.[60] In another study that pooled results of two open-label studies, tolterodine LA was associated with significantly greater patient-perceived improvement in bladder control and fewer withdrawals due to adverse effects than oxybutynin XL.

However, the treatments were similar in patients' or physicians' perception of benefit over baseline and proportions of withdrawals due to lack of efficacy. However, the lack of blinding may have introduced patient and observer bias.[61]

Oxybutynin XL, available only in a tablet formulation, is administered once daily, with or without food, and should not be crushed or chewed (see Table 83–4). Like oxybutynin IR, the dosage does not require adjustment in patients of advanced age, or in patients with renal or hepatic impairment. However, treatment should still be initiated at the smallest recommended dosage in the elderly (5 mg once daily).[32,53]

TABLE 83–5. Efficacy of First-Choice Drugs for Bladder Overactivity in Placebo-Controlled Trials[a]

Drug	Decreased Incontinence Episodes	Restored Continence	Decreased Frequency of Micturitions	Increased Volume per Void
Oxybutynin IR	24–52	16–67	−2 to −63	9–24
Oxybutynin XL	47	37	1	13
Oxybutynin TDS	10–20	6–17	4–6	12–14
Tolterodine	16–33	9	4–19	11–20
Tolterodine LA	23	NR	6	14

[a]All values constitute mean or median drug effect (drug response minus placebo response in percent), predominantly using poled data from multiple independent studies.

IR, immediate-release; LA, long-acting; NR, not reported; XL, extended-release; TDS, transdermal system.

The maximum benefit of oxybutynin XL may not be realized for up to 4 weeks after starting therapy or after dose escalation. No known clinically relevant drug-drug interactions with either oxybutynin XL or oxybutynin IR have been identified. However, other drugs with anticholinergic activity may increase overall anticholinergic effects (i.e., produce an additive or synergistic pharmacodynamic interaction), as would be expected.[53] Another potential pharmacodynamic interaction involves the mutual antagonism of anticholinergic agents and cholinergic stimulants such as the acetylcholinesterase inhibitors used to treat dementia.

Extended-Release Transdermal Oxybutynin

The oxybutynin transdermal system (Oxytrol), which delivers 3.9 mg per day, is applied twice weekly (every 3 or 4 days). Transdermal absorption of oxybutynin from this formulation bypasses first-pass hepatic and gut metabolism, resulting in similar oxybutynin but lower plasma N-desethyloxybutynin concentrations than after administration of an equivalent dose via the oral route.[50,62] Similar findings have been noted for the active R-enantiomer of N-desethyloxybutynin.[63] No dosage adjustment of the TDS product for advancing age is necessary.[44]

Oxybutynin TDS is superior to placebo in reducing incontinence episodes and number of micturitions and increasing the volume voided per micturition.[43,44] It is also similar to oxybutynin IR in reducing the frequency of UUI episodes and improving patient-perceived urinary leakage.[64] Oxybutynin TDS and tolterodine LA are significantly superior to placebo and similar to each other in reducing the frequency of UUI episodes, increasing the volume voided per micturition, attaining complete continence, and improving quality of life.[43]

The commonest adverse effects with the TDS formulation are pruritus (15%) and erythema (9%) at the application site. The events of dry mouth (11%), constipation (5%), dizziness (5%), and abnormal vision (<5%) occur less frequently with the TDS formulation than with the IR formulation, and similarly in frequency to those with oxybutynin XL and tolterodine IR/LA.[39,40,42–44,47,60,64]

Immediate-Release Tolterodine

Tolterodine (Detrol) is a competitive muscarinic receptor antagonist that can be considered first-line therapy of UI in patients with symptoms of urinary frequency, urgency, or urge incontinence (see Tables 83–4 and 83–5).[33]

Controlled studies demonstrated that tolterodine was significantly more effective than placebo and as effective as oxybutynin IR in decreasing the mean daily number of micturitions and increasing the mean volume voided per micturition (see Table 83–5).[27,34–38,65,6] However, while three controlled trials showed significant decreases in the mean number of incontinence episodes per 24 hours as compared to placebo, most studies have not and the manufacturer's package insert does not claim a significant improvement in this parameter (see Table 83–5).[28,34–38,66] The only controlled study of the ability of tolterodine to restore urinary continence reported an insignificant effect rate of 9% over placebo.[34]

Extended-Release Tolterodine

In a controlled study of 1529 adult outpatients with urinary frequency and UUI, tolterodine LA, an extended-release formulation of tolterodine tartrate, significantly decreased the mean number of weekly incontinence episodes (23% effect rate over placebo and 7% effect rate over tolterodine IR). Patient withdrawal rates did not differ significantly between the two active treatments, but dry mouth was observed significantly less often in patients taking the LA formulation than among those patients receiving the IR formulation.[40]

Tolterodine LA was significantly superior to placebo and similar in elderly and young patient populations in reducing the frequencies of incontinence episodes and micturitions, increasing the volume voided per micturition and ability to complete tasks before voiding, and enhancing the patient perception of benefit. Adverse effect types and frequencies were also similar in the two age groups.[67]

A major consideration in using tolterodine is its pharmacokinetics, specifically its metabolism. The agent is predominantly eliminated by hepatic metabolism, and it exhibits genetic polymorphism.[33] The principal metabolic pathway in extensive metabolizers involves oxidation of the parent drug by the CYP450 isoenzyme 2D6 to the active 5-hydroxymethyl metabolite (DD01), followed by further oxidation and dealkylation.

In poor metabolizers who lack CYP450 isoenzyme 2D6 (approximately 7% of the U.S. population), the principal metabolic pathway involves CYP450 isoenzyme 3A4, with dealkylation of the amino group, oxidation to a dealkylated hydroxy metabolite, and further oxidation to a dealkylated acid metabolite that undergoes glucuronidation. Since tolterodine is principally metabolized by CYP450 isoenzyme 3A4 in this case, its elimination may be impaired by inhibitors of this isoenzyme (e.g., fluoxetine, sertraline, fluvoxamine, macrolide antibiotics, imidazoles, and grapefruit juice). For example fluoxetine, an inhibitor of CYP450 isoenzymes 2D6 and 3A4, decreases he metabolism of tolterodine to DD01, resulting in a 4.8-fold increase in tolterodine AUC with a 52% decrease in the peak plasma concentration and a 20% decrease in the AUC of DD01.[33] Whether tolterodine significantly alters the pharmacokinetics of drugs metabolized by CYP450 isoenzyme 2D6 is unknown, so caution is advised with concurrent use of these agents.

Single-dose interaction studies have demonstrated that concurrent administration of tolterodine LA with antacid leads to a rapid release of drug (70% within 4 hours) and results in a 1.5-fold elevation in tolterodine peak plasma concentration compared with placebo. The clinical implications of this interaction and whether a similar interaction exists with gastric acid suppressants such as the histamine H₂-receptor antagonists and proton pump inhibitors are unclear. In the same study, the pharmacokinetics of oxybutynin XL were unaltered by antacid administration.[68]

Although one of two phase I pharmacokinetic studies comparing healthy elderly volunteers (aged 64 to 80 years) with healthy volunteers younger than 40 years of age found no difference in pharmacokinetic parameters between the groups, the other study noted that the mean serum concentrations of tolterodine and DD01 were 20% and 50% greater in elderly volunteers than in young healthy volunteers, respectively. Despite possibly altered pharmacokinetics in elderly individuals, no differences in the incidence and severity of adverse effects between these age groups have been noted in clinical trials, and therefore no dosage adjustment is recommended on the basis of age alone.[33]

Tolterodine elimination is diminished in patients with impaired hepatic function. Patients with hepatic cirrhosis who are extensive metabolizers exhibit a higher mean AUC of DD01, higher serum tolterodine and DD01 concentrations, and a longer terminal disposition half-life of tolterodine and DD01 than do healthy subjects who are extensive metabolizers. The tolterodine AUC was higher in cirrhotic patients who were poor metabolizers than in healthy poor metabolizers.[33] If the use of tolterodine cannot be avoided in patients with hepatic impairment or in those receiving inhibitors of CYP450 isoenzyme 3A4 (and possibly inhibitors of CYP450 isoenzyme 2D6), the initial dose should be reduced by 50% to tolterodine IR 1 mg twice daily or tolterodine LA 2 mg once daily (see Table 83–4).[33] No formal tolterodine dosage recommendation is possible based on available information for individuals who concurrently have hepatic impairment and are taking a CYP450 isoenzyme 3A4 inhibitor; intuitively, the initial dose should not exceed 1 mg twice daily (IR) or 2 mg once daily (LA).

The elimination of tolterodine has not been evaluated in patients with impaired renal function, and therefore the drug should be used more cautiously in such individuals (i.e., starting dose of the IR product of 1 mg twice daily with gradual dose escalation, if needed, to a maximum of 2 mg twice daily, or a starting dose of the LA formulation of 2 mg once daily with gradual dose escalation, if needed, to 4 mg once daily).[33]

Tolterodine is better tolerated than oxybutynin IR, with about 8% of patients discontinuing treatment (compared with approximately 27% of individuals taking oxybutynin IR).[26,28,34,35,37,45,69] The most common adverse effects of tolterodine are dry mouth, dyspepsia, headache, constipation, and dry eyes.[33]

Tolterodine, available only as a tablet formulation, can be administered with or without food, and the LA product should not be crushed or chewed or taken less than 2 hours before or 4 hours after an antacid. The maximum benefit from tolterodine may not be realized for up to 8 weeks after starting therapy or dose escalation.

Trospium Chloride

Trospium chloride (Sanctura) is a quaternary ammonium anticholinergic approved in 2004 by the U.S. Food and Drug Administration (FDA) for the management of OAB. However, it has been available for many years in other countries. This agent has been comprehensively reviewed, and the data provided below come from that publication.[70]

Preclinical studies have demonstrated that trospium chloride is an antimuscarinic agent in bladder and gastrointestinal tract tissues. It is poorly absorbed after oral administration (<10%), and food reduces bioavailability by 70% to 80%. It is principally cleared by the renal route (70%), with 80% of urinary excretion being accounted for by the parent compound. The mean half-life in the presence of normal renal function is 10 to 12 hours. Advancing age and mild to moderate hepatic impairment do not affect trospium chloride pharmacokinetics to a clinically significant degree. In contrast, renal impairment does significantly reduce drug clearance. When creatinine clearance is below 30 mL/min, AUC is increased by a mean of 4.5-fold, C_{max} by a mean of twofold, and half-life by a mean of two- to threefold. In this patient population, the daily dose should be reduced by 50%.

Nine English language efficacy/tolerability papers are available for trospium chloride in UUI. With the exception of the two trials described in the product information (one is published), trials have emphasized cystometric and not clinical endpoints. The paucity of clinical outcome data makes it difficult to evaluate this drug compared to other approved and investigational anticholinergics. Although statistically superior to placebo, the absolute differences in results between trospium chloride and placebo calls into question the clinical relevance of such differences. In the three trials with active controls, results with trospium chloride were statistically equivalent to those with oxybutynin IR and tolterodine IR. No comparative data with long-acting formulations of these two agents are available.

The expected anticholinergic adverse effects occur with trospium chloride as well. Of interest, the frequency of these events is increased in patients 75 years old and older compared to younger subjects. This is believed to be pharmacodynamic in nature (i.e., increased sensitivity) and not pharmacokinetic. There are no data at present to support the hypothesis that trospium chloride is less neurotoxic than non-quaternary-ammonium anticholinergics (based on the hypothesis of reduced transit across the blood-brain barrier of trospium chloride due to its positive electrical charge on the quaternary nitrogen). Available drug-drug interaction data are clearly inadequate.

The usual dosage regimen is 20 mg twice daily. The drug should be taken on an empty stomach. Dosage reduction (by 50% of the daily dose) is recommended when creatinine clearance is below 30 mL/min. In patients 75 years old and older, dose reduction to 20 mg once daily should be considered based upon tolerability. At this time, trospium chloride does not appear to be a significant advance over oxybutynin and tolterodine in managing UUI.

Anticholinergic Agents Under Development

Solifenacin succinate (Vesicare) was approved in late 2004 by FDA for the treatment of OAB with urge incontinence, urgency, and urinary frequency. This agent was comprehensively reviewed and the data provided below come principally from that publication.[71]

Preclinical studies have demonstrated that solifenacin is an antagonist at M_1, M_2, and M_3 muscarinic cholinergic receptors. Based on comparative ex vivo and animal studies with solifenacin and oxybutynin, it was felt that solifenacin was a "uroselective" agent. The drug is well absorbed (mean absolute bioavailability = 88%) and food has no clinically relevant effect on absorption.[72,73] It is principally eliminated via metabolism and renal excretion of metabolites, with renal excretion of parent compound being less than 10% of the dose. With a mean half-life of 50 to 60 hours, the drug can be dosed once daily.[74] Results of two placebo-controlled and two placebo- and active (tolterodine)-controlled clinical trials in UUI are available. Like oxybutynin and tolterodine, solifenacin significantly reduced the number of incontinence episodes, urge episodes and micturitions per day and increased the volume voided per micturition in a dose-dependent fashion compared to placebo. In the active-controlled trials, solifenacin was statistically superior to tolterodine in these effects. Surprisingly, the effect of tolterodine in these trials was no better than that of placebo. No comparative efficacy/tolerability data with oxybutynin are available. The effect sizes (solifenacin effect minus placebo effect) in these studies were similar to those noted earlier with oxybutynin and tolterodine. The recommended dose of solifenacin is 5 mg once daily. If well tolerated and the effectiveness is not optimal, the dose can be increased to 10 mg once daily. Solifenacin can be administered with or without food. For patients with severe renal impairment (creatinine clearance less than 30 mL/min) or moderate hepatic impairment (Child–Pugh class B), the daily dosage should not exceed 5 mg. If the patient has severe hepatic impairment (Child–Pugh class C), the drug should not be used. If the patient is receiving concurrent therapy with one or more potent CYP 3A4 inhibitors, the daily dose should not exceed 5 mg. In contrast to the preclinical studies, solifenacin behaves like a nonselective anticholinergic in humans, causing dry mouth, constipation, blurred vision, and other anticholinergic effects to a similar extent compared to tolterodine in the clinical trials and oxybutynin in the pharmacokinetic trials. At this time, solifenacin does not appear to be a significant advance over existing anticholinergics in managing UUI.

Darifenacin (Enablex) is another recently approved anticholinergic drug. This agent has also been comprehensively reviewed, and the data provided below come from that publication.[75]

Preclinical studies have demonstrated that darifenacin is an antagonist at M_1, M_3, and M_5 muscarinic cholinergic receptors. As with solifenacin, darifenacin was also felt to be "uroselective" on the basis of preclinical data. The mean absolute bioavailabilities of the 7.5, 15, and 30 mg extended-release (ER) formulations are 15%, 19%, and 25%, respectively. Bioavailability is affected by formulation, CYP2D6 genotype, dose, and race. Bioavailability is enhanced using an ER formulation (70–110% higher than IR) in heterozygous extensive metabolizers (EM), poor metabolizers (2D6, 40–90% higher than homozygous EM), and Caucasian race (56% higher than Japanese). This agent is extensively metabolized, with urinary excretion of parent compound being less than 10%. The 2D6 and 3A4 isozymes of CYP450 are responsible for darifenacin metabolism. With a mean half-life of 3 to 5 hours (depending on 2D6 metabolizer status), an ER formulation is needed to allow once-daily dosing. Results of four placebo-controlled clinical trials (one published) in UUI are available. Once-daily darifenacin was significantly superior to placebo in reducing the numbers of micturitions, urinary urges, incontinence episodes, and urge severity and in increasing the volume voided per micturition. No comparative efficacy/tolerability data with other anticholinergics are available. The recommended daily dose of darifenacin is 7.5 to 15 mg once daily of an ER oral formulation. Again, as with solifenacin, darifenacin behaves like a nonselective anticholinergic in humans, causing dry mouth, constipation, and other well-known anticholinergic adverse effects. At this time, darifenacin does not

appear to be a significant advance over existing anticholinergics in managing UUI.

CLINICAL CONTROVERSY

Should anticholinergic pharmacotherapy be used to treat UUI in patients with mild or moderate dementia?

Other Anticholinergics and Antispasmodics

Other drugs for treating UUI are less effective, no safer, or have not been adequately studied (see Table 83–4);[24,76] hence their use is not recommended. Tricyclic antidepressants are generally no more effective than oxybutynin IR and exhibit a high incidence of bothersome and potentially serious adverse effects (e.g., orthostatic hypotension, cardiac conduction abnormalities, dizziness, confusion, and they can be life-threatening in overdose). Therefore their use should be limited to those individuals who have one or more additional medical indications for these agents (e.g., depression or neuropathic pain); to patients with mixed UI (because of their effect of decreasing bladder contractility and increasing outlet resistance); and possibly to those with nocturnal incontinence associated with altered sleep patterns.[24,76–79] Because of the lower incidence of adverse effects, desipramine and nortriptyline may be preferred over imipramine and doxepin. However, because of their lower anticholinergic activity, they may also not be as effective.

Propantheline, a quaternary ammonium anticholinergic and potential treatment, produces a high incidence of adverse effects and is only modestly effective for UUI.[80–84] When used, propantheline appears to be best tolerated at a dose of no more than 15 mg three times daily plus 60 mg at bedtime.[80]

Flavoxate, a tertiary amine that relaxes smooth muscle in vitro, is not recommended for treating UUI because four controlled trials have revealed that it is no more effective than placebo.[24]

Dicyclomine hydrochloride, an anticholinergic agent that relaxes smooth muscle, produced minimal benefit as well as bothersome adverse effects in two small studies.[85,86]

Hyoscyamine, an anticholinergic and antispasmodic drug related to atropine, has also been suggested for treating UUI, but data are insufficient to recommend its use.[24]

In a systematic review and pooled analysis of 32 controlled trials of anticholinergic therapy for overactive bladder (January 2002 database), the above agents were found to be modestly effective clinically and urodynamically. While the clinical relevance of the small improvements in clinical and urodynamic parameters were questioned, the effects of these agents were still considered positive.[87]

It is hoped that an improved understanding of the pathophysiology of UUI will lead to the development of safer and more effective pharmacotherapy.

CLINICAL CONTROVERSY

Which anticholinergic agent should be used as first-line pharmacotherapy of UUI (oxybutynin, tolterodine, trospium chloride, solifenacin, or dorifenacin) and which formulation of oxybutynin (oral IR, oral XL, or topical) or tolterodine (oral IR, oral LA) is unclear. Financial considerations currently favor generic oxybutynin IR, and this is the initial choice of many clinicians.

Catheterization Combined with Medications

Patients with UUI and an elevated postvoid residual urine volume due to retention may require intermittent self-catheterization along with frequent voiding between catheterizations.

If intermittent catheterization is not possible, surgical placement of a suprapubic catheter may be necessary. The use of a chronic indwelling catheter should be avoided because of the increased occurrence of urinary tract infections and nephrolithiasis.

Regardless of catheterization status, patients may experience symptom relief with oxybutynin (IR, XL, or TDS formulations), tolterodine (IR or LA formulations), trospium chloride, or solifenacin or darifenacin, as these relax the detrusor muscle and enhance bladder storage. Patients with UUI and symptoms of retention may also benefit from an α-adrenergic receptor antagonist that relaxes the internal bladder sphincter (e.g., prazosin, terazosin, doxazosin, tamsulosin, and alfuzosin). Although theoretically of benefit, bethanechol, a cholinergic agonist, has not been demonstrated effective in improving bladder emptying in well-done trials. In addition, it causes numerous bothersome (e.g., muscle and abdominal cramping and diarrhea) and potentially life-threatening adverse effects, and should not be used in patients with asthma or heart disease.[24]

URETHRAL UNDERACTIVITY

Urethral underactivity, or SUI, may be aggravated by agents with α-adrenergic receptor blocking activity, including prazosin, terazosin, doxazosin, tamsulosin, alfuzosin, methyldopa, clonidine, guanfacine, guanadrel, and labetalol. The goal of therapy is to improve the urethral closure mechanism by either stimulating α-adrenergic receptors in the smooth muscle of the bladder neck and proximal urethra, enhancing the supportive structures underlying the urethral epithelium, or enhance the positive effects of serotonin and norepinephrine in the afferent and efferent pathways of the micturition reflex. There is no role for medications in the management of SUI after radical prostatectomy.[88]

Estrogens

Local and systemic estrogens have been considered the mainstays of pharmacologic management of SUI since the 1940s. Estrogens are believed to work via several mechanisms, including enhancement of the proliferation of urethral epithelium, local circulation, and numbers and/or sensitivity of urogenital α-adrenergic receptors.[89] However, a recent trial has questioned whether estrogens exert a stimulatory effect on vaginal collagen production, at least over the short term.[90]

Open trials support the use of a variety of estrogens in the management of SUI: transdermal estradiol, conjugated estrogen vaginal cream, Estring, oral-conjugated estrogen, oral quinestradol, oral estriol, intramuscular estrogens, estriol vaginal suppositories, and oral estradiol.[91] Variable effects of estrogen treatment on urodynamic parameters, such as maximum urethral closure pressure, functional urethral length, and pressure transmission ratio, have been noted in these studies.

Unfortunately, results of four placebo-controlled comparative trials have not been as favorable, finding no significant clinical or urodynamic effects for oral estrogen as compared with placebo (see Table 83–4).[92–95] In fact, observational studies have documented that

estrogen use is associated with an increased risk of UI compared to that in nonusers.[96–99] Systemic estrogen therapy is associated with numerous adverse effects, including mastodynia, uterine bleeding, nausea, thromboembolism, cardiac and cerebrovascular ischemic events, and enhancement of the risk of certain cancers.[76] If estrogens are to be used in the treatment of SUI, only topical products should be administered. Estrogen use is best justified when SUI exists together with urethritis or vaginitis due to estrogen deficiency.

α-Adrenergic Receptor Agonists

Numerous open trials have supported the use of a variety of α-adrenergic receptor agonists in SUI, including ephedrine, norfenefrine, phenylpropanolamine, and midodrine.[86] Phenylpropanolamine was withdrawn from the U.S. market in late 2000 because of a risk of stroke in women using the agent.[100] Some patients may have leftover supplies of this agent or may obtain it from international sources. If so, those with the contraindications listed below—especially coronary artery disease and/or cardiac arrhythmias—should be warned against self-treatment with this or other α-adrenergic receptor agonists.

Placebo-controlled comparative trials with phenylpropanolamine, norfenefrine, and norephedrine support the modest efficacy of these agents in mild or moderate SUI.[91] These agents have been found to variably affect maximum urethral closure pressure and functional urethral length.

Adverse effects include hypertension, headache, dry mouth, nausea, insomnia, and restlessness.[76] Contraindications to the use of these agents include the presence of hypertension, tachyarrhythmias, coronary artery disease, myocardial infarction, cor pulmonale, hyperthyroidism, renal failure, and narrow-angle glaucoma.

Usual doses are ephedrine 25 to 50 mg four times daily (25 mg twice daily in elders) and pseudoephedrine 60 mg three times daily (15 to 30 mg three times daily in elders; see Table 83–4).

Several studies have evaluated whether the clinical and urodynamic effects of a combination of estrogen and an α-adrenergic receptor agonist exceed those of the individual therapies in SUI.[101–105] In general, combination therapy has resulted in somewhat superior clinical and urodynamic responses compared with monotherapy, including severity of complaints, amount of urine lost per episode, number of daily voluntary micturitions, number of leakage episodes per day, patient preference, pad use, maximum urethral closure pressure, functional urethral length, and pressure transmission ratio.

Duloxetine

Duloxetine, a dual inhibitor of serotonin and norepinephrine reuptake, was approved in 2004 for the treatment of depression and painful diabetic neuropathy (Cymbalta).[106] Its use in SUI (which was in early 2005 awaiting FDA approval under the trade name Yentreve) is based on studies in rats and cats which demonstrated that central serotoninergic and noradrenergic regions are involved in ascending and descending control of urethral smooth muscle and the external urethral sphincter. These mechanisms facilitate the bladder-to-sympathetic reflex pathway, increasing urethral and external urethral sphincter muscle tone during the storage phase. Data documenting this control mechanism in humans are currently very limited. The mean half-life, clearance, and volume of distribution of duloxetine in healthy volunteers are 10 to 12 hours, 114 to 119 L/h, and 1787 to 1943 L, respectively. The drug is extensively metabolized to inactive metabolites (via oxidation at the 4, 5, and/or 6 positions in the naphthyl ring followed by further oxidation or via methylation) with elimination in the urine as conjugated metabolites. CYP450 isoenzymes 2D6 and 1A2 are involved in the ring oxidations. This was demonstrated in studies involving the interaction of duloxetine with the 2D6 substrate desipramine (wherein desipramine's maximum concentration, AUC, and half-life were increased 1.7-, 2.9-, and 1.9-fold, respectively; and clearance fell by 66% during concurrent therapy) and the 2D6 inhibitor paroxetine (wherein duloxetine's maximum concentration, AUC, and half-life increased 1.6-, 1.6-, and 1.3-fold, respectively; and clearance fell 37% during concurrent therapy). Fluvoxamine, a 1A2 inhibitor, increased duloxetine's maximum concentration, AUC, and half-life by over 5-fold, 2.5-fold, and 3-fold, respectively. Thus clinicians will have to be careful when duloxetine is to be used concurrently with 2D6 and 1A2 substrates or inhibitors. The effect of advancing age on duloxetine pharmacokinetics is not clinically significant. Moderate hepatic dysfunction (Child–Pugh class B) significantly affects duloxetine disposition, increasing mean AUC and half-life 5-fold and 3-fold, respectively, and reducing clearance 85% compared with controls. Mild renal impairment does not affect drug disposition, and no data are available for moderate renal impairment. In hemodialysis patients, mean maximum concentration and AUC are each increased 100% while metabolite concentrations are increased up to 900%.

Results of six large clinical trials with duloxetine in SUI have been published. All were double-blind, randomized, placebo-controlled, and parallel group in design. Compared with placebo, duloxetine therapy produced significant reductions in incontinent episode frequency and number of micturitions per day, improvement in Incontinence Quality of Life questionnaire scores and patient self-assessment, and increase in mean micturition interval. Results were independent of baseline UI severity (based on incontinent episode frequency). Significant intergroup differences were seen by week 4. However, cure rates were generally not improved by duloxetine. When evaluating the absolute differences between treatments, the actual benefit of duloxetine was generally quite modest.

Although duloxetine is an encouraging development in the pharmacologic management of SUI, its adverse event profile may make adherence problematic. In the SUI trials, treatment-emergent adverse events occurred in 68% to 93% of duloxetine and 50% to 72% of placebo recipients. Premature study withdrawal rates (due to adverse events) were 12% to 33% for duloxetine and 2% to 8% for placebo. The frequencies of individual events in duloxetine recipients were as follows: nausea, 9% to 46%; headache, 7% to 27%; insomnia, 13% to 14%; constipation, 4% to 27%; dry mouth, 4% to 22%; dizziness, 8% to 16%; fatigue, 10% to 18%; somnolence, 8% to 13%; vomiting, 6% to 13%; and diarrhea 4% to 6%. Of additional interest, the drug may be associated with small increases in blood pressure (like venlafaxine, another dual reuptake inhibitor) and withdrawal symptoms (sleep disturbances).

Despite these negatives, duloxetine would be the first drug approved by the FDA for treating SUI. Based on studies conducted to date, a dosage regimen of 40 to 80 mg/day (in 1 or 2 doses) appears reasonable.

OVERFLOW INCONTINENCE

Overflow incontinence secondary to benign or malignant prostatic hyperplasia may be amenable to pharmacotherapy. For management of malignant prostatic disease, the reader is referred to Chap. 128. The pharmacotherapy of BPH is described in Chap. 82.

CURRENT CONTROVERSY

The optimal approach to the pharmacotherapy of SUI, is unclear. Although not supported by evidence-based medicine, many clinicians will initiate a trial of topical estrogen initially, followed by addition of an α-adrenergic receptor agonist in estrogen nonresponders unless contraindicated. Once duloxetine is approved, it will probably be the drug of choice in SUI, providing that it is tolerated.

SURGICAL TREATMENT

Only rarely does surgery play a role in the initial management of UI.[109] In the absence of secondary complications from UI (e.g., skin breakdown or infection), the decision to surgically treat symptomatic UI should be based on the premise that the degree of bother or lifestyle compromise to the patient is great enough to warrant an elective operation, and that nonoperative therapy is either undesired or has been ineffective.

Successful application of surgery depends most on defining the underlying abnormalities responsible for UI (bladder vs. urethra, underactivity vs. overactivity). Once the underlying factors are clear, other considerations come into play: renal function, sexual function, severity of the leakage, history of prior abdominal or pelvic surgery, the presence of concurrent abdominal or pelvic pathology requiring surgical correction, and finally the patient's suitability for, and willingness to accept the risks of, surgery.

When patients with uncomplicated SUI become dissatisfied with the initial management approaches of pelvic floor exercises, medications, and/or behavioral modification,[109] surgical treatment assumes the primary role.

Surgical correction of female SUI (urethral underactivity) is directed toward either: (1) repositioning the urethra and/or creating a backboard of support, or otherwise stabilizing the urethra and bladder neck in a well-supported retropubic (intra-abdominal) position that is receptive to changes in intra-abdominal pressure; or (2) creating coaptation and/or compression or otherwise augmenting the urethral resistance provided by the intrinsic sphincteric unit, with (i.e., sling) or without (i.e., periurethral collagen and other injectables) urethral and bladder neck support.

In men, SUI may be treated surgically with collagen or the artificial urinary sphincter. The vast majority of collagen injections in men are performed in a retrograde fashion under direct vision through a cystoscope. However, a transabdominal, transvesical, suprapubic antegrade approach has also been used.[110] The artificial urinary sphincter is generally considered to be the gold standard for the treatment of male SUI. Placement of this manually operated silicone device has been associated with very high long-term success and satisfaction rates.[111]

Most patients with UUI are managed nonsurgically with a combination of behavioral modification, pelvic floor exercises, and pharmacologic therapy. Only rarely is surgery applied to the problem of UUI.[101] When employed, surgery may involve bladder denervation, implantation of a sacral nerve stimulator, or augmentation (enlargement) cystoplasty.

Currently there are no effective surgical treatments for bladder underactivity. After an appropriate evaluation is performed for reversible causes, the most effective management for this condition is intermittent self-catheterization performed by the patient or a caregiver.

ree or four times per day. Alternative methods of management that re less satisfactory are indwelling urethral or suprapubic catheters nd urinary diversion.

Urethral overactivity is most commonly caused by anatomic bstruction. Anatomic obstruction in men is most often aused by benign prostatic enlargement, which is discussed in 'hap. 82.

Rarely, bladder outlet obstruction may be caused by a functional obstruction at the level of the bladder neck. Hypertrophy of the smooth muscle fibers at the level of the bladder neck in men and women may result in obstruction to the flow of urine. In those patients who fail pharmacologic therapy with α-adrenergic receptor antagonists, endoscopic incision using the cystoscope is highly effective in treating this very uncommon condition.

EVALUATION OF THERAPEUTIC OUTCOMES

In the long-term management of UI, the patient-specific clinical signs and symptoms of most distress ("bother") to the individal need to be monitored. Use of a daily diary may be very useful n this regard. Some of the short-form instruments used in incontience research for measuring symptom impact and condition-specific uality-of-life can be used in clinical monitoring. In addition, quantating the use of ancillary supplies such as pads may be useful. The oal of therapy is to minimize those signs and symptoms of most other to the patient, as well as the use of pads and other ancillary upplies or devices. Total elimination of UI signs and symptoms may ot be possible, and patients and practitioners need to mutually estabish realistic goals of therapy. As the therapies for UI frequently have uisance adverse effects, such as anticholinergic effects like xerostoia, xerophthalmia, and constipation, that may compromise regimen dherence, the presence and severity of adverse effects need to be arefully elicited at each visit to the health care practitioner. Emerence of adverse effects may necessitate drug dosage adjustment or se of alternative strategies (e.g., chewing sugarless gum, sucking on ard sugarless candy, or the use of saliva substitutes in xerostomia) r even drug discontinuation.

ABBREVIATIONS

\UC: area under the plasma or serum concentration-versus-time curve

3PH: benign prostatic hyperplasia

'YP450: cytochrome P450

)D01: 5-hydroxymethyl metabolite of tolterodine

)EO: N-desethyloxybutynin

EF: incontinence episode frequency

R: immediate-release

_A: long-acting

;UI: stress urinary incontinence

'DS: transdermal system

JI: urinary incontinence

JUI: urge urinary incontinence

XL: extended-release

Review Questions and other resources can be found at vww.pharmacotherapyonline.com.

REFERENCES

1. Abrams P, Cardozo L, Fall M, et al. The standardization of terminology of lower urinary tract function: Report from the standardization subcommittee of the International Continence Society. Neurourol Urodyn 2002;21:167–178.
2. Arnold EP, Burgio K, Diokno AC, et al. Epidemiology and natural history of urinary incontinence (UI). In: Abrams P, Khoury S, Wein AJ, eds. Incontinence. Plymouth, U.K., Plymbridge Distributors, 1999: 199–226.
3. Simeonova Z, Milsom I, Kullendorff AM, et al. The prevalence of urinary incontinence and its influence on the quality of life in women from an urban Swedish population. Acta Obstet Gynecol Scand 1999;78: 546–551.
4. Kobelt F, Kirchberger I, Malone-Lee J. Quality-of-life aspects of the overactive bladder and the effect of treatment with tolterodine. BJU Int 1999;83:583–590.
5. DuBeau CF, Kiely DK, Resnick NM. Quality of life impact of urge incontinence in older persons: A new measure and conceptual structure. J Am Geriatr Soc 1999;47:989–994.
6. Diokno AC, Brock BM, Brown MB, et al. Prevalence of urinary incontinence and other urological symptoms in the noninstitutionalized elderly. J Urol 1986;136:1022–1025.
7. Brown JS, Nyberg LM, Kusek JW, et al. Proceedings of the National Institute of Diabetes, Digestive and Kidney Diseases International Symposium on Epidemiologic Issues in Urinary Incontinence in Women. Am J Obstet Gynecol 2003;188:S77–S88.
8. Ouslander JG, Kane RL, Abrass IB. Urinary incontinence in elderly nursing home patients. JAMA 1982;248:1194–1198.
9. Bump RC. Racial comparisons and contrasts in urinary incontinence and pelvic organ prolapse. Obstet Gynecol 1993;81:421–425.
10. Burgio KL, Matthews KA, Engel BT. Prevalence, incidence and correlates of urinary incontinence in healthy, middle-aged women. J Urol 1991;146:1255–1259.
11. Fliegner JR, Glenning PP. Seven years experience in the evaluation and management of patients with urge incontinence of urine. Aust N Z J Obstet Gynecol 1979;19:42–44.
12. Breakwell SL, Walker SN. Differences in physical health, social interaction and personal adjustment between continent and incontinent homebound aged women. J Community Health Nurs 1988;5:19–31.
13. Malmsten UG, Milsom I, Molander U, Norlen LJ. Urinary incontinence and lower urinary tract symptoms: An epidemiological study of men aged 45–99 years. J Urol 1997;158:1733–1737.
14. Andersson K-E. The overactive bladder: Pharmacologic basis of drug treatment. Urology 1997;50(6A Suppl):74–84.
15. Blaivas JG, Heritz DM. Classification, diagnostic evaluation and treatment overview. In: Blaivas JG, ed. Topics in Clinical Urology—Evaluation and Treatment of Urinary Incontinence. New York, Igaku-Shoin, 1996:22–45.
16. Kuh D, Cardozo L, Hardy R. Urinary incontinence in middle-aged women: Childhood enuresis and other lifetime risk factors in a British prospective cohort. J Epidemiol Community Health 1999;53: 453–458.
17. Groutz A, Gordon D, Keidar R, et al. Stress urinary incontinence: Prevalence among nulliparous compared with primiparous and grand multiparous premenopausal women. Neurourol Urodyn 1999;18:419–425.
18. deGroat WC. A neurologic basis for the overactive bladder. Urology 1997;50(6A Suppl):36–52.
19. Brading AF. A myogenic basis for the overactive bladder. Urology 1997;50(6A Suppl):57–67.
20. Turner WH, Brading AF. Smooth muscle of the bladder in the normal and the diseased state: Pathology, diagnosis and treatment. Pharmacol Ther 1997;75:77–110.
21. Resnick NM, Yalla S. Detrusor hyperactivity with impaired contractile function. An unrecognized but common cause of incontinence in the elderly patient. JAMA 1987;257:3076–3081.

22. Rovner ES, Wein AJ. Today's treatment of overactive bladder and urge incontinence. Womens Health Prim Care 2000;3:179–192.

23. James M, Jackson S, Shepard A, Abrams P. Pure stress leakage symptomatology: Is it safe to discount detrusor instability? Br J Obstet Gynaecol 1999;106:1255–1258.

24. Abrams P, Cardozo L, Khoury S, Wein A, eds. Incontinence. Second International Consultation on Incontinence, 2nd ed. Plymouth, U.K., Health Publications Ltd., 2002.

25. Ouslander JG, Schnelle JF, Uman G, et al. Does oxybutynin add to the effectiveness of prompted voiding for urinary incontinence among nursing home residents? A placebo-controlled trial. J Am Geriatr Soc 1995;43:610–617.

26. Burgio KL, Locher JL, Goode PS, et al. Behavioral vs drug treatment for urge urinary incontinence in older women: A randomized controlled trial. JAMA 1998;280:1995–2000.

27. Drutz HP, Appell RA, Gleason D, et al. Clinical efficacy and safety of tolterodine compared to oxybutynin and placebo in patients with overactive bladder. Int Urogynecol 1999;10:283–289.

28. Abrams P, Freeman R, Anderstrom C, Mattiasson A. Tolterodine, a new antimuscarinic agent: As effective but better tolerated than oxybutynin in patients with an overactive bladder. Br J Urol 1998;81:801–810.

29. Tapp AJ, Cardozo LD, Versi E, Cooper D. The treatment of detrusor instability in post-menopausal women with oxybutynin chloride: A double blind placebo controlled study. Br J Obstet Gynaecol 1990;97:1063–1064.

30. Riva D, Casolati E. Oxybutynin chloride in the treatment of female idiopathic bladder instability. Clin Exp Obstet Gynecol 1984;11:37–42.

31. Schmidt RA, The Oxybutynin XL Study Group. Efficacy of controlled-release, once-a-day oxybutynin chloride for urge urinary incontinence. Jerusalem, International Continence Society, Sept. 14–17, 1998:188.

32. ALZA Corporation. Ditropan XL (oxybutynin chloride) extended-release tablets. Data on file. Palo Alto, CA, 1999.

33. Pharmacia & Upjohn. Detrol (tolterodine) package insert. Kalamazoo, MI, March 1998.

34. Pharmacia & Upjohn. Detrol (tolterodine). Data on file. Kalamazoo, MI, 1998.

35. Appell RA. Clinical efficacy and safety of tolterodine in the treatment of overactive bladder: A pooled analysis. Urology 1997;50(Suppl 6A):90–96.

36. Chancellor M, Freedman S, Mitcheson HD, et al. Tolterodine, an effective and well tolerated treatment for urge incontinence and other overactive bladder symptoms. Clin Drug Invest 2000;19:83–91.

37. Rentzhog L, Stanton SL, Cardozo L, et al. Efficacy and safety of tolterodine in patients with detrusor instability: A dose-ranging study. Br J Urol 1998;81:42–48.

38. Millard R, Tuttle J, Moore K, et al. Clinical efficacy and safety of tolterodine compared to placebo in detrusor overactivity. J Urol 1999;161:1551–1555.

39. Appell RA, Sand P, Dmochowski R, et al. Prospective randomized controlled trial of extended-release oxybutynin chloride and tolterodine tartrate in the treatment of overactive bladder: Results of the OBJECT study. Mayo Clin Proc 2001;76:358–363.

40. Van Kerrebroeck P, Kreder K, Jonas U, et al. Tolterodine once daily: Superior efficacy and tolerability in the treatment of the overactive bladder. Urology 2001;57:414–421.

41. Malone-Lee JG, Walsh JB, Maugourd M-F. Tolterodine: A safe and effective treatment for older patients with overactive bladder. J Am Geriatr Soc 2001;49:700–705.

42. Dmochowski RR, Sand PK, Zinner NR, et al. Comparative efficacy and safety of transdermal oxybutynin and oral tolterodine versus placebo in previously treated patients with urge and mixed urinary incontinence. Urology 2003;62:237–242.

43. Dmochowski RR, Davila GW, Zinner NR, et al. Efficacy and safety of transdermal oxybutynin in patients with urge and mixed urinary incontinence. J Urol 2002;168:580–586.

44. Watson Pharma, Oxytrol (oxybutynin transdermal system) package insert. Morristown, NJ, 2003.

45. Nilsson CG, Lukkari E, Haarala M, et al. Comparison of a 10-mg controlled release oxybutynin tablet with a 5-mg oxybutynin tablet in urge incontinent patients. Neurourol Urodyn 1997;16:533–542.

46. Birns J, Malone Lee JG, and the Oxybutynin CR Study Group. Controlled-release oxybutynin maintains efficacy with a 43% reduction in side effects compared with conventional oxybutynin treatment. Neurourol Urodyn 1997;16:429–430.

47. Anderson RU, Mobley D, Blank B, et al. Once daily controlled versus immediate-release oxybutynin chloride for urge urinary incontinence. OROS Oxybutynin Study Group. J Urol 1999;161:1809–1812.

48. Katz IR, Sands LP, Bilker E, et al. Identification of medications that cause cognitive impairment in older people: The case of oxybutynin chloride. J Am Geriatr Soc 1998;46:8–13.

49. Kelleher CJ, Cardozo LD, Khullar S. A medium term analysis of the subjective efficacy of treatment for women with detrusor instability and low bladder compliance. Obstet Gynecol 1997;104:988–993.

50. Appell RA, Chancellor MB, Zobrist RH, et al. Pharmacokinetics, metabolism, and saliva output during transdermal and extended release oxybutynin administration in healthy subjects. Mayo Clin Proc 2003;78:696–702.

51. Hughes KM, Lang JCT, Lazare R, et al. Measurement of oxybutynin and its N-desethyl metabolite in plasma and its application to pharmacokinetic studies in young, elderly and frail elderly volunteers. Xenobiotica 1992;22:859–869.

52. Amarenco G, Marquis P, McCarthy C, Richard F. Efficacy of oxybutynin on health related quality of life (HRQL) in 1701 women suffering from urinary urge incontinence (UUI). Eur Urol 1998;33(Suppl 1):32–38.

53. ALZA Corporation. Ditropan XL (oxybutynin chloride) extended release tablets package insert. Palo Alto, CA, 1999.

54. Paine MF, Khalighi M, Fisher JM, et al. Characterisation of interintestinal and intraintestinal variations in human CYP3A-dependent metabolism. J Pharmacol Exp Ther 1997;283:1552–1562.

55. Gupta SK, Sathyan G. Pharmacokinetics of an oral once-a-day controlled-release oxybutynin formulation compared with immediate release oxybutynin. J Clin Pharmacol 1999;39:289–296.

56. Buyse G, Waldeck K, Ver C, et al. Intravesical oxybutynin for neurogenic bladder: Less systemic side effects due to reduced first-pass metabolism. J Urol 1998;160:892–896.

57. Gleason DM, Susset J, White C. Evaluation of a new once-daily formulation of oxybutynin for the treatment of urinary urge incontinence. Urology 1999;54:420–423.

58. Susset JG, Gleason DM, White CF, et al. Open-label safety and dose conversion/determination of once-daily OROS oxybutynin chloride for urge urinary incontinence. J Urol 1998;159(Suppl):36.

59. Moore KH, Hay DM, Imrie AE, et al. Oxybutynin hydrochloride (3 mg) in the treatment of women with idiopathic detrusor instability. Br J Urol 1990;66:479–485.

60. Diokno AC, Appell RA, Sand PK, et al. Prospective, randomized, double blind study of the efficacy and tolerability of the extended-release formulations of oxybutynin and tolterodine for overactive bladder: Results of the OPERA trial. Mayo Clin Proc 2003;78:687–695.

61. Sussman D, Garely A. Treatment of overactive bladder with once daily extended-release tolterodine or oxybutynin: The Antimuscarinic Clinical Effectiveness Trial (ACET). Curr Med Res Opin 2002;18:177–184.

62. Guay DRP. Clinical pharmacokinetics of drugs used to treat urge incontinence. Clin Pharmacokinet 2003;42:1243–1285.

63. Zobrist RH, Schmid B, Feick A, et al. Pharmacokinetics of the R- and S-enantiomers of oxybutynin and N-desethyloxybutynin following oral and transdermal administration of the racemate in healthy volunteers. Pharm Res 2001;18:1029–1034.

64. Davila GW, Daugherty CA, Sanders SW. A short-term, multicenter, randomized double-blind dose titration study of the efficacy and anticholinergic side effects of transdermal compared to immediate release oral oxybutynin treatment of patients with urge urinary incontinence. J Urol 2001;166:140–145.

65. Leung HY, Yip SK, Cheon C, et al. A randomized trial of tolterodine and oxybutynin on tolerability and clinical efficacy for treating Chinese women with an overactive bladder. BJU Int 2002;90:375–380.

66. Malone-Lee J, Shaffu B, Anand C, Powell C. Tolterodine: Superior tolerability than and comparable efficacy to oxybutynin in individuals 50 years old or older with overactive bladder. A randomized controlled trial. J Urol 2001;165:1452–1456.

67. Zinner NR, Mattiason A, Stanton SL. Efficacy, safety, and tolerability of extended-release once-daily tolterodine treatment for overactive bladder in older versus younger patients. J Am Geriatr Soc 2002;50:799–807.

68. Dmochowski R, Sathyan G, Ye C, et al. The pH effect of drug release from extended-release formulations of oxybutynin and tolterodine. Proceedings of the Second International Consultation on Incontinence. Paris, France, July 2001.

69. Jonas U, Hofner K, Madersbacher H. Efficacy and safety of two doses of tolterodine versus placebo in patients with detrusor overactivity and symptoms of frequency, urge incontinence, and urgency: Urodynamic evaluation. World J Urol 1997;15:144–151.

70. Guay DRP. Trospium chloride: An update on a quaternary anticholinergic for treatment of urge urinary incontinence. Ther Clin Risk Manage 2004 (invited, in press).

71. Guay DRP. Drug forecast: Solifenacin: An investigational anticholinergic for overactive bladder. Consult Pharm 2004;19:437–444.

72. Kuipers ME, Krauwinkel WJ, Mulder H, Visser N. Solifenacin demonstrates high absolute bioavailability in healthy men. Drugs R D 2004;5:73–81.

73. Uchida T, Krauwinkel WJ, Mulder H, Smulders RA. Food does not affect the pharmacokinetics of solifenacin, a new muscarinic receptor antagonist: Results of a randomized crossover trial. Br J Clin Pharmacol 2004;58:4–7.

74. Smulders RA, Krauwinkel WJ, Swart PJ, Huang M. Pharmacokinetics and safety of solifenacin succinate in healthy young men. J Clin Pharmacol 2004;44:1023–1033.

75. Guay DRP. Drug forecast: Darifenacin: Another investigational antimuscarinic for overactive bladder. Consult Pharm 2004 (invited, in press).

76. Owens RG, Karram MM. Comparative tolerability of drug therapies used to treat incontinence and enuresis. Drug Saf 1998;2:123–139.

77. Milner G, Hills NF. A double-blind assessment of antidepressants in the treatment of 212 enuretic patients. Med J Aust 1968;1:943–947.

78. Castleden CM, George CF, Renwick AG, Asher MJ. Imipramine—A possible alternative to current therapy for urinary incontinence in the elderly. J Urol 1981;125:318–320.

79. Lose G, Jorgenson L, Thuriedborg P. Doxepin in the treatment of female detrusor overactivity: A randomized double-blind crossover study. J Urol 1989;142:1042–1026.

80. Deguecker J. Drug treatment of urinary incontinence in the elderly: Controlled trial with vasopressin and propantheline bromide. Gerontol Clin 1965;7:311–317.

81. Zorzitto ML, Jewett MAS, Fernie GR, et al. Effectiveness of propantheline bromide in the treatment of geriatric patients with detrusor instability. Neurourol Urodyn 1986;5:133–140.

82. Blaivas JG, Labib AB, Michalik SJ, Zayed AAH. Cystometric response to propantheline in detrusor hyperreflexia: Therapeutic implications. J Urol 1980;124:259–262.

83. Holmes DM, Montz FJ, Stanton SL. Oxybutynin versus propantheline in the management of detrusor instability: A patient-regulated variable dose trial. Br J Obstet Gynaecol 1989;96:607–612.

84. Thuroff JW, Bunke B, Ebner A, et al. Randomized, double-blind, multicentre trial on treatment of frequency, urgency and incontinence related to detrusor hyperactivity: Oxybutynin versus propantheline versus placebo. J Urol 1991;145:813–817.

85. Beck RP, Arnusch D, King C. Results in treating 210 patients with detrusor overactivity incontinence of urine. Am J Obstet Gynecol 1976;125:593–596.

86. Castleden CM, Duffin HM, Millar AW. Dicyclomine hydrochloride in detrusor instability: A controlled clinical pilot study. J Clin Exp Gerontol 1987;9:265–270.

87. Herbison P, Hay-Smith J, Ellis G, Moore K. Effectiveness of anticholinergic drugs compared with placebo in the treatment of overactive bladder: systematic review. BMJ 2003;326:841–844.

88. Peyromaure M, Ravery V, Boccon-Gibod L. The management of stress urinary incontinence after radical prostatectomy. BJU Int 2002;90:155–161.

89. Schreiter F, Fuchs P, Stockamp K. Estrogenic sensitivity of α-receptors in the urethral musculature. Urol Int 1976;31:13–19.

90. Jackson S, James M, Abrams P. The effect of oestradiol on vaginal collagen metabolism in postmenopausal women with genuine stress incontinence. BJOG 2002;109:339–344.

91. Guay DRP. Incontinence. Clin Trends Pharm Prac 2002;June:entire issue.

92. Samsioe G, Jansson I, Mellstrom D, Svanborg A. Occurrence, nature, and treatment of urinary incontinence in a 70-year-old female population. Maturitas 1985;7:335–342.

93. Wilson PD, Faragher B, Butler B, et al. Treatment with oral piperazine oestrone sulphate for genuine stress incontinence in postmenopausal women. Br J Obstet Gynecol 1987;94:568–574.

94. Jackson S, Shepherd A, Brookes S, Abrams P. The effect of oestrogen supplementation on post-menopausal urinary stress incontinence: A double-blind placebo-controlled trial. Br J Obstet Gynecol 1999;106:711–718.

95. Jackson S, Shepherd A, Abrams P. Does oestrogen supplementation improve the symptoms of postmenopausal urinary stress incontinence? Neurourol Urodyn 1997;16:350–351 (Abstract).

96. Brown JS, Seeley DG, Fong J, et al. Urinary incontinence in older women: Who is at risk? Study of Osteoporotic Fractures Research Group. Obstet Gynecol 1996;87:715–721.

97. Thom DH, van den Eeden SK, Brown JS. Evaluation of parturition and other reproductive variables as risk factors for urinary incontinence in later life. Obstet Gynecol 1997;90:983–989.

98. Diokno AC, Brock BM, Herzog AR, Bromberg J. Medical correlates of urinary incontinence. Urology 1990;36:129–138.

99. Grady D, Brown JS, Vittinghoff E, et al, and HERS Research Group. Postmenopausal hormones and incontinence: The Heart & Estrogen/Progestin Replacement Study. Obstet Gynecol 2001;97:116–120.

100. Kernan WN, Viscoli CM, Brass LM, et al. Phenylpropanolamine and the risk of hemorrhagic stroke. N Engl J Med 2000:343:1826–1832.

101. Ahlstrom K, Sandahl B, Sjoberg B, et al. Effect of combined treatment with phenylpropanolamine and estriol, compared with estriol treatment alone, in postmenopausal women with stress urinary incontinence. Gynecol Obstet Invest 1990;30:37–43.

102. Kinn A-C, Lindskog M. Estrogens and phenylpropanolamine in combination for stress urinary incontinence in postmenopausal women. Urology 1988;32:273–280.

103. Ek A, Andersson K-E, Gullberg B, Ulmsten U. Effects of oestradiol and combined norephedrine and oestradiol treatment on female stress incontinence. Zentralbl Gynakol 1980;102:839–844.

104. Kiesswetter H, Hennrich F, Englisch M. Clinical and urodynamic assessment of pharmacologic therapy of stress incontinence. Urol Int 1983;38:58–63.

105. Beisland HO, Fossberg E, Moer A, Sander S. Urethral sphincteric insufficiency in postmenopausal females: Treatment with phenylpropanolamine and estriol separately and in combination. Urol Int 1984;39:211–216.

106. Guay DRP. Duloxetine—the first therapy licensed for stress urinary incontinence? Am J Geriatr Pharmacother 2004 (invited, in press).

107. Urinary Incontinence Guideline Panel. Urinary Incontinence in Adults: Clinical Practice Guideline. AHCPR Pub. No. 92–0038. Rockville, MD, Agency for Health Care Policy and Research, Public Health Service, U.S. Department of Health and Human Services, March 1992.

108. Klutke CG, Tiemann DD, Nadler RB, Andriole GL. Early results with antegrade collagen injection for post-radical prostatectomy stress urinary incontinence. J Urol 1996;156:1703–1706.

109. Litwillwer SE, Kim KB, Fone PD, et al. Post-prostatectomy incontinence and the artificial urinary sphincter: A long-term study of patient satisfaction and criteria for success. J Urol 1996;156:1975–1980.

84

FUNCTION AND EVALUATION OF THE IMMUNE SYSTEM

Philip D. Hall and Mary S. Hayney

Learning Objectives and other resources can be found at *www.pharmacotherapyonline.com.*

KEY CONCEPTS

❶ After activation, dendritic cells express higher concentrations of MHC class II molecules B7-1, B7-2, and CD40 and, ICAM-1 and LFA-3 molecules than other antigen-presenting cells. They also produce more interleukin 12 (IL-12). This may explain why in vitro dendritic cells are the most efficient antigen-presenting cells.

❷ A T-lymphocyte expresses hundreds of T-cell receptors (TCRs). All the TCRs expressed on the surface of an individual T-lymphocyte have the same antigen specificity.

❸ A B-lymphocyte can simultaneously express membrane immunoglobulin as IgM (monomeric) or IgD with the same variable region (i.e., antigen-binding site). The B-lymphocyte then can secrete different isotypes [e.g., IgM

(pentamer), IgA, IgG, or IgE] with the same variable region as the membrane immunoglobulin.

❹ A serum protein electrophoresis determines the total concentration of circulating immunoglobulins (i.e., IgG, IgA, IgM, IgD, and IgE). If one wishes to determine the concentration of the individual isotypes, one needs to order isotype quantification. The vast majority of clinical laboratories quantitate only IgG, IgM, and IgA because they are the most prevalent isotypes in the bloodstream. In patients with allergic disorders, quantification of IgE may be useful. Depending on the clinical laboratory, results may be measured in International Units per milliliter or milligrams per deciliter for IgE.

The immune system encompasses a wide range of components, including mechanical immunodefenses, soluble mediators, ands cellular and humoral immune responses. Cells involved in the immune response, from granulocytes to antigen-presenting cells to lymphocytes, develop from a common pluripotent stem cell. Please refer to Chap. 98 for a review of normal hematopoiesis. The human immune system evolved to protect the body against infectious pathogens and cancer. To accomplish this task, the immune system exhibits specificity, memory, mobility, and replicability. *Specificity* indicates that the immune system can distinguish between non-cross-reacting antigens. *Memory* ensures a quicker and more vigorous response to subsequent pathogenic invasion. *Mobility* of the elements of the immune system enables local reactions to provide systemic protection. *Replication* of the cellular components of the immune system amplifies the immune response. In addition, the immune response normally distinguishes "self" from "non-self" to prevent damage to the host. This discrimination between "self" and "nonself" is done by the adaptive or specific arm of the immune response. The immune system includes two functional divisions: *innate* (nonspecific) and *adaptive* (specific)[1] (Table 84–1). Despite this simple separation, these divisions interact heavily.[2]

The innate arm provides the first line of defense against pathogens. One of the most frequently overlooked methods of host

defense is the body's ability to provide a physical and chemical defense against invading pathogens. The skin, the largest organ of the body, has the primary role of providing a physical defense. Alterations in the skin, such as burns or abrasions, allow an easy portal of entry for pathogens. The gastrointestinal tract also plays an important role in providing a physical defense against pathogenic invasion. The low pH of the stomach (pH 1–2) kills many organisms. The rapid turnover of intestinal cells also limits systemic infection because cells, including infected cells, are sloughed frequently. Drugs such as cell-cycle-specific antineoplastics that disrupt the sloughing process leave the patient at an increased risk of infection. Likewise, the respiratory tract has its forms of physical defense. The mucus coating the epithelial cells serves in part to prevent microorganisms from adhering to cell surfaces, and the cilia lining the epithelium of the lungs help to repel inhaled organisms. The combination of cilia, mucus, and reactive coughing provides a natural barrier to invasion via the respiratory tract. Other examples of mechanical or nonspecific defenses include normal urine flow, lysozymes in tears and saliva, and the normal flora in the throat, the lower gastrointestinal tract, and the genitourinary tract. It is these physical and chemical defenses that often form the first line of defense against infectious pathogens. It is well known that conditions or devices that allow microorganisms to transgress these normal barriers predispose patients to infections. As

TABLE 84–1. Functional Divisions of the Immune System

	Innate	Adaptive
Exterior defenses	Skin, mucus, cilia, normal flora, saliva, low pH of the stomach, skin, and genitourinary tract	None
Specificity	Limited and fixed	Extensive
Memory	None	Yes
Time to response	Hours	Days
Soluble factors	Lysozymes, complement, C-reactive protein, interferons, mannose binding lectin	Antibodies, cytokines
Cells	Neutrophils, monocytes, macrophages, NK cells, eosinophils	B-lymphocytes, T-lymphocytes

NK, natural killer.

such, patients with a substantial loss of the skin from a burn or those requiring mechanical ventilation, bladder catheterization, or central venous access are at increased risk of infection.

THE IMMUNE RESPONSE

When an infectious pathogen eludes the exterior defenses of the body, an immune response involving both leukocytes and soluble mediators then attacks the pathogen.

INNATE RESPONSE

Innate immunity is present from birth and uses a preexisting but limited repertoire of receptors to recognize pathogens and destroy them. The innate leukocytes include monocytes, macrophages, neutrophils, basophils, mast cells, and eosinophils. All except basophils act as phagocytes, while mast cells and basophils secrete inflammatory mediators when stimulated. The phagocytes recognize, internalize, and destroy invading pathogens. These cells use either opsonin-dependent phagocytosis or opsonin-independent phagocytosis. For opsonin-dependent phagocytosis, antibody (e.g., IgG), complement (e.g., C3b), or lectin (e.g., C-reactive protein) coats the infectious pathogens in a process termed *opsonization;* then the antibody, complement, or lectin binds to the receptors on the innate leukocyte (Fig. 84–1), thereby activating the phagocytic process. For opsonin-independent phagocytosis, innate leukocytes utilize pattern recognition receptors. Pattern-recognition receptors focus on highly conserved structures present on a large group of microorganisms and essential for survival of the microorganisms or pathogenicity. These receptors include the macrophage mannose receptor, the macrophage scavenger receptor, and members of the toll-like receptor family. Pattern-recognition receptors on phagocytes directly recognize ligands (e.g., lipoteichoic acid from gram-positive organisms, lipopolysaccharide from gram-negative organisms, or mannoses on the surfaces of infectious pathogens (see Fig. 84–1). The macrophage mannose receptor recognizes a variety of gram-positive bacteria, gram-negative bacteria, and fungi based on their overexpression of mannoses. The macrophage scavenger receptor recognize

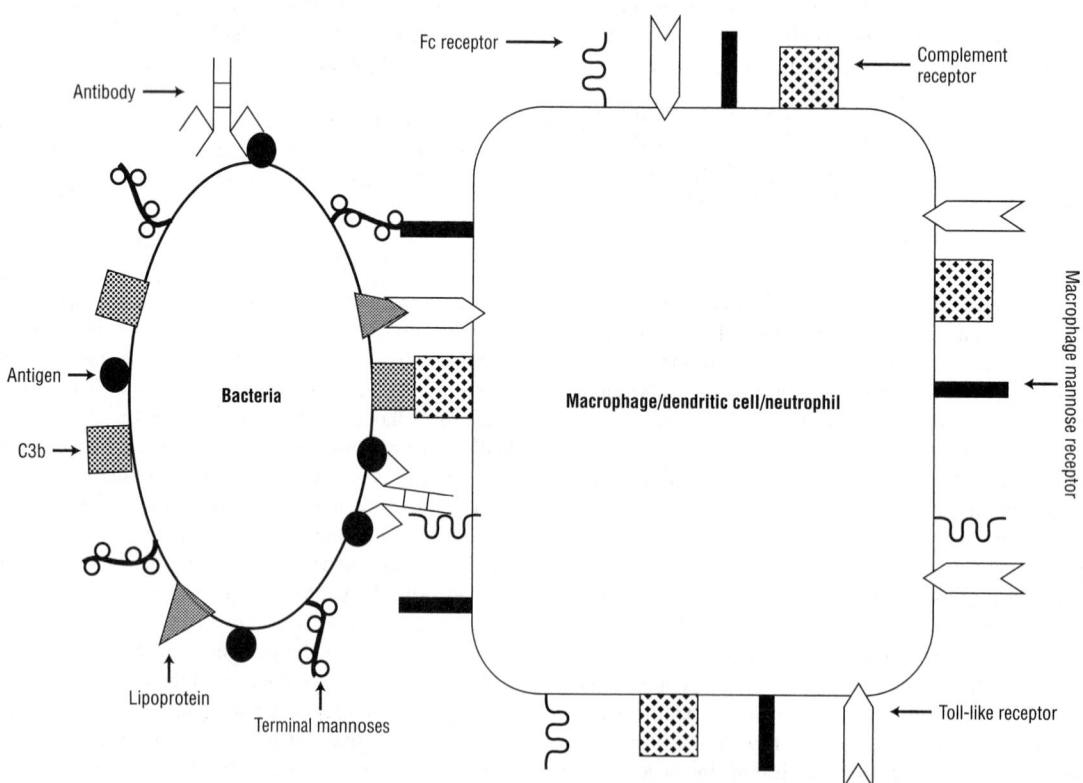

FIGURE 84–1. Phagocytosis of bacteria by macrophages, dendritic cells, and neutrophils. Macrophages, dendritic cells, and neutrophils recognize bacteria that are opsonized and coated with antibody or complement (C3b). On the surfaces of the macrophages, dendritic cells, and neutrophils reside receptors for antibody (Fc receptor) and complement (CR1, CR3, CR4). In addition, these cells may recognize the bacteria by pattern-recognition receptors on the surfaces of the macrophages, dendritic cells, and neutrophils. Pattern-recognition receptors include the toll-like receptors, scavenger receptors, and mannose receptors.

e lipopolysaccharide from bacteria and double-stranded RNA from RNA viruses. The major function of these receptors is phagocytosis of the pathogen. Other pattern-recognition receptors that mediate phagocytosis include MARCO and DEC205. Toll-like receptors are another family of pattern-recognition receptors on the cell surface of innate leukocytes. To date, 10 toll-like receptors have been identified in humans. They recognize a broad spectrum of antigens ranging from lipopolysaccharide and flagellin on bacteria to zymosan on yeast to double-stranded RNA from RNA viruses. Binding of the ligand to the toll-like receptors results in the secretion of chemokines, inflammatory cytokines, and antimicrobial peptides, as well as the increased expression of costimulatory proteins (e.g., B7) and the major histocompatibility complex (MHC) proteins. This leads to the recruitment and activation of antigen-specific lymphocytes.[2-4]

The granulocytes include neutrophils, eosinophils, and basophils. The cytoplasmic granules of these cells often contain inflammatory mediators or digestive enzymes. Neutrophils are polymorphonuclear cells, often denoted as PMNs for this reason, that serve as the primary human defense against invasive bacteria and comprise the majority of leukocytes in the bloodstream. Neutrophils migrate from the bloodstream into infected or inflamed tissue in response to chemotactic factors such as IL-8 and C3a and C5a, breakdown products of complement. This migration of neutrophils to sites of infection is termed *chemotaxis,* whereupon they recognize, adhere to, and phagocytose pathogens. Neutrophils can only recognize pathogens opsonized or coated with complement or IgG (antibody) via the complement and antibody receptors located on the surface of the neutrophil. They also can recognize pathogens via toll-like receptors. Once bound, the neutrophil then releases its granular contents into lysosome and generates the release of oxidative metabolites, thereby killing engulfed pathogens.[5]

Eosinophils are also granulocytic cells involved in innate immunity. They exhibit motility and migrate from the blood into the tissues. They play a less significant role in combating bacterial infections, but eosinophils play a major role against nonphagocytable multicellular pathogens such as parasites. After activation via a high-affinity receptor for IgE (i.e., Fcε), granule exocytosis releases the granule contents (e.g., major basic protein, reactive oxygen metabolites) into the microenvironment to lyse the parasite. Besides Fcε receptors, eosinophils express lower levels of complement receptor 3 and Fcγ for IgG than neutrophils. Because of their ability to bind IgE, eosinophils contribute to the pathogenesis of allergic disorders (i.e., allergic asthma).[6]

Macrophages and monocytes are mononuclear cells capable of phagocytosis. Tissue macrophages arise from the migration of monocytes from the bloodstream into the tissues. Macrophages differ from monocytes by possessing an increased number of Fc and complement receptors. Macrophages are found within specific tissues such as the liver, spleen, gastrointestinal tract, lymph nodes, brain, and others. These specific types of macrophages are often called *histiocytes* or referred to by a specialized name depending on the site where they are found (Kupffer cells in the liver, osteoclasts in the bone, microglial cells in the central nervous system, etc. The term *reticuloendothelial system* (RES) was used commonly to refer to macrophages found in reticular connective tissue, but the preferred term is now the *mononuclear phagocyte system.*[7]

Despite the first description of Langerhans cells, a type of dendritic cell found in the skin, in 1868, our understanding of the biologic function of dendritic cells did not develop until the past decade. Before encountering a pathogen, most dendritic cells are in an immature/resting state with limited ability to activate T-lymphocytes; however, they express numerous receptors (e.g., Fc receptors of IgG

and IgE, macrophage mannose receptor, toll-like receptors) to capture antigen. After taking up antigen, they become activated, which leads to a dramatic increase in their expression of MHC class II, B7, CD40, and adhesion molecules. Dendritic cells then begin to migrate through the tissues toward lymphoid organs (e.g., spleen, lymph nodes) to present antigen to T-lymphocytes to initiate the activation process.[8]

In addition to phagocytosing pathogens, macrophages and dendritic cells act as antigen-presenting cells (APCs) to stimulate the adaptive (specific) system. Macrophages and dendritic cells internalize the organism, digest it into small peptide fragments, and then combine these antigenic fragments together with MHC proteins. Once the APC has formed the antigen-MHC complex, the APC places the complex on its surface. This surface complex then can be recognized by the T-cell receptor on the surface of a T-lymphocyte. Recognition of the antigen-MHC complex by the T-cell receptor is the first step in the activation of the T-lymphocyte (Fig. 84–2). Other cells, B-lymphocytes and mast cells, can act as APCs[7-9] (Fig. 84–3).

Mast cells and basophils act primarily by releasing inflammatory mediators. Mast cells are tissue cells predominately associated with IgE-mediated inflammation. They are especially abundant in the skin, lungs, and nasal mucosa. Granules within the mast cells contain large amounts of preformed mediators that include histamine, heparin, serotonin, etc. Mast cells can phagocytize, destroy, and present bacterial antigens to T-lymphocytes.[10] Basophils are similar to mast cells because they contain granules filled with histamine, but they typically are found circulating in the blood and are not found in connective tissue. Like mast cells, basophils also express high-affinity IgE Fc receptors (Fcε). IgE-mediated anaphylaxis (type I hypersensitivity; see Chap. 86) is caused by the stimulation of mast cells and/or basophil degranulation and the release of preformed mediators after allergen binds to IgE bound to the Fcε receptor on the surface of mast cells or basophils.[11]

Soluble mediators of innate immunity include the complement system, mannose-binding lectin, and C-reactive protein (CRP).[1] The complement system consists of more than 30 proteins in the plasma and on cell surfaces that play a key role in immune defense. The four major functions of the complement system include (1) the ability to lyse certain microorganisms and cells, (2) the ability to stimulate the chemotaxis of phagocytic cells, (3) the ability to coat or opsonize foreign pathogens, which allows phagocytosis of the pathogen by leukocytes expressing complement receptors, and (4) the clearance of immune complexes. Complement factors (C3a, C5a) act as chemotactic factors for phagocytic cells.[12] Two different pathways stimulate the complement cascade. In the *classic pathway,* antibody binds to its target antigen and activates the first component of complement (C1), thereby initiating the complement cascade. The *alternative complement pathway* relies on the inability of microorganisms to clear spontaneously produced C3b, the active form of third complement protein, from their surfaces. Patients with hereditary deficiencies of complement have recurrent bacterial infections or immune-complex disease. Both mannose-binding lectin and C-reactive protein are acute-phase reactants produced by the liver during the early stages of an infection that bind to infectious pathogens and then activate the lectin or minor pathway of the complement system. Mannose-binding lectin binds to mannose-rich glycoconjugates on microorganisms, whereas C-reactive protein binds to phosphorylcholine on bacterial surfaces.[1,12]

Chemokines play an essential role in linking the innate and adaptive immune responses by orchestrating leukocyte trafficking. The chemokine system consists of a group of small polypeptides and their receptors. Chemokines possess four conserved cysteines. Based on

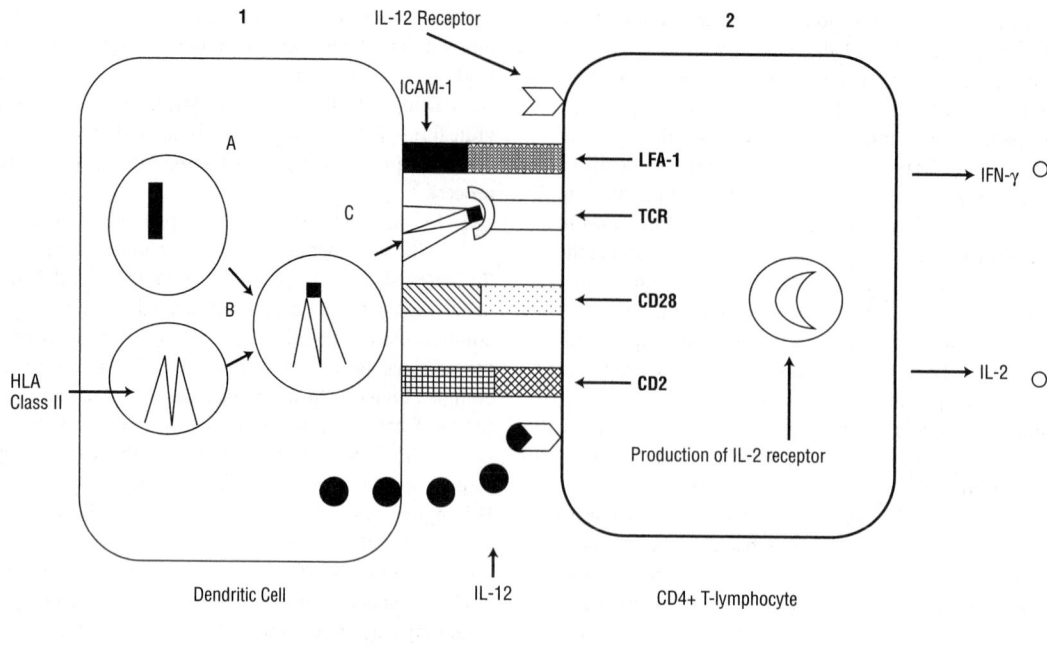

FIGURE 84–2. Induction of TH$_1$ response. The antigen- presenting cell, in this case a dendritic cell, engulfs the pathogen by any of numerous cell surface receptors (see Fig. 84–1). (1) After phagocytosis of the bacteria by the dendritic cell (*A*), the pathogen is digested into small peptides and becomes associated with MHC class II within the endosome (*B*). Finally, the MHC class II plus peptide is expressed on the surface of the dendritic cell (*C*). The activated dendritic cell also secretes IL-12. (2) The naïve CD4$^+$ T-lymphocyte activation requires the T-cell receptor (TCR) to recognize the antigenic peptide in association with MHC class II as well as the B7-1 (CD80) binding to CD28. The binding of CD2––CD58 and LFA-1 (CD11a/CD18) allows the adherence between the T-lymphocyte and dendritic cell. Upon activation, the TH$_1$ CD4$^+$ T-lymphocyte secretes IL-2 and γ-interferon and increases the production and the expression of the IL-2 receptor.

the positions of the cysteines, almost all chemokines fall into one of two categories: (1) the CC group, in which the conserved cysteines are contiguous, or (2) the CXC subgroup, in which the cysteines are separated by some other amino acid (X). As with all ligand-receptor interactions, a cell can only respond to a chemokine if it possesses a receptor that recognizes it. Chemokine receptors are unique in that they traverse the membrane seven times. CC receptors (CCR) and CXC receptors (CXCR) bind CC ligands (CCL) and CXC ligands (CXCL), respectively (Table 84–2).

Binding of infectious pathogens to pattern-recognition receptors stimulates the release of macrophage inflammatory protein (MIP) 1α, MIP-1β, MIP-3α, and IP-10 from macrophages and dendritic cells

embedded in the tissues. These chemokines attract more immature dendritic cells to the site of inflammation/infection. Immature dendritic cells constitutively express CCR1, CCR5, and CCR6. The interaction between pattern-recognition receptors on the dendritic cell and the infectious pathogen causes the activation and maturation of the dendritic cell. After activation, dendritic cells downregulate the expression of CCR1, CCR5, and CCR6 and upregulate the expression of CCR7. This switch in chemokine-receptor expression results in the antigen-loaded dendritic cell leaving the tissue and migrating toward the lymph nodes.[13]

ADAPTIVE RESPONSE

To amplify the immune response, activation of the adaptive immune system is required. The adaptive immune response differs from the innate immune response in two critical areas: specificity and memory. T- and B-lymphocytes comprise the cells of the adaptive response. These cells have surface receptors specific for the invading organism. In a manner that uses genetic rearrangement of their DNA, it is estimated that lymphocytes have the ability to recognize over 10^{15} different types of antigens. Generally, the body will employ both the innate and adaptive immune responses to kill foreign pathogens.[1]

The adaptive immune response can be divided into two major arms: humoral and cellular-mediated. The B-lymphocytes and plasma cells, activated B-lymphocytes that secrete antibody, comprise the humoral arm of the adaptive immune response. The humoral response is so denoted because it was found that the factors that provided the

TABLE 84–2. Common Chemokines

Receptor	Cell Expression	Ligand
CCR1	Immature DC	MIP-1α, MIP-1β, MCP-2, RANTES
CCR3	Eosinophils, basophils	Eotaxin-1, -2, -3, MCP-4
CCR6	Immature DC	Exodus-1
CCR7	Activated DC	CCL21 (SLC), CCL19 (ELC)
CXCR1/2	Neutrophils	IL-8
CXCR3	NK cells, activated T-lymphocytes	IP-10

DC, dendritic cell; MCP, monocyte chemoattractant protein; RANTES, regulated upon activation normal T-lymphocyte expressed and secreted.

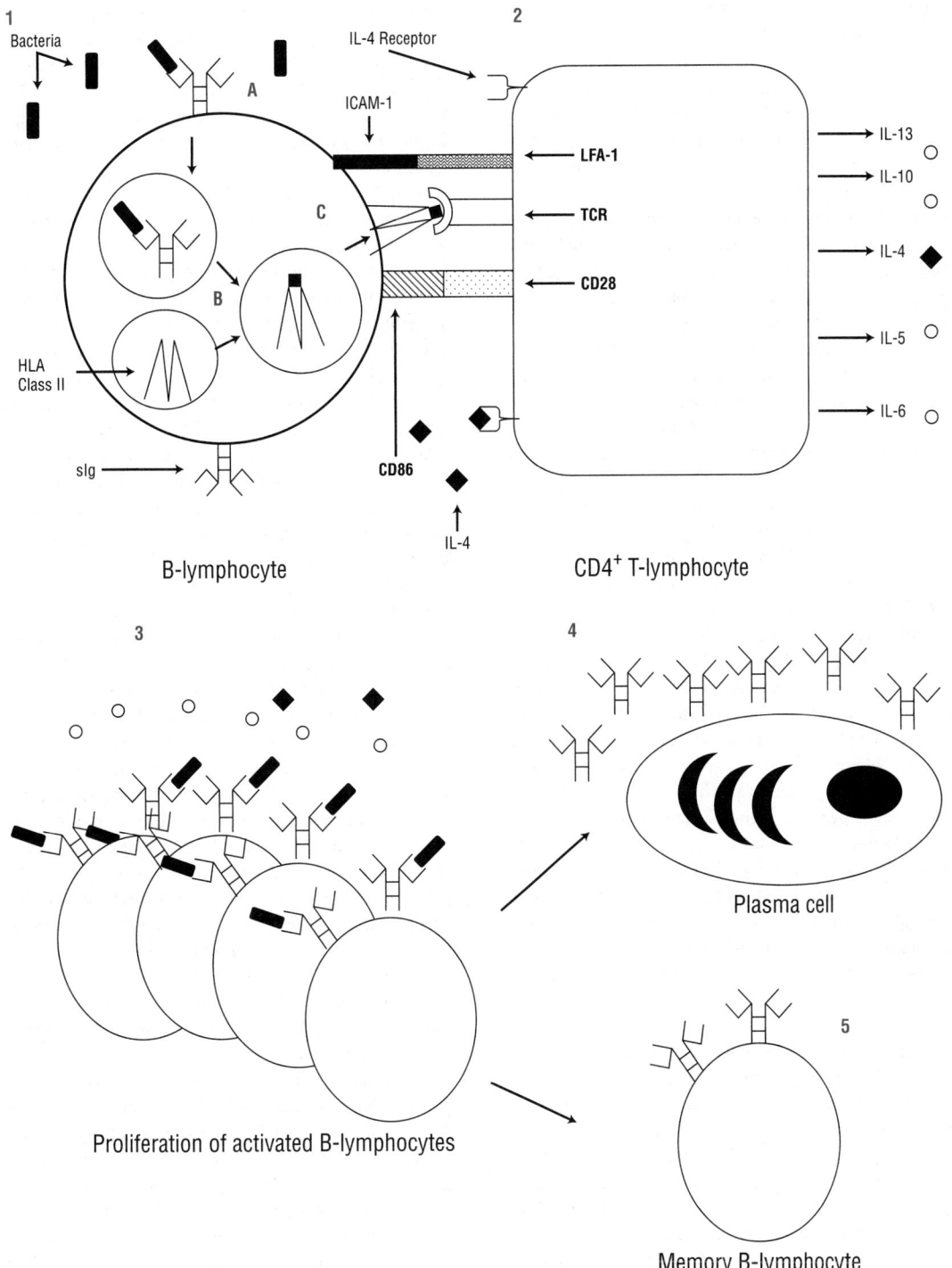

FIGURE 84–3. Induction of a TH₂ response. (*1A*) A B-lymphocyte recognizes an invading bacteria via its surface immunoglobulin (sIg) (*B*). (*1B*) The bound bacteria is then phagocytosed into an endosome, where the bacteria is broken down into small peptide fragments (*B*). (*1C*) The small peptide fragments are then placed within MHC class II molecules and transported to the surface of the B-lymphocyte for antigen presentation to a CD4⁺ T-lymphocyte (*C*). (*2*) CD4⁺ T-lymphocyte recognition requires antigen recognition within the MHC class II peptide groove by the T-lymphocyte receptor (TCR) and a secondary signal from B7 from the antigen presenting cell, in this case a B-lymphocyte, binding to CD28 on the T-lymphocyte. When both signals are delivered to the CD4⁺ T-lymphocyte, it becomes activated. In the TH₂ environment (see text), the naïve CD4⁺ T-lymphocyte develops into a TH₂ subtype and secretes IL-4, IL-5, IL-6, IL-10, and IL-13 that promote a TH₂ response. (*3*) In the presence of these cytokines plus antigen binding to the its sIg, the B-lymphocyte becomes activated. The activated B-lymphocyte becomes a plasma cell (*4*) that produces and secretes immunoglobulin or becomes a memory B-lymphocyte (*5*). The minority of B-lymphocytes become memory B-lymphocytes.

immune protection could be found in the blood humor or serum. The cell-mediated arm is mediated by T-lymphocytes. The immune protection provided by these cells could not be transferred by serum alone. Rather, it is essential to actually have T-lymphocytes present, thus the term *cell-mediated immunity*. T-lymphocytes are specially tailored to defend against infections that are intracellular, such as virally infected cells, whereas B-lymphocytes secrete antibodies that can neutralize pathogens prior to their entry into host cells.

T-lymphocytes do not recognize intact antigen. T-lymphocytes recognize processed antigen in association with the MHC. APCs (e.g., macrophages and dendritic cells) phagocytize the pathogen and then break down the pathogen and express peptide fragments of the processed antigen in association with the MHC on their surface. T-lymphocytes express a specific antigen receptor, the TCR. The TCR is comprised of two chains, with each chain having a variable and a constant region. The variation in the amino acid sequence within the variable domain of the TCR gives the cell its unique antigen specificity. Linked to the TCR is a complex of single chains known as the *CD3 complex*.[1,9]

Naïve T-lymphocytes, cells that have not been exposed previously to an antigen specific for their TCR, require two signals for activation. The first signal for activation involves the T-lymphocyte recognizing both the processed antigen and the MHC-molecule complex. The second signal involves the interaction of the B7-1 (CD80) or B7-2 (CD86) molecule on the APC with the CD28 molecule on the surface of the T-lymphocyte (see Figs. 84–2 and 84–3). Without the second signal, the T-lymphocyte becomes anergic or inactive. Memory T-lymphocytes are less dependent on the second signal than are naïve T-lymphocytes. CD28 is expressed on both resting and activated T-lymphocytes, whereas CTLA-4, a second ligand for B7 on T-lymphocytes, is expressed only on activated T-lymphocytes. CTLA-4 binding B7 transduces a negative signal so that it plays a role in downregulating a T-lymphocyte response.[14] After the two activation signals, a message is sent through the TCR to the CD3 complex into the cell. Then a calcium influx occurs with subsequent activation of the T-lymphocyte. Activated CD4$^+$ T-lymphocytes release various soluble factors (e.g., IL-2) to stimulate T-lymphocytes and other cells of the immune system (see Fig. 84–2) and to express high-affinity IL-2 receptor. Autocrine stimulation by IL-2 leads to the proliferation of the activated T-lymphocyte.

Cell surface markers or functional activity delineate T-lymphocyte populations. All T-lymphocytes express the CD3 protein. Typically, T-lymphocytes are further divided into helper cells (CD4$^+$), suppressor cells (CD8$^+$), and cytotoxic cells (CD8$^+$). Each of the subclasses appears to play a distinct role in the cell-mediated immune response. Naïve T-lymphocytes express CD45RA, a high-molecular-weight isoform of CD45, while memory T-lymphocytes express CD45RO, a lower-molecular-weight isoform of CD45.[15] The primary role of CD4$^+$ cells is to stimulate other cells in the immune response. Functionally, CD4$^+$ cells can be divided into TH$_1$ and TH$_2$. This functional system was first described in mice. TH$_1$ cells secrete IL-2 and γ-interferon and stimulate CD8$^+$ cytotoxic cells, while TH$_2$ cells secrete IL-4, IL-5, and IL-10 and stimulate B-lymphocyte production of antibody.[16] Multiple factors determine whether a naïve CD4$^+$ T-lymphocyte develops into a TH$_1$ or a TH$_2$ cell. The cytokine microenvironment plays an important role in this development. IL-12 secreted by the APCs promotes TH$_1$, whereas IL-4 promotes TH$_2$ development. Other factors that promote TH$_1$ development include B7-1 (CD80), high affinity of the TCR for the antigen, γ-interferon, and α-interferon. Factors that promote TH$_2$ development include B7–2 (CD86), low affinity of the TCR for the antigen, IL-10, and IL-1.[17]

CD8$^+$ T-lymphocytes recognize antigen in association with MHC class I. CD8$^+$ cytotoxic cells are instrumental in killing cells

recognized as foreign, such as those which have become infected by a virus. These cells also play an important beneficial role in the eradication of tumor cells but also are responsible for rejection of transplanted organs.[9] Classically, a second type of CD8$^+$ T-lymphocyte was a suppressor cell. It is clear that some T-lymphocytes help to suppress the immune responses, but whether this subset is CD8$^+$ is debatable. Emerging evidence is leading away from CD8$^+$ T-lymphocytes toward CD4$^+$ and CD25$^+$ T-lymphocytes in maintaining self-tolerance. The preferred term for these suppressive T-lymphocytes is *regulatory T-lymphocytes*.[18]

To fully activate the CD8$^+$ cytotoxic T-lymphocyte requires CD4$^+$ T-lymphocyte activation, namely, the TH$_1$ subset, and its subsequent secretion of IL-2 (Fig. 84–4A). This model of CD8$^+$ cytotoxic T-lymphocyte activation requires the close proximity of two rare- antigen-specific T-lymphocytes. In addition, some CD8$^+$ cytotoxic T-lymphocyte responses can occur in the absence of CD4$^+$ T-lymphocytes. New data suggest that CD4$^+$ T-lymphocytes can activate/prime APCs through CD40. This interaction primes the APC (e.g., dendritic cell) to fully activate CD8$^+$ cytotoxic T-lymphocytes[19] (see Fig. 84–4B). It is important to remember that the classification of CD4$^+$ lymphocytes as T-helper lymphocytes and CD8$^+$ lymphocytes as T-cytotoxic lymphocytes is not an absolute. Some CD8$^+$ T-lymphocytes secrete cytokines similar to a T-helper lymphocyte, and some CD4$^+$ T-lymphocytes can act as cytotoxic cells.

Unlike neutrophils and macrophages, cytotoxic T-lymphocytes are unable to ingest their targets. They destroy target cells by two different mechanisms: the *perforin system* and the *Fas ligand pathway*. After recognition by the cytotoxic T-lymphocyte, cytoplasmic granules containing perforins and granzymes are oriented rapidly toward the target cell, and the contents of the granules are released into the intracellular space. Like the membrane-attack complex formed after complement activation, perforins form a pore in the target cell membrane. Besides a direct cytotoxic effect on the target cell, the pores produced by perforins allow the granzymes to penetrate into the target cell to induce apoptosis. The second mechanism of cytotoxicity involves the binding of Fas ligand on the cytotoxic T-lymphocyte to the Fas receptor on the target cell. The Fas ligand is predominately expressed on CD8$^+$ cytotoxic T-lymphocytes and natural killer (NK) cells, and its expression increases after activation. After killing by either mechanism, the cytotoxic T-lymphocyte detaches from the target cell and attacks other targets.[20]

B-lymphocytes recognize antigen via its antibody or immunoglobulin located on the surface of the B-lymphocyte (see Fig. 84–3). The antibody on the surface can recognize an intact pathogen, such as bacteria, and present antigen to T-lymphocytes (i.e., acting as APC). However, the major function of B-lymphocytes is to produce antibody to bind to the invading pathogen, a process that first entails activation of the lymphocyte. The activation of B-lymphocytes also requires two steps: (1) recognition of antigen by the surface immunoglobulin and (2) the presence of B-lymphocyte growth factors (IL-4, IL-5, and IL-6) secreted by activated CD4$^+$ T-lymphocytes. Once activated, the B-lymphocyte becomes a plasma cell, a differentiated cell capable of producing and secreting antibody. A fraction of activated B-lymphocytes does not differentiate into plasma cells but rather forms a pool of memory cells. The memory cells will respond to subsequent encounters with the pathogen, generating a quicker and more vigorous response to the pathogen. Some B-lymphocytes can become activated without help from T-lymphocytes, but these responses generally are weak and do not invoke memory.[1,9]

When binding of a specific antigen to the surface immunoglobulin receptor of B-lymphocytes occurs, the B-lymphocyte matures into a plasma cell and produces large quantities of antibodies that have the ability to bind to the inciting antigen. The secreted

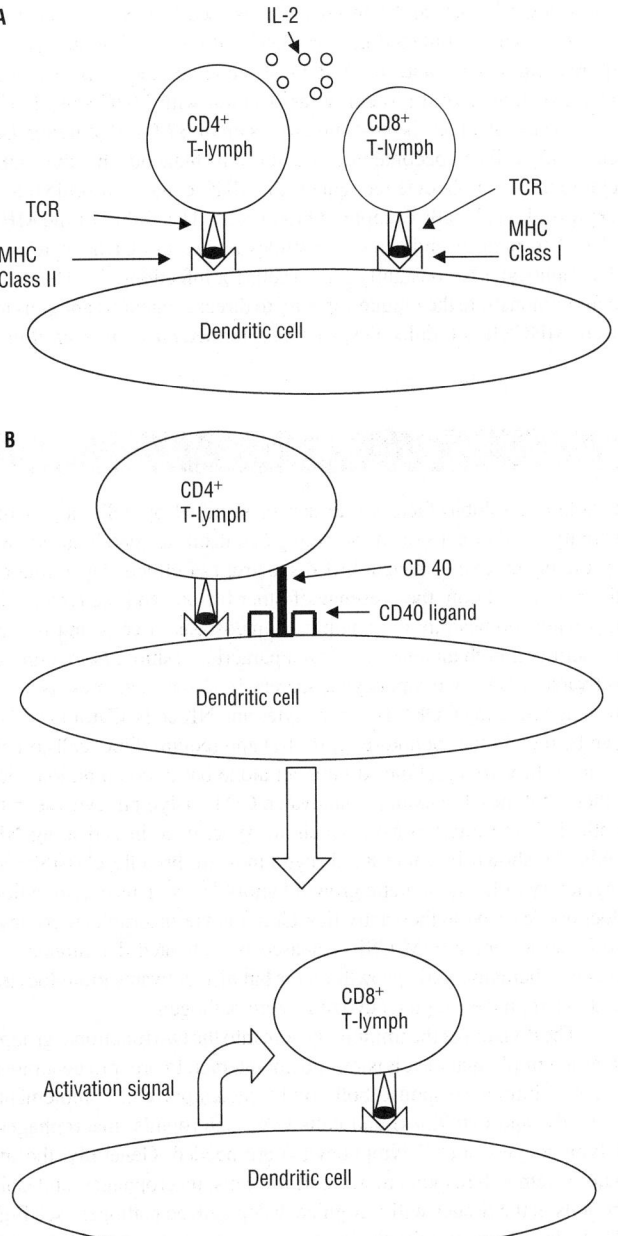

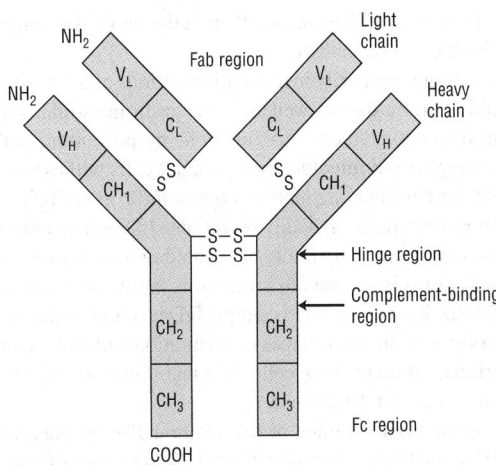

FIGURE 84–5. Schematic structure of the immunoglobulin G (IgG) molecule. An IgG molecule consists of two heavy (H) and two light (L) chains covalently linked by disulfide bonds. Each chain is comprised of variable (V) and constant (C) regions. A light chain consists of one variable (VL) and one constant (CL) region. Heavy chains consist of one variable (VH) and three or four constant (CH) regions, depending on the isotype. The variable regions (VL and VH) comprise the antigen-binding region of the IgG molecule, or fragment antigen binding (Fab). The constant regions provide the structure to the IgG molecule as well as binding the first component of complement (CH2) and binding to Fc receptors via the Fc portion of the molecule (CH3).

FIGURE 84–4. In the classic model of CD8+ T-lymphocyte activation (A), the CD4+ and CD8+ T-lymphocytes recognize antigen on the same dendritic cell. In the presence of IL-2 from the activated CD4+ T-lymphocyte and the recognition of antigen in association with MHC class I, the CD8+ T-lymphocyte becomes activated. In the new model (B), activated CD4+ T-lymphocytes activate dendritic cells via CD40 ligand binding to CD40. The activated dendritic cell then migrates through the tissues to present antigen to CD8+ T-lymphocytes. If recognition via the TCR on the CD8+ T-lymphocyte occurs, the dendritic cell can fully activate the CD8+ T-lymphocyte without the presence of CD4+ T-lymphocytes.

antibodies may be of five different isotypes. On primary exposure to the pathogen, the plasma cell will secrete IgM, but eventually there is a switch to predominately IgG during the first exposure. On second exposure, the memory B-lymphocytes will predominately produce IgG. Isotype switching from IgM to IgG, IgA, or IgE is controlled by T-lymphocytes.

An antibody or immunoglobulin is a glycoprotein consisting of two different chains, heavy and light (Fig. 84–5). The basic structure of every immunoglobulin consists of four peptide chains: two identical

heavy chains and two identical light chains held together by disulfide bonds. The basic structure of the antibody is a Y-shaped figure. Each arm of the Y is formed by the linkage of the end of the light chain to its heavy-chain partner. These arms contain the portions described as the *fragments of antigen binding (Fab fragment)*. The stem of the Y contains the heavy chains that comprise the *fragment crystallizable (Fc fragment)* portion of the antibody. It is within the Fc portion that complement is activated once the antibody has bound its target. Likewise, it is the Fc portion of the antibody that is recognized by Fc receptors on the surface of phagocytes (see Fig. 84–1). The amino acid composition of the same isotype is homogeneous except in the variable regions of the light (V_L) and heavy chains (V_H). The variation in amino acid composition of the variable region gives the antibody its unique specificity (see Fig. 84–5)

IgG, the most prevalent of the antibody classes, comprises approximately 80% of serum antibody. IgG is usually the second isotype of antibody to be produced in an initial humoral immune response. IgG is the only isotype of antibody that can cross the placenta. Therefore, early maternal humoral protection of neonates is primarily due to maternal IgG that crossed the placenta in utero.

Four different subclasses of IgG have been described: IgG_1, IgG_2, IgG_3, and IgG_4. These subclasses differ slightly in their constant amino acid sequences. IgG_1 constitutes the majority (60%) of the subclasses. It appears that different subclasses recognize different types of antigen. IgG_1 and IgG_3 are principally responsible for recognition of protein antigens. Whereas IgG_2 and IgG_4 commonly bind to carbohydrate antigens. Another difference in the subclasses is the ability to activate complement, with IgG_3 and IgG_1 being the most efficient but IgG_4 unable to to do so.

IgM can be found on the surfaces of B-lymphocytes as a monomeric Y-shaped structure. In contrast, IgM is a pentamer in which five of the monomers are joined together by a joining chain (*J-chain*). IgM is the first class of antibody to be produced on initial exposure to an antigen. Because the pentameric form of IgM has no Fc portions exposed, phagocytic cells cannot bind pathogens opsonized by IgM. However, IgM is an excellent activator of the complement cascade by the classic pathway.

IgA is found primarily in the fluid secretions of the body—tears, saliva, and nasal fluids—as well as in the gastrointestinal, genitourinary, and respiratory tracts. IgA functions by preventing pathogens from adhering to and infecting the epithelial cells at these sites. IgA is also secreted in a nursing mother's breast milk, as are IgG and IgM in lower concentrations. In bodily secretions, IgA is in a dimeric form in which a J-chain and a secretory chain hold two monomers together. The dimeric form is resistant to proteolysis in mucosal secretions.

IgD is the least understood isotype. IgD is found on the surface of B-lymphocytes at different stages of maturation and may be involved in the differentiation of these cells. The main function of circulating IgD has not yet been determined.

IgE is the least common of the serum antibody isotypes. Most of the IgE in the body is bound to the IgE Fc receptors on mast cells. When the IgE on the surface of mast cells binds antigen, it causes the release of various inflammatory substances (e.g., histamine) from the mast cell. The overall effect is the stimulation of inflammation. Asthma and hay fever are a few examples of allergic reactions primarily due to antigen binding to IgE.[21]

NK cells, often referred to as *large granular lymphocytes,* are defined functionally by their ability to lyse target cells without prior sensitization and without restriction by MHC. Resting NK cells express the intermediate-affinity IL-2 receptor CD122. Upon exposure to IL-2, NK cells exhibit greater cytotoxic activity against a wide variety of tumors. NK cells recognize target cells by two mechanisms. First, NK cells express an IgG Fc receptor, CD16, that allows recognition of IgG-coated cells. Second, NK cells express killer-activating and killer-inhibiting receptors. The killer-activating receptors recognize multiple targets on normal cells; however, the binding of MHC class I to the killer-inhibitor receptor blocks release of perforins and granzymes. Therefore, cells (e.g., tumor cells, virally infected cells) that downregulate MHC class I expression are susceptible to NK cell cytolysis. NK cells play important roles in surveillance against tumors and virally infected host cells, as well as in the regulation of hematopoiesis.[1,22]

MAJOR HISTOCOMPATIBILITY COMPLEX (MHC)

The MHC, a cluster of genes found on chromosome 6 in humans, is also known as the *human leukocyte antigen (HLA) complex.* The genes from this complex encode for molecules that play a pivotal role in immune recognition and response. The MHC complex is divided into three different classes: I, II, and III. The molecules encoded by class I HLA genes include HLA-A, HLA-B, and HLA-C antigens. These molecules can be found on all nucleated cells within the body, as well as on platelets. Class I antigens are not found on mature red blood cells. Molecules encoded by class II HLA genes include HLA-DP, HLA-DQ, and HLA-DR. The expression of these molecules is more restricted and can be found primarily on APCs such as macrophages, dendritic cells, B-lymphocytes, etc. The class III HLA antigens encode for soluble factors, complement, and tumor necrosis factors.[23]

In order for a CD4[+] T-lymphocyte to become activated, CD4[+] T-lymphocyte must recognize the antigenic peptide in association with MHC class II (see Figs. 84–2 and 84–3). CD8[+] T-lymphocytes recognize antigenic peptide in association with class I molecules. Class I molecules generally contain endogenous peptides from within the cell, such as those derived from viruses, whereas class II molecules contain exogenous peptides from antigen that has been phagocytized

and digested, such as bacterial peptides (see Fig. 84–2). For it to destroy a virally infected cell, a CD8[+] cytotoxic T-lymphocyte requires two steps. First, its TCR must recognize the antigenic fragment, such as a viral protein, in association with MHC class I. The second step involves the costimulatory step of B7-CD28 binding. Because any cell can become infected, it is advantageous that the CD8[+] cytotoxic T-lymphocyte recognizes the MHC class I molecule that is expressed on all cells except red blood cells. The ability of the MHC class I to present endogenous peptides allows the CD8[+] cytotoxic T-lymphocytes to constantly screen cells for infections.[23,24] Dendritic cells demonstrate the unique capacity to direct exogenous antigens toward MHC class I molecules, a process termed *cross-presentation.*[2]

CYTOKINES

Cytokines, soluble factors released or secreted by cells, affect the activity of other cells or the secreting cell itself. Research has shown that many cytokines have a broad spectrum of effects depending on their concentration, the presence of other factors, and the target cell. Cytokines orchestrate the complex homeostasis of cells and tissues by acting in both an autocrine and a paracrine fashion. For example, activated CD4[+] T-lymphocytes secrete IL-2 that activates itself as well as activating CD8[+] T-lymphocytes and NK cells. Cytokines also can be membrane- bound (e.g., IL-1α) and require direct cell-to-cell contact. In vivo, cytokines do not act alone but in combination with other cytokines. For example, activated CD4[+] T-lymphocytes secrete both IL-2 and interferon-γ, which are synergistic in activating NK cells. As shown in Table 84–3, cytokines are broadly classified as regulatory or hematopoietic growth factors.[9,26–30] This classification does not describe all their activities. Granulocyte-macrophage colony-stimulating factor (GM-CSF) released by activated T-lymphocytes acts as a hematopoietic growth factor but also activates granulocytes and macrophages to phagocytize foreign pathogens.

The division of the immune system into the two functional groups does not imply that the divisions do not interact. In order to generate a vigorous immune response, both soluble mediators (e.g., complement, antibody, and cytokines) and cells (e.g., neutrophils, macrophages, T-lymphocytes, and B-lymphocytes) are needed. Generally, the innate system will respond first. Dendritic cells, macrophages, and neutrophils in the tissues will recognize the opsonized pathogen (see Fig. 84–1). In order to amplify the immune response, the APCs will present antigen to CD4[+] T-lymphocytes (see Figs. 84–2 and 84–3). The activated CD4[+] T-lymphocytes then will secrete cytokines to activate B-lymphocytes, CD8[+] T-lymphocytes, NK cells, macrophages, and neutrophils. The next section of this chapter discusses evaluation of the immune system.

EVALUATION OF COMPONENTS OF THE IMMUNE SYSTEM

Assessment of a patient's immune function requires consideration of multiple components, including mechanical defenses, cell phenotypes and cell numbers, and soluble components. Recent developments in biotechnology made possible extraordinary progress in the characterization of immune function. Despite the technological advances, careful patient evaluations are required to assess the structure and function of the immune system accurately. Specific methods for assessment of patient immune status are discussed below.

TABLE 84–3. Cytokines

Cytokines	Sources	Principal Effects
Regulatory		
IL-1	Macrophages, fibroblasts, endothelial cells	Activation of T- and B-lymphocytes, hematopoietic growth factor, and induction of inflammatory events
IL-2	CD4$^+$ T-lymphocytes (TH$_1$ subset)	Activation of T- and B-lymphocytes and NK cells
IL-4	CD4$^+$ T-lymphocytes (TH$_2$ subset), mast cells, basophils, eosinophils	B- and T-lymphocytic growth factor, activation of macrophages, promotes IgE production, proliferation of bone marrow precursors
IL-5	CD4$^+$ T-lymphocytes (TH$_2$ subset), mast cells	Activation of B-lymphocytes and eosinophils, promotes IgE production
IL-6	CD4$^+$ T-lymphocytes (TH$_2$ subset), macrophages, mast cells, fibroblasts	T- and B-lymphocytic growth factor, hematopoietic growth factor, augments inflammation
IL-8	T-lymphocytes, monocytes, endothelial cells, fibroblasts	Neutrophil, basophil, and T-lymphocyte chemotaxis
IL-10	T- and B-lymphocytes, macrophages	Cytokine synthesis inhibitory factor, growth of mast cells
IL-12	Macrophages, neutrophils, dendritic cells	Induce TH$_1$ cells, ⇑ NK cell activity, ⇑ generation of cytotoxic T-lymphocytes
IL-13	Activated T-lymphocytes	Proliferation of B-lymphocytes, suppression of proinflammatory cytokines, directs IgE isotype switching
IL-14	T-lymphocytes	Induces B-lymphocyte proliferation, inhibits secretion of Igs
IL-15	Macrophages, fibroblasts, dendritic cells, epithelial cells	T-lymphocyte proliferation and activation of NK cells
IL-16	CD8$^+$ T-lymphocytes, epithelial cells	Chemoattractant for CD4$^+$ T-lymphocytes and eosinophils; stimulation of secondary cytokine secretion from and proliferation of CD4$^+$ T-lymphocytes
IL-18	Macrophages	Induces γ-interferon production
TNF-α	Macrophages, NK cells, T-lymphocytes, B-lymphocytes, mast cells	Activation of neutrophils, endothelial cells, lymphocytes, and liver cells to produce acute-phase proteins
TNF-β	T-lymphocytes	Tumoricidal
IFN-α	Monocytes, other cells	Antiviral, activation of NK cells and macrophages, upregulation MHC class I
IFN-γ	T-lymphocytes, NK cells	Activation of macrophages, NK cells, upregulation of MHC classes I and II
Hematopoietic Growth Factors		
IL-3	T-lymphocytes, macrophages	Maturation and differentiation of hematopoietic and mast cells
IL-7	Bone marrow stromal cells	Lymphopoietin
IL-9	T-lymphocytes	Maturation and proliferation of T-lymphocytes and mast cells
IL-11	Bone marrow stromal cells	Maturation of B-lymphocytes and megakaryocytes
G-CSF	Macrophages, endothelial cells, fibroblasts	Maturation and activation of neutrophils
GM-CSF	T-lymphocytes, macrophages, endothelial cells, fibroblasts	Maturation and activation of granulocytes dendritic cells, monocytes-macrophages, and eosinophils
M-CSF	Macrophages, endothelial cells, fibroblasts	Maturation and activation of monocytes-macrophages
Erythropoietin	Kidney, liver	Maturation of red blood cells
Stem cell factor	Bone marrow stromal cells, hepatocytes	Activation of mast cells, early-acting growth factor for myeloid and lymphoid precursors
c-MPL ligand (thrombopoietin)	Bone marrow stromal cells, liver, kidney	Lineage-specific growth factor for megakaryocytes (platelets)
FLT3 ligand	Bone marrow stromal cells	Early-acting growth factor

MECHANICAL AND NONSPECIFIC IMMUNODEFENSES

As discussed earlier, the mechanical aspects of host defense are extremely important in protection from infection; therefore, assessment of mechanical defenses is critical. Much of the assessment of mechanical immunodefense is accomplished by recognition of situations where such defense is compromised. Careful patient examination usually reveals the extent of compromise, and laboratory tests generally are not necessary for evaluation of this component. To assess the extent of compromise in mechanical immunodefenses, the clinician should examine the patient carefully and identify the specific types of risks present. Specific examples of altered mechanical defenses are listed in Table 84–4.

TABLE 84–4. Examples of Alteration in Mechanical Immunodefenses That Result in Impaired Immune Status

Reduced gastric pH
  Achlorhydria
  Use of histamine-2 blockers and proton pump inhibitors
  Patients with acquired immunodeficiency syndrome (AIDS)
Break in skin barrier
  Burns
  Surgical incision
  Penetrating trauma
  Vascular access devices
Impaired mucociliary function of the lungs
  Smoking
Impaired esophageal or epiglottal function
  Endotracheal intubation
  Stroke
  Recumbent position
Altered urine flow
  Urinary stones
  Anatomic deformities obstructing flow
  Bladder catheter
Anatomic alterations of the heart resulting in turbulent blood flow
  and endocarditis

CELLULAR ASPECTS OF IMMUNE FUNCTION

A major aspect of the assessment of immune function relates to the cells of the immune system. Assessment of cells in the clinical setting includes determination of cell type, cell number, and/or function. Generally, determination of the cell types and quantification of the cell numbers are performed first because of the ease of obtaining these results and the common correlation with the clinical situation.

QUANTIFICATION

To quickly screen cell numbers, a white blood cell (WBC) count with differential is performed. Normal cell counts are shown in Table 84–5.[31] This simple test often steers the differential diagnosis. In interpreting a WBC count with differential, several factors must be considered. A normal cell count does not mean that a leukocyte disorder does not exist. For example, in chronic granulomatous disease, a child has a normal neutrophil count, but the neutrophils are unable to

TABLE 84–5. Leukocytes in Adults

Cell	Absolute Count (Range)[a]	Percent (Range)
White blood cells	7.5 (4.5–11.0)	100
Neutrophils	4.5 (2.3–7.7)	60 (50–70)
Eosinophils	0.2 (0.0–0.45)	3 (0–5)
Basophils	0.04 (0.0–0.2)	1 (0–2)
Monocytes	0.3 (0.0–0.8)	4 (0–10)
Lymphocytes	2.1 (1.6–2.4)	32 (28–39)
T-lymphocytes	1.4 (1.1–1.7)	72 (67–76)[b]
CD4+	0.8 (0.7–1.1)	42 (38–46)[b]
CD8+	0.7 (0.5–0.9)	35 (31–40)[b]
B-lymphocytes	0.3 (0.2–0.4)	13 (11–16)[b]
NK cells	0.3 (0.2–0.4)	14 (10–19)[b]
CD4:CD8 ratio	1.2 (1.0–1.5)	

[a]Times 10^3 cells/mm^3.
[b]Percentage of lymphocyte subpopulations expressed as percentage of total lymphocyte population.

destroy the bacteria. Second, a differential is reported as a percentage of the WBC count; therefore, one must assess the absolute number as well as the percentage of WBC subtypes. For example, a patient admitted to the hospital with pneumonia has an elevated WBC count (15.0×10^3 cells/mm^3) that is predominantly neutrophils (segs + bands × $100 = 80\%$). The percentage of lymphocytes appears low at 15%, but the absolute number of lymphocytes is actually normal, 2250 cells/mm^3. A third factor to consider is that the majority of lymphocytes are in secondary lymphoid organs (e.g., lymph nodes, spleen), and changes in peripheral blood lymphocytes do not always mirror changes in the secondary lymphoid organs. Additionally, the majority of granulocytes, macrophages, and mast cells are in the tissues, not the bloodstream.

Generally, the numbers of granulocytes (neutrophils, basophils, eosinophils) and monocytes are assessed by a WBC count with differential. It has long been recognized that the lower the absolute neutrophil count, the greater is the risk of infection. Drugs (e.g., chemotherapy) and diseases (e.g., collagen-vascular disorders) may lower the neutrophil count and make the patient more susceptible to infections. Patients with a neutrophil count below 1500 cells/mm^3 are considered to have neutropenia. Functional analysis of these cell types is done rarely in routine clinical practice. Patients with functional deficits in these cell types generally are referred to tertiary medical centers for evaluation and treatment.

A routine WBC count with differential can determine the total lymphocyte count. Total lymphocyte count has been used as a measure of nutritional status because this changes rapidly with nutrient loss or repletion. This is a relatively gross measure of a patient's immune status, although it has been correlated with patient outcome and risk of infection.

Lymphocyte populations with different functions or in various stages of activation can be enumerated based on their cell surface markers. These cell surface markers are known as *clusters of differentiation* (CDs). The CD is usually a protein or glycoprotein on the surface of the cell. CD followed by a number designates the marker. Hundreds of monoclonal antibodies have been designed to recognize these cell surface markers. Monoclonal antibodies can be coupled with a fluorescent marker. The labeled monoclonal antibodies are incubated with the lymphocytes. Antibodies will recognize and bind to the cells expressing the CD of interest. The cells are then counted with flow cytometry. For flow cytometry, the cell suspension is put under pressure such that the cells flow past a laser in a stream of single cells. The laser will excite the fluorescently-labeled antibodies bound to the lymphocytes. A light detector is able to count the labeled cell as the fluorescent tag emits light and determines the size of the cell based on its light scatter. These evaluations are valuable for assessment of patients with immune-deficiency states such as AIDS or leukemias and for patients who have received organ transplants. Quantification of CD3+ and CD4+ cells is used to monitor muromonab immunosuppression and in the clinical management of patients with human immunodeficiency virus (HIV) infection, respectively. Some of the more common CD antigens and their respective cellular distribution are listed in Table 84–6.[32] Flow cytometry can be used for leukocyte phenotyping, tumor cell phenotyping, and some types of DNA analysis.

FUNCTIONAL EVALUATION OF IMMUNE RESPONSE

In Vivo

The most common in vivo assay of lymphocyte function is the delayed hypersensitivity skin test. This test specifically evaluates the presence

TABLE 84–6. Cluster of Differentiation (CD) Guide: Characterization of Human Leukocyte Antigens

CD	Predominant Cellular Distribution
CD3	All T-lymphocytes
CD4	Helper T-lymphocytes either TH_1 or TH_2
CD5	T-lymphocytes, B-lymphocyte subset
CD8	Cytotoxic/suppressor T-lymphocytes
CD14	Monocytes, macrophages
CD20	B-lymphocytes
CD25	Activated T-lymphocytes, B-lymphocytes IL-2-receptor alpha chain (Tac)
CD33	Committed myeloid progenitor cells
CD34	Hematopoietic progenitor cells that include the stem cell
CD56	NK cells
CD83	Dendritic cells

NK, natural killer.

delayed-type hypersensitivity or memory T-lymphocytes. By injecting a small amount of test material, antigen to which the patient has been exposed previously, into the patient's skin, a visual assessment can be made of the patient's ability to react to the antigen.

When an antigen to which a normal patient has been exposed previously is injected into the skin, the area of the injection becomes infiltrated with lymphocytes within a few hours. In the next stage, additional lymphocytes and phagocytes (e.g., macrophages, neutrophils) infiltrate. The maximal intensity of the inflammatory reaction occurs by 24 to 72 hours. This reaction is often referred to as *type IV hypersensitivity* (i.e., cell-mediated; see Chap. 86). In type I hypersensitivity, positive skin reaction is evident usually within 15 minutes and always within 24 hours. Type I hypersensitivity involves the release of histamine from basophils and mast cells when antigen binds to the IgE on the surfaces of these cells.

A delayed-type hypersensitivity reaction is a test of cell-mediated immunity. The most common method is to administer intradermally a panel of recall antigens. Commonly used antigens include *Candida albicans*, mumps, *Trichophyton*, tetanus toxoid, and purified protein derivative of tuberculin (PPD).[33] Measurements in millimeters of induration at the site of injection should be taken 48 to 72 hours after placement of the antigens. A reaction is considered positive if the diameter of induration is 2 mm or greater. The degree of sensitivity correlates with the area of induration.[32] Reaction to even a single antigen indicates a functioning cell-mediated immunity. The majority of immunocompetent individuals will show a positive reaction to at least one of these antigens. Possible reasons for not mounting a response to these antigens include congenital T-lymphocyte deficiency, cancer, HIV infection, or immunosuppressive drug therapy.[33] Sometimes, no response is mounted because the individual being tested has not been exposed previously to a particular test antigen, although this is rare.

The accepted indications for delayed hypersensitivity skin testing include evaluation of immune disorders or chronic diseases that cause cellular immune dysfunction (e.g., uremia, cancer, AIDS, etc), exposure to infectious pathogens (e.g., *Mycobacterium tuberculosis*), evaluation of nutritional status (because malnutrition can result in cell-mediated immune deficiency), and in some cases, assessment of immune senescence.

In vivo assessment of B-lymphocyte function involves immunizing the patient with a protein (e.g., tetanus toxoid) and a polysaccharide (e.g., pneumococcal polysaccharide vaccine) antigen to elicit and measure antibody responses after immunization. After two to three weeks, the patient's serum is tested for antibodies specific for the immunized antigen. This test measures B-lymphocyte responsiveness to the inoculated antigens but is reserved for patients who are suspected to have impaired B-lymphocyte function.[32]

In Vitro

There are a number of specific lymphocyte functional assays that are used in the research setting. A few assays are performed at specialized clinical laboratories. One of these tests is the lymphocyte proliferation assay. In this assay, lymphocytes are obtained from a patient's peripheral blood and cultured in vitro. The cells are exposed to nonspecific mitogens such as pokeweed mitogen, phytohemagglutin, or concanavalin A. Then the cells are incubated in growth media containing tritium-labeled [^{3}H]thymidine, a nucleotide used in the synthesis of DNA. Normally, in the presence of the mitogens, lymphocytes will be stimulated to proliferate. Proliferating lymphocytes will incorporate [^{3}H]thymidine as they replicate DNA. The level of radioactivity of the cells can be measured on a β-scintillation counter and is proportional to the degree of proliferation. The patient sample would be compared with samples from normal, healthy controls. Patients with immune deficiencies (AIDS, cancer, etc.) have fewer active or less active lymphocytes, as detected by this test.

A modification of the lymphocyte proliferation assay is used in allogeneic hematopoietic stem cell transplantation to evaluate how closely a donor and host are "matched" in order to predict a patient's risk for developing graft-versus-host disease. A mixed-lymphocyte culture (MLC) can be used to assess the potential of the donor cells to attack the host cells (see Chap. 134). In this test, donor cells and host cells are incubated in vitro. The host lymphocytes are irradiated prior to the incubation so that they cannot proliferate. In vitro, [^{3}H]thymidine is provided to the cells, and uptake is measured. The degree of uptake correlates with the level of proliferation of donor lymphocytes. If the cells are well matched, proliferation is minimal. If the cells are mismatched, proliferation will be noted, with the level of proliferation predictive of the risk of graft-versus-host disease. With the introduction of DNA-based molecular typing of HLA antigens, the clinical utility of the MLC appears less important. However, the MLC may play a role in selecting not completely histocompatible donors.[34]

In addition to the test just described, a number of other tests have been devised to evaluate the function of CD8$^+$ T-lymphocytes, NK cells, and monocytes/macrophages. Although these evaluations are not performed commonly, they may be helpful in some specific diseases. A thorough discussion of these tests is available.[35]

HUMORAL ASPECTS OF HUMORAL FUNCTION

The humoral components of the immune system (e.g., immunoglobulins, complement, and cytokines) are often assessed. Assays of humoral components may be either quantitative to determine the absolute concentration of the factor or qualitative to determine the function of the component.

IMMUNOGLOBULINS

The most common evaluation of immunoglobulins is the estimation of total immunoglobulin. This is approximated by subtracting the albumin concentration from the total protein concentration in serum. This difference gives a gross estimation of the total immunoglobulin concentration. Actual determination of the total immunoglobulin

TABLE 84–7. Potential Indications for Measurement of Antigen-specific Antibody

Environmental or drug allergy
Exposure to or infection with bacteria
    Streptococci (ASO titer)
    Staphylococcus aureus (teichoic acid antibody)
    Neisseria gonorrhoeae
    Legionella pneumophila
Exposure to or infection with viruses
    Human immunodeficiency virus
    Cytomegalovirus
    Epstein-Barr virus
    Hepatitis A, B, or C
    Rubella
Exposure to or infection with other pathogens
    Syphilis
    Lyme disease
    Typhoid
    Chlamydia
Immune disorders
    Rheumatoid factor antibody, rheumatoid arthritis
    Anti-nuclear antibodies, systemic lupus erythematosus
    Platelet-associated IgG, idiopathic thrombocytopenia purpura (ITP)
Blood typing and crossmatching
Transplantation
    HLA antibodies

concentration is done by serum protein electrophoresis (SPEP). Five separate zones are detected by this method: albumin, α_1-globulin, α_2-globulin, β-globulin, and γ-globulin.

The γ-globulin fraction contains the five isotypes of immunoglobulin (i.e., IgG, IgA, IgM, IgE, and IgD). A normal total immunoglobulin or γ-globulin concentration ranges from 0.8 to 1.6 g/dL. This test is used to determine if patients have hypogammaglobulinemia (i.e., primary and secondary immunodeficiencies), a monoclonal peak (e.g., multiple myeloma, Waldenstrom's macroglobulinemia), or a polyclonal hypergammaglobulinemia (e.g., chronic inflammatory conditions such as systemic lupus erythematosus or chronic active hepatitis). Total immunoglobulin or γ-globulin concentrations cannot be used to measure antigen-specific antibodies or specific isotypes, although other evaluations can.

In a patient suspected of having humoral immune deficiency or B-lymphocyte failure (i.e., primary and secondary immunodeficiency), specific immunoglobulin isotypes in the plasma should be measured.

There are many indications for the measurement of antigen-specific antibody. Some common indications are listed in Table 84–7. Methods to perform these measurements include enzyme-linked immunosorbent assay (ELISA), radioimmunoassay (RIA), and radioallergosorbent test (RAST) (Fig. 84–6). The most common reason to measure antigen-specific antibody is to determine whether or not a patient has been exposed to an infectious agent. Generally, IgM antibodies directed against the pathogen indicate an active or recent infection, whereas IgG antibodies directed against the pathogen indicate prior exposure. Initially, plasma cells produce IgM in response to an infection, but subsequently, memory B-lymphocytes produce IgG. Therefore, IgM antibodies will be present during an active infection and shortly after recovery from the infection, but IgG concentrations will go up in a second exposure. Other uses of antigen-specific antibody include determining if a patient has had exposure and is likely to be protected from infection (e.g., hepatitis A virus) or to determine adequate response to vaccination (e.g. hepatitis vaccine).

Antigen-specific IgE is commonly measured in patients with allergies. Because the presence of antigen-specific IgE is related to clinical allergy, measurement of these antibodies can be helpful in diagnosing allergies and determining offending substances. A standard method for determination of allergen-specific IgE is the RAST. The basic technique involves adding the antigen of interest, which is bound to beads or disks, to the patient's serum. After precipitation and several washings, the antibody bound to the bead or disk is isolated. Finally, a radiolabeled antibody that binds to IgE is added. After further washings, the radiolabeled antibody bound to IgE, which is bound to the antigen on the bead or disk, is counted on a gamma counter.

Antigen skin testing is the preferred method to determine the presence of allergen-specific IgE. When it is produced, IgE binds to high-affinity IgE Fc receptors on basophils or mast cells. Contact of an allergen with the specific IgE on the basophil or mast cell surface causes activation of these cells and the release of inflammatory mediators (e.g., histamine). When this occurs systemically, it can cause anaphylaxis. When it occurs in a confined area such as the skin, erythema and induration are observed within a few minutes of allergen injection. This is the principle used for detection of penicillin allergy as well as for environmental or food allergies. A positive skin reaction (5 mm or greater of induration) within 15 to 20 minutes is indicative of the presence of allergen-specific IgE.

IgG SUBCLASSES

There are four subclasses of IgG: IgG_1, IgG_2, IgG_3, and IgG_4, that make up 65%, 20%, 10%, and 5% of total plasma IgG, respectively. Concentrations of the subclasses are often measured in patients with primary and secondary immunodeficiencies. IgG_2 and IgG_4 deficiencies are associated with chronic infections. IgG_4 deficiencies are also associated with autoimmune disorders.

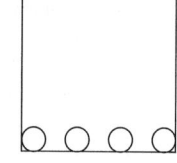 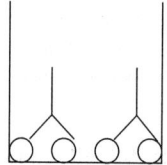 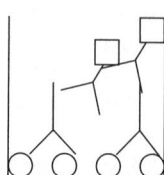 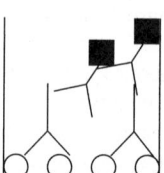

FIGURE 84–6. Enzyme-linked immunosorbant assay (ELISA). ELISA is a commonly used method to measure concentrations of a wide variety of substances. To measure the concentration of antibodies to a particular antigen, the antigen is coated onto a solid phase, such as a microtiter plate, beads, etc. If the purpose of the assay is to measure the concentration of antigen in solution, an antibody to the antigen is coated on the solid phase. The biologic fluid, often sera, is added to the wells. An enzyme-labeled antihuman antibody is added next. Finally, the chromogenic substrate for the enzyme is added. The intensity of the color as measured spectrophotometrically is proportional to the concentration of the antibody in the biologic fluid.

COMPLEMENT SYSTEM

The complement system consists of a group of over 30 different proteins involved in lysing and opsonizing invading pathogens, as well as serving as chemotactic factors. Numbers following the letter C (e.g., C1, C2) name the various proteins of the complement system. A test for the global assessment of the complement system is the CH_{50}, the total hemolytic complement test. This test is based on the premise that complement is needed for a rabbit anti-sheep antibody to lyse sheep red blood cells. The source of the complement is the patient's serum. Each laboratory standardizes the test, so normal ranges vary, but a standard curve is developed by adding titrated amounts of sera and measuring the amount of hemolysis. The hemolysis is determined with a spectrophotometer to measure the amount of hemoglobin released. The patient's serum is then tested, and the amount of serum that is needed to lyse 50% of the red blood cells is reported as the CH_{50}. This test does not provide an indication of the function of any specific complement component but is used as a screening test for any complement system defects. If a defect is found, individual complement proteins then can be evaluated by functional or immunochemical methods. Assessment of the complement system is important in patients suspected of having humoral immune deficiencies (i.e., recurrent infections).[32]

Several disease states can alter complement concentrations. Complement concentrations frequently are found to be lower than normal during states of acute inflammation. Low complement concentrations often are associated with systemic lupus erythematosus, rheumatoid arthritis, collagen-vascular disorders, poststreptococcal glomerulonephritis, and subacute bacterial endocarditis. These states of apparent low complement concentrations generally are due to high rates of complement utilization that cannot be compensated for by increased complement synthesis.[12]

The liver is the primary source of several components of the complement system (i.e., C2, C3, C4, and factors B and D); therefore, in severe liver failure, a global decrease in complement factors occurs. Inherited complement deficiencies have been described in patients with systemic lupus erythematosus, autoimmune diseases, recurrent gonococcal and meningococcal infections, membranoproliferative glomerulonephritis, and hereditary angioedema.[12]

CYTOKINES

Cytokines are an important means of communication among cells of the immune system and other organ systems. Multiple cytokines with overlapping and redundant functions have been identified. Methods to detect and measure cytokines in biologic samples have been developed. For nearly all the currently identified cytokines, commercial kits are available to measure endogenous and exogenously administered cytokines. The most common and preferable methods to measure cytokines are ELISAs and RIAs. ELISAs and RIAs are easy to run and measure immunoactivity but not biologic activity (see Fig. 84–6). Bioassays measure biologic activity but are cumbersome and extremely variable. Using ELISA, we are able to measure only how much cytokine was produced by the cells in the culture. An ELISPOT is an enzyme-linked assay for detecting and enumerating cytokine-producing leukocytes.[36] In contrast to conventional ELISA, ELISPOT allows the user to detect absolute numbers and frequencies of cytokine-secreting leukocytes.

We are still at the very early stages of interpreting the clinical relevance of endogenous cytokine concentrations. Not only is the immune system affected by cytokines such as IL-1, IL-6, and tumor necrosis factor α (TNF-α), but other systems (skeletal, endocrine, central nervous system) are also affected. Therefore, measurement of cytokine concentrations may be important in the evaluation of other systems as well as the immune system.

Administering cytokines in clinical practice may change not only the concentration of that particular cytokine but also the resulting concentration of other cytokines. For example, systemic administration of GM-CSF to patients increases concentrations not only of GM-CSF but also of TNF-α, IL-6, IL-8, macrophage colony-stimulating factor, and erythropoietin.[37,38] Secondary endogenous cytokine release should be taken into account when considering the therapeutic effects of these agents and when monitoring cytokine concentrations.

In the future, tissue concentrations as well as blood concentrations may be measured. For example, while most centers currently measure cyclosporine concentrations to estimate the potential for immunosuppressive effects, it may be advantageous to monitor IL-2 concentrations. One of the primary actions of cyclosporine is the inhibition of IL-2 production. Furthermore, perhaps it would be beneficial to measure tissue concentrations of IL-2 in the transplanted organ to get a better estimate of the extent of immunologic suppression.

SOLUBLE CYTOKINE RECEPTORS AND RECEPTOR ANTAGONISTS

The inflammatory response is highly regulated. The activity of cytokines, their receptors, and their antagonists is in a delicate balance. Although cytokine receptors typically are thought of as being found on the target cell, soluble cytokine receptors can modulate the activity of a cytokine in at least two ways: (1) acting as anti-inflammatory agents by binding the cytokine with high affinity but without biologic activity[39] and (2) augmenting cytokine activity by prolonging the cytokine's plasma half-life and even maintaining agonist activity on cells that do not inherently respond to the cytokine.[40] Finally, antagonists to cytokine receptors have been identified.

TNF-α plays a central role in the inflammatory response by both increasing the expression of adhesion molecules in the tissues and stimulating production of proinflammatory cytokines (e.g., IL-2, IL-8), prostaglandins, and nitric oxide. Soluble tumor necrosis factor receptors (sTNFRs) act primarily as inhibitors of TNF by preventing TNF from binding to the membrane-bound TNFRs or by causing the cells to shed the receptor from the surface of the cell so that it can no longer serve as a signaling molecule.[41] Monoclonal antibodies against both TNF (e.g., infliximab and adalimumab) and sTNFRs (e.g., etanercept) have been shown to modulate the activity of TNF and are used clinically for the treatment of autoimmune diseases.

The best-characterized receptor-binding antagonist is the IL-1 receptor antagonist (IL-1RA). IL-1RA blocks the binding of IL-1 to its receptor by competing for the same binding site, but IL-1RA does not possess agonist activity.[42] A recombinant IL-1RA, anakinra, is used clinically for the treatment of severe rheumatoid arthritis.[43]

Our developing understanding of soluble receptors and receptor antagonists allows us to better mimic natural mechanisms for minimizing the toxicity of exogenously administered cytokines (e.g., IL-1, IL-2, TNF-α, etc.), as well as for immunomodulating of various diseases (e.g., solid organ transplant rejection, collagen-vascular disorders, sepsis, etc).

MODULATION OF THE IMMUNE RESPONSE

IMMUNOSUPPRESSION

Glucocortiocoids, cytotoxic drugs, and antibody preparations have been employed in the control of transplant rejection and to modulate the inflammatory process in autoimmune diseases. As our understanding of the pathogenesis of transplant immunology and autoimmune diseases has improved, more directed therapy at the underlying pathogenesis has been developed.

Since the 1980s, two mainstays in the transplant armamentarium have been: (1) a polyclonal antibody preparation, equine antithymocyte globulin, and (2) a murine monoclonal antibody, muromonab CD3. Clinically, these products lead to destruction of host T-lymphocytes. Since both products are animal proteins, patients can develop a humoral response to the products [e.g., serum sickness to the equine antithymocyte product or a human antimurine antibody (HAMA) response to muromonab CD3]. To overcome the immune response to foreign proteins, several humanized monoclonal antibodies were developed and are now being used clinically. Humanized monoclonal antibodies consist of the murine hypervariable regions incorporated into a human IgG molecule.[44]

A second concern with equine antithymocyte globulin and muromonab CD3 is that they are directed against all T-lymphocytes. By eliminating all T-lymphocytes, the patient's risk of developing a cytomegalovirus infection and/or posttransplant lymphoproliferative disease increases. The alpha chain of the IL-2 receptor is an ideal target for a humanized monoclonal antibody because it is selectively expressed on activated T-lymphocytes. Chimeric and humanized monoclonal antibodies directed against the alpha chain of the IL-2 receptor offer the advantages of selective immunosuppression and decreased adverse effects. Basiliximab and daclizumab in combination with other maintenance immunosuppressants are highly effective for the prevention of acute rejection in patients with renal transplants (see Chap. 87).[45] Their use is also being investigated in other types of transplants, for reversal of acute rejection episodes, and for the treatment of autoimmune diseases.

IMMUNOPOTENTIATION

In an attempt to restore normal immune system function or to activate the immune system, immunopotentiators often are used. The best example of immunopotentiation of the immune system is the practice of immunizations. Active immunization with a vaccine or toxoid induces the host's immune system to confer protection against a pathogen (e.g., hepatitis A, hepatitis B, diphtheria toxoid, etc.). This process requires the uptake of the immunogenic epitope by APCs, followed by presentation to CD4$^+$ T-lymphocytes, and the subsequent development of either a cellular or humoral immune response.

In contrast to active immunization, passive immunity entails the administration of human immunoglobulin to provide short-term protection to individuals who will be or have been exposed to a pathogen. Intravenous immunoglobulin (IVIG) consists of more than 90% polyclonal IgG that is prepared from donated plasma. In patients with primary or secondary immunodeficiencies, IVIG restores circulating IgG concentrations, thus decreasing the incidence of infections in these patients. In addition to restoring IgG concentrations, IVIG potentially can immunomodulate the immune response. For example, in immune thrombocytopenic purpura (ITP), an autoantibody directed against the platelets leads to the destruction of platelets by antibody-dependent cellular cytotoxicity (ADCC). IVIG saturates the Fc receptors on phagocytic cells, thereby preventing the engulfment of autoantibody-opsonized platelets. IVIG also can contain anti-idiotype antibodies to immunomodulate an immune response. Anti-idiotype antibodies are directed against the idiotype or hypervariable region of a native antibody. After administration of IVIG, the anti-idiotypes bind to the hypervariable region of the autoantibody and prevent the autoantibody from opsonizing circulating platelets. In addition, the anti-idiotypes directed against the autoantibody can bind to the surface immunoglobulin on the B-lymphocyte, producing the autoantibody that leads to destruction of the B-lymphocyte.[46]

There is an inverse relationship between the absolute neutrophil count (ANC) and the risk of infection. As the ANC falls, the risk of infection increases, with a dramatic rise in the incidence of infection when the ANC falls below 500 cells/mm^3. Filgrastim (and pegfilgrastim) and sargramostim are myeloid growth factors that accelerate neutrophil recovery after chemotherapy. Filgrastim (and pegfilgrastim) and sargramostim administered after myelosuppressive chemotherapy reduce the severity and duration of neutropenia compared with placebo. In addition to accelerating neutrophil recovery, these myeloid growth factors also enhance the activity (e.g., phagocytosis, superoxide production) of mature neutrophils. Currently, both filgrastim (and pegfilgrastim) and sargramostim are being investigated as adjunct to antibiotics in patients with bacterial and/or fungal diseases and as immunotherapy in patients with sepsis. Sargramostim or GM-CSF plays a critical role in the maturation and proliferation of dendritic cells. Because of the essential role of dendritic cells in antigen presentation, sargramostim is also being investigated as an adjunct to vaccines.[47,48]

CONCLUSION

Our understanding of the immune system has increased dramatically over the last decade. An immune response encompasses dynamic events involving both immunologic cells (e.g., phagocytes, lymphocytes) and soluble mediators (e.g., complement, cytokines, antibodies). A better understanding of the normal immune response allows us to investigate the pathophysiology of diseases in which the immune response is inappropriate. All clinicians need a basic understanding of the immune system and a familiarity with parameters to monitor immune system function in order to refine the development of immunologic treatments for diseases ranging from diabetes mellitus to collagen-vascular disorders to cancer.

Review Questions and other resources can be found at *www.pharmacotherapyonline.com*.

REFERENCES

1. Delves PJ, Roitt IM. The immune system, first of two parts. New Engl Med 2000;343:37–49.
2. Medzhitov R, Janeway C. Innate immunity. New Engl J Med 2000;343: 338–344.
3. Modlin RL. Mammalian toll-like receptors. Ann Allergy Asthma Immunol 2002;88:543–548.
4. Janeway CA, Medzhitov R. Innate immune recognition. Annu Rev Immunol 2002;20:197–216.
5. Witko-Sarsat V, Rieu P, Descamps-Latscha B, et al. Neutrophils Molecules, functions, and pathophysiological aspects. Lab Invest 2000;80 617–653.
6. Wardlaw AJ, Moqbel R, Kay AB, Weller PF. Eosinophils: biology and role in disease. Adv Immunol 1995;60:151–266.
7. Aderem A, Underhill DM. Mechanisms of phagocytosis in macrophages Annu Rev Immunol 1999;17:593–623.
8. Bancherau J, Steinman RM. Dendritic cells and the control of immunity. Nature 1998;392:245–252.
9. Delves PJ, Roitt IM. The immune system, second of two parts. New Engl J Med 2000;343:108–117.
10. Mecheri S, David B. Unravelling the mast cell dilemma: Culprit or victim of its generosity? Immunol Today 1997;18:212–215.

. Falcone FH, Haas H, Gibbs BF. The human basophil: A new appreciation of its role in immune responses. Blood 2000;96:4028–4038.

. Walport MJ. Complement, first of two parts. New Engl J Med 2001;344: 1058–1066.

. Luster AD. The role of chemokines in linking innate and adaptive immunity. Curr Opin Immunol 2002;14:129–135.

. Reiser H, Stadecker MJ. Costimulatory B7 molecules in the pathogenesis of infectious and autoimmune diseases. New Engl J Med 1996;335: 1369–1377.

. Dutton RW, Bradley LM, Swain SL. T cell memory. Annu Rev Immunol 1998;16:201–223.

. Farrar JD, Asnagli H, Murphy KM. T-helper subset development: Role of instruction, selection, and transcription. J Clin Invest 2002;109:431–435.

. Constant SL, Bottomly K. Induction of TH$_1$ and TH$_2$ CD4+ T cell responses: The alternative approaches. Annu Rev Immunol 1997;15: 297–322.

. Bach JF. Regulatory T cells under scrutiny. Nature Rev Immunol 2003; 3:189–198.

. Lanzavecchia A. License to kill. Nature 1998;393:413–414.

. Liu CC, Young LHY, Young JDE. Lymphocyte-mediated cytolysis and disease. New Engl J Med 1996;335:1651–1659.

. Anonymous. Antibodies: Structure and function. In: Goldsby RA, Kindt TH, Obsborne BA, Kuby J, eds. Immunology. New York, Freeman, 2003: 76–102.

. Lanier LL. NK cell receptors. Annu Rev Immunol 1998;16:359–393.

. Klein J, Sato A. The HLA system, first of two parts. New Engl J Med 2000;343:702–709.

. Klein J, Sato A. The HLA system, second of two parts. New Engl J Med 2000;343:782–786.

. Hartgers FC, Figdor CG, Adema GJ. Towards a molecular understanding of dendritic cell immunobiology. Immunol Today 2000;21:542–545.

. Anonymous. Cytokines. In: Goldsby RA, Kindt TH, Obsborne BA, Kuby J, eds. Immunology. New York, Freeman, 2003:277–298.

. Trinchieri G. Interleukin-12: A cytokine at the interface of inflammation and immunity. Adv Immunol 1998;70:83–243.

. Wynn TA. IL-13 effector functions. Annu Rev Immunol 2003;21: 425–456.

. Kennedy MK, Park LS. Characterization of interleukin-15 (IL-15) and the IL-15 receptor complex. J Clin Immunol 1996;16:134–143.

. Okamura H, Tsutsui J, Kashiwamura SI, et al. Interleukin-18: A novel cytokine that augments both innate and acquired immunity. Adv Immunol 1998;70:281–312.

. Elliott MB. Interpretation of clinical laboratory test results. In: Boh LE, ed. Pharmacy Practice Manual: A Guide to the Clinical Experience. Baltimore, Lippincott Williams & Wilkins, 2001:136–212.

32. Fleisher TA, Tomar RH. Introduction to diagnostic laboratory immunology. JAMA 1997; 278:1823–1834.

33. Folds JD, Schmitz JL. Clinical and laboratory assessment of immunity. J Allergy Clin Immunol 2003;111:S702–711.

34. Jeras M. The role of in vitro alloreactive T-cell functional tests in the selection of HLA matched and mismatched haematopoietic stem cell donors. Transplant Immunol 2002;10:205–214.

35. Lowell C. Immunological laboratory tests. In: Parslow TG, Stites DP, Terr AI, Imboden JB, eds. Medical Immunology. New York, Lange Medical/McGraw-Hill Medical, 2001.

36. Helms T, Boehm BO, Asaad RJ, et al. Direct visualization of cytokine-producing recall antigen-specific CD4 memory T cells in healthy individuals and HIV patients. J Immunol 2000;164:3723–3732.

37. Rabinowitz J, Petros W, Stuart A, Peters W. Characterization of endogenous cytokine concentrations after high-dose chemotherapy with autologous bone marrow support. Blood 1993;81:2452–2459.

38. van Pelt L, Huisman M, Weening R, et al. A single dose of granulocyte-macrophage colony-stimulating factor induces systemic interleukin-8 release and neutrophil activation in healthy volunteers. Blood 1996;87: 5305–5313.

39. Opal SM, DePalo VA. Anti-inflammatory cytokines. Chest 2000;117: 1162–1172.

40. Jones SA, Horiuchi S, Topley N, et al. The soluble interleukin 6 receptor: Mechanisms of production and implications in disease. FASEB J 2001; 15:43–58.

41. Dinarello CA. Proinflammatory cytokines. Chest 2000;118:503–508.

42. Choy EH, Panayi GS. Cytokine pathways and joint inflammation in rheumatoid arthritis. New Engl J Med 2001;344:907–916.

43. Cohen S, Hurd E, Cush J, et al. Treatment of rheumatoid arthritis with anakinra, a recombinant human interleukin-1 receptor antagonist, in combination with methotrexate: Results of a twenty-four-week, multicenter, randomized, double-blind, placebo-controlled trial. Arthritis Rheum 2002;46:614–624.

44. Ballow M, Nelson R. Immunopharmacology: Immunomodulation and immunotherapy. JAMA 1997;278:2008–2017.

45. Adu D, Cockwell P, Ives NJ, et al. Interleukin-2 receptor monoclonal antibodies in renal transplantation: Meta-analysis of randomised trials. Br Med J 2003;326:789–793.

46. Kazatchkine MD, Kaveri SV. Immunomodulation of autoimmune and inflammatory diseases with intravenous immune globulin. New Engl J Med 2001;345:747–755.

47. Hotchkiss RS, Karl IE. The pathophysiology and treatment of sepsis. New Engl J Med 2003;348:138–150.

48. Armitage JO. Emerging applications of recombinant human granulocyte-macrophage colony-stimulating factor. Blood 1998;92:4491–4508.

85

SYSTEMIC LUPUS ERYTHEMATOSUS AND OTHER COLLAGEN-VASCULAR DISEASES

Jeffrey C. Delafuente and Kimberly A. Cappuzzo

Learning Objectives and other resources can be found at *www.pharmacotherapyonline.com.*

KEY CONCEPTS

1. Systemic lupus erythematosus (SLE) is a disease predominately in women.

2. The hallmark of SLE is the development of autoantibodies to cellular nuclear components, resulting in chronic inflammatory autoimmune disease. Symptoms and organ involvement depend on the nature of the autoantibodies.

3. SLE has a large spectrum of symptoms and organ system involvement, making therapy highly patient-specific. In addition, the signs and symptoms will fluctuate over time.

4. The large spectrum of symptoms and organ system involvement makes pharmacotherapy difficult because therapy must be individualized based on each patient's disease activity.

5. There is a paucity of quality evidence for the treatment of SLE except for lupus nephritis.

6. Almost all classes of medications, including anti-inflammatory and immunosuppressive agents, have been reported to cause vasculitis in most major organ systems.

The collagen-vascular diseases are a heterogeneous group of diseases that can involve the musculoskeletal system, integument, and blood vessels. Each collagen-vascular disease has its own set of diagnostic criteria, although diagnosis can be difficult because of overlapping and nonspecific clinical presentations. The etiology of the various collagen-vascular diseases is often unknown, although the immune system usually is involved in mediation of disease. Therefore, pharmacotherapy usually includes anti-inflammatory agents with or without immunosuppressive drugs.

Although the prevalence of other collagen-vascular diseases may be greater than that of SLE (e.g., polymyalgia rheumatica), SLE is discussed most extensively in this chapter because it is a major collagen-vascular disease with numerous clinical manifestations, its pharmacotherapy can be complex, and a plethora of data is available on the therapy of SLE. Since all the diseases discussed in this chapter have an immune-mediated pathogenesis, the therapeutic principles of SLE can be applied to other autoimmune collagen-vascular diseases. The collagen-vascular diseases discussed include systemic sclerosis, polymyositis/dermatomyositis, polymyalgia rheumatica, and drug-induced vasculitis; these were chosen because they are seen in general practice.

SYSTEMIC LUPUS ERYTHEMATOSUS

SLE is a fluctuating multisystem disease with a diversity of clinical presentations. Abnormal immunologic function and formation of antibodies against "self" antigens underlie the pathogenesis of SLE.

The term *lupus erythemateux* was first used in 1851 by Cazenave, a Frenchman who described an illness in a patient with manifestations occurring in the skin. It is not surprising that SLE was first recognized

as a skin disorder because cutaneous manifestations constitute one of the most common clinical features of the disease. Further descriptions by Kaposi in 1872 and Osler in 1895 led to the concept of a multisystem disease as it became recognized that patients developed complications in other organ systems.[1,2]

The hallmark of SLE is the development of autoantibodies to cellular nuclear components that leads to a chronic inflammatory autoimmune disease. Recognition of SLE as an autoimmune disease of multisystemic nature led the American College of Rheumatology (ACR) to develop criteria for identifying lupus patients (Table 85–1). These criteria were developed in 1971, revised in 1982, and modified slightly in 1997. The criteria do not include all the clinical manifestations of the disease and are used primarily for distinguishing SLE from other collagen-vascular diseases.[3] If 4 or more of the 11 criteria are documented at any time in a patient's medical history, the diagnosis of SLE can be made with about 95% specificity and 85% sensitivity.[4] Although these criteria may be helpful, diagnosis requires additional serologic, immunopathologic, and clinical evaluations.

EPIDEMIOLOGY

1. The incidence of SLE in the United States is estimated to be 5.6 to 7.3 per 100,000 persons per year, with a prevalence of between 124 and 130 cases per 100,000 persons.[5–7] International studies report similar ranges.[8,9] The disease occurs predominantly in women, with a reported female-to-male ratio approaching 10:1. Those afflicted with SLE are usually diagnosed between the ages of 15 and 45.[9,10] SLE is reported to be less prevalent in whites than in other ethnic groups, including blacks, Hispanics, Native Americans, and Asians.[8–11] Although the most typical SLE patient is a young

TABLE 85–1. Revised Criteria for Classification of Systemic Lupus Erythematosus[a]

Criterion	Definition
Malar rash	Fixed erythema, flat or raised, over the malar eminences, tending to spare the nasolabial folds
Discoid rash	Erythematous raised patches with adherent keratotic scaling and follicular plugging; atrophic scarring may occur older lesions
Photosensitivity	Skin rash as a result of unusual reaction to sunlight, by patient history or physician observations
Oral ulcers	Oral or nasopharyngeal ulceration, usually painless, observed by a physician
Arthritis	Nonerosive arthritis involving two or more peripheral joints, characterized by tenderness, swelling, or effusion
Serositis	Pleuritis—convincing history of pleuritic pain or rub heard by a physician or evidence of pleural effusion *or* Pericarditis—documented by ECG or rub or evidence of pericardial effusion
Renal disorder	Persistent proteinuria greater than 0.5 g/day or greater than 3+ if quantitation not performed *or* Cellular casts—may be red cell, hemoglobin, granular, tubular, or mixed
Neurologic disorder	Seizures—in the absence of offending drugs or known metabolic derangements, e.g., uremia, ketoacidosis, or electrolyte imbalance *or* Psychosis—in the absence of offending drugs or known metabolic derangements, e.g., uremia, ketoacidosis, or electrolyte imbalance
Hematologic disorder	Hemolytic anemia—with reticulocytosis *or* Leukopenia—fewer than 4000/mm^3 total on two or more occasions *or* Lymphopenia—fewer than 1500/mm^3 on two or more occasions *or* Thrombocytopenia—fewer than 100,000/mm^3 in the absence of offending drugs
Immunologic disorder	Anti-DNA; antibody to native DNA in abnormal titer *or* Anti-Sm; presence of antibody to Sm nuclear antigen *or* Positive finding of antiphospholipid antibodies based on (1) an abnormal serum level of IgG or IgM anticardiolipi antibodies, (2) a positive test result for lupus anticoagulant using a standard method, or (3) a false-positive serologic test for syphilis known to be positive for at least 6 months and confirmed by *Treponema pallidum* immobilization or fluorescent treponemal antibody absorption test.
Antinuclear	An abnormal titer of antinuclear antibody by immunofluorescence or an antibody equivalent assay at any point ir time in the absence of drugs known to be associated with "drug-induced lupus" syndrome

[a]The proposed classification is based on 11 criteria. For the purpose of identifying patients in clinical studies, a person shall be said to have systemic lupus erythematosus any 4 or more of the 11 criteria are present, serially or simultaneously, during any interval of observation.
From Tan EM, Cohen AS, Fries JF, et al. The 1982 revised criteria for the classification of systemic lupus erythematosus. Arthritis Rheum 1982;25:1274; and Hochbe MC. Updating the American College of Rheumatology Revised Criteria for the Classification of Systemic Lupus Erythematosus, Arthritis Rheum 1997;40;1725, w permission.

adult woman, the disease can occur in people of any age or race and either gender.

ETIOLOGY

The etiology of abnormal autoantibody production and development of SLE is still unknown. Genetic, environmental, and hormonal factors all may play a role in loss of "self" tolerance and expression of disease. A popular theory is that autoimmune disease such as SLE develops in genetically susceptible individuals after exposure to a triggering agent, possibly something in the environment.[10,12,13]

Genetic analysis shows that at least four susceptibility genes are required for the expression of lupus in humans.[13] Familial and twin studies indicate a genetic predisposition for the development of SLE. First-degree relatives of SLE patients are approximately 20 times more likely to develop SLE than the general population; more than 5% of cases are familial. The concordance rate among identical twins ranges from 24% to 58% compared with 3% to 10% for nonidentical twins.[14] Multiple genes contribute to SLE susceptibility, and at least 100 genes have been linked to SLE in humans. Evidence indicates that

major histocompatibility complex (MHC) genes, particularly sever. human leukocyte antigen (HLA) genes, may be important in lupu However, non-MHC genes, such as immunoglobulin receptor gene and mannose-binding protein genes, also may contribute to diseas susceptibility.[13,14] Environmental agents that may have a role in ir duction or activation of SLE include sunlight (i.e., ultraviolet light drugs, chemicals such as hydrazine (found in tobacco) and aromati amines (found in hair dyes), diet, environmental estrogens, and ir fection with viruses or bacteria.[13] A number of viruses have bee implicated as causative agents in genetically susceptible people, b much of the evidence is circumstantial.[15] Additionally, androgen ma inhibit and estrogen enhance the expression of autoimmunity, an elevated circulating prolactin levels have been associated with lupu in males and females.[12,13]

PATHOPHYSIOLOGY

 SLE represents a clinical syndrome rather than a discrete dis ease with a unique pathogenesis.[16] SLE has a large spectrum o symptoms and organ system involvement. A major event in the development of SLE is excessive and abnormal autoantibody production and the formation of immune complexes. Patients may develop autoantibodies against multiple nuclear, cytoplasmic, and surface components of multiple types of cells in various organ systems in addition to soluble markers such as immunoglobulin G (IgG) and coagulation factors; this fact underlines the multiple organ system involvement of the disease.[13]

Excessive autoantibody production results from hyperactive B-lymphocytes. Multiple mechanisms likely lead to B-cell hyperactivity, including loss of immune "self" tolerance and high antigenic load consisting of environmental and self antigens presented to B cells by other B cells or specific antigen presenting cells (APCs), a shift of T-helper 1 (Th$_1$) cells to Th$_2$ cells that further enhance B-cell antibody production, and defective B-cell suppression. Impairment in other immune regulatory processes involving T-lymphocytes (suppressor T cells), cytokines (e.g., interleukins, interferon-γ, tumor necrosis factor α, transforming growth factor β), and natural killer cells also may be involved.[13,17]

Many autoantibodies are directed against nuclear constituents of the cell and are called collectively *antinuclear antibodies*. Several antinuclear antibodies are important because their presence or absence may aid in the diagnostic and clinical evaluation of patients with SLE. The SLE patient usually has more than one antigen-specific antinuclear antibody in his or her serum and tissues.[18] These are antibodies against such nuclear constituents as double-stranded, or native, DNA (dsDNA); single-stranded, or denatured, DNA (ssDNA); and RNA. Four RNA-associated antigens frequently occurring in SLE are the Smith (Sm) antigen, the small nuclear ribonucleoprotein (snRNP), the Ro (SS-A) antigen, and the La (SS-B) antigen.[19,20] Histone, a basic component of chromatin and nucleosomes, is another important

nuclear component against which antinuclear antibodies are formed in lupus patients. Antibodies to Ro, La, Sm, or RNP antigens plus antibodies to dsDNA will detect most patients with SLE.[19] Antibodies also may be directed against the phospholipid moiety of the prothrombin activator complex (lupus anticoagulant) and against cardiolipin. The lupus anticoagulant and anticardiolipin antibodies constitute the two main types in a group of autoantibodies called *antiphospholipid antibodies*.

These autoantibodies often are present many years before the diagnosis of SLE.[21] The appearance of these autoantibodies follows a predictable pattern, with accumulation of specific autoantibodies before the onset of clinical illness. For instance, antinuclear, anti-La, anti-Ro, and antiphospholipid antibodies often precede the onset of SLE by many years, whereas anti-Sm and anti-snRNP antibodies appear only months before diagnosis, usually when clinical symptoms begin to manifest.

Immune dysregulation leading to B-cell hyperactivity and subsequent production of pathogenic autoantibodies, coupled with defective clearance of apoptotic cells, followed by immune-complex formation, complement activation, and defective clearance of immune complexes all lead to inflammatory reactions that ultimately result in tissue injury and damage. An overview of the pathogenesis[13] of SLE is illustrated in Fig. 85–1.

CLINICAL PRESENTATION

As mentioned previously, SLE is a multisystem disease. Below are many of the signs and symptoms and incidences in patients with SLE.[22–24] Although certain of these may be more common than others, each patient presents differently, and the course of the disease is highly unpredictable. Furthermore, SLE is not static, and

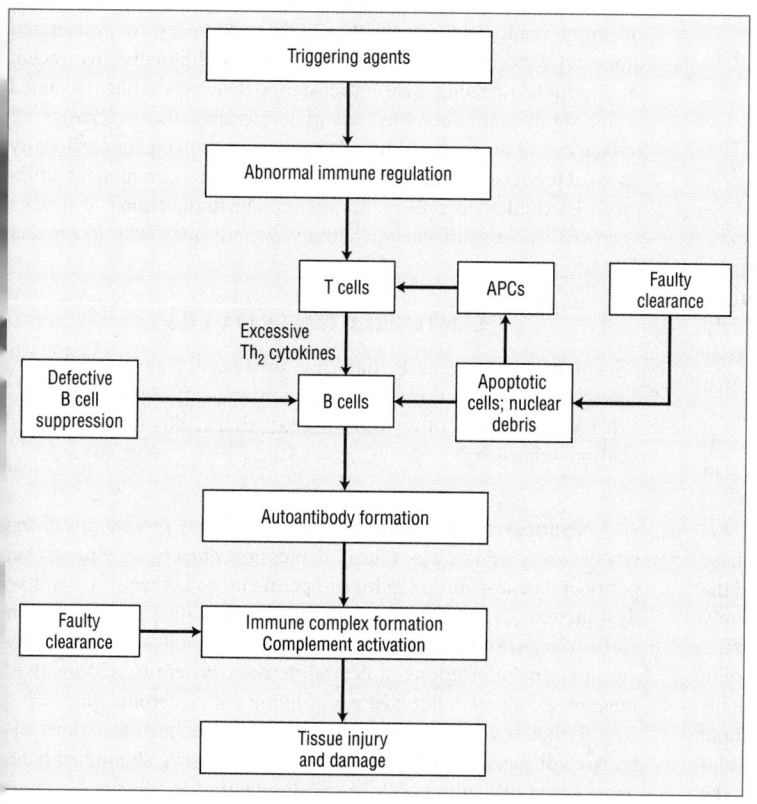

FIGURE 85–1. Pathogenesis of systemic lupus erythematosus. Environmental factors, such as infectious organisms, drugs, and chemicals, serve as triggering agents in genetically and hormonally susceptible individuals to induce a state of immune dysregulation. These abnormal immune responses lead to hyperactive T-helper-2 lymphocyte and B-lymphocyte function. Suppressor T-lymphocyte function, cytokine production, faulty clearance mechanisms, and other immune regulatory mechanisms also are abnormal and fail to downregulate autoantibody formation from hyperactive B-lymphocytes. The autoantibodies formed from this immune dysregulation become pathogenic, form immune complexes, and activate complement that leads to damage of host tissue.

most patients have fluctuations or flare-ups during the course of the disease.

CLINICAL PRESENTATION OF SLE

Sign/Symptom	Incidence (%)
Musculoskeletal:	
Arthritis and arthralgia	53–95
Consitutional	
Fatigue	81
Fever	41–86
Weight loss	31–71
Mucocutaneous	55–85
Butterfly rash	10–61
Photosensitivity	11–45
Raynaud's phenomenon	10–44
Discoid lesions	9–29
Central nervous system	13–59
Psychosis	5–37
Seizures	6–26
Pulmonary	
Pleuritis	31–57
Pleural effusion	12–40
Cardiovascular	
Pericarditis	2–45
Myocarditis	3–40
Heart murmur	1–44
Hypertension	23–46
Renal	13–65
Gastrointestinal	
Nausea	7–53
Abdominal pain	8–34
Bowel hemorrhage (vasculitis)	1–6
Hematologic	
Anemia	30–78
Leukopenia	35–66
Thrombocytopenia	7–30
Lymphadenopathy	10–59

Nonspecific signs and symptoms such as fatigue, fever, anorexia, and weight loss are seen frequently in patients with active disease. Musculoskeletal involvement (e.g., arthralgia, myalgia, and arthritis) is very common in SLE,[22,24,25] with arthritis and arthralgia frequently the chief complaint on initial presentation of the disease.[24] All major and minor joints may be affected, and the pattern of arthritis is often recurrent and of short duration, presenting mainly as joint stiffness, pain, and sometimes inflammation.[26] Objective evidence of musculoskeletal disease often is missing, although a few patients may present with deforming arthritis or subcutaneous nodules.

Manifestations in the skin are nearly as common as those involving the musculoskeletal system.[2,22,24] The most well known of these is the butterfly rash, which occurs over the bridge of the nose and the malar eminences. The classic butterfly rash is seen in approximately one-half of patients and often is observed after sun exposure. In fact, photosensitivity is common to many SLE patients who present with cutaneous manifestations. Skin lesions characteristic of discoid lupus occur in 10% to 20% of patients with SLE and may occur without other clinical or serologic evidence of lupus.[22,23,27] Some individuals are said to develop *subacute cutaneous lupus erythematosus,* the nature of whose lesions falls between discoid (one type of *chronic*

cutaneous lupus erythematosus) and the butterfly rash (an example of *acute cutaneous lupus erythematosus).*[27] Other cutaneous manifestations include vasculitis (which may be ulcerative), livedo reticularis, periungual erythema, Raynaud's phenomenon, and alopecia.[2,24]

Another common source of symptomatology in SLE is the pulmonary system, with manifestations such as pleurisy, coughing, and dyspnea. Pleurisy may present as pleuritic pain, a pleural rub, or a pleural effusion that usually is exudative in nature. Lupus pneumonitis may present acutely with fever, dyspnea, tachypnea, cough, rales, and patchy infiltrates or chronically with interstitial fibrosis. Lupus pneumonitis is an uncommon manifestation of SLE and can be difficult to distinguish from infectious pneumonia, which is more common in SLE patients and should be the primary consideration when evaluating new pulmonary infiltrates.[28] Pulmonary hypertension associated with SLE is more common than previously thought, which is likely due to the fact that asymptomatic increases in pulmonary arterial pressures are more common than symptomatic increases. Patients with SLE-associated pulmonary hypertension have a poor prognosis. Pulmonary embolism also should be ruled out in any SLE patient presenting with pleuritic chest pain and dyspnea.

Cardiac manifestations of SLE often present as pericarditis, myocarditis, electrocardiographic (ECG) changes, or valvular heart disease, including the classic cardiac lesion of Libman-Sacks endocarditis (nonbacterial verrucous endocarditis).[28] Coronary artery disease (CAD) is being seen in SLE with increasing frequency as the life expectancy of SLE patients increases.[29] It is thought that the development of heart disease in these patients is multifactorial. Traditional CAD risk factors are common in patients with SLE.

Corticosteroid therapy and underlying renal disease are also believed to be contributing factors in the development of these cardiac risk factors.[28] Although hypertension, obesity, and hyperlipidemia are common in SLE patients, these traditional risk factors do not account for the strikingly high cardiovascular event rate found in some recent studies.[30,31] Other SLE-related risk factors highlight the importance of autoimmunity and inflammation in the pathogenesis of accelerated atherosclerotic cardiovascular disease.[31,32] Additionally, two recent studies found that long-term corticosteroid therapy was not associated with a significantly increased risk of accelerated atherosclerosis.[33,34] In fact, one of the studies[33] found that patients with higher mean daily doses of prednisone and more frequent use of other common therapies for SLE exhibited less plaque formation. The implication is that more aggressive control of disease activity actually may help to prevent CAD.[32,33]

CLINICAL CONTROVERSY

Some research suggests that long-term corticosteroid therapy is responsible for the increased incidence of coronary heart disease, whereas other data suggest that it has no effect on atherosclerosis.

Neuropsychiatric manifestations of SLE may present in a diversity of ways, including psychosis, depression, anxiety, seizure, stroke, peripheral neuropathy, cognitive impairment, and others.[35] Cognitive dysfunction is seen in 12% to 87% of patients with SLE. Depression and anxiety are common among SLE patients, but it is unclear if they are direct manifestations of central nervous system (CNS) involvement or secondary to the distress of living with a chronic illness.[36]

Symptoms associated with gastrointestinal manifestations often are nonspecific for lupus and include dyspepsia, abdominal pain, nausea, and difficulty swallowing. Mesenteric vasculitis and venous occlusion owing to thrombosis may be problematic if not diagnosed

TABLE 85–2. Antinuclear Antibody Test: Patterns, Antigens, and Specificities

Pattern	Antigen	Disease
Peripheral	dsDNA	SLE
Speckled	Acidic nuclear protein	Rheumatoid arthritis
	Ribonucleoprotein	SLE
	Extractable nuclear antigen	Scleroderma
		Mixed connective tissue disease
Homogeneous	dsDNA, ssDNA	Rheumatoid arthritis
	Histones	SLE, drug-induced lupus
Nucleolar	Nucleolar RNA	Progressive systemic sclerosis

ds = double-stranded; ss = single-stranded.

nd treated promptly. Hepatitis and pancreatitis also may be present nd may be secondary to drugs used to treat SLE or the disease self.[37]

HEMATOLOGIC MANIFESTATIONS

Anemia is found in many patients with SLE. It is usually an anemia of chronic inflammation, with a mild normochromic, normocytic smear nd low serum iron concentration but adequate iron stores. Some patients may develop a hemolytic anemia with a positive Coombs' test.[38] Leukopenia, usually mild, is present in approximately half of SLE patients. Both granulocytes and lymphocytes may be affected, but there s usually a larger decrease in lymphocytes.[2,24] Thrombocytopenia may occur in SLE, often during disease exacerbation, but is usually mild and does not increase bleeding tendency.[38] Another significant finding associated with SLE is the presence of antiphospholipid antibodies such as the lupus anticoagulant (LA) and anticardiolipin antibodies. Although the LA is directed against the prothrombin activator complex and implies potential bleeding complications, this is not the case. In fact, the presence of LA, anticardiolipin, or other antiphospholipid antibodies may be associated with thrombosis, neurologic disease, thrombocytopenia, and fetal loss.[25,39] Thrombotic events occur in more than 10% of patients with SLE.[39] Not all patients with antiphospholipid syndrome have lupus. If a patient has no concomitant autoimmune disease, the syndrome is *primary*. If a patient has accompanying SLE, the syndrome is *secondary*.[40,41]

LUPUS NEPHRITIS

Clinical evidence of renal involvement, such as a rising serum creatinine or proteinuria level, generally is associated with a poorer outcome compared with patients without renal involvement. Progression to end-stage renal disease is a major cause of morbidity and mortality in SLE. However, the extent and course of renal disease are quite variable, and many lupus nephritis patients do very well. The World Health Organization (WHO) has classified lupus nephritis on the basis of histologic characteristics observed following renal biopsy. This system, revised in 1995, identifies lupus nephritis as normal (class I), mesangial (classes IIA and IIB), focal proliferative (class IIIA–C), diffuse proliferative (class IVA–D), diffuse membranous (class VA and VB),

or advanced sclerosing (class VI) glomerulonephritis.[42] Many patients progress from one form of nephritis to another during the course of the disease. Predictors of poorer outcome in proliferative lupus nephritis include African-American race, increased serum creatinine level, poor initial response to immunosuppressive drugs, hypertension, and persistent nephrotic syndrome.[43]

DIAGNOSIS

As mentioned earlier, the diagnostic criteria listed in Table 85–1 should not be the primary means for diagnosing SLE, although many of the criteria may be valuable in the diagnostic process. Epidemiologic characteristics, clinical signs and symptoms, and common laboratory abnormalities all are used in the diagnosis of SLE.

Once the disease is suspected, serologic tests may be helpful in making the diagnosis. A serologic test used extensively to aid in the diagnosis of SLE is the fluorescent antinuclear antibody (ANA) test. Nearly all SLE patients are ANA-positive, but other diseases also can be associated with a positive test (Table 85–2); however, in other diseases, many of the positive ANA tests are of a lower titer. The pattern of immunofluorescence of the ANA test also may be of diagnostic value (see Table 85–2), with a peripheral (also called *rim*) pattern being specific for SLE. Detecting antibodies to specific nuclear constituents also may be useful diagnostically. Antibodies to native DNA (dsDNA) and to Sm antigen are quite specific for and are considered diagnostic of SLE.[13,19,44,45]

PROGNOSIS

In earlier years, SLE was associated with a poor prognosis. For example, the classic report of patients diagnosed between 1949 and 1953 showed a 5-year survival rate of less than 50%.[46] Today, as a result of improved treatment and improved diagnostic techniques that allow earlier diagnosis, the 5-year survival exceeds 96%, and 20-year survival rates approach 70%.[47,48] The natural course of SLE has changed dramatically since the 1970s not only because of improved therapies but also because of improvement in ability to manage patients with kidney disease (e.g., dialysis), infection, and CAD.[8,43,48,49] However, CAD and infection are still among the leading causes of death among SLE patients.[8]

▶ TREATMENT: Systemic Lupus Erythematosus

Desired treatment outcomes for the patient with SLE are twofold: (1) management of symptoms and induction of remission during times of disease flare and (2) maintenance of remission for as long as possible between disease flares. An approach to the management of the

patient with SLE is outlined in Fig. 85–2. Because of the variability in clinical presentation of disease, treatment will vary accordingly and should be highly individualized. Optimal care of the patient with SLE will offer education and support services in addition to

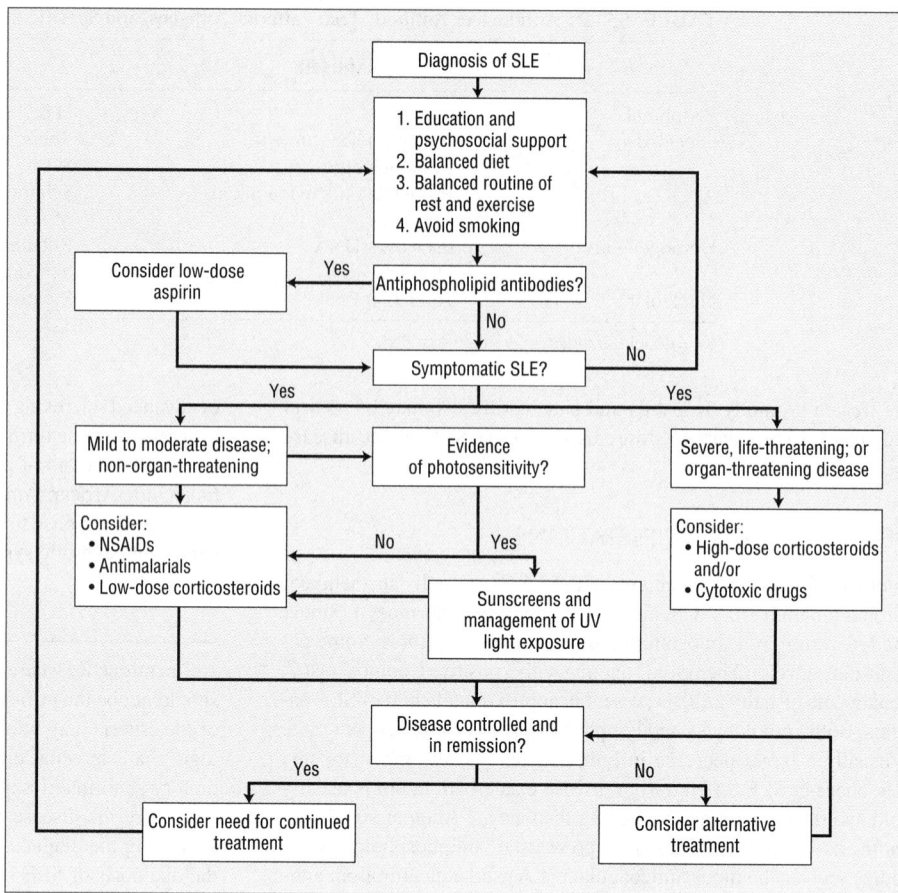

FIGURE 85–2. General approach to the management of SLE.

the nonpharmacologic and pharmacologic treatments discussed below. Numerous lupus organizations exist throughout the world and can be located by contacting the Lupus Foundation of America[50] (*www.lupus.org*), the Arthritis Foundation[51] (*www.arthritis.org*), and Lupus Canada[52] (*www.lupuscanada.org*).

NONPHARMACOLOGIC THERAPY

Several nonpharmacologic measures can be employed to manage symptoms and help maintain remission. Fatigue is a common symptom in patients with lupus.[47] A balanced routine of rest and exercise, while avoiding overexertion, is essential in managing fatigue.[53] Avoidance of smoking may be particularly important because hydrazines in tobacco smoke may be an environmental trigger of lupus and likely contribute to accelerated CAD.[13] Smoking also has been associated with increased disease activity in SLE patients.[54] No specific dietary measures are known to clearly affect the clinical course of lupus. However, fish-oil derivatives might prevent miscarriages in pregnant women with antiphospholipid antibodies,[53] but alfalfa sprouts should be avoided because they contain the amino acid L-canavanine, which has been linked to the development of lupus-like symptoms in numerous case reports.[13] Many patients with SLE will need to limit exposure to sunlight and use sunscreens to block the possible exacerbating effects of ultraviolet light.[55] The amount of sunlight exposure limitation should be individualized.

PHARMACOLOGIC THERAPY

Drug therapy for SLE is often designed to suppress the immune response and inflammation. Except for lupus nephritis, large controlled clinical trials comparing treatment options for SLE are needed. Table 85–3 lists common agents and doses used to control SLE. In general, the choice of drug therapy depends on the extent and severity of disease. Table 85–4 describes selected monitoring parameters and adverse events for many of the drugs used to treat collagen-vascular diseases.

NONSTEROIDAL ANTI-INFLAMMATORY DRUGS

As discussed earlier, signs and symptoms such as fever, arthritis, and serositis are among the most common in patients with active disease. Therefore, in many patients with mild disease, initial treatment with a nonsteroidal anti-inflammatory drug (NSAID) is a logical choice. The choice of NSAIDs in SLE is empirical. The dose used should be adequate to provide anti-inflammatory effects, although low-dose aspirin may be useful in the management of patients with antiphospholipid syndrome.[39]

Nonselective cyclooxygenase NSAIDs significantly increase the risk of gastric irritation and peptic ulceration. Coprescribing with a gastroprotective agent such as a proton pump inhibitor may be beneficial.[41] Patients with SLE taking NSAIDs may experience

TABLE 85–3. Drug Treatment of Systemic Lupus Erythematosus

Drug Class	Drug and Dose	Indication
NSAID	Various agents Anti-inflammatory dose	Mild disease: fever, arthritis, skin rash, serositis
Antimalarial	Hydroxychloroquine, 200–400 mg PO daily Chloroquine, 250–500 mg PO daily	Mild disease: arthritis, skin rash, serositis
Corticosteroid	Prednisone, 1–2 mg/kg/d PO (or equivalent) <1 mg/kg/d (or equivalent)	Initial control of severe disease Control of mild disease or maintenance after disease suppression with higher doses
	Methylprednisolone, 500–1000 mg IV daily × 3–6 d	Life-threatening disease
Cytotoxic	Cyclophosphamide, 0.5–1.0 g/m² IV monthly for 6 months; then, every 3 months for 2 years or for 1 year after remission Azathioprine, 1–3 mg/kg PO daily Cyclophosphamide, 1–3 mg/kg PO daily Mycophenolate mofetil, 1–3 g PO daily	Most commonly used in severe lupus nephritis; may be necessary for other severe disease manifestations

TABLE 85–4. Monitoring Adverse Effects of Drugs Commonly Used in SLE

Drug	Toxicities to Monitor	Baseline Evaluation	Monitoring System Review	Monitoring Laboratory
Salicylates, NSAIDs	Gastrointestinal bleeding, hepatic toxicity, renal toxicity, hypertension	CBC, creatinine, urinalysis, AST, ALT	Dark/black stool, dyspepsia, nausea/vomiting, abdominal pain, shortness of breath, edema	CBC yearly, creatinine yearly
Corticosteroids	Hypertension, hyperglycemia, hyperlipidemia, hypokalemia, osteoporosis, avascular necrosis, cataract, weight gain, infections, fluid retention	Blood pressure, bone densitometry, glucose, potassium, cholesterol, triglycerides (HDL, LDL)	Polyuria, polydipsia, edema, shortness of breath, blood pressure, visual changes, bone pain	Urinary dipstick for glucose every 3–6 months, total cholesterol yearly, bone densitometry yearly to assess osteoporosis
Hydroxychloroquine	Macular damage	None unless patient is over 40 years of age or has previous eye disease	Visual changes	Funduscopic and visual fields every 6–12 months
Azathioprine	Myelosuppression, hepatoxicity, lymphoproliferative disorders	CBC, platelet count, creatinine, AST or ALT	Symptoms of myelosuppression	CBC and platelet count every 1–2 weeks with changes in dose (every 1–3 months thereafter), AST yearly, Pap test at regular intervals
Cyclophosphamide	Myelosuppression, myeloproliferative disorders, malignancy, immunosuppression, hemorrhagic cystitis, secondary infertility	CBC and differential and platelet count, urinalysis	Symptoms of myelosuppression, hematuria, infertility	CBC and urinalysis monthly, urine cytology and Pap test yearly for life
Mycophenolate mofetil	Myelosuppression, hepatotoxicity, lymphoproliferative disorders, malignancy	CBC, hepatic function tests, renal function tests	Symptoms of myelosuppression, diarrhea, nausea/vomiting, dyspepsia, abdominal pain, dark/black stool or blood in stool	CBC weekly during first month, twice monthly during the second and third months, then monthly through the first year

NSAIDs = nonsteroidal anti-inflammatory drugs; CBC = complete blood count; AST = aspartate transaminase; ALT = alanine transaminase; HDL = high density lipoprotein; LDL = low density lipoprotein.

Modified from American College of Rheumatology Ad Hoc Committee on Systemic Lupus Erythematosus Guidelines. Guidelines for referral and management of systemic lupus erythematosus in adults. Arthritis Rheum 1999; 42:1790 (with permission). Other refs. 25, 110, and 111.

a decline in renal function because of drug effects and not the underlying disease. NSAIDs can decrease renal blood flow and glomerular filtration rates. This may be particularly important for patients with nephritis. Awareness of this effect is important because declining renal function may be attributed mistakenly to progression of lupus nephritis. Patients with SLE have a higher incidence of hepatotoxicity than other patients taking traditional NSAIDs. There also exist reports of an association between aseptic meningitis in SLE patients and the use of NSAIDs.[4,25,55]

ANTIMALARIAL DRUGS

Antimalarial agents such as chloroquine and hydroxychloroquine have been used successfully in the management of discoid lupus and SLE. A few controlled trials provide evidence for the role of antimalarial therapy in controlling disease exacerbations and as steroid-sparing agents.[56–58] In general, the manifestations of SLE that can be managed with antimalarials are cutaneous manifestations, arthralgia, pleuritis, mild pericardial inflammation, fatigue, and leukopenia.[25,41] Because these drugs are not effective immediately, they are best used in long-term management. Response to chloroquine occurs within 1 to 3 months, while the maximal effect of hydroxychloroquine may not occur for 3 to 6 months.[25] Hydroxychloroquine is probably safer than chloroquine and is considered the antimalarial of first choice.

The mechanism of action of the antimalarial drugs is uncertain. It has been proposed that antimalarials interfere with T-lymphocyte activation.[25] Other effects of antimalarials that may benefit patients with SLE include inhibition of cytokines, decreased sensitivity to ultraviolet light, anti-inflammatory activity, antiplatelet effects, and antihyperlipidemic activity.[25,32]

Dosage and duration of therapy depend on patient response, tolerance of side effects, and development of retinal toxicity, which is a potentially irreversible adverse reaction associated with long-term therapy, especially with chloroquine. Current recommended doses of antimalarials in SLE are hydroxychloroquine 200–400 mg/day and chloroquine 250–500 mg/day. After 1 or 2 years of treatment, gradual tapering of dosage can be attempted. Some patients may require only one or two tablets per week to suppress cutaneous manifestations.[25,59]

Side effects of these drugs include CNS effects (e.g., headache, nervousness, insomnia, and others), rashes, dermatitis, pigmentary changes of the skin and hair, gastrointestinal disturbance (e.g., nausea), and reversible ocular toxicities such as cycloplegia and corneal deposits. Potentially serious retinal toxicity is uncommon when the currently recommended doses are used and is least common with hydroxychloroquine.[60] However, because of the possibility of permanent damage associated with the retinopathy, an ophthalmologic evaluation should be done at baseline and every 3 months when chloroquine is used and every 6 to 12 months when hydroxychloroquine is used. If retinal abnormalities are noted, antimalarial therapy should be discontinued or the dose reduced.[25]

CORTICOSTEROIDS

Corticosteroid therapy is commonplace in therapeutic regimens for SLE. Although evidence for improved survival with corticosteroid therapy is inadequate, these agents are known to be effective for suppressing the clinical expression of disease and are considered by many to be a major factor in the improved prognosis in recent years. Although most controlled trials of corticosteroid therapy have been conducted in patients with severe lupus nephritis, evidence suggests that corticosteroids are also effective in the management of severe cases of

CNS disease, pneumonitis, polyserositis, vasculitis, thrombocytopenia, and other clinical manifestations.[25]

A patient with the diagnosis of SLE does not automatically require corticosteroid therapy. Mild disease with such manifestations as fever, arthralgia, pleuritis, or skin manifestations may respond adequately to NSAIDs or antimalarials, but patients with clinical manifestations that are more serious or unresponsive to other drugs may require corticosteroids. Some patients with lupus dermatitis may benefit from topical or intralesional administration of corticosteroids.

The goal of treatment when using corticosteroids in SLE is to suppress and maintain suppression of active disease with the lowest dose possible. In patients with mild disease, low-dose therapy (prednisone 10–20 mg/day) is adequate,[41,45] but in patients with more severe disease (severe hemolytic anemia or cardiac involvement), high doses, such as prednisone 1–2 mg/kg daily, may be required. Once adequate suppression of disease is achieved, the dose should be tapered to the minimum amount required for continued disease suppression. When analyzing the need to treat with corticosteroids, the clinician should consider other conditions that may increase the risk of corticosteroid therapy, such as infection, hypertension, atherosclerotic disease, diabetes, obesity, osteoporosis, and psychiatric disease.[4,25]

Steroid pulse therapy is the administration of short-term, high-dose intravenous corticosteroids with the goal of inducing remission in SLE patients with serious, life-threatening disease, such as severe active nephritis, CNS involvement, or hemolytic disease. A standard pulse regimen consists of intravenous methylprednisolone 500–1000 mg for 3 to 6 consecutive days. Pulse therapy usually is followed by high-dose prednisone (1–1.5 mg/kg per day) therapy that is tapered rapidly to low-dose maintenance therapy.[25] Potential advantages of pulse therapy over high-dose oral steroids include a quicker response and avoidance of side effects associated with the longer duration of therapy required with oral steroids. Although generally well tolerated, methylprednisolone pulse therapy may result in significant adverse effects, including infection, gastrointestinal disturbances, rapid increases in blood pressure, arrhythmias, seizures, and sudden death. Furthermore, there are insufficient data from controlled clinical trials to clearly define the role of pulse steroids in the management of SLE. Thus pulse therapy represents an alternative mode of treatment for patients with life-threatening disease or disease unresponsive to other pharmacotherapy.

CYTOTOXIC DRUGS

A considerable amount of literature exists describing the use of cytotoxic and immunosuppressive drugs in SLE, although few of these are reports of controlled clinical trials. Included in this category are the alkylating agent cyclophosphamide and the antimetabolite azathioprine. These agents, usually used in combination with corticosteroids, have been the mainstays of immunosuppressive therapy. Although both are known to suppress and stabilize extrarenal disease activity, much of the evaluation of these agents has focused on lupus nephritis, a major factor associated with morbidity and mortality in SLE.

Evidence supporting the use of cyclophosphamide in lupus nephritis has been collected over the last several decades. Controlled clinical trials have shown that cyclophosphamide improved the long-term outcomes in lupus nephritis.[41,61,62] Based on controlled trials, combination prednisone and cyclophosphamide has become standard treatment for focal and diffuse proliferative lupus nephritis (WHO class III/IV) and is superior to prednisone alone.[16] There are no studies examining cyclophosphamide in earlier stages of nephritis (WHO class II/III), and therefore, corticosteroids remain the treatment of choice for these less severe forms of nephritis.[61] A meta-analysis of clinical trials revealed that pulse intravenous cyclophosphamide plus prednisone was more effective at increasing patient survival and renal function than prednisone only.[63] Cyclophosphamide plus corticosteroids preserves renal function and decreases the risk of developing end-stage renal failure requiring dialysis and renal transplantation.[16] Intermittent pulse administration of intravenous cyclophosphamide is preferred over daily oral therapies because of reduced adverse effects. However, pulse cyclophosphamide plus prednisone is not always effective. Other cytotoxic combinations have been examined, but none has been found to be significantly better than any other at reducing the risk of death or renal failure.[16]

When used in combination with corticosteroids, cyclophosphamide is dosed at 1–3 mg/kg for oral therapy and 0.5–1.0 g/m² of body surface area for intravenous therapy. The most common route of cyclophosphamide administration is intravenous, although there is little evidence that this is better than oral administration.[61,62] Likewise, there is no evidence to suggest the optimal duration of treatment. Based on empirical experience, cyclophosphamide generally is dosed monthly for 6 months and then every 3 months for a period of either 2 years or for 1 year after the nephritis is in remission.[43,61,64] Of course, cyclophosphamide therapy is not without risk. Serious toxic effects include suppression of hematopoiesis, opportunistic infections, bladder complications (e.g., hemorrhagic cystitis and cancer), sterility, and teratogenesis. White blood cell counts must be monitored during cyclophosphamide therapy, and if the nadir is less than 1500/mm³, the dose must be adjusted to keep the white cell count above 1500/mm³. Nausea and vomiting associated with cyclophosphamide can be controlled with oral ondansetron plus dexamethasone.[61]

Azathioprine can be used as a "steroid-sparing" agent, allowing for the reduction of corticosteroid doses.[41,45] Azathioprine has not been studied as extensively as cyclophosphamide for lupus nephritis. Additionally, azathioprine is only slightly more effective than prednisone alone.[43] Azathioprine may find usefulness in treating early-onset and less severe nephritis.[41,43] Long-term maintenance azathioprine therapy also may be beneficial in preventing renal flares after successful induction with cyclophosphamide.[62] Azathioprine is given orally in doses of 1 to 3 mg/kg per day, often in combination with corticosteroids for severe disease.[25] Azathioprine generally is less toxic than cyclophosphamide, but adverse reactions may be serious and include suppression of hematopoiesis, opportunistic infections including herpes zoster, cancer, hepatotoxicity, and ovarian failure.

Cyclophosphamide often is administered intravenously in intermittent pulse doses to minimize toxicity. To decrease the risk of bladder toxicity, patients should be well hydrated with oral or intravenous fluids, and urinary output should be monitored. Mesna may be used to prevent hemorrhagic cystitis. Mesna is administered as a bolus of 25 mg/kg 30 minutes before cyclophosphamide therapy and 3, 6, and 9 hours after therapy.[44]

Cyclophosphamide may be of benefit to some patients with other serious, refractory manifestations of lupus, including neurologic manifestations.[65] Reports of the use of other cytotoxic drugs for lupus in recent years include methotrexate,[25] mycophenolate mofetil,[7,25,41,62] mechlorethamine (nitrogen mustard), chlorambucil, and cyclosporine.[7,25,41,62]

Mycophenolate mofetil is a new immunosuppressive agent now rapidly establishing its role in the treatment of severe renal and nonrenal lupus refractory to conventional cytotoxic agents.[41,62] Mycophenolate mofetil showed equal efficacy at 12 months in a randomized, controlled trial comparing mycophenolate mofetil with sequential oral cyclophosphamide followed by azathioprine in proliferative lupus nephritis.[62,66] However, the extended follow-up for 36 months demonstrated higher renal relapse rates in the mycophenolate mofetil–treated group.[62,67] Additionally, in an ongoing randomized, controlled trial, mycophenolate mofetil maintenance therapy thus far has proven to be more effective in preventing renal flares than quarterly intravenous pulse cyclophosphamide or daily azathioprine with fewer adverse events.[62,68]

Cytotoxic therapy is useful in combination with corticosteroids, allowing for lower steroid doses and improved efficacy compared with steroids alone. However, cytotoxic therapy must be monitored closely for adverse effects, and maximum response may take 6 months or longer in some patients. No data from controlled trials are available to support the combination of two or more cytotoxic agents; however, this approach has been used in patients refractory to standard therapies.[16,61]

ALTERNATIVE AND EXPERIMENTAL TREATMENTS

As the pathogenesis of SLE continues to be elucidated, new and promising treatments are being developed. Several alternative treatments reportedly successful in managing various manifestations of SLE[53,69–73] are listed in Table 85–5. However, many of these are reports of uncontrolled trials. Furthermore, in addition to reports of success, the literature contains reports of unsuccessful or controversial treatments for many of these therapies (e.g., plasmapheresis or immune globulin for lupus nephritis). A number of newer agents are being examined and include various biologic therapies that interfere with immune response, ablative chemotherapy with stem cell transplantation, and combination chemotherapy.[16,55,74,75]

TABLE 85–5. Alternative and Experimental Treatments for SLE

Treatment	Symptom	Reference
Cyclosporine	Nephritis	69
	Multiple symptoms—anemia, leukopenia, thrombocytopenia, nephritis	53
Dehydroepiandrosterone (DHEA)	Multiple symptoms	70
LJP 394	Reduction in anti-dsDNA titers	71
	Nephritis	72
Anti-CD20 monoclonal antibody (Rituximab)	Multiple symptoms	73
Thalidomide	Cutaneous lesions	75
Cladaribine	Nephritis	75

SPECIAL POPULATIONS

PREGNANCY AND SLE

Pregnancy in SLE patients has been associated with exacerbation of disease during pregnancy, exacerbation during the early postpartum period, a greater incidence of spontaneous abortion, and a greater chance of developing preeclampsia or pregnancy-induced hypertension (particularly in patients with nephritis).

Lupus flares during pregnancy are associated with prematurity. Whether there is an increased risk for lupus flares during pregnancy versus those who are not pregnant is controversial, but exacerbation of lupus during pregnancy seems to be less likely if the disease is in remission at conception.[7,76,77] Disease exacerbations can be managed aggressively with corticosteroids, if needed, with little concern about harm to the fetus.[76] The decision to use other classes of drug therapy to control disease exacerbation should be highly individualized, although hydroxychloroquine has been shown to be safe during pregnancy.[64,78,79] In fact, it may be safer to continue hydroxychloroquine during pregnancy than to discontinue it.[41,76] The decision to use cytotoxic drugs during pregnancy should be made with extreme caution because of potential harmful effects (e.g., teratogenesis, fetal loss) to the fetus.[80] Azathioprine may be the safest of the cytotoxic drugs if needed during pregnancy.[64,76]

Antiphospholipid antibodies may be associated with a greater likelihood of spontaneous abortion.[7,41] Corticosteroids, intravenous immuoglobulin, aspirin, and heparin, alone and in various combinations, have been used to try to improve fetal outcome.[45] Fetal survival increases with all these therapies, and none has been shown to be superior.[25] The optimal treatment regimen for pregnant patients with antiphospholipid antibodies is yet to be determined, although it has been recommended that women with antiphospholipid antibodies and no prior fetal losses should receive low-dose daily aspirin. High-risk women with a history of recurrent fetal loss should be treated with low-dose subcutaneous heparin with or without aspirin.[25,76] Low-molecular-weight heparin may be an effective alternative to low-dose heparin in the treatment of antiphospholipid syndrome-related pregnancy loss.[7,25,76]

Although there is an increased chance of a high-risk pregnancy in women with SLE, appropriate planning and disease management will result in a high likelihood of a successful pregnancy and a healthy child.

ANTIPHOSPHOLIPID SYNDROME AND THROMBOSIS

As mentioned earlier, the presence of antiphospholipid antibodies may result in several clinical manifestations, including thrombosis. There is no agreement on prophylaxis of patients with antiphospholipid antibodies without a history of thromboembolism.[39] In such patients, low-dose aspirin (100–325 mg/day) may be used prophylactically, although efficacy has not been established.[39] Patients with an acute thrombotic event should receive standard treatment with anticoagulants (e.g., heparin). Follow-up treatment with warfarin to prevent recurrence may require an international normalized ratio (INR) of 3 or greater in patients with antiphospholipid syndrome.[7,45] However, currently, there is no consensus on the intensity of anticoagulation or duration of secondary prophylaxis, but since recurrence is common, patients usually are treated with oral anticoagulants indefinitely.[45]

CLINICAL CONTROVERSY

The optimal dose of aspirin and the intensity of anticoagulation therapy have not been well established, and clinicians will use various strategies for prevention of thrombosis in the presence of antiphospholipid antibodies.

DRUG-INDUCED LUPUS

One of the earliest descriptions of a drug-induced SLE-like syndrome was reported in 1945 and was associated with the use of sulfadiazine.[81] Today, procainamide and hydralazine are associated most commonly with drug-induced lupus (DIL), although numerous other drugs have been implicated[41,81–83] (Table 85–6). A consensus on diagnostic criteria for DIL does not exist. To meet criteria for DIL, a patient should have exposure to a suspected drug, no prior history of idiopathic SLE prior to the use of the drug, development of ANAs (usually antihistone antibodies) and at least one clinical feature of SLE, and rapid improvement of symptoms with a gradual decline in ANAs following drug discontinuation.[81,82,84] The epidemiologic characteristics of DIL are different from those of idiopathic SLE. In general, patients with procainamide- or hydralazine-induced lupus develop the disease much later in life compared with idiopathic SLE probably because the majority of people who use these drugs are older. There is also an absence of female predominance when compared with idiopathic SLE.[85]

Patients of the slow acetylator phenotype may have a greater risk for developing DIL, particularly with procainamide and hydralazine.[13,81,85] Procainamide-induced lupus can present as early as 1 month or even after years of therapy. Hydralazine-induced lupus is related to dose and appears in patients receiving 100 mg/day or more.[81,85]

Musculoskeletal symptoms are the most common clinical manifestations, whereas renal manifestations and CNS involvement are rare. Other common features of DIL include fever, fatigue, pericarditis, pleurisy, and weight loss.[84] Although the classic malar rash is

TABLE 85–6. Medications Implicated in Drug-Induced Lupus

Acebutolol	Interleukin 2	Pindolol
Amiodarone	**Isoniazid**	Primidone
Anti-TNF therapies	Labetalol	**Procainamide**
Atenolol	Lisinopril	Propranolol
Captopril	Lithium	Propylthiouracil
Carbamazepine	Mephenytoin	**Quinidine**
Chlorpromazine[a]	Methimazole	Reserpine
Ciprofloxacin	**Methyldopa**	Simvastatin
Clobazam	Metoprolol	Streptomycin
Clonidine	Minocycline	Sulfasalazine
Clozapine	Nifedipine	Tetracycline
Diltiazem	Oral contraceptives	Thiazide diuretics
Ethosuximide	Para-aminosalicylate	Ticlopidine
Gold salts	Penicillamine	Timolol
Griseofulvin	Penicillin	Tocainide
Hydralazine	Phenytoin	Valproate
Hydroxyurea	Phenylbutazone	Verapamil
Interferon (α, γ)	Phenelzine	Zafirlukast

[a]Drugs in boldface represent those with best evidence of association.
Adapted from refs. 81–83.

rare in DIL, skin manifestations are seen in 25% to 53% of patients with DIL.[81,84] A positive ANA test is found in nearly all (~90%) hydralazine-induced cases and in 50% to 90% of procainamide-induced disease. The immunofluorescence pattern usually is homogeneous, and antibodies are primarily against ssDNA and not dsDNA as in idiopathic SLE. Antihistone antibodies are specific for DIL but might be found in only 20% of patients with idiopathic SLE.[81]

If signs and symptoms of SLE appear in a patient and are thought to be drug-related, the drug should be discontinued. If the lupus is drug-induced, the clinical manifestations should disappear in days to weeks, although it may take up to 1 year or longer for symptoms and serologic abnormalities to resolve completely.[41] A NSAID might be useful in treating musculoskeletal manifestations. Other, more aggressive drug therapy should not be necessary unless manifestations are deemed more serious.

PHARMACOECONOMIC CONSIDERATIONS

Treating patients with SLE is costly, requiring frequent visits to physician offices for monitoring therapy and treating adverse reactions from therapy and hospitalization for disease exacerbation and adverse drug effects. Therefore, it is particularly important in the management of a potentially debilitating chronic disease such as SLE to achieve desired treatment outcomes in an optimal manner to minimize the impact on use of health care resources. Costs of treating patients with SLE are similar in the United States, Canada, and the United Kingdom.[86] In one study, the average total annual costs in 1997 were approximately $3800 per patient with SLE, with medication costing approximately $880 per patient.[86]

Lupus patients with poor physical or poor psychological functioning have been shown to incur higher direct medical costs, whereas patients with the poorest psychological functioning and those with the most severe pain incur higher indirect costs (costs associated with loss of productivity such as days of work missed).[87] Higher direct, indirect, and total costs also have been associated with higher education level, greater disease activity, and lower physical functioning in another study.[87] Specific treatment strategies that incorporate therapies to improve physical and psychological functioning, as well as reduce disease activity and end-organ damage, might reduce use of health care resources.

One study targeting a cohort of patients with severe lupus nephritis found that compared with prednisone alone, combined treatment with intravenous cyclophosphamide and prednisone resulted in slightly higher costs early in therapy (0–4 years) but substantial savings later (5–10 years) as a result of less need for dialysis and transplantation and increased productivity of patients.[88] Another study examined antiemetic therapy in patients with lupus nephritis receiving pulse cyclophosphamide and found that a regimen of combined oral ondansetron plus dexamethasone was completely effective in preventing emesis and was less expensive than a conventional intravenous regimen in patients who had previously failed conventional antiemetic therapy.[89]

As the field of pharmacoeconomics grows, and as clinicians and researchers attempt to define the optimal management of patients in our cost-conscious environment, additional examination of the economics of treating patients with lupus will be needed.

SYSTEMIC SCLEROSIS

CLINICAL MANIFESTATIONS

Systemic sclerosis is characterized by alteration of the microvasculature and by massive deposition of collagen. This disease can present as a spectrum of differing manifestations depending on affected areas and the extent of disease. Sclerosis of the skin is a hallmark for this disease. There can be a proximal diffuse (truncal) sclerosis, with skin tightness and marked skin thickening involving most of the body. There also can be internal organ involvement, such as the gastrointestinal tract, lung, kidney, or heart, which can result in death. *Scleroderma* refers to patients with only skin involvement. Disease that affects only the fingers and toes is referred to as *sclerodactyly*.

> ### CLINICAL PRESENTATION OF SYSTEMIC SCLEROSIS
>
> **GENERAL**
>
> - Sclerosis of the skin
>
> **SYMPTOMS**
>
> - Raynaud's phenomenon
> - Dyspepsia
> - Constipation
> - Diarrhea
> - Steatorrhea
> - Esophageal dysmotility

Most patients with systemic sclerosis have Raynaud's phenomenon, where the digits turn white, followed by a bluish color, which is then followed by reddening in response to an appropriate stimulus. Usually the precipitating event is cold temperature or emotion. The pallor is due to vasospasm, the bluish color is from ischemia, and the reddish color is caused by a reactive hyperemia. Raynaud's phenomenon is a common manifestation of other syndromes, and most patients with Raynaud's phenomenon do not have systemic sclerosis. Approximately 50% to 80% of patients with systemic sclerosis have gastrointestinal symptoms, and 75% to 90% of patients have esophageal dysmotility.[90,91]

Survival rates are highly variable depending on the extent of disease presentation, organ involvement, and other factors. In general, the 5-year survival rate is greater than 60%, which diminishes to approximately 50% at 10 years.[92,93]

ETIOLOGY AND PREVALENCE

The cause of systemic sclerosis is unknown. Ninety-five percent of patients have identifiable autoantibodies. There are two major subsets of the disease, limited cutaneous and diffuse systemic sclerosis. Patients with limited cutaneous involvement often have the CREST syndrome (*c*alcinosis, *R*aynaud's, *e*sophageal dysmotility, *s*clerodactyly, and *t*elangiectasias), whereas patients with diffuse systemic sclerosis have a more aggressive disease with renal, cardiac, or pulmonary involvement. The prevalence of the disease is estimated to be between 138 and 286 cases per 1 million population.[93] The wide range may be due to differences in diagnostic criteria, regional variation, or sample sizes used to estimate the prevalence.

▶ TREATMENT: Systemic Sclerosis

Treatment often is empirical because there are no well-controlled trials evaluating and comparing various forms of therapy. Available data are difficult to interpret because of the heterogeneity of the disease and spontaneous remissions that can occur. There is also a lack of objective measures to assess changes in clinical status. D-Penicillamine is used most often for skin involvement. When started within the first 2 years of the disease, this drug does seem to improve the skin manifestations and prolong survival.[94] The initial dose of D-penicillamine is 250 mg/day, with gradual increases in dose every 2 to 3 months to an optimal dose of 750–1000 mg/day. Response occurs over many months, and the drug is not always effective. The high incidence of severe adverse events and the increased dropout rates for D-penicillamine limit its usefulness. Anti-inflammatory agents and corticosteroids have not been effective in systemic sclerosis.

Angiotensin-converting enzyme (ACE) inhibitors have improved survival dramatically in patients with renal involvement and improve outcomes in patients with disease-associated pulmonary hypertension or myocardial involvement.[95,96] Patients with sclerosis of the kidneys develop hypertension, leading to a renal crisis. In these patients, plasma renin activity and angiotensin concentrations can be more than twice normal. Renal involvement should be anticipated in all systemic sclerosis patients who develop hypertension. Patients with systemic sclerosis and hypertension should be treated and maintained with an ACE inhibitor regardless of renal involvement. ACE inhibitors have allowed some dialysis-dependent systemic sclerosis patients to discontinue dialysis.[95] Treatment of Raynaud's phenomenon requires patient education and sometimes drug therapy. Patients must maintain their peripheral extremity and core body temperatures. Wearing appropriate clothing in cold environments is essential. Reaching into a freezer with unprotected hands should be avoided. Drugs that can cause peripheral vasoconstriction, such as pseudoephedrine and β-blockers, should be avoided in patients with Raynaud's or systemic sclerosis. Smoking causes cutaneous vasoconstriction and should be eliminated, including passive smoke. When preventive measures are not sufficient, calcium channel blocking agents have become the agents of choice for Raynaud's phenomenon. Nifedipine (10–20 mg three or four times per day) decreases the frequency and duration of attacks. Diltiazem (60 mg three or four times per day) also can be used. The sustained-release formulations of these agents may enhance patient compliance. Although there are limited data, other agents that may be beneficial for Raynaud's are selective serotonin reuptake inhibitors and angiotensin II receptor antagonists.[91]

POLYMYOSITIS AND DERMATOMYOSITIS

CLINICAL MANIFESTATIONS

Polymyositis (PM) and dermatomyositis (DM) are chronic inflammatory diseases of skeletal muscle and skin of unknown etiology. DM is distinguished from PM by a typical rash, which is red, scaly, and plaquelike over the knuckles, wrists, elbows, and knees. A blue-purple discoloration on the upper eyelids with edema also can occur in dermatomyositis.

There is an increase in serum creatine kinase concentration and electromyography abnormalities. Other serum enzymes, such as the alanine transaminase, aspartate transaminase, and lactate dehydrogenase, also may be increased.[97] Muscle biopsies show a necrotizing inflammatory process. The skin lesions of dermatomyositis show an immune-complex-mediated necrosis of the microvasculature. PM appears to be related to cytotoxic T-cell activity, and up to 20% of patients with inflammatory myopathies have ANAs and cytoplasmic antibodies.

CLINICAL PRESENTATION OF POLYMYOSITIS AND DERMATOMYOSITIS

GENERAL

- Inflammation of skeletal muscle and skin

SYMPTOMS

- Muscle weakness in shoulder and hip girdles and trunk
- Insidious onset
- Arthritis, Raynaud's phenomenon, and other symptoms of connective tissue diseases

▶ TREATMENT: Polymyositis and Dermatomyositis

Large controlled trials of drug therapy have not been conducted. The goal of therapy is to increase muscle strength so as to improve function in activities of daily living (e.g., bathing, dressing, feeding, and toileting). Treatment consists of physical therapy during periods of remission and rest during periods of disease activity. Prednisone is the first line of drug therapy for PM and DM. There is no consensus as to the optimal dose of prednisone to use. Most clinicians use prednisone at a starting dose of 60–100 mg/day or approximately 1 mg/kg per day as a single morning dose.[97–99] Higher prednisone doses of 1.5 mg/kg per day can be used if needed.[100] The initial dose of prednisone is continued for 1 to 2 months or until maximum benefit is achieved or a remission is induced. The full effect of prednisone may not be evident for several months. Approximately 85% of patients treated with prednisone will have normal muscle strength after 4 months of treatment. The prednisone dose is tapered when muscle strength improves and serum creatine kinase concentrations decrease. If the prednisone is working and there are no serious side effects, the drug is tapered slowly. Again, there is no consensus on how to accomplish this. One expert advocates using prednisone for 3 to 4 weeks and then tapering the dose over 10 weeks to an every-other-day regimen.[97] The dose that maintains a good clinical response can be used as maintenance. Tapering too quickly can cause an exacerbation of disease activity. Monitoring serum creatine kinase concentrations is useful because they tend to increase several weeks before clinical symptoms become apparent. Some clinicians will treat patients with daily prednisone for 1 or more years, whereas others may use every-other-day therapy for many years.

One complication from corticosteroid use is the development of a myopathy. Based on symptoms, it is difficult to know if increased muscle weakness is due to the corticosteroid or to worsening disease tus. Lowering the prednisone dose may be useful. If patients get tter on a lower dose of prednisone, then most likely the muscle eakness was due to the drug. It may take 2 to 8 weeks for this to come evident clinically. Use of serum creatine kinase concentration so may be helpful because this does not increase with steroid my-pathy. It is possible that a steroid myopathy and worsening disease n coexist.

Although most patients with PM or DM improve with pred-sone, some will not, and some will develop corticosteroid resistance. these patients, azathioprine has been used at a dose of 2–3 mg/kg per day in divided doses, with a maintenance dose of 0.5 mg/kg per day.[99] Clinical response may take 3 to 6 months. Another alternative is methotrexate at a dose of 5–20 mg once weekly.[99] In patients resistant to these therapies, cyclophosphamide, cyclosporine, or chlorambucil can be tried. Intravenous γ-globulin at a dose of 2 g/kg per month for 3 months may be effective in patients with refractory disease.[100] There are no large series of data available on clinical outcomes in patients on alternative therapies for PM or DM. These alternative therapies also may be beneficial in patients who cannot take corticosteroids because of serious adverse effects.

POLYMYALGIA RHEUMATICA AND GIANT CELL ARTERITIS

CLINICAL MANIFESTATIONS

olymyalgia rheumatica (PMR) and giant cell arteritis are closely lated diseases, and some experts consider them to be different phases the same disease.[101, 102]

Giant cell arteritis is a vasculitis of large and medium-sized ves-ls. The most frequent symptom is headache, with pain usually in the mporal or occipital areas, and signs of systemic inflammation also ually are present.[101, 103] Giant cell arteritis was referred to previously "temporal arteritis" or "granulomatous arteritis." Both PMR and ant cell arteritis occur in people over 50 years of age, and the inci-nce increases with age, peaking between 70 and 80 years.[101] Some tients go from exhibiting no symptoms to overt clinical manifes-tions overnight, whereas others have a gradual onset of symptoms er a number of weeks. The etiology is unknown.

CLINICAL PRESENTATION OF PMR AND GIANT CELL ARTERITIS

GENERAL

- Aching and morning stiffness of neck, shoulder, and pelvic girdle musculature and torso.

SYMPTOMS

- Pain and morning stiffness lasting 1–6 hours
- Fatigue, malaise, weight loss usually present
- Anorexia
- Headache in giant cell arteritis

SIGNS

- Low-grade fever

LABORATORY TESTS

- ESR is generally >40 mm/h and often >100 mm/h

▶ TREATMENT: Polymyalgia Rheumatica and Giant Cell Arteritis

ne treatment of choice for PMR is prednisone at a dose of 10–) mg/day, and giant cell arteritis requires doses of 40–60 mg/day. ılse therapy with intravenous methylprednisolone, 1000 mg/day for days, may be used in patients experiencing visual loss.[101,102] Corti-osteroid therapy is so effective that if improvement does not occur ithin a week, another diagnosis should be considered. The erythro-yte sedimentation rate (ESR) should decrease by 2 weeks and be ormal after 4 weeks of therapy. The prednisone should be tapered eginning several weeks following control of symptoms. The rate of pering is based on clinical response. A taper of 2.5 mg/day at 2- to -week intervals to 5–10 mg/day followed by a slower tapering of mg/day at monthly intervals has been suggested.[104,105] The lowest ose of prednisone that controls symptoms should be used for main-nance, which is usually between 7 and 15 mg/day. Maintaining the

ESR and C-reactive protein concentration in the normal range is a good monitoring approach. For elderly patients, the normal ESR may be slightly higher than that usually given as a reference value by the clinical laboratory. PMR is a self-limited disease, and patients usually continue maintenance therapy for 2 to 5 years. Patients may experi-ence a relapse when the prednisone is discontinued and may require prednisone therapy for up to 15 years.[106] Every-other-day prednisone has not been as successful as daily therapy. Since these are diseases of the elderly, it is particularly important to use calcium and vitamin D supplements to prevent corticosteroid-induced osteoporosis. Prophy-lactic bisphosphonate therapy also should be considered. Unlike most other autoimmune diseases, other forms of immunosuppressive ther-apy are not as effective as corticosteroids in PMR and giant cell arteritis.[102]

DRUG-INDUCED VASCULITIS

CLINICAL MANIFESTATIONS

Drugs are common causes of vasculitis, often occurring in the skin, but other organ involvement can occur. The pathogenesis of flammation of small and medium-sized blood vessel walls caused by rugs is poorly understood.[107] Even drugs used to treat inflammatory id immune-mediated disease, such as NSAIDs, sulfasalazine, and anercept, can cause vasculitis.

CLINICAL PRESENTATION OF DRUG-INDUCED VASCULITIS

GENERAL

- Signs and symptoms depend on organ involvement

SYMPTOMS

- Rash
- Glomerulonephritis

- Hepatitis
- Fatigue
- Myalgias
- Arthralgias

SIGNS

- Fever

Symptoms can occur within hours of drug administration or after more than 15 years of using a drug.[108] Most classes of medications have been reported to cause vasculitis. There are no specific diagnostic tests for drug-induced vasculitis. Antineutrophil cytoplasmic autoantibodies have been identified in many cases of drug-induced vasculitis.[107,108] Eosinophilia, leukocytosis, and elevated ESR also may occur.

▶ TREATMENT: Drug-Induced Vasculitis

The first step in therapy of drug-induced vasculitis is to discontinue the suspected inducing agent. This may be all that is necessary to abate symptoms in mild cases. For more serious cases, corticosteroids may be used, and where life-threatening organ involvement occurs, immunosuppressive therapy with agents such as cyclophosphamide may be used.[108] Following therapy, symptoms resolve within a few weeks to a few months.

EVALUATION OF THERAPEUTIC OUTCOMES

The diversity of clinical features and disease severity associated with the collagen-vascular diseases leads to a number of possible clinical outcomes with a broad range of desired therapeutic outcomes. Achieving desired therapeutic outcomes for most of the collagen-vascular diseases is highly variable. Currently, it is not possible to predict which patients will have a satisfactory therapeutic response and which will have unrelenting progressive disease. These diseases often have fluctuating courses, necessitating frequent changes in drug therapy and drug doses.

Evaluation of drug therapy of several of the collagen-vascular diseases often only requires monitoring for resolution of symptoms such as rash or muscle pain. However, patients with life-threatening disease receiving aggressive pharmacotherapy may require intensive monitoring and evaluation of therapy. For example, the patient receiving cytotoxic drug therapy for severe lupus nephritis requires close monitoring of laboratory indices of renal function, as well as monitoring of symptomatology and laboratory indices for possible bone marrow suppression, infection, cystitis, or other undesired therapeutic outcomes.

Evaluation of therapeutic outcomes also should include an awareness of the possibility of drug therapy mimicking signs and symptoms of disease, such as the lupus patient receiving NSAID therapy and presenting with renal insufficiency or the patient with PM receiving prednisone and presenting with an exacerbation of muscle weakness.

As patients live longer, as is the case with SLE, outcome measures other than mortality will be needed to assess the effect of treatment. Clinicians and researchers working with lupus patients have developed and continue to refine some of these alternative outcome measures. Three important domains for assessing lupus patients include disease activity, accumulated damage, and quality of life.[10] Several instruments useful for assessing patients with SLE are listed in Table 85–7. Increased use of these and similar instruments for assessment of treatment outcomes in patients with SLE can be expected.

CONCLUSION

SLE is a disease that affects multiple organ systems and consists of abnormal immunologic function and the development of autoantibodies. The disease is quite variable in clinical presentation and progression. The cause of lupus is unknown, although several factors (e.g., genetics, environment, and hormones) may predispose an individual to the development of the disease. Although SLE was once thought to be rapidly fatal, today nearly 90% of patients survive 10 years.

Drug therapy is nonspecific and is aimed at suppressing the inflammation and abnormal immune response associated with active disease. Clinical trials with various agents often have been inadequate and contradictory, and the therapeutic management of lupus is not optimal. Nevertheless, drug therapy of recent years probably has contributed significantly to the improved survival of these patients. As the understanding of SLE progresses and advances in biotechnology occur, we can expect to see the development of more specific and optimal treatment and further improvement in survival.

Each of the collagen-vascular diseases has its own recommended form of therapy. For most of these diseases, there are few well controlled clinical trials evaluating pharmacotherapy. Treatment of most of these diseases requires anti-inflammatory or immunosuppressive drugs. Monitoring therapeutic outcomes is essential because drugs and drug doses may need to be modified frequently.

TABLE 85–7. Instruments Used for Assessing Outcome Measures in Patients with SLE

Outcome Domain	Instrument
Disease activity	Systemic Lupus Activity Measure (SLAM)/Revised SLAM (SLAM-R)
	Systemic Lupus Erythematosus Disease Activity Index (SLEDAI)
	British Isles Lupus Activity Group (BILAG)
Accumulated damage	Systemic Lupus International Collaborating Clinics/American College of Rheumatology (SLICC/ACR) damage index
Quality of life	Health Assessment Questionnaire (HAQ) functional ability index
	Medical Outcome Survey short form (MOS SF-20) and (MOS SF-36)

From ref. 109.

ABBREVIATIONS

ACE: angiotensin-converting enzyme
ACR: American College of Rheumatology
ANA: antinuclear antibodies

APCs: antigen-presenting cells
CAD: coronary artery disease
DIL: drug-induced lupus
DM: dermatomyositis
DNA: deoxyribonucleic acid
dsDNA: double-stranded DNA
ECG: electrocardiograph
ESR: erythrocyte sedimentation rate
HLA: human leukocyte antigen
INR: international normalized ratio
LA: lupus anticoagulant
MHC: major histocompatibility complex
NSAID: nonsteroidal anti-inflammatory drug
PM: polymyositis
PMR: polymyalgia rheumatica
RNP: ribonucleoprotein
SLE: systemic lupus erythematosus
ssDNA: single-stranded DNA
RNA: ribonucleic acid
Th: T-helper cell
WHO: World Heath Organization

Review Questions and other resources can be found at *www.pharmacotherapyonline.com.*

REFERENCES

1. Benedek TG. Historical background of discoid and systemic lupus erythematosus. In: Wallace DJ, Hahn BH, eds. Dubois' Lupus Erythematosus, 6th ed. Philadelphia, Lippincott Williams & Wilkins, 2002:3–16.
2. Edworthy SM. Clinical manifestations of systemic lupus erythematosus. In: Ruddy S, Harris ED, Sledge CB, eds. Kelley's Textbook of Rheumatology, 6th ed. Philadelphia, Saunders, 2001:1105–1123.
3. Tan EM, Cohen AS, Fries JF, et al. The 1982 revised criteria for the classification of systemic lupus erythematosus. Arthritis Rheum 1982;25:1271–1277.
4. Hochberg MC, for the Diagnostic and Therapeutic Criteria Committee of the American College of Rheumatology. Updating the American College of Rheumatology revised criteria for the classification of systemic lupus erythematosus (Letter). Arthritis Rheum 1997;40:1725.
5. Uramoto KM, Michet CJ, Thumboo J, et al. Trends in the incidence and mortality of systemic lupus erythematosus, 1950–1992. Arthritis Rheum 1999;42:46–50.
6. Jacobson DL, Gange SJ, Rose NR, Graham NMH. Epidemiology and estimated population burden of selected autoimmune diseases in the United States. Clin Immunol Immunopathol 1997;84:223–243.
7. Ruiz-Irastorza G, Khamashta MA, Castellino G, Hughes GRV. Systemic lupus erythematosus. Lancet 2001;357:1027–1032.
8. Petri M. Epidemiology of systemic lupus erythematosus. Best Pract Res Clin Rheumatol 2002;16:847–858.
9. The Lupus Site. Lupus incidence within the community. Available at *www.uklupus.co.uk/aslera.html;* accessed January 2004.
10. Lupus Foundation of America. Statistics about lupus. Available at *www.lupus.org/index.html;* accessed January 2004.
11. Alarcon GS, Rodriguez JL, Benavides G Jr, et al. Systemic lupus erythematosus in three ethnic groups: V. Acculturation, health-related attitudes and behaviors, and disease activity in Hispanic patients from the LUMINA cohort. LUMINA Study Group. Lupus in Minority Populations, Nature versus Nurture. Arthritis Care Res 1999;12:267–276.
12. Cooper GS, Dooley MA, Treadwell EL, et al. Hormonal, environmental, and infectious risk factors for developing systemic lupus erythematosus. Arthritis Rheum 1998;41:1714–1724.
13. Mok CC, Lau CS. Pathogenesis of systemic lupus erythematosus. J Clin Pathol 2003;56:481–490.
14. Perdriger A, Werner-Leyval S, Rollot-Elamrani K. The genetic basis for systemic lupus erythematosus. Joint Bone Spine 2003;70:103–108.
15. Denman AM. Systemic lupus erythematosus: Is a viral aetiology a credible hypothesis? J Infect 2000;40:229–233.
16. Balow JE, Boumpas DT, Austin HA III. New prospects for treatment of lupus nephritis. Semin Nephrol 2000;20:32–39.
17. Lauwerys BR, Houssiau FA. Involvement of cytokines in the pathogenesis of systemic lupus erythematosus. Adv Exp Med Biol 2003;520:237–251.
18. Olhoffer IH, Peng SL, Craft J. Revisiting autoantibody profiles in systemic lupus erythematosus. J Rheumatol 1997;24:297–302.
19. Enger W. The use of laboratory tests in the diagnosis of SLE. J Clin Pathol 2000;53:424–432.
20. Shmerling RH. Autoantibodies in systemic lupus erythematosus: There before you know it. New Engl J Med 2003;349:1499–1500.
21. Arbuckle MR, McClain MT, Rubertone MV, et al. Development of autoantibodies before the clinical onset of systemic lupus erythematosus. New Engl J Med 2003;349:1526–1533.
22. Lupus Foundation of America. Lupus fact sheet. Available at *www.lupus.org/index.html;* accessed January 2004.
23. National Institute of Arthritis and Musculoskeletal and Skin Diseases. Lupus: A Patient Care Guide for Nurses and Other Health Professionals, Chapter 1, Lupus Erythematosus, May 2001. Available at *www.niams.nih.gov/hi/topics/lupus/lupusguide/chp1.htm;* accessed January 2004.
24. Wallace DJ. The clinical presentation of systemic lupus erythematosus. In: Wallace DJ, Hahn BH, eds. Dubois' Lupus Erythematosus, 6th ed. Philadelphia, Lippincott Williams & Wilkins, 2002:621–628.
25. Hahn BH. Management of systemic lupus erythematosus. In: Ruddy S, Harris ED, Sledge CB, eds. Kelley's Textbook of Rheumatology, 6th ed. Philadelphia, Saunders, 2001:1125–1143.
26. Wallace DJ. The musculoskeletal system. In: Wallace DJ, Hahn BH, eds. Dubois' Lupus Erythematosus, 6th ed. Philadelphia, Lippincott Williams & Wilkins, 2002:629–644.
27. Patel P, Werth V. Cutaneous lupus erythematosus: A review. Dermatol Clin 2002;20:373–385.
28. Kao AH, Manzi S. How to manage patients with cardiopulmonary disease? Best Pract Res Clin Rheumatol 2002;16:211–227.
29. Manzi S, Meilahn EN, Rairie JE, et al. Age-specific incidence rates of myocardial infarction and angina in women with systemic lupus erythematosus: Comparison with the Framingham Study. Am J Epidemiol 1997;145:408–415.
30. Esdaile JM, Abrahamowicz M, Grodzicky T, et al. Traditional Framingham risk factors fail to fully account for accelerated atherosclerosis in systemic lupus erythematosus. Arthritis Rheum 2001;44:2331–2337.
31. Shattner A, Liang MH. The cardiovascular burden of lupus: A complex challenge. Arch Intern Med 2003;163:1507–1510.
32. Hahn BH. Systemic lupus erythematosus and accelerated atherosclerosis. New Engl J Med 2003;349:2379–2380.
33. Roman MJ, Shanker B, Davis A, et al. Prevalence and correlates of accelerated atherosclerosis in systemic lupus erythematosus. New Engl J Med 2003;349:2399–2406.
34. Asanuma Y, Oeser A, Shintani AK, et al. Premature coronary-artery atherosclerosis in systemic lupus erythematosus. New Engl J Med 2003;349:2407–2415.
35. ACR Ad Hoc Committee on Neuropsychiatric Lupus Nomenclature. The American College of Rheumatology nomenclature and case definitions for neuropsychiatric lupus syndromes. Arthritis Rheum 1999;42:599–608.
36. Harrison MJ, Ravdin LD. Cognitive dysfunction in neuropsychiatric systemic lupus erythematosus. Curr Opin Rheumatol 2002;14:510–514.
37. Hallegua DS, Wallace DJ. Gastrointestinal manifestations of systemic lupus erythematosus. Curr Opin Rheumatol. 2000;12:379–385.
38. Quismorio FP. Hematologic and lymphoid abnormalities in systemic lupus erythematosus. In: Wallace DJ, Hahn BH, eds. Dubois' Lupus Erythematosus, 6th ed. Philadelphia, Lippincott Williams & Wilkins, 2002:793–819.
39. Wahl DG, Bounameaux H, de Moerlosse P, Sarasin FP. Prophylactic antithrombotic therapy for patients with systemic lupus erythematosus

with or without antiphospholipid antibodies: Do the benefits outweigh the risks? Arch Intern Med 2000;160:2042–2048.

40. Lockshin MD, Sammaritano LR, Schwartzman S. Validation of the Sapporo criteria for antiphospholipid syndrome. Arthritis Rheum 2000;43:440–443.

41. Ioannou Y, Isenberg DA. Current concepts for the management of systemic lupus erythematosus in adults: A therapeutic challenge. Postgrad Med J 2002;78:599–606.

42. Cameron JS. Lupus nephritis. J Am Soc Nephrol 1999;10:413–424.

43. Austin HA, Balow JE. Treatment of lupus nephritis. Semin Nephrol 2000;20:265–276.

44. Pisetsky DS, Gilkeson G, St Clair EW. Systemic lupus erythematosus: Diagnosis and treatment. Med Clin North Am 1997;81:113–129.

45. Brasington RD Jr, Kahl LE, Ranganathan P, et al. Immunologic rheumatic disorders. J Allergy Clin Immunol 2003;111:S593–601.

46. Merrell M, Shulman LE. Determination of prognosis in chronic disease, illustrated by systemic lupus erythematosus. J Chron Dis 1955;1:12–32.

47. Urowitz MD, Gladman DD. How to improve morbidity and mortality in systemic lupus erythematosus. Rheumatology 2000;39:238–244.

48. Manger K, Manger B, Repp R, et al. Definition of risk factors for death, end stage renal disease, and thromboembolic events in a monocentric cohort of 338 patients with systemic lupus erythematosus. Ann Rheum Dis 2002;61:1065–1070.

49. Petri M. Hopkins lupus cohort: 1999 update. Rheum Dis Clin North Am 2000;26:199–213.

50. Lupus Foundation of America, Inc., 1300 Picard Drive, Suite 200, Rockville, MD, 301-670-9292 or 800-558-0121.

51. Arthritis Foundation, 1330 West Peachtree Street, Atlanta, GA, 404-872-7100.

52. Lupus Canada, Box 64034 5512-4 ST NW, Calgary, Alberta, Canada T2K 6J1, 800-661-1468.

53. Wallace DJ. Principles of therapy and local measures. In: Wallace DJ, Hahn BH, eds. Dubois' Lupus Erythematosus, 6th ed. Philadelphia, Lippincott Williams & Wilkins, 2002:1131–1140.

54. Ghaussy NO, Sibbitt WL, Bankhurst AD, Qualls CR. Cigarette smoking and disease activity in systemic lupus erythematosus. J Rheumatol 2003;30:1215–1221.

55. Solsky MA, Wallace DJ. New therapies in systemic lupus erythematosus. Best Pract Res Clin Rheumatol 2002;16:293–312.

56. The Canadian Hydroxychloroquine Study Group. A randomized study of the effect of withdrawing hydroxychloroquine sulfate in systemic lupus erythematosus. New Engl J Med 1991;324:150–154.

57. Williams HJ, Egger MJ, Singer JZ, et al. Comparison of hydroxychloroquine and placebo in the treatment of the arthropathy of mild systemic lupus erythematosus. J Rheumatol 1994;21:1457–1462.

58. Meinao IM, Sato EI, Andrade LE, et al. Controlled trial with chloroquine diphosphate in systemic lupus erythematosus. Lupus 1996;5:237–241.

59. Wallace DJ. Antimalarial therapies. In: Wallace DJ, Hahn BH, eds. Dubois' Lupus Erythematosus, 6th ed. Philidelphia, Lippincott Williams & Wilkins, 2002:1149–1172.

60. Rynes RI. Antimalarial drugs. In: Ruddy S, Harris ED, Sledge CB, eds. Kelley's Textbook of Rheumatology, 6th ed. Philadelphia, Saunders, 2001:859–867.

61. Ortmann RA, Klippel JH. Update on cyclophosphamide for systemic lupus erythematosus. Rheum Dis Clin North Am 2000;26:363–375.

62. Mok CC, Wong RWS, Lai KN. Treatment of severe proliferative lupus nephritis: the current state. Ann Rheum Dis 2003;62:799–804.

63. Bansal VK, Beto JA. Treatment of lupus nephritis: A meta-analysis of clinical trials. Am J Kidney Dis 1997;29:193–199.

64. Mosca M, Ruiz-Irastorza G, Khamashta MA, Hughes GRV. Treatment of systemic lupus erythematosus. Int Immunopharmacol 2001;1:1065–1075.

65. Gold R, Fontana A, Zierz S. Therapy of neurological disorders in systemic vasculitis. Semin Neurol 2003;23:207–214.

66. Chan TM, Li FK, Tang CS, et al. Efficacy of mycophenolate mofetil in patients with diffuse proliferative lupus nephritis. Hong Kong-Guangzhou Nephrology Study Group. New Engl J Med 2000;343:1156–1162.

67. Chan TM, Wong RWS, Lau CS, et al. Prolonged follow-up of patien with diffuse proliferative lupus nephritis treated with prednisolone a mycophenolate mofetil (abstract). J Am Soc Nephrol 2001;12:A1010

68. Contreras G, Pardo V, Leclercq B, et al. Maintenance therapy for pr liferative forms of lupus nephritis: A randomized clinical trial comp ing quarterly intravenous cyclophosphamide versus oral mycophenola mofetil or azathioprine (abstract). J Am Soc Nephrol 2002;13:15A.

69. Fu LW, Yang LY, Chen WP, Lin CY. Clinical efficacy of cyclosporin a n oral in the treatment of paediatric lupus nephritis with heavy proteinur Br J Rheumatol 1998;37:217–221.

70. Van Vollenhoven RF, Park JL, Genovese MC, et al. A double-bli placebo-controlled trial of dehydroepiandrosterone in severe system lupus erythematosus. Lupus 1999;8:181–187.

71. Furie RA, Cash JM, Cronin ME, et al. Treatment of systemic lup erythematosus with LJP 394. J Rheumatol 2001;28:257–265.

72. Alarcon-Segovia D, Tumlin JA, Furie RA, et al. LJP 394 for the pr vention of renal flare in patients with systemic lupus erythematosus: R sults form a randomized, double-blind, placebo-controlled study. Arth tis Rheum 2003;48:442–454.

73. Leandro MJ, Edwards JC, Cambridge G, et al. An open study B lymphocyte depletion in systemic lupus erythematosus. Arthri Rheum 2002;46:2673–2677.

74. Gescuk BD, Davis JC Jr. Novel therapeutic agents for systemic lup erythematosus. Curr Opin Rheumatol 2002;14:515–521.

75. Strand V. New therapies for systemic lupus erythematosus. Rheum D Clin North Am 2000;26:389–406.

76. Mok CC, Wong RWS. Pregnancy in systemic lupus erythematosus. Pos grad Med J 2001;77:157–165.

77. Cervera R, Font J, Carmona F, Balasch J. Pregnancy outcome in system lupus erythematosus: Good news for the new millennium. Autoimm Rev 2002;1:354–359.

78. Costedoat-Chalumeau N, Amoura Z, Duhaut P, et al. Safety of hydrox chloroquine in pregnant patients with connective tissue diseases: A stu of one hundred thirty-three cases compared with a control group. Arth tis Rheum 2003;48:3207–3211.

79. Levy RA, Vilela VS, Cataldo MJ, et al. Hydroxychloroquine (HCC in lupus pregnancy: Double-blind and placebo-controlled study. Lup 2001;10:401–404.

80. Petri M. Immunosuppressive drug use in pregnancy. Autoimmun 2003;36:51–56.

81. Pramatarov KD. Drug-induced lupus erythematosus. Clin Dermat 1998;16:367–377.

82. Brogan BL, Olsen NJ. Drug-induced rheumatic syndromes. Curr Op Rheumatol 2003;15:76–80.

83. Spiera RF, Berman RS, Werner AJ, Spiera H. Ticlopidine-induced lup A report of 4 cases. Arch Intern Med 2002;162:2240–2243.

84. di Fazano CS, Berrin P, Vergne P, et al. The pharmacological ma agement of drug-induced rheumatic disorders. Exp Opin Pharmacoth 2001;2:1623–1631.

85. Sameri RM, Self TH. Drug-induced lupus: Focus on hydralazine ar procainamide. J Crit Ill 2001;16:298–299.

86. Clarke AE, Petri MA, Manzi S, et al. An international perspective c the well-being and health care costs for patients with systemic lup erythematosus. J Rheumatol 1999;26:1500–1511.

87. Sutcliffe N, Clarke AE, Taylor R, et al. Total costs and predictors costs in patients with systemic lupus erythematosus. Rheumatolog 2001;40:37–47.

88. McInnes PM, Schuttinga J, Sanslone WR, et al. The economic impa of treatment of severe lupus nephritis with prednisone and intravenou cyclophosphamide. Arthritis Rheum 1994;37:1000–1006.

89. Yarboro CH, Wesley R, Amantea MA, et al. Modified oral ondansetro regimen for cyclophosphamide-induced emesis in lupus nephritis. An Pharmacother 1996;30:752–755.

90. Cossio M, Menon Y, Wilson W, deBoisblanc BP. Life-threatening con plications of systemic sclerosis. Crit Care Clin 2002;18:819–839.

91. Leighton C. Drug treatment of scleroderma. Drugs 2001;61:419–427.

92. Steen VD, Medsger TA Jr. Severe organ involvment in systemic scleros with diffuse scleroderma. Arthritis Rheum 2000;43:2437–2444.

93. Mayers MD, Lacey JV Jr, Beebe-Dimmer J, et al. Prevalence, incidence, survival, and disease characteristics of systemic sclerosis in a large US population. Athritis Rheum 2003;48:2246–2255.

94. Steen VD, Medsger TA Jr. Improvement in skin thickening in systemic sclerosis associated with improved survival. Athritis Rheum 2001;44:2828–2835.

95. Lin ATH, Clements PJ, Furst DE. Update on disease-modifying antirheumatic drugs in the treatment of systemic sclerosis. Rheum Dis Clin North Am 2003;29:409–426.

96. Maddison P. Prevention of vascular damage in scleroderma with angiotensin-converting enzyme (ACE) inhibition. Rheumatology 2002;41:965–971.

97. Dalakas MC, Hohlfeld R. Polymyositis and dermatomyositis. Lancet 2003;362:971–982.

98. Choy EHS, Isenberg DA. Treatment of dermatomyositis and polymyositis. Rheumatology 2002;41:7–13.

99. Ghate J, Katsambas A, Augerinou G, Jorizzo JL. A therapeutic update on dermatomyositis/polymyositis. Int J Dermatol 2000;39:81–87

00. Koler RA. Dermatomyositis. Am Fam Phys 2001;64:1565–1572.

01. Salvarani C, Cantini F, Boiardi L, Hunder GG. Polymyalgia rheumatica and giant-cell arteritis. New Engl J Med 2002;347:261–271.

102. Weyand CM, Goronzy JJ. Giant-cell arteritis and polymyalgia rheumatica. Ann Intern Med 2003;139:505–515.

103. Weyand CM, Goronzy JJ. Medium- and large-vessel vasculitis. New Engl J Med 2003;349:160–169.

104. Epperly TD, Moore KE, Harrover JD. Polymyalgia rheumatica and temporal arteritis. Am Fam Phys 2000;62:789–796, 801.

105. Evans JM, Hunder GG. Polymyalgia rheumatica and giant cell arteritis. Rheum Dis Clin North Am 2000;26:493–515.

106. Brooks RC, McGee SR. Diagnostic dilemmas in polymyalgia rheumatica. Arch Intern Med 1997;157:162–168.

107. Merkel PA. Drug-induced vasculitis. Rheum Dis Clin North Am 2001;27:849–862.

108. tan Holder SM, Joy MS, Falk RJ. Cutaneous and systemic manifestations of drug-induced vasculitis. Ann Pharmacother 2002;36:130–147.

109. Strand V, Gladman D, Isenberg D, et al. Outcome measures to be used in clinical trials in systemic lupus erythematosus. J Rheumatol 1999;26:490–497.

110. Stein CM. Immunoregulatory drugs. In: Ruddy S, Harris ED, Sledge CB, eds. Kelley's Textbook of Rheumatology, 6th ed. Philadelphia, Saunders, 2001:879–898.

111. Package insert. Cellcept (mycophenolate mofetil). Nutley, NJ, Roche Laboratories, March, 2003.

86

ALLERGIC AND PSEUDOALLERGIC DRUG REACTIONS

Joseph T. DiPiro and Dennis R. Ownby

Learning Objectives and other resources can be found at *www.pharmacotherapyonline.com*.

KEY CONCEPTS

1 Allergic reactions are responsible for 6% to 10% of adverse reactions to medications. Although some reactions are relatively well defined, the majority are due to mechanisms that are either unknown or poorly understood.

2 The following criteria suggest that a drug reaction may be immunologically mediated: (a) The reaction occurs in a small percentage of patients receiving the drug, (b) the observed reaction does not resemble the drug's pharmacologic effect, (c) the type of manifestation is similar to that seen with other allergic reactions (anaphylaxis, urticaria, serum sickness), (d) there is a lag time between first exposure of the drug and reaction, (e) the reaction is reproduced even by minute doses of the drug, (f) the reaction is reproduced by agents with similar chemical structures, (g) eosinophilia is present, and (h) the reaction resolves after the drug has been discontinued. Exceptions to each of these criteria are observed commonly.

3 Factors that influence the likelihood of allergic drug reactions are the dose of the allergen, the route of exposure, and the sensitivity of the individual as determined by age, genetics, or environmental factors. For many drugs, the severity of a reaction is determined by the dose and duration of exposure.

4 Anaphylaxis is an acute, life-threatening allergic reaction involving multiple organ systems that generally begins within 30 minutes but almost always within 2 hours after exposure to the inciting allergen. Anaphylaxis requires prompt treatment to restore respiratory and cardiovascular function. Epinephrine is administered as primary treatment to counteract bronchoconstriction and vasodilatation. Intravenous fluids should be administered to restore intravascular volume.

5 Patients with a history of a reaction to penicillin are advised not to receive cephalosporins if they can be avoided. Patients who have negative penicillin skin tests or experienced only mild cutaneous reactions, such as maculopapular rashes, have a low risk of serious reactions to cephalosporins.

6 Less than 1% of patients receiving nonionic radiocontrast agents experience some type of adverse reaction. Of the variety of reactions reported, approximately 90% are allergic-like, mostly urticarial, with severe reactions occurring as infrequently as 0.02%.

7 Aspirin and other nonsteroidal anti-inflammatory drugs (NSAIDs) can produce two general types of reactions, urticaria/angioedema and rhinosinusitis/asthma, in susceptible patients. Approximately 20% of asthmatics are sensitive to aspirin and other NSAIDs.

8 Adverse reactions to trimethoprim-sulfamethoxazole have been observed to occur much more frequently in AIDS patients compared with those without AIDS (50% to 80% of AIDS patients compared with 10% in other immunocompromised patients).

9 The basic principles of management of allergic reactions to drugs or biologic agents include (a) discontinuation of the medication or agent when possible, (b) treatment of the adverse clinical signs and symptoms, and (c) substitution, if necessary, of another agent.

10 One of the most helpful tests to evaluate risk of penicillin allergy is the skin test. Skin testing can demonstrate the presence of penicillin-specific IgE and predict a relatively high risk of immediate hypersensitivity reactions. Skin testing does not predict the risk of delayed or most dermatologic reactions.

Allergic drug reactions are adverse medication effects that involve immunologic mechanisms. Adverse drug effects not proven to be immune mediated but resembling allergic reactions in their clinical presentation are referred to as *allergic-like* or *pseudoallergic reactions*.[1] Immunologically mediated adverse drug reactions account for 6% to 10% of all adverse drug reactions.[2]

The true frequency of allergic drug reactions is difficult to determine because many reactions may not be reported, and others may be difficult to distinguish from nonallergic adverse events. Dermatologic reactions represent the most frequently recognized and reported form of allergic drug reaction.[3]

TABLE 86–1. Classification of Allergic Drug Reactions

Type	Descriptor	Characteristics	Typical Onset	Drug Causes
I	Anaphylactic (IgE mediated)	Allergen binds to IgE on basophils or mast cells resulting in release of inflammatory medicators	Within 30 min	Penicillin immediate reaction Blood products Polypeptide hormones Vaccines Dextran
II	Cytotoxic	Cell destruction occurs because of cell-associated antigen that initiates cytolysis by antigen-specific antibody (IgG or IgM). Most often involves blood elements.	Typically 5–12 h	Penicillin, quinidine, phenylbutazone, thiouracils, sulfonamides, methyldopa
III	Immune complex	Antigen–antibody complexes form and deposit on blood vessel walls and activate complement. Result is a serum-sickness-like syndrome.	3–8 h	May be caused by penicillins, sulfonamides, radiocontrast agents, hydantoins
IV	Cell mediated (delayed)	Antigens cause activation of lymphocytes, which release inflammatory mediators.	24–48 h	Tuberculin reaction

MECHANISMS OF ALLERGIC DRUG REACTIONS

Drugs can cause allergic reactions by a variety of immunologic mechanisms. Although some reactions are relatively well defined, the majority are due to mechanisms that are either unknown or poorly understood.[4]

The following criteria suggest that a drug reaction may be immunologically mediated[5]: (1) The reaction occurs in a small percentage of patients receiving the drug, (2) the observed reaction does not resemble the drug's pharmacologic effect, (3) the manifestations are similar to those seen with other allergic reactions (e.g., anaphylaxis, urticaria, serum sickness), (4) there is a lag time between first exposure of the drug and reaction unless the recipient has been sensitized by prior exposure to the drug, which can lead to immediate reactions, (5) the reaction is reproduced even by minute doses of the drug, (6) the reaction may be reproduced by agents with similar chemical structures, (7) peripheral blood eosinophilia is present, and (8) the reaction resolves after the drug has been discontinued. Exceptions to each of these criteria are observed commonly.

Many allergic reactions can be classified into one of four immunopathologic categories: types I, II, III, and IV[6,7] (Table 86–1 and Fig. 86–1). Some drug reactions suspected of being mediated immunologically are considered possibly allergic. Examples include drug-associated skin eruptions, drug fever, drug-induced hepatitis, and interstitial nephritis. Other drug reactions can be classified as *pseudoallergic* or *idiosyncratic*. Examples include anaphylactoid (anaphylaxis-like) reactions to radiocontrast media, sulfite sensitivity, and reactions to local anesthetics.

EFFECTORS OF ALLERGIC DRUG REACTIONS

Allergic drug reactions can involve most of the major components of the immune system, including the cellular elements, immunoglobulins, complement, and cytokines. Most immunoglobulin isotypes have been implicated in immunologically mediated drug reactions.

Immunoglobulin E (IgE) bound to basophils or mast cells mediates immediate (anaphylactic-type) reactions. IgG or IgM antibodies also may be involved in allergic reactions, resulting in destruction of cells and tissues.

CELLULAR ELEMENTS

A variety of cells may be involved in immunologic drug reactions. Basophils, mast cells, eosinophils, and lymphocytes are involved most

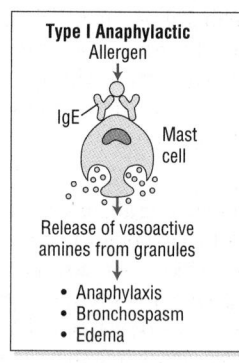
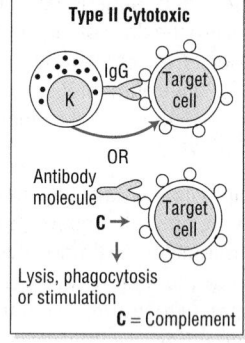
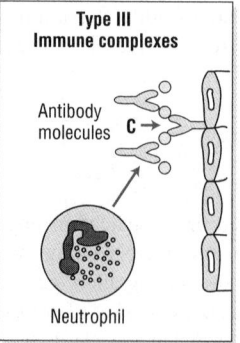
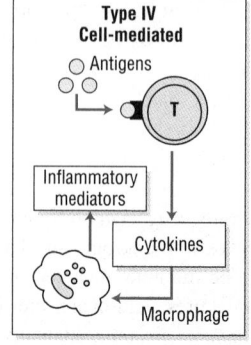

FIGURE 86–1. Types of hypersensitivity reactions.

equently. Platelets and vascular endothelial cells are also important because they also can release a number of inflammatory mediators. Most cells of the body, including nerve cells, can become involved directly or indirectly in allergic drug reactions.[8]

MEDIATORS OF ALLERGIC REACTIONS

The release of a number of preformed, pharmacologically active chemical mediators (e.g., histamine, serotonin, eosinophil chemotactic factor, neutrophil chemotactic factor, and bradykinin-generating factor, also known as *basophil kalikrein of anaphylaxis*) is triggered by antigen cross-linking IgE molecules on the surface of circulating basophils and tissue mast cells. Newly generated mediators include platelet-activating factor and arachidonic acid metabolites (e.g., prostaglandins, thromboxanes, and leukotrienes). Each of these mediators is discussed in the following sections.

Histamine is a low-molecular-weight amine compound formed by decarboxylation of histidine and is stored in basophil and mast cell granules.[9] The release of histamine from these cells is triggered by antigen cross-linking IgE bound to specific receptors on the surface membranes of mast cells and basophils. The tissue effects of histamine are evident within 1 to 2 minutes, but it is rapidly metabolized within 10 to 15 minutes. The major effects of histamine on target tissues include increased capillary permeability, contraction of bronchial and vascular smooth muscle, and hypersecretion of mucus glands.

Serotonin is also a low-molecular-weight amine stored in and released from platelets and mast cells with effects similar to histamine. It may cause vasoconstriction or vasodilatation in some animal species but has no clear role in human anaphylaxis. Eosinophil chemotactic factors are a group of preformed cellular tetrapeptides and dodecapeptides released by stimulated mast cells. They attract eosinophils to inflammatory sites and participate in phagocytosis. Neutrophil chemotactic factor is a high-molecular-weight protein that enhances neutrophil migration to areas of mast cell activation. Bradykinin-generating factor is a series of proteases that activate Hageman factor, resulting in the production of kinins, including bradykinin, which is more potent than histamine on a molar basis in causing vascular permeability and contraction of smooth muscle.

Platelet-activating factor (PAF) is a glyceride-derived substance that is released by mast cells, alveolar macrophages, neutrophils, platelets, and other cells but not by basophils. It has potent bronchoconstrictor effects and also causes platelet aggregation and lysis. It attracts neutrophils and causes their activation. Also, PAF enhances vascular permeability and can cause pain, pruritus, and erythema.

The leukotrienes (LTs) are metabolites of arachidonic acid produced through the 5-lipoxygenase pathway that have potent effects on bronchial and vascular smooth muscle. Three important leukotrienes, LTC_4, LTD_4, and LTE_4, are produced by basophils or mast cells. These three substances are also referred to as *cystinyl leukotrienes* and in older literature as *slow-reacting substances of anaphylaxis*. The LTs have more potent and longer-lasting bronchoconstrictor effects than histamine and also can increase vascular permeability and cause arteriolar vasoconstriction followed by vasodilatation. Their effects are slower in onset but longer lasting than those of histamine. Another product, LTB_4, is a potent chemoattractant, particularly for neutrophils. It is also produced by neutrophils, macrophages, and monocytes.

Prostaglandins (PGs) and thromboxanes are metabolites of arachidonic acid produced through the cyclooxygenase pathway. Some PGs have vasoconstrictive and/or bronchodilatory properties, whereas others are vasodilatory (e.g., PGD_2) and/or bronchoconstric-

tive (e.g., $PGF_{2\alpha}$). PGD_2 is the major prostaglandin product of mast cells. It is a potent inhibitor of platelet aggregation. Thromboxanes cause platelet aggregation and are important regulators of coagulation.

The complement system consists of approximately 30 plasma proteins and is involved in hypersensitivity through a variety of immunologic responses, including enhancement of phagocytosis (opsonization of target cells), cell lysis, and generation of anaphylatoxins (C3a, C4a, and C5a), which can cause non-IgE-mediated activation of mast cells and release of inflammatory mediators.

CLASSIFICATION OF IMMUNOPATHOLOGIC DRUG REACTIONS

Immunologic mechanisms have been identified for some drug reactions. Many can be classified into one of four immunopathologic reactions, as described below. In general, small-molecular-weight molecules (<10,000 MW) are not immunogenic. Most drugs are less than 1000 MW. To become immunogenic, these small compounds must first combine with carrier proteins in plasma or tissue. The combination of the drug bound to a carrier protein can be recognized as foreign, leading to an immune response. The more likely that large amounts of the drug become chemically bound to a protein, the greater is the risk that it will produce an allergic reaction. Penicillin G (356 MW) is an example of a drug that binds covalently to serum proteins through amide or disulfide linkages. For drugs such as the sulfonamides, the parent compound first must be converted to a metabolite before it can combine with the macromolecule. The species that combines with the carrier macromolecule is referred to as a *hapten* or an *incomplete antigen*.[10] Some macromolecular drugs such as insulin are referred to as *complete antigens* because they are large enough to initiate an immune response without binding to another protein.

TYPE I

Type I reactions require the presence of IgE specific for the drug or the portion of the drug that becomes a hapten. IgE specific for the drug allergen is produced on initial exposure to the drug, and then it binds to basophils and mast cells through high-affinity receptors. On repeat exposure to the drug, two or more IgE molecules on the basophil or mast cell surface may bind to one multivalent antigen molecule (referred to as *cross-linking;* see Fig.86–1), initiating an activation of the cell. Activation causes the extracellular release of granules with preformed inflammatory mediators, including histamine, serotonin, heparin, proteases (tryptase in the mast cell), bradykinin-generating factor, eosinophil chemotactic factors, and neutrophil chemotactic factor, as well as generation of newly formed mediators, as previously discussed, such as LTs, prostaglandins, thromboxanes, and PAF, among others.

Generation of a type I reaction can be evident as an immediate hypersensitivity reaction, or anaphylaxis. Immediate reactions may be limited to single organs, typically in the nasal mucosa (rhinitis), respiratory tract (acute asthma), skin, or gastrointestinal tract, or can involve multiple organs simultaneously, termed *analphylaxis.*

TYPE II

Type II immunopathologic reactions involve destruction of host cells (usually blood cells) through cytotoxic antibodies by one of two mechanisms (see Fig. 86–1). First, the drug binds to the cell as a hapten (e.g., the platelet or red blood cell). Antibodies (IgG or IgM) specific for the bound drug or to a component of the cell surface that has been altered by the drug then bind, initiating a cytolytic reaction. The cell destruction may be mediated by complement or by phagocytic cells that have Fc receptors on their surfaces. Activation of complement near the cell surface can result in loss of cell membrane integrity and cell death. Alternatively, neutrophils, monocytes, or macrophages may bind to an antibody-coated cell through IgG Fc receptors on their cell surfaces, and this binding results in phagocytosis of the target cell. The process of enhancement of phagocytosis by antibody binding to cell surfaces or other particles is referred to as *opsonization.* In addition, cell-bound IgG may direct the nonphagocytic action of T cells or natural killer cells, which results in cell destruction by a process called *antibody-dependent cellular cytotoxicity.* This process can proceed in a nonspecific fashion as T cells bind to the target cell through IgG Fc receptors on the T-cell surface. Contact is necessary between the target and effector cells.

Cells commonly affected by these types of reactions include erythrocytes, leukocytes, and platelets, resulting in hemolytic anemia, agranulocytosis, or thrombocytopenia, respectively. This process may be initiated by drugs such as penicillin, quinidine, quinine, phenacetin, cephalosporins, and sulfonamides.

Another type of reaction that may affect the formed elements in blood is the "innocent bystander" reaction. With this type of reaction, antigen-antibody complexes formed in blood adhere nonspecifically to cells. Complement is then activated, resulting in cell lysis.

TYPE III

Type III immunologic reactions are caused by antigen-antibody complexes that are formed in blood. The complexes form with drug allergen and antibody in varying ratios and may deposit in tissues, resulting in local or disseminated inflammatory reactions. Antigen-antibody complex formation can result in platelet aggregation, complement activation, or macrophage activation. Chemotactic substances such as C4a are also produced, and they cause the influx of neutrophils and result in the release of a number of toxic substances from the neutrophil (e.g., proteinases, collagenases, kinin-generating enzymes, and reactive oxygen and nitrogen substances), which can cause local tissue destruction.

Platelet aggregation may occur as a result of immune-complex formation, resulting in the formation of microthrombi and the release of vasoactive mediators. Also, insoluble complexes may be phagocytized by macrophages and activate these cells.

The formation of antigen-antibody complexes can lead to clinical syndromes such as the Arthus reaction. In this model, a high level of preformed specific IgG antibody combines with antigen to produce a localized edematous, erythematous reaction within 5 to 8 hours. The reaction involves local formation of insoluble antigen-antibody complexes, complement activation with release of C3a and C5a collectively referred to as *anaphylatoxins,* mast cell degranulation, and influx of polymorphonuclear cells.

TYPE IV

Type IV reactions are delayed hypersensitivity reactions that typically are demonstrated as dermatologic reactions and are mediated by T cells (CD4$^+$ or CD8$^+$).[11] Type IV reactions require memory T cells specific for the antigen in question. On exposure to the antigen, T cells become activated and produce an inflammatory response. Although these reactions may be associated with adverse effects (e.g., contact dermatitis, maculopapular exanthemas, bullous exanthemas, eczema, or pustular exanthemas), they also may be useful for diagnostic pur-

poses. Examples of the latter include the purified protein derivative (PPD) antigen from *Mycobacterium tuberculosis* used in the tuberculin skin test and other recall skin test antigens, such as mumps. After intradermal injection, these antigens produce a local reaction (erythema and induration) within 48 to 72 hours. Delayed contact hypersensitivity also can be caused by a wide variety of chemicals and drugs.

OTHER ALLERGIC REACTIONS

The precise mechanisms of many drug reactions are not known, although the reactions are believed to be immune mediated. Perhaps most common are the delayed dermatologic reactions that occur with a variety of drugs (especially penicillins and sulfonamides).[11] These reactions may be evident as macropapular, morbilliform, or erythematous rashes; exfoliative dermatitis; photosensitivity reactions; or eczema. These reactions also may be manifest as pruritus, urticaria, and angioedema.

Other serious dermatologic syndromes may be the result of immunologic reactions. Erythema multiforme is an acute syndrome characterized by a variety of skin lesions. The skin lesions typically start as a maculopapular eruption that may progress to irregular lesions with central clearing (target lesions) mostly on the extremities. The rash may be accompanied by bullous lesions that break down into erosions involving more of the body, especially mucous membranes. This more extensive disease usually associated with fever and extensive purpura is called *erythema multiforme major* or *Stevens-Johnson syndrome* (SJS). Some have termed these types of reactions *febrile mucocutaneous syndromes.* If the skin lesions progress to sloughing of large portions of the skin, resembling third-degree burns, the term *toxic epidermal necrolysis* (TEN) is applied. Mortality from TEN can be as high as 30%. Drugs commonly associated with these syndromes include the penicillins, sulfonamides, and anticonvulsants such as phenytoin and phenobarbital, as well as a number of other agents. Drug-induced fever also may involve immunologic mechanisms. Other general types of reactions believed to be immune mediated in some cases include hepatic drug reactions (cholestatic or hepatocellular) and pulmonary reactions, e.g., interstitial pneumonitis, which has been associated with nitrofurantoin.

ANAPHYLACTOID REACTIONS

Various drugs and other substances can produce anaphylactoid (anaphylaxis-like) reactions that are similar to anaphylaxis in clinical signs and symptoms. The substances causing these reactions can produce the direct release of inflammatory mediators from cells by a pharmacologic or physical effect rather than through cell-bound IgE. These reactions are sometimes referred to as *pseudoallergic,* but not all pseudoallergic reactions are anaphylactoid. Drugs that can produce anaphylactoid reactions include vancomycin, opiates, iodinated radiocontrast agents, amphotericin, and D-tubocurarine. The "red man syndrome" is a common example of an anaphylactoid reaction from vancomycin. If vancomycin is infused too rapidly, it can cause the direct release of histamine and other mediators from cutaneous mast cells. This produces a typical clinical picture of itching, flushing, and hives first around the neck and face and then progressing to the chest and other parts of the body usually beginning shortly after the infusion has begun. Most patients who have had "red man syndrome" will tolerate vancomycin if the rate of infusion is slowed. A number of other agents (including aspirin) may produce anaphylactoid reactions by altering the metabolism of inflammatory mediators such as PGs or kinins.

CLINICAL MANIFESTATIONS OF ALLERGIC AND ALLERGIC-LIKE REACTIONS

ANAPHYLAXIS

Anaphylaxis is an acute, life-threatening allergic reaction involving multiple organ systems.[12] Approximately 1500 deaths occur annually in the United States from anaphylaxis.[13] From 1.2% to 5% of the U.S. population may be at risk of anaphylactic reactions.[14] Although many drugs may cause anaphylaxis (or anaphylactoid) reactions, those reported most commonly are aspirin and other NSAIDs, penicillins, and insulins.[15] The manifestations of anaphylaxis may include signs and symptoms referable to the skin, gastrointestinal tract, respiratory tract, and cardiovascular system or any combination of these systems. Common dermatologic manifestations include urticaria, angioedema, and pruritus.[15] Urticaria is a dermatologic reaction noted by elevated, erythematous patches that are pruritic. Gastrointestinal manifestations include nausea, abdominal pain, vomiting, and diarrhea. With respiratory tract involvement, the patient may experience stridor, dyspnea, or wheezing. The major cardiovascular manifestations include hypotension, tachycardia, and arrhythmias.

Anaphylactic reactions generally begin within 30 minutes but almost always within 2 hours of exposure to the inciting allergen. The risk of fatal anaphylaxis is greatest within the first few hours. After apparent recovery, anaphylaxis may recur 6 to 8 hours after antigen exposure. Because of the possibility of these "late phase" reactions, patients should be observed for at least 12 hours after an anaphylactic reaction. Fatal anaphylaxis most often results from asphyxia due to airway obstruction either at the larynx or within the lungs. Cardiovascular collapse may occur as a result of asphyxia in some cases, whereas in others cases cardiovascular collapse may be the dominant manifestation from the release of mediators within the heart muscles and coronary blood vessels.

SERUM SICKNESS

Serum sickness is a clinical syndrome resulting from the effects of soluble circulating immune complexes that form under conditions of antigen excess. The reaction commonly results from the use of antisera containing foreign (donor) antigens such as equine serum in the form of antitoxins or antivenins. The onset of serum sickness usually occurs 7 to 14 days after antigen administration. The onset may be more rapid with reexposure to the same agent in an individual with prior serum sickness. Fever, malaise, and lymphadenopathy are the most common clinical manifestations. Arthralgias, urticaria, and morbilliform skin eruption also may be present. Although often associated with administration of heterologous antisera, serum sickness also may be caused by drugs, including sulfonamides, hydantoins, penicillins, minocycline, and cephalosporins (especially cefaclor). In addition, immune-complex-mediated systemic lupus erythematosus-like syndrome has been attributed to reactions from drugs such as hydralazine, procainamide, isoniazid, and phenytoin.

DRUG FEVER

Fever may occur in response to an inflammatory process or develop as a manifestation of a drug reaction. Drug fever occurs in as many as 10% of hospital inpatients.[16] A large number of drugs have been reported to cause fever, including methyldopa, procainamide, phenytoin, barbiturates, quinidine, and a variety of antibiotics. These drugs may affect the central nervous system directly to alter temperature regulation or stimulate the release of endogenous pyrogens (e.g.,

interleukin 1 and tumor necrosis factor) from white blood cells. Drugs also may cause fever as a result of their pharmacologic effects on tissues, e.g., fever resulting from massive tumor cell destruction caused by chemotherapy. However, the mechanism of drug fever remains unknown for agents such as amphotericin B and radiographic contrast agents.

The temperature pattern of drug-induced fever is quite variable and therefore of little help in the diagnosis. It may be low grade and continuous or spiking and intermittent. A temporal relationship between drug administration and occurrence of fever has been noted for some medications. Generally, withdrawal of the causative agent results in prompt defervescence as soon as the drug is eliminated completely. Fever usually recurs on readministration of the causative agent.

DRUG-INDUCED AUTOIMMUNITY

Autoimmune diseases have been associated with drugs and may involve a variety of tissues and organs. A commonly recognized drug-related autoimmune disorder is systemic lupus erythematosus (SLE) induced by procainamide, hydralazine, or isoniazid. Other drugs associated with SLE include methyldopa, β-adrenergic blockers, penicillamine, quinidine, interferon-γ, and sulfasalazine.[17] Exposure of susceptible persons to these agents appears to alter normal body proteins, RNA, or DNA in such a way as to make these components antigenic, leading to the formation of autoreactive antibodies and cells. The most common clinical manifestations include arthralgias, myalgias, and polyarthritis. Facial rash, ulcers, and alopecia occur less frequently. Renal or pulmonary involvement also may occur. These reactions typically develop several months after beginning the drug and generally resolve soon after it is discontinued.[18]

Other syndromes believed to involve autoimmune mechanisms include drug-induced hemolytic anemia owing to methyldopa, renal interstitial nephritis produced by methicillin, and hepatitis caused by phenytoin and halothane. Interstitial nephritis is characterized by fever, rash, and eosinophilia associated with proteinuria and hematuria. Hepatic damage due to drugs generally is manifested as either hepatocellular necrosis or cholestatic hepatitis. Drug-induced hepatitis has been associated with phenothiazines, sulfonamides, halothane, phenytoin, and isoniazid (see Chap. 38). Hepatocellular destruction is evidenced by elevations in serum transaminases. Hepatomegaly and jaundice sometimes may be evident. Cholestasis may be manifested by jaundice and elevations in serum alkaline phosphatase and sometimes by rash, fever, and eosinophilia.

VASCULITIS

Vasculitis is a clinicopathologic process characterized by inflammation and necrosis of blood vessels walls. The vasculitic process may be limited to the skin or may involve multiple organs, including the liver or kidney, joints, or central nervous system. Characteristically, cutaneous vasculitis is manifested by purpuric lesions that vary in size and number. Vasculitis also may be manifested as papules, nodules, ulcerations, or vesiculobullous lesions, generally occurring on the lower extremities, but the upper extremities, including the hands, also may be involved. Drugs associated with vasculitis include allopurinol, β-lactam antibiotics, sulfonamides, thiazide diuretics, and phenytoin.

DERMATOLOGIC REACTIONS

A wide variety of dermatologic drug reactions has been reported to have an immunologic basis (see Chap. 94).[4,19] As noted previously,

TABLE 86–2. Top 10 Drugs or Agents Reported to Cause Skin Reactions

	Reactions per 1000 Recipients
Amoxicillin	51.4
Trimethoprim-sulfamethoxazole	33.8
Ampicillin	33.2
Iopodate	27.8
Blood	21.6
Cephalosporins	21.1
Erythromycin	20.4
Dihydralazine hydrochloride	19.1
Penicillin G	18.5
Cyanocobalamin	17.9

Adapted from Ref. 19.

cutaneous reactions are the most common manifestations of allergic drug reactions. Although most dermatologic reactions are mild and resolve promptly after discontinuing the drug, some may progress to serious or even life-threatening reactions (e.g., toxic epidermal necrolysis or Stevens-Johnson syndrome). Stevens-Johnson syndrome is a serious dermatologic reaction characterized by blistering of the mucous membranes (mouth, eyes, vagina) with patchy rashes that can cover most of the body. Patients also may experience fever, headache, and cough. Toxic epidermal necrolysis is a syndrome similar to Stevens-Johnson syndrome characterized by blistering of skin and mucous membranes in response to administration of a drug. Large areas of skin may peel off.

Cutaneous adverse reactions were reported to occur in 2.7% of hospitalized patients.[20] Serious dermatologic drug reactions are estimated to occur in 1.9 cases per 1 million people per year and can have a mortality rate as high as 40%.[21,22] Table 86–2 lists drugs and agents associated most commonly with cutaneous reactions.[23] Antimicrobials are implicated most frequently with reaction rates ranging from 1% to 8%. In a report of almost 6000 children, about 12% developed rashes with cefaclor compared with 7.4% with penicillins and 8.5% with sulfonamides.[24]

RESPIRATORY REACTIONS

Drugs also may produce upper or lower respiratory tract reactions, including rhinitis and asthma. Respiratory tract manifestations may result from direct injury to the airways or may occur as a component of a systemic reaction (e.g., anaphylaxis). Asthma may be induced by aspirin and other NSAIDs or by sulfites used as preservatives in foods and medications. Other pulmonary drug reactions believed to be immunologic include acute infiltrative and chronic fibrotic pulmonary reactions. The latter is often caused by antineoplastic agents such as bleomycin. For a more detailed discussion of drug-induced pulmonary disease, see Chap. 29.

HEMATOLOGIC REACTIONS

Most formed elements and soluble components of the hematopoietic system may be affected by immunologic drug reactions. Eosinophilia is a common manifestation of drug hypersensitivity and may be the only presenting sign. Hemolytic anemia may result from hypersensitivity to drugs. Other hematologic reactions include thrombocytopenia, granulocytopenia, and agranulocytosis. For a detailed discussion of hematologic drug reactions, see Chap. 102.

FACTORS RELATED TO THE OCCURRENCE OR SEVERITY OF ALLERGIC DRUG REACTIONS

Among the factors that influence the likelihood of allergic drug reactions are the dose of the drug, how the drug is metabolized, and the degree to which the drug and metabolites bind to human proteins, the route of exposure, and the sensitivity of the individual as determined by age, genetics, and environmental factors. For many drugs, the severity of a reaction is determined by the dose and the duration of exposure. A relatively larger dose or longer duration of treatment encourages development of drug sensitivity. The route of administration also influences drug sensitivity. The topical route of drug administration appears to be the most likely to sensitize and predispose to drug reactions. The oral route is the safest, and the parenteral route is the most hazardous for administration of drugs in sensitive individuals. There are relatively few reported cases of immediate hypersensitivity-associated deaths with oral β-lactam antimicrobials. Although intravenous administration is more likely to result in severe immediate reactions in a sensitized individual, it may be the least likely route for initially inducing sensitivity. One possible explanation is that intravenous administration results in systemic drug exposure for the shortest period of time.

Individual host factors are also important in determining drug sensitivity. There may be a genetic predisposition for some types of allergic reactions. Slow acetylators of procainamide and hydralazine are at increased risk for SLE.

Drug allergies appear to develop with equal frequency in atopic and nonatopic individuals.[4] In addition, patients with a history of drug allergy appear to be at increased risk of adverse reactions to other pharmacologic agents. Age seems to be related to the risk of allergic reactions because they occur less frequently in children. This may be related to immaturity of the immune system or decreased exposure. The presence of some concurrent diseases predisposes to drug reactions. Examples include the morbilliform rash that occurs after ampicillin administration to patients with infectious mononucleosis and the reactions that occur with trimethoprim-sulfamethoxazole in AIDS patients.

DRUGS COMMONLY CAUSING ALLERGIC OR ALLERGIC-LIKE DRUG REACTIONS

β-LACTAM ANTIMICROBIALS

Allergic reactions to penicillin occur in 0.7% to 8% of treatment courses but was as high as 15% in one retrospective report of hospitalized patients treated with penicillin.[25,26] While most patients reporting penicillin allergy do not have allergy, a reported history is associated with a higher likelihood of positive skin test reactivity.[27] Only 10% to 20% of patients reporting penicillin allergy are found to be allergic by skin testing.[27]

The most common reactions to penicillin include urticaria, pruritus, and angioedema. All four of the major types of hypersensitivity reactions have been reported with penicillin, as well as some reactions that do not fit into these categories. A wide variety of idiopathic reactions occurs, e.g., maculopapular eruptions, eosinophilia, Stevens-Johnson syndrome, and exfoliative dermatitis. Cutaneous reactions can occur in up to 4.4% of treatment courses of penicillin[28] and in up to 8% with aminopenicillins.[29] The incidence of ampicillin rash is 69% to 100% in patients with Epstein-Barr virus infection, cytomegalovirus infection, or acute lymphocytic leukemia.[30]

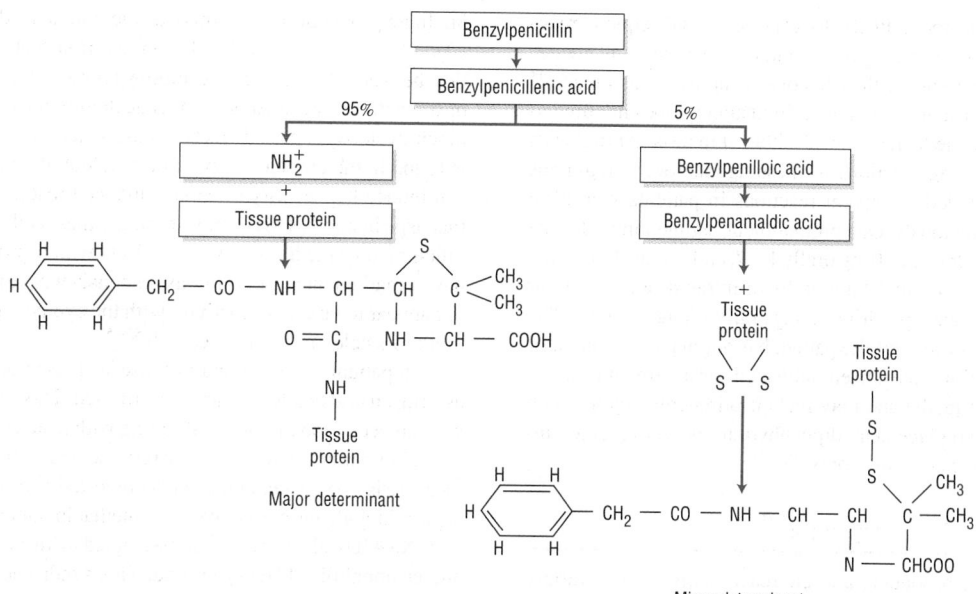

FIGURE 86–2. Formation of a benzyl penicilloyl hapten–protein complex.

Some aspects of the mechanism of penicillin immunogenicity have been determined. Because benzylpenicillin is a relatively small molecule (MW 356), it must combine with macromolecules (presumably proteins) to elicit an immune response. Penicillin may bind covalently to the lysine residues of proteins such as albumin through an amide linkage involving the β-lactam ring (Fig. 86–2). This is the penicilloyl-protein conjugate and is referred to as the *major antigenic determinant*. In addition, a number of other penicillin metabolites may bind covalently to proteins. These are referred to as *minor antigenic determinants*. The terms *major* and *minor* refer to the relative proportions of these conjugates that are formed and not to the clinical severity of the reactions generated. Immediate hypersensitivity reactions may be mediated by IgE for both minor and major determinants. In fact, the minor antigenic determinants are more likely to cause life-threatening anaphylactic reactions.

Patients who are allergic to penicillins also may be sensitive to other β-lactams.[31] The exact incidence of cross-reactivity between cephalosporins and penicillins is not known, although it is believed to be low. Patients who report penicillin allergy and are penicillin-skin-test-positive have an eightfold greater risk of allergic reaction to cephalosporins compared with patients not reporting penicillin allergy. In contrast, patients with reported penicillin allergy and negative skin test are at no greater risk.[32]

Most allergists would not administer cephalosporins to patients who had a history of hives or other immediate hypersensitivity reactions from penicillin, although some studies have suggested that there is little risk of an allergic response to a cephalosporin even in a person with a positive skin test to penicillin.[33–35] One post-marketing surveillance report states that there was no increase in allergic reactions to second- and third-generation cephalosporins in patients with histories of penicillin allergy.[36] Results of skin testing with cephalosporins are not reliable because the mechanism of cephalosporin sensitivity has not been clearly defined. A study from France has suggested that skin tests are predictive of hypersensitivity to a number of β-lactam antibiotics, but this study only performed oral challenges on skin-test-negative children.[35] At present, patients with positive penicillin skin tests are advised not to receive cephalosporins if they can be avoided. Patients who have negative penicillin skin tests

or experienced only mild cutaneous reactions, such as maculopapular rashes, may receive cephalosporins with caution.

Other β-lactam derivatives (e.g., monobactams and carbapenems) have been studied for potential cross-reactivity with penicillins. In vitro and in vivo studies have demonstrated that aztreonam only weakly cross-reacts with penicillin and that it may be administered safely to most patients who are penicillin-allergic.[37] In contrast, there is considerable cross-reactivity between imipenem (a carbapenem) and penicillin. Therefore, imipenem (and other carbapenems) should not be administered to patients who have positive penicillin skin tests.

RADIOCONTRAST MEDIA

Radiocontrast agents frequently cause allergic-like reactions because these agents are used commonly in medical practice and are administered as large, rapidly infused intravenous boluses. Fewer than 1% of patients receiving nonionic radiocontrast agents experience some type of adverse reaction.[38] Of the variety of reactions reported, approximately 90% are allergic-like, mostly urticarial, and severe reactions occur as infrequently as 0.02%. In addition, radiocontrast agents may cause dose-dependent toxic reactions that can produce cardiovascular effects, arrhythmias, changes in renal blood flow, diuresis, or proteinuria.[39,40] The older, high-osmolar agents that are now used less commonly have a greater frequency of reactions compared with the newer, low-osmolar agents.

The mechanism of reactions to radiocontrast agents is not clearly understood. Histamine release and mast cell triggering have been documented in severe immediate reactions, suggesting an IgE-mediated mechanism.[41] The older, high-osmolar radiocontrast agents can activate mast cells and basophils directly (IgE-independent mechanism), resulting in the release of inflammatory mediators.[42] The low-osmolar contrast agents appear to result in fewer anaphylactoid reactions. The adverse reaction rate for ionic iodinated contrast media was as high as 6% to 8%.[38] The relative risk of having a reaction to a lower-osmolarity, nonionic agent is estimated to be at least five times lower than with the ionic agents.[43]

Patients at risk of reactions to radiocontrast agents are difficult to identify. History is helpful because a patient who has experienced previous reactions is more likely to experience subsequent reactions. The risk of allergic reactions to radiocontrast media is greater in women and in patients with a history of atopy or asthma.[43,44] Despite a common misconception, a seafood allergy does not predispose to radiocontrast media reactions. Neither skin tests nor oral tests are useful for predicting reactions to these agents. Some regimens have been recommended to prevent reactions in patients who have experienced them previously. One pretreatment regimen includes the administration of prednisone 50 mg orally 13, 7, and 1 hours before the procedure; diphenhydramine 50 mg orally or intramuscularly 1 hour before the procedure; and ephedrine 25 mg orally 1 hour before.[45] The ephedrine should be omitted if the patient has angina, arrhythmia, or hypertension. Guidelines have been published for treatment of acute reactions to contrast media and may include adrenergic agents such as epinephrine, fluid replacement, diphenhydramine, H_2-receptor antagonist, and systemic corticosteroids.[40]

INSULIN

Insulin is capable of producing allergic reactions through a variety of immunologic mechanisms. A protein molecule, insulin is a complete antigen. Allergic reactions have been reported with beef, pork, and recombinant human insulin, although the frequency of reactions with human insulin appears low. Reactions to insulin may involve the insulin molecule itself or other substances that have been added to insulin (e.g., protamine). Most patients have anti-insulin IgG antibodies after a few months of therapy.

Insulin reactions may be limited to the site of injection, or they may produce systemic reactions. Local reactions present most often as a wheal and flare at the injection site and may occur immediately after injection or up to 8 to 12 hours later. Generally, these reactions are mild, do not require treatment, and resolve with continued insulin administration. If a patient does not tolerate the local reaction well, antihistamines may be given or a different insulin source (or product of higher purity) may be substituted. Rarely, systemic reactions to insulin (e.g., urticaria or anaphylaxis) occur. IgE-mediated reactions to insulin allergy appear to be declining with greater use of human insulins.[46] Skin testing with various products can aid in selecting the type of insulin least likely to cause a systemic reaction. Human insulin appears to be least allergenic but occasionally may cause reactions. In some patients, insulin desensitization may be indicated.

ASPIRIN AND NSAIDs

◀**7** Aspirin and other NSAIDs can produce two general types of reactions, urticaria/angioedema or rhinosinusitis/asthma, in susceptible patients.[47] Approximately 20% of asthmatics are sensitive to aspirin and other NSAIDs.[48,49]

The rhinosinusitis/asthma syndrome typically develops in middle-aged patients who are nonatopic and have no history of aspirin intolerance. Generally, it progresses from rhinitis to sinusitis with nasal polyps and steroid-dependent asthma. It is uncommon in children and young adults. However, children with asthma may be aspirin-sensitive. Aspirin-sensitive asthma appears to be an inherited disorder characterized by overexpression of LTC_4 synthase in airways.[50] In aspirin-sensitive asthmatics, administration of aspirin and NSAIDs may provoke severe and sometimes fatal asthmatic attacks. Ketorolac can cause severe, life-threatening bronchospasm in aspirin-sensitive asthmatics.[51] The mechanism of aspirin sensitivity is not completely understood. One suspected mechanism of aspirin and NSAID sensitivity is cyclooxygenase-1 blockade, which may

facilitate production of alternative arachidonic acid metabolites (e.g. LTs). This is supported by the observation that there is a correlation between the degree of cyclooxygenase-1 blockade and the risk of a reaction; thus agents such as acetaminophen, which minimally block cyclooxygenase-1, rarely cause reactions. Additional support is found in the clinical observation that leukotriene-modifying drugs can reduce the severity of aspirin-induced reactions.[49] It is possible that aspirin and NSAIDs may stimulate mast cells directly to release inflammatory mediators. Also, subjects with aspirin-induced asthma have a marked increase in airway responsiveness to LTs.[52] There does not appear to be cross-reactivity with the cyclooxygenase-2-selective inhibitors celecoxib and rofecoxib.[53-55]

In patients with asthma or those suspected of being sensitive to aspirin, an oral challenge can be performed. This should be performed with great caution in a hospital setting with resuscitation equipment at hand. For patients known to be aspirin-sensitive, the major preventive measure is avoidance. Other agents reported to be cross-reactive with aspirin include tartrazine dye, indomethacin, and phenylbutazone.

NSAIDs also have been associated with pulmonary infiltrates and eosinophilia (PIE) syndrome. This syndrome is associated with fever, cough, dyspnea, infiltrates on chest roentgenogram, and a peripheral eosinophilia that develop 2 to 6 weeks after initiating treatment. PIE syndrome occurs more frequently for naproxen compared with other NSAIDs and is noted to resolve rapidly after discontinuation of the offending agent.[56]

SULFONAMIDES

Sulfonamide drugs, including antimicrobials, diuretics, oral hypoglycemics, and carbonic anhydrase inhibitors, are a common cause of allergic reactions. Allergic reactions were recognized in 4.8% of 20,226 patients who received a sulfonamide antibiotic and in 2.0% of patients who received a nonantibiotic sulfonamide.[57] Although immediate IgE-mediated reactions such as anaphylaxis can occur, sulfonamides typically cause delayed cutaneous reactions, often beginning with fever and then followed by a rash (e.g., morbilliform eruptions, erythema multiforme, or less frequently, Stevens-Johnson syndrome/toxic epidermal necrolysis).[2] Other reactions to sulfonamides may include mucocutaneous, gastrointestinal, hepatic, renal, or hematologic complications, which may be fatal. Immune-mediated sulfonamide reactions involve the production of reactive metabolites (hydroxylamines).[58] Patients with the slow acetylator phenotype may be at increased risk of these reactions.[3]

While allergic reactions to sulfonamides can occur with a wide variety of chemical entities, there appears to be a low level of cross-reactivity between sulfonamide antibiotics and nonantibiotics (about 10%). The occurrence of allergic reactions after receipt of nonantibiotic sulfonamides may reflect a predisposition to allergic reactions rather than cross-reactivity with sulfonamide antibiotics.[57]

◀**8** Trimethoprim-sulfamethoxazole is used frequently for preventive or active treatment of *Pneumocystis carinii* pneumonia in patients with the AIDS. Adverse reactions to trimethoprim-sulfamethoxazole have been observed to occur much more frequently in these patients compared with those without AIDS. Adverse effects to trimethoprim-sulfamethoxazole occur in 50% to 80% of AIDS patients compared with 10% of other immunocompromised patients.[59] Trimethoprim-sulfamethoxazole was associated with an adverse-event rate of 26.3 per 100 person-years and hypersensitivity events at 22 per 100 person-years. Adverse-event rate was related to lower $CD4^+$ cell count. When the $CD4^+$ cell count was less than $100/mm^3$, the adverse drug event rate was 31 per 100 person-years.[60]

PHARMACEUTICAL EXCIPIENTS AND ADDITIVES

Pharmaceutical products contain a number of "inert" additives (e.g., dyes, fillers, buffers, and stabilizers) in addition to the therapeutic ingredients. These additives are not always inert and may cause adverse effects, including allergic reactions.

The azo dye tartrazine (FD&C Yellow No. 5) is associated with anaphylactoid reactions, acute bronchospasm, urticaria, rhinitis, and contact dermatitis.[61,62] Although the immunologic mechanisms are unclear, approximately 10% of aspirin-sensitive asthmatics are also intolerant to tartrazine,[63,64] suggesting a role for tartrazine as a cyclooxygenase inhibitor. As little as 0.85 mcg or as much as 25 mg tartrazine has provoked positive responses.[63]

Sulfites (including sulfur dioxide, sodium sulfite, sodium and potassium bisulfite, and sodium and potassium metabisulfite) are used commonly as antioxidants in pharmaceutical products and some foods. Over 250 cases of adverse reactions associated with ingestion of sulfites (usually in foods) have been reported to the Food and Drug Administration (FDA),[65] including wheezing, dyspnea, chest tightness, urticaria, angioedema, flushing, weakness, nausea, anaphylaxis, and death.

IgE-mediated and nonimmunologic sulfite hypersensitivity has been demonstrated in children with a history of chronic asthma. Adverse reactions to sulfite-preserved injectables, such as gentamicin, metoclopramide, lidocaine, and doxycycline, have been reported. In contrast to reactions caused by foods, these reactions do not occur more frequently in steroid-dependent asthmatics and do not always coincide with a positive oral sulfite challenge.[65,66] Blunted bronchodilation may be observed in asthmatics following inhalation of sulfite-containing nebulizer solutions. Although many nebulizer solutions contain sulfites, metered-dose inhalers do not. Many aqueous epinephrine products also contain sulfites. The FDA labeling states that in emergency situations when sulfite-free preparations are not available, sulfite-containing epinephrine should not be withheld from a sulfite-intolerant individual because small subcutaneous doses of sulfites usually are well tolerated. However, an increased risk of anaphylaxis exists after subcutaneous injection in rare patients with a positive oral challenge to 5 to 10 mg sulfite.

Parabens (including methyl-, ethyl-, propyl-, and butylparaben) are used widely in pharmaceutical products as a biocidal agent. The majority of allergic reactions to parabens are observed after topical exposure.[67] Delayed hypersensitivity contact dermatitis occurs more often in individuals with preexisting dermatitis.[63] Immediate hypersensitivity after parenteral administration is rare. Although these agents are chemically related to benzoic acid and *p*-aminobenzoic acid, the evidence for cross-sensitivity is lacking.[63]

CANCER CHEMOTHERAPY AGENTS

Chemotherapy agents are implicated in hypersensitivity reactions in 5% to 15% of patients who receive them.[68] Up to 65% of patients receiving L-asparaginase experience immediate hypersensitivity reactions such as urticaria and anaphylaxis.[69]

The combination regimen of paclitaxel (or docetaxel) and carboplatin frequently is responsible for producing hypersensitivity reactions. Each agent precipitates a distinct reaction, allowing for differentiation between causative factors. Hypersensitivity reactions have been observed with paclitaxel and docetaxel as frequently as 34% of patients.[2,70,71] The reaction, typically occurring shortly after initiation of the first dose, is due to Cremophor EL, the polyoxyethylated castor oil vehicle for paclitaxel. Severe reactions are characterized by dyspnea, bronchospasm, urticaria, and hypotension. Minor reactions include flushing and rashes. In patients receiving a 3-hour infusion, the incidence of severe reactions is reduced to 1.3%, and the incidence of minor reactions is 42%.[72] To reduce the risk of hypersensitivity reaction, patients are routinely premedicated with corticosteroids and H_1- and H_2-receptor antagonists. Carboplatin hypersensitivity develops after six or more courses of carboplatin or its parent compound, cisplatin.[73] Reactions typically develop shortly after completing the infusion or up to 3 days after therapy.[74] Symptoms of severe reaction include tachycardia, dyspnea, facial swelling, rigors, and hypotension. Mild reactions include itching, erythema, and facial flushing. Desensitization with carboplatin usually is not successful owing to previous prolonged exposure. Skin testing is useful because a negative test has a high predictive value for nonreactivity.[75]

ANTICONVULSANTS

Many anticonvulsant drugs produce a variety of hypersensitivity reactions and pseudoallergic reactions. Drugs such as phenytoin, phenobarbital, carbamazepine, and lamotrigine can cause a "anticonvulsant hypersensitivity syndrome" characterized by fever, rash, lymphadenopathy, and internal organ involvement. Eosinophilia is frequently present. The onset is usually several weeks into therapy.[2,76] In some cases, morbilliform rash develops in exfoliative dermatitis. Concomitant use of valproate significantly increases the risk of hypersensitivity owing to reduced lamotrigine metabolism, leading to a prolonged elimination half-life.[77]

▶ TREATMENT: Allergic Reactions

9 The basic principles for management of allergic reactions to drugs or biologic agents include (1) discontinuation of the medication or agent when possible, (2) treatment of the adverse clinical signs and symptoms, and (3) substitution, if necessary, of another agent.[1]

Identification of patients at high risk for allergic drug reactions requires a careful history and, where appropriate, performance of specific tests to evaluate sensitivity.[78] One of the most helpful tests to evaluate risk is the allergen skin test. For some drugs, skin testing can demonstrate the presence of drug-specific IgE and predict a relatively high risk of immediate hypersensitivity reactions. Note that skin testing does not predict the risk of delayed or most dermatologic reactions.

A higher proportion of patients report an "allergic reaction" to penicillin than actually experience a reaction. However, patients with a history of penicillin allergy are recognized to have a four- to sixfold greater risk of subsequent reactions.[25] In addition, a negative history of penicillin allergy does not eliminate the risk of immediate reactions because many serious and even fatal allergic reactions to β-lactam antibiotics occur in patients who have no history of penicillin allergy.[25]

10 Skin testing can reduce the uncertainty of penicillin sensitivity and should be performed in all patients who have a history of penicillin allergy and require treatment with these agents. Penicillin skin testing in advance of need for penicillin treatment in patients with a history of penicillin allergy does not appear to induce sensitization.[79] Testing for the major penicillin determinant is accomplished with

TABLE 86–3. Procedure for Performing Penicillin Skin Testing

A. Percutaneous (prick) skin testing

Materials	Volume
Pre-Pen 6×10^6M	1 drop
Penicillin G 10,000 U/mL	1 drop
β-Lactam drug 3 mg/mL	1 drop
0.03% albumin-saline control	1 drop
Histamine control (1 mg/mL)	1 drop

1. Place a drop of each test material on the volar surface of the forearm.
2. Prick the skin with a sharp needle inserted through the drop at a 45° angle gently tenting the skin in an upward motion.
3. Interpret skin responses after 15 minutes.
4. A wheal at least 2 × 2 mm with erythema is considered positive.
5. If the prick test is nonreactive, proceed to the intradermal test.
6. If the histamine control is nonreactive, the test is considered uninterpretable.

B. Intradermal skin testing

Materials	Volume
Pre-Pen 6×10^6M	0.02 mL
Penicillin G 10,000 U/mL	0.02 mL
β-Lactam drug 3 mg/mL	0.02 mL
0.03% albumin-saline control	0.02 mL
Histamine control (0.1 mg/mL)	0.02 mL

1. Inject 0.02–0.03 mL of each test material intradermally (amount sufficient to produce a small bleb).
2. Interpret skin responses after 15 minutes.
3. A wheal at least 6 × 6 mm with erythema and at least 3 mm greater than the negative control is considered positive.
4. If the histamine control is nonreactive, the test is considered uninterpretable.

Antihistamines may blunt the response and cause false-negative reactions.

From Sullivan TJ. Current Therapy in Allergy. St Louis, Mosby, 1985:57–61.

penicilloyl-polylysine (PPL; Pre-Pen). If this agent is used alone, patients reacting only to minor determinants will be missed. At present, there is no commercially available product that can be used to test for most of the minor determinants. Benzylpenicillin (at a concentration of 10,000 units/mL) has been used; however, some reactive patients still will be missed. Penicillin skin testing can facilitate the safe use of penicillin in 90% of patients with a history of penicillin allergy.[80] Even in patients who report a history of penicillin allergy, if they are skin-test-negative, penicillin treatment does not appear to cause resensitization.[81] The procedure for performing penicillin skin testing is presented in Table 86–3.

The National Institute of Allergy and Infectious Diseases reported a collaborative trial to test the predictive value of skin testing with major and minor penicillin derivatives.[82] The frequency of IgE-mediated reactions to penicillin was 1.2% and 0% in patients with a positive and negative history of penicillin allergy, respectively, in subjects who were skin-test-negative. Of skin-test-positive patients who received penicillin, 22% experienced immediate or accelerated penicillin allergy. Of skin test-positive patients, 84% had dermal reactions to skin testing with the major determinant (benzylpenicilloyl-octalysine), whereas 16% reacted only to an experimental minor determinant mixture of benzylpenicillin, benzylpenicilloate, and benzylpenicilloyl-N-propylamine.

Immediate hypersensitivity reactions to penicillin are rare after a properly performed negative skin test when both major and minor determinants are used. Dermatologic reactions occur in 1% of skin-test-negative patients.[25] A negative penicillin skin test indicates

that the risk of life-threatening reactions is extremely low with administration of penicillin or other β-lactams. Occasionally, patients may experience systemic reactions after skin testing. Also, certain types of patients (e.g., those with dermatographism or taking antihistamines) may be unsuitable for skin testing because a false-positive or false-negative test may result. Penicillin is the only drug for which the predictive value of skin testing has been well established. The value of skin testing for evaluating the risk of adverse reactions to other drugs is largely unknown, but these tests are recommended in selected patients with histories of immediate reactions to nonpenicillin antibiotics.[81]

ANAPHYLAXIS

Anaphylaxis requires prompt treatment to minimize the risk of serious morbidity or death. On presentation, attention should be given first to stopping the likely offending agent, if possible, and restoring respiratory and cardiovascular function. A protocol for the treatment of anaphylaxis is presented in Table 86–4. Epinephrine is administered as primary treatment to counteract bronchoconstriction and vasodilatation. Epinephrine should be administered intramuscularly in the lateral aspect of the thigh.[83] If blood pressure is not restored by epinephrine, crystalloids should be administered intravenously to restore intravascular volume. Typically, 1 L of 0.9% sodium chloride or lactated Ringer's solution will be administered over 10 to 15 minutes. This may be repeated if the patient is still believed to be volume-depleted. Intravenous fluids should be given early in the course in an attempt to prevent shock. A maintenance intravenous fluid then will be initiated. An immediate priority is establishment and maintenance of an airway. This should be achieved by the use of endotracheal intubation if necessary. When a patient with anaphylaxis is hypotensive, vasopressors also will be needed in addition to crystalloids. Norepinephrine is the vasoconstrictor agent of choice for treatment of anaphylactic shock, although dopamine also may be useful.

A number of other agents may be required for the treatment of anaphylactic reactions. Corticosteroids (hydrocortisone sodium succinate intravenously) are recommended to reduce the risk of late phase reactions. Aminophylline may be used as adjunctive therapy for bronchospasm. Histamine (H_1) receptor blockers (such as diphenhydramine) may be administered to reduce some of the symptoms associated with anaphylaxis; however, these agents are not effective as primary therapy.

DESENSITIZATION

For some patients allergic to penicillin, no reasonable alternatives exist, and penicillin therapy may be necessary for treatment of severe life-threatening infection. In this situation, penicillin desensitization should be considered. Desensitization can reduce the risk of anaphylaxis but does not influence the likelihood of other types of reactions such as exfoliative dermatitis or Stevens-Johnson syndrome.

Penicillin desensitization should be performed in a hospital setting where resuscitation equipment is readily available by a physician experienced in the risks and management of severe allergic reactions. The potential risks and benefits should be discussed with the patient. Prior to initiating the protocol, the patient should be stabilized and fluid, pulmonary, and cardiovascular function optimized. The use of

TABLE 86–4. Treatment of Anaphylaxis

1. Place patient in recumbent position and elevate extremities.
2. Monitor vital signs often (or continuously if possible).
3. Apply tourniquet proximal to site of antigen injection; remove every 10–15 min.
4. Administer epinephrine 1:1000 into nonoccluded site: 0.3–0.5 mL subcutaneously or intramuscularly in adults and 0.01 mL/kg subcutaneously or intramuscularly in children.
5. Administer aqueous epinephrine 1:1000 into site of antigen injection; 0.15–0.25 mL subcutaneously in adults and 0.005 mL/kg subcutaneously in children.
6. Establish and maintain airway with oropharyngeal airway device, endotracheal intubation, transtracheal catheterization, or cricothyrotomy.
7. Administer oxygen at 6–10 L/min.
8. Institute rapid fluid replacement with 0.9% sodium chloride, lactated Ringer's, or colloid solution (e.g., 5% albumin or 4% hetastarch).
9. For hypotension in adults, administer norepinephrine, 32 mcg/min (use 8 mg in 500 mL dextrose 5%) with the rate adjusted to maintain low-normal blood pressure. Alternatively, administer dopamine at 2–10 mcg/kg/min intravenously.
10. If refractory hypotension is present, administer cimetidine 300 mg or ranitidine 50 mg, intravenously over 3–5 min.
11. If bronchospasm is present, administer aminophylline 6 mg/kg intravenously over 20 min.
12. Administer hydrocortisone sodium succinate 100 mg intravenously (push) and 100 mg intravenously in saline every 2–4 h to block the late-phase reaction.
13. Administer diphenhydramine 1–2 mg/kg intravenously (up to 50 mg) over 3 min to block histamine-1 receptors.
14. For adults taking a β-adrenergic blocker, administer atropine (0.5 mg intravenously) every 5 min until heart rate is greater than 60 beats/min, or isoproterenol 2–20 mcg/min intravenously titrated to heart rate of 60 beats/min, or glucagon 0.5 mg/kg intravenously (push) followed by 0.07 mg/ kg/h continuously intravenously.

From Weiss ME, Adkinson NF, Clin Allergy 1988;18:515–540.

premedicants (antihistamines or corticosteroids) is controversial because these agents may mask the early signs of acute reactions and do not reliably reduce the severity of acute reactions. About one-third of patients who have undergone desensitization experience mild, transient allergic reaction either during the desensitization procedure or during penicillin therapy.[25] Patients who can take oral medication should undergo desensitization with oral penicillin. Protocols for oral and intravenous penicillin desensitization are presented in Tables 86–5 and 86–6. It is important that once the desensitization protocol is begun it not be interrupted except for severe reactions. Antihistamines

or epinephrine may be administered to treat reactions. In addition, if the patient completes the desensitization regimen and then undergoes penicillin treatment, a lapse between doses of as little as 24 hours can allow for reemergence of sensitivity.

Desensitization of trimethoprim-sulfamethoxazole can be achieved within 2 days in most AIDS patients.[2,84] This can be accompanied by use of the following schedule of doses (milligrams of sulfamethoxazole-trimethoprim): day 1: 9 A.M., 4 and 0.8 mg; 11 A.M., 8 and 1.6 mg; 1 P.M., 20 and 4 mg; 5 P.M., 40 and 8 mg; day 2:9 A.M., 80 and 16 mg; 3 P.M., 160 and 32 mg; 9 P.M., 200 and 40 mg; day 3:9 A.M.,

TABLE 86–5. Protocol for Oral Desensitization

| Step[a] | Phenoxymethyl Penicillin | | | |
	Concentration (units/mL)	Volume (mL)	Dose (units)	Cumulative Dose (units)
1	1000	0.1	100	100
2	1000	0.2	200	300
3	1000	0.4	400	700
4	1000	0.8	800	1500
5	1000	1.6	1600	3100
6	1000	3.2	3200	6300
7	1000	6.4	6400	12,700
8	10,000	1.2	12,000	24,700
9	10,000	2.4	24,000	48,700
10	10,000	4.8	48,000	96,700
11	80,000	1.0	80,000	176,700
12	80,000	2.0	160,000	336,700
13	80,000	4.0	320,000	656,700
14	80,000	8.0	640,000	1,296,700
Observe for 30 min				
15	500,000	0.25	125,000	
16	500,000	0.5	250,000	
17	500,000	1.0	500,000	
18	500,000	2.25	1,125,000	

[a]The interval between steps is 15 min.
From Ref. 78.

TABLE 86–6. Parenteral Desensitization Protocol

Injection No.	Benzylpenicillin Concentration (units)	Volume (mL)	(Route)
1[a,b]	100	0.1	ID
2	100	0.2	SC
3	100	0.4	SC
4	100	0.8	SC
5[b]	1000	0.1	ID
6	1000	0.3	SC
7	1000	0.6	SC
8[b]	10,000	0.1	ID
9	10,000	0.2	SC
10	10,000	0.4	SC
11	10,000	0.8	SC
12[b]	100,000	0.1	ID
13	100,000	0.3	SC
14	100,000	0.6	SC
15[b]	1,000,000	0.1	ID
16	1,000,000	0.2	SC
17	1,000,000	0.2	IM
18	1,000,000	0.4	IM
19	Continuous IV infusion at 1,000,000 U/h		

[a]Administer doses at intervals of not less than 20 min.
[b]Observe and record skin wheal-and-flare response.
From Ref. 78.

400 and 80 mg, and 400 and 80 mg daily thereafter. Other investigators have described a 6-hour graded challenge in HIV-infected patients.[85]

Skin tests often become negative during and shortly after desensitization. The mechanism by which desensitization is protective is unclear. It does not seem to be that penicillin-specific IgE is neutralized or that IgG as "blocking antibody" is produced. One possible explanation is that basophils and mast cells attain some degree of tolerance on exposure to the antigen.

ABBREVIATIONS

IgE: immunoglobulin E
LT: leukotriene
PAF: platelet activating factor
PG: prostaglandin
PIE: pulmonary infiltrates and eosinophilia
SLE: systemic lupus erythematosus

Review Questions and other resources can be found at *www.pharmacotherapyonline.com.*

REFERENCES

1. Anderson JA. Allergic reactions to drugs and biologic agents. JAMA 1992; 268:2845–2857.
2. Gruchalla RS. Drug allergy. J Allerg Clin Immunol 2003;111:S548–559.
3. Svensson CK, Cowen EW, Gaspari AA. Cutaneous drug reactions. Pharmacol Rev 2000;53:357–379.
4. Borish L, Tilles SA. Immune mechanisms of drug allergy. Immunol Clin North Am 1998;18:717–729.
5. DeSwarte RD. Drug allergy. In: Patterson R, ed. Allergic Diseases, 4th ed. Philadelphia, Lippincott, 1993.
6. Roitt I, Brastoff J, Male D. Immunology, 4th ed. London, Mosby, 1996.
7. Anonymous. Disease management of drug hypersensitivity: A practical approach. Ann Allerg Asthma Immunol 1999;83:665–700.
8. Schwartz LB, Austen KF. The mast cell and mediators of immediate hypersensitivity. In: Samter M, Talmage DW, Frank MM, et al, eds. Immunologic Diseases, 5th ed. Boston, Little, Brown, 1995.
9. MacGlashan D. Histamine: A mediator of inflammation. J Allerg Clin Immunol 2003;112:S53–59. [Winbery SL, Lieberman PL. Histamine and antihistamines in anaphylaxis. Clin Allergy Immunol. 2002;17:287–317.]
10. Solensky R, Mendelson LM. Systemic reactions to antibiotics. Immunol Allergy Clin North Am. 2001;21:679–697.
11. Pichler WJ. Delayed drug hypersensitivity reactions. Ann Intern Med. 2003;139:683–693.
12. Bochner BS, Lichtenstein LM. Anaphylaxis. New Engl J Med 1991;324: 1785–1790.
13. Matasar MJ, Neugut AI. Epidemiology of asthma. Curr Allerg Asthma Reports 2003;3:30–35.
14. Neuqut AI, Ghatak AT, Miller RL. Anaphylaxis in the United States: An investigation into its epidemiology. Ann Intern Med 2001;161:15–21.
15. Kemp SF, Lockey RF, Wolf BL, Lieberman P. Anaphylaxis: A review of 266 cases. Arch Intern Med 1995;155:1749–1754.
16. Johnson DH, Cuhna BA. Drug fever. Infect Dis Clin North Am 1996; 10:85–91.
17. Prince EJ, Venables PJ. Drug-induced lupus. Drug Saf 1995;12:283–290.
18. Rich MW. Drug-induced lupus: The list of culprits grows. Postgrad Med 1996;100:299–302.
19. Roujeau JC, Stern RS. Severe adverse cutaneous reactions to drugs. New Engl J Med 1994;331:1272–1285.
20. Hunziker T, Kunzi U, Braunschweig S, et al. Comprehensive hospital drug monitoring: Adverse drug reactions—A 20-year survey. Allergy 1997; 52:388–393.
21. Mockenhaupt M, Schopf E. Epidemiology of drug-induced severe skin reactions. Semin Cutan Med Surg 1996;15:236–243.
22. Stern RS, Steinberg LA. Epidemiology of adverse cutaneous reactions to drugs. Dermatoepidemiology 1995;13:681–688.
23. Bigby M. Rates of cutaneous reactions to drugs. 2001;137:765–770.
24. Ibia EO, Schwartz RH, Wiederman BL. Antibiotic rashes in children: A survey in a private practice setting. Arch Dermatol 2000;136:849–854.
25. Weiss ME, Adkinson NF. Immediate hypersensitivity reactions to penicillin and related antibiotics. Clin Allergy 1988;18:515–540.
26. Lee CE, Zembower TR, Fotis MA, et al. The incidence of antimicrobial allergies in hospitalized patients. Arch Intern Med 2000;160:2819–2822.
27. Salkind AR, Cuddy PG, Foxworth JW. Is this patient allergic to penicillin? An evidence-based analysis of the likelihood of penicillin allergy. JAMA 2001;285:2498–2505.
28. Hunziker T, Kunzi UP, Braunschweig S, et al. Comprehensive hospital drug monitoring (CHDM): Adverse skin reactions, a 20-year survey. Allergy 1997;52:388–393.
29. Bigby M. Rates of cutaneous reactions to drugs. Arch Dermatol 2001;137 765–770.
30. Weiss ME. Drug allergy. Clin Allergy 1992;76:857–882.
31. Baldo BA. Penicillins and cephalosporins as allergens: Structural aspects of recognition and cross-reactions. Clin Exp Allergy 1999;29:744–749.
32. Kelkar PS, Lu JT. Cephalosporin allergy. New Engl J Med 2001;345 804–809.
33. Anne S, Reisman RE. Risk of administering cephalosporin antibiotics to patients with histories of penicillin allergy. Ann Allergy Asthma Immunol 1995;74:167–170.
34. Wickern GM, Nish WA, Bitner AS, Freeman TM. Allergy to β-lactams A survey of current practices. J Allerg Clin Immunol 1994;94:725–731.
35. Ponvert C, Le Clainche L, de Blic J, et al. Allergy to β-lactam antibiotics in children. Pediatrics 1999;104:45.
36. Anne S, Reisman RE. Risk of administering cephalosporin antibiotics to patients with histories of penicillin allergy. Ann Allergy Asthma Immunol 1995;74:167–170.
37. Kishiyama JL, Adelman DC. The cross-reactivity of β-lactam antibiotics. Drug Saf 1994;10:318–327.
38. Cochran ST, Bomyea K, Sayre JW. Trends in adverse events after intravenous administration of contrast media. AJR 2002;178:765–766.
39. Bush WH, Swanson DP. Acute reactions to intravascular contrast media: Types, risk factors, recognition, and specific treatment. AJR 1991;157:1153–1161.
40. Lang DM, Alpeen MB, Visitainer PF, et al. Gender risk for anaphylactoid reaction to radiographic contrast media. J Allergy Clin Immunol 1995;95:813.
41. Laroche D, Aimone-Gastin I, Dubois F, et al. Mechanisms of severe, immediate reactions to iodinated contrast material. Radiology 1998;209: 183–190.
42. Greenberger PA, Patterson R. The prevention of immediate generalized reactions to radiocontrast media in high-risk patients. J Allergy Clin Immunol 1991;87:867–872.
43. Murphy KJ, Brunberg JA, Cohan RH. Adverse reactions to gadolinium contrast media. AJR 1996;167:847–849.
44. Marshall GD, Lieberman PL. Anaphylactoid reactions to radiocontrast agents. Immunol Allergy Clin North Am 1998;18:799–807.
45. Cohan RH, Leder RA, Ellis JH. Treatment of adverse reactions to radiographic contrast media in adults. Radiol Clin North Am 1996;34: 1055–1076.
46. Patterson R, Roberts M, Grammer LC. Insulin allergy: Reevaluation after two decades. Ann Allergy 1990;64:459–462.
47. Samter M, Stevenson DD. Reactions to aspirin and aspirin-like drugs. In: Samter M, Talmage DW, Frank MM, et al, eds. Immunologic Diseases, 5th ed. Boston, Little, Brown, 1995.
48. Babu KS, Salvi SS. Aspirin and asthma. Chest. 2000;118:1470–1466.
49. Stevenson DD, Simon RA, Zuraw BL. Sensitivity to aspirin and nonsteroidal anti-inflammatory drugs. In: Adkinson NF Jr, Yunginger JW, Busse WW, et al, eds. Allergy: Principles and Practice, Vol 2, 6th ed. 2003: 1695–1710.

50. Sanak M, Szczeklik. Genetics of aspirin induced asthma. Thorax 2000; 55(suppl 2):S45–47.

51. Vicks SD, Dean JR, Tenholder MF. Ketorolac-induced respiratory failure in an aspirin-sensitive asthmatic. Immunol Allergy Pract 1991;13:23–25.

52. Lee TH. Mechanisms of aspirin sensitivity. Am Rev Respir Dis 1992;145: S34–36.

53. Stevenson DD, Simon RA. Lack of cross-reactivity between rofecoxib and aspirin in aspirin-sensitive patients with asthma. J Allergy Clin Immunol 2001;108:47–51.

54. Woessner KM, Simon RA, Stevenson DD. The safety of celecoxib in patients with aspirin-sensitive asthma. Arthritis Rhematism. 2002;46: 2201–2206.

55. Gyllfors P, Bochenek G, Overholt J, et al. Biochemical and clinical evidence that aspirin-intolerant asthmatic subjects tolerate the cyclo-oxygenase 2-selective analgesic celecoxib. J Allerg Clin Immunol 2003; 111:1116–1121.

56. Goodwin SD, Glenny RW. Nonsteroidal anti-inflammatory drug–associated pulmonary infiltrates with eosinophilia. Arch Intern Med 1992; 152:1521–1524.

57. Strom BL, Schinnar R, Apter AJ, et al. Absense of cross-reactivity between sulfonamide antibiotics and sulfonamide nonantibiotics. New Engl J Med. 2003;349:1628–635.

58. Reider MJ, Uetrecht J, Shear NH, et al. Diagnosis of sulfonamide hy-persensitivity reactions by in vitro "rechallenge" with hydroxylamine metabolites. Ann Intern Med 1989;110:286–289.

59. Santomauro JT, Stover DE. Pneumocystis carinii pneumonia. Med Clin North Am 1997;81:299–318.

60. Moore RD, Fortgang I, Keruly J, Chaisson RE. Adverse events from drug therapy for human immunodeficiency virus disease. Am J Med 1996;101: 34–40.

61. Bhatia MS. Allergy to tartrazine in psychotropic drugs. J Clin Psychiatry 2000;61:473–476.

62. Ardern KD, Ram FS. Tartrazine exclusion for allergic asthma. Cochrane Database of Systemic Reviews 2001;4:CD000460.

63. American Academy of Pediatrics Committee on Drugs. "Inactive" ingre-dients in pharmaceutical products. Pediatrics 1985;76:635–642.

64. Stevenson DD, Simon RA. Sensitivity to ingested metabisulfites in asth-matic subjects. J Allergy Clin Immunol 1981;68:26–32.

65. Smolinski SC. Review of parenteral sulfide reactions. J Toxicol Clin Toxicol 1992;30:597–606.

66. Campbell JR, Maestrello CL, Campbell RL. Allergic responses to metabisulfite in lidocaine anesthetic solution. Anesth Prog 2001;48: 21–26.

67. Mowad CM. Allergic contact dermatitis caused by parabens: Two case reports and a review. Am J Contact Dermatitis 2000;11:53–56.

68. Weiss RB. Hypersensitivity reactions. Semin Oncol 1992;19:458–477.

69. Koppel RA, Boh EE. Cutaneous reactions to chemotherapeutic agents. Am J Med Sci 2001;321:327–335.

70. Markman M, Kennedy A, Webster K, et al. Combination chemotherapy with carboplatin and docetaxel in the treatment of cancers of the ovary and fallopian tube and primary carcinoma of the peritoneum. J Clin Oncol 2001;19:1901–1905.

71. Bookman MA, Kloth DD, Kover PE, et al. Intravenous prophylaxis for paclitaxel-related hypersensitivity reactions. Semin Oncol 1997;24: S19-13–19-15.

72. Eisenhauer EA, ten Bokkel Huinink WW, Swenerton KD, et al. European-Canadian randomized trial of paclitaxel in relapsed ovarian cancer: High-dose versus low-dose and long versus short infusion. J Clin Oncol 1994; 12:2654–2666.

73. Hendrick AM, Simmons D, Cantwell BMJ. Allergic reactions to carbo-platin. Ann Oncol 1992;3:239–240.

74. Markman M, Kennedy A, Webster K, et al. Clinical features of hy-persensitivity reactions to carboplatin. J Clin Oncol 1999;17:1141–1145.

75. Zanotti K, Rybicki L, Kennedy A, et al. Carboplatin skin testing: A skin-testing protocol for predicting hypersensitivity to carboplatin chemother-apy. J Clin Oncol 2001;19:3126–3129.

76. Sullivan JR, Shear NH. The drug hypersensitivity syndrome: What is the pathogenesis? Arch Dermatol 2001;137:357–364.

77. Schlienger RG, Knowles SR, Shear NH. Lamotrigine-associated anticonvulsant hypersensitivity syndrome. Neurology 1998;51:1172–1175.

78. Weiss ME, Adkinson NF. Diagnostic testing for drug hypersensitivity. Immunol Allerg Clin North Am 1998;18:731–734.

79. Macy E, Mangat R, Burchetts RJ. Penicillin skin testing in advance of need: Multiyear follow-up in 568 test result-negative subjects exposed to oral penicillins. J Allerg Clin Immunol 2003;111:1111–1115.

80. Gadde J, Spence M, Wheeler B, Adkinson NF. Clinical experience with penicillin skin testing in a large inner-city STD clinic. JAMA 1993;270:2456–2463.

81. Solensky R, Earl HS, Gruchalla RS. Lack of penicillin resensitization in patients with a history of penicillin allergy after receiving repeated penicillin courses. Arch Intern Med 2002;162:822–826.

82. Sogn DD, Evans R, Shepherd GM, et al. Results of the National Institute of Allergy and Infectious Diseases collaborative clinical trial to test the predictive value of skin testing with major and minor penicillin derivatives in hospitalized patients. Arch Intern Med 1992;152:1025–1032.

83. Lieberman P. Use of epinephrine in the treatment of anaphylaxis. Curr Opin Allerg Clin Immunol 2003;3:313–318.

84. Caumes E, Guermonprez G, Lecomte C, et al. Efficacy and safety of desen-sitization with sulfamethoxazole and trimethoprim in 48 previously hy-persensitive patients infected with human immunodeficiency virus. Arch Dermatol 1997;133:465–469.

85. Demoly P, Messaad D, Sahla H, et al. Six-hour trimethoprim-sulfamethoxazole-graded challenge in HIV-infected patients. J Allerg Clin Immunol 1998;102:1033–1036.

87

SOLID-ORGAN TRANSPLANTATION

Heather J. Johnson and Kristine S. Schonder

Learning Objectives and other resources can be found at *www.pharmacotherapyonline.com.*

KEY CONCEPTS

❶ T cells are the primary component of the immune system responsible for acute allograft rejection. The activity of T cells in acute rejection is mediated, to a large degree, by interleukin 2 (IL-2).

❷ Immunosuppressive protocols use a multidrug approach to target various levels of the immune cascade to prevent allograft rejection.

❸ The goals of immunosuppression are to decrease the incidence of acute and chronic rejection while minimizing adverse events associated with immunosuppressive medications.

❹ Calcineurin inhibitors (CIs), such as cyclosporine and tacrolimus, block T-cell activity by inhibiting the production of IL-2. They are associated with significant adverse effects, namely, nephrotoxicity and neurotoxicity.

❺ CI-induced nephrotoxicity often manifests clinically in the same manner as acute or chronic rejection. A biopsy is the definitive diagnostic tool.

❻ Glucocorticoids inhibit the initial steps in allograft rejection. They also aid in reversing the clinical symptoms associated with rejection.

❼ Antiproliferative agents such as azathioprine and mycophenolate mofetil inhibit T-cell proliferation by altering purine synthesis to prevent acute rejection. Bone marrow suppression is the most significant adverse effect associated with these agents.

❽ Sirolimus exerts its activity by inhibiting T-cell response to IL-2. The adverse effects associated with sirolimus include thrombocytopenia, anemia, and hyperlipidemia.

❾ Antibody preparations target specific receptors on the surface of T cells. The effect on T cells and adverse effects depend on the receptor targets.

❿ Long-term allograft and patient survival is limited by chronic rejection, cardiovascular disease, and long-term immunosuppressive complications, such as malignancy.

Solid-organ transplantation provides a lifesaving treatment for patients with end-stage cardiac, kidney, liver, lung, and intestinal disease. In 2003, 25,463 transplants were performed. Of these, the most common were kidney (8667 cadaveric donors, 6468 living donors), liver (5348 cadaveric donors, 322 living donors), and heart (2056).[1] Despite the demand for transplantation, the number of cadaveric donors has remained relatively stable during the past decade. In 2004, almost 87,000 persons in the United States were waiting for transplantation (kidney > 60,000; liver > 17,000; heart > 3200). Median waiting time for a cadaveric kidney is over 3 years. For liver transplantation the median time to transplant is over 2 years, whereas for heart transplantation it is approximately 6 months. For both heart and liver transplantation, clinical status is an important factor affecting waiting times, with the sickest patients receiving priority for available organs.

In order to increase the number of organs available for transplantation, several strategies have been employed. The use of living donors for renal transplantation represents almost half of all kidney transplants. Between 1998 and 2001, the number of living liver transplants increased over 700%. Efforts to expand the cadaveric donor pool include relaxation of age restrictions, development of better preservations solutions, use of "marginal" and non-heart beating donors, and the use of split livers. Procurement of donor hearts with longer ischemic times, those with borderline left ventricular function, and even those with mild coronary artery disease amenable to bypass grafting

have all been considered in an effort to increase the supply.[2] The use of heart donors older than 45 years of age is associated with a higher risk for 1-year mortality, but this must be viewed in the context of the higher risk of death with longer time on the waiting list if only younger donors are used.[1]

Despite all these efforts, patients continue to die awaiting transplant. In 2001, over 6000 people died on transplant waiting lists. While renal dialysis may be used for an extended period of time to partially replace the function of the kidneys, such options are not readily available for all liver and heart transplant candidates. Hepatocyte transplantation and artifical liver support are areas of research as alternatives or bridges to liver transplantation.[3] Left-ventricular assist devices (LVADs) are now used commonly as a bridge to transplantation for many heart transplant candidates.

Patient and graft survival rates following transplantation have improved significantly over the past 30 years as a result of advances in pharmacotherapy, surgical techniques, organ preservation, and the postoperative management of patients. (Table 87–1). In this chapter the epidemiology of endstage kidney, liver and heart disease is presented, the pathophysiology of organ rejection is reviewed, the pharmacotherapeutic options for the generation of individualized immunosuppressive regimens are critiqued and the unique complications of these regimens along with the therapeutic challenges they present are discussed.

TABLE 87–1. Organ-Specific Waiting Times for Transplant and Patient and Graft Survival Rates

Organ	Median Waiting Time (days)	Patient Survival (%)		Graft Survival (%)	
		1 Year	5 Years	1 Year	5 Years
Kidney	1,144[a]				
Living donor		97.5	90.1	94.3	78.6
Cadaveric donor		94.2	80.7	88.7	65.7
Liver	412				
Living donor		86.9	84.2	79.3	78.1
Cadaveric donor		86.3	72.1	80.6	64.1
Heart	141	85.6	72	85.3	70.6

[a]Based on data from 1999; inadequate follow-up for 2002 data.
From ref. 1.

EPIDEMIOLOGY AND ETIOLOGY

KIDNEY

The number of people diagnosed with end-stage kidney disease (ESKD) in 2002 exceeded 400,000. There were over 100,000 new cases of ESKD in 2002. The primary therapeutic options for these individuals are hemodialysis, peritoneal dialysis, and/or renal transplantation. Renal transplantation is the preferred long-term therapeutic option for most patients with ESKD because it provides patients with the greatest potential improvement in overall quality of life. Dialysis catheter–related infections, update peritoneal dialysis–associated peritonitis, and scheduled dialysis treatments are avoided, and dietary restrictions are fewer. While the analysis of quality of life is complex, patients generally report improved quality of life following transplantation as compared with patients on maintenance dialysis.[4]

The most commonly reported causes of ESKD, diabetes mellitus, hypertension, and glomerulonephritis account for about 80% of all kidney transplants (see Chap. 44).[5] Patients with medical conditions such as unstable cardiac disease or recently diagnosed malignancy, for whom the risk of surgery or chronic immunosuppression would be greater than the risks associated with chronic dialysis, are excluded from consideration for transplantation.

LIVER

Noncholestatic cirrhosis (hepatitis C, alcoholic cirrhosis, hepatitis B, cryptogenic cirrhosis, and autoimmune hepatitis) accounts for approximately 60% of liver transplant recipients (see Chap. 37).[1] Other indications for liver transplantation include primary biliary cirrhosis, primary sclerosing cholangitis, acute hepatic failure, primary liver cancer, and inborn errors of metabolism such as α_1-antitrypsin deficiency, Wilson's disease, tyrosinemia, types I, III, and IV glycogen storage disease, type I hyperoxaluria, and hemophilia A and B. Pediatric liver transplantation has been performed primarily for biliary atresia and inborn errors of metabolism. Timing of the transplant is critical for correction of the metabolic disease in order to prevent irreversible damage to the end organ (e.g., central nervous system in ornithine transcarbamylase deficiency) or to prevent hepatocellular carcinoma (e.g., tyrosinemia). In an effort to better allocate the available livers, a system based on the MELD (Model for End-stage Liver Disease) score has been adapted by the United Network for Organ Sharing (UNOS). This score, based on serum creatinine concentration, total serum bilirubin concentration, international normalization ratio (INR), and etiology of cirrhosis, is useful in predicting mortality.

There are few absolute contraindications to liver transplantation. Patients should have a reasonable life expectancy after transplantation. While hepatitis B and C can recur in the transplanted liver, these are not absolute contraindications to liver transplantation.[3,6] However, retransplant for hepatitis B or C is highly controversial.

HEART

Heart failure affects an estimated 4.9 million Americans, and approximately 400,000 new case are diagnosed each year (see Chap. 14).[7] Cardiac transplant candidates typically are patients with end-stage heart failure who have New York Heart Association (NYHA) class III or IV symptoms despite maximal medical management and have an expected 1-year mortality risk of 25% or greater without a transplant.[8] Idiopathic cardiomyopathy and ischemic heart disease account for heart failure in almost 90% heart transplant recipients.[1] Other less common etiologies include valvular disease (4%), retransplantation for graft atherosclerosis or dysfunction (2%), and congenital heart disease (1.5%).

Absolute contraindications to orthotopic cardiac transplantation include the presence of an active infection (except in the case of an infected ventricular assist device, which is an indication for urgent transplantation) or the presence of other diseases (i.e., malignancy) that may limit survival and/or rehabilitation and severe, irreversible pulmonary hypertension.

SURGICAL PROCEDURES

Kidney transplantation is generally performed by placing the allograft retroperitoneally in the right iliac fossa. The renal artery and vein are anastamosed to the external iliac artery and vein, respectively, and the donor ureter is connected directly to the bladder. If the donor kidney has not undergone prolonged ischemia, the production of urine immediately follows revascularization. For the most part, native kidneys are not removed.[9]

The transplanted liver, in contrast to kidney, is placed orthotopically; the recipient's own liver must be removed. Liver transplant occurs in several phases: removal of recipient liver, donor graft revascularization, and biliary reconstruction. During the anhepatic phase, the patient is placed on venovenous bypass to preserve venous return from the kidney and lower extremities. Size may be a limiting factor in liver transplantation. Donor and recipient are usually matched for size (±20%) to prevent splinting of the diaphragm and pulmonary complications that would result from transplantation of an excessively large liver.[10]

Heart transplantation is usually an orthotopic procedure. Leaving most of the atria and septum of the recipient, the patient is placed on cardiopulmonary bypass. The donor heart is implanted by anastamosis of the left atrium to the residual left atrial wall and joining the right atrial wall and septum. The main pulmonary artery is connected to the ascending aorta.[11]

PHYSIOLOGIC CONSEQUENCES OF TRANSPLANTATION

Transplantation is truly lifesaving for heart and liver transplant recipients, whereas renal transplantation is associated with improved quality of life and survival when compared with dialysis.[12] Most heart transplant patients return to NYHA functional class I following transplantation. In fact, 89.9% of patients consider themselves to have no limitations on activity at 1-year follow-up; however, not all have returned to work.[13] The specific physiologic consequences of kidney, liver, and heart transplantation are discussed below.

KIDNEY TRANSPLANTATION

The glomerular filtration rate (GFR) of a successfully transplanted kidney may be near normal almost immediately after transplantation. In some patients, however, the concentration of standard biochemical indicators of renal function, such as serum creatinine and blood urea nitrogen (BUN), may remain elevated for several days. Standard formulas used to predict drug dosing rely on a stable serum creatinine and may be inaccurate immediately following transplantation (see Chap. 41).

Although the allograft is able to remove uremic toxins from the body, it may take several weeks for other physiologic complications of chronic renal failure, such as anemia, calcium and phosphate imbalance, and altered lipid profiles, to resolve. The renal production of erythropoietin and 1-hydroxylation of vitamin D may return toward normal early in the postoperative period. Because the onset of physiologic effects may be delayed, continuation of pretransplant calcitriol, calcium supplementation, and/or phosphate binders may be warranted in some patients.

Primary nonfunction of a renal allograft or delayed graft function (DGF) is characterized by the need for dialysis in the first 7 postoperative days or the failure of the serum creatinine to fall below 4 mg/dL or by 30% of the pretransplant value. The incidence of DGF in primary cadaveric renal transplantation ranges from 8% to 50% and results in a slower return of the kidney's excretory, metabolic, and synthetic functions. DGF is associated with prolonged hospital stays, higher costs, difficult management of immunosuppressive therapy, slower patient rehabilitation, and poor graft survival. Urinary complications such as ureteral obstruction, thrombosis, or leak or vascular complications, including arterial or venous stenosis or thrombosis, also may result in early graft dysfunction.

The primary cause of DGF is acute tubular necrosis (ATN). The incidence of ATN increases when kidneys are harvested from donors following cardiac arrest, from donors who are hypotensive or on vasopressors, or from older donors. Prolonged periods of ischemia can increase the risk of ATN. The management of patients with ATN may be difficult (see Chap. 42). Cyclosporine and tacrolimus may be implicated in the prolongation of ATN, but a clear cause-and-effect relationship has not been established.

Persistently elevated serum creatinine and BUN levels confound the perioperative management of renal transplant recipients.

Among the differential diagnoses are acute rejection, ATN, and/or cyclosporine or tacrolimus toxicity (see Chap. 46). These processes are not mutually exclusive. Definitive diagnosis is made by renal biopsy. In the presence of an elevated serum creatinine level, clinicians may reduce the dose of cyclosporine or tacrolimus to minimize the potential for drug nephrotoxicity and hasten the recovery from ATN. This practice may result in subtherapeutic immunosuppressant concentrations and hasten the occurrence of acute rejection. DGF predisposes patients to acute rejection. Induction therapy (e.g., using antibody preparations) and delaying the initiation of cyclosporine or tacrolimus administration may be useful in this setting.

LIVER TRANSPLANTATION

The physiologic consequences of liver transplantation are complex, involving changes in both metabolic and synthetic function. Postoperatively, the liver transplant recipient likely will have many fluid, electrolyte, and nutritional abnormalities. Biliary tract dysfunction may alter the absorption of fats and fat-soluble drugs.[14] The poor absorption of the lipid-soluble drug cyclosporine improves after successful liver transplantation and reestablishment of bile flow. Vitamin E deficiency and its neurologic complications in liver failure patients are reversed after successful liver transplantation in pediatric patients. In stable adult liver transplant patients, the concentrations of retinol and tocopherol are similar to those seen in normal healthy subjects, indicating recovery of transplanted liver production and excretion of bile salts needed for fat-soluble vitamin absorption. The effects of liver metabolism on drug disposition and elimination are summarized in Table 87–2.

Failure of the newly transplanted liver occurs in 10% to 15% of cases and can result from several different mechanisms. Early graft failure can result from preexisting disease in the donor, and even coagulation defects have been acquired through donor organs. The technical complexity of the operation can produce flaws in revascularization that also lead to graft nonfunction. Surgical complications occur in about 25% of cases and result in a doubling of the hospital expense for the patient.[15] Portal vein thrombosis, hepatic artery thrombosis, and bile duct leaks are all technical problems that have been encountered. Ischemic injury to the donor liver through preservation is difficult to predict and can produce early graft dysfunction. Perioperative immune events rarely lead to the classic picture of hyperacute rejection in liver transplantation, but graft failure in the first 2 postoperative weeks still may indicate antibody-mediated graft destruction.

HEART TRANSPLANTATION

The orthotopically transplanted heart is denervated and no longer responds to physiologic stimuli in a normal manner. Patients, for example, do not experience classic angina. In situations requiring an increased heart rate (e.g., exercise or hypotension), the denervated heart is unable to acutely increase heart rate but instead relies on increasing the stroke volume. Later in the course of exercise or hypotension, heart rate increases in response to circulating catecholamines. While the maximum exercise capacity of heart transplant recipients is below normal, most patients are able to resume normal lifestyles and reasonably vigorous activity levels. Partial reinnervation may occur over time, thereby facilitating more normal physiologic (e.g., presence of classic angina) and pharmacologic responses and better exercise capacity.[16]

In the acute postoperative phase (0–6 weeks), responses present in the normal heart are interrupted or blunted. In the acutely

TABLE 87–2. Changes in Drug Disposition and Elimination Following Liver Transplantation

	Result	Comment
Serum Proteins		
↓ Albumin	↑ Free fraction of drugs usually bound to albumin	Diazepam, salicylic acid binding greater in liver transplant than chronic liver disease due to endogenous binding inhibitors (up to 45 days posttransplant)
↑ Alpha-acid glycoprotein	Lower free fraction of drugs-lidocaine	
Metabolism/Elimination		
Microsomes		
	↑ CYP2E1 activity	Increased drug metabolism (induction)
	↔ CYP2D6	Unaffected
	↓ P450 enzymes activity	Decreased drug elimination (inhibition)
Oxidation	Stable	
Conjugation	Normalizes after transplant	Renal elimination of metabolites limited
Biliary dysfunction	↓ Absorption of lipophilic compounds	
	↑ CSA metabolites in blood	
Renal elimination	Elimination of gentamicin, vancomycin, cephalosporins less than predicted by serum creatinine	

CYP = cytochrome P450 liver enzyme system.
From ref. 14.

denervated heart, changes in cardiac output (heart rate × stroke volume) largely depend on heart rate changes engendered by circulating catecholamines. The donor sinus node function may be impaired by preservation injury, direct surgical trauma at excision, the presence of long-acting antiarrhythmics (e.g., amiodarone) taken prior to transplant by the recipient, and a lack of "conditioning" responsiveness to catecholamines.[16] Therefore, the transplanted heart generally requires chronotropic support with either milrinone or pacing in the early posttransplant period to maintain a heart rate of 90 to 110 beats per minute and satisfactory hemodynamics (i.e., blood pressure, urine output, and tissue perfusion). Approximately 10% to 20% of transplant patients will have persistent chronotropic incompetence requiring either cardiac pacing or pharmacologic manipulation of the heart with theophylline or terbutaline after hospital discharge; however, few patients who receive a pacemaker use it permanently. Anatomic variables may further compromise optimal hemodynamic function and complicate hemodynamic assessment of the patient.

Right ventricular function frequently is impaired, presumably as a result of preservation injury and elevated pulmonary vascular resistance. A "restrictive" hemodynamic pattern may be present initially, but it usually improves over the 6 weeks following transplantation. Donor-recipient size mismatch may contribute to early posttransplantation hemodynamic abnormalities characterized by higher right and left ventricular end-diastolic pressures. Supraventricular arrhythmias in the early posttransplant period usually are transient and may result from overvigorous use of catecholamines or milrinone; later, they should raise suspicion for acute rejection.

Myocardial depression frequently occurs and generally requires inotropic support with agents such as dobutamine, milrinone, and epinephrine. On occasion, intra- or postoperative administration of vasodilators, including nitric oxide, and inotropic agents may be necessary to treat right-sided failure in the transplant patient; milrinone and isoproterenol are the preferred inodilators in this setting.

Persistent abnormalities of diastolic function are noted in the transplanted heart such that intracardiac pressures increase in an exaggerated fashion with response to exercise and/or volume infusion.[16] These abnormalities of diastolic function are due, at least in part, to

denervation but also to acute rejection or to the scarring secondary to previously treated rejection episodes, hypertension, or cardiac allograft vasculopathy.

Hypertension often occurs following surgery secondary to the elevated catecholamine levels and systemic vascular resistance associated with end-stage heart failure on a healthy heart. Systolic blood pressure is maintained at 110 to 120 mm Hg to enhance cardiac function. Initial treatment may include nitroprusside or nitroglycerin; hydralazine and amlodipine are used later.

The pharmacologic implications of the physiologic consequences of the transplanted heart are summarized in Table 87–3.[2]

PATHOPHYSIOLOGY OF REJECTION

GENERAL CONCEPTS

Allograft rejection depends on activation of alloreactive T cells and antigen-presenting cells (APCs) such as B-lymphocytes, macrophages, and dendritic cells. Acute allograft rejection is caused primarily by the infiltration of T cells into the allograft, which triggers inflammatory and cytotoxic effects on the graft. Complex interactions between the allograft and cellular cytokines, cell-to-cell interactions, CD4+ and CD8+ T cells, and B cells ultimately lead to chronic rejection and graft loss if adequate immunosuppression is not maintained.[17]

The sequence of events that underlies graft rejection is recognition of the donor's histocompatibility differences by the recipient's immune system, recruitment of activated lymphocytes, initiation of immune effector mechanisms, and finally graft destruction.

Class I and II antigens of the major histocompatibility complex (MHC) are important for histocompatibility in transplantation.[17] Class I antigens are present on virtually all nucleated cells in the body, whereas the class II antigens are located primarily on B-lymphocytes, APCs, and vascular endothelium.[17] T helper (TH) cells, specialized to direct the immune system, can only recognize foreign antigen in the presence of MHC type II. Cytotoxic T cells, specialized to destroy, can only recognize antigen in the presence of MHC type I antigens.

TABLE 87–3. Effect of Denervation on Cardiac Pharmacology

Drug	Effect	Mechanism	Comment
Digitalis	Normal inotropic effect Minimal effect on AV node	Direct mycocardial effect Denervation	
Atropine	No effect on AV node	Denervation	

Adrenaline/
    noradrenaline
	Increased contractility
	Increased chronotropy
		Denervation
		Hypersensitivity
			Increased cardiac output mediated by
			    increased heart rate

Isoproterenol	Normal increase in contractility; normal increase in chronotropy	No neuronal uptake	
Quinidine	No vagolytic effect	Denervation	
Verapamil	AV block	Direct effect	
Nifedipine	No reflex tachycardia	Denervation	
Hydralazine	No reflex tachycardia	Denervation	
β-Blocker	Increased antagonist effect	Denervation	Impair HR response, use sparingly

Adenosine	Negative chronotropic effect	Hypersensitivity
		Effect on sinus node of denervated heart
			Life-threatening asystole (>0.5 min) may
			    occur if used to treat supraventricular
			    arrhythmia or stress testing

Acetylcholine	Negative chronotropic effect	Hypersensitivity Effect on sinus node of denervated heart	

AV = atriovenous node.
From ref. 2.

Lymphocytes are the only cells in the body that can recognize specific antigens and are central to allograft rejection.

◄ T-cell activation is caused by interactions between T-cell receptors, the MHC, cellular adhesion molecues, and costimulatory molecules. Among the series of events is calcineurin activation, which ultimately promotes interleukin 2 (IL-2) proliferation. After initial T-cell activation, the process of clonal expansion and immunologic progression is mediated by cytokines. IL-2 is released from T cells and activates T-lymphocytes locally and in other regions of the body. Undifferentiated T-helper cells can be induced to develop along two lines: TH_1 cells secrete IL-2, interferon-γ, and IL-12 and favor cytotoxicity, while TH_2 cells secrete IL-4, -5, -10, and 13, which stimulate B-cell and immunoglobulin development. A predominance of TH_2 cells has been associated with tolerance (the ability of the body to recognize the transplanted allograft as "self") in some experiemental models. The complex nature of these cytokine interactions makes it very difficult to design drugs with exclusive actions (see Fig. 87–1). Allograft inflammation results from these processes

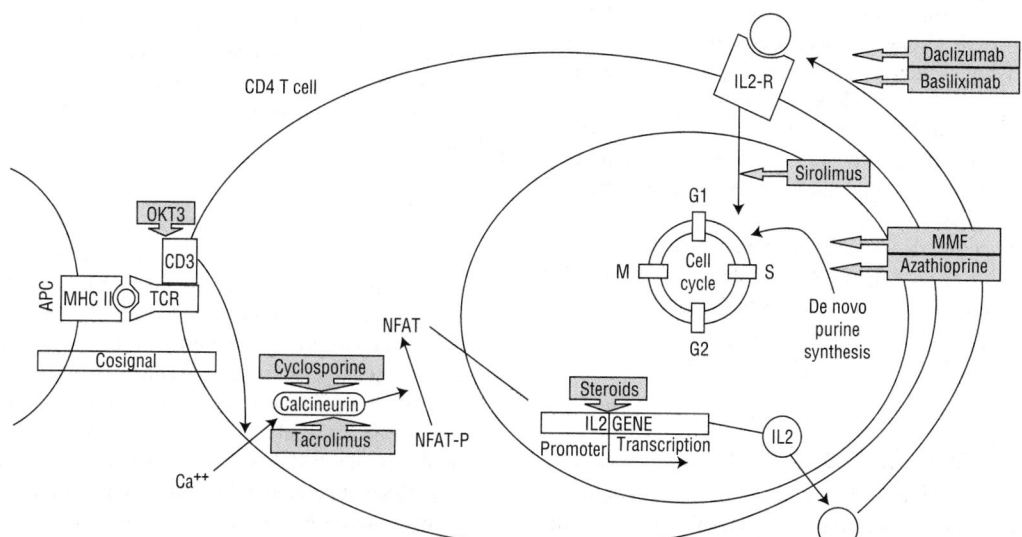

FIGURE 87–1. Stages of CD4 T-cell activation and cytokine production with identification of the sites of action of different immunosuppressive agents. Antigen-major histocompatibility complex (MHC) II molecule complexes are responsible for initiating the activation of CD4 T cells. These MHC-peptide complexes are recognized by the T-cell recognition complex (TCR). A costimulatory signal initiates signal transduction with activation of second messengers, one of which is calcineurin. Calcineurin removes phosphates from the nuclear factors (NFAT-P) allowing them to enter the nucleus. These nuclear factors specifically bind to an interleukin-2 (IL-2) promoter gene facilitating IL-2 gene transcription. Interaction of IL-2 with the IL-2 receptor (IL-2R) on the cell membrane surface induces cell proliferation and production of cytokines specific to the T cell. APC = antigen-producing cells; MMF = mycophenolate mofetil. (With permission from ref. 17.)

acting through specific (T-cell interactions with APCs) and nonspecific immunologic mechanisms (natural killer cell chemotaxis, release of vasoactive substances). Rejection of the transplanted tissue can take place at any time following surgery and is classified clinically as hyperacute rejection, acute cellular rejection, humoral rejection or chronic rejection.

Efforts are made to allocate well-matched (HLA-A, -B, -DR) kidneys to improve overall rejection and survival rates. However, the benefit of having no recipient donor mismatches may be negated by excessive cold ischemia time (>36 hours) and donor age older than 60 years. Because of greater organ availability and more restricted cold ischemia times for livers and hearts, HLA tissue matching is not performed routinely before transplantation. However, if the potential recipient is reactive against a panel of random donor antigens (i.e., patient has a positive panel reactive antibody [PRA] > 10% to 20%), then a negative T-cell crossmatch is required prior to transplantation. Transplanted organs must be matched for ABO blood group compatibility with the recipient. ABO mismatching will result in hyperacute rejection. Liver transplantation may be carried out in emergency situations across ABO blood groups, but survival is lower than for ABO compatible liver transplants.

HYPERACUTE REJECTION

Hyperacute rejection may occur when preformed donor-specific antibodies are present in the recipient at the time of the transplant and may be evident within minutes of the transplant procedure. Hyperacute rejection can be induced by immunoglobulin G (IgG) antibodies that bind to antigens on the vascular endothelium, such as class I MHC, ABO, and vascular endothelial cell antigens. Tissue damage can be mediated through antibody-dependent, cell-mediated cytotoxicity or through activation of the complement cascade. The ischemic damage to the microvasculature rapidly produces tissue necrosis.

Hyperacute rejection has become uncommon in kidney and heart transplants because transplant donors are matched for ABO blood groups and crossmatch testing is done to determine the presence of donor-specific lymphocytotoxic antibodies. A positive crossmatch presents a serious risk for graft failure even if hyperacute rejection does not occur. A negative lymphocytotoxicity crossmatch does not entirely rule out the possibility of hyperacute rejection because non-MHC antigens on the vascular endothelium can serve as targets of donor-specific antibodies.

Hyperacute rejection rarely occurs in patients receiving a liver transplant. The liver's special status for transplantation is not fully understood, but the local release of cytokines may alter the immunologic reaction taking place in the liver. Early graft dysfunction is treated with supportive care and retransplantation if possible.

ACUTE CELLULAR REJECTION

Acute rejection is most common in the first few months following transplantation but can occur at any time during the life of the allograft. Acute rejection generally is reversible, especially if treated. While most cases of acute rejection can be treated effectively, none of the currently available therapies prevents or changes the course of chronic rejection.

Cellular rejection is mediated by alloreactive T-lymphocytes that appear in the circulation and infiltrate the allograft through the vascular endothelium. After the graft is infiltrated by lymphocytes, the cytotoxic cells can specifically kill allograft targets, whereas the local release of lymphokines will attract and stimulate macrophages to produce tissue damage through a delayed hypersensitivity-like mechanism. These immunologic and inflammatory events lead to the nonspecific signs and symptoms of acute rejection: pain and tenderness, fever, and lethargy.

KIDNEY

Acute rejection which may affect 20% of patients during the first 6 months following transplantation is evidenced by an abrupt rise in serum creatinine concentration of ≥30%. A specific histologic diagnosis can be obtained via biopsy of the allograft and often is used to guide therapy for rejection. A biopsy specimen with a diffuse infiltrate of lymphocytes is consistent with acute cellular rejection. After the diagnosis of rejection has been confirmed, the potential risks and benefits of specific antirejection therapies must be evaluated. Hypertension often worsens during an episode of rejection. Patients may experience edema and weight gain as a result of sodium and fluid retention. Symptomatic azotemia also may develop in severe cases. Appropriate adjustments in pharmacotherapy are warranted in the face of diminished renal function.

LIVER

The liver appears to be less immunogenic and more likely to promote immunologic tolerance than the other vascularized organs. An immunologic explanation for graft dysfunction becomes more probable as time passes in a patient with an initially functioning liver graft. Initial episodes of acute cellular rejection often occur between 6 days and 6 weeks post-transplantation but also can occur earlier or later. The clinical signs of acute cellular rejection include leukocytosis and a change in the color or quantity of bile. An increased serum bilirubin concentration and increases in hepatic enzymes are the most common biochemical parameters monitored and are sensitive markers of rejection. The liver biopsy is used as definitive evidence of the diagnosis of rejection, but response to antirejection medication also has been used in differentiating rejection from other causes of hepatic dysfunction in a liver transplant patient. Other reasons for graft dysfunction include defects in bile duct reconstruction, opportunistic infections, and toxicity from parenteral nutrition, sepsis, or drug-induced hepatotoxicity.

HEART

Acute rejection is a major determinant of survival following cardiac transplantation and accounts for approximately 17% of all deaths.[18] The incidence of rejection is substantially higher during the early months following transplantation, with 90% of all rejections occurring within the first 6 months. Because the incidence of acute rejection is highest during this time period, surveillance endomyocardial biopsies are performed at regularly scheduled intervals following transplantation. A typical schedule would be to perform weekly biopsies for the first postoperative month, biweekly biopsies for the next 2 months, monthly biopsies for the next 4 to 6 months, and bimonthly biopsies for the next 7 to 12 months. Biopsy frequency subsequently decreases to every 3 to 12 months. In addition, the severity of rejection tends to be greater when it occurs early in the postoperative period. Although a minority of patients (37%) remain rejection-free, most will experience at least one episode of rejection during the first year. Rejection of the cardiac allograft is not necessarily accompanied by overt clinical signs or symptoms. Nonspecific findings may include low-grade fever, malaise, and mild reduction in exercise capacity, whereas heart failure or atrial arrhythmias may reflect more severe rejection. The "gold standard" for detection of rejection is histologic confirmation using endomyocardial specimens obtained by transvenous biopsy of the right ventricle. Cardiac function is assessed by either echocardiography or measurement of right-sided heart and pulmonary wedge pressures and cardiac output by pulmonary artery catheterization at the time of each biopsy. The majority of rejection episodes are characterized histologically by lymphocytic infiltrates with or without myocyte degeneration. The treatment of rejection is based on a number of factors, including type, histologic grade, clinical symptoms, hemodynamic changes, noninvasive findings, and duration of time post-transplantation. Mild degrees of acute cellular rejection usually are not treated unless the patient is symptomatic, whereas the presence of moderate to severe rejection with or without necrosis mandates treatment.[19]

HUMORAL REJECTION

Humoral rejection, sometimes referred to as *vascular rejection,* is an antibody-mediated process directed against HLA antigens present on the donor vascular endothelium. It can be characterized by capillary deposition of immunoglobulins (IgG), complement, and fibrinogen on immunofluorescence staining. Circulating immune complexes often precede humoral rejection. This form of rejection is less common than cellular rejection and generally occurs in the first 3 months after transplantation. It is associated with an increased fatality rate and appears to be more common when antilymphocyte antibodies are used for rejection prophylaxis. An increased risk of humoral rejection has been linked to females, recipients with elevated PRA, cytomegalovirus seropositivity, a positive crossmatch, and prior sensitization to OKT3.[20] Strategies to reverse humoral rejection include plasmapheresis, often in combination with intravenous immunoglobulin (IVIG), high-dose intravenous glucocorticoids, antithymocyte globulin, cyclosphosphamide, rituximab, and mycophenolate mofetil.

CHRONIC REJECTION

Chronic rejection is a major cause of late graft loss and is one of the most important problems that remains to be resolved. While chronic rejection simply may be a slow and indolent form of acute cellular rejection, the involvement of the humoral immune system and antibodies against the vascular endothelium appear to play a role. Persistent perivascular and interstitial inflammation is a common finding in kidney, liver, and heart transplantation. Owing to the complex interaction of multiple drugs and diseases over time, it is difficult to delineate the true nature of chronic rejection. For example, cytomegalovirus is associated with the development of chronic rejection in both liver and heart transplant recipients. Unlike acute rejection, chronic rejection is not reversible.

KIDNEY

Advances in the management of acute rejection, has increased the duration of functioning grafts from living and cadaveric donors by more than 70%.[21] Chronic rejection remains the most common cause of graft loss in the late post-transplant period (>1 year). Although acute rejection is a strong predictor of chronic rejection, it is unclear why the reduction in the incidence of acute rejection associated with the widespread adoption of cyclosporine and tacrolimus has not had an impact on the incidence of chronic rejection. The current tendency to decrease doses of cyclosporine and tacrolimus in the face of "good" graft function without dynamic measurement of immunologic factors may lead to subclinical rejection. Hypertension, proteinuria, and a progressive decline in renal function represent the classic triad of chronic rejection. Manifestations of chronic rejection generally depend on the degree of renal insufficiency and hypoalbuminemia. Classic symptoms of uremia occur as end-stage kidney disease develops.

LIVER

Chronic rejection of the liver is characterized by an obliterative arteriopathy and the loss of bile ducts, which has been referred to as the *vanishing bile duct syndrome.* These patients experience an asymptomatic rise in the canalicular liver enzymes (alkaline phosphatase and γ-glutamyl transpeptidase) and become jaundiced. These changes are considered the result of immunologic and ischemic injury and can be seen in patients who have not responded adequately to therapy for acute rejection.

HEART

Chronic rejection is the leading cause of graft failure and death in heart transplant recipients.[22] It manifests as a vasculopathy that is characterized by accelerated intimal thickening or development of atherosclerotic plaques, similar to those seen in the general population with coronary artery disease (CAD). Endothelial injury is the first step in the process, which can be caused by both cell-mediated and humoral responses to the transplanted allograft. Vasculopathy can affect both the arterial and venous vessels but is restricted to the transplanted allograft and rarely affects the recipient's native vessels. Lipid abnormalities, immunosuppressants, and cytomegalovirus have been linked to the development of vasculopathy. Routine surveillance with coronary angiography, intravascular ultrasound, or other procedures can aid in the diagnosis of vasculopathy. HMG-CoA reductase inhibitors and angiotensin-converting enzyme inhibitors (ACEIs) have been used to decrease the incidence of vasculopathy.[22] Percutaneous transluminal coronary angioplasty (PTCA) and coronary artery bypass grafting (CABG) have been used in severe cases of vasculopathy; these procedures, however, are limited by significantly increased mortality compared with the general population.[22]

▶ TREATMENT: Solid-Organ Rejection

■ DESIRED OUTCOME

Transplant immunosuppression must be balanced in terms of graft and patient survival (the prevention of rejection versus the risk of adverse effects associated with therapy, including life-threatening infection or malignancy). A multidrug approach is rational from the immunomechanistic viewpoint because the agents may have overlapping and potentially synergistic mechanisms. Furthermore, multidrug immunosuppression may allow the use of lower doses of individual agents associated with different side-effect profiles to minimize the severity of expected adverse effects.

The goals of immunosuppression vary depending on the time interval since transplantation. Immediately following surgery, the primary goal of therapy is to prevent hyperacute and acute rejection. The high doses of immunosuppressants required to achieve this goal may result in serious complications (e.g., nephrotoxicity, infection, thrombocytopenia, and drug-induced diabetes) if maintained long term. Rapid dosage reductions may minimize these effects.

■ GENERAL APPROACH TO TREATMENT

■ INDUCTION THERAPY

Induction therapy involves the use of a high level of immunosuppression at the time of transplantation with or without the immediate introduction of cyclosporine or tacrolimus (see Fig. 87–2). While induction historically consisted of the use of polyclonal or monoclonal antibodies in addition to triple therapy of azathioprine, high-dose corticosteroids, and a calcineurin inhibitor (e.g., cyclosporine

or tacrolimus) at the time of transplantation, the term is used more recently to define two perioperative immunosuppressive strategies: (1) the provision of a highly intense level of immunosuppression, either universally or on the basis of patient-specific risk factors such as age and race, or (2) the use of antibody therapy to provide enough immunosuppression to delay the administration of the nephrotoxic calcineurin inhibitors cyclosporine and tacrolimus. The rationale for delayed calcineurin inhibitor administration varies slightly depending on the type of transplant. In renal transplantation, the newly transplanted kidney is susceptible to nephrotoxic injury, whereas in liver and heart transplantation, the idea is to protect patients with preexisting renal insufficiency from further insults during the perioperatiave period. Additionally, cyclosporine and tacrolimus dosage adjustment to maintain target concentrations may be difficult in the perioperative period.

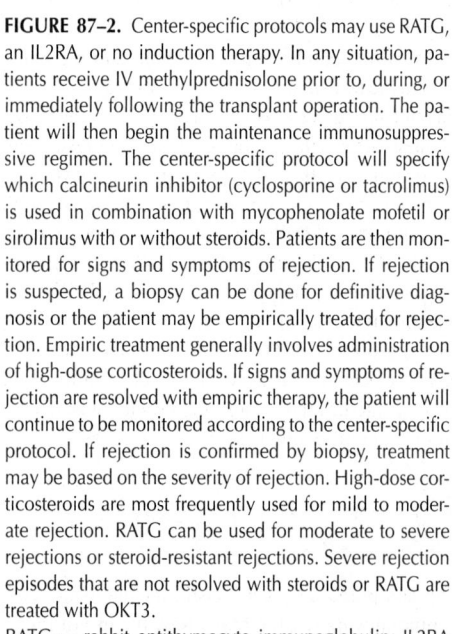

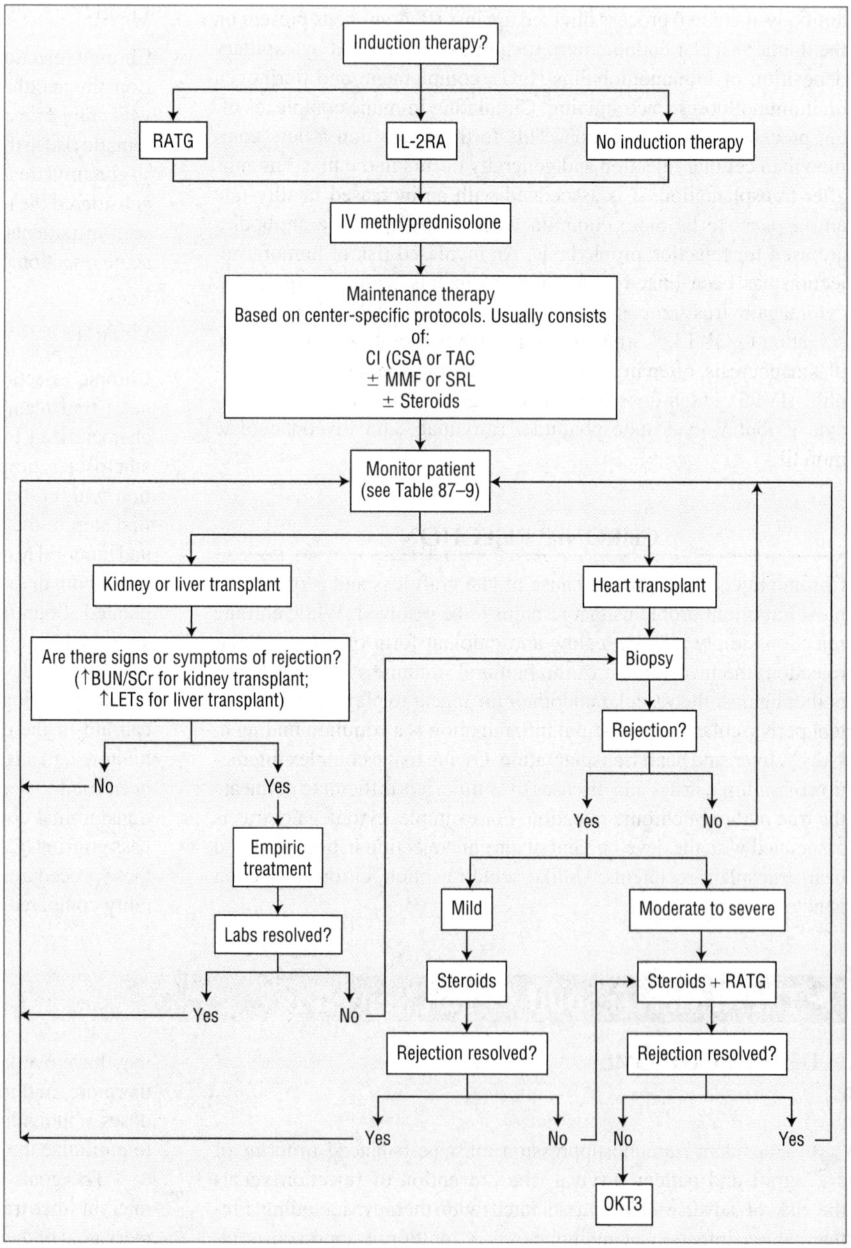

FIGURE 87–2. Center-specific protocols may use RATG, an IL2RA, or no induction therapy. In any situation, patients receive IV methylprednisolone prior to, during, or immediately following the transplant operation. The patient will then begin the maintenance immunosuppressive regimen. The center-specific protocol will specify which calcineurin inhibitor (cyclosporine or tacrolimus) is used in combination with mycophenolate mofetil or sirolimus with or without steroids. Patients are then monitored for signs and symptoms of rejection. If rejection is suspected, a biopsy can be done for definitive diagnosis or the patient may be empirically treated for rejection. Empiric treatment generally involves administration of high-dose corticosteroids. If signs and symptoms of rejection are resolved with empiric therapy, the patient will continue to be monitored according to the center-specific protocol. If rejection is confirmed by biopsy, treatment may be based on the severity of rejection. High-dose corticosteroids are most frequently used for mild to moderate rejection. RATG can be used for moderate to severe rejections or steroid-resistant rejections. Severe rejection episodes that are not resolved with steroids or RATG are treated with OKT3.
RATG = rabbit antithymocyte immunoglobulin; IL2RA = interleukin-2 receptor antagonist; CI = calcineurin inhibitor; CSA = cyclosporine; TAC = tacrolimus; MMF = mycophenolate mofetil; SRL = sirolimus; BUN =blood urea nitrogen; SCr = serum creatinine; LFTs = liver function tests; OKT3 = muromonab CD3.

CLINICAL CONTROVERSY

Some clinicians use induction therapy with IL2RAs or RATG for all transplant recipients. Others reserve induction therapy for patients who are at a higher risk for rejections, such as those who have a high PRA, had previous transplants or multiple pregnancies, or are of non-Caucasian race.

ACUTE REJECTION

The primary goal of acute rejection therapy is to minimize the intensity of the immune response and prevent irreversible injury to the allograft. The available options may include (1) increasing the doses of current immunosuppressive drugs such as cyclosporine or tacrolimus, (2) "pulse" steroids with subsequent dose taper, (3) addition of an additional immunosuppressant indefinitely, or (4) short-term treatment with antirejection therapy such as OKT3 or antithymocyte globulin. The treatment of acute rejection varies among transplant centers and by type of allograft, but most always begins with "pulse" steroid therapy for several days (oral or intravenous). Recent data in renal transplantation indicate, however, that African-Americans do not respond as well to glucocorticoids as non-African-Americans. Other therapies, such as antithymphocyte globulin, thus may be preferable for this patient population.[23]

If biopsy results are available, these findings also may guide therapy in favor of other approaches such as antilymphocyte preparations. Cytolytic agents generally are reserved for steroid-resistant rejection, signs of hemodynamic compromise (heart), or more severe rejections. For the treatment of acute allograft rejection, antithymocyte globulin is better tolerated than and preferred over OKT3. Other innovative forms of therapy for persistent or intractable rejection have been investigated, including mycophenolate mofetil, tacrolimus, low-dose methotrexate, sirolimus, total lymphoid irradiation, and photopheresis (e.g., immune-modulating therapy, which involves apheresis with isolation of peripheral blood leukocytes, treatment of the leukocytes ex vivo with 8-methoxypsoralen and ultraviolet light, and subsequent reinfusion into the patient).[24,25]

The dosages of other immunosuppressant drugs often are decreased while administering corticosteroids, OKT3, or antithymocyte globulin therapy. Prophylactic agents such as valganciclovir, nystatin, trimethoprim-sulfamethoxazole, H_2-receptor antagonists or proton-pump inhibitors, and/or antacids may be used to minimize adverse effects associated with intensive immunosuppression.

MAINTENANCE THERAPY

The goal of maintenance immunosuppression is to prevent acute and chronic rejection while minimizing drug-related toxicity. In the long-term management of the transplant patient, the doses of immunosuppressants are reduced gradually (over 6 to 12 months) in an effort to minimize adverse effects. Many institutions may withdraw specific immunosuppressives completely in select patients to reduce long-term toxicity as well as cost. It is important to recognize that while the goals of transplant immunosuppression are universal, protocols for immunosuppressive therapy vary widely among institutions.

Maintenance therapy can involve numerous combinations of the various available immunosuppressive agents. Transplant organ and type (cadaveric versus living-related), the degree of HLA mismatch, time post-transplant, post-transplant complications (including the number of acute rejections), previous immunosuppressive adverse reactions, compliance, and financial considerations are among the patient-specific factors considered in individualizing maintenance immunosuppression. Calcineurin inhibitors (CIs) generally are a central component in most maintenance regimens, although CI-free immunosuppression remains the "Holy Grail" of transplant immunology. Transplant patients may receive mono-, dual-, or triple-drug therapy during the maintenance phase. As patients progress through the posttransplant course, the risk of acute rejection decreases; accordingly, maintenance immunosuppression is tapered, and in some cases, certain agents may be discontinued.

The changes seen with chronic rejection are not reversible with current immunosuppressive therapies. Some strategies for managing chronic rejection include increasing immunosuppression or changing immunosuppression to prevent further progression of chronic rejection. However, often this strategy provides little clinical benefit. Ideally, immunosuppression should be optimized to prevent acute rejection episodes to minimize the occurrence of chronic rejection.

CALCINEURIN INHIBITORS (CIs)

CYCLOSPORINE (CSA)

The introduction of CSA has improved the outcomes of transplantation significantly. Patient and graft survival rates have improved secondary to a lower incidence of acute rejection episodes and severe infectious complications.[26] Despite these improvements in survival, concerns regarding its long-term use include late rejection episodes, frequency of hypertension, drug cost, and quality of kidney function.

Pharmacology/Mechanism of Action

CSA inhibits T-cell proliferation by inhibiting the production of IL-2 and other cytokines by T cells (see Fig. 87–1). CSA binds to cyclophilin, a cytoplasmic immunophilin. The CSA-cyclophilin complex inhibits the action of calcineurin, an enzyme that activates the nuclear factor of activated T cells (NF-AT), which is, in turn, responsible for the transcription of several key cytokines necessary for T-cell activity, including IL-2. IL-2 is a potent growth factor for T cells, responsible for activation and clonal expansion.

Pharmacokinetics

CSA is highly lipophilic and depends on bile for intestinal absorption. Following oral administration, the absorption of CSA is incomplete and erratic, especially in liver recipients with T-tube diversion of bile. CSA is associated with clinically significant interpatient and intrapatient variability in pharmacokinetic parameters owing to unpredictable bioavailability, which averages 30% (range 3% to 60%). Bowel function and bile flow play a major role in intestinal absorption. Because of the significant variability in absorption, peak concentrations are reached within 2 to 6 hours of oral administration. CSA is distributed widely into tissues and body fluids, resulting in a large and variable volume of distribution. The mean terminal half-life with normal liver function is 19 hours.

TABLE 87–4. Summary of Immunosuppressant Adverse Effects

Adverse Effects	AZA	MMF	Steroids	CSA	TAC	SIR	IL2RA	ATG	OKT3	Management
Adrenal suppression			+							Taper doses slowly; administer every other day; patient identification card
Cataracts/glaucoma			+							Annual eye examinations or as indicated
Hypertension			++	++	++					Monitor blood pressure; sodium restriction and antihypertensive medications as needed
Tremor				++	++					Adjust dose as needed
Gastrointestinal abnormalities	++ Nausea, vomiting	++ Diarrhea, nausea, abdominal pain	+ GI bleeding	+	++ Diarrhea, nausea, vomiting, anorexia					AZA: administer after meals; MMF: decrease or divide dose, administer with food; TAC/PRED: administer with food; ulcer prophylaxis
Respiratory abnormalities					++				+	TAC: pleural effusion, dyspnea; OKT3: pulmonary edema
Nephrotoxicity				++	++	+				Monitor serum creatinine/BUN; adjust dose and discontinue as needed
Headache				+	++					Check drug concentration; adjust dose
Hepatotoxicity	+			+	++					Monitor liver enzymes; AZA-associated toxicity is reversible and usually occurs within the first 6 months of therapy; adjust dose and discontinue as needed
Hyperlipidemia			++	++	+	++				Dietary counseling; pharmacotherapy as needed
Glucose alterations			++	+	++					Monitor glucose; adjust doses of hypoglycemics or immunosuppressants
Osteoporosis/aseptic necrosis			+/++							Annual bone examinations; weight bearing exercise
Personality changes			++							Patient and family education
Weight gain			++							Patient education; exercise
Acne			+	+						Dose reduction; increased hygiene; topical agents (e.g. retinoic acid)
Gingival hyperplasia				++						Patient education; appropriate dental hygiene; consider TAC
Hirsutism				++						Patient education; consider TAC
Pruritis					++					Treatment when appropriate
Thrombocytopenia	++	+			+	++				Monitor platelets
Leukocytosis				++	++					Monitor WBCs
Leukopenia	++	++		+				++		Monitor WBCs; dose-dependent and reversible with AZA/MMF
Hyperkalemia				+	++					Monitor serum electrolytes
Hypokalemia								+		
Hypomagnesemia				+	++					Monitor serum magnesium

++ indicates >10% risk; + indicates <10% risk.

AZA = azathioprine; MMF = mycophenolate mofetil; CSA = cyclosporine; TAC = tacrolimus; SIR = sirolimus; IL2RA = interleukin 2 receptor antagonist; ATG = antithymocyte globulin; OKT3 = muromonab CD3; PRED = prednisone; BUN = blood urea nitrogen; WBC = white blood cells.

To overcome the pharmacokinetic problems of CSA, a micro-emulsion formulation was developed. Both forms are available commercially in the United States, referred to as "cyclosporine, USP" and "cyclosporine, USP [MODIFIED]." The two formulations are not bioequivalent and should not be used interchangeably. The microemulsion formulation is self-emulsifying and forms a microemulsion spontaneously with aqueous fluids in the gastrointestinal tract, making it less dependent on bile for absorption. The result is a significantly greater rate and extent of absorption and decreased intraindividual variability in pharmacokinetic parameters. Bioavailability is enhanced owing to better dispersion and absorption and does not require bile excretion. The relative bioavailability of the microemulsion formulation is 60%. Peak concentrations generally are reached within 1.5 to 2 hours after oral administration. The terminal half-life is 8.4 hours.

Following oral absorption, 90% to 97% of CSA is bound to lipoproteins in the blood. CSA is metabolized by the cytochrome P450 3A4 (CYP 3A4) system in both the gut and the liver, which accounts for both its poor bioavailability and numerous drug interactions. Children have a shorter half-life as a result of an increased rate of metabolism.

Efficacy

The introduction of CSA significantly improved the outcomes of transplantation. Since its approval and widespread use, patient and graft survival rates have improved secondary to a lower incidence of acute rejection episodes and severe infectious complications. In heart transplant recipients, for example, 1-year survival rates increased from 56% to 85%, and 5-year survival rates increased from 31% to 75%.[27] The efficacy of CSA is well established in all types of solid-organ transplants. Currently, CSA is approved for use in kidney, liver, and heart transplantation.

When compared with the standard formulation, the microemulsion formulation has demonstrated equivalent or superior efficacy in kidney, liver, and heart transplant recipients. Other areas of research include CSA as monotherapy and as rescue therapy for patients who are unable to tolerate tacrolimus.

The efficacy of CSA monotherapy has been described.[28] The avoidance of long-term steroids is the primary advantage of CSA monotherapy, whereas the primary disadvantage is the higher incidence of rejection. As a result, CSA is used rarely as monotherapy.

Patients who are unable to tolerate tacrolimus owing to side effects can be switched to CSA as rescue therapy. CSA rescue therapy was studied in a group of kidney and liver transplant recipients who were unable to tolerate tacrolimus. The initial dose of CSA was based on organ function, tacrolimus levels, and the reason for tacrolimus intolerance and generally began 24 hours after tacrolimus was discontinued. Symptoms improved or resolved in more than 70% of patients within 3 months of conversion to CSA. However, 27% of patients who were switched to CSA experienced an episode of acute rejection.[29] Jain and colleagues[30] reported similar results with a 39% rejection rate but noted that many patients were able to be converted back to tacrolimus without recurrence of the original complication.

Adverse Effects

The adverse effects of CSA and other immunosuppressants are summarized in Table 87–4. The magnitude of adverse effects is often related to the dose and duration of exposure to CSA. Neurotoxicity typically manifests as tremors, headache, and peripheral neuropathy but can be as severe as seizures. Nephrotoxicity is displayed as increased serum creatinine concentration, decreased glomerular filtration rate, and hyperkalemia. Hypertension can be uncontrollable and may warrant drug discontinuation in some cases. Often, additional drug therapy is required to manage the adverse effects of CSA. Cosmetic changes such as hirsutism and gingival hyperplasia often are managed by converting from CSA to tacrolimus or by proper hygiene in patients who cannot be switched to tacrolimus.

Drug-Drug and Drug-Food Interactions

Drug interactions occur frequently with CSA since it extensively metabolized by CYP 3A4 in both the gut and the liver. CSA is also a substrate for p-glycoprotein, which contributes to its drug interactions.[31,32] Inhibition of CYP 3A4 by drugs such as diltiazem or ketoconazole can increase drug concentrations significantly, whereas induction by drugs such as phenytoin or rifampin can decrease drug concentrations significantly. Some centers take advantage of these interactions by routinely using CSA-sparing agents to reduce the dosage and cost of therapy while maintaining the same therapeutic concentrations.[33]

While most drug interactions with CSA result from the effects of the CYP 3A4 on CSA, it is important to remember that CSA is also an inhibitor of CYP 3A4 (Table 87–5). The inhibitory effects of CSA on CYP 3A4 can be seen with weaker substrates, such as the HMG-CoA reductase inhibitors. Concomitant administration of CSA with HMG-CoA reductase inhibitors results in an increase in the HMG-CoA reductase inhibitor levels, which increases the risk of HMG-CoA reductase inhibitor adverse effects, most notably myopathy.[35] Myopathy associated with this reaction usually is reversible with discontinuation of the HMG-CoA reductase inhibitor.

Consistency in administration of CSA with regard to meals and food intake is important to minimize alterations in CSA absorption and pharmacokinetics. High-fat meals can enhance both plasma clearance and the volume of distribution by more than 60%.[36] Grapefruit juice increases CSA concentrations significantly. Furancoumarins found in grapefruit juice, such as quercetin, naringin, and bergamottin, are potent inhibitors of CYP 3A4. The area under the concentration-time curve (AUC) and C_{max} of CSA have been reported to be increased by more than 55%, and CSA peak concentration levels were 35% higher when CSA was taken with grapefruit juice.[37] Commonly administered drugs which are known to result in clinically significant alterations of CSA levels are listed in Table 87–6.

Dosing and Administration

Initiation of oral CSA therapy generally begins with a dose of 8–18 mg/kg per day divided into two doses administered every 12 hours. Higher CSA doses are used more commonly in two-drug regimens, whereas lower doses are part of triple-drug regimens. Some immunosuppressive strategies use lower doses of CSA (e.g., 1 to 3 mg/kg per day) until day 3 or 4 to decrease potential nephrotoxicity in the immediate postoperative period. Since the risk for acute rejection decreases with time, oral CSA doses are reduced and may be as low as 3 to 5 mg/kg per day or less during maintenance therapy. If oral administration is not possible, CSA may be administered intravenously at one-third the oral dosage, usually 2 to 5 mg/kg per day.

CSA is excreted in the bile and is nephrotoxic; therefore, dosage adjustments should be made when hepatic dysfunction is present.

TABLE 87–5. Substrates, Inducers and Inhibitors of Cytochrome P450 (CYP) Enzymes

CYP1A	CYP2C	CYP2D6		CYP3A	
Substrates	*Substrates*	*Substrates*		*Substrates*	
Acetaminophen	Amitriptyline	Amitriptyline	Thioridazine	ABT-378	Lovastatin
Amitriptyline	Benzphetamine	Bufuralol	Timolol	Alfentanil	Mephenytoin
Antipyrine	Celecoxib	Captopril	Tramadol	Alprazolam	Methadone
Caffeine	Citalopram	Carvedilol	Trazodone	Amiodarone	Miconazole
Chlorotriansene	Clomipramine	Citalopram	Triazolam	Amlodipine	Midazolam
Chlorzoxazone	Cyclophosphamide	Chlorpheniramine	Trifluperidol	Antipyrine	Nefazodone
Clarithromycin	Dapsone	Chlorpromazine	Trimipramine	Astemizole	Nelfinavir
Clomipramine	Diazepam	Clomipramine	Venlafaxine	Atorvastatin	Nicardipine
Clozapine	Diclofenac	Clozapine	Vinblastine	Benzphetamine	Nifedipine
Cyclobenzaprine	Ethosuximide	Codeine	Zonisamide	Buspirone	Nisoldipine
Dantrolene	Fluoxetine	Debrisoquine		Caffeine	Nitrendipine
Diethylstilbestrol	Fluvastatin	Desipramine		Carbamazepine	Omeprazole
Estradiol	Glipizide	Dextromethorphan		Cerivastatin	Ondansetron
Flutamine	Glyburide	Doxepin		Chlorpheniramine	Paclitaxel
Fluvoxamine	Hexobarbital	Encainide		Chlorpromazine	Paracetamol
Haloperidol	Ibuprofen	Ethylmorphine		Cisapride	Pimozide
Imipramine	Imipramine	Flecainide		Clarithromycin	Prednisone
Lidocaine	Indomethacin	Fluoxetine		Cocaine	Progesterone
Methadone	Irbesartan	Fluvoxamine		Cortisol	Propranolol
Mexiletine	Lansoprazole	Fluphenazine		Cyclophosphamide	Quinidine
Naproxen	Losartan	Haloperidol		Cyclosporine	R-warfarin
Olanzapine	Mephenytoin	Imipramine		Dantrolene	Ritonavir
Ondansetron	Naproxen	Indoramin		Dapsone	Saquinavir
Paracetamol	Nelfinavir	Labetolol		Delavirdine	Sertraline
Paraxathine	Nifedipine	Lidocaine		Dextromethorphan	Sildenafil
Phenacetin	Omeprazole	Maprotiline		Diazepam	Simvastatin
Procarbazine	Pantoprazole	R-methadone		Digitoxin	Sirolimus
Propafenone	Phenylbutazone	Metoclopramide		Diltiazem	Tacrolimus
Propranolol	Phenytoin	Metoprolol		Disopyramide	Tamoxifen
Prostaglandins	Piroxicam	Mexiletine		Enalapril	Taxol
R-warfarin	Primidone	Morphine		Erythromycin	Terfenadine
Ritonavir	Progesterone	Nelfinavir		Estradiol	Testosterone
Ropivicaine	Proguanil	Nortriptyline		Estrogen	Trazodone
Tacrine	Propranolol	Omeprazole		Ethosuximide	Triazolam
Tamoxifen	Ritonavir	Ondansetron		Ethylmorphine	Verapamil
Theobromine	Rosiglitazone	Paroxetine		Etoposide	Vinblastine
Theophylline	S,R-warfarin	Perphenazine		Felodipine	Vincristine
Toltrazuril	Sulfinpyrazone	Phenformin		Fentanyl	Zaleplon
Verapamil	Sullfaphenazole	Propafenone		Finasteride	Zolpidem
Zileuton	Sulfonamides	Propranolol		Flutamide	
Zolmitriptan	Tamoxifen	Quinidine		Gleevec	
	Taxol	Retinoic acid		Haloperidol	
	Tenoxicam	Risperidone		Hydrocortisone	
	Testosterone	Ritonavir		Indinavir	
	Tetrahydrocannabinol	RU486		Irinotecan	
	Tolbutamide	Sparteine		Itraconazole	
	Torsemide	Tamoxifen		Ketoconazole	
	Tricyclics	Taxol		Lidocaine	
	Trimethadione	Teniposide		Lopinavir	
	Valproic acid	Testosterone		Loratidine	
Inducers	*Inducers*	*Inducers*		*Inducers*	
Broccoli	For CYP2C9/10:	**Dexamethasone**		Carbamazepine	
Brussels sprouts	**Dexamethasone**	Rifampin		Dexamethasone	
Charbroiled food	Phenobarbital			DMP-266	
Cigarette smoke	Rifampicin			Isoniazid	
Cruciferous	For CYP2C19:			Nevirapine	
vegetables	**Carbamazepine**			Phenobarbital	
Insulin	Prednisone			Phenytoin	
Modafinil	Rifampin			Prednisone	
Omeprazole				Rifabutin/rifampicin	
Phenobarbital					
Phenytoin					
Tobacco					

TABLE 87-5. (Continued)

CYP1A	CYP2C	CYP2D6	CYP3A	
Inhibitors	*Inhibitors*	*Inhibitors*	*Inhibitors*	
Amiodarone	Amiodarone (2C9/10)	Amiodarone	Amiodarone	Saquinavir
Cimetidine	Chloramphenicol	Bupropion	Chloramphenicol	Sertraline
Enoxacin	Cimetidine	Celecoxib	Cimetidine	Verapamil
Fluvoxamine	Disulfiram	Chlorpromazine	Ciprofloxacin	
Nalidixic acid	Fluconazole	Chlorpheniramine	Clarithromycin	
Norfloxacin	Fluoxetine	Cimetidine	Clotrimazole	
Ticlopidine	Fluvastatin	Clomipramine	Delavirdine	
	Fluvoxamine	Cocaine	Diltiazem	
	Indomethacin	Desipramine	Erythromycin	
	Isoniazid	Doxorubicin	Fluconazole	
	Ketoconazole (2C9/10)	Fluoxetine	Fluoxetine	
	Lansoprazole	Fluvoxamine	Fluvoxamine	
	Lovastatin	Haloperidol	Grapefruit juice	
	Modafinil	Metoclopramide	Indinavir	
	Omeprazole (2C9/10)	Methadone	Itraconazole	
	Paroxetine	Mibefradil	Ketoconazole	
	Probenacid	Moclobemide	Lopinavir	
	Ritonavir	Norfluoxetine	Miconazole	
	Sertraline	Paroxetine	Nefazodone	
	Sulfamethoxazole	Perphenazine	Nelfinavir	
	Teniposide	Quinidine	Nifedipine	
	Ticlopidine	Ranitidine	Norfloxacin	
	Topiramate	Ritonavir	Omeprazole	
	Trimethoprim	Sertraline	Paroxetine	
	Zafirlukast	Terbinafine	Propoxyphene	
		Thioridazine	Ritonavir	

Liver transplant recipients with T-tube diversion of bile require increased doses because of decreased absorption. Children require higher doses of CSA to maintain therapeutic drug concentrations, up to 14 to 18 mg/kg per day.

CSA blood concentrations are measured routinely in an attempt to optimize therapy. Radioimmunoassay (RIA) and fluorescence polarization immunoassay are the most commonly used methods; however, high-performance liquid chromatography (HPLC) is recognized as the reference procedure.[38] It is important to determine which assay methodology the laboratory is using because target ranges vary between nonspecific (which quantitates parent plus metabolite concentration, such as RIA) and specific (which quantitates parent CSA, such as HPLC using mass spectrometry) assays. The therapeutic range for whole-blood RIA is 375 to 400 ng/mL versus 100 to 300 ng/mL

TABLE 87-6. Effect of Concomitant Drug Administration on Cyclosporine, Tacrolimus and Sirolimus[a]

Cyclosporine Levels		Tacrolimus Levels		Sirolimus Levels	
Increase[b]	*Decrease[c]*	*Increase[b]*	*Decrease[c]*	*Increase[b]*	*Decrease[c]*
Ketoconazole	Rifampicin	Ketoconazole	Rifampin	Ketoconazole	Rifampin
Fluconazole	Phenytoin	Fluconazole	Dexamethasone	Fluconazole	Phenytoin
Itraconazole	Phenobarbital	Itraconazole	Phenytoin	Erythromycin	
Erythromycin	Carbamazepine	Voriconazole		Clarithromycin	
Diltiazem	Sulfadimidine	Erythromycin		Diltiazem	
Verapamil	Trimethoprim	Diltiazem		Verapamil	
Danazol		Verapamil		Cyclosporine	
Nicardipine		Danazol		Protease inhibitors	
Metoclopramide		Cimetidine			
Methylprednisolone		Omeprazole			
Norethisterone		Clotrimazole			
Sirolimus		Nefazodone			
Tacrolimus		Corticosteroids			
Protease inhibitors		Cyclosporine			
		Basiliximab			
		Protease inhibitors			

[a]This is not a complete list of all drug interactions.
[b]Medications known to inhibit the cytochrome P450 3A4 enzyme system can increase levels of cyclosporine, tacrolimus, and sirolimus.
[c]Medications known to induce the cytochrome P450 3A4 enzyme system can decrease levels of cyclosporine, tacrolimus, and sirolimus.
From refs. 31,32,33, and 34.

for HPLC. In serum or plasma, the therapeutic range for RIA or HPLC is 150 to 250 ng/mL and 75 to 150 ng/mL, respectively.

The most common and practical method of CSA monitoring is the measurement of trough blood concentrations. CSA trough concentrations are measured frequently (daily or three times per week) following initiation of the drug and during the stabilization period after transplantation. However, studies have revealed lack of predictive value of trough concentrations and rejection.[39] Alternative strategies have been proposed to better correlate CSA levels with rejection. Proposed strategies include pharmacokinetic profiling to determine the area under the concentration curve and peak concentration, which are suggested to correlate with graft function.[40] AUC monitoring can be problematic because of the need for sequential CSA levels throughout the dosing interval. Limited sampling techniques using two to five blood samples within the first 4 hours after an oral dose have been used. AUC levels >440 mcg/L per hour have been shown to correlate with rejection.[40] Peak concentrations measured 2 hours after an oral dose (C_2) have been shown to have a better predictive value in terms of rejection compared with trough concentrations.[39] Some transplant centers have adopted this strategy to manage CSA levels because of the convenience of a single blood sample. The suggested therapeutic range for C_2 CSA levels is 1.5 to 2 mcg/mL for the first few months after transplant and 0.8 mcg/mL after 6 to 12 months.[40,41]

TACROLIMUS (TAC)

TAC is a macrolide antibiotic with immunosuppressive activity via inhibition of calcineurin. It was thought originally that TAC may decrease the risk of chronic allograft rejection, but experience has demonstrated that this is not the case. However, it should be noted that up to this point, TAC traditionally has been used in high-risk patients. Today, TAC is used more commonly than CSA by most transplant centers in all transplant patients, regardless of risk category.

Pharmacology/Mechanism of Action

TAC inhibits T-cell activity by inhibiting the production of IL-2 and other cytokines by T cells (See Fig. 87–1). TAC binds to a cytoplasmic immunophilin called *FK-binding protein-12* (FKBP12). Like CSA, the TAC-FKBP12 complex inhibits calcineurin, ultimately inhibiting NF-AT and the transcription of cytokines necessary for T-cell activity, most notably IL-2.

Pharmacokinetics

TAC is a highly lipophilic compound; however, it does not rely on bile for absorption. Following oral administration, the bioavailability of TAC ranges from 5% to 67%, with a mean of 29%.[42] FKBP12 is found in high concentrations in red blood cells, which causes extensive binding of TAC to erythrocytes. TAC is also metabolized primarily by CYP 3A4, although other cytochrome P450 enzymes have been reported.[42] The elimination half-life of TAC is 8.7 hours. Increased metabolism in children results in a shorter half-life.

Efficacy

Currently, TAC is approved for use in kidney and liver transplants. However, it has been studied extensively and is used widely in all types of solid-organ transplants. Studies comparing CSA with TAC

as primary immunosuppression demonstrate equal efficacy of the two agents in kidney, liver, and heart transplants.

The potency and effectiveness of TAC have prompted studies to investigate withdrawal of corticosteroids or other concomitant immunosuppressants. A large randomized, controlled trial compared triple-drug therapy, consisting of TAC, corticosteroids, and mycophenolate mofetil, with early withdrawal of corticosteroids or mycophenolate in kidney transplant recipients. The results demonstrated equal efficacy in the three arms with no difference in acute rejection rate after 6 months of therapy.[43] Furthermore, TAC has demonstrated equal efficacy to CSA, each in combination with azathioprine, with regard to corticosteroid withdrawal.[44]

Adverse Effects

The adverse effects associated with TAC include neurologic toxicity, nephrotoxicity, and electrolyte disturbances such as hyperkalemia and hypomagnesemia[42] (see Table 87–4). The incidence of post-transplant diabetes is approximately 8% to 10% but is often reversible when doses of TAC and/or steroids are reduced.[45] As observed with CSA, most adverse effects related to TAC improve with dosage reduction or discontinuation.

In comparison with CSA, TAC may be associated with increased occurrence of neurologic complications, including tremor, paresthesias, headache, and insomnia. On the contrary, TAC is associated with less hypercholesterolemia and hypertension.[45–47] The occurrence of nephrotoxocity appears to be similar to CSA. TAC also has been reported to cause alopecia, which is usually self-limiting and reversible.

Drug-Drug and Drug-Food Interactions

Because of their common metabolic pathways, CSA and TAC share the same drug interaction profile (see Table 87–6). CYP 3A4 inhibitors increase TAC concentrations, whereas CYP 3A4 inducers decrease blood levels. One distinct drug interaction with TAC that differs from CSA is an interaction with antacids. In vitro data suggest that drugs that increase the pH of the gastrointestinal tract, such as magnesium-aluminum- or calcium-containing antacids, sodium bicarbonate, and magnesium oxide, can cause a pH-mediated degradation of TAC or physical adsorption to TAC in the gastrointestinal tract.[48,49] Such compounds should be separated from TAC administration by at least 2 hours to prevent the physical interaction.

Reversible myopathy has been reported with concomitant administration of TAC with HMG-CoA reductase inhibitors.[50] TAC is also an inhibitor of CYP 3A4 but much weaker than CSA.[51] The number of reported cases of myopathy with HMG-CoA reductase inhibitors in patients treated with TAC is fewer than with CSA. Nonetheless, patients should be monitored for clinical signs of myopathy when receiving HMG-CoA reductase inhibitors in combination with TAC.

It is also important to maintain consistency with administration of TAC with regard to meals and food intake to minimize alterations in TAC absorption and pharmacokinetics. One study in healthy volunteers indicates that the C_{max}, AUC, and t_{max} of TAC were significantly higher when administered after a 10-hour fast compared with either a high-fat or low-fat/high-carbohydrate meal. Administration of TAC with food decreased C_{max} by 77% for the high-fat meal and 64.7% for the low-fat meal. AUC also was decreased by 33.5% and 26.1%, respectively, and t_{max} was increased 4.72- and 2.34-fold, respectively. The authors concluded that food reduces both the rate and extent of TAC absorption and that a high-fat meal may further delay gastric mptying, further reducing TAC concentrations.[52] As with CSA, rapefruit juice also significantly increases TAC concentrations.

Dosing and Administration

initial intravenous TAC doses range from 0.05 to 0.1 mg/kg per day and are administered by continuous infusion. Oral doses range from .1 to 0.3 mg/kg per day given in two divided doses every 12 hours. AC doses are then adjusted according to trough blood levels, clinical response, and adverse effects. A review of the role of TAC in renal ransplantation suggests that target 12-hour whole-blood trough concentrations are 15 to 20 ng/mL (0 to 1 month after transplantation), 0 to 15 ng/mL (1 to 3 months after transplantation), and 5 to 12 ng/mL >3 months after transplantation).[44] Because TAC is highly bound to ed blood cells, plasma levels are much lower than whole blood concentrations. Therapeutic plasma levels of TAC range from 0.5 to 2 g/mL. Pediatric transplant patients clear the drug more rapidly and equire doses two- to fourfold higher than adults on a milligram per ilogram basis to maintain equivalent therapeutic concentrations. A nodified release formulation of TAC that will allow for once-daily dministration is currently in phase III clinical trials.

CALCINEURIN INHIBITOR NEPHROTOXICITY

One of the most common side effects observed in all transplant recipients receiving maintenance CSA or TAC therapy is ephrotoxicity. Two types of toxicity can occur. Acute nephrotoxicity frequently is seen early and is dose-dependent and reversible, ut chronic nephropathy is more common. Clinical manifestations of CI nephrotoxicity include elevated serum creatinine and blood urea itrogen levels, hyperkalemia, hyperuricemia, mild proteinuria, and decreased fractional excretion of sodium. CI nephrotoxicity is rec-gnized as the leading cause of renal dysfunction following nonrenal olid-organ transplant. One study looked at more than 69,000 liver, eart, lung, and intestinal transplant recipients and found a combined ncidence of 16.5% of newly diagnosed chronic renal failure after a nean follow-up of 46 months. A total of 28.9% of these patients with hronic renal failure went on to develop ESRD, requiring dialysis or kidney transplant. Patients with no history of CI use had a lower elative risk of developing nephropathy compared with those who did eceive CI. Furthermore, CSA was associated with a higher risk of leveloping nephropathy compared with TAC (RR 1.25, $p < 0.001$).[53]

The predominant mechanism for CI nephrotoxicity is renal vaso-constriction, primarily of the afferent arteriole, resulting in increased renal vascular resistance, decreased renal blood flow by up to 40%, re-duced glomerular filtration rate by up to 30%, and increased proximal tubular sodium reabsorption with a reduction in urinary sodium and potassium excretion. A number of other mechanisms have been impli-cated, including changes in the renin-angiotensin-aldosterone system, prostaglandin synthesis, nitrous oxide production, sympathetic ner-vous system activation, and calcium handling.[54]

Measures to reduce CI nephrotoxicity include delaying adminis-tration immediately postoperatively in patients at high risk for nephro-toxicity (using alternative induction protocols including an IL-2 re-ceptor antagonist or antilymphocyte globulin), monitoring CI trough blood levels and reducing the CI dosage if the vasoconstrictive ef-fects are problematic, and avoiding other nephrotoxins (e.g., amino-glycosides, amphotericin B, and NSAIDs) when possible. When us-ing these agents, drug concentrations of CI and those of the other drugs, if available, should be monitored closely. In addition, the con-comitant administration of drugs known to elevate CI levels requires intentional dosage reductions to avoid unnecessary renal and other toxicity[31] (see Table 87–6). Currently, no proven therapies consis-tently prevent or reverse the nephrotoxic effects of CSA; however, a number of agents have been studied, including prostaglandin ana-logues, pentoxyphylline, and fish oils.[55]

In kidney transplants, it is often difficult to differentiate CI nephrotoxicity from renal allograft rejection. Because the clini-cal features of acute renal allograft rejection and CI nephrotoxicity may overlap considerably, a renal biopsy continues to be the diagnos-tic "gold standard" (Table 87–7). However, differentiating between chronic renal allograft rejection and CI nephrotoxicity may be more difficult because, in addition to clinical signs and symptoms, biopsy findings also may be similar.

CLINICAL CONTROVERSY

Although CIs are the mainstay of immunosuppressive pro-tocols, some clinicians attempt to use CI-sparing protocols to avoid the significant adverse effects associated with CIs. Others will delay the initiation of CIs to avoid the dose-related adverse effects associated with early use of CIs post-transplantation.

GLUCOCORTICOIDS

Corticosteroids have been used since the beginning of the mod-ern transplantation era. Despite their many adverse events, they

TABLE 87–7. Differential Diagnosis of Acute Rejection and CSA or TAC Nephrotoxicity

	Acute Rejection	CSA or TAC Nephrotoxicity
History	Often <4 weeks postoperatively	Often >6 weeks postoperatively
Clinical	Fever	Afebrile
presentation	Hypertension	Hypertension
	Weight gain	Graft nontender
	Graft swelling/tenderness	Good urine output
	Decreased daily urine volume	
Laboratory	Rapid rise in serum Cr (0.3 mg/dL/day)	Gradual rise in serum Cr (>0.15 mg/dL/day)
Biopsy	Normal CSA or TAC concentration	Elevated CSA or TAC concentration
	Interstitial lymphocytic infiltrates	Interstitial fibrosis, tubular atrophy, glomerular thrombosis, arterial inflammation

CSA = cyclosporine; TAC = tacrolimus; Cr = creatinine.

continue to be a cornerstone of immunosuppression regimens in many transplant centers. The most commonly used corticosteroids in transplantation are methylprednisolone and prednisone.

PHARMACOLOGY/MECHANISM OF ACTION

Corticosteroids block cytokine activation by binding to glucocorticoid response elements, thereby inhibiting IL-1, -2, -3, and -6, γ-interferon, and tumor necrosis factor α (TNF-α) synthesis (See Fig. 87–1). Additionally, steroids interfere with cell migration, recognition, and cytotoxic effector mechanisms.[56]

PHARMACOKINETICS

Prednisone is converted to active prednisolone in the body and has multiple effects on the immune system. Prednisone is very well absorbed from the gastrointestinal (GI) tract and has a long biologic half-life, so it can be dosed once daily.

EFFICACY

Animal models of transplantation in the 1950's and 1960's used steroids empirically in combination with azathioprine.[57] Steroids subsequently became a part of the immunosuppressive regimens used in the first human transplants[58] and continue to be used in immunosuppressive protocols today. The efficacy of steroids is irrefutable based on the decades of clinical experience. Systematic studies comparing steroid-free immunosuppressive agent combinations with conventional therapy are difficult to perform due to the hundreds of potential combinations that now exist. However, recent studies of steroid-free immunosuppressive agent combinations with newer, more specific immunosuppressants suggests that steroids may in the future have less of a role in maintenance immunosuppression.[43,44]

ADVERSE EFFECTS

Adverse effects of prednisone that occur in more than 10% of patients include increased appetite, insomnia, indigestion (bitter taste), and mood changes. Side effects that occur less commonly but which are seen with high doses or prolonged therapy include cataracts, hyperglycemia, hirsutism, bruising, acne, sodium and water retention, hypertension, bone growth suppression, and ulcerative esophagitis (see Table 87–4).

DRUG-DRUG AND DRUG-FOOD INTERACTIONS

Barbiturates, phenytoin, and rifampin induce hepatic metabolism of prednisone and thus decrease the effectiveness of prednisone. Prednisone decreases the effectiveness of vaccines and toxoids.[56]

DOSING AND ADMINISTRATION

An intravenous corticosteroid, commonly high-dose methylprednisolone, is given during the perioperative period. The dose of methylprednisolone is tapered rapidly and discontinued within days and oral prednisone is initiated. Prednisone doses are tapered progressively over time depending on the type of additional immunosuppression and organ function. As doses are tapered, it is preferable to administer steroids every other day and between 7 and 8 A.M. to mimic the body diurnal release of cortisol. Although conversion to alternate-day regimens or complete withdrawal of prednisone in patients with stable posttransplant courses has been used with success in some transplant centers, steroids often are continued for the entire life of the functioning graft. Long-term steroid use and its associated deleterious effects are well recognized and particularly troublesome in transplant patients (see Table 87–4).

The first-line therapy for the treatment of acute graft rejection is high-dose intravenous methylprednisolone (250 to 1000 mg) daily for 3 days or oral prednisone (200 mg). Doses of oral prednisone are then tapered over 5 days to 20 mg/day. Prednisone should be taken with food to minimize GI upset. The dose of prednisone varies with the transplant center's protocol but usually is highest immediately following transplant and during treatment for acute rejection. It is becoming frequent practice to taper prednisone with the goal of discontinuation over a period of months. Corticosteroids never should be discontinued abruptly; tapering should be gradual because of suppression of the hypothalamic-pituitary-adrenal axis. Corticosteroids slow the growth rates in children, prompting clinicians to use alternate-day dosing or to withhold steroids until rejection occurs.

Because of the many detrimental effects associated with chronic steroid therapy, dose minimization has been the goal of therapy. The availability of CSA, TAC, and mycophenolate mofetil has permitted complete withdrawal of corticosteroids in some patients. Steroid withdrawal protocols use either a rapid taper of steroids within days of the transplant or a slower taper, whereby patients are weaned gradually from steroids over months to years after transplant. Factors to consider when evaluating studies of these alternative strategies in transplant patients include patient selection criteria, timing and rapidity of withdrawal, and duration of follow-up.

ANTIPROLIFERATIVE AGENTS

MYCOPHENOLATE MOFETIL (MMF)

Mycophenolic acid (MPA) was first isolated from the *Penicillium glaucum* mold. It was first studied as an antibiotic but later was found to have immunosuppressive properties. Mycophenolate mofetil (MMF) the morpholinoethyl ester of MPA appears to be a specific immunosuppressant for lymphocytes, resulting in fewer adverse effects than azathioprine, making it the preferred agent over azathioprine.

Pharmacology/Mechanism of Action

MMF is rapidly and completely converted to MPA by first-pass metabolism. MPA exerts its immunosuppressive effect through noncompetitive binding to inosine monophosphate dehydrogenase (IMPDH). IMPDH is the key enzyme responsible for guanosine nucleotide synthesis via the de novo pathway. Inhibition of IMPDH results in decreased nucleotide synthesis and diminished DNA polymerase activity, ultimately reducing lymphocyte proliferation.[59] The actions of MPA are more specific for T and B cells, which use only the de novo pathway for nucleotide synthesis (see Fig. 87–1). Other cells within the body have a salvage pathway by which they can synthesize nucleotides, making them less susceptible to the action of MPA and thereby reducing, but not eliminating, the potential for the hematologic adverse effects seen with azathioprine, which affect both the de novo and salvage pathways. In addition to the decreasing mphocyte proliferation, MPA also may downregulate activation of mphocytes.[60]

Pharmacokinetics

ollowing oral administration, bioavailability of MMF is 94%, and ak concentrations of MPA are reached within 1 hour. A total of 97% MPA is bound to albumin in the blood. MPA is eliminated by the dney and also undergoes glucuronidation in the liver to an inactive ucuronide metabolite (MPAG) that is excreted in the bile and urine. nterohepatic cycling of MPAG can undergo deconjugation, thereby circulating MPA into the bloodstream. The half-life of MPA is 3 hours.

Efficacy

urrently, MMF is approved for use in kidney, liver, and heart trans- ants. A recent analysis of 5599 patients in the Joint International ociety for Heart and Lung Transplantation (ISHLT) and UNOS horacic Registry showed a statistically significant survival advan- ge for MMF compared with azathioprine (1 year, 96% versus 93%; years, 91% versus 86%).[61] Efficacy has been demonstrated in com- ination with both CSA and TAC.

MMF also has demonstrated efficacy in the treatment of acute ejection. Kidney transplant recipients converted to MMF after the rst acute rejection episode had fewer subsequent rejections compared ith those who continued with azathioprine after rejection treatment. he change in therapy was associated with no increase in adverse ffects or malignancies and a trend toward better graft function and urvival.[62]

Monotherapy with MMF can decrease the risk of nephrotoxicity ssociated with CIs. Clinical trials have evaluated the benefits of CI ithdrawal from MMF-based immunosuppression in stable kidney nd liver transplants. Withdrawal of CIs resulted in improved renal unction and lower blood pressure, lipid, and uric acid levels. These enefits, however, were offset by an unacceptable increase in organ ejection in all the studies.[63–65] Monotherapy with MMF generally is ot used in clinical practice.

Adverse Effects

Jnlike CSA and TAC, MMF is not associated with nephrotoxicity, eurotoxicity, or hypertension. GI side effects such as nausea, vomit- ng, diarrhea, and abdominal pain, however, occur more frequently in MMF-treated patients compared with those receiving azathioprine or lacebo[66] (see Table 87–4). In addition, GI symptoms occur with simi- ar frequency during intravenous and oral therapy. Clinically, however, ose reduction, dividing the total daily dose into three, administration ith food, and upward titration from lower doses during initial therapy ay alleviate some of these GI symptoms. MMF also has hemato- ogic effects resulting in leukopenia and anemia, particularly with igher doses. Tissue-invasive cytomegalovirus (CMV) also was more ommon in MMF-treated patients,[66] although this may be related to ifferenes in the use of CMV prophylaxis within the studies. Ma- gnancy and post-transplant lymphoproliferative disease (PTLD) are f significant concern with greater amounts of immunosuppression. onger follow-up of patients receiving MMF is required to charac- rize the lifelong risk of malignancy. Because peripheral intravenous MMF administration is associated with local edema and inflamma- on, central venous administration may be the preferred route.

Drug-Drug and Drug-Food Interactions

Food delays the absorption and decreases MPA C_{max} by 25% but has no effect on MPA AUC. As a result, prescribing information indicates that MMF should be taken on an empty stomach; however, MMF is often given with food in clinical practice to minimize GI adverse effects. Administration with aluminum- and magnesium-containing antacids or cholestyramine, significantly decreases the AUC of MPA and should be avoided.[59] It has been suggested that administration of iron may produce similar results, but this has not been tested.

Acyclovir, commonly used in renal transplant recipients for the treatment and prevention of viral infections, competes with MPAG for renal tubular secretion. $AUCs$ of both entities are increased with concomitant acyclovir and MMF administration.[59] Single-dose intra- venous ganciclovir in combination with MMF produced no change in the disposition of ganciclovir, MPA, or MPAG.[67] Although no pharmacokinetic interaction in a single-dose study was demonstrated, there is potential for additive pharmacodynamic effects such as bone marrow suppression.

Decreased MPA trough concentrations have been reported when MMF is administered with CSA compared with those achieved when MMF is given with TAC or sirolimus. This interaction is most likely due to CSA interference with the enterohepatic recycling of MPAG, which results in decreased MPA concentrations.[68] To achieve equiv- alent MPA and MPAG concentrations, it is necessary to administer MMF 3 g/day with CSA compared with MMF 2 g/day with TAC.

Dosing and Administration

MMF is currently available in both oral and intravenous formulations. Although intravenous administration of equal doses closely mimics oral administration, the two cannot be considered bioequivalent.[69] Unlike other immunosuppressive agents, there is no compelling in- dication that MMF should be dosed in adult patients on a milligram per kilogram basis given the weak correlation between MPA AUC and body weight.[59] The dose of MMF for optimizing immunosuppression and minimizing adverse effects is 2 g/day administered in two divided doses given every 12 hours. The dose of MMF in heart transplantation is 3 g/day in two divided doses to achieve the necessary higher levels of immunosuppression. Pediatric doses of MMF are approximately 40 mg/kg per day in two doses. The total daily dose may be separated into three or four dosing intervals if patients are unable to tolerate the GI side effects.

With regard to therapeutic drug monitoring, plasma appears to be the most appropriate medium for measuring MPA. Better outcomes are associated with MPA AUC levels of greater than 42.8 mcg/mL per hour (by HPLC)[70] although a reference range of 30 to 60 mcg/mL per hour has been proposed.[71] However, the correlation between MPA AUC levels and adverse effects is low. Further studies are required to determine the best modality to monitor MPA levels (AUC versus trough concentrations), the acceptable targets for each, and the ap- propriate strategy to monitor MPA levels.[70,71]

MYCOPHENOLATE SODIUM

Mycophenolate sodium is an enteric-coated formulation of the sodium salt of mycophenolic acid designed to reduce the GI side effects of MMF. This formulation allows for mycophenolic acid to be released directly in the small intestine for absorption rather than in the stomach. Because mycophenolic acid is the activated form of MMF, the actions are identical between the two. Likewise, the adverse effects are similar between the two, including the incidence of GI toxicity, despite the enteric coating. Clinical trials have demonstrated similary efficacy between MMF and mycophenolate sodium in kidney transplants both immediately following transplantation[72] and in patients who were switched from MMF to mycophenolate sodium.[73] Mycophenolate sodium 1.44 g/day is therapeutically equivalent to MMF 2 g/day.[74]

AZATHIOPRINE

Azathioprine, a prodrug for 6-mercaptopurine, has been used as an immunosuppressant in combination with glucocorticoids since the earliest days of the modern transplant era. It is associated with substantial toxicities, however, and its use has dramatically declined with the availability of newer, less toxic immunosuppressants.

Pharmacology/Mechanism of Action

Azathioprine is an inactive compound that is converted rapidly to 6-mercaptopurine (6-MP) in the blood and is subsequently metabolized by three different enzymes. Xanthine oxidase (XO), found in the liver and GI tract, converts 6-MP to the inactive final end product, 6-thiouric acid. Thiopurine methyltransferase (TPMT), found in hematopoietic tissues and red blood cells, methylates 6-MP to an inactive product, 6-methylmercaptopurine. Finally, hypoxanthine-guanine phophoribosyltransferase (HGPRT) is the first step responsible for converting 6-MP to 6-thioguanine nucleotides (TGNs), the active metabolites, which are incorporated into nucleic acids, ultimately disrupting both the salvage and de novo pathways of DNA, RNA, and protein synthesis. This process is toxic to the cell and renders the cell unable to proliferate (see Fig. 87–1). TGNs eventually are catabolized by XO and TPMT to inactive products.

Pharmacokinetics

Oral bioavailability of azathioprine is approximately 40%. Metabolism of 6-MP is primarily by xanthine oxidase to inactive metabolites, which are excreted by the kidneys. The half-life of azathioprine, the parent compound, is very short, approximately 12 minutes. The half-life of 6-MP is longer, ranging from 0.7 to 3 hours. However, it is the activity of the TGNs that determines the pharmacodynamic half-life of the drug. The half-life of TGNs has been estimated to be 9 days once therapy has been stopped.[75]

Adverse Effects

Dose-limiting adverse effects of azathioprine are often hematologic (see Table 87–4). Leukopenia, anemia, and thrombocytopenia can occur within the first few weeks of therapy and can be managed by dose reduction or discontinuation of azathioprine. Other common adverse effects include nausea and vomiting, which can be minimized by taking azathioprine with food. Alopecia, hepatotoxicity and pancreatitis are less common adverse effects of azathioprine; they generally are reversible on dose reduction or discontinuation.[26]

Drug-Drug and Drug-Food Interactions

Allopurinol inhibits xanthine oxidase and can increase the bioavailability of azathioprine and 6-MP concentrations by as much as fourfold. The metabolic pathways shift to favor production of TGNs which ultimately results in increased bone marrow suppression and panctopenia. Doses of azathioprine should be reduced by 50% to 75% wh allopurinol is added. Additional clinically significant drug interactic include other bone marrow–suppressing agents such as gancicloy sulfamethoxazole-trimethoprim, and sirolimus and other drugs tl irritate the GI tract.

Dosing and Administration

Initial doses of azathioprine are 3 to 5 mg/kg per day intravenous or orally. Individualization to maintain the white blood cell cou between 3500 and 6000 cells/mm may be accomplished in some w doses as low as 0.25 mg/kg per day.[3] Patients often are instructed take azathioprine in the evening when initiating or titrating therapy allow for dose adjustments based on morning determinations of th white blood cell count.

SIROLIMUS (SRL)

Sirolimus (SRL), also known as rapamycin, is another immun suppressive macrolide antibiotic that is structurally similar TAC. It represents the first in the newest class of immunosuppre sants, with a unique mechanism of action. The potential of SRL decrease the incidence of chronic rejection remains to be seen.

PHARMACOLOGY/MECHANISM OF ACTION

The mechanism of action of SRL is distinct from CSA or TAC. SR binds to FKBP12, but the resulting complex does not inhibit the a tivity of calcineurin. Whereas CSA and TAC inhibit cytokine pr duction, SRL appears to inhibit the response to these cytokines. Tl SRL-FKBP12 complex binds to the mammalian target of rapamyc (mTOR) (see Fig. 1). IL-2 stimulates mTOR to activate kinases th ultimately advance the cell cycle from G_1 to the S phase. Thus tl SRL-FKBP12 complex inhibits T-cell proliferation by inhibiting tl cellular response to IL-2 and progression of the cell cycle.[76]

PHARMACOKINETICS

SRL is a lipophilic compound. Bioavailability after oral administr tion is low, only 15%, with peak concentrations being reached with 1 to 2 hours.[76] SRL has a high volume of distribution, readily di tributing into most tissues of the body. SRL binds extensively to er throcytes because of the high FKBP12 concentration found in re blood cells (RBCs). Metabolism occurs primarily by CYP 3A4 bo in the gut and in the liver. The half-life is reported to be 60 hours b can range up to 110 hours in patients with liver dysfunction.[77]

EFFICACY

Currently, SRL is only approved for the prevention of rejection in ki ney transplants in combination with corticosteroids and CSA or aft withdrawal of CSA in patients with low to moderate immunolog risk.

Two concurrent clinical trials evaluated the use of SRL in kidne transplants. All patients in both studies received CSA and steroic and were randomly assigned to one of three groups. The U.S. tri compared patients randomly assigned to receive SRL in a fixed do of a 6-mg loading dose followed by 2 mg daily (I), a fixed dose of

5-mg loading dose followed by 5 mg daily (II), or azathioprine (III). The global trial used the same SRL administration arms (I and II) but compared patients with placebo (III). The results of both studies showed similar patient and graft survival in all groups at 12 months but lower rates of acute rejection in the SRL arms compared with azathioprine and placebo.[78,79]

Studies evaluating early CSA withdrawal in SRL-based immunosuppressive protocols enrolled patients 3 months after transplant who were receiving SRL, which was adjusted based on trough blood concentrations, who did not have a recent or severe rejection episode and adequate renal function. Patients were randomly assigned to continue triple-drug therapy with SRL (adjusted to trough concentrations of greater than 5 ng/mL), CSA, and steroids or to double-drug therapy with SRL (adjusted to trough concentrations of 20 to 30 ng/mL) and steroids. The results showed a low risk of acute rejection following CSA discontinuation (5.6%) and no difference in graft survival. Long-term follow-up (2 years) showed improved renal function and blood pressure without an increase in acute rejection or graft loss in patients who discontinued CSA.[80]

Currently, since the safety and efficacy of SRL has not been established in liver or lung transplants, it is recommended that its use be avoided in these populations immediately following transplant. In contrast, limited data on the use of SRL in heart transplantation indicate benefit in reversing acute rejection in patients who do not respond to antilymphocyte therapy.[81] Furthermore, SRL may slow the progression of vasculopathy, which may have an impact on chronic rejection and long-term patient survival after heart transplantation.[82]

Use of SRL and TAC concomitantly was avoided in early studies because it was thought that the two would compete for FKBP12 receptor binding sites. However, clinical experience has demonstrated that this is not the case, and literature now substantiates the efficacy of SRL in combination with TAC.[83,84] SRL has also demonstrated efficacy in combination with MMF in kidney transplants to avoid the use of CIs and decrease the risk of nephrotoxicity.[85,86]

ADVERSE EFFECTS

Myelosuppression associated with SRL appears to be dose-related. Thrombocytopenia is usually seen within the first 2 weeks of SRL therapy but generally improves with continued treatment. Leukopenia and anemia caused by SRL typically are transient.[87] SRL levels greater than 15 ng/mL have been correlated with thrombocytopenia and leukopenia.[88] Hypercholesterolemia and hypertriglyceridemia are quite common in patients receiving SRL. It is postulated that the mechanism of this adverse effect is related to an overproduction of lipoproteins or inhibition of lipoprotein lipase. Peak cholesterol and triglyceride levels are often seen within 3 months of starting SRL but usually decrease after 1 year of therapy and can be managed by reducing the dose, discontinuing SRL, or by starting therapy with a HMG-CoA reductase inhibitor or fibric acid derivative. One recent study suggests that the dyslipidemia associated with SRL is not a major risk factor for early cardiovascular complications following kidney transplant.[89] Reports of delayed wound healing and wound dehiscence could be due to inhibition of smooth muscle proliferation and intimal thickening.[90] Mouth ulcers also have been reported with SRL, more commonly with the oral solution. The cause may be a direct effect of the drug or secondary to activation of herpes simplex virus.[91] Interstitial pneumonitis has been described in kidney, liver, and heart-lung transplant recipients that is reversible after discontinuing SRL.[77] Other adverse effects reported with SRL include increased liver enzymes, hypertension, rash, acne, diarrhea, and arthralgia (see Table 87–4).

DRUG-DRUG AND DRUG-FOOD INTERACTIONS

CYP 3A4 is the major metabolic pathway for SRL; thus the drug interactions mediated by induction or inhibition of the CYP 3A4 enzyme system are similar to those seen with CSA and TAC (see Table 87–6). Administration of the microemulsion formulation of CSA with SRL significantly increases the *AUC* and trough SRL levels. The same is not seen with the standard formulation of CSA. Conversely, CSA concentrations and *AUC* are also increased by SRL. The mechanism is proposed to be competitive binding to CYP 3A4 and *p*-glycoprotein.[77] It is recommended that patients separate the dose of SRL and CSA by 4 hours to minimize the interaction.[92] Concomitant administration of TAC does not affect SRL levels.[93]

As with CSA and TAC, grapefruit juice produces increases in SRL levels. Administration of SRL with a high-fat meal was associated with a delayed rate of absorption, decreased C_{max}, and increased AUC, indicating an increase drug exposure, whereas the half-life remained unchanged.[94] The clinical significance of this is unknown.

DOSING AND ADMINISTRATION

A fixed SRL dosing regimen is approved for concomitant use with CSA that includes a loading dose of 6- or 15-mg followed by 2 or 5 mg daily, respectively. Therapeutic monitoring of SRL is advocated using whole blood concentrations measured by HPLC, which is specific for the parent compound to a target level of 10 to 15 ng/mL when used in combination with a CI or, 15 to 25 ng/mL, when used in regimens that include CSA withdrawal. When RIA is used, which measures the parent compound and metabolites, reference ranges of 15 to 20 ng/mL and 20 to 30 ng/mL should be used, respectively.

> ### CLINICAL CONTROVERSY
>
> Routine therapeutic drug monitoring of SRL therapy is not recommended in patients who are receiving triple-drug therapy with CSA and steroids. However, many clinicians now feel that SRL drug levels should be monitored in all patients, although there is no accepted therapeutic range.

POLYCLONAL ANTIBODIES (ANTITHYMOCYTE GLOBULINS)

There are currently two antithymocyte globulins available in the United States: ATG (ATGAM®), an equine polyclonal antibody, and RATG (Thymoglobulin®), a rabbit polyclonal antibody. The rabbit preparation is less immunogenic and may have other advantages over the equine preparation. Both ATG and RATG are currently approved only for the treatment of rejection; however, the drugs are used often as induction therapy to prevent acute rejection.

PHARMACOLOGY/MECHANISM OF ACTION

Because of their polyclonal antibody nature, both ATG and RATG exert their immunosuppressive effect by binding to a wide array of lymphocyte receptors, including CD2, CD3, CD4, CD8, CD25, and CD45, among others. Binding of ATG or RATG to the various receptors results in complement-mediated lysis and subsequent lymphocyte depletion. T cells are the major lymphocytic target for the compounds; however, other blood cell components are also affected, including B cells and other leukocytes (see Fig. 87–1). Damaged T cells are removed subsequently by the spleen, liver, and lungs.

PHARMACOKINETICS

ATG is poorly distributed into lymphoid tissue and binds primarily to circulating lymphocytes, granulocytes, and platelets. The terminal half-life of ATG is 5.7 days. RATG has a volume of distribution of 0.12 L/kg. The terminal half-life in renal transplant recipients is significantly longer than ATG at 30 days.[95] Peak plasma concentrations are reached after 5 to 7 days of ATG or RATG infusions. Antiequine antibodies can form in up to 78% of patients receiving ATG therapy. Similarly, antirabbit antibodies can form in up to 68% of patients receiving RATG therapy. The effects of preformed antibodies on the efficacy and safety of these preparations has not been studied adequately.

EFFICACY

ATG and RATG are used most commonly for the treatment of acute allograft rejection or as induction therapy to prevent acute rejection. ATG is currently approved for both indications in kidney transplants. RATG, however, is approved only for the treatment of acute allograft rejection in kidney transplants. However, both drugs have been studied extensively for both indications.

The efficacy of ATG and RATG induction therapy has been described in liver and heart transplant recipients. Use of RATG as part of quadruple therapy in liver transplant is associated with similar rates of patient and graft survival and acute rejection compared with dual therapy; however, a significant increase in the number of CMV infections was noted. The clinical usefulness of quadruple therapy is questionable in light of the increased cost.[96] Quadruple-drug therapy results in similar rates of patient and graft survival and malignancy in heart transplants, but a significantly lower rate of acute rejection and infection episodes is seen at 1 year compared with triple-drug therapy.[97]

ADVERSE EFFECTS

Most adverse effects reported with ATG and RATG are related to the lack of specificity for T cells owing to their polyclonal nature. Dose-limiting myelosuppression, including leukopenia, anemia, and thrombocytopenia, occurs frequently. Other adverse effects include anaphylaxis, hypotension, hypertension, tachycardia, dyspnea, urticaria, and rash (see Table 87–4). Serum sickness is seen more frequently with ATG than RATG. Nephrotoxicity has been reported but is rare in the absence of serum sickness. Infusion-related febrile reactions are most common with the first few doses and can be managed by premedicating the patient with acetaminophen, diphenhydramine, and steroids. Finally, as with any immunosuppressive agent, ATG and RATG are associated with an increased risk of infections, particularly viral infections, and malignancy.

DRUG-DRUG AND DRUG-FOOD INTERACTIONS

Administration of ATG or RATG can interfere with the immune response to live vaccines, such as varicella vaccine. Immune globulins, including ATG and RATG, should not be administered within 2 months of receiving a live vaccine.

DOSING AND ADMINISTRATION

ATG doses range from 10 to 30 mg/kg per day as a single dose for 7 to 14 days. RATG is a more potent compound and is administered at doses of 1 to 1.5 mg/kg per day as a single dose for 7 to 14 days for rejection or for 5 to 10 days for induction of immunosuppression. It is recommended that both ATG and RATG be administered centrally through a high-flow vein with an in-line 0.22-micron filter over at least 4 hours to minimize phlebitis and thrombosis. However, literature supports peripheral administration of both agents.[98,99]

MONOCLONAL ANTIBODIES

INTERLEUKIN 2 RECEPTOR ANTAGONISTS (IL2RA)

There are currently two available interleukin 2 receptor antagonists: basilixmab, a chimeric monoclonal antibody (25% murine), and daclizumab, a humanized monoclonal antibody (90% human, 10% murine). Daclizumab contains a greater proportion of human sequences, making it theoretically less immunogenic. The percentage of murine component determines the antibody's affinity for the epitope. Therefore, the chimeric antibody basiliximab has a higher affinity than daclizumab.[100]

Pharmacology/Mechanism of Action

Both basiliximab and daclizumab exert their immunosuppressive effect by specifically binding to the alpha chain (CD25) on the surface of activated T-lymphocytes (see Fig. 87–1). Binding of either basiliximab or daclizumab to the IL-2 receptor prevents IL-2-mediated activation and proliferation of T cells, a critical step in clonal expansion of T cells and the development of allograft rejection. Saturation of the IL-2 receptor occurs rapidly and confers immunosuppressive effect immediately.[100]

Pharmacokinetics

Most of the pharmacokinetic data available for both basiliximab and daclizumab are in renal transplant patients. Caution must be used when extrapolating these data to non-renal-transplant recipients. Daclizumab has a small volume of distribution, approximately 5.3 L. The system clearance is highly variable and depends on body weight. The terminal half-life of daclizumab is about 20 days in renal transplant patients compared with 3 to 4 days in bone marrow transplant recipients. Specific data on the pharmacokinetics of daclizumab in liver transplant patients are lacking, but the half-life appears to be significantly lower compared with renal transplant recipients. It has been suggested that the increased elimination rate seen in liver transplant recipients may be due to significant intraoperative blood losses as well as loss via ascites. Therapeutic concentrations are 5 to 10 mg/L. Adjustments are not required on the basis of weight, race, gender, or degree of proteinuria.

Basiliximab has a slightly higher volume of distribution, 8 L, and a shorter half-life, approximately 7 days. Additionally, the half-life of basiliximab appears to be lower in liver transplant recipients. Increased blood loss did not account for this difference in elimination, but losses via ascites accounted for about 20% of basiliximab elimination. It has been recommended that patients with volumes of ascites greater than 10 L receive an additional dose of basiliximab on postoperative day 8.[101] While drug elimination is enhanced in liver transplants, receptor suppression with the two-dose regimen seems to be long lasting.[102] Both basiliximab and daclizumab saturate CD25 in vivo at serum concentrations of 0.2 and 1 mg/L or greater, respectively.[103]

Efficacy

Induction therapy with IL-2 receptor antagonists has been studied extensively in kidney, liver, and heart transplants.[102–107] A meta-analysis of daclizumab and basiliximab in renal transplantation evaluated the result of eight randomized, controlled trials involving more than 1800 patients. IL-2 receptor antagonists reduced the risk of rejection significantly (odds ratio 0.51) in CSA-based regimens at 6 months. No increases in graft loss, infectious complications, malignancy, or death were noted.[104] Review of the daclizumab trials continued to show less biopsy-proven rejection at 1 year, 28% versus 43% ($p < 0.0001$) in the daclizumab (both double- and triple-therapy combined) and standard-therapy arms, respectively. No graft or patient survival advantage was found for daclizumab-treated patients, but the studies were not powered to detect this difference.[103]

A large multicenter, randomized trial of 381 liver transplant recipients compared basiliximab with CSA and steroids alone. The results showed a decrease in acute rejection in the basiliximab group regardless of hepatitis C virus (HCV) status, although only the HCV-negative cohort was statistically significant.[102] Other investigators have reported higher rates of HCV recurrence in patients receiving daclizumab (54% versus 15%).[103] The most effective IL-2 receptor antagonist regimens remain to be defined, particulary for those with HCV.

In heart transplantation, induction with daclizumab produced favorable results with a lower incidence of acute rejection: 18% in the daclizumab-treated patients compared with 63% in the group receiving CSA, MMF, and prednisone with no induction therapy ($P = 0.04$). The time to occurrence of the first rejection episode also was significantly longer in the daclizumab-treated patients.[106] There were no adverse reactions to daclizumab and no significant differences between the groups in the incidence of infection or cancer during follow-up. Data for basiliximab in heart transplant recipients are lacking.

IL-2 receptor antagonists offer a reasonable addition to CI- or steroid-sparing protocols. In renal transplant recipients, 40% to 50% of patients receiving daclizumab with no initial CI required the eventual addition of CSA.[103] Alternative protocols using low-dose CSA in conjunction with daclizumab, MMF, and steroids showed similar results to matched controls[107] and lower rejection rates compared with OKT3 induction.[100] Basiliximab has been used in combination with low-dose TAC in patients with early evidence of DGF. Similar rates of rejection and steroid-resistant rejection were seen in patients who received basiliximab (20 mg at the time of diagnosis of DGF and again 5 days later) in conjunction with lower TAC doses compared with patients without DGF who received standard TAC doses and no IL2RA induction.[100]

Adverse Effects

Few adverse effects have been reported with basiliximab and daclizumab (see Table 87–4). In clinical trials, these drugs were associated with no increased risk of infectious complications or malignancy when compared with standard immunosuppression. In contrast to polyclonal antibody preparations and OKT3, basiliximab and daclizumab have not been associated with infusion-related reactions. However, since the marketing of basiliximab, an increased number of hypersensitivity reactions have been reported. Of note, only one patient developed anti-idiotypic antibodies to the murine portion during clinical trials.[100] The manufacturer of basiliximab reported an increase in mortality in a placebo-controlled trial, which was associated with an increase in severe infections.

Drug-Drug and Drug-Food Interactions

Reports of increased CSA and TAC levels in patients receiving concomitant basiliximab have recently been published.[109,110] Both authors hypothesized a potential interaction with the cytochrome P450. No drug interactions have been reported with daclizumab.

Dosing and Administration

Basiliximab is administered as two 20-mg intravenous doses: intraoperatively and again on postoperative day 4. Basiliximab is compatible with both 0.9% sodium chloride and 5% dextrose and can be administered either centrally or peripherally over 20 to 30 minutes in a solution of 50 mL. This regimen results in saturation of the IL-2 receptor for 30 to 45 days. The daclizumab approved dosing regimen for renal transplantation is 1 mg/kg every 2 weeks from the time of transplant for a total of five doses. Daclizumab should be diluted in 50 mL sterile 0.9% sodium chloride and administered peripherally or centrally over 15 minutes. This regimen saturates the IL-2 receptors for approximately 90 to 120 days after renal transplantation.[56,100]

Alternative dosing regimens have been proposed for daclizumab in combination with TAC, MMF, and steroids: 1 mg/kg every 2 weeks for five doses or, daclizumab 2 mg/kg every 2 weeks for two doses. At 6 months, the probability of kidney or pancreas allograft rejection and patient survival was similar in the daclizumab groups. This is an important finding because the two-dose regimen may have considerable implications for posthospital adminstration.[108] Eckhoff and colleagues[111] compared liver transplant recipients at risk for renal dysfunction who recieved daclizumab 2 mg/kg on day 0 followed by daclizumab 1 mg/kg on day 5 with a group who received conventional immunosuppression without daclizumab. There were fewer rejection episodes in the daclizumab group, and graft and patient survival were similar.[111]

MUROMONAB-CD3 (OKT3)

Pharmacology/Mechanism of Action

Muromonab-CD3 (OKT3) is a murine monoclonal antibody to the CD3 receptor on mature human T cells (see Fig. 87–1). Minutes following the administration of OKT3, T-cell concentrations decrease dramatically, as measured by CD3 levels. Cells reappear after a few days but bear no CD3 receptors. After cessation of OKT3 therapy, T-cell function normalizes in a week.[112]

Pharmacokinetics

OKT3 has a volume of distribution of 6.5 L and half-life of about 18 hours. Concentrations above 0.9 mcg/mL are considered therapeutic. OKT3 concentrations of 800 ng/mL or greater in combination with a CD3+ T cell counts of <25 cells/mL is also a reasonable therapeutic target. If CD3 levels begin to rise, this may signify the presence of antimurine antibodies antagonizing OKT3. Administration of MMF has been suggested to reduce the formation of antimurine antibodies during OKT3 administration. While T-cell depletion is achieved within minutes of administration, resolution of rejection takes 3 to 4 days.

Efficacy

OKT3 generally is reserved for steroid-resistant rejection, but it also has been used as induction therapy. Induction with the conventional OKT3 dose (5 mg/day for 7 to 14 days) effectively prevents rejection in renal transplant recipients. OKT3 can be used safely and successfully as rejection therapy in patients who have undergone previous OKT3 induction.[112] Specifically, these studies confirm that the presence of low anti-OKT3 antibody titers (≤1:100) does not preclude successful retreatment with OKT3 for rejection.

A sequential induction protocol using OKT3 is more cost-effective than conventional therapy in renal transplantation.[113] Furthermore, low-dose administration of OKT3 in this setting additionally may enhance cost-effectiveness. The exact role of OKT3 in induction therapy needs to be further defined (i.e., high- versus low-risk patients and conventional versus reduced dosing).

In addition to maintenance therapy, a number of heart transplant centers use either monoclonal or polyclonal induction agents including the IL2RAs (e.g., basiliximab or daclizumab), OKT3, or the antithymocyte globulins (e.g., ATG or RATG) for short periods of time immediately after transplantation in high-risk patients (e.g., high PRA, retransplants) or to spare the kidney from exposure to the nephrotoxicity of CSA or TAC.[112] To date, pooled data series show no clearcut survival advantages with induction therapy, although it appears that a higher percentage of patients may be weaned from prednisone, thereby reducing the incidence of steroid-associated complications.[112] Controversy exists as to whether prophylactic therapy with these cytolytic agents confers any added benefit other than delaying the onset of the first rejection episode.[112] In addition, this combination therapy is very expensive, inconvenient to administer, possibly alters the incidence and character of infectious complications, and may result in a higher incidence of malignancy.

Adverse Effects

OKT3 administration is associated with significant first-dose adverse reactions. The cytokine-release syndrome related to OKT3, including fever, chills, rigors, pruritus, and alterations in blood pressure, may occur with the first several doses. Methylprednisolone, acetaminophen, diphenhydramine, indomethacin, and pentoxifylline may be used as premedications. Other adverse effects include capillary leak syndrome and pulmonary edema, which may be particularly associated with OKT3 use in fluid overloaded patients (see Table 87–4). It is recommended that patients be within 3% of their dry weight and have chest x-rays evaluated prior to administration. Aseptic meningitis is another potential complication of OKT3 therapy. If encephalitic symptoms develop, OKT3 should be discontinued and appropriate care initiated. Other adverse effects include encephalopathy, nephrotoxicity, infection, and posttransplant lymphoproliferative disorder.[56]

Drug-Drug and Drug-Food Interactions

No drug or food interactions have been reported with OKT3.

Dosing and Administration

OKT3 should be filtered with a 0.2- to 0.22-micron filter and then administered as intravenous push over 1 minute. The dose of OKT3 usually is 5 mg/day for 5 to 14 days. Induction with 2.5 mg also has been used effectively.[112] Vital signs should be assessed frequently during the first few doses, and it is advisable to have a physician present for the first dose. A high proportion of patients treated with OKT3 form antibodies to one of the components of OKT3 and may not be able to receive or adequately respond to retreatment.[112]

INVESTIGATIONAL AGENTS

ALEMTUZUMAB

Alemtuzumab is a humanized monoclonal antibody directed at cells that express the CD52 surface antigen which is found on both T- and B-lymphocytes, as well as macrophages, monocytes, and natural killer (NK) cells. When alemtuzumab binds to the CD52 surface antigen, antibody-dependent lysis occurs, which removes T cells from the blood, bone marrow, and organs, resulting in T-cell depletion.

The adverse effects of alemtuzumab include infusion-related reactions, hematologic effects, and infections. Infusion-related reactions include rigors, hypotension, fever, shortness of breath, bronchospasms, and chills. The potential for developing these reactions can be reduced by administering premedications, including steroids, diphenhydramine, and acetaminophen or by administering smaller doses and escalating the dose gradually. Hematologic effects include pancytopenia, neutropenia, thrombocytopenia, and lymphopenia. Dose modifications are recommended based on the degree of thrombocytopenia.

Several dosing regimens have been proposed for alemtuzumab in solid-organ transplantation. For induction therapy, the most commonly reported doses in the literature are 0.3 mg/kg per dose, as a single or multiple dose regimen 20 mg times two doses given on days 0 and 1, 30 mg given on day 0 or 30 mg times two once on day 0 and once again between day 1–5.[113–117] The latter dosing scheme is currently recommended for use in most patient situations.[117] Early experience indicates that monotherapy with CSA, TAC, or SRL may be used following alemtuzumab induction.[114–118]

> ### CLINICAL CONTROVERSY
>
> New immunosuppressive protocols are being used to promote tolerance in transplant recipients to avoid long-term use of immunosuppressants. These protocols typically use high doses of RATG or alemtuzumab before transplantation and low-dose immunosuppression after transplantation with gradual weaning.

EVEROLIMUS

Everolimus, also knows as SDZ-RAD or RAD, is a rapamycin derivative (RAD) with similar immunosuppressive activity as SRL. Everolimus binds to FKBP12 and inhibits mTOR and the cellular response to IL-2, ultimately preventing progression of the cell cycle.

a lipophilic compound that readily distributes into RBCs, as well as to tissues. The half-life of everolimus is shorter than SRL at 16 to hours, lending itself to twice-daily dosing as compared with once-ly dosing with SRL.[119]

Adverse effects of everolimus are similar to SRL. Thrombotopenia and leukopenia are common within the first 2 months of erapy. Both total cholesterol and triglyceride levels also increase th everolimus use and generally peak within the first month of erapy.[120] Increases in cholesterol values appear to plateau after 2 to nonths of therapy, most likely as the result of the initiation of antihy-lipidemic agents. The hematologic and cholesterol adverse effects ve been reported to occur when RAD concentrations are within the cepted therapeutic range of 7–15 ng/mL.[121] Significant increases in um creatinine were note in phase III studies using everolimus with l-dose CSA. This is believed to be caused by CSA. Improved re-l function has been noted in trials investigating reduced-dose CSA, ich are ongoing.[122]

Phase III clinical trials currently are evaluating doses of 0.75 mg ice daily and 1.5 mg twice daily in combination with CSA and roids. Favorable preliminary results in kidney and heart transplant cipients are suggested by the decrease allograft loss and death.[123]

LEFLUNOMIDE

flunomide is a prodrug the active metabolite of which inhibits novo pyrimidine synthesis and tyrosine kinase activity in T- and B-lymphocytes. It is currently approved for use in rheumatoid arthritis. Bioavailability is 80% after oral administration. Leflunomide is metabolized in the liver to the active metabolite A77,1726. Biliary recirculation of A77,1726 contributes to the long half-life of 15 to 18 days. Adverse effects noted with leflunomide in solid-organ transplantation studies include skin rash, anemia, and elevated liver enzymes.

Studies of leflunomide in kidney and liver transplant recipients utilized a loading dose of 200 mg daily for 7 days, followed by a maintenance dose of 40 to 60 mg daily. The target concentration appears to be 50 to 80 mcg/mL, which also allows for lower doses of steroids and CIs.[124] A small open-label pilot study reported potential benefit with leflunomide in reversing chronic renal allograft dysfunction.[125]

FTY-720

FTY-720 is a novel immunosuppressant that alters lymphocyte migration via alteration of adhesion molecules. The resulting effect is a transient sequestration of T cells into lymphoid organs away from the allograft. Preliminary data from clinical trials indicate that FTY-720 is effective in reducing CSA doses in renal transplant recipients. FTY-720 has shown promise in preventing and reversing chronic rejection in animal models.[126] Early experience in clinical trials indicated that FTY-720 is associated with bradycardia compared with other immunosuppressants, namely, MMF,[127] but the effects are reported to be transient and usually occur following the first dose.[128] Phase III human trials in kidney transplantation are currently underway.

EVALUATION OF THERAPEUTIC OUTCOMES

The success of transplantation can be measured in terms of length of graft and patient survival or quality of life. Several nor and recipient factors have been identified that have an impact graft and patient survival (Table 87–8). Estimated half-lives for kid-ys are 26.9 years for HLA-identical grafts and 12.2 and 10.8 years, spectively, for grafts from a sibling or parent who are 1-haplotype atches. The estimated half-life for HLA-matched grafts was .3 and 7.8 years for mismatched kidneys.[21] The overall median rvival time for heart transplant recipients is 9.8 years, and for pa-nts surviving the first year after transplantation, the median survival 12 years.[1] The highest rate of mortality occurs within the first year after liver transplantation owing to the risks of surgery and early post-operative complications but progressively decline after the first year. A typical post-transplantation laboratory monitoring plan is depicted in Table 87–9.

IMMUNOSUPPRESSION-RELATED COMPLICATIONS

Comorbidities such as cardiovascular disease and malignancy, re-current disease, drug toxicities (namely nephrotoxicity), and chronic rejection are the primary causes of mortality in patients beyond year five after transplantation.[1] Special considerations for therapy in transplant patients are discussed below and are summarized in Table 87–10.

TABLE 87–8. Factors Affecting Allograft and Patient Survival

	Kidney	Liver	Heart
Donor factors	HLA matching	Size mismatch	Size mismatch
	Age	Age (youngest, oldest)	Age
	Serum creatinine		
	Cardiac instability		
	Prolonged ischemia time		Ischemia time
	History of hypertension		
Recipient factors	Age <15, >50 years	Age	Age <5, >60 years
	Retransplantation	Retransplantation	ICU pretransplant
	African race	African race	Mechanical ventilation
	PRA	ICU pretransplant	LVAD
	Multiparous women	ABO blood type	IABP
	Drug compliance	Drug compliance	Drug compliance

HLA = human leukocyte antigens; PRA = panel of reactive antibodies; LVAD = left ventricular assist device; IABP = intraaortic balloon pump.

TABLE 87–9. Laboratory Monitoring After Transplantation and Example of Frequency Parameters

	1–2 weeks	1 month	2–4 months	4–12 months	>12 months
SCr/BUN	Daily	1–2 times per week	Every 1–2 weeks	Monthly	Every 1–2 months
Chemistries	Daily	1–2 times per week	Every 1–2 weeks	Monthly	Every 1–2 months
Liver function tests					
Kidney or heart recipient	Once	Once	Monthly	Every 1–3 months	Every 1–3 months
Liver recipient	Daily	1–3 times per week	Every 1–2 weeks	Monthly	Every 1–2 months
Immunosuppressant level	Daily	1–2 times per week	Every 1–2 weeks	Monthly	Every 1–2 months
Complete blood count	Daily	1–2 times per week	Every 1–2 weeks	Monthly	Every 1–2 months
Lipid panel	Once	Every 3 months	Every 3 months	Every 3 months	Every 3 months
HbA1c	Once	Every 3 months	Every 3 months	Every 3 months	Every 3 months

Chemistries include sodium, potassium, chloride, CO_2 content, magnesium, calcium, phosphorus and blood glucose.
Liver function tests include total bilirubin, aspartate transaminase (AST), alanine transaminase (ALT), gamma glutamyl transpeptidase (GGTP), alkaline phosphatase.
Complete blood count includes white blood cells (WBC), red blood cells (RBC), platelets and/or differential.
Lipid panel includes total cholesterol, low-density lipoprotein (LDL), high-density lipoprotein (HDL), triglyceride and/or very low-density lipoprotein (VLDL).
SCr = serum creatinine; BUN = blood urea nitrogen; HbA1c = hemoglobin A1c.

CARDIOVASCULAR DISEASE

Cardiovascular disease is a leading cause of morbidity and mortality in transplant patients.[129] Preexisting cardiovascular disease, which is common in end-stage organ failure, is not reversed with transplantation. Additionally, hypertension, hyperlipidemia, and diabetes are common complications in transplant recipients and are independent risk factors that contribute significantly to cardiovascular disease. Chronic rejection has been linked to hypertension and hyperlipidemia.[130,131]

HYPERTENSION

Corticosteroids, CSA, TAC, and impaired kidney graft function may cause post-transplant hypertension. The primary mechanism of CI-associated hypertension in heart transplant recipients may be related to the CI-induced stimulation of intact renal sympathetic nerves and the absence of reflex cardiac inhibition of the sympathetic nervous system, but a number of other mechanisms, including decreased prostacyclin and nitric oxide production, also have been proposed.[54,132,133] In addition to the propensity to cause peripheral vasoconstriction, CIs promote sodium retention, resulting in extracellular fluid volume expansion. TAC appears to have less potential to induce hypertension following transplantation than CSA.[134] Most classes of antihypertensive medications effectively reduce blood pressure in transplant patients (see Chap. 13).[135]

Calcium channel blockers traditionally have been the first-line agents to treat hypertension after transplantation.[136] In addition to their ability to control blood pressure, calcium channel blockers may ameliorate the nephrotoxic effects of CSA, improve renal hemodynamics, decrease the incidence of delayed graft function and development of allograft atherosclerosis, and provide some immunosuppression. Calcium channel blockers, however, also may contribute to gingival hyperplasia that is often associated with CSA-based immunosuppression.[130] CYP 3A4 interactions with CSA and TAC are of concern with this class of medications, particularly with diltiazem, verapamil, and nicardipine, and CSA or TAC concentrations must be monitored to ensure proper dosage adjustments.

ACEIs and angiotensin II receptor blockers (ARBs) traditionally have been avoided in kidney transplant recipients because of the potential for hyperkalemia and decreased glomerular filtration rate. ACEIs and ARBs are now considered to be an equivalent alternative to calcium channel blockers for the treatment of hypertension in all transplant recipients. When ACEIs or ARBs are used in patients after transplantation, serum creatinine and potassium levels should be monitored closely. If the increase in serum creatinine is greater than 30% within 1–2 weeks after initiating ACEIs or ARBs, the drug should be discontinued and other measures used to control blood pressure (see Chap. 46).

CLINICAL CONTROVERSY

Many clinicians avoid using ACEIs in kidney transplant recipients because of the potential to decrease the glomerular filtration rate by promoting efferent arteriole vasodilation in the presence of CI-induced afferent arteriole vasoconstriction. Emerging evidence suggests that this situation does not occur. ACEIs should be avoided in recipients with renal artery stenosis or discontinued in recipients who have an acute significant elevation in serum creatinine after ACEI initiation.

Multiple antihypertensive agents usually are necessary to achieve the goal blood pressure in transplant recipients. Therefore, the addition of β-blockers, diuretics, or centrally acting antihypertensives usually is necessary. β-blockers generally are considered to be second-line therapy in solid-organ transplant recipients, because of the potential to worsen metabolic disturbances caused by immunosuppressants such as hyperkalemia and dyslipidemia. CI-induced hypertension is often salt-sensitive, making it very responsive to diuretics. Centrally acting agents (e.g., clonidine) are used often as adjunctive therapy in transplant recipients who are not able to achieve blood pressure control with calcium channel blockers or ACEIs.

HYPERLIPIDEMIA

Hyperlipidemia may be exacerbated by corticosteroids, CIs, diuretics, and β-blockers.[137] Corticosteroids promote insulin resistance and a decrease in lipoprotein lipase activity, as well as excessive triglyceride production. The mechanism of CI-induced hyperlipidemia is not well understood. CIs may decrease the activity of the low-density lipoprotein (LDL) receptor or lipoprotein lipase, altering LDL catabolism.[131] TAC appears to have less potential to induce hyperlipidemia than CSA.[44,45,138] Post-transplant hyperlipidemia is characterized by elevated LDL, very-low-density lipoprotein (VLDL), triglyceride apolipoprotein B, and lipoprotein(a) levels.[131] It is controversial whether the management of hyperlipidemia in transplant recipients should be more aggressive than current guidelines for the general population established by the National Cholesterol Education Program (NCEP).[139] Aggressive lipid lowering may not only

TABLE 87–10. Special Pharmacotherapy Considerations in Transplant Recipients

Problem	Pharmacotherapy	Special Considerations
Infection		
Perioperative prophylaxis		Donor culture results
		Penicillin allergy: vancomycin
	Bowel decontamination	
Pneumocystis carinii pneumonia prophylaxis	TMP/SMX 400/80 qd or tiw	Sulfa allergy
	Pentamidine 300 mg inhaled q mo	
	OR Dapsone 50–100 mg po qd	
Fungal		
Prophylaxis	Nystatin, clotrimazole	
Treatment	Fluconazole, itraconazole, ketoconazole	Inhibit P450 3A4; monitor CSA and TAC levels; decrease doses
	Amphotericin B	Consider liposomal products; decrease or stop CSA or TAC to minimize nephrotoxicity
		Remember to adjust doses of renally eliminated drugs, e.g., acyclovir, ganciclovir, TMP-SMX
Hyperkalemia	Restrict dietary intake; dialysis	May be exacerbated by CSA or TAC or ACEIs, acidosis or RI; fludrocortisone acetate 0.1 mg PO qd–bid for refractory hyperkalemia
Hyperglycemia		
Diabetes pretransplant	Insulin	Glucocorticoids, TAC, and CSA also increase hypoglycemic requirements
	Oral hypoglycemics	Insulin requirements will increase with improving renal function
	Metformin	Avoid in those with RI
Post-transplant diabetes	Insulin	Risk factors: Obesity, family history, African-American race, cadaveric kidney, TAC > CSA
	Oral hypoglycemics	May resolve/improve as immunosuppressive doses decrease
Ulcer Prophylaxis	H$_2$-receptor antagonists	Adjust dose in those with RI
	Sucralfate	Decreased TAC absorption
		If RI: Caution aluminum content
		No RI: Caution hypophosphatemia
	Proton pump inhibitors	
Hyperlipidemia	Diet	CSA > TAC; consider switch to TAC; discontinue or hold SRL
	HMG-CoA reductase inhibitors ("statins")	CSA/TAC may increase "statin" levels; start at lowest dose
		Monitor for muscle cramps, CPK levels and LFTs
	Gemfibrozil	Adjust dose in those with RI
		Caution with concomitant "statin"
Hypertension	Calcium channel blockers	Diltiazem, verapamil inhibit CSA/TAC metabolism
		Dihydropyridines may potentiate CSA-gingival hyperplasia
	ACE inhibitors; angiotensin II receptor antagonists	May exacerbate hyperkalemia
		Monitor K$^+$, S_{Cr} to assess for renal allograft vascular disease; may be useful in post-transplant erythrocytosis (HCT > 55%)
Osteoporosis	Oral calcium supplementation (1000–1500 mg/day)	If daily intake <1000 mg elemental calcium
	Oral vitamin D	Documented deficiency
	Calcifediol (1000 IU/day)	If kidney functioning
	Calcitriol (0.5 mcg/day)	If kidney not functioning
	Hormone-replacement therapy	Postmenopausal women without contraindications
	Calcitonin or oral bisphophonates	Documented loss in bone mineral density > 3%
		Data lacking for bisphosphonates in patients with RI
Malignancy		
Prevention	Minimize immunosuppressant doses; avoid sun exposure (sun block, hats, clothing); routine self-examinations (skin, lymph nodes); yearly gynecologic/prostate exams	AZA particularly associated with skin cancers
		CSA/TAC may be associated with lymphoproliferative disorders (lymphomas)
Treatment	Discontinue or minimize immunosuppressants	Do not abruptly withdraw corticosteroids
	Surgical, radiologic, or anti-neoplastic therapy	

TMP-SMX = trimethoprim-sulfamethoxazole; CSA = cyclosporine; TAC = tacrolimus; ACEI = ACE inhibitor; RI = renal insufficiency; CMV = cytomegalovirus; SRL = sirolimus; CPK = creatinine phosphokinase enzymes; LFTs = liver function tests; K$^+$ = potassium; S_{Cr} = serum creatinine; HCT = hematocrit.

arrest the progress or prevent the complications of atherosclerosis but also may promote graft survival in the kidney and heart transplant population. With the use of lipid-lowering agents, potential interactions with immunosuppressive regimens must be considered.

Dietary intervention, although safe, may be relatively ineffective for the treatment of hyperlipidemia in the transplant population. Along with dietary modification, dose reduction or withdrawal of CSA and/or steroids may assist in minimizing hyperlipidemia. For most patients, the combination of dietary intervention and an HMG-CoA reductase inhibitor should be considered the treatment of choice. HMG-CoA reductase inhibitors are highly effective in the treatment of hyperlipidemia, especially increased LDL, in transplant patients. HMG-CoA reductase inhibitors as a class have been shown to have immunomodulatory effects on MHC expression and T-cell activation and have been shown to reduce cardiac allograft rejection.[131,140]

HMG-CoA reductase inhibitors should be used with caution in transplant recipients because of several reports of rhabdomyolysis when these agents are combined with CIs.[35,50,140] Safety measures, including the use of low HMG-CoA reductase inhibitor doses and avoiding inappropriately high CSA or TAC concentrations. The concurrent use of medications known to increase the risk of myopathy (such as gemfibrozil) should be avoided.[131] Patients should be informed of the signs and symptoms of rhabdomyolysis. Baseline and follow-up creatine phosphokinase (CPK) measurements (every 6 months) have been used to identify patients who develop subclinical rhabdomyolysis when cholesterol-lowering therapy is used. Pravastatin may be preferred as a result of its lower interactive potential with CIs because it is not metabolized by CYP 3A4. The potential for hepatotoxicity from HMG-CoA reductase inhibitors warrants close monitoring of liver function in all transplant recipients.[137]

Bile acid–binding resins may be used to lower cholesterol in transplant patients, but adequate doses are difficult to achieve without the development of GI adverse effects. Because the absorption of CSA is dependent on the presence of bile in the GI tract, patients should be instructed to separate dosing of bile acid–binding resins and CSA by at least 2 hours. Bile acid–binding resins also should be separated from other immunosuppressants by at least 2 hours to avoid physical adsorption in the GI tract. For transplant patients who have hypertriglyceridemia refractory to dietary intervention, fish oil and fibric acid derivatives are well-tolerated, effective alternatives (see Chap. 21). Fibric acid derivatives are most effective in lowering serum triglyceride concentrations.

POST-TRANSPLANT DIABETES MELLITUS (PTDM)

Corticosteroids and CIs can impair glucose control in previously diabetic patients, as well as cause new-onset post-transplant diabetes mellitus (PTDM) in 4% to 20% of patients. Corticosteroids induce insulin resistance and impair peripheral glucose uptake, whereas CIs appear to inhibit insulin production.[142] TAC seems to be more diabetogenic than CSA, although recent studies have failed to show a statistical difference.[44] Other possible risk factors that have been identified for PTDM include ethnicity (African-American or Hispanic), age (>40 years), pretransplant diabetes status, family history, and weight.[143]

Patients with PTDM should be referred for nutritional counseling and advised on the merits of weight loss (if appropriate). There are, however, some special considerations in transplant patients. Up to 40% of patients with PTDM will require insulin therapy.[142] In diabetic patients who can be managed with an oral hypoglycemic agent, glipizide, which is metabolized extensively by the liver, may be preferred over renally eliminated agents such as glyburide. Metformin should

be used with extreme caution because of the risk of accumulation and lactic acidosis in those with moderate renal impairment. Regardless of therapy, frequent blood glucose monitoring is imperative in the early postoperative phase both to improve glucose control and identify those with PTDM. Changes in renal function secondary to CI nephrotoxicity or delayed graft function or acute rejection in kidney transplant recipients affects the elimination of many hypoglycemic agents, including insulin, and may result in hyper- or hypoglycemia. Patients and clinicians also should be aware that dose changes in immunosuppressant drugs also affect glycemic control. Tapering of immunosuppressive medications may result in reduced insulin requirements, whereas steroid pulses for the treatment of rejection may result in increased insulin requirements.

INFECTION

Both the severity and incidence of infections and deaths due to infections have decreased dramatically since the introduction of CSA and the use of lower steroid dosages. Nonetheless, infection and rejection remain the most frequently encountered complications associated with immunosuppression in the first year after transplantation.[144] The risk of infection is related directly to the overall level of immunosuppression and is greatest during the first 3 postoperative months, as well as following treatment of acute rejection episodes.[145] Infectious complications following transplantation generally are classified according to the causative organism, site of infection, and time of appearance following surgery. Bacterial infections occur most frequently within the first month after transplantation and generally affect the urinary tract, wound, or vascular access sites. Viral infections are caused most commonly by herpes simplex (early transplant), herpes zoster (late post-transplant), or cytomegalovirus (CMV). Chapter 120 discusses the treatment of infection in the immunocompromised host. Special considerations of therapy in transplant patients for CMV, herpes, and *Pneumocystis carinii* infections are described in the following paragraphs.

Cytomegalovirus (CMV) is the most important viral pathogen affecting transplant patients; 50% to 60% of patients have been infected with the virus. Following transplantation, patients may develop symptomatic primary or secondary CMV infections. A previously CMV-seronegative patient who receives an organ or blood product from a CMV-seropositive donor is considered to have primary CMV infection. A secondary infection is characterized by reactivation of the latent virus or reinfection in a previously seropositive patient. Patients with primary infections generally are more symptomatic than patients with secondary infections.

The incidence and severity of CMV infections in transplant recipients are related to the intensity of immunosuppression required to prevent graft rejection. Patients treated on multiple occasions with high-dose steroids or patients receiving OKT3 or antilymphocyte preparations[146] and patients with poor HLA matching, cadaveric allografts, and CMV-positive donor serology have more severe CMV disease. Transplant centers use different strategies for managing CMV, which often are based on the risk of CMV infection. Prophylactic strategies use oral or intravenous antiviral or immunoglobulin preparations to prevent the reactivation or emergence of CMV. Prophylaxis is used most often in high-risk patients (i.e., donor-recipient CMV serology mismatch or use of antilymphocyte preparations). Some centers routinely screen transplant recipients for CMV via blood tests (i.e., pp65 antigenemia, polymerase chain reaction [PCR]) and use preemptive therapy in patients who have a positive test. Treatment is given to all patients who have evidence of active CMV infection. Ganciclovir and valganciclovir have been used prophylactically and emptively in transplant patients. Other treatment strategies include ntravenous immunoglobulins (IVIGs) and CMV hyperimmune immunoglobulin (CMVIG). Ganciclovir and CMVIG are the mainstays r treatment of CMV infection. CMV has been linked to chronic jection and cardiac allograft vasculopathy.

CLINICAL CONTROVERSY

Some clinicians will use CMV prophylaxis for all patients receiving transplants. Others will reserve prophylaxis for only those patients who are at a higher risk for CMV infection, such as those with donor-recipient CMV serology mismatch or recipients who have received induction therapy or rejection treatment with antithymocyte globulin. A third strategy is to preemptively treat patients who have laboratory evidence of CMV infection.

Herpes simplex virus (HSV) infections in transplant patients are ost commonly the result of reactivation of a previous infection. ymptomatic HSV infection usually presents as labial or oral lesions the first 1 to 3 months after transplantation, but patients also may esent with reactivation of varicella-zoster as "shingles." Prophylac- therapy with low-dose oral acyclovir delays the development of SV infections in patients following transplantation.

The incidence of *Pneumocystis carinii* pneumonia (PCP) within e first year after transplantation is reported to be 3% to 5%.[147] ow-dose trimethoprim-sulfamethoxazole (TMP-SMX 400 mg/) mg three times weekly) is effective in the prevention of PCP in- ctions. Alternative agents include aerosolized pentamidine (300 mg very month), dapsone, and atovaquone. The duration of PCP prophy- xis is unclear. The risk of infection caused by *P. carinii* is likely to crease as immunosuppression is reduced; therefore, prophylaxis in tients requiring treatment for acute rejection may be appropriate.

MALIGNANCY

dvances in immunosuppression have decreased the incidence of ute rejection and increased patient survival, thus increasing the pa- nt's lifetime exposure to immunosuppression. While the precise echanism is unclear, post-transplant malignancy seems to be related the overall level of immunosuppression, as evidenced by a differ- ce in the rates of malignancy associated with quadruple versus triple rsus dual immunosuppressant regimens. The risk of malignancy in ansplant recipients is increased three- to fourfold over the general pulation. While the risk of lung, breast, colon, and prostate cancers es not appear to increased, a number of cancers that are uncom- on in the general population often occur with a higher prevalence in ansplant recipients: post-transplant lymphomas and lymphoprolif- ative disorders (PTLD), Kaposi's sarcoma, renal carcinoma, in situ rcinomas of the uterine cervix, hepatobiliary tumors, and anogeni- l carcinomas. Skin cancers are the most common tumors, account- g for 38% of all malignancies. Factors that may predispose trans- ant recipients to skin cancers include copious sun exposure and erapy with azathioprine, possibly due to azathioprine's metabolite, troimidazole, which causes significant photosensitivity.[148] Azathio- ine therapy is associated with a 2:1 predominance of squamous over asal cell carcinomas, whereas basal cell carcinoma occurs more fre- ently in the general population. Azathioprine-induced cutaneous quamous cell carcinoma is also associated with more metastatic dis- se and accounts for 6% of all deaths in comparison with less than % with CSA. Patients must be encouraged to use effective techniques reduce sun exposure.[148]

PTLD encompasses a broad spectrum of disorders ranging from benign polyclonal hyperplasias to malignant monoclonal lymphomas. Factors that predispose patients to PTLD include Epstein-Barr virus seronegativity at transplant and intense immunosuppression, particularly with OKT3 and antithymocyte globulin. Non-renal-transplant recipients are more likely to develop PTLD secondary to the heavy immunosuppression used to reverse rejection. Administration of ganciclovir or acyclovir preemptively during antilymphocyte therapy may decrease the risk of eventual PTLD. Treatment of life-threatening PTLD generally includes severe reduction or cessation of immunosuppression. Other options include systemic chemotherapy or rituximab.[149]

Post-transplant malignancies appear an average of 5 years after transplantation and increase with the length of follow-up. As many as 72% of patients surviving greater than 20 years may be affected. Malignancy accounts for 11.8% of deaths after cardiac transplantation and is the single most common cause of death in the sixth to the tenth posttransplant years.[147]

CONCLUSION

Transplantation is a lifesaving therapy for several types of end-organ failure. Advances in the understanding of transplant immunology have produced an unprecedented number of choices in terms of immunosuppression. The increasing number of effective immunosuppressive medications and therapies offer clinicians diverse ways to prevent allograft rejection in a patient-specific manner. However, the vast array and efficacy of currently available immunosuppressive agents make it increasingly difficult to evaluate their long-term efficacy. Clinicians must be keenly aware of the adverse effects of immunosuppressive medications and their treatment in order to optimize the care of the transplanted patient.

ABBREVIATIONS

6-MP: 6-mercaptopurine
ACE: angiotensin-converting enzyme
ARB: angiotensin II receptor blocker
ATG: antithymocyte globulin
ATN: acute tubular necrosis
AUC: area under the concentration curve
AZA: azathioprine
BUN: blood urea nitrogen
CABG: coronary artery bypass grafting
CAD: coronary artery disease
CI: calcineurin inhibitor
C_{max}: peak concentration
CMV: cytomegalovirus
CPK: creatinine phosphokinase
CSA: cyclosporine
CYP: cytochome P450 liver enzyme system
DGF: delayed graft function
ESRD: end-stage renal disease
FKBP: FK-binding protein
GI: gastrointestinal
HCT: hematocrit
HLA: human leukocyte antigen
HPLC: high-performance liquid chromatography
HSV: herpes simplex virus
IABP: intraaortic balloon pump

IgG: immunoglobulin G

IL-2: interleukin 2

IL2RA: interleukin 2 receptor antagonist

IMPDH: inosine monophosphate dehydrogenase

ISHLT: International Society of Heart and Lung Transplantation

LDL: low-density lipoprotein

LVAD: left ventricular assist device

MELD: model for end-stage liver disease

MHC: major histocompatibility complex

MMF: mycophenolate mofetil

MPA: mycophenolic acid

MPAG: mycophenolic acid glucuronide

mTOR: mammalian target of rapamycin

NFAT: nuclear factor of activated T cells

NYHA: New York Heart Association

OKT3: muromonab-CD3

PCP: *Pneumocystis carinii* pneumonia

PRA: panel of reactive antibodies

PTCA: percutaneous transluminal coronary angioplasty

PTDM: posttransplant diabetes mellitus

PTLD: posttransplant lymphoproliferative disorder

RBC: red blood cell

RIA: radioimmunoassay

SIR: sirolimus

TAC: tacrolimus

TGN: 6-thioguanine nucleotides

t_{max}: time to peak concentration

TMP-SMX: trimethoprim-sulfamethoxazole

TNF: tumor necrosis factor

TPMT: thiopurine methyltransferase

UNOS: United Network for Organ Sharing

VLDL: very-low-density lipoprotein

WBC: white blood cells

XO: xanthine oxidase

Review Questions and other resources can be found at *www.pharmacotherapyonline.com.*

REFERENCES

1. U.S. Organ Procurement and Transplantation Network and the Scientific Registry of Transplant Recipients: Transplant Data 2004. http://www.optn.org; accessed 1/5/05.
2. Deng MC. Heart failure: cardiac transplantation. Heart 2002;87: 177–184.
3. Wiesner RH, Rakela J, Ishitani MB, et al. Recent advances in liver transplantation. Mayo Clin Proc 2003;78:197–210.
4. Pablo R, Ortega F, Baltar JM, et al. Health-related quality of life (HRQOL) of kidney transplanted patients: Variables that influence it. Clin Transplant 2000;14:199–207.
5. U.S. Renal Data System. USRDS 2004 Annual Data Report. Bethesda, MD, National Institutes of Health, National Institute of Diabetes and Digestive and Kidney Diseases, 2004.
6. Saab S, Wang V. Recurrent hepatitis C following liver transplant: Diagnosis, natural history and therapeutic options. J Clin Gastroenterol 2003; 37:155–163.
7. American Heart Association. 1998 Heart and Stroke Statistical Update. Dallas, AHA, 1998.
8. Keck BM, Bennett LE, Rosendale J, et al. Worldwide Thoracic Organ Transplantation: A report from the UNOS/ISHLT International Registry for Thoracic Organ Transplantation. In: JM Cecka, PI Terasaki, eds. Clinical Transplants 1999. Los Angeles, UCLA Immunogenetics Center, 1999;35–49.

9. Merion RM, Magee JC. Renal transplantation. In: Greenfield LJ, e Surgery: Scientific Principles and Practice. Philadelphia, Lippinco Williams & Wilkins, 2001:568–576.
10. Campbell DA, Magee JC, Rudich SM, Punch JD. Hepatic transplant tion. In: Greenfield LJ, ed. Surgery: Scientific Principles and Practic Philadelphia, Lippincott Williams & Wilkins, 2001:577–597.
11. Pierson RN. Cardiac transplantation. In: Greenfield LJ, ed. Surger Scientific Principles and Practice. Philadelphia, Lippincott Williams Wilkins, 2001:597–608.
12. Wolfe RA, Ashby VB, Milford EL, et al. Comparison of mortality all patients on dialysis, patients on dialysis awaiting transplantation ar recipients of a first cadaveric transplant. New Engl J Med 1999;34 1725–1730.
13. Hosenpud JD, Bennett LE, Keck BM, et al. The Registry of the Inte national Society for Heart and Lung Transplantation: Fifteenth Offici Report—1998. J Heart Lung Transplant 1998;17:656–668.
14. Venkataramanan R, Habucky K, Burckart GJ, et al. Clinical pharma cokinetics in organ transplant patients. Clin Pharmacokinet 1989;1 134–161.
15. Brown RS, Ascher NL, Lake JR, et al. The impact of surgical com plications after liver transplantation on resource utilization. Arch Su 1997;132:1098–1103.
16. Braith RW, Edwards DG. Exercise following heart transplantation. Spor Med 2000;30:171–192.
17. Mueller XM. Drug immunosuppresive therapy for adult heart transplan tation. Part I: Immune response to allograft and mechanism of action immunosuppressants. Ann Thorac Surg 2004;77:354–362.
18. Kobashigawa JA, Kirklin JK, Naftel DC, et al. Pretransplantation ri factors for acute rejection after heart transplantation: A multiinstitution study. The Transplant Cardiologists Research Database Group. J Hea Lung Transplant 1993;12:355–366.
19. Winters GL, Marboe CC, Billingham ME. The International Socie for Heart and Lung Transplantation grading system for heart transpla biopsy specimens: Clarification and commentary. J Heart Lung Tran plant 1998;17:754–760.
20. Michaels PJ, Espejo ML, Kobashigawa J, et al. Humoral rejection cardiac transplantation: Risk factors, hemodynamic consequences an relationship to transplant coronary artery disease. J Heart Lung Tran plant 2003;22:58–69.
21. Hariharan S, Johnson CP, Bresnahan BA, et al. Improved graft surviv after renal transplantation in the US, 1988 to 1996. N Engl J Med 200 342:605–612.
22. Behrendt D, Ganz P, Fang JC. Cardiac allograft vasculopathy. Curr Op Cardiol 2000;15:422–429.
23. Vasquez EM, Benedetti E, Pollak R. Ethnic differences in clinical r sponse to corticosteroid treatment of acute allograft rejection. Transpla 2001;71:229–233.
24. Ross HJ, Gullestad L, Pak J, et al. Methotrexate or total lymphoid radia tion for treatment of persistent or recurrent allograft cellular rejectio A comparative study. J Heart Lung Transplant 1997;16:179–189.
25. Bodmer JG, Marsh SG, Albert ED, et al. Nomenclature for factors of th HLA system, 1991. Hum Immunol 1992;34:4–18.
26. Najarian JS, Fryd DS, Strand M, et al. A single institution, randomize prospective trial of cyclosporine versus azathioprine-antilymphocy globulin for immunosuppression in renal allograft recipients. Ann Su 1985;201:142–157.
27. Valentine H. Neoral use in the cardiac transplant recipient. Transplar Proc 2000;32(suppl 1):27–44.
28. Andreu J, Campistol JM, Oppenheimer F, et al. Cyclosporine mono therapy as primary immunosuppression in renal transplantation: Five year experience. Transplant Proc 1994;26:337–340.
29. Abouljoud MS, Kumar A, Brayman KL, et al. Neoral rescue therap in transplant patients with intolerance to tacrolimus. Clin Transpla 2002;16:168–172.
30. Jain A, Brody D, Hamad I, et al. Conversion to Neoral for neurotoxicit after primary adult liver transplantation under tacrolimus. Transplanta tion 2000;69:172–177.
31. Kahan BD. Cyclosporine. N Engl J Med 1989;321:1725–1738.

2. Lake KD, Canafax DM. Important interactions of drugs with immunosuppressive agents used in transplant recipients. J Antimicrob Chemother 1995;36:11–22.

3. Jones TE. The use of other drugs to allow a lower dosage of cyclosporine to be used: Therapeutic and pharmacoeconomic considerations. Clin Pharmacokinet 1999;32:357–367.

4. van Gelder T. Drug interactions with tacrolimus. Drug Saf 2002;25:707–712.

5. Asberg A. Interactions between cyclosporin and lipid-lowering drugs: implications for organ transplant recipients. Drugs 2003;63:367–378.

6. Gupta SK, Benet LZ. High-fat meals increase the clearance of cyclosporine. Pharm Res 1990;7:46–68.

7. Edwards DJ, Fitzsimmons ME, Schuetz EG, et al. 6',7'-Dihydroxybergamottin in grapefruit juice and Seville orange juice: Effects on cyclosporine disposition, enterocyte CYP3A4, and p-glycoprotein. Clin Pharmacol Ther 1999;65:237–244.

8. Dumont RJ, Ensom MH. Methods for clinical monitoring on cyclosporin in transplant patients. Clin Pharmacokinet 2000;38:427–447.

9. Morris RG, Russ GR, Cervelli MJ, et al. Comparison of trough, 2-hour, and limited AUC blood sampling for monitoring cyclosporin (Neoral) at day 7 post-renal transplantation and incidence of rejection in the first month. Ther Drug Monit 2002;4:479.

50. Keown PA. New concepts in cyclosporine monitoring. Curr Opin Nephrol Hypertens 2002;11:61.

51. Levy G, Thervet E, Lake J, et al. Patient management by Neoral C$_2$ monitoring: An international consensus statement. Transplantation 2002;73:S12.

52. Kelly PA, Burckart GJ, Venkataramanan R. Tacrolimus: A new immunosuppressive agent. Am J Health Syst Pharm 1995;52:1521.

53. Squifflet JP, Vanrenterghem Y, van Hooff JP, et al. Safe withdrawal of corticosteroids or mycophenolate mofetil: Results of a large, prospective, multicenter, randomized study. Transplant Proc 2002;34:1584–1586.

54. Scott LJ, McKeage K, Keam SJ, Plosker GL. Tacrolimus: A further update of its use in the management of organ transplantation. Drugs 2003;63:1247–1297.

55. Laskow DA, Neylan JF III, Shapiro RS, et al. The role of tacrolimus in adult kidney transplantation: A review. Clin Transplant 1998;12:489–503.

56. Hohage H, Arlt M, Brückner D, et al. Effects of cyclosporin A and FK 506 on lipid metabolism and fibrinogen in kidney transplant recipients. Clin Transplant 1997;11:225–230.

57. Chan MCY, Kwok BW, Shiba N, et al. Conversion of cyclosporine to tacrolimus for refractory or persistent myocardial rejection. Transplant Proc 2002;34:1850–1852.

58. Steeves M, Abdallah HY, Venkataramanan R, et al. In-vitro interaction of a novel immunosuppressant, FK506, and antacids. J Pharm Pharmacol 1991;43:574–577.

59. Mignat C. Drug interactions with new immunosuppressive agents. Drug Saf 1997;16:267–278.

60. Kotanko P, Kirisits W, Skrabal F. Rhabdomyolysis and acute renal graft impairment in a patient treated with simvastatin, tacrolimus, and fusidic acid (letter). Nephron 2002;90:234–235.

61. Christians U, Jacobsen W, Benet LZ, Lampen A. Mechanisms of clinically relevant drug interactions associated with tacrolimus. Clin Pharmacokinet 2002;41:813–851.

62. Bekersky I, Dressler D, Mekki QA. Effect of low- and high-fat meals on tacrolimus absorption following 5 mg single oral doses to healthy human subjects. J Clin Pharmacol 2001;41:176–182.

63. Ojo AO, Held PJ, Port FK, et al. Chronic renal failure after transplantation of a nonrenal organ. N Engl J Med 2003;349:931–940.

64. Sturrock ND, Struthers AD. Hormonal and other mechanisms involved in the pathogenesis of cyclosporin-induced nephrotoxicity and hypertension in man (editorial). Clin Sci 1994;86:1–9.

65. Rodicio JL. Calcium antagonists and renal protection from cyclosporine nephrotoxicity: Long-term trial in renal transplantation patients. J Cardiovasc Pharm 2000;35:S7–11.

66. Bush WW. Overview of transplantation immunology and the pharma-

cotherapy of adult solid organ transplant recipients: Focus on immunosuppression. Adv Pract Acute Crit Care 1999;10:253–269.

57. Kahan BD, Ghobiral R. Immunosuppressive agents. Surg Clin North Am 1994;74:1029–1054.

58. Halloran PF. Immunosuppressive drugs for kidney transplantation. N Engl J Med 2004;351:2715–2729.

59. Bullingham RES, Nicholls AJ, Kamm BR. Clinical pharmacokinetics of mycophenolate mofetil. Clin Pharmacokinet 1998;34:429–455.

60. Weigel G, Griesmacher A, Karimi A, et al. Effect of mycophenolate mofetil therapy on lymphocyte activation in heart transplant recipients. J Heart Lung Transplant 2002;21:1074–1079.

61. Hosenpud JD, Bennett LE. Mycophenolate mofetil compared to azathioprine improves survival in patients surviving the initial cardiac transplant hospitalization: An analyisis of the joint ISHLT/UNOS Thoracic Registry. J Heart Lung Transplant 2000;19:72.

62. The Mycophenolate Mofetil Acute Renal Rejection Study Group. Mycophenolate mofetil for the treatment of a first acute renal allograft rejection: three-year follow-up. Transplantation 2001;71:1091–1097.

63. Abramowicz D, Manas D, Lao M, et al. Cyclosporine withdrawal from a mycophenolate mofetil–containing immunosuppressive regimen in stable kidney transplant recipients: A randomized, controlled study. Transplantation 2002;74:1725–1734.

64. Stewart SF, Hudson M, Talbot D, et al. Mycophenolate mofetil monotherapy in liver transplantation. Lancet 2001;357:609–610.

65. Schlitt HJ, Barkmann A, Böker HHJ, et al. Replacement of calcineurin inhibitors with mycophenolate mofetil in liver-transplant patients with renal dysfunction: A randomized, controlled study. Lancet 2001;357:587–591.

66. Sievers TM, Rossi SJ, Ghobiral RM, et al. Mycophenolate mofetil. Pharmacotherapy 1997;17:1178–1197.

67. Wolfe EJ, Mathur V, Tomlanovich S, et al. Pharmacokinetics of mycophenolate mofetil and intravenous ganciclovir alone and in combination in renal transplant recipients. Pharmacotherapy 1997;17:591–598.

68. van Gelder T, Klupp J, Barten MJ, et al. Comparison of the effects of tacrolimus and cyclosporine on the pharmacokinetics of mycophenolic acid. Ther Drug Monit 2001;23:119–128.

69. Pescovitz MD, Conti D, Dunn J, et al. Intravenous mycophenolate mofetil: Safety, tolerability, and pharmacokinetics. Clin Transplant 2000;14:179–188.

70. Cox VC, Ensom MHH. Mycophenolate mofetil for solid organ transplantation: Does the evidence support the need for clinical pharmacokinetic monitoring? Ther Drug Monit 2003;25:137–157.

71. Shaw LM, Korecka M, Venkataramanan R, et al. Mycophenolic acid pharmacodynamics and pharmacokinetics provide a basis for rational monitoring strategies. Am J Transplant 2003;3:534–542.

72. Salvadori M, Holzer H, de Mattos A, et al. Enteric-coated mycophenolate sodium is therapeutically equivalent to mycophenolate mofetil in de novo renal transplant patients. Am J Transplant 2003;4:231–236.

73. Budde K, Curtis J, Knoll G, et al. Enteric-coated mycophenolate sodium can be safely administered in maintenance renal transplant patients: Results of a 1-year study. Am J Transplant 2003;4:237–243.

74. Granger DK. Enteric-coated mycophenolate sodium: Results of two pivotal global multicenter trials. Transplant Proc 2001;33:3241–3244.

75. Lancaster DL, Patel N, Lennard L, Lilleyman JS. 6-Thioguanine in children with acute lymphoblastic leukemia: Influence of food on parent drug pharmacokinetics and 6-thioquanine nucleotide concentrations. Br. J Clin Pharmacol 2001;51:531–539.

76. Ingle GR, Sievers TM, Hold CD: Sirolimus: Continuing the evolution of transplant immunosuppression. Ann Pharmacother 2000;34:1044.

77. Kahan BD, Camardo JS. Rapamycin: Clinical results and future opportunities. Transplantation 2001;72:1181.

78. Kahan BD. Efficacy of sirolimus compared with azathioprine for reduction of acute renal allograft rejection: A randomized multicentre study. Lancet 2000;356:194–202.

79. MacDonald AS. A worldwide, phase III, randomized, controlled, safety and efficacy study of a sirolimus/cyclosporine regiment for prevention of acute rejection in recipients of primary mismatched renal allografts. Transplantation 2001;71:271–280.

80. Oberbauer R, Kreis H, Johnson RWG, et al. Long-term improvement in renal function with sirolimus after early cyclosporine withdrawal in renal transplant recipients: 2-year results of the Rapamune maintenance regimen study. Transplantation 2003;76:364–370.

81. Ankersmit HJ, Roth G, Zuckermann A, et al. Rapamycin as rescue therapy in a patient supported by biventricular assist device to heart transplantation with consecutive ongoing rejection. Am J Transplant 2003;3: 231–234.

82. Mancini D, Pinney S, Burkhoff D, et al. Use of rapamycin slows progression of cardiac transplantation vasulopathy. Circulation 2003;108:48–53.

83. van Hooff JP, Squifflett JP, Wlodarczyk Z, et al. A prospective, randomized multicenter study of tacrolimus in combination with sirolimus in renal transplant receipients. Transplantation 2003;75:1934–1939.

84. Pham SM, Qi XS, Mallon SM, et al. Sirolimus and tacrolimus in clinical cardiac transplantation. Transplant Proc 2002;34:1839–1842.

85. Flechner SM, Goldfard D, Moldin C, et al. Kidney transplantation without calcineurin inhibitor drugs: A prospective, randomized trial of sirolimus versus cyclosporine. Transplantation 2002;74:1070–1076.

86. Kreis H, Cisterne JM, Land W, et al. Sirolimus in association with mycophenolate mofetil induction for the prevention of acute graft rejection in renal allograft recipients. Transplantation 2000;69:1252–1260.

87. Saunders RN, Metcalfe MS, Nicholson ML. Rapamycin in transplantation: A review of the evidence. Kidney Int 2001;59:3.

88. Kahan BD, Napoli KL, Kelly PA, et al. Therapeutic drug monitoring of sirolimus: Correlations with efficacy and toxicity. Clin Transplant 2000; 14:97–109.

89. Chueh SCJ, Kahan BD. Dyslipidemia in renal transplant recipients treated with a sirolimus and cyclosporine-based immunosuppressive regimen: Incidence, risk factors, progression, and prognosis. Transplantation 2003;76:375–382.

90. Guilbeau JM. Delayed wound healing with sirolimus after liver transplant. Ann Pharmacother 2002;36:1391–1395.

91. van Gelder T, ter Meulen CG, Hené R, et al. Oral ulcers in kidney transplant recipients treated with sirolimus and mycophenolate mofetil. Transplantation 2003;75:788–791.

92. Kaplan B, Meier-Kriesche HU, Napoli KL, Kahan BD. The effects of relative timing of sirolimus and cyclosporine microemulsion formulation coadministration on the pharmacokinetics of each agent. Clin Pharmacol Ther 1998;63:48.

93. McAlister VC, Mahalati K, Peltekian KM, et al. A clinical pharmacokinetic study of tacrolimus and sirolimus combination immunosuppression comparing simultaneous to separated administration. Ther Drug Monit 2002;23:346–350.

94. Zimmerman JJ, Ferron GM, Lim HK, Parker V. The effect of a high-fat meal on the oral bioavailability of the immunosuppressant sirolimus (rapamycin). J Clin Pharmacol 1999;39:1155–1161.

95. Bunn D, Lea CK, Bevan DJ, et al. The pharmacokinetics of antithymocyte globulin (ATG) following intravenous infusion in man. Clin Nephrol 1996;45:29–32.

96. Neuhaus P, Klupp J, Langrehr JM, et al. Quadruple tacrolimus-based induction therapy including azathioprine and ALG does not significantly improve outcome after liver transplantation when compared with standard induction with tacrolimus and steroids: Results of a prospective, randomized trial. Transplantation 2000;69:2343–2353.

97. Carrier M, White M, Perrault LP, et al. A 10-year experience with intravenous Thymoglobuline in induction of immunosuppression following heart transplantation. J Heart Lung Transplant 1999;18:1218–1223.

98. Marvin MR, Drogan C, Sawinski D, et al. Administration of rabbit antithymocyte globulin (Thymoglobulin) in ambulatory renal-transplant patients. Transplantation 2003;75:488–489.

99. Rahman GF, Hardy MA, Cohen DJ. Administration of equine antithymocyte globulin via peripheral vein in renal transplant recipients. Transplantation 2000;69:1958–1960.

100. Cibrik DM, Kaplan B, Meier-Kriesche H. Role of anti-interleukin-2 receptor antibodies in kidney transplantation. BioDrugs 2001;15:655–666.

101. Kovarik J, Breidenbach T, Gerveau C, et al. Disposition and immunodynamics of basiliximab in liver allograft recipients. Clin Pharmacol Ther 1998;64:66–72.

102. Moser, MAJ. Options for induction immunosuppression in liver transplant recipients. Drugs 2002;62:995–1011.

103. Carswell CI, Plosker GL, Wagstaff AJ. Daclizumab: A review of its use the management of organ transplantation. BioDrugs 2001;15:745–77

104. Adu D, Cockwell P, Ives NJ, et al. Interleukin-2 receptor monoclon antibodies in renal transplantation: Meta-analysis of randomized tria Br Med J 2003;326:789–794.

105. Neuhaus P, Clavien PA, Kittur D, et al. Improved treatment respon with basiliximab immunoprophylaxis after liver transplantation: Resu from a double-blind randomized placebo-controlled trial. Liver Trans 2002;8:132–142.

106. Beniaminovitz A, Itescu S, Letiz K, et al. Prevention of rejection cardiac transplantation by blockade of the interleukin-2 receptor wi a monoclonal antibody (see comments). N Engl J Med 2000;34 613–619.

107. Leitz K, John R, Beniaminovitz A, et al. Interleukin-2 receptor blocka in cardiac transplanation: Influence of HLA-DR locus incompatibili on treatment efficacy. Transplantation 2003;75:781–787.

108. Stratta RJ, Alloway RR, Lo A, Hodge E. Two-dose daclizumab reg men in simultaneous kidney-pancreas transplant recipients: Primary en point analysis of a multicenter, randomized study. Transplanation 200 75:1260–1266.

109. Strehlau J, Pape L, Offner G, et al. Interleukin-2 receptor antibod induced alterations of ciclosporin dose requirements in paediatric trar plant recipients. Lancet 2000;356:1327–1328.

110. Sifontis NM, Benedetti E, Vasquez EM. Clinically significant drug inte action between basiliximab and tacrolimus in renal transplant recipien Transplant Proc 2002;34:1730–1732.

111. Eckhoff DE, McGuire G, Sellers M, et al. The safety and efficacy a two-dose daclizumab (Zenapax) induction therapy in liver transpla recipients. Transplantation 2000;69:1867–1872.

112. Wilde MI, Goa KL. Muromonab-CD3: A reappraisal of it pharmaco ogy and use as prophylaxis of solid organ transplant rejection. Dru 1996;51:865–894.

113. Shield CF III, Jacobs RJ, Wyant S, Da A. A cost-effective analys of OKT3 induction therapy in cadaveric kidney transplantation. Am Kidney Dis 1996;27:855–864.

114. Calne R, Moffatt SD, Friend PJ, et al. Campath-IH allows low-dose c closporine monotherapy in 31 cadaveric renal allograft recipients. Tran plant 1999;68:1613.

115. Knechtle SJ, Pirsch JD, Becher BN, et al. Campath-1H induction pl rapamycin monotherapy in renal transplantation (abstract). Am J Tran plant 2002;2:S459.

116. Tzakis AG, Kato T, Nishida S, et al. Preliminary experience with car path 1H (C1H) in intestinal and liver transplantation. Transplantatio 2003;75:1227.

117. Reams BD, Davis RD, Curl J, Palmer SM. Treatment of refractory acu rejection in a lung transplant recipient with campath 1H. Transplanatic 2002;74:903.

118. Marcos A, Eghtesad G, Fung JJ, et al. Use of alemtuzumab and tacrolim monotherapy for cadaveric liver transplantation: With particular refe ence to Hepatitis C virus. Transplantation 2004;78:966–971.

119. Kahan BD, Wong RL, Carter C, et al. A phase I study of a 4-week cour of SDZ-RAD (RAD) quiescent cyclosporine-prednisone-treated ren transplant recipients. Transplantation 1999;68:1100.

120. Kovarik JM, Kahan BD, Kaplan B, et al. Longitudinal assessment everolimus in de novo renal transplant recipients over the first pos transplant year: Pharmacokinetics, exposure-response relationships, a influence on cyclosporine. Clin Pharmacol Ther 2001;69:48–56.

121. Nashan B. Early clinical experience with a novel rapamycin derivativ Ther Drug Monit 2002;24:53–58.

122. Kirchner GI, Meier-Wiedenbach I, Manns MP. Clinical pharmacoki etics of everolimus. Clin Pharmacokinet 2004;43:83–95.

123. Eisen HJ, Tuzcu EM, Dorent R, et al. Everolimus for the preventio of allograft rejection and vasculopathy in cardiac-transplant recipient N Engl J Med 2003;349:847–858.

124. Williams JW, Mital D, Chong A, et al. Experiences with leflunomide solid organ transplantation. Transplantation 2002;73:358–366.

135. Hardinger KL, Wang CD, Schnitzler MA, et al. Prospective, pilot, open-label, short-term study of conversion to leflunomide reverses chronic renal allograft dysfunction. Am J Transplant 2002;2:867–871.

136. Koshiba R, van Damme B, Rutgeerts O, et al. FTY720, an immunosuppressant that alters lymphocyte trafficking, abrogates chronic rejection in combination with cyclosporine A. Transplantation 2003;75:945–952.

137. Ferguson RM, Mulgaonkar S, Tedesco H, et al. High efficacy of FTY720 with reduced cyclosporine dose in preventing rejection in renal transplantation: 12-month preliminary results (abstract 624). Am J Transplant 2003;3(suppl 5):311.

138. Tedesco H, Kahan B, Maurad G, et al. FTY720 combined with Neoral and corticosteroids is effective and safe in prevention of acute rejection in renal allograft recipients (interim data) (abstract 429). Am J Transplant 2001;1(suppl 1):243.

139. Bostom AD, Brown RS, Chavers BM, et al. Prevention of post-transplant cardiovascular disease: Report and recommendations of an ad hoc group. Am J Transplant 2002;2:491–500.

140. Zhang R, Leslie B, Boudreaux P, et al. Hypertension after kidney transplantation: Impact, pathogenesis and therapy. Am J Med Sci 2003;325:202–208.

141. Moore R, Hernandez D, Valantine H. Calcineurin inhibitors and post-transplant hyperlipidemias. Drug Saf 2001;24:755–766.

142. Textor SC, Taler SJ, Canzanello VJ, Schwartz L. Cyclosporine, blood pressure and atherosclerosis. Cardiol Rev 1997;5:141–151.

143. Ventura HO, Malik FS, Mehra MR, et al. Mechanisms of hypertension in cardiac transplantation and the role of cyclosporine. Curr Opin Cardiol 1997;12:375–381.

144. Taylor DO, Varr ML, Radovancevic B, et al. A randomized, multicenter comparison of tacrolimus and cyclosporine immunosuppressive regimens in cardiac transplantation: Decreased hyperlipidemia and hypertension with tacrolimus. J Heart Lung Transplant 1999;18:336–345.

145. Chobanian AV, Bakris GL, Black HR, et al. The seventh report of the Joint National Committee on Prevention, Detection, Evaluation, and Treatment of High Blood Pressure: the JNC 7 report. JAMA 2003:289;2560–2572.

136. Tylicki L, Habicht A, Watchinger B, Hörl WH. Treatment of hypertension in renal transplant recipients. Curr Opin Urol 2003;13:91–98.

137. Massy ZA, Kasiske BL. Post-transplant hyperlipidemia: Mechanisms and management. J Am Soc Nephrol 1996;7:971–977.

138. Vincenti F, et al. Tacrolimus (FK506) in kidney transplantation: Five-year survival results of the U.S. multicenter, randomized, comparative trial. Transplant Proc 2001;33:1019–1020.

139. Executive Summary of the Third Report of the National Cholesterol Education Program (NCEP). Expert Panel on Detection, Evaluation, and Treatment of High Blood Cholesterol in Adults (Adult Treatment Panel III). JAMA 2001;285:2486–2497.

140. Mach F. Statins as immunomodulators. Transplant Immunol 2002;9:197–200.

141. Asberg A. Interactions between cyclosporin and lipid-lowering drugs: implications for organ transplant recipients. Drugs 2003;63:367–378.

142. Jindal RM, Sidner RA, Milgrom ML. Post-transplant diabetes mellitus: The role of immmunosuppression. Drug Saf 1997;16:242–257.

143. Reisæter AV, Hartmann A. Risk factors and incidence of post-transplant diabetes mellitus. Transplant Proc 2001;33:8–18S.

144. Fishman JA, Rubin RH. Infection in organ-transplant recipients. N Engl J Med 1998;338:1741–1751.

145. Thaler SJ, Rubin RH. Opportunistic infections in the cardiac transplant patients. Curr Opin Cardiol 1996;11:191–203.

146. Hebart H, Kanz L, Jahn G, Einsel H. Management of cytomegalovirus infection after solid-organ or stem-cell transplantation. Drugs 1998;55:59–72.

147. Higgins RM, Bloom SL, Hopkin JM, Morris PJ. The risks and benefits of low-dose cotrimoxazole prophylaxis for *Pneumocystis* pneumonia in renal transplantation. Transplantation 1989;47:558–560.

148. Penn I. Post-transplant malignancy: The role of immunosuppression. Drug Saf 2000;23:101–113.

149. Berney T, Delis S, Kato T, et al. Successful treatment of post-transplant lymphoproliferative disease with prolonged rituximab treatment in intestinal transplant recipients. Transplantation 2002;74:1000–1006.

88

OSTEOPOROSIS AND OSTEOMALACIA

Mary Beth O'Connell and Terry L. Seaton

Learning Objectives and other resources can be found at *www.pharmacotherapyonline.com.*

KEY CONCEPTS

❶ Women and men over age 50 should be assessed for factors that increase the risk of developing osteoporosis and related fractures. Patients with premature or severe osteoporosis should be evaluated for secondary causes of bone loss.

❷ Bone density testing can establish the degree of bone health, predict fracture risk, and influence prevention and treatment decisions. Portable equipment can be used as a preliminary screening method in the community to determine the need for further testing.

❸ All people, regardless of age, should incorporate a healthy lifestyle beginning at birth that emphasizes regular exercise, nutritious diet, and tobacco avoidance to prevent and treat osteoporosis.

❹ To ensure adequate calcium intake, most Americans will need supplementation with 500 mg of elemental calcium once or twice daily. Most elderly patients require vitamin D supplementation of 400 to 1000 units/day, from sources such as beverages, multivitamins, and combination calcium and vitamin D products.

❺ Bisphosphonates are the cornerstone for osteoporosis treatment. They are the drugs of choice because they prevent both nonvertebral (especially hip) and vertebral fractures.

❻ Raloxifene is an alternative treatment option to prevent vertebral fractures, particularly in women who cannot tolerate or will not take bisphosphonates. It may also be useful for women who have a history of breast cancer or a significant risk for developing breast cancer (investigational).

❼ Although estrogens increase bone mineral density and decrease fractures, they are no longer recommended for osteoporosis prevention because of toxicity concerns. When used to treat menopausal symptoms, they will have a positive bone effect.

❽ Male osteoporosis is often secondary to specific diseases and drugs and responds well to bisphosphonate therapy and lifestyle changes including diet.

❾ Patients chronically taking glucocorticoids need to be identified and started on bisphosphonate therapy to prevent osteoporosis-related fractures.

❿ Osteomalacia, although less common than osteoporosis, can be insidious and coexist with osteoporosis. A serum 25-hydroxyvitamin D concentration should be obtained in anyone with decreased oral vitamin D intake, limited or no sun exposure, or unexplained muscle weakness or pain.

Despite being an essentially preventable condition, osteoporosis remains a disturbingly common health problem. As such, the U.S. president declared 2002–2011 to be the "Decade of the Bone and Joint," and the U.S. Surgeon General in 2004 released a report, "Bone Health and Osteoporosis." This report has activities for patients and health professionals to use in promoting bone health and preventing complications of osteoporosis (www.hhs.gov/surgeongeneral/library/bonehealth/). Decreased bone mass, quality, and strength contribute to increased osteoporosis and fracture risk. Osteoporosis-related fractures commonly cause pain, kyphosis, disability, and death. Because a perfect bone formation therapy remains elusive, clinicians must actively promote a bone-healthy lifestyle beginning at birth in all people to prevent bone loss. Osteomalacia, or deficient bone mineralization, is less common but also leads to skeletal muscle weakness, fractures, and other complications. This chapter reviews bone physiology, pathophysiol-ogy, and assessment, and offers nonpharmacologic and pharmacologic prevention and treatment strategies for these skeletal diseases.

OSTEOPOROSIS

EPIDEMIOLOGY

The exact prevalence is unknown, but experts estimate that nearly half of Americans aged 50 years or older, or approximately 44 million people, have low bone mass. This number is expected to rise to over 60 million people during the next 15 years. The incidence varies widely among subpopulations and depends on many risk factors, the skeletal site measured, and the radiologic technology used. In the late 1990s, based on peripheral bone mineral density (BMD) measurements, 40% of postmenopausal women had osteopenia and 7% had osteoporosis.[1]

When World Health Organization BMD classifications are applied to central BMD (femoral neck) data from the third National Health and Nutrition Examination Survey (NHANES III, conducted from 1988 to 1994), the respective osteopenia and osteoporosis prevalences among American subgroups are as follows:[2]

- Non-Hispanic white women: 52% and 20%
- Mexican-American women: 49% and 10%
- Non-Hispanic black women: 35% and 5%
- Men of all races: 47% and 6%, using the mean young male BMD
- Men of all races: 33% and 4%, using the mean young female BMD

Osteoporosis increases with age. Osteoporosis prevalences are even higher for nursing home residents.

Hundreds of thousands of fractures occur each year in the United States. The lifetime risk of a white woman experiencing a fracture is approximately 50%.[3] Fracture risk increases with age and lower BMD.

ETIOLOGY AND RISK FACTORS

Many modifiable and nonmodifiable factors are associated with an increased risk of developing osteoporosis and related bone fractures (Table 88–1).[3–8] The magnitude and significance of these risk factors varies by gender, ethnicity, age, and the duration of risk factor presence. After accounting for confounders, the four strongest factors that predict fracture risk are low BMD, prior fragility fracture, age, and family history of osteoporosis.[7] The largest trial, the Study of Osteoporotic Fractures, revealed that women with five or more risk factors were at increased risk of hip fracture compared to women with two or fewer risk factors.[9] While the existence of multiple risk factors incurs greater fracture risk, the absence of risk factors does not necessarily eliminate fracture risk.

PHYSIOLOGY

BONE FUNCTION AND COMPOSITION

The skeleton provides structural support, protects vital organs and the hematopoietic system, and maintains homeostasis of calcium and other ions. The two types of bone, trabecular (cancellous) and cortical (compact) bone, occur in varying amounts at different anatomic sites:

- Distal radius: 75% cortical and 25% trabecular
- Lumbar spine: 34% cortical and 66% trabecular
- Femoral neck: 75% cortical and 25% trabecular
- Trochanter: 50% cortical and 50% trabecular.[10]

Trabecular bone is a meshwork of struts giving it a large surface area that is in close contact with the bone marrow cavity for bone turnover and metabolic activity. Cortical bone is formed in layers and is highly calcified (about 80% to 90%). Because of these different structures and environments, trabecular bone is more metabolically active and cortical bone is more structurally strong and protective.

Bone comprises minerals (50% to 70%), an organic matrix (20% to 40%), water (5% to 10%), and lipids (<3%).[10] The predominant mineral is hydroxyapatite $[3Ca_3(PO_4)_2(OH)_2]$. Bone contains 99% of the body's calcium and 85% of its phosphorus. The organic matrix is primarily protein; 90% type I collagen and 10% to 15% noncollagenous proteins (proteoglycans, glycosylated proteins [e.g., osteonectin], and γ-carboxylated proteins [e.g., osteocalcin]); and cells (osteoclasts, osteoblasts, and osteocytes). The mineral provides strength and rigidity while the proteins provide elasticity and flexibility.

Bone Remodeling and Its Control

The skeleton undergoes constant remodeling throughout life. Peak bone mass is achieved by age 20 to 30 years, long after maximum bone length has been achieved. Men achieve higher peak bone mass than women. For 5 to 10 years after menopause, women have accelerated bone loss, up to 3% per year. Age-related bone loss, about 0.5% per year, begins 10 to 15 years after menopause in women and in men at about age 55 years.[10]

Bone is a dynamic tissue. The majority of the skeleton is replaced approximately every 7 to 10 years. Remodeling repairs microfractures, prepares bone for weight bearing, and provides access to mineral stores. Teams of osteoclasts and osteoblasts, termed *basic multicellular units* (BMUs), perform this remodeling process. Steps in remodeling are resorption, reversal, formation, and quiescence (Fig. 88–1). This process begins with activation of osteoclasts, causing bone resorption. Osteoclasts attach to bone by an integrin, $\alpha V\beta 3$, and create a leakproof seal. The osteoclast's ruffled border secretes acid and proteases, such as H^+ and cathepsin K, to dissolve bone. Osteoclasts create tunnels in cortical bone and pits (Howship lacunae) in trabecular bone. By-products of collagen degradation include hydroxyproline, and N-terminal and C-terminal collagen peptides, which can also serve as biomarkers of resorption. When excavation is complete, reversal begins by osteoclasts undergoing apoptosis or moving to a new section. Resorption takes 3 to 4 weeks. Formation begins with osteoblasts making osteoid that is mineralized over the ensuing 3 to 4 months. Osteoblasts then either line the bone (lining cells) or become part of the bone as osteocytes. Quiescence follows mineralization.

Numerous agents control mesenchymal stem cell derivation and differentiation of osteoblasts (Fig. 88–2).[10,11] Adipocytes can be converted to osteoblasts under the control of Runx2 and peroxisome proliferator-activated receptor-$\gamma 2$ (PPAR $\gamma 2$). Osteoclasts are derived from the myeloid/monocyte cell line with derivation and differentiation also under the control of numerous agents, some of which are expressed from osteoblasts.[10,12]

A complex array and timing of cytokines and hormones control osteoblasts and osteoclasts during bone remodeling (see Fig. 88–2).[10] Intensive investigation continues to define the complete process. Although the triggers to begin remodeling are not completely understood, osteocytes may act as mechanosensors, reacting to bone strain and sensing fatigue and damage. Osteocytes communicate with lining cells via a homing signal, which is thought to summon osteoclast precursors to initiate resorption. Osteoblasts regulate osteoclastic activity by secreting colony-stimulating factors (macrophage colony-stimulating factor [MCSF]; CSF-1) to promote differentiation of osteoclast precursors, receptor activator of nuclear factor κB ligand (RANKL) to promote osteoclast differentiation and maturation, and osteoprotegerin (OPG) to compete with RANKL and prevent osteoclastic differentiation. Regulation of osteoblast secretion of CSF-1, RANKL, and OPG is complex, involving parathyroid hormone (PTH), 1α-25-dihydroxyvitamin D, leptin, estrogen, and other agents. Transforming growth factor-β (TGF-β), platelet-derived growth factor (PDGF), insulin-like growth factor-1 (IGF-1), PTH, growth hormone, and other factors promote bone formation.

Bone mineral density peaks between the ages of 20 and 30 in men and women. Peak bone mass and rate of bone loss is controlled partly by genetics. Polymorphisms of collagen type 1, vitamin D receptor, estrogen receptor, and other genes are being investigated as contributors to this variance. Under normal conditions in adults, resorption equals formation for no net loss or gain of bone mass. Aging, menopause, and certain diseases and drugs can create an imbalance between formation and resorption and result in bone loss.

TABLE 88–1. Risk Factors Affecting Bone Health

Factors associated with clinical bone fractures	Prior fragility fracture Low bone mineral density Advanced age Family history of osteoporosis or fragility fracture

Factors associated with low bone mass	Gender (female)
	Ethnicity (Caucasian or Asian)
	Lifestyle (sedentary)
	Immobility
	Low body weight (<125 pounds)
	Low calcium intake (anytime in life; lactose intolerance)
	Smoking (tobacco)
	Weight loss (>10% of weight at age 25)
	Alcohol (excessive intake)
	Malnutrition (eating disorders)
	Low sun exposure
	Nulliparity
	Medical problems
	  Rheumatoid arthritis
	  Hyperthyroidism
	  Hyperparathyroidism
	  Cushing's syndrome
	  Gastrointestinal disorders (gastrectomy, malabsorption syndromes, inflammatory bowel disease, sprue)
	  Genetic bone disorders
	  Cancers (multiple myeloma, lymphoma, leukemia)
	  Diabetes (type 1)
	  Pernicious anemia
	  Human immunodeficiency virus infection
	  Transplantation
	  Cystic fibrosis
	  Hypophosphatasia
	  Scoliosis
	  Severe liver disease (especially primary biliary cirrhosis)
	  Sex hormone deficiency (hypogonadism, menopause [natural, premature, oophorectomy], female athlete triad)
	  Amyloidosis
	  Ankylosing spondylitis
	  Chronic obstructive pulmonary disease
	Medications (usually long-term)
	  Glucocorticoids (systemic exposure >3 months)
	  Anticonvulsants (phenytoin, phenobarbital)
	  Heparin
	  Parenteral nutrition
	  Thyroid supplements
	  Aluminum
	  Medroxyprogesterone (acetate contraceptive implant)
	  Lithium
	  Immunosuppressants
	  Diuretics (loop)
	  Cancer chemotherapy
	  Gonadotropin-releasing hormone agonists

Factors associated with falls	Prior fall or fear of falling
	Impaired senses (vision or hearing)
	Physical disabilities (deconditioning/decreased strength, ambulation difficulties)
	Environmental (obstacles, lack of handrails, poor lighting, slippery floors)
	Orthostatic hypotension
	Visual impairment
	Environmental obstacles and hazards
	Cognitive impairment
	Medications
	  Antidepressants (tricyclic agents or selective serotonin reuptake inhibitors)
	  Benzodiazepines (especially long-acting)
	  Diuretics (any)
	  Hypotensive agents (any)

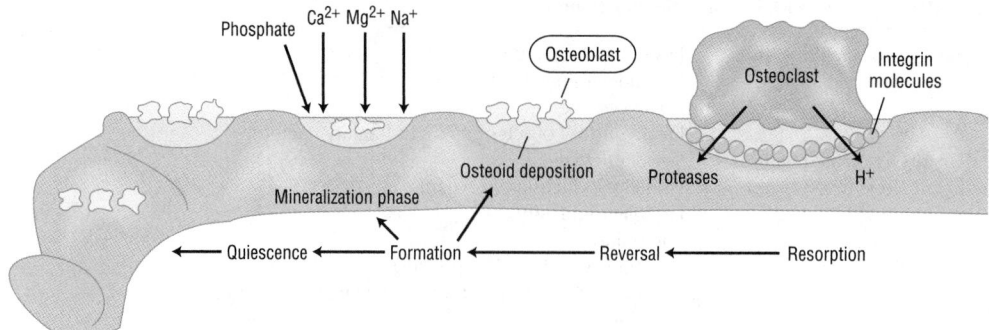

FIGURE 88–1. Steps in bone remodeling: resorption, reversal, formation, and quiescence. See text for details.

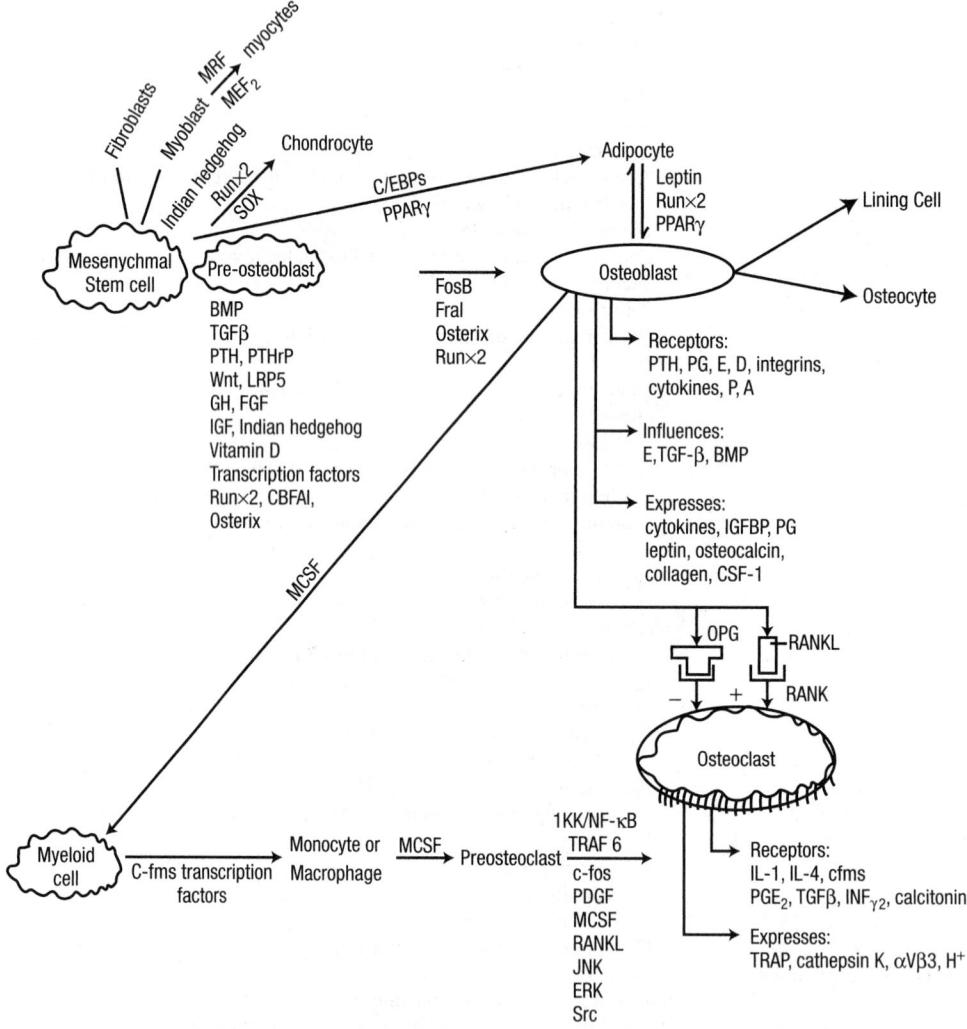

FIGURE 88–2. Differentiation and feedback control of osteoblasts and osteoclasts. $\alpha V\beta 3$, integrin; A, androgen; BMP, bone morphogenetic proteins; C/EBP, IGFBP, insulin-like growth factor binding protein; CCAAT-enhancer binding protein; cfms, transcription factor; CSF, colony-stimulating factor; cFOS, activator protein; D, vitamin D; E, estrogen; ERK, extracellular signal-regulated kinase; FGF, fibroblast growth factor; fos B, regulatory protein; Fral, regulatory protein; GH, growth hormone; H^+, hydrogen ion; IGF, insulin-like growth factor; CBFAI, transcription factor; IKK, inhibitor of NF-κB kinase; IL, interleukins; INF, interferon; JNK, c-Jun N-terminal kinase; LRP, Wnt co-receptor; MCSF, macrophage colony-stimulating factor; MRF, myogenic regulatory factors; MEF, myocyte-enhancer factor; NF-κB, nuclear factor κB; OPG, osteoprotegerin; osterix, transcription factor; P, progestin; PDGF; platelet-derived growth factor; PG, prostaglandin; PPAR, peroxisome proliferator-activated receptor; PTH, parathyroid hormone; PTHrP, PTH-related peptide; RANK, receptor activator of nuclear factor κB; RANKL, receptor activator of nuclear factor κB ligand; Runx2, rnt-related transcription factor 2; Src, tyrosine kinase; SOX, transcription factor; TGF, transforming growth factor; TNF, tumor necrosis factor; TRAF6, TNF receptor associated factor 6; TRAP, tartrate-resistant acid phosphatase; Wnt, protein.

Serum Calcium and Phosphate Regulation and Vitamin D Metabolism

Vitamin D and PTH maintain calcium homeostasis (Fig. 88–3).[10,13,14] The sun (ultraviolet B, 290 to 315 nm) converts 7-dehydrocholesterol in the skin to vitamin D_3. Sunscreens inhibit vitamin D skin production. In northern climates, during the winter months the angle of the sun limits the ability to create vitamin D. Significant seasonal variations lead to fluctuations in 25(OH) vitamin D concentrations. Nadirs occur in February and March and peaks occur in August.[15,16] Although a few foods naturally contain vitamin D_3 (e.g., cholecalciferol from fish oils) or vitamin D_2 (e.g., ergocalciferol from plants), most dietary intake is from foods fortified with vitamin D (Table 88–2). Because both vitamin D_3 and D_2 work similarly in the body, they are referred to here as vitamin D. Vitamin D undergoes hepatic conversion to 25(OH) vitamin D (calcidiol) via D-25-hydroxylase (cytochrome P450 27A1). PTH stimulates renal conversion of 25-hydroxyvitamin D to the active form, 1α-25-dihydroxyvitamin D (calcitriol), via 25(OH)D-1α-hydroxylase (cytochrome P450 27B1).

Decreased serum calcium concentrations lead to increased serum PTH concentrations, which lead to elevated calcitriol concentrations (see Fig. 88–3). Calcitriol promotes intestinal calcium absorption, and calcitriol and PTH work together to release calcium from bone to restore homeostasis. Polymorphisms with the intestinal vitamin D receptor (*Bsm*I, *Apa*I, *Taq*I, and *Fok*I) have been inconsistently associated with low bone density.[17] Vitamin D receptors are found in many tissues, such as bone, intestine, brain, heart, stomach, pancreas, lymphocytes, skin, and gonads.[14]

Serum phosphorus is less tightly regulated than serum calcium. Excess ingested phosphorus is absorbed and adjusted by the kidney.

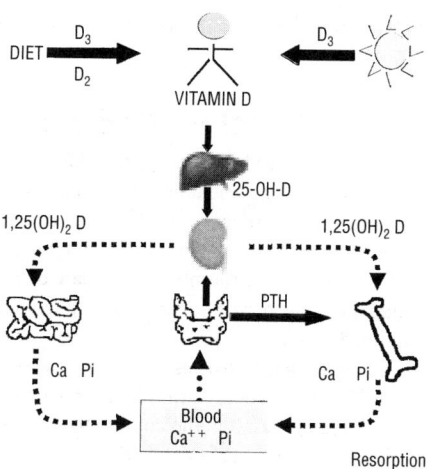

FIGURE 88–3. Effects of vitamin D and parathyroid hormone on calcium balance. See text for details. PTH, parathyroid hormone, Ca, calcium, Pi, phosphorus.

TABLE 88–2. Dietary Sources of Calcium and Vitamin D[a]

Food	Serving Size	Calcium Content (mg)	Vitamin D Content (units)
Milk	1 cup	300	100
Powdered nonfat milk	1 teaspoon	50	
Ice cream	1 cup	200	
Yogurt, fortified	1 cup	240–415	60
American cheese	1 oz	150	
Cheddar cheese	1 oz	211	
Cottage cheese	1/2 cup	100	
Swiss cheese	1 oz	250	
Parmesan cheese	1 tablespoonful	70	
Cheese pizza	1 slice	150	
Macaroni and cheese	1 cup	360	
Slim Fast	11 oz	400	140
Orange juice, fortified	1 cup	350	100
Soymilk, fortified	1 cup	80–300	100
Bread, fortified	1 slice	100	
Cereals, fortified	1 cup	100–250	60
Sardines with bones	3 oz	370	230
Salmon with bones	3 oz	170–210	310
Catfish	3 oz		570
Halibut	3 oz		680
Tuna	4 oz		260
Almonds	1 oz	80	
Bok choy	1/2 cup	125	
Broccoli	1 cup	130–160	
Collards	1/2 cup	180	
Cornbread	1 slice	85	
Egg, medium	1	55	25
Figs, dried	5 medium	125	
Kale	1/2 cup	95	
Orange	1	52	
Soybeans	1 cup	130	
Spinach	1/2 cup	110	
Tofu	4 oz	140	
Turnip greens	1/2 cup	125	

[a]To calculate calcium content, multiply precentage on package by 1000. To calculate vitamin D content, multiply percentage on package by 400.

PTH also controls the kidney "set point" and decreases renal phosphorus reabsorption.

PATHOPHYSIOLOGY OF OSTEOPOROSIS

Osteoporosis is "characterized by low bone mass and microarchitectural deterioration of bone tissue leading to enhanced bone fragility and a consequent increase in fracture risk."[3] Bone loss results when resorption exceeds formation. The World Health Organization classifies bone mass based on T-score (number of standard deviations from the mean compared to bone mass of average young women). Normal bone mass is defined as a T-score greater than −1, osteopenia as a T-score of −1 to −2.5, and osteoporosis as a T-score of less than −2.5.[3,7] In addition to low BMD, high bone turnover, poor bone strength, and impaired bone architecture result in the bone's increased susceptibility to fracture. Severe osteoporosis is defined as a history of a fragility fracture plus a T-score <−2.5. Women with osteopenia have a 1.8-fold increase in fracture rate, and women with osteoporosis have a fourfold increase in fracture rate, compared to women with normal BMD.[1]

Clinically, osteoporosis is categorized as postmenopausal, age-related, or secondary. Postmenopausal osteoporosis affects primarily trabecular bone in the decade following menopause, with fractures occurring predominantly at vertebral and distal forearm sites. Within a few years after peak BMD is attained, usually in the mid- to late-30s, bone loss slowly begins. The cumulative effect over time can translate into age-related osteoporosis that affects both cortical and trabecular bone and leads to vertebral, hip, and wrist fractures. Secondary osteoporosis is caused by either diseases or medications and afflicts both bone types. Secondary causes can be found in 11% to 31% of women and 30% to 54% of men.[4]

POSTMENOPAUSAL

The rate of bone loss commonly accelerates at menopause due to a decline in trophic sex hormone production, especially when a bone-healthy lifestyle is not practiced. In older studies, approximately 10% to 25% of bone loss was documented in the decade after menopause. Bone loss then slows to 8% to 12% per decade, a rate that was similar to that of older men.[18] This accelerated loss has not been demonstrated in most of the placebo groups who were taking calcium and vitamin D supplements in recently conducted randomized controlled trials.

Estrogen deficiency increases bone resorption more than formation. This process appears to depend on tumor necrosis factor (TNF), interleukin-1 (IL-1), interleukin-11, interleukin-6, MCSF, and prostaglandin E_2, which stimulate osteoclastic activity through the OPG/RANK/RANKL system (see Fig. 88-2). Reduced TGF-β, associated with estrogen loss, enhances osteoclast action through decreased apoptosis. Osteocytes also may play a role. Normally, with more weight bearing, osteocytes trigger increased BMD. With menopause, osteocyte apoptosis blunts this response. With the resetting of the mechanostat set point at menopause, increased loading is required to maintain bone. After menopause, some estrogen is still synthesized by aromatization in adipose tissue.

AGE-RELATED

Bone resorption increases with age, but changes in bone formation are not observed consistently. Increased osteocyte apoptosis may decrease responses to mechanical strain and hinder bone repair. Cortical porosity from years of remodeling and decreased trabecular connectivity, particularly of horizontal struts, promotes microarchitectural deterioration of bone that is not always reflected in BMD. Aging also increases fracture risk in other ways that are independent of BMD.

Comorbid conditions, cognitive impairment, medications, and deconditioning can increase falls. Some falls lead to fractures, usually of the hip.

Inadequate calcium, vitamin D, and nutritional intake also contribute to bone loss and fractures. Vitamin D insufficiency results from poor sun exposure, decreased cutaneous production, insufficient dietary intake, and decreased absorption. Calcium and vitamin D insufficiency promotes secondary hyperparathyroidism and associated bone loss (see Fig. 88-3).

MEN

For many reasons, men experience fewer osteoporosis-related fractures than women.[19] Men comprise only approximately 20% of all persons with osteoporosis. This is likely attributable to men attaining a 20% to 40% higher peak BMD than women and losing BMD at a slower rate after the peak. Men's bones also have a mechanical advantage because the larger bone diameter makes them more fracture-resistant. Finally, men have a shorter life expectancy and experience fewer falls than women. Male osteoporosis remains an underrecognized problem. Although fewer men than women have osteoporosis, men still suffer up to 30% of all hip fractures and are more likely than women to die within 1 year after fracture.[20]

Hypogonadism, secondary to age-related decreased testosterone and increased sex hormone–binding globulin (SHBG), endocrine dysfunction, or androgen ablation, can also cause bone loss. Estrogen, synthesized from testosterone by the enzyme aromatase, appears more important than testosterone in men for bone maintenance, with greater bone density seen in men with higher estradiol concentrations. Secondary causes often contribute to male osteoporosis. Other factors are listed in Table 88-1.

SECONDARY CAUSES

Numerous diseases and drugs can decrease bone mass (see Table 88-1). Secondary causes are suspected when osteoporosis occurs in premenopausal women, men younger than age 70, those with no risk factors, multiple low trauma fractures (especially at a young age), a Z-score less than −2.0 (see section below on quantification of BMD), or bone loss despite adequate drug treatment and calcium supplementation.[4] Patients suspected of having secondary causes should undergo careful evaluation that includes a comprehensive physical exam and laboratory assessment. Both the osteoporosis and contributing disorders should be treated.

DRUG-INDUCED

Unfortunately, several medications (see Table 88-1) can cause bone loss by a variety of mechanisms. Examples include systemic glucocorticoids (see section on glucocorticoid-induced osteoporosis, below),[21,22] thyroid hormone replacement, some antiepileptic drugs, and heparin use. Thyroid dose adjustment is needed to keep the thyroid-stimulating hormone (TSH) in the upper half of the normal range to minimize bone loss. Some anticonvulsants, like phenobarbital and phenytoin, hasten vitamin D metabolism and the resultant effects can lead to osteomalacia (see section later in the chapter on osteomalacia).[23] Those at higher risk include people who take multiple anticonvulsants, are institutionalized, or have multiple comorbidities. Heparin therapy, in excess of 15,000 to 30,000 units daily for greater than 3 to 6 months, is associated with bone loss and vertebral fractures. Low-molecular-weight heparins such as enoxaparin may pose less risk of bone loss. A black-box warning has been added to the product labeling of medroxyprogesterone acetate injectable contraceptive warning that it significantly decreases bone loss that increases

TABLE 88–3. Clinical Presentation of Osteoporosis

General

Many patients are unaware they have osteoporosis and only present after fracture.

Fractures can occur after bending, lifting, or falling, or independent of any activity.

Symptoms

Pain

Immobility

Bruising

Depression and lower self-esteem can result from pain and physical changes.

Signs

Shortened stature, kyphosis, or lordosis

Vertebra, hip, or forearm fracture

Laboratory tests

25(OH) vitamin D

Other tests to identify secondary causes (e.g., thyroid-stimulating hormone, parathyroid hormone, complete blood count)

Other diagnostic tests

Central or peripheral bone density measurement

---

with longer durations of therapy. Thus, this contraceptive product should be used only when other medications prove inadequate.

CLINICAL PRESENTATION

Osteopenia and asymptomatic osteoporosis are generally diagnosed only by bone density measurement. Osteoporosis is frequently diagnosed after a fragility fracture or after a work-up of pain or curvature in the spine (Table 88–3). Although fractures can occur after any minimal activity, such as bending, lifting, or twisting, the shearing force from a fall is the greatest contributor to fracture, especially nonvertebral fracture. Multiple vertebral fractures, even clinically unrecognizable ones, may lead to dorsal kyphosis and exaggerated cervical lordosis, frequently referred to as *dowager* or *widow's hump.* Subsequent chest wall changes can lead to pulmonary and cardiovascular complications. Collapsed vertebrae rarely lead to spinal cord compression. Recurrent fractures are common. Nonvertebral fractures are almost always evident because of severe pain at the fracture site, inability to bear weight, and obvious deformity. Depression and lower self-esteem can result from pain, physical changes, and dependence on others for activities of daily living.

FRACTURE OUTCOMES

Fractures can be devastating. While acute fracture pain usually resolves within 2 to 3 months, chronic fracture pain can occur, and is manifested as a deep, dull, nagging pain near the fracture site. Up to 50% of hip fracture patients do not regain their prefracture function by up to 1 year following hip fracture.[3,8] About 25% of women will spend some time in a nursing home after a hip fracture. Between 10% and 20% of hip fracture patients die within 1 year following the fracture. In the late 1990s, 51% of women and 96% of men were not screened for osteoporosis nor did they receive treatment after a fracture.[24]

PATIENT ASSESSMENT

Patient assessment should begin with identifying risk factors for osteoporosis and fractures (see Table 88–1). Important points include age, history of nontraumatic adult fractures, family history of osteoporosis or fragility fractures, comorbid medical and mental illnesses, lifestyle habits (diet, physical activity, smoking, and alcohol use), menstrual history, fall risk, prior and current medications (especially

glucocorticoid use), and calcium and vitamin D supplements. Lateral spine radiographs to detect vertebral fractures are reasonable in patients with acute or chronic severe back pain. For patients in whom a diagnosis of osteoporosis is made, secondary causes (see Table 88–1) should be sought if the degree of bone loss is severe or unexplained.[4] Surveys and questionnaires are used in research and for screening and sometimes for prediction and treatment evaluation. For patients with established osteoporosis, the validated Mini Osteoporosis Quality of Life tool, which takes 2 to 3 minutes to administer, can evaluate the impact of osteoporosis on daily physical and emotional functioning.[25] A risk factor checklist can be developed to help direct care plans for lifestyle changes to prevent and treat osteoporosis.

QUANTIFICATION OF BONE MINERAL DENSITY

BMD remains a very strong predictor of fracture risk.[3,7,8,10] The gold standard method of bone density assessment is to measure central skeletal BMD (hip and spine) by dual-energy x-ray absorptiometry (DXA). DXA uses minimal radiation and has the greatest precision (reproducibility on repeat examinations). Quantitative computed tomography measures trabecular and cortical bone separately, but is not ideal for routine use because it is expensive, not widely available, and uses more radiation. Measurements at peripheral sites (forearm, heel, and phalanges) with ultrasound or DXA are currently just used for screening purposes and to determine the need for further testing. Portable units are easy to transport.

Variability exists with BMD measurements. A T-score is the number of standard deviations an individual's BMD is away from the mean BMD for normative reference databases for young women or men. The Z-score compares bone mass to a group matched for age, sex, weight, and race. Different central and peripheral T-scores can be measured. The lowest T-score is used for decision making. Differences also depend on the technology used, thus only the same machine's T-scores can be compared. Most machines use a different normal reference population to calculate the T- and Z-scores. Consensus does not exist regarding what peripheral T-score should be used as a threshold for obtaining a central DXA measurement, but –1 or –1.6 has been suggested. T-score adjustments need to be made for children and thin adults.

Medicare patients are eligible for BMD testing.[3] In the United States, the Centers for Medicare & Medicaid Services regulations provide reimbursement to providers every 2 years for BMD measurement for patients with estrogen-deficiency or clinical risk for osteoporosis, those with vertebral abnormalities or primary hyperparathyroidism, and those on long-term glucocorticoid therapy (>7.5 mg prednisone/day for >3 months) or FDA-approved osteoporosis therapy. Knowledge of low BMD can encourage prevention and lead to positive lifestyle changes.

BIOCHEMICAL AND BIOPSY EVALUATION

A complete blood count, chemistry panel (with calcium corrected for albumin), erythrocyte sedimentation rate, PTH concentration, and 24-hour urine for calcium and creatinine are occasionally ordered to determine secondary causes.[4] Measurement of 25(OH) vitamin D is becoming more common. Measurement of TSH, free T_4 (thyroxine) and free T_3 (triiodothyronine) can be used to rule out hyperthyroidism from endogenous disease or thyroid replacements.

In the past, biochemical markers have been considered as research tools only.[7,10] Now that increased bone turnover independently predicts fracture risk and more automated and precise assays exist, these tests may become more common for drug selection and monitoring.[10] Response to drug therapy can be measured more quickly than bone density measurements, 1 to 3 months vs. 6 to 12 months, respectively.[4,10] A decrease of bone resorption tests of at least 20% is considered a positive response. Until assay variability is further improved, these tests should not be used for diagnosis. Commonly used markers of bone resorption include urine and serum *C*-terminal or *N*-terminal telopeptides and urine deoxypyridinoline, and of bone

formation include bone-specific alkaline phosphatase and osteocal cin. When possible, these tests should be performed at similar time due to circadian rhythms.

Bone biopsy is rarely useful for osteoporosis, but can be used t identify other conditions such as osteomalacia.

▶ PREVENTION AND TREATMENT: Osteoporosis

■ DESIRED OUTCOMES

The goal from birth to around 20 to 30 years of age is to achieve the highest peak bone mass as possible. Beyond this age, the goals are to maintain BMD and minimize age-related and postmenopausal bone loss. In women and men with osteopenia, prevention of osteoporosis is the goal. For a variety of reasons, osteoporosis prevention is not always possible. For those at significant risk of developing an osteoporosis-related fracture, the aims are to increase bone mineral density, prevent further bone loss, and to prevent falls and fractures and their associated sequelae. For those who experience an osteoporosis-related fracture, the goals are to achieve adequate pain control, maximize rehabilitation

to restore independence and quality of life, and prevent subsequen fractures or death.

■ GENERAL APPROACH TO TREATMENT

A bone-healthy lifestyle beginning at birth is advocated for all peo ple throughout life. Calcium and vitamin D supplements are use for everyone when diet is insufficient. Treatment of osteopenia re mains controversial (see clinical controversy below). Prescriptio medications, with bisphosphonates being the drugs of choice, ar used for treating patients with a T-score of –2.5 or lower. Figure 88–

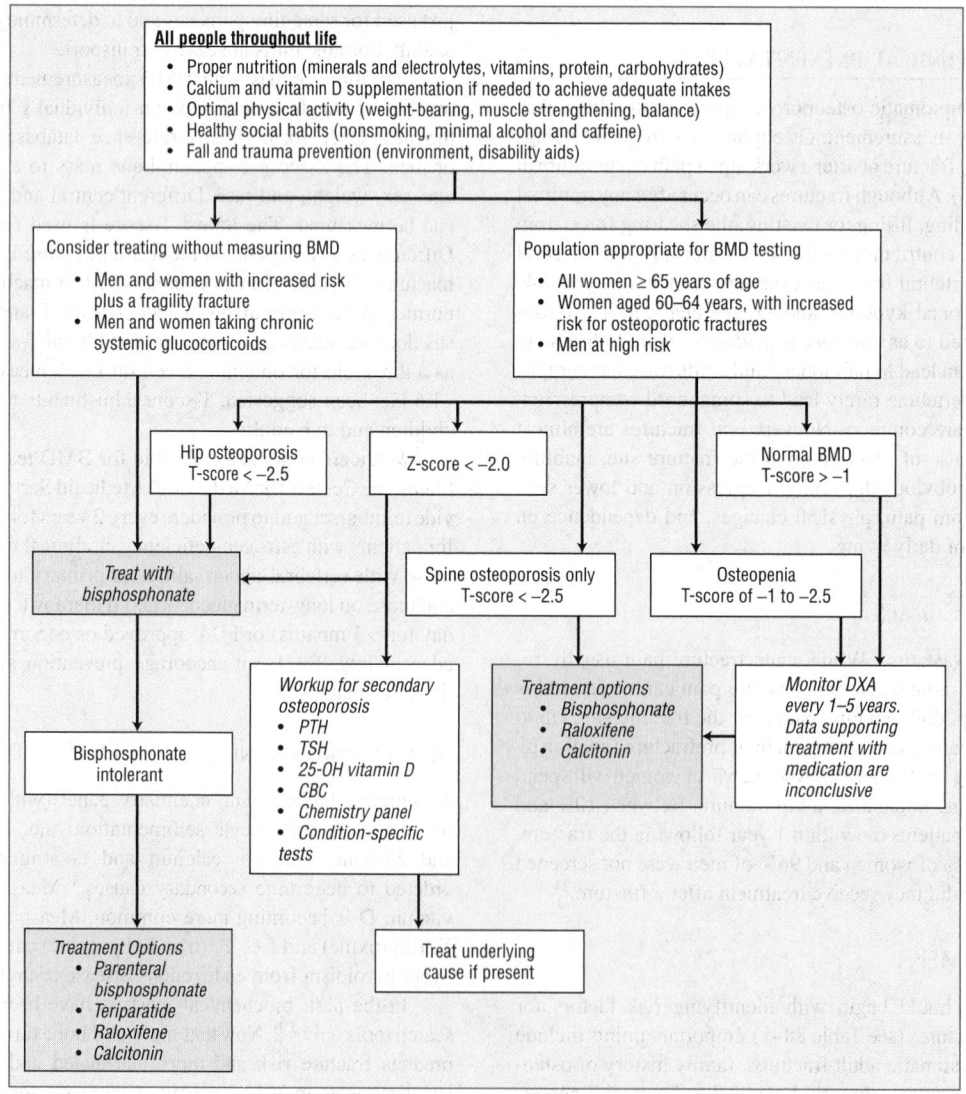

FIGURE 88–4. Bone health therapeutic algorithm. BMD, bone mineral density; CBC, complete blood count; DXA, dual-energy x-ray absorptiometry; PTH, parathyroid hormone; TSH, thyroid-stimulating hormone.

rovides an osteoporosis management algorithm that incorporates oth nonpharmacologic and pharmacologic approaches.

CLINICAL CONTROVERSY

Not all clinicians believe that women and men with osteopenia, especially premenopausal women, should receive osteoporosis prevention beyond instituting bone-healthy lifestyle and calcium and vitamin D supplementation. Although some statistically significant findings exist, the absolute clinical value of treatment is very small. Women with osteopenia have a 1.8-fold greater risk for developing a fracture than women with normal BMD, but the absolute risk difference is very low (0.86 fractures/100 person-years with normal BMD vs. 1.55 fractures/100 person-years with osteopenia).[1] The FOSIT study investigators report reduced fracture risk in 1 year with alendronate in patients with either osteopenia or osteoporosis, but in a trial that was only designed to assess BMD change.[130] Furthermore, the patients with osteopenia were not analyzed separately. Reanalysis of the Multiple Outcomes of Raloxifene Evaluation (MORE) trial[72] found that postmenopausal women with osteopenia had a 75% reduction in new clinical vertebral fractures compared with the placebo group (16 vs. 4 new fractures, respectively).[131] Because long-term data on treating osteopenia in younger premenopausal, perimenopausal, or postmenopausal women or men with osteoporosis prescription medications are not known, the benefit-risk profile for early or lifelong use is also not known. Until clinical data are sufficiently collected, an adequate guideline cannot be established and a pharmacoeconomic analysis cannot be conducted.

NONPHARMACOLOGIC PREVENTION AND TREATMENT

DIET CHANGES

For all individuals, a well-balanced diet with adequate calcium and vitamin D is essential for healthy bones (see Table 88–2). Dairy products account for most dietary calcium intake. Americans, specially seniors and those with lactose intolerance, ingest insufficient dietary calcium. Serum calcium does not reflect dietary intake because calcium homeostasis is tightly controlled. A practical pproach is to count calcium contributions from certain key foods: milk, yogurt, cheese, ice cream, cottage cheese, and fortified orange uice or soy products. Most vitamin D comes from sun-induced skin onversion, except in northern climates or people with minimal to no un exposure. Besides fatty fish, few unfortified foods contain subtantial amounts of vitamin D (see Table 88–2). In the United States, milk and orange juice are fortified with 400 units/quart of vitamin D; however, quantities are quite variable and the process is not well egulated. If adequate intakes[26] (Table 88–4) cannot be achieved with ood, calcium and vitamin D supplements are needed (Table 88–5).

Many observational studies have found an association between igh caffeine intake and decreased BMD. This finding, however, could e a surrogate marker for decreased calcium-containing beverage and ood intake.[27] Although 2 to 5 cups of caffeine produce small increases n calcium excretion (about 4 to 5 mg calcium per cup of coffee), the ffect can be offset with adequate calcium intake.

Phosphorus is part of bone hydroxyapatite $[3Ca_3(PO_4)_2(OH)_2]$. Normally the body has sufficient phosphorus and bone resorption is ot required. Insufficient intake (e.g., carbonated beverages replacng milk) or increased phosphorous-bound calcium complexes (e.g.,

TABLE 88–4. Daily Calcium and Vitamin D Requirements

	Adequate Calcium Intake (mg)	Adequate Vitamin D Intake (units)
Infant		
Birth to 6 months	210	200
6 months–1 year	270	200
Children		
1–3 years	500	200
4–8 years	800	200
9–13 years	1300	200
Adolescents		
14–18 years	1300	200
Adults		
19–50 years	1000	200
51–70 years	1200	400
≥71 years	1200	600

Adapted from Institute of Medicine Dietary Reference Intakes.[26]

calcium ingested with food) can produce hypophosphatemia and a corresponding rise in PTH.[28] A growing concern now exists for approximately 10% to 15% of seniors who are hypophosphatemic, and also during teriparatide administration, when the need for phosphorus is large. Drinking some milk or orange juice, eating some meals without supplemental calcium, or occasionally using a calcium phosphate supplement may help. Phosphorus supplementation is not routinely recommended.

Magnesium is found in bone and is required for enzymatic reactions. Fruits and vegetables contain magnesium and may be important for healthy bone.[29] No data currently exist to support supplementation.

Vitamin A can increase production and action of osteoclasts and impair osteoblasts. Excessive vitamin A intake (≥1.5 to 2 mg/day) from foods or supplements has been associated with decreased BMD and increased fracture risk in women[30] and men.[31] Patients should be educated to avoid consuming excessive amounts of vitamin A.

Vitamin C positively influences collagen production, and increases osteoblast formation and osteoclast formation and survival. Some, but not all, observational studies showed that vitamin C supplementation (1000 mg or more) was associated with higher BMD than that of nonusers.[32] Again, it is premature to suggest routine supplementation.

Vitamin K is required for γ-carboxylation of osteocalcin before incorporation into bone matrix.[33] Low-vitamin-K diets are associated with high amounts of uncarboxylated osteocalcin, lower BMD, and higher hip fracture rates. Early research suggests added vitamin K, especially when combined with other antiresorptive agents, has a positive effect on bone health. Currently, however, supplements are not recommended. Although warfarin decreases clotting factor production by antagonizing vitamin K, it alone probably does not cause bone loss.

Protein intake can increase IGF-1, low-protein diets can increase PTH, and high-protein diets can increase urinary calcium excretion.[34] Many observational studies reported higher BMD with higher protein intakes; however, most observational studies also found low protein intake to be associated with a lower fracture rate.[35] Moderate protein intake is recommended.

SOCIAL HABIT CHANGES

Smoking cessation and minimal alcohol use should be advocated. Smoking causes bone loss and increases hip fracture risk by several mechanisms. Smoking is associated with early menopause,

TABLE 88–5. Calcium and Vitamin D Product Selection[a]

Product[b]	Calcium (mg)	Vitamin D (units)
Calcium carbonate (40%)		
Trade and generic products	200–600	
Generic suspension	500/5 mL	
Titralac Liquid	400/5 mL	
Titralac Chewable	168	
Titralac Extra Strength	300	
Tums Chewable	200	
Tums E-X	300	
Tums Ultra	500	
Other chewable brands	168–500	
Mylanta Soothing Lozenges	240	
Cal Carb-HD powder	2.4 g/7-g packet	
Calcium carbonate with vitamin D		
Generic + vitamin D	600	125
Calcilyte + vitamin D[d]	500	200
Calel-D + vitamin D	500	200
Caltrate + vitamin D	600	200
Os-Cal + vitamin D	500	125
Viactiv chews[c]	500	100
Caltrate 600 plus[e]	600	200
Olay Vitamins		
Essential Bone		
Health Formulation[f]	600	200
Calcium citrate (24%)		
Generic	240	
Citracal	200	
Citracal Liquitab[d]	500	
Citracal + vitamin D	316	200
Calcium phosphate tribasic (39%)		
Posture	600	
Posture-D	600	125
Dical-D chewable wafers + vitamin D	232	200
Multivitamin (D₃)	40	400
Vitamin A (5000 units)		
Cod liver oil (D₃)		500
5 mL: vitamin A (4000 units),		130–270
Gel caps: vitamin A (1250–2500 units)		
Ergocalciferol (D₂)		
Drops (per mL)		8000
Tablets		50,000

[a]Only calcium products with 500–600 mg per tablet or with an alternative dosage form (i.e., chewable, liquid, or dissolvable tablet) are listed.
[b]Many products beginning to add magnesium, boron, zinc, copper, and manganese, and adding "Plus" or "Ultra" to name.
[c]Also contains vitamin K.
[d]Tablet for solution.
[e]Also contains magnesium, zinc, copper, boron, and manganese.
[f]Also contains phosphorus and magnesium.

decreased body weight, enhanced estrogen metabolism, increased PTH concentrations, and decreased vitamin D concentrations. Excessive alcohol use has been associated with low BMD and subsequent fracture in some, but not all, studies. The effects are greater with chronic heavy drinking early in life. Malnutrition associated with alcoholism could also play a role. Alcohol use also may increase the risk of falls.

EXERCISE

Bones adapt to handle the workload to which they are subjected. Long-term exercise (likely many years) during youth increases peak BMD. Physical activity, especially aerobics, weight bearing, and resistance exercise and walking, preserves BMD in post-menopausal women.[36] Continued activity appears necessary to maintain benefit. Exercise also enhances calcium and estrogen therapy.[3] In addition to the positive bone effects, physical activity likely reduces fracture risk by reducing falls (from improved balance, posture, flexibility, range of motion, muscle strength, and endurance). Physical activity, as tolerated, should be encouraged for all patients with osteoporosis. Before starting an exercise program for an elderly patient or one with severe osteoporosis, a medical examination is recommended. Referral to a physical therapist may be helpful.

Excessive exercise in a premenstrual woman, however, can lead to amenorrhea and estrogen deficiency with consequent bone loss and increased fracture risk.[38]

FALL PREVENTION

Exercises to improve muscle strength, gait, balance, and flexibility should be employed whenever possible. Tai chi also reduces fall risk.[39] The need for ambulation-assistive devices (canes and walkers) and assistance with transferring from various positions or for toileting should be assessed. Vision should be assessed and corrected when necessary. The living environment should be evaluated and modified to minimize falls. Loose rugs and extension cords should be eliminated, grab bars mounted in the bathroom, handrails installed on stairs, nonskid tape placed in bathtubs, and adequate lighting ensured. Although the use of hip protectors decreases fractures from falls, most patients do not like to wear them.

Medications should be reviewed and those that may cause falls should be eliminated when possible. Examples include psychotropics, sedative-hypnotics, antidepressants, antihypertensives, and diuretics. Sedative-hypnotic use should be limited or discontinued. When benzodiazepines must be used, shorter-acting ones are recommended, but are still not risk-free. Other drugs altering balance and lowering blood pressure and blood glucose changes should be carefully monitored. Patients should be warned about medications that contribute to orthostasis and should be warned about abrupt postural changes.

PHARMACOLOGIC PREVENTION AND TREATMENT

Nonpharmacologic interventions alone are not always sufficient to prevent osteoporosis-related fractures, and drug therapy is often necessary. Table 88–6 describes the important aspects of the commonly prescribed medications for osteoporosis. The choice of pharmacotherapy depends on many individual patient-specific characteristics and preferences. Regardless of the medication selected, all patients should receive adequate calcium and vitamin D intake. In order to optimally reduce fracture risk, all people should also implement lifestyle modifications that reduce fall risk.

The two FDA-approved indications for osteoporosis medications—prevention and treatment—were created before enhanced understanding of the disease. The "prevention" of osteoporosis indication applies to drugs that demonstrate maintenance of BMD above the osteoporosis threshold (T-score >–2.5) compared to placebo over a 3-year period in patients with low bone mass (T-score <–1.0). Although commonly misinterpreted by clinicians, this indication does not infer a fracture risk reduction, the primary therapeutic end point. The "treatment" indication, however, is based on a drug's ability to demonstrate fracture risk reduction, either at the vertebral or nonvertebral sites, compared to placebo.

TREATMENT GUIDELINES

No single, widely accepted treatment guideline exists for osteoporosis. Several organizations have suggested various treatment approaches, most of which are based more on consensus opinion than evidence-based medical data.

The updated 2003 National Osteoporosis Foundation (NOF) guidelines, created in collaboration with nine specialty physician professional organizations, encourage a healthy lifestyle, including adequate calcium and vitamin D, exercise, and tobacco avoidance.[3] The NOF favors BMD testing in all women 65 years and older as well as younger postmenopausal white women with at least one risk factor. Their recommendations for testing all postmenopausal women with a

fragility fracture and the initiation of therapy for those with osteopenia (T-score <–2.0 without risk factors and <–1.5 with one or more risk factors) are not data-based. They currently consider all approved medications as appropriate pharmacotherapy. A specific monitoring approach is not articulated. No recommendations exist for men. Unfortunately, the guidelines often lack sufficient detail and supporting clinical evidence and rationale.

For postmenopausal women, the 2002 U.S. Preventive Services Task Force addressed screening and only recommends routine screening beginning at age 65, with earlier screening suggested at age 60 for women who are at increased risk.[40] A companion document provides discussion of the specific evidence.[41]

The 2002 Canadian osteoporosis guidelines for women and men were developed using an evidence-based process.[7] This comprehensive document cites levels of supporting evidence and grades its recommendations. They identify four key risk factors for osteoporosis: low BMD, prior fragility fracture, age, and positive family history of osteoporosis. The guidelines also advocate treating patients with a clinical diagnosis of osteoporosis (BMD <–2.5, but history of atraumatic fracture).

The 2002 North American Menopause Society's position statement on the management of postmenopausal osteoporosis reviews pertinent literature pertaining to the pathophysiology, identification, and treatment of osteoporosis.[8]

ANTIRESORPTIVE THERAPY

Calcium

Hypocalcemia can result from inadequate dietary intake, decreased fractional calcium absorption (as seen with increasing age), or enhanced calcium excretion. To restore calcium homeostasis after hypocalcemia, PTH concentrations rise, and vitamin D metabolism increases to enhance intestinal calcium absorption (see Fig. 88–3), renal calcium reabsorption, and bone resorption. Fracture risk is greatest with low calcium intake and low fractional calcium absorption.[42]

Clinical Effectiveness. Although a few studies have found calcium to decrease fractures,[43] most well-conducted studies do not.[44,45] When fracture prevention was documented, concomitant vitamin D therapy was usually given. Over 150 studies have evaluated calcium's effect on BMD, with almost all trials and observational studies showing higher calcium intake in children and adults produced greater increases or maintenance of BMD compared to BMD losses with placebo.[46] During the first 5 years following menopause, calcium is less effective, when estrogen deficiency is the predominant cause of accelerated bone loss. Calcium's effects are augmented when combined with exercise or antiresorptive drugs.[43] Thus adequate calcium intake (see Table 88–4) is considered standard for osteoporosis prevention and treatment for all people.

Nonbone benefits of high calcium intake include reduced colorectal cancer risk and decreased blood pressure.[43]

Administration. Most children and adults do not ingest sufficient dietary calcium and require supplements (see Tables 88–5 and 88–6). Individuals with certain characteristics or conditions—such as lactose intolerance; nondairy vegetarian diet; malnutrition; low-fat diets; and glucocorticoid, antiresorptive, or parathyroid therapy—also require evaluation for calcium supplementation. To ensure adequate calcium absorption, 25(OH) vitamin D concentrations should be maintained in the normal range.[47]

TABLE 88–6. Medications Used to Prevent and Treat Osteoporosis

Drug	Dosage	Pharmacokinetics	Adverse Effects	Drug Interactions
Calcium	200–1500 mg/day; see Tables 88–3 and 88–5; divided doses	Absorption: predominantly active transport with some passive diffusion; fractional absorption 10–60%; fecal elimination for the unabsorbed and renal elimination for the absorbed calcium	Constipation, gas, upset stomach, rare kidney stones	• Absorption is decreased with proton pump inhibitors • Decreases absorption of iron, tetracycline, quinolones, alendronate, risedronate, etidronate, phenytoin, and fluoride when given concomitantly • May antagonize verapamil • May induce hypercalcemia with thiazide diuretics • Fiber laxatives, oxalates, phytates, and sulfates decrease calcium absorption if given concomitantly
Vitamin D_2 or D_3	200–1000 units/day; if malabsorption or on multiple anticonvulsants, may require higher doses (~4000 units/day or more); for vitamin D deficiency, 50,000 units once weekly or once monthly can be used; monitor serum calcium	Hepatic and renal metabolism to active compound 1,25 (OH) vitamin D; active and inactive metabolites	Hypercalcemia, (weakness, headache, somnolence, nausea, cardiac rhythm disturbance); hypercalciuria	• Phenytoin, barbiturates, carbamazepine, rifampin increase vitamin D metabolism • Cholestyramine, colestipol, orlistat, or mineral oil decrease vitamin D absorption • May induce hypercalcemia with thiazide diuretics in hypoparathyroid patients
Bisphosphonates Alendronate (Fosamax) Risedronate (Actonel) Ibandronate (Boniva)	5 mg daily (prevention); 10 mg daily; 70-mg tablet or 75-mL single-use oral dose weekly (treatment) 5 mg daily, 35 mg weekly 2.5 mg daily,[a] 100–150 mg monthly,[b] 3 mg IV every 3 months[c]	Poorly absorbed <1%, decreasing to zero with food or beverage intake; long half-lives (2–10 years); renal elimination (of absorbed) and fecal elimination (of unabsorbed)	Nausea; GI irritation, perforation, ulceration, and/or bleeding	• Do not coadminister with any other medication, including calcium
Selective estrogen receptor modulators Raloxifene (Evista)	60 mg daily	Hepatic metabolism	Hot flushes, leg cramps, venous thromboembolism	None
Calcitonin (Miacalcin)	200 units daily, intranasally (alternating nares every other day)	3% nasal availability; renal elimination	Rhinitis, epistaxis	None
Teriparatide (Forteo)	20 mcg subcutaneously daily for up to 2 years	95% bioavailability; T_{max}: ~30 minutes; half-life ~60 minutes; hepatic metabolism	Pain at injection site, dizziness, leg cramps	None
Testosterone (used in men) Androderm Testoderm TTS Androgel Testim gel Injectable products Pellets	 2.5–5 mg daily 5-mg patch/day 5 mg/day 5 mg/day 10–400 mg IM every 2–4 weeks 150–450 mg/implant every 3–6 months	Hepatic metabolism; highly protein bound to SHBG	Weight gain, acne, hirsutism, dyslipidemia, hepatotoxicity, gynecomastia, priapism, prostate disorders, testicular atrophy, sleep apnea, aggressive behavior, erythrocytosis, skin reaction to patches, drug absorption by sex partner	• Potentiation of oral anticoagulants • Can increase or decrease glucose, necessitating monitoring of antidiabetic medications at start of therapy

T_{max}, time to maximum concentration; SHBG, sex hormone–binding globulin; IV, intravenous; IM, intramuscular; FDA, Food and Drug Administration.
[a]FDA approved at time chapter was prepared.
[b]Filed for FDA review, May 2004.
[c]Filed for FDA review, December 2004.

Calcium carbonate is the salt of choice because it contains the highest amount of elemental calcium and is the least expensive (see Table 88–5). The fraction of calcium absorbed is dose-limited, so maximum single doses of 600 mg or less of elemental calcium are recommended. Calcium carbonate tablets should be taken with meals to enhance absorption. Calcium citrate absorption is acid-independent and need not be administered with meals. Although tricalcium phosphate contains 39% calcium, nonabsorbable calcium-phosphorus complexes may limit overall calcium absorption compared to other products. This product may be required for up to 10% of seniors with hypophosphatemia that cannot be resolved with increased dietary intake.[28] Disintegration and dissolution rates vary significantly between products and lots. Products with good disintegration and dissolution rates and lead contents of less than 1 mcg/day should be recommended.

Calcium's most common adverse reaction, constipation, can be treated with increased water intake, dietary fiber (given separately from calcium), and exercise. Calcium carbonate can create gas, causing stomach upset, or absorb acid and relieve stomach upset. Food sources may be better tolerated. In some cases, the dosage may need to be lowered and reinstated slowly over time.

Diuretics

Thiazide diuretics increase urinary calcium resorption. A 10-year retrospective study of 83,728 women demonstrated fewer fractures among patients currently taking thiazides.[48] A prospective trial demonstrated maintenance of BMD at the spine and hip over a 3-year period with low-dose hydrochlorothiazide, with a greater effect seen in women.[49] Prescribing thiazide diuretics solely for osteoporosis is not recommended, but is a reasonable choice for the patient with osteoporosis who requires a diuretic.

Vitamin D and Its Metabolites

Vitamin D is responsible for maintaining calcium homeostasis. Low calcium concentrations lead to hyperparathyroidism and bone resorption. Vitamin D insufficiency (11 to 20 ng/mL) and deficiency (<10 ng/mL) [25(OH) vitamin D measurement, 10 ng/mL = 25 mcmol/L] is becoming more commonly recognized in all age groups,[50–52] especially malnourished individuals, northerners, women wearing veiled dresses, African-Americans, seniors, and long-term care residents. Low vitamin D concentrations result from insufficient intake, decreased sun exposure, decreased skin production, decreased liver and renal metabolism, and winter residence in northern climates.

Clinical Effectiveness. Product and dose influence outcomes. Observational data suggested daily vitamin D intakes of 12.5 mcg or greater are associated with decreased hip fracture.[45] A meta-analysis of eight studies evaluating vertebral fractures found vitamin D to be protective, with a relative risk of 0.63 (95% confidence interval [CI] 0.45 to 0.88).[53] Seven of the eight studies evaluated calcitriol. The relative risk for nonvertebral fractures was 0.78 (95% CI 0.55 to 1.09) for the one standard vitamin D study and 0.87 (95% CI 0.29 to 2.59) for hydroxylated vitamin D studies. Combined calcium and vitamin D (700 to 800 units/day) supplementation reduced nonvertebral fractures in elderly community dwellers and nursing home residents.[43] Higher doses of vitamin D are associated with improved BMD. Vitamin D 400 units with calcium 500 mg twice daily increased spine and hip BMD in seniors with vitamin D deficiency.[54] Vitamin D's effect on maintaining muscle function[55] and decreasing pain are also important in the prevention and treatment of osteoporosis and falls. Because vitamin D receptors are found in intestine, brain, heart, stomach, pancreas, lymphocytes, skin, and gonads, vitamin D is being explored for effects on hypertension and certain cancers.[14]

Orally administered vitamin D_3, in a dosage of 100,000 units once every 4 months for 5 years, reduced the risk of fracture by 22% to 33% in a population of men and women.[56]

Doxercalciferol (1α-hydroxyvitamin D_2) is under investigation for osteoporosis treatment.

Administration. Although the Institute of Medicine adequate intakes (see Table 88–4) are usually recommended,[26] many experts feel that adult daily vitamin D intake should be 800 to 1000 units.

Given the relatively low cost and safety of vitamin D, no patient should have hypovitaminosis D. Sunlight exposure of 5% of skin equates to 435 units and whole-body exposure to sunlight to cause slight pinkness of the skin equates to 10,000 to 25,000 units of vitamin D.[10,13] Within 20 minutes for whites and 60 to 120 minutes for blacks, the skin reaches maximum production for that day.[13] In addition to milk, more foods—such as orange juice, soymilk, and cereals—are being fortified with vitamin D (see Table 88–2). Multivitamins, cod liver oil, combination calcium and vitamin D supplements, and single source products contain vitamin D (see Tables 88–5 and 88–6). Daily intake of more than one multivitamin or large doses of cod liver oil are no longer advocated to reduce the risk of hypervitaminosis A.

In patients with vitamin D deficiency, oral vitamin D 50,000 units daily for 10 days[57] or once weekly for 8 weeks, or 50,000 to 500,000 units intramuscularly[10] is recommended. Serum calcium and 25(OH) vitamin D should be monitored periodically. Once replete, daily intakes of 600 to 1000 units are usually required. In the community or nursing home, vitamin D 100,000 units once per quarter is reasonable.[56] In patients with vitamin D malabsorption (e.g., gluten-sensitive celiac sprue), 25(OH) vitamin D (calcidiol) administration is needed. In patients with severe hepatic or renal disease, calcitriol therapy may be required. This drug requires careful titration and serum calcium and creatinine monitoring because of its hypercalcemic potential and the limited calciuric ability of the dysfunctional kidney.

When monitoring therapy, 25(OH) vitamin D concentrations, reflective of stores, should be used instead of 1,25(OH) vitamin D. Pharmacokinetics and season need to be taken into account. Since the half-life of vitamin D is about 1 month, minimally 1 to 4 months of therapy are required before the new steady state is achieved.[13]

CLINICAL CONTROVERSY

Although the Institute of Medicine recommends 400 units daily if under 71 years old and 600 units daily if 71 years or older,[26] many prescribers recommend higher doses since Institute of Medicine–recommended doses do not prevent hyperparathyroidism in everyone, which requires attaining 25(OH) vitamin D concentrations of 30 to 40 ng/mL.[13] The relationship between intake and 25(OH) vitamin D concentration is curvilinear. Vitamin D 400 units produced average 25(OH) vitamin D concentrations of 18 ng/mL.[132] Vitamin D 1000 units per day for more than 3 months produced 25(OH) vitamin D concentrations of at least 30 ng/mL in 35% of subjects (range among all patients, 16 to 40 ng/mL), and 4000 units of vitamin D daily produced these concentrations in 88% of subjects (range, 28 to 50 ng/mL). Vitamin D

800 units per day with calcium increased 25(OH) vitamin D concentrations by 22 ng/mL, decreased parathyroid hormone concentrations, and increased bone density in seniors with vitamin D deficiency,[54] whereas 400 units a day did not. Furthermore, fracture prevention with vitamin D was seen with $1,25(OH)_2$ vitamin D products or standard vitamin D of 800 units or greater.[43,45,53]

Bisphosphonates

Bisphosphonates mimic endogenous pyrophosphate. By binding to hydroxyapatite in bone, they decrease resorption by inhibiting osteoclast adherence to bone surfaces. The estimated terminal half-lives of bisphosphonates reflect the slow rates of bone turnover (many years). Etidronate may also inhibit bone mineralization that could lead to osteomalacia. Alendronate, risedronate, and ibandronate are currently FDA-approved for the prevention and treatment of postmenopausal osteoporosis. Risedronate and alendronate are indicated in glucocorticoid-induced osteoporosis, and alendronate is approved for osteoporosis in men.

Clinical Effectiveness. Bisphosphonates reduce the risk of fracture by 45% to 55% at all skeletal sites: vertebral, nonvertebral, and hip. Of the antiresorptive agents, bisphosphonates consistently provide the greatest BMD increases and fracture risk reductions at all skeletal sites. The effect demonstrated in large clinical studies is dose-dependent. The respective BMD increases range from 5% to 8% at the lumbar spine and 2% to 4% at the femoral neck. BMD increases are greatest in the first year of therapy, continue for at least 2 to 3 years, and then plateau for the duration of therapy. After discontinuation, the increased BMD is sustained for at least 1 year and remains higher than that of nonusers. BMD increases are seen in all subsets of patients (women, men, and seniors) but are not as pronounced in patients taking glucocorticoids. Although combination therapy with bisphosphonates plus either estrogen therapy (ET) or raloxifene produces greater BMD increases than either agent alone, alendronate appears to blunt the effects of teriparatide.[58,59]

Alendronate is the most widely studied agent. Data generated from 10 years of therapy support its long-term benefit.[60] The Fracture Intervention Trial studied two populations of patients with low bone mass. First, alendronate demonstrated a robust and early (1 year) fracture risk reduction in a group with severe osteoporosis and pre-existing fractures at study entry.[61] This was the first trial specifically showing a reduction in hip fractures. A second study arm evaluated the effects in patients with either osteopenia or osteoporosis, but without prevalent fractures. Although alendronate significantly reduced fracture risk in those with osteoporosis (T-score <−2.5), it did not reduce the risk of fractures in patients with osteopenia (T-score between −1.0 and −2.5) over a 3-year period.

The second bisphosphonate approved, risedronate, has also demonstrated significant fracture risk reduction in several North American and multinational studies.[62,63] A pre-planned analysis revealed that risedronate reduced the risk of vertebral fractures by approximately 63% within the first year of therapy. Risedronate also reduced the risk of hip fractures.[64]

Because ibandronate is the newest approved agent in the class, fewer published studies exist to support its beneficial effects on fracture rates. One 3-year pivotal efficacy trial, the BONE trial, demonstrated a 52% relative reduction (4.7% with daily doses, 4.9% with intermittent doses, and 9.6% with placebo) in new vertebral fractures in postmenopausal women.[65] The MOBILE trial evaluated once-

monthly ibandronate, but results had not been published when this chapter was finalized.

Oral etidronate, the first bisphosphonate to demonstrate a benefit, is rarely used because up to 33% of patients develop osteomalacia. Etidronate is administered intermittently as quarterly cycles of 400 mg daily for 2 weeks followed by calcium and vitamin D for 11 weeks. It increases vertebral BMD and decreases vertebral fracture risk, but not nonvertebral fracture risk.[66] When given with ET for 4 years, additive vertebral and hip BMD effects were seen without osteomalacia.

Some patients cannot tolerate oral bisphosphonates. Zoledronic acid is not FDA-approved for osteoporosis treatment, but is sometimes administered intravenously once yearly in patients for whom bisphosphonates are indicated. It improved BMD similarly to oral bisphosphonates,[67] but the impact on fracture rates is under investigation. Quarterly administration of intravenous pamidronate[68] or ibandronate[69] also improves BMD.

Administration. Even under optimal conditions, all bisphosphonates are poorly absorbed (bioavailability = 1% to 5%). Bisphosphonates must be administered carefully to optimize the clinical benefit and minimize the risk of adverse GI effects. Each oral tablet should be taken with at least 4 ounces of plain tap water (not coffee, juice, mineral water, or milk) at least 30 minutes before consuming any food or any other supplement or medication. The weekly oral solution needs to be taken with only 2 ounces of water. The patient should remain upright (either sitting or standing) for at least 30 minutes after bisphosphonate administration. When calcium and vitamin D dietary consumption are insufficient, supplementation is needed to ensure the beneficial effects of bisphosphonates.

Most patients prefer once-weekly bisphosphonate administration (see Table 88–6). This dosing schedule lowers GI tract drug exposure. Because the turnover rate of the cells lining the GI tract is about 5 days, any cells damaged during drug exposure are theoretically replaced before the next week's dose is taken. Once-weekly alendronate administration achieved similar BMD results, had similar GI adverse effects, and did not impair mineralization, compared with daily doses of 10 mg.[70]

The most common bisphosphonate adverse effects are nausea, abdominal pain, and dyspepsia. They occur in 10% to 20% of women taking alendronate 10 mg daily, a rate that is similar to placebo in clinical trials. GI event rates are not significantly higher in bisphosphonate users who take nonsteroidal anti-inflammatory drugs. Increased perforations, ulcerations, and bleeding have been seen in the oldest women in studies, but the frequencies were not significantly different from events for similarly aged women in the placebo group. Perforations, ulcerations, and bleeding can also result when administration directions are not followed or when bisphosphonates are prescribed for patients with contraindications. Patients should be encouraged to discuss GI complaints with a health care provider. Risedronate, a pyridinyl bisphosphonate, may have fewer GI effects than alendronate, an amino bisphosphonate, but long-term comparisons are not available.

Selective Estrogen Receptor Modulators

Raloxifene, the first selective estrogen receptor modulator (SERM) approved for prevention and treatment of postmenopausal osteoporosis, is an estrogen agonist in bone tissue but an antagonist in the breast and uterus. Although tamoxifen, a SERM that is approved for breast cancer prevention, also inhibits bone loss, it is an agonist in the uterus and thus can cause endometrial cancer.[71] Investigational SERMs include arzoxifene, bazedoxifene, lasofoxifene, and ospemifene.

Clinical Effectiveness. Raloxifene increases spine and hip BMD by 2% to 3%, a response less than that seen with bisphosphonates or estrogen therapy.[71] From the Multiple Outcomes of Raloxifene Evaluation (MORE) 4-year trial, raloxifene reduced vertebral fractures by 68% within the first year,[72] with prevention persisting throughout the study duration (4-year relative risk, 0.64; 95% CI 0.53 to 0.76).[73] Although fracture prevention was associated with increased BMD, this surrogate outcome only accounted for 4% of the fracture prevention.[74] Raloxifene improved bone quality by increasing heterogeneous bone mineralization.[75] Nonvertebral fractures were not prevented by raloxifene.[73]

Raloxifene combined with alendronate[76] produced greater BMD effects than raloxifene alone, but not greater than alendronate alone. The impact on fracture outcomes, however, is not yet known. Contrary to bisphosphonate discontinuation—in which the achieved BMD is maintained or decreased much more slowly than among those in the placebo group—raloxifene discontinuation results in BMD decreasing immediately at a rate similar to that of placebo.[77]

Like tamoxifen, raloxifene is associated with decreased breast cancer risk. In the MORE trial, raloxifene users developed an estrogen-dependent first breast cancer 70% less often than those in the placebo group, but differences were not statistically significant with regard to estrogen-negative breast cancers.[78] Greater prevention was seen in women with pretreatment estrogen concentrations greater than 10 pmol/L. Raloxifene is not approved yet for breast cancer prevention or treatment. In the Study of Tamoxifen and Raloxifene trial, these SERMs are being compared for breast cancer prevention in high-risk women.

Despite seemingly positive lipid effects (decreased total and LDL cholesterol, neutral effect on HDL cholesterol, but slightly increased triglycerides) with SERMs, beneficial cardiovascular effects have not yet been clinically demonstrated. Coronary and cerebrovascular outcomes as well as safety end points were similar to placebo in the 4-year MORE trial, even within the first year.[79]

For women with severe osteoporosis, particularly when hip fracture risk reduction is desired, a bisphosphonate is likely a better choice than a SERM.

Administration. Overall, raloxifene therapy is well tolerated, but hot flushes occasionally cause women to discontinue therapy (see Table 88–6). Raloxifene use is associated with a threefold increased risk of venous thromboembolism,[73] similar to the increased risk seen in women taking estrogens. Raloxifene is contraindicated for those with active thromboembolic disease. Therapy should be stopped if a patient anticipates a significant period (several hours or more) of immobility. Raloxifene does not induce endometrial bleeding.

Calcitonin

Calcitonin is released from the thyroid gland when serum calcium is elevated. Salmon calcitonin is used clinically because it is more potent and longer lasting than the mammalian form. Pharmacologic doses decrease bone resorption. Calcitonin is indicated for osteoporosis treatment for women at least 5 years past menopause. Although the agent is also used in men, it is not approved for this indication. Because calcitonin reduces fracture risk to a lesser extent than other osteoporosis medications, calcitonin is reserved for second-line treatment.

Clinical Effectiveness. The largest calcitonin study, the PROOF study, randomized 1255 osteoporotic women, most with prevalent vertebral fractures, to intranasal calcitonin or placebo for up to 5 years.[80] The 200-unit daily regimen increased spine BMD and reduced new vertebral fractures by 36%. A dose-response relationship did not exist and the dropout rate was 59%. Calcitonin does not consistently affect hip BMD and does not decrease hip fracture risk.

Calcitonin may provide pain relief to some patients with acute vertebral fractures, but this effect is minimal. Calcitonin should not be used in place of other more effective and much less expensive analgesics.[81,82]

Administration. The intranasal dose of calcitonin is sprayed in alternating nares every other day (see Table 88–6). Other than minor nasal adverse effects, calcitonin is well tolerated. Subcutaneous administration at 100 units daily is available but rarely used.

Estrogen and Hormonal Therapy

Estrogen receptors exist on osteoblasts, osteoclasts, macrophage cells, intestinal cells, and many other tissues. Estrogens decrease osteoclast recruitment and activity, inhibit PTH peripherally, increase calcitriol concentrations and intestinal calcium absorption, and decrease renal calcium excretion. They also decrease cytokine concentrations and decrease the activity of the OPG/RANK/RANKL pathway, inhibiting bone resorption. Response to estrogen deficiency and replacement may be related to estrogen receptors and polymorphisms.

Clinical Effectiveness. Hormonal therapy (HT) was shown to statistically decrease vertebral, hip, and all fractures by 34%, 34%, and 24%, respectively; however, this effect become insignificant when analyzed as a secondary finding in the Women's Health Initiative.[83] The estrogen-alone arm of the Women's Health Initiative (WHI) trial also found decreased hip fractures in estrogen therapy (ET) users.[84] Meta-analyses using various study inclusion criteria also found ET/HT to decrease vertebral and nonvertebral fractures by 33% to 40% and 13% to 27%, respectively.[85,86]

BMD effects from ET or HT are less than for bisphosphonates or teriparatide, but greater than for raloxifene, tibolone, and phytoestrogens. Pooled results from prevention studies showed that ET and HT increased lumbar spine BMD by 4.9% and 7.0%, femoral neck BMD by 2.3% and 4.1%, and forearm BMD by 3% and 4.5% in the first and second years, respectively.[86] Both younger and older postmenopausal women achieve increased BMD with ET and HT. Oral and transdermal estrogens at equivalent doses and continuous or cyclic HT regimens have similar BMD effects. ET implants and intrauterine impregnated devices and creams have shown positive bone effects. Effect on BMD is dose-dependent, with benefit seen with doses as low as 0.025 mg transdermal estradiol, 0.3 mg conjugated equine estrogen,[87] and 0.3 mg esterified estrogen. Most BMD gains were seen within the first few years of treatment, with slight increases or a plateau thereafter. Longer duration of use is associated with greater BMD effects. Women who continuously used ET or HT since menopause or those with long-term use beginning in their senior years had the highest BMD.[41] ET and HT is not protective for all women; thus women who have or are receiving ET or HT should be monitored for effectiveness. BMD effects are increased when ET or HT is combined with bisphosphonates[10] and parathyroid hormone.[88] Progestins added to ET resulted in no change or a slight increase in BMD. When ET or HT was discontinued, bone loss was accelerated for a short period, compared with placebo, in most[77] but not all studies.

The bone benefits of ET and HT documented in observational and clinical trials are not greater than the negative effects. Contrary to observational studies, ET and HT do not prevent primary or secondary cardiovascular disease, and may even increase events within the first years of use.[83,85] For every 10,000 woman-years of HT, 5 hip fractures and 6 colorectal cancers were prevented, while 7 coronary heart disease events, 8 strokes, 8 breast cancer cases, and 8 pulmonary emboli were caused.[83] The net balance for HT prevention in the WHI trial would be an additional 19 negative events per 10,000 woman-years, which is not considered acceptable by most. Of note, mortality was not changed with HT. None of the subgroups of patients at high risk for osteoporotic fractures had a positive overall effect from HT.[89] Increased strokes were the reason for the ET WHI arm to be stopped early.[84] For every 10,000 woman-years of ET, the net balance between benefit and risk was 2 additional negative events, which was not significant. Like the HT arm, ET did not change overall mortality. Reasons why the WHI trial refutes the large volume of supportive literature may be due to selection biases such as higher socioeconomic status, greater literacy, better access to health care, more preventive health behaviors, earlier detection of conditions with better survival rates, and less baseline cardiovascular disease and mortality of women who chose to use ET or HT.

Thus ET and HT are not advocated for prevention of osteoporosis and fractures since other better and safer medications exist.[90,83] Even though the WHI trial only assessed one ET and HT dose, most clinicians are extrapolating the results to all estrogen replacement therapies until data exist to document the contrary. The lowest effective dose of ET and HT should still be used for preventing and controlling menopausal symptoms, with use discontinued with symptom abatement.

Administration. The risks and benefits of beginning or continuing ET and HT must be discussed with all women. Numerous contraindications to ET and HT exist and must be identified before initiation. For women with an intact uterus, a progestin (e.g., medroxyprogesterone 2.5 to 5 mg daily or the equivalent) should also be used to decrease the risk of endometrial cancer. The lowest estrogen dose to maintain BMD is advocated (see menopause chapter for other ET product doses, specific use, and adverse effects information). Vaginal administration from creams or rings results in significant systemic absorption, but concentrations are much lower than normal oral dosing of ET products, and thus effects on BMD are minimal.

▨ Tibolone

Tibolone, a synthetic steroid, and its metabolites are weak estrogen-, progesterone-, and androgen-receptor agonists. They relieve hot flushes and increase BMD, but have no effect on the endometrium. In younger and older postmenopausal women, tibolone increased spine and hip BMD after 1 to 10 years of 1.25 or 2.5 mg daily.[91] Effects on fractures and cardiovascular disease are still unknown. Adverse effects are less than with estrogen/progestin regimens. Currently used in Europe, tibolone is not yet FDA-approved for use in the United States.

▨ Phytoestrogens

The isoflavonoids (soy proteins) and lignans (flaxseed) are the most common forms of phytoestrogens. Isoflavones are metabolized to genistein and daidzein, ligands for both estrogen α and β receptors, with a greater affinity for β receptors.[92] Bone effects may be related to bone estrogen receptor agonist activity or potentially direct or indirect effects on osteoblasts and osteoclasts. A red clover–derived supplement decreased lumbar spine but not hip bone loss in a large, placebo-controlled clinical trial.[93] No fracture outcome data are available. Bone density results are difficult to analyze due to different phy-

toestrogen products, quantities, and preparations; differing age and race of the study samples; small samples; and suboptimal study design. Overall, isoflavone pharmaceuticals or food studies using large doses have reported decreased bone resorption markers and small increases in bone density; however, inconsistencies and negative results have been reported as well.[92,94] Thus these products can be used for preventive bone-sparing effects, but are probably not sufficient alone for treatment.

Although ipriflavone, a synthetic isoflavone available in health food stores, is partially metabolized to daidzein, it is void of estrogenic activity outside of bone. Increased to no change in BMD were measured in 2-year or shorter studies.[92,95] A 4-year study with 474 postmenopausal women showed no effect of ipriflavone 200 mg three times daily on vertebral fractures or BMD.[96] Subclinical lymphocytopenia developed in 13% of the sample, with 19% of these women's lymphocyte counts not returning to normal after 2 years off therapy. Therefore ipriflavone's use, especially long-term use, should be discouraged.

▨ Testosterone and Anabolic Steroids

Decreased testosterone concentrations are seen with certain gonadal diseases, eating disorders, glucocorticoid therapy, oophorectomy, and menopause, and in aging men with hypogonadism. In a few studies, women receiving methyltestosterone 1.25 or 2.5 mg oral daily or testosterone implants 50 mg every 3 months had increased BMD.[9] Testosterone, in various salt forms, was associated with increased BMD in some studies when given to hypogonadal men and senior men with normal hormone levels or mild hormonal deficiency.[19] Transdermal gel, oral, intramuscular, and pellet testosterone products are available. Testosterone products are generally prescribed only by specialist physicians. Anabolic steroids (nandrolone decanoate) have shown minimal to no effect on BMD, but do increase muscle strength.

The virilizing and estrogenic adverse effects of these products are listed in Table 88–6.[97,98] Patients using these products should be evaluated within 1 to 2 months of onset and then every 3 to 6 months thereafter.

▨ BONE-FORMATION THERAPY

▨ Teriparatide (Parathyroid Hormone)

Teriparatide contains the first 34 amino acids in human parathyroid hormone and represents a novel approach to osteoporosis treatment. Although hyperparathyroidism leads to bone loss (see Fig. 88–3), therapeutic doses (for shorter periods of time) conversely improve BMD and reduce fracture risk. Parathyroid hormone is currently the only approved osteoporosis medication that works by stimulating bone formation. Because of adverse effects and cost concerns, teriparatide is reserved for treating those at high risk of osteoporosis-related fractures who cannot or will not take or have failed bisphosphonate therapy.

Recombinant human parathyroid hormone (1-84) and once-weekly PTH administration are being evaluated.

Clinical Effectiveness. Teriparatide works equally well in women and men with osteoporosis. Teriparatide has reduced the risk of new vertebral fractures by 65% compared with placebo (actual fracture incidence 5% vs. 14%, respectively) in postmenopausal women with osteoporosis and pre-existing fractures.[99] New nonvertebral fracture risk was reduced by 53% (3% fractures with teriparatide vs. 6% fractures with placebo) with the 20-mcg/day dosage. Teriparatide can increase lumbar spine BMD by 9% to 13% and femoral neck BMD by 2.8%. In men with osteoporosis, teriparatide increased BMD, but its impact on fracture rate remains undetermined.[100] In a small study, when parathyroid hormone 25 mcg/day was added to established HT, spine BMD increased by 13.4% and total hip BMD increased by 4.4%, and resulted in a corresponding 75% to 100% reduction of vertebral fractures.[88] Teriparatide should not be used in combination with alendronate because the bisphosphonate may blunt the teriparatide's beneficial effects.[58,59]

Administration. Teriparatide is contraindicated in patients with Paget's disease of the bone, unexplained elevations in alkaline phosphatase, or a history of previous skeletal radiation therapy (a black-box warning from the manufacturer). Osteosarcoma was seen in a small number of rats, but the incidence in humans is unknown but of potential concern.

Teriparatide is commercially available as a prefilled 3-mL pen-type delivery device that administers subcutaneous injections in the thigh or abdominal area (see Table 88–6). The initial dose should be administered with the patient either sitting or lying down in case orthostatic hypotension occurs. Health care providers should re-educate patients about syringe use with each refill, and the patient or caregiver should also re-read the user's manual each month. The pen should be refrigerated and can be used for up to 28 days following the initial injection. Teriparatide is also the most expensive of the approved osteoporosis therapies.

Strontium

Strontium stimulates bone formation and decreases bone resorption. In a preliminary study of postmenopausal women with severe osteoporosis, strontium ranelate 1 g twice daily or 2 g once daily reduced new vertebral fractures by 41%, and increased lumbar spine BMD by 14% and femoral neck BMD by 8% compared with placebo.[101] Nonvertebral fracture rates were similar. Diarrhea was more common in the strontium group. Small decreases in serum calcium and PTH, small increases in serum phosphate, and transient increases in creatine kinase were measured.

HMG-CoA Reductase Inhibitors (Statins)

In the search for agents to increase bone formation through bone morphogenetic proteins, 3-hydroxymethyl-4-glutaryl CoA reductase inhibitors (statins) were discovered to increase bone density in animal models. Interest in the potential skeletal benefits of statins was heightened by the discovery that bisphosphonates may also affect cholesterol biosynthesis, but at a different step than statins. Although observational studies have linked statin use with decreased fracture risk, a large case-control study did not demonstrate reduction in fracture risk for statin-treated patients. A meta-analysis casts doubt on a protective effect of statins (odds ratio for hip fracture, 0.87; 95% CI 0.48 to 1.58).[102]

Growth Hormones and Factors

Growth hormone (GH) and IGF-1 play important roles in bone turnover and remodeling, with multiple effects on other tissues. Their serum concentrations decline with age and frequently are decreased in osteoporosis. Growth hormone injections have been found to increase or cause no change in BMD in patients with osteoporosis and normal GH concentrations, and patients with GH deficiency.[103] Short-term studies showed a negative effect, while the longer-term studies showed a positive effect that continued to increase for 1 to 2 years after discontinuation of GH therapy.[103,104] Growth hormone–releasing hormone and other GH secretagogues, some of which are oral, are undergoing extensive research.[103,105] Recombinant IGF-1 injections, with or without IGF-3 binding protein, increased both bone formation and resorption.[106]

Adverse effects reported for GH and for IGF-1 include skin irritations, alterations in glucose utilization, joint stiffness, and peripheral edema.

Fluoride

Although fluoride increases osteoblastic activity and bone formation through intracellular signaling pathways involving tyrosine phosphatases and mitogen-activated protein kinases, it remains an unapproved therapy despite 30 years of clinical study. Early studies, in fact, demonstrated an increased risk of cortical bone fractures. Although men and women given fluoride monophosphate and women given lower-dose, slow-release sodium fluoride had fewer vertebral fractures, these findings were not validated in two other studies. A meta-analysis also determined that fluoride lacked antifracture efficacy.[107] Fluoride is currently not recommended for use.

Investigational Agents

In addition to the above drugs, new classes of medications are beginning to show promise.[108] Osteoprotegerin (OPG), a competitive inhibitor of RANKL, blocks osteoclastic differentiation and has decreased bone resorption biomarkers (phase I and II). As it is a large protein, administration is via injection. Agents to enhance endogenous OPG, decrease RANKL production, or block RANKL binding to RANK are being developed. Agents to block osteoclast attachment ($\alpha V\beta 3$ integrin receptor antagonists, in preclinical testing), inhibit bone matrix degradation (cathepsin K inhibitors, in phase I studies, and nitrosylated nonsteroidal anti-inflammatory drugs, in phase II studies), or change osteoclast cell structure (Src inhibitors, in preclinical studies) have been initially effective.

VERTEBROPLASTY AND KYPHOPLASTY

The percutaneous injection of polymethylmethacrylate (PMMA) bone cement into a compressed vertebral fracture confers significant pain relief for many patients. Under local anesthetic, with computed tomography scanning or fluoroscopic guidance, PMMA is injected under slight pressure during vertebroplasty. The procedure stabilizes the damaged vertebrae and reduces pain in 70% to 92% of patients. Pain scores usually improve by approximately 50% at 1 month following the treatment.[109]

Kyphoplasty is a newer procedure that requires drilling into the vertebral body and inflating a balloon to re-expand the fracture. The process is followed by the injection of about 7 mL of the PMMA cement. The patient remains in a supine position for 1 to 2 hours to allow the cement to cure. Because this curing process creates an exothermic reaction, surrounding tissue is slightly damaged. It remains unclear whether this is an unwanted side effect or in fact the mechanism by which pain is relieved. Cement leakage into the spinal column can result in complicating nerve damage.[110]

SPECIAL POPULATIONS

WOMEN WITH AMENORRHEA

Adolescents and women with primary or secondary amenorrhea, due to diet,[111] excessive exercise,[38] or hypothalamus-pituitary-ovarian axis disorders,[112] have lower BMD than other age-equivalent individuals.

Although predominantly attributed to hypoestrogenemia, diet has a significant impact, since BMD is lower in those with amenorrhea from anorexia than in those whose conditions result from excessive exercise. Anorexia's effect is greatest if it occurs before peak bone mass achievement. After 6 months of amenorrhea, a bone density test should be performed and then repeated yearly while amenorrheic. BMD measurements may be inaccurate in small-boned people and children, requiring the use of Z-scores, especially before peak bone mass achievement, or corrections for age and sexual maturity. For those with amenorrhea or anorexia, higher calcium intakes of 1200 to 1500 mg and adequate vitamin D are recommended.

In anorexia, the primary therapy is normal diet, weight gain, and return of normal menses. Of note, BMD improves but never returns to the level of age-matched controls.

The American Academy of Pediatrics recommends low-dose estrogen supplementation for amenorrhea if age is greater than 16 until normal menses returns.[38] Most studies do not find that oral contraceptives improve BMD.[38,111] Bisphosphonates are not approved for children. Hormone therapy and bisphosphonates may be used in adults. Recombinant IGF-I and dehydroepiandrosterone are being explored as possible for treatments for women with osteoporosis.

MEN

Some men with osteoporosis possess clearly identifiable risk factors. In others, further investigation for secondary causes is warranted (see above patient assessment section). Men 70 years and older should have DXA tests to screen for osteoporosis. DXA standards state T-scores should be compared with a white male normative reference database, regardless of ethnicity. BMD determination should also be considered for men with a low-trauma fracture, prevalent vertebral deformity, glucocorticoid use, hypogonadism, alcoholism, or poor overall health. Measurement of serum free or total testosterone can also determine if hypogonadism is contributing to bone loss.

Management of male osteoporosis is similar to that of women except that neither estrogens nor SERMs are used. Lifestyle modifications (see above) are important interventions in men. Bisphosphonates are the drugs of first choice. Although alendronate is FDA-approved for men and reduces the risk of vertebral fractures, other available bisphosphonates are also clinically used.[113] Osteoporosis due to secondary causes should include treatment of the underlying cause plus a bisphosphonate. Bisphosphonates also appear to have beneficial BMD effects in men receiving androgen deprivation therapy for prostate cancer.[113]

For the man with symptomatic hypogonadism (decreased libido, energy loss, and erectile dysfunction), a normal prostate examination, and a normal serum prostate-specific antigen, testosterone can be considered as adjunctive therapy. Testosterone patches (2.5–5 mg daily), intramuscular injections (10 to 400 mg every 2 to 4 weeks), 1% topical gel, pellet implants (150–450 mg every 3–6 months), and a buccal formulation are available (see Table 88–6). Testosterone replacement increases bone density in men. The benefits of therapy need to be weighed against a higher risk of prostate cancer and benign prostatic hyperplasia. Adverse effects are listed in Table 88–6.

SENIORS

Even though therapies exist, many seniors are not evaluated or treated for osteoporosis, including those who have had a fracture.[114] In these patients, fall prevention plus BMD optimization is necessary to optimally reduce fracture risk. Functional status impairment is also an important contributor to fractures in seniors.[115]

Adequate calcium and vitamin D intake (see Table 88–4) should be assured. For seniors with severe osteoporosis, a 25(OH) vitamin D concentration should be used to guide vitamin D supplementation. Centenarians have a particularly high rate of hypovitaminosis D.[116] Smoking cessation and exercise begun late in life still have positive bone effects.

For most seniors, bisphosphonates are the preferred agents. Esophageal dysfunction should be clinically ruled out, and the patient's ability to adhere to the complex administration process must be assured before beginning therapy. Once-weekly dosing is usually preferred. Although bisphosphonates are not recommended in patients with renal insufficiency (creatinine clearance <35 mL/min), some clinicians are using lower-dose (alendronate 35 mg once weekly) therapy. Because many seniors do not have medication coverage, cost issues need to be addressed.

Raloxifene, nasal calcitonin, or parenteral teriparatide are treatment options for seniors who will not or cannot take an oral bisphosphonate. Hormone therapy is no longer advocated because of the WHI trial results. Current ET or HT use still confers a bone benefit, but benefits from past hormone use are lost after discontinuation. Seniors have a greater incidence of ET and HT adverse effects (especially breast tenderness). Most seniors should be tapered off ET and HT if they are still using either one. When used, lower ET/HT doses (0.3 mg conjugated equine estrogen or equivalent) should be prescribed. Clinical guidelines for the diagnosis and management of osteoporosis in the long-term setting have been created.[117,118] Patients and family may help decide if pharmacotherapy for bone health is wanted.

TRANSPLANT RECIPIENTS

Underlying diseases that necessitate solid organ or bone marrow transplantation can cause bone loss prior to surgery. After the transplant, bone loss may accelerate during the first 6 months. Decreased physical activity and glucocorticoid use are major contributors to this phenomenon (see below).[119] After transplantation, fractures are greater and Z- and T-scores are lower in transplant recipients. During the early posttransplant period, resorption decreases and formation increases, but later after transplantation, both formation and resorption increase. Additional causes for bone loss include other medications (loop diuretics, aluminum-containing phosphate binders, and heparin), hyperparathyroidism, hypogonadism, hypovitaminosis D, decreased calcium intake or absorption, hepatic congestion, prerenal azotemia, and cystic fibrosis. Animal, but not human, research showed cyclosporine and tacrolimus decreased BMD.

Before transplant, BMD should be measured and vitamin D and gonadal status assessed. Bone-healthy lifestyle changes and therapy should be instituted as needed (see Fig. 88–4) and hypogonadism corrected before and after transplant. Intermittent pamidronate has decreased bone loss in most transplant recipients.[119] Use of bisphosphonates in children and when creatinine clearance is less than 30 mL/min is being explored. Glucocorticoid doses should be reduced as quickly as possible. Estrogen enhances hepatic metabolism of cyclosporine. Ovulation and testosterone production may increase after transplantation and hormone supplementation may no longer be needed. Calcitriol may be needed instead of vitamin D, depending on the severity of renal or liver dysfunction. A multidisciplinary clinic may be best suited to identify and ensure appropriate therapy for transplant recipients.[120]

HIV/AIDS

Although the connection between the human immunodeficiency virus (HIV), its therapy, and osteoporosis is still being studied, current data suggest that both the virus and its medical treatments can decrease BMD. The effects are greater if other osteoporosis risk factors exist.[121] Potential mechanisms include direct and indirect effect on osteoblasts and osteoclasts such as HIV invasion of cells and changes in cytokines and hormone concentrations, inhibition of 1α hydroxylase metabolism of 25(OH) vitamin D, lipodystrophy, and lactic acidosis. Other medications to treat HIV complications such as foscarnet, trimethoprim-sulfamethoxazole, and certain antibiotics can cause hypocalcemia. BMD measurements are only warranted if additional risk factors, long-term HIV, or long-term HIV medication use are present. Screening recommendations do not yet exist. Standard treatment, usually consisting of a bisphosphonate plus calcium and vitamin D supplementation, should be used once osteoporosis is diagnosed, although no specific population data yet exist.

ARTHRITIS

In most studies, patients with rheumatoid arthritis have lower BMD and more fractures than do age-matched controls.[122] Common disease pathways, including proinflammatory cytokines and the OPG/RANK/RANKL system, may be responsible along with increased glucocorticoid use, hypogonadism, decreased activity, and increased fall risk. Patients taking glucocorticoids should be managed with calcium and vitamin D supplementation plus a bisphosphonate. Otherwise, standard osteoporosis prevention and treatment interventions are recommended.

CYSTIC FIBROSIS

Osteoporosis and fractures may develop in patients with cystic fibrosis from vitamin D deficiency, glucocorticoid use, calcium malabsorption, hypogonadism, inactivity, increased cytokines, and lung transplantation.[123] Bone density monitoring is done for patients at high risk, including those with malnutrition and glucocorticoid use. BMD testing corrections for children need to be made.

Prevention and treatment efforts usually include adequate calcium and vitamin D intake, adherence to pancreatic enzymes, correction of hypogonadism, exercise, potential use of GH in children whose height is below the tenth percentile, and when possible, reductions in glucocorticoid use. Calcitriol may be needed to overcome vitamin D malabsorption problems, but needs to be monitored for hypercalcemia. Bisphosphonates are generally not recommended for children.

GASTROINTESTINAL DISEASE

Recently, comprehensive reviews have been written on the lower BMD and higher fracture rates seen with inflammatory bowel disease,[124] celiac disease,[124] postgastrectomy,[124] and liver disease.[125] Mechanisms include malabsorption, glucocorticoid use, increased inflammatory cytokines, and decreased metabolism. In patients with these diseases, and especially with other osteoporosis risk factors, bone density and secondary cause evaluations may be warranted. Prevention and treatment options currently reflect those for children, postmenopausal women, and men, and when applicable, for glucocorticoid use.

DIABETES

Patients with type 1 and type 2 diabetes have increased fracture rates in some studies.[126] Increased fall risk may contribute to this increased fracture risk. Standard assessment and prevention and treatment regimens are employed. In many studies, ET and HT have beneficial effects on glucose homeostasis and overall positive lipid effects, except for the increased triglycerides, which might be problematic.[127] Testosterone may cause hypoglycemia. Although one study with alendronate documented decreased insulin requirements, further data are needed.[126]

PHARMACOECONOMIC CONSIDERATIONS

Annual direct costs for osteoporotic fractures were estimated to be $17 billion (in 2001 dollars).[3,128] A hip fracture costs about $40,000 (in 2001 dollars). Health care costs for women aged 45 and older indicate that osteoporosis accounts for 6.9% of direct medical expenditures, with one-half of these expenses borne by Medicare. Direct costs in the year following hip fracture range from $16,000 to $36,000. Indirect costs of hip fracture, including lost quality of life, add at least $20,000 per fracture. Appreciation of these costs and availability of preventive therapies have established osteoporosis as a significant public health priority.

The estimated cost for each quality-adjusted life year (QALY) for treating women with T-scores below −2 is $51 to $8,447, varying by age, with the lowest cost for the oldest women.[128] This analysis assumed a drug treatment cost of $300/year and a hip fracture cost of $30,000. The National Osteoporosis Foundation estimated that for women with average fracture risks, age-specific costs of osteoporosis prevention or treatment per QALY were $13,794 for a 50-year-old, $6,884 for a 60-year-old, $2,924 for a 70-year-old, and $949 for a 80-year-old. These estimates conservatively assume a 33% fracture risk reduction and annual treatment costs of $500. The adjusted cost values are lower for women at greater risk. To put these pharmacoeconomic figures into perspective, the average cost per QALY saved approximates $2,800 for Papanicolaou smears done every 3 years after age 65, $34,000 for lovastatin for men 45 to 54 with total cholesterol equal to 300 mg/dL or higher, $32,000 for hypertension treatment for those 40 and older with diastolic blood pressures of 95 to 104 mm Hg; and $62,000 for annual mammography for women 40 to 49 years of age.[129] Based on this economic analysis, the National Osteoporosis Foundation indicated that treatment could be appropriate for postmenopausal women with T-scores less than −2 and in those with T-scores below −1.5 who also have increased risk.

Key pharmacoeconomic issues are the human and economic burden from an expanding elderly population, development of new, more effective, but potentially more expensive medications, enhanced screening and identification of patients at risk, and targeting of high-risk populations.

EVALUATION OF THERAPEUTIC OUTCOMES

Patients receiving pharmacotherapy for low bone mass should be examined at least annually. Because the primary therapeutic outcome is fracture prevention, patients should be asked about possible fracture symptoms (primarily bone pain or disability) at each visit. Routine bone x-ray films are not warranted. Patients should be questioned about medication adherence and tolerability at each visit. Collecting a detailed history, according to the pertinent review of systems, should identify commonly occurring or potentially serious side effects unique to each medication.

Two approaches of monitoring BMD exist in clinical practice. Some clinicians choose to measure BMD every 1 to 2 years following the commencement of therapy. They argue that this tactic identifies patients with medication nonadherence or secondary osteoporosis. Others advocate no subsequent BMD measurement because of expense and lack of correlation to fracture risk reduction. The optimal strategy has not yet been determined.

GLUCOCORTICOID-INDUCED OSTEOPOROSIS

9 The drug class most commonly associated with drug-induced osteoporosis is glucocorticoids.[22] Oral daily doses greater than 7.5 mg of prednisone or equivalent generally constitute significant risk. Inhaled daily doses greater than 800 to 1200 mcg for beclomethasone, 800 to 1000 mcg for budesonide, 750 mcg for fluticasone, and 1000 mcg for flunisolide[133] are generally required for significant bone loss. Bone loss and fractures rarely occur with lower inhaled doses.[21]

PATHOPHYSIOLOGY

Glucocorticoids decrease muscle strength and bone formation and increase bone resorption.[134] Glucocorticoids decrease calcium absorption, increase renal calcium excretion, and result in secondary hyperparathyroidism. Glucocorticoid effects on vitamin D are variable. Differentiation, replication, and life span of osteoblasts are reduced, as is osteoid synthesis. Osteoblasts change in their sensitivity to prostaglandins, PTH, cytokines, growth factors, and calcitriol. Changes at the pituitary and gonadal level decrease synthesis of estrogen and testosterone. Myopathy can decrease mobility and lead to further bone loss. Although bone loss is continuous throughout steroid therapy, the greatest loss is experienced during the first 6 to 12 months of therapy. Trabecular bone (ribs, vertebrae, and pelvis) is affected more than cortical bone. Women, men, and children are susceptible. Although low BMD found in steroid users is a good predictor of fracture risk, patients with osteopenia and even normal BMD still develop fractures because of impaired bone quality, which is difficult to measure. For each 1 standard deviation decrease in T-score prior to therapy, the relative risk of fracture is 1.85.[135] Similarly, the relative risk is 1.62 for each 10-mg prednisone dosage equivalent. Compared to nonusers, the overall relative risk of fracture is 5.67 and the risk is present whether or not osteoporosis (T-score <–2.5) exists.

DIAGNOSIS

Patients taking long-term glucocorticoids represent a challenging group in which to diagnose osteoporosis. Because bone quality is compromised, at any level of BMD, some clinicians choose to treat without BMD testing. However, guidelines for the management of glucocorticoid-induced osteoporosis recommend measuring BMD at the beginning of chronic therapy, defined as ≥5 mg prednisone or equivalent daily for 3 months, and follow-up monitoring with a DXA in up to 6–12 months, and measurement of BMD in those on chronic therapy whose baseline values were not measured.[133,136]

▶ PREVENTION AND TREATMENT: Glucocorticoid-Induced Osteoporosis

Although the best means of preventing glucocorticoid-induced osteoporosis and related fracture would be discontinuing glucocorticoids, this is not always clinically feasible. Using the lowest possible dose for the shortest duration minimizes glucocorticoid exposure. The bone effects of alternate-day therapy and pulse (intermittent) therapy are not completely known, but some data suggest that these regimens also have negative bone effects.

All patients receiving chronic or recurrent glucocorticoid therapy should adopt bone-healthy lifestyle changes (see above) and ingest adequate amounts of calcium and vitamin D.[137] According to the American College of Rheumatology guidelines, calcium intakes should be higher: 800 mg for children between 1 and 5 years, 1200 mg for children between 6 and 10 years, and 1500 mg for other patients.[133] All children should receive 400 units and adults 800 units vitamin D per day.

Bisphosphonates are the best therapeutic choice for patients with glucocorticoid-induced osteoporosis. Bisphosphonates generally produce greater BMD increases than do other agents used to treat osteoporosis. They increase spine (4.3%) and femoral neck (2.1%) BMD, but to a lesser extent than in bisphosphonate users who do not take glucocorticoids.[138] They also likely reduce the risk of vertebral fractures by approximately 50%.[139]

Data using calcitonin for glucocorticoid-induced osteoporosis do not support its routine use.[140]

OSTEOMALACIA

10 Osteomalacia results from defective osteoid mineralization. Defective mineralization in the infant or child produces rickets. In the adult, the syndrome is called osteomalacia.

EPIDEMIOLOGY

The incidence of osteomalacia is not known precisely, but is lower in the United States because foods are supplemented with vitamin D. However, hypovitaminosis D in the United States is still identified in young, old, and new immigrants.[50–52,141] Osteomalacia is more prevalent in countries with little sun exposure, minimal dietary supplementation, malnutrition, or traditional clothing covering most of the skin. Dark-skinned individuals synthesize less vitamin D cutaneously and can be at risk for hypovitaminosis D.[14]

PATHOPHYSIOLOGY

Mechanisms leading to osteomalacia include low serum calcium or phosphorus, chronic acidosis, hypophosphatemia, liver or renal disease, and drug-induced mineralization defects.[10,23,142,143] The most common cause is vitamin D deficiency secondary to inadequate intake, decreased sun exposure, malabsorption, or decreased metabolism. Renal disease is associated with decreased 25(OH) vitamin D 1α-hydroxylase, with consequently decreased calcitriol and poor calcium absorption. In vitamin D–dependent rickets type I, a genetic defect exists in 25(OH) vitamin D 1α-hydroxylase. Vitamin D–dependent rickets type II results from defects in the vitamin D receptor or its activity. In vitamin D–resistant rickets, renal phosphate reabsorption is defective, and 25(OH) vitamin D 1α-hydroxylase activity is inadequate. A genetic defect in the *PHEX* gene may allow inappropriate activity of an undefined inhibitor of phosphate reabsorption that also lowers serum calcitriol concentrations. Pancreatitis, chronic hepatobiliary disease, Crohn's disease, gastrectomy, and celiac sprue are also risk factors for vitamin D deficiency.

Other chronic disorders cause osteomalacia.[10,142,143] Phosphate depletion from low dietary intake, phosphate-binding antacids, and oncogenic osteomalacia (potentially phosphaturic effect) can cause osteomalacia. Hypophosphatasia is an inborn error of metabolism in which deficient activity of alkaline phosphatase causes impaired mineralization of bone matrix. Acidosis from renal dysfunction, distal renal tubular acidosis, hypergammaglobulinemic states (e.g., multiple myeloma), and drugs (e.g., chemotherapy) compromises bone mineralization. Renal tubular disorders secondary to Fanconi's syndrome, hereditary diseases (e.g., Wilson's disease, a defect in copper metabolism), acquired disease (e.g., myeloma), and toxins (e.g., lead) cause osteomalacia to varying degrees. Chronic wastage of phosphorus and/or calcium limits mineralization, which may be further compromised by acidosis and secondary hyperparathyroidism.

DRUG-INDUCED OSTEOMALACIA

Drugs induce osteomalacia through various mechanisms.[23] Phenytoin, primidone, phenobarbital, carbamazepine, rifampin, and some hypnotic medications may cause osteomalacia, potentially through hepatic microsomal cytochrome P450 induction and increased vitamin D metabolism. Anticonvulsant-associated osteomalacia usually occurs only in patients living in an institution or those receiving multiple anticonvulsant drugs. Cholestyramine may decrease vitamin D absorption. Long-term hyperalimentation may also result in osteomalacia. Defective mineralization can result from continuous or intermittent etidronate treatment or sodium fluoride. Aluminum accumulation in patients with severe renal impairment or in patients undergoing hemodialysis may lead to osteomalacia, potentially through insoluble complexes with phosphates and inhibition of mineral deposition.

CLINICAL PRESENTATION

Adult osteomalacia often has an insidious presentation.[10,142,143] The underlying disorder may be more apparent than skeletal defects (e.g., diarrhea in sprue). Diffuse skeletal pain, bony tenderness, and proximal muscle weakness may occur. Pain on movement and muscle weakness may result in a characteristic waddling gait. Hypophosphatemia and secondary hyperparathyroidism may contribute to these symptoms. Tetany can result from sufficiently depressed serum ionized calcium. Skeletal deformities (infrequent in adults) include leg bowing, pigeon chest, scoliosis, kyphosis, and shortening of the spine.

Findings on x-ray films depend on the cause and age of the patient.[143] Radiographic changes include changes in the growth plate bone areas, bone erosion, osteopenia, and pseudofractures (Looser's zones).

Various etiologies produce differing biochemical pictures.[143] Determination of serum content of calcium (albumin corrected), phosphorus, alkaline phosphatase, urea nitrogen, creatinine, PTH, 25(OH) vitamin D, and calcitriol, as well as urinary calcium, creatinine, and phosphorus, can help in determining the cause, deciding on treatment, and monitoring efficacy of therapy. Definitive diagnosis is by bone biopsy.

▶ PREVENTION AND TREATMENT: Osteomalacia

Treatment of osteomalacia depends on the underlying cause.[10,142,143] Management may be difficult and may require a renal, bone, or endocrine specialist.

Treatment of osteomalacia from vitamin D deficiency is vitamin D therapy, with dose depending on severity. Supplements of 800 to 4000 units/day or 50,000 units weekly for 8 weeks may be necessary. For sprue, a gluten-free diet is necessary. With intestinal malabsorption, high oral doses (50,000 to 100,000 units/day) or daily intramuscular injections of 10,000 units of vitamin D may be initially required. With disordered vitamin D metabolism caused by anticonvulsants or rifampin, supplemental vitamin D (4000 units/day) can be effective. Sun exposure can also be useful. Serum calcium and 25(OH) vitamin D monitoring is necessary with high vitamin D doses.

Renal disease with deficient 1,25(OH) vitamin D synthesis can be treated with calcitriol, with careful monitoring of serum calcium and creatinine. This compound has a 6-hour half-life and a rapid onset of action. Patients with renal dysfunction should decrease oral phosphate ingestion, use a phosphate binder, and avoid aluminum-containing antacids.

Vitamin D–dependent rickets type I can be treated with calcitriol (0.25 to 1 mcg/day) to achieve physiologic levels. Vitamin D–dependent rickets type II can be treated with high vitamin D doses or calcitriol if necessary. Often, maintenance of serum calcitriol above the physiologic level is required, with doses of calcitriol up to 30 to 60 mcg/day.

For vitamin D–resistant rickets, patients can be treated with calcitriol and phosphate supplements. For oncogenic osteomalacia, tumor resection is best. Otherwise, pharmacologic doses of calcitriol (1.5 to 3 mcg/day) and phosphate supplementation may help.

For osteomalacia with renal tubular acidosis, acidosis is corrected with oral bicarbonate. For osteomalacia from Fanconi's syndrome, treatment depends on the underlying disorder, but often includes phosphate supplements and vitamin D analogues.

No established treatment exists for hypophosphatasia. Intramedullary rods can help prevent fractures. Bone marrow transplant is being considered.

CONCLUSIONS

Osteoporosis can be prevented or minimized through a healthy diet and an active lifestyle throughout life. Postmenopausal estrogen deficiency, aging, and various diseases and medications can lead to osteoporosis. Although teriparatide can increase bone formation, only short-term therapy is used. Thus prevention is the key. Prevention of osteoporosis includes adequate calcium and vitamin D intake, exercise, smoking cessation, and minimal alcohol use. For osteopenia, preventive therapy with bisphosphonates or raloxifene is sometimes used, even though convincing data continue to be lacking. For osteoporosis treatment, bisphosphonates are the mainstay of therapy. Raloxifene, calcitonin, and teriparatide are alternative therapies in those who will not or cannot take an oral bisphosphonate. Fall prevention and pain control after fracture are important.

Osteomalacia is a disease of decreased bone mineralization with multiple etiologies, involving calcium, phosphorus, or vitamin D homeostasis. Vitamin D insufficiency and deficiency are becoming common again. Adequate intake of vitamin D is essential for everyone. Eliminating or treating any underlying causes of osteomalacia is the first step. In most cases, pharmacologic doses of vitamin D or treatment with calcitriol are also required.

ABBREVIATIONS

BMD: bone mineral density
BMU: basic multicellular unit
CSF-1: colony-stimulating factor-1
DXA: dual-energy x-ray absorptiometry
ET: estrogen therapy
GH: growth hormone
HIV: human immunodeficiency virus
HMG-CoA reductase: 3-hydroxymethyl-4-glutaryl CoA reductase
HT: hormonal therapy (estrogen plus progestin)
IGF-1: insulin-like growth factor-1
IL-1, IL-6, IL-11: interleukins-1, -6, and -11
MCSF: macrophage colony-stimulating factor
MORE: Multiple Outcomes of Raloxifene Evaluation trial
NOF: National Osteoporosis Foundation
OPG: osteoprotegerin
PDGF: platelet-derived growth factor
PMMA: polymethylmethacrylate
PPARγ2: peroxisome proliferator-activated receptor-γ2
PTH: parathyroid hormone
QALY: quality-adjusted life year
RANK: receptor activator of nuclear factor κB
RANKL: receptor activator of nuclear factor κB ligand
SERM: selective estrogen receptor modulator
TGF-β: transforming growth factor-β
TNF: tumor necrosis factor
TSH: thyroid-stimulating hormone
WHI: Women's Health Initiative trial

Review Questions and other resources can be found at *www.pharmacotherapyonline.com.*

REFERENCES

1. Siris ES, Miller PD, Barrett-Connor E, et al. Identification and fracture outcomes of undiagnosed low bone mineral density in postmenopausal women: Results from the National Osteoporosis Risk Assessment. JAMA 2001;286:2815–2222.
2. Looker AC, Orwoll ES, Johnston CC Jr., et al. Prevalence of low femoral bone density in older U.S. adults from NHANES III. J Bone Miner Res 1997;12:1761–1768.
3. National Osteoporisis Foundation. Physician's Guide to Prevention and Treatment of Osteoporosis. 2003. www.nof.org/physguide/table_of_contents.htm.
4. Becker C. Clinical evaluation for osteoporosis. Clin Geriatr Med 2003;19:299–320.
5. Espallargues M, Sampietro-Colom L, Estrada MD, et al. Identifying bone-mass-related risk factors for fracture to guide bone densitometry measurements: A systematic review of the literature. Osteoporos Int 2001;12:811–822.
6. U.S. Preventive Services Task Force. Screening for osteoporosis in postmenopausal women: Recommendations and rationale. Ann Intern Med 2002;137:526–528.
7. Brown JP, Josse RG. 2002 clinical practice guidelines for the diagnosis and management of osteoporosis in Canada. CMAJ 2002;167(10 Suppl):S1–S34.
8. Management of postmenopausal osteoporosis: position statement of the North American Menopause Society. Menopause 2002;9:84–101.
9. Cummings SR, Nevitt MC, Browner WS, et al. Risk factors for hip fracture in white women. Study of Osteoporotic Fractures Research Group. N Engl J Med 1995;332:767–773.
10. Favus M, ed. Primer on the Metabolic Bone Diseases and Disorders of Mineral Metabolism, 5th ed. Washington, Cadmus Professional Communications, 2003.
11. Harada S, Rodan GA. Control of osteoblast function and regulation of bone mass. Nature 2003;423:349–355.
12. Boyle WJ, Simonet WS, Lacey DL. Osteoclast differentiation and activation. Nature 2003;423:337–342.
13. Vieth R. Vitamin D supplementation, 25-hydroxyvitamin D concentrations, and safety. Am J Clin Nutr 1999;69:842–856.
14. Holick MF. Vitamin D: A millennium perspective. J Cell Biochem 2003;88:296–307.
15. Kapuri PB, Kinyamu HK, Gallagher JC, Haynatzka V. Seasonal changes in calciotropic hormones, bone markers, and bone mineral density in elderly women. J Clin Endocrinol Metab 2002;87:2024–2032.
16. Vieth R, Cole DE, Hawker GA, et al. Wintertime vitamin D insufficiency is common in young Canadian women, and their vitamin D intake does not prevent it. Eur J Clin Nutr 2001;55:1091–1097.
17. Uitterlinden AG, Fang Y, Bergink AP, et al. The role of vitamin D receptor gene polymorphisms in bone biology. Mol Cell Endocrinol 2002;197:15–21.
18. Hannan MT, Felson DT, Dawson-Hughes B, et al. Risk factors for longitudinal bone loss in elderly men and women: The Framingham Osteoporosis Study. J Bone Miner Res 2000;15:710–720.
19. Olszynski WP, Shawn Davison K, Adachi JD, et al. Osteoporosis in men: Epidemiology, diagnosis, prevention, and treatment. Clin Ther 2004;26:15–28.
20. Campion JM, Maricic MJ. Osteoporosis in men. Am Fam Physician 2003;67:1521–1526.
21. Jones A, Fay JK, Burr M, et al. Inhaled corticosteroid effects on bone metabolism in asthma and mild chronic obstructive pulmonary disease. Cochrane Database Syst Rev 2002;1:CD003537.
22. Boling EP. Secondary osteoporosis: Underlying disease and the risk for glucocorticoid-induced osteoporosis. Clin Ther 2004;26:1–14.
23. Lawson J. Drug-induced metabolic bone disorders. Semin Musculoskelet Radiol 2002;6:285–297.
24. Feldstein A, Elmer PJ, Orwoll E, et al. Bone mineral density measurement and treatment for osteoporosis in older individuals with fractures: A gap in evidence-based practice guideline implementation. Arch Intern Med 2003;163:2165–2172.
25. Cook DJ, Guyatt GH, Adachi JD, et al. Development and validation of the mini-osteoporosis quality of life questionnaire (OQLQ) in osteoporotic women with back pain due to vertebral fractures. Osteoporosis Quality of Life Study Group. Osteoporos Int 1999;10:207–213.
26. Institute of Medicine. Dietary Reference Intakes for Calcium, Phosphorus, Magnesium, Vitamin D, and Fluoride. Washington, National Academy Press, 1997.
27. Heaney RP. Effects of caffeine on bone and the calcium economy. Food Chem Toxicol 2002;40:1263–1270.
28. Heaney RP. Phosphorus nutrition and the treatment of osteoporosis. Mayo Clin Proc 2004;79:91–97.
29. Tucker KL, Hannan MT, Chen H, et al. Potassium, magnesium, and frui

and vegetable intakes are associated with greater bone mineral density in elderly men and women. Am J Clin Nutr 1999;69:727–736.

30. Feskanich D, Singh V, Willett WC, Colditz GA. Vitamin A intake and hip fractures among postmenopausal women. JAMA 2002;287:47–54.

31. Michaelsson K, Lithell H, Vessby B, Melhus H. Serum retinol levels and the risk of fracture. N Engl J Med 2003;348:287–294.

32. Morton DJ, Barrett-Connor EL, Schneider DL. Vitamin C supplement use and bone mineral density in postmenopausal women. J Bone Miner Res 2001;16:135–140.

33. Weber P. Vitamin K and bone health. Nutrition 2001;17:880–887.

34. Dawson-Hughes B. Interaction of dietary calcium and protein in bone health in humans. J Nutr 2003;133:852S–854S.

35. Kerstetter JE, O'Brien KO, Insogna KL. Low protein intake: The impact on calcium and bone homeostasis in humans. J Nutr 2003;133:855S–861S.

36. Bonaiuti D, Shea B, Iovine R, et al. Exercise for preventing and treating osteoporosis in postmenopausal women. Cochrane Database Syst Rev. 2002;3:CD000333.

37. Going S, Lohman T, Houtkooper L, et al. Effects of exercise on bone mineral density in calcium-replete postmenopausal women with and without hormone replacement therapy. Osteoporos Int 2003;14:637–643.

38. Kazis K, Iglesias E. The female athlete triad. Adolesc Med 2003;14:87–95.

39. Gillespie L, Gillespie W, Robertson M, et al. Interventions for preventing falls in elderly people. Cochrane Database Syst Rev 2003;4:CD000340.

40. Screening for osteoporosis in postmenopausal women: Recommendations and rationale. Ann Intern Med 2002;137:526–528.

41. Nelson HD, Rizzo J, Harris E, et al. Osteoporosis and fractures in postmenopausal women using estrogen. Arch Intern Med 2002;162:2278–2284.

42. Ensrud KE, Duong T, Cauley JA, et al. Low fractional calcium absorption increases the risk for hip fracture in women with low calcium intake. Study of Osteoporotic Fractures Research Group. Ann Intern Med 2000;132:345–353.

43. The role of calcium in peri- and postmenopausal women: Consensus opinion of The North American Menopause Society. Menopause 2001;8:84–95.

44. Shea B, Wells G, Cranney A, et al. Meta-analyses of therapies for postmenopausal osteoporosis. VII. Meta-analysis of calcium supplementation for the prevention of postmenopausal osteoporosis. Endocr Rev 2002;23:552–559.

45. Feskanich D, Willett WC, Colditz GA. Calcium, vitamin D, milk consumption, and hip fractures: A prospective study among postmenopausal women. Am J Clin Nutr 2003;77:504–511.

46. Heaney RP. Calcium, dairy products and osteoporosis. J Am Coll Nutr 2000;19(2 Suppl):83S–99S.

47. Heaney RP, Dowell MS, Hale CA, Bendich A. Calcium absorption varies within the reference range for serum 25-hydroxyvitamin D. J Am Coll Nutr 2003;22:142–146.

48. Feskanich D, Willett WC, Stampfer MJ, Colditz GA. A prospective study of thiazide use and fractures in women. Osteoporos Int 1997;7:79–84.

49. LaCroix AZ, Ott SM, Ichikawa L, et al. Low-dose hydrochlorothiazide and preservation of bone mineral density in older adults. A randomized, double-blind, placebo-controlled trial. Ann Intern Med 2000;133:516–526.

50. Harris SS, Dawson-Hughes B. Seasonal changes in plasma 25-hydroxyvitamin D concentrations of young American black and white women. Am J Clin Nutr 1998;67:1232–1236.

51. Harris SS, Soteriades E, Coolidge JA, et al. Vitamin D insufficiency and hyperparathyroidism in a low income, multiracial, elderly population. J Clin Endocrinol Metab 2000;85:4125–4130.

52. Guzel R, Kozanoglu E, Guler-Uysal F, et al. Vitamin D status and bone mineral density of veiled and unveiled Turkish women. J Womens Health Gend Based Med 2001;10:765–770.

53. Papadimitropoulos E, Wells G, Shea B, et al. Meta-analyses of therapies for postmenopausal osteoporosis. VIII. Meta-analysis of the efficacy of vitamin D treatment in preventing osteoporosis in postmenopausal women. Endocr Rev 2002;23:560–569.

54. Grados F, Brazier M, Kamel S, et al. Effects on bone mineral density of calcium and vitamin D supplementation in elderly women with vitamin D deficiency. Joint Bone Spine 2003;70:203–208.

55. Pfeifer M, Begerow B, Minne HW. Vitamin D and muscle function. Osteoporos Int 2002;13:187–194.

56. Trivedi DP, Doll R, Khaw KT. Effect of four monthly oral vitamin D3 (cholecalciferol) supplementation on fractures and mortality in men and women living in the community: Randomised double blind controlled trial. BMJ 2003;326:469.

57. Wu F, Staykova T, Horne A, et al. Efficacy of an oral, 10-day course of high-dose calciferol in correcting vitamin D deficiency. N Z Med J 2003;116:U536.

58. Black DM, Greenspan SL, Ensrud KE, et al. The effects of parathyroid hormone and alendronate alone or in combination in postmenopausal osteoporosis. N Engl J Med 2003;349:1207–1215.

59. Finkelstein JS, Hayes A, Hunzelman JL, et al. The effects of parathyroid hormone, alendronate, or both in men with osteoporosis. N Engl J Med 2003;349:1216–1226.

60. Bone HG, Hosking D, Devogelaer JP, et al. Ten years' experience with alendronate for osteoporosis in postmenopausal women. N Engl J Med 2004;350:1189–1199.

61. Black DM, Cummings SR, Karpf DB, et al. Randomised trial of effect of alendronate on risk of fracture in women with existing vertebral fractures. Fracture Intervention Trial Research Group. Lancet 1996;348:1535–1541.

62. Fogelman I, Ribot C, Smith R, et al. Risedronate reverses bone loss in postmenopausal women with low bone mass: Results from a multinational, double-blind, placebo-controlled trial. BMD-MN Study Group. J Clin Endocrinol Metab 2000;85:1895–1900.

63. Harris ST, Watts NB, Genant HK, et al. Effects of risedronate treatment on vertebral and nonvertebral fractures in women with postmenopausal osteoporosis: A randomized controlled trial. Vertebral Efficacy With Risedronate Therapy (VERT) Study Group. JAMA 1999;282:1344–1352.

64. McClung MR, Geusens P, Miller PD, et al. Effect of risedronate on the risk of hip fracture in elderly women. Hip Intervention Program Study Group. N Engl J Med 2001;344:333–340.

65. Chestnut CH, Skag A, Christiansen C, et al. Effects of oral ibandronate administered daily or intermittently on fracture risk in postmenopausal osteoporosis. J Bone Miner Res 2004;19:1241–1249.

66. Cranney A, Welch V, Adachi JD, et al. Etidronate for treating and preventing postmenopausal osteoporosis. Cochrane Database Syst Rev 2001;4:CD003376.

67. Reid IR, Brown JP, Burckhardt P, et al. Intravenous zoledronic acid in postmenopausal women with low bone mineral density. N Engl J Med 2002;346:653–661.

68. Krieg MA, Seydoux C, Sandini L, et al. Intravenous pamidronate as treatment for osteoporosis after heart transplantation: A prospective study. Osteoporos Int 2001;12:112–116.

69. Thiebaud D, Burckhardt P, Kriegbaum H, et al. Three monthly intravenous injections of ibandronate in the treatment of postmenopausal osteoporosis. Am J Med 1997;103:298–307.

70. Schnitzer T, Bone HG, Crepaldi G, et al. Therapeutic equivalence of alendronate 70 mg once-weekly and alendronate 10 mg daily in the treatment of osteoporosis. Alendronate Once-Weekly Study Group. Aging (Milano) 2000;12:1–12.

71. Fontana A, Delmas PD. Selective estrogen receptors modulators in the prevention and treatment of postmenopausal osteoporosis. Endocrinol Metab Clin North Am 2003;32:219–232.

72. Maricic M, Adachi JD, Sarkar S, et al. Early effects of raloxifene on clinical vertebral fractures at 12 months in postmenopausal women with osteoporosis. Arch Intern Med 2002;162:1140–1143.

73. Delmas PD, Ensrud KE, Adachi JD, et al. Efficacy of raloxifene on vertebral fracture risk reduction in postmenopausal women with osteoporosis: Four-year results from a randomized clinical trial. J Clin Endocrinol Metab 2002;87:3609–3617.

74. Sarkar S, Mitlak BH, Wong M, et al. Relationships between bone mineral density and incident vertebral fracture risk with raloxifene therapy. J Bone Miner Res 2002;17:1–10.

75. Boivin G, Lips P, Ott SM, et al. Contribution of raloxifene and calcium and vitamin D3 supplementation to the increase of the degree of mineralization of bone in postmenopausal women. J Clin Endocrinol Metab 2003;88:4199–4205.

76. Johnell O, Scheele WH, Lu Y, et al. Additive effects of raloxifene and alendronate on bone density and biochemical markers of bone remodeling in postmenopausal women with osteoporosis. J Clin Endocrinol Metab 2002;87:985–992.

77. Neele SJ, Evertz R, De Valk-De Roo G, et al. Effect of 1 year of discontinuation of raloxifene or estrogen therapy on bone mineral density after 5 years of treatment in healthy postmenopausal women. Bone 2002; 30:599–603.

78. Cummings SR, Duong T, Kenyon E, et al. Serum estradiol level and risk of breast cancer during treatment with raloxifene. JAMA 2002;287: 216–220.

79. Barrett-Connor E, Grady D, Sashegyi A, et al. Raloxifene and cardiovascular events in osteoporotic postmenopausal women: four-year results from the MORE (Multiple Outcomes of Raloxifene Evaluation) randomized trial. JAMA 2002;287:847–857.

80. Chesnut CH 3rd, Silverman S, Andriano K, et al. A randomized trial of nasal spray salmon calcitonin in postmenopausal women with established osteoporosis: the prevent recurrence of osteoporotic fractures study. PROOF Study Group. Am J Med 2000;109:267–276.

81. Lyritis GP, Paspati I, Karachalios T, et al. Pain relief from nasal salmon calcitonin in osteoporotic vertebral crush fractures. A double blind, placebo-controlled clinical study. Acta Orthop Scand Suppl 1997; 275:112–114.

82. Pun KK, Chan LW. Analgesic effect of intranasal salmon calcitonin in the treatment of osteoporotic vertebral fractures. Clin Ther 1989;11: 205–209.

83. Rossouw JE, Anderson GL, Prentice RL, et al. Risks and benefits of estrogen plus progestin in healthy postmenopausal women: principal results from the Women's Health Initiative randomized controlled trial. JAMA 2002;288:321–333.

84. The Women's Health Initiative Steering Committee. Effects of conjugated equine estrogen in postmenopausal women with hysterectomy. The Women's Health Initiative randomized controlled trial. JAMA 2004;291:1701–1712.

85. Nelson HD, Humphrey LL, Nygren P, et al. Postmenopausal hormone replacement therapy: scientific review. JAMA 2002;288:872–881.

86. Wells G, Tugwell P, Shea B, et al. Meta-analyses of therapies for postmenopausal osteoporosis. V. Meta-analysis of the efficacy of hormone replacement therapy in treating and preventing osteoporosis in postmenopausal women. Endocr Rev 2002;23:529–539.

87. Lindsay R, Gallagher JC, Kleerekoper M, Pickar JH. Effect of lower doses of conjugated equine estrogens with and without medroxyprogesterone acetate on bone in early postmenopausal women. JAMA 2002; 287:2668–2876.

88. Cosman F, Nieves J, Woelfert L, et al. Parathyroid hormone added to established hormone therapy: Effects on vertebral fracture and maintenance of bone mass after parathyroid hormone withdrawal. J Bone Miner Res 2001;16:925–931.

89. Cauley JA, Robbins J, Chen Z, et al. Effects of estrogen plus progestin on risk of fracture and bone mineral density: The Women's Health Initiative randomized trial. JAMA 2003;290:1729–1738.

90. Postmenopausal hormone replacement therapy for primary prevention of chronic conditions: Recommendations and rationale. Ann Intern Med 2002;137:834–839.

91. Berning B, Bennink HJ, Fauser BC. Tibolone and its effects on bone: A review. Climacteric 2001;4:120–136.

92. Fitzpatrick LA. Phytoestrogens—mechanism of action and effect on bone markers and bone mineral density. Endocrinol Metab Clin North Am 2003;32:233–252, viii.

93. Atkinson C, Compston JE, Day NE, et al. The effects of phytoestrogen isoflavones on bone density in women: A double-blind, randomized, placebo-controlled trial. Am J Clin Nutr 2004;79:326–333.

94. Setchell KD, Lydeking-Olsen E. Dietary phytoestrogens and their effect on bone: Evidence from in vitro and in vivo, human observational, and dietary intervention studies. Am J Clin Nutr 2003;78(3 Suppl):593S–609S.

95. Scheiber MD, Rebar RW. Isoflavones and postmenopausal bone health: A viable alternative to estrogen therapy? Menopause 1999;6:233–241.

96. Alexandersen P, Toussaint A, Christiansen C, et al. Ipriflavone in the treatment of postmenopausal osteoporosis: A randomized controlled trial. JAMA 2001;285:1482–1488.

97. Rohr UD. The impact of testosterone imbalance on depression and women's health. Maturitas 2002;41(Suppl 1):S25–S46.

98. Rhoden EL, Morgentaler A. Risks of testosterone-replacement therapy and recommendations for monitoring. N Engl J Med 2004;350:482–492.

99. Neer RM, Arnaud CD, Zanchetta JR, et al. Effect of parathyroid hormone (1-34) on fractures and bone mineral density in postmenopausal women with osteoporosis. N Engl J Med 2001;344:1434–1441.

100. Orwoll ES, Scheele WH, Paul S, et al. The effect of teriparatide [human parathyroid hormone (1-34)] therapy on bone density in men with osteoporosis. J Bone Miner Res 2003;18:9–17.

101. Meunier PJ, Roux C, Seeman E, et al. The effects of strontium ranelate on the risk of vertebral fracture in women with postmenopausal osteoporosis. N Engl J Med 2004;350:459–468.

102. Bauer DC, Mundy GR, Jamal SA, et al. Use of statins and fracture: Results of 4 prospective studies and cumulative meta-analysis of observational studies and controlled trials. Arch Intern Med 2004;164:146–152.

103. Svensson J. The importance of growth hormone (GH) and GH secretagogues for bone mass and density. Curr Pharm Des 2002;8:2023–2032.

104. Landin-Wilhelmsen K, Nilsson A, Bosaeus I, Bengtsson BA. Growth hormone increases bone mineral content in postmenopausal osteoporosis: A randomized placebo-controlled trial. J Bone Miner Res 2003;18: 393–405.

105. Ehlers MR. Recombinant human GHRH(1-44)NH2: Clinical utility and therapeutic development program. Endocrine 2001;14:137–141.

106. Geusens PP, Boonen S. Osteoporosis and the growth hormone-insulin-like growth factor axis. Horm Res 2002;58(Suppl 3):49–55.

107. Haguenauer D, Welch V, Shea B, et al. Fluoride for treating postmenopausal osteoporosis. Cochrane Database Syst Rev 2000;4: CD002825.

108. Biskobing DM. Novel therapies for osteoporosis. Expert Opin Investig Drugs 2003;12:611–621.

109. Eck JC, Hodges SD, Humphreys SC. Vertebroplasty: A new treatment strategy for osteoporotic compression fractures. Am J Orthop 2002; 31:123–127, discussion 128.

110. Watts NB, Harris ST, Genant HK. Treatment of painful osteoporotic vertebral fractures with percutaneous vertebroplasty or kyphoplasty. Osteoporos Int 2001;12:429–437.

111. Misra M, Klibanski A. Evaluation and treatment of low bone density in anorexia nervosa. Nutr Clin Care 2002;5:298–308.

112. Csermely T, Halvax L, Schmidt E, et al. Occurrence of osteopenia among adolescent girls with oligo/amenorrhea. Gynecol Endocrinol 2002; 16:99–105.

113. Orwoll E, Ettinger M, Weiss S, et al. Alendronate for the treatment of osteoporosis in men. N Engl J Med 2000;343:604–610.

114. Feldstein AC, Nichols GA, Elmer PJ, et al. Older women with fractures: Patients falling through the cracks of guideline-recommended osteoporosis screening and treatment. J Bone Joint Surg Am 2003;85-A:2294–2302.

115. Colon-Emeric CS, Pieper CF, Artz MB. Can historical and functional risk factors be used to predict fractures in community-dwelling older adults? Development and validation of a clinical tool. Osteoporos Int 2002;13:955–961.

116. Passeri G, Pini G, Troiano L, et al. Low vitamin D status, high bone turnover, and bone fractures in centenarians. J Clin Endocrinol Metab 2003;88:5109–5115.

117. Dragon C, Baran R, Lindsay R, et al. Diagnosis and management of osteoporosis in the long-term setting: Part 2—pharmacologic treatment. Long-Term Care Interface 2000;1:54–60.

118. Dragon C, Baran R, Lindsay R, et al. Diagnosis and management of osteoporosis in the long-term setting: Part 1—risk assessment. Long-Term Care Interface 2000;1:51–62.

119. Cohen A, Shane E. Osteoporosis after solid organ and bone marrow transplantation. Osteoporos Int 2003;14:617–630.

120. Joy MS, Neyhart CD, Dooley MA. A multidisciplinary renal clinic for corticosteroid-induced bone disease. Pharmacotherapy 2000;20: 206–216.

121. Thomas J, Doherty SM. HIV infection—a risk factor for osteoporosis. J Acquir Immune Defic Syndr 2003;33:281–291.

122. Bijlsma JW, Jacobs JW. Hormonal preservation of bone in rheumatoid arthritis. Rheum Dis Clin North Am 2000;26:897–910.

123. Lambert JP. Osteoporosis: A new challenge in cystic fibrosis. Pharmacotherapy 2000;20:34–51.

124. Bernstein CN, Leslie WD, Leboff MS. AGA technical review on osteoporosis in gastrointestinal diseases. Gastroenterology. 2003;124: 795–841.

125. Leslie WD, Bernstein CN, Leboff MS. AGA technical review on osteoporosis in hepatic disorders. Gastroenterology 2003;125:941–966.

126. Chau DL, Edelman SV, Chandran M. Osteoporosis and diabetes. Curr Diab Rep 2003;3:37–42.

127. Cefalu WT. The use of hormone replacement therapy in postmenopausal women with type 2 diabetes. J Womens Health Gend Based Med 2001; 10:241–255.

128. Tosteson A. The Economic Impact of Osteoporosis. Osteoporosis Prevention, Diagnosis, and Therapy. NIH Consensus Statement No. 111, Vol. 17. Bethesda, MD, 2000:1–36.

129. Tengs TO, Adams ME, Pliskin JS, et al. Five-hundred life-saving interventions and their cost-effectiveness. Risk Anal 1995;15:369–390.

130. Pols HA, Felsenberg D, Hanley DA, et al. Multinational, placebo-controlled, randomized trial of the effects of alendronate on bone density and fracture risk in postmenopausal women with low bone mass: Results of the FOSIT study. Fosamax International Trial Study Group. Osteoporos Int 1999;9:461–468.

131. Kanis JA, Johnell O, Black DM, et al. Effect of raloxifene on the risk of new vertebral fracture in postmenopausal women with osteopenia or osteoporosis: A reanalysis of the Multiple Outcomes of Raloxifene Evaluation trial. Bone 2003;33:293–300.

132. Vieth R, Chan PC, MacFarlane GD. Efficacy and safety of vitamin D3 intake exceeding the lowest observed adverse effect level. Am J Clin Nutr 2001;73:288–294.

133. Recommendations for the prevention and treatment of glucocorticoid-induced osteoporosis: 2001 update. American College of Rheumatology Ad Hoc Committee on Glucocorticoid-Induced Osteoporosis. Arthritis Rheum 2001;44:1496–1503.

134. McIlwain HH. Glucocorticoid-induced osteoporosis: Pathogenesis, diagnosis, and management. Prev Med 2003;36:243–249.

135. Van Staa TP, Laan RF, Barton IP, et al. Bone density threshold and other predictors of vertebral fracture in patients receiving oral glucocorticoid therapy. Arthritis Rheum 2003;48:3224–3229.

136. Compston J. US and UK guidelines for glucocorticoid-induced osteoporosis: Similarities and differences. Curr Rheumatol Rep 2004;6: 66–69.

137. Homik J, Suarez-Almazor ME, Shea B, et al. Calcium and vitamin D for corticosteroid-induced osteoporosis. Cochrane Database Syst Rev 2000;2:CD000952.

138. Homik J, Cranney A, Shea B, et al. Bisphosphonates for steroid induced osteoporosis. Cochrane Database Syst Rev 2000;2:CD001347.

139. Adachi JD, Saag KG, Delmas PD, et al. Two-year effects of alendronate on bone mineral density and vertebral fracture in patients receiving glucocorticoids: A randomized, double-blind, placebo-controlled extension trial. Arthritis Rheum 2001;44:202–211.

140. Cranney A, Welch V, Adachi JD, et al. Calcitonin for the treatment and prevention of corticosteroid-induced osteoporosis. Cochrane Database Syst Rev 2000;2:CD001983.

141. Plotnikoff GA, Quigley JM. Prevalence of severe hypovitaminosis D in patients with persistent, nonspecific musculoskeletal pain. Mayo Clin Proc 2003;78:1463–1470.

142. Berry JL, Davies M, Mee AP. Vitamin D metabolism, rickets, and osteomalacia. Semin Musculoskelet Radiol 2002;6:173–182.

143. Dresner M. Osteomalacia and rickets. In: Goldman L, Bennett JC, ed. Cecil Textbook of Medicine. Philadelphia, WB Saunders, 2000:1391–1398.

89
RHEUMATOID ARTHRITIS

Arthur A. Schuna

Learning Objectives and other resources can be found at *www.pharmacotherapyonline.com.*

KEY CONCEPTS

1 Rheumatoid arthritis is a systemic disease characterized by symmetrical inflammation of joints, yet may involve other organ systems.

2 Control of inflammation is the key to slowing or preventing disease progression as well as managing symptoms.

3 Drug therapy should be only part of a comprehensive program for patient management, which would also include physical therapy, exercise, and rest. Assistive devices and orthopedic surgery may be necessary in some patients.

4 Disease-modifying antirheumatic drugs (DMARDs) or biological agents should be started within 3 months of the diagnosis of rheumatoid arthritis.

5 When DMARDs used singly are ineffective or not adequately effective, combination therapy with two or more DMARDs or a DMARD plus biological agents may be used to induce a response.

6 Nonsteroidal anti-inflammatory drugs (NSAIDs) and/or corticosteroids should be considered adjunctive therapy early in the course of treatment and as needed if symptoms are not adequately controlled with DMARDs.

7 Patients require careful monitoring for toxicity and therapeutic benefit for the duration of treatment.

Rheumatoid arthritis is the most common systemic inflammatory disease, and is characterized by symmetrical joint involvement. Extra-articular involvement including rheumatoid nodules, vasculitis, eye inflammation, neurologic dysfunction, cardiopulmonary disease, lymphadenopathy, and splenomegaly are manifestations of the disease. Although the usual disease course is chronic, some patients will enter a remission spontaneously.

EPIDEMIOLOGY

Rheumatoid arthritis is estimated to have a prevalence of 1% to 2% and does not have any racial predilections. It can occur at any age, with increasing prevalence up to the seventh decade of life. The disease is three times more common in women. In people aged 15 to 45 years, women predominate by a ratio of 6:1; the sex ratio is approximately equal among patients in the first decade of life and in those more than 60 years old.

Epidemiologic data suggest that a genetic predisposition and exposure to unknown environmental factors may be necessary for expression of the disease. The major histocompatibility complex (MHC) molecules, located on T lymphocytes, appear to have an important role in most patients with rheumatoid arthritis. These molecules can be characterized using human lymphocyte antigen (HLA) typing. A majority of patients with rheumatoid arthritis have HLA-DR4, HLA-DR1, or both antigens found in the MHC region. Patients with HLA-DR4 antigen are 3.5 times more likely to develop rheumatoid arthritis than those who have other HLA-DR antigens.[1] Although the MHC region is important, it is not the sole determinant, because patients can have the disease without these HLA types. Rheumatoid arthritis is six times more common among dizygotic twins and nontwin children of parents with rheumatoid factor–positive erosive rheumatoid arthritis when compared with children whose parents do not have the disease. If one of a pair of monozygotic twins is affected, the other twin has a 30 times greater risk of developing the disease.[2,3]

PATHOPHYSIOLOGY

1 Chronic inflammation of the synovial tissue lining the joint capsule results in the proliferation of this tissue. The inflamed, proliferating synovium characteristic of rheumatoid arthritis is called *pannus* (Fig. 89–1). This pannus invades the cartilage and eventually the bone surface, producing erosions of bone and cartilage and leading to destruction of the joint. The factors that initiate the inflammatory process are unknown.

The immune system is a complex network of checks and balances designed to discriminate self from nonself (foreign) tissues. It helps rid the body of infectious agents, tumor cells, and products associated with the breakdown of cells. In rheumatoid arthritis this system no longer can differentiate self from nonself tissues and attacks the synovial tissue and other connective tissues.

The immune system has both humoral and cell-mediated functions (Fig. 89–2). The humoral component is necessary for the formation of antibodies. These antibodies are produced by plasma cells. Most patients with rheumatoid arthritis form antibodies called *rheumatoid factors*. Rheumatoid factors have not been identified as pathogenic, nor does the quantity of these circulating antibodies always correlate with disease activity. Seropositive patients tend to have a more aggressive course of their illness than do seronegative patients. Immunoglobulins can activate the complement system. The complement system amplifies the immune response by encouraging

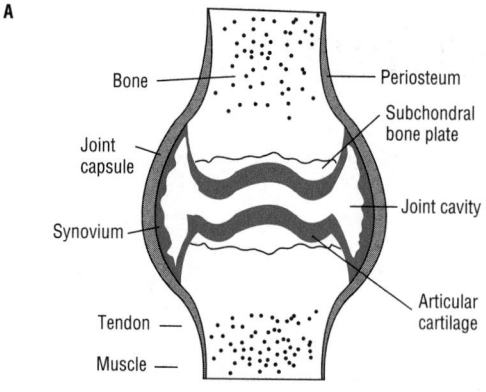

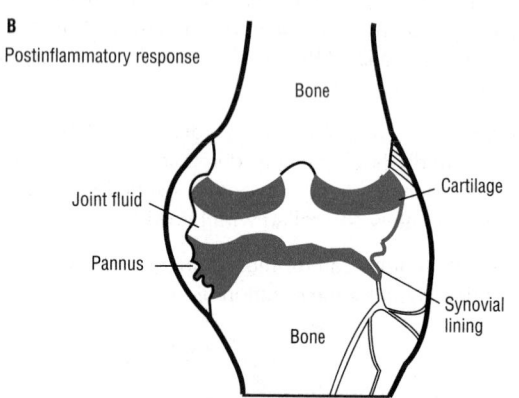

FIGURE 89–1. *A.* Schematic diagram of a normal diarthrodial joint. *B.* Schematic diagram of a knee joint with active rheumatoid arthritis showing pannus invading and destroying the cartilage and bone. (Adapted from the Arthritis Foundation Allied Health Professions Teaching Slide Collection, Copyright ©1980, with permission.)

chemotaxis, phagocytosis, and the release of lymphokines by mononuclear cells, which are then presented to T lymphocytes. The processed antigen is recognized by MHC proteins on the lymphocyte, which activates it to stimulate the production of T and B cells. The proinflammatory cytokines tumor necrosis factor (TNF), interleukin-1 (IL-1), and interleukin-6 (IL-6) are key substances in the initiation and continuance of rheumatoid inflammation. Lymphocytes may be either B cells (derived from bone marrow) or T cells (derived from thymus tissue). T cells may be either T-helper (which promote inflammation) or T-suppressor cells (which attenuate the inflammatory response). Activated T cells produce cytotoxins, which are directly toxic to tissues, and cytokines, which stimulate further activation of inflammatory processes and attract cells to areas of inflammation. Macrophages are stimulated to release prostaglandins and cytotoxins. Activated B cells produce plasma cells, which form antibodies. These antibodies in combination with complement result in the accumulation of polymorphonuclear leukocytes (PMNs). These PMNs release cytotoxins, oxygen free radicals, and hydroxyl radicals that promote cellular damage to synovium and bone. Patients with rheumatoid arthritis appear to have an excessive amount of T-helper cell activity in synovial tissues.

Vasoactive substances also play a role in the inflammatory process. Histamine, kinins, and prostaglandins are released at the site of inflammation. These substances increase both blood flow to the site of inflammation and the permeability of blood vessels. These substances cause the edema, warmth, erythema, and pain associated with joint inflammation and make it easier for granulocytes to pass from blood vessels to the site of inflammation.

The end results of the chronic inflammatory changes are variable. Loss of cartilage may result in a loss of the joint space. The formation of chronic granulation or scar tissue can lead to loss of joint motion or bony fusion (called *ankylosis*). Laxity of tendon structures can result in a loss of support to the affected joint, leading to instability or subluxation. Tendon contractures also may occur, leading to chronic deformity.[1,3–6]

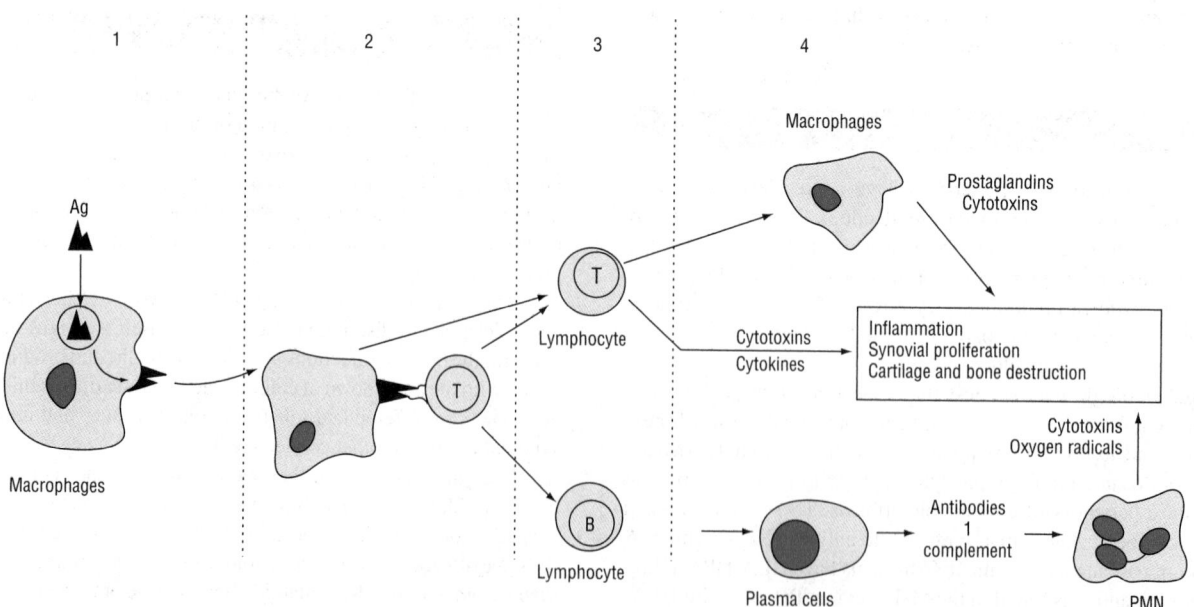

FIGURE 89–2. Pathogenesis of the inflammatory response. Phase 1: Antigen-presenting cell phagocytizes antigen. Phase 2: Antigen is presented to a T lymphocyte. The T lymphocyte attaches to antigen at the MHC portion of cell wall, causing activation. Phase 3: An activated T cell stimulates T- and B-lymphocyte production, promoting inflammation. Phase 4: Activated T cells and macrophages release factors that promote tissue destruction, increase blood flow, and result in cellular invasion of synovial tissue and joint fluid. Ag, antigen; PMN, polymorphonuclear leukocyte.

CLINICAL PRESENTATION OF RHEUMATOID ARTHRITIS

SYMPTOMS

Joint pain and stiffness of more than 6 weeks' duration. May also experience fatigue, weakness, low-grade fever, and loss of appetite. Muscle pain and afternoon fatigue may also be present. Joint deformity is generally seen late in the disease.

SIGNS

Tenderness with warmth and swelling over affected joints usually involving hands and feet. Distribution of joint involvement is frequently symmetrical. Rheumatoid nodules may also be present.

LABORATORY TESTS

Rheumatoid factor detectable in 60% to 70%.
Elevated erythrocyte sedimentation rate and C-reactive protein are markers for inflammation.
Normocytic normochromic anemia is common, as is thrombocytosis.

OTHER DIAGNOSTIC TESTS

Joint fluid aspiration may show increased white blood cell counts without infection, and crystals.
Joint radiographs may show periarticular osteoporosis, joint space narrowing, or erosions.

CLINICAL PRESENTATION

The symptoms of rheumatoid arthritis usually develop insidiously over the course of several weeks to months. Prodromal symptoms include fatigue, weakness, low-grade fever, loss of appetite, and joint pain. Stiffness and muscle aches (myalgias) may precede the development of joint swelling (synovitis). Fatigue may be more of a problem in the afternoon. During disease flares, the onset of fatigue begins earlier in the day and subsides as disease activity lessens. Most commonly, joint involvement tends to be symmetrical; however, early in the disease some patients present with an asymmetrical pattern involving one or a few joints that eventually develops into the more classic presentation. About 20% of patients develop an abrupt onset of their illness with fevers, polyarthritis, and constitutional symptoms (e.g., depression, anxiety, fatigue, anorexia, and weight loss).[2,3] No single test or physical finding can be used to make the diagnosis of rheumatoid arthritis.

JOINT INVOLVEMENT

The joints affected most frequently by rheumatoid arthritis are the small joints of the hands, wrists, and feet (Fig. 89–3). In addition, elbows, shoulders, hips, knees, and ankles may be involved. Patients usually experience joint stiffness that typically is worse in the morning. The duration of stiffness tends to be correlated directly with disease activity, usually exceeds 30 minutes, and may persist all day. Chronic inflammation with lack of an adequate exercise program results in loss of range of motion, atrophy of muscles, weakness, and deformity.

On examination, the swelling of the joints may be visible or may be apparent only by palpation. The swelling feels soft and spongy because it is caused by proliferation of soft tissues or fluid accumulation within the joint capsule. The swollen joint may appear erythematous and feel warmer than nearby skin surfaces, especially early in the course of the disease. In contrast, the swelling associated with osteoarthritis usually is bony (caused by osteophytes) and infrequently is associated with signs of inflammation.

Involvement of the hands and wrists is common in rheumatoid arthritis. Hand involvement is manifested by pain, swelling, tenderness, and grip weakness during the acute phase, and by subluxation, instability, deformity, and muscle atrophy in the chronic phase of the disease. Functional difficulties with clasp, grasp, and pinch alter both strength and fine motor movement.

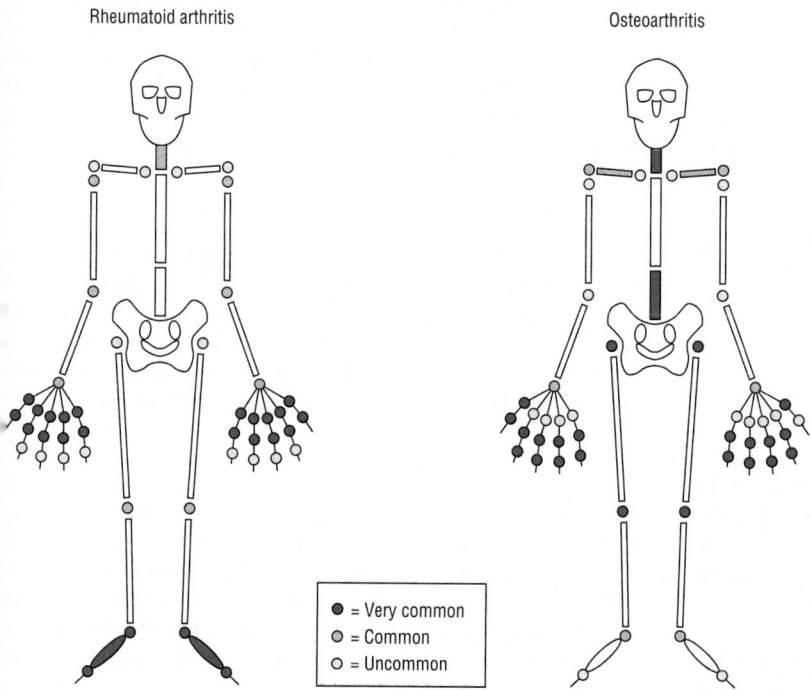

Rheumatoid arthritis

Osteoarthritis

● = Very common
◐ = Common
○ = Uncommon

FIGURE 89–3. Patterns of joint involvement in rheumatoid arthritis and osteoarthritis.

Deformity of the hand may be seen with chronic inflammation. These changes may alter the mechanics of hand function, reducing grip strength and making it difficult to perform usual daily activities.

Swelling at the elbow is most evident at the radiohumeral joint. Shoulder pain may result from involvement of the joint itself or from tendon inflammation (tendinitis) or inflammation of the bursa (bursitis) near the deltoid muscle.

The knee also can be involved, with loss of cartilage, instability, and joint pain. Synovitis of the knee may cause the formation of a cyst behind the knee called a popliteal or Baker's cyst. These cysts may become painful as they get tense, or they may rupture, producing a clinical picture similar to thrombophlebitis secondary to the release of inflammatory components into the area of the calf muscle. Chronic joint pain leads to muscle atrophy, which can result in a laxity of the ligamentous structures that support the knee, causing instability. Maintenance of an adequate range of motion of the knee is essential to normal gait.

Foot and ankle involvement in rheumatoid arthritis is common. The metatarsophalangeal joints are involved commonly in rheumatoid arthritis, making walking difficult. Subluxation of the metatarsal heads leads to "cock-up" or hammer-toe deformities. Subluxation also may cause a flexion deformity at the proximal interphalangeal joint of the toe, leading to pressure necrosis of the skin over the joint secondary to irritation caused by shoes. Hallux valgus (lateral deviation of the digit) and bunion or callus formation may occur at the great toe. A widening of the foot occurs commonly with long-standing disease.

Involvement of the spine usually occurs in the cervical vertebrae; lumbar vertebral involvement is rare. Involvement of the first and second cervical vertebrae can lead to instability of this joint. Patients with this problem are at a greater risk for spinal cord compression, although this complication is rare.

The temporomandibular joint (jaw) can be affected, resulting in malocclusion and difficulty in chewing food. Inflammation of cartilage in the chest can lead to chest wall pain. Hip pain may occur as a result of destructive changes in the hip joint, soft-tissue inflammation (e.g., bursitis), or referred pain from nerve entrapment at the lumbar vertebrae.

EXTRA-ARTICULAR INVOLVEMENT

RHEUMATOID NODULES

Rheumatoid nodules occur in 20% of patients with rheumatoid arthritis. These nodules are seen most commonly on the extensor surfaces of the elbows, forearms, and hands, but also may be seen on the feet and at other pressure points. They also may develop in the lung or pleural lining of the lung, and rarely in the meninges. Rheumatoid nodules usually are asymptomatic and do not require any special intervention. Nodules are observed more commonly in patients with erosive disease.[7]

VASCULITIS

Vasculitis usually is seen in patients with long-standing rheumatoid arthritis. Vasculitis may result in a wide variety of clinical presentations. Invasion of blood vessel walls by inflammatory cells results in an obliteration of the vessel, producing infarction of tissue distal to the area of involvement. Most commonly, small-vessel vasculitis produces infarcts near the ends of the fingers or toes, especially around the nail beds. These infarcts are usually of little consequence.

Vasculitis also may cause the breakdown of skin, especially in the lower extremities, producing ulcers that may be indistinguishable in appearance from stasis ulcers. However, these ulcers do not heal with the usual modes of treatment used for stasis ulcers. Involvement of larger vessels with vasculitis can result in life-threatening complications. Infarction of vessels supplying blood to nerves can cause irreversible motor deficits. Involvement of vessels supplying other organ systems can lead to visceral involvement and a polyarteritis nodosa–like illness. Aggressive treatment of the inflammatory process is necessary in these patients. Fortunately, the more serious vasculitic picture is seen rarely.

PULMONARY COMPLICATIONS

Rheumatoid arthritis may involve the pleura of the lung, which is often asymptomatic, although pleural effusions may result. Pulmonary fibrosis also may develop as a result of rheumatoid involvement; smoking appears to increase the risk of this complication. Rheumatoid nodules may develop in lung tissue and appear similar to neoplasms on chest x-ray films. Interstitial pneumonitis and arteritis are rare, potentially life-threatening complications of rheumatoid arthritis.

OCULAR MANIFESTATIONS

Ocular manifestations include keratoconjunctivitis sicca and inflammation of the sclera, episclera, and cornea. Atrophy of the lacrimal duct may result in a decrease in tear formation, causing dry and itchy eyes, termed *keratoconjunctivitis sicca*. When this is observed in association with rheumatoid arthritis, it is referred to as Sjögren's syndrome. Artificial tears may be used to relieve symptoms. Inflammation of the superficial layers of the sclera (episcleritis) is generally self-limiting. Involvement of deeper tissues (scleritis) usually results in a more serious, painful, and chronic inflammation. Rheumatoid nodules may develop on the sclera.

CARDIAC INVOLVEMENT

The heart is sometimes affected by rheumatoid arthritis. Rheumatoid arthritis is associated with an increased risk of cardiovascular mortality. This risk appears to be higher in those with more active inflammation and is reduced with treatment, particularly with methotrexate.[8,9] Pericarditis may occur, resulting in the accumulation of fluid. Although many patients show evidence of previous pericarditis at autopsy, the development of clinically evident pericarditis with tamponade is a rare complication. Cardiac conduction abnormalities and aortic valve incompetence, caused by aortic root dilatation, may occur. Myocarditis is a rare complication of rheumatoid arthritis.

FELTY'S SYNDROME

Rheumatoid arthritis in association with splenomegaly and neutropenia is known as Felty's syndrome. Thrombocytopenia also may be a manifestation of the syndrome. Patients with Felty's syndrome and severe leukopenia are more susceptible to infection. The decrease in granulocytes appears to be mediated by the immune system because splenectomy does not result in improvement of the patient.[7]

OTHER COMPLICATIONS

Lymphadenopathy may occur in patients with rheumatoid arthritis, particularly in nodes proximal to more actively involved joints. Renal involvement is rare but can be associated with treatment, including nonsteroidal anti-inflammatory drugs (NSAIDs), gold salts, and penicillamine. Amyloidosis is a rare complication of long-standing rheumatoid arthritis. It appears to be more common in Europe than in the United States.

LABORATORY FINDINGS

Hematologic tests often reveal a mild to moderate anemia with normocytic, normochromic indices. The hematocrit may fall as low as 30%. The anemia is usually inversely related to inflammatory disease activity and is referred to as an *anemia of chronic disease*. This type of anemia does not respond to iron therapy and can present a diagnostic dilemma because NSAIDs may induce gastritis and chronic blood loss, leading to iron-deficiency anemia. Laboratory tests useful in differentiating these anemias include stool guaiac (or other stool tests for occult blood), serum iron:iron-binding capacity ratio (decreased in iron deficiency), and mean corpuscular volume (more likely to be decreased in iron deficiency). Other causes of anemia also must be considered in the differential diagnosis (see anemias, Chap. 99).

Thrombocytosis is another common hematologic finding with active rheumatoid arthritis. Platelet counts rise and fall in direct correlation with disease activity in many patients. Thrombocytopenia may result from toxicity of gold salts, penicillamine, or immunosuppressive therapy. Thrombocytopenia also may be observed in Felty's syndrome or vasculitis.

Although leukopenia is associated with Felty's syndrome, it also may result from toxicity of gold, sulfasalazine, penicillamine, immunosuppressive drugs, and biologic agents. Leukocytosis is seen commonly as a result of corticosteroid treatment.

The erythrocyte sedimentation rate is usually elevated in patients with rheumatoid arthritis and other inflammatory diseases. This test is very nonspecific, and although the erythrocyte sedimentation rate usually falls as patients respond to therapy, there is a large variability among patients in response to treatment. C-reactive protein is another nonspecific marker for inflammatory arthritis when it is elevated. This protein is produced by the liver in response to certain cytokines.

Rheumatoid factor is present in 60% to 70% of patients with rheumatoid arthritis. The usual laboratory test for rheumatoid factor is an antibody specific for IgM rheumatoid factor. Patients with rheumatoid arthritis and a negative test for rheumatoid factor may have IgG or IgA rheumatoid factors, but tests for these are not routinely available. Rheumatoid factor tests may be reported positive at a specific serum dilution. Serum is diluted to a standard series of dilutions; the greatest dilution that yields a positive test result will be reported (e.g., rheumatoid factor positive at 1:640). Some laboratories quantify rheumatoid factor rather than using titers. Higher dilutional titers or serum concentrations of rheumatoid factors usually indicate a more severe disease, but like the erythrocyte sedimentation rate, the large interpatient variability makes this test unreliable as a means of assessing patient progress. Rheumatoid factor may be positive in patients without rheumatoid arthritis (Table 89–1).

Antinuclear antibodies are detected in 25% of patients with rheumatoid arthritis. These antibodies usually have a diffuse pattern of immunofluorescence. Tests for antibodies to double-stranded DNA (usually positive in systemic lupus erythematosus) are negative. Serum complement is usually normal, although complement concentrations of joint fluid often are depressed from consumption secondary

TABLE 89–1. Diseases Associated with a Positive Rheumatoid Factor

Rheumatic diseases
  Rheumatoid arthritis
  Sjögren's syndrome (with or without arthritis)
  Systemic lupus erythematosus
  Progressive systemic sclerosis
  Polymyositis/dermatomyositis
Infectious diseases
  Bacterial endocarditis
  Tuberculosis
  Syphilis
  Infectious mononucleosis
  Infectious hepatitis
  Leprosy
Other causes
  Aging
  Interstitial pulmonary fibrosis
  Cirrhosis of the liver
  Chronic active hepatitis
  Sarcoidosis

to the inflammatory process. In patients with vasculitis, serum complement concentrations may be low.

Synovial fluid usually is turbid because of the large number of leukocytes in inflammatory fluid. White cell counts of 5000 to 50,000/mm³ are not uncommon in inflamed joints. The fluid is usually less viscous than that in normal joints or in fluid associated with osteoarthritis. Glucose concentrations of joint fluid are normal or low compared with those in serum drawn at the same time as synovial aspirates. The decrease is not as profound as the decrease associated with joint infection or systemic lupus erythematosus.

Radiologic manifestations of rheumatoid arthritis include soft-tissue swelling and osteoporosis near the joint (periarticular osteoporosis). Erosions tend to occur later in the course of the disease and usually are seen first in the metacarpophalangeal and proximal interphalangeal joints of the hands and the metatarsophalangeal joints of the feet. Periodic joint radiographs are a useful way of evaluating disease progression.

SERONEGATIVE INFLAMMATORY ARTHRITIS

Although rheumatoid arthritis may have a negative rheumatoid factor titer, a number of other systemic inflammatory arthritic conditions exist, including psoriatic arthritis, ankylosing spondylitis, and arthritis associated with inflammatory bowel disease. These conditions often tend to be less aggressive than those typically seen with rheumatoid arthritis. Detailed discussion about these conditions is beyond the scope of this chapter, but further information may be found elsewhere.[3] Management principles are similar to those for rheumatoid arthritis.

▶ TREATMENT: Rheumatoid Arthritis

DESIRED OUTCOME

❷ The primary objective is to improve or maintain functional status, thereby improving quality of life. Treatment of rheumatoid arthritis is a multifaceted approach that includes pharmacologic and nonpharmacologic therapies. Recent emphasis has been placed on aggressive treatment early in the disease course. The ultimate goal is to achieve complete disease remission, although this goal is seldom achieved. Additional goals of treatment include controlling disease activity and joint pain, maintaining the ability to function in daily activities or work, improving the quality of life, and slowing destructive joint changes.

NONPHARMACOLOGIC THERAPY

◀3 Rest, occupational therapy, physical therapy, use of assistive devices, weight reduction, and surgery are the most useful types of nonpharmacologic therapy used in patients with rheumatoid arthritis. Rest is an essential component of a nonpharmacologic treatment plan. It relieves stress on inflamed joints and prevents further joint destruction. Rest also aids in alleviation of pain. Too much rest and immobility, however, may lead to decreased range of motion, and ultimately muscle atrophy and contractures.

Occupational and physical therapy can provide the patient with skills and exercises necessary to increase or maintain mobility. These disciplines also may provide patients with supportive and adaptive devices such as canes, walkers, and splints.

Other nonpharmacologic therapeutic options include weight loss and surgery. Weight reduction helps to alleviate stress on inflamed joints. This should be instituted and monitored with close supervision of a health care professional. Tenosynovectomy, tendon repair, and joint replacements are surgical options for patients with rheumatoid arthritis. Such management usually is reserved for patients with severe disease.[10,11]

PHARMACOLOGIC THERAPY

◀4 A disease-modifying antirheumatic drug (DMARD) should be started within the first 3 months of onset of symptoms of rheumatoid arthritis[10] (Fig. 89–4). Early introduction of DMARDs results in a more favorable outcome.[12–17] NSAIDs and/or corticosteroids may be used for symptomatic relief if needed. They provide relatively rapid improvement in symptoms compared with DMARDs, which may take weeks to months before benefit is seen; however, NSAIDs

have no impact on disease progression, and corticosteroid use carries a long-term risk of complications that makes them less desirable.[17]

Early treatment with DMARDs can reduce mortality. Patients with rheumatoid arthritis have increased mortality compared to people without the disease. In one trial, methotrexate reduced risk of mortality.[8] Early treatment with DMARDs in patients followed for up to 10 years had mortality rates similar to patients without the disease.[18]

DMARDs—including biologic agents—should be used in all patients except those with limited disease or those with class IV disease, in whom little reversibility of disease is expected. Commonly used DMARDs include methotrexate, hydroxychloroquine, sulfasalazine, and leflunomide. The biologic agents that have also been demonstrated to have disease-modifying activity include the anti-TNF drugs (etanercept, infliximab, and adalimumab) and the interleukin-1–receptor antagonist, anakinra. Less frequently used are azathioprine, d-penicillamine, gold (including auranofin), minocycline, cyclosporine, and cyclophosphamide. This is due to either less efficacy, high toxicity, or both. The order in which the first-line agents are used is not clearly defined, though methotrexate is often chosen in more severe cases due to long-term data suggesting superior outcomes than those with other DMARDs, and lower cost than biologic agents. Leflunomide appears to have similar long-term efficacy as that of methotrexate.[19]

The biologic agents have proven effective for patients who fail treatment with other DMARDs. Infliximab should be given in combination with methotrexate to prevent development of antibodies that may reduce drug efficacy or induce allergic reactions.

◀5 Combination therapy with two or more DMARDs may be effective when single-DMARD treatment is unsuccessful.[17,20–26] The combinations of cyclosporine plus methotrexate and methotrexate plus sulfasalazine and hydroxychloroquine have been shown to be particularly effective.[25]

Corticosteroids can be used in various ways. They are valuable in controlling symptoms before the onset of action of DMARDs. A burst of corticosteroids can be used in acute flares. Continuous low doses may be adjuncts when DMARDs do not provide adequate disease control. Corticosteroids may be injected into joints and soft tissues to control local inflammation. Steroids seldom should be used as monotherapy. There are data to suggest they have disease-modifying activity;[27,28] however, it is preferable to avoid chronic use when possible to avoid long-term complications. NSAIDs and DMARDs have steroid-sparing properties that permit reductions of steroid doses.

For monitoring parameters and dosing guidelines for DMARDs and NSAIDs used in rheumatoid arthritis, see Tables 89–2 and 89–3.

> ### CLINICAL CONTROVERSY
>
> For patients with rheumatoid arthritis, the order of DMARD or biological agent choice is not clearly defined. In addition, some advocate trials of combination DMARD therapy before courses of biological agents are tried.

NONSTEROIDAL ANTI-INFLAMMATORY DRUGS

◀6 NSAIDs should seldom be used as monotherapy for rheumatoid arthritis. NSAIDs possess both analgesic and anti-inflammatory properties and reduce stiffness associated with rheumatoid arthritis. NSAIDs mainly inhibit prostaglandin synthesis, which is only a small

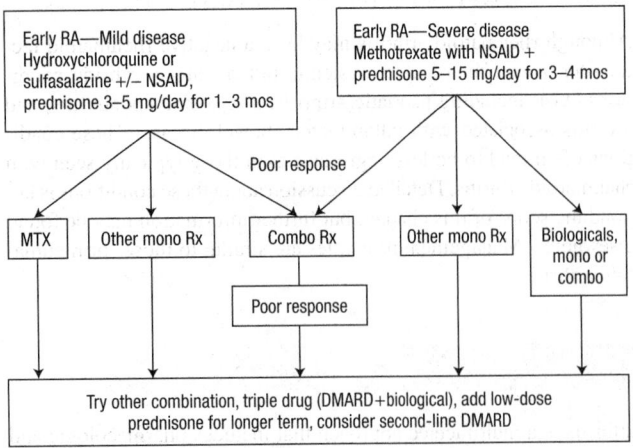

FIGURE 89–4. Algorithm for treatment of rheumatoid arthritis. RA, rheumatoid arthritis; NSAID, nonsteroidal anti-inflammatory drugs; Rx, therapy; DMARD, disease-modifying antirheumatic drug.

TABLE 89–2. Usual Doses and Monitoring Parameters for Antirheumatic Drugs

Drug	Usual Dose	Initial Monitoring Tests	Maintenance Monitoring Tests
NSAIDs	See Table 90–4 in the osteoarthritis chapter	S_{Cr} or BUN, CBC every 2–4 weeks after starting therapy for 1–2 months; *salicylates:* serum salicylate levels if therapeutic dose and no response	Same as initial plus stool guaiac every 6–12 months
Methotrexate	Oral or IM: 7.5–15 mg per week	Baseline: AST, ALT, ALK-P, albumin, total bilirubin, hepatitis B and C studies, CBC with platelets, S_{Cr}	CBC with platelets, AST, albumin every 1–2 months
Leflunomide	Oral: 100 mg daily for 3 days, then 10–20 mg daily	Baseline: ALT	ALT monthly initially, and then periodically when stable
Hydroxychloroquine	Oral: 200–300 mg twice daily; after 1–2 months may increase to 200 mg once or twice daily	Baseline: color fundus photography and automated central perimetric analysis	Ophthalmoscopy every 9–12 months and Amsler grid at home every 2 weeks
Sulfasalazine	Oral: 500 mg twice daily, then increase to 1 g twice daily max	Baseline: CBC with platelets, then every week for 1 month	Same as initial every 1–2 months
Etanercept	25 mg SC twice weekly or 50 mg every 7 days	None	None
Infliximab	3 mg/kg IV at 0, 2, and 6 weeks, then every 8 weeks	None	None
Adalimumab	40 mg SC every 2 weeks	None	None
Anakinra	100 mg SC daily	None	None
Auranofin	Oral: 3 mg once or twice daily	Baseline: UA, CBC with platelets	Same as initial every 1–2 months
Gold thiomalate	IM: 10-mg test dose, then weekly dosing 25–50 mg; after response may increase dosing interval	Baseline and until stable: UA, CBC with platelets preinjection	Same as initial every other dose
Azathioprine	Oral: 50–150 mg daily	CBC with platelets, AST every 2 weeks for 1–2 months	Same as initial every 1–2 months
D-Penicillamine	Oral: 125–250 mg daily, may increase by 125–250 mg every 1–2 months; max 750 mg/day	Baseline: UA, CBC with platelets, then every week for 1 month	Same as initial every 1–2 months, but every 2 weeks if dose changes
Cyclophosphamide	Oral: 1–2 mg/kg per day	UA, CBC with platelets every week for 1 month	Same tests as initial but every 2–4 weeks
Cyclosporine	Oral: 2.5 mg/kg per day	S_{Cr}, blood pressure every month	Same as initial
Corticosteroids	Oral, IV, IM, IA, and soft-tissue injections: variable	Glucose; blood pressure every 3–6 months	Same as initial

ALK-P, alkaline phosphatase; ALT, alanine aminotransferase; AST, aspartate aminotransferase; BUN, blood urea nitrogen; CBC, complete blood cell count; IA, intra-articular; IM, intramuscular; IV, intravenous; SC, subcutaneously; S_{Cr}, serum creatinine; UA, urinalysis.

portion of the inflammatory cascade (see Fig. 89–2). Cyclooxygenase-2–specific NSAIDs have a better gastrointestinal safety profile and similar therapeutic efficacy as conventional NSAIDs.[29,30] For discussion of the mechanism of action, adverse effects, and drug interactions, see osteoarthritis, Chap. 90. Dosing information for NSAIDs is provided in Table 90–4.

METHOTREXATE

Methotrexate is now considered the DMARD of choice by many rheumatologists for treating rheumatoid arthritis. In psoriatic arthritis it not only treats the joint symptoms, but also improves the skin disease for most patients. Methotrexate is contraindicated in pregnant and nursing women. It is also contraindicated in patients with chronic liver disease, immunodeficiency, pleural or peritoneal effusions, leukopenia, thrombocytopenia, pre-existing blood disorders, and a creatinine clearance of less than 40 mL/min.

Absorption of methotrexate is variable and averages about 70% of an oral dose. Methotrexate is 35% to 50% bound to albumin; it may be displaced by highly protein-bound drugs such as NSAIDs, but the clinical importance of this interaction is not known. Methotrexate is extensively metabolized intracellularly to polyglutamated derivatives. It is excreted by the kidney, 80% unchanged, by glomerular filtration and active transport. Some methotrexate may be reabsorbed, but this transport process may be saturated even with low doses, resulting in increased renal clearance.

Methotrexate inhibits cytokine production, inhibits purine biosynthesis, and may stimulate release of adenosine, all of which may lead to its anti-inflammatory properties. The drug has a fairly rapid onset of action; results may be seen as early as 2 to 3 weeks after starting therapy. Some 45% to 67% of patients remain on methotrexate therapy in studies ranging from 5 to 7 years.[31,32] Methotrexate may be given intramuscularly, subcutaneously, or orally. Doses greater than 15 mg per week generally are given parenterally because of decreased oral bioavailability of larger doses.

The toxicities of methotrexate therapy are mainly gastrointestinal, hematologic, pulmonary, and hepatic. Stomatitis occurs in 3% to 10% of patients and may be painful or painless. Diarrhea, nausea, and vomiting may occur in up to 10% of patients. The most common

TABLE 89–3. Clinical Monitoring of Drug Therapy in Rheumatoid Arthritis

Drug	Toxicities Requiring Monitoring	Symptoms to Inquire About[a]
NSAIDs and salicylates	GI ulceration and bleeding, renal damage	Blood in stool, black stool, dyspepsia, nausea/vomiting, weakness, dizziness, abdominal pain, edema, weight gain, shortness of breath
Corticosteroids	Hypertension, hyperglycemia, osteoporosis[b]	Blood pressure if available, polyuria, polydipsia, edema, shortness of breath, visual changes, weight gain, headaches, broken bones or bone pain
Azathioprine	Myelosuppression, hepatotoxicity, lymphoproliferative disorders	Symptoms of myelosuppression (extreme fatigue, easy bleeding or bruising, infection), jaundice
Gold (intramuscular or oral)	Myelosuppression, proteinuria, rash, stomatitis	Symptoms of myelosuppression, edema, rash, oral ulcers, diarrhea
Hydroxychloroquine	Macular damage, rash, diarrhea	Visual changes including a decrease in night or peripheral vision, rash, diarrhea
Methotrexate	Myelosuppression, hepatic fibrosis, cirrhosis, pulmonary infiltrates or fibrosis, stomatitis, rash	Symptoms of myelosuppression, shortness of breath, nausea/vomiting, lymph node swelling, coughing, mouth sores, diarrhea, jaundice
Leflunomide	Hepatitis, GI distress, alopecia	Nausea/vomiting, gastritis, diarrhea, hair loss, jaundice
Penicillamine	Myelosuppression, proteinuria, stomatitis, rash, dysgeusia	Symptoms of myelosuppression, edema, rash, diarrhea, altered taste perception, oral ulcers
Sulfasalazine	Myelosuppression, rash	Symptoms of myelosuppression, photosensitivity, rash, nausea/vomiting
Etanercept, adalimumab, anakinra	Local injection-site reactions, infection	Symptoms of infection
Infliximab	Immune reactions, infection	Postinfusion reactions, symptoms of infection

[a]Altered immune function increases infection, which should be considered, particularly in patients taking azathioprine, methotrexate, corticosteroids, or other drugs that may produce myelosuppression.
[b]Osteoporosis is not likely to manifest early in treatment, but all patients should be taking appropriate steps to prevent bone loss.
NSAID, nonsteroidal anti-inflammatory drug.
Adapted from American College of Rheumatology Ad Hoc Committee on Clinical Guidelines. Guidelines for monitoring drug therapy in rheumatoid arthritis. Arthritis Rheum 1996;39:723–731.

TABLE 89–4. Dosage Regimens and Durations of Antiplatelet Effect for Nonsteroidal Anti-Inflammatory Drugs

Drug	Recommended Total Daily Anti-Inflammatory Dosage		Dosing Schedule	Approximate Duration of Antiplatelet Effect
	Adult	Children		
Aspirin	2.6–5.2 g	60–100 mg/kg	Four times daily	14 days
Celecoxib	200–400 mg	–	Once or twice daily	None
Diclofenac	150–200 mg	–	Three to four times daily Extended release: twice daily	5–10 h
Diflunisal	0.5–1.5 g	–	Twice daily	2–7 days
Etodolac	0.2–1.2 g (max. 20 mg/kg)	–	Three to four times daily	36 h
Fenoprofen	0.9–3.0 g	–	Four times daily	15–24 h
Flurbiprofen	200–300 mg	–	Two to four times daily	24–48 h
Ibuprofen	1.2–3.2 g	20–40 mg/kg	Three to four times daily	5–10 h
Indomethacin	50–200 mg	2–4 mg/kg (max. 200 mg)	Two to four times daily Extended release: once daily	24–48 h
Ketoprofen	150–300 mg	–	Three to four times daily Extended release: once daily	5–10 h
Meclofenamate	200–400 mg	–	Three to four times daily	24–48 h
Meloxicam	7.5–15 mg	–	Once daily	Uncertain
Nabumetone	1–2 g	–	Once or twice daily	4–7 days
Naproxen	0.5–1.0 g	10 mg/kg	Twice daily Extended release: once daily	4 days
Naproxen sodium	0.55–1.1 g	–	Twice daily	4 days
Nonacetylated salicylates	1.2–4.8 g	–	Two to six times daily	None
Oxaprozin	0.6–1.8 g (max. 26 mg/kg)	–	One to three times daily	8–10 days
Piroxicam	10–20 mg	–	Once daily	7–20 days
Sulindac	300–400 mg	–	Twice daily	4 days
Tolmetin	0.6–1.8 g	15–30 mg/kg	Three to four times daily	8–16 h
Valdecoxib	10 mg	–	Once daily	None

ematologic toxicity is thrombocytopenia in 1% to 3% of patients. eukopenia also may occur, but in a smaller number of patients. Al_ough pulmonary fibrosis and pneumonitis can be severe adverse _fects, they are rare.

Elevated liver enzymes may occur in up to 15% of patients; cir_osis is rare. Liver function tests, aspartate aminotransferase (AST) _ alanine aminotransferase (ALT), should be performed periodically. _ethotrexate should be discontinued if these test values show sus_ined results greater than twice the upper limits of normal. Serum _bumin levels also should be checked periodically, as signs of liver _xicity in some patients may not have liver inflammation manifested _y AST or ALT elevation. Liver biopsy is now recommended before _eginning methotrexate therapy only for patients with a history of ex_essive alcohol use, ongoing hepatitis B or C infection, or recurring _evation of AST. Biopsies during methotrexate therapy are recom_ended only for patients who develop consistently abnormal liver _nction tests.[10]

Since the drug is teratogenic, patients should use contraception _ avoid pregnancy and discontinue the drug if conception is planned.

Because it is a folic acid antagonist, methotrexate can induce a _lic acid deficiency. This deficiency is thought to be partly responsi_le for methotrexate toxicity, and supplementation with folic acid has _een shown to alleviate some adverse effects. Addition of folic acid to _ methotrexate regimen for rheumatoid arthritis does not compromise _rug efficacy.[10,33,34]

LEFLUNOMIDE

_eflunomide is a DMARD that inhibits pyrimidine synthesis, leading _ a decrease in lymphocyte proliferation and modulation of inflam_ation. It is given as a loading dose of 100 mg daily for 3 days, _ollowed by a maintenance dose of 20 mg daily. Lower doses may _e used if patients have gastrointestinal intolerance, complain of hair _oss, or have other signs of dose-related toxicity. The loading dose al_ows the patient to achieve a therapeutic response, usually within _e first month. The long elimination half-life of the drug (14 to _6 days) would require the patient to take the drug for months to _chieve steady state without a loading dose.

Leflunomide has efficacy similar to that of methotrexate for treat_ng rheumatoid arthritis. The drug may cause liver toxicity and is _ontraindicated in patients with pre-existing liver disease. Patients _aking the drug should have ALT monitored monthly initially, and _eriodically thereafter as long as they continue treatment.

The drug is teratogenic, and appropriate contraceptive measures _re recommended to avoid pregnancy for all sexually active male and _emale patients taking leflunomide. If conception is desired, lefluno_ide must be discontinued. Because leflunomide undergoes entero_epatic circulation, the drug takes many months to drop to a plasma _oncentration considered safe during pregnancy (<0.02 mcg/mL). _holestyramine may be used to rapidly clear the drug from plasma. _nlike many DMARDs, leflunomide bone marrow toxicity is reported _ rarely that blood cell monitoring is not necessary.[19,35,36]

HYDROXYCHLOROQUINE

_he pharmacokinetics of hydroxychloroquine are poorly understood. _t is well absorbed orally and widely distributed to body tissues. _ydroxychloroquine is partially metabolized in the liver and is ex_reted by the kidney. The onset of action of hydroxychloroquine may

be delayed up to 6 weeks, but the drug is considered a therapeutic failure only when 6 months of therapy without a response has elapsed.

The main advantage of hydroxychloroquine is the lack of myelosuppressive, hepatic, and renal toxicities that may be seen with other DMARDs, which simplifies monitoring. Short-term toxicities of hydroxychloroquine include gastrointestinal effects such as nausea, vomiting, and diarrhea, which can be managed by taking doses with food. Ocular toxicity includes accommodation defects, benign corneal deposits, blurred vision, scotomata (small areas of decreased or absent vision in the visual field), and night blindness. Although the risk of true retinopathy with hydroxychloroquine approaches zero, preretinopathy may occur in 2.7% of patients. All patients must understand the importance of adhering to hydroxychloroquine monitoring guidelines as delineated in Table 89–2. Any visual change must be reported immediately. Dermatologic toxicities include rash, alopecia, and increased skin pigmentation; neurologic adverse effects such as headache, vertigo, and insomnia usually are mild.[26,37,38]

SULFASALAZINE

Sulfasalazine, a prodrug, is cleaved by bacteria in the colon into sulfapyridine and 5-aminosalicylic acid. It is believed that the sulfapyridine moiety is responsible for the agent's antirheumatic properties, although the exact mechanism of action is not known. Once the colonic bacteria have cleaved sulfasalazine, sulfapyridine and 5-aminosalicylic acid are absorbed rapidly from the gastrointestinal tract. Sulfapyridine distributes rapidly throughout the body, but higher concentrations are found in certain tissues such as serous fluid, liver, and intestines. Both sulfasalazine and its metabolites are excreted in the urine. Antirheumatic effects should be seen within 2 months.

Use of sulfasalazine is often limited by its adverse effects. Gastrointestinal adverse effects such as nausea, vomiting, diarrhea, and anorexia are the most common. These can be minimized by initiating therapy with low doses and titrating gradually to higher doses, dividing the dose more evenly throughout the day, or using enteric-coated preparations. Rash, urticaria, and serum sickness–like reactions can be managed with antihistamines, and if indicated, corticosteroids. If a hypersensitivity reaction occurs, therapy should be stopped immediately and another DMARD substituted. Sulfasalazine has been associated with leukopenia, alopecia, stomatitis, and elevated hepatic enzymes. It also may cause the patient's urine and skin to turn a yellow-orange color which is of no clinical consequence; however, patients should be educated about this to avoid premature discontinuance.

Sulfasalazine's absorption can be decreased when antibiotics are used that destroy the colonic bacteria. Sulfasalazine also binds iron supplements in the gastrointestinal tract that can lead to a decreased absorption of sulfasalazine. The administration of these two agents should be separated temporally to avoid this interaction. Sulfasalazine can potentiate warfarin's effects by displacing it from protein-binding sites. Close monitoring of the patient's International Normalized Ratio is indicated.[39,40]

OTHER DMARDS

Gold salts, azathioprine, d-penicillamine, cyclosporine, cyclophosphamide, and minocycline have all been used to treat rheumatoid arthritis. Although these drugs can be effective and they may be of value in certain clinical settings, they are used less frequently today due to toxicity, lack of long-term benefit, or both. See Tables 89–2 and 89–3 for dosing and toxicity information.

BIOLOGIC AGENTS

Biologic agents are genetically engineered protein molecules that block proinflammatory cytokines. These drugs may be effective when other DMARDs fail to achieve adequate responses, but they are considerably more expensive to use. They have no toxicity that requires laboratory monitoring, but have a small increased risk for infection. There is an increased incidence of tuberculosis in patients treated with these agents. Tuberculin skin testing is recommended before treatment with these drugs.[41–44] Patients with a history of significant tuberculosis exposure or recurrent infection may not be good candidates for these drugs. Those who develop infections while on biologic agents should at least temporarily discontinue them until the infection is cured. Additionally, congestive heart failure is a relative contraindication for infliximab and etanercept. Increased cardiac mortality has been seen in patients treated with infliximab, and etanercept-associated heart failure exacerbations have been documented.[45,46] TNF inhibitors may predispose patients to increased cancer risk, as TNF plays a role in ridding the body of cancer cells. The reported incidence of malignancy is similar to that of patients with rheumatoid arthritis who are not on these drugs; however, long-term surveillance studies are lacking.[47,48]

Etanercept

Etanercept is a fusion protein consisting of two p75 soluble TNF receptors linked to an Fc fragment of human IgG_1. The drug binds to TNF, making it biologically inactive and preventing it from interacting with the cell-surface TNF receptors and thereby activating cells.

The drug is given by subcutaneous injection, 25 mg twice weekly or 50 mg once weekly, usually through self-injections or administration by a caregiver. Aside from local injection-site reactions, adverse effects are rare. There have been case reports of pancytopenia and neurologic demyelinating syndromes like multiple sclerosis that have prompted Food and Drug Administration (FDA) warnings, but the incidence of these complications is not known at this time. The infection and congestive heart failure precautions are discussed above. No laboratory monitoring is required.

Most clinical trials have used etanercept in patients who failed DMARDs. Response was seen in 60% to 75% of patients. The drug also has been shown to be useful in juvenile rheumatoid arthritis and psoriatic arthritis, for which it is approved by the FDA, and ankylosing spondylitis and other inflammatory arthropathies, for which it is not approved. It has been shown in clinical trials to slow erosive disease progression to a greater degree than oral methotrexate therapy in patients with inadequate response to methotrexate monotherapy.[49–54]

Infliximab

Infliximab is a chimeric antibody combining portions of mouse and human IgG_1. An anti-TNF antibody was created by exposing mice to human TNF. The binding portion of that antibody was fused to a human constant-region IgG_1 to reduce the antigenicity of the foreign protein. This antibody, when injected in humans, binds to TNF and prevents its interaction with TNF receptors on inflammatory cells.

Infliximab is given by intravenous infusion at a dose of 3 mg/kg at 0, 2, and 6 weeks, and then every 8 weeks. To prevent the formation of antibodies to this foreign protein, methotrexate should be given orally in doses typically used to treat rheumatoid arthritis for as long as the patient continues on infliximab. The clinical significance of these antibodies in rheumatoid arthritis has not been demonstrated, but in Crohn's disease they are associated with infusion reactions and reduce the duration of response.[55] Infusion reactions may occur in any patient treated with the drug. Loss of response may be seen in patients with rheumatoid arthritis who have initial good response which requires increased doses or shorter intervals between doses to maintain response.

The drug may increase risk of infection as noted above. An acute infusion reaction with symptoms including fever, chills, pruritus, and rash may occur within 1 to 2 hours after giving the drug. Autoantibodies and lupus-like syndrome also have been reported. In clinical trials, the combination of methotrexate plus infliximab halted progression of joint damage in patients and was superior to methotrexate monotherapy.[53,56–58]

Adalimumab

Adalimumab is a human IgG_1 antibody to TNF. Since it has no foreign protein components, it is less antigenic than infliximab. The drug is provided as a premixed syringe containing 40 mg, which is administered by subcutaneous injection every 14 days. It has similar response rates to those seen with the other TNF inhibitors. Local injection-site reactions were the most common adverse reactions noted in clinical trials. It has the same precautions regarding tuberculosis and other infections as the other biologics. To date, congestive heart failure exacerbations have not been reported.[59,60]

Anakinra

Anakinra is an interleukin-1–receptor antagonist (IL-1ra) which is a naturally occurring anti-inflammatory. By binding to IL-1 receptors on target cells, it prevents the interaction between IL-1 and the cell.

IL-1 is very important in the pathogenesis of rheumatoid arthritis. It stimulates release of chemotactic factors and adhesion molecules, and these promote migration of inflammatory leukocytes to tissues. It also causes release of factors known to dilate blood vessels and direct cytotoxins that produce connective tissue damage.

In a double-blind, placebo-controlled trial, anakinra 150 mg given by daily subcutaneous injection had a response rate of 43% compared with 27% for placebo-treated patients. Less radiographic progression of joint damage was noted in those receiving anakinra. Injection-site reactions were the most common adverse effect noted. Infection risk and precautions are similar to those for the TNF inhibitors.[61–64]

CORTICOSTEROIDS

Corticosteroids are used in rheumatoid arthritis for their anti-inflammatory and immunosuppressive properties. They interfere with antigen presentation to T lymphocytes, inhibit prostaglandin and leukotriene synthesis, and inhibit neutrophil and monocyte super-oxide radical generation. Corticosteroids also impair cell migration and cause redistribution of monocytes, lymphocytes, and neutrophils, thus blunting the inflammatory and autoimmune responses.

Oral corticosteroids are absorbed rapidly and completely from the gastrointestinal tract. They are metabolized and inactivated primarily by the liver and excreted in the urine. The elimination half-life of most corticosteroids is sufficiently long that once-daily dosing is possible.

Oral corticosteroids can be used in several ways. They can be used in bridging therapy, continuous low-dose therapy, and short-term high-dose bursts to control flares. Oral steroids (e.g., prednisone and methylprednisolone) can be used to control pain and synovitis while DMARDs are taking effect. This is termed *bridging therapy* and is often used in patients with debilitating symptoms when DMARD therapy is initiated. Patients with difficult-to-control disease may be placed on low-dose, long-term corticosteroid therapy to control their symptoms. Prednisone doses below 7.5 mg daily are well tolerated, but are not devoid of the long-term adverse effects associated with corticosteroids. The lowest dose of corticosteroid that controls symptoms should be used to reduce adverse effects. Alternate-day dosing of low-dose oral corticosteroids usually is ineffective in rheumatoid arthritis; symptoms usually flare on days without medication. High-dose corticosteroid bursts often are used to suppress disease flares. High doses are sustained for several days until symptoms are controlled, followed by a taper to the lowest effective dose.

Corticosteroids also may be delivered by injection. The intramuscular route is preferable in patients with compliance problems, since a depot effect is achieved. Depot forms of corticosteroids include triamcinolone acetonide, triamcinolone hexacetonide, and methylprednisolone acetate. This provides the patient with 2 to 8 weeks of symptomatic control. The depot effect provides a physiologic taper, avoiding withdrawal reaction associated with hypothalamic-pituitary axis suppression. It should be noted that the onset of effect via this route may be delayed by several days. Intravenous corticosteroids may be used to provide the patient with large amounts of drug during a steroid burst to control severe symptoms. Intra-articular injections of depot forms of corticosteroids can be useful in treating synovitis and pain when a small number of joints are affected. The onset and duration of symptomatic relief are similar to those of intramuscular injection. The intra-articular route often is preferred because it is associated with the fewest number of systemic adverse effects. If efficacious, intra-articular injections may be repeated every 3 months. No one joint should be injected more than two to three times per year because of the risk of accelerated joint destruction and atrophy of tendons. Soft tissues such as tendons and bursae also may be injected. This may help control the pain and inflammation associated with these structures. The onset and duration of symptomatic relief are similar to those of intramuscular and intra-articular injections.

The major limitation to the long-term use of corticosteroids is adverse effects. They include hypothalamic-pituitary-adrenal suppression, Cushing's syndrome, osteoporosis, myopathies, glaucoma, cataracts, gastritis, hypertension, hirsutism, electrolyte imbalances, glucose intolerance, skin atrophy, and increased susceptibility to infections. To minimize these effects, use the lowest effective corticosteroid dose and limit the duration of use. Patients on long-term therapy should be given calcium and vitamin D (and estrogen supplements for postmenopausal women) to minimize bone loss. Alendronate has been shown to be effective in preventing the bone loss and might be considered prophylactically for patients when long-term corticosteroid use is anticipated, particularly for patients at high risk (e.g., postmenopausal females and the elderly).[65,66] There is no evidence that corticosteroids alone increase the risk of gastrointestinal ulcerations, even though they have been implicated often. Therefore gastrointestinal protective measures usually are not indicated.[67]

CLINICAL CONTROVERSY

Even the best therapy currently available does not completely eliminate all signs and symptoms of rheumatoid arthritis for most patients. Clinicians struggle with determining how much treatment is enough. Also, some patients show evidence of disease progression despite apparent control of clinical symptoms. How can these patients be identified and the treatment course changed before progression occurs?

PHARMACOECONOMIC CONSIDERATIONS

The total cost of treating a patient with rheumatoid arthritis is estimated to be between $5000 and $7300 annually (1991 dollars). Of this, drugs account for roughly 10% of the total, excluding monitoring costs. These costs are approximately three times the cost of medical care for patients of similar age and gender without rheumatoid arthritis. However, if biologic agents are used, the cost of this drug therapy alone may be as much as $12,000. The costs must be balanced against the high cost of disability to earning potential in these patients. Men with rheumatoid arthritis have average annual wages that are 50% lower than those of men of similar age without rheumatoid arthritis. In women with the disease, average annual wages are only 25% of those without. The costs of disability make treatment worth the price if disability can be prevented or delayed, and patients can continue to function as productive members of society.[68]

EVALUATION OF THERAPEUTIC OUTCOMES

The evaluation of therapeutic outcomes is based primarily on improvements of clinical signs and symptoms of rheumatoid arthritis. Clinical signs of improvement include a reduction in joint swelling, decreased warmth over actively involved joints, and decreased tenderness to joint palpation. Improvement in rheumatoid arthritis symptoms includes reduction in perceived joint pain and morning stiffness, longer time to onset of afternoon fatigue, and improvement in ability to perform activities of daily living. Improvement of activities of daily living may be assessed objectively using a health assessment questionnaire. Joint radiographs may be of some benefit in assessing the progression of the disease and should show little or no evidence of disease progression if treatment is effective.

Laboratory monitoring is of little value in monitoring individual patient response to therapy. Monitoring of toxicity of drugs is shown in Tables 89–2 and 89–3. Routine monitoring of patients is essential to the safe use of these drugs. In addition, patients should be questioned about symptoms of the adverse effects outlined in the drug section of this chapter.

CONCLUSION

Rheumatoid arthritis is the most common inflammatory arthritis, affecting approximately 1% of the population. The disease is characterized by symmetrical swelling and stiffness of the involved joints. The stiffness is usually more prominent in the morning. Extraarticular features of rheumatoid arthritis include rheumatoid nodules, vasculitis, and ocular, cardiac, and pulmonary complications. The course of the disease is highly variable. Treatment is aimed at relieving pain and inflammation and maintaining and preserving joint function. Nondrug therapy, including exercise and adequate rest periods, should also be used early in the course of treatment. Early use of a DMARD or biologic agent has been shown to result in better patient outcomes. Methotrexate, sulfasalazine, and hydroxychloroquine are often considered for initial therapy. Biologic agents have also been shown to be effective in these patients, but may be considered secondline agents due to cost considerations and lack of long-term outcome documentation. Combination DMARDs or biologicals may be considered in those who fail adequate trials of single-agent therapy. Corticosteroids and NSAIDs may be useful adjuncts for treatment, but because of adverse effects and limited impact on long-term outcomes, they should not be considered as sole treatment for most patients.

ABBREVIATIONS

ALT: alanine aminotransferase
AST: aspartate aminotransferase
DMARD: disease-modifying antirheumatic drug
HLA: human lymphocyte antigen
IL-1, IL-6: interleukins-1, and -6
IL-1ra: interleukin-1–receptor antagonist
MHC: major histocompatibility complex
NSAID: nonsteroidal anti-inflammatory drugs
PMN: polymorphonuclear leukocyte
TNF: tumor necrosis factor

Review Questions and other resources can be found at *www.pharmacotherapyonline.com.*

REFERENCES

1. Smith JB, Haynes MK. Rheumatoid arthritis—a molecular understanding. Ann Intern Med 2002;136:908–922.
2. Harris ED. The clinical features of rheumatoid arthritis. In: Ruddy S, Harris ED, Sledge CB, eds. Textbook of Rheumatology, 6th ed. Philadelphia, Saunders, 2001:967–1000.
3. Klippel JH, Crawford L, Stone JH, Weyand CM, eds. Primer on the Rheumatic Diseases, 12th ed. Atlanta, Arthritis Foundation, 2001:209.
4. Firestein GS. Etiology and pathogenesis of rheumatoid arthritis. In: Ruddy S, Harris ED, Sledge CB, eds. Textbook of Rheumatology, 6th ed. Philadelphia, Saunders, 2001:921–926.
5. Weyand CM, Goronzy JJ. Pathogenesis of rheumatoid arthritis. Med Clin North Am 1997;81:29–55.
6. Choy EH, Panayi GS. Cytokine pathways and joint inflammation in rheumatoid arthritis. N Engl J Med 2001;344:907–916.
7. Hard ER. Extraarticular manifestations of rheumatoid arthritis. Semin Arthritis Rheum 1979;8:151–176.
8. Choi HK, Hernan MA, Seeger JD, et al. Methotrexate and mortality in patients with rheumatoid arthritis: A prospective study. Lancet 2002;359: 1173–1177.
9. Wallberg-Jonsson S, Johansson H, Ohman ML, Rantapaa-Dahlqvist S. Extent of inflammation predicts cardiovascular disease and overall mortality in seropositive rheumatoid arthritis. A retrospective cohort study from disease onset. J Rheumatol 1999;26:2562–2571.
10. American College of Rheumatology Subcommittee on Rheumatoid Arthritis G. Guidelines for the management of rheumatoid arthritis: 2002 update. Arthritis Rheum 2002;46:328–346.
11. Genovese MC, Harris ED. The treatment of rheumatoid arthritis. In: Ruddy S, Harris ED, Sledge CB, eds. Textbook of Rheumatology, 6th ed. Philadelphia, Saunders, 2001:1079–1100.
12. Anderson JJ, Wells G, Verhoeven AC, Felson DT. Factors predicting response to treatment in rheumatoid arthritis: The importance of disease duration. Arthritis Rheum 2000;43:22–29.
13. Fries JF. Current treatment paradigms in rheumatoid arthritis. Rheumatology 2000;39(Suppl 1):30–35.
14. Mottonen T, Hannonen P, Korpela M, et al. Delay to institution of therapy and induction of remission using single-drug or combination-disease-modifying antirheumatic drug therapy in early rheumatoid arthritis. Arthritis Rheum 2002;46:894–898.
15. Tsakonas E, Fitzgerald AA, Fitzcharles MA, et al. Consequences of delayed therapy with second-line agents in rheumatoid arthritis: A 3 year followup on the hydroxychloroquine in early rheumatoid arthritis (HERA) study. J Rheumatol 2000;27:623–629.
16. Verstappen SM, Jacobs JW, Bijlsma JW, et al. Five-year followup of rheumatoid arthritis patients after early treatment with disease-modifying antirheumatic drugs versus treatment according to the pyramid approach in the first year. Arthritis Rheum 2003;48:1797–1807.
17. Goldbach-Mansky R, Lipsky PE. New concepts in the treatment of rheumatoid arthritis. Ann Rev Med 2003;54:197–216.
18. Kroot EJ, VanLeeuwen MA, VanRijswijk MH, et al. No increased mortality in patients with rheumatoid arthritis: Up to 10 years of follow up from disease onset. Ann Rheum Dis 2000;59:954–958.
19. Kalden JR, Schattenkirchner M, Sorensen H, et al. The efficacy and safety of leflunomide in patients with active rheumatoid arthritis: A five-year followup study. Arthritis Rheum 2003;48:1513–1520.
20. Bingham S, Emery P. Combination therapy in rheumatoid arthritis. Springer Semin Immunopathol 2001;23(1-2):165–183.
21. Calguneri M, Pay S, Caliskaner Z, et al. Combination therapy versus monotherapy for the treatment of patients with rheumatoid arthritis. Clin Exp Rheumatol 1999;17:699–704.
22. Dougados M, Combe B, Cantagrel A, et al. Combination therapy in early rheumatoid arthritis: A randomised, controlled, double blind 52 week clinical trial of sulphasalazine and methotrexate compared with the single components. Ann Rheum Dis 1999;58:220–225.
23. O'Dell JR. Combinations of conventional disease-modifying antirheumatic drugs. Rheum Dis Clin North Am 2001;27:415–426, x.
24. Pincus T, O'Dell JR, Kremer JM. Combination therapy with multiple disease-modifying antirheumatic drugs in rheumatoid arthritis: A preventive strategy. Ann Intern Med 1999;131:768–774.
25. Verhoeven AC, Boers M, Tugwell P. Combination therapy in rheumatoid arthritis: Updated systematic review [comment]. Br J Rheumatol 1998; 37:612–619.
26. Kremer JM. Rational use of new and existing disease-modifying agents in rheumatoid arthritis. Ann Intern Med 2001;134:695–706.
27. Bijlsma JW, Van Everdingen AA, Huisman M, et al. Glucocorticoids in rheumatoid arthritis: Effects on erosions and bone. Ann N Y Acad Sci 2002;966:82–90.
28. Rau R, Wassenberg S, Zeidler H. Low dose prednisolone therapy (LDPT) retards radiographically detectable destruction in early rheumatoid arthritis—preliminary results of a multicenter, randomized, parallel, double blind study. Z Rheumatol 2000;59(Suppl 2):II/90–96.
29. Langman MJ, Jensen DM, Watson DJ, et al. Adverse upper gastrointestinal effects of rofecoxib compared with NSAIDs. JAMA 1999;282:1929–1933.
30. Silverstein FE, Faich G, Goldstein JL, et al. Gastrointestinal toxicity with celecoxib versus nonsteroidal anti-inflammatory drugs for osteoarthritis and rheumatoid arthritis. JAMA 2000;284:1247–1255.
31. Pincus T, Ferraccioli G, Sokka T, et al. Evidence from clinical trials and long-term observational studies that disease-modifying anti-rheumatic drugs slow radiographic progression in rheumatoid arthritis: Updating a 1983 review. Rheumatology 2002;41:1346–1356.
32. Wolfe F, Hawley DJ, Cathey MA. Termination of slow acting antirheumatic therapy in rheumatoid arthritis: A 14-year prospective evaluation of 1017 consecutive starts. J Rheumatol 1990;17:994–1002.

33. Kremer JM. Methotrexate and emerging therapies. Rheum Dis Clin North Am 1998;24:651–658.

34. O'Dell JR. Methotrexate use in rheumatoid arthritis. Rheum Dis Clin North Am 1997;23:779–796.

35. Prakash A, Jarvis B. Leflunomide: A review of its use in active rheumatoid arthritis. Drugs 1999;58:1137–1164.

36. Strand V, Cohen S, Schiff M, et al. Treatment of active rheumatoid arthritis with leflunomide compared with placebo and methotrexate. Leflunomide Rheumatoid Arthritis Investigators Group. Arch Intern Med 1999; 159:2542–2550.

37. Maturi RK, Folk JC, Nichols B, et al. Hydroxychloroquine retinopathy. Arch Ophthalmol 1999;117:1262–1263.

38. Suarez-Almazor ME, Belseck E, Shea B, et al. Antimalarials for treating rheumatoid arthritis [update of Cochrane Database Syst Rev 2000;2: CD000959; PMID: 10796401]. Cochrane Database Syst Rev 2000;4: CD000959.

39. Weinblatt ME, Reda D, Henderson W, et al. Sulfasalazine treatment for rheumatoid arthritis: A metaanalysis of 15 randomized trials. J Rheumatol 1999;26:2123–2130.

40. Rains CP, Noble S, Faulds D. Sulfasalazine: A review of its pharmacological properties and therapeutic efficacy in the treatment of rheumatoid arthritis. Drugs 1995;50:137–156.

41. Gomez-Reino JJ, Carmona L, Valverde VR, et al. Treatment of rheumatoid arthritis with tumor necrosis factor inhibitors may predispose to significant increase in tuberculosis risk: A multicenter active-surveillance report. Arthritis Rheum 2003;48:2122–2127.

42. Keane J, Gershon S, Wise RP, et al. Tuberculosis associated with infliximab, a tumor necrosis factor alpha-neutralizing agent [comment]. N Engl J Med 2001;345:1098–1104.

43. Myers A, Clark J, Foster H. Tuberculosis and treatment with infliximab. N Engl J Med 2002;346:623–626.

44. Weisman MH. What are the risks of biologic therapy in rheumatoid arthritis? An update on safety. J Rheumatol Suppl 2002;65:33–38.

45. Chung ES, Packer M, Lo KH, et al. Randomized, double-blind, placebo-controlled, pilot trial of infliximab, a chimeric monoclonal antibody to tumor necrosis factor-alpha, in patients with moderate-to-severe heart failure: Results of the anti-TNF Therapy Against Congestive Heart Failure (ATTACH) trial. Circulation 2003;107:3133–3140.

46. Kwon HJ, Cote TR, Cuffe MS, et al. Case reports of heart failure after therapy with a tumor necrosis factor antagonist. Ann Intern Med 2003; 138:807–811.

47. Beauparlant P, Papp K, Haraoui B. The incidence of cancer associated with the treatment of rheumatoid arthritis. Semin Arthritis Rheum 1999; 29:148–158.

48. Cohen RB, Dittrich KA. Anti-TNF therapy and malignancy—a critical review. Can J Gastroenterol 2001;15:376–384.

49. Bathon JM, Martin RW, Fleischmann RM, et al. A comparison of etanercept and methotrexate in patients with early rheumatoid arthritis [comment] [erratum appears in N Engl J Med 2001;344:240]. N Engl J Med 2000;343:1586–1593.

50. Genovese MC, Bathon JM, Martin RW, et al. Etanercept versus methotrexate in patients with early rheumatoid arthritis: Two-year radiographic and clinical outcomes. Arthritis Rheum 2002;46:1443–1450.

51. Moreland LW. Inhibitors of tumor necrosis factor for rheumatoid arthritis. J Rheumatol 1999;26(Suppl 57):7–15.

52. Moreland LW, Schiff MH, Baumgartner SW, et al. Etanercept therapy in rheumatoid arthritis. A randomized, controlled trial. Ann Intern Med 1999; 130:478–486.

53. Maini RN, Taylor PC. Anti-cytokine therapy for rheumatoid arthritis. Ann Rev Med 2000;51:207–229.

54. Jarvis B, Faulds D. Etanercept: A review of its use in rheumatoid arthritis. Drugs 1999;57:945–966.

55. Baert F, Noman M, Vermeire S, et al. Influence of immunogenicity on the long-term efficacy of infliximab in Crohn's disease. N Engl J Med 2003; 348:601–608.

56. Blumenauer B, Judd M, Wells G, et al. Infliximab for the treatment of rheumatoid arthritis. Cochrane Database Syst Rev 2002;3:CD003785.

57. Maini R, St Clair EW, Breedveld F, et al. Infliximab (chimeric anti-tumour necrosis factor alpha monoclonal antibody) versus placebo in rheumatoid arthritis patients receiving concomitant methotrexate: A randomised phase III trial. ATTRACT Study Group. Lancet 1999;354:1932–1939.

58. Lipsky PE, van der Heijde DM, St Clair EW, et al. Infliximab and methotrexate in the treatment of rheumatoid arthritis. Anti-Tumor Necrosis Factor Trial in Rheumatoid Arthritis with Concomitant Therapy Study Group [comment]. N Engl J Med 2000;343:1594–1602.

59. den Broeder A, van de Putte L, Rau R, et al. A single dose, placebo controlled study of the fully human anti-tumor necrosis factor-alpha antibody adalimumab (D2E7) in patients with rheumatoid arthritis. J Rheumatol 2002;29:2288–2298.

60. Weinblatt ME, Keystone EC, Furst DE, et al. Adalimumab, a fully human anti-tumor necrosis factor alpha monoclonal antibody, for the treatment of rheumatoid arthritis in patients taking concomitant methotrexate: The ARMADA trial [erratum appears in Arthritis Rheum 2003;48:855]. Arthritis Rheum 2003;48:35–45.

61. Calabrese LH. Anakinra treatment of patients with rheumatoid arthritis. Ann Pharmacother 2002;36:1204–1209.

62. Cohen S, Hurd E, Cush J, et al. Treatment of rheumatoid arthritis with anakinra, a recombinant human interleukin-1 receptor antagonist, in combination with methotrexate: Results of a twenty-four-week, multicenter, randomized, double-blind, placebo-controlled trial [comment]. Arthritis Rheum 2002;46:614–624.

63. Fleischmann RM, Schechtman J, Bennett R, et al. Anakinra, a recombinant human interleukin-1 receptor antagonist (r-metHuIL-1ra), in patients with rheumatoid arthritis: A large, international, multicenter, placebo-controlled trial. Arthritis Rheum 2003;48:927–934.

64. Jiang Y, Genant HK, Watt I, et al. A multicenter, double-blind, dose-ranging, randomized, placebo-controlled study of recombinant human interleukin-1 receptor antagonist in patients with rheumatoid arthritis. Arthritis Rheum 2000;43:1001–1009.

65. Adachi JD, Saag KG, Delmas PD, et al. Two-year effects of alendronate on bone mineral density and vertebral fracture in patients receiving glucocorticoids: A randomized, double-blind, placebo-controlled extension trial. Arthritis Rheum 2001;44:202–211.

66. McIlwain HH. Glucocorticoid-induced osteoporosis: Pathogenesis, diagnosis, and management. Prev Med 2003;36:243–249.

67. Morand EF. Corticosteroids in the treatment of rheumatologic diseases. Curr Opin Rheumatol 1998;10:179–183.

68. Gabriel SE, Coyle D, Moreland LW. A clinical and economic review of disease-modifying antirheumatic drugs. Pharmacoeconomics 2001;19: 715–728.

90

OSTEOARTHRITIS

Karen E. Hansen and Mary Elizabeth Elliott

Learning Objectives and other resources can be found at *www.pharmacotherapyonline.com.*

KEY CONCEPTS

1 The most common form of arthritis is osteoarthritis (OA). It affects individuals in the middle to later years of life, with women more commonly affected than men after age 45 years.

2 OA is primarily a disease of cartilage that reflects a failure of the chondrocyte to maintain proper balance between cartilage formation and destruction.

3 The most common symptom associated with OA is pain, which leads to decreased function and motion, and pain relief is the primary objective of medication therapy.

4 Patients have bony proliferation of affected joints that should be differentiated from the swelling of rheumatoid or inflammatory arthritis. OA is not a systemic disease such as rheumatoid arthritis. The joint distribution often involves the knees, hips, and hands, although other joints also can be affected.

5 Nonpharmacologic therapy is the foundation of the pharmaceutical care plan and should be initiated before, or simultaneously with, initiation of pharmacologic therapy.

6 Based upon efficacy, safety, and cost considerations, scheduled acetaminophen, up to 4 g/day, should be tried initially for pain relief in OA.

7 Failure with acetaminophen warrants a trial with a nonsteroidal anti-inflammatory drug (NSAID).

8 NSAIDs are associated with GI, renal, liver, or central nervous system toxicity. Appropriate monitoring with complete blood count, serum creatinine, and hepatic transaminase levels is valuable in detecting potential toxicity. Cyclooxygenase-2 (COX-2)–specific inhibitors carry a lower risk of GI bleeding or platelet inhibition, and may be appropriate in selected patients.

9 Prevention of NSAID-induced GI toxicity includes the use of nonacetylated salicylates, COX-2 inhibitors, or use of protective agents with NSAIDs. Misoprostol reduces both gastric and duodenal ulcers, while histamine (H_2)-receptor antagonists are effective in preventing duodenal ulcers but not gastric ulcers. Proton pump inhibitors may have comparable effects to misoprostol and are also recommended for reducing GI toxicity.

10 Glucosamine, alone or with chondroitin sulfate, warrants further study for its potential to relieve OA symptoms and possibly slow disease progression.

Osteoarthritis (OA) is the most common joint disease, affecting nearly 50% of those over 65 years of age and almost all individuals over age 75.[1–4] OA ranks second only to cardiovascular disease in causing chronic disability, making this condition of substantial importance to public health. Appreciation of the human and economic costs of this disease has prompted exciting advances concerning etiology and treatment.

OA affects primarily the weight-bearing joints of the axial and peripheral skeleton, causing pain, limitation of motion, deformity, progressive disability, and decreased quality of life.[1–5] Other names for OA include *degenerative joint disease* and *hypertrophic arthritis*, but these terms have shortcomings. OA implies lack of inflammation and excess materials in the joint, degenerative joint disease suggests a wearing out of the joint, and hypertrophic arthritis describes the overgrowth of bone and cartilage that is only one aspect of OA. Thus the term "osteoarthritis" best reflects the degenerative changes that occur in the metabolically active cartilage and bone within a joint.

OA is characterized by increased destruction of cartilage and subsequent proliferation of adjacent bone. The regenerated articular surfaces do not possess the same qualities and architecture as the original joint, and this change in structure leads to pain, decreased or altered motion, crepitus, and possibly local inflammation.[2] The pain of OA typically worsens with use and improves with rest. Morning stiffness lasting less than 1 hour and "gelling" of the joints after inactivity are also common. The inflammation associated with OA is usually mild or localized, in contrast to that of rheumatoid arthritis or other inflammatory diseases affecting the joints.

The major goals of OA therapy are to educate the patient, alleviate pain and other symptoms, and improve function.[1,6–8] Nonpharmacologic therapy is the foundation of OA management and includes patient education, strengthening and range-of-motion exercises, and use of assistive devices, joint protection, and weight loss as necessary.[8–11] Pharmacologic therapy begins with nonopioid analgesics such as acetaminophen, followed by nonsteroidal anti-inflammatory drugs (NSAIDs), inhibitors specific for the cyclooxygenase-2 (COX-2) enzyme when indicated, and topical analgesic creams containing capsaicin or methylsalicylate.[1,6–8] Intra-articular glucocorticoid or hyaluronic acid injections and opioid analgesics play an important role in management of pain related to OA, with use of the latter in those unresponsive to other therapies. New therapeutic approaches are being developed based on recent information about chondrocyte metabolism and the control of proteases that contribute to cartilage destruction.

EPIDEMIOLOGY

◁ OA is the most prevalent of the rheumatic diseases, and is responsible for enormous disability and loss of productivity.[1-4] Prevalence increases with age, and radiographic data show that OA at some skeletal site occurs in the majority of people over 65 years of age, and in nearly everyone over 75 years of age. Despite intense epidemiologic study, the exact prevalence of OA is unknown, owing to the uncertainties and variations of diagnostic definition and reporting mechanisms. Another confounder is that many patients with radiographically apparent OA do not have symptoms that lead them to medical care.

PREVALENCE BY AGE, SEX, AND RACE

Based on prevalence data from the National Centers for Health Statistics, an estimated 15.8 million adults, or 12% of those between 25 and 74 years of age, have signs and symptoms of OA.[4] The prevalence of OA increases with age. In those under age 45, about one-fifth have OA of the hands, while for those aged 75 to 79 years, 85% have OA of the hands. OA of the knee occurs in less than 0.1% of those aged 25 to 34 years, but in 10% to 20% of those aged 65 to 74 years.

OA severity also increases with age.[1-4] For those between 65 and 74 years of age, 33% have moderate to severe knee OA, and 50% have moderate to severe hip OA. The National Arthritis Data Workgroup, using National Health and Nutrition Examination Survey and other data, has projected that by the year 2020, 18.2% of Americans (59.4 million people) will be affected by OA. In the United States, women are more often affected by OA; older women are twice as likely as men to have OA of the knee and hands.[2,4] Women are also more likely to have inflammatory OA of the proximal and distal interphalangeal joints of the hands, giving rise to the formation of Bouchard's and Heberden's nodes, respectively. Knee OA appears to be twice as prevalent in black as opposed to white women. Chinese, East Indian, and Native American people have lower incidences of hip OA than do Caucasians.

INCIDENCE

The overall incidence of hip or knee OA is approximately 200 per 100,000 person-years. The incidence of hip OA is greater in women than in men, whereas the rate for knee OA is similar between genders. In men, rates of knee and hip OA increase with age, but in women rates remain stable. Based on these population data, one-half million symptomatic cases of idiopathic OA are estimated to occur annually in the U.S. white population.

ETIOLOGY

OBESITY

Increased body weight is strongly associated with hip, knee, and hand OA.[3,12,13] Obesity often precedes OA and contributes to its development, rather than occurring as a result of inactivity from joint pain. In

a three-decade Framingham Study, the highest quintile of body mass was associated with a higher relative risk of knee OA (relative risk of 1.5 to 1.9 for men and 2.1 to 3.2 for women). Another study of 1,108 men in their twenties also showed that high body mass index was associated with later development of knee OA.[13] The risk of developing OA increases by about 10% with each additional kilogram of weight, and in obese persons without OA, weight loss of even 5 kg decreases the risk of future knee OA by one-half. In addition to being a risk factor for OA, obesity is also a predictor for eventual prosthetic joint replacement.

OCCUPATION, SPORTS, AND TRAUMA

Those participating in activities involving repetitive motion or injury are at increased risk for developing OA.[14] Workers exposed to repetitive stress of the hands or lower limbs are at higher risk for OA of the stressed joints. Lower-extremity OA in some professional sports is also increased, likely secondary to repetitive motion, trauma to the joint, loss of ligament integrity, or damage to the meniscus. Risk for OA depends on the type and intensity of physical activity. The Framingham Study showed that heavy physical activity increases knee OA risk, especially in the obese, whereas moderate or light activity does not.[15] Interestingly, long-distance runners are not at higher risk of developing OA. Age at injury does matter, because older individuals who damage ligaments tend to develop OA more rapidly than young people with a similar injury.

Finally, there are interesting inverse associations between quadriceps strength and knee OA and disability. Quadriceps weakness, once thought to result from disuse atrophy in OA patients, may precede and even contribute to the development of OA, possibly through decreased knee stability.[16]

GENETIC FACTORS

Heredity plays a role in osteoarthritis.[3,17] Heberden's nodes are 10 times more prevalent in women than in men, with a twofold higher risk if the woman's mother had them. Genetic links also have been shown with OA of the first metatarsophalangeal joint and with generalized OA. Premature development of OA is associated with a defect in type II procollagen. The discovery of a genetic link between the cartilage matrix and OA may shed light on disease development, and has the potential to aid in screening and treatment strategies in certain groups of patients.

OSTEOPOROSIS

An inverse correlation between OA and osteoporosis has been demonstrated, and both men and women with OA have increased bone mineral density at numerous skeletal sites.[2,18] This relationship may derive from the influence of body weight on both diseases, because heavy individuals have higher bone density as well as increased risk of OA. Despite their lower risk of osteoporosis, individuals with OA are not protected against fracture. OA patients tend to be less posturally stable and more likely to fall, so despite the higher bone density, their fracture rates are similar to those of patients without OA.

PATHOPHYSIOLOGY

◁ OA falls into two major etiologic classes. *Primary (idiopathic) OA,* the most common type, has no identifiable cause. Subclasses of primary OA are *localized OA,* involving one or two sites, and

TABLE 90–1. Classification of Osteoarthritis

Primary (Idiopathic)	Secondary
Localized	Trauma—acute/chronic
Generalized	Underlying joint disorder
	Local (fracture/infection)
	Diffuse (rheumatoid arthritis)
Erosive	Systemic metabolic or endocrine disorders
	Wilson's disease
	Acromegaly
	Hyperparathyroidism
	Hemochromatosis
	Paget's disease
	Diabetes mellitus
	Obesity
	Crystal deposition disease
	Basic calcium phosphate crystal disease
	Calcium pyrophosphate dihydrate
	Hydroxyapatite
	Other calcium-containing crystals
	Monosodium urate monohydrate
	Neuropathic disorders
	Intra-articular corticosteroid overuse
	Avascular necrosis
	Bone dysplasia

Data from Felson et al[3] and Mankin et al.[20]

generalized OA, affecting three or more sites. *Erosive osteoarthritis* is used to describe the presence of erosion and marked proliferation in the proximal and distal interphalangeal joints of the hands. *Secondary OA* is that associated with a known cause such as rheumatoid or another inflammatory arthritis, trauma, metabolic or endocrine disorders, and congenital factors (Table 90–1).[2,19–21]

To aid uniform reporting of rheumatic diseases, a classification scheme and criteria for OA of the hip, knee, and hand were devised by the American College of Rheumatology (ACR). Criteria include the presence of pain, bony changes on examination, a normal erythrocyte sedimentation rate, and characteristic radiographs.[1,2,22] For hip OA, a patient must have hip pain plus two of the following: an erythrocyte sedimentation rate of less than 20 mm/h, radiographic femoral or acetabular osteophytes, or radiographic joint space narrowing. For knee OA, a patient must have knee pain and radiographic osteophytes plus one of the following: age greater than 50 years, morning stiffness of 30 minutes' or less duration, or crepitus on motion.

Improved understanding of articular cartilage physiology has transcended the wear-and-tear theory of OA. Some changes in the

OA joint may reflect compensatory processes to maintain function in the face of ongoing joint destruction. As such, the pathogenesis of OA involves not only biomechanical forces, but also inflammatory, biochemical, and immunologic factors.[19–21,23–26] To understand the pathophysiology of OA, familiarity with the normal joint is essential. To this end, a review of the biochemistry and function of normal cartilage and of the diarthrodial joint is provided.

NORMAL CARTILAGE

FUNCTION

In the diarthrodial joint (Fig. 90–1), cartilage provides a low-friction surface covering the concave and convex ends of the bone. Cartilage has viscoelastic properties that provide lubrication with motion, shock absorbency during rapid movements, and load support. The major functions of cartilage are to (1) enable movement within the required range of motion, (2) distribute loading across joint tissues, thereby preventing damage, and (3) stabilize the joint during use. Cartilage is avascular, aneural, and alymphatic, with a calcified base over a thin layer of cortical bone, the subchondral plate. It is easily compressed, losing up to 40% of its original height when a load is applied. Compression increases the area of contact and disperses force more evenly to underlying bone, tendons, ligaments, and muscles.

STRUCTURE AND BIOCHEMICAL COMPOSITION OF CARTILAGE

Articular cartilage is a hydrated (75% to 80% water), complex extracellular matrix (ECM) with a small number of chondrocytes (<5%). The remaining 20% to 25% of matrix contains three types of molecules: collagens, large aggregates of proteoglycans, and noncollagenous proteins. Orientation of collagen fibers is critical: superficial fibers are parallel to the surface, reducing friction and allowing forces to be dissipated; basal layer collagen fibers are perpendicular to the surface to anchor cartilage to the calcified zone or subchondral bony end plate.

Cartilage undergoes continual biochemical and structural remodeling controlled by chondrocytes, which synthesize collagen and proteoglycans, and also play a role in their degradation. Because adult articular cartilage is avascular, chondrocytes are nourished by synovial fluid. With the cyclic movement and loading of joints, nutrients flow into the cartilage, whereas immobilization reduces nutrient supply.

Recent research has highlighted the role of peptides and proteins regulating chondrocyte function and cartilage metabolism.[19–21,23–26]

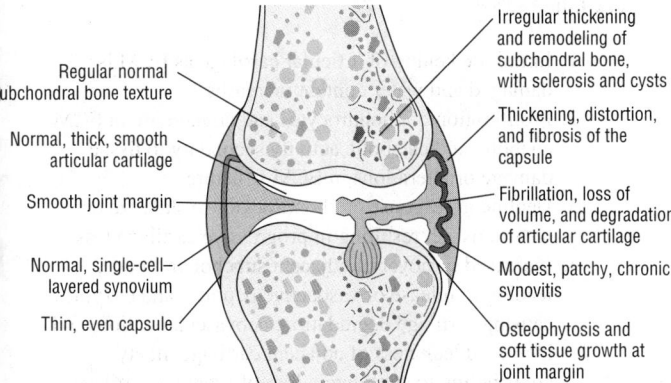

Regular normal subchondral bone texture

Normal, thick, smooth articular cartilage

Smooth joint margin

Normal, single-cell–layered synovium

Thin, even capsule

Irregular thickening and remodeling of subchondral bone, with sclerosis and cysts

Thickening, distortion, and fibrosis of the capsule

Fibrillation, loss of volume, and degradation of articular cartilage

Modest, patchy, chronic synovitis

Osteophytosis and soft tissue growth at joint margin

FIGURE 90–1. Characteristics of osteoarthritis in the diarthrodial joint.

Insulin-like growth factor, epidermal growth factor, fibroblast growth factor, and other agents enhance chondrocyte proliferation and proteoglycan synthesis. By contrast, interleukin-1 and tumor necrosis factor-α promote chondrocyte secretion of matrix metalloproteinases (MMPs), including collagenase (MMP-1) and stromelysin (MMP-2). These proteinases in turn degrade matrix proteins. Interleukin-1 and tumor necrosis factor-α also suppress proteoglycan and collagen synthesis in the ECM. Biomechanical factors, including load and strain, also affect chondrocyte function, and joint loading increases proteoglycan synthesis. The following sections will review the components of the joint matrix, and the pathologic changes in this matrix leading to OA.

Collagen

Five types of collagen (II, IX, X, XI, and VI) are located in cartilage. Type II collagen accounts for 90% to 95% of the total collagen in articular cartilage.[19-21,23-26] Type VI appears to attach chondrocytes to the matrix. Type IX collagen, a proteoglycan, may link matrix molecules together. The cross-linked network of type II collagen fibrils with other ECM proteins provides tensile strength and maintains cartilage volume and shape.

Proteoglycans

The cartilage matrix is comprised of large proteoglycan (PG) aggregates within a collagen network. PGs combine with long hyaluronate molecules in hydrophilic and anionic aggregates that maintain the high water content of cartilage. PGs within the collagen network, coupled with the high water content, endow cartilage with the viscoelastic properties required for resiliency and load bearing. Under pressure, PGs release water and enhance solute flux and chondrocyte nutrition; with removal of pressure, the matrix regains water.

The structure of the PG molecule renders it vulnerable to degradation by MMPs, since cleavage of only one or two peptide bonds can destroy its function.[23-26] As a result, PG turns over more rapidly than collagen. When protease degradation of PGs is induced experimentally, cartilage maintains its shape but loses elasticity.

With degradation of the ECM, collagen and PG fragments are released into the synovial fluid, eventually reaching the blood and urine. Identification and quantitation of these fragments could potentially aid in diagnosis or monitoring of disease, and also may provide insights into metabolic changes in OA.

OSTEOARTHRITIC CARTILAGE

BIOCHEMICAL CHANGES

Numerous compositional differences have been noted between cartilage in OA and normal individuals (Table 90–2).[19-21,23-26] Early in OA, cartilage water content increases, possibly as a result of a

TABLE 90–2. Changes in Osteoarthritic Cartilage

Increase in water content
Increase in chondroitin sulfate-4:chondroitin sulfate-6 ratio
Increase in proteases, especially neutral metalloproteinases
Decrease in glycosaminoglycans—chondroitin sulfate and keratan sulfate
Decrease in proteoglycan aggregation
Decrease in proteoglycan monomer size
Minimal change in collagen content

Data from Kraus,[19] Mankin et al,[20] Lajeunesse et al,[21] and Mansell et al.[26]

damaged collagen network that is unable to constrain PGs, which subsequently gain water. As osteoarthritis progresses, cartilage PG content decreases, possibly through the action of MMPs. Increased collagen synthesis and altered distribution and diameter of the fibers are seen, but collagen content does not appear to change until severe disease is present.

Earlier theories suggested that cartilage was passively eroded in OA, but in fact, there is increased metabolic activity, suggesting a reparative response to damage.[19-21,23-26] Despite the increased matrix synthesis by chondrocytes, there is a net loss of PG, as degradation proceeds faster than synthesis.

Intense research efforts are directed toward understanding the roles of MMPs and other collagen-degrading enzymes. MMPs are zinc-containing proteinases falling into five related subgroups. MMPs are normally held in check by tissue inhibitors of metalloproteinases (TIMPs), but there are also substances produced by chondrocytes that activate MMPs.[23-26] Imbalance between activators and inhibitors of MMPs in synovial fluid or local tissues can lead to proteolysis of the ECM, promoting osteoarthritic changes. Recent work showed that cartilage from osteoarthritic human joints exhibited increased collagen-degrading activity colocalized with increased levels of MMP mRNA.[24]

The subchondral bone adjacent to articular cartilage also undergoes pathologic changes that may precede, coincide with, or follow damage to the articular cartilage. Nevertheless, this damage to subchondral bone is required and appears to permit continued damage to articular cartilage, leading to progression to OA.[25] This subchondral bone demonstrates increased bone turnover, with both increased osteoclast and osteoblast activity. There is an associated release of vasoactive peptides and matrix metalloproteinases, neovascularization, and subsequent increased permeability of the adjacent cartilage.[25,26] This sequence of events leads to continued cartilage degradation, and eventually substantial loss of cartilage, leading to a painful, deformed joint.

In summary, the slow progressive changes in OA consist of an increase in water content, loss of PG, and reduction of PG aggregates of cartilage. The cartilage is subsequently unable to repair itself. Alterations in metabolism of subchondral bone adjacent to articular cartilage appear necessary for continued cartilage destruction. Eventually, progressive loss of articular cartilage and increasing subchondral sclerosis lead to an abnormal and painful joint.

PATHOLOGIC CHANGES

Pathologic changes in bone and cartilage accompany the biochemical changes just described. These changes are noted in both weight-bearing and non–weight-bearing joints, and in both primary and secondary OA. A summary of the biochemical changes in cartilage in OA follows.[19,20]

1. Initial thickening of articular cartilage as ECM is damaged and water content increases
2. Proliferation of chondrocytes and an increase in ECM anabolic and catabolic activity secondary to tissue damage or alterations in ECM structure
3. Decline in response of chondrocytes to stabilize or restore tissue, resulting in progressive cartilage loss
4. Increased turnover of adjacent subchondral bone, leading to release of vasoactive peptides and enzymes, causing cartilage degradation, neovascularization, and increased leakiness of adjacent cartilage, likely contributing to subsequent loss of articular cartilage

5. Fibrillation or splitting of the noncalcified cartilage, likely related to the biochemical changes described earlier; loss of cartilage exposes the underlying subchondral bone and may lead to microfractures

As cartilage is destroyed and the adjacent subchondral bone undergoes pathologic changes, cartilage is eroded completely, leaving denuded subchondral bone to become dense, smooth, and glistening (eburnation). A more brittle, stiffer bone results, with decreased weight-bearing ability and development of sclerosis and microfractures.[19,20] Microfractures lead to callus and osteoid production. New bone formations at the joint margins distant from cartilage destruction are referred to as *osteophytes,* and may be an attempt to stabilize the joint.

The joint capsule and synovium also show pathologic changes in OA. Inflammation, noted clinically as synovitis, may result from release of inflammatory mediators from chondrocytes, such as prostaglandins.[19–21,23–26] Inflammation is localized to the affected joint, in contrast to that seen in rheumatoid or other inflammatory arthritides.

The pain of OA is not related to the destruction of cartilage, but arises from the activation of nociceptive nerve endings within the joint by mechanical and chemical irritants.[27] OA pain may result from distention of the synovial capsule by increased joint fluid, microfracture, periosteal irritation, or damage to ligaments, synovium, or the meniscus.[2,27]

CLINICAL PRESENTATION

Key aspects of the clinical presentation of OA are provided in Table 90–3.[2,28] Presentation of OA depends on duration and severity of disease, and the number of joints affected.

If several joints are involved or if systemic symptoms are present, another form of arthritis or connective tissue disease should be considered. Pain caused by bursitis, tendinitis, or muscular pain

---

TABLE 90–3. Presentation of Osteoarthritis

Age
  Usually elderly
Gender
  Age <45 more common in men
  Age >45 more common in women
Symptoms
  Pain
    Deep, aching character
    Pain on motion
    Pain with motion early in disease
    Pain with rest late in disease
  Stiffness in affected joints
    Resolves with motion, recurs with rest
      ("gelling" phenomenon)
    Usually <30 minutes' duration
    Often related to weather
    Limited joint motion
    May result in limitations activities
      of daily living
  Instability of weight-bearing joints
Signs, history, and physical examination
  Monarticular or oligoarticular;
    asymmetrical involvement
  Hands
    Distal interphalangeal joints
      Heberden's nodes (osteophytes
      or bony enlargements)
    Proximal interphalangeal joints
      Bouchard's nodes (osteophytes)
    First carpometacarpal joint
      Osteophytes give characteristic square
        appearance of the hand (shelf sign)
  Knees
    Patellofemoral compartment involvement
      Pain related to climbing stairs
    Medial compartment involvement
      Genu varum (bowlegged deformity)
    Lateral compartment involvement
      Genu valgum (knock-knee deformity)
    Transient joint effusions
      Typically noninflammatory
        synovial fluid (WBC <2000/mm³)

Hips
  Groin pain during weight-bearing activities
  Stiffness, especially after inactivity
  Limited joint motion
Spine
  L3 and L4 involvement is most common in
    the lumbar spine
  Signs and symptoms of nerve root compression
    Radicular pain
    Paresthesias
    Loss of reflexes
    Muscle weakness associated with
      the affected nerve root
Feet
  Typically involves the first metatarsophalangeal
    joint
Other sites, less commonly involved
  Shoulder, elbow, acromioclavicular,
    sternoclavicular, and temporomandibular joints
Observation on joint examination
  Bony proliferation or occasional synovitis
  Local tenderness
  Crepitus
  Muscle atrophy
  Limited motion with passive/active movement
  Deformity
Radiologic evaluation
  Early mild OA
    Radiographic changes often absent
  Progression of OA
    Joint space narrowing
    Subchondral bone sclerosis
    Marginal osteophytes
  Late OA
    Abnormal alignment of joints
    Effusions
Characteristics of synovial fluid
  High viscosity
  Mild leukocytosis (<2000 WBC/mm³)
Laboratory values
  No specific test
  Erythrocyte sedimentation rate and hematologic
    and chemistry survey are normal

may complicate the clinical presentation and requires an accurate diagnosis.

PHYSICAL EXAMINATION

❹ Examination of the affected joints reveals tenderness, crepitus, and joint enlargement.[2,7,19,22] Crepitus is a crackling or grating sound heard with joint movement that is caused by irregularity of joint surfaces. Joint enlargement is related to bony proliferation or to thickening of the synovium and joint capsule. Joint deformity may be present in the later stages of OA as a result of subluxation, collapse of subchondral bone, formation of bone cysts, or bony overgrowth. The presence of a warm, red, tender joint may indicate the presence of an inflammatory arthritis such as gout.

HANDS

Hand OA is associated with pain in specific joints and often with development of bony enlargements (osteophytes). These usually develop slowly and painlessly, appear on lateral and medial aspects of the joint, and are about 10 times more common in women than in men.[2,22] Occasionally, these nodes become red, warm, swollen, and painful, usually as a result of trauma or use.

KNEES

The knee is commonly affected in OA. It is important to localize the symptoms because the joint has three separate articulations. Knee OA is associated with pain, tenderness, crepitus, and limited range of motion. Limited joint motion occurs from loss of articular surfaces, muscle spasm, capsular contracture, or mechanical blockage secondary to osteophytes (bony enlargements). Weakness or instability (the joint "gives way") is frequently noted by patients with knee OA. Such joint instability may lead to decreased activity and muscle atrophy.

HIPS

Hip OA is common in the elderly, with a characteristic presentation as shown in Table 90-3. However, pain located on the lateral hip typically represents trochanteric bursitis, while pain in the buttock region may indicate lumbar spine OA or iliopsoas bursitis.

SPINE

Degenerative changes involving the spine may occur in the interve■ tebral disks, vertebral bodies, or posterior apophyseal articulation■ Aside from pain and limitation of motion, nerve root compression ■ a potential complication of arthritis (see Table 90–3).

LABORATORY FINDINGS

No specific laboratory abnormalities occur in *primary* OA.[2] If sec ondary OA is suspected, specific laboratory tests can help identify th■ cause.

RADIOLOGIC EVALUATION

Radiologic evaluation is an absolute necessity in the diagnosis o■ OA (see Table 90–3). Bone erosions and unequivocal radiographi■ osteopenia are uncommon except in erosive or secondary OA. Finally■ many patients who do not have clinical OA and do not have pain ma■ nonetheless exhibit radiologic changes typical of OA.[28]

Newer techniques—computed tomography, magnetic resonanc■ imaging, and ultrasound—have been used, but are not suitable fo■ routine use in diagnosing OA.[2,19,20,28]

DIAGNOSIS

The diagnosis of OA is easily made by history, physical examinatio■ and characteristic radiographic findings.[2,6,22,28] The major diagnosti■ goals are (1) to discriminate between primary and secondary OA■ and (2) to clarify the joints involved, severity of joint involvement■ and response to prior therapies, providing a basis for a treatmen■ plan.

PROGNOSIS

The prognosis for patients with primary OA is variable and depend■ on the joint involved. If a weight-bearing joint or the spine is involved■ considerable morbidity and disability are possible. In the case of sec ondary OA, the prognosis depends on the underlying cause. Treatmen■ of OA may relieve pain or prevent further progression, but does no■ reverse pre-existing damage to the articular cartilage.

▶ TREATMENT: Osteoarthritis

▥ DESIRED OUTCOME AND GOALS OF TREATMENT

Management of the patient with OA begins with a diagnosis based on a careful history, physical examination, radiographic findings, and an assessment of the extent of joint involvement. Treatment should be tailored to each individual. Goals are (1) to educate the patient, caregivers, and relatives; (2) to relieve pain and stiffness; (3) to maintain or improve joint mobility; (4) to limit functional impairment; and (5) to maintain or improve quality of life.[1,6–8]

▥ GENERAL APPROACH TO TREATMENT

Treatment for each OA patient depends on the distribution and severity of joint involvement, comorbid disease states, concomitant medications, and allergies (Fig. 90–2). Management for all individuals with

OA should begin with patient education, and physical and/or occupa tional therapy, and weight loss or assistive devices if appropriate.

The primary objective of medication is to alleviate pain.[1,6–■ Scheduled acetaminophen, up to 4 g/day, should be tried initially■ If this is ineffective, NSAIDs are prescribed, with specific COX-2 inhibitors preferable for some patients. Application of capsaicin o■ methyl salicylate topical creams over specific joints can sometime■ be helpful adjuncts for pain control. Many patients have turned t■ glucosamine or chondroitin, and evidence is accumulating that thes■ agents may have benefit in OA.[29–30] Joint aspiration followed by glu■ cocorticoid or hyaluronate injection can relieve pain, and is offere■ concomitantly with oral analgesics or after their lack of efficacy, de■ pending on the practitioner's style. Narcotic analgesics are a fina■ medication to prescribe if other therapies are unsuccessful. When symptoms are intractable or there is significant loss of function, join■ replacement may be appropriate if the patient is a surgical candidate■

Finally, for patients interested in clinical trials, investigationa■ strategies with oral doxycycline, matrix metalloproteinase inhibitors

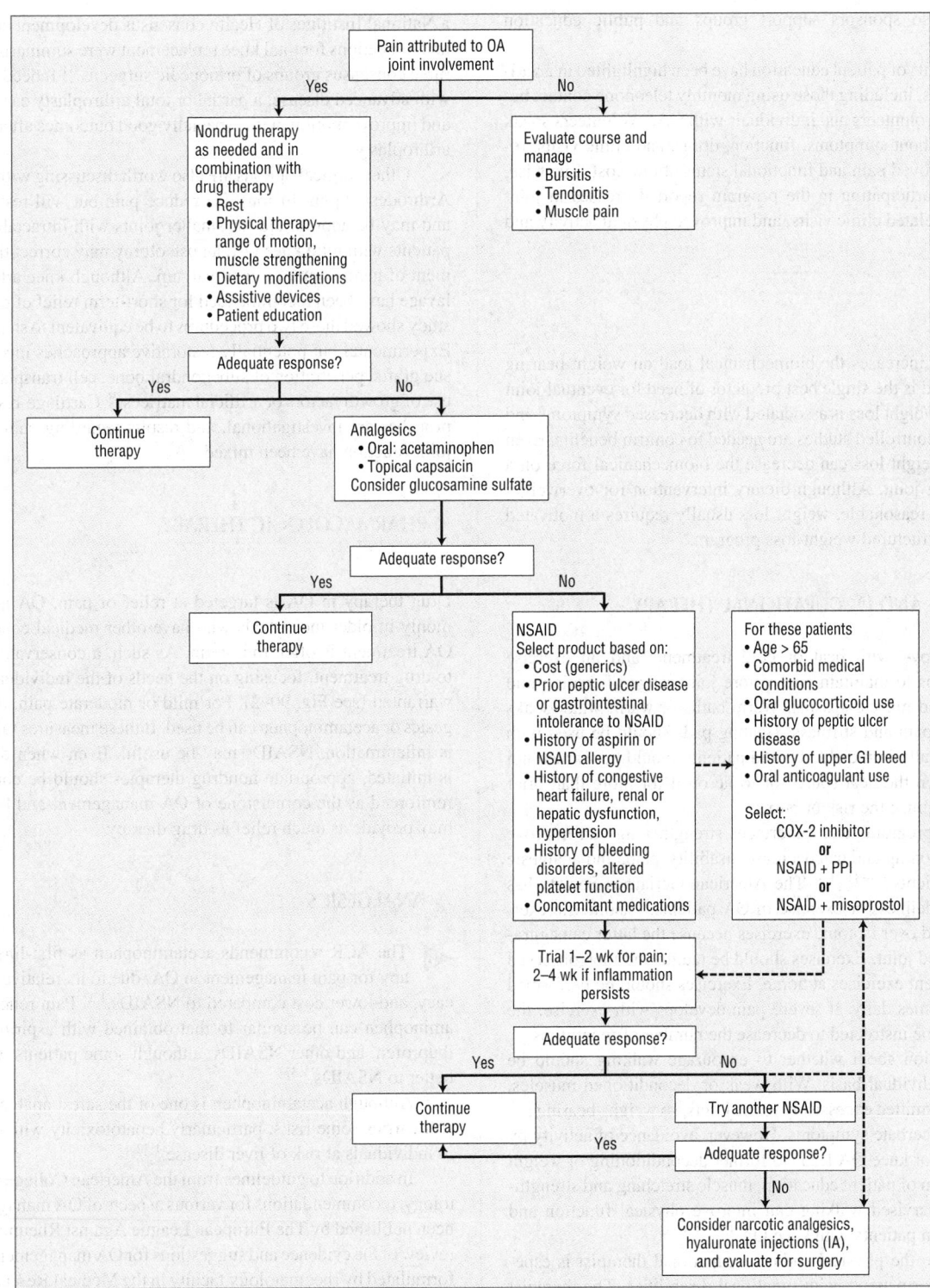

FIGURE 90–2. Treatment for osteoarthritis.

tramuscular injection of pentosan polysulfate and polysulfated gly-osaminoglycans, or cartilage transplants may be considered.

NONPHARMACOLOGIC THERAPY

5 The first step in OA treatment is patient education about the disease process, the extent of OA, the prognosis, and treatment

options. Education is paramount, in that OA is often seen as a "wear and tear" disease, an inevitable consequence of aging for which nothing helps. Even worse, patients may resort to the use of alternative but unproven medications or quackery. Patients should be warned about these and encouraged to access information from local or national units of the Arthritis Foundation or at http://www.arthritis.org. The Arthritis Foundation provides literature about OA and OA medications, as well as information about local clinics and agencies offering physical and economic assistance. The Arthritis

Foundation also sponsors support groups and public education programs.

The benefits of patient education have been highlighted in a variety of programs, including those using monthly telephone contact between trained volunteers and individuals with OA.[1] Volunteers speak with patients about symptoms, function, drugs, and clinic visits, resulting in improved pain and functional status at low cost. Likewise, OA patients participating in the program report decreases in joint pain and OA-related clinic visits, and improved physical activity and quality of life.[1]

DIET

Excess weight increases the biomechanical load on weight-bearing joints,[3,12,13] and is the single best predictor of need for eventual joint replacement. Weight loss is associated with decreased symptoms and disability, but controlled studies are needed to confirm benefits. Even 5 pounds of weight loss can decrease the biomechanical force on a weight-bearing joint. Although dietary intervention for overweight OA patients is reasonable, weight loss usually requires a motivated patient and a structured weight-loss program.

PHYSICAL AND OCCUPATIONAL THERAPY

Physical therapy—with heat or cold treatments and an exercise program—helps to maintain and restore joint range of motion and reduce pain and muscle spasms. Warm baths or warm water soaks may decrease pain and stiffness. Heating pads should be used with caution, especially in the elderly, and patients should be warned not to fall asleep on the heat source or to lie on it for more than brief periods to minimize the risk of burns.

Exercise programs and quadriceps strengthening can improve physical functioning and can decrease disability, pain, and analgesic use by OA patients.[1,9–11,31,32] The American Geriatrics Society has developed guidelines for exercise in OA patients.[11] Isometric exercise is preferred over isotonic exercises because the latter can aggravate the affected joint. Exercises should be taught and then observed before the patient exercises at home. Exercises should be performed three to four times daily. If severe pain develops with exercise, the patient should be instructed to decrease the number of repetitions.

The decision about whether to encourage walking should be made on an individual basis. With weak or deconditioned muscles, the load is transmitted excessively to the joints, so weight-bearing activities can exacerbate symptoms. However, avoidance of activity by those with hip or knee OA leads to further deconditioning or weight gain. A program of patient education, muscle stretching and strengthening, and supervised walking can improve physical function and decrease pain in patients with knee OA.[1,9–11,31,32]

Referral to the physical and/or occupational therapist is especially helpful for patients with functional disabilities. The therapist can assess muscle strength and joint stability, and recommend exercises and methods of protecting the affected joint from excessive forces. The therapist can also provide assistive and orthotic devices, such as canes, walkers, braces, heel cups, splints, or insoles for use during exercise or daily activities.

SURGERY

Surgery can be recommended for OA patients with functional disability and/or severe pain that is unresponsive to conservative therapy.[33–35] Indications for total hip replacement were developed by a National Institutes of Health consensus development conference,[33] and indications for total knee replacement were summarized based on three consensus groups of orthopedic surgeons.[34] Indeed, for patients with advanced disease, a partial or total arthroplasty can relieve pain and improve motion, with especially good outcomes after hip or knee arthroplasty.

Other surgical options are also worth discussing with the patient. Arthrodesis (joint fusion) can reduce pain but will restrict motion, and may be appropriate for smaller joints with intractable pain. For patients with mild knee OA, an osteotomy may correct the misalignment of genu varum or genu valgum. Although knee arthroscopy or lavage have been recommended for short-term relief of pain, a recent study showed these two procedures to be equivalent to sham surgery.[35] Experimental but potentially restorative approaches involve soft tissue grafts, penetration of subchondral bone, cell transplantation, and use of growth factors or artificial matrices.[36] Cartilage-restoration approaches are investigational, and results regarding pain control and joint function have been mixed.

PHARMACOLOGIC THERAPY

Drug therapy in OA is targeted at relief of pain. OA is seen commonly in older individuals who have other medical conditions, and OA treatment is often long-term. As such, a conservative approach to drug treatment, focusing on the needs of the individual patient, is warranted (see Fig. 90–2). For mild or moderate pain, topical analgesics or acetaminophen can be used. If these measures fail, or if there is inflammation, NSAIDs may be useful. Even when drug therapy is initiated, appropriate nondrug therapies should be continued and reinforced as the cornerstone of OA management and because they may provide as much relief as drug therapy.

ANALGESICS

The ACR recommends acetaminophen as first-line drug therapy for pain management in OA, due to its relative safety, efficacy, and lower cost compared to NSAIDs.[1,37] Pain relief with acetaminophen can be similar to that obtained with aspirin, naproxen, ibuprofen, and other NSAIDs, although some patients will respond better to NSAIDs.[1,37]

Although acetaminophen is one of the safest analgesics, its use still carries some risks, particularly hepatotoxicity with overdose or in individuals at risk of liver disease.[1,38]

In addition to guidelines from the American College of Rheumatology, recommendations for various aspects of OA management have been published by The European League Against Rheumatism, and a review of the evidence and suggestions for OA management have been formulated by rheumatology faculty in the Medical Research Council (UK) Environmental Epidemiology Unit.[1,6,7] These guidelines stress the importance of acetaminophen as first-line drug therapy for OA.

The ACR recommends NSAID use for pain management in OA patients in whom acetaminophen is ineffective. NSAIDs have analgesic properties at lower doses and anti-inflammatory effects at higher doses. The various NSAIDs all display comparable analgesic and anti-inflammatory efficacy and are similarly beneficial in OA (Table 90–4).[39] Although some studies have shown comparable efficacy for acetaminophen and NSAIDS, others have reported that patients experienced better pain control with NSAIDs than with acetaminophen, and that OA patients preferred NSAIDs to acetaminophen.[37,39,40]

ABLE 90—4. Medications Commonly Used in the Treatment of Osteoarthritis

Medication	Dosage and Frequency	Maximum Dosage (mg/day)
Oral analgesics		
Acetaminophen	325–650 mg every 4–6 hours or 1 g 3–4 times/day	4000
Tramadol	50–100 mg every 4–6 hours	400
Topical analgesics		
Capsaicin 0.025% or 0.075%	Apply to affected joint 3–4 times per day	—
Nutritional supplements		
Glucosamine sulfate	500 mg 3 times/day or 1500 mg once daily	1500
Nonsteroidal anti-inflammatory drugs (NSAIDs)		
Carboxylic acids		
Acetylated salicylates		
Aspirin, plain, buffered, or enteric-coated	325–650 mg every 4–6 hours for pain; anti-inflammatory doses start at 3600 mg/day in divided doses	3600[a]
Nonacetylated salicylates		
Salsalate	500–1000 mg 2–3 times a day	3000[a]
Diflunisal	500–1000 mg 2 times a day	1500
Choline salicylate[b]	500–1000 mg 2–3 times a day	3000[a]
Choline magnesium salicylate	500–1000 mg 2–3 times a day	3000[a]
Acetic acids		
Etodolac	800–1200 mg/day in divided doses	1200
Diclofenac	100–150 mg/day in divided doses	200
Indomethacin	25 mg 2–3 times a day; 75 mg SR once daily	200; 150
Ketorolac[c]	10 mg every 4–6 hours	40
Nabumetone[d]	500–1000 mg 1–2 times a day	2000
Propionic acids		
Fenoprofen	300–600 mg 3–4 times a day	3200
Flurbiprofen	200–300 mg/day in 2–4 divided doses	300
Ibuprofen	1200–3200 mg/day in 3–4 divided doses	3200
Ketoprofen	150–300 mg/day in 3–4 divided doses	300
Naproxen	250–500 mg twice a day	1500
Naproxen sodium	275–550 mg twice a day	1375
Oxaprozin	600–1200 mg daily	1800
Fenamates		
Meclofenamate	200–400 mg/day in 3–4 divided doses	400
Mefenamic acid[e]	250 mg every 6 hours	1000
Oxicams		
Piroxicam	10–20 mg daily	20
Meloxicam	7.5 mg daily	15
Coxibs[f]		
Celecoxib	100 mg twice daily or 200 mg daily	200 (400 for RA)
Valdecoxib	10 mg daily	10 (40 for dysmenorrheic pain)

Monitor serum salicylate levels over 3–3.6 g/day.
Only available as a liquid; 870 mg salicylate/5 mL.
Not approved for treatment of OA for more than 5 days.
Nonorganic acid but metabolite is an acetic acid.
Not approved for treatment of OA.
ee note at end of text regarding cardiovascular problems with coxibs.
A, rheumatoid arthritis; SR, sustained-release.

The most common adverse effects of NSAIDs involve the gastrointestinal tract. Minor complaints (nausea, dyspepsia, norexia, and abdominal pain) are common (up to 60% of patients). erious GI complications associated with NSAIDs including perforations, gastric outlet obstruction, and GI bleeding, occur in 1.5% to % of patients per year.

NSAIDs may cause renal dysfunction, characterized by increased serum creatinine and blood urea nitrogen, hyperkalemia, elevated blood pressure, peripheral edema, and weight gain. Hypersensitivity reactions may also occur in response to NSAIDs.

Alternative drug treatments include topical agents such as apsaicin and methyl salicylate, injections with glucocorticoids, and other oral agents (narcotic analgesics and chondroitin sulfate/glucosamine).[29,30,41]

ACETAMINOPHEN

Pharmacology and Mechanism of Action

Acetaminophen is thought to work within the central nervous system to inhibit the synthesis of prostaglandins, agents that enhance pain sensations. Acetaminophen prevents prostaglandin synthesis by blocking the action of central cyclooxygenase. Acetaminophen is well absorbed after oral administration (bioavailability is 60% to 98%), achieves peak concentrations within 1 to 2 hours, is inactivated in the liver by conjugation with sulfate or glucuronide, and its metabolites are renally excreted.

Efficacy

Comparable relief of mild to moderate OA pain has been demonstrated for acetaminophen at 2.6 to 4 g/day, aspirin 650 mg four times daily, ibuprofen at 1200 or 2400 mg daily, and naproxen 750 mg/day, as well as other NSAIDs.[1]

Adverse Effects

Although acetaminophen is one of the safest analgesics, its use carries some risks, primarily hepatotoxicity, and possibly renal toxicity with long-term use.[1,38,42] Serious and potentially fatal hepatotoxicity with overdose is well documented. It should be used with caution in patients with liver disease or those who chronically abuse alcohol. The FDA has recommended that chronic alcohol users (three or more drinks daily) should be warned regarding an increased risk of liver damage or GI bleeding with acetaminophen. Other individuals do not appear to be at increased risk of GI bleeding.

The National Kidney Foundation strongly discourages the use of over-the-counter combination analgesic products (e.g., acetaminophen and NSAIDs) because this is associated with an increased prevalence of renal failure.[38] Finally, patients should be warned about potential toxicity if they inadvertently ingest more than the recommended dose when using both nonprescription and prescription products containing acetaminophen.

Drug-Drug Interactions and Drug-Food Interactions

Drug interactions with acetaminophen can occur; for example, isoniazid can increase the risk of hepatotoxicity. Chronic ingestion of maximal doses of acetaminophen may intensify the anticoagulant effect in patients taking warfarin, so that such individuals may require closer monitoring. Food decreases the maximum serum concentration of acetaminophen by approximately one-half.

Dosing and Administration

When used for chronic OA, acetaminophen should be administered in a scheduled manner. It may be taken with or without food. The dose of acetaminophen is 325 to 650 mg taken up to four times daily, or to a maximum dose of 4 g daily.

NONSTEROIDAL ANTI-INFLAMMATORY DRUGS

Pharmacology and Mechanism of Action

Blockade of prostaglandin synthesis through inhibition of cyclooxygenase (both COX-1 and COX-2 enzymes) is believed to be the principal mechanism by which NSAIDs relieve pain and inflammation[43-46] (Fig. 90–3). Given the similar efficacy of nonspecific NSAIDs and COX-2 inhibitors, toxicity and cost play major roles in determining the medication chosen for a given patient. To understand the differences between nonspecific NSAIDs and COX inhibitors, the next section will review the COX-2 paradigm.[44-50]

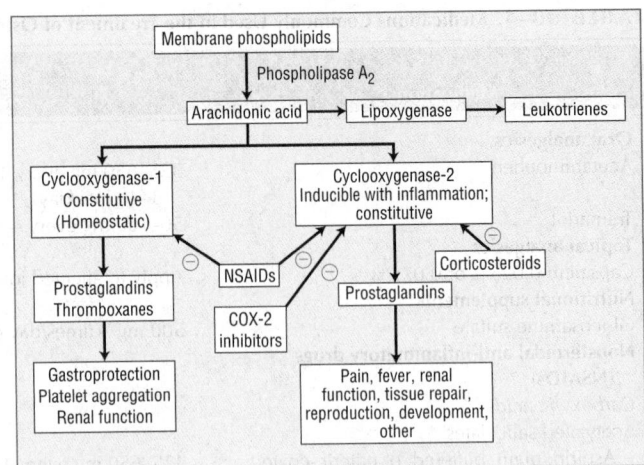

FIGURE 90–3. Pathway of synthesis for prostaglandins and leukotrienes. COX-1 and COX-2 are cyclooxygenase 1 and 2 enzymes.

The COX-2 Paradigm

Table 90–5 depicts basic facts about cyclooxygenase enzymes and their inhibition.[43-50] The COX-1 enzyme is involved in "housekeeping" or routine physiologic functions such as generation of gastroprotective prostaglandins to promote gastric blood flow and bicarbonate generation. COX-1 is expressed constitutively in gastric mucosa, vascular endothelial cells, platelets, and renal collecting tubules, so that COX-1–generated prostaglandins also participate in hemostasis and renal blood flow.

In contrast, the COX-2 enzyme is not normally expressed in most body tissues, but is rapidly induced by inflammatory mediators, local injury, and cytokines including interleukins, interferon, and tumor necrosis factor (see Fig. 90–3 and Table 90–5). COX-1 blockade (which occurs with nonspecific NSAIDs) is potentially undesirable and may lead to GI ulcers and increased bleeding risk due to inhibition of platelet aggregation. Specific COX-2 inhibition is considered desirable for the potential lack of such toxicities while exerting anti-inflammatory and analgesic effects.

Nonspecific NSAIDs and COX-2 inhibitors exhibit mechanistic differences. The former penetrate the enzyme active site for both COX-1 and COX-2 and block entry of the enzyme's usual substrate, arachidonic acid. By contrast, COX-2 inhibitors are much more potent at inhibiting COX-2; they tightly interact in a time-dependent manner with a side pocket within the active site of COX-2. This high-affinity binding to COX-2 provides excellent COX-2 inhibition with virtually no effect on COX-1.

Although the COX-2 paradigm has merit, several issues and observations regarding COX enzymes and NSAIDs require further scrutiny and could carry implications for COX-2 inhibitor safety.[44-55] These observations and issues include the following:

1. Gastroprotection by COX-1 and gastropathy via COX-1 blockade may not be as simple as originally thought. Knockout mice lacking COX-1 do not develop spontaneous gastropathy, but they do develop ulcers when given nonspecific NSAIDs.

2. COX-2 activity in the gastric mucosa may be helpful in some situations. COX-2 is induced with gastric injury and is seen at the rim of ulcers in humans, and COX-2 inhibitors retard ulcer healing in humans and animals and angiogenesis in experimental systems.[47,53,54]

TABLE 90–5. Characteristics of Cyclooxygenase-1 (COX-1) and Cyclooxygenase-2 (COX-2) Enzymes

	COX-1 Enzyme	COX-2 Enzyme
Location in genome	Chromosome 9	Chromosome 1
Molecular weight (kDa)	69,054	69,093
Cellular location	Integral membrane protein in ER and nuclear envelope	Integral membrane protein in ER and nuclear envelope
Tissue location	Gastric mucosa, intestine, kidney, platelets, endothelial cells, other	Macrophages, fibroblasts, chondrocytes, epithelial cells, endothelial cells, synoviocytes, CNS, bone, kidney, reproductive tract, other
Control of expression	Constitutive	Rapidly inducible: inflammation, IL-1, TNF TGF-β mitogens, lipopolysaccharides
		Constitutive in some tissues
Effect of glucocorticoids	Unaffected	Inhibited (transcriptional level)
Enzymologic function	Arachidonic acid $\rightarrow$ PGG$_2$ $\rightarrow$ PGH$_2$. (PGH$_2$ $\rightarrow$ final products [PGs, PGI$_2$, TX] depends on tissue)	Arachidonic acid $\rightarrow$ PGG$_2$ $\rightarrow$ PGH$_2$ PGH$_2$ $\rightarrow$ final products (PGs, PGI$_2$) depends on tissue
Biologic function	Gastrointestinal mucosal integrity, platelet aggregation; renal function; other	Inflammation, development, renal function, reproduction, bone metabolism, other
Kinetics of inhibition by NSAIDs	Immediate, competitive inhibition (strong for COX-1 inhibitors, weak for COX-2 inhibitors)[a]	COX-2 inhibitors: noncompetitive (irreversible?), time-dependent COX-1 inhibitors: competitive, immediate

[a]Aspirin inhibition is irreversible.
CNS, central nervous system; ER, endoplasmic reticulum; IL-1, interleukin-1; kDa, kilodalton;
NSAID, nonsteroidal anti-inflammatory drug; PG, prostaglandin; PGG$_2$, prostaglandin G$_2$;
PGH$_2$, prostaglandin H$_2$; PGI$_2$, prostaglandin I$_2$; TNF, tumor necrosis factor; TGF-β, transforming growth factor-β; TX, thromboxane.
Data from Hawkey,[44] Golden et al,[45] Garavito et al,[46] Jones et al,[47] Wolfe et al,[48] Lichtenstein et al,[49] and Crofford et al.[50]

3. COX-2 activity is beneficial in renal function. COX-2 has some constitutive expression in the kidney, and its intrarenal distribution and its upregulation in salt depletion suggest that it helps regulate renal hemodynamics in some situations.

4. A COX-2 inhibitor's analgesic mechanism may not be as simple as sometimes thought, because COX-2 inhibitors reduce pain, even in noninflammatory conditions.

5. There may be a tendency to overprescribe COX-2 inhibitors, especially in patients who are frail, if the potential toxicities of these agents are unappreciated.

6. Since aspirin blocks the COX-1 enzyme, the GI safety advantage of COX-2–specific inhibitors is blunted by the concomitant use of aspirin, even at low doses.[55]

CLINICAL CONTROVERSY

Controversy has arisen regarding whether or not COX-2 inhibitors may increase cardiovascular risk in some patients.[51,52] Concern has arisen about the possible prothrombotic potential of the available COX-2 inhibitors. Patients taking rofecoxib had more thrombotic events than did patients taking naproxen in the Vioxx Gastrointestinal Outcomes Research Study (VIGOR), which led to an FDA labeling change for rofecoxib regarding cardiovascular risk. However, since naproxen may possess antiplatelet effects, and some subjects normally taking low-dose aspirin were asked to stop aspirin to participate in the study, it is unclear whether thrombotic events resulted from rofecoxib toxicity, antiplatelet effects of naproxen, discontinuation of aspirin, or a combination of these factors. Patients given rofecoxib also had higher rates

of hypertension and congestive heart failure. (See Note at end of chapter.)

Despite these complexities, COX-2–specific inhibitors relieve pain in many OA patients with a lower risk of GI adverse events than nonspecific NSAIDs. COX-2 inhibitors, members of the "coxib" class newly created by the World Health Organization,[49] have become extremely widely used over a short period of time. These agents continue to be studied intensely not only for their efficacy and toxicity profile in rheumatic disease, but also for exciting potential applications such as the prevention of Alzheimer's disease and colorectal cancer.

Pharmacokinetics

The various NSAIDs exhibit several pharmacokinetic similarities, including high oral availability, high protein binding, and absorption as active drugs (except for sulindac and nabumetone, which require hepatic conversion for activity). The most important difference in NSAIDs is a serum half-life ranging from 1 hour for tolmetin to 50 hours for piroxicam, impacting the frequency of dosing and potentially, compliance with therapy.[43] Elimination of NSAIDs largely depends on hepatic inactivation, with a small fraction of active drug being renally excreted. NSAIDs penetrate joint fluid, reaching about 60% of blood levels.[43]

Efficacy

Prescription-strength NSAIDs are often prescribed for OA patients after treatment with acetaminophen proves ineffective, or for patients with inflammatory OA. All NSAIDs and aspirin have similar analgesic and anti-inflammatory effects.[39,43,56] Analgesic effects begin within hours, whereas anti-inflammatory benefits may require 2 to 3 weeks of continuous therapy.

A systematic review of studies of NSAIDs for OA found no evidence to support a definitive ranking of NSAID efficacy.[56] However, individual patient response does differ among NSAIDs. The prescriber often relies on personal experience in choosing an NSAID. To assess efficacy in the individual patient, a trial that is adequate in time (2 to 3 weeks) and dose is needed. If the first trial fails, another NSAID in the same or another chemical class can be tried until an effective agent is found. Thus if a trial with one NSAID fails, the clinician should try a different NSAID (see Table 90-4).[39,43,56] Patients must understand this approach, appreciate the necessity of adherence to medication therapy throughout the trial, and actively participate in assessment of drug efficacy. Combining two NSAIDs increases adverse effects without providing additional benefit.

COX-2 inhibitors demonstrate similar analgesic benefits when compared to traditional NSAIDs.[57] For example, 748 subjects randomized to rofecoxib (12.5 or 25 mg daily) or diclofenac (50 mg three times daily) showed similar improvements in pain, stiffness, physical function, and other measures of efficacy.[58] In a 12-week trial of 1003 subjects with knee OA, celecoxib at 100 or 200 mg twice daily was more effective than placebo and comparable to naproxen 500 mg twice daily for relief of pain, stiffness, and limitation of physical function.[59]

Valdecoxib, a more recently marketed coxib, has been studied in 14 clinical studies involving more than 4000 patients, for OA, rheumatoid arthritis, or pain associated with dysmenorrhea or surgery. Valdecoxib 10 mg once daily was as effective as naproxen 500 mg twice daily for pain relief from knee OA and for hip OA.[60]

▨ Adverse Effects

▨ *Gastrointestinal Effects of NSAIDs.* The most common adverse effects of NSAIDs involve the GI tract, contributing to many treatment failures.[48] Minor complaints—nausea, dyspepsia, anorexia, abdominal pain, flatulence, and diarrhea—affect 10% to 60% of patients. To minimize these symptoms, NSAIDs should be taken with food or milk, except for enteric-coated products, which should *not* be taken with milk or antacids.

All NSAIDs have the potential to cause GI bleeding.[48] Unionized NSAIDs enter gastric mucosal cells, release hydrogen ions, and are concentrated ("ion trapped") within cells, with cell death or damage. Gastric mucosal injury can also result from NSAID inhibition of gastroprotective prostaglandins.

The most common sites of GI injury are the gastric and duodenal mucosae.[48] The incidence of gastric ulcers with NSAID use is approximately 11% to 13%, and that for duodenal ulcers is 7% to 10%. Serious GI complications associated with NSAIDs, including perforations, gastric outlet obstruction, and GI bleeding, occur in 1.5% to 4% of patients per year. NSAIDs are so widely used that these small percentages translate into substantial morbidity and mortality.[1,48] Moreover, the risk increases to 9% per year for patients with the risk factors of advanced age, history of peptic ulcer or GI bleeding, or cardiovascular disease. Consequently, about 16,500 deaths are associated annually with NSAID use in rheumatoid arthritis or OA patients.

Notably, there is a poor correlation between GI ulceration and GI symptoms, with 50% of dyspeptic patients having a normal-appearing mucosa, and 40% of asymptomatic persons having endoscopically evident erosive gastritis. Approximately 80% of those who develop serious GI complications have no preceding dyspepsia.[61] The ACR

has thus recommended a complete blood count yearly to detect a silent bleeding ulcer by means of an asymptomatic decline in hematocrit.[62] Fecal occult blood is an unreliable predictor of complications.

◀▨ H2-receptor antagonists prevent NSAID-induced *duodenal* ulcers, and at high dose may prevent *gastric* ulcers.[1] Misoprostol protects against both gastric and duodenal NSAID-induced ulcers, and more importantly, their associated complications.[1] Unfortunately, misoprostol frequently causes diarrhea and abdominal cramps. Because of its abortifacient properties, misoprostol is contraindicated in pregnancy and in women of childbearing age who are not maintaining adequate contraception. It must be dispensed in its original container, which carries a warning for these individuals. Misoprostol is also available in a combination product with diclofenac, which bears the same restrictions as misoprostol alone.

Other agents have been evaluated in attempts to prevent NSAID-induced gastropathy. Among 935 NSAID users with baseline gastric or duodenal erosions, omeprazole and misoprostol were similarly effective in the treatment of ulcers and their symptoms, but omeprazole maintenance therapy conferred a lower rate of relapse.[63] Thus several medications are available for the treatment or prevention of ulcers in high-risk patients.

▨ *Gastrointestinal Effects of COX-2 Inhibitors.* For treatment of OA patients at high risk for GI complications of NSAIDs, the ACR recommends either a COX-2 inhibitor or an NSAID in combination with either a proton pump inhibitor or misoprostol. Studies of both rofecoxib and celecoxib, using endoscopy to assess appearance of gastric ulcers, demonstrated little or no increase in ulcers with these agents. Among 1149 patients with RA randomized to receive placebo, celecoxib (100, 200, or 400 mg twice daily), or naproxen (500 mg twice daily), the incidence of endoscopically-determined gastroduodenal ulcers after 12 weeks was significantly higher with naproxen (26%) than celecoxib at any dose (4% to 8%) or placebo (4%).[64] Similarly, in comparing rofecoxib (25 or 50 mg daily), ibuprofen (800 mg three times daily), or placebo, fewer endoscopic ulcers were detected in subjects taking rofecoxib than ibuprofen, while results were similar for rofecoxib and placebo.[65]

The incidence of endoscopically observed gastroduodenal ulcers in RA patients taking valdecoxib 20 mg daily (6%) and valdecoxib 40 mg daily (4%) was reduced compared to that in patients receiving diclofenac 75 mg sustained-release twice daily (16%; $p < 0.001$). Valdecoxib 20 mg daily was also associated with significantly improved GI tolerability ($p = 0.035$) compared with diclofenac.[66] Four safety studies and two reviews of clinical trials indicated decreased rates of gastroduodenal ulceration with valdecoxib versus ibuprofen, naproxen, and diclofenac ($p < 0.001$ to < 0.05).[67]

To study effects on clinically important GI complications with celecoxib, the CLASS study used celecoxib (400 mg twice daily, or twice the highest FDA-approved dose) compared to diclofenac and ibuprofen at standard dose. Celecoxib use was reported to be associated with a reduced incidence for the combined end point of symptomatic ulcers and ulcer complications (perforations, gastric outlet obstruction, or bleeding).[55] Some subjects also used aspirin for cardioprotection, but there is concern that GI safety of COX-2 inhibitors is blunted with use of concomitant aspirin (even 30 mg of aspirin can suppress gastric prostaglandin production).[43] For patients taking aspirin and celecoxib, ulcer complications were higher than with celecoxib only, but lower than with traditional NSAIDs.

Concerns have been raised by the FDA and others with regard to the CLASS study design and whether the published results, based on 6 months, clearly reflect the overall GI safety profile, as these patients were actually followed for a longer time period.[68,69] The

FDA concluded that although there were trends favoring celecoxib, this drug did not show clear statistical superiority over nonspecific NSAIDs for clinically significant upper GI events.

To further assess whether COX-2 inhibitors cause fewer serious GI events (perforations, bleeding, and gastric outlet obstruction), a meta-analysis of eight double-blind studies was performed. These studies used rofecoxib and either ibuprofen, diclofenac, nabumetone, or placebo.[70] The risk of serious adverse GI events was lowest for placebo, intermediate for rofecoxib, and highest with NSAID therapy. The VIGOR study, a large study included in this meta-analysis, randomized 8076 rheumatoid arthritis patients to receive rofecoxib 50 mg daily or naproxen 500 mg twice daily; use of concomitant aspirin was prohibited. Subjects randomized to rofecoxib experienced a 50% lower risk of serious GI events.[71] FDA-approved labeling for rofecoxib states that the VIGOR study showed a significant reduction in the risk of development of peptic ulcer bleeding (symptomatic ulcers, upper GI perforation, obstruction, major or minor upper GI bleeding), including complicated peptic ulcer bleeding in patients taking rofecoxib compared to naproxen.

Aside from consideration of the relatively uncommon but serious GI adverse effects described above, fewer overall GI complaints from patients are found for COX-2 inhibitors compared to nonspecific NSAIDs.[55,59,65,70] Moreover, celecoxib use was associated with decreased outpatient physician claims for upper GI symptoms compared with other prescription nonspecific NSAIDs.[72] Finally, celecoxib was comparable to a combination of diclofenac and misoprostol in reducing the risk of recurrent GI bleeding in patients who had a prior GI bleed.[73]

In summary, there is evidence that COX-2 inhibitors pose a decreased risk of GI toxicity compared to nonspecific NSAIDs, an especially important consideration when treating those at risk for clinically significant GI adverse effects. Rofecoxib decreases the extent of clinically significant GI complications. Celecoxib likely decreases these events, although the proof is less rigorous and still debated. For valdecoxib, its effect on clinically significant GI events awaits further study.

Other Toxicities Associated with NSAIDs. NSAIDs may cause kidney diseases, including acute renal insufficiency, tubulointerstitial nephropathy, hyperkalemia, and renal papillary necrosis.[74] Clinical features of these NSAID-induced renal syndromes include increased serum creatinine and blood urea nitrogen, hyperkalemia, elevated blood pressure, peripheral edema, and weight gain. Mechanisms of NSAID injury include direct toxicity, and inhibition of local prostaglandins that promote vasodilation of renal blood vessels and preserve renal blood flow. Patients at high risk have conditions associated with decreased renal blood flow, including chronic renal insufficiency, congestive heart failure, severe hepatic disease, nephrotic syndrome, advanced age, or diuretic therapy (Fig. 90–4).[74] Close monitoring is advisable for high-risk patients taking an NSAID, with monitoring of serum creatinine at baseline and within 3 to 7 days of drug initiation. For those with impaired renal function, the National Kidney Foundation recommends acetaminophen as the drug of choice.[38]

COX-2 inhibitors also have potential for renal toxicity; COX-2 activity has been demonstrated in a variety of sites in the kidney and is upregulated in salt-depleted states[74,75] (see Fig. 90–4). Importantly, COX-2 inhibitors decrease urinary prostaglandins and cause sodium and potassium retention, as do nonspecific NSAIDs. Postmarketing surveillance of coxibs has confirmed the risk of renal dysfunction. Therefore coxibs should be prescribed with the same caution as NSAIDs in patients at increased risk for renal dysfunction.

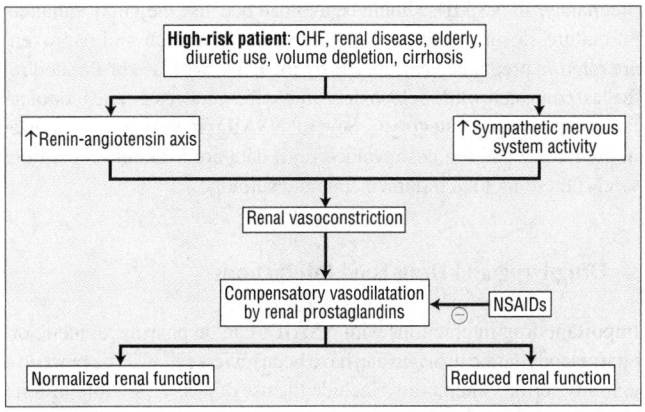

FIGURE 90–4. Mechanisms implicated in NSAID-induced renal injury.

Recent evidence has indicated the potential for cardiovascular risk with coxibs, particularly rofecoxib.[51,52]

Coxibs and NSAIDs uncommonly cause drug-induced hepatitis; the two NSAIDs most frequently implicated are diclofenac and sulindac. Patient monitoring should include periodic liver enzymes (aspartate aminotransferase and alanine aminotransferase), with cessation of therapy if these values exceed two to three times the normal range.

Other toxic effects of NSAIDs include hypersensitivity reactions, rash, and central nervous system complaints of drowsiness, dizziness, headaches, depression, confusion, and tinnitus.[43] Although NSAIDs are generally avoided in patients with asthma who are aspirin-intolerant, studies indicate that celecoxib and rofecoxib are well tolerated in aspirin-sensitive asthma, providing a viable option for these patients.[76–78] Celecoxib and valdecoxib are sulfonamides and are thus contraindicated for those with sulfa allergies.

All nonspecific NSAIDs inhibit COX-1–dependent thromboxane production in platelets and thus increase bleeding risk. Importantly, aspirin inhibition is irreversible, and bleeding time requires 5 to 7 days to normalize after cessation of therapy, as new platelets enter the circulation. Other nonspecific NSAIDs inhibit thromboxane formation reversibly, with normalization of platelet function 1 to 3 days after the drug is stopped. The nonacetylated salicylate products and nabumetone, which have partial COX-2 selectivity, may be preferable to nonspecific NSAIDs.[43] COX-2 inhibitors do not block thromboxane synthesis and pose even less bleeding risk. Among subjects treated with supratherapeutic doses of celecoxib (600 mg twice daily) and regular doses of naproxen (500 mg twice daily), a substantial decrease in platelet aggregation and thromboxane production occurred with naproxen but not with celecoxib. However, because warfarin and celecoxib are metabolized by the cytochrome P450 (CYP450) isoenzyme CYP2C9, and since postmarketing interactions between warfarin and both celecoxib and rofecoxib have been noted, patients receiving warfarin and COX-2 inhibitors should be followed closely.

In a study of healthy adults, valdecoxib (40 mg twice a day), did not affect platelet function, whereas naproxen 500 mg twice a day or diclofenac 75 mg twice a day significantly reduced the platelet aggregation response. In elderly subjects (65 to 85 years), valdecoxib (40 mg twice daily) had no platelet effects (platelet aggregation, bleeding time, and serum thromboxane B_2 levels), whereas ibuprofen (800 mg three times a day) significantly decreased platelet aggregation, significantly increased bleeding time, and significantly decreased thromboxane B_2 levels.[79]

Finally, NSAIDs should be used cautiously during pregnancy because of the risk to the fetus posed by the bleeding problems. In late pregnancy, all NSAIDs should be avoided because they may enhance premature closure of the ductus arteriosus. Ibuprofen and naproxen are rated as pregnancy category B by the FDA, with use prohibited in the last trimester, while celecoxib, rofecoxib, valdecoxib, and etodolac fall into pregnancy category C. Several NSAIDs have no rating for use in pregnancy and are best avoided until data are available regarding safety; these include indomethacin and sulindac.

Drug-Drug and Drug-Food Interactions

Important drug interactions with NSAIDs can be pharmacokinetic or pharmacodynamic in origin and have been reviewed.[43,80] The most potentially serious interactions include the use of NSAIDs with lithium, warfarin, oral hypoglycemics, high-dose methotrexate, antihypertensives, angiotensin-converting enzyme inhibitors, β-blockers, and diuretics. Anticipation and careful monitoring often can prevent serious events when these drugs are used together.

Celecoxib metabolism is primarily via cytochrome P450 2C9.[80] In clinical studies, increased celecoxib levels were seen with fluconazole administration. Cytochrome P450 inducers such as rifampin, carbamazepine, and phenytoin have the potential to reduce celecoxib levels. However, no clinically significant interactions have been documented with celecoxib and methotrexate, glyburide, ketoconazole, phenytoin, or tolbutamide. Because celecoxib inhibits CYP450 2D6, it has the potential to increase concentrations of a variety of agents, including antidepressants. Celecoxib increases lithium levels, as do other NSAIDs, thus caution is needed when using coxibs or NSAIDs with lithium.

Rofecoxib is metabolized in the liver, primarily by cytosolic enzymes, with little renal excretion of unchanged drug. Rofecoxib at 75 mg daily modestly increased methotrexate concentrations, and at 50 mg daily modestly elevated the International Normalized Ratios (INRs) of warfarin patients. Additionally, rifampin can decrease rofecoxib concentrations. Clinically significant interactions were not observed when rofecoxib was administered with cimetidine, digoxin, oral contraceptives, or ketoconazole. Rofecoxib inhibits CYP450 1A2 and may increase serum theophylline area under the curve.

Valdecoxib undergoes metabolism in hepatic microsomes (primarily by CYP450 3A4 and CYP450 2C9) and by other pathways, including glucuronidation. Inhibitors of CYP450 3A4 and CYP450 2C9 such as fluconazole and ketoconazole may increase valdecoxib plasma levels. Valdecoxib moderately inhibits CYP450 2C19 and weakly inhibits CYP450 3A4 and CYP450 2C9. Valdecoxib modestly increases concentrations of R and S warfarin, slightly increases INR, and increases INR variability. Valdecoxib increases lithium plasma concentrations by an unknown mechanism. Coxibs may decrease the antihypertensive effects of angiotensin-converting enzyme inhibitors and may interfere with the natriuretic effect of diuretics by affecting renal prostaglandin production.[74,80]

Dosing and Administration

Administration of NSAIDs must be tailored to the individual patient with OA. For the OA patient who has failed an adequate trial of acetaminophen, trial with an NSAID is warranted. Selection of an NSAID depends on the prescriber's experience, medication cost, patient preference, allergies, toxicities, and adherence issues. Individual patient response differs among NSAIDs (see Table 90-4), so if an inadequate response is obtained with one NSAID, another NSAID may yet provide benefit.[1,39,43]

TOPICAL THERAPIES

Topical products can be used alone or in combination with oral analgesics or NSAIDs. Capsaicin, isolated from hot peppers, releases and ultimately depletes substance P from afferent nociceptive nerve fibers. Substance P has been implicated in the transmission of pain in arthritis, and capsaicin cream has been shown in four controlled studies to provide pain relief in OA when applied over affected joints.[1,41]

To be effective, capsaicin must be used regularly, and it may take up to 2 weeks to work. It is well tolerated, except that some patients experience a temporary burning sensation at the site of application. Patients should be warned not to get the cream in their eyes or mouth and to wash their hands after application. Although use is recommended four times a day, a twice-daily application may enhance long-term adherence and still provide adequate pain relief.[41]

GLUCOSAMINE AND CHONDROITIN

Interest in chondroitin and glucosamine was spurred initially by anecdotal reports of benefit in animals and humans, and by the fact that these substances stimulate proteoglycan synthesis from articular cartilage in vitro and have an excellent safety profile. Enthusiasm for these agents continues.[81–85]

A total of 17 double-blind, placebo-controlled trials have subsequently shown that chondroitin and glucosamine are superior to placebo in alleviating pain from knee or hip OA. In one study, chondroitin sulfate showed similar analgesic benefits to diclofenac.[82]

A recent meta-analysis of glucosamine and chondroitin indicated that both agents had efficacy in reducing pain and improving mobility, and that glucosamine reduced joint space narrowing.[83] Use of glucosamine or chondroitin sulfate was associated with slower loss of cartilage than placebo, in knees affected by OA.[29,84] Further support for the structural benefits of these compounds comes from a follow-up survey 5 years after completion of a 3-year study comparing glucosamine and placebo. In this survey, rates of lower limb joint replacement were twofold higher in subjects given placebo, compared with subjects given glucosamine. In addition, subjects treated with glucosamine had lower rates of pain, joint space narrowing, and limitations of physical function.[85] If the positive findings with these compounds are confirmed by an ongoing study sponsored by the National Institutes of Health, this would represent an important advance in the treatment of OA.

Because glucosamine and chondroitin are marketed in the United States as dietary supplements, neither the products nor their purity is adequately regulated by the FDA. Some reliable products include Cosamin DS, Condrosulf, and Dona.[29,86]

CORTICOSTEROIDS

Intra-articular glucocorticoid injections can provide excellent pain relief, particularly when a joint effusion is present.[1,87] Aspiration of the effusion and injection of glucocorticoid are carried out aseptically and examination of the aspirate to exclude crystalline arthritis or infection is recommended. After injection, the patient should minimize activity and stress on the joint for several days. The risk of infection is estimated at 1 in 50,000 joint injections.

A recent randomized, placebo-controlled, double-blind study showed that intra-articular triamcinolone 40 mg every 3 months was superior to placebo in alleviating knee pain and stiffness due to OA during a 2-year trial.[87] The potential risk of cartilage destruction with steroid injections was not substantiated, as the rate of cartilage loss was similar in both groups. The therapy is generally limited to three or four injections per year because of the potential systemic effects of steroids, and because the need for more frequent injections indicates little response to the therapy.

Systemic corticosteroid therapy is not recommended in OA, given the lack of proven benefit and the well-known adverse effects with long-term use.

HYALURONATE INJECTIONS

Agents containing hyaluronic acid (HA) (sodium hyaluronate) are available for intra-articular injection for treatment of knee OA.[88–90] High-molecular-weight HA is an important constituent of normal cartilage, with viscoelastic properties providing lubrication with motion and shock absorbency during rapid movements. Endogenous HA also may have anti-inflammatory effects. Because the concentration and molecular size of synovial HA decrease in OA, administration of exogenous HA products has been studied, with the theory that this could reconstitute synovial fluid and reduce symptoms. Injections temporarily and modestly increase viscosity. Although HA injections were reported to decrease pain, many studies were short term and poorly controlled, and placebo injections also reduced OA pain dramatically.

HA products are injected once weekly for either 3 or 5 weeks. Injections are well tolerated, although acute joint swelling and local skin reactions, including rash, ecchymoses, and pruritus have been reported.

HA injections may be beneficial for patients unresponsive to other therapies. These agents are expensive because the treatment includes both drug costs and administration costs. As a result, HA injections are often used after less expensive therapies have demonstrated lack of efficacy.

DISEASE-MODIFYING DRUGS

Disease-modifying drugs are targeted not at pain relief but at preventing, retarding, or reversing damage to articular cartilage.[91] Most products have been tested in animal models, and limited human data are available.

Thus far, OA is a disease whose symptoms can be alleviated, but whose progress is impossible to stop. Because of this, clinicians were very interested to learn that both chondroitin and glucosamine show disease-modifying potential in patients with OA (see above information on these agents).

Another approach is that of pharmacologic agents that could mimic TIMPs and thus potentially decrease cartilage destruction. Some studies have explored the use of tetracycline or doxycycline, which appear to inhibit the degradative MMPs.[19,92] Preliminary data indicate that doxycycline delays loss of articular cartilage in humans when compared with placebo.[93] Other studies using heparinoid products that contain glycosaminoglycans, sodium pentosan polysulfate, and calcium pentosan polysulfate show promise in preliminary work limited largely to animal models and in vitro studies.[94] There is also recent interest in the potential of cyclooxygenase-inhibiting nitric oxide–donor compounds to relieve OA while sparing GI adverse effects.[95] Thus ongoing research with several agents may identify new treatment options to delay OA progression, thereby improving outcomes for people with OA.

NARCOTIC ANALGESICS

Low-dose narcotic analgesics may be very useful in patients who experience no relief with acetaminophen, NSAIDs, intra-articular injections, or topical therapy. These agents are particularly useful in patients who cannot take NSAIDs due to renal failure, or for patients in whom all other treatment options have failed and who are at high surgical risk, precluding joint arthroplasty. Low-dose narcotics are the initial intervention, usually given in combination with acetaminophen.

Sustained-release compounds usually offer better pain control throughout the day, and are used when simple narcotics are ineffective. A recent randomized double-blind placebo-controlled study showed that extended-release oxymorphone (40 to 50 mg twice daily) was superior to placebo in reducing pain and improving both function and quality of life.[96]

If pain is intolerable and limits activities of daily living, and the patient has sufficiently good cardiopulmonary health to undergo a major surgery, joint replacement may be preferable to continued reliance on narcotics.

PHARMACOECONOMIC CONSIDERATIONS

Economic considerations in the treatment of OA are of considerable import, since the disease is extremely common, ranking second in causes of disability in the United States.[97–99]

One of the largest costs associated with OA is hospitalization for joint replacement or treatment of NSAID-related complications, particularly serious GI adverse events. To provide perspective on patient care costs for GI complications of NSAIDs, a 1997 report on more than 10,000 OA patients followed in a managed-care setting showed that the mean annual cost of care per patient was $543, with hospital costs accounting for 46%, medications 32%, and ambulatory care 22%.[100] Consequently, intense focus has emerged on the cost:benefit ratio of medications to prevent ulcer complications, and the use of coxibs, which cause fewer ulcer complications.

For example, analysis of the cost effectiveness of misoprostol was reported, based on data from a study of RA patients taking NSAIDs.[55,97] Misoprostol was shown to be cost-effective if reserved for high-risk patients. The cost of avoiding one serious GI complication would be $94,766 if all NSAID patients were given misoprostol, but only $4,101 if misoprostol were limited to high-risk patients. A problem with misoprostol, however, is its low tolerability because it often causes diarrhea. Cost-effectiveness of a different strategy, that of using COX-2–specific inhibitors rather than NSAIDs, is still being debated.[101–103]

Pharmacoeconomic considerations for OA involve the selection of therapy for the initial treatment of patients with OA. Use of the nonprescription analgesic acetaminophen as initial therapy has greatly reduced medication costs in comparison with the use of NSAIDs, many of which are by prescription only. NSAID costs range from $20 to $100 per month, depending on the medication, daily dose, and regimen selected. Since NSAIDs as a class are therapeutically equivalent, use of less expensive NSAIDs, such as nonprescription ibuprofen or naproxen, may minimize the cost of medicine to the patient. More expensive NSAIDs can be prescribed if neither of these offers benefit after a 2-week trial at sufficient doses.

Although use of nonprescription medications can be viewed as a reduction in the cost of prescription medications, cost shifting to "out of pocket" expense greatly affects patients on fixed incomes. Many elderly patients, who are most likely to need OA drugs, have little or no prescription reimbursement. Careful attention to affordability of medication should be given for all patients receiving drug therapy for OA.

CLINICAL CONTROVERSY

COX-2 inhibitors are recommended by ACR guidelines for those at high risk of adverse GI events, and controversy has arisen regarding cost-effectiveness of this recommendation. For patients without risk factors, 500 patients would need treatment with a COX-2 inhibitor, costing $400,000, to avoid one serious GI complication from a nonspecific NSAID. For high-risk individuals, the number needed to treat would be 40, costing $30,000.[101] Another study indicated that, without regard to risk factors, it would be cost-effective to provide rofecoxib or celecoxib for those over age 76 and 81, respectively.[102] Another report examined the cost-utility of COX-2 inhibitors in a model system including RA and OA patients, and found costs of $275,809 per quality-adjusted life year gained when using coxibs in average-risk patients. If costs as low as $150,000 per quality-adjusted life year were to be obtained, it would be necessary to restrict coxib use to the 4.2% of patients at highest risk.[103] These findings are being debated, based on the many assumptions that had been made in the model. Debates about cost effectiveness are likely to continue. However, with existing evidence of increased GI safety, coupled with huge patient demand, coxibs are heavily used despite these cost concerns.

EVALUATION OF THERAPEUTIC OUTCOMES

Pharmacotherapy monitoring in OA is patient-specific, focusing on patient age, concomitant medications and comorbidities, and the therapy selected. To monitor efficacy, the patient's baseline pain can be assessed with a visual analogue scale, and range of motion for affected joints can be assessed, providing baseline measures to monitor the success of therapy. Baseline radiographs are helpful to document the extent of joint involvement and follow progression of disease with therapy. Additional tests of OA severity may include measurement of grip strength, 50-foot walking time, patient and physician global assessment of OA severity, and the Western Ontario and McMaster Universities Arthrosis Index or Stanford Health Assessment Questionnaire to monitor ability to perform activities of daily living. A decrease in the use of analgesics or NSAIDs would suggest a beneficial effect of nonpharmacologic interventions. Lastly, disease-specific quality of life is valuable in assessing clinical response to interventions.[5]

When assessing toxicity of therapy, patients should be asked first if they are having any "problems" with their medications. This open-ended question can be followed with more direct questions relating to the most common adverse effects associated with the respective medication. Symptoms of abdominal pain, heartburn, nausea, or change in stool color provide valuable clues to the presence of GI complications. Patients also should be monitored for the development of hypertension, weight gain, edema, skin rash, and central nervous system adverse effects such as headaches and drowsiness. Baseline serum creatinine, complete blood count, and serum transaminases are repeated at 6- to 12-month intervals to identify GI, renal, hepatic, and hematologic toxicities.

CONCLUSIONS

OA is a very common, slowly progressive disorder that affects diarthrodial joints and is characterized by progressive deterioration of articular cartilage, subchondral sclerosis, and osteophyte production. Clinical manifestations include gradual onset of joint pain, stiffness, and limitation of motion. The primary treatment goals are to reduce pain, maintain function, and prevent further destruction. An individualized approach based on education, rest, exercise, weight loss as needed, and analgesic medication can succeed in meeting these goals. Recommended drug treatment starts with acetaminophen <4 g/day and topical analgesics as needed. If acetaminophen is ineffective, NSAIDs may be used, often providing satisfactory relief of pain and stiffness. Individuals at increased risk for toxicity from NSAIDs, especially for GI, cardiovascular, or renal events, deserve special attention. Experimental therapy aimed at preventing the progression of OA requires further clinical investigation before entering widespread clinical use.

NOTE ADDED IN PROOF

On September 30, 2004, rofecoxib was withdrawn from the worldwide market by the manufacturer, based on results obtained from the APPROVe (Adenomatous Polyp Prevention on Vioxx) trial. For those on rofecoxib 25 mg daily compared with placebo, risk for confirmed cardiovascular events, including myocardial infarction and stroke, was approximately doubled, beginning after 18 months of treatment.

In addition, on December 9, 2004, the FDA announced a new boxed warning for valdecoxib, stating that serious, at times fatal, skin reactions, including Steven-Johnson syndrome and toxic epidermal necrolysis, have been reported for patients taking valdecoxib. There is also a new bolded warning specifically contraindicating valdecoxib for treating pain following coronary artery bypass graft (CABG) surgery. This was based on a study of more than 1500 patients treated after CABG, where increased cardiovascular risk (myocardial infarction, stroke, and deep vein thrombosis) was seen in those receiving valdecoxib compared with placebo. In addition, reports of problems with celecoxib and naproxen emerged later that month.

Although new coxibs are in development, and valdecoxib and celecoxib remain on the market as this chapter went to press, it appears that all these agents will be the focus of increased scrutiny with regard to their potential cardiovascular and other risks.

ABBREVIATIONS

ACR: American College of Rheumatology
COX-2: cyclooxygenase-2
CYP450: cytochrome P450
ECM: extracellular matrix
HA: hyaluronic acid
INR: International Normalized Ratio
MMP: matrix metalloproteinase
NSAID: nonsteroidal anti-inflammatory drug
OA: osteoarthritis
PG: proteoglycan
TIMP: tissue inhibitor of metalloproteinases
VIGOR: Vioxx Gastrointestinal Outcomes Research Study

Review Questions and other resources can be found at *www.pharmacotherapyonline.com.*

REFERENCES

1. ACR Subcommittee on Osteoarthritis Guidelines. Recommendations for the medical management of osteoarthritis of the hip and knee: 2000 update. Arthritis Rheum 2000;43:1905–1915.

2. Solomon L. Clinical features of osteoarthritis. In: Kelly WN, Harris ED, Ruddy S, Sledge CB, eds. Textbook of Rheumatology, 6th ed. Philadelphia, Saunders, 2001:1409–1418.

3. Felson DT, Lawrence RC, Dieppe PA, Hirsch R, et al. Osteoarthritis: New insights. Part 1: The disease and its risk factors. Ann Intern Med 2000;133:635–646.

4. Lawrence RC, Helmick CG, Arnett FC, et al. Estimates of the prevalence of arthritis and selected musculoskeletal disorders in the United States. Arthritis Rheum 1998;41:778–799.

5. Jakobsson U, Hallberg IR. Pain and quality of life among older people with rheumatoid arthritis and/or osteoarthritis: A literature review. J Clin Nurs 2002;11:430–443.

6. Walker-Bone K, Javaid K, Arden N, Cooper C. Regular review: Medical management of osteoarthritis. BMJ 2000;321:936–940.

7. Pendleton A, Arden N, Dougados M, et al. EULAR recommendations for the management of knee osteoarthritis: Report of a task force of the Standing Committee for International Clinical Studies Including Therapeutic Trials (ESCISIT). Ann Rheumc Dis 2000;59:936–944.

8. Manek NJ. Medical management of osteoarthritis. Mayo Clinic Proc 2001;76:533–539.

9. Fransen M, McConnell S, Bell M. Exercise for osteoarthritis of the hip or knee. Cochrane Database Syst Rev 2003;3:CD004286.

10. Bischoff HA, Roos EM. Effectiveness and safety of strengthening, aerobic, and coordination exercises for patients with osteoarthritis. Curr Opin Rheumatol 2003;15:141–144.

11. American Geriatrics Society Panel on Exercise and Osteoarthritis. Exercise prescription for older adults with osteoarthritis pain: Consensus practice recommendations. J Am Geriatr Soc 2001;49:808–823.

12. Lievense AM, Bierma-Zeinstra SM, Verhagen AP, et al. Influence of obesity on the development of osteoarthritis of the hip: A systematic review. Rheumatology 2002;41:1155–1162.

13. Gelber AC, Hochberg MC, Mead LA, et al. Body mass index in young men and the risk of subsequent knee and hip osteoarthritis. Am J Med 1999;107:542–548.

14. Schouten JS, de Bie RA, Swaen G. An update on the relationship between occupational factors and osteoarthritis of the hip and knee. Curr Opin Rheumatol 2002;14:89–92.

15. McAlindon TE, Wilson PWF, Aliabadi P, et al. Level of physical activity and the risk of radiographic and symptomatic knee osteoarthritis in the elderly: The Framingham study. Am J Med 1999;106:151–157.

16. Hurley MV. The role of muscle weakness in the pathogenesis of osteoarthritis. Rheum Dis Clin North Am 1999;25:283–298.

17. Scott Simonet W. Genetics of primary generalized osteoarthritis. Mol Genet Metab 2002;77:31–34.

18. Lane NE, Nevitt MC. Osteoarthritis, bone mass, and fractures: How are they related? Arthritis Rheum 2002;46:1–4.

19. Kraus VB. Pathogenesis and treatment of osteoarthritis. Med Clin North Am 1997;81:85–112.

20. Mankin HJ, Brandt KD. Pathogenesis of osteoarthritis. In: Kelly WN, Harris ED, Ruddy S, Sledge CB, eds. Textbook of Rheumatology, 6th ed. Philadelphia, Saunders, 2001:1391–1408.

21. Lajeunesse D, Reboul P. Subchondral bone in osteoarthritis: A biologic link with articular cartilage leading to abnormal remodeling. Curr Opin Rheumatol 2003;15:628–633.

22. Mazzuca S. Plain radiography in the evaluation of knee osteoarthritis. Curr Opin Rheumatol 1997;9:263–267.

23. Yoshihara Y, Nakamura H, Obata K, et al. Matrix metalloproteinases and tissue inhibitors of metalloproteinases in synovial fluids from patients with rheumatoid arthritis or osteoarthritis. Ann Rheum Dis 2000;59:455–461.

24. Freemont AJ, Byers RJ, Taiwo YO, et al. In situ zymographic localisation of type II collagen degrading activity in osteoarthritic human articular cartilage. Ann Rheum Dis 1999;58:357–365.

25. Burr DA, Schaffler MB. The involvement of subchondral mineralized tissues in osteoarthritis: Quantitative microscopic evidence. Microsc Res Tech 1997;37:343–357.

26. Mansell JP, Bailey AJ. Abnormal cancellous bone collagen metabolism in osteoarthritis. J Clin Invest 1998;101:1596–1603.

27. Creamer P. Osteoarthritis pain and its treatment. Curr Opin Rheumatol 2000;12:450–455.

28. Ravaud P, Dougados M. Radiographic assessment in osteoarthritis. J Rheumatol 1997;24:786–791.

29. Reginster JY, Deroisy R, Rovati LC, et al. Long-term effects of glucosamine sulphate on osteoarthritis progression: A randomised, placebo-controlled clinical trial. Lancet 2001;357:251–256.

30. McAlindon TE, LaValley MP, Gulin JP, et al. Glucosamine and chondroitin for treatment of osteoarthritis: A systematic quality assessment and meta-analysis. JAMA 2000;283:1469.

31. Penninx BW, Messier SP, Rejeski WJ, et al. Physical exercise and the prevention of disability in activities of daily living in older persons with osteoarthritis. Arch Intern Med 2001;161:2309–2316.

32. O'Reilly SC, Muir KR, Doherty M. Effectiveness of home exercise on pain and disability from osteoarthritis of the knee: A randomised controlled trial. Ann Rheum Dis 1999;58:15–19.

33. National Institutes of Health. Total hip replacement. NIH Consensus Statement 1994;12:1–31.

34. Dieppe P, Basler H-D, Chard J, et al. Knee replacement surgery for osteoarthritis: Effectiveness, practice variations, indications and possible determinants of utilization. Rheumatology 1999;38:73–38.

35. Moseley JB, O'Malley K, Petersen NJ, et al. A controlled trial of arthroscopic surgery for osteoarthritis of the knee. N Engl J Med 2002;347:81–88.

36. Jorgensen C, Noel D, Apparailly F, Sany J. Stem cells for repair of cartilage and bone: The next challenge in osteoarthritis and rheumatoid arthritis. Ann Rheum Dis 2001;60:305–309.

37. Towheed TE, Judd MJ, Hochberg MC, Wells G. Acetaminophen for osteoarthritis. Cochrane Database Syst Rev 2003;2:CD004257.

38. Henrich WL, Agodoa LE, Barrett B, et al. Analgesics and the kidney: Summary recommendations to the Scientific Advisory Board of the National Kidney Foundation from an ad hoc committee of the National Kidney Foundation. Am J Kidney Dis 1996;27:162–165.

39. Eccles M, Freemantle N, Mason J, for the North of England Non-Steroidal Anti-Inflammatory Drug Guideline Development Group. North of England Evidence Based Guideline Development Project: Summary guideline for nonsteroidal anti-inflammatory drugs versus basic analgesia in treating the pain of degenerative arthritis. Br Med J 1998;317:526–530.

40. Pincus T, Swearingen C, Cummins P, et al. Preference for nonsteroidal anti-inflammatory drugs versus acetaminophen and concomitant use of both types of drugs in patients with osteoarthritis. J Rheumatol 2000;27:1020–1027.

41. Schnitzer TJ. Non-NSAID pharmacologic treatment options for the management of chronic pain. Am J Med 1998;105:45S–52S.

42. Fored CM, Ejerblad E, Lindblad P, et al. Acetaminophen, aspirin, and chronic renal failure. N Engl J Med 2001;345:1801–1808.

43. Pepper GA. Nonsteroidal anti-inflammatory drugs: New perspectives on a familiar drug class. Rheumatology 2000;35:223–244.

44. Hawkey CJ. COX-2 inhibitors. Lancet 1999;353:307–314.

45. Golden BD, Abramson SB. Selective cyclooxygenase-2 inhibitors. Rheum Dis Clin North Am 1999;25:359–378.

46. Garavito RM, DeWitt DL. The cyclooxygenase isoforms: Structural insights into the conversion of arachidonic acid to prostaglandins. Biochim Biophys Acta 1999;1441:278–287.

47. Jones MK, Wang H, Peskar BM, et al. Inhibition of angiogenesis by nonsteroidal anti-inflammatory drugs: Insight into mechanisms and implications for cancer growth and ulcer healing. Nature Med 1999;5:1418–1423.

48. Wolfe MM, Lichenstein DR, Singh G. Medical progress: Gastrointestinal toxicity of nonsteroidal anti-inflammatory drugs. N Engl J Med 1999;340:1888–1899.

49. Lichtenstein DR, Wolfe MM. COX-2-selective NSAIDs: New and improved? JAMA 2000;284:1297–1299.

50. Crofford LJ, Lipsky PE, Brooks P, et al. Basic biology and clinical application of specific cyclooxygenase-2 inhibitors. Arthritis Rheum 2000; 43:4–13.

51. Mukherjee D, Nissen SE, Topol EJ. Risk of cardiovascular events associated with selective COX-2 inhibitors. JAMA 2001;286:954–959.

52. Anonymous. Vioxx lack of cardioprotection may offset GI benefit in at-risk group. FDC Reports 2001;63:3–4.

53. Berenguer B, Alarcon de la Lastra C, Moreno FJ, Martin MJ. Chronic gastric ulcer healing in rats subjected to selective and nonselective cyclooxygenase-2 inhibitors. Eur J Pharmacol 2002;442:125–135.

54. Brzozowski T, Konturek PC, Konturek SJ, et al. Role of prostaglandins generated by cyclooxygenase-1 and cyclooxygenase-2 in healing of ischemia-reperfusion-induced gastric lesions. Eur J Pharmacol 1996; 385:47–61.

55. Silverstein FE, Faich G, Goldstein JL, et al. Gastrointestinal toxicity with celecoxib vs nonsteroidal anti-inflammatory drugs for osteoarthritis and rheumatoid arthritis: The CLASS study. A randomized, controlled trial. JAMA 2000;284:1247–1255.

56. Towheed T, Shea B, Wells G, et al. Analgesia and nonaspirin, nonsteroidal anti-inflammatory drugs of osteoarthritis of the hip. Cochrane Database of Systematic Reviews. (2) CD000517, 2000.

57. Hochberg MC. New directions in symptomatic therapy for patients with osteoarthritis and rheumatoid arthritis. Semin Arthritis Rheum 2002; 32(3 Suppl 1):4–14.

58. Cannon GW, Caldwell JR, Holt P, et al. Rofecoxib, a specific inhibitor of cyclooxygenase 2, with clinical efficacy comparable with that of diclofenac sodium: Results of a one-year, randomized, clinical trial in patients with osteoarthritis of the knee and hip. Arthritis Rheum 2000;43: 978–987.

59. Bensen WG, Fiechtner JJ, McMillen JI, et al. Treatment of osteoarthritis with celecoxib, a cyclooxygenase-2 inhibitor: A randomized controlled trial. Mayo Clin Proc 1999;74:1095–1105.

60. Ormrod D, Wellington K, Wagstaff AJ. Valdecoxib. Drugs 2002;62: 2059–2071, discussion 2072–2073.

61. Singh G, Ramey DR, Morfeld D, et al. Gastrointestinal tract complications of nonsteroidal anti-inflammatory drug treatment in rheumatoid arthritis: A prospective observational cohort study. Arch Intern Med 1996;156:1530–1536.

62. American College of Rheumatology Ad Hoc Committee on Clinical Guidelines. Guidelines for monitoring drug therapy in rheumatoid arthritis. Arthritis Rheum 1996;39:723–731.

63. Hawkey CJ, Karrasch JA, Szczepanski L, et al. Omeprazole compared with misoprostol for ulcer associated with nonsteroidal anti-inflammatory drugs. N Engl J Med 1998;338:727–734.

64. Simon LS, Weaver AL, Graham DY, et al. Anti-inflammatory and upper gastrointestinal effects of celecoxib in rheumatoid arthritis: A randomized controlled trial. JAMA 1999;282:1921–1928.

65. Hawkey C, Laine L, Simon T, et al, for the Rofecoxib Osteoarthritis Endoscopy Multinational Study Group. Comparison of the effect of rofecoxib (a cyclooxygenase 2 inhibitor), ibuprofen, and placebo on the gastroduodenal mucosa of patients with osteoarthritis. Arthritis Rheum 2000;43:370–377.

66. Pavelka K, Recker DP, Verburg KM. Valdecoxib is as effective as diclofenac in the management of rheumatoid arthritis with a lower incidence of gastroduodenal ulcers: Results of a 26-week trial. Rheumatology 2003;42:1207–1215.

67. Chavez ML, DeKorte CJ. Valdecoxib: A review. Clin Ther 2003;25: 817–851.

68. Wright JM. The double-edged sword of COX-2 selective NSAIDs. Can Med Assoc J 2002;167:1131–1137.

69. Witter J. Celebrex capsules (Celecoxib) NDA 20-998/S-009 Medical Officer Review. September 20, 2000. http://www.fda.gov/ohrms/dockets/ac/01/briefing/3677b1_03_med.pdf, accessed February 24, 2004.

70. Langman JM, Jensen DM, Watson DJ, et al. Adverse upper gastrointestinal effects of rofecoxib compared with NSAIDs. JAMA 1999;282: 1929–1933.

71. Bombardier C, Laine L, Reicin A, et al. Comparison of upper gastrointestinal toxicity of rofecoxib and naproxen in patients with rheumatoid arthritis. N Engl J Med 2000;343:1520–1528.

72. Goldstein JL, Zhao SZ, Burke TA, et al. Incidence of outpatient physician claims for upper gastrointestinal symptoms among new users of celecoxib, ibuprofen, and naproxen in an insured population in the United States. Am J Gastroenterol 2003;98:2627–2634.

73. Chan FK, Hung LC, Suen BY, et al. Celecoxib versus diclofenac and omeprazole in reducing the risk of recurrent ulcer bleeding in patients with arthritis. N Engl J Med 2002;347:2104–2110.

74. Whelton A. Nephrotoxicity of nonsteroidal anti-inflammatory drugs: Physiologic foundations and clinical implications. Am J Med 1999;106: 13S–24S.

75. Rossat J, Maillard M, Nussberger J, et al. Renal effects of selective cyclooxygenase-2 inhibition in normotensive salt-depleted subjects. Clin Pharmacol Ther 1999;66:76–84.

76. Martin-Garcia C, Hinjosa M, Berges P, et al. Safety of cyclooxygenase-2 inhibitor in patients with aspirin-sensitive asthma. Chest 2002;121: 1812–1817.

77. Woessner KM, Simon RA, Stevenson DD. The safety of celecoxib in patients with aspirin-sensitive asthma. Arthritis Rheum 2002;8: 2201–2206.

78. Dahlen B, Szczeklik A, Murray JJ. Celecoxib in patients with asthma and aspirin intolerance. N Engl J Med 2001;344:142.

79. Leese PT, Recker DP, Kent JD. The COX-2 selective inhibitor, valdecoxib, does not impair platelet function in the elderly: Results of a randomized controlled trial. J Clin Pharmacol 2003;43:504–513.

80. Garnett WR. Clinical implications of drug interactions with coxibs. Pharmacotherapy 2001;21:1223–1232.

81. Reginster JY, Bruyere O, Lecart MP, Henrotin Y. Naturocetic (glucosamine and chondroitin sulfate) compounds as structure-modifying drugs in the treatment of osteoarthritis. Curr Opin Rheumatol 2003;15: 651–655.

82. Morreale P, Manopulo R, Galati M, et al. Comparison of the anti-inflammatory efficacy of chondroitin sulfate and diclofenac sodium in patients with knee osteoarthritis. J Rheumatol 1996;23:1385–1391.

83. Richy F, Bruyere O, Ethgen O, et al. Structural and symptomatic efficacy of glucosamine and chondroitin in knee osteoarthritis: A comprehensive meta-analysis. Arch Intern Med 2003;163):1514–1522.

84. Uebelhart D, Thonar E, Delmas DP, et al. Effects of oral chondroitin sulfate on the progression of knee osteoarthritis: A pilot study. Osteoarthritis Cartilage 1998;6(Suppl A):39–46.

85. Bruyere O, Compere S, Rovati LC, et al. Five-year follow up of patients from a previous 3-year randomized, controlled trial of glucosamine sulfate in knee osteoarthritis. Arthritis Rheum 2003;48:S80.

86. Volpi N. Oral bioavailability of chondroitin sulfate (Condrosulf) and its constituents in healthy male volunteers. Osteoarthritis Cartilage 2002;10:768–777.

87. Raynauld JP, Buckland-Wright C, Ward R, et al. Safety and efficacy of long-term intraarticular steroid injections in osteoarthritis of the knee. Arthritis Rheum 2003;48:370–377.

88. Hochberg MC. Role of intra-articular hyaluronic acid preparations in medical management of osteoarthritis of the knee. Semin Arthritis Rheum 2000;30(2 Suppl 1):2–10.

89. Uthman I, Raynauld JP, Haraoui B. Intra-articular therapy in osteoarthritis. Postgrad Med J 2003;79:449–453.

90. Hammesfahr JF, Knopf AB, Stitik T. Safety of intra-articular hyaluronates for pain associated with osteoarthritis of the knee. Am J Orthop 2003;32:277–283.

91. Brandt KD. Second-line drug therapy for osteoarthritis. Clin Med 2001; 1:110–112.

92. Smith GN Jr, Yu LP Jr, Brandt KD, et al. Oral administration of doxycycline reduces collagenase and gelatinase activities in extracts of human osteoarthritic cartilage. J Rheumatol 1998;25:532–535.

93. Brandt KD, Mazzuca SA, Katz BP, Lane KA. Doxycycline (Doxy) Slows the Rate of Joint Space Narrowing (JSN) in Patients with Knee Osteoarthritis (OA). American College of Rheumatology 68th Annual Meeting, San Antonio, Texas, October 21–28, 2003. Abstract LB22.

94. Ghosh P. The pathobiology of osteoarthritis and the rationale for the use of pentosan polysulfate for its treatment. Semin Arthritis Rheum 1999; 28:211–267.

95. Skelly MM, Hawkey CJ. Potential alternatives to COX 2 inhibitors. BMJ 2002;324:1289–1290.

96. Kivitz A, Ma C, Ahdieh H. Oxymorphone extended release improves pain and quality of life in patients with osteoarthritis: Results of a dose-ranging study. Arthritis Rheum 2003;48:S485 (abstract).

97. Ferraz MB, Maetzel A, Bombardier C. A summary of economic evaluations published in the field of rheumatology and related disciplines. Arthritis Rheum 1997;40:1587–1593.

98. Gabriel SE, Crowson CS, Campion ME, et al. Indirect and nonmedical costs among people with rheumatoid arthritis and osteoarthritis compared with nonarthritic controls. J Rheumatol 1997;24:43–48.

99. Maetzel A, Ferraz MB, Bombardier C. The cost-effectiveness of miso-prostol in preventing serious gastrointestinal events associated with the use of nonsteroidal anti-inflammatory drugs. Arthritis Rheum 1998; 41:16–25.

100. Lanes SF, Lanza LL, Radensky PW, et al. Resource utilization and cost of care for rheumatoid arthritis and osteoarthritis in a managed care setting: The importance of drug and surgery costs. Arthritis Rheum 1997;40:1475–1481.

101. Peterson WL, Cryer B. COX-1-sparing NSAIDs: Is the enthusiasm justified? JAMA 1999;282:1961–1963.

102. Maetzel A, Krahn M, Naglie G. The cost effectiveness of rofecoxib and celecoxib in patients with osteoarthritis or rheumatoid arthritis. Arthritis Rheum 2003;49:283–292.

103. Spiegel BM, Targownik L, Dulai GS, Gralnek IM. The cost-effectiveness of cyclooxygenase-2 selective inhibitors in the management of chronic arthritis. Ann Intern Med 2003;138:795–806.

91

GOUT AND HYPERURICEMIA

David W. Hawkins and Daniel W. Rahn

Learning Objectives and other resources can be found at *www.pharmacotherapyonline.com.*

KEY CONCEPTS

◀1 Asymptomatic hyperuricemia discovered incidentally requires no therapy.

◀2 Acute gouty arthritis may be treated effectively with short courses of high-dose nonacetylated nonsteroidal anti-inflammatory drugs (NSAIDs) or colchicine.

◀3 Intravenous colchicine is rapidly effective but cannot be administered to individuals with renal impairment or extrahepatic biliary obstruction. A single intravenous dose should not exceed 2 to 3 mg, with a cumulative total dose not exceeding 4 to 5 mg per episode.

◀4 Individuals with contraindications to NSAIDs (e.g., active peptic ulcer disease, renal impairment, heart failure, or history of hypersensitivity) or individuals who cannot ingest medications orally may be treated with intravenous corticosteroids or intra-articular corticosteroids.

◀5 Recurrent attacks of gouty arthritis can be prevented effectively through administration of uric acid–lowering therapy.

◀6 Treatment with urate-lowering drugs is considered cost effective for acute gouty arthritis in patients having two or more attacks of gout per year.

◀7 When allopurinol is used for prophylaxis, start with a low dose (100 mg/day) after the acute attack has settled, and adjust the dose every 4 weeks until the goal is reached (serum urate of <6 mg/dL). Give colchicine (0.5 mg twice daily) during the first 3 months of therapy, and stop allopurinol if rash develops or liver function tests become abnormal.

◀8 Uricosuric agents should be avoided in patients with renal impairment (a creatinine clearance below 50 mL/min), a history of renal calculi, and overproduction of uric acid.

◀9 Uric acid nephrolithiasis should be treated with adequate hydration (2 to 3 L/day), a daytime urine-alkalinizing agent, and a 250-mg bedtime dose of acetazolamide.

◀10 Individuals with tophaceous deposits have a large uric acid pool and benefit from allopurinol administration.

The term *gout* describes a disease spectrum including hyperuricemia, recurrent attacks of acute arthritis associated with monosodium urate crystals in leukocytes found in synovial fluid, deposits of monosodium urate crystals in tissues (tophi), interstitial renal disease, and uric acid nephrolithiasis.[1]

Hyperuricemia may be an asymptomatic condition with an increased serum uric acid level as the only apparent abnormality. Statistically, hyperuricemia is defined as serum urate concentrations greater than two standard deviations above the population mean. However, for determination of the risk for gout, hyperuricemia is defined as a supersaturated urate concentration.[2] By this definition, a urate concentration greater than 7.0 mg/dL is abnormal and is associated with an increased risk for gout. This corresponds to a measured value greater than 7.5 mg/dL by most autoanalyzers.

EPIDEMIOLOGY

Population studies have shown that serum urate concentration (and consequently the risk of gout) correlates with age, serum creatinine level, blood urea nitrogen level, male gender, blood pressure, body weight, and alcohol intake. Serum urate concentrations are normally distributed with slight skewing toward higher values. In gout, mean serum urate concentration values are 6.8 mg/dL for men and 6.0 mg/dL for women.

There is a direct correlation between the serum uric acid concentration and both the incidence and prevalence of gout. The incidence of gout varies from 20 to 35 per 100,000 persons, with an overall prevalence of 1.6 to 13.6 per thousand. Prevalence increases with age, especially in men.[1] Men are affected by gout approximately 10 times more often than women. Although no genetic marker has been isolated for gout, the familial nature of gout strongly suggests an interaction between genetic and environmental factors.

ETIOLOGY AND PATHOPHYSIOLOGY

In humans, uric acid is the end product of the degradation of purines. Uric acid serves no known physiologic purpose and therefore is regarded as a waste product. In lower animals, the enzyme uricase breaks down uric acid to the more soluble allantoin, and thus uric acid does not accumulate. Gout occurs exclusively in humans in whom a miscible pool of uric acid exists. Under normal conditions, the amount of accumulated uric acid is about 1200 mg in men and about 600 mg in women. The size of the urate pool is increased severalfold in individuals with gout. This excess accumulation may result from either overproduction or underexcretion.

OVERPRODUCTION OF URIC ACID

The purines from which uric acid is produced originate from three sources: dietary purine, conversion of tissue nucleic acid to purine nucleotides, and de novo synthesis of purine bases. The purines derived from these three sources enter a common metabolic pathway leading to the production of either nucleic acid or uric acid. Under normal circumstances, uric acid may accumulate excessively if production exceeds excretion. The average human produces about 600 to 800 mg of uric acid each day.

Several enzyme systems regulate purine metabolism. Abnormalities in these regulatory systems can result in overproduction of uric acid.[3] Uric acid also may be overproduced as a consequence of increased breakdown of tissue nucleic acids, as with myeloproliferative and lymphoproliferative disorders. Dietary purines play an unimportant role in the generation of hyperuricemia in the absence of some derangement in purine metabolism or elimination.

Two enzyme abnormalities resulting in an overproduction of uric acid have been well described (Fig. 91–1). The first is an increase in the activity of phosphoribosyl pyrophosphate (PRPP) synthetase, which leads to an increased concentration of PRPP. PRPP is a key determinant of purine synthesis and thus uric acid production. The second is a deficiency of hypoxanthine guanine phosphoribosyl transferase (HGPRT).

HGPRT is responsible for the conversion of guanine to guanylic acid and hypoxanthine to inosinic acid. These two conversions require PRPP as the cosubstrate and are important reutilization reactions involved in the synthesis of nucleic acids. A deficiency in the HGPRT enzyme leads to increased metabolism of guanine and hypoxanthine to uric acid, and more PRPP to interact with glutamine in the first step of the purine pathway.[4] Complete absence of HGPRT results in the childhood Lesch-Nyhan syndrome, characterized by choreoathetosis, spasticity, mental retardation, and markedly excessive production of uric acid. A partial deficiency of the enzyme may be responsible for marked hyperuricemia in otherwise normal, healthy individuals.

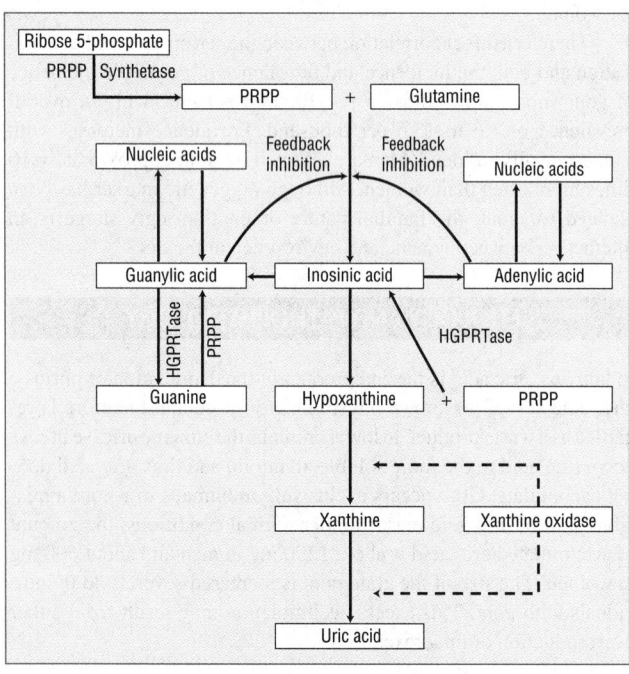

FIGURE 91–1. Purine metabolism.

TABLE 91–1. Conditions Associated with Hyperuricemia

Primary gout	Obesity
Diabetic ketoacidosis	Sarcoidosis
Myeloproliferative disorders	Congestive heart failure
Lactic acidosis	Renal dysfunction
Lymphoproliferative disorders	Down syndrome
Starvation	Lead toxicity
Chronic hemolytic anemia	Hyperparathyroidism
Toxemia of pregnancy	Acute alcoholism
Pernicious anemia	Hypoparathyroidism
Glycogen storage disease type 1	Acromegaly
Psoriasis	Hypothyroidism

UNDEREXCRETION OF URIC ACID

Uric acid does not accumulate as long as uric acid production is balanced with elimination. Uric acid is eliminated in two ways. About two-thirds of the uric acid produced each day is excreted in the urine. The rest is eliminated through the gastrointestinal tract after enzymatic degradation by colonic bacteria.

A decline in the urinary excretion of uric acid to a level below the rate of production leads to hyperuricemia and an increased miscible pool of sodium urate. Almost all the urate in plasma is freely filtered across the glomerulus. The concentration of uric acid appearing in the urine is determined by multiple renal tubular transport processes in addition to the filtered load. Evidence favors a four-component model including glomerular filtration, tubular reabsorption, tubular secretion, and postsecretory reabsorption.[2]

Approximately 90% of filtered uric acid is reabsorbed in the proximal tubule, probably by both active and passive transport mechanisms. There is a close linkage between proximal tubular sodium reabsorption and uric acid reabsorption, so states that enhance sodium reabsorption (e.g., dehydration) also lead to increased uric acid reabsorption. The exact site of tubular secretion of uric acid has not been determined; this too appears to involve an active transport process. Postsecretory reabsorption occurs somewhere distal to the secretory site.

Factors that decrease uric acid clearance or increase its production will result in an increase in serum urate concentration. Some of these factors are listed in Table 91–1. Drugs that decrease renal clearance of uric acid through modification of filtered load or one of the tubular transport processes are listed in Table 91–2. By enhancing renal urate reabsorption, insulin resistance is also associated with gout.[5]

The pathophysiologic approach to the evaluation of hyperuricemia requires determining whether the patient is overproducing or underexcreting uric acid. This can be accomplished by placing the patient on a purine-free diet for 3 to 5 days and then measuring the amount of uric acid excreted in the urine in 24 hours. Normal individuals produce 600 to 800 mg of uric acid daily and excrete less than 600 mg in urine. Individuals who excrete more than 600 mg on a purine-free diet may be considered overproducers. Hyperuricemic individuals who excrete less than 600 mg of uric acid per 24 hours

TABLE 91–2. Drugs Capable of Inducing Hyperuricemia and Gout

Diuretics	Ethanol	Ethambutol
Nicotinic acid	Pyrazinamide	Cytotoxic drugs
Salicylates (<2 g/day)	Levodopa	Cyclosporine

n a purine-free diet may be classified as underexcretors of uric acid. However, it is very difficult in clinical practice to maintain someone on a purine-free diet for several days. On a regular diet, excretion of greater than 1000 mg per 24 hours reflects overproduction; less than this is probably normal.

PRESENTATION OF ACUTE GOUTY ARTHRITIS

GENERAL
Gout typically involves acute attacks of arthritis, nephrolithiasis, gouty nephropathy, and aggregated deposits of sodium urate (tophi) in cartilage, tendons, synovial membranes, and elsewhere.

SIGNS AND SYMPTOMS
Fever; intense pain, erythema, warmth, and swelling of involved joints
Excruciating pain, swelling, and inflammation involving one or more joints, most commonly starting in the great toe, but sometimes involving other joints of the extremities

LABORATORY TESTS
Elevated serum uric acid levels; leukocytosis

OTHER DIAGNOSTIC TESTS
None

CLINICAL PRESENTATION

Gout is a disease diagnosed by symptoms rather than laboratory tests of uric acid. In fact, asymptomatic hyperuricemia discovered incidentally generally requires no therapy.

ACUTE GOUTY ARTHRITIS

Acute attacks of gouty arthritis are characterized by rapid onset of excruciating pain, swelling, and inflammation. The attack typically is nonarticular at first, most often affecting the first metatarsophalangeal joint (great toe) and then, in order of frequency, the insteps, ankles, heels, knees, wrists, fingers, and elbows. In one-half of initial attacks, the first metatarsophalangeal joint is affected. Of gouty patients, 90% experience attacks in the great toe at some point in their disease.

The predilection of acute gout for peripheral joints of the lower extremity is probably related to the low temperature of these joints combined with high intra-articular urate concentration. Synovial effusions are postulated to occur transiently in weight-bearing joints in the course of a day with routine activity. At night, water is reabsorbed from the joint space, leaving behind a supersaturated solution of monosodium urate, which can precipitate attacks of acute arthritis. Attacks generally begin at night with the patient awakening from sleep in excruciating pain.

The development of crystal-induced inflammation involves a number of chemical mediators causing vasodilation, increased vascular permeability, and chemotactic activity for polymorphonuclear leukocytes.[6] Phagocytosis of urate crystals by the leukocytes results in rapid lysis of cells and a discharge of proteolytic enzymes into the cytoplasm. The ensuing inflammatory reaction is associated with intense joint pain, erythema, warmth, and swelling. Fever is common, as is leukocytosis. Untreated attacks may last from 3 to 14 days before spontaneous recovery.

Although acute attacks of gouty arthritis may occur without apparent provocation, a number of conditions may precipitate an attack. These include stress, trauma, alcohol ingestion, infection, surgery, rapid lowering of serum uric acid by ingestion of uric acid–lowering agents, and ingestion of certain drugs known to elevate serum uric acid concentrations. The diagnosis is best accomplished by aspiration of synovial fluid from the affected joint and identification of intracellular crystals of monosodium urate monohydrate in synovial fluid leukocytes. Other crystal-induced arthropathies that may resemble gout on clinical presentation are caused by calcium pyrophosphate dihydrate crystals (pseudogout) and calcium hydroxyapatite crystals, which are associated with calcific periarthritis, tendinitis, and arthritis.[7,8]

URIC ACID NEPHROLITHIASIS

Nephrolithiasis occurs in 10% to 25% of patients with gout.[9] Factors that predispose individuals to uric acid nephrolithiasis include excessive urinary excretion of uric acid, an acidic urine, and a highly concentrated urine. The risk of renal calculi approaches 50% in individuals whose renal excretion of uric acid exceeds 1100 mg/day. In addition to pure uric acid stones, hyperuricosuric individuals are at increased risk for mixed uric acid–calcium oxalate stones and pure calcium oxalate stones. Uric acid stones are usually small, round, and radiolucent. Uric acid stones containing calcium are radiopaque.[9]

Uric acid has a negative logarithm of the acid ionization constant of 5.5. Therefore when the urine is acidic, uric acid exists primarily in the un-ionized, less soluble form. At a urine pH of 5.0, urine is saturated at a uric acid level of 15 mg/dL. When the urine pH is 7.0, the solubility of uric acid in urine is increased to 200 mg/dL.[10] In patients with uric acid nephrolithiasis, urinary pH typically is less than 6.0 and frequently less than 5.5. When an acidic urine is saturated with uric acid, spontaneous precipitation of stones may occur.

GOUTY NEPHROPATHY

There are two types of gouty nephropathy: acute uric acid nephropathy and chronic urate nephropathy.[11] In acute uric acid nephropathy, acute renal failure occurs as a result of blockage of urine flow secondary to massive precipitation of uric acid crystals in the collecting ducts and ureters. This syndrome is a well-recognized complication in patients with myeloproliferative or lymphoproliferative disorders and is a result of massive malignant cell turnover, particularly after initiation of chemotherapy.

Chronic urate nephropathy is caused by the long-term deposition of urate crystals in the renal parenchyma. Microtophi may form, with a surrounding giant cell inflammatory reaction. A decrease in the kidney's ability to concentrate urine and the presence of proteinuria may be the earliest pathophysiologic disturbances. Hypertension and nephrosclerosis are common associated findings. Although renal failure occurs in a higher percentage of gouty patients than expected, it is not clear that hyperuricemia per se has a harmful effect on the kidney. The chronic renal impairment seen in individuals with gout may result largely from the co-occurrence of hypertension, diabetes mellitus, and atherosclerosis.

TOPHACEOUS GOUT

Tophi (urate deposits) are uncommon in the general population of gouty subjects and are a late complication of hyperuricemia. The most common sites of tophaceous deposits in patients with recurrent acute gouty arthritis are the base of the great toe, helix of the ear, olecranon bursae, Achilles tendon, knees, wrists, and hands.[2] Eventually, even the hips, shoulders, and spine may be affected. In addition to causing obvious deformities, tophi may damage surrounding soft tissue, cause joint destruction and pain, and even lead to nerve compression syndromes including carpal tunnel syndrome.

▶ TREATMENT: Gout and Hyperuricemia

The goals in the treatment of gout are to terminate the acute attack, prevent recurrent attacks of gouty arthritis, and prevent complications associated with chronic deposition of urate crystals in tissues.[12] Patients should be advised to reduce their dietary intake of saturated fats and meats high in purines (e.g., organ meats).[13]

■ ACUTE GOUTY ARTHRITIS

Acute attacks of gouty arthritis may be treated successfully with colchicine or any of a variety of nonsteroidal anti-inflammatory drugs (NSAIDs) (Fig. 91–2).

Colchicine can be given orally or parenterally. Unless contraindications exist or the patient has renal insufficiency, the usual oral dose is 1 mg initially, followed by 0.5 mg every 2 hours until the joint symptoms subside, until the patient develops abdominal discomfort or diarrhea, or until a total dose of 8 mg has been administered.[14] About 75% to 95% of patients with acute gouty arthritis respond favorably to colchicine when ingestion of the drug is begun within 24 to 48 hours of the onset of joint symptoms.[15] If the initiation of colchicine is delayed longer than 48 hours after the onset of acute symptoms, the probability of success with the drug diminishes substantially.

The major problem associated with the use of oral colchicine is that it causes gastrointestinal side effects in 50% to 80% of patients before the relief of the attack.

This high incidence of gastrointestinal side effects may be circumvented by administering colchicine intravenously. Except in patients with renal insufficiency, the initial intravenous dose of colchicine is 2 mg. If relief is not obtained, an additional 1-mg dose may be given at 6 and 12 hours to a total dose of 4 mg for a specific attack. The colchicine should be diluted with 20 mL normal saline before administration to minimize sclerosis of the vein. The intravenous administration of colchicine eliminates most of the gastrointestinal symptoms associated with the oral dose, but subjects the patient to the risk of local extravasation, which can cause inflammation in and necrosis of the surrounding tissue. Very small, difficult-to-inject veins and renal impairment represent relative contraindications to intravenous colchicine therapy.

Because of the risk of bone marrow toxicity, colchicine should be discontinued for 7 days following initial therapy with either oral or intravenous administration. Colchicine should not be used intravenously in individuals who are neutropenic, have severe renal impairment (a creatinine clearance of <10 mL/min), or have combined renal and hepatic insufficiency. The dose should be decreased by 50% in individuals with renal insufficiency (a creatinine clearance of 10 to 50 mL/min) and limited to a total dose of 2 mg in patients receiving oral maintenance colchicine.[16]

Indomethacin is as effective as colchicine in the treatment of acute gouty arthritis. Because acute gastrointestinal toxicity occurs far less frequently with indomethacin than with colchicine, it is preferred. Side effects unique to indomethacin include headache and dizziness. All NSAIDs have been implicated in the cause of gastric ulceration and bleeding, but with short-term therapy, this is not likely.

For treatment of acute gouty arthritis, indomethacin may be begun with a relatively large dose for the first 24 to 48 hours and then tapered over 3 to 4 days to minimize the risk of recurrent attacks. For example, 75 mg of indomethacin should be given initially, followed by 50 mg every 6 hours for 2 days and then 50 mg every 8 hours for 1 or 2 days.

A number of other NSAIDs (e.g., naproxen, fenoprofen, ibuprofen, and piroxicam) are also effective in relieving the inflammation of acute gout. There is no evidence that any given NSAID is superior to all the others in the management of acute gout.[17] All NSAIDs should be used with caution in individuals with a history of acid peptic disease, heart failure, chronic renal failure, or coronary artery disease. Selective cyclooxygenase-2 inhibitors, such as celecoxib and valdecoxib, can be used as an alternative for patients who cannot tolerate nonselective cyclooxygenase inhibitors (see note at end of Chap. 90 for information on problems with these agents that emerged while this chapter was in production).[18]

Corticosteroids may be used to treat acute attacks of gouty arthritis, but they are reserved primarily for resistant cases or for patients with a contraindication to colchicine and NSAID therapy.[17] Doses of 40 to 80 USP units of adrenocorticotropic hormone gel are given intramuscularly every 6 to 8 hours for 2 to 3 days, and then the doses are reduced in stepwise fashion and discontinued. Intraarticular administration of triamcinolone hexacetonide in a dose of 20 to 40 mg may be useful in treating acute gout limited to one or two joints.[19] Prednisone may be administered orally in doses of 30 to 60 mg for 3 to 5 days in patients with multiple-joint involvement. Because rebound attacks may occur on steroid withdrawal, the dose should be tapered gradually by 5-mg decreases over 10 to 14 days and discontinued.

■ NEPHROLITHIASIS

The medical management of uric acid nephrolithiasis includes hydration sufficient to maintain a urine volume of

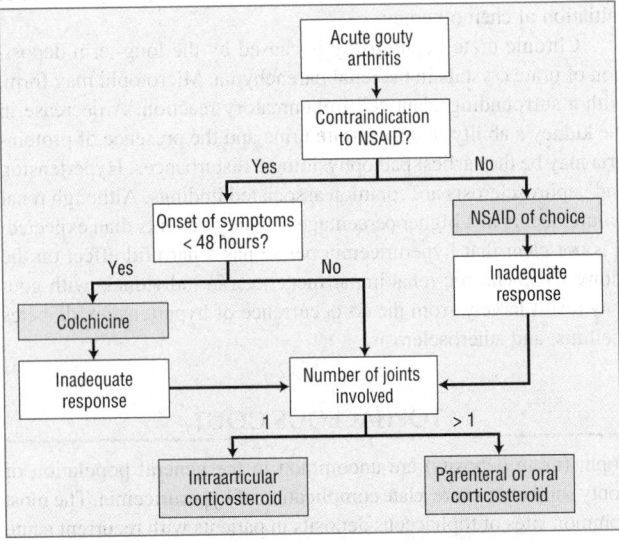

FIGURE 91–2. Treatment algorithm for acute gouty arthritis.

to 3 L/day, alkalinization of urine, avoidance of purine-rich foods, moderation of protein intake, and reduction of urinary uric acid excretion.

Maintenance of a 24-hour urine volume of 2 to 3 L with an adequate intake of fluids is desirable for all gouty patients, but especially for those with excessive (>1 g/day) uric acid excretion. Alkalinizing agents should be used with the objective of making the urine less acidic. Urine pH should be maintained at 6 to 6.5. In this pH range, up to 85% of uric acid will be in the form of the soluble urate ion.

Reduction of urine acidity can be accomplished by the administration of sodium bicarbonate or Shohl's solution (40 g citric acid and 98 g sodium citrate per liter). With the former, 2 to 6 g/day is given in equally divided doses at 6- to 8-hour intervals. A dose of 20 to 60 mL of Shohl's solution per day, given in three or four divided doses, provides an equivalent amount of alkali. If use of a sodium salt is contraindicated, potassium citrate may be used instead.

One must keep in mind that older patients with uric acid kidney stones also may have hypertension, congestive heart failure, or renal insufficiency, and obviously should not be exposed to overload with alkalinizing sodium salts or unlimited fluid intake. Acetazolamide, a carbonic anhydrase inhibitor, produces rapid and effective urinary alkalinization and sometimes is used in conjunction with alkali therapy. When a 250-mg dose of acetazolamide is given at bedtime, the excretion of an acidic urine in the early morning hours is avoided. The usual tachyphylaxis (rapid tolerance) to this drug is obviated by a daily repletion dose of bicarbonate.

Since the advent of allopurinol, a low-purine, low-protein diet in the patient with uric acid lithiasis is no longer as critical as it once was; however, it is still advisable to instruct the patient to avoid foods rich in purine and to limit protein to no more than 90 g/day. Such a diet is still palatable and reduces appreciably the amount of uric acid in the urine.

The mainstay of drug therapy for recurrent uric acid lithiasis is allopurinol. It is effective in reducing both serum and urinary uric acid levels, thus preventing the formation of calculi. Allopurinol is also recommended as prophylactic treatment in patients who will receive cytotoxic agents for the treatment of lymphoma or leukemia. The marked increase in uric acid production associated with cytolysis of a neoplasm predisposes a patient to the development of uric acid nephrolithiasis.

PROPHYLACTIC THERAPY

After the first attack of acute gouty arthritis or after the passage of the first renal stone, a decision to institute prophylactic therapy must be entertained. If the first episode was mild and responded promptly to treatment, the patient's serum urate concentration was elevated only minimally, and the 24-hour urinary uric acid excretion was not excessive (<1000 mg/24 hours on a regular diet), then prophylactic treatment can be withheld. Some patients never have a second attack or a second stone. Others may not experience a second gouty episode for 5 to 10 years. Therefore a wait-and-see attitude seems justified in patients who meet these conditions.[7]

On the other hand, if the patient had a severe attack of gouty arthritis, a complicated course of uric acid lithiasis, a substantially elevated serum uric acid level (>10 mg/dL), or a 24-hour urinary excretion of uric acid of more than 1000 mg, then prophylactic treatment should be instituted immediately after resolution of the acute episode. Prophylactic therapy is also appropriate for patients with frequent attacks (more than two or three per year) of gouty arthritis,

even if the serum uric acid concentration is normal or only minimally elevated.

Recurrences of acute gouty arthritis may be prevented with continuous low-dose daily oral colchicine or by uric acid–lowering therapy with either uricosuric agents or inhibition of xanthine oxidase with allopurinol. Combination therapy consisting of colchicine plus a uricosuric agent or allopurinol may be employed in resistant cases. The choice of treatment depends on the serum urate concentration, the amount of uric acid excreted in a 24-hour period, and the renal function status of the patient.

Prophylactic therapy with low-dose oral colchicine, 0.5 to 0.6 mg twice daily, may be effective in preventing recurrent arthritis in patients with no evidence of visible tophi and a normal or slightly elevated serum urate concentration.[14] Patients do not become resistant to or tolerant of daily colchicine, and if they sense the beginning of an acute attack, they should increase the dose to 1 mg every 2 hours; in most instances the attack will abort after 1 or 2 mg of colchicine. If the serum urate concentration is within the normal range and the patient has been symptom-free for 1 year, maintenance colchicine may be discontinued. The patient should be advised, however, that discontinuation of the treatment program may be followed by an exacerbation of acute gouty arthritis.

Patients with a history of recurrent acute gouty arthritis and a significantly elevated serum uric acid concentration probably are best managed with uric acid–lowering therapy. Colchicine at a dose of 0.5 mg twice daily should be administered during the first 6 to 12 months of antihyperuricemic therapy to minimize the risk of acute attacks that may occur during initiation of uric acid–lowering therapy. The therapeutic objective of antihyperuricemic therapy is to reduce the serum urate concentration below 6 mg/dL, well below the saturation point.

Reduction of the serum urate concentration can be accomplished pharmacologically by increasing the renal excretion of uric acid or by decreasing its synthesis. The drugs used most widely to increase uric acid excretion are probenecid and sulfinpyrazone. Several other uricosuric drugs are available in Europe, but they have not been approved for use in the United States.

URICOSURIC DRUGS

Uricosuric drugs increase the renal clearance of uric acid by inhibiting the renal tubular reabsorption of uric acid. Therapy with uricosuric drugs should be started at a low dose to avoid marked uricosuria and possible stone formation. The maintenance of adequate urine flow and alkalinization of the urine with sodium bicarbonate or Shohl's solution during the first several days of uricosuric therapy further diminish the possibility of uric acid stone formation. Probenecid is given initially at a dose of 250 mg twice a day for 1 to 2 weeks and then 500 mg twice a day for 2 weeks. Thereafter the daily dose is increased by 500-mg increments every 1 to 2 weeks until satisfactory control is achieved or a maximum dose of 2 g is reached. The initial dose of sulfinpyrazone is 50 mg twice a day for 3 to 4 days and then 100 mg twice a day, increasing the daily dose by 100-mg increments each week up to 800 mg/day.

The major side effects associated with uricosuric therapy are gastrointestinal irritation, rash and hypersensitivity, precipitation of acute gouty arthritis, and stone formation. These drugs are contraindicated in patients who are allergic to them and in patients with impaired renal function (a creatinine clearance <50 mL/min), a history of renal calculi, and in patients who are overproducers of uric acid; for such patients, allopurinol should be used.

XANTHINE OXIDASE INHIBITOR

Currently, allopurinol is the only drug approved for use in inhibiting uric acid synthesis. Both allopurinol and its major metabolite, oxypurinol, are xanthine oxidase inhibitors and thus impair the conversion of hypoxanthine to xanthine and xanthine to uric acid. Allopurinol also lowers the intracellular concentration of PRPP. Because of the long half-life of its metabolite, allopurinol can be given once daily. An oral daily dose of 300 mg usually is sufficient. Occasionally, as much as 600 to 800 mg/day may be necessary.

Allopurinol is the antihyperuricemic drug of choice in patients with a history of urinary stones or impaired renal function, in patients who have lymphoproliferative or myeloproliferative disorders and need pretreatment with a xanthine oxidase inhibitor before initiation of cytotoxic therapy to protect against acute uric acid nephropathy, and in patients with gout who are overproducers of uric acid. The major side effects of allopurinol are skin rash, leukopenia, occasional gastrointestinal toxicity, and increased frequency of acute gouty attacks with the initiation of therapy. An allopurinol hypersensitivity syndrome characterized by fever, eosinophilia, dermatitis, vasculitis, and renal and hepatic dysfunction is a rare side effect, but is associated with a 20% mortality rate.[18]

CLINICAL CONTROVERSY

To reduce the risk of developing the allopurinol hypersensitivity syndrome, some experts believe that the dose of allopurinol should be adjusted based on the patient's creatinine clearance.

ASYMPTOMATIC HYPERURICEMIA

Questions are often raised regarding the indications for drug therapy for asymptomatic hyperuricemia. The purported benefits from treatment include prevention of acute gouty arthritis, tophi formation, nephrolithiasis, and chronic urate nephropathy. The first three complications are easily controlled should they develop; therefore antihyperuricemic therapy is not warranted to prevent these conditions.

The prevention of urate nephropathy might be a stronger indication because it is irreversible even with proper treatment. Available data indicate, however, that gouty nephropathy is extremely rare in the absence of clinical gout, and evidence that elevation of uric acid by itself may cause renal disease is weak and inconclusive.[20,21] As discussed previously, renal impairment is very rare in the absence of concurrent hypertension and atherosclerosis. In addition, it is unclear whether uric acid–lowering therapy protects renal function in such individuals. Available data thus do not justify therapy for most patients with asymptomatic hyperuricemia.

CLINICAL CONTROVERSY

While asymptomatic hyperuricemia is not generally treated, some clinicians have begun recommending treatment to reduce the risk of coronary artery disease. Hyperuricemia is associated with both hypertension and coronary artery disease, and patients with elevated uric acid levels and hypertension are at increased risk of cardiovascular morbidity and mortality.

PHARMACOECONOMIC CONSIDERATIONS

Assuming no treatment of asymptomatic hyperuricemia, pharmacoeconomic considerations apply only to the management of the acute and chronic clinical manifestations of gout.

In a cost-effectiveness analysis in patients with nontophaceous recurrent gouty arthritis, urate-lowering therapy was found to reduce costs if patients experienced two or more recurrent attacks per year.[2] Generic allopurinol was associated with a lower incremental cost-effectiveness ratio than were either probenecid or sulfinpyrazone.

In the case of chronic tophaceous gout, a need to continue long-term therapy with a urate-lowering drug clearly exists. Allopurinol generally is less expensive than uricosuric therapy and may be more effective. Comparative trials are lacking. For severe cases, combination therapy may be indicated. Many clinicians will add colchicine to the regimen to reduce the likelihood of precipitating acute gouty arthritis, but this does not appear to be a cost-effective measure.

CONCLUSION

Hyperuricemia may lead to acute arthritis, chronic gout, or kidney stones or remain asymptomatic. Asymptomatic hyperuricemia need not be treated, especially if the serum urate concentration remains below 10 mg/dL.

Acute gouty arthritis requires either colchicine or an NSAID to treat the underlying inflammatory condition. The management of uric acid kidney stones includes hydration and alkalinization of the urine. Prevention of recurrent gouty arthritis or recurrent nephrolithiasis and treatment of chronic gout require hypouricemic therapy with either a uricosuric drug or allopurinol. Allopurinol is the hypouricemic drug of choice in patients with a history of uric acid stones or renal insufficiency and in patients known to be overproducers of uric acid.

ABBREVIATIONS

HGPRT: hypoxanthine guanine phosphoribosyl transferase
NSAID: nonsteroidal anti-inflammatory drug
PRPP: phosphoribosyl pyrophosphate (synthetase)

Review Questions and other resources can be found at *www.pharmacotherapyonline.com*.

REFERENCES

1. Kelley WN, Worthman RL. Gout and hyperuricemia. In: Kelley WN, Harris EP, Ruddy S, Sledge CB, eds. Textbook of Rheumatology. Philadelphia, Saunders, 1997:1313–1351.
2. Levinson DJ, Becker MA. Clinical gout and the pathogenesis of hyperuricemia. In: Koopman WJ, ed. Arthritis and Allied Conditions, 13th ed. Baltimore, Williams & Wilkins, 1997:2041–2071.
3. Wortmann RL. Gout and hyperuricemia. Curr Opin Rheumatol 2002;14:281–286.
4. Wilson JM, Young AB, Kelley WN. Hypoxanthine-guanine phosphoribosyltransferase deficiency. N Engl J Med 1983;309:900–910.
5. Agedelo CA, Wise CM. Gout: Diagnosis, pathogenesis, and clinical manifestations. Curr Opin Rheumatol 2001;13:234–239.
6. Beutler A, Schumacher HR. Gout and "pseudogout": When are arthritis symptoms caused by crystal deposition? Postgrad Med 1994;95:103–116.
7. McGill NW. Gout and other crystal arthropathies. Med J Aust 1997;166:33–38.

8. Schumacher HR. Crystal-reduced arthritis: An overview. Am J Med 1996; 100(Suppl 2A):46S–52S.

9. Yu T. Nephrolithiasis in patients with gout. Postgrad Med 1978;63: 164–170.

10. Worthman RL. Management of hyperuricemia. In: Koopman WJ, ed. Arthritis and Allied Conditions, 13th ed. Baltimore, Williams & Wilkins, 1997:2073–2083.

11. Klineberg JR. Role of the kidneys in the pathogenesis of gout. Postgrad Med 1978;63:145–150.

12. Star VL, Hochberg MC. Prevention and management of gout. Drugs 1993; 45:212–222.

13. Davis JC. A practical approach to gout: Current management of an "old" disease. Postgrad Med 1999;106:115–123.

14. Emmerson BT. The management of gout. N Engl J Med 1996;334: 445–451.

15. Tan N, Lertratanakul Y, Barr WG. Acute gouty arthritis. Postgrad Med 1993;94:73–87.

16. Evans TI, Wheeler MT, Small RE, et al. A comprehensive investigation of inpatient intravenous colchicine use shows more education is needed. J Rheumatol 1996;23:143–148.

17. Rott KT, Agudelo CA. Gout. JAMA 2003;289:2857–2860.

18. Terkeltaub RA. Gout. N Engl J Med 2003;349:1647–1655.

19. Schlesinger N, Schumacher HR. Gout: Can management be improved? Curr Opin Rheumatol 2001;13:240–246.

20. Dykman D, Simon EE, Avioli W. Hyperuricemia and uric acid nephropathy. Arch Intern Med 1987;147:1341–1345.

21. Harris MD, Siegel LB, Alloway JA. Gout and hyperuricemia. Am Fam Physician 1999;59:925–934.

22. Ferrgz MB, O'Brien B. A cost effectiveness analysis of urate lowering drugs in nontophaceous recurrent gouty arthritis. J Rheumatol 1995; 22:908–914.

92
GLAUCOMA

Timothy S. Lesar, Richard G. Fiscella, and Deepak Edward

Learning Objectives and other resources can be found at *www.pharmacotherapyonline.com.*

KEY CONCEPTS

◀1 Primary open-angle glaucoma (POAG) or ocular hypertension (OHT) is more prevalent than closed- or narrow-angle glaucoma.

◀2 In any form of glaucoma, reduction of intraocular pressure (IOP) is essential.

◀3 IOP is a very important risk factor for glaucoma, but the most important considerations are progression of glaucomatous changes in the back of the eye (optic disk and nerve fiber layer) and visual field changes when diagnosing and monitoring for POAG or OHT.

◀4 Fundus changes often occur before visual field changes are exhibited.

◀5 Recent studies have demonstrated that reduction in IOP will prevent progression or even onset of glaucoma.

◀6 Newer medications have simplified treatment regimens for patients. Prostaglandin analogs are considered the most potent topical medications for reducing IOP and flattening diurnal variations.

◀7 Local adverse events are common with topical glaucoma medications, but patient education and reinforcing adherence are essential to prevent glaucoma progression.

The glaucomas are a group of ocular disorders that lead to an optic neuropathy characterized by changes in the optic nerve head (optic disk) that is associated with loss of visual sensitivity and field. Increased intraocular pressure (IOP), a traditional diagnostic criterion for glaucoma, is thought to play an important role in the pathogenesis of glaucoma, but is no longer a diagnostic criterion for glaucoma.[1-10] Two major types of glaucoma have been identified: open angle and closed angle. Open-angle glaucoma accounts for the great majority of cases. Either type can be a primary inherited disorder, congenital, or secondary to disease, trauma, or drugs, and can lead to serious complications.[11-16] Both primary and secondary glaucomas may be caused by a combination of open-angle and closed-angle mechanisms (Table 92–1).

BASIC CONCEPTS

AQUEOUS HUMOR DYNAMICS AND IOP

An understanding of IOP and aqueous humor dynamics will assist the reader in understanding the drug therapy of glaucoma.[1,2,17-19]

Aqueous humor is formed in the ciliary body and its epithelium (Figs. 92–1 and 92–2) through both filtration and secretion. Because ultrafiltration depends on pressure gradients, blood pressure and IOP changes influence aqueous humor formation. Osmotic gradients produced by active secretion of sodium and bicarbonate, and possibly other solutes such as ascorbate from the ciliary body epithelial cells into the aqueous humor, result in movement of water from the pool of ciliary stromal ultrafiltrate into the posterior chamber, forming aqueous humor. Carbonic anhydrase (primarily isoenzyme type II), α- and β-adrenergic receptors, and sodium- and potassium-activated ATPases are found on the ciliary epithelium and appear to be involved in this secretion of the solutes sodium and bicarbonate.

Receptor systems controlling aqueous inflow have not been elucidated fully. Pharmacologic studies suggest that β-adrenergic agents increase inflow, whereas α_2-adrenergic-blocking, α-adrenergic-blocking, β-adrenergic-blocking, dopamine-blocking, carbonic anhydrase–inhibiting, and adenylate cyclase–stimulating agents decrease aqueous inflow. Aqueous humor produced by the ciliary body is secreted into the posterior chamber at a rate of approximately 2 to 3 μL/min. The pressure in the posterior chamber produced by the constant inflow pushes the aqueous humor between the iris and lens and through the pupil into the anterior chamber of the eye[1,2,17-22] (see Fig. 92–2).

Aqueous humor in the anterior chamber leaves the eye by two routes: (1) filtration through the trabecular meshwork (conventional outflow) to Schlemm's canal (80% to 85%) and (2) through the ciliary body and the suprachoroidal space (uveoscleral outflow or unconventional outflow). Cholinergic agents such as pilocarpine increase outflow by physically opening the meshwork pores secondary to ciliary muscle contraction. The uveoscleral outflow of aqueous humor is also increased by prostaglandin analogs, and β- and α_2-adrenergic agonists. Constant inflow of aqueous humor from the ciliary body and resistance to outflow result in an IOP great enough to produce an outflow rate equal to the inflow rate (see Fig. 92–2).

TABLE 92–1. General Classification of Glaucoma

I. Primary glaucoma
   A. Open-angle
   B. Angle closure
      1. With pupillary block
      2. Without pupillary block
II. Secondary glaucoma
   A. Open-angle
      1. Pretrabecular
      2. Trabecular
      3. Posttrabecular
   B. Angle closure
      1. Without pupillary block
      2. With pupillary block
III. Congenital glaucoma

The median IOP measured in large populations is 15.5 ± 2.5 mm Hg; however, the distribution of pressures around the mean is skewed to the right (toward higher readings). IOP is not constant and changes with pulse, blood pressure, forced expiration or coughing, neck compression, and posture. IOP is measured by tonometry: indentation tonometry, applanation tonometry, or a noncontact method using an air pulse. These methods may result in slightly different pressure readings. IOPs consistently greater than 21 mm Hg are found in 5% to 8% of the general population. The incidence increases with age such that "abnormal" (i.e., >22 mm Hg) IOP is found in 15% of those 70 to 75 years of age. Intermittently high IOP (>40 mm Hg) is found in patients with closed-angle glaucoma (CAG). The increased IOP in all types of glaucoma results from the decreased facility for aqueous humor outflow through the trabecular meshwork. Aqueous humor production in primary open-angle glaucoma (POAG) is normal.[1,2,17–19]

IOP demonstrates considerable circadian variation (often referred to as *diurnal* IOP or the IOP during the daily 24-hour cycle) primarily because of changes in the rate of aqueous humor formation.

This circadian variation results in a minimum IOP at approximately 6 PM and a maximum IOP at awakening, although some studies have suggested that both healthy and glaucoma patients may have their highest IOP at night after falling asleep.[20] Low systemic blood pressure in conjunction with high IOPs (decreased ocular perfusion pressure) at night can result in optic nerve head damage.[20] Generally, the circadian IOP variation is usually less than 3 to 4 mm Hg; however, it may be greater in patients with glaucoma. This circadian variation and the poor relationship of IOP with visual loss make measurement of IOP a poor screening test for glaucoma.

Although increased IOP within any range is associated with a higher risk of glaucomatous damage, it is both an insensitive and nonspecific diagnostic and monitoring tool. Of individuals with IOP between 21 and 30 mm Hg, only 0.5% to 1% per year will develop optic disk changes and visual field loss (i.e., glaucoma) over 5 to 15 years. However, more subtle retinal damage, such as alteration of color vision or decreased contrast sensitivity, occurs in a higher percentage of patients with IOPs greater than 21 mm Hg, and the incidence of visual field defects increases to as high as 28% in individuals with IOPs above 30 mm Hg. For a given abnormal IOP, the incidence of glaucoma increases with age. In patients with pre-existing optic nerve damage, the worse the existing damage, the more sensitive the eye is to a given IOP. As many as 20% to 30% of patients with glaucomatous visual field loss have an IOP of less than 21 mm Hg (called *normal-tension glaucoma,* referring to the normal IOP). Thus the absolute IOP is a less precise predictor of optic nerve damage. More direct measurements of therapeutic outcome such as optic disk examination and visual-field evaluation also must be used as monitors of disease progression.[1–7,17–24] Taking the above factors into consideration, glaucoma medications that provide maximal reduction of IOP over 24 hours and have minimal influence on blood pressure may be advantageous in treating glaucoma patients.

OPTIC DISK AND VISUAL FIELDS

The optic disk is the portion of the optic nerve ophthalmoscopically visible as it leaves the eye. It consists of approximately one million retinal ganglion nerve cell axons, blood vessels, and supporting connective tissue structures (lamina cribrosa). The small depression within the disk is termed the *cup* (Fig. 92–3). A normal physiologic cup does not extend beyond the optic nerve rim and has a varying diameter of less than one-third to one-half that of the disk (cup:disk ratio 0.33 to 0.5). The common alterations of the optic disk found in glaucoma are listed in Table 92–2. These disk changes result from optic nerve axonal degeneration and remodeling of the supporting structures. As the nerve axons die, the cup becomes larger in relation to the whole disk. A loss of retinal nerve fiber layer visibility might be visualized in glaucoma patients with detectable visual field loss. This pattern of changes is consistent with visual field losses and loss of visual sensitivity seen in glaucoma.[1,2,17–24]

Determination of the visual field allows assessment of optic nerve damage and is an important monitoring parameter in treatment. However, visual field changes lag behind optic disk changes, and a loss of 25% to 35% of retinal ganglion cells is usually required before detectable visual field defects are noted. The peripheral visual field is measured using a visual field instrument called a *perimeter.* Characteristic visual field loss occurs in glaucoma (Fig. 92–4; see also Table 92–2), but loss of central visual acuity usually does not occur until late in the disease. Other indicators such as color vision changes and contrast sensitivity may allow earlier and more sensitive detection of glaucomatous changes.[1,2]

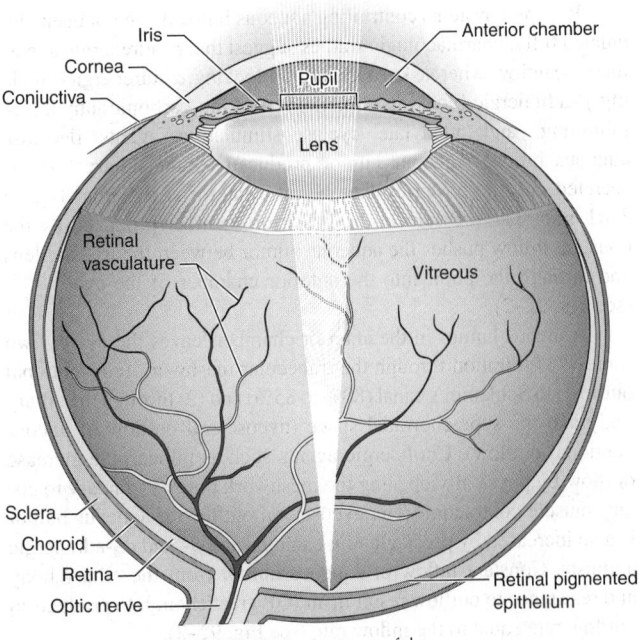

Iris
Cornea
Conjuctiva
Pupil
Anterior chamber
Lens
Retinal vasculature
Vitreous
Sclera
Choroid
Retina
Optic nerve
Retinal pigmented epithelium

FIGURE 92–1. Anatomy of the eye.

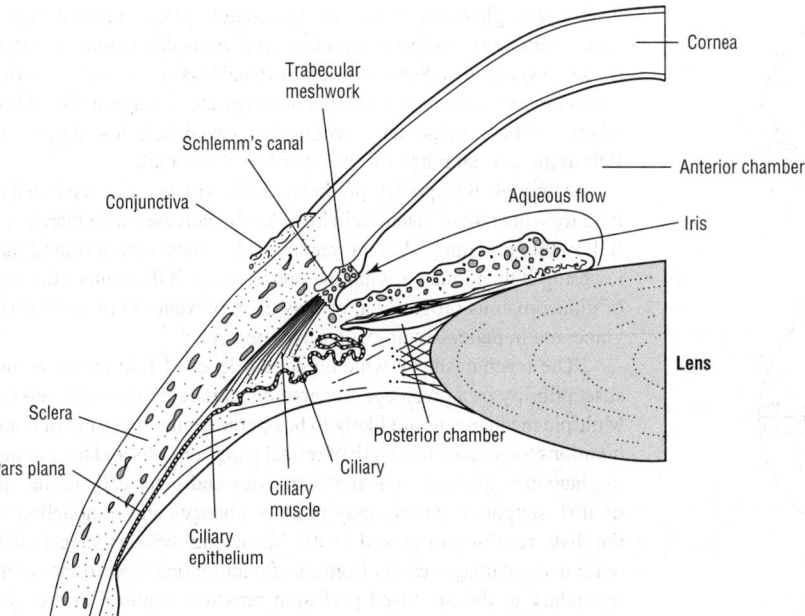

FIGURE 92–2. Anterior chamber of the eye and aqueous humor flow.

GENETICS

A number of major gene loci associated with POAG have been identified. The molecular mechanism of how mutations in any of these genes result in increased IOP with loss of visual field has not been elucidated. One gene, *GLC1A,* codes for the trabecular meshwork–induced glucocorticoid response protein, also commonly known as *myocilin,* in the trabecular meshwork. Its function and role in POAG is under active investigation. Discovery of mutations in the optineurin gene were reported in about 17% of patients in families with autosomal-dominant inherited normal-tension glaucoma patients, but the mutation is likely responsible for less than 0.1% of all glaucomas.[25–26] It is hoped that improved understanding of the genetic origins of POAG will lead to new diagnostic tools and therapies that target the underlying causes of the disease.[1,2,25,26]

EPIDEMIOLOGY OF OPEN-ANGLE GLAUCOMA

Glaucoma affects up to 3 million individuals in the United States and 66.8 million individuals worldwide, of whom 135,000 in the United States and 6.7 million worldwide will have bilateral blindness as a result. The prevalence rate varies with age, race, diagnostic criteria, and other factors. In the United States, open-angle glaucoma occurs in 1.5% of the population over 30 years of age, 1.3% of whites and 3.5% of blacks. The incidence of open-angle glaucoma increases with increasing age. The incidence of the disease in patients 80 years of age is 3% in whites and 5% to 8% in blacks.

ETIOLOGY OF OPEN-ANGLE GLAUCOMA

The specific cause of glaucomatous optic neuropathy is presently unknown. Previously, increased IOP was considered to be the sole cause of the damage; however, it is now recognized that IOP is only one of many factors associated with the development

TABLE 92–2. Optic Disk and Visual Field Findings

Optic disk findings
Cup:disk ratio >0.5
Progressive increase in cup size
Cup:disk ratio asymmetry >0.2
Vertical elongation of the cup
Excavation of the cup
Increased exposure of lamina cribosa
Pallor of the cup
Splinter hemorrhages
Cupping to edge of disk
Notching of the cup (usually superior or inferior)
Nerve fiber defects
Visual field findings
General peripheral field constriction
Isolated scotomas (blind spots)
Nasal visual field depression ("nasal step")
Enlargement of blind spot
Large arclike scotomas
Reduced contrast sensitivity
Reduced peripheral acuity
Altered color vision

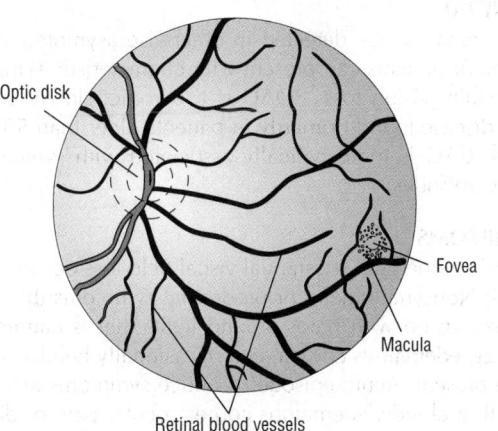

FIGURE 92–3. Normal fundus of the eye and optic disk and cup.

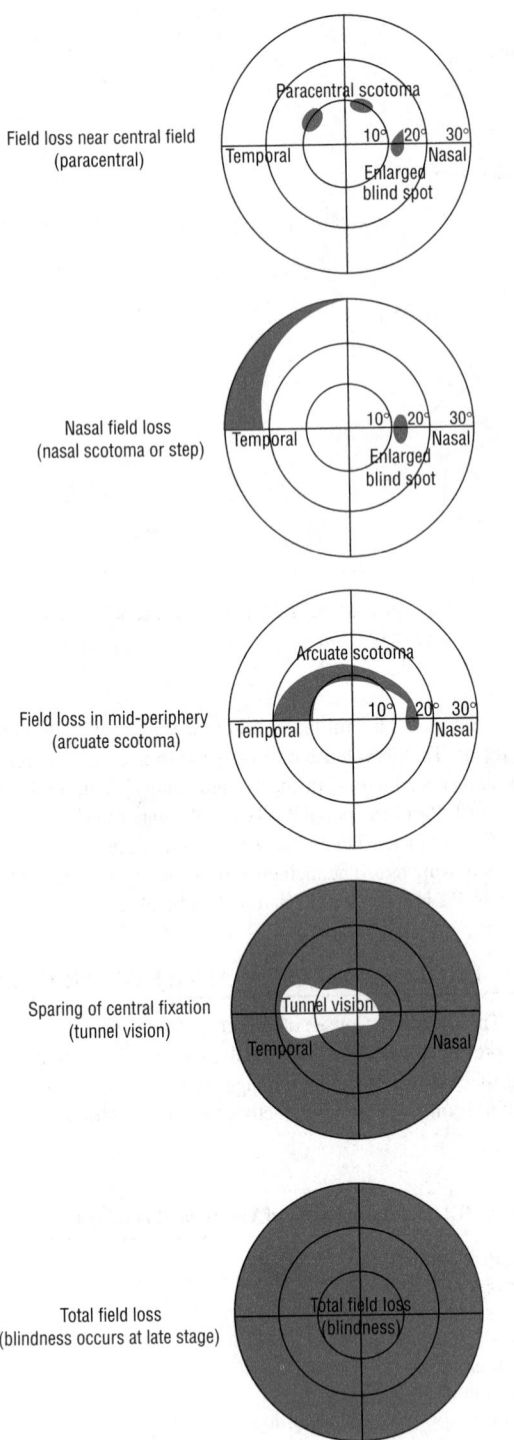

Field loss near central field
(paracentral)

Nasal field loss
(nasal scotoma or step)

Field loss in mid-periphery
(arcuate scotoma)

Sparing of central fixation
(tunnel vision)

Total field loss
(blindness occurs at late stage)

FIGURE 92–4. Schematic representation of the progression of visual field loss in glaucoma.

and progression of glaucoma.[1–10] Increased susceptibility of the optic nerve to ischemia, a reduced or dysregulated blood flow, excitotoxicity, autoimmune reactions, and other abnormal physiologic processes are likely additional contributory factors. The final outcome of these processes is believed to be apoptosis of the retinal ganglion cells, which results in axonal degeneration, and finally permanent loss of vision.[11–16] Interestingly enough, there appears to be a fair amount of similarity between neuronal cell death by apoptosis in Alzheimer's

disease and glaucoma.[13] Indeed, open-angle glaucoma may represent a number of distinct diseases or conditions that simply manifest the same symptoms. Susceptibility to visual loss at a given IOP varies considerably; some patients do not demonstrate damage at high IOPs, whereas other patients have progressive visual field loss despite an IOP in the normal range (normal-tension glaucoma).

Although IOP poorly predicts which patients will have visual field loss, the risk of visual field loss clearly increases with increasing IOP within any range. In fact, recent studies have demonstrated that lowering IOP, no matter what the pretreatment IOP, reduces the risk of glaucomatous progression or may even prevent the onset to early glaucoma in patients with ocular hypertension.[3–7]

The mechanism by which a certain level of IOP increases the susceptibility of a given eye to nerve damage remains controversial. Multiple mechanisms are likely to be operative in a spectrum of combinations to produce the death of retinal ganglion cells and their axons in glaucoma. Pressure-sensitive astrocytes and other cells in the optic disk supportive matrix may produce changes and remodeling of the disk, resulting in axonal death. Vasogenic theories suggest that optic nerve damage results from insufficient blood flow to the retina secondary to the increased perfusion pressure required in the eye, dysregulated perfusion, or vessel wall abnormalities, and results in degeneration of axonal fibers of the retina. Another theory suggests that the IOP may disrupt axoplasmic flow at the optic disk.

Recently, focus on the mechanisms of the retinal ganglion cell apoptosis and the role of excessive glutamate and nitric oxide found in glaucoma patients has broadened the focus of drug therapy research to include evaluation of agents that act as neuroprotectants.[12–15] Such agents may be particularly useful in patients with normal-pressure glaucoma, in whom pressure-independent factors may play a relatively larger role in disease progression. These agents would target risk factors and underlying pathophysiologic mechanisms of disease other than IOP.[11–16]

PATHOPHYSIOLOGY OF OPEN-ANGLE GLAUCOMA

As stated previously, optic nerve damage in POAG can occur at a wide range of intraocular pressures, and the rate of progression is highly variable. Patients may exhibit pressures in 20 to 30 mm Hg range for years before any disease progression is noticed in the optic disk or visual fields. That is why open-angle glaucoma is often referred to as the "sneak thief of sight."

CLINICAL PRESENTATION OF GLAUCOMA

GENERAL
Glaucoma can be detected in otherwise asymptomatic patients, or patients can present with characteristic symptoms, especially vision loss. POAG is a chronic, slowly progressive disease found primarily in patients older than 50 years, while CAG is more typically associated with symptomatic acute episodes.

SYMPTOMS
POAG: None until substantial visual field loss occurs
CAG: Nonsymptomatic or prodromal symptoms (blurred or hazy vision with halos around lights that is caused by a hazy, edematous cornea, and occasionally headache) may be present. Acute episodes produce symptoms associated with a cloudy, edematous cornea, ocular pain or discomfort, nausea, vomiting, abdominal pain, and diaphoresis.

SIGNS

POAG: Disk changes and visual field loss (see Table 94-2); IOP can be normal or elevated (>21 mm Hg)

CAG: Hyperemic conjunctiva, cloudy cornea, shallow anterior chamber, and occasionally an edematous and hyperemic optic disk; IOP is generally elevated markedly (40 to 90 mm Hg) when symptoms are present.

LABORATORY TESTS

None

OTHER DIAGNOSTIC TESTS

Emerging tests include retinal nerve fiber analyzers or confocal scanning laser tomography of the optic nerve.

CLINICAL PRESENTATION OF OPEN-ANGLE GLAUCOMA

POAG is a bilateral, genetically determined disorder constituting 60% to 70% of all glaucomas and 90% to 95% of primary glaucomas (see clinical presentation box). An increased IOP is not required for diagnosis of POAG. Symptoms do not present until substantial visual field constriction occurs. Central visual acuity typically is maintained, even in the late stages of the disease. Even though POAG is a bilateral disease, it may have greater progression and severity in one eye.

Detection and diagnosis involve evaluation of the optic disk and retinal nerve fiber layer, assessment of the visual fields, and measurement of IOP. The presence of characteristic disk changes and visual field loss with or without increased IOP confirms the diagnosis of glaucoma. Typical disk changes and field loss occurring at an IOP of less than 21 mm Hg account for 20% to 30% of patients and are referred to as *normal-tension glaucoma*. Elevated IOP (>21 mm Hg) without disk changes or visual field loss is observed in 5% to 7% of individuals (known as *glaucoma suspects*) and is referred to as *ocular hypertension* (OHT). New technologies such as retinal nerve fiber analyzers or confocal scanning laser tomography of the optic nerve head may allow early identification of signs of glaucomatous retinal changes in ocular hypertensives, thus allowing for earlier initiation of therapy.[1-3,17]

Secondary open-angle glaucoma has many causes, including systemic diseases, trauma, surgery, rubeosis, lens changes, ocular inflammatory diseases, and medications. A system for classifying secondary glaucomas into pretrabecular, trabecular, and posttrabecular forms has been proposed. This classification allows drug therapy to be chosen on the basis of the pathogenic mechanism involved. In pretrabecular forms, a normal meshwork is covered that does not permit aqueous humor outflow. Trabecular forms of secondary glaucoma result from either an alteration of meshwork or an accumulation of material in the intertrabecular spaces. The posttrabecular forms result primarily from disorders causing increased episcleral venous blood pressure.[1,2,15-17]

PROGNOSIS OF OPEN-ANGLE GLAUCOMA

In most cases of POAG, the overall prognosis is excellent when it is discovered early and treated adequately. Even patients with advanced visual field loss can have continued visual field loss reduced if the IOP is maintained at low enough pressures (often <10 to 12 mm Hg). Progression of visual field loss still occurs in 8% to 20% of patients despite reaching standard therapy IOP goals. However, in untreated patients or in those failing to achieve target IOP reduction, up to 80% have continued visual field loss. Estimates of progression to bilateral blindness in treated patients range from 4% to 22%. Thus the keys to medical treatment of POAG are an effective, well-tolerated drug regimen, close monitoring of therapy, and adherence. Medications will control IOP successfully in 60% to 80% of patients over a 5-year period. Availability of newer, highly effective, well-tolerated agents may improve the prognosis further.[1,2,5,17-19,23-28]

EPIDEMIOLOGY OF CLOSED-ANGLE GLAUCOMA

The incidence of closed-angle glaucoma varies by ethnic group, with higher incidence in individuals of Inuit, Chinese, and Asian-Indian descent. Incidence rates of 1% to 4% have been reported in these populations.[1,2]

ETIOLOGY OF CLOSED-ANGLE GLAUCOMA

Primary CAG accounts for 5% or less of primary glaucomas; however, when CAG occurs, it may need to be treated as an emergency to avoid visual loss. CAG results from mechanical blockage of the (usually normal) trabecular meshwork by the peripheral iris. Partial or complete blockage of the meshwork occurs intermittently, resulting in extreme fluctuations between normal IOP with no symptoms, and very high IOP with symptoms of acute CAG. Between attacks of CAG, the IOP is usually normal unless the patient has concomitant open-angle glaucoma or nonreversible blockage of the meshwork with synechiae ("creeping" angle closure) that develops over time in the narrow-angle eye. Primary CAG occurs in patients with inherited shallow anterior chambers, which produce a narrow angle between the cornea and iris or tight contact between the iris and lens (pupillary block). The presence of a narrow angle is determined mainly by visualization of the angle by gonioscopy. Other tests for CAG involve provocation of an angle-closure–induced IOP increase. These tests, which attempt to produce angle closure through mydriasis (darkroom test or mydriasis test), or gravity (prone test), are rarely performed in the clinical setting.

Two major types of classic, reversible primary CAG have been described: CAG with pupillary block and CAG without pupillary block. CAG with pupillary block results when the iris is in firm contact with the lens. This produces a relative block of aqueous flow through the pupil to the anterior chamber (pupillary block), resulting in a bowing forward of the iris, which blocks the trabecular meshwork. CAG with pupillary block occurs most commonly when the pupil is in mid-dilation. In this position, the combination of pupillary block and relaxed iris allows the greatest bowing of the iris; however, angle closure may occur during miosis or mydriasis.

CAG without pupillary block occurs in patients with an abnormality called a *plateau iris*. The ciliary processes in these cases are situated anteriorly, which indent the iris forward and cause closure of the trabecular meshwork, especially during mydriasis. The mydriasis produced by anticholinergic drugs or any other drug results in precipitation of both types of CAG glaucoma, whereas drug-induced miosis may produce pupillary block.

PATHOPHYSIOLOGY OF CLOSED-ANGLE GLAUCOMA

The mechanism of IOP elevation in CAG is clearer than that of POAG. In CAG, a physical blockage of trabecular meshwork is present. In many cases, single or multiple episodes of excessively high IOP (>40 mm Hg) result in optic nerve damage. Very high IOP (>60 mm Hg) may result in permanent loss of visual field within a matter of hours to days.

One type of CAG, known as "creeping" angle closure, occurs in patients with narrow angles in which the iris adheres to the trabecular meshwork and may result in continuously increased IOP in ranges more similar to those of POAG, and the clinical behavior is similar to POAG, with individuals differing in the degree and rapidity of visual loss from any given elevated IOP.[1]

CLINICAL PRESENTATION OF CLOSED-ANGLE GLAUCOMA

Patients with untreated CAG typically experience intermittent non-symptomatic or prodromal symptoms brought on by precipitating events (see clinical presentation box). Increased IOP during such pro-dromal episodes is not great enough or long enough to produce the other symptoms of a full-blown attack. Such prodromal attacks last 1 to 2 hours, at which time pupillary block is broken by further my-driasis or miosis; or when miosis or mydriasis occurs in patients with plateau iris. The rate at which IOP increases may be a determinant of when full-blown symptoms occur. Visual fields demonstrate gen-eralized constriction or typical glaucomatous defects. In prolonged attacks, total loss of vision may occur if the IOP is high enough. Tonometry reveals IOPs as high as 40 to 90 mm Hg. Patients who have developed adhesions between the iris and meshwork (anterior synechiae) may have chronic IOP elevation with intermittent spikes of high IOP when angle closure occurs.

DRUG-INDUCED GLAUCOMA

A number of medications have been associated with increased IOP or carry labeling that cautions against use of the medication in glau-coma patients. The potential for a medication to produce or worsen glaucoma depends on the type of glaucoma and whether or not the patient is treated adequately.[25]

Patients with treated, controlled POAG are at minimal risk of in-duction of an increase in IOP by systemic medications with anticholin-ergic properties or vasodilators; however, in patients with untreated glaucoma or uncontrolled POAG, the potential of these medications to increase IOP should be considered. Topical anticholinergic agents used to produce mydriasis may result in an increase in IOP. Potent an-ticholinergic agents such as atropine or homatropine are most likely to increase IOP. Weaker anticholinergics, such as tropicamide, that produce less cycloplegia are less likely to increase IOP and are fa-vored, along with phenylephrine, when mydriasis is desired in POAG patients. Inhaled, nasal, topical, or systemic glucocorticoids may in-crease IOP in both normal individuals and patients with POAG.

Patients with POAG appear to be particularly susceptible to glucocorticoid-induced increases in IOP. Glucocorticoids reduce the facility of aqueous humor outflow through the trabecular meshwork. The decreased facility of outflow appears to result from the accu-

TABLE 92–3. Drugs That May Induce or Potentiate Increased Intraocular Pressure

Open-angle glaucoma
Ophthalmic corticosteroids (high risk)
Systemic corticosteroids
Nasal/inhaled corticosteroids
Fenoldopam
Ophthalmic anticholinergics
Succinylcholine
Vasodilators (low risk)
Cimetidine (low risk)
Closed-angle glaucoma
Topical anticholinergics
Topical sympathomimetics
Systemic anticholinergics
Heterocyclic antidepressants
Low-potency phenothiazines
Antihistamines
Ipratropium
Benzodiazepines (low risk)
Theophylline (low risk)
Vasodilators (low risk)
Systemic sympathomimetics (low risk)
Central nervous system stimulants (low risk)
Serotonin selective reuptake inhibitors
Imipramine
Venlafaxine
Topiramate
Tetracyclines (low risk)
Carbonic anhydrase inhibitors (low risk)
Monoamine oxidase inhibitors (low risk)
Topical cholinergics (low risk)

mulation of extracellular material blocking the trabecular channels. The potential of a glucocorticoid to increase IOP is related to its anti-inflammatory potency and intraocular penetration. Thus patients should be treated with the lowest potency and dose and for the shortest time possible when steroids are indicated.

In patients predisposed to CAG (i.e., narrow anterior chambers), angle closure may be produced by any drug that causes mydriasis (e.g., anticholinergics). A wide range of sulfa compounds cause id-iosyncratic reactions that result in anterior choroidal effusions with anterior movement of the iris and lens, resulting in angle closure. The topical use of anticholinergics or sympathomimetic agents most likely will result in angle closure. Systemic and inhaled anticholin-ergic and sympathomimetic agents also must be used with caution in such patients. As discussed previously, potent miotic agents such as echothiophate may produce angle closure by increasing pupillary block. Drugs associated with potentiation of glaucoma are listed in Table 92–3.

▶ TREATMENT: Ocular Hypertension

Treatment of the patient with possible glaucoma (ocular hyperten-sion; i.e., patients with IOP >22 mm Hg) is less controversial than it was in the past, with the recent results of the Ocular Hyperten-sive Treatment Study (OHTS).[3] The OHTS helped to identify risk factors for treatment. Patients with intraocular pressures higher than 25 mm Hg, vertical cup:disk ratio of more than 0.5, and central corneal thickness of less than 555 micrometers are at greater risk for develop-ing glaucoma. Risk factors such as family history of glaucoma, black ethnicity, severe myopia, and patients with only one eye must also

be taken into consideration when deciding which individuals need treatment.

Patients without risk factors typically are not treated and are mon-itored for the development of glaucomatous changes. Patients with significant risk factors usually will be treated with a well-tolerated top-ical agent such as a β-blocking agent, an α_2-agonist (brimonidine), a topical carbonic anhydrase inhibitor (CAI), or a prostaglandin analog, depending on individual patient characteristics. Optimally, therapy is initiated in one eye to assess efficacy and tolerance. Use of second- or third-line agents (e.g., pilocarpine or epinephrine) when first-line agents fail to reduce IOP depends on the risk-benefit assessment of each patient. The cost, inconvenience, and frequent adverse effects of combination therapies, anticholinesterase inhibitors, and oral CAIs result in an unfavorable risk-benefit ratio in patients with possible glaucoma.[29]

The goal of therapy is to lower the IOP to a level associated with a decreased risk of optic nerve damage, usually at least a 20% if not a 25% to 30% decrease from the baseline IOP. Greater decreases may be required in high-risk patients or those with higher initial IOPs. Drug therapy should be monitored by measurement of IOP, examination of the optic disk, assessment of the visual fields, and evaluation of the patient for drug adverse effects and compliance with therapy. Patients who are unresponsive to or intolerant of a drug should be switched to an alternative agent rather than given an additional drug. Many clinicians prefer to discontinue all medications in patients failing to respond adequately to simple topical therapy, closely monitor for development of disk changes or visual field loss, and treat again when such changes occur.[1,2,17–19,29]

▶ TREATMENT: Open-Angle Glaucoma

All patients with elevated IOP and characteristic optic disk changes and/or visual field defects not due to other factors (i.e., glaucoma by definition) should be treated. Recent findings that one in five patients with "normal" IOP and glaucomatous retinal nerve findings (i.e., normal-tension glaucoma) do not have progression of visual field loss if left untreated have prompted recommendations to monitor normal-tension glaucoma patients without immediate threat of loss of central vision, and treat only when progression is documented. Some controversy exists as to whether the initial therapy of glaucoma should be surgical trabeculectomy (filtering procedure), argon laser trabeculectomy, or medical therapy.[1,2,17,18] Presently, drug therapy remains the most common initial treatment modality.

Drug therapy of patients with documented glaucomatous change with either elevated or normal IOP is initiated in a stepwise manner (Fig. 92–5), starting with lower concentrations of a single well-tolerated topical agent. The goal of therapy is to prevent further visual loss. A "target" IOP is chosen based on a patient baseline IOP and the amount of existing visual field loss. Typically, an initial target IOP reduction of 30% is desired. Greater reductions may be desired in patients with very high baseline IOPs or advanced visual field loss. Patients with normal baseline IOPs (normal-tension glaucoma) may have target IOPs of less than 10 to 12 mm Hg.

CLINICAL CONTROVERSY

How much should the IOP be reduced in patients who may have POAG? Although the major clinical trial (OHTS[3]) required a 20% reduction in IOP for patients with ocular hypertension, many clinicians believe a further lowering of IOP may be more beneficial in preventing the progression of ocular hypertension to glaucoma. The American Academy of Ophthalmology (AAO) Preferred Practice Guidelines suggest 20% to 30% IOP lowering. It remains to be seen if a more aggressive approach earlier in the treatment of the POAG suspect would be more beneficial.

PHARMACOTHERAPEUTIC APPROACH

❻ Medications most commonly used to treat glaucoma are the nonselective β-blockers, the prostaglandin analogs (latanoprost, travoprost, and bimatoprost), brimonidine (an α_2-agonist), and the fixed combination product of timolol and dorzolamide.[21–22]

Before 1996, a β-blocker was used provided no contraindications existed, because this class of drugs has a long history of successful use, providing a combination of clinical efficacy and tolerability. The newer agents, in particular the prostaglandin analogs, brimonidine, and topical CAIs, are also considered suitable first-line therapy or alternative initial therapy in patients with contraindications to or other concerns with β-blockers (see Fig. 92–5). Pilocarpine and epinephrine (or dipivefrin) are used commonly as third-line therapies because of their increased frequency of adverse effects or reduced efficacy.

Therapy optimally is started as a single agent in one eye (except in patients with very high IOP or advanced visual field loss) to evaluate drug efficacy and tolerance. Monitoring of therapy should be individualized: Initial response to therapy is typically done 4 to 6 weeks after the medication is started. A monocular trial of medication is recommended when possible. Once IOPs reach acceptable levels, the IOP is monitored every 3 to 4 months (more frequently after any change in drug therapy).

Visual fields and disk changes are typically monitored annually, or earlier if the glaucoma is unstable or there is suspicion of disease worsening. Patients should always be questioned regarding adherence to and tolerance of prescribed therapy. Initial IOP response does not predict long-term IOP control. Using more than one drop per dose does not improve response, but increases the likelihood of adverse effects and the cost of therapy. When using more than one medication, separation of drop instillation of each agent by at least 5 to 10 minutes is suggested to provide optimal ocular contact for each agent.

The value of an agent with which the patient has shown a drop in IOP following an initial response can be measured by discontinuing the medication completely and determining if an increase in IOP occurs. Patients responding to but intolerant of initial therapy may be switched to another drug or to an alternative dosage form of the same medication. For patients failing to respond to the highest tolerated concentrations of an initial drug, a switch to an alternative agent after 1 day of concurrent therapy should be considered. Alternatively, if only a partial response occurs, addition of another topical drug to be used in combination is a possibility. A number of drugs or drug combinations may need to be tried before an effective and well-tolerated regimen is identified. Because of the frequency of adverse effects, carbachol, topical cholinesterase inhibitors, and oral CAIs are considered last-line agents to be used in patients who fail less toxic combination topical therapy.

CLINICAL CONTROVERSY

The AAO has not designated any agent as the drug of choice for initiation of glaucoma treatment. Many clinicians in recent years have used the prostaglandin analogs because they are dosed once daily and achieve the best pressure reduction. However, others believe that even though the β-blockers are less potent in reducing IOP, they should still be used as initial agents because they are dosed once or twice daily, and are available as generic products and are therefore more cost effective.

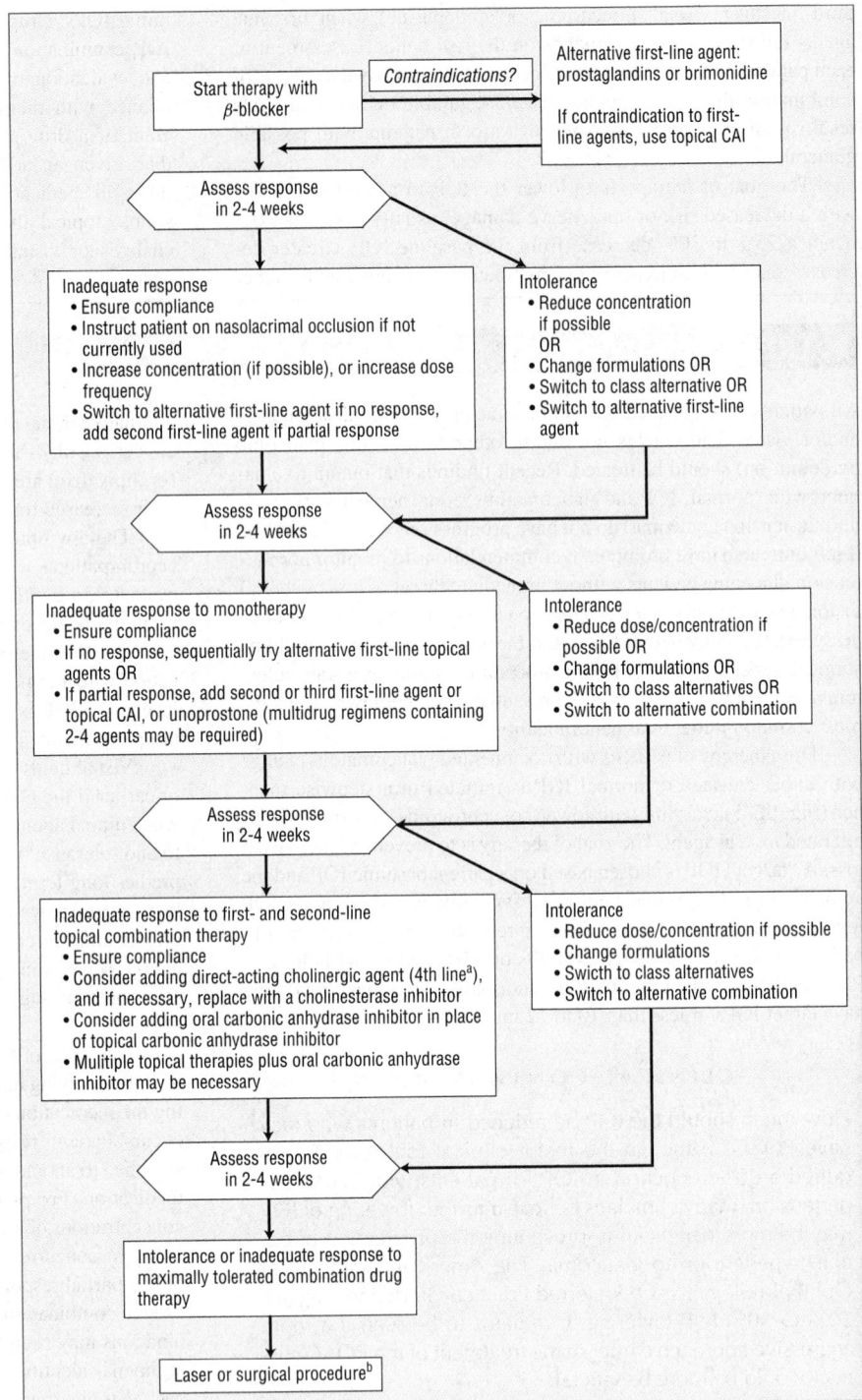

FIGURE 92–5. Algorithm for the pharmacotherapy of open-angle glaucoma.
[a] Fourth-line agents not commonly used any longer.
[b] Most clinicians believe laser procedure should be performed earlier (e.g., after 3 drug maximum, poorly adherent patient).

■ NONPHARMACOLOGIC THERAPY: LASER AND SURGICAL PROCEDURES

When drug therapy fails, is not tolerated, or is excessively complicated, surgical procedures such as laser trabeculoplasty (argon [ALT] or selective [SLT]) or a surgical trabeculectomy (filtering procedure) may be performed to improve outflow. Laser trabeculoplasty is usually an intermediate step between drug therapy and trabeculectomy. Procedures with higher complication rates, such as those involving place-

ment of draining tubes or destruction of the ciliary body (cyclodestruction), may be required when other methods fail[1,2,25] (see Fig. 92–2).

Surgical methods for reduction of IOP involve the creation of a channel through which aqueous humor can flow from the anterior chamber to the subconjunctival space (filtering bleb), where it is reabsorbed by the vasculature. A major reason for failure of the procedure is healing and scarring of the site.

Modification of the healing process to maintain patency is possible with the use of antiproliferative agents. The antiproliferative agents 5-fluorouracil and mitomycin C are used in patients undergoing aucoma-filtering surgery to improve success rates by reducing e inflammatory response and fibroblast proliferation. Although sed most commonly in patients with increased risk for suboptimal

surgical outcome (after cataract surgery and a previous failed filtering procedure), use of these agents also improves success in low-risk patients.[30–33]

► TREATMENT: Closed-Angle Glaucoma

he goal of initial therapy for acute CAG with high IOP is rapid reduction of the IOP to preserve vision and to avoid surgical or laser idectomy on a hypertensive, congested eye. Iridectomy (laser or irgical) is the definitive treatment of CAG; it produces a hole in ie iris that permits aqueous humor flow to move directly from the osterior chamber to the anterior chamber, opening up the block at ie trabecular meshwork. Drug therapy of an acute attack typically ivolves administration of pilocarpine, hyperosmotic agents, and a seretory inhibitor (a β-blocker, α_2-agonist, prostaglandin $F_{2\alpha}$ analog, r a topical or systemic CAI). With miosis produced by pilocarpine, ie peripheral iris is pulled away from the meshwork. Although traitionally the drug of choice, pilocarpine used as initial therapy is ontroversial. Miotics may worsen angle closure by increasing pupilry block and producing anterior movement of the lens because of rug-induced accommodation.

At IOPs greater than 60 mm Hg, the iris may be ischemic and nresponsive to miotics; as the pressure drops and the iris responds, iiosis occurs. During this time, the urge to use excessive amounts of ilocarpine must be resisted. The dose of pilocarpine commonly used a 1% or 2% solution instilled every 5 minutes for two or three doses nd then every 4 to 6 hours. However, many practitioners withhold pplication of pilocarpine until the IOP has been reduced by other

agents, and then apply a single drop of 1% to 2% pilocarpine to produce miosis. In either case, the unaffected contralateral eye should be treated with the miotic every 6 hours to prevent development of angle closure. An osmotic agent also commonly is administered because these drugs produce the most rapid decrease in IOP. Oral glycerin 1 to 2 g/kg can be used if an oral agent is tolerated; if not, intravenous mannitol 1 to 2 g/kg should be used. Osmotic agents reduce IOP by withdrawing water from the eye secondary to the osmotic gradient between the blood and the eyes. These drugs are among the first-line agents in the short-term treatment of CAG or other forms of acute very high IOP elevations. Topical corticosteroids often are used to reduce the ocular inflammation and reduce the development of synechiae in CAG eyes. In classic CAG, once the IOP is controlled, pilocarpine may be given every 6 hours until iridectomy is performed. Patients failing therapy altogether will require an emergency iridectomy.

Peripheral iridectomy essentially "cures" primary CAG without significant synechiae. Long-term drug therapy is not used unless IOP remains high due to the presence of synechiae blocking the trabecular meshwork or concurrent POAG. In such cases, the pharmacotherapeutic approach is essentially identical to that for the POAG patient, or laser or surgical procedures are performed.[1,2]

PHARMACOLOGIC AGENTS USED IN GLAUCOMA

β-BLOCKING DRUGS

he topical β-blocking agents are one of the most commonly used ntiglaucoma medications (Table 92–4). β-Blockers lower IOP by 0% to 30% with a minimum of local ocular adverse effects. These re commonly the agents of first choice in treating POAG if no conraindications exist.[1,2,17–19,34–36]

The β-blocking agents produce ocular hypotensive effects by decreasing the production of aqueous humor by the ciliary body withut producing substantial effects on aqueous humor outflow facilty. The mechanism by which β-blockers decrease aqueous humor nflow remains controversial, but it is most frequently attributed to β_2-adrenergic receptor blockade in the ciliary body.

Five ophthalmic β-blockers are presently available: timool, levobunolol, metipranolol, carteolol, and betaxolol. Timolol, evobunolol, and metipranolol are nonspecific β-blocking agents, vhereas betaxolol is a relatively β_1-selective agent. Carteolol is a ionspecific blocker with intrinsic sympathomimetic activity (ISA). Despite differences in potency, selectivity, lipophilicity, and ISA, the ive agents reduce IOP to a similar degree, although betaxolol has een reported to produce somewhat less lowering of IOP than timlol and levobunolol. Levobunolol may be more effective than timlol and betaxolol in reducing post–cataract surgery IOP increases. evobunolol solution is more effective in controlling IOP than other gents when given as aqueous solutions on a once-daily schedule up to 70% of patients). Timolol in the form of a gel-forming soluion (Timoptic-XE) provides equivalent IOP control with once-daily dministration when compared with the same concentration of the

aqueous solution administered twice daily. The choice of a specific β-blocking agent generally is based on differences in adverse-effect potential, individual patient response, and cost. Long-term treatment with topical β-blockers results in tachyphylaxis in 20% to 25% of patients. The mean IOP reduction from baseline may be smaller in patients receiving topical β-blockers with concurrent systemic β-blockers.[29]

Local adverse effects with β-blockers usually are tolerable, although stinging on application occurs commonly, particularly with betaxolol solution (less with betaxolol suspension) and metipranolol. Other local effects include dry eyes, corneal anesthesia, blepharitis, blurred vision, and rarely, conjunctivitis, uveitis, and keratitis. Some local reactions may be a result of preservatives used in the commercially available products. Switching from one agent to another or switching the type of formulation may improve tolerance in patients experiencing local adverse effects.

Systemic effects are the most important adverse effects of β-blockers. Drug absorbed systematically may produce decreased heart rate, reduced blood pressure, negative inotropic effects, conduction defects, bronchospasm, central nervous system effects, and alteration of serum lipids, and may block the symptoms of hypoglycemia. The β_1-specific agents betaxolol and possibly carteolol (due to ISA) are less likely to produce the systemic adverse effects caused by β-adrenergic blockade, such as the cardiac effects and bronchospasm, but a real risk still exists. The use of timolol as a gel-forming liquid or betaxolol as a suspension allows for administration of less drug per day, and therefore reduces the chance for systemic adverse effects compared with the aqueous solutions.

Because of their systemic adverse effects, all ophthalmic β-blockers should be used with caution in patients with pulmonary

TABLE 92–4. Topical Drugs Used in the Treatment of Open-Angle Glaucoma

Drug	Pharmacologic Properties	Common Brand Names	Dose Form	Strength (%)	Usual Dose[a]	Mechanism of Action
β-Adrenergic blocking agents						
Betaxolol	Relative β_1-selective	Generic	Solution	0.5	1 drop twice a day	All reduce aqueous production of ciliary body
		Betoptic-S	Suspension	0.25	1 drop twice a day	
Carteolol	Nonselective, ISA	Generic	Solution	1	1 drop twice a day	
Levobunolol	Nonselective	Betagan	Solution	0.25, 0.5	1 drop twice a day	
Metipranolol	Nonselective	OptiPranolol	Solution	0.3	1 drop twice a day	
Timolol	Nonselective	Timoptic, Betimol	Solution	0.25, 0.5	1 drop every day—one to two times a day	
		Timoptic-XE	Gelling solution	0.25, 0.5	1 drop every day[a]	
Nonspecific adrenergic agonists						
Dipivefrin	Prodrug	Propine	Solution	0.1	1 drop twice a day	Increased aqueous humor outflow
α_2-Adrenergic agonists						
Apraclonidine	Specific α_2-agonists	Iopidine	Solution	0.5, 1	1 drop two to three times a day	Both reduce aqueous humor production; brimonidine known to also increase uveoscleral outflow
Brimonidine		Alphagan P	Solution	0.15	1 drop two to three times a day	
Cholinergic agonists						
Direct-acting						
Carbachol	Irreversible	Carboptic, Isopto Carbachol	Solution	0.75, 1.5, 2.25, 3	1 drop two to three times a day	All increase aqueous humor outflow through trabecular meshwork
Pilocarpine	Irreversible	Isopto Carpine, Pilocar	Solution	0.25, 0.5, 1, 2, 4, 6, 8, 10	1 drop two to three times a day 1 drop four times a day	
		Pilopine HS	Gel	4	Every 24 h at bedtime	
Cholinesterase inhibitors						
Echothiophate		Phospholine iodide	Solution	0.125	Once or twice a day	
Carbonic anhydrase inhibitors						
Topical						
Brinzolamide	Carbonic anhydrase type II inhibition	Azopt	Suspension	1	Two to three times a day	All reduce aqueous humor production of ciliary body
Dorzolamide		Trusopt	Solution	2	Two to three times a day	
Systemic						
Acetazolamide		Generic	Tablet	125 mg, 250 mg	125–250 mg two to four times a day	
			Injection	500 mg/vial	250–500 mg	
		Diamox Sequels	Capsule	500 mg	500 mg twice a day	
Dichlorphenamide		Daranide	Tablet	50 mg	25–50 mg one to three times a day	
Methazolamide		Generic	Tablet	25 mg, 50 mg	25–50 mg two to three times a day	
Prostaglandin analogs						
Latanoprost	Prostaglandin $F_{2\alpha}$ analog	Xalatan	Solution	0.005	1 drop every night	Increases aqueous uveoscleral outflow and to a lesser extent trabecular outflow
Bimatoprost	Prostamide analog	Lumigan	Solution	0.03	1 drop every night	
Travoprost		Travatan	Solution	0.004	1 drop every night	
Combinations						
Timolol-dorzolamide		Cosopt	Solution	Timolol 0.5% Dorzolamide 2%	1 drop twice daily	

[a]Use of nasolacrimal occlusion will increase number of patients successfully treated with longer dosage intervals.

ISA, *Intrinsic sympathomimetic activity.*

diseases, sinus bradycardia, second- or third-degree heart block, congestive heart failure, atherosclerosis, diabetes, and myasthenia gravis, as well as in patients receiving oral β-blocker therapy. Use of nasolacrimal occlusion (NLO; see section on patient education for description) technique during administration reduces the risk or severity of systemic adverse effects as well as optimizes response. Overall, β-adrenergic blocking agents are well tolerated by most patients, and most potential problems can be avoided by appropriate patient evaluation, drug choice, and monitoring of drug therapy. In patients failing or having an inadequate response to single-drug therapy with a

β-blocking agent, the addition of a CAI, parasympathomimetic agent, prostaglandin analog, or an α_2-adrenergic receptor agonist usually will result in additional IOP reduction. Epinephrine or dipivefrin added to a β-blocking agent (particularly nonspecific β-blockers) usually results in only minimal additional IOP reduction.[1–3,17–19,29]

α_2-ADRENERGIC AGONISTS

Brimonidine and the less lipid-soluble and less receptor-selective apraclonidine are α_2-adrenergic agonists structurally similar to clonidine. Apraclonidine is indicated and brimonidine is effective for prevention or control of postoperative or postlaser treatment increases in IOP, and both are indicated in the treatment of open-angle glaucoma. Brimonidine is considered a first-line or adjunctive agent in the therapy of POAG, and apraclonidine is seen as a second-line or adjunctive therapy.

Use of apraclonidine has fallen dramatically because of a high incidence of loss of control of IOP (tachyphylaxis) and a more severe and prevalent ocular allergy rate.

α_2-Agonists reduce IOP by decreasing the rate of aqueous humor production (some increase in uveoscleral outflow also occurs with brimonidine). The drugs reduce IOP by 18% to 27% at peak (2 to 5 hours) and by 10% at 8 to 12 hours. Comparative trials demonstrate a reduction in IOP similar to that obtained with 0.5% timolol. Use of brimonidine 0.2% every 8 to 12 hours appears to provide maximum IOP-lowering effects in long-term use. Use of NLO (see section on patient education, below) may improve response and allow the longer dosing frequency (i.e., every 12 hours). Combinations of α_2-agonists with β-blockers, prostaglandin analogs, or CAIs produce additional IOP reduction.

An allergic-type reaction characterized by lid edema, eye discomfort, foreign-object sensation, itching, and hyperemia occurs in approximately 30% of patients with apraclonidine. Brimonidine produces this adverse effect in up to 8% of patients. This reaction commonly necessitates drug discontinuation. Systemic adverse effects with brimonidine include dizziness, fatigue, somnolence, dry mouth, and possibly a slight reduction in blood pressure and pulse. α_2-Agonists should be used with caution in patients with cardiovascular diseases, renal compromise, cerebrovascular disease, and diabetes, as well as in those taking antihypertensives and other cardiovascular drugs, monoamine oxidase inhibitors, and tricyclic antidepressants.

Brimonidine is also contraindicated in infants because of apneic spells and hypotensive reactions. In terms of overall efficacy and tolerability, brimonidine approximates that achieved with β-blockers.[1,2,17–19,29]

Brimonidine-purite 0.15% is a formulation of brimonidine in a lower concentration than the original product, and it contains a less toxic preservative than the most commonly employed benzalkonium chloride. The newer formulation is as effective as the original because the more neutral pH of brimonidine-purite allows for higher concentrations of brimonidine in the aqueous humor.[29]

CLINICAL CONTROVERSY

Many animal trials demonstrate that brimonidine has excellent neuroprotective properties.[12–15] Some clinicians believe that one of the major advantages of using brimonidine lies in its potential neuroprotective properties. However, neuroprotection has not been demonstrated in human trials.

PROSTAGLANDIN ANALOGS

The prostaglandin analogs, including latanoprost, travoprost, bimatoprost, and unoprostone, reduce IOP by increasing the uveoscleral and to a lesser extent trabecular outflow of aqueous humor. Some differences in receptor sites and mechanisms of action may exist between the two prostaglandins (latanoprost and travoprost), the prostamide (bimatoprost), and the docosanoid (unoprostone) classes. Bimatoprost may be slightly more effective in lowering IOP, getting a larger percentage of patients to lower IOPs, and in patients unresponsive to latanoprost.[29,37–39]

Reduction in IOP with once-daily doses of prostaglandin $F_{2\alpha}$ analogs (a 25% to 35% reduction) is often greater than that seen with timolol 0.5% twice daily. In addition, nocturnal control of IOP is improved compared with timolol. Interestingly, administration of prostaglandin $F_{2\alpha}$ analogs twice daily may reduce the IOP comparably to once-daily dosing. The drugs are administered at nighttime, although they are probably as effective if given in the morning.

Unoprostone 0.15% reduces IOP somewhat less than prostaglandin analogs and requires twice-daily administration. Prostaglandin analogs are well tolerated and produce fewer systemic adverse effects than timolol. Local ocular tolerance generally is good, but ocular reactions such as punctate corneal erosions and conjunctival hyperemia do occur. Local intolerance occurs in 10% to 25% of patients with these agents.

With prostaglandin analogs, altered iris pigmentation occurs in 15% to 30% of patients, particularly those with mixed-color irises (blue-brown, green-brown, blue-gray-brown, or yellow-brown eyes), which become more brown in color over 3 to 12 months. The change in iris pigmentation will often appear within 2 years, and long-term consequences of this pigment change appear to be mostly cosmetic. Hypertrichosis and increased eyelash pigmentation also have been reported.

These agents have been associated with uveitis, and caution is recommended in patients with ocular inflammatory conditions. Cystoid macular edema also has been reported. Cases of worsening of herpetic keratitis have been reported.

Prostaglandin analogs can be used in combination with other antiglaucoma agents for additional IOP control, due to their unique mechanism of action. Given their excellent efficacy and side-effect profile, prostaglandin analogs provide effective monotherapy or adjunctive therapy in patients not responding to or tolerating other agents. Many glaucoma experts have advocated the use of prostaglandin analogs as first-line therapy in POAG. Long-term studies of these agents are ongoing, but they appear to be safe, efficacious, and well tolerated in glaucoma therapy. The present role of unoprostone is not well delineated.[17–19,29,37,38]

CARBONIC ANHYDRASE INHIBITORS

TOPICAL AGENTS

CAIs reduce IOP by decreasing ciliary body aqueous humor secretion. CAIs appear to inhibit aqueous production by blocking active secretion of sodium and bicarbonate ions from the ciliary body to the aqueous humor.[1,2,29] Topical CAIs such as dorzolamide and brinzolamide are well tolerated and are indicated for monotherapy or adjunctive therapy of open-angle glaucoma and ocular hypertension. Relatively specific inhibitors of carbonic anhydrase enzyme II such as dorzolamide and brinzolamide reduce IOP by 15% to 26%.

Topical CAIs generally are well tolerated. Local adverse effects include transient burning and stinging, ocular discomfort and transient blurred vision, tearing, and rarely, conjunctivitis, lid reactions, and photophobia. A superficial punctate keratitis occurs in 10% to 15% of patients. Brinzolamide produces more blurry vision but is less stinging than dorzolamide. Systemic adverse effects are unusual despite the accumulation of drug in red blood cells. Because of their favorable adverse-effect profile, topical CAIs provide a useful alternative agent for monotherapy or adjunctive therapy in patients with inadequate response to or who are unable to use other agents. The drugs may add additional IOP reduction in patients using other single or multiple topical agents. The usual dose of a topical CAI is one drop every 8 to 12 hours. Administration every 12 hours produces somewhat less IOP reduction than administration every 8 hours. Use of NLO should optimize response to CAI given at any interval.[1,2,17–19,29,34,36] The combination product timolol 0.5% and dorzolamide 2% (Cosopt) is dosed twice daily and produces equivalent IOP lowering to each product dosed separately.

SYSTEMIC AGENTS

Systemic CAIs are indicated in patients failing to respond to or tolerate maximum topical therapy. Systemic and topical CAIs should not be used in combination because no data exist concerning improved IOP reduction, and the risk for systemic adverse effects is increased. Oral CAIs reduce aqueous humor inflow by 40% to 60% and IOP by 25% to 40%. The available systemic CAIs (see Table 92–4) produce equivalent IOP reduction but differ in potency, adverse effects, dosage forms, and duration of action. Despite their excellent effects on elevated IOP of any etiology, the systemic CAIs frequently produce intolerable adverse effects. As a result, CAIs are considered third-line agents in the treatment of POAG.

On average, only 30% to 60% of patients are able to tolerate oral CAI therapy for prolonged periods. Intolerance to CAI therapy results most commonly from a symptom complex attributable to systemic acidosis and including malaise, fatigue, anorexia, nausea, weight loss, altered taste, depression, and decreased libido. Other adverse effects include renal calculi, increased uric acid, blood dyscrasias, diuresis, and myopia. Elderly patients do not tolerate CAIs as well as younger patients. The three available CAIs produce the same spectrum of adverse effects; however, the drugs differ in the frequency and severity of the adverse effects listed. Acetazolamide (standard or sustained-release capsules) and methazolamide are considered the best-tolerated CAIs.

CAIs should be used with caution in patients with sulfa allergies (all CAIs, topical or systemic, contain sulfonamide moieties), sickle-cell disease, respiratory acidosis, pulmonary disorders, renal calculi, electrolyte imbalance, hepatic disease, renal disease, diabetes mellitus, or Addison's disease. Concurrent use of a CAI and a diuretic may rapidly produce hypokalemia. High-dose salicylate therapy may increase the acidosis produced by CAIs, whereas the acidosis produced by CAIs may increase the toxicity of salicylates.[1,2,17–19,21,29,34,35]

PARASYMPATHOMIMETIC AGENTS

The parasympathomimetic (cholinergic) agents reduce IOP by increasing aqueous humor trabecular outflow. The increase in outflow is a result of physically pulling open the trabecular meshwork secondary to ciliary muscle contraction, thereby reducing resistance to outflow. These agents may reduce uveoscleral outflow. Cholinergics agents work well to decrease IOP, but their use as primary or even adjunctive agents in the treatment of glaucoma has decreased

significantly because of local ocular adverse effects and/or frequent dosing requirements.

Pilocarpine, the parasympathomimetic agent of choice in POAG, is available as an ophthalmic solution, an ocular insert, and a hydrophilic polymer gel (see Table 92–4). Pilocarpine produces similar (20% to 30%) reductions in IOP as those seen with β-blocking agents. Pilocarpine in POAG or "glaucoma suspects" is initiated as 0.5% or 1% solution, one drop three to four times daily. The use of NLO improves response and reduces the need for an every-6-hour dosing frequency. Use of one drop of 2% pilocarpine every 6 to 12 hours and NLO provides optimal response in many patients. Both drug concentration and frequency may be increased if IOP reduction is inadequate. Patients with darkly pigmented eyes frequently require higher concentrations of pilocarpine than patients with lightly pigmented eyes. Concentrations of pilocarpine above 4% rarely improve IOP control in patients other than those with darkly pigmented eyes.

Pilocarpine 4% gel (Pilopine HS) once daily is equivalent to treatment with pilocarpine solution 4% four times daily or timolol 0.5% twice daily. When using every-24-hour dosing of pilocarpine gel, the adequacy of IOP control late in the dosing interval should be confirmed. Ocular adverse effects of pilocarpine include miosis, which decreases night vision and vision in patients with central cataracts. Visual field constriction may be seen secondary to miosis and should be considered when evaluating visual field changes in a glaucoma patient. Pilocarpine ciliary muscle contraction produces accommodative spasm, particularly in young patients still able to accommodate (prepresbyopic). Pilocarpine also may produce frontal headache, brow ache, periorbital pain, eyelid twitching, and conjunctival irritation or injection early in therapy, which tends to decrease in severity over 3 to 5 weeks of continued therapy.

Cholinergics produce a breakdown of the blood–aqueous humor barrier and may result in a worsening of an ocular inflammatory reaction or condition. Systemic cholinergic adverse effects of pilocarpine—such as diaphoresis, nausea, vomiting, diarrhea, cramping, urinary frequency, bronchospasm, and heart block—are rare but may be seen in patients using products with high pilocarpine concentrations (6% to 8%), or those using such products overzealously in treatment of acute angle closure. Other adverse effects associated with direct-acting miotics include retinal tears or detachment, allergic reaction, permanent miosis, cataracts, precipitation of CAG, and rarely, miotic cysts of the pupillary margin.

Carbachol is a potent direct-acting miotic agent; its duration of action is longer than that of pilocarpine (8 to 10 hours) because of resistance to hydrolysis by cholinesterases. This drug also may act as a weak inhibitor of cholinesterase. Patients with an inadequate response to or intolerance of pilocarpine as a result of ocular irritation or allergy frequently do well on carbachol. The ocular and systemic adverse effects of carbachol are similar to but more frequent, constant, and severe than those of pilocarpine.[1,2,17–19,29,34,35]

The cholinesterase inhibitors used most commonly in the treatment of POAG are the long-acting, relatively irreversible agents demecarium and echothiophate (limited commercial availability; see Table 92–4). These agents are potent inhibitors of pseudocholinesterase, but they also inhibit true cholinesterase. Because of the serious ocular and systemic toxic effects of these agents, the cholinesterase inhibitors are reserved primarily for patients not responding to or those intolerant of other therapy. Because of their cataractogenic properties, most ophthalmologists use these agents only in patients without lenses (aphakia) or those with artificial lenses (pseudophakia). The ocular and periocular parasympathomimetic adverse effects are more common and more severe than with pilocarpine or carbachol.

In addition to the parasympathomimetic effects, the cholinesterase inhibitors may produce severe fibrinous iritis (particularly with the irreversible inhibitors), synechiae, iris cysts, conjunctival thickening, and occlusion of the nasolacrimal ducts. Cataracts occur at high frequency with the use of cholinesterase inhibitors, particularly echothiophate, after about 10 to 18 months of therapy. The incidence of cataracts appears to increase with increasing concentration, with up to 60% of patients developing cataracts at higher concentrations. The inhibition of systemic pseudocholinesterase by these agents decreases the rate of succinylcholine hydrolysis, resulting in prolonged muscle paralysis. Cholinesterase inhibitors should be discontinued at least 2 weeks before procedures in which succinylcholine is to be used.

The role of cholinesterase inhibitors in glaucoma is limited by the frequency and potential toxicity of these agents. In phakic patients, cholinesterase inhibitors should be administered only if intolerance or failure results with other antiglaucoma medications. Cholinesterase inhibitors have been shown to provide additional IOP-lowering effects when used with β-blockers, CAIs, and sympathomimetic (adrenergic) agents. As with all agents for glaucoma, therapy should be initiated with lower concentrations of these agents. A once-daily administration frequency should be used in most patients unless very high IOP is present.

Use of NLO likely improves response and reduces systemic adverse effects and should be performed by all patients administering cholinesterase inhibitors. These agents should be used with caution in patients with asthma, retinal detachments, narrow angles, bradycardia, hypotension, heart failure, Down's syndrome, epilepsy, parkinsonism, peptic ulcer, and ocular inflammation, as well as in those receiving cholinesterase inhibitor therapy for myasthenia gravis or exposure to carbamate or organophosphate insecticides and pesticides.[1,2,17–19,29,34,35]

EPINEPHRINE AND DIPIVEFRIN

The mechanism of action by which epinephrine lowers IOP has not been fully elucidated; however, a β_2-receptor–mediated increase in outflow facility through the trabecular meshwork and the uveoscleral route appears to be the primary mechanism. Compared with β-blockers or miotics, epinephrine and dipivefrin reduce IOP less. With the advent of the better tolerated and more efficacious agents to treat glaucoma, the clinical use of epinephrines has decreased dramatically.

Epinephrine is available as epinephrine hydrochloride and epinephryl borate solutions. The various salts of epinephrine produce equivalent IOP-lowering effects and adverse reactions. Patients with minor ocular irritation from one salt of epinephrine occasionally may benefit from use of another salt because of differences in pH of the commercial solutions.

Use of the prodrug dipivefrin allows use of lower concentrations secondary to improved intraocular absorption (10- to 15-fold higher). The 0.1% dipivefrin produces equivalent IOP reduction to 1% to 2% epinephrine. Dipivefrin therefore may be tolerated by patients unable to tolerate epinephrine solutions, and it is often chosen over other epinephrine products when this class of drugs is indicated.

A factor limiting the usefulness of epinephrine is the high frequency of local ocular adverse effects. Tearing, burning, ocular discomfort, brow ache, conjunctival hyperemia, punctate keratopathy, allergic blepharoconjunctivitis, rare loss of eyelashes, stenosis of the nasolacrimal duct, and blurred vision may occur. Prolonged use (>1 year) may result in deposition of pigment (adrenochrome) in the conjunctiva and cornea. Pigment also may deposit in soft contact lenses, turning them black. These adverse effects occur less frequently with dipivefrin. Epinephrine may produce mydriasis (particularly when combined with a β-blocker) and may precipitate acute CAG in patients with narrow anterior chambers. A transient increase in IOP may occur with initial therapy, particularly in patients not using other antiglaucoma medications. A relative contraindication to the use of epinephrine (and dipivefrin) is aphakia (i.e., after cataract removal) or lens dislocation because of the development of swelling of the macular portion of the retina. The edema is dose dependent and disappears with drug discontinuation.

Systemic adverse effects of epinephrine include headache, faintness, increased blood pressure, tachycardia, arrhythmias, tremor, pallor, anxiety, and increased perspiration. Epinephrine should be used with caution in patients with cardiovascular diseases, cerebrovascular diseases, aphakia, CAG, hyperthyroidism, and diabetes mellitus, as well as in patients undergoing anesthesia with halogenated hydrocarbon anesthetics. Using NLO with epinephrine and dipivefrin will improve therapeutic response and reduce the risk of systemic adverse effects.[1,2,17–19,29,34,35]

FUTURE DRUG THERAPIES

It is hoped that new agents, improved formulations, and novel approaches to the reduction of IOP and other methods of prevention of glaucomatous visual field loss will provide more effective and better-tolerated therapies.

Agents that are neuroprotective and act through mechanisms other than IOP reduction are likely to be part of glaucoma therapy in the future.[13–15,40]

EVALUATION OF THERAPEUTIC OUTCOMES

The ultimate goal of drug therapy in the patient with glaucoma is to preserve visual function through reduction of IOP to a level at which no further optic nerve damage occurs. Because of the poor relationship between IOP and optic nerve damage, no specific target IOP exists. Indeed, drugs used to treat glaucoma may act in part to halt visual field loss through mechanisms separate from or in addition to IOP reduction, such as improvements in retinal or choroidal blood flow. Often a 25% to 30% reduction is desired, but greater reductions (40% to 50%) may be desired in patients with initially high IOPs. For patients with glaucoma, an IOP of less than 21 mm Hg generally is desired, with progressively lower target pressures needed for greater levels of glaucomatous damage. Even lower IOPs (possibly even below 10 mm Hg) are required in patients with very advanced disease, those showing continued damage at higher IOPs, and those with normal-tension glaucoma and pretreatment pressures in the low to middle teens. The IOP considered acceptable for a patient is often a balance of desired IOP and acceptable treatment-related toxicity and patient quality of life.

PATIENT EDUCATION

An important consideration in patients failing to respond to drug therapy is adherence. Poor adherence or nonadherence occurs in 25% to 60% of glaucoma patients.

A large percentage of patients also fail to use topical ophthalmic drugs correctly. Patients should be taught the following procedure:

1. Wash and dry the hands; shake the bottle if it contains a suspension.
2. With a forefinger, pull down the outer portion of the lower eyelid to form a "pocket" to receive the drop.

3. Grasp the dropper bottle between the thumb and fingers with the hand braced against the cheek or nose and the head held upward.
4. Place the dropper over the eye while looking at the tip of the bottle; then look up and place a single drop in the eye.
5. The lids should be closed (but not squeezed or rubbed) for 1 to 3 minutes after instillation. This increases the ocular availability of the drug.
6. Recap bottle and store as instructed.

Note that many patients are physically unable to administer their own eyedrops without assistance. NLO also should be used to improve ocular bioavailability and reduce systemic absorption.[1,2,17–19,29,34,35] The patient induces NLO for 1 to 3 minutes by closing the eyes and placing the index finger over the nasolacrimal drainage system in the inner corner of the eye. This maneuver, as well as eyelid closure itself, decreases nasolacrimal drainage of drug, thereby decreasing the amount of drug available for systemic absorption by the nasopharyngeal mucosa. The use of NLO may improve drug response significantly, reduce adverse effects, and allow less frequent dosing intervals and the use of lower drug concentrations.

Use of more than one drop per dose increases costs, does not improve response significantly, and may increase adverse effects. When two drugs are to be administered, instillations should be separated by at least 3 to 5 minutes (preferably 10 minutes) to prevent the drug administered first from being washed out. The patient should be taught not to touch the dropper bottle tip with eye, hands, or any surface.

Adherence to glaucoma therapy commonly is inadequate, and it always should be considered as a possible cause of drug therapy failure. Assessment of adherence by health care providers generally is poor, so all patients should be encouraged continually to administer prescribed therapy diligently as instructed. To improve adherence, the patient, family, and care providers should be fully informed of the expectations of therapy and the need to continue therapy despite a lack of symptoms. Possible adverse effects of the medication and ways to reduce them should be discussed. Adherence will be improved by good communication, close monitoring, and use of well-tolerated and convenient drug regimens.[1,2,17–19,29]

CONCLUSIONS

The glaucomas are a group of primary and secondary diseases, the management of which presents a considerable challenge to the clinician. Successful therapy requires rational use of antiglaucoma medications and patient adherence to the selected regimen, combined with conscientious monitoring for adverse effects and disease progression. The reward for successful therapy is considerable: the maintenance of vision. The overview of the clinical findings, pathology, and drug therapy presented in this chapter provides the clinician with the fundamentals necessary to understand and treat glaucoma.

ABBREVIATIONS

AAO: American Academy of Ophthalmology
ALT: argon laser trabeculoplasty
CAG: closed-angle glaucoma
CAI: carbonic anhydrase inhibitor
IOP: intraocular pressure
ISA: intrinsic sympathomimetic activity

NLO: nasolacrimal occlusion
OHT: ocular hypertension
OHTS: Ocular Hypertensive Treatment Study
POAG: primary open-angle glaucoma
SLT: selective laser trabeculoplasty

Review Questions and other resources can be found a *www.pharmacotherapyonline.com.*

REFERENCES

1. Coleman AL. Glaucoma. Lancet 1999;354:1803–1810.
2. Infield DA, O'Shea J. Glaucoma: Diagnosis and management. Postgra Med J 1998;74:709–715.
3. Kass MA, Heuer DK, Higginbotham EJ, et al. The ocular hypertensio treatment study: A randomized trial determines that topical ocular hy potensive medication delays or prevents the onset of primary open-angl glaucoma. Arch Ophthalmol 2002;120:701–713, discussion 829–830.
4. Leske MC, Heijl A, Hussein M, et al. Factors for glaucoma progressio and the effect of treatment: The early manifest glaucoma trial. Arch Ophthalmol 2003;121:48–56.
5. Van Veldhuisen PC, Schwartz AL, Gaasterland DE, et al. The advance glaucoma intervention study (AGIS): 7. The relationship between contro of intraocular pressure and visual field deterioration. Am J Ophthalmo 2000;130:429–440.
6. Janz NK, Wren PA, Lichter PR, et al. Quality of life in newly diagnose glaucoma patients: The collaborative initial glaucoma treatment study Ophthalmology 2001;108:887–897.
7. Collaborative Normal-Tension Glaucoma Study Group. Comparison o glaucomatous progression between untreated patients with normal-tensio glaucoma and patients with therapeutically reduced intraocular pressures Am J Ophthalmol 1998;126:487–497.
8. Khaw PT, Cordiero MF. Towards better treatment of glaucoma. Br Med 2000;320:1619–1620.
9. Dreyer FB, Lipton SA. New perspectives in glaucoma. JAMA 1999 281:306–308.
10. Stewart WC. Perspectives in the medical treatment of glaucoma. Cur Opin Ophthalmol 1999;10:99–108.
11. Chung HS, Harris A, Evans DW, et al. Vascular aspects in the patho physiology of glaucomatous optic neuropathy. Surv Ophthalmol 1999 43(Suppl 1):S43–50.
12. Levin LA. Retinal ganglion cells and neuroprotection for glaucoma. Surv Ophthalmol 2003;48(Suppl 1):S21–24.
13. Tatton W, Chen D, Chalmers-Redman R, et al. Hypothesis for a commo basis for neuroprotection in glaucoma and Alzheimer's disease: Anti apoptosis by alpha-2-adrenergic receptor activation. Surv Ophthalmo 2003;48(Suppl 1):S25–37.
14. Levin LA. Extrapolation of animal models of optic nerve injury to clinica trial design. J Glaucoma 2004;13:1–5.
15. Kaushik S, Pandav SS, Ram J. Neuroprotection in glaucoma. J Postgrad Med 2003;49:90–95.
16. Yu DY, Su EN, Cringle SJ, et al. Systemic and ocular vascular roles of th antiglaucoma agents beta-adrenergic antagonists and Ca^{2+} entry blockers Surv Ophthalmol 1999;43(Suppl 1):S214–222.
17. Alward WL. Medical management of glaucoma. N Engl J Med 1998;339 1298–1307.
18. King A, Migdal C. Clinical management of glaucoma. J R Soc Med 2000 93:175–177.
19. Hoyng PF, van Beek LM. Pharmacological therapy for glaucoma: A re view. Drugs 2000;59:411–434.
20. Wax MB, Camras CB, Fiscella RG, et al. Emerging perspectives in glau coma: Optimizing 24-hour control of intraocular pressure. Am J Ophthal mol 2002;133:S1–S10.
21. Kooner KS. New agents in glaucoma therapy. Int Ophthalmol Clin 1999 39:1–15.
22. Kaufman PL, Gabelt B, Tian B, Liu X. Advances in glaucoma diagnosis

and therapy for the next millennium: New drugs for trabecular and uveoscleral outflow. Semin Ophthalmol 1999;14:130–143.

23. Caprioli J. The treatment of normal-tension glaucoma. Am J Ophthalmol 1998;126:578–581.

24. Kamal D, Hitchings R. Normal-tension glaucoma: A practical approach. Br J Ophthalmol 1998;82:835–840.

25. Triptahi RC, Tripathi BJ, Haggerty C. Drug-induced glaucomas. Drug Saf 2003;26:749–767.

26. Rezaie T, Child A, Hitching R, et al. Adult-onset primary open-angle glaucoma caused by mutations in optineurin. Science 2002;295:1077–1079.

27. Hattenhaurr MG, Johnson DH, Ing HH. The probability of blindness from open angle glaucoma. Ophthalmology 1998;105:2099–2104.

28. Quigley HA. Proportion of those with open angle glaucoma who become blind. Ophthalmology 1999;106:2039–2041.

29. Cantor L. Achieving low target pressures with today's glaucoma medications. Surv Ophthalmol 2003;48(Suppl 1):S8–16.

30. Cooper R. Surgical management of the glaucomas. Aust N Z J Ophthalmol 1999;27:352.

31. Cordeiro MF, Siriwardena D, Chang L, Khaw PT. Wound healing modulation after glaucoma surgery. Curr Opin Ophthalmol 2000;11:121–126.

32. Donohue EK, Cioffi GA. Glaucoma surgery: Are there new perspectives in perioperative pharmacology? Curr Opin Ophthalmol 1999;10:93–98.

33. Loon SC, Chew PT. A major review of antimetabolites in glaucoma therapy. Ophthalmologica 1999;213:234–245.

34. Schuman JS. Antiglaucoma medications: A review of safety and tolerability issues related to their use. Clin Ther 2000;22:167–208.

35. Vogel R, Strahlman E, Rittenhouse KD. Adverse events associated with commonly used glaucoma drugs. Int Ophthalmol Clin 1999;39:107–124.

36. Stewart WC, Garrison PM. Beta-blocker-induced complications and patients with glaucoma. Arch Intern Med 1998;158:221–226.

37. Noecker R, Dirks M, Choplin N. A six-month randomized clinical trial comparing the IOP lowering efficacy of bimatoprost and latanoprost in patients with ocular hypertension or glaucoma. Am J Ophthalmol 2003;135:55–63.

38. Parrish RK, Palmberg P, Sheu W, et al. A comparison of latanoprost, bimatoprost, and travoprost in patients with elevated intraocular pressure: A 12 week, randomized, masked-evaluator multicenter study. Am J Ophthalmol 2003;135:688–703.

39. Gandolfi SA, Cimino L. Effect of bimatoprost on patients with primary open-angle glaucoma or ocular hypertension who are nonresponders to latanoprost. Ophthalmology 2003;110:609–614.

40. Naskar R, Vorwerk CK, Dreyer EB. Saving the nerve from glaucoma: Memantine to caspaces. Semin Ophthalmol 1999;14:152–158.

93

ALLERGIC RHINITIS

J. Russell May and Philip H. Smith

Learning Objectives and other resources can be found at *www.pharmacotherapyonline.com.*

KEY CONCEPTS

◀ **1** Allergic rhinitis is one of the most common diseases. Treatment is justified in most cases because of the potential for complications.

◀ **2** An immune response to allergens results in release of inflammatory mediators that cause allergic rhinitis symptoms. Therefore patients must be thoroughly knowledgeable about the proper timing and administration of prophylactic regimens.

◀ **3** Proven therapeutic modalities include avoidance of allergens and pharmacologic management with antihistamines, topical and systemic decongestants, topical steroids, cromolyn sodium, and immunotherapy.

◀ **4** Immunotherapy can be highly successful, offering long-term benefits, but expense, potential risks, and a major time commitment makes proper patient selection critical.

Rhinitis is inflammation of the nasal mucous membrane. In a sensitized individual, allergic rhinitis occurs when mucous membranes are exposed to inhaled allergenic materials that elicit a specific response mediated by immunoglobulin E (IgE). This response involves the release of inflammatory mediators and is characterized by sneezing, nasal itching, and watery rhinorrhea, often associated with nasal congestion. Itching of the throat, eyes, and ears frequently accompanies allergic rhinitis.

Allergic rhinitis may be regarded as seasonal allergic rhinitis, commonly known as hay fever, or perennial allergic rhinitis (increasingly called "intermittent" and "persistent"). Seasonal rhinitis occurs in response to specific allergens usually present at predictable times of the year, during the plants' blooming seasons (typically the spring or fall). Seasonal allergens include pollen from trees, grasses, and weeds. Perennial allergic rhinitis is a year-round disease caused by nonseasonal allergens, such as house dust mites, animal dander, and molds, or multiple allergic sensitivities. It typically results in subtle, chronic symptoms. Many patients have a combination of these two types of allergic rhinitis, with symptoms year-round and seasonal exacerbations. About one-third to one-half of sufferers have recognizable seasonal disease with the remainder having perennial or a combination of both.[1]

EPIDEMIOLOGY AND ETIOLOGY

◀ **1** Allergic rhinitis is one of the most common medical disorders found in humans. An estimated 20% to 30% of the American adult population and up to 40% of children are affected, with some believing the percentage to be much higher.[2,3] It ranks as the sixth most prevalent chronic illness in the United States.[1] Patients are limited in their ability to carry out normal daily functions: higher levels of general fatigue, mental fatigue, anxiety, and depressive disorders are seen.[4,5]

In addition, the impact of allergic rhinitis goes well beyond these central nervous system issues. Allergic rhinitis is associated with several other serious medical conditions, including asthma, rhinosinusitis, otitis media, nasal polyposis, respiratory infections, and orthodontic malocclusions.[2]

PREDISPOSING FACTORS

The development of allergic rhinitis is likely influenced by genetics, allergen exposure, and the presence of other risk factors. Allergic rhinitis has a strong genetic predisposition. A family history of allergic rhinitis, atopic dermatitis, or asthma suggests that rhinitis is allergic. The risk of developing allergic disease is approximately 50% for children with one atopic parent and 66% for those with two allergic parents.[3]

Allergen exposure is another predisposing factor. For allergic rhinitis to occur, an individual must be exposed to a protein that elicits the allergic response in that individual. Many potential sufferers never develop symptoms because they do not come into contact with the allergen that would produce symptoms in them.

Recent evidence suggests microbial exposure in the first years of life could help prevent allergic disease by developing a non-atopic immune response.[6] Farm children are exposed to higher concentrations of endotoxin, derived from cell walls of gram-negative bacteria, in stables and in dust around the farmhouse. Consumption of non-pasteurized farm milk may cause further exposure. This concept has led to the idea that allergic disease could be prevented by proactively increasing exposure to harmless bacteria early in life (see alternative treatment section below). This could explain why positive skin tests indicating allergen sensitization have been observed more frequently in people in higher socioeconomic classes and people who live in suburban areas.[7]

Other predisposing factors include an elevated serum IgE (>100 international units/mL) before the age of 6 years, eczema, and heavy exposure to second-hand cigarette smoke.[8]

ALLERGENS

Allergens that produce seasonal rhinitis are the protein components of airborne pollen grains, often enzymes, from a variety of trees, grasses, and weeds. Ragweed and grass pollen are the most common offenders in the United States; however, this changes with the geographic region. In general, tree pollens cause symptoms in the spring, grass pollens cause symptoms in the late spring to summer, and weed pollens are the culprits in the late summer to early fall. Patients who are hypersensitive to all three may have overlapping problem periods, and may be described as having perennial rhinitis, when they are actually experiencing prolonged seasonal rhinitis. For this reason and the fact that most patients with seasonal problems are sensitive to at least some of the perennial allergens, many allergists are less often distinguishing between the two types of allergic rhinitis.

To complicate matters further, the antigenic components of many grasses—including fescue, Kentucky bluegrass, orchard, redtop, and timothy—are similar, resulting in cross-allergenicity. Fortunately, most trees that produce many of the offending airborne pollens produce antigenically distinct pollens. These trees include ash, beech, birch, cedar, hickory, maple, oak, poplar, and sycamore. Flowering plants that depend on insect pollination usually do not cause allergic rhinitis.

Mold spores are also important allergens. Spores are present year-round; however, mold growth on decaying vegetation increases seasonally. Just walking through uncut fields or raking leaves can increase exposure. Thus mold spores can be responsible for both perennial and seasonal allergies.

Indoor allergens usually are present perennially; most important among these are house dust mite fecal proteins, animal dander, cockroaches, and certain mold species. Dust mite levels are on the rise, possibly due to the improved construction of energy-efficient homes and offices that result in reduced ventilation and increased humidity, use of wall-to-wall carpeting, and the popularity of cool water detergents and cold water washing.[3]

PHYSIOLOGY AND PATHOPHYSIOLOGY

NASAL PHYSIOLOGY

Knowledge of nasal physiology aids in the understanding of allergic rhinitis. The nose performs three "air conditioning" functions to prepare incoming gases and their contents for the lungs. During the fraction of a second that air is in the nose, it is heated, humidified, and cleaned. The cleaning process plays a role in the development of allergic rhinitis. As the air passes through the nose, the turbulence throws particulate matter against a mucous blanket. The rhythmic movements of the nasal cilia cause the mucous blanket to move posteriorly at approximately 9 mm/min, where it is eventually swallowed; therefore foreign particles are removed via the gastrointestinal tract and do not reach the lungs.

The vascular tissue in the nose is erectile. Stimulation of sympathetic fibers causes vasoconstriction, reduction in erectile tissue size, and airway widening. Parasympathetic stimulation causes vasodilatation, an increase in erectile tissue size, and airway narrowing.

Located in the nasal mucosa are the mast cells, which participate in the regulation of nasal patency by releasing such mediators as histamine. These are described below.

IMMUNE RESPONSE TO ALLERGENS

Allergic reactions in the nose are mediated by antigen-antibody responses, during which allergens interact with specific IgE molecules bound to nasal mast cells and basophils. In allergic people, these cells are increased in both number and reactivity. During inhalation, airborne allergens enter the nose and are processed by lymphocytes, which produce antigen-specific IgE, thereby sensitizing genetically predisposed hosts to those agents. Upon nasal re-exposure, IgE bound to mast cells interacts with airborne allergen, triggering release of inflammatory mediators (Fig. 93–1).[9]

Both immediate and late-phase reactions are observed after allergen exposure. The immediate reaction occurs within minutes, resulting in the rapid release of preformed mediators and newly generated mediators from the arachidonic acid cascade as the mast cell membrane is disturbed (Table 93–1). These mediators of immediate hypersensitivity include histamine, leukotrienes (LTs) C_4, LTD_4, LTE_4, prostaglandin D_2, tryptase, and kinins.[9] In addition, the mast

A

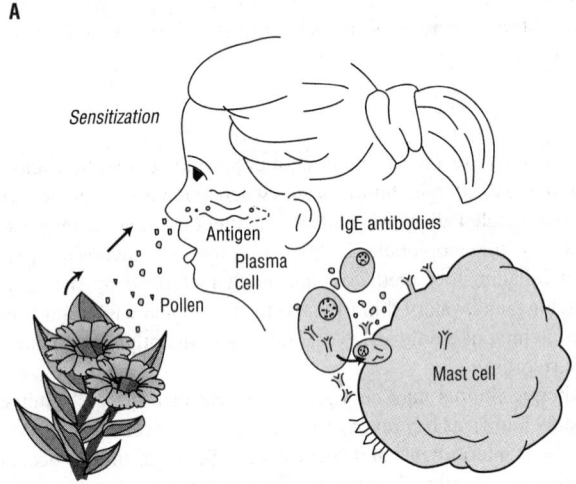

B

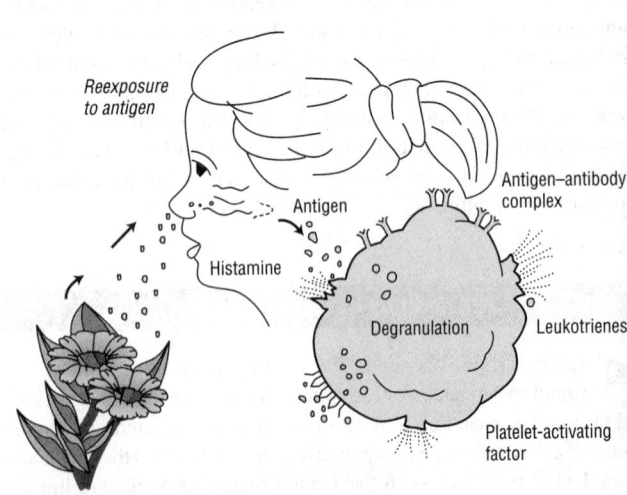

FIGURE 93–1. Allergen sensitization and the allergic response. *A.* Exposure to antigen stimulates IgE production and sensitization of mast cells with antigen-specific IgE antibodies. *B.* Subsequent exposure to the same antigen produces an allergic reaction when mast cell mediators are released.

TABLE 93–1. Mast Cell Mediators

Mediator	Effect
Preformed and rapidly released	
Histamine	Stimulates irritant receptors
	Pruritus
	Vascular permeability
	Mucosal permeability
	Smooth muscle contraction
Neutrophil chemotactic factor	Influx of inflammatory cells
Eosinophil chemotactic factor	Influx of inflammatory cells
Kinins	Vascular permeability
N-α-tosyl L-arginine methyl esterase	Vascular permeability
Newly generated	
Leukotrienes	Smooth muscle contraction
	Vascular permeability
	Mucus secretion
	Chemotaxis
	Neutrophil chemotaxis
Thromboxanes	Smooth muscle spasm
Platelet-activating factor	Mucus secretion
	Airway permeability
	Chemotaxis
	Vascular permeability
Granule matrix contents	
Heparin	Anti-inflammatory
Tryptase	Protein hydrolysis
Kallikrein	Protein hydrolysis

cell has been found to be a source of several cytokines that probably are relevant to the chronicity of the mucosal inflammation that characterizes allergic rhinitis.[10] Sensory nerve stimulation produces itching, and sneezing occurs via reflex stimulation of efferent vagal pathways. Neuropeptides substance P and calcitonin gene-related peptide from nonadrenergic, noncholinergic nerves affect vascular engorgement directly and via modulation of sympathetic tone. Histamine produces rhinorrhea, itching, sneezing, and obstruction, with the obstruction only partially blocked by H_1- or H_2-blocking agents.[11] Nasal obstruction is also caused by kinins, prostaglandin D_2, and LTC_4/LTD_4, and kinins, when directly administered, produce pain rather than itching.[12] These inflammatory mediators also produce vasodilation, increased vascular permeability, and production of nasal secretions.[13]

Four to eight hours after the initial exposure to an allergen, a late-phase reaction occurs in 50% of allergic rhinitis patients.[14] This response, thought to be due to cytokines released primarily by mast cells and thymus-derived helper lymphocytes, is characterized by profound infiltration and activation of migrating cells. This inflammatory response likely is responsible for the persistent, chronic symptoms of allergic rhinitis, including nasal congestion. The inflamed mucosa become hyperresponsive, a state characterized by exacerbation of nasal reactions to nonspecific or irritant triggers. In this state the patient also reacts to increasingly lower amounts of the same allergen.[15]

CLINICAL PRESENTATION

SYMPTOMS AND DIAGNOSIS

The patient with allergic rhinitis typically complains of clear rhinorrhea, paroxysms of sneezing, nasal congestion, postnasal drip, and pruritic eyes, ears, nose, or palate. Symptoms of allergic conjunctivitis are associated more frequently with seasonal than perennial allergic rhinitis, since a majority of the perennial allergens, such as dust mites and molds, are indoors, where air velocity is too low for substantial deposition of allergenic particles on the conjunctivae. However, with heavy exposure from animal or mold allergens, allergic conjunctivitis can be pronounced.

Symptoms secondary to the late-phase reaction, predominantly nasal congestion, begin 3 to 5 hours after antigen exposure and peak at 12 to 24 hours. Subsequent symptoms, both allergic and irritant, are elicited more easily because of the priming effect. For instance, a ragweed-sensitive patient, when exposed to ragweed pollen out of season, responds with modest symptoms and may be very tolerant of irritants such as air pollution or tobacco smoke. During the ragweed season, however, when the nasal mucosa is already inflamed, exposure to small doses of pollen or to irritants to which the patient is usually tolerant elicits a response clinically indistinguishable from his allergy.

Allergic rhinitis is differentiated from other causes of rhinitis by a thorough history, physical examination, and certain diagnostic tests. The medical history consists of a careful description of symptoms, environmental factors and exposures, results of previous therapy, use of other medications, previous nasal injuries, previous nasal or sinus surgery, family history, and the presence of other medical problems. Identification of specific causative allergens may be difficult. For example, a reaction induced by mowing the lawn may not be caused by grass pollens, but by the disturbance of various weeds, molds, or other plants in the lawn. With perennial allergic rhinitis, the cause-effect and temporal relationships are less clear, making the diagnosis more difficult, especially with such covert allergens as house dust mites and molds.

Physical examination may reveal allergic shiners, a transverse nasal crease caused by repeated rubbing of the nose, and adenoidal breathing. Pale, bluish, edematous nasal turbinates coated with thin, clear secretions are characteristic of a purely allergic reaction. Tearing, conjunctival injection and edema, and periorbital swelling may be present. Physical findings are generally less clear-cut in adults.

Nasal scrapings will provide a representative sample of cells infiltrating the nasal mucosa and can be helpful in supporting the diagnosis.[16] Microscopic examination of the nasal smear from an allergic individual typically will show numerous eosinophils. The blood eosinophil count may be elevated in allergic rhinitis, but it is nonspecific and has limited usefulness.[17]

Allergy testing can help determine whether a patient's rhinitis is caused by an allergic response to allergens. Immediate-type hypersensitivity skin tests are commonly used for the diagnosis of allergic rhinitis. These skin tests can be performed by the percutaneous route, where the diluted allergen is pricked or scratched into the skin surface, or by the intradermal route, where a small volume (0.01 to 0.05 mL) of diluted allergen is injected between the layers of skin. Percutaneous tests are more commonly performed and are safer and more generally accepted, with intradermal tests reserved for patients requiring confirmation.

In percutaneous testing, a positive control (histamine) and a negative control are essential for correct interpretation. After 15 minutes of the application of the allergen, the site is examined for a positive reaction (defined as a wheal and flare reaction). Because correct testing is done with extremely minute doses, undetectable by nonsensitized individuals, this reaction is evidence of the presence of mast cell–bound IgE specific to the allergen tested. Common allergens are available as standardized allergenic extracts.

Antihistamines and a few other medications interfere with the wheal and flare reaction. First-generation antihistamines should be stopped 3 days before testing, while second-generation, nonsedating antihistamines should be stopped for 10 days.[18] Medications with antihistamine properties (e.g., sympathomimetic agents, phenothiazines, and tricyclic antidepressants) and H_2-receptor antagonists (e.g., cimetidine, ranitidine, and famotidine) should be discontinued before skin testing. The radioallergosorbent test (RAST) was the first commonly used method for detecting IgE antibodies in the blood that are specific for a given allergen. Several other quantitative assays that include a reference curve calculated against standardized IgE are available.[19] These tests are highly specific but less sensitive than percutaneous tests.

COMPLICATIONS

Not only is allergic rhinitis aggravating, it also frequently leads to further complications, particularly if the patient does not receive adequate treatment. Symptoms of untreated rhinitis may lead to inability to sleep, chronic malaise, fatigue, and poor work or school efficiency. Patients often are plagued by loss of smell or taste, with sinusitis or polyps underlying many cases of allergy-related hyposmia. Postnasal drip with cough, hoarseness, and even vocal polyps also can be bothersome.

The role of allergic rhinitis in the development of acute otitis media or chronic middle ear effusion remains controversial. Children with allergic rhinitis appear to be at greater risk of these conditions because of nasal obstruction, insufflation of nasal secretions into the middle ear via eustachian tube obstruction, and negative middle ear pressure. Hearing problems in children related to middle ear effusion may lead to delayed development of language in young children school problems in older children.

Structural facial and dental problems can result from chronic allergic rhinitis.[20,21] The chronic edema and venous stasis may contribute to the development of a high-arched, V-shaped palate. Mouth breathing caused by nasal obstruction can be responsible for dental malocclusion and orthodontic problems. Constant upward rubbing of the nose (allergic salute) can cause a lasting transverse crease across the lower nose; nasal congestion leads to venous pooling and dark circles under the eyes known as *allergic shiners*.

Allergic rhinitis is clearly a risk factor for asthma. As many as 78% of asthma patients have nasal symptoms, while about 38% of allergic rhinitis patients have asthma.[3] Asthma is more common in those with perennial than seasonal allergic rhinitis, and it is less likely to be "outgrown" when associated with allergic rhinitis.[22]

Recurrent and chronic sinusitis are relatively common complications of allergic rhinitis. The structure of the mucus blanket breaks down, with a severe decrease of water production by serous glands leaving hair cells trapped in the larger mucus layer. This greatly reduces the clearance of trapped bacteria. This offers ideal breeding grounds and greatly increased growing time for the bacteria. Nasal polyps are less common but nonetheless bothersome; they require specific therapy but may improve with management of the underlying allergic state. Epistaxis also can be a problem; it is related to mucosal hyperemia and inflammation.

▶ TREATMENT: Allergic Rhinitis

DESIRED OUTCOME

The therapeutic goal for patients with allergic rhinitis is to minimize or prevent symptoms. This goal should be accomplished with no or minimal adverse medication effects and reasonable medication expenses. The patient should be able to maintain a normal lifestyle, including participating in outdoor activities, yard work, and playing with pets as desired.

GENERAL APPROACH TO TREATMENT

Once the causative allergens and the specific symptoms are identified, management consists of three possible approaches: (1) allergen avoidance, (2) pharmacotherapy for prevention or treatment of symptoms, and (3) specific immunotherapy. The pharmacotherapy for symptoms approach includes several options that are based on patient-specific information (Table 93–2). Figure 93–2 depicts an algorithm for treatment options.

AVOIDANCE

Avoidance of offending allergens is the most direct method of preventing allergic rhinitis, but it is often the most difficult to accomplish, especially for perennial allergens. Mold growth can be reduced by maintaining household humidity below 50% and removing obvious growth with bleach or disinfectant. Patients sensitive to animals will benefit most by removing pets from the home; however, most animal lovers are reluctant to comply with this approach. Cats may be more of a problem than dogs. Cat allergen is so prevalent and persistent in the air that in one survey 25% of cat-free houses contained detectable cat allergen.[23] Washing cats weekly may reduce allergens but studies have been inconclusive.[24] Some dogs display more profuse antigen than do others; clinically, a sensitized person may tolerate one animal better than another.

Efforts to eliminate dust mites should be rigorous, particularly in the bedroom. Exposure to dust mites can be reduced by encasing mattresses and pillows with impermeable covers and washing bed linens in hot water. Washable area rugs are preferable to wall-to-wall carpeting. Acaricide treatment of carpets has been shown to denature the dust mite allergen, but must be done repeatedly, resulting in inconvenience and expense. Atopic infants who are exposed to high levels of dust mites are at increased risk for developing asthma. Environmental control of these allergens may be helpful in forestalling further rhinitis and preventing later asthma.

Older central air-filtration systems for houses were expensive and minimally effective. High-efficiency particulate air (HEPA) filters have minimal effect on the dust mite allergens because these allergens are heavy and heavily charged electrically and are not typically floating in the air in the first place. These filters are effective in removing lightweight airborne particulates, including pollen, mold spores, and cat allergen, thus reducing allergic respiratory symptoms.[26]

Patients with seasonal allergic rhinitis should keep windows closed and minimize time spent outdoors during pollen season. Immediate hair washing and change of clothes are recommended upon returning indoors. Use of fans that direct outside air into the

TABLE 93–2. Pharmacotherapeutic Options For Allergic Rhinitis

Medication Class	Symptoms Controlled	Comments
Antihistamines		
Systemic	Sneezing, rhinorrhea, itching, conjunctivitis	For seasonal allergic rhinitis, begin treatment before allergen exposure. Nonsedating agents should be tried first. If ineffective or too expensive for the patient, the older agents may be used. For perennial allergic rhinitis, use an intranasal steroid as an alternative to or in combination with systemic antihistamines.
Ophthalmic	Conjunctivitis	Logical addition to nasal steroids if ocular symptoms are present.
Intranasal	Sneezing, rhinorrhea, nasal pruritus	Option for seasonal allergic rhinitis. Warn patients of potential drowsiness.
Decongestants		
Systemic	Nasal congestion	Only needed when nasal congestion is present.
Topical	Nasal congestion	Only needed when nasal congestion is present. Do not exceed 3–5 days.
Intranasal corticosteroids	Sneezing, rhinorrhea, itching, nasal congestion	For seasonal allergic rhinitis, an option when congestion is present. Must begin therapy before allergen exposure. Excellent choice for perennial rhinitis.
Mast cell stabilizers	See comments	Prevents symptoms; therefore, for seasonal allergic rhinitis, use before offending allergen's season starts. For perennial rhinitis, improvement may not be seen for up to 1 month.
Intranasal anticholinergics	Rhinorrhea	Reserve for use when above therapies fail or cannot be tolerated.

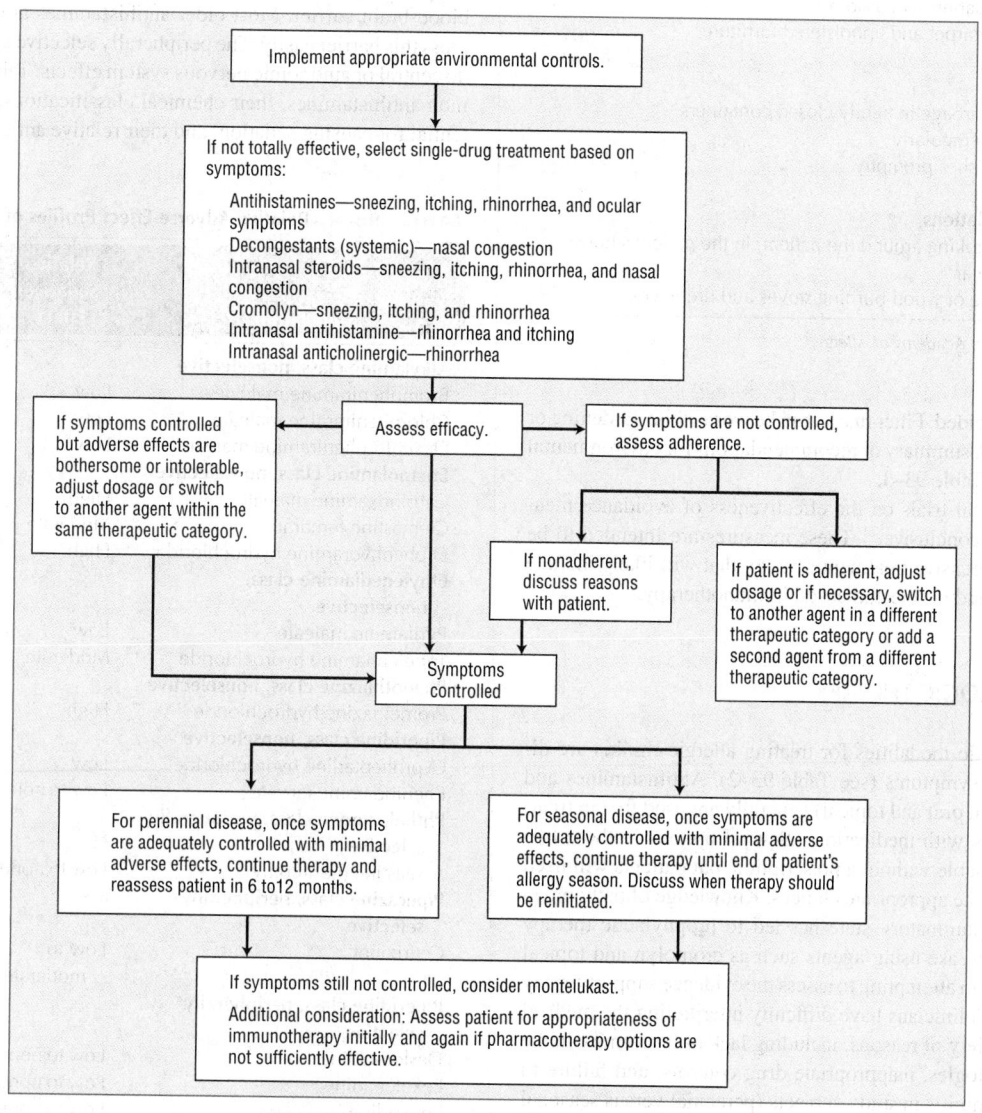

FIGURE 93–2. Treatment algorithm for allergic rhinitis.

TABLE 93–3. Environmental Controls to Prevent Allergic Rhinitis

Pollens
- Keep windows and doors closed during pollen season
- Avoid fans that draw in outside air
- Use air conditioning
- If possible, eliminate outside activities during times of high pollen counts
- Shower, shampoo, and change clothes following outdoor activity
- Use a vented dryer rather than an outside clothesline

Molds
- Use similar controls as above
- Avoid walking through uncut fields, working with compost or dry soil, and raking leaves
- Clean indoor moldy surfaces
- Fix all water leaks in home
- Reduce indoor humidity to <50% if possible

House dust mites
- Encase mattress, pillow, and box springs in an allergen-impermeable cover
- Wash bedding in hot water weekly
- Remove stuffed toys from bedroom
- Minimize carpet use and upholstered furniture
- Reduce indoor humidity to <50% if possible

Animal allergens (if removal of pet is not acceptable)
- Keep pet out of patient's bedroom
- Isolate pet from carpet and upholstered furniture
- Wash pet weekly

Cockroaches
- Keep food and garbage in tightly closed containers
- Take out garbage regularly
- Clean up dirty dishes promptly
- Use roach traps

Other recommendations
- Do not allow smoking around the patient, in the patient's house, or in the family car
- Minimize the use of wood-burning stoves and fireplaces

Adapted from American Academy of Allergy.[3]

house should be avoided. Filter masks can be worn while gardening or mowing the lawn. A summary of recommendations for environmental control is given in Table 93–3.

The few clinical trials on the effectiveness of avoidance measures have been inconclusive.[24] These measures are intended to be a part of a comprehensive treatment strategy that will likely include pharmacotherapy and in selected cases, immunotherapy.

PHARMACOLOGIC THERAPY

First-line therapeutic modalities for treating allergic rhinitis are directed at relief of symptoms (see Table 93–2). Antihistamines and decongestants (both oral and topical) generally are used first in treating allergic rhinitis with medications. Several options in these two categories are available without a prescription, but patients will need sound advice to make appropriate choices. Knowledge of pathophysiology and the inflammatory state has led to prophylactic therapy for more severe disease using agents such as cromolyn and topical steroids. However, in attempting to assess the evidence supporting any particular therapy, clinicians have difficulty interpreting the medical literature for a variety of reasons, including lack of uniformity in the research methodologies, inappropriate drug controls, and failure to identify types of rhinitis in study subjects (perennial versus seasonal and allergic versus nonallergic).

Antihistamines

Histamine (H_1)-receptor antagonists are competitive antagonists to histamine. They bind to H_1 receptors without activating them, preventing histamine binding and action. Newer antihistamines may also affect components of the inflammatory response such as histamine release, generation of adhesion molecules, and influx of inflammatory cells. While it was once thought that the older antihistamines had no anti-inflammatory action, some were shown to have these effects as early as the 1950s.[27] Antihistamines are available in oral, ophthalmic, and intranasal dosage forms.

The oral antihistamines are the most commonly used and can be divided two major categories: nonselective (first-generation) and peripherally selective (second-generation). Nonselective agents are commonly referred to as *sedating antihistamines*, and peripherally selective agents are referred to as *nonsedating antihistamines*. These generalizing terms can be misleading. Individual agents should be judged on their specific characteristics because variation within these broad categories exists. Also, the nonsedating claim is only valid when the newer agents are used at recommended doses.[28] This is of particular concern since some of these antihistamines are now available without a prescription. The mechanism for sedation is not well understood, but its central effect depends on the drugs' ability to cross the blood-brain barrier. Most older antihistamines are lipid-soluble and cross this barrier easily. The peripherally selective agents have little or no central or autonomic nervous system effects. Table 93–4 lists common antihistamines, their chemical classifications, their relative potential for causing sedation, and their relative anticholinergic effects.

TABLE 93–4. Relative Adverse-Effect Profiles of Antihistamines

Medication	Relative Sedative Effect	Relative Anticholinergic Effect
Alkylamine class, nonselective		
Brompheniramine maleate	Low	Moderate
Chlorpheniramine maleate	Low	Moderate
Dexchlorpheniramine maleate	Low	Moderate
Ethanolamine class, nonselective		
Carbinoxamine maleate	High	High
Clemastine fumarate	Moderate	High
Diphenhydramine hydrochloride	High	High
Ethylenediamine class, nonselective		
Pyrilamine maleate	Low	Low to none
Tripelennamine hydrochloride	Moderate	Low to none
Phenothiazine class, nonselective		
Promethazine hydrochloride	High	High
Piperidine class, nonselective		
Cyproheptadine hydrochloride	Low	Moderate
Phenindamine tartrate	Low to none	Moderate
Phthalazinone class, peripherally selective		
Azelastine (nasal only)	Low to none	Low to none
Piperazine class, peripherally selective		
Cetirizine	Low to moderate	Low to none
Piperidine class, peripherally selective		
Desloratadine	Low to none	Low to none
Fexofenadine	Low to none	Low to none
Loratadine	Low to none	Low to none

Antihistamines are more effective in preventing the actions of histamines than in reversing these actions once they have taken place. Reversal of symptoms is, at least in part, caused by the anticholinergic properties of these drugs. This activity is responsible for the drying effect of antihistamines, which reduces the problem of nasal, salivary, and lacrimal gland hypersecretion. Antihistamines antagonize increased capillary permeability, wheal-and-flare formation, and itching.

In general, the antihistamines are well absorbed, have large volumes of distribution, and are metabolized by the liver. Serum half-lives vary considerably between patients. Also, the therapeutic effects of these agents are more prolonged than might be predicted by their half-lives.

Drowsiness is usually the chief complaint of patients who take antihistamines. It can interfere with a patient's ability to drive a car or operate machinery and may interfere with the patient's ability to function adequately at the workplace. Remember that these problems can also be a reflection of the disease itself. For this reason, many recommend the use of peripherally selective agents as first-line treatment for any patients at high risk for the development of adverse events. This includes patients with renal or hepatic impairment, those with small weights (for whom adult doses may provide larger-than-recommended doses on a milligram per kilogram basis), patients with pre-existing central nervous system or cardiac disorders, patients who require higher doses, and patients who have shown tendencies to overuse nonprescription or prescription medications.[27]

The sedative effects of antihistamines can be useful in patients who suffer from sleeplessness caused by the symptoms of allergic rhinitis. In these patients, a bedtime dose may prove beneficial. However, they may cause residual daytime sedation, decreased alertness, and performance impairment.[24]

The logic of preferentially using the newer agents is not clear cut. A recent meta-analysis of performance-impairment trials did not show a clear and consistent distinction between diphenhydramine and the peripherally selective agents.[29] Another study showed that tolerance to sedation secondary to diphenhydramine developed by day 4 of treatment, becoming indistinguishable from placebo,[30] but sedation must be distinguished from impairment, as the two are not equivalent.

Anticholinergic (drying) effects contribute to the agents' therapeutic efficacy, but they also cause most adverse effects. Dry mouth, difficulty in voiding urine, constipation, and potential cardiovascular effects may be troublesome. Keep in mind that the differences may be small. Patients with a predisposition to urinary retention (e.g., elderly men and those on concurrent anticholinergic therapy) should use antihistamines with caution. Caution also should be used in patients with increased intraocular pressure, hyperthyroidism, and cardiovascular disease.

Other adverse effects of oral antihistamines include loss of appetite (and paradoxically, weight gain with increased appetite), nausea, vomiting, and epigastric distress.

Antihistamines are only fully effective when taken approximately 1 to 2 hours before anticipated exposure to the offending allergen. If tolerance develops to the therapeutic effect, a change to an agent in a different chemical class may be effective.

Patients should be counseled about the proper use of antihistamines. Adverse effects, especially drowsiness, should be emphasized. Patients should be warned against taking other central nervous system depressants, including the use of alcohol. Patients should be told not to take a double dose when a dose is missed. Taking the antihistamine with meals or at least a full glass of water will help prevent gastrointestinal adverse effects such as nausea, vomiting, and epigastric distress. Patients should check with their health care professional and read labels before taking nonprescription medications. Many cold products and sleep aids contain antihistamines. Patients should be instructed not to use more than one antihistamine at a time. Table 93–5 lists the recommended dosages of the commonly used agents with their prescription status.

TABLE 93–5. Oral Dosages of Commonly Used Oral Antihistamines and Decongestants

Medication	Availability	Dosage and Interval[a]	
		Adults	*Children*
Nonselective (First-generation) antihistamines			
Chlorpheniramine maleate, plain[b]	OTC	4 mg every 6 h	6–12 y: 2 mg every 6 h 2–5 y: 1 mg every 6 h
Chlorpheniramine maleate, sustained-release	OTC	8–12 mg daily at bedtime or 8–12 mg every 8 h	6–12 y: 8 mg at bedtime <6 y: Not recommended
Clemastine fumarate[b]	OTC	1.34 mg every 8 h	6–12 y: 0.67 mg every 12 h
Diphenhydramine hydrochloride[b]	OTC	25–50 mg every 8 h	5 mg/kg per day divided every 8 h (up to 25 mg per dose)
Peripherally selective (second-generation) antihistamines			
Loratadine[b]	OTC	10 mg once daily	6–12 y: 10 mg once daily 2–5 y: 5 mg once daily
Fexofenadine	RX	60 mg twice daily or 180 mg once daily	6–11 y: 30 mg twice daily
Cetirizine[b]	RX	5–10 mg once daily	>6 y: 5 mg once daily Infants 6–11 mo[c]
Oral decongestants			
Pseudoephedrine, plain	OTC	60 mg every 4–6 h	6–12 y: 30 mg every 4–6 h 2–5 y: 15 mg every 4–6 h
Pseudoephedrine, sustained-release[d]	OTC	120 mg every 12 h	Not recommended

[a]Dosage adjustment may be needed in renal/hepatic dysfunction. Refer to manufacturers' prescribing information.
[b]Available in liquid form.
[c]0.25 mg/kg orally demonstrated to be safe.[31]
[d]Controlled-release product available: 240 mg once daily (60-mg immediate-release with 180-mg controlled-release).

Many patients respond to and tolerate the older agents quite well. Because many of the older agents are available generically, they are much less expensive. Patient cost for many of the older nonprescription agents is less than $5 for a 30-day supply, compared with more than $20 for some of the nonprescription selective agents, and more than $70 dollars for the selective prescription-only products. While cost is a concern, patient safety should be the first consideration. Interestingly, in a 2003 survey, the most frequently recommended nonprescription antihistamine to adults by pharmacists was diphenhydramine.[32] This may change with the heavy promotion of competing brands of nonprescription loratadine. Loratadine in combination with pseudoephedrine did show up in the survey as the top pharmacists' pick in the "adult multisymptom allergy" category in that 2003 survey.

For seasonal allergic rhinitis, an intranasal antihistamine, azelastine, is available. Azelastine has been used successfully in patients who did not respond to loratadine.[33] Using the nasal route offers an alternative to switching to another oral antihistamine. Patient satisfaction has been varied because while the product produces rapid symptom relief, patients complain of drying effects, headache, and diminished effectiveness over time. Patients should be warned of the medication's potential to produce drowsiness, as its systemic availability is approximately 40%.[34]

Allergic conjunctivitis, often associated with allergic rhinitis, can be treated with an ophthalmic antihistamine such as levocabastine. Since systemic antihistamines usually are also effective for allergic conjunctivitis, levocabastine is a logical addition to nasal steroids when ocular symptoms occur, and is an acceptable approach in patients whose only symptoms involve the eyes.

CLINICAL CONTROVERSY

While many clinicians strongly prefer a peripherally selective agent as the first antihistamine choice, economic considerations still result in the first-line choice of the less expensive and more sedating products by some prescription plans and clinicians.

Decongestants

Topical and systemic decongestants are sympathomimetic agents that act on adrenergic receptors in the nasal mucosa, producing vasoconstriction. Decongestants shrink swollen mucosa and improve ventilation. When nasal congestion is part of the clinical picture, decongestants work well in combination with antihistamines.

Topical Decongestants. Topical decongestants are applied directly to swollen nasal mucosa via drops or sprays. Table 93–6 lists the common topical decongestants and their durations of action. The use of these agents results in little or no systemic absorption.

Because these agents are extremely effective and are available to patients without a prescription, they are widely used. However, prolonged use of these agents (for more than 3 to 5 days) can result in a condition known as *rhinitis medicamentosa*, or *rebound vasodilation*, with associated congestion. Patients who develop this condition use more spray more often with less response. While the methods used to treat this "addiction" have not been studied formally, several are used commonly. Abrupt cessation works, but it is difficult because of rebound congestion that may leave the patient congested for several days or weeks. Sleeping may become difficult. Nasal steroids have been used successfully, but they take several days to work. Weaning the patient off topical decongestants can be accomplished by decreasing the dosing frequency or the concentration over several weeks. Combining the weaning process with nasal steroids may prove useful.

Other adverse effects of topical decongestants include burning, stinging, sneezing, and dryness of the nasal mucosa.

Patients should be counseled on the use of topical decongestants to prevent rhinitis medicamentosa. Patients should be instructed to use as small a dose as possible as infrequently as possible and only when absolutely necessary (e.g., at bedtime to aid in falling asleep). Duration of therapy always should be limited to 3 to 5 days.

Systemic Decongestants. Oral decongestants are not as effective on an immediate basis as the topical agents, but their effects sometimes last longer and they cause less local irritation.

Also, rhinitis medicamentosa is not a problem with older agents. The most commonly used agent is pseudoephedrine. Usual doses for the regular and sustained-release version are given in Table 93–5. An oral form of phenylephrine is available by prescription only.

Concerns of safety have greatly limited the systemic decongestant options. Pseudoephedrine continues to be the most frequently used and the safest choice. Doses of 180 mg have been shown to produce no measurable change in blood pressure or heart rate.[35] In higher doses (210 to 240 mg), pseudoephedrine has raised both blood pressure and heart rate.[36] Pseudoephedrine can cause mild central nervous system stimulation, even at therapeutic doses. Stroke, related to oral decongestant use including pseudoephedrine, can occur in patients with hypertension and/or vasospasm.[37] Although stroke complications seem to be associated with higher-than-recommended doses, there is also a stroke risk when these agents are taken properly. Severe hypertensive reactions can occur when pseudoephedrine is given concomitantly with monoamine oxidase inhibitors.[38] Hypertensive patients should, unless absolutely necessary, avoid systemic decongestants.

Combination Products

Numerous products combine an antihistamine with a decongestant. The combination is rational because of the different mechanisms of action. Both nonselective and peripherally selective antihistamines are available in such combinations. As mentioned previously, patients should read labels to avoid therapeutic duplication.

Nasal Steroids

Nasal steroids are an excellent choice for treating perennial rhinitis and can be useful in seasonal rhinitis, especially if dosed in advance

TABLE 93–6. Duration of Action of Topical Decongestants

Medication	Duration (h)
Short-acting	
Phenylephrine hydrochloride	Up to 4
Intermediate-acting	
Naphazoline hydrochloride	4–6
Tetrahydrozoline hydrochloride	
Long-acting	
Oxymetazoline hydrochloride	Up to 12
Xylometazoline hydrochloride	

ABLE 93–7. Dosage of Nasal Steroids

Medication	Dosage and Interval
Beclomethasone dipropionate	>12 y: 1 inhalation (42 mcg) per nostril 2–4 times a day (maximum, 336 mcg/day) 6–12 y: 1 inhalation per nostril 3 times per day
Beclomethasone dipropionate, monohydrate	>12 y: 1–2 inhalations once daily 6–12 y: 1 inhalation per nostril (42 mcg) twice daily to start
Budesonide	>6 y: 2 sprays (64 mcg) per nostril in AM and PM or 4 sprays per nostril in AM (maximum, 256 mcg)
Flunisolide	Adults: 2 sprays (50 mcg) per nostril twice daily (maximum, 400 mcg) Children: 1 spray per nostril 3 times a day
Fluticasone	Adults: 2 sprays (100 mcg) per nostril once daily; after a few days decrease to 1 spray per nostril Children >4 y and adolescents: 1 spray per nostril once daily (maximum, 200 mcg/day)
Mometasone furoate	>12 y: 2 sprays (100 mcg) per nostril once daily
Triamcinolone acetonide	>12 y: 2 sprays (110 mcg) per nostril once daily (maximum, 440 mcg/day)

symptoms. Nasal steroids appear to be effective with minimal adverse effects. Some believe that nasal steroids should be recommended as initial therapy over antihistamines because of their high level of efficacy when used properly and along with avoidance of allergens.[39] Multiple mechanisms are involved with the effects of nasal steroids on the nasal mucosa: reducing inflammation by reducing mediator release, suppressing neutrophil chemotaxis, reducing intracellular edema, causing mild vasoconstriction, and inhibiting mast cell–mediated late-phase reactions.[40] Table 93–7 lists the available nasal steroids and their usual doses.

Topical steroids produce only minor adverse effects, most commonly sneezing, stinging, headache, and epistaxis. Despite concerns about safety of systemic steroids, nasal steroids have been found to have no significant association with hypothalamic-pituitary axis suppression, cataract formation, glaucoma, or bone mineral density changes in the doses used for allergic rhinitis. Growth suppression remains a question with some evidence showing that nasal steroids with higher bioavailability (e.g., beclomethasone) may have a greater growth suppression effect than less bioavailable agents.[41] These findings require more study. Most likely, all currently available nasal steroids are safe in the majority of patients and their clinical benefits outweigh any small growth suppressive effect. Other concerns include local infections with *Candida albicans*, which have occurred rarely.

The therapeutic benefits of topical steroids are not immediate. Patients need to understand this to ensure cooperation and continuation of therapy. Some patients notice improvement in a few days, but peak responses may not be observed for 2 to 3 weeks. Once a response is achieved the dosage may be reduced. Blocked nasal passages should be cleared with a decongestant before administration to ensure adequate penetration of the spray. Patients should be advised to avoid sneezing or blowing their noses for at least 10 minutes after administration. Topical steroids should not be used in patients with nasal septum ulcers or recent nasal surgery or trauma.

One additional benefit of nasal steroids in treating allergic rhinitis in individuals with asthma and upper airway conditions is that they

may confer some protection against exacerbations of asthma, leading to fewer emergency room visits. The overall relative risk for an emergency visit among asthma patients who received intranasal steroids was 0.7.[42] No effect was seen in patients receiving antihistamines.

Other Inhalant Medications

Cromolyn sodium and ipratropium bromide offer two additional approaches for treating allergic rhinitis. Cromolyn sodium is a mast cell stabilizer. Increased interest in this product has resulted from it becoming available without a prescription. Ipratropium bromide is an anticholinergic agent useful in perennial allergic rhinitis.

Cromolyn sodium nasal spray is used for the symptomatic prevention and treatment of allergic rhinitis. It curtails antigen-triggered mast cell degranulation and release of the mediators of allergic reactions, including histamine. Cromolyn sodium has no direct antihistaminic, anticholinergic, or anti-inflammatory properties. Similarly to topical steroids, the most common adverse effects—sneezing and nasal stinging—result from local irritation. The dose in adults and children at least 2 years of age is one spray in each nostril three to four times per day at regular intervals every 4 to 6 hours. Cromolyn sodium must cover the entire nasal lining; therefore patients should be instructed to clear nasal passages before administration. Inhaling through the nose during administration aids in this process. Dosing must be repeated at 6-hour intervals to maintain the effect.

For seasonal rhinitis, treatment with cromolyn sodium should be initiated just before the usual start of the offending allergen's season and continued throughout the season. In perennial rhinitis, the effects may not be seen for 2 to 4 weeks; therefore antihistamines or decongestants may be needed during this initial phase of therapy. As cromolyn sodium begins to work, the need for these medications should decrease.

Ipratropium nasal spray is an anticholinergic agent that exhibits antisecretory properties when applied locally. It provides symptomatic relief of rhinorrhea associated with allergic and other forms of chronic rhinitis. The 0.03% solution is given as two sprays (42 mcg) two to three times daily. The optimal dose should be determined based on the specific patient's symptoms and response. Adverse effects are mild, with the most common being headache, nosebleeds, and nasal dryness.

IMMUNOTHERAPY

The first report of the successful use of grass pollen extract injections to treat allergic rhinitis was published in 1911 by Noon.[43] The therapy was first called *desensitization*; however, this did not seem appropriate because skin reactivity sometimes remained. The name was later changed to *hyposensitization*. While this term is still used today, *immunotherapy* is used more commonly and is less confusing.

Immunotherapy is the slow, gradual process of injecting increasing doses of antigens responsible for eliciting allergic symptoms in a patient with the hope of inducing tolerance to the allergen when natural exposure occurs. Several mechanisms have been proposed to explain the beneficial effects of immunotherapy, including: induction of IgG antibodies, reduction in specific IgE (long-term), reduced recruitment of effector cells, altered T-cell cytokine balance (a shift from Th1 to Th2), T-cell anergy, and induction of regulatory T cells.[44]

Immunotherapy is expensive, has significant potential risks, and requires a major time commitment from the patient. For these reasons, it should be considered only in a select group of patients. Candidates for immunotherapy should have a strong history of severe symptoms unsuccessfully controlled by avoidance and pharmacotherapy, or stand to achieve more benefit in other significant ways, such as with asthma. Immunotherapy may postpone the onset of asthma or possibly even prevent it.[45] Patients who have been unable to tolerate the adverse effects of properly managed drug therapy also should be considered. Patients must be committed to the necessary regular office visits required to complete this long course of therapy.

The effectiveness of immunotherapy for seasonal allergic rhinitis appears to be better than that seen with perennial rhinitis, in part because it is more difficult to determine which allergen is responsible for perennial symptoms, and it is more due to multiple sensitizations. Effectiveness has been shown in a number of clinical studies using a variety of pollen extracts, even in patients with severe disease resistant to pharmacotherapy.[44] Specific immunotherapy for house dust mites has had good results in appropriately selected patients, while several studies have described marked improvement in patients with allergy to cats. Data indicate that in some patients 3 years of immunotherapy may be sufficient to give lasting benefit.[46]

The selection of antigens should be based on patient history and skin test results. Numerous regimens for administration of selected allergens have been suggested. In general, very dilute solutions are given initially one to two times per week. The concentration is increased until the maximum tolerated dose is achieved. This maintenance dose is continued every 2 to 6 weeks, depending on clinical response. In light of the present understanding of the immunologic results of immunotherapy, it should be given year-round rather than seasonally.

Adverse reactions can occur with immunotherapy and range from mild to life-threatening. Among the most common are mild local reactions, consisting of induration and swelling at the site of the injection. These may be immediate or delayed. Other more serious reactions (e.g., generalized urticaria, bronchospasm, laryngospasm, and vascular collapse) occur rarely; deaths can result from anaphylactic reactions. Severe reactions are treated with epinephrine. Antihistamines and systemic corticosteroids may also be used as adjunctive therapy, and in rare circumstances glucagon may be necessary.

Several patient types have been identified as poor candidates for immunotherapy, including: patients with any medical condition that would compromise the ability to tolerate an anaphylactic-type reaction, patients with impaired immune systems, and patients with a history of nonadherence to therapy.[47]

NEW AND ALTERNATIVE TREATMENT OPTIONS

Montelukast is the first leukotriene receptor antagonist that has received approved labeling for the treatment of seasonal allergic rhinitis. Leukotriene receptor antagonists inhibit the cysteinyl leukotriene receptor. The cysteinyl leukotrienes are among the inflammatory mediators released from mast cells. Montelukast is effective alone or in combination with an antihistamine.[48] Dosage regimens are given in Table 93–8. While this class represents a therapeutic alternative,

TABLE 93–8. Dosage Regimens for Montelukast in Treatment of Allergic Rhinitis

Age	Dosage[a]
Adults and adolescents >15 years	One 10-mg tablet daily
Children 6–14 years	One 5-mg chewable tablet daily
Children 2–5 years	One 4-mg chewable tablet or oral granule packet daily

[a]The timing of drug administration can be individualized. If the patient has combined asthma and seasonal allergic rhinitis, the dose should be given in the evening.

studies published to date show them to be no more effective than peripherally selective antihistamines, and less effective than intranasal steroids.[49]

The recent development of monoclonal antibodies directed against the binding site of IgE points to a potentially exciting new way to treat allergic respiratory diseases. Omalizumab, a recombinant humanized anti-IgE monoclonal antibody, is the first to show efficacy in allergic rhinitis.[50] The actual mechanism of how this agent is thought to work is quite complex.[51] Anti-IgE antibodies bind to the site on the IgE molecule that recognizes the IgE receptor, thereby preventing the IgE molecule from binding to mast cells or basophils. The half-life of IgE antibodies on the mast cell surface is about 6 weeks, and as the antibodies turn over they become available for binding to anti-IgE antibodies. Therefore, by giving repeated doses of omalizumab, the number of IgE antibodies on the mast cell surface can be significantly reduced over time. These new IgE molecules are not eliminated, but remain in circulation as small immune complexes. IgE receptor numbers on basophils and mast cells may be decreased as a result of downregulation. Because of the expensive nature of this therapy, omalizumab's role has not been defined. Some promising results have been described when it is used in combination with immunotherapy.[52]

CLINICAL CONTROVERSY

Omalizumab may offer significant long-term benefits to allergic rhinitis patients, but it may prove to be too expensive to gain widespread acceptance.

As mentioned earlier in this chapter, microbial exposure in the early years of life could help prevent allergic disease by developing a non-atopic immune response.[6] This concept was further studied by administering *Lactobacillus rhamnosus* prenatally to mothers who had at least one first-degree relative or partner with atopic disease (eczema, allergic rhinitis, or asthma) and postnatally for 6 months to their infants.[53]

CLINICAL CONTROVERSY

Recent evidence shows that probiotics might be useful in preventing the onset of allergic disease, but more research needs to be conducted before use of these products is recommended.

PHARMACOECONOMIC CONSIDERATIONS

The economic impact of allergic rhinitis is enormous. The direct costs have grown significantly over the past few years because of the increasing use of peripherally selective antihistamines and nasal steroids. The most recent detailed review estimated expenditures of $3.4 billion annually in the United States, with the majority of this cost attributed to prescription medications and outpatient visits.[5] Of prescribed medications, 51% were peripherally selective antihistamines, 25% intranasal steroids, and 5% were older antihistamines.

tal of 58% of patients received one or more agents. The mean prescription medication expenditure was $103 per patient for those on Medicaid, $155 with private insurance, and $69 for patients with no insurance. These figures do not include expenditures for nonprescription medications. With various brands and generic equivalents of nonprescription nonsedating products being heavily marketed to consumers, one would guess that usage of these agents would greatly increase. How this will affect the prescription market is unknown.

Direct-to-consumer advertising for prescription-only allergic rhinitis treatment options has also increased significantly. Indirect costs related to missed school or work days and loss of productivity may approach the amount for the direct costs.[55]

The most cost-effective choice of treatment for allergic rhinitis an individualized decision. Seasonal allergic rhinitis patients who see improvement and can tolerate nonprescription and/or generic antihistamines will experience the least impact on out-of-pocket medical and drug expenses. If these are not effective, the economic picture becomes more complicated. Choices should follow the logical path based on symptoms, tolerance, and efficacy, as described earlier in this chapter.

EVALUATION OF THERAPEUTIC OUTCOMES

With allergic rhinitis, the major outcomes issues include the effect of the disease on a patient's life, the efficacy and tolerability of treatment, and patient satisfaction. Consideration must be given to how the condition is affecting the patient's job or school performance, family and social interactions, and other aspects of quality of life. The drug therapy should prevent or minimize symptoms with minimal or no adverse effects. The patient should not have difficulty obtaining needed medication for financial or other reasons. Patients should be questioned about their satisfaction with the management of their allergic rhinitis. The management should result in minimal disruption to their lives.

Both the Medical Outcomes Study 36-Item Short Form Health Survey and the Rhinoconjunctivitis Quality of Life Questionnaire have been used to evaluate outcomes of treatment for seasonal and perennial allergic rhinitis.[56–58] These tools go beyond measuring improvement in symptoms and include such items as sleep quality, nonallergic symptoms (e.g., fatigue, poor concentration, and others), emotions, and participation in a variety of activities. How well each of the current treatment modalities performs and how they compare in improving patient outcomes remain to be determined.

Clinicians caring for allergic rhinitis patients should develop a comprehensive pharmaceutical care plan that addresses several areas. Discuss and agree on therapeutic end points for allergic rhinitis, including the patient's acceptable level of symptom relief, onset of symptom relief expectations, and seasonal starts and stops. Discuss adverse drug reaction self-monitoring and prevention based on treatment selection. Assess patient attitude toward adherence to and persistence with oral, ocular, intranasal, or immunologic therapies. Ensure proper matching of treatment to symptoms and intervene with the prescriber if necessary. Conduct seasonal or annual review with patient.

The therapeutic goal for all patients with allergic rhinitis is to minimize or prevent symptoms. Evaluation of success is accomplished primarily through the discussions with the patient, in whom both relief of symptoms and tolerance of drug therapy must be discussed.

ABBREVIATIONS

HEPA: high-efficiency particulate air (filter)
IgE: immunoglobulin E
LT: leukotriene
RAST: radioallergosorbent test

Review Questions and other resources can be found at *www.pharmacotherapyonline.com*.

REFERENCES

1. McCrory DC, Williams JW, Dolor RJ, et al. Management of Allergic Rhinitis in the Working-Age Population. Evidence Report/Technology Assessment No. 67. Prepared by Duke Evidence-based Practice Center under Contract No. 290-97-0014. Agency for Healthcare Research and Quality, January 2003.
2. Spector SL. Supplement: New insights into allergic rhinitis: Quality of life, associated airway diseases, and antihistamine potency. Overview of comorbid associations of allergic rhinitis. J Allergy Clin Immunol 1997; 99:S773–780.
3. The American Academy of Allergy, Asthma, and Immunology Inc. The Allergy Report. Available at http://www.aaaai.org/ar/. Accessed October 31, 2003.
4. Marshall PS, O'Hara C, Steinberg P. Effects of seasonal allergic rhinitis on fatigue levels and mood. Psychosom Med 2002;64:684–691.
5. Sauder A, Kovacs M. Anxiety symptoms in allergic patients: Identification and risk factors. Psychosom Med 2003;65:816–823.
6. Riedler J, Braun-Fahrlander C, Eder W, et al. Exposure to farming early in life and development of asthma and allergy: A cross-sectional survey. Lancet 2001;358:1129–1133.
7. Crimi P, Boidi M, Minale P, et al. Differences in prevalence of allergic sensitization in urban and rural school children. Ann Allergy Asthma Immunnol 1999;83:252–256.
8. Skoner DP. Allergic rhinitis: Definition, epidemiology, pathophysiology, detection, and diagnosis. J Allergy Clin Immunol 2001;8:S2–S8.
9. Wilson SJ, Shute JK, Holgate ST, et al. Localization of interleukin (IL)-4 but not 5 to human mast cell secretory granules by immunoelectron microscopy. Clin Exp Allergy 2000;30:493–500.
10. Riccio AAM, Tosco MA, Cosentino C, et al. Cytokine pattern in allergic and non-allergic chronic rhinosinusitis in asthmatic children. Clin Exp Allergy 2002;32:422–426.
11. Wood-Baker R, Lau L, Howarth PH. Histamine and the nasal vasculature: the influence of H1 and H2-histamine receptor antagonism. Clin Otolaryngol 1996;21:348–352.
12. Howarth PH. Mediators of nasal blockage in allergic rhinitis. Allergy 1997;52(40 Suppl):12–18.
13. Howarth PH. Leukotrienes in rhinitis. Am J Resp Crit Care Med 2000; 161(2 Pt 2):S133–136.
14. Clark RR, Baroody FM. What drives the symptoms of allergic rhinitis? J Respir Dis 1998;19:S6–15.
15. Gerth van Wijk R. Perennial allergic rhinitis and nasal hyperreactivity. Am J Rhinol 1998;12:33–35.
16. Klaewsongkram J, Ruxrungtham K, Wannakrairot P, et al. Eosinophil count in nasal mucosa is more suitable than the number of ICAM-1-positive nasal epithelial cells to evaluate the severity of house dust mite-sensitive allergic rhinitis: A clinical correlation study. Int Arch Allergy Immunol 2003;132:68–75.
17. Braunstahl GJ, Fokkens WJ, Overbeek SE, et al. Mucosal and systemic inflammatory changes in allergic rhinitis and asthma: A comparison between upper and lower airways. Clin Exp Allergy 2003;33:579–587.
18. Lasley MV, Shapiro GG. Testing for allergy. Pediatr Rev 2000;21:39–43.
19. Li JT. Allergy testing. Am Fam Physician 2002;66:621–626.
20. Trask G, Shapiro G, Shapiro P. The effects of perennial allergic rhinitis on dental and skeletal development: A comparison of sibling pairs. Am J Orthod Dentofacial Orthop 1987;92:286–293.

21. Shapiro G, Shapiro P. Nasal airway obstruction and facial development. Clin Rev Allergy 1984;2:225–236.

22. Verdiani P, Di CS, Baronti A. Different prevalence and degree of nonspecific bronchial hyperreactivity between seasonal and perennial rhinitis. J Allergy Clin Immunol 1990;86:576–582.

23. Ferguson BJ. Allergic rhinitis: Recognizing signs, symptoms and triggering allergens. Postgrad Med 1997;101:110–116.

24. Rosenwasser LJ. Treatment of allergic rhinitis. Am J Med 2002;113: 17S–24S.

25. Sporik S, Holgate S, Platts-Mills T. Exposure to house dust mite allergen and the development of asthma in childhood: A prospective study. N Engl J Med 1990;323:502.

26. Reisman R, Mauriello P, Davis G, et al. A double-blind study of the effectiveness of a high efficiency particulate air (HEPA) filter in the treatment of patients with perennial allergic rhinitis and asthma. J Allergy Clin Immunol 1990;85:1050–1057.

27. Casale TB, Blaiss MS, Gelfand E, et al. First do no harm: Managing antihistamine impairment in patients with allergic rhinitis. J Allergy Clin Immunol 2003;111:S835–842.

28. Sansgiry SS, Shringarpure GS. Springtime confusion: Are consumers getting the right information on how to treat seasonal allergies? J Allergy Clin Immunol 2003;112:627–628.

29. Bender BG, Berning S, Dudden R, et al. Sedation and performance impairment of diphenhydramine and second-generation antihistamines: A meta-analysis. J Allergy Clin Immunol 2003;111:770–776.

30. Richardson GS, Roehrs TA, Rosenthal L, et al. Tolerance to daytime sedative effects of H1 antihistamines. J Clin Psychopharmacol 2002;22: 511–515.

31. Simons FE, Silas P, Portnoy JM, et al. Safety of cetirizine in infants 6 to 11 months of age: A randomized, double-blind, placebo-controlled study. J Allergy Clin Immunol 2003;111:1244–1248.

32. 2003 Survey Pharmacist Survey of OTC Products. Pharmacy Today 2003 (October Supplement):22–26.

33. Berger WE, White MV. Efficacy of azelastine nasal spray in patients with an unsatisfactory response to loratadine. Ann Allergy Immunol 2003; 91:205–211.

34. Astelin product information. Wallace Laboratories, Cranbury, NJ, 1997.

35. Empey DE, Young GA, Letley E, et al. Dose response study of the nasal decongestant and cardiovascular effects of pseudoephedrine. Br J Clin Pharmacol 1980;9:351–358.

36. Drew CDM, Knight GT, Hughes DTD, et al. Comparison of the effects of D-(−)-ephedrine and L-(+)-pseudoephedrine on the cardiovascular and respiratory systems in man. Br J Clin Pharmacol 1978;6:221–225.

37. Cantu C, Arauz A, Murilla-Bonilla LM, et al. Stroke associated with sympathomimetics contained in over-the-counter cough and cold drugs. Stroke 2003;34:1667–1673.

38. Drug interaction facts. In: Tatro DS, ed. Facts and Comparisons. St. Louis, Facts and Comparisons, 1999:679.

39. Weiner JM, Abramson MJ, Puy RM. Intranasal corticosteroids versus oral H1 receptor antagonists in allergic disease: Systematic review of randomized controlled trials. Br Med J 1998;317:1624–1629.

40. Quintiliani R. Hypersensitivity and adverse reactions associated with the use of newer intranasal corticosteroids for allergic rhinitis. Curr Ther Res 1996;57:478–488.

41. Mehle ME. Are nasal steroids safe? Curr Opin Otolaryngol Head Neck Surg 2003;11:201–205.

42. Adams RJ, Fuhlbrigge AL, Finkelstein JA, Weiss ST. Intranasal steroids and the risk of emergency department visits for asthma. J Allergy Clin Immunol 2002;109:636–642.

43. Noon L. Prophylactic inoculation against hay fever. Lancet 1911;1: 1572–1573.

44. Frew AJ. Immunotherapy of allergic disease. J Allergy Clin Immunol 2003;111:S712–S719.

45. Moller C, Dreborg S, Ferdousi HA, et al. Pollen immunotherapy reduces the development of asthma in children with seasonal rhinoconjunctivitis (the PAT-study). J Allergy Clin Immunol 2002;109:251–256.

46. Durham SR, Walker SM, Varga EM, et al. Long term clinical efficacy of grass pollen immunotherapy. N Engl J Med 1999;341:468–475.

47. Schoenwetter WF. Safe allergen immunotherapy. Postgrad Med 1996; 100:123–135.

48. Meltzer EO, Malmstrom K, Lu S, et al. Concomitant montelukast and loratadine as treatment for seasonal allergic rhinitis: A randomized placebo controlled clinical trial. J Allergy Clin Immunol 2000;105:917–922.

49. Casale TB, Condemi J, LaForce C, et al. Effect of omalizumab on symptoms of seasonal allergic rhinitis. JAMA 2001;286:2956–2967.

50. Nathan RA. Pharmacotherapy of allergic rhinitis: A critical review of leukotriene receptor antagonists compared with other treatments. Ann Allergy Asthma Immunol 2003:90:182–190.

51. Frew AJ. Anti-IgE and asthma. J Allergy Asthma Immunol 2003;91: 117–118.

52. Kuehr J, Brauburger J, Zielen S, et al. Efficacy of combination treatment with anti-IgE plus immunotherapy in polysensitized children and adolescents with seasonal allergic rhinitis. J Allergy Clin Immunol 2002;109: 274–280.

53. Kalliomaki M, Salminen S, Arvilommi H, et al. Probiotics in primary prevention of atopic disease: A randomized placebo-controlled trial. Lancet 2001;357:1076–1079.

54. Law AW, Reed SD, Sundy JS, Schulman KA. Direct costs of allergic rhinitis in the United States: Estimates from the 1996 medical expenditure survey. J Allergy Clin Immunol 2003;111:296–300.

55. Rossoff LJ, Stempel DA, Alam R, et al. The health and economic impact of allergic rhinitis. Am J Manage Care 1997;3:S8–S18.

56. Bousquet J, Duchateau J, Pignat JC, et al. Improvement of quality of life by treatment with cetirizine in patients with perennial allergic rhinitis as determined by a French version of the SF-36 questionnaire. J Allergy Clin Immunol 1996;98:309–316.

57. Meltzer EO, Nathan RA, Selner JC, Storms W. Quality of life and rhinitic symptoms: Results of a nationwide survey with the SF-36 and RQLQ questionnaires. J Allergy Clin Immunol 1997;99:S815–S819.

58. Harvey RP, Comer C, Sanders B, et al. Model for outcomes assessment of antihistamine use for seasonal allergic rhinitis. J Allergy Clin Immunol 1996;97:1233–1241.

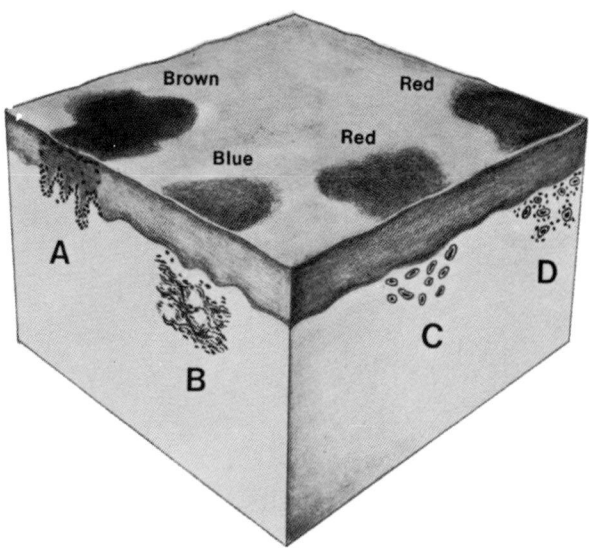

A.

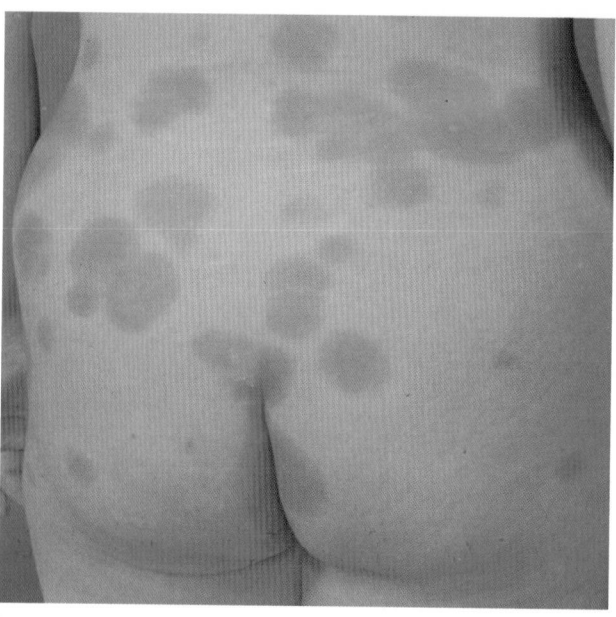

B.

PLATE 1. *Macules* are circumscribed, flat lesions of any shape or size that differ from surrounding skin because of their color. *A.* Macules may be the result of hyperpigmentation (*A*), hypopigmentation, dermal pigmentation (*B*), vascular abnormalities, capillary dilatation (erythema) (*C*), or purpura (*D*). *B.* The clinical appearance of a drug reaction that has produced an eruption consisting of multiple, well-defined red macules of varying size that blanch upon pressure (diascopy) and are thus due to inflammatory vasodilation. (Reprinted with permission from Freedberg IM, et al, eds. Fitzpatrick's Dermatology in General Medicine, 6th ed. New York, McGraw-Hill, 2003, p 14.)

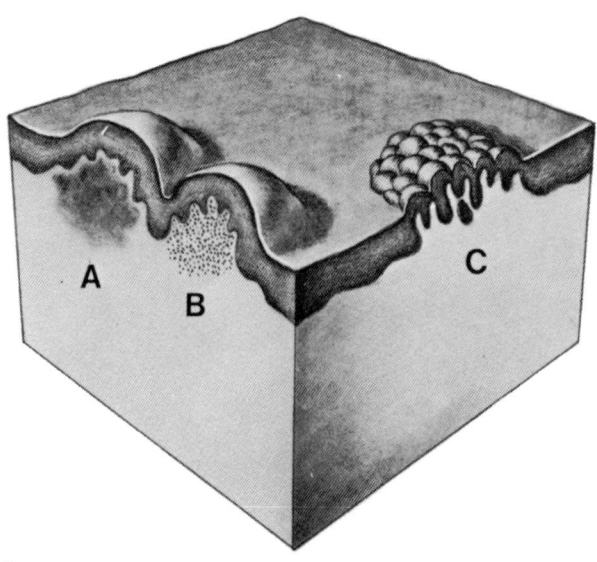

A.

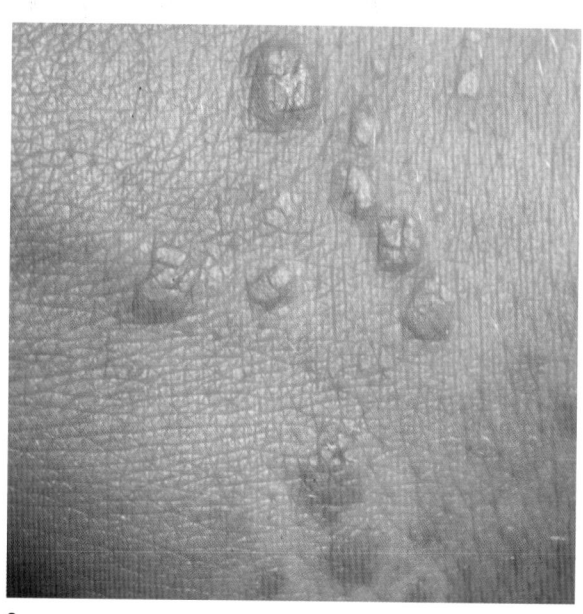

C.

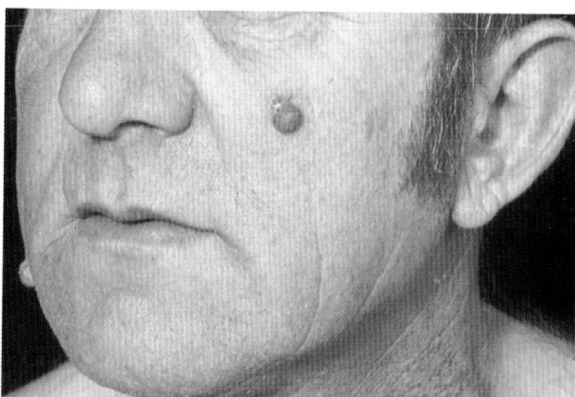

B.

PLATE 2. *Papules* are small, solid, elevated lesions that are less than 1 cm in diameter. The major portion of a papule projects above the plane of the surrounding skin. *A.* Papules may result, for example, from metabolic deposits in the dermis (*A*), from localized dermal cellular infiltrates (*B*), and from localized hyperplasia of cellular elements in the dermis and epidermis (*C*). Papules with scaling are referred to as *papulosquamous lesions*, as in psoriasis (see Chap. 96). *B.* Clinical examples of papules. *C.* Two well-defined and dome-shaped papules of firm consistency and brownish color, which are dermal melanocytic nevi; multiple, well defined, and coalescing papules of varying size are seen. Their violaceous color, glistening surface, and flat tops are characteristic of lichen planus. (Reprinted with permission from Freedberg IM, et al, eds. Fitzpatrick's Dermatology in General Medicine, 6th ed. New York, McGraw-Hill, 2003, p 15.)

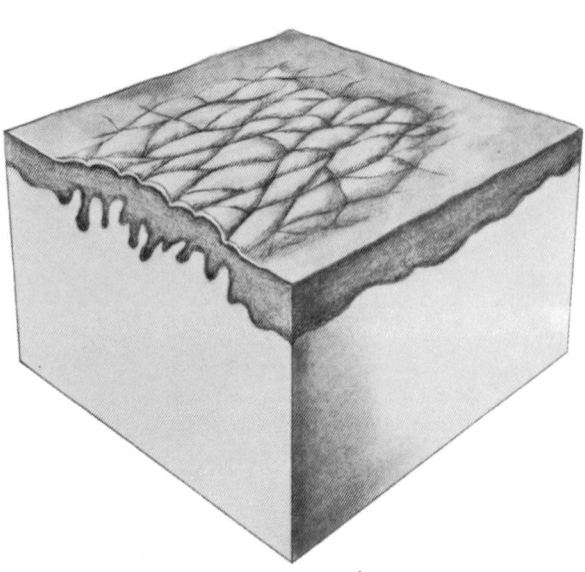

A.

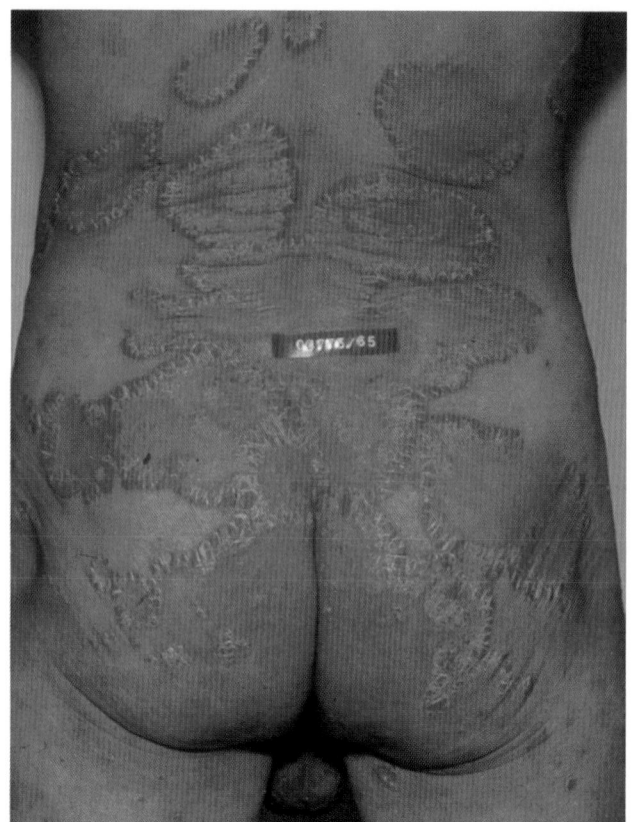

B.

PLATE 3. *A. Plaque* is a mesa-like elevation that occupies a relatively large surface area in comparison with its height above the skin surface. *B.* Well-defined, reddish, scaling plaques can coalesce to cover large areas of the back and buttocks, with some regression in the center as is common in psoriasis (see Chap. 96). *C. Lichenification*, a thickening of the skin and accentuation of skin, can result from repeated rubbing. It develops frequently in patients with atopy, and also occurs in eczematous dermatitis or other conditions associated with pruritus. Lesions of lichenification are not as well defined as most plaques and often show signs of scratching, such as in excoriations and crusts. (Reprinted with permission from Freedberg IM, et al, eds. Fitzpatrick's Dermatology in General Medicine, 6th ed. New York, McGraw-Hill, 2003, p 16.)

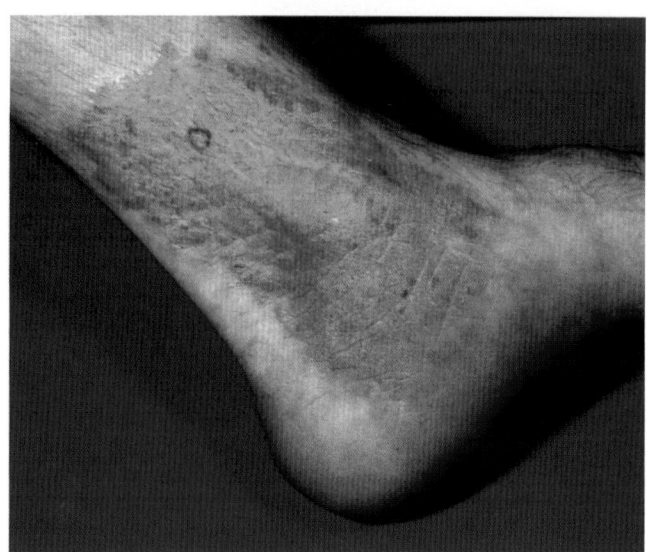

C.

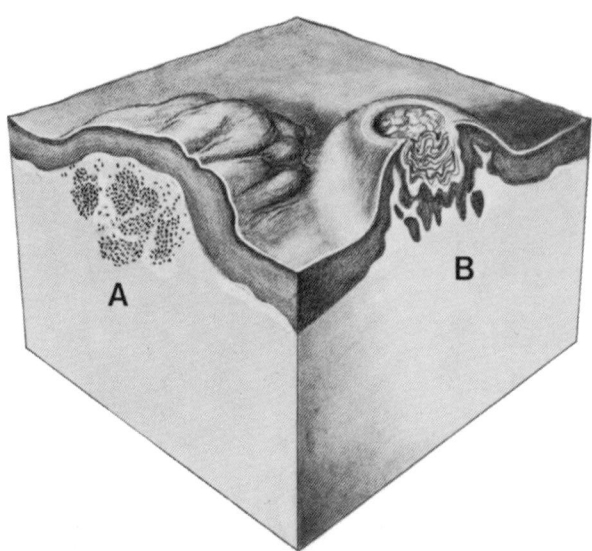

A.

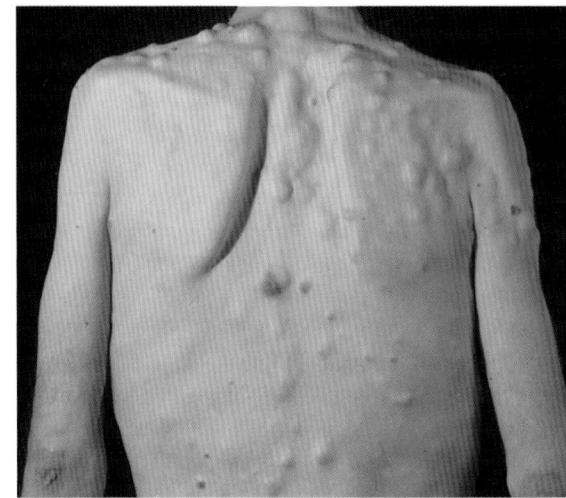

C.

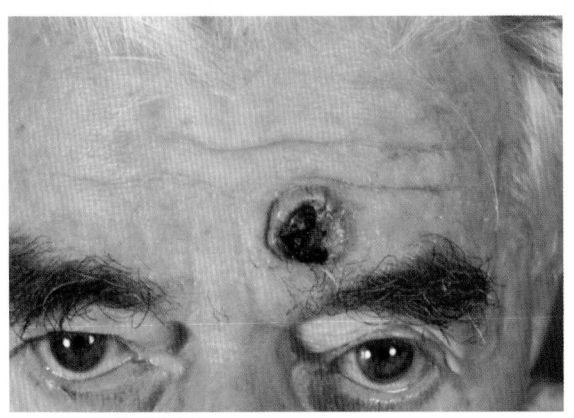

B.

PLATE 4. *Nodules* are palpable, solid, round or ellipsoidal lesions. Depth of involvement and/or substantive palpability rather than diameter differentiates a nodule from a papule. *A.* Nodules may be located in the epidermis (*B*) or extend into the dermis or subcutaneous tissue (*A*). *B.* This photograph shows a well-defined, firm nodule with a smooth and glistening surface through which telangiectasia (dilated capillaries) can be seen; there is central crusting indicating tissue breakdown and thus incipient ulceration (nodular basal cell carcinoma). *C.* Multiple nodules of varying size can be seen (melanoma metastases). (Reprinted with permission from Freedberg IM, et al, eds. Fitzpatrick's Dermatology in General Medicine, 6th ed. New York, McGraw-Hill, 2003, p 17.)

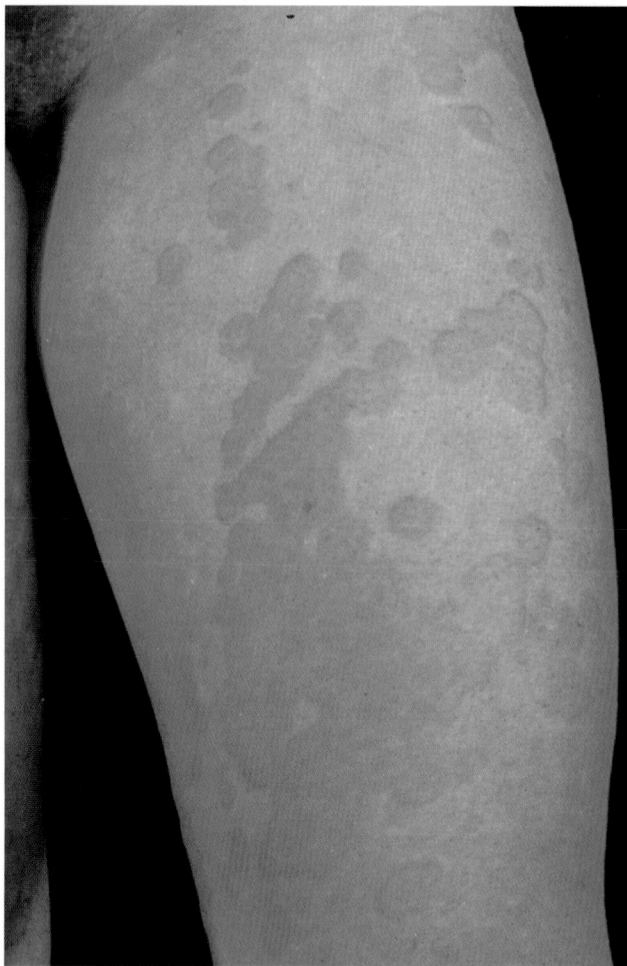

C.

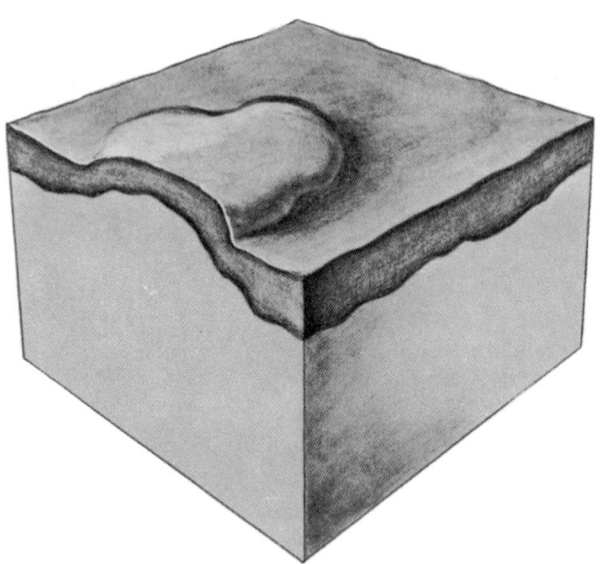

A.

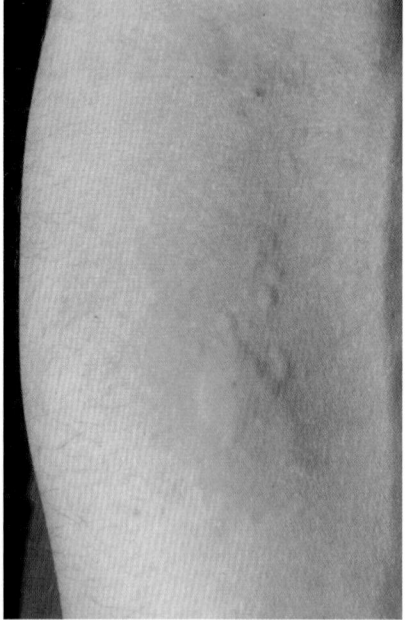

B.

PLATE 5. A. *Wheals* are rounded or flat-topped papules or plaques that are characteristically evanescent, disappearing within hours. An eruption consisting of wheals is termed *urticaria* and usually itches. B. Wheals may be tiny papules 3 to 4 mm in diameter, as in cholinergic urticaria. C. Alternatively, wheals may present as large coalescing plaques, as in allergic reactions to penicillin, other drugs, or alimentary allergens. (Reprinted with permission from Freedberg IM, et al, eds. Fitzpatrick's Dermatology in General Medicine, 6th ed. New York, McGraw-Hill, 2003, p 18.)

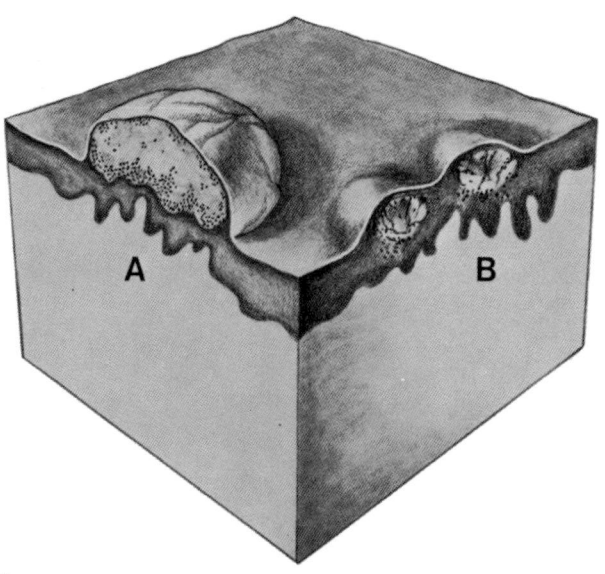

A.

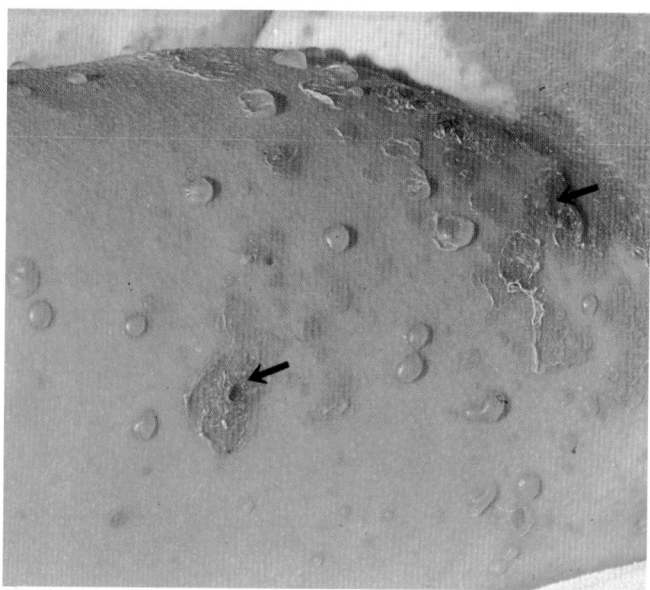

B.

PLATE 6. *Vesicles* and *bullae* are the technical terms for blisters. Vesicles are circumscribed lesions that contain fluid, while bullae are vesicles that are larger than 0.5 cm in diameter. *A. Subcorneal vesicles* (A) result from fluid accumulation just below the stratum corneum, while *spongiotic vesicles* (B) result from intercellular edema. *B.* Multiple translucent subcorneal vesicles are extremely fragile, collapse easily, and thus lead to crusting (*arrows*). These lesions are staphylococcal impetigo. (Reprinted with permission from Freedberg IM, et al, eds. Fitzpatrick's Dermatology in General Medicine, 6th ed. New York, McGraw-Hill, 2003, p 18.)

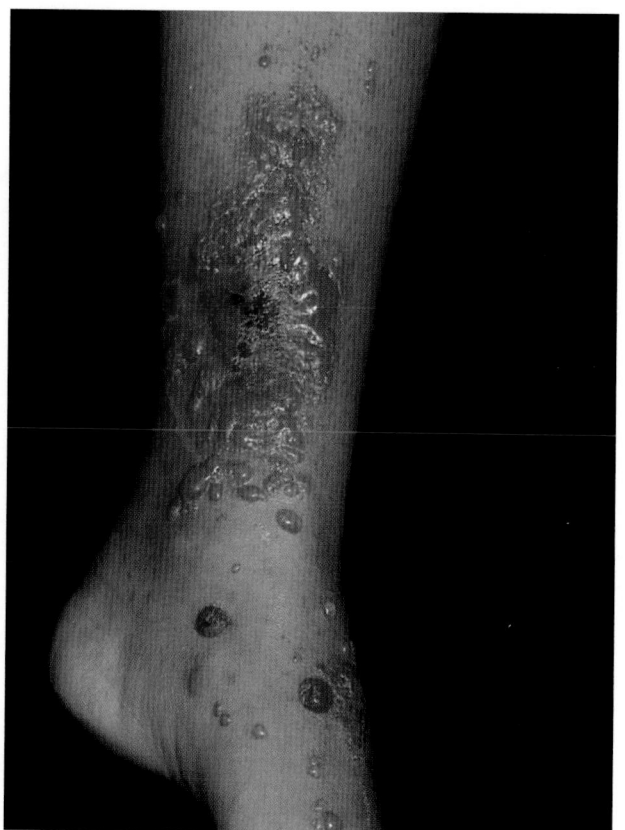

PLATE 7. Acute dermatitis caused by poison ivy. Note the linear arrangement of lesions typical of phytodermatitis acquired by inadvertent contact with the plant. The severe vesiculobullous reaction is typical for urushiol, an oily poisonous irritant found in plants of the genus *Toxicodendron.* (Reprinted with permission from Freedberg IM, et al, eds. Fitzpatrick's Dermatology in General Medicine, 6th ed. New York, McGraw-Hill, 2003, p 1167.)

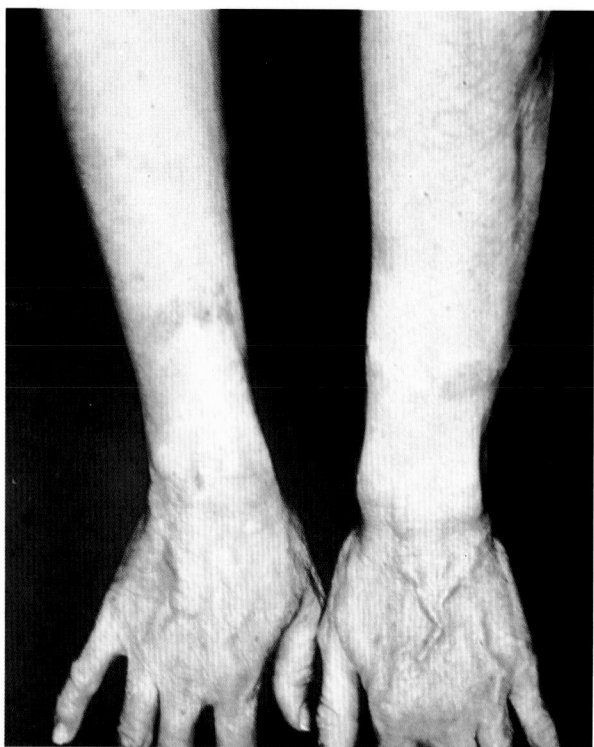

A.

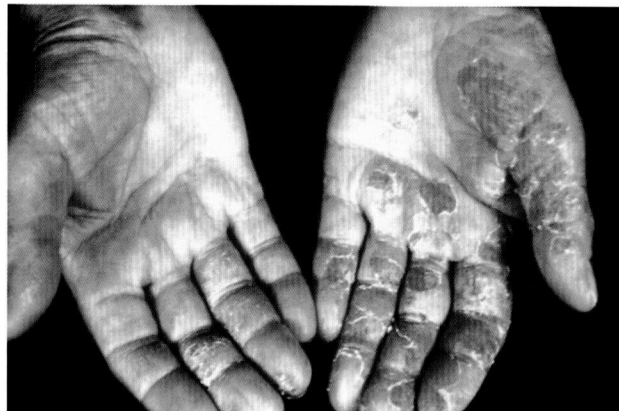

B.

PLATE 8. *A.* This patient has allergic chronic dermatitis involving the dorsal aspects of the hands and the distal forearms, but with minimal involvement of the palms. In this case, contact dermatitis is secondary to use of thiuram present in rubber gloves, prescribed for treatment of an irritant hand dermatitis. *B.* This patient, a florist, has allergic contact dermatitis due to exposure to tuliposide A, the allergen in Peruvian lilies (*Alstroemeria* spp.). Note the more prominent involvement of the palms of the dominant hand. (Reprinted with permission from Freedberg IM, et al, eds. Fitzpatrick's Dermatology in General Medicine, 6th ed. New York, McGraw-Hill, 2003, p 1169.)

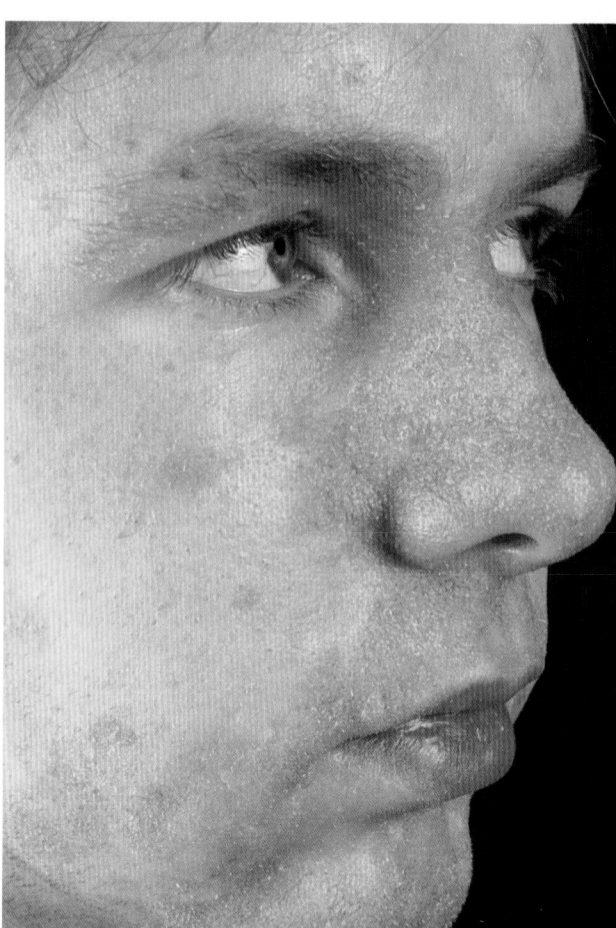

PLATE 9. Seborrheic dermatitis with involvement of the nasolabial folds, cheeks eyebrows, and nose. (Reprinted with permission from Freedberg IM, et al, eds Fitzpatrick's Dermatology in General Medicine, 6th ed. New York, McGraw-Hill 2003, p 1199.)

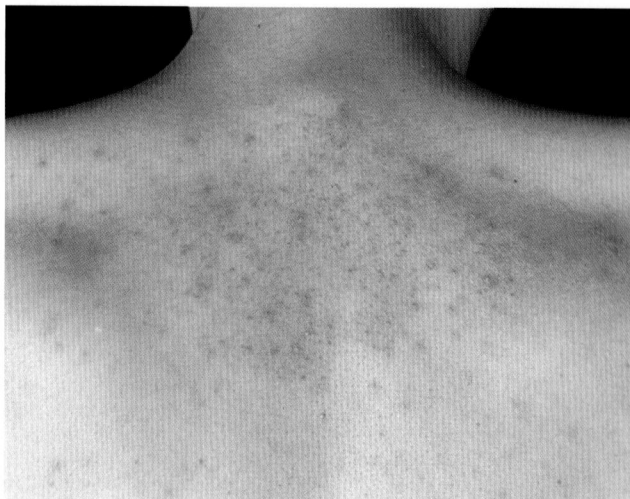

PLATE 10. Seborrheic dermatitis of the upper back. (Reprinted with permission from Freedberg IM, et al, eds. Fitzpatrick's Dermatology in General Medicine 6th ed. New York, McGraw-Hill, 2003, p 1200.)

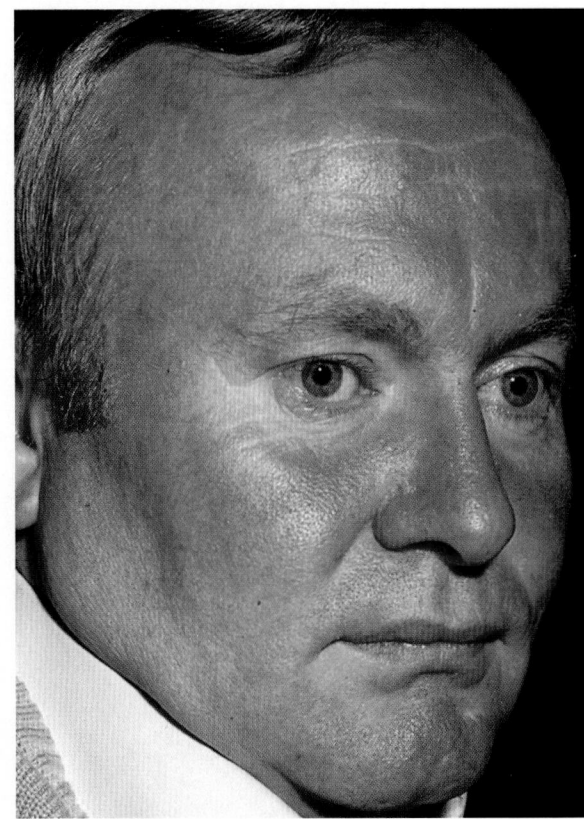

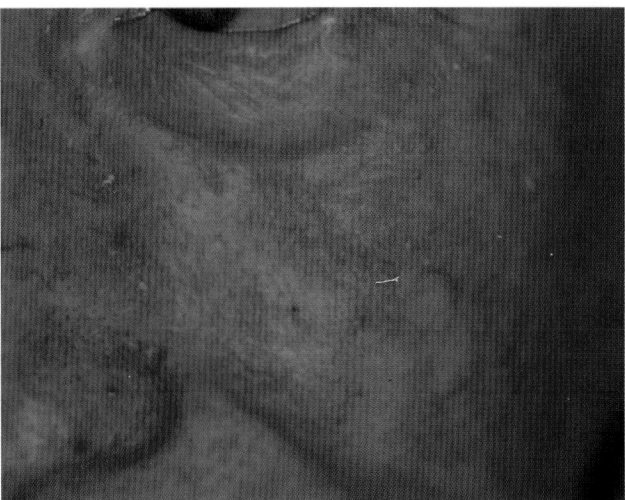

PLATE 12. Severe solar damage of the face revealing telangiectasias as well as actinic keratoses at different stages in development, including the flat, pink macules and hyperkeratotic papules. (Reprinted with permission from Freedberg IM, et al, eds. Fitzpatrick's Dermatology in General Medicine, 6th ed. New York, McGraw-Hill, 2003, p 722.)

PLATE 11. This patient exhibits a striking amiodarone-induced, slate-gray pigmentation of the face. The blue color (ceruloderma) is caused by deposition in the dermis of a brown pigment, which is contained in macrophages and endothelial cells. (Reprinted with permission from Freedberg IM, et al, eds. Fitzpatrick's Dermatology in General Medicine, 6th ed. New York, McGraw-Hill, 2003, p 876.)

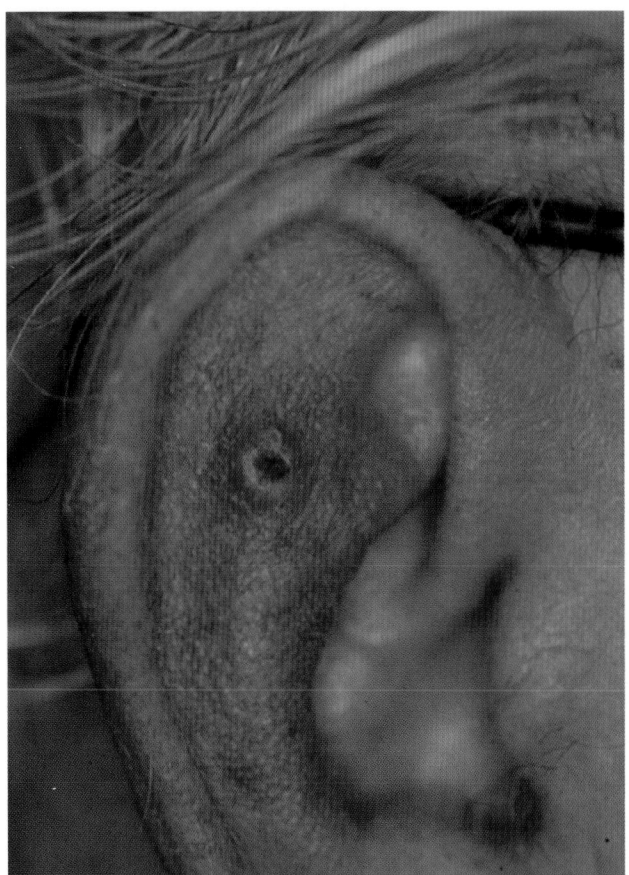

PLATE 13. This case of squamous cell carcinoma must be differentiated in diagnosis from chondrodermatitis nodularis helicis, which unlike the carcinoma, is painful. (Reprinted with permission from Freedberg IM, et al, eds. Fitzpatrick's Dermatology in General Medicine, 6th ed., New York, McGraw-Hill, 2003, p 738.)

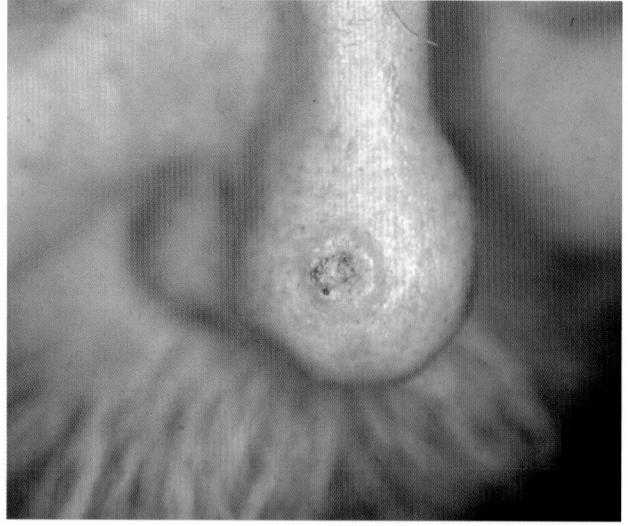

A.

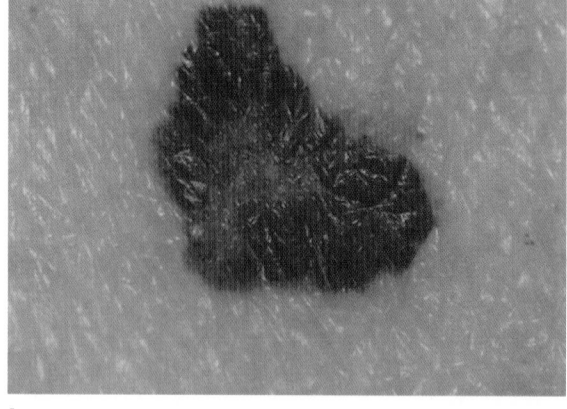

A.

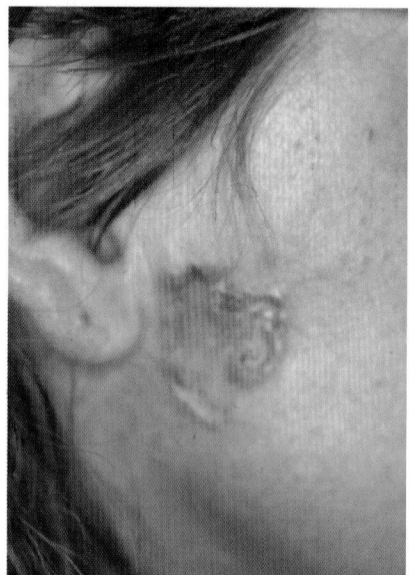

B.

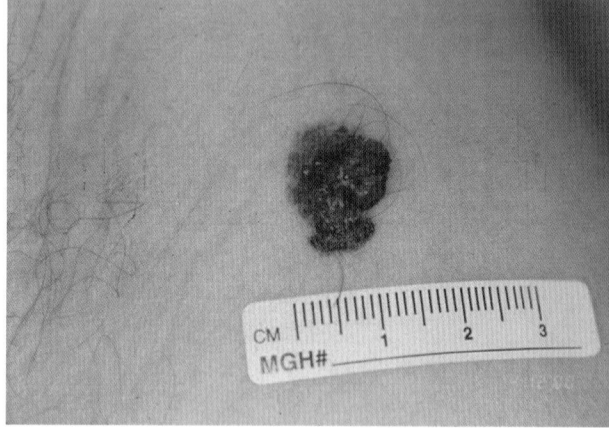

B.

PLATE 14. *A.* Basal cell carcinoma, nodular type. *B.* An ulcerated nodular basal cell carcinoma. (Reprinted with permission from Freedberg IM, et al, eds. Fitzpatrick's Dermatology in General Medicine, 6th ed. New York, McGraw-Hill, 2003, p 749.)

PLATE 15. These two superficial spreading melanomas illustrate the ABCDs of melanoma. *A,* asymmetry: The lesions are not symmetrical and often have irregular borders. *B,* border: Note the highly irregular, uneven, and notched border. *C,* color: The color is variegated with different shades of brown, black, and tan. *D,* diameter: The diameter is usually (but not always) more than 6 mm in melanomas. (Reprinted with permission from Freedberg IM, et al, eds. Fitzpatrick's Dermatology in General Medicine, 6th ed. New York, McGraw-Hill, 2003, p 925.)

94

DERMATOLOGIC DRUG REACTIONS, SELF-TREATABLE SKIN DISORDERS, AND SKIN CANCER

Nina H. Cheigh

Learning Objectives and other resources can be found at *www.pharmacotherapyonline.com*.

As the largest organ of the body, the skin, also known as the integumentary system, is the site of a vast number of pathologic conditions. Patients present with insults to and infections of the skin in a variety of primary care settings, ranging from community pharmacies to emergency departments, requesting evaluation of and advice about skin lesions.

In a survey of patients about the sources of advice they use for skin conditions, pharmacists ranked second, just behind physicians. Interestingly, the advice sought seemed to depend on the nature of the condition, in that patients sought more pharmacist advice on conditions such as dermatitis, psoriasis, skin cancer, and acne.[1] To properly assess a patient, pharmacists and other primary care providers must not only understand clinical presentations of common skin disorders, but they must also be able to quickly identify patients that may need referral for further evaluation by a physician.

In this chapter skin disorders that are self-treatable and dermatologic reactions to medications are presented from a primary care perspective of a pharmacist or other health professional who commonly recommends nonprescription therapies, or refers patients to prescribers or physician specialists. Skin infections are mentioned here, but covered in detail in Chap. 108, on skin and soft tissue infections.

SKIN STRUCTURE AND FUNCTION

The skin has many important functions. Its three layers—the epidermis, dermis, and hypodermis (subcutaneous tissue)—provide a barrier, prevent dehydration, protect from external injury or microorganisms, maintain body temperature, and even express emotions through dilation or constriction of blood vessels. The dermal layer contains most of the structural components of skin, such as mast cells, fibroblasts, collagen, elastic fibers, sweat glands, sebaceous glands, pigment-producing melanin cells, and vasculature.

The hair and nails are considered appendages of the skin. Hair, comprising keratinized epithelial cells, is protein bound and grows in cycles. Scalp hair grows at a rate of approximately 35 mm/day, but this can be affected by various medications and hormones. The nails, also comprised of keratinized cells, have different anatomic components. The nail plate is the main part of the nail, and is highly adherent to the

nail bed, which grows underneath. Generally, toenails tend to grow at a much slower rate than fingernails. Several factors affect the growth of the nails, including genetics, age, and weather.[2]

PATIENT ASSESSMENT

Before a treat-or-refer recommendation can be made, the pharmacist or other health professional must make a reasoned assessment of the problem and make a presumptive diagnosis (or at least rule out some of the many skin disorders). Several factors affect this decision, including patient age and hormonal status, patient complaint and history, and lesion assessment.

AGE AND HORMONAL STATUS

A primary factor to consider in evaluation is the age of the patient. Changes in the anatomy and physiology of skin and its appendages relate closely to patient age, and for women hormonal status also affects the evaluation.

GERIATRIC CONSIDERATIONS

In addition to wrinkling and dryness, expected age-related skin changes include an increase in uneven pigmentation and thinning of the protective layers, thus predisposing the skin to external injuries. Langerhans cells are reduced by 50% in number, reducing natural immunity to skin cancers. The vascularity of the skin declines, and thus older patients tend to look pale (pallor), feel cold to the touch, and have an increased predisposition to develop certain conditions such as psoriasis, seborrhea, pemphigoid, and candidiasis. Changes in the skin appendages can also occur in the elderly, such as thinning and graying of the hair on the scalp. Women can develop facial hair due to the reduction of estrogen levels. The thickness of the nails is reduced, and nails change in color.

PEDIATRIC CONSIDERATIONS

Certain dermatologic conditions, such as atopic dermatitis, are most likely to occur in children. Also, the rate and amount of absorption of medications through the skin is higher in children. Infants may not be able to safely metabolize or excrete medications because of immaturity of their hepatic and renal systems. They also have immature sebaceous gland activity, and thus present frequently with seborrheic dermatitis of the scalp, also known as "cradle cap."

In adolescence, hair appears in new places: the face in boys, and the pubic and other areas in both boys and girls. Sweating and sebaceous gland activity is greater, thus resulting in increased body odor and skin conditions such as acne (see Chap. 96).

HORMONE-RELATED CONSIDERATIONS

Variations in progesterone and estrogen can result in dermatologic disorders as women go through changes and events of their lives.

Menopausal women tend to develop brown hyperpigmentation, or melasma. Women who are on hormone replacement therapy or oral contraceptives also develop these nonspecific brown discolorations on their skin.

Pregnant women develop many changes, including hyperpigmentation of the areola and genitalia. These women can also develop melasma, otherwise commonly known as the "mask of pregnancy." Most pregnant women develop stretch marks, or striae gravidarum, around the abdomen, thighs, breasts, and buttocks. They can also develop disorders such as pruritic urticarial papules and plaques of pregnancy (PUPPPS). Women who are pregnant also typically notice changes in their hair, as it becomes thinner or thicker, or straighter or curlier.

PATIENT HISTORY

In addition to clues offered by patient age and special conditions such pregnancy, several key questions can provide insights into the patient's skin disorder or injury. Getting an accurate history and other information from the patient is critical for ensuring optimal treatment and avoiding undue complications.

THE INTERVIEW

When interviewing the patient, the health care professional should make careful notes of the interaction. Questions that are helpful in assessment include:

- *Are you having other symptoms, such as difficulty breathing, fever, or nausea and vomiting?* When patients present with a rash or skin lesion, the first consideration should be for any potential anaphylaxis or angioedema. Many medications can be responsible for these reactions, and these must be ruled out. If a patient has a severe reaction with difficulty breathing, the patient may require immediate or even emergent referral to an emergency care facility to obtain proper care. Epinephrine, intravenous corticosteroids, or oral prednisone may be needed immediately.
- *Where did the problem first appear? Where are you affected? Did it spread?* Asking where the skin lesions are is important, as it is likely that the entire skin surface is not visible to the health care professional, and the source of the infection may be concealed. For example, although the arms and legs can demonstrate a rash, it would be pertinent to determine if the trunk is also affected, indicating a more systemic cause, as

opposed to an unaffected trunk, which would likely indicate a nonsystemic cause.
- *If they are not visible, what do the lesions took like?* The patient can be asked whether the lesion is painful or itchy, and can thus can be assessed for any infection requiring immediate treatment. For example, if the area is oozing, erythematous, and warm to the touch, it is most likely infected. Alternatively, if the lesion is not painful and no other symptom are present, other conditions are likely present. If appropriate, the lesions can be assessed by the clinician for color, texture, size, and temperature. Also, it is important to note any asymmetry (e.g., the lesion is present on only one side of the body).
- *How long have the lesions been present?* Some patients present after having had a skin condition for quite sometime without seeking any advice. This information is also helpful if the lesions appeared soon after the start of a certain suspected medication.
- *Have the lesions changed in size, shape, color, or consistency?* This question is important in determining any changes that might have occurred with the condition. Most importantly, this question enables evaluation of the patient's melanoma risk. Typically, any skin lesion that changes in these elements should be further examined by a physician.
- *What do you think the problem may be?* Many patients have some idea as to what the source of their problem may be, so it is helpful to ask this question, and get their opinions and observations.
- *Obtain a general medical and allergy history.* After questioning the patient, the clinician or other health care professional may be able to rule out recently started drugs or new diseases as causes of the patient's reaction.

LESION ASSESSMENT

If appropriate and acceptable to the patient, the health professional should make a quick visual assessment of the skin lesions. The skin surface should be closely examined, preferably in natural light. A proper diagnosis is based on pattern recognition, the pharmacist or other health professional must understand and demonstrate competence in assessing the lesions (Figs. 94–1 through 94–6, Plate 1 through 6).[3] In addition, when referral is needed, the clinician or other health care professional should describe lesions to dermatologists or other physicians in a consistent manner.

SITE DISTRIBUTION AND ARRANGEMENT

Note the area involved (e.g., face, trunk, arms, or legs) and the number of lesions present (single or multiple). The arrangement of the lesion is also helpful, such as stating that the lesions are linear (in a line), grouped, annular (ring-shaped), or serpiginous (resembling a snake). Symmetry or asymmetry should be noted; in skin cancer, lesions are typically asymmetrical.

SURFACE TEXTURE

Unless the lesions are oozing or appear to be infectious (see Fig. 94–6B), they should be palpated with caution. Palpation helps the health care professional determine whether the lesion is smooth or rough, firm or soft, or scaly or crusting.

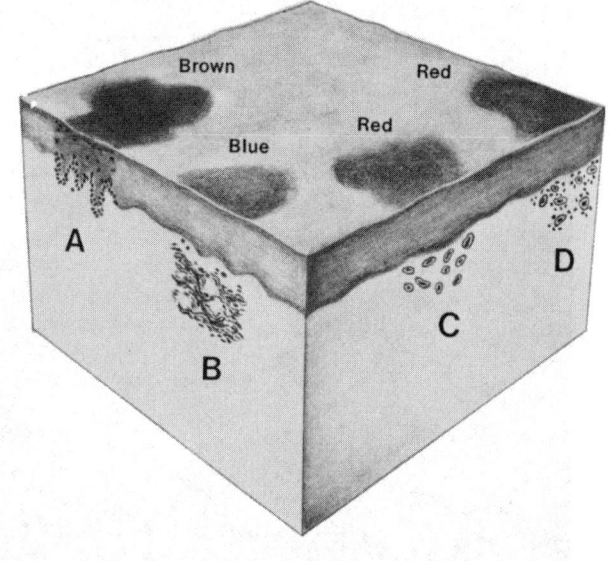

A

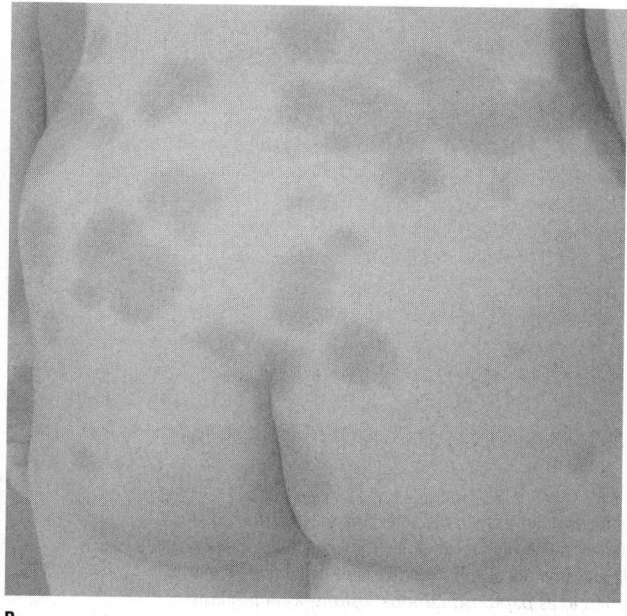

B

FIGURE 94–1. *Macules* are circumscribed, flat lesions of any shape or size that differ from surrounding skin because of their color. A. Macules may be the result of hyperpigmentation (A), hypopigmentation, dermal pigmentation (B), vascular abnormalities, capillary dilatation (erythema) (C), or purpura (D). B. The clinical appearance of a drug reaction that has produced an eruption consisting of multiple, well-defined red macules of varying size that blanch upon pressure (diascopy) and are thus due to inflammatory vasodilation. See Plate 1. (Reprinted with permission from Freedberg IM, et al, eds. Fitzpatrick's Dermatology in General Medicine, 6th ed. New York, McGraw-Hill, 2003, p 14.)

TYPE OF LESIONS

The size of lesions should be measured. Typically, lesions are described as being less than or greater than 0.5 cm in diameter. A *macule* (see Fig 94–1A) or a *papule* (see Fig. 94–2A) is typically 1 cm or less in diameter, while the term *patch* is sometimes used for larger flat macules (see Fig. 94–1B).

BORDER

Poorly circumscribed lesions are those for which it is hard to tell where the normal skin begins and ends (see Fig. 94–5B), while well-defined lesions have clearer demarcations between healthy skin and lesions (see Fig. 94–5B).

LESIONS AND SKIN COLOR

Lesions should be examined for variations from the patient's predominant skin color. Increased pigmentation (brownish color), loss of pigmentation, redness (erythema), pallor, cyanosis, and yellowing should be noted. Color can be very indicative when underlying systemic diseases are involved. For example, anemia and reduced blood flow can result in decreased skin redness. Cyanosis can indicate reduced cardiac blood flow or lung disease. Jaundice can suggest liver disease.

OTHER FEATURES

An assessment of the nails, hair, and mucous membranes should also be performed as needed and appropriate.

Once the health care professional identifies the specific questions to ask and can provide a reasonable description of the lesion, referral or appropriate therapies can be recommended. As there are hundreds of varieties of dermatologic disorders, here we will focus on common conditions most frequently encountered by the pharmacist and other primary care professionals, with an emphasis on skin disorders that are often treated with nonprescription medications, and on drug-induced skin disorders. Infectious skin conditions are covered in detail in Chap. 108, on skin and soft tissue infections.

ALLERGIC, IRRITANT, AND INFECTION-RELATED SKIN DISORDERS

DERMATITIS

The word *dermatitis* is a general term denoting an inflammatory erythematous rash. Many types of dermatitis have been described, with the most common being atopic dermatitis (see Chap. 97 for a complete discussion) and contact dermatitis. Although atopic dermatitis can occur at any age, it is most common in infants and children, and thus age can be a critical identifier in distinguishing between atopic and contact dermatitis. Atopic dermatitis is also frequently associated with elevated IgE levels and family history of atopic disease, such as dermatitis, allergic rhinitis, and asthma.[4]

CONTACT DERMATITIS

Contact dermatitis is an acute (Fig. 94–7, Plate 7) or chronic (Fig. 94–8, Plate 8) inflammatory skin condition that results from contact of an inciting factor with the skin. Typically, contact dermatitis can be further divided into two major subgroups, allergic or irritant, depending on whether the cause is an antigen (allergen), or irritant, such as an organic substance. In allergies, the antigenic substance triggers the Langerhans cells, and their immunologic responses produce the allergic skin reaction, sometimes several days later. Irritant contact dermatitis is more likely to be the result of a reaction within a few hours of exposure. Although symptoms of either type of contact dermatitis (erythematous vesicles with pruritus) are generally similar, the allergic type can result in more serious erosions or oozing pustules. Common offending agents for contact dermatitis are listed in Table 94–1.[5]

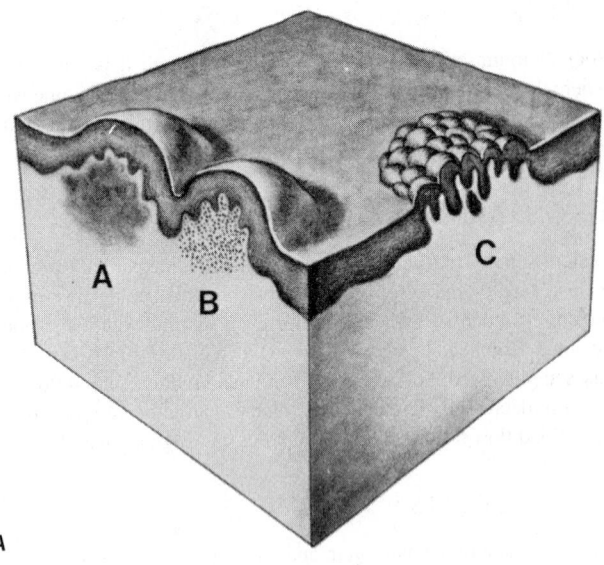

A

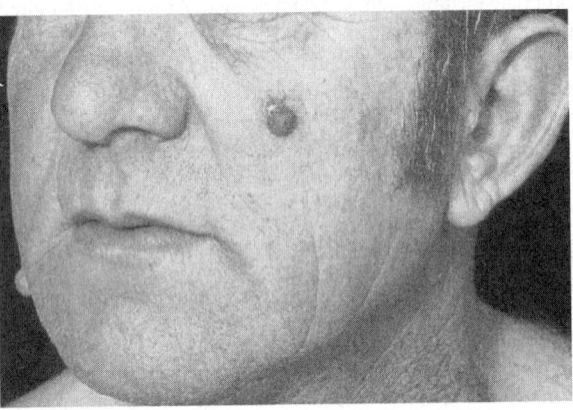

B

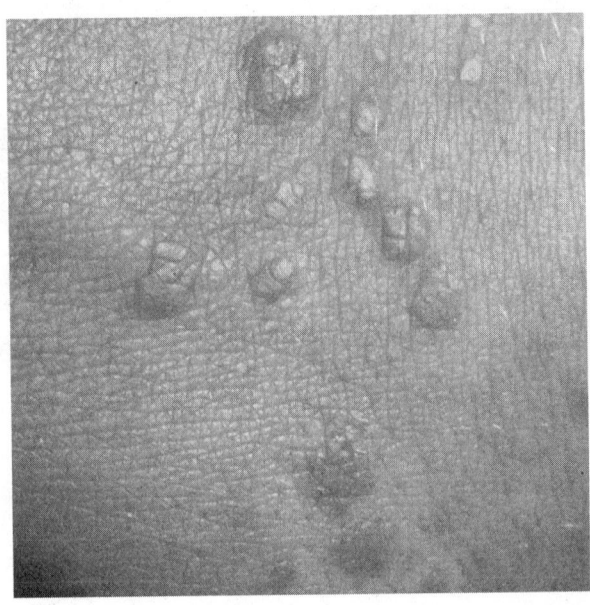

C

FIGURE 94–2. *Papules* are small, solid, elevated lesions that are less than 1 cm in diameter. The major portion of a papule projects above the plane of the surrounding skin. *A.* Papules may result, for example, from metabolic deposits in the dermis (*A*), from localized dermal cellular infiltrates (*B*), and from localized hyperplasia of cellular elements in the dermis and epidermis (*C*). Papules with scaling are referred to as *papulosquamous lesions*, as in psoriasis (see Chap. 96). *B.* Clinical examples of papules. *C.* Two well-defined and dome-shaped papules of firm consistency and brownish color, which are dermal melanocytic nevi; multiple, well defined, and coalescing papules of varying size are seen. Their violaceous color, glistening surface, and flat tops are characteristic of lichen planus. See Plate 2. (Reprinted with permission from Freedberg IM, et al, eds. Fitzpatrick's Dermatology in General Medicine, 6th ed. New York, McGraw-Hill, 2003, p 15.)

TABLE 94–1. Common Allergens Producing Contact Dermatitis Among People in the United States.

Fragrance	Formaldehyde
Flavorings	Lanolin (wool)
Rubber	Neomycin sulfate
Metals	Nickel
Adhesives	Paraben mix
Glues	Thimerosal
Plastics	

When patients present with symptoms of contact dermatitis, pharmacists and other primary care providers should initially ask key questions about exposure to potentially offending substances. Initial treatment of contact dermatitis should always focus on identification and removal of the offending agent. When this is not possible, the patient should be advised to avoid exposure to those agents considered most likely to be responsible. The second goal of treatment is the relief of symptoms. Products that relieve itching, rehydrate the skin, and decrease weeping of the lesions will provide some immediate relief. The dosage form of topical preparations is determined by the stage of inflammation. In the acute stage, wet dressings are preferred because ointments and creams further irritate the tissue. Astringents such as aluminum acetate, Burow solution, or witch hazel decrease

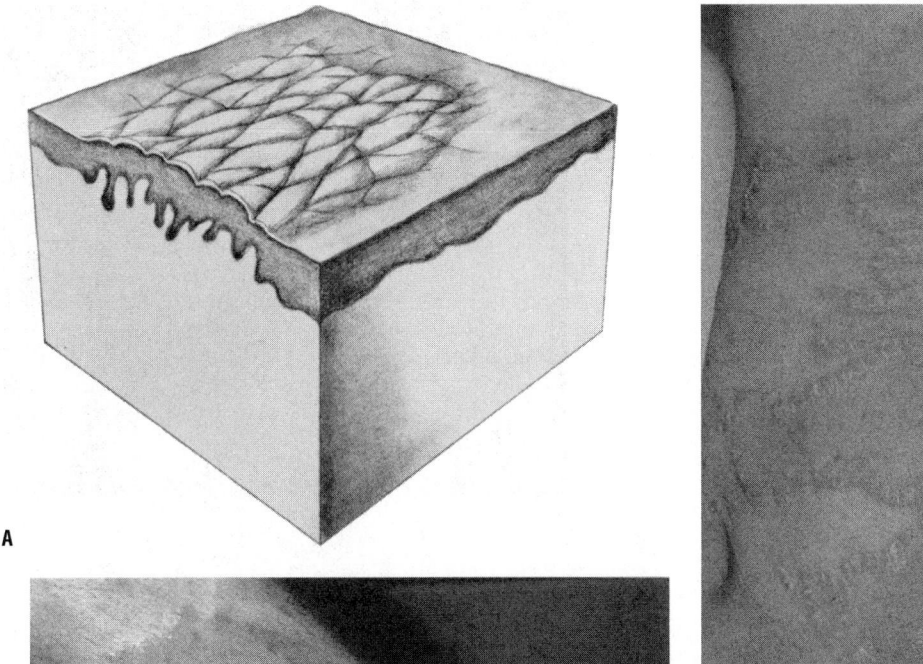

A

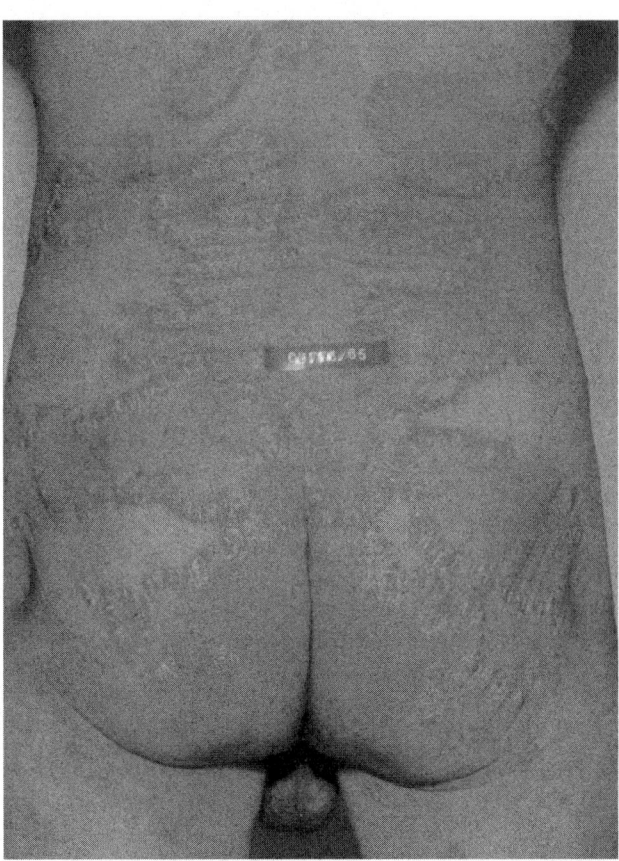

B

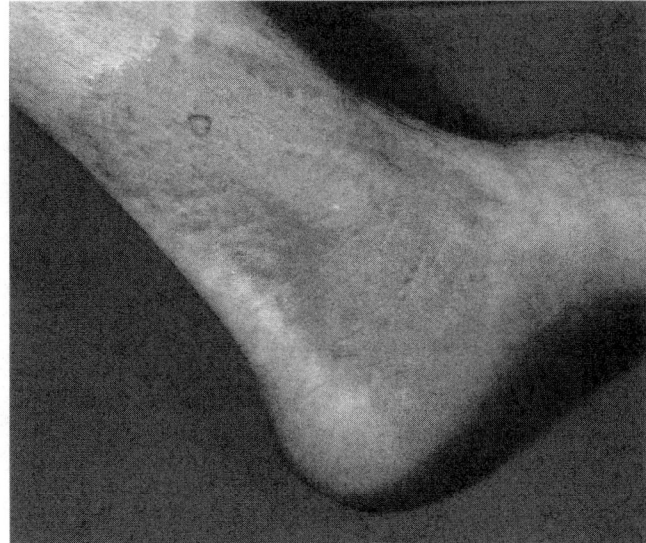

C

FIGURE 94–3. *A. Plaque* is a mesa-like elevation that occupies a relatively large surface area in comparison with its height above the skin surface. *B.* Well-defined, reddish, scaling plaques can coalesce to cover large areas of the back and buttocks, with some regression in the center as is common in psoriasis (see Chap. 96). *C. Lichenification*, a thickening of the skin and accentuation of skin, can result from repeated rubbing. It develops frequently in patients with atopy, and also occurs in eczematous dermatitis or other conditions associated with pruritus. Lesions of lichenification are not as well defined as most plaques and often show signs of scratching, such as in excoriations and crusts. See Plate 3. (Reprinted with permission from Freedberg IM, et al, eds. Fitzpatrick's Dermatology in General Medicine, 6th ed. New York, McGraw-Hill, 2003, p 16.)

weeping from lesions, "dry out" the skin, and provide relief from itching. These agents are applied as wet dressings and should not be used for more than 7 days.

For chronic dermatitis, lubricants, emollients, or moisturizers should be applied after bathing. Soap-free (or mild) cleansers and products containing colloidal oatmeal also contribute to alleviating itch and soothing the skin. If the patient's reaction does not subside within a few days, or further spread occurs, the patient should be referred for specialist follow-up and for prescription therapy with stronger topical corticosteroids and possibly oral corticosteroid therapy.

SEBORRHEIC DERMATITIS

The prevalence of *seborrheic dermatitis* peaks during infancy, and then again during the fourth to seventh decades of life, affecting 3% to 5% of adults in the United States. In infants, seborrheic dermatitis is commonly referred to as "cradle cap." Typically, this condition occurs around the areas of skin rich in sebaceous follicles, such as the face (Fig. 94–9, Plate 9), ears, scalp, and upper trunk (Fig. 94–10, Plate 10), although it is not classified as a disease of the sebaceous glands per se.[6]

Therapy of seborrheic dermatitis has four major goals: to loosen and remove scales, prevent yeast colonization, control any secondary

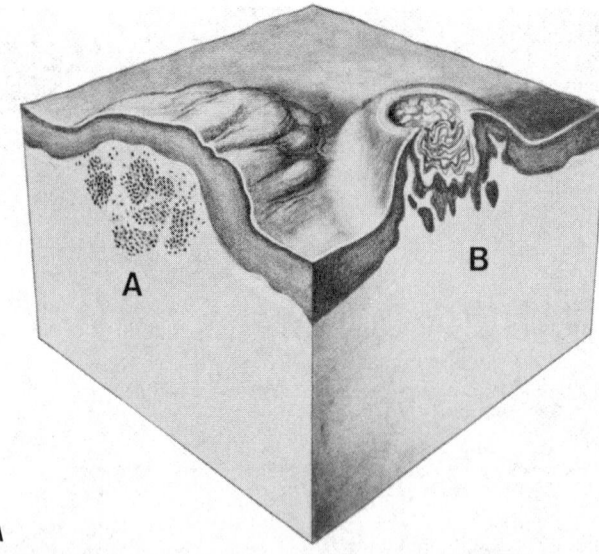

A

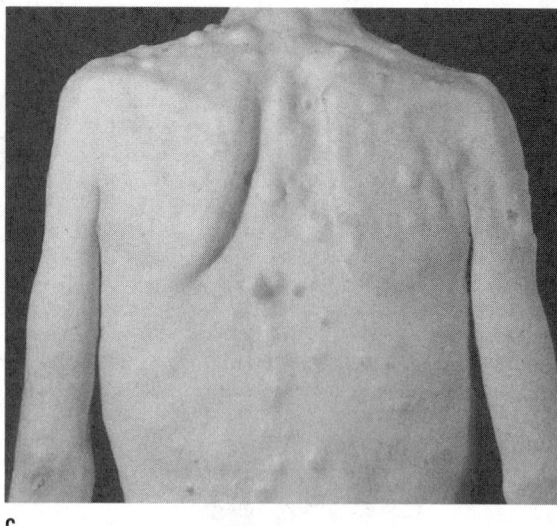

C

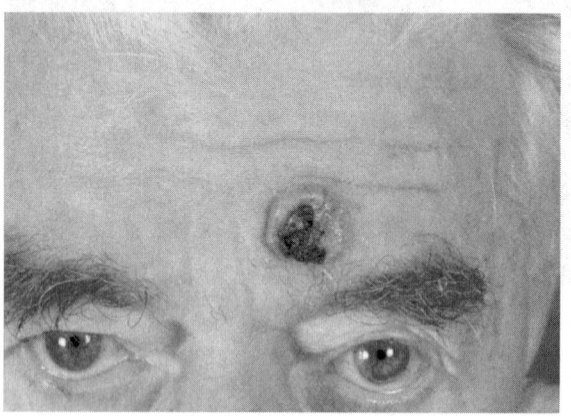

B

FIGURE 94-4. *Nodules* are palpable, solid, round or ellipsoidal lesions. Depth of involvement and/or substantive palpability rather than diameter differentiates a nodule from a papule. *A.* Nodules may be located in the epidermis (*B*) or extend into the dermis or subcutaneous tissue (*A*). *B.* This photograph shows a well-defined, firm nodule with a smooth and glistening surface through which telangiectasia (dilated capillaries) can be seen; there is central crusting indicating tissue breakdown and thus incipient ulceration (nodular basal cell carcinoma). *C.* Multiple nodules of varying size can be seen (melanoma metastases). See Plate 4. (Reprinted with permission from Freedberg IM, et al, eds. Fitzpatrick's Dermatology in General Medicine, 6th ed. New York, McGraw-Hill, 2003, p 17.)

infections, and reduce itching and erythema. Interestingly, the disease typically seems to improve with warmer weather and worsens when the air is colder.

Many topical agents are used to manage seborrheic dermatitis. Depending on what area of the body is affected, the pharmacist or other health professional can assist in selection of proper vehicles (i.e., solutions or shampoos for the scalp). Ingredients such as selenium sulfide, salicylic acid, and coal tar can help soften and remove the scales. Seborrheic dermatitis responds very quickly to low-potency topical corticosteroid preparations, but judicious use is important to avoid long-term adverse effects. Topical ketoconazole 2% can also be used to help control the yeast colonization.[7]

DIAPER DERMATITIS

Diaper dermatitis, or diaper rash, is an acute, inflammatory dermatitis of the buttocks and genital and perineal region. Commonly seen in infants in diapers, this condition, which results in erythematous patches, erosion of skin, vesicles, and ulcerations, can be seen in adults who wear diapers for incontinence. This reaction is a type of contact dermatitis, as it results from direct fecal and moisture contact with the skin in an occlusive environment.

Treatment of diaper dermatitis includes frequent diaper changes and keeping the area dry. Lukewarm water and mild soap can be used to cleanse the area thoroughly, which should then be allowed to dry. Occlusive agents—such as zinc oxide, titanium dioxide, petrolatum, or any combination of these—should be generously applied to the area before the diaper is applied.

DRUG-INDUCED SKIN DISORDERS

Approximately 2% to 3% of hospitalized patients experience an adverse cutaneous drug reaction, with a higher incidence in older individuals. Almost every commonly used drug has been implicated in producing local and/or systemic drug reactions (Table 94–2).

TABLE 94–2. Types of Drug-Induced Skin Eruptions

Clinical Presentation	Pattern and Distribution of Skin Lesions	Mucous Membrane Involvement	Implicated Drugs	Treatment
Erythema multiforme	Target lesions, limbs	Absent	Anticonvulsants (including lamotrigine), sulfonamide antibiotics, allopurinol, NSAIDs, dapsone	Supportive[a]
Stevens-Johnson syndrome	Atypical targets, widespread	Present	As above	Intravenous immunoglobulins, cyclosporine
Toxic epidermal necrolysis	Epidermal necrosis with skin detachment	Present	As above	Supportive[a]
Pseudoporphyria	Skin fragility, blister formation in photodistribution	Absent	Tetracycline, furosemide, naproxen	Supportive[a]
Linger IgA disease	Bullous dermatosis	Present or absent	Vancomycin, lithium, diclofenac, piroxicam, amiodarone	Supportive[a]
Pemphigus	Flaccid bullae, chest	Present or absent	Penicillamine, captopril, piroxicam, penicillin, rifampin	Supportive[a]
Bullous pemphigoid	Tense Bullae, widespread	Present or absent	Furosemide, penicillamine, penicillins, sulfasalazine, captopril	Supportive[a]

[a]Supportive care includes administration of systemic glucocorticoids until all symptoms of active disease disappear.
NSAIDs, nonsteroidal anti-inflammatory drugs.
Reprinted with permission from Freedberg IM, et al, eds. Fitzpatrick's Dermatology in General Medicine, 6th ed. New York, McGraw-Hill, 2003, p 1335.

Typically, these reactions are unpredictable, ranging from mild, self-limiting episodes, to more severe, life-threatening ones. Some reactions are nonallergic, but drug-induced skin reactions tend to be immunologic in origin and relate to hypersensitivity.

Pharmacists and other primary care providers should develop an organized and thorough approach to evaluation of patients with potential drug-induced skin disorders. This process begins with a comprehensive drug history, including episodes of previous drug allergies, and is based on an understanding of the mechanisms involved in drug reactions.

CUTANEOUS DRUG REACTIONS

Maculopapular eruptions are the most common manifestation of drug-induced skin reactions. Lesions tend to resemble those of measles, often involving the trunk or pressure areas, and are frequently symmetrical. These eruptions are classified as either early, appearing within a few hours to 3 days after ingestion of the drug, or late, appearing up to 9 days after the exposure. Most reactions disappear within a few days after discontinuing the agent, and thus symptomatic control of the affected area is the primary intervention. Topical corticosteroids and oral antihistamines can relieve pruritus. In severe eruptions, a short course of systemic corticosteroids may be warranted.

A fixed-drug reaction, typically presenting as an erythematous or hyperpigmented round or oval lesion, usually ranges from a few millimeters to 20 cm in diameter.[8] Although the lesion can appear anywhere, the oral mucosa or genitalia are the most common sites. If the patient takes the agent again, the drug reaction tends to recur within 30 minutes to 8 hours after rechallenge, in the exact same location, and this is highly indicative of the fixed-drug reaction (lesions may also occur in other locations).[9] The pathogenesis of fixed-drug reactions is not well understood.

Treatment of fixed-drug reactions involves removal of the offending agent. Rechallenge should be avoided when possible. Other therapeutic measures include the use of corticosteroids, antihistamines to relieve itching, and perhaps cool water compresses on the affected area.[9]

Sun-induced drug eruptions tend to appear similar to a sunburn, and present with erythema, papules, edema, and sometimes vesicle formation. They also appear in areas that tend to be most exposed to sunlight, such as the ears, nose, cheeks, forearms, and hands. Photosensitivity is subdivided into *phototoxicity*, which is defined as a nonimmunologic reaction, and a *photoallergic reaction*, which involves an immunologic mechanism and is far less common.[10] Common medications associated with photosensitivity reactions include fluoroquinolones, nonsteroidal anti-inflammatory drugs, phenothiazines, antihistamines, estrogens, progestins, sulfonamides, sulfonylureas, thiazide diuretics, and tricyclic antidepressants.[2] Typically, patients can achieve symptom resolution by discontinuing the medication.

Patients with photosensitivity reactions should be treated much the same as burn victims would be; management of the "burn" is of primary importance. Some patients benefit from topical corticosteroids and oral antihistamines, but these are relatively ineffective. Systemic corticosteroids, typically oral prednisone at 1 mg/kg per day tapered over 3 weeks, is more effective for these patients. Pharmacists and other health care professionals should encourage the proper use of sunscreen, and recommend a protective product that protects against ultraviolet A and B rays.[11]

HYPERPIGMENTATION

Many medications can cause changes in skin color. These can be caused by the medication, or may be due to disturbances in melanin production or formation. Depending on the medication, the site of hyperpigmentation can vary. For example, patients receiving

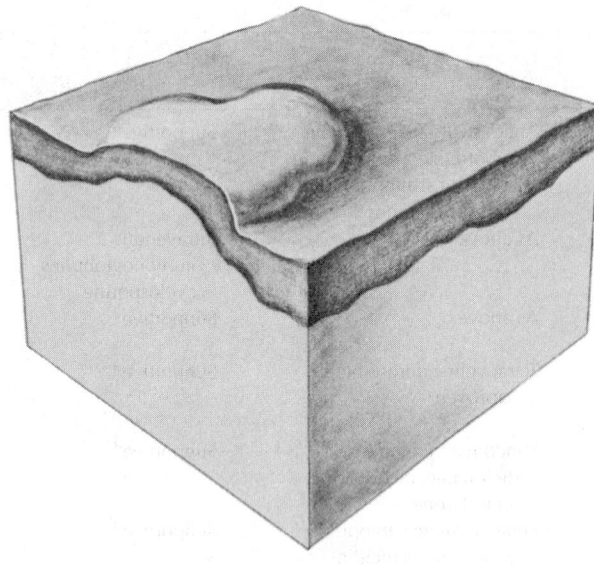

A

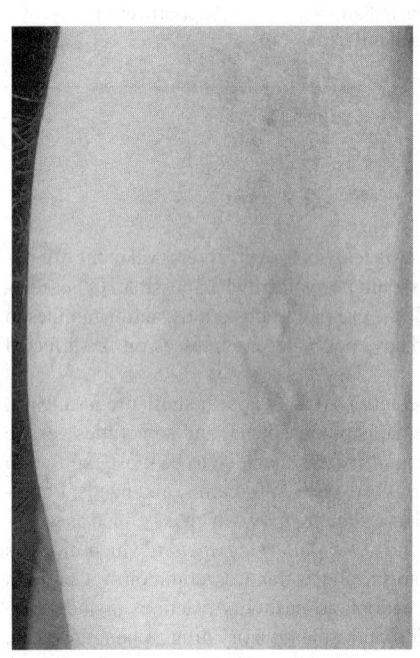

B

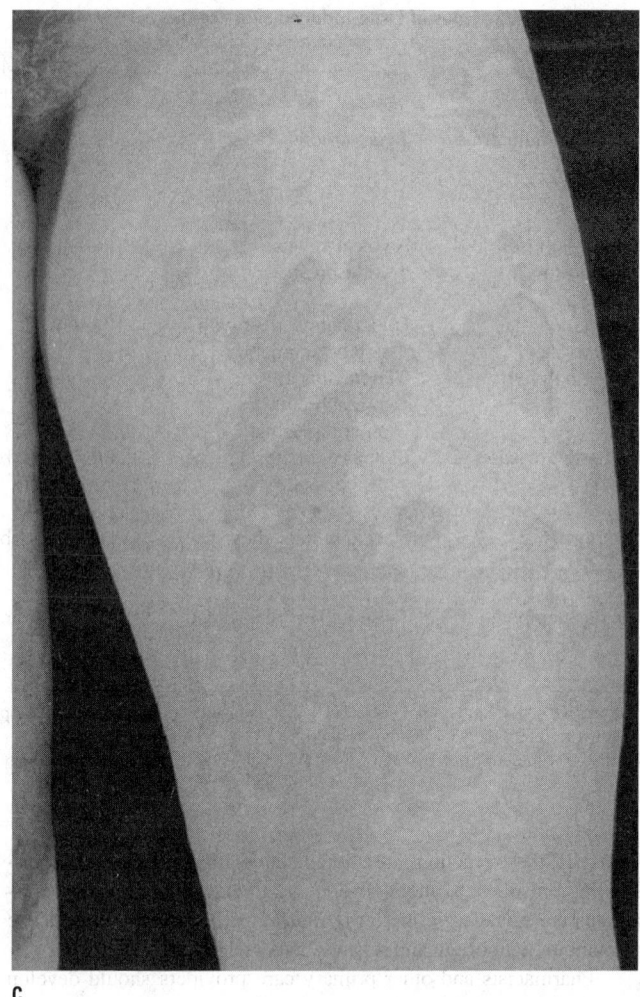

C

FIGURE 94–5. A. *Wheals* are rounded or flat-topped papules or plaques that are characteristically evanescent, disappearing within hours. An eruption consisting of wheals is termed *urticaria* and usually itches. *B*. Wheals may be tiny papules 3 to 4 mm in diameter, as in cholinergic urticaria. *C*. Alternatively, wheals may present as large, coalescing plaques, as in allergic reactions to penicillin, other drugs, or alimentary allergens. See Plate 5. (Reprinted with permission from Freedberg IM, et al, eds. Fitzpatrick's Dermatology in General Medicine, 6th ed. New York, McGraw-Hill, 2003, p 18.)

anticonvulsants such as phenytoin, phenobarbital, and carbamazepine report a brown patchy lesion in sun-exposed areas.[8] Patients who receive anticonvulsant therapy for more than 1 year are at a 10% risk of developing some form of hyperpigmentation related to the medication.[12] Women on oral contraceptives frequently report melasma, or brown, irregularly-shaped macules on the cheeks, forehead, or upper lip. Hormonal changes in estrogen and progesterone as well as sun exposure may cause the increase in melanin deposition.[13] Other medications commonly associated with skin hyperpigmentation include antimalarial agents, phenothiazines, tetracyclines,[14] and amiodarone (Fig. 94–11, Plate 11).[15]

Patients with drug-induced hyperpigmentation can use skin bleaching creams and/or cosmetic agents that help to even out skin tone. Many such products have been marketed. Hydroquinone or kojic acid are most commonly found in cosmetic agents to aid in bleaching the darkened area of skin. Many times these agents are formulated in conjunction with such agents as α-hydroxy acids, which help to slowly slough off the outermost layer of skin. These patients using bleaching

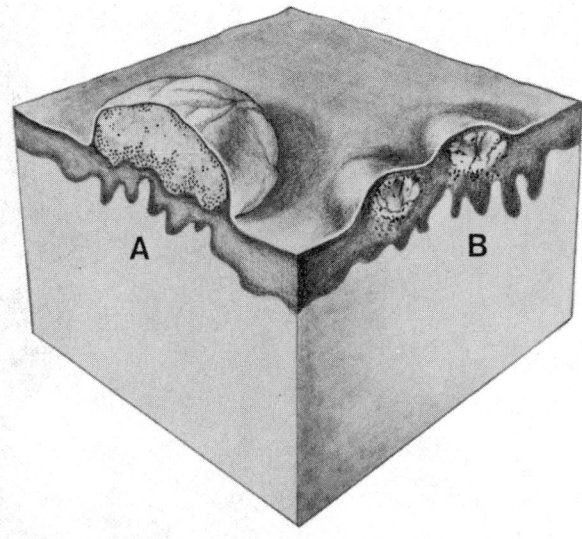

A

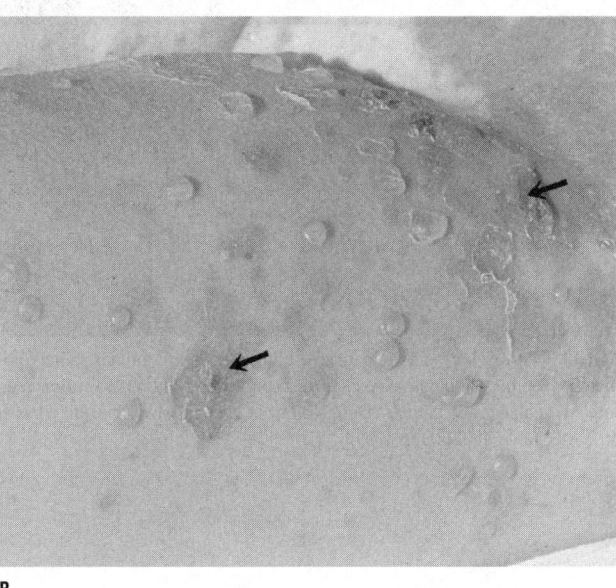

B

FIGURE 94–6. *Vesicles* and *bullae* are the technical terms for blisters. Vesicles are circumscribed lesions that contain fluid, while bullae are vesicles that are larger than 0.5 cm in diameter. *A. Subcorneal vesicles* (*A*) result from fluid accumulation just below the stratum corneum, while *spongiotic vesicles* (*B*) result from intercellular edema. *B.* Multiple translucent subcorneal vesicles are extremely fragile, collapse easily, and thus lead to crusting (*arrows*). These lesions are staphylococcal impetigo. See Plate 6. (Reprinted with permission from Freedberg IM, et al, eds. Fitzpatrick's Dermatology in General Medicine, 6th ed. New York, McGraw-Hill, 2003, p 18.)

creams absolutely must use sunscreen, as areas being treated with these creams tend to be even more sun-sensitive.

SKIN CANCERS

Actinic keratoses (AKs) are abnormal keratinocytes that develop in response to prolonged exposure to ultraviolet radiation. These lesions can develop into squamous cell or basal cell carcinomas, and the

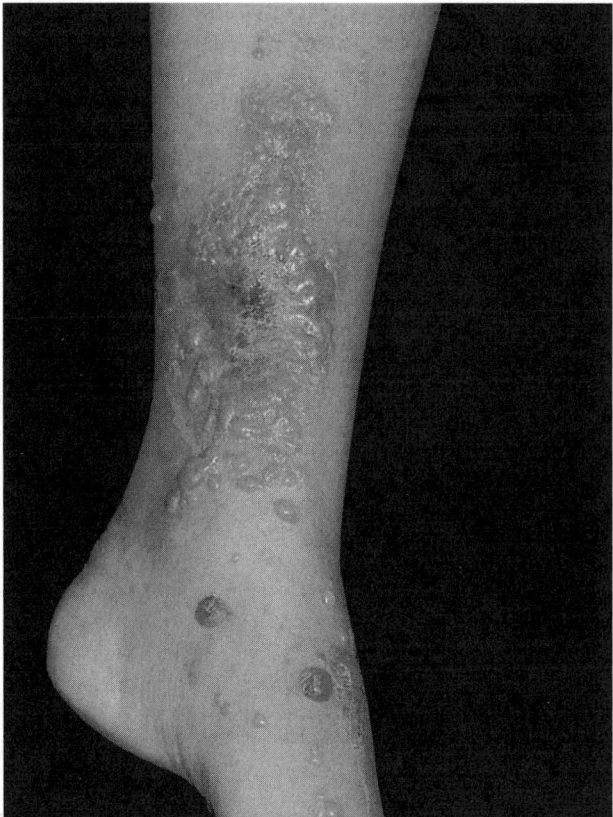

FIGURE 94–7. Acute dermatitis caused by poison ivy. Note the linear arrangement of lesions typical of phytodermatitis acquired by inadvertent contact with the plant. The severe vesiculobullous reaction is typical for urushiol, an oily poisonous irritant found in plants of the genus *Toxicodendron*. See Plate 7. (Reprinted with permission from Freedberg IM, et al, eds. Fitzpatrick's Dermatology in General Medicine, 6th ed. New York, McGraw-Hill, 2003, p 1167.)

presence of suspicious lesions is one of the top reasons that patients seek medical attention for dermatologic disorders.

AK usually presents as a small (2 to 6 mm), erythematous papule that feels flat, rough, or scaly when palpated (Fig. 94–12, Plate 12). It tends to be found in chronically sun-exposed areas, such as the top of the hands, head, neck, and forearms. Typically, patients with AKs are elderly and have fair skin, light-colored eyes, freckles, and a history of significant sun exposure and tend to sunburn easily. Because AKs are likely caused by ultraviolet radiation, sun-preventive measures, particularly in childhood, are of utmost importance.[16] Most commonly, AKs are treated with liquid nitrogen, which will remove the lesion. Another frequently used therapy is topical 5-fluorouracil. Patients who are prescribed topical 5-fluorouracil should be properly counseled, as significant erythema, erosion, crusting, and even ulceration normally occur during treatment.

Squamous cell carcinoma (SCC) is a cutaneous malignancy with estimates of approximately 200,000 cases in the United States in 2001. SCC seems to be more common in advanced age, and twice as common in men as in women. Because of their susceptibility to the negative effects of long-term sun exposure, patients of Celtic ancestry and those with blue or green eyes, red hair, and fair complexion are at the greatest risk of developing SCC.[17] Other risk factors include precursor lesions such as AKs, long-term immunosuppression, and ultraviolet radiation. SCC can appear in many areas, but mainly occurs

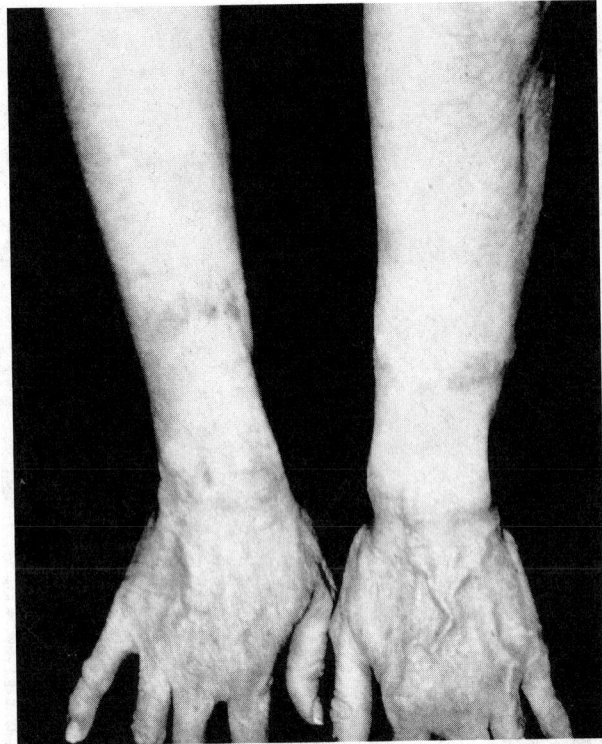

A

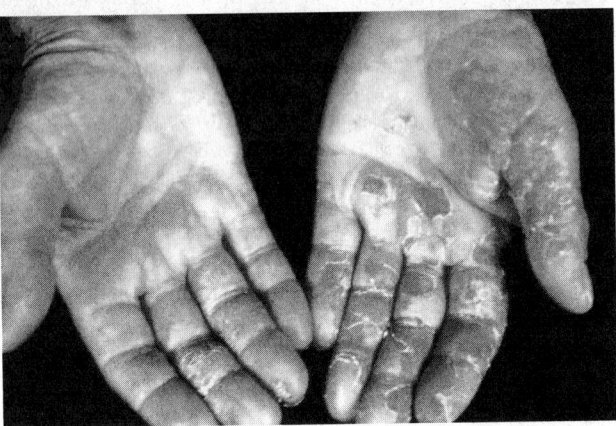

B

FIGURE 94–8. *A.* This patient has allergic chronic dermatitis involving the dorsal aspects of the hands and the distal forearms, but with minimal involvement of the palms. In this case, contact dermatitis is secondary to use of thiuram present in rubber gloves, prescribed for treatment of an irritant hand dermatitis. *B.* This patient, a florist, has allergic contact dermatitis due to exposure to tuliposide A, the allergen in Peruvian lilies (*Alstroemeria* spp.). Note the more prominent involvement of the palms of the dominant hand. See Plate 8. (Reprinted with permission from Freedberg IM, et al, eds. Fitzpatrick's Dermatology in General Medicine, 6th ed. New York, McGraw-Hill, 2003, p 1169.)

in sun-exposed areas such as the head, neck, and dorsal aspect of the hands. Most SCCs appear as a firm, flesh-colored, or erythematous papule or plaque (Fig. 94–13, Plate 13). Some resemble an ulcer. Treatment for SCC is determined by the tumor's risk for metastasis, but commonly involves some form of surgical excision.

Basal cell carcinoma (BCC) is the most common cancer in humans, with an estimated 900,000 cases per year in the United States.[17]

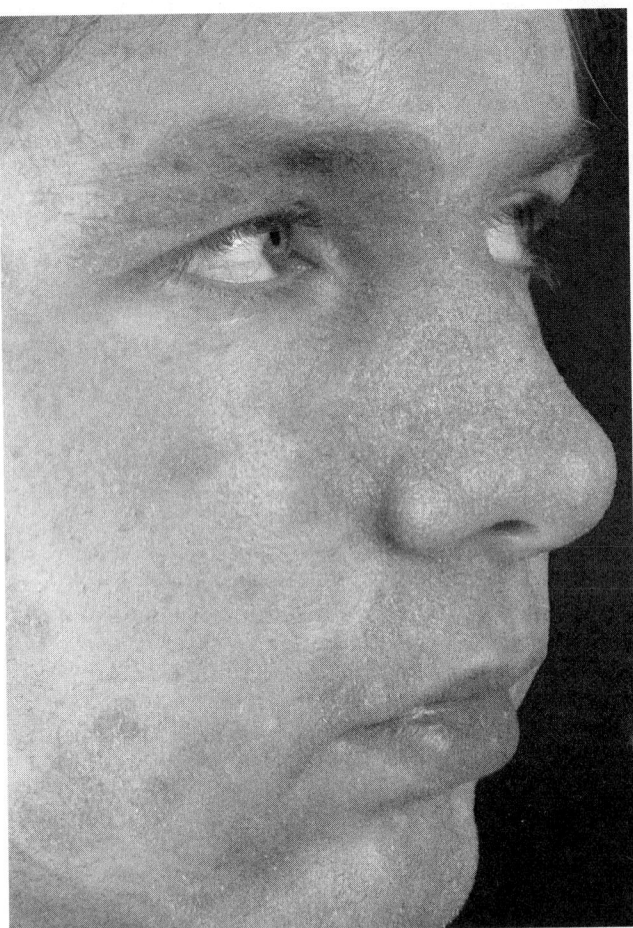

FIGURE 94–9. Seborrheic dermatitis with involvement of the nasolabial folds, cheeks, eyebrows, and nose. See Plate 9. (Reprinted with permission from Freedberg IM, et al, eds. Fitzpatrick's Dermatology in General Medicine, 6th ed. New York, McGraw-Hill, 2003, p 1199.)

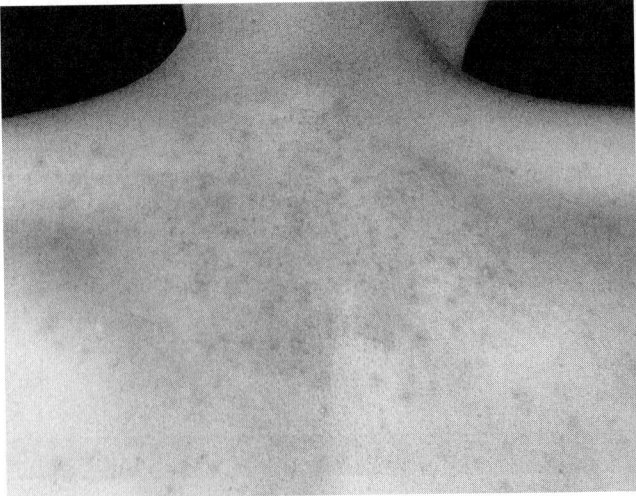

FIGURE 94–10. Seborrheic dermatitis of the upper back. See Plate 10. (Reprinted with permission from Freedberg IM, et al, eds. Fitzpatrick's Dermatology in General Medicine, 6th ed. New York, McGraw-Hill, 2003, p 1200.)

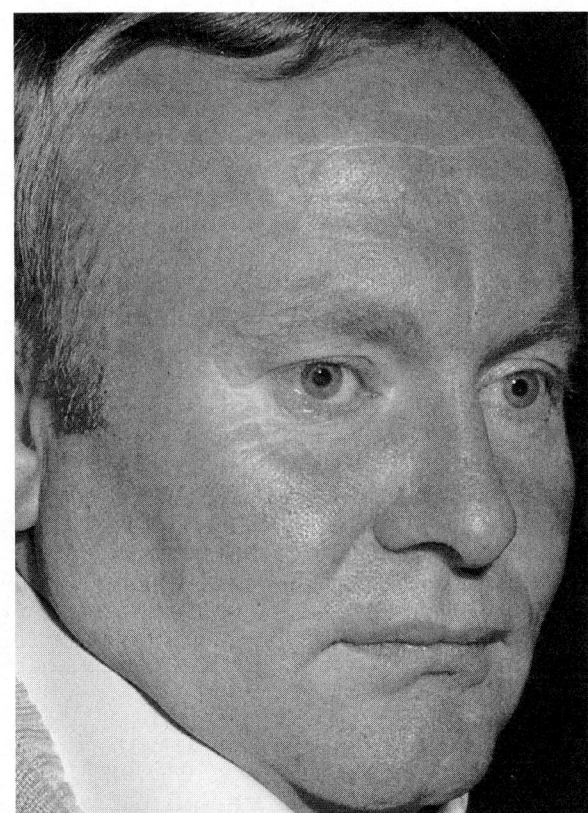

FIGURE 94–11. This patient exhibits a striking amiodarone-induced, slate-gray pigmentation of the face. The blue color (ceruloderma) is caused by deposition in the dermis of a brown pigment, which is contained in macrophages and endothelial cells. See Plate 11. (Reprinted with permission from Freedberg IM, et al, eds. Fitzpatrick's Dermatology in General Medicine, 6th ed. New York, McGraw-Hill, 2003, p 876.)

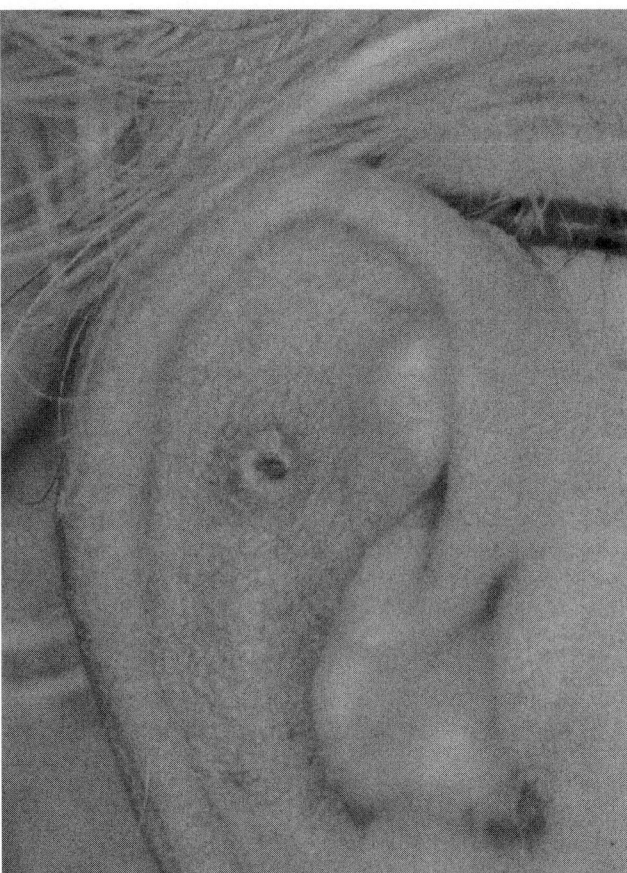

FIGURE 94–13. This case of squamous cell carcinoma must be differentiated in diagnosis from chondrodermatitis nodularis helicis, which unlike the carcinoma, is painful. See Plate 13. (Reprinted with permission from Freedberg IM, et al, eds. Fitzpatrick's Dermatology in General Medicine, 6th ed., New York, McGraw-Hill, 2003, p 738.)

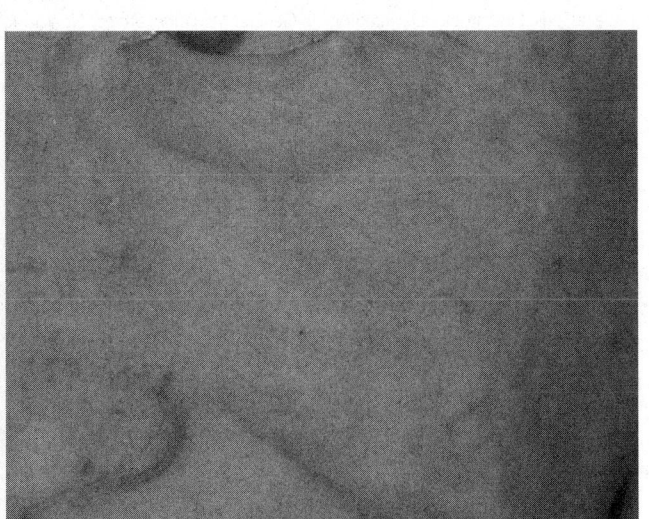

FIGURE 94–12. Severe solar damage of the face revealing telangiectasias as well as actinic keratoses at different stages in development, including the flat, pink macules and hyperkeratotic papules. See Plate 12. (Reprinted with permission from Freedberg IM, et al, eds. Fitzpatrick's Dermatology in General Medicine, 6th ed. New York, McGraw-Hill, 2003, p 722.)

BCCs can occur anywhere on the body, but they appear most commonly on the head and neck, usually as a nodular, pigmented lesion (Fig. 94–14, Plate 14). Treatment varies depending on the histology of the lesion, but frequently requires Mohs micrographic surgery, surgical excision, and possible use of topical agents. Topical imiquimod is approved by the Food and Drug Administration for treating BCC of areas other than the face, and this agent resulted in some clearances in a phase II study.[18] Topical 5-fluorouracil has also been used, but needs further evaluation to warrant routine use.

The risk of malignant melanoma is increasing, with a prediction that prevalence could reach 1 in 50 by 2010.[19] Most frequently, melanoma occurs on the back and extremities of white males and females, while in Asians and blacks, it tends to appear on mucous membranes and soles and palms. Risk factors include skin type, sun exposure and response to the sun (i.e., ability to tan), family history, and change in the appearance of moles. The presence of any nonhealing lesion should raise the suspicion of skin cancer. In addition to assessing these risk factors, pharmacists can play a key role in examining the questionable lesion(s) and by assessing the lesion's asymmetry, border, color, diameter, and history, as when a mole changed and led to the appearance of the lesion (Fig. 94–15, Plate 15). Patients who fit these criteria should be further evaluated by a dermatologist.

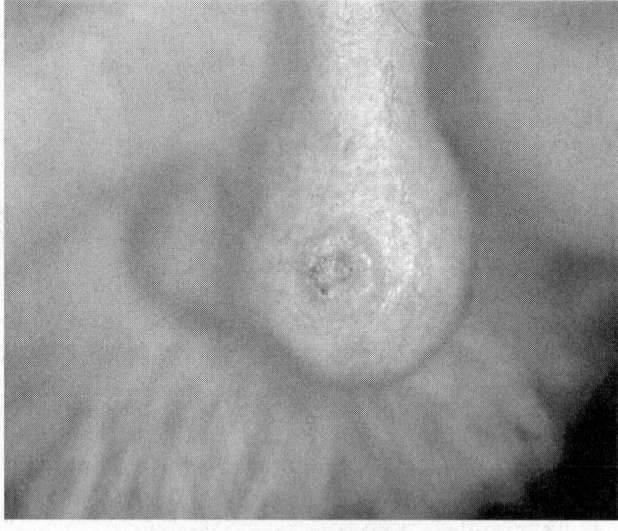

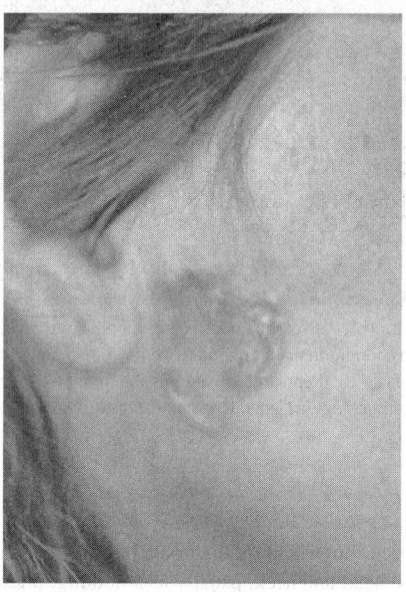

FIGURE 94–14. *A.* Basal cell carcinoma, nodular type. *B.* An ulcerated nodular basal cell carcinoma. See Plate 14. (Reprinted with permission from Freedberg IM, et al, eds. Fitzpatrick's Dermatology in General Medicine, 6th ed. New York, McGraw-Hill, 2003, p 749.)

ABBREVIATIONS

AK: actinic keratosis
BCC: basal cell carcinoma
PUPPPS: pruritic urticarial papules and plaques of pregnancy
SCC: squamous cell carcinoma

Review Questions and other resources can be found at *www.pharmacotherapyonline.com.*

REFERENCES

1. Kilkenny M, Stathakis V, Jolley D, et al. Maryborough skin health survey: Prevalence and sources of advice for skin conditions. Austral J Dermatol 1998;39:235–237.

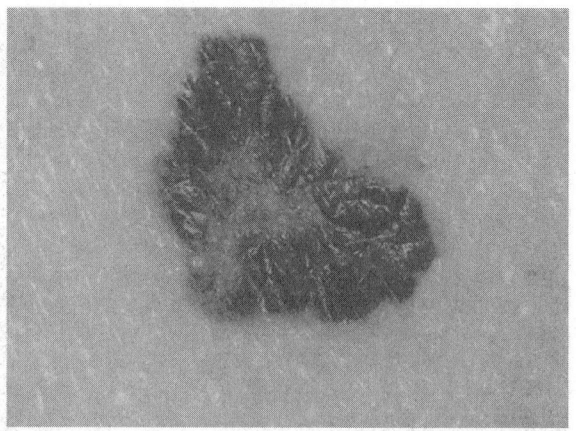

FIGURE 94–15. These two superficial spreading melanomas illustrate the ABCDs of melanoma. *A,* asymmetry: The lesions are not symmetrical and often have irregular borders. *B,* border: Note the highly irregular, uneven, and notched border. *C,* color: The color is variegated with different shades of brown, black, and tan. *D,* diameter: The diameter is usually (but not always) more than 6 mm in melanomas. See Plate 15. (Reprinted with permission from Freedberg IM, et al, eds. Fitzpatrick's Dermatology in General Medicine, 6th ed. New York, McGraw-Hill, 2003, p 925.)

2. DeSimone II EM. Skin, hair and nails. In: Jones RM, Rospond RM, eds. Patient Assessment in Pharmacy Practice. Baltimore, Lippincott Williams & Wilkins, 2003:102–128.

3. Ashton RE. Teaching non-dermatologists to examine the skin: a review of the literature and some recommendations. Br J Dermatol 1995;132: 221–225.

4. Leung DYM, Eichenfield LF, Boguniewicz M. Atopic dermatitis (atopic eczema). In: Freedberg IM, Eisen AZ, Wolff K, et al, eds. Dermatology in General Medicine, 6th ed. New York, McGraw-Hill, 2003:1180–1194.

5. Belsito DV. Allergic contact dermatitis. In: Freedberg IM, Eisen AZ, Wolff K, et al, eds. Dermatology in General Medicine, 6th ed. New York, McGraw-Hill, 2003:1164–1180.

6. Burton JL, Pye PJ. Seborrhea is not a feature of seborrheic dermatitis. Br Med J 1983;286:1169.

7. Katsambas A, et al. A double-blind trial of treatment of seborrheic dermatitis with 2% ketoconazole cream compared with 1% hydrocortisone cream. Br J Dermatol 1989;353:121.

8. Bruinsma W. A Guide to Drug Eruptions, 6th ed. Oosthuizen, Netherlands, DeZwaluw, 1995.

9. Korkij W, Soltani K. Fixed drug eruption. Arch Dermatol 1984;120: 520–524.

10. Gamis-Jones S. Dermatologic side effects of psychopharmacologic agents. Dermatol Clin 1996;14:503–507.

11. Mammen L, Schmidt CP. Photosensitivity reactions: a case report involving NSAIDS. Am Fam Physician 1995;52:575–578.

12. Moller R. Pigmentary disturbances due to drugs. Acta Derm Venereol (Stockh) 1966;46:423–431.

13. Jelinek JE. Cutaneous side effects of oral contraceptives. Arch Dermatol 1970;101:181–186.

14. Granstein RD, Sober AJ. Drug and heavy metal-induced hyperpigmentation. J Am Acad Dermatol 1981;5:1–18.

15. Trimble JW, Mendelson DS, Fetter BF, et al. Cutaneous pigmentation secondary to amiodarone therapy. Arch Dermatol 1983;119:914–918.

16. Salasche S. Epidemiology of actinic keratoses and squamous cell carcinoma. J Am Acad Dermatol 200;42:S4.

17. Miller DI, Weinstock MA. Nomnelanoma skin cancer in the United States: incidence. J Am Acad Dermatol 1994;30:774.

18. Marks R, et al. Imiquimod 5% cream in the treatment of superficial basal cell carcinoma: results of a multicenter 6-week dose-response trial. J Am Acad Dermatol 2001;44:807.

19. Rigel DS. Melanoma update: 2001. Skin Cancer Found J 2001;19:13.

95

ACNE VULGARIS

Dennis P. West, Lee E. West, Maria Letizia Musumeci, and Giuseppe Micali

Learning Objectives and other resources can be found at *www.pharmacotherapyonline.com.*

KEY CONCEPTS

1 In the United States, acne vulgaris is the most common skin disorder, affecting 40 to 50 million people.

2 Four primary factors are identified as being involved in the formation of acne lesions: increased sebum production, sloughing of keratinocytes, bacterial growth, and inflammation.

3 Acne vulgaris is a disease of the pilosebaceous unit (i.e., the sebaceous glands and adjacent hair follicle).

4 Several types of lesions present at the same time in various stages of development, including noninflammatory and inflammatory lesions, scars, and residual hyperpigmentation.

5 Most therapeutic interventions function primarily to prevent the formation of new acne lesions and have minimal impact on existing lesions.

6 Because most treatments for acne reduce or prevent new eruptions, they may take up to 8 weeks for visible results.

7 *Mild acne* usually is managed with topical retinoids alone or with topical antimicrobials, salicylic acid, or azelaic acid. *Moderate acne* may be managed with topical retinoids in combination with oral antibiotics, and if indicated, benzoyl peroxide. *Severe acne* is often managed with oral isotretinoin.

8 Minocycline has more adverse effects than the other tetracyclines.

Acne is a common, chronic inflammatory disorder of the pilosebaceous unit in which a microcomedo develops as the initial condition. The most common form of acne is acne vulgaris. Other variants of acne are neonatal acne, adult acne, acne cosmetica, and acne mechanica. These descriptors refer to age of onset or causative factors.

Localization of acne vulgaris on the facial area, especially in an adolescent population, significantly impacts self-esteem. Although acne is self-limiting, it can persist for years and can result in disfigurement and scarring.[1] Acne may also be associated with anxiety, depression, and higher-than-average unemployment rates.[2] As the emotional impact of acne is not always easy to assess clinically,[3,4] it is important for the health care professional to educate patients on causes of acne, discussing treatment regimens, and counseling on proper medication use.

EPIDEMIOLOGY

1 In the United States, acne vulgaris is the most common skin disorder, affecting between 40 and 50 million people.[3] Acne vulgaris affects approximately 80% of the population between the age of 12 and 25 years,[5] with no gender, race, or ethnicity prevalence.[3,6]

Acne age of onset varies, but usually begins at puberty. A form of acne called *adult acne* may first occur after the mid-20s,[7] affecting females more than males, and with lesions generally distributed in the lower facial area around the mouth, chin, and jaw line.[8]

ETIOLOGY

2 Four primary factors are identified as being involved in the formation of acne lesions: increased sebum production, sloughing of keratinocytes, bacterial growth, and inflammation.[9–11]

INCREASED SEBUM PRODUCTION

Androgen stimulation is enhanced at puberty and sebaceous glands actively produce sebum. Testosterone, the predominant androgen, and its metabolites along with androstenedione, dehydroepiandrosterone, and dehydroepiandrosterone sulfate, are all increased in acne and apparently capable of enhancing sebaceous gland activity. Anatomic sites for acne tend to be more metabolically active in converting androgens to dihydrotestosterone.

Androgenic activity drives sebum production in the sebaceous glands; however, most acne patients do not have an endocrine abnormality. Acne-affected pilosebaceous units apparently have a hyperresponsiveness to circulating androgens.[9] Increased sebum production per se is not necessarily responsible for acne, but may rather be viewed as an underlying factor.

SLOUGHING OF KERATINOCYTES

A primary factor in the development of acne is the process of follicular keratinization. Sloughing of keratinocytes within the hair follicle is a normal process, but in acne, follicular keratinization more readily involves keratinocyte clumping and subsequent plugging of the hair follicle pore. Increased sloughing of keratinocytes correlates with comedo formation and may be related to influences such as local cytokine modulation, a decrease in sebaceous linoleic acid, and androgen stimulation.[9,12] Abnormal follicular keratinization may be a primary event, or may be a secondary response to irritation or other factors.

BACTERIAL GROWTH AND COLONIZATION

The mix of "trapped" keratinocytes and sebum provide an environment for the normally-occurring bacteria *Propionibacterium acnes* to flourish.[13] Although *P. acnes,* a partial anaerobe, resides in the follicle as normal flora, it triggers immune responses such that titers of antibodies to *P. acnes* are higher in patients with severe acne than in non-acne control subjects.

INFLAMMATION AND IMMUNE RESPONSE

Inflammation may be a consequence of increased sebum production, keratinocyte sloughing, and bacterial growth. Also, *P. acnes* may trigger inflammatory acne lesions by producing biologically active mediators and promoting proinflammatory cytokine release.[14–16]

PATHOPHYSIOLOGY

3 Acne vulgaris is a disease of the pilosebaceous unit (i.e., the sebaceous gland and adjacent hair follicle). Sebaceous glands, predominant on the face, chest, and upper back, respond to androgen stimulation. These glands provide sebum to the follicular canal and eventually to the skin surface through the follicular opening (the pore). Follicular canal contents include keratinocytes, *Propionibacterium acnes* (*P. acnes*), and free fatty acids.

Formation of the primary lesion, the comedo, may be thought of as a plugging of the pilosebaceous follicle. In acne, the follicular canal widens and an increase in cell production may be seen. Sebum mixes with excess loose cells in the follicular canal to form a keratinous plug. The resulting lesion appears as a "blackhead," or open comedo. The brown or black color is not a result of dirt accumulation, but that of melanin (pigment). Inflammation or trauma to the follicle may lead to formation of a "whitehead," or closed comedo. If the follicular wall is damaged or ruptured, the contents of the follicle may extrude into dermis and present clinically as a pustule. Closed comedones are of clinical importance since they may become larger, inflammatory lesions secondary to local *P. acnes* activity (Fig. 95–1).[9] Acne lesions may take months to heal completely, and fibrosis associated with healing may lead to permanent scarring.[17]

4 CLINICAL PRESENTATION OF ACNE VULGARIS

Acne lesions typically occur on the face, back, upper chest, and shoulder area. Severity of the disease varies from a mild comedonal form to severe inflammatory necrotic acne.[18] Acne vulgaris is described as mild, moderate, or severe, depending on the type and severity of lesions present. See Table 95–1 for descriptions of mild, moderate, and severe acne.

SYMPTOMS

Generally, the diagnosis of acne vulgaris consists of findings that include a mixture of lesions of acne (e.g., comedones,

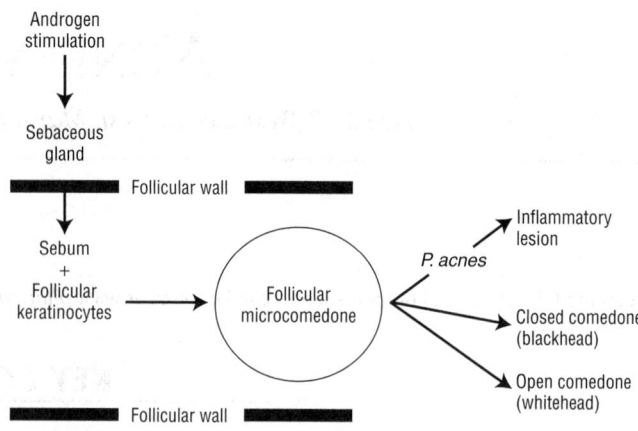

FIGURE 95–1. Principal influences in formation of acne lesions.

pustules, papules, nodules, and cysts) on the face, back, or chest. Although there is no precise definition for acne, many practitioners consider the presence of 5 to 10 comedones to be diagnostic.

SIGNS

There may be more than one morphologic type of lesion present (see Table 95–1), in various stages of development, including noninflammatory and inflammatory lesions, scars, and residual hyperpigmentation.[18]

NONINFLAMMATORY LESIONS

An open comedo or blackhead is a plug of sebum, keratinocytes, and microorganisms blocking a *dilated* hair follicle opening, whereas a closed comedone or whitehead is a similar plug blocking a *closed* hair follicle opening to the surface of the skin.

INFLAMMATORY LESIONS

- A papule is a well-defined, elevated, palpable, distinct area of skin generally less than 1 cm in diameter involving the epidermis and/or dermis. Papules may not have a change in skin color, but are always raised and may have variable textures.
- A pustule is an elevated, distinct, superficial cavity filled with purulent fluid, typically surrounding a hair follicle.
- A nodule is an elevated, firm, distinct, palpable, round or oval lesion up to 1 cm in diameter which occurs in the dermis and/or hypodermis.

SCARS

Permanent scars may occur as a result of inflammatory acne lesions.

RESIDUAL HYPERPIGMENTATION

Inflammatory acne lesions may trigger noticeable hyperpigmentation that may persist weeks to months after resolution of the lesion.[1]

LABORATORY TESTS

There are no laboratory tests to diagnose acne vulgaris. Diagnosis is based on clinical signs. Other dermatologic conditions, such as folliculitis, acne rosacea, and other various acneiform disorders, sometimes may be confused with acne vulgaris.[19]

TABLE 95–1. Predominance of Acne Lesion Type by Acne Severity

Acne Severity	Predominant Lesions	Typical Frequency of Lesion Type						
		Closed Comedones	Open Comedones	Papules	Pustules	Nodules	Scarring
Mild	Noninflammatory lesions (open and closed comedones)	Few to numerous	Few to numerous	Possible	Possible	None	None
Moderate	Inflammatory papules and pustules with some noninflammatory lesions	Few to numerous	Few to numerous	Numerous	Numerous	Few	Possible
Severe	Inflammatory lesions and scarring with some noninflammatory lesions	Few to numerous	Few to numerous	Extensive	Extensive	Extensive	Extensive

▶ TREATMENT: Acne Vulgaris

5 Most therapeutic interventions function primarily to prevent the formation of new acne lesions and have minimal impact on existing lesions. Among the factors that may affect acne are genetics, climate, diet, environment, stress, and physical activity.

Stress seems to aggravate, but not induce, acne.[20] In response to stress, immunoreactive nerve fibers may stimulate sebaceous gland activity and provoke inflammatory reactions via mast cells.[21]

The ingestion of iodine may exacerbate acne or induce acneiform lesions.[10] Dietary factors in acne are controversial.

CLINICAL CONTROVERSY

An observational study has concluded that the incidence of acne in Western and non-Western societies is greatly different and suggests that it is not due to genetic influence alone, but most likely occurs due to differences in diet. These authors felt that a non-westernized diet, representing a substantially low glycemic index, influenced a dramatically lower incidence of acne.[22] It is disputed whether this conclusion is accurate, since acne is influenced by multiple factors and there are no data to support an effect of glycemic index on acne.[23,24] Whether proven or not, some clinicians feel that diet is a factor in skin conditions, including acne, and needs to be further addressed.[25]

GENERAL APPROACH TO TREATMENT

6 Severity, lesion types,[18] scarring, and skin discoloration, as well as previous treatment history, helps to determine a treatment approach to acne vulgaris (see Table 95–1).[9,11,26,27] Most treatments reduce or prevent new eruptions and may take up to 8 weeks to produce visible results. During the first few weeks of therapy, acne may appear to worsen as existing acne lesions may resolve more rapidly. Patients must understand the need to continue therapy for optimal outcome.

7 Patient education with emphasis on goals, realistic expectations, and dangers of overtreatment is important to optimize therapeutic outcomes. Treatment regimens are targeted to types of lesions and acne severity.[9,18] Mild acne usually is managed with topical retinoids alone or with topical antimicrobials, salicylic acid, or azelaic acid. Moderate acne may be managed with topical retinoids in combination with oral antibiotics, and if indicated, benzoyl peroxide.[27] Severe acne is often managed with oral isotretinoin.

Initial treatment is aimed at reducing lesion count and will vary in duration from a few months to a few years, depending on severity and response to treatment. Once control is achieved, chronic indefinite treatment may be required. Therapy with both topical and systemic antibiotics should be for the minimum duration necessary to achieve control of acne, in order to minimize the likelihood of resistance.[9,26,27]

Topical treatment forms include creams, lotions, solutions, gels, and disposable wipes. Responses to different formulations may be dependent on skin type and individual preferences:

- Oily to normal skin types may tolerate gels, solutions, and lotions.
- Normal skin may tolerate gels, solutions, lotions, and creams.
- Normal to dry skin may tolerate lotions and creams.

Ointments are not typically included in topical acne therapy due to their occlusive nature and possible induction of acne cosmetica.

Systemic treatment is required in patients with moderate to severe acne, especially when acne scarring is a possibility.[28]

Antibiotics such as tetracyclines and macrolides are the agents of choice for papulopustular acne. In severe papulopustular and nodulocystic/conglobate acne, oral isotretinoin is the treatment of choice. Hormonal therapy represents an alternative effective regimen in female patients.

NONPHARMACOLOGIC THERAPY

Scrubbing the skin with abrasive scrubs or excessive face washing does not necessarily open or cleanse pores. Follicular plugging originates too deeply to be affected by superficial epidermal scrubbing, which often leads to skin irritation.

Since surface cleansing with soap and water primarily affects sebum and bacteria on the surface of the skin and has minimal impact within the follicle, cleansing has a relatively small impact on the treatment of acne.

To avoid skin irritation and dryness during some acne therapies, it is important to use gentle, nondrying cleansing agents.

PHARMACOLOGIC THERAPY

Recently, worldwide consensus statements regarding management and treatment of acne have been widely distributed to improve and optimize outcomes. See Table 95–2 for highlights of consensus statements from The Global Alliance to Improve Outcomes in Acne.[9] Figure 95–2 provides acne treatment algorithms based on acne severity. See Table 95–3 for the action spectra of selected acne treatments.

TABLE 95–2. Treatment Guidelines for Acne Vulgaris

Therapy	Recommendations
Topical retinoids	• Should be primary treatment for most forms of acne vulgaris • Use early for best results • Should be applied to the entire affected area • Combine with antimicrobial therapy when inflammatory lesions are present • Essential part of maintenance therapy
Hormonal therapy	Excellent choice for women who also need oral contraceptives for gynecologic reasons • Use early in female patients with moderate to severe acne or with symptoms of seborrhea, acne, hirsutism, or alopecia • Useful as part of combination therapy in women with or without endocrine abnormalities • Sometimes used in women with late-onset acne
Oral isotretinoin	*Indications:* • Severe nodulocystic acne • Severe acne variants • Inflammatory acne with scarring, after conventional therapy has failed • Moderate to severe acne, especially frequently relapsing cases • Acne with severe psychological distress *Typical dose:* • 0.5–1.0 mg/kg daily in two divided doses, with cumulative dose of 120–150 mg/kg per treatment course (4–6 months) • A lower dose (<0.5 mg/kg) may be used but is associated with a higher relapse rate • Patient counseling is critical
Combination therapy	• Should be used when inflammatory lesions are present • Speeds clearing and provides greater resolution of both inflammatory lesions and comedones • Topical retinoid should be started at the initiation of antimicrobial therapy • Antibiotic should be discontinued when inflammatory lesions resolve adequately • If this is not possible, then switch to a combination agent with benzoyl peroxide plus an antibiotic • Continue use of topical retinoid to maintain remission of new acne lesions when antibiotic therapy is discontinued

From the consensus recommendations from The Global Alliance to Improve Outcomes in Acne.[9]

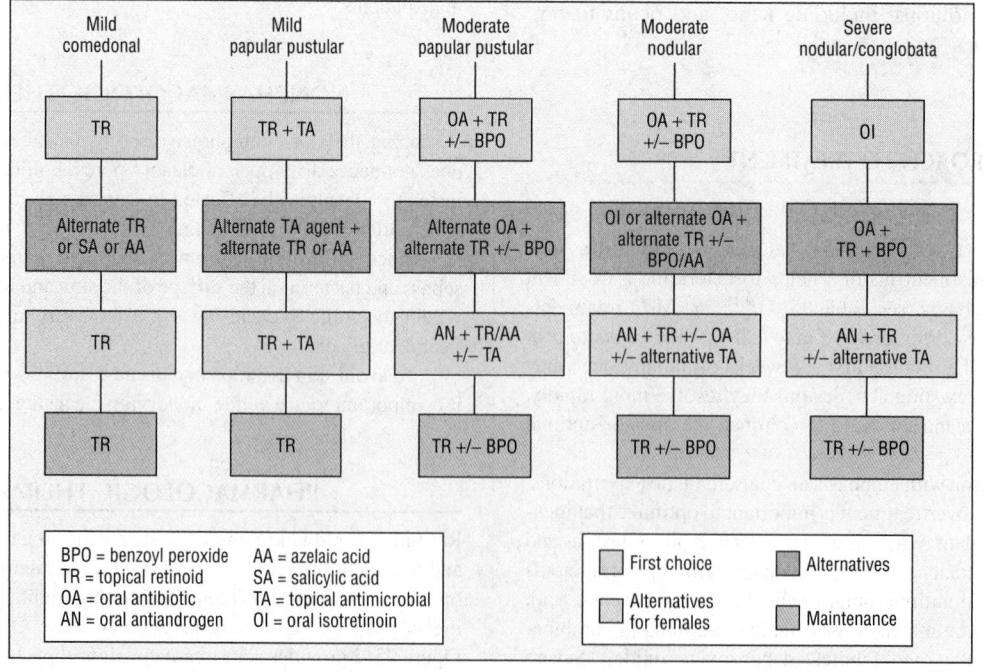

FIGURE 95–2. Algorithms for acne treatment.

TABLE 95-3. Mechanism of Action of Selected Pharmacotherapeutic Agents in Acne

Treatment	Antimicrobial	Anti-Inflammatory	Decreased Sebum Production	Keratolytic/Comedolytic
Adapalene	+	++	−	+++
Antibacterial oral agents	+++	++	−	+
Antibacterial topical agents	+++	+	−	+
Azelaic acid	++	+	−	++
Benzoyl peroxide	+++	++	−	+
Oral isotretinoin	++	++	+++	+++
Oral contraceptives	−	−	+++	++
Salicylic acid	−	−	−	+
Spironolactone	−	++	++	−
Topical retinoids	−	+	−	+++

−, No activity; +, low activity; ++, moderate activity; +++, high activity.

TOPICAL AGENTS: FIRST-LINE THERAPIES

Benzoyl Peroxide

Superficial inflammatory acne is typically treated with benzoyl peroxide (BPO), a nonantibiotic antibacterial agent that is rapidly bacteriostatic and possibly bactericidal against *P. acnes.*[29] Its antibacterial mechanism of action is uncertain, although BPO is decomposed on the skin by cysteine, liberating free oxygen radicals that oxidize bacterial proteins.[30] BPO increases the sloughing rate of epithelial cells, loosens the follicular plug structure, and thus possesses some degree of comedolytic activity. An advantage to using topical BPO is that *P. acnes* resistance is not known to develop.[9,27]

BPO is available in soaps, lotions, creams, washes, and gels, in concentrations ranging from 1% to 5%;[9] 10% concentrations are not significantly more efficacious, but may be more irritating. Gel formulations have better stability and are usually most potent, while lotions, creams, and soaps are weaker. Gels are usually based on alcohol, propylene glycol, or water; the alcohol-based preparations generally cause more dryness and irritation. Fair or moist skin usually is more sensitive to irritation from BPO; thus patients should be advised to apply medication to dry skin (at least 30 minutes after washing) to decrease irritation.

Cleansing dosage forms (washes) that contain antiacne ingredients such as α-hydroxy acids, BPO, or salicylic acid are available. BPO cleansers may be considered for adolescent boys, both to enhance compliance and to cover large skin areas such as the chest and back.[9]

Dryness and irritation from a primary irritant such as BPO may limit therapy in some patients; allergic contact dermatitis (delayed-type hypersensitivity reaction) has also been reported.[31]

To limit irritation and increase patient tolerance of BPO, one may initiate therapy with a low-potency formulation (2.5%), and increase either strength (5% to 10%) or application frequency (every other day, each day, and then twice a day). To minimize irritation potential, BPO should be applied to cool, clean, dry skin, no more frequently than twice daily. Use should be discontinued if excessive irritation or allergy occurs. One disadvantage is that BPO may bleach or discolor some fabrics (clothing, bed linen, or towels). Tolerability and effectiveness are enhanced when used in combination with other agents such as topical retinoids, clindamycin, and erythromycin.[9,27,29,32]

Retinoids

Topical retinoids—tretinoin, adapalene, tazarotene, and in some countries topical isotretinoin, motretinide, retinaldehyde, and retinoyl-β-glucuronide[9]—should be used as first-line therapy for mild to moderate inflammatory acne and comedonal acne. They are also preferred agents for maintenance therapy to minimize antibiotic use in acne therapy.[9] To optimize efficacy in moderate inflammatory acne, topical retinoids should be combined with topical antibiotics or BPO.[27,33]

Tretinoin

Tretinoin, a topical vitamin A analogue, is a comedolytic agent that increases cell turnover in the follicular wall and decreases cohesiveness of cells, leading to extrusion of existing comedones and inhibition of the formation of new comedones,[30] and may reduce the number of inflammatory acne lesions.[27] Tretinoin significantly decreases the number of cell layers in the stratum corneum from about 14 to about 5.[30]

In a 12-week study of tretinoin, the reduction of lesion counts ranged from 32% to 81% for noninflammatory lesions, and 17% to 71% for inflammatory lesions (22% to 83% for the total lesion count).[27] Comparing tretinoin 0.025% gel or 0.025% cream with vehicles only in a once-daily application regimen, tretinoin was significantly more effective in reducing both inflammatory and noninflammatory lesions.[34,35]

Tretinoin is available as 0.05% solution (most irritating), 0.01% and 0.025% gels, and 0.025%, 0.05%, and 0.1% creams (least irritating).[9] Treatment initiation with 0.025% cream usually is recommended for mild acne in patients with easily irritated and nonoily skin, 0.01% gel for moderate acne in easily irritated skin with oily complexion, and 0.025% gel for moderate acne with nonsensitive and oily skin. A "flare" of acne may appear suddenly after initiation of treatment, followed by clinical clearing in about 8 to 12 weeks.[30]

Once control is established, therapy should be continued at the lowest effective concentration and at the maximum effective interval sufficient to minimize acne exacerbations.

Concomitant use of an antibacterial agent with tretinoin can decrease keratinization, inhibit *P. acnes*, and decrease inflammation. In addition, both BPO and tretinoin have shown additive or synergistic effects in the treatment of inflammatory acne.[36] A regimen of BPO each morning and tretinoin at bedtime may enhance efficacy and be less irritating than either agent used alone.[36] By slowly increasing application frequency from every other day, to daily, and then twice daily, tolerance to tretinoin may be increased. Increased sensitivity to sun exposure, wind, cold, and other irritants may also be evident in patients using tretinoin.

Two reformulations of tretinoin include a porous bead (0.01% gel) (microspheres) and liquid polymer (0.025% cream and 0.025% gel). These are less irritating than standard vehicles for tretinoin. In the topical gel formulation containing polyolprepolymer-2, tretinoin penetration was significantly reduced while epidermal deposition was enhanced, compared with a commercially available gel preparation at the same concentration. Polyolprepolymer-2 promotes retention of drug molecules on the skin surface and in the upper layers of the skin.[37]

In a double-blind 12-week study, tretinoin microsphere gel demonstrated faster onset of action than adapalene, including a greater reduction in comedone counts at week 4; yet reductions in acne lesions at 12 weeks were similar with the two drugs, and an increased incidence of dryness and peeling was associated with tretinoin.[38]

Another formulation is a microsponge delivery system consisting of macroporous beads 10 to 15 micrometers in diameter that are loaded with tretinoin. Gradual release of active ingredient after topical application depends on mechanical rubbing, temperature, pH, and other factors.[39] Tretinoin 0.1% gel microsponge, tretinoin 0.025% gel, tazarotene 0.1% gel, and adapalene 0.1% gel all showed equivalent facial tolerability in a split-face study.[39] In another variation, a formulation of liposomally encapsulated tretinoin showed potentially better tolerance than gel dosage forms, yet demonstrated equivalent efficacy.[40]

Adverse reactions to tretinoin—such as skin irritation, erythema, and peeling—will vary depending on individual skin type and dosage form used. Allergic contact dermatitis is rare and much less common than with BPO. Teratogenicity risk with topical retinoids remains controversial.

CLINICAL CONTROVERSY

During treatment with topical tretinoin, plasma tretinoin concentrations are typically less than endogenous levels, and apparently do not affect endogenous levels of tretinoin or its metabolites or alter plasma vitamin A levels. However, controversy continues with regard to teratogenicity and embryotoxicity risk versus benefit issues in the use of topical retinoids during pregnancy.[41,42]

Adapalene

Adapalene, a third-generation retinoid,[9] is a retinoid-mimetic compound (a naphthoic acid derivative), available as 0.1% gel, cream, alcoholic solution, and pledgets. It has selective affinity for retinoic acid receptor (RAR) subtypes RAR-β and RAR-γ found in the epidermis,[43,44] and has comedolytic, keratolytic, and anti-inflammatory activity.[11,44,45] Vehicle-controlled and comparative studies have demonstrated the utility of adapalene in treatment of acne.[43,45,46]

Adapalene is indicated for mild to moderate acne vulgaris. Adapalene 0.1% gel may be used as an alternative to tretinoin 0.025% gel to achieve better tolerability in some patients.[46,47] Adapalene coadministered with a topical or oral antibiotic represents a rational therapy for moderate forms of acne.[11]

In a double-blind 12-week study, tretinoin microsphere gel demonstrated faster onset of action than adapalene, including a greater reduction in comedone counts at week 4. Yet reductions in acne lesions at 12 weeks were similar with the two drugs, and an increased incidence of dryness and peeling was associated with tretinoin.[38]

Adapalene may also be an alternative in treating some patients of color since it produces less skin irritation and subsequent discoloration than the first-generation topical tretinoin products.[11]

Tazarotene

Tazarotene, a prodrug and a synthetic acetylenic retinoid, is converted to its active form, tazarotenic acid, after topical application. This new-generation retinoid also selectively binds to RARs and can alter expression of genes involved in cell proliferation, cell differentiation, and inflammation.[44]

Tazarotene is used in the treatment of mild to moderate acne vulgaris and has comedolytic, keratolytic, and anti-inflammatory action. Tazarotene 0.1% and 0.05% gel and cream have been shown to be more effective than vehicle in the treatment of acne vulgaris.[48,49] The 0.1% gel was slightly more effective than the 0.05% gel in decreasing lesion counts, with treatment success rates of 68% and 51% of patients, respectively.[3]

Once-daily tazarotene gel may be more effective than once-daily tretinoin in reducing papules and open comedones, with equal efficacy against closed comedones.[50,51] Efficacy is comparable to adapalene, but its local tolerance by daily application is similar to tretinoin. In addition, tazarotene was studied for its efficacy with short contact application. Once-daily short contact applications significantly reduced irritation potential, yet maintained therapeutic equivalency to standard application regimens.[52]

Both 0.1% and 0.05% concentrations had acceptable tolerability profiles, with no serious adverse events.[49] Dose-related local adverse effects include erythema, pruritus, stinging, and burning.[4]

Erythromycin

Erythromycin in topical form in concentrations of 1% to 4% with or without the addition of zinc is effective against inflammatory acne. Zinc combination products possibly enhance penetration of erythromycin into the pilosebaceous unit.[53]

Combinations of erythromycin and BPO have shown greater efficacy in treating acne than a combination of erythromycin and tretinoin.[33] Development of P. acnes resistance to erythromycin may be reduced by combination therapy with BPO.

Topical erythromycin, usually applied twice daily, is formulated as a gel, lotion, solution, and disposable pad. Reduction of the percentage of free fatty acids in sebum has been noted with the use of topical erythromycin.[53]

Clindamycin

Topical clindamycin inhibits P. acnes and provides comedolytic as well as anti-inflammatory activity.[54] It is available in gel, lotion, solution, and disposable pad formulations, and is usually applied twice daily. Combination with BPO increases efficacy.[55] Though rare, diarrhea and pseudomembranous colitis may occur secondary to topical clindamycin.[56]

Azelaic Acid

Azelaic acid has a dicarboxylic acid structure that confers antibacterial, anti-inflammatory, and comedolytic activity.[54] Azelaic acid is useful for treating mild to moderate acne in patients who do not tolerate BPO. It is useful in treating postinflammatory hyperpigmentation since it also has skin-lightening properties.[57]

Azelaic acid has no likelihood of bacterial resistance, systemic adverse effects, or photosensitivity reactions. Although uncommon, adverse effects, usually transient, include burning, pruritus, stinging, and tingling.[9,27]

Azelaic acid is available in a 20% cream formulation. Application is usually twice daily on clean, dry skin.

TOPICAL AGENTS: SECOND-LINE THERAPIES

Motretinide

Motretinide, also available outside the U.S., is a topical aromatic ester retinoid with an efficacy profile similar to low-dose tretinoin concentrations, but with somewhat less irritant potential.[27]

Retinaldehyde

Retinaldehyde is biotransformed into all-*trans*-retinoic acid and induces biologic effects including comedolytic activity[58] similar to those of topical tretinoin when administered at comparatively lower concentrations.[9]

After topical application of retinaldehyde 0.1% gel or its vehicle every morning and erythromycin 4% lotion every evening in the treatment of acne for 8 weeks, comedones and microcysts were significantly improved with retinaldehyde combined with erythromycin, but not with erythromycin alone. In both treatment groups, papules and pustules were reduced significantly. Local tolerance is satisfactory.[59]

Retinoyl-β-Glucuronide

Retinoyl-β-glucuronide is a naturally occurring, biologically active metabolite of vitamin A. A 0.16% retinoyl-β-glucuronide cream has been shown to be effective against inflammatory and noninflammatory acne lesions[60] with comparable efficacy to tretinoin, but with less irritation potential and comparatively fewer other adverse effects than with tretinoin.

Isotretinoin

Isotretinoin is available outside the U.S. as a gel formulation; it does not reduce sebum secretion as does oral isotretinoin. Used topically, the effectiveness of isotretinoin is similar to that of other topical retinoids, but it causes somewhat less skin irritation.[23] It reduces noninflammatory lesions from 46% to 78% and inflammatory lesions from 24% to 55% after 12 to 14 weeks of treatment.[27]

Keratolytic Agents

In addition to keratolytic activity, salicylic acid, sulfur, and resorcinol are mildly antibacterial.

Salicylic acid has comedolytic and anti-inflammatory action.[26] Also known as β-hydroxy acid, it is deemed a more effective comedolytic than most α-hydroxy acids.[13] In addition, it increases penetration of other substances, and in low concentrations is bacteriostatic and fungistatic.[27]

Although evidence for efficacy in the treatment of acne is conflicting, each agent has been classified as safe and effective by an advisory review panel of the FDA. Some combinations of these agents may be considered synergistic (e.g., sulfur and resorcinol, salicylic acid, BPO). Keratolytic products, in the concentration allowed, may be less irritating than BPO and tretinoin; however, they are not considered as effective comedolytic agents, as are BPO and tretinoin.

Disadvantages of these agents include the odor created by hydrogen sulfide on reaction of sulfur with the skin, the brown scale from use of resorcinol, and the possibility of salicylism from repeated and widespread use of sufficient concentrations of salicylic acid on highly permeable (inflamed and/or abraded) skin.[56]

Corticosteroids

Topical corticosteroids can be applied in very selected patients with very inflammatory acne for short periods of time. They may play a role in reducing flare-up reactions in severe conglobate acne and for reduction of granuloma pyogenicum–like lesions under systemic isotretinoin treatment.[27]

Chemical Peeling

Light chemical peels may be useful in some acne patients to reduce superficial scarring and hyperpigmentation.[61] Chemical peeling targets the interfollicular epidermis.[27]

Some currently available substances for chemical peeling include: α-hydroxy acids (glycolic acid), salicylic acid, and trichloroacetic acid.[61] Salicylic acid is lipid soluble and may penetrate into sebum-laden follicles more readily than water-soluble α-hydroxy acids. Salicylic acid may also have some ability to reduce the inflammatory component of acne.[9,26] Patients with sensitive skin types tolerate salicylic acid peels.[62]

Dapsone

Topical dapsone, exhibiting antibacterial and anti-inflammatory properties, is being investigated for effectiveness in the treatment of acne.[63]

SYSTEMIC AGENTS: FIRST-LINE THERAPY—SEVERE NODULAR/CONGLOBATA

Isotretinoin

As an oral retinoid, isotretinoin is the most effective sebosuppressive agent that affects all of the etiologic factors involved in inflammatory acne, including induction of atrophy of the sebaceous gland with decreased sebum production and change in sebum composition, inhibition of *P. acnes* growth within follicles, inhibition of inflammation, and altered patterns of keratinization within follicles (decreased size and increased differentiation).[64,65] These characteristics make it the treatment of choice in severe nodulocystic acne.[66] It may be used

TABLE 95–4. Principal Adverse Effects of Oral Isotretinoin

Adverse Effect	Response
Teratogenicity	Contraindicated during pregnancy
Depression	Patient monitoring and counseling; antidepressants
Dryness	
Mouth	Hard candy
Eyes	Eyedrops; avoid contact lenses if possible during treatment course
Nose	Lubricant
Skin	Nondrying gentle skin cleansers; non-comedolytic moisturizers
Lips	Lip moisturizer with sunscreen
Muscle and joint pain	Nonsteroidal anti-inflammatory drugs
Alopecia	Reversible when drug discontinued or dose decreased
Hypertriglyceridemia	Reversible when drug discontinued or dose decreased
Acne flare at start of therapy	Continue therapy
Photosensitivity	Use sunscreens (moisturizing), protective clothing, and sun avoidance

in patients who have failed conventional treatment, those who have scarring acne, those who have chronic relapsing acne, and those who have acne with severe psychological distress.[67]

Adverse effects from orally administered isotretinoin are numerous, frequent, and often dose related.[68] About 90% of patients receiving isotretinoin therapy suffer from mucocutaneous effects. Drying of the mucosa of the mouth, nose, and eyes is the most common problem, with relatively rare involvement of the genito-anal mucosa. Cheilitis and skin desquamation occurs in more than 80% of patients. Less frequently, the conjunctiva and nasal mucosa are affected. Table 95–4 shows selected responses to some of the adverse effects of oral isotretinoin.

Disturbances in lipid metabolism also may occur, resulting in transitory increase of blood values for cholesterol and triglycerides.[67] Liver function and serum lipids should initially be monitored, typically at baseline and at weeks 4 and 8.[69] Serious adverse effects of isotretinoin therapy include: increased creatine phosphokinase and blood glucose, as well as photosensitivity, pseudotumor cerebri, excess granulation tissue, hepatomegaly with abnormal liver function tests, bone abnormalities, arthralgias, muscle stiffness, and headaches.[70]

Hyperlipidemia, diabetes mellitus, and severe osteoporosis are relative contraindications for oral isotretinoin. The drug may very occasionally produce significant mood changes, depression, and other significant psychiatric adverse effects. Although relationship to drug therapy is controversial, current recommendations are that patients be counseled about and screened for depression during therapy.[71,72]

Isotretinoin dosing guidelines range from 0.5 to 1 mg/kg per day, but the cumulative dose taken by patients during a treatment course may be the major factor influencing long-term outcome.[73] Optimal results generally have occurred when cumulative doses have attained a range of 120 to 150 mg/kg.[73]

A 6-month course of therapy is sufficient for most patients, but it has been observed that an initial dose of 1 mg/kg per day for 3 months, then reduced to 0.5 mg/kg per day, and if possible, to 0.2 mg/kg per day for 3 to 9 additional months will optimize the therapeutic outcome.[28] Generally, after 2 to 4 weeks of treatment, a 50% reduction of the pustules can be expected. Pustules clear more rapidly than papules or nodules. Improvement continues during the posttreatment period. In female patients contraception is required because of teratogenicity,[68] recommended to begin 1 month before therapy, continuing during the entire period of treatment, and for up to 3 months after discontinuation of isotretinoin.[68]

Although costs of therapy with isotretinoin are greater in the first year, isotretinoin can be more cost effective than long-term antibiotic treatment.[74]

SYSTEMIC AGENTS: FIRST-LINE THERAPY—MODERATE PAPULAR PUSTULAR/NODULAR

Macrolide Antibiotics

The macrolide antibiotics (erythromycin, azithromycin, and clindamycin) exhibit anti-inflammatory properties in patients with acne.

Erythromycin can be used for patients who require systemic antibiotics, but cannot tolerate tetracyclines, or who acquire bacterial strains resistant to tetracyclines.[75,76] The dosage is usually 1 g/day with meals to minimize gastrointestinal intolerance. Zinc combination products possibly enhance penetration of erythromycin into the pilosebaceous unit.[53] Erythromycin's efficacy is similar to tetracycline, but it induces higher rates of bacterial resistance.[75,76] Development of erythromycin resistance by P. acnes may be reduced by combination therapy with BPO.

Azithromycin, an azalide antibiotic and derivative of erythromycin, is a safe and effective alternate treatment of moderate to severe inflammatory acne. With a half-life of 68 hours, it may be intermittently dosed three times a week.[77] One study using pulse therapy, 500 mg daily for 3 to 4 consecutive days every week for 4 weeks, demonstrated efficacy similar to other systemic antibacterial agents.[78] Adherence is high with this regimen, and phototoxicity and resistance have not been reported.[78]

Clindamycin is very effective in the treatment of acne, but has disadvantages for long-term therapy due to the possible induction of pseudomembranous colitis. For this reason, its use in acne is uncommon.

Tetracyclines

The tetracyclines are effective in reducing P. acnes.[79] In addition to their antibacterial effects, they reduce the amount of keratin in sebaceous follicles and inhibit chemotaxis, phagocytosis, complement activation (by the alternate pathway), and cell-mediated immunity.[80] Tetracyclines also appear to have an affinity for inflammatory cells and bacteria, resulting in higher drug concentration in areas of inflamed skin.

Adverse reactions involving the gastrointestinal tract may occur with the tetracyclines. Drawbacks to the use of tetracyclines include hepatotoxicity and predisposition to superinfections (vaginal candidiasis), and very rarely benign intracranial hypertension. All tetracyclines are photosensitizing, and a sun protection plan should be used. Also, these agents should not be used in children under 10 years of age or in pregnant women because the risk of tooth discoloration when used in children and inhibition of skeletal growth in the developing fetus. Emergence of resistant strains of *P. acne,*[75] adverse events, and adherence issues associated with long-term systemic tetracycline use have led to new treatment approaches.

Adverse effects of tetracyclines include resistant bacteria, folliculitis, candidiasis, gastrointestinal upset, and phototoxic effects. Tetracyclines must not be combined with systemic retinoids because of the increased probability for development of intracranial hypertension. Tetracycline is used in the treatment of moderate to severe acne vulgaris. It is the least expensive of the tetracyclines and therefore often prescribed for initial therapy.[30] A common initial approach includes tetracycline 1 g daily (500 mg twice daily), 1 hour before meals; after 1 or 2 months, when marked improvement of inflammatory lesions is observed, the dose may be decreased to 500 mg every day, for another 1 or 2 months.[75] Drawbacks to the use of tetracycline include also a drug–food interaction with dairy products.

Doxycycline is commonly used in the treatment of moderate to severe acne vulgaris. It is more effective and produces less resistance than tetracycline. The initial dosage is usually 100 or 200 mg daily, followed after improvement by 50 mg/day as a maintenance dose; it may be taken with food even though it is more effective when taken 30 minutes before meals. Subantimicrobial-dose doxycycline (20 mg) has been investigated in a double-blind, placebo-controlled trial in the treatment of moderate facial acne. Positive outcomes were achieved with no development of resistant organisms or change in normal skin flora.[81,82] Adverse effects include resistant bacteria, folliculitis, candidiasis, gastrointestinal upset, and phototoxic effects such as photoonycholysis.[83]

Minocycline is another commonly prescribed oral antibiotic used in the treatment of moderate to severe acne vulgaris. It is more effective than tetracycline because of greater lipid solubility and enhanced penetration into tissue and sebaceous follicles.[84] It is dosed similarly to doxycycline (100 mg/day or 50 mg twice daily) and on an indefinite basis in selected patients.

Of the tetracyclines, minocycline has the most reported adverse effects.[85] Neither tetracycline nor doxycycline contain an amino acid side chain found in minocycline that has potential to form a reactive metabolite. Perhaps related to this, in addition to usual tetracycline adverse effects, minocycline may cause vestibular toxicity, discoloration of skin and visceral tissues,[86] discoloration of the gums, drug-induced lupus erythematosus,[86] interstitial nephritis/hepatic failure/systemic eosinophilia,[86] hypersensitivity syndromes,[85] serum sickness–like illness,[85] severe fever,[87] depersonalization symptoms,[88] and cutaneous hyperpigmentation of at least four distinct types:[89]

1. Blue-black pigmentation confined to sites of scarring or inflammation on the face
2. Blue-gray circumscribed pigmentation of normal skin of the lower legs and forearms
3. Diffuse muddy brown pigmentation of normal skin accentuated in sun-exposed areas
4. Circumscribed blue-gray pigmentation within acne scars confined to the back

SYSTEMIC AGENTS: SECOND-LINE THERAPY

Cotrimoxazole

Cotrimoxazole (trimethoprim-sulfamethoxazole) or trimethoprim alone may be used for treating patients who do not tolerate tetracycline and erythromycin or in cases of resistance to these antibiotics.[90] The adult dosage is usually 800 mg sulfamethoxazole and 160 mg trimethoprim twice daily.

Hormonal Therapy

Hormonal therapy is useful in treating acne in women with elevated or normal serum androgens. It may also be warranted for female patients with severe seborrhea, clinically apparent androgenic alopecia, seborrhea/acne/hirsutism/alopecia syndrome, late-onset acne, and with proven ovarian or adrenal hyperandrogenism.[91]

Hormonal therapy is absolutely contraindicated in women who want to become pregnant due to the risk of sexual organ malformation in a developing fetus.[28]

Antiandrogens, or androgen-receptor blockers, should be avoided during pregnancy.[9] Both cyproterone and spironolactone should be used for acne only in women, because they lead to feminization in men.[92]

Cyproterone Acetate

Cyproterone acetate (CPA), the most widely used antiandrogen compound, is not available in the United States. It is a progestational agent that blocks the androgen receptors and also inhibits the synthesis of adrenal androgens. In Europe and Canada, CPA is widely used in women for the treatment of acne, with or without signs of hyperandrogenism, and as an oral contraceptive formulation (CPA 2 mg with ethinyl estradiol 35 mcg or 50 mcg).[93]

Adverse effects include menstrual abnormalities, breast tenderness and enlargement, nausea and vomiting, fluid retention, leg edema, headache, and melasma.

Chlormadinone Acetate

Chlormadinone acetate (2 mg), alone or in combination with 50 mcg ethinyl estradiol or 50 mcg mestranol in a contraceptive pill, is available in several European countries and is slightly less efficacious than CPA.[94]

Spironolactone

Spironolactone, an antiandrogen and inhibitor of 5α-reductase, reduces sebum production and improves acne at dosages of 50 to 200 mg twice daily in patients with acne resistant to conventional therapy.[91] Most commonly, it is used in countries where other antiandrogen drugs are not available.

Adverse effects are dose dependent and can be lessened by initiating therapy with doses as low as 25 mg/day. They include potential hyperkalemia, irregular menses, breast tenderness, headache, and fatigue.[26]

Drospirenone

Drospirenone, a derivative of spironolactone, has been introduced in Europe as another antiandrogen agent that may prove to be useful in some patients.[93]

Flutamide

Flutamide, a drug approved for treatment of prostate cancer, blocks the androgen receptor. It is used in combination with oral contraceptives in seborrhea and acne therapy for females.[92] The dose is usually 250 to 500 mg twice daily over 6 months.

Flutamide use is limited due to reports of fatal hepatitis requiring monitoring of liver function during therapy.[92] Pregnancy must be avoided due to the risk of feminization of a male fetus.[9]

Estrogens

Estrogens are indicated in female patients with clinical evidence of hyperandrogenism. They suppress the ovarian production of androgens. They are of limited use because the dose of estrogen required for suppression of sebum production is greater than that required to suppress ovulation. Response to 0.035 to 0.050 mcg of ethinyl estradiol or its esters occurs in some women, but higher doses are often required.[95] Breast examinations and Pap smears may be recommended in women receiving long-term estrogen therapy; other serious adverse effects such as clotting and hypertension are possible but very rare in young healthy females.

Oral Contraceptives

Oral contraceptives containing two agents, an estrogen and a progestin, are used as an alternate treatment for moderate acne in women.[95]

Oral contraceptives decrease free testosterone levels by increasing sex hormone–binding globulin, leading to a decrease in sebum production,[12,95] and they inhibit the ovarian production of androgens by suppressing ovulation.

Common adverse effects of oral contraceptives include nausea and vomiting, breast tenderness, headache, spotting and breakthrough bleeding, edema of the venous system of the lower extremities, decreased libido, increased appetite, and weight gain. A transient flare of inflammatory acne may also accompany the initiation of therapy. The most serious adverse effect of oral contraceptives, thromboembolism, has been greatly reduced by the use of lowered doses of estrogens.[91]

Gonadotropin-Releasing Hormone Agonists

Gonadotropin-releasing hormone agonists (buserelin, nafarelin, and leuprolide), available as injectable drugs or nasal spray, suppress the production of ovarian androgens and are efficacious in acne. By reducing estrogen, they can produce menopausal symptoms (headache and bone loss). They have not been approved for treatment of acne.[91]

Corticosteroids

Low-dose corticosteroids (prednisone, prednisolone, or dexamethasone) are indicated in patients with adrenal hyperandrogenism or acne fulminans.

Dapsone

Oral dapsone, a sulfone, has been used for treatment of acne conglobata (a rare condition that is highly inflammatory; onset usually occurs in adults) and acne inversa (chronic lesions in the axillary and groin areas).[63]

PHARMACOECONOMIC CONSIDERATIONS

Although costs of therapy with oral isotretinoin are greater than with other therapeutic choices in the first year, this option can be more cost-effective than long-term antibiotic treatment.[74]

EVALUATION OF THERAPEUTIC OUTCOMES

See Tables 95–5 through 95–9 for prototypical examples of pharmaceutical care plans in the evaluation of therapeutic outcomes for each grade of acne severity.

TABLE 95–5. Typical Pharmaceutical Care Plan for Mild Comedonal Acne

Mild comedonal	Baseline	2 wk	1 mo	2 mo	3 mo	4 mo	5 mo	6 mo	9 mo	12 mo	Every 12 mo
First choice											
TR	PA PT		PA		PA			PA		PA	PA
Alternatives											
Alternate TR, SA, or AA	PA		PA		PA			PA		PA	PA
Alternatives for females											
TR	PA		PA		PA			PA		PA	PA
Maintenance											
TR											PA

AA, azelaic acid; blank, N/A; PA, physical assessment; PT, pregnancy test; SA, salicylic acid; TR, topical retinoid.

TABLE 95–6. Typical Pharmaceutical Care Plan for Mild Papular Pustular Acne

Mild Papular Pustular	Baseline	2 wk	1 mo	2 mo	3 mo	4 mo	5 mo	6 mo	9 mo	12 mo	Every 12 mo
First choice											
TR + TA	PA PT		PA		PA			PA		PA	PA
Alternatives											
Alternate TA agent + alternate TR or AA	PA PT		PA		PA			PA		PA	PA
Alternatives for females											
TR + TA	PA PT		PA		PA			PA		PA	PA
Maintenance											
TR											PA

AA, azelaic acid; blank, N/A; PA, physical assessment; PT, pregnancy test; TA, topical antimicrobial; TR, topical retinoid.

TABLE 95–7. Typical Pharmaceutical Care Plan for Moderate Papular Pustular Acne Moderate

Papular Pustular Acne	Baseline	2 wk	1 mo	2 mo	3 mo	4 mo	5 mo	6 mo	9 mo	12 mo	Every 12 mo
First choice											
OA + TR ± BPO	PA PT lab		PA		PA lab			PA	PA	PA lab	PA lab
Alternatives											
Alternate OA + alternate TR ± BPO	PA PT lab		PA		PA lab			PA	PA	PA lab	PA lab
Alternatives for females											
AN + TR/AA ± TA	PA PT lab		PA		PA lab			PA		PA lab	PA lab
Maintenance											
TR ± BPO											PA lab

AA, azelaic acid; AN, oral antiandrogen; blank, N/A; BPO, benzoyl peroxide; lab, CBC, chem screen, urinalysis; OA, oral antibiotic; PA, physical assessment; PT, pregnancy test; TA, topical antimicrobial; TR, topical retinoid.

TABLE 95–8. Typical Pharmaceutical Care Plan for Moderate Nodular Acne

Moderate Nodular Acne	Baseline	2 wk	1 mo	2 mo	3 mo	4 mo	5 mo	6 mo	9 mo	12 mo	Every 12 mo
First choice											
OA + TR ± BPO	PA PT lab		PA		PA lab			PA	PA	PA lab	PA lab
Alternatives											
OI or alternate OA + alternate TR ± BPO/AA	PA PT lab SLA	PA PT lab SLA	PA PT lab SLA	PA PT	PA PT lab SLA	PA PT	PA PT	PA PT lab SLA			
Alternatives for females											
AN + TR ± OA ± alternate TA	PA PT lab		PA lab		PA lab			PA		PA lab	PA lab
Maintenance											
TR ± BPO ± OA											PA lab

AA, azelaic acid; AN, oral antiandrogen; blank, N/A; BPO, benzoyl peroxide; lab, CBC, chem screen, urinalysis; OA, oral antibiotic; OI, oral isotretinoin; PA, physical assessment; PT, pregnancy test; SLA, serum lipid analysis; TA, topical antimicrobial; TR, topical retinoid.

TABLE 95–9. Typical Pharmaceutical Care Plan for Severe Nodular/Conglobata Acne

Severe Nodular Acne	Baseline	2 wk	1 mo	2 mo	3 mo	4 mo	5 mo	6 mo	9 mo	12 mo	Every 12 mo
First choice OI	PA PT lab SLA	PA PT lab SLA	PA PT lab SLA	PA PT	PA PT lab SLA	PA PT	PA PT	PA PT lab SLA			
Alternatives OA + TR + BPO	PA PT lab		PA lab		PA lab			PA	PA	PA lab	PA lab
Alternatives for females AN + TR ± alternate TA	PA PT lab		PA lab		PA lab			PA		PA lab	PA lab
Maintenance TR ± BPO											PA

AN, oral antiandrogen; blank, N/A; BPO, benzoyl peroxide; lab, CBC, chem screen, urinalysis; OA, oral antibiotic; OI, oral isotretinoin; PA, physical assessment; PT, pregnancy test; SLA, serum lipid analysis; TA, topical antimicrobial; TR, topical retinoid.

ABBREVIATIONS

BPO: benzoyl peroxide
CPA: cyproterone acetate
RAR: retinoic acid receptor

Review Questions and other resources can be found at *www.pharmacotherapyonline.com.*

REFERENCES

1. Layton AM, Seukeran D, Cunliffe WJ. Scarred for life? Dermatology 1997;195:15–21.
2. Hanna S, Sharma J, Klotz J. Acne vulgaris: more than skin deep. Dermatol Online J 2003;9:8.
3. Berson DS, Chalker DK, Harper JC, et al. Current concepts in the treatment of acne: report from a clinical roundtable. Cutis 2003;72:5–13.
4. Mallon E, Newton JN, Klassen A, et al. The quality of life in acne: a comparison with general medical conditions using generic questionnaires. Br J Dermatol 1999;140:672–676.
5. Goulden V, Stables GI, Cunliffe WJ. Prevalence of facial acne in adults. J Am Acad Dermatol 1999;41:577–580.
6. Purdy S, Langston J, Tait L. Presentation and management of acne in primary care: a retrospective cohort study. Br J Gen Pract 2003;53: 525–529.
7. Fitzpatrick TB, Johnson RA, Wolff K, et al. Disorders of apocrine and sebaceous glands. In: Color Atlas and Synopsis of Clinical Dermatology, Common & Serious Diseases, 4th ed. New York, McGraw-Hill, 2001:2–7.
8. White GM. Recent findings in the epidemiologic evidence, classification, and subtypes of acne vulgaris. J Am Acad Dermatol 1998;39:S34–S37.
9. Gollnick H, Cunliffe W, Berson D, et al. Management of acne, a report from a Global Alliance to Improve Outcomes in Acne. J Am Acad Dermatol 2003;49:S1–S37.
10. Hunter JAA, Savin JA, Dahl MV. Sebaceous and sweat gland disorders. In: Clinical Dermatology, 3rd ed. Malden, MA, Blackwell Science, 2002:148–161.
11. Leyden JJ. A review of the use of combination therapies for the treatment of acne vulgaris. J Am Acad Dermatol 2003;49:S200–S210.
12. Lucky AW, Henderson TA, Olson WH, et al. Effectiveness of norgestimate and ethinyl estradiol in treating moderate acne vulgaris. J Am Acad Dermatol 1997;37:746–754.
13. Baumann L. Acne. In: Cosmetic Dermatology, Principles & Practice. New York, McGraw-Hill, 2002:55–61.
14. Jappe U. Pathological mechanisms of acne with special emphasis on *Propionibacterium acnes* and related therapy. Acta Derm Venereol 2003; 83:241–248.
15. Burkhart CN, Gottwald L. Assessment of etiologic agents in acne pathogenesis. Skinmed 2003;2:222–228.
16. Burkhart CN, Burkhart CG. Microbiology's principle of biofilms as a major factor in the pathogenesis of acne vulgaris. Int J Dermatol 2003; 42:925–927.
17. Holland DB, Jeremy AH, Roberts SG, et al. Inflammation in acne scarring: a comparison of the responses in lesions from patients prone and not prone to scar. Br J Dermatol 2004;150:72–81.
18. Gollnick H, Schramm M. Topical therapy in acne. J Eur Acad Dermatol Venereol 1998;11(Suppl 1):S8–S12.
19. White GM. Recent findings in the epidemiologic evidence, classification, and subtypes of acne vulgaris. J Am Acad Dermatol 1998;39:S34–S37.
20. Chiu A, Chon SY, Kimball AB. The response of skin disease to stress: changes in the severity of acne vulgaris as affected by examination stress. Arch Dermatol 2003;139:897–900.
21. Toyoda M, Morohashi M. New aspects in acne inflammation. Dermatology 2003;206:17–23.
22. Cordain L, Lindeberg S, Hurtado M, et al. Acne vulgaris, a disease of Western civilization. Arch Dermatol 2002;138:1584–1590.
23. Thiboutot DM, Strauss JS. Diet and acne revisited. Arch Dermatol 2002; 138:1591–1592
24. Bershad S. The unwelcome return of the acne diet. Arch Dermatol 2003; 139:940–941.
25. Treloar V. Diet and acne redux. Arch Dermatol 2003;139:941.
26. Longshore SJ, Hollandsworth K. Acne vulgaris: one treatment does not fit all. Cleve Clin J Med 2003;70:670–680.
27. Gollnick HP, Krautheim A. Topical treatment in acne: current status and future aspects. Dermatology 2003;206:29–36.
28. Zouboulis CC, Piquero-Martin J. Update of future of systemic acne treatment. Dermatology 2003;206:37–53.
29. Tan HH. Antibacterial therapy for acne: a guide to selection and use of systemic agents. Am J Clin Dermatol 2003;4:307–314.
30. Arndt KA, Bowers KE. Acne. In: Manual of Dermatologic Therapeutics, 6th ed. Philadelphia, Lippincott Williams & Wilkins, 2002:3–20.
31. Shwereb C, Lowenstein EJ. Delayed type hypersensitivity to benzoyl peroxide. J Drugs Dermatol 2004;3:197–199.
32. Rodriguez D, Davis MW. The BEST study: results according to prior treatment. Cutis 2003;71:27–34.

33. Gupta AK, Lynde CW, Kunynetz RA, et al. A randomized, double-blind, multicenter, parallel group study to compare relative efficacies of the topical gels 3% erythromycin/5% benzoyl peroxide and 0.025% tretinoin/erythromycin 4% in the treatment of moderate acne vulgaris of the face. J Cutan Med Surg 2003;7:31–37.

34. Lucky A, Cullen S, Funicella T, et al. Double-blind, vehicle-controlled, multicenter comparison of two 0.025% tretinoin creams in patients with acne vulgaris. J Am Acad Dermatol 1998;38:S24–S30.

35. Lucky A, Cullen S, Jarratt M, Quigley JW. Comparative efficacy and safety of two 0.025% tretinoin gels: results from a multicenter, double-blind, parallel study. J Am Acad Dermatol 1998;38:S17–S23.

36. Shalita AR, Rafal ES, Anderson DN, et al. Compared efficacy and safety of tretinoin 0.1% microsphere gel alone and in combination with benzoyl peroxide 6% cleanser for the treatment of acne vulgaris. Cutis 2003;72: 167–172.

37. Quigley JW, Bucks DA. Reduced skin irritation with tretinoin containing polyolprepolymer-2, a new topical tretinoin delivery system: a summary of preclinical and clinical investigations. J Am Acad Dermatol 1998;38: S5–S10.

38. Nyirady J, Grossman RM, Nighland M, et al. A comparative trial of two retinoids commonly used in the treatment of acne vulgaris. J Dermatol Treat 2001;12:149–157.

39. Leyden J, Grove GL. Randomized facial tolerability studies comparing gel formulations of retinoids used to treat acne vulgaris. Cutis 2001;67: 17–27.

40. Patel VB, Misra A, Marfatia YS. Clinical assessment of the combination therapy with liposomal gels of tretinoin and benzoyl peroxide in acne. AAPS PharmSci Tech 2001;2:E-TN4.

41. van Hoogdalem EJ, Baven TL, Spiegel-Melsen I, Terpstra IJ. Transdermal absorption of clindamycin and tretinoin from topically applied anti-acne formulations in man. Biopharm Drug Dispos 1998;19:563–569.

42. Latriano L, Tzimas G, Wong F, Wills RJ. The percutaneous absorption of topically applied tretinoin and its effect on endogenous concentrations of tretinoin and its metabolites after single doses or long-term use. J Am Acad Dermatol 1997;36:S37–S46.

43. Brogden RN, Goa KE. Adapalene: A review of its pharmacological properties and clinical potential in the management of mild to moderate acne. Drugs 1997;53:511–519.

44. Thiboutot DM. Acne: An overview of clinical research findings. Dermatol Clin 1997;15:97–109.

45. Millikan LE. Adapalene: an update on newer comparative studies between the various retinoids. Int J Dermatol 2000;39:784–788.

46. Wolf JE. An update of recent clinical trials examining adapalene and acne. J Eur Acad Venereol 2001;15:23–29.

47. Cunliffe WJ, Poncet M, Loesche C, Verschoore M. A comparison of the efficacy and tolerability of adapalene 0.1% gel versus tretinoin 0.025% gel in patients with acne vulgaris: a meta-analysis of five randomized trials. Br J Dermatol 1998;139(Suppl 52):48–56.

48. Foster RH, Brogden RN, Benfield P. Tazarotene. Drugs 1998;55:705–711.

49. Shalita AR, Chalker DK, Griffith RF, et al. Tazarotene gel is safe and effective in the treatment of acne vulgaris: a multicenter, double-blind, vehicle-controlled study. Cutis 1999;63:349–354.

50. Bershad S, Poulin YP, Berson, et al. Topical retinoids in the treatment of acne vulgaris. Cutis 1999;64:8–23.

51. Kakita L. Tazarotene versus tretinoin or adapalene in the treatment of acne vulgaris. J Am Acad Dermatol 2000;43:S51–S54.

52. Bershad S, Kranjac Singer GK, Parente JE, et al. Successful treatment of acne vulgaris using a new method: results of a randomized vehicle-controlled trial of short-contact therapy with 0.1% tazarotene gel. Arch Dermatol 2002;138:481–489.

53. Tan HH. Topical antibacterial treatments for acne vulgaris: comparative review and guide to selection. Am J Clin Dermatol 2004;5:79–84.

54. Gollnick H. Current concepts of the pathogenesis of acne: implications for drug treatment. Drugs 2003;63:1579–1596.

55. Tschen E, Jones T. A new treatment for acne vulgaris combining benzoyl peroxide with clindamycin. J Drugs Dermatol 2002;1:153–157.

56. Akhavan A, Bershad S. Topical acne drugs: review of clinical properties, systemic exposure, and safety. Am J Clin Dermatol 2003;4:473–492.

57. White GM. Acne therapy. In: James WD, Cockerell CJ, Dzubow LM, et al, eds. Advances in Dermatology. St. Louis, Mosby, 1999:29–59.

58. Fort-Lacoste L, Verscheure Y, Tisne-Versailles J, Navarro R. Comedolytic effect of topical retinaldehyde in the rhino mouse model. Dermatology 1999;199:33–35.

59. Morel P, Vienne MP, Beylot C, et al. Clinical efficacy and safety of a topical combination of retinaldehyde 0.1% with erythromycin 4% in acne vulgaris. Clin Exp Dermatol 1999;24:354–357.

60. Goswami BC, Baishya B, Barua AB, Olson JA. Topical retinoyl beta-glucuronide is an effective treatment of mild to moderate acne vulgaris in Asian-Indian patients. Skin Pharmacol Appl Skin Physiol 1999;12: 167–173.

61. Monheit GD. Chemical peels. Skin Therapy Lett 2004;9:6–11.

62. Lee HS, Kim IH. Salicylic acid peels for the treatment of acne vulgaris in Asian patients. Dermatol Surg 2003;29:1196–1199.

63. Kaminsky A. Less common methods to treat acne. Dermatology 2003; 206:68–73.

64. Zaenglein AL, Thiboutot DM. Acne vulgaris. In: Horn TD, Mancini AJ, Mascaro JM, et al, eds. Dermatology. London, Mosby, 2003:531–544.

65. Ortonne JP. Oral isotretinoin treatment policy: Do we all agree? Dermatology 1997;195(Suppl):34–37.

66. Goulden V. Guidelines for the management of acne vulgaris in adolescents. Paediatr Drugs 2003;5:301–313.

67. Cooper AJ, Australian Roaccutane Advisory Board. Treatment of acne with isotretinoin: recommendations based on Australian experience. Australas J Dermatol 2003;44:97–105.

68. Charakida A, Mouser PE, Chu AC. Safety and side effects of the acne drug, oral isotretinoin. Expert Opin Drug Saf 2004;3:119–129.

69. Altman RS, Altman LJ, Altman JS. A proposed set of new guidelines for routine blood tests during isotretinoin therapy for acne vulgaris. Dermatology 2002;204:232–235.

70. Kunynetz RA. A review of systemic retinoid therapy for acne and related conditions. Skin Therapy Lett 2004;9:1–4.

71. Bremner JD. Does isotretinoin cause depression and suicide? Psychopharmacol Bull 2003;37:64–78.

72. Hersom K, Neary MP, Levaux HP, et al. Isotretinoin and antidepressant pharmacotherapy: a prescription sequence symmetry analysis. J Am Acad Dermatol 2003;49:424–432.

73. Meigel WN. How safe is oral isotretinoin? Dermatology 1997;195(Suppl 1):22–28.

74. Newton JN. How cost-effective is oral isotretinoin? Dermatology 1997;195(Suppl 1):10–14.

75. Ross JI, Snelling AM, Carnegie E, et al. Antibiotic-resistant acne: lessons from Europe. Br J Dermatol 2003;148:467–478.

76. Eady EA, Gloor M, Leyden JJ. Propionibacterium acnes resistance: a world wide problem. Dermatology 2003;206:54–56.

77. Fernandez-Obregon AC. Azithromycin for the treatment of acne. Int J Dermatol 2000;39:45–50.

78. Gruber F, Grubisic-Greblo H, Kastelan M, et al. Azithromycin compared with minocycline in the treatment of acne comedonica and papulopustulosa. J Chemother 1998;10:469–473.

79. Golub LM, Lee HM, Ryan ME, et al. Tetracyclines inhibit connective tissue breakdown by multiple non-antimicrobial mechanisms. Adv Dent Res 1998;12:12–26.

80. Sadick NS. Antibiotics: unapproved uses or indications. Clin Dermatol 2000;18:11–16.

81. Bikowski JB. Subantimicrobial dose doxycycline for acne and rosacea. Skinmed 2003;2:234–245.

82. Skidmore R, Kovach R, Walker C, et al. Effects of subantimicrobial-dose doxycycline in the treatment of moderate acne. Arch Dermatol 2003;139:459–464.

83. Carroll LA, Laumann AE. Doxycycline-induced photo-onycholysis. J Drugs Dermatol 2003;2:662–663.

84. Chosidow O, Poli F, Naline E, et al. Comedonal diffusion of minocycline in acne. Dermatology 1998;196:162.

85. Sturkenboom MCJM, Meier CR, Jick H, Stricker BHC. Minocycline and lupuslike syndrome in acne patients. Arch Intern Med 1999;159:493–497.

86. Shapiro LE, Knowles SR, Shear NH. Comparative safety of tetracycline, minocycline, and doxycycline. Arch Dermatol 1997;133:1224–1230.

87. Grim SA, Romanelli F, Jennings PR, Ofotokun I. Late-onset drug fever associated with minocycline: case report and review of the literature. Pharmacotherapy 2003;23:1659–1662.

88. Cohen PR. Medication-associated depersonalization symptoms: report of transient depersonalization symptoms induced by minocycline. South Med J 2004;97:70–73.

89. Mouton RW, Jordaan HF, Schneider JW. A new type of minocycline-induced cutaneous hyperpigmentation. Clin Exp Dermatol 2004;29:8–14.

90. Tan HH. Antibacterial therapy for acne: a guide to selection and use of systemic agents. Am J Clin Dermatol 2003;4:307–314.

91. Thiboutot D, Chen W. Update and future of hormonal therapy in acne. Dermatology 2003;206:57–67.

92. Shaw JC. Hormonal therapies in acne. Expert Opin Pharmacother 2002;3:865–874.

93. van Vloten WA, van Haselen CW, van Zuuren EJ, et al. The effect of 2 combined oral contraceptives containing either drospirenone or cyproterone acetate on acne and seborrhea. Cutis 2002;69:2–15.

94. Worret I, Arp W, Zahradnik HP, et al. Acne resolution rates: results of a single-blind, randomized, controlled, parallel phase III trial with EE/CMA (Belara) and EE/LNG (Microgynon). Dermatology 2001;203:38–44.

95. Redmond GP, Olson WH, Lippman JS, et al. Norgestimate and ethinyl estradiol in the treatment of acne vulgaris: a randomized, placebo-controlled trial. Obstet Gynecol 1997;89:615–622.

96

PSORIASIS

Dennis P. West, Lee E. West, Laura Scuderi, and Giuseppe Micali

arning Objectives and other resources can be found at *www.pharmacotherapyonline.com.*

KEY CONCEPTS

1 Exogenous trigger factors such as climate, stress, alcohol, smoking, infection, trauma, and drugs may aggravate psoriasis.

2 As a result of pathogenic T-cell production and activation, psoriatic epidermal cells proliferate at a rate sevenfold faster than normal epidermal cells.

3 In general, psoriatic lesions are characterized by sharply demarcated, erythematous papules and plaques often covered with silver-white scales.

4 Goals of treatment are usually directed at skin normalization: reduction or clearing of erythema, papules, and plaques, as well as scales.

5 A variety of topical (most commonly salicylic acid, corticosteroids, anthralin, and/or vitamin D analogues)

and systemic (most often acitretin but also cyclosporine, tacrolimus, methotrexate, mycophenolate mofetil, sulfasalazine, 6-thioguanine, and/or hydroxyurea) pharmacotherapeutic agents can be used for treating psoriasis, with treatment determined by the severity of a patient's condition and the probability of controlling long-term symptoms with minimal adverse effects. Biologic therapies (infliximab, etanercept, alefacept, or efalizumab) and photochemotherapy (photochemotherapy using ultraviolet A light; PUVA) provide additional options, especially for patients with severe or refractory cases.

6 Combination, rotational, and sequential therapy is commonly used in treatment of psoriasis to achieve a response, increase effectiveness of treatment, or enable lowering of doses of individual agents.

oriasis is a common chronic inflammatory skin disorder characterzed by recurrent exacerbations and remissions of thickened, erythe-atous, and scaling plaques. The clinical appearance of psoriasis ay be cosmetically disfiguring, and the disease may be physilly and emotionally debilitating, especially for patients with severe sease.

EPIDEMIOLOGY

oriasis is universal in occurrence and affects up to 3% of the Amer-an population. Approximately 25% of affected patients have se-re conditions.[1] The disorder occurs in all racial groups but is most evalent in Caucasians. It is equally common in males and females. vo peaks of age of onset have been described: the greatest inci-nce is between 20 and 30 years, and a smaller peak occurs be-een 50 and 60 years of age;[2] however, the age of onset is widely riable from infancy to old age. Although rarely life-threatening, oriasis has an adverse physical and emotional impact on quality of e.[3,4]

ETIOLOGY

oriasis is a complex and multifactorial disease due to the interaction tween environmental factors (exogenous or endogenous antigens) d a specific genetic background. The antigens involved in disease velopment are not completely known or understood.[5]

GENETIC FACTORS

There is a significant genetic component in psoriasis, but the exact mode of inheritance is uncertain.[6] Most patients with psoriasis have at least one immediate relative with the disorder.[7] Some studies have shown that the development and severity of psoriasis is influenced by gender of the contributing parent. One study showed an earlier age of onset when the disease was inherited from the father.[8]

Monozygotic twins have a higher concordance for psoriasis than dizygotic twins.

A number of genetic loci have been identified by genome-wide linkage scans and two loci have been replicated: *PSORS1* on chromosome 6, within the major histocompatibility complex, and *PSORS2* on chromosome 17q. *PSORS1* accounts for an estimated 30% to 50% of the genetic contribution to psoriasis.[9]

Studies of histocompatibility antigens in psoriatic patients indicate statistically significant associations on the B, C, and D loci, more specifically, HLA-B13, HLA-B17, and HLA-B37.[2]

The most significant association is with HLA-Cw6, where the relative likelihood for developing psoriasis is 9 to 15 times normal.[2] Identification of multiple loci for psoriasis susceptibility indicates that psoriasis is a genetically heterogeneous disease with different genetic causes.

EXOGENOUS TRIGGER FACTORS

1 Factors such as climate, stress, alcohol, smoking, infection, trauma, and drugs may aggravate psoriasis. Warm seasons and

sunlight reportedly improve psoriasis in 80% of patients, whereas 90% report worsening in cold weather. In addition, stress worsens psoriasis in up to 40% of patients; however, the exact role stress plays in exacerbation of psoriasis is uncertain. Alcohol seems to have a greater influence on the progression of psoriasis in men, and the association between smoking and psoriasis seems to be stronger in women.[10]

Infection has been identified retrospectively as a common precipitating factor in psoriasis.[11] About 25% of patients have initial onset of the disease after clinically documented infections, and more than one half have exacerbations within 3 weeks after an upper respiratory infection. A variant known as guttate (small drop-like plaques) psoriasis is often associated with infections of group A β-hemolytic streptococci.[11]

Psoriatic lesions may develop at the site of injury on normal-appearing skin (Koebner response). This response may be induced by a variety of trauma that includes rubbing, venipuncture, bites, surgery, and mechanical pressure. The mechanism for a Koebner response is unknown, is not unique to psoriasis, and yet occurs in a majority of psoriatic patients. Duration of time between injury and lesion development may vary from a day to several weeks.

Lithium carbonate, β-adrenergic blocking agents, some antimalarial agents, nonsteroidal anti-inflammatory drugs, angiotensin-converting enzyme inhibitors, tetracyclines, and interferons are among the most commonly reported drugs to exacerbate psoriasis or to trigger psoriasiform lesions.[12]

PATHOPHYSIOLOGY

IMMUNOLOGIC MECHANISMS

Recently, much attention has been directed to cell-mediated immune mechanisms in psoriasis. A central role for activated T cells has been demonstrated by response to drugs that block T-cell activation, migration, or cytokine secretion in psoriasis.[13]

Cutaneous inflammatory T-cell–mediated immune activation requires two T-cell signals that are mediated via cell-cell interactions by surface proteins and by antigen-presenting cells (APC) such as dendritic cells or macrophages.

The "first signal" is the interaction of the T-cell receptor with antigen presented by the APC. Table 96–1 lists cell surface proteins important to this first signal.

The "second signal," also called *costimulation*, is mediated through various surface interactions. Both signals are essential for initial activation of T cells in psoriasis.[14]

Once T cells are activated, they migrate from lymph nodes and the circulation into skin. Specific cell surface proteins on T cells and vascular endothelium including selectins, integrins, and other adhesion molecules mediate this movement. The best understood cellular interaction is the relationship between LFA-1 on T cells and intercellular adhesion molecule-1 on endothelial cells. Once in the skin, activated T cells secrete various cytokines that induce the pathologic changes of psoriasis.[15] Cytokines are proteins secreted by immune cells that bind to very specific receptors on the cell surface, influencing keratinocytes and other cells to produce pathologic changes characteristic of psoriasis.

The cytokine profile in psoriasis is known as a T-helper cell type 1 (Th1) response; this subset of T cells produces primarily interferon-γ (IFN-γ) and interleukin (IL)-2.[16] Other local cells, including keratinocytes and local neutrophils, are induced to produce other cytokines, including tumor necrosis factor-α (TNF-α)[17] and interleukin

TABLE 96–1. Cell Surface Proteins Mediating Cell-Cell Interactions via the First Signal Prior to Costimulation (Second Signal

Protein Abbreviation	Protein
Anti-CD11a	Monoclonal antibody toward the α chain (CD11a) of LFA-1
APC	Antigen-presenting cells
CD2	Cluster of differentiation 2
CD3	Cluster of differentiation 3
CD4	Cluster of differentiation 4
CD28	Cluster of differentiation 28
CTCL	Cutaneous T-cell lymphoma
DAB	β Subunit of diphtheria toxin
Fab	Fraction antibody binding
Fc	Fraction crystallizable
ICAM	Intercellular adhesion molecule
ICAM-1	Intercellular adhesion molecule-1
IFN-α	Interferon-α
IFN-γ	Interferon-γ
IL-2	Interleukin-2
IL-2/DAB	Interleukin-2 combined with diphtheria to× β subunit
IL-4	Interleukin-4
IL-8	Interleukin-8
IL-10	Interleukin-10
LFA-1	Lymphocytic function-associated antigen-1
LFA-3	Lymphocytic function-associated antigen-3
LFA-3/TIP	Recombinantly-engineered LFA-3/Ig G1 human fusion protein
MHC	Major histocompatibility complex
PASI	Psoriasis activity and severity index
Th1	T-helper cells type 1
Th2	T-helper cells type 2
TNF-α	Tumor necrosis factor-α

(IL)-8,[18] which are believed to be important in the pathophysiolog of psoriasis. All of these cytokines are important in the developme of psoriasis and represent possible targets of biologic therapies.

Cytokines and chemokines with a currently recognized potenti role in psoriasis include: granulocyte-macrophage colony-stimulati factor; regulated on activation, normal T-cell expressed and secrete (RANTES; causes keratinocyte proliferation); epidermal growth fa tor and monokine induced by interferon-γ (MIG; increases neutroph migration); IL-8 and inducible protein-10 (increases differentiatic of type 1 T cells); IL-12 and macrophage inflammatory protein-3 (MIP-3α; produces angiogenesis); IL-1 and thymus- and activatio regulated chemokine (TARC; produces epidermal hyperplasia); IL (increases other chemokine release); INF-γ (increases upregulatic of adhesion molecules on endothelial cells); TNF-α; and vascul endothelial growth factor (VEGF).

DEFECTS IN THE EPIDERMAL CELL CYCLE

As a result of pathogenic T-cell production and activation, psor atic epidermal cells proliferate at a rate sevenfold faster than norm epidermal cells. The germinative cell population increases in psor atic skin, and duration of the epidermal cell cycle is calculated 37.5 hours (versus 300 hours in normal skin). Lesion-free skin psoriatic patients generally is considered to be involved because ep dermal proliferation is elevated in apparently normal skin of psoriat patients.[19]

CLINICAL PRESENTATION OF PSORIASIS

GENERAL

Although psoriasis is a nonmalignant, hyperproliferative epidermal cell disorder, it results in accumulated, immature, excessively thickened skin that is manifested as plaques.

SYMPTOMS

Psoriatic lesions are relatively asymptomatic; however, pruritus is a complaint in about 25% of patients. Severe, widespread psoriasis may involve symptomatology similar to that of exfoliative dermatitis, which may include fever and chills. Psoriatic arthritis is a distinct clinical entity in which both psoriatic lesions and inflammatory arthritis-like symptoms occur. Classically, distal interphalangeal joints and adjacent nails are involved, but knees, elbows, wrists and ankles also may be involved.

SIGNS

In general, psoriatic lesions are characterized by sharply demarcated, erythematous papules and plaques often covered with silver-white scales. Initial lesions are usually small papules that enlarge over time and coalesce into plaques, sometimes as serpiginous or geographic forms. If the covering scale is removed, a salmon-pink to erythematous lesion is exposed, perhaps with punctate bleeding from prominent dermal capillaries (Auspitz sign).

Psoriatic lesions vary in appearance depending on the anatomic site and the variant of psoriasis. The most common type of psoriasis is psoriasis vulgaris. Scalp involvement may vary from diffuse scaling on an erythematous scalp to thickened plaques with exudation, microabscesses and fissures. Trunk, back, arm, and leg lesions may appear as generalized, scattered, discrete, guttate (resembling drops or spots), or large plaques. Palms, soles, face, and genitalia may be commonly involved. Affected nails often are pitted with subungual keratotic material. Yellowing under the nail plate also may be seen.

LABORATORY TESTS

Skin biopsy of lesional skin is useful in confirming the diagnosis.

OTHER DIAGNOSTIC TESTS

None

▶ TREATMENT: Psoriasis

4 Goals of treatment of psoriasis are directed at skin normalization: reduction or clearing of erythema, papules, and plaques, as well as scales. Reduction or clearing of skin signs as a treatment objective leads to normalized cosmesis and improvement in quality of life. A goal of therapy is to achieve resolution of lesions, but partial clearing is sometimes acceptable when using regimens with decreased toxicity and increased patient acceptability.

The Psoriasis Area and Severity Index (PASI) serves as a uniform method to determine the amount of body surface area affected, along with the degree of erythema, induration, and scaling. Mild psoriasis is considered to have a PASI score of less than 12, moderate involvement is PASI 12 to 18, and severe psoriasis is PASI greater than 18.

The National Psoriasis Foundation advocates that PASI 50 (50% decrease from baseline) is a clinically relevant end point when assessing efficacy of treatment. As a new class of agents, the biologic agents were required to demonstrate a PASI 75 decrease for approval by the Food and Drug Administration. No prior nonbiologic agents were required to meet such a high standard to be approved.

GENERAL APPROACH TO TREATMENT

Although the exact cause of psoriasis is unknown, in a majority of patients, pharmacotherapy is usually effective in establishing good clinical control. Psoriasis may be a lifelong relapsing and remitting disease, so therapy should be selected with careful consideration of long-term adverse effects. Major points for consideration include the extent and site of disease involvement, the patient's age, and concurrent associated diseases.

5 Drug treatments for psoriasis, discussed in detail below, include the following:

Topical therapy:

Keratolytics

- Coal tar
- Corticosteroids
- Anthralin
- Vitamin D analogues (calcipotriene and calcitriol)
- Tazarotene
- Immunomodulators (tacrolimus and pimecrolimus)

Systemic therapy:

- Acitretin
- Cyclosporine
- Tacrolimus
- Methotrexate
- Mycophenolate mofetil
- Sulfasalazine
- 6-Thioguanine
- Hydroxyurea

Biologic therapy:

- Infliximab
- Etanercept
- Alefacept
- Efalizumab

Photochemotherapy:

- PUVA

NONPHARMACOLOGIC THERAPY

EMOLLIENTS

Emollients are frequently used during therapy-free periods to minimize skin dryness that may lead to early recurrence. These agents hydrate stratum corneum and minimize cutaneous transepidermal water loss (evaporation). Hydration causes the stratum corneum to swell and flattens the surface contour. Emollients effective as moisturizers decrease binding forces within the horny layer, enhance desquamation, and eliminate scaling. Emollients also may increase pliability of the skin, have antipruritic activity, and possess mild vasoconstrictor activity.

As lotions, creams, or ointments, emollients often need to be applied several times per day (about four times per day) to achieve a beneficial response. Adverse effects of emollients include folliculitis and allergic or irritant contact dermatitis.

BALNEOTHERAPY

Balneotherapy (and climatotherapy) is a therapeutic approach that consists of bathing in waters containing certain salts, often combined with natural exposure to the sun. Certain areas around the world have been targeted as excellent places to receive balneotherapy (or climatotherapy); the Dead Sea is salt filled, located below sea level, and capable of enhancing exposure to a natural ultraviolet A (UVA) light source. The Kangal hot spring in Turkey and the Blue Lagoon in Iceland are also notable salt-containing waters. The salts in these waters are a mixture of salts that reduce activated T cells in skin and are remittive for psoriasis. Reduction in serum manganese and lithium levels is significant after bathing with Dead Sea salt, an effect believed to be related to effectiveness of the salts.[20]

ULTRAVIOLET B PHOTOTHERAPY

Ultraviolet B (UVB) light (290 to 320 nm) continues to be an important phototherapeutic intervention for psoriasis.

Exposure to UV light by natural sunlight has been used to treat psoriasis for centuries. At the beginning of the twentieth century patients were treated with topical, occlusive coal tar all day and night, removing the tar just before exposure to a hot quartz mercury vapor lamp (Goeckerman therapy).[7] Subsequent development of various forms of UVB phototherapy have led to the use of more precise wavelengths within the UVB range in order to achieve an optimal therapeutic benefit for psoriasis.

The most effective wavelength of UVB for treatment of psoriasis is 310 to 315 nm, and this has led to the development of a UVB "narrow-band" (NB) light source, in which 83% of the UVB emission is at 310 to 313 nm.[21] Numerous clinical trials have demonstrated efficacy of NB-UVB for the treatment of plaque-type psoriasis.[22]

Numerous topical and systemic psoriatic therapies (discussed individually below) are used adjunctively to hasten and improve the response to UVB phototherapy. Several studies showed an advantage to combining short-contact anthralin with UVB.[23] The addition of calcipotriene also improved results compared to UVB alone.[24] Emollients enhance efficacy of UVB and may be applied to the skin just before treatments for this purpose.[23] UVB phototherapy has also produced more effective results when added to systemic psoriatic treatments, such as methotrexate and retinoids.[25]

EXCIMER LASER PHOTOTHERAPY

Lasers have been used for the treatment of psoriasis with variable results. Most laser therapy has been ineffective, while excimer lasers which generate a 308-nm UVB wavelength, have some efficacy at clearing psoriasis and inducing moderately prolonged remissions.[26,2] Unfortunately, this approach to therapy is limited to treatment of individual, isolated plaques. The excimer laser has some advantage over traditional NB-UVB phototherapy, including the capability to successfully treat psoriatic plaques with fewer treatments and with a smaller UV radiation dose. Moreover, it may have a lower risk of carcinogenicity and photoaging.[28]

PHARMACOLOGIC THERAPY

Topical treatments of first choice for mild to moderate psoriasis include keratolytics, corticosteroids, vitamin D analogues (calcipotriene, calcitriol, and tacalcitol), and tazarotene. The systemic treatment of first choice for moderate to severe psoriasis is acitretin. See Tables 96–2 and 96–3 for topical and systemic psoriasis treatment guidelines.

Multiple pharmacotherapeutic approaches to psoriasis management include first-line therapy for mild to moderate psoriasis with topical agents. In severe psoriasis, photochemotherapy and

TABLE 96–2. Selected Topical Psoriasis Treatment Guidelines

Active Ingredient	Regimen	Selected Adverse Effects
Emollients	About 4 times/day	Folliculitis, allergic or irritant contact dermatitis
Salicylic acid	2–3 times/day	Irritation, salicylism with symptoms of nausea, vomiting, tinnitus, or hyperventilation
Coal tar	Apply in the evening, allowing to remain through the night	Irritation, photoreactions, unpleasant odor, staining skin and clothing
Corticosteroids	2–4 times/day	Local tissue atrophy, degeneration, and striae; epidermal thinning; acneiform eruptions; bacterial or fungal skin infections; glucocorticoid systemic effects
Calcipotriene	1–2 times/day, no more than 100 g/wk	Burning and stinging (10% of patients), irritant contact dermatitis
Anthralin	Usually applied in the evening, allowed to remain overnight; short-contact regimens may also be used	Stains skin and clothing; irritation
Tazarotene	1 time/day, usually in the evening	Pruritus, burning, stinging, and erythema

TABLE 96–3. Selected Systemic Psoriasis Treatment Guidelines

Active Ingredient	Regimen	Selected Adverse Effects
Acitretin	25–50 mg/day until lesions have resolved	Hypervitaminosis A (dry lips/cheilitis, dry mouth, dry nose, dry eyes/conjunctivitis, dry skin, pruritus, scaling, and hair loss), hepatotoxicity, skeletal changes, hypercholesterolemia, hypertriglyceridemia
Cyclosporine	2.5–4 mg/kg per day in 2 divided doses; may increase to 5 mg/kg per day in 1 month if no response	Nephrotoxicity, malignancies, hypertension, hypomagnesemia, hyperkaliemia, alterations in liver function tests, elevations of serum lipids, gastrointestinal intolerance, paresthesias, hypertrichosis, gingival hyperplasia
Methotrexate	7.5–15 mg per week, increased incrementally by 2.5 mg every 2 to 4 weeks until response; maximal doses are approximately 25 mg/wk	Anemia, leukopenia, thrombocytopenia, hepatotoxicity, gastrointestinal upset, nausea, vomiting, mucosal ulceration, stomatitis, malaise, headaches, pulmonary toxicity
Tacrolimus	0.05 mg/kg daily, with increases to 0.10 mg/kg daily at 3 weeks and to 0.15 mg/kg daily at 6 weeks, depending on results	Nephrotoxicity, immunosuppression, gastrointestinal upset, diarrhea, nausea, paresthesias, hypertension, tremor, insomnia
Mycophenolate mofetil	500 mg 4 times a day, up to maximum of 4 g/day	Gastrointestinal toxicity (diarrhea, nausea, vomiting), hematologic effects (anemia, neutropenia, thrombocytopenia), viral and bacterial infections; lymphoproliferative disease or lymphoma can occur
Sulfasalazine	3–4 g/day for 8 weeks	Gastrointestinal upset
6-Thioguanine	80 mg twice weekly, increased by 20 mg every 2–4 weeks; maximum dose 160 mg/3 times week	Bone marrow suppression; gastrointestinal complications including nausea and diarrhea; elevation of liver function tests
Hydroxyurea	1 g/day; may increase to 2 g/day	Bone marrow toxicity with leukopenia or thrombocytopenia, cutaneous reactions, leg ulcers, megaloblastic anemia
Infliximab	5 or 10 mg/kg for 3 intravenous infusions at weeks 0, 2, and 6	Headaches, fever, chills, fatigue, diarrhea, pharyngitis, upper respiratory and urinary tract infections; hypersensitivity reactions (urticaria, dyspnea, hypotension); lymphoproliferative disorders
Etanercept	50 mg subcutaneously twice a week	Local reaction at the injection site (20% of patients); respiratory tract and gastrointestinal infections, abdominal pain, nausea and vomiting, headaches, rash; serious infections (including tuberculosis) and malignancies are rare
Alefacept	15 mg intramuscularly once weekly	Pharyngitis, influenza-like symptoms, chills, dizziness, nausea, headache, injection site pain and inflammation, and nonspecific infection; opportunistic infections and malignancy are rare
Efalizumab	1 mg/kg subcutaneously once weekly	Headache, nausea, chills, nonspecific infection, pain, fever, and asthenia; no evidence drug causes organ toxicity, serious infection, or malignancy

systemic agents, including biologic therapies, are used. Psoriasis treatment regimens now include combination, rotational, and sequential therapy.

COMBINATION, ROTATIONAL, AND SEQUENTIAL THERAPY

Frequently, monotherapy with a systemic agent does not provide optimal outcomes. Combination therapy of systemic agents with other modalities may enhance therapeutic benefit. In addition, the dose of each agent may often be reduced when used in combination that may result in lower toxicity.[29]

Combinations may include:

- Acitretin + UVB
- Acitretin + photochemotherapy using ultraviolet A light (PUVA)
- Methotrexate + UVB
- PUVA + UVB
- Methotrexate + cyclosporine

Although combination therapies with biologic agents may be clinically useful, they are still being evaluated for safety and efficacy.

In addition to combination therapy, biologic agents may also be used in rotational therapy. Patients may receive a biologic regimen for a limited period of time and are then switched to a nonbiologic regimen, continuing on a rotational basis. One objective of rotational therapy is to minimize cumulative drug toxicity.

Sequential therapy is another treatment strategy designed to optimize therapeutic outcome. It involves rapid clearing of psoriasis with aggressive therapy by an agent such as cyclosporine, followed by a transitional period in which a safer drug such as acitretin is introduced at maximal dosing. Subsequently, a maintenance period with acitretin in lower doses, or if necessary, acitretin in combination with UVB or PUVA, may be continued.[30]

Pharmacotherapeutic approaches to the treatment of psoriasis are shown in the treatment algorithm (Fig. 96–1).

TOPICAL THERAPY: FIRST-LINE AGENTS

Keratolytics

Keratolytic agents are used to remove scale, smooth the skin, and decrease hyperkeratosis. The mechanism of action of salicylic acid, one of the most commonly used keratolytics, is disruption in corneocyte-to-corneocyte cohesion in the abnormal horny layer of psoriatic skin.

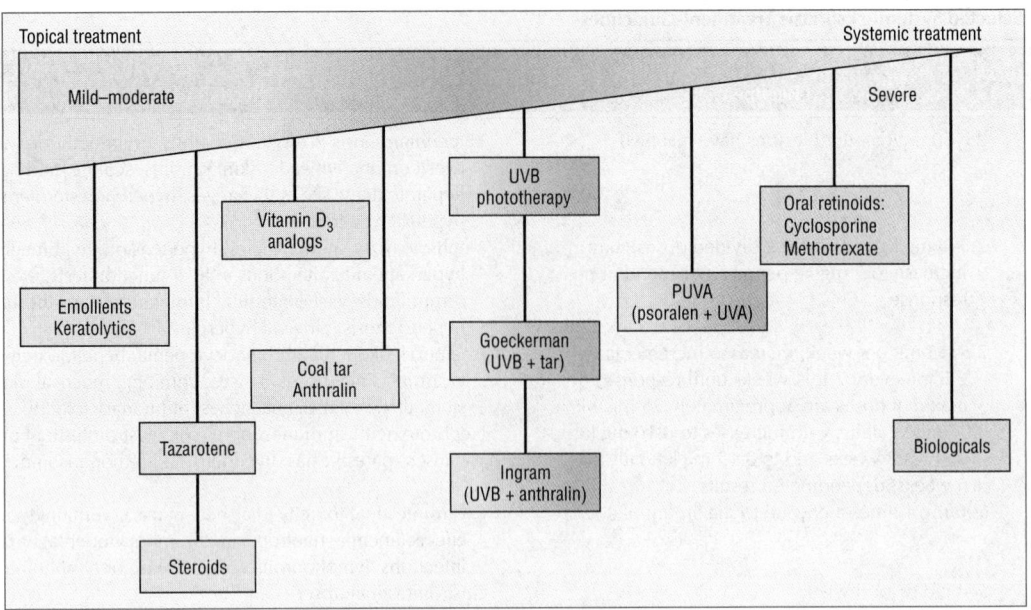

FIGURE 96–1. Psoriasis treatment spectrum.

For this reason, salicylic acid is especially useful at anatomic sites where thick scales are present.[31]

When applied to large, inflamed areas of skin, salicylic acid may induce salicylism, with symptoms of nausea, vomiting, tinnitus, and hyperventilation. Salicylate poisoning in small children is potentially more serious than in older people because they are at higher risk of developing metabolic acidosis. Several fatal cases of percutaneous salicylate intoxication have been reported in children under 3 years of age.[32]

The keratolytic effect of salicylic acid enhances penetration and efficacy of some other topical agents such as corticosteroids.[5]

Salicylic acid, as a gel or lotion, is usually applied two to three times a day in concentrations of 2% to 10%.

Corticosteroids

Topical corticosteroids are the most widely used agents in the treatment of psoriasis in the United States. They are often used to decrease erythema, scaling, and pruritus. Topical vasoconstricting potencies of corticosteroids are ranked by the Stoughton-Cornell classification in seven classes (Table 96–4). Class I steroids are very high-potency products such as clobetasol propionate 0.05%, halobetasol propionate, and betamethasone dipropionate.[23]

High-potency agents are used primarily as alternatives to systemic adrenocorticoid therapy when local therapy is feasible. Examples of conditions for which very-high-potency products are used include thick, chronic psoriatic plaques. They should be used for finite periods of time (as short as possible) and on relatively small body surface areas.

Class VII steroids are agents with the lowest level of vasoconstricting potency (e.g., hydrocortisone 1%). They have a weak anti-inflammatory effect and are safest for long-term application. These products are also the safest products for use on the face and intertriginous areas, in infants and young children, and with occlusion when necessary and appropriate.

Intermediate classes include products with a medium-potency ranking and are used in moderate inflammatory dermatoses. Medium-potency preparations may be used on the face and intertriginous areas for limited periods of time.[23]

The mechanism of action of corticosteroids in psoriasis is not fully understood.[33] Topical corticosteroids appear to inhibit phospholipase A, and to thus reduce levels of arachidonic acid, prostaglandins, and leukotrienes in skin. Moreover, steroid receptors have been identified in skin, with synthesis and mitosis of DNA in epidermal cells being inhibited by topical corticosteroids as demonstrated by decreased epidermal proliferation.[34]

Topical corticosteroid adverse reactions are not uncommon. Local tissue atrophy, epidermal and dermal degeneration, and striae are manifestations of corticosteroid effect on collagen synthesis and fibroblast growth. If detected early, atrophy and striae may be reversible on drug discontinuation, but in numerous cases of prolonged therapy with high-potency agents, these atrophic changes may be long lasting. Thinning of the epidermis may result in visibly distended capillaries (telangiectasias) and purpura. Acneiform eruptions and masking of symptoms of bacterial or fungal skin infections also have been reported with topical corticosteroid use.

Systemic consequences of topical corticosteroid use include risk of suppression of the hypothalamic-pituitary-adrenal axis, hyperglycemia, and development of cushingoid features. Avoidance of prolonged therapy with very-high-potency agents minimizes the risk of these adverse effects. Tachyphylaxis and rebound flare of psoriasis after abrupt cessation of topical corticosteroid therapy may also occur. With proper monitoring, topical corticosteroids are a safe and effective adjunctive approach to psoriasis treatment.[35]

Topical corticosteroids are available in ointments, creams, lotions, gels, sprays, shampoos, and mousses. An ointment is considered the most clinically effective dosage form in psoriasis treatment because it consists of an oily phase that is occlusive and conveys a hydrating effect. Due to the lipophilicity of ointments, penetration of corticosteroid into dermis is enhanced, resulting in increased vasoconstriction.

Ointments are not suitable for use in areas such as the axilla, groin, or other intertriginous areas where maceration and folliculitis may develop secondary to the occlusive effect. Creams—typically emulsified products with an aqueous phase—are preferred by some

TABLE 96–4. Selected Corticosteroid Products Useful for Treating Psoriasis

Corticosteroids	Dosage Forms	Strength (%)	USP Potency Ratings[a]	Vasoconstrictive Potency Rating[b]
Alclometasone dipropionate	Cream	0.05	Low	VI
	Ointment	0.05	Low	V
Amcinonide	Lotion, ointment	0.1	High	II
	Cream	0.1	High	III
Beclomethasone dipropionate	Cream, lotion, ointment	0.025	Medium	—
Betamethasone benzoate	Cream, gel	0.025	Medium	III
	Ointment	0.025	Medium	IV
Betamethasone dipropionate	Cream AF (optimized vehicle)	0.05	Very high	I
	Cream	0.05	High	III
	Gel, lotion, ointment (optimized vehicle)	0.05	Very high	I
	Lotion	0.05	High	V
	Ointment	0.05	High	II
	Topical aerosol	0.1	High	—
Betamethasone valerate	Cream	0.01, 0.05, 0.1	Medium	V
	Lotion, ointment	0.05, 0.1	Medium	III
	Foam	0.12	Medium	IV
Clobetasol propionate	Cream, ointment, solution, foam	0.05	Very high	I
Clobetasol butyrate	Cream, ointment	0.05	Medium	—
Clocortolone pivalate	Cream	0.1	Low	—
Desonide	Cream, lotion, ointment	0.05	Low	VI
Desoximetasone	Cream	0.05	Medium	II
	Cream, ointment	0.25	High	II
	Gel	0.05	High	II
Dexamethasone	Gel	0.1	Low	VII
	Topical aerosol	0.01, 0.04	Low	VII
Dexamethasone sodium phosphate	Cream	0.1	Low	VII
Diflorasone diacetate	Cream	0.05	High	III
	Ointment	0.05	High	II
	Ointment (optimized vehicle)	0.05	Very high	II
Diflucortolone valerate	Cream, ointment	0.1	Medium	—
Flumethasone pivalate	Cream, ointment	0.03	Low	—
Fluocinolone acetonide	Cream	0.01	Medium	VI
	Cream	0.025	Medium	V
	Cream	0.2	High	—
	Ointment	0.025	Medium	IV
	Solution	0.01	Medium	VI
Fluocinonide	Gel, cream, ointment	0.05	High	II
	Solution	0.05	High	II
Flurandrenolide	Cream, ointment	0.0125	Low	—
	Ointment	0.05	Medium	IV
	Cream, lotion	0.05	Medium	V
	Tape	4 mcg/cm^2	Medium	I
Fluticasone propionate	Cream	0.05	Medium	IV
	Ointment	0.05	Medium	III
Halcinonide	Cream	0.025, 0.1	High	II
	Ointment	0.1	High	III
	Solution	0.1	High	—
Halobetasol propionate	Cream, ointment	0.05	Very high	I
Hydrocortisone	Cream, lotion, ointment	All strengths	Low	VII
Hydrocortisone acetate	Cream, lotion, ointment	All strengths	Low	VII
Hydrocortisone butyrate	Cream	0.1	Medium	V
	Ointment	0.1	Medium	—
Hydrocortisone valerate	Cream	0.2	Medium	V
	Ointment	0.2	Medium	IV
Methylprednisolone acetate	Cream, ointment	0.25	Low	VII
	Ointment	1	Low	VII
Mometasone furoate	Cream	0.1	Medium	IV
	Lotion, ointment	0.1	Medium	II
Triamcinolone acetonide	Cream, ointment	0.1	Medium	IV
	Cream, lotion, ointment	0.025	Medium	—
	Cream (Aristocort)	0.1	Medium	VI
	Cream (Kenalog)	0.1	High	IV
	Lotion	0.1	Medium	V
	Ointment (Aristocort, Kenalog)	0.1	High	III
	Cream, ointment	0.5	High	III
	Topical aerosol	0.015	Medium	—

USP ratings are low, medium, high, and very high.
Vasoconstriction potency scale is I (highest) to VII (lowest)—denotes unknown vasoconstrictive properties.

patients as more cosmetically desirable. They may be used in intertriginous areas even though their lower oil content makes them more drying than ointments.

Topical corticosteroids are applied 2 to 4 times daily during long-term therapy.

Vitamin D Analogues

Vitamin D, important in cellular and systemic calcium metabolism, also inhibits keratinocyte differentiation and proliferation, suggesting a role in the treatment of hyperkeratotic skin disease. Vitamin D and its analogues provide anti-inflammatory benefits by inducing a shift towards Th2 cytokine expression, with a decrease in IL-8 and increase in IL-10.[36] Moreover, it induces inhibition of nuclear factor-κB protein in lymphocytes, leading to a reduced transcription of IL-2.[19]

However, use of vitamin D has been limited by its propensity to cause hypercalcemia. This has driven the development of analogues of vitamin D with less effect on calcium homeostasis. Calcipotriene binds to vitamin D receptors as does vitamin D, but it is 100 times less active on systemic calcium metabolism because of its rapid local metabolism. Its long-term effect on altered calcium homeostasis is unknown. On average, improvement is seen within 2 weeks of treatment with calcipotriene, with approximately 70% of patients demonstrating marked improvement after 8 weeks of therapy. Adverse effects of calcipotriene include lesional and perilesional irritation, occurring in approximately 10% of treated patients and consisting of mild burning and stinging. Irritant contact dermatitis is reported to occur more commonly on the face.[37] Calcipotriene, available in a 0.005% concentration as a cream, ointment, and solution, is generally applied 1 to 2 times/day (no more than 100 g/wk).

Calcitriol (1,25-dihydroxyvitamin D_3) is another analogue used in the treatment of mild to moderate plaque psoriasis. As demonstrated in several open-label or randomized, double-blind, controlled trials, calcitriol is effective in improving or clearing psoriatic plaques. A 0.03% formulation showed clearance or considerable improvement in 89% of patients.[38]

Tacalcitol (1α, 24-dihydroxyvitamin D_3) is a biologically active hormone derived from vitamin D. In a study of 157 patients with chronic plaque psoriasis, tacalcitol ointment applied once daily during a 6-month treatment period decreased mean PASI score by 67% and body area affected from 13.3% to 8.8%. Reported adverse effects of tacalcitol are limited to local, transient, mild irritation.[39]

Tazarotene

Tazarotene, a synthetic retinoid, is a prodrug that exerts its pharmacologic activity when hydrolyzed to its active metabolite, tazarotenic acid. Like other topical retinoids, it modulates keratinocyte proliferation and differentiation.[40,41]

Treatment with 0.1% gel, applied once daily, results in substantial reduction in the severity of scaling and plaque thickness during 12-week treatments. The 0.1% gel is somewhat more efficacious, but the 0.05% formulation is associated with less irritation.[40,41] Based on the results of clinical trials, tazarotene is effective for the treatment of mild to moderate plaque psoriasis.[40,42]

Predominant treatment-related adverse effects are mild to moderate pruritus, burning, stinging, or erythema. These local reactions have been shown to be dose- and frequency-related.[42,43] Tazarotene is often used in combination with topical corticosteroids to decrease the incidence of local adverse events and to increase efficacy.[7] Application of the gel to eczematous skin or to more than 20% of body surface area is not recommended because this may lead to extensive systemic absorption.[42]

Tazarotene is available as a 0.05 or 0.1% gel and cream, and is applied once a day, usually in the evening.

TOPICAL THERAPY: SECOND-LINE AGENTS

Coal Tar

The use of tar as coal tar, shale tar, or wood tar has a long history in antipsoriatic therapy. In recent years, wood and shale tars have fallen out of use because they demonstrate relatively less efficacy than coal tar. Coal tar contains numerous hydrocarbon compounds formed from distillation of bituminous coal.

Although the mechanism of action is not fully understood, coal tar, when applied to normal skin, stimulates transient epidermal hyperplasia followed by a cytostatic effect with epidermal thinning. There is evidence that UVB light–activated topical coal tar forms photoadducts with epidermal DNA, thereby inhibiting DNA synthesis. This downregulated epidermal proliferation rate approaches a normal rate of proliferation and leads to reduction in plaque elevation.[44]

Coal tar treatment is a burdensome, time-consuming treatment with disadvantages that include local irritation, unpleasant odor, staining of skin and clothing, and increased sensitivity to UV light, including the sun. The risk of carcinogenicity is low; however, there are cases indicating a higher rate of nonmelanoma skin cancers in patients chronically exposed to tar and UV light.[45]

Coal tar preparations of 2% to 5% tar are available in lotions, creams, shampoos, ointments, gels, and solutions. It also may be used in bath water. It is generally applied in the evening and allowed to remain in skin contact through the night.

Anthralin

Anthralin, an anthrone derivative of chrysarobin, was introduced under the name dithranol in Great Britain decades ago. Chronic plaque-type and guttate psoriasis respond better than other variants to anthralin treatment. Topical anthralin, particularly with UV light, is long established as an effective approach to the treatment of psoriasis.[19]

Anthralin possesses antiproliferative activity on human keratinocytes, inhibiting DNA synthesis by intercalation between DNA strands.[46] It induces nuclear factor-κB (NF-κB) in murine keratinocytes. Since NF-κB is involved in the transcription of proinflammatory cytokines such as IL-6, IL-8, and TNF-α, these findings may be helpful in explaining the irritant properties of anthralin. Other hypotheses support the role of anthralin-generated free radicals in producing both antipsoriatic effects and irritation.

The patient must apply anthralin products only to affected areas of skin because contact with uninvolved skin may result in excessive and unwanted irritation and staining. Skin staining usually disappears within 1 to 2 weeks of discontinuation. Staining of affected plaques is a positive response sign because cell turnover has been slowed enough to take up the stain.

Inflammation, irritation, and staining of skin and clothing (via oxidation and binding to keratins) are often therapy-limiting effects.

Fortunately, anthralin exerts its clinical effects at low cellular concentrations; classic anthralin therapy starts with low concentrations (0.1% to 0.25%) and gradually proceeds to higher concentrations (0.5% to 1%). Short-contact anthralin therapy regimens are alternative modes of application with decreased local adverse effects. Higher concentrations of anthralin (1% to 5%) in water-soluble vehicles are applied to lesions for a short period of time (application for 10 to 20 minutes).[19]

Anthralin traditionally was formulated in stiff paste bases to provide adherence to plaques. Subsequently, cream and ointment formulations have been developed that are more cosmetically appealing and appear to be equivalent in efficacy. Usually it is applied in the evening and allowed to remain overnight.

Immunomodulators

Pimecrolimus and tacrolimus are calcineurin inhibitors capable of exerting a local immunomodulating effect that may serve to normalize hyperproliferation of epidermis. As topical agents, tacrolimus and pimecrolimus are approved for the treatment of atopic dermatitis; however, regulatory approval regarding the efficacy of these agents in psoriasis is yet to be completed.

SYSTEMIC THERAPY: FIRST-LINE AGENTS

Acitretin

Acitretin, an oral retinoid, is the active metabolite of etretinate and has demonstrated clinical effects similar to etretinate, but with fewer adverse effects.[29] Acitretin is indicated for the treatment of severe psoriasis, including erythrodermic and generalized pustular types, but is more useful as an adjunct in the treatment of plaque psoriasis. In contrast to the fast-acting cyclosporine and methotrexate, acitretin resolves psoriatic lesions more slowly.

Acitretin has a shorter half-life than etretinate. Its mechanism of action is not completely understood; it may achieve benefits by acting on retinoid receptors in the keratinocyte nucleus to correct abnormal cell differentiation.[47]

Acitretin has shown good results when combined with other psoriatic therapies, including PUVA and UVB, cyclosporine, and methotrexate.[48] The combination of acitretin and PUVA is highly effective and provides faster and more complete clearance, as well as allowing a decrease in the doses of both agents, thereby limiting the risk of adverse effects.[29]

Adverse effects are dose dependent. They include hypervitaminosis A (i.e., dry lips/cheilitis, dry mouth, dry nose, dry eyes/conjunctivitis, dry skin, pruritus, scaling, and hair loss), hepatoxicity, skeletal changes, hypercholesterolemia, and hypertriglyceridemia. To counteract hyperlipidemic effects, gemfibrozil has been studied for concomitant use with acitretin. In addition, acitretin is a known teratogen and thus is contraindicated in females who are pregnant or who plan pregnancy within the 3 years following drug discontinuation.[49]

Absorption is enhanced when taken with food. Concurrent ingestion of alcohol converts acitretin to etretinate, which has a longer half-life.

An initial recommended dose of acitretin is 25 to 50 mg once daily, with therapy continued until lesions have resolved. A dosage of 50 mg/day is typically required for plaque psoriasis, and even at this relatively high dose, acitretin is only moderately effective. It is better tolerated when taken in conjunction with a meal.

SYSTEMIC THERAPY: SECOND-LINE AGENTS

Cyclosporine

An effective immunosuppressive agent that inhibits the first phase of T-cell activation, cyclosporine is used in the treatment of both cutaneous and arthritic manifestations of severe psoriasis.[50] It also inhibits the release of inflammatory mediators from mast cells, basophils, and polymorphonuclear cells.[51]

A meta-analysis of 579 patients with severe psoriasis treated with either 2.5 or 5 mg/kg per day of cyclosporine for 10 to 12 weeks found that the PASI decreased by 70% and 72%, respectively.[52] An oral microemulsion formulation of cyclosporine has shown a better pharmacokinetic profile, resulting in a more consistent and predictable rate of absorption than the original formulation.[5,53]

Cyclosporine is nephrotoxic with prolonged use. Published studies have demonstrated interstitial fibrosis and renal tubular atrophy on kidney biopsy specimens in patients treated for more than 2 years with cyclosporine. To decrease the risk of nephrotoxicity, the dose of cyclosporine should be kept below 5 mg/kg per day.[54,55] In addition, use for more than 2 years of cumulative treatment may increase the risk of malignancy, including skin cancers and lymphoproliferative disorders.[29] One study has suggested that cyclosporine renders malignancies more aggressive. Other complications include hypertension, hypomagnesemia, hyperkalemia, decreased liver function, elevation of serum lipids, gastrointestinal intolerance, paresthesias, hypertrichosis, and gingival hyperplasia.[51,54]

See Chap. 87 on solid organ transplantation for a discussion of drug interactions involving cyclosporine.

The typical dose of cyclosporine is usually between 2.5 and 5 mg/kg per day.

Tacrolimus

Tacrolimus is a macrolide immunosuppressive agent indicated for the prevention of organ transplant rejection and useful as an alternative treatment in severe recalcitrant psoriasis. Tacrolimus, like cyclosporine, inhibits T-cell activation.[7]

Adverse effects include diarrhea, nausea, paresthesias, hypertension, tremor, and insomnia. Other toxicities with topical tacrolimus—including renal insufficiency and immunosuppression—have been rarely reported.[56]

See Chap. 87 on solid organ transplantation for a discussion of drug interactions involving tacrolimus.

In recalcitrant plaque-type psoriasis, patients receive tacrolimus at oral doses of 0.05 mg/kg per day (increased up to 0.15 mg/kg per day as needed).[57]

Methotrexate

Methotrexate, a common antimetabolite, was introduced several decades ago for the treatment of psoriasis and remains an effective therapeutic approach. It is a synthetic analogue of folic acid that acts as a competitive inhibitor of the enzyme dihydrofolate reductase, that is responsible for the conversion of dihydrofolate to tetrahydrofolate. Tetrahydrofolate is an essential cofactor for the synthesis of thymidylate and purine nucleotides required for DNA and RNA synthesis.[58]

Methotrexate inhibits replication and function of T and B cells and suppresses secretion of various cytokines such as IL-1, IFN-γ, and TNF-α. It also suppresses epidermal cell division. Methotrexate is indicated in patients with moderate to severe psoriasis.

Methotrexate is particularly beneficial for patients with psoriatic arthritis. It is also indicated for patients that are refractory to topical or ultraviolet therapy.[29] Methotrexate should be avoided in patients with active infections because of its immunosuppressive activity.[59]

Methotrexate is associated with nausea and vomiting as well as mucosal ulceration, stomatitis, malaise, headaches, macrocytic anemia, and pulmonary toxicity. Nausea and macrocytic anemia can be ameliorated by administering oral folic acid in doses of 1 to 5 mg/day.

Bone marrow toxicity that leads to leukopenia, anemia, and thrombocytopenia has been shown to be induced by methotrexate. A serious long-term adverse effect is hepatotoxicity. Consequently, methotrexate should typically be avoided in patients with liver disease. Risk factors for hepatotoxicity include a history of excessive alcohol consumption, hepatitis, persistent elevated liver function tests, and family history of inheritable liver disease.[58]

Malignant lymphomas have been reported in several patients treated with methotrexate. In some cases, lymphomas regressed when methotrexate was discontinued, strongly suggesting a causal relationship.[60] Methotrexate is contraindicated in pregnant women because it is teratogenic.[58]

Drug interactions may potentiate methotrexate toxicity. For example nonsteroidal anti-inflammatory drugs can reduce renal clearance of methotrexate, resulting in toxic levels.[61] Table 96–5 lists selected drugs that interact with, and increase toxicity of, methotrexate.

The starting methotrexate dose is 7.5 to 15 mg per week, and this is increased incrementally by 2.5 mg every 2 to 4 weeks until a response is evident. Maximal doses are typically about 25 mg per

TABLE 96–5. Interacting Drugs that Increase the Toxicity of Methotrexate

Mechanism	Drug
Additive or synergistic toxicity	Ethanol
	Pyrimethamine
	Trimethoprim-sulfamethoxazole
Decreased renal elimination of methotrexate	Aminoglycosides
	Cephalothin
	Colchicines
	Cyclosporine
	Nonsteroidal anti-inflammatory drugs (naproxen and ibuprofen)
	Penicillins
	Phenylbutazone
	Probenecid
	Salicylates
	Sulfonamides
Displacement of methotrexate from protein binding	Barbiturates
	Phenytoin
	Probenecid
	Retinoids
	Salicylates
	Sulfonamides
	Sulfonylureas
	Tetracycline
Hepatotoxicity	Ethanol
	Retinoids
Intracellular accumulation of methotrexate	Dipyridamole

week.[56] It can be administered orally, subcutaneously, or intramuscularly. It is renally excreted and should therefore not be administered to patients with impairment of kidney function.

Mycophenolate Mofetil

Mycophenolate mofetil, a semisynthetic morpholinoester of mycophenolic acid, initially was used to prevent acute rejection after renal and cardiac transplantation, but it is now used as part of combination therapy in moderate to severe psoriasis and other autoimmune dermatoses. It reversibly blocks de novo synthesis of guanine nucleotides required for DNA and RNA synthesis. The drug has been shown to have a specific lymphocyte antiproliferative effect.[62,63] Oral mycophenolate mofetil, as well as topical mycophenolic acid, must undergo further clinical studies to establish efficacy in the treatment of patients with severe psoriasis.[64]

Commonly reported adverse effects of mycophenolate mofetil include gastrointestinal toxicity (diarrhea, nausea, and vomiting), hematologic effects (anemia, neutropenia, and thrombocytopenia), and an increased incidence of viral and bacterial infections. Lymphoproliferative disease or lymphoma has developed in up to 1% of patients who received mycophenolic acid with other immunosuppressive agents.

See Chap. 87 on solid organ transplantation for a discussion of drug interactions involving mycophenolate mofetil.

Mycophenolate mofetil is usually administered in 500-mg doses four times a day; the dosage can be increased up to 4 g/day.

Sulfasalazine

Sulfasalazine, commonly used in the treatment of inflammatory bowel disease and rheumatoid arthritis, is selectively used as an alternative treatment, particularly in patients with concurrent psoriatic arthritis. Sulfasalazine is an anti-inflammatory agent that inhibits 5-lipoxygenase. When used as a single agent in the treatment of psoriasis, it is not as effective as is therapy with methotrexate, PUVA, or acitretin. One possible advantage of sulfasalazine therapy compared with other systemic treatments is its relatively high margin of safety. The usual dose of oral sulfasalazine is 3 to 4 g/day for 8 weeks.[7]

See Chap. 89 on rheumatoid arthritis for a discussion of drug interactions involving sulfasalazine.

6-Thioguanine

A purine analog that acts as an antimetabolite in the S-phase of cell division, 6-thioguanine is approved for treatment of leukemia, but has been used as an alternative treatment for psoriasis for decades when conventional therapies have failed.[65] It appears to be less hepatotoxic than methotrexate and therefore may be more useful in treating hepatically-compromised patients with severe psoriasis.

Adverse effects of 6-thioguanine include bone marrow suppression, gastrointestinal complications including nausea and diarrhea, and elevation of liver function tests.

See Chap. 124 on cancer treatment and chemotherapy, for a discussion of drug interactions involving 6-thioguanine.

The typical dose of 6-thioguanine is 80 mg twice weekly, increased by 20 mg every 2 to 4 weeks. Its maximum dose is considered to be 160 mg three times a week.

Hydroxyurea

Hydroxyurea inactivates the enzyme ribonucleotide reductase, inhibiting cell synthesis in the S-phase of the DNA cycle. An antimetabolite that is primarily used to treat hematologic malignancies, it has been used for the treatment of psoriasis for more than 3 decades.[29] It is selectively used, particularly in those with liver disease who would be at risk of adverse effects with other antipsoriatic agents. However, hydroxyurea is less effective than methotrexate.[7]

Adverse effects of hydroxyurea are bone marrow toxicity with leukopenia or thrombocytopenia, cutaneous reactions, leg ulcers, and megaloblastic anemia.

See Chap. 124 on cancer treatment and chemotherapy for a discussion of drug interactions involving hydroxyurea.

The typical dose of hydroxyurea is 1 g/day, with gradual increase to 2 g/day as needed as tolerated. Improvement is gradual, usually seen after 4 weeks of therapy.[7]

BIOLOGIC THERAPY

The field of biologic therapy is expanding rapidly as a result of advances in recombinant DNA technology, microbiology, and immunology. In dermatology, biologic therapies—primarily immunomodulating agents designed to alter immune responses—are the basis for treatment of cutaneous diseases such as psoriasis and atopic dermatitis. These agents, produced in vitro through recombinant DNA technology, fall into three categories: (1) recombinant human cytokines, (2) humanized monoclonal antibodies, and (3) molecular receptors that can bind target molecules.[66]

The biologic agents currently used in moderate to severe psoriasis treatment are infliximab, etanercept, alefacept, and efalizumab.

CLINICAL CONTROVERSY

While some authors seem to successfully argue the advantages of remittive therapy in a potentially lifelong disorder,[67] others hypothesize the notion that biologic agents are excessively costly and that less expensive alternatives need development.[68] Despite the annual cost, given careful oversight, patient quality of life can be dramatically improved with an acceptable risk:benefit ratio if remittive therapy is accomplished with a biologic agent.

In psoriasis, biologic agents typically act through one or more of the following mechanisms: (1) elimination of activated T cells, (2) inhibition of T-cell activation, (3) interference with T-cell trafficking to the skin, (4) neutralization of the effects of Th1-type cytokines, and (5) induction of immune deviation by introducing Th2-type cytokines.[66]

Infliximab

Infliximab is a chimeric monoclonal antibody (immunoglobulin G_1; IgG_1) directed against TNF-α. It binds with high affinity to the soluble and transmembranous forms of TNF-α and inhibits binding of TNF-α with its receptors. TNF-α is believed to play an important role in the pathogenesis of psoriasis. Increased amounts of TNF-α have been found in psoriatic lesions. The proposed mechanism of action

of TNF-α includes stimulation of synthesis of numerous cytokines and induction of the expression of intracellular adhesion molecules on endothelial cells and keratinocytes.[69]

Infliximab is approved for treatment of rheumatoid arthritis and Crohn's disease, but has been studied for use in psoriasis. One double-blind, randomized, placebo-controlled clinical trial studied the effectiveness and safety of infliximab in patients with moderate to severe psoriasis. A good response was seen in 82% and 91% of patients treated with infliximab 5 mg/kg or 10 mg/kg, respectively. Median time to response for all patients receiving infliximab was 4 weeks. The investigators concluded that patients treated with infliximab had a high degree of clinical improvement with rapid response rate, similar to that observed with cyclosporine therapy.[70]

The most common adverse effects of infliximab are headaches, fever, chills, fatigue, diarrhea, pharyngitis, upper respiratory and urinary tract infections, and hypersensitivity reactions (urticaria, dyspnea, and hypotension). Infliximab has been also associated with infections and lymphoproliferative disorders. It is not associated with end-organ toxicity, and blood counts, liver enzyme levels, kidney function, and complement values can be expected to remain normal during treatment. This gives it a major advantage over other systemic psoriasis treatments.

Infliximab is administered in three doses at weeks 0, 2, and 6, of 5 mg/kg or 10 mg/kg by slow intravenous infusion.[70]

Etanercept

Etanercept, another TNF-α blocker, is a genetically engineered fusion protein that combines the extracellular domain of the TNF-α receptor with the Fc region of human IgG_1. Etanercept binds free and membrane-bound TNF-α, competitively interfering with the interaction of TNF-α with cell-bound receptors, and inhibits the effects of this cytokine on target cells. Unlike the chimeric infliximab, etanercept is fully humanized, thereby minimizing the risk of immunogenicity.[71]

Etanercept has been approved in several countries for subcutaneous treatment of rheumatoid arthritis and psoriatic arthritis. Safety and efficacy of etanercept for psoriatic arthritis and psoriasis were demonstrated in a 12-week randomized, double-blind, placebo-controlled trial of twice-weekly subcutaneous injections of etanercept 25 mg. The median reduction in PASI in the treatment group was 46%, compared with 8.7% in the placebo group.[72]

Adverse effects of etanercept include a local reaction at the injection site (20% of patients), respiratory tract and gastrointestinal infections, abdominal pain, nausea and vomiting, headaches, and rash. Serious infections (including tuberculosis) and malignancies have rarely been observed.

Etanercept is usually given in doses up to 50 mg subcutaneously twice a week.

Alefacept

Alefacept is a dimeric fusion protein that combines the first extracellular domain of human LFA-3 with the Fc portion of human IgG_1. The LFA-3 segment of alefacept binds specifically to CD2 on T cells to prevent costimulatory signals delivered by LFA-3 and thereby inhibit cutaneous T-cell activation and proliferation. Alefacept also induces selective apoptosis of memory-effector T cells and produces a dose-dependent decrease in circulating total lymphocytes.[7,73]

TABLE 96–6. Skin Classification Based on Reaction to Sun Exposure

Skin Type	Description	Generalized Characteristics
1	Always burns easily, never tans	Light skin color, often blue eyes, very light skin
2	Usually burns easily, tans minimally	Light skin color, often blue eyes, fair skin
3	Burns moderately, tans gradually	Light brown skin
4	Burns minimally, tans readily	Moderate brown skin or olive skin
5	Rarely burns, tans profusely	Deeply pigmented, dark olive skin
6	Never burns	Darkly pigmented, brown or black skin

From Lindelof et al.[83]

Alefacept is approved for treatment of moderate to severe plaque psoriasis in patients and is also effective for the treatment of psoriatic arthritis.[74] Significant clinical response is achieved after about 3 months of therapy, and improvements are relatively long lasting.

Alefacept is well tolerated and its safety profile is equivalent to that of placebo. The most common adverse events are mild and include pharyngitis, influenza-like symptoms, chills, dizziness, nausea, headache, injection site pain and inflammation, and nonspecific infection; the frequency of these effects is low. Also, the drug produces no increase in the rate of opportunistic infections or malignancies.[75] Weekly visits to a physician's office for drug administration and CD4 T-cell monitoring are required, and not all patients respond to treatment.

Alefacept is administered by intramuscular injection in once-weekly doses of 15 mg for 12 weeks.

Efalizumab

Efalizumab is a humanized monoclonal antibody (IgG_1) against CD11-α integrin. CD11-α/CD18 comprise subunits of LFA-1, a T-cell surface molecule important in T-cell activation, T-cell migration into skin, and cytotoxic T-cell function.[76]

Clinical studies with efalizumab have shown efficacy with few adverse effects. In an open-label, multicenter, dose-escalating study of repeated intravenous infusions of efalizumab over 7 weeks in 39 subjects with moderate to severe psoriasis, the individuals who were exposed to the optimum dose (1 mg/kg weekly) showed a mean decrease in PASI of 47%.[77] A subcutaneous formulation is under investigation.

The most frequent adverse effects of efalizumab are mild to moderate influenza-like complaints such as headache, nausea, chills, nonspecific infection, pain, fever, and asthenia; however, organ toxicity, serious infections, and malignancies have not been reported.[78]

The usual dose is 1 mg/kg subcutaneously once weekly.

PHOTOCHEMOTHERAPY

UVA combined with oral methoxsalen is a photochemotherapeutic approach to treatment of psoriasis. Although burdensome, photochemotherapy is an important treatment consideration for patients with moderate to severe psoriasis, when time needed to treat and risk factors are balanced with potential benefit.

The mechanism of action of both UVB and PUVA in treating psoriasis is thought to be immunomodulatory. Phototherapy apparently modulates expression of cellular adhesion molecules and induce T-cell apoptosis.[79]

Candidates for PUVA therapy usually have moderate to severe incapacitating psoriasis unresponsive to conventional topical and systemic therapies. A recent comparison of PUVA and NB-UVB involve 100 patients, 51 treated with NB-UVB and 49 receiving PUVA, wit the results clearly favoring PUVA. Of these patients, 84% cleare with 16 PUVA treatments, whereas 63% cleared with 25 treatment of NB-UVB.[80]

Adverse effects from oral methoxsalen include nausea, dizzi ness, and headache. Long-term adverse effects from combined pso ralen (methoxsalen) and UV light include actinic skin damage, sola elastosis, dry and wrinkled skin, and hyperpigmentation or hypopig mentation. An increased risk of skin cancers, both squamous ce carcinoma and melanoma, exists after PUVA therapy, and is corre lated with the cumulative UVA exposure.[81] Although the proportio of patients with malignant melanoma has remained small, an increas in malignant melanoma has been observed in patients who receive more than 250 PUVA sessions.

Oral methoxsalen is usually dosed with milk or food to minimiz risk of nausea and gastrointestinal upset.

Systemic PUVA is approved for the treatment of psoriasis. It con sists of oral ingestion of a potent photosensitizer such as methoxsale (8-methoxypsoralen) at a constant dose (0.6 to 0.8 mg/kg) and variabl doses of UVA, depending on patient skin type and history of previ ous response to ultraviolet radiation[7] (see Table 96–6 for skin typ classifications[83]). Approximately 2 hours after ingesting psoralen, th patient is exposed to UVA light. Photochemotherapy is performed tw or three times a week. In most patients, control and partial clearin occurs by the twenty-fifth treatment.

Another method—one that may have less carcinogeni potential—is to topically deliver the photosensitizer (methoxsalen to the skin by addition to the bath water (bath PUVA) instead o through systemic administration.[83] Major advantages of this therap are minimal risk of systemic effects and the overall reduction of UVA dose to one-fourth that required with conventional PUVA. A reductio in the risk of nonmelanoma skin cancer has also been demonstrated

CLINICAL CONTROVERSY

Although PUVA is apparently not responsible for any increased incidence of internal malignancy,[84] risk:benefit considerations with regard to melanoma and nonmelanoma skin cancers indicate an increased risk for melanoma,[85] but no increase for nonmelanoma skin cancers, according to some authors,[86] despite development of increased numbers of lentigines. Other investigators report an increased incidence of nonmelanoma skin cancers in association with PUVA.[87]

PHARMACOECONOMIC CONSIDERATIONS

Outpatient costs for a patient with mild to moderate psoriasis may run as high as $4,000 per patient per year. Psoriasis is a chronic disease with patients either requiring treatment or being in remission. Patients with severe psoriasis may be disabled. A patient with early onset of psoriasis may require treatment for more than 50 years.

By effectively controlling psoriasis, costs to patients, lost work days, and health plan costs may be reduced.

EVALUATION OF THERAPEUTIC OUTCOMES

See Tables 96–2 and 96–3 for pharmaceutical care guidelines and Fig. 96–1 for treatment algorithm based on severity of psoriasis.

ABBREVIATIONS

APC: antigen-presenting cell
IFN-γ: interferon-γ
IgG$_1$: immunoglobulin G$_1$
IL-2: interleukin-2
IL-8: interleukin-8
IL-10: interleukin-10
MIG: monokine induced by interferon-γ
MIP-3α: macrophage inflammatory protein-3α
NB-UVB: narrow-band ultraviolet B
NF-κB: nuclear factor-κB
PASI: Psoriasis Area and Severity Index
PUVA: photochemotherapy using ultraviolet A light
RANTES: regulated on activation, normal T-cell expressed and secreted
TARC: thymus- and activation-regulated chemokine
Th1: T-helper cell type 1
TNF-α: tumor necrosis factor-α
UVA: ultraviolet A
UVB: ultraviolet B
VEGF: vascular endothelial growth factor

Review Questions and other resources can be found at www.pharmacotherapyonline.com.

REFERENCES

1. Christophers E. Psoriasis—epidemiology and clinical spectrum. Clin Exp Dermatol 2001;26:314–320.
2. Bowcock AM, Barker JN. Genetics of psoriasis: the potential impact on new therapies. J Am Acad Dermatol 2003;49(2 Suppl):S51–56.
3. Krueger G, Koo J, Lebwohl M, et al. The impact of psoriasis on quality of life: results of a 1998 National Psoriasis Foundation patient-membership survey. Arch Dermatol 2001;137:280–284.
4. Weiss SC, Kimball AB, Liewehr DJ, et al. Quantifying the harmful effect of psoriasis on health-related quality of life. J Am Acad Dermatol 2002;47:512–518.
5. Koo J, Lee E, Lee CS, Lebwohl M. Psoriasis. J Am Acad Dermatol 2004;50:613–622.
6. Elder JT, Nair RP, Henseler T, et al. The genetics of psoriasis 2001: the odyssey continues. Arch Dermatol 2001;137:1447–1454.
7. Mendonca CO, Burden AD. Current concepts in psoriasis and its treatment. Pharmacol Ther 2003;99:133–147.
8. Burden AD, Javed S, Bailey M, et al. Genetics of psoriasis: paternal inheritance and a locus on chromosome 6p. J Invest Dermatol 1998;110:958–960.
9. Trembath RC, Clough RL, Rosbotham JL, et al. Identification of a major susceptibility locus on chromosome 6p and evidence for further disease loci revealed by a two stage genome-wide search in psoriasis. Hum Mol Genet 1997;6:813–820.
10. Higgins E. Alcohol, smoking and psoriasis. Clin Exp Dermatol 2000;25:107–110.
11. Rasmussen JE. The relationship between infection with group A beta hemolytic streptococci and the development of psoriasis. Pediatr Infect Dis J 2000;19:153–154.
12. Tsankov N, Kazandjieva J, Drenovska K. Drugs in exacerbation and provocation of psoriasis. Clin Dermatol 1998;16:333–351.
13. Nickoloff BJ, Wrone-Smith T, Bonish B, Porcelli SA. Response of murine and normal human skin to injection of allogeneic blood-derived psoriatic immunocytes: detection of T cells expressing receptors typically present on natural killer cells, including CD94, CD158, and CD161. Arch Dermatol 1999;135:546–552.
14. Mehlis SL, Gordon KB. The immunology of psoriasis and biologic immunotherapy. J Am Acad Dermatol 2003;49:S44–S50.
15. Bonifati C, Ameglio F. Cytokines in psoriasis. Int J Dermatol 1999;38:241–251.
16. Ferenczi K, Burack L, Pope M, et al. CD69, HLA-DR and the IL-2R identify persistently activated T cells in psoriasis vulgaris lesional skin: blood and skin comparisons by flow cytometry. J Autoimmun 2000;14:63–78.
17. Mussi A, Bonifati C, Carducci M, et al. Serum TNF-alpha levels correlate with disease severity and are reduced by effective therapy in plaque-type psoriasis. J Biol Regul Homeost Agents 1997;11:115–118.
18. Biasi D, Carletto A, Caramaschi P, et al. Neutrophil functions and IL-8 in psoriatic arthritis and in cutaneous psoriasis. Inflammation 1998;22:533–543.
19. Christophers E, Morwietz U: Psoriasis. In: Freedberg IM, Eisen AZ, Wolff K, et al, eds. Dermatology in General Medicine. New York, McGraw Hill, 2003:407–427.
20. Hodak E, Gottlieb AB, Segal T, et al. Climatotherapy at the Dead Sea is a remittive therapy for psoriasis: combined effects on epidermal and immunologic activation. J Am Acad Dermatol 2003;49:451–457.
21. Langan SM, Heerey A, Barry M, Barnes L. Cost analysis of narrow-band UVB phototherapy in psoriasis. J Am Acad Dermatol 2004;50:623–626.
22. Larko O. Treatment of psoriasis with a new UVB-lamp. Acta Derm Venereol 1989;69:357–359.
23. Lebwohl M, Ali S. Treatment of psoriasis. Part 1. Topical therapy and phototherapy. J Am Acad Dermatol 2001;45:487–498.
24. Molin L. Topical calcipotriol combined with phototherapy for psoriasis. The results of two randomized trials and a review of the literature. Calcipotriol-UVB Study Group. Dermatology 1999;198:375–381.
25. Lebwohl M. Acitretin in combination with UVB or PUVA. J Am Acad Dermatol 1999;41:S22–S24.
26. Bonis B, Kemeny L, Dobozy A, et al. 308 nm UVB excimer laser for psoriasis. Lancet 1997;350:1522.
27. Asawananda P, Anderson RR, Chang Y, Taylor CR. 308-nm excimer laser for the treatment of psoriasis: a dose-response study. Arch Dermatol 2000;136:619–624.
28. Spann CT, Barbagallo J, Weinberg JM. A review of the 308-nm excimer laser in the treatment of psoriasis. Cutis 2001;68:351–352.
29. Lebwohl M, Ali S. Treatment of psoriasis. Part 2. Systemic therapies. J Am Acad Dermatol 2001;45:649–661.
30. Koo J. Systemic sequential therapy of psoriasis: a new paradigm for improved therapeutic results. J Am Acad Dermatol 1999;41:S25–S28.
31. Scott SA, Martin III RW. Scaly dermatoses. In: Berardi RR, McDermott J, Newton GD, et al, eds. Handbook of Nonprescription Drugs, 14th ed. Washington, American Pharmacists Association, 2004:831–848.
32. Micali G, West DP. Poisoning and paediatric skin. In: Harper J, Oranje A, Prose N, eds. Textbook of Pediatric Dermatology. Oxford, Blackwell, 2000:1753–1763.

33. Travis L, Weinberg JM. Medical backgrounder: psoriasis. Drugs Today 2002;38:847–865.

34. Lange K, Kleuser B, Gysler A, et al. Cutaneous inflammation and proliferation in vitro: differential effects and mode of action of topical glucocorticoids. Skin Pharmacol Appl Skin Physiol 2000;13:93–103.

35. Gilbertson EO, Spellman MC, Piacquadio DJ, Mulford MI. Super potent corticosteroid use associated with adrenal suppression: clinical considerations. J Am Acad Dermatol 1998;38:318–321.

36. Kang S, Yi S, Griffiths CE, et al. Calcipotriene-induced improvement in psoriasis is associated with reduced interleukin-8 and increased interleukin-10 levels within lesions. Br J Dermatol 1998;138:77–83.

37. Fisher DA. Allergic contact dermatitis to propylene glycol in calcipotriene ointment. Cutis 1997;60:43–44.

38. Langner A, Stapor W, Ambroziak M. Efficacy and tolerance of topical calcitriol 3 microg g(-1) in psoriasis treatment: a review of our experience in Poland. Br J Dermatol 2001;144(Suppl 58):11–16.

39. Lambert J, Trompke C. Tacalcitol ointment for long-term control of chronic plaque psoriasis in dermatological practice. Dermatology 2002; 204:321–324.

40. Duvic M, Nagpal S, Asano AT, Chandraratna RA. Molecular mechanisms of tazarotene action in psoriasis. J Am Acad Dermatol 1997;37:S18–S24.

41. Chandraratna RA. Tazarotene: the first receptor-selective topical retinoid for the treatment of psoriasis. J Am Acad Dermatol 1997;37:S12–S17.

42. Weinstein GD, Krueger GG, Lowe NJ, et al. Tazarotene gel, a new retinoid, for topical therapy of psoriasis: vehicle-controlled study of safety, efficacy, and duration of therapeutic effect. J Am Acad Dermatol 1997;37:85–92.

43. Marks R. Clinical safety of tazarotene in the treatment of plaque psoriasis. J Am Acad Dermatol 1997;37:S25–32.

44. Thami GP, Sarkar R. Coal tar: past, present and future. Clin Exp Dermatol 2002;27:99–103.

45. Vlajinac HD, Adanja BJ, Lazar ZF, et al. Risk factors for basal cell carcinoma. Acta Oncol 2000;39:611–616.

46. Farkas A, Kemeny L, Szony BJ, et al. Dithranol upregulates IL-10 receptors on the cultured human keratinocyte cell line HaCaT. Inflamm Res 2001;50:44–49.

47. Nguyen EH, Wolverton SE. Systemic retinoids. In: Wolverton SE, ed. Comprehensive Dermatologic Drug Therapy. Philadelphia, Saunders, 2001:269–310.

48. Bleiker TO, Bourke JF, Graham-Brown RA, Hutchinson PE. Etretinate may work where acitretin fails. Br J Dermatol 1997;136:368–370.

49. Katz HI, Waalen J, Leach EE. Acitretin in psoriasis: an overview of adverse effects. J Am Acad Dermatol 1999;41:S7–S12.

50. Tourne L, Durez P, Van Vooren JP, et al. Alleviation of HIV-associated psoriasis and psoriatic arthritis with cyclosporine. J Am Acad Dermatol 1997;37:501–502.

51. Olivieri I, Salvarani C, Cantini F, et al. Therapy with cyclosporine in psoriatic arthritis. Semin Arthritis Rheum 1997;27:36–43.

52. Faerber L, Braeutigam M, Weidinger G, et al. Cyclosporine in severe psoriasis. Results of a meta-analysis in 579 patients. Am J Clin Dermatol 2001;2:41–47.

53. Erkko P, Granlund H, Nuutinen M, Reitamo S. Comparison of cyclosporin A pharmacokinetics of a new microemulsion formulation and standard oral preparation in patients with psoriasis. Br J Dermatol 1997;136:82–88.

54. Zachariae H, Kragballe K, Hansen HE, et al. Renal biopsy findings in long-term cyclosporin treatment of psoriasis. Br J Dermatol 1997;136: 531–535.

55. Shupack J, Abel E, Bauer E, et al. Cyclosporine as maintenance therapy in patients with severe psoriasis. J Am Acad Dermatol 1997;36:423–432.

56. Yamauchi PS, Rizk D, Kormeili T, et al. Current systemic therapies for psoriasis: where are we now? J Am Acad Dermatol 2003;49(2 Suppl): S66–77.

57. Skaehill PA. Tacrolimus in dermatologic disorders. Ann Pharmacother 2001;35:582–588.

58. Roenigk HH Jr, Auerbach R, Maibach H, et al. Methotrexate in psoriasis: consensus conference. J Am Acad Dermatol 1998;38:478–485.

59. Saporito FC, Menter MA. Methotrexate and psoriasis in the era of new biologic agents. J Am Acad Dermatol 2004;50:301–309.

60. Kono H, Inokuma S, Matsuzaki Y, et al. Two cases of methotrexate induced lymphomas in rheumatoid arthritis: an association with increased serum IgE. J Rheumatol 1999;26:2249–2253.

61. Kremer JM. Toward a better understanding of methotrexate. Arthriti Rheum 2004;50:1370–1382.

62. Kirby B, Yates VM. Mycophenolate mofetil for psoriasis. Br J Dermato 1998;139:357.

63. Geilen CC, Arnold M, Orfanos CE. Mycophenolate mofetil as a systemic antipsoriatic agent: positive experience in 11 patients. Br J Dermato 2001;144:583–586.

64. Kitchin JE, Pomeranz MK, Pak G, et al. Rediscovering mycophenoli acid: a review of its mechanism, side effects and potential uses. J A Acad Dermatol 1997;37:445–449.

65. Murphy FP, Cover TR, Burack LH, et al. Clinical clearing of psoriasis b 6-thioguanine correlates with cutaneous T-cell depletion via apoptosi evidence for selective effects on activated T lymphocytes. Arch Dermato 1999;135:1495–1502.

66. Gordon KB, West DP. Biologic therapy in dermatology. In: Wolverton SI ed. Comprehensive Dermatologic Drug Therapy. Philadelphia, Saunder 2001:928–942.

67. Rich SJ. Considerations for assessing the cost of biologic agents in th treatment of psoriasis. J Manag Care Pharm 2004;10:S38–S41.

68. Elias AN. Anti-thyroid thioureylenes in the treatment of psoriasis. Me Hypotheses 2004;62:431–437.

69. Gottlieb AB. Infliximab for psoriasis. J Am Acad Dermatol 2003;4 S112–S117.

70. Chaudhari U, Romano P, Mulcahy LD, et al. Efficacy and safety of infli imab monotherapy for plaque-type psoriasis: a randomised trial. Lance 2001;357:1842–1847.

71. Sobell JM, Hallas SJ. Systemic therapies for psoriasis: understandin current and newly emerging therapies. Semin Cutan Med Surg 2003;2 187–195.

72. Mease PJ, Goffe BS, Metz J, et al. Etanercept in the treatment of psoriati arthritis and psoriasis: a randomised trial. Lancet 2000;356:385–390.

73. Krueger GG, Ellis CN. Alefacept therapy produces remission for patien with chronic plaque psoriasis. Br J Dermatol 2003;148:784–788.

74. Kraan MC, van Kuijk AW, Dinant HJ, et al. Alefacept treatment in psoriati arthritis: reduction of the effector T cell population in peripheral bloo and synovial tissue is associated with improvement of clinical signs c arthritis. Arthritis Rheum 2002;46:2776–2784.

75. Ellis CN, Krueger GG, Alefacept Clinical Study Group. Treatmer of chronic plaque psoriasis by selective targeting of memory effectc T lymphocytes. N Engl J Med 2001;345:248–255.

76. Leonardi CL. Efalizumab: an overview. J Am Acad Dermatol 200 49(2 Suppl):S98–S104.

77. Gottlieb AB, Krueger JG, Wittkowski K, et al. Psoriasis as a model fc T-cell-mediated disease: immunobiologic and clinical effects of treatmer with multiple doses of efalizumab, an anti-CD11a antibody. Arch Derma tol 2002;138:591–600.

78. Kanitakis J, Butnaru AC, Claudy A. Novel biological immunotherapie for psoriasis. Expert Opin Investig Drugs 2003;12:1111–1121.

79. Krutmann J. Therapeutic photoimmunology: photoimmunological mech anisms in photo(chemo)therapy. J Photochem Photobiol B 1998;4 159–164.

80. Gordon PM, Diffey BL, Matthews JN, Farr PM. A randomized compariso of narrow-band TL-01 phototherapy and PUVA photochemotherapy fc psoriasis. J Am Acad Dermatol 1999;41:728–732.

81. Stern RS, Nichols KT, Vakeva LH. Malignant melanoma in patien treated for psoriasis with methoxsalen (psoralen) and ultraviolet A ra diation (PUVA). The PUVA Follow-Up Study. N Engl J Med 199 336:1041–1045.

82. Arndt KA, Bowers KE. Sun reactions and sun protection. In: Manual c Dermatologic Therapeutics, 6th ed. Philadelphia, Lippincott Williams Wilkins, 2002:221–229.

83. Lindelof B, Sigurgeirsson B, Tegner E, et al. PUVA and cancer risk: th Swedish follow-up study. Br J Dermatol 1999;141:108–112.

84. Gach JE, Madrigal AM, Hutton JL, Charles-Holmes R. Retrospectiv

analysis of the occurrence of internal malignancy in patients treated with PUVA between 1986 and 1999 in South Warwickshire. Clin Exp Dermatol 2004;29:154–155.

Stern RS, Nichols KT, Vakeva LH. Malignant melanoma in patients treated for psoriasis with methoxsalen (psoralen) and ultraviolet A radiation (PUVA). The PUVA Follow-Up Study. N Engl J Med 1997; 336:1041–1045.

86. Takashima A, Matsunami E, Yamamoto K, et al. Cutaneous carcinoma and 8-methoxypsoralen and ultraviolet A (PUVA) lentigines in Japanese patients with psoriasis treated with topical PUVA: a follow-up study of 214 patients. Photodermatol Photoimmunol Photomed 1990;7: 218–221.

87. Lindelof B, Sigurgeirsson B, Tegner E, et al. PUVA and cancer risk: the Swedish follow-up study. Br J Dermatol 1990;141:108–112.

97

ATOPIC DERMATITIS

Nina H. Cheigh

Learning Objectives and other resources can be found at *www.pharmacotherapyonline.com.*

KEY CONCEPTS

❶ Atopic dermatitis has increased in prevalence in recent years by two- to threefold, particularly in industrialized countries, along with an associated increase in prevalence of other IgE-mediated diseases such as allergic rhinitis and asthma.

❷ Atopic dermatitis most often initially presents during infancy but can occur at any age.

❸ Clinical presentation differs according to age. Infants typically have face, trunk, and neck involvement, while older children and adults present with lesions in the antecubital and popliteal fossa and on the hands and face.

❹ Patients with atopic dermatitis are extremely susceptible to allergens and other triggering factors, including aeroallergens (dander, grass, mold, and pollen), food (eggs, peanuts, soy, and milk), detergents and soaps, chemicals, varying humidities, temperature, and emotional stress.

❺ Most patients with atopic dermatitis have elevated serum IgE levels as well as eosinophilia. But pathogenesis also involves a complex process of interactions among lymphocytes, macrophages, and mast cells.

❻ Control of atopic dermatitis flare-ups includes identification and elimination of trigger allergens, as well as maintenance of skin patency.

❼ Topical corticosteroids and emollients are the mainstay for treatment of atopic dermatitis.

❽ Topical immunomodulators, tacrolimus, and pimecrolimus provide new options for patients with mild to severe cases of atopic dermatitis.

❾ In severe, refractory cases, atopic dermatitis can be treated with ultraviolet radiation, oral corticosteroids, cyclosporine, azathioprine, methotrexate, and interferon-γ.

Atopic dermatitis (AD), a common pervasive inflammatory skin condition, is notorious for creating a vicious cycle of itching and scratching. Chronic, relapsing, itchy and inflamed skin is the hallmark symptom of AD (also known as atopic eczema).[1] The condition is characterized by an itch so unbearable that patients often find that they must scratch until the itch is replaced by pain. Although the term "atopy" is widely accepted throughout clinical medicine to describe a person's susceptibility to hay fever, asthma, and atopic dermatitis, there is no precise definition or marker of atopy.[2] Certainly there is an association among these chronic conditions, as some 80% of children with AD eventually develop allergic rhinitis or asthma, or have a family history of one or both of these conditions.[3,4]

EPIDEMIOLOGY

❶ A recent and substantial increase in prevalence of AD has been well documented over a wide variety of age groups and geographic locations.[5,6] Approximately 10% to 15% of children under the age of 5 years have been afflicted with AD at some stage in more developed countries.[6] Levels of air pollution, industrialization and urbanization, dietary modifications, and higher socioeconomic class are some of the factors that have been attributed to this increase in prevalence.[5] Although approximately one-half of AD cases are diagnosed during the first year of life, AD typically is a long-term condition, with one third of patients having symptoms that continue into

adulthood.[7] However, those with severe symptoms and early onset have a greater likelihood for a more pervasive course of disease.

Many times, AD is not perceived as a major illness and is frequently dismissed as a minor skin condition. However, studies have demonstrated considerable financial, emotional, and social impact on families of those with moderate or severe AD.[8] An Australian study reported results of significantly more stress in taking care of a child with moderate or severe AD than that involved with care of a child with insulin-dependent diabetes.[9] Disturbed or lack of sleep has also been reported.[10] In the United States, AD accounts for 4% of emergency department visits. The health systems of all countries are burdened with the economic load of AD's direct and indirect costs of treatment and social morbidity.[11]

ETIOLOGY

Despite important contributions of research into the cause of AD, the complicated genetic, environmental, and immunologic mechanisms that produce AD are not completely understood. The hereditary component of AD's etiology is particularly strong, as children with one affected parent have a 60% likelihood of having an atopic disease. If both parents are afflicted, the child has an 80% chance of developing an atopic condition.[12] Paternal AD and asthma are stronger contributors to this risk, in contrast to maternal history. Most patients with AD are found to have elevated eosinophils and serum immunoglobulin (Ig) E levels—findings commonly found in patients with allergic rhinitis or asthma—and 80% of children with AD eventually develop one of these other immunologic/allergic diseases. Children with AD more frequently develop severe asthma than do asthmatic children without AD.[5]

Almost every immunocyte—including Langerhans cells, monocytes, macrophages, lymphocytes, mast cells, and keratinocytes—have some demonstrated abnormality in patients with AD.[13] In addition, AD skin is characterized by an elevated transepidermal water loss and lower skin barrier functions, and for this reason patients must use proper cleansing and moisturizing techniques to maintain skin integrity.

PATHOPHYSIOLOGY AND CLINICAL PRESENTATION

Intense itching (pruritus) and skin reactivity are the hallmarks of AD.[14] Typically, three different types of skin lesions are associated with AD: acute, subacute, and chronic.

The acute rash lesions are intensely pruritic, erythematous papules and vesicles over erythematous skin. These itchy lesions are subsequently associated with scratching that results in excoriations and exudates. Subacute lesions are typically thicker, paler, scaly, erythematous, and excoriated plaques. Chronic lesions are characterized by thickened plaques, accentuated skin markings (lichenification), and fibrotic papules. Most patients exhibit all three lesion types. At all phases, the atopic skin usually has a dry luster.[1]

AD, often referred to as infantile eczema, commonly involves the extensor surfaces of the extremities, trunk, face, scalp, and neck.[15] Although infantile eczema commonly subsides in severity, it often causes the adult to develop a tendency for inflammatory, erythematous, pruritic reactions when exposed to irritants. When AD presents in older children or adults, the lesions are present in the flexural areas of the antecubital (inside the elbow) and popliteal (behind the knee) fossae. Atopic skin is associated with xerosis, which is recognized as a fine scaling, noninflamed skin involving large areas of the body. Atopic skin has a genetically determined decreased ability for keratinocytes to bind water, thus producing dry skin regardless of the weather.[16] The atopic epidermis not only triggers pruritus, but also results in an abnormal protective layer, predisposing the patients to irritation from allergens.

DIAGNOSIS

Hanifin and Rajka[14] published the first major and minor diagnostic criteria for AD in 1980. These diagnostic criteria include the presence of pruritus, with three of more of the following:

1. History of flexural dermatitis, or dermatitis of the face in children younger than 10 years of age
2. History of asthma or allergic rhinitis in the child or a first-degree relative
3. History of generalized xerosis (dry skin) within the past year
4. Visible flexural eczema
5. Onset of rash before 2 years of age

If a diagnosis of AD cannot be made, the presenting symptoms can be indicative of a wide array of other conditions and differential diagnoses, and thus referral to a specialist is warranted.[17] Although elevated IgE and peripheral eosinophilia are found in most patients with AD, no single laboratory test can be relied upon for diagnosis of

AD, as some patients do not present with such abnormalities.[17] Skin prick tests or enzyme-linked immunosorbent assay tests can be used to aid in identification and exclusion of allergic triggers, but these are not specific or sensitive enough to be diagnostic.

Not only is there a lack of absolute diagnoses or laboratory tests, a lack of standardization in objective severity scales hampers classification of the disease. Of the systems available, the SCORAD index, adapted by the European Task Force on Atopic Dermatitis,[18] was previously the most often used, but it demonstrated interobserver variation. As such, research is continuing to identify a better system for classifying patients.[19]

ALLERGEN TRIGGERS

Immunologic triggers that contribute to AD development include food allergens and aeroallergens. A variety of allergens cause approximately 85% of AD patients to demonstrate an immediately positive skin test of serum IgE antibody.[1] However, AD is not a purely IgE-type of condition, as this would indicate presence of an immediate hypersensitivity mast-cell mechanism.

Instead, type 2 T-helper (Th2) cells, found in atopic individuals, play an important role in the condition.[20] Studies have demonstrated flaring of AD on exposure to various aeroallergens such as horse dander, grass, and ragweed pollen.[1] Although variation in performance and evaluation of these tests is difficult to avoid, patch tests with allergens can result in eczematous reactions.[3]

The most common household aeroallergens are dust mites, cat dander, and molds. Dust mites, a commonly encountered allergen, occur in more than 45% of American homes in a concentration exceeding that needed for sensitization.[20] Even so, simple steps can reduce the amount of dust mites in homes.

Food allergy is also a contributing factor to AD, and generally, the more severe the AD and younger the patient, the more likely food allergy is the cause of the symptoms.[21] Egg, milk, peanut, soy, and wheat are noted to account for almost 90% of food allergy in children with AD.[22] Even so, almost one-third of the children with AD and food allergies will "outgrow" the condition over 1 to 3 years.[23] But given this, it is essential that patients (parents) are properly instructed on how to read labels for "hidden sources" of allergenic foods. Patients should be rechallenged at certain times to determine whether they have truly outgrown their food allergy.[22]

The question remains as to whether breast-feeding helps prevent allergy, but this cannot be ethically studied. Human breast milk is the most hypoallergenic substance that can be used to nourish infants, but no evidence shows that either prolonged breast-feeding or manipulations of a mother's diet during lactation protects in the development of AD in infants with a family history of atopy.[24] In infants with a strong family history of AD, thus putting them at high risk, occurrence of AD may be decreased during the first 4 years of life by prolonged breast-feeding (4 to 6 months), and introduction of solid foods at a later point in development (after 4 months of age).[25]

In stressful situations, in which the patient is frustrated or embarrassed, itching, sweating, and scratching are more likely.[1] Stress itself does not cause AD, but it can exacerbate the condition.[26] Stress management, relaxation, and behavioral modification may be important.

Knowing that atopic patients are more susceptible to irritants, there should be an attempt to identify and remove the common irritants. Soaps, detergents, abrasive clothing, smoke, and exposure to extremes in temperature and humidity can be aggravating factors. Although UV light may be beneficial to some patients, sunscreen should be used to avoid sunburns. Care should be used in selection, as many chemical sunscreens can cause contact dermatitis. In addition, as modernization and "Westernization" occurs, people spend the majority of their time in modern buildings with reduced ventilation. This has resulted in an increased load of chemical vapors and gases, along with indoor house dust mites and mold.[25]

COMPLICATIONS

Atopic skin also has a predisposition for increased microbial organisms, namely *Staphylococcus aureus*, which is found in more than 90% of AD skin lesions.[13] Patients with AD are also more prone to herpes simplex infections than the general population.[27] These viral infections can spread locally or become generalized. In addition, fungal pathogens, particularly *Malassezia furfur* or *Pityrosporum ovale*, have been identified.

Patients with AD can also present with eyelid dermatitis, nipple dermatitis, and cheilitis of the lips.[28] Eyelid dermatitis and chronic blepharitis are commonly associated with AD, and can result in visual impairment from corneal scarring. Other ocular complications include atopic keratoconjunctivitis, vernal conjunctivitis, and keratoconus.[1]

▶ TREATMENT: Atopic Dermatitis

Currently, AD cannot be cured. As such, this condition requires a management plan, including identification and avoidance of external triggers, maintenance of skin patency, and use of several therapeutic options for symptomatic relief. Therapy should be individualized, and a multipronged approach should be initiated. Reduction of symptoms, prevention of recurrent flares, and modification of the course of the disease is the best long-term strategy for managing AD (Fig. 97–1).

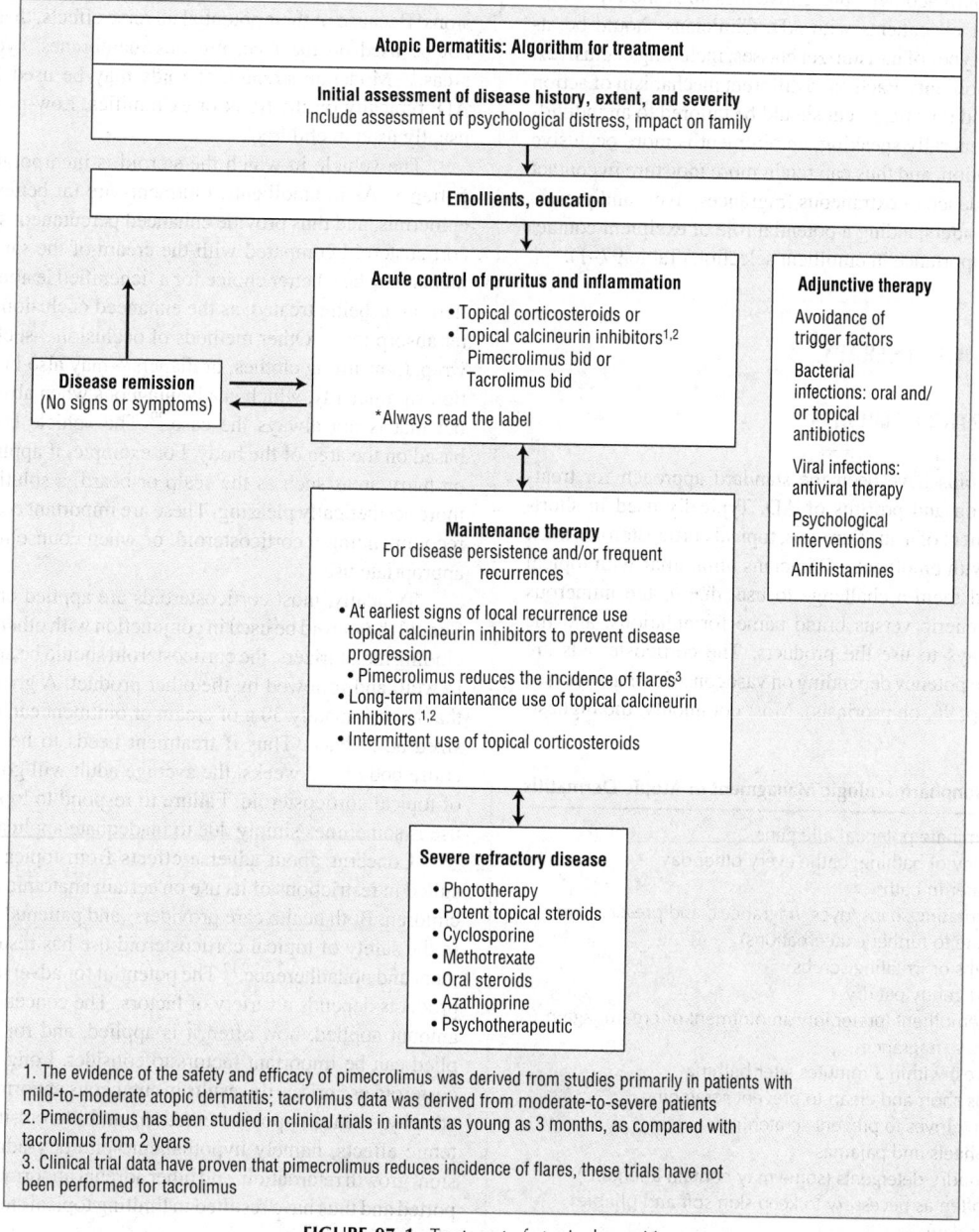

FIGURE 97–1. Treatment of atopic dermatitis

NONPHARMACOLOGIC THERAPY

Given that patients with AD are more susceptible to irritants than normal individuals, possible aggravating factors that may trigger a flare-up should be identified. Recommendations can include avoiding extraneous perfumed or dyed soaps and detergents, using a second rinse cycle for laundry, avoiding extremes of temperature fluctuations, and otherwise being cognizant of potential allergens. Sunscreens should be used in patients with AD, but judicious use of nonchemical agents (e.g., physical sunscreens such as titanium or zinc oxide products) are probably less likely to cause further irritation or contact dermatitis.[1]

The epidermis of atopic skin has a reduced capability of holding moisture. This inherently dry skin is also exacerbated by external changes, including variations in weather and allergen exposures. Thus the importance of maintaining proper skin patency cannot be overstressed, as slight irritations to atopic skin can result in microfissures, which act as portals of entry for various pathogens.[17]

Simple, nonpharmacologic, preventive measures should be recommended for all patients with AD. Clinicians should be attuned to the various types of moisturizer classes, including occlusives, humectants, and emollients. Each has a different mechanism of action on the epidermis, and thus treatment should be tailored to an individual patient need. Generally speaking, an ointment is more occlusive than a cream or a lotion, and thus can retain more moisture in contact with the skin. Avoidance of extraneous fragrances, dyes, and preservatives, as well as understanding a potential role of excipient contact allergy is also of importance in emollient selection (Table 97–1).

PHARMACOLOGIC THERAPY

TOPICAL CORTICOSTEROIDS

Topical corticosteroids have been the standard approach for treating the inflammation and pruritus of AD. Typically used in short-term reactive treatment of acute flare-ups, topical corticosteroids must be supplemented with emollients. Clinicians unfamiliar with topical corticosteroids find them a challenge to use, due to the numerous types, strengths, generic versus brand name formulations, and the wide variety of ways to use the products. The corticosteroids are ranked according to potency depending on vasoconstrictor assays (see Table 96–4 in Chap. 96, on psoriasis). Most commonly, the highest-

---

TABLE 97–1. Nonpharmacologic Managment of Atopic Dermatitis

- Identify and eliminate potential allergens
- Reduce frequency of bathing; bathe every other day
- Use of tepid water in baths
- Avoidance of irritating soaps (dyes, fragrances, and preservatives can all contribute to further exacerbations)
- Avoid washcloths or irritating scrubs
- Air dry skin and gently pat dry
- Application of emollient (preferably an ointment or cream, again watching for dyes, fragrances, and preservatives) within 3 minutes after bathing
- Keep fingernails short and clean to prevent scratching
- Consider cotton gloves to prevent scratching at night
- Use of cotton sheets and pajamas
- Avoid harsh laundry detergents (some may contain allergens)
- Moisturize as often as necessary to keep skin soft and pliable (at least twice a day)

TABLE 97–2. Topical Corticosteroid Use in Atopic Dermatitis

Potency of the steroid depends upon the vasoconstrictive properties
- Typically, with high-potency steroids:
  Use no longer than 3 weeks
  Use on thickened lesions
  Not for use on face, skinfolds, or mucous membranes

The vehicle is as important as the steroid concentration
- Occlusives can increase percutaneous absorption
- Ointments are stronger than creams, which are stronger than lotions
- Gels may be beneficial for hairy or oily areas

Use with moisturizers
- Apply corticosteroid first
- The goal is to increase moisturizers while decreasing corticosteriod use

---

potency steroids are used for short periods of time (generally less than 3 weeks) for acute flare-ups of AD or for lichenified (thickened) lesions. Because of their potential adverse effects, these steroids should not be used on the face, mucous membranes, eyelids, or skinfold areas.[17] Moderate-strength steroids may be used for more chronic AD, typically on the trunk or extremities. Low-potency steroids are usually used in children.

The vehicle in which the steroid is incorporated is also of importance. As in emollients, ointments are far better at occluding the epidermis, and thus provide enhanced percutaneous absorption of the corticosteroid compared with the cream of the same strength. Ointments may be a better choice for a lichenified lesion or when an acute flare-up is being treated, as the enhanced occlusion will result in better absorption.[17] Other methods of occlusion—such as use of plastic wrap, tight-fitting clothes, or diapers—may also increase the absorption significantly, which is advantageous when absorption is desired but that is not always the case.[29] The vehicle can also be chosen based on the area of the body. For example, if application is required on hairy areas such as the scalp or beard, a solution or gel may be more aesthetically pleasing. These are important considerations when recommending a corticosteroid, or when counseling a patient on its appropriate use.

Typically, most corticosteroids are applied once to twice daily. Should the steroid be used in conjunction with other topical agents, including moisturizers, the corticosteroid should be applied first, rubbed in well, and followed by the other product. A good rule of thumb is that approximately 30 g of cream or ointment can cover the average sized adult once. Thus if treatment needs to be twice daily to the entire body for 2 weeks, the average adult will go through 2 pounds of topical corticosteroid. Failure to respond to topical corticosteroid use is sometimes simply due to inadequate application.[1]

Concerns about adverse effects from topical steroids have resulted in restrictions of its use on certain anatomic areas and its use in children. Both health care providers' and patients' lack of confidence in the safety of topical corticosteroid use has resulted in undertreatment and nonadherence.[17] The potential for adverse effects with these products depends a variety of factors. The concentration applied, the amount applied, how often it is applied, and for how long it is applied can be important factors to consider. Long-term topical corticosteroid use primarily results in cutaneous abnormalities such as skin atrophy, striae, hypopigmentation, and steroid-induced acne. Systemic effects, namely hypothalamic-pituitary-adrenal axis suppression, growth retardation, and other adrenal abnormalities have been reported and thus have resulted in limiting topical steroid use in children (Table 97–2).[7,17]

ANTIHISTAMINES

Antihistamines are used to attempt to break the itch-scratch cycle that results from the pruritus of AD. Despite frequent use of antihistamines, few clinical studies support their efficacy, most likely because not all pruritus is mediated by histamine.[1,17] Because pruritus is worse at night, the sedating antihistamines (i.e., hydroxyzine or diphenhydramine) can offer an advantage by facilitating sleep, whereas the newer nonsedating antihistamines have shown variable results.

One tricyclic antidepressant, doxepin, inhibits both H_1 and H_2 receptors, and it has been used for treating adults with AD in doses of 10 to 75 mg at night and up to 75 mg twice daily. This may be beneficial in those atopic patients who have some depression as well.[1,17,30] Topical antihistamines, such as 5% doxepin cream or diphenhydramine cream, also have demonstrated neutral results, but are generally not recommended because of high cutaneous sensitization from excipient ingredients in the formulation.[17]

TOPICAL IMMUNOMODULATORS

Topical calcineurin inhibitors, including tacrolimus and pimecrolimus, have added a new dimension to treatment of AD. Unlike corticosteroids, these agents offer a more long-term option, as they can be used on all parts of the body for prolonged periods without fear of corticosteroid-induced adverse effects. These agents form a complex that results in inhibition of calcineurin, which normally initiates T-cell activation. Through inhibition, the complex subdues the inflammatory component of AD (Table 97–3).[31]

Although the structures of both of these compounds are similar, pimecrolimus is more lipophilic than tacrolimus, and this reduces its cutaneous penetration.[31,32] Studies show that both compounds can be used long-term without skin atrophy occurring.[33,34]

A number of studies have demonstrated the short-term and long-term effectiveness of topical tacrolimus 0.03% and 0.1% ointment in AD for children and adults.[31] When used twice daily, tacrolimus significantly reduced pruritus, cleared lesions, and otherwise improved quality of life. Since the 0.1% formulation is no more effective than the 0.03% concentration, the lower strength is preferred in children with moderate or severe AD,[35] but both strengths are used in adults with AD in those severity categories.[31]

The most common patient complaints with topical tacrolimus therapy are transient itching and burning at the site of application. Although no data support the practice, many clinicians recommend pretreatment with topical corticosteroids to prevent or reduce tacrolimus-induced burning and erythema. Systemic adverse effects of tacrolimus, while well documented with oral therapy, have not been observed in patients using the topical ointment for AD.[36] Patients who receive long-term systemic immunosuppressants are prone to developing actinic keratoses, viral warts, and nonmelanoma skin cancers. Although there are no such reports from topical use, the judicious use of adequate sun protection should be stressed in patients receiving topical tacrolimus for AD.

Topical pimecrolimus 1% cream is safe and effective for treating long-term AD.[31] Preliminary evidence also indicates a potential for use in the treatment of allergic and irritant contact dermatitis.[37] Topical pimecrolimus has been evaluated in both children and infants as young as 3 months of age. These multicenter, randomized, double-blind trials found that flare-ups were prevented and overall disease severity reduced.[38,39] When pimecrolimus is used as first-line therapy for acute AD, the need for corticosteroids can be reduced or eliminated. Even when steroids are needed for flare-ups, the duration of steroid use can be significantly shortened.[40] Thus pimecrolimus is increasingly accepted as a first-line therapy and effective means of reducing the amount of corticosteroid needed for managing AD.[41]

Pharmacokinetic studies have evaluated the systemic concentrations of pimecrolimus when the agent is administered topically in children. These studies concluded that pimecrolimus is well tolerated locally, and systemic effects were not seen.[42,43] Currently, the FDA has approved pimecrolimus cream 1% twice daily for use in mild to moderate AD in children older than 2 years of age and adults.

Although no direct comparative data exist, tacrolimus may be more effective in clearing severe cases of AD than is pimecrolimus.[31] However, increased transient local burning with topical tacrolimus, possibly reflecting its higher immunosuppressant activity, might indicate an increased possibility of skin cancers, as these are more common when skin immunity is impaired. Other areas that require further study are the use of each of these agents in combination regimens and use of these calcineurin inhibitors as maintenance therapy for AD supplemented with corticosteroids during acute flare-ups.[7,31]

TAR PREPARATIONS

Coal tar preparations reduce itching and inflammation of the skin.[1] These products have been used in combination with topical corticosteroids, as adjuncts so that lower strengths of corticosteroid can be used effectively, and in conjunction with ultraviolet light therapies. These preparations are available as crude coal tar (1% to 3%), or liquor carbonis detergens (5% to 20%). At times, coal tar is compounded by pharmacists into various concentrations and sometimes with topical corticosteroids.

Coal tar preparations should not be used on acute oozing lesions, as this would result in stinging and irritation.[44] The strong odor of coal tar products and their staining of clothing are limiting factors. Patients can be instructed to use the product at bedtime and wash it off in the morning. In addition, folliculitis and photosensitivity have been reported.

THERAPIES FOR REFRACTORY CONDITIONS

WET DRESSINGS WITH OCCLUSION

Cool wet dressings or total body wraps placed directly onto the skin can be effective in relieving itching, particularly at night. Wet wraps used in conjunction with topical corticosteroids can be used for acute flares or chronic, lichenified lesions.[44] Skin maceration, fissures, and subsequent infections can occur, and thus these occlusive dressings should be limited to severe, chronic lesions. Tepid compresses applied to skin for 20 minutes four to six times daily can aid in drying out the oozing lesions.

TABLE 97–3. Topical Immunomodulator Use in Atopic Dermatitis

- Tacrolimus (Protopic) 0.1% ointment: for moderate to severe AD in adults not responding adequately to other therapies
- Tacrolimus 0.03% ointment: for moderate to severe AD in children over 2 years old
- Pimecrolimus (Elidel) 1% cream: for mild to moderate AD in children and adults (it has been studied in infants as young as 3 months)

    Applied twice daily
    May be used for longer term
    Can result in reduction in flare-ups

ULTRAVIOLET LIGHT

Ultraviolet light can have phototherapeutic benefits to patients with severe AD. Though natural sunlight can be a source, ensuring that the sunlight is not associated with high heat or humidity (which can exacerbate the condition further) is difficult. Thus short-wave UVB therapies can be useful as adjunctive therapy in chronic recalcitrant AD.[45] At times, higher-intensity UVA therapy has been therapeutic in acute exacerbations, and the mechanism indicates that eosinophils and epidermal Langerhans cells may be targets for high-intensity UVA.[46] Photochemotherapy with oral methoxypsoralen followed by UVA may be indicated in patients with severe, widespread AD, particularly in corticosteroid failure.[47] Adverse effects, ranging from erythema and pigmentation to premature photoaging and cutaneous malignancies are possible, and thus caution should be used in assessing risks versus benefits of therapy.

SYSTEMIC IMMUNOSUPPRESSANTS

If aggressive topical therapy and phototherapy fail to control AD symptoms, the systemic immunosuppressant agents can play a role. Given that AD is a T-cell–mediated disease with involvement from Langerhans cells, eosinophils, and mast cells, immunosuppressant agents are logical agents to use in treatment of severe, refractory, or extensive disease. However, because of their possible adverse effects, judicious use of systemic immunosuppressants is warranted.[48]

Systemic Corticosteroids

Oral corticosteroids, such as prednisone, may be indicated in the treatment of severe chronic AD.[1,17] Typically, a short course can be used to control a severe flare. Proper tapering is necessary, as misuse of the medications can result in dramatic improvement of symptoms, followed by a significant rebound flare upon discontinuation of the medication.[17] Long-term use can cause the well-recognized adverse effects of systemic corticosteroids, including hypertension, growth stunting and developmental delays, and cushingoid features. Thus use of these agents, particularly in children, should be limited to severe conditions that do not respond to safer treatments.[48] Concomitant and proper use of intensified skin care, particularly of topical corticosteroid and emollient use during therapy, is also of utmost importance.

Cyclosporine

Although cyclosporine is not currently approved by the FDA for use in psoriasis, it has been effective in treating many other immunologically based skin diseases.[48] Similarly to systemic corticosteroids, rebound flare-ups of AD are possible with cyclosporine use. Oral cyclosporine can be used on a short-term basis for severe, recalcitrant disease in adults at a dose of 5 mg/kg per day,[48,49] and slightly lower doses, 3 mg/kg per day, can be used with caution in children.

Tolerability in children is good, and most common adverse effects are limited to abdominal pain and headaches.[50] Adverse effects such as renal toxicity were mild and reversible in a long-term multicenter study of safety of cyclosporine use in adults.[51] Even so, appropriate monitoring parameters—electrolytes, renal function, complete blood counts, fasting lipid profiles, and uric acid levels—should be measured at baseline and periodically. Cyclosporine is also involved in many drug-drug interactions, and careful monitoring is required (see Chap. 87 on solid organ transplantation).

Azathioprine

Azathioprine, a purine analogue, is another systemic immunosuppressant that may be helpful in severe cases of AD. Its main disadvantage, compared with cyclosporine, is a delayed onset of action of 4 to 6 weeks. Most reports of azathioprine use have been in uncontrolled, open, retrospective trials, and the use of inconsistent regimens in these trials makes determination of dosing schedules difficult. Despite numerous adverse effects—including myelosuppression, hepatotoxicity, and gastrointestinal disturbances—azathioprine can be helpful in reduction of AD disease activity.[48]

Antimetabolites

Mycophenolate mofetil (MMF), an immunosuppressant used in organ transplant, has cleared refractory symptoms of AD in short-term open-label studies.[1] Since dose finding and well-controlled studies are not available for MMF use in AD, the agent should be used with caution and discontinued if the patient does not respond within 4 to 8 weeks of therapy.[1,48]

Methotrexate, an antimetabolite, is a folic acid antagonist that is primarily used as an antineoplastic agent and in the treatment of psoriasis and rheumatoid arthritis. Although no controlled studies have examined its use in AD, anecdotal evidence supports its effectiveness at a dosage of 2.5 mg/day given four times a week.[1,48,52] Because of its myelosuppressive effects, patient hematologic parameters should be closely monitored. Other adverse effects include hepatotoxicity, pulmonary toxicity, and gastrointestinal toxicity. Folic acid supplementation should also be instituted during methotrexate therapy, and addition of this nutrient does not compromise methotrexate effectiveness.

Interferon-γ

Interferon-γ, a known inhibitor of Th2 cells, has been considered a logical choice in suppressing the IgE responses in AD, and several multicenter, double-blind, placebo-controlled trials have demonstrated clinical improvement with its use in AD.[1,48] However, interferon injections are expensive and may be associated with flu-like symptoms such as fever, chills, headache, myalgia, arthralgia, nausea, vomiting, and diarrhea.[53] Further controlled studies are warranted before its routine use for AD patients can be recommended.

CLINICAL CONTROVERSY

AD and contact dermatitis (both the irritant and allergic types) are eczematous diseases with very similar pathologies. Although AD, unlike contact dermatitis, maintains an important genetic component, evidence is increasing that these diseases are closely related. The current consensus is that atopic and acute contact dermatitis are both immune-mediated, and AD increases one's susceptibility to irritant contact dermatitis. More investigations are needed, but understanding the possible links between AD and contact dermatitis can aid clinicians in understanding the pathophysiology, diagnosis, and treatment of patients who are ailing from these diseases.[54]

EVALUATION OF THERAPEUTIC OUTCOMES

⌐e overall goal for managing patients with AD is to control the con-
⌐tion by preventing flare-ups and to produce a better quality of life
⌐thout disease- or treatment-related complications. Patients with AD
⌐d their caregivers should consult with health care practitioners for
⌐sistance with identifying and eliminating trigger factors and aller-
⌐ns and nonpharmacologic management of the disease. All patients
⌐th AD should be counseled on the importance of emollient use and
⌐her measures for proper skin care.

Depending on the severity of AD, some patients may need
⌐aintenance treatment with low-strength topical corticosteroids. Cur-
⌐ntly, topical corticosteroids are the mainstay for treatment of flare-
⌐s associated with AD. However, patients can be quite concerned
⌐out use of corticosteroids. One recent study showed that 73% of
⌐tients worried about using topical corticosteroids for fear of adverse
⌐fects; 24% of the patients were concerned enough that they did not
⌐here to recommendations for corticosteroid treatment.[55]

Patients older than 16 years who present with AD should be
⌐tch tested for possible contact dermatitis.[17] Health care practi-
⌐ners should also inform patients of the possibility of problematic
⌐cterial, viral, or herpetic skin infections with AD and during its
⌐eatment.

ABBREVIATIONS

⌐D: atopic dermatitis
⌐: immunoglobulin
⌐MF: mycophenolate mofetil
⌐2: type 2 T-helper cells

⌐eview Questions and other resources can be found at
⌐ww.pharmacotherapyonline.com.

REFERENCES

. Leung DYM, Eichenfield LF, Boguniewicz M. Atopic dermatitis (atopic
eczema). In: Freedberg IM, Eisen AZ, et al, eds. Fitzpatrick's Dermatology in General Medicine, 6th ed. New York, McGraw-Hill, 2003:1180–
1194.

. Rocken M, Schallreuther K, et al. What exactly is atopy? Exp Dermatol
1998;7:97–104.

. Leung DYM. Atopic dermatitis: New insights and opportunities for therapeutic intervention. J Allergy Clin Immunol 2000;105:860–876.

. Bleiker TO, Shahidullah H, et al. The prevalence and incidence of atopic
dermatitis in a birth cohort: the importance of a family history of atopy.
Arch Dermatol 2000;136:274–275.

. Levy RM, Gelfand JM, Yan AC. The epidemiology of atopic dermatitis.
Clin Dermatol 2003;21:109–115.

. Hanafin JM. Epidemiology of atopic dermatitis. Immunol Allergy Clin
North Am 2002;22:1–24.

. The International Study of Asthma and Allergies in Childhood (ISAAC)
Steering Committee. International consensus conference on atopic der-
matitis II (ICCAD II): clinical update and current treatment strategies.
Br J Dermatol 2003;148(Suppl 63):3–10.

. Kemp AS. Atopic eczema: its social and financial costs. J Paediatr Child
Health 1999;35:229–231.

. Su JC, Kemp AS, et al. Atopic eczema: its impact on the family and
financial cost. Arch Dis Child 1997;76:159–162.

. Reid P, Lewis-Jones MS. Sleep difficulties and their management in
preschoolers with atopic eczema. Clin Exp Dermatol 1995;20:38–41.

11. Lapidus CS, Schwarz DF, et al. Atopic dermatitis in children: Who cares?
Who pays? J Am Acad Dermatol 1993;28:699–703.

12. Uehara M, Kimura C. Descendant family history of atopic dermatitis. Acta
Derm Venereol 1993;73:62–63.

13. Kang K, Stevens SR. Pathophysiology of atopic dermatitis. Clin Dermatol
2003;21:116–121.

14. Hanifin JM, Rajka G. Diagnostic features of atopic dermatitis. Acta Derm
Venereol 1980;92:44–47.

15. Leung DYM. Pathogenesis of atopic dermatitis. J Allergy Clin Immunol
1999;104(3 Pt 2):S99–S108.

16. Werner Y, Lindberg M. Transepidermal water loss in dry and clinically
normal skin in patients with atopic dermatitis. Acta Derm Venereol 1985;
65:102–105.

17. Leung DY, Hanifin JM, the Work Group on Atopic Dermatitis, et al. Disease management of atopic dermatitis: a practice parameter. Ann Allergy
Asthma Immunol 1997;79:197–209.

18. European Task Force on Atopic Dermatitis. Severity scoring of atopic
dermatitis: the SCORAD index. Dermatology 1993;186:23–31.

19. Charman, C, Williams HC. Outcome measures of disease severity in atopic
eczema. Arch Dermatol 2000;136:763–769.

20. Beltrani VS. The role of house dust mites and other aeroallergens in atopic
dermatitis. Clin Dermatol 2003;21:177–182.

21. Guillet G, Guillet MH. Natural history of sensitizations in atopic dermatitis. Arch Dermatol 1992;128:187–192.

22. Sampson HA. The evaluation and management of food allergy in atopic
dermatitis. Clin Dermatol 2003;21:183–192.

23. Sampson HA, Scanlon SM. Natural history of food hypersensitivity in
children with atopic dermatitis. J Pediatr 1989;115:23–27.

24. Charman C. Clinical evidence: atopic eczema. BMJ 1999;318:1600–1604.

25. Halken S, Host A. The lessons of noninterventional and interventional
prospective studies on the development of atopic disease during childhood.
Allergy 2000;55:793–802.

26. Ginsburg IH et al. Role of emotional factors in adults with dermatitis. Int
J Dermatol 1993;32:656.

27. Leyden JJ, Baker DA. Localized herpes simplex infections in atopic dermatitis. Arch Dermatol 1979;115:311–312.

28. Beltrani VS. The clinical spectrum of atopic dermatitis. J Allergy Clin
Immunol 1999;104:S87–S98.

29. Drake LA, Dinehart SM et al. Guidelines of care for the use of topical
glucocorticosteroids. J Am Acad Dermatol 1996;35:615–619.

30. Klein PA, Clark RAF. An evidence-based review of the efficacy of antihistamines in relieving pruritus in atopic dermatitis. Arch Dermatol 1999;
135:1522–1525.

31. Tomi NS, Luger TA. The treatment of atopic dermatitis with topical immunomodulators. Clin Dermatol 2003;21:215–224.

32. Stuetz A, Grassberger M, Meingassner JG. Pimecrolimus (Elidel, SDZ
ASM 981): preclinical pharmacological profile and skin selectivity. Semin
Cutan Med Surg 2001;20:233–241.

33. Queille-Roussel C, Paul C, Duteil L, et al. The new topical ascomycin
derivative SDZ ASM 981 does not induce skin atrophy when applied to
normal skin for 4 weeks: a randomized, double-blind controlled study.
Br J Dermatol 2001;144:507–513.

34. Reitamo S, Rissanen C, Paul C, et al. Tacrolimus ointment does not affect
collagen synthesis: results of a single-center randomized trial. J Invest
Dermatol 1998;111:396–398.

35. Boguniewicz M, Fiedler VC, Raimer S, et al. A randomized, vehicle-
controlled trial of tacrolimus ointment for treatment of atopic dermatitis in
children: Pediatric tacrolimus study group. J Allergy Clin Immunol 1998;
102(4 Pt 1):637–644.

36. Plosker GL, Foster RH. Tacrolimus: a further update of its pharmacology
and therapeutic use in the management of organ transplantation. Drugs
2000;59:323–389.

37. Queille-Roussel C, Graeber M, et al. SDZ ASM 981 is the first non-steroid
that suppresses established nickel contact dermatitis elicited by allergen
challenge. Contact Derm 2000;42:349–350.

38. Papp K, Ho V, Halber A, et al. Pimecrolimus (Elidel, SDZ ASM 981)
cream 1% is effective and safe in infants aged 3–23 months with atopic
dermatitis. Pediatr Dermatol 2001;18(Suppl):76 (Abstract).

39. Kapp A, Papp K, Bingham A, et al. Long-term management of atopic dermatitis in infants with topical pimecrolimus, a nonsteroid anti-inflammatory drug. J Allergy Clin Immunol 2002;10:277–284.

40. Wahn U, Bos JD, Goodfield M, et al. Efficacy and safety of pimecrolimus cream in the long-term management of atopic dermatitis in children. Pediatrics 2002;110(1 Pt. 1):e2.

41. Boguniewicz M. Treatment options and new therapeutic approaches in atopic dermatitis. Dermatol Nurs 2003;8(Suppl):12–18.

42. Lakhanpaul M, Wahn U, Pariser D, et al. Pimecrolimus (Elidel, SDZ ASM 981) cream 1%: minimal systemic absorption in infants with extensive atopic dermatitis. Pediatr Dermatol 2001;18(Suppl):78 (Abstract).

43. Harper J, Green A, Scott G, et al. First experience of topical SDZ ASM 981 in children with atopic dermatitis. Br J Dermatol 2001;144:781–787.

44. Raimer SS. Managing pediatric atopic dermatitis. Clin Pediatr 2000;39:1–14.

45. George SA et al. Narrow band (TL-O1) UVB phototherapy for chronic severe adult atopic dermatitis. Br J Dermatol 1993;128:49.

46. Krutmann J, et al. High-dose UVA1 phototherapy: a novel and highly effective approach for the treatment of acute exacerbation of atopic dermatitis. Acta Derm Venereol Suppl (Stockh) 1992;176:120.

47. Morison WL, et al. Oral psoralen photochemotherapy of atopic eczema. Br J Dermatol 1978;98:25.

48. Akhavan A, Rudikoff D. The treatment of atopic dermatitis with systemic immunosuppressive agents. Clin Dermatol 2003;21:225–240.

49. Sowden JM, Berth-Jones J, Ross JS, et al. Double-blind, controlled crossover study of cyclosporin in adults with severe refractory atopic dermatitis. Lancet 1991;338:137–140.

50. Berth-Jones J, Finlay AY, Zaki I, et al. Cyclosporine in severe childhood atopic dermatitis: a multicenter study. J Am Acad Dermatol 1996;3:1016–1021.

51. Berth-Jones J, Graham-Brown RA, Marks R, et al. Long term efficacy and safety of cyclosporin in severe adult atopic dermatitis. Br J Dermatol 1997;136:76–81.

52. Sidbury R, Hanifin JM. Systemic therapy of atopic dermatitis. Clin Exp Dermatol 2000;25:559–566.

53. Actimmune (Interferon γ-1b) injection (package insert). Brisbane, CA: InterMune, Inc, 2001.

54. Akhavan A, Cohen SR. The relationship between atopic dermatitis and contact dermatitis. Clin Dermatol 2003;21:158–162.

55. Charman CR, Morris AD, Williams HC. Topical corticosteroid phobia in patients with atopic eczema. Br J Dermatol 2000;142:931–936.

98
HEMATOPOIESIS

William P. Petros and Solveig Ericson

Learning Objectives and other resources can be found at *www.pharmacotherapyonline.com.*

KEY CONCEPTS

◀1 Leukocytes are subdivided into specific cell types which have important functional differences.

◀2 All hematopoietic cells are thought to be generated from one common type of cell (stem cell).

◀3 Blood concentrations of some hematopoietic cell types may not be reflective of total body content.

◀4 Cytokines such as colony-stimulating factors are important regulators of hematopoiesis.

◀5 The kinetics of hematopoietic cells vary with cell type, maturity, pathophysiology, and external stimuli.

◀6 Both the number of cells and other cofactors determine the clinical consequences of neutropenia or anemia.

Hematopoiesis is defined as the formation and maturation of blood cells and their derivatives. There is a tremendous daily turnover rate of cells in this system, with more than 6 billion cells produced per kilogram of body weight every 24 hours.[1] These accelerated processes result in vastly exaggerated and rapid responses to the slightest perturbation.

In humans, hematopoiesis takes place primarily in the bone marrow. Hematopoietic cells were among the first to be evaluated for their biologic function and pattern of maturation, and recent identification of the protein molecules (cytokines) that regulate this system has yielded an extraordinary amount of new information regarding its control. The process of continual hematopoietic cell production is complicated, involving interactions between immature cells, the surrounding microenvironment, and cytokines.

HEMATOPOETIC SYSTEM

The hematopoietic system consists of three primary cell components: leukocytes, platelets, and erythrocytes. The first group encompasses a functionally diverse group of cells that includes neutrophils, eosinophils, basophils, monocytes/macrophages, lymphocytes, and plasma cells. Typical concentrations of mature hematopoietic cells found in the peripheral blood of adults are shown in Table 98–1.

LEUKOCYTES

NEUTROPHILS (SEGS AND BANDS)

◀ The major functions of neutrophils (also known as polymorphonuclear leukocytes) are to prevent pathogenic microorganism invasion and to localize and kill these microorganisms if they

do invade the body. These effects are mediated by a series of events, including migration to the site (chemotaxis), recognition/attachment to the invader, phagocytosis, lysosomal fusion, degranulation, and local generation of oxidants (respiratory burst) and degrading enzymes (Fig. 98–1).[2] A neutrophil is attracted to the site of infection by chemotactic factors. Once migration to the site has occurred, the neutrophil ingests the opsonized microorganism. (Opsonization is the process whereby antibody and complement coat the microorganism, allowing for increased neutrophil recognition.) Following ingestion or phagocytosis, the cytoplasmic granules within the neutrophil fuse with the phagosome or phagocytosed microorganism, thereby initiating degranulation and release of enzymes. These degrading enzymes kill the microorganism through oxygen reduction. Secretion of these enzymes may also result in localized host tissue injury. The actions of cytokines such as granulocyte colony-stimulating factor (G-CSF) and granulocyte-macrophage colony-stimulating factor (GM-CSF) may intensify neutrophil activity.[3]

EOSINOPHILS

Although eosinophils are less efficient than neutrophils, they elicit similar effector functions. Eosinophil activity is directed primarily against large invaders, such as helminths and other parasites that cannot be phagocytized. During an allergic reaction, activated mast cells secrete chemicals that attract and stimulate eosinophils, which in turn produce substances that neutralize or degrade the reaction products of mast cells. Unfortunately, the eosinophil constituents may also damage normal tissue and cause secondary histamine release. High concentrations of eosinophils for prolonged periods may result in damage to the cardiac and central nervous systems, with possible pulmonary and dermatologic involvement.[4]

TABLE 98–1. Average (Normal Range) Adult Blood Cell Concentrations

White cell count ($\times 10^9$/L)		7.8 (4.4–11.3)
Red cell count ($\times 10^{12}$/L)	Male	5.21 (4.52–5.90)
	Female	4.60 (4.10–5.10)
Hemoglobin[a] (g/dL)	Male	15.7 (14.0–17.5)
	Female	13.8 (12.3–15.3)
Hematocrit	Male	0.46 (0.42–0.50)
	Female	0.40 (0.36–0.45)
Mean corpuscular volume (fL/red cell)		88.0 (80.0–96.1)
Platelet count ($\times 10^9$/L)		311 (172–450)

[a]May be 0.5–1.0 g/dL lower in black patients.

BASOPHILS AND MAST CELLS

Through a massive release of their granule contents upon stimulation, basophils and mast cells function as mediators of inflammatory processes. The released chemicals include heparin, histamine, and other substances. The mediator may be vasoactive, bronchoconstrictive, and/or chemotactic (attractive) for eosinophils.[5,6]

MONOCYTES/MACROPHAGES

Derived from the granulocyte-monocyte colony-forming unit, monocytes are peripheral cells in transit from the bone marrow to tissues. Once in the tissues, under the influence of local factors, monocytes become macrophages. Macrophages exist in the liver (Kupffer cells),

spleen, lymph nodes, microglial (CNS) cells, skin (Langerhans cells), and bone.

Monocytes and macrophages perform a variety of functions, including initiation of immune responses for recognition by lymphocytes, regulation of immune response intensity, phagocytosis of foreign invaders, tumor cytotoxicity, degradation of cellular debris, and secretion of peptide molecules called monokines (a subclassification of cytokines).[7] Examples of monokines include interferons, tumor necrosis factor, and interleukin-1 (IL-1). Monokines and other cytokines regulate the activity of these cells.

LYMPHOCYTES

The primary functions of lymphocytes are to control and be the effector cells for the immune system. Many of these cells also are important synthetic sites for various cytokines. Lymphocytes can be functionally divided into cells that display cell-mediated immunity (T cells) and those that are responsible for humoral immunity (B cells; Table 98–2). Several different T-cell subtypes are found in peripheral blood. These include the cytotoxic suppressor T cells (CD8), which attack intracellular pathogens and regulate the size and duration of the immune response, as well as helper T cells (CD4). The latter cells are responsible for delayed hypersensitivity, stimulation of B-cell differentiation (maturation), and antibody production, in addition to regulation of inflammatory reactions. B lymphocytes ultimately become plasma cells, which produce immunoglobulin specific for an antigen attached to the cell's surface.

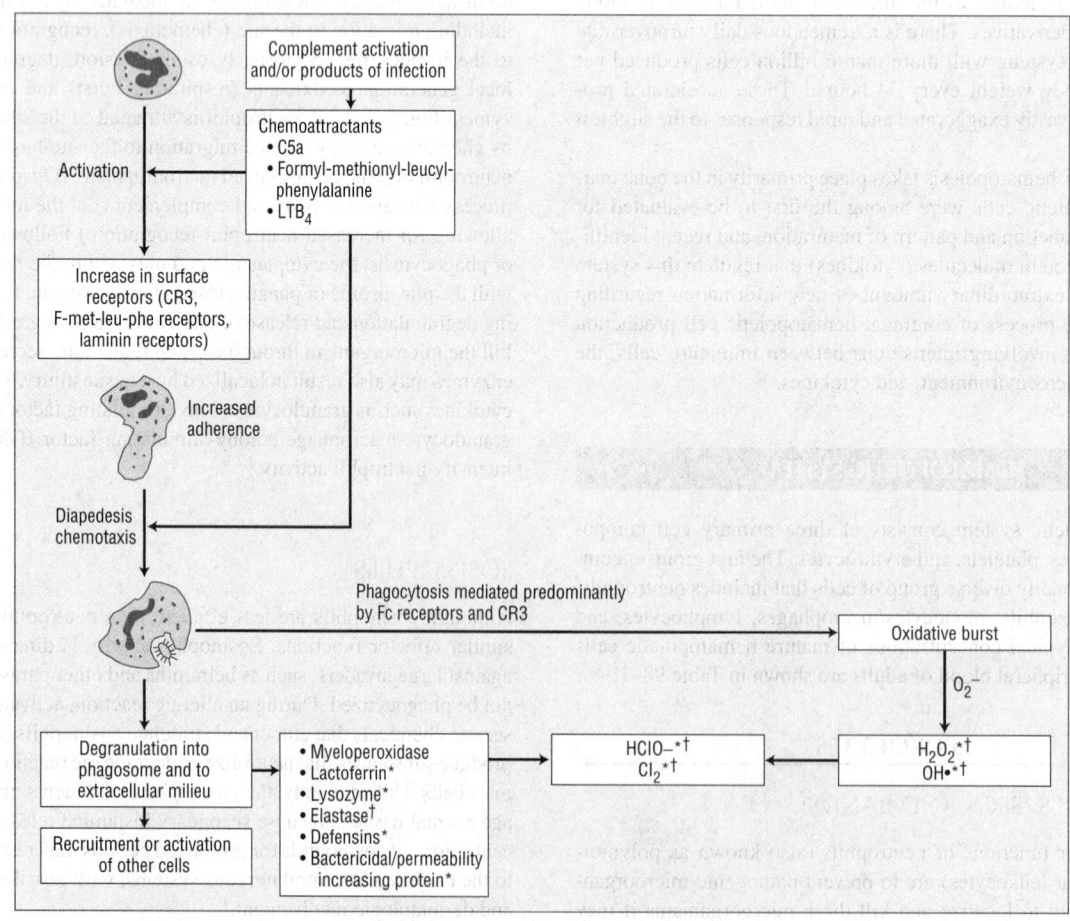

FIGURE 98–1. Neutrophil responses to infection or inflammation. *Microbicidal. †Damage to host tissues.

TABLE 98–2. Lymphocyte-Mediated Immune Function

Cellular immunity (T cells)
1. Provides resistance against intracellular pathogens such as viruses, protozoa, fungi, and bacteria
2. Mediates allogeneic transplant rejection
3. Responsible for contact dermatitis
4. Provides autologous reaction to tumor cells

Humoral immunity (B cells)
1. Serves as major component of allergic reactions and other autoimmune diseases
2. Aids in eradication of encapsulated bacteria
3. Inactivates circulating toxins
4. May play role in antitumor reactions

Null cells are a separate subset of lymphocytes that lack surface markers of B or T origin. These cells, also referred to as large granular lymphocytes, are thought to perform functions such as direct cytotoxicity to foreign entities, and they act either alone (natural killer cells) or in concert with immunoglobulin (antibody-dependent cellular cytotoxicity).[8,9] (Further details regarding lymphocytes are found in Chap. 84, on the immune system.)

PLATELETS

There are several mechanisms by which platelets (thrombocytes) interact to facilitate blood coagulation. These include localization of the thrombus and provision of a specific receptor site for clotting factors, as well as the necessary phospholipid surface for the conversion of prothrombin to thrombin, and protection of thrombin from antithrombin. The process begins with a vascular injury that causes platelets to adhere to the exposed collagen fibers of the damaged wall as blood flows out. These events require the presence of other plasma proteins, namely von Willebrand factor. Platelets then aggregate through a process that is calcium dependent. Following aggregation, various platelet mediators are released (thromboxane, serotonin, and platelet factor V), resulting in the formation of an irreversible platelet aggregate with subsequent formation of a stable fibrin cross-linked clot.[10,11]

ERYTHROCYTES

The primary function of the erythrocyte is to carry oxygen from the lungs to the peripheral tissues. Its optimal design enables efficient oxygen transport via the hemoglobin molecule. The general metabolic state of the patient and local factors control oxygen release.

Some drugs selectively accumulate in erythrocytes, resulting in substantial differences when comparing blood to plasma drug concentrations. In a few instances, enzymes found in erythrocytes (e.g., aldehyde dehydrogenase) may impact on the systemic metabolism of drugs.

HEMATOPOIETIC STRUCTURE AND COMPARTMENTS

Embryonic development of hematopoietic tissue occurs in the yolk sac mesenchyme, with fetal transition occurring in the liver and spleen. Very immature hematopoietic cells can also appear in umbilical cord blood, but not many are evident in the peripheral blood of adults.[12] The ultimate location of immature hematopoietic cells is in the bone marrow. The average adult has approximately 1.7 L of bone marrow, which provides an optimal environment for the development and proliferation of hematopoietic cells.

The hematopoietic bone marrow is located primarily in the central portion of the pelvis, ribs, vertebrae, skull, and femoral and humeral epiphyses. The anatomic structure of the bone marrow is characterized by the central venous marrow sinus, which is linked by coarse vascular sinusoids that intertwine a reticulin mesh where the cells are suspended. Thus hematopoiesis occurs in the extravascular marrow spaces, which also contain endothelial cells, fibroblasts, macrophages, and adipocytes, collectively termed bone marrow stroma.[13] Stromal cells are thought to be important hematopoietic components, providing growth factors, collagen, and cell adhesion proteins.[14] When these cells are combined with accessory cells (lymphocytes/monocytes) and cytokines, the mixture is referred to as the hematopoietic microenvironment.

Egress of more mature cells from the bone marrow occurs through the endothelial cell barrier. Release of cells such as neutrophils may be stimulated by complement, steroids, or endotoxin. Immature (progenitor) cells that may ultimately become any one of the blood cellular components can be mobilized from the bone marrow into peripheral blood by the administration of a cytotoxic chemotherapy drug (e.g., cyclophosphamide)[15] or a colony-stimulating factor (G-CSF or GM-CSF).[16] This process is commonly referred to as "priming" the bone marrow for peripheral blood progenitor or stem cell transplantation (see Chap. 134).

The least mature hematopoietic cell, accounting for only a fraction of a percentage of bone marrow cells, is referred to as the stem cell. Because these cells have the unique potential to ultimately become any of the mature hematopoietic cells, they are termed pluripotent. Importantly, they have self-renewal capacity (Fig. 98–2).[17] Extensive research has been conducted describing the morphologic and immunologic characteristics indicative of the earliest stem cell, but investigators have yet to arrive at a consensus model. Only a small percentage of these cells is likely to be dividing at any one time, and thus most are dormant in the cell cycle.

Stem cell renewal and differentiation occur within the bone marrow under the influence of the marrow microenvironment. Stromal endothelial cells, fibroblasts, and fat cells (adipocytes) are necessary to support stem cell proliferation and division by providing anchorage for adhesion and secreting various hematopoietic growth factors necessary for differentiation. It is the characteristics of the local microenvironment (cellular matrix and growth factor concentrations) that influence the differentiation of a particular hematopoietic lineage, favoring it over another.

The next step in hematopoietic cell differentiation is thought to be represented by committed pluripotent stem cells that can still differentiate into any cell line (red blood cells [RBCs], white blood cells [WBCs], and platelets); however, they have a limited capacity for self-renewal (see Fig. 98–2).

Cells that differentiate can proceed to either myeloid or lymphoid cell precursors (oligopotent progenitors). These cells may ultimately become B or T lymphocytes in the case of lymphoid cells. Myeloid progenitors may become granulocytes, erythrocytes, macrophages, or megakaryocytes, as displayed in Fig. 98–2. Nomenclature for immature hematopoietic cells often uses terms developed during in vitro experiments of cell proliferation. Thus the term *burst-forming unit* (BFU) or *colony-forming unit* (CFU) is added to the suffix of the cell lines ultimately produced by the specific cell.

Leukocytes found in the peripheral blood can generally be classified into neutrophils (the most frequently occurring blood leukocyte, subdivided into the more mature segs and less mature bands), lymphocytes, monocytes, eosinophils, basophils, and the tissue derivative of basophils, mast cells. Immature neutrophils such as metamyelocytes are rarely seen in peripheral blood. Strictly speaking, the group of

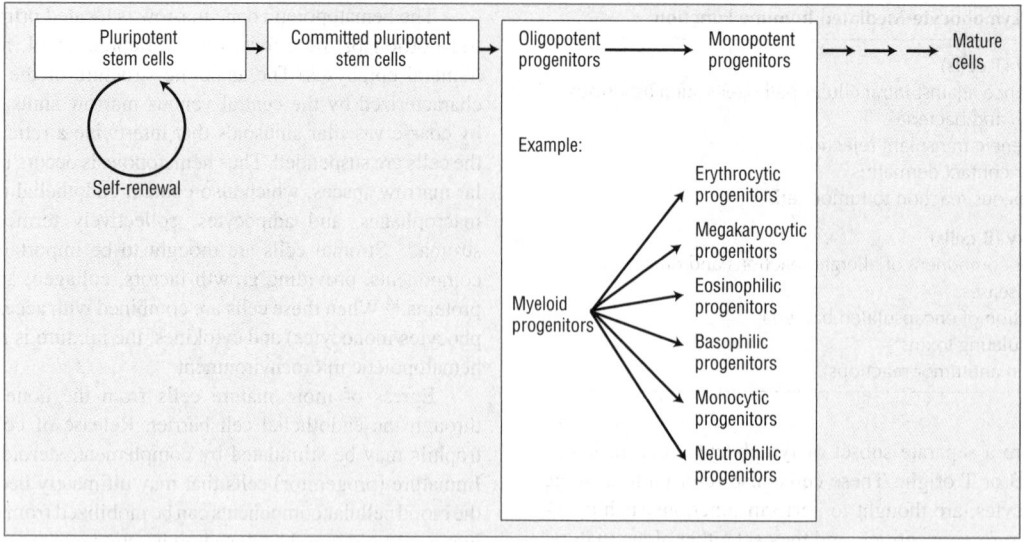

FIGURE 98–2. Rudimentary model of hematopoiesis, displaying the basic steps a cell may take from its inception as a stem cell in the bone marrow, through stages in which it can become multiple (oligopotent) or only one specific (monopotent) type of mature blood cell.

cells referred to as granulocytes includes neutrophils, eosinophils, and basophils, although common use tends to include only the neutrophils. The terminally differentiated leukocytes, which are usually not seen in blood, include the macrophage or histiocyte (derived from monocytes) and plasma cells (derived from B lymphocytes).

Most of the body's neutrophils and neutrophilic precursors reside in the bone marrow (approximately 9 billion cells) in contrast to the circulation (approximately 700 million). Similarly, only 1% of the eosinophils in the body are found in peripheral blood, whereas the skin, lungs, and gastrointestinal tract are the preferred sites of residence.[4] There is no marrow reserve pool of monocytes. Neutrophil development in the bone marrow begins with the stem cell and proceeds through intermediate precursors, such as the myeloblast, promyelocyte, myelocyte, and metamyelocyte.

Only a small fraction of the total body pool of lymphocytes resides in the blood. Immature T cells are evident in the circulation on their way to full maturation in the thymus. Mature B lymphocytes express surface immunoglobulin, which functions as an antigen receptor. Most of these cells migrate from the bone marrow to areas such as the lymph nodes (dense collections of lymphocytes, plasma cells, and macrophages that are supplied by postcapillary venules and drained by a system of efferent lymphatics) and spleen, where antigenic stimulation results in specific immunoglobulin production.[13] Approximately 75% of blood lymphocytes are T cells; 15% null cells, and 10% B cells. Various antigens expressed on the surface of leukocytes, depending on the degree of cell maturity and function, are termed clusters of differentiation (CD).

Progenitor cells that give rise to platelets are referred to as colony-forming unit megakaryocytes. Megakaryocytes account for only 0.05% to 0.02% of marrow cells. Morphologic changes in both the cytoplasm and nucleus accompany the maturation of megakaryocytes. Therefore, at differing stages of maturation, it is possible to see granules, organelles, and increasing segmentation of the nucleus. Cells in this lineage progress through three stages of development: commitment, proliferation, and differentiation, similar to that of leukocytes.[18,19] Receptors for the cytokine thrombopoietin (TPO) are expressed on both megakarocytes and platelets, as well as hematopoietic stem cells.

The term *erythron* has been used to describe collectively the erythropoietic cellular pathway, composed of all cells involved in erythropoiesis, starting with the earliest committed erythroid progenitor and ending with the mature circulating RBC. The earliest cell committed to the erythroid lineage is known as a BFU-E (erythroid)

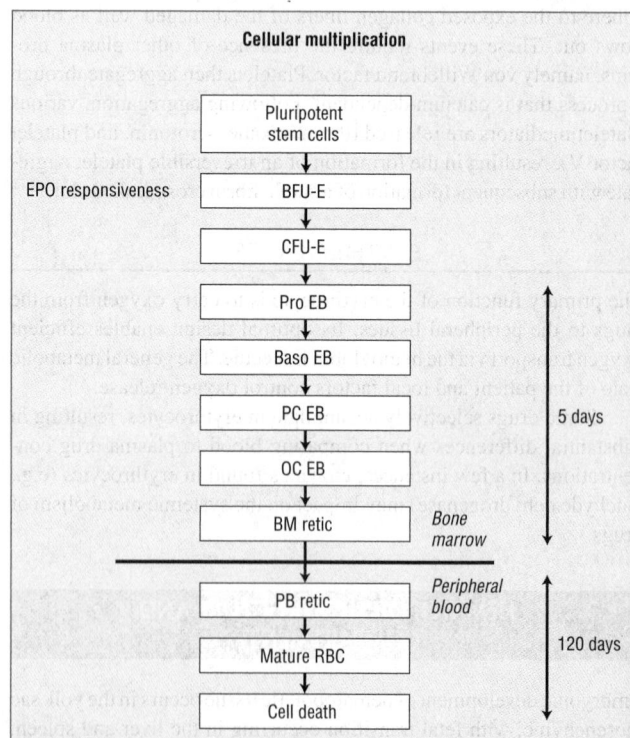

FIGURE 98–3. Proposed differentiation pattern of cells into mature erythrocytes with identification of various immature cell types. In addition, the cells that may be stimulated by the cytokine erythropoietin (EPO) are identified. BM, bone marrow; BFU, burst-forming unit; CFU, colony-forming unit; E, erythroid; EB, erythroblast; OC, orthochromatophilic; PB, peripheral blood; PC, polychromatophilic; RBC, red blood cell; retic, reticulocyte.

Through in vitro culture systems, one BFU-E can proliferate into several hundred progeny. These cells are followed in differentiation by the CFU-E cell, and subsequently by the nucleated normoblast and the immediate RBC precursor, the circulating anuclear reticulocyte as outlined in Fig. 98–3. The remaining RNA is typically lost from the RBC within 2 days of its appearance in the peripheral blood; thus the mature cell does not synthesize new proteins such as enzymes.[20]

The erythrocyte precursor cell types display a continuum of changes in shape, hemoglobin concentration, Rh antigen, and erythropoietin (EPO) receptor expression with maturity. However, mature erythrocytes express significantly lower EPO receptor density than do proerythroblasts.[21]

Neonatal RBCs contain primarily fetal hemoglobin. Adult hemoglobin, 85% of which is synthesized in the erythropoietic marrow, replaces the fetal hemoglobin within a few months. Heme-synthesizing cells must have mitochondria; therefore its synthesis cannot occur in the mature erythrocyte. Genetic alterations in hemoglobin structure may dramatically alter the stability or solubility of the hemoglobin and also cell confirmation. The characteristic biconcave-disk shape of the normal RBC is approximately 8×2 mcm. Pathologic alterations in plasma lipids may affect the outer phospholipid membrane of the RBC, thus changing the cell's shape and survival. Blood types are characterized by the antigenic structure of the external surface of the cell membrane. The interactions of antibodies with RBC surface antigens affect the membrane function, integrity, and phagocytosis of the cells.

NATURAL REGULATION OF CELL PROLIFERATION AND DIFFERENTIATION

The generic model of cell maturation presented in Fig. 98–2 includes a population of stem cells, thought to be capable of self-renewal, that provides the initial cell (committed progenitor) for subsequent maturation, differentiation (i.e., commitment to a cell line), and expansion into all blood cell types. This is followed by an initial differentiation step when a cell is produced (oligopotent progenitor) that will ultimately become one of only several mature blood cell types. Finally, monopotent progenitors are noted in which differentiation is restricted to one cell type. The latter cells then undergo a series of maturation steps, ultimately resulting in a mature cell.

STEM CELLS

The action of a stem cell in self-renewing rather than differentiating and the selection of lineage by a multipotential progenitor cell during the differentiation process are thought to be stochastic (random) events. Conversely, the survival and proliferation of the subsequent progenitor cells are thought to be regulated by the group of cytokines referred to as colony-stimulating factors (also known as CSFs, hematopoietins, hematopoietic cytokines, or hematopoietic growth factors).[22] Receptors for a variety of CSFs are present on the surface of stem cells, which agrees with in vitro studies demonstrating stimulatory activity for cytokines such as stem cell factor (SCF), IL-1, IL-6, G-CSF, IL-10, IL-11, IL-12, IL-13, TPO, basic fibroblast growth factor, and leukemia inhibitory factor, when present in combinations. Whether or not the therapeutic use of a CSF that is thought to act primarily on more mature cells will exhaust (deplete) the stem cell pool over the course of multiple cycles of therapy is under active debate and study.[23] Proposed "cascades" of hematopoiesis are represented in Fig. 98–3 through 98–6. Inserted within some figures are the

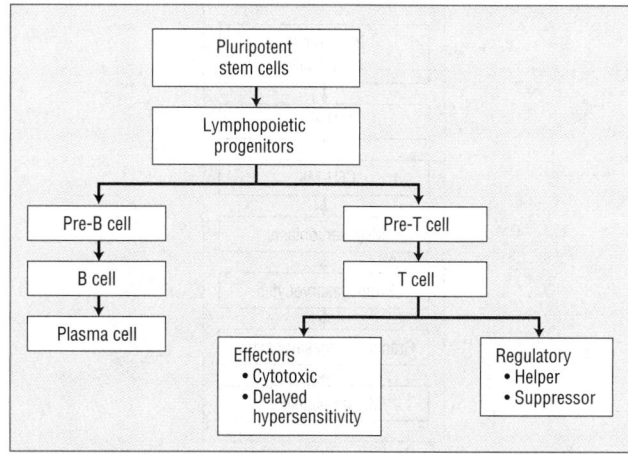

FIGURE 98–4. Pattern of lymphocyte maturation and differentiation into T and B cells. The plasma cell is a factory for antibodies, whereas the T cells have both effector and regulatory functions on the immune system.

suspected sites in the process where CSFs are thought to interact by promoting the production, proliferation, and survival of hematopoietic cells. These schema are simple representations of a system of complex interactions between stimulatory and inhibitory cytokines that may not be adequately described by the in vitro models used thus far to define them. (Details regarding the clinical pharmacology of individual CSFs are presented in Chap. 124.)

Immature bone marrow precursor cells such as the myeloblast (first recognizable cell of granulocytic differentiation), promyelocyte, myelocyte, and erythroblast are thought to be capable of replication. This is in contrast to most mature hematopoietic cells, which are incapable of division. Exceptions to the latter statement include monocytes, macrophages, and tissue mast cells. Evaluation of reasons for

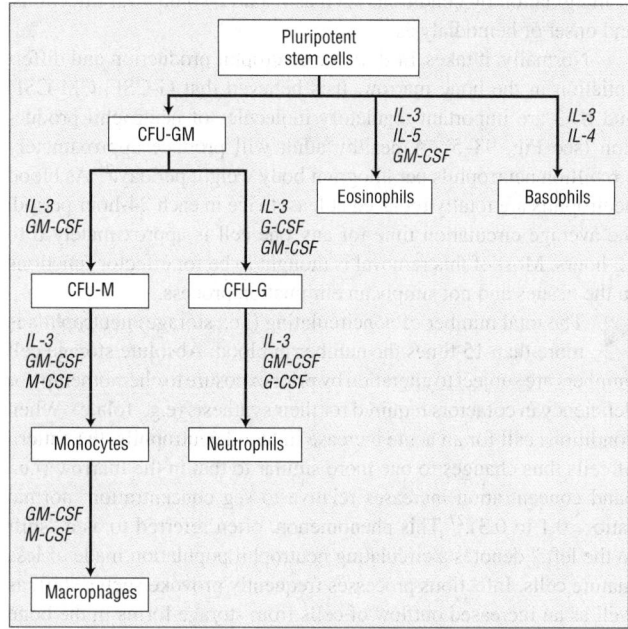

FIGURE 98–5. Maturation of precursor cells into granulocytes and macrophages, including some intermediate precursor cells (CFU-GM, G, and M). The colony-stimulating factors (CSFs) that affect the more terminal (mature) pathways are also shown. (CSFs that regulate immature cell types are not displayed.) CFU, colony-forming unit; G, granulocyte; M, monocyte.

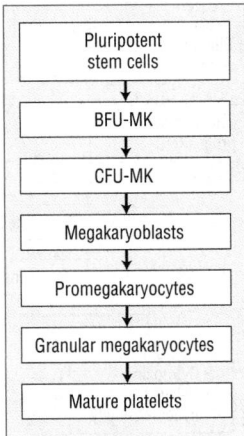

FIGURE 98–6. Maturation steps of megakaryocyte precursors prior to becoming mature platelets. BFU, burst-forming unit; CFU, colony-forming unit; MK, megakaryocyte.

a change in hematopoietic cellular concentration over time must be conducted with a thorough knowledge of the mechanisms of both cellular production and destruction.

NEUTROPHILS

Blood neutrophils are in constant exchange with an equal number of "marginated" cells. The latter are stuck to the walls of vessels in the peripheral blood, liver, lungs, and spleen. Therefore, demargination or the opposite, increased adhesion, can dramatically change the peripheral neutrophil concentration, even though cell production remains constant. A variety of stimuli can result in demargination, including infection, exercise, epinephrine, corticosteroids, and sickle cell anemia.[24] Conversely, transient neutropenia can occur via stimulation of margination by conditions such as malaria, some viral infections, and onset of hemodialysis.[25]

Normally, it takes 14 days for neutrophil production and differentiation in the bone marrow. It is believed that G-CSF, GM-CSF, and IL-3 are important regulatory molecules of neutrophil production (see Fig. 98–5). A healthy adult will produce approximately 1.6 billion neutrophils per kilogram body weight per day.[26] As blood neutrophils are totally replaced at least twice in each 24-hour period, the average circulation time for any one cell is approximately 6 to 12 hours. Most of this removal is thought to be for effector functions in the tissues and not simply an elimination process.

The total number of noncirculating (i.e., storage) neutrophils is more than 15 times the number in blood. Absolute storage cell numbers are subject to alteration by prior exposure to chemotherapy or deficiency in cofactors required for their synthesis (e.g., folate). When conditions call for an acute increase in blood neutrophils, the pattern of cells thus changes to one more similar to that in the marrow (i.e., band concentration increases relative to seg concentration; normal ratio <0.1 to 0.3).[27] This phenomenon, often referred to as a "shift to the left," denotes a circulating neutrophil population made of less mature cells. Infectious processes frequently provoke such a shift, as well as an increased outflow of cells from storage forms in the bone marrow, but extreme cases may require so many granulocytes at the infection site that marrow pools are depleted, resulting in neutropenia. Cytokine expression, and thus hematopoiesis, may be impaired in the elderly, resulting in a reduced ability to tolerate myelosuppressive chemotherapy.[28]

EOSINOPHILS

The typical blood circulation time for an eosinophil is approximately 6 hours, but it may survive weeks within tissues. Cytokines thought to be important in eosinophil production or function include IL-1, IL-3, GM-CSF, G-CSF, and perhaps most important, IL-5. Corticosteroids cause a transient margination of eosinophils and inhibit release of mature cells from the bone marrow.[4]

MONOCYTES AND MACROPHAGES

Both macrophages and T lymphocytes secrete cytokines that stimulate monocytopoiesis.[29] Examples of cytokines that act on relatively mature monocytes include macrophage colony-stimulating factor (M-CSF) and GM-CSF. Blood monocytes have a shorter marrow transit time than neutrophils (6 vs. 13 days, respectively), and there is no monocyte reserve in the marrow.[27] The peripheral blood turnover of these cells is much slower (circulation half-life, 3 days) than for neutrophils; similarly, tissue macrophages are thought to be very long-lived. Macrophages may be able to produce their own progeny as well as attract additional monocytes for differentiation in the local environment.

LYMPHOCYTES

Immature T cells produced in the bone marrow ultimately migrate to the thymus, where they both expand and mature into immunologically competent cells (see Fig. 98–4). A variety of cytokines, including IL-2, IL-4, and IL-7, facilitate lymphopoiesis, whereas others such as transforming growth factor-β may decelerate this process.[30] T lymphocytes are probably the longest lived hematopoietic cell, as there is experimental evidence that the life span of some is more than 10 years.

The term *lymphokine* is used to describe cytokines secreted by T cells. Lymphokines such as IL-2 are important in both activation and proliferation of the immune response, while monokines are also important regulators of lymphocyte development. T and B lymphocytes have important interactions with each other in both lymphocyte development and activation, which seem necessary for immunocompetence. There is some evidence for age-associated reductions in circulating helper and suppressor T cells and B cells.[31]

PLATELETS

Thrombopoiesis is the term used to describe the process of platelet production. The bone marrow manufactures 40,000 platelets/mL of blood each day. Proliferation and differentiation of platelet precursors are thought to be primarily influenced by cytokines such as IL-6, IL-11, leukemia inhibitory factor, and perhaps most specifically, by thrombopoietin (TPO or megakaryocyte growth and development factor; see Fig. 98–6).[32,33] Other hematopoietins that may act in concert producing synergistic effects include IL-3, IL-1, GM-CSF, EPO, and SCF.[34] The platelet survival time is a clinical test that can estimate the rate of platelet turnover.[35] In healthy individuals, this time is 9.5 ± 0.6 days.[36]

ERYTHROCYTES

The normal life span of a RBC is approximately 100 to 120 days, with a circulating cell turnover rate of 1% per day. Thus a typical adult produces approximately 200 billion reticulocytes every day. Condition such as anemia or hypoxemia primarily stimulate the renal peritubula interstitial cells to produce EPO by interaction with the renal oxygen sensor. The degree of elevation in blood EPO concentrations is dependent on the severity of anemia or hypoxemia. This in turn recruits RBC precursors and shortens the normal time for differentiation if adequate cofactors such as iron, folate, and vitamin B_{12} are present. Although the overall time for differentiation is shortened (as is the duration of time that a reticulocyte spends in the marrow), the RBC's blood maturation time is lengthened. The increase in EPO concentrations is relatively quick (within hours), but the effects on marrow transpire over several days. The ultimate increase in RBC mass occurs at an even slower pace, generally over weeks to months (see Fig. 98–3). Multiple other endogenous cytokines are also thought to play a role in either stimulating or inhibiting erythropoiesis by acting on the early progenitors. These include GM-CSF, G-CSF, IL-1, IL-3, IL-6, IL-9, SCF, and some stromal proteins.[21]

Adequate production of RBCs for a degree of anemia is best assessed by evaluation of the number of circulating reticulocytes. Although the normal range is approximately 0.4% to 1.7% of the RBCs, this percentage would obviously be higher in anemic patients with adequate productive capacity. The calculation of a corrected reticulocyte count involves multiplying the percentage of circulating reticulocytes by the hemoglobin concentration and dividing the result by the normal hemoglobin level expected for a healthy patient with similar characteristics. Additional correction accounts for the increased life span of reticulocytes in the peripheral blood, depending directly on the patient's degree of anemia. Figure 98–7 displays correction factors that can be used to accommodate these changes.[37]

Direct assessment of erythropoiesis in the bone marrow can be performed by estimating the myeloid:erythroid cell ratio from a marrow aspirate. The range of the normal adult ratio is 3:1 to 5:1, but changes in erythroid or myeloid production can obviously influence the ratio. RBCs lose flexibility with age and eventually undergo lysis or are phagocytized and removed by the monocyte-macrophage system (primarily via the spleen). Accelerated red cell destruction can be grossly quantitated by determining increases in plasma concentrations of bilirubin and lactate dehydrogenase.[37]

Although clinical laboratories measure RBC concentrations with excellent accuracy, the most useful tool for assessment of the blood's

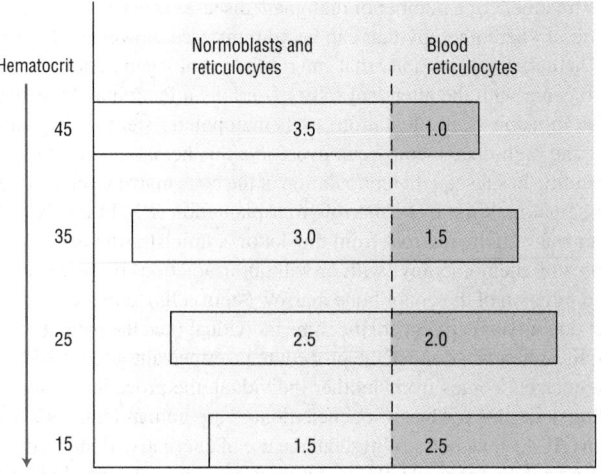

FIGURE 98–7. Correction of hematocrit with the marrow and blood reticulocyte maturation times. With a hematocrit of 45, the blood reticulocytes circulate for 1 day, whereas reduction in hematocrit to 15 results in a 2.5-day circulation time. The numbers found under the blood reticulocyte concentrations can be used as a correction factor in evaluation of reticulocyte concentrations. (From Hillman et al.[37])

oxygen-carrying capacity is the hemoglobin concentration because of the variability in RBC size. The average RBC and hemoglobin concentrations in healthy adult male and female patients are approximately 5.21 and $4.60 \times 10^6/mm^3$, respectively; and 15.7 and 13.8 g/dL, respectively. Variations in normal concentrations will also be evident, depending on age, menstruation status, race, environmental factors, and pregnancy.[38]

DISEASE-ASSOCIATED HEMATOPOIETIC CHANGES

NEUTROPHILS

The usual definition of neutropenia is an absolute neutrophil count below $1,800/mm^3$ in white patients, $1,400/mm^3$ in black patients, and $1,500/mm^3$ for children 1 month to 10 years old. Clinical manifestations of neutropenia (i.e., infection) are not typically evident without other cofactors until the concentration drops below $1,000/mm^3$.[39] Accompanying factors that may influence the risk of infection for a particular patient include skin and mucous membrane integrity; vascular tissue supply; nutritional status; and lymphocytopenia, monocytopenia, or hypogammaglobulinemia. Persistent agranulocytosis ($<500/mm^3$ or no measurable neutrophils) is almost uniformly fatal without the use of supportive antibiotics.

Disorders resulting in defective granulopoiesis can be subdivided into those that result in marrow aplasia or diseases that replace the normal neutrophilic component (see Chap. 102 for drug-induced neutropenia). Diseases associated with granulopoietic suppression include viral infection, tuberculosis, anorexia, autoimmune diseases (e.g., systemic lupus erythematosus), Felty's syndrome (rheumatoid arthritis, splenomegaly, and leukopenia), myelodysplastic syndromes, and leukemias.[39,40] A congenital form of severely defective neutrophil production (Kostmann's syndrome) has been described that is possibly a result of defective regulation of the late-acting hemopoietin G-CSF.[41] Patients with the rare disorder of cyclic neutropenia display periodic wide fluctuations in the WBCs at approximately 3-week intervals that last for 3 to 6 days. Other forms of chronic neutropenias may occur with adequate marrow stores and can be relatively benign in symptomatology.

Neutrophilia is typically defined as an absolute neutrophil count greater than $7,500/mm^3$ of blood and is sometimes referred to as a leukemoid reaction, if extreme.[24] Acute neutrophilia may be a result of emotional or physical stimuli (e.g., exercise, seizures, labor, pain, or temperature changes), infections, inflammation or tissue necrosis, or drugs or toxins (e.g., CSFs, epinephrine, corticosteroids, lithium, vaccines, or endotoxin). Chronic causes of increased neutrophilia include persistent infections, inflammation, malignancies, drugs, metabolic or endocrine disorders, cigarette smoking, hereditary or congenital abnormalities, and myeloproliferative diseases such as polycythemia vera.[24]

EOSINOPHILS

Eosinophilia (absolute count greater than $700/mm^3$) may result from neoplastic processes, parasitic or fungal infections, gastrointestinal disorders, malignancies, dermatitis, granulomatous disorders (e.g., sarcoidosis or Wegener's granulomatosis), or collagen-vascular diseases in addition to the more typical cause, allergic reactions.[42] One mechanism that may be common to several of these etiologic factors is antigenic stimulation of T cells, which produces a cytokine (IL-5) that mediates eosinophil proliferation.[43] Infections may cause eosinopenia; however, its significance is not thought to be of concern in that setting.

BASOPHILS

Basophilia occurs frequently in patients with myeloproliferative disorders and in association with inflammatory reactions and diseases. Viral infections, iron deficiency, or lung cancer can sometimes increase basophil counts. Mastocytosis is usually evident only on analysis of tissue or bone marrow mast cells. Causes include hypersensitivity reactions, malignancy, osteoporosis, and chronic liver or renal disease.

MONOCYTES

Monocytosis ($>800/mm^3$ of blood) occurs with some infections (e.g., tuberculosis, histoplasmosis, toxoplasmosis, bacterial endocarditis, and salmonellosis), collagen vascular diseases (rheumatoid arthritis and systematic lupus erythematosus), gastrointestinal disorders (ulcerative colitis and alcoholic liver disease), leukemias, and up to 60% of nonhematologic malignancies, whereas abnormally low monocyte concentrations occur in patients with hairy cell leukemia or aplastic anemia.[44]

LYMPHOCYTES

Significant reductions in lymphocyte concentration ($<1000/mm^3$ of blood) can be evident without apparent cause or in a variety of diseases, including acute inflammatory disorders, severe uremia, immune deficiency diseases such as systemic lupus erythematosus, chronic infections such as tuberculosis or human immunodeficiency virus (HIV) infection, malignancies, and connective tissue diseases.[45] Lymphocytosis ($>4000/mm^3$) may occur with mononucleosis, pertussis, measles, or chickenpox, and in lymphoid malignancies. A progressive increase in mature lymphocytes may be indicative of chronic lymphocytic leukemia. Increased levels of atypical lymphocytes may occur in patients with infections (e.g., mononucleosis, hepatitis, or cytomegalovirus), allergic reactions, or lymphomas.[46]

PLATELETS

Both qualitative and quantitative platelet disorders have important pathophysiologic consequences. Thrombocytopenia, defined as a platelet count less than 150,000 cells/mm^3, may result from a defect in production, increased sequestration, or accelerated destruction.[47]

Certain stimuli may damage the marrow by reducing the number of megakaryocytes available. Drugs, chemicals, radiation, and infection are among the potential causes of marrow injury. Diseases that produce general bone marrow failure or those that invade the bone marrow may result in thrombocytopenia. Examples of the latter include cancers such as leukemia, lymphoma, myelofibrosis, myelodysplasia, and metastatic solid tumors (breast and prostate cancer), and infections such as those caused by mycobacteria. Suboptimal platelet production may also result from defects in maturation seen with vitamin B_{12} and/or folate deficiency or in congenital syndromes.[48]

Alteration in platelet distribution may also result in thrombocytopenia. Splenomegaly is the most frequent cause of increased platelet sequestration.

Owing to its accelerated destruction of platelets, idiopathic thrombocytopenic purpura (ITP) is a common cause of thrombocytopenia. Antiplatelet antibodies combine with platelets in ITP, thus sensitizing them to removal by the immune system. Accelerated platelet destruction can also occur in patients with connective tissue disorders. Approximately 14% of patients with systemic lupus erythematosus experience thrombocytopenia similar to ITP.

ERYTHROCYTES

Suboptimal erythropoiesis can be classified by changes in the size of RBCs noted on examination of the peripheral blood. Because the excretory and endocrine functions of the kidney usually mirror each other, renal dysfunction can lead to anemia by reduction in EPO production, resulting in a normochromic, normocytic pattern. Other causes of insufficient erythropoiesis include replacement of bone marrow by fibrosis, solid tumors, or leukemia, as well as defects in erythroid maturation. Relative deficiencies in the cofactors required for heme-RBC synthesis such as iron, folate, and vitamin B_{12} may also be important contributors. Structurally, RBC macrocytosis denotes defects in the maturation of the nucleus, whereas microcytosis is indicative of cytoplasmic defects (reduced hemoglobin synthesis). (A detailed description regarding the pathogenesis and treatment of anemic disorders is found in Chap. 99.)

Exaggerated erythropoiesis with increased RBC mass (polycythemia) can be mistaken for a reduction in plasma volume. Symptoms are not always immediately evident, but may progress to reduced tissue oxygenation, thrombosis, and congestive heart failure. The most common cause is hypoxia; alternative causes can be grouped according to their ability to stimulate EPO production. EPO (or a similar cytokine) may be produced in response to genetic alterations or a variety of malignancies, including angioblastoma, hepatomas, and hypernephroma.[49] Polycythemia vera, a malignancy of the bone marrow stem cells, results in an increased sensitivity of RBC precursors to stimulation by EPO and is accompanied in many patients by thrombocytosis and leukocytosis.

CLINICAL USES OF HEMATOPOIETIC CELLS

HEMATOPOIETIC STEM CELL TRANSPLANTATION

High-dose chemotherapy with or without irradiation is beneficial in the treatment of a number of malignant diseases (see Chap. 134). The dose of chemotherapy that can be administered, however, is limited by hematopoietic toxicity that can result in prolonged periods of pancytopenia with the attendant risks of serious infection and bleeding. The infusion (transplantation) of hematopoietic stem cells following the high-dose therapy can overcome this hematopoietic toxicity, resulting in subsequent repopulation of the bone marrow and recovery of hematopoiesis. Bone marrow transplantation (BMT) involves the removal of bone marrow from the donor, administration of intensive doses of chemotherapy (with or without irradiation) to the recipient, and infusion of the donor bone marrow (stem cells) to the recipient. If the donor and recipient are the same individual (i.e., the patient serves as his or her own donor), the procedure is termed autologous BMT. If the marrow comes from another individual, the procedure is termed allogeneic BMT. Most allogeneic donors are human leukocyte antigen (HLA)-matched siblings, but the use of alternative donors such as HLA-matched related volunteer donors or umbilical cord blood cells is increasing.

Allogeneic transplantation is complicated by the immune recognition of host tissues by donor T lymphocytes, resulting in a syndrome called graft-versus-host disease (GVHD). Because immune recognition of tumor cells also occurs (graft-versus-tumor effect), the relapse rates associated with allogeneic transplants are lower than those associated with autologous transplants for similar disease stages. Allogeneic transplantation is commonly used for diseases primarily involving the bone marrow, such as acute and chronic leukemias, aplastic anemia, thalassemia, and severe combined immunodeficiency syndrome.

Autologous transplantation is commonly used in non-Hodgkin's lymphoma, Hodgkin's disease, multiple myeloma, and a relatively small subset of patients with solid tumors. A number of laboratory techniques are evolving to allow the bone marrow harvested for autologous transplantation to expand in the laboratory prior to infusion and to cleanse the marrow of potential malignant cell contamination.

Small numbers of hematopoietic progenitor (stem) cells capable of reconstituting hematopoiesis circulate in the blood under normal circumstances.[50] Commonly referred to as peripheral blood progenitor cells (PBPCs), these circulating progenitor cells increase in number during recovery from myelosuppressive chemotherapy or after treatment with cytokines such as G-CSF or GM-CSF.[16,51] These cells can be collected by a process called leukapheresis and stored for reinfusion following high-dose chemotherapy. Hematopoietic recovery is generally more rapid following rescue with PBPCs as compared with rescue with bone marrow. Potential tumor cell contamination may also be less with PBPC transplants. The use of PBPCs has essentially replaced the use of autologous bone marrow, and allogeneic transplants of PBPCs are becoming more common.

Cytokine-mobilized PBPC transplants from allogeneic donors have been shown to result in more rapid white cell and platelet engraftment and shorter hospital stays than bone marrow transplants.[52] The incidence of acute GVHD is not increased, but there is a significant increase in the incidence of chronic GVHD with PBPC. Relapse rates and overall survival rates are similar with the use of allogeneic PBPC or bone marrow.

Only about one-third of patients who would otherwise be eligible for allogeneic BMT have HLA-matched related donors. One alternative is the use of closely HLA-matched, unrelated donor marrow. The National Marrow Donor Program (NMDP) is a registry of volunteer marrow donors now containing more than 4 million members. By coordinating the activities of a network of donor, collection, and transplant centers, the NMDP facilitates the identification of potential donors and the procurement of marrow. Unrelated donor marrow transplants are associated with an increased incidence of GVHD compared to related donor transplants; however, recent advances in tissue typing and donor matching and GVHD prophylaxis have resulted in comparable overall survival rates for many diseases.

Grafts of PBPCs from unrelated donors are also increasingly used for transplantation. The cells are collected by leukapheresis after mobilization of PBPCs by giving the donor G-CSF. This spares the donor from potential complications related to general or spinal anesthesia and pain associated with bone marrow harvest. Unrelated PBPC transplants are associated with more rapid engraftment compared to unrelated BMT, with no increase in GVHD or relapse rates.[53]

Many patients do not have HLA-matched family members or unrelated donors in the marrow registries. An alternative for these patients is the use of human umbilical cord blood, which contains hematopoietic stem cells capable of reconstituting bone marrow function following high-dose chemotherapy.[54] An almost unlimited number of cord blood donors is potentially available, because the cord and its associated blood are commonly discarded following delivery.

There are cord blood banks in which cord blood cells are HLA-typed, cryopreserved, and made available for transplantation for appropriate recipients. To date, the majority of cord blood progenitor cell transplantations performed have been in children because of the relatively small number of cells available from a cord blood unit, although the number of cord blood transplantations performed in adults is increasing. A major problem with cord blood transplants is a more prolonged period of neutropenia (often greater than 1 month.) This leads to additional infectious complications and associated morbidity. Laboratory methods to expand the number of progenitor cells in cord blood units are under investigation. Cord blood transplants are thought to lead to less GVHD than transplants from matched unrelated bone marrow donors with similar degrees of matching, and they may prove to be an important source of progenitor cells for transplantation in the near future.

The application of allogeneic transplantation has been limited to younger patients without comorbid conditions secondary to the toxicity of the myeloablative preparative regimen and the allogeneic bone marrow graft. Recently, a number of centers have reported successful allogeneic engraftment following nonmyeloablative, immunosuppressive conditioning regimens.[55,56] The goal of this approach is to establish donor hematopoiesis and a graft-versus-tumor effect while minimizing toxicity. These transplants can be offered to older patients and to patients with diminished end-organ function. This approach has also been used for patients with disorders that may be responsive to immune-based therapy, such as renal cell carcinoma.

ADOPTIVE IMMUNOTHERAPY

Experiments involving the administration of immune system cells for the purpose of cancer treatment (adoptive immunotherapy) have been conducted for well over a decade; however, the clinical benefit has only recently been substantiated. As described earlier, nonspecific, total depletion of donor T cells following high-dose chemotherapy and stem cell reinfusion produces fewer graft-versus-host effects, but attenuated anticancer responses. However, it has been shown that careful attention to the T-cell dose and timing of infusion may maximize the potential for beneficial immunologic responses and minimize graft-versus-host effects. It has been found that the administration of allogeneic donor lymphocyte infusions to patients with leukemia relapse following myeloablative stem cell transplantation has anticancer efficacy in diseases such as chronic myelogenous leukemia (65% complete response), acute nonlymphocytic leukemia, or myelodysplastic syndrome (25% complete response).[57] Some of these remissions have prolonged durability. Similar strategies have been utilized in nonmyeloablative stem cell transplantation. The complications of donor lymphocyte infusions include the obvious risk of GVHD, but the condition does not develop in all patients who have clinical benefit. This mode of therapy can also result in marrow aplasia for approximately 20% of patients; however, it is self-limiting or treatable with G-CSF in most cases.

GENE THERAPY

Hematopoietic progenitor cells are the focus of intense research in gene therapy. The self-renewal capacity of these cells makes them an obvious target for delivering corrective genetic information for a variety of both hematologic and metabolic inherited disorders, such as sickle cell anemia, thalassemia, immunodeficiency syndromes, and glycogen storage diseases.

TRANSFUSION AND BLOOD PRODUCT SUPPORT

Advances in blood banking and transfusion support have been critical to the improved outcome of therapy for patients with hematologic and malignant diseases. Platelet transfusions are indicated for the prevention and treatment of bleeding. In general, prophylactic platelet transfusions are not indicated for platelet counts above 10,000 cells/mm^3 unless the patient is febrile or actively bleeding. Platelets are available as pooled random donor concentrates obtained from RBC donations (six to eight donors per transfusion) or single-donor platelets collected by apheresis.

Administration of multiple platelet transfusions increases the risk of developing a platelet-refractory state termed alloimmunization. This effect is thought to be an immune-mediated reaction to HLA antigens on donor platelets or WBC contaminants. A common method of identifying such patients is evaluation of platelet counts within an hour of transfusion. For example, a 1-m^2 person should obtain an increase in platelet concentration between 7,000 and 11,000/mm^3 for each unit of platelet concentrate administered (in the absence of other risk factors such as infection, splenomegaly, etc). The diagnosis can be confirmed by in vitro demonstration of platelet antibodies. The use of leukocyte filters prior to storage of donated platelets or UV irradiation of the product has been shown to decrease the development of alloimmunization and refractoriness to platelet transfusions. Leukocyte filters also decrease the risk of transmission of cytomegalovirus and febrile transfusion reactions. Treatment of alloimmunized patients often entails use of platelets obtained from single donors (to lessen exposure to HLA), or use of HLA-compatible or platelet cross-match–compatible donors. Unfortunately, such approaches are not always effective and additional therapies (plasma exchange or intravenous immunoglobulin) have been added with some limited success.

Packed RBC transfusions are indicated to keep hemoglobin levels above 7 to 8 g/dL to maintain adequate oxygen-carrying capacity. Each unit of packed RBCs should increase the hemoglobin level by approximately 1 g/dL unless active blood loss is evident. RBCs should also be filtered to reduce the risk of nonhemolytic, febrile transfusion reactions. Patients who are candidates for bone marrow transplantation should receive blood products that have been irradiated with 2,500 cGy to prevent transfusion-associated GVHD.

Fresh frozen plasma contains the components of the coagulation system and is indicated for the replacement of deficient coagulation factors II, V, VII, X, XI, and XIII. Factor VIII and IX deficiencies are treated with specific factor concentrates. Fresh frozen plasma is also used for the rapid reversal of warfarin anticoagulation and in the treatment of disseminated intravascular coagulation. Thrombotic thrombocytopenic purpura is treated by means of therapeutic plasma exchange with fresh frozen plasma as the replacement fluid. Cryoprecipitate, which contains factor VIII, von Willebrand's factor, and fibrinogen, is indicated for the treatment of von Willebrand's disease that does not respond to desmopressin acetate, and for fibrinogen replacement (see Chap. 100).

INTRAVENOUS IMMUNOGLOBULIN

Pharmaceutical products containing immunoglobulin for intravenous use in humans are pooled from blood collection in over 1,000 donors for each lot of drug. The high number of donors provides a wide diversity in the capability of the antibodies to react with antigenic targets. Products are similar in content of each IgG subclass; however, the titers against specific antigens vary between manufacturers (as do other pharmaceutical characteristics, such as osmolarity).

The IV administration of immunoglobulin has been used in a variety of hematologic disorders, but for most of these situations, it is still considered experimental or indicated only when other therapeutic options have been exhausted. Patients with deficient immunoglobulin production (e.g., agammaglobulinemia or hypogammaglobulinemia) or function (e.g., chronic lymphocytic leukemia, multiple myeloma, and children with HIV) may benefit from this therapy, with the goal of raising the immunoglobulin G level such that there is less chance for bacterial infection (>500 mg/dL). This approach has other pharmacologic properties as well, including blockade of Fc receptors, modification of complement activation, and modulation of the immune response by anti-idiotypic antibodies.[58] It is also beneficial for patients with ITP who are at high bleeding risk or need higher platelet counts prior to surgery.[59] Posttransplant prophylaxis (approximately 3 months) with Ig given IV is also sometimes used in patients receiving allogeneic hematopoietic stem cell transplantation for prevention of bacterial sepsis and acute GVHD. The IV treatment with Ig may benefit patients whose platelet counts do not increase substantially despite transfusions, owing to the formation of alloantibodies. A number of immunoglobulin products are available that provide more specific immunity toward selected antigens. These pharmaceuticals are generated from individuals who have been exposed to the antigen and thus developed antibody "titers" more specific to the infectious agent. Products include: botulism immunoglobulin, cytomegalovirus immunoglobulin, hepatitis B immunoglobulin, rabies immunoglobulin, respiratory syncytial virus immunoglobulin, tetanus immunoglobulin, and varicella-zoster immunoglobulin.

ABBREVIATIONS

BFU: burst-forming unit
BMT: bone marrow transplantation
CD: cluster of differentiation
CFU: colony-forming unit
CSF: colony-stimulating factor
EPO: erythropoietin
G-CSF: granulocyte colony-stimulating factor
GM-CSF: granulocyte-macrophage colony-stimulating factor
GVHD: graft-versus-host disease
HIV: human immunodeficiency virus
HLA: human leukocyte antigen
IL: interleukin
ITP: idiopathic thrombocytopenic purpura
MCSF: macrophage colony-stimulating
NMDP: National Marrow Donor Program
PBPC: peripheral blood progenitor cell
RBC: red blood cell
SCF: stem cell factor
TPO: thrombopoietin
WBC: white blood cells

Review Questions and other resources can be found at *www.pharmacotherapyonline.com*.

REFERENCES

1. Abboud EN, Lichtman MA. Structure of the marrow and the hematopoietic microenvironment. In: Beutler E, Lichtman MA, Coller BS, et al, eds. Williams Hematology, 6th ed. New York, McGraw-Hill, 2001:29.

2. Lehrer RI, Ganz T, Selsted ME, et al. Neutrophils in human diseases. N Engl J Med 1987;317:687–694.

3. Lieschke GJ, Burgess AW. Granulocyte colony-stimulating factor and granulocyte-macrophage colony-stimulating factor. N Engl J Med 1992;327:28–35.

4. Weller PF. The immunobiology of eosinophils. N Engl J Med 1991;324:1110–1118.

5. Kitamura Y, Kasugai T, Arizono N, Matsuda H. Development of mast cells and basophils: processes and regulation mechanisms. Am J Med Sci 1993;306:185–191.

6. Bainton DF. Morphology of neutrophils, eosinophils and basophils. In: Beutler E, Lichtman MA, Coller BS, et al, eds. Williams Hematology, 6th ed. New York, McGraw-Hill, 2001:729.

7. Johnston RB. Monocytes and macrophages. N Engl J Med 1988;318:747–752.

8. Kipps TJ. Functions of B lymphocytes and plasma cells in immunoglobulin production. In: Beutler E, Lichtman MA, Coller BS, et al, eds. Williams Hematology, 6th ed. New York, McGraw-Hill, 2001:937.

9. Kipps TJ. Functions of T lymphocytes: T-cell receptors for antigen. In: Beutler E, Lichtman MA, Coller BS, et al, eds. Williams Hematology, 6th ed. New York, McGraw-Hill, 2001:949.

10. Thompson AR, Harker LA. Manual of Hemostasis and Thrombosis, 3rd ed. Philadelphia, FA Davis, 1983:47.

11. Mustard JF, Packham MA, Kinlough-Rathbone RL. Platelets, blood flow, and the vessel wall. Circulation 1990;81(Suppl 1):I40–I41.

12. Gordon MY. Physiological mechanisms in BMT and haematopoiesis-revisited. Bone Marrow Transplant 1993;11:193–197.

13. Verfaillie CM. Anatomy and physiology of hematopoiesis. In: Hoffman R, Benz EJ, Shattil SJ, et al, eds. Hematology—Basic Principles and Practice. New York, Churchill Livingstone, 2000:139.

14. Greenberger J. The hematopoietic microenvironment. Crit Rev Oncol Hematol 1991;11:65–84.

15. To LB, Shepperd KM, Haylock DN, et al. Single high doses of cyclophosphamide enable the collection of high numbers of hematopoietic stem cells from the peripheral blood. Exp Hematol 1990;18:442–447.

16. Peters WP, Rosner G, Ross M, et al. Comparative effects of granulocyte-macrophage colony-stimulating factor (GM-CSF) and granulocyte colony-stimulating (G-CSF) factor on priming peripheral blood progenitor cells for use with autologous bone marrow after high-dose chemotherapy. Blood 1993;81:1709–1719.

17. Spangrude GJ, Heimfeld S, Wessman IL. Purification and characterization of mouse hematopoietic stem cells. Science 1988;241:58–62.

18. Williams N, Levine RF. The origin, development, and regulation of megakaryocytes. Br J Hematol 1982;52:173–180.

19. Hoffman R. Regulation of megakaryocytopoiesis. Blood 1989;74:1196–1212.

20. Papayannopoulou T, Abkowitz J, D'Andrea A. Biology of erythropoiesis, erythroid differentiation, and maturation. In: Hoffman R, Benz EJ, Shattil SJ, et al, eds. Hematology—Basic Principles and Practice. New York, Churchill Livingstone, 2000:202.

21. McGuire MJ, Spivak JL. Erythropoiesis. In: Anderson KC, Ness PM, eds. Scientific Basis of Transfusion Medicine—Implications for Clinical Practice. Philadelphia, WB Saunders, 1994:1.

22. Ogawa M. Differentiation and proliferation of hematopoietic stem cells. Blood 1993;81:2844–2853.

23. Moore MAS. Does stem cell exhaustion result from combining hematopoietic growth factors with chemotherapy? If so, how do we prevent it? Blood 1992;80:3–7.

24. Dale DC. Neutrophilia and neutrophilia. In: Beutler E, Lichtman MA, Coller BS, et al, eds. Williams Hematology, 6th ed. New York: McGraw-Hill, 2001:823.

25. Coates T, Baehner R. Leukocytosis and leukopenia. In: Hoffman R, Benz EJ, Shattil SJ, et al, eds. Hematology—Basic Principles and Practice. New York, Churchill Livingstone, 1991:552.

26. Gabrilove J. Granulopoiesis. In: Anderson KC, Ness PM, eds. Scientific Basis of Transfusion Medicine—Implications for Clinical Practice. Philadelphia, WB Saunders, 1994:17.

27. Rosenthal DS. Hematologic manifestations of infectious disease. In: Hoffman R, Benz EJ, Shattil SJ, et al, eds. Hematology—Basic Principles and Practice. New York: Churchill Livingstone, 1991:2420.

28. Rothstein G. Hematopoiesis in the aged: a model of hematopoietic dysregulation? Blood 1993;82:2601–2604.

29. Bagby GC, Heinrich MC. Growth factors, cytokines, and the control of hematopoiesis. In: Hoffman R, Benz EJ, Shattil SJ, et al, eds. Hematology—Basic Principles and Practice. New York, Churchill Livingstone, 2001:154.

30. Jordan SC. Cytokines and lymphocytes. In: Kunkel SL, Remick DG, eds. Cytokines in Health and Disease. New York, Marcel Dekker, 1992:309.

31. Yamashiki M, Nishimura A, Kosaka Y, James SP. Two-color analysis of peripheral lymphocyte surface antigens in inherently healthy adults. J Clin Lab Anal 1994;8:22–26.

32. Du XX, Williams DA. Interleukin-11: a multifunctional growth factor derived from the hematopoietic microenvironment. Blood 1994;83:2023–2030.

33. Metcalf D. Thrombopoietin—at last. Nature 1994;369:519–520.

34. Gordon MS, Hoffman R. Growth factors affecting human thrombocytopoiesis: potential agents for the treatment of thrombocytopenia. Blood 1992;80:302–307.

35. Shulman NR, Jordan JV Jr. Platelet kinetics. In: Colman RW, Hirsh J, Marder VJ, Saltzman EW, eds. Hemostasis and Thrombosis. Basic Principles and Clinical Practice, 2nd ed. Philadelphia, JP Lippincott, 1987:341–351.

36. Harker LA, Finch CA. Thrombokinetics in man. J Clin Invest 1969;48:963–974.

37. Hillman RS, Finch CA. Red Cell Manual. Philadelphia, FA Davis, 1996:59.

38. Glassman AB. Anemia: diagnosis and clinical considerations. In: Harmening DM, ed. Clinical Hematology and Fundamentals of Hemostasis, 2nd ed. Philadelphia, FA Davis, 1992:54.

39. Lichtman MA. Classification and clinical manifestations of neutrophil disorders. In: Beutler E, Lichtman MA, Coller BS, et al, eds. Williams Hematology, 6th ed. New York, McGraw-Hill, 2001:817.

40. Malech HL, Gallin JI. Neutrophils in human disease. N Engl J Med 1987;317:687–694.

41. Dong F, Hoefsloot LH, Schelen AM, et al. Identification of a nonsense mutation in the G-CSF receptor in severe congenital neutropenia. Proc Natl Acad Sci USA 1994;91:4480–4484.

42. Wardlaw AJ, Kay AB. Eosinophils and their disorders. In: Beutler E, Lichtman MA, Coller BS, et al, eds. Williams Hematology, 6th ed. New York, McGraw-Hill, 2001:785.

43. Sanderson CJ. Interleukin-5, eosinophils and disease. Blood 1992;79:3101–3109.

44. Lichtman MA. Classification and clinical manifestations of disorders of monocytes and macrophages. In: Beutler E, Lichtman MA, Coller BS, et al, eds. Williams Hematology, 6th ed. New York, McGraw-Hill, 2001:877.

45. Williams WJ. Lymphocytosis and lymphocytopenia. In: Beutler E, Lichtman MA, Coller BS, et al, eds. Williams Hematology, 6th ed. New York, McGraw-Hill, 2001:969.

46. Gay JC, Athens JW. Variations of leukocytes in disease. In: Lee GR, Foerster J, Lukens J, et al, eds. Wintrobe's Clinical Hematology, 10th ed. Baltimore, Williams & Wilkins, 1999:1836.

47. Rutherford CJ, Frenkel EP. Thrombocytopenia: issues in diagnosis and therapy. Med Clin North Am 1994;78:555–575.

48. Seligsohn U, Coller BS. Classification, clinical manifestations, and evaluation of disorders of hemostasis. In: Beutler E, Lichtman MA, Coller BS, et al, eds. Williams Hematology, 6th ed. New York, McGraw-Hill, 2001:1471.

49. Tabbara IA. Erythropoietin biology and clinical applications. Arch Intern Med 1993;153:298–304.

50. Kessinger A, Armitage JO, Landmark JD, et al. Autologous peripheral hematopoietic stem cell transplantation restores hematopoietic function following marrow ablative therapy. Blood 1988;71:723–727.

51. To LB, Shepperd KM, Haylock DN, et al. Single high doses of cyclophosphamide enable the collection of high numbers of hematopoietic cells from the peripheral blood. Exp Hematol 1990;18:442–447.

52. Champlin RE, Schmitz N, Horowitz MM, et al. Blood stem cells compared with bone marrow as a source of hematopoietic cells for allogeneic transplantation. Blood 2000;95:3702–3709.

53. Ringden O, Remberger M, Runde V, et al. Peripheral blood stem cell transplantation from unrelated donors: a comparison with marrow transplantation. Blood 1999;94:455–464.

54. Auerbach AD, Liu Q, Ghosh R, et al. Prenatal identification of potential donors for umbilical cord blood transplantation for Fanconi anemia. Transfusion 1990;30:682–687.

55. Slavin S, Nagler A, Naparstek E, et al. Nonmyeloablative stem cell transplantation and cell therapy as an alternative to conventional bone marrow transplantation with lethal cytoreduction for the treatment of malignant and nonmalignant hematologic diseases. Blood 1998;91:756–763.

56. Khouri IF, Keating M, Korbing M, et al. Transplant-lite: induction of graft-versus-malignancy using fludarabine-based nonablative chemotherapy and allogeneic blood progenitor-cell transplantation as treatment for lymphoid malignancies. J Clin Oncol 1999;16:2817–2824.

57. Baron F, Beguin Y. Adoptive immunotherapy with donor lymphocyte infusions after allogeneic HPC transplantation. Transfusion 2000;4: 468–476.

58. Otten A, Bossuyt PMM, Vermeulen M, Brand A. Intravenous immunoglobulin treatment in hematological diseases. Eur J Haematol 1998; 60:73–85.

59. George JN, Woolf SH, Gary E, et al. Idiopathic thrombocytopenic purpura: a practice guideline developed by explicit methods for the American Society of Hematology. Blood 1996;88:3–40.

99

ANEMIAS

Beata Ineck, Barbara J. Mason, and E. Gregory Thompson

Learning Objectives and other resources can be found at *www.pharmacotherapyonline.com.*

KEY CONCEPTS

1 Anemias are a group of diseases characterized by a decrease in either the hemoglobin (Hgb) or the volume of red blood cells (RBCs), which results in decreased oxygen-carrying capacity of the blood.

2 Anemias are often a sign of underlying pathology. Therefore a rapid diagnosis of the cause of the anemia is essential.

3 Patients with acute-onset anemias are most likely to present with tachycardia, light-headedness, and dyspnea; those with chronic anemia often present with weakness, fatigue, headache, vertigo, faintness, sensitivity to cold, pallor, and loss of skin tone.

4 Iron deficiency anemia (IDA) is characterized by decreased levels of ferritin (most sensitive marker) and serum iron, as well as decreased transferrin saturation; the Hgb and hematocrit (Hct) fall late in the disease. Total iron-binding capacity (TIBC) is increased. RBC morphology includes hypochromia and microcytosis. Most patients with IDA are adequately treated with oral ferrous (Fe^{2+}) sulfate therapy, although parenteral iron therapy is necessary in select patient populations.

5 Vitamin B_{12} deficiency, a macrocytic anemia, can be due to inadequate intake, decreased absorption, or inadequate utilization. Anemia caused by a lack of intrinsic factor, resulting in decreased vitamin B_{12} absorption, is called pernicious anemia. Vitamin B_{12} levels and the reticulocyte count are usually low. Neurologic symptoms are often present. Oral or parenteral therapy may be used for replacement therapy.

6 Folic acid deficiency, a macrocytic anemia, results from inadequate intake, decreased absorption, hyperutilization, or inadequate utilization. Treatment consists of the oral administration of folic acid, even in patients with absorption problems. Adequate folic acid intake is essential in women of childbearing years to decrease the risk of neural tube defects in their children.

7 Anemia of chronic disease (ACD) is a diagnosis of exclusion. It results from chronic inflammation, infection, or malignancy, and can occur as early as 1 to 2 months after the onset of these processes. The serum iron level is usually decreased, but in contrast to IDA, the serum ferritin concentration is normal or increased and TIBC is usually decreased. Treatment is aimed at correcting the underlying pathology.

8 Anemia is a common complication in critically ill patients and is almost universally found in this patient population. Contributing factors include sepsis, frequent blood samples, surgical blood loss, immune-mediated functional iron deficiency, decreased erythropoietin (EPO) production, reduced RBC life span, and gastrointestinal bleeding. Low serum iron, TIBC, and a low iron:TIBC ratio result. Serum ferritin is normal to high. The role of EPO in treatment is yet to be defined.

9 One of the most prevalent clinical problems observed in the elderly is anemia, although it is not an inevitable outcome of aging. The anemia is associated with an increased risk of mortality, poor health, and decreased physical functioning. Those with iron deficiency may have concurrent folic acid or vitamin B_{12} deficiency.

10 IDA is a leading cause of infant morbidity and mortality in the world. The age of the child can yield some clues to the etiology of the anemia. Age- and sex-adjusted norms need to be utilized in interpretation of lab results in pediatric patients. Primary prevention of IDA is the goal. A therapeutic trial of oral iron is the standard of care. EPO may be used in anemia of prematurity (AOP).

11 Hemolytic anemia results in decreased survival time of RBCs secondary to destruction in the spleen or circulation. Hemolytic anemias are normocytic and normochromic, with increased levels of reticulocytes, lactate dehydrogenase, and indirect bilirubin. Treatment is directed towards correcting or controlling the underlying pathology.

This chapter will provide an overview of anemia. This first section will present definitions and classification systems. A review of basic aspects of erythropoiesis, followed by laboratory evaluation of the anemia patient will then be discussed. The general similarities in the clinical presentation of the anemic patient will be presented in the text.

INTRODUCTION

According to the World Health Organization, anemia is second only to tuberculosis as the world's most prevalent and costly public health issue. Anemia defined as Hgb <13 g/dL in men or <12 g/dL in women (as recommended by the World Health Organization) occurs in

TABLE 99–1. Classification Systems for Anemias

I. Morphology
  Macrocytic anemias
    Megaloblastic anemias
      Vitamin B_{12} deficiency
      Folic acid deficiency anemia
  Microcytic, hypochromic anemias
    Iron deficiency anemia
    Genetic anomaly
      Sickle cell anemia
      Thalassemia
      Other hemoglobinopathies (abnormal hemoglobins)
  Normocytic anemias
    Recent blood loss
    Hemolysis
    Bone marrow failure
    Anemia of chronic disease
    Renal failure
    Endocrine disorders
    Myeloplastic anemias
II. Etiology
  Deficiency
    Iron
    Vitamin B_{12}
    Folic acid
    Pyridoxine
  Central—caused by impaired bone marrow function
    Anemia of chronic disease
    Anemia of the elderly
    Malignant bone marrow disorders
  Peripheral
    Bleeding (hemorrhage)
    Hemolysis (hemolytic anemias)
III. Pathophysiology
  Excessive blood loss
    Recent hemorrhage
    Trauma
    Peptic ulcer

  Gastritis
  Hemorrhoids
Chronic hemorrhage
  Vaginal bleeding
  Peptic ulcer
  Intestinal parasites
  Aspirin and other nonsteroidal anti-inflammatory agents
Excessive RBC destruction
  Extracorpuscular (outside the cell) factors
    RBC antibodies
    Drugs
    Physical trauma to RBC (artifical valves)
    Excessive sequestration in the spleen
  Intracorpuscular factors
    Heredity
    Disorders of hemoglobin synthesis
Inadequate production of mature RBCs
  Deficiency of nutrients (B_{12}, folic acid, iron, protein)
  Deficiency of erythroblasts
    Aplastic anemia
    Isolated (often transient) erythroblastopenia
    Folic acid antagonists
    Antibodies
  Conditions with infiltration of bone marrow
    Lymphoma
    Leukemia
    Myelofibrosis
    Carcinoma
  Endocrine abnormalities
    Hypothyroidism
    Adrenal insufficiency
    Pituitary insufficiency
  Chronic renal disease
  Chronic inflammatory disease
    Granulomatous diseases
    Collagen vascular diseases
  Hepatic disease

RBC, red blood cell.

approximately 3.4 million Americans based on self-reported data from the National Center for Health Statistics. The highest prevalence is in women, African-Americans, the elderly, and low-income persons. Laboratory data from the second National Health and Nutrition Examination Survey (NHANES) reports anemia prevalence as 5.7% in infants, 5.9% in teenage girls, 5.8% in young women, and 4.4% in elderly men.[1] Prevalence data is confounded by the lack of a standardized definition of anemia. Since no guidelines for screening for the presence of anemia in the elderly exist, the incidence of anemia may be even greater than suspected.[2]

There is increasing evidence that anemia is not an innocent by-stander. It appears to have an impact on both length and quality of life.[3] Retrospective and observational studies in hemodialysis patients and congestive heart failure patients suggest that anemia is an independent risk factor for mortality.[4] In addition, anemia significantly influences morbidity, as shown in patients with end-stage renal disease, chronic kidney disease, and congestive heart failure.[5] The data regarding quality of life in anemic patients stems mainly from cancer patients.[6] The effect of treatment of anemia on patient outcomes needs to be the focus of research with each specific type of anemia. Global goals of treatment for anemic patients are to alleviate signs and symptoms, correct the underlying etiology, and prevent recurrence of anemia.

Anemias are a group of diseases characterized by a decrease in either Hgb or RBCs, resulting in reduced oxygen-carrying capacity of the blood. Anemias can result from inadequate RBC production, increased RBC destruction, accelerated loss of RBC mass, or they can be a manifestation of a host of systemic disorders such as infection, chronic renal disease, or malignancy. Since anemias are often a sign of underlying pathology, a rapid diagnosis of the cause of the anemia is essential.

Anemias can be classified on the basis of the morphology of the RBCs, etiology, or pathophysiology. Table 99–1 gives some examples of anemias in these classifications. IDA, ACD, and anemias associated with vitamin B_{12} and folic acid deficiency will be the emphasis of this chapter. Characteristic changes in the size of the RBC seen in erythrocyte indices can be the first step in the morphologic classification and understanding of the anemia.

Anemias are classified by RBC size as macrocytic, normocytic, or microcytic. Vitamin B_{12} deficiency and folic acid deficiency are both macrocytic anemias. An example of a microcytic anemia is iron deficiency, whereas a normocytic anemia may be the result of recent blood loss or chronic disease. In many patients more than one anemia and etiology may occur at the same time. Inclusion of the underlying cause of the anemia makes diagnostic terminology easier to understand (e.g., microcytic anemia secondary to iron deficiency).

Microcytic anemias are pathogenically a result of a quantitative deficiency in Hgb synthesis, usually due to iron deficiency or impaired iron utilization. This results in the formation of erythrocytes containing insufficient Hgb. Microcytosis and hypochromia are the morphologic abnormalities that provide evidence of impaired Hgb synthesis. Macrocytic anemias can be divided into megaloblastic and nonmegaloblastic anemias. The type of macrocytic anemia can be distinguished microscopically with a peripheral blood smear examination. Megaloblasts are distinctive cells that express a biochemical abnormality of retarded DNA synthesis, resulting in unbalanced cell growth. Megaloblastic anemias affect all hematopoietic cell lines. The most common cause of megaloblastic anemia is vitamin B_{12} and/or folate deficiency. Nonmegaloblastic macrocytic anemias may be due to membrane cholesterol defects, so white blood cells and platelets may look normal. Nonmegaloblastic anemias do not have a common pathogenic mechanism and may be macrocytic or normocytic. This type of macrocytic anemia may be due to etiologies such as liver disease, hypothyroidism, hemolytic anemia, and alcoholism.

MATURATION AND DEVELOPMENT OF RED BLOOD CELLS

In adults, RBCs are formed in the marrow of the vertebrae, ribs, sternum, clavicle, pelvic (iliac) crest, and the proximal epiphyses of the long bones. In children, most bone marrow space is hematopoietically active to meet increased RBC requirements.

In normal RBC formation, a pluripotent stem cell yields an erythroid burst-forming unit. EPO and cytokines such as interleukin-3 and granulocyte-macrophage colony-stimulating factor stimulate this cell to form an erythroid colony-forming unit in the marrow. The erythroid colony-forming unit is very sensitive to EPO and produces proerythroblasts. Subsequent divisions yield basophilic erythroblasts, polychromatic erythroblasts, pyknotic erythroblasts, reticulocytes, and finally an erythrocyte. During this process, the nucleus becomes smaller with each division, finally disappearing in the normal erythrocyte (Fig. 99–1). Hgb and iron are incorporated into the gradually maturing RBC, which is eventually released from the marrow into the circulating blood as a reticulocyte. The maturation process usually takes about 1 week. Several days are then necessary for the reticulocyte to lose its nucleus and become an erythrocyte. The circulating erythrocyte is a non-nucleated, nondividing cell. More than 90% of the protein content of the erythrocyte consists of the oxygen-carrying molecule Hgb. Erythrocytes compose 40% to 50% of the total blood volume and have a normal survival time of 120 days.

STIMULATION OF ERYTHROPOIESIS

The hormone EPO, 90% of which is produced by the kidneys, initiates and stimulates the production of RBCs. Erythropoiesis is driven by a feedback loop. The main mechanism of action of EPO is to prevent apoptosis, or programmed cell death, of erythroid precursor cells and to allow their proliferation and subsequent maturation. A decrease in tissue oxygen concentration signals the kidneys to increase the production and release of EPO into the plasma, which (1) stimulates stem cells to differentiate into proerythroblasts, (2) increases the rate of mitosis, (3) increases the release of reticulocytes from the marrow, and (4) induces Hgb formation. In normal circumstances, the RBC mass is kept at an almost constant level by EPO matching new erythrocyte production to the natural rate of loss of RBCs. Accelerated Hgb synthesis makes it possible to achieve the critical Hgb concentration necessary for RBCs to mature more rapidly, and a feedback mechanism stops further RBC nucleic acid synthesis, causing an earlier release of reticulocytes. Early appearance of large quantities of reticulocytes in the peripheral circulation (reticulocytosis) is another indication of increased RBC production.

SYNTHESIS OF HEMOGLOBIN

Hgb consists of a protein component with two α and two β chains; each chain is linked to a heme group consisting of a porphyrin ring structure with an iron atom chelated at its center, which is capable of binding oxygen. The initial step in the synthesis of heme from the substrate succinyl CoA and glycine requires the presence of pyridoxine phosphate (vitamin B_6) as a catalyst. Following its synthesis in the cytoplasmic mitochondria of the RBC, heme diffuses into the extra-mitochondrial space, combines with the completed α and β chains, and forms Hgb.

Under normal conditions, the body produces approximately 6.25 g of Hgb daily. If the bone marrow functions at maximal capacity, the normal RBC survival time of 120 days can decrease to 18 to 20 days before an anemia develops. When hemolytic destruction of RBCs exceeds marrow production capacity and anemia develops, the Hgb value decreases to a steady-state level at which production is equal to destruction. Hgb values in these hemolytic anemias, such as sickle cell anemia, (see Chap. 101 on sickle cell anemia) will remain stable unless other factors further shorten the RBC life span.

The affinity of Hgb for oxygen is influenced by three intracellular components and by temperature. Increasing hydrogen ion concentration (decreasing pH), carbon dioxide, and 2,3-bisphosphoglycerate, together with increased temperature, all enhance the ability of Hgb to release oxygen into tissue by decreasing oxygen affinity. This physiologic compensation also increases plasma volume which can increase tissue perfusion.

BODY IRON

The normal iron content of the body is about 3 to 4 g. Approximately 2.5 g of the iron exists in the form of Hgb, whereas about 400 mg

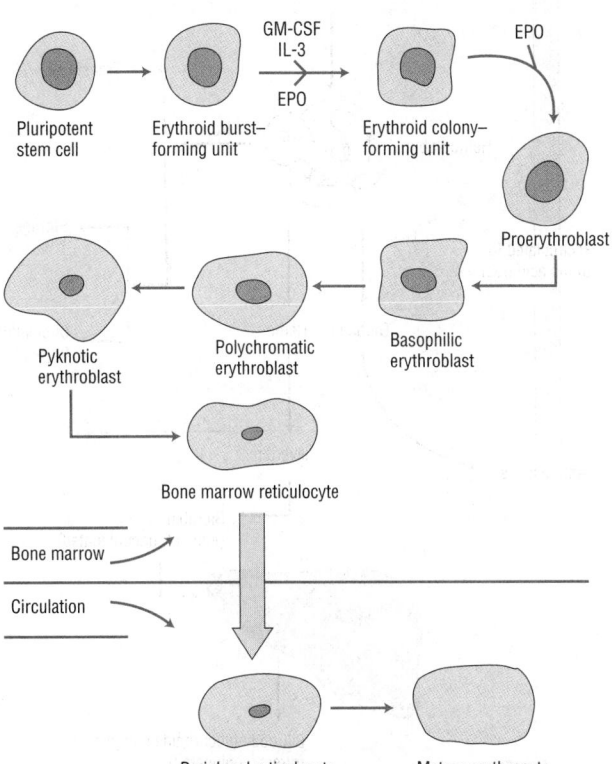

FIGURE 99–1. Erythrocyte maturation sequence. EPO, erythropoietin; GM-CSF, granulocyte-macrophage colony-stimulating factor; IL-3, interleukin-3.

exists as iron-containing proteins such as myoglobin and cytochromes. Another 3 to 7 mg of iron is bound to transferrin in plasma, while the remaining iron exists as storage iron in the form of ferritin or hemosiderin. Due to the toxicity of inorganic iron, the body has an intricate system for iron absorption, transport, storage, assimilation, and elimination.

ABSORPTION OF IRON

Iron is best absorbed in its ferrous (Fe^{2+}) form. The normal daily Western diet contains approximately 12 to 15 mg of iron, mainly in the ferric (Fe^{3+}) nonabsorbed form. After being ionized by stomach acid and then reduced to the Fe^{2+} state, iron is absorbed primarily in the duodenum, and to a smaller extent in the jejunum, via intestinal mucosal cell uptake. Subsequently, it is transferred across the cell into the plasma.[7] Iron absorption is not directly correlated to iron intake. As physiologic iron levels decrease, gastrointestinal absorption of iron increases.

The daily recommended dietary allowance for iron is 8 mg in adult males and postmenopausal females, and 18 mg in menstruating females. Children require more iron due to growth-related increases in blood volume, and pregnant women have an increased iron demand brought about by fetal development. However, iron overload does not occur, as only the amount of iron lost per day is absorbed. The amount of iron absorbed from food depends on the body stores, the rate of RBC production, the type of iron provided in the diet, and the presence of any substances that may enhance or inhibit iron absorption.

Heme iron, found in meat, fish, and poultry, is about three times more absorbable than the nonheme iron found in vegetables and dietary supplements. Forty percent of iron from animal sources is in the heme form.[7] Heme and nonheme iron are absorbed by different receptors on the intestinal mucosa. The iron content of some foods high in iron is shown in Table 99–2. Gastric acid and other dietary components such as ascorbic acid increase the absorption of nonheme iron. Dietary components that form insoluble complexes with iron (phytates, tannates, and phosphates) decrease absorption.[8] Phytates, a natural component of grains, brans, and some vegetables, can form poorly absorbed complexes and partially explain the increased prevalence of IDA in poorer countries, where grains and vegetables compose a disproportionate amount of the normal diet, with the more readily absorbable heme iron lacking in the diet. Though the mechanism is unknown, calcium inhibits absorption of both heme and nonheme iron. Epidemiologic studies show a correlation between milk intake and prevalence of iron deficiency.[9] Finally, because gastric acid improves iron absorption, patients who have undergone a gastrectomy or have achlorhydria will have decreased iron absorption.

INCORPORATION OF IRON INTO HEME

A specific plasma transport protein called transferrin delivers iron to the bone marrow for incorporation into the Hgb molecule. Transferrin enters cells by binding to transferrin receptors, which circulate and then attach to cells needing iron. Conversely, there are fewer transferrin receptors on the surface of cells not currently in need of iron, thus preventing iron-replete cells from receiving excess iron.[10]

Circulating transferrin is normally about 30% saturated with iron. Transferrin delivers extra iron to other body storage sites, such as the liver, marrow, and spleen, for later use. This iron is stored within macrophages as ferritin or hemosiderin. Ferritin consists of a Fe^{3+} hydroxyphosphate core surrounded by a protein shell called apoferritin. Hemosiderin can be described as compacted ferritin molecules with an even greater iron:protein shell ratio. Physiologically it is a more stable, but less available, form of storage iron.

NORMAL DESTRUCTION OF RED BLOOD CELLS

Phagocytic breakdown destroys older blood cells, primarily in the spleen, but also in the marrow (Fig. 99–2). Amino acids from the globin chains return to an amino acid pool; heme oxygenase acts on the porphyrin heme structure to form biliverdin and to release its iron. Iron returns to the iron pool to be reused while biliverdin is further catabolized to bilirubin. The bilirubin is then released into the

TABLE 99–2. Good Sources of Iron

Food	Serving Size	Amount (mg)
Total cereal	1 cup	18
Grape-nuts cereal	1 cup	18
Instant Cream of Wheat	1 cup	8.2
Instant plain oatmeal	1 cup	6.7
Wheat germ	1 oz.	2.6
Broccoli	1 medium stalk	2.1
Baked potato	1 medium	2.7
Raw tofu	1/2 cup	4
Lentils	1/2 cup	3.3
Beef chuck	3 ounces	3.2

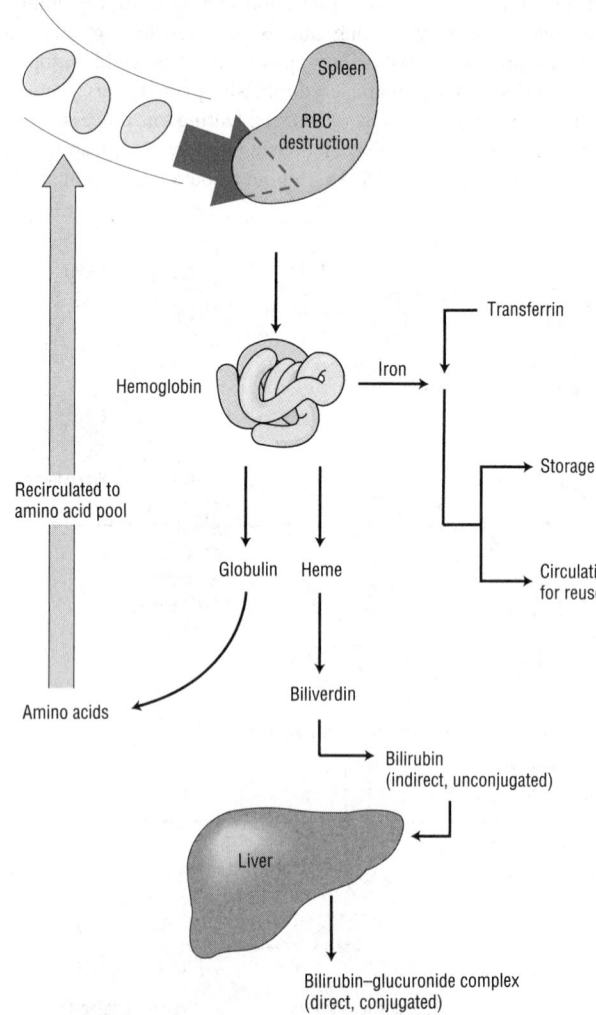

FIGURE 99–2. Destruction of red blood cells (RBCs).

plasma where it binds to albumin and is transported to the liver for glucuronide conjugation and excretion via bile. If the liver is unable to perform the conjugation, as seen with intrinsic liver disease or oversaturation of conjugation enzymes by excessive cell hemolysis, the result is an elevated indirect (unconjugated) bilirubin. Should there be an obstruction in the biliary excretion pathway for the already conjugated bilirubin, an elevated direct bilirubin would result. Comparison of direct and indirect bilirubin values helps to determine if the defect in bilirubin clearance occurs before or after bilirubin enters the liver. The Hgb in RBCs, which is destroyed by intravascular hemolysis, becomes attached to haptoglobin and is carried back to the marrow for processing in the normal manner.

DIAGNOSIS OF ANEMIA

GENERAL PRESENTATION

History, physical examination and laboratory testing are utilized in the evaluation of the anemic patient. The work-up determines if the patient is bleeding, if there is evidence for increased RBC destruction, if the bone marrow is suppressed, or if the patient is iron deficient and if so why. A previous abnormal blood exam may suggest a congenital problem. Occupation, social habits, travel history, and diet are all important in identifying causes of anemia. Additionally, information about concurrent nonhematologic disease states and a drug ingestion history are essential when evaluating the cause of the anemia (see Chap. 102, on drug-induced hematologic disorders). Past history of blood transfusions, liver disease, and exposure to toxic chemicals should also be obtained.

Anemias are a sign of disease, so clinical presentation may relate to the underlying pathology. The presenting signs and symptoms of anemias depend on the rate of development and the age of the patient, as well as the cardiovascular status of the patient. Severity of symptoms does not always correlate with the degree of the anemia.[11] If the myocardium is healthy and the anemia evolves slowly, the combined effects of the shift in the oxygen dissociation curve and increased cardiac output may allow acclimatization at very low Hgb concentrations. Mild anemia is often associated with no clinical symptoms and is often found incidentally upon obtaining a complete blood count (CBC) for other reasons. The signs and symptoms in elderly patients with anemia may be attributed to their age or concomitant disease states. Levels of Hgb tolerated by younger persons may not be tolerated by the elderly. Premature infants with anemia may be asymptomatic or have tachycardia, poor weight gain, increased supplemental oxygen needs, or increased episodes of apnea or bradycardia.

PRESENTATION OF ANEMIA

GENERAL

- Patients may be asymptomatic or have vague complaints.
- Patients with vitamin B_{12} deficiency may develop neurologic consequences.
- In ACD, the signs and symptoms of the underlying disorder often overshadow those of the anemia.

SYMPTOMS

- Decreased exercise tolerance
- Fatigue
- Dizziness
- Irritability
- Weakness
- Palpitations
- Vertigo
- Shortness of breath
- Chest pain
- Neurologic symptoms such as numbness and paresthesias often present in vitamin B_{12} deficiency.

SIGNS

- Tachycardia
- Pale appearance (most prominent in conjunctivae)
- Decreased mental acuity
- Increased intensity of some cardiac valvular murmurs
- Diminished vibratory sense in vitamin B_{12} deficiency

LABORATORY TESTS

- Hemoglobin, hematocrit, and RBC indices may remain normal early in the disease and then decrease as the anemia progresses.
- Low serum iron in IDA and ACD
- Ferritin levels are low in IDA and normal to increased in ACD.
- High TIBC in IDA, low TIBC in ACD
- MCV elevated in vitamin B_{12} deficiency and /folate deficiency
- Vitamin B_{12} and folate levels are low in their respective types of anemia.
- Homocysteine elevated in vitamin B_{12} deficiency and folate deficiency
- Methylmalonic acid elevated in vitamin B_{12} deficiency

OTHER DIAGNOSTIC TESTS

- Schilling test determines deficiency in intrinsic factor.
- Bone marrow testing with iron staining can indicate low iron levels in IDA and an abundance of iron in ACD.

Anemia of rapid onset is most likely to present with cardiorespiratory symptoms such as tachycardia, palpitations, angina, hypotension, light-headedness, and breathlessness due to decreased oxygen delivery to tissues or from hypovolemia in those with acute bleeding. With severe intravascular blood volume loss, peripheral vasoconstriction and central vasodilation preserve blood flow to vital organs. Over time systemic small vessel dilation increases tissue oxygenation. Vascular compensation results in decreased systemic vascular resistance, increased cardiac output, and tachycardia. With acute hemolysis and fall in RBC mass, there is some decrease in blood volume, but not in plasma volume.

If the onset is more chronic in nature, the presenting symptoms may include fatigue, weakness, headache, symptoms of heart failure, vertigo, faintness, sensitivity to cold, pallor, and loss of skin tone. Traditional anemia signs such as pallor have limited sensitivity and specificity and may be misinterpreted. In chronic bleeding there is time for equilibration with extravascular space and total blood volume will remain normal. Some of these physiologic effects, such as effects on respiratory function demonstrated by measurements of maximal oxygen consumption, may serve as end points of clinical benefit of treating anemia.

Manifestations of IDA include glossal pain, smooth tongue, reduced salivary flow, pica (compulsive eating of nonfood items), and pagophagia (compulsive eating of ice). These symptoms usually do

TABLE 99–3. Normal Hematologic Values

Test	Reference Range (y)			
	2–6	6–12	12–18	18–49
Hemoglobin (g/dL)	11.5–15.5	11.5–15.5	M 13.0–16.0 F 12.0–16.0	M 13.5–17.5 F 12.0–16.0
Hematocrit (%)	34–40	35–45	M 37–49 F 36–46	M 41–53 F 36–46
MCV (fL)	75–87	77–95	M 78–98 F 78–102	80–100
MCHC (%)	—	31–37	31–37	31–37
MCH (pg)	24–30	25–33	25–35	26–34
RBC (million/mm^3)	3.9–5.3	4.0–5.2	M 4.5–5.3	M 4.5–5.9
Reticulocyte count, absolute (%)				0.5–1.5
Serum iron (mcg/dL)		50–120	50–120	M 50–160 F 40–150
TIBC (mcg/dL)	250–400	250–400	250–400	250–400
RDW (%)				11–16
Ferritin (ng/mL)	7–140	7–140	7–140	M 15–200 F 12–150
Folate (ng/mL)				1.8–16.0[a]
Vitamin B$_{12}$ (pg/mL)				100–900[a]
Erythropoietin (mU/mL)				0–19

[a]Varies by assay method.

F, female; M, male; MCHC, mean corpuscular hemoglobin concentration; MCH, mean corpuscular hemoglobin; MCV, mean corpuscular volume; RDW, red blood cell distribution; TIBC, total iron-binding capacity.

not appear until the Hgb concentration falls below 8 or 9 g/dL. IDA has negative effects on psychomotor and mental development in infants, children, and adolescents.[12] Additionally, maternal IDA can result in low birth weight infants and preterm delivery.[13]

Clinically, patients with vitamin B$_{12}$ deficiency may be pale and mildly icteric, and they may develop gastric mucosal atrophy. Neurologic findings in vitamin B$_{12}$ deficiency, which often precede hematologic findings, may be partly due to the impairment of the conversion of homocysteine to methionine, as methionine is necessary for the production of choline and choline-containing phospholipids.[14] Neurologic findings are found in 75% to 95% of individuals with clinically apparent vitamin B$_{12}$ deficiency. The occurrence of neurologic findings is inversely correlated with the degree of anemia.[15] The neurologic findings include numbness and paresthesias as the earliest findings, then peripheral neuropathy, ataxia, diminished vibratory sense, increased deep tendon reflexes, decreased proprioception, imbalance, and demyelination of the dorsal columns and corticospinal tract develop.[16] Psychiatric findings include irritability, personality changes, memory impairment, dementia, depression, and infrequently, psychosis. Other reported symptoms include glossitis, muscle weakness, dysphagia, and anorexia.

Symptoms associated with folate deficiency are similar to those seen in patients with vitamin B$_{12}$ deficiency, with the absence of neurologic symptoms. Although the symptoms of anemia will improve with folate replacement and a partial hematologic response will occur, the neurologic manifestations of vitamin B$_{12}$ deficiency will not be reversed with folic acid replacement therapy and consequently may become irreversible if not treated.

LABORATORY EVALUATION

The initial evaluation of anemia involves a CBC, including RBC indices; a reticulocyte index; examination of a peripheral blood smear; and examination of a stool sample for occult blood. The results from the preliminary evaluation determine the need for other studies.

Table 99–3 shows normal hematologic values. By definition, anemia is present in males if the Hct is less than 41% or the Hgb is less than 13 g/dL, while females have a Hct less than 36% or a Hgb less than 12 g/dL.

Figure 99–3 provides a broad, general algorithm for the diagnosis of anemias based on laboratory data. There are many exceptions and additions to this algorithm, but it can serve as a guide to the typical presentation of the most common types and causes of anemia. Algorithms such as this are less useful in the presence of more than one cause of anemia.

HEMOGLOBIN

Values given for Hgb represent the amount of Hgb per volume of whole blood. The higher values seen in males are due to stimulation of RBC production by androgenic steroids, and to a lesser extent due to the decrease in Hgb in females caused by blood loss during menstruation. The level of Hgb can be used as a very rough estimate of the oxygen-carrying capacity of blood. Hgb levels may be diminished because of a decreased quantity of Hgb per RBC or because of a decrease in the actual number of RBCs.

HEMATOCRIT

Expressed as a percentage, Hct is the actual volume of RBCs in a unit volume of whole blood. In general, it is about three times the Hgb value. An alteration in this ratio may occur with abnormal cell size or shape and often indicates the pathology. A low Hct indicates a reduction in either the number or size of RBCs, or an increase in plasma volume.

RED BLOOD CELL COUNT

The RBC count is an indirect estimate of the Hgb content of the blood as it is an actual count of RBCs per unit of blood.

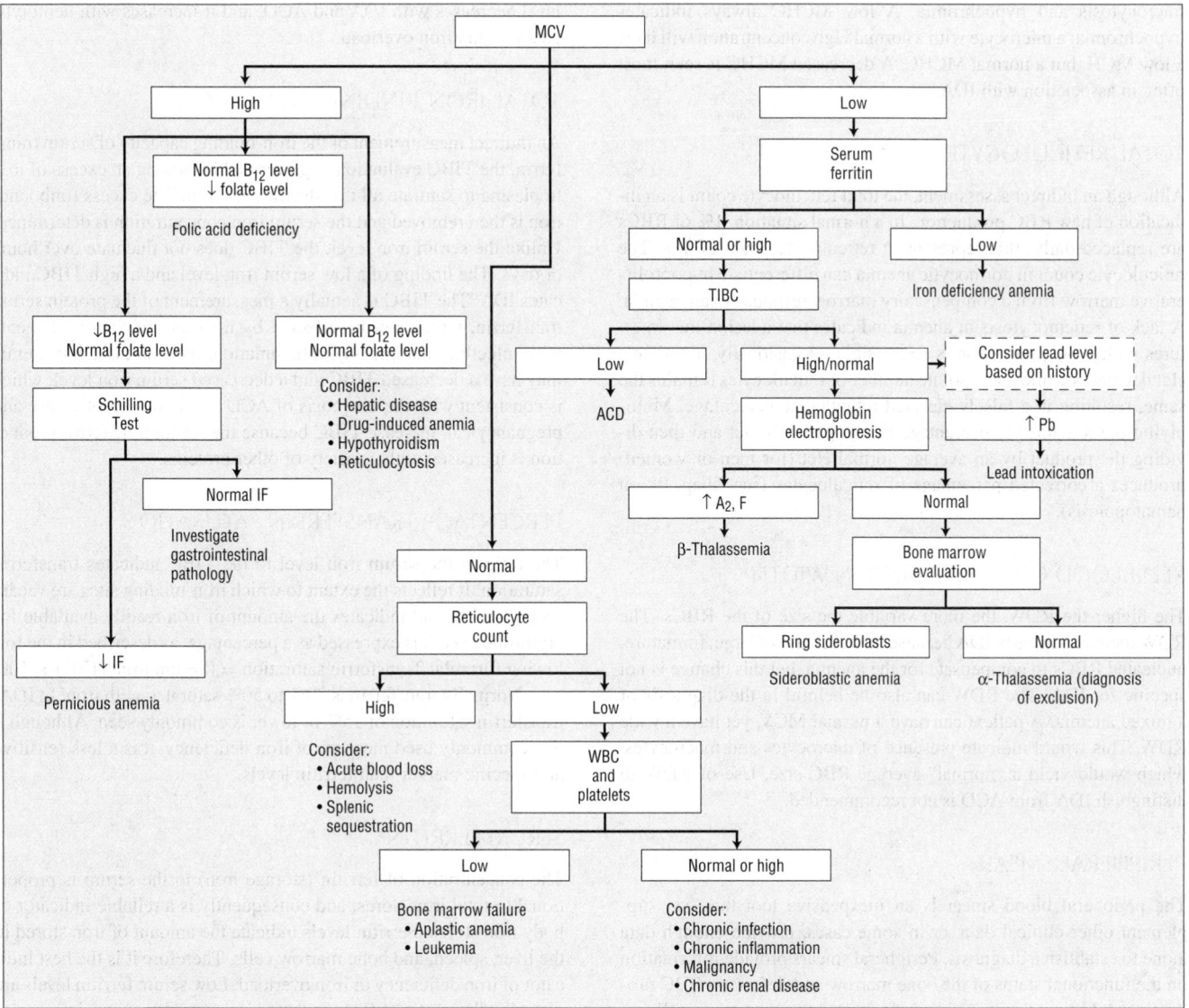

FIGURE 99–3. General algorithm for the diagnosis of anemias. ↑, increased; ↓, decreased; ACD, anemia of chronic disease; A_2, hemoglobin A_2; F, hemoglobin F; IF, intrinsic factor; MCV, mean corpuscular volume; Pb, lead; TIBC, total iron-binding capacity; WBC, white blood cells.

RED BLOOD CELL INDICES

Wintrobe indices describe the size and Hgb content of the RBCs, and are calculated from the Hgb, Hct, and RBC count. RBC indices, such as mean corpuscular volume (MCV) or mean corpuscular hemoglobin (MCH) for example, are single mean values that do not express the variation that may occur in cells.

Mean Corpuscular Volume (Hct/RBC Count)

MCV represents the average volume of RBCs. Cells are said to be macrocytic if they are larger than normal, microcytic if they are smaller than normal, and normocytic if their size falls within normal limits. Folic acid and vitamin B_{12} deficiency anemias yield macrocytic morphology, whereas iron deficiency and thalassemia are examples of microcytic anemias. A falsely elevated MCV occurs with reticulocytosis because reticulocytes are larger than erythrocytes. The MCV is also falsely elevated in the presence of cold agglutinins and hyperglycemia. When IDA (decreased MCV) is accompanied by folate deficiency (increased MCV), failure to understand that the MCV rep-

resents an average RBC size creates the potential for overlooking the real cause of the anemia.

Mean Corpuscular Hemoglobin (Hgb/RBC Count)

The percent volume of Hgb in an RBC is the MCH. Two morphologic changes, microcytosis or hypochromia, can reduce the MCH. A microcytic cell contains less Hgb because it is a smaller cell, whereas a hypochromic cell has a low MCH because of the decreased amount of Hgb present in a normocytic cell. Cells can be both microcytic and hypochromic, as seen with IDA, and the MCH alone cannot distinguish between microcytosis and hypochromia. The most common cause of an elevated MCH is macrocytosis (e.g., vitamin B_{12} or folate deficiency).

Mean Corpuscular Hemoglobin Concentration (Hgb/Hct)

The weight of Hgb per volume of cells is the mean corpuscular Hgb concentration (MCHC). Because the MCHC is independent of cell size, it is more useful than the MCH in distinguishing between microcytosis and hypochromia. A low MCHC always indicates hypochromia; a microcyte with a normal Hgb concentration will have a low MCH, but a normal MCHC. A decreased MCHC is seen most often in association with IDA.

TOTAL RETICULOCYTE COUNT

Although an indirect assessment, the total reticulocyte count is an indication of new RBC production. In a normal situation, 1% of RBCs are replaced daily; this represents a reticulocyte count of 1%. The reticulocyte count in normocytic anemia can differentiate hypoproliferative marrow from a compensatory marrow response to an anemia. A lack of reticulocytosis in anemia indicates that a lesion that interferes with RBC production is responsible. Occasionally, a patient's Hct decreases while the absolute number of reticulocytes remains the same, resulting in a falsely elevated reticulocyte percentage. Multiplying the reticulocyte percentage by the patient's Hct and then dividing the product by an average normal Hct (for men or women) produces a corrected percentage of reticulocytes (see Chap. 98 on hematopoiesis).

RED BLOOD CELL DISTRIBUTION WIDTH

The higher the RDW, the more variable the size of the RBCs. The RDW increases in early IDA because of the release of large, immature, nucleated RBCs to compensate for the anemia, but this change is not specific for IDA. The RDW can also be helpful in the diagnosis of a mixed anemia. A patient can have a normal MCV, yet have a wide RDW. This would indicate presence of microcytes and macrocytes, which would yield a "normal" average RBC size. Use of RDW to distinguish IDA from ACD is not recommended.

PERIPHERAL SMEAR

The peripheral blood smear is an inexpensive tool that can supplement other clinical data, or in some cases, provide enough data alone to establish a diagnosis. Peripheral smears provide information on the functional status of the bone marrow and defects in RBC production. Additionally, it provides information on variations in cell size (anisocytosis) and shape (poikilocytosis). Automated blood counters, used for the complete blood count, can flag specific RBC changes which can be confirmed on a peripheral blood smear. Blood smears are placed on a microscope slide following precise preparation techniques and stained as appropriate. Morphologic examination includes assessment of size, shape, and color. The extent of anisocytosis correlates with increased range of cell sizes, and poikilocytosis suggests a defect in the maturation of RBC precursors in the bone marrow. The detected abnormalities can then suggest pathology.

SERUM IRON

The level of serum iron is the concentration of iron bound to transferrin. Normally, transferrin is about one-third bound (saturated) to iron. Unfortunately, the serum iron level of many patients with IDA remains within the lower limits of normal, as it takes a considerable amount of time to deplete iron stores, giving a false-negative test result. There is also a 20% to 30% diurnal variation in serum iron levels (higher in the morning, lower in the afternoon) as well as a 20% to 25% day-to-day variation among individuals.[17] Variability results from technical and physiologic influences. Serum iron levels are decreased by infection and inflammation. Consequently, as a diagnostic tool, serum iron levels are best interpreted in conjunction with the TIBC. The serum iron

level decreases with IDA and ACD, and it increases with hemolytic anemias and iron overload.

TOTAL IRON-BINDING CAPACITY

An indirect measurement of the iron-binding capacity of serum transferrin, the TIBC evaluation is performed by adding an excess of iron to plasma to saturate all transferrin with iron. The excess (unbound) iron is then removed and the serum iron concentration is determined. Unlike the serum iron level, the TIBC does not fluctuate over hours or days. The finding of a low serum iron level and a high TIBC indicates IDA. The TIBC is actually a measurement of the protein serum transferrin, which can be affected by a variety of factors. Patients with infection, malignancy, inflammation, liver disease, and uremia may have a decreased TIBC and a decreased serum iron level, which is consistent with the diagnosis of ACD. Oral contraceptive use and pregnancy can increase TIBC because the serum transferrin production is increased with a variety of other proteins.

PERCENTAGE TRANSFERRIN SATURATION

The ratio of the serum iron level to the TIBC indicates transferrin saturation. It reflects the extent to which iron-binding sites are vacant on transferrin and indicates the amount of iron readily available for erythropoiesis. It is expressed as a percentage, as described in the following formula: Transferrin saturation = (Serum iron/TIBC) × 100.

Normally transferrin is 20% to 50% saturated with iron. In IDA, transferrin saturation of 15% or lower is commonly seen. Although it is a commonly used measure of iron deficiency, it is a less sensitive and specific marker than ferritin levels.

SERUM FERRITIN

The concentration of ferritin (storage iron) in the serum is proportional to total iron stores, and consequently is a reliable indicator of body iron stores. Ferritin levels indicate the amount of iron stored in the liver, spleen, and bone marrow cells. Therefore it is the best indicator of iron deficiency or iron overload. Low serum ferritin levels are virtually diagnostic of IDA, as they decrease only in association with IDA. In contrast, serum iron levels may decrease both in IDA and in ACD. Serum ferritin is an acute phase reactant, so chronic infection or inflammation can raise its concentration independent of iron status, masking depleted tissue stores. This limits the specificity and the utility of the serum ferritin if it is normal or high in a chronically ill patient.

FOLIC ACID

The results of folic acid measurements may vary depending on the assay method used. Decreased serum folic acid levels indicate a folate deficiency megaloblastic anemia that may coexist with a vitamin B_{12} deficiency anemia. An erythrocyte folic acid level is less volatile than serum levels, as it is slow to decrease in an acute process such as drug-induced folic acid deficiency, and slow to increase with oral folic acid replacement. However, the clinical utility of determining the erythrocyte folic acid level is questionable, and the procedure should be reserved for cases in which the clinician suspects folic acid depletion and the serum folic acid may be falsely elevated or depleted.

VITAMIN B_{12}

Low levels of vitamin B_{12} (cyanocobalamin) indicate vitamin B_{12} deficiency. However, a deficiency may exist prior to the recognition of low serum levels, as serum values are maintained at the expense of vitamin B_{12} tissue stores. Since vitamin B_{12} deficiency and folate deficiency may overlap, it is recommended to determine serum level of both vitamins. Vitamin B_{12} levels may be falsely low with folate deficiency, pregnancy, use of oral contraceptives, congenital deficiency of serum haptocorrins, and in multiple myeloma.[18]

SCHILLING TEST

The purpose of the rarely used Schilling urinary excretion test is to diagnose vitamin B_{12} deficiency anemia caused by a B_{12} absorption defect resulting from a lack of intrinsic factor (pernicious anemia). The patient first receives an oral dose of radiolabeled vitamin B_{12}. Two hours later, the patient receives a large intramuscular dose of nonlabeled vitamin B_{12} to saturate plasma transport proteins. Any excess vitamin B_{12} that is not taken up by the transport proteins or stored in the liver will be excreted in the urine. A 24-hour urine collection is then measured for radioactivity. If sufficient gastrointestinal intrinsic factor is being produced, the radiolabeled B_{12} will be absorbed.

If oral absorption is impaired, part 2 of the test is conducted 5 to 7 days later. The second stage of the Schilling test differentiates inadequate secretion of intrinsic factor by the stomach from an abnormality in absorption by the ileum. Radiolabeled vitamin B_{12} is administered orally with a sufficient amount of intrinsic factor. Results within the normal range indicate that the defect is in the production of intrinsic factor as opposed to other causes of vitamin B_{12} deficiency such as dietary deficiency or small bowel pathology. Generally, abnormal results for stage 1 followed by a normal result in stage 2 is consistent with pernicious anemia.

If the results in part 2 are still low, then the third stage of the test is conducted to determine whether the cause of the deficiency is due to bacterial overgrowth or ileal disease. The patient is given 250 mg of tetracycline four times daily for 10 days. Tetracycline reduces the intestinal bacteria in blind loop syndrome. Blind loops occur when a segment of the intestine is not contiguous with the rest of the gastrointestinal tract, which necessarily occurs with some surgical procedures. The loops are subject to bacterial overgrowth that may lead to malabsorption. If the excretion of radiolabeled vitamin B_{12} improves after the tetracycline, a malabsorptive syndrome related to intestinal bacteria is confirmed.

HOMOCYSTEINE

Vitamin B_{12} and folate are both required for conversion of homocysteine to methionine. Increased serum homocysteine may help define vitamin B_{12} or folate deficiency. Homocysteine levels can also be elevated in vitamin B_6 deficiency, renal failure, hypothyroidism, and in persons with a genetic defect in cystathionine β-synthase.[19] Additionally, elevated levels have been caused by medications including nicotinic acid, theophylline, methotrexate, and L-dopa.

METHYLMALONIC ACID

A vitamin B_{12} coenzyme is needed to convert methylmalonyl coenzyme A to succinyl co-enzyme A. Patients with vitamin B_{12} deficiency almost always have increased urinary excretion of methylmalonic acid (MMA). MMA is a more specific marker for vitamin B_{12} deficiency compared to homocysteine. MMA levels are not elevated in folate deficiency, as folate does not participate in MMA metabolism. Levels of both MMA and homocysteine are usually elevated prior to the development of hematologic abnormalities and reductions in serum vitamin B_{12} levels.[18] MMA levels need to be interpreted cau-

tiously in patients with renal disease and hypovolemia, as it may be elevated due to decreased urinary excretion.

COOMBS TEST

Antiglobulin tests, also called Coombs tests, indicate hemolytic anemia caused by an immune response. A direct Coombs test detects antibodies bound to erythrocytes, whereas an indirect Coombs test measures antibodies present in the serum. A positive finding in a direct Coombs test is usually indicative of antibody-mediated hemolysis.

ERYTHROPOIETIN LEVELS

Healthy individuals require 10 to 30 milliunits/mL of EPO to maintain normal Hgb and Hct concentrations. Endogenous EPO levels can increase 100- to 1,000-fold during hypoxia or anemia. This marked increase does not occur in patients with end-stage renal disease, patients receiving chemotherapy, and patients with acquired immunodeficiency syndrome (AIDS), especially those taking azidothymidine. These patients will have an EPO response that is insufficient to correct their anemia.

SPECIFIC ANEMIAS

IRON DEFICIENCY ANEMIA

EPIDEMIOLOGY

Iron deficiency is the most common nutritional deficiency in developing and developed countries and it is estimated that over 500 million people worldwide have IDA.[1,20] Data from the Third NHANES indicates IDA is prevalent in 1% to 2% of adults.[21]

Prevalence data varies because screening uses a simple Hgb test, arbitrary normals are used, and selection of samples in population surveys tends to lead to errors. The normal ranges for Hgb and Hct are so wide that a patient may lose up to 15% of their RBC mass and still have a Hct within the normal range.

ETIOLOGY

Iron deficiency results from prolonged negative iron balance or failure to meet increased physiologic iron need. The speed of iron deficiency development depends on an individuals initial iron stores and balance between iron absorption and loss. Multiple etiologic factors are usually involved.

In less industrialized nations, the risks for developing IDA are largely related to dietary factors. Diets limited in meat or fresh fruits and vegetables or diets high in substances that form complexes with iron may result in IDA. Other causes of IDA include chronic illnesses, inflammatory conditions like rheumatoid arthritis, and malabsorptive syndromes. Situations that increase the demand for iron are frequent blood donations, endurance sports, menstruation, pregnancy and lactation, infancy, and adolescence.[22] Iron deficiency in pregnant women is so common that the Centers for Disease Control (CDC) and Prevention guidelines recommend low-dose iron supplements (30 mg/day) to be initiated at the woman's first prenatal visit for the primary prevention of IDA. At diagnosis, the cause of IDA must be considered a consequence of blood loss until proven otherwise. More than 50% of adults with IDA have some form of gastrointestinal bleeding. Blood loss may occur as a result of many disorders, including trauma, hemorrhoids, peptic ulcers, gastritis, gastrointestinal malignancies, diverticular disease, copious menstrual flow, nosebleeds, or postpartum bleeding. Occult blood loss from a single gastrointestinal lesion has been shown to be a frequent cause of "idiopathic" IDA.[23] Diseases contributing to the development of IDA include various malignancies, usually in the gastrointestinal tract, and renal disease. Additionally, the possibility of multifactorial causes must always be considered. Medication history, specifically about use of recent or past iron or hematinics, alcohol, corticosteroids, aspirin, and nonsteroidal anti-inflammatory drugs is a vital part of the history. Other possible causes of hypochromic, microcytic anemia include ACD, thalassemia, sideroblastic anemia, and heavy metal (mostly lead) poisoning (see Fig. 99–3). Patients with a past medical history significant for IDA should be periodically re-evaluated for iron deficiency.

PATHOPHYSIOLOGY

Iron is vital to the function of all cells. It is a critical element in iron-containing enzymes such as the mitochondria's cytochrome system.[24] Without iron, cells lose their capacity for electron transport and energy metabolism. IDA is associated with abnormal neurotransmitter function and altered immunologic and inflammatory defenses. This is because in addition to iron's role in oxygen transport and delivery, iron is a cofactor for oxidative metabolism, dopamine and DNA synthesis, and free radical function in neutrophils.[25] The balance of iron metabolism is designed to conserve iron for reutilization. The margin between the amount of iron available for absorption and the body's iron requirement is narrow for growing infants and female adults, which explains why IDA prevalence is highest in these populations. Risk of iron deficiency is related to levels of iron loss, iron intake, iron absorption, and physiologic demands. Iron deficiency is usually the result of a long period of negative iron balance. Manifestations of iron deficiency occur in several stages and three stages have been described: prelatent, latent, and IDA. Prelatent refers to a reduction in iron stores without reduced serum iron levels, and can be assessed with serum ferritin measurement. In this first stage, iron stores can be depleted without causing anemia. The stores allow iron to be utilized when there is an increased need for Hgb synthesis. Once stores are depleted, there is still adequate iron from the daily RBC turnover for Hgb synthesis. Further iron losses would make the patient vulnerable to anemia development. Latent iron deficiency occurs when iron

stores are depleted, but Hgb is above the lower limit of normal for the population, yet may be reduced for a given patient. This can be determined by serial CBC measurements. Findings would include reduced transferrin saturation and increased TIBC. IDA occurs when the Hgb falls to less than normal values. Deficiency progresses to the classic hypochromia and microcytosis of iron-deficient erythropoiesis.

LABORATORY FINDINGS

Abnormal laboratory findings in patients with IDA generally include low serum iron and ferritin levels and a high TIBC.[26] The first apparent sign of iron deficiency is the increased RDW, although it is not specific to IDA. In the early stages of IDA, the RBC size is not changed. Low ferritin concentration is the earliest and most sensitive indicator of iron deficiency. The disadvantage of using ferritin to evaluate iron stores is that renal or liver disease, malignancies, infection, or inflammatory processes may elevate the measured values, and these values may not correlate with iron stores in the bone marrow.[27] The Hgb, Hct, and RBC indices usually remain normal.

In the later stages of IDA, the Hgb and Hct fall below normal values, and a microcytic, hypochromic anemia develops. Microcytosis may precede hypochromia, as erythropoiesis is programmed to maintain normal Hgb concentration in deference to cell size. As a consequence, even slightly abnormal Hgb and Hct levels may indicate significant depletion of iron stores and should not be ignored. In terms of RBC indices, MCV reduction occurs earlier in iron-deficient hematopoiesis than reduction in Hgb concentration.

As noted earlier, transferrin saturation (i.e., serum iron level divided by the TIBC) is also useful in assessing IDA. Low values likely indicate IDA, although low serum transferrin saturation values may also be present in inflammatory disorders. Fortunately, the TIBC usually helps to differentiate the diagnosis in these patients: a TIBC greater than 400 mcg/dL suggests IDA, whereas values below 200 mcg/dL usually represent inflammatory disease. With continued progression of IDA, anisocytosis occurs and poikilocytosis develops, as seen on peripheral smear and indicated by increased RDW. In rare cases, a bone marrow examination can be performed to assess bone marrow iron stores. Bone marrow examination reveals absent iron stores in IDA. Documenation of decreased hemosiderin can confirm the diagnosis of IDA. In microcytic anemias due to all other causes, iron stores are detectable.

▶ TREATMENT: Iron Deficiency Anemia

The severity and cause of IDA determines the approach to treatment.

Treatment is focused on replenishing iron stores. Since iron deficiency can be an early sign of other illnesses, treatment of the underlying disease may aid in the correction of the iron deficiency.

■ DIETARY SUPPLEMENTATION AND THERAPEUTIC IRON PREPARATIONS

Treatment of IDA usually consists of dietary supplementation and administration of therapeutic iron preparations. As discussed earlier, iron is poorly absorbed from vegetables, grain products, dairy products, and eggs; it is best absorbed from meat, fish, and poultry. Beverages have also been shown to affect iron absorption. It is recommended that meat, orange juice, and other ascorbic acid–rich foods be included in meals, while milk and tea be consumed in moderation between meals.

In most cases of IDA, oral administration of iron therapy with soluble Fe^{2+} iron salts is appropriate.[28]

CLINICAL CONTROVERSY

Daily Fe^{2+} sulfate is not tolerated by all and can be difficult to administer in populations of developing nations. Weekly rather than daily supplements have been used with conflicting efficacy results. The weekly approach follows the natural pattern of mucosal cell iron turnover.

Fe^{2+} sulfate, succinate, lactate, fumarate, glycine sulfate, glutamate, and gluconate are all about equally absorbed. The addition of copper, cobalt, molybdenum, or other minerals, as well as hematinics provides no advantage but adds expense. The carbonyl iron may be advantageous because of lower risk of death in cases of accidental overdose. Iron is best absorbed in the reduced Fe^{2+} form, with maximal absorption occurring in the duodenum, primarily due

TABLE 99–4. Oral Iron Products

Salt	Elemental Iron Percentage	Elemental Iron Provided
Ferrous sulfate	20%	60–65 mg/324–325 mg tablet 18 mg iron/5 mL syrup 44 mg iron/5 mL elixir 15 mg iron/0.6 mL drop
Ferrous sulfate (exsiccated)	30%	65 mg/200 mg tablet 60 mg/187 mg tablet 50 mg/160 mg tablet
Ferrous gluconate	12%	36 mg/325 mg tablet 27 mg/240 mg tablet
Ferrous fumarate	33%	33 mg/100 mg tablet 63–66 mg/200 mg tablet 106 mg/324–325 mg tablet 15 mg/0.6 mL drop 33 mg/5 mL suspension
Polysaccharide iron complex	100%	150 mg capsule 50 mg tablet 100 mg/5 mL elixir
Carbonyl iron	100%	50 mg caplet

to the acidic medium of the stomach. The presence of mucopolysaccharide chelator substances prevent the iron from precipitating and maintains the iron in a soluble form. In the alkaline environment of the small intestines, iron tends to form insoluble complexes that are unavailable for absorption. Slow-release or sustained-release iron preparations do not undergo sufficient dissolution until reaching the small intestines, which significantly reduces iron absorption and can attenuate the hematinic effects.[29] This is especially true when enteric-coated preparations are used in achlorhydric patients. The dose of iron replacement therapy depends on the patient's ability to tolerate the administered iron. Tolerance of iron salts improves with a small initial dose and gradual escalation to the full dose. In patients with IDA, it is generally recommended that approximately 200 mg of elemental iron be administered daily, usually in two or three divided doses to maximize tolerability.[30] However, if patients cannot tolerate this daily dose of elemental iron, smaller amounts of elemental iron, such as a single 325-mg tablet of Fe^{2+} sulfate, is usually sufficient to replace iron stores, albeit at a slower rate. Table 99–4 shows the percentage of elemental iron of commonly available iron salts. The percentage of iron absorbed progressively decreases as the dose increases, but the absolute amount absorbed increases. Iron should be preferably administered at least 1 hour prior to meals, as food interferes with its absorption. Many patients must take their iron with food, as they experience nausea and diarrhea when iron is administered on an empty stomach. Gastrointestinal side effects are usually dose-related and are similar among iron salts when equivalent amounts of elemental iron are administered. Administration of smaller amounts of iron with

each dose may minimize these adverse effects. H_2-blockers or proton pump inhibitors that reduce gastric acidity may impair iron absorption (see Table 99–5 for drug interactions with iron).

Adverse reactions to therapeutic doses of iron are primarily gastrointestinal in nature and consist of a dark discoloration of feces, constipation or diarrhea, nausea, and vomiting. Failure to develop at least some of these symptoms, even mildly, may indicate noncompliance. If these side effects become intolerable, the total daily dose may be decreased to 110 to 120 mg of elemental iron or the dose may be taken with meals. As noted, however, the administration of iron with meals reduces the amount of iron absorbed by more than one-half.

Failure to respond to appropriate treatment regimens necessitates re-evaluation of the patient's condition. Occasionally a "therapeutic trial of iron" approach will be used to confirm a presumptive diagnosis of IDA. Common causes of treatment failure include poor patient compliance, inability to absorb iron, incorrect diagnosis, continued bleeding, or a concurrent condition that blocks full reticulocyte response. Even when iron deficiency is present, response may be impaired when a coexisting cause for anemia exists. Rarely, patients may not be able to absorb iron, most often due to previous gastrectomy or celiac disease. Malabsorption can be ruled out by the iron test, in which plasma iron levels are determined at half-hour intervals for 2 hours following the administration of 50 mg of elemental iron as liquid Fe^{2+} sulfate. If plasma iron levels increase by more than 50 mcg during this time, absorption is satisfactory. Regardless of the form of oral therapy used, treatment must be continued 3 to 6 months after the

TABLE 99–5. Iron Salt–Drug Interactions

Drugs that Decrease Iron Absorption	Object Drugs Affected by Iron
Al-, Mg-, and Ca^{+2}-containing antacids	Levodopa ↓ (chelates with iron)
Tetracycline and doxycycline	Methyldopa ↓ (decreases efficacy of methyldopa)
H_2 antagonists	Levothyroxine ↓ (decreased efficacy of levothyroxine)
Proton pump inhibitors	Penicillamine ↓ (chelates with iron)
Cholestyramine	Fluoroquinolones ↓ (forms ferric ion-quinolone complex)
	Tetracycline and doxycycline ↓ (when administered within 2 hours of iron salt)
	Mycophenolate ↓ (decreases absorption)

TABLE 99–6. Comparison of Parenteral Iron Preparations

	Sodium Ferric Gluconate	Iron Dextran	Iron Sucrose
Amount of elemental iron	62.5 mg iron/5 mL	50 mg iron/mL	20 mg iron/mL
Molecular weight	Ferrlecit: 289,000–444,000 daltons	InFeD: 165,000 daltons DexFerrum: 267,000 daltons	Venofer: 34,000–60,000 daltons
Composition	Ferric oxide hydrate bonded to sucrose chelates with gluconate in a molar rate of 2 iron molecules to 1 gluconate molecule	Complex of ferric hydroxide and dextran	Complex of polynuclear iron hydroxide in sucrose
Preservative	Benzyl alcohol 9 mg/5 mL 20% (975 mg in 62.5 mg iron)	None	None
Indication	Treatment of iron deficiency anemia in patients undergoing chronic hemodialysis who are receiving supplemental erythropoietin therapy	Treatment of patients with documented iron deficiency in whom oral therapy is unsatisfactory or impossible	Treatment of iron deficiency anemia in patients undergoing chronic hemodialysis who are receiving supplemental epoetin alfa therapy
Warning	No black box warning; hypersensitivity reactions	Black box warning: anaphylactic-type reactions	Black box warning: anaphylactic-type reactions
IM injection	No	Yes	No
Usual dose	125 mg (10 mL) diluted in 100 mL normal saline, infused over 60 minutes; may also be administered as a slow IV injection (rate of 12.5 mg/min).	100 mg undiluted at a rate not to exceed 50 mg (1 mL) per min	100 mg into the dialysis line at a rate of 1 mL (20 mg of iron) undiluted solution per minute
Treatment	8 doses × 125 mg = 1,000 mg	10 doses × 100 mg = 1,000 mg	Up to 10 doses × 100 mg = 1,000 mg
Common adverse effects	Cramps, nausea and vomiting, flushing, hypotension, rash, pruritus	Pain and brown staining at injection site, flushing, hypotension, fever, chills, myalgia, anaphylaxis	Leg cramps, hypotension

anemia is resolved to allow for repletion of iron stores and to avoid relapse.

PARENTERAL IRON THERAPY

When there is evidence of iron malabsorption or intolerance to orally administered iron, or when long-term noncompliance is a problem, parenteral iron therapy may be warranted. Patients with significant blood loss who refuse transfusions and in whom oral iron therapy is not possible may also require parenteral iron therapy. Parenteral iron does not lead to a quicker hematologic response than oral iron.[31] The ideal parenteral iron supplement would be safe, efficacious, convenient, and maintain consistent patient outcomes. There are currently three different parenteral iron preparations available in the U.S.: iron dextran, sodium ferric gluconate, and iron sucrose (Table 99–6). They differ in their molecular size, degradation kinetics, bioavailability, and side-effect profiles. Although toxicity profiles of these agents differ, clinical studies indicate that each is efficacious.[32] Most of the recent IV iron research has been done in hemodialysis patients.[33] The dextran parenteral preparation(s) have been associated with deaths due to anaphylactic reactions. These reactions may be related to immune reactions to the iron-carbohydrate or iron-dextran complex. Another theory for the anaphylaxis may be the high-molecular-weight dextran component, which may be antigenic even when not complexed to iron. The safety profile of iron is largely assessed by spontaneous reports to the Food and Drug Administration, as well as via retrospective and open-label prospective studies. Data suggests that Fe^{3+} gluconate and iron sucrose are safer than iron dextran.[34] The concern with parenteral iron is that iron may be released too quickly and overload the ability of transferrin to bind it, leading to free iron reactions resulting in interference with neutrophil function.

Iron dextran, a complex of Fe^{3+} hydroxide and the carbohydrate dextran, contains 50 mg of iron/mL and may be given via the IM or IV route. Different brands of iron dextran are available and differ in their molecular weight. They are not substitutable.[35]

Iron dextran must be processed by macrophages for the iron to be biologically available. The absorption and metabolism varies with the route and amount of drug given. Absorption of an IM dose of iron dextran occurs in two phases. During the first 72 hours, iron dextran is absorbed primarily through the lymphatics into the left superior vena cava. A smaller amount is absorbed directly through the IM capillary network into the blood.[36] A second, slower phase involves uptake of the iron dextran complex by macrophages, with subsequent transport through the lymphatics into the blood. The macrophages phagocytize the iron dextran complex and cleave the dextran moiety, making free iron available to the body as circulating iron, transferrin-bound iron, or storage iron (ferritin and hemosiderin). Iron dextran can remain within these cells for many months. About 60% of an IM dose of iron dextran is absorbed after 3 days, and up to 90% is absorbed within 3 weeks.[37] The remainder is absorbed slowly over several months or longer.

When iron dextran is given IV, the iron is taken up immediately by the reticuloendothelial system.[38] Small to intermediate IV doses (50 to 500 mg of elemental iron) can be cleared from the plasma within 3 days of administration. In contrast, larger IV doses of iron dextran (500 mg of elemental iron) are processed by the reticuloendothelial system at a constant rate of 10 to 20 mg/h.[39] Doses this large are associated with increased plasma concentrations of iron dextran for as long as 3 weeks.

The iron dextran package insert carries a black box warning regarding the risk of anaphylaxis and requires a test dose before administration of the repletion dose. Methods of IV administration include multiple slow injections of undiluted iron dextran solution or an infusion of a diluted preparation. This latter method is often referred

TABLE 99–7. Equations for Calculating Doses of Parenteral Iron

In patients with iron deficiency anemia:

Adults + children over 15 kg

Dose (mL) = 0.0442 (desired Hgb − observed Hgb)

$\times$ LBW + (0.26 $\times$ LBW)

LBW males = 50 kg + (2.3 $\times$ inches over 5 ft)

LBW females = 45.5 kg + (2.3 $\times$ inches over 5 ft)

Children 5–15 kg

Dose (mL) = 0.0442 (desired Hgb − observed Hgb)

$\times$ W + (0.26 $\times$ W)

Hgb = hemoglobin
mL = milliliter
W = weight
LBW = lean body weight

In patients with anemia secondary to blood loss (hemorrhagic diathesis or long-term dialysis):

mg of iron = blood loss $\times$ hematocrit

where blood loss is in milliliters and hematocrit is expressed as a decimal fraction.

to as total dose infusion. The IM administration of iron dextran should take place via Z-tract injection technique (a technique to handle IM injections of irritating substances with minimal tracking of the medication through surrounding tissues) to minimize staining of the skin. Because each IM dose is limited to 2 mL (100 mg of iron), multiple injections are often required. Daily IM doses should not exceed 25 mg in patients less than 5 kg, 50 mg in patients less than 10 kg, and 100 mg in all other patients. Problems with IM administration include patient discomfort, sterile abscesses, tissue necrosis, or atrophy. In addition, up to 30% of an administered dose remains physiologically unavailable. For these reasons, the IV route is the preferred parenteral route of administration.

Equations for calculating the appropriate dose of parenteral iron in patients with IDA or those with anemia secondary to blood loss can be found in Table 99–7. When given by IV administration, the dose should not exceed 50 mg of iron per minute (1 mL/min). It is suggested that all patients considered for an iron dextran injection receive a test dose of 25 mg IM or IV, or a 5- to 10-minute infusion of the diluted solution. Patients should then be observed for more than 1 hour for untoward reactions. If an anaphylaxis-like reaction were to occur, it generally responds to IV epinephrine, diphenhydramine, and corticosteroids. Patients receiving total dose infusions can have the remaining solution infused during the next 2 to 6 hours if the test dose is tolerated.

Total replacement doses of IV iron dextran have been given as a single dose, diluted in 250 to 1000 mL normal saline or 5% dextrose in water and infused over 4 to 6 hours. A test dose is still required. The ability to give a total dose infusion is a benefit of iron dextran over the other parenteral iron products. Iron dextran is best utilized when smaller frequent doses of sodium ferric gluconate or iron sucrose are impractical, such as with peritoneal dialysis.

If the patient receives a total dose infusion, there is an increased possibility of adverse reactions such as arthralgias, myalgias, flushing, malaise, and fever. Other adverse reactions of iron dextran include staining of the skin, pain at the injection site, allergic reactions, and rarely anaphylaxis. Patients most likely to experience adverse effects with iron dextran include individuals with a history of allergies, asthma, or inflammatory diseases. Patients with pre-existing immune-mediated diseases such as active rheumatoid arthritis or systemic lupus erythematosus are considered at high risk for adverse reactions because of their hyperreactive immune response capabilities.

Sodium ferric gluconate is a complex of iron bound to one gluconate and four sucrose molecules in a repeating pattern. The molecular weight is 289,000 to 440,000 daltons and it is available in an aqueous solution. Pharmacokinetically, there is no direct transfer of iron from the Fe^{3+} gluconate to the transferrin. It is taken up quickly by the reticuloendothelial system and has a half-life of about 1 hour in the bloodstream. It is supplied in 5-mg ampules containing 62.5 mg of elemental iron. It has been available in Europe since 1959, but was recently introduced in the U.S. It is FDA-indicated for iron supplementation in hemodialysis patients. The parenteral drug exposure differences between countries makes it difficult to compare allergy and anaphylaxis reports for sodium ferric gluconate complex and iron dextran. Sodium ferric gluconate appears to produce fewer anaphylactic reactions than does iron dextran. According to the package insert, a test dose of sodium ferric gluconate is not required; however, when utilized, it is given as 2 mL IV (25 mg elemental iron) in 50 mL normal saline over 60 minutes. Although sodium ferric gluconate may be administered undiluted as a slow IV injection (up to 12.5 mg/min), it is most commonly administered 10 mL IV (125 mg elemental iron) in 100 mL normal saline over 1 hour. Most hemodialysis patients require a minimum total of 1 g of elemental iron over eight dialysis sessions to replete their stores. Side effects for sodium ferric gluconate include cramps, nausea, vomiting, flushing, hypotension, loin pain, intense upper gastric pain, rash, and pruritus.

Iron sucrose is a polynuclear iron (III) hydroxide in sucrose complex with a molecular weight of about 34,000 to 60,000 daltons, and is available in 5-mL single-dose vials. Each vial contains 100 mg (20 mg/mL) of iron sucrose. Following IV administration of iron sucrose, the iron is released directly from the circulating iron sucrose to the transferrin, and is taken up in the reticuloendothelial system and metabolized. The half-life is approximately 6 hours with a volume of distribution similar to that of iron dextran. For adults on hemodialysis, it is administered at an IV dose of 100 mg one to three times per week to a total dose of 1000 mg in 10 doses. It can be given IV directly into the dialysis line by slow injection (20 mg iron [1 mL] per minute) or infusion without the requirement for a test dose. For infusion, it needs to be diluted in normal saline (maximum 100 mL) immediately prior to use and infused over a minimum of 15 minutes. Iron sucrose injection should not be administered concomitantly with oral iron preparations, as it will reduce the absorption of oral iron. Adverse effects include leg cramps and hypotension. Iron sucrose has been shown to be well tolerated, but with less-than-expected efficacy at maintaining Hgb levels above 11 g/dL and transferrin saturation above 25%.[40] Also, about 50% of patients studied experienced serum ferritin levels greater than 1,100 ng/mL, suggesting iron overload. The reduced hematologic response and development of high serum ferritin levels may be due to oversaturation of transferrin and the release of free iron. Varying doses of iron sucrose may not produce these results. Overall, iron sucrose has been shown to be safe and efficacious.[41]

■ TRANSFUSIONS

Another form of IDA treatment involves blood transfusions. The decision to manage anemia with blood transfusions is based on the evaluation of risks and benefits.[42] This form of therapy requires extreme caution with existing cardiovascular compromise. Once Hct decreases to less than 30%, the oxygen-carrying capacity in older patients drops precipitously, predisposing them to ischemia. Tachycardia, angina, ischemic patterns on electrocardiogram, cerebrovascular insufficiency, postural hypotension, and prerenal azotemia are strong indications that transfusions are necessary to maintain the Hct above 30%. An exception to this treatment option relates to the patient who has developed low Hct values over extended time periods. These patients often demonstrate cardiac compromise after transfusion despite Hct levels

in the 20s. Therapy in these patients should consist of iron therapy, followed by transfusion only if necessary. Guidelines for transfusion in perisurgical anemias exist.[43] They suggest 6 to 8 g/dL of Hgb as a threshold for treatment, with no benefit above 10 g/dL.

EVALUATION OF THERAPEUTIC OUTCOMES

A positive response to a trial of oral iron therapy would result in a modest reticulocytosis in 5 to 7 days, with an increase in Hgb at a rate of about 2 to 4 g/dL every 3 weeks until Hgb is normalized. As the Hgb level approaches normal, the rate of increase slows progressively. A Hgb response of less than 2 g over a 3-week period is unacceptable and warrants further evaluation. If the patient does not develop reticulocytosis, it is necessary to re-evaluate the diagnosis or iron replacement therapy.

Iron therapy should continue for a period sufficient for complete restoration of iron stores. Serum ferritin concentrations should return to the normal range prior to iron discontinuation. The time interval required to accomplish this goal varies, although at least 3 to 6 months of therapy is usually warranted.[44] Patients with negative iron balances caused by bleeding may require iron replacement therapy for only 1 month after correction of the underlying lesion, whereas patients with recurrent negative balances may require long-term treatment. This latter group may require as little as 30 to 60 mg of elemental iron daily.

When large amounts of parenteral iron are administered, either by total dose infusion or by multiple IM or IV doses, the patient's iron status should be closely monitored. Patients receiving regular IV iron should be monitored for clinical or laboratory evidence of iron toxicity or overload. Iron overload may be indicated by abnormal liver function tests, serum ferritin greater than 800 ng/mL or a transferrin saturation greater than 50%. Serum ferritin and transferrin saturation should be measured in the first week after doses of 100 to 200 mg, and at 2 weeks after larger IV iron doses. Hgb and Hct should be measured weekly, and serum iron and ferritin levels should be measured at least monthly. Serum iron values may be obtained reliably 48 hours after IV dosing.

MEGALOBLASTIC ANEMIAS

Macrocytic anemias are divided into megaloblastic and nonmegaloblastic anemias. Macrocytosis, as seen in megaloblastic anemias, is due to abnormalities in DNA metabolism resulting from a deficiency in vitamin B_{12} or folate, as well as due to various drugs such as hydroxyurea, zidovudine, cytosine arabinoside, methotrexate, azathioprine, 6-mercaptopurine, or cladribine.

In vitamin B_{12} or folate deficiency anemia, megaloblastosis results from interference in folic acid–and vitamin B_{12}–interdependent nucleic acid synthesis in the immature erythrocyte. The rate of RNA and cytoplasm production exceeds the rate of DNA production. The maturation process is retarded, resulting in immature large RBCs (macrocytosis). Synthesis of the RNA and DNA necessary for cell division depends on a series of reactions catalyzed by vitamin B_{12} and folic acid, as they have a role in the conversion of uridine to thymidine. As shown in Fig. 99–4, dietary folates are absorbed in this process and converted (A) to 5-methyl tetrahydrofolate, which is then converted via a B_{12}-dependent reaction (B) to tetrahydrofolate (C). After gaining a carbon, tetrahydrofolate is converted to a folate cofactor (D), 5,10-methyl-tetrahydrofolate, used by thymidylate synthetase (E) in the

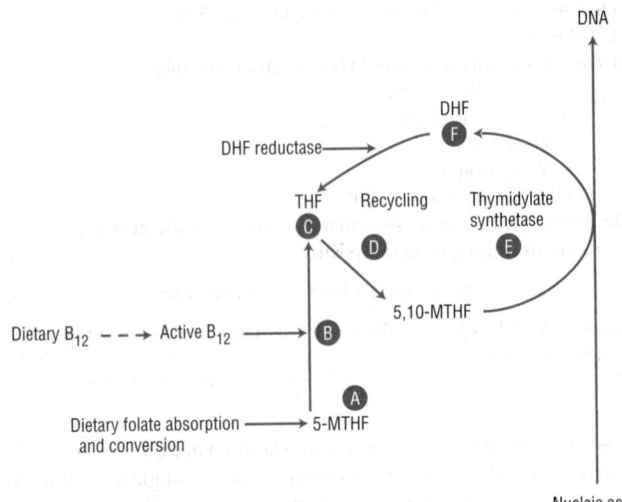

FIGURE 99–4. Drug induced megaloblastosis. DHF, dihydrofolate; 5-MTHF, 5-methyl-tetrahydrofolate; 5,10-MTHF, 5,10-methyl-tetrahydrofolate THF; THF, tetrahydrofolate.

biosynthesis of nucleic acids. The 5,10-methyl-tetrahydrofolate cofactor is converted to dihydrofolate (F) during biosynthesis. Normally, dihydrofolate reductase reduces dihydrofolate back to tetrahydrofolate (C), which can again pick up a carbon and be recycled to produce more 5,10-methyl-tetrahydrofolate (D).

Although vitamin B_{12} deficiency and folate deficiency are the most common causes of macrocytosis, other factors need to be considered if these deficiencies are not found to exist. Other causes of macrocytosis include: (1) a shift to immature or stressed RBCs as seen in reticulocytosis, aplastic anemia, and pure RBC aplasia; (2) a primary bone marrow disorder such as myelodysplastic syndromes, congenial dyserythropoietic anemias, and large granular lymphocyte leukemia; (3) lipid abnormalities as seen with liver disease, hypothyroidism, or hyperlipidemia, and lastly; (4) unknown mechanisms resulting from alcohol abuse and multiple myeloma. Alcoholism is a common cause of macrocytosis, as approximately 90% of alcoholics have macrocytosis prior to the appearance of an anemia.[45] Even with adequate folate and vitamin B_{12} levels plus the absence of liver disease, patients may present with an alcohol-induced macrocytosis. Cessation of alcohol ingestion results in resolution of the macrocytosis within a couple of months.

VITAMIN B_{12} DEFICIENCY ANEMIA

Epidemiology

Adult-onset pernicious anemia has an estimated annual incidence of 100 per 1 million population in the United States, and is slightly more common in women. However, the incidence may be underestimated due to the aging population and universal use of gastric acid–suppressing agents, as these agents may inhibit vitamin B_{12} absorption. Older adults have an estimated prevalence reaching 40%.[46]

Etiology

5 The three major causes of vitamin B_{12} deficiency are inadequate intake, malabsorption syndromes, and inadequate utilization. Inadequate dietary consumption of vitamin B_{12} is rare. It usually occurs only in patients who are strict vegans and their breast-fed infants, chronic alcoholics, or elderly patients with a "tea and toast" diet due to financial limitations or poor dentition. Decreased absorption of vitamin B_{12} is seen in patients with pernicious anemia. It is caused by the absence of intrinsic factor due to either autoimmune destruction of the gastric parietal cells or atrophy of the gastric mucosa. It is most commonly seen in Europeans of northern descent and African-Americans. A deficiency in intrinsic factor limits vitamin B_{12} absorption, but is rarely diagnosed in patients less than 35 years of age. Another cause accounting for up to 50% of deficiencies later in life is the inability of vitamin B_{12} to be cleaved and released from the proteins in food due to inadequate gastric acid production.[47] Conditions leading to this phenomenon include subtotal gastrectomy, atrophic gastritis resulting in decreased acid pepsin production, and prolonged use of acid suppression therapy. Supplemental cobalamin is well absorbed in these individuals, as it is not protein bound. Additionally, the treatment of *Helicobacter pylori* may improve vitamin B_{12} status, as it is a cause of chronic gastritis.[48] Vitamin B_{12} deficiency may also result from overgrowth of bacteria in the bowel that utilizes vitamin B_{12}, or from injury or removal of ileal receptor sites where vitamin B_{12} and the intrinsic factor complex are absorbed. Blind loop syndrome, Whipple's disease, Zollinger-Ellison syndrome, tapeworm infestations, intestinal resections, tropical sprue, surgical resection of the ileus, pancreatic insufficiency, inflammatory bowel disease, advanced liver disease, tuberculosis, and Crohn's disease may all contribute to the development of vitamin B_{12} deficiency.[49]

Pathophysiology

Vitamin B_{12} is necessary for DNA synthesis, is important in metabolic reactions involving folic acid, and is essential in maintaining the integrity of the neurologic system. It is a water-soluble vitamin obtained exogenously by ingestion of meat, fish, poultry, dairy products, and fortified cereals. Body stores, which are found primarily in the liver, range from 2 to 5 mg. The recommended daily allowance is 2.4 mcg in adults and is slightly higher in pregnant or breast-feeding women. The average Western diet contains 5 to 30 mcg of vitamin B_{12}, of which 1 to 5 mcg is absorbed. It takes several years for a vitamin B_{12} deficiency to develop following vitamin deprivation, due to efficient enterohepatic circulation of the vitamin.

After the stomach's acidic environment facilitates the breakdown of vitamin B_{12} bound to food, the vitamin B_{12} binds to the intrinsic factor released by the stomach's parietal cells. The secretion of intrinsic factor generally corresponds to the release of hydrochloric acid and serves as a cell-directed carrier protein similar to transferrin for iron. This complex, resistant to degradation, forms in the duodenum and allows for subsequent absorption of vitamin B_{12} in the terminal ileum. The cobalamin-intrinsic factor complex is taken up into the ileal mucosal cell, the intrinsic factor is discarded, and the cobalamin is transferred to transcobalamin II, which serves as a transport protein. This complex is secreted into the circulation and is taken up by the liver, bone marrow, and other cells. Transcobalamin II has a short half-life of 1 hour and is rapidly cleared from the blood. Consequently, most circulating cobalamin is bound to serum haptocorrins (formerly transcobalamin I and transcobalamin III) whose function is unknown. However, it should be noted that an alternate pathway for vitamin B_{12} absorption independent of intrinsic factor or an intact ter-

minal ileum accounts for a small amount of vitamin B_{12} absorption.[50] This alternate pathway involves passive diffusion and accounts for approximately 1% absorption of the ingested vitamin B_{12}.

Cobalamin is also a crucial cofactor in the conversion of homocysteine to methionine. When this reaction is impaired, folate metabolism is disturbed, resulting in folate-deficient tissues, and consequently, megaloblastic erythropoiesis.

Laboratory Findings

In macrocytic anemias, the MCV is usually elevated to 110 to 140 fL, but some patients deficient in vitamin B_{12} may have a normal MCV. Mild leukopenia and thrombocytopenia are often present, as DNA synthesis derangements affect all cells in the bone marrow. Advanced cases of vitamin B_{12} deficiency may result in pancytopenia. A peripheral blood smear demonstrates macrocytosis accompanied by hypersegmented polymorphonuclear leukocytes (one of the earliest and most specific indications of this disease), oval macrocytes, anisocytosis, and poikilocytosis. Serum lactate dehydrogenase and indirect bilirubin levels may be elevated as a result of hemolysis or ineffective erythropoiesis. Serum iron concentrations and transferrin saturation are usually elevated, although iron levels may be low in some patients with pernicious anemia.[51] Other laboratory findings include a low reticulocyte count, low serum vitamin B_{12} level (<100 pg/mL), and low Hct (sometimes as low as 10% to 15%).[51] If a bone marrow biopsy is performed, marked erythroid hyperplasia and megaloblastic changes in the cells of erythroid lineage will be observed.

In the early stages of vitamin B_{12} deficiency, classic signs and symptoms of megaloblastic anemia may not be evident and serum levels of vitamin B_{12} may be within normal limits. Therefore measurement of MMA and homocysteine is useful, as these parameters are often the first to change.[52] Increased levels of serum MMA and homocysteine may be evident, as both of these are involved in enzymatic reactions dependent on vitamin B_{12}, and a deficiency in vitamin B_{12} allows for accumulation of these precursors. Elevations in MMA are more specific for vitamin B_{12} deficiency, while elevated homocysteine can be indicative of either vitamin B_{12} or folic acid deficiency, but offers greater specificity for folate plasma levels. Low levels of vitamin B_{12} result in hyperhomocysteinemia, which the majority of data suggest is an independent risk factor for cerebrovascular, peripheral vascular, coronary, and venous thromboembolic disease. Hyperhomocysteinemia may also be linked to dementia and Alzheimer's disease.[53]

All patients with a suspected low vitamin B_{12} level should be screened. Vitamin B_{12} values below 150 pg/mL in a patient with macrocytosis, hypersegmented polymorphonuclear leukocytes, peripheral neuropathy, or dementia, is diagnostic of B_{12} deficiency, even though the Schilling test results may be normal. About one-third of patients with pernicious anemia will not demonstrate macrocytosis if their condition is complicated by iron deficiency, thalassemia, or a predominant neurologic involvement.

Vitamin B_{12} values of 200 to 300 pg/mL are suggestive of depletion, and the patient should undergo repeated testing in 1 to 3 months. A Schilling test may be performed to diagnose pernicious anemia, but the utility of this test is questionable and rarely alters the clinical management of the vitamin B_{12} deficiency. The Schilling test was once performed to determine whether vitamin B_{12} needed to be replaced via an oral or parenteral route, but evidence now suggests oral replacement is as efficacious as parenteral supplementation due to the vitamin B_{12} absorption pathway independent of intrinsic factor. Limitations to the test include its complicated protocol, the need for a 24-hour urine collection, difficulty in obtaining radiolabeled vitamin B_{12}, and difficulty in interpreting results in patients with renal insufficiency.[50]

Other potentially useful tests include antibody testing and serum gastrin levels. Positive anti–intrinsic factor antibodies may be present in approximately half of patients with pernicious anemia, but is highly specific for the disease.[18] Additionally, an estimated 85% of patients have anti–parietal cell antibodies, but they are nonspecific, as 3% to 10% of healthy patients have these antibodies.[18] Fasting serum gastrin levels are elevated in more than 70% of patients with cobalamin deficiency and may be useful in assessing patients with borderline

serum cobalamin levels.[54] If the results of the Schilling test are normal and the serum gastrin level is elevated, this is suggestive of food-cobalamin malabsorption. When evaluating low serum vitamin B_{12} levels, one should rule out other causes besides dietary deprivation and malabsorption. For example, levels may be falsely low in patients receiving antibiotics, anticonvulsants, cytotoxic agents, oral contraceptives, and high-dose vitamin C. In addition, conditions that can result in falsely low vitamin B_{12} levels include multiple myeloma, malignancy, aplastic anemia, a deficiency in serum haptocorrins, gastrectomy, the third trimester of pregnancy, and radioisotope exposure studies.

▶ TREATMENT: Vitamin B_{12} Deficiency Anemia

The goals of treatment for vitamin B_{12} deficiency include reversal of hematologic manifestations, replacement of body stores, and the prevention or reversal of neurologic manifestations. Early treatment is of paramount importance to reverse any neurologic symptoms present, as they may be irreversible if the deficiency is not detected for 6 to 12 months. Permanent disabilities may range from mild paresthesias and numbness to memory loss and outright psychosis. In addition to replacement therapy, any underlying etiology that is treatable, such as bacterial overgrowth, should be remedied. In the rare cases of nutritional deficiency, the oral or parenteral administration of vitamin B_{12} is beneficial. Patients should also be counseled on the types of foods high in vitamin B_{12} content (Table 99–8). The oral administration of vitamin B_{12} can also be used effectively to treat pernicious anemia or cobalamin deficiency due to ileal resection, but in much larger doses than those used to treat other causes of vitamin B_{12} deficiency. Oral replacement therapy can be utilized due to the aforementioned alternate pathway, independent of intrinsic factor. Oral doses may be initiated at 1 to 2 mg daily for 1 to 2 weeks, followed by 1-mg daily, since doses less than 0.5 mg may result in variable absorption.[55] The 1-mg cobalamin tablets are available over

the counter. The only contraindications to oral replacement therapy include inability to take medications orally, diarrhea, or vomiting. A commonly used initial parenteral vitamin B_{12} regimen consists of daily injections of 1,000 mcg of cyanocobalamin for 1 week to saturate vitamin B_{12} stores in the body and to resolve clinical manifestations of the deficiency. Afterwards, it can be given weekly for 1 month and monthly thereafter for maintenance. Hydroxocobalamin is a less popular formulation of parenteral vitamin B_{12} that is available. Its low utilization rate may be due to the possibility of antibody development to the hydroxocobalamin-transcobalamin II complex in some patients. Parenteral therapy is preferred for patients exhibiting neurologic symptoms until resolution of symptoms and hematologic indices, since the most rapid-acting therapy is necessary.[56] If converting patients from the parenteral to the oral form of cobalamin, 1 mg of oral cobalamin daily can be initiated on the due date of the next injection.

In addition to the oral and parenteral form, vitamin B_{12} is available in an intranasal gel formulation. This form may be advantageous for patients who are homebound, have cognitive impairment, or are experiencing dysphagia. Intranasal administration should be avoided in patients with nasal diseases or those receiving medications intranasally in the same nostril. Additionally, patients should avoid administering the gel 1 hour before or after the ingestion of hot foods or beverages, as cobalamin absorption may be impaired. The efficacy of the nasal gel formulation has not been well studied and it should only be used for maintenance therapy once hematologic parameters have normalized.

Potential adverse effects with vitamin B_{12} replacement therapy are rare. Uncommon side effects include hyperuricemia and hypokalemia. Rebound thrombocytosis may precipitate thrombotic events. Another side effect of vitamin B_{12} therapy is sodium retention. This effect is more likely to occur in the patient with compromised cardiovascular status, because of an expansion in intravascular volume secondary to the sudden increase in the production of RBCs. Rare cases of anaphylaxis with parenteral administration of cobalamin have been reported.

TABLE 99–8. Good Sources of Vitamin B_{12}

Food	Serving Size	Amount (mcg)
Beef liver, cooked	3 oz	60
Breakfast ceral, fortified (100%)	3/4 cup	6
Rainbow trout, cooked	3 oz	5.3
Sockeye salmon, cooked	3 oz	4.9
Beef, cooked	3 oz	2.1
Breakfast cereal, fortified (25%)	3/4 cup	1.5
Haddock, cooked	3 oz	1.2
Clams, breaded and fried	3/4 cup	1.1
Oysters, breaded and fried	6 pieces	1
Tuna, canned in water	3 oz	0.9
Milk	1 cup	0.9
Yogurt	8 oz	0.9

Evaluation of Therapeutic Outcomes

Most patients respond rapidly to vitamin B_{12} therapy. The patient will experience an improvement in strength and well-being within a few days. If glossitis is present, improvement is seen within 24 hours. Bone marrow becomes normoblastic after 24 hours, but is not evident in the plasma for another 7 days. Reticulocytosis is evident in 2 to 5 days and peaks around day 7. Hgb begins to rise after the first week and the leukocyte and platelet counts normalize

after about 7 days. Hypersegmented neutrophils persist for about 2 weeks. A CBC count and a serum cobalamin level is usually drawn 1 to 2 months after the initiation of therapy and 3 to 6 months thereafter for surveillance monitoring. Homocysteine and MMA levels should be repeated 2 to 3 months after the initiation of replacement therapy to evaluate for normalization of levels, although levels begin to decrease in 1 to 2 weeks. Failure to observe these findings usually indicates an incorrect diagnosis or other factors contributing to the anemia such as iron deficiency or thalassemia trait. The neuropsychiatric signs and symptoms can be reversible if they are of less than 6 months' duration, but 6 months of replacement therapy or longer may be necessary before improvement is noted.[44] If permanent neurologic damage has resulted, progression should cease with replacement therapy. Demands for iron may be greater during the initiation of therapy as a result of increased erythropoiesis.[57]

FOLIC ACID DEFICIENCY ANEMIA

Epidemiology

Folic acid deficiency is one of the most common vitamin deficiencies in the United States, largely due to its association with excessive alcohol intake and pregnancy. Requirements for folate in pregnancy are about five times higher than normal daily requirements.

Etiology

⬖ **6**   Major causes of folic acid deficiency include inadequate intake, decreased absorption, hyperutilization, and inadequate utilization. Since folic acid deficiency is associated with poor eating habits, it is common in elderly patients, alcoholics, food faddists, the poverty stricken, and those who are chronically ill or in demented states. Folic acid absorption may decrease in patients who have malabsorption syndromes or those who have received certain drugs. In addition to poor dietary habits associated with alcoholics, alcohol also interferes with folic acid absorption, interferes with folic acid utilization at the cellular level, and decreases hepatic stores of folic acid.

Hyperutilization of folic acid may occur when the rate of cellular division is increased as is seen during pregnancy; hemolytic anemia; myelofibrosis; malignancy; chronic inflammatory disorders such as Crohn's disease, rheumatoid arthritis, or psoriasis; long-term dialysis; burn patients; and growth spurts seen in adolescence and infancy. This can lead to anemia, particularly when the daily intake of folate is borderline, resulting in inadequate replacement of folate stores.

Several drugs (e.g., sulfasalazine, trimethoprim-sulfamethoxazole, and methotrexate) have been reported to cause a folic acid deficiency megaloblastic anemia. These drugs either interfere with folate absorption or inhibit the dihydrofolate reductase enzyme necessary for conversion of dihydrofolate to its active tetrahydrofolate form (see Chap. 102, on drug-induced blood dyscrasias).

Phenytoin may induce a megaloblastic anemia, as the levels of serum folic acid decrease up to 40% in about half of all patients treated with the anticonvulsant. The progression to overt megaloblastic anemia occurs in less than 1% of patients. Since folic acid doses as low as 1 mg/day may affect serum phenytoin levels, routine supplementation is not generally advised. This decline in phenytoin concentration is usually evidenced within the first 10 days and may diminish the phenytoin levels by 15% to 50%.[58]

Pathophysiology

Folic acid is a water-soluble vitamin readily destroyed by cooking or processing. It is necessary for the production of nucleic acids, proteins, amino acids, purines, and thymine, and hence DNA and RNA. It acts as a methyl donor to form methylcobalamin, which is used in the remethylation of homocysteine to methionine. Because humans are unable to synthesize total daily folate requirements, they depend on a dietary source of this vitamin. Major dietary sources of folate include fresh, green, leafy vegetables, citrus fruits, yeast, mushrooms, dairy products, and such animal organs as liver and kidney. Most folate in food is present in the polyglutamate form, which needs to be broken down into the monoglutamate form prior to absorption in the small intestine. Once absorbed, dietary folate must be converted to tetrahydrofolate through a cobalamin-dependent reaction in order to achieve its active state. Additionally, in 1997 the U.S. government mandated the fortification of grain products with folic acid with the desire to increase the dietary intake of folate by 100 mcg of folate per person daily. This amount of supplementation was chosen to decrease the incidence of neural tube defects without masking occult vitamin B_{12} deficiency. Even though body demands for folate are high, owing to high rates of RBC synthesis and turnover, the minimum daily requirement is 50 to 100 mcg. In the general population, the recommended daily allowance for folate is 400 mcg in nonpregnant females, 600 mcg for pregnant females, and 500 mcg for lactating females.[59] On average, Americans ingest 200 to 300 mcg of folate per day. The body stores approximately 5 to 10 mg of folate, primarily in the liver; therefore cessation of dietary folate intake results in depletion of body stores in a relatively short period of time. Folate is distributed to the other tissues primarily via enterohepatic recirculation. The methylated form of folate is reabsorbed from the bile into the serum. As it enters the tissues, including erythrocytes, it endures for the remaining life span of the cell.

Laboratory Findings

It is of paramount importance to rule out vitamin B_{12} deficiency when folate deficiency is detected, as symptoms are similar. Laboratory changes associated with folate deficiency are similar to those seen in vitamin B_{12} deficiency, except vitamin B_{12} levels are normal. Decreases occur in the serum folate level (<3 ng/mL) within a few days of dietary folate limitations. The RBC folate level (<150 ng/mL) also declines and may be a better indicator of deficiency, as levels remain constant throughout the life span of the erythrocyte. Serum folate levels are sensitive to short-term changes such as dietary restrictions or alcohol intake, which may result in a short-term decline in serum levels with adequate tissue stores. It should be noted that an estimated 60% of patients with pernicious anemia have falsely low RBC folate levels, in all probability due to the requirement of cobalamin for the normal transfer of methyltetrahydrofolate from plasma to cells.[18] Additionally, if serum or erythrocyte folate levels are borderline, serum homocysteine is usually increased with a folic acid deficiency. If serum MMA levels are also elevated, vitamin B_{12} deficiency needs to be ruled out.

▶ TREATMENT: Folic Acid Deficiency Anemia

Therapy for folic acid deficiency consists of the administration of exogenous folic acid in order to induce hematologic remission, replace body stores, and resolve signs and symptoms. In the majority of cases, 1 mg daily is sufficient to replace stores except in cases of deficiency due to malabsorption, in which case doses up to 5 mg daily may be necessary. Synthetic folic acid is almost completely absorbed by the gastrointestinal tract and is converted to tetrahydrofolate without cobalamin. Therapy should continue for approximately 4 months if the underlying cause of the deficiency can be identified and corrected. This treatment period allows a sufficient amount of time for all folate-deficient RBCs to be cleared from the circulation. Long-term folate administration may be necessary in chronic conditions associated with increased folate requirements as listed previously. It is also recommended that patients with a folic acid deficiency be placed on diets containing foods high in folate (Table 99–9). Low-dose folate therapy (500 mcg daily) may be administered when anticonvulsant drugs produce a megaloblastic anemia and may make it unnecessary to discontinue the anticonvulsant. Adverse effects have not been reported with folic acid doses used for replacement therapy.

Although megaloblastic anemia during pregnancy is rare, the most common cause is folate deficiency. The condition usually manifests itself as an underweight, premature infant and suboptimal health for the mother. Folic acid supplementation (800 to 1,000 mcg daily) prior to conception and during pregnancy reduces the incidence of neural tube defects in the general population.[60] Women who have previously given birth to offspring with neural tube defects or those with a family history of neural tube defects should ingest 4 mg of folic acid daily.[58] Finally, it has been suggested that supplementation with 10 mg of folic acid daily may reduce the incidence of cleft lip.[61] It is clearly essential that women in their childbearing years maintain adequate folic acid intake.

TABLE 99–9. Good Sources of Folate

Food	Serving	Amount (mcg)
Chicken liver	3.5 oz	770
Cereal	$\frac{1}{2}$ to $1\frac{1}{2}$ cups	100–400
Lentils, cooked	$\frac{1}{2}$ cup	180
Chickpeas	$\frac{1}{2}$ cup	141
Asparagus	$\frac{1}{2}$ cup	132
Spinach, cooked	$\frac{1}{2}$ cup	131
Black beans	$\frac{1}{2}$ cup	128
Pasta	2 oz	100–120
Kidney beans	$\frac{1}{2}$ cup	115
Lima beans	$\frac{1}{2}$ cup	78
White rice, cooked	$\frac{3}{4}$ cup	60
Tomato juice	1 cup	48
Brussels sprouts	$\frac{1}{2}$ cup	47
Orange	1 medium	47

Evaluation of Therapeutic Outcomes

Symptomatic improvement, as evidenced by increased alertness, appetite, and cooperation, often takes place early during the course of treatment. Reticulocytosis occurs within 2 to 3 days and peaks within 5 to 8 days after beginning therapy. Hct begins to rise within 2 weeks and should reach normal levels within 2 months. The MCV initially increases because of an increase in reticulocytes, but then gradually decreases to normal.

ANEMIA OF CHRONIC DISEASE

EPIDEMIOLOGY

ACD is one of the most common forms of anemia seen clinically and is especially important in the differential diagnosis of iron deficiency. Since ACD, as the name implies, is associated with other prominent disease states, the usual signs and symptoms are often overshadowed. The diagnosis of ACD is usually one of exclusion, with particular emphasis on the possibility of IDA as the primary anemia or as a coexistent anemia with ACD because of chronic disease–associated conditions (e.g., gastrointestinal blood loss from aspirin, other nonsteroidal anti-inflammatory agents, or steroids) or malignancy-associated bleeding. ACD is often observed in patients with diseases that last longer than 1 to 2 months, although it can occur in conditions with a fairly rapid onset of several weeks, such as a pneumonia. It can also coexist with anemia of renal disease, IDA, chemotherapy-induced anemia, and AIDS-related anemia. Anemia is the most common hematologic abnormality associated with human immunodeficiency virus (HIV), and the yearly incidence of developing anemia increases with disease progression.[62] Table 99–10 lists common diseases associated with ACD.

ETIOLOGY

ACD is one response to the stimulation of the cellular immune system by various underlying disease processes. ACD commonly develops in AIDS patients, especially those with opportunistic infections or malnutrition, and is associated with increased morbidity and mortality. It may also be due to drugs used to treat AIDS and associated illness.[63] HIV contributes to abnormalities of hematopoiesis. Infection of progenitor cells is just one factor involved in HIV-induced bone marrow suppression.

PATHOPHYSIOLOGY

ACD is a hypoproliferative anemia that has traditionally been associated with infectious or inflammatory processes, tissue injury, or conditions associated with the release of proinflammatory cytokines. Alternative names include anemia of inflammation and cytokine-mediated anemia. The pathogenesis of the anemia of chronic disorders is based on three abnormalities: shortened erythrocyte survival, impaired marrow response, and disturbance of iron metabolism. Pathologically, the RBCs have a shortened life span, and the bone marrow's capacity to respond to EPO is inadequate to maintain normal Hgb concentration. The cause of this defect is still uncertain, but appears to involve a block in the release of iron from the reticuloendothelial cells of the marrow. Various cytokines, such as interleukin-1, interferon-γ, and tumor necrosis factor released during these illnesses may inhibit the production or action of EPO or the production of RBCs.[64]

TABLE 99–10. Diseases Causing Anemia of Chronic Disease

Common causes
  Chronic infections
    Tuberculosis
    Other chronic lung infections
    Human immunodeficiency virus
    Subacute bacterial endocarditis
    Osteomyelitis
    Chronic urinary tract infections
  Chronic inflammation
    Rheumatoid arthritis
    Systemic lupus erythematosus
    Rheumatoid (collagen vascular) diseases
    Inflammatory osteoarthritis
    Gout
    Chronic inflammatory liver diseases
  Malignancies
    Carcinoma
    Lymphoma
    Leukemia
    Multiple myeloma
Less common causes
  Alcoholic liver disease
  Congestive heart failure
  Thrombophlebitis
  Chronic obstructive lung disease
  Ischemic heart disease

LABORATORY FINDINGS

No definitive test will confirm a diagnosis of ACD, and the diagnosis is often overlooked.[27] The practitioner should maintain a high index of suspicion in any patient with a chronic disease. ACD may coexist with IDA and folic acid deficiency, as many of these patients will have poor dietary intake or gastrointestinal blood loss. Examination of the bone marrow reveals an abundance of iron, suggesting the release mechanism for iron is the central defect. Patients with ACD usually have a decreased serum iron level, but unlike those with IDA, their serum ferritin level is normal or increased and their TIBC decreased. Generally, ACD is normocytic and normochromic. With ACD, hypochromia usually precedes microcytosis, with the opposite finding in IDA. Erythrocyte survival may be reduced in patients with ACD, but a compensatory erythropoietic response usually does not occur.

▶ TREATMENT: Anemia of Chronic Disease

The treatment of ACD is somewhat less specific than the treatment of other anemias. Focus should be on treating the underlying disorder and correcting reversible causes of anemia. Direct approaches to correction of anemia may not be needed. During inflammation, oral or parenteral iron therapy is ineffective. Transfusions of RBCs are effective, but should be limited to situations in which oxygen transport is inadequate due to concomitant medical problems. The Hgb level necessitating a RBC transfusion varies from 8 to 10 g/dL based on factors such as cost, convenience, and risk of infectious complications. Assessment of the symptomatic state should always be considered before blood products are administered.

Exogenous EPO (or epoetin alfa) has been used to stimulate erythropoiesis in patients with ACD, as a relative EPO deficiency exists for the degree of anemia. Use should be considered in patients with compromised cardiovascular status, although patients with chronic disease may have a relatively impaired response to epoetin alfa. The dosage is 50 to 100 units per kilogram three times a week. The dosage can be increased to 150 units per kilogram per dose if no increase in Hgb concentration occurs after 6 to 8 weeks. Response to EPO varies depending on dose and cause of the anemia. EPO treatment is effective when the marrow has an adequate supply of iron, cobalamin, and folic acid.

Treatment of anemia in HIV-infected patients starts with therapy of HIV and correction of reversible causes of anemia.[65] For zidovudine-treated HIV-infected patients, an initial IV or subcutaneous dose of 100 units/kg, three times per week for 8 weeks is suggested. If response is not satisfactory based on decreased transfusion requirements or increased Hct after 8 weeks of therapy, the dose is increased by 50 to 100 units/kg, three times per week. Dosage adjustments in increments of 50 to 100 units/kg three times a week can be made to a maximum of 300 units/kg per dose three times a week. The dose should be discontinued when the Hct is greater than 40%. Treatment should then be restarted at a 25% dosage reduction when Hct decreases to 36%. A simplified weekly regimen of 40,000 units of subcutaneously administered EPO has been given successfully to some patients with HIV-associated anemia.[66]

Most patients tolerate EPO therapy well. Iron deficiency can occur in patients treated with EPO and close monitoring of iron levels is necessary. Oral iron supplementation should be given if transferrin saturation drops to 20% or the serum ferritin level drops below 100 ng/mL. Some patients develop "functional" iron deficiency, in which the iron stores are normal, but the supply of iron to the erythroid marrow is less than that necessary to support the demand for RBC production. Therefore many practitioners routinely supplement EPO therapy with oral iron therapy. The hypertension commonly seen in end-stage renal disease patients on EPO is far less common in AIDS patients. More common toxicities of EPO administration include nausea, headache, fever, bone pain, and fatigue. Other adverse effects to monitor include seizures, thrombotic events, and allergic reactions such as rash or local reactions at the injection site.

EVALUATION OF THERAPEUTIC OUTCOMES

An easy way to monitor the immediate effect of increased endogenous or exogenous EPO is an increase in blood reticulocyte count in the first few days. Baseline iron status should be checked before and during treatment, as many patients on EPO require supplemental iron therapy. The optimal form and schedule of iron supplementation is not known. A fall in Hgb during EPO therapy usually signifies development of an infection or iron depletion. Baseline and periodic monitoring of iron, TIBC, transferrin saturation, or ferritin levels may be useful in maximizing iron repletion and limiting the need for epoetin. EPO patients who do not respond clinically by 12 weeks should not be continued on EPO.

ANEMIA OF CRITICAL ILLNESS

EPIDEMIOLOGY

Anemia is a common complication in critically ill patients and is almost universally found in this patient population.[67,68]

ETIOLOGY

Factors that may contribute to anemia in critically ill patients include sepsis, frequent blood samples, surgical blood loss, immune-mediated functional iron deficiency, decreased production of endogenous EPO, reduced RBC life span, and gastrointestinal bleeding. Deleterious effects of anemia may include increased risk of cardiac-related morbidity and mortality, and decreased oxygen-carrying capacity with risk of multiple organ deterioration. Consequences of anemia in critically ill patients may be enhanced due to increased metabolic demands of critical illness. Additionally, it is difficult to wean anemic patients from mechanical ventilation.

PATHOPHYSIOLOGY

In anemia of critical illness, alteration in the mechanism for RBC replenishment and homeostasis occurs. The effect of cytokines on EPO may partly explain anemia of critical illness, as they are associated with a blunting of the erythropoietic response in this population.[69] In addition, the cytokines seem to directly inhibit RBC production and stimulate iron binding proteins that sequester iron and limit RBC production.[69] Impaired RBC production by the bone marrow contributes to the development and persistence of anemia.

LABORATORY FINDINGS

Anemia of critical illness is similar to ACD. Lab findings frequently seen in anemia of critical illness are low serum iron, TIBC, and iron:TIBC ratio. Serum ferritin is normal to high and EPO levels are usually slightly decreased despite the presence of anemia, with minimal reticulocyte response.[67,69] This differs from patients with IDA who generally have elevated EPO concentrations in response to a low Hct.

▶ TREATMENT: Anemia of Critical Illness

Patients with anemia of critical illness need the necessary substrates of iron, folic acid, and vitamin B_{12} for RBC production in order for the physiologic response for anemia correction to occur. Iron stores are usually insufficient to meet physiologic demands, hence the administration of supplemental iron in the oral or parenteral form is necessary to support erythropoiesis. Parenteral iron is often utilized in this population, as often patients are on enteral therapy or there are concerns regarding inadequate iron absorption. The disadvantage of parenteral therapy is the theoretical risk of infection.[70] The low iron concentrations in critically ill patients may be a defense mechanism, as microbes require iron for sustenance. Therefore diminished iron levels may inhibit bacterial growth.

The pathophysiology of anemia of critical illness would lead to the hypothesis that treatment with pharmacologic doses of EPO might be beneficial. Few randomized, controlled trials have evaluated the role of EPO in critically ill patients, and these have resulted in mixed findings regarding EPO's ability to decrease transfusion requirements.[69] A recently published literature review found that EPO cannot be recommended to reduce the need for RBC transfusions in critically ill patients with anemia.[71] Even though EPO administration may reduce the need for transfusions, improved clinical outcomes may not result. Further investigation is necessary to define the role of EPO in critically ill patients, as well as to better define optimal dosing and end points for therapy.

Many critically ill patients receive RBC transfusions, although the actual benefits of increasing Hgb in this patient population has not been clearly established. Stored RBCs may not function as well as endogenous blood. Although RBC transfusions may increase oxygen delivery to tissues, the cellular oxygen may or may not increase.[72] Transfusion practices vary in intensive care units, with clinicians using different Hgb concentrations as thresholds for administering transfusions. Recent data have suggested that RBC transfusions may decrease the likelihood of survival in some subgroups of critically ill patients.[73] Decisions to use transfusions must include a discussion of the risks of transfusions, including immunosuppression, immunosaturation, microthrombosis, and virus transmission. Additional immediate risks of transfusions include infections, infusion reactions, and transfusion-related acute lung injury. Lastly, the clinician must take into consideration administrative, logistic, and economic factors.[74]

EVALUATION OF THERAPEUTIC OUTCOMES

Treatment of anemia of critical illness has nonspecific goals of therapy. The role of monitoring RBCs, Hgb, Hct, EPO levels, and reticulocyte counts remains to be determined. Outcomes used in EPO studies are transfusion requirements and transfusion independence. Morbidity, mortality, and length of stay are also assessed. Adverse effects such as risk of thrombotic events must be monitored. More research is needed to determine whether reduction in RBC transfusions and increases in Hgb will result in improved clinical outcomes.

ANEMIA IN THE ELDERLY

EPIDEMIOLOGY

9 One of the most common clinical problems observed in the elderly is anemia. Anemia is a prevalent and increasing problem in the elderly, with approximately 12% of people aged 60 and over affected.[75] The number of cases increases with age with the highest prevalence in men 85 and older.[2] Prior to the age of 55, the incidence of anemia is higher in women (3% in men vs. 6% in women aged 50 to 54), whereas after this point the prevalence appears to be higher in men (at 65 years of age, prevalence is found to be 21% in men and 16% in women).[76] Elderly patients with the highest incidence of anemia are those that are hospitalized, followed by residents of nursing homes and institutions at an estimated rate of 31% to 40%.[54] The lowest incidence is seen in elderly patients that are community dwellers. Although the incidence of anemia is high in the elderly, it should not be alleged as an inevitable outcome of aging, as an underlying cause can be identified in approximately 80% of patients.[75] Undiagnosed and untreated anemia can have severe ramifications and is affiliated with an increased risk of mortality, poor health, and decreased physical function. Additionally, it can cause neurologic, cognitive, and cardiovascular complications. Anemia may also be an indication of serious diseases such as gastrointestinal cancer. Various studies have indicated the risk of mortality is increased among elderly with anemia.[75]

PATHOPHYSIOLOGY

Data have indicated that aging is associated with a progressive reduction in hematopoietic reserve, which makes individuals more susceptible to developing anemia in times of hematopoietic stress.[77] Although Hgb levels may remain normal, the diminished marrow reserve leaves the elderly patient more susceptible to other causes of anemia. Additionally, renal insufficiency is common in elderly patients and this may reduce the ability of the kidneys to produce EPO. Patients often have a normal creatinine level but a diminished glomerular filtration rate. It has been suggested that a deficiency in endogenous EPO develops when the GFR falls below 50% of the normal range.

ETIOLOGY

In the acute ward setting, the top three causes of anemia in the elderly have been identified as chronic disease (35%), unexplained cause (17%), and iron deficiency (15%), whereas in community-based outpatient clinics the most prevalent causes are unexplained (36%), infection (23%), and chronic disease (17%).[76] Risk factors for the development of anemia in the elderly include race and ethnicity with the highest prevalence in elderly blacks, those with serum albumin and serum creatinine abnormalities, and recent hospitalization or placement in an institution.[54]

In general, the anemia is hyporegenerative and represents an inability of the older hematopoietic system to replace the peripheral blood loss. The unexplained causes may be due to inadequate diagnostic evaluation or due to absolute or relative EPO deficiency. Absolute deficiency may be associated with renal insufficiency, whereas relative deficiency may be due to the body's inability to provide adequate response to declining Hgb levels.[76]

Another common problem in the elderly is vitamin B_{12} deficiency, with the most common causes of clinically overt deficiency due to pernicious anemia, small bowel disease, and food-cobalamin malabsorption. A preclinical deficiency in vitamin B_{12} is seen in 5% to 30% of all seemingly healthy elderly patients and is predominantly metabolic in expression, although subtle neurologic and cognitive defects may be present.[54]

One often-overlooked major factor that may contribute to anemia in the older population is nutritional status. Cross-sectional studies demonstrate a higher prevalence of anemia in low socioeconomic populations, as well as a high prevalence of other nutritional deficiencies. Thus nutritional deficiencies not usually severe enough to affect the hematopoietic system in the younger population may account for anemia in the aged. Edentulous or infirm elderly who may be too ill to prepare their meals are at risk for nutritional folate deficiency. However, unlike cobalamin levels, it has been demonstrated that folate levels increase rather than decline with age.[78] This may be due to the dramatic increase in folate supplements used by the elderly, especially in white women, as well as the fortification of the American diet with folic acid.[79]

Other common anemias in the elderly include IDA and ACD. Iron malabsorption may occur after total gastrectomy. Bleeding with resultant iron deficiency in the elderly may be due to carcinoma, ulcer, atropic gastritis, drug-induced gastritis, postmenopausal vaginal bleeding, or bleeding hemorrhoids. Elderly women have a much lower incidence of IDA as compared to younger, menstruating women. Until proven otherwise, iron deficiency in the elderly should be considered a sign of chronic blood loss. ACD is more common in the elderly, as diseases that contribute to ACD such as cancer, infection, and rheumatoid arthritis are more prevalent in this population.

LABORATORY FINDINGS

Elderly males may have lower Hgb levels, but it is not known if this is secondary to physiologic reasons or increased prevalence of anemia. Low levels may be due to decreased androgen secretion in men or age-related changes in stem cells. For practical purposes, it is best to use usual adult reference values for labs in the elderly and realize that some mild anemias may go unexplained.

A CBC, including a peripheral smear and reticulocyte count, should be performed in any elderly patient with symptoms that may be attributed to anemia, along with a physical exam to look for signs of renal or hepatic failure as well as to evaluate for gastrointestinal or genitourinary blood loss. If the reticulocyte count is adequate, blood loss or RBC destruction should be suspected, whereas a low level will indicate decreased RBC production. With a low reticulocyte count, RBC indices should be evaluated and if the MCV is >100 fL, further evaluation should be performed to discern vitamin B_{12} deficiency and folate deficiency as possible causes. A vitamin B_{12} deficiency may be present even when plasma levels of vitamin B_{12} are within normal range, but elevated levels of MMA will detect the deficiency. A refractory macrocytic anemia in the elderly should raise suspicion of a myelodysplastic or leukemic syndrome.

If the MCV is <100 fL, further studies should be evaluated to determine if possible causes are iron deficiency or ACD.

With IDA, laboratory abnormalities are similar to those discussed above in the microcytic anemia section. However, serum iron and TIBC decrease with age, making the transferrin saturation ratio less useful in the elderly. MCVs and mean cell Hgb concentrations may appear normal even in the presence of IDA, as patients may have concurrent vitamin B_{12} or folate deficiency anemias.

▶ TREATMENT: Anemia in the Elderly

Depending on the type of anemia unveiled, treatment in the elderly is the same as that specified for each type of anemia previously discussed in this chapter. With IDA it is essential to treat the underlying cause if known (i.e., bleeding) as well as with iron supplementation in the dose of 50 to 100 mg of elemental iron three times a day if tolerated. Vitamin B_{12} deficiency is treated with parenteral or oral vitamin B_{12} supplementation, while folic acid deficiency is treated with folic acid, generally at a dose of 1 mg daily. ACD does not have any specific treatment except to resolve the underlying cause. EPO is helpful in some patients with ACD at a dosage of 50 to 100 units/kg three times a week and adjusted upwards if response is inadequate.

EVALUATION OF THERAPEUTIC OUTCOMES

Reticulocytosis usually starts within 1 week of oral supplementation with iron. If the reticulocyte count rises but the anemia does not improve, inadequate absorption of iron or continued blood loss needs to be considered. Also, with any form of anemia, symptomatic improvement should be evident shortly after starting therapy. Additionally, Hgb/Hct should begin to rise within a few weeks of initiating therapy.

ANEMIA IN PEDIATRIC POPULATIONS

EPIDEMIOLOGY

IDA is a leading cause of infant morbidity and mortality in the world. In the United States, the prevalence of IDA among children is declining due to improved iron supplementation.[1] Data from the third NHANES indicated that 9% of children ages 12 to 36 months in the United States had iron deficiency and 3% had IDA.[80] Another source states that as many as 20% of children in the United States and 80% of children in developing countries will have anemia prior to the age of 18 years.[13] Peak requirements for iron absorption occur during puberty. The prevalence of iron deficiency is highest among premature or low-birth-weight infants; children living below the poverty level; African-American and Mexican-American children; and infants fed only non–iron fortified formulas. An anemia of prematurity can occur 3 to 12 weeks after birth in infants less than 32 weeks' gestation and spontaneously resolves by 3 to 6 months. The prevalence of vitamin B_{12} deficiency has been identified as 1 in 1,255 for levels <100 pg/mL and 1 in 200 for levels of <200 pg/mL, with the lowest levels in non-Hispanic whites.[81]

PATHOPHYSIOLOGY

In contrast to anemias in adults, which tend to be manifestations of some broader underlying pathology, anemias in the pediatric population are more often due to a primary hematologic abnormality.[82] The amount of iron present at birth depends on gestational length and weight. Erythropoiesis normally decreases after birth. A concurrent decrease in EPO production results in a physiologic anemia at 2 to 9 weeks of age. Iron stores are mostly depleted by age 6 months, while the blood volume is doubling from 4 to 12 months.

ETIOLOGY

The age of the child can yield some clues about the etiology of the anemia. The optimal amount of nutritional iron and folate required varies in an individual, based on life cycle stages. Two peak periods place children at risk of developing IDA, with the first being during late infancy and early childhood, when children undergo rapid body growth, have low levels of dietary iron, and exhaust stores accumulated during gestation. The second peak period is recognized during adolescence, when rapid growth, poor diets, and onset of menses occurs.[83]

During the first 5 to 6 months, the normal term infant is iron replete. Conditions in the newborn period that can lead to IDA may include prematurity, administration of EPO for AOP, or insufficient dietary intake. Premature infants are at increased risk of IDA because of a smaller total blood volume, increased blood loss through phlebotomy, and poor gastrointestinal absorption. However, iron deficiency can only occur after the birth weight has doubled in premature infants.[13] Factors leading to unbalanced iron metabolism in infants include insufficient iron intake, decreased absorption, early introduction of cow's milk, cow milk intolerance, medications, and malabsorption. However, dietary deficiency of iron in the first 6 to 12 months of life is less common today because of the increased use of iron supplementation during breast-feeding and use of iron-fortified formulas. Iron deficiency becomes more prominent when children change to regular diets. Blood loss and hemolysis are other common causes of anemia in neonates.

Day care attendance at an earlier age may result in a higher incidence of anemia due to frequent infections. Anorexia associated with infection can lead to decreased ingestion of iron-containing foods and infection can also decrease erythropoiesis. When screening for iron deficiency in young children, a careful dietary history can help identify children at risk. Dietary deficiency has been defined as one or more of the following: less than five servings each of meat, grains, vegetables, and fruit per week; more than 16 oz of milk per day; or daily intake of fatty snacks, sweets, or more than 16 oz of soft drinks. High iron needs and the tendency to eat fewer iron-containing foods contribute to the etiology of iron deficiency during adolescence.[84]

Other causes of microcytic anemia include thalassemia, lead poisoning, and sideroblastic anemia. Homeopathic or herbal medication use may place children at risk for lead exposure, as may exposure to paint or certain cooking materials. Normocytic anemias in children include infection with human parvovirus B19 and glucose-6-phosphate dehydrogenase deficiency, while macrocytic anemias are caused by deficiencies in vitamin B_{12} and folate, chronic liver disease, hypothyroidism, and myelodysplastic disorders. Folic acid deficiency is usually due to inadequate dietary intake; however, human and cow's milk provide adequate sources. Folic acid deficiency may be seen in infants and children who primarily consume goat's milk or health food milk alternatives, as well as in children with insufficient intake of green leafy vegetables.[83] Vitamin B_{12} deficiency due to nutritional reasons is rare, but may occur due to a congenital pernicious anemia.

LABORATORY FINDINGS

When evaluating lab values in pediatric patients, it is imperative to use age- and sex-adjusted norms. It is also important to know that many blood samples are capillary samples, such as heel- or fingersticks, that may have slightly different results than venous samples.

In regular well child checks for infants, screening of the Hgb or Hct level is obtained between 6 and 12 months of age, and further testing is not pursued unless an abnormality is found.[13] If an abnormality is found, a CBC should be ordered to evaluate the MCV to determine whether the anemia is microcytic, normocytic, or macrocytic. Additionally, a peripheral smear and reticulocyte count is recommended for further differentiation if necessary. The peripheral smear can indicate the etiology based on RBC morphology, and the reticulocyte count helps differentiate between decreased RBC production and increased RBC destruction. More complete studies would include serum iron, ferritin, TIBC, and transferrin saturation. Mild hereditary anemias may produce a mild hypochromic, microcytic anemia which can be confused with IDAs. The RDW may be high with iron deficiency and is more likely to be normal with thalassemia. Lab features of AOP include normocytic normochromic cells, low reticulocyte count, and decreased RBC presence in bone marrow. Serum concentrations of EPO are low. Laboratory diagnosis of vitamin B_{12} deficiency in children is similar to that of adults, and includes a CBC, measurement of vitamin B_{12}, and MMA and homocysteine levels. Serum or erythrocyte folate levels would also be measured if a folic acid deficiency anemia is suspected.

▶ TREATMENT: Anemia in Pediatric Populations

Primary prevention of IDA in infants, children, and adolescents is the most appropriate goal since delays in mental and motor development are potentially irreversible. In April of 1998, the CDC published revised recommendations to prevent and control iron deficiency in the United States, focusing on children and women of childbearing age.[85]

Interventions likely to prevent anemia include diverse foods with bioavailable forms of iron, food fortification for infants and children, and individual supplementation. Routine screening for iron deficiency in nonpregnant adolescents is only recommended for those with risk factors. These include significant physical activity (especially adolescent female athletes), vegetarian diets, malnutrition, low body weight, chronic illness, or history of heavy menstrual blood loss. Utilizing the four questions listed in Table 99–11 can identify patients at risk for the development of IDA.[7] Patients answering "no" to one of the first three questions may be at risk for iron deficiency.

TABLE 99–11. Questions to Assess Adequacy of Dietary Iron Intake

1. Do you consume two or more portions of meat, fish, chicken, nuts, seeds, or legumes per day?
2. Do you eat at least six servings of grain per day?
3. Do you generally eat at least one serving of fruits or vegetables at the same meal that includes grains or beans?
4. Do you take a calcium supplement at every meal?

From Ross.[7]

AOP is usually treated with red blood cell transfusions. Premature infants fed human milk need 2 mg/kg per day iron supplementation. EPO may be used in AOP, keeping in mind that EPO pharmacokinetics are influenced by the developmental age of the infant. EPO has limited efficacy in decreasing the requirement for transfusions, making it a controversial treatment approach. Infants on full enteral feedings treated with EPO need iron supplements in doses of 6 mg/kg per day.

For infants aged 9 to 12 months with a mild microcytic anemia, it may be most cost effective to give a therapeutic trial of iron. Fe^{2+} sulfate at a dose of 3 mg/kg of elemental iron once or twice daily between meals for 4 weeks is recommended as the standard of care. In children that respond, iron should be continued for 2 to 3 months to replace storage iron pools, along with dietary intervention and patient education. If the anemia recurs, the work-up should include sources of occult blood loss. Higher doses of oral iron (6 mg/kg per day of elemental iron divided into two or three daily doses) are administered to older children. Parenteral iron therapy has a limited role and is rarely necessary.

For the macrocytic anemias in children, parenteral or oral folate may be administered in a dose of 1 to 3 mg daily, while vitamin B_{12} deficiency due to congenital pernicious anemia would require lifelong vitamin B_{12} supplementation.[82] Dose and frequency need to be titrated according to clinical response and laboratory values. No data are currently available regarding the use of oral vitamin B_{12} supplementation in children.

EVALUATION OF THERAPEUTIC OUTCOMES

Children with anemia as identified by labs are usually treated with further evaluation performed only if treatment response is inadequate. Therapeutic outcomes are assessed in children by checking Hgb, Hct, and RBC indices at 6 to 8 weeks after initiation of iron therapy. In premature infants, Hgb or Hct should be monitored weekly. Reticulocyte counts should be checked at 4 to 6 weeks after birth. Reticulocyte count, Hct, and absolute neutrophil counts are measured before and 1 to 2 weeks after starting EPO treatment. EPO is held for an absolute neutrophil count of less than 1,000 units/L. Serum ferritin levels may help evaluate infants not responding. Use of EPO in premature infants is not associated with the side effects frequently seen in adults.

HEMOLYTIC ANEMIA

PATHOPHYSIOLOGY

⏴11 Hemolytic anemia results from decreased survival time of RBCs secondary to destruction in the spleen or circulation. The severity of hemolytic anemia varies with the mechanism. Hemolysis may be mild, chronic, and compensated, or lifelong or acute, severe, and life-threatening.

The normal 120-day life span of a RBC comes from its inherent flexibility in passing through the microvasculature and spleen without disruption of the cell membrane or sequestration and phagocytosis by reticuloendothelial cells. Hemolysis, as defined by an RBC life span of less than 120 days, results from one of three primary defects that are intrinsic or extrinsic in origin: (1) membrane defects, (2) alterations in Hgb solubility or stability, and (3) changes in intracellular metabolic processes. Intrinsic defects are intracorpuscular changes and are often genetically determined; extrinsic defects, or extracorpuscular changes, are usually the cause of acquired hemolytic anemia. Acquired disorders result mainly from a direct effect on the membrane and less often from alterations in Hgb or metabolism. Table 99–12 lists examples of the different classes of hemolytic anemias.

Causes of hemolytic anemia in the younger patient differ from those in the elderly patient. Most younger patients exhibit congenital disease, whereas older patients most often experience autoimmune hemolytic anemia. A positive Coombs test is diagnostic in the latter group.

Alterations in Hgb solubility or stability, as seen with sickle cell anemia and the thalassemias, cause cell deformations leading to hemolysis (see Chap. 101 on sickle cell disease).

Finally, alterations in cell metabolism (enzymopathies) lead to hemolytic disease by changing cell dimensions and Hgb solubility.

The two major metabolic pathways necessary for normal RBC metabolism are the hexose monophosphate shunt pathway, with its associated enzyme systems, and the Embden-Myerhof pathway of anaerobic glycolysis. The former is responsible primarily for maintaining Hgb in the reduced state and thus preventing the formation of methemoglobin, while the latter metabolizes glucose to lactic acid, which leads to adenosine triphosphate formation.

The most common metabolic abnormality resulting in a hemolytic syndrome is glucose-6-phosphate dehydrogenase (G6PD) deficiency in the hexose monophosphate shunt pathway (see Chap. 102 on drug-induced hematologic disorders). Hgb is oxidized to methemoglobin and then to sulfhemoglobin. Heinz bodies of denatured Hgb form, resulting in damage to the RBC membrane. Hemolysis results from the action of the spleen and reticuloendothelial system, which normally removes damaged cells. The disease more typically occurs in whites of Mediterranean descent upon exposure to oxidant drugs (e.g., sulfamethoxazole and dapsone) and chemicals or with infection.

Some drugs and ingested toxins such as nitrofurantoin, cancer chemotherapy agents, phenazopyridine, sulfones, amyl nitrate, mothballs, paraquat, and hydrogen peroxide can cause direct oxidative damage to erythrocytes (see Chap. 102 on drug-induced hematologic disorders).

LABORATORY FINDINGS

Hemolytic anemias tend to be normocytic and normochromic. An increased reticulocyte count is evidence of an attempt to maintain RBC mass. A peripheral blood smear may reveal sickle cells, target cells, spherocytes, elliptocytes, and fragmented RBCs. Decreased haptoglobin is seen, caused by increased hemoglobin-haptoglobin

TABLE 99–12. Common Classes of Hemolytic Anemias

Intrinsic (intracorpuscular; usually genetically inherited)
  Membrane defect
    Spherocytosis and elliptocytosis
  Hemoglobin defect
    Sickle cell anemia
    Thalassemia syndrome
  Metabolic defect
    Glucose-6-phosphate dehydrogenase (G6PD) deficiency
    Many other enzyme deficiencies
Extrinsic
  Membrance defect
    Autoimmune hemolytic anemias
    Oxidants, may cause unstable hemoglobin to clump

complex formation. Lactate dehydrogenase increases secondary to release from RBCs; however, this is a very nonspecific enzyme.

Hemoglobinuria may result and an increase in indirect bilirubin often occurs.

▶ TREATMENT: Hemolytic Anemia

Therapy for hemolytic anemia consists of managing the underlying cause of the anemia. Clearly, avoidance of precipitating oxidant medications and chemicals in patients with G6PD deficiency is essential. Currently, there is no specific therapy that compensates for this enzyme deficiency. Steroids and other immunosuppressive agents have been used for management of autoimmune hemolytic anemias. In some instances, a splenectomy is indicated in an attempt to reduce RBC destruction.

ANEMIAS CAUSED BY ABNORMAL HEMOGLOBIN SYNTHESIS

A defect in Hgb synthesis, as well as acquired defects in EPO precursor cell metabolism, may cause changes in iron incorporation, producing a cell with an excess of nonheme iron within the cytoplasm. Called sideroblasts, these cells cause sideroblastic anemia, which is usually microcytic. Sideroblastic anemia can be congenital (hereditary, sex-linked in males) or acquired. The acquired forms can be either primary or secondary to drugs, toxins (e.g., lead or alcohol), or other disease states. Reduced copper content of the blood, known as hypocupremia, has long been associated with sideroblastosis. Excess zinc intake causes sideroblastic anemia by binding preferentially to copper, impairing copper absorption and leading to hypocupremia.[86] Primary acquired sideroblastic anemia is usually classified as myelodysplastic syndrome and may eventually transform into acute myeloblastic leukemia in some patients.

Other hereditary defects in heme synthesis can lead to an overproduction of heme precursors resulting in porphyria. The most common form, acute intermittent porphyria (AIP), results from a hereditary (autosomal dominant) partial deficiency in the enzyme uroporphyrinogen I synthetase, which is responsible for converting porphobilinogen to uroporphyrinogen. This deficiency inhibits the normal feedback mechanism of porphyrin synthesis, leading to an excess production of the heme intermediate pigments uroporphyrin I and coproporphyrin I. These products can be detected in abnormal amounts in urine and feces to confirm the diagnosis of AIP.

Neuropsychiatric, neuromuscular, autonomic dysfunction, and intense abdominal pain characterize AIP. In the liver, this enzyme deficiency results in the increased inducibility of abnormal heme intermediates by certain drugs. Drugs and agents known to induce hepatic cytochrome P450 enzymes or to increase hepatic heme turnover are theoretically capable of precipitating porphyria. Barbiturates, estrogens, alcohol, and heavy metals such as lead have been documented to induce porphyria in genetically susceptible people.[87–89]

Genetic expression of an abnormal amino acid substitution in either the α or β globin chains can lead to a variety of hemoglobinopathies causing hemolytic diseases such as sickle cell anemia and thalassemia (see Chap. 101 on sickle cell disease). Four genes control α-chain production, and two genes regulate β-chain production. Thalassemias result when these genes are defective. If three or four α genes or both β genes are not functioning properly, a major thalassemia, which is often incompatible with life, develops. Fortunately, thalassemia minor (trait) is more common. The trait results from deficiencies in one or two α genes or one β gene. For example, if α genes are affected, normal β chains would accumulate in the cell and damage the membrane. This cell would then be prematurely cleared from the circulation, exacerbating the anemia. Surviving cells have inadequate Hgb and are microcytic and hypochromic.

The thalassemias are widely disseminated throughout parts of Africa, the Mediterranean region, the Middle East, the Indian subcontinent, and southeast Asia, but occur sporadically in all racial groups.[90] Specifically, β-thalassemia is well recognized in persons of Greek and Italian descent while the α-thalassemic syndromes have an increased prevalence in African-American, American Indian, and Asian groups. It is frequently asymptomatic and requires no treatment. It is unusual for patients to need transfusions or EPO and the use of iron supplementation is not needed unless the patient has excessive blood loss and confirmed iron deficiency. It is important to distinguish thalassemia from IDA to avoid inappropriate iron therapy, as the excess iron may be deleterious and lead to possible organ damage. Although both are microcytic, the MCV tends to be much lower with thalassemia than with IDA. Also, target cells may be seen on the peripheral smear in patients with thalassemia. Finally, in contrast to patients with IDA, ferritin levels are normal or increased in patients with thalassemia. Hundreds of these abnormal Hgb diseases exist and are best diagnosed by Hgb electrophoresis.

PHARMACOECONOMIC CONSIDERATIONS

Anemia has an independent impact on many clinical, functional, and economic indicators, and evidence suggests that treatment can improve patient outcomes. The implications of treating anemia are becoming increasingly recognized and the elderly are one subset of patients where this can be appreciated.[91] The cost of the comorbidities associated with anemia in the elderly is significant, as it has been linked to an increased risk of falls, dementia, depression, and general functional disability that increases the demand for long-term care services.[92] However, the causal link between anemia and the costs of the above diseases is not known. Data to date have indicated that the treatment of anemia in elderly patients with renal failure and congestive heart failure is beneficial.[92] However, more research is needed to assess the costs and benefits of therapies in individuals and in groups, especially when treatment of mild anemia is considered.[93]

Although the direct medical costs of anemia are unknown, the direct costs of drug treatment must be weighed with the indirect costs associated with anemia.[94] The costs of laboratory tests used to diagnose anemia, the role of screening for anemia, and the prevention of anemia are all components that necessitate consideration in the pharmacoeconomic analysis. Anemia practice guidelines within medical subspecialties must take pharmacoeconomics into consideration as they are developed. Additionally, the frequency of blood transfusions must be considered, as it impacts cost and therapeutic decision making in patients.

For IDA, IV iron, though costly, has superior bioavailability compared with oral preparations. In select individuals the bioavailability advantage of parenteral iron over oral iron can be the difference in the achievement of a successful outcome. The benefits of using combination oral iron products designed to enhance absorption is probably not warranted.

In regard to vitamin B_{12} deficiency, the average wholesale price for oral cyanocobalamin tablets and the IM injections is inexpensive. However, significant costs are added to the parenteral route, including the cost of a physician or nurse's visit for injection or home health visit. Additionally, many elderly patients may have difficulties attending additional clinic appointments due to transportation difficulties. An IM injection of cyanocobalamin costs between $10 and $25 for an in-office visit and between $60 and $100 for administration via home health care provider. A 90-day supply of 1-mg oral tablets can be purchased over the counter for approximately $5. The disadvantage of the nasal gel is its cost as compared to the oral or parenteral route, with a 2-month supply costing approximately $60.

For ACD, EPO is effective and safe, but expensive. Cost of IV iron is low compared with the cost of EPO. Since most patients are not symptomatic from this type of anemia, patients may actually feel no improvement with therapy. Symptom severity should be considered in the decision to use EPO. One study in patients with heart failure found use of erythropoietin to be highly cost-effective.[95] Transfusion use for ACD as an alternative to EPO must take into consideration cost, convenience, and risk of complications.

Total costs associated with EPO have not been evaluated for anemia of critical illness. Doses used for anemia of critical illness have been 40,000 units weekly, which costs approximately $400. The cost of an RBC unit transfusion is about $400, and two or three doses of EPO are needed to avoid one RBC transfusion. Future studies may need to assess the cost per unit of RBC saved, since these variables differ from institution to institution.

Other pharmacoeconomic factors to consider include morbidity and mortality of transfusion reactions, related infections, potential for medical errors, and availability of RBCs as a resource. Length of ICU and total hospital stay and length of time on mechanical ventilation are also key factors.

ABBREVIATIONS

ACD: anemia of chronic disease
AIDS: acquired immunodeficiency syndrome
AIP: acute intermittent porphyria
AOP: anemia of prematurity
CBC: complete blood count
CDC: Centers for Disease Control and Prevention
EPO: erythropoietin
Fe^{2+}: ferrous iron
Fe^{3+}: ferric iron
G6PD: glucose-6-phosphate dehydrogenase
Hct: hematocrit
Hgb: hemoglobin
HIV: human immunodeficiency virus
IDA: iron deficiency anemia
MCHC: mean corpuscular hemoglobin concentration
MCH: mean corpuscular hemoglobin
MCV: mean corpuscular volume
MMA: methylmalonic acid
NHANES: National Health and Nutrition Examination Survey
RBC: red blood cell
RDW: red blood cell distribution width
TIBC: total iron-binding capacity
WBC: white blood cells

Review Questions and other resources can be found at *www.pharmacotherapyonline.com.*

REFERENCES

1. Gleason G. Iron deficiency anemia finally reaches the global stage of public health. Nutr Clin Care 2002;5:217–219.
2. Ania BJ, Suman VJ, Fairbanks VF, et al. Incidence of anemia in older people: An epidemiologic study in a well defined population. J Am Geriatr Soc 1997;45:825–831.
3. Silverberg DS, Wexler D, Blum M, et al. The use of subcutaneous erythropoietin and intravenous iron for the treatment of the anemia of severe, resistant congestive heart failure improves cardiac and renal function and functional cardiac class and markedly reduces hospitalizations. J Am Coll Cardiol 2000;35:1737–1744.
4. Nissenson A. Anemia not just an innocent bystander. Arch Intern Med 2003;163:1400–1404.
5. Mozaffarian D. Anemia predicts mortality in severe heart failure: The prospective randomized amlodipine survival evaluation (PRAISE). J Am Coll Cardiol 2003;41:1933–1939.
6. Bottomley A, Thomas R, Van SK, et al. Human recombinant erythropoietin and quality of life: A wonder drug or something to wonder about? Lancet Oncol 2002;3:1145–1153.
7. Ross E. Evaluation and treatment of iron deficiency in adults. Nutr Clin Care 2002;5:220–224.
8. Davidsson L. Approaches to improve iron bioavailability from complementary foods. J Nutr 2003;133:1560S–1562S.
9. Zlotkin S. Clinical Nutrition: 8. The role of nutrition in the prevention of IDA in infants, children and adolescents. Can Med Assoc J 2003;168:59–63.
10. Wians FH, Urban JE, Keffer JH, Kroft SH. Discriminating between iron deficiency anemia and anemia of chronic disease using traditional indices of iron status vs transferrin receptor concentration. Am J Clin Pathol 2001;115:112–118.
11. Ludwig H, Strasser K. Symptomatology of anemia. Semin Oncol 2001;28(2 Suppl 18):7–14.
12. Gran Ham-McGregor S, Ani C. A review of studies on the effect of iron deficiency on cognitive development in children. J Nutr 2001;131:649S–668S.
13. Irwin JJ, Kirchner JT. Anemia in children. Am Fam Physician 2001;64:1379–1386.
14. Adamson JW. Iron deficiency and other hypoproliferative anemias. In: Braunwald E, Fauci AS, Isselbacher KJ, et al, eds. Harrison's Online [Internet], McGraw-Hill, 2001–2004. Available from: *http://harrisons.accessmedicine.com.*
15. Baik HW, Russell RM. Vitamin B_{12} deficiency in the elderly. Annu Rev Nutr 1999;19:357–377.
16. Healton EB, Savage DG, Brust JC. Neurologic aspects of cobalamin deficiency. Medicine 1991;70:229–245.
17. Andrews NC. Iron metabolism and absorption. Rev Clin Exp Hematol 2000;4:283–301.
18. Snow CF. Laboratory diagnosis of vitamin B_{12} and folate deficiency. Arch Intern Med 1999;159:1289–1298.
19. Dharmarajan TS, Norkus EP. Approaches to vitamin B_{12} deficiency. Early treatment may prevent devastating complications. Postgrad Med 2001;110:99–105.
20. Iron deficiency—United States, 1999–2000. Morb Mortal Wkly Rep 2002;51:897–899.
21. Institute of Medicine. Dietary Reference Intakes (DRI) for Vitamin A, Vitamin K, Arsenic, Boron, Chromium, Copper, Iodine, Iron, Manganese, Molybdenum, Nickel, Silicon, Vanadium, and Zinc. Washington, National Academy Press, 2002:18–19.
22. Marx JJM. Iron deficiency in developed countries: prevalence, influence of lifestyle factors and hazards of prevention. Eur J Clin Nutr 1997;51:491–494.
23. Annibale B, Chistolin A, D'Ambra G, et al. Gastrointestinal causes of refractory iron deficiency anemia in patients without gastrointestinal symptoms. Am J Med 2001;111:439–445.
24. Tapiero H, Gate L, Tew KD. Iron: deficiency and requirements. Biomed Pharmacother 2001;55:324–332.

25. Haas JD, Brownlie T. Iron deficiency and diminished work capacity: A critical review of the research to determine a causal relationship. J Nutr 2001;131:676S–690S.

26. Guyatt GH, Oxman AD, Ali M, et al. Laboratory diagnosis of iron-deficiency anemia: An overview. J Gen Intern Med 1992;7:145–153.

27. Tefferi A. Anemia in adults: A contemporary approach to diagnosis. Mayo Clin Proc 2003;78:1274–1280.

28. Provan D. Mechanisms and management of iron deficiency anemia. Br J Haematol 1999;105:19–26.

29. Rudinskas L, Paton TW, Walker SE, et al. Poor clinical response to enteric-coated iron preparations. Can Med Assoc J 1989;141:565–566.

30. Walker SE, Paton TW, Cowen DH, et al. Bioavailability of iron in oral ferrous sulfate preparations in healthy volunteers. Can Med Assoc J 1989;141:543–547.

31. MacDougall IC. Strategies for iron supplementation: Oral versus intravenous. Kidney Int Suppl 1999;69:S61–S66.

32. Van Wyck DB, Cavallo G, Spinowitz BS, et al. Safety and efficacy of iron sucrose in patients sensitive to iron dextran: North American clinical trial. Am J Kidney Dis 2000;36:88–97.

33. Matzke GR. Intravenous iron supplementation in end-stage renal disease patients. Am J Kidney Dis 1999;33:595–597.

34. Faich G, Strobos J. Sodium Fe^{3+} gluconate complex in sucrose: safer IV iron therapy than iron dextrans. Am J Kidney Dis 1999;33:464–470.

35. Coyne DW, Adkinson NF, Nissenson AR, et al. Sodium Fe^{3+} gluconate complex in hemodialysis patients. Adverse reactions in iron dextran-sensitive and dextran-tolerant patients. Kidney Int 2003;63:217–224.

36. Beresford CR, Goldberg L, Smith JP. Local effects and mechanism of absorption of iron preparations administered intramuscularly. Br J Pharmacol 1957;12:107–114.

37. Will G. The absorption, distribution and utilization of intramuscularly administered iron-dextran: a radioisotope study. Br J Haematol 1968;14:395–406.

38. Grime AJ, Hutt MSR. Metabolism of 59Fe-dextran complex in human subjects. Br J Med 1957;2:1074–1077.

39. Henderson PA, Hillman RS. Characteristics of iron dextran utilization in man. Blood 1969;34:357–375.

40. Chandler G, Harchowal J, Macdougall IC. Intravenous iron sucrose: Establishing a safe dose. Am J Kidney Dis 2001;38:988–991.

41. Kosch M, Bahner U, Bettger H, et al. A randomized, controlled parallel-group trial on efficacy and safety of iron sucrose vs iron gluconate in hemodialysis patients treated with rHu Epo. Nephrol Dial Transplant 2001;16:1239–1244.

42. Practice guidelines for blood component therapy. A report by the American Society of Anethesiologists Task Force on Blood Component Therapy. Anesthesiology 1996;84:732–747.

43. Goodnough LT, Brecher ME, Kamter MH, Aubuchon JP. Transfusion medicine, part 1; blood transfusions. N Engl J Med 1999;340:438–444.

44. Little DR. Ambulatory management of common forms of anemia. Am Fam Physician 1999;59:1598–1604.

45. Savage D, Lindenbaum J. Anemia in alcoholics. Medicine 1986;65:322–338.

46. Lindenbaum J, Rosenberg IH, Wilson PWF, et al. Prevalence of cobalamin deficiency in the Framingham elderly population. Am J Clin Nutr 1994;60:2–11.

47. Dharmarajan TS, Adiga GU, Norkus EP. Vitamin B_{12} deficiency. Recognizing subtle symptoms in older adults. Geriatrics 2003;58:30–38.

48. Kaptan K, Beyan C, Ural AU, et al. *Helicobacter pylori*—is it a novel causative agent in vitamin B_{12} deficiency? Arch Intern Med 2000;160:1349–1353.

49. Clementz GL, Schade SG. The spectrum of vitamin B_{12} deficiency. Am Fam Physician 1990;41:150–162.

50. Oh RC, Brown DL. Vitamin B_{12} deficiency. Am Fam Physician 2003;67:979–986, 993–994.

51. Christensen DJ. Diagnosis of anemia: clues to greater precision. Postgrad Med J 1983;73:293–297, 300.

52. Kapadia CR. Gastric atrophy, metaplasia, and dysplasia: a clinical perspective. J Clin Gastroenterol 2003;36(5 Suppl):S29–36.

53. Aronow WS. Homocysteine. The association with atherosclerotic vascular disease in older persons. Geriatrics 2003;58:22–28.

54. Carmel R, Aurangzeb I, Qian D. Associations of food-cobalamin malabsorption with ethnic origin, age, *Helicobacter pylori* infection, and serum markers of gastritis. Am J Gastroenterol 2001;96:63–70.

55. Lederle FA. Oral cobalamin for pernicious anemia. Medicine's best kept secret? JAMA 1991;265:94–95.

56. Lane LA, Rojas-Fernandez. Treatment of vitamin B_{12}-deficiency anemia: oral versus parenteral therapy. Ann Pharmacother 2002;36:1268–1272.

57. Carmel R, Weiner JM, Johnson CS. Iron deficiency occurs frequently in patients with pernicious anemia. JAMA 1987;257:1081–1083.

58. Yerby MS. Clinical care of pregnant women with epilepsy: neural tube defects and folic acid supplementation. Epilepsia 2003;44(Suppl 3):33–40.

59. Institute of Medicine. Food and Nutrition Board. Dietary Reference Intakes: Thiamin, riboflavin, niacin, vitamin B6, folate, vitamin B12, pantothenic acid, biotin, and choline. Washington, National Academy Press, 1998.

60. Cziezel AE, Dudas I. Prevention of the first occurrence of neural tube defects by periconceptual vitamin supplementation. N Engl J Med 1992;327:1832.

61. Tobarova M. Periconceptual supplementation with vitamins and folic acid to prevent recurrence of cleft lip. Lancet 1982;2:217.

62. Volberding P. Consensus statement: Anemia in HIV infection—current trends, treatment options, and practice strategies. Anemia in HIV Working Group. Clin Ther 2000;22:1004–1020.

63. Moore RD. Anemia and human immunodeficiency virus disease in the era of highly active antiretroviral therapy. Semin Hematol 2000;37:18–23.

64. Means RT, Krantz SB. Progress in understanding the pathogenesis of the anemia of chronic disease. Blood 1992;80:1639–1647.

65. Brokering KL, Quqish RB. Management of anemia of chronic disease in patients with the human immunodeficiency virus. Pharmacotherapy 2003;23:1475–1485.

66. Ifudu O. Maximizing response to erythropoietin in treating HIV-associated anemia. Clev Clin J Med 2001;68:643–648.

67. Corwin HL, Gettinger A, Pearl RG, et al. The CRIT Study: Anemia and blood transfusion in the critically ill—current clinical practice in the United States. Crit Care Med 2004;32:39–52.

68. Eckardt KU. Anaemia of critical illness—implications for understanding and treating rHuEPO resistance. Nephrol Dial Transplant 2002;17:48–55.

69. Rudis M, Jacobi J, Hassan E, Dasta J. Managing anemia in the critically ill patient. Pharmacotherapy 2004;24:229–247.

70. Patruta SL, Horl WH. Iron and infection. Kidney Int 1999;55(Suppl 69):S125–S130.

71. Darveau M, Notebaert E, Denault AY, et al. Recombinant human erythropoietin use in intensive care. Ann Pharmacother 2002;36:1068–1074.

72. Hébert PC, Wells G, Martin C, et al. Do blood transfusions improve outcomes related to mechanical ventilation? Chest 2001;119:1850–1857.

73. Hebert PC, Wells G, Blajchman MA, et al, for the transfusion requirements in critical care investigators, Canadian critical care trials group. A multicenter, randomized, controlled clinical trial of transfusion requirements in critical care. N Engl J Med 1999;340:409–417.

74. Vincent JL, Baron J-F, Reinhart K, et al. Anemia and blood transfusion in critically ill patients. JAMA 2002;288:1499–1507.

75. Lipschitz D. Medical and functional consequences of anemia in the elderly. J Am Geriat Soc 2003;51:S10–S13.

76. Balducci L. Epidemiology of anemia in the elderly: information on diagnostic evaluation. J Am Geriatr Soc 2003;51:S2–S9.

77. Balducci L, Hardy CL, Lyman GH. Hematopoietic growth factors in the older cancer patient. Current Opin Hematol 2001;8:170–187.

78. Selhub J, Jacques PR, Rosenberg IH, et al. Serum total homocysteine concentrations in the Third National Health and Nutrition Survey (1991–1994): population reference ranges and contribution of vitamin status to high serum concentrations. Ann Intern Med 1999;131:331–339.

79. Ford ES, Bowman BA. Serum and red blood cell folate concentrations, race, and education: findings from the third National Health and Nutrition Examination Survey. Am J Clin Nutr 1999;69:476–481.

80. Recommendations to prevent and control iron deficiency in the United States. Morb Mortal Wkly Rep 1998;47:1–36.

81. Wright JD, Bialostosky K, Gunter EW, et al. Blood folate and vitamin B12: United States, 1988–94. Vital Health Stat 1998;11:1–78.

82. Schwartz E. Anemias of inadequate production. In: Behrman RE, Kliegman RM, Jenson HB, eds. Nelson Textbook of Pediatrics, 16th ed. Philadelphia, Saunders, 2000:1463–1472.

83. Hermiston ML, Mentzer WC. A practical approach to the evaluation of the anemic child. Pediatr Clin North Am 2002;49:877–891.

84. Jacobs P, Wood L. Hematology of malnutrition, Part One. Disease-a-Month 2003;49:564–588.

85. Morey SS. CDC issues guidelines for prevention, detection and treatment of iron deficiency. Am Fam Physician 1998;58:1475–1477.

86. Ramadurai J, Shapiro C, Kozloff M, Telfer M. Zinc abuse and sideroblastic anemia. Am J Hematol 1993;42:227–228.

87. Hryhorczuk DO, Hogan MM. Variegate porphyria and heavy metal poisoning from ingestion of moonshine. South Med J 1983;76:1027–1031.

88. McKenzie AW, Acharya U. Oestrogen-induced familial porphyria. Br J Dermatol 1975;92:707–709.

89. Doss M, Baumann H, Sixel F. Alcohol in acute porphyria. Lancet 1982;1:1307.

90. Weatherall DJ, Provan AB. Red cells I: inherited anaemias. Lancet 2000; 355:1169–1175.

91. Smith DL. Anemia in the elderly. Am Fam Physician 2000;62:1565–1572.

92. Robinson B. Cost of anemia in the elderly. J Am Geriatr Soc 2003;51: S14–S17.

93. Cogswell M, Kettel-Khan L, Ramakrishnan V. Iron supplement use among women in the United States: science, policy and practice. J Nutr 2003;133:1974S–1977S.

94. Tice JA, Ross E, Coxson PG, et al. Cost-effectiveness of vitamin therapy to lower plasma homocysteine levels for the prevention of coronary heart disease. JAMA 2001;286:936–943.

95. Caro J, Klittich W, Caro G. The health economic implications of treating anemia in patients with congestive heart failure (abstr). Value Health 2002;5:487.

100

COAGULATION DISORDERS

Betsy Bickert and Janet L. Kwiatkowski

Learning Objectives and other resources can be found at *www.pharmacotherapyonline.com.*

KEY CONCEPTS

❶ Hemophilia is an inherited bleeding disorder resulting from a congenital deficiency in factor VIII or IX.

❷ The goal of therapy for hemophilia is to arrest bleeding when it occurs and to prevent bleeding episodes and their long-term complications.

❸ Recombinant factor concentrates are usually first-line treatment for moderate and severe hemophilia because they have the lowest risk of infection.

❹ The goal of therapy for von Willebrand disease is to improve von Willebrand factor and factor VIII levels.

❺ Factor VIII concentrates that contain von Willebrand factor are the agents of choice for the treatment of type 3 von Willebrand disease, some type 2 von Willebrand disease, and for serious bleeding in type 1 von Willebrand disease.

❻ Desmopressin acetate is often effective for the treatment of type 1 von Willebrand disease. It may also be effective for the treatment of some forms of type 2 von Willebrand disease.

❼ The optimal approach for patients with disseminated intravascular coagulation remains to be determined. The goal of treatment is to diagnose and treat the underlying disease.

❽ Prophylactic use of phytonadione can effectively prevent vitamin K–dependent bleeding in the newborn.

Coagulation disorders result from a decreased number of platelets, decreased function of platelets, coagulation factor deficiency, or enhanced fibrinolytic activity. A series of complex actions and reactions of procoagulant and anticoagulant events regulate blood flow. Maintenance of blood flow involves the interplay of four major components: (1) the vessel wall, (2) platelets, (3) the coagulation system, and (4) the fibrinolytic system.

The traditional view of the coagulation cascade consisted of intrinsic, extrinsic, and common pathways. Coagulation could be initiated via either the intrinsic or extrinsic pathways as depicted in Fig. 100–1. The extrinsic pathway is initiated by the exposure of tissue during trauma. The intrinsic pathway is initiated when circulating factor XII comes in contact with the subendothelial membrane. These two pathways converge at the activation of factor X, forming the common pathway. While the historical model in Fig. 100–1 shows the basic dependency of the various coagulation factors, it does not reflect the interactions with platelets and the endothelium. Thus it has been replaced by the cell-based model depicted in Fig. 100–2 that more accurately describes these interactions. This is known as the tissue factor pathway because it recognizes the central role of tissue factor in coagulation.

REGULATION OF HEMOSTASIS

COAGULATION FACTORS

Twelve plasma proteins are considered coagulation factors (Table 100–1). The coagulation factors can be divided into three groups on the basis of biochemical properties. These groups include vitamin K–dependent factors (II, VII, IX, and X), contact activation factors (XI and XII, prekallikrein, high-molecular-weight kininogen), and thrombin-sensitive factors (V, VIII, XIII, and fibrinogen).

Coagulation factors circulate as inactive precursors (zymogens). Coagulation of blood entails a cascading series of proteolytic reactions. At each step, a clotting factor undergoes limited proteolysis and becomes an active protease (designated by a lowercase "a," as in Xa). These coagulation factors play key roles in the coagulation pathway.

VESSEL WALL AND PLATELETS

Blood vessel walls and activated platelets play central roles in primary hemostasis. Damage to a vessel wall initiates vasoconstriction and the exposure of collagen and tissue factor to blood. This exposure initiates coagulation via the tissue factor pathway.

Platelet function in response to vascular injury includes four phases: (1) adhesion, (2) secretion, (3) aggregation, and (4) elaboration of procoagulant activity. Release of von Willebrand factor from activated platelets and fibrinogen from the endothelium causes adhesion of platelets at the site. Platelets release granular contents, such as adenosine diphosphate and thromboxane A_2 that lead to platelet aggregation. A platelet plug is formed that occludes the blood vessel lesion. Activated coagulation factors are generated at the site of bleeding on the activated platelets. Factor XIIIa cross-links fibrin and stabilizes the clot.[1]

Unbound factors IIa, IXa, Xa, XIa, and XIIa are inactivated by antithrombin when they migrate to the endothelial cell surface. Heparin and heparin-like substances present on the surface of endothelial cells enhance the inhibitory capacity of antithrombin.[1] Thrombomodulin binds thrombin and activates protein C. Activated protein C and its cofactor, protein S, are vitamin K–dependent proteins

INTRINSIC PATHWAY

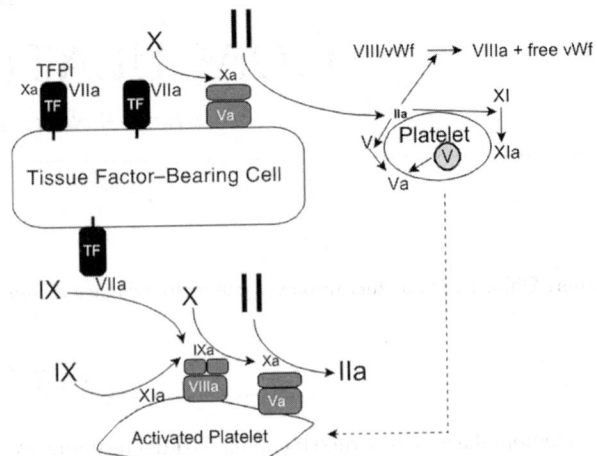

FIGURE 100–1. Cascade model of coagulation demonstrates activation via the intrinsic or extrinsic pathway. This model shows successive activation of coagulation factors proceeding from the top to the bottom where thrombin and fibrin are generated. PK, Prekallikrein; HK, high-molecular, weight kininogen; TF, tissue factor. (*Reproduced from Roberts HR et al. Molecular biology and biochemistry of the coagulation factors and pathways of hemostasis. In: Beutler et al. Williams Hematology, 6th ed. New York, McGraw-Hill, 2001, pp 1409–1434.*)

that inactivate factor Va and VIIIa on the endothelial cell surface. These interactions localize the clotting to the site of injury and prevent clotting in the intact vascular system.

TISSUE FACTOR PATHWAY

Tissue factor is a membrane protein found in organs and surrounding the vasculature. Tissue factor is exposed to blood as a consequence of vessel wall damage or inflammatory cytokine release from vascular cells or monocytes.[2] Coagulation is initiated when factor VIIa binds to exposed or expressed tissue factor (see Fig. 100–2). The factor VIIa–tissue factor complex activates factors IX and X. Activated platelets form complexes with factor IXa-factor VIIIa (tenase) and factor

FIGURE 100–2. Cell-based model of hemostasis. TF, tissue factor; TFPI, tissue factor pathway inhibitor; vWF, von Willebrand factor. (*Reproduced from Roberts HR et al. Molecular biology and biochemistry of the coagulation factors and pathways of hemostasis. In: Beutler et al. Williams Hematology, 6th ed. New York, McGraw-Hill, 2001, pp 1409–1434.*)

Xa-factor Va (prothrombinase).[2] Tenase activates factor X and prothrombinase converts prothrombin to thrombin. Thrombin activates platelets and catalyzes the conversion of fibrinogen to fibrin. Thrombin also amplifies coagulation by activating factors V, VIII, and XI.

FIBRINOLYSIS

The coagulation system regulates fibrin clot formation, whereas the fibrinolytic system dissolves the polymerized clot and restores blood flow. As a regulatory mechanism to maintain blood flow, the fibrinolytic system removes fibrin deposits and prevents formation of unnecessary fibrin clots. It also contributes to the localized repair of damaged endothelium.

Plasminogen is the primary compound of the fibrinolytic enzyme system. Plasminogen activators (tissue plasminogen activator and urokinase plasminogen activator) are released in response to thrombin, venous stasis, physical exercise, or ischemia.[3] Activators convert plasminogen to plasmin in the presence of fibrin. Plasmin enzymatically digests fibrin, dissolves the clot, and releases a number of fibrin degradation products. The interaction between plasminogen activators, plasminogen, and fibrin restricts the fibrinolytic activity to the site of the clot. Plasminogen-activator inhibitor type 1 (PAI-1) blocks the plasminogen activators while antiplasmin directly inhibits circulating plasmin to prevent systemic fibrinolysis.[3]

TABLE 100–1. Blood Coagulation Factors

Factor[a]	Synonym	Biologic Half-life	Blood Product Source
I	Fibrinogen	100–150 h	Cryoprecipitate (200–300 mg/bag)
II	Prothrombin	50–80 h	FFP, plasma, PCC
V	Proaccerlerin	24 h	FFP
VII	Proconvertin	6 h	Recombinant VIIa, FFP, plasma, PCC
VIII	Antihemophilic factor	12 h	FFP, PCC, factor concentrates, cryoprecipitate
IX	Christmas factor	24 h	FFP, PCC, factor concentrates
X	Stuart-Power factor	25–60 h	FFP, plasma, PCC
XI	Plasma thromboplastin antecedent	40–80 h	FFP, plasma
XII	Hageman factor	50–70 h	
XIII	Fibrin-stabilizing factor	150 h	FFP, plasma, cryoprecipitate

[a]Coagulation factors are numbered with roman numerals in order of their discovery. The most common synonyms are listed. Factor III (tissue factor) and factor IV (calcium ions) have been omitted. There is no factor VI.
FFP, fresh frozen plasma; PCC, prothrombin complex concentrate.

SIMPLE LABORATORY TESTS

The diagnosis of coagulation disorders can be established from a detailed clinical history, a physical examination, and laboratory test results. The most common screening tests include bleeding time, prothrombin time, activated partial thromboplastin time, thrombin time, and platelet count.[1] The results of these standard laboratory procedures can distinguish bleeding disorders caused by defects in the intrinsic, extrinsic, and common coagulation pathways (see Fig. 100–1), or from alterations in the number of functioning platelets. Specific assays of individual coagulation factors and platelet function tests can be performed after abnormalities are identified by initial screening tests. The following is a brief review of widely available tests. These tests are summarized in Table 100–2.

BLEEDING TIME

Bleeding time assesses platelet and capillary function. Bleeding time reflects the time to cessation of bleeding following a standardized skin cut. Patients with an abnormal bleeding time but a normal platelet count are arbitrarily designated as having qualitative abnormalities of platelet function. Such patients include those with von Willebrand disease, those who have recently ingested various antiplatelet drugs (i.e., aspirin), those with renal failure, those with fibrinogen disorders or with abnormal blood vessels.

PROTHROMBIN TIME

The prothrombin time (PT) assesses the function of the extrinsic system and common pathway of the coagulation system.[4] In particular, the test measures the activity of the vitamin K–dependent proteins (factors II, VII, IX, and X, and proteins C and S). Prothrombin time reflects the time required for fibrin strands to appear after the addition of tissue thromboplastin to a patient's plasma. Thus the PT yields evidence about the current synthetic capacity of the liver, the adequacy of vitamin K absorption, and the inhibition of clotting factor synthesis by warfarin. Prothrombin time is expressed as an International Normalized Ratio to normalize the values due to variability of the test reagents.[4]

ACTIVATED PARTIAL THROMBOPLASTIN TIME

The activated partial thromboplastin time (aPTT) measures the activity of the intrinsic system and common pathway (factors II, V, X, VIII, IX, XI, XII, high-molecular-weight kininogen, prekallikrein, and fibrinogen). aPTT reflects the time required for a fibrin clot to form after a partial thromboplastin, calcium, and an activating agent are added to the patient's plasma. aPTT is widely used for monitoring heparin therapy.

THROMBIN TIME

The thrombin time measures the conversion of fibrinogen to fibrin and is affected by quantitative and qualitative abnormalities of fibrinogen and the presence of thrombin inhibitors or fibrinogen degradation products. The thrombin time measures the time required for the formation and the appearance of the fibrin clot after thrombin is added to plasma. It may be used to monitor the effect of systemic fibrinolytic therapy and can be modified for monitoring heparin therapy.

TABLE 100–2. Laboratory Procedures

Procedure	Identifies	Cause of Prolonged Value	Clinical Manifestations
Bleeding time	Platelet number and function	Thrombocytopenia Inherited qualitative platelet defects von Willebrand disease Antiplatelet drugs Factor V or XI deficiency Afibrinogenemia	Bleeding from the gums Easy bruising Bleeding following surgery or tooth extraction Epistaxis Menorrhagia
Prothrombin time (PT)	Factors I, II, V, VII, X	Newborn Vitamin K deficiency Inherited factor deficiencies Warfarin Liver disease Lupus anticoagulant[a] Afibrinogenemia	Bleeding following surgery, trauma, etc Easy bruising
Activated partial thromboplastin time (aPTT)	Factors I, II, V, VIII, IX, X	Inherited factor deficiencies Lupus anticoagulant[a] Heparin therapy Liver disease Afibrinogenemia	Joint and muscle bleeding Bleeding after surgery, trauma, etc
	HMWK Prekallikrein Factor XII		No bleeding manifestations Increased incidence of thrombotic disease possible with factor XII deficiency
	Factor XI		Variable bleeding tendency Bleeding following surgery, trauma, etc
Thrombin time (TT)	Fibrinogen Inhibitors of fibrin aggregation	Afibrinogenemia Heparin therapy	Lifelong hemorrhagic disease

[a]Bleeding manifestations dependent on factor levels.
HMWK, high-molecular-weight kininogen.

CONGENITAL COAGULATION DISORDERS

HEMOPHILIA

◄ Hemophilia is a bleeding disorder that results from a congenital deficiency in a plasma coagulation protein. Hemophilia A (classic hemophilia) is caused by a deficiency of factor VIII, while hemophilia B (Christmas disease) is caused by a deficiency of factor IX. The incidence of hemophilia A is approximately 1 in 5,000 male births.[5-7] Hemophilia B occurs less commonly, with only one-fourth the incidence of hemophilia A.[5,7] There are no significant racial differences in the incidence of hemophilia.

Thirty percent of severe hemophilia patients have a negative family history, presumably representing a spontaneous mutation. Both hemophilia A and hemophilia B are recessive X-linked diseases; that is, the defective gene is located on the X chromosome. In general, the disease affects only males, while females are carriers. Affected males have the abnormal allele on their X chromosome and no matching allele on their Y chromosome. Thus their sons would be normal (assuming the mother is not a carrier), and their daughters would be obligatory carriers. Female carriers have one normal allele, and therefore do not usually have a bleeding tendency. Sons of a female carrier and a normal male have a 50% chance of being hemophiliacs, whereas daughters have a 50% chance of being carriers. Thus there is a "skipped generation" mode of inheritance in which the female carriers, who are the children of hemophiliacs, do not express the disease, but can pass it on to the next male generation.

Hemophilia has been observed in a small number of females. This can occur if both factor VIII or IX genes are defective, if a female patient has only one X chromosome, as in Turner's syndrome,[8] or if the normal X chromosome is excessively inactivated through a process called lyonization.

In 1984, researchers isolated and cloned the human factor VIII gene.[9,10] It is a large gene, consisting of 186 kilobases (kb).[5,10] More than 800 unique mutations in the factor VIII gene, including point mutations, deletions, and insertions, have been reported (*http://europium. csc.mrc.ac.uk*). Deletions and nonsense mutations are often associated with the more severe forms of factor VIII deficiency, because no functional factor VIII is produced. In 1993, researchers identified an inversion in the factor VIII gene at intron 22 that accounts for about 45% of severe hemophilia A gene abnormalities.[11] That discovery has greatly simplified carrier detection and prenatal diagnosis for families with this gene mutation. A more recently discovered inversion mutation involving intron 1 of the factor VIII gene accounts for an additional 5% of severe hemophilia mutations.[12]

The factor IX gene, cloned and sequenced in 1982,[13] consists of only 34 kb and thus is significantly smaller than the factor VIII gene.[5,9] Unlike the factor VIII gene in patients with severe hemophilia A, the factor IX gene in patients with hemophilia B has no predominant mutation. Direct gene mutation analysis is simpler in hemophilia B because of the smaller gene size, and to date more than 800 different mutations have been reported (*www.kcl.ac.uk/ip/ petergreen/haemBdatabase.html*). Most of these mutations are single base pair substitutions. Approximately 3% of factor IX gene mutations are deletions or complex rearrangements, and the presence of these mutations is associated with a severe phenotype.[10]

Hemophilia B Leiden is a rare variant in which factor IX levels are initially low, but rise at puberty. This phenotype results from a mutation in the promoter region of the gene that is apparently ameliorated by the action of testosterone.[5,14] The identification of this genotype is clinically important, because it confers a better prognosis.

CLINICAL PRESENTATION

The characteristic bleeding manifestations of hemophilia include ecchymoses, bleeding into joint spaces (hemarthroses), muscle hemorrhages, and excessive bleeding after surgery or trauma. The severity of clinical bleeding generally correlates with the degree of deficiency of factor VIII or factor IX. Factor VIII and factor IX activity levels are usually measured in units per milliliter with 1 unit/mL representing 100% of the factor found in 1 mL of normal plasma. Normal plasma levels range from 0.5 to 1.5 units/mL.[5] Patients with less than 0.01 unit/mL (1%) of either factor are classified as severe hemophiliacs; those with 0.01 to 0.05 unit/mL (1% to 5%) are moderate hemophiliacs, and those with greater than 0.05 unit/mL (5%) are mild hemophiliacs (Table 100–3). Patients with severe disease often experience frequent spontaneous hemorrhages and joint space bleeding, while those with moderate disease have excessive bleeding following trauma and rarely experience spontaneous hemarthroses. Patients with mild hemophilia may have so few symptoms that their condition is undiagnosed for many years, and they usually have excessive bleeding only after significant trauma or surgery. Occasionally those with severe disease (less than 1% factor activity) may not display a severe phenotype; conversely, some with milder forms of the disease may have more severe bleeding symptomatology. Patients with hemophilia usually present with clinical manifestations after the age of 1 year, when they begin to walk and increase their risk of bleeding.

TABLE 100–3. Laboratory and Clinical Manifestations of Hemophilia

	Severe (<0.01 units/mL)	Moderate (0.01–0.05 units/mL)	Mild (>0.05 units/mL)
Age at onset	≤1 year	1–2 years	2 years–adult
Neonatal symptoms			
PCB:	Usually	Usually	Rare
ICH:	Occasionally	Uncommonly	Rare
Muscle/joint hemorrhage	Spontaneous	Minor trauma	Minor trauma
CNS hemorrhage	High risk	Moderate risk	Rare
Postsurgical hemorrhage (without prophylaxis)	Frank bleeding, severe	Wound bleeding, common	Wound bleeding, with factor <0.3 units/mL
Oral hemorrhage following trauma, tooth extraction	Usual	Common	Often

Normal range of factor VIII/IX activity level is 0.5–1.5 units/mL (50%–150%). 1 unit/mL corresponds to 100% of the factor found in 1 mL of normal plasma. CNS, central nervous system; ICH, intracranial hemorrhage; PCB, postcircumceisional bleeding.

CLINICAL PRESENTATION OF HEMOPHILIA

SIGNS AND SYMPTOMS
Ecchymoses
Hemarthrosis (especially knee, ankle, and elbow)
Joint pain
Joint swelling and erythema
Decreased range of motion
Muscle hemorrhage
Swelling
Pain with motion of affected muscle
Signs of nerve compression
Potential life-threatening blood loss, especially with thigh
  bleeding
Mouth bleeding with dental extractions or trauma
Genitourinary bleeding
Hematuria
Intracranial hemorrhage (spontaneous or following trauma),
  with headache, vomiting, change in mental status, and focal
  neurologic signs
Excessive bleeding with surgery

LABORATORY TESTING
Prolonged aPTT
Decreased factor VIII/factor IX level
Normal PT
Normal platelet count
Normal von Willebrand factor antigen and activity

DIAGNOSIS

The diagnosis of hemophilia should be considered in any male with unusual bleeding. A family history of bleeding is also helpful in the diagnosis, but this is absent in up to one-third of patients.[15] Brothers of patients with hemophilia should be screened; sisters should have carrier testing.

Recent advances in molecular genetic analysis have greatly improved the accuracy of carrier status evaluation. Thus female relatives of patients with hemophilia who are at risk of being carriers for the disorder should be tested. Additionally, the appropriate factor level should be measured in female carriers to identify those with levels less than 0.3 units/mL (30%) who might themselves be at risk of bleeding.

Patients with severe hemophilia A should be tested for the common factor VIII gene inversions. If the patient has this mutation, family members should undergo testing to determine if they also have the mutation and thus are carriers. In those patients with hemophilia A who lack the inversion mutation, other methods to determine the carrier status of their family members are available.[16] Techniques to determine carrier status in families with hemophilia B are similar, although no predominant mutation like the factor VIII inversion has been found. The smaller size of the factor IX gene facilitates direct DNA mutational analysis.[16]

Hemophilia can be diagnosed prenatally by chorionic villus sampling in the tenth to eleventh gestational week or by amniocentesis after 15 weeks' gestation.[5,17] Fetal blood can be sampled and assayed directly for factor VIII levels by the eighteenth to twentieth week of gestation.[5,17] This procedure is less useful for diagnosing factor IX deficiency, because factor IX levels are physiologically low in fetuses and infants.[5]

▶ TREATMENT: Hemophilia

The comprehensive care of hemophilia requires a multitude of health care professionals. The patient is best managed in specialized centers with trained personnel and appropriate laboratory, radiologic, and pharmaceutical services. The health care team includes hematologists, orthopedic surgeons, nurses, physical therapists, dentists, genetic counselors, psychologists, pharmacists, case managers, and social workers.

Patients with hemophilia should receive routine immunizations, including immunization against hepatitis B. Hepatitis A vaccine is also recommended for patients with hemophilia because of the risk (albeit small) of transmitting the causative agent through factor concentrates.[18] The use of a small-gauge needle can prevent excessive bleeding. Some health care providers advocate giving immunizations subcutaneously rather than intramuscularly to decrease the risk of hematoma formation.

A few special considerations apply to the perinatal care of male infants of hemophilia carriers. Intracranial or extracranial hemorrhage has been estimated to occur in 1% to 4% of newborns with hemophilia.[19,20] Vacuum extraction and forceps delivery increase the risk of cranial bleeding. Elective cesarean section has not prevented intracranial bleeding. There is no clear consensus on the optimal mode of delivery or the use of prophylactic factor replacement in male infants of hemophilia carriers.[19] Circumcision should be postponed until a diagnosis of hemophilia is excluded. Factor levels can be assayed from cord blood samples or from peripheral venipuncture. Arterial puncture should be avoided because of the risk of hematoma formation.

Intravenous factor replacement therapy to treat or prevent bleeding is the mainstay of treatment for hemophilia. It is common for families to learn how to treat patients with factor concentrate at home. Parents may learn to infuse factor for younger children, and older children and adult patients may learn self-administration. Home health care nursing support may also be helpful, particularly for the youngest patients in whom venous access may be difficult. Administration of factor at home is more convenient for families and allows for earlier treatment of acute bleeding episodes. However, serious bleeding episodes always require medical evaluation.

■ HISTORY OF HEMOPHILIA TREATMENT

Therapy for hemophilia has undergone dramatic advances over the past few decades. Fifty years ago, the administration of fresh frozen plasma was the only available treatment. The introduction of cryoprecipitate in the early 1960s allowed more specific therapy for hemophilia A.[5,7] Intermediate-purity factor VIII and IX concentrates became available in the 1970s.[5,7] Plasma-derived factor concentrates are made from the donations of thousands of people. Contamination of plasma pools with hepatitis B, hepatitis C, and the human immunodeficiency virus (HIV) during the late 1970s and early 1980s resulted in transmission to most patients with severe hemophilia. Since the mid-1980s, plasma-derived concentrates have been manufactured with a variety of virus-inactivating techniques including dry heat, pasteurization, and treatment with chemicals (e.g., solvent detergent mixtures).[7] Since 1986, no transmission of HIV through factor concentrates to patients with hemophilia in the United States has been reported.[5,7]

Protein purification, introduced in the 1990s, produced high-purity concentrates with increased amounts of factor VIII or factor IX relative to the product's total protein content. Recombinant factor VIII and then factor IX also became available.[5] The first-generation recombinant factor VIII products utilize human and animal proteins in culture and add human albumin as a protein stablilizer.[7] Second-generation recombinant factor VIII concentrates removed albumin as a protein stabilizer, and the third-generation products lack human and animal proteins in the culture media.[21] Finally, gene therapy for the treatment of hemophilia is now in the early stages of clinical trials.

HEMOPHILIA A

Table 100–4 summarizes the factor VIII products currently available in the United States. Most patients are treated with high-purity products. In general, products that have the lowest risk of transmitting infectious disease should be used. Thus recombinant products are generally used when available, rather than plasma-derived products.

RECOMBINANT FACTOR VIII

Derived from cultured Chinese hamster ovary cells or baby hamster kidney cells transfected with the human factor VIII gene,[22] recombinant factor VIII is produced from DNA technology. Because it is not derived from blood donations, the risk of transmitting infections through the administration of recombinant factor VIII is low. For this reason, recombinant products are generally favored over plasma-derived products. There is still a small risk of viral infection of the cell lines used to produce the clotting factor.[23] Furthermore, human and/or animal proteins are utilized in the production process of some recombinant products.[21] Therefore these products have a theoretical risk of transmitting infection, although hepatitis and HIV infection have never been reported with their use.[5] The presence of parvovirus B19 DNA has been reported in recombinant factor VIII products.[24] First-generation recombinant factor VIII products contain human albumin as a stabilizing protein.[7] Second-generation recombinant factor VIII products add sucrose instead of human albumin as a stabilizer, but human albumin is utilized in the culture process. One second-generation product (ReFacto) has the B domain of the factor VIII gene

TABLE 100–4. Factor Concentrates

Brand Name	Product Type	Viral Inactivation or Exclusion Method	Other Contents
Factor VIII concentrates			
Alphanate	Plasma	Solvent detergent, dry heat	Albumin, heparin, vWF
Hemophil M	Plasma	Solvent detergent, monoclonal antibody	Albumin
Humate-P	Plasma	Pasteurization	Albumin, vWF
Koāte-DVI	Plasma	Solvent detergent, dry heat	Albumin, heparin, vWF
Monarc-M	Plasma	Solvent detergent, monoclonal antibody	Albumin
Monoclate P	Plasma	Pasteurization, monoclonal antibody	Albumin
Advate	Recombinant	None	
Bioclate	Recombinant	None	Albumin
Helixate FS	Recombinant	Solvent detergent	Albumin (fermentation only); sucrose
Kogenate	Recombinant	Monoclonal antibody	Albumin
Kogenate FS	Recombinant	Solvent detergent, monoclonal antibody	Albumin (fermentation only); sucrose
Recombinate	Recombinant	Monoclonal antibody	Albumin
ReFacto	Recombinant B domain deleted	None	Albumin (fermentation only); sucrose
Factor IX concentrates			
AlphaNine SD	Plasma	Solvent detergent, filtered	Heparin
Mononine	Plasma	Monoclonal antibody, ultrafiltration	Heparin
Benefix	Recombinant	None	
APCC			
Autoplex T	Plasma	Dry heat	Heparin, IIa, VIIa, trace VIIIa, IXa, Xa
Feiba VH Immuno	Plasma	Vapor heat	IIa, VIIa, VIIIa, IXa, Xa
PCC			
Bebulin VH	Plasma	Vapor heat	Heparin, II, IX, X
Profilnine SD	Plasma	Solvent detergent	II, VII, IX, X
Proplex T	Plasma	Dry heat	Heparin, II, VII, IX, X
Other			
NovoSeven	Recombinant VII	None	
Hyate:C	Porcine VIII	Freeze-dried	Citrate

APCC, activated prothrombin complex concentrate; PCC, prothrombin complex concentrate; vWF, von Willebrand factor.

deleted, yielding a smaller protein product.[25] This B domain does not appear to be necessary for coagulation function. Third-generation recombinant factor VIII products contain no human protein in either the culture or in the stabilization processes.[21]

Clinical trials have demonstrated that recombinant factor VIII products are comparable in effectiveness to the plasma-derived products.[25] The risk of developing an inhibitory antibody to factor VIII in patients with severe hemophilia A with the use of recombinant factor VIII is 28% to 33%.[25] This risk is higher than that reported with plasma-derived products. The difference may be partly attributable to more frequent screening for inhibitors in the recombinant product trials, with the detection of transient inhibitors that might have been missed in the trials with plasma-derived products.[26] However, the incidence of high-responding inhibitors, which are clinically significant, was higher in trials with the use of recombinant factor VIII compared with the use of a single plasma-derived product.[26]

PLASMA-DERIVED FACTOR VIII PRODUCTS

Several different plasma-derived factor VIII products are available (see Table 100–4). These products are derived from the plasma of thousands of donors, and therefore potentially can transmit infection. Donor screening, testing plasma pools for evidence of infection, viral reduction through purification steps, and viral inactivation procedures (e.g., dry heat, pasteurization, and solvent detergent treatment) have all resulted in a safer product.[21] No cases of HIV transmission from factor concentrates have been reported since 1986.[5] However, there have been isolated reports of hepatitis C infection with the use of plasma-derived products.[5] Additionally, there have been outbreaks of hepatitis A viral infections associated with plasma-derived products, likely because solvent detergent treatment does not inactivate this nonenveloped virus.[18] Parvovirus has also been reported to be present in both plasma-derived and recombinant factor VIII products.[24,27] Finally, there remains concern about the possibility for infection with as yet unidentified viruses that currently used methods would not inactivate.

Factor VIII concentrates can be classified according to their level of purity, which refers to the specific activity of factor VIII in the product. Cryoprecipitate is a low-purity product, containing a specific factor VIII activity level of less than 5 units/mg of protein.[5] This product is no longer considered a primary treatment for factor VIII deficiency in countries where factor VIII concentrates are available, because cryoprecipitate does not undergo a viral inactivation process. Intermediate-purity products have a specific activity of factor VIII of 1 to 10 units/mg of protein, while high-purity products have a specific activity of 50 to 1,000 units/mg of protein.[5] Ultrahigh-purity plasma-derived products are prepared with monoclonal antibody purification steps and have a specific activity of 3,000 units/mg of protein prior to the addition of albumin as a stabilizer.

FACTOR VIII CONCENTRATE REPLACEMENT

Appropriate dosing of factor VIII concentrate depends on several considerations, including the half-life of the infused factor, the patient's body weight, and the volume of distribution. The presence or absence of an inhibitory antibody to factor VIII and the titer of this antibody also influence treatment. Recovery studies, which measure the immediate postinfusion factor level, and survival studies, which assess the half-life of the factor, can establish patient-specific pharmacokinetics. The location and magnitude of the bleeding episode determine the

percent correction to target, as well as the duration of treatment. Serious or life-threatening bleeding requires peak factor levels of greater than 0.75 to 1 unit/mL (75% to 100%), while less severe bleeding may be treated with a goal of 0.3 to 0.5 unit/mL (30% to 50%) peak plasma levels. Table 100–5 provides general guidelines for the management of bleeding in different locations.

Factor VIII is a large molecule that remains in the intravascular space. Therefore the plasma volume, approximately 50 mL/kg, can be used to estimate the volume of distribution.[28] In general, each unit of factor VIII concentrate infused per kilogram of body weight yields a 2% rise in plasma factor VIII levels. The following equation may be used to calculate an initial dose of factor VIII:

$$\text{Factor VIII (units)} = (\text{desired level} - \text{baseline level})$$
$$\times\ 0.5 \times (\text{weight in kilograms})$$

The baseline level is usually omitted from the equation because it is negligible compared to the desired level. The half-life of factor VIII ranges from 8 to 15 hours.[28] It is generally necessary to administer half of the initial dose approximately every 12 hours to sustain the desired level of factor VIII. A single treatment may be adequate for minor bleeding such as mouth bleeding or slight muscle hemorrhages. However, because of the potential for long-term joint damage with hemarthroses, 2 or 3 days of treatment are often recommended for these bleeds. Serious bleeding episodes may require maintenance of 70% to 100% factor activity for a week or longer. As previously mentioned, factor VIII dosing depends on several variables and each case must be considered individually. Individual pharmacokinetics may help guide treatment, particularly for serious bleeding episodes.

Alternatively, factor VIII may be administered as a continuous infusion when prolonged treatment is required, such as in the perioperative period or for serious bleeding episodes. Infusion rates ranging from 2 to 4 units/kg per hour are usually employed in fixed dose continuous infusion protocols, with the aim of maintaining a steady-state level of 60% to 100%.[29,30] The administration of factor concentrate via continuous infusion may reduce factor requirements by 20% to 50%, because unnecessarily high peaks of factor VIII that occur with bolus injections are avoided.[30] A gradual decrease in factor VIII clearance during the first 5 to 6 days of treatment contributes to the lower factor concentrate requirements.[29] Daily factor level monitoring can help determine the appropriate rate of infusion.

The administration of factor VIII concentrate via continuous infusion has been shown to be safe and effective,[29] and it may be more convenient than bolus therapy for hospitalized patients. The advantages of continuous infusion include the maintenance of a steady-state plasma level, with avoidance of potentially subtherapeutic trough levels, and a reduction in cost associated with decreased factor requirements. A potential side effect with continuous infusion is thrombophlebitis at the delivery site. Concomitant infusion of saline or the addition of heparin (2 to 5 units/mL) to the infusion bag can minimize this risk.[29,30] Bacterial contamination of the concentrate is another theoretical concern. However, studies have shown that the products can remain sterile for more than a week if prepared and kept under appropriate conditions.[29] Finally, concerns about the stability of the formulations appear to be unwarranted in that most of the high-purity factor VIII concentrates have been shown to remain stable for at least 7 days after reconstitution.[30]

OTHER PHARMACOLOGIC THERAPY

Treatment with 1-desamino-8-D-arginine vasopressin (desmopressin acetate) is often adequate for minor bleeding episodes in patients with

TABLE 100–5. Guidelines for Factor Replacement Therapy for Hemorrhage in Hemophilia A and B

Site of Hemorrhage	Desired Hemostatic Factor Level (% of Normal)	Comments
Joint	50%–70%	Rest/immobilization/physical therapy rehabilitation following bleed; several doses may be necessary to prevent or treat target joint
Muscle	30%–50% for most sites 70%–100% for thigh, iliopsoas, or nerve compression	Risk of significant blood loss with femoral/retroperitoneal bleed; bed rest for iliopsoas or other retroperitoneal bleeding
Oral mucosa	30%–50%	May try antifibrinolytic or topical thrombin prior to factor replacement for minor bleeding; higher factor levels may be needed for tongue swelling or risk of airway compromise; antifibrinolytic therapy should be used following factor replacement; do not use with APCCs or PCCs
Gastrointestinal	Initially 100%, then 30% until healing occurs	Endoscopy is highly recommended; antifibrinolytic therapy may be useful
Hematuria	30% if no trauma 70%–100% if traumatic	If no pain or trauma, consider bed rest and fluids for 24 hours; factor should be given if hematuria persists; evaluate if hematuria persists; if trauma to abdomen or back, perform imaging and give aggressive factor replacement
Central nervous system	Initially 100%, then 50%–100% for 10–14 days	Anticonvulsants may be given preventively with neurologic follow-up; lumbar puncture requires prophylactic factor coverage
Trauma or surgery	Initially 100%, then 50% until wound healing complete	Perioperative and postoperative management plan must be in place preoperatively; evaluation for inhibitors is crucial prior to elective surgery

APCC, activated prothrombin complex concentrate; PCC, prothrombin complex concentrate.

mild hemophilia A. A synthetic analog of the antidiuretic hormone vasopressin, desmopressin causes release of von Willebrand factor and factor VIII from endogenous storage sites. It appears to be most effective in those with higher baseline factor VIII levels (0.1 to 0.15 units/mL).[31] The recommended dose of desmopressin is 0.3 mcg/kg diluted in 50 mL of normal saline and infused IV over 15 to 30 minutes.[5,31] Patients with mild or moderate hemophilia A should have a desmopressin trial performed to determine their response to this medication. At least a twofold rise in factor VIII to a minimal level of 0.3 units/mL within 60 minutes is considered an adequate response.[32] In adults with mild hemophilia A, the response rate to desmopressin has been reported to be 80% to 90%.[32] One study reported a lower response rate of 57% in pediatric patients with mild hemophilia A.[32] Furthermore, the response rate was related to age; the mean age of those who responded to desmopressin was 5.2 years compared with 3 years for those who failed to respond. Seven of the eleven children who failed to respond to desmopressin initially demonstrated an adequate response when the desmopressin challenge was repeated at an older age.

The infusion of desmopressin may be repeated daily for up to 2 to 3 days. Tachyphylaxis, an attenuated response with repeated dosing, may develop after that. The factor increase after the second dose of desmopressin is approximately 30% lower than after the initial dose.[31]

Factor concentrate therapy may be necessary if the patient requires further treatment. Factor levels should be measured to ensure that an adequate response has been achieved. Treatment with desmopressin will not result in hemostasis for patients who have severe hemophilia and for those who are only marginally responsive. Also, it should not be used as primary therapy for life-threatening bleeding episodes such as intracranial hemorrhage or for major surgical procedures when a minimum factor VIII concentration of 0.7 to 1 unit/mL is required.[31]

Desmopressin may be administered intranasally via a concentrated nasal spray.[31] It effectively increases factor VIII levels, but its peak effect occurs 60 to 90 minutes after administration, somewhat longer than with desmopressin administered intravenously.[5,31,33] The dosage is one spray (150 mcg) for children who weigh less than 50 kg and two sprays (300 mcg) for those who weigh more than 50 kg.[33] The nasal spray may serve as an alternative to the intravenous formulation, especially in patients with mild bleeding episodes.

Very few adverse effects are associated with desmopressin. The most commonly observed side effect is facial flushing.[31] Less frequently reported side effects include mild headaches, increased heart rate, and decreased blood pressure. Thrombosis is a rare complication associated with desmopressin.[5] Because of its antidiuretic effects, desmopressin also has the potential to cause water retention, which may lead to severe hyponatremia. This may be a particular problem in children less than 1 to 2 years old, in whom hyponatremic seizures have been reported.[5,31] Therefore desmopressin should be used with caution in this age group.[31,32] Patients with congestive heart failure may also be at increased risk of developing hyponatremia with the use of desmopressin.[31] Mild fluid restriction and monitoring of urine output are also recommended with desmopressin administration.[5]

Antifibrinolytic therapy inhibits clot lysis and therefore is a useful adjunctive therapy in the treatment of hemophilia. These antifibrinolytic agents are particularly beneficial in the treatment of oral bleeding because of the high concentration of fibrinolytic enzymes present in saliva. Two currently available antifibrinolytics are aminocaproic acid and tranexamic acid. Aminocaproic acid is given at a dosage of 100 mg/kg (maximum 6 g) every 6 hours and may be administered orally or intravenously.[5] The dosage of tranexamic acid is 25 mg/kg (maximum 1.5 g) orally every 8 hours or 10 mg/kg (maximum 1 g) intravenously every 8 hours.[5,34]

HEMOPHILIA B

Therapeutic options for hemophilia B have improved greatly over the past several years, first with the development of monoclonal antibody–purified plasma-derived products, and then with the licensure of recombinant factor IX. Products that are currently available in the United States for treatment of hemophilia B are listed in Table 100–4.

RECOMBINANT FACTOR IX

First marketed in the United States in 1996,[5,7] recombinant factor IX is produced in Chinese hamster ovary cells transfected with the factor IX gene. Blood and plasma products are not used to produce recombinant factor IX nor to stabilize the final product; thus recombinant factor IX has an excellent viral safety profile.[35] Clinical trials have shown the product to be safe and efficacious in the treatment of acute bleeding episodes and in the management of bleeding associated with surgical procedures.[36,37] Although the half-life of recombinant factor IX is similar to that of the plasma-derived products, recovery is approximately 28% lower.[37] As a result, doses of recombinant factor IX concentrate must be higher than those of plasma-derived products to achieve equivalent plasma levels. Because individual pharmacokinetics may vary, recovery and survival studies should be performed to determine optimal treatment. Recombinant factor IX is often considered the treatment of choice for hemophilia B.

PLASMA-DERIVED FACTOR IX PRODUCTS

High-purity factor IX plasma concentrates have been available in the United States since the early 1990s.[5] These products are derived from plasma through biochemical purification and monoclonal immunoaffinity techniques. Other viral inactivation measures, such as solvent detergent or chemical treatment, are also employed.

Before the high-purity products were approved for use, hemophilia B patients had been treated with factor IX concentrates that also contained other vitamin K–dependent proteins (factors II, VII, and X), known as prothrombin complex concentrates (PCCs). These products contain small amounts of activated factors generated during processing, and their use has been associated with thrombotic complications, including deep venous thrombosis, pulmonary embolism, myocardial infarction, and disseminated intravascular coagulation (DIC).[38,39] The risk of such complications is highest in patients who are receiving high or repeated doses of PCCs, in those who have liver disease, in neonates, and in patients who have experienced crush injuries or who are undergoing major surgery.[39] Concomitant use of PCCs and antifibrinolytics should be avoided because of the risk of thrombosis.

Because of the lower purity of PCCs and their thrombogenic potential, these products are not first-line treatment for hemophilia B, although they are still used in the treatment of patients with hemophilia A or B who have developed inhibitory antibodies against factor VIII or factor IX, respectively. High-purity factor IX concentrates have excellent efficacy in the treatment of bleeding episodes and in the control of bleeding associated with surgical procedures.[40] Their viral safety profile has also been reported to be excellent,[40] and the risk of thromboembolic complications is low.[5]

FACTOR IX CONCENTRATE REPLACEMENT

Factor IX is a relatively small protein. Unlike factor VIII, it is not limited to the intravascular space, but also passes into the extravascular compartment.[28] This results in a volume of distribution that is approximately twice that of factor VIII. In general, for plasma-derived factor IX concentrates, each unit of factor IX infused per kilogram of body weight yields a 1% rise in the plasma level of factor IX (range, 0.67% to 1.28%).[28] The following equation can be used to calculate the initial dose:

$$\text{Plasma-derived factor IX (units)} = (\text{desired level} - \text{baseline level})$$
$$\times (\text{weight in kilograms})$$

As with the similar calculation for factor VIII dosing, the baseline level term can be omitted from the formula. Because the recovery of recombinant factor IX is approximately 20% lower than that of the plasma-derived products, the following adjustment is made:

$$\text{Recombinant factor IX (units)} = (\text{desired level} - \text{baseline level})$$
$$\times 1.2 \times (\text{weight in kilograms})$$

A recovery study to determine optimal dosing is recommended for patients who receive recombinant factor IX because of the wide interpatient variability in pharmacokinetics.

Because the half-life of factor IX is approximately 24 hours, dosing can be less frequent than with factor VIII. Table 100–5 provides general guidelines for dosing factor IX, based on the site and severity of the bleeding episode. As with factor VIII replacement therapy, individual pharmacokinetics may vary, and monitoring the patient's factor IX levels helps optimize therapy.

PROPHYLACTIC REPLACEMENT THERAPY

Traditionally, factor concentrates for hemophilia patients have been given on demand, as the bleeding episode occurs. However, recurrent joint bleeding can damage the joint and lead to the development of severe physical disability. Thus it would be preferable to prevent bleeding episodes and avoid the resultant damage. Known as prophylactic factor replacement therapy, this approach entails the regular infusion of concentrate to maintain the deficient factor at a minimum of 0.01 unit/mL (1%).

In effect, prophylactic replacement therapy converts severe hemophilia into a milder form of the disease. The rationale for this approach is that patients with moderate hemophilia rarely experience spontaneous hemarthroses, and they have a much lower incidence of chronic arthropathy. Patients with hemophilia A usually require 25 to 40 units of factor VIII per kilogram of body weight, given every other day or three times a week.[41] For hemophilia B, the usual dosage is 25 to 40 units/kg of factor IX given twice weekly instead of three times weekly because of the longer half-life of factor IX.[5,42]

Primary prophylaxis is regular replacement therapy started at a young age (usually before the patient is 2 years old), prior to the onset of joint bleeding.[41] The results of primary prophylaxis have been very promising. In the Swedish experience, children who began prophylaxis at 1 to 2 years of age experienced almost no bleeding episodes and had normal joint examinations and radiographs over a 5-year period.[41–43] Secondary prophylaxis begins after significant joint bleeding has already occurred. It is associated with a significant reduction in the number of joint bleeding episodes and a better clinical and orthopedic outcome.[41,44] However, radiographic evidence of joint disease rarely improves and often progresses despite the institution of secondary prophylaxis.[5] Therefore it may not be possible to avoid chronic arthropathy when prophylaxis is initiated after significant joint bleeding has already occurred; this supports a need for earlier intervention.

CLINICAL CONTROVERSY

Hemophilia patients may receive prophylactic factor concentrate therapy to prevent or decrease bleeding episodes or they may receive on-demand factor concentrate therapy in response to a bleeding episode. In addition, prophylaxis may be primary on secondary. Controversy exists over whether the benefits of prophylaxis justify the cost, as well as the appropriate time to initiate prophylaxis.

Prophylactic replacement therapy is now in widespread use in Europe. Although the Medical and Scientific Advisory Council of the National Hemophilia Foundation of the United States has recommended primary prophylaxis beginning at 1 to 2 years of age for children with severe hemophilia,[5] this therapeutic approach has not yet been widely accepted in the United States. There are several disadvantages associated with prophylactic regimens that may be responsible for this lack of acceptance. Perhaps most important is the high cost of prophylactic replacement therapy. Factor requirements have been estimated to be two- to threefold higher with prophylactic regimens than with treatment on demand.[41,45] The use of individual pharmacokinetics to titrate dosage may help to lessen costs.[41] Other issues to consider are the inconvenience to families and the possible difficulties with compliance. Central venous lines may be necessary for the frequent administration of factor concentrates, particularly in children less than 3 to 5 years old, the age targeted for initiation of primary prophylaxis regimens. Potential complications of central venous access include surgical risks, infection, and catheter-related deep venous thrombosis.[46,47] Catheter-related sepsis has been reported to occur in up to 50% of patients with hemophilia who have central lines.[47] Catheter-related infectious complications appear to be more common in hemophilia patients who have developed inhibitory antibodies.[46] Finally, there are concerns that the routine use of primary prophylaxis may overtreat some patients with severe hemophilia who do not have a severe clinical phenotype. Prospective, randomized studies and more formal cost-effectiveness analyses are needed to determine the relative benefits and optimal timing of prophylactic factor replacement therapy.

TREATMENT OF INHIBITORS IN HEMOPHILIA

Neutralizing antibodies to factor VIII and IX, known as inhibitors, develop in a subset of patients with hemophilia, challenging the management of these patients. The development of inhibitors is probably the most common serious complication of factor replacement therapy. The reported incidence of inhibitor development has varied considerably, depending on the population studied, the study design, the method of detection, and the frequency and duration of testing. Inhibitor formation has been reported to occur in 4% to 20% of patients with factor VIII deficiency, and in up to 52% of patients with severe factor VIII deficiency.[48] The reported prevalence of inhibitors is much lower in hemophilia B, occurring in only 1% to 4% of patients.[48]

Most inhibitors develop in childhood, often after relatively few exposure days.[26] Patients with severe hemophilia are much more likely to develop inhibitors than those with milder forms of the disease.[26] A possible explanation is that the low levels of factor produced in patients with mild and moderate hemophilia may induce immune tolerance in these individuals. In contrast, factor levels are undetectable in patients with severe hemophilia, and infused factor VIII, regarded as a foreign protein, may provoke an antibody response. Similarly, in patients with severe hemophilia there is a higher rate of inhibitor development (23% to 40%) in those with mutations that result in undetectable plasma factor VIII levels than in those with missense mutations and small deletions (3% to 13%) when circulating, albeit abnormal, protein is present.[49] The rate of inhibitor formation varies even among patients with identical mutations, which suggests that host factors modify the risk. One possibility is that HLA genotype may influence the risk of inhibitor formation, but studies have been inconclusive.[26]

Inhibitors are usually immunoglobulins of the IgG subclass that are directed against the factor coagulant portion of the complex. The presence of an inhibitor is suspected when there is a decreased clinical response to factor replacement. It may also be discovered incidentally on routine laboratory screening. Inhibitors are measured with the Bethesda assay, and titers are reported in Bethesda units (BU). One BU is the amount of inhibitor needed to inactivate half of the factor VIII or factor IX in a mixture of inhibitor-containing plasma and pooled normal plasma.[48] Patients with inhibitors to factor VIII or factor IX are divided into two groups: low responders, who have low levels of inhibitors (<10 BU/mL) and generally have little or no rise in antibody titers after exposure to the factor; and high responders, who have higher inhibitor levels (>10 BU/mL) and develop an increase in antibody titer after exposure (anamnestic response).[48]

The treatment of patients with inhibitors is twofold, involving treatment of acute bleeding episodes as well as treatment directed at eradicating the inhibitor. The inhibitor titer, the site and magnitude of bleeding, and the patient's past response to therapy determine the approach to treatment. For patients with a low inhibitor titer, administration of high doses of the specific factor can often control bleeding episodes. Two to three times the usual replacement dose and more frequent dosing intervals are often necessary to overcome the antibody. Factor level monitoring and clinical assessments help to evaluate the adequacy of treatment. Additional supportive measures, such as immobilization and the administration of antifibrinolytic agents, should be employed, where appropriate.

In the presence of a high-titer inhibitor, it may be impossible to administer enough factor VIII or factor IX to neutralize the antibody and achieve a hemostatic plasma level. Therefore the approach to treatment of bleeding episodes in these patients is to use agents that bypass the factor to which the antibody is directed. These include PCCs, activated PCCs, and recombinant activated factor VII.

PCCs contain the vitamin K–dependent factors II, VII, IX, and X. Small quantities of activated factors VII and IX are present in these products. Activated PCCs (aPCCs) contain greater quantities of the activated factors.[50] The usual dosage is 50 to 100 units/kg administered every 12 to 24 hours, depending on the severity of the bleeding episode.[48] The maximum dose should not exceed 200 units/kg per day. The use of PCCs and aPCCs, when not restricted to one or two doses, is effective in obtaining hemostasis in approximately 80% of bleeding episodes in patients with inhibitors, and aPCCs appear to be more effective than PCCs.[50] As previously mentioned, there is a risk of serious thrombotic complications including pulmonary emboli, deep venous thrombosis, and myocardial infarction associated with the use of PCCs and aPCCs.[50] Additionally, because these products contain trace amounts of factor VIII and larger amounts of factor IX, they can stimulate an anamnestic response in patients with hemophilia A, and more commonly, in those with hemophilia B.[38,50] Other minor side effects include dizziness, nausea, hives, flushing, and headaches.[50] Patients with factor IX inhibitors may occasionally develop severe allergic reactions in response to infusion of factor IX–containing products; therefore these patients should be monitored closely.[51]

A newer bypassing agent, recombinant factor VIIa, is thought to be hemostatically active only at the site of tissue injury where tissue factor is present; thus the risk of systemic thrombotic events associated with this agent is minimal.[52] Additionally, because recombinant VIIa is not a plasma-derived product, both viral transmission and anamnestic responses to factor VIII or factor IX are unlikely.[38,50] The initial dose for bleeding episodes ranges from 35 to 120 mcg/kg.[50,52] Doses of 70 mcg/kg or higher are more effective, and often a dose of 90 to 120 mcg/kg is used for the treatment of patients with hemophilia and inhibitors.[52] A drawback is the product's short half-life, which necessitates dosing every 2 hours. The continuous infusion of recombinant factor VIIa, which may be more convenient and cost-effective, has been successful, although studies are limited.[50] Recombinant factor VIIa appears to be efficacious in controlling bleeding episodes and in managing hemophilia during surgical procedures.[50] Patients treated with bypassing agents must be monitored clinically, because there are no laboratory tests that directly measure the effectiveness of the treatment.

Porcine factor VIII is an alternative therapeutic option for patients who have hemophilia A and inhibitors. In general, porcine factor VIII is most useful when the inhibitor titer is less than 50 BU.[28,48] The recommended initial dose is 50 to 100 units/kg for those with inhibitor titers less than 50 BU.[28] The rationale is that porcine factor VIII is enough like human factor VIII to participate in the coagulation cascade, yet most factor VIII inhibitors have absent or only weak neutralizing activity against nonhuman factor VIII. However, cross-reactivity with porcine factor VIII does occur, and there is also the potential for developing a high titer of antibody against porcine factor VIII. Although the rise in antibody titer is generally lower than that seen with the administration of human factor VIII,[48] anamnestic rises in inhibitor titers to both porcine and human factor VIII may occur and can limit future use.[38,50] Other potential side effects include severe allergic reactions and thrombocytopenia.[38,48,50] Supply problems may limit the availability of this product. Because of these limitations, porcine factor VIII is usually indicated only after recombinant factor VIIa and PCC have failed or when hemorrhages are severe.[48] An advantage to porcine factor VIII is that treatment response may be monitored with factor VIII levels.

The ideal therapy for patients with hemophilia and inhibitors is to eradicate the inhibitor so that future treatment with factor VIII or factor IX concentrates is possible. Immune tolerance therapy, which involves the regular infusion of high doses of the factor to which the antibody is directed, may accomplish this eradication. A variety of different dosing regimens, ranging from 25 units/kg every other day to more than 200 units/kg every day have been employed. Some treatment protocols include adjunctive immunomodulatory therapy, such as the administration of cyclophosphamide, prednisone, and intravenous immune globulin.[53] The overall success rate is 50% to 70% and it is best in patients with low inhibitor titers and in those whom the inhibitor has recently developed.[5,54] Weeks to years of therapy may be required to eradicate the antibody. Unfortunately, immune tolerance therapy is costly, time-consuming, and often requires the placement of a central venous catheter.[5] Once achieved, however, immune tolerance facilitates the management of bleeding episodes with specific factor replacement therapy. Rituximab, an anti-CD20 monoclonal antibody, has been used in a few patients with acquired factor VIII inhibitors with some success.[55] The mechanism of action involves the rapid depletion of circulating B cells, which produce antibodies, including the anti–factor VIII antibody. The use of rituximab in patients with hemophilia and inhibitors has yet to be tested on a large scale.

Figure 100–3 summarizes the therapeutic options in the management of hemophilia A patients with inhibitors. The same algorithm can be applied to the management of hemophilia B patients, except that factor IX should be substituted for factor VIII. The use of porcine factor VIII is not indicated for the inhibitors in hemophilia B.

GENE THERAPY IN HEMOPHILIA

The use of gene therapy for hemophilia A and B is currently under investigation. A number of different viral and nonviral vectors have been used to transfer the recombinant factor gene to human cells, such as liver and muscle cells.[56,57] Even low levels of factor expression through gene therapy should reduce bleeding episodes in patients with severe hemophilia, a rationale for gene therapy similar to that for prophylactic factor replacement. Furthermore, given that there is a broad range of physiologically normal factor levels, very tight regulation of gene expression is not necessary. The safety and efficacy of this approach to treatment remain to be determined. Potential benefits to gene therapy include patient convenience, viral safety, and decreased cost. Possible drawbacks to gene therapy include a risk of inhibitor formation, tumorigenesis related to integration of the viral vector, possible germline transmission, and concerns about long-term gene expression.[56,57]

PAIN MANAGEMENT IN HEMOPHILIA

Pain, both acute and chronic, can be a common occurrence for patients with hemophilia. The likely cause of acute pain is bleeding, and control of the bleeding episode should ease the pain. Chronic pain may be the result of permanent joint changes. Surgical intervention may help to alleviate the pain, as may an intensive physical therapy program.[58] The intra-articular administration of dexamethasone may also be useful.[59] Acetaminophen may be used, although narcotic analgesia may be required for more severe pain. Nonsteroidal anti-inflammatory drugs impair platelet function and may increase the risk of bleeding in patients with hemophilia, although these drugs have been used for the management of chronic arthropathy.

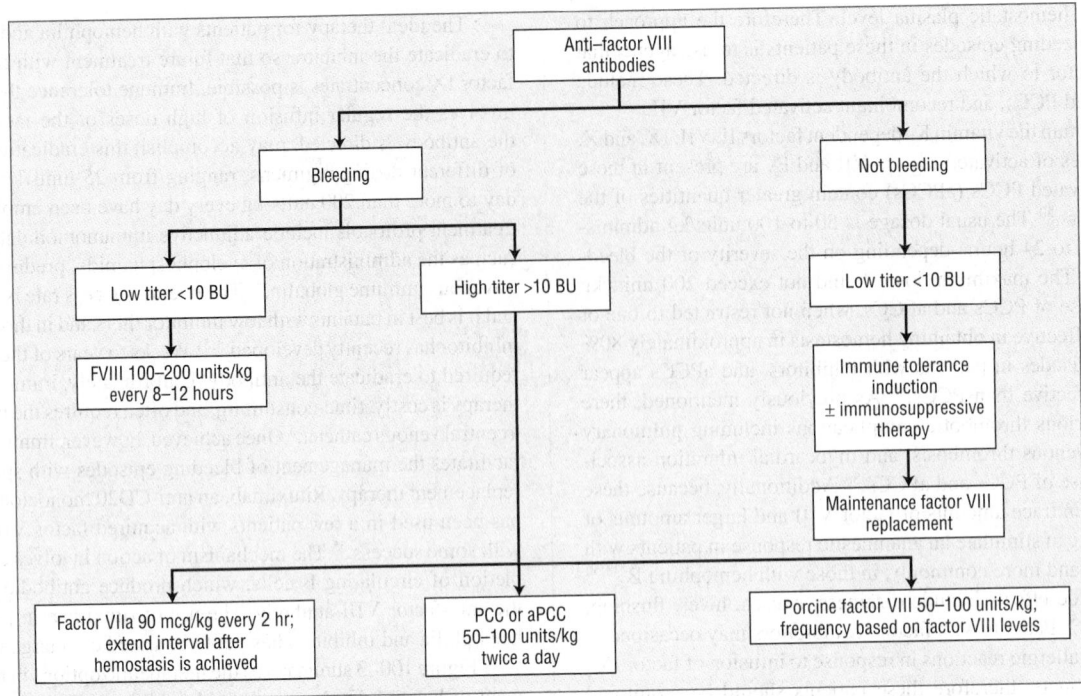

FIGURE 100–3. Treatment algorithm for the management of patients with hemophilia A and factor VIII antibodies. BU, Bethesda unit; PCC, prothrombin complex concentrate; aPCC, activated prothrombin complex concentrate.

Cyclooxygenase-2 inhibitors have less antiplatelet activity and may be an option for pain management.

SURGERY IN HEMOPHILIA

The goal of treatment of the patient with hemophilia undergoing a surgical procedure is to maintain factor levels of at least 0.5 to 0.7 unit/mL (50% to 70%) during surgery and in the postoperative period in order to prevent excessive bleeding. Intermittent dosing or continuous infusion factor replacement may accomplish this goal. Before surgery, factor concentrate is usually infused to obtain a plasma level of 1 unit/mL (100%).[60] Replacement therapy is continued to maintain plasma levels greater than 0.5 unit/mL (50%) for 5 to 7 days or longer, depending on the type of surgery. Preoperative evaluation for elective procedures should include the measurement of an inhibitor titer and assessment of the recovery and half-life of infused factor in the patient. Elective surgery should not proceed unless therapeutic plasma levels can be obtained.

EVALUATION OF THERAPEUTIC OUTCOMES

The main goal in the treatment of hemophilia is to control and prevent bleeding episodes and their long-term sequelae, such as chronic arthropathies. Pharmacologic and nonpharmacologic interventions should be aimed at achieving this goal. Treatment response can be monitored through clinical parameters, such as cessation of bleeding and resolution of symptoms. It may also be useful to determine plasma factor levels, particularly for severe bleeding episodes. Home therapy for the administration of factor concentrates is common among these patients, because this approach can lead to earlier treatment and more independence for the patient. Diaries in which the patient documents symptoms, the dose of factor replacement, adjuvant therapies used, and treatment response can help the caregiver evaluate the success of home therapy. Monitoring the number and type of bleeding episodes and measuring trough plasma factor levels makes it possible to evaluate the adequacy of prophylactic regimens. Physical examination with evaluation of joint range of motion and radiographs of target joints indicates the long-term success of preventing and treating arthropathies.

Clinicians should check for the development of inhibitors, especially in patients with severe disease and exposure to factor concentrates, at least yearly and with any suspicion of poor treatment

response. The development of inhibitors challenges the management and control of bleeding episodes. A full understanding of the clinical situation and the titer of the inhibitor are mandatory to address all treatment options for each patient. Because there is no laboratory test to measure the effectiveness of therapy in this scenario, close clinical monitoring for worsening or resolution of the symptoms is essential to optimize the outcome.

VON WILLEBRAND DISEASE

The most common congenital bleeding disorder, von Willebrand disease has a prevalence of 1% to 2%.[61] It refers to a family of disorders caused by a quantitative and/or qualitative defect of von Willebrand factor, a glycoprotein that plays a role in both platelet aggregation and coagulation. Unlike hemophilia, von Willebrand disease has an autosomal inheritance pattern, resulting in an equal frequency of disease in males and females.

The gene for von Willebrand factor is located on chromosome 12 and is 178 kb in length.[61] Transcription and translation produce a large primary product that subsequently undergoes complex modifications, resulting in von Willebrand factor multimers of various sizes with molecular weights ranging from 500 to 20,000 kd.[61] Von Willebrand factor is synthesized in endothelial cells where it is either stored in Weibel-Palade bodies or secreted constitutively. It is also synthesized in megakaryocytes and stored in alpha granules, from which it is released following platelet activation.[61]

Von Willebrand factor is important for both primary and secondary hemostasis. In response to vascular injury, it promotes platelet adhesion by interacting with the glycoprotein Ib receptor on platelets.[61,62] It can also facilitate platelet aggregation by binding to the platelet glycoprotein IIb/IIIa receptor, although fibrinogen is the main ligand for this receptor.[61,62] The highest-molecular-weight von Willebrand factor multimers appear to be the most important in platelet adhesion because their large surface area contains numerous binding sites for various ligands and receptors. An additional function of von Willebrand factor is that it is the carrier molecule for circulating factor VIII, protecting it from premature degradation and removal.[61] A deficiency of von Willebrand factor thus reduces the half-life of factor VIII, causing decreased plasma factor VIII levels as well. Therefore von Willebrand factor plays a dual role in hemostasis, affecting both platelet function and coagulation.

CLASSIFICATION OF VON WILLEBRAND DISEASE

As shown in Table 100–6, von Willebrand disease consists of a heterogeneous group of disorders that can be classified into three major subtypes. Types 1 and 3 are associated with quantitative defects in von Willebrand factor, while type 2 mutations refer to functional abnormalities in von Willebrand factor. The determination of the disease subtype is important, because it influences treatment.

Type 1 von Willebrand disease is the most common type, accounting for 59% to 76% of cases.[61] It is characterized by a mild to moderate reduction in the level of von Willebrand factor (although its multimeric structure is normal) and a similar reduction in the level of factor VIII. It is usually inherited in an autosomal dominant fashion with variable penetrance and expression.[63] Bleeding symptoms are often only very mild to moderate.[61]

Type 2 von Willebrand disease, diagnosed in 9% to 30% of affected patients, is characterized by a qualitative abnormality of von Willebrand factor.[61] Bleeding manifestations may be more severe than with type 1 disease. Inheritance is most often autosomal dominant, but may be recessive.[63] Type 2 von Willebrand disease may be further subdivided into four variants. Type 2A is the most frequent subtype and is characterized by a reduced von Willebrand factor–platelet interaction and an absence of high- and intermediate-molecular-weight factor multimers. Type 2B is a less common variant in which there is an abnormal von Willebrand factor that has an increased affinity for the platelet glycoprotein Ib receptor. This is associated with thrombocytopenia, which is usually mild. In addition, there are usually no high-molecular-weight forms of von Willebrand factor.[63] Type 2M

arises from a qualitative defect in von Willebrand factor that impairs its binding to platelets; it is similar to type 2A, except that there is no measurable reduction in the high-molecular-weight multimers.[63] Finally, type 2N von Willebrand disease (Normandy) is a rare form of the disease in which von Willebrand factor has a markedly reduced affinity for factor VIII. This leads to a moderate to severe reduction of factor VIII plasma levels with normal von Willebrand factor levels.[63]

Type 3 von Willebrand disease refers to a severe quantitative variant of the disease in which von Willebrand factor is nearly undetectable and factor VIII levels are very low. It is often inherited in an autosomal recessive fashion.[61] The clinical phenotype is severe, reflecting major deficits in primary hemostasis and coagulation. There is also a platelet-type pseudo–von Willebrand disease in which von Willebrand factor is normal, but there is a defect in the platelet glycoprotein Ib receptor that causes an increased affinity for normal von Willebrand factor.[61] As a result, it is phenotypically similar to type 2B disease, but should be distinguished from it because the treatment is different.

Acquired von Willebrand disease is a rare bleeding disorder that is similar to the congenital form of the disease. It has been reported primarily in association with autoimmune disorders, such as systemic lupus erythematosus, lymphoproliferative disorders, and neoplastic disease.[61] Certain medications also have been associated with acquired von Willebrand disease, including valproic acid, dextran, and ciprofloxacin.[64] Bleeding manifestations vary from mild to severe, and the condition often resolves with treatment of the underlying disease. In the acquired disease, von Willebrand factor appears to be synthesized in normal amounts, but then is rapidly removed from plasma by anti–von Willebrand factor antibodies, adsorption to tumor cells, or other mechanisms.[61,64]

> ## CLINCAL PRESENTATION OF VON WILLEBRAND DISEASE
>
> Clinical manifestations are variable; some patients are asymptomatic.
> Mucocutaneous bleeding: epistaxis, gingival bleeding with minor manipulation, menorrhagia
> Easy bruising
> Postoperative bleeding

DIAGNOSIS

When a patient has a lifelong history of mucocutaneous bleeding and a family history of abnormal bleeding, the clinician should suspect von Willebrand disease. Several different laboratory tests are helpful in the diagnosis of the hemostatic abnormality. Initial screening tests include determinations of PT, aPTT, and bleeding time, as well as a platelet count. The PT is normal, whereas the aPTT may be prolonged in relation to the reduction in plasma factor VIII levels. The platelet count is usually normal, although thrombocytopenia is common in type 2B and platelet-type pseudo–von Willebrand disease. The bleeding time, which measures platelet function, is often prolonged, but may be normal in patients with milder forms of the disease.

Specific laboratory tests to investigate the possible presence of von Willebrand disease include measurement of von Willebrand factor antigen (vWF:Ag) level, factor VIII assay, determination of ristocetin cofactor activity, and von Willebrand factor multimer analysis. Plasma concentrations of von Willebrand factor increase with cigarette smoking, exercise, pregnancy, and infection, as well as with the use of certain medications, such as corticosteroids, birth control pills, and desmopressin.[65] Repeated test measurements may be

TABLE 100–6. Von Willebrand Disease

von Willebrand factor (vWF)
The large multimeric glycoprotein that is necessary for normal platelet adhesion, a normal bleeding time, and stabilizing factor VIII.
von Willebrand factor antigen (vWF:Ag)
The antigenic determinant(s) on vWF measured by immunoassays; usually low in types 1 and 2; virtually absent in type 3.
Ristocetin cofactor activity
Functional assay of vWF activity based on platelet aggregation with ristocetin. Reduced by the same degree as vWF:Ag in types 1 and 3, but to a greater extent in type 2 disease (except 2B).

necessary to make the diagnosis because of physiologic variations in plasma levels.

Electroimmunoassay, immunoradiometric assay, or enyzme-linked immunosorbent assay can be used to quantify vWF:Ag.[61] Because vWF:Ag levels are known to vary with different ABO blood types,[66] interpretation requires reference to values specific for the patient's blood type. The vWF:Ag level is usually low in types 1 and 2 von Willebrand disease and virtually absent in type 3 disease. Factor VIII levels are normal or mildly decreased in patients with type 1 or 2 disease and very low (<10%) in those with type 3 disease.[61] Ristocetin, an antibiotic that causes platelet aggregation in the presence of functional von Willebrand factor, is used to measure von Willebrand factor activity. The assay is performed by mixing platelet-free patient plasma, normal formalin-fixed platelets, and ristocetin, and then quantitating the extent of platelet agglutination. Ristocetin cofactor activity is usually reduced in parallel to vWF:Ag levels in types 1 and 3, and decreased to a greater extent than vWF:Ag in type 2 disease (except type 2B).[63] Ristocetin-induced platelet agglutination is useful to further distinguish type 2B disease, as a low concentration of ristocetin induces excessive aggregation in type 2B disease.

Von Willebrand factor multimers can be analyzed by separating them by size on an agarose gel. All multimer sizes are present in type 1 disease, while a reduction in intermediate- and high-molecular-weight multimers is characteristic of type 2 disease. Type 3 patients lack all types of von Willebrand factor multimers. A summary of the laboratory findings in the various types of von Willebrand disease is provided in Table 100–6.

▶ TREATMENT: von Willebrand Disease

4 The specific type of von Willebrand disease, as well as the location and severity of bleeding, determine the approach to treatment. Local measures, including pressure, ice, and topical thrombin, can often control superficial bleeding. Systemic treatment is used for bleeding that cannot be controlled in this manner and for the prevention of bleeding with surgery. The goal of systemic therapy is to correct the platelet adhesion and coagulation defects. This may be accomplished by stimulating the release of endogenous von Willebrand factor or by administering products that contain von Willebrand factor and factor VIII. General guidelines for the treatment of von Willebrand disease are shown in Fig. 100–4.

■ REPLACEMENT THERAPY

5 The treatment of choice for patients with types 2B, 2M, and 3 von Willebrand disease and for patients with type 1 or 2A von Willebrand disease who are unresponsive to desmopressin is replacement therapy with plasma-derived von Willebrand factor–containing products.[60] Several virus-inactivated, intermediate- or high-purity factor VIII concentrates contain sufficient amounts of functional von Willebrand factor.[60] Ultrahigh-purity (monoclonal antibody-derived) plasma-derived products and recombinant factor VIII products

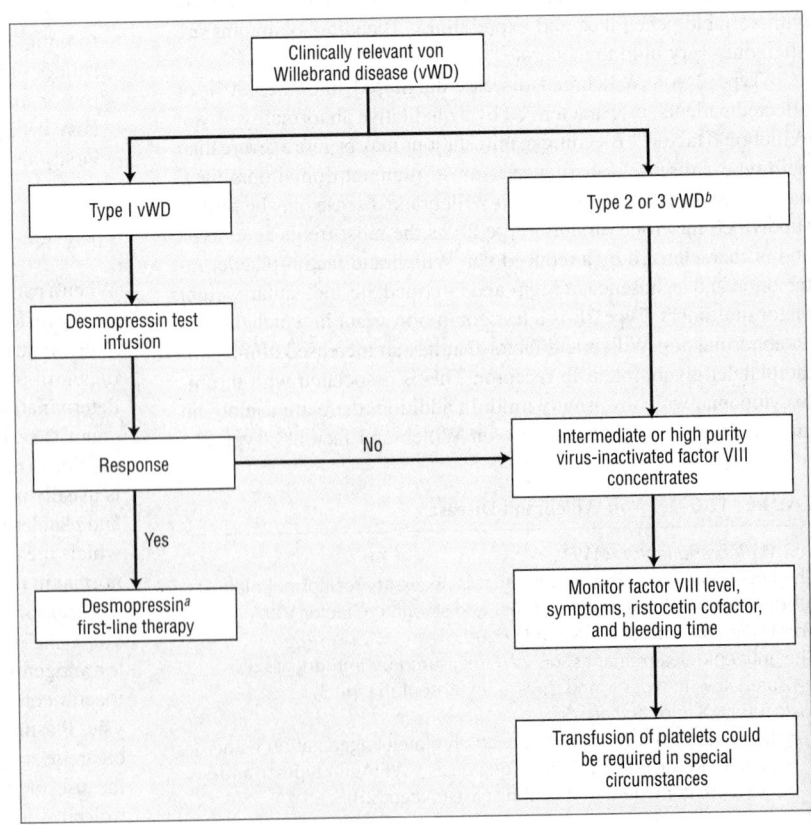

FIGURE 100–4. Guidelines for the treatment of von Willebrand disease. [a]Use factor VIII concentrate for life-threatening bleeding. [b]Some patients with type 2 or 3 von Willebrand disease may respond to desmopressin.

TABLE 100–7. Replacement Therapy in von Willebrand Disease[a]

Condition	Therapy
Major surgery	Maintain factor VIII level ≥50% for 1 week Prolonged treatment in type 3 patients (>7 days)
Minor surgery	Maintain factor VIII level ≥50% for 1–3 days Maintain factor VIII level >20%–30% for an additional 4–7 days
Dental extraction	Single infusion to achieve factor VIII level >50% Desmopressin prior to procedure for type I
Spontaneous or posttraumatic bleeding	Usually single infusion of 20–40 units/kg

[a]The yield of factor VIII after first infusion is similar to that observed in hemophilia A (about 2% increment over baseline amount for every 1 unit/kg of factor VIII infused).

contain only negligible amounts of von Willebrand factor and are inadequate for the treatment of von Willebrand disease. A very high-purity plasma-derived von Willebrand factor concentrate and a recombinant von Willebrand factor product are currently in clinical trials.[62] Because these von Willebrand factor concentrates do not contain appreciable factor VIII, concomitant administration of a factor VIII–containing product may be necessary for patients with severe disease and low levels of factor VIII.[62] Cryoprecipitate contains approximately 80 to 100 units of von Willebrand factor per unit, and it was the mainstay of therapy for von Willebrand disease in the past.[61] However, because cryoprecipitate is not virally inactivated, it is seldom used as first-line treatment. General guidelines for the dosing of replacement therapy in patients with von Willebrand disease unresponsive to desmopressin are provided in Table 100–7.

OTHER PHARMACOLOGIC THERAPY

6 Desmopressin stimulates the endothelial cell release of von Willebrand factor and factor VIII.[60] It is effective for patients with von Willebrand disease who have adequate endogenous stores of functional von Willebrand factor. This group includes most patients with type 1 disease and some patients with type 2A disease. Conversely, desmopressin is not appropriate for patients with type 3 disease, who lack stores of von Willebrand factor.

CLINICAL CONTROVERSY

Some hematologists find desmopressin beneficial in treating patients with type 2B von Willebrand disease, while others feel it may exacerbate thrombocytopenia.

Desmopressin also is not usually recommended for the treatment of type 2B disease, because the release of additional abnormal von Willebrand factor may exacerbate thrombocytopenia.[61] However, desmopressin has been reported to be beneficial in some patients with type 2B disease.[61] If desmopressin is used for type 2B disease, close monitoring is necessary.

The dose of desmopressin for von Willebrand disease is identical to that used in the treatment of mild factor VIII deficiency, 0.3 mcg/kg diluted in 30 to 50 mL of normal saline and given intravenously over 15 to 30 minutes.[60] In general, patients with von Willebrand disease have a better response to desmopressin than those with hemophilia, with an average three- to fivefold rise in von Willebrand factor and factor VIII levels.[61] These levels remain elevated for about 6 to 8 hours. The response to desmopressin in a given patient is usually consistent, and a trial of desmopressin should establish if the medication is likely to be effective for the individual. Desmopressin is preferable to the use of plasma-derived products for patients who have an adequate response because desmopressin does not carry a risk of viral transmission. An added benefit is that desmopressin is substantially less costly than the plasma-derived products. (For a discussion of the side effects of desmopressin, see the section on the treatment of hemophilia A.)

Desmopressin can be administered every 12 to 24 hours, but the response diminishes with repeated treatment. After three to four doses, desmopressin is often no longer effective, and alternative replacement therapy may be necessary if prolonged treatment is required. Laboratory monitoring, including vWF:Ag measurements, factor VIII assays, ristocetin cofactor activity assessments, and clinical examinations, will help determine the adequacy of treatment.

The intranasal administration of desmopressin, at the same dosage as that used in mild factor VIII deficiency, can be useful in the treatment of mild bleeding episodes. One or two doses administered at the start of menses may be helpful in controlling menorrhagia.[62] Oral contraceptives may be very effective in controlling this symptom as well.[61,62] Inhibitors of the fibrinolytic system may be of special value in those tissues rich in plasminogen activators, such as the mouth, especially with tooth extractions.[61] Antifibrinolytic agents may also be used in the management of epistaxis, gastrointestinal bleeding, and menorrhagia. However, these agents should be avoided in urinary tract bleeding, because of the risk of thrombosis and obstruction.[62]

OTHER CONGENITAL FACTOR DEFICIENCIES

In addition to deficiencies in factors VIII and IX, congenital deficiencies in fibrinogen; in factors II, V, VII, X, XI, and XIII; as well as combinations of factor deficiencies have been reported.[67] Contact factor abnormalities, including deficiencies in factor XII and prekallikrein, prolong the aPTT, but do not lead to any bleeding diathesis. It is important to identify these disorders so that treatment is not inappropriate. The only contact factor deficiency associated with bleeding symptoms is factor XI deficiency. Also known as hemophilia C, this deficiency is particularly common in people of Ashkenazi Jewish descent.[67,68] Bleeding manifestations are variable. Bleeding does not usually occur spontaneously, but there may be excessive bleeding after trauma or surgery. Most other deficiencies are inherited as autosomal recessive disorders and are rare. Some patients with abnormal molecules,

such as fibrinogen, may have an increased tendency to develop thromboembolic disease. Most of these deficiencies are treated with fresh frozen plasma, although newer specific concentrates are becoming available. Cryoprecipitate, which is rich in fibrinogen, may be used to treat patients with fibrinogen deficiency or dysfunctional fibrinogen (dysfibrinogenemias).

COMPLICATIONS OF REPLACEMENT THERAPY

Transmission of blood-borne viruses is always a concern when blood and blood-derived products are used. The infection of a large number of hemophiliac patients with hepatitis viruses and HIV during the 1980s prompted the development of virucidal methods to inactivate infectious agents.[5,7] All currently available plasma-derived factor concentrates come from screened donors and undergo viral inactivation procedures in an effort to reduce the risk of viral transmission. Heat treatment, which includes dry and wet heat, is one method of viral inactivation. Wet heat is applied while the concentrate is in suspension or in solution (pasteurization) and appears to be more effective than dry heat.[5,7] Other methods of viral inactivation include chemical (solvent detergent) and affinity chromatography with monoclonal antibodies. Solvent detergent treatment inactivates lipid-coated viruses such as HIV and hepatitis B and C, but it is not effective against nonenveloped viruses, including hepatitis A.[5,7,69,70] Outbreaks of hepatitis A associated with factor concentrates have occurred.[69,70] Another nonenveloped virus that has been identified in plasma-derived products, parvovirus B19,[15] may be particularly important for patients with hemophilia and HIV infection because it can cause chronic anemia in patients with immune deficiency.[69] Although concern has arisen, to date there has been no evidence of transmission of variant Creutzfeldt-Jakob disease from plasma-derived products.[15]

Other complications associated with factor administration include allergic reactions, fever, chills, urticaria, and nausea. PCCs and aPCCs also have the potential to cause thromboembolic complications, including deep vein thrombosis, pulmonary embolism, myocardial infarction, and DIC, likely related to the presence of activated factors.[39] Antifibrinolytic agents should be avoided in patients receiving PCCs or aPCCs to avoid thrombotic complications.

Porcine factor VIII, used in the treatment of patients with inhibitors to factor VIII, is not known to transmit human viruses. However, allergic-type reactions (e.g., fever, chills, skin rashes, nausea, and headaches) have been reported.[38,48] Patients who experience these reactions may be treated with hydrocortisone and/or diphenhydramine. Thrombocytopenia is another potential complication of porcine factor VIII use.[38,48]

Recombinant factor VIII has a low risk of viral transmission. Adverse effects of these products include metallic taste, mild dizziness, mild rash, burning at the infusion site, and a small drop in blood pressure.[22]

PHARMACOECONOMIC CONSIDERATIONS

Treatment of severe hemophilia is often expensive, with a substantial portion of the cost related to the expense of factor concentrates.[71] The highly purified plasma-derived products and recombinant factor concentrates are considerably more expensive than the low- and intermediate-purity products. However, the viral safety of recombinant products must be weighed against the added cost. Recombinant products are often used, particularly for children with hemophilia. With prophylactic factor replacement regimens to prevent chronic arthropathy becoming more widespread, factor usage and cost of treatment have greatly increased over that for on-demand therapy.[72] The positive impact on patient lifestyle must be weighed against the drawbacks of cost, the potential need for permanent venous access, and patient compliance. Finally, the use of immune tolerance therapy is associated with extremely high factor usage and cost, but with the potential benefit of eradicating an inhibitor. A formal cost-benefit analysis has suggested that this therapy may be cost-effective over the patient's lifetime.[71]

As noted earlier, the optimal management of von Willebrand disease starts with adequate identification of the patient's disease type. Desmopressin is considerably less expensive than plasma-derived factor VIII concentrates.[61] It should be the treatment of choice for all patients responsive to the test dose because of its viral safety, reduced cost, and ease of administration.

ACQUIRED COAGULATION DISORDERS

DISSEMINATED INTRAVASCULAR COAGULATION

The systemic activation of coagulation that results from DIC leads to clot formation in the microvasculature, often with compensatory bleeding owing to biodegradation of coagulation factors and platelets. Although the causes for DIC can be diverse, the pathophysiology leading to DIC is the same once the triggering event occurs (Fig. 100–5).

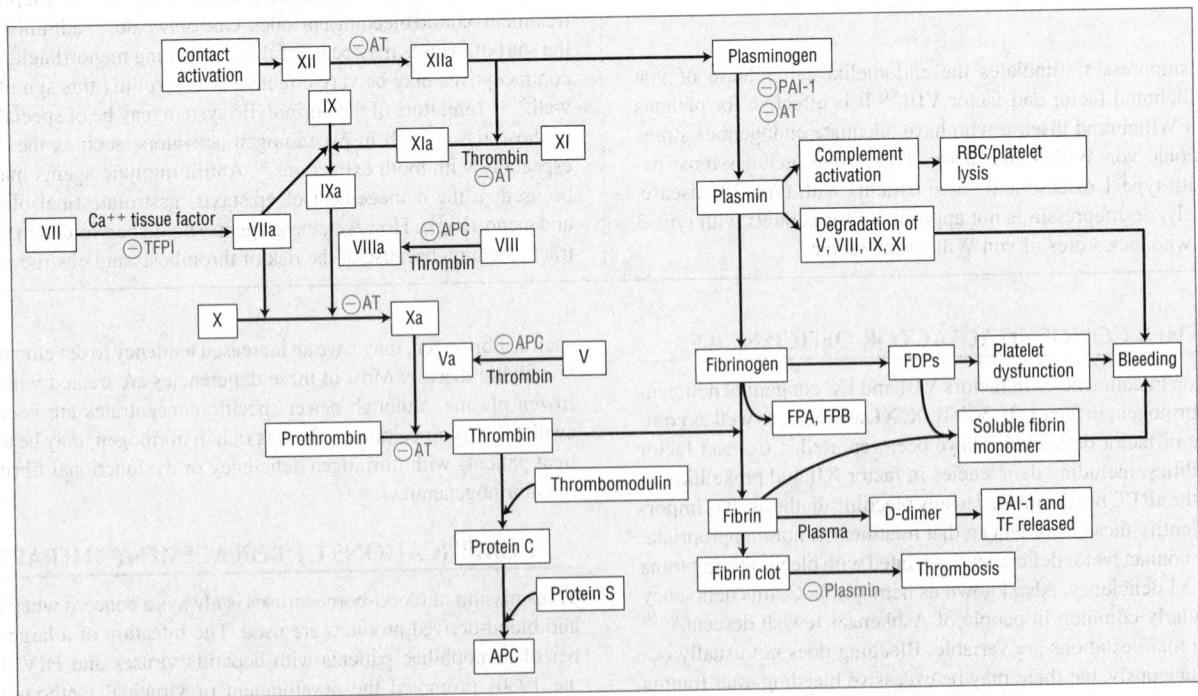

FIGURE 100–5. Pathophysiology of disseminated intravascular coagulation. APC, activated protein C; AT, antithrombin; FDP, fibrin degradation products; FPA, FPB, fibrinopeptides A and B; PAI-1, plasminogen activator type 1; RBC, red blood cell; TFPI, tissue factor pathway inhibitor.

An overwhelming insult leads to the formation of thrombin and plasmin beyond the control of the regulatory systems. Once thrombin is formed, it leads to the cleavage of fibrinopeptide A and B from fibrinogen, leaving a fibrin monomer. The monomer polymerizes into a clot, leading to microvascular and macrovascular thrombosis while consuming platelets by trapping them in the clots. Thrombosis will ultimately decrease blood flow to multiple organs, leading to organ damage. Plasmin cleaves fibrinogen into fibrin(ogen) degradation products (FDP), which can combine with the fibrin monomer before polymerization. This forms a soluble fibrin monomer, impairing hemostasis and leading to hemorrhage. Also, some of the FDPs may adhere to platelets, causing platelet dysfunction that may contribute to clinically significant hemorrhage. In addition, plasmin is a proteolytic enzyme that can degrade factors V, VIII, IX, XI, and other plasma proteins. Circulation of plasmin can activate the complement system, leading to red blood cell and platelet lysis. The activated complement system also increases vascular permeability that can cause hypotension and shock.[73]

Complicating this process is an intricate web of feedback systems. Thrombin induces activation of factors V and XI, while it also activates protein C that inhibits the activation of the same. Antithrombin is a serine protease that mediates the antithrombotic effect of heparin. It also inhibits the activation of thrombin, plasmin, and factors IXa, Xa, XIa, and XIIa.[74] Acute DIC is characterized by a rapid and extensive depletion of coagulation factors and inhibitors, as well as excessive fibrinolysis in an attempt to compensate for microvascular clotting. Normally, a balanced dynamic process of clotting and fibrinolysis operates to prevent organ dysfunction, bleeding, or clotting. In acute DIC, excessive intravascular coagulation overcomes the normal inhibitory processes. In subacute or chronic DIC, the balance between depletion and synthesis of coagulation factors in the circulation may make the diagnosis difficult, as patients may be asymptomatic, bleeding, and/or forming thromboses.

In summary, bleeding problems observed during DIC can be the result of the consumption of coagulation factors during clotting, the depletion or dysfunction of platelets, interference in fibrin formation by FDPs, and lysis of clots by plasmin. In parallel with the bleeding process, thrombosis is occurring, and the extent of microvascular obstruction will determine the degree of organ damage.

CLINICAL PRESENTATION OF DISSEMINATED INTRAVASCULAR COAGULATION

GENERAL
Underlying illness as described in Table 100–8

SIGNS AND SYMPTOMS
Bleeding, thrombosis or both
Petechiae and purpura
Peripheral cyanosis
Hemorrhagic bullae

LABORATORY TESTS
Elevated D-dimer
Decreased antithrombin
Decreased fibrinogen
Thrombocytopenia
Decreased protein C and protein S
Increased fibrinopeptides A and B
Elevated prothrombin fragments 1 and 2
Evidence of end-organ dysfunction or failure

TABLE 100–8. Conditions Associated with Disseminated Intravascular Coagulation

Cardiovascular	**Obstetrics (Continued)**
Acute myocardial infarction	Fatty liver of pregnancy
Angiopathy	Placental abruption
Aortic aneurysm	Preeclampsia/eclampsia
Aortic balloon assist devices	Retained fetus syndrome
Giant hemangiomas	**Pulmonary**
Peripheral vascular disease	syndrome
Postcardiac arrest	syndrome
Prosthetic devices	Empyema
Raynaud's syndrome	Hyaline membrane disease
Infectious	Pulmonary embolism
Arbovirus	Pulmonary infarction
Aspergillus	**Tissue injury**
Candida albicans	Burns
Cytomegalovirus	Crush injuries
Ebola virus	Extensive surgery
Gram-negative bacteria	Head trauma
Gram-positive bacteria	Multiple trauma
Herpesvirus	**Miscellaneous**
Histoplasma	Acid-base imbalance
Human immunodeficiency	Acute liver failure
virus	Amphetamines
Influenza	Anaphylaxis
Kala-azar	Autoimmune diseases
Malaria	Cholestasis
Mycobacteria	Chronic inflammatory diseases
Mycoplasma	Collagen vascular disease
Paramyxoviruses	Craniotomy
Rocky Mountain spotted fever	Extracorporeal circulation
Rubella	Extracorporeal membrane
Typhoid	oxygenation
Varicella	Fat embolism
Variola	Heat stroke
Intravascular hemolysis	Hemorrhagic telangiectasia
Hemolytic transfusion	Hepatitis
reaction	Leukemia
Hemolytic uremic syndrome	Lightening strikes
Minor hemolysis	Near drowning
Massive transfusion	Organic solvent poisoning
Newborn	Paroxysmal nocturnal
Birth asphyxia	hemoglobinuria
Hypothermia	Peritoneovenous or pleurovenous
Meconium or amniotic fluid	shunts
aspiration	Polycythemia rubra vera
Necrotizing enterocolitis	Renal vascular disorders
Respiratory distress syndrome	Severe anoxia
Shock	Snake bite
Obstetrics	Solid tumors
Abortion	Transplant rejection
Amniotic fluid embolism	

LABORATORY DIAGNOSIS

The basis for a diagnosis of DIC is a combination of laboratory test results in the setting of a known causative clinical disorder.[73,75] The relative importance of any particular laboratory test is controversial. Routine tests of blood coagulation, including prothrombin time and aPTT, are unreliable and of minimal use. The PT and aPTT are usually prolonged, but may be decreased or normal.[73] The thrombin time is usually prolonged because of the absolute decrease in fibrinogen as well as the presence of FDPs, which inhibit the conversion of fibrinogen to fibrin.[73]

Liver disease may cause a decreased synthesis of coagulation factors, and the subsequent abnormal laboratory results can be difficult to differentiate from DIC. Increased levels of FDPs are not specific to DIC, but elevated levels occur in 85% to 100% of patients with DIC.[73] Because FDPs are metabolized in the liver and excreted by the kidney, organ damage may increase the level of FDPs.[76] However, an increased FDP level may help to identify compensated DIC, as it may be the only abnormal laboratory result. D-dimer is formed when plasmin digests cross-linked fibrin; thus the level of D-dimer is a more specific measure of FDPs and should be elevated only in DIC.[77]

Fibrinogen levels and platelet counts are usually decreased in patients with DIC. Fifty percent of patients have schistocytes (red blood cell fragments) in fulminant DIC.[73] Unfortunately, these findings may also be evident in patients with severe liver disease with hypersplenism. Depressed antithrombin, protein C, and protein S levels are seen in most patients. Severe initial decreases in antithrombin levels occur in septic DIC. Activity levels below 50% to 60% correlate with poor outcome.[74]

Since thrombin cleaves fibrinopeptides A and B from fibrinogen, the levels of fibrinopeptides A and B should be elevated in patients with DIC. Initial studies have shown a good correlation between an elevated level of fibrinopeptide A and DIC, but other inflammatory conditions such as systemic lupus erythematosus, infections, and thrombosis may also result in elevated levels, thus decreasing the specificity of this test. Elevated prothrombin 1 and 2 indicates factor Xa generation, and is a reliable DIC marker, indicating procoagulant activation.[73]

Factor VIII and V levels should be decreased in DIC, but results of these tests may be quite variable because of the systemic activation of the coagulation system. The most specific findings of DIC are a low platelet count associated with an elevated D-dimer level, fibrinopeptide A, and prothrombin 1 and 2, along with depressed antithrombin and fibrinogen levels.

▶ TREATMENT: Disseminated Intravascular Coagulation

If unrecognized and left untreated, DIC may lead to death as a result of hemorrhage or thrombosis. However, because of the different mechanisms and clinical manifestations that can occur with DIC, there is some controversy regarding optimal treatment. Even so, there is a consensus that the most important step in the treatment of DIC is treatment of the underlying disease.[73,75,77,78] In a pregnant woman with placental abruption or retained placenta in whom the disease is self-limited, delivery of the fetus with the products of conception usually returns hemostasis to normal. In those patients who have overwhelming sepsis or shock, antibiotics and treatment of hypotension are the mainstays of therapy. In patients who are receiving maximum treatment for the underlying condition, but in whom the process is worsening or in whom bleeding develops, additional treatments may be used.

The efficacy of transfusing fresh frozen plasma or platelets has not been proven in randomized clinical trials, but is rational for patients who are bleeding or require invasive procedures.[75] Fresh frozen plasma replaces clotting factors, fibrinogen, protein S, protein C, and antithrombin. If hypofibrinogenemia is severe, cryoprecipitate may be useful as a concentrated source of fibrinogen. Although it has been argued that replacement of coagulation factors may worsen the situation, in practice this does not appear to make the situation worse, and it frequently improves hemostasis.

Trials of antithrombin concentrate in the treatment of DIC from various causes show some beneficial effect on improving DIC score, decreasing duration of DIC, or improving end-organ function.[74,75] A meta-analysis of a number of well-designed studies demonstrated a trend toward decreased mortality (from 56% to 44%).[75] In addition to variable efficacy, antithrombin is an expensive product with only intermittent availability. Therefore restricting its use to patients at high risk for morbidity and mortality should be considered.

CLINICAL CONTROVERSY

Heparin use in patients with disseminated intravascular coagulation may prevent the formation of new blood clots. The most common complication of heparin therapy is bleeding, so some clinicians find it too risky to justify its use.

Anticoagulation is controversial in patients with DIC.[75,77] The main pathogenic factor of DIC is considered to be the generation of intravascular thrombin. Interference of thrombin activity by an agent such as heparin appears to be a logical therapeutic step. The main advantage of heparin is that it can prevent further thrombosis and consumption of hemostatic factors, but it has no influence on an already established microthrombus within the vasculature. Because the major complication of heparin therapy is bleeding, some experts argue against its use in patients with an existing bleeding disorder. There are numerous anecdotal reports of improvement in individual patients, but controlled clinical studies are lacking. Heparin has not been shown to reduce morbidity or mortality in uncontrolled series.[75] Heparin rarely restores the coagulopathy to normal, although both the deficiency of coagulation factors and the thrombocytopenia may improve. If the patient does not respond to the replacement of coagulation factors, the addition of heparin may improve the coagulopathy by forming the heparin-antithrombin complex to inhibit thrombin.

Heparin is given subcutaneously or as a continuous IV infusion. The dosage of heparin for DIC is controversial, ranging anywhere from full-dose to low-dose heparin.[75,77] Full-dose heparin in adults requires that 5,000 units be administered as an IV bolus, followed by a continuous infusion at 1,000 units per hour or according to a weight-based heparin-dosing regimen. Some experts advocate low-dose heparin, such as an infusion of 500 units per hour in adults, and adjusting the dose based on clinical and laboratory data. Low-dose heparin given subcutaneously has been used with success. Monitoring of heparin therapy is difficult because the aPTT is often elevated before the initiation of heparin therapy. Therefore it is best to follow D-dimer and fibrinogen levels.

Anticoagulation is contraindicated in patients with life-threatening or serious bleeding (e.g., intracranial, retroperitoneal, or pericardial). Patients with symptomatic thromboemboli, extensive fibrin deposition, persistent coagulation abnormalities despite replacement of hemostatic factors, solid tumors, or chronic DIC may benefit from heparin therapy.[75,79] Historically, an infusion of low-dose heparin, 7.5 units/kg per hour, has been used in patients with acute promyelocytic leukemia (APML), along with the administration of platelets, fresh frozen plasma, and cryoprecipitate.[79] The availability of differentiating agents may decrease or prevent the need for anticoagulation of these patients.[77] Patients with solid tumors who are symptomatic from a thrombosis should receive an infusion of heparin, 15 units/kg per hour. Once asymptomatic, heparin can be administered subcutaneously.

In two uncontrolled trials, patients tolerated the use of low-molecular-weight heparin well, and this approach showed a possible beneficial outcome.[75] A randomized, double-blind study compared the efficacy of dalteparin with that of low-dose heparin. Dalteparin was more effective at improving bleeding symptoms, but there was no difference in mortality.[75]

Antifibrinolytics, such as aminocaproic acid, have been used in patients in whom the dominant clinical picture is one of excessive fibrinolysis.[75] Because aminocaproic acid can increase fibrin deposition, many experts believe that it is usually contraindicated. In patients with chronic liver disease who manifest dominant fibrinolysis, attempts to inhibit the fibrinolytic system have generally been unsuccessful. Patients with APML may benefit from an antifibrinolytic, as hyperfibrinolysis is the dominant clinical feature of their condition. Tranexamic acid and aminocaproic acid have shown benefits in patients with APML.[75]

Critically ill patients may develop vitamin K deficiency. In addition, patients with DIC may consume vitamin K and may need supplementation to replenish stores. Other treatment modalities may include the use of protein C concentrate; lepirudin; anti–tissue factor antibody; recombinant tissue factor pathway inhibitor; thrombomodulin; or thrombin inhibitors such as dermatan sulfate, anti–plasminogen activator inhibitor type 1, and dithiocarbamates.[75,77,80,81]

Activated protein C modulates coagulation as shown in Fig. 100–5. The activation of protein C may be impaired during sepsis. Drotrecogin alfa (activated protein C) administration resulted in an absolute reduction in mortality of 6.1% from severe sepsis without undue bleeding in carefully chosen adult patients.[82] Strategies for use in adults have been developed to target appropriate patients[83] while pediatric data are forthcoming. Patients must be carefully chosen to minimize bleeding complications and optimize benefits.

EVALUATION OF THERAPEUTIC OUTCOMES

The management of DIC is surrounded by controversy, and the optimal approach to these patients is still to be determined. Diagnosis and treatment of the underlying disease should be the goal in all cases. Determination, if possible, of the dominant process (i.e., hemorrhage vs. thrombosis) can help focus the treatment approach. This is often impossible, however, so clinicians institute replacement therapy of the deficient clotting factors and attempt to control the clotting problems with agents such as heparin.

Risk versus benefit, as well as any contraindications, should be considered at the start of any given therapy for each patient. Monitoring therapy for DIC with laboratory tests can be difficult, because the underlying process can cause a variety of laboratory abnormalities. For example, monitoring the effect of heparin by using the aPTT can be a complex task, especially when the patient has an abnormal baseline aPTT; in this case, monitoring fibrinogen and D-dimer may be more useful in detecting any need to adjust therapy. In addition, it is important to combine laboratory parameters with clinical assessment to make rational treatment adjustments. Aggressive hemodynamic stabilization and other supportive measures to prevent organ failure are also important in the overall management and prognosis of patients with DIC.

VITAMIN K DEFICIENCY

Vitamin K is a cofactor for the activation of factors II, VII, IX, and X.[84] When vitamin K deficiency occurs, the inactive precursors of these coagulation factors that do not bind calcium accumulate in the plasma. Vitamin K is also necessary for the active forms of proteins C and S, which inhibit factor Va and VIIIa. In most clinical situations, vitamin K deficiency causes a bleeding diathesis as a result of the marked deficiency of factors II, VII, IX, and X.

Vitamin K is a fat-soluble vitamin. Vitamin K_1, phytonadione, is found in green vegetables. Bacteria in the large intestine produce vitamin K_2, the menaquinones, which require bile salts to be solubilized and absorbed.[84]

HEMORRHAGIC DISEASE OF THE NEWBORN

Newborns are vitamin K–deficient at birth, although not completely because some maternal vitamin K crosses the placenta.[85] The level may continue to fall during the neonatal period because the infant's gut has not had sufficient time to undergo bacterial colonization. Breast milk contains a low vitamin K content in comparison to infant formulas, and therefore breast-fed infants are more vulnerable to developing vitamin K deficiency. In addition, the plasma concentrations of the vitamin K–dependent factors are physiologically low in infants.[86] Vitamin K deficiency in neonates can cause intracranial hemorrhage and bleeding from the umbilical cord or the gastrointestinal tract.[85]

Bleeding within 24 hours of birth, early vitamin K–dependent bleeding, is usually the result of maternal ingestion of anticonvulsants, warfarin, rifampin, or isoniazid. Treatment of these women prior to delivery with vitamin K may decrease the incidence of hemorrhagic disease of the newborn among their offspring.[85] Classic vitamin K–dependent bleeding usually appears during the first week of life, and it results from the lack of prophylactic vitamin K administration at birth. Risk factors identified for late vitamin K–dependent bleeding, which occurs at 2 to 12 weeks, include cholestatic liver disease, exclusive breast-feeding, and failure to give adequate vitamin K at birth.[85] The use of oral vitamin K at birth is also associated with a higher incidence of late vitamin K–dependent bleeding. It has been suggested that the intramuscular route of administration allows the vitamin K to act as a depot preparation, and may explain the lower rate of late vitamin K–dependent bleeding with this route.[85]

The levels of vitamin K–dependent coagulation factors are low at birth. Without adequate vitamin K, these levels may fall even further. In this situation, the PT and the aPTT are prolonged, but the thrombin time, fibrinogen level, and platelet count are normal. Most infants achieve adult levels by 3 months of age if intramuscular phytonadione was received at birth.[85]

In the United States, infants usually receive 1 mg of phytonadione intramuscularly at birth for prophylaxis. Most infants build up vitamin K_1 and K_2 stores in the liver during the first month of life. The speed of repletion depends on the amount of milk or formula received. Oral supplementation results in late vitamin K–dependent bleeding if not given for a prolonged course. Controversy has arisen over whether the high plasma vitamin K levels achieved with intramuscular injection may lead to an increased incidence of childhood cancer. This risk has not been substantiated and the benefits of widespread use outweigh the minimal risk.[87] Fresh frozen plasma is used to treat hemorrhages.

MALABSORPTION

Patients may become vitamin K–deficient because of poor nutrition or malabsorption. A careful dietary history is important in this regard. Broad-spectrum antibiotics may sterilize the large intestine and prevent vitamin K_2 production.[88]

Vitamin K absorption depends on both bile acids and pancreatic enzymes to create micelles. Malabsorption resulting from diseases of the small intestine or pancreas—such as cystic fibrosis, Crohn's disease, ulcerative colitis, cholestatic liver disease, celiac disease, amyloidosis, Whipple's disease, and short-bowel syndrome—may cause abnormal development in children, weight loss, muscle wasting, steatorrhea, vitamin deficiencies, and anemia. Significant malabsorption can occur even without the symptoms of diarrhea or steatorrhea.

▶ TREATMENT: Vitamin K Deficiency

Phytonadione is used to treat vitamin K deficiency. The dose, frequency, and duration of vitamin K depend on the severity of the deficiency and the patient's response. Vitamin K may be administered orally, intramuscularly, subcutaneously, or intravenously. After an oral dose of vitamin K_1, the blood coagulation factors increase within 6 to 12 hours. When administered parenterally, the PT may take 12 to 24 hours to normalize, although improvement usually occurs within 1 to 2 hours. Failure to correct the PT after 48 hours should raise suspicion about the etiology of the coagulation abnormality (e.g., liver disease).

The appropriate route of administration depends on the severity and the cause of the vitamin K deficiency. For instance, in patients with severe hypoprothrombinemia, it is best to avoid the intramuscular route because of the risk of forming a hematoma. Because of the rare anaphylactic reaction associated with the intravenous route of administration, this route is often restricted to patients who are thrombocytopenic or unable to absorb the drug via the gastrointestinal tract.[89] Vitamin K can be administered subcutaneously to those patients without intravenous access. Bleeding patients should receive fresh frozen plasma as a source of vitamin K–dependent factors to ensure immediate correction.

Patients with malabsorption or obstructive jaundice may require the parenteral administration of vitamin K. Phytonadione 10 mg weekly is usually sufficient in adults. Patients on long-term total parenteral nutrition should receive it daily in the multivitamin additive.

COAGULOPATHY AND LIVER DISEASE

Bleeding disorders can be associated with acute or chronic liver disease. The degree of coagulopathy correlates with the degree of hepatocellular disease. The liver synthesizes the blood coagulation factors and inhibitors of coagulation (e.g., antithrombin and proteins C and S). All clotting factors except factor VIII are decreased in liver failure.[90] The ability of the liver to clear activated clotting factors and their degradation products is reduced with liver failure.[90] Primary fibrinolysis occurs due to a decline in the level of the inhibitors of plasmin activation.[90] Platelet count and function are decreased in patients with liver disease. The development of DIC may potentially worsen the coagulopathy.

The PT, the aPTT, and the thrombin time are useful in screening for a deficiency of liver-dependent factors. The PT is sensitive to deficiencies in the vitamin K–dependent factors. The aPTT helps to determine deficiencies in factor IX, as well as some other factors. The thrombin time can help to detect hypofibrinogenemia, dysfibrinogenemia, and the presence of FDPs that interfere with fibrin polymerization. Because defects in polymerization may occur before severe hypofibrinogemia, this may be an indication of the degree of liver dysfunction. The level of D-dimer should be normal unless DIC is present.

Factor V is synthesized by hepatic cells, but is not dependent on vitamin K. Therefore it may be useful in distinguishing vitamin K deficiency from liver disease. Deficiency of antithrombin occurs with severe hepatocellular disease and may contribute to the development of DIC. In acute hepatic failure, the level of plasminogen may be low, reflecting decreased synthesis or increased catabolism associated with DIC. The level of factor VIII is usually normal or elevated in liver disease, whereas it is decreased in DIC.

▶ TREATMENT: Coagulopathy and Liver Disease

Treatment of the coagulopathy associated with liver disease is recommended for overt bleeding or for the correction of coagulation parameters (e.g., PT and aPTT) prior to an invasive procedure. Major bleeding may occur with normal coagulation parameters secondary to esophageal varices or peptic ulcer disease. To ensure that vitamin K deficiency is not contributing to the abnormalities, adults may receive 10 mg of vitamin K for one or more days.

When a patient bleeds in association with a coagulopathy, replacement therapy with platelets and fresh frozen plasma may decrease bleeding. Fresh frozen plasma supplies all of the missing coagulation factors, but fluid overload may be a serious problem. If fluid overload becomes an issue, plasma exchange may be considered. If the patient has ascites, the half-life of many of these factors is decreased, and it is difficult to correct the coagulopathy. PCCs can be given, but they may increase the risk of intravascular coagulation and cause DIC if it is not already present. In general, the use of these concentrates is not recommended. Only when the administration of fresh frozen plasma does not correct the coagulopathy and the patient continues to have serious bleeding should PCCs be considered.

The use of heparin and antifibrinolytic drugs is controversial. The administration of aminocaproic acid may be successful, especially with mucosal bleeding. Heparin has not been demonstrated to improve survival in acute liver failure and may exacerbate bleeding. Antithrombin concentrates have been evaluated in fulminant liver failure. They had no benefit on mortality, clinical complications, or coagulation laboratory findings. Desmopressin may decrease the bleeding time in patients with liver failure.[90] The administration of recombinant factor VIIa has successfully corrected coagulation parameters and stopped bleeding in patients with liver disease.[91]

ABBREVIATIONS

aPCC: activated prothrombin complex concentrate
APML: acute promyelocytic leukemia
aPTT: activated partial thromboplastin time
BU: Bethesda unit
DIC: disseminated intravascular coagulation
FDP: fibrin degradation products
HIV: human immunodeficiency virus
kb: kilobase
PAI-1: plasminogen-activator inhibitor type 1
PCC: prothrombin complex concentrate
PT: prothrombin time
vWF:Ag: von Willebrand factor antigen

Review Questions and other resources can be found at
www.pharmacotherapyonline.com.

REFERENCES

1. Dahlback B. Blood coagulation. Lancet 2000;355:1627–1632.
2. Mann KG. Biochemistry and physiology of blood coagulation. Thromb Haemost 1999;82:165–174.
3. Wiman B. The fibrinolytic enzyme system. Basic principles and links to arterial and venous thrombosis. Hematol Oncol Clin North Am 2000;14:325–338.
4. Ens GE, Fristma GA, Jensen R, et al. Coagulation Handbook. Jensen R, ed. Tuscon, AZ, Hemostasis Resources, 1998.
5. DiMichele D, Neufeld EJ. Hemophilia. A new approach to an old disease. Hematol Oncol Clin North Am 1998;12:1315–1344.
6. Soucie JM, Evatt B, Jackson D. Occurrence of hemophilia in the United States. Am J Hematol 1998;59:288–294.
7. Mannucci PM, Tuddenham EGD. The hemophilias: progress and problems. Semin Hematol 1999;36(Suppl 7):104–117.
8. Chuansumrit A, Sasanakul W, Goodeve A, et al. Inversion of intron 22 of the factor VIII gene in a girl with severe hemophilia A and Turner's syndrome. Thromb Haemost 1999;82:1379.
9. Bowen DJ. Haemophilia A and haemophilia B: molecular insights. Mol Pathol 2002;55:1–18.
10. Lillicrap D. Molecular diagnosis of inherited bleeding disorders and thrombophilia. Semin Hematol 1999;36:340–351.
11. Lakich D, Kazazian H, Antonarakis SE. Inversions disrupting the factor VIII gene are a common cause of severe hemophilia A. Nat Genet 1993;5:236–241.
12. Bagnall RD, Waseem N, Green PM, et al. Recurrent inversion breaking intron 1 of the factor VIII gene is a frequent cause of severe hemophilia A. Blood 2002;99:168–174.
13. Kurachi K, Davie EW. Isolation and characterization of a cDNA coding for human factor IX. Proc Natl Acad Sci U S A 1982;79:6461–6464.
14. Crossley M, Ludwig M, Stowell KM, et al. Recovery from hemophilia B Leyden: an androgen-responsive element in the factor IX promoter. Science 1992;257:377–379.
15. Bolton-Maggs PHB, Pasi KJ. Haemophilias A and B. Lancet 2003;361:1801–1809.
16. Goodeve AC. Advances in carrier detection in haemophilia. Haemophilia 1998;4:358–364.
17. Tedgard U. Carrier testing and prenatal diagnosis of haemophilia—utilisation and psychological consequences. Haemophilia 1998;4:365–369.
18. Richardson LC, Evatt BL. Risk of hepatitis A infection in persons with hemophilia receiving plasma-derived products. Transfus Med Rev 2000;14:64–73.
19. Kulkarni R, Lusher J. Perinatal management of newborns with haemophilia. Br J Haematol 2001;112:264–274.
20. Kulkarni R, Lusher JM. Intracranial and extracranial hemorrhages in newborns with hemophilia: A review of the literature. J Pediatr Hematol Oncol 1999;21:289–295.
21. United Kingdom Haemophilia Centre Doctors' Organisation (UKHCDO). Guidelines on the selection and use of therapeutic products to treat haemophilia and other hereditary bleeding disorders. Haemophilia 2003;9:1–23.
22. Bray GL, Gomperts ED, Courter S, et al. A multicenter study of recombinant factor VIII (Recombinate): Safety, efficacy, and inhibitor risk in previously untreated patients with hemophilia A. The Recombinate study group. Blood 1994;83:2428–2435.
23. Minor PD. Are recombinant products really infection risk free? Haemophilia 2001;7:114–116.
24. Eis-Hubinger AM, Sasowski U, Brackmann HH, et al. Parvovirus B19 DNA is frequently present in recombinant coagulation factor VIII products. Thromb Haemost 1996;76:1120.
25. Lusher JM. First and second generation recombinant factor VIII concentrates in previously untreated patients: recovery, safety, efficacy, and inhibitor development. Semin Thromb Hemostas 2002;28:273–276.
26. Wight J, Paisley S. The epidemiology of inhibitors in haemophilia A: a systematic review. Haemophilia 2003;9:418–435.
27. Cohen AJ. Treatment of inherited coagulation disorders. Am J Med 1995;99:675–682.
28. Shord SS, Lindley CM. Coagulation products and their uses. Am J Health Syst Pharm 2000;57:1403–1420.
29. Batorova A, Martinowitz U. Continuous infusion of coagulation factors. Haemophilia 2002;8:170–177.
30. Varon D, Martinowitz U. Continuous infusion therapy in haemophilia. Haemophilia 1998;4:431–435.
31. Lethagen S. Desmopressin in mild hemophilia A: indications, limitations, efficacy, and safety. Sem Thromb Hemostas 2003;29:101–105.
32. Revel-Vilk S, Blanchette VS, Sparling C, et al. DDAVP challenge tests in boys with mild/moderate haemophilia A. Br J Haematol 2002;117:947–951.
33. Mannucci PM. Desmopressin (DDAVP) in the treatment of bleeding disorders: the first 20 years. 1997;90:2515–2521.
34. Mannucci PM. Hemostatic drugs. N Engl J Med 1998;339:245–253.
35. Adamson S, Charlebois T, O'Connell B, et al. Viral safety of recombinant factor IX. Semin Hematol 1998;35:22–27.
36. Roth DA, Kessler CM, Pasi KJ, et al. Human recombinant factor IX: safety and efficacy studies in hemophilia B patients previously treated with plasma-derived factor IX concentrates. Blood 2001;98:3600–3606.
37. White G, Shapiro A, Ragni M, et al. Clinical evaluation of recombinant factor IX. Semin Hematol 1998;35(2 Suppl 2):33–38.
38. Green D. Complications associated with the treatment of haemophiliacs with inhibitors. Haemophilia 1999;5(Suppl 3):11–17.
39. Kohler M. Thrombogenicity of prothrombin complex concentrates. Thromb Res 1999;95(4 Suppl 1):S13–S17.
40. Shapiro AD, Ragni MV, Lusher JM, et al. Safety and efficacy of monoclonal antibody purified factor IX concentrate in previously untreated patients with hemophilia B. Thrombo Haemost 1996;75:30–35.
41. Ljung RC. Prophylactic infusion regimens in the management of hemophilia. Thromb Haemost 1999;82:525–530.
42. Lofqvist T, Nilsson IM, Berntorp E, et al. Haemophilia prophylaxis in young patients: A long-term follow-up. J Intern Med 1997;241:395–400.
43. Lusher JM. Prophylaxis in children with hemophilia: Is it the optimal treatment? Thromb Haemost 1997;78:726–729.
44. Panicker J, Warrier I, Thomas R, et al. The overall effectiveness of prophylaxis in severe haemophilia. Haemophilia 2003;9:272–278.
45. Fischer K, Van den Berg M. Prophylaxis for severe haemophilia: clinical and economical issues. Haemophilia 2003;9:376–381.
46. Ljung R. Central venous lines in haemophilia. Haemophilia 2003;9(Suppl 1):88–93.
47. Bollard CM, Teague LR, Berry EW, et al. The use of central venous catheters (portacaths) in children with haemophilia. Haemophilia 2000;6:66–70.

48. Manno CS. Treatment options for bleeding episodes in patients undergoing immune tolerance therapy. Haemophilia 1999;5(Suppl 3):33–41.

49. Hay CRM. Why do inhibitors arise in patients with haemophilia A? Br J Haematol 1999;105:584–590.

50. Jones ML, Wight J, Paisley S, et al. Control of bleeding in patients with hemophilia A with inhibitors: a systematic review. Haemophilia 2003; 9:464–520.

51. Warrier I, Ewenstein BM, Koerper MA, et al. Factor IX inhibitors and anaphylaxis in hemophilia B. J Pediatr Hematol Oncol 1997;19:23–27.

52. Hedner U. Treatment of patients with factor VIII and factor IX inhibitors with special focus on the use of recombinant factor VIIa. Thromb Haemost 1999;82:531–539.

53. Paisley S, Wight J, Currie E, et al. The management of inhibitors in haemophilia A: introduction and systematic review of current practice. Haemophilia 2003;9:405–417.

54. Wight J, Paisley S, Knight C. Immune tolerance induction in patients with haemophilia A with inhibitors: a systematic review. Haemophilia 2003; 9:436–463.

55. Wiestner A, Cho HJ, Asch AS, et al. Rituximab in the treatment of acquired factor VIII inhibitors. Blood 2002;100:3426–3428.

56. White GC. Gene therapy in hemophilia: Clinical trials update. Thromb Haemost 2001;86:172–177.

57. Walsh CE. Gene therapy progress and prospects: gene therapy for the hemophilias. Gene Ther 2003;10:999–1003.

58. Beeton K, Cornwell J, Alltree J. Muscle rehabilitation in haemophilia. Haemophilia 1998;4:532–537.

59. Fernandez-Palazzi F, Caviglia HA, Salazar JR, et al. Intraarticular dexamethasone in advanced chronic synovitis in hemophilia. Clin Orthop Rel Res 1997;343:25–29.

60. Hemophilia of Georgia, U.S.A. Protocols for the treatment of haemophilia and von Willebrand disease. Haemophilia 2000;6(Suppl 1):84–93.

61. Federici AB, Castaman G, Mannuci PM. Guidelines for the diagnosis and management of von Willebrand disease in Italy. Haemophilia 2002;8: 607–621.

62. Phillips MD, Santhouse A. von Willebrand disease: Recent advances in pathophysiology and treatment. Am J Med Sci 1998;316:77–86.

63. Federici AB, Mannuci PM. Advances in the genetics and treatment of von Willebrand disease. Curr Opin Pediatr 2002;14:23–33.

64. Nitu-Whalley IC, Lee CA. Acquired von Willebrand syndrome—report of 10 cases and review of the literature. Haemophilia 1999;5:318–326.

65. Batlle J, Torea J, Rendal E, et al. The problem of diagnosing von Willebrand's disease. J Int Med 1997;242(Suppl 740):121–128.

66. Gill JC, Endres-Brooks J, Bauer PJ, et al. The effect of ABO blood group on the diagnosis of von Willebrand disease. Blood 1987;69:1691–1695.

67. Peyvandi F, Duga S, Akhavan S, et al. Rare coagulation deficiencies. Haemophilia 2002;8:308–321.

68. Bolton-Maggs PHB. Factor XI deficiency and its management. Haemophilia 2000;6(Suppl 1):100–109.

69. Ludlam CA. Viral safety of plasma-derived factor VIII and IX concentrates. Blood Coagul Fibrinolysis 1997;8(Suppl 1):S19–S23.

70. Giangrande PL. Hepatitis in haemophilia. Br J Haematol 1998;103:1–9.

71. Colowick AB, Bohn RL, Avorn J, et al. Immune tolerance induction in hemophilia patients with inhibitors: costly can be cheaper. Blood 2000; 96:1698–1702.

72. Miners AH, Sabin CA, Tolley KH, et al. Assessing the effectiveness and cost-effectiveness of prophylaxis against bleeding in patients with severe haemophilia and severe von Willebrand's disease. J Intern Med 1998; 244:515–522.

73. Bick RL. Disseminated intravascular coagulation: Current concepts of etiology, pathophysiology, diagnosis, and treatment. Hematol Oncol Clin North Am 2003;17:149–176.

74. Bucur SZ, Levy JH, Despotis GJ, et al. Uses of antithrombin III concentrate in congenital and acquired deficiency states. Transfusion 1998;38: 481–497.

75. Levi M, de Jonge E, van der Poll T, et al. Disseminated intravascular coagulation. Thromb Haemost 1999;82:695–705.

76. Muller-Berghaus G, ten Cate H, Levi M. Disseminated intravascular coagulation: Clinical spectrum and established as well as new diagnostic approaches. Thromb Haemost 1999;82:706–712.

77. Carey MJ, Rodgers GM. Disseminated intravascular coagulation: clinical and laboratory aspects. Am J Hematol 1998;59:65–73.

78. Levi M, deJong E, van der Poll T, et al. Novel approaches to the management of disseminated intravascular coagulation. Crit Care Med 2000; 28:S20–S24.

79. Arkel YS. Thrombosis and cancer. Semin Oncol 2000;27:362–374.

80. Maruyama I. Recombinant thrombomodulin and activated protein C in the treatment of disseminated intravascular coagulation. Thromb Haemost 1999;82:718–721.

81. Pernerstorfer T, Hollenstein U, Hansen JB, et al. Lepirudin blunts endotoxin-induced coagulation activation. Blood 2000;95:1729–1734.

82. Bernard GR, Vincent J-L, Laterre P-F, et al. Efficacy and safety of recombinant human activated protein C for severe sepsis. N Engl J Med 2001;344: 699–709.

83. Cohen H, Welage LS. Strategies to optimize drotrecogin alfa (activated) use: guidelines and therapeutic controversies. Pharmacotherapy 2002;22: 223S–235S.

84. Vermeer C, Schurgers LG. A comprehensive review of vitamin K and vitamin K antagonists. Hematol Oncol Clin North Am 2000;14: 339–353.

85. Zipursky A. Prevention of vitamin K deficiency bleeding in newborns. Br J Haematol 1999;104:430–437.

86. Andrew M. Developmental hemostasis: Relevance to hemostatic problems during childhood. Semin Thromb Hemost 1995;21:341–356.

87. Ross JA, Davies SM. Vitamin K prophylaxis and childhood cancer. Med Pediatr Oncol 2000;34:434–437.

88. Beker LT, Ahrens RA, Fink RJ, et al. Effect of vitamin K1 supplementation on vitamin K status in cystic fibrosis patients. J Pediatr Gastroenterol Nutr 1997;24:512–517.

89. Riegert-Johnson DL, Volcheck GW. The incidence of anaphylaxis following intravenous phytonadione (Vitamin K1): a 5-year retrospective review. Ann Allergy Asthma Immunol 2002;89:400–406.

90. Lisman T, Leebeek FW, deGroot PG. Haemostatic abnormalities in patients with liver disease. J Hepatol 2002;37:280–287.

91. Erhardtsen E. Ongoing Novoseven trials. Intensive Care Med 2002; 28(Suppl):S248–S255.

101
SICKLE CELL DISEASE

C.Y. Jennifer Chan and Reginald Moore

Learning Objectives and other resources can be found at *www.pharmacotherapyonline.com.*

KEY CONCEPTS

◄1 Sickle cell disease is an inherited disorder caused by a defect in the gene for hemoglobin. Patients may have one defective gene (sickle cell trait) or two defective genes (sickle cell disease).

◄2 Although most often seen in persons of African ancestry, other ethnic groups can be affected.

◄3 Sickle cell disease involves multiple organ systems.

◄4 Prophylaxis against pneumococcal infection reduces death during childhood.

◄5 Hydroxyurea has been shown to decrease the incidence of painful crises. However, the patient population that receives hydroxyurea should be carefully monitored.

◄6 Chronic transfusion therapy programs have been shown to be beneficial in decreasing the occurrence of stroke in children with sickle cell disease.

◄7 Patients with fever greater than 38.5°C should be evaluated and appropriate antibiotics should include coverage for encapsulated organisms, especially pneumococcal.

◄8 Pain episodes can usually be managed at home. Hospitalized patients usually require parenteral analgesics. Analgesic options include opioids, nonsteroidal anti-inflammatory agents, and acetaminophen. The patient characteristics and the severity of the crisis should determine the choice of agent and regimen.

◄1 Sickle cell syndromes, which can be divided into sickle cell disease (SCD) and sickle cell trait (SCT), are a group of hereditary disorders characterized by the presence of sickle hemoglobin (HbS) in red blood cells. SCT is the heterozygous inheritance of one normal and one sickle hemoglobin (HbAS) gene. Individuals with SCT are usually asymptomatic. SCD can be of homozygous or compounded heterozygous inheritance. Homozygous HbS (HbSS) is called sickle cell anemia (SCA); whereas heterozygous inheritance of HbS compounded with another mutation results in sickle-hemoglobin C (HbSC), sickle β-thalassemia (HbSβ^+-thal and HbSβ^0-thal), and some other rare phenotypes such as sickle O-Arab.

This complex disorder was first described in the literature by Herrick in 1910. Since then, much progress has been made in identifying the molecular and functional defects, as well as understanding the relationship between genotypes and clinical severity of the disease.[1,2]

SCD is a chronic illness with significant burden for family and society.[3] Frequent crisis episodes can interrupt schooling and result in employment difficulties. Acute complications of the disease can be unpredictable, rapidly progressive, and life-threatening. Later in life, chronic organ damage may develop. Due to the complexity and seriousness of the illness, it is essential that comprehensive care is available and that providers involved must have a good understanding of the disease and its management options.[4]

EPIDEMIOLOGY

More than 50,000 Americans have sickle cell disease and approximately 2000 infants with SCD are identified each year in the United States. In addition, for every 1 infant with SCD, about 50 infants are identified as carriers. The most common SCD genotype is HbSS ($\sim$45%), followed by HbSC ($\sim$25%), HbSβ^+-thalassemia ($\sim$8%), and HbSβ^0-thalassemia ($\sim$2%). Other variants account for less than 1% of patients.[5,6]

Sickle cell gene mutation offers partial protection against serious malarial infection. Abnormal red blood cells (RBCs) are less easily parasitized by *Plasmodium falciparum* than normal RBCs. Consequently, persons with heterozygous sickle gene (SCT) have a selective advantage in regions (tropical areas) where malaria is endemic. The incidence of the sickle gene in a population correlates with the historical incidence of malaria.

◄2 SCD is most common in people with African heritage, with a frequency of about 1 in 400 for SCD and 8% for SCT in African-Americans. The prevalence is higher in Africa, where an estimated 120,000 babies are born with SCD each year. The prevalence rate of SCT in Africa varies across regions, with a higher rate in western, central, and eastern Africa (10% to 30%) but lower in northern and southern Africa (0% to 5%). Hemoglobin C (HbC) appears primarily in the inhabitants of western and northern Africa or in descendants of people from this area. About 2% to 3% of African-Americans carry HbC gene (HbC-trait).[5–8]

Other areas with sickle mutation are the Arabian Peninsula, Indian subcontinent, and the Mediterranean region. HbS has been reported in up to 25% in certain Middle Eastern populations and greater than 30% in Greece and Cyprus. Genetic analysis shows that the mutation found in Arabic patients is different from those of African descent. Sickle gene mutation variants have been associated with different geographic locations and may be responsible for variations in clinical manifestations. In Africa, the variants are Senegal (Atlantic West Africa), Benin (Central West Africa), Bantu (Central African

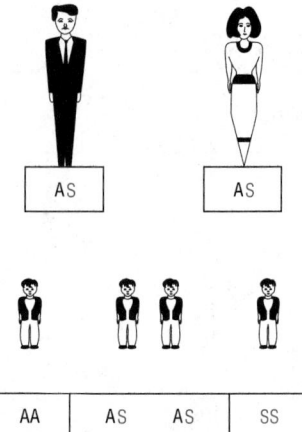

FIGURE 101–1. Sickle gene inheritance scheme for both parents with sickle cell trait (SCT). A, normal hemoglobin; S, sickle hemoglobin. Possibilities with each pregnancy: 25% normal (AA); 50% SCT (AS); 25% sickle cell anemia (SS).

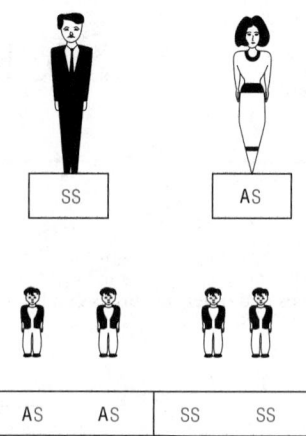

FIGURE 101–3. Sickle gene inheritance scheme for 1 parent with sickle cell trait (SCT) and 1 parent with sickle cell anemia (SCA). A, normal hemoglobin; S, sickle hemoglobin. Possibilities with each pregnancy: 50% SCA (SS); 50% SCT (AS).

Republic), and Cameroon. The Arab-Indian haplotype is seen in certain areas of Saudi Arabia and India.[8–10]

ETIOLOGY

Normal hemoglobin (HbA) is composed of two α chains and two β chains ($\alpha_2\beta_2$). The biochemical defect that leads to the development of HbS involves the substitution of valine for glutamic acid as the sixth amino acid in the β-polypeptide chain. Another type of abnormal hemoglobin, hemoglobin C (HbC), is produced by the substitution of lysine for glutamic acid as the sixth amino acid in the β-chain. Structurally, the α-chains of HbS, HbA, and HbC are identical. Therefore it is the chemical differences in the β-chain that explain sickling and its related sequelae.[2,7]

Sickle cell anemia (SCA) is a form of SCD in which the patient has inherited both genes that code for formation of HbS, one from each parent (HbSS). Figures 101–1, 101–2, 101–3, and 101–4 illustrate the possibility of inheritance with each pregnancy for the offspring of parents with normal hemoglobin (HbA), SCT, and SCA. If both parents are carriers, the offspring will have a 25% risk of having SCD and 50% risk of being a carrier (see Fig. 101–1). β-Thalassemia can

be found in conjunction with HbS. Since patients with HbSS and HbSβ^0-thalassemia do not have normal β-globulin production, they usually have a more severe course than those with HbSC and HbSβ^+-thalassemia. As discussed earlier, several haplotypes characterize the sickle gene, resulting in differing clinical and hematologic courses. Included among these types are the three most commonly found in the United States: the Bantu haplotype, characterized by severe disease; the Senegal haplotype, characterized by mild disease; and the Benin haplotype, characterized by a course intermediate to that of the other two haplotypes. Although there are a number of other haplotypes seen around the world, the remaining major types include Saudi Arabian and Cameroon. Both of these types usually follow milder courses of illness.[2,7–11]

PATHOPHYSIOLOGY

To understand the pathophysiology of SCD, one must understand the normal physiology of RBC production. Normal adult RBCs contain 33 to 35 g/dL hemoglobin, predominantly HbA (96%). Other forms of hemoglobin are HbA$_2$ (2% to 3%) and fetal hemoglobin (<2%). Fetal

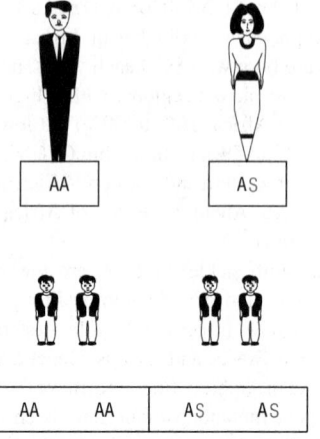

FIGURE 101–2. Sickle gene inheritance scheme for 1 parent with sickle cell trait (SCT) and 1 parent with no sickle cell gene. A, normal hemoglobin; S, sickle hemoglobin. Possibilities with each pregnancy: 50% normal (AA); 50% SCT (AS).

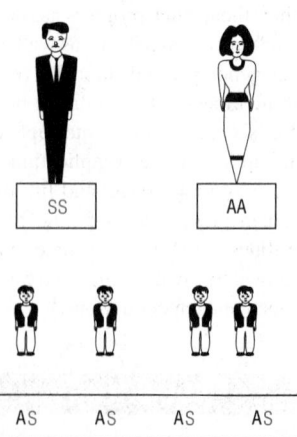

FIGURE 101–4. Sickle inheritance scheme for 1 parent without sickle cell gene and 1 parent with sickle cell anemia (SCA). A, normal hemoglobin; S, sickle hemoglobin. Possibilities with each pregnancy: 100% SCT (AS).

hemoglobin (HbF) is present predominantly in fetal RBCs. Instead of β chains in HbA or HbS, HbF contains 2 gamma chains ($\alpha_2\gamma_2$). The switch from production of γ chains to β chains occurs shortly before birth. A few red cell clones remain to produce HbF postnatally. Increased production of HbF is seen under severe erythroid stress, such as anemia, hematopoietic stem cell transplant or chemotherapy. Both water and hemoglobin content in the RBCs determine the mean corpuscular hemoglobin concentration (MCHC). Passive diffusion and active transport regulate intracellular cation and volume contents, which determine the intracellular viscosity of RBC. Normal RBCs are biconcave shape and able to deform to squeeze through capillaries (Fig. 101–5). As RBCs age, MCHC increases, deformability decreases, and the cells are removed by the reticuloendothelial system.[12]

In the pathogenesis of SCD, three known problems are primarily responsible for various clinical manifestations: impaired circulation, destruction of RBCs, and stasis of blood flow. These three problems probably relate directly to two major disturbances involving RBCs: polymerization and membrane damage (Fig. 101–6).

The solubility of HbS and HbA are the same when oxygenated. Due to increased hydrophobicity as a result of valine substituting glutamic acid, solubility of deoxygenated HbS is reduced to 17 g/dL. Saturation of deoxy-HbS leads to intermolecular binding and formation of thin bundles of fibers, which initially are unstable but with

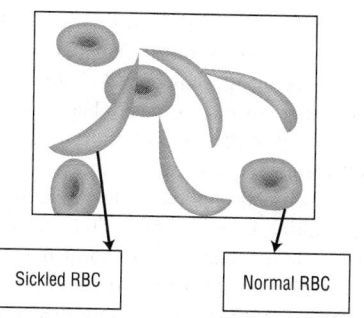

FIGURE 101–5. Elongated sickle and normal discoid shaped red blood cells.

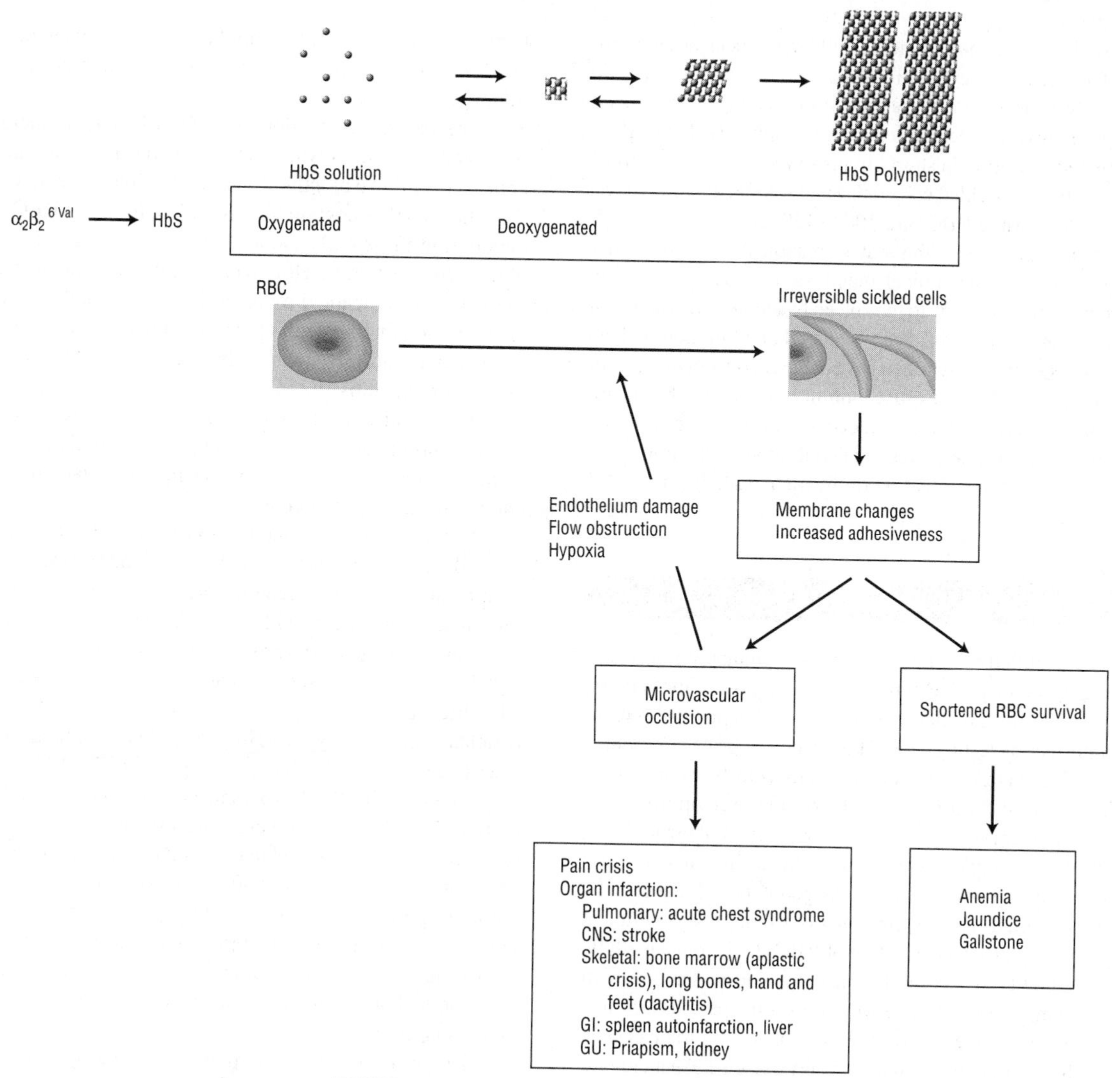

time, increased binding of deoxy-HbS results in cross-linking fibers and stable polymers. This process is influenced by MCHC, temperature, intracellular pH, and the amount of HbS. Polymerization allows deoxygenated hemoglobin molecules to exist as a semisolid gel that protrudes into the cell membrane, leading to distortion of RBCs (sickled shape) and loss of deformability. The presence of sickled RBCs increases blood viscosity and encourages sludging in the capillaries and small venous vessels. Such obstructive events lead to local tissue hypoxia, which tends to accentuate the pathologic process.

$\alpha_2\beta_2{}^{6\,Val} \longrightarrow$ HbS

HbS solution

HbS Polymers

Oxygenated   Deoxygenated

RBC

Irreversible sickled cells

Endothelium damage
Flow obstruction
Hypoxia

Membrane changes
Increased adhesiveness

Microvascular
occlusion

Shortened RBC survival

Pain crisis
Organ infarction:
    Pulmonary: acute chest syndrome
    CNS: stroke
    Skeletal: bone marrow (aplastic
        crisis), long bones, hand and
        feet (dactylitis)
    GI: spleen autoinfarction, liver
    GU: Priapism, kidney

Anemia
Jaundice
Gallstone

FIGURE 101–6. Pathophysiology of sickle cell disease.

When reoxygenated, polymers within the RBCs are lost, and the RBCs eventually return to normal shape. This process contributes to the vaso-occlusive manifestation in that HbS is able to squeeze into microvasculature when oxygenated, but becomes sickled when deoxygenated. The cycle of sickling and unsickling results in damage to the cell membrane, loss of membrane flexibility, and rearrangement of surface phospholipids. Membrane damage also alters ion transport, resulting in loss of potassium and water, which lead to a dehydrated state that enhances the formation of sickled forms. After continual repetitions of the process, the RBC membrane develops into a more rigid form, irreversibly sickled cells (ISC). Unlike the reversible sickle cells, which have normal morphology when oxygenated, ISCs are elongated cells and remain sickled when oxygenated. More rigid membranes of HbS-containing RBC retard their flow, particularly through the microcirculation. In addition, sickled RBCs tend to adhere to vascular endothelial cells, which further increases polymerization and obstruction.

Intermolecular binding and polymer formation are reduced by fetal hemoglobin (HbF) and to a lesser degree by HbA_2. RBCs that contain HbF sickle less readily than cells without. ISCs, not surprisingly, have a low HbF level. Increased levels of HbF, as in the case of the Saudi Arabian genotype, results in more benign forms of SCD. The amount of HbF and HbA_2 in relation to HbS influences clinical manifestations and explains the variability in severity among different SCD genotypes.

Intravascular destruction of sickle cells may occur at an accelerated rate. The stresses of circulation, and repetitive sickle-unsickle cycles are likely to lead to cell fragmentation. Damage to the cell membrane promotes cell recognition by macrophages. Rigid ISCs are easily trapped, resulting in short circulatory survival and chronic hemolysis. The typical sickled cell survives for about 10 to 20 days, while life spans of normal RBCs are 100 to 120 days.

Factors in addition to sickling may be responsible for the pathogenesis of a number of the clinical manifestations associated with SCD. Obstruction of blood flow to the spleen by sickle cells can result in functional asplenia, defined as the loss of splenic function with an intact spleen. These patients may also have deficient opsonization. Impaired splenic function increases susceptibility to infection by encapsulated organisms, particularly pneumococcal disease. Coagulation abnormalities in SCD may be the result of continuous activation of the hemostatic system or disorganization of the membrane layer.[7,9,12–14]

CLINICAL PRESENTATION

SCD is usually identified by routine neonatal screening programs. The sensitivity and specificity of screening methods, most commonly by isoelectric focusing, are excellent. For infants with a positive screening result, confirmation testing should be performed prior to 2 months of age. Even with universal screening, infants with SCD are sometimes not identified at birth because of extreme prematurity, prior blood transfusion, inability to contact family, or clerical errors.[4]

SCD involves multiple organ systems and its clinical manifestations vary greatly between and among genotypes (Table 101–1). Persons with SCT are usually asymptomatic, although some clinical signs and symptoms can occur. Sickling of RBCs in the renal medulla results in loss of ability to maximally concentrate urine. Patients with such impairment may be at risk of dehydration during periods in which the body normally conserves water. Microscopic hematuria has been seen and gross hematuria can occur after heavy exercise. An increased incidence of urinary tract infection in women, especially during pregnancy, has been reported. In general, trait carriers are not considered

TABLE 101–1. Clinical Features of Sickle Cell Trait and Common Sickle Cell Disease

Type	Clinical Features
Sickle cell trait (SCT)	Rare painless hematuria; normal Hgb level; heavy exercise under extreme conditions may provoke gross hematuria and complications
Sickle cell anemia (SCA)	Pain crises, microvascular disruption of organs (spleen, liver, bone marrow, kidney, brain, and lung), gallstone, priapism, leg ulcers; anemia (Hgb 7–10 g/dL)
Sickle hemoglobin C	Painless hematuria and rare aseptic necrosis of bone; vaso-occlusive crises are less common and occur later in life; other complications are ocular disease and pregnancy-related problems; mild anemia (Hgb 10–12 g/dL)
Sickle β^+-thalassemia	Rare crises; milder severity than sickle cell disease because production of HbA; Hgb 10–14 g/dL with microcytosis
Sickle β^0-thalassemia	No HbA production; severity similar to SCA; Hgb 7–10 g/dL with microcytosis

to have clinical disease, but should be cautious when participating in exercise under extreme conditions, such as high altitude or military training.[5,13]

The feature presentations of SCD are hemolytic anemia and vaso-occlusion. In patients who are homozygous for HbS, anemia usually appears from 4 to 6 months after birth. Symptoms are delayed because the infant's RBCs contain mainly HbF at birth. As RBC turnover occurs during those early months, cells containing HbS gradually replace those containing HbF, which typically leads to attacks of pain frequently accompanied by fever. Pneumonia and splenomegaly are also common findings. Infants can also present with pain and swelling of the hands and feet, commonly referred to as "hand-and-foot syndrome" or dactylitis.[4,5]

The usual clinical signs and symptoms associated with SCA include chronic anemia; fever and pallor; arthralgia; scleral icterus; abdominal pain; weakness; anorexia; fatigue; enlargement of the liver, spleen, and heart; and hematuria.

Laboratory findings include low hemoglobin (Hgb) level and increased reticulocyte, platelet, and white blood cell (WBC) counts. The peripheral blood smear demonstrates sickle forms (see Fig. 101–5). Presentation of patients with HbSC disease is less severe than that of SCA, and is characterized primarily by mild anemia (Hgb levels above 9 g/dL), infrequent episodes of pain, persistence of splenomegaly into adult life, and excessive target cells in the peripheral blood smear. In patients with heterozygous HbS and β-thalassemia gene, severity of disease depends on the thalassemia gene involved.[5,7,13]

Patients with SCD experience delayed growth and sexual maturation. Both height and weight are usually below average, and the poor growth cannot be explained by nutritional factors alone. Fertility problems tend to occur more often, and some menstrual abnormalities are more prevalent in female SCD patients than in normal women. Other typical physical characteristics include a protuberant abdomen with exaggerated lumbar lordosis, usually an asthenic appearance with rather long extremities and tapered fingers, and frequently a barrel-shaped chest.[4,5]

The previously high mortality rate of early childhood has been reduced for patients with SCD with availability of public health programs and comprehensive care.[4] The median survival rate is estimated

TABLE 101–2. Acute Complications of Sickle Cell Disease (SCD)

Infection[a]

Clinical features: SCD carries a high risk for overwhelming sepsis due to functional asplenia and failure to make antibodies against encapsulated organisms; patients should be evaluated for temperature greater than 38.5°C. A low threshold for empiric therapy is recommended.

Pathogens: Streptococcus pneumoniae (most common), *Haemophilus influenzae, Salmonella, Mycoplasma pneumoniae, Chlamydia*, and viruses (parvovirus B19)

Evaluation: Physical examination, complete blood count (CBC) with reticulocyte, urinalysis, chest x-ray, and cultures (blood, urine, and throat); lumbar puncture if toxic-looking or presenting with signs of meningitis; needle aspirate in patients with findings suggestive of osteomyelitis

Cerebrovascular accidents (stroke)[b]

Clinical features: Incidence is four times higher for HbSS than HbSC. Initial episode most often occurs during the first 10 years of life. "Silent infarcts" as evidenced by changes on magnetic resonance imaging (MRI) have been reported in 21.8% of HbSS and may be associated with increased risk of stroke and decreased neurocognitive function.

Cause: Most common is cerebrovascular occlusion. Other causes include intracranial hemorrhage, cardiac embolism, infection, and clotting disorders.

Signs and symptoms: Headache, vomiting, stupor, hemiparesis, aphasia, visual disturbances, and seizure; transient ischemic attack is a strong predictor for stroke. Behavioral and performance changes may be present in patients with asymptomatic infarction.

Evaluation: Perform computed tomography (CT) scan and MRI for evaluation of acute event. Perform magnetic resonance angiography for asymptomatic infarction. Perform transcranial Doppler to detect abnormal velocity and identify high-risk patients. Perform electroencephalography if there is a history of seizure.

Acute chest syndrome (ACS)[c]

Clinical features: ACS occurs in 15% to 43% of patients and is responsible for up to 25% of deaths. Risk factors include young age, low HbF level, high Hgb and WBCs, winter seasons, and reactive airway disease. Recurrences are up to 80% and can lead to chronic lung diseases in adulthood.

Signs and symptoms: New infiltration on X-ray accompanied by fever, cough, dyspnea, chest pain, hypoxia, leukocytosis. Can progress to acute respiratory distress syndrome and death.

Cause: Exact cause remains unknown but pulmonary sickling resulting in infraction is the key element. Proposed etiologies include: infectious (*S. pneumoniae, H. influenzae, Chlamydia, Mycoplasma*, and viral) and noninfectious (fat embolization from bone infarction, hypoventilation secondary to pain, narcotics, etc).

Evaluation: Close monitoring of pulmonary status, blood gases (if indicated), oxygen saturation, chest x-ray, blood and sputum cultures, CBC, bronchoscopy with lavage (if needed)

Priapism[d]

Clinical features: Priapism is defined as a painful and unwanted erection, which is classified as stuttering (less than 3 hours, often multiple episodes) or prolonged (more than 3 hours). Up to 89% of males with SCD will have at least one episode by age 20. The mean age of the initial episode is 12 years of age. Repeated episodes can cause fibrosis and impotence.

Cause: Sickling in the sinusoids of the penis

Signs and symptoms: Prepubertal children often present with stuttering priapism. Older males can present with prolonged episodes that last for days and should be managed as medical emergencies. Urinary obstruction can occur in severe cases.

Evaluation: Physical examination; monitor duration of episode and for signs of urinary retention.

---

[a]From Fixler et al,[1] National Institutes of Health,[5] Dover et al,[13] Hord et al,[18] and Smithy-Whitley et al.[19]

[b]From Fixler et al,[1] Dover et al,[13] Pegelow et al,[20] Kral et al,[21] and Miller et al.[22]

[c]From Dean et al,[23] Siddiqui et al,[24] Vichinsky et al,[25] Neumayr et al,[26] and Vichinsky et al.[27]

[d]From Fixler et al,[1] National Institutes of Health,[5] and Dover et al.[13]

HbF, fetal hemoglobin; HbSC, sickle-hemoglobin C; HbSS, homozygous sickle hemoglobin; Hgb, hemoglobin; WBC, white blood cell.

---

to be 42 years for males and 48 years for females for HbA, and 60 years for males and 68 years for females for HbSC.[5] Predictors for severe disease in children who are less than 10 years of age include dactylitis before 1 year of age, an average Hgb level less than 7 g/dL in the second year of life, and WBC count greater than 13,700/mm³ in the absence of infection. Risk factors for early death in adults with SCD include acute complications such as pain crisis, anemic events, acute chest syndrome, renal failure, and pulmonary disease (Tables 101–2 and 101–3).[5,15–17] Today, with longer survival for SCD, chronic manifestations of the disease contribute to the morbidity later in life (Table 101–4).

COMPLICATIONS

ACUTE COMPLICATIONS

For acute complications of SCD, see Table 101–2.

FEVER AND INFECTION

Functional asplenia and failure to make antibodies against encapsulated organisms contribute to the high risk of overwhelming sepsis in patients with SCD. The most common pathogen is *Streptococcus pneumoniae*. Other encapsulated organisms are *Haemophilus influenzae* and *Salmonella*, and the latter has been known to cause osteomyelitis and pneumonia in SCD. *Mycoplasma pneumoniae* should be considered in older children with infiltrates on chest x-ray. Viral infections (e.g., influenza and parvovirus B19) can result in severe morbidity.[1,5,18,19]

All SCD patients with fever greater than 38.5°C must be evaluated to determine the extent of sepsis; work-up may include physical examination, complete blood count with reticulocyte count, blood culture, chest x-ray, urinalysis, and urine culture. Lumbar puncture may be needed, especially in young children and toxic-looking children. A low threshold for empiric therapy compared to that in the general population is recommended.[1,5,13]

NEUROLOGIC

Neurologic abnormalities can occur in both adults and children. Vaso-occlusive processes occasionally lead to cerebrovascular occlusion that manifests itself as the signs and symptoms of stroke, such as drowsiness, paralysis, transitory or permanent blindness, aphasia, visual disturbances, spinal cord infarction, and convulsions. The onset

TABLE 101–3. Sickle Cell Crisis

Vaso-occlusive Pain Crisis[a]

Clinical features: Acute painful infarction without changes in Hgb; almost all patients with SCA will have episodes of acute pain. Recurrent acute crises result in bone, joint, and organ damage and chronic pain. Vaso-occlusive crisis most commonly involves the bones, liver, spleen, brain, lungs, and penis. Acute long bone pains may be accompanied by signs of inflammation, making it difficult to differentiate from osteomyelitis. Abdominal involvement may resemble a surgical abdomen. Precipitating factors include infection, extreme weather conditions, dehydration, and stresses.

Signs and symptoms: Deep throbbing pain; local tenderness, erythema, and swelling may be seen. Fever and leukocytosis are common. Dactylitis usually occurs in young infants. Jaundice and increased transaminases present if liver is involved.

Evaluation: Frequent physical examination, complete blood count (CBC), reticulocyte, and urinalysis; based on symptomatology, the following may be needed: needle aspiration to rule out osteomyelitis, abdominal studies (x-ray, computed tomography scan, etc), liver function tests, bilirubin, culture, and chest x-ray.

Aplastic crisis[b]

Clinical features: Acute decrease in Hgb with decreased reticulocyte count (usually less than 1%); transient suppression of RBC production in response to bacterial or viral infection, most common being parvovirus B19

Signs and symptoms: Headache, fatigue, dyspnea, pallor, and tachycardia; may also present with fever, upper respiratory or gastrointestinal infection symptoms.

Evaluation: CBC, reticulocyte count, x-ray, cultures (blood, urine, and throat), parvovirus titers

Acute splenic sequestration crisis[c]

Clinical features: Acute exacerbation of anemia due to sequestration of large blood volume by the spleen. More commonly seen in patients with functioning spleens (e.g., infants and adults with HbSC disease); onset often is associated with viral or bacterial infections; recurrences are common and can be fatal.

Signs and symptoms: Sudden onset of fatigue, dyspnea, and distended abdomen; rapid decrease in Hgb and Hct with elevated reticulocyte count, abdominal pain, splenomegaly, vomiting, hypotension, and shock

Evaluation: Close monitoring of vital signs, spleen size, and oxygen saturation, CBC, reticulocyte, and cultures

[a]From Fixler et al,[1] National Institutes of Health,[5] Dover et al,[13] and Yale.[28]
[b]From Fixler et al,[1] National Institutes of Health,[5] Dover et al,[13] and Kellermayer et al.[28]
[c]From Fixler et al,[1] National Institutes of Health,[5] and Dover et al.[13]
HbSC, sickle-hemoglobin C; Hgb, hemoglobin; RBC, red blood cell; SCA, sickle cell anemia.

TABLE 101–4. Chronic Complications of Sickle Cell Disease (SCD)

System	Complications
Auditory	Sensorineural hearing loss due to sickling in cochlear vasculature with hair cell damage
Cardiovascular	Cardiomegaly, myocardial ischemia, murmurs, and abnormal electrocardiogram; patients with SCD have lower blood pressure (BP) than the normal population; normal BP values for SCD should be used for diagnosis of hypertension ("relative" hypertension); heart failure usually is related to fluid overload
Dermatologic	Painful leg ulcers; failure to heal occurs in 50% of patients; recurrences are common
Genitourinary	Renal papillary necrosis, hematuria, hyposthenuria, proteinuria, nephritic syndrome, tubular dysfunction, chronic renal failure, impotence
Growth and development	Delay in growth (weight and height) and sexual development; decreased fertility; increased complications during pregnancy; depression may be more prevalent than in general population, especially in patients with unstable disease
Hepatic and biliary	Cholelithiasis, biliary sludge, acute and chronic cholecystitis, and cholestasis (can be progressive and life-threatening)
Neurologic	"Silent" brain lesions on magnetic resonance imaging are associated with poor cognitive and fine motor functions; pseudotumor cerebri (case report)
Ocular	Retinal or vitreous hemorrhage, retinal detachment, transient or permanent visual loss; central retinal vein occlusion
Pulmonary	Pulmonary fibrosis, pulmonary hypertension, cor pulmonale
Renal	Hematuria, hyposthenuria (inability to concentrate urine maximally), tubular dysfunction, enuresis during early childhood, acute renal failure can also occur
Skeletal	Aseptic necrosis of ball-and-socket joints (shoulder and hip); prostheses may be needed due to permanent damage; bone marrow hyperplasia resulting in growth disturbances of maxilla and vertebrae
Spleen	Asplenia (autosplenectomy or surgical splenectomy)

From Fixler et al,[1] National Institutes of Health,[5] Dover et al,[13] Kral et al,[21] Vichinsky et al,[27] Gladwin et al,[30] Henry et al,[31] Mukisi-Mukaza et al,[32] Hasan et al,[33] Babalola et al,[34] de Montalembert et al,[35] Hassan et al,[36] and Schatz et al.[37]

is usually sudden, but occasionally may be gradual. Milder symptoms may occur as a result of vascular stasis. Some patients recover rapidly and completely, while others are left with permanent neurologic deficits. In addition, some patients who have SCA with no prior history of stroke have been found to have changes on magnetic resonance imaging of the brain that suggests infarction or ischemia. These "silent infarcts" have been reported to occur in up to 21.8% of HbSS patients and may be associated with increased risk of stroke and decreased neurocognitive functions.[1,13,20–22]

ACUTE CHEST SYNDROME

Acute chest syndrome (ACS) is the leading cause of death among patients with SCD. It is characterized by acute new pulmonary infiltrate, other respiratory symptoms (such as cough, dyspnea, chest pain, fever, and wheezing), and an equivocal response to antibiotic therapy. As many as one-half of patients with SCD develop ACS at least once. Pulmonary infarcts often involve the lower lobes of the lungs and are a frequent cause of pleural effusions. Pneumonia occurs most often in the middle and upper lobes. These pulmonary manifestations must be recognized early and managed aggressively because the patient may rapidly progress to pulmonary failure and death.[23–27]

PRIAPISM

Sickling in the sinusoids of the penis can cause priapism, a sustained painful erection that may last several hours or days. Impotence has been reported after repeated episodes. ASPEN (association of sickle cell disease, priapism, exchange transfusion, and neurological events) syndrome has occurred in some patients with priapism after partial exchange transfusion. The syndrome can range from headaches and seizures to obtundation requiring ventilation.[1,5,13]

SICKLE CELL CRISIS

Chronic hemolytic anemia in the SCD patient is periodically interrupted by crises, particularly in childhood (see Table 101–3). Patients with HbSS disease experience crises more often than do patients with HbSC disease or some other variants. Although fever, infections, dehydration, hypoxia, acidosis, and sudden temperature alterations can precipitate crises, multiple factors often contribute to development of a crisis.

Vaso-Occlusive Pain Crisis

The most common type of crisis is the vaso-occlusive crisis, which is usually characterized by pain affecting the involved areas, without changes in hemoglobin. Laboratory changes that may be seen include leukocytosis, increased serum levels of fibrinogen, and decreased serum pH and bicarbonate level. Dactylitis (hand-and-foot syndrome) occurs in infancy and early childhood, and is characterized by redness and swelling of the dorsal aspects of the hands, feet, fingers, and toes. The episodes are painful, but there usually is no permanent damage. Children most likely to develop severe SCD later in life are those who experience dactylitis, along with severe anemia and noninfectious leukocytosis during the first 2 years of life.[1,5,13,28]

Aplastic Crisis

Aplastic crisis is characterized by a decrease in the reticulocyte count and a rapidly developing severe anemia. The bone marrow is hypoplastic. There may be associated pain. The crisis is thought to be caused by a viral infection, particularly B19 parvovirus.[1,5,13,29]

Splenic Sequestration Crisis

This is a sudden massive enlargement of the spleen resulting from the sequestration of blood from the reticuloendothelial system. There is a dramatic fall in hematocrit and hemoglobin concentration, with no evidence of marrow failure or accelerated hemolysis. The trapping of the sickled RBCs by the spleen also leads to a drop in circulating blood volume, which can result in hypotension and shock. The condition is most often seen in infants and children, as their spleens are intact. These crises can cause sudden death in young children. Repeated infarctions lead to autosplenectomy as the disease progresses; therefore the incidence declines as adolescence approaches.[1,5,13]

CHRONIC COMPLICATIONS

SCD manifests in a variety of chronic problems involving multiple organs (see Table 101–4). Pulmonary hypertension has been reported to be a risk factor for death in adult patients with SCD.[30] Headache is a symptom associated with acute neurologic events; however, pseudotumor cerebri presenting with severe headache and blurred vision was recently reported.[31] Destructive bone and joint problems are common. Aseptic necrosis, particularly of the femoral or humeral heads, causes permanent damage and disability. Patients with SCD also have an increased incidence of osteomyelitis; the organism most often responsible is *Salmonella*. In addition to necrosis of joints, chronic leg ulcers can become a difficult skeletal problem. The inner aspect of the lower leg just above the ankle is the site most often affected. Ulcers are often seen after trauma or infection; they are usually slow to heal, taking several weeks to a year.[1,5,32]

Ocular problems seen in patients with SCD include transient monocular blindness, visual field defects from retinal hemorrhage, retinal detachment, vitreous hemorrhage, venous microaneurysms, and neovascularization. The incidence of proliferative retinopathy in SCD patients varies from 5% to 10%. Vaso-occlusion in the eye can occur as early as 20 months and clinically detectable retinal diseases usually occur during adolescence and early adulthood. Despite the less systemic manifestations, patients with HbSC develop serious retinal complications more often and earlier. Annual examination with retinal evaluation is recommended for patients with SCD to prevent blindness from retinopathy and other complications.[5,33,34]

Cholelithiasis is a common occurrence in the SCD patient. It is the result of the chronic hemolysis that results in increased bilirubin production, leading to biliary sludge and/or stone formation. Cholecystitis, exemplified by pain in the right iliac fossa, can be confused with abdominal pain crisis.[1,5]

As with any anemia, cardiovascular abnormalities, including cardiac enlargement and various murmurs, can occur in patients with SCD. Patients complain of various degrees of exertional dyspnea, tachycardia, and palpitation owing to the decreased oxygen-carrying capacity of the blood.[5,35]

Renal complications include unilateral hematuria and hyposthenuria (inability to concentrate urine maximally). Enuresis, as a result of increased urine production, is a common complaint. Death from renal disease is unusual among younger patients, but does occur among older patients with SCD.[1,5]

Depression may be more prevalent than in the general population, especially in patients with unstable disease.[36,37] Delay in growth and sexual development are seen in patients with SCD. Adults with SCD have decreased fertility. Finally, pregnancy introduces an increased risk for the mother with SCD and for the fetus. The anemia of SCD may lead to intrauterine growth retardation. Preterm labor and premature delivery are common occurrences in mothers with SCD, and the risk of spontaneous abortion is increased. The incidence of preeclampsia is also higher than in mothers who do not have SCD. The periodicity of past pain crisis is predictive of the likely events during pregnancy, although some patients may experience increased frequency of pain crisis during pregnancy. The presentation of such patients is similar to that of nonpregnant patients—severe localized or generalized pain, low-grade fever, and mild leukocytosis.[1,5]

CONTINUING CARE AND SUPPORT

Patients with SCD require lifelong multidisciplinary care. All patients with SCD should receive regularly scheduled comprehensive medical evaluations. The goals of the comprehensive care are reduction of hospitalizations, complications, and mortality. Due to the complexity of the disease, a multidisciplinary team is needed to provide medical care, education, counseling, and psychosocial support. Appropriate comprehensive care can have a positive impact on both longevity and general quality of life. This care includes the use of traditional prophylactic and general symptomatic supportive care, as well as the use of newer, more specific therapies aimed at altering hematologic capacity and function.[1,5]

Treatment for patients with SCD involves the use of general measures to meet the unique demands for increased erythropoiesis. Additional interventions may be aimed at preventing or treating complications of the disease. When crises occur, the type and severity of the crisis determines the appropriate therapeutic plan. A treatment overview is shown in Table 101–5.[1,5,13,20,26–28,38–79]

TABLE 101–5. Management of Sickle Cell Disease

	Options and Comments
Health maintenance	
Infection prophylaxis	• Pneumococcal vaccines (PCV 7 and PPV 23) • Penicillin prophylaxis for children less than 5 years old • Annual influenza vaccine
Induction of fetal hemoglobin	• Hydroxyurea is the primary agent • Other agents are butyrates (arginine butyrate and sodium phenylbutyrate), decitabine, clotrimazole, and erythropoietin • Combination HbF inducers have been proposed
Chronic transfusion therapy	• Primary indication: stroke prevention in pediatric patients • May also reduce pain crisis and acute chest syndrome • Goal: maintain HbS less than 30%
Future prospects	
Transplantation	• May potentially cure the disease • Most experience is with HLA-matched donors; umbilical cord blood transplantation is being evaluated
Crises and complications	
Fever and infection	• Broad-spectrum antibiotic: cefotaxime or ceftriaxone (clindamycin for cephalosporin allergy); vancomycin for staphylococcal and resistant pneumococcal organisms • Fluids • Acetaminophen or ibuprofen for fever
Stroke	• Exchange transfusion • Initiate chronic transfusion therapy to prevent recurrent strokes
Acute chest syndrome	• Broad-spectrum antibiotics (include *Mycoplasma* coverage) • Bronchodilator if wheezing or history of reactive airway disease • Fluids • Pain management • Transfusion
Priapism	• Hydration • Pain management • Urology consult for other options (intrapenile injection or surgery)
Aplastic crisis	• Supportive care • Transfusion for severe symptomatic anemia
Sequestration crisis	• Transfusion • Broad-spectrum antibiotic • Splenectomy in severe cases
Pain crises	• Hydration • Analgesics

HbF, fetal hemoglobin; HbS, sickle hemoglobin; HLA, human leukocyte antigen.
From Fixler et al,[1] National Institutes of Health,[5] Dover et al,[13] Pegelow et al,[20] Neumayr et al,[26] Vichinsky et al,[27] Yale,[28] Adamikiewicz et al,[38] Advisory Committee on Immunization Practices,[39] Committee on Infectious Diseases,[40] Sickle Cell Disease Care Consortium,[41] Falletta et al,[42] Kennedy et al,[43] Rodriguez-Cortes,[44] Rabb et al,[45] Charache et al,[46] Nathan,[47] Cokic et al,[48] Gladwin et al,[49] Charache et al,[50] Steinbert et al,[51] National Heart, Lung and Blood Institute,[52] National Heart, Lung and Blood Institute,[53] Zimmerman et al,[54] Wilson,[55] Najean et al,[56] Atweh et al,[57] Resar et al,[58] Saunthararajah et al,[59] Scothorn et al,[60] Pegelow et al,[61] Russell et al,[62] Adams et al,[63] Harmatz et al,[64] Walters et al,[65] Atkins et al,[66] Brachet et al,[67] Baron et al,[68] Walters,[69] Knight-Madden et al,[70] Sullivan et al,[71] Li et al,[72] Mantadakis et al,[73] Dahm et al,[74] Jacob et al,[75] Berde et al,[76] Stinson et al,[77] Christensen et al,[78] and Elander et al.[79]

TABLE 101–6. Pneumococcal Immunization for Children with Sickle Cell Disease

	Recommended Schedule
Previously unvaccinated	
Age 2–6 months	**PCV 7 (Prevnar):** 3 doses 6–8 wk apart; then 1 dose at 12–15 months
Age 7–11 months	**PCV 7 (Prevnar):** 2 doses 6–8 wk apart; then 1 dose at 12–15 months
Age ≥12–23 months	**PCV 7 (Prevnar):** 2 doses 6–8 wk apart
Age 24–59 months	**PCV 7 (Prevnar):** 2 doses 6–8 wk apart
	PPV 23 (Pneumovax): 2 doses; first dose at least 6–8 wk after last PCV 7 dose; second dose 3–5 years after the first PPV 23 dose
Age 5 years or older	**PCV 7 (Prevnar):** 1 dose
	PPV 23 (Pneumovax): 2 doses; first dose at least 6–8 wk after last PCV 7 dose; second dose 3–5 years (for those age 10 years or younger) or more than 5 years (for those age 10 years or older) after the first PPV 23 dose
Previously vaccinated	
Age 12–23 months, incomplete PCV 7 series	**PCV 7 (Prevnar):** 2 doses 6–8 wk apart
Age 24–59 months, received four doses of PCV 7	**PPV 23 (Pneumovax):** 2 doses; first dose at least 6–8 wk after last PCV 7 dose; second dose 3–5 years after the first PPV 23 dose
Age 24–59 months, three doses PCV 7 given before 24 months of age	**PCV 7 (Prevnar):** 1 dose **PPV 23 (Pneumovax):** 2 doses; first dose at least 6–8 wk after last PCV 7 dose; second dose 3–5 y after the first PPV 23 dose
Age 24–59 months, 1 dose PPV 23 given	**PCV 7 (Prevnar):** 2 doses 6–8 wk apart; first dose at least 8 wk after PPV 23 dose **PPV 23 (Pneumovax):** second dose 3–5 years after first PPV 23
Age 5 years or older, received PPV 23	**PCV 7 (Prevnar):** 1 dose 6–8 wk after PPV 23 **If only received 1 dose of PPV 23 (Pneumovax):** Second dose 6–8 wk after PCV 7 *and* 3–5 years (for those age 10 years or less) or more than 5 years (for those age 10 years or older) after the first PPV 23 dose

PCV 7, 7-valent pneumococcal conjugated vaccine; PPV 23, 23-valent pneumococcal polysaccharide vaccine.
From Advisory Committee on Immunization Practices,[39] *Committee on Infectious Diseases,*[40] *and Sickle Cell Disease Care Consortium.*[41]

HEALTH MAINTENANCE

IMMUNIZATIONS

Administration of routine immunizations as recommended by the American Academy of Pediatrics is crucial. In addition to the routine immunizations, SCD patients 6 months and older should also receive influenza vaccine annually. Meningococcal vaccine is also recommended for patients greater than 2 years of age undergoing splenectomy.[38–40]

Patients with SCD have impaired splenic function, which increases their susceptibility to infection by encapsulated organisms, particularly pneumococci. Prior to the routine use of penicillin prophylaxis and the development of pneumococcal vaccines, invasive pneumococcal disease was 20- to 100-fold more common in children with SCD than in healthy children. Even with these interventions, some groups of children with SCD continue to have a high rate of invasive pneumococcal infections.[18,38]

Two different pneumococcal vaccines are available. The 7-valent pneumococcal conjugate vaccine (PCV 7; Prevnar) induces good antibody responses in infants. Immunization with the PCV 7 is recommended for all children less than 24 months of age. Infants should receive the first dose between 6 weeks and 6 months. Two additional doses should be given at approximately 2-month intervals, followed by a fourth dose at age 12 to 15 months. The 23-valent pneumococcal polysaccharide vaccine (PPV 23; Pneumovax 23) was not recommended for use in children less than 2 years of age because

of poor antibody response. To cover for different serotypes, the immunization schedule for children with sickle cell disease should include both pneumococcal vaccines. PPV 23 should be given at 2 years of age or older, administered approximately 2 months after the last dose of the PCV 7. An additional dose of the PPV 23 administered 3 to 5 years later should be considered. The recommended immunization schedule and catch-up schedule for PCV 7 and PPV 23 are presented in Table 101–6.[39–41]

CLINICAL CONTROVERSY

Some sickle cell centers administer a third dose of PPV 23. Meningococcal vaccine is recommended by the American Academy of Pediatrics for asplenic patients, but its routine use for nonsurgical asplenic patients varies among centers.

PENICILLIN

Penicillin prophylaxis until at least 5 years of age is also recommended in children with SCD, even if they have been immunized with the 7-valent vaccine as prophylaxis against pneumococcal infections. Prophylactic treatment should begin at 2 months of age or earlier. An effective regimen that yields an 84% decrease in observed incidence of pneumococcal infections is penicillin V potassium at a dosage of 125 mg orally twice daily until the age of 3 years, followed by 250 mg twice daily until the age of 5 years. An alternate regimen is benzathine penicillin, 600,000 units given intramuscularly every 4 weeks for children age 6 months to 6 years, and 1.2 million units every 4 weeks for those over 6 years of age for whom continued therapy is warranted. Patients who are allergic to penicillin can be given erythromycin 20 mg/kg per day twice daily. Penicillin prophylaxis is not routinely needed in older children, based on a study demonstrating no benefit over placebo beyond the age of 5. However, continuation of oral pneumococcal prophylaxis should be handled on a case-by-case basis, especially in patients with a history of invasive pneumococcal infection or surgical splenectomy.[1,5,13,39–42]

CLINICAL CONTROVERSY

Routine penicillin prophylaxis is controversial in HbSβ^+-thalassemia patients.

FOLIC ACID

Patients with SCD have an increased demand for folic acid because of accelerated erythropoiesis. Megaloblastic changes have been reported, but the actual incidence of megaloblastic anemia in association with SCD is unknown. Conflicting data on serum folate levels have been reported. In children and adolescents, one study reported normal folate stores in SCD patients without receiving supplemental folic acid, and another study reported that 15% of patients had low folate levels despite daily supplementation. A trial of folate supplementation in infants and young children has not shown any beneficial effect on growth or acute events. In general, folic acid supplementation at a dose of 1 mg/day is recommended in adult patients, women who are contemplating pregnancy, and patients of all ages with chronic hemolysis.[5,13,43–45]

FETAL HEMOGLOBIN INDUCERS

Fetal hemoglobin (HbF) has a direct effect on polymer formation. Increases in HbF levels significantly decrease RBC sickling and RBC adhesion. Epidemiologic studies have demonstrated the direct relationship between HbF concentration and severity of the disease. Patients with low HbF levels have more frequent crises and higher mortality. Based on these observations, HbF induction has become a treatment modality for patients with SCD.[6,13]

HYDROXYUREA

Hydroxyurea, a chemotherapeutic agent, stimulates the production of HbF, resulting not only in increased HbF levels, but also increases in the number of HbF-containing reticulocytes and intracellular HbF. Its antineoplastic activity involves prevention of DNA synthesis by blocking ribonucleoside conversion to deoxyribonucleotides. The exact mechanism on HbF production is unknown, but it may be directly or indirectly related to erythropoiesis in that cytoreduction in the bone marrow results in alteration of RBC differentiation toward macrocytosis and HbF production. Recent studies show that hydroxyurea increases nitric oxide (NO) levels, which suggests its effect on HbF may be mediated by stimulation of NO-dependent guanylyl cyclase, which induces γ-globin expression.[46–48] This new finding provides the rationale for the development of NO as a treatment modality for SCD.[49] In addition to increased HbF, hydroxyurea has other beneficial effects, including reduction of neutrophils and monocytes, possession of antioxidant properties, alteration of RBC membrane properties, increased red cell deformability by increased intracellular water content, decreased red cell adhesion to endothelium, and increased NO, a regulator involved in physiologic disturbances.[5,46–48,50]

Hydroxyurea is useful in the prevention of painful crises and has been approved by the FDA for adult patients based on a double-blind, placebo-controlled study called the Multicenter Study of Hydroxyurea in Sickle Cell Anemia (MSH). In this study of 299 adult SCD patients, hydroxyurea significantly reduced the frequency of painful episodes, the incidence of ACS, the need for blood transfusions, and the number of hospitalizations.[50] The number of crises was 44% lower in those who received hydroxyurea, declining from an average of 4.5 to an average of 2.5 crises per year. The incidence of severe crises, defined as those requiring hospitalization, was also lower, with a median rate of 2.4 severe crises per year in the placebo group versus 1 severe crisis in the hydroxyurea group. The risk of ACS was also significantly reduced in patients receiving hydroxyurea. Of the 152 patients in the hydroxyurea group, 25 (16.4%) developed ACS, as compared with 51 (34.7%) of the 147 patients in the placebo group. Blood transfusion requirements were decreased by 34% in the hydroxyurea group. The study was terminated early after interim analyses revealed the significant benefits. The incidence of death, stroke, and hepatic sequestration in the hydroxyurea and placebo groups was not significantly different during the 29-month evaluation period. However, a follow-up study of 233 of the 299 patients reported a 40% reduction in mortality with hydroxyurea over a 9-year period.[51] The patients enrolled in the study were adult populations with moderate to severe SCD in adult populations. Therefore its benefits may not be applicable to patients with milder disease, such as HbSC.

Although not FDA approved, hydroxyurea is also used in selected children and adolescents with SCD. A phase I/II study of hydroxyurea in pediatric patients (Pediatric Hydroxyurea in Sickle Cell Anemia) reported similar benefits as in adults with no adverse effects on growth and development. A pilot study in infants demonstrated that the agent is well tolerated. Both studies involved smaller number of pediatric patients. Another study, BABY HUG, supported by the National Heart, Lung and Blood Institute will be available to evaluate if hydroxyurea therapy is effective in prevention of chronic end-organ damage in young children with SCA.[5,52–54]

The most common side effect of hydroxyurea is bone marrow suppression. In the MSH trial, 14 of 152 patients in the hydroxyurea group and 6 of 147 patients in the placebo group required permanent discontinuation of treatment due to medical reasons. Temporary discontinuation of therapy occurred in almost all patients because of bone marrow suppression, which usually recovered within 2 weeks.[50] Long-term side effects of hydroxyurea therapy in patients with SCD are not fully known. Myelodysplasia, acute leukemia, and chronic opportunistic infection associated with T-lymphocyte abnormalities have been reported.[13,41,55] In the 9-year follow-up study, 3 of 233 patients who received hydroxyurea have developed cancer.[51] However, only 23 of those patients received more than 8 years therapy, a duration that had been associated with an increased risk of acute leukemia.[56] Therefore longer follow-up is needed to determine its carcinogenic or leukemogenic effects. Teratogenicity is another concern, as high-dose hydroxyurea has been shown to be teratogenic in animals. Normal pregnancies resulting in no birth defects have been reported in at least 15 women receiving hydroxyurea.[13,41]

Clinical indications for hydroxyurea use include frequent painful episodes, severe symptomatic anemia, a history of ACS, or other severe vaso-occlusive complications.[13,41] It has not been proved that hydroxyurea will prevent organ damage or reverse previous damage. Splenic regeneration, however, has been reported in adult patients who received the agent. Hydroxyurea does not appear to prevent neurologic complications, but preserved cognitive performance has been

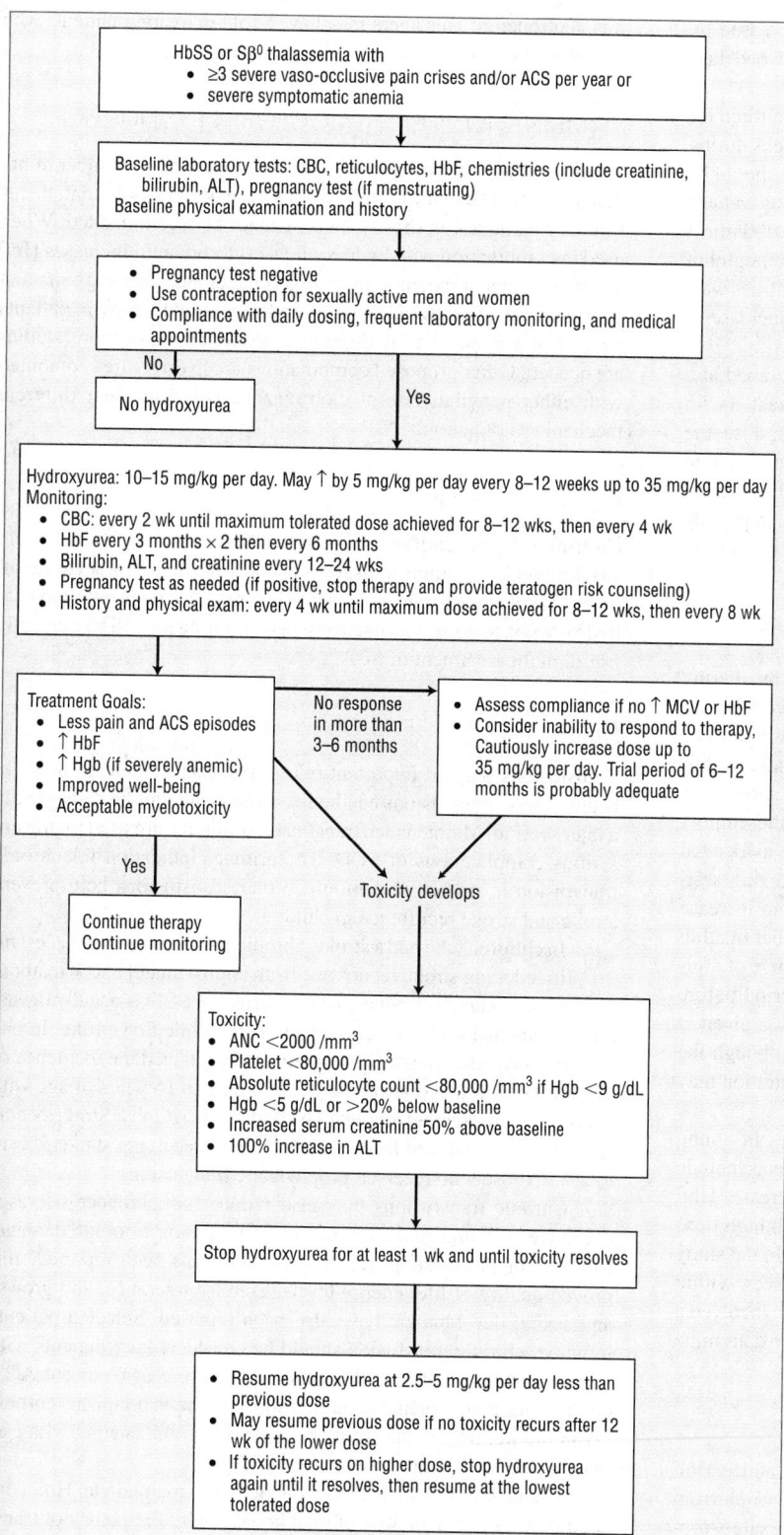

FIGURE 101–7. Hydroxyurea use in sickle cell disease. ACS, acute chest syndrome; ALT, alanine aminotransferase; ANC, absolute neutrophil count; CBC, complete blood cell count; HbF, fetal hemoglobin; Hgb, hemoglobin; HbSS, homozygous sickle hemoglobin; MCV, mean corpuscular volume. *(From Dover et al[13] and Sickle Cell Disease Care Consortium.[41])*

reported. As mentioned previously, decreases in mortality have been reported in adult sickle cell patients in a 9-year follow-up study.[30,51]

Hydroxyurea is available in 200-, 300-, 400-, and 500-mg capsules. For children who are unable to swallow capsules, liquid preparations (100 mg/mL) can be prepared extemporaneously. The starting dose for hydroxyurea is 10 to 15 mg/kg per day as a single daily dose (Fig. 101–7). The dosage can be increased after 8 to 12 weeks if the patient has not experienced intolerable adverse effects and blood counts are stable. Hydroxyurea dosage should be individualized based on response and toxicity. In general, 3 to 6 months of daily administration are required before improvement is observed. Compliance with medication use can be an issue. Since the mean corpuscular volume (MCV) generally increases as the level of HbF increases, monitoring the MCV is an inexpensive and convenient method of monitoring response. With close monitoring, hydroxyurea can be increased by 5 mg/kg per day up to 35 mg/kg per day, the maximal prescribed dose in the MSH study.[13,50]

Patients receiving hydroxyurea should be closely monitored for toxicity. Blood counts should be checked every 2 weeks during dose titration and every 4 to 6 weeks thereafter. Treatment should be interrupted if hematologic indices fall below the following values: absolute neutrophil count, 2000/mm³; platelet count, 80,000/mm³; hemoglobin, 5 g/dL; or reticulocytes, 80,000/mm³ if the hemoglobin concentration is less than 9 g/dL. Other laboratory abnormalities warranting temporary discontinuation of therapy are a 50% increase in serum creatinine and a 100% increase in transaminase.

After recovery has occurred, treatment should be resumed at a dose that is 2.5 to 5 mg/kg per day lower than the dose associated with toxicity. If no toxicity occurs after 12 weeks with the lower dose, the dose may be increased by 2.5 to 5 mg/kg per day. A given dose that twice produces a toxic hematologic response should not be tried again. Failure to see an increase in the MCV with hydroxyurea therapy may indicate that the marrow is unable to respond, the hydroxyurea dose is inadequate, or the patient is noncompliant.[13,41]

BUTYRATE

Butyrate, a naturally occurring fatty acid, increases HbF by altering gene expression, which leads to increased gamma globin chain production. Unlike hydroxyurea, butyrate does not appear to be cytotoxic.

Butyrate has been studied in small number of adult patients. Initial trials administering butyrate by continuous infusion showed an increase not only in HbF, but also in total Hgb and in the number of cells containing HbF. However, a sustained effect or an associated clinical benefit has not been observed. A later study utilizing arginine butyrate as a pulse regimen demonstrated a sustained increase in HbF and reduction of hospitalized days in a small number of adult patients. In that study, adult patients received a 4-day course of arginine butyrate, followed by a 10- to 24-day drug-free period before the administration of the next dose. Arginine butyrate was given at a daily dose of 250 to 500 mg/kg over 6 to 12 hours. Although the results are encouraging, the need for intravenous administration may prevent wide use of the regimen.[57]

Oral sodium penylbutyrate has been used for years in young children with urea cycle disorders. At high doses, side effects include transient fluid retention, rashes, and unusual body odor. Increased HbF levels were seen in patients with SCA who received both high-dose (15 to 20 g/day) and low-dose (1 to 11 g/day) regimens. In the study of low-dose sodium penylbutyrate, increased HbF was seen within 5 weeks, but may not be sustained. The studies of butyrate involved a small number of patients. More clinical trials are needed to determine the optimal dosage and regimen.[5,58]

5-AZA-2'-DEOXYCYTIDINE (DECITABINE)

5-Azacytidine and 5-aza-2'-deoxycytidine (decitabine) induce HbF by inhibiting methylation of DNA, thus preventing the switch from γ- to β-globin production. Decitabine has a more favorable safety profile and is a more potent methylation inhibitor than 5-azacytidine. Virtually abandoned in the past because of concerns regarding the cytotoxicity of 5-azacytidine, decitabine has now been studied in a small number of patients with SCD who did not respond to hydroxyurea. In one study, 5-aza-2'-deoxycytidine was given at a dose of 0.2 mg/kg one to three times a week subcutaneously to eight adult patients resistant or intolerant to hydroxyurea. An increase in fetal hemoglobin was seen in all patients. In addition, reduction of adhesion was reported with the RBC adhesion study. The only significant toxicity reported was neutropenia. This agent may have a role in treating patients who fail to respond to hydroxyurea.[5,59]

COMBINATIONS OF HEMOGLOBIN F INDUCERS

Erythropoietin therapy has been used in only a limited number of patients with SCD and the clinical results have been inconsistent; therefore its routine use in these patients cannot be recommended. When used in combination with hydroxyurea, erythropoietin increases HbF levels to a greater extent than hydroxyurea alone. This suggests that there may be a role for addition of erythropoietin therapy in patients who do not respond to hydroxyurea alone, although more studies are needed. Other proposed combinations are hydroxyurea combined with either penylbutyrate or clotrimazole, based on their different mechanisms of action.[13,47,58]

CLOTRIMAZOLE

Clotrimazole, an antifungal agent, causes a decrease in cell density by blocking cation transport channels in the erythrocyte membrane. The decrease seen, however, is less than that demonstrated with hydroxyurea therapy. It is unclear whether this agent will be clinically useful in the treatment of SCA.[47]

CHRONIC TRANSFUSION THERAPY

Transfusions play an important role in the management of SCD. In acute illness, transfusions can be life-saving and will be discussed in a later section. Maintenance transfusion programs are used to prevent serious complications of SCD. The primary indication for chronic transfusion is stroke prevention. Chronic transfusions help prevent stroke and stroke recurrence in children.

In children who had a stroke, chronic transfusions are successful in reducing stroke recurrence from approximately 50% to about 10% over 3 years.[60-62] Since the first stroke in SCD is usually devastating, transfusions have been used to prevent the first stroke. In one trial, prophylactic transfusions significantly reduced the incidence of first stroke over a 2-year period in children 2 to 16 years of age with abnormal transcranial Doppler (TCD) ultrasonography. Stroke occurrence rate was reduced from 16% in patients receiving standard care to 2% in those who received prophylactic transfusions.[63]

Chronic transfusions may also reduce the incidence of vaso-occlusive pain and ACS, and prevent progression of organ damage. Reversal of pre-existing organ dysfunction has been reported. Improved quality of life, energy levels, exercise tolerance, and growth and sexual development have also been reported. Selected patients in whom chronic transfusion should be considered are patients with transient ischemic attack, abnormal TCD, severe or recurrent ACS, debilitating pain, splenic sequestration, recurrent priapism, chronic organ failure, intractable leg ulcers, severe chronic anemia with cardiac failure, and complicated pregnancies.[5,41]

The goal of transfusions is to achieve and maintain an HbS concentration of less than 30% of total hemoglobin. Frequency of transfusions is adjusted to maintain the desired HbS levels and is usually every 3 to 4 weeks. After 4 years of therapy without development of complications, many clinicians give transfusions less frequently and allow the HbS concentration to rise to 50% of total hemoglobin.[4,5,41] The optimal duration of chronic transfusion therapy is not known. For secondary prevention, current recommendations are to continue transfusion for at least 5 years or until age 18. A study is underway to determine when transfusions can be safely stopped for primary stroke prevention.[5]

Although the benefits of transfusion therapy are relatively clear in some clinical situations, the usefulness of this therapy in other situations remains controversial. Therefore the risks of transfusion therapy must be weighed against possible benefits. The risks associated with transfusion therapy include alloimmunization (sensitization to the blood received), hyperviscosity, viral transmission, volume overload, iron overload, and transfusion reactions. Alloimmunization occurs in 18% to 36% of SCD patients who receive blood transfusions. The use of leukocyte-reduced RBC transfusions or HLA-matched units in chronically transfused patients may reduce the risk of alloimmunization. Transfusion-related infections also remain a concern. All patients should be immunized with hepatitis A and B vaccines. Presently, hepatitis C is considered the most serious risk associated with transfusion therapy, with an infection rate of approximately 1 in every 100,000 transfusions. The risk of contracting acquired immunodeficiency syndrome from blood transfusions, while still of concern, has decreased with routine blood screening. Iron overload is another complication of transfusions and patients should be counseled to avoid excess dietary iron. Abnormal liver biopsy results showing mild to moderate inflammation or fibrosis have been reported. Chelation therapy with deferoxamine should be considered after more than 1 year of chronic transfusions or when serum ferritin is greater than 1500 to 2000 ng/mL. Deferoxamine has been associated with oto- and ocular toxicity and growth failure. Therefore patients receiving chelation therapy should have yearly ophthalmologic and auditory examinations.[5,13,41,64]

Unique to the population with SCD is a constellation of features that may occur in response to blood transfusion; this is often referred to as the sickle cell hemolytic transfusion reaction syndrome. This syndrome includes manifestations of an acute or delayed transfusion reaction due to alloimmunization. Delayed reaction can occur 5 to 20 days after transfusion. During the hemolytic reaction, the patient develops symptoms suggestive of a pain crisis, or symptoms worsen if the patient is already in crisis. The patient may also develop an anemia posttransfusion that is more severe than previously observed because of the rapid drop in hemoglobin and hematocrit, accompanied by a suppression of erythropoiesis. Alloantibodies and autoantibodies that formed as a result of past transfusions can serve as a trigger, causing a return of symptoms in the postrecovery period. Subsequent transfusions may further worsen the clinical situation due to the presence of autoimmune antibodies. There may be no serologic explanation for the hemolytic transfusion reaction. Recovery, as evidenced by reticulocytosis with a gradual increase in the hemoglobin level, may occur only after the withholding of further transfusions. Although some patients tolerate further transfusions after recovery, others may experience a recurrence of the hemolytic transfusion reaction.[3,5,13,41]

FUTURE PROSPECTS

ALLOGENEIC HEMATOPOIETIC STEM CELL TRANSPLANTATION

Currently, allogeneic hematopoietic stem cell transplantation (HSCT) is the only therapy that provides a cure for patients with SCD. A report of a multicenter trial of allogeneic HSCT in 50 patients with SCD showed a 94% survival rate and 84% event-free survival. All of the patients in the study were less than 16 years of age, had symptomatic SCD, and had an HLA-identical sibling donor. Two patients died from chronic graft-versus-host disease, and one died of intracranial hemorrhage. Of the 47 surviving patients, 5 experienced graft rejection and recurrent SCD. These rejections occurred a median of 5.1 months after transplantation.[65,66] One recent study in 24 children with severe SCD reported that pretransplant use of hydroxyurea appeared to be associated with a lower incidence of rejection or failure of engraftment.[67] Based on these data and worldwide experience, it appears that a stable engraftment of donor cells can eradicate or arrest the clinical manifestations of SCD.

The best candidates for allogeneic HSCT are SCD patients who are younger than 16 years of age; have severe complications such as refractory pain, stroke, or recurrent ACS; and have an HLA-matched donor. Although allogeneic HSCT in young children before organ damage and alloimmunization occur may be associated with an increased success rate, disease progression is unpredictable, making it difficult to determine the optimal time for transplantation. The risks associated with allogeneic HSCT must be carefully considered, as the transplant-related mortality rate is about 5% to 10% and graft rejection is about 10%. Approximately 5% of patients developed grade III–IV acute or extensive chronic graft-versus-host disease. Other risks associated with allogeneic HSCT are secondary malignancies, and recently there was a case of transmission of chronic myeloid leukemia to a peripheral blood stem cell recipient who was a sickle cell patient. Efforts to decrease the posttransplant risk of seizures or intracranial bleeding include prophylactic anticonvulsant therapy, aggressive platelet support, and stringent patient selection.[5,41,66,68,69]

Experience with unrelated or HLA-mismatched related donor transplant is very limited. Data on transplantation in thalassemia patients do not support the use of these alternate sources at this point. Umbilical cord blood is another donor source. Its advantages include a lower incidence of severe graft-versus-host disease and the potential of using umbilical cord blood from unrelated donors; however, such advantages are balanced by longer duration for engraftment and a higher rate of graft rejection.[5,41,69]

▶ TREATMENT: Sickle Cell Disease

■ GENERAL MANAGEMENT

Parents and older children should be educated on the signs and symptoms of complications and conditions that require urgent evaluation. During acute illness, patients should be evaluated promptly, as deterioration can occur rapidly. Keeping a balanced fluid status is essential because both dehydration and fluid overload can worsen complications associated with SCD. Oxygen saturation by pulse oximetry should be maintained at least 92% or at baseline. New or increasing supplemental oxygen requirements should be investigated.[5,13,41]

■ EPISODIC TRANSFUSIONS FOR ACUTE COMPLICATIONS

Indications for red cell transfusions include (1) acute exacerbation of baseline anemia, such as aplastic crisis if the anemia is severe, hepatic or splenic sequestration, or severe hemolysis; (2) severe vaso-occlusive episodes, such as ACS, stroke, or acute multiorgan failure; and (3) preparation for procedures that require the use of general anesthesia or ionic contrast. Other patients in whom transfusions may be useful include patients with complicated obstetric problems, refractory leg ulcers, or refractory and protracted painful episodes or severe priapism. Transfusion can be done by simple transfusion or partial exchange transfusion. If simple transfusion is used, volume overload leading to congestive heart failure can occur if anemia is corrected too rapidly in patients with severe anemia. In addition, increases in Hgb levels to greater than 10 to 11 g/dL may cause hyperviscosity and should be avoided.[5,41]

■ INFECTION AND FEVER

Patients with SCD should be evaluated as soon as possible for any fever greater than 38.5°C. Evaluation should be initiated as outlined in Table 101–2. Criteria for hospitalization include an infant less than 1 year old, history of previous bacteremia or sepsis, temperature greater than 40°C, WBC greater than 30,000/mm^3 or less than 5000/mm^3 and/or platelets less than 100,000/mm^3, and evidence of other acute complications or toxic appearance. Outpatient management can be considered in older nontoxic children with reliable family caregivers. Antibiotic choice should provide adequate coverage for encapsulated organisms.

◁ Ceftriaxone should be used for outpatient management because it provides coverage for 24 hours. If admitted, cefotaxime can also be used. For patients with cephalosporin allergy, clindamycin may be used. Vancomycin should be considered for toxic-appearing children or if *Staphylococcus* is suspected. A macrolide antibiotic should be added if mycoplasma pneumonia is suspected. Penicillin prophylaxis should be discontinued while receiving broad-spectrum antibiotics. Acetaminophen or ibuprofen may be used for fever control. Increased fluid requirements may be needed due to dehydration and/or increased insensible loss.[1,4,5,13,41]

■ CEREBROVASCULAR ACCIDENTS

Patients with acute neurologic events must be hospitalized and monitored closely. Physical and neurologic examination should be performed every 2 hours. Acute treatment for children should include exchange transfusion or simple transfusion to maintain Hgb at approximately 10 g/dL and HbS less than 30%, anticonvulsants for patients with a history of seizure, and therapy for increased intracranial pressure if needed. Chronic transfusion therapy should be initiated for children with ischemic stroke as discussed above. In adults presenting with ischemic stroke, thrombolytic therapy should be considered if less than 3 hours since onset of symptoms.[1,4,5,13,41]

■ ACUTE CHEST SYNDROME

Patients with ACS should use incentive spirometry frequently (e.g., at least every 2 hours). In incentive spirometry, the patient tries to take long, slow, deep breaths. A visual indicator on the spirometer indicates when the patient achieves the targeted flow rate or volume. In addition to spirometry, proper management of pain is important. The goal is to provide relief while avoiding analgesic-induced hypoventilation. Appropriate fluid therapy is important as overhydration may cause pulmonary edema and exacerbate respiratory distress. Early use of broad-spectrum antibiotics, including a macrolide or quinolone, is also recommended. Studies indicate that infection is common with ACS, and may involve gram-positive, gram-negative, or atypical bacteria. Oxygen therapy is indicated for all patients who are hypoxic or in acute distress. In a patient with a history of reactive airway disease or wheezing on examination, a trial of bronchodilators is appropriate. Transfusions are often used in the treatment of acute lung disease.[5,13,27,70]

Steroids may decrease inflammation and endothelial cell adhesion. Use of glucocorticoids has been associated with decreases in hospital stay, transfusions, and need for other supportive care. However, higher readmission rates for SCA-related complications was also reported. Another promising therapy is the use of NO. NO inhalation relaxes and dilates blood vessels. Its hematologic effects include inhibition of platelet aggregation and reduced polymerization tendency of HbS. Marked improvement of pulmonary status and cardiac output have been reported in a patient with ACS. Both inhaled NO and oral L-arginine, the precursor of NO, are being evaluated for management of ACS.[27,71]

■ PRIAPISM

Stuttering priapism, episodes that last a few minutes to 2 hours, resolve spontaneously. Prolonged episodes lasting more than 2 to 3 hours require prompt medical attention. The initial goals of treatment are to provide appropriate analgesic therapy, reduce anxiety, produce detumescence, and preserve testicular function and fertility. Treatment given within 4 to 6 hours can usually reduce erection. Aggressive hydration and adequate pain control should be initiated. Use of ice packs is not recommended. Although transfusions have been given to these patients, the usefulness of this therapeutic intervention has not been established.[1,5,72]

CLINICAL CONTROVERSY

Some clinicians transfuse patients to maintain an HbS level less than 30% to prevent recurrent priapism. Duration of such regimens should be limited to 6 to 12 months.

Clinicians have used both vasoconstrictors and vasodilators in the treatment of priapism. Vasoconstrictors, such as phenylephrine or epinephrine, are thought to work by forcing blood out of the corpus cavernosum into the venous return. Epinephrine use has been associated with increases in heart rate and blood pressure. In one prospective nonrandomized unblinded study, aspiration followed by intrapenile irrigation with epinephrine was effective and well tolerated. In that study, as much blood as possible was aspirated from the corpus cavernosum, and the area was irrigated with a 1:1,000,000 solution of epinephrine.[73] The priapism resolved in 37 of the 39 occasions in which it was used. The therapy was well tolerated with no serious immediate or long-term side effects. On two occasions, a small intrapenile hematoma formed after treatment.

Vasodilators, such as terbutaline and hydralazine, induce relaxation of the smooth muscle of the vasculature. It is suggested that this relaxation allows oxygenated arterial blood to enter the corpus cavernosum, which displaces or washes out the damaged sickle cells that are stagnant in the corpus cavernosum. Terbutaline has been used to treat priapism, but it has not been formally studied in patients with SCA. Surgical interventions used in severe refractory priapism have included a variety of shunt procedures. These surgical procedures have been successful in some cases, but they have a high failure rate and serious complications, which include skin sloughing, cellulitis, and urethral fistulas.[5]

Modalities to prevent priapism are limited and not well studied. Pseudoephedrine (30 or 60 mg/day given orally at bedtime) and leuprolide, a gonadotropin-releasing hormone, have been used to decrease the number of recurrent episodes of priapism. Hydroxyurea therapy may also be useful. Recently, low-doses of an antiandrogen, bicalutamide, have been used in two patients with SCD and one patient with spinal cord injury for treatment of recurrent and refractory priapism without major side effects.[5,13,41,74]

MANAGEMENT OF CRISES

APLASTIC CRISIS

Treatment of aplastic crisis is primarily supportive and most patients recover spontaneously. The patient may need blood transfusions if anemia is severe or symptomatic. Reticulotye count helps to determine if there is red cell production and the need for transfusions. The most common cause for aplastic crisis is acute infection with human parvovirus B19. Parvovirus is contagious; therefore infected patients should be placed in isolation. In addition, contact with pregnant health care providers should be avoided because parvovirus infection during the midtrimester of pregnancy may result in hydrops fetalis and stillbirth.[4,5,13,41]

SEQUESTRATION CRISIS

Splenic sequestration crisis is a major cause of mortality in young patients with SCD. The sequestration of RBCs in the spleen may result in a rapid drop of hematocrit, leading to hypovolemia, shock, and death. Immediate treatment is red cell transfusion to correct hypovolemia. Broad-spectrum antibiotic therapy, which includes coverage for pneumococci and *H. influenzae,* may also be beneficial, because infection may precipitate crises.[4,5,13,41]

Recurrent episodes are common; approximately 50% in one study, and are associated with mortality. Options for management of recurrence include observation, chronic transfusion, and splenectomy. Observation is common in adults because they tend to have milder episodes. Increased risk of invasive infection after splenectomy is a concern in young children. Chronic transfusion may allow delaying splenectomy and temporarily restore splenic function, but it is associated with its own risks. Splenectomy is probably indicated, even after a single sequestration crisis, if that event is life-threatening. Splenectomy should be considered after repetitive episodes, even if they are less serious. For children less than 2 years of age, chronic blood transfusions have been recommended to prevent sequestration and to delay splenectomy until the age of 2, when the risk of post-splenectomy septicemia is less. Finally, splenectomy should also be considered for patients with chronic hypersplenism.[1,4,5,13]

VASO-OCCLUSIVE PAIN CRISIS

Hydration and analgesia are the mainstays of treatment for vaso-occlusive (painful) crises (Table 101–7). Mild pain crisis may be treated on an outpatient basis with rest, increased fluid intake, warm compresses, and oral analgesics. Hospitalization is necessary for moderate to severe crisis. Since infection can precipitate crises, an infectious etiology should be ruled out and appropriate empiric therapy should be initiated in patients with fever or patients who are critically ill. In patients who are anemic, transfusion to maintain the Hgb level

at baseline may be needed. Fluid replacement given intravenously or orally at 1.5 times the maintenance requirement is recommended. Close monitoring of fluid status is essential as aggressive hydration, particularly with sodium-containing fluids, may lead to volume overload, ACS, and heart failure.[4,5,13,41]

There is great variability in the frequency and severity of acute pain episodes associated with SCD. Thus the pain should be assessed and analgesic therapy should be tailored for each patient. Pain scales can be useful to quantify the degree of pain. Several pain assessment tools are available. Unfortunately, they have not been validated for sickle cell pain. The health care provider should choose one tool appropriate for age and use it routinely to assess pain. Other useful information to guide choice of analgesics should include previous effective agents and their dosages, response to therapy and previous clinical course, and duration of pain crisis.[28,75–77]

8 Aggressive therapy to relieve pain and enable the patient to attain maximum functional ability should be initiated in patients with pain crisis. Treatment of mild to moderate pain should include the use of nonsteroidal anti-inflammatory drugs (NSAIDs) or acetaminophen, unless there are contraindications to their use. Ketorolac is the only injectable NSAID available and is useful for patients requiring intravenous therapy. Due to concerns about gastrointestinal bleeding, it is recommended to limit the duration of therapy to 5 days or less. When acetaminophen is used, it is important to review the total dose of acetaminophen administered in patients who may also be receiving the agent for fever or other acetaminophen-containing product for pain. If mild to moderate pain persists, an opioid should be added. Effective combination therapy, such as an NSAID combined with an opioid, may enhance analgesic efficacy while decreasing side effects.[28,75–77]

Severe pain should be treated aggressively until the pain is tolerable. Commonly used opioids include morphine, hydromorphone, fentanyl, and methadone. The weak opioids, codeine and hydrocodone, are used to manage moderate pain. Meperidine has no advantages as an analgesic. Its duration of action is short compared to the half-life of the metabolite, normeperidine. The accumulation of normeperidine can cause central nervous system side effects, ranging from dysphoria to seizures. Therefore it is recommended that meperidine should only be used for a very brief duration in patients who are allergic or intolerant to other opioids.[28,75–77]

Both prior history and current assessment are important considerations when managing pain crisis. For patients whose typical crisis improves in a short time, preparations with a short duration of action are appropriate. For patients whose crises require many days to resolve, sustained-release preparations combined with a short-acting product for breakthrough pain are more appropriate. If the patient has been on long-term opioid therapy at home, tolerance may develop. In these cases, the pain of acute crises can be treated with a different potent opioid or a larger dose of the same medication. Intravenous administration provides a rapid onset of action and therefore is preferred for severe pain. Intramuscular injections should be avoided. Children may actually deny pain because of fear of injections. Analgesics should be titrated to pain relief. In patients with continuous pain, the analgesic should be given as a scheduled dose or continuous infusion. Continuous infusion has the advantage of less fluctuation of blood levels between dosing intervals. As-needed dosing is only appropriate for breakthrough pain. Patient-controlled analgesia (PCA) is commonly utilized. When used properly, PCA allows patients (or their families) to have control over pain therapy and minimizes the lag time between perception of pain and administration of analgesics. The transdermal fentanyl patch has also been used successfully. Its role in sickle cell pain crisis remains uncertain due to its long duration of 12 to 16 hours to achieve therapeutic effect and

TABLE 101–7. Management of Acute Pain of SCD

Principles
- Treat underlying precipitating factors
- Avoid delays in analgesia administration
- Use pain scale to assess severity
- Choice of initial analgesic should be based on previous pain crisis pattern, history of response, current status, and other medical conditions
- Schedule pain medication; avoid as-needed dosing
- Provide rescue dose for breakthrough pain
- If adequate pain relief can be achieved with one or two doses of morphine, consider outpatient management with a weak opioid; otherwise hospitalization is needed for parenteral analgesics
- Frequently assess to evaluate pain severity and side effects; titrate dose as needed
- Treating adverse effects of opioids is part of pain management
- Consider nonpharmacologic intervention
- Transition to oral analgesics as the patient improves; choose an oral agent based on previous history, anticipated duration, and ability to swallow tablets; if sustained-release products are used, a fast-release product is also needed for breakthrough pain

Analgesic regimens

Mild to moderate pain:

Acetaminophen with codeine
    Dose based on codeine—children: 1 mg/kg per dose every 6 h; adult: 30–60 mg/dose

Hydrocodone + acetaminophen
    Dose based on hydrocodone—children: 0.2 mg/kg per dose every 6 h; adults: 5–10 mg/dose

Anti-inflammatory agents
    Use with caution in patients with renal failure (dehydration) and bleeding
    Ibuprofen—children: 10 mg/kg every 6–8 h; adult: 200–400 mg/dose
    Naproxen: 5 mg/kg every 12 h; adult 250–500 mg/dose
    Ibuprofen + hydrocodone: Each tablet contains 200 mg ibuprofen and 7.5 mg hydrocodone per tablet; only for older children who can swallow tablets

Moderate to severe pain:

Morphine: 0.1–0.15 mg/kg per dose every 3–4 h for children; 5–10 mg/dose for adults
    Continuous infusion: 0.04–0.05 mg/kg per h; titrate to effect

Hydromorphone: 0.015 mg/kg per dose every 3–4 h for children; 1.5–2 mg/dose for adults
    Continuous infusion: 0.004 mg/kg per h; titrate to effect

Intravenous anti-inflammatory agents:
    Ketorolac: 0.5 mg/kg up to 30 mg/dose every 6 h

Patient-controlled analgesics:
    Morphine: 0.01–0.03 mg/kg per h basal; demand 0.01–0.03 mg/kg every 6–10 min; 4 h lock out 0.4–0.6 mg/kg
    Hydromorphone: 0.003–0.005 mg/kg per h basal; demand 0.03–0.05 mg/kg every 6–10 min; 4 h lock out 0.06–0.08 mg/kg

Rescue therapy:
    For breakthrough, give 1/4 to 1/2 of the scheduled dose as bolus every 1–2 h; assess amount of rescue dose used in 8–12 h and readjust scheduled dose or infusion rate as needed

Other adjunct therapy:
    Hydration, heating pads, relaxation, and distraction
    Stool softener and/or stimulants for constipation
    Antihistamine for itching
    Antiemetics for nausea or vomiting

From Yale,[28] Jacob et al,[75] Berde et al,[76] Stinson et al,[77] Christensen et al,[78] and Elander et al.[79]

fixed dosage form, which makes it difficult to titrate the dose. Other alternative pain management techniques such as physical therapy and relaxation therapy can be helpful as adjunct therapy.[28,75–78]

The most common issue leading to suboptimal pain control in children with SCA is the suspicion of addiction. This obstacle is especially common in adolescents. In one study, 53% of emergency physicians believed that 20% of SCD patients are addicted to analgesics. Elander and associates interviewed 51 SCD patients and utilized symptoms described in the *Diagnostic and Statistical Manual of Mental Disorders, Fourth Edition* to assess substance dependence.[79] They reported that when pain-related symptoms are included, 31% met criteria for substance dependence, but when symptoms are restricted those that are not pain-related, only 2% met the criteria for substance dependence. Another barrier for effective pain control is the difference in perception between patients, family, and health care providers. Patients with SCD often suffer from chronic pain and they may cope with the pain by being inactive. Patients who have inad-

equate pain control may exhibit anxiety and drug-seeking behavior for fear of pain. Tolerance to narcotics can also be misinterpreted as drug addiction by health care providers and families. Aggressive pain control, frequent monitoring of pain during crises, and tapering medication according to response are factors that minimize physical dependence.[28,75–79]

Agents Under Development: Purified Poloxamer 188

Poloxamer 188 (Flocor), a highly purified poloxamer, is an agent currently being evaluated under orphan drug status for the management of vaso-occlusive pain crisis in SCD. It acts as a surfactant and normalizes the RBC to its nonadhesive state. In addition, it enhances blood flow in ischemic areas by blocking RBC aggregation. The antiadhesive and hemorheologic properties result in improved blood flow, increased oxygen delivery, and decreased cell injury. A Phase II inical study conducted in adults and children aged 8 to 65 years d with vaso-occlusive crises reported a faster resolution. Patients ounger than 15 years and those who were receiving hydroxyurea

therapy were two groups that appeared to have the most beneficial effect.[80] Another Phase III study in patients younger than 15 years with vaso-occlusive crisis has been planned.[81]

PHARMACOECONOMIC CONSIDERATIONS

eing a chronic condition, SCD has a significant impact on health re costs. Pharmacoeconomic considerations should include new- orn screening, cost of managing acute and chronic complications, nd the economic impact of new treatment modalities. Early peni- llin prophylaxis prevents pneumococcal sepsis in infants. Newborn creening targeted at African-Americans has been shown to be cost- ffective. Whether it is cost-effective to screen all infants depends on e prevalence of high-risk infants in the area. The estimated annual ost through universal screening programs ranged from $1,402 in Mississippi to $304,215 in Vermont per case identified. In general, niversal screening identifies more infants with disease, prevents more eaths, and may provide for a certain degree of cost-effectiveness nce targeted screening may not detect all infants with the disease.[8,82]

Hospitalization is an important societal financial burden. A 1996 ational estimate reported the average cost per hospitalization to be 6300, which totals a cost of $475 million per year. Studies conducted various regions have shown that a small number of patients consume disproportionate amount of care as a result of severe illness, and most f the total cost results from hospitalization. Patients who are not be- g followed in settings that provide comprehensive medical care tend acquire higher costs for emergency room and hospital visits. An- her study examining relationships between socioeconomic factors nd geographic distribution in Alabama reported that utilization of omprehensive care was lower for those living in rural areas. Using mathematical model and data available from studies, researchers stimated lifetime costs for SCA and other hemoglobinopathies to e $83,200 for patients with early diagnoses and $78,400 for late iagnosis.[3,8,83–85]

Newer therapies, diagnostic methods such as TCD, and chronic ansfusions further increase cost. The cost of a year of hydroxyurea erapy has been estimated to be $2000. Utilizing the data from the MSH trial, Moore and colleagues reported that the average annual cost r medical care was lower in the hydroxyurea group as compared with e placebo group ($12,160 vs. $22,020). Hospitalization due to pain risis accounted for the highest cost in both groups and was lower r the hydroxyurea group ($12,160 vs. $17,290). Allogeneic HSCT an potentially cure the disease, and if successful can reduce long- rm costs, but it requires a high up-front cost. The new therapies, lthough expensive, may keep patients out of emergency departments nd inpatient beds, improving the cost-effectiveness of those therapies ver a patient's lifetime.[7,86]

EVALUATION OF THERAPEUTIC OUTCOMES

CD is a complex disorder that requires multidisciplinary compre- ensive care. All patients should be medically evaluated regularly to stablish baseline, monitor changes, and provide education appropri- te for age. For infants less than a year old, medical evaluations every to 4 months are needed. Beyond 1 year of age, evaluation can be xtended to every 6 to 12 months with modifications depending on everity of the illness.[41]

It is important to establish baseline laboratory values and imag- ng studies. Routine laboratory evaluation includes complete blood

cell counts and reticulocyte counts every 3 months up to 2 years of age, then every 6 months; HbF level should be taken every 6 months until 2 years of age, then annually. Evaluation of renal, hepatobiliary, and pulmonary function should be done annually. TCD screening is recommended to start at age 2, then annually. Ophthalmologic exam- ination to screen for retinopathy is recommended at around age 10. In patients with recurrent ACS, pulmonary function tests should be done to establish baseline and identify declines in lung function.

It is essential to ensure that prophylactic immunizations and anti- biotics are being given. When infections do occur, appropriate antibi- otic therapy should be initiated and the patient should be monitored for laboratory and clinical improvement. The efficacy of hydroxyurea can best be assessed in terms of the decrease in number, severity, and duration of sickle cell pain crises. Fetal hemoglobin concentrations or MCV values may also provide some indication of the patient's re- sponse to therapy. When painful crises do occur, the evaluation of the effectiveness of analgesics depends mainly on the subjective assess- ments made by the patient, family, and health care practitioners. The success of poststroke blood transfusions can be measured by clinical progression or the occurrence of subsequent strokes.

CONCLUSION

The goals of the general management of SCA are to decrease the num- ber of sickle cell crises, to decrease the complications arising from the disease, and to improve the overall quality of the patient's life. The general care of SCA patients still includes early penicillin prophy- laxis and appropriate immunization. HbF inducers such as hydroxy- urea may decrease the frequency and severity of painful episodes. Continued studies of other possible agents and treatment modalities that may reduce crises or reverse organ damage are warranted.

ABBREVIATIONS

ACS: acute chest syndrome
ASPEN syndrome: association of sickle cell disease, priapism, exchange transfusion, and neurologic events
HbAS: one normal and one sickle hemoglobin gene
HbC: hemoglobin C
HbF: fetal hemoglobin
HbSβ^+-thal, HbSβ^0-thal: hemoglobin sickle β^+-thalassemia and hemoglobin sickle β^0-thalassemia
HbSC: sickle-hemoglobin C
HbSS: homozygous sickle hemoglobin
HbS: sickle hemoglobin
HSCT: hematopoietic stem cell transplantation
ISC: irreversibly sickled cell
MCHC: mean corpuscular hemoglobin concentration
MCV: mean corpuscular volume
MSH: Multicenter Study of Hydroxyurea in Sickle Cell Anemia
NO: nitric oxide
NSAID: nonsteroidal anti-inflammatory drug
PCA: patient-controlled analgesia
PCV 7: 7-valent pneumococcal conjugate vaccine

PPV 23: 23-valent pneumococcal polysaccharide vaccine
RBC: red blood cell
SCA: sickle cell anemia
SCD: sickle cell disease
SCT: sickle cell trait
TCD: transcranial Doppler
WBC: white blood cell

Learning Objectives and other resources can be found at *www.pharmacotherapyonline.com.*

REFERENCES

1. Fixler J, Styles L. Sickle cell disease. Pediatr Clin North Am 2002;49:1193–1210.
2. Eaton WA. Linus Pauling and sickle cell disease. Biophys Chem 2003;100:109–116.
3. Davis H, Moore RM, Gergen PJ. Cost of hospitalizations associated with sickle cell disease in the United States. Public Health Rep 1997;112:40–43.
4. Ad Hoc writing Committee, American Academy of Pediatrics. Health supervision for children with sickle cell disease. Pediatrics 2002;109:526–535.
5. National Institutes of Health. The Management of Sickle Cell Disease. NIH Pub. No. 02-2117. Bethesda, MD, Division of Blood Diseases and Resources, Public Health Service, U.S. Department of Health and Human Services, June 2002:1–88.
6. Ashley-Koch A, Yang Q, Olney RS. Sickle hemoglobin (HbS) allele and sickle cell disease: A huge review. Am J Epidemiol 2000;151:839–844.
7. Benz EJ. Hemoglobinopathies 2001–2003. Available at *http://www.harrisonsonline.com*. Accessed July 16, 2003.
8. Nietert PJ, Silverstein MD, Abboud MR. Sickle cell anaemia epidemiology and cost of illness. Pharmacoeconomics 2002;20:357–366.
9. Steensma DP, Hoyer JD, Fairbanks VF. Hereditary red blood cell disorders in Middle Eastern patients. Mayo Clin Proc 2001;76:285–293.
10. Nagel RL, Fleming AF. Genetic epidemiology of the beta s gene. Baillieres Clin Haematol 1992;5:331–365.
11. El-Hazmi MA, Warsy AS, Bashir N, et al. Haplotypes of beta-globin gene as prognostic factors in sickle-cell disease. East Mediterr Health J 1999;5:1154–1158.
12. Schrier SL. Hemoglobinopathies and Hemolytic Anemias. WebMD Scientific American Medicine. Available at *http://www.samed.com*. Accessed August 3, 2003.
13. Dover GJ, Platt OS. Sickle cell disease. In: Nathan DG, Orkin SH, Ginsburg D, Lock AT, eds. Nathan and Oski's Hematology and Infancy and Childhood, 6th ed. Philadelphia, WB Saunders, 2003:790–841.
14. Parise LV, Telen MJ. Erythrocyte adhesion in sickle cell disease. Cur Hematol Rep 2003;2:102–108.
15. Quinn CT, Rogers ZR, Buchanan GR. Survival of children with sickle cell disease. Blood 2004;103:4023–4027.
16. Miller ST, Sleeper LA, Pegelow CH, et al. Prediction of adverse outcomes in children with sickle cell disease. N Engl J Med 2000;342:83–89.
17. Prasad R, Hasan S, Castro O, et al. Long-term outcomes in patients with sickle cell disease and frequent vaso-occlusive crises. Am J Med Sci 2003;325:107–109.
18. Hord J, Byrd R, Stowe L, et al. *Streptococcus pneumoniae* sepsis and meningitis during the penicillin prophylaxis era in children with sickle cell disease. J Pediatr Hematol Oncol 2002;24:470–472.
19. Smithy-Whitley K, Zhao H, Hodinka RL, et al. The epidemiology of human parvovirus B 19 in children with sickle cell disease. Blood 2004;103:422–427.
20. Pegelow CH, Mackoin EA, Moser FG, et al. Longitudinal changes in brain magnetic resonance imaging findings in children with sickle cell disease. Blood 2002;15:3014–3018.
21. Kral MC, Brown RT, Nietert PJ, et al. Transcranial Doppler ultrasonography and neurocognitive functioning in children with sickle cell disease. Pediatrics 2003;112:324–331.
22. Miller ST, Macklin EA, Pegelow CH, et al. Silent infarction as a risk factor for overt stroke in children with sickle cell anemia: A report from the Cooperative Study of Sickle Cell Disease. J Pediatr 2001;139:385–390.
23. Dean D, Neumayr L, Kelly DM, et al. *Chlamydia pneumoniae* and acute chest syndrome in patients with sickle cell disease. J Pediatr Hematol Oncol 2003;25:46–55.
24. Siddiqui AK, Ahmed S. Pulmonary manifestations of sickle cell disease. Postgrad Med J 2003;79:384–390.
25. Vichinsky EP, Neumayr LD, Earles AE, et al. Causes and outcomes of the acute chest syndrome in sickle cell disease. N Engl J Med 2000;342:1855–1865.
26. Neumayr L, Lennette E, Kelly D, et al. Mycoplasma disease and acute chest syndrome in sickle cell disease. Pediatrics 2003;112:87–95.
27. Vichinsky E. Novel therapeutic approaches in sickle cell disease: Understanding the pathophysiology and treatment of pulmonary injury in sickle cell disease. Hematology (Am Soc Itematol Educ Program) 2002;16–22.
28. Yale SH. Approach to the vaso-occlusive crisis in adults with sickle cell disease. Am Fam Physician 2000;61:1349–1356, 1363–1364.
29. Kellermayer R, Faden H, Grossi M. Clinical presentation of parvovirus B19 infection in children with aplastic crisis. Pediatr Infect Dis J 2003;22:1100–1101.
30. Gladwin MT, Sachdev V, Jison ML, et al. Pulmonary hypertension as a risk factor for death in patients with sickle cell disease. N Engl J Med 2004;350:886–895.
31. Henry M, Driscoll CM, Miller M, et al. Pseudotumor cerebri in children with sickle cell disease: a case series. Pediatrics 2004;113:e265–269.
32. Mukisi-Mukaza M, Samuel-Leborge Y, Keclard L, et al. Prevalence, clinical features and risk factors of osteonecrosis of the femoral head among adults with sickle cell disease. Orthopedics 2000;23:357–363.
33. Hasan S, Elbedawi M, Castro O, et al. Central retinal vein occlusion in sickle cell disease. South Med J 2004;97:202–204.
34. Babalola OE, Wambebe CO. When should children and young adults with sickle cell disease be referred for eye assessment? Afr J Med Med Sci 2001;30:261–263.
35. de Montalembert M, Maunoury C, Acar P, et al. Myocardial ischaemia in children with sickle cell disease. Arch Dis Child 2004;89:359–362.
36. Hassan SP, Hashmi S, Alhassen M, et al. Depression in sickle cell disease. J Natl Med Assoc 2003;95:533–537.
37. Schatz J, Finke RL, Kellett JM, Kramer JH. Cognitive functioning in children with sickle cell disease: a metaanalysis. J Pediatr Psychol 2002;27:739–748.
38. Adamkiewicz TV, Sarnaik S, Buchanan GR, et al. Invasive pneumococcal infections in children with sickle cell disease in the era of penicillin prophylaxis antibiotic resistance and 23-valent pneumococcal polysaccharide vaccination. J Pediatr 2003;143:438–444.
39. Advisory Committee on Immunization Practices, CDC. Preventing pneumococcal disease among infants and young children. Morb Mortal Wkly Rep 2000;49:1–38.
40. Committee on Infectious Diseases, American Academy of Pediatrics. Policy Statement: Recommendations for the prevention of pneumococcal infections, including the use of pneumococcal conjugate vaccine (Prevnar) pneumococcal polysaccharide vaccine, and antibiotic prophylaxis. Pediatrics 2000;106:362–366.
41. Sickle Cell Disease Care Consortium. Sickle cell disease in children and adolescents: diagnosis, guidelines for comprehensive care, and care paths and protocols for management of acute and chronic complications, November 2001. Available at *http://www.tdh.texas.gov/newborn/sedona02.htm*. Accessed August 26, 2003.
42. Falletta JM, Woods RM, Verter JI, et al. Discontinuing penicillin prophylaxis in children with sickle cell anemia. J Pediatr 1995;127:685–690.
43. Kennedy TS, Fung EB, Kawchak DA, et al. Red blood cell folate and serum vitamin B12 status in children with sickle cell disease. J Pediatr Hematol Oncol 2001;23:165–169.
44. Rodriguez-Cortes HM, Griener JC, Hyland K, et al. Plasma homocysteine levels and folate status in children with sickle cell anemia. J Pediatr Hematol Oncol 1999;21:219–223.
45. Rabb LM, Grandision Y, Mason K, et al. A trial of folate supplementation in children with homozygous sickle cell disease. Br J Hematol 1983;54:589–594.

46. Charache S, Barton FB, Moore RD, et al. Hydroxyurea and sickle cell anemia: clinical utility of a myelosuppressive "switching" agent. Medicine 1996;75:300–326.

47. Nathan DG. Search for improved therapy of sickle cell anemia. J Pediatr Hematol Oncol 2002;24:700–703.

48. Cokic VP, Smith RD, Beleslin-Cokic BB, et al. Hydroxyurea induces fetal hemoglobin by the nitric oxide-dependent activation of soluble guanylyl cyclase. J Clin Invest 2003;111:231–239.

49. Gladwin MT, Schechter AN. Nitric oxide therapy in sickle cell disease. Semin Hematol 2001;38:333–342.

50. Charache S, Terrin ML, Moore RD, et al. Effect of hydroxyurea on the frequency of painful crises in sickle cell anemia. N Engl J Med 1995;332:1317–1322.

51. Steinbert MH, Bartin F, Castro O, et al. Effect of hydroxyurea on mortality and morbidity in adult sickle cell anemia. Risks and benefits up to 9 years of treatment. JAMA 2003;289:1645–1651.

52. National Heart, Lung and Blood Institute (NHLBI). Hydroxyurea in pediatric patients with sickle cell disease: fact sheet. *http://www.nhlbi.nih.gov/health/public/blood/sickle/hydrox.htm*, June 1998. Accessed September 2003.

53. National Heart, Lung, and Blood Institute (NHLBI). Pediatric hydroxyurea in sickle cell anemia (BABY HUG). Study details. *http://www.clinicaltrials.gov*. Accessed September 2003.

54. Zimmerman SA, Schultz WH, Davis JS, et al. Sustained long-term hematological efficacy of hydroxyurea at maximal tolerated dose in children with sickle cell disease. Blood 2004;103:2039–2045.

55. Wilson S. Acute leukemia in a patient with sickle cell anemia treated with hydroxyurea (Letter). Ann Intern Med 2000;133:925–926.

56. Najean Y, Rain JD. Treatment of polycythemia vera: Use of 32P alone or in combination with maintenance therapy using hydroxyurea in 461 patients greater than 65 years of age. Blood 1997;89:2319–2327.

57. Atweh GF, Sutton M, Nassif I, et al. Sustained induction of fetal hemoglobin by pulse butyrate therapy in sickle cell disease. Blood 1999;93:1790–1797.

58. Resar LMS, Segal JB, Fitzpatric LK, et al. Induction of fetal hemoglobin synthesis in children with sickle cell anemia on low-dose oral sodium phenylbutyrate therapy. J Pediatr Hematol Oncol 2002;24:737–741.

59. Saunthararajah Y, Hillery CA, Lavelle D, et al. Effects of 5-aza-2-deoxycytidine on fetal hemoglobin levels, red cell adhesion and hematopoietic differentiation in patients with sickle cell disease. Blood 2003;102:3865–3870.

60. Scothorn DJ, Price C, Schawartz D, et al. Risk of recurrent stroke in children with sickle cell disease receiving blood transfusion therapy for at least five years after initial stroke. J Pediatr 2002;140:348–354.

61. Pegelow CH, Adams RJ, McKie V, et al. Risk of recurrent stroke in patients with sickle cell disease treated with erythrocyte transfusions. J Pediatr 1995;126:896–899.

62. Russell MO, Goldberg HI, Hodson A, et al. Effect of transfusion therapy on arteriographic abnormalities and on recurrence of stroke in sickle cell disease. Blood 1984;63:162–169.

63. Adams RJ, McKie VC, Hsu L, et al. Prevention of a first stroke by transfusions in children with sickle cell anemia and abnormal results on transcranial doppler ultrasonography. N Engl J Med 1998;339:5–11.

64. Harmatz P, Butensky E, Quirolo K, et al. Severity of iron overload in patients with sickle cell disease receiving chronic red blood cell transfusion therapy. Blood 2000;96:76–79.

65. Walters MC, Storb R, Patience M, et al. Impact of bone marrow transplan-

66. Atkins RC, Walters MC. Haematopoietic cell transplantation in the treatment of sickle cell disease. Expert Opin Biol Ther 2003;3:1215–1224.

67. Brachet C, Azzi N, Demulder A, et al. Hydroxyurea treatment for sickle cell disease: Impact on haematopoietic stem cell transplantation's outcome. Bone Marrow Transplant 2004;33:779–803.

68. Baron F, Dresse MF, Beguin Y. Transmission of chronic myeloid leukemia through peripheral-blood stem-cell transplantation. N Engl J Med 2003;349:913–914.

69. Walters MC. Novel therapeutic approaches in sickle cell disease: Stem cell transplantation for sickle cell disease: How and when to intervene? Hematology (Am Soc Itematol Edu Program) 2002;22–29.

70. Knight-Madden J, Hambleton I. Inhaled bronchodilators for acute chest syndrome in people with sickle cell disease. Cochrane Database Syst Rev 2003;3:CD003733.

71. Sullivan KJ, Goodwin SR, Evangelist J, et al. Nitric oxide successfully used to treat acute chest syndrome of sickle cell disease in a young adolescent. Crit Care Med 1999;27:2563–2568.

72. Li M, Fogarty J, Whitney KD, Stone P. Repeated testicular infarction in a patient with sickle cell disease: A possible mechanism for testicular failure. Urology 2003;62:551.

73. Mantadakis E, Ewalt DH, Cavender JD, et al. Outpatient penile aspiration and epinephrine irrigation for young patients with sickle cell anemia and prolonged priapism. Blood 2000;95:78–82.

74. Dahm P, Rao DS, Donatucci CF. Antiandrogens in the treatment of priapism, case report. Urology 2002;59:138.

75. Jacob E, Miaskowski C, Savedra M, et al. Management of vaso-occlusive pain in children with sickle cell disease. J Pediatr Hematology Oncology 2003;25:307–311.

76. Berde CB, Sethna NF. Analgesics for the treatment of pain in children. N Engl J Med 2002;347:1094.

77. Stinson J, Naser B. Pain management in children with sickle cell disease. Paediatr Drugs 2003;5:229–238.

78. Christensen ML, Wang WC, Harris S, et al. Transdermal fentanyl administration in children and adolescents with sickle cell pain crisis. J Pediatr Hematol Oncol 1996;18:372–376.

79. Elander J, Lusher J, Bevan D, et al. Pain management and symptoms of substance dependence among patients with sickle cell disease. Soc Sci Med 2003;7:1683–1696.

80. Orringer EP, Casella JF, Ataga KI, et al. Purified poloxamer 188 for treatment of acute vaso-occlusive crisis of sickle cell disease, a randomized controlled trial. JAMA 2001;286:2099–2106.

81. Flocor overview. CytRx Corporation. Available at *http://www.cytrx.com*. Accessed April 25, 2004.

82. Panepinto JA, Magid D, Rewers MJ, Lane PA. Universal versus targeted screening of infants for sickle cell disease: a cost effectiveness analysis. J Pediatr 2000;136:201–208.

83. Woods K, Karrison T, Koshy M, et al. Hospital utilization patterns and costs for sickle cell patients in Illinois. Public Health Rep 1997;112:44–51.

84. Nietert PJ, Abboud MR, Zoller JS, Silverstein MD. Costs, charges and reimbursements for persons with sickle cell disease. J Pediatr Hematol Oncol 1999;21:389–396.

85. Telfair J, Haque A, Etienne M, et al. Rural/urban difference in access to and utilization of services among people in Alabama with sickle cell disease. Public Health Rep 2003;118:27–36.

86. Moore RD, Charache S, Errin ML, et al. Cost-effectiveness of hydroxyurea in sickle cell anemia. Am J Hematol 2000;64:26–31.

102

DRUG-INDUCED HEMATOLOGIC DISORDERS

S. Jay Weaver and Thomas E. Johns

Learning Objectives and other resources can be found at *www.pharmacotherapyonline.com.*

KEY CONCEPTS

◀1 Drug-induced hematologic disorders are, in general, rare adverse effects associated with drug therapy.

◀2 The most common drug-induced hematologic disorders include aplastic anemia, agranulocytosis, megaloblastic anemia, thrombocytopenia, and hemolytic anemia.

◀3 Reporting during postmarketing surveillance of a drug is usually the method by which the incidence of rare adverse drug reactions is established.

◀4 Because drug-induced blood disorders are dangerous, rechallenging a patient with a suspected agent in an attempt to confirm a diagnosis may not be ethical.

◀5 The mechanisms of drug-induced hematologic disorders are thought to be the result of direct toxicity or an immune reaction.

◀6 The primary treatment of drug-induced hematologic disorders is removal of the drug in question and symptomatic support of the patient.

◀7 Frequent laboratory monitoring may be warranted for agents commonly demonstrating severe hematologic reactions.

Hematologic disorders have long been a potential risk of modern pharmacotherapy. Granulocytopenia (agranulocytosis) was reported in association with one of medicine's early therapeutic agents, sulphanilamide, in 1938.[1] Some agents cause predictable hematologic disease (e.g., antineoplastics), but others induce idiosyncratic reactions not directly related to the drugs' pharmacology. Such drug-induced hematologic disorders may include aplastic anemia, agranulocytosis, megaloblastic anemia, thrombocytopenia, and hemolytic anemia.[2]

◀1 By most reports, idiosyncratic drug-induced hematologic disorders are rare. Relatively few epidemiologic studies have addressed the actual incidence of these adverse reactions. A report from The Netherlands estimated the incidence of drug-associated agranulocytosis as 1.6 to 2.5 cases per million inhabitants per year.[3] Similar results were found in epidemiologic studies conducted in Thailand and Brazil.[4,5] Older data from a study conducted in Europe and Israel estimated the incidences of aplastic anemia and agranulocytosis to be 0.5 and 3.1 cases per million per year, respectively.[6]

◀2 Although rare, drug-induced hematologic disorders are important because they are associated with significant morbidity and mortality. An epidemiologic study held in the United States estimated that 4490 deaths in 1984 were attributable to blood dyscrasias from all causes. Aplastic anemia was the leading cause of death, followed by thrombocytopenia, agranulocytosis, and hemolytic anemia.[7] Like most other adverse drug reactions, drug-induced hematologic disorders are more common in the elderly than in the young; the risk of death also appears to be greater with increasing age. The risk of agranulocytosis has been reported to be higher in women than in men.[4]

◀3 Because of the seriousness of drug-induced hematologic disorders, it is necessary to track the development of these disorders in order to predict their occurrence and to estimate their incidence.

Reporting during postmarketing surveillance of a drug is the most common method of establishing the incidence of adverse drug reactions. The MedWatch program supported by the Food and Drug Administration is one such program.[8] Many facilities have similar drug-reporting programs to follow adverse drug reaction trends and to determine whether an association between a drug and an adverse drug reaction is causal or coincidental. In the case of drug-induced hematologic disorders, these programs can enable practitioners to confirm that an adverse event is indeed the result of drug therapy rather than one of many other potential causes; general guidelines are readily available.[9,10]

◀4 Because drug-induced blood disorders are dangerous, rechallenging a patient with a suspected agent in an attempt to confirm a diagnosis may not be ethical. In vitro studies with the offending agent and cells or plasma from the patient's blood can be performed to determine causality.[11] These methods are often expensive, however, and require facilities and expertise that are not generally available. One study demonstrated that only 19% of the cases with suspected drug-induced agranulocytosis could be documented by in vitro testing.[12]

The rarity and seriousness of drug-induced hematologic disorders make it extremely important that clinicians be able to evaluate suspect drugs quickly and to interrupt therapy when necessary. Throughout the past decades, lists of drugs that have been associated with adverse events have been developed to help clinicians identify possible causes of adverse events. Unfortunately, these lists are comprehensive and include commonly used drugs, making it difficult to elicit the root cause of any abnormality. Furthermore, the absence of a drug from such a list should not discourage the investigation and reporting of an agent associated with an adverse event. It is imperative that clinicians use a rational approach to determine causality and identify the agents associated with a reaction. Focusing on the issue, performing a high-quality investigation, developing appropriate criteria, using levels of evidence to grade the response, and having a quantifiable summary can all help to ensure the validity of the findings. A systematic approach to evaluate the information available in the literature also helps the clinician to focus and intervene in the cause of the disorder.

A common tool employed by clinicians to rate the likelihood of causality in adverse drug reaction (ADR) investigations is an ADR probability scale (algorithm). One such scale was developed and tested by Naranjo and colleagues.[13] This tool provides a series of scored questions that lead an investigator to the likelihood that an ADR was caused by the suspected medication. Depending on the aggregate score, the causality is rated as Doubtful, Possible, Probable, or Definite. The scale gives the most weight to the temporal relationship of the reaction with relation to administration of the drug, observations following a rechallenge of the patient with the suspected medication, and alternate explanations for the ADR. As mentioned above, it is often unethical to rechallenge patients who experience severe hematologic toxicities. Thus without a rechallenge it is difficult to achieve a causality rating of "definite" using such an algorithm.

In determining the likelihood that an observed reaction is due to a particular medication, clinicians should review the medical literature for past reports supporting the observation. Using an evidence-based approach such as that proposed by Sackett,[14] the investigator assigns greater weight to prospective study designs such as clinical trials or cohort studies than to case reports or expert opinion. This will provide a framework for the investigator's confidence in published literature describing ADRs.

In this chapter, we use both methods described to review and present published information on hematologic drug toxicities. When only case reports were available, the Naranjo algorithm was applied to the cases (if not already used). This algorithm was used for two reasons. First, the algorithm has been validated for interrater reliability.[13] The algorithm was also the most commonly applied algorithm by authors of the case reports evaluated for this chapter. Drugs rated as "Definite" and those rated as "Probable" when only a lack of rechallenge prevented a rating of "Definite" were included in the lists. An evidence-based approach was incorporated through a review of the medical literature for prospective and retrospective studies of the adverse reactions and medications of interest. Drugs significantly associated with an adverse reaction of interest through studies were also deemed to have a causal relationship to the reaction.

The understanding of drug-induced hematologic disorders requires a basic understanding of hematopoiesis (see Chap. 98 on hematopoiesis). The pluripotential hematopoietic stem cells in the bone marrow, which have the ability to self-reproduce, maintain the blood. These pluripotential hematopoietic stem cells are further differentiated to intermediate precursor cells, which are also called "progenitor cells" or "colony-forming cells." Committed to a particular cell line, these intermediate stem cells differentiate into colonies of each type of blood cell in response to a particular colony-stimulating factor (Fig. 102–1).

Drug-induced hematologic disorders can affect any cell line, including white blood cells (WBCs), red blood cells (RBCs), and platelets. When a drug causes decreases in all three cell lines accompanied by a hypoplastic bone marrow, the result is drug-induced

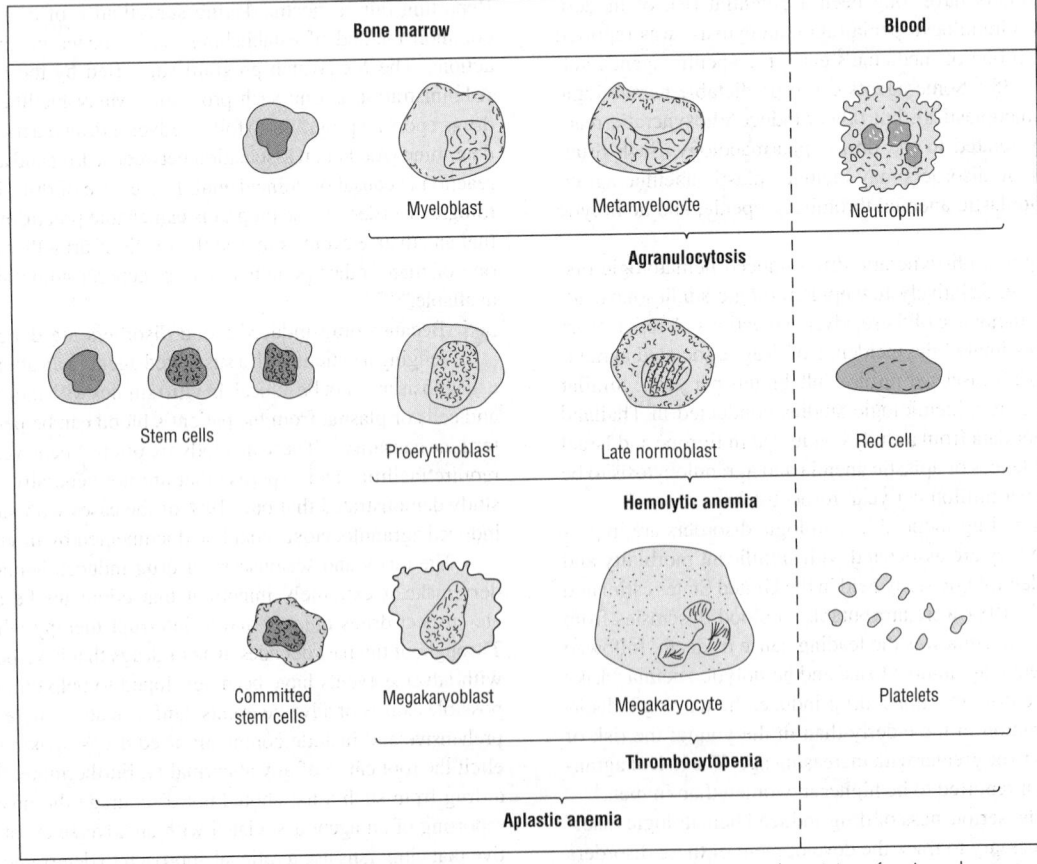

FIGURE 102–1. Differentiation of the stem cell into committed cell lines, illustrating the origins of various drug-induced hematologic disorders.

aplastic anemia. The decrease in WBC count alone by a medication is drug-induced agranulocytosis. Drugs can affect RBCs by causing a number of different anemias, including drug-induced immune hemolytic anemia, drug-induced oxidative hemolytic anemia, or drug-induced megaloblastic anemia. A drug-induced decrease in platelet count is drug-induced thrombocytopenia.

DRUG-INDUCED APLASTIC ANEMIA

Ehrlich first described aplastic anemia in 1888 following an episode of failed hematopoiesis identified during the autopsy of a pregnant woman.[15] Since then there have been 500 to 2500 cases reported annually, with up to 33% diagnosed in patients greater than 60 years of age.[15] A number of variables can incite immune destruction of the bone marrow; the most common are drugs, chemicals, toxins, viruses, and radiation.

Drug-induced aplastic anemia is classified as an acquired form of the disorder and accounts for 7% to 86% of cases of aplastic anemia.[16] It is considered the most serious drug-induced blood dyscrasia because of the associated high mortality rate, often exceeding 50% of treated cases.[17] It is characterized by pancytopenia (presence of anemia, neutropenia, and thrombocytopenia) with a hypocellular or "fatty" bone marrow and no gross evidence of increased peripheral blood cell destruction.[2] A diagnosis of aplastic anemia can be made by the presence of two of the following criteria: a WBC count of 3500/mm^3 or less, a platelet count of 55,000/mm^3 or less, or a hemoglobin value of 10 g/dL or less with a reticulocyte count of 30,000/mm^3 or less.[16] Severe aplastic anemia is defined by at least two of the following three peripheral blood findings: neutrophil count of less than 500/mm^3, platelet count of less than 20,000/mm^3, and anemia with a corrected reticulocyte index of less than 1%.[17,18] The prognosis is extremely poor if the neutrophil count declines to less than 200/mm^3.[19] A bone marrow aspirate and biopsy are required to exclude other causes of pancytopenia, including neoplastic infiltration or significant myelofibrosis.[20] There must also be no history of iatrogenic exposure to cytotoxic chemotherapy that is known to cause transient bone marrow suppression or to intensive radiation.

The onset of drug-induced aplastic anemia is variable and insidious. Symptoms appear on the average about 6.5 weeks after the initiation of the offending agent,[19] sometimes after the drug has been discontinued. Clinical features of drug-induced aplastic anemia depend on the degree to which each cell line is suppressed, similarly to idiopathic disease. Symptoms of anemia include pallor, fatigue, and weakness, while fever, chills, pharyngitis, or other infection may characterize neutropenia. Thrombocytopenia, often the initial clue to diagnosis, is manifest by easy bruisability, petechiae, and bleeding.

The incidence of drug-induced aplastic anemia is estimated at 2.5 to 7.8 cases per 1 million population per year.[6,21,22] Higher rates of occurrence have been seen in patients taking antirheumatic drugs such as indomethacin, penicillamine, and gold compounds.[17] Table 102–1 lists drugs that have been associated with drug-induced aplastic anemia.

The cause of drug-induced aplastic anemia is damage to the pluripotential hematopoietic stem cells, before their differentiation to committed stem cells. This damage effectively reduces the normal levels of circulating erythrocytes, neutrophils, and platelets. Three mechanisms have been proposed as causes of damage to the pluripotent hematopoietic stem cells.[23] The most common proposed mechanism is direct, dose-dependent drug toxicity. This type of injury leads to transient marrow failure secondary to direct sup-

TABLE 102–1. Drugs Associated with Aplastic Anemia

Observational study evidence	Case report evidence ("probable" or "definite" causality rating)
Carbamazepine	Acetazolamide
Diclofenac	Aspirin
Furosemide	Captopril
Gold salts	Chloramphenicol
Indomethacin	Chloroquine
Methimazole	Chlorothiazide
Oxyphenbutazone	Chlorpromazine
Penicillamine	Dapsone
Phenobarbital	Felbamate
Phenothiazines	Interferon-alfa
Phenytoin	Lisinopril
Propylthiouracil	Lithium
Sulfonamides	Pentoxifylline
Tocainide	Quinidine
	Sulindac
	Ticlopidine

pression of proliferating cell lines, and hematopoietic suppression continues with dose escalation. Most often caused by chemotherapy or radiotherapy, this injury is frequently iatrogenic. The second mechanism is idiosyncratic and operates through toxic metabolites. Furthermore, individual variations in the pharmacokinetics of the suspected agent or a hypersensitivity of the stem cells to the destructive effects of the implicated drug may increase the potential for apoptosis. The third mechanism is a drug- or metabolite-induced immune reaction specific to the stem cell population. It is proposed that immunologically mediated, tissue-specific organ destruction occurs following exposure to an inciting antigen (drug) that activates cells and cytokines of the immune system, leading to the death of stem cells.[23] There is little evidence that drug-induced aplastic anemia results from the destruction of the microenvironment of the bone marrow.[20]

The antineoplastic agents exemplify the dose-dependent mechanism for the development of aplastic anemia. Many of these agents have the ability to suppress one or more cell lines in a reversible manner. The degree of suppression and the cell line involved depend on the nature of the particular drug and its potential for inhibiting marrow proliferation. Chloramphenicol, an antimicrobial agent, also causes a bone marrow depression that is dose-dependent and reversible. In this reaction, chloramphenicol affects primarily the erythroid cell line due to an injury of the mitochondria, resulting in inhibition of protein synthesis with a subsequent reduction in reticulocytes and hematocrit.[24]

Idiosyncratic drug-induced aplastic anemia secondary to direct toxicity may be characterized by dose independence, a latent period prior to the onset of anemia, and continuance of the marrow injury following drug discontinuation.[25] Drugs that cause aplastic anemia in a minority of patients suggest an abnormal metabolism or excretion. Chloramphenicol, already known to cause a dose-dependent reaction, is the prototype drug for the idiosyncratic mechanism, with an approximate incidence of 1 case per 20,000 patients treated;[19] however, the overall prevalence has fallen with decreased use of this agent.[25] The idiosyncratic mechanism is believed to result from abnormal metabolism of chloramphenicol. The nitrobenzene ring on chloramphenicol is thought to be reduced to form a nitroso group on the chloramphenicol molecule.[24] The nitroso group may then interact with DNA in the stem cell, causing damage to the chromosomes, and eventually cell death. Other investigators have hypothesized that bacteria from the gastrointestinal tract may metabolize chloramphenicol to marrow-toxic metabolites.[26] There appears to be no relationship between the dose-dependent and idiosyncratic reactions seen with chloramphenicol.

Other drugs thought to induce aplastic anemia through toxic metabolites include phenytoin and carbamazepine. Investigators have theorized that metabolites from phenytoin and carbamazepine bind covalently to macromolecules in the cell, and then cause cell death either by exerting a direct toxic effect on the stem cell or by causing the death of lymphocytes involved in regulating hematopoiesis.[27]

Of the three potential mechanisms, the most common cause of drug-induced aplastic anemia is the development of an immune reaction. Early laboratory observations revealed that the removal of T lymphocytes from samples of patients with aplastic anemia improved in vitro colony formation.[28] Furthermore, overproduction of cytokines (e.g., tumor necrosis factor and interferon-γ) from activated T lymphocytes appears to be responsible for hematopoietic failure, as well as for the initiation of apoptosis.[29] Clinical evidence supporting this hypothesis revolves around improved hematopoiesis in patients who receive a conditioning regimen with antithymocyte globulin and cyclophosphamide prior to allogeneic bone marrow transplantation.[30] After the initiation of immunosuppressive therapy, bone marrow concentrations of interferon-γ decreased, while all cell lines improved.[31] Inciting agents (i.e., drugs) are suspected to affect the function of suppressor T cells, which could inhibit stem cell production.[19]

Inconsistencies in the identification of antibodies to medication have made it difficult to implicate drugs as the main determinant for the development of hematologic disease. Rather, clinical history and exposure history determine the assignment of causality. Additional supporting evidence for an immunologic basis as a mechanism of aplastic anemia comes from a prospective, randomized, placebo-controlled trial evaluating the efficacy of antilymphocyte globulin and methylprednisolone, with or without cyclosporine, in patients with severe aplastic anemia.[32] The primary response variable was an improvement in blood counts (i.e., platelets, erythrocytes, and leukocytes) at 3 months. Patients receiving therapy with antilymphocyte globulin, methylprednisolone, and cyclosporine had a response rate of 65% versus a response rate of 39% in the group not receiving cyclosporine. This finding lends support to the fact that patients receiving aggressive immunotherapy are more likely to recover from a hematologic disorder and further implicates immunomodulation as a cause of disease.

Genetic predisposition may also influence the development of drug-induced aplastic anemia. Studies in animals and a case report of chloramphenicol-induced aplastic anemia in identical twins suggest a genetic predisposition to the development of drug-induced aplastic anemia.[19,24] Furthermore, pharmacogenetic research that focuses on patients who may be slow or normal metabolizers of drugs may increase the clinician's ability to predict the development of aplastic anemia. Initial case-control studies have not had the power necessary to identify a statistical difference between controls and cases, but continued research may establish the role of altered metabolism in this population.[33]

► TREATMENT: Drug-Induced Aplastic Anemia

Because of an extremely high mortality rate among patients with this disorder, it is imperative that drug-induced aplastic anemia be diagnosed quickly and therapy initiated immediately. It must be emphasized that prognosis, response to therapy, and management of drug-induced aplastic anemia are similar to that of idiopathic disease.[34] The goals of therapy are to improve peripheral blood counts so that patients do not require transfusions and are not at risk for opportunistic infections.

As with all cases of drug-induced hematologic disorders, the first step is to remove the suspected offending agent. Early withdrawal of the agent may allow for reversal of the aplastic anemia.[19] The next step is to provide adequate supportive care, including symptomatic treatment of infection and transfusion support with erythrocytes and platelets. Appropriate supportive care is essential, as the major causes of mortality in patients with aplastic anemia are infections and bleeding. One study showed that 62% of deaths were due to infections, consisting mostly of bacterial and fungal pathogens.[35] Current treatment guidelines do not include chemoprophylaxis, except in patients undergoing hematopoietic stem cell transplantation (HSCT). Therefore, in patients receiving immunotherapy, fever of unknown origin should be aggressively managed.

The two major treatment options for patients with drug-induced aplastic anemia are HSCT and immunosuppressive therapy.

A retrospective analysis reviewing the outcomes of patients who underwent allogeneic HSCT for severe aplastic anemia between 1978 and 1991 showed an 89% response rate (including complete and partial responses).[36] The 15-year survival rate for complete and partial responders to HSCT was 75% and 64%, respectively. Improvement in supportive care, prevention of graft-versus-host disease, and improved engraftment have further enhanced survival benefits. Considerations in deciding to treat patients with HSCT are the availability of a donor, the age of the patient, the absolute neutrophil count, and the number of transfusions received prior to transplantation.[36]

An alternative to HSCT is immunosuppressive therapy. Current options for this approach include antithymocyte globulin, antilymphocyte globulin, cyclosporine, and glucocorticoids. Antithymocyte globulin is a polyclonal immunoglobulin that disrupts cell-mediated immune responses and may have some immunosuppressive effects.[37] Antithymocyte globulin monotherapy may achieve response rates up to 50% of patients.[38] Recommended dosing of antithymocyte globulin has varied from 40 mg/kg per day for 4 days to 15 to 20 mg/kg per day for 8 to 14 days. Shorter, more intense regimens are preferred, as they are associated with fewer adverse events (i.e., serum sickness).[39] Corticosteroids (i.e., methylprednisolone) have long been used in conjunction with antithymocyte globulin for the management of drug-induced aplastic anemia, but their efficacy is questionable.[18] They have minimal effects on hematopoiesis, although they benefit patients by decreasing the incidence of serum sickness. Methylprednisolone dosing is 1 mg/kg per day for 4 weeks. Cyclosporine blocks T-lymphocyte proliferation and function through alterations in interleukin-2 production. Cyclosporine dosing has varied from 4 to 6 mg/kg per day to 10 to 12 mg/kg per day with response rates equivalent to those of antithymocyte globulin monotherapy. Recommended dosing of cyclosporine is 5 mg/kg per day and titrated to a target blood concentration of 200 to 400 ng/mL. Adverse effects of cyclosporine include hypertension, renal failure, tremors, electrolyte abnormalities, and opportunistic infections.

The optimal immunosuppressive regimen is a combination of antithymocyte globulin, glucocorticoids, and cyclosporine. Three-year survival rates can approach 90%,[32,40] which is comparable to that for HSCT, and makes immunosuppressive therapy a possible option for patients who are elderly (age >50 years), those who lack an eligible donor, and those who have less severe disease. A study comparing survival following immunosuppressive therapy or HSCT in patients with severe aplastic anemia found no significant difference between the treatment modalities at 6 years.[41] These data provide additional support for the aggressive management of all patients with aplastic anemia, regardless of age. Long-term complications of immunosuppressive therapy include relapse and conversion to other stem cell disorders (e.g., myelodysplastic syndrome, acute myelogenous leukemia, and paroxysmal nocturnal hemoglobinuria), which have occurred with relatively high incidence.[19,36]

Granulocyte colony-stimulating factor (G-CSF),[42] granulocyte-macrophage colony-stimulating factor (GM-CSF),[43] and interleukin-1[44] have also been investigated in the treatment of aplastic anemia. G-CSF, in combination with aggressive immunotherapy, may improve trilineage hematopoietic reconstitution, but it is unclear whether current data support a positive effect on outcomes (i.e., infectious complications and improved survival).[42] Therefore prospective evaluations are required to further delineate the role of G-CSF in aplastic anemia. If long-term bone marrow suppression continues after initial treatment with optimal immunosuppression, the only viable option at present is allogeneic HSCT. Otherwise, aggressive immunosuppressive therapy plays a distinct role in treating patients with drug-induced aplastic anemia and provides a viable alternative to patients ineligible for HSCT.

DRUG-INDUCED AGRANULOCYTOSIS

It is possible to define drug-induced agranulocytosis as a drug-mediated reduction in the number of mature myeloid cells in the blood (granulocytes and immature granulocytes [bands]) to a total count of 500/mm^3 or less. Symptoms of agranulocytosis include sore throat, fever, malaise, weakness, and chills. It occurs more frequently in females than in males,[45] with an overall estimated incidence of 1.6 to 3.4 million persons per year.[3,17] The overall mortality rate in agranulocytosis is 16%; the rate increases among patients with agranulocytosis when they develop bacteremia or renal failure.[46] The symptoms can appear rapidly, within 7 to 14 days after the initiation of the offending agent. In contrast, patients with phenothiazine-induced agranulocytosis can be asymptomatic at the time of diagnosis, probably because they have a milder form of the disorder.[47] In the large majority of cases, drug-induced agranulocytosis will resolve over time.[46] Table 102–2 provides a list of medications that have been associated with drug-induced agranulocytosis.

A number of different mechanisms may lead to drug-induced agranulocytosis. Initially, it was thought that drugs affected only the mature granulocytes, causing a "maturation arrest." More recent studies have demonstrated that drugs may have a toxic effect on the myeloid colony-forming unit in the bone marrow (either a direct toxic effect or an antibody-mediated effect);[48,49] this may be the most frequent mechanism of drug-induced agranulocytosis.[45]

Drug-induced agranulocytosis can be classified into three types (i.e., types I, II, and III).[50] The type I reaction is immune-mediated and involves the drug or drug metabolite, antibodies, and neutrophils. A type II reaction is associated with accumulated drug toxicity in hypersensitive individuals. The final type, type III, results from a combination of both immune and toxic mechanisms.

It has been postulated that drug-induced immune agranulocytosis (type I) develops by one of four different mechanisms.[51] The first mechanism involves drug adsorption on the membrane of the neutrophil. The drug-membrane complex then acts as a hapten to stimulate antibody formation. The antibodies produced attach to the drug-membrane complex, causing WBC destruction through complement activation and removal by the phagocytic system (Fig. 102–2). This hapten-type reaction is often seen when drugs, such as the penicillin derivatives, are given in large doses. The dose at which this immune-mediated reaction occurs is higher than 150 mg/kg per day with the majority of penicillin derivatives, but it has occurred at lower doses.[49,52,53]

The second mechanism of immune-mediated agranulocytosis is called the "innocent bystander phenomenon." In this reaction, the drug combines with a drug-specific antibody. The complex is

TABLE 102–2. Drugs Associated with Agranulocytosis

Observational study evidence	Case report evidence ("probable" or "definite" causality rating)
β-Lactam antibiotics	Acetaminophen
Carbamazepine	Acetazolamide
Carbimazole	Captopril
Clomipramine	Chloramphenicol
Digoxin	Chlorpropamide
Dipyridamole	Chlorpheniramine
Ganciclovir	Clindamycin
Glyburide	Clozapine
Gold salts	Colchicine
Imipenem-cilastatin	Dapsone
Indomethacin	Desipramine
Macrolide antibiotics	Ethacrynic acid
Methimazole	Ethosuximide
Mirtazapine	Gentamicin
Phenobarbital	Griseofulvin
Phenothiazines	Hydralazine
Phenytoin	Hydroxychloroquine
Prednisone	Imipramine
Procainamide	Levodopa
Propranolol	Meprobamate
Propylthiouracil	Methazolamide
Spironolactone	Methyldopa
Sulfonamides	Metronidazole
Sulfonylureas	NSAIDs
Ticlopidine	Olanzapine
Valproic acid	Penicillamine
Zidovudine	Pentazocine
	Primidone
	Pyrimethamine
	Quinine
	Rifampin
	Streptomycin
	Terbinafine
	Tocainide
	Tolbutamide
	Vancomycin

NSAID, nonsteroidal anti-inflammatory drug.

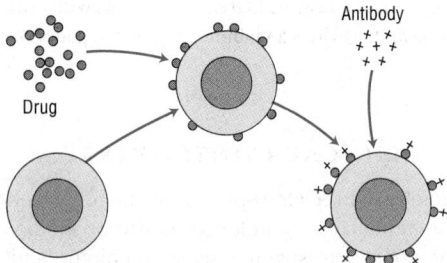

FIGURE 102–2. Drug adsorption mechanism. The drug binds to the membrane of the blood cell. Antibodies are formed to the drug-membrane complex (hapten). The antibodies then attach to the complex, and cell toxicity occurs. (*Reproduced with permission from Petz LD. Drug-induced haemolytic anaemia. Ballieres Clin Haematol 1980;91:455–482.*)

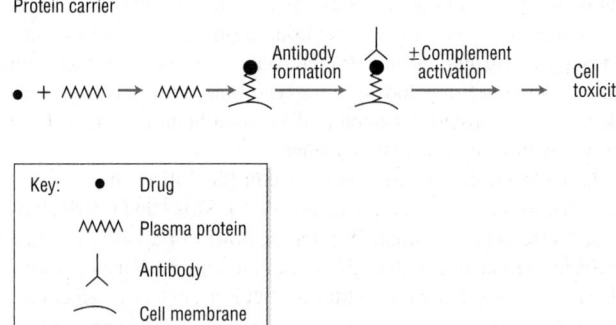

FIGURE 102–4. Protein carrier mechanism. The drug combines with a plasma protein. The complex then attaches to the cell membrane, and antibody formation is stimulated. Antibodies later attach to the complex and activate complement. The cell is then lysed by the complement. (*Reproduced with permission from Young et al.[51]*)

nonspecifically adsorbed to the neutrophil membrane, resulting in complement activation. The activated complement then destroys the cell (Fig. 102–3). Quinidine has been associated with this type of reaction.

Functioning in a manner somewhat similar to that of the second mechanism, the third mechanism of immune response involves a protein carrier that combines with the drug and then attaches to the cell membrane. This in turn causes antibody formation. The antibodies attach to the drug protein carrier–membrane complex and activate complement. The cells are then cleared by the phagocytic system (Fig. 102–4).

The final mechanism for an immune-mediated reaction is the production of autoantibodies to a "spoiled membrane." The offending drug alters the neutrophil membrane, which induces the formation of autoantibodies (antibodies that attach directly to the neutrophil). Their attachment to the neutrophil causes cellular destruction by the phagocytic system.

The onset of symptoms associated with immune-mediated mechanisms is rapid, occurring within 7 to 15 days of drug exposure. In the case of penicillin-induced agranulocytosis, the patient can often begin taking penicillin again, at a lower dosage, after the neutropenia has resolved without any relapse of drug-induced agranulocytosis.[52,53] Because of the rapid onset of symptoms and the dose-related phenomenon, a second mechanism (type II) could possibly be involved with penicillin-induced agranulocytosis. This mechanism involves an accumulation of drug to toxic concentrations in hypersensitive individuals. Researchers have shown with in vitro cell cultures that

penicillin derivatives in high concentrations inhibit the growth of myeloid colony-forming units in patients recovering from drug-induced agranulocytosis.[54] Penicillin derivatives, therefore, may suppress WBCs by several mechanisms.

Antithyroid medications such as propylthiouracil and methimazole produce agranulocytosis in about 0.3% to 0.6% of patients.[55,56] The mechanism by which antithyroid agents cause agranulocytosis is unknown, but antibodies to granulocytes have been demonstrated.[57,58] In a study by Cooper and coworkers,[55] agranulocytosis occurred more frequently in older patients (>40 years old), and it appeared within 2 months after the initiation of therapy. The investigators also reported a possible dose-response relationship with methimazole.[55] For patients receiving less than 30 mg/day of methimazole, no agranulocytosis occurred, but in patients receiving higher doses, neutropenia was evident.[55] There appeared to be no dose-response relationship with conventional doses of propylthiouracil. However, another study demonstrated no relationship between age or dose and the incidence of thionamide-induced agranulocytosis.[59]

Ticlopidine is an antiplatelet agent indicated for the treatment of cerebrovascular disease and the prevention of reocclusion associated with stent placement. It produces agranulocytosis in approximately 2.4% of patients,[60] reportedly by inhibiting myeloid colony growth.[61] This evidence supports a potential direct toxic effect of ticlopidine on the bone marrow. In addition, ticlopidine is associated with an increase in prostaglandin E_1 concentrations, a known myelosuppressant.[62] Other factors associated with the development of agranulocytosis include poor medullary reserve and age. Agranulocytosis occurs within 1–3 months from the initiation of therapy. Removal of the agent is the best treatment option, with counts returning to normal within 2 to 4 weeks.

The phenothiazines as a group are known to cause a type I drug-induced agranulocytosis. The onset of phenothiazine-induced agranulocytosis is approximately 2 to 15 weeks after the initiation of therapy.[51] Although there is one report of acute agranulocytosis in a child who accidentally ingested a large quantity of chlorpromazine,[48] patients usually have ingested 10 to 20 g of a phenothiazine before the onset of neutropenia. Phenothiazine-induced agranulocytosis occurs most frequently in females older than 50 years of age.[47] The mechanism by which phenothiazines cause the drug-induced agranulocytosis has been studied primarily with chlorpromazine,[47] which is thought to affect cells in the cell cycle phase that manufacture enzymes needed for DNA synthesis (G_1 phase), or the phase in which cells are resting and not committed to cell division (G_0 phase).[4]

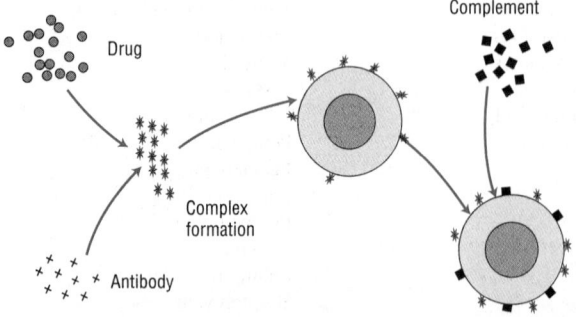

FIGURE 102–3. Innocent bystander mechanism. The drug induces antibody formation. The antibodies and drug form a complex in the serum, and the complex nonspecifically binds to the cell membrane. Complement is activated, and the cell is lysed. (*Reproduced with permission from Petz LD. Drug-induced haemolytic anaemia. Ballieres Clin Haematol 1980;91:455–482.*)

he antipsychotic agents are known to precipitate proteins and may precipitate polynucleotides so they can no longer participate in cleic acid synthesis. Chlorpromazine also increases the loss of acromolecules from the intracellular pools that are essential for llular replication.[47] When the bone marrow from a patient with enothiazine-induced agranulocytosis is examined, it initially appears to have no cellularity (aplastic), but over time it becomes hyperplastic. It is believed that toxic effects of the phenothiazines are ot seen in all patients taking the medications because the majority patients have enough bone marrow reserve to overcome the toxic fects.[47]

Clozapine, an antipsychotic agent, has demonstrated an approximately 10-fold higher incidence of agranulocytosis compared with other antipsychotics.[63] The incidence of clozapine-induced agranulocytosis increases with age and occurs more frequently in female patients, but does not appear to be dose-related.[64] The agranulocytosis is reversible if detected early in therapy; therefore close monitoring of the WBC count is warranted. An in vitro study has suggested that the formation of a free radical metabolite may be responsible for clozapine-induced agranulocytosis.[65] The resulting oxidative stress caused by this metabolite may cause cytotoxicity or an immune reaction.[65]

▶ TREATMENT: Drug-Induced Agranulocytosis

The primary treatment of drug-induced agranulocytosis is the removal of the offending drug. Following discontinuation of the ug, most cases of neutropenia resolve over time, and only symptomatic treatment (e.g., antimicrobials for infections) is necessary. argramostim (GM-CSF) and filgrastim (G-CSF) have been used shorten the duration of neutropenia with varying degrees of success. A review of 118 cases of non–chemotherapy-induced agranulocytosis treated with colony-stimulating factors revealed a decrease

in the duration of neutropenia with a trend toward improved mortality, especially in patients with granulocyte counts of less than 100/mm^3.[66] The time to recovery of the granulocyte count ranged from 3 to 15 days.[67–69] A case series was published describing several schizophrenic patients who developed clozapine-induced agranulocytosis and were subsequently successfully treated with concomitant clozapine and G-CSF.[70]

DRUG-INDUCED HEMOLYTIC ANEMIA

ollowing their release from the bone marrow, normal RBCs have 20 days before they are removed by phagocytic cells of the spleen d liver. The process of premature RBC destruction is referred to as emolysis, which can occur either because of defective RBCs or abormal changes in the intravascular environment. Drugs can promote emolysis by both processes.

The causes of drug-induced hemolytic anemia can be divided to two categories: immune or metabolic. Those in the first category ay operate much like the process that leads to immune-regulated granulocytosis, or they may suppress regulator cells, which allows e production of autoantibodies. The second category involves the duction of hemolysis by metabolic abnormalities in the RBCs. Paents with drug-induced hemolytic anemia can present with signs of travascular or extravascular hemolysis. Intravascular hemolysis, the sis of RBCs in the circulation, can result from trauma, complement xation to the RBC, or exogenous toxic factors. Extravascular hemolsis refers to the ingestion of RBCs by macrophages in the spleen and ver, a process that requires the existence of surface abnormalities on BCs, such as bound immunoglobulin.[71] The onset of drug-induced emolytic anemia is variable and depends on the drug and mechanism f the hemolysis. Table 102–3 provides a list of drugs that have been ssociated with drug-induced immune hemolytic anemia.

DRUG-INDUCED IMMUNE HEMOLYTIC ANEMIA

laboratory test called the direct Coombs test (or direct anti–human obulin test), which identifies foreign immunoglobulins either in the atient's serum or on the RBCs themselves, is the best means to lentify drug-induced immune hemolytic anemia. The Coombs test egins with the antiglobulin serum, which is produced by injecting bbits with preparations of human complement, Fc fragments, or munoglobulins. The rabbits produce antibodies that are foreign to uman immunoglobulins and complement. The direct Coombs test volves combining the patient's RBCs with the antiglobulin serum. the patient's RBCs are coated with antibody or complement (as a

result of a drug-induced process), the antibodies in the serum (produced by the rabbit) will attach to the Fc regions of the autoimmune globulins on two separate RBCs, creating a lattice formation called agglutination.[72] This agglutination is considered positive for the presence of immunoglobulin G (IgG) or complement on the cell surfaces.

An indirect Coombs test can identify antibodies in a patient's serum. This test is performed by combining the patient's serum with normal RBCs, then subjecting them to the direct Coombs test. Antibodies that have attached to the normal RBCs will be identified. This process is important in blood bank procedures.

The mechanisms that have been proposed to explain how drugs can induce immune hemolytic anemia are similar to the mechanisms that produce drug-induced agranulocytosis. The first mechanism is the adsorption of the drug to the RBC membrane to form a hapten,

TABLE 102–3. **Drugs Associated with Hemolytic Anemia**

Observational study evidence	Levofloxacin
Phenobarbital	Methyldopa
Phenytoin	Minocycline
	NSAIDs
Case report evidence ("probable"	Omeprazole
or "definite" causality rating)	p-Aminosalicylic acid
Acetaminophen	Phenazopyridine
Angiotensin-coverting enzyme	Probenecid
inhibitors	Procainamide
β-Lactam antibiotics	Quinidine
Cephalosporins	Rifabutin
Ciprofloxacin	Rifampin
Erythromycin	Streptomycin
Hydrochlorothiazide	Sulfonamides
Indinavir	Sulfonylureas
Interferon-alfa	Tacrolimus
Ketoconazole	Tolbutamide
Lansoprazole	Tolmetin
Levodopa	Triamterene

NSAID, nonsteroidal anti-inflammatory drug.

and subsequently, an antibody. The antibody attaches to the drug without direct interaction with the erythrocyte. The extravascular anemia that follows is usually caused by IgG, and generally there is no complement activation. The anemia usually develops gradually over 7 to 10 days and reverses over a couple of weeks after discontinuation of the offending drug. The direct Coombs test may remain positive for several weeks. The penicillin and cephalosporin derivatives given in high doses are mainly associated with this type of immune reaction.[73] Other drugs that have been reported to cause drug-induced immune hemolytic anemia by this process include minocycline, tolbutamide, and semisynthetic penicillins.[73] Streptomycin is also associated with this type of reaction and is associated with activation of the complement system.[74]

Like drug-induced agranulocytosis, immune hemolytic anemia has been associated with the formation of immune complexes in a reaction formally known as the "innocent bystander phenomenon." Quinidine and phenacetin are the prototype drugs of this reaction, but many other drugs have been implicated, including quinine and several sulfonamides. Drugs that induce this reaction form a "neoantigen" with a specific alloantigen on the RBC. This neoantigen, in turn, forms complexes with drug-specific antibodies (IgG or IgM) that adhere to the RBC membrane. Complement then lyses the RBC membrane.[73] Interestingly, the trimolecular complex is attached very loosely to the RBC.[73] As soon as complement is activated, the complex can detach and move on to other RBCs, and to leukocytes or platelets. Because of this low affinity, only a small amount of drug is needed to cause the reaction, and the direct Coombs test is positive for complement only. RBCs are essentially victims or "innocent bystanders" of the immunologic reaction. This type of mechanism is associated with acute intravascular hemolysis that can be severe, sometimes leading to hemoglobinuria and renal failure. Following discontinuation and clearance of the drug from the circulation, the direct Coombs test will be negative.

A third type of immune-mediated mechanism has occurred with cephalosporin derivatives. The cephalosporins can combine with nonspecific proteins, including albumin, IgG, IgA, and fibrinogen, and adhere to the RBC; when this happens, a Coombs test will have a positive result. The binding is not immunologic in origin, and hemolytic anemia has not been associated with this reaction (Fig. 102–5). However, the nonspecific binding of antibodies to the RBC membrane can cause difficulties in cross-matching patients for blood transfusions.[73]

The fourth mechanism is best described. Methyldopa, like a few other drugs, is known to induce true autoantibodies to RBCs; the antibodies can be identified without the presence of the offending drug or its metabolites. About 20% of patients receiving methyldopa have a positive finding on Coombs test, but less than 1% of these patients experience hemolysis. The result of a Coombs test usually becomes positive 3 to 6 months after the beginning of therapy, but hemolysis develops from 4 to 6 months to more than 2 years after the start of therapy. After the withdrawal of the drug, results of the Coombs test can remain positive for many months.[74]

The mechanism by which methyldopa induces antibody production is not completely known, but there are several hypotheses. One suggests that methyldopa inhibits suppressor T-lymphocyte function, resulting in uncontrolled autoantibody formation by B cells.[75] However, some data contradict this concept.[76] An alternative hypothesis suggests that the offending drug may bind to immature RBCs, altering the membrane antigens and inducing autoantibodies.[77]

Overall, however, the reason that only some patients develop autoantibodies, and that only some of those have hemolytic disease, is not known. In an effort to explain why patients may have a positive result from a Coombs test and no hemolysis, Kelton demonstrated that methyldopa impairs the ability of these patients to remove antibody-sensitized cells.[78] In Coombs-positive patients receiving methyldopa, patients with impairment of the reticuloendothelial system could not clear the RBCs coated with autoantibodies from their bloodstream, and therefore hemolysis did not occur. Patients with hemolysis had no impairment of the reticuloendothelial system. Procainamide has also been reported to cause a positive result on the direct anti–human globulin test and hemolytic anemia.[79] Other drugs that have been reported to cause autoimmune hemolytic anemia include levodopa, mefenamic acid, and diclofenac.[77]

DRUG-INDUCED OXIDATIVE HEMOLYTIC ANEMIA

A hereditary condition, drug-induced oxidative hemolytic anemia, most often accompanies a glucose-6-phosphate dehydrogenase (G6PD) enzyme deficiency, but it can occur because of other enzyme defects (reduced nicotinamide adenine dinucleotide phosphate [NADPH] methemoglobin reductase or reduced glutathione peroxidase). A G6PD deficiency is a disorder of the hexose monophosphate shunt, which is responsible for producing NADPH in erythrocytes, which in turn keeps glutathione in a reduced state. Reduced glutathione is a substrate for glutathione peroxidase, an enzyme that removes peroxide from erythrocytes, thus protecting them from oxidative stress.[80] Without reduced glutathione, oxidative drugs may oxidize the sulfhydryl groups of hemoglobin, removing them prematurely from the circulation (i.e., causing hemolysis).

A G6PD deficiency is the most common of all enzyme defects, affecting millions of people. Because the G6PD gene is located on the X chromosome, the disorder is consequently inherited via a sex-linked mode. There are many G6PD variants, but the most common types occur in American and African blacks (about 10%), people from Mediterranean areas (e.g., Greeks, Sardinians, and Khurdic and Sephardic Jews), and Asians.[74,80] The Mediterranean variety tends to be more severe, and those with this defect also may experience hemolysis from the ingestion of fava beans ("favism").[80]

The degree of hemolysis depends on the severity of the enzyme deficiency and the amount of oxidative stress. However, the dose

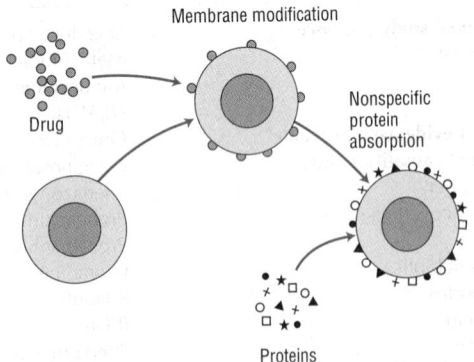

FIGURE 102–5. Nonspecific binding of proteins mechanism. The drug combines with the cell membrane, which in turn causes a nonspecific binding of serum protein. This reaction is seen primarily with the cephalosporins, and no cell lysis or toxicity occurs. (*Reproduced with permission from Petz LD. Drug-induced haemolytic anaemia. Ballieres Clin Haematol 1980;91:455–482.*)

Membrane modification

Drug

Nonspecific protein absorption

Proteins

required for hemolysis to occur is often less than prescribed quantities of the suspected agent.[80] Although severe hemolysis is rare, any drug that places oxidative stress on the RBC will cause drug-induced oxidative hemolytic anemia. There was one case of drug-induced oxidative hemolytic anemia that occurred in a child when dapsone (an oxidizing agent) was transferred through the breast milk of the mother, who was taking the drug.[81] For a list of agents associated with drug-induced oxidative hemolytic anemia, refer to Table 102–4. An additional form of drug-induced anemia is pure red-cell aplasia. Patients with this disorder have a normochromic, normoblastic anemia and an absence of reticulocytes.[82] Although this disorder is thought to have a directly toxic etiology, there is also evidence supporting an immune-mediated etiology. One case series described a group of 13 chronic renal failure patients who developed immune pure red-cell aplasia associated with recombinant erythropoietin injections.[83]

TABLE 102–4. Drugs Associated with Oxidative Hemolytic Anemia

Observational study evidence
Dapsone
Case report evidence ("probable" or "definite" causality rating)
Ascorbic acid
Metformin
Methylene blue
Nalidixic acid
Nitrofurantoin
Phenazopyridine
Primaquine
Sulfacetamide
Sulfamethoxazole
Sulfanilamide

▶ TREATMENT: Drug-Induced Hemolytic Anemia

The severity of drug-induced immune hemolytic anemia is usually a function of the rate of hemolysis. Hemolytic anemia caused by drugs via the hapten/adsorption and autoimmune mechanisms tend to be slower in onset and mild to moderate in severity. Conversely, hemolysis prompted via the neoantigen mechanism (innocent bystander) phenomenon may have a sudden onset, lead to severe hemolysis, and result in renal failure. The treatment of drug-induced immune hemolytic anemia includes the removal of the offending agent and supportive care. Glucocorticoids are usually unnecessary, and practitioners have questioned their efficacy.[77]

A recent development in the treatment of autoimmune hemolytic anemia is the use of the chimeric, human anti-CD20 monoclonal antibody rituximab.[84] The role of immunoglobulin treatments in drug-induced hemolytic anemia has yet to be clearly defined.

■ DRUG-INDUCED OXIDATIVE HEMOLYTIC ANEMIA

Removal of the offending drug is the primary treatment for drug-induced oxidative hemolytic anemia. No other therapy is usually necessary, as most cases of drug-induced oxidative hemolytic anemia are mild in severity. Patients with these enzyme deficiencies should be advised to avoid medications capable of inducing the hemolysis.

DRUG-INDUCED MEGALOBLASTIC ANEMIA

In drug-induced megaloblastic anemia, the development of RBC precursors called megaloblasts in the bone marrow is abnormal. Deficiencies in either B_{12} or folate are responsible for the impaired proliferation and maturation of hematopoietic cells, resulting in cell arrest and subsequent sequestration. Examination of peripheral blood shows a rise in the mean corpuscular hemoglobin concentration. These megaloblastic changes are due to the direct or indirect effects of the drug on DNA synthesis. Some patients may have a normal-appearing cell line, and diagnosis must be made through alterations in B_{12} and folate concentrations. The abnormality can be seen in any portion of the replication process, including DNA assembly, base precursor metabolism, or RNA synthesis.[86]

Because of their pharmacologic action on DNA replication, the antimetabolite chemotherapeutic agents are most frequently associated with drug-induced megaloblastic anemia. Methotrexate, an irreversible inhibitor of dihydrofolate reductase, causes megaloblastic anemia in 3% to 9% of patients.[87] Dihydrofolate reductase is an enzyme responsible for generating tetrahydrofolate, an essential factor in making deoxythymidine triphosphate, which is necessary for DNA synthesis. Other drugs such as cotrimoxazole, phenytoin, or the barbiturates have also been implicated in megaloblastic anemia. Cotrimoxazole, for example, has been reported to cause drug-induced megaloblastic anemia with both low and high doses,[88,89] particularly in patients with a partial B_{12} or folate deficiency.[86] Because the drug's affinity for human dihydrofolate reductase is low, patients with adequate stores of these vitamins are at low risk of developing drug-induced megaloblastic anemia if they are taking cotrimoxazole. It has been postulated that phenytoin, primidone, and phenobarbital cause drug-induced megaloblastic anemia by either inhibiting folate absorption or by increasing folate catabolism. In both instances, the patient develops a relative deficiency of folate. Table 102–5 provides a list of drugs that have been suggested as causative factors in drug-induced megaloblastic anemia.

TABLE 102–5. Drugs Associated with Megaloblastic Anemia

Case report evidence ("probable" or "definite" causality rating)	
Azathioprine	Methotrexate
Chloramphenicol	Oral contraceptives
Colchicine	p-Aminosalicylate
Cyclophosphamide	Phenobarbital
Cytarabine	Phenytoin
5-Fluorodeoxyuridine	Primidone
5-Fluorouracil	Pyrimethamine
Hydroxyurea	Sulfasalazine
6-Mercaptopurine	Tetracycline
	Vinblastine

▶ TREATMENT: Drug-Induced Megaloblastic Anemia

When drug-induced megaloblastic anemia is related to chemotherapy, no real therapeutic option is available, and the anemia becomes an accepted side effect of therapy. If drug-induced megaloblastic anemia results from cotrimoxazole, a trial course of folinic acid, 5 to 10 mg up to four times a day, may correct the anemia.[88,89]

Folic acid supplementation of 1 mg every day often corrects the drug-induced megaloblastic anemia produced by either phenytoin or phenobarbital, but some clinicians suggest that supplementation of folic acid may decrease the effectiveness of the antiepileptic medications.[90]

DRUG-INDUCED THROMBOCYTOPENIA

Thrombocytopenia is defined as a platelet count below 150,000/mm³. There are three types of drug-induced thrombocytopenia: direct toxicity reactions, hapten-type immune reactions, and innocent bystander–type immune reactions. Direct toxicity reactions, resulting in suppressed thrombopoiesis, produce a decrease in the number of megakaryocytes in the bone marrow. In contrast, immune reactions result in an increased peripheral destruction of platelets and an increased number of megakaryocytes. Early symptoms of drug-induced thrombocytopenia include increased bruising, petechiae, ecchymoses, and epistaxis. Bleeding from mucous membranes and severe purpura can appear later in the disorder. A list of medications associated with drug-induced thrombocytopenia can be found in Table 102–6. Several comprehensive reviews are available.[91,92]

Drugs that induce thrombocytopenia by their toxic effects are primarily cancer chemotherapy agents; however, organic solvents, pesticides, and inamrinone (formally named amrinone) have also been implicated. Orally administered inamrinone has been shown to cause thrombocytopenia in up to 18.6% of patients.[93] The only commercially available formulation of inamrinone in the United States is to be given IV, and it is associated with a 2% to 4% incidence of thrombocytopenia, possibly reflecting the short-term nature of IV administration compared to the oral route. Although investigators have demonstrated an inamrinone-dependent antibody, it is believed that because of the rapid onset, the dose-related response, and the absence of amnestic effect, a non–immune-mediated peripheral destruction of platelets may be responsible for the thrombocytopenia.[93] Additional data suggest that this toxic effect may be due to the inamrinone metabolite, N-acetylamrinone.[94]

In the majority of patients, drug-induced thrombocytopenia develops through an immunologic mechanism. The agents most commonly implicated are quinine, quinidine, gold salts, sulfonamide antibiotics, and heparin.[92] Study of these agents has revealed extensive information regarding the mechanism of drug-induced immune thrombocytopenia. In hapten-type reactions, the offending drug binds to certain platelet glycoproteins, most commonly Ib/IX, V, and IIb/IIIa.[95] Antibodies are generated that bind to these drug-bound glycoprotein epitopes. After the binding of drug-dependent antibodies to the platelet surface, lysis occurs through complement activation or through clearance from the circulation by macrophages.

Hapten-mediated immune thrombocytopenia usually occurs at least 7 days after the initiation of the drug, although it may occur much sooner if the exposure is actually a re-exposure to a previously administered drug. It occurs frequently in patients receiving large doses of the medication (e.g., penicillin derivatives >150 mg/kg).[96,97] The recovery period, once the suspected drug is discontinued, is often short in duration.[98]

Rare cases of acute profound thrombocytopenia (i.e., platelet count <20,000/mm³) have been reported with the glycoprotein IIb/IIIa receptor antagonist abciximab.[99–101] Although the mechanism is unknown, it is thought that abciximab binding to the glyco-

protein IIb/IIIa receptor may induce the expression of ligand-induced binding sites. These new binding sites may react with antibodies, leading to an increased clearance of platelets.[101,102] In a report that does not support this immunologic hypothesis, Peter and associates describe a patient with demonstrated platelet activation and subsequent thrombocytopenia.[103] In clinical trials with abciximab plus heparin, the incidence of thrombocytopenia with platelet count less than 50,000/mm³ ranged from 1.3% to 1.6%. In comparison, in patients

TABLE 102–6. Drugs Associated with Thrombocytopenia

Observational study evidence	Indomethacin
Carbamazepine	Interferon-alfa
Phenobarbital	Isoniazid
Phenytoin	Isotretinoin
Valproic acid	Itraconazole
	Levamisole
Case report evidence ("probable" or "definite" causality rating)	Linezolid
	Lithium
	Low-molecular-weight heparins
Abciximab	Measles, mumps, and rubella vaccine
Acetaminophen	Meclofenamate
Acyclovir	Mesalamine
Albendazole	Methyldopa
Aminoglutethimide	Minoxidil
Aminosalicylic acid	Morphine
Aminodarone	Nalidixic acid
Amphotericin B	Naphazoline
Ampicillin	Naproxen
Aspirin	Nitroglycerin
Atorvastatin	Octreotide
Captopril	Oxacillin
Chlorothiazide	p-Aminosalicylic acid
Chlorpromazine	Penicillamine
Chlorpropamide	Pentoxifylline
Cimetidine	Piperacillin
Clarithromycin	Primidone
Clopidogrel	Procainamide
Danazol	Pyrazinamide
Deferoxamine	Quinidine
Diazepam	Quinine
Diazoxide	Ranitidine
Diclofenac	Recombinant hepatitis B vaccine
Diethylstilbestrol	Rifampin
Digoxin	Simvastatin
Ethambutol	Sirolimus
Felbamate	Sulfasalazine
Fluconazole	Sulfonamide antibiotics
Gold salts	Sulindac
Haloperidol	Tamoxifen
Heparin	Tolmetin
Hydrochlorothiazide	Trimethoprim
Ibuprofen	Vancomycin
Inamrinone	
Indinavir	

who received placebo plus heparin, thrombocytopenia ranged from 0.3% to 0.7%.[101] Published case reports indicate that the incidence of acute profound thrombocytopenia with abciximab is less than 1%, and that nadir platelet counts of 1000 to 4000/mm³ occurred from 2 to 31 hours following bolus infusion.[101] This time course contrasts with that of other hapten-type thrombocytopenias; the decrease in platelet count can occur within hours of first drug exposure.

Because abciximab is coadministered with heparin, it is important to distinguish between abciximab-induced and heparin-induced thrombocytopenia. Performing a heparin-induced platelet aggregation study is helpful in making this differentiation.

CLINICAL CONTROVERSY

Profound thrombocytopenia (i.e., platelet count less than 20,000/mm³) has been reported with the glycoprotein IIb/IIIa receptor antagonist abciximab. Before this effect was fully appreciated, clinicians were inclined to attribute this event to heparin, which was coadministered with abciximab. The current challenge for clinicians is to distinguish between abciximab-induced and heparin-induced thrombocytopenia, so that the patient's adverse event is documented properly. Thrombocytopenia associated with abciximab may present with a nadir of platelet counts of 1000 to 4000/mm³ occurring from 2 to 31 hours following bolus infusion. This is much sooner than the 5 to 10 days observed with initial heparin exposure. However, re-exposure to heparin can produce profound thrombocytopenia within hours, much like abciximab. The ubiquity of heparin use for flushing catheters renders it difficult to determine previous exposure in many cases. Clinicians can choose from several types of assays to aid in the diagnosis of heparin-induced thrombocytopenia, including platelet activation assays, platelet aggregation studies, and enzyme-linked immunosorbent assay methods, each with varying sensitivity, specificity, and availability.

Pseudothrombocytopenia, defined as in vitro platelet aggregation in blood anticoagulated with ethylenediaminetetraacetic acid (EDTA), is clinically insignificant, but it must also be differentiated from thrombocytopenia induced by abciximab. In this case, microscopic examination of a peripheral blood smear, along with repeated platelet counts in citrate-anticoagulated blood samples, makes the distinction possible.[104]

Heparin can cause at least two types of thrombocytopenia.[105] The first is a mild, reversible, non–immune-mediated reaction that occurs 2 to 4 days after the initiation of therapy. The platelet count slowly returns to normal following an initial decline, despite continued heparin therapy. This benign condition is thought to result from weak activation of platelets, leading to sequestration.[105] No major sequelae develop from this type of heparin-induced thrombocytopenia.

The second type of heparin-induced thrombocytopenia is severe and may be associated with a platelet count below 100,000/mm³ and thrombosis.[105,106] The platelet count generally begins to decline 5 to 10 days after the start of heparin therapy (sooner in patients previously treated with heparin). Thrombocytopenia and thrombosis may develop with low-dose heparin,[105,107] heparin-coated catheters,[108] or even heparin flushes. Historically, the reaction was thought to be mediated by the formation of antibodies to the platelet-heparin complex. However, evidence suggests a complex interaction between heparin, platelet factor 4 (PF4), platelet membrane Fc receptors, and possibly heparin-like molecules on the surface of endothelial cells (Fig. 102–6). Circulating heparin reacts with PF4 to produce a

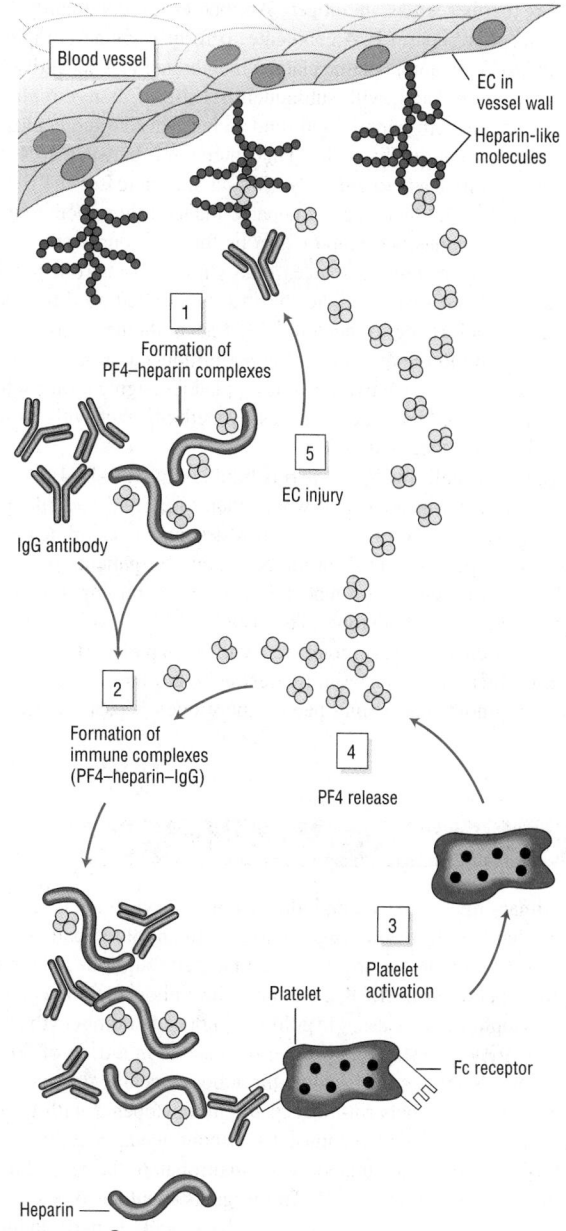

FIGURE 102–6. Proposed explanation for the presence of both thrombocytopenia and thrombosis in heparin-sensitive patients who are treated with heparin. Injected heparin reacts with platelet factor 4 (PF4), which is normally present on the surface of endothelial cells (ECs) or released in small quantities from circulating platelets, to form PF4-heparin complexes (1). Specific IgG antibodies react with these conjugates to form immune complexes (2) that bind to Fc receptors on circulating platelets. Fc-mediated platelet activation (3) releases PF4 from α-granules in platelets (4). Newly released PF4 binds to additional heparin, and the antibody forms more immune complexes, establishing a cycle of platelet activation. PF4 released in excess of the amount that can be neutralized by available heparin binds to heparin-like molecules (glycosaminoglycans) on the surface of ECs to provide targets for antibody binding. This process leads to immune-mediated EC injury (5) and heightens the risk of thrombosis and disseminated intravascular coagulation. (*Reproduced with permission from Bell et al.*[111])

complex that is seen as an antigen. Antibodies, predominantly IgG, react with this heparin-PF4 conjugate to form immune complexes that bind to Fc receptors on the platelet membrane. Platelet activation and aggregation occur, with subsequent release of more circulating PF4 to interact with heparin and bind to heparin-like molecules on the surface of endothelial cells. This interaction between PF4 and endothelial cells leads to antibody binding and increases the risk of thrombosis.[109] The incidence of heparin-induced thrombocytopenia with thrombosis has been reported to be three to four times higher with heparin from bovine sources than with heparin from porcine sources,[110,111] but several studies have demonstrated no differences between animal sources of heparin.[111-114] Several types of assays are available to aid in the diagnosis of heparin-induced thrombocytopenia, including platelet activation assays, platelet aggregation studies, and enzyme-linked immunosorbent assay methods, each with varying sensitivities and specificities.[115]

Low-molecular-weight heparins bind less well to PF4 than unfractionated heparin does, and would therefore seem less likely to produce thrombocytopenia.[115] In a study designed to examine the incidence of heparin-induced thrombocytopenia in patients receiving prophylaxis for venous thromboembolism following hip surgery, it was found that thrombocytopenia occurred in 2.7% of patients treated with unfractionated heparin compared with 0% of patients treated with low-molecular-weight heparin. Interestingly, 2.2% of those who received low-molecular-weight heparin developed heparin-dependent

antibodies.[116] Therefore, low-molecular-weight heparin should not be expected to eliminate the risk of thrombocytopenia, and should not be considered an alternative to unfractionated heparin in patients with heparin-induced thrombocytopenia because of the potential for cross-reactivity with heparin-dependent antibodies.[117]

The thrombocytopenia induced by gold salts is related to antibody formation to platelets.[118,119] The incidence of gold-induced thrombocytopenia ranges from 1% to 3%, and the condition often has an abrupt and severe onset.[118] The autoantibody formed to the platelets appears to be associated with the human leukocyte antigens (HLAs), which are located on the platelet membrane and on a number of other different cells in the body.[118,119] An interaction between the gold salts and the HLAs causes the platelets to be recognized as nonself, thus inducing destruction of the platelets. The most commonly reported HLA associated with induction of the autoantibodies is DR-3, but DR-4 may also interact with the antibodies.[118-121] The exact mechanism by which gold causes the formation of the autoantibody to regulated DR-3 and DR-4 antigens has not been elucidated. In addition to gold, autoantibodies have been identified for α-methyldopa.[91]

The third mechanism described for drug-induced thrombocytopenia is the innocent bystander–type immune response. The most commonly implicated drug is quinidine, and the drug-induced thrombocytopenia is frequently related to higher doses of the drug.[121] Quinidine may also form a hapten with the platelet membrane to produce thrombocytopenia.[122]

▶ TREATMENT: Drug-Induced Thrombocytopenia

The primary treatment of drug-induced thrombocytopenia is removal of the offending drug and symptomatic treatment of the patient. The use of corticosteroid therapy in the treatment of drug-induced thrombocytopenia is controversial, although some authors recommend it in severe symptomatic cases.[123] In gold salt–induced thrombocytopenia, however, some investigators believe prednisone in a dose of 60 mg daily is beneficial in correcting the thrombocytopenia.[118]

In the case of heparin-induced thrombocytopenia with thrombosis, all forms of heparin must be discontinued, including heparin flushes, and anticoagulation with argatroban or the recombinant hirudin lepirudin initiated.[122,124] These agents should also be considered for the treatment of patients who have acute heparin-induced thrombocytopenia without thrombosis because of the increased risk

of thrombosis occurring in these patients. Because of the increased risk of venous limb gangrene, warfarin should not be used alone to treat acute heparin-induced thrombocytopenia complicated by deep vein thrombosis.[124] The relatively high risk of continued thrombocytopenia with thrombosis is a contraindication for the use of low-molecular-weight heparin in the treatment of acute heparin-induced thrombocytopenia. Abciximab-induced acute profound thrombocytopenia is effectively treated with platelet transfusion, if clinically indicated.[95]

It is important for clinicians to avoid using heparin products for these patients. Several options now exist for the appropriate anticoagulation of patients prior to surgical procedures. These agents include argatroban, tirofiban, fondaparinux, and bivalirudin.

SUMMARY

Drug-induced hematologic disorders are rare but potentially life-threatening conditions. Clinicians should be cognizant of medications with the potential of causing hematologic disorders, and educate patients to recognize the symptoms associated with such events. Frequent laboratory monitoring of patients taking medications associated with severe hematologic events can facilitate diagnosis and treatment. Identifying the etiology of the event and documenting the causative agents may serve to prevent a recurrence secondary to the use of a related medication. Reporting such an event to national adverse event reporting services and in the peer-reviewed medical literature can serve to improve the understanding of the prevalence and risk factors for such a disorder.

ABBREVIATIONS

ADR: adverse drug reaction
G-CSF: granulocyte colony-stimulating factor
GM-CSF: granulocyte-macrophage colony-stimulating factor
G6PD: glucose-6-phosphate dehydrogenase
HLA: human leukocyte antigen
HSCT: hematopoietic stem cell transplantation
IgG: immunoglobulin G
NADPH: reduced nicotinamide adenine dinucleotide phosphate
PF4: platelet factor 4
RBC: red blood cell
WBC: white blood cell

Review Questions and other resources can be found at *www.pharmacotherapyonline.com.*

REFERENCES

1. Johnston FD. Granulocytopenia following the administration of sulphanilamide compounds. Lancet 1938;2:1044–1047.
2. Council for International Organizations of Medical Sciences. Standardization of definitions and criteria of assessment of adverse drug reactions: Drug-induced cytopenia. Int J Clin Pharmacol Toxicol 1990;29:75–81.
3. van der Klauw MM, Goudsmit R, Halie MR. A population-based case cohort study of drug-associated agranulocytosis. Arch Intern Med 1999;159:369–374.
4. Shapiro S, Surapol I, Kaufman DW, et al. Agranulocytosis in Bangkok, Thailand: A predominantly drug-induced disease with an unusually low incidence. Am J Trop Med Hyg 1999;60:573–577.
5. Maluf EM, Pasquini R, Eluf JN, et al. Aplastic anemia in Brazil: Incidence and risk factors. Am J Hematol 2002;71:268–274.
6. Patton WN, Duffull SB. Idiosyncratic drug-induced haematologic abnormalities. Drug Saf 1994;11:445–462.
7. Hine LK, Gerstman BB, Wise RP, Song YT. Mortality resulting from blood dyscrasia in the United States. Am J Med 1990;88:151–153.
8. Kessler DA. Introducing MEDWatch: A new approach to reporting medication and device adverse effects and product problems. JAMA 1993;269:2765–2768.
9. ASHP reports. ASHP guidelines on adverse drug reaction monitoring or reporting. Am J Hosp Pharm 1989;46:336–337.
10. Rieder MJ. In-vivo and in-vitro testing for adverse drug reactions. Pediatr Clin North Am 1997;44:93–111.
11. Parent-Mussin DM, Sensebe L, Leqlise MC, et al. Relevance of in-vitro studies of drug-induced agranulocytosis: report of 14 cases. Drug Saf 1993;9:463–469.
12. Claas FHJ. Drug-induced immune granulocytopenia. Baillieres Clin Immunol Allergy 1987;1:357–368.
13. Naranjo CA, Busto U, Sellers EM, et al. A method of estimating the probability of adverse drug reactions. Clin Pharmacol Ther 1981;30:239–245.
14. Sackett DA. Clinical Epidemiology: A Basic Science for Clinical Medicine, 2nd ed. Boston, Little, Brown, 1991.
15. Gale RP, Champlin RE, Feig SA, et al. Aplastic anemia: Biology and treatment. UCLA conference. Ann Intern Med 1981;95:477–494.
16. Heimpel H. Epidemiology and etiology of aplastic anemia. In: Schrezenmeier H, et al, eds. Aplastic Anemia: Pathophysiology and Treatment. Cambridge, UK, Cambridge University Press, 2000:97–116.
17. International Agranulocytosis and Aplastic Anemia Study. Risk of agranulocytosis and aplastic anemia: A first report of their relation to drug use with special reference to analgesics. JAMA 1986;256:1749–1757.
18. Camitta BM, Thomas ED, Nathan DG. A prospective study of androgens and bone marrow transplantation for treatment of severe aplastic anemia. Blood 1979;53:504–514.
19. Shadduck RK. Aplastic anemia. In: Williams WJ, et al, eds. Hematology, 5th ed. New York, McGraw-Hill, 1995:238–251.
20. Vincent PC. In vitro evidence of drug action in aplastic anemia. Blood 1984;49:3–12.
21. Modan B, Segal S, Shani M, et al. Aplastic anemia in Israel: Evaluation of the etiological role of chloramphenicol on a community wide basis. Am J Med Sci 1975;270:441–445.
22. Lubran MM. Hematologic side effects of drugs. Ann Clin Lab Sci 1989;19:114–121.
23. Young NS, Maciejewski J. The pathophysiology of acquired aplastic anemia. N Engl J Med 1997;336:1365–1372.
24. Yunis AA, Miller AM, Salem Z, et al. Chloramphenicol toxicity: Pathogenetic mechanisms and the role of the p–NO2 in aplastic anemia. Clin Toxicol 1980;17:359–373.
25. Malkin D, Koren G, Saunders EF. Drug-induced aplastic anemia pathogenesis and clinical aspects. Am J Pediatr Hematol Oncol 1990;12:402–410.
26. Jimenez JJ, Arimura GK, Abou-Khalil WH, et al. Chloramphenicol-induced bone marrow injury: Possible role of bacterial metabolites of chloramphenicol. Blood 1987;70:1180–1185.
27. Gerson WT, Fine DG, Spielberg SP, et al. Anticonvulsant-induced aplastic anemia: increased susceptibility to toxic drug metabolites in vitro. Blood 1983;61:889–893.
28. Kagan WA, Ascensao JA, Pahwa RN, et al. Aplastic anemia: Presence in human bone marrow of cells that suppress myelopoiesis. Proc Natl Acad Sci U S A 1985;82:188–192.
29. Selleri C, Sato T, Anderson S, et al. Interferon-γ and tumor necrosis factor-α suppress both early and late stages of hematopoiesis and induce programmed cell death. J Cell Physiol 1995;165:538–546.
30. Mathe G, Amiel JL, Schwarzenberg L, et al. Bone marrow graft in man after conditioning by antilymphocytic serum. BMJ 1970;2:131–136.
31. Platanias L, Gascon P, Bielory L, et al. Lymphocyte phenotype and lymphokines following anti-lymphocyte globulin therapy in patients with aplastic anemia. Br J Haematol 1987;66:437–443.
32. Frickhofen N, Kaltwasser J, Schrezenmeier H, et al. Treatment of aplastic anemia with antilymphocyte globulin and methylprednisolone with or without cyclosporine. N Engl J Med 1991;324:1297–1304.
33. Marsh JC, Chowdry J, Parry-Jones N, et al. Study of the association between cytochromes P450 2D6 and 2E1 genotypes and the risk of drug and chemical induced idiosyncratic aplastic anemia. Br J Haemotol 1999;104:266–270.
34. Marin-Fernandez P. Clinical presentation, natural course, and prognostic factors. In: Schrezenmeier H, et al, eds. Aplastic Anemia: Pathophysiology and Treatment. Cambridge, UK, Cambridge University Press, 2000:117–133.
35. Weinberger M, Elattar I, Marshall D, et al. Patterns of infection in patients with aplastic anemia and the emergence of *Aspergillus* as a major cause of death. Medicine 1992;71:24–43.
36. Doney K, Leisenring W, Storb R, et al. Primary treatment of acquired aplastic anemia: outcomes with bone marrow transplantation and immunosuppressive therapy. Ann Intern Med 1997;126:107–115.
37. Colby C, Stoukides CA, Spitzer TR. Antithymocyte immunoglobulin in severe aplastic anemia and bone marrow transplantation. Ann Pharmacother 1996;30:1164–1174.
38. Young N, Speck B. Antithymocyte and antilymphocyte globulins: Clinical trials and mechanism of action. In: Young S, et al, eds. Aplastic Anemia. Stem Cell Biology and Advances in Treatment. New York, Alan R Liss, 1984:221–226.
39. Tichelli A, Schrezenmeier H, Bacigalupo A. Immunosuppressive treatment of aplastic anemia. In: Schrezenmeier H, et al, eds. Aplastic Anemia: Pathophysiology and Treatment. Cambridge, UK, Cambridge University Press, 2000:154–196.
40. Bacigalupo A, Broccia G, Codra G, et al. Antilymphocyte globulin, cyclosporin, and granulocyte colony-stimulating factor in patients with acquired severe aplastic anemia (SAA): A pilot study of the EBMT SAA Working Party. Blood 1995;85:1348–1353.
41. Ahn MJ, Choi JH, Lee YY, et al. Outcome of adult severe or very severe aplastic anemia treated with bone marrow transplantation: A multicenter trial. Int J Hematol 2003;78:133–138.
42. Schrezenmeier H. Role of cytokines in the treatment of aplastic anemia. In: Schrezenmeier H, et al, eds. Aplastic Anemia: Pathophysiology and Treatment. Cambridge, UK, Cambridge University Press, 2000:197–229.
43. Antin JH, Smith BR, Holmes W, et al. Phase I/II study of recombinant human granulocyte-macrophage colony-stimulating factor in aplastic anemia and myelodysplastic syndrome. Blood 1988;72:705–713.
44. Walsh CE, Liu JM, Anderson SM, et al. A trial of recombinant human interleukin-I in patients with severe refractory aplastic anaemia. Br J Haematol 1992;80:106–110.
45. Heit W, Heimpel H, Fischer A, et al. Drug-induced agranulocytosis: Evidence for the commitment of bone marrow haematopoiesis. Scand J Haematol 1985;35:459–468.

46. Julia A, Olona M, Bueno J, et al. Drug-induced agranulocytosis: Prognostic factors in a series of 168 episodes. Br J Haematol 1991;79:366–371.

47. Pisciotta V. Drug-induced agranulocytosis. Drugs 1978;15:132–143.

48. Burckart GJ, Snidow J, Bruce W. Neutropenia following acute chlorpromazine ingestion. Clin Toxicol 1981;18:797–801.

49. Neftel KA, Muller MR, Hauser SD, et al. More on penicillin-induced leukopenia. N Engl J Med 1983;308:901.

50. Heit WF. Hematologic effects of antipyretic analgesics: Drug-induced agranulocytosis. Am J Med 1983;75:65–68.

51. Young GA, Vincent PC. Drug-induced agranulocytosis. Baillieres Clin Haematol 1980;9:483–504.

52. Kirkwood CF, Smith LL, Rustagi PK, et al. Neutropenia associated with beta-lactam antibiotics. Clin Pharm 1983;2:569–578.

53. Homayouni H, Gross PA, Setia V, et al. Leukopenia due to penicillin and cephalosporin homologues. Arch Intern Med 1979;139:827–828.

54. Neftel KA, Hauser SP, Muller MR. Inhibition of granulopoiesis in vivo and in vitro by beta-lactam antibiotics. J Infect Dis 1985;152:90–98.

55. Cooper DS, Goldmiriz D, Lewin AA, et al. Agranulocytosis associated with antithyroid drug. Ann Intern Med 1983;98:26–29.

56. Tajiri J, Noguchi S, Murakami T, et al. Antithyroid drug-induced agranulocytosis: The usefulness of routine white blood cell count monitoring. Arch Intern Med 1990;150:621–624.

57. Toth AL, Mant MJ, Shivji S, et al. Propylthiouracil-induced agranulocytosis: An unusual presentation and a possible mechanism. Am J Med 1988;85:725–727.

58. McIntyre PA, Laleli YR, Hodkinson BA, et al. Evidence for antileukocyte antibodies as a mechanism for drug-induced agranulocytosis. Trans Assoc Am Phys 1971;84:217–225.

59. Werner MC, Romaldini JH, Bromberg N, et al. Adverse effects related to thionamide drugs regimen. Am J Med Sci 1989;297:216–219.

60. Hass WK, Easton JD, Adams HP, et al, for the Ticlopidine Aspirin Study Group. A randomized trial comparing ticlopidine hydrochloride with aspirin for the prevention of stroke in high-risk patients. N Engl J Med 1989;321:501–507.

61. Quaglino D, Venturoni L, Cretara G, et al. Reversible bone marrow suppression primarily involving granulopoiesis following the use of ticlopidine. Haematologica 1982;67:940–941.

62. Resegotti L, Pistone MA, Testa D, et al. Bone marrow culture in patients treated with ticlopidine. Nouv Rev Fr Hematol 1985;27:19–22.

63. Krupp P, Barnes P. Leponex-associated granulocytopenia: A review of the situation. Psychopharmacology 1989;99(Suppl):S118–121.

64. Alvir JM, Lieberman JA, Safferman AZ, et al. Clozapine-induced agranulocytosis: Incidence and risk factors in the United States. N Engl J Med 1993;329:162–167.

65. Fischer V, Haar JA, Greiner L, et al. Possible role of free radical formation in clozapine (Clozaril) induced agranulocytosis. Mol Pharmacol 1991;40:846–853.

66. Beauchesne MF, Shalansky SJ. Nonchemotherapy drug-induced agranulocytosis: A review of 118 patients treated with colony-stimulating factors. Pharmacotherapy 1999;19:299–305.

67. Teitelbaum AH, Bell AJ, Brown SL. Filgrastim (r-metHuG-CSF) reversal of drug-induced agranulocytosis. Am J Med 1993;95:245–246.

68. Nielsen H. Recombinant human granulocyte colony-stimulating factor (rhG-CSF): Filgrastim treatment of clozapine-induced agranulocytosis. J Intern Med 1993;234:529–531.

69. Bjorkholm M, Pisa P, Arver S, Beran M. Haematologic effects of granulocyte-macrophage colony-stimulating factor in a patient with thiamazole-induced agranulocytosis. J Intern Med 1992;232:443–445.

70. Hagg S, Rosenius S, Spigset O. Long-term combination treatment with clozapine and filgrastim in patients with clozapine-induced agranulocytosis. Int Clin Psychopharmacol 2003;18:173.

71. Tabbara IA. Hemolytic anemias: diagnosis and management. Med Clin North Am 1992;76:649–669.

72. McKenzie SB. Hemolytic anemias due to extrinsic factors. In: Balado D, ed. Textbook of Hematology, 2nd ed. Baltimore, Williams & Wilkins, 1996:245–257.

73. Thomas AT. Autoimmune hemolytic anemias. In: Lee RG, et al, ed. Wintrobe's Clinical Hematology, 10th ed. Baltimore, Williams Wilkins, 1999:1233–1263.

74. Jandl JH. Immunohemolytic anemias. In: Strangis JT, ed. Blood, Textbook of Hematology, 2nd ed. Boston, Little, Brown, 1996:421–518.

75. Kirtland HH, Mohler DN, Horwitz DA. Methyldopa inhibition of suppressor-lymphocyte function: A proposed cause of autoimmune hemolytic anemia. N Engl J Med 1980;302:825–832.

76. Garratty G, Arndt P, Prince HE, Schulman IA. The effect of methyldopa and procainamide on suppressor cell autoantibody production. Br Haematol 1993;84:310.

77. Packman CH, Leddy JP. Drug-related immune hemolytic anemia. In Williams WJ, et al, eds. Hematology, 5th ed. New York, McGraw-Hill 1995:691–697.

78. Kelton JG. Impaired reticuloendothelial function in patients treated with methyldopa. N Engl J Med 1985;313:596–600.

79. Kleinman S, Nelson R, Smith L, et al. Positive direct antiglobulin tests and immune hemolytic anemia in patients receiving procainamid N Engl J Med 1984;311:809–812.

80. Beutler E. G6PD deficiency. Blood 1994;84:3613–3636.

81. Sanders SW, Zone JJ, Foltz RR, et al. Hemolytic anemia induced dapsone transmitted through breast milk. Ann Intern Med 1981;9 465–466.

82. Djaldetti M, Blay A, Bergman M, et al. Pure red cell aplasia—a rar disease with multiple causes. Biomed Pharmacother 2003;57:326–33.

83. Casadevall N, Nataf J, Viron B, et al. Pure red-cell aplasia and antierythro poietin antibodies in patients treated with recombinant erythropoieti N Engl J Med 2002;346:469–475.

84. Ahrens N, Kingreen D, Seltsam A, Salama A. Treatment of refractory a toimmune haemolytic anaemia with anti-CD (rituximab). Br J Haemate 2001;114:244–245.

85. Flores G, Cunningham-Rundles C, Newland AC, et al. Efficacy of intr venous immunoglobin in the treatment of autoimmune hemolytic an mia: results in 73 patients. Am J Hematol 1993;44:237–242.

86. Scott JM, Weir DG. Drug-induced megaloblastic change. Clin Haemat 1980;9:587–606.

87. Weinblatt ME. Toxicity of low dose methotrexate in rheumatoid arthriti J Rheumatol 1985;12(Suppl 12):S35–S39.

88. Magee F, O'Sullivan H, McCann SR. Megaloblastosis and low-dos trimethoprim-sulfamethoxazole. Ann Intern Med 1981;95:657.

89. Kobrinsky NL, Ramsay NK. Acute megaloblastic anemia induced b high-dose trimethoprim-sulfamethoxazole. Ann Intern Med 1981;9 780–781.

90. Rivey MP, Schotteluis DD, Berg MJ. Phenytoin-folic acid: A review Drug Intell Clin Pharm 1984;18:292–301.

91. George JN, Raskob GE, Rizvi R, et al. Drug-induced thrombocytopeni A systematic review of published case reports. Ann Intern Med 1998;12 886–890.

92. George JN, El-Harake MA, Aster RH. Thrombocytopenia due to e hanced platelet destruction by immunologic mechanisms. In: Beutler Lichtman MA, Coller BS, Kipps TJ, eds. Williams Hematology, 5th e New York, McGraw-Hill, 1995:1315–1355.

93. Ansell J, Tiarks C, McCue J, et al. Amrinone-induced thrombocytopeni Arch Intern Med 1984;144:949–952.

94. Ross MP, Allen-Webb EM, Pappas JB, et al. Amrinone-associated throm bocytopenia: Pharmacokinetic analysis. Clin Pharmacol Ther 1993;5 661–667.

95. Kiefel V. Differential diagnosis of acute thrombocytopenia. I Warkentin TE, Greinacher A, eds. Heparin-induced Thrombocytopeni 2nd ed. New York, Marcel Dekker, 2001:17–41.

96. Murphy MF, Riordant T, Minchinton RM, et al. Demonstration of immune-mediated mechanism of penicillin-induced neutropenia an thrombocytopenia. Br J Haematol 1983;55:155–160.

97. Salamon DJ, Nusbacher J, Stroupe T, et al. Red cell and platelet-boun IgG penicillin antibodies in a patient with thrombocytopenia. Transfusi 1984;24:395–398.

98. Miescher PA, Graf J. Drug-induced thrombocytopenia. Clin Haemat 1980;9:505–519.

99. Berkowitz SD, Harrington RA, Rund MM, et al. Acute profound thrombocytopenia after c7E3 Fab (abciximab) therapy. Circulation 1997;95: 809–913.

100. Joseph T, Marco J, Gregorini L. Acute profound thrombocytopenia after abciximab therapy during coronary angioplasty. Clin Cardiol 1998; 21:851–852.

101. Jubelirer SJ, Koenig BA, Bates MC. Acute profound thrombocytopenia following c7E3 Fab (abciximab) therapy: Case reports, review of the literature and implications for therapy. Am J Hematol 1999;61:205–208.

102. Cines DB. Glycoprotein IIb/IIIa antagonists: Potential induction and detection of drug-dependent antiplatelet antibodies. Am Heart J 1998;135: S152–S159.

103. Peter K, Straub A, Kohler B, et al. Platelet activation as a potential mechanism of GP IIb/IIIa inhibitor-induced thrombocytopenia. Am J Cardiol 1999;84:519–524.

104. Stiegler H, Fischer Y, Steiner S, et al. Sudden onset of EDTA-dependent pseudothrombocytopenia after therapy with the glycoprotein IIb/IIIa antagonists c7E3 Fab. Ann Hematol 2000;79:161–164.

105. Johnson RA, Lazarus KH, Henry DH. Heparin-induced thrombocytopenia prospective study. Am J Hematol 1984;17:349–353.

106. Cines DB, Kaywin P, Bina M, et al. Heparin-associated thrombocytopenia. N Engl J Med 1980;303:788–795.

107. Cheng TC. Thrombocytopenia associated with minidose heparin therapy. Postgrad Med 1981;70:73–78.

108. Laster JL, Nichols WK, Silver D. Thrombocytopenia associated with heparin-coated catheters in patients with heparin-associated antiplatelet antibodies. Arch Intern Med 1989;149:2285–2287.

109. Aster RH. Heparin-induced thrombocytopenia and thrombosis. N Engl J Med 1995;332:1374–1376.

110. King DJ, Kelton JG. Heparin-associated thrombocytopenia. Ann Intern Med 1984;100:535–540.

111. Bell WR, Royall RM. Heparin-associated thrombocytopenia: A comparison of three heparin preparations. N Engl J Med 1980;303:902–907.

112. Green D, Martin GJ, Shoichet SH, et al. Thrombocytopenia in a prospective, randomized, double-blind trial of bovine and porcine heparin. Am J Med Sci 1984;288:60–64.

113. Rao AK, White GC, Sherman L, et al. Low incidence of thrombocytopenia with porcine mucosal heparin: A prospective multicenter study. Arch Intern Med 1989;149:1285–1288.

114. Bailey RT, Ursick JA, Heim KL, et al. Heparin-associated thrombocytopenia: A prospective comparison of bovine lung heparin, manufactured by a new process, and porcine intestinal heparin. Drug Intell Clin Pharm 1986;20:374–378.

115. Warkentin TE, Barkin RL. Newer strategies for the treatment of heparin-induced thrombocytopenia. Pharmacotherapy 1999;19:181–195.

116. Warkentin TE, Levine MN, Hirsh J, et al. Heparin-induced thrombocytopenia in patients treated with low-molecular-weight heparin or unfractionated heparin. N Engl J Med 1995;332:1330–1335.

117. Kikta MJ, Keller MP, Humphrey PV, et al. Can low molecular weight heparins and heparinoids be safely given to patients with heparin-induced thrombocytopenia syndrome? Surgery 1993;114:705–710.

118. Armstrong RD, Faith A, Panayi GS, et al. Gold-induced thrombocytopenia: Detection of anti-platelet antibody. Clin Rheumatol 1983;2: 183–188.

119. Adachi JD, Bensen WG, Singal DP, et al. Gold induced thrombocytopenia: platelet associated IgG and HLA typing in three patients. J Rheumatol 1984;11:355–357.

120. Coblyn JS, Weinblatt M, Holdsworth D, et al. Gold-induced thrombocytopenia: A clinical and immunogenic study of twenty-three patients. Ann Intern Med 1981;95:178–181.

121. Kelton JG, Meltzer D, Moore J, et al. Drug-induced thrombocytopenia is associated with increased binding of IgG to platelets both in vivo and in vitro. Blood 1981;58:524–529.

122. Chong BH, Berndt MC, Koutts J, et al. Quinidine-induced thrombocytopenia and leukopenia: Demonstration and characterization of distinct antiplatelets and antileukocyte antibodies. Blood 1983;62:1218–1223.

123. Pedersen-Bjergaard U, Andersen M, Hansen PB. Drug-induced thrombocytopenia: Clinical data on 309 cases and the effect of corticosteroid therapy. Eur J Clin Pharmacol 1997;52:183–189.

124. Hirsh J, Warkentin TE, Raschke R, et al. Heparin: Mechanism of action, pharmacokinetics, dosing considerations, monitoring, efficacy, and safety. Chest 1998;114:489S–510S.

103

LABORATORY TESTS TO DIRECT ANTIMICROBIAL PHARMACOTHERAPY

Michael J. Rybak and Jeffrey R. Aeschlimann

Learning Objectives and other resources can be found at *www.pharmacotherapyonline.com.*

KEY CONCEPTS

1. Familiarity with normal host flora and typical pathogens will help to determine whether a patient is truly infected or merely colonized.

2. Direct examination of tissue and body fluids by Gram stain provides simple and rapid information about the potential pathogen.

3. Isolation of the offending organism by culture assists in the diagnosis of infection and allows for more definitive directed treatment.

4. The development of molecular testing systems has improved our ability to diagnose infection and determine the antimicrobial susceptibilities for numerous fastidious or slow-growing pathogens, such as mycobacteria and viruses.

5. Although highly standardized, in vitro antimicrobial susceptibility testing has limitations and often cannot truly mimic the conditions found at the site of an infection. This may have implications for discordance between in vitro susceptibility results and in vivo response to therapy.

6. The laboratory evaluation of antimicrobial activity is an important component of the pharmacotherapeutic management of infectious diseases.

7. Antimicrobial pharmacodynamics have become a crucial consideration for the clinician during the selection of both empirical and pathogen-directed therapy in the current era of antimicrobial resistance.

8. When used appropriately, rapid automated susceptibility test systems appear to improve therapeutic outcomes of patients with infection, especially when they are linked with other clinical information systems.

9. Although not performed routinely during the clinical management of patients with infections, data from certain laboratory tests (e.g., minimal bactericidal concentration tests, timed-kill tests, post-antibiotic-effect tests, and antimicrobial combination testing) are important for the clinician to understand because they help to determine an antimicrobial's pharmacodynamic properties.

10. Routine monitoring of serum concentrations is currently used for a select few antimicrobials (e.g., aminoglycosides, chloramphenicol, and vancomycin) in an attempt to minimize toxicity and maximize efficacy.

11. Appropriate timing for the collection of serum samples is crucial to ensure that proper data are generated on the pharmacokinetics of antimicrobials.

12. The monitoring of serum concentrations of aminoglycosides and the use of extended-interval doses of aminoglycosides can help to maximize the probability of therapeutic success and minimize the probability of aminoglycoside-related toxicity.

13. Vancomycin serum concentration monitoring can either be minimized or avoided entirely for many patients who are treated with this antimicrobial.

14. Optimization of antimicrobial pharmacodynamic parameters such as the ratio of the peak serum concentration to minimum inhibitory concentration or the time that the serum concentration remains above the minimum inhibitory concentration can improve infection treatment outcomes.

Appropriate antimicrobial pharmacotherapy for a given infectious disease requires knowledge of the infecting pathogen, host characteristics, and the drug's expected activity against the pathogen. The most fundamental aspect of therapy starts with an appropriate diagnosis.

A vast array of laboratory tests is available to assist the clinician in verifying the presence of infection and for monitoring the response to therapy. Although useful, these tests are subject to interpretation and cannot be substituted for sound clinical judgment. Organism susceptibility to a given group of antimicrobials is key to determining the patient's therapy. Host characteristics, however, such as immune status, infection-site location, and body organ function, play a significant role in selecting the most appropriate antimicrobial for a given individual.[1] This chapter reviews the routine laboratory tests that are used to assist in the diagnosis and treatment of infection.

LABORATORY TESTS CONFIRMING THE PRESENCE OF INFECTION

NONSPECIFIC TESTS

A number of tests are used by clinicians to determine whether a patient has an infection. Although no single test can prove that a patient is infected, when used in combination with clinical findings, tests are helpful to establish the diagnosis of infection. Because many tests are nonspecific, there are often factors other than infection that can cause a test to be reported as positive when no infection exists. Therefore, the importance of careful interpretation and sound clinical judgment cannot be overemphasized. This chapter reviews the commonly employed tests and their interpretation and application for the diagnosis and management of infection.

WHITE BLOOD CELL COUNT AND DIFFERENTIAL

◀ Understanding the role of the white blood cell (WBC) in fighting infection is important in the diagnosis of infection, the selection of drug therapy, and the monitoring of patient progress. The major role of the WBC is to defend the body against invading organisms such as bacteria, viruses, and fungi. The normal range of the WBC is 4500 to 10,000 cells/mm³. WBCs usually are elevated in response to infection. The WBC count can become elevated in response to a number of noninfectious causes, including stress, inflammatory conditions such as rheumatoid arthritis, and leukemia or in response to certain drugs (e.g., corticosteroids).

WBCs are divided into two groups: the granulocytes, which have prominent cytoplasmic granules, and the agranulocytes, which lack granules. Polymorphonuclear granulocytes PMNs) are made up of neutrophils, basophils, and eosinophils. The two other classes of WBCs are the monocytes and lymphocytes. Neutrophils are the most common type of WBCs in the blood, comprising approximately 70% of the total WBC count. In response to infection, they leave the bloodstream and enter the tissue to interact with and phagocytize offending pathogens. Mature neutrophils sometimes are referred to as *segs* because of their segmented nucleus, which usually consists of two to five lobes. Immature neutrophils lack this segmented feature and are referred to as *bands*. During an acute infection, immature neutrophils, such as bands (single-lobed nucleus), are released from the bone marrow into the bloodstream at an increased rate, and the percentage of bands (usually 5%) may increase in relationship to mature cells. The change in the ratio of mature to immature cells is often referred to as a *shift to the left* because of the way the cells were counted by hand with a microscope and charted from immature to mature cells.

Leukocytosis is a normal host defense to infection and is an important adjunct to antimicrobial therapy. Unfortunately, bacterial infection is a common complication of neutropenia from cancer chemotherapy. These patients are incapable of increasing their WBCs in response to infection. In fact, susceptibility to infection in these patients is highly dependent on their WBC status. Patients with neutrophil counts of less than 500 cells/mm³ are at high risk for the development of bacterial or fungal infections. The absence of leukocytosis also occurs in the elderly and in severe cases of sepsis.[2,3]

Lymphocytes comprise 15% to 40% of all WBCs and are of central importance to the immune system. Two functional types of lymphocytes are the T cell, which is involved in cell-mediated immunity, and the B cell, which produces antibodies involved in humoral immunity. Lymphocytosis frequently is associated with acute viral infections such as Epstein-Barr virus infection (mononucleosis) and cytomegalovirus in fection and rarely with unusual bacterial infections (i.e., *Brucella* spp. infections).

T-lymphocytes are characterized on the basis of function (type 1 or type 2) and on the basis of surface antigen. Most type 1 and type 2 T cells carry a T4 (CD4) marker that recognizes class II major histocompatibility complex (MHC) antigens, and most cytoxic T cells carry a T8 (CD8) marker that recognizes class I MHC antigens. A severe deficiency of CD4 cells is associated with human immunodeficiency virus (HIV) infection.[4] Malignancies also may adversely affect cellular immunity. Patients with Hodgkin's disease and other types of lymphoma exhibit defective cell-mediated immunity that predisposes them to a variety of infections, notably fungal diseases and infections by the *Listeria* spp. Drug treatment with cytotoxic chemotherapy and corticosteroids also may have profound deleterious effects on cell-mediated immunity.[5] Defects in cell-mediated immune function can be demonstrated by a variety of simple laboratory tests, including quantification of lymphocytes on a routine complete blood cell count and skin testing for anergy. A more detailed investigation includes quantitative measurements of CD4+ and CD8+ cells. Monocytosis is correlated less frequently with acute bacterial infection, although its presence has been associated with the response of certain infections (e.g., tuberculosis) to chemotherapy. Eosinophilia may result from parasitic infection.[6] Figure 103–1 describes a number of cell types and their biologic function.

OTHER TESTS

There are a number of nonspecific laboratory tests that are useful to support the diagnosis of infection. The inflammatory process initiated by an infection sets up a complex of host responses. Activation of complements, such as C3a and C5a, initiates inflammation and sets off a cascade of changes and the subsequent release of mediators, all of which can be measured and monitored. Serum complement concentrations, particularly C3, usually are consumed as part of the host defense mechanism and subsequently are reduced during the early stages of an acute infectious process.[7] Acute-phase reactants, such as the erythrocyte sedimentation rate (ESR) and the C-reactive protein concentration, are elevated in the presence of an inflammatory process but do not confirm the presence of infection because they are often elevated in noninfectious conditions, such as collagen-vascular diseases and arthritis. Large elevations in ESR are associated with infections such as endocarditis, osteomyelitis, and intraabdominal infections.[8]

Changes in endothelial membranes and the presence of a foreign pathogen and its endotoxins cause certain cytokines, such as interleukin 1 (IL-1), IL-6, and IL-8 and tumor necrosis factor α (TNF-α), to be produced by macrophages or lymphocytes. Fluctuations in cytokine levels occur during the course of an infection, which may be useful in staging and monitoring the response to therapy. Although abnormally high levels of TNF have been associated with a variety of noninfectious causes, spiked elevations in TNF are found in patients with serious infections, such as sepsis. Studies of the relationship of circulating mediators to patient outcome have determined the value of endotoxin and cytokine measurements in patients with sepsis. Although the combination of elevations in endotoxin and individual cytokines has correlated well with the mortality rate, measurement

Cell type	Cellular function	
Macrophage/monocyte	Antigen presenting cell Surveillance of antigens	
Neurophils	Defense against bacteria and fungus	
Eosinophils	Defense against parasite Response against allergic reactions	
Basophil	Allergic response	
B lymphocyte	Antibody production Antigen presenting cell	
T lymphocytes	Cellular immunity against virus and tumors Regulation of the immune system	

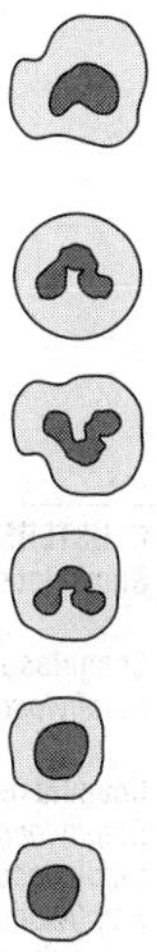

FIGURE 103–1. Various cell types and their biologic functions.

IL-6 was by far the best individual cytokine that predicted patient outcome.[9] More recent information has demonstrated a significant relationship between monocyte human leukocyte antigen (HLA) DR expression and the risk of mortality in patients with community-acquired severe infections.[10] Understanding the balance between these proinflammatory and anitinflammatory processes likely will lead to interventions that may have a direct impact on the outcome of patients with sepsis.[11]

LABORATORY IDENTIFICATION OF PATHOGENS

COLONIZATION VERSUS INFECTION

Pathogens are organisms that are capable of damaging host tissues and that elicit specific host responses and symptoms that are consistent with an infectious process. These organisms are transferred from patient to patient, vector to patient (animals, insects, and so on), environment to patient (e.g., hospital settings) or are derived from the patient's own flora. On the other hand, the human body contains a vast variety of microorganisms that colonize body systems and make up the so-called normal flora. These organisms occur naturally in the tissues of the host and provide some benefits, including defense by occupying space, competing for essential nutrients, stimulating cross-protective antibodies, and suppressing the growth of potentially pathogenic bacteria and fungi (Table 103–1).

Organisms that comprise the normal flora can become pathogenic when host defenses become impaired or if they are translocated to other body sites during trauma. The identification of an organism considered to be normal flora in a wound or otherwise sterile body cavity or fluid often becomes a dilemma for the clinician in deciding whether or not a patient is infected and whether or not the patient requires treatment. Such is the case with *Staphylococcus epidermidis* when it is identified in the blood of a hospitalized patient. *S. epidermidis* is considered normal skin flora and commonly colonizes intravenous catheters. In these conditions, identification of the organism must be taken in light of the patient circumstances (signs and symptoms, laboratory indices supporting infection) and the probability of the organism being responsible for the infection. Often the simple removal of the catheter may eliminate the organism from the bloodstream, thereby preventing misdiagnosis and unnecessary application of antimicrobials.[12]

DIRECT EXAMINATION

Direct examination of tissue or body fluids believed to be infected can provide simple, rapid information to the clinician. Microscopic examination of wet-mount specimen preparations can provide valuable information regarding potential pathogens. Applications of this procedure with or without staining preparations include direct examination of sputum, bronchial aspirates, scrapings of mucosal lesions, and urinary sediment. The Gram stain is one of the

TABLE 103–1. Examples of Normal Bacterial Flora

	Gram-Positive		Gram-Negative		
	Cocci	*Rods*	*Cocci*	*Rods*	*Other*
Skin	*Staphylococcus* spp. (e.g., *S. epidermidis*) *Streptococcus* spp.	*Corynebacterium* spp. *Propionibacterium* spp.		Enteric bacilli (some sites) *Acinetobacter* spp. (Coccobacilli)	
Oropharynx	Streptococci—viridans group Micrococcus	*Corynebacterium* spp.	Neisseria	*Hemophilus* spp.	Spirochetes
Gastrointenstinal tract	*Enterococcus* spp. *Peptostreptococcus* spp.	*Lactobacillus, Clostridium*		*Bacteroides* spp. Enteric bacilli (*E. coli, Klebsiella* spp.)	
Genital tract	*Streptococcus* spp. *Staphylococcus* spp.	*Lactobacillus* *Corynebacterium* spp.		Enterobacteriaceae *Prevotella* spp.	*Mycoplasma*

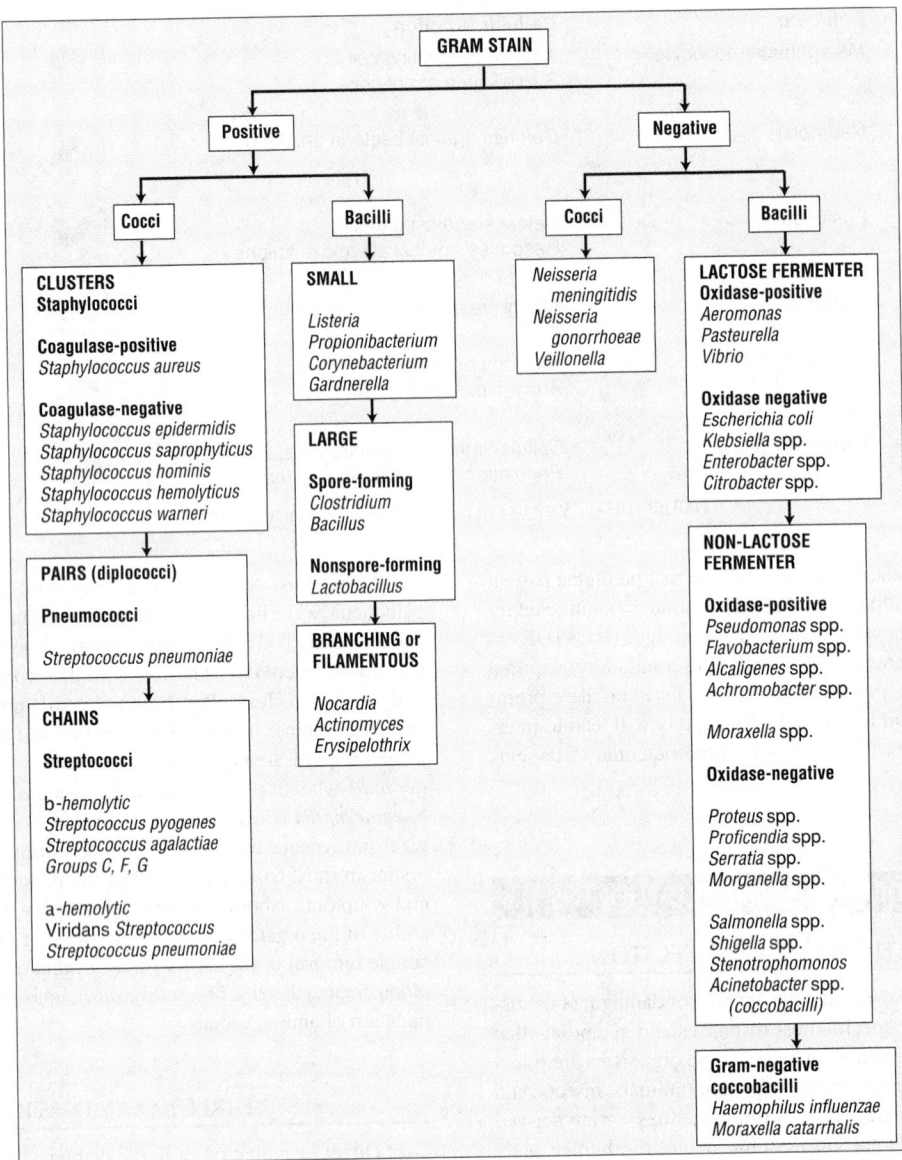

FIGURE 103–2. Important bacterial pathogens classified according to Gram stain and morhologic characteristic.

first identification tests run on a specimen brought to the laboratory. For this procedure, crystal violet is applied as the primary stain, with iodine added to enhance the staining process and to form a crystal violet–iodine complex. Alcohol decolorization is the next step in the procedure. Gram-negative cells are decolorized by the addition of alcohol, and they take in a red color when counterstained by safranin. Gram-positive cells are not decolorized by alcohol and retain the crystal violet color and appear purple. Gram staining in conjunction with microscopic examination may provide a presumptive diagnosis and some indication of the organism's characteristics (gram-positive, gram-negative, gram-variable, bacillus, or cocci). This is extremely useful information for the selection of empirical antibiotic therapy.

Gram stains are performed routinely on cerebrospinal fluid (CSF) in cases of suspected meningitis, on urethral smears for venereal diseases, and on abscess or effusion specimens. They are helpful in identifying organisms that may not grow on culture and which otherwise would be missed. Although Gram stains of sputum are performed routinely when respiratory tract infections are suspected, there is controversy regarding the usefulness of this test because the sputum is often contaminated with mixed or normal flora. The predominance of

one particular organism, the overall number of organisms present, the amount of PMNs present, and the presence or absence of a significant amount of squamous epithelial cells (<10 per low-power field) may improve the significance of the sputum Gram stain specimen. Figure 103–2 lists some common infecting pathogens grouped according to Gram stain and other characteristics.

A number of other staining techniques are used to identify pathogens. In particular, staining procedures are used for pathogens that are best identified microscopically because of their poor growth characteristics in the laboratory setting. The best examples of these are the Ziehl-Neelsen stain for acid-fast bacilli, which is used for the identification of mycobacteria, and the india ink, potassium hydroxide (KOH), and Giemsa stains, which are useful for detecting certain fungi.[13]

CULTURES

Isolation of the etiologic agent by culture is the most definitive method available for the diagnosis and eventual treatment of infection. Although suspicion of a specific pathogen or group pathogens is helpful to the laboratory for the selection of a specific cultivating medium, the more common procedure for the laboratory is to screen for the presence of any potential pathogen. After receipt of a clinical specimen, the laboratory will inoculate the specimen in a variety of artificial media. Some culture media are designed to differentiate various organisms on the basis of biochemical characteristics or to select specific organisms on the basis of resistance to certain antimicrobials. Other media are employed commonly for the isolation of more fastidious organisms, such as *Listeria, Legionella, Mycobacterium,* or *Chlamydia.* Cultures for viruses are more difficult to perform and are undertaken primarily by larger institutions or outside laboratories because of the technical expense and time involved in processing samples.

When a culture is obtained, careful attention must be paid to ensuring that specimens are collected and transported appropriately to the laboratory. Every effort should be made to avoid contamination with normal flora and to ensure that the specimen is placed in the appropriate transport medium. Culture specimens should be transported to the laboratory as soon as possible because organisms may perish from prolonged exposure to air or drying. This is especially important for swab specimen preparations. Transport media may not be ideal for all organisms. Specimens that contain fastidious organisms or anaerobes require special transport media and should be forwarded immediately to the laboratory for processing. Finally, the source of the specimen should be clearly recorded and forwarded along with the culture to the laboratory. This process will aid the laboratory in differentiating true pathogens from the expected normal flora, and it will help in the selection of the appropriate culture media.

Detection of microorganisms in the bloodstream by standard culturing techniques is difficult because of the inherently low yield of organisms diluted by blood, humoral factors with bactericidal activity, and the potential of antimicrobial pretreatment affecting organism growth. Newer automated systems employing the use of medium-containing culture bottles and innovative organism-detection techniques have improved this situation. Most blood collection bottles dilute the blood specimen 1:10 with growth medium to neutralize the bactericidal properties of blood and antimicrobials. The addition of a polyanionic anticoagulant abolishes the effect of complement and antiphagocytic activity in the specimen. Some laboratories also add β-lactamase to their blood collection bottles. Antibiotic-binding resin bottles, such as Bactec 16 B, are also commercially available.

Rapid detection of bacteria or fungi within a few hours of specimen collection is now possible by the use of automated culturing systems, such as Bactec (Becton Dickinson Diagnostic Instruments, Sparks, MD), that use bottles of growth medium containing a fluorescent sensor to monitor culture bottles for the presence of CO_2 every 10 minutes as a by-product of microorganism growth. Computers monitoring the system alert laboratory personnel of positive culture results by both audible and visual alarms. Once detected, a battery of testing can be performed rapidly that shortens the reporting time and that enables clinicians to obtain preliminary information about the organism.[13,14]

The initial identity of the organism can be determined by a variety of testing procedures. General schemes differentiate organisms into primary groups, such as gram-positive and gram-negative bacteria. This can be accomplished by simple Gram staining, as described previously, by evaluating organism growth patterns on selective media, and by testing for the presence or absence of specific enzymes and chemical characteristics, such as hemolytic and fermentation properties. For example, non-lactose-fermenting gram-negative bacilli that

are oxidase-positive may suggest *Pseudomonas aeruginosa* as opposed to a variety of other potential gram-negative organisms. This preliminary information, which is readily obtainable from the laboratory, may greatly assist the clinician in choosing the appropriate empirical therapy.

Definitive identification of organisms requires more complex testing procedures and devices that can further differentiate the organism on the basis of specific fermentation and biochemical reactive properties. Commercially available automated systems can inoculate the test organism into a series of panels containing a variety of test media, sugars, and other reagents. The system can then photometrically determine the results and compare the findings to a library of organism characteristics to produce a definitive identification.[14]

Viral agents may be detected by direct observation of inoculated culture cells for cytopathic effects or by detection of antigens after incubation by immunofluorescent methods. The culture method is most useful for organisms such as cytomegalovirus (CMV) or herpes simplex virus because these viral agents are rapidly propagated in culture cells, making them easily detected.[15]

DIAGNOSIS OF INFECTION USING IMMUNOLOGIC AND MOLECULAR METHODS

ANTIBODY AND ANTIGEN DETECTION

5 The use of immunologic methods for the diagnosis and monitoring of human host immune response to infection has become an indispensable laboratory tool. This is especially important in the detection of microorganisms, such as bacteria, fungi, and viruses, that otherwise would elude detection or severely delay results from conventional culturing techniques. These methods have the advantage of a rapid turnaround time and an acceptable level of sensitivity and specificity. Some tests (e.g., identification of group A streptococci) are simple to use, can be performed conveniently in the physician's office, and often may be used to decide whether antibiotics should be administered for a suspected upper respiratory infection.

The primary immunologic methods involve the detection and quantification of antibodies directed against a specific pathogen or its components (i.e., surface proteins of HIV, such as p24 antigen). The commercial availability of specific monoclonal antibodies in a variety of testing formats has led to an increased use of these methods for direct pathogen detection. Although pathogen antigenic proteins may be increased and, therefore, detected easily during acute infection, detection of past or asymptomatic infection may be difficult because of undetectable levels of antigen and, therefore, low antibody titers. Continued advancement in test sensitivity (the capability to detect a true-positive state) and specificity (the capability to detect a negative state), as well as the use of amplification techniques, likely will improve these tests in the near future.

Antibody or antigen detection may be accomplished by a variety of techniques, including immunofluorescence, which has been used routinely for the detection of cytomegalovirus, respiratory syncytial virus, varicella-zoster virus, *Treponema pallidum* (syphilis), *Borrelia burgdorferi* (Lyme's disease), and *Chlamydia trachomatis.* Latex agglutination is useful for detecting meningococcal capsular antigens in CSF of patients suspected of having bacterial meningitis and as an aid in the diagnosis of *Legionella pneumophila.* Enzyme-linked immunosorbent assay (ELISA) is a commonly employed method for detecting HIV, herpes simplex virus, respiratory syncytial virus, pneumococcal serum antibody, *Neisseria gonorrhoeae,* and *Haemophilus pylori.*[15]

MOLECULAR TECHNIQUES FOR THE DETECTION OF MICROORGANISMS

HYBRIDIZATION DNA PROBES

Highly sensitive and specific molecular methods are now available for the rapid detection and identification of a variety of pathogens. The two primary molecular techniques used commonly are nucleic acid hybridization, which involves the binding of a specific DNA or RNA probe to its target, and DNA amplification schemes. Probe-based methods require the extraction of DNA or RNA from a clinical specimen (i.e., body fluid, tissue, or WBC) or directly from a microorganism culture. The extract is then tested for the presence of pathogen DNA or RNA using a probe that contains a specific oligonucleic acid–based sequence for the organism. For example, a probe with a sequence of ACTGTT would bind to the complementary organism nucleic acid sequence of TGACAA. Because the probe is labeled with a signal-emitting molecule (i.e., radiolabeled, colorimetric, or chemoluminescent), a match would be detected. The primary means for detection involves the use of separation of the organism DNA into specific fragments (gel electrophoresis), transfer and fixation of the mixture to specialized paper or nylon membranes (Southern or Northern blotting), the mixing of the DNA fragments with the labeled probe (hybridization), and transfer to radiographic or photographic film for processing. These techniques have been used for many years and are fairly standardized methods for the detection of a variety of organisms. Hybridization probes are useful for a variety of diagnostic and clinical applications, including the direct examination of organisms in tissue, which enables the evaluation and documentation of organism infestation, location, distribution, and host response. The use of hybridization probes is particularly helpful for the detection of slow-growing organisms such as *Mycobacterium tuberculosis, N. gonorrhoeae,* and certain species of fungi. This technique is also used to document the presence or absence of antimicrobial-resistant genes in a cell culture and to track the spread of resistant microorganisms in hospital and outpatient settings.

Although employed widely, the use of hybridization probes is often limited by their lack of sensitivity. Probe amplification methods are available that improve the sensitivity of these assays. The principle of these probe-amplification schemes is to boost the probe's signal-emitting molecule to make it more easily detected. The most advanced signal-amplification system available is the branched DNA (bDNA) probe system (Chiron Corp., Emeryville, CA). This system uses multiple probes and multiple signal-emitting molecules (reporters). The target-binding probe contains two hybridization regions. One region is complementary to the target, and the other region is capable of binding with the bDNA amplification multimer. The amplification multimer binds multiple reporter molecules (as many as 3000), which provides a significant boost in the probe's signal. Branched DNA probe systems are being developed for rapid detection of hepatitis B and C, HIV-1, and CMV. Because of the system's high specificity and quantitative ability, bDNA probe assays may be useful for therapeutic monitoring, such as in the case of monitoring the response to antiretroviral therapy in acquired immunodeficiency syndrome (AIDS).[16,17]

NUCLEIC ACID AMPLIFICATION METHODS

Nucleic acid amplification methods are now considered a standard laboratory tool. They have had a tremendous impact on the diagnosis and treatment of infectious diseases. These highly sensitive methods have the capability to detect and quantitate minute amounts of target nucleic acid in a rapid manner. The polymerase chain reaction (PCR) is based on the capability of a DNA polymerase to copy and elongate a targeted strand of DNA. This is accomplished by the use of short oligonucleotide primers (20 to 25 nucleotides long) that correspond to the DNA targeted to be expanded. After an excess of primers and heat-stable DNA polymerases are added to the targeted DNA mixture, the targeted DNA is denatured and separated by a process of cycling hot and cool temperatures. The heat-stable DNA polymerase elongates the primers on the two separate strands of DNA, thereby generating two new strands of targeted DNA. The process of cycling typically is repeated 20 to 35 times. Each cycle doubles the amount of DNA originally present at the start of the cycle, thereby exponentially increasing the overall number of DNA copies. In theory, more than 1 million copies of the original DNA can be generated from as few as 20 cycles.

Although this amplification technique is very sensitive and has tremendous application potential, it is not without problems. The powerful amplification procedure may yield false-positive results when samples are contaminated by nucleic acid left over from previously amplified DNA. Other problems include primer artifact formation and nonspecific hybridization of primers to DNA samples. Several modifications to the original PCR technology have been made over the years to improve the sensitivity and application potential for PCR, including the use of multiple sets of amplification primers, multiplex PCR, PCR amplification of RNA by converting targeted RNA with reverse transcriptase to complementary DNA templates (which are then suitable for DNA amplification by traditional PCR techniques), and real-time quantitative PCR.

The cost-benefit ratio of PCR as compared with traditional microbiologic methods must be evaluated. Molecular amplification schemes such as PCR have become routine in situations in which rapid turnaround time is essential to improve patient diagnosis and outcome, e.g., real-time universal screening for acute HIV infection and routine testing and monitoring of patients receiving treatment for HIV infection, and the isolation and detection of fastidious or slow-growing organisms such as *M. tuberculosis, B. burgdorferi,* and *Helicobacter pylori.* Another potential application for this technology is the early detection of multidrug-resistant organisms. Amplification of resistant gene markers would aid in rapid selection of the most appropriate therapy in the treatment of organisms in which days or weeks traditionally are required for culturing and determining basic susceptibility. Examples fitting this description include the rapid detection of isoniazid and rifampin gene markers for *M. tuberculosis,* early detection of the *mec* gene responsible for methicillin resistance in *S. aureus,* and identification of resistant genes responsible for production of β-lactamase capable of destroying specific cephalosporins and multidrug resistant *H. pylori.*[17–20]

EVALUATION OF ANTIMICROBIAL ACTIVITY AND DETERMINATION OF ANTIMICROBIAL PHARMACODYNAMICS

The laboratory evaluation of antimicrobial activity is an important component of the pharmacotherapeutic management of infectious diseases. The integration of this activity with various pharmacokinetic properties of the antimicrobial agent determines the drug's pharmacodynamic characteristics. Antimicrobial pharmacodynamics have become a crucial consideration for the clinician during the selection of both empirical and pathogen-directed therapy in the current era of antimicrobial resistance. Antimicrobial activity and pharmacodynamics also weigh heavily in contemporary formulary decision-making processes, the development of antimicrobial streamlining programs, and for intravenous-to-oral antimicrobial switch protocols.[21]

Most antimicrobial susceptibility tests used in the clinical laboratory are well characterized and have been standardized by the National Committee for Clinical Laboratory Standards (NCCLS). However, controversies still exist surrounding the exact test methods, interpretation and reporting of test results, and application of the results to the treatment of patients.[22] Nevertheless, there are many investigations that show that the general antimicrobial susceptibility or resistance profile of an infecting organism correlates with clinical and/or microbiologic responses to therapy.

Most of the standardized and well-accepted test methods evaluate the susceptibility of aerobic, nonfastidious bacteria. However, substantial progress has been made in the past decade toward the development of sensitive, specific, reproducible, and clinically useful susceptibility tests for anaerobic bacteria, yeasts, mycobacteria, and viruses. Continued advances in technology should further improve test methods and the rapidity with which the results can be applied to the management of patients. Although these newer systems are often very expensive, the increased quality and decreased overall costs of patient care may determine their cost-effectiveness.

QUANTITATIVE ANTIMICROBIAL SUSCEPTIBILITY TESTING

MINIMAL INHIBITORY CONCENTRATIONS

The *minimal inhibitory concentration* (MIC) is defined as the lowest antimicrobial concentration that prevents visible growth of an organism after approximately 24 hours of incubation in a specified growth medium. The MIC quantitatively determinates in vitro antibacterial activity. Classically, MICs were determined via the macrotube dilution method, which uses liquid growth medium (broth), doubling serial dilutions of antimicrobials in test tubes, and a standard inoculum of bacteria (approximately 10^5 colony-forming units [CFU]/mL). The tubes (up to 10 mL) are incubated at approximately 35°C (95°F) for 18 to 24 hours and then examined for visible bacterial growth (Fig. 103–3). Since macrodilution MIC testing is laborious and supply-intensive, it is not used often in the contemporary clinical microbiology laboratory. However, one advantage of this method is that it tests a large inoculum of bacteria—a factor that can improve the detection of small numbers of resistant subpopulations or document the presence of inducible resistance.[23]

The development and use of 96-well microtiter plates enabled the increased use of broth-dilution MIC testing in the clinical

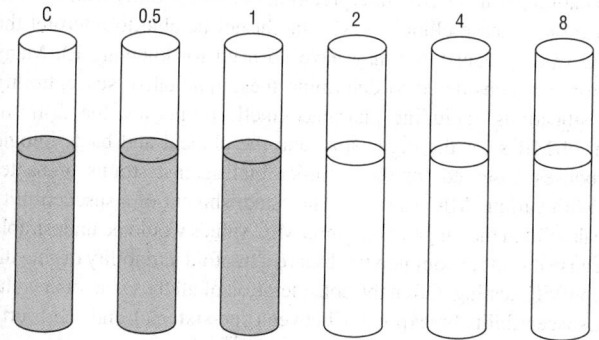

FIGURE 103–3. Macrotube minimal inhibitory concentration (MIC) determination. The growth control (*C*), 0.5 mg/dL, and 1 mg/dL tubes are visibly turbid, indicating bacterial growth. The MIC is read as the first clear test tube (2 mg/dL).

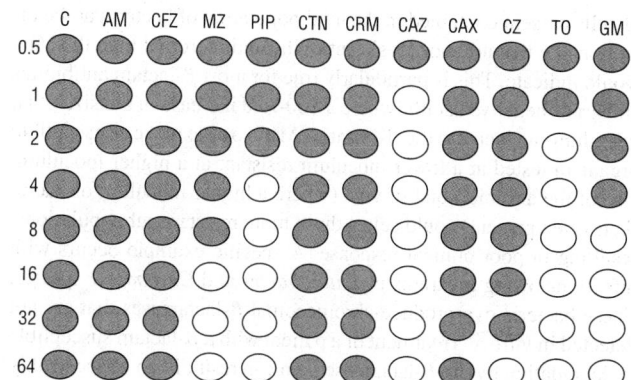

FIGURE 103–4. A prepared microtiter minimal inhibitory concentration (MIC) panel represents antibiotics tested commonly against gram-negative pathogens. This tray indicates that the organism is resistant to ampicillin (AM), cefazolin (CFZ), cefotetan (CTN), cefuroxime (CRM), ceftriaxone (CAX), and gentamicin (GM). The isolate is sensitive to mezlocillin (MZ), piperacillin (PIP), ceftazidime (CAZ), and tobramycin (TO). The isolate would be considered intermediately susceptible to cefizoxime (CZ).

laboratory owing to significant reductions in the amount of labor and medium needed. Volumes of 100 to 200 microliters (mcL) or less of medium are used, and multichannel pipets, automated preparation/test interpretation systems, and/or the combination of both can allow efficient preparation of numerous tests (Fig. 103–4). The microdilution MIC test method (or adaptations of this test) is the most commonly used susceptibility test method in the clinical microbiology laboratory.[19] Although microdilution MIC testing is a vast improvement over macrodilution MIC testing, it still has important shortcomings. These include both limitations in the numbers and various types of antimicrobials to use in the test (especially with premade or premanufactured trays) and a decreased ability to detect some forms of antimicrobial resistance (e.g., inducible β-lactamses) as compared with the macrodilution MIC method.[18,19]

The MIC also can be determined using solid agar. For the agar dilution MICs, the test antimicrobial is added to the molten agar at the desired concentration just prior to its solidification. After the agar has hardened, suspensions of test bacteria are applied to the agar. As with broth MICs, the agar dilution MIC is defined as the lowest concentration that prevents the visible growth of the organism after an overnight incubation period. The primary advantages of the agar dilution MICs are the ability to test many bacteria on the same agar plate and the flexibility to choose specific antimicrobials, but these advantages often are outweighed by the need to prepare agar plates manually and the instability of the antimicrobial in the agar as compared with commercially prepared microtiter MIC trays. Although agar dilution MIC once was considered the standard susceptibility test for many bacteria and for certain slow-growing organisms such as *M. tuberculosis*, its use has declined in most clinical laboratories with the advent of more rapidly performed and less cumbersome susceptibility testing methods (microtiter MICs, PCR, radiometric, and/or fluorometric tests).[24]

LIMITATIONS AND PROBLEMS WITH MIC TESTING

Some limitations and problems of MIC testing are academic in nature, whereas others may have important implications for the clinician's everyday management of patients with serious infections. For example, because the MIC only represents the concentration of antimicrobial that is needed to inhibit visual growth of the most resistant cells within the tested bacterial population, there actually may be small numbers of cells present contained in the total population of bacteria at the infection site that are more resistant to the antimicrobial than the MIC would indicate. This is particularly true for most β-lactam antibiotics and gram-negative bacilli, where a 100-fold increase in the size of an inoculum can increase the β-lactam's MIC so as to make a susceptible organism tested at a lower inoculum resistant at a higher inoculum. Use of the antimicrobial in vivo (where a higher inoculum of bacteria is often present) could select these more resistant subpopulations, resulting in poor clinical response. A specific example occurs with infections owing to strains of *Enterobacter* and *Citrobacter* species. These bacteria overproduce chromosomal β-lactamases that are not detected in vitro.[25] Treatment of a patient with a β-lactam susceptible to degradation by the β-lactamase then can result in an unacceptably high frequency of resistance development and treatment failure.

Many other factors also can influence the in vitro MIC value obtained and its subsequent application to the in vivo situation. The bacterial growth medium used and cation content can affect the activity of many drugs significantly. For example, aminoglycosides are less active against *P. aeruginosa* in a medium supplemented with physiologic concentrations of magnesium and calcium (NCCLS standardized method) than in a medium without these cations. MIC values of antibiotics that are highly bound to plasma proteins are significantly higher when the test medium contains human serum. Since testing of these drugs in a serum-supplemented medium has not gained widespread acceptance, their in vivo activity may be overestimated by in vitro MIC test results. Fortunately, the standardized guidelines for testing and quality assurance procedures proposed by the NCCLS attempt to minimize the impact of these problems and are followed by most clinical and research laboratories.[26] However, when a patient infected with an apparently susceptible organism fails therapy, it is important for the clinician to consider these potential confounding factors as possibly being related to the observed failure. In such situations, consideration of antimicrobial pharmacokinetics and pharmacodynamics also often can help to better predict therapeutic response as compared with organism susceptibility alone.

QUALITATIVE ANTIMICROBIAL SUSCEPTIBILITY TEST METHODS

DISK DIFFUSION ASSAY

The disk diffusion assay method for susceptibility testing (Bauer-Kirby method) was developed in the 1960s by Bauer and coworkers as a way to reduce the labor needed for tube dilution susceptibility testing.[27] It still remains one of the more common susceptibility test methods used in the clinical microbiology laboratory owing to its high degree of standardization, reliability, flexibility, low cost, and simplicity of test interpretation.[25] Up to 12 user-selected antibiotic-impregnated disks are placed on an agar plate previously streaked with a standard suspension of bacteria ($1-2 \times 10^8$ CFU/mL). The drug contained in the disk diffuses in a concentration gradient out into the agar. The plate is incubated (18 to 24 hours at 35°C [95°F]), and visual bacterial growth occurs only in areas in which the drug concentrations are below those required for growth inhibition. The diameters of the zones of inhibition are measured via calipers or automated scanners and are compared with standard zone size ranges that determine susceptibility, intermediate susceptibility, or resistance to the antimicrobials that were tested (Fig. 103–5). Although factors such as agar composition, incubation temperature, bacterial inoculum, and antibiotic paper disk composition can influence results, the standards for testing conditions and interpretive zone sizes are well defined by the NCCLS.

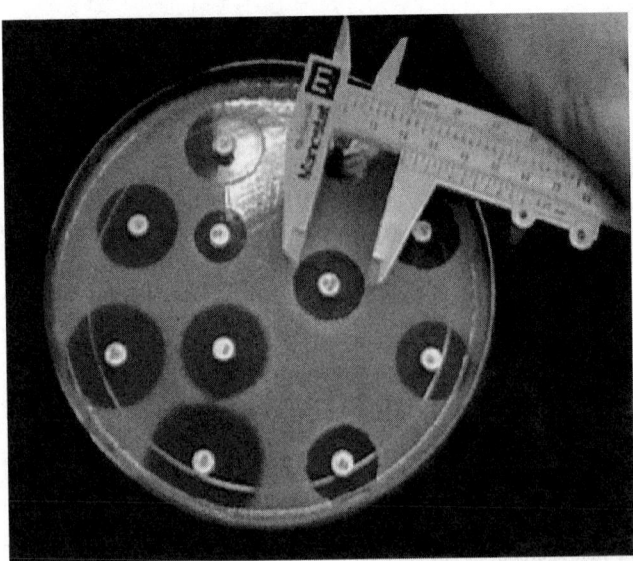

FIGURE 103–5. Disk diffusion susceptibility test. Antibiotic-impregnated disks are placed on the surface of a plate previously inoculated with the test organism. The plate is incubated for 18 hours, and the subsequent zones of inhibition are measured. The zone size correlates with the sensitivity of the organism. The larger the zone, the more sensitive is the organism to the specific antibiotic. On the basis of predetermined zone breakpoints, organisms may be classified as susceptible, resistant, or intermediately susceptible to the antibiotic. (*Photograph courtesy of the Anti-Infective Research Laboratory, Wayne State University, Detroit, Michigan.*)

Although a survey that was conducted of clinical microbiology laboratories in the 1990s indicated that only approximately one-quarter of laboratories performed disk diffusion as the primary susceptibility test (the remainder used primarily microdilution methods/automated testing systems), the lack of realization of substantial cost savings from automated susceptibility testing systems (discussed in more detail below), along with the emergence of more difficult-to-detect resistance mechanisms, may result in an increased use of this time-proven susceptibility testing method, especially for smaller clinical laborotories.[23,28]

QUALITATIVE VERSUS QUANTITATIVE SUSCEPTIBILITY TESTING OF MICROORGANISMS

MIC data often are reported qualitatively by deeming an organism "susceptible," "intermediate or indeterminate" or "moderately susceptible," or "resistant" to the given antimicrobial agent. This simplification permits easier interpretation of susceptibility data by non-infectious-disease clinicians who might not be able to interpret the MIC value properly (or may have no need for knowing it). Many factors are considered to determine these qualitative susceptibility classifications, including pharmacokinetic properties, the distribution of MICs for the organisms, and the clinical and bacteriologic responses observed for the antimicrobial against strains of bacteria with various MIC values.[19] The establishment of a susceptibility breakpoint in the range of common MIC values would be undesirable because it is quite common to observe a twofold variability during dilution MIC testing. Often the consideration of all these factors results in a susceptibility breakpoint of between one-sixteenth and one-fourth the achievable peak serum concentration.[28]

Pathogens classified as susceptible to an antibiotic are those with the lowest MICs, and they are the most likely to be eradicated during therapy of infections using typical drug doses. Conversely, resistant organisms are bacteria with significantly higher MICs that will result in a less-than-optimal clinical response, even at the highest doses. Responses to therapy for organisms that are moderately susceptible/intermediately susceptible/indeterminate are less clearly defined. These organisms may be less likely to be treated effectively with typical doses of the antimicrobial but may respond to treatment with maximal doses or when the drug is known to be concentrated in the site of infection (e.g., urinary tract). The indeterminate classification exists when the number of strains with MICs in the given range is too small to derive robust conclusions on susceptibility or resistance to the antimicrobial.

There are concerns that the "user friendly" susceptible/resistant classification system may oversimplify the decision-making process in the treatment of infectious diseases. For example, a critically ill patient may not respond to the antimicrobial therapy of a susceptible organism at the usual doses. If serum concentrations or concentrations at the site of infection could be assayed (not practically done), one might discover suboptimal concentrations as a result of inadequate tissue perfusion. Likewise, a patient with severe vascular insufficiency and a diabetic foot infection may fail a course of therapy with normal doses of an antimicrobial and a susceptible organism because of inadequate drug delivery. Additionally, some investigators have shown that different outcomes can be achieved for susceptible organisms with different MIC values[29,30] and also that substantial (although not clinically acceptable) clinical and/or microbiologic cure rates can occur for infections that are caused by resistant organisms.[31] These reports emphasize that susceptibility does not correlate unequivocally with clinical success and that resistant organisms do not always equate with impending clinical failure.

Similarities in the spectrum of activity for classes of antibiotics have led to the concept of *class testing.* Thus cephalothin susceptibility results are extrapolated to other first-generation cephalosporins, such as cephalexin or cefazolin. Likewise, susceptibility to an antibiotic that typically has minimal activity usually ensures that other more potent agents in its class will have activity as well. However, many gram-negative organisms have developed extended-spectrum β-lactamases (ESBLs) that often have different activity against members of the same drug class. These developments limit the utility of class testing to reduce susceptibility testing workload. In the setting of an inadequately responding infection with a common ESBL-producing organism (e.g., *Klebsiella pneumoniae*), the pathogen may be susceptible to a class testing antibiotic but actually may be resistant to the antimicrobial agent being administered to the patient.

CLINICAL CONTROVERSY

Some clinicians believe that the MICs of all antimicrobials for which susceptibility testing was performed should be reported in order to allow for proper selection of the best antimicrobial for a given infection in a patient. However, other clinicians argue that the additional information may be misapplied or that the nonselective reporting of all antimicrobial susceptibility data will result in the increased use of more costly broad-spectrum antimicrobials.

OTHER SUSCEPTIBILITY TESTS

EPSILOMETER TEST

The Epsilometer test (E-test; AB Biodisk, Solna, Sweden) combines the benefits of quantitative MIC test methods with the ease of agar diffusion testing. The E-test is a plastic strip impregnated with

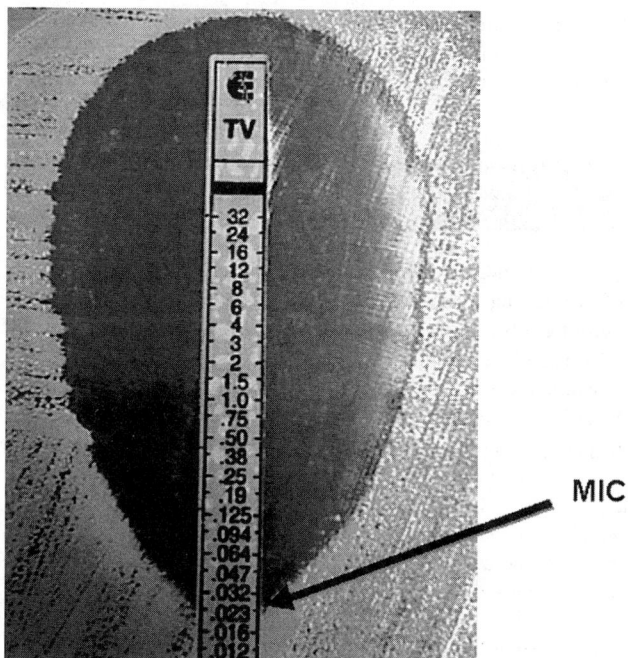

FIGURE 103–6. Photograph of E-strip susceptibility test. The minimal inhibitory concentration (MIC) is determined from the point where the zone of inhibition intersects with the numerical scale. *(Photograph courtesy of the Anti-Infective Research Laboratory, Wayne State University, Detroit, Michigan.)*

a known, prefixed concentration gradient of antibiotic that is placed on an agar plate streaked with a suspension of known bacterial inoculum. The drug instantly diffuses from the plastic strip to form an effective concentration gradient within the agar. After overnight incubation, elliptical zones of inhibition are formed; the point where the bottom of the ellipse crosses the plastic strip is correlated with an MIC value printed on the strip (Fig. 103–6). Many investigators have analyzed the E-test's correlation with standard susceptibility methods and assessed its potential clinical use. In general, values obtained with E-test methods are comparable with or even more consistent and accurate than standard methods. In fact, the E-test method is the recommended method for susceptibility testing of *Streptococcus pneumoniae*. In addition, good correlation with more laborious agar or broth dilution methods is documented for other fastidious or difficult-to-test organisms, such as *H. influenzae,* anaerobes, *Bartonella, Flavobacterium, Legionella,* and nutritionally variant streptococci.[24] However, the widespread clinical use of the E-test has been limited primarily by the excessive costs of the test strips (nearly 10 times more costly than antibiotic-impregnated disks) in relation to the benefits that may be gained from their use.

SPIRAL GRADIENT MINIMAL INHIBITORY CONCENTRATION DETERMINATIONS

The spiral gradient MIC is performed using an apparatus that applies a liquid sample of antimicrobial from the center of an agar plate to its periphery. Because of the exponential deposition of the sample, an antimicrobial gradient is formed. Bacterial inocula are streaked radially on the plate, and the distance of growth toward the center is measured after proper incubation. The distance of growth is measured and correlated with an MIC based on predetermined drug concentrations at various distances. This method has proven useful for the testing of anaerobic bacteria and for susceptibility testing in the research setting and has correlated well with agar dilution MIC test results.[32]

However, as with the E-test, its use in the clinical microbiology laboratory has been limited because of the high costs of the testing apparatus and costs of operation as compared with more traditional methods.

AUTOMATED ANTIMICROBIAL SUSCEPTIBILITY TESTING

Various degrees of automation have been applied to susceptibility testing. Early advances included automated preparation of microtiter trays, instrument-assisted readers, and computer-assisted result databases.[24] Although these improvements helped to decrease preparation and interpretation times, these methods still required an 18- to 24-hour lag period for bacterial growth to evaluate susceptibility. Rapid automated susceptibility tests became available in the 1980s, and their use has increased substantially in the two subsequent decades. These systems often incorporate microprocessors, robotics, and microcomputers to produce susceptibility test results in as few as 3 hours.[24] These systems permit the rapid identification of organisms through the use of biochemical test batteries.

There are two rapid automated susceptibility test systems in common use in clinical microbiology laboratories. The Vitek system (bioMerieux Vitek, Hazelwood, MO) uses technology originally developed for use in spacecraft to rapidly identify and test organisms for antimicrobial susceptibility.[24] This system uses small plastic reagent "cards" that contain 30 or 45 wells for the testing of various antimicrobials or indicator chemicals. Bacterial test suspensions (25 mcL total, providing 1×10^5 CFU/well) enter the wells by capillary diffusion, and growth is monitored automatically via photometric assessment of turbidity every hour for up to 15 hours. When the growth control reaches a specified turbidity level, growth curves for all wells are calculated and compared with the growth control curve for slope normalization. Computerized linear regression and the use of best-fit line coefficients produce an algorithm-derived MIC. The clinical laboratory can control the result output that is generated (qualitative susceptibility, quantitative susceptibility, or both).

The MicroScan WalkAway system (Dade Microscan, West Sacramento, CA) is a rapid test system that uses fluorogenic substrate hydrolysis as an indicator of bacterial growth.[24] This system uses standard microdilution test trays and a computer-controlled incubator and reader unit that can perform robotic manipulations, such as reagent addition and tray rotation, to allow for spectrophotometric or fluorometric growth assessments. Bacterial inocula (approximately 6×10^4 CFU/well for gram-negative organisms and approximately 10^5 CFU/well for gram-positive organisms are added to the wells), and growth is detected by the production of fluorophores from hydrolysis of amidomethylcoumarin or methyl umbelliferyl fluorogenic substrates. Although this method is a more sensitive assessment of growth as compared with turbidity, its indirect nature allows for the possibility of bacterial growth without hydrolysis of the fluorophores; this occurrence is rare, however. As with the Vitek system, growth curves are generated and algorithms applied for the determination of MICs; output is via computer or video display.

CONSIDERATIONS FOR THE USE OF RAPID AUTOMATED SUSCEPTIBILITY SYSTEMS

With integration and mergers being commonplace in health care systems around the country, correlation between the susceptibility results obtained from these different systems is important to enable different institutions to compare data reliably. Such correlation between the Vitek and MicroScan WalkAway systems has been shown, with acceptable rates for the categories "very major" and "major discrepancies" shown between the two systems.[36]

Both the Vitek and WalkAway systems also contain information management systems that allow for the storage and rapid retrieval of susceptibility data. Both systems are also capable of producing chartable patient data reports, antibiograms, and epidemiologic reports. Importantly, these systems can be interfaced with other clinical information systems, such as the pharmacy, infection control, or other laboratory data systems, which may help to improve clinical outcomes.[24,34] Although the use of a rapid susceptibility testing system was associated with more rapid modification to appropriate antimicrobial therapy and also was associated with significantly lower antimicrobial and total hospitalization costs, these results also depended on aggressive result reporting strategies (which are less likely to occur in a nonstudy clinical environment).[24,35] This factor, when coupled with disadvantages such as limitations on test drug flexibility and the need to perform confirmatory testing for certain difficult-to-detect resistance mechanisms, has resulted in lower-than-expected cost savings with these systems.[24]

ADVANCES IN SUSCEPTIBILITY TESTING FOR MYCOBACTERIA, FUNGI, AND VIRUSES

Impressive advances have been made in the past decade in the areas of mycobacterial, fungal, and viral susceptibility testing. The use of radiometric techniques, such as the Bactec TB460 system (Becton Dickinson Biosciences, Sparks, MD), has revolutionized the analysis of antimicrobial susceptibility for *M. tuberculosis* and other slow-growing mycobacteria. Radiometric susceptibility testing involves the incubation of *M. tuberculosis* in liquid medium containing ^{14}C-labeled growth substrate. As organisms grow, respiration causes the release of ^{14}C, which is then detected. The growth indices for antimicrobial-containing bottles are compared with those of a control bottle with the calculation of an MIC. Use of this method, when coupled with the rapid processing of samples, can reduce the time to susceptibility result generation to approximately 1 week. A newer mycobacterial susceptibility testing method (the Bactec Mycobacteria Growth Indicator Tube [MGIT 960], Becton Dickinson Diagnostic Instruments, Sparks, MD) that is fully automated and that employs detection of fluorescence related to growth also has been developed; it produces results in a similar time frame and with similar reliability as the radiometric method. Primary advantages of this system are its automation, the elimination of radioactivity, and the elimination of needle use. Although the slower agar proportion susceptibility method (generating results in approximately 1 month) is still considered the reference standard for mycobacterial susceptibility testing by the NCCLS, the group now recommends the use of a rapid susceptibility testing method to ensure that the Centers for Disease Control and Prevention (CDC) guidelines for reporting susceptibility results for *M. tuberculosis* infections within 28 days of specimen receipt in the laboratory can be met.[36,39]

Antimicrobial susceptibility testing for *M. avium* complex is less standardized owing to such factors as its intrinsic antimicrobial resistance and the presence of different colony variants that have differing antimicrobial susceptibilities. Nonetheless, the broth radiometric method appears to be the most consistent and reproducible method for quantitative MIC determination, and it has been advocated for use by the NCCLS and leading experts in mycobacteriology.[35,3] In the future, the use of molecular probes for mycobacterial resistance genes most likely will become a more important component of mycobacterial susceptibility determinations, especially in light of the increasing problems with antimicrobial resistance. Probes or PCR techniques for the *katG* gene (which is needed to cause isoniazid susceptibility) and the *rpoB* gene (which alters the β subunit of RNA polymerase causing rifampin resistance) have been evaluated in the research laboratory and hold promise for eventual clinical application.[40]

There has been a substantial increase in the prevalence of fungal infections in the past two decades. An increase in the use and development of newer antifungal agents has followed.[48] Historically, antifungal susceptibility testing was imprecise and fraught with many inconsistencies. However, pioneering research in the past decade has resulted in the development of NCCLS guidelines for the antifungal susceptibility testing methods of both yeasts and filamentous fungi (molds).[41-43] Use of these techniques can result in greater than 90% inter- and intralaboratory reproducibility. Although routine antifungal testing of every isolate is not generally necessary for most clinical microbiology laboratories, periodic batch testing for antibiograms and surveillance of resistance and/or antifungal testing of patients with such infections as cryptococcal meningitis or oropharyngeal candidiasis refractory to therapy are warranted.[44] Future research should further define the relationship between in vitro antifungal susceptibility test results and clinical outcomes of serious fungal infections.

FUTURE METHODS FOR EVALUATION OF ANTIMICROBIAL ACTIVITY

There are many innovative methods still under investigation for providing both qualitative and quantitative assessments of antimicrobial activity. Flow cytometry is a technique that has been well described as a means of assessing human cell lines for abnormalities. It has been studied increasingly in the past decade as a means of determining the antimicrobial susceptibility of bacteria, fungi, and viruses. It has the added advantages of providing quantitative information on the diversity of susceptibility to antimicrobials (commonly found in a large population of microorganisms) and also provides data on the effects of the antimicrobial on the morphology of the treated cells. It also has the potential advantages of (1) rapid determination of susceptibility (data can be obtained within one to two cell growth cycles—as quick as 10 minutes for some organisms), (2) quantification of the subinhibitory and postantibiotic effects of antimicrobials, (3) the ability to investigate cellular changes related to the mechanism of antimicrobial action, and (4) the ability to evaluate the effects of both concentration and time on cellular changes.[45] Although additional standardization and the development of cost-effective apparatus are still ongoing, it is likely that flow cytometry will become a component of antimicrobial susceptibility testing in the clinical laboratory in the future.

DETECTION OF RESISTANCE FACTORS

There are a number of methods in use that directly detect the production of antimicrobial resistance in pathogens. β-Lactamase production can be detected rapidly and easily in the clinical laboratory with the use of nitrocephin disks. Nitrocephin is a chromogenic cephalosporin derivative that changes color on hydrolysis by β-lactamase. Colonies from a growing bacterial culture can be touched to a disk, with β-lactamase production noted within a few minutes. Although rapid and reliable, this method is limited to the assessment of strains of staphylococci, enterococci, *H. influenzae, Moraxella catarrhalis,* and *N. gonorrhoeae.* The nitrocephin disk also cannot detect β-lactam

resistance caused by altered penicillin-binding proteins or by some of the newer ESBLs.[23] The use of PCR or DNA probes for detection of β-lactamases improves sensitivity/specificity but is still limited to the research setting. In the years to come, these molecular biologic techniques should become more refined and more prominent in the clinical microbiology laboratory.

The detection of methicillin resistance in *Staphylococcus* is particularly difficult because of the heterogeneous expression of the phenotype—it is common for only 1 in 10^{4-6} tested cells to express methicillin resistance (even though all cells may have the genetic ability to do so). Methicillin resistance is the result of the *mecA* gene, which encodes for an altered penicillin-binding protein (penicillin-binding protein 2a) that has a low binding affinity for β-lactams. Screening via oxacillin disks or by oxacillin-containing agar (6 mcg/mL) was once considered the "gold standard" for resistance detection prior to the development of PCR and DNA probes that were specific for *mecA.* The *mecA* PCR test is available for clinical use, is 99% sensitive and specific, and allows for the rapid (within 6 hours) determination of the presence of methicillin resistance. Although the *mecA* PCR test has been available for many years, many laboratories do not use it commonly because of its high costs relative to screening with oxacillin-containing agar (which still has acceptable sensitivity/specificity).

The detection of decreased vancomycin susceptibility in grampositive organisms has become more important with the increased prevalence of both vancomycin-resistant enterococci (VRE) and vancomycin-intermediate and vancomycin-resistant *S. aureus* (VISA and VRSA). The vancomycin agar screening method (Brain-Heart Infusion agar containing 6 mcg/mL of vancomycin) is an inexpensive and reliable way to detect vancomycin resistance for both of these problem pathogens.[23] With this test, the growth of any colonies from a sample of the test organism (10^5–10^6 CFU) after 24 hours of incubation indicates the presence of decreased vancomycin susceptibility (VISA) or vancomycin resistance (VRE, VRSA) within the test strain. Most MIC test methods used in the clinical laboratory that incorporate at least a 16-hour incubation period also appear to reliably detect strains of VRE, VISA, and VRSA.[46]

The use of PCR has now become a standard method to quantify the replication of the HIV and hepatitis viruses in infected patients (the *viral load,* described as copies per milliliter).[47] Similar methods are used to determine the presence of genetic mutations in the HIV that are associated with increased resistance to one or more of the many antiretroviral medications available for clinical use. The use of these genotyping methods as an aid to select an optimized antiretroviral regimen has been correlated with an improved clinical response to therapy, as well as with a more potent reduction in the viral load.[47] Guidelines for the use of these assays have been developed by a consensus panel of HIV therapy experts owing their the exceptionally high costs (often in excess of $1000 per test), as well as the complexity of interpretation of the test results.[47]

SPECIAL IN VITRO TESTS OF ANTIMICROBIAL ACTIVITY

MINIMAL BACTERICIDAL CONCENTRATION

In certain infections (e.g., meningitis and endocarditis), the bactericidal (killing) activity may be more predictive of a favorable infection outcome than the MIC. The minimal bactericidal concentration (MBC) can performed in conjunction with the broth microtiter MIC test by taking aliquots of broth from microtiter wells that demonstrate no visible growth and plating the samples onto antibiotic-free agar plates for subsequent incubation. The MBC is defined as the lowest concentration of drug that kills 99.9% of the total initially viable cells (representing a 3 $\log_{10}$ CFU/mL or greater reduction in the starting inoculum).

For certain antibiotic classes such as the aminoglycosides and the quinolones, the MIC often approximates the MBC. However, for β-lactam antibiotics and glycopeptides, the MBC may exceed the MIC substantially, resulting in an overestimation of in vivo bactericidal activity. When the MBC exceeds the MIC by 32-fold or more, an organism is said to be *tolerant* to the antimicrobial's killing activity. Although the phenomenon of tolerance has been documented for β-lactams and glycopeptides against certain staphylococci, streptococci, and enterococci, its impact on the outcome of infections caused by organisms other than those just mentioned appears to be limited.

TIMED-KILL CURVE TESTS

Timed-kill curve tests are not performed routinely in the clinical laboratory but can provide important additional data on the effects of an antimicrobial on bacteria. For timed-kill curve tests, a standard inoculum of bacteria (10^6 CFU/mL) is placed in a test tube containing liquid growth medium with or without desired test concentrations of antimicrobial. Samples are removed periodically to determine the number of living cells at the given time points. The viable cell counts are plotted versus time to construct the timed-kill profile of the antimicrobial. By standard convention, the tested concentration of antimicrobial is considered to be bactericidal if it causes at least a 3 $\log_{10}$ CFU/mL reduction in viable inoculum.[49] Comparisons of the relative rates of bacterial killing also can be performed in timed-kill curve experiments. Additionally, the presence of concentration-dependent killing activity (where killing increases with increasing drug concentrations above the MIC) versus concentration-independent killing activity can be determined from a timed-kill curve experiment. An example of results from a timed-kill curve experiment is depicted in Fig. 103–7. These data can help to predict the best way to administer an antimicrobial to maximize activity (e.g., lower-dose continuous infusions for concentration-independent antibiotics versus higher-dose intermittent administrations for concentration-dependent antibiotics).

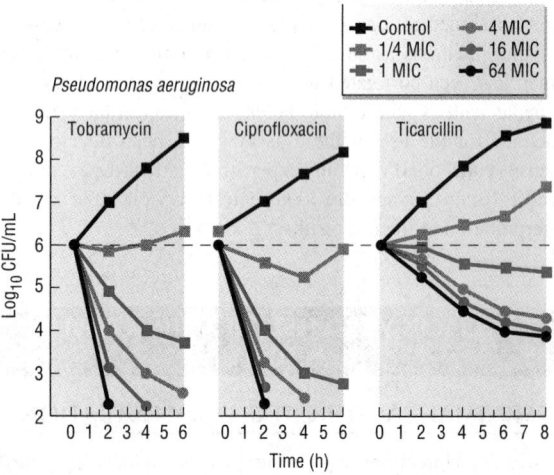

FIGURE 103–7. Killing curve depicting the effect of concentration on antibiotic bactericidal activity. CFU = colony-forming units; MIC = minimal inhibitory concentration. 0.25–64 times the MIC; the organism tested was *P. aeruginosa* ATCC 27853. *(From ref 51.)*

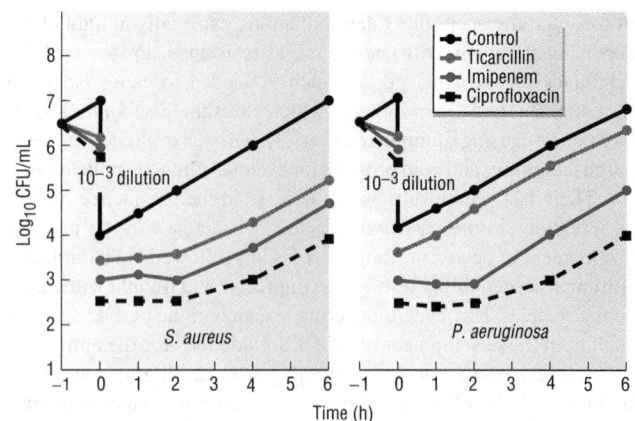

FIGURE 103–8. Postantibiotic effect. In this experiment, fixed inocula of *S. aureus* and *P. aeruginosa* are exposed to ticarcillin, imipenem, and ciprofloxacin at a set concentration of four times the MIC. The organism and the antibiotic are then diluted 1000-fold to a point where the antibiotic concentration is far below the MIC of the organism. Growth supression of *S. aureus* following exposure to the three drugs (PAE) occurs for approximately 2 hours. Growth suppression of *P. aeruginosa*, however, is only demostrated for imipenem and ciprofloxacin. The β-lactam ticarcillin has no effect on the growth of *P. aeruginosa*. *(From refs, 51 and 51.)*

POSTANTIBIOTIC EFFECT

The *postantibiotic effect* (PAE) is defined as the persistent suppression of an organism's growth after a brief exposure to an antibiotic.[45] A PAE experiment is performed by exposing a fixed inoculum of organism to a set concentration of antibiotic (typically some multiple of the MIC) (Fig. 103–8). The antibiotic is then removed either by inactivation (e.g., inactivation by a β-lactamase or binding the antibiotic to a resin) or by filtration/centrifugation of the mixture. The cells are resuspended in antibiotic-free growth medium, and samples are removed frequently (every 0.5 to 2 hours) to determine resumption of normal growth. The PAE is quantified as the difference in time that it takes the organism exposed to the antibiotic to demonstrate a 10-fold increase in viable cells per milliliter as compared with a separate culture of organism not subjected to the antibiotic. A PAE equal to or greater than 1 hour has been demonstrated for most antibiotics against gram-positive bacteria. As a general rule, antibiotics that inhibit DNA or protein synthesis (e.g., quinolones and aminoglycosides) demonstrate significant PAEs against gram-negative organisms. An exception to this rule are the carbapenem cell wall synthesis inhibitors (e.g., ertapenem, imipenem, and meropenem), which demonstrate PAEs against selected strains of gram-negative organisms. The primary clinical application of the PAE is to allow for less frequent administration of antimicrobials while still maintaining adequate antibacterial activity (e.g., extended-interval aminoglycoside administration).[50]

ANTIMICROBIAL COMBINATION EFFECT TESTS

Antimicrobial combination therapy is used frequently to treat serious infections. Combination therapy may be used prior to knowing the pathogen or antibiotic susceptibility for the treatment of infections in neutropenic patients and in patients with enterococcal endocarditis or bacteremia, sepsis, or pneumonia caused by *P. aeruginosa*. In these cases, it is important to know whether the combination will have beneficial (or detrimental) effects on the overall antibacterial activity of the regimen. For example, the combination may result in activity that is significantly greater than the sum of activity of either agent alone (i.e., synergy). Conversely, the combination may result in activity that is worse than either agent alone (i.e., antagonism). Combination activity that is neither synergistic nor antagonistic is said to be *indifferent* or *additive*.[52]

Two methods are used to determine the expected effects of combination antibiotic therapy. For the most part, both methods are not used commonly in the clinical microbiology laboratory owing to the substantial labor involved with these tests and the lack of strong correlation with clinical outcome in the majority of infections. The first method is the microtiter fractional inhibitory concentration (FIC, or "checkerboard" method). The FIC is performed in a similar manner to the microtiter broth MIC except that two antibiotics are tested in the same microtiter plate. Twofold serial dilutions of one antibiotic are made in one direction on the plate (e.g., from right to left), whereas dilutions of the second antibiotic are made from the other direction on the same plate (e.g., from top to bottom). This method produces all possible combinations of twofold concentrations for the two drugs being tested. An inoculum of test bacteria is added to all wells, and the results are read in a similar manner as the MIC test. The FIC is expressed mathematically by calculation of the FIC index. The FIC index is calculated as

$$\text{FIC index} = \frac{A}{\text{MIC}_A} + \frac{B}{\text{MIC}_B}$$

where A or B is the lowest concentration of the drug that is inhibitory in the presence of the second drug, and the MIC is the minimal inhibitory concentration of each drug tested alone. Synergism is defined as an FIC index of 0.5 or less, indifference is defined as an FIC index of between 0.6 and 4.0, and antagonism is defined as an FIC index of greater than 4.0.[53] The microtiter FIC methods have been adapted to allow the use of E-test antibiotic-susceptibility test strips.[54] In this method, two antibiotic E-test strips are crossed at the individual MIC of each antibiotic; an extension of the zone of inhibition beyond that from either antibiotic alone is considered additive or synergistic activity, and an FIC index can be calculated in a similar manner as the microtiter method.

The second most common method to determine the effects of antibiotic combinations is an adaptation of timed-kill curve tests. Two antibiotics are added to the same test tube at fixed concentration fractions of the MIC for each drug, and killing is quantified. With this method, synergism is defined as a 100-fold decrease in viable organisms at 24 hours for the combination as compared with the most potent antibiotic tested alone. Antagonism is defined as a 100-fold or greater increase in viable organism count[53] (Fig. 103–9). It is important to note that although antagonism has been demonstrated for several combinations in vitro (e.g., penicillin plus tetracycline, chloramphenicol and an aminoglycoside, fluoroquinolones and rifampin), antagonism in vivo has been demonstrated only infrequently.

Although the methods for testing the effects of antimicrobial combinations are well described, the results from these tests have not been adequately studied in the context of infection outcome. There is little debate that the combination of a β-lactam antibiotic and an aminoglycoside is required for successful treatment of enterococcal endocarditis.[52] For enterococci, susceptibility to high concentrations of aminoglycosides (e.g., gentamicin, 500 mg/mL) is evaluated in the clinical laboratory because it correlates closely with synergy when the drug is combined with β-lactam antibiotics.

The concept of combination therapy is not universally accepted for the treatment of other infections. There is ongoing debate as to whether the combination of a broad-spectrum β-lactam and an aminoglycoside is needed (versus the β-lactam alone) for the therapy of such infections as gram-negative bloodstream infections or infections in neutropenic patients.[55,56] Although the data are conflicting, combination therapy usually has resulted in improved outcomes in patients with severe illness and in patients with *P. aeruginosa* bloodstream infections.[52,56]

LABORATORY MONITORING OF ANTIMICROBIAL THERAPY

10 The clinician should have an understanding of in vivo antimicrobial agent disposition in order to select the most appropriate therapy for a given infection and to help monitor for clinical or bacteriologic efficacy. Serum concentration monitoring is the most common method used to attempt to maximize efficacy and minimize toxicity of antimicrobials. Since most antimicrobials are well tolerated at their usual doses, only a select few agents (e.g., aminoglycosides, chloramphenicol, and vancomycin) are monitored routinely in the current clinical environment. There are a number of direct and indirect methods that are used to quantify the concentration of antimicrobial in an experimental sample.

METHODS OF ANTIMICROBIAL CONCENTRATION DETERMINATION IN CLINICAL SAMPLES

FLUORESCENCE POLARIZATION IMMUNOASSAY

The fluorescence polarization immunoassay (FPIA) technique involves the application of the principles of fluorescence when molecules are exposed to light. A fluorescein-labeled drug and antibody that is directed against the drug are added in constant amounts to samples with unknown drug concentrations and to concentration standards. When the fluorescein-labeled drug complexes with the antibody, a quantifiable change in the fluorescence polarization occurs. When a sample containing non-fluorescein-labeled drug (i.e., a patient's serum sample) is mixed with the standard mixture, competition for antibody binding occurs. Comparison of the change caused by the patient's sample to the changes caused by standard concentrations determines the specific drug concentration in the patient sample.

FPIA is the most commonly used assay method for the determination of aminoglycoside and vancomycin serum concentrations in the clinical laboratory setting. Advantages of this technique include its automation through the use of the TDx system (Abbott Laboratories, North Chicago, IL). Disadvantages include the expenses for reagents and the cost for the purchase of the automated system.

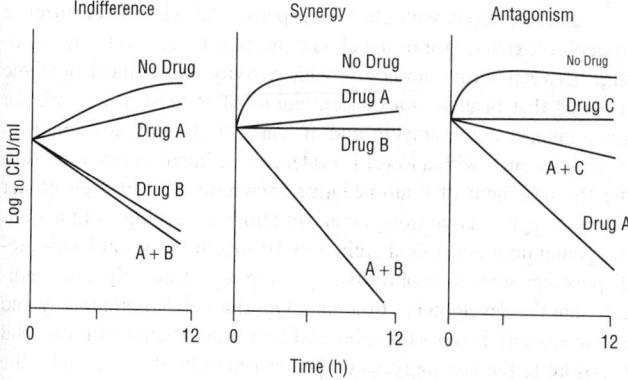

FIGURE 103–9. Timed-kill curve illustrating indifference, synergy, and antagonism.

RADIOIMMUNOASSAY

Radioimmunoassay (RIA) uses a radiolabeled drug and an antibody directed against the specific drug to determine the concentration contained in an unknown sample. The theory behind the assay is similar to FPIA because radiolabeled antibiotic and unlabeled antibiotic (in the patient's serum sample) are equilibrated with the antibody. The amount of free radiolabeled drug is measured and compared with the values obtained with standard concentrations of the radiolabeled drug alone to determine the concentration in the patient sample. Although RIA has good sensitivity and specificity, its main disadvantage compared with FPIA is the expense and hassle of handling and disposal of the radioactive waste generated during the test.

HIGH-PRESSURE LIQUID CHROMATOGRAPHY

High-pressure liquid chromatography (HPLC) permits the separation of different molecular species by passing a mobile solvent phase over a stationary phase. Drugs with a polarity similar to that of the stationary phase are retained for a time on the chromatographic column and then released after various retention times. Detection can be accomplished via fluorescence, electrochemical, or radiometric methods. The detector signal is proportional to the amount of molecules present. Standard curves are generated from known concentrations of the drug (usually recorded as peak area or peak height). Advantages of HPLC include a rapid turnaround time, precision, and an ability to detect the test drug in the presence of its metabolites and/or other drugs. Disadvantages include the high cost of HPLC instruments and the expertise required to perform the assays. These disadvantages usually relegate HPLC drug assay to the experimental and/or research settings.

SERUM INHIBITORY/BACTERICIDAL TITERS

Serum inhibitory titers (SITs) and serum bactericidal titers (SBTs) sometimes are used to monitor the antimicrobial therapy of certain serious infections (e.g., osteomyelitis and endocarditis). SITs and SBTs for antimicrobials are determined in a similar standardized manner as microdilution MICs and MBCs, but dilutions of the patient's serum are used instead of known concentrations of antimicrobial.[53] Patient serum can be collected near the expected peak, midpoint, and/or trough concentration(s) of the antimicrobial dose. The SIT is the highest twofold dilution of the serum sample that inhibits the visible growth of the patient's infecting organism, whereas the SBT is defined as the highest dilution of serum that kills 99.9% of the original bacterial inoculum is the SBT. Values for the SIT and SBT are expressed as the number of twofold serial dilutions relative to the original serum sample (e.g., SIT = 1:32, SBT = 1:8). A peak SBT of greater than 1:32 predicted successful outcome for endocarditis, whereas a trough SBT of greater than 1:2 predicted success for osteomyelitis.[59,60]

MICROBIOLOGIC ASSAY

Microbioassay of antimicrobial agents can be performed by several methods. The most common method is a modification of the disk diffusion antimicrobial-susceptibility technique. Typically, paper disks are placed on agar that contains an inoculum of a bacterium known to be highly susceptible to the antimicrobial agent to be assayed. Fixed volumes (usually 10 mcL) of a range of prepared concentration standards of the test drug are placed on the disks. The zones of growth inhibition are measured and plotted versus the drug concentration to generate a standard curve. Zone sizes from samples containing the unknown concentrations of the test drug are measured, and the concentrations are determined from the plotted curve; the drug concentration in unknown samples is determined from the standard curve generated from the known concentrations of the drug. The advantages of this method include its relative ease of performance and the minimal cost for equipment. The disadvantages of this method include interference from other antibiotics that may be present in the unknown sample, a lack of sensitivity/specificity for certain antimicrobials, and a slow turnaround time (usually 24 to 48 hours) for generation of results.

TIMING OF COLLECTION OF SERUM SAMPLES

Peak and/or trough concentrations are monitored routinely for only a select few antimicrobials (e.g., aminoglycosides and vancomycin) during the contemporary management of infections. It is crucial for the health care team to ensure that the antimicrobial's administration time and serum sample time(s) are meticulously recorded because even small errors in recording these (e.g., 1 hour) may have a substantial impact on the calculation of pharmacokinetics for antibiotics such as the aminoglycosides, which have relatively short elimination half-lives.

Samples ideally should be obtained after steady state is achieved (usually defined as the passage of at least 3 to 4 anticipated half-lives), but in certain situations, this may not be possible (e.g., critically ill patients with fluctuations in drug elimination owing to fluctuating hemodynamics, kidney function, and/or liver function). Generally, the timing of the peak serum sample collection is usually more critical than the trough concentration because adequate time must elapse to allow for completion of the distribution phase and to avoid underestimating the drug's volume of distribution. Since the distribution half-life may even vary between different dosage regimens of the same antibiotic (e.g., traditional versus extended-interval aminoglycoside dosing),[61] clinicians always should plan peak serum sample collections carefully with this variability in mind.

SPECIFIC AGENTS

The aminoglycosides (i.e., amikacin, gentamicin, and tobramycin) and vancomycin remain the most common agents for which serum concentrations are monitored. A summary of the recommendations for serum concentration monitoring of these agents is shown in Table 103-2.

AMINOGLYCOSIDES

There are many studies that have linked serum aminoglycoside concentrations with clinical response and with the occurrence of nephrotoxicity. One of the classic investigations into the relationship between serum aminoglycoside activity and clinical outcome revealed that peak serum concentrations of at least 5 mcg/mL for gentamicin and tobramycin and at least 20 mcg/mL for amikacin were associated with a lower prevalence of clinical failure rates during the treatment of gram-negative bacteremia.[62] Although earlier studies suggested that trough concentrations exceeding 2-4 mcg/mL for gentamicin and tobramycin and 10 mcg/mL for amikacin predisposed patients to nephrotoxicity, more recent investigations indicate that the development of aminoglycoside-related ototoxicity and nephrotoxicity is more complex and also is associated with the total exposure to the aminoglycoside (as measured by the area under the concentration-time curve [AUC]) and/or the total duration of aminoglycoside therapy.[58-60] The specific recommended serum peak and

TABLE 103–2. Suggested Therapeutic Serum Concentrations for Selected Antimicrobial Agents

Drug	Time of Collection	Target Concentrations (mg/L)	Comments
Aminoglycosides[70,71]	Peak (1 h after the start of a 15- to 45-min infusion)	<5	Urinary tract infections
Traditional dosage regimens			
Gentamicin		>5	Bacteremia
Tobramycin		>6	Bacterial pneumonia
		>12	Endocarditis caused by *Pseudomonas aeruginosa*
	Trough	<2–3	High trough concentrations are most likely a result and not a cause of nephrotoxicity
Amikacin	Peak	>15	Urinary tract infections
		>20	Bacteremia
		>24	Bacterial pneumonia, other serious infections
	Trough	>9–10	See comments regarding trough gentamicin/tobramycin concentrations
Single daily dosage regimens[76]			
Gentamicin	8 h postdose	1.5–6	Concentrations above this range associated with nephrotoxicity in one study with netilmicin
Netilmicin			
Tobramycin			
Vancomycin[80,81]	Peak (1–2 h after a 30- to 60–min infusion)	20–50	Recommendations should be considered tentative, as definitive data are not available
	Trough	<10	Therapeutic monitoring is probably not necessary for most patients

trough concentrations for the various aminoglycosides are described in Table 103–2.

Newer regimens of once-daily or extended-interval aminoglycoside administration have gained widespread acceptance for use in the clinical setting. These regimens exploit the pharmacodynamic properties of these agents (i.e., concentration-dependent bacterial killing and a substantial PAE) to maximize activity while also attempting to minimize drug nephrotoxicity by reducing the total aminoglycoside exposure time for the patient's kidneys. The doses employed for extended-interval treatment typically range from 5–7 mg/kg of lean body weight (administered every 24 to 48 hours), with the dose and/or interval adjusted based on renal function or observed mid-dose serum concentrations.[66,67] Although many prospective studies have been performed to evaluate the safety and efficacy of once-daily aminoglycoside dosing, substantial controversy still exists.[66–70] Most of these studies have revealed equivalent rates of efficacy and toxicity or trends toward improved efficacy and reduced toxicity for once-daily dosage regimens as compared with traditional (thrice daily) regimens. Meta-analyses also have been performed on these study data.[79] However, since the individual studies are heterogeneous and possess many weaknesses, these meta-analyses subsequently have inherited many these scientific study flaws.[68,69]

CLINICAL CONTROVERSY

Although some clinicians believe that the clinical data are sufficient to support widespread use of once-daily aminoglycoside dosing without determination of individualized patient pharmacokinetics, other clinicians believe that the data from investigations on once-daily aminoglycosides are incomplete and that patients still should receive individualized pharmacokinetic assessments and dosage adjustments.

Traditional methods of aminoglycoside serum concentration monitoring (evaluating peak and trough serum concentrations) cannot be applied to extended-interval dosing because the serum concentrations 24 hours after a dose ideally should be undetectable. If desired, pharmacokinetic assessment during extended-interval aminoglycoside regimens should be accomplished by obtaining a peak sample at least 1 hour after the end of the infusion [owing to a longer distribution phase compared with traditional (1 mg/kg) doses].[56] A midinterval serum sample can be taken approximately 6 to 12 hours after the dose to allow for use of first-order pharmacokinetic equations. A single-point nomogram-based dosing method that uses midinterval serum samples also is used frequently in the clinical setting.[66]

VANCOMYCIN

Convincing data do not exist that definitively relate the specific recommended vancomycin peak (20–40 mcg/mL) or trough (5–15 mcg/mL) serum concentrations to efficacy and/or toxicity.[71,72] Although intravenous vancomycin has been associated with oto- and nephrotoxicity in humans, most of these reports occurred with older, impure formulations of the drug, with extremely high concentrations uncommon with contemporary dosing regimens, or when vancomycin was combined with known nephrotoxic agents.[84] A recent investigation revealed that continuous infusions of vancomycin that resulted in constant serum vancomycin concentrations of 20–25 mcg/mL caused no substantial nephrotoxicity when compared with intermittent regimens that targeted the "accepted" serum trough concentration range.[73]

Because vancomycin appears to possess a time-dependent killing-activity profile, it has been recommended that vancomycin concentrations remain above the organism's MIC during the entire dosing interval. Most methods of empirical vancomycin dosing result in peak concentrations of between 20 and 50 mcg/mL and trough concentrations of between 5 and 15 mcg/mL. Since the vast majority of organisms have vancomycin MICs of 2 mcg/mL or less, weight-based dosage regimens and/or nomogram-based dosage methods can be used with minimal monitoring of serum concentrations (e.g., evaluation of vancomycin trough concentration every 5 days of therapy) for the vast majority of patients.[74]

INTEGRATING ORGANISM SUSCEPTIBILITY WITH SERUM CONCENTRATION DATA TO IMPROVE ANTIMICROBIAL THERAPY

7 **14** We have advanced our understanding substantially of the importance of considering both antimicrobial pharmacokinetics and organism susceptibility when selecting therapy for the treatment of infections. Antimicrobial regimens should be selected and/or designed to maximize the probability that bacterial killing is optimized and that the probability of resistance is minimized. For example, the activity of antimicrobials such as the fluoroquinolones and the aminoglycosides can be maximized if the ratio of the peak serum concentration to the organism MIC (peak-to-MIC ratio) is greater than or equal to 10.[77,78] Similarly, the probability of clinical and/or microbiologic infection cure can be maximized if a fluoroquinone is chosen that achieves an area under the concentration-time curve to MIC ratio (*AUC*-to-MIC ratio) of 100 to 125 or greater for gram-negative bacteria (e.g., *P. aeruginosa*) and 30 to 40 or greater for gram positive bacteria (e.g., *S. pneumoniae*).[79,80] The clinical application of these principles to aminoglycoside dosage regimen optimization is depicted in Fig. 103–10.

The maintenance of concentrations above the infecting organism's MIC (the time above the MIC) best predicts the clinical efficacy of the β-lactam antimicrobials and glycopeptides, although the *AUC*-to-MIC ratio also has been suggested as a predictor for treatment outcome for certain organisms and in certain clinical situations.[75,76] In the setting of bacterial otitis media, for example, a time above the MIC of approximately 40% to 50% correlated with rates of response of greater than 90%.[31]

It is important to recognize that most of the data on optimization of antimicrobial pharmacodynamics have been generated in in vitro models of infection, in animal models of infection, within the context of controlled clinical trials, or through mathematical modeling of small data sets. However, research continues on the best ways to apply these valuable data to the everyday management of patients in the clinical setting. The recognition of the importance of antimicrobial pharmacodynamics already has resulted in the expansion of serum concentration monitoring for select antimicrobials (e.g., antiretroviral agents), the suggested revisions of breakpoint values that define antimicrobial susceptibility and/or resistance, the development of nomograms or computer programs that can suggest optimal drugs and doses for a given infection, and/or the development of newer antimicrobial agents that minimize the probability of suboptimal pharmacodynamics.[77–82] These developments present exciting opportunities for health care providers to improve the outcomes of patients with infections in a variety of different health care settings.

ABBREVIATIONS

AIDS: acquired immunodeficiency syndrome
AUC: area under the plasma concentration versus time curve
bDNA: branched DNA
CDC: Centers for Disease Control and Prevention
CFU: colony-forming unit
CMV: cytomegalovirus
ELISA: enzyme-linked immunosorbent assay
ESBL: extended-spectrum β-lactamase
ESR: erythrocyte sedimentation rate
FIC: fractional inhibitory concentration
FPIA: fluorescence polarization immunoassay
HIV: human immunodeficiency virus
HPLC: high-performance liquid chromatography
KOH: potassium hydroxide
MBC: minimum bactericidal concentration
MHC: major histocompatibility complex
MIC: minimum inhibitory concentration
NCCLS: National Committee for Clinical Laboratory Standards
PAE: postantibiotic effect
PCR: polymerase chain reaction
PMN: polymorphonuclear leukocyte
RIA: radioimmunoassay
SBT: serum bactericidal titer
SIT: serum inhibitory titer
TNF: tumor necrosis factor
VISA: vancomycin-intermediate *Staphylococcus aureus*
VRE: vancomycin-resistant enterococci
VRSA: vancomycin-resistant *Staphylococcus aureus*

Review Questions and other resources can be found a *www.pharmacotherapyonline.com.*

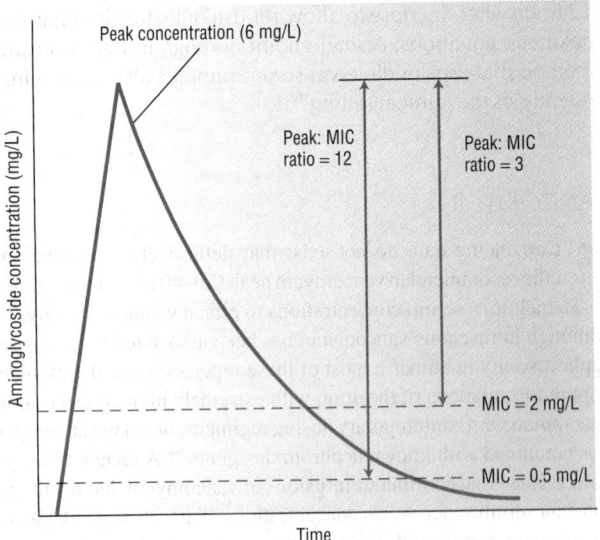

FIGURE 103–10. Illustration of the concept of peak concentration to the minimal inhibitory concentration (MIC) ratio for aminoglycosides. The MIC for the given organism to gentamicin is 2 mg/L, whereas the tobramycin MIC is 0.5 mg/L. Administration of gentamicin would result in a suboptimal peak:MIC ratio (<10), which could increase the chances for development of resistance or an inadequate response. Administration of tobramycin would result in a peak:MIC ratio of 12, which should improve efficacy. Note that modification of the gentamicin regimen to produce peak serum concentrations of 20 mg/L or more (as commonly done with once-daily administration) also would result in a peak:MIC ration of 10 or grester.

REFERENCES

1. Reese RE, Betts RF. Principles of Antibiotic Use. In: Betts RF, Chapma SW, Penn RL, eds. A Practical Approach to Infectious Diseases, 5th ed Philadelphia, Lippincott Williams & Wilkins, 2003:969–988.

2. andro V, Cainelli F. Infections in patients with cancer undergoing chemotherapy: Aetiology, prevention, and treatment. Lancet Oncol 2003;595–604.

3. Crawford J, Dale DC, Lyman GH. Chemotherapy-induced neutropenia: Risks, consequences, and new directions for its management. Cancer 2003;100:228–237.

4. Day CL, Walker BD. Progress in defining CD4 helper cell responses in chronic viral infections. J Exp Med 2003;198:1773–1777.

5. Smith JM, Nemeth TL, McDonald RA. Current immunosuppressive agents: Efficacy, side effects and ultilization. Pediatr Clin North Am. 2003;6:1283–1300.

6. Penn RL, Betts RF. Lower respiratory tract infections (including tuberculosis). In: Betts RF, Chapman SW, Penn RL, eds. A Practical Approach to Infectious Diseases, 5th ed. Philadelphia, Lippincott Williams & Wilkins, 2003:295–371.

7. Lannergard A, Larsson A, Kragsbjerg P, Friman G. Correlation between serum amyloid A protein and C-reactive protein in infectious diseases. Scand J Clin Lab Invest 2003;4:267–272.

8. Brigden ML. Clinical utility of the erythrocyte sedimentation rate. Am Fam Phys 1999;9:1443–1450.

9. Cavaillon JM, Adib-Conquy M, Fitting C, et al. Cytokine cascade in sepsis. Scand J Infect Dis 2003;35:535–544.

10. Lekkou A, Karakantza M, Mouzaki A, et al. Cytokine production and moncyte HLH-DR expression as predictors of outcome for patients with community-acquired severe infections. Clin Diagn Lab Immunol. 2004;11:161–167.

11. Dorman NJ. Sepsis. In: Betts RF, Chapman SW, and Penn RL, eds. A Practical Approach to Infectious Diseases, 5th ed. Philadelphia, Lippincott Williams & Wilkins, 2003:19–66.

12. Safdar N, Kluger DM, Maki DG. A review of risk factors for catheter-related bloodstream infection caused by percutaneoulsy inserted, non-cuffed central venous catheters: Implications for preventive strategies. Medicine 2002;86:466–479.

13. Graman PS, Menegus MA. Microbiology laboratory tests In: Betts RF, Chapman SW, and Penn RL., eds. A Practical Approach to Infectious Diseases, 5th ed. Philadelphia, Lippincott Williams & Wilkins, 2003:929–956.

14. O'Hara CM, Weinstein MP, Miller JM. Manual and automated systems for detection and identification of microorganisms. In:Murry PR, Baron EJ, Jorgensen JH, et al, eds. Manual of Clinical Microbiology, 8th ed. Washington, ASM Press, 2003:185–207.

15. Constantine NT, Lana DP. Immunoassays for the diagnosis of infectious diseases. In: Murray PR, Baron EJ, Jorgensen JH, et al, eds. Manual of Clinical Microbiology, 8th ed. Washington, ASM Press, 2003:218–256.

16. Gill VJ, Fedorko DP, Witebsky FG. The clinician and the microbiology laboratory. In: Mandell GL, Bennet JE., Dolin R, eds. Principles and Practice of Infectious Diseases, 5th ed. New York, Churchill-Livingstone, 2000:184–221.

17. Nolte FS, Caliendo AM. Molecular detection and identification of microorganisms. In: Murry PR, Baron EJ, Jorgensen JH., et al, eds. Manual of Clinical Microbiology, 8th ed. Washington, ASM Press, 2003:234–256.

18. Pilcher CD, McPherson JD, Leone PA, et al. Real-time, universal screening for actue HIV infection in a routine HIV counseling and testing population. JAMA 2002;288:216–221.

19. Bryant P, Venter D, Robins-Browne R, Curtis N. Chips with everything: DNA microarrays in infectious diseases. Lancet Infect Dis. 2004;4:100–111.

20. Owen RJ. Molecular testing for antibiotic resistance in *Helicobacter pylori*. Gut 2002;50:285–289.

21. Hitt CM, Nightingale CH, Quintiliani R, Nicolau DP. Streamlining antimicrobial therapy for lower respiratory tract infections. Clin Infect Dis 1997;24(suppl 2):S231–237.

22. Varaldo PE. Antimicrobial resistance and susceptibility testing: an evergreen topic. J Antimicrob Chemother 2002;50:1–4.

23. Jorgensen JH, Ferraro MJ. Antimicrobial susceptibility testing: Special needs for fastidious organisms and difficult-to-detect resistance mechanisms. Clin Infect Dis 2000:30:799–808.

24. Jorgensen JH, Ferraro MJ. Antimicrobial susceptibility testing: General principles and contemporary practices. Clin Infect Dis 1998;26:973–980.

25. Sanders CC, Thomson KS, Bradford PA. Problems with detection of β-lactam resistance among nonfastidious gram-negative bacilli. Infect Dis Clin North Am 1993;7:411–424.

26. National Committee for Clinical Laboratory Standards (NCCLS). Methods for Dilution Antimicrobial Susceptibility Tests for Bacteria that Grow Aerobically—Approved Standard, 6th ed. NCCLS document M7-A6. Wayne, PA, National Committee for Clinical Laboratory Standards, 2003.

27. Bauer AW, Kirby MM, Sherris JC, et al. Antibiotic susceptibility testing by a standardized, single-disk method. Am J Clin Pathol 1966;45:493–496.

28. Hessen MT, Kaye D. Principles of selection and use of antimicrobial agents. Infect Dis Clin North Am 1995;9:531–545.

29. Moore RD, Lietman PS, Smith CR. Clinical response to aminoglycoside therapy: Importance of peak concentration to minimal inhibitory concentration. J Infect Dis 1987;155:93–99.

30. Peloquin CA, Cumbo TJ, Nix DE, et al. Evaluation of intravenous ciprofloxacin in patients with nosocomial lower respiratory tract infections. Arch Intern Med 1989;149:2269–2273.

31. Craig WA. Does the dose matter? Clin Infect Dis 2001;33(suppl 3):S233–237.

32. Wexler HM, Molitoris E, Murray PR, et al. Comparison of spiral gradient endpoint and agar dilution methods for susceptibility testing of anaerobic bacteria: A multilaboratory collaborative evaluation. J Clin Microbiol 1996;34:170–174.

33. Rittenhouse SF, Miller LA, Utrup LJ, Poupard JA. Evaluation of 500 gram-negative isolates to determine the number of major susceptibility interpretation discrepancies between the Vitek and Microscan Walkaway for 9 antimicrobial agents. Diagn Microbiol Infect Dis 1996;26:1–6.

34. Pestotnik SL, Classen DC, Evans RS, Burke JP. Implementing antibiotic practice guidelines through computer-assisted decision support: Clinical and financial outcomes. Ann Intern Med 1996;124:884–890.

35. Doern GV, Vautour R, Gaudet M, Levy B. Clinical impact of rapid in vitro susceptibility testing and bacterial identification. J Clin Microbiol 1994;32:1757–1762.

36. Woods GL. Susceptibility testing for mycobacteria. Clin Infect Dis 2000;31:1209–1215.

37. Heifets L. Susceptibility testing of *Mycobacterium avium* complex isolates. Antimicrob Agents Chemother 1996;40:1759–1767.

38. Ardito F, Posteraro B, Sanguinetti M, et al. Evaluation of Bactec Mycobacteria Growth Indicator Tube (MGIT 960) automated system for drug susceptibility testing of *Mycobacterium tuberculosis*. J Clin Microbiol. 2001;38:4440–4444.

39. National Committee for Clinical Laboratory Standards (NCCLS). Susceptibility Testing for Mycobacteria, Nocardiae, and other aerobic Actinomycetes—Approved Standard. NCCLS Document M24-A. Wayne, PA, National Committee for Clinical Laboratory Standards, 2003.

40. Garcie de Viedma D. Rapid detection of resistance in *Mycobacterium tuberculosis*: A review discussing molecular approaches. Clin Microbiol Infect 2003;9:349–59.

41. National Committee for Clinical Laboratory Standards (NCCLS). Reference Method for Broth Dilution Antifungal Susceptibility Testing of Yeasts; Approved Standard, 2d ed. NCCLS Document M27-A2. Wayne, PA, National Committee for Clinical Laboratory Standards, 2002.

42. National Committee for Clinical Laboratory Standards (NCCLS). Reference Method for Broth Dilution Antifungal Susceptibility Testing of Filamentous Fungi—Approved Standard. NCCLS Document M38-A. Wayne, PA, National Committee for Clinical Laboratory Standards, 2002.

43. Rex JH, Pfaller MA, Galgiani JN, et al. Development of interpretive breakpoints for antifungal susceptibility testing: Conceptual framework and analysis of in vitro–in vivo correlation data for fluconazole, itraconazole, and candidal infections. Clin Infect Dis 1997;24:235–247.

44. Rex JH, Pfaller MA, Walsh TJ, et al. Antifungal susceptibility testing: practical aspects and current challenges. Clin Microbiol Rev 2001;14:643–658.

45. Alvarez-Barrientos A, Arroyo J, Canton R, et al. Applications of flow cytometry to clinical microbiology. Clin Microbiol Rev 2001;13:167–195.

46. Tenover FC, Lancaster MV, Hill BC, et al. Characterization of staphylococci with reduced susceptibilities to vancomycin and other glycopeptides. J Clin Microbiol 1998;36:1020–1027.

47. Dybul M, Fauci AS, Bartlett JG, et al. Guidelines for using antiretroviral agents among HIV-infected adults and adolescents: Recommendations of the Panel on Clinical Practices for Treatment of HIV. MMWR 2002;51:1–56.

48. Voorn GP, Kuyvenhoven J, Goessens WHF, et al. Role of tolerance in treatment and prophylaxis of experimental *Staphylococcus aureus* endocarditis with vancomycin, teicoplanin, and daptomycin. Antimicrob Agents Chemother 1994;38:487–493.

49. Amsterdam D. Susceptibility testing of antimicrobials in liquid media. In: Lorian V, ed. Antibiotics in Laboratory Medicine, 4th ed. Baltimore, Williams & Wilkins, 1996:52–111.

50. Craig WA, Gudmundsson S. Postantibiotic effect. In: Lorian V, ed. Antibiotics in Laboratory Medicine, 4th ed. Baltimore, Williams & Wilkins, 1996:296–329.

51. Li RC, Zhu M, Schentag JJ. Achieving an optimal outcome in the treatment of infections: The role of clinical pharmacokinetics and pharmacodynamics of antimicrobials. Clinl Pharmacokinet 1999;37:1–16.

52. Rybak MJ, McGrath BJ. Combination antimicrobial therapy for bacterial infections: Guidelines for the clinician. Drugs 1996;52:390–405.

53. Elipoulos G, Moellering RC Jr. Antimicrobial combinations. In: Lorian V, ed. Antibiotics in Laboratory Medicine, 4th ed. Baltimore, Williams & Wilkins, 1996:330–397.

54. White RL, Burgess DS, Manduru M, Bosso JA. Comparison of three different in vitro methods of detecting synergy: Time-kill, checkerboard, and E test. Antimicrob Agents Chemother 1996;40:1914–1918.

55. Ramphal R, Gucalp R, Rotstein C, et al. Clinical experience with single-agent and combination regimens in the management of infection in the febrile neutropenic patient. Am J Med 1996;100(suppl 6A):83–89S.

56. Chow JW, Yu VL. Combination antibiotic therapy versus monotherapy for gram-negative bacteraemia: A commentary. Int J Antimicrob Agents 1999;11:7–12.

57. Cappelletty DM, Rybak MJ. Comparison of methodologies for synergism testing of drug combinations against resistant strains of *Pseudomonas aeruginosa*. Antimicrob Agents Chemother 1996;40:677–683.

58. National Committee for Clinical Laboratory Standards (NCCLS). Methodology for the Serum Bactericidal Test—Approved Standard. NCCLS Document M21-A. Wayne, PA, National Committee for Clinical Laboratory Standards, 1999.

59. Weinstein MP, Stratton CW, Acklery A, et al. Multicenter collaborative evaluation of a standardized serum bactericidal test as a prognostic indicator in infective endocarditis. Am J Med 1985;78:262–269.

60. Weinstein MP, Stratton CW, Hawley HB, et al. Multicenter collaborative evaluation of a standardized serum bactericidal test as a predictor of therapeutic efficacy in acute and chronic osteomyelitis. Am J Med 1987;83:218–222.

61. Demczar DJ, Nafziger AN, Bertino JS. Pharmacokinetics of gentamicin at traditional versus high doses: Implications for once-daily dosing. Antimicrob Agents Chemother 1997;41:1115–1119.

62. Moore RD, Smith CR, Lietman PS. The association of aminoglycoside plasma levels with mortality in patients with gram-negative bacteremia. J Infect Dis 1984;149:443–448.

63. Bertino JS, Booker LA, Franck PA, et al. Incidence of and significant risk factors for aminoglycoside-associated nephrotoxicity in patients dosed by using individualized pharmacokinetic monitoring. J Infect Dis 1993;167:173–179.

64. Blaser J, Konig C, Simmen H-P, Thurnheer U. Monitoring serum concentrations for once-daily netilmicin dosing regimens. J Antimicrob Chemother 1994;33:341–348.

65. Rybak MJ, Abate BJ, Kang SL, et al. Prospective evaluation of the effect of an aminoglycoside dosing regimen on rates of observed nephrotoxicity and ototoxicity. Antimicrob Agents Chemother 1999;43:1549–1555.

66. Nicolau DP, Freeman CD, Belliveau PP, et al. Experience with a once-daily aminoglycoside program administered to 2,184 adult patients. Antimicrob Agents Chemother 1995;39:650–655.

67. Gilbert DN, Lee BL, Dworkin RJ, et al. A randomized comparison of the safety and efficacy of once-daily gentamicin or thrice-daily gentamicin in combination with ticarcillin-clavulanate. Am J Med 1998;105:182–191.

68. Bertino JS, Rotschafer JC. Single daily dosing of aminoglycosides: A concept whose time has not yet come. Clin Infect Dis 1997;24:820–823.

69. Gilbert DN. Meta-analyses are no longer required for determining the efficacy of single daily dosing of aminoglycosides. Clin Infect Dis 1997;24:816–819.

70. Ali MZ, Goetz MB. A meta-analysis of the relative efficacy and toxicity of single daily dosing versus multiple daily dosing of aminoglycosides. Clin Infect Dis 1997;24:796–809.

71. Cantu TG, Yamanaka-Yuen NA, Lietman PS. Serum vancomycin concentrations: Reappraisal of their clinical value. Clin Infect Dis 1994;18:533–543.

72. Moellering RC Jr. Monitoring serum vancomycin levels: Climbing the mountain because it is there? Clin Infect Dis 1994;18:544–546.

73. Wysocki M, Delatour F, Faurisson F, et al. Continuous versus intermittent infusion of vancomycin in severe staphylococcal infections: Prospective, multicenter randomized study. Antimicrob Agents Chemother. 2001;45:2460–2467.

74. Karam CM, McKinnon PS, Neuhauser MM, et al. Outcome assessment of minimizing vancomycin monitoring and dosing adjustments. Pharmacotheraoy 1999;19:257–266.

75. Moise PA, Forrest A, Bhavnani SM, et al. Area under the inhibitory curve and a pneumonia scoring system for predicting outcomes of vancomycin therapy for respiratory infections by *Staphylococcus aureus*. Am J Health Syst Pharm 2000;57:S4–9.

76. Aeschlimann JR, Allen GP, Hershberger E, Rybak MJ. Activities of LY333328 and vancomycin administered alone or in combination with gentamicin against three strains of vancomycin-intermediate *Staphylococcus aureus* in an in vitro pharamacodynamic infection model. Antimicrob Agents Chemother 2000;44:2991–2998.

77. Kashuba A, Nafziger A, Drusano G, Bertino J. Optimizing aminoglycoside therapy for nosocomial pneumonia caused by gram-negative bacteria. Antimicrob Agents Chemother 1999;43:623–629.

78. Preston S, Drusano G, Berman A, et al. Pharmacodynamics of levofloxacin: A new paradigm for early clinical trials. JAMA 1998;279:125–129.

79. Forrest A, Nix DE, Ballow CH, et al. Pharmacodynamics of intravenous ciprofloxacin in seriously ill patients. Antimicrob Agents Chemother 1993;37:1073–1081.

80. Ambrose P, Grasela, D, Grasela T, et al. Pharmacodynamics of fluoroquinolones against *Streptococcus pneumoniae* in patients with community-acquired respiratory tract infections. Antimicrob Agents Chemother 2001;45:2793–2797.

81. Department of Health and Human Service Panel on Clinical Practices for Treatment of HIV Infection. Guidelines for the use of antiretroviral agents in HIV-1-Infected adults and adolescents, Atkanta, Centers for Disease Control and Prevention; accessed January 15, 2004.

82. Schentag J. Antimicrobial action and pharmacokinetics/pharmacodynamics: The use of AUIC to improve efficacy and avoid resistance. J Chemother 1999;11:426–39.

104

ANTIMICROBIAL REGIMEN SELECTION

David S. Burgess and Betty J. Abate

Learning Objectives and other resources can be found at *www.pharmacotherapyonline.com*.

KEY CONCEPTS

1 Every attempt should be made to obtain specimens for culture and sensitivity testing prior to initiating antibiotics.

2 Empirical antibiotic therapy should be based on knowledge of likely pathogens for the site of infection, information from patient history (e.g., recent hospitalizations, work-related exposure, travel, and pets), and local susceptibility.

3 Patients with delayed reactions to penicillin (skin rash) generally can receive cephalosporins. Patients with type I hypersensitivity reactions to penicillins (anaphylaxis) should not receive cephalosporins or carbapenems (alternatives include aztreonam, quinolones, sulfa drugs, or vancomycin based on type of coverage indicated).

4 Estimated renal function should be calculated for every patient who is to receive antibiotics and the antibiotic dose interval adjusted accordingly. Hepatic function should be considered for drugs eliminated through the hepatobiliary system, such as clindamycin, erythromycin, and metronidazole.

5 All concomitant drugs and nutritional supplements should be reviewed when an antibiotic is added to a patient's therapy.

6 Combination antibiotic therapy may be indicated for polymicrobial infections (abdominal, gynecologic infections), to produce synergistic killing (β-lactam plus aminoglycoside versus *Pseudomonas aeruginosa*), or to prevent the emergence of resistance.

7 All patients receiving antibiotics should be monitored for resolution of infectious signs and symptoms (e.g., decreasing temperature and WBC count) and adverse drug events.

8 Agents with the narrowest spectrum of activity that is effective are preferred. Antibiotic route of administration should be evaluated daily, and conversion from intravenous to oral therapy should be attempted as signs of infection improve for patients with functioning gastrointestinal tracts (general exceptions are bloodstream and central nervous system infections).

9 Patients not responding to an appropriate antibiotic treatment in 2 to 3 days should be reevaluated to ensure (a) the correct diagnosis, (b) that therapeutic drug concentrations are being achieved, (c) that the patient is not immunosuppressed, (d) that the patient does not have isolated infection (i.e., abscess, foreign body), or (e) that resistance has not developed.

Choosing an antimicrobial agent to treat an infection is far more complicated than matching a drug to a known or suspected pathogen.[1] Most clinicians generally follow a systematic approach to select an antimicrobial regimen (Table 104–1). Problems arise when this systematic approach is replaced by prescribing broad-spectrum therapy to cover as many organisms as possible. Consequences of not using the systematic approach include the use of more expensive and potentially more toxic agents, which may, in turn, lead to widespread resistance and difficult-to-treat superinfections. Another abuse of antimicrobial agents is administration when they are not needed. An example of this is prescribing antibacterials for self-limited clinical conditions that are most likely viral in origin (i.e., the common cold).

Initial selection of antimicrobial therapy is nearly always empirical, which is the initiation of antimicrobials sometimes prior to documentation of the presence of infection and before the offending organism is identified. Infectious diseases generally are acute, and a delay in antimicrobial therapy may result in serious morbidity or even mortality. An example is the rapidly lethal nature of various forms of meningitis. Thus empirical antimicrobial therapy selection is based on information gathered from the patient's history and physical examination and results of Gram stains or of rapidly performed tests on specimens from the infected site. This information, combined with knowledge of the most likely offending organism(s) and an institution's local susceptibility patterns, should result in a rational selection of antibiotics to treat the patient.

This chapter introduces a systematic approach to the selection of antimicrobial therapeutic regimens.

CONFIRMING THE PRESENCE OF INFECTION

FEVER

The presence of a temperature greater than the expected 98.6°F (37°C) "normal" body temperature is considered a hallmark of infectious diseases. Body temperature is controlled by the hypothalamus. In addition, the circadian rhythm, a built-in temperature cycle, is also operational. The daily temperature rhythm may vary for each individual. In a healthy person, the internal thermostat is set between the

TABLE 104–1. Systematic Approach for Selection of Antimicrobials

Confirm the presence of infection
  Careful history and physical
  Signs and symptoms
  Predisposing factors
Identification of the pathogen (see Chap. 103)
  Collection of infected material
  Stains
  Serologies
  Culture and sensitivity
Selection of presumptive therapy considering every infected site
  Host factors
  Drug factors
Monitor therapeutic response
  Clinical assessment
  Laboratory tests
  Assessment of therapeutic failure

morning low temperature and the afternoon peak as controlled by the circadian rhythm. During fever, the hypothalamus is reset at a higher temperature level.[2]

Fever is defined as a controlled elevation of body temperature above the normal range. The average normal body temperature range taken orally is 98.0 to 98.6°F (36.7 to 37°C). Body temperatures obtained rectally generally are 1°F (0.6°C) higher and axillary temperatures are 1°F (0.6°C) lower than oral temperatures, respectively. Skin temperatures are also less than the oral temperature but may vary depending on the specific measurement method. Fever can be a manifestation of disease states other than infection. Collagen-vascular (autoimmune) disorders and several malignancies may have fever as a manifestation. Fever of unknown or undetermined origin is a diagnostic dilemma and is reviewed extensively elsewhere.[3]

Many drugs have been identified as causes of fever.[4] *Drug-induced fever* is defined as persistent fever in the absence of infection or other underlying condition. The fever must coincide temporally with the administration of the offending agent and disappear promptly on its withdrawal, after which the temperature remains normal. Possible mechanisms of drug-induced fever are either a hypersensitivity reaction or development of antigen-antibody complexes that result in the stimulation of macrophages and the release of interleukin 1 (IL-1). Although this is not a common drug effect (accounting for no more than 5% of all drug reactions), it should be suspected when obvious reasons for fever are not present. Almost any medication can produce fever, but certain ones appear to be responsible more often than others. These include β-lactam antibiotics, anticonvulsants, allopurinol, hydralazine, nitrofurantoin, sulfonamides, phenothiazines, and methyldopa.[4]

Noninfectious etiologies of fever may be referred to as "false-positives." Although these certainly may confuse the clinician, even more troublesome are false-negatives: the absence of fever in a patient with signs and symptoms consistent with an infectious disease. Careful questioning of the patient or family is vital to assess the ingestion of any medication that can mask fever (e.g., aspirin, acetaminophen, nonsteroidal anti-inflammatory agents, and corticosteroids). The use of antipyretics should be discouraged during the treatment of infection unless absolutely necessary because they may mask a poor therapeutic response. Moreover, elevated body temperature, unless very high [>105°F (40.5°C)], is not harmful and may be beneficial.[2]

SIGNS AND SYMPTOMS

WHITE BLOOD CELL COUNT

Most infections result in elevated white blood cell (WBC) counts (leukocytosis) because of the increased production and mobilization of granulocytes (neutrophils, basophils, and eosinophils), lymphocytes, or both to ingest and destroy invading microbes. The generally accepted range of normal values for WBC counts is between 4000 and 10,000 cells/mm³. Values above or below this range hold important prognostic and diagnostic value.

Bacterial infections are associated with elevated granulocyte counts, often with immature forms (band neutrophils) seen in peripheral blood smears. Mature neutrophils are also referred to as *segmented neutrophils* or *polymorphonuclear leukocytes* (PMNs). The presence of immature forms (left shift) is an indication of an increased bone marrow response to the infection. With infection, peripheral WBC counts may be very high, but they are rarely higher than 30,000 to 40,000 cells/mm³. Because leukocytosis indicates the normal host response to infection, low leukocyte counts after the onset of infection indicate an abnormal response and generally are associated with a poor prognosis.

The most common granulocyte defect is neutropenia, a decrease in absolute numbers of circulating neutrophils. A thorough description of the consequences of neutropenia is given in Chap. 120. Lymphocytosis, even with normal or slightly elevated total WBC counts, generally is associated with tuberculosis and viral or fungal infections. Increases in monocytes may be associated with tuberculosis or lymphoma, and increases in eosinophils may be associated with allergic reactions to drugs or infections caused by metazoa. Many types of infections may be accompanied by a completely normal WBC count and differential.

LOCAL SIGNS

The classic signs of pain and inflammation may manifest as swelling, erythema, tenderness, and purulent drainage. Unfortunately, these are only visible if the infection is superficial or in a bone or joint. The manifestations of inflammation in deep-seated infections (e.g., meningitis, pneumonia, endocarditis, and urinary tract infection) must be ascertained by examining tissues or fluids. For example, the presence of neutrophils in spinal fluid, lung secretions (sputum), or urine is highly suggestive of a bacterial infection.

Symptoms referable to an organ system must be sought out carefully because not only do they help in establishing the presence of infection, but they also aid in narrowing the list of potential pathogens. For example, a febrile patient with complaints of flank pain and dysuria may well have pyelonephritis. In this situation, enteric gram-negative bacilli, especially *Escherichia coli*, are the predominant pathogens. If a febrile patient has no symptoms suggestive of an organ system but only constitutional complaints, the list of possible infectious diseases is lengthy.[3] A febrile individual with cough and sputum production probably has a pulmonary infection. What is not so evident, however, is the etiologic organism in this situation, because it may be caused by bacteria, mycobacteria, viruses, chlamydia, or mycoplasmas.[5] In this situation, attention to the patient's history and background disease states is important. Even more important is a careful examination of the infected material (in this case sputum) in order to ascertain the identity of the pathogen.

IDENTIFICATION OF THE PATHOGEN

MICROBIOLOGY ISSUES

◀1 Infected body materials must be sampled, if at all possible or practical, before institution of any antimicrobial therapy for two reasons. First, a Gram stain of the material rapidly may reveal bacteria, or an acid-fast stain may detect mycobacteria or actinomycetes. Second, a delay in obtaining infected fluids or tissues until after antimicrobial therapy is started may result in false-negative culture results or alterations in the cellular and chemical composition of infected fluids. This is particularly true in patients with urinary tract infections, meningitis, and septic arthritis.[6]

Blood cultures usually should be performed in the acutely ill febrile patient. Blood culture collection should coincide with sharp elevations in temperature, suggesting the possibility of microorganisms or microbial antigens in the bloodstream. Ideally, blood should be obtained from peripheral sites as two sets (one set consists of an aerobic bottle and one set an anaerobic bottle) from two different sites approximately 1 hour apart. In selected infections, bacteremia is qualitatively continuous (e.g., endocarditis), so cultures may be obtained at any time.[7]

In addition to the infected materials produced by the patient (e.g., blood, sputum, urine, stool, and wound or sinus drainage), other less accessible fluids or tissues must be obtained based on localized signs or symptoms (e.g., spinal fluid in meningitis and joint fluid in arthritis). Abscesses and cellulitic areas also should be aspirated.

INTERPRETING RESULTS

After a positive Gram stain, culture results, or both are obtained, the clinician must be cautious in determining whether the organism recovered is a true pathogen, a contaminant, or a part of the normally expected flora (see Chap. 103). This latter consideration is especially problematic with cultures obtained from the skin, oropharynx, nose, ears, eyes, throat, and perineum. These surfaces are heavily colonized with a wide variety of bacteria, some of which may be pathogenic in certain settings. For example, coagulase-negative staphylococci are found in cultures of all the aforementioned sites yet are seldom regarded as pathogens unless recovered from blood, venous access catheters, or prosthetic devices.

Importantly, cultures of specimens from purportedly infected sites that are obtained by sampling from or through one of these contaminated areas may contain significant numbers of the normal flora. In the case of urine cultures, the urinalysis should be used in combination with culture results to assess the presence of WBCs, nitrite, and leukocyte esterase to help confirm infection and rule out colonization.

Particularly problematic are expectorated sputum specimens that must be evaluated carefully by determination of the presence of squamous epithelial cells and leukocytes.[5] A predominance of epithelial cells in sputum specimens reduces the likelihood that recovered bacteria are pathogenic, especially when multiple types of organisms are seen on Gram stain. In contrast, the discovery of leukocytes in large numbers with one predominant type of organism is a more reliable indicator of a valid collection. In general, however, sputum evaluation has poor sensitivity and specificity as a diagnostic test.[5]

Caution also must be used in the evaluation of positive culture results from normally sterile sites (e.g., blood, cerebrospinal fluid, or joint fluid). The recovery of bacteria normally found on the skin in large quantities (e.g., coagulase-negative staphylococci or diphtheroids) from one of these sites may be a result of contamination of the specimen rather than a true infection. These organisms may be pathogenic in certain settings.

Gram-staining techniques, culture methods, and serologic identification, as well as susceptibility testing, are discussed in detail in Chap. 103. Emphasis must be placed on the proper collection and handling of specimens and careful assessment of Gram stain or other test results in guiding the clinician toward appropriate selection of initial antimicrobial therapy.[8]

SELECTION OF PRESUMPTIVE THERAPY

◀2 To select rational antimicrobial therapy for a given clinical situation, a variety of factors must be considered. These include the severity and acuity of the disease, host factors, factors related to the drugs used, and the necessity for using multiple agents. In addition, there are generally accepted drugs of choice for the treatment of most pathogens (see Appendix 104–1).

Drugs of choice are compiled from a variety of sources and are intended as guidelines rather than as specific rules for antimicrobial use. These choices are influenced by local antimicrobial susceptibility data rather than information published by other institutions or national compilations. Each institution should publish an annual summary of antibiotic susceptibilities (antibiogram) for organisms cultured from patients. Antibiograms contain both the number of nonduplicate isolates for common species and the percentage susceptible to the antibiotics tested. To further guide empirical antibiotic therapy, some hospitals publish unit-specific antibiograms in unique patient care areas, such as intensive care units or burn units.

Susceptibility of bacteria may differ substantially among hospitals within a community. For example, the prevalence of methicillin-resistant *Staphylococcus aureus* (MRSA) in some centers is quite high, whereas in other centers the problem may be nonexistent. This particular situation will influence the selection of therapy for possible *S. aureus* infection, where the clinician must choose either a β-lactam or vancomycin. The problem of differing susceptibilities is limited not only to gram-positive bacteria but also to gram-negative organisms, and all drug classes are affected.

Empirical therapy is directed at organisms that are known to cause the infection in question. These organisms for different sites of infection are discussed in Chap. 105 to 123. To define the most likely infecting organisms, a careful history and physical examination must be performed. The place where the infection was acquired should be determined, e.g., the home (community-acquired), nursing home environment, or hospital-acquired (nosocomial). Nursing home patients may be exposed to potentially more resistant organisms because they are often surrounded by ill patients who may be receiving antibiotics. Other important questions to ask infected patients regarding the history of the present illness include

1. Are any other people sick at home, especially children?
2. Are any unusual pets kept in the home such as pigeons?
3. Where are you employed (i.e., are you exposed to contaminated meat or infectious biohazards)?
4. Has there been any recent travel, for example, to endemic areas of fungal infections or developing countries?

HOST FACTORS

Several host factors should be considered when evaluating a patient for antimicrobial therapy. The most important factors are drug allergies, age, pregnancy, genetic or metabolic abnormalities, renal and hepatic function, site of infection, concomitant drug therapy, and underlying disease states.

ALLERGY

3 Allergy to an antimicrobial agent generally precludes its use. Careful assessment of allergy histories must be performed because many patients confuse common adverse drug effects (i.e., gastrointestinal disturbance) with true allergic reactions.[9] Among the most commonly cited antimicrobial allergies are those to penicillin, penicillin-related compounds, or both. In the absence of complete penicillin skin testing capabilities, a rule of thumb for giving cephalosporins or carbapenems to patients allergic to penicillin is to avoid giving them to patients who give a good history for immediate or accelerated reactions (e.g., anaphylaxis, laryngospasm) and to give them under close supervision in patients with a history of delayed reactions, such as a rash.[10] If gram-negative infection is suspected or documented, therapy with a monobactam may be appropriate because cross-reactivity with other β-lactams is virtually nil.[11]

AGE

The patient's age is an important factor both in trying to identify the likely etiologic agent and in assessing the patient's ability to detoxify or eliminate the drug(s) to be used. The best example of an age determinant of organisms is in bacterial meningitis, where the pathogens differ as the patient grows from the neonatal period through infancy and childhood and into adulthood.[12]

In the case of the neonate, hepatic and liver functions are not well developed. The use of chloramphenicol can lead to shock and cardiovascular collapse (gray baby syndrome) caused by the inability of the newborn's liver to metabolize and detoxify the drug.[13] Serum concentrations of chloramphenicol must be monitored to ensure that concentrations of the drug do not exceed 20–25 mcg/mL. Neonates (especially when premature) may develop kernicterus when given sulfonamides. This results from displacement of bilirubin from serum albumin.[14] Additional special drug considerations for pediatric patients include low frequency of adverse effects and compliance-enhancing features (e.g., absorption not affected by food, once- to twice-daily dosing, and good taste).[15,16]

The major physiologic change in persons older than 65 years of age is a decline in the number of functioning nephrons that, in turn, results in decreased renal function.[17] This is usually manifested by an increased incidence of side effects caused by antimicrobials that are eliminated renally. For example, renal toxicity caused by aminoglycosides may be apparent much sooner during therapy than in younger patients. Oral absorption is also decreased in the elderly; in most cases, however, this has not proved to be significant clinically. Furthermore, in many cases, no identifiable cause of adverse drug effects can be determined other than "old age"; thus increased monitoring is warranted in the elderly.

PREGNANCY

During pregnancy, not only is the fetus at risk for drug teratogenicity (see Chap. 76), but also the pharmacokinetic disposition of certain drugs may be altered.[18] Penicillins, cephalosporins, and aminoglyco-

sides are cleared from the peripheral circulation more rapidly during pregnancy. This is probably a result of marked increases in intravascular volume, glomerular filtration rate, and hepatic and metabolic activities. The net result is that maternal serum antimicrobial concentrations may be as much as 50% lower during this period than in the nonpregnant state. Increased dosages of certain compounds may be necessary to achieve therapeutic levels during late pregnancy.

METABOLIC ABNORMALITIES

Inherited or acquired metabolic abnormalities will influence the therapy of infectious diseases in a variety of ways. For example, patients with impaired peripheral vascular flow may not absorb drugs given by intramuscular injection. In addition, certain metabolic states may predispose patients to enhanced drug toxicity. For example, patients who are phenotypically slow acetylators of isoniazid are at greater risk for peripheral neuropathy.[19] Patients with severe deficiency of glucose-6-phosphate dehydrogenase may develop significant hemolysis when exposed to such drugs as sulfonamides, nitrofurantoin, nalidixic acid, antimalarials, dapsone, and perhaps, chloramphenicol.[20] Although mild deficiencies are found in African-Americans, the more severe forms of the disease generally are confined to persons of eastern Mediterranean origin.

ORGAN DYSFUNCTION

4 Patients with diminished renal or hepatic function or both will accumulate certain drugs unless the dosage is adjusted.[21,22] Recommendations for dosing antibiotics in patients with liver dysfunction are not as formalized as guidelines for patients with renal dysfunction.[22] Antibiotics that should be adjusted in severe liver disease include chloramphenicol, clindamycin, erythromycin, metronidazole, and rifampin. Significant accumulation may occur when both liver dysfunction and renal dysfunction are present for these drugs: cefotaxime, nafcillin, piperacillin, and sulfamethoxazole.

CONCOMITANT DRUGS

5 Any concomitant therapy that the patient is receiving may influence the drug selection, dose, and monitoring. For example, administration of isoniazid to a patient who is also receiving phenytoin may result in phenytoin toxicity secondary to inhibition of phenytoin metabolism by isoniazid. Furthermore, drugs that possess similar adverse-effect profiles may increase the risk for effects, e.g., two drugs that cause nephrotoxicity or neutropenia. Lists of potentially severe drug-drug interactions are provided in Tables 104–2 and 104–3.

CONCOMITANT DISEASE STATES

Concomitant disease states may influence the selection of therapy. Certain diseases will predispose patients to a particular infectious disease or will alter the type of infecting organism. For example, patients with diabetes mellitus and the resulting peripheral vascular disease often develop infections of the lower extremity soft tissue. Moreover, the alterations in peripheral blood flow associated with the disease and perhaps altered immunity make such infections more difficult to treat than in nondiabetics. Patients with chronic lung disease or cystic fibrosis develop frequent pulmonary infections that may be caused by somewhat different microorganisms than are found in otherwise normal hosts.

Patients with immunosuppressive diseases, such as malignancies or acquired immunologic deficiencies, are highly predisposed to

TABLE 104–2. Major Drug Interactions with Antimicrobials

Antimicrobial	Other Agent(s)	Mechanism of Action/Effect	Clinical Management
Aminoglycosides	Neuromuscular blocking agents	Additive adverse effects	Avoid
	Nephrotoxins (N) or ototoxins (O) (e.g., amphotericn B (N) cisplatin (N/O), cyclosporine (N), furosemide (O), NSAIDs (N), radio contrast (N), vancomycin (N)	Additive adverse effects	Monitor aminoglycoside SDC and renal function
Amphotericin B	Nephrotoxins (e.g., aminoglycosides, cidofovir, cyclosporine, foscarnet, pentamidine)	Additive adverse effects	Monitor renal function
Azoles	See Chap. 119		
Chloramphenicol	Phenytoin, tolbutamide, ethanol	Decreased metabolism of other agents	Monitor phenytoin SDC, blood glucose
Foscarnet	Pentamidine IV	Increased risk of severe nephrotoxicity/hypocalcemia	Monitor renal function/serum calcium
Isoniazid	Carbamazepine, phenytoin	Decreased metabolism of other agents (nausea, vomiting, nystagmus, ataxia)	Monitor drug SDC
Macrolides/azalides	Digoxin	Decreased digoxin bioavailability and metabolism	Monitor digoxin SDC; avoid if possible
	Theophylline	Decreased metabolism of theophylline	Monitor theophylline SDC
Metronidazole (also cefamandole, cefoperazone)	Ethanol (drugs containing ethanol)	Disulfiram-like reaction	Avoid
Penicillins and cephalosporins	Probenecid, aspirin	Blocked excretion of β-lactams	Use if prolonged high concentration of β-lactam desirable
Ciprofloxacin/norfloxacin	Theophylline	Decreased metabolism of theophylline	Monitor theophylline
Quinolones	Class Ia and III Antiarrhythmics	Increased Q-T interval	Avoid
	Multivalent cations (antacids, iron, sucralfate, zinc, vitamins, dairy, citric acid) didanosine	Decreased absorption of quinolone	Separate by 2 hours
Rifampin	Azoles, cyclosporine, methadone propranolol, protease inhibitors (PI), oral contraceptives, tacrolimus, warfarin	Increased metabolism of other agent	Avoid if possible
Sulfonamides	Sulfonylureas, phenytoin, warfarin	Decreased metabolism of other agent	Monitor blood glucose, SDC, PT
Tetracyclines	Antacids, iron, calcium, sucralfate	Decreased absorption of tetracycline	Separate by 2 hours
	Digoxin	Decreased digoxin bioavailability and metabolism	Monitor digoxin SDC; avoid if possible

Azalides: azithromycin; azoles: fluconazole, itraconazole, ketoconazole, and voriconazole; macrolides: erythromycin, clarithromycin; protease inhibitors: aprenavir, indinavir, lopinavir/ritonavir, nelfinavir, ritonavir, and saquinavir; quinolones: ciprofloxacin, gatifloxacin, levofloxacin, moxifloxacin. SDC = serum drug concentrations.

infections, and the types of organisms may be vastly different from what would be expected (see Chap. 120). For example, patients undergoing chemotherapy for acute forms of leukemia often are profoundly granulocytopenic and are predisposed to infections caused by bacteria and fungi.[23] Patients with the acquired immunodeficiency syndrome (AIDS) often become infected with an enormous variety of organisms[24] (see Chap. 123).

Many factors predisposing to infection are related to disruption of the host's integumentary barriers. For example, trauma, burns, and iatrogenic wounds induced in surgery may lead to a substantial risk of infection depending on the severity and location of the injury or disruption. For a complete discussion of the various risks involved in surgical procedures, see Chap. 121.

DRUG FACTORS

PHARMACOKINETIC AND PHARMACODYNAMIC CONSIDERATIONS

Integration of both pharmacokinetic and pharmacodynamic properties of an agent is important when choosing antimicrobial therapy to ensure efficacy and to prevent resistance.[25] Early researchers relied solely on pharmacokinetic properties such as area under the drug concentration curve (AUC), maximum observed concentration (peak), and drug half-life to optimize therapy. Pharmacodynamics is the study of the relationship between drug concentration and the effects on the microorganism (see Chap. 103). Researchers now realize the

TABLE 104–3. **Major Drug Interactions with Antiretroviral (AR) Agents**

Antiretroviral	Other Agent(s)	Mechanism of Action/Effect	Clinical Management
Groups of Antiretrovirals with Similar Drug Interactions			
PI[a]/delavirdine/ Efavirenz	Ergot alkaloids midazolam/triazolam/ alrpazolam	Decreased metabolism of other agents	Avoid
	Phenobarbital/phenytoin/carbamazepine	Increased metabolism of AR Decreased metabolism of anticonvulsants	Monitor anticonvulsant SDC
PI[a]/delavirdine	Lovastatin/simvastatin	Decreased metabolism of statin drug	Avoid
	Rifabutin	Increased metabolism of AR Decreased metabolism of rifabutin	Avoid Avoid
	Rifampin	Increased metabolism of AR	Avoid
	Sildenafil	Decreased metabolism of sildenafil	Max dose of sildenafil 25 mg/48 h
PI[a]/nevirapine	Oral contraceptives (OC)	Increased metabolism of OC	Use alternative method
Individual Agents in Alphabetical Order by Generic Name			
Delavirdine[b]	Antacids/didanosine	Decreased absorption of delavirdine	Separate by 1 h
	Clarithromycin	Decreased metabolism of clarithromycin	Dose adjust in renal failure
	Dapsone/warfarin/quinidine	Decreased metabolism of the other agent	Monitor warfarin/avoid others
	Dihydropyridine Ca^{++} channel antagonists		
	H$_2$ blockers/proton pump inhibitors	Decreased absorption of delavirdine	Avoid
	Indinavir	Increased metabolism of indinavir	Indinavir 1000 mg tid
	Ketoconazole	Decreased metabolism of delavirdine	Avoid
Didanosine	Allopurinol	Decreased metabolism of didanosine	Avoid
	Drugs requiring low pH; dapsone, indinavir, itra/ketoconazole	Decreased absorption of the other agent	Separate by 2 h
	Pyrimethamine		For quinolones: 6 h before or 2 h after
	Tetracycline/quinolones		
	Methadone	Decreased didanosine SDC	Increase didanosine
	Ritonavir	Formulation incompatibility	Separate by 2.5 h
Efavirenz[b]	Clarithromycin	Decreased clarithromycin SDC	Avoid: use azithromycin
	Indinavir	Increased metabolism of indinavir	Indinavir 1000 mg tid
	Rifabutin	Increased metabolism of rifabutin	Rifabutin 450 mg qd
Indinavir[b]	Delavirdine/efavirenz/nevirapine	Increased metabolism of indinavir	Indinavir 1000 mg tid
	Itra/ketoconazole	Decreased metabolism of indinavir	Indinavir 600 mg tid
Nevirapine[b]	Indinavir	Increased metabolism of indinavir	Indinavir 1000 mg tid
	Methadone/opiates/warfarin	Increased metabolism of other agents	Titrate to response/monitor warfarin
	Phenobarbital/phenytoin/carbamazepine	Unknown	Monitor anticonvulsant SDC
	Ketoconazole/Rifampin/Tacrolimus	Increased metabolism of other agents	Avoid
Ritonavir[b]	Amiodarone/flecainide propafenone/quinidine	Decreased metabolism of other agents	Avoid
	Ca^{++} channel antagonists		
	Clarithromycin	Decreased metabolism of clarithromycin	Dose adjust in renal failure
	Didanosine	Formulation incompatibility	Separate by 2.5 h
	Desipramine	Decreased metabolism of desipramine	Reduce dose of desipramine
	Ketoconazole	Decreased metabolism of ketoconazole	Max dose of ketoconazole 200 mg qd
	Meperidine/methadone	Increased metabolism of other drug	Titrate to response
	Theophylline	Increased metabolism of theophylline	Monitor theophylline
	Warfarin	Increased metabolism of warfarin	Monitor warfarin
Zidovudine	Ribavirin	Ribavirin inhibits phosphorylation of zidovudine	Avoid

[a]PI: Protease inhibitors amprenavir, indinavir, lopinavir, nelfinavir, ritonavir, saquinavir
[b]Also note additional drug interactions above.
SDC = serum drug concentration.
Note: This list is meant to include major interactions and is not exhaustive. Individual package inserts along with the primary literature should be consulted because new interactions continue to be studied and reported. Avoid combinations of drugs with overlapping toxicities whenever possible.

important relationship between both pharmacokinetic and microbiologic parameters that has resulted in new measurements such as *AUC*:minimal inhibitory concentration (MIC) ratio, peak:MIC ratio, and time *T* the concentration is above MIC ($T > $ MIC).

Aminoglycosides exhibit concentration-dependent bactericidal effects.[25] An example of the integration of pharmacokinetics and microbiological activity is the use of high-dose, once-daily aminoglycosides. For these regimens, the drug is given as a single large daily dose to maximize the peak:MIC ratio. Aminoglycosides also possess a postantibiotic effect (persistent suppression of organism growth after concentrations fall below the MIC) that appears to contribute to the success of high-dose, once-daily administration.[26] Fluoroquinolones exhibit concentration-dependent killing activity, but optimal killing appears to be characterized by the *AUC*:MIC ratio.[27,28]

β-Lactams and vancomycin display time-dependent bactericidal effects. Killing activity is enhanced only marginally if drug concentration exceeds the MIC. Therefore, the important pharmacodynamic relationship for these antimicrobials is the duration that drug concentrations exceed the MIC ($T > $ MIC). Effective dosing regimens require serum drug concentrations to exceed the MIC for at least 40% to 50% of the dosing interval.[25] Frequent small doses or a continuous infusion of β-lactams appears to be correlated with positive outcomes.[29]

The ability of bacteriostatic antimicrobial agents to eradicate infections is reliant on host immune function and a postantibiotic effect. Examples include clindamycin, macrolides, and tetracyclines.[25]

TISSUE PENETRATION

The importance of tissue penetration varies with site of infection. Some of the difficulties in interpreting data include a lack of correlation with clinical outcomes and poor understanding of whether the antimicrobial agents are present in a biologically active form.[30] An example of the former problem is the recognized efficacy of drugs with low biliary fluid concentrations in the treatment of cholecystitis, cholangitis, or both and the absence of the enhanced efficacy of drugs whose primary route of elimination is biliary excretion of active drug. An example of the latter difficulty is with penetration to deep infections, such as abscesses, where various factors such as acid pH, WBC products, and various enzymes may inactivate even high concentrations of certain drugs.

The central nervous system (CNS) is one body site where antimicrobial penetration is relatively well defined, and correlations with clinical outcomes are established.[31] Cerebrospinal fluid (CSF) concentrations of antimicrobial agents necessary to cure bacterial meningitis have been defined, and drugs that do not reach significant concentrations in the CSF should either be avoided or instilled directly, if feasible.

Caution must be exercised when selecting an antimicrobial agent for clinical use on the basis of tissue or fluid penetration. Body fluids where drug concentration data are clinically relevant include CSF, urine, synovial fluid, and peritoneal fluid. Apart from these areas, more attention should be paid to clinical efficacy, antimicrobial spectrum, toxicity, and cost than to comparative data on penetration into a given body site.

The proper route of administration for an antimicrobial depends on the site of infection. Parenteral therapy is warranted when patients are being treated for febrile neutropenia or deep-seated infections such as meningitis, endocarditis, and osteomyelitis. Severe pneumonia often is treated initially with intravenous antibiotics and switched to oral therapy as clinical improvement is evident.[5,32,33] Patients treated in the ambulatory setting for upper respiratory tract infections (e.g., pharyngitis, bronchitis, sinusitis, and otitis media), lower respiratory tract infections, skin and soft tissue infections, uncomplicated urinary tract infections, and selected sexually transmitted diseases may receive oral therapy.

DRUG TOXICITY

It is incumbent on health professionals to avoid toxic drugs whenever possible. Antibiotics associated with CNS toxicities, usually when not dose-adjusted for renal function, include penicillins, cephalosporins, quinolones, and imipenem. Hematologic toxicities generally are manifested with prolonged use of nafcillin (neutropenia), piperacillin (platelet dysfunction), cefotetan (hypoprothrombinemia), chloramphenicol (bone marrow suppression, both idiosyncratic and dose-related toxicity), and trimethoprim (megaloblastic anemia). Reversible nephrotoxicity classically is associated with aminoglycosides

and vancomycin. Reversible ototoxicity can occur with aminoglycosides or erythromycin. In the outpatient setting, patients must be counseled regarding photosensitivity with azithromycin, quinolones, tetracyclines, pyrazinamide, sulfamethoxazole, and trimethoprim. Lastly, all antibiotics have been implicated in causing diarrhea and colitis secondary to *Clostridium difficile*[34] (see Chap. 36).

Aside from consideration of drug toxicity, some antimicrobial use requires more intensive risk-benefit analysis. An example of this is the decision to use isoniazid prophylactically to prevent tuberculosis. Because the hepatotoxicity of isoniazid increases in frequency with age, older persons (>45 years) who are candidates for isoniazid prophylaxis (positive skin test) must have additional risk factors for tuberculosis to balance the potential toxic effects. These include evidence of recent skin-test conversion, immunosuppression, or previous gastrectomy. Older patients without additional risk factors are more likely to suffer toxicity from isoniazid than derive benefit from its use.[35]

COST

The costs of drug therapy are increasing dramatically, especially as new products, derived from biotechnology, are introduced. Greater attention is being paid to the pharmacoeconomics of drug therapy, where patient outcomes are valued and the costs to arrive at those outcomes are estimated. With increasing numbers of patients enrolled in managed-care organizations, understanding the true cost of antimicrobial therapy is more important than ever. The total cost of antimicrobial therapy includes much more than just the acquisition cost of the drugs.[36]

Many ancillary costs and factors affect the true cost of therapy. These include factors such as storage, preparation, distribution, and administration, as well as all the costs incurred from monitoring for adverse effects and factors such as length of hospitalization, readmissions, and all directly provided health care goods and services. More difficult to value but equally as important are indirect costs such as patient quality-of-life issues. Pharmacoeconomic and outcomes analyses are becoming more widely applied and used in order to derive values such as cost-benefit ratios and the cost-effectiveness of various products as compared with other products. A detailed review of pharmacoeconomic analyses is beyond the scope of this chapter, but excellent reviews of the subject are available.[37] A great deal more research in this area is needed, and multidisciplinary, collaborative efforts with the involvement of pharmacy, medicine, nursing, and microbiology are essential.[38]

Many new oral antimicrobials have been approved, including cephalosporins, linezolid, and fluoroquinolones, that can be used in place of more expensive parenteral therapy. These agents offer extended-spectrum killing activity, increased tissue penetration, and excellent safety and pharmacokinetic profiles. Many older, less expensive oral agents also remain appropriate choices. When oral therapy is being considered, the choice between convenient once-a-day expensive agents versus multiple-dose inexpensive agents arises. It is easy to calculate the difference in acquisition cost; however, the overall cost between agents is more difficult to determine. Factors to weigh include safety, effectiveness, tolerability, patient compliance, and potential drug-drug interactions. In some instances, more expensive agents may be warranted to avoid adverse outcomes.[39]

COMBINATION ANTIMICROBIAL THERAPY

In selecting a drug regimen for a given patient, consideration must be given to the necessity of using more than one drug. Combinations of antimicrobials generally are used to broaden the spectrum of coverage for empirical therapy, achieve synergistic activity against the infecting organism, and prevent the emergence of resistance.[40]

BROADENING THE SPECTRUM OF COVERAGE

Increasing the coverage of antimicrobial therapy generally is necessary in mixed infections where multiple organisms are likely to be present. This is the case in intraabdominal and female pelvic infections, in which a variety of aerobic and anaerobic bacteria may produce disease.[41] Traditionally, a combination of a drug active against aerobic gram-negative bacilli, such as an aminoglycoside, and a drug active against anaerobic bacteria, such as metronidazole or clindamycin, is selected. Newer β-lactam compounds, which possess good activity against both these types of organisms, such as the cephamycins, carbapenems, or the β-lactam/β-lactamase inhibitor combinations, may be adequate to replace the combination and thereby reduce the cost of therapy. The other clinical situation in which an increased spectrum of activity is desirable is with nosocomial infections.[32]

SYNERGISM

The achievement of synergistic antimicrobial activity is advantageous for infections caused by enteric gram-negative bacilli in immunosuppressed patients. Laboratory tests to identify synergy between antibiotic combinations are described in Chap. 103. Traditionally, combinations of aminoglycosides and β-lactams have been used because these drugs together generally act synergistically against a wide variety of bacteria. The data supporting superior efficacy of synergistic over nonsynergistic combinations are weak, however. At best, it would appear that synergistic combinations produce better results in infections caused by *P. aeruginosa*, in certain infections caused by *Enterococcus* spp., and perhaps in patients with profound, persistent neutropenia.[42,43]

The most obvious example of the use of synergy is the treatment of enterococcal endocarditis. The causative organism is usually only inhibited by penicillins, but it is killed rapidly by the addition of streptomycin or gentamicin to a penicillin.[42] The need for bactericidal activity in the treatment of endocarditis underscores the need for these synergistic combinations.

PREVENTING RESISTANCE

The use of combinations to prevent the emergence of resistance is applied widely but not often realized. The only circumstance where this has been clearly effective is in the treatment of tuberculosis. The prevalence of resistance to a first-line drug such as isoniazid or rifampin in a population of organisms may be as high as 1 in 10^6 to 10^8. Because the bacterial load in a patient with active tuberculosis often exceeds this, two drugs are given to reduce the likelihood of encountering resistance to less than 1 in 10.[35] There is ample evidence from in vitro data and experimental bacterial infections that combinations of drugs with different mechanisms are effective in the prevention of the emergence of resistance. Data from clinical trials, however, are either conflicting or do not convincingly support this concept.[44]

DISADVANTAGES OF COMBINATION THERAPY

Although there are potentially beneficial effects from combining drugs, there also are potential disadvantages. Examples include additive nephrotoxicity from drugs such as aminoglycosides,

amphotericin, and possibly vancomycin.[45] Inactivation of aminoglycosides by penicillins may be clinically significant when excessive doses of penicillin are given to a patient in renal failure.[46]

The combination of two or more antibiotics may result in antagonistic effects. Clinically, the effect of antagonism may be evident when one drug induces β-lactamase production and another drug is β-lactamase unstable.[47] Cefoxitin and imipenem are examples of drugs capable of inducing β-lactamases and may result in more rapid inactivation of penicillins when used together.

MONITORING THERAPEUTIC RESPONSE

After antimicrobial therapy has been instituted, the patient must be monitored carefully for a therapeutic response. Culture and sensitivity reports from specimens sent to the microbiology laboratory must be reviewed and the therapy changed accordingly. Use of agents with the narrowest spectrum of activity against identified pathogens is recommended. If anaerobes are suspected, even if they are not identified, anaerobic therapy should be continued.

Patient monitoring should include many of the same parameters used to diagnose the infection. The WBC count and temperature should start to normalize. Physical complaints from the patient also should diminish (i.e., decreased pain, shortness of breath, cough, or sputum production). Appetite should improve. Radiologic improvement may lag behind clinical improvement. Determinations of serum (or other fluid) levels of antimicrobials may be useful in ensuring outcome, preventing toxicity, or both. There are only a few antimicrobials that require serum concentration monitoring and then only in selected situations. These include the aminoglycosides, flucytosine, and chloramphenicol. Achievement of adequate aminoglycoside concentrations within the first few days of therapy of gram-negative infection has been correlated with better therapeutic outcome.[48] In addition, ensuring that excessive concentrations of flucytosine or chloramphenicol (in neonates) are avoided will prevent toxicity.

Changes in the volume of distribution may have a significant impact on the efficacy, safety, or both of therapy. An unexpectedly low volume of distribution (such as in the dehydrated patient) will result in higher, potentially toxic drug concentrations, whereas a larger-than-expected volume of distribution (such as in patients with edema or ascites) will result in low, potentially subtherapeutic concentrations. The most effective methods use measured serum concentrations of the drugs rather than estimations from renal function tests to assess true drug clearance from the body.

As patients improve clinically, the route of administration should be reevaluated. Streamlining therapy from parenteral to oral (switch therapy) has become an accepted practice for many infections outside the bloodstream and CNS.[33,49] Criteria that should be present to justify a switch to oral therapy include (1) overall clinical improvement, (2) lack of fever for 24 to 48 hours, (3) decreased WBC count, and (4) a functioning gastrointestinal tract. Drugs that exhibit excellent oral bioavailability when compared with intravenous formulations include ciprofloxacin, clindamycin, doxycycline, gatifloxacin, levofloxacin, metronidazole, moxifloxacin, linezolid, and trimethoprim-sulfamethoxazole.

FAILURE OF ANTIMICROBIAL THERAPY

A variety of factors may be responsible for an apparent lack of response to therapy.[50] Patients who fail to respond over 2 to 3 days require a thorough reevaluation. It is possible that the disease is not infectious or is nonbacterial in origin, or there is an undetected pathogen in a polymicrobial infection. Other factors include those directly related to drug selection, the host, or the pathogen. Laboratory error in identification, susceptibility testing, or both (presence of inoculum effect or resistant subpopulations) is a rare cause of antimicrobial failure.

FAILURES CAUSED BY DRUG SELECTION

Factors related directly to the drug selection include an inappropriate drug selection or dosage or route of administration. Malabsorption of a drug product because of gastrointestinal (GI) disease, such as a short-bowel syndrome, or a drug interaction, such as complexation of fluoroquinolones with multivalent cations resulting in reduced absorption, may lead to potentially subtherapeutic serum concentrations. Accelerated drug elimination is also possible. This may occur in patients with cystic fibrosis or during pregnancy, when more rapid clearance or larger volumes of distribution may result in low serum concentrations, particularly for aminoglycosides. A common cause of failure of therapy is poor penetration into the site of infection. This is especially true for sites such as the CNS, eye, and prostate gland. Drug failure also can result from drugs that are highly protein bound or that are chemically inactivated at the site of infection.

FAILURES CAUSED BY HOST FACTORS

Host defenses must be considered when evaluating a patient who is not responding to antimicrobial therapy. Patients who are immunosuppressed (e.g., granulocytopenia from chemotherapy or AIDS) may respond poorly to therapy because their defenses are inadequate to eradicate the infection despite seemingly adequate drug regimens. A good example is the poor response of infection in granulocytopenic patients that is seen when their WBC counts remain low during therapy. This contrasts with a much better response when granulocyte counts rise during therapy.[51]

Other host factors are related to the need for surgical drainage of abscesses or removal of foreign bodies, necrotic tissue, or both. If these situations are not corrected, they result in persistent infection and, occasionally, bacteremia despite adequate antimicrobial therapy.

FAILURES CAUSED BY MICROORGANISMS

Factors related to the pathogen include the development of drug resistance during therapy.[52] *Primary resistance* refers to the intrinsic resistance of the pathogens producing the infection. Several infections are more likely to result in drug resistance because of drug inaccessibility (e.g., pneumonia, endocarditis, abdominal and deep-seated skin and soft tissue infections). It has become increasingly obvious that despite the development and introduction of numerous new antimicrobial agents, bacterial resistance has continued to increase both within and across different bacterial genera.

Organisms in which resistance has increased most dramatically include enterococci, pneumococci, and *Mycobacterium tuberculosis*. Enterococci have been isolated with multiple resistance patterns. They may be resistant to β-lactams (by virtue of β-lactamase production, altered penicillin-binding proteins [PBPs], or both), vancomycin (via alterations in peptidoglycan synthesis), and high levels of aminoglycosides (via enzymatic degradation).

Pneumococci resistant to penicillins, certain cephalosporins, and macrolides are increasingly common. These organisms generally are susceptible to vancomycin, the new fluoroquinolones, and cefotaxime or ceftriaxone. *M. tuberculosis* resistant to one or more first-line antitubercular agents (e.g., isoniazid, rifampin, ethambutol, streptomycin, and pyrazinamide) have increased in frequency as well. This has been observed principally in populations of prison inmates and patients with AIDS.

The increase in resistance among these organisms is believed to be a result of continued overuse of antimicrobials in the community, as well as in hospitals, and the increasing prevalence of immunosuppressed patients receiving long-term suppressive antimicrobials for the prevention of infections. These resistance patterns are regionally variable, and susceptibility patterns in the community (or hospital) should be monitored closely to promote rational antimicrobial selection.[53]

Recently approved antimicrobial agents such as quinupristin-dalfopristin and linezolid have been targeted at resistant gram-positive bacteria. Numerous other drugs currently in development also have enhanced activity against these bacteria.

The emergence of resistance during antimicrobial therapy is reported most frequently in pulmonary or other deep-seated infections caused by *P. aeruginosa*. This occurs in 20% to 30% of cases and with all the available antibacterial agents, including imipenem. This organism and a group of enteric gram-negative bacilli (*Enterobacter aerogenes, E. cloacae, Citrobacter freundii, Serratia marcescens*, and a few others) can produce a β-lactamase that is capable of hydrolyzing broad-spectrum cephalosporins and, to a lesser extent, penicillins.[53] These enzymes are categorized as Bush group I, and their genetic code is found on the chromosome. Resistant mutants of these aforementioned organisms that produce large quantities of these enzymes may be present within an infection and may be responsible for the emergence of resistance during therapy. The mutants occur at a frequency of 1 in 10^6 to 1 in 10^8 bacteria, the numbers of bacteria commonly encountered in clinical infections.[53] Because only 10^4 to 10^5 bacteria are tested for susceptibility in the microbiology laboratory, however, this potential resistance may not be detected.

Treatment of an infection caused by *Enterobacter, Citrobacter, Serratia*, or *P. aeruginosa* with a third-generation cephalosporin or aztreonam may produce an initial clinical response by eradicating all the susceptible bacteria in the population. Within a few days, however, the highly resistant subpopulations have a selective advantage and may overgrow the infection site to produce a relapse.[53] These bacteria usually retain susceptibility to aminoglycosides, carbapenems, and fluoroquinolones but are resistant to all other β-lactams. Host defenses are extremely important in this scenario. Debilitated patients with pulmonary infections, abscesses, or osteomyelitis are at high risk for drug failure. In these situations, a combination regimen to prevent the emergence of resistance or the use of carbapenem or a fluoroquinolone may be warranted for empirical therapy.

ANTIMICROBIAL USE MANAGEMENT

ANTIBIOTIC FORMULARY

Institutions must decide which antibiotics to include on their formularies. The actual decision to have a formulary remains controversial; however, restricting choices does encourage familiarity with a core of antibiotics for residents and attending physicians. Open formularies allow the empirical use of any commercially available antibiotics, with recommended guidelines for changes when culture and sensitivity results are finalized. Many institutions have organized an antibiotic subcommittee to the pharmacy and therapeutics committee that meets to discuss trends in resistance and review new agents. The subcommittee is generally a multidisciplinary group including representation from microbiology, infection control, pharmacy, and physicians from several disciplines, including infectious disease. The actual implementation of the guidelines and restrictions recommended by such groups requires the cooperation of the entire medical staff. Education is vital to the success of the antibiotic formulary.[54]

ANTIMICROBIAL CYCLING

An interesting topic in formulary management that continues to gain interest despite little scientific research is *antimicrobial cycling*. Antimicrobial cycling is a predetermined change in an antimicrobial recommendation for empirical therapy of a specific infection at a predetermined time.[55] It also has been called *rotation of antimicrobials*. This strategy should not be confused with *antimicrobial switch therapy*, which involves changes in the route of administration of antimicrobial therapy (i.e., intravenous to oral).

Antimicrobial cycling is employed as a mechanism to reduce or prevent antimicrobial resistance. *Proactive cycling* is a planned switch to preempt resistance at a predetermined point or series of points with a predetermined schedule. *Reactive cycling* is a response to high or unacceptable resistance and is often a one-time switch. Most programs incorporate aspects of both types of cycling. Cycling implies returning to the original drug after other choices have been used. Rotation implies several planned changes.

Antimicrobial cycling is based on the assumptions that the resistance problem is (1) caused by the overuse of a particular agent or class of agents and (2) that discontinuation of the particular agent or class of agents will restore susceptibility. These assumptions correlate best with nosocomial gram-negative organisms that can rapidly develop resistance. Theoretically, antimicrobial agents should be sequenced in such an order that mechanisms of resistance do not overlap (i.e., changing drug classes).[55] Experts have expressed the need for further well-controlled long-term studies. The Centers for Disease Control and Prevention is currently funding several antimicrobial cycling programs.

KEEPING CURRENT

Attention must be paid to the literature on antimicrobials to assist in the selection of therapy. The results from prospective, controlled, randomized clinical trials should be evaluated whenever possible when considering appropriate antimicrobial therapy. Results from prelicensing open trials offer only limited information that may be useful in this regard because patients in these trials generally are not seriously ill and are not infected with multiple resistant bacteria and other confounding factors found in most clinical situations are excluded by virtue of the study design. Therefore, comparative data in more seriously ill patients are essential for the appropriate application of new agents.[56]

Postmarketing trials are also important because results may demonstrate superiority of one regimen over another, either in efficacy, safety, or cost-effectiveness. Appropriate antimicrobial therapy may change as new organisms are discovered, susceptibility patterns change, new drugs become available, and new clinical trial results are published. Classical thinking in the treatment of infectious diseases will continue to change and evolve to maintain antimicrobial efficacy. Optimal use of modern antimicrobials is just beginning to be defined.[57]

ABBREVIATIONS

AUC: area under the curve
IL: interleukin
MIC: minimal inhibitory concentration

PBP: penicillin-binding protein
PMN: polymorphonuclear leukocytes
WBC: white blood cell

Review Questions and other resources can be found at *www.pharmacotherapyonline.com.*

REFERENCES

1. Hessen TM, Kaye D. Principles of selection and use of antibacterial agents: In vitro activity and pharmacology. Infect Dis Clin North Am 2000;14:265–279.
2. Dinarello CA, Cannon JG, Wolff SM. New concepts on the pathogenesis of fever. Rev Infect Dis 1988;10:168–189.
3. Mackowiak PA, Durach DT. Fever of unknown origin. In: Mandell GL, Bennett JE, Dolin R, eds. Mandell, Douglas and Bennett's Principles and Practice of Infectious Diseases, 5th ed. New York, Churchill-Livingstone, 2000:622–633.
4. Johnson DH, Cunha BA. Drug fever. Infect Dis Clin North Am 1996;10:85–91.
5. Official ATS statement. Guidelines for the management of adults with community-acquired pneumonia: Diagnosis, assessment of severity, antimicrobial therapy, and prevention. Am J Respir Crit Care Med 2001;163:1730–1754.
6. Andes DR, Craig WA. Pharmacokinetics and pharmacodynamics of antibiotics in meningitis. Infect Dis Clin North Am 1999;13:595–618.
7. Mylonakis E, Calderwwod SB. Infective endocarditis in adults. N Engl J Med 2001;345:1318–1320.
8. Thomson RB Jr, Miller JM. Specimen collection, transport, and processing: Bacteriology. In: Murray PR, Baroon EJ, Jorgensen JH, et al, eds. Manual of Clinical Microbiology, 8th ed. Washington, ASM Press, 2003:286–330.
9. Weiss ME. Drug allergy. Med Clin North Am 1992;76:857–882.
10. Kelkar PS, Li JTC. Cephalosporin allergy. N Engl J Med 2001;345:804–809.
11. Saxon A, Swabb EA, Adkinson NF. Investigation into the immunologic cross-reactivity of aztreonam with other beta-lactam antibiotics. Am J Med 1985;78(suppl 2A):19–26.
12. Heath PT, Nik Yusoff NK, Baker CJ. Neonatal meningitis. Arch Dis Child Fetal Neonatal Ed 2003;88:F173–178.
13. Kasten MJ. Clindamycin, metronidazole, and chloramphenicol. Mayo Clinic Proc 1999;74:825–833.
14. Kantor HI, Sutherland DA, Leonard JT, et al. Effect of bilirubin metabolism in the newborn of sulfisoxazole administered to the mother. Obstet Gynecol 1961;17:494–500.
15. San Joaquin VH, Stull TL. Antibacterial agents in pediatrics. Infect Dis Clin North Am 2000;14:341–355.
16. Pichichero ME. Empiric antibiotic selection criteria for respiratory infections in pediatric practice. Pediatr Infect Dis J 1997;16:S60–64.
17. Stalam M, Kaye D. Antibiotic agents in the elderly. Infect Dis Clin North Am 2000;14:357–369.
18. Duff P. Antibiotic selection in obstetric patients. Infect Dis Clin North Am 1997;11:1–12.
19. Weinshilboum R. Inheritance and drug response. N Engl J Med 2003;348:529–537.
20. Tabbara IA. Hemolytic anemias: Diagnosis and management. Med Clin North Am 1992;76:649–668.
21. Livornese LL, Slavin D, Benz RL, et al. Use of antibacterial agents in renal failure. Infect Dis Clin North Am 2000;14:371–389.
22. Tschida SJ, Vance-Bryan K, Zaske DE. Anti-infective agents in hepatic disease. Med Clin North Am 1995;79:895–917.
23. Hughes WT, Armstrong D, Bodey GP, et al. 2002 Guidelines for the use of antimicrobial agents in neutropenic patients with cancer. Clin Infect Dis 2002;34:730–751.
24. Guidelines for preventing opportunistic infections among HIV-infected persons—2002. Recommendations of the U.S. Public Health Service and

the Infectious Diseases Society of America. MMWR 2002;51(RR-08): 1–46.

35. Levison ME. Pharmacodynamics of antibacterial agents. Infect Dis Clin North Am 2000;14:281–291.

36. Craig WA, Gudmundsson S. Postantibiotic effect. In: Lorian V, ed. Antibiotics in Laboratory Medicine, 4th ed. Baltimore, Williams & Wilkins, 1996,296–329.

37. Forest A, Nix DE, Ballow CH, et al. Pharmacodynamics of intravenous ciprofloxacin in seriously ill patients. Antimicrob Agents Chemother 1993;37:1073–1081.

38. Thomas JK, Forest A, Bhavnani SM, et al. Pharmacodynamic evaluation of factors associated with the development of bacterial resistance in acutely ill patients during therapy. Antimicrob Agents Chemother 1998;42: 521–527.

39. MacGowan AP, Bowker KE. Continuous infusion of beta-lactam antibiotics. Clin Pharmacokinet 1998;35:391–402.

40. Nix DE, Goodwin SD, Peloquin CA, et al. Antibiotic tissue penetration and its relevance: Impact of tissue penetration on infection response. Antimicrob Agents Chemother 1991;35:1953–1959.

41. Quagliarello VJ, Scheld WM. Treatment of bacterial meningitis. N Engl J Med 1997;336:708–716.

42. Campbell GD, Niederman MS, Broughton WA, et al. Official ATS statement: Hospital-acquired pneumonia in adults: Diagnosis, assessment of severity, initial antimicrobial therapy and preventative strategies. Am J Respir Crit Care Med 1995;153:1711–1725.

43. Bartlett JG, Dowell SF, Mandell LA, et al. Infectious Diseases Society of America. Practice guidelines for the management of community-acquired pneumonia. Clin Infect Dis 2000;31:347–382.

44. Johnson S, Gerding DN. Clostridium difficile–associated diarrhea. Clin Infect Dis 1998;26:1027–1034.

45. American Thoracic Society, Centers for Disease Control and Prevention, and Infectious Diseases Society of America. Treatment of tuberculosis. Am J Respir Crit Care Med 2003;167:603–662.

46. McNabb J, Quintiliani R, Nicolau DP, et al. Cost-effectiveness in the use of antibiotics. Curr Clin Top Infect Dis 2002;20:24–42.

47. McGhan WF. Pharmacoeconomics and the evaluation of drugs and services. Hosp Formul 1993;28:365–378.

48. Scott RD 2d, Solomon SL, McGowan JE Jr. Applying economic principles to health care. Emerg Infect Dis 2001;7:282–285.

49. Nightingale CH, Quintiliani R. Cost of oral antibiotic therapy. Pharmacotherapy 1997;17:302–307.

40. Rybak MJ, McGrath BJ. Combination antibacterial therapy for bacterial infections: Guidelines for the clinician. Drugs 1996;52:390–405.

41. Solomkin JS, Mazuski JE, Baron EJ, et al. Guidelines for the selection of anti-infective agents for complicated intra-abdominal infections. Clin Infect Dis 2003;37:997–1005.

42. Murray BE. Vancomycin-resistant enterococcal infections. N Engl J Med 2000;342:710–721.

43. Giamarellou H, Antoniadou A. Antipseudomonal antibiotics. Med Clin North Am 2001;85:19–42.

44. Chow JW, Yu JL. Combination antibiotic therapy versus monotherapy for gram-negative bacteraemia: A commentary. Intern J Infect Dis 1999;11: 7–12.

45. Rybak MJ, Abate BJ, Kang SL, et al. Prospective evaluation of the effect of an aminoglycoside dosing regimen on rates of observed nephrotoxicity and ototoxicity. Antimicrob Agents Chemother 1999;43:1549–1555.

46. Wright AJ. The penicillins. Mayo Clinic Proc 1999;74:290–307.

47. Pitout JD, Sanders CC, Sanders WE Jr. Antimicrobial resistance with focus on beta-lactam resistance in gram-negative bacilli. Am J Med 1997;103:51–59.

48. Moore RD, Smith CR, Lietman PS. Association of aminoglycoside plasma levels with therapeutic outcome in gram-negative pneumonia. Am J Med 1984;77:657–662.

49. Cunha BA. Intravenous-to-oral antibiotic switch therapy. Postgrad Med 1997;101:111–128.

50. Cunha BA, Ortega AM. Antibiotic failure. Med Clin North Am 1995;79:663–672.

51. Pizzo PA. Fever in immunocompromised patients. N Engl J Med 1999; 341:893–900.

52. Kaye KS, Fraimiw HS, Abrutyn E. Pathogens resistant to antimicrobial agents: Epidemiology, molecular mechanisms, and clinical management. Infect Dis Clin North Am 2000;14:293–319.

53. Shlaes DM, Gerding DN, John JF Jr, et al. Society for Healthcare Epidemiology of America and Infectious Diseases Society of America Joint Committee on the Prevention of Antimicrobial Resistance: Guidelines for the prevention of antimicrobial resistance in hospitals. Infect Control Hosp Epidemiol 1997;18:275–291.

54. John JF Jr, Fishman NO. Programmatic role of the infectious diseases physician in controlling antimicrobial costs in the hospital. Clin Infect Dis 1997;24:471–485.

55. McGowan JE Jr. Strategies for study of the role of cycling on antimicrobial use and resistance. Infect Control Hosp Epidemiol 2000;21:S36–43.

56. Gilbert DN. Guidelines for evaluating new antimicrobial agents. J Infect Dis 1987;156:934–941.

57. Polk R. Optimal use of modern antibiotics: Emerging trends. Clin Infect Dis 1999;29:264–274.

GRAM-POSITIVE COCCI

Enterococcus faecalis (generally not as resistant to antibiotics as
E. faecium)

Serious infection (endocarditis, meningitis, pyelonephritis with
bacteremia)

Ampicillin (or penicillin G) + (gentamicin or streptomycin)

Vancomycin + (gentamicin or streptomycin), linezolid

Urinary tract infection (UTI)

Ampicillin, amoxicillin

Doxycycline,[a] fosfomycin, or nitrofurantoin

E. faecium (generally more resistant to antibiotics than *E. faecalis*)

Recommend consultation with infectious disease specialist.

Linezolid, quinupristin/dalfopristin

Staphylococcus aureus/Staphylococcus epidermidis

Methicillin (oxacillin)-sensitive

PRP[c] (penicillinase resist PCN) - nafloxac

*FGC,[d,e] trimethoprim-sulfamethoxazole, clindamycin,[f]
ampicillin-sulbactam, amoxicillin-clavulante, or
fluoroquinolone*

Methicillin (oxacillin)–resistant

Vancomycin + (gentamicin or rifampin)

Linezolid, quinupristin-dalfopristin, daptomycin

*Per sensitivities: Trimethoprim-sulfamethoxazole,
doxycycline,[a] or clindamycin*

Streptococcus (groups A, B, C, G, and *S. bovis*)

Penicillin G[h] or V[i] or ampicillin

FGC,[d,e] erythromycin, azithromycin, clarithromycin,[j]

S. pneumoniae

Penicillin-sensitive (MIC < 0.1 mcg/mL)

Penicillin G or V or ampicillin

Erythromycin, FGC,[d,e] azithromycin, or clarithromycin[j]

Penicillin intermediate (MIC 0.1–1.0 mcg/mL)

High-dose penicillin (12 million units/day for adults) or
ceftriaxone[e] or cefotaxime[e]

Gatifloxacin,[b] levofloxacin,[b] moxifloxacin,[b] or vancomycin

Penicillin-resistant (MIC ≥ 1.0 mcg/mL)

Recommend consultation with infectious disease specialist.

Vancomycin ± rifampin

*Per sensitivities: TGC,[e,k] levofloxacin,[b] gatifloxacin,[b] or
moxifloxacin[b]*

Streptococcus, viridans group

Penicillin G ± gentamicin[l]

*TGC,[d,e] erythromycin, azithromycin, clarithromycin,[j] or
vancomycin ± gentamicin*

GRAM-NEGATIVE COCCI

Moraxella (Branhamella) catarrhalis

Amoxicillin-clavulanate, ampicillin-sulbactam

*Trimethoprim-sulfamethoxazole, erythromycin, azithromycin,
clarithromycin,[j] doxycycline,[a] SGC,[e,m] TGC,[e,k] or TGCpo[e,n]*

Neisseria gonorrhoeae (also give concomitant treatment for
Chlamydia trachomatis)

Disseminated gonococcal infection

Ceftriaxone[e] or cefotaxime[e]

*Oral follow-up: Cefixime,[e] cefpodoxime,[e] ciprofloxacin,[b] or
ofloxacin[b]*

Uncomplicated infection

Ceftriaxone[e] or cefotaxime,[e] cefixime,[e] or cefpodoxime[e]

Ciprofloxacin[b] or ofloxacin[b]

N. meningitides

Penicillin G

TGC[e,k]

GRAM-POSITIVE BACILLI

Clostridium perfringens

Penicillin G ± clindamycin

*Metronidazole, clindamycin, doxycycline,[a] cefazolin,[e]
imipenem,[o] meropenem,[o] or ertapenem[o]*

C. difficile

Oral metronidazole

Oral vancomycin

GRAM-NEGATIVE BACILLI

Acinetobacter spp.

Imipenem or meropenem either ± aminoglycoside[p] (amikacin
usually most effective)

*Ciprofloxacin,[b] trimethoprim-sulfamethoxazole, or
ampicillin-sulbactam*

Bacteroides fragilis (and others)

Metronidazole

BLIC,[g] clindamycin, cephamycin,[e,q] or carbapenem[o]

Enterobacter spp.

Imipenem, meropenem, ertapenem, or cefepime ±
aminoglycoside[p]

*Ciprofloxacin,[b] levofloxacin,[b] piperacillin-tazobactam,
ticarcillin-clavulanate, or trimethoprim-sulfamethoxazole*

Escherichia coli

Meningitis

TGC[e,k] or meropenem

Systemic infection

TGC[e,k]

*Ampicillin-sulbactam, FGC,[d,e] BL/BLI,[g]
trimethoprim-sulfamethoxazole, SGC,[e,m]
fluoroquinolone,[b,o,r] imipenem,[o] meropenem[o]*

Urinary tract infection

Most oral agents: Check sensitivities.

Ampicillin, amoxicillin-clavulanate,
trimethoprim-sulfamethoxazole, or cephalexin[e]

Aminoglycoside, FGC[d,e] nitrofurantoin, fluoroquinolone[b,o,r]

Gardnerella vaginalis

Metronidazole

Clindamycin

Hemophilus influenzae

Meningitis

Cefotaxime[e] or ceftriaxone[e]

Meropenem[o] or chloramphenicol[r]

Other infections

BLIC,[g] or if β-lactamase-negative, ampicillin or amoxicillin

Trimethoprim-sulfamethoxazole, cefuroxime,[e] erythromycin,
   azithromycin, clarithromycin,[j] or fluoroquinolone[b,o,r]
Klebsiella pneumoniae
   TGC[e,k] (if UTI only: Aminoglycoside[p])
   Trimethoprim-sulfamethoxazole, cefuroxime,[e]
      fluoroquinolone,[b,r] BLIC,[g] imipenem,[o] or meropenem[o]
Legionella spp.
   Erythromycin ± rifampin or fluoroquinolone[b,r]
   Trimethoprim-sulfamethoxazole, clarithromycin,[j]
      azithromycin, or doxycycline[a]
Pasteurella multocida
   Penicillin G, ampicillin, amoxicillin
   Doxycycline,[a] BLIC,[g] trimethoprim-sulfamethoxazole or
      ceftriaxone[e,k]
Proteus mirabilis
   Ampicillin
   Trimethoprim-sulfamethoxazole, most antibiotics except PRP[c]
Proteus (indole-positive) (including Providencia rettgeri,
   Morganella morganii, and Proteus vulgaris)
   TGC[e,k] or fluoroquinolone[b,r]
   Trimethoprim-sulfamethoxazole, BLIC,[g] aztreonam,[t]
      imipenem,[o] or TGCpo[e,n]
Providencia stuartii
   TGC[e,k] or fluoroquinolone[b,r]
   Trimethoprim-sulfamethoxazole, aztreonam,[t] imipenem,[o] or
      meropenem[o]
Pseudomonas aeruginosa
   Cefepime, ceftazidime, piperacillin-tazobactam, or
      ticarcillin-clavulanate plus aminoglycoside[p]
   Ciprofloxacin,[b] levofloxacin,[b] aztreonam,[t] imipenem,[o] or
      meropenem[o]
   UTI only: Aminoglycoside[p]
   Ciprofloxacin,[b] levofloxacin,[b] or gatifloxacin[b]
Salmonella typhi
   Ciprofloxacin,[b] levofloxacin,[b] ceftriaxone,[e] or cefotaxime[e]
   Trimethoprim-sulfamethoxazole
Serratia marcescens
   Piperacillin-tazobactam, ticarcillin-clavulanate, or TGC[e,k] ±
      gentamicin
   Trimethoprim-sulfamethoxazole, ciprofloxacin,[b] levofloxacin,[b]
      aztreonam,[t] imipenem,[g] meropenem,[o] or ertapenem
Stenotrophomonas (Xanthomonas) maltophilia
   Trimethoprim-sulfamehtoxazole
   Generally very resistant to all antimicrobials; check
      sensitivities to ceftazidime,[e] ticarcillin-clavulanate,
      doxycycline,[a] and minocycline[a]

MISCELLANEOUS MICROORGANISMS

Chlamydia pneumoniae
   Doxycycline[a]
   Erythromycin, azithromycin, clarithromycin,[j] or
      fluoroquinolone[b,r]
C. trachomatis
   Doxycycline[a] or azithromycin
   Levofloxacin[b] or ofloxacin[b]
Mycoplasma pneumoniae
   Erythromycin, azithromycin, clarithromycin[j]
   Doxycycline[a] or fluoroquinolone[b,r]

SPIROCHETES

Treponema pallidum
   Neurosyphilis
   Penicillin G
   Ceftriaxone[e]
   Primary or secondary
   Benzathine penicillin G
   Doxycycline[a] or ceftriaxone[e]
Borrelia burgdorferi (choice depends on stage of disease)
   Ceftriaxone[e] or cefuroxime axetil,[e] doxycycline,[a] amoxicillin
   High-dose penicillin, cefotaxime,[e] azithromycin, or
      clarithromycin[j]

[a] *Not for use in pregnant patients or children younger than 8 years old.*
[b] *Not for use in pregnant patients or children younger than 18 years old.*
[c] *Penicillinase-resistant penicillin: nafcillin or oxacillin.*
[d] *First-generation cephalosporins—IV: cefazolin; PO: cephalexin, cephradine, or cefadroxil.*
[e] *Some penicillin-allergic patients may react to cephalosporins.*
[f] *Not reliably bactericidal; should not be used for endocarditis.*
[g] *β-Lactamase inhibitor combination—IV: ampicillin-sulbactam, piperacillin-tazobactam, ticarcillin-clavulante; PO: amoxicillin-clavulanate.*
[h] *Either aqueous penicillin G or benzathine penicillin G (pharyngitis only).*
[i] *Only for soft tissue infections or upper respiratory infections (pharyngitis, otitis media).*
[j] *Do not use in pregnant patients.*
[k] *Third-generation cephalosporins—IV: cefotaxime, ceftriaxone.*
[l] *Gentamicin should be added if tolerance or moderately susceptible (MIC > 0.1 g/mL) organisms are encountered; streptomycin is used but may be more toxic.*
[m] *Second-generation cephalosporins—IV: cefuroxime; PO: cefaclor, cefditoren, cefprozil, cefuroxime axetil, and loracarbef.*
[n] *Third-generation cephalosporins—PO: cefdinir, cefixime, cefetamet, cefpodoxime proxetil, and ceftibuten.*
[o] *Reserve for serious infection.*
[p] *Aminoglycosides: gentamicin, tobramycin, and amikacin; use per sensitivities.*
[q] *Cefoxitin, cefotetan.*
[r] *IV/PO: ciprofloxacin, ofloxacin, levofloxacin, gatifloxacin, and moxifloxacin.*
[s] *Reserve for serious infection when less toxic drugs are not effective.*
[t] *Generally reserved for patients with hypersensitivity reactions to penicillin.*

105

CENTRAL NERVOUS SYSTEM INFECTIONS

Elizabeth D. Hermsen and John C. Rotschafer

Learning Objectives and other resources can be found at *www.pharmacotherapyonline.com.*

KEY CONCEPTS

1 The three most likely pathogens of bacterial meningitis in the United States are *Streptococcus pneumoniae, Neisseria meningitidis,* and *Hemophilus influenzae,* although routine vaccination may cause a change in the epidemiology in the years to come.

2 In cases of meningitis, initial findings can include (a) *presenting signs and symptoms:* fever, headache, nuchal rigidity, Brudzinski's or Kernig's sign, and altered mental status, and (b) *abnormal cerebrospinal fluid (CSF) chemistries:* elevated white blood cell (WBC) count (>100 cells/mm^3), elevated protein (>50 mg/dL), and decreased glucose levels (<40 mg/dL).

3 Two main microbiologic tests that should be obtained include a Gram stain of the CSF and CSF cultures.

4 Three primary goals of treatment in meningitis include (a) *amelioration* of signs and symptoms, (b) *eradication* of infection, and (c) *prevention* of the development of neurologic sequelae, such as seizures, deafness, coma, and death.

5 When selecting antibiotics, the clinician must consider the antibiotic concentration at the site of infection, as well as the spectrum of antibacterial activity. Empirical choices should be based on age and predisposing conditions. (a) *Ceftriaxone* or *cefotaxime* and *vancomycin* are reasonable initial choices for empirical coverage of community-acquired meningitis in adult patients. (b) *Listeria monocytogenes*

is a common pathogen in infants and elderly. Therefore, *ampicillin* should be added empirically to antimicrobial coverage.

6 Empirical coverage with an appropriate antibiotic should be started as soon as possible when clinical suspicion of meningitis exists. If there is a delay in doing a lumbar puncture (even 30 to 60 minutes), the first dose of an antibiotic *should not* be withheld. Changes in the CSF after initiation of antibiotics usually take 12 to 24 hours.

7 In contrast to the treatment of other infectious diseases, antibiotic dosages in the treatment of meningitis should be maximized to optimize CNS penetration.

8 The duration of antibiotic treatment for meningitis has not been standardized; however, the duration of antibiotic therapy generally is based on the causative organism and the individual case and may range from 7 to 21 days.

9 Close contacts and relatives of the index case should be assessed for appropriate prophylaxis, particularly with *N. meningitidis* and *H. influenzae* meningitis.

10 Steroid treatment includes dexamethasone 0.15 mg/kg per dose to be given four times daily for 4 days in infants and children older than 2 months of age with proven or strongly suspected bacterial meningitis. Steroids should be given prior to antibiotics.

Central nervous system (CNS) infections are caused by various pathogens, including bacteria, viruses, fungi, and parasites. Infections are the result of hematogenous spread from a primary infection site, seeding from a parameningeal focus, reactivation from a latent site, trauma, or congenital defects in the CNS. Newer diagnostic techniques have enabled more rapid and definitive diagnoses, thus diminishing the number of unknown "aseptic meningitis" diagnoses and improving targeted therapy. Bacteria resistant to multiple antibiotics present new challenges in the management of meningitis. This chapter presents the etiologies, pathophysiology, therapy, and prophylaxis of these infections but will concentrate predominantly on bacterial meningitis.

EPIDEMIOLOGY

Approximately 1.2 million cases of acute bacterial meningitis, excluding epidemics, occur every year around the globe, resulting in

135,000 deaths.[1] Overall mortality rates for patients with meningitis range from 2% to 30%.[2] Neurologic sequelae frequently associated with meningitis include seizures, sensorineural hearing loss, and hydrocephalus. Risk for the development of neurologic sequelae depends on the infecting organism. Generally, 30% to 50% of patients who survive meningitis may develop neurologic disabilities.[3,4] Despite the availability of antimicrobial therapy against the most common CNS pathogens, CNS infections continue to have significant morbidity and mortality.

Two recent findings have the potential for great epidemiologic impact on bacterial meningitis. First, both passive and active exposures to cigarette smoke were shown to be risk factors for bacterial meningitis, especially meningococcal disease.[4a] Second, children with cochlear implants that include a positioner are at increased risk of bacterial meningitis, specifically pneumococcal meningitis. A recent study demonstrated an incidence of meningitis due to *Streptococcus pneumoniae* that was more than 30 times the incidence in a similar cohort of the U.S. population.[5]

ETIOLOGY

◀ CNS infections are caused by a variety of microorganisms. Historically, CNS infections were primarily community acquired; however, an increasing number are now nosocomial.[6] Surveillance studies of bacterial meningitis in the United States were conducted in 1986 and, in a smaller study, again in 1995.[7,8] In 1986, *Hemophilus influenzae* was the most commonly identified cause of bacterial meningitis (45%), followed by *S. pneumoniae* (18%) and *Neisseria meningitidis* (14%). In 1995, approximately 5 years after introduction of the *H. influenzae* type b conjugate (Hib) vaccine, *S. pneumoniae* was the most commonly identified cause of bacterial meningitis (47%), followed by *N. meningitidis* (25%), *Listeria monocytogenes* (8%), and *H. influenzae* (7%).

The incidence of invasive *H. influenzae* infections has decreased by more than 90% since the introduction of the Hib vaccine.[8] Mass immunization with the Hib vaccine also has resulted in alterations in the age distribution of bacterial meningitis. While the median age was 15 months in 1986, by 1995 that age increased to 25 years. Accordingly, the proportion of cases in those 18 years of age and older increased from 20.8% to 51.5%.[8] However, many developing countries have not adopted the Hib vaccine as part of the standard vaccines offered to children owing to cost. Thus approximately 350,000 to 700,000 children die each year worldwide owing to invasive *H. influenzae* infections.[1]

Similar to the Hib vaccine, the introduction of the conjugate pneumococcal vaccine and the implementation of uniform vaccination have resulted in near-total elimination of invasive pneumococcal disease in young children in the United States.[1] To our knowledge, no studies have been published to date regarding the incidence of pneumococcal meningitis owing to *S. pneumoniae* since the introduction of the conjugate vaccine. However, the near-total elimination of pneumococcal meningitis appears to be possible with uniform vaccination. Uniform vaccination was problematic beginning in 2001, when a shortage of the conjugate vaccine resulted in interim vaccination recommendations from the Centers for Disease Control and Prevention (CDC), calling for withholding the vaccine from healthy children over the age of 2 years. Clinicians should be aware that the shortage may have caused an interruption in many vaccination schedules. As discussed for the Hib vaccine, cost will be the rate-limiting factor in developing countries.

ANATOMY AND PHYSIOLOGY OF THE CENTRAL NERVOUS SYSTEM

MENINGES

The skull and vertebrae protect the CNS from blunt or penetrating trauma (Fig. 105–1). The brain is suspended in these structures by cerebrospinal fluid (CSF) and is surrounded by the meninges. The meninges are made up of three separate membranes: dura mater, arachnoid, and pia mater.[9] Dura mater, or pachymeninges, lies directly beneath and is adherent to the skull. The other two membranes are referred to collectively as *leptomeninges*. Pia mater lies directly over brain tissue. Arachnoid, the middle layer, lies between the dura mater and the pia mater. The subarachnoid space, located between the arachnoid and the pia mater, is the conduit for CSF. By definition, meningitis refers to inflammation of the subarachnoid space or spinal fluid, whereas encephalitis is an inflammation of the brain

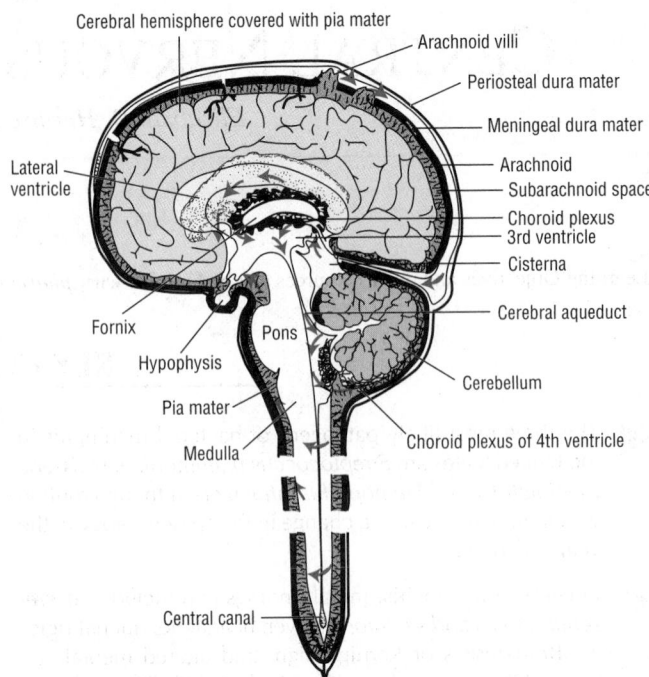

FIGURE 105–1. Diagram of the central nervous system.

itself. Since infectious microorganisms frequently are an underlying cause of these inflammatory processes, the terms *meningitis* and *encephalitis* frequently are used to denote an infectious process. The decision regarding the diagnosis of meningoencephalitis depends on radiographic, laboratory, and clinical information but would refer to inflammation of both tissue and fluid.

CEREBROSPINAL FLUID

Approximately 85% of the CSF is produced within the third, fourth, and lateral ventricles by the choroid plexus (see Fig. 105–1). CSF volume in the CNS is related to patient age: Infants have approximately 40 to 60 mL of CSF, older children have 60 to 100 mL, and adults have 110 to 160 mL. Normally, CSF is produced at the rate of approximately 500 mL/day and flows unidirectionally downward through the spinal cord. The CSF is removed by the arachnoid villi and vertebral venous plexus located in the spinal cord and does not recommunicate with the point of production.[9]

The CSF normally is clear, with a protein content of less than 50 mg/dL, a glucose concentration of approximately 50% to 66% of the simultaneous peripheral serum glucose concentration, and a pH of approximately 7.4; also, it typically contains fewer than five white blood cells (WBCs) per cubic millimeter, all of which should be lymphocytes (Table 105–1). As meninges become inflamed, the constituency of the CSF will change, and these changes can be used diagnostically as markers of infection.

BLOOD-BRAIN BARRIER/BLOOD-CSF BARRIER

Natural barriers to the exchange of drugs and endogenous compounds among the blood, brain, and CSF are the blood-brain barrier (BBB) and the blood-CSF barrier (BCSFB) (Fig. 105–2). The BBB consists of tightly joined capillary endothelial cells. Drug entry into brain tissue is accomplished by direct passage through the capillary

TABLE 105–1. Mean Values of the Components of Normal and Abnormal Cerebrospinal Fluid

Type	Normal	Bacterial	Viral	Fungal	Tuberculosis
WBC (cells/mm^3)	<5	1000–5000	100–1000	40–400	100–500
Differential (%)	>90[a]	≥80 PMNs	50[b,c]	>50[b]	>80[b,c]
Protein (mg/dL)	<50	100–500	30–150	40–150	≤40–150
Glucose (mg/dL)	50–66% simultaneous serum value	<40 (<60% simultaneous serum value)	<30–70	<30–70	<30–70

[a]Monocytes.
[b]Lymphocytes.
[c]Initial cerebrospinal fluid (CSF), while blood cell (WBC) count may reveal a predominance of polymorphonuclear neutrophils (PMNs).
From refs. 9 and 92.

endothelial cells and further penetration of the glial cells that envelop the capillary structure.[9]

Passage of drugs into the CSF is controlled by the BCSFB. This barrier is created by ependymal cells of the choroid plexus, which function as an active transport system similar to the renal tubular epithelial cells. The inflammatory process associated with meningitis inhibits the active transport system of the choroid plexus.[10] As in the active transport system in the kidney, the secretion of substances out of the choroid plexus also can be inhibited by the administration of probenecid.[9]

PATHOPHYSIOLOGY OF THE CNS INFECTION

The development of bacterial meningitis occurs following bacterial invasion of the host and CNS, bacterial multiplication with subsequent inflammation of the CNS, specifically the subarachnoid space and the ventricular space, pathophysiologic alterations owing to progressive inflammation, and the resulting neuronal damage.[11] The critical first step in the acquisition of acute bacterial meningitis is nasopharyngeal colonization of the host. Immunoglobulins (Igs) such as secretory IgA are found in high concentrations within nasopharyngeal secretions and work to inhibit bacterial colonization. However, the mucus barrier is deteriorated by IgA proteases secreted by the bacteria, which then extend pili that allow adherence to the host cell surface receptors.[12] Bacterial pathogens attach themselves to nasopharyngeal epithelial cells and are phagocytized into the host's bloodstream. After accessing the patient's bloodstream, bacteria must overcome the host's defense mechanisms.[1] Commonly, CNS bacterial pathogens will produce an extensive polysaccharide capsule resistant to neutrophil phagocytosis and complement opsonization. *H. influenzae, Escherichia coli,* and *N. meningitidis* strains lacking polysaccharide capsules are unable to cause meningitis. Capsular polysaccharides activate the alternate complement pathway, which promotes phagocytosis and clearance of infecting pathogens. Patients unable to activate the alternative complement pathway, such as asplenic and sickle cell patients, are predisposed to bacterial infections caused by encapsulated microorganisms and therefore are at risk for meningitis.

Although the exact site and mechanism of bacterial invasion into the CNS is unknown, studies suggest that invasion into the subarachnoid space occurs by continuous exposure of the CNS to large bacterial inocula. Bacteremia with inoculum densities of at least 10^3 colony-forming units (CFU)/mL appears to be essential for subarachnoid space invasion.[4] Although several sites of bacterial invasion have been theorized, the most plausible sites are the choroid plexus and/or the cerebral microvasculature. Recent studies have delineated the pathophysiology of *E. coli* meningitis, showing that successful translocation of *E. coli* across the BBB requires a high bacterial inoculum, *E. coli* binding to and invading the brain microvascular endothelial cells through specific ligand-receptor interactions, host cytoskeletal reorganization, and activation of various signaling pathways.[4] Host defense mechanisms within the subarachnoid space are inadequate to combat bacterial pathogens; bacteria, therefore, replicate freely within the CSF until either overgrowth occurs or an effective antibiotic regimen is administered that terminates the process.

The effects of meningitis, namely, inflammation within the subarachnoid space and the ensuing neurologic damage, are not a direct result of the pathogens themselves. The neurologic sequelae occur owing to the activation of the host's inflammatory pathways, which is induced by the pathogens or their products.[2] Bacterial cell death can cause the release of cell wall components, such as lipopolysaccharide (LPS), lipid A (endotoxin), lipoteichoic acid, teichoic acid, and peptidoglycan, depending on whether the pathogen is gram-positive or gram-negative (Fig. 105–3). These cell wall components cause

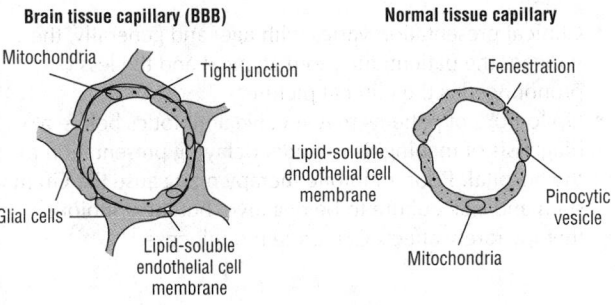

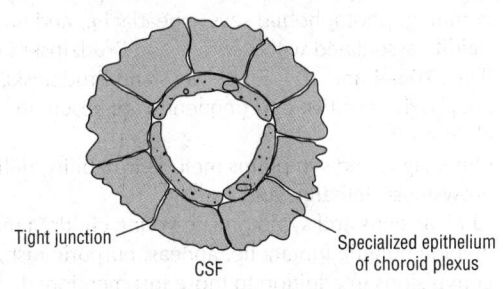

FIGURE 105–2. Schematic representation of a blood–cerebrospinal fluid barrier capillary, brain tissue capillary, and normal tissue capillary (*below*).

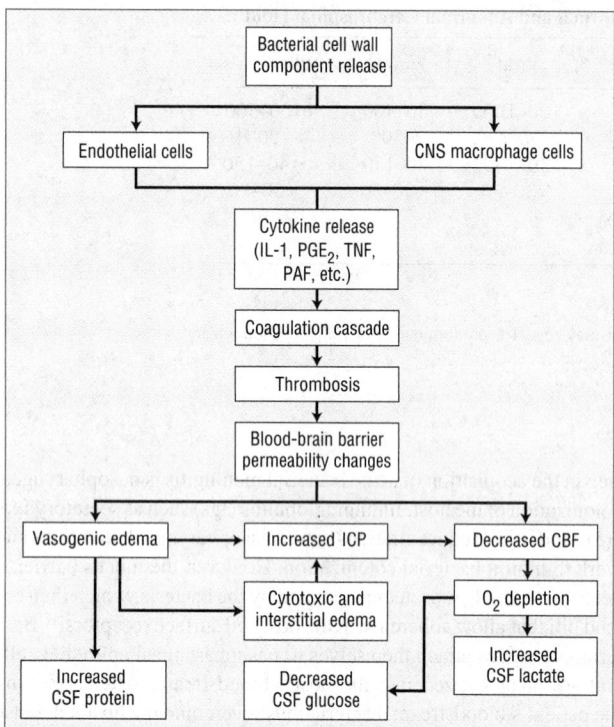

FIGURE 105–3. Hypothetical schema of pathophysiologic events that occur during bacterial meningitis. IL-1 = interleukin 1; TNF = tumor necrosis factor; PAF = platelet-activating factor; CBF = cerebral blood flow; CSF = cerebrospinal fluid; PGE_2 = prostaglandin E_2; ICP = intracranial pressure.

capillary endothelial cells and CNS macrophages to release cytokines (interleukin 1 [IL-1] and tumor necrosis factor [TNF]) and other inflammatory mediators (IL-6, IL-8, platelet-activating factor [PAF], nitric oxide, arachadonic acid metabolites [e.g., prostaglandin and prostacycline], and macrophage-derived proteins). Proteolytic products and toxic oxygen radicals are released from the capillary endothelium, causing an alteration in the permeability of the BBB. PAF activates the coagulation cascade, and arachidonic acid metabolites stimulate vasodilation. These events propagate other sequential events that lead to cerebral edema, elevated intracranial pressure (ICP), CSF pleocytosis, decreased cerebral blood flow, cerebral ischemia, and death.[2]

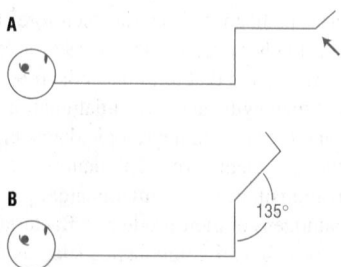

FIGURE 105–5. Kernig's sign. (*A*) Knees are raised to form a 90-degree angle relative to the trunk, and the examiner attempts to extend the knees. (*B*) Once the knee angle reaches approximately 135 degrees, contracture or extensor spasm occurs.

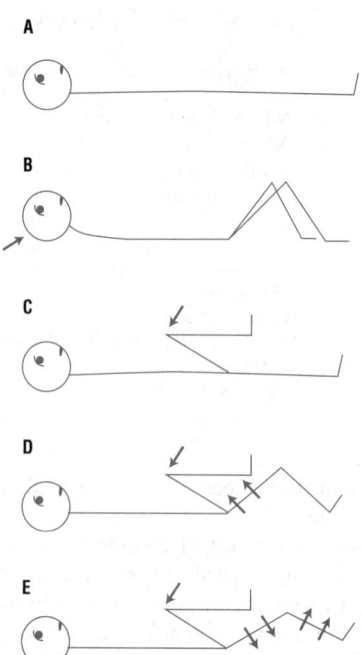

FIGURE 105–4. (*A,B*) Brudzinski's neck signs. Hip and knee flexion occurs as a result of flexion of the neck (*B*). (*C–E*) Brudzinski's leg signs. (*C*) Patient leg is flexed by examiner (*arrow*). (*D*) The contralateral leg begins to flex—identical contralateral sign (*arrows*). (*E*) The contralateral leg now begins to extend spontaneously, resembling a little kick (*arrows*).

CLINCAL PRESENTATION AND DIAGNOSIS

CLINICAL PRESENTATION OF ACUTE MENINGITIS

GENERAL

- Clinical presentation varies with age, and generally, the younger the patient, the more atypical and the less pronounced is the clinical picture.
- Up to 50% of patients may receive antibiotics before a diagnosis of meningitis is made, delaying presentation to the hospital. Prior antibiotic therapy may cause the Gram stain and CSF culture to be negative, but the antibiotic therapy rarely affects CSF protein or glucose.[13]

SIGNS AND SYMPTOMS

- Classic signs and symptoms include fever, chills, vomiting, photophobia, severe headache, and nuchal rigidity associated with Kernig's and Brudzinski's signs (Figs. 105–4 and 105–5). Kernig's and Brudzinski's signs are poorly sensitive and frequently are absent in children.[13,14]
- Other signs and symptoms include irritability, delirium, drowsiness, lethargy, and coma.
- Clinical signs and symptoms in young children may include bulging fontanelle, apneas, purpuric rash, and convulsions in addition to those just mentioned.[13]
- Seizures occur more commonly in children (20% to 30%) than in adults (0% to 12%).[15]

DIFFERENTIAL SIGNS AND SYMPTOMS[2]

- Purpuric and petechial skin lesions typically indicate meningococcal involvement, although the lesions may be present with *H. influenzae* meningitis. Rashes rarely occur with pneumococcal meningitis.
- Waterhouse-Friderichsen syndrome, a rapid eruption of multiple hemorrhagic lesions associated with a shocklike state, is associated with meningococcal meningitis.
- *H. influenza* meningitis and meningococcal meningitis both can cause involvement of the joints during the illness.
- A history of head trauma with or without skull fracture or presence of a chronically draining ear is associated with pneumococcal involvement.

LABORATORY TESTS

- Several tubes of CSF are collected via lumbar puncture for chemistry, microbiology, and hematology tests. Theoretically, the first tube has a higher likelihood of being contaminated with both blood and bacteria during the puncture, although the total volume is more important in practice than the tube cultured. CSF should not be refrigerated or stored on ice.[16]
- Analysis of CSF chemistries typically includes measurement of glucose and total protein concentrations. An elevated CSF protein of 100 mg/dL or greater and a CSF glucose concentration of less than 50% of the simultaneously obtained peripheral value suggest bacterial meningitis (see Table 105–1).
- The values for CSF glucose, protein, and WBC concentrations found with bacterial meningitis overlap significantly with those for viral, tuberculous, and fungal meningitis (see Table 105–1) Therefore, CSF WBC counts and CSF glucose and protein concentrations cannot always distinguish the different etiologies of meningitis.

OTHER DIAGNOSTIC TESTS[16]

- Blood and other specimens should be cultured according to clinical judgment because meningitis frequently can arise via hematogenous dissemination or can be associated with infections at other sites. A minimum of 20 mL of blood in each of two to three separate cultures per each 24-hour period is necessary for the detection of most bacteremias.
- ❸ Gram stain and culture of the CSF are the most important laboratory tests performed for bacterial meningitis. The Gram stain continues to be the most rapid and accurate method of presumptively diagnosing acute bacterial meningitis. When performed before antibiotic therapy is initiated, Gram stain is both rapid and sensitive and can confirm the diagnosis of bacterial meningitis in 75% to 90% of cases. The sensitivity of the Gram stain decreases to 40% to 60% in patients receiving prior antibiotic therapy. Culture is required to differentiate the various bacterial etiologies.
- Polymerase chain reaction (PCR) techniques can be used to diagnose meningitis caused by *N. meningitidis, S. pneumoniae,* and Hib. PCR is considered to be highly sensitive, but use of this diagnostic approach is limited owing to expense.
- Latex fixation, latex coagglutination, and enzyme immunoassay (EIA) tests provide for the rapid identification of several bacterial causes of meningitis, including *S. pneumoniae, N. meningitidis,* and Hib.[13] Rapid-identification latex tests work by bringing potential capsular antigens of the pathogen causing meningitis in contact with a specific antibody, causing an antigen-antibody reaction. This capsular antigen-antibody reaction can be observed visually and quickly without waiting for culture results. The rapid antigen tests should be used in situations in which the Gram stain is negative.[15] The sensitivity and specificity of latex fixation and coagglutination tests can vary with the manufacturer of the antibody, density of the antigen present in the CSF, and pathogen being tested.
- Diagnosis of tuberculosis meningitis employs acid-fast staining, culture, and PCR of the CSF.
- PCR testing of the CSF is the preferred method of diagnosing most viral meningitis infections.
- The standard diagnostic tests for fungal meningitis include culture, direct microscopic examination of stained and unstained specimens of CSF, antigen detection of cryptococcal or histoplasmal antigens, and antibody assay of serum and/or CSF.

▶ TREATMENT: CNS Infections

■ DESIRED OUTCOME

The importance of supportive care, particularly early in the course of treatment, cannot be emphasized enough. Administration of fluids, electrolytes, antipyretics, analgesics, and other supportive measures is indicated for patients presenting with acute bacterial meningitis. Although supportive care is important initially, appropriate antibiotic therapy (empirical or definitive) should be started as soon as possible. ❹ Understanding antibiotic selection and the issues surrounding antibiotic penetration will assist in meeting the goals of treatment, which include eradication of infection with amelioration of signs and symptoms and prevention of neurologic sequelae, such as seizures, deafness, coma, and death.

■ APPROACH TO TREATMENT

This section discusses issues surrounding the approach to treatment, such as antibiotic penetration within the CNS, duration of antibiotic therapy, and the use of adjunctive steroids. Until a pathogen is identified, prompt empirical antibiotic coverage is often needed. ❺ Based on the patient's profile (i.e., allergies, age, and concurrent medical conditions), extent of antibiotic CNS penetration, and spectrum of activity, appropriate recommendations can be made, and therapy should last at least 48 to 72 hours or until the diagnosis of ❻ bacterial meningitis can be ruled out (Tables 105–2 and 105–3). The first dose of antibiotics should not be withheld even if there is a delay in doing a lumbar puncture. Changes in the

TABLE 105–2. Bacterial Meningitis: Most Likely and Empirical Therapy by Age Group

Age Commonly Affected	Most Likely Organisms	Empirical Therapy	Risk Factors for All Age Groups
Newborn–1 month	Gram-negative enterics[a] Group B Streptococcus Listeria monocytogenes	Ampicillin + cefotaxime or ceftriaxone or aminoglycoside	Respiratory tract infection Otitis media Mastoiditis Head trauma Alcoholism High-dose steroids
1 month–4 years	H. influenzae N. meningitidis S. pneumoniae	Cefotaxime or ceftriaxone and vancomycin[b]	Splenectomy Sickle cell disease Immunoglobulin deficiency
5–29 years	N. meningitidis S. pneumoniae H. influenzae	Cefotaxime or ceftriaxone and vancomycin[b]	Immunosuppression
30–60 years	S. pneumoniae N. meningitidis	Cefotaxime or ceftriaxone and vancomycin[b]	
>60 years	S. pneumoniae Gram-negative enterics L. monocytogenes	Ampicillin + cefotaxime or ceftriaxone or aminoglycoside and vancomycin[b]	

[a]Escherichia coli, Klebsiella spp., Enterobacter spp. common.
[b]Vancomycin use should be based on local incidence of penicillin-resistant S. pneumoniae and until cefotaxime or ceftriaxone minimum inhibitory concentration results are available.

TABLE 105–3. Penetration of Antimicrobial Agents into the Cerebrospinal Fluid

Therapeutic Levels in CSF with or without Inflammation

Sulfonamides	Trimethoprim
Choramphenicol	Isoniazid
Rifampin	Pyrazinamide
Ethionamide	Cycloserine
Metronidazole	

Therapeutic Levels in CSF with Inflammation of Meninges

Penicillin G	Ampicillin ± sulbactam
Carbenicillin	Ticarcillin ± clavulanic acid
Nafcillin	Mezlocillin
Piperacillin	Cefuroxime
Cefotaxime	Ceftizoxime
Ceftriaxone	Ceftazidime
Imipenem	Aztreonam
Meropenem	Ofloxacin
Vancomycin	Ciprofloxacin
Vidarabine	Ethambutol
Flucytosine	Fluconazole
Pyrimethamine	Ganciclovir
Acyclovir	Foscarnet
Linezolid	Quinupristin/dalfopristin
Colistin	

Nontherapeutic Levels in CSF with or without Inflammation

Aminoglycosides	First-generation cephalosporins
Cefoperazone	Second-generation cephalosporins[a]
Clindamycin[b]	Ketoconazole
Amphotericin B	Itraconazole[c]

[a]Cefuroxime is an exception.
[b]Achieves therapeutic brain tissue concentrations.
[c]Achieves therapeutic concentrations for Cryptococcus neoformans therapy.
CSF = cerebrospinal fluid.

CSF after antibiotic administration usually take 12 to 24 hours. Continued therapy should be based on the assessment of clinical improvement, cultures, and susceptibility testing results. Once a pathogen is identified, antibiotic therapy should be tailored toward the specific pathogen (Tables 105–4 and 105–5). Throughout the course of treatment, various efficacy parameters, such as signs and symptoms, microbiologic findings, and CSF examination, should be followed to evaluate the success of meeting the desired outcomes.

Several factors influence the transfer of antibiotic from capillary blood into the CNS, including inflammation of the meninges, which increases antibiotic penetration through damage to tight junctions between capillary endothelial cells and decreases the activity of an energy-dependent efflux pump in the choroid plexus responsible for movement of penicillins and, to a much lesser extent, fluoroquinolones and aminoglycosides (see Table 105–3). Antibiotics having low molecular weights are passed more easily through biologic barriers than compounds of higher molecular weight. Only antibiotics that are nonionized at physiologic or pathologic pH are capable of diffusion. Highly lipid-soluble compounds penetrate more readily than water-soluble compounds. Antibiotics not extensively protein bound in the serum provide a larger free fraction of drug capable of passing into the CSF. Passage of large, polar antibiotics into the CSF may be assisted, however, by a carrier transport system. Unlike the treatment of many other infections, antibiotic dosages in the treatment of CNS infections must be maximized to optimize penetration to the site of infection.

Problems of CSF penetration may be overcome by direct instillation of antibiotics intrathecally, intracisternally, or intraventricularly (Table 105–6). Advantages of direct instillation, however, must be weighed against the risks of invasive CNS procedures. Intrathecal administration of antibiotics is unlikely to produce therapeutic concentrations in the ventricles possibly owing to the unidirectional flow of CSF.[17] Although intraventricular administration from a

TABLE 105–4. Antimicrobial Agents of First Choice and Alternative Choice in the Treatment of Meningitis Caused by Gram-Positive Microorganisms

Organism	Antibiotic of First Choice[a]	Alternative Antibiotics[a]
Streptococcus pneumoniae		
Penicillin susceptible	Penicillin G 200,000–300,000 units/kg/day every 4 h IV; max: 4 million units every 4 h IV	Cefotaxime 200 mg/kg/day every 4–6 h IV; max: 2 g every 4 h
		Ceftriaxone 100 mg/kg/day every 24 h IV[b]; max: adults 2 g every 12 h
		Chloramphenicol[e] 100 mg/kg/day every 6 h; max: 1.5 g every 6 h
Penicillin resistant[c]	Cefotaxime or ceftriaxone and vancomycin[e] 30–40 mg/kg/day IV (60 mg/kg/day IV every 6 h[b])	Cefepime 50 mg/kg/dose every 12 h[b]; max: adult 2 g every 8 h IV
		Or meropenem 40 mg/kg every 8 h IV[b]; max: adults 1 g every 8 h IV with vancomycin[e]
		Linezolid 600 mg every 12 h IV[d]
Group B *Streptococcus*	Penicillin ± gentamicin[e]	Ampicillin ± gentamicin[e]
		Cefotaxime
		Ceftriaxone
		Chloramphenicol[e]
Staphylococcus aureus		
Penicillin resistant	Nafcillin 200 mg/kg/day every 4 h IV; max: 2 g every 4 h IV	Vancomycin[e]
Methicillin resistant	Vancomycin[e]	Linezolid[d]
Staphylococcus epidermidis		
Penicillin resistant	Nafcillin	Vancomycin[e]
Methicillin resistant	Vancomycin[e]	Linezolid[d]
Listeria monocytogenes	Ampicillin 220–400 mg/kg/day, every 6 h IV or penicillin G max: 2 g every 4 h IV plus gentamicin[e]	Trimethoprim 10 mg/kg/day and sulfamethoxazole 50 mg/kg/day, every 6 h
Bacillus anthracis	A consensus regarding recommended agents for the treatment of CNS infections caused by anthrax or other biologic warfare agents has not been reached. Optimal treatment must be tailored to the particular pathogen and/or genetic variants of the pathogen.	

[a]Recommended doses for adults and pediatric patients with normal renal and/or hepatic function.
[b]Pediatrics.
[c]Incidence of resistance is 20% to 45% worldwide.
[d]Clinical data are lacking, but linezolid may offer an alternative for the treatment of such infections.
[e]Monitor drug levels in serum.

therapeutic standpoint may be preferred over intrathecal administration, the former requires neurosurgical placement of a subcutaneous reservoir. Intraventricular delivery may be necessary when bacteria that require treatment with aminoglycosides, such as *L. monocytogenes*, *Pseudomonas aeruginosa* or enterococci, are isolated. In a review of antibiotic-induced endotoxin release, children receiving both parenteral antibiotics and intrathecal gentamicin had higher CSF endotoxin levels, higher CSF IL-1β levels, and higher mortality than children receiving only parenteral antibiotics.[18] Interestingly, the differences were attributed to direct CSF administration of gentamicin, which generally is thought to blunt the endotoxin release caused by β-lactam antibiotics.[18]

Although the length of treatment for bacterial meningitis generally is based on the causative organism, there is no universally accepted standard. Traditionally, meningitis caused by *S. pneumoniae* and *H. influenzae* has been treated successfully with 10 to 14 days of antibiotic therapy. Meningitis caused by *N. meningitidis* usually can be treated with a 7-day course of antibiotics. In contrast, a longer duration of 14 to 21 days has been recommended for patients infected with *L. monocytogenes* or group B streptococci because of a high probability of relapse. Likewise, a minimum of 3 weeks of treatment is recommended for meningitis caused by gram-negative bacilli.[13] Therapy should be individualized, and some patients may require longer courses.

CAUSATIVE AGENTS

N. MENINGITIDIS (MENINGOCOCCUS)

N. meningitidis is the leading cause of bacterial meningitis in children and young adults in the United States, with the highest prevalence in those aged less than 2 years.[19] The source of infection usually is an asymptomatic carrier. Most cases occur in the winter or spring at a time when viral meningitis is relatively uncommon. Five serogroups of *N. meningitidis* (A, B, C, Y, and W-135) are primarily responsible. Clusters of meningococcal disease, defined as two or more cases of the same serogroup that are closer in time and space than expected for the population or group under observation, generally are associated with schools.[20] Although some of these clusters have been due to serogroup B, the majority have been due to serogroup C. Serogroup A, although associated with meningococcal outbreaks in Africa and Asia, is a rare cause of disease in the United States.[21] Serogroup Y, although frequently associated with pneumonia, is emerging as an important cause of invasive meningococcal disease in select areas.[22,23] Overall, *N. meningitidis* accounts for 25% of all meningitis cases, 60% of cases in persons aged 2 to 18 years, and carries a case-fatality rate of approximately 10%.[8,22]

Initially, patients are colonized and, at some point, develop a bacteremia, which most likely occurs prior to hospital admission.

TABLE 105–5. Antimicrobial Agents of First Choice and Alternative Choice in the Treatment of Meningitis Caused by Gram-Negative Microorganisms

Organism	Antibiotic of First Choice[a]	Alternative Antibiotics[a]
Neisseria meningitis (meningococcal)	Penicillin G 200,000–300,000 units/kg/day	Cefotaxime 200 mg/kg/day every 4 h; max: 2 g IV every 4 h Ceftriaxone 100 mg/kg/day every 24 h[b]; max: adults 2 g IV every 12 h Chloramphenicol[e] 100 mg/kg/day every 6 h; max: 1.5 g IV every 6 h
Escherichia coli	Cefotaxime or ceftriaxone	Cefepime 50 mg/kg/dose every 12 h[b]; max: adult 2 g every 8 h IV Meropenem 40 mg/kg every 8 h IV[b]; max: adults 1 g every 8 h IV
Hemophilus influenzae		
β-Lactamase positive	Cefotaxime	Ceftriaxone
β-Lactamase negative	Ampicillin 200–400 mg/kg/day every 6 h IV; max: 2 g every 4 h IV	Cefotaxime Ceftriaxone
Pseudomonas aeruginosa	Ceftazidime 85 mg/kg/day; max: 2 g IV every 6 h plus tobramycin[e] 5–7.5 mg/kg/day IV[c]	Meropenem Piperacillin 200–300 mg/kg/day; max: 3 g every 4 h IV plus tobramycin[e] Colistin sulfomethate[e] 5 mg/kg/day IV[d]
Enterobacteriaceae	Cefotaxime	Ceftriaxone Piperacillin plus aminoglycoside[e] Meropenem

[a]Recommended doses for adults and pediatric patients with normal renal and/or hepatic function.
[b]Pediatrics.
[c]Direct central nervous system administration may be added; see Table 105–6 for dosage.
[d]Should be reserved for multidrug-resistant pseudomonal or *Actinetobacter* infections for which all other therapeutic options have been exhausted.
[e]Monitor drug levels in serum.

Meningitis occurs after the bacteria seeds into the meninges, which can occur in 50% of the cases of meningococcal disease.[24] After the acute phase of meningitis has resolved, there is a unique immune reaction that distinguishes meningococcal meningitis from other bacterial causes. The patient develops a characteristic immunologic reaction of fever, arthritis (usually involving large joints), and pericarditis approximately 10 to 14 days after the onset of disease and despite successful treatment.[25] At this time, examination of the synovial fluid will reveal a large number of polymorphonuclear cells, elevated protein concentrations, normal glucose concentrations, and sterile cultures. The reaction may last a week or longer, and no additional antibiotic therapy is required. Patients, however, may benefit from nonsteroidal anti-inflammatory agents and supportive care.[25]

Seizures and coma are uncommon with meningococcal meningitis. Patients may behave aggressively, however, and often are maniacal. Patients may develop deafness and transiently impaired ocular movements. Deafness unilaterally or, more commonly, bilaterally may develop early or late in the disease course.[25] Hearing loss secondary to sensory nerve damage (sensorineural hearing) is usually permanent, whereas conductive hearing impairment, such as damage to the tympanic membrane, often is reversible.

The presence of petechiae may be the primary clue that the underlying pathogen is *N. meningitidis*. Approximately 50% of patients with meningococcal meningitis have purpuric lesions, petechiae, or both. Patients may have an obvious or subclinical picture of disseminated intravascular coagulation (DIC), which may progress to

TABLE 105–6. Intraventricular and Intrathecal Antibiotic Dosage Recommendation

Antibiotic	Dose (mg)	Expected CSF Concentration[a] (mg/L)	Reference
Ampicillin	10–50	60–300	104–106
Methicillin	25–100	160–600	104–106
Nafcillin	75	500	105
Cephalothin	25–100	160–600	104–106
Chloramphenicol	25–100	160–600	104, 106, 107
Gentamicin	1–10	6–60	104–108
Quinupristin/dalfopristin	1–2	7–13	109
Tobramycin	1–10	6–60	108
Vancomycin	5	30	110–112
Amphotericin B	0.05–0.25 mg/d to 0.05–1 mg 1–3 times weekly	—	113

[a]Assumes adult CSF volume = 150 mL. CSF = cerebrospinal fluid.

farction of the adrenal glands and renal cortex and cause widespread thrombosis.

Aggressive, early intervention with high-dose intravenous crystalline penicillin G, 50,000 units/kg every 4 hours, is usually recommended for the treatment of *N. meningitidis* meningitis. Chloramphenicol is bactericidal for *N. meningitidis* and may be used in place of penicillin G. However, chloramphenicol has unpredictable metabolism in young infants and several drug-drug interactions and is used rarely in developed countries.[2] Chloramphenicol frequently is used as initial empirical therapy for meningitis in developing countries owing to the low cost. Several third-generation cephalosporins (i.e., cefotaxime, ceftazidime, ceftizoxime, ceftriaxone, and cefuroxime) have indications for the treatment of meningitis and are acceptable alternatives to penicillin G (see Table 105–5).

Cases of meningitis caused by relatively (minimun inhibitory concentration [MIC] 0.1–1 mg/L) and highly (MIC $\geq$ 256 mg/L) penicillin-resistant meningococci have been reported. Prevalence varies geographically, ranging from 0.4% to 42.6%.[26] Isolated reports of treatment failure with penicillin have surfaced in recent years.[27,28] Completely resistant strains produce β-lactamase, whereas relatively resistant strains have an alteration of penicillin-binding proteins. In 1991, strains with altered penicillin-binding proteins represented approximately 4% of meningococcal isolates in the United States.[21] Resistance patterns of meningococci may necessitate a change away from penicillin as the antibiotic treatment of choice for meningococcal meningitis, and some authorities recommend using a third-generation cephalosporin (cefotaxime or ceftriaxone) instead of penicillin for meningococcal meningitis.[29]

N. meningitidis is spread by direct person-to-person close contact, including respiratory droplets and pharyngeal secretions.[24] Close contacts of patients contracting *N. meningitidis* meningitis are at an increased risk of developing meningitis. Close contacts include day-care center contacts, members of the household, or anyone who has been exposed to respiratory or oral secretions through activities such as coughing, sneezing, or kissing.[24] Household contacts of people who have sporadic disease are estimated to have an incidence of meningococcal meningitis that is 500 to 800 times greater than that of the overall population.[24] Secondary cases of meningitis usually develop within the first week following exposure, but they may take up to 60 days after contact with the index case.[30] Young children are at the greatest risk of contracting *N. meningitidis;* however, all ages are at risk, especially close contacts exposed via household, day-care, or military contact.

Prophylaxis of close contacts should be started only after consultation with the local health department. In general, rifampin is given as prophylaxis for 2 days.[21] The adult dose is 600 mg every 12 hours, whereas children aged 1 month and older should receive 10 mg/kg, and children younger than 1 month should receive 5 mg/kg. Intramuscular ceftriaxone (250 mg in adults, 125 mg in children younger than 12 years of age) and oral ciprofloxacin (500 mg in adults and children older than 12 years) are alternatives to rifampin.[13] Further discussion of who should receive prophylaxis is beyond the scope of this chapter; interested readers can refer to the recommendations of the U.S. Centers for Disease Control and Prevention for that information.[31]

S. PNEUMONIAE (PNEUMOCOCCUS OR DIPLOCOCCUS)

S. pneumoniae is the leading cause of meningitis in adults. Moreover, *S. pneumoniae* is the most common cause of bacterial meningitis in children younger than 2 years of age, accounting for 45 to 145 cases per 100,000 of this population, and the second most common cause in children older than 2 years of age.[32] Case-fatality rates in children are highest with this organism and approach 20%. Approximately 50% of cases are secondary infections resulting from primary infections of parameningeal foci, such as the ear or paranasal sinuses. Pneumonia, endocarditis, CSF leak secondary to head trauma, splenectomy, alcoholism, sickle cell disease, and bone marrow transplantation may predispose the patient to the development of pneumococcal meningitis.

Neurologic complications, such as coma and seizures, are common with pneumococcal meningitis. Children with pneumococcal meningitis have lower mortality rates (4% to 17%) compared with the mortality rates in adults (20% to 30%), but children who survive suffer from a high rate of neurologic sequelae (29% to 56%).[33,34] Risk factors for recurrent pneumococcal meningitis include traumatic tears of the dura, fracture of the cribriform plate or paranasal sinuses, nasal meningoceles, repeated episodes of otitis media, basilar skull fractures, and CSF leaks. The prognosis of pneumococcal meningitis depends on a variety of factors, including the number of WBCs in the CSF, the number of WBCs in the periphery, the CSF glucose concentration, the CSF protein concentration, the serum sodium concentration, and the presence of a comatose state and/or shock.[35]

Treatment with intravenous crystalline penicillin G (50,000 units/kg every 4 hours) in adult patients with a penicillin-susceptible isolate and normal renal function usually results in a favorable outcome. However, the frequency of penicillin-resistant pneumococcal strains (MIC $\geq$ 2 mg/L) in the United States increased from 14% in 1994 to 25% in 1997 and continues to rise.[29] Based on these resistance patterns and the fact that sufficient CSF concentrations of penicillin are difficult to achieve with standard intravenous doses, penicillin should not be used as empirical therapy if *S. pneumoniae* is a suspected pathogen. Furthermore, appropriate National Committee for Clinical Laboratory Standards (NCCLS)–approved testing of all CSF isolates for penicillin resistance is recommended. Ceftriaxone and cefotaxime have served as alternatives to penicillin in the treatment of penicillin intermediate- and high-resistant pneumococci. Of note, treatment failures with third-generation cephalosporins in the management of penicillin-resistant pneumococci have been reported.[29] Therapeutic approaches to cephalosporin-resistant pneumococcus include the addition of vancomycin and rifampin, which have demonstrated synergistic activity with ceftriaxone. However, no data from controlled clinical trials supporting the use of rifampin are available. Therefore, the combination of vancomycin and ceftriaxone has been suggested as empirical treatment until the results of antimicrobial susceptibility testing are available.[2,29] Some investigators have suggested that the addition of vancomycin to the initial empirical regimen may not be necessary because the prevalence of β-lactam–resistant pneumococci has been reduced greatly as a result of the pneumococcal vaccines.[2]

Ceftriaxone and vancomycin are the agents of choice to treat presumed pneumococcal meningitis empirically until the susceptibility is known. Penicillin may be used for drug-susceptible isolates with MICs of 0.06 mg/L or less, but for intermediate isolates, ceftriaxone is used, and for highly drug resistant isolates, a combination of ceftriaxone and vancomycin should be used. Vancomycin should not be used as monotherapy.[29] In especially severe cases, therapeutic drug monitoring of the CSF and possibly even direct antibiotic instillation may be necessary.

Recent reports of the isolation of pneumococcal strains exhibiting tolerance to vancomycin are of great concern, but the clinical significance is unknown.[36,37] Based on concern about the limited therapeutic options for penicillin- and cephalosporin-resistant pneumococcal meningitis, newer agents have been evaluated. Meropenem is approved by the Food and Drug Administration (FDA) for the treatment of bacterial meningitis in children aged 3 months and older and has shown similar clinical and microbiologic efficacy to cefotaxime or ceftriaxone. Some concern is warranted with the use of imipenem for CNS infections because of the possibility of drug-induced seizures, especially if the dose is not adjusted for renal function. Of note, seizures may be caused by meningitis itself or by imipenem, and the cause is difficult to differentiate. The newer fluoroquinolones represent another therapeutic option owing to favorable activity against multidrug-resistant pneumococci and good penetration into the CSF.[38] However, clinical data to date regarding fluoroquinolone treatment of pneumococcal meningitis are limited mainly to animal models. Comparative, controlled clinical efficacy trials in patients with meningitis will be necessary before routine use of the fluoroquinolones is viable. Interestingly, some of the newer fluoroquinolones act synergistically with vancomycin and β-lactam antibiotics against penicillin-resistant pneumococcal meningitis in an animal model, but this claim has not been substantiated in humans.[29,39] Quinupristin-dalfopristin, linezolid, and daptomycin have emerged as therapeutic options for treating multidrug-resistant gram-positive infections. However, limited data are available, and these agents cannot be recommended for use in the treatment of pneumococcal meningitis.

CLINICAL CONTROVERSY

Some investigators believe that the use of vancomycin in the empirical treatment of pneumococcal meningitis is no longer necessary owing to the great reduction in the prevalence of β-lactam–resistant pneumococci because of the widespread use of the pneumococcal vaccines. However, because the infecting organism is rarely known initially, most clinicians still use the combination of a third-generation cephalosporin and vancomycin for empirical treatment.

The available pneumococcal vaccines help in reducing the risk of invasive pneumococcal disease. Virtually all serotypes of *S. pneumoniae* exhibiting intermediate or complete resistance to penicillin are found in the 23-serotype pneumococcal polysaccharide vaccine. However, in 1997, surveillance data indicated that only 30% of people 65 years of age and older had been immunized against pneumococcal disease.[40] Therefore, the CDC issued stronger recommendations for the use of the pneumococcal polysaccharide vaccine, calling for vaccination of the following high-risk groups: persons over the age of 65 years; persons aged 2 to 64 years who have a chronic illness, who live in high-risk environments (e.g., Alaskan Natives and residents of long-term care facilities), and who lack a functioning spleen (e.g., sickle cell disease and splenectomy); and immunocompromised persons over the age of 2 years, including those with HIV infection. Additionally, the question of whether or not college students living in dormitories, a possible high-risk environment, should be vaccinated remains debatable. Unfortunately, owing to variability in the host's ability to mount an immune response to the vaccine, the efficacy of this product in children younger than 2 years of age and immunocompromised adults limits the usefulness of the vaccine as a solution to the problem of penicillin-resistant pneumococci.

In 2000, a heptavalent pneumococcal conjugate vaccine (Prevnar) was approved for use in children 2 months of age and older. Use of the vaccine has been associated with a reduction of more than 90% in invasive pneumococcal infections, including sepsis and meningitis.[41] Moreover, the vaccine is safe and effective in low-birth-weight and preterm infants.[42,43] Widespread vaccination is expected to have a significant impact on the prevalence of pneumococcal meningitis, including infection caused by antibiotic-resistant strains. A cohort study of 3.8 million healthy infants projected that vaccination would prevent more than 12,000 cases of invasive disease for each U.S. birth cohort, resulting in substantial decreases in morbidity and mortality, as well as possible dollar savings.[44] Current recommendations are for all healthy infants younger than 2 years of age to be immunized with the heptavalent vaccine at 2, 4, 6, and 12 to 15 months. The recommendations are extended to include Alaskan Native, Native American, and African-American children between the ages of 2 and 5 years. Recently, owing to the recognition that children with cochlear implants are at increased risk for the development of pneumococcal meningitis, the CDC has issued a recommendation that all persons with cochlear implants receive age-appropriate vaccination with the pneumococcal conjugate vaccine, pneumococcal polysaccharide vaccine, or both.[45]

H. INFLUENZAE

In the past, *H. influenzae* was the most common cause of meningitis in children 6 months to 3 years of age. Since the introduction of effective vaccines, however, the incidence of *H. influenzae* type B disease in the United States has declined dramatically. Widespread vaccination of infants and children has decreased the incidence of bacterial meningitis due to *H. influenzae* in children between the ages of 1 month and 5 years by 87%, resulting in a 55% decline in all cases of bacterial meningitis.[12] Worldwide, in countries that have adopted universal immunization, the incidence of bacterial meningitis caused by *H. influenzae* type b has decreased more than 99%.[2] In children older than 3 years and adults, meningitis caused by *H. influenzae* may indicate a parameningeal focus of infection such as middle ear infection, paranasal sinus infection, or CSF leakage. Spread of the organism occurs either through direct spread from infected sinuses, draining of these areas via the veins, or bacteremia originating from the local focus of infection.[46]

In the past, ampicillin and chloramphenicol were the drugs of choice to treat pediatric meningitis. However, since approximately 30% to 40% of *H. influenzae* are now ampicillin-resistant, many clinicians use a third-generation cephalosporin or the combination of chloramphenicol and ampicillin for initial antimicrobial therapy. If the organism is sensitive to ampicillin, the patient then can be switched from the third-generation cephalosporin to ampicillin, and chloramphenicol, if used initially, can be discontinued. Most clinicians regard third-generation cephalosporins as the drugs of choice for meningitis caused by *H. influenzae*. Third-generation cephalosporins (cefotaxime and ceftriaxone) are active against β-lactamase–producing and non–β-lactamase–producing strains of *H. influenzae,* are relatively free of toxicity, and do not require serum concentration monitoring. Serum concentration monitoring is required for chloramphenicol to avoid toxicity and subtherapeutic levels.

Secondary cases resulting from close contact with an index case occur within 30 days of the onset of disease. Close contacts, which include household members, individuals sharing sleeping quarters, day-care attendees, nursing home residents, and crowded, confined populations, may be at 200 to 1000 times the risk of the general population for acquiring *H. influenzae* meningitis.[47] The risk of acquiring *H. influenzae* meningitis is low without intimate contact with the index patient's respiratory secretions.[47]

Prophylaxis is to protect close contacts from the index case by eliminating nasopharyngeal and oropharyngeal carriage of *H. influenzae*. Invasive disease should be reported to the local public health department and the CDC. Prophylaxis of close contacts should be started only after consultation with the local health department. In general, children should receive rifampin 20 mg/kg per day (maximum 600 mg) and adults 600 mg/day in one dose for days.[13] Any unvaccinated children between the ages of 12 and 48 months should receive one dose of the vaccine, whereas those between the ages of 2 and 11 months should be given three doses of the vaccine.[13] Individuals fully vaccinated are not recommended to receive prophylaxis.[21] Further discussion of who should receive prophylaxis is beyond the scope of this chapter; interested readers can refer to the recommendations of the American Academy of Pediatrics for that information.[48]

Vaccination includes a series of doses and usually is begun in children at 2 months of age. In addition to pediatric immunization, the vaccine also should be considered in patients older than 5 years of age with the following underlying conditions: sickle cell disease, asplenia, and immunocompromising diseases. Refer to the Chap. 122 for further information on dosing and administration.

L. MONOCYTOGENES

L. monocytogenes is a gram-positive diphtheroid-like organism responsible for 8% of all reported cases of meningitis.[8] This disease primarily affects neonates, alcoholics, immunocompromised adults, and the elderly. Infections caused by *Listeria* in healthy individuals are extremely rare. *L. monocytogenes* is implicated in 20% of meningitis cases in those older than 60 years of age and carries a case-fatality rate of approximately 15%.[8]

Transmission usually involves colonization of the patient's gastrointestinal (GI) tract with the organisms, which then penetrate the gut lumen. Coleslaw, unpasteurized milk, Mexican-style soft cheese, ready-to-eat foods, and raw beef and poultry all have been identified as sources of this food-borne pathogen.[21] If a sufficient cell-mediated immune response (T-lymphocytes, macrophages) is not produced, bacteremia, meningitis, meningoencephalitis, or cerebritis may develop.[49] Infection of the CNS may be diffuse or localized, possibly involving the cerebral hemispheres, thalamus, and brain stem. In immunocompromised hosts, approximately 75% of *L. monocytogenes* infections result in transmission into the CNS.[49]

Incidence of *L. monocytogenes* meningitis tends to peak in the summer and early fall. As with gram-negative meningitis, presentation may be subtle and insidious, and clinical suspicion should prompt lumbar puncture. *L. monocytogenes* produces primarily a mononuclear CSF response.[49] One common laboratory error seen with *L. monocytogenes* is a tendency to misidentify the organism on Gram stain as a diphtheroid, streptococcus, or a poorly staining gram-negative rod.

Treatment of *L. monocytogenes* meningitis with penicillin G or ampicillin may result in only a bacteriostatic effect and possible persistence of infection. Usually the combination of penicillin G or ampicillin with an aminoglycoside results in a bactericidal effect. Patients should be treated for 2 to 3 weeks after defervescence.[13] Combination therapy usually is employed for at least 10 days, with the remaining course of therapy completed with penicillin G or ampicillin alone. Trimethoprim-sulfamethoxazole may be an effective alternative because adequate CSF penetration is achieved. Chloramphenicol and vancomycin both possess in vitro activity against *Listeria*, but they are not be recommended for use in meningitis caused by *L. monocytogenes* owing to unacceptably high failure rates.[29] None of the cephalosporins is effective for *L. monocytogenes*.

GRAM-NEGATIVE MENINGITIS

During the last several years, the incidence of gram-negative bacillary meningitis, excluding *H. influenzae,* has been increasing in both children and adults. Enteric gram-negative organisms are the fourth leading cause of meningitis, with only *S. pneumoniae, H. influenzae,* and *N. meningitidis* having a higher incidence.

Several factors predispose patients to the development of gram-negative meningitis: congenital defects involving the CNS, accidental cranial trauma, neurosurgery, the use of antimicrobial agents with exclusive gram-positive activity preoperatively in neurosurgery, any form of communication between the skin and subarachnoid space (such as a dermal sinus), diabetes, malignancy, urinary tract infection in neonates, cirrhosis, parameningeal infection, spinal anesthesia, advanced age, immunosuppression, and hospitalization in general.

Elderly debilitated patients are at an increased risk of gram-negative meningitis but typically lack the classic signs and symptoms of the disease. Nuchal rigidity may be difficult to detect secondary to cervical arthritis. Presence of a low-grade fever and changes in mental status without other obvious cause should prompt consideration of meningitis and a lumbar puncture. Neonates are also at risk for gram-negative meningitis with *E. coli* and *Klebsiella pneumoniae,* which are responsible for 60% to 70% of cases.

Optimal antimicrobial therapies for gram-negative bacillary meningitis have not been fully defined. The therapy of gram-negative meningitis is complex owing to the variety of organisms that can infect the CNS. The treatment of meningitis due to *P. aeruginosa* remains a unique problem because antibiotics showing good antibacterial activity against *P. aeruginosa,* such as antipseudomonal penicillins and aminoglycosides, penetrate the CSF poorly. Furthermore, many isolates of *P. aeruginosa* are resistant to multiple, if not all, commonly used agents, and this trend in resistance is increasing. Initially, cases of *P. aeruginosa* meningitis should be treated with an extended-spectrum β-lactam such as ceftazidime, cefepime, piperacillin, or meropenem plus an aminoglycoside, usually tobramycin.[2] Since aminoglycosides penetrate the CSF poorly, their inclusion is predominantly to aid in the treatment of extracerebral infections. If multidrug-resistant *Pseudomonas* is suspected initially, intraventricular administration of aminoglycoside should be considered along with intravenous administration. Preservative-free forms of gentamicin and tobramycin are available and should be used for direct administration into the CSF. Intraventricular aminoglycoside dosages should be adjusted to the estimated CSF volume (0.03 mg tobramycin or gentamicin per milliliter of CSF and 0.1 mg amikacin per milliliter of CSF every 24 hours). Since CSF flows unidirectionally with gravity, intraventricular aminoglycoside administration is more likely to produce therapeutic concentrations throughout the CSF than intrathecal administration.[17] While intraventricular administration of aminoglycosides is considered for treatment of *P. aeruginosa* meningitis, this method produced higher mortality in a sample of infants treated for gram-negative bacillary meningitis.[17] Thus intraventricular administration of aminoglycosides to infants is not recommended routinely. Ventricular levels of aminoglycoside should be monitored every 2 or 3 days, just prior to the next intraventricular dose, and should approximate 2–10 mg/L. Interpretation of drug levels may be difficult because determinations often are contaminated with residual aminoglycoside from the preceding dose.

A recent case report exhibited favorable effects of high-dose intravenous ciprofloxacin (400 mg every 8 hours) plus intravenous ceftazidime for pseudomonal meningitis.[50] However, this information must be evaluated in a controlled clinical trial before high-dose ciprofloxacin can be recommended for use.

Multidrug-resistant *Pseudomonas* and *Acinetobacter* infections are of concern to clinicians because of the limited therapeutic options available for the treatment of such infections. This concern has led to the reemergence of older antibiotics, such as colistin. Limited data exist suggesting that colistin can be used, both intravenously and intrathecally, in the treatment of multidrug-resistant *Pseudomonas* or *Acinetobacter* CNS infections.[51–53] Furthermore, recent in vitro data have suggested synergistic activity with the combination of colistin and ceftazidime against multidrug-resistant *P. aeruginosa*.[54] The use of colistin should be reserved for only the most severe cases.

Other gram-negative organisms causing meningitis, excluding *P. aeruginosa* and *Acinetobacter* spp., most likely can be treated with a third-generation cephalosporin, such as cefotaxime, ceftriaxone, or ceftazidime. Ceftazidime, however, may not be the best choice of empirical antibiotic for situations where the offending organism is not known initially because CSF antibiotic concentrations greater than 10 times the minimal bactericidal concentration (MBC) may not be produced reliably for gram-positive organisms. In adults, daily doses of 8 to 12 g/day of third-generation cephalosporins (2 g twice a day of ceftriaxone) should produce CSF concentrations of 5–20 mg/L. Ceftriaxone is not recommended for use in the neonatal period because of the potential for the displacement of bilirubin from albumin-binding sites.[2]

Trimethoprim-sulfamethoxazole is useful in the management of the Enterobacteriaceae family and also may be useful in the management of *L. monocytogenes*.[2,6] One advantage of trimethoprim-sulfamethoxazole is that its penetration into the CSF does not depend on meningeal inflammation. Trimethoprim-sulfamethoxazole is not, however, bactericidal. Trimethoprim-sulfamethoxazole produces CSF levels of 1.9–5.7 mg/L for the former and 20–63 mg/L for the latter when given parenterally in doses of 10 mg/kg per day (trimethoprim) and 50 mg/kg per day (sulfamethoxazole).

Fluoroquinolones are not approved for the treatment of gram-negative bacterial meningitis, and clinical experience is minimal. Animal data have shown similar effectiveness between select newer fluoroquinolones and third-generation cephalosporins. Fluoroquinolones should be considered only when multidrug-resistant gram-negative rods are suspected.[29] Cefepime and meropenem represent other therapeutic options for the treatment of gram-negative bacterial meningitis, as does aztreonam.[2,29]

CSF cultures may remain positive for several days or more with a regimen that eventually will be curative. Therapeutic efficacy can be monitored through bacterial colony counts every 2 or 3 days, which should decrease progressively over the period of therapy. Therapy for gram-negative meningitis should be continued for a minimum of 21 days from the start of treatment.[13]

■ BACILLUS ANTHRACIS

B. anthracis is a large, endospore-forming, aerobic, gram-positive bacteria capable of producing infection via the cutaneous, pulmonary, or GI routes. Cases of meningitis have been reported following both cutaneous and inhalational infection. Prior to the bioterrorism-related outbreak of 11 inhalational and 12 suspected or confirmed cases of cutaneous anthrax in 2001, a total of only 18 sporadic cases had occurred in the United States in the twentieth century, with the last occurrence in 1976.[55] However, since the terrorist attack on the United States on September 11, 2001, heightened awareness of biologic warfare agents, which include *B. anthracis*, has percolated throughout the United States.

The major neurologic complication of anthrax infection is fulminant, rapidly fatal hemorrhagic meningoencephalitis. The inhalational form of anthrax seems to be a potent inducer of neurologic symptoms, and death usually occurs within a week for those with neurologic complications.[55] Neurologic manifestations may be the initial symptoms leading to the diagnosis of anthrax. An index case of fatal inhalational anthrax owing to bioterrorism developed acute fever, emesis, disorientation, and confusion. A head computed tomographic (CT) scan showed no abnormalities, but a Gram stain exhibited cloudy CSF, low CSF glucose concentration, high CSF protein concentration, increased leukocytes in the CSF, and large gram-positive bacilli in chains. Shortly thereafter, the patient developed a generalized seizure and died on the third hospital day.[56]

Consistent findings in the CSF of anthrax meningitis cases include a low CSF glucose level, marked infiltration of WBCs into the CSF, and the presence of gram-positive bacilli in chains. High suspicion of anthrax meningitis is warranted in the additional presence of grossly visible blood or elevated red blood cell counts with hemorrhagic changes on a CT scan.[55] Recent molecular advances can aid in the rapid diagnosis of *B. anthracis* infections. Rapid PCR techniques, such as the Light Cycler (Roche Applied Science, Indianapolis, IN.), can produce molecular confirmation for the presence of anthrax within 1 hour.[55] Extreme caution is warranted for diagnosis without the use of molecular techniques because *B. anthracis* can be confused easily with *B. cereus*, which is found commonly in soil and often considered a contaminant if identified.

B. anthracis typically is susceptible to penicillin, amoxicillin, erythromycin, doxycycline, ciprofloxacin, and chloramphenicol. The bioterrorism-related strain was susceptible to the fluoroquinolones, rifampin, tetracycline, vancomycin, imipenem, meropenem, chloramphenicol, clindamycin, and the aminoglycosides. However, the strain was resistant to third-generation cephalosporins and trimethoprim-sulfamethoxazole.[55] Ciprofloxacin or doxycycline plus one or two of the aforementioned antibiotics is the currently recommended regimen for the treatment of inhalational anthrax, but doxycycline is not recommended for the treatment of anthrax meningitis owing to poor CNS penetration and recent in vitro resistance.[55]

Clinicians must be aware that what we know now about biologic weapons may be helpful, but knowledge of natural disease may not reflect what could happen in biologic attacks. First, antibiotic susceptibility is a function of how the organism may or may not have been altered genetically. For example, anthrax could be manipulated genetically to be resistant to the commonly used agents. Second, the antibiotics used for biologic attacks may not have FDA indications for such uses, and many physicians may be placed under pressure to prescribe. Additionally, security issues may emerge for pharmacists and pharmacies and their antibiotic supply. Third, patient compliance will be important to ensure proper treatment and the prevention of resistance. Fourth, most metropolitan areas have a response plan, and clinicians should be aware of their role, if any. Lastly, be watchful, because many health care workers will be the first line of defense. Of note, the Web site of the Center for Infectious Disease Research and Policy (*www.cidrap.umn.edu*) provides a wealth of information regarding bioterrorism and is an up-to-date resource for clinicians.

■ Dexamethasone as an Adjunctive Treatment for Meningitis

In addition to antibiotics, dexamethasone has become a commonly used therapy for the treatment of pediatric meningitis.[12] Corticosteroids inhibit the production of both TNF and IL-1. A series of clinical studies assessing the efficacy of corticosteroid therapy for the initial treatment of bacterial meningitis has reported conflicting results.[57–6] The majority of trials were conducted on small sample populations, each with different pathogenic bacterial causes and treatment modalities. The findings of several studies have shown significant improvement in markers of active infection, such as CSF levels of proinflammatory cytokines, as well as CSF protein, glucose, and lactate concentrations, after corticosteroid administration as adjunctive treatment.[12]

Trials consistently detected a significantly lower incidence of neurologic sequelae commonly associated with bacterial meningitis with corticosteroid use. In trials that measured inflammatory mediators, lower levels of TNF, PAF, or IL-1 were detected in patients treated with dexamethasone.[57,58,61] No study, however, has detected a significant difference in time to bacterial eradication. Only one study has detected a significant difference in mortality between patients treated with dexamethasone plus antibiotics and antibiotic therapy alone, favoring use of the corticosteroid.[59] Based on these investigations, some authors advocate all infants (>2 months of age) and children with suspected bacterial meningitis receive dexamethasone.[57,58,60–62]

Data suggesting the use of corticosteroids in adults with meningitis is scarce. A recent prospective, randomized, double-blind multicenter study evaluated the use of adjuvant therapy plus dexamethasone compared with adjuvant therapy plus placebo in adults with acute bacterial meningitis.[63] The results showed that early treatment with dexamethasone improved clinical outcome in adults with bacterial meningitis, reducing the risk of both unfavorable outcome and death. However, the study did not show a beneficial effect of dexamethasone on neurologic sequelae, including hearing loss.

Routine use of dexamethasone in meningitis is not without controversy. A potential concern is that adjunctive dexamethasone therapy might reduce the penetration of antibiotics into the CSF by inhibiting meningeal inflammation. In experimental models of meningitis, steroids decreased the CSF concentrations of ampicillin, rifampin, vancomycin, and gentamicin.[61,64] Ceftriaxone penetration into CSF was unaffected by concurrent dexamethasone administration in pediatric patients.[65]

A fundamental problem with corticosteroid investigations to date is that the majority of patients in the trials had *H. influenzae* meningitis. While *H. influenzae* was the most commonly identified causative pathogen responsible for bacterial meningitis in the United States in 1986, the incidence of *H. influenzae* meningitis has decreased dramatically because of the introduction of polysaccharide conjugate vaccines. Additionally, the majority of studies examining dexamethasone use for pneumococcal meningitis were conducted before the widespread problem of penicillin-resistant pneumococcus had emerged. Whether or not steroids are beneficial in meningitis caused by penicillin-resistant *S. pneumoniae, N. meningitidis,* and group B streptococci is unclear at this time. A retrospective analysis of pediatric patients with pneumococcal meningitis and one unblinded, noncontrolled trial suggested that adjunctive steroids may decrease the neurologic sequelae and mortality associated with *S. pneumoniae* meningitis.[57,66] A meta-analysis suggests that with the possible exception of hearing loss, dexamethasone does not protect against neurologic sequelae.[67] The protective effect of dexamethasone was observed to be strongest in those with meningitis due to *H. influenzae.*

The use of dexamethasone interferes with the interpretation of clinical response to treatment. For example, corticosteroid use interferes with the resolution of fever. Thus all infants and children are recommended to undergo a repeat lumbar puncture after 24 to 48 hours of treatment to verify CSF sterilization.[12]

The American Academy of Pediatrics suggests that dexamethasone be considered for infants and children 2 months of age or older with pneumococcal meningitis and be given to those with *H. influenzae* meningitis.[48,68] The commonly used intravenous dose is 0.15 mg/kg every 6 hours for 4 days. Alternatively, prospective, randomized, double-blind studies have found dexamethasone 0.15 mg/kg

every 6 hours for 2 days or dexamethasone 0.4 mg/kg every 12 hours for 2 days to be equally effective and potentially less toxic.[61,69] Dexamethasone should be administered prior to or with the first antibiotic dose and not after antibiotics already have been started.[12] Additionally, serum hemoglobin and stool guaiac should be monitored for evidence of GI bleeding.[58,60,66,69] Dexamethasone should not be used in neonates or any infant younger than 6 weeks of age.[12,17] The dose used for adults in the recent multicenter trial was 10 mg every 6 hours for 4 days.[63]

MYCOBACTERIUM TUBERCULOSIS

M. tuberculosis is the primary cause of tuberculous meningitis. Tuberculous meningitis is associated with significant morbidity and mortality and is difficult to diagnose in a timely manner. The most life-threatening form of extrapulmonary tuberculosis is tuberculous meningitis.[70] The epidemiology of tuberculous meningitis as a cause of extrapulmonary tuberculosis has changed. Between the years 1997 and 1990, an average of 193 cases of tuberculous meningitis were reported to the CDC, representing 4.7% of extrapulmonary cases.[71] The number of cases reported in 1990 was 284, or 6.2% of extrapulmonary cases.[71] This change is most likely secondary to HIV/AIDS and rising rates among minority adults leading to increased tuberculosis in their children.[71] The incidence of tuberculosis in general has increased 15% since 1985, and the increase is more substantial in children than in adults.[70]

The most useful clue to diagnose tuberculous meningitis is the presence of inflammation of the CSF in an individual who is at epidemiologic risk for tuberculosis. Although up to 40% of patients may present with evidence of pulmonary involvement with hilar adenopathy, tuberculous meningitis still may exist in the absence of disease in the lung or extrapulmonary sites. The tuberculin skin test (purified protein derivative [PPD]) is also negative in 5% to 50% of cases.[72]

On initial examination, CSF usually contains from 100 to 1000 WBCs/mm^3, which may be 75% to 80% polymorphonuclear cells.[72,73] Over time, the pattern of WBCs in the CSF will shift to lymphocytes and monocytes (see Table 105–1). CSF glucose concentration may be normal initially but gradually decreases as the disease progresses.[72,73] Protein concentration within the CSF may be normal or elevated, with high protein levels shown to correlate with advanced disease.[72–74] CSF cultures often are positive for *M. tuberculosis* even if the patient is asymptomatic.

One potentially useful diagnostic sign unique to tuberculous meningitis is paralysis of the VI cranial nerve, which initially is unilateral and then progresses to bilateral.[25] Initial acid-fast bacilli (AFB) smears are approximately 37% sensitive and as high as 87% sensitive following subsequent smears. Sensitivity of the AFB smear is enhanced by the examination of multiple CSF specimens collected on consecutive days. Cultures of CSF are positive in 45% to 90% of cases depending on the quantity of CSF used in the culture, pathogen density, and experience of the laboratory in culturing *M. tuberculosis.*

Some clinicians will obtain fluid from the base of the brain or the ventricles in an attempt to increase the yield. Positive culture results may take up to 8 weeks, providing little help with the initial diagnosis.[72,73] Several systems employing rapid broth culture (Organon Teknika MB/BacT, Organon Teknika, Durham, NC; ESP system, Trek Diagnostic Systems, Inc., Westlake, OH; and Bactec 9000 TB series or Bactec 460, Becton Dickinson Diagnostic Instruments, Sparks, MD) have considerably shortened the time to detection and are able to detect organisms in less than 3 weeks.[16] Nucleic acid amplification products, such as Amplicor (Roche) and MTD (Genprobe), allow for the direct identification of *M. tuberculosis* within 48 hours and yield higher sensitivity than a smear.

Unfortunately, the incidence of multidrug-resistant strains of *M. tuberculosis* has increased, necessitating the use of at least three antitubercular agents to treat active pulmonary disease. The CDC recommends an initial regimen of four drugs for empirical treatment of *M. tuberculosis*.[75] This regimen consists of isoniazid, rifampin, pyrazinamide, and ethambutol 15 to 20 mg/kg per day (maximum 1.6 g/day) for the first 2 months, generally followed by isoniazid plus rifampin for the remaining duration of therapy. The recommended therapy for HIV-positive individuals is the same as for immunocompetent patients, although rifabutin may be considered in place of other rifamycins in an effort to minimize drug interactions with protease inhibitors and nonnucleoside reverse-transcriptase inhibitors. Therapy in HIV-negative and HIV-positive patients should be individualized based on susceptibility patterns and guidelines from the CDC and the American Thoracic Society, which are updated frequently and available on the Internet (*www.cdc.gov/nchstp/tb/pubs/mmwrhtml/maj_guide.htm*). Patients with *M. tuberculosis* meningitis should be treated for a duration of 9 months or longer with multiple-drug therapy, and patients with rifampin-resistant strains should receive 18 to 24 months of therapy.

Isoniazid, the mainstay in virtually any regimen to treat *M. tuberculosis*, penetrates the CSF with or without meningeal inflammation and achieves concentrations of more than 30 times the MIC of *M. tuberculosis* (MICs of 0.05 to 0.2 mg/L).[49,72,73] Rifampin's penetration of CSF approximates only 20% of serum concentrations in the presence of meningeal inflammation. *M. tuberculosis* typically is so exquisitely sensitive to rifampin, however, that the low penetration ratio is of little clinical significance.[72,73,76] However, the incidence of *M. tuberculosis* resistance to rifampin has increased, necessitating empirical multiple-antibiotic regimens.

Pyrazinamide is a small molecule that penetrates the CSF well in the presence or absence of meningeal inflammation. Streptomycin, an aminoglycoside, penetrates the CSF poorly, even in the presence of meningeal inflammation. The incidence of resistance to streptomycin is increasing, and this drug should not be recommended unless susceptibility is known. Ethambutol is a weak antitubercular agent that reaches the CSF in moderate concentrations. Ethambutol's use is also limited by a high incidence of dose-related optic neuritis. Ethionamide and cycloserine are two other agents that sometimes are used to treat tuberculous meningitis. These agents both penetrate the CSF well in the absence of meningeal inflammation.[72,73]

The usual dose of isoniazid in children is 10 to 15 mg/kg per day (maximum 300 mg/day), and adults usually receive 5 mg/kg per day or a daily dose of 300 mg.[75] Supplemental doses of pyridoxine hydrochloride (vitamin B_6) 50 mg/day are recommended to prevent the peripheral neuropathy associated with isoniazid administration.[72,73] Concurrent administration of rifampin is recommended at doses of 10 to 20 mg/kg per day (maximum 600 mg/day) for children and 600 mg/day for adults.[75] The addition of pyrazinamide (children and adults 15 to 30 mg/kg per day; maximum in both 2 g/day) to the regimen of isoniazid and rifampin is recommended.[75] Duration of concomitant pyrazinamide therapy generally should be limited to 2 months to avoid hepatotoxicity.

The role of steroids in the management of tuberculous meningitis remains unclear. The administration of oral prednisone 60 to 80 mg/day or 0.2 mg/kg per day of intravenous dexamethasone for adults and prednisone 1 to 2 mg/kg per day for children, tapered over 4 to 8 weeks, has been used in clinical practice. Corticosteroids improve neurologic sequelae and survival in adults and decrease mortality, long-term neurologic complications, and permanent sequelae in children.[77,78] Concerns regarding the use of steroids include a possible interference with CSF chemistry studies and decreased penetration of antitubercular agents because of a decrease in inflammation. Despite the controversy, the trend toward an improved outcome generally supports their use for tuberculous meningitis.[77,78]

Tuberculous meningitis has a mortality rate of 10% to 50% despite early diagnosis and treatment.[72,73,79] The level of patient consciousness at the start of therapy is the most useful prognostic indicator. Patients who are comatose at the beginning of therapy have a mortality rate of approximately 75%.[73] Other negative prognostic factors include old age, poor nutrition, evidence of miliary disease, high initial CSF protein concentrations, presence of hydrocephalus, and evidence of elevated ICP.[73] Bewteen 10% and 30% of patients surviving the disease have physical or mental sequelae, including deafness, vertigo, and short-term memory loss.[72,73]

CRYPTOCOCCUS NEOFORMANS

Cryptococcal meningitis is the most common form of fungal CNS infection in the United States and is a major cause of morbidity and mortality in immunosuppressed patients. In the United States, 85% of cases occur in HIV-infected patients. *C. neoformans* is a soil fungus acquired by inhalation of spores from the environment leading to a pneumonia, which is usually asymptomatic. Most patients present initially with disseminated disease, especially meningoencephalitis. The incubation period in AIDS patients may be very short, as opposed to a relatively normal host, in whom it may be very long.

Symptoms of cryptococcal meningitis are insidious and may be present for varying periods, depending on the host involved, before the definitive diagnosis is made. Fever and a history of headaches are the most common symptoms, although altered mentation and evidence of focal neurologic deficits may be present. Examination of the CSF usually reveals small numbers of WBCs ($<150/mm^3$), which are primarily lymphocytes (see Table 105–1). Diagnosis is based on the presence of a positive CSF, blood, sputum, or urine culture for *C. neoformans*. The CSF cultures are positive in more than 90% of cases. Organisms may be seen by microscope when stained with india ink and are more likely to be seen in AIDS patients compared with other hosts. An additional rapid test helpful in diagnosis is latex agglutination, which detects the presence of cryptococcal antigens.[80] Latex agglutination is positive in more than 90% of culture-positive cases. A cryptococcal antigen test can be used to follow the prognosis of non-AIDS patients, but cryptococcal antigen titers do not correlate well with treatment efficacy in AIDS patients.[81] A cryptococcal antigen detection test needs to be considered in any patient presenting initially with meningitis. Risk factors predictive of a poor outcome include lethargy at presentation, high CSF cryptococcal antigen titer, and low CSF WBC count.[82]

Despite poor penetration into the CSF, amphotericin B has long been the drug of choice for the treatment of acute *C. neoformans* meningitis. Amphotericin B 0.5 to 1 mg/kg per day combined with flucytosine 100 mg/kg per day is more effective than amphotericin alone, with successful outcomes in 75% of non-AIDS patients and

0% in AIDS patients.[83] Unfortunately, in the AIDS population, flucytosine is often poorly tolerated, causing bone marrow suppression and GI distress. Amphotericin B alone, although less effective, has been used in AIDS patients with preexisting granulocytopenia.[83,84] Because of the high acute mortality rate of up to 40% and a relapse rate of 50% in AIDS patients receiving therapy, many new agents and regimens are being investigated in this population.[82] A small, noncomparative open study evaluating the safety and efficacy of liposomal amphotericin B (AmBisome) found the product to be well tolerated and moderately effective.[85] A second study found high-dose liposomal amphotericin B (4 mg/kg) to clear CSF cultures more rapidly relative to standard amphotericin B, although clinical efficacy was not significantly different.[86]

Azole therapy is the most studied alternative regimen for the treatment of *C. neoformans* meningitis in AIDS patients. Fluconazole at doses of 200 mg/day was compared with amphotericin B alone (0.4 mg/kg per day) with no significant difference in overall mortality between groups.[87] However, patients receiving fluconazole had a higher 2-week mortality rate and time to CSF conversion.[87] High-dose fluconazole therapy (800 mg/day) was tried as salvage therapy in eight AIDS patients who failed previous antifungal therapy, but success was limited.[88] Itraconazole 200 mg orally twice daily was less effective than amphotericin B plus flucytosine in a small nonblinded study.[89]

Patients with AIDS often require lifelong maintenance or suppressive therapy because of high relapse rates following acute therapy for *C. neoformans*. A large multicenter, controlled trial compared fluconazole (200 mg/day) and amphotericin B (1 mg/kg per week) in the prevention of relapse.[90] Two percent of patients receiving fluconazole versus 18% of patients on amphotericin B relapsed. In addition, the amphotericin B group had significantly more frequent bacterial infections, bacteremias, and drug-related toxicity.[90] Fluconazole is superior to itraconazole in the prevention of relapse.[91] Therefore, patients with AIDS-associated cryptococcal meningitis should receive primary therapy generally using amphotericin B, with or without flucytosine, followed by maintenance therapy with fluconazole for the life of the patient unless a sustained (>6 months) immune reconstitution occurs as a result of highly active antiretroviral therapy. However, treatment recommendations are controversial, and treatment needs to be individualized. Guidelines for the prevention of opportunistic infections in HIV-infected persons are updated frequently and can be found at *www.aidsinfo.nih.gov*.

VIRAL ENCEPHALITIS

The epidemiology of viral encephalitis in the United States has changed dramatically since the mid-1960s because of the introduction of large-scale polio and mumps immunization programs. In the United States, the incidence of mumps has decreased 98% between 1967 and 1985. Worldwide, mumps remains a causative agent of viral encephalitis in countries with low vaccination rates. Poliomyelitis, once a significant cause of encephalitis, is now confined to only a few less developed countries and likely soon will be eradicated as an infectious agent.

Nonpolio enteroviruses such as coxsackieviruses A and B, echoviruses, and enteroviruses 70 and 71 cause approximately 85% of all viral encephalitis cases.[92,93] The remaining 10% to 15% of viral encephalitis cases are caused by a variety of pathogens, such as arboviruses, adenoviruses, influenzae virus A and B, rotavirus, corona virus, cytomegalovirus, varicella-zoster, herpes simplex virus, Epstein-Barr virus, and lymphocytic choriomeningitis.[16,92] In the past, the St. Louis and LaCrosse viruses have been the most common cause

of arbovirus encephalitis.[16] However, in 2002, the largest arboviral meningoencephalitis epidemic in the western hemisphere was caused by the West Nile Virus, accounting for 4156 human cases of West Nile disease in 44 states and the District of Columbia.[94]

Viral encephalitis is acquired primarily by hematogenous spread or, alternatively, by neuronal spread of the causative pathogen.[95] After entry into the host, viral replication occurs, resulting in dissemination through the reticuloendothelial system or vasculature. Infection of the capillary endothelial cells and choroid plexus may provide a conduit for CNS infections.[95] Viruses such as polio, herpes, and varicella-zoster virus also may gain access to the CNS by axonal retrograde transmission from peripheral nerve endings.[95] Once a virus gains access to the CNS, the course of infection depends on the virulence of the particular virus and the host immune response. Host response to aseptic CNS infections is mediated by a complex cascade of inflammatory cytokines in a manner similar to purulent meningitis. In contrast with purulent meningitis, host response to viral encephalitis is mediated primarily through cytotoxic T-lymphocytes. Although TNF is a prominent mediator in purulent bacterial meningitis, TNF concentrations are not increased in viral encephalitis, whereas increases in concentrations of IL-1 and interferon (INF) α and γ occur.[96] TNF concentrations have been suggested as a diagnostic tool for differentiating between bacterial meningitis and viral encephalitis.[96] While cytokine assays are available for investigational use, they are not used routinely in the clinical diagnosis of viral encephalitis.

The clinical syndrome associated with viral encephalitis generally is independent of viral etiology and may vary depending on the patient's age. Common signs in adults include headache, mild fever (<40°C), nuchal rigidity, malaise, drowsiness, nausea, vomiting, and photophobia. Only fever and irritability may be evident in the infant, and meningitis must be ruled out as a cause of fever when no other localized findings are observed in a child. Duration of symptoms generally is 1 to 2 weeks, and specific manifestations outside the meninges also can occur depending on the viral etiology.

Laboratory examination of the CSF usually reveals a pleocytosis with 100 to 1000 WBCs/mm^3, which are primarily lymphocytic; however, 20% to 75% of patients with viral encephalitis may have a predominance of polymorphonuclear cells on initial examination of the CSF, especially in enteroviral meningitis.[92] On repeat lumbar puncture, 90% of patients presenting initially with a predominance of neutrophils experience a shift to a predominance of mononuclear cells. Other laboratory findings include normal to mildly elevated protein concentrations and normal or mildly reduced glucose concentrations[92] (see Table 105–1).

Historically, pathogens responsible for viral encephalitis were not identified.[97] Poor laboratory recovery of viral pathogens and limited treatment options for viral encephalitis made the need for specific identification of pathogens of questionable value. Advances in diagnostic laboratory techniques and the potential for decreased costs associated with longer duration of hospitalization for patients with unconfirmed viral encephalitis have led to a reevaluation of the need for confirmatory pathogen diagnosis.[98] When clinical signs warrant pathogen identification, appropriate laboratory diagnostic techniques, including PCR, should be undertaken. Molecular methods are preferred to conventional laboratory tests in the diagnosis of viral encephalitis owing to the ability to detect a specific virus in 30% to 70% of cases as compared with the 14% to 24% sensitivity of viral culture.[16]

Although there are numerous pathogenic causes of viral encephalitis, much of the clinical presentation, diagnosis, and treatment are similar. The most commonly isolated viral etiologies are described next.

Nonpolio enteroviruses are unenveloped single-strand RNA viruses. Commonly, the incidence of enteroviral encephalitis peaks in late summer and continues into early fall. Enteroviruses are transmitted in the host via the fecal-oral route. Clinical presentation of enteroviral infection frequently is nonspecific and characterized by fever, nausea, vomiting, and malaise; however, GI symptoms may not be present. Following a prodrome of 1 to 2 days, headache, photophobia, and neck stiffness develop. Diagnosis can be confirmed by cell culture from the CSF, where the incidence of successful isolation has ranged from 40% to 80%.[96] In addition, enterovirus can be isolated from throat swabs (60%) and stool cultures (80%), but they are not necessarily diagnostic because the virus is shed in the stool for 1 to 2 weeks following infection.[97] Conversely, an enterovirus-specific reverse-transcriptase polymerase chain reaction (EV-PCR) test can provide prompt results within 24 hours with a sensitivity and a specificity of 100%.[99] Treatment for enteroviral encephalitis consists of supportive care, fluids, antipyretics, and analgesics. Generally, disease progression is self-limiting, and the patient recovers fully without long-term neurologic complications.

Both herpes simplex virus types 1 and 2 have been associated with infections of the CNS. Herpes simplex type 1 (HSV1) is associated with encephalitis in adults, whereas herpes simplex type 2 (HSV2) is associated predominantly with encephalitis in newborns.[93] An HSV infection of the CNS most likely is spread via retrograde movement from the dorsal root ganglion. Sexually active adults acquire herpes simplex meningitis during or after an attack of genital or rectal herpes. Although HSV2 frequently can be cultured from CSF, HSV1 cannot. As such, PCR may be more useful than culture in detecting infection with HSV; diagnosis is usually made by PCR, culture, or a fourfold rise in complement-fixing antibody to the virus. Establishing the correct diagnosis as early as possible is paramount because mortality rates are between 50% and 85% without treatment, and unlike other viral encephalitides, specific and effective therapy is available. As a result, empirical therapy of suspected HSV encephalitis while laboratory results are pending is necessary. Additionally, a clinical decision to treat may need to be made regardless of test results.

Acyclovir is the drug of choice for herpes simplex encephalitis. In patients with normal renal function, acyclovir is usually administered as 10 mg/kg intravenously every 8 hours for 2 to 3 weeks.[93] Herpes virus resistance to acyclovir has been reported with increasing incidence, particularly from immunocompromised patients with prior or chronic exposures to acyclovir.[100] The alternative treatment for acyclovir-resistant herpes simplex virus is foscarnet.[93] The major toxicity of foscarnet is renal impairment, and doses must be individualized for renal function.[101] The dose for patients with normal renal function is 40 mg/kg infused over 1 hour every 8 to 12 hours for 2 to 3 weeks. Ensuring adequate hydration is imperative. In addition, patients receiving foscarnet should be monitored for seizures related to alterations in plasma electrolyte levels.

Historically, the four most important arboviral pathogens in the United States were the St. Louis virus, the La Crosse virus, and the eastern and western equine viruses. However, the West Nile virus has been recognized as an emerging pathogen and has been implicated in an epidemic occurring in the United States since 1999. Transmission of these viruses occurs through the bites of mosquitoes. Typically, an incubation period of 2 to 14 days precedes the onset of clinical symptoms. Infection of the brain tissue results in fever, headache, paralysis, and coma. While many patients have a benign presentation, symptomatic cases are associated with a higher degree of mortality. Mortality rates of 50% to 75% have been reported for eastern equine virus, whereas mortality rates for western equine and St. Louis viruses are 3% to 4% and 10% to 20%, respectively.[93,95] Treatment is supportive, including treatment for seizures and increased ICP, and in the majority of cases, the disease is self-limiting.[95]

Because of the recent epidemic in the United States, a separate discussion of the West Nile virus is warranted. Although West Nile virus is transmitted primarily by mosquitoes, transmission of the virus via blood products, organ transplantation, transplacental transfer, and breast milk has been documented recently.[94] Similar to the other arboviruses, the incubation period for West Nile virus ranges from 3 days to 2 weeks. West Nile virus infection is asymptomatic in most adults or causes a mild flulike syndrome characterized by fever, malaise, myalgia, and lymphadenopathy. Typically, less than 1% of patients develop neurologic disease, and approximately two-thirds have encephalitis, with the remainder having meningitis without encephalitis.[12] Many patients develop a maculopapular, erythematous rash, which is more common in children than in adults and is uncommon in other forms of viral encephalitis.[12] The other neurologic manifestations include fever, nausea, vomiting, headache, altered mental status, movement disorders, and/or a syndrome much like poliomyelitis.[12,102,103] The primary risk factor for this manifestation seems to be advanced age. The poliomyelitis syndrome is characterized by an early prodromic phase of fevers and weakness followed by the sudden onset of flaccid paralysis. Among patients hospitalized with West Nile virus, the mortality rate is approximately 10% to 15%, whereas patients with encephalitis and weakness have a mortality rate of 30%.[12] CSF examination of West Nile virus encephalitis typically shows pleocytosis and a slightly elevated CSF protein concentration.[12] Several diagnostic methods have been developed for West Nile virus, including a PCR assay and ELISA tests. However, serologic tests (ELISA) can cross-react with other flaviviruses causing a false-positive result. Moreover, the IgM antibodies for West Nile virus can persist for up to 1 year, leading to confusion regarding whether the infection is an acute or previous infection.[12] Ribavirin has shown inhibitory effects on the West Nile virus in neural tissue cultures, but this has not been studied in controlled trials.

HIV encephalitis is the most common CNS complication associated with AIDS. Frequently, patients may complain of headache, photophobia, or stiff neck at the time of presumed seroconversion. As the disease progresses, however, neurologic symptoms are reported frequently secondary to other opportunistic infections. Diagnosis of viral encephalitis is difficult because mental status and neurologic examinations are not sensitive enough to detect early changes. Direct evidence of HIV encephalitis can be obtained through CSF culture, p24 antigen testing, or qualitative or quantitative PCR for HIV RNA. Diagnostic workup of other potential copathogens, such as herpes simplex virus (HSV), *Toxoplasma gondii*, *M. tuberculosis*, *Aspergillus* spp., and *Cryptococcus* also should be performed. Refer to Chap. 126 for a complete discussion of infectious complications in HIV-positive individuals.

EVALUATION OF THERAPEUTIC OUTCOMES

SIGNS AND SYMPTOMS

Because of the potential for rapid deterioration associated with meningitis, signs and symptoms of fever, headache, meningismus (e.g., nuchal rigidity, Brudzinski's sign, or Kernig's sign), vital signs, and signs of cerebral dysfunction should be evaluated every 4 hours for the initial 3 days and then daily thereafter. The Glasgow Coma Scale should be used in severely ill patients. Trends in improvement and resolution rather than single evaluations in time are more important in monitoring the signs and symptoms of meningitis.

MICROBIOLOGIC FINDINGS

CSF and blood samples for Gram stain, cultures, and sensitivity testing should be taken prior to starting antibiotic therapy. If lumbar puncture is delayed, however, antibiotics should be started. Although the CSF cultures may be negative, antibiotic therapy rarely interferes with the protein and/or glucose concentrations in the CSF.[13] Furthermore, if the laboratory is made aware of the antibiotic therapy, steps can be taken to diminish the effects of the antibiotic during the detection process.[16] Gram stain results can be obtained immediately and can guide empirical antibiotic treatment. Identification of the organism can be made within 24 hours, and sensitivities should be available within 48 hours. Repeat cultures should be performed to help determine if sterilization is achieved. A second tube of blood should be taken to allow for latex agglutination tests of antigens to common meningeal pathogens (*H. influenzae, S. pneumoniae, N. meningitidis, E. coli,* and group B streptococcus) if the Gram stain has not been helpful.

CSF EXAMINATION

In bacterial meningitis, the CSF WBC count usually is greater than 1000 cells/mm^3, the CSF protein concentration is elevated, and the CSF glucose concentration (hypoglycorachia) is often low (<50 mcg/dL or 50% to 60% of a simultaneous blood glucose value). Viral encephalitis, in contrast, results in relatively normal CSF protein and glucose levels and typically does not result in greater than 90% polymorphonuclear neutrophils (PMNs) in the CSF (see Table 105–1).

ABBREVIATIONS

AFB: acid-fast bacilli
AIDS: acquired immunodeficiency syndrome
BBB: blood-brain barrier
BCSFB: blood–cerebrospinal fluid barrier
CBF: cerebral blood flow
CDC: Centers for Disease Control and Prevention
CFU: colony forming unit
CNS: central nervous system
CSF: cerebrospinal fluid
CT: computed tomographic
DIC: disseminated intravascular coagulation
EV-PCR: enterovirus-specific reverse-transcriptase polymerase chain reaction
FDA: Food and Drug Administration
GI: gastrointestinal
Hib: *H. influenzae* type b
HIV: human immunodeficiency virus
ICP: intracranial pressure
IL-1: interleukin 1
INF: interferon
LPS: lipopolysaccharide
MBC: minimum bactericidal concentration
MIC: minimum inhibitory concentration
NCCLS: National Committee for Clinical Laboratory Standards
PAF: platelet-activating factor
PCR: polymerase chain reaction
PGE$_2$: prostaglandin E$_2$
PPD: purified protein derivative
TNF: tumor necrosis factor
WBC: white blood cell

Review Questions and other resources can be found at *www.pharmacotherapyonline.com*.

REFERENCES

1. Scheld WM, Koedel U, Nathan B, Pfister HW. Pathophysiology of bacterial meningitis: Mechanism(s) of neuronal injury. J Infect Dis 2002; 186(suppl 2):S225–233.
2. Saez-Llorens X, McCracken Jr GH. Bacterial meningitis in children. Lancet 2003;361:2139–2148.
3. Meli DN, Christen S, Leib SL, Tauber MG. Current concepts in the pathogenesis of meningitis caused by *Streptococcus pneumoniae*. Currt Opin Infect Dis 2002;15:253–257.
4. Kim KS. Pathogenesis of bacterial meningitis: From bacteraemia to neuronal injury. Nature Rev Neurosci 2003;4:376–385.
4a. Gold R. Epidemiology of bacterial meningitis. Infect Dis Clin N Am 1999;13:515–525.
5. Reefhuis J, Honein MA, Whitney CG, et al. Risk of bacterial meningitis in children with cochlear implants. N Engl J Med 2003;349:435–445.
6. Parodi S, Lechner A, Osih R, et al. Nosocomial enterobacter meningitis: Risk factors, management, and treatment outcomes. Clin Infect Dis 2003;37:159–166.
7. Wenger JD, Hightower AW, Facklam RR, et al. Bacterial meningitis in the United States, 1986: Report of a multistate surveillance study. The Bacterial Meningitis Study Group. J Infect Dis 1990;162:1316–1323.
8. Schuchat A, Robinson K, Wenger JD, et al. Bacterial meningitis in the United States in 1995. Active Surveillance Team. N Engl J Med 1997;337:970–976.
9. Greenlee J. Anatomic considerations in central nervous system infections. In: Mandell GL, Bennett JE, Dolin R, eds. Principles and Practice of Infectious Diseases, 4th ed. New York: Churchill-Livingstone; 1995: 821–831.
10. Spector R, Lorenzo AV. Inhibition of penicillin transport from the cerebrospinal fluid after intracisternal inoculation of bacteria. J Clin Invest 1974;54:316–325.
11. Leib SL, Tauber MG. Pathogenesis of bacterial meningitis. Infect Dis Clin North Am 1999;13:527–548.
12. Bonthius DJ, Karacay B. Meningitis and encephalitis in children: An update. Neurol Clin North Am 2002;20:1013–1038.
13. Bashir HE, Laundy M, Booy R. Diagnosis and treatment of bacterial meningitis. Arch Dis Child 2003;88:615–620.
14. Thomas KE, Hasbun R, Jekel J, Quagliarello VJ. The diagnostic accuracy of Kernig's sign, Brudzinski's sign, and nuchal rigidity in adults with suspected meningitis. Clin Infect Dis 2002;35:46–52.
15. Kaplan SL. Clinical presentations, diagnosis, and prognostic factors of bacterial meningitis. Infect Dis Clin North Am 1999;13:579–593.
16. Thomson RB, Bertram H. Laboratory diagnosis of central nervous system infections. Infect Dis Clin North Am 2001;15:1047–1071.
17. Heath PT, Yusoff NK, Baker CJ. Neonatal meningitis. Arch Dis Child Fetal Neonatal Ed 2003;88:F173–178.
18. Prins JM, van Deventer SJ, Kuijper EJ, Speelman P. Clinical relevance of antibiotic-induced endotoxin release. Antimicrob Agents Chemother 1994;38:1211–1218.
19. Shepard CW, Rosenstein NE, Fischer M. Neonatal meningococcal disease in the United States, 1990 to 1999. Pediatr Infect Dis J 2003;22: 418–422.
20. Gold R. Epidemiology of bacterial meningitis. Infect Dis Clin North Am 1999;13:515–525, v.
21. Spach DH, Jackson LA. Bacterial meningitis. Neurol Clin 1999;17: 711–735.
22. Moura AS, Mendez AP, Layton M, Weiss D. Epidemiology of meningococcal disease, New York City, 1989–2000. Emerg Infect Dis 2003;9:355–361.
23. Rosenstein NE, Perkins BA, Stephens DS, et al. The changing epidemiology of meningococcal disease in the United States. J Infect Dis 1999;180:1894–1901.
24. Kelleher JA, Raebel MA. Meningococcal vaccine use in college students. Ann Pharmacother 2002;36:1776–1784.

25. Weinstein L. Bacterial meningitis: Specific etiologic diagnosis on the basis of distinctive epidemiologic, pathogenetic, and clinical features. Med Clin North Am 1985;69:219–229.

26. Klugman KP, Madhi SA. Emergence of drug resistance: Impact on bacterial meningitis. Infect Dis Clin North Am 1999;13:637–646, vii.

27. Glodani LZ. Inducement of *Neisseria meningitidis* resistance to ampicllin and penicillin in a patient with meningococcemia treated with high doses of ampicillin. Clin Infect Dis 1998;26:772.

28. Casado-Flores J, Osona B, Domingo P, Barquet N. Meningococcal meningitis during penicillin therapy for meningococcemia. Clin Infect Dis 1997;25:1479.

29. Chowdhury MH, Tunkel AR. Antibacterial agents in infections of the central nervous system. Infect Dis Clin North Am 2000;14:391–407.

30. Schwartz B. Chemoprophylaxis for bacterial infections: Principles of and application to meningococcal infections. Rev Infect Dis 1991; 13(suppl 2):S170–173.

31. Anonymous. Prevention and control of meningococcal disease: Recommendations of the Advisory Committee on Immunization Practices (ACIP). MMWR 2000;49(RR-7):1–10.

32. Kaplan SL. Management of pneumococcal meningitis. Pediatr Infect Dis J 2002;21:589–591.

33. Aronin SI. Current pharmacotherapy of pneumococcal meningitis. Expert Opin Pharmacother 2002;3:121–129.

34. Kastanbauer S, Pfister HW. Pneumococcal meningitis in adults. Brain 2003;126:1015–1025.

35. Kaplan SL. Clinical presentations, diagnosis, and prognostic factors of bacterial meningitis. Infect Dis Clin North Am 1999;13:579–594, vi–vii.

36. Mitchell L, Tuomanen E. Vancomycin-tolerant *Streptococcus pneumoniae* and its clinical significance. Pediatr Infect Dis J 2001;20:531–533.

37. Novak R, Henriques B, Charpentier E, et al. Emergence of vancomycin tolerante in *Streptococcus pneumoniae*. Nature 1999;399:590–593.

38. Ross GH, Wright DH, Ibrahim KH, et al. Use of fluoroquinolones in central nervous system infections. J Infect Dis Pharmacother 2001;4: 47–72.

39. Cottagnoud P, Tauber MG. Fluoroquinolones in the treatment of meningitis. Curr Infect Dis Rep 2003;5:329–336.

40. CDC. Prevention of pneumococcal disease: Recommendations of the Advisory Committee on Immunization Practices. MMWR 1997; 46(RR-08):1–24.

41. Black S, Shinefield H, Fireman B, et al. Efficacy, safety and immunogenicity of heptavalent pneumococcal conjugate vaccine in children. Northern California Kaiser Permanente Vaccine Study Center Group (see comments). Pediatr Infect Dis J 2000;19:187–195.

42. Shinefield H, Black S, Ray P, et al. Efficacy, immunogenicity and safety of heptavalent pneumococcal conjugate vaccine in low-birth-weight and preterm infants. Pediatr Infect Dis J 2002;21:182–186.

43. Black S, Shinefield H. Safety and efficacy of the seven-valent pneumococcal conjugate vaccine: Evidence from northern California. Eur J Pediatr 2002;161(suppl 2):S127–131.

44. Lieu TA, Ray GT, Black SB, et al. Projected cost-effectiveness of pneumococcal conjugate vaccination of healthy infants and young children. JAMA 2000;283:1460–1468.

45. CDC. Pneumococcal vaccination for cochlear implant candidates and recipients: Updated recommendations of the Advisory Committee on Immunization Practices. MMWR 2003;52:739–740.

46. Tang LM, Chen ST, Wu YR. *Hemophilus influenzae* meningitis in adults. Diagn Microbiol Infect Dis 1998;32:27–32.

47. Lieberman JM, Greenberg DP, Ward JI. Prevention of bacterial meningitis: Vaccines and chemoprophylaxis. Infect Dis Clin North Am 1990;4:703–729.

48. Pediatrics AAo. *Hemophilus influenzae* infections. In: Pickering LK, ed. 2000 Red Book: Report of the Committee on Infect Diseases, 25th ed. Elk Grove Village, IL, American Academy of Pediatrics, 2000:262–272.

49. Rubin RH, Hooper DC. Central nervous system infection in the compromised host. Med Clin North Am 1985;69:281–296.

50. Lipman J, Allworth A, Wallis SC. Cerebrospinal fluid penetration of high doses of intravenous ciprofloxacin in meningitis. Clin Infect Dis 2000;31:1131–1133.

51. Levin AS, Barone AA, Penco J, et al. Intravenous colistin therap for nosocomial infections caused by multidrug-resistant *Pseudomona aeruginosa* and *Acinetobacter baumannii*. Clin Infect Dis 1999;2 1008–1011.

52. Jimenez-Mejias ME, Pichardo-Guerrero C, Marquez-Rivas FJ, et a Cerebrospinal fluid penetration and pharmacokinetic/pharmacodynami parameters of intravenously administered colistin in a case of multidrug resistant *Acinetobacter baumannii* meningitis. Eur J Clin Microbiol Ir fect Dis 2002;21:212–214.

53. Vasen W, Desmery P, Ilutovich S, Di Martino A. Intrathecal use c colistin. J Clin Microbiol 2000;38:3523.

54. Gunderson BW, Ibrahim KH, Hovde LB, et al. Synergistic activity c colistin and ceftazidime against multiantibiotic-resistant *Pseudomona aeruginosa* in an in vitro pharmacodynamic model. Antimicrob Agen Chemother 2003;47:905–909.

55. Meyer MA. Neurologic complications of anthrax. Arch Neurol 2003;6 483–488.

56. Bush LM, Abrams BH, Beall A, Johnson CC. Index case of fatal inhal tional anthrax due to bioterrorism in the United States. N Engl J Me 2001;345:1607–1610.

57. Girgis NI, Farid Z, Mikhail IA, et al. Dexamethasone treatment for bac terial meningitis in children and adults. Pediatr Infect Dis J 1989;8 848–851.

58. Lebel MH, Freij BJ, Syrogiannopoulos GA, et al. Dexamethasone the apy for bacterial meningitis: Results of two double-blind, placebc controlled trials. N Engl J Med 1988;319:964–971.

59. Lebel MH, Hoyt MJ, Waagner DC, et al. Magnetic resonance imagin and dexamethasone therapy for bacterial meningitis. Am J Dis Chil 1989;143:301–306.

60. Odio CM, Faingezicht I, Paris M, et al. The beneficial effects of early dex amethasone administration in infants and children with bacterial menir gitis (see comments). N Engl J Med 1991;324:1525–1531.

61. Schaad UB, Lips U, Gnehm HE, et al. Dexamethasone therapy for bacte rial meningitis in children. Swiss Meningitis Study Group. Lancet 199 342:457–461.

62. Quagliarello VJ, Scheld WM. New perspectives on bacterial meningiti Clin Infect Dis 1993;17:603–608.

63. De Gans J, Van De Beek D. Dexamethaxone in adults with bacteri meningitis. N Engl J Med 2002;347:1549–1556.

64. Paris MM, Hickey SM, Uscher MI, et al. Effect of dexamethasone o therapy of experimental penicillin- and cephalosporin-resistant pneumo coccal meningitis. Antimicrob Agents Chemother 1994;38:1320–1324

65. Gaillard JL, Abadie V, Cheron G, et al. Concentrations of ceftriaxone i cerebrospinal fluid of children with meningitis receiving dexamethason therapy. Antimicrob Agents Chemother 1994;38:1209–1210.

66. Kennedy WA, Hoyt MJ, McCracken GH Jr. The role of corticosteroi therapy in children with pneumococcal meningitis. Am J Dis Child 1991 145:1374–1378.

67. McIntyre PB, Berkey CS, King SM, et al. Dexamethasone as adjunctiv therapy in bacterial meningitis: A meta-analysis of randomized clinica trials since 1988. JAMA 1997;278:925–931.

68. Pediatrics AAo. Pneumococcal infections. In: Pickering LK, ed. 200 Red Book: Report of the Committee on Infectious Diseases. 25 ed. El Grove Village, IL, American Academy of Pediatrics, 2000:452–460.

69. Syrogiannopoulos GA, Lourida AN, Theodoridou MC, et al. Dexam ethasone therapy for bacterial meningitis in children: 2- versus 4-da regimen. J Infect Dis 1994;169:853–858.

70. Tung YR, Lai MC, Lui CC, et al. Tuberculous meningitis in infancy Pediatr Neurol 2002;27:262–266.

71. Iseman MD. Extrapulmonary Tuberculosis in Adults: A Clinician Guide to Tuberculosis. Philadelphia, Lippincott Williams & Wilkins 2000:145–197.

72. Leonard JM, Des Prez RM. Tuberculous meningitis. Infect Dis Cli North Am 1990;4:769–787.

73. Holdiness MR. Management of tuberculosis meningitis. Drugs 1990;39 224–233.

74. Kent SJ, Crowe SM, Yung A, et al. Tuberculous meningitis: A 30-yea review (see comments). Clin Infect Dis 1993;17:987–994.

75. CDC. Treatment of tuberculosis. MMWR 2003;52(RR-11):1–77.

76. Ellard GA, Humphries MJ, Allen BW. Cerebrospinal fluid drug concentrations and the treatment of tuberculous meningitis. Am Rev Respir Dis 1993;148:650–655.

77. Byrd T, Zinser P. Tuberculosis meningitis. Curr Treat Options Neurol 2001;3:427–432.

78. Waecker NJ. Tuberculosis meningitis in children. Curr Treat Options Neurol 2002;4:249–257.

79. Alzeer AH, FitzGerald JM. Corticosteroids and tuberculosis: risks and use as adjunct therapy (see comments). Tubercle Lung Dis 1993;74:6–11.

80. Sugar AM, Stern JJ, Dupont B. Overview: Treatment of cryptococcal meningitis. Rev Infect Dis 1990;12(suppl 3):S338–348.

81. Powderly WG, Cloud GA, Dismukes WE, Saag MS. Measurement of cryptococcal antigen in serum and cerebrospinal fluid: Value in the management of AIDS-associated cryptococcal meningitis. Clin Infect Dis 1994;18:789–792.

82. Powderly WG. Therapy for cryptococcal meningitis in patients with AIDS. Clin Infect Dis 1992;14(suppl 1):S54–59.

83. Bennett JE, Dismukes WE, Duma RJ, et al. A comparison of amphotericin B alone and combined with flucytosine in the treatment of cryptoccal meningitis. N Engl J Med 1979;301:126–131.

84. Chuck SL, Sande MA. Infections with *Cryptococcus neoformans* in the acquired immunodeficiency syndrome. N Engl J Med 1989;321:794–799.

85. Coker RJ, Viviani M, Gazzard BG, et al. Treatment of cryptococcosis with liposomal amphotericin B (AmBisome) in 23 patients with AIDS. AIDS 1993;7:829–835.

86. Leenders AC, Reiss P, Portegies P, et al. Liposomal amphotericin B (AmBisome) compared with amphotericin B both followed by oral fluconazole in the treatment of AIDS-associated cryptococcal meningitis. AIDS 1997;11:1463–1471.

87. Saag MS, Powderly WG, Cloud GA, et al. Comparison of amphotericin B with fluconazole in the treatment of acute AIDS-associated cryptococcal meningitis. The NIAID Mycoses Study Group and the AIDS Clinical Trials Group (see comments). N Engl J Med 1992;326:83–89.

88. Berry AJ, Rinaldi MG, Graybill JR. Use of high-dose fluconazole as salvage therapy for cryptococcal meningitis in patients with AIDS. Antimicrob Agents Chemother 1992;36:690–692.

89. de Gans J, Portegies P, Tiessens G, et al. Itraconazole compared with amphotericin B plus flucytosine in AIDS patients with cryptococcal meningitis. AIDS 1992;6:185–190.

90. Powderly WG, Saag MS, Cloud GA, et al. A controlled trial of fluconazole or amphotericin B to prevent relapse of cryptococcal meningitis in patients with the acquired immunodeficiency syndrome. The NIAID AIDS Clinical Trials Group and Mycoses Study Group. N Engl J Med 1992;326:793–798.

91. Saag MS, Cloud GA, Graybill JR, et al. A comparison of itraconazole versus fluconazole as maintenance therapy of AIDS-associated crytococcal meningitis. Clin Infect Dis 1999;28:291–296.

92. Maxson S, Jacobs RF. Viral meningitis. Tips to rapidly diagnose treatable causes. Postgrad Med 1993;93:153–156, 159–160, 163–166.

93. Roos KL. Encephalitis. Neurol Clin 1999;17:813–833.

94. CDC. Epidemic/Epizootic West Nile Virus in the United States: Guidelines for Surveillance, Prevention, and Control. Atlanta, National Center for Infectious Diseases, Division of Vector-Borne Infectious Diseases, 2003.

95. Rubeiz H, Roos RP. Viral meningitis and encephalitis. Semin Neurol 1992;12:165–177.

96. Glimaker M. Enteroviral meningitis: Diagnostic methods and aspects on the distinction from bacterial meningitis. Scand J Infect Dis Suppl 1992;85:1–64.

97. Overall JC Jr. Is it bacterial or viral? Laboratory differentiation. Pediatr Rev 1993;14:251–261.

98. Dalton M, Newton RW. Aseptic meningitis. Dev Med Child Neurol 1991;33:446–451.

99. Sawyer MH, Holland D, Aintablian N, et al. Diagnosis of enteroviral central nervous system infection by polymerase chain reaction during a large community outbreak. Pediatr Infect Dis J 1994;13:177–182.

100. Gateley A, Gander RM, Johnson PC, et al. Herpes simplex virus type 2 meningoencephalitis resistant to acyclovir in a patient with AIDS. J Infect Dis 1990;161:711–715.

101. Astra USA I. Package insert: Foscavir Injection, 1999.

102. Kelley TW, Prayson RA, Ruiz AI, et al. The neuropathology of West Nile virus meningoencephalitis. Am J Clin Pathol 2003;119:749–753.

103. Sejvar JJ, Haddad MB, Tierney BC, et al. Neurologic manifestations and outcome of West Nile virus infection. JAMA 2003;290:511–515.

104. Salmon JH. Ventriculitis complicating meningitis. Am J Dis Child 1972;124:35–40.

105. Wald SL, McLaurin RL. Cerebrospinal fluid antibiotic levels during treatment of shunt infections. J Neurosurg 1980;52:41–46.

106. McLaurin RL. Infected cerebrospinal fluid shunts. Surg Neurol 1973;1:191–195.

107. Sells CJ, Shurtleff DB, Loeser JD. Gram-negative cerebrospinal fluid shunt-associated infections. Pediatrics 1977;59:614–618.

108. Kaiser AB, McGee ZA. Aminoglycoside therapy of gram-negative bacillary meningitis. N Engl J Med 1975;293:1215–1220.

109. Williamson JC, Glazier SS, Peacock JE. Successful treatment of ventriculostomy-related meningitis caused by vancomycin-resistant *Enterococcus* with intravenous and intraventricular quinupristin/dalfopristin. Clin Neurol Neurosurg 2002;104:54–56.

110. Congeni B, Tan J, Salstrom S. Kinetics of vancomycin after intraventricular and intravenous adminsitration. Pediatr Res 1979;13:459–463.

111. Pau AK, Smego RA, Jr., Fisher MA. Intraventricular vancomycin: Observations of tolerance and pharmacokinetics in two infants with ventricular shunt infections. Pediatr Infect Dis 1986;5:93–96.

112. Visconti EB, Peter G. Vancomycin treatment of cerebrospinal fluid shunt infections: Report of two cases. J Neurosurg 1979;51:245–246.

113. Wen DY, Bottini AG, Hall WA, Haines SJ. Infections in neurologic surgery: The intraventricular use of antibiotics. Neurosurg Clin North Am 1992;3:343–354.

106

LOWER RESPIRATORY TRACT INFECTIONS

Mark L. Glover and Michael D. Reed

Learning Objectives and other resources can be found at *www.pharmacotherapyonline.com.*

KEY CONCEPTS

❶ Respiratory infections remain the major cause of morbidity from acute illness in the United States and likely represent the most common reasons why patients seek medical attention.

❷ The majority of pulmonary infections follow colonization of the upper respiratory tract with potential pathogens, whereas microbes less commonly gain access to the lungs via the blood from an extrapulmonary source or by inhalation of infected aerosol particles. The competency of a patient's immune status is an important factor influencing the susceptibility to infection, etiologic cause, and disease severity.

❸ An appropriate treatment regimen for the patient with uncomplicated lower respiratory tract infection usually can be established by patient history, physical examination, chest radiograph, and properly collected sputum for culture interpreted in light of current knowledge of the most common lung pathogens and their antibiotic susceptibility patterns within one's community.

❹ Acute bronchitis is caused most commonly by respiratory viruses and almost always is self-limiting with therapy targeting associated symptoms, such as lethargy, malaise, or fever (ibuprofen or acetaminophen), fluids for rehydration, and in some patients cough suppressants. The routine use of antibiotics should be avoided.

❺ Chronic bronchitis is a result of several contributing factors; the most prominent of these are cigarette smoking and exposure to occupational dusts, fumes, environmental pollution, and bacterial (and possibly viral) infection. The hallmark of this disease is a chronic cough with resulting sputum production and the persistent presence of microorganisms in the patient's sputum.

❻ The treatment of acute exacerbations of chronic bronchitis includes attempts to mobilize and enhance sputum expectoration (chest physiotherapy, humidification of inspired air), oxygen if needed, aerosolized bronchodilators (al-buterol) in select patients with demonstrated benefit, and antibiotics.

❼ Respiratory syncytial virus is the most common cause of acute bronchiolitis, an infection that mostly affects infants during their first year of life. In the well infant, bronchiolitis is usually a self-limiting viral illness, whereas in the child with underlying respiratory or cardiac disease or both, the child may develop severe respiratory compromise (failure) necessitating in-hospital treatment, such as rehydration, oxygen, and in select patients, bronchodilators, ribavirin aerosol, or both.

❽ The most prominent pathogens causing community-acquired pneumonia in otherwise healthy adults are *Streptococcus pneumoniae* (70%) and *Mycoplasma pneumoniae* (10% to 20%), whereas the most common pathogens causing hospital-acquired pneumonia (including in nursing home residents) are *Staphylococcus aureus* and gram-negative aerobic bacilli. Anaerobic bacteria are the most common etiologic agents in pneumonia that follows aspiration of gastric or oropharyngeal contents.

❾ The treatment of community-acquired pneumonia may consist of humidified oxygen for hypoxemia, bronchodilators (albuterol) when bronchospasm is present, rehydration fluids, and chest physiotherapy for marked accumulation of retained respiratory secretions. Antibiotic regimens should be selected based on presumed causative pathogens and pulmonary distribution characteristics and should be adjusted to provide optimal activity against pathogens identified by culture (sputum or blood).

❿ The treatment of nosocomial pneumonia requires aggressive therapy with careful consideration of the dominance and susceptibility patterns of the pathogens present within the institution. The epidemiology of these common pathogens should be evaluated on a regular basis to identify changing resistance patterns and subsequent alternation of treatment guidelines.

❶ Respiratory tract infections remain the major cause of morbidity from acute illness in the United States and most likely represent the single most common reason patients seek medical attention. This chapter focuses on bacterial and viral infections involving the lower respiratory tract, which includes the tracheobronchial tree and lung parenchyma.

❷ The respiratory tract has an elaborate system of host defenses, including humoral immunity, cellular immunity, and anatomic mechanisms.[1–4] When functioning properly, the host defenses of the respiratory tract are markedly effective in protecting against pathogen invasion and removing potentially infectious agents from the lungs.[2–4] For the most part, infections in the lower respiratory tract occur only when these defense mechanisms are impaired, such as with dysgammaglobulinemia or compromised ciliary function caused by the chronic inflammation that accompanies cigarette smoking. In addition, local defenses may be overwhelmed when a particularly virulent microorganism or excessive inoculum invades lung parenchyma. The majority of pulmonary infections follow colonization of the upper respiratory tract with potential pathogens, which, after achieving sufficiently high concentrations, gain access to the lung via aspiration of oropharyngeal secretions. Less commonly, microbes enter the lung via the blood from an extrapulmonary source or by the inhalation of infected aerosolized particles. The specific type of pulmonary infection caused by an invading microorganism is determined by a variety of host factors, including age, anatomic features of the airway, and specific characteristics of the infecting agent.

The most common infections involving the lower respiratory tract include bronchitis, bronchiolitis, and pneumonia. Lower respiratory tract infections in children and adults are most commonly a result of either viral or bacterial invasion of lung parenchyma. The diagnosis of viral infections rests primarily on the recognition of a characteristic constellation of clinical signs and symptoms. Because treatment is largely supportive, only occasionally does the diagnosis require laboratory confirmation; this is achieved through serologic tests or identification of the organism by culture or antigen detection in respiratory secretions. New laboratory techniques employing

polymerase chain reaction (PCR) technology have emerged as a means to identify specific pathogens rapidly and accurately.

In contrast, because bacterial pneumonia usually necessitate expedient, effective, and specific antibiotic therapy, its management depends, in large part, on isolation of the etiologic agent by culture from lung tissue or secretions. The pharynx is colonized with many organisms that potentially can cause pneumonia; therefore, culture of expectorated sputum can be misleading unless the specimen is examined to ensure that it has originated from the lower respiratory tract. The Gram stain provides the easiest method to distinguish lower from upper respiratory tract secretions; moreover, through determination of the shape and color of the bacteria, the Gram stain frequently narrow the microbiologic differential diagnosis sufficiently to allow accurate initial therapy. Scanned under low-power microscopy, Gram-stained expectorated upper respiratory tract secretions contain many irregularly shaped epithelial cells with little evidence of inflammation. Microorganisms of a variety of morphologies are present (Fig. 106–1). In contrast, a lower-tract specimen from a patient with bacterial pneumonia usually contains multiple neutrophils per high-powered field and a single or predominant bacterial species. Culture of specimen confirmed to originate from the lower tract by Gram stain provides valuable diagnostic information in the majority of patients with bacterial pneumonia.[6,7]

◀3 An appropriate treatment regimen for the patient with an uncomplicated lower respiratory tract infection usually can be

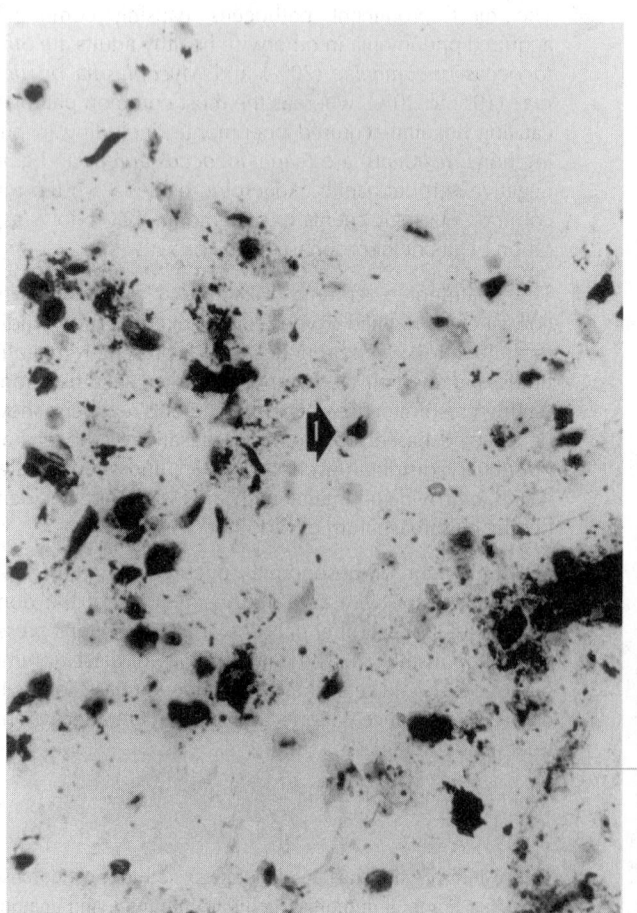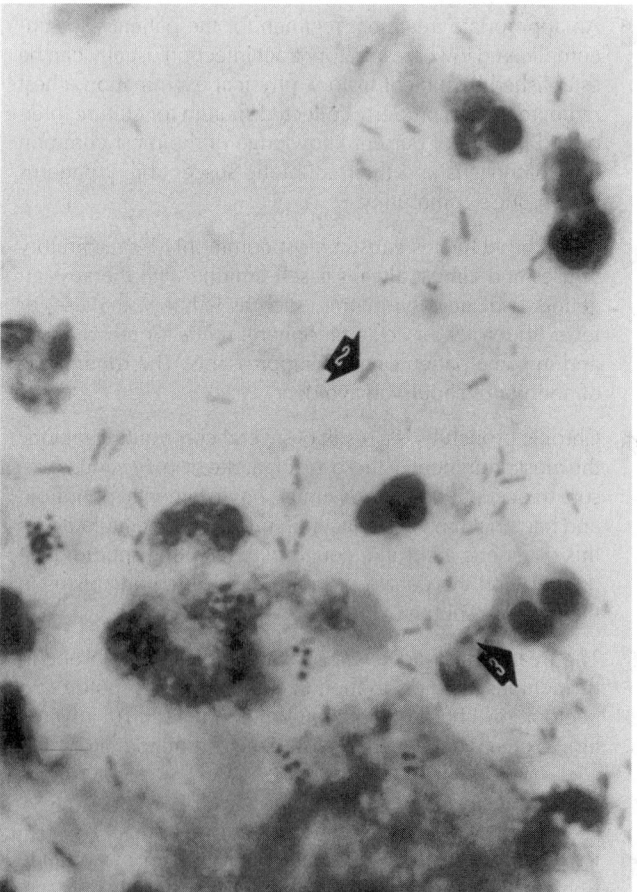

FIGURE 106–1. Gram stain of sputum. *(Left panel)* Scanned under low power (10×), this sample contains many irregularly shaped epithelial cells *(arrow 1)* and no inflammatory cells, indicating that the specimen was derived from the upper respiratory tract. *(Right panel)* Under oil immersion (100×), this specimen contains a predominance of gram-negative rods *(arrow 2)* and many polymorphonuclear cells *(arrow 3)* per high-power field, confirming that this specimen was derived from the lower respiratory tract. The sample grew *Klebsiella pneumoniae.*

stablished by history, physical examination, chest radiograph, and properly collected sputum cultures interpreted in light of the most common lung pathogens and their antibiotic susceptibility patterns within one's community. More sophisticated or invasive diagnostic methods (such as computed tomography, bronchoscopy, and lung biopsy)[8–11] should be reserved for very ill patients who are unable to expectorate sputum or who are not responding to empirical therapy or for pulmonary infections occurring in immunocompromised patients.

BRONCHITIS

Bronchitis and bronchiolitis are inflammatory conditions of the large and small elements, respectively, of the tracheobronchial tree. The inflammatory process does not extend to the alveoli. Bronchitis frequently is classified as acute or chronic. Acute bronchitis occurs in all ages, whereas chronic bronchitis primarily affects adults. Bronchiolitis is a disease of infancy.

ACUTE BRONCHITIS

EPIDEMIOLOGY AND ETIOLOGY

Acute bronchitis occurs most commonly during the winter months, following a pattern similar to those of other acute respiratory tract infections. Cold, damp climates, the presence of high concentrations of irritating substances, such as air pollution or cigarette smoke, or both may precipitate attacks.[12,13]

Respiratory viruses are by far the most common infectious agents associated with acute bronchitis. The common cold viruses, rhinovirus and coronavirus, and lower respiratory tract pathogens, including influenza virus and adenovirus, account for the majority of cases. In children, similar pathogens are observed with the addition of the parainfluenza viruses. While the true incidence remains to be defined, *Mycoplasma pneumoniae* also appears to be a frequent cause of acute bronchitis. Additionally, *Chlamydia pneumoniae*[14] and *Bordetella pertussis* (the agent responsible for whooping cough) have been associated with acute respiratory tract infections. Although a variety of bacteria, including *Streptococcus pneumoniae, Streptococcus* spp., *Staphylococcus* spp., and *Hemophilus* spp., may be isolated from throat or sputum culture, it is probable that these organisms represent contamination by normal flora of the upper respiratory tract rather than true pathogens. Although a primary bacterial etiology for acute bronchitis appears rare, secondary bacterial infection may be involved.

PATHOGENESIS

Because acute bronchitis is primarily a self-limiting illness and rarely a cause of death, few data are available to describe the pathology. In general, infection of the trachea and bronchi yields

TABLE 106–1. Clinical Presentation of Acute Bronchitis

Signs and Symptoms
Cough
Coryza, sore throat, malaise, headache
Fever rarely exceeds 39°C
Physical Examination
Rhonchi or coarse, moist, bilateral rales
Chest Radiograph
Normal

hyperemic and edematous mucous membranes with an increase in bronchial secretions. Destruction of respiratory epithelium can range from mild to extensive and may affect bronchial mucociliary function. In addition, the increase in bronchial secretions, which can become thick and tenacious, further impairs mucociliary activity. The probability of permanent damage to the airways as a result of acute bronchitis remains unclear; however, epidemiologic evaluations support the belief that recurrent acute respiratory infections may be associated with increased airway hyperreactivity and possibly the pathogenesis of asthma or chronic obstructive pulmonary disease (COPD).[13,15]

CLINICAL PRESENTATION

Acute bronchitis usually begins as an upper respiratory infection with nonspecific complaints (Table 106–1). Cough is the hallmark of acute bronchitis and occurs early. The onset of cough may be insidious or abrupt, and the symptoms persist despite resolution of nasal or nasopharyngeal complaints. Frequently, the cough is initially nonproductive, but progresses, yielding mucopurulent sputum. In older children and adults, the sputum is raised and expectorated; in the young child, sputum is often swallowed and can result in gagging and vomiting. Substantial discomfort may result from the coughing. Dyspnea, cyanosis, or signs of airway obstruction are observed rarely unless the patient has underlying pulmonary disease, such as emphysema or COPD. Fever, when present, rarely exceeds 39°C (102.2°F) and appears most commonly with adenovirus, influenza virus, and *M. pneumoniae* infections. The diagnosis typically is made on the basis of a characteristic history and physical examination. Bacterial cultures of expectorated sputum generally are of limited use because of the inability to avoid normal nasopharyngeal flora by the sampling technique. In routine cases, viral cultures are unnecessary and frequently unavailable. Viral antigen-detection tests, developed to identify respiratory viral antigens from nasal secretions rapidly, can be obtained in many hospital laboratories and in some practice settings when a specific diagnosis is necessary for clinical or epidemiologic reasons.[16] Cultures or serologic diagnosis of *M. pneumoniae* and culture or direct fluorescent antibody detection for *B. pertussis* should be obtained in prolonged or severe cases when epidemiologic considerations would suggest their involvement.[17]

▶ TREATMENT: Acute Bronchitis

■ DESIRED OUTCOME

In the absence of a complicating bacterial superinfection, acute bronchitis is almost always self-limiting. The goals of therapy, therefore, are to provide comfort to the patient and, in the unusually severe case, to treat associated dehydration and respiratory compromise.

■ GENERAL APPROACH TO TREATMENT

The treatment of acute bronchitis is symptomatic and supportive in nature. Reassurance and antipyretics frequently are all that are needed. Bed rest for comfort may be instituted as desired. Patients should be encouraged to drink fluids to prevent dehydration and possibly to decrease the viscosity of respiratory secretions. Mist therapy, the use of a vaporizer, or both may further promote the thinning and loosening of respiratory secretions.

PHARMACOLOGIC THERAPY

Mild analgesic-antipyretic therapy is often helpful in relieving the associated lethargy, malaise, and fever. Aspirin or acetaminophen (650 mg in adults or 10–15 mg/kg per dose in children; maximum daily pediatric dose 60 mg/kg; maximum daily adult dose 4 g) or ibuprofen (200–800 mg in adults or 10 mg/kg per dose in children; maximum daily pediatric dose 40 mg/kg; maximum daily adult dose 3.2 g) should be administered every 4 to 6 hours. In children, aspirin should be avoided and acetaminophen used as the preferred agent because of the possible association between aspirin use and the development of Reye's syndrome.[18]

The use of ibuprofen as an antipyretic has increased. The drug's antipyretic efficacy appears identical to that of aspirin or acetaminophen, although its duration of antipyretic effect may be slightly longer (e.g., 3 to 4 hours for aspirin and acetaminophen versus 5 to 6 hours for ibuprofen). Caution should be exercised in the administration of ibuprofen in those younger than 3 months of age and elderly patients and individuals with poor renal function. Aspirin and ibuprofen inhibit prostaglandin synthesis and may adversely influence renal function in these predisposed patient populations.

Patients suffering from acute bronchitis frequently medicate themselves with over-the-counter (OTC) cough and cold remedies containing various combinations of antihistamines, sympathomimetics, and antitussives despite the lack of definitive evidence supporting their effectiveness.[19] In fact, the tendency of these agents to dehydrate bronchial secretions potentially could aggravate and prolong the recovery process. Persistent, mild cough, which may be bothersome, can be treated with dextromethorphan; more severe coughs may require intermittent codeine or other similar agents. In severe cases, cough may be persistent enough to disrupt sleep, and the use of a mild sedative-hypnotic, concomitantly with a cough suppressant, may be desirable; however, antitussives should be used cautiously when the cough is productive. The primary or supplemental use of expectorants is questionable because their clinical effectiveness has not been well established.

Routine use of antibiotics in the treatment of acute bronchitis should be discouraged[20,21]; however, in patients who exhibit persistent fever or respiratory symptoms for more than 4 to 6 days, the possibility of a concurrent bacterial infection should be suspected. When possible, antibiotic therapy should be directed toward anticipated respiratory pathogen(s) (*S. pneumoniae*, *H. influenzae*). *M. pneumoniae*, if suspected by history or positive cold agglutinins (titers > 1:32) or if confirmed by culture or serology, may be treated with erythromycin or its analogues (clarithromycin, azithromycin). Alternatively and empirically, a fluoroquinolone with activity against these pathogens (e.g., gatifloxacin or levofloxacin) may be used. During known epidemics involving the influenza A virus, amantadine or rimantadine may be effective in minimizing associated symptoms if administered early in the course of the disease.[22] The recently marketed neuraminidase inhibitors (zanamivir and oseltamivir) are active against both influenza A and B viral infections and may reduce the severity and duration of the influenza episode if administered promptly during the onset of the viral infection.[23,24]

CHRONIC BRONCHITIS

EPIDEMIOLOGY AND ETIOLOGY

Chronic bronchitis is a nonspecific disease that primarily affects adults. Between 10% and 25% of the adult population 40 years of age or older suffer from chronic bronchitis, resulting in substantial health care dollar expenditures and lost wages.[25–27] This disease is so common that acute bronchitis and acute exacerbations of chronic bronchitis result in approximately 14 million physician visits per year in the United States. Similar to acute bronchitis, cold, damp climates and the presence of elevated airborne concentrations of irritating substances may favor this disease.[25–27] Chronic bronchitis occurs more commonly in men than in women.

Chronic bronchitis is a result of several contributing factors; the most prominent of these include cigarette smoking; exposure to occupational dusts, fumes, and environmental pollution; and bacterial (and possibly viral) infection. The influence that each of these factors and others, either alone or in combination, contributes to chronic bronchitis is unknown. Cigarette smoke is a well-known airway irritant and is believed to be the predominant factor in the etiology of chronic bronchitis. Studies of lungs from smoking and nonsmoking individuals clearly have demonstrated a substantial increase in the number of alveolar macrophages, as well as the presence of bronchial inflammation, in individuals who smoke cigarettes. Although the majority of patients who suffer from chronic bronchitis have a positive smoking history, no history of smoking can be identified in as many as 10% of patients. These findings suggest that additional airway irritants, either alone or more probably in combination, are responsible for the pathogenesis of chronic bronchitis. The only known genetic abnormality leading to COPD is α_1-antitrypsin deficiency, which occurs in less than 1% of COPD patients in the United States.

In addition, the influence of recurrent respiratory tract infections during childhood or young adult life on the later development of chronic bronchitis remains obscure. Recurrent respiratory infections at a young age may predispose individuals to the development of chronic bronchitis[15,28]; however, it is unclear whether these recurrent respiratory tract infections are a result of unrecognized anatomic abnormalities of the airways or impaired pulmonary defense mechanisms.

PATHOGENESIS

The chronic inhalation of an irritating noxious substance compromises the normal secretory and mucociliary function of bronchial mucosa. In chronic bronchitis, the bronchial wall is thickened, and the number of mucus-secreting goblet cells in the surface epithelium of both larger and smaller bronchi is increased markedly.[29] In contrast, goblet cells generally are absent from the smaller bronchi of normal individuals. In addition to the increased number of goblet cells, hypertrophy of the mucous glands and dilation of the mucous gland ducts are also observed. As a result of these changes, chronic bronchitics have substantially more mucus in their peripheral airways, further impairing normal lung defenses. This increased quantity of tenacious secretions within the bronchial tree frequently causes mucous plugging of the smaller airways. Accompanying these changes are squamous cell metaplasia of the surface epithelium, edema and increased vascularity of the basement membrane of larger airways, and variable chronic inflammatory cell infiltration. Continued progression of this pathology an result in residual scarring of small bronchi, augmenting airway obstruction and weakening of bronchial walls.

CLINICAL PRESENTATION

The hallmark of chronic bronchitis is a cough that may range from a mild "smoker's cough" to severe, incessant coughing productive of purulent sputum. Coughing may be precipitated by multiple stimuli, including simple, normal conversation. Expectoration of the largest quantity of sputum usually occurs on arising in the morning, although many patients expectorate sputum throughout the day. The expectorated sputum usually is tenacious and can vary in color from white to yellow-green. As a result, many patients complain of a frequent bad taste in their mouth and of halitosis.

The diagnosis of chronic bronchitis is based primarily on clinical assessment and history. Any patient who reports the coughing up of sputum on most days for at least 3 consecutive months each year for 2 consecutive years presumptively has chronic bronchitis.[26,27] The diagnosis of chronic bronchitis is made only when the possibilities of bronchiectasis, cardiac failure, cystic fibrosis, and lung carcinoma have been effectively excluded. In an attempt to be more specific in the diagnosis, some investigators have added lost wages for 3 or more weeks to the criteria. In addition, many clinicians attempt to subdivide their patients into one of three subgroups: (1) those with simple chronic bronchitis, (2) those with chronic or recurrent mucopurulent bronchitis (based on the presence of mucopurulent sputum confirmed by microscopic analysis), and (3) those with chronic obstructive bronchitis (based on the clinical history and presence of airway obstruction documented by pulmonary function testing). More recently, an ad hoc international committee comprised of pulmonary and infectious disease physicians developed a classification system that can serve as a practical guide for initial patient assessment and management (Table 106–2) for patients with chronic bronchitis.[27]

TABLE 106–3. Clinical Presentation of Chronic Bronchitis

Signs and Symptoms
Cyanosis (advanced disease)
Obesity

Physical Examination
Chest auscultation usually reveals inspiratory and expiratory rales, rhonchi, and mild wheezing with an expiratory phase that is frequently prolonged. There is hyperresonance on percussion with obliteration of the area of cardiac dullness
Normal vesicular breathing sounds are diminished
Clubbing of digits (advanced disease)

Chest Radiograph
Increase in the anteroposterior diameter of the thoracic cage (observed as a barrel chest)
Depressed diaphragm with limited mobility

Laboratory Tests
Erythrocytosis (advanced disease)

Pulmonary Function Tests
Decreased vital capacity
Prolonged expiratory flow

Typical clinical presentation of chronic bronchitis is found in Table 106–3.

In more progressed stages of chronic bronchitis, physical findings associated with cor pulmonale, including cardiac enlargement, hepatomegaly, and edema of the lower extremities, are observed. In general, chronic bronchitics tend to maintain at least normal body weight and are commonly obese. Radiographic studies are of limited value either in the diagnosis or as a means of sequentially following a patient. The microscopic and laboratory assessment of sputum is considered an important component in the overall evaluation of patients with chronic bronchitis. A fresh sputum specimen obtained

TABLE 106–2. Classification System for Patients with Chronic Bronchitis and Initial Treatment Options[27]

Baseline Status	Criteria or Risk Factors	Usual Pathogens	Initial Treatment Options
Class I Acute tracheobronchitis	No underlying structural disease	Usually a virus	1. None unless symptoms persist 2. Amoxicillin; amoxicillin-clavulanate; or a macrolide/azalide
Class II Chronic bronchitis	FEV$_1$ > 50% predicted value, increased sputum volume and purulence	*Hemophilus influenzae, Hemophilus* spp., *Moraxella catarrhalis, Streptococcus pneumoniae* (β-lactam resistance possible)	1. Amoxicillin, or fluoroquinolone if prevalence of *H. influenzae* resistance to amoxicillin is >20% 2. Fluoroquinolone, amoxicillin-clavulanate, azithromycin, tetracycline, or trimethoprim-sulfamethoxazole
Class III Chronic bronchitis with complications	FEV$_1$ < 50% predicted value, increased sputum volume and purulence, advanced age, at least four flares per year, or significant comorbidity	Same as class II; also *Klebsiella pneumoniae, Pseudomonas aeruginosa, K. pneumoniae,* and other gram-negative organisms (β-lactam resistance common)	1. Fluoroquinolone 2. Expanded spectrum cephalosporin, amoxicillin-clavulanate, or azithromycin
Class IV Chronic bronchial Infection	Same as for class III plus yearlong production of purulent sputum	Same as class III	1. Oral or parenteral fluoroquinolone, carbapenem or expanded spectrum cephalosporin

1 = preferred therapy; 2 = alternative treatment options. Fluoroquinolone: ciprofloxacin, gatifloxacin, levofloxacin; tetracycline: tetracycline HCL, doxycycline; carbapenem: imipenem-cilastatin, meropenem; expanded-spectrum cephalosporin: ceftazidime, cefepime.

as an early-morning sample is preferred. Comparison of the cellular constituents of chronic bronchitic sputum with those of normal sputum can provide insight into the degree of activity of the disease processes.[25] An increased number of polymorphonuclear granulocytes often suggests continual bronchial irritation, whereas an increased number of eosinophils suggests an allergic component that should be further investigated. Gram staining of the sputum often reveals a mixture of both gram-positive and gram-negative bacteria, reflecting normal oropharyngeal flora and tracheal colonization by *S. pneumoniae*, *H. influenzae*, and *Moraxella catarrhalis*. Table 106–4 outlines the most common bacterial isolates identified from sputum culture in patients experiencing an acute exacerbation of chronic bronchitis.

TABLE 106–4. Common Bacterial Pathogens Isolated from the Sputum of Patients with an Acute Exacerbation of Chronic Bronchitis

Pathogen	Percent of Cultures
Hemophilus influenzae[a]	24–26
Hemophilus parainfluenzae	20
Streptococcus pneumoniae[b]	15
Moraxella catarrhalis[a]	15
Klebsiella pneumoniae	4
Serratia marcescens	2
Neisseria meningitidis[a]	2
Pseudomonas aeruginosa	2

[a]Often β-lactamase–positive.
[b]As many as 25% of strains may be intermediate or highly resistant to penicillin.

▶ TREATMENT: Chronic Bronchitis

■ DESIRED OUTCOME

The goals of therapy for chronic bronchitis are twofold: to reduce the severity of the chronic symptoms and to ameliorate acute exacerbations and achieve prolonged infection-free intervals.

■ GENERAL APPROACH TO TREATMENT

The approach to the treatment of chronic bronchitis is multifactorial. First and foremost, attempts must be made to reduce the patient's exposure to known bronchial irritants (e.g., smoking). A complete occupational and environmental history for the determination of exposure to noxious, irritating gases, as well as preference toward cigarette smoking, must be assessed. Often easier discussed than accomplished, honest, yet reasonable attempts should be made with the patient to reduce or eliminate completely the number of cigarettes smoked daily and to reduce exposure to secondhand smoke. In an organized, coordinated smoking-cessation program, which includes counseling and hypnotherapy, the adjunctive use of nicotine substitutes, such as a nicotine gum or patch, may promote the reduction or complete withdrawal from cigarette smoking. Often just as difficult is the modification of exposure to irritating substances within the home and workplace.

⬦ 6 Additionally, measures to provide pulmonary toilet can be instituted. During acute pulmonary exacerbations of the disease, a patient's ability to mobilize and expectorate sputum may be reduced dramatically. In these instances, attempts at postural drainage techniques, with instruction, active participation, or both from a respiratory therapist, may assist in promoting clearance of pulmonary secretions. In addition, humidification of inspired air may promote the hydration (liquefaction) of tenacious secretions, allowing for more productive removal. The use of mucolytic aerosols, such as *N*-acetylcysteine and DNAse, is of questionable therapeutic value, particularly considering their propensity to induce bronchospasm (*N*-acetylcysteine) and their excessive cost. Oral or aerosolized bronchodilators may benefit some patients during acute pulmonary exacerbations. Finally, in the face of an acute exacerbation, a trial of antibiotics directed against the most likely underlying pathogens may be initiated.

■ PHARMACOLOGIC THERAPY

For patients who consistently demonstrate clinical limitation in airflow, a therapeutic challenge of bronchodilators (such as albuterol aerosol) should be considered. Pulmonary function tests can be performed before and after β_2-agonist aerosol administration to determine more objectively a patient's propensity to benefit from supplemental aerosol therapy. However, this laboratory assessment, often performed at times of better health, may not accurately predict a patient's potential benefit from β_2 aerosols during an acute exacerbation of chronic bronchitis.

Although chronic theophylline administration has been used extensively in the past, this therapy is being employed with decreasing frequency in favor of aerosolized β_2-receptor agonists. Albuterol is used most commonly, one to two puffs of the metered-dose inhaler three to four times daily.[26] The role of aerosolized surfactant also has been assessed in patients with stable chronic bronchitis and has demonstrated encouraging results with respect to improvement in pulmonary function and sputum transport by cilia (i.e., clearance).[30] The role of surfactant as a carrier vehicle for other aerosol medications also appears promising and most likely will continue to be evaluated.

The use of antimicrobials for chronic bronchitis is controversial. Numerous comparative evaluations, including placebo-controlled studies of antibiotic administration with acute and chronic treatment of chronic bronchitics, have suggested definite clinical benefit, whereas other similar studies have not.[26,27,31–33] The antibiotics selected most frequently possess variable in vitro activity against the common sputum isolates *H. influenzae*, *S. pneumoniae*, *M. catarrhalis*, and *M. pneumoniae*.

In general, these conflicting results appear independent of which antibiotic was used or regimen compared. The wide disparity that exists in the results from these studies, combined with the difficulties in recognition and lack of standardized diagnostic criteria for acute exacerbation of chronic bronchitis,[31] serves as the basis for the enormous controversy surrounding the use of antibiotics in this condition.[34,35]

Further complicating antibiotic selection is the increasing resistance of the common bacterial pathogens to first-line agents. As many as 30% to 40% of *H. influenzae* and 95% of *M. catarrhalis* produce β-lactamase. Moreover, up to 30% of *S. pneumoniae* isolates demonstrate resistance to penicillin (minimum inhibitory concentration [MIC] = 0.1–2 mg/L), with approximately 14% of isolates being highly resistant (MIC > 2 mg/L).[36,37] In addition, concern for *pneumoniae* resistance is increasing because the incidence of macrolide resistance is approximately 20%.[33,38] Despite these changes in bacterial susceptibility, it is recommended to initiate therapy with first-line agents in less severely affected patients. The scheme outlined in Table 106–2 can be used as an initial guide in the selection of antibiotics based on disease severity (classes I through IV). These guidelines are quite consistent with those recently published by the Canadian Thoracic and Infectious Disease Societies.[39]

Regardless of which antibiotic is selected, careful attention to predetermined outcome measures should be monitored closely in each patient to determine the success or failure of the therapeutic intervention.[35] Oral antibiotics with broader antibacterial spectra (e.g., cefixime, amoxicillin-clavulanate, fluoroquinolones, or azalides) that possess more potent in vitro activity against sputum isolates generally are not needed as initial therapy because clinical response often appears independent of the pathogen's in vitro susceptibility for many patients.[26,27,32,33]

An important clinical outcome variable directing drug selection and criteria for beginning antibiotics in individual patients is the infection-free period when chronic bronchitics are off antibiotics. The actual length of the infection-free time period, as well as the change in the number of physician office visits and hospital admissions with a particular antibiotic regimen, are extremely important to identify, whenever possible, for each patient. The antibiotic regimen that results in the longest infection-free period defines the "regimen of choice" for specific patients for future acute exacerbations of their disease.

Antibiotics should be selected that are effective against responsible pathogens, that demonstrate the least risk of drug interactions, and that can be administered in a manner that promotes compliance. Antibiotics commonly used in the treatment of these patients and their respective adult starting doses are outlined in Table 106–5. Doses of antibiotics should be adjusted as needed to the desired clinical effect and the lowest incidence of acceptable side effects. A frequently used clinical strategy to enhance the duration of symptom-free periods incorporates higher-dose antibiotic regimens using the upper limit of the recommended daily antibiotic dose for a period of 10 to 14 days.[33]

Traditionally, ampicillin has been considered the drug of choice for the treatment of acute exacerbations of chronic bronchitis. Unfortunately, the need for multiple repeat daily doses (four times daily), increased incidence of gastrointestinal side effects, and the increasing incidence of penicillin-resistant β-lactamase–producing strains of bacteria (see Tables 106–2 and 106–4) have limited the usefulness of this safe and very cost-effective antibiotic. As stated earlier, the proposed classification system outlined in Table 106–2 offers first- and second-line treatment options for acute exacerbations of chronic bronchitis that are directed by the baseline clinical status of the patient. These treatment recommendations can be used to initiate therapy in patients with class I through IV disease.

The value of the erythromycins when *Mycoplasma* is involved is unquestionable, whereas the value, if any, of the newer erythromycin analogues azithromycin or clarithromycin as first-line agents in the

TABLE 106–5. Oral Antibiotics Commonly Used for the Treatment of Acute Respiratory Exacerbations in Chronic Bronchitis

Antibiotic	Usual Adult Dose (g)	Dose Schedule (doses/day)
Preferred Drugs		
Ampicillin	0.25–0.5	4
Amoxicillin	0.5	3
Cefprozil	0.5	2
Cefuroxime	0.5	2
Ciprofloxacin	0.5–0.75	2
Gatifloxacin	0.4	1
Levofloxacin	0.5–0.75	1
Doxycycline	0.1	2
Minocycline	0.1	2
Tetracycline HCl	0.5	4
Amoxicillin-clavulanate	0.5	3
Trimethoprim-sulfamethoxazole	1 DS[a]	2
Supplemental Drugs		
Azithromycin	0.25–0.5	1
Erythromycin	0.5	4
Clarithromycin	0.25–0.5	2
Cefixime	0.4	1
Cephalexin	0.5	4
Cefaclor	0.25–0.5	3

[a]DS = double-strength tablet (160 mg trimethoprim/800 mg sulfamethoxazole).

treatment of these patients is unknown. Azithromycin should be considered as the macrolide/azalide of choice when considering the drug's in vitro antibacterial spectrum of activity, tissue distribution characteristics, and lack of metabolic-based drug-drug interactions.[40] In contrast, the fluoroquinolones have emerged as effective alternative agents, particularly when gram-negative pathogens are involved or in more clinically or severely ill patients (see Table 106–2). The increasing resistance of selected pathogens to ciprofloxacin may necessitate the use of newer analogues with greater in vitro antibacterial activity, including penicillin-tolerant or -resistant *S. pneumoniae* (e.g., gatifloxacin). The increased cost of fluoroquinolones may be outweighed by the possible superiority of fluoroquinolones in their apparent initial success rate and more prolonged infection-free time period.[26,27]

In the patient whose history suggests recurrent exacerbations of disease that might be attributable to specific events (i.e., it is seasonal or related to the winter months), a trial of prophylactic antibiotics might be beneficial. If no clinical improvement is noted over an appropriate time period (2 to 3 months per year for 2 to 3 years), further attempts at prophylactic therapy could be discontinued. Similarly, patient-specific antibiotic trials could be performed in individuals experiencing acute exacerbations, focusing on defining the infection-free period. Although less than desirable, this method of clinical assessment may distinguish patients who will benefit from prophylactic antibiotic therapy from those who will not.

BRONCHIOLITIS

EPIDEMIOLOGY AND ETIOLOGY

Bronchiolitis is an acute viral infection of the lower respiratory tract most commonly affecting infants during the first year of life, with peak attack rates occurring in infants between the ages of 2 and 10 months. Infectious bronchiolitis is unusual in children older than 2 years of age. The occurrence of bronchiolitis peaks during the winter months and persists through early spring. Bronchiolitis remains a major reason why infants younger than 6 months of age require hospitalization. The hospitalization rate for infants younger than 6 months of age for bronchiolitis approximates 6 per 1000 children per year. The incidence of bronchiolitis appears to be more common in males than in females.[12,13,41]

Respiratory syncytial virus (RSV) is the most common cause of bronchiolitis, accounting for 45% to 60% of all cases. During epidemic periods, the incidence of RSV-induced bronchiolitis can exceed 80% of cases. Parainfluenza viruses type 3 (10% to 15%), type 1 (5% to 10%), and type 2 (1% to 5%) are the second most common pathogens, constituting as a group nearly 25% of cases. Bacteria serve as secondary pathogens in a minority of cases.

CLINICAL PRESENTATION

A prodrome suggesting an upper respiratory tract infection, usually lasting from 2 to 7 days, precedes the onset of clinical symptoms (Table 106–6). As a result of limited oral intake because of coughing combined with fever, vomiting, and diarrhea, infants frequently are dehydrated. The increased work of breathing and tachypnea most likely further increases fluid loss. In most cases, this clinical picture persists between 3 and 7 days. Although the hospital course of bronchiolitic children is often variable, substantial clinical improvement usually is observed within the first 2 days, with gradual improvement and resolution over the next 7 to 21 days.

The diagnosis of bronchiolitis is based primarily on history and clinical findings. It is important for the clinician to attempt to differentiate between bronchiolitis and a host of other clinical entities affecting infants, which may produce a similar picture of dyspnea and wheezing. Asthma, congestive heart failure, anatomic airway abnormalities, cystic fibrosis, foreign bodies, and gastroesophageal reflux are the primary disease entities that may present with wheezing on physical examination in children. The isolation of a viral pathogen in the respiratory secretions of a wheezing child establishes a presumptive diagnosis of infectious bronchiolitis. The ability to identify specific viral pathogens is, however, often hindered by the limited availability of special virology laboratories. The proliferation of commercial enzyme-linked immunosorbent assays (ELISA) and fluorescent antibody staining techniques of nasopharyngeal secretions has increased the ability to identify viral antigens within several hours.[16]

TABLE 106–6. **Clinical Presentation of Bronchiolitis**

Signs and Symptoms
Prodrome with irritability, restlessness, and mild fever
Cough and coryza
Vomiting, diarrhea, noisy breathing, and an increase in respiratory rate as symptoms progress
Labored breathing with retractions of the chest wall, nasal flaring, and grunting
Physical Examination
Tachycardia and respiratory rate of 40–80 per minute in hospitalized infants
Wheezing and inspiratory rales
Mild conjunctivitis in one third of patients
Otitis media in 5–10% of patients
Laboratory Examinations
Peripheral white blood cell count normal or slightly elevated
Abnormal arterial blood gases (hypoxemia and, rarely, hypercarbia)

Identification of RSV by PCR should be available routinely from most clinical laboratories, but its relevance to the clinical management of bronchiolitis remains obscure.

Multiple clinical laboratory determinations have been used to assist in the management of cases of bronchiolitis. Roentgenographic evaluation of the chest in children with bronchiolitis yields variable findings, but may help to distinguish this illness from other entities characterized by wheezing.[28] In children requiring hospitalization, abnormalities in blood gas tensions are frequent and appear to relate to disease severity. Hypoxemia is common and increases the respiratory drive, whereas hypercarbia is seen only in the most severe cases. Despite the presence of moderate degrees of hypoxemia, clinical cyanosis is unusual.

▶ TREATMENT: Bronchiolitis

▦ DESIRED OUTCOME

⏴ In the well infant, bronchiolitis is usually a self-limiting illness, and reassurance and antipyretics are usually all that are necessary while waiting for resolution of the underlying viral infection. In-hospital support is necessary for the child suffering from respiratory failure or dehydration; underlying cardiac and pulmonary diseases potentiate these conditions.

▦ GENERAL APPROACH TO TREATMENT

⏴ Almost all otherwise healthy babies with bronchiolitis can be followed as outpatients. Such infants are treated for fever, provided generous amounts of oral fluids, and observed closely for evidence of respiratory deterioration. In severely affected children, the mainstays of therapy for bronchiolitis are oxygen therapy and intravenous fluids. In a subset of patients, aerosolized bronchodilators may have a role. In selected infants, particularly those with underlying pulmonary or cardiac disease or both, with severe acute infection, therapy with the antiviral agent ribavirin may be considered.

▦ PHARMACOLOGIC THERAPY

⏴ Aerosolized β_2-adrenergic therapy appears to offer little benefit for the majority of patients and may even be detrimental.[13,41,42] However, this therapy may offer some benefit to the child with a predisposition toward bronchospasm. In hospitalized patients, bronchodilator therapy may be offered initially, but should not be pursued in the absence of a clearcut clinical benefit. Similarly, controlled trials of corticosteroids have failed to reveal any therapeutic benefit (or harmful effect) when administered to bronchiolitic infants.[41,42] As a result, the routine use of systemically administered corticosteroids is discouraged. Although it has been common practice to place children with bronchiolitis in mist tents, there are no data to document the effectiveness of this practice.

CLINICAL CONTROVERSY

Because bacteria do not represent primary pathogens in the etiology of bronchiolitis, antibiotics should not be administered routinely. Despite this, many clinicians frequently administer antibiotics initially while awaiting culture results because the clinical and radiographic findings in bronchiolitis are often suggestive of a possible bacterial pneumonia.[43]

Ribavirin may offer benefit to a subset of infants with bronchiolitis. Although ribavirin, a synthetic nucleoside, possesses in vitro antiviral properties against a variety of RNA and DNA viruses, including influenza A, influenza B, parainfluenza, and adenovirus,[44] it is approved only in aerosolized form against RSV.[45] Use of the drug requires special equipment (small-particle aerosol generator) and specially trained personnel for administration via oxygen hood or mist tent.[13] Special care must be taken to avoid drug particle deposition and the resulting clogging of respiratory tubing and valves in mechanical ventilators.[46]

Among hospital admissions for RSV infection, ribavirin therapy failed to decrease length of hospital stay, number of days in the intensive care unit, or number of days receiving mechanical ventilation.[47] Consequently, the American Academy of Pediatrics has modified its recommendation for the use of ribavirin from "should be used" to "may be considered."[48] In light of this and because of the requirement for special aerosolization equipment and the cost of the drug itself, most experts recommend reserving use of ribavirin for severely ill patients, especially those with chronic lung disease (particularly bronchopulmonary dysplasia), congenital heart disease, prematurity, and immunodeficiency (especially severe combined immunodeficiency and human immunodeficiency virus [HIV] infection).[49,50] Ribavirin also may be considered in otherwise healthy patients with severe distress because of RSV infection.

In infants with underlying pulmonary or cardiovascular disease, prophylaxis against RSV may be warranted. When administered monthly during the RSV season, both respiratory syncytial virus immune globulin (RSVIG)[51] and palivizumab[52] (a monoclonal antibody for RSV) may decrease the number of RSV episodes and the need for hospitalization. Among the two, palivizumab appears to be preferred, given its ease of administration, lack of administration-related adverse effects, and noninterference with select immunizations.

PNEUMONIA

EPIDEMIOLOGY

Pneumonia is the most common infectious cause of death in the United States, where approximately 4 million cases are diagnosed annually at a cost of $23 billion redundant to the health care system. Pneumonia occurs throughout the year, with the relative prevalence of disease resulting from different etiologic agents varying with the seasons. It occurs in persons of all ages, although the clinical manifestations are most severe in the very young, the elderly, and the chronically ill.

PATHOGENESIS

Microorganisms gain access to the lower respiratory tract by three routes. They may be inhaled as aerosolized particles, or they may enter the lung via the bloodstream from an extrapulmonary site of infection; however, aspiration of oropharyngeal contents, a common occurrence in both healthy and ill persons during sleep, is the major mechanism by which pulmonary pathogens gain access to the normally sterile lower airways and alveoli. When pulmonary defense mechanisms are functioning optimally, aspirated microorganisms are cleared from the region before infection can become established[1-4]; however, aspiration of potential pathogens from the oropharynx can result in pneumonia if lung defenses are impaired. Factors that promote aspiration, such as altered sensorium and neuromuscular disease, may result in an increase in the size of the inoculum delivered to the lower respiratory tract, thereby overwhelming local defense mechanisms. Lung infections with viruses suppress the antibacterial activity of the lung by impairing alveolar macrophage function and mucociliary clearance, thus setting the stage for secondary bacterial pneumonia. Mucociliary transport is also depressed by ethanol and narcotics and by obstruction of a bronchus by mucus, tumor, or extrinsic compression. All these factors can severely impair the pulmonary clearance of aspirated bacteria.[1-4]

The most prominent pathogens causing community-acquired pneumonia in otherwise healthy adults are S. pneumoniae (pneumococcus) and M. pneumoniae. Pneumococcus is the most common cause of bacterial pneumonia in all age groups and accounts for up to 70% of all acute bacterial pneumonias in the United States. M. pneumoniae is believed to account for 10% to 20% of cases. Legionella, C. pneumoniae, and a variety of viruses also cause pneumonia among otherwise healthy persons.[53] Community-acquired pneumonias caused by S. aureus and gram-negative rods are observed primarily in the elderly, especially those residing in nursing homes, and in association with alcoholism and other debilitating conditions.[54] The term atypical may be applied to pneumonia to indicate that the pneumonia may be caused by an atypical pathogen. Although this is older terminology that is slowly fading, a reference to atypical pneumonia or atypical pathogens refers to pneumonia (i.e., bilateral lobar pneumonia with a negative Gram stain) caused by M. pneumoniae, C. pneumoniae, or Legionella.

Gram-negative aerobic bacilli and S. aureus are the leading causative agents in hospital-acquired pneumonia.[55] Anaerobic bacteria are the most common etiologic agents in pneumonia that follows the gross aspiration of gastric or oropharyngeal contents.

Pneumonia in infants and children is caused by a wider range of microorganisms, and unlike in adults, nonbacterial pathogens predominate. Most pneumonias in the pediatric age group are caused by viruses, especially RSV, parainfluenza, and adenovirus. M. pneumoniae is an important pathogen in older children. Beyond the neonatal period, pneumococcus is the major bacterial pathogen in childhood pneumonia, followed by group A Streptococcus and S. aureus. H. influenzae type b, once a major childhood pathogen, has become an infrequent cause of pneumonia since the introduction of active vaccination against this organism in the late 1980s.

CLINICAL PRESENTATION

BACTERIAL PNEUMONIA

Bacterial pneumonia is caused most commonly by gram-positive streptococci and staphylococci and gram-negative organisms that normally inhabit the gastrointestinal tract (enterics) and soil and water (nonenterics). In addition, Legionella pneumophila, itself a weakly staining gram-negative nonenteric organism, accounts for a small percentage of community- and hospital-acquired bacterial pneumonia. Finally, Mycobacterium tuberculosis, an acid-fast staining bacillus, has reemerged as an important cause of pneumonia in urban centers throughout the United States.

Although a wide array of gram-positive and gram-negative organisms can cause pneumonia, they usually present a similar clinical appearance (Table 106–7). Pneumococcus, Staphylococcus, the enteric gram-negative rods, and occasionally other organisms may produce local irritation or destruction of blood vessels leading to rust-colored sputum or hemoptysis. Pleural effusions, both sterile

TABLE 106–7. Clinical Presentation of Pneumonia

Signs and Symptoms
Abrupt onset of fever, chills, dyspnea, and productive cough
Rust-colored sputum or hemoptysis
Pleuritic chest pain

Physical Examination
Tachypnea and tachycardia
Dullness to percussion
Increased tactile fremitus, whisper pectoriloquy, and egophony
Chest wall retractions and grunting respirations
Diminished breath sounds over the affected area
Inspiratory crackles during lung expansion

Chest Radiograph
Dense lobar or segmental infiltrate

Laboratory Examination
Leukocytosis with a predominance of polymorphonuclear cells
Low oxygen saturation on arterial blood gas or plus oximetry

and empyematous, may be associated with many of these entities, evidenced by distant breath sounds and a wide area of dulled percussion. The chest radiograph and sputum examination and culture are the most useful diagnostic tests in gram-positive and gram-negative bacterial pneumonia. Typically, the chest radiograph reveals a dense lobar or segmental infiltrate. Patchy consolidation may be seen occasionally, however, with virtually all these pathogens. Occasionally, pneumonia resulting from hematogenous spread of the organisms results in a diffuse, alveolar pattern on chest radiograph. Gram stain of the expectorated sputum demonstrates many polymorphonuclear cells per high-powered field in the presence of a predominant organism (see Fig. 106–1), which is reflected in heavy growth of a single species on culture. Other laboratory tests are less sensitive or specific. Blood cultures may be helpful in identifying the offending organism, but are positive in only a minority of patients. The complete blood count usually reflects a leukocytosis with a predominance of polymorphonuclear cells; in some instances, particularly with pneumococcus, the elevation of the white blood cell (WBC) count may be pronounced. Normal or mildly elevated WBC counts, however, do not exclude bacterial pneumonic disease. The patient also may be hypoxic, as reflected by low oxygen saturation on arterial blood gas or pulse oximetry.

Although the clinical appearance of the gram-positive and gram-negative pneumonias is similar, there are epidemiologic and clinical clues that render one more likely than the other.

Gram-Positive Bacteria

Pneumococcus is the most common community-acquired bacterial pneumonia, accounting for 25% to 70% of cases. It is particularly prevalent and severe in patients with splenic dysfunction, diabetes mellitus, chronic cardiopulmonary or renal disease, or HIV infection. *S. aureus* pneumonia occurs in both the community and hospital settings.[55] Community-acquired disease with *S. aureus* is identified most frequently in young infants, patients with early cystic fibrosis, and those recovering from an antecedent respiratory viral infection. *S. aureus* is a prominent cause of nosocomial pneumonia and may result from hematogenous spread from a distant source. In both settings, it is characteristically severe and accompanied by the formation of pneumatoceles (air-containing cavities within the lung). Group B *Streptococcus*, although rare in adults, is the most common cause of bacterial pneumonia among neonates, where it typically causes a clinical and radiographic picture nearly indistinguishable from hya-

line membrane disease.[56] Group A *Streptococcus* is an uncommon cause of community-acquired pneumonia and frequently occurs after a viral respiratory tract infection. Only occasionally is it associated with streptococcal pharyngitis. The organism is pyogenic and the presentation can be severe.

Enteric Gram-Negative Bacteria

Community-acquired enteric gram-negative pneumonia is identified most frequently among patients with chronic illness, especially alcoholism and diabetes mellitus. The enteric gram-negative bacteria are also leading causes of nosocomial pneumonia because the upper respiratory tract becomes rapidly colonized with gram-negative organisms after hospitalization, particularly among critically ill patients and those receiving antibiotics. Outbreaks of nosocomial disease may be caused occasionally by contaminated respiratory therapy equipment. *Klebsiella pneumoniae* is the most frequently encountered pathogen among the gram-negative enteric bacteria, although the relative prominence of these organisms varies from hospital to hospital. The gram-negative bacilli are associated with high mortality, sometimes exceeding 50%; their potential to produce significant morbidity and mortality also has been enhanced by the emergence of highly antibiotic-resistant organisms in some hospital settings.[57]

Nonenteric Gram-Negative Bacteria

The most prominent nonenteric gram-negative rods associated with pneumonia include *Pseudomonas, Hemophilus,* and *Moraxella.* Like the enteric gram-negative organisms, *Pseudomonas aeruginosa* is a frequent cause of hospital-acquired pneumonia and is particularly prominent among neutropenic and burn patients.[57] In addition, cystic fibrosis patients suffer from chronic, multilobar infections with *P. aeruginosa,* as well as other *Pseudomonas* spp.; these infections are punctuated with acute exacerbations.[58] *H. influenzae* type b historically has been a prominent pathogen in childhood pneumonia. Since the introduction of the conjugated *Hemophilus* vaccines in the late 1980s, however, there has been a dramatic drop in the incidence of all invasive disease owing to this organism in the pediatric age group. Two different clinical presentations of *H. influenzae* pneumonia are still seen in adults, however. The most common by far is the bronchopneumonia form, which develops most frequently in patients with underlying chronic lung disease and is believed to represent, in most patients, an exacerbation of chronic bronchitis. In the second form of *H. influenzae* pneumonia, segmental or lobar involvement predominates. The course of this illness is more acute, with sudden onset of cough, fever, and pleuritic chest pain. Finally, *M. catarrhalis,* an important cause of otitis media and sinusitis, has been found to be an increasingly important cause of lower respiratory tract infections in immunoincompetent and hospitalized patients.

Legionella pneumophila

Of the several *Legionella* spp. known to cause pneumonia in humans, *L. pneumophila* is by far the most important and accounts for 2% to 15% of all community-acquired pneumonias in North America and Europe.[59] *Legionella* is a water and soil organism and most probably is transmitted by the inhalation of aerosols containing the organism or by microaspiration of contaminated water. Outbreaks of illness caused by *L. pneumophila* have been linked to excavation sites and to contaminated water from air conditioners and showers. Person-to-person transmission has not been demonstrated. In addition to epidemics, *L. pneumophila* causes sporadic illness that peaks in summer and fall. Individuals who are male, middle-aged or older, immunocompromised, chronic bronchitics, or cigarette smokers are at increased risk.

Infection with *L. pneumophila* is characterized by multisystem involvement, including rapidly progressive pneumonia. It has a gradual onset, with prominent constitutional symptoms, such as malaise, lethargy, weakness, and anorexia, occurring early in the course of the illness. A dry, nonproductive cough is present initially that becomes productive of mucoid or purulent sputum over several days. Fevers exceeding 40°C (104°F) develop in more than half of patients and typically are unremitting and associated with a relative bradycardia. Pleuritic chest pain and progressive dyspnea may be seen. Extrapulmonary symptoms remain evident throughout the course of the illness, particularly diarrhea, nausea, and vomiting. Myalgias and arthralgias also occur. Substantial changes in a patient's mental status, often out of proportion to the degree of fever, are seen in approximately one-fourth of patients. Obtundation, hallucinations, grand mal seizures, and focal neurologic findings are also associated with this illness. Chest roentgenograms initially reveal patchy alveolar infiltrates that may be bilateral. Progression to lobar or multilobar consolidation is frequent, as are small pleural effusions.

Laboratory findings include leukocytosis with a predominance of mature and immature granulocytes in 50% to 75% of patients. Urinalysis may reveal proteinuria, hematuria, and casts; liver function tests may be abnormal. Hyponatremia and hypophosphatemia also have been reported frequently. Because *L. pneumophila* stains poorly with commonly used stains, routine microscopic examination of sputum is of little diagnostic value. While it exhibits slow growth and has highly selective growth requirements, *L. pneumophila* has been isolated successfully from tissue using a specialized medium. Direct fluorescent antibody examination of respiratory tract secretions, lung tissue, or pleural fluid is the most rapid means of establishing the diagnosis. The sensitivity of this method approaches 70% for sputum and 90% for lung tissue, and diagnostic specificity is high for both.[59] Commercially available urine antigen tests have been developed for *L. pneumophila;* these tests are 70% sensitive and remain positive for weeks, even after effective antibiotics have been started. Because these diagnostic tests are unavailable in many clinical laboratories, the diagnosis of Legionnaire's disease often is presumptive and based on a suggestive clinical presentation.

Anaerobic Pneumonia

Anaerobic pneumonitis is most likely to occur in individuals predisposed to aspiration by impaired consciousness and may be more prevalent in those with periodontal disease or dysphagia. In addition, bronchogenic carcinoma is an associated underlying condition. A variety of gram-positive and gram-negative anaerobic bacteria indigenous to the upper airway may cause pneumonitis when large quantities of oropharyngeal secretions are aspirated into the lower airways. The organisms most frequently implicated are *Peptostreptococcus* spp., *Fusobacteria, Bacteroides melaninogenicus, Bacteroides fragilis,* and *Peptococcus* spp.; polymicrobial infections with anaerobes and aerobes, such as *S. aureus, S. pneumoniae,* and gram-negative bacilli, are common.[60]

The course of illness typically is indolent, with cough, low-grade fever, and weight loss, although an acute presentation may occur. Rigors are notably absent and bacteremia is rare. Putrid sputum, when present, is highly suggestive of the diagnosis. Chest radiographs reveal infiltrates typically located in dependent lung segments, and lung abscesses develop in 20% of patients 1 to 2 weeks into the course of the illness.[60]

Tuberculosis

The acid-fast bacillus *M. tuberculosis* causes tuberculosis. After years of steady decline, the number of cases of pneumonia caused by

M. tuberculosis in the United States began to increase in the middle to late 1980s. The new epidemic was a consequence of an increased incidence in prison inmates, intravenous drug abusers, immigrants, and most prominently, HIV-infected patients[61] and is most prominent in urban neighborhoods afflicted with crowded conditions and poor access to health care. Unlike previous eras in which tuberculosis was seen most frequently in elderly men, infection currently is identified in increasing numbers of young minority adults.[62] As mentioned, the resurgence of tuberculosis is at least partially related to coinfection with HIV; HIV-infected patients are more likely to develop symptomatic disease with its associated fits of coughing than their immunocompetent counterparts, and this enables further spread of infection.[63] Other groups prone to tuberculosis include the homeless and patients in chronic care facilities and homes for the elderly. Fortunately, since 1992, the incidence of tuberculosis in the United States has declined, reaching a record low. However, worldwide, the incidence continues to increase. Both this sustained worldwide increase in tuberculosis and the past reemergence of tuberculosis in the United States are important reasons for the development of multiple-drug resistance, that is, mycobacteria that are resistant to two or more of the first-line antituberculosis drugs. Infection caused by these organisms is poorly responsive to alternative therapy and is associated with mortality rates exceeding 50% (see Chap. 110).

Tuberculosis is spread person-to-person through the inhalation of droplet nuclei generated by vigorous coughing. Most patients who become infected with *M. tuberculosis* remain asymptomatic despite lifelong infection and have a normal chest radiograph. Infection in these patients is detected only through routine skin testing. Less frequently, particularly in those with poor immunity, the infection cannot be contained by local macrophages, and the tuberculous burden grows sufficiently to cause clinical manifestations.

Adult disease (from adolescence onward) begins with constitutional complaints, followed by a prominent chronic, troublesome cough productive of mucopurulent material. The infection appears initially in the lung apices with little or no hilar adenopathy and, in advanced disease, results in lung necrosis, producing a cavity containing enormous numbers of organisms. With sufficient cough, the cavitary contents are mobilized and aspirated into other areas of the lung, where additional cavities may be formed.

In contrast, pediatric tuberculosis commonly is associated with little cough even in the presence of extensive pulmonary infection. Instead, the child presents with a subacute course of poor appetite, weight loss, lethargy, fever, and sweats. The chest radiograph reveals a widened mediastinum representing enlarged hilar lymph nodes reacting to the tuberculin inoculum. In progressive cases, the nodes impinge on or erode through a large bronchus, resulting in a dense consolidation of the segment distal to the lesion. Cavitary disease is uncommon.

Nonbacterial Pneumonia

Viruses, *Mycoplasma* spp., *Chlamydia* spp., and fungi are recognized causes of pneumonia syndromes in all age groups. The designation *atypical pneumonia,* distinct from the typical bacterial pneumonia seen most commonly in adults, has been used to describe the illness caused by many of these agents.[64]

Mycoplasma Pneumonia

Taxonomically, the mycoplasmas are included in their own class labeled Mollicutes. Although their small size and filterability are similar to viruses, the structure of their ribosomal RNA indicates that they have evolved from bacteria, and unlike any virus, they contain cytoplasm and can replicate in an extracellular environment. They are distinguished from eubacteria by their low genetic content; in addition, the mycoplasmas lack a cell wall and are surrounded instead by a lipid membrane.[64]

M. pneumoniae causes human disease throughout the year, with a slightly increased incidence in fall and early winter. During the summer months when other causes of pneumonia are less common, *M. pneumoniae* is responsible for a greater proportion of cases. Both infection and disease from *M. pneumoniae* are common, with two-thirds of children ages 2 to 5 years and 97% of persons older than 17 years of age having detectable serum antibody to the organism. Overall, *M. pneumoniae* is responsible for approximately 20% of pneumonia cases, although in enclosed populations, such as military recruits and college dormitory residents, it may cause more than 50%. Infection is spread by close person-to-person contact, and the incubation period is 2 to 3 weeks. *M. pneumoniae* infections are unusual in children younger than 5 years of age and show a peak incidence in older children and young adults. Only 3% to 10% of persons infected with *M. pneumoniae* develop pneumonia, with the majority of respiratory tract involvement being manifested as pharyngitis and tracheobronchitis. Asymptomatic infection is common.

M. pneumoniae presents with a gradual onset of fever, headache, and malaise, with the appearance 3 to 5 days after the onset of illness of a persistent, hacking cough that initially is nonproductive. Sore throat, ear pain, and rhinorrhea often are present. Chills are seen only occasionally, and pleuritic pain is uncommon. Lung findings generally are limited to rales and rhonchi; findings of consolidation are present rarely. Nonpulmonary manifestations are extremely common and include nausea, vomiting, diarrhea, myalgias, arthralgias, polyarticular arthritis, skin rashes, myocarditis and pericarditis, hemolytic anemia, meningoencephalitis, cranial neuropathies, and Guillain-Barré syndrome. Systemic symptoms generally clear in 1 to 2 weeks, whereas respiratory symptoms may persist for up to 4 weeks. Although the course of mycoplasmal pneumonia usually is benign and self-limited, severe respiratory disease may develop in patients with sickle cell disease, agammaglobulinemia, and COPD.[64]

Radiographic findings generally are more impressive than the patient's physical findings and include patchy or interstitial infiltrates, which are seen most commonly in the lower lobes. Small unilateral, transient pleural effusions are common, but large effusions and empyema are rare. Roentgenographic abnormalities resolve slowly, and 4 to 6 weeks may be required for complete resolution.

Sputum Gram stain may reveal mononuclear or polymorphonuclear leukocytes, with no predominant organism. Although *M. pneumoniae* can be cultured from respiratory secretions using specialized medium, its growth is slow, and 2 to 3 weeks may be necessary for culture identification. Indirect evidence of infection by *M. pneumoniae* is the presence of elevated levels of serum cold hemagglutinins. These immunoglobulin M (IgM) antibodies develop in approximately half of patients with mycoplasmal pneumonia and can be elevated in other illnesses, especially viral infection. A definitive diagnosis also can be made by demonstrating a fourfold or greater rise in serum antibodies to *M. pneumoniae;* however, because this test also requires 2 to 4 weeks for results, the diagnosis of mycoplasmal pneumonia during the acute phase of the illness must be based on the characteristic history, appropriate clinical setting, and typical physical findings.

Chlamydia Pneumonia

C. pneumoniae, formally designated the *TWAR agent,* after the laboratory designations for the first two isolates, is a relatively recently identified pathogen antigenically similar to *C. psittaci. C. pneumoniae* infection is ubiquitous worldwide, but only a small percentage of

infections result in clinically apparent pneumonia.[65] Conversely, approximately 5% to 15% of pneumonia is associated with this pathogen. Primary-infection *Chlamydia* pneumonia typically occurs in young adults and is characterized by mild respiratory symptoms with a gradual onset. Constitutional manifestations, particularly fever and headache, are common. The radiographic findings are nonspecific and usually consist of multilobular interstitial infiltrates. Immunity is incomplete and reinfection with *C. pneumoniae* is common, particularly among the elderly. The definitive diagnosis of *C. pneumoniae*–associated pneumonia depends on identification of the organism in sputum. Culture of this organism is difficult, and antigen-detection systems, though available commercially, are insensitive.

Viral Pneumonia

Viruses are an uncommon cause of pneumonia in adults except in the immunosuppressed. Influenza virus, usually type A, is the most common cause of pneumonia in the adult civilian population, whereas adenoviruses cause most cases in military trainees. In contrast, viruses are by far the most common agents producing pneumonia in infants and young children, with RSV, parainfluenza, and adenovirus producing most cases.

All viral respiratory tract infections occur more commonly in the winter, and rapid person-to-person spread through susceptible populations is typical. Underlying cardiac or pulmonary disease predisposes to an increased incidence and severity of viral lower respiratory tract infection, especially with influenza virus in adults and RSV in children. Radiographic findings are nonspecific and include bronchial wall thickening and perihilar and diffuse interstitial infiltrates. Pleural effusions may be seen, especially in adenovirus and parainfluenza pneumonia.

The clinical pictures produced by respiratory viruses are sufficiently variable and overlap to such a degree that an etiologic diagnosis cannot be made confidently on clinical grounds alone. Although virus isolation in tissue culture is possible, 7 or more days are often required for virus identification; thus this method usually cannot be relied on for definitive diagnosis during the acute phase of illness. Serologic tests for virus-specific antibodies are used often in the diagnosis of viral infections. The diagnostic fourfold rise in titer between acute and convalescent phase sera may require 2 to 3 weeks to develop. Same-day diagnosis of viral infections is now possible through the use of indirect immunofluorescence tests on exfoliated cells from the respiratory tract. The immunofluorescence technique frequently employs a battery of monoclonal antibodies, including those against influenza A and B, RSV, parainfluenza, and adenovirus, to provide rapid diagnosis of a range of viral infections.[16]

PNEUMONIA IN SPECIAL CLINICAL CIRCUMSTANCES

Pneumonia in the HIV-Infected Patient

HIV infects and destroys helper T-lymphocytes bearing the CD4 surface molecule; these cells are critical for orchestrating a wide variety of immunologic responses. Their depletion consequently results in the dysfunction of both cell-mediated and humoral immunity. As a result, a broad range of pathogens can cause pneumonia in HIV infection[66–68] (Table 106–8). The HIV-infected patient may be afflicted with pneumonia multiple times in his or her lifetime, particularly in the advanced stages of the disease, and a given episode may be caused by more than one species.

The clinical presentation of pneumonia in HIV-infected persons is frequently not helpful in distinguishing one pathogen from another.

TABLE 106–8. Pulmonary Complications of Human Immunodeficiency Virus Infection

Infections
  Viruses
    Cytomegalovirus
    Herpes simplex virus
    Varciella-zoster virus
    Respiratory syncytial virus and other common respiratory
      pathogens (parainfluenza virus, adenovirus)
    Measles virus
  Bacteria
    Pyogenic organisms (especially *Streptococcus pnuemoniae,*
      Hemophilus influenzae; in late disease, *S. aureus* and
      gram-negatives)
    Mycobacterium tuberculosis
    Mycobacterium avium complex and other nontuberculous
      mycobacteria
  Fungi
    Histoplasma capsulatum
    Coccidioides immitis
    Cryptococcus neoformans
    Candida spp.
    Aspergillus spp.
  Parasites
    Pneumocystis carinii
    Toxoplasma gondii
    Cryptosporidia
    Strongyloides stercoralis
Malignancies
  Kaposi's sarcoma
  Non-Hodgkin's lymphoma
  Smooth muscle tumors
Lymphocytic interstitial pneumonitis
Nonspecific interstitial pneumonitis
Drug-induced pneumonitis

From ref. 61.

The pneumonia usually is subacute in onset and consists of fever, nonproductive cough, and dyspnea. Radiographically, most of these entities produce a multilobular or diffuse pattern. Some practitioners initially treat the HIV-infected patient with pneumonia empirically, covering the most common entities (bacteria and *Pneumocystis carinii*). More frequently, however, given the wide array of possible pathogens, a specific microbiologic diagnosis is aggressively pursued early in the patient's course through sputum induction or bronchoalveolar lavage to allow a rational choice of an antimicrobial regimen.[66–68] The diagnosis and treatment of HIV-infected patients with pulmonary disease is discussed in detail in Chap. 123.

Pneumonia in the Neutropenic Host

Neutropenia in the cancer patient is a common complication of aggressive chemotherapy, but occasionally can result from the cancer itself. The risk of infection in the cytopenic patient is increased significantly when the absolute neutrophil count falls below 500 cells/mm³ and the neutropenia persists for longer than 7 days.[69–71] In many patients, the duration of chemotherapy-induced cytopenia can be reduced by the judicious application of colony-stimulating factors.[72]

The organisms that cause pneumonia in the cytopenic cancer patient include a broad range of bacteria and fungi. Prominent among these are enteric and nonenteric (particularly *Pseudomonas*) gram-negative rods, streptococci, and staphylococci, as well as the fungi *Candida, Aspergillus,* and *Mucor.*[69–71] The chest radiograph may reveal the lobar pattern typical of bacterial infection in the normal host, or it may exhibit a diffuse pattern; sometimes the pneumonia remains invisible by chest radiograph until the neutropenia resolves. Noninfectious entities also may cause pulmonary symptoms; these include toxicity from radiation or chemotherapy or infiltration of the lung parenchyma by the tumor itself.

Nosocomial Pneumonia

After the urinary tract and the bloodstream, the lungs are the most frequent site of infection acquired in the hospital.[57,73] Nosocomial pneumonia is seen most commonly in critically ill patients. Several factors that predispose to the development of nosocomial pneumonia include the severity of illness, duration of hospitalization, and prior antibiotic exposure. The strongest predisposing factor, however, is mechanical ventilation (intubation), which bypasses the natural airway defenses against the migration of upper respiratory tract organisms into the lower tract. This situation is exacerbated by the wide use of H_2-receptor blocking agents in the intensive care unit.[57,74] Such use increases the pH of gastric secretions and may promote the proliferation of microorganisms in the upper gastrointestinal tract. Subclinical microaspirations are events that occur routinely in intubated patients resulting in the inoculation of bacteria-contaminated gastric contents into the lung and a higher incidence of nosocomial pneumonia. Ventilator-associated pneumonia can be diagnosed accurately by any one of multiple standard criteria, including histopathologic examination of lung tissue obtained by open-lung biopsy, rapid cavitation of a pulmonary infiltrate in the absence of cancer or tuberculosis, positive pleural fluid culture, and same species with an identical antibiogram for a pathogen(s) isolated from blood and respiratory secretions without another identifiable source of bacteremia.[75]

The organisms most commonly associated with nosocomial pneumonia are *S. aureus* and enteric (e.g., *Klebsiella* or *Escherichia coli*) and nonenteric (e.g., *Pseudomonas*) gram-negative bacilli, organisms that colonize the pharynx of the hospitalized, critically ill patient. The diagnosis of nosocomial pneumonia usually is established by the presence of a new infiltrate on chest radiograph, fever, worsening respiratory status, and the appearance of thick, neutrophil-laden respiratory secretions. In actuality, the diagnosis is often difficult to make in the intensively ill patient with underlying lung pathology that can itself be associated with an abnormal, changing radiograph, such as congestive heart failure or chronic lung disease. Broad-spectrum antibiotics frequently are started empirically even in equivocal circumstances, with bronchoscopy reserved for poorly responsive patients.[74,76]

Severe Acute Respiratory Syndrome

In November 2002, an extremely contagious atypical pneumonia manifested in China that since has been termed *severe acute respiratory syndrome* (SARS).[77] The etiology of SARS is an enveloped RNA virus, a coronavirus, referred to as SARS-CoV. The virus is transmitted primarily via large-droplet spread; however, surface contamination and airborne and fecal spread are also possible. Signs and symptoms associated with SARS include high fever, myalgias, headache, diarrhea, and a dry, nonproductive cough. The respiratory symptoms may progress to shortness of breath and hypoxemia, necessitating the need for intubation and mechanical ventilation. Diagnostic tests for patients suspected of contracting SARS should include chest x-ray, blood cultures, sputum cultures and Gram stain, pulse oximetry, and identification of other potential pathogens, including influenza A and B, *Legionella,* and RSV. For unclear reasons, SARS appears to be less severe in pediatric patients.

▶ TREATMENT: Pneumonia

▉ DESIRED OUTCOME

Eradication of the offending organism through the selection of the appropriate antibiotic and complete clinical cure are the goals of therapy for bacterial pneumonia. Therapy should minimize associated morbidity, including either one or both of these: reversible or irreversible disease and drug-induced organ toxicity (e.g., renal, lung, or hepatic dysfunction). Most cases of viral pneumonia are self-limiting, although therapy of influenza pneumonia with specific antiviral agents (amantadine or rimantadine) may hasten recovery. All efforts should focus on the design of the most cost-effective approach to therapy. Whenever possible, the oral (versus parenteral) route for drug administration should be selected, encouraging outpatient management rather than hospitalization.

▉ GENERAL APPROACH TO TREATMENT

⑨ The first priority in assessing the patient with pneumonia is to evaluate the adequacy of respiratory function and to determine whether there are signs of systemic illness, specifically dehydration or sepsis with resulting circulatory collapse. Oxygen or, in severe cases, mechanical ventilation and fluid resuscitation should be provided as necessary. Further supportive care of the patient with pneumonia includes humidified oxygen for hypoxemia, administration of bronchodilators (albuterol) when bronchospasm is present, and chest physiotherapy with postural drainage if there is evidence of retained secretions. Additional therapeutic adjuncts include adequate hydration (intravenously if necessary), optimal nutritional support, and control of fever. Appropriate sputum samples may be obtained to determine the microbiologic etiology. Rehydration should be provided to replace losses that may have occurred because of fever, poor intake, associated vomiting, or all these. Finally, selection of an appropriate antimicrobial must be made based on the patient's probable or documented microbiology, distribution in the respiratory tract, side effects, and cost.

▉ PHARMACOLOGIC THERAPY

▉ ANTIBIOTIC CONCENTRATIONS

Antibiotic concentrations in respiratory secretions in excess of the pathogen MIC are necessary for successful treatment of pulmonary infections.[78,79] The concept of a blood-bronchus barrier, analogous but dissimilar to the blood-brain barrier, has been used to assess the characteristics of drug penetration into pulmonary secretions. The ability of a drug to penetrate respiratory secretions depends on multiple physicochemical factors, including molecular size, lipid solubility, and degree of ionization at serum and biologic fluid pH and extent of protein binding. Studies performed in animals and cystic fibrosis patients suggest that larger molecular size favors the accumulation of drugs in bronchial secretions. This finding contrasts with data on drug penetration of other physiologic compartments, such as the cerebrospinal fluid, and may be a result of the trapping of lower-molecular-weight compounds in mucin pores. Nevertheless, the rate at which a drug may accumulate in certain respiratory secretions would

appear to remain an important factor relative to the drug's clinical efficacy in treating pulmonary infections. The un-ionized form of a drug and lipid solubility also appear to favor drug penetration. It should be noted that the pH of the infected bronchi is often more acidic than that of normal tissue and blood.[79-81]

Fewer data are available for assessing the influence of drug protein binding on the rate and amount of respiratory secretion penetration. Clearly, it is the free antibiotic fraction reaching the infected site capable of binding to the bacterial cell target that is responsible for antibacterial activity. Since the degree of protein binding influences a drug's ability to traverse membranes, a similar relationship would be expected within the lung. However, focusing on the absolute amount for which an antibiotic is bound to plasma/tissue proteins without accounting for the drug's overall antibacterial potency is errant. To completely assess an antibiotic's therapeutic potential in the treatment of pneumonia, or any infectious process, it is prudent to assess the antibiotic's integrated pharmacokinetic-pharmacodynamic characteristics (i.e., bacterial killing may be concentration-dependent or time-dependent) that account for the drug's degree of binding to serum proteins, tissue distribution, and in vitro potency. Thus, simply focusing on a drug's degree of protein binding is an errant, overly simplistic approach that does not account for the drug's inherent antibacterial activity or distribution characteristics.

The concepts relating to antibiotic activity and overall drug penetration of respiratory secretions just outlined have supported the clinical practice of administering certain antibiotics (aminoglycosides) to achieve high peak serum concentrations on the assumption that higher (and possibly more effective) biologic fluid concentrations of the drug will be achieved. The aminoglycosides are large, polar molecules that diffuse poorly into tissue and respiratory secretions; however, with increasing concentrations as obtained with once-daily dosing, increased target-tissue concentrations would be expected with increasing individual doses. Substantial clinical experience supports this practice for treating pulmonary infections with certain antibiotics (i.e., concentration-dependent antimicrobials), although more data are needed to describe the relationships between these variables and clinical response (see Chap. 103).

CLINICAL CONTROVERSY

Prior to the availability of newer β-lactam and fluoroquinolone antibiotics possessing consistently potent activity against multiple gram-negative pathogens, the administration of antibiotics by direct endotracheal instillation was promoted by some investigators.[79,81] This method of drug administration is an attempt to provide increased topical concentrations of antibiotics that do not appear to penetrate respiratory secretions effectively while reducing the likelihood of systemic toxicity. In addition, greater local concentrations of antibiotics, particularly for the polymyxins and aminoglycosides, are believed to overcome partially the substantial decrease in antibiotic bioactivity observed when these agents interact with the purulent material present in infectious foci.[79-81] Despite these potential theoretical advantages, the role of antibiotic aerosols or direct endotracheal instillation in clinical practice remains controversial.

Sputum is frequently assessed as possibly representing the pharmacodynamic interface for pulmonary infections. However, sputum represents only one of many pulmonary fluids and secretions, although sputum may serve as a reservoir for pathogen growth. These beliefs have led many investigators to assess antibiotic concentrations in sputum, frequently describing sputum drug concentrations as a ratio of serum to sputum drug concentration. Although sputum drug concentrations provide us with some insight into the characteristics of drug penetration of respiratory secretions, caution should be exercised in the interpretation of these data. Data describing sputum drug concentrations are often difficult to interpret because of differences in analytic techniques, method of sputum sampling, and random nature of sampling times relative to drug dose. Moreover, representation of sputum drug concentrations as a ratio of serum drug concentration can be misleading and most probably should be described relative to absolute drug concentration or apparent area under the drug concentration versus time curve in sputum. To more accurately describe the distribution characteristics of antimicrobial agents in sputum, research studies should be designed to allow sequential repeated sputum sampling over a dosage interval under both first-dose and steady-state conditions. Thus, until greater sophistication is realized in our understanding of the relationships between antibiotic concentrations in specific anatomic sites, plasma (blood)–based integrated pharmacokinetic-pharmacodynamic correlates should be used for antibiotic and dose selection.

SELECTION OF ANTIMICROBIAL AGENTS

The treatment of bacterial pneumonia, like the treatment of most infectious diseases, initially involves the empirical use of a relatively broad-spectrum antibiotic that is effective against probable pathogens after appropriate cultures and specimens for laboratory evaluation have been obtained.[82] Therapy should be narrowed to cover specific pathogens after the results of cultures are known. Multiple factors that help to define the potential pathogens involved include patient age, previous and current medication history, underlying disease(s), major organ function, and present clinical status. These factors must be evaluated to select an appropriate and effective empirical antibiotic regimen, as well as the most appropriate route for drug administration (oral or parenteral). For a more detailed discussion on the principles of antibiotic selection, see Chap. 104.

Numerous antibiotics are available, and the majority are effective in the treatment of bacterial pneumonia. Superiority of one antibiotic over another when both demonstrate similar in vitro activity and tissue distribution characteristics is difficult to define. Our opinions on appropriate empirical choices for the treatment of bacterial pneumonias relative to a patient's underlying disease are shown in Table 106–9 for adults and Table 106–10 for children. A complete listing of antimicrobial agents for specific pathogens is beyond the scope of this chapter and is presented in Chap. 104.

Table 106–11 lists dosages for the treatment of bacterial pneumonia. The list of commercially available antimicrobial agents with documented bacterial and clinical effectiveness in the treatment of pneumonia appears endless. The large number of expensive drugs mandates critical evaluation for formulary selection and clinical use. Similarities of in vitro activity, resistance to bacterial-inactivating enzymes, and overall effectiveness often make rational therapeutic decisions difficult and even appear random. Some general principles, however, may be applied to guide rational antibiotic choice, including direct comparison of the antibiotic's likely attainment of the defined pharmacokinetic-pharmacodynamic target correlate for specific bacterial species within the infected site. For the treatment of bacterial pneumonia with concentration-independent antimicrobials (e.g., β-lactams and carbapenems), a plasma drug concentration exceeding the pathogen MIC for more than 50% of the dosing interval correlates with

TABLE 106–9. Empirical Antimicrobial Therapy for Pneumonia in Adults[a]

Clinical Setting	Usual Pathogen(s)	Presumptive Therapy
Previously healthy, ambulatory patient	Pneumococcus, *Mycoplasma pneumoniae*	Macrolide/azalide,[b] tetracycline[c]
Elderly	Pneumococcus, gram-negative bacilli (such as *Klebsiella pneumoniae*); *Staphylococcus aureus, Hemophilus influenzae*	Piperacillin/tazobactam, cephalosporin[d]; carbapenem[e]
Chronic bronchitis	Pneumococcus, *H. influenzae, M. catarrhalis*	Amoxicillin, tetracycline,[c] TMP-SMZ,[f] cefuroxime, amoxicillin/clavulanate, macrolide-azalide,[b] fluoroquinolone
Alcoholism	Pneumococcus, *K. pneumoniae, S. aureus, H. influenzae*, possibly mouth anaerobes	Ticarcillin-clavulanate, piperacillin-tazobactam, plus aminoglycoside; carbapenem,[e] fluoroquinolone[g]
Aspiration		
Community	Mouth anaerobes	Penicillin or clindamycin
Hospital/residential care	Mouth anaerobes, *S. aureus*, gram-negative enterics	Clindamycin, ticarcillin-clavulanate, piperacillin-tazobactam, plus aminoglycoside
Nosocomial pneumonia	Gram-negative bacilli (such as *K. pneumoniae, Enterobacter* spp., *Pseudomonas aeruginosa*), *S. aureus*	Piperacillin-tazobactam, carbapenem,[e] or expanded spectrum cephalosporin[h] plus aminoglycoside, fluoroquinolone[g]

[a]See section on treatment of bacterial pneumonia.
[b]Macrolide/azalide: erythromycin, clarithromycin-azithromycin.
[c]Tetracycline: tetracycline HCl, doxycycline.
[d]Cephalosporin: cefuroxime, ceftriaxone, cefotaxime.
[e]Carbapenem: imipenem-cilastatin, meropenem.
[f]TMP-SMZ: trimethoprim-sulfamethoxazole.
[g]Fluroquinolone: ciprofloxacin, gatifloxacin, or levofloxacin.
[h]Expanded-spectrum cephalosporin: ceftazidime, cefepime.

TABLE 106–10. Empirical Antimicrobial Therapy for Pneumonia in Pediatric Patients[a]

Age	Usual Pathogen(s)	Presumptive Therapy
1 month	Group B streptococcus, *Hemophilus influenzae* (nontypable), *Escherichia coli*, *Staphylococcus aureus*, *Listeria*, CMV, RSV, adenovirus	Ampicillin-sulbactam, cephalosporin[b] carbapenem[c] Ribavirin for RSV
1–3 months	*Chlamydia*, possibly *Ureaplasma*, CMV, *Pneumocystis carinii* (afebrile pneumonia syndrome) RSV Pneumococcus, *S. aureus*	Macrolide-azalide,[d] trimethoprim-sulfamethoxazole Ribavirin Semisynthetic penicillin[e] or cephalosporin[f]
3 months–6 years	Pneumococcus, *H. influenzae*, RSV, adenovirus, Parainfluenza	Amoxicillin or cephalosporin[f] Ampicillin-sulbactam, amoxicillin-clavulanate Ribavirin for RSV
>6 years	Pneumococcus, *Mycoplasma pneumoniae*, adenovirus	Macrolide/azalide[d] cephalosporin,[f] amoxicillin-clavulanate

CMV = cytomegalovirus; RSV = respiratory syncytial virus.
[a]See section on treatment of bacterial pneumonia.
[b]Third-generation cephalosporin: ceftriaxone, cefotaxime, cefepime. Note that cephalosporins are not active against *Listeria*.
[c]Carbapenem: imipenem-cilastatin, meropenem.
[d]Macrolide/azalide: erythromycin, clarithromycin-azithromycin.
[e]Semisynthetic penicillin: nafcillin, oxacillin.
[f]Second-generation cephalosporin: cefuroxime, cefprozil.
See text for details regarding ribavirin treatment for RSV infection.

bacteriologic cure. For concentration-dependent antimicrobials (e.g., aminoglycosides and fluoroquinolones), a peak drug concentration to pathogen MIC ratio of greater than 8 to 10 or the ratio of the pathogen MIC to antibiotic area under the curve (*AUC*) of greater than 25 to 40 for gram-positive pathogens and greater than 100 for gram-negative pathogens correlates with bacteriologic cure. An understanding and application of these inherent drug characteristics would appear to be of the utmost importance for the selection of an optimal therapeutic regimen. Thus, whenever possible, identification of the causative pathogen and expected/defined antibiotic activity

(i.e., MIC) is of paramount importance to the selection/design of the optimal antibiotic regimen.

■ COMMUNITY-ACQUIRED PNEUMONIA

For community-acquired pneumonia, the bacterial causes are relatively constant, even across geographic areas and patient populations. Unfortunately, pathogen resistance to standard antimicrobials is increasing (e.g., penicillin-resistant pneumococci), necessitating

TABLE 106–11. Antibiotic Doses for the Treatment of Bacterial Pneumonia

Antibiotic Class	Antibiotic	Daily Antibiotic dose	
		Pediatric (mg/kg/day)	Adult (total dose/day)
Macrolide	Clarithromycin	15	0.5–1 g
	Erythromycin	30–50	1–2 g
Azalide	Azithromycin	10 mg/kg × 1 day, then 5 mg/kg/day × 4 days	500 mg day 1, then 250 mg/day × 4 days
Tetracycline[a]	Tetracycline HCL	25–50	1–2 g
	Oxytetracycline	15–25	0.25–0.3 g
Penicillin	Ampicillin	100–200	2–6 g
	Amoxicillin/amoxicillin-clavulanate[b]	40–90	0.75–1 g
	Piperacillin-tazobactam	200–300	12 g
	Ampicillin-sulbactam	100–200	4–8 g
Extended-spectrum cephalosporins	Ceftriaxone	50–75	1–2 g
	Ceftazidime	150	2–6 g
	Cefepime	100–150	2–4 g
Fluoroquinolones	Gatifloxacin[c]	10–20	0.4 g
	Levofloxacin	10–15	0.5–0.75 g
	Ciprofloxacin	20–30	0.5–1.5 g
Aminoglycosides	Gentamicin	7.5	3–6 mg/kg
	Tobramycin	7.5	3–6 mg/kg

Note: Doses may be increased for more severe disease and may require modification in patients with organ dysfunction.
[a]Tetracyclines are rarely used in pediatric patients, particularly in those younger than 8 years of age because of tetracycline-induced permanent tooth discoloration.
[b]Higher dose amoxicillin, amoxicillin-clavulanate (e.g., 90 mg/kg/day) is used for penicillin resistant *S. pneumoniae*.
[c]Fluoroquinolones are avoided in pediatric patients because of the potential for cartilage damage; however, their use in pediatrics is emerging. Doses shown are extrapolated from adults and will require further study.

TABLE 106–12. Guidelines for the Empirical Treatment of Community-Acquired Pneumonia

Clinical Setting	Empirical Therapy
Outpatients	Macrolide/azalide, doxycycline, or fluoroquinolone
Inpatients, general medical ward	Extended-spectrum cephalosporin + macrolide/azalide or β-lactam/β-lactamase inhibitor + macrolide/azalide or fluoroquinolone
Inpatients, intensive care unit	Extended-spectrum cephalosporin or β-lactam/β-lactamase inhibitor + fluoroquinolone or macrolide/azalide

careful attention by the clinician to local and regional bacterial susceptibility patterns.[83] Thus, whenever possible, initial therapy should be based on presumed antibacterial susceptibility and consist of older, less-expensive agents, with newer and more expensive antibiotics reserved for unresponsive illness or special circumstances. The indiscriminate use of recently introduced agents increases health care costs and, in some instances (such as with the widespread use of fluoroquinolones), induces resistance among a significant percentage of community-acquired organisms.[84,85] It must be emphasized, however, that the rapidly evolving epidemiology of bacterial resistance, including the increasing emergence of penicillin-resistant pneumococcus in many areas of the United States and Europe,[86] forces the clinician to be vigilant and knowledgeable about antibiotic sensitivity patterns in each community. The indiscriminate use of antimicrobials for the treatment of pneumonia has contributed to the problem of antimicrobial resistance, underscoring the need for defining the optimal antibiotic regimen for each patient.[82,83]

Recommended empirical therapy differs among outpatients, hospitalized patients, and hospitalized patients admitted to an intensive care unit[82] (Table 106–12). Additionally, antimicrobial therapy should be initiated in hospitalized patients with acute pneumonia within 8 hours of admission because an increase in mortality has been demonstrated when therapy was delayed beyond 8 hours of admission.

NOSOCOMIAL PNEUMONIA

Antibiotic selection within the hospital environment demands greater care because of constant changes in antibiotic resistance patterns in vitro and in vivo. Ironically, some β-lactam antibiotics, which were developed to treat multiple-antibiotic–resistant hospital-acquired organisms, can themselves induce broad-spectrum bacterial β-lactamases and thereby lead to even greater problems with resistance.[86] These facts underscore the importance of regularly documenting the epidemiology of pathogens and infectious diseases within a specific practice or institution. As a result, an antimicrobial agent for a specific infectious disease favored in one practice site may not be the most desirable selection in another despite similarities in size and patient profile. Strict and careful control and, possibly, rotation of empirical antibiotics in the hospital environment may help to limit the emergence of resistant organisms. Newer antibiotics developed to treat resistant, hospital-acquired pathogens are, however, costly; therefore, their use must be moderated to some extent in an era where capitated hospital costs and mandated budget cuts will not tolerate careless antibiotic use.

SEVERE ACUTE RESPIRATORY SYNDROME

The treatment of SARS involves primarily supportive care and procedures to prevent transmission to others.[77] Owing to the uncertainty associated with the diagnosis of SARS, empirical therapy with broad-spectrum antibiotics should be employed. To date, fluoroquinolones or macrolides typically have been used. Although its efficacy is unproven, patients also have been treated with ribavirin. Owing to the potential benefit of corticosteroids in the presence of progressive pulmonary disease, methylprednisolone also has been used in doses ranging from 80 to 500 mg/day.

FLUOROQUINOLONE ANTIBIOTICS

The in vitro spectrum of antibacterial activity of systemically absorbed fluoroquinolone antibiotics, such as ciprofloxacin, levofloxacin, moxifloxacin, and gatifloxacin, suggests that these drugs have an important role in the treatment of bacterial infections of the lower respiratory tract. Numerous clinical studies describe the efficacy of these drugs for the treatment of purulent bronchitis, acute exacerbations of chronic bronchitis, pneumonia, and cystic fibrosis.[87] The widespread use of earlier analogues (ciprofloxacin) by primary care physicians has led, however, to pathogen resistance and treatment failures, including, perhaps most important, isolates of *S. pneumonia*. Although newer fluoroquinolones are more active against common respiratory tract pathogens than older agents, this experience renders it difficult to recommend their indiscriminate use for routine community-acquired pneumonia. Nevertheless, these drugs may be effective alternative agents for the treatment of community-acquired pneumonia or in the initial treatment of nosocomial pneumonia for hospitalized patients and patients residing in extended-care facilities. The availability of newer analogues with broad spectra of antibacterial activity, including *S. pneumoniae* (e.g., gatifloxacin), further enhances the desirability of a fluoroquinolone as a first-line agent, expanding the therapeutic armamentarium for both community-acquired and nosocomially acquired pneumonia.

At present, fluoroquinolone use in pediatrics remains restricted and limited because of possible fluoroquinolone-induced destructive lesions of growing cartilage primarily of the weight-bearing joints. These fluoroquinolone-associated arthritic lesions were determined in animals following large doses, but have not been reflected in the human experience. The need for fluoroquinolones for the treatment of selected infections arising in pediatric patients continues, and their continued safety in these patients has served as the foundation for ongoing controlled clinical efficacy and safety trials in pediatric patients.

MACROLIDE-AZALIDE ANTIBIOTICS

Among the more recently introduced classes of oral antibiotics, the newer macrolide-azalide antibiotics (clarithromycin-azithromycin) possess excellent activity against most *S. pneumoniae* and *Mycoplasma* and appear to offer viable alternatives to erythromycin, particularly in patients who are intolerant of erythromycin analogues (e.g., gastrointestinal upset) and, with azithromycin, in patients who are taking medications that may result in a clinically significant drug-drug interaction (e.g., erythromycin with carbamazepine or theophylline).[40] Azithromycin offers the added advantage of once-daily dosing and short-course therapy because of the drug's extensive tissue distribution characteristics and prolonged elimination half-life.[40]

PREVENTION

Prevention of some cases of pneumonia is possible through the use of vaccines and medications against selected infectious agents. Polyvalent polysaccharide vaccines are available for two of the leading causes of bacterial pneumonia, pneumococcus and *H. influenzae* type b. Inactivated influenza virus vaccines formulated annually to contain antigens representative of expected prevalent strains are widely available and generally well tolerated. Recently, a newly developed cold-adapted live influenza virus vaccine available as a nasal spray (Flumist) was approved.[88] Immunization is recommended for individuals likely to experience serious complications from influenza infection, such as patients with underlying heart or lung disease or chronic renal disease and the elderly. For a detailed description of the use of these vaccines, see Chap. 122. Although they should not replace active immunization, the tricyclic amines amantadine hydrochloride and rimantadine hydrochloride may be administered for prevention and treatment of influenza A infection.[89] When therapy is initiated to healthy individuals within 48 hours of the onset of symptoms, both drugs have been proved to decrease the severity and shorten the course of illness by approximately 1 day. The recommended dose for each drug is 5 mg/kg per day in one or two doses not to exceed 150 mg/day in children 1 to 9 years of age and 200 mg/day in two divided doses in patients 9 years of age or older. Additionally, the discovery of the importance of neuraminidase to the viability of the influenza A and B virus has led to the development of the most effective drugs available for the prevention and treatment of influenza disease. Oseltamivir and zanamivir are the first of a new class of neuraminidase inhibitors. Zanamivir is available for aerosol administration, leading to some concern over aerosolization in patients with disease-induced hyperactive airways, whereas oseltamivir is available for oral administration. Both agents are effective in preventing disease, particularly if therapy is begun within 30 hours of symptom onset or exposure (e.g., epidemics) and for treatment in febrile individuals.[90,91]

EVALUATION OF THERAPEUTIC OUTCOMES

After therapy has been instituted, appropriate clinical parameters should be monitored to ensure efficacy and safety of the therapeutic regimen. In patients with bacterial infections of the upper or lower respiratory tract, the time to resolution of initial presenting symptoms and the lack of appearance of new associated symptomatology is important to determine. In patients with community-acquired pneumonia or pneumonia from any source of mild to moderate clinical severity, the time to resolution of cough, decreasing sputum production, and fever, as well as other constitutional symptoms of malaise, nausea, vomiting, and lethargy, should be noted. If the patient requires supplemental oxygen therapy, the amount and need also should be assessed regularly. A gradual and persistent improvement in the resolution of these symptoms and therapies should be observed. Initial resolution should be observed within the first 2 days, progressing to complete resolution within 5 to 7 days, but usually in no more than 10 days. In patients with nosocomial pneumonia or substantial underlying diseases or both, additional parameters can be followed, including the magnitude and character of the peripheral blood WBC count, chest radiograph, and blood gas determinations. Similar to patients with less severe disease, some resolution of symptoms should be observed within 2 days of instituting antibiotic therapy. If within 2 days of starting seemingly appropriate antibiotic therapy no resolution of symptoms is observed, or if the patient's clinical status is

deteriorating, the appropriateness of initial antibiotic therapy should be critically reassessed. The patient should be evaluated carefully for deterioration in underlying concurrent disease(s). Additionally, the caregiver should consider the possibility of changing the initial antibiotic therapy to expand antimicrobial coverage not included in the original regimen (e.g., *Mycoplasma, Legionella,* and anaerobes). Furthermore, the possible need for antifungal therapy (amphotericin B) should be considered. Some resolution of symptoms should be observed within 2 days of starting proper antibiotic therapy, with complete resolution expected within 10 to 14 days.

ABBREVIATIONS

AUC: area under the curve
COPD: chronic obstructive pulmonary disease
ELISA: enzyme-linked immunosorbent assay
MIC: minimum inhibitory concentration
PCR: polymerase chain reaction
RSV: respiratory syncytial virus
RSVIG: repiratory syncytial virus immune globulin
SARS: severe acute respiratory syndrome

Review Questions and other resources can be found at *www.pharmacotherapyonline.com.*

REFERENCES

1. DeLong PA, Kotloff RM. An overview of pulmonary host defenses. Semin Roentgenol 2000;35:118–123.
2. Ward PA. Role of complement, chemokines and regulatory cytokines in acute lung injury. Ann NY Acad Sci 1996;796:104–112.
3. Brandtzaeg P. The role of humoral mucosal immunity in the induction and maintenance of chronic airway infections. Am J Respir Crit Care Med 1995;151:2081–2087.
4. Standiford TJ. Cytokines and pulmonary defenses. Curr Opin Pulm Med 1997;3:81–88.
5. Yungbluth M. The laboratory diagnosis of pneumonia: The role of the community hospital pathologist. Clin Lab Med 1995;15:209–234.
6. Griffin JJ, Meduri GU. New approaches in the diagnosis of nosocomial pneumonia. Med Clin North Am 1994;78:1091–1122.
7. Cook DJ, Brun-Buisson C, Guyatt GH, et al. Evaluation of new diagnostic technologies: Bronchoalveolar lavage and the diagnosis of ventilator associated pneumonia. Crit Care Med 1994;22:1314–1322.
8. Galvin JR, Gingrich RD, Hoffman E, et al. Ultrafast computed tomography of the chest. Radiol Clin North Am 1994;32:775–793.
9. Marik PE, Brown WJ. A comparison of bronchoscopic vs blind protected specimen brush sampling in patients with suspected ventilator-associated pneumonia. Chest 1995;108:203–207.
10. Kirtland SH, Corley DE, Winterbauer RH, et al. The diagnosis of ventilator-associated pneumonia: A comparison of histologic, microbiologic, and clinical criteria. Chest 1997;112:445–457.
11. Jimenez P, Saldias F, Meneses M, et al. Diagnostic bronchoscopy in patients with community-acquired pneumonia: Comparison between bronchoalveolar lavage and telescoping plugged catheter cultures. Chest 1993;103:1023–1027.
12. Stark JM. Lung infections in children. Curr Opin Pediatr 1993;5:273–280.
13. Everard ML. Bronchiolitis: Origins and optimal management. Drugs 1995;49:885–896.
14. Falck G, Gnarpe J, Gnarpe H. Prevalence of *Chlamydia pneumoniae* in healthy children and in children with respiratory tract infections. Pediatr Infect Dis J 1997;16:549–554.

5. Rodriguez WJ. Management strategies for respiratory syncytial virus infections in infants. J Pediatr 1999;135(suppl 2):S45–50.

6. Adcock PM, Stout GG, Hauck MA, Marshall GS. Effect of rapid viral diagnosis on the management of children hospitalized with lower respiratory tract infection. Pediatr Infect Dis J 1997;16:842–846.

7. Black S. Epidemiology of pertussis. Pediatr Infect Dis J 1997;16(suppl 4):S85–89.

8. Visentin M, Salmona M, Tacconi MT. Reye's and Reye-like syndromes: Drug-related diseases? Drug Metab Rev 1995;27:517–539.

9. Katcher ML. Cold, cough, and allergy medications: Uses and abuses. Pediatr Rev 1996;17:12–17.

20. MacKay DN. Treatment of acute bronchitis in adults without underlying lung disease. J Gen Intern Med 1996;11:557–562.

21. O'Brien KL, Dowell SF, Schwartz B, et al. Cough illness/bronchitis: Principles of judicious use of antimicrobial agents. Pediatrics 1998;101:178–181.

22. Nicholson KG. Use of antivirals in influenza in the elderly: Prophylaxis and therapy. Gerontology 1996;42:280–289.

23. Treanor JJ, Hayden FG, Vrooman PS, et al. Efficacy and safety of the oral neuraminidase inhibitor oseltamivir in treating acute influenza: A randomized, controlled trial. JAMA 2000;283:1016–1024.

24. Monto AS, Webster A, Keene O. Randomized, placebo-controlled studies of inhaled zanamivir in the treatment of influenza A and B: Pooled efficacy analysis. J Antimicrob Chemother 1999;44(suppl B):23–29.

25. Adams SG, Anzueto A. Antibiotic therapy in acute exacerbations of chronic bronchitis. Semin Respir Infect 2000;15:234–247.

26. American Thoracic Society. Standards for the diagnosis and care of patients with chronic bronchitis. Am J Respir Crit Care Med 1995;152(suppl):S78–122.

27. Grossman RF. Acute exacerbations of chronic bronchitis. Hosp Pract 1997;132:85–94.

28. Godfrey S. Bronchiolitis and asthma in infancy and early childhood. Thorax 1996;51(suppl 2):S60–64.

29. Wilson R, Wilson CB. Defining subsets of patients with chronic bronchitis. Chest 1997;112:303S–309.

30. Anzueto A, Jubran M, Ohan JA, et al. Effects of aerosolized surfactant in patients with stable bronchitis: A prospective, randomized, controlled trial. JAMA 1997;278:957–960.

31. Wilson R, Tillotson G, Ball P. Clinical studies in chronic bronchitis: A need for better definition and classification of severity. J Antimicrob Chemother 1996;37:205–208.

32. Saint S, Bent S, Vittinghoff E, Grady D. Antibiotics in chronic obstructive pulmonary disease exacerbations: A meta-analysis. JAMA 1995;273:957–960.

33. Russo RL, D'Aprile MD. Role of antimicrobial therapy in acute exacerbations of chronic obstructive pulmonary disease. Ann Pharmacother 2001;35:576–581.

34. Ball P. Epidemiology and treatment of chronic bronchitis and its exacerbations. Chest 1995;108:43S–52.

35. Wilson R. Outcome predictors in bronchitis. Chest 1995;108(suppl):53S–57.

36. Lund BC, Ernst EJ, Klepser ME. Strategies in the treatment of penicillin-resistant *Streptococcus pneumoniae*. Am J Health Syst Pharm 1998;55:1987–1994.

37. Harwell JI, Brown RB. The drug-resistant pneumococcus: Clinical relevance, therapy, and prevention. Chest 2000;117:530–541.

38. Campbell GD, Silberman R. Drug-resistant *Streptococcus pneumoniae*. Clin Infect Dis 1998;26:1188–1195.

39. Balter MS, La Forge J, Low DE, et al. Canadian guidelines for the management of acute exacerbations of chronic bronchitis. Can Respir J 2003;10(suppl B):3B–32.

40. Reed MD, Blumer JL. Azithromycin: A critical review of the first azilide antibiotic and its role in pediatric practice. Pediatr Infect Dis J 1997;16:1069–1083.

41. Klassen TP. Recent advances in the treatment of bronchiolitis and laryngitis. Pediatr Clin North Am 1997;44:249–261.

42. Klassen TP, Sutcliffe T, Watters LK, et al. Dexamethasone in salbutamol-treated inpatients with acute bronchiolitis: A randomized, controlled study. J Pediatr 1997;130:191–196.

43. Muller NL, Miller RR. Diseases of the bronchioles: CT and histopathologic findings. Radiology 1995;196:3–12.

44. Ottolini MG, Hemming VG. Prevention and treatment recommendations for respiratory syncytial virus infection. Drugs 1997;54:867–884.

45. McCarthy CA, Hall CB. Recent approaches to the management and prevention of respiratory syncytial virus infection. Curr Clin Top Infect Dis 1998;18:1–18.

46. Englund JA, Piedra PA, Ahn YM, et al. High-dose, short-duration ribavirin aerosol therapy compared with standard ribavirin therapy in children with suspected respiratory syncytial virus infection. J Pediatr 1994;125:635–641.

47. Darville T, Yamauchi T. Respiratory syncytial virus. Pediatr Rev 1998;19:55–61.

48. Committee on Infectious Diseases. Reassessment of the indications for ribavirin therapy in respiratory syncytial virus infections. Pediatrics 1996;97:137–140.

49. Committee on Infectious Diseases. 1997 Redbook: Report of the Committee on Infectious Diseases, 24th ed. Elk Grove Village, IL, American Academy of Pediatrics, 1997:445.

50. Meert KL, Sarnaik AP, Gelmini MJ, et al. Aerosolized ribavirin in mechanically ventilated children with respiratory syncytial virus lower respiratory tract disease: A prospective, double-blind, randomized trial. Crit Care Med 1994;22:566–572.

51. The Prevent Study Group. Reduction of respiratory syncytial virus hospitalizations among premature infants and infants with bronchopulmonary dysplasia using respiratory syncytial virus immune globulin prophylaxis. Pediatrics 1997;99:93–99.

52. The Impact-RSV Study Group. Palivizumab, a humanized respiratory syncytial virus monoclonal antibody, reduces hospitalization from respiratory syncytial virus infection in high-risk infants. Pediatrics 1998;102:531–537.

53. Cunha BA. Community-acquired pneumonia: Diagnostic and therapeutic approach. Med Clin North Am 2001;85:43–77.

54. Mandell LA. Community-acquired pneumonia: Etiology, epidemiology and treatment. Chest 1995;108(suppl):35S–42.

55. Cunha BA. Nosocomial pneumonia: Diagnostic and therapeutic considerations. Med Clin North Am 2001;85:79–114.

56. Baker CJ, Edwards MS. Group B streptococcal infections. In: Remington JS, Klein JO, eds. Infectious Diseases of the Fetus and Newborn Infant, 4th ed. Philadelphia, Saunders, 1995:980–1054.

57. American Thoracic Society. Hospital-acquired pneumonia in adults: Diagnosis, assessment of severity, initial antimicrobial therapy, and preventative strategies. Am J Respir Crit Care Med 1996;153:1711–1725.

58. Beringer PM. New approaches to optimizing antimicrobial therapy in patients with cystic fibrosis. Curr Opin Pulm Med 1999;5:371–377.

59. Stout JE, Yu VL. Legionellosis. N Engl J Med 1997;337:682–687.

60. Bartlett JG. Anaerobic bacterial infections of the lung and pleural space. Clin Infect Dis 1993;16(suppl 4):S248–255.

61. Martin G, Lazarus A. Epidemiology and diagnosis of tuberculosis. Postgrad Med 2000;108:42–54.

62. McCray E, Weinbaum CM, Braden CR, et al. The epidemiology of tuberculosis in the United States. Clin Chest Med 1997;18:99–113.

63. Telzak EE. Tuberculosis and human immunodeficiency virus infection. Med Clin North Am 1997;81:345–360.

64. Plouffe J. Importance of typical pathogens of community acquired pneumonia. Clin Infect Dis 2000;31(suppl 2):S35–39.

65. File TM, Tan JS, Plouffe JF. The role of atypical pathogens: *Mycoplasma pneumoniae, Chlamydia pneumoniae* and *Legionella pneumophila* in respiratory infection. Infect Dis Clin North Am 1998;12:569–592.

66. Ashley EA, Johnson MA, Lipman MC. Human immunodeficiency virus and respiratory infection. Curr Opin Pulm Med 2000;6:240–245.

67. Schneider RF, Rosen MJ. Pulmonary complications of HIV infection. Curr Opin Pulm Med 1997;3:151–158.

68. Noskin GA, Glassroth J. Bacterial pneumonia associated with HIV-1 infection. Clin Chest Med 1996;17:713–723.

69. Pizzo PA. Management of fever in patients with cancer and treatment-induced neutropenia. N Engl J Med 1993;328:1323–1332.

70. Hughes WT, Armstrong D, Bodey GP, et al. 1997 guidelines for the use of antimicrobial agents in neutropenic patients with unexplained fever. Clin Infect Dis 1997;25:551–573.

71. Whimbey E, Goodrich J, Bodey GP. Pneumonia in cancer patients. Cancer Treat Rep 1995;79:185–210.

72. Mayhall CG. Ventilator-associated pneumonia or not? Contemporary diagnosis. Emerg Infect Dis 2001;7:200–204.

73. ASCO Ad Hoc Colony-Stimulating Factor Guidelines Expert Panel. Update of recommendations for the use of hematopoietic colony-stimulating factors: Evidence-based clinical practice guidelines. J Clin Oncol 1996;14:1957–1960.

74. Gallego M, Valles J, Rello J. New perspectives in the diagnosis of nosocomial pneumonia. Curr Opin Pulm Med 1997;3:116–119.

75. Young PJ, Ridley SA. Ventilator-associated pneumonia: Diagnosis and prevention. Anaesthesia 1999;54:1183–1197.

76. Estes RJ, Meduri GU. The pathogenesis of ventilator-associated pneumonia: I. Mechanisms of bacterial transcolonization and airway inoculation. Intensive Care Med 1995;21:365–383.

77. Sampathkumar P, Temesgen Z, Smith TF, Thompson RL. SARS: Epidemiology, clinical presentation, management, and infection control measures. May Clin Proc 2003;78:882–890.

78. Amsden GW, Duran JM. Interpretation of antibacterial susceptibility reports: In vitro clinical breakpoints. Drugs 2001;61:163–166.

79. Honeybourne D. Antibiotic penetration in the respiratory tract and implications. Curr Opin Pulm Med 1997;3:170–174.

80. Bodem CR, Lampton LM, Miller DP, et al. Endobronchial pH: Relevance to aminoglycoside activity in gram-negative bacillary pneumonia. Am Rev Resp Dis 1983;127:39–41.

81. Smaldone GC, Palmer LB. Aerosolized antibiotics: Current and future. Respir Care 2000;45:667–675.

82. Barlett JG, Dowell SF, Mandell LA, et al. Practice guidelines for the management of community-acquired pneumonia in adults. Clin Infec Dis 2000;31:347–382.

83. Heffelfinger JD, Dowell SF, Jorgensen JH. Management of community acquired pneumonia in the era of pneumococcal resistance: A report from the Drug-Resistant Streptococcus pneumoniae Therapeutic Working Group. Arch Intern Med 2000;160:1399–1408.

84. Jacoby GA. Prevalence and resistance mechanisms of common bacteria respiratory pathogens. Clin Infect Dis 1994;18:951–957.

85. Collignon P, Turnidge JD. Antibiotic resistance in Streptococcus pneumoniae. Med J Aust 2000;173(suppl):S58–64.

86. Shlaes DM, Gerding DN, John JF, et al. Society for Healthcare Epidemiology of America and Infectious Diseases Society of America Joint Committee on the Prevention of Antimicrobial Resistance: Guidelines for the prevention of antimicrobial resistance in hospitals. Clin Infect Dis 1997;25:584–599.

87. Aminimanizani A, Beringer P, Jelliffe R. Comparative pharmacokinetics and pharmacodynamics of the newer fluoroquinolone antibacterials. Clin Pharmacokinet 2001;40:169–187.

88. Gruber WC. The role of live influenza vaccines in children. Vaccine 2002;20(suppl 2):S66–73.

89. Committee on Infectious Diseases, American Academy of Pediatrics. Reduction of the influenza burden in children. Pediatrics 2002;110: 1246–1252.

90. Gubareva LV, Kaiser L, Hayden FG. Influenza virus neuraminidase inhibitors. Lancet 2000;355:827–835.

91. McNicholl IR, McNicholl JJ. Neuraminidase inhibitors: Zanamivir and oseltamivir. Ann Pharmacother 2001;35:57–70.

107
UPPER RESPIRATORY TRACT INFECTIONS

Yasmin Khaliq, Sarah Forgie, and George Zhanel

Learning Objectives and other resources can be found at *www.pharmacotherapyonline.com.*

KEY CONCEPTS

◀ Most nonspecific upper respiratory tract infections have a viral, not bacterial, etiology and tend to resolve spontaneously.

◀ Each time antibiotics are administered for an upper respiratory tract infection, the recipient is at increased risk of selection and carriage of resistant organisms that can be passed to others. This can lead to future antibiotic failure.

◀ Amoxicillin is the drug of choice for acute otitis media. For patients who are suspected of having infection or who are at high risk for infection with drug-resistant *Streptococcus pneumoniae*, high-dose amoxicillin should be administered.

◀ Vaccination against influenza and pneumococcus may decrease the risk of acute otitis media, especially in those with recurrent episodes.

◀ Viral and bacterial sinusitis are difficult to differentiate because their clinical presentations are similar. Viral infections, however, tend to resolve by 7 to 10 days. Persistence of symptoms beyond this time likely indicates a bacterial infection.

◀ Amoxicillin is first-line treatment for acute bacterial sinusitis. Since there is no difference in clinical outcome among antibiotics, the advantages of amoxicillin include proven efficacy and safety, a relatively narrow spectrum that minimizes emergence of resistance, good tolerability, and low cost.

◀ Group A β-hemolytic *Streptococcus* (*S. pyogenes*) is the most common bacterial cause of pharyngitis, and despite representing a small percentage of causes of pharyngitis, it is the only commonly occurring form of acute pharyngitis for which antimicrobial therapy is indicated.

◀ Antimicrobial treatment of pharyngitis should be limited to those who have clinical and epidemiologic features of group A streptococcal pharyngitis with a positive laboratory test. Penicillin is first-line treatment. Amoxicillin can be used for children because of its better taste.

◀ The evidence that treatment of group A streptococcal pharyngitis prevents rheumatic fever comes solely from studies using depot intramuscular penicillin. Penicillin administered by other routes has been assumed to be equally efficacious. The ability of other antibiotics to eradicate group A *Streptococcus* has led to extrapolation that these agents also will prevent rheumatic fever.

Upper respiratory tract infections include otitis media, sinusitis, pharyngitis, laryngitis (croup), rhinitis, and epiglottitis. These infections are responsible for the majority of antibiotics prescribed in ambulatory practice in the United States.[1] In 1998, the estimated cost of otitis media was $3 to $4 billion in the United States and $600 million in Canada.[2]

◀ Most nonspecific upper respiratory tract infections have a viral, not bacterial, etiology and tend to resolve spontaneously.[3,4] Strategies for limiting unnecessary antibiotic use have been developed[1,3,5] in an effort to address the problem of increased bacterial resistance that is associated with antibiotic use. This is particularly important for *Streptococcus pneumoniae*, the leading bacterial cause of meningitis, pneumonia, otitis media, and sinusitis.[1] In Canada, an average of 15 deaths per year due to *S. pneumoniae* are reported in children younger than 5 years of age.[6]

This chapter will focus primarily on otitis media, pharyngitis, and sinusitis because these infectious entities are frequently bacterial in origin, and apprpriate antibiotic treatment can minimize morbidity and potentially prevent complications.

OTITIS MEDIA

Otitis media is inflammation of the middle ear. The diagnosis of acute otitis media includes signs and symptoms of infection of the middle ear, such as otalgia, fever, and irritability, as well as the presence of fluid in the middle ear.[7-11] In otitis media with effusion, middle ear fluid is present, but signs and symptoms of infection are absent. Otitis media is most common in infants and children, 75% of whom have had at least one episode by the age of 1 year.[12] About 20% of otitis cases occur in adults, particularly in those with a history of these infections as a child.[13] Table 107–1 lists the risk factors for otitis media. Risk factors for otitis media owing to resistant pathogens include (1) daycare attendance, (2) prior antibiotic exposure, and (3) age younger than 2 years.[14]

PATHOPHYSIOLOGY

Acute otitis media usually follows a viral upper respiratory tract infection that causes Eustachian tube dysfunction and mucosal swelling in

TABLE 107–1. Risk Factors for Otitis Media

Winter season/outbreaks of respiratory syncytial or influenza virus
Attendance of day care centers
Lack of breastfeeding in infants
Native American or Inuit origin
Early age of first diagnosis
Nasopharyngeal colonization with middle ear pathogens
Genetic predisposition
Siblings in the home
Lower socioeconomic status
Exposure to tobacco smoke
Use of a pacifier
Male gender
Immunodeficiency
Allergy
Urban population

From refs. 11, 12, and 14.

the middle ear.[12,14] Bacteria and viruses that colonize the nasopharynx thus enter the middle ear and are not cleared properly by the mucociliary system.[7] In the presence of effusion, the bacteria proliferate and cause infection.[7,14] Children tend to be more susceptible to otitis media than adults because the anatomy of their Eustachian tube is shorter and more horizontal, facilitating bacterial entry into the middle ear.[14]

MICROBIOLOGY

S. pneumoniae is the most common bacterial cause of acute otitis media, with an incidence of 20% to 35%.[6,8,15] Nontypeable *Haemophilus influenzae* and *Moraxella catarrhalis* are each responsible for 20% to 30% and 20% of cases, respectively. Bacterial organisms that have been associated less frequently with otitis media include *Staphylococcus aureus*, *S. pyogenes,* and gram-negative bacilli such as *Pseudomonas aeruginosa.*[14] In 20% to 30% of cases, no bacterial pathogen is found, and in up to 44%, a viral etiology is found with or without concomitant bacteria.[7]

BACTERIAL RESISTANCE

Bacterial resistance to antimicrobial therapy for acute otitis media is of growing concern, particularly in view of the increasing levels of drug resistant *S. pneumoniae.* Data from the United States (1999–2000) indicate that 8.3% to 34.2% of all *S. pneumoniae* isolates are penicillin-nonsusceptible (minimum inhibitory cincentration [MIC] = 0.12–1 mcg/mL), that 12.2% to 21.5% are highly penicillin-resistant (MIC $\geq$ 2 mcg/mL), and that these rates are highly variable based on regional differences.[16,17] Canadian data from isolates collected between 1997 and 2002 indicate that 20.2% of *S. pneumoniae* isolates are penicillin-nonsusceptible.[18] High-level penicillin resistance increased from 2.4% to 13.8% from 1999 to 2002, and multidrug resistance was reported at 8.8% in 2002. Multidrug resistance in the United States is reported as 12.2% to 22.4% of *S. pneumoniae* isolates.[16,17] *Multidrug resistance* is defined as concomitant resistance to at least three different antibiotic classes. Antibiotic resistance rates with other β-lactams (penicillins other than penicillin, as well as cephalosporins), macrolides (azithromycin and clarithromycin), clindamycin, trimethoprim-sulfamethoxazole, tetracyclines, and fluoroquinolones also must be considered. In oti-

tis media, non–β-lactam antibiotic treatment is mostly considered when penicillin-allergic patients are treated or when treatment failure occurs.

S. pneumoniae resistance to amoxicillin with or without clavulanate is reported to range from 1% to 14%.[17,18] The second-generation cephalosporins that were most active were cefuroxime and cefprozil, followed by cefixime and cefaclor, with resistance rates of 6% to 12% in Canada and about 25% to 50% in the United States. The approximate rates of resistance for individual classes are clarithromyin (8% to 26%), trimethoprim-sulfamethoxazole (16% to 30%), doxycycline (4%), and levofloxacin (1%).

β-Lactamase–producing *H. influenzae* and *M. catarrhalis* are found in 23% to 35% and up to 100% of infected patients, respectively.[17,19] It is important to note that susceptibilities vary by geographic region, particularly for *H. Influenzae.*[20] While these organisms tend to cause infection that is more likely to resolve spontaneously as compared with *S. pneumoniae,* they are still pathogens that must be accounted for, particularly in treatment failures.

Bacterial resistance increases with antibiotic usage such that it is difficult to achieve an appropriate balance between antibiotic prescribing and minimizing resistance. Each time antibiotics are administered, the recipient is at increased risk of selection and carriage of resistant organisms that can be passed to others. This can lead to future antibiotic failure. Without antibiotic therapy, however, acute otitis media secondary to *S. pneumoniae* is less likely to resolve spontaneously than that from other causes. *S. pneumoniae* is increasingly resistant to penicillin, and penicillin-resistant *S. pneumoniae* is more likely to be resistant to multiple antibiotics.[15,16,18]

CLINICAL PRESENTATION AND DIAGNOSIS

Acute otitis media presents as an acute onset of signs and symptoms of middle ear infection such as otalgia, irritability, and tugging on the ear, following cold symptoms of runny nose, nasal congestion, or cough (Table 107–2).

Resolution of the symptoms of acute otitis media occurs over 1 week. Pain and fever tend to resolve after 2 to 3 days, with most children becoming asymptomatic at 7 days. Over a period of 1 week, changes in the eardrum normalize, and the pus becomes serous

TABLE 107–2. Clinical Presentation of Acute Otitis Media

General

The acute onset of signs and symptoms of middle ear infection
  following cold symptoms of runny nose, nasal congestion, or cough

Signs and Symptoms

Pain that can be severe (more than 75% of patients)
Children may be irritable, tug on the involved ear, and have difficulty
  sleeping
Fever is present in less than 25% of patients and, when present, is more
  often in younger children
Examination shows a discolored, thickened, bulging eardrum
Pneumatic otoscopy or tympanometry demonstrates an immobile
  eardrum; 50% of cases are bilateral
Draining middle ear fluid occurs (less than 3% of patients) that usually
  reveals a bacterial etiology

Laboratory Tests

Gram stain, culture, and sensitivies of draining fluid or aspirated fluid
  if tympanocentesis is performed

From ref. 7.

...iid. Air-fluid levels are apparent behind the eardrum, at which the ...age is now referred to as *otitis media with effusion*. This does not ...present ongoing infection, nor are additional antibiotics required.[12] ...titis media with effusion also can occur de novo and is thought to ...e a result of respiratory viruses. Otitis media with effusion usu-...ly occurs in spring or autumn, not winter, and may be a result ...f allergens or viruses common at these times. It also differs from ...ute otitis media in that pain is not present, nor a bulging eardrum. ...ffusions resolve slowly. At 3 months, 90% have disappeared.[10,12] ...ounger children or those with a history of recurrent infections have

a further delay in resolution.[7,12,21] Because of symptoms of viral upper respiratory tract infection (the "common cold"), antibiotics frequently are prescribed for otitis media with effusion but are not needed if duration is less than 3 months.[8] Limiting antibiotic use to documented acute otitis media would save up to $8 million annually in the United States.[8,20] Unfortunately the longer the time spent with otitis media with effusion, the higher is the likelihood of poor linguistic performance.[22,23] Complications of otitis media are infrequent but include mastoiditis, bacteremia, meningitis, and auditory sequelae.

▶ TREATMENT: Acute Otitis Media

■ DESIRED OUTCOME

...he goals of treatment of acute otitis media are the reduction in signs ...nd symptoms, eradication of the infection, and prevention of com-...lications. Avoidance of unnecessary antibiotic prescribing is another ...oal in view of the increasing problem of *S. pneumoniae* resistance.

■ GENERAL APPROACH TO TREATMENT [8]

...he management of acute otitis media is not without controversy. ...or example, a systematic review of studies demonstrated that an-...microbial therapy provides resolution of symptoms in about 95% of ...atients, whereas about 80% of placebo-treated patients also have a ...esolution of symptoms.[21,24] Although only a small benefit has been ...ound, antimicrobial treatment is still considered an appropriate man-...gement strategy.[15] However, the choices of which patient should re-...eive antimicrobials, which antimicrobial regimen, and at what point ...ntibiotics should be given after diagnosis require further evalua-...on. Generally, otitis media is treated empirically without laboratory ...ests.

■ NONPHARMACOLOGIC THERAPY

...cetaminophen or a nonsteroidal anti-inflammatory agent such as ...buprofen can be used to relieve pain and malaise in acute otitis media. ...Decongestants, antihistamines, topical corticosteroids, and expecto-...ants have not been proved effective for acute otitis media.[10,26] Side ...ffects associated with these treatments also may be unpleasant. ...   Surgical insertion of tympanostomy tubes (T-tubes) is an ef-...ective method for the prevention of recurrent otitis media. These ...mall tubes are placed through the inferior portion of the tympanic ...nembrane under general anesthesia and aerate the middle ear. Chil-...lren with recurrent otitis who have more than three episodes in ...months or four or more episodes (one of which is recent) in a year ...hould be considered for T-tube placement. If these children have ...noderate to severe nasal obstruction in addition to recurrent otitis, ...denoidectomy may be of benefit. Tonsillectomy, however, is not in-...licated for the treatment of otitis media. Although T-tube insertion is ...ffective for many, some children may require subsequent surgeries. ...Repeat T-tube placement with adenoidectomy (regardless of adenoid ...ize) should be considered if the child continues to have episodes of ...cute otitis media after extrusion of the original T-tubes.

■ PHARMACOLOGIC THERAPY

■ ANTIMICROBIAL THERAPY

Acute otitis media must be distinguished from otitis media with effusion. Antimicrobials are indicated only in the former unless the effusion persists beyond 3 months in otitis media with effusion. Middle ear effusion in acute otitis media tends to continue after antimicrobial therapy is completed but does not require retreatment.

Studies have not demonstrated any one antimicrobial agent to be superior in the treatment of acute uncomplicated otitis media.[21] Amoxicillin is considered the drug of choice regardless of the prevalence of drug resistant *S. pneumoniae*.[6,15] Amoxicillin has the best pharmacodynamic profile (time above the minimum inhibitory concentration [MIC_{90}] in the middle ear fluid for more than 40% of the dosing interval) against drug-resistant *S. pneumoniae* of all available oral agents, it has a long record of safety, it possesses a narrow spectrum, and it is inexpensive.[20] Its excellent efficacy against *S. pneumoniae* outweighs the issue of β-lactamase–producing *H. influenzae* and *M. catarrhalis*, against which amoxicillin may not be effective. This is so because *H. influenzae* and *M. catarrhalis* are both more likely to lead to a spontaneous resolution of the infection compared with *S. pneumoniae*.

❸   Amoxicillin is the drug of choice for acute otitis media. High-dose amoxicillin (80–90 mg/kg per day) is recommended if drug-resistant *S. pneumoniae* is suspected or a patient is at high risk for a resistant infection. Treatment recommendations for acute otitis media are found in Table 107–3. Patients who have received a course of antibiotics within the last 3 months are considered high risk. Higher middle ear fluid concentrations of amoxicillin as a result of higher dosing should overcome drug-resistant *S. pneumoniae* even with its increased MIC.[27] Some clinicians have expressed concerns, however, about the increased risk of adverse effects and patient noncompliance associated with high-dose amoxicillin.

If treatment failure occurs with amoxicillin, an agent should be chosen with activity against β-lactamase–producing *H. influenzae* and *M. catarrhalis*, as well as drug-resistant *S. pneumoniae*.[14,20] Examples include amoxicillin-clavulanate, cefuroxime, and intramuscular ceftriaxone. Second-generation cephalosporins, while β-lactamase–stable, are expensive, have an increased incidence of side effects, and may increase selective pressure for resistant bacteria. They also are less effective against drug-resistant *S. pneumoniae*. Consideration also must be given to the fact that most cephalosporins do not achieve adequate middle ear fluid concentrations against drug-resistant *S. pneumoniae* for the desired duration over the dosing interval. Oral cephalosporins that may be tried include cefuroxime (as advocated by the Centers for Disease Control and Prevention [CDC]

TABLE 107–3. Acute Otitis Media Treatment Recommendations[a,b]

Antibiotic Therapy in Prior Month	Day 0	Clinically Defined Treatment Failure Day 3	Clinically Defined Treatment Failure Days 10 to 28
No	Amoxicillin usual dose 40–45 mg/kg/day	Amoxicillin-clavulanate high dose[d] Amoxicillin component 80–90 mg/kg/day clavulanate component 6.4 mg/kg/day	Same as day 3
	Amoxicillin high dose 80–90 mg/kg/day (high-risk patients)	Cefuroxime axetil Suspension: 30 mg/kg/day divided twice daily (max: 1 g) Tablets: 250 mg twice daily Intramuscular ceftriaxone 1 g (50 mg/kg) daily for 3 days	
Yes	Amoxicillin high dose 80–90 mg/kg/day	Intramuscular ceftriaxone 1 g (50 mg/kg) daily for 3 days	Amoxicillin-clavulanate high dose[d] Amoxicillin component 80–90 mg/kg/day Clavulanate component 6.4 mg/kg/day
	Amoxicillin-clavulanate high dose[d] Amoxicillin component 80–90 mg/kg/day Clavulanate component 6.4 mg/kg/day Cefuroxime axetil Suspension: 30 mg/kg/day divided twice daily (max: 1 g) Tablets: 250 mg twice daily	Clindamycin[c] 10–30 mg/kg/day divided every 6–8 hours (max: 1.8 g/day) Tympanocentesis	Cefuroxime axetil Suspension: 30 mg/kg/day divided twice daily (max: 1 g) Tablets: 250 mg twice daily Intramuscular ceftriaxone 1 g (50 mg/kg) daily for 3 days Tympanocentesis

[a]These recommendations are made by a group convened by the Centers for Disease Control.
[b]The recommended duration of treatment for oral therapy is 7 to 10 days.
[c]Clindamycin is only recommended in cases of documented *S. pneumoniae*. It is not effective against *H. influenzae* or *M. catarrhalis*.
[d]Higher doses of clavulanate produce a significant increase in diarrhea.
From refs. 8 and 15.

guidelines), as well as cefprozil or cefpodoxime.[11,15] Intramuscular ceftriaxone is the only agent other than amoxicillin that achieves middle ear fluid concentrations above the MIC for more than 40% of the dosing interval.[20] While single doses have been used, daily doses for 3 days are recommended to optimize clinical outcomes.[14,15] Ceftriaxone should be reserved for severe and unresponsive infections or for patients in whom oral medication is inappropriate because of vomiting, diarrhea, or possible nonadherence. Ceftriaxone is an expensive agent, and the intramuscular injections generally are not appealing to young patients. Tympanocentesis also can be considered for treatment failure. It has a therapeutic effect of relieving pain and pressure and can be used to collect fluid to identify the causative agent. This procedure, however, is not frequently performed in practice.[9,14]

CLINICAL CONTROVERSY

It is not clear when antibiotics should be prescribed for acute otitis media—at the onset of signs and symptoms or after 48 to 72 hours to allow assessment for a spontaneous resolution. In general, the North American approach is to institute empirical treatment immediately. In some European countries such as the Netherlands, the practice is not to initiate treatment initially, but rather to treat a child 6 months to 2 years of age only if he or she does not improve by 24 hours or an older child by 72 hours.

Patients with penicillin allergy can be treated with several alternative antibiotics. Some clinicians feel that the incidence of cross-reaction is sufficiently low that use of a cephalosporin is warranted in patients who have not experienced immediate penicillin hypersensitivity reactions. Others prefer to use a macrolide such as azithromycin or clarithromycin, erythromycin-sulfisoxazole, trimethoprim-sulfamethoxazole, or if *S. pneumoniae* is documented, clindamycin as alternative agents. However, the incidence of resistance is much higher with these agents,[9,14] and of these agents, only clindamycin is recommended by the CDC guidelines.[15]

◼ DELAYED ANTIMICROBIAL THERAPY

It is difficult to identify who will benefit from antimicrobial therapy. With or without treatment, about 60% of children who have acute otitis media are symptom-free within 24 hours. In almost 40% of the remaining children, antibiotic use reduces the duration of symptoms by about 1 day.[28,29] A trial of 315 children (6 months to 10 years of age) compared immediate antibiotic treatment with a 72-hour delay in treatment that was to be given only if the child had not improved. Symptoms continued for 1 extra day in 10% to 20% of the delayed-therapy group, but 10% fewer also experienced diarrhea. At 3 days, there was no difference in symptoms. In the delayed-therapy group, only 24% of children eventually received antibiotics, and 77% of parents reported being satisfied with this approach.[30]

Delayed treatment decreases antibiotic use by 31% (and associated side effects) and minimizes bacterial resistance to rates as low as 30% to 50% of that in countries that do not delay antimicrobial therapy.[31,32] Some clinicians feel that delayed treatment is not dvisable in children younger than 2 years of age, those with recent ntimicrobial exposure, or when underlying conditions exist because hese patients are at increased risk of susceptibility to invasive disease nd resistant bacerial infections.[11]

If delayed therapy is tried, use of appropriate pain medi-ation, such as oral ibuprofen or acetaminophen, should be ad-ised. If a child 6 months to 2 years of age does not improve by 4 hours or an older child by 72 hours, antibiotic treatment should be nitiated.[31]

In addition to the desire for immediate symptom improvement, revention of mastoiditis and meningitis has been suggested as a rea-on to prescribe immediate antibiotic treatment for acute otitis media. he rates of mastoiditis in the Netherlands, Norway, and Denmark all countries in which delayed therapy has been adopted) and those n Canada, the United States, Australia, and the United Kingdom vere compared.[32] The delay of antibiotic use resulted in an in-rease from about 2 to 4 cases of mastoiditis per 100,000 children er year, accompanied by about 1600 fewer children per 100,000 xperiencing antibiotic side effects. Of note, in the Netherlands, nly 1.1% of infections caused by *S. pneumoniae* are penicillin-esistant.

SHORT COURSES OF THERAPY

2 A meta-analysis of 32 trials[33] reported no difference in effect (cure rates) after short (<7 days) and usual durations (≥7 days) of antibiotic therapy in children. The authors suggest that 5 days of therapy is effective in acute uncomplicated otitis media. The advan-tages of short-term therapy are an increased likelihood the patient will adhere to the full course of treatment and decreased bacterial selective pressure for both the individual and the community. The disadvan-tages are that the data are not well established for complicated or recurrent acute otitis media, and there are inadequate data to support short treatment courses in children younger than 2 years of age.[34]

CLINICAL CONTROVERSY

The optimal duration of antimicrobial therapy for otitis media has not been established. Some studies have demonstrated efficacy with 3 to 5 days of therapy in acute uncomplicated otitis media. However, high-risk populations, e.g., children younger than 3 years of age and those with resistant or recur-rent infections, were not studied.

EVALUATION OF THERAPEUTIC OUTCOMES

Treatment failure is a lack of clinical improvement after 3 days n the signs and symptoms of infection, including pain, fever, and edness/bulging of the tympanic membrane. Early reevaluation of he eardrum when signs and symptoms are improving can be mis-eading because effusions persist. A concern that requires evalua-tion after otitis infections is hearing loss resulting from persis-ent middle ear effusions. Examination of an asymptomatic child nay be delayed until 3 months after the infection began, at which ime the continued presence of fluid should prompt a hearing valuation.[10]

ANTIBIOTIC PROPHYLAXIS OF RECURRENT INFECTIONS

Recurrent otitis media is defined as at least three episodes in 6 months or at least four episodes in 12 months. Recurrent infections are of con-ern because patients younger than 3 years of age are at high risk for earing loss and language and learning disabilities.[11] Data from stud-es generally do not favor prophylaxis. A meta-analysis demonstrated hat prophylaxis against these infections leads to a reduction of 0.11 episodes per month.[35] This translates into one infection prevented each time one child is treated for 9 months. Prophylaxis is even less effective in those with effusion. Amoxicillin 20 mg/kg per day and ulfisoxazole 75 mg/kg per day have been evaluated. Success with ulfizoxazole generally is thought to be better because it results in ess carriage of resistant organisms; however, side effects are much vorse (i.e., rash, mouth sores, and potential for blood dyscrasias). Of further concern is antibiotic resistance as a result of continued use of these antibiotics. For this reason, treatment can be delayed until he onset of symptoms of an upper respiratory tract infection (viral symptoms). Another approach is to limit antibiotic prophylaxis dura-ion to 6 months and during the winter months.[11] T-tube placement, denoidectomy, and tonsillectomy may be of value in children with ecurrent treatment failure.

VACCINATION

4 Vaccination against influenza and pneumococcus may decrease the risk of acute otitis media, especially in those with recurrent episodes. Immunization with the influenza vaccine has been associ-ated with up to a 36% reduction in the incidence of acute otitis me-dia infection.[36] Others have described a benefit during the influenza season.[12,37] The influenza vaccine can be administered to any healthy person without contraindications, especially individuals with chronic disease who are at least 6 months of age.[6,15] Some clinicians feel that the data do not justify universal influenza vaccination but that it is warranted for high-risk patients, including those younger than 2 years of age.[25]

A conjugate pneumococcal vaccine that is indicated in infants and children has become available and provides a 6% reduction in the frequency of acute otitis media and a 20% reduction in the need for placement of a T-tube.[38] Also, vaccine use has demonstrated an 8% decrease in office visits, as well as a 10% to 26% decrease in otitis media episodes in children who experienced 3 to 10 infections per year.[39] Pneumococcal congugate vaccine is recommended for all children aged 2 to 23 months; it is also recommended for those 24 to 59 months of age who are at high risk of invasive disease.[6,40] Previ-ously unvaccinated children older than age 1 who have had recurrent otitis media infections do not benefit from later vaccination.[41]

SINUSITIS

Sinusitis is an inflammation and/or infection of the paranasal sinus mucosa.[42–44] The term *rhinosinusitis* is used by some specialists be-cause sinusitis typically also involves the nasal mucosa.[42,44–46] The majority of these infections are viral in origin; nevertheless, antimi-crobials are prescribed frequently. It is thus important to differentiate between viral and bacterial sinusitis to aid in optimizing treatment decisions.

5 Viral sinusitis and bacterial sinusitis are difficult to differ-entiate because their clinical presentations are similar. Viral

TABLE 107–4. Clinical Presentation and Diagnosis of Bacterial Sinusitis[42–44,46–49]

General

A nonspecific upper respiratory tract infection that persists beyond 7 to 14 days

Signs and Symptoms

Acute

  Adults:

Nasal discharge/congestion

Maxillary tooth pain, facial or sinus pain that may radiate (unilateral in particular) as well as deterioration after initial improvement

Severe or persistent (beyond 7 days) signs and symptoms are most likely bacterial and should be treated with antimicrobials

  Children:

    Nasal discharge and cough for greater than 10 to 14 days or severe signs and symptoms such as temperature above 39°C or facial swelling or pain are indications for antimicrobial therapy

Chronic

  Symptoms are similar to acute sinusitis but more nonspecific

  Rhinorrhea is associated with acute exacerbations

  Chronic unproductive cough, laryngitis, and headache may occur

  Chronic/recurrent infections occur 3 to 4 times a year and are unresponsive to steam and decongestants

From refs. 42–44 and 46–49.

infections, however, tend to resolve by 7 to 10 days. Persistence of symptoms beyond this time likely indicates a bacterial infection. Bacterial sinusitis can be categorized into acute and chronic disease. Acute disease lasts less than 30 days with complete resolution of symptoms.[42–44,47] Chronic sinusitis is defined as episodes of inflammation lasting more than 3 months with persistence of respiratory symptoms.[42,43,48]

Sinusitis is diagnosed more frequently in children than in adults. Typical clinical presentation and diagnosis of bacterial sinusitis are illustrated in Table 107–4. Between 5% and 13% of viral upper respiratory tract infections in children are complicated by bacterial sinusitis,[46,47] whereas only 0.5% to 2% of viral upper respiratory tract infections in adults are complicated by sinusitis.[42–44,4] Factors associated with the development of bacterial sinusitis include viral respiratory tract infections and, less commonly, allergic inflammation.[46] Other factors that can be associated with sinus disease include systemic diseases, trauma, environmental exposures, and anatomic abnormalities.[44,46,49]

PATHOPHYSIOLOGY

Similar to acute otitis media, acute sinusitis usually is preceded by a viral respiratory tract infection that causes mucosal inflammation.[43,45] This can lead to obstruction of the sinus ostia—the pathways that drain the sinuses. Mucosal secretions become trapped, local defenses are impaired, and bacteria from adjacent surfaces begin to proliferate.[42,44] The pathogenesis of chronic sinusitis has not been well studied. Whether it is caused by more persistent pathogens or there is a subtle defect in the host's immune function, some patients develop chronic symptoms after their acute infection.[44,46,51,52]

MICROBIOLOGY

Viruses are responsible for most cases of acute sinusitis; however, when symptoms are persistent (≥7 days) or severe, bacteria may be a primary cause or the cause of secondary infection.[42] Acute sinusitis that is bacterial in origin is caused most often by the same bacteria implicated in acute otitis media: *S. pneumoniae* and *H. influenzae*.[1,43–46,50] These organisms are responsible for about 70% of bacterial causes of acute sinusitis in both adults and children.[45,48] *M. catarrhalis* is also frequently implicated in children (25%).[44–46] *Streptococcus pyogenes, Staphylococcus aureus,* fungi, and anaerobes have been associated less frequently with acute sinusitis.[42,47] Chronic sinusitis can be polymicrobial with an increased prevalence of anaerobes, as well as less common pathogens, including gram-negative bacilli and fungi.[44] Issues of bacterial resistance are similar to those found with otitis media and are further addressed in that section of this chapter.

▶ TREATMENT: Sinusitis

■ DESIRED OUTCOME

The goals of treatment of acute sinusitis are the reduction in signs and symptoms, achieving and maintaining patency of the ostia, limiting antimicrobial treatment to those who may benefit, eradication of bacterial infection with appropriate antimicrobial therapy, minimizing the duration of illness, prevention of complications, and prevention of progression from acute disease to chronic disease.[43–45,47,51]

■ GENERAL APPROACH TO TREATMENT

Approximately 40% to 60% of patients with acute sinusitis will recover spontaneously (these are likely patients with viral sinusitis).[45,48] When the decision to treat with antimicrobials thus is made, the choice must be effective and safe, and cost must be considered.

CLINICAL CONTROVERSY

Is antimicrobial treatment warranted in bacterial sinusitis? Since most studies have not used sinus aspiration to diagnose bacterial sinusitis, many patients with viral infections likely have diluted the results of studies of antimicrobial therapy. It is recommended that patients with mild acute sinusitis can be given decongestants and reassurance, whereas those with moderate to severe disease for 7 days or more and those with severe disease should be given antimicrobial therapy.

■ NONPHARMACOLOGIC THERAPY

Data regarding supportive therapy are limited, but such therapy may be useful. Nasal decongestant sprays such as phenylephrine and oxymetazoline that reduce inflammation by vasoconstriction are used often in sinusitis.[42,44,46] Use should be limited to the recommended duration of the product to prevent rebound congestion. Oral decongestants also may aid in nasal/sinus patency.[48] To reduce mucociliary function, irrigation of the nasal cavity with saline and steam inhalation may be used to increase mucosal moisture, and mucolytics (e.g., guaifenesin) may be used to decrease the viscosity of nasal secretions.[42,46]

Antihistamines should not be used for acute bacterial sinusitis in view of their anticholineric effects that can dry mucosa and disturb clearance of mucosal secretions.[48] Second-generation antihistamines may play a role in chronic sinusitis where allergy is a component.[49] Glucocorticoids intranasally decrease tissue inflammation and edema[44]; however, delayed onset limits their usefulness in acute sinusitis.

PHARMACOLOGIC THERAPY

ANTIMICROBIAL THERAPY

Two meta-analyses have demonstrated that antimicrobial therapy is superior to placebo in reducing or eliminating symptoms, although the benefit is small.[46,54] Two randomized, controlled, double-blind studies reported conflicting results as to the value of antimicrobial therapy.[30,55] Neither used sinus aspiration for diagnosis. The study that showed no benefit with antibiotic treatment had two major flaws.[55] Radiography was used for diagnosis of sinusitis, and duration of illness was not specified. Viral infection thus was likely present in a number of patients, complicating evaluation of antimicrobial usefulness. The second study[50] demonstrated the effectiveness of penicillin and amoxicillin in patients with at least 7 days of illness and findings of sinusitis on computed tomography. Because of more rigorous inclusion criteria and better diagnostic tools, patients with bacterial sinusitis were included, and those with viral sinusitis were more likely excluded.

Amoxicillin is first-line treatment for acute bacterial sinusitis. Since there is no difference in clinical outcome among antibiotics, the advantages of amoxicillin include proven efficacy and safety, a relatively narrow antibacterial spectrum that minimizes emergence of resistance, good tolerability, and low cost. Most consensus reports and reviews consider amoxicillin as first-line treatment for acute bac-

TABLE 107–5. Approach to Treatment of Acute Bacterial Sinusitis

Uncomplicated Sinusitis	Amoxicillin
Uncomplicated sinusitis, penicillin-allergic patient	Immediate-type hypersensitivity: Clarithromycin or azithromycin or trimethoprim-sulfamethoxazole Nonimmediate-type hypersensitivity: β-Lactamase–stable cephalosporin
Treatment failure or prior antibiotic therapy in past 4 to 6 weeks	High-dose amoxicillin with clavulanate or β-lactamase–stable cephalosporin
High suspicion of penicillin-resistant S. pneumoniae	High-dose amoxicillin or clindamycin

From refs. 43–48.

terial sinusitis (Table 107–5). It is cost-effective in acute uncomplicated disease, and intial use of newer broad-spectrum agents is not justified.[43,46–48,56,57] If a patient is penicillin-allergic, azithromycin or clarithromycin may be used. In adults, a quinolone such as levofloxacin is an alternative in the penicillin-allergic patient. If the penicillin allergy is not a true IgE-mediated reaction (e.g., hives or anaphylaxis), a second-generation cephalosporin may be used (e.g., cefprozil, cefuroxime, or cefpodoxime).[47,58]

If drug-resistant S. pneumoniae is highly suspected (day-care attendance, recent antibiotic use, age younger than 2 years), high-dose amoxicillin should be given. Some recommend clindamycin, but it is important to note that this drug is not active against H. influenzae and M. catarrhalis.[43,47]

In the case of treatment failure with amoxicillin (i.e., no improvement in symptoms 72 hours after starting therapy) or in patients who have received antimicrobial therapy in the prior 4 to 6 weeks, improved coverage of H. influenzae and M. catarrhalis with either high-dose amoxicillin plus clavulanate or a β-lactamase–stable cephalosporin that covers S. pneumoniae (e.g., cefprozil, cefuroxime, or cefpodoxime[IS1]) is suggested.[45,47] Other alternatives include[IS2][IS3] cefdinir, azithromycin, clarithromycin, and trimethoprim-sulfamethoxazole.[44,47] Clinical cure rates are similar among antimicrobial agents,[56,57] although local-area resistance rates also must be considered. Increasing resistance of S. pneumoniae,

TABLE 107–6. Dosing Guidelines for Acute Bacterial Sinusitis

Drug	Adult Dosage	Pediatric Dosage
Amoxicillin	500 mg three times daily High dose = 1 g three times daily	Low dose: 40–50 mg/kg/day divided in 3 doses High dose: 80–100 mg/kg/day divided in 3 doses
Amoxicillin-clavulanate	500/125 mg three times daily	40–50 mg/kg/day divided in 3 doses High dose: Can add 40–50 mg/kg/day amoxicillin
Cefuroxime	250–500 mg twice daily	15 mg/kg/day divided in 2 doses
Cefaclor	250–500 mg three times daily	20 mg/kg/day divided in 3 doses
Cefixime	200–400 mg twice daily	8 mg/kg/day in 1 dose or divided in 2 doses
Cefdinir	600 mg daily or divided in 2 doses	14 mg/kg/day in 1 dose or divided in 2 doses
Cefpodoxime	200 mg twice daily	10 mg/kg/day in 2 divided doses (max: 400 mg daily)
Cefprozil	250–500 mg twice daily	15–30 mg/kg/day divided in 2 doses
Trimethoprim-sulfamethoxazole	160/800 mg every 12 hours	6–8 mg/kg/day trimethoprim, 30–40 mg/kg/day sulfamethoxazole divided in 2 doses
Clindamycin	150–450 mg every 6 hours	30–40 mg/kg/day divided in 3 doses
Clarithromycin	250–500 mg twice daily	15 mg/kg/day divided in 2 doses
Azithromycin	500 mg day 1, then 250 mg/day × 4 days	10 mg/kg day 1, then 5 mg/kg/day × 4 days
Levofloxacin	500 mg daily	N/A

N/A = not applicable.
From refs. 44, 47, 48, 58, and 59.

H. influenzae, and *M. catarrhalis* to trimethoprim-sulfamethoxazole and resistance of *S. pneumoniae* to macrolides must be taken into consideration. See Table 107–6 for dosing guidelines.

Duration of therapy for treatment of sinusitis is not well established. Most trials have used 10- to 14-day antimicrobial courses, although some trials also have investigated courses as short as 3 days.[60] In one placebo-controlled comparision of 3- versus 10-day treatment with trimethoprim-sulfamethoxazole and decongestant, a similar number in each group were cured or improved at 14 days. Since the publication of this study, however, rates of resistant *S. pneumoniae* have increased dramatically, and trimethprim-sulfamethoxazole is not an effective agent against resistant *S. pneumoniae.* Furthermore, extrapolation of these results to other antimicrobials is not appropriate. Therefore, the current recommendations are 10 to 14 days of antimicrobial therapy or at least 7 days after signs and symptoms are under control.[43–45,48]

EVALUATION OF THERAPEUTIC OUTCOMES

Antimicrobial therapy reduces the median duration of illness from 17 to 9 to 11 days.[50] A patient with persistence or worsening of symptoms 72 hours after initiating antimicrobial therapy may be considered a treatment failure.[45] Referral to a specialist should be considered in patients who have not responded to first- or second-line therapy, those with recurrent and chronic disease, and patients at risk for complications. Surgery may be considered in more complicated patients.

PHARYNGITIS

Pharyngitis is an acute infection of the oropharynx or nasopharynx.[61] It results in 1% to 2% of all outpatient visits.[62] While viral causes are most common, group A β-hemolytic *Streptococcus,* or *S. pyogenes,* is the primary bacterial cause and is the focus of this section.[61,63] In the pediatric population, group A *Streptococcus,* or "strep throat," causes 15% to 30% of cases of pharyngitis. In adults, it is the cause of 5% to 15% of all symptomatic episodes of pharyngitis.[61–64]

MICROBIOLOGY

Viruses cause most of the cases of acute pharyngitis. Specific etiologic agents include rhinovirus (20%), coronavirus (≥5%), adenovirus (5%), influenza virus (2%), parainfluenza virus (2%), and Epstein-Barr virus (>1%).[61,63] A bacterial etiology for acute pharyngitis is far less likely. Out of all the bacterial causes, group A *Streptococcus* is the most common (15% to 30% of persons of all ages with pharyngitis[52]), and it is the the only commonly occurring form of acute pharyngitis for which antimicrobial therapy is indicated.[52,61]

Other less common causes of acute pharyngitis include groups C and G Streptococcus, *Corynebacterium diphtheriae, Neisseria gonorrhoeae, M. pneumoniae, Arcanobacterium haemolyticum, Yersinia enterocolitica,* and *Chlamydia pneumoniae.* Treatment options for these organisms will not be addressed in this chapter.[61,63]

PATHOPHYSIOLOGY

The mechanism by which group A *Streptococcus* causes pharyngitis is not well defined.[52] Asymptomatic pharyngeal carriers of the organism may have an alteration in host immunity (e.g., a breach in the pharyngeal mucosa) and the bacteria of the oropharynx, allowing colonization to become infection. Pathogenic factors associated wtih the organism itself also may play a role. These include the antiphagocytic M protein, erythrogenic toxins, hemolysins, streptokinase, and proteinase.

Group A streptococcal pharyngitis is difficult to differentiate from viral pharyngitis based on history and clinical findings. However, although all age groups are susceptible, epidemiologic data show that certain groups are at higher risk for group A streptococcal pharyngitis. Children aged 5 to 15 years old are most susceptible, and parents of school-age children and those who work with children are also at increased risk. Pharyngitis in a child younger than 3 years of age is rarely due to group A *Streptococcus.*[52]

Seasonal outbreaks occur, and the occurrence of group A streptococcal pharyngitis is highest in winter and early spring.[61,65] The incubation period is 2 to 5 days, and the illness often occurs in clusters.[62,6] Spread occurs via direct contact with droplets of saliva or nasal secretions, and transmission is thus worse in institutions, schools, families, and areas of crowding.[64,66] See Table 107–7 for clinical presentation and diagnosis of pharyngitis.

Nonsuppurative complications such as acute rheumatic fever, acute glomerulonephritis, and reactive arthritis may occur, as well as suppurative complications, such as peritonsillar abcess, retropharyngeal abscess, cervical lymphadenitis, mastoiditis, otitis media, sinusitis, and necrotizing fasciitis.

Acute rheumatic fever is seen rarely in developed countries. Acute rheumatic fever secondary to group A streptococcal infection was a cause of concern in the 1950s and was the major reason for penicillin therapy, but the incidence of this disease today is extremely rare (>1 in 1 million). However, the risk remains. Outbreaks have been reported in the United States as recently as the late 1980s and early 1990s. Furthermore, acute rheumatic fever is widespread in developing countries (e.g., it is estimated that there are 50,000 cases of acute rheumatic fever per year in India).

TABLE 107–7. Clinical Presentation and Diagnosis of Group A Streptococcal Pharyngitis

General
A sore throat of sudden onset that is mostly self-limited
Fever and constitutional symptoms resolving in about 3 to 5 days
Clinical signs and symptoms are similar for viral causes as well as nonstreptococcal bacterial causes

Signs and Symptoms
Sore throat
Pain on swallowing
Fever
Headache, nausea, vomiting, and abdominal pain (especially children)
Erythema/inflammation of the tonsils and pharynx with or without patchy exudates
Enlarged, tender lymph nodes
Red swollen uvula, petechiae on the soft palate, and a scarlatiniform rash
Several symptoms that are not suggestive of group A *Streptococcus* are cough, conjunctivitis, coryza, and diarrhea

Laboratory Tests
Throat swab and culture or rapid antigen detection testing

From refs. 52, 61–65, 67, and 68.

DIAGNOSIS

For a patient presenting with pharyngitis, the most important clinical decision that needs to be made is whether the pharyngitis is caused by group A *Streptococcus*. Diagnosis is essential because it it directs management.

Clinical scoring systems such as the Centor criteria[69] have been advocated for diagnosis in adults to overcome the lack of sensitivity and specificity of clinician judgment and to avoid laboratory testing of all patients.[62,64] These criteria include history of fever, tonsillar exudates, absence of cough, and presence of enlarged lymph nodes. However, there is concern that use of these criteria will lead to over-prescribing because they give physicians the option of a "no test" strategy, where prescriptions can be written based purely on the clinical criteria.[61,63] Guidelines from the Infectious Disease Society of America, the American Academy of Pediatrics, and the American Heart Association suggest that testing be done in all patients with signs and symptoms. Only those with a positive test for group A *Streptococcus* require antibiotic treatment.[61,65,70]

A combined approach would take into account the prevalence of group A streptococcal disease (which differs by age group and geography) and history of a close contact of a well-documented case, along with clinical criteria, to aid in assessing a patient's risk of the disease. If the diagnosis cannot be excluded at this point,

laboratory testing is recommended to confirm or exclude group A *Streptococcus* as the cause of pharyngitis. It is important to note that laboratory testing should not be used without consideration of clinical criteria. This is so because a positive test does not necessarily indicate disease. A positive test may indicate carriage (but not active infection) with group A *Streptococcus*. The incidence of carriage in children is 5% to 20% and is considerably lower in adults.[52,65]

There are several options to test for group A streptococcal pharyngitis. A throat swab can be sent for culture or used for rapid antigen-detection testing (RADT). RADT is more practical in that it gives results quickly, it can be done at the bedside, and it is less expensive than culture. Cultures are the "gold standard" and have a 90% sensitivity but require 24 to 48 hours for results.[63] Cultures are recommended for children, adolescents, parents, and schoolteachers with negative RADT tests (which have a sensitivity below 80%), as well as in situations of outbreak or to monitor resistance.[64,65,67] Delaying therapy while awaiting test results does not affect the risk of complications (although some argue that symptomatic benefit is postponed), and patients must be educated as to the value of waiting. Newer RADT tests use optical immunoassay and chemiluminescent DNA probes, but the cost of such tests may be prohibitive, and results of individual tests should be compared with cultures to validate their sensitivity in practice.[65]

▶ TREATMENT: Pharyngitis

DESIRED OUTCOME

The goals of treatment of pharyngitis are to improve clinical signs and symptoms, minimize adverse drug reactions, prevent transmission to close contacts, and prevent acute rheumatic fever and suppurative complications, such as peritonsillar abscess, cervical lymphadenitis, and mastoiditis.[61,62]

GENERAL APPROACH TO TREATMENT

Antimicrobial therapy should be limited to those who have clinical and epidemiologic features of group A streptococcal pharyngitis with a positive laboratory test.

NONPHARMACOLOGIC THERAPY

Since pain is often the primary reason for visiting a physician, emphasis on analgesics such as acetaminophen and nonsteroidal anti-inflammatory drugs (NSAIDs) to aid in pain relief is strongly recommended.[71] However, acetaminophen is a better option because there is some concern that NSAIDs may increase the risk for necrotizing fasciitis/toxic shock syndrome. Toxic shock syndrome has been linked to GAS pharyngitis. Either systemic or topical analgesics can be used, as well as antipyretics and other supportive care, including rest, fluids, lozenges, and saltwater gargles. Symptoms may resolve 1 to 2 days sooner with such interventions.[62–64]

PHARMACOLOGIC THERAPY

ANTIMICROBIAL THERAPY

Antimicrobial therapy decreases the duration of signs and symptoms by 1 to 2 days.[62,72] Therapy also decreases the severity of symptoms when initiated within 2 to 3 days of onset in patients with proven group A *Streptococcus*. Microbiological eradication will occur in 48 to 72 hours, which aids in decreasing transmission.[62]

Antimicrobial treatment should be limited to those who have clinical and epidemiologic features of group A streptococcal pharyngitis with a positive laboratory test. Penicillin is the drug of choice in the treatment of group A streptococcal pharyngitis[61,62] (Table 107–8). It has the narrowest spectrum of activity, and it is effective, safe, and inexpensive. The only controlled studies that have demonstrated that antimicrobial therapy prevents rheumatic fever were done with procaine penicillin, which was later replaced with benzathine penicillin.[73,74]

The evidence that treatment of group A streptococcal pharyngitis prevents rheumatic fever comes solely from studies using depot intramuscular penicillin. Penicillin given by other routes has been assumed to be equally efficacious. The ability of other antibiotics to eradicate group A *Streptococcus* has led to extrapolation that these agents also will prevent rheumatic fever.[64] Amoxicillin can be used in children because the suspension has a better taste than that of penicillin.[61,66] Gastrointestinal side effects and rash, however, are more common. In patients allergic to penicillin, a macrolide such as erythromycin or a first-generation cephalosporin such as cephalexin (if the reaction is non–IgE-mediated hypersensitivity with hives or anaphylaxis) can be used.[61] Newer macrolides such as azithromycin and clarithromycin are equally effective as erythromycin and cause fewer gastrointestinal adverse effects.

TABLE 107–8. Dosing Guidelines for Pharyngitis

Drug	Adult Dosage	Pediatric Dosage	Duration
Penicillin VK	250 three times daily or four times daily or 500 mg twice daily	50 mg/kg/day divided in 3 doses	10 days
Penicillin benzathine	1.2 million units intramuscularly	0.6 million units for under 27 kg (50,000 units/kg)	One dose
Penicillin G procaine and benzathine mixture	Not recommended in adolescents and adults	1.2 million units (benzathine 0.9 million units, procaine 0.3 million units)	One dose
Amoxicillin	500 mg three times daily	40–50 mg/kg/day divided in 3 doses	10 days
Erythromycin			10 days
Estolate	20–40 mg/kg/day divided two to four times daily (max: 1 g/day)	Same as adults	
Stearate	1 g daily divided two to four times daily (adolescents, adults)	—	
Ethylsuccinate	40 mg/kg/day divided two to four times daily (max: 1 g/day)	Same as adults	
Cephalexin	250–500 mg PO four times daily	25–50 mg/kg/day divided in 4 doses	10 days

From refs. 61, 63, 65, and 79.

Second-generation cephalosporins, such as cefuroxime and cefprozil, or third-generation cephalosporins, such as cefpodoxime and cefdinir, which are β-lactamase–stable, have been advocated for clinical failures with penicillin. In cases of documented macrolide resistance (owinng to low-level macrolide resistance—erythromycin MIC 1–8 mcg/mL—caused by expression of the *mefA/E* gene leading to efflux of macrolide out of the bacterial cell), clindamycin is an alternative. The new ketolides such as telithromycin also may have a role to play, especially in regions with a high prevalence of macrolide-resistant strains. If patients are unable to take oral medications, intramuscular benzathine penicillin can be given, although it is painful and is no longer available in Canada.[61] Amoxicillin-clavulanate or clindamycin may be considered for recurrent episodes to maximize bacterial eradication in potential carriers and to counter copathogens that produce β-lactamases.[61,65,67] Tables 107–8 and 107–9 outline dosing for acute and recurrent episodes of pharyngitis.

To date, no resistance of group A *Streptococcus* to penicillin has been reported in clinical isolates.[61,62,65,75] Macrolide resistance is low (>5%) and is not widespread.[75,76] However, there have been reports of an outbreak of macrolide-resistant group A streptococcal pharyngitis in the United States. The concern is that if macrolide use continues to increase, macrolide resistance rates also will increase.[77,78] Therefore, use of newer macrolides as first-line therapy is discouraged in febrile patients with upper respiratory tract infections. Group A *Streptococcus* resistance rates to tetracyclines and sulfonamides are high; therefore, use of these agents is no longer recommended.[61]

CLINICAL CONTROVERSY

The duration of therapy for group A streptococcal pharyngitis is 10 days to maximize bacterial eradication.[61] Short-course therapy has been advocated to help overcome compliance issues that lead to bacteriologic failure.[80] A 6-day course of amoxicillin shows promising results, as well as other recent studies with newer broad-spectrum agents (e.g., azithromycin, cefuroxime, cefprozil, cefdinir, cefixime, cefpodoxime, and telithromycin) that have demonstrated durations of 5 days to be effective. However, confounding factors from these studies, such as lack of strict entry criteria or differentiation between new or failed infections, limit the widespread application of short antibiotic courses at this time.[61] Furthermore, newer agents are more expensive and may be more likely to lead to resistance in light of their broad spectra of activity.[63]

CLINICAL CONTROVERSY

Once-daily amoxicillin given at a dose of 750 mg is as effective as penicillin 250 mg three times daily (duration 10 days each) in children aged 4 to 18 years with group A streptococcal pharyngitis.[81] This dosing regimen has not yet been endorsed by expert panels but may gain support in the future if the results are reproducible.[61,62,64]

TABLE 107–9. Antibiotics and Dosing for Recurrent Episodes of Pharyngitis

Drug	Adult Dosage	Pediatric Dosage
Clindamycin	600 mg orally divided in 2–4 doses	20 mg/kg/day in 3 divided doses (max: 1.8 g/day)
Amoxicillin-clavulanate	500 mg twice daily	40 mg/kg/day in 3 divided doses
Penicillin benzathine	1.2 million units intramuscularly for one dose	0.6 million units for under 27 kg (50,000 units/kg)
Penicillin benzathine with rifampin	As above	As above
	20 mg/kg/day orally in 2 divided doses × last 4 days of treatment with penicillin	Rifampin dose same as adults

From refs. 61, 63, 65, and 79.

Overprescribing is a large concern that requires consideration. Antibiotics are prescribed in 73% of patients who visit their physician with a complaint of sore throat.[82] This is well above the incidence of group A *Streptococcus*. For those who receive antibiotics, 68% of prescriptions are described as being nonrecommended treatments, e.g., extended-spectrum macrolides (e.g., azithromycin and clarithromycin) or fluoroquinolones (e.g., ciprofloxacin, gatifloxacin, levofloxacin, and moxifloxacin). Cost and resistance are factors that should discourage this practice.

EVALUATION OF THERAPEUTIC OUTCOMES/CONTACT CASES

Most cases of pharyngitis are self-limited; however, antimicrobial therapy will hasten resolution when given early to proven cases of group A *Streptococcus*.[52,61] Fever generally resolves by 3 to 5 days and most other acute symptoms by 1 week.[52] Tonsils and lymph nodes may take a few weeks to return to baseline. Children should be kept home from day care or school until afebrile and for the first 24 hours after antimicrobial treatment is initiated, after which time transmission is unlikely.[64–66]

Follow-up testing generally is not necessary for index cases or in asymptomatic contacts of the index patient.[61,63,65] Symptomatic contacts may be treated without cultures.[66] In epidemics or in cases of severe infection, follow-up testing may be prudent. The incidence of invasive group A streptococcal infection in household contacts is rare, and routine chemoprophylaxis is not recommended by the CDC,[83] although testing is advocated and guides management.[61,65] Twenty-five percent of household contacts are carriers, but treatment would only be required in persons with signs and symptoms of disease or contacts of severe or resistant disease.[61]

ABBREVIATIONS

MIC: minimal inhibitory concentration
MIC_{90}: minimal inhibitory concentration for 90% of isolates
RADT: rapid antigen-detection testing

Review Questions and other resources can be found at *www.pharmacotherapyonline.com.*

REFERENCES

1. Snow V, Mottur-Pilson C, Gonzales R, for the American College of Physicians-American Society of Internal Medicine. Principles of appropriate antibiotic use for treatment of nonspecific upper respiratory tract infections in adults. Ann Intern Med 2001;134:487–489.
2. Elden LM, Coyte PC. Socioeconomic impact of otitis media in north America. J Otolaryngol 1998;27(suppl 2):9–16.
3. Gonzales R, Bartlett JG, Besser RE, et al. Principles of appropriate antibiotic use for treatment of nonspecific upper respiratory tract infections in adults: Background. Ann Intern Med 2001;134:490–494.
4. Turnidge J. Responsible prescribing for upper respiratory tract infections. Drugs 2001;61:2065–2077.
5. Gonzales R, Bartlett JG, Besser RE, et al. Principles of appropriate antibiotic use for treatment of acute respiratory tract infections in adults: Background, specific aims, and methods. Ann Intern Med 2001;134:479–486.
6. Canadian Immunization Guide, 6th ed. Ottawa, Health Canada, 2002.
7. Hendley JO. Otitis media. New Engl J Med 2002;347:1169–1174.
8. Dowell SF, Marcy SM, Phillips WR, et al. Otitis media: Principles of judicious use of antimicrobial agents. Pediatrics 1998;101(suppl): 165–171.
9. Canadian Pediatric Society (CPS). Antibiotic management of acute otitis media. Pediatr Child Health 1998;3:265–267.
10. American Academy of Pediatrics. Managing otitis media with effusion: Practice guideline. Pediatrics 1994;94:5.
11. Bitnum A, Allen UD. Medical therapy of otitis media: Use, abuse, efficacy, and morbidity. J Otolaryngol 1998;27(suppl 2):26–35.
12. Faden H, Duffy L, Boeve M. Otitis media: Back to the basics. Pediatr Infect Dis J 1998;17:1103–1113.
13. Culpepper L, Froom J, Grob P, et al. Acute otitis media in adults: A report from the International Primary Care Network. J Am Board Fam Pract 1993;6:333–339.
14. Hoberman S, Marchant CD, Kaplan SL, et al. Treatment of acute otitis media consensus recommendations. Clin Pediatr 2002;41:373–390.
15. Dowell SF, Butler JC, Giebink GS, et al. Acute otitis media: Management and surveillance in an era of pneumococcal resistance. A report from the Drug-Resistant *Streptococcus pneumoniae* Therapeutic Working Group. Pediatr Infect Dis J 1999;18:1–9.
16. Doern GV, Heilmann KP, Huynh HK, et al. Antimicrobial resistance among clinical isolates of *Streptococcus pneumoniae* in the United States during 1999–2000, including a comparison of resistance rates since 1994–1995. Antimicrob Agents Chemother 2001;45:1721–1729.
17. Thornsberry C, Sahm DF, Kelly LJ, et al. Regional trends in antimicrobial resistance among clinical isolates of *Streptococcus pneumoniae*, *Haemophilus influenzae*, and *Moraxella catarrhalis* in the United States: Results from the TRUST surveillance program, 1999–2000. Clin Infect Dis 2002;34(suppl 1):S4–16.
18. Zhanel GG, Palatnick L, Nichol KA, et al. Five year incidence of antimicrobial resistance in respiratory tract isolates of *Streptococcus pneumoniae*: Results of the Canadian Respiratory Organism Susceptibility Study (CROSS), 1997–2002. Antimicrob Agents Chemother 2003;47:1867–1874.
19. Zhanel GG, Palatnick L, Nichol KA, et al. Five year incidence of antimicrobial resistance in respiratory tract isolates of *Haemophilus influenzae* and *Moraxella catarrhalis*: Results of the Canadian Respiratory Organism Susceptibility Study (CROSS), 1997–2002. Antimicrob Agents Chemother 2003;47:1875–1881.
20. McCracken GH. Prescribing antimicrobial agents for treatment of acute otitis media. Pediatr Infect Dis J 1999;18:1141–1146.
21. Rosenfeld RM, Vertrees JE, Carr J, et al. Clinical efficacy of antimicrobial drugs for acute otitis media: Metaanalysis of 5400 children from thirty-three randomized trials. J Pediatr 1994;124:355–367.
22. Teele DW, Klein JO, Chase C, et al. Otitis media in infancy and intellectual ability, school achievement, speech, and language at age 7 years. J Infect Dis 1990;162:685–694.
23. Luotonen M, Uhari M, Aitola L, et al. Recurrent otitis media during infancy and linguistic skills at the age of nine years. Pediatr Infect Dis J 1996;15:854–858.
24. Takata GS, Chan LS, Morphew T, et al. Evidence assessment of the accuracy of methods of diagnosing middle ear effusion in children with otitis media with effusiom. Pediatrics 2003;112:1379–1387.
25. American Academy of Pediatrics. Policy statement: Reduction of the influenza burden in children. Pediatrics 2002;110:1246–1252.
26. Flynn CA, Griffin G, Tudiver F. Decongestants and antihistamines for acute otitis media in children. Cochrane Database Syst Rev 2002; D001727.
27. Seikel K, Shelton S, McCracken G. Middle ear fluid concentrations of amoxicillin after large dosages in children with acute otitis media. Pediatr Infect Dis J 1997;16:710–711.
28. Del Mar CB, Glasziou P, Hayem M. Are antibiotics indicated as intial treatment for children with acute otitis media? A meta analysis. Br Med J 1997;314:1526.

29. Culpepper L, Froom J. Routine antimicrobial treatment of acute otitis media: Is it necessary? JAMA 1997;278:1643–1645.

30. Little P, Gould C, Williamson I, et al. Pragmatic randomised, controlled trial of two prescribing strategies for childhood acute otitis media. Br Med J. 2001;322:336–342.

31. Froom J, Culpepper L, Jacobs M, et al. Antimicrobials for acute otitis media? A review from the international primary care network. Br Med J 1997;315:98–102.

32. van Zuijlen DA, Schilder AG, van Balen FA. National differences in incidence of acute mastoiditis: Relationship to prescribing patterns of antibiotics for acute otitis media? Pediatr Infect Dis J 2001;20:140–144.

33. Korzyrskyj AL, Hildes-Ripstein E, Longstaffe SEA, et al. Treatment of acute otitis media with shortened courses of antibiotics: A meta-analysis. JAMA 1998;279:1736–1742.

34. Cohen R, Levy C, Boucherat M, et al. A multicentre, randomized, double-blind trial of 5 versus 10 days of antibiotic therapy for acute otitis media in young children. J Pediatr 1998;133:634–639.

35. Williams RL, Chalmers TC, Stange KC, et al. Use of antibiotics in preventing recurrent otitis media and in treatinn otitis media wtih effusion: A meta-analytic attempt to resolve the brouhaha. JAMA 1993;270:1344–1351.

36. Heikkinen T, Ruuskanen O, Waris M, et al. Influenza vaccination in the prevention of acute otitis media in children. Am J Dis Child 1991;145:445–448.

37. Clements DA, Langdon L, Bland C, et al. Influenza A vaccine decreases the incidence of otitis media in 6- to 30-month-old children in day care. Arch Pediatr Adolesc Med 1995;149:1113–1117.

38. Eskola J, Kilpi T, Palmu A, et al. Efficacy of a pneumococcal conjugate vaccine against acute otitis media. N Engl J Med 2001;344:403–409.

39. Fireman B, Black SB, Shinefield HR, et al. Impact of the pneumococcal conjugate vaccine on otitis media. Pediatr Infect Dis J 2003;22:10–15.

40. Recommendations of the Advisory Committee on Immunization Practices (ACIP) Advisory Committee on Immunization Practices. Preventing pneumococcal disease among infants and young children. MMWR 2000;43(RR-09):1–38.

41. Vennhoven R, Bogaert D, Uiterwaal C, et al. Effect of conjugate penumococcal vaccine followed by polysaccharide penumococcal vaccine on recurrent acute otitis media: A randomised study. Lancet 2003;361:2189–2195.

42. Hickner JM, Bartlett JG, Besser RE, et al. Principles of appropriate antibiotic use for acute rhinosinusitis in adults: Background. Ann Intern Med 2001;134:498–505.

43. O'Brien KL, Dowell SF, Schwartz B, et al. Acute sinusitis: Principles of judicious use of antimicrobial agents. Pediatrics 1998;101(suppl):174–77.

44. Noyek A, Brodovsky D, Coyle S, et al. Classification, diagnosis and treatment of sinusitis: Evidence-based clinical practice guidelines. Can J Inf Dis 1998;9(suppl B):3–24B.

45. Sinus and Allergy Health Partnership. Antimicrobial treatment guidelines for acute bacterial rhinosinusitis. Otolaryngol Head Neck Surg Suppl 2000;123:S1–32.

46. Agency for Health Care Policy and Research. Diagnosis and Treatment of Acute Bacterial Rhinosinusitis: Summary—Evidence Report/Technology Assessment, Number 9, March 1999. Rockville, MD, Agency for Health Care Policy and Research; available at *www.ahrq.gov/clinic/epcsums/sinussum.htm.*

47. American Academy of Pediatrics. Clinical practice guidelines: Management of sinusitis. Pediatrics 2001;108:798–808.

48. Low DE, Desrosiers M, McSherry J, et al. A practical guide for the diagnosis and treatment of acute sinusitis. Can Med Assoc J 1997;156(suppl 6):S1–14.

49. Evans KL. Recognition and management of sinusitis. Drugs 1998;56:59–71.

50. Lindbaek M, Hjortdahl P, Johnsen ULH. Randomised, double-blind, placebo-controlled trial of penicillin V and amoxycillin in treatment of acute sinus infections. Br Med J 1996;313:325–329.

51. Wald E. Microbiology of acute and chronic sinusitis. In: Lusk RP, ed. Pediatric Sinusitis. New York, Raven Press, 1992:43–47.

52. Mandell GL, Bennett JE, Dolin R, eds. Principles and Practice of Infectious Diseases, 4th ed. New York, Churchill-Livingstone, 2000.

53. Gwaltney JM. Acute community acquired bacterial sinusitis: To treat or not to treat. Can Respir J 1999;6(suppl A):46–50A.

54. Williams JW Jr, Aguilar CCCC, Cornell J, et al. Antibiotics for acute maxillary sinusitis. Cochrane Rev 2003;3.

55. van Buchem FL, Knottnerus JA, Schrijnemaekers VJJ, et al. Primary-care-based randomised, placebo-controlled trial of antibiotic treatment in acute maxillary sinusitis. Lancet 1997;349:683–687.

56. Piccirillo JF, Mager DE, Frisse ME, et al. Impact of first-line vs second-line antibiotics for the treatment of acute uncomplicated sinusitis. JAMA 2001;286:1849–1856.

57. de Bock GH, Dekker FW, Stolk J, et al. Antimicrobial treatment in acute maxillary sinusitis: A meta-analysis. J Clin Epidemiol 1997;50:881–890.

58. Canadian Pharmacists Association. Compendium of Pharmaceutical Specialties. Ottawa, Canadian Pharmacists Association, 2003.

59. Gilbert DN, Moellering RC, Sande MA, eds. The Sanford Guide to Antimicrobial Therapy 2003. Hyde Park, NY, Antimicrobial Therapy, Inc., 2003.

60. Williams JW Jr, Holleman DR Jr, Samsa GP, et al. Randomized controlled trial of 3 vs 10 days of trimethoprim-sulfamethoxazole for acute maxillary sinusitis. JAMA 1995;273:1015–1021.

61. Bisno AL, Gerber MA, Gwaltney JM, et al. Practice guidelines for the diagnosis and management of group A streptococcal pharyngitis (IDSA guidelines). Clin Infect Dis 2002;35:113–125.

62. Snow V, Mottur-Pilson C, Cooper RJ, et al, for the American College of Physicians, American Society of Internal Medicine. Principles of appropriate antibiotic use for acute pharyngitis in adults. Clinical practice guideline, part I. Ann Intern Med 2001;134:506–508.

63. Bisno A. Acute pharyngitis. N Engl J Med 2001;344:205–211.

64. Cooper RJ, Hoffman JR, Bartlett JG, et al. Principles of appropriate antibiotic use for acute pharyngitis in adults: Background. Clinical practice guideline, part II (endorsed by the Center for Disease Control, American Academy of Family Physicians, and the American College of Physicians-American Society of Internal Medicine). Ann Intern Med 2001;134:509–517.

65. American Academy of Pediatrics. Group A streptococcal infections. In: Pickering LK, ed. Red Book 2003: Report of the Committee on Infectious Diseases, 26th ed. Elk Grove Village, IL, American Academy of Pediatrics 2003:526–536.

66. Hayes CS, Williamson HW. Management of group A beta-hemolytic streptococcal pharyngitis. Am Fam Phys 2001;63:1557–1565.

67. Schwartz B, Marcy M, Phillips WR, et al. Pharyngitis: Principles of judicious use of antimicrobial agents. Pediatrics 1998;101;171–174.

68. Summary of notifiable diseases, United States, 1998. MMWR 1998; 47:1.

69. Centor RM, Witherspoon JM, Dalton HP, et al. The diagnosis of strep throat in adults in the emergency room. Med Decision Making 1981;1:239–246.

70. Dajani A, Taubert K, Ferrieri P, et al. Treatment of acute streptococcal pharyngitis and prevention of rheumatic fever: A statement for health professionals. Committee on Rheumatic Fever, Endocarditis, and Kawasaki Disease of the Council on Cardiovascular Disease in the Young, the American Heart Association. Pediatrics 1995;96:758–764.

71. Dickinson JA. Acute pharyngitis (letter). N Engl J Med 2001;344: 1479–1480.

72. Del Mar CB, Glasziou PP, Spinks AB. Antibiotics for sore throat. Cochrane Rev 2003;2.

73. Chamovitz R, Catanzaro FJ, Stetson CA, et al. Prevention of rheumatic fever by treatment of previous streptococcal infections. N Engl J Med 1954;251:466–471.

74. Denny FW, Wannamaker LW, Brink WR, et al. Prevention of rheumatic fever. JAMA 1950;143:151–153.

75. Kaplan EL, Johnson DR, del Rosario MC, et al. Susceptibility of group A beta-hemolytic streptococci to thirteen antibiotics: Examination of 301 strains isolated in the United States between 1994 and 1997. Pediatr Infec Dis J 1999;18:1069–1072.

76. De Azavedo JCS, Yeung RH, Bast DJ, et al. Prevalence and mechanisms of macrolide resistance in clinical isolates of group A streptococci from Ontario, Canada. Antimicrob Agents Chemother 1999;43: 2144–147.

77. Martin JM, Green M, Barbadora KA, et al. Erythromycin-resistant group A streptococcus in schoolchildren in Pittsburgh. N Engl J Med 2002;346:1200–1206.

78. Seppala H, Klaukka T, Vuopio-Varkila J, et al. The effect of changes in the consumption of macrolide antibiotics on erythromycin resistance in group A streptococci in Finland. N Engl J Med 1997;337:441–446.

79. Bacterial diseases. In: Beers MH, Berkow R., *eds.* The Merck Manual of Diagnosis and Therapy, 17th ed. Whitehouse Station, NJ, Merck & Co., Inc., 1995–2003. Accessed on November 29th, 2003 at *www.merck.com/ mrkshared/mmanual/section13/chapter157/157a.jsp.*

80. Guay DRP. Short-course antimicrobial therapy of respiratory tract infections. Drugs 2003;63:2169–2184.

81. Feder HMJ, Gerber MA, Randolph MF, et al. Once daily therapy for streptococcal pharyngitis with amoxicillin. Pediatrics 1999;103:47–51.

82. Linder JA, Stafford RS. Antibiotic treatment of adults with sore throat by community primary care physicians: A national survey, 1989–1999. JAMA 2001;286:1181–1186.

83. Robinson KA, Rothcock G, Phan Q, et al. Risk for severe group A streptococcal disease among patients' household contacts. Emerg Infect Dis 2003;9; found at *www.medscape.com/viewarticle/45281'print.*

108

SKIN AND SOFT TISSUE INFECTIONS

Susan L. Pendland, Douglas N. Fish, and Larry H. Danziger

Learning Objectives and other resources can be found at *www.pharmacotherapyonline.com*.

KEY CONCEPTS

❶ Folliculitis, furuncles (boils), and carbuncles begin around hair follicles and are caused most often by *Staphylococcus aureus*. Folliculitis generally can be treated with local measures such as warm, moist compresses or topical antibiotics. Small furuncles usually are treated with warm, moist heat to promote drainage; large furuncles and carbuncles are treated most often with an antistaphylococcal antibiotic such as dicloxacillin. Lesions often drain spontaneously; if not, surgical incision may be necessary.

❷ Erysipelas is a superficial skin infection with extensive lymphatic involvement that is caused by *Streptococcus pyogenes* and is treated with penicillin. Serious infections should be treated with intravenous antibiotics.

❸ Impetigo, a superficial skin infection characterized by fluid-filled vesicles that develop rapidly into pus-filled blisters that rupture to form golden-yellow crusts, is caused by *S. aureus* and/or *S. pyogenes* and occurs most commonly in children. Dicloxacillin is used commonly for treatment, although topical antibiotics such as mupirocin are also effective.

❹ Lymphangitis is an infection of the subcutaneous lymphatic channels generally caused by *S. pyogenes*. Acute lymphangitis is characterized by the rapid development of fine red linear streaks extending from the initial infection site toward the regional lymph nodes, which are usually enlarged and tender. Penicillin is the drug of choice.

❺ Cellulitis is an infection of the epidermis, dermis, and superficial fascia. Lesions generally are hot, painful, and erythematous, with nonelevated, poorly defined margins. The most common causes of cellulitis are *S. pyogenes* and *S. aureus*. Treatment generally consists of a penicillinase-resistant penicillin for 7 to 10 days.

❻ Necrotizing fasciitis is a rare but life-threatening infection of subcutaneous tissue that results in progressive destruction of superficial fascia and subcutaneous fat. Early and aggressive surgical débridement is an essential part of therapy for treatment of necrotizing fasciitis.

❼ Diabetic foot infections are managed with a comprehensive treatment approach that includes both proper wound care and antimicrobial therapy. Antimicrobial regimens for diabetic foot infections should include broad-spectrum coverage of staphylococci, streptococci, enteric gram-negative bacilli, and anaerobes. Outpatient therapy with oral antimicrobials should be used whenever possible.

❽ Prevention is the single most important aspect in the management of pressure sores. After a sore develops, successful local care includes a comprehensive approach consisting of relief of pressure, proper cleaning (débridement), disinfection, and appropriate antimicrobial therapy if an infection is present. Good wound care is crucial to successful management.

❾ All bite wounds (either animal or human) should be irrigated thoroughly with large volumes of sterile normal saline, and the injured area should be immobilized and elevated. Infections developing within the first 24 hours after a dog or cat bite are caused most often by *Pasteurella multocida* and should be treated with penicillin or amoxicillin for 10 to 14 days. Infections developing more than 36 to 48 hours after an animal bite are most likely caused by staphylococci or streptococci and should be treated with an antistaphylococcal penicillin or cephalosporin.

❿ While antimicrobial prophylaxis of dog or cat bites is not recommended routinely, patients with noninfected human bite injuries of the hand should be given prophylactic antimicrobial therapy with penicillin plus dicloxacillin for 3 to 5 days. Infected wounds of the hand, particularly clenched-fist injuries, should be treated with penicillin plus dicloxacillin or amoxicillin-clavulanate for 7 to 14 days.

The skin serves as a barrier between humans and their environment and therefore functions as a primary defense mechanism against infections. The skin consists of the epidermis, the dermis, and subcutaneous fat. The epidermis is the outermost, nonvascular layer of the skin. It varies in thickness from approximately 0.1 mm on most areas of the body to a maximum of 1.5 mm on the soles of the feet.

Although extremely thin, the epidermis is composed of several layers. The innermost layer consists of continuously dividing cells. The outer layers are renewed as cells are gradually pushed outward. As the cells approach the surface, they become flattened, lose their nuclei, and are filled with keratin. The outermost layer, the stratum corneum, is composed of flattened, cornified, nonnucleated cells. The dermis is the layer of skin directly beneath the epidermis. It consists of connective tissue and contains blood vessels and lymphatics, sensory nerve endings, sweat and sebaceous glands, hair follicles, and smooth muscle fibers. Beneath the dermis is a layer of loose connective tissue containing primarily fat cells. This subcutaneous fat layer is of variable thickness over the body. Beneath the subcutaneous fat lies the fascia, which separates the skin from underlying muscle. It is generally divided into superficial fascia, which is located immediately beneath the skin, and deep fascia, which forms sheaths for muscles.

Skin and soft tissue infections (SSTIs) may involve any or all layers of the skin, fascia, and muscle. They also may spread far from the initial site of infection and lead to more severe complications, such as endocarditis, Gram-negative sepsis, or streptococcal glomerulonephritis. The treatment of SSTIs at times may necessitate both medical and surgical management. This chapter presents details of the pathogenesis and management of some of the most common infections involving the skin and soft tissues. The first part of the chapter discusses a variety of SSTIs that range in severity from superficial to life-threatening. The remainder of the chapter discusses diabetic foot infections, pressure sores, and human and animal bites.

EPIDEMIOLOGY

A number of classification schemes have been developed to describe SSTIs. Bacterial infections of the skin can be classified as primary or secondary (Table 108–1). Primary bacterial infections usually involve areas of previously healthy skin and typically are caused by a single pathogen. In contrast, secondary infections occur in areas of previously damaged skin and are frequently polymicrobic. SSTIs are also classified as complicated or uncomplicated. Infections are considered complicated when they involve deeper skin structures (e.g., fascia, muscle layers, etc), require significant surgical intervention, or occur in patients with compromised immune function (e.g., diabetes mellitus, human immunodeficiency virus [HIV] infection, etc).[1]

The classification system recently developed by Eron divides SSTIs into four classes based on severity of signs and symptoms, as well as the presence and stability of any comorbidities.[2] The classification was used to develop an algorithm to help with admission and treatment decisions. Class 1 includes patients who are afebrile and otherwise healthy. These patients generally can be managed on an outpatient basis with topical or oral antimicrobials. Class 2 includes patients who are febrile and ill-appearing but have no unstable comorbid conditions. Some class 2 patients may be treated with oral antimicrobials, but most likely will require some parenteral therapy, either as an outpatient or with short-term hospitalization. Patients having a toxic appearance, at least one unstable comorbidity, or a limb-threatening infection are grouped into class 3. Class 4 includes patients with sepsis syndrome or other life-threatening infection, such as necrotizing fasciitis. Patients in classes 3 and 4 require hospitalization and parenteral antimicrobial therapy initially but may be candidates for oral or outpatient parenteral therapy once their condition has stabilized. Patients in class 4 also generally require some type of surgical intervention.

SSTIs are among the most common infections seen in both community and hospital settings. However, data on the exact incidence of SSTIs are lacking. Most infections are believed to be mild and therefore treated in an outpatient setting, making it difficult to quantify community-acquired SSTIs. One description of office visits among health plan members listed cellulitis and impetigo as the primary diagnosis for 2.2% and 0.3% of patients, respectively.[3] According to the most recent Healthcare Cost and Utilization Project Nationwide Inpatient Sample, SSTIs are the twenty-eighth most common diagnosis of patients in community hospitals.[4] Approximately 0.1% of the adult population in the United States required hospitalization for SSTIs in 1995.[2]

While the exact incidence of SSTIs is unknown, the frequency of infection caused by invasive group A streptococci and drug-resistant gram-positive cocci have been increasing.[1] Group A streptococci (*Streptococcus pyogenes*) are among the most common etiologic agents of SSTIs. While they may be found in many mild, superficial skin infections, they are also responsible for life-threatening cases of necrotizing fasciitis.[1] A dramatic increase in necrotizing fasciitis due

TABLE 108–1. Bacterial Classification of Important Skin and Soft Tissue Infections

Primary Infections	
Erysipelas	Group A streptococci
Impetigo	*Staphylococcus aureus*, group A streptococci
Lymphangitis	Group A streptococci; occasionally *S. aureus*
Cellulitis	Group A streptococci, *S. aureus;* occasionally other gram-positive cocci, gram-negative bacilli, and/or anaerobes
Necrotizing fasciitis	
Type I	Anaerobes (*Bacteroides* spp., *Peptostreptococcus* spp.) and facultative bacteria (streptococci, Enterobacteriaceae)
Type II	Group A streptococci
Secondary Infections	
Diabetic foot infections	*S. aureus*, streptococci, Enterobacteriaceae, *Bacteroides* spp., *Peptostreptococcus* spp., *Pseudomonas aeruginosa*
Pressure sores	*S. aureus*, streptococci, Enterobacteriaceae, *Bacteroides* spp., *Peptostreptococcus* spp., *Pseudomonas aeruginosa*
Bite wounds	
Animal	*Pasteurella multocida, S. aureus*, streptococci, *Bacteroides* spp.
Human	*Eikenella corrodens, S. aureus*, streptococci, *Corynebacterium* spp., *Bacteroides* spp., *Peptostreptococcus* spp.
Burn wounds	*Pseudomonas aeruginosa*, Enterobacteriaceae, *S. aureus*, streptococci

TABLE 108–2. Predominant Microorganisms of Normal Skin

Bacteria
Gram-positive
  Coagulase-negative staphylococci
  Micrococci (*Micrococcus luteus*)
  Corynebacterium species (diphtheroids)
  Propionibacterium species
Gram-negative
  Actinetobacter species
Fungi
  Malassezia species
  Candida species

to *S. pyogenes* is a major concern because of the high morbidity and mortality associated with these infections.

Another worrisome trend is the increased in vitro resistance reported for many gram-positive bacteria.[1] Of greatest concern is the increasing incidence of methicillin-resistant *Staphylococcus aureus* (MRSA).[5] Treatment choices for SSTIs have been further complicated by the increased incidence of macrolide-resistant strains of *S. aureus* and *S. pyogenes*.[1]

ETIOLOGY

The majority of SSTIs are caused by gram-positive organisms and, less commonly, gram-negative bacteria present on the skin surface.[1] Gram-positive bacteria (coagulase-negative staphylococci, diphtheroids) are the predominant flora of the skin, with gram-negative organisms (*Escherichia coli* and other Enterobacteriaceae) being relatively uncommon[6] (Table 108–2). *S. aureus*, as well as a variety of gram-negative bacteria, can be found in moist intertriginous areas (e.g., axilla, groin, and toe webs) of the body. *Acinetobacter* species have been cultured from these moister areas in 25% of the population.[6,7] *S. aureus* also inhabits the anterior nares of approximately 30% of healthy individuals.[6] Colonization, whether transient or permanent, provides a nidus for infection should the integrity of the epidermis be compromised.

S. aureus and *S. pyogenes* account for the majority of community-acquired SSTIs.[1] Data from the most recent SENTRY Antimicrobial Surveillance Program showed *S. aureus* to also be the most common cause (45.9%) of nosocomial SSTIs.[5] Also of note in this study was the 30% incidence of methicillin resistance among strains of *S. aureus*. Other common nosocomial pathogens included *Pseudomonas aeruginosa* (11%), enterococci (8%), and *E. coli* (7%).[5]

PATHOPHYSIOLOGY

The skin and subcutaneous tissues normally are extremely resistant to infection but may become susceptible under certain conditions. Even when high concentrations of bacteria are applied topically or injected into the soft tissue, resulting infections are rare.[8] Several host factors act together to confer protection against skin infections. The surface of the skin is relatively dry, has a pH of approximately 5.6, and therefore is not conducive to bacterial growth.[6] Continuous renewal of the epidermal layer results in the shedding of keratocytes, as well as skin bacteria. In addition, sebaceous secretions are

hydrolyzed to form free fatty acids that strongly inhibit the growth of many bacteria and fungi.[8] The conditions that may predispose a patient to the development of skin infections include (1) a high concentration of bacteria ($>10^5$ microorganisms), (2) excessive moisture of the skin, (3) inadequate blood supply, (4) availability of bacterial nutrients, and (5) damage to the corneal layer allowing for bacterial penetration.[7,8]

The majority of SSTIs result from the disruption of normal host defenses by processes such as skin puncture, abrasion, or underlying diseases (e.g., diabetes). The nature and severity of the infection depends on both the type of microorganism present and the site of inoculation.

FOLLICULITIS, FURUNCLES, AND CARBUNCLES

Folliculitis is inflammation of the hair follicle and can be caused by physical injury, chemical irritation, or infection.[3] Infection occurring at the base of the eyelid is referred to as a stye. Furuncles and carbuncles occur when a follicular infection extends from around the hair shaft to involve the deeper areas of the skin. A furuncle, commonly known as an *abscess* or *boil*, is a walled-off mass of purulent material arising from a hair follicle.[3] The lesions are called *carbuncles* when they coalesce and extend to the subcutaneous tissue. This aggregate of infected hair follicles forms deep masses that generally open and drain through multiple sinus tracts.[3] *S. aureus* is the most common cause of folliculitis, furuncles, and carbuncles. Inadequate chlorine levels in whirlpools, hot tubs, and swimming pools have been responsible for outbreaks of folliculitis caused by *P. aeruginosa*.[9]

CLINICAL PRESENTATION

FOLLICULITIS

* Pruritic, erythematous papules typically appear within 48 hours (range 6–72 hours) of exposure to large numbers of organisms.
* Papules evolve into pustules that generally heal in several days.
* Systemic signs such as fever and malaise are uncommon, although they have been reported in cases caused by *P. aeruginosa*.

FURUNCLES

* Furuncles can occur anywhere on hairy skin but generally develop in areas subject to friction and perspiration.
* Furuncles are discrete lesions, whether occurring as singular or multiple nodules.
* The lesion starts as a firm, tender, red nodule that becomes painful and fluctuant.
* Lesions often drain spontaneously.

CARBUNCLES

* Carbuncles are broad, swollen, erythematous, deep, and painful follicular masses.
* Unlike folliculitis and furuncles, carbuncles are commonly associated with fever, chills, and malaise.
* Bacteremia with secondary spread to other tissues is common.

▶ TREATMENT: Folliculitis, Furuncles, and Carbuncles

Treatment of folliculitis generally requires only local measures, such as warm saline compresses or topical therapy (e.g., clindamycin, erythromycin, mupirocin, or benzoyl peroxide).[10] Topical agents generally are applied two to four times daily for 7 days. Small furuncles generally can be treated with moist heat, which promotes localization and drainage of pus.[10] Large and/or multiple furuncles and carbuncles generally are treated with a penicillinase-resistant penicillin (dicloxacillin 250 mg orally every 6 hours for 7 to 10 days). An alternative agent for penicillin-allergic patients is clindamycin (150–300 mg orally every 6 hours). Surgical incision is indicated for large and fluctuant lesions that do not drain spontaneously.[10]

EVALUATION OF THERAPEUTIC OUTCOMES

Many follicular infections resolve spontaneously without medical or surgical intervention. Lesions may need to be incised if they do not respond to a few days of moist heat and over-the-counter topical agents. Following drainage, most lesions begin to heal within several days.

ERYSIPELAS

Erysipelas is an infection of the more superficial layers of the skin and cutaneous lymphatics.[11] The intense red color and burning pain associated with this skin infection led to the common name of St. Anthony's fire. The infection is almost always caused by β-hemolytic streptococci, with the organisms gaining access via small breaks in the skin. While group A streptococci (*S. pyogenes*) are responsible for most infections, group G streptococci also have been implicated in a considerable number of infections.[12,13] Infections are more common in infants, young children, the elderly, and patients with nephrotic syndrome.[10] Erysipelas also commonly occurs in areas of preexisting lymphatic obstruction or edema.[10] Diagnosis is made on the basis of the characteristic lesion.

CLINICAL PRESENTATION

GENERAL

- The lower extremities are the most common sites for erysipelas.

SYMPTOMS

- Patients often experience flulike symptoms (fever, malaise) prior to the appearance of the lesion.
- The infected area is described as painful or as a burning pain.

SIGNS

- The lesion is bright red and edematous, often with lymphatic streaking.
- Temperature is often mildly elevated.
- The clinical presentation differs from cellulitis in that the lesion has clearly demarcated raised margins.

LABORATORY TESTS

- Cultures should be considered.
- The causative organism usually cannot be cultured from the surface skin but sometimes may be aspirated from the edge of the advancing lesion.

OTHER DIAGNOSTIC TESTS

- A complete blood count is often performed because leukocytosis is common.
- C-reactive protein is also generally elevated.

▶ TREATMENT: Erysipelas

The goal of treatment of erysipelas is rapid eradication of the infection. Mild to moderate cases of erysipelas are treated with procaine penicillin G 600,000 units intramuscularly twice daily or penicillin VK 250–500 mg orally four times daily (in children 1–18 years of age, 25,000–90,000 units/kg per day divided into four doses) for 7 to 10 days.[10,14,15] Penicillin-allergic patients can be treated with clindamycin 150–300 mg orally every 6 to 8 hours (in children, 10–30 mg/kg per day in three to four divided doses). For more serious infections, the patient should be hospitalized, and aqueous penicillin G 2–8 million units daily should be administered intravenously.[10,11] Marked improvement usually is seen within 48 hours, and the patient often may be switched to oral penicillin to complete the course of therapy. One randomized, double-blind, placebo-controlled study showed that the median time for cure, intravenous antibiotics, and hospital stay was reduced in patients receiving prednisolone in addition to antibiotics. Further studies are needed, however, before corticosteroids can be recommended for routine use.[13]

EVALUATION OF THERAPEUTIC OUTCOMES

Erysipelas generally responds quickly to appropriate antimicrobial therapy. Temperature and white blood count should return to normal within 48 to 72 hours. Erythema, edema, and pain also should resolve gradually.

IMPETIGO

Impetigo is a superficial skin infection that is seen most commonly in children and is transmitted easily from person to person.[16] The infection generally is classified as bullous or nonbullous ased on clinical presentation.[3] Impetigo is most common during hot, umid weather, which facilitates microbial colonization of the skin.[10] Minor trauma, such as scratches or insect bites, then allows entry of organisms into the superficial layers of skin, and infection ensues.[10] Impetigo is highly communicable and readily spreads through close contact, especially among siblings and children in day-care centers and schools.[10,11]

Most cases of impetigo were caused by *S. pyogenes*, but *S. aureus* either alone or in combination with *S. pyogenes* has emerged more recently as the principal cause of impetigo.[16] The bullous form is caused by strains of *S. aureus* capable of producing exfoliative toxins.[16] The bullous form most frequently affects neonates and accounts for approximately 10% of all cases of impetigo.[10,16]

CLINICAL PRESENTATION

GENERAL

- Exposed skin, especially the face, is the most common site for impetigo.

SYMPTOMS

- Pruritus is common, and scratching of the lesions may further spread infection through excoriation of the skin.
- Other systemic signs of infection are minimal.
- Weakness, fever, and diarrhea sometimes are seen with bullous impetigo.

SIGNS

- Nonbullous impetigo manifests initially as small, fluid-filled vesicles.
- These lesions rapidly develop into pus-filled blisters that rupture readily.
- Purulent discharge from the lesions dries to form golden-yellow crusts that are characteristic of impetigo.
- In the bullous form of impetigo, the lesions begin as vesicles and turn into bullae containing clear yellow fluid.
- Bullae soon rupture, forming thin, light brown crusts.
- Regional lymph nodes may be enlarged.

LABORATORY TESTS

- Cultures should be collected.
- Crusted tops of lesions should be raised so that purulent material at the base of the lesion can be cultured.
- Cultures should not be collected from open, draining skin pustules because they may be colonized with staphylococci and other normal skin flora.

OTHER DIAGNOSTIC TESTS

- A complete blood count is often performed because leukocytosis is common.

▶ TREATMENT: Impetigo

Although impetigo may resolve spontaneously, antimicrobial treatment is indicated to relieve symptoms, prevent formation of new lesions, and prevent complications, such as cellulitis. Penicillinase-resistant penicillins (dicloxacillin 12.5 mg/kg orally daily in four divided doses for children) are preferred for treatment because of the increased incidence of infections caused by *S. aureus*. First-generation cephalosporins are also effective, although they are generally more expensive. Cephalexin (25–50 mg/kg orally daily in two divided doses for children) and cefadroxil (30 mg/kg orally daily in two divided doses for children) are used commonly. Penicillin, administered as either a single intramuscular dose of benzathine penicillin G (300,000–600,000 units in children, 1.2 million units in adults) or as oral penicillin VK, is effective for infections caused by *S. pyogenes*. Penicillin-allergic patients can be treated with clindamycin (adults 150–300 mg orally every 6 to 8 hours; children 10–30 mg/kg per day in three to four divided doses). The duration of therapy is 7 to 10 days. Topical antibiotics, such as mupirocin and bacitracin, have been used to treat nonbullous impetigo. Mupirocin ointment (applied three times daily for 7 days) is as effective as erythromycin.[17] With proper treatment, healing of skin lesions generally is rapid and occurs without residual scarring. Removal of crusts by soaking in soap and warm water also may be helpful in providing symptomatic relief.[10,14]

EVALUATION OF THERAPEUTIC OUTCOMES

Clinical response should be seen within 7 days of initiating antimicrobial therapy for impetigo. Treatment failures could be due to noncompliance or antimicrobial resistance. A follow-up culture of exudates should be collected for culture and sensitivity, with treatment modified accordingly.[16]

LYMPHANGITIS

Acute lymphangitis is an inflammation involving the subcutaneous lymphatic channels. Lymphangitis usually occurs secondary to puncture wounds, infected blisters, or other skin lesions. Most infections are caused by *S. pyogenes*.[14,18]

CLINICAL PRESENTATION

GENERAL

- Lymphadenitis (acute or chronic inflammation of the lymph nodes) also may occur when microorganisms reach the lymph nodes and elicit an inflammatory response.

SYMPTOMS

- Systemic manifestations of infection (i.e., fever, chills, malaise, and headache) often develop rapidly before any sign of infection is evident at the initial site of inoculation or even after the initial lesion has subsided.
- Systemic symptoms often are more profound than would be expected based on examination of the cutaneous lesion.

SIGNS

- Identification of a peripheral lesion associated with proximal red linear streaks directed toward the regional lymph nodes is diagnostic of acute lymphangitis.
- Lymph nodes usually are enlarged and tender.
- Peripheral edema of the involved extremity often is present.
- Thrombophlebitis and acute lymphangitis in the lower extremities may be confused because both are associated with red linear streaking and tender areas; however, in thrombophlebitis, no portal of entry is identifiable.

LABORATORY TESTS

- Cultures of the affected lesions often yield negative results because the infection resides within the lymphatic channels.
- Offending pathogens often can be identified by Gram stain of the initial lesion if done early in the course of the disease.

OTHER DIAGNOSTIC TESTS

- A complete blood count frequently is performed because leukocytosis is common.

► TREATMENT: Lymphangitis

The goal of therapy for lymphangitis is rapid eradication of infection and prevention of further systemic complications. Penicillin is the antibiotic of choice. Because these infections are potentially serious and rapidly progressive, initial treatment should be with intravenous penicillin G. Parenteral treatment should be continued for 48 to 72 hours, followed by oral penicillin VK for a total of 10 days.[14,18,19] Nondrug therapy includes immobilization and elevation of the affected extremity and warm-water soaks every 2 to 4 hours.[14] For penicillin-allergic patients, clindamycin may be used.

EVALUATION OF THERAPEUTIC OUTCOMES

Lymphangitis usually responds rapidly to appropriate therapy; signs and symptoms often are decreased markedly or absent within 24 hours of starting antibiotics.

CELLULITIS

5 Cellulitis is an acute, infectious process that represents a more serious type of SSTI. Cellulitis initially affects the epidermis and dermis and may spread subsequently within the superficial fascia. Cellulitis is considered a serious disease because of the propensity of the infection to spread through lymphatic tissue and to the bloodstream. *S. pyogenes* and *S. aureus* are the most frequent etiologic agents. However, a number of bacteria have been implicated in various types of cellulitis (see Table 108–1). The rising incidence of infections due to MRSA is a major concern in both the community and hospital settings.

Injection drug users are predisposed to a number of infectious complications, including abscess formation and cellulitis at the site of injection.[20] These SSTIs are located most frequently on the upper extremities and often are polymicrobic in nature.[21] Infecting organisms are believed to originate from the skin and/or oropharynx, as well as from contaminated needles, syringes, and diluents.[21] *S. aureus* and streptococci are the most common pathogenic organisms isolated from these infections. Anaerobic bacteria, especially oropharyngeal anaerobes, are also found commonly, particularly in polymicrobic infections.[21]

Acute cellulitis with mixed aerobic and anaerobic flora generally occurs in diabetics, where the skin is adjacent to some site of trauma, at sites of surgical incisions to the abdomen or perineum, or where host defenses have been otherwise compromised (vascular insufficiency). In older patients, cellulitis of the lower extremities also may be complicated by thrombophlebitis. Other complications of cellulitis include local abscess, osteomyelitis, and septic arthritis.[14,15]

CLINICAL PRESENTATION

GENERAL

- There is usually a history of an antecedent wound from a minor trauma, abrasion, ulcer, or surgery.
- Because these infections occur often in patients with alterations in host defense mechanisms, poor nutrition, or both, systemic findings such as hypotension, dehydration, and altered mental status are common.

SYMPTOMS

- Patients often experience fever, chills, or malaise and complain that the affected area feels hot and painful.

SIGNS

- Cellulitis is characterized by erythema and edema of the skin.
- Lesions, which may be extensive, are nonelevated and have poorly defined margins.
- Affected areas generally are warm to touch.
- Inflammation generally is present with little or no necrosis or suppuration of soft tissue.
- Tender lymphadenopathy associated with lymphatic involvement is common.

LABORATORY TESTS

- Cultures should be collected when possible.
- A Gram stain of fluid obtained by injection and aspiration of 0.5 mL of saline (using a small 22-gauge needle) into the advancing edge of the lesion may aid the microbiologic diagnosis but often yields negative results.
- Diagnosis usually is made on clinical grounds, i.e., the appearance of the lesion.

OTHER DIAGNOSTIC TESTS

- A complete blood count frequently is performed because leukocytosis is common.

Bacteremia may be present in as many as 30therefore, blood cultures may be useful for diagnosis in some patients.

▶ TREATMENT: Cellulitis

The goal of therapy of acute bacterial cellulitis is rapid eradication of the infection and prevention of further complications. Antimicrobial therapy of bacterial cellulitis is directed against the type of bacteria either documented or suspected to be present based on the clinical presentation. Local care of cellulitis includes elevation and immobilization of the involved area to decrease swelling. Cool sterile saline dressings can decrease pain and can be followed later with moist heat to aid in localization of the cellulitis. Surgical intervention (incision and drainage) as a mode of therapy is rarely indicated in the treatment of cellulitis.

Since staphylococcal and streptococcal cellulitis are indistinguishable clinically,[11] administration of a semisynthetic penicillin (nafcillin or oxacillin) is recommended until a definitive diagnosis, by skin or blood cultures, can be made[10,14,15] (Table 108–3). Mild to moderate infections not associated with systemic symptoms may be treated orally with dicloxacillin. If documented to be a mild cellulitis secondary to streptococci, oral penicillin VK or intramuscular procaine penicillin may be administered. More severe infections, either staphylococcal or streptococcal, should be treated initially with intravenous antibiotic regimens. Ceftriaxone 50–100 mg/kg as a single daily dose is efficacious in the treatment of cellulitis in pediatric patients.[22] The usual duration of therapy for cellulitis is 7 to 10 days.[10,14,15]

In penicillin-allergic patients, oral or parenteral clindamycin may be used.[1,2] Alternatively, a first-generation cephalosporin, such as cefazolin (1–2 g intravenously every 8 hours), may be used cautiously for patients who have not experienced immediate or anaphylactic penicillin reactions and are negative for a penicillin skin test. In mild cases in which an oral cephalosporin can be used, cefadroxil 500 mg twice daily or cephalexin 250–500 mg four times daily is recommended. Other oral cephalosporins, such as cefaclor, cefprozil, and cefpodoxime proxetil, are also effective in the treatment of cellulitis but are considerably more expensive.[14] In severe cases in which cephalosporins cannot be used because of documented methicillin-resistant staphylococci or severe β-lactam allergies, vancomycin should be administered.

Alternative agents for documented infections with resistant gram-positive bacteria such as MRSA and vancomycin-resistant enterococci (VRE) include linezolid, quinupristin-dalfopristin, and daptomycin.[1,2,23–26] The excellent activity of these drugs against resistant gram-positive pathogens and significantly higher cost make them most appropriate for treatment of complicated or refractory infections or those caused by multidrug-resistant pathogens.

The carbapenems (i.e., imipenem, meropenem, and ertapenem) and the β-lactamase inhibitor combination antibiotics (ampicillin-sulbactam, ticarcillin–lavulanic acid, and piperacillin-tazobactam) also appear to be equivalent to standard therapies in adults.[1,27–30] The greater cost of these newer agents without increased efficacy compared with other reliable regimens, however, makes them less desirable.

CLINICAL CONTROVERSY

Oral fluoroquinolones have demonstrated efficacy similar to parenteral cephalosporins in the treatment of soft tissue infections caused by gram-positive organisms.[1,31,32] Caution is warranted when treating SSTIs with ciprofloxacin owing to the unreliable activity of this agent against streptococci.[1] Lower eradication rates of streptococci also have been reported with moxifloxacin when compared with cephalexin in the treatment of uncomplicated SSTIs.[33] The newer fluoroquinolones (i.e., levofloxacin, gatifloxacin, and moxifloxacin) are all effective treatment for uncomplicated SSTIs, but their role in complicated infections has not been elucidated.[1,33–35] The use of fluoroquinolones is of concern, however, because of increasing reports of resistance among both gram-positive and gram-negative bacteria.[36] Sensitivity testing is recommended when a fluoroquinolone is to be used. Also, fluoroquinolones are not approved for use in children because of toxicity concerns.

For cellulitis caused by gram-negative bacilli or a mixture of microorganisms, immediate antimicrobial chemotherapy, as determined by Gram stain, is essential (see Table 108–3). Surgical excision of necrotic tissue and drainage also may be appropriate. Gram-negative cellulitis may be treated appropriately with an aminoglycoside or first- or second-generation cephalosporin. If gram-positive aerobic bacteria are also present, penicillin G or a semisynthetic penicillin should be added to the regimen. Ceftazidime and the fluoroquinolones are effective in the treatment of cellulitis caused by both gram-negative and gram-positive bacteria.[1,31]

Since some infections may be polymicrobic in nature, antibiotic therapy may need to be broadened to include agents with good activity against anaerobic bacteria. Many different treatment regimens are possible depending on the bacteriology of the lesion (see Table 108–3). Usually an aminoglycoside combined with an antianaerobic cephalosporin, extended-spectrum penicillin, or clindamycin is used. Second- or third-generation cephalosporins have been suggested as single-agent therapy in certain instances.[37,38] Monotherapy with a β-lactam plus β-lactamase inhibitor combination antibiotic or a carbapenem also may be appropriate in seriously ill patients. Therapy should be 10 to 14 days in duration.

Because gram-negative and mixed aerobic-anaerobic cellulitis can progress quickly to serious tissue invasion, therapeutic intervention should be immediate. If treated early, a quick response can be seen. Unfortunately, because these infections often occur in patients with compromised immune defenses, they may still progress, even with therapeutic intervention. If the infectious process is secondary to a systemic cause (e.g., diabetes), the treatment course often is prolonged and may be associated with high morbidity and mortality.

Infections in injection drug users generally are treated similarly to those in other types of patients.[21] It is important that

TABLE 108–3. Initial Treatment Regimens for Cellulitis Caused by Various Pathogens

Antibiotic	Adult Dose and Route	Pediatric Dose and Route
Staphylococcal or Unknown Gram-Positive Infection		
Mild infection	Dicloxacillin 0.25–0.5 g PO every 6 h[a,b]	Dicloxacillin 25–50 mg/kg/day PO in four divided doses[a,b]
Moderate–severe infection	Nafcillin or oxacillin 1–2 g IV every 4–6 h[a,b]	Nafcillin or oxacillin 150–200 mg/kg/day (not to exceed 12 g/24 h) IV in four to six equally divided doses[a,b]
Streptococcal (Documented)		
Mild infection	Penicillin VK 0.5 g PO every 6 h[a] or procaine penicillin G 600,000 units IM every 8–12 h[a]	Penicillin VK 125–250 mg PO every 6–8 h, or procaine penicillin G 25,000–50,000 units/kg (not to exceed 600,000 units) IM every 8–12 h[a]
Moderate–severe infection	Aqueous penicillin G 1–2 million units IV every 4–6 h[a,c]	Aqueous penicillin G 100,000–200,000 units/kg/day IV in four divided doses[a]
Gram-Negative Bacilli		
Mild infection	Cefaclor 0.5 g PO every 8 h[d] or cefuroxime axetil 0.5 g PO every 12 h[d]	Cefaclor 20–40 mg/kg/day (not to exceed 1 g) PO in three divided doses or cefuroxime axetil 0.125–0.25 g (tablets) PO every 12 h
Moderate–severe infection	Aminoglycoside[e] or IV cephalosporin (first- or second-generation depending on severity of infection or susceptibility pattern)[d]	Aminoglycoside[e] or intravenous cephalosporin (first- or second-generation depending on severity of infection or susceptibility pattern)
Polymicrobic Infection without Anaerobes		
	Aminoglycoside[e] + penicillin G 1–2 million units every 4–6 h or a semisynthetic penicillin (nafcillin 1–2 g every 4–6 h) depending on isolation of staphylococci or streptococci[b]	Aminoglycoside[e] + penicillin G 100,000 to 200,000 units/kg/day IV in four divided doses or a semisynthetic penicillin (nafcillin 150–200 mg/kg/day [not to exceed 12 g/24 h] IV in four to six equally divided doses) depending on isolation of staphylococci or streptococci[b]
Polymicrobic Infection with Anaerobes		
Mild infection	Amoxicillin/clavulanate 0.875 g PO every 12 h *or* A fluoroquinolone (ciprofloxacin 0.4 g PO every 12 h or levofloxacin 0.5–0.75 g PO every 24 h) plus clindamycin 0.3–0.6 g PO every 8 h or metronidazole 0.5 g PO every 8 h	Amoxicillin/clavulanic acid 20 mg/kg/day PO in three divided doses
Moderate–severe infection	Aminoglycoside[e,f] + clindamycin 0.6–0.9 g IV every 8 h or metronidazole 0.5 g IV every 8 h *or* Monotherapy with second- or third-generation cephalosporin (cefoxitin 1–2 g IV every 6 h or ceftizoxime 1–2 g IV every 8 h) *or* Monotherapy with imipenem 0.5 g IV every 6–8 h, meropenem 1 g IV every 8 h, or extended-spectrum penicillins with a β-lactamase inhibitor (piperacillin/tazobactam 4.5 g IV every 6 h)	Aminoglycoside[e] plus clindamycin 15 mg/kg/day IV in three divided doses or metronidazole 30–50 mg/kg/day IV in three divided doses

[a]For penicillin-allergic patients, use clindamycin 150–300 mg orally every 6–8 h (pediatric dosing: 10–30 mg/kg/day in 3–4 divided doses).

[b]For methicillin-resistant staphylococci, use vancomycin 0.5–1 g every 6–12 h (pediatric dosing 40 mg/kg/day in divided doses) with dosage adjustments made for renal dysfunction.

[c]For type II necrotizing fasciitis, use clindamycin 0.6–0.9 g IV every 8 h (in children, clindamycin 15 mg/kg/day IV in 3 divided doses) should be added.

[d]For penicillin-allergic adults, use a fluoroquinolone (ciprofloxacin 0.5–0.75 g PO every 12 h or 0.4 g IV every 12 h; levofloxacin 0.5–0.75 g PO or IV every 24 h; gatifloxacin 0.4 g PO or IV every 24 h; or moxifloxacin 0.4 g PO or IV every 24 h).

[e]Gentamicin or tobramycin, 2 mg/kg loading dose, then maintenance dose determined by serum concentrations.

[f]A fluoroquinolone or aztreonam 1 g IV every 6 h may be used in place of the aminoglycoside in patients with severe renal dysfunction or other relative contraindications to aminoglycoside use.

blood cultures be obtained because 25% to 35% of patients may be bacteremic.[21,39] Also, patients should be assessed for the presence of abscesses; incision, drainage, and culture of these lesions are of extreme importance.[10] Initial antimicrobial therapy while awaiting culture results of abscesses should include coverage for anaerobic organisms, in addition to *S. aureus* and streptococci.[21] In areas where MRSA is prevalent, treatment with vancomycin plus metronidazole is preferred.[21]

EVALUATION OF THERAPEUTIC OUTCOMES

If treated promptly with appropriate antibiotics, the majority of patients with cellulitis are cured rapidly. Culture and sensitivity results should be evaluated carefully both for the adequacy of culture material and the presence of resistant organisms. Additional high-quality samples for culture may be needed for microbiologic analysis. Failure to respond to therapy also may be indicative of an underlying local or systemic problem or a misdiagnosis.

NECROTIZING SOFT TISSUE INFECTIONS

Necrotizing soft tissue infections consist of a group of highly lethal infections that require early and aggressive surgical débridement in addition to appropriate antibiotics and intensive supportive care.[40] A number of different descriptive terms have been used to classify necrotizing infections. These have been based on factors such as predisposing conditions, onset of symptoms, pain, skin appearance, etiologic agent, gas production, muscle involvement, and systemic toxicity. While many of the necrotizing soft tissue infections have been designated as unique infectious processes, they all share similar pathophysiologies, clinical features, and treatment approaches.[40] The major clinical entities of necrotizing infections are *necrotizing fasciitis* and *clostridial myonecrosis* (gas gangrene).[40]

❻ Necrotizing fasciitis is a rare but very severe infection of the subcutaneous tissue that may be caused by aerobic and/or anaerobic bacteria and results in progressive destruction of the superficial fascia and subcutaneous fat. It is generally characterized as one of two different types based on bacterial etiology. Type I necrotizing fasciitis generally occurs after trauma and surgery and involves a mixture of anaerobes (*Bacteroides, Peptostreptococcus*) and facultative bacteria (streptococci and members of Enterobacteriaceae) that act synergistically to cause destruction of fat and fascia. In type I infections, the skin may be spared, and the speed at which the infection spreads is somewhat slower than type II. Necrotizing fasciitis affecting the male genitalia has been termed *Fournier's gangrene.* Type II necrotizing fasciitis is caused by virulent strains of *S. pyogenes* and is more commonly referred to as *streptococcal gangrene.* This type of infection has received considerable attention in recent years because of reports of "flesh-eating bacteria" by the lay press. Unlike previous reports of streptococcal gangrene that affected older individuals with underlying diseases, recent reports have occurred primarily in young, previously healthy adults following some type of minor trauma. It differs from the polymicrobial type I infections in its clinical presentation. Type II infections have rapidly extending necrosis of subcutaneous tissues and skin, gangrene, severe local pain, and systemic toxicity.[11] Type II infections are also highly associated with an early onset of shock and organ failure and are present in approximately half the cases of streptococcal toxic shock-like syndrome.[11]

Clostridial myonecrosis is a necrotizing infection that involves the skeletal muscle. Gas production and muscle necrosis are prominent features of this infection, which readily explains why this infection is commonly referred to as *gas gangrene.*[40] The infection advances rapidly, often over a matter of a few hours.[40] Most infections occur after surgery or trauma, with *Clostridium perfringens* identified as the most common etiologic agent.

CLINICAL PRESENTATION

GENERAL

- These infections may occur in almost any anatomic location but most frequently involve the abdomen, the perineum, and the lower extremities.
- Patients often have predisposing factors such as diabetes mellitus, local trauma or infection, or recent surgery.

SYMPTOMS

- Systemic symptoms generally are marked (e.g., fever, chills, and leukocytosis) and may include shock and organ failure, especially in patients with type II infections.
- In general, pain in the affected area and systemic toxicity are more pronounced than would be expected with cellulitis.

SIGNS

- At the beginning of an infection, it may be difficult to differentiate between necrotizing fasciitis and cellulitis.
- Like cellulitis, the affected area is initially hot, swollen, and erythematous without sharp margins.
- The affected area is often shiny, exquisitely tender, and painful.
- Diffuse swelling of the area is followed by the appearance of bullae filled with clear fluid.
- The infectious process progresses rapidly, with the skin taking on a maroon or violaceous color after several days.
- Without appropriate intervention, the infection will evolve rapidly into a frank cutaneous gangrene, sometimes with myonecrosis (involvement of skin and muscle).
- Because of the aggressive nature and high mortality (20% to 50%) associated with these infections, a rapid diagnosis is critical.

LABORATORY TESTS

- Although computed tomography and magnetic resonance imaging studies can distinguish these infections, the best and most rapid diagnosis of necrotizing infections is obtained via surgical exploration.
- Intraoperative samples should be collected for culture and sensitivity, as well as for histologic examination.
- Unlike necrotizing fasciitis, clostridial myonecrosis shows little inflammation on histologic examination.

OTHER DIAGNOSTIC TESTS

- Because marked systemic symptoms are seen commonly in necrotizing infections, blood samples should be collected for complete blood count and chemistry profile, as well as for bacterial culture.

▶ TREATMENT: Necrotizing Soft Tissue Infections

After the diagnosis is made, immediate and aggressive surgical débridement of all necrotic tissue is essential.[40] Broad-spectrum antibiotics should be administered, with coverage against streptococci, Enterobacteriaceae, and anaerobes. A number of antibiotic regimens have been used successfully to treat necrotizing soft tissue infections; these are generally similar to those used for severe polymicrobic cellulitis involving anaerobes (see Table 108–3). Other combina-

tion antibiotic regimens that may be used prior to obtaining bacteriologic data include ampicillin, gentamicin, and clindamycin (or metronidazole); ampicillin-sulbactam and gentamicin; or imipenem and metronidazole.[10]

Antibiotic therapy can be modified after Gram stain and culture reports are available. If a diagnosis of type II necrotizing fasciitis is established, the broad-spectrum empirical therapy should be replaced with the combination of penicillin and clindamycin.[11] While *S. pyogenes* remains susceptible to penicillin, clindamycin has been shown experimentally to be more effective.[11] A number of factors have been postulated to explain the higher efficacy of clindamycin. These include the mechanism of action (inhibition of protein synthesis), which is not affected by the size of the inoculum or the stage of bacterial growth.[11] In addition, clindamycin has immunomodulatory properties that may account for the higher efficacy.[11] The combination of penicillin and clindamycin is also recommended for treatment of clostridial myonecrosis.[40] In addition, hyperbaric oxygen is of some benefit for clostridial myonecrosis.[40]

EVALUATION OF THERAPEUTIC OUTCOMES

Because of the high mortality associated with necrotizing infections, rapid and complete débridement of all devitalized and necrotic tissue is essential. Surgical débridement, coupled with appropriate antimicrobial therapy and typical supportive measures for management of shock and organ failure, should stabilize the patient. Vital signs and laboratory tests should be monitored carefully for signs of resolution of the infection. Change in antimicrobial therapy or additional surgical débridement may be needed in patients who do not show signs of improvement.

DIABETIC FOOT INFECTIONS

Three major types of foot infections are seen in diabetic patients: deep abscesses, cellulitis of the dorsum, and mal perforans ulcers.[41] Most deep abscesses involve the central plantar space (arch) and are caused by minor penetrating trauma or by an extension of infection of a nail or web space of the toes. Skin infections of the dorsal area generally arise from infections in the toes that are related to routine care of the nails, nailbeds, and calluses of the toes. Mal perforans ulcer is a chronic ulcer of the sole of the foot. The ulcer develops on thickened, hardened calluses over the first or fifth metatarsal. Mal perforans ulcers are associated with neuropathy, which is responsible for the misalignment of the weight-bearing bones of the foot.[41] Osteomyelitis is one of the most serious complications of foot problems in diabetic patients and may occur in 30% to 40% of infections.[42–44]

EPIDEMIOLOGY

Disorders of the foot are among the most common complications of diabetes, accounting for as many as 20% of all hospitalizations in diabetic patients at an annual cost of $200 to $350 million.[42,45] Approximately 25% of diabetic patients experience significant soft tissue infection at some time during the course of their lifetime. Approximately 55,000 lower extremity amputations, often sequelae of uncontrolled infection, are performed each year on diabetic patients; this represents 50% of all nontraumatic amputations in the United States.[45] Between 10% and 20% of diabetics will undergo additional surgery or amputation of a second limb within 12 months of the initial amputation.[46] By 5 years, this increases to 25% to 50%, with death reported in as much as two-thirds of patients.[46]

ETIOLOGY

Diabetic foot infections begin with local bacterial invasion and typically involve a number of different bacterial pathogens.[46] The infections are polymicrobic in nature, with an average of 4.1 to 5.8 isolates per culture[47] (Table 108–4). Staphylococci (especially *S. aureus*) and streptococci are the most common pathogens, although gram-negative bacilli and/or anaerobes occur in approximately 50% of cases.[48] Common gram-negative bacilli isolated include *E. coli, Klebsiella* spp., *Proteus* spp., and *P. aeruginosa. Bacteroides fragilis* and *Peptostreptococcus* spp. are among the most common anaerobes isolated.

The optimum technique for obtaining culture material from ulcerated lesions is still debated.[41] Routine swab cultures of ulcerative lesions are difficult to interpret because of organisms that colonize the surface of the wounds. Cultures of material from sinus tracts are also unreliable. The correlation between these superficial cultures and true deep cultures (via biopsy or needle aspiration of drainage or abscess fluid) is poor.[43,47,48] Therefore, cultures and sensitivity tests should be done with specimens obtained from a deep culture whenever possible. Before the wound is cultured, it should be scrubbed vigorously with saline-moistened sterile gauze to remove any overlying necrotic debris.[49] Cultures then can be obtained from the wound base, preferably from expressed pus.[49] Specimens obtained from curettage of the base of the ulcer correlate best with results from deep-tissue or bone biopsies.[49]

PATHOPHYSIOLOGY

Three key factors are involved in the development of diabetic foot problems: (1) neuropathy, (2) angiopathy and ischemia, and (3) immunologic defects. Any of these disorders can occur in isolation; however, they frequently occur together.

Neuropathic changes to the autonomic nervous system as a consequence of diabetes may affect the motor nerve supply of small intrinsic muscles of the foot, resulting in muscular imbalance, abnormal stresses on tissues and bone, and repetitive injuries.[50] Diminished sensory perception causes an absence of pain and unawareness of minor injuries and ulceration. Also, the sympathetic nerve supply may be damaged and can result in an absence of sweating; this leads to dry cracked skin, which can become secondarily infected.[42]

TABLE 108–4. Bacterial Isolates from Foot Infections in Diabetic Patients

Organisms	Percentage of Isolates
Aerobes	69%
Gram-positive	45%
Staphylococcus aureus	13%
Streptococcus spp.	11%
Enterococcus spp.	8%
Coagulase-negative staphylococci	7%
Gram-negative	24%
Proteus spp.	5%
Enterobacter spp.	3%
Escherichia coli	3%
Klebsiella spp.	2%
Pseudomonas aeruginosa	2%
Other gram-negative bacilli	7%
Anaerobes	31%
Peptostreptococcus spp.	13%
Bacteroides fragilis group	5%
Other Bacteroides spp.	4%
Clostridium spp.	2%
Other anaerobes	7%

From Ref. 34 with permission.

Atherosclerosis is more common, appears at a younger age, and progresses more rapidly in the diabetic than in the nondiabetic. Diabetics may have problems with both small vessels (microangiopathy) and large vessels (macroangiopathy) that can result in varying degrees of ischemia, ultimately leading to skin breakdown and infection.

Diabetic patients typically have normal humoral immunity, normal levels of immunoglobulins, and normal antibody responses. Patients with diabetes, however, have impaired phagocytosis and intracellular microbicidal function as compared with nondiabetics; this may be related to angiopathy and low tissue levels of oxygen.[42] These defects in cell-mediated immunity make patients with diabetes more susceptible to certain types of infection and impair the patients' ability to heal wounds adequately.[50]

CLINICAL PRESENTATION

GENERAL

- Infections are often much more extensive than they appear initially.

SYMPTOMS

- Patients with peripheral neuropathy often do not experience pain but seek medical care for swelling or erythema in the foot.

SIGNS

- Clinical signs of infection in the diabetic foot may not be present secondary to the angiopathy and neuropathy.
- When present, lesions vary in size and clinical features (e.g., erythema, edema, warmth, presence of pus, draining sinuses, pain, and tenderness).
- A foul-smelling odor suggests the presence of anaerobic organisms.
- Temperature may be mildly elevated or normal.

LABORATORY TESTS

- Specimens for culture and sensitivities should be collected.
- If possible, deep intraoperative samples should be obtained during surgical débridement.
- Because of the complex microbiology of these infections, wounds must be cultured for both aerobic and anaerobic organisms.

OTHER DIAGNOSTIC TESTS

- The presence of osteomyelitis also must be assessed via radiograph, bone scan, or both, as appropriate.

▶ TREATMENT: Diabetic Foot Infections

The goal of therapy of diabetic foot infections is preservation of as much normal limb function as possible while preventing additional infectious complications. Up to 90% of these infections can be treated successfully with a comprehensive treatment approach that includes both wound care and antimicrobial therapy.[43] After carefully assessing the extent of the lesion and obtaining necessary cultures, necrotic tissue must be thoroughly débrided, with wound drainage and amputation as required. Wounds must be kept clean and dressings changed frequently (two to three times daily). Because of the relationship between hyperglycemia and immune system defects, glycemic control must be maximized to ensure optimal wound healing. In addition, the patient's activities should be restricted initially to bed rest for leg elevation and control of edema, if present. Finally, appropriate antimicrobials must be initiated.[42–45] However, the optimal antimicrobial therapy for diabetic foot infections has yet to be defined.

The majority of mild, uncomplicated infections can be managed successfully on an outpatient basis with oral antimicrobials and good wound care. Many different agents have been studied, including cefaclor, cephalexin, fluoroquinolones, clindamycin, and amoxicillin–clavulanic acid; these agents provide clinical cure rates of 60% to 85% in published studies.[44,48,50,51] However, significant failure rates and/or relapse rates have been reported with the use of oral agents. In addition, the development of resistance was problematic in some infections involving *P. aeruginosa* and staphylococci.[52] Many clinicians consider amoxicillin–clavulanic acid to be the preferred agent because of its broad spectrum of activity, which includes staphylococci, streptococci, enterococci, and many Enterobacteriaceae and anaerobes.[48] However, this agent does not have activity against *P. aeruginosa*. Fluoroquinolones, which provide coverage against *P. aeruginosa,* have been studied extensively as monotherapy, but they are perhaps most appropriately used in combination with metronidazole or clindamycin to provide anaerobic activity.[2] Oral antimicrobials should be used cautiously in serious infections, especially those complicated by osteomyelitis, extensive ulceration, areas of necrosis, or a combination of these.

Initial therapy for patients requiring hospitalization for moderate to severe infections is similar to that for polymicrobic cellulitis with anaerobes (see Table 109–3). Monotherapy with broad-spectrum parenteral antimicrobials, along with appropriate medical or surgical management, or both, is often effective in treating these infections, including those in which osteomyelitis is present.[53,54] Monotherapy is particularly attractive because of the potential advantages of convenience, cost, and avoidance of toxicities. Microbiologic and clinical cure rates ranging from 60% to 90% may be expected from any of these agents; selection of a specific regimen is determined primarily by cost. In penicillin-allergic patients, metronidazole or clindamycin plus either a fluoroquinolone, aztreonam, or possibly a third-generation cephalosporin is appropriate.[2,44,48,50] Vancomycin also is used frequently in severe infections because of its excellent activity against gram-positive pathogens. With the increased incidence of MRSA, linezolid, quinupristin-dalfopristin, and daptomycin are alternatives for treatment of these resistant organisms.[1,2] Because these patients already may have some degree of diabetic nephropathy that may place them at higher risk of nephrotoxicity, strong recommendations have been made for the avoidance of aminoglycoside antibiotics unless no alternative agents are available.[42] When an aminoglycoside is used, care must be taken to avoid further compromising renal function. All antibiotic regimes should be adjusted as necessary for renal dysfunction.

Empirical therapy that is totally comprehensive in its coverage of all possible pathogens may not be necessary unless the infection is life-threatening.[48,53,54] No differences were reported in the efficacy of ampicillin-sulbactam versus imipenem-cilastatin for treatment of limb-threatening diabetic foot infections despite the higher incidence of potential pathogens resistant to the ampicillin-sulbactam regimen.[53]

Mild infections can be treated with oral agents and generally should be treated for at least 10 to 14 days, whereas more severe infections dictate initial parenteral therapy and often require up to 21 days or more of antibiotic therapy. In cases of underlying osteomyelitis, treatment should continue for 6 to 12 weeks.[42,44,48,50] After healing of the infection has occurred, a well-designed program for prevention of further infections should be instituted.

EVALUATION OF THERAPEUTIC OUTCOMES

Therapy should be reevaluated carefully after 48 to 72 hours to assess favorable response. Change in therapy (or route of administration, if oral) should be considered if clinical improvement is not observed at this time. For optimal results, drug therapy should be appropriately modified according to information from deep tissue culture and the clinical condition of the patient. Infections in diabetic patients often require extended courses of therapy because of impaired host immunity and poor wound healing.

PRESSURE SORES

The terms *decubitus ulcer, bed sore,* and *pressure sore* are used interchangeably. The decubitus ulcer and the bed sore are types of pressure sores. The term *decubitus ulcer* is derived from the Latin word *decumbere,* meaning "lying down." Pressure sores, however, can develop regardless of a patient's position.

Numerous systems for classification of pressure sores have been described. The two most frequently used systems are those of Shea[55] and the 1989 National Pressure Ulcer Advisory Panel.[56] These classification systems define the various stages of progression through which a pressure sore may pass (Table 108–5).

Complications of pressure sores are not uncommon and may be life-threatening. Infection is one of the most serious and most frequently encountered complications of pressure ulcers. Bacterial colonization must be differentiated from true bacterial infection. While most pressure sore wounds are colonized, the majority of these eventually heal.[57] When the tissue is infected, there is bacterial invasion of previously healthy tissue. Without treatment, an initial small, localized area of ulceration can progress rapidly to 5 to 6 cm within days. The visible ulcer is just a small portion of the actual wound; up to 70% of the total wound is below the skin. A pressure-gradient phenomenon is created by which the wound takes on a conical nature; the smallest point is at the skin surface, and the largest portion of the defect is at the base of the ulcer (Fig. 108–1).

EPIDEMIOLOGY

Pressure sores are seen most frequently in chronically debilitated persons, the elderly, and persons with serious spinal cord injury. Generally, patients who are at risk for pressure sores are elderly or chronically ill young patients who are immobilized either in bed or a wheelchair and who may have altered mental status and/or incontinence.

ETIOLOGY

Similar to diabetic foot infections, a large variety of aerobic gram-positive and gram-negative organisms, as well as anaerobes, frequently are isolated from wound cultures.[58] Curettage of the ulcer base after débridement provides more reliable culture information than does needle aspiration.[57] Biopsy specimens give the most reliable data but may not be practical to obtain. Deep-tissue cultures from different sites may give different results. Cultures collected from pressure ulcers reveal polymicrobial growth. A culture collected by swab is likely to identify surface bacteria colonizing the wound rather than to diagnose the infection.[59]

PATHOPHYSIOLOGY

Many factors are thought to predispose patients to the formation of pressure sores: paralysis, paresis, immobilization, malnutrition, anemia, infection, and advanced age. Four factors thought to be most critical to their formation are pressure, shearing forces, friction, and moisture; however, there is still debate as to the exact pathophysiology of pressure sore formation.

Pressure is the essential element in the formation of pressure sores. The areas of highest pressure are generated most often over the bony prominences. Studies show that when the pressure is relieved intermittently within a 2-hour period, only minimal changes

TABLE 108–5. Pressure Sore Classification[48]

Stage 1	Pressure sore is generally reversible, is limited to the epidermis, and resembles an abrasion. It is best described as an irregularly shaped area of soft tissue swelling with induration and heat.
Stage 2	A stage 2 sore may also, be reversible; it extends through the dermis to the subcutaneous fat along with extensive undermining.
Stage 3*	In this instance, the sore or ulcer extends further into subcutaneous fat along with extensive undermining.
Stage 4*	The sore or ulcer is characterized by penetration into deep fascia involving both muscle and bone.

*Stage 3 and 4 lesions are unlikely to resolve on their own and often require surgical intervention.

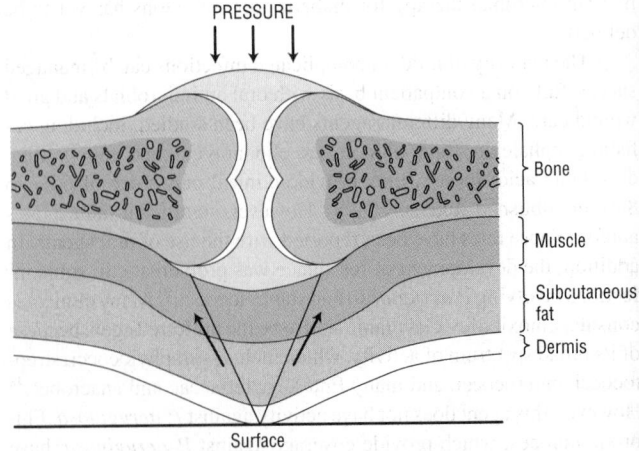

FIGURE 108–1. Distribution of forces involved with sore formation in a conical fashion.

occur in soft tissue and skin structures.[60] Therefore, both the degree of pressure and the length of time that the pressure is applied are important.

Shearing forces are caused by the sliding of adjacent parallel surfaces of soft tissues in an unequal fashion. This situation can occur when the head of a bed is raised, causing the upper torso to slide downward, transmitting pressure to the sacrum and other areas. This effect results in occlusion or distortion of vessels, leading to compromise of the dermis. At the same time, sitting and gravity create shearing forces; the posterior sacral skin area can become fixed secondary to friction with the bed. The effects of friction and shearing forces combine, resulting in transmission of force to the deep portion of the superficial fascia and leading to further damage of soft tissue structures.

Compounding the problems of shearing and friction forces are the macerating effects of excessive moisture in the local environment, resulting from incontinence and perspiration. This factor is of critical importance because when combined with the other forces, it increases the risk of pressure sore formation fivefold.[61]

CLINICAL PRESENTATION

GENERAL

- Pressure sores can occur anywhere on the body.
- However, more than 95% of all pressure sores are located on the lower part of the body (65% in the region of the pelvis and 3.4% on the lower extremities) (Fig. 108–2).
- The most common sites on the lower portion of the body are the sacral and coccygeal areas, ischial tuberosities, and greater trochanter.

SYMPTOMS

- Patients with pressure sores commonly have other medical problems that may mask the typical signs and symptoms of infection.

SIGNS

- Clinical infection is recognized by the presence of surrounding redness, heat, and pain.
- Purulent discharge, foul odor, and systemic signs (e.g., fever and leukocytosis) of infection may be present.

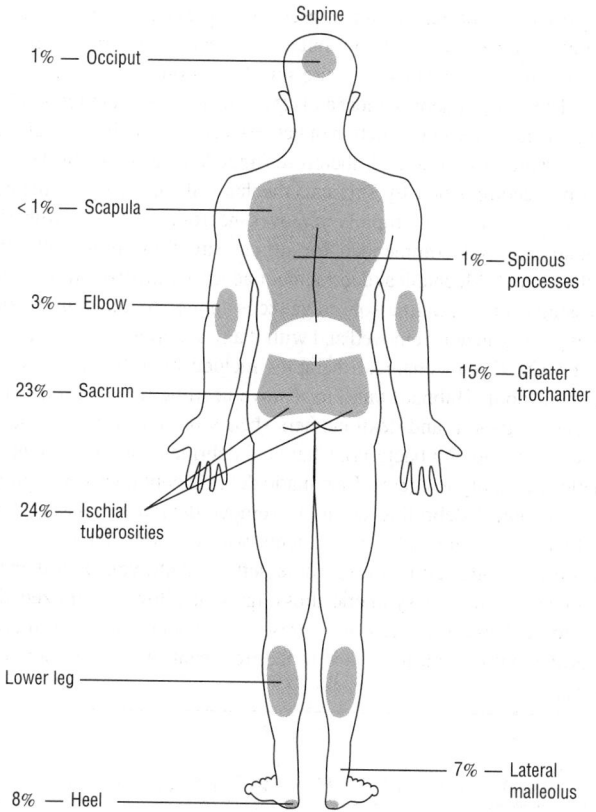

FIGURE 108–2. Supine view of areas where pressure sore formation tends to occur.

LABORATORY TESTS

- Cultures should be collected from either a biopsy or fluid obtained by needle aspiration.

OTHER DIAGNOSTIC TESTS

- Clinicians also must be aware of the possibility of underlying osteomyelitis; therefore, magnetic resonance imaging or other radiographic procedures should be considered.

▶ TREATMENT: Pressure Sores

8 Prevention is the single most important aspect in the management of pressure sores. Prevention is far easier and less costly than the intensive care necessary for the healing and eventual closure of pressure sores. Of primary importance, then, is the ability to identify patients who are at high risk so that preventive measures may be instituted.

The medical approach to the treatment of pressure sores depends on the stage of the disease. Medical management generally is indicated for lesions that are of moderate size and relatively shallow depth (stage 1 or 2 lesions) and are not located over a bony prominence. Depending on their location and severity, from 30% to 80% of these ulcers will heal without an operation. Surgical intervention is almost always necessary for ulcers that extend through superficial fascia or into bone (stage 3 and 4 lesions).

The goal of therapy is to clean and decontaminate the ulcer to promote wound healing by permitting the formation of healthy granulation tissue or to prepare the wound for an operative procedure. The main factors to be considered for successful topical therapy (local care) are (1) relief of pressure, (2) débridement of necrotic tissue as needed, (3) wound cleansing, (4) dressing selection, and (5) prevention, diagnosis, and treatment of infection.[62]

Friction and shearing forces can be minimized with proper positioning. Skin care and prevention of soilage are important, with the intent being to keep the surface relatively free of moisture. Patients with problems of incontinence should be cleaned frequently, and efforts should be made to keep the involved areas dry. Natural sheepskin is believed to be useful in minimizing the effects of moisture, shearing forces, and friction. Relief of pressure is probably the single most important factor in preventing pressure sore formation. Relief for a period of only 5 minutes once every 2 hours is believed to give protection against pressure sore formation.[60]

The goals of débridement and cleansing measures are removal of devitalized tissue and reduction of bacterial contamination, which can slow granulation time and, therefore, impede healing. Débridement can be accomplished by surgical, mechanical, or chemical means. Surgical débridement rapidly removes necrotic material from the wound and is recommended for urgent situations (e.g., cellulitis and sepsis).[62] Mechanical débridement generally involves wet-to-dry dressing changes. Saline-soaked gauze is applied to the wound; after drying, the gauze is removed and with it any adherent necrotic tissue. Other effective mechanical therapies include hydrotherapy (use of the whirlpool [Hubbard tank] to remove necrotic tissue and debris), wound irrigation, and dextranomers (beads placed in the wound to absorb exudate and bacteria). Chemical débridement includes enzymatic and autolytic agents. Enzymatic débridement involves application of topical débriding agents to remove devitalized tissue. This method is recommended for patients who cannot tolerate surgery or are in a long-term care or home setting. Autolytic débridement involves the use of synthetic dressings that allow devitalized tissue to self-digest via enzymes present in wound fluids. Autolytic débridement is contraindicated in the treatment of infected pressure sores.

Pressure sore wounds should be cleaned with normal saline. Cleansing agents that are cytotoxic, such as povidone-iodine, iodophor, sodium hypochlorite solution, hydrogen peroxide, and acetic acid, should be avoided.[62] Many of these agents impair healing. Many different types of dressings are available for pressure sores. Wound dressing materials should keep the wound moist, allow free exchange of air, act as a physical barrier to bacteria, and prevent physical damage. Controlled studies of the various types of wound dressings have shown no significant differences in healing outcomes.[62] Occlusive dressings should be avoided if infection is present.[59] If occlusive dressings are used, any infection should be controlled or the dressing frequency increased.

Systemic treatment (see Table 108–3) of an infected pressure ulcer should be guided by results from appropriately collected cultures. Systemic antibiotics generally are reserved for treatment of bacteremia, sepsis, cellulitis, or osteomyelitis.[59] However, a 2-week trial of topical antibiotics (silver sulfadiazine or triple antibiotic) is recommended for a clean ulcer that is not healing or is producing a moderate amount of exudate despite appropriate care.[59]

Other nonpharmacologic approaches to shortening the healing time have included the use of hyperbaric oxygenation, hydrotherapy, high-frequency/high-intensity sound waves, and electrotherapy.[57,63] Electrical stimulation is the only adjunctive therapy that has been shown to be effective.[57,63]

EVALUATION OF THERAPEUTIC OUTCOMES

With appropriate wound care and antimicrobial therapy, infected pressure sores can heal. A reduction in erythema, warmth, pain, and other signs and symptoms should be seen in 48 to 72 hours.

BITE WOUNDS

Bite wounds have a substantial potential for infectious complications. If left untreated, complications such as soft tissue infection and osteomyelitis may occur, possibly requiring extensive débridement or amputation. Approximately half the population in the United States will be bitten by either an animal or another human sometime during their lifetimes.[64]

ANIMAL BITES

EPIDEMIOLOGY

Dog bites account for approximately 80% of all animal bite wounds requiring medical attention. A survey of U.S. emergency departments reported an annual adjusted total of 333,687 visits from 1992 to 1994 for new dog bite–related injuries.[65] Based on the data gathered in this study, approximately 914 new dog bite injuries are seen in emergency departments every day. Dog bites commonly occur in individuals younger than 20 years of age (52.2% of reported cases) who are most often male (57.8%). More than 70% of bites are to the extremities.[64] Occasionally, facial bites may occur, and these are seen most often in children younger than 15 years of age and can be a lethal event via exsanguination. From 1979 through 1994, 279 deaths were the result of attacks by dogs.[66]

Patients at greatest risk of acquiring an infection after a bite have had a puncture wound (usually the hand), have not sought medical attention within 12 hours of the injury, and are older than 50 years of age.[67,68]

Cat bites, with an estimated incidence of 5% to 15% of all animal bites, are the second most common cause of animal bite wounds in the United States.[69] Bites and scratches occur most commonly on the upper extremities, with most injuries reported in women.[64] Infection rates, estimated at 30% to 50%, are more than double those seen with dog bites.[64,69]

ETIOLOGY

Infections from dog bite wounds are caused predominantly by organisms documented to be from the dog's oral flora.[68,70] Most infections are polymicrobial, with approximately five bacterial isolates per culture.[71] Pasteurella species are the most frequent isolates. Other common aerobes include streptococci, staphylococci, Moraxella, and Neisseria. The most common anaerobes are Fusobacterium, Bacteroides, Porphyromonas, and Prevotella.[71] Wound-site cultures in both infected and noninfected patients have similar bacteria present, with aerobic organisms isolated from 74% to 90% and anaerobic organisms isolated from 41% to 49%.[71–73]

Infections arising from cat bites or scratches are frequently (75%) caused by P. multocida, which has been isolated in the oropharynx of 50% to 70% of healthy cats.[67] Mixed aerobic and anaerobic infections have been reported in 63% of cat bite wounds, whereas approximately one-third of cultures grow aerobes only.[71] Both tularemia (Pasteurella tularensis) and rabies also have been transmitted by cat bites.[67]

PATHOPHYSIOLOGY

The potential for infection from an animal bite is great owing to the pressure that can be exerted during the bite and the vast number of potential pathogens that make up the normal oral flora.[70] Cats' teeth are slender and extremely sharp. Their teeth easily penetrate into bones and joints, resulting in a higher incidence of septic arthritis and osteomyelitis.[64] While a dog's teeth may not be as sharp, they can exert a pressure of 200 to 450 lb/in^2 and therefore result in a serious crush injury with much devitalized tissue.[70] Known human pathogens such as *S. aureus*, *P. multocida*, and anaerobes are among the more than 64 species of bacteria that are harbored in the average dog mouth.[70] In addition, the polymicrobic (aerobic and anaerobic) nature of animal bites provides a synergistic relationship, thus making an infection harder to eradicate.[70]

CLINICAL PRESENTATION

GENERAL

- Health care providers see two distinct groups of patients seeking medical attention for dog bites.
- The first group presents within 12 hours of the injury; these patients require general wound care, repair of tear wounds, or rabies and/or tetanus treatment.
- The second group of patients presents more than 12 hours after the injury has occurred; these patients usually have clinical signs of infection and seek medical attention for infection-related complaints.

SYMPTOMS

- Patients seek medical care for infection-related complaints (i.e., pain, purulent discharge, and swelling).

SIGNS

- Patients with infected dog bite wounds generally present with a localized cellulitis and pain at the site of injury.
- Cellulitis usually spreads proximally from the initial site of injury, and a gray malodorous discharge may be encountered.
- If *P. multocida* is present, a rapidly progressing cellulitis is observed, with pain and swelling developing within 24 (70%) to 48 (90%) hours of initial injury.
- Fever is uncommon.
- Fewer than 20% of patients have a concomitant adenopathy or lymphangitis.

LABORATORY TESTS

- Samples for bacterial cultures (aerobic and anaerobic) should be obtained.
- Wounds seen less than 8 hours or more than 24 hours after injury that show no signs of infection may not need to be cultured.

OTHER DIAGNOSTIC TESTS

- A roentgenogram of the affected part should be considered when infection is documented in proximity to a bone or joint.

▶ TREATMENT: Dog and Cat Bites (see Table 108–3)

Cultures obtained from early, noninfected bite wounds are not of great value in predicting the subsequent development of infection. Documentation of the mechanism of injury is important; if possible, an immunization history of the animal should be obtained. It is also important for the patient's tetanus immune status to be determined.

Wounds should be irrigated thoroughly with a copious volume (>150 mL) of sterile normal saline. Proper irrigation will reduce the bacterial count in the wound. Antibiotic or iodine solutions do not offer any advantage over saline and actually may increase tissue irritation. Several management techniques used in the treatment of bite wounds remain controversial; these include the extent and type of débridement,[74] the use of primary closure within 24 hours of the injury,[73] and indications for the use of antibiotics.

The role of prophylactic antimicrobial therapy for the early, non-infected bite wound remains controversial.[64,75] Unfortunately, suggestions concerning the use of prophylactic antibiotics are based on minimal data because few clinical trials have been performed. Most reports are of retrospective studies or observations of complicated cases. A meta-analysis of eight randomized trials of dog-bite wounds evaluated the use of antibiotics for prophylaxis for the prevention of infectious complications.[76] The overall occurrence of infectious complications ranged from 3.2% to 45.8%. All studies used oral antibiotics, with six of the eight using either penicillin or a penicillinase-resistant penicillin. Five of the eight studies documented a reduced risk of infection in patients receiving antimicrobial prophylaxis.

Controlled studies have not shown benefits definitively with prophylactic antibiotics for noninfected bites. Because up to 20% of bite wounds may become infected, a 3- to 5-day course of antimicrobial therapy generally is recommended.[64] This is especially important for patients at greater risk for infection (patients older than 50 years of age and those with puncture wounds and wounds to the hands, and

those who are immunocompromised).[77,78] Treatment should be directed at the typical aerobic and anaerobic oral flora of dogs, as well as at potential pathogens from the skin flora of the bite victim.

CLINICAL CONTROVERSY

To date, there is no single, universally agreed on treatment regimen for bite wounds. Penicillin provides excellent coverage for *P. multocida* but not for *S. aureus* and most of the other staphylococci that are commonly isolated from bite wounds. Although penicillinase-resistant penicillins, first-generation cephalosporins, erythromycin, and clindamycin have excellent activity against staphylococci, these agents are not active against most strains of *P. multocida*.

Antibiotic regimens suggested for empirical therapy of dog bite wounds include (1) a combination of a β-lactam antibiotic and a β-lactamase inhibitor, (2) a second-generation cephalosporin with anaerobic activity, or (3) penicillin in combination with a first-generation cephalosporin or clindamycin. Tetracyclines (e.g., doxycycline) and trimethoprim-sulfamethoxazole have activity against *P. multocida* and often are recommended as an alternative form of therapy for patients who are allergic to penicillins. However, tetracyclines should not be used in children and/or pregnant women; trimethoprim-sulfamethoxazole also should be avoided during pregnancy. Erythromycin may be considered an alternative in growing children or pregnant women. If erythromycin is selected, bacterial sensitivities should be obtained and clinical response monitored carefully because most strains of *P. multocida* are resistant.

In addition to irrigation and antibiotics, when indicated, the injured area should be immobilized and elevated. Clinical failures due to edema have occurred despite appropriate antibiotic therapy.[64] Therefore, it is important to stress to patients that the affected area should be elevated for several days or until edema has resolved.

Infections developing within the first 24 hours of a bite are caused most often by *P. multocida* and should be treated with penicillin VK 500 mg orally four times daily (in children, 80,000–90,000 units/kg per day orally divided into four doses) or amoxicillin 500 mg orally three times daily (in children, 40 mg/kg per day orally divided into three doses). Tetracycline is an alternative for penicillin-allergic children and nonpregnant adults (500 mg orally four times daily; in children, 50 mg/kg per day orally divided into four doses).[77] For severe infections, IV penicillin (1.2 million units every 4 to 6 hours) therapy should be started and followed by oral therapy when the signs of cellulitis have subsided. Treatment should be given for 10 to 14 days.

For infections developing more than 36 to 48 hours after the bite, the risk of *P. multocida* being involved decreases dramatically. In these patients, staphylococci or streptococci are the most likely causative pathogens. Therapy in this instance includes a penicillinase-resistant penicillin (dicloxacillin 250–500 mg orally four times daily; in children, 25–50 mg/kg per day orally divided into four doses) or a cephalosporin (cefuroxime axetil 500 mg orally twice daily; in children, 20–30 mg/kg per day orally divided into two doses) and should be given for a full 10 to 14 days.[77]

The fluoroquinolones are highly active in vitro against *Pasteurella* and other common aerobic isolates found in these bite wounds. Some of the newer fluoroquinolones also have activity against anaerobes commonly isolated in these infections. However, clinical data on the use of fluoroquinolones with enhanced anaerobic activity are lacking, and the role of these agents in the therapy of bite wounds has yet to be defined.[79]

Tetanus does not occur commonly after dog bites; however, it is a theoretical possibility. If the immunization history of a patient with anything other than a clean, minor wound is unknown, tetanus-diphtheria (TD) toxoids and tetanus immune globulin (TIg) should be administered.[80] Patients with wounds that do not require immunization with TD toxoids are those who have had three or more immunization doses of TIg within the past 5 years. Patients who have received three or more doses of TIg within the last 10 years or patients who received two doses of TIg within the first 24 hours of injury do not require additional TIg therapy.[80]

Because the rabies virus can be transmitted via saliva, rabies may be a potential complication of a bite. When the symptoms of rabies develop after a bite, the prognosis for survival is poor. Roughly 3% of rabies cases documented in animals were in dogs (the most frequent vectors are skunks, raccoons, and bats).

After a patient has been exposed to rabies, the treatment objectives consist of thorough irrigation of the wound, tetanus prophylaxis, antibiotic prophylaxis, if indicated, and immunization. Prompt, thorough irrigation of the wound with soap or iodine solution may reduce the development of rabies.[69] Postexposure prophylaxis immunization consists of the administration of both passive antibody and vaccine. The only exceptions to antibody administration are patients who have been immunized previously and have the appropriate degree of documented rabies antibody titers.

The management of cat bites is similar to that discussed for dog bites. Cat scratches typically involve the same organisms as bites and should be treated accordingly. Antibiotic therapy with penicillin is the mainstay, and therapy is as described for dog bites.

EVALUATION OF THERAPEUTIC OUTCOMES

Results of a Gram stain should be used to confirm the appropriateness of therapy. If signs and symptoms are not reduced within 24 hours, then surgical débridment may be needed.

HUMAN BITES

EPIDEMIOLOGY

Human bites are the third most frequent type of bite. Infected human bites can occur as bites from the teeth or from blows to the mouth (clenched-fist injuries). Human bites generally are more serious than animal bites and carry a higher likelihood of infection than do most animal bites. Infectious complications occur in 10% to 50% of patients with human bites.[69,81,82]

Self-inflicted bites most commonly occur on the lips or around the fingernails (from sucking or biting the nails). Bites by others can occur to any part of the body, but most often involve the hands. Bites to the hand are most serious and become infected more frequently. The clenched-fist injury is a traumatic laceration caused by one person hitting another in the mouth and is a very serious bite wound. The areas most commonly affected by this injury are the third and fourth metacarpophalangeal joints.

ETIOLOGY

Infections caused by these injuries are similar and are caused most often by the normal oral flora, which include both aerobic and anaerobic microorganisms. *Streptococcus* spp. (especially *S. anginosus*) are the most common isolates, followed by *Staphylococcus* spp. (predominately *S. aureus*).[79] *Eikenella corrodens* is isolated from human bite wounds approximately 30% of the time.[69,79] Anaerobic microorganisms have been isolated in approximately 40% of human bites and 55% of clenched-fist injuries.[60] Common anaerobes recovered from human bite infections include *Prevotella*, *Fusobacterium*, *Veillonella*, and *Peptostreptococcus* species.[79]

PATHOPHYSIOLOGY

Human bites generally are more serious and more prone to infection than animal bites, particularly clenched-fist injuries.[70] While the force of a punch may sever a tendon or nerve or break a bone, it most often causes a breach in the capsule of the metacarpophalangeal joint, leading to direct inoculation of bacteria into the joint or bone.[64] When the hand is relaxed, the tendons carry bacteria into deeper spaces of the hand, resulting in more extensive infection.[64]

CLINICAL PRESENTATION

GENERAL

- Most clenched-fist injuries are already infected by the time patients seek medical care, and most require hospitalization.

SYMPTOMS

- Patients with infected bites to the hand may develop a painful, throbbing, swollen extremity.

- Wounds often have a purulent discharge, and the patient complains of a decreased range of motion.

SIGNS

- Signs of infection include erythema, swelling, and clear or pussy discharge.
- Adjacent lymph nodes may be enlarged.
- In clenched-fist injuries, edema may limit the ability of tendons to glide in their sheaths, thereby limiting a joint's range of motion.

LABORATORY TESTS

- Samples for bacterial cultures (aerobic and anaerobic) should be collected as per animal bites.
- In severe infections, a peripheral leukocytosis of 15,000 to 30,000 cells/mm^3 may be seen; therefore, the white blood count should be monitored for resolution of infection.

OTHER DIAGNOSTIC TESTS

- If damage to a bone or joint is suspected, radiographic evaluation should be undertaken.

▶ TREATMENT: Human Bites (see Table 108–4)

9 Management of bite wounds consists of aggressive irrigation, surgical débridement, and immobilization of the affected area. Primary closure for human bites generally is not recommended. Tetanus toxoid and antitoxin may be indicated. Transmission of viruses has been documented through human bites; therefore, information about the biter is important. Although the possibility of acquiring the human immunodeficiency virus (HIV) through bites is believed to be unlikely, the presence of the virus in the saliva makes disease transmission possible. If the biter is HIV-positive, the victim should have a baseline blood specimen drawn to determine preexposure HIV status and then be retested in 3 months and 6 months.[82] The bite wound should be irrigated thoroughly and vigorously with a virucidal agent such as povidone-iodine.[69] Bite victims exposed to blood-tainted saliva should be offered antiretroviral chemoprophylaxis.

10 Patients with noninfected hand bite injuries should be given prophylactic antibiotic therapy. Initial therapy should consist of a penicillinase-resistant penicillin (dicloxacillin 250–500 mg orally four times daily; in children, 25–50 mg/kg per day orally divided into four doses) in combination with penicillin VK 250–500 mg orally four times daily (in children, 40,000–90,000 units/kg per day orally divided into four doses). Prophylactic therapy should be given for

3 to 5 days as for dog bites.[83] A first-generation cephalosporin or macrolide is not recommended because the sensitivity of these agents to *E. corrodens* is variable.[84]

For infected bite wounds, penicillin and a penicillinase-resistant penicillin or amoxicillin–clavulanic acid 875 mg/125 mg orally twice daily (40 mg/kg per day orally of the amoxicillin component divided into two doses) should be started empirically pending the culture results. Tetracyclines or a combination of clindamycin plus a fluoroquinolone or trimethoprim-sulfamethoxazole may be used as an alternative therapy for the penicillin-allergic patient. Hospitalization for minor wounds is not necessary if surgical repair of vital structures has not been performed. Patients suffering serious injuries or clenched-fist injuries should be started on intravenous antibiotics. Duration of therapy for infected bite injuries should be 7 to 14 days.

Antibiotic therapy always should be used in clenched-fist injuries. Therapy should include penicillin (or ampicillin) plus a penicillinase-resistant penicillin until the final cultures are available. Therapeutic failures have been documented when either first-generation cephalosporins or penicillinase-resistant penicillins have been used alone, most likely because of their poor and variable activity against *E. corrodens*.[85,86] Therapy should be continued from 7 to 14 days.[83]

EVALUATION OF THERAPEUTIC OUTCOMES

Results of a Gram stain should be used to confirm the appropriateness of therapy. Surgical débridement may be necessary if signs and symptoms are not reduced within 24 hours.

ABBREVIATIONS

HIV: human immunodeficiency virus
MRSA: methicillin-resistant *Staphylococcus aureus*
SSTI: skin and soft tissue infection
TD: tetanus-diphtheria
TIg: tetanus immune globulin
VRE: vancomycin-resistant enterococci

Review Questions and other resources can be found at *www.pharmacotherapyonline.com.*

REFERENCES

1. Fung HB, Chang JY, Kuczynski S. A practical guide to the treatment of complicated skin and soft tissue infections. Drugs 2003;63:1459–1480.

2. Eron LJ, Lipsky BA, Low DE, et al. Managing skin and soft tissue infections: Expert panel recommendations on key decision points. J Antimicrob Chemother 2003;52(suppl. S1):i3–i17.

3. Stulberg DL, Penrod MA, Blatny RA. Common bacterial skin infections. Am Fam Phys 2002;66:119–124.

4. Elixhauser A, Steiner CA. Most Common Diagnoses and Procedures in U.S. Community Hospitals, 1996: Summary. HCUP Research Note. Rockville, MD, Agency for Health Care Policy and Research, 1996; available at *http://www.ahrq.gov/data/hcup/commdx/commdx.htm.*

5. Rennie RP, Jones RN, Mutnick AH, and the SENTRY Program Study Group (North America). Occurrence and antimicrobial susceptibility patterns of pathogens isolated from skin and soft tissue infections: report from the SENTRY Antimicrobial Surveillance Program (United States and Canada, 2000). Diagn Microbiol Infect Dis 2003;45:287–293.

6. Granato PA. Pathogenic and indigenous microorganisms of humans. In: Murray PR, Baron EJ, Jorgensen JH, et al, eds. Manual of Clinical Microbiology, 8th ed. Washington, ASM Press, 2003:44–54.

7. Ducan WC, McBride ME, Knox JM. Experimental production of infection in humans. J Invest Dermatol 1970;54:319–323.

8. Yagupski P. Bacteriologic aspects of skin and soft tissue infections. Pediatr Ann 1993;22:217–224.

9. Centers for Disease Control and Prevention. *Pseudomonas* dermatitis/folliculitis associated with pools and hot tubs: Colorado and Maine, 1999–2000. MMWR 2000;49:1087–1091.

10. Swartz MN. Cellulitis and subcutaneous tissue infections. In: Mandell GL,

Bennett JE, Dolin R, eds. Principles and Practice of Infectious Diseases, 5th ed. New York, Churchill-Livingstone, 2000:1037–1057.

11. Bisno AL, Stevens DL. Streptococcal infections of skin and soft tissues. New Engl J Med 1996;334:240–245.

12. Eriksson B, Jorup-Ronstrom C, Karkkonen K, et al. Erysipelas: Clinical and bacteriologic spectrum and serological aspects. Clin Infect Dis 1996;23:1091–1098.

13. Bergkvist P, Sjobeck K. Antibiotic and prednisolone therapy of erysipelas: A randomized, double-blind, placebo-controlled study. Scand J Infect Dis 1997;29:377–382.

14. Sadick NS. Current aspects of bacterial infections of the skin. Dermatol Clin 1997;15:341–349.

15. Ben-Amitai D, Ashkenazi S. Common bacterial skin infections in childhood. Pediatr Ann 1993;22:225–233.

16. Brown J, Shriner DL, Schwartz RA, Janniger CK. Impetico: An update. Int J Dermatol 2003;42:251–255.

17. Britton JW, Fajardo JE, Krafte-Jacobs B. Comparison of mupirocin and erythromycin in the treatment of impetigo. J Pediatr 1990;117:827–829.

18. Swartz MN. Lymphadenitis and lymphangitis. In: Mandell GL, Bennett JE, Dolin R, eds. Principles and Practice of Infectious Diseases, 5th ed. New York, Churchill-Livingstone, 2000:1066–1075.

19. Bass JW. Treatment of skin and skin structure infections. Pediatr Infect Dis J 1992;11:152–155.

20. Binswanger IA, Kral AH, Bluthenthal RN, et al. High prevalence of abscesses and cellulitis among community-recruited injection drug users in San Francisco. Clin Infect Dis 2000;30:579–581.

21. Ebright JR, Pieper B. Skin and soft tissue infections in injection drug users. Infect Dis Clin North Am 2002;16:697–712.

22. Dagan R, Moshe P, Watemberg N, et al. Outpatient treatment of serious community-acquired pediatric infections using once daily intramuscular ceftriaxone. Pediatr Infect Dis J 1987;6:1080–1084.

23. Stevens DL, Herr D, Lampiris H, et al, and the Linezolid MRSA Study Group. Linezolid versus vancomycin for the treatment of methicillin-resistant *Staphylococcus aureus* infections. Clin Infect Dis 2002;34:1481–1490.

24. Stevens DL, Smith LG, Bruss JB, et al. Randomized comparison of linezolid (PNU-100766) versus oxacillin-dicloxacillin for treatment of complicated skin and soft tissue infections. Antimicrob Agents Chemother 2000;44:3408–3413.

25. Tedesco KL, Rybak MJ. Daptomycin. Pharmacotherapy 2004;24:41–57.

26. Nichols RL, Graham DR, Barriere SL, et al. Treatment of hospitalized patients with complicated gram-positive skin and skin structure infections: Two randomized, multicentre studies of quinupristin/dalfopristin versus cefazolin, oxacillin or vancomycin. Synercid Skin and Skin Structure Infection Group. J Antimicrob Chemother 1999;44:263–273.

27. Gould IM, Hudson M, Morris J, et al. Imipenem versus standard therapy in the treatment of serious soft tissue infection. Drugs Exp Clin Res 1988;14:555–558.

28. Graham DR, Lucasti C, Malafaia O, et al. Ertapenem once daily versus piperacillin-tazobactam four times per day for treatment of complicated skin and skin-structure infections in adults: Results of a prospective, randomized, double-blind multicenter study. Clin Infect Dis 2002;34:1460–1468.

29. Kulhanjian J, Dunphy M, Hamstra S, et al. Randomized comparative study of ampicillin/sulbactam vs ceftriaxone for treatment of soft tissue and skeletal infections in children. Pediatr Infect Dis J 1989;8:605–610.

30. Tan JS, Wishnow RM, Talan DA, et al. Treatment of hospitalized patients with complicated skin and skin structure infections: Double-blind, randomized, multicenter study of piperacillin-tazobactam versus ticarcillin-clavulanate. Antimicrob Agents Chemother 1993;37:1580–1586.

31. Gentry LO, Ramirez-Ronda CH, Rodriquez-Noriega E, et al. Oral ciprofloxacin vs parenteral cefotaxime in the treatment of difficult skin and skin structure infections. Arch Intern Med 1989;148:2579–2583.

32. Gentry LO. Therapy with newer oral β-lactam and quinolone agents for infections of the skin and skin structures: A review. Clin Infect Dis 1992;14:285–297.

33. Parish LC, Routh HB, Miskin B, et al. Moxifloxacin versus cephalexin in the treatment of uncomplicated skin infections. Int J Clin Pract 2000;54:497–503.

34. Nichols RL, Smith JW, Gentry LO, et al. Multienter randomized study comparing levofloxacin and ciprofloxacin for uncomplicated skin and skin structure infections. South Med J 1997;90:1193–1200.

35. Tarshis GA, Miskin BM, Jones TM, et al. Once daily oral gatifloxacin verus oral levofloxacin in treatment of uncomplicated skin and soft tissue infections: Double-blind multicenter randomized study. Antimicrob Agents Chemother 2001;45:2358–2362.

36. Zervos MJ, Hershberger E, Nicolau DP, et al. Relationship between fluoroquinolone use and changes in susceptibility to fluoroquinolones of selected pathogens in 10 United States teaching hospitals, 1991–2000. Clin Infect Dis 2003;37:1643–1648.

37. LeFrock J, Blais F, Schell R, et al. Cefoxitin in the treatment of diabetic patients with lower extremity infections. Infect Surg 1983;2:361–374.

38. Hughes C, Johnson C, Bamberger D, et al. Treatment and long-term follow-up of foot infections in patients with diabetes or ischemia: A randomized, prospective, double-blind comparison of cefoxitin and ceftizoxime. Clin Ther 1987;10(suppl A):36–49.

39. Crane L, Levine D, Aervos M, et al. Bacteremia in narcotic addicts at Detroit Medical Center: Microbiology, epidemiology, risk factors, and empiric therapy. Rev Infect Dis 1986;8:364–373.

40. Urschel JD. Necrotizing soft tissue infections. Postgrad Med J 1999;75:645–649.

41. Gentry LO. Diagnosis and management of the diabetic foot ulcer. J Antimicrob Chemother 1993;32(suppl A):77–89.

42. Lipsky BA, Pecoraro RE, Wheat LJ. The diabetic foot: Soft tissue and bone infection. Infect Dis Clin North Am 1990;4:409–432.

43. Caputo GM, Cavanagh PR, Ulbrecht JS, et al. Assessment and management of foot disease in patients with diabetes. New Engl J Med 1994;331:854–860.

44. Smith AJ, Daniels T, Bohnen JMA. Soft tissue infections and the diabetic foot. Am J Surg 1996;172(suppl 6A):7S–12S.

45. Levin ME. Foot lesions in patients with diabetes mellitus. Endocrinol Metab Clin North Am 1996;25:447–462.

46. Slovenkai MP. Foot problems in diabetes. Med Clin North Am 1998;82:949–971.

47. Gerding DN. Foot infections in diabetic patients: The role of anaerobes. Clin Infect Dis 1995;20(suppl 2):S283–288.

48. Grayson ML. Diabetic foot infections: Antimicrobial therapy. Infect Dis Clin North Am 1995;9:143–161.

49. Shea KW. Antimicrobial therapy for diabetic foot infections. Postgrad Med 1999;106:85–94.

50. West NJ. Systemic antimicrobial treatment of foot infections in diabetic patients. Am J Health Syst Pharm 1995;52:1199–207.

51. Parish LC, Aten EM. Treatment of skin and skin structure infections: A comparative study of augmentin and cefaclor. Cutis 1984;34:567–570.

52. Eron LJ, Harvey L, Hixon DL, et al. Ciprofloxacin therapy of infections caused by *Pseudomonas aeruginosa* and other resistant bacteria. Antimicrob Agents Chemother 1985;28:308–310.

53. Grayson ML, Gibbons GW, Habershaw GM, et al. Use of ampicillin-sulbactam versus imipenem-cilastatin in the treatment of limb-threatening foot infections in diabetic patients. Clin Infect Dis 1994;18:683–693.

54. Lipsky BA, Baker PD, Landon GC, et al. Antibiotic therapy for diabetic foot infections: Comparison of two parenteral-to-oral regimens. Clin Infect Dis 1997;24:643–648.

55. Shea JD. Pressure sores: Classification and management. Clin Orthop 1975;112:89–100.

56. National Pressure Ulcer Advisory Panel. Pressure ulcers: Incidence, economics, risk. Consensus Development Conference Statement. Decubitus 1989;2:24–29.

57. Kanj LF, Wilking SVB, Phillips TJ. Pressure ulcers. J Am Acad Dermatol 1998;38:517–536.

58. Gradon J, Adamsom C. Infections of pressure ulcers: Management and controversies. Infect Dis Clin Pract 1995;1:11–16.

59. Findlay D. Practical management of pressure ulcers. Am Fam Phys 1996;54:1519–1528.

60. Goode PS, Allman RM. The prevention and management of pressure sores. Med Clin North Am 1989;73:1511–1524.

61. Reuler JB, Cooney TG. The pressure sore: Pathophysiology and principles of management. Ann Intern Med 1981;94:661–666.

62. Cervo FA, Cruz AC, Posillico JA. Pressure ulcers: Analysis of guidelines for treatment and management. Geriatrics 2000;55:55–60.

63. Cuddigan J, Frantz RA. Pressure ulcer research: Pressure ulcer treatment. A monograph from the National Pressure Ulcer Advisory Panel. Adv Wound Care 1998;2:294–300.

64. Goldstein E. Bite wounds and infection. Clin Infect Dis 1992;14:633–640.

65. Weiss HB, Friedman DI, Coben JH. Incidence of dog bite injuries treated in emergency departments. JAMA 1998;279:51–53.

66. Anonymous. Dog bite related fatalities—United States, 1995–1996. MMWR 1997;46:463–467.

67. Rest JG, Goldstein EJC. Management of human and animal bite wounds. Emerg Med Clin North Am 1985;3:117–126.

68. Goldstein EJC, Citron DM, Finegold SM. Role of anaerobic bacteria in bite wound infections. Rev Infect Dis 1984;6(suppl 1):S177–183.

69. Griego RD, Rosen T, Orengo IF, et al. Dog, cat, and human bites: A review. J Am Acad Dermatol 1995;33:1019–1029.

70. Brooks I. Microbiology and management of human and animal bite wound infections. Primary Care Clin Office Pract 2003;30:1–11.

71. Talan DA, Citron DM, Abrahamian FM, et al. Bacteriologic analysis of infected dog and cat bites. New Engl J Med 1999;340:85–92.

72. Wiggins ME, Akelamn E, Weiss AP. The management of dog bites and dog bite infections to the hand. Orthopedics 1994;17:617–623.

73. Goldstein EJC, Citron DM, Finegold SM. Dog bite wounds and infection: A prospective clinical study. Ann Emerg Med 1980;9:508–512.

74. Callaham ML. Treatment of common dog bites: Infection risk factors. J Am Coll Emerg Phys 1978;7:83–87.

75. Elenbass RM, McNaoney WK, Robinson WA. Prophylactic oxacillin in dog bite wounds. Ann Emerg Med 1982;11:248–251.

76. Cummings P. Antibiotics to prevent infections in patients with dog bite wounds: A meta-analysis of randomized trials. Ann Emerg Med 1994;23:535–540.

77. Elliot DL, Tolle SW, Goldberg L, et al. Pet-associated illness. New Engl J Med 1985;313:985–995.

78. Goldstein E, Citron DM, Richwals GA. Lack of in vitro efficacy of oral forms of certain cephalosporins, erythromycin, and oxacillin against *Pasteurella multocida.* Antimicrob Agents Chemother 1988;32:213–215.

79. Talan DA, Abrahamian FM, Moran GJ, et al. Clinical presentation and bacteriologic analysis of infected human bites in patients presenting to emergency departments. Clin Infect Dis 2003;37:1481–1489.

80. Goldstein EJ, Reinhardt JF, Murray PM, et al. Outpatient therapy of bite wounds: Demographic data, bacteriology, and a prospective, randomized trial of amoxicillin–clavulanic acid versus penicillin (dicloxacillin). Int J Dermatol 1987;26:123–127.

81. Mann RJ, Hoffield TA, Farmer CB. Human bites of the hand: Twenty years of experience. J Hand Surg 1977;2:97–99.

82. Bunzli WF, Wright DH, Hoang AD, et al. Current management of human bites. Pharmacotherapy 1998;18:227–234.

83. Talan D. Infectious disease issues in the emergency department. Clin Infect Dis 1996;23:1–14.

84. Goldstein E, Gombert M, Agyare E. Susceptibility of *Eikenella corrodens* to newer beta-lactam antibiotics. Antimicrob Agents Chemother 1980; 18:832–833.

85. Goldstein E, Miller T, Citron D, et al. Infections following clenched-fist injury: A new perspective. J Hand Surg 1978;3:455–459.

86. Goldstein E, Barene M, Miller TA. *Eikenella corrodens* in hand infections. J Hand Surg 1983;8:563–566.

109

INFECTIVE ENDOCARDITIS

Michael A. Crouch and Angie Veverka

Learning Objectives and other resources can be found at *www.pharmacotherapyonline.com*.

KEY CONCEPTS

① Infective endocarditis (IE) is an uncommon infection usually occurring in persons with preexisting cardiac valvular abnormalities (e.g., prosthetic heart valves) or with other specific risk factors (e.g., intravenous drug abuse).

② Three groups of organisms cause a majority of IE cases: streptococci (55% to 62% of cases), staphylococci (25% to 35%), and enterococci (5% to 18%).

③ The clinical presentation of IE is highly variable and nonspecific, although a fever and murmur usually are present. Classic peripheral manifestations (Osler nodes) may or may not occur.

④ The diagnosis of IE requires the integration of clinical, laboratory, and echocardiographic findings. The two major diagnostic criteria are bacteremia and echocardiographic changes (e.g., valvular vegetation).

⑤ Treatment of IE involves isolation of the infecting pathogen and determination of antimicrobial susceptibilities, followed by high-dose, parenteral, bactericidal antibiotics for an extended period.

⑥ Surgical replacement of the infected heart valve is an important adjunct to endocarditis treatment in certain situations (e.g., patients with acute heart failure).

⑦ β-Lactam antibiotics, such as penicillin G, nafcillin, and ampicillin, remain the drugs of choice for streptococcal, staphylococcal, and enterococcal endocarditis, respectively.

⑧ Aminoglycosides are essential to obtain a synergistic bactericidal effect in the treatment of enterococcal endocarditis. Adjunctive aminoglycosides also may decrease the emergence of resistant organisms (e.g., prosthetic valve endocarditis caused by coagulase-negative staphylococci) and hasten the pace of clinical and microbiologic response (e.g., some streptococcal and staphylococcal infections).

⑨ Vancomycin is reserved for patients with immediate β-lactam allergies and the treatment of resistant organisms.

⑩ Antimicrobial prophylaxis is used as an attempt to prevent IE in patients at high risk (such as persons with prosthetic heart valves) before a bacteremia-causing procedure (e.g., dental extraction).

Endocarditis is an inflammation of the endocardium, the membrane lining the chambers of the heart and covering the cusps of the heart valves.[1,2] More commonly, *endocarditis* refers to infection of the heart valves by various microorganisms. Although it typically affects native valves, it also may involve nonvalvular areas or implanted mechanical devices (e.g., mechanical heart valves). Bacteria primarily cause endocarditis, but fungi and other atypical microorganisms can lead to the disease; thus the more encompassing term *infective endocarditis* (IE) is preferred.

Endocarditis is often referred to as acute or subacute depending on the pace and severity of the clinical presentation. The acute, fulminating form is associated with high fevers and systemic toxicity. Virulent bacteria, such as *Staphylococcus aureus,* frequently cause this syndrome, and if untreated, death occurs within a few days to weeks. On the other hand, subacute IE is more indolent and is caused by less invasive organisms, such as viridans streptococci, usually occurring in preexisting valvular heart disease. IE is best classified based on the etiologic organism, the anatomic site of infection, and pathogenic risk factors.[2] Infection also may follow surgical insertion of a prosthetic heart valve, resulting in prosthetic valve endocarditis (PVE).[3]

EPIDEMIOLOGY AND ETIOLOGY

IE is an uncommon but not rare infection affecting about 10,000 to 20,000 persons annually in the United States. The infection accounts for approximately 1 in every 1000 hospital admissions.[1] Yet the incidence of IE may be increasing, and it is now the fourth leading cause of infectious disease syndromes that are life threatening, after urosepsis, pneumonia, and intraabdominal sepsis.[4] The male-to-female ratio is 1.7:1. Overall, most cases occur in individuals older than 50 years of age, and it is uncommon in children.[1,2] PVE accounts for 7% to 25% of cases of IE.[5] As the population ages, and as valve replacement surgery becomes more common, the mean age of patients with IE increases. However, those with a history of intravenous drug abuse (IVDA), who tend to be younger males, are also at high risk of IE. Other conditions associated with a higher incidence of IE include diabetes, long-term hemodialysis, and poor dental hygeine.

① Most persons with IE have risk factors, such as preexisting cardiac valvular abnormalities. Many types of structural heart disease result in turbulence of blood flow that increases the risk for IE.

TABLE 109–1. Etiologic Organisms in Infective Endocarditis

Agent	Percentage of Cases
Streptococci	55–62
Viridans streptococci	30–40
Other streptococci	15–25
Staphylococci	20–35
Coagulase-positive	10–27
Coagulase-negative	1–3
Enterococci	5–18
Gram-negative aerobic bacilli	1.5–13
Fungi	2–4
Miscellaneous bacteria	<5
Mixed infections	1–2
"Culture negative"	<5–24

Adapted from ref. 1.

A predisposing factor, however, may be absent in up to 25% of cases. Some of the more important risk factors include[5]

- Presence of a prosthetic valve (400-fold increased risk)
- Previous endocarditis (400-fold increased risk)
- Complex cyanotic congenital heart disease (e.g., single-ventricle states)
- Surgically constructed systemic pulmonary shunts or conduits
- Acquired valvular dysfunction (e.g., rheumatic heart disease)
- Hypertrophic cardiomyopathy
- Mitral valve prolapse with regurgitation
- Intravenous drug abuse

In the past, rheumatic heart disease was a prevalent risk factor for IE, but the incidence of this disease continues to decline. The risk of IE in persons with mitral valve prolapse and regurgitation is small; however, because the condition is prevalent, it is an important contributor to the overall number of IE cases.[5] Prosthetic valve endocarditis occurs in 1% to 4% of patients undergoing valve replacement surgery.[3]

Nearly every organism causing human disease has been reported to cause IE (Table 109–1), but three groups of organisms result in a majority of cases: streptococci (55% to 62% of cases), staphylococci (25% to 35%), and enterococci (5% to 18%).[1] The incidence of staphylococci, particularly *S. aureus,* has increased, and staphylococci have surpassed viridans streptococci as the leading cause of IE.[5] In general, streptococci cause IE in patients with underlying cardiac abnormalities, such as mitral valve prolapse or rheumatic heart disease. Staphylococci (*S. aureus* and coagulase-negative staphylococci) are the most common cause of PVE within the first year after valve surgery, and *S. aureus* is common in those with a history of IVDA. Although polymicrobial IE is uncommon, it is encountered most often in association with IVDA.[5] Enterococcal endocarditis tends to follow genitourinary manipulations (older men) or obstetric procedures (younger women). There are many exceptions to the preceding generalizations; thus isolation of the causative pathogen and determination of its antimicrobial susceptibilities offer the best chance for successful therapy.

The mitral and aortic valves are affected most commonly in cases involving a single valve. Subacute endocarditis tends to involve the mitral valve, whereas acute disease often involves the aortic valve. Up to 35% of cases involve concomitant infections of both the aortic and the mitral valves. Infection of the tricuspid valve is less common, with a majority of these cases occurring in patients with a history of IVDA. It is rare for the pulmonary valve to be infected.[1,2]

PATHOPHYSIOLOGY

The development of IE via hematogenous spread, the most common route, requires the sequential occurrence of several factors. These components are complex and not fully elucidated[1,2]:

- *The endothelial surface of the heart is damaged.* This injury occurs with turbulent blood flow associated with the valvular lesions previously described.
- *Platelet and fibrin deposition occurs on the abnormal epithelial surface.* These platelet-fibrin deposits are referred to as *nonbacterial thrombotic endocarditis* (NBTE).
- *Bacteremia gives organisms access to and results in colonization of the endocardial surface.* Bacteremia is the result of trauma to a mucosal surface with a high concentration of resident bacteria, such as the oral cavity and gastrointestinal tract. Transient bacteremia commonly follows certain dental, gastrointestinal, urologic, and gynecologic procedures. Staphylococci, viridans streptococci, and enterococci are most likely to adhere to NBTE, probably because of production of specific adherence factors, such as dextran by some oral streptococci and glycocalyx for staphylococci.[2,8] Gram-negative bacteria rarely adhere to heart valves and are uncommon causes of IE.
- *After colonization of the endothelial surface, a "vegetation" of fibrin, platelets, and bacteria forms.* The protective cover of fibrin and platelets allows unimpeded bacterial growth to concentrations as high as 10^9 to 10^{10} organisms per gram of tissue.

The pathogenesis of early PVE differs from the IE acquired by the hematogenous route in that surgery may directly inoculate the valve with bacteria from the patient's skin or operating room personnel. The recently placed nonendothelialized valve is more susceptible to bacterial colonization than native valves. Bacteria also may colonize the new valve from contaminated bypass pumps, cannulas, and pacemakers or from a nosocomial bacteremia subsequent to an intravascular catheter.[3,6,7] The mechanism of bacterial colonization and pathogenesis in late PVE is similar to native-valve endocarditis.[3]

The vegetations seen in IE may be single or multiple and vary in size from a few millimeters to centimeters. Bacteria within the vegetation grow slowly and are protected from antibiotics and host defenses. The adverse effects of IE and the resulting lesions can be far-reaching and include (1) local perivalvular damage, (2) embolization of septic fragments with potential hematogenous seeding of remote sites, and (3) formation of antibody complexes.

Formation of vegetations may destroy valvular tissue, and continued destruction can lead to acute heart failure via perforation of the valve leaflet, rupture of the chordae tendineae or papillary muscle, or in the patient with PVE, valve dehiscence. Occasionally, valvular stenosis may occur. Abscesses can develop in the valve ring or in myocardial tissue itself. Even with resolution of the process, fibrosis of tissue with some residual dysfunction is possible.

Vegetations may be friable, and fragments may be released downstream. These infected particles, termed *septic emboli,* can result in organ abscess or infarction. Septic emboli from right-sided endocarditis commonly lodge in the lungs, causing pulmonary abscesses. Emboli from left-sided vegetations commonly affect organs with high blood flow, such as the kidneys, spleen, and brain.

Circulating immune complexes consisting of antigen, antibody, and complement may deposit in organs, producing local inflammation and damage (e.g., glomerulonephritis in the kidneys). Other potential pathologic changes that result from immune-complex deposition or septic emboli include the development of "mycotic" aneurysms (although the aneurysm is usually bacterial in origin, not fungal), cerebral infarction, splenic infarction and abscess, and skin manifestations such as petechiae, Osler nodes, and Janeway lesions.

CLINICAL PRESENTATION

The clinical presentation of IE is highly variable and nonspecific. Fever is the most common finding and is often accompanied by other vague symptoms (Table 109–2). The fever may be relatively low grade, particularly in subacute cases. Heart murmurs are found in a majority of patients, most often preexisting, with some documented as new or changing. Infective endocarditis usually begins insidiously and worsens gradually. Patients may present with nonspecific findings, such as fever, chills, weakness, dyspnea, night sweats, weight loss, or malaise. In contrast, patients with acute disease, such as those with a history of IVDA with *S. aureus* IE, may appear with classic signs of sepsis.

Splenomegaly is a frequent finding in patients with prolonged endocarditis. Other important clinical signs especially prevalent in subacute illness may include the following peripheral manifestations ("stigmata") of endocarditis[1,2]:

- *Osler nodes.* Purplish or erythematous subcutaneous papules or nodules on the pads of the fingers and toes. These lesions are 2 to 15 mm in size and are painful and tender. These nodes are not specific for IE and may be the result of embolism, immunologic phenomena, or both.
- *Janeway lesions.* Hemorrhagic, painless plaques on the palms of the hands or soles of the feet. These lesions are believed to be embolic in origin.
- *Splinter hemorrhages.* Thin, linear hemorrhages found under the nailbeds of the fingers or toes. These lesions are not specific for IE and more commonly are the result of traumatic injuries.

TABLE 109–2. Clinical Presentation of Infective Endocarditis

General
The clinical presentation of IE is highly variable and nonspecific.
Symptoms
The patient may complain of fever, chills, weakness, dyspnea, night sweats, weight loss, and/or malaise.
Signs
Fever is common as well as a heart murmur (sometimes new or changing). The patient may or may not have embolic phenomenon, splenomegaly, or skin manifestations (e.g., Osler nodes, Janeway lesions).
Laboratory Tests
The patient's WBC count may be normal or only slightly elevated.
Nonspecific findings include anemia (normocytic, normochromic), thrombocytopenia, an elevated erythrocyte sedimentation rate or C-reactive protein, and altered urinary analysis (proteinuria/microscopic hematuria).
The hallmark laboratory finding is continuous bacteremia; three sets of blood cultures should be collected over 24 hours.
Other Diagnostic Tests
An electrocardiogram, chest radiograph, and echocardiogram are commonly performed. Echocardiography to determine the presence of valvular vegetations plays a key role in the diagnosis of IE; it should be performed in all suspected cases.

Distal lesions are more likely the result of trauma, whereas proximal lesions tend to be associated with IE.

- *Petechiae.* Small (usually 1 to 2 mm in diameter), erythematous, painless, hemorrhagic lesions. These lesions appear anywhere on the skin but more frequently on the anterior trunk, buccal mucosa and palate, and conjunctivae. Petechiae are nonblanching and resolve after a few days.
- *Clubbing of the fingers.* Proliferative change in the soft tissues about the terminal phalanges observed in long-standing endocarditis.
- *Roth spots.* Retinal infarct with central pallor and surrounding hemorrhage.
- *Emboli.* Embolic phenomena occur in up to one-third of cases and may result in significant complications. Left-sided endocarditis can result in renal artery emboli causing flank pain with hematuria, splenic artery emboli causing abdominal pain, and cerebral emboli, which may result in hemiplegia or alteration in mental status. Right-sided endocarditis may result in pulmonary emboli, causing pleuritic pain with hemoptysis.

Patients with IE typically have laboratory abnormalities; however, none of these changes is specific for the disease.[7] Anemia (normocytic, normochromic), leukocytosis, and thrombocytopenia may be present. The white blood cell (WBC) count is often normal or only slightly elevated, sometimes with a mild left shift. Acute bacterial endocarditis, however, may present with an elevated WBC count, consistent with a fulminant infection. The erythrocyte sedimentation rate (ESR) is elevated in 90% to 100% of patients, and the level of C-reactive protein also may be elevated.[1] Often the urinary analysis is abnormal, with proteinuria and microscopic hematuria occurring in approximately 50% of individuals.

The hallmark of IE is a continuous bacteremia caused by bacteria shedding from the vegetation into the bloodstream; more than 95% of patients with IE have positive blood cultures.[1,2] Three sets of blood cultures, each from separate venipuncture sites, should be collected over 24 hours, and antibiotics should be withheld until adequate blood cultures are obtained. On the other hand, if a patient has a toxic appearance, several blood cultures should be collected promptly, followed by immediate empirical antimicrobial treatment. The blood cultures in patients who have received previous antibiotics should be monitored more closely because pathogen growth may be suppressed. "Culture negative" endocarditis describes a patient in whom a clinical diagnosis of IE is likely but blood cultures do not yield a pathogen.[8] This condition is often the consequence of previous antibiotic therapy, improperly collected blood cultures, or unusual organisms.[4] When blood cultures from patients suspected of having IE show no growth after 48 to 72 hours, the laboratory should be advised and cultures held for up to a month to detect growth of fastidious organisms.

An electrocardiogram (ECG), chest radiograph, and echocardiogram are performed commonly in patients suspected of endocarditis. The ECG rarely shows important diagnostic findings but may reveal heart block suggesting extension of the infection. The chest radiograph may provide more diagnostic information, especially in a patient with right-sided endocarditis. Septic pulmonary emboli may occur, leading to multiple lung foci. The echocardiogram is the most important test and should be performed in all patients suspected of this infection.

Echocardiography using the transthoracic (TTE) or transesophageal (TEE) technique plays an important role in the diagnosis and management of IE.[4] The TEE technique is more sensitive for detecting vegetations (90% to 100%) as compared with TTE (58%

to 63%), and TEE maintains good specificity (85% to 95%).[2] TEE is preferred in high-risk patients such as those with a prosthetic heart valve, congenital heart disease, previous endocarditis, a new murmur, or stigmata of endocarditis.[4,9,10] TTE appears reasonable in the evaluation of those with native valves who are good candidates for imaging.[5,11] The lack of vegetation on echocardiogram does not exclude infection even if the transesophageal approach is used. Conversely, the test may reveal an unsuspected large vegetation, extension of the disease into surrounding tissue, valvular defects, abscess formation, cordial rupture, or an intracardiac fistula. Thus, in addition to helping in the diagnosis of IE, the echocardiogram allows the physician to evaluate hemodynamic stability and the need for urgent surgical intervention; it also provides a rough estimate of the likelihood of embolism.[12,13]

CLINICAL CONTROVERSY

Some clinicians argue that the cost and invasiveness of TEE warrant performing a TTE first and obtaining a TEE only if TTE images are inconclusive. There are currently no prospective, randomized, controlled trials comparing the cost-effectiveness of either strategy.

DIAGNOSIS

The signs and symptoms of IE are not specific, and the diagnosis is often unclear. The diagnosis of IE requires the integration of clinical, laboratory, and echocardiographic findings. The most

TABLE 109–3. Diagnosis of Infective Endocarditis According to the Modified Duke Criteria

Criteria	Comments
Major Criteria	
Microbiologic	
Typical microorganism isolated from two separate blood cultures: *Streptococcus viridans, Streptococcus bovis,* HACEK group, *Staphylococcus aureus,* or community-acquired enterococcal bacteremia without a primary focus *or* Microorganism consistent with IE isolated from persistently positive blood cultures *or*	In patients with possible IE, at least two sets of cultures of blood collected by separate venipunctures should be obtained within the first 1–2 hours of presentation. Patients with cardiovascular collapse should have three cultures of blood obtained at 5–10-minute intervals and thereafter receive empirical antibiotic therapy.
Single positive blood culture for *Coxiella burnetii* or phase IIgG antibody titer to *C. burnetii* > 1:800	*C. burnetii* is not readily cultivated in most clinical microbiology laboratories.
Evidence of endocardial involvement	
New valvular regurgitation (increase or change in preexisting murmur not sufficient) *or*	Three echocardiographic findings qualify as major criteria: a discrete, echogenic, oscillating intracardiac mass located at a site of endocardial injury; a periannular abscess; and a new dehiscence of a prosthetic valve
Positive echocardiogram (transesophageal echocardiography recommended in patients who have a prosthetic valve, who are rated as having at least possible IE by clinical criteria, or who have complicated IE)	
Minor Criteria	
Predisposition to IE that includes certain cardiac conditions and IV drug use	Cardiac abnormalities that are associated with IE are classified into three groups: *High-risk conditions:* Previous IE, aortic valve disease, rheumatic heart disease, prosthetic heart valve, coarctation of the aorta, and complex cyanotic congenital heart diseases *Moderate-risk conditions:* Mitral valve prolapse with valvular regurgitation or leaflet thickening, isolated mitral stenosis, tricuspid-valve disease, pulmonary stenosis, and hypertrophic cardiomyopathy *Low- or no-risk conditions:* Secundum atrial septal defect, ischemic heart disease, previous coronary artery bypass graft surgery, and mitral valve prolapse with thin leaflets in the absence of regurgitations
Fever	Temperature >38°C (100.4°F)
Vascular phenomena	Petechiae and splinter hemorrhages are excluded. None of the peripheral lesions are pathognomonic for IE
Immunologic phenomena	Presence of rheumatoid factor, glomerulonephritis, Osler's nodes, or Roth spots
Microbiologic findings	Positive blood cultures that do not meet the major criteria Serologic evidence of active infection; single isolates of coagulase-negative staphylococci, and organisms that very rarely cause IE are excluded from this category

Note: Cases are defined clinically as definite if they fulfill two major criteria, one major criterion plus three minor criteria, or five minor criteria; they are defined as possible if they fulfill one major and one minor criterion or three minor criteria. HACEK denotes *Haemophilus* species (*H. parainfluenzae, H. aphrophilus, H. paraphrophilus, Actinobacillus actinomycetemcomitans, Cardiobacterium hominis, Eikenella corrodens,* and *Kingella kingae*).
Adapted from ref. 15.

recent diagnostic criteria (the Duke criteria) include major and minor variables[14,15] (Table 109–3). Based on the number of major and minor criteria that are fulfilled, patients suspected of IE are divided into three separate categories: definite IE, possible IE, or IE rejected[15] (see Table 109–3).

PROGNOSIS

The outcome for endocarditis is improved with rapid diagnosis, appropriate treatment (i.e., antimicrobial therapy, surgery, or both), and prompt recognition of complications should they arise. Factors associated with increased mortality include (1) heart failure, (2) culture-negative endocarditis, (3) endocarditis caused by resistant organisms such as fungi or gram-negative bacteria, (4) left-sided endocarditis caused by *S. aureus,* and (5) prosthetic-valve endocarditis.[1,16] The presence of heart failure has the greatest negative impact on the short-term prognosis.[4] For native-valve IE, mortality rates range from 16% to 27%; lower rates occur with viridans streptococci (4% to 9%), and higher rates occur with left-sided IE caused by enterococci (15% to 20%) and staphylococci (25% to 47%). Even higher rates of mortality are seen with unusually encountered organisms (e.g., mortality greater than 50% for *Pseudomonas aeruginosa*). The mortality rate for right-side IE associated with IVDA is generally low (e.g., 10%).[4] For those who relapse after treatment for IE, most will do so within the first 2 months after discontinuation of antimicrobials. Relapse rates for viridans streptococcus are generally low (2%), whereas relapse is more likely in those with enterococcal infection (8% to 20%) and PVE (10% to 15%).[5] After appropriate treatment and recovery, the risk of morbidity and mortality following IE persist for years, although it declines gradually annually. Morbidity remains elevated because of a greater likelihood of recurrent IE, heart failure, and embolism or, if a valve is replaced, the risk of anticoagulation, valve thrombosis, or additional valve surgery.[17]

▶ TREATMENT: Infective Endocarditis

DESIRED OUTCOMES

The desired outcomes for treatment and prophylaxis of IE are to

- Relieve the signs and symptoms of the disease.
- Decrease morbidity and mortality associated with the infection.
- Eradicate the causative organism with minimal drug exposure.
- Provide cost-effective antimicrobial therapy determined by the likely or identified pathogen, drug susceptibilities, hepatic and renal function, drug allergies, and anticipated drug toxicities.
- Prevent IE from occurring or recurring in high-risk patients with appropriate prophylactic antimicrobials.

GENERAL APPROACH TO TREATMENT

The most important approach in the treatment of IE is isolation of the infecting pathogen and determination of antimicrobial susceptibilities, followed by high-dose, parenteral, bactericidal antibiotics for an extended period.[1,2] Treatment usually is started in the hospital, but in selected patients it is often completed in the outpatient setting so long as defervescence has occurred and follow-up blood cultures show no growth. Large doses of parenteral antimicrobials usually are necessary to achieve bactericidal concentrations within vegetations. An extended duration of therapy is required, even for susceptible pathogens, because microorganisms are enclosed within valvular vegetations and fibrin deposits. These barriers impair host defenses and protect microbes from phagocytic cells. In addition, the high bacterial concentrations within vegetations may result in an inoculum effect that further resists killing (see Chap. 103 for additional discussion). Many bacteria are not actively dividing, further limiting the rate of bacterial death. For most patients, 4 to 6 weeks of therapy is required.

Pharmacodynamic investigations in the IE animal model allow quantitation of bacterial densities within vegetations over time as a function of antibiotic concentration. These models empirically confirm many of the observed IE treatment principles.[18,19] The antibiotic concentration in serum that is needed to kill bacteria within vegetations may be many times the minimal bactericidal concentration (MBC) of the infecting pathogen depending on additional characteristics. The most effective antibiotics have a rapid and homogeneous distribution into the vegetation, kill bacteria rapidly, and are least susceptible to a large inoculum. Aminoglycosides have the most favorable characteristics, followed by β-lactams, and then glycopeptides.[19]

NONPHARMACOLOGIC THERAPY

Surgery is an important adjunct in the management of endocarditis. In most surgical cases, valvectomy and valve replacement are performed to remove infected tissue and to restore hemodynamic function. Echocardiographic features that suggest the need for surgery include persistent vegetation or an increase in vegetation size after prolonged antibiotic treatment, valve dysfunction, or perivalvular extension (e.g., abscess).[4] Surgery also may be considered in cases of PVE endocarditis caused by resistant organisms (e.g., fungi or gram-negative bacteria), or if there is persistent bacteremia or other evidence of failure despite appropriate antimicrobial therapy.[3,21] The major indications for surgical intervention in the past have been heart failure in left-sided IE and persistent infection in right-sided IE.[1]

PHARMACOLOGIC THERAPY

Specific treatment recommendations from the American Heart Association (AHA) provide guidance for the management of the more common causes of IE.[22] These guidelines were last updated in 1995, with expected revision to be initiated in 2005. β-Lactam antibiotics, such as penicillin G, nafcillin, and ampicillin, remain the drugs of choice for streptococcal, staphylococcal, and enterococcal endocarditis, respectively. These recommendations are summarized in Tables 109–4 through 109–9 and are discussed in more detail in the following sections. Because these guidelines address only common causes of endocarditis, readers are referred to other references for more in-depth discussion of unusually encountered organisms.[4]

TABLE 109–4. Suggested Regimens for Therapy of Native-Valve Endocarditis Due to Penicillin-Susceptible Viridans Streptococci and *Streptococcus bovis* (Minimum Inhibitory Concentration ≤0.1 mcg/mL)[a]

Antibiotic	Dosage and Route	Duration (wks)	Comments
Aqueous crystalline penicillin G sodium	12–18 million units/24 h IV either continuously or in six equally divided doses	4	Preferred in most patients older than 65 years and in those with impairment of the eighth nerve or renal function
or			
Ceftriaxone sodium	2 g once daily IV or IM[b]	4	
Aqueous crystalline penicillin G sodium	12–18 million units/24 h IV either continuously or in six equally divided doses	2	
With gentamicin sulfate[c]	1 mg/kg IM or IV every 8 h	2	When obtained 1 h after a 20–30 min IV infusion or IM injection, serum concentration of gentamicin of approximately 3 mcg/mL is desirable; trough concentration should be <1 mcg/mL.
Vancomycin hydrochloride[d]	30 mg/kg per 24 h IV in two equally divided doses, not to exceed 2 g/24 h unless serum levels are monitored	4	Vancomycin therapy is recommended for patients allergic to β-lactams (see text regarding drug levels); according to the guidelines, serum concentrations of vancomycin should be obtained 1 h after completion of the infusion and should be in the range of 30–45 mcg/mL for twice-daily dosing

[a]Dosages recommended are for patients with normal renal function. For nutritionally variant streptococci, see Table 109–8.
[b]Patients should be informed that IM injection of ceftriaxone is painful.
[c]Dosing of gentamicin on a mg/kg basis will produce higher serum concentrations in obese patients than in lean patients. Therefore, in obese patients, dosing should be based on ideal body weight. (Ideal body weight for men is 50 kg + 2.3 kg per inch over 5 feet, and ideal body weight for women is 45.5 kg + 2.3 kg per inch over 5 feet.) Relative contraindications to the use of gentamicin are age > 65 years, renal impairment, or impairment of the eighth nerve. Other potentially nephrotoxic agents (e.g., nonsteroidal anti-inflammatory drugs) should be used cautiously in patients receiving gentamicin.
[d]Vancomycin dosage should be reduced in patients with impaired renal function. Each dose of vancomycin should be infused over at least 1 h to reduce the risk of the histamine-release "red man" syndrome.
IV = intravenous; IM = intramuscular.
From Wilson WR, Karchmer AW, Dajani AS, et al. Antibiotic treatment of adults with infective endocarditis due to streptococci, enterococci, and staphylococci, and HACEK microorganisms. JAMA 1995;274:1706–1713, with permission. Copyright 1995–1997, American Medical Association.

8 For some pathogens, such as enterococci, the use of synergistic antimicrobial combinations (including an aminoglycoside) is essential to obtain a bactericidal effect. Combination antibiotics also may decrease the emergence of resistant organisms during treatment (e.g., PVE caused by coagulase-negative staphylococci) and hasten the pace of clinical and microbiologic response (e.g., some streptococcal and staphylococcal infections). Occasionally, combination treatment will result in a shorter treatment course.

CLINICAL CONTROVERSY

The AHA guidelines recommend traditional aminoglycoside dosing whenever clinicians use these antibiotics. Extended-interval dosing (once-daily administration) is an intriguing dosing strategy, but data only support this approach for the treatment of streptococcal IE, and it is not recommended routinely.

TABLE 109–5. Therapy for Native-Valve Endocarditis Due to Strains of Viridans Streptococci and *Streptococcus bovis* Relatively Resistant to Penicillin G (Minimum Inhibitory Concentration > 0.1 mcg/mL and < 0.5 mcg/mL)[a]

Antibiotic	Dosage and Route	Duration (wks)	Comments
Aqueous crystalline penicillin G sodium	18 million units/24 h IV either continuously or in six equally divided doses	4	Cefazolin or other first-generation cephalosporins may be substituted for penicillin in patients whose penicillin hypersensitivity is not of the immediate type
With gentamicin sulfate[b]	1 mg/kg IM or IV every 8 h	2	
Vancomycin hydrochloride[c]	30 mg/kg per 24 h IV in two equally divided doses, not to exceed 2 g/24 h unless serum levels are monitored	4	Vancomycin therapy is recommended for patients allergic to β-lactams

[a]Dosages recommended are for patients with normal renal function.
[b]For specific dosing adjustment and issues concerning gentamicin, see Table 109–4 footnotes.
[c]For specific dosing adjustment and issues concerning vancomycin, see Table 109–4 footnotes.
IV = intravenous; IM = intramuscular.
From Wilson WR, Karchmer AW, Dajani AS, et al. Antibiotic treatment of adults with infective endocarditis due to streptococci, enterococci, and staphylococci, and HACEK microorganisms. JAMA 1995;274:1706–1713, with permission. Copyright 1995–1997, American Medical Association.

TABLE 109–6. Therapy for Endocarditis Due to *Staphylococcus* in the Absence of Prosthetic Material[a]

Antibiotic	Dosage and Route	Duration (wks)	Comments
Methicillin-Susceptible Staphylococci			
Regimens for non-β-lactam-allergic patients			
Nafcillin sodium or oxacillin sodium	2 g IV every 4 h	4–6	Benefit of additional aminoglycosides has not been established
With optional addition of gentamicin sulfate[†]	1 mg/kg IM or IV every 8 h	3–5 days	
Regimens for β-lactam-allergic patients			
Cefazolin (or other first-generation cephalosporins in equivalent dosages)	2 g IV every 8 h	4–6	Cephalosporins should be avoided in patients with immediate type hypersensitivity to penicillin
With optional addition of gentamicin[b]	1 mg/kg IM or IV every 8 h	3–5 days	
Vancomycin hydrochloride[c]	30 mg/kg per 24 h IV in two equally divided doses, not to exceed 2g/24 h unless serum levels are monitored	4–6	Recommended for patients allergic to penicillin
Methicillin-Resistant Staphylococci			
Vancomycin hydrochloride[c]	30 mg/kg per 24 h IV in two equally divided doses, not to exceed 2 g/24 h unless serum levels are monitored	4–6	

[a]For treatment of endocarditis due to penicillin-susceptible staphylococci (minimum inhibitory concentration ≤0.1 mcg/mL), aqueous crystalline penicillin G sodium (Table 109-4, first regimen) can be used for 4 to 6 wk instead of nafcillin or oxacillin. Shorter antibiotic courses have been effective in some drug addicts with right-sided endocarditis due to *Staphylococcus aureus* (see text). See text for comments on use of rifampin.
[b]For specific dosing adjustment and issues concerning gentamicin, see Table 109–4 footnotes.
[c]For specific dosing adjustment and issues concerning vancomycin, see Table 109–4 footnotes.
IV = intravenous; IM = intramuscular.
From Wilson WR, Karchmer AW, Dajani AS, et al. Antibiotic treatment of adults with infective endocarditis due to streptococci, enterococci, and staphylococci, and HACEK microorganisms. JAMA 1995;274:1706–1713, with permission. Copyright 1995–1997, American Medical Association.

Subsequent to the most recent publication of the AHA guidelines (1995), the British Society for Antimicrobial Chemotherapy (BSAC) has published treatment recommendations.[23] Although derived separately, these recommendations are quite similar to those of the AHA with regard to organism-specific treatment. The only major difference in these two guidelines pertains to empirical treatment of endocarditis. After appropriate blood cultures are obtained, the BSAC guidelines suggest empirical therapy with penicillin plus gentamicin for most patients, but when staphylococcal infection is suspected, they recommend vancomycin plus gentamicin. Although community-acquired staphylococcal infections rarely are methicillin-resistant, the BSAC guidelines recommend vancomycin for all suspected staphylococcal infections in an attempt to simplify recommendations, at least during the initial phase of treatment. While not specifically mentioned in the BSAC guidelines, a penicillinase-resistant penicillin (e.g., nafcillin) is a reasonable alternative to vancomycin during the short-term empirical treatment of community-acquired infection suspected to be staphylococci while identification and susceptibilities are obtained.

TABLE 109–7. Treatment of Staphylococcal Endocarditis in the Presence of a Prosthetic Valve or Other Prosthetic Material[a]

Antibiotic	Dosage and Route	Duration (wks)	Comments
Regimen for Methicillin-Resistant Staphylococci			
Vancomycin hydrochloride[b]	30 mg/kg per 24 h IV in 2 or 4 equally divided doses, not to exceed 2 g/24 h unless serum levels are monitored	≥6	
With rifampin[c]	300 mg orally every 8 h	≥6	Rifampin increases the amount of warfarin sodium required for antithrombotic therapy.
And with gentamicin sulfate[d,e]	1 mg/kg IM or IV every 8 h	2	
Regimen for Methicillin-Susceptible Staphylococci			
Nafcillin sodium or oxacillin sodium	2 g IV every 4 h	≥6	First-generation cephalosporins or vancomycin should be used in patients allergic to β-lactam.
With rifampin[c]	300 mg orally every 8 h	≥6	
And with gentamicin sulfate[d,e]	1 mg/kg IM or IV every 8 h	2	Cephalosporins should be avoided in patients with immediate-type hypersensitivity to penicillin or with methicillin-resistant staphylococci.

[a]Dosages recommended are for patients with normal renal function.
[b]For specific dosing adjustment and issues concerning vancomycin, see Table 109–4 footnotes.
[c]Rifampin plays a unique role in the eradication of staphylococcal infection involving prosthetic material (see text); combination therapy is essential to prevent emergence of rifampin resistance.
[d]For specific dosing adjustment and issues concerning gentamicin, see Table 109–4 footnotes.
[e]Use during initial 2 weeks.
IV = intravenous; IM = intramuscular.
From Wilson WR, Karchmer AW, Dajani AS, et al. Antibiotic treatment of adults with infective endocarditis due to streptococci, enterococci, and staphylococci, and HACEK microorganisms. JAMA 1995; 274:1706–1713, with permission. Copyright 1995–1997, American Medical Association.

TABLE 109–8. Standard Therapy for Endocarditis Due to Enterococci[a]

Antibiotic	Dosage and Route	Duration (wks)	Comments
Aqueous crystalline penicillin G sodium	18–30 million units/24 h IV either continuously or in six equally divided doses	4–6	Four-week therapy recommended for patients with symptoms <3 months in duration; 6-week therapy recommended for patients with symptoms >3 months in duration
With gentamicin sulfate[b]	1 mg/kg IM or IV every 8 h	4–6	
Ampicillin sodium	12 g/24 h IV either continuously or in six equally divided doses	4–6	
With gentamicin sulfate[b]	1 mg/kg IM or IV every 8 h	4–6	
Vancomycin hydrochloride[c]	30 mg/kg per 24 h IV in two equally divided doses, not to exceed 2 g/24 h unless serum levels are monitored	4–6	Vancomycin therapy is recommended for patients allergic to β-lactams; cephalosporins are not acceptable alternatives for patients allergic to penicillin
With gentamicin sulfate[b]	1 mg/kg IM or IV every 8 h	4–6	

[a]All enterococci causing endocarditis must be tested for antimicrobial susceptibility in order to select optimal therapy (see text). This table is for endocarditis due to gentamicin- or vancomycin-susceptible enterococci, viridans streptococci with a minimum inhibitory concentration of >0.5 mcg/mL, nutritionally variant viridans streptococci, or prosthetic valve endocarditis caused by viridans streptococci or *Streptococcus bovis*. Antibiotic dosages are for patients with normal renal function.
[b]For specific dosing adjustment and issues concerning gentamicin, see Table 109–4 footnotes.
[c]For specific dosing adjustment and issues concerning vancomycin, see Table 109–4 footnotes.
IV = intravenous; IM = intramuscular.
From Wilson WR, Karchmer AW, Dajani AS, et al. Antibiotic treatment of adults with infective endocarditis due to streptococci, enterococci, and staphylococci, and HACEK microorganisms. JAMA 1995; 274:1706–1713, with permission. Copyright 1995–1997, American Medical Association.

▓ STREPTOCOCCAL ENDOCARDITIS

Streptococci cause a majority of IE cases, with most isolates being viridans streptococci. *Viridans streptococci* refer to a large number of different species, such as *S. mutans, S. sanguis,* and *S. mitis.* These bacteria are common inhabitants of the human mouth and gingiva, and they are especially common causes of endocarditis involving native valves.[1,24] During dental surgery and even when brushing the teeth, these organisms can cause a transient bacteremia. In susceptible individuals, this potentially can result in IE. Streptococcal endocarditis is usually subacute, and the response to medical treatment is good. *S. bovis* is not a viridans streptococcus, but it is included in this group because it is penicillin sensitive and requires the same treatment as viridans streptococci. *S. bovis* is a group D *Streptococcus* that resides in the gastrointestinal tract. IE caused by this organism is often associated with a gastrointestinal pathology, especially colon carcinoma. Endocarditis caused by *S. pneumoniae, S. pyogenes,* and groups B, C, and G streptococci are relatively uncommon, and their treatment is not well defined.[1]

Antimicrobial regimens for viridans streptococci are well studied, and in uncomplicated cases, response rates as high as 98% can be expected. Viridans streptococci are penicillin-susceptible, although some are more susceptible than others. Most are exquisitely sensitive to penicillin G and have minimal inhibitory concentrations (MICs) of less than 0.1 mcg/mL.[22,24] Approximately 10% to 20% are moderately susceptible (MIC 0.1–0.5 mcg/mL). This difference in in vitro susceptibility led to recommendations that the MIC be determined for all viridans streptococci and that the results be used to guide therapy. Some streptococci are deemed tolerant to the killing effects of penicillin, where the MBC exceeds the MIC by 32 times. A tolerant organism is inhibited but not killed by an antibiotic normally considered bactericidal.[25] Bactericidal activity is required for successful treatment of IE; therefore, infections with a tolerant organism may relapse after treatment. Despite some animal studies of endocarditis suggesting that tolerant strains do not respond as readily to β-lactam therapy as nontolerant ones, this phenomenon is primarily a laboratory finding with little clinical significance.[26] Treatment for tolerant strains is identical to that for nontolerant organisms, and measurement of the MBC is not recommended.[22,23]

An assortment of regimens can be used to treat uncomplicated endocarditis caused by fully susceptible viridans streptococci (see Table 109–4). Two single-drug regimens consist of either

TABLE 109–9. Therapy for Endocarditis Due to HACEK Microorganisms (*Haemophilus parainfluenzae, Haemophilus aphrophilus, Actinobacillus actinomycetemocomitans, Cardiobacterium hominis, Eikenella corrodens,* and *Kingella kingae*)[a]

Antibiotic	Dosage and Route	Duration (wks)	Comments
Ceftriaxone sodium	2 g once daily IV or IM[b]	4	Cefotaxime sodium or other third-generation cephalosporins may be substituted
Ampicillin sodium[c]	12 g/24 h IV either continuously or in six equally divided doses	4	
With gentamicin sulfate[d]	1 mg/kg IM or IV every 8 h	4	

[a]Antibiotic dosages are for patients with normal renal function.
[b]Patients should be informed that IM injection of ceftriaxone is painful.
[c]Ampicillin should not be used if laboratory tests show β-lactamase production.
[d]For specific dosing adjustment and issues concerning gentamicin, see Table 109–4 footnotes.
IV = intravenous; IM = intramuscular.
From Wilson WR, Karchmer AW, Dajani AS, et al. Antibiotic treatment of adults with infective endocarditis due to streptococci, enterococci, and staphylococci, and HACEK microorganisms. JAMA 1995; 274:1706–1713, with permission. Copyright 1995–1997, American Medical Association.

high-dose parenteral penicillin G or ceftriaxone for 4 weeks. If a shorter course of therapy is desired, the guidelines suggest high-dose parenteral penicillin G plus an aminoglycoside.[22] When used in select patients, this combination is equally effective to 4 weeks of penicillin alone. Although streptomycin was listed in previous guidelines, gentamicin is the preferred aminoglycoside because serum drug concentrations are obtained easily, clinicians are more familiar with its use, and the few strains of streptococci resistant to the effects of streptomycin-penicillin remain susceptible to gentamicin-penicillin. Other aminoglycosides are not recommended.

The decision of which regimen to use depends on the perceived risk versus benefit. For example, a 2-week course of gentamicin in an elderly patient with renal impairment may be associated with ototoxicity, worsening renal function, or both. Furthermore, the 2-week regimen is not recommended for patients with complications such as extracardiac foci. On the other hand, a 4-week course of penicillin alone generally entails greater expense, especially if the patient remains in the hospital. Monotherapy with once-daily ceftriaxone offers ease of administration, facilitates home health care treatment, and may be cost-effective.[27]

The BSAC guidelines suggest that all the following conditions be present to consider a 2-week treatment regimen for penicillin-sensitive streptococcal endocarditis[23,28]:

- Penicillin-sensitive viridans streptococcus or *S. bovis* (penicillin MIC < 0.1 mcg/mL)
- No cardiovascular risk factors such as heart failure, aortic insufficiency, or conduction abnormalities
- No evidence of thromboembolic disease
- Native-valve infection
- No vegetation of greater than 5 mm diameter on echocardiogram
- Clinical response within 7 days (The temperature should return to normal, the patient should feel well, and the patient's appetite should return to normal.)

When a patient has a history of an immediate-type hypersensitivity to penicillin, vancomycin is the drug of choice for IE caused by viridans streptococci. When vancomycin is chosen, the addition of gentamicin is not recommended.[22] First-generation and some third-generation cephalosporins (ceftriaxone) are alternatives in patients with a history of delayed penicillin reactions. Most patients who report a penicillin allergy have a negative penicillin skin test and consequently are at low risk of anaphylaxis.[29] The published experience with penicillin is more extensive than with alternative regimens; therefore, a thorough allergy history must be obtained before a second-line therapy is administered.

In patients with complicated infections (e.g., extracardiac foci) or when the streptococcus has an MIC of 0.1–0.5 mcg/mL, combination therapy with an aminoglycoside and penicillin (higher dose preferred) for the first 2 weeks, followed by penicillin alone for an additional 2 weeks, is recommended[22] (see Table 109–5). Some viridans streptococci have biologic characteristics that complicate diagnosis and treatment. For example, a few bacteria have nutritional deficiencies that hinder growth in routine culture media.[2] These organisms require special broth supplemented with pyridoxal hydrochloride or cysteine. For patients infected with nutritionally variant streptococc,i or when the *Streptococcus* has an MIC of more than 0.5 mcg/mL, treatment should follow the enterococcal endocarditis treatment guidelines[22] (see Table 109–8).

The rationale for combination therapy of penicillin-susceptible viridans streptococci is that enhanced activity against these organisms usually is observed when cell wall active agents are combined with aminoglycosides in vitro.[22,26] Combined treatment results in quicker sterilization of vegetations in animal models of endocarditis and probably explains the high response rates observed in patients treated for a total of 2 weeks.[22] The combined treatment, however, is not superior to penicillin alone. For IE caused by streptococci relatively resistant to penicillin (MIC of 0.1–0.5 mcg/mL), combination therapy for 2 weeks is recommended, followed by penicillin alone for 2 additional weeks.[22,24] Some authors question the need for combination therapy for such relatively resistant streptococci, emphasizing that few human data suggest that patients with endocarditis caused by these organisms respond less well to penicillin alone.[30]

Whether or not extended-interval aminoglycoside dosing has a role in IE is controversial. This dosing approach, as compared with thrice-daily dosing, appears to have an equal and possibly greater efficacy in streptococcal endocarditis.[31–34] One study specifically evaluated the combination of ceftriaxone (2 g daily) with gentamicin (3 mg/kg daily) for 2 weeks compared with ceftriaxone (2 g daily) alone for 4 weeks for penicillin-sensitive streptococci. Both regimens were safe and effective with similar clinical cure rates at 3 months following treatment.[35]

STAPHYLOCOCCAL ENDOCARDITIS

Endocarditis caused by staphylococci is becoming more prevalent, mainly because of increased IVDA, more frequent use of peripheral and central venous catheters, and increased frequency of valve replacement surgery.[36,37] *Staphylococcus aureus* is the most common organism causing IE among those with IVDA and persons with venous catheters. Coagulase-negative staphylococci (usually *S. epidermidis*) are prominent causes of PVE.

Staphylococcal endocarditis is not a homogeneous disease; appropriate management requires consideration of several questions, such as, Is the organism methicillin resistant? Should combination therapy be used? Is the infection on a native or prosthetic valve? Does the patient have a history of IVDA? Is the infection on the left or right side of the heart? Another consideration in staphylococcal endocarditis is that some organisms may exhibit tolerance to antibiotics. However, similar to streptococci, the concern for tolerance among staphylococci should not affect antibiotic selection.[22]

Any patient who develops staphylococcal bacteremia is at risk for endocarditis. Many investigators have attempted to develop criteria that identify the bacteremic patient likely to have IE.[37] In hospitalized patients with *S. aureus* bacteremia and an identified focus of infection, such as a vascular catheter, the risk of concomitant IE is low, and treatment of the bacteremia can be reduced to 2 weeks. This approach applies only if the patient does not have a prosthetic valve or additional clinical evidence for endocarditis.[36,37] On the other hand, the following parameters predict higher risk of IE in patients with *S. aureus* bacteremia: (1) the absence of a primary site of infection, (2) community acquisition of infection, (3) metastatic signs of infection, and (4) valvular vegetations detected by echocardiography.[1,4]

The recommended therapy for patients with left-sided IE caused by methicillin-sensitive *S. aureus* (MSSA) is 4 to 6 weeks of nafcillin or oxacillin, often combined with a short course of gentamicin (see Table 109–6). From in vitro studies, the combination of an aminoglycoside and penicillinase-resistant penicillin or vancomycin enhances the activity of these drugs toward MSSA. In animal models of endocarditis, combinations of penicillin with an aminoglycoside eradicate organisms from vegetations more rapidly than penicillins alone.[36] In human studies, the addition of an aminoglycoside to nafcillin for the first week of therapy hastens the resolution of fever and bacteremia, but it does not affect survival or relapse rates.[38] Traditional thrice-daily dosing of aminoglycosides is recommended when administered for staphlococcal IE, albeit initial data have evaluated gentamicin given once a day.[39]

If a patient has a mild, delayed allergy to penicillin, first-generation cephalosporins (such as cefazolin) are effective alternatives, but they should be avoided in patients with a history of immediate-type hypersensitivity reactions to penicillins (see Table 109–6). The potential for a true immediate-type allergy should be assessed carefully, and a penicillin skin test should be conducted before giving antibiotic treatment to any patient claiming an allergy.[40] In a patient with a positive skin test or a history of immediate hypersensitivity to penicillin, vancomycin is the agent of choice. Vancomycin, however, kills *S. aureus* slowly and is regarded as inferior to penicillinase-resistant penicillins for MSSA.[37] Rifampin as an adjunctive therapy is controversial; however, this agent, added to vancomycin in refractory or complicated infections in patients with left-sided IE may result in dramatic patient improvement.[36,37] Generally, antibiotic therapy should be continued for 4 to 6 weeks. Unfortunately, left-sided IE caused by *S. aureus* continues to have a poor prognosis, with a mortality rate of 25% to 47%.[16,22] For reasons discussed in the following section, those with IE associated with IVDA have a more favorable response to therapy.

During the past decade, greater numbers of staphylococci became resistant to penicillinase-resistant penicillins (e.g., methicillin). Vancomycin is the drug of choice for these resistant organisms because most MRSAs and coagulase-negative staphylococci are susceptible to it (see Table 109–6). The presence or lack of a prosthetic heart valve in patients with a methicillin-resistant organism guides therapy and determines whether vancomycin should be used alone or, if a prosthetic valve is present, whether combination therapy is necessary[3,22] (see Table 109–7).

Staphylococcus Endocarditis: Intravenous Drug Abuser

Infective endocarditis in those with IVDA is frequently (60% to 70%) caused by *S. aureus,* although other organisms may be common in certain geographic locations.[41] In this setting, the tricuspid valve is frequently infected, resulting in right-sided IE. Most patients have no history of valve abnormalities, are usually otherwise healthy, and have a good response to medical treatment. Nonetheless, surgery may be required.

Standard treatment for MSSA endocarditis is 4 weeks of monotherapy with a penicillinase-resistant penicillin (see Table 109–6). In the intravenous drug abuser, however, the clinical response with right-sided MSSA endocarditis is usually excellent. Emerging data suggest that these patients may be treated effectively (clinical and microbiologic cure exceeding 90%) with a 2-week course of nafcillin or oxacillin plus an aminoglycoside.[41-47] Short-course vancomycin, in place of nafcillin or oxacillin, appears to be ineffective.[45] Another trial suggested that a 2-week regimen of a penicillinase-resistant penicillin alone, without the addition of an aminoglycoside, is as effective as combined therapy in MSSA tricuspid valve endocarditis.[48] Although these data suggest that an aminoglycoside is unnecessary for short-course treatment in the intravenous drug abuser with right-sided IE, most clinicians are uncomfortable with monotherapy and choose combination treatment in this situation so long as there are

no reasons to avoid an aminoglycoside. Short-course therapy should not be used in left-sided endocarditis, and it is inappropriate in patients with underlying acquired immunodeficiency syndrome (AIDS) or substantial pulmonary complications, such as lung abscess from right-sided IE.[22]

An intriguing therapeutic approach for staphylococcal endocarditis in those with IVDA is oral treatment. Preliminary data have suggested that short-course intravenous treatment (primarily nafcillin, mean 16 days) followed by oral treatment (dicloxacillin or oxacillin, mean 26 days) might be effective for tricuspid valve MSSA endocarditis.[49] The positive results of this trial can be explained by the duration of intravenous antibiotics (>2 weeks), which may be a sufficient treatment course in this patient population. Yet two other studies that predominantly used oral therapy (ciprofloxacin and rifampin) found this approach to be effective (cure rates exceeding 90%) in addicts with uncomplicated right-sided endocarditis caused by MSSA.[50,51] At this time, concerns with resistance (e.g., ciprofloxacin) and limited published data preclude routine use of oral antibacterial regimens for the treatment of IE in the intravenous drug abuser.

> ### CLINICAL CONTROVERSY
>
> Oral antibiotics for the treatment of IE have been assessed primarily in those with IVDA. Although treating IE with oral antibiotics would decrease adverse events associated with prolonged use of intravenous catheters (e.g., infection, septic thrombus), the paucity of data preclude this being a routine treatment.

Staphylococcal Endocarditis: Prosthetic Valves

PVE accounts for approximately 15% of all IE cases.[52] An episode of PVE occurring within 2 months of surgery strongly suggests that the cause is staphylococci implanted during the procedure.[3] Yet the risk of staphylococcal endocarditis remains elevated for up to 12 months after valve replacement. Because this type of IE is typically a nosocomial infection, methicillin-resistant organisms are common, and vancomycin is the cornerstone of therapy. Combination antimicrobials are recommended because of the high morbidity and mortality associated with PVE and its refractoriness to therapy.[3,22] Although the addition of rifampin to a penicillinase-resistant penicillin or vancomycin does not result in predictable bacterial synergism, rifampin may have unique activity against staphylococcal infection that involves prosthetic material, where its addition results in a higher microbiologic cure rate.[2] Combination therapy also decreases the emergence of resistance to rifampin, which frequently occurs when it is used alone. For methicillin-resistant staphylococci (both MRSA and coagulase-negative staphylococci), vancomycin is recommended with rifampin for 6 weeks or more (see Table 109–7). An aminoglycoside is added for the first 2 weeks if the organism is aminoglycoside-susceptible. For MSSA, a penicillinase-resistant penicillin is administered in place of vancomycin. PVE responds poorly to medical treatment and has a higher mortality compared with native-valve endocarditis. Valve dehiscence and incompetence can result in acute heart failure, and surgery is often a component of treatment.[3]

After 12 months, the likely organism for PVE parallels that of native-valve endocarditis. As with native-valve endocarditis, antimicrobial therapy should be based on the identified organism and in vitro susceptibility. If an organism is identified other than staphylococci, the treatment regimen should be guided by susceptibilities and should be at least 6 weeks in duration.[3,23] Additionally, a concomitant aminoglycoside is recommended if streptococci or enterococci are identified. Once-daily aminoglycoside regimens have not been evaluated in PVE and are not recommended.[3]

The use of anticoagulation is controversial in PVE. Those who require anticoagulation for prosthetic valves should continue the anticoagulant cautiously during endocarditis therapy, unless a contraindication to therapy exists.

ENTEROCOCCAL ENDOCARDITIS

Enterococci are normal inhabitants of the human gastrointestinal tract and, occasionally, of the anterior urethra. These organisms are usually of low virulence but can become a pathogen in predisposed patients following genitourinary manipulations (older men) or obstetric procedures (younger women).[2] Historically, enterococci were considered group D streptococci, but they have been reclassified into the genus *Enterococcus* (*E. faecalis* and *E. faecium*). *E. faecalis* is the most common clinical isolate (approximately 90%) of the two species. Enterococci cause 5% to 18% of endocarditis cases, but they are more resistant to therapy than staphylococci and streptococci. Enterococci are noteworthy for these reasons: (1) no single antibiotic is bactericidal, (2) MICs to penicillin are relatively high (1–25 mcg/mL), (3) intrinsic resistance occurs to all cephalosporins and relative resistance occurs to aminoglycosides (e.g., "low level" aminoglycoside resistance), (4) combinations of a cell wall active agent such as a penicillin or vancomycin and an aminoglycoside are necessary for killing, and (5) resistance to all available drugs is increasing.[1,22,53]

Monotherapy with penicillin for IE caused by enterococci results in relapse rates of 50% to 80%. When used alone, penicillins are only bacteriostatic against enterococci, and combination therapy is always recommended for susceptible strains.[53] The relapse rate following penicillin-gentamicin therapy for susceptible strains is less than 15%.[13] The killing of enterococci by the bactericidal combination of an aminoglycoside and a penicillin is the best clinical example of antibiotic synergy. Because the aminoglycoside cannot penetrate the bacterial cell in the absence of the penicillin, enterococci usually will appear to be resistant to aminoglycosides by routine susceptibility testing (low-level resistance). However, in the presence of an agent that disrupts the cell wall such as penicillin, the aminoglycoside can gain entry, attach to bacterial ribosomes, and cause rapid cell death. An aminoglycoside-vancomycin combination is also synergistic against enterococci and is appropriate therapy for the penicillin-allergic patient.[54]

Enterococcal endocarditis ordinarily requires 4 to 6 weeks of high-dose penicillin G or ampicillin plus an aminoglycoside for cure (see Table 109–8). Ampicillin has greater in vitro activity than penicillin G, although there are no clinical data to document differences in efficacy. A 6-week course is recommended for patients with symptoms lasting longer than 3 months, recurrent cases, and those with mitral valve involvement. Streptomycin has been the most extensively studied aminoglycoside, but gentamicin is presently favored. Other aminoglycosides cannot be substituted routinely. In the treatment of enterococcal endocarditis, relatively low serum concentrations of aminoglycosides appear adequate for successful therapy, such as a gentamicin peak concentration of approximately 3 mcg/mL.[55] Even though the most recent treatment guidelines advocate this

low-peak-concentration approach, it is debated as to whether this is suitable because it has not been well documented to be equally or more efficacious than higher-serum-concentration approaches.[56] Treatment of enterococcal endocarditis does not have the high success rate seen with IE caused by viridans streptococci presumably because the organism is more resistant to killing.

Although some data support the use of extended-interval aminoglycoside dosing for other types of endocarditis (i.e., streptococci), the data are more vague regarding this strategy in enterococcal IE.[57] While some studies suggest that extended-interval aminoglycoside dosing and short-interval (traditional) dosing are clinically equivalent,[58–60] discordant studies imply otherwise.[61,62] The paucity of human data precludes routine use of extended-interval aminoglycoside dosing in this setting.

Resistance among enterococci to penicillins and aminoglycosides is increasing.[53] Enterococci that exhibit high-level resistance to streptomycin (MIC > 2000 mcg/mL) are not synergistically killed by penicillin and streptomycin because the aminoglycoside either no longer binds to the ribosome or is inactivated by an aminoglycoside-modifying enzyme, streptomycin adenylase. Because enterococci will appear resistant to aminoglycosides on routine susceptibility testing, the only way to distinguish high-level from low-level resistance is by performing special susceptibility tests using 500–2000 mcg/mL of the aminoglycoside. High-level streptomycin-resistant enterococci occur with a frequency of 40% to 50%, and high-level resistance to gentamicin is now found in 10% to 50% of isolates. Although most gentamicin-resistant enterococci are resistant to all aminoglycosides (including amikacin), 30% to 50% remain susceptible to streptomycin.[53] High-level gentamicin resistance is mediated by a bifunctional aminoglycoside-modifying enzyme, 6′-acetyltransferase/2′-phosphotransferase, and most strains also possess streptomycin adenylase. These organisms do not commonly cause IE; data on appropriate therapy are sparse, and therapeutic options are few. Case reports indicate that some patients will respond to high doses of ampicillin, as observed in the early trials of penicillin monotherapy.[63]

In addition to isolates with high-level aminoglycoside resistance, β-lactamase-producing enterococci (especially *E. faecium*) have been reported.[64] If these organisms are discovered, use of vancomycin or ampicillin-sulbactam should be considered. VRE are reported increasingly, primarily with *E. faecium*. Vancomycin resistance occurs when the bacterium replaces the normal vancomycin target with a peptidoglycan precursor that does not bind vancomycin.[65] Combination therapies including teicoplanin, quinupristin-dalfopristin, or linezolid appear to be the most promising treatments.

LESS COMMON TYPES OF INFECTIVE ENDOCARDITIS
HACEK Group

Gram-negative bacteria from the HACEK group (*Hemophilus parainfluenzae, H. aphrophilus, Actinobacillus actinomycetemcomitans, Cardiobacterum hominis, Eikenella corrodens,* and *Kingella kingae*) are unusual causes of IE. Frequently, these types of IE present as subacute illnesses with large vegetations and emboli.[66] These oropharyngeal organisms typically are slow growing and should be considered as possible causes of "culture negative" endocarditis. Ceftriaxone or high-dose ampicillin with gentamicin for 4 weeks is the recommended therapy, although ceftriaxone may be preferred[22] (see Table 109–9). Valve replacement is required occasionally.

Culture-Negative Endocarditis

Sterile blood cultures are reported in up to 5% of patients with IE if strict diagnostic criteria are used.[1,5,67] This type of IE may occur as a result of unidentified subacute right-sided IE, previous antibiotic therapy, slow-growing fastidious organisms, nonbacterial etiologies (e.g., fungi), and improperly collected blood cultures. When blood cultures from patients suspected of IE show no growth after 48 to 72 hours, the laboratory should be advised and cultures held for up to a month to detect growth of fastidious organisms.

Clinicians should individualize therapy for culture-negative IE. In patients without a history of IVDA, culture-negative IE treatment usually will follow an approach that encompasses treatment for enterococci, the HACEK group, and nutritionally variant streptococci. Although controversial, one source recommends penicillin or ampicillin, an aminoglycoside (e.g., gentamicin), and ceftriaxone. In the intravenous drug abuser in whom staphylococci are suspected, a penicillinase-resistant penicillin or a cephalosporin with activity against staphylococci could be added to the preceding regimen.[1] Therapy for PVE often includes at least vancomycin and gentamicin.[5] Irrespective of the treatment chosen, extended antimicrobial therapy is required (e.g., 6 weeks), although the aminoglycoside may be removed after 2 weeks if clinical improvement is observed. The preceding empirical approaches to culture-negative IE highlight the need for proper collection and monitoring of blood cultures and an extensive medication history.

Other Atypical Microorganisms

Endocarditis caused by organisms such as *Coxiella burnetii; Brucella, Candida,* and *Aspergillus* spp.; *Legionella;* and gram-negative bacilli (e.g., *Pseudomonas*) is relatively uncommon. Medical therapy for IE caused by these organisms is usually unsuccessful.[5] Readers are referred elsewhere for an in-depth discussion regarding the management of unusually encountered organisms.[4] Consultation with an infectious disease expert is warranted when these microorganisms are identified.

Patients at higher risk of gram-negative bacilli IE include intravenous drug abusers and those with prosthetic heart valves. In addition to *Pseudomonas* spp., other gram-negative bacilli that have been implicated include *Salmonella* spp., *Escherichia coli, Citrobacter* spp., *Klebsiella-Enterobacter* spp., *S. marcescens, Proteus* spp., and *Providencia* spp.[1] Generally, these infections have a poor prognosis, with mortality rates as high as 60% to 80%.[16] Valve replacement is considered mandatory for left-sided pseudomonal IE.[4] If medical management is implemented, large doses of a penicillin with activity toward *Pseudomonas* (e.g., piperacillin 18 g/day) with an aminoglycoside are necessary for an extended period (e.g., 6 weeks).[1,4] Higher doses of the aminoglycoside (e.g., 8 mg/kg per day) may improve the survival rates of *Pseudomonas* IE, especially when combined with surgery.[66,68]

All cases of *Legionella* IE have had an extended febrile course over months and high anti-*Legionella* antibody titers and have occurred in patients with prosthetic valves.[4] When special media are used, blood cultures will reveal this organism. Prolonged parenteral therapy with either doxycycline or erythromycin, with prolonged oral therapy (e.g., 6 to 17 months), has elicited cure in some patients.[4] Most patients require concomitant valve replacement.

Fungi cause between 2% and 4% of endocarditis cases; most patients with fungal endocarditis have undergone recent cardiovascular surgery, are intravenous drug abusers, have received prolonged treatment with intravenous catheters or antibiotics, or are immunocompromised.[1,2,69] *Candida* spp. and *Aspergillus* spp. are most commonly involved, and the mortality rate is high for these reasons: (1) large, bulky vegetations that often form, (2) systemic septic embolization that may occur, (3) the tendency for fungi to invade the myocardium, (4) poor penetration of vegetations by antifungals, (5) the low toxic:therapeutic ratio of agents such as amphotericin B, and (6) the lack of consistent fungicidal activity of available antifungal agents.[1,70] When fungal IE is identified, the combined medical-surgical approach is recommended. Because these infections occur infrequently, scant clinical data are available to make solid treatment recommendations; however, the use of antifungal agents alone has been globally unsuccessful. Amphotericin B is the mainstay pharmacologic approach with the possible addition of flucytosine. The usefulness of fluconazole and itraconazole remains unknown at this time, although high-dose itraconazole may be of worth in *Aspergillus* endocarditis, and fluconazole has had limited success in *Candida* IE.

Coxiella burnetii (Q fever) just recently has been recovered from blood cultures, but infection is more likely to be identified via serologic tests. It is a common cause of IE in certain areas of the world where goat, cattle, and sheep farming are widespread. The most favorable therapy for Q fever is unknown but may include doxycycline with trimethoprim-sulfamethoxazole, rifampin, or fluoroquinolones.[4]

Brucella are facultative intracellular gram-negative bacilli. Humans are infected by this organism after ingesting infected unpasteurized milk or undercooked meat, inhalation of infectious aerosols, or contact with infected tissues. This type of IE is more common in veterinarians and livestock handlers. Cure requires valve replacement and antimicrobial agents including doxycycline with streptomycin or gentamicin or doxycycline with trimethoprim-sulfamethoxazole or rifampin for an extended period (8 weeks to months).[4]

PHARMACOECONOMIC CONSIDERATIONS

IE remains an uncommon disease, but the cost of treatment can be substantial. In the past, the long duration of hospitalization required to administer intravenous antimicrobials was the major expense. In selected cases, abbreviated, outpatient, and possibly in the future oral antimicrobial therapy may appreciably reduce the cost of care.

Shorter-course antimicrobial regimens are advocated when possible. For instance, in exquisitely sensitive streptococcal endocarditis (MICs < 0.1 mcg/mL), a 2-week regimen of high-dose parenteral penicillin G in combination with an aminoglycoside is as effective as 4 weeks of penicillin alone.[22,23] Uncomplicated right-sided MSSA endocarditis in the intravenous drug abuser also may be treated with a 2-week course. Treatment with nafcillin or oxacillin in combination with an aminoglycoside appears to be cost-effective.

The initiation of outpatient parenteral antibiotics should be considered early in the treatment of IE, after the patient is stable clinically and responds favorably to initial antibiotics. Outpatient treatment has been demonstrated to be safe and effective in select situations.[71] Patients considered for home therapy must be hemodynamically stable, compliant with therapy, have careful medical monitoring, understand the potential complications of the disease, and have immediate access to medical care. Advances in technology allow for the outpatient administration of complex antibiotic regimens that significantly reduce the cost of therapy. Simple regimens, such as single daily doses of ceftriaxone for streptococcal IE, are particularly attractive. Although endocarditis is common in those with a history of IVDA, and home health care would substantially reduce the cost of treatment, many clinicians are uncomfortable with outpatient intravenous therapy because central venous access is required. Sudden cardiac decompensation in an outpatient setting is also of concern.

EVALUATION OF THERAPEUTIC OUTCOMES

The evaluation of patients treated for IE includes assessment of disease signs and symptoms, blood cultures, microbiologic tests, serum drug concentrations, and other tests that evaluate organ function.

SIGNS AND SYMPTOMS

Fever usually subsides within 1 week of initiating therapy.[1,2] Persistence of fever may indicate ineffective antimicrobial therapy, emboli, infections of intravascular catheters, or drug reactions. In some patients, low-grade fever may persist even with appropriate antimicrobial therapy. With defervescence, the patient should begin to feel better, and other symptoms, such as lethargy or weakness, should subside.

BLOOD CULTURES

Blood cultures should be negative within a few days, although microbiologic response to vancomycin may be slower.[1,2] If bacteria continue to be isolated from blood beyond the first few days of therapy, it may indicate that the antimicrobials are inactive against the pathogen or that the doses are not producing adequate concentrations at the site of infection. After the initiation of therapy, blood cultures should be rechecked until negative. During the remainder of therapy, frequent blood culturing is not necessary. Additional blood cultures should be rechecked after successful treatment (e.g., once or twice within the 8 weeks after treatment) to ensure cure.

MICROBIOLOGIC TESTS

For all isolates from blood cultures, MICs should be determined; MBCs are no longer recommended.[22,23] The agent currently being used should be tested, as well as alternatives that may be required if intolerance, allergy, or resistance occurs. Occasionally, it is useful to determine whether synergy exists for antimicrobial combinations, although synergistic regimens usually can be predicted from the literature. Methods for in vitro determinations of synergy are summarized in Chap. 103.

Serum bactericidal titers (SBTs; also called *Schlicter tests*) have been used in the past in association with a number of infectious diseases.[72,73] The SBT is the greatest dilution of a patient's serum sample that is obtained while receiving antimicrobial treatment that kills greater than 99.9% of an inoculum of the infecting pathogen in vitro over 18 to 24 hours. In animal models of endocarditis, studies suggest that an SBT of 1:8 is predictive of response.[18] In humans with endocarditis, however, the correlation with SBTs and outcome is not clear. One investigation found peak and trough SBT ratio of 1:64 or greater and 1:32 predicted cure, although a lower titer did not predict failure.[74] Serum bactericidal titers of 1:32 are achieved easily for most streptococci causing endocarditis because the MBC is low relative to achievable concentrations of penicillin; however, for enterococci, methicillin-resistant staphylococci, and gram-negative bacilli, high SBTs may be difficult to achieve.

At present, SBTs have little value in monitoring treatment of common types of IE and should not be recommended routinely.[22,23]

This test may be useful when the causative organisms are only moderately susceptible to antimicrobials, when less well-established regimens are used, or when response to therapy is suboptimal and dosage escalation is being considered.

SERUM DRUG CONCENTRATIONS

Of the agents used commonly for IE, measurement of serum drug concentrations is routinely available for aminoglycosides (except streptomycin) and vancomycin. Few data, however, support attaining any specific serum concentrations in patients with IE. In general, serum concentrations of the antimicrobial should exceed the MBC of the organisms, but in practice, this principle is usually not helpful in monitoring patients with endocarditis. Aminoglycoside concentrations rarely exceed the MBC for certain organisms, such as streptococci and enterococci, and concentrations have not been correlated with response, such as aminoglycosides and vancomycin for staphylococci.[74,75]

When aminoglycosides are administered for IE caused by gram-positive cocci with a traditional thrice-daily regimen, peak serum concentrations are recommended to be on the low side of the traditional ranges (3 mcg/mL for gentamicin). If extended-interval dosing is used, which is not a standard practice at this time, the most appropriate method of monitoring has not been determined. When vancomycin is administered, the most recent treatment guidelines (1995) recommend serum drug monitoring.[22] Although the guidelines recommend to obtain peak serum concentrations when using vancomycin, measuring peak concentrations has limited applicability. The primary goal of serum vancomycin monitoring clinically is to ensure that there are adequate trough concentrations when treating resistant organisms.

TABLE 109–10. Cardiac Conditions Associated with Endocarditis

Endocarditis Prophylaxis Recommended
High-risk category
  Prosthetic cardiac valves, including bioprosthetic and homograft valves
  Previous bacterial endocarditis
  Complex cyanotic congenital heart disease (e.g., single ventricle states, transposition of the great arteries, tetralogy of Fallot)
  Surgically constructed systemic pulmonary shunts or conduits
Moderate-risk category
  Most other congenital cardiac malformations (other than above and below)
  Acquired valvular dysfunction (e.g., rheumatic heart disease)
  Hypertrophic cardiomyopathy
  Mitral valve prolapse with valvar regurgitation and/or thickened leaflets
Endocarditis Prophylaxis Not Recommended
Negligible-risk category (no greater risk than the general population)
  Isolated secundum atrial septal defect
  Surgical repair of atrial septal defect, ventricular septal defect, or patent ductus arteriosus (without residua beyond 6 mo)
  Previous coronary artery bypass graft surgery
  Mitral valve prolapse without valvar regurgitation
  Physiologic, functional, or innocent heart murmurs
  Previous Kawasaki disease without valvar dysfunction
  Previous rheumatic fever without valvar dysfunction
  Cardiac pacemakers (intravascular and epicardial) and implanted defibrillators

From Dajani AS, Taubert KA, Wilson W, et al. Prevention of bacterial endocarditis: Recommendations by the American Heart Association. JAMA 1997;277:1794–1801, with permission. Copyright 1995–1997, American Medical Association.

TABLE 109–11. Dental Procedures and Endocarditis Prophylaxis

Endocarditis Prophylaxis Recommended[a]
  Dental extractions
  Periodontal procedures including surgery, scaling and root planing,
    probing, and recall maintenance
  Dental implant placement and reimplantation of avulsed teeth
  Endodontic (root canal) instrumentation or surgery only beyond the
    apex
  Subgingival placement of antibiotic fibers or strips
  Initial placement of orthodontic bands but not brackets
  Intraligamentary local anesthetic injections
  Prophylactic cleaning of teeth or implants where bleeding is
    anticipated

Endocarditis Prophylaxis Not Recommended
  Restorative dentistry[b] (operative and prosthodontic) with or without
    retraction cord[c]
  Local anesthetic injections (nonintraligamentary)
  Intracanal endodontic treatment; after placement and buildup
  Placement of rubber dams
  Postoperative suture removal
  Placement of removable prosthodontic or orthodontic appliances
  Taking of oral impressions
  Fluoride treatments
  Taking of oral radiographs
  Orthodontic appliance adjustment
  Shedding of primary teeth

[a]Prophylaxis is recommended for patients with high- and moderate-risk cardiac
conditions.
[b]This includes restoration of decayed teeth (filling cavities) and replacement of
missing teeth.
[c]Clinical judgment may indicate antibiotic use in selected circumstances that may
create significant bleeding.
*From Dajani AS, Taubert KA, Wilson W, et al. Prevention of bacterial endocarditis:
Recommendations by the American Heart Association. JAMA 1997;277:1794–
1801, with permission. Copyright 1995–1997, American Medical Association.*

TABLE 109–12. Other Procedures and Endocarditis Prophylaxis

Endocarditis Prophylaxis Recommended
Respiratory tract
  Tonsillectomy and/or adenoidectomy
  Surgical operations that involve respiratory mucosa
  Bronchoscopy with a rigid bronchoscope
Gastrointestinal tract[a]
  Sclerotherapy for esophageal varices
  Esophageal stricture dilation
  Endoscopic retrograde cholangiography with biliary obstruction
  Biliary tract surgery
  Surgical operations that involve intestinal mucosa
Genitourinary tract
  Prostatic surgery
  Cystoscopy
  Urethral dilation

Endocarditis Prophylaxis Not Recommended
Respiratory tract
  Endotracheal intubation
  Bronchoscopy with a flexible bronchoscope, with or without
    biopsy[b]
  Tympanostomy tube insertion
Gastrointestinal tract
  Transesophageal echocardiography[b]
  Endoscopy with or without gastrointestinal biopsy[b]
Genitourinary tract
  Vaginal hysterectomy[b]
  Vaginal delivery[b]
  Cesarean section
  In uninfected tissue
    Urethral catheterization
    Uterine dilation and curettage
    Therapeutic abortion
    Sterilization procedures
    Insertion or removal of intrauterine devices
Other
  Cardiac catheterization, including balloon angioplasty
  Implanted cardiac pacemakers, implanted defibrillators, and
    coronary stents
  Incision or biopsy of surgically scrubbed skin
  Circumcision

[a]Prophylaxis is recommended for high-risk patients; optional for medium-risk
patients.
[b]Prophylaxis is optional for high-risk patients.
*From Dajani AS, Taubert KA, Wilson W, et al. Prevention of bacterial endocarditis:
Recommendations by the American Heart Association. JAMA 1997;277:1794–
1801, with permission. Copyright 1995–1997, American Medical Association.*

PREVENTION

Antimicrobial prophylaxis is used as an attempt to prevent IE in patients at high risk.[76,77] The use of antimicrobials for this purpose requires consideration of (1) cardiac conditions associated with endocarditis, (2) procedures causing bacteremia, (3) organisms likely to cause endocarditis, and (4) pharmacokinetics, spectrum, cost, adverse effects, and ease of administration of available antimicrobial agents. The objective of prophylaxis is to diminish the likelihood of IE in high-risk individuals (Table 109–10) who are undergoing procedures that cause transient bacteremia (Tables 109–11 and 109–12). Although there are no prospective, controlled human trials demonstrating that prophylaxis in high-risk individuals protects against the development of endocarditis during bacteremia-induced procedures, animal studies suggest possible benefit.[78] Most causes of IE, however, appear not to be secondary to an invasive procedure. Bacteremia as a consequence of daily activities in fact may be the major culprit, and the value of antibiotic prophylaxis before bacteremia-causing procedures has been questioned.[79] Retrospective human studies, though, support that a reduction of endocarditis occurs in selected patients following dental surgery where prophylaxis is employed.[80] The common practice of using antimicrobal therapy in this setting remains controversial. The mechanism of a beneficial effect in humans is unclear, but antibiotics may decrease the number of bacteria at the surgical site, kill bacteria after they are introduced into the blood, and prevent adhesion of bacteria to the valve. Studies have found that prophylaxis does not reduce the frequency of bacteremia immediately following tooth extraction as compared with a control group, suggesting that a reduction in adhesion or effects after the bacteria adhere to the endocardium are more likely mechanisms.[81,82] Other studies have further questioned the benefit of antibiotic prophylaxis.[83]

CLINICAL CONTROVERSY

The common practice of administering antibiotics to high-risk individuals before a bacteremia-causing procedure is controversial. Despite limited data supporting this approach and the fact that 100% compliance with AHA preventative guidelines would have only a modest benefit, the use of single-dose antibiotics for the prevention of endocarditis remains a standard of care.

TABLE 109–13. Prophylactic Regimens for Dental, Oral, Respiratory Tract, or Esophageal Procedures

Situation	Agent	Regimen[a]
Standard general prophylaxis	Amoxicillin	Adults: 2 g; children: 50 mg/kg orally 1 h before procedure
Unable to take oral medications	Ampicillin	Adults: 2 g intramuscularly (IM) or intravenously (IV); children: 50 mg/kg IM or IV within 30 min before procedure
Allergic to penicillin	Clindamycin *or*	Adults: 600 mg; children: 20 mg/kg orally 1 h before procedure
	Cephalexin[b] or cefadroxil[b] *or*	Adults: 2 g; children: 50 mg/kg orally 1 h before procedure
	Azithromycin or chlarithromycin	Adults: 500 mg; children: 15 mg/kg orally 1 h before procedure
Allergic to penicillin and unable to take oral medications	Clidamycin *or*	Adults: 600 mg; children: 20 mg/kg IV within 30 min before procedure
	Cefazolin[b]	Adults 1 g; children: 25 mg/kg IM or IV within 30 min before procedure

[a]Total children's dose should not exceed adult dose.

[b]Cephalosporins should not be used in individuals with immediate-type hypersensitivity reaction (urticaria, angioedema, or anaphylaxis) to penicillins.

From Dajani AS, Taubert KA, Wilson W, et al. Prevention of bacterial endocarditis: Recommendations by the American Heart Association. JAMA 1997;277:1974–1801, with permission. Copyright 1995–1997, American Medical Association.

PATIENTS AT RISK

Patients with certain cardiac lesions, particularly those with prosthetic heart valves or a history of bacterial endocarditis, are at high risk for developing IE (see Table 109–10). Nevertheless, only 15% to 25% of patients who develop IE are in a definable high-risk category.[76] Few cases of IE are preventable with antibiotic prophylaxis, even with 100% effectiveness.[84] The concern of antibiotic resistance also questions the routine use of antimicrobials in this setting. Despite the low probability that IE will develop, prophylaxis is recommended for some dental, respiratory, gastrointestinal, and genitourinary pro-

cedures (see Tables 109–11 and Tables 109–12) because of the significant morbidity associated with the disease. Patients undergoing valve implant surgery are at a much greater risk for IE than are those patients undergoing dental surgery.

PROCEDURES CAUSING BACTEREMIA

Bacteremia accompanies many everyday events, such as brushing the teeth and chewing, although certain medical and surgical procedures are more likely to cause a transient bacteremia (see Tables 109–11 and

TABLE 109–14. Prophylactic Regimens for Genitourinary Gastrointestinal (Excluding Esophageal) Procedures

Situation	Agent[a]	Regimen[b]
High-risk patients	Ampicillin plus gentamicin	Adults: Ampicillin 2 g intramuscularly (IM) or intravenously (IV) plus gentamicin 1.5 mg/kg (not to exceed 120 mg) within 30 min of starting the procedure; 6 h later, ampicillin 1 g IM/IV or amoxicillin 1 g orally.
		Children: Ampicillin 50 mg/kg IM or IV (not to exceed 2 g) plus gentamicin 1.5 mg/kg within 30 min of starting the procedure; 6 h later, ampicillin 25 mg/kg IM/IV or amoxicillin 25 mg/kg orally.
High-risk patients allergic to ampicillin/amoxicillin	Vancomycin plus gentamicin	Adults: Vancomycin 1 g IV over 1–2 h plus gentamicin 1.5 mg/kg IV/IM (not to exceed 120 mg); complete injection/infusion within 30 min of starting the procedure.
		Children: Vancomycin 20 mg/kg IV over 1–2 h plus gentamicin 1.5 mg/kg IV/IM; complete injection/infusion within 30 min of starting the procedure.
Moderate-risk patients	Amoxicillin or ampicillin	Adults: Amoxicillin 2 g orally 1 h before procedure, or ampicillin 2 g IM/IV within 30 min of starting the procedure.
		Children: Amoxicillin 50 mg/kg orally 1 h before procedure, or ampicillin 50 mg/kg IM/IV within 30 min of starting the procedure.
Moderate-risk patients allergic to ampicillin/amoxicillin	Vancomycin	Adults: Vancomycin 1 g IV over 1–2 h; complete infusion within 30 min of starting the procedure.
		Children: Vancomycin 20 mg/kg IV over 1–2 h; complete infusion within 30 min of starting the procedure.

[a]Total children's dose should not exceed adult dose.

[b]No second dose of vancomycin or gentamicin is recommended.

From Dajani AS, Taubert KA, Wilson W, et al. Prevention of bacterial endocarditis: Recommendations by the American Heart Association. JAMA 1997;277:1794–1801, with permission. Copyright 1995–1997, American Medical Association.

109–12). Antibiotic prophylaxis is recommended in patients at risk undergoing a bacteremia-causing procedure. For dental procedures of the gums and oral structures that cause bleeding, viridans streptococci frequently cause bacteremia, whereas instrumentation and surgery of the gastrointestinal and genitourinary tracts more often result in enterococcal bacteremia.[1]

ANTIBIOTIC REGIMENS

The AHA routinely publishes guidelines regarding the prevention of IE, with the most recent revision occurring in 1997.[78] A single 2-g dose of amoxicillin is recommended for adult patients at risk, given 1 hour before undergoing procedures associated with bacteremia (see Table 109–13). Because the duration of antimicrobial prophylaxis appears to be relatively short, these guidelines do not advocate a second oral dose of amoxicillin, which was recommended previously. Alternative prophylaxis regimens for patients allergic to penicillins or those unable to take oral medications and regimens for genitourinary and gastrointestinal procedures are provided (Tables 109–13 and 109–14). One report highlights the need to educate physicians and patients regarding these guidelines because overuse of IE prophylaxis occurs in low-risk patients, and underuse is common in moderate-risk patients.[85]

ABBREVIATIONS

AHA: American Heart Association
BSAC: British Society for Antimicrobial Chemotherapy
IE: infective endocarditis
IVDA: intravenous drug abuse
MBC: minimal bactericidal concentration
MIC: minimal inhibitor concentration
MRSA: methicillin-resistant *S. aureus*
MSSA: methicillin-sensitive *S. aureus*
NBTE: nonbacterial thrombotic endocarditis
PVE: prosthetic valve endocarditis
SBT: serum bactericidal titers
TEE: transesophageal echocardiogram
TTE: transthoracic echocardiogram

Review Questions and other resources can be found at *www.pharmacotherapyonline.com.*

REFERENCES

1. Bayer AS, Scheld WM. Endocarditis and intravascular infections. In: Mandell GL, Bennett JE, Dolin R, eds. Principles and Practice of Infectious Diseases, 5th ed. New York, Churchill-Livingstone, 2000:857–902.
2. Karchmer AW. Infective endocarditis. In: Braunwald E, ed. Heart Disease: A Textbook of Cardiovascular Medicine, 6th ed. Philadelphia, Saunders, 2001:1723–1748.
3. Karchmer AW. Infections of prosthetic valves and intravascular devices. In: Mandell GL, Bennett JE, Dolin R, eds. Principles and Practice of Infectious Diseases, 5th ed. New York, Churchill Livingstone, 2000: 903–917.
4. Bayer AS, Bolger AF, Taubert KA, et al. Diagnosis and management of infective endocarditis and its complications. Circulation 1998;98: 2936–2948.
5. Mylonakis E, Calderwood SB. Infective endocarditis in adults. N Engl J Med 2001;345:1318–1320.
6. Guoello JP, Asfar P, Brenet O. Nosocomial endocarditis in the intensive care unit: An analysis of 22 cases. Crit Care Med 2000;28:377–382.
7. Whitener C, Caputo GM, Weitekamp MR, Karchmer AW. Endocarditis due to coagulase-negative staphylococci: Microbiologic, epidemiologic, and clinical considerations. Infect Dis Clin North Am 1993;7: 81–96.
8. Werner M, Andersson R, Olaison L. A clinical study of culture-negative endocarditis. Medicine 2003;82:263–273.
9. Sachdev M, Peterson GE, Jollis JG. Imaging techniques for diagnosis of infective endocarditis. Cardiol Clin 2003;21:185–195.
10. Kupferwasser LI, Darius H, Mulller AM, et al. Diagnosis of culture-negative endocarditis: The role of the Duke criteria and the impact of transesophageal echocardiography. Am Heart J 2001;142:146–152.
11. Cheitlin MD, Armstrong WF, Aurigemma GP, et al. AHA/ACC/ASE 2003 guideline update for the clinical application of echocardiography. A report of the American College of Cardiology/American Heart Association Task Force on Practice Guidelines. 2003. American College of Cardiology Web site; available at *www.acc.org/clinical/guidelines/echo/index/.pdf.*
12. Mugge A. Echocardiographic detection of cardiac valve vegetations and prognostic implications. Infect Dis Clin North Am 1993;7:877–898.
13. Flachskampf FA, Daniel WG. Role of transoesophageal echocardiography in infective endocarditis. Heart 2000;84:3–4.
14. Durack DT, Lukes AS, Bright DK. New criteria for diagnosis of infective endocarditis: Utilization of specific echocardiographic findings. Am J Med 1994;96:200–209.
15. Li JS, Sexton DJ, Mick N, et al. Proposed modifications to the Duke criteria for the diagnosis of infective endocarditis. Clin Infect Dis 2000;30: 633–638.
16. Gold MJ. Cure rates and long-term prognosis. In: Kaye D, ed. Infective Endocarditis, 2d ed. New York, Raven Press, 1992:455–464.
17. Pokorski RJ. Long-term survival of patients with infective endocarditis. J Insur Med 1998;30:76–87.
18. Tunkel AR, Scheld WM. Experimental models of endocarditis. In: Kaye D, ed. Infectious Endocarditis, 2d ed. New York, Raven Press, 1992: 37–56.
19. Carbon C, Cremieux A-C, Fantin B. Pharmacokinetics and pharmacodynamic aspects of therapy of experimental endocarditis. Infect Dis Clin North Am 1993;7:37–51.
21. Ferguson E, Reardon MJ, Letsou GV. The surgical management of bacterial valvular endocarditis. Curr Opin Cardiol 2000;15:82–85.
22. Wilson WR, Karchmer AW, Dajani AS, et al. Antibiotic treatment of adults with infective endocarditis due to streptococci, enterococci, staphylococci, and HACEK microorganisms. JAMA 1995;274:1706–1713.
23. Simmons NA, Ball AP, Eykyn SJ, et al. Antibiotic treatment of streptococcal, enterococcal, and staphylococcal endocarditis. Heart 1998;79: 207–210.
24. Hoen B. Special issues in the management of infective endocarditis caused by gram-positive cocci. Infect Dis Clin North Am 2002;16:437–452.
25. Levison ME. In vitro assays. In: Kaye D, ed. Infectious Endocarditis, 2d ed. New York, Raven Press, 1992:151–167.
26. Baldassarre JS, Kaye D. Principles and overview of antibiotic therapy. In: Kaye D, ed. Infectious Endocarditis, 2d ed. New York, Raven Press, 1992: 169–190.
27. Francioli PB. Ceftriaxone and outpatient treatment of infective endocarditis. Infect Dis Clin North Am 1993;7:97–116.
28. Shanson DC. New guidelines for the antibiotic treatment of streptococcal, enterococcal and staphylococcal endocarditis. J Antimicrob Chemother 1998;42:292–296.
29. Weiss ME, Adkinson NF. Beta-lactam allergy. In: Mandell GL, Bennett JE, Dolin R, eds. Principles and Practice of Infectious Diseases, 5th ed. New York, Churchill-Livingstone, 2000:299–305.
30. DiNubile MJ. Treatment of endocarditis caused by relatively resistant nonenterococcal streptococci: Is penicillin enough? Rev Infect Dis 1990; 12:112–115.
31. Blatter M, Fluckiger U, Entenza J, et al. Simulated human serum profiles of one daily dose of ceftriaxone plus netilmicin in treatment of experimental streptococcal endocarditis. Antimicrob Agents Chemother 1993;37: 1971–1976.
32. Francioli PB, Glauser MP. Synergistic activity of ceftriaxone combined with netilmicin administered once daily for treatment of experimental

streptococcal endocarditis. Antimicrob Agents Chemother 1993;37: 207–212.

3. Gavalda J, Pahissa A, Almirante B, et al. Effect of gentamicin dosing interval on therapy of viridans streptococcal experimental endocarditis with gentamicin plus penicillin. Antimicrob Agents Chemother 1995;39: 2098–2103.

4. Francioli P, Ruch W, Stamboulian D, et al. Treatment of streptococcal endocarditis with a single daily dose of ceftriaxone and netilmicin for 14 days: A prospective multicenter study. Clin Infect Dis 1995;21: 1406–1410.

5. Sexton DJ, Tenenbaum MJ, Wilson WR, et al. Ceftriaxone once daily for 4 weeks compared to ceftriaxone plus gentamicin once daily for 2 weeks for treatment of penicillin-susceptible streptococcal endocarditis. Clin Infect Dis 1998;27:1470–1474.

6. Karchmer A. Staphylococcal endocarditis. In: Kaye D, ed. Infectious Endocarditis, 2d ed. New York, Raven Press, 1992:225–249.

7. Petti CA, Fowler VG. Staphylococcus aureus bacteremia and endocarditis. Cardiol Clin 2003;21:219–233.

8. Korzeniowski O, Sande MA. The National Collaborative Endocarditis Study Group: Combination antimicrobial therapy for Staphylococcus aureus endocarditis in patients addicted to parenteral drugs and in nonaddicts. Ann Intern Med 1982;97:496–503.

9. Gavalda J, Lopez P, Martin T, et al. Efficacy of ceftriaxone and gentamicin given once a day using human-like pharmacokinetics in treatment of experimental staphylococcal endocarditis. Antimicrob Agents Chemother 2002;46:378–384.

10. Dodek P, Phillip P. Questionable history of immediate-type hypersensitivity to penicillin in staphylococcal endocarditis: Treatment based on skin test results versus empirical alternative treatment—A decision analysis. Clin Infect Dis 1999;29:1251–1256.

11. Miro JM, del Rio A, Mestres CA. Infective endocarditis and cardiac surgery in intravenous drug abusers and HIV-1 infected patients. Cardiol Clin 2003;21:167–184.

12. Chambers HF. Short-course combination and oral therapies of Staphylococcus aureus endocarditis. Med Clin North Am 1993;7:69–80.

13. DiNubile MJ. Abbreviated therapy for right-sided Staphylococcus aureus endocarditis in injection drug users: The time has come? Eur J Clin Microbiol Infect Dis 1994;13:533–534.

14. DiNubile MJ. Short-course antibiotic therapy for right-sided Staphylococcus aureus endocarditis in injection drug users. Ann Intern Med 1994; 121:873–876.

15. Chambers HF, Miller T, Newman MD. Right-sided endocarditis in intravenous drug abusers: Two-week combination therapy. Ann Intern Med 1988;109:619–624.

16. Espinosa FJ, Valdes M, Martin-Luengo M, et al. Right sided endocarditis caused by Staphylococcus aureus in parenteral drug addicts: Evaluation of a combined therapeutic scheme for 2 weeks versus conventional treatment. Enferm Infec Microbiol Clin 1993;11:235–240.

17. Torres-Tortosa M, de Cueto M, Vergara A, et al. Prospective evaluation of a two-week course of intravenous antibiotics in intravenous drug addicts with infective endocarditis. Eur J Clin Microbiol Infect Dis 1994;13: 559–564.

18. Ribera E, Gomez-Jimenez J, Cortes E, et al. Effectiveness of cloxacillin with and without gentamicin in short-term therapy for right-sided Staphylococcus aureus endocarditis: A randomized, controlled trial. Ann Intern Med 1996;125:969–974.

19. Parker RH, Fossieck BE. Intravenous followed by oral antimicrobial therapy for staphylococcal endocarditis. Ann Intern Med 1980;93: 832–834.

50. Dworkin RJ, Lee BL, Sande MA, Chambers HF. Treatment of right-sided Staphylococcus aureus endocarditis in intravenous drug abusers with ciprofloxacin and rifampin. Lancet 1989;2:1071–1073.

51. Heldman AW, Hartert TV, Ray SC, et al. Oral antibiotic treatment of right-sided staphylococcal endocarditis in injection drug users: Prospective, randomized comparison with parenteral therapy. Am J Med 1996;101: 68–76.

52. Berlin JA, Abrutyn E, Strom BL, et al. Incidence of infective endocarditis in the Delaware Valley, 1988–1990. Am J Cardiol 1995;76:933–936.

53. Eliopolis GM. Enterococcal endocarditis. In: Kaye D, ed. Infective Endocarditis, 2d ed. New York, Raven Press, 1992:209–223.

54. Murray BE. The life and times of the enterococcus. Clin Microbiol Rev 1990;3:46–65.

55. Wilson WR, Wilkowske CJ, Wright AJ, et al. Treatment of streptomycin-susceptible and streptomycin resistant enterococcal endocarditis. Ann Intern Med 1984;100:816–823.

56. Eliopolis GM. Aminoglycoside resistant enterococcal endocarditis. Infect Dis Clin North Am 1993;7:117–133.

57. Tam VH, Preston SL, Briceland LL. Once-daily aminoglycosides in the treatment of gram-positive endocarditis. Ann Pharmacother 1999;33: 600–606.

58. Houlihan HH, Stokes DP, Rybak MJ. Pharmacodynamics of vancomycin and ampicillin alone and in combination with gentamicin once daily or thrice daily against Enterococcus faecalis in an in vitro infection model. J Antimicrob Chemother 2000;46:79–86.

59. Gavalda J, Cardona PJ, Almirante B, et al. Treatment of experimental endocarditis due to Enterococcus faecalis using profiles of ampicillin in human serum. Antimicrob Agents Chemother 1996;40: 173–178.

60. Schwank S, Blaser J. Once versus thrice-daily netilmicin combined with amoxicillin, penicillin, or vancomycin against Enterococcus faecalis in a pharmacodynamic in vitro model. Antimicrob Agents Chemother 1996; 40:2258–2261.

61. Fantin B, Carbon C. Importance of the aminoglycoside dosing regimen in the penicillin-netilmicin combination for treatment of Enterococcus faecalis–induced experimental endocarditis. Antimicrob Agents Chemother 1990;34:2387–2391.

62. Marangos MN, Nicolau DP, Quintiliani R, Nightingale CH. Influence of gentamicin dosing interval on the efficacy of penicillin-containing regimens in experimental Enterococcus faecalis endocarditis. J Antimicrob Chemother 1997;39:519–522.

63. Lipman ML, Silva J. Endocarditis due to Streptococcus faecalis with high-level resistance to gentamicin. Rev Infect Dis 1989;11:325–328.

64. Wells VD, Wong ES, Murray BE, et al. Infections due to beta-lactamase-producing, high-level gentamicin-resistant Enterococcus faecalis. Ann Intern Med 1992;116:285–292.

65. Tailor SA, Bailey EM, Rybak MJ. Enterococcus: An emerging pathogen. Ann Pharmacother 1993;27:1231–1242.

66. Hessen MT, Abrutyn E. Gram-negative bacterial endocarditis. In: Kaye D, ed. Infective Endocarditis, 2d ed. New York, Raven Press, 1992: 251–264.

67. Tunkel AR, Kaye D. Endocarditis with negative blood cultures. N Engl J Med 1992;326:1215–1217.

68. Reyes MP, Lerner AM. Current problems in the treatment of infective endocarditis due to Pseudomonas aeruginosa. Rev Infect Dis 1983;5: 314–321.

69. Moyer DV, Edwards JE. Fungal endocarditis. In: Kaye D, ed. Infective Endocarditis, 2d ed. New York, Raven Press, 1992:299–312.

70. Pierrotti LC, Baddour LM. Fungal endocarditis, 1995–2000. Chest 2002; 122:302–310.

71. Rehm SJ. Outpatient intravenous antibiotic therapy for endocarditis. Infect Dis Clin North Am 1998;12:879–901.

72. Santoro J, Ingerman M. Response to therapy: Relapse and reinfections. In: Kaye D, ed. Infective Endocarditis, 2d ed. New York, Raven Press, 1992:423–433.

73. Levinson ME. In vitro assays. In: Kaye D, ed. Infective Endocarditis, 2d ed. New York, Raven Press, 1992:151–167.

74. Weinstein MP, Stratton CW, Ackley A, et al. Multicenter collaborative evaluation of a standardized serum bactericidal test as a prognostic indicator in infective endocarditis. Am J Med 1985;78:262–269.

75. McCormack JP, Jewesson PJ. A critical reevaluation of the "therapeutic range" of aminoglycosides. Clin Infect Dis 1992;14:320–339.

76. Durack DT. Prophylaxis of infective endocarditis. In: Mandell GL, Bennett JE, Dolin R, eds. Principles and Practice of Infectious Diseases, 5th ed. New York, Churchill-Livingstone, 2000:917–925.

77. Durack DT. Prevention of infective endocarditis. N Engl J Med 1995; 332:38–44.

78. Dajani AS, Taubert KA, Wilson W, et al. Prevention of bacterial endocarditis: Recommendations by the American Heart Association. JAMA 1997; 277:1794–1801.

79. Roberts GJ. Dentist are innocent! "Everyday" bacteremia is real culprit: A review and assessment of the evidence that dental surgical procedures are a principal cause of bacterial endocarditis. Pediatr Cardiol 1999;20: 317–325.

80. Greenman RL, Bisno AL. Prevention of bacterial endocarditis. In: Kaye D, ed. Infective Endocarditis, 2d ed. New York, Raven Press, 1992:465–481.

81. Hall G, Hedstrom SA, Heimdahl A, Nord CE. Prophylactic administration of penicillins for endocarditis does not reduce the incidence of postextraction bacteremia. Clin Infect Dis 1993;17:188–194.

82. Van der Meer JT, Van Wijk W, Thompson J, et al. Efficacy of antibiotic prophylaxis for prevention of native-valve endocarditis. Lancet 1992; 339:135–139.

83. Strom BL, Abrutym E, Berlin JA, et al. Risk factors for infective endocarditis: oral hygiene and nondental exposures. Circulation 2000;102: 2842–2848.

84. Strom BL, Abrutyne E, Berlin JA, et al. Dental and cardiac risk factors for infective endocarditis: A population-based, case-control study. Ann Intern Med 1998;129:761–769.

85. Seto TB, Kwiat D, Taira DA, et al. Physicians' recommendations to patients for use of antibiotic prophylaxis to prevent endocarditis. JAMA 2000;284:68–71.

110

TUBERCULOSIS

Charles A. Peloquin

Learning Objectives and other resources can be found at www.pharmacotherapyonline.com.

KEY CONCEPTS

1 Tuberculosis (TB) is the most prevalent communicable infectious disease on earth and remains out of control in many developing nations. These nations require medical and financial assistance from developed nations in order to control the spread of TB globally.

2 In the United States, TB disproportionately affects ethnic minorities as compared with whites, reflecting greater ongoing transmission in ethnic minority communities. Additional TB surveillance and preventive treatment are required within these communities.

3 Coinfection with human immunodeficiency virus (HIV) and TB accelerates the progression of both diseases, thus requiring rapid diagnosis and treatment of both diseases.

4 Mycobacteria are slow growing organisms; in the laboratory, they require special stains, special growth media, and long periods of incubation to isolate and identify.

5 TB can produce atypical signs and symptoms in infants,

the elderly, and immunocompromised hosts, and it can progress rapidly in these patients.

6 Latent TB infection (LTBI) can lead to reactivation disease years after the primary infection occurred.

7 The patient suspected of having active TB disease must be isolated until the diagnosis is confirmed and he or she is no longer contagious. Often, isolation takes place in specialized "negative pressure" hospital rooms to prevent the spread of TB.

8 Isoniazid and rifampin are the two most important TB drugs; organisms resistant to both these drugs (multidrug-resistant TB [MDR-TB]) are much more difficult to treat.

9 *Never add a single drug to a failing regimen!*

10 Directly observed treatment (DOT) should be used whenever possible to reduce treatment failures and the selection of drug-resistant isolates.

1 Tuberculosis (TB) remains a leading infectious killer globally. TB is caused by *Mycobacterium tuberculosis*, which can produce either a silent, latent infection or a progressive, active disease.[1] Left untreated or improperly treated, TB causes progressive tissue destruction and eventually death. Because of renewed public health efforts, TB rates in the United States continue to decline. In contrast, TB remains out of control in many developing countries—to the point that one-third of the world's population currently is infected.[1] Estimates suggest that 1 person dies of TB in India each minute (*Times of India*, August 29, 2003). Given increasing drug resistance, it is critical that a major effort be made to control TB before the most effective drugs are lost permanently.

M. tuberculosis preferentially infects humans, and the closely related *M. bovis* causes a similar disease in cattle and other livestock. Although uncommon today, humans frequently developed TB by drinking milk contaminated with *M. bovis*—a threat that spurred the development of pasteurization. Today, airborne *M. tuberculosis* is the main threat to humans.

Evidence of TB has been found in ancient human remains, and ancient texts describe it.[1-3] TB commonly was known as "consumption" because of the pronounced weight loss that it caused.[1] Other common names included "wasting disease" and the "white plague." As the term *plague* implies, TB had a profound impact on human

history, most notably in Europe. (*Note:* The "black plague," or bubonic plague, is a separate disease caused by *Yersinia pestis*.)

TB rates generally have risen with increasing urbanization and overcrowding because it is easier for an airborne disease to spread when people are packed closely together.[3] Hence TB became a significant pathogen in Europe during the Middle Ages and peaked during the Industrial Revolution, when it caused about 25% of all deaths in Europe and in the United States.[1-3] This dire threat led to the rise of public health departments and to procedures such as the isolation of infected patients. Thus TB was directly responsible for many of the health care practices that we take for granted today. Unfortunately, in developing nations, some of these practices are not widely available, and TB continues to rage unabated.

EPIDEMIOLOGY

Globally, roughly 2 billion people are infected by *M. tuberculosis*, and roughly 2 to 3 million people die from active TB each year despite the fact that it is curable.[1,2,4] In the United States, about 13 million people are latently infected with *M. tuberculosis*, meaning that they are not currently sick but that they could fall ill with TB at any time. The United States had over 15,000 new cases of active

2015

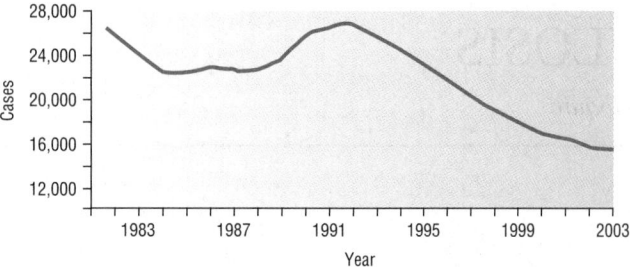

FIGURE 110–1. Reported TB cases in the United States, 1982–2003.

TB in 2002 and about 1500 deaths.[5] (For detailed data analysis, visit the Centers for Disease Control and Prevention (CDC) Web site at *www.cdc.gov/nchstp/tb.*)

The annual incidence of TB in the United States declined by about 5% per year from 1953 to 1983[6] (Fig. 110–1). In 1984, this decline slowed, and then the incidence of TB rose from 1988 to 1992, reaching 10.5 cases per 100,000 population. Since 1992, more effective infection control practices and treatment protocols have reduced TB rates to 5.2 per 100,000 population as of 2002.[5] Despite this good news, the eradication of TB from the United States will remain very difficult. One reason is that we continue to import new cases from countries where TB remains out of control.[4,5]

RISK FACTORS FOR INFECTION

LOCATION AND PLACE OF BIRTH

TB can infect anyone, but the risk is not evenly distributed across the U.S. population. The major points of entry into the United States have the most TB cases. California, Florida, Illinois, New York, and Texas accounted for over 50% of all TB cases in 2002.[5] Within these states, TB is most prevalent in large urban areas.[4]

The percentage of foreign-born TB patients in the United States has increased annually since 1986, reaching 51% in 2002.[5] Nearly two-thirds of these patients came from only seven countries, in order of highest to lowest: Mexico, the Philippines, Vietnam, India, China, Haiti, and South Korea.[5] Therefore, health care workers must "think TB" when caring for patients from these countries who experience symptoms such as cough, fever, and weight loss.

Close contacts of pulmonary TB patients are most likely to become infected.[2-4] These include family members, coworkers, or coresidents in places such as prisons, shelters, or nursing homes. The more prolonged the contact, the greater is the risk, with infection rates as high as 30%.[5,6] Although many circumstances exist, TB patients frequently have limited access to health care, live in crowded conditions, or are homeless.[2,4] Many patients have histories of alcohol abuse or illicit drug use, and many are coinfected with hepatitis B or human immunodeficiency virus (HIV). These concurrent social and health problems make treating some TB patients particularly difficult.

RACE, ETHNICITY, AGE, AND GENDER

In the United States, TB disproportionately affects ethnic minorities. In 2002, non-Hispanic blacks accounted for 30% of all TB cases, followed by Hispanics at 27%.[6] Asians and Pacific Islanders accounted for 22%, whereas non-Hispanic whites accounted for only 20% of the new TB cases.[6]

TB is most common among people 25 to 44 years of age (35% of all U.S. cases in 2002).[6] They are followed by those 45 to 64 years of age (28%) and 65+ years of age (21%). TB is more common in older whites and Asians compared with younger people from these groups. This reflects reactivation of latent infection acquired many years earlier when TB was very common. Older blacks and Hispanics also have more TB than younger folks, but the differences by age are not as pronounced.[6] This reflects a greater amount of recent transmission among younger blacks and Hispanics compared with younger whites and Asians. Until the age of 15, TB rates are similar for males and females, but after that, the male predominance increases with each decade of life.[6]

COINFECTION WITH HUMAN IMMUNODEFICIENCY VIRUS (HIV)

HIV is the most important risk factor for active TB, especially among people 25 to 44 years of age.[2,4,6,7] TB and HIV seem to act synergistically within patients and across populations, making each disease worse than it might otherwise be. Roughly 10% of U.S. TB patients are coinfected with HIV, and roughly 20% of TB patients ages 25 to 44 years are coinfected.[5,6] HIV coinfection may not increase the risk of acquiring *M. tuberculosis* infection, but it does increase the likelihood of progression to active disease.[1,7] Further, TB and HIV patients share a number of behavioral risk factors that contribute to the high rates of coinfection.[2,8,9]

RISK FACTORS FOR DISEASE

Once infected with *M. tuberculosis*, a person's lifetime risk of active TB is about 10%.[2,4,7] The greatest risk for active disease occurs during the first 2 years after infection. Children younger than 2 years and adults over 65 years of age have 2 to 5 times greater risk for active disease compared with other age groups. Patients with underlying immune suppression (e.g., renal failure, cancer, and immunosuppressive drug treatment) have 4 to 16 times greater risk than other patients. Finally, HIV-infected patients with *M. tuberculosis* infection are 100 times more likely to develop active TB than normal hosts.[4,10] HIV-infected patients have an annual risk of active TB of about 10% rather than a lifetime risk at that rate. Therefore, all patients with HIV infection should be screened for tuberculous infection, and those known to be infected with *M. tuberculosis* should be tested for HIV infection.

ETIOLOGY

M. tuberculosis is a slender bacillus with a very waxy outer layer.[2,7] It is 1 to 4 microns in length, and under the microscope, it is either straight or slightly curved in shape.[1,11,12] It does not stain well with Gram's stain, so the Ziehl-Neelsen stain (ZN) or the fluorochrome stain must be used instead.[1,2,7] After ZN staining with carbol-fuchsin, mycobacteria retain the red color despite acid-alcohol washes. Hence they are called *acid-fast bacilli* (AFB).[11] After staining, microscopic examination ("smear") detects about 8000 to 10,000 organisms per milliliter of specimen, so a patient can be "smear negative" but still grow *M. tuberculosis* on culture. Microscopic examination also cannot determine which of the 80+ mycobacterial species is present or whether the organisms in the original samples were alive or dead.[1,11,12] On smear, they are all dead. On culture, *M. tuberculosis* grows slowly, doubling about every 20 hours. This is very slow compared with gram-positive and gram-negative bacteria, which double about every 30 minutes.

Among the mycobacteria, only *M. tuberculosis* is a frequent human pathogen. Some nontuberculous mycobacteria (NTM) such as *M. kansasii, M. fortuitum,* and *M. avium* complex (MAC) cause nfections in patients with other medical problems, especially the acquired immunodeficiency syndrome (AIDS). The treatment of these infections is discussed in Chap. 123.

CULTURE AND SUSCEPTIBILITY TESTING

◄ Direct susceptibility testing involves inoculating specialized media with organisms taken directly from a concentrated, smear-positive specimen.[1,11,12] This approach produces susceptibility results in 2 to 3 weeks. Indirect susceptibility testing involves inoculating the test media with organisms obtained from a pure culture of the organisms, which can take several more weeks. The most common agar method, known as the *proportion method,* uses the ratio of colony counts on drug-containing agar to that on drug-free agar.[1,12] In the United States, the critical proportion for resistance is 1%. That means that if a drug-containing plate shows only 2% of the growth seen on a drug-free plate, some of the organisms from the specimen were resistant to that drug. Therefore, it is likely that many of the organisms in the patient also are resistant to that drug, and it should not be used to treat that patient.

The proportion method's limitations include many weeks to obtain results, drug degradation during the incubation, and a qualitative result (susceptible or resistant). The Bactec system (Becton-Dickinson, Sparks, MD) uses liquid medium (7H12 broth) and detects live mycobacteria based on the release of radiolabeled CO_2.[11] Advantages of the Bactec system include reduced incubation time (as few as 9 to 14 days), reduced drug loss in the medium, and when multiple concentrations are tested, a truly quantitative end point (minimal inhibitory concentration [MIC]).[1,11,12] Newer, nonradiometric rapid methods such as the MIGIT system are now being marketed.[13]

Rapid-identification tests are now available.[13] Nucleic acid probes such as the AccuProbe (Gen-Probe, San Diego) use DNA probes to identify the presence of complementary rRNA for several mycobacterial species.[7,11,14] DNA fingerprinting using restriction-fragment-length polymorphism (RFLP) analysis has been used to identify clusters of cases.[1,11,14] Amplification of the genetic material can be achieved through polymerase chain reaction (PCR; Roche Molecular Systems, Branchburg, NJ), the amplified *M. tuberculosis* direct test (MTD; Gen-Probe), and strand-displacement amplification (SDA; Becton-Dickinson, Sparks, MD).[11,15] Thin-layer chromatography (TLC), high-performance liquid chromatography (HPLC) for mycolic acid identification, and gas chromatography (GC) for short-chain fatty acids (methyl esters) have been used to speciate mycobacterial isolates.[1,11,14] Other tests are designed to detect common genetic changes associated with drug resistance, such as changes in the *katG* gene associated with isoniazid resistance and the *rpoB* gene associated with rifampin resistance.[7,16–18] These tests offer clinicians a chance to know rapidly what organism they are treating and what drugs might be good initial choices.

TRANSMISSION

M. tuberculosis is transmitted from person-to-person by coughing or sneezing.[2,7,13] This produces "droplet nuclei" that are dispersed in the air. Each droplet nuclei contains one to three organisms. Riley and colleagues[19] showed that air circulated from a hospital TB ward could cause disease in guinea pigs. When this air was filtered or treated with ultraviolet radiation, the animals were not infected. About 30% of individuals who experience prolonged contact with an infectious TB patient will become infected.

A person with cavitary, pulmonary TB and a cough may infect roughly one person per month until he or she is treated effectively,

although this number can vary significantly. A person with the uncommon laryngeal form of TB can spread organisms even when talking, so the transmission rates can be very high. HIV-infected patients acquire the organisms through the lungs just like normal hosts, but their weakened immune system puts them at very high risk for active disease.[2,4,7,13]

PATHOPHYSIOLOGY

IMMUNE RESPONSE

Good T-lymphocyte responses are essential to controlling *M. tuberculosis* infections.[2,7,20,21] In the mouse model, two different T-cell responses—the type 1 T-helper (TH_1) response and the type 2 T-helper (TH_2) response—have been described. The TH_1 response is the preferred response to TB, and the TH_2 response, including the potentially subversive influence of interleukin 4 (IL-4), is undesirable.[2,20,21] Some workers have argued that this dichotomy is clearer in the mouse model, and in many humans, the T-cell response may be classified as TH_0 (elements of both TH_1 and TH_2).[20] In either case, T-lymphocytes activate macrophages that, in turn, engulf and kill mycobacteria. T-lymphocytes also destroy immature macrophages that harbor *M. tuberculosis* but are unable to kill the invaders.[20,21] CD4+ cells are the primary T cells involved, with contributions by gamma-delta T cells and CD8+ T cells.[20] CD4+ T cells produce interferon-γ (IFN-γ) and other cytokines, including IL-2 and IL-10, that coordinate the immune response to TB.[20] Because CD4+ cells are depleted in HIV-infected patients, these patients are unable to mount an adequate defense to TB.[20,21]

Although B-cell responses and antibody production can be demonstrated in TB-infected mammals, these humoral responses do not appear to contribute much to the control of TB within the host.[2,7,20] T cells are responding to certain mycobacterial antigens, but the key antigen(s) invoking the immune response have not been identified.[20] Tumor necrosis factor (TNF-α) and IFN-γ important cytokines involved in coordinating the host's cell-mediated response. Rheumatoid arthritis patients treated with TNF-α inhibitors (infliximab) have high rates of reactivation TB.[22] Therefore, patients known to be deficient in the activity of TNF-α or IFN-γ should be screened for TB infection and offered appropriate treatment.

M. tuberculosis has several ways of evading or resisting the host immune response.[20,21] In particular, *M. tuberculosis* can inhibit the fusion of lysosomes to phagosomes inside macrophages. This prevents the destructive enzymes found in the lysosomes from getting to the bacilli captured in the phagosomes. This stay of execution allows time for *M. tuberculosis* to escape into the cytoplasm. Virulent *M. tuberculosis* are able to multiply in the macrophage cytoplasm, thus perpetuating their spread. Finally, lipoarabinomannan (LAM), the principal structural polysaccharide of the mycobacterial cell wall, inhibits the host immune response.[20,21] LAM induces immunosuppressive cytokines, thus blocking macrophage activation, and LAM scavenges O_2, thus preventing attack by superoxide anions, hydrogen peroxide, singlet oxygen, and hydroxyl radicals.[20,21] These survival mechanisms make *M. tuberculosis* a particularly difficult organism to control. Any defects in the host immune system make it likely that *M. tuberculosis* will not be controlled and that active disease will ensue.

PRIMARY INFECTION

Primary infection usually results from inhaling airborne particles that contain *M. tuberculosis*.[2,7,21] These particles, called *droplet nuclei,* contain one to three bacilli and are small enough (1 to 5 mm) to reach the alveolar surface. Ingestion (swallowing) and inoculation (puncture wound) are other rare pathways to acquire *M. tuberculosis* infection.[21]

The progression to clinical disease depends on three factors: (1) the number of *M. tuberculosis* organisms inhaled (infecting dose), (2) the virulence of these organisms, and (3) the host's cell-mediated immune response.[2,5,7,13,21,23] At the alveolar surface, the bacilli that were delivered by the droplet nuclei are ingested by pulmonary macrophages.[21] If these macrophages inhibit or kill the bacilli, infection is aborted.[21] If the macrophages cannot do this, the organisms continue to multiply. The macrophages eventually rupture, releasing many bacilli, and these mycobacteria are then phagocytized by other macrophages. This cycle continues over several weeks until the host is able to mount a more coordinated response.[21] During this early phase of infection, *M. tuberculosis* multiplies logarithmically.[21]

Some of the intracellular organisms are transported by the macrophages to regional lymph nodes in the hilar, mediastinal, and retroperitoneal areas. The cycle of phagocytosis and cell rupture continues. During lymph node involvement, the mycobacteria may be held in check. More frequently, *M. tuberculosis* spreads throughout the body through the bloodstream.[2,7,21] When this intravascular dissemination occurs, *M. tuberculosis* can infect any tissue or organ in the body. Most commonly, *M. tuberculosis* infects the posterior apical region of the lungs. This may be so because of the high oxygen content, and it may be due to a less-vigorous immune response in this area.

After about 3 weeks of infection, T-lymphocytes are presented with *M. tuberculosis* antigens. These T cells become activated and begin to secrete IFN-γ and the other cytokines noted earlier. The processes described in the immune response section earlier then begin to occur. First, T-lymphocytes stimulate macrophages to become bactericidal.[21] Large numbers of activated microbicidal macrophages surround the solid caseous (cheeselike) tuberculous foci (the necrotic area of infection).[21] This process of creating activated microbicidal macrophages is known as *cell-mediated immunity* (CMI).[21]

At the same time that CMI occurs, delayed-type hypersensitivity (DTH) also develops through the activation and multiplication of T-lymphocytes. DTH refers to the cytotoxic immune process that kills nonactivated immature macrophages that are permitting intracellular bacillary replication.[21] These immature macrophages are killed when the T-lymphocytes initiate Fas-mediated apoptosis (programmed cell death).[21] The bacilli released from the immature macrophages then are killed by the activated macrophages.[21]

By this time (>3 weeks), macrophages have begun to form granulomas to contain the organisms. In a typical tuberculous granuloma, activated macrophages accumulate around a caseous lesion and prevent its further extension.[21] At this point, the infection is largely under control, and bacillary replication falls off dramatically. Depending on the inflammatory response, tissue necrosis and calcification of the infection site plus the regional lymph nodes may occur.

Over 1 to 3 months, activated lymphocytes reach an adequate number, and tissue hypersensitivity results. This is shown by a positive tuberculin skin test. Any remaining mycobacteria are believed to reside primarily within granulomas or within macrophages that have avoided detection and lysis, although some residual bacilli have been found in various types of cells.[2,7,20]

Approximately 90% of infected patients have no further clinical manifestations. Most patients only show a positive skin test (70%), whereas some also have radiographic evidence of stable granulomas (about 20%). This radiodense area on chest x-ray is called a *Ghon complex*. About 5% of patients (usually children, the elderly, or the immunocompromised) experience "progressive primary" disease that occurs before skin test conversion.[24,25] This presents as a progressive pneumonia, usually in the lower lobes. Disease frequently spreads, leading to meningitis and other severe forms of TB.[24,25] Because of this risk of severe disease, very young, elderly, and immunocompromised patients, including those with HIV, should be evaluated and treated for latent or active TB.

REACTIVATION DISEASE

❻ Roughly 10% of infected patients develop reactivation disease at some point in their lives. Nearly half of these cases occur within 2 years of infection.[2,7,13] In the United States, most cases of TB are believed to result from reactivation. Reinfection is uncommon in the United States because of the low rate of exposure and because previously sensitized individuals possess some degree of immunity to reinfection.[2,21] Exceptions include patients coinfected with HIV who live in areas of higher exposure to *M. tuberculosis*.

The apices of the lungs are the most common sites for reactivation (85% of cases).[2] This reflects the fact that *M. tuberculosis* prefers areas with high oxygen content and possibly because the immune response may not be as effective in this region.[2,21] For reasons that are not entirely known (waning cellular immunity, loss of specific T-cell clones, blocking antibody), organisms within granulomas emerge and begin multiplying extracellularly.[24] The inflammatory response produces caseating granulomas, which eventually will liquefy and spread locally, leading to the formation of a hole (cavity) in the lungs.

The immune response contributes to the severity of the lung damage. There is targeted killing of immature macrophages that are allowing mycobacterial multiplication (DTH).[20,21] In addition, there is "innocent bystander" killing of host cells and locally thrombosed blood vessels.[21] The killing of mycobacteria, macrophages, and neutrophils that have entered the battle releases cytokines and lysozymes into the infectious foci. This toxic mixture can be too much for the surrounding alveoli and airway cells, causing regional necrosis and structural collapse.[2,21] These unstable foci liquefy, spreading the infection to neighboring areas of the lung, creating a cavity. Some of this necrotic material is coughed out, producing droplet nuclei. Bacterial counts in the cavities can be as high as 10^8 per milliliter of cavitary fluid. Partial healing may result from fibrosis, but these lesions remain unstable and may continue to expand.[2,21] If left untreated, pulmonary TB continues to destroy the lungs, resulting in hypoxia, respiratory acidosis, and eventually death.

EXTRAPULMONARY AND MILIARY TUBERCULOSIS

Caseating granulomas at extrapulmonary sites can undergo liquefaction, releasing tubercle bacilli and causing symptomatic disease.[2,7] Extrapulmonary TB without concurrent pulmonary disease is uncommon in normal hosts but more common in HIV-infected patients. Because of these unusual presentations, the diagnosis of TB is difficult and often delayed in immunocompromised hosts.[2,4,7] Lymphatic and pleural diseases are the most common forms of extrapulmonary TB, followed by bone, joint, genitourinary, meningeal, and other forms.[2,7] Left untreated, these forms will spread to other organs and may result in death.

Occasionally, a massive inoculum of organisms enters the bloodstream, causing a widely disseminated form of the disease known as *miliary TB*. It is named for the millet seed appearance of the small granulomas seen on chest radiographs, and it can be rapidly fatal.[20] Miliary TB is a medical emergency requiring immediate treatment.

INFLUENCE OF HIV INFECTION ON PATHOGENESIS

HIV infection is the largest risk factor for active TB.[2,7,20] As CD4+ lymphocytes multiply in response to the mycobacterial infection, HIV multiplies within these cells and selectively destroys them. In turn, the TB-fighting lymphocytes are depleted.[20] This vicious cycle puts HIV-infected patients at 100 times the risk of active TB compared with HIV-negative people.[25] In addition, the combination of HIV infection and certain social behaviors increases the risk of newly acquired TB. In selected areas of the United States, up to 50% of new TB cases are the result of recent infection, particularly among HIV-infected individuals.[26–28]

While mycobacteria are spreading throughout the body, HIV replication accelerates in lymphocytes and macrophages. This leads to progression of HIV disease.[20,29] HIV-infected patients infected with TB deteriorate more rapidly unless they receive antimycobacterial chemotherapy.[30,31] Most clinicians elect to begin TB treatment first, and once this is under control, begin HIV treatment as well. Starting both treatments at the same time can lead to paradoxical worsening of the TB.[13,32] This appears to result from a reinvigorated inflammatory response to TB. Because TB can be very dangerous in HIV-positive patients, they should be screened for tuberculous infection or disease soon after they are shown to be HIV-positive.[2,4,7,20]

CLINICAL PRESENTATION

The classical presentation of TB is shown below. The onset of TB may be gradual, and the diagnosis may not be considered until a chest radiograph is performed. Unfortunately, many patients do not seek medical attention until more dramatic symptoms, such as frank hemoptysis, occur. At this point, patients typically have large cavitary lesions in the lungs. These cavities are loaded with *M. tuberculosis*. Expectoration or swallowing of infected sputum may spread the disease to other areas of the body.[1,2,7,23] Physical examination is nonspecific but suggestive of progressive pulmonary disease.

CLINICAL PRESENTATION OF TUBERCULOSIS

SIGNS AND SYMPTOMS

- Patients typically present with weight loss, fatigue, a productive cough, fever, and night sweats[1,2,7,23]
- Frank hemoptysis

PHYSICAL EXAMINATION

- Dullness to chest percussion, rales, and increased vocal fremitus are observed frequently on auscultation

LABORATORY TESTS

- Moderate elevations in the white blood cell (WBC) count with a lymphocyte predominance

CHEST RADIOGRAPH

- Patchy or nodular infiltrates in the apical areas of the upper lobes or the superior segment of the lower lobes[2,7,23]
- Cavitation that may show air-fluid levels as the infection progresses

Patients coinfected with HIV may have atypical presentations.[1,2,7,23,33] As their CD4+ counts decline, HIV-positive patients are less likely to have positive skin tests, cavitary lesions, or fever. Pulmonary radiographic findings may be minimal or absent. HIV-positive patients have a higher incidence of extrapulmonary TB and are more likely to present with progressive primary disease. Because their symptoms are not specific to TB, a thorough work-up for TB is essential.[2,7,20,23]

Extrapulmonary TB typically presents as a slowly progressive decline in organ function.[2,7,23] Patients may have low-grade fever and other constitutional symptoms. Patients with genitourinary TB may present with sterile pyuria and hematuria. Lymphadenitis often involves the cervical and supraclavicular nodes and may appear as a neck mass with spontaneous drainage. Tuberculous arthritis and osteomyelitis occur most commonly in the elderly and usually affect the lower spine and weight-bearing joints. TB of the spine is known as *Pott's disease*.[2] Abnormal behavior, headaches, or convulsions suggest tuberculous meningitis. Involvement of the peritoneum, pericardium, larynx, and adrenal glands also occurs.[2,7,23]

THE ELDERLY

TB in the elderly is easily confused with other respiratory diseases. Many clinical findings are muted or absent altogether. Compared with younger patients, TB in the elderly is far less likely to present with positive skin tests, fevers, night sweats, sputum production, or hemoptysis.[2,23,34,35] Weight loss may occur but is nonspecific. In contrast, mental status changes are twice as common in the elderly, and mortality is six times higher.[2,23,34] TB is a preventable cause of death in the elderly that should not be overlooked.

CHILDREN

TB in children, especially those younger than 12 years of age, may present as a typical bacterial pneumonia and is called *progressive primary TB*.[23–25] Clinical disease often begins 1 to 2 months after exposure and precedes skin-test positivity. Unlike adults, pulmonary TB in children often involves the lower and middle lobes.[23–25] Dissemination to the lymph nodes, gastrointestinal and genitourinary tracts, bone marrow, and meninges is fairly common. Because of delays in recruitment of cellular immunity, cavitary disease is infrequent, and the number of organisms present typically is smaller than in an adult. Because cavitary lesions are uncommon, children do not spread TB readily. However, TB can be rapidly fatal in a child, and it requires prompt chemotherapy.

DIAGNOSIS

SKIN TESTING

The key to stopping the spread of TB is early identification of infected individuals.[1,2,7,23] Populations most likely to benefit from skin testing are listed in Table 110–1 (column 1 patients are at highest risk for TB, followed by those in column 2). Members of these high-risk groups should be tested for TB infection and educated about the disease.

The Mantoux test is the preferred TB skin test. It uses tuberculin purified protein derivative (PPD), and unlike the Heaf or tine test, the Mantoux test is quantitative. The standard 5 tuberculin unit PPD dose is placed intracutaneously on the volar aspect of the forearm with a 26- or 27-gauge needle.[2,23,30] This injection should produce a small, raised, blanched wheal. An experienced professional should

TABLE 110–1. Criteria for Tuberculin Positivity, by Risk Group

Reaction ≥5 mm of Induration	Reaction ≥10 mm of Induration	Reaction ≥15 mm of Induration
Human immunodeficiency virus (HIV)-positive persons	Recent immigrants (i.e., within the last 5 yr) from high prevalence countries	Persons with no risk factors for TB
Recent contacts of tuberculosis (TB) case patients	Injection drug users	
Fibrotic changes on chest radiograph consistent with prior TB	Residents and employees[b] of the following high-risk congregate settings: prisons and jails, nursing homes and other long-term facilities for the elderly, hospitals and other health care facilities, residential facilities for patients with acquired immunodeficiency syndrome (AIDS), and homeless shelters	
Patients with organ transplants and other immunosuppressed patients (receiving the equivalent of ≥15 mg/d of prednisone for 1 mo or more)[a]	Mycobacteriology laboratory personnel	
	Persons with the following clinical conditions that place them at high risk: silicosis, diabetes mellitus, chronic renal failure, some hematologic disorders (e.g., leukemias and lymphomas), other specific malignancies (e.g., carcinoma of the head or neck and lung), weight loss of ≥10% of ideal body weight, gastrectomy, and jejunoileal bypass	
	Children younger than 4 yr of age or infants, children, and adolescents exposed to adults at high-risk	

[a]Risk of TB in patients treated with corticosteroids increases with higher dose and longer duration.
[b]For persons who are otherwise at low risk and are tested at the start of employment, a reaction of ≥15 mm induration is considered positive.
Adapted from Centers for Disease Control and Prevention. Screening for tuberculosis and tuberculosis infection in high-risk populations: recommendations of the Advisory Council for the Elimination of Tuberculosis. MMWR 1995;44(No. RR-11):19–34.

read the test in 48 to 72 hours. The area of induration (the "bump") is the important end point, not the area of redness. Criteria for interpretation are listed in Table 110–1.[1,2,7,23,30] The CDC does not recommend the routine use of anergy panels.[30,36] Aplisol and Tubersol 5 tuberculin unit products are available commercially, but because of more predictable results, Tubersol appears to be the preferred product.

The "booster effect" occurs in patients who do not respond to an initial skin test but show a positive reaction if retested about a week later.[23,36] Patients with past *M. tuberculosis* infection and some patients with past immunization with bacillus Calmette-Guérin (BCG) vaccine or past infection with other mycobacteria may "boost" with a second skin test. Individuals who require periodic skin testing, such as health care workers, should receive a two-stage test initially.[23,36,37] Once they are shown to be skin-test–negative, any positive skin test later shows recent infection, and this requires treatment.

The PPD skin test is an imperfect diagnostic tool. Up to 20% of patients with active TB are falsely skin-test–negative presumably because their immune systems are overwhelmed.[20,36] False-positive results are more common in low-risk patients and those recently vaccinated with BCG. Despite BCG vaccination, one should not ignore a positive PPD result. These patients require careful evaluation for active disease, and they may be offered preventive treatment because many come from areas where TB infection is common.

ADDITIONAL TESTS

When active TB is suspected, attempts should be made to isolate *M. tuberculosis* from the site of infection.[2,7,23,36] Sputum collected in the morning usually has the highest yield.[2,11,23] Daily sputum collections over three consecutive days is recommended.

For patients unable to expectorate, sputum induction with aerosolized hypertonic saline may produce a diagnostic sample. Bronchoscopy, or aspiration of gastric fluid via a nasogastric tube, may be attempted in selected patients.[23] For patients with suspected extrapulmonary TB, samples of draining fluid, biopsies of the infected site, or both may be attempted. Blood cultures are positive occasionally, especially in AIDS patients.[23,33,38]

▶ TREATMENT: Tuberculosis

The desired outcomes for the treatment of tuberculosis are

1. Rapid identification of a new TB case
2. Isolation of the patient with active disease to prevent spread of the disease
3. Collection of appropriate samples for smears and cultures
4. Initiation of specific antituberculosis treatment
5. Prompt resolution of the signs and symptoms of disease
6. Achievement of a noninfectious state in the patient, thus ending isolation
7. Adherence to the treatment regimen by the patient
8. Cure of the patient as quickly as possible (generally at least 6 months of treatment)

Secondary goals are identification of the index case that infected the patient, identification of all persons infected by both the index case and the new case of TB, and completion of appropriate treatments for those individuals.

GENERAL APPROACHES TO TREATMENT

Drug treatment is the cornerstone of TB management.[2,7,13,39] Monotherapy can be used only for infected patients who do not have active TB (latent infection, as shown by a positive skin test). Once active disease is present, a minimum of two drugs and generally three or four drugs must be used simultaneously.[2,7,13,39] The duration of treatment depends on the condition of the host, extent of disease, presence of drug resistance, and tolerance of medications. The shortest duration of treatment generally is 6 months, and 2 to 3 years of treatment may be necessary for cases of multidrug-resistant TB (MDR-TB).[2,7,13,39] Because the duration of treatment is so long, and because many patients feel better after a few weeks of treatment, careful follow-up is required. Directly observed therapy (DOT) by a health care worker is a cost-effective way to ensure completion of treatment.[2,7,13,39–41]

PRINCIPLES FOR TREATING INFECTION AND TREATING DISEASE

Asymptomatic patients with tuberculous infection have a bacillary load of about 10^3 organisms, compared with 10^{11} organisms in a patient with cavitary pulmonary TB.[2,7,42] As the number of organisms increases, the likelihood of naturally occurring drug-resistant mutants also increases. Naturally occurring mutants are found at rates of 1 in 10^6 to 1 in 10^8 organisms for the antituberculosis drugs.[2,39,42] When treating asymptomatic latent infection with isoniazid monotherapy, the risk of selecting out isoniazid-resistant organisms is low. The isoniazid mutation rate is about 1 in 10^6, but only about 10^3 organisms are present in the body. In contrast, the risk of selecting out isoniazid-resistant organisms is unacceptably high in patients with cavitary TB. One can prevent selection of these resistant mutants by adding more drugs because the rates for resistance mutations to multiple drugs are additive functions of the individual rates. For example, only 1 in 10^{13} organisms would be naturally resistant to both isoniazid (1 in 10^6) and rifampin (1 in 10^7).[2,39,42] It is unlikely that such rare organisms are present in a previously untreated patient.

Combination chemotherapy is required for treating active TB disease. The patient should receive at least two drugs to which the isolate is susceptible, and generally four drugs are given at the outset of treatment. Rifampin and isoniazid are the best drugs for preventing drug resistance, followed by ethambutol, streptomycin, and pyrazinamide.[2,7,39,42,43]

Three subpopulations of mycobacteria are proposed to exist within the body, and each appears to respond to certain drugs.[2,39,42] Most numerous are the extracellular, rapidly dividing bacteria, often found within cavities (about 10^7 to 10^9 organisms). These are killed most readily by isoniazid, followed by rifampin, streptomycin, and the other drugs. A second group resides within caseating granulomas (possibly 10^5 to 10^7 organisms). These organisms appear to be in a semidormant state, with occasional bursts of metabolic activity. Pyrazinamide, through its conversion within *M. tuberculosis* to pyrazinoic acid, appears most active against these organisms. Rifampin and isoniazid also may be active against this subpopulation. The third subset is the intracellular mycobacteria present within macrophages (10^4 to 10^6). Rifampin, isoniazid, and the quinolones appear to be most active against intracellular *M. tuberculosis*. While these theories appear to explain what happens during the treatment of TB, there is no practical way to quantitate these populations within a given patient.

NONPHARMACOLOGIC THERAPY

Nonpharmacologic interventions aim to (1) prevent the spread of TB, (2) find where TB has already spread using contact investigation, and (3) replenish the weakened (consumptive) patient to a state of normal weight and well-being. Items 1 and 2 are performed by public health departments. Clinicians involved in the treatment of TB should verify that the local health department has been notified of all new cases of TB.

Workers in hospitals and other institutions must prevent the spread of TB within their facilities.[2,4,13,30] All such workers should learn and follow each institution's infection control guidelines. This includes using personal protective equipment, including properly fitted respirators, and closing doors to "negative pressure" rooms. These hospital isolation rooms draw air in from surrounding areas rather than blowing air (and *M. tuberculosis*) into these other areas. The air from the isolation room may be treated with ultraviolet lights and then vented safely outside. However, these isolation rooms work properly only if the door is closed.

Debilitated TB patients may require therapy for other medical problems, including substance abuse and HIV infection, and some may need nutritional support. Therefore, clinicians involved in substance abuse rehabilitation and nutritional support services should be familiar with the needs of TB patients.

Surgery may be needed to remove destroyed lung tissue, space-occupying infected lesions (*tuberculomas*), and certain extrapulmonary lesions.[2,13,39] Vaccines against TB include BCG and *M. vaccae*.[39] However, these vaccines are of limited value, and neither can prevent infection by *M. tuberculosis*. BCG (discussed below) may prevent extreme forms of TB in infants, whereas *M. vaccae* cannot be recommended.[39,44]

PHARMACOLOGIC THERAPY

TREATING LATENT INFECTION

Isoniazid is the preferred drug for treating latent TB infection.[2,7,13,39] Generally, isoniazid alone is given for 9 months. The treatment of latent TB infection (LTBI) reduces a person's lifetime risk of active TB from about 10% to about 1%. Because TB is spread easily through the air, each case prevented also prevents a second wave of cases that each prevented case would have produced. Historically, the treatment of LTBI has been called *prophylaxis, chemoprophylaxis,* or *preventive treatment*. By any name, it is one of the primary mechanisms for reducing TB in the United States. The LTBI treatment options are listed in Table 110–2.

Because young children, the elderly, and HIV-positive patients are at greater risk of active disease once infected with *M. tuberculosis*, they require careful evaluation. Once active TB is ruled out, they should receive treatment for latent infection.[2,22,23,39]

The keys to successful treatment of LTBI are (1) infection by an isoniazid-susceptible isolate, (2) adherence to the 9-month regimen, and (3) no exogenous reinfection.[2] Isoniazid adult doses are usually 300 mg daily (5–10 mg/kg of body weight)[52] (see Table 110–2). Lower doses are less effective.[2,49] Isoniazid should be

TABLE 110–2. Recommended Drug Regimens for Treatment of Latent Tuberculosis (TB) Infection in Adults

Drug	Interval and Duration	Comments	Rating[a] (Evidence)[b] HIV−	HIV+
Isoniazid	Daily for 9 mo[c,d]	In human immunodeficiency virus (HIV)-infected patients, isoniazid may be administered concurrently with nucleoside reverse transcriptase inhibitors (NRTIs), protease inhibitors, or non-nucleoside reverse transcriptase inhibitors (NNRTIs)	A (II)	A (II)
	Twice weekly for 9 mo[c,d]	Directly observed therapy (DOT) must be used with twice-weekly dosing	B (II)	B (II)
Isoniazid	Daily for 6 mo[d]	Not indicated for HIV-infected persons, those with fibrotic lesions on chest radiographs, or children	B (I)	C (I)
	Twice weekly for 6 mo[d]	DOT must be used with twice-weekly dosing	B (II)	C (I)
Rifampin	Daily for 4 mo	For persons who cannot tolerate pyrazinamide	B (II)	B (III)
		For persons who are contacts of patients with isoniazid-resistant, rifampin-susceptible TB who cannot tolerate pyrazinamide		

[a]Strength of recommendation: A = preferred; B = acceptable alternative; C = offer when A and B cannot be given.
[b]Quality of evidence: I = randomized clinical trial data; II = data from clinical trials that are not randomized or were conducted in other populations; III = expert opinion.
[c]Recommended regimen for children younger than 18 yr of age.
[d]Recommended regimens for pregnant women. Some experts would use rifampin and pyrazinamide for 2 mo as an alternative regimen in HIV-infected pregnant women, although pyrazinamide should be avoided during the first trimester.
Adapted from Centers for Disease Control and Prevention. Targeted tuberculin testing and treatment of latent tuberculosis infection. MMWR 2000;49(RR-6):31.

given on an empty stomach, and antacids should be avoided within 2 hours of dosing. When adherence is an issue, twice-weekly isoniazid (900 mg in an adult) can be given using DOT. Nine months of treatment is recommended, but 6 months still provides considerable benefit.

Rifampin 600 mg daily for 4 months can be used when isoniazid resistance is suspected or when the patient cannot tolerate isoniazid.[2,25,48,49] Rifabutin 300 mg daily might be substituted for rifampin for patients at high risk of drug interactions. The combination of pyrazinamide plus rifampin is no longer recommended because of higher than expected rates of hepatotoxicity. When resistance to isoniazid and rifampin is suspected in the isolate causing infection, there is no regimen proved to be effective.[2,39] Regimens that *might* be effective include ethambutol plus levofloxacin, but data regarding efficacy are lacking.

For recent skin-test converters of all ages, the risk of active TB outweighs the risk for drug toxicity.[30,39] Pregnant women, alcoholics, and patients with poor diets who are treated with isoniazid should receive pyridoxine (vitamin B_6) 10–50 mg daily to reduce the incidence of central nervous system (CNS) effects or peripheral neuropathies. All patients who receive treatment of LTBI should be monitored monthly for adverse drug reactions and for possible progression to active TB.

TREATING ACTIVE DISEASE

The treatment of active TB requires the use of multiple drugs. There are two primary antituberculosis drugs, isoniazid and rifampin, with the rest of the drugs having specific roles.[39,42,43] Isoniazid and rifampin should be used together whenever possible. Typically, *M. tuberculosis* is either very susceptible or very resistant to a given drug. This contrasts with *M. avium*, where moderately resistant organisms are a frequent occurrence. Theoretically, minimal inhibitory concentration (MIC) results could be used to guide dosing in the treatment of moderately resistant *M. tuberculosis*, but this remains to be studied prospectively.[2,13,39]

Drug-susceptibility testing should be done on the initial isolate for all patients with active TB. These data should guide the selection of drugs over the course of treatment.[2,7,13,39] However, some patients are unable to provide a suitable specimen for laboratory testing. If susceptibility data are not available for a given patient, the drug-susceptibility data for the suspected source case or regional susceptibility data should be used.[2,39]

Drug resistance should be expected in patients presenting for the retreatment of TB. These patients require retesting of drug susceptibility using freshly collected specimens. It is imperative to learn what drugs the patient received and for how long the patient received them.[2,13,39] A treatment history, often called a "drug-o-gram," shows the start and stop dates of all antimycobacterial drugs on a horizontal bar graph.[2,39] A "drug-o-gram" should be constructed for all retreatment patients.

The standard TB treatment regimen is isoniazid, rifampin, pyrazinamide, and ethambutol for 2 months, followed by isoniazid and rifampin for 4 months, for a total of 6 months of treatment.[2,13,39] If susceptibility to isoniazid, rifampin, and pyrazinamide is shown, ethambutol can be stopped at any time. Without pyrazinamide, a total of 9 months of isoniazid and rifampin treatment is required. Table 110–3 shows the recommended treatment regimens. When intermittent therapy is used, DOT is essential. Doses missed during an intermittent TB regimen decrease its efficacy and increase the relapse rate. Note that Table 110–3 shows recommendations that differ for HIV-negative and HIV-positive patients. HIV-positive patients should not receive highly intermittent regimens. In general, regimens given daily five times each week or three times weekly can be used for HIV-positive patients. Less frequent dosing has been associated with higher failure and relapse rates and the selection of rifampin-resistant organisms.[39]

CLINICAL CONTROVERSY

The recommended duration of treatment often is the same for HIV-negative and HIV-positive patients. However, some clinicians believe that thereapy should be extended for patients with weakened immune systems. These clinicians treat HIV-positive patients with drug-susceptible TB for 9 months rather than the usual 6 months.

TABLE 110–3. Drug Regimens for Culture-Positive Pulmonary Tuberculosis Caused by Drug-Susceptible Organisms

Initial Phase			Continuation Phase			Range of Total Doses (Minimal Duration)	Rating[a] (Evidence)[b]	
Regimen	Drugs	Interval and Doses[c] (Minimal Duration)	Regimen	Drugs	Interval and Doses[c,d] (Minimal Duration)		HIV⁻	HIV⁺
1	INH RIF PZA EMB	Seven days per week for 56 doses (8 wk) or 5 d/wk for 40 doses (8 wk)[c]	1a	INH/RIF	Seven days per week for 126 doses (18 wk) or 5 d/wk for 90 doses (18 wk)[c]	182–130 (26 wk)	A (I)	A (II)
			1b	INH/RIF	Twice weekly for 36 doses (18 wk)	92–76 (26 wk)	A (I)	A (II)[f]
			1c[g]	INH/RPT	Once weekly for 18 doses (18 wk)	74–58 (26 wk)	B (I)	E (I)
2	INH RIF PZA EMB	Seven days per week for 14 doses (2 wk), then twice weekly for 12 doses (6 wk) or 5 d/wk for 10 doses (2 wk)[e] then twice weekly for 12 doses (6 wk)	2a	INH/RIF	Twice weekly for 36 doses (18 wk)	62–58 (26 wk)	A (II)	B (II)[f]
			2b[g]	INH/RPT	Once weekly for 18 doses (18 wk)	44–40 (26 wk)	B (I)	E (I)
3	INH RIF PZA EMB	Three times weekly for 24 doses (8 wk)	3a	INH/RIF	Three times weekly for 54 doses (18 wk)	78 (26 wk)	B (I)	B (II)
4	INH RIF EMB	Seven days per week for 56 doses (8 wk) or 5 d/wk for 40 doses (8 wk)[c]	4a	INH/RIF	Seven days per week for 217 doses (31 wk) or 5 d/wk for 155 doses (31 wk)[e]	273–195 (39 wk)	C (I)	C (II)
			4b	INH/RIF	Twice weekly for 62 doses (31 wk)	118–102 (39 wk)	C (I)	C (II)

Definition of abbreviations: EMB = Ethambutol; INH = isoniazid; PZA = pyrazinamide; RIF = rifampin; RPT = rifapentine.
[a]Definitions of evidence ratings: A = preferred; B = acceptable alternative; C = offer when A and B cannot be given; E = should never be given.
[b]Definition of evidence ratings: I = randomized clinical trial; II = data from clinical trials that were not randomized or were conducted in other populations; III = expert opinion.
[c]When DOT is used, drugs may be given 5 days/week and the necessary number of doses adjusted accordingly. Although there are no studies that compare five with seven daily doses, extensive experience indicates this would be an effective practice.
[d]Patients with cavitation on initial chest radiograph and positive cultures at completion of 2 months of therapy should receive a 7-month (31 week; either 217 doses [daily] or 62 doses [twice weekly]) continuation phase.
[e]Five-day-a-week administration is always given by DOT. Rating for 5 day/week regimens is AIII.
[f]Not recommended for HIV-Infected patients with CD4⁺ cell counts <100 cells/μL.
[g]Options 1c and 2b should be used only in HIV-negative patients who have negative sputum smears at the time of completion of 2 months of therapy and who do not have cavitation on initial chest radiograph (see text). For patients started on this regimen and found to have a positive culture from the 2-month specimen, treatment should be extended an extra 3 months.
From Centers for Disease Control and Prevention. Treatment of tuberculosis. MMWR 2003;52 (RR-11).

When the patients' sputum smears convert to a negative, the risk of them infecting others is greatly reduced, but it is not zero.[2,21,39] Such patients can be removed from respiratory isolation, but they must be careful not to cough on others and should meet only in well-ventilated places. Smear-negative patients still may be culture-positive, so they still can transmit TB to others.

Patients who are slow to respond clinically, those who remain culture-positive at 2 months of treatment, those with cavitary lesions on chest radiograph, and perhaps HIV-positive patients should be treated for a total of 9 months and for at least 6 months from the time that they convert to smear and culture negativity.[2,7,13,39] Some authors recommend therapeutic drug monitoring for such patients.[2,39,43,45] When isoniazid and rifampin cannot be used, treatment durations become 2 years or more regardless of immune status.[2,13,39,43]

Adjustments to the regimen should be made once the susceptibility data are available.[2,13,39] If the organism is drug-resistant, careful consideration of the remaining therapeutic options must be made. Two or more drugs with in vitro activity against the patient's isolate and that the patient has not received previously should be added to the regimen, as needed.[2,13,39] TB specialists should be consulted regarding cases of drug-resistant TB.[2,13,39]

There is no standard regimen for MDR-TB.[2,13,39] Each patient's exposure history, previous treatment history (including toxicity and adherence issues), and current susceptibility data must be considered simultaneously. *It is critical to avoid monotherapy, and it is critical to avoid adding a single drug to a failing regimen.*[2,13,39] Adding one drug at a time leads to the sequential selection of drug resistance until there are no drugs left. The treatment of MDR-TB

should be managed by TB specialists. It may take several months for a patient with MDR-TB to become culture-negative because the drugs used lack the potency of isoniazid and rifampin.[2,42,43] Therefore, prolonged respiratory isolation may be required.

Drug resistance should be suspected in the following situations:

- Patients who have received prior therapy for TB
- Patients from areas with a high prevalence of resistance (New York City, Mexico, Southeast Asia, the Baltic countries, and the former Soviet states)
- Patients who are homeless, institutionalized, intravenous drug abusers, or infected with HIV
- Patients who still have AFB-positive sputum smears after 1 to 2 months of therapy
- Patients who still have positive cultures after 2 to 4 months of therapy
- Patients who fail treatment or relapse after treatment
- Patients known to be exposed to MDR-TB cases

The patients just listed should be considered infected with drug-resistant TB until proved otherwise. Empirical therapy with four or more drugs may be needed for acutely ill patients.[2,13,39] These regimens may be altered when the susceptibility pattern becomes known. If the index case is known, then the same effective regimen should be employed for the new case. Again, MDR-TB cases should be referred to specialists.

TABLE 110–4. Evidence-Based[a] Guidelines for the Treatment of Extrapulmonary Tuberculosis and Adjunctive Use of Corticosteriods[b]

Site	Length of Therapy (mo)	Rating (Duration)	Corticosteroids[c]	Rating (Corticosteroids)
Lymph node	6	AI	Not recommended	DIII
Bone and joint	6–9	AI	Not recommended	DIII
Pleural disease	6	AII	Not recommended	DI
Pericarditis	6	AII	Strongly recommended	AI
CNS tuberculosis including meningitis	9–12	BII	Strongly recommended	AI
Disseminated disease	6	AII	Not recommended	DIII
Genitourinary	6	AII	Not recommended	DIII
Peritoneal	6	AII	Not recommended	DIII

[a]For rating system, see Table 110–3.
[b]Duration of therapy for extrapulmonary tuberculosis caused by drug-resistant organisms is not known.
[c]Corticosteroid preparations vary among studies.
See Table 110–3.

SPECIAL POPULATIONS

Tuberculous Meningitis and Extrapulmonary Disease

Patients with CNS tuberculosis usually are treated for longer periods (9 to 12 months instead of 6 months)[2,13,39] (Table 110–4). In general, isoniazid, pyrazinamide, ethionamide, and cycloserine penetrate the cerebrospinal fluid (CSF) readily, but rifampin, ethambutol, and streptomycin have variable CNS penetration.[46] Of the quinolones, levofloxacin may be preferred based on current data. Extrapulmonary TB of the soft tissues can be treated with conventional regimens.[2,13,39] TB of the bone typically is treated for 9 months, occasionally with surgical débridement.[2,13,39]

Children

TB in children may be treated with regimens similar to those used in adults, although some physicians still prefer to extend treatment to 9 months.[2,13,23,24,39,47,48] Pediatric doses of isoniazid and rifampin on a milligram per kilogram basis are higher than those used in adults[39] (Table 110–5).

Pregnancy

Women with TB should be cautioned against becoming pregnant because the disease poses a risk to the fetus and to the mother. If already pregnant, the usual treatment is isoniazid, rifampin, and ethambutol for 9 months.[39] Isoniazid or ethambutol are relatively safe for use in pregnant women.[2,39,46–48] B vitamins are particularly important during pregnancy and should be provided to women being treated for TB. Rifampin has been associated rarely with birth defects, including limb reduction and CNS lesions.[46] In general, rifampin is used in pregnant women with TB. Pyrazinamide has not been studied in large numbers of pregnant women, but anecdotal data suggest that it may be safe.[39]

Streptomycin use during pregnancy may lead to hearing loss in the newborn, including complete deafness. Streptomycin and the other aminoglycosides must be reserved for critical situations where alternatives do not exist.[2,39] Although the polypeptide capreomycin has not been studied, it probably carries the same risks.

Ethionamide may cause premature delivery and congenital deformities when used during pregnancy.[39,46] Mongolism also has been reported, so it cannot be recommended in this setting. *p*-Aminosalicylic acid has been used safely in pregnancy, but specific data are lacking.[39,46] Cycloserine is known to cross the placenta, but the effects on the developing fetus are not known. Therefore, cycloserine generally cannot be recommended during pregnancy.[46]

Ciprofloxacin, levofloxacin, moxifloxacin, and the other quinolones have been associated with permanent damage to cartilage in the weight-bearing joints of immature animals, especially dogs and rabbits.[39,46] While these drugs have not been shown to cause joint problems frequently in humans, other antituberculosis agents should be used during pregnancy.

Pregnant women with LTBI are not at the same level of risk compared with those with active disease. Therapy with isoniazid for LTBI may be delayed until after pregnancy or, if recent skin-test conversion has occurred, started during the second trimester of pregnancy.[39,46–48] Although most antituberculosis drugs are excreted in breast milk, the amount of drug received by the infant through nursing is insufficient to cause toxicity. Quinolones should be avoided in nursing mothers, if possible.

HIV Infection

Patients with AIDS and other immunocompromised hosts may be managed with chemotherapeutic regimens similar to those used in immunocompetent individuals, although treatment is often extended to 9 months[2,13,39] (see Table 110–3). The precise duration to recommend remains a matter of debate. Highly intermittent regimens (twice or once weekly) are not recommended for HIV-positive TB patients. Prognosis has been particularly poor for HIV-infected patients infected with MDR-TB. Differentiation must be made between infection with *M. tuberculosis* and NTM, such as MAC, because the drugs used are different. While awaiting laboratory results, the patient can be treated empirically for TB if there is any doubt about the causative organism. Some patients with AIDS malabsorb their oral medications; this is discussed under therapeutic drug monitoring later.[2,39,43,45] The major issue of drug interactions is discussed further below under rifampin.

Renal Failure

In nearly all patients, isoniazid and rifampin do not require dose modification in renal failure. They are eliminated primarily by the liver.[43,46,49] In the unlikely event that peripheral neuropathies develop, the frequency of isoniazid dosing may be reduced. Pyrazinamide and ethambutol typically require a reduction in dosing frequency from daily to three times weekly[39,49] (Table 110–6).

Renally cleared TB drugs include the aminoglycosides (amikacin, kanamycin, and streptomycin), capreomycin, ethambutol, cycloserine, and levofloxacin.[39,46,49,50] Dosing intervals need to

TABLE 110–5. Doses[a] of Antituberculosis Drugs for Adults and Children[b]

Drug	Preparation	Adults/Children	Doses			
			Daily	*11×/wk*	*2×/wk*	*3×/wk*
First-Line Drugs						
Isoniazid	Tablets (50 mg, 100 mg, 300 mg); elixir (50 mg/5 ml); aqueous solution (100 mg/mL) for intravenous or intramuscular injection	Adults (max.) Children (max.)	5 mg/kg (300 mg) 10–15 mg/kg (300 mg)	15 mg/kg (900 mg) —	15 mg/kg (900 mg) 20–30 mg/kg (900 mg)	15 mg/kg (900 mg) —
Rifampin	Capsule (150 mg, 300 mg); powder may be suspended for oral administration; aqueous solution for intravenous injection	Adults[c] (max.) Children (max.)	10 mg/kg (600 mg) 10–20 mg/kg (600 mg)	— 	10 mg/kg (600 mg) 10–20 mg/kg (600 mg)	10 mg/kg (600 mg) —
Rifabutin	Capsule (150 mg)	Adults[c] (max.) Children	5 mg/kg (300 mg) Appropriate dosing for children is unknown	— Appropriate dosing for children is unknown	5 mg/kg (300 mg) Appropriate dosing for children is unknown	5 mg/kg (300 mg) Appropriate dosing for children is unknown
Rifapentine	Tablet (150 mg, film coated)	Adults	—	10 mg/kg (continuation phase) (600 mg)	—	—
		Children	The drug is not approved for use in children	The drug is not approved for use in children	The drug is not approved for use in children	The drug is not approved for use in children
Pyrazinamide	Tablet (500 mg, scored)	Adults	1000 mg (40–55 kg) 1500 mg (56–75 kg) 2000 mg (76–90 kg)[k]	— — —	2000 mg (40–55 kg) 3000 mg (56–75 kg) 4000 mg (76–90 kg)[k]	1500 mg (40–55 kg) 2500 mg (56–75 kg) 3000 mg (76–90 kg)[k]
		Children (max.)	15–30 mg/kg (2.0 g)	—	50 mg/kg (2 g)	—
Ethambutol	Tablet (100 mg, 400 mg)	Adults	800 mg (40–55 kg) 1200 mg (56–75 kg) 1600 mg (76–90 kg)[k]	— — —	2000 mg (40–55 kg) 2800 mg (56–75 kg) 4000 mg (76–90 kg)[k]	1200 mg (40–55 kg) 2000 mg (56–75 kg) 2400 mg (76–90 kg)[k]
		Children[d] (max.)	15–20 mg/kg daily (1.0 g)	—	50 mg/kg (2.5 g)	—
Second-Line Drugs						
Cycloserine	Capsule (250 mg)	Adults (max.)	10–15 mg/kg/day (1.0 g in two doses), usually 500–750 mg/d in two doses[e]	There are no data to support intermittent administration	There are no data to support intermittent administration	There are no data to support intermittent administration
		Children (max.)	10–15 mg/kg/day (1.0 g/day)	—	—	—
Ethionamide	Tablet (250 mg)	Adults[f] (max.)	15–20 mg/kg/day (1.0 g/day), usually 500–750 mg/day in a single daily dose or two divided doses[f]	There are no data to support intermittent administration	There are no data to support intermittent administration	There are no data to support intermittent administration
		Children (max.)	15–20 mg/kg/day (1.0 g/day)	There are no data to support intermittent administration	There are no data to support intermittent administration	There are no data to support intermittent administration
Streptomycin	Aqueous solution (1-g vials) for intravenous or intramuscular administration	Adults (max.) Children (max.)	g 20–40 mg/kg/day (1 g)	g —	g 20 mg/kg	g —
Amikacin/ kanamycin	Aqueous solution (500-mg and 1-g vials) for intravenous or intramuscular administration	Adults (max.) Children (max.)	g 15–30 mg/kg/day (1 g) intravenous or intramuscular as a single daily dose	g —	g 15–30 mg/kg	g —
Capreomycin	Aqueous solution (1-g vials) for intravenous or intramuscular administration	Adults (max.) Children (max.)	g 15–30 mg/kg/day (1 g) as a single daily dose	g —	g 15–30 mg/kg	g —

(*continued*)

TABLE 110–5. (Continued)

Drug	Preparation	Adults/Children	Daily	11×/wk	2×/wk	3×/wk
p-Aminosalicylic acid (PAS)	Granules (4-g packets) can be mixed with food; tablets (500 mg) are still available in some countries, but not in the United States; a solution for intravenous administration is available in Europe	Adults	8–12 g/day in two or three doses	There are no data to support intermittent administration	There are no data to support intermittent administration	There are no data to support intermittent administration
		Children	200–300 mg/kg/day in two to four divided doses (10 g)	There are no data to support intermittent administration	There are no data to support intermittent administration	There are no data to support intermittent administration
Levofloxacin	Tablets (250 mg, 500 mg, 750 mg); aqueous solution (500-mg vials) for intravenous injection	Adults	500–1000 mg daily	There are no data to support intermittent administration	There are no data to support intermittent administration	There are no data to support intermittent administration
		Children	h	h	h	h
Moxifloxacin	Tablets (400 mg); aqueous solution (400 mg/250 mL) for intravenous injection	Adults	400 mg daily	There are no data to support intermittent administration	There are no data to support intermittent administration	There are no data to support intermittent administration
		Children	i	i	i	i
Gatifloxacin	Tablets (400 mg); aqueous solution (200 mg/20 mL; 400 mg/40 mL) for intravenous injection	Adults	400 mg daily	There are no data to support intermittent administration	There are no data to support intermittent administration	There are no data to support intermittent administration
		Children	j	j	j	j

[a]Dose per weight is based on ideal body weight. Children weighing more than 40 kg should be dosed as adults.

[b]For purposes of this document adult dosing begins at age 15 years.

[c]Dose may need to be adjusted when there is concomitant use of protease inhibitors or nonnucleoside reverse transcriptase inhibitors.

[d]The drug can likely be used safely in older children but should be used with caution in children less than 5 years of age, in whom visual acuity cannot be monitored. In younger children EMB at the dose of 15 mg/kg per day can be used if there is suspected or proven resistance to INH or RIF.

[e]It should be noted that, although this is the dose recommended generally, most clinicians with experience using cycloserine indicate that it is unusual for patients to be able to tolerate this amount. Serum concentration measurements are often useful in determining the optimal dose for a given patient.

[f]The single daily dose can be given at bedtime or with the main meal.

[g]Dose: 15 mg/kg per day (1 g), and 10 mg/kg in persons more than 59 years of age (750 mg). Usual dose: 750–1000 mg administered intramuscularly or intravenously, given as a single dose 5–7 days/week and reduced to two or three times per week after the first 2–4 months or after culture conversion, depending on the efficacy of the other drugs in the regimen.

[h]The long-term (more than several weeks) use of levofloxacin in children and adolescents has not been approved because of concerns about effects on bone and cartilage growth. However, most experts agree that the drug should be considered for children with tuberculosis caused by organisms resistant to both INH and RIF. The optimal dose is not known.

[i]The long-term (more than several weeks) use of moxifloxacin in children and adolescents has not been approved because of concerns about effects on bone and cartilage growth. The optimal dose is not known.

[j]The long-term (more than several weeks) use of gatifloxacin in children and adolescents has not been approved because of concerns about effects on bone and cartilage growth. The optimal dose is not known.

[k]Maximum dose regardless of weight.

be extended for these drugs (see Table 110–6). Ciprofloxacin is about 50% cleared by the kidneys but may not require a change in dose from once daily, as it is used for TB. The metabolites of isoniazid, pyrazinamide, and p-aminosalicylic acid are cleared primarily by the kidneys. The role of these metabolites in causing toxicity is unknown, so their accumulation in renal failure may carry some risk.

Ethionamide and its sulfoxide metabolite are cleared hepatically, so dosing is unchanged.[39,50] p-Aminosalicylic acid is converted largely to metabolites prior to renal elimination; these metabolites may accumulate in renal failure.[50] For patients on hemodialysis, the usual 12-hour dosing interval for p-aminosalicylic acid granules seems to be safe. Dialysis will remove the metabolites. Serum concentration monitoring must be performed for cycloserine to avoid dose-related toxicities in renal failure patients.[43,45,50]

Hepatic Failure

Antituberculosis drugs that rely on hepatic clearance for most of their elimination include isoniazid, rifampin, pyrazinamide, ethionamide,

and p-aminosalicylic acid.[46] Ciprofloxacin is about 50% cleared by the liver. Elevations of serum transaminase concentrations generally are not correlated with the residual capacity of the liver to metabolize drugs, so these markers cannot be used as guides for drug dosing. Further, isoniazid, rifampin, pyrazinamide, and to a lesser degree, ethionamide, p-aminosalicylic acid, and rarely, ethambutol may cause hepatotoxicity.[39,43,46] For some patients with drug-susceptible TB, a "liver sparing" regimen may be used, at least temporarily. It consists of streptomycin, levofloxacin, and ethambutol.[39,43,46] Note that this regimen would require 18 or more months of treatment to be successful. Therefore, patients usually are switched to isoniazid- and rifampin-containing regimens as soon as they are able.

Morbid Obesity

Data are not available for dosing the TB drugs in patients with morbid obesity.[46] Relatively hydrophilic drugs (isoniazid, pyrazinamide, the aminoglycosides, capreomycin, ethambutol, p-aminosalicylic acid, and cycloserine) can be dosed initially based on ideal body weight

TABLE 110–6. Dosing Recommendations for Adult Patients with Reduced Renal Function and for Adult Patients Receiving Hemodialysis

Drug	Change in Frequency?	Recommended Dose and Frequency for Patients with Creatinine Clearance <30 mL/min or for Patients Receiving Hemodialysis
Isoniazid	No change	300 mg once daily, or 900 mg three times per week
Rifampin	No change	600 mg once daily, or 600 mg three times per week
Pyrazinamide	Yes	25–35 mg/kg per dose three times per week (not daily)
Ethambutol	Yes	15–25 mg/kg per dose three times per week (not daily)
Levofloxacin	Yes	750–1000 mg per dose three times per week (not daily)
Cycloserine	Yes	250 mg once daily, or 500 mg/dose three times per week[a]
Ethionamide	No change	250–500 mg/dose daily
p-Aminosalicylic acid	No change	4 g/dose, twice daily
Streptomycin	Yes	12–15 mg/kg per dose two or three times per week (not daily)
Capreomycin	Yes	12–15 mg/kg per dose two or three times per week (not daily)
Kanamycin	Yes	12–15 mg/kg per dose two or three times per week (not daily)
Amikacin	Yes	12–15 mg/kg per dose two or three times per week (not daily)

Standard doses are given unless there is intolerance.
The medications should be given after hemodialysis on the day of hemodialysis.
Monitoring of serum drug concentrations should be considered to ensure adequate drug absorption, without excessive accumulation, and to assist in avoiding toxicity. Data currently are not available for patients receiving peritoneal dialysis. Until data become available, begin with doses recommended for patients receiving hemodialysis and verify adequacy of dosing, using serum concentration monitoring.
[a]The appropriateness of 250-mg daily doses has not been established. There should be careful monitoring for evidence of neurotoxicity.

(IBW). Very low or very high serum concentrations can be avoided by checking the serum concentrations.

THE TB DRUGS

The interested reader is referred to several other publications for more detailed information regarding these drugs.[2,12,39,42,43,45,46,51–53] Note that although the ATS/CDC guidelines recommend "maximum" doses, I disagree with this approach to therapy[39] (see Table 110–5). In my view, the "maximum" dose for a given patient is the dose that produces the desired response with an acceptable level of toxicity.[43,45] This can only be determined on a case-by-case basis. Artificially capping doses may deprive patients of needed drug.

Primary Antituberculosis Drugs

Isoniazid. Isoniazid is one of the two most important TB drugs. It is highly specific for mycobacteria, with an MIC against *M. tuberculosis* of 0.01 to 0.25 mcg/mL. Most NTM such as *M. avium* are resistant to isoniazid, although *M. kansasii* and *M. xenopi* are susceptible. The most common mechanism of resistance results from mutations in the *katG* gene leading to the loss of catalase-peroxidase activity and the failure to produce the toxic isoniazid derivatives.

Isoniazid is readily absorbed from the gastrointestinal tract and from intramuscular injection sites. It also can be given as a short intravenous infusion over 5 minutes if diluted in about 20 mL of normal saline.[54] Isoniazid should be given on an empty stomach whenever possible.[55] N-acetyltransferase 2 (NAT2) forms the principal metabolite, acetylisoniazid, which lacks antimycobacterial activity. The rate at which humans acetylate isoniazid is determined genetically; slow acetylation is an autosomal recessive trait and reflects a relative lack of NAT2. Fast acetylators have isoniazid half-lives of less than 2 hours. Approximately 50% of whites and blacks and 80% to 90% of Asians and Eskimos are rapid acetylators. Slow acetylators have isoniazid half-lives of 3 to 4 hours and may be at an increased risk of neurotoxicity. The association of acetylator status and risk of hepatotoxicity, however, appears to be weak.[56] Poor absorption and rapid clearance of isoniazid in patients receiving highly intermittent therapy have been associated with poor clinical outcomes.[57]

Transient elevations of the serum transaminases occur in 12% to 15% of patients receiving isoniazid and usually occur within the first 8 to 12 weeks of therapy.[39] Overt hepatotoxicity, however, occurs in only 1% of cases. Risk factors for hepatotoxicity include patient age, preexisting liver disease, excessive alcohol intake, pregnancy, and the postpartum state. Isoniazid also may result in neurotoxicity, most frequently presenting as peripheral neuropathy or, in overdose, as seizures and coma. Patients with pyridoxine deficiency, such as pregnant women, alcoholics, children, and the malnourished, are at increased risk. Isoniazid may inhibit the metabolism of phenytoin, carbamazepine, primidone, and warfarin.[43] Patients who are being treated with these agents should be monitored closely, and appropriate dose adjustments should be made when necessary.

Rifampin. The introduction of rifampin into routine use during the 1970s allowed for true short-course treatment of TB (6 to 9 months).[2,13,39] Without rifampin, treatment is generally 18 months or longer. Drug resistance to rifampin is an ominous prognostic factor because it is frequently associated with isoniazid resistance and leaves the patient with few good therapeutic options. Clinicians *must* take care to protect susceptibility to rifampin by carefully treating their patients.

Rifampin shows bactericidal activity against *M. tuberculosis* and several other mycobacterial species, including *M. bovis* and *M. kansasii*.[58] Other NTM, including MAC, show variable susceptibility to rifampin. Rifampin also is active against a broad array of other bacteria. Alteration of the target site on RNA polymerase, primarily through changes in the *rpoB* gene, leads to most forms of rifampin resistance.[39,58]

Rifampin usually is given orally, but it also can be given as a 30-minute intravenous infusion.[51,58] Oral doses are best given on an empty stomach.[59] Patients with AIDS, diabetes, and other gastrointestinal problems appear to have difficulty absorbing rifampin after oral doses, and this has been associated with therapeutic failures in some cases.[43,45] Rifampin is metabolized to 25-desacetylrifampin, which retains most of rifampin's activity; most of rifampin and its metabolite are cleared in the bile. Rifampin generally is given at 600 mg daily or intermittently, although this dose does not take full advantage of rifampin's concentration-dependent killing.[43,45] Higher doses should be tested in humans within the context of clinical trials.

Elevations in hepatic enzymes have been attributed to rifampin in 10% to 15% of patients, with overt hepatotoxicity occurring in less than 1%.[39,58] More frequent adverse effects of rifampin include rash, fever, and gastrointestinal distress. Allergic reactions to rifampin have been reported and occur more frequently with intermittent rifampin doses 900 mg or more twice weekly. These reactions may take the form of a flulike syndrome with development of fever, chills, headache, arthralgias, and rarely, hypotension and shock.[39,52] Alternatively, hemolytic anemia or acute renal failure may occur, requiring permanent discontinuation.

Rifampin's potent induction of hepatic enzymes, especially cytochrome P450 (CYP) 3A4, may enhance the elimination of many other drugs, most notably the protease inhibitors used to treat HIV (Table 110–7). HIV-positive patients may benefit from the use of rifabutin instead of rifampin (see below).[39,60–63] Also, women who use oral contraceptives must use another form of contraception during therapy because increased clearance of the hormones may lead to unexpected pregnancies. Patient records should be reviewed for potential drug interactions before dispensing rifampin.[51] Rifampin may turn urine and other secretions orange-red and may permanently stain some types of contact lenses.

▓ *Other Rifamycins.* Rifabutin is used for disseminated *M. avium* infection in AIDS patients and is quite active against *M. tuberculosis*. Most rifampin-resistant organisms are resistant to rifabutin. Because rifabutin is a less potent enzyme inducer than rifampin, it may be used in patients receiving protease inhibitors.[39,60–63] For HIV-positive patients, the American Thoracic Society (ATS)/CDC recommends regimens with three or more doses of the TB drugs per week (see Table 110–3). Rifapentine is a long-acting rifamycin that can be used once weekly in the continuation phase of treatment (after the first 2 months) in carefully selected HIV-negative patients. Rifapentine is about 85% as potent an enzyme inducer as rifampin, so similar drug interactions are likely.[39,60–63]

▓ *Pyrazinamide.* Adding pyrazinamide to the first 2 months of treatment with isoniazid and rifampin shortens the duration to 6 months for most patients.[2,39] It is usually well absorbed and displays a fairly long half-life.[64,65] The most common toxicities of pyrazinamide are gastrointestinal distress, arthralgias, and elevations in the serum uric acid concentrations.[39,52] Most patients do not experience true gout. Hepatotoxicity is the major limiting adverse effect and is dose-related when pyrazinamide is given daily.

A fixed-combination product (Rifater, Aventis) of rifampin 120 mg, isoniazid 50 mg, and pyrazinamide 300 mg is designed to prevent drug resistance by keeping the self-medicating patient from using only one drug at a time. If the patient is receiving DOT, there is no particular advantage to this product. The typical dose of Rifater will be five to six tablets daily. When pyrazinamide is discontinued after 2 months of treatment, the combination product Rifamate (isoniazid 150 mg and rifampin 300 mg) can be substituted.

▓ *Ethambutol.* Ethambutol replaced *p*-aminosalicylic acid as a first-line agent in the 1960s because it was better tolerated by patients.[2,39] Ethambutol is used as a fourth drug for TB while awaiting susceptibility data.[39] If the organism is susceptible to isoniazid, rifampin, and pyrazinamide, ethambutol can be stopped. Ethambutol is active against most mycobacteria, including *M. tuberculosis* and *M. avium*, but it is generally bacteriostatic.

Ethambutol should not be given with antacids.[66] The ethambutol dose should be reduced to three times per week in patients with renal failure.[49,67] Retrobulbar neuritis is the major adverse effect. Patients may complain of a change in visual acuity, the inability to see the color green, or both. They should be monitored monthly while on the drug using Snellen wall charts for visual acuity and Ishihara red-green color discrimination cards.[39,51,52]

▓ Second-Line Antituberculosis Drugs

▓ *Streptomycin.* Streptomycin is one of three aminoglycoside antibiotics (along with amikacin and kanamycin) that are active against mycobacteria. Streptomycin is quite active against MAC and several other mycobacteria, *Enterococci, Brucella, Yersinia*, and various other bacteria. Although labeled only for intramuscular dosing, streptomycin can be given safely as intravenous infusions (100 mL of dextrose 5% water or normal saline) over 30 minutes, similar to the other aminoglycosides.[68] Streptomycin, like other aminoglycosides, is cleared renally by glomerular filtration and must be given less often in patients with renal dysfunction.[39,43,51]

Streptomycin occasionally causes nephrotoxicity, although it tends to be mild and reversible. It also is capable of causing ototoxicity (vestibular and cochlear), which may become permanent with continued use.[39,52] Older patients and those receiving long durations of treatment are most likely to experience hearing loss, whereas vestibular toxicity is highly unpredictable.

Resistance to amikacin and kanamycin is frequently linked but independent of resistance to streptomycin and independent of resistance to capreomycin. Therefore, susceptibility tests should guide the selection of these injectable drugs.

▓ *p-Aminosalicylic Acid.* In the United States, only the enteric-coated, sustained-release granule form (Paser) is available.[69–71] Gastrointestinal disturbances are the most common adverse effects from *p*-aminosalicylic acid. Diarrhea is usually self-limited, with symptoms improving after the first 1 to 2 weeks of therapy. Occasionally, a few doses of an opiod will resolve the problem. It is also important to tell the patient that the empty granules will appear in the stool. Although FDA approved for three daily doses, pharmacokinetic data support twice-daily dosing.[70]

Various types of malabsorption, including steatorrhea, were reported with previous dosage forms of *p*-aminosalicylic acid. Hypersensitivity may occur and, rarely, severe hepatitis. *p*-Aminosalicylic acid is known to produce goiter, with or without myxedema, that seems to occur more frequently with concomitant ethionamide therapy.

▓ *Cycloserine.* Cycloserine is only used to treat MDR-TB. It is well absorbed orally and is best taken on an empty stomach.[72] It is cleared primarily through the kidneys by glomerular filtration and requires dosage reduction in renal failure. Cycloserine can produce

TABLE 110–7. Clinically Significant Drug-Drug Interactions Involving the Rifamycins

Drug Class	Drugs Whose Concentrations Are Substantially Decreased by Rifamycins (References)	Comments
Antiinfectives	HIV-1 protease inhibitors (saquinavir, indinavir, nelfinavir, amprenavir, ritonavir, lopinavir/ritonavir)	Can be used with rifabutin. Ritonavir, 400–600 mg twice daily, probably can be used with rifampin. The combination of saquinavir and ritonavir can also be used with rifampin.

	Nonnucleoside reverse transcriptase inhibitors
	  Delavirdine
	  Nevirapine
	  Efavirenz
		Delavirdine should not be used with any rifamycin. Doses of nevirapine and efavirenz need to be increased if given with rifampin, no dose increase needed if given with rifabutin.

	Macrolide antibiotics (clarithromycin, erythromycin)	Azithromycin has no significant interaction with rifamycins.
	Doxycycline	May require use of a drug other than doxycycline.
	Azole antifungal agents (ketoconazole, itraconazole, voriconazole)	Itraconazole, ketoconazole, and voriconazole concentrations may be subtherapeutic with any of the rifamycins. Fluconazole can be used with rifamycins, but the dose of fluconazole may have to be increased.
	Atovaquone	Consider alternate form of *Pneumocystis carinii* treatment or prophylaxis.
	Chloramphenicol	Consider an alternative antibiotic.
	Mefloquine	Consider alternate form of malaria prophylaxis.
Hormone therapy	Ethinylestradlol, norethindrone	Women of reproductive potential on oral contraceptives should be advised to add a barrier method of contraception when taking a rifamycin.
	Tamoxifen	May require alternate therapy or use of a nonrifamycin-containing regimen.
	Levothyroxine	Monitoring of serum TSH recommended; may require increased dose of levothyroxine.
Narcotics	Methadone	Rifampin and rifapentine use may require methadone dose increase; rifabutin infrequently causes methadone withdrawal.
Anticoagulants	Warfarin	Monitor prothrombin time; may require two- to threefold dose increase.
Immunosuppressive agents	Cyclosporine, tacrolimus	Rifabutin may allow concomitant use of cyclosporine and a rifamycin; monitoring of cyclosporine serum concentrations may assist with dosing.
	Corticosteroids	Monitor clinically; may require two- to threefold increase in corticosteroid dose.
Anticonvulsants	Phenytoin, lamotrigine	Therapeutic drug monitoring recommended; may require anticonvulsant dose increase.
Cardiovascular agents	Verapamil, nifedipine, diltiazem (a similar interaction is also predicted for felodipine and nisoldipine)	Clinical monitoring recommended; may require change to an alternate cardiovascular agent.
	Propranolol, metoporol	Clinical monitoring recommended; may require dose increase or change to an alternate cardiovascular drug.
	Enalapril, losartan	Monitor clinically; may require a dose increase or use of an alternate cardiovascular drug.
	Digoxin (among patients with renal insufficiency), digitoxin	Therapeutic drug monitoring recommended; may require digoxin or digitoxin dose increase.
	Quinidine	Therapeutic drug monitoring recommended; may require quinidine dose increase.
	Mexilitine, tocainide, propafenone	Clinical monitoring recommended; may require change to an alternate cardiovascular drug.
Bronchodilators	Theophylline	Therapeutic drug monitoring recommended; may require theophylline dose increase.
Sulfonylurea hypoglycemics	Tolbutamide, chlorpropamide, glyburide, glimepiride, repaglinide	Monitor blood glucose; may require dose increase or change to an alternate hypoglycemic drug.
Hypolipidemics	Simvastatin, fluvastatin	Monitor hypolipidemic effect; may require use of an alternate hypolipidemic drug.
Psychotropic drugs	Nortriptyline	Therapeutic drug monitoring recommended; may require dose increase or change to alternate psychotropic drug.
	Haloperidol, quetiapine	Monitor clinically; may require a dose increase or use of an alternate psychotropic drug.
	Benzodiazepines (e.g., diazepam, triazolam), zolpidem, buspirone	Monitor clinically; may require a dose increase or use of an alternate psychotropic drug.

dose-related CNS toxicity, including lethargy, confusion, or unusual behavior. Seizures, although reported, are exceedingly rare.[2,39,51] Therapy is vastly improved by maintaining 2-hour postdose serum concentrations between 20 and 35 mcg/mL.[43,45] Most patients reach a maximum dose of 750 mg daily, divided unevenly into two doses. This can be achieved by starting with 250 mg daily for 2 days, followed by 250-mg increments over 2-day intervals. This dose of cycloserine can be maintained if the patient complains of only occasional mild CNS effects, such as difficulty concentrating. Serum concentrations can be checked 1 to 2 weeks into therapy. The addition of pyridoxine 50 mg daily may improve patient tolerance of cycloserine.

Ethionamide.
Ethionamide shares structural features with two other antimycobacterial agents, isoniazid and, more distantly, thiacetazone, a drug not used in the United States. Prothionamide, the *n*-propyl derivative of ethionamide, is used in Europe. Ethionamide is only active against organisms of the genus *Mycobacterium*, and it should be considered primarily bacteriostatic because it is difficult to achieve serum concentrations that would be bactericidal.[39,43,45]

Gastrointestinal toxicity is the dose-limiting adverse effect. The drug should be introduced gradually in 250-mg increments, as described earlier for cycloserine. Rarely will a patient tolerate more than 1000 mg daily in divided oral doses. Ethionamide may be administered with a light snack or prior to bedtime to minimize gastrointestinal intolerance. Food does not affect absorption significantly.[73] Little ethionamide is recovered in the urine, so doses remain the same in renal failure. Ethionamide may cause goiter, with or without hypothyroidism (especially when given with *p*-aminosalicylic acid), gynecomastia, alopecia, impotence, menorraghia, photodermatitis, and acne. The management of diabetes also may be more difficult in patients receiving ethionamide. Because of these problems, ethionamide is only used when absolutely necessary.

Clofazimine.
Clofazimine is a drug with good activity against *M. leprae* and weak activity against *M. tuberculosis* and *M. avium*. It is used in doses of 100 to 200 mg daily in advanced cases of MDR-TB or MAC, especially when therapeutic options are limited.[39,43] The drug has a terminal elimination half-life that is weeks long. Gastrointestinal distress and skin discoloration are the most important adverse reactions. Although uncommon, severe gastrointestinal pain may occur because of deposition of clofazimine crystals within the intestines; this may require surgical correction.

Thiacetazone.
Thiacetazone is a weak agent used rarely in parts of the developing world because of its low cost. Skin reactions, including rash and Stevens-Johnson syndrome, may occur. Thiacetazone must be discontinued permanently as soon as a rash appears. Similar to trimethoprim-sulfamethoxazole, the incidence of skin reactions is much higher in AIDS patients.[74]

Quinolones.
Levofloxacin, ciprofloxacin, and moxifloxacin are sometimes used to treat MDR-TB. Moxifloxacin also is being studied as a possible replacement for certain first line agents, but data are not available at this time.[2,13,39,43] Quinolones are useful because most are available in oral and intravenous dosage forms, so they can be used in critically ill patients.

β-Lactam and β-Lactamase Inhibitor Combinations.
The β-lactams have limited activity against mycobacteria because of β-lactamases and because β-lactams fail to enter macrophages.[39,43,75] Cefoxitin, a β-lactamase-stable cephalosporin, has useful activity against rapidly growing mycobacteria, such as *M. fortuitum* and *M. chelonae*. Combinations of β-lactams with β-lactamase inhibitors have been used in salvage regimens for TB patients with no other options but are not used routinely to treat TB.

Macrolides/Azalides.
The macrolide clarithromycin and azalide azithromycin represent substantial advances in the treatment of MAC but demonstrate limited activity against *M. tuberculosis* and are not used frequently for TB.[2,13,39,43]

New Drugs and Delivery Systems.
The nitroimidazopyran PA 824, which is chemically related to metronidazole and tinidazole, has activity against *M. tuberculosis* in vitro.[76] This class, along with the oxazolidinones, may produce useful agents for TB. Linezolid has been used in a few patients with TB.[96] Long-term use of linezolid requires careful monitoring of hematologic indices for potential anemia and thrombocytopenia. Although not proved conclusively, it may be possible to reduce the incidences of these toxicities by giving linezolid 600 mg daily for the slow-growing *M. tuberculosis* rather than the usual twice-daily dose used for gram-positive organisms. Chemical modification of existing compounds, such as pyrazinamide, may produce new TB drugs. Finally, continuing research on the construction of the mycobacterial cell wall and intracellular pathways may lead to agents with unique activity against this genus.

Liposomes have been investigated as delivery systems for various agents against mycobacteria, including isoniazid, rifampin, and the aminoglycosides. Liposomes also could be used to deliver β-lactams or other agents that generally are excluded from macrophages. By changing the pharmacokinetic profile of such agents, their use in the treatment of mycobacterial infections could be enhanced greatly. Currently, no such product is licensed for use against TB.

Corticosteroids.
Adjunctive therapy with corticosteroids may be of benefit in some patients with tuberculous meningitis or pericarditis to relieve inflammation and pressure[2,39] (see Table 110–4). They should be avoided in most other circumstances because they detract from the immune response to TB.

Bacille Calmette-Guérin Vaccine (BCG).
The BCG vaccine is an attenuated, hybridized strain of *M. bovis*. It was developed in 1921 and is used as a prophylactic vaccine against TB. Administration of BCG vaccine is compulsory in many developing countries and is officially recommended in many others. Vaccination with BCG produces a subclinical infection resulting in sensitization of T-lymphocytes and cross-immunity to *M. tuberculosis*, as well as cutaneous hypersensitivity and, in many cases, a positive tuberculin skin test.

In the published clinical trials, several different BCG preparations were used, and the efficacy of these vaccinations ranged from negative 56% (some patients did worse with the vaccine) to positive 80%.[2,39] Trials within the United States and Puerto Rico have shown efficacy rates of 6% to 29%. The primary benefit of BCG vaccination appears to be the prevention of severe forms of TB in children. Data from the BCG trials show that the incidence of tuberculous meningitis and miliary TB is 52% to 100% lower and that the incidence of pulmonary TB is 2% to 80% lower in vaccinated children younger than 15 years of age than it was in unvaccinated controls.

Unfortunately, BCG does not appear to be very reliable in preventing disease by *M. tuberculosis* in other segments of the population. Side effects occur in 1% to 10% of vaccinated persons and usually include severe or prolonged ulceration at the vaccination site, lymphadenitis, and lupus vulgaris. It is recommended that pregnant women and patients with impaired immune systems, including those with HIV infection, avoid vaccination. The World Health Organization (WHO) has recommended, however, that in populations where the risk of TB is high, HIV-infected infants who are asymptomatic should receive BCG vaccine at birth or as soon as possible there-after. Because BCG infection has occurred in AIDS patients given the vaccine, individuals with symptomatic HIV infection should not be vaccinated.[2,39]

In the United States, BCG vaccination is recommended only for uninfected children who are at unavoidable risk of exposure to TB and for whom other methods of prevention and control have failed or are not feasible.[2,39] Its use is very limited.

PHARMACOECONOMIC CONSIDERATIONS

The WHO and the World Bank agree that the control of TB is one of the most cost-effective health interventions any nation can pursue. Early identification of TB cases and the effective use of isoniazid, rifampin, and pyrazinamide (plus ethambutol) while the isolate is still drug-susceptible always should be the primary goals of public health departments. Contact investigation and treatment of those infected but without disease are important secondary goals to reduce the number of future cases.

Patients who complete all their treatment for drug-susceptible TB have cure rates approaching 100%. Noncompliance (nonadherence), drug resistance, extrapulmonary disease, and concomitant disease states reduce the overall effectiveness of chemotherapy of TB to about 75%.

The treatment of TB is not particularly expensive, especially if hospitalization is not required.[77] Further, TB is quite curable. Because the various TB drugs each have a role to play in the treatment of TB or MDR-TB, all the antituberculosis drugs approved by the Food and Drug Administration should be on institutional formularies. Centers that see little MDR-TB need not keep stocks of the second-line drugs, provided that they are readily available should the need arise. Because the treatment of MDR-TB is difficult, and because missteps are potentially disastrous, such patients should be referred to centers experienced in the management of MDR-TB.[2,39,78,79]

EVALUATION OF THERAPEUTIC OUTCOMES

MONITORING OF THE PHARMACEUTICAL CARE PLAN

The most serious problem with TB therapy is patient nonadherence to the prescribed regimens.[80,81] Unfortunately, there is no reliable way to identify such patients a priori. In the study by Brudney and Dobkin,[80] 89% of the patients were noncompliant with therapy. It is critical to the control of TB that such adherence rates be improved dramatically. The most effective way to achieve this end is with DOT.[2,13,39] Despite criticisms that it will cost more money, it is far cheaper in the long run to prevent the further spread of disease with DOT than to track down and treat additional cases of TB continuously.

The homeless and other underprivileged individuals are assumed to constitute the group of patients considered "unreliable," and DOT should be reserved for them; it is also assumed that "responsible" patients cared for by private physicians may be treated with daily, unsupervised therapy. A study conducted in Baltimore, however, compared outcomes (sputum culture conversion to negative at 3 months) in patients with pulmonary TB who were treated by private physicians with outcomes in patients treated via DOT in a city-run clinic. Surprisingly, 3-month culture conversion occurred in only 40% of the private-care patients compared with 90% in the city clinic-care

patients.[82] Clearly, expansion of the use of DOT to nearly all patients with TB may be of benefit.

For patients who are AFB smear positive, they should have sputum samples sent for AFB stains every 1 to 2 weeks until two consecutive smears are negative. This provides early evidence of a response to treatment.[39] Once on maintenance therapy, sputum cultures can be performed monthly until two consecutive cultures are negative, which generally occurs over 2 to 3 months. If sputum cultures continue to be positive after 2 months, drug susceptibility testing should be repeated, and serum concentrations of the drugs should be checked.

Serum chemistries, including blood urea nitrogen, creatinine, aspartate transaminase (AST), and alanine transaminase (ALT) and a complete blood count with platelets should be performed at baseline and periodically thereafter, depending on the presence of other factors that may increase the likelihood of toxicity (e.g., advanced age, alcohol abuse, pregnancy).[2,39] Hepatotoxicity should be suspected in patients whose transaminases exceed five times the upper limit of normal or whose total bilirubin concentration exceeds 3 mg/dL and in patients with symptoms such as nausea, vomiting, or janudice. At this point, the offending agent(s) should be discontinued. Sequential reintroduction of the drugs with frequent testing of liver enzymes is often successful in identifying the offending agent; other agents may be continued. Alternative agents should be selected as needed. Audiometric testing should be performed at baseline and monthly in patients who must receive streptomycin for more than 1 to 2 months. Vision testing (Snellen visual acuity charts and Ishihara color discrimination plates) should be performed on all patients who receive ethambutol. All patients diagnosed with TB should be tested for HIV infection.

THERAPEUTIC DRUG MONITORING

Therapeutic drug monitoring (TDM) or applied pharmacokinetics is the use of serum drug concentrations to optimize therapy.[39,43,45] Non-AIDS patients with drug-susceptible TB generally do well, and TDM generally should be used if they are failing appropriate DOT (no clinical improvement after 2 to 4 weeks or smear-positive after 4 to 6 weeks). On the other hand, patients with AIDS, diabetes, cystic fibrosis, and various gastrointestinal disorders often fail to absorb these drugs properly and are candidates for TDM. Also, patients with hepatic or renal disease should be monitored, given their potential for overdoses.

In the treatment of MDR-TB, the differences between the maximum serum concentration (C_{max}) and the minimal inhibitory concentration (MIC) for the second-line agents are much smaller that with isoniazid and rifampin. Therefore, alterations in the absorption of these drugs can have significant impact on the outcome of therapy.[43,45] Although the optimal serum concentrations for TB are not known, target serum peak concentrations have been proposed.[43,45] Blood samples collected at 2 and 6 hours after a dose have been used with some success, although they may not be the optimal sampling times for all the drugs. Long-half-life drugs (e.g., pyrazinamide and cycloserine) can be sampled at 2 and 10 hours if an estimate of the half-life is desired. Finally, TDM of the TB and HIV drugs is perhaps the most logical way to untangle the complex drug interactions that take place[83] (see Table 110–7).

CLINICAL CONTROVERSY

Some TB centers employ TDM for many of their patients at the outset of treatment in order to identify drug-delivery problems early. Other centers wait to see how the patient responds and perform TDM only if problems arise. An argument can be made for either approach. The latter can save money, but delays in effective treatment can affect the patient's outcome adversely. Most otherwise healthy TB patients will absorb their drugs adequately. Patients who are critically ill or who have MDR-TB can benefit from early TDM.

CONCLUSIONS

Good patient adherence to treatment regimens is the cornerstone to effective antimycobacterial chemotherapy. Pharmacists should monitor TB therapy with particular interest in drug-drug interactions, drug malabsorption, and avoiding the error of adding a single drug to a failing regimen. They should educate patients on the importance of continuing their chemotherapy despite symptomatic improvement. Pharmacists should become part of a multidisciplinary team (with nurses, physicians, social workers) devoted to successful chemotherapy of TB patients and their families.

ABBREVIATIONS

AFB: acid-fast bacillus
ALT: alanine transaminase
AST: aspartate transaminase
ATS: American Thoracic Society
BCG: bacillus Calmette-Guérin
CDC: Centers for Disease Control and Prevention
CMI: cell-mediated immunity
CYP: cytochrome P450
DOT: directly observed treatment
DTH: delayed-type hypersensitivity
GC: gas chromatography
HPLC: high-pressure liquid chromatography
IBW: ideal body weight
IFN: interferon
LTBI: latent tuberculosis infection
MAC: *Mycobacterium avium* complex
MDR: multidrug resistance
MIC: minimal inhibitory concentration
NTM: nontuberculosis mycobacterium
PPD: purified protein derivative
RFLP: restriction-fragment-length polymorphism
TB: tuberculosis
TDM: therapeutic drug monitoring
TLC: thin-layer chromatography
TNF: tumor necrosis factor
WHO: World Health Organization
ZN: Ziehl-Neelsen strain

Review Questions and other resources can be found at *www.pharmacotherapyonline.com.*

REFERENCES

1. World Health Organization Report on the Global Tuberculosis Epidemic. Geneva, WHO, 1998.
2. Iseman MD. A Clinician's Guide to Tuberculosis. Philadelphia, Lippincott Williams & Wilkins, 2000.
3. Stead WW. The origin and erratic global spread of tuberculosis. Clin Chest Med 1997;18:65–77.
4. McCray E, Weinbaum CM, Braden CR, Onorato IM. The epidemiology of tuberculosis in the United States. Clin Chest Med 1997;18: 99–113.
5. Centers for Disease Control and Prevention. Trends in tuberculosis morbidity—United States, 1992–2002. MMWR 2003;52:222–224.
6. Centers for Disease Control and Prevention. Tuberculosis in the United States, 2002. Atlanta, CDC, September 2003.
7. Haas DW. *Mycobacterium tuberculosis.* In: Mandell GL, Bennett JE, Dolin R, eds. Principles and Practice of Infectious Diseases, 5th ed. New York, Churchill-Livingstone, 2000:2576–2607.
8. Small PM, Shafer RW, Hopewell PC, et al. Exogenous reinfection with multidrug-resistant *Mycobacterium tuberculosis* in patients with advanced HIV infection. N Engl J Med 1993;328:1137–1144.
9. Beck-Sague C, Dooley SW, Hutton MD, et al. Hospital outbreak of multidrug-resistant *Mycobacterium tuberculosis* infections: Factors in transmission to staff and HIV-infected patients. JAMA 1992;268:1280–1286.
10. Centers for Disease Control and Prevention. Meeting the challenge of multidrug-resistant tuberculosis: Summary of a conference. MMWR 1992;41:51–71.
11. Heifets L. Mycobacteriology laboratory. Clin Chest Med 1997;18: 35–53.
12. Heifets LB. Drug susceptibility tests in the management of chemotherapy of tuberculosis. In: Heifets LB, ed. Drug Susceptibility in the Chemotherapy of Mycobacterial Infections. Boca Raton, FL, CRC Press, 1991: 89–122.
13. Daley CL, Chambers HF. *Mycobacterium tuberculosis* complex. In: Yu VL, Weber R, Raoult D, eds. Antimicrobial Therapy and Vaccines, Vol I: Microbes, 2d ed. New York, Apple Trees Productions, 2002: 841–865.
14. Roberts GD, Böttger EC, Stockman L. Methods for the rapid identification of macybacterial species. Clin Lab Med 1996;16:603–615.
15. Sandin RL. Polymerase chain reaction and other amplification techniques in mycobacteriology. Clin Lab Med 1996;16:617–39.
16. Blanchard JS. Molecular mechanisms of drug resistance in *Mycobacterium tuberculosis.* Annu Rev Biochem 1996;65:215–239.
17. Somoskovi A, Parsons LM, Salfinger M. The molecular basis of resistance to isoniazid, rifampin, and pyrazinamide in *Mycobacterium tuberculosis.* Respir Res 2001;2:164–168.
18. Marin M, Garcia de Viedma D, Ruiz-Serrano MJ, Bouza E. Rapid direct detection of multiple rifampin and isoniazid resistance mutations in Mycobacterium tuberculosis in respiratory samples by real-time PCR. Antimicrob Agents Chemother 2004;48:4293–4300.
19. Riley RL, Mills CC, Nyka W, et al. Aerial dissemination of pulmonary tuberculosis: A two-year study of contagion in a tuberculosis ward. Am J Hygiene 1959;70:185–196.
20. Daniel TM, Boom WH, Ellner JJ. Immunology of tuberculosis. In: Reichman LB, Hershfield ES, eds. Tuberculosis: A Comprehensive International Approach, 2d ed. New York, Marcel Dekker, 2000:157–185.
21. Piessens WF, Nardell EA. Pathogenesis of tuberculosis. In: Reichman LB, Hershfield ES, eds. Tuberculosis: A Comprehensive International Approach, 2d ed. New York, Marcel Dekker, 2000: 241–260.
22. Long, R, Gardam, M. Tumour necrosis factor-α inhibitors and the reactivation of latent tuberculosis infection. Can Med Assoc J 2003;168:1153–1156.
23. American Thoracic Society/Centers for Disease Control and Prevention. Diagnostic standards and classification of tuberculosis in adults and children. Am J Respir Crit Care Med 2000;161:1376–1395.

24. Peloquin CA, Berning SE. Tuberculosis and multi-drug resistant tuberculosis in children. Pediatr Nurs 1995;21:566–572.

25. Correa AG. Unique aspects of tuberculosis in the pediatric population. Clin Chest Med 1997;18:89–98.

26. Alland D, Kalkut GE, Moss AR, et al. Transmission of tuberculosis in New York City: An analysis of DNA fingerprinting and conventional epidemiologic methods. N Engl J Med 1994;330:1710–1716.

27. Small PM, Hopewell PC, Singh SP, et al. The epidemiology of tuberculosis in San Francisco: A population-based study using conventional and molecular methods. N Engl J Med 1994;330:1703–1709.

28. Daley CL, Small PM, Schecter GF, et al. An outbreak of tuberculosis with accelerated progression among persons infected with the human immunodeficiency virus: An analysis using restricted-fragment-length polymorphisms. N Engl J Med 1992;326:231–235.

29. Wallis RS, Vjecha M, Amir-Tahmasseb M, et al. Influence of tuberculosis on human immunodeficiency virus (HIV-1): Enhanced cytokine expression and elevated β_2-microglobulin in HIV-1-associated tuberculosis. J Infect Dis 1993;167:43–48.

30. American Thoracic Society/Centers for Disease Control and Prevention. Targeted tuberculin skin testing and treatment of latent tuberculosis infection. Am J Respir Crit Care Med 2000;161:S221–247.

31. Pape JW, Jean SS, Ho JL, et al. Effect of isoniazid prophylaxis on incidence of active tuberculosis and progression of HIV infection. Lancet 1993;342:268–272.

32. Narita M, Ashkin D, Hollender ES, Pitchenik AE. Paradoxical worsening of tuberculosis following antiretroviral therapy in patients with AIDS. Am J Respir Crit Care Med 1998;158:157–161.

33. Barnes PF, Bloch AB, Davidson PT, Snider DE. Tuberculosis in patients with human immunodeficiency virus infection. N Engl J Med 1991;324:1644–1650.

34. Alvarez S, Shell C, Berk SL. Pulmonary tuberculosis in elderly men. Am J Med 1987;82:602–606.

35. Umeki S. Comparison of younger and elderly patients with pulmonary tuberculosis. Respiration 1989;55:75–83.

36. Centers for Disease Control and Prevention. Anergy skin testing and preventive therapy for HIV-infected persons: Revised recommendations. MMWR 1997;46:1–10.

37. Rosenberg T, Manfreda J, Hershfield ES. Two-step tuberculin testing in staff and residents of a nursing home. Am Rev Resp Dis 1993;148:1537–1540.

38. Bouza E, Diaz-Lopez MD, Moreno S, et al. Mycobacterium tuberculosis bacteremia in patients with and without human immunodeficiency virus infection. Arch Intern Med 1993;153:496–500.

39. American Thoracic Society/Centers for Disease Control/Infectious Disease Society of America. Treatment of tuberculosis. Am J Respir Crit Care Med 2003;167:603–662.

40. Fujiwara PI, Larkin C, Frieden TR. Directly observed therapy in New York City. Clin Chest Med 1997;18:135–148.

41. Weis SE. Universal directly observed therapy. Clin Chest Med 1997;18:155–163.

42. Mitchison DA. Basic mechanisms of chemotherapy. Chest 1979;76(suppl):771–781.

43. Peloquin CA. Pharmacological issues in the treatment of tuberculosis. Ann NY Acad Sci 2001;953:157–164.

44. Fourie PB, Ellner JJ, Johnson JL. Whither Mycobacterium vaccae—encore. Lancet 2002;360:1032–1033.

45. Peloquin CA. Therapeutic drug monitoring in the treatment of tuberculosis. Drugs 2002;62:2169–2183.

46. Peloquin CA. Antituberculosis drugs: Pharmacokinetics. In: Heifets LB, ed. Drug Susceptibility in the Chemotherapy of Mycobacterial Infections. Boca Raton, FL, CRC Press, 1991:59–88.

47. Hamadeh MA, Glassroth J. Tuberculosis and pregnancy. Chest 1992;101:1114–1120.

48. Vallejo JG, Starke JR. Tuberculosis and pregnancy. Clin Chest Med 1992;13:693–707.

49. Malone RS, Fish DN, Spiegel DM, et al. The effect of hemodialysis on isoniazid, rifampin, pyrazinamide, and ethambutol. Am J Respir Crit Care Med 1999;159:1580–1584.

50. Malone RS, Fish DN, Spiegel DM, et al. The effect of hemodialysis on cycloserine, ethionamide, para-aminosalicylate, and clofazimine. Chest 1999;116:984–990.

51. McEvoy GK, ed. AHFS Drug Information. Bethesda, MD, American Society of Health-Systems Pharmacists, 2003.

52. Girling DJ. Adverse effects of antituberculous drugs. Drugs 1982;23:56–74.

53. Holdiness MR. Clinical pharmacokinetics of the antituberculosis drugs. Clin Pharmacokinet 1984;9:511–544.

54. Crabbe SJ. Drug infosearch—intravenous isoniazid. P&T 1990;15:1483–1484.

55. Peloquin CA, Namdar R, Dodge AA, Nix DE. Pharmacokinetics of isoniazid under fasting conditions, with food, and with antacids. Intl J Tuberculosis Lung Dis 1999;3:703–710.

56. Berning SE, Peloquin CA. Antimycobacterial agents: Isoniazid. In: Yu VL, Merigan TC, Barriere S, White NJ, eds. Antimicrobial Chemotherapy and Vaccines. Baltimore, Williams & Wilkins, 1998:654–663.

57. Weiner M, Burman W, Vernon A, et al and the Tuberculosis Trials Consortium. Low isoniazid concentration associated with outcome of tuberculosis treatment with once-weekly isoniazid and rifapentine. Am J Respir Crit Care Med 2003;167:1341–1347.

58. Morris AB, Kanyok TP, Scott J, et al. Rifamycins. In: Yu VL, Merigan TC, Barriere S, White NJ, eds. Antimicrobial Chemotherapy and Vaccines. Baltimore, Williams & Wilkins, 1998:901–963.

59. Peloquin CA, Namdar R, Singleton MD, Nix DE. Pharmacokinetics of rifampin under fasting conditions, with food, and with antacids. Chest 1999;115:12–18.

60. CDC. Prevention and treatment of tuberculosis among patients infected with human immunodeficiency virus: Principles of therapy and revised recommendations. MMWR 1998;47:1–58.

61. CDC. Updated guidelines for the use of rifabutin or rifampin for the treatment and prevention of tuberculosis among HIV-infected patients taking protease inhibitors on nonnucleoside reverse transcriptase inhibitors. MMWR 2000;49:185–189.

62. Burman WJ, Gallicano K, Peloquin CA. Therapeutic implications of drug interactions in the treatment of HIV-related tuberculosis. Clin Infect Dis 1999;28:419–430.

63. Burman WJ, Gallicano K, Peloquin CA. Comparative pharmacokinetics and pharmacodynamics of the rifamycin antibiotics. Clin Pharmacokinet 2001:40:327–341.

64. Peloquin CA, Jaresko GS, Yong CL, et al. Population pharmacokinetic modeling of isoniazid, rifampin, and pyrazinamide. Antimicrob Agents Chemother 1997;41:2670–2679.

65. Peloquin CA, Bulpitt AE, Jaresko GS, et al. Pharmacokinetics of pyrazinamide under fasting conditions, with food, and with antacids. Pharmacotherapy 1998;18:1205–1211.

66. Peloquin CA, Bulpitt AE, Jaresko GS, et al. Pharmacokinetics of ethambutol under fasting conditions, with food, and with antacids. Antimicrob Agents Chemother 1999;43:568–572.

67. Summers KK, Hardin TC. Treatment of tuberculosis in hemodialysis patients. J Infect Dis Pharmacother 1996;2:37–55.

68. Peloquin CA, Berning SE. Comment: Intravenous streptomycin. Ann Pharmacother 1993;27:1546–1547.

69. Peloquin CA, Henshaw TL, Huitt GA, et al. Pharmacokinetic evaluation of p-aminosalicylic acid granules. Pharmacotherapy 1994;14:40–46 (and correction: Pharmacotherapy 1994;14:2).

70. Peloquin CA, Berning SE, Huitt GA, et al. Once-daily and twice-daily dosing of p-aminosalicylic acid (PAS) granules. Am J Respir Crit Care Med 1999;159:932–934.

71. Peloquin CA, Zhu M, Adam RD, et al. Pharmacokinetics of p-aminosalicylate under fasting conditions, with orange juice, food, and antacids. Ann Pharmacother 2001;35:1332–1338.

72. Zhu M, Nix DE, Adam RD, et al. Pharmacokinetics of cycloserine under fasting conditions, with orange juice, food, and antacids. Pharmacotherapy 2001;21:891–897.

73. Zhu M, Namdar R, Stambaugh JJ, et al. Population pharmacokinetics of ethionamide in patients with tuberculosis. Tuberculosis 2002;82:91–96.

74. Elliott AM, Foster SD. Thiacetazone: Time to call a halt? Tubercle Lung Dis 1996;77:27–29.

75. Zhang Y, Steingrube VA, Wallace RJ. Beta-lactamase inhibitors and the inducibility of the beta-lactamase of *Mycobacterium tuberculosis*. Am Rev Respir Dis 1992;145:657–660.

76. Stover CK, Warrener P, VanDevanter DR, et al. A small-molecule nitroimidazopyran drug candidate for the treatment of tuberculosis. Nature 2000;405:962–966.

77. Reves R, Burman W, Dalton C, et al. A cost-effectiveness analysis of directly-observed therapy versus self-administered therapy for treatment of tuberculosis. Am J Respir Crit Care Med 1997;155(suppl):A33.

78. Goble M, Iseman MD, Madsen LA, et al. Treatment of 171 patients with pulmonary tuberculosis resistant to isoniazid and rifampin. N Engl J Med 1993;328:527–532.

79. Iseman MD. Treatment of multidrug-resistant tuberculosis. N Engl J Med 1993;329:784–791.

80. Brudney K, Dobkin J. Resurgent tuberculosis in New York City: Human immunodeficiency virus, homelessness, and the decline of tuberculosis control programs. Am Rev Respir Dis 1991;144:745–749.

81. Mahmoudi A, Iseman MD. Pitfalls in the care of patients with tuberculosis: Common errors and their association with the acquisition of drug resistance. JAMA 1993;270:65–68.

82. Chaulk CP, Bartlett JG, Chaisson RE. 15 years of directly observed therapy for TB (abstract 181). In: Program and Abstracts, 32d Annual Meeting, Infectious Diseases Society of America, Orlando, FL, October 7–9, 1994.

83. Peloquin CA. Agents for tuberculosis. In Piscitelli SC, Rodvold KA, eds. Drug Interactions in Infectious Diseases. Totowa, NJ, Humana Press, 2001:109–120.

111

GASTROINTESTINAL INFECTIONS AND ENTEROTOXIGENIC POISONINGS

Steven Martin and Rose Jung

Learning Objectives and other resources can be found at *www.pharmacotherapyonline.com.*

KEY CONCEPTS

❶ The etiology of infectious diarrhea includes bacteria, viruses, and protozoans. Viral infections are the leading cause of diarrhea in the world.

❷ Fluid and electrolyte replacement is the cornerstone of therapy. Oral rehydration therapy is preferred in most cases of mild and moderate diarrhea. The necessary components of oral replacement therapy are glucose, sodium, potassium, chloride, and water.

❸ Antimicrobial therapy often is not indicated for enteritis because many cases are mild and self-limited or are viral in nature.

❹ When antimicrobials are used for enteritis, they should be active against the most likely pathogen based on clinical symptoms, epidemiologic patterns, and resistance patterns in the area.

❺ The most common pathogens for traveler's diarrhea include enterotoxigenic *Escherichia coli*, *Shigella*, *Campylobacter*, *Salmonella*, and viruses.

❻ Patient education and prevention strategies are important in preventing and treating traveler's diarrhea. Prophylaxis with antibiotics is appropriate in certain situations.

❼ Common pathogens responsible for food poisoning include *Staphylococcus*, *Salmonella*, *Shigella*, and *Clostridium*.

Gastrointestinal (GI) infections encompass a wide variety of syndromes from mild gastroenteritis to life-threatening systemic infections. Dehydration from GI infections is the second leading cause of morbidity and mortality worldwide, especially in infants and children younger than 5 years of age. From 1992 to 2000, the median incidence of diarrhea for all children younger than 5 years of age was 3.2 episodes per child-year. The incidence of diarrhea was higher in younger children, with 4.8 episodes per child per year among children aged 6 to 11 months in comparison with 1.4 episodes per child per year for 4-year-olds. Younger children also had a higher risk for death from acute dehydrating diarrhea. For children younger than 1 year of age and those aged 1 to 4 years, the median mortality rates were 8.5 and 3.8 per 1000 children per year, respectively. Overall, the median mortality for children younger than 5 years of age was 4.9 per 1000 per year.[1] Although this was a decrease from 13.6 per 1000 per year during 1955–1979 and 5.6 per 1000 per year during 1980–1989, diarrhea remains a severe disease in children, especially in those younger than 1 year of age.[2,3]

In the developing world, the risk of death is highest among young children, but in developed countries such as the United States, most of those who die of diarrheal illness are elderly. According to data from the National Center for Health Statistics, for the 9-year period from 1979 to 1987, there were an average of 3171 deaths per year from diarrheal disease, of which 51% were among patients over 74 years of age, 27% were 55 to 74 years old, and 11% were younger than 5 years of age.[4] Similarly, a study of the McDonnell-Douglas Health Information System database revealed that 25% of all hospitalizations and 85% of all mortality associated with diarrhea involved the elderly ($\geq$60 years old).[5] Other groups at risk for GI infections include travelers and campers, immunocompromised patients such as those with the acquired immunodeficiency syndrome (AIDS), patients in chronic care facilities, and military personnel assigned overseas.

❶ A variety of pathogens can be responsible for acute infectious diarrhea. Viruses are the most common cause of gastroenteritis in children. Bacterial species that are commonly associated with infectious diarrhea in the United States are *Shigella* spp., *Salmonella* spp., *Campylobacter* spp., *Yersinia* spp., *Escherichia* spp., *Clostridium* spp., and *Staphylococcus* spp. Although not a major cause in North America, *Vibrio* spp. is a leading cause of bacterial gastroenteritis on a global scale. This chapter focuses on the bacterial and viral etiologies of GI infections such as *Vibrio cholerae*, *Escherichia coli*, *Salmonella*, *Shigella*, *Campylobacter jejuni*, rotaviruses, Norwalk-like viruses, astrovirus, and enteric adenovirus.

EPIDEMIOLOGY

Several U.S. population–based studies have estimated the prevalence of acute GI infections and the burden of illness resulting from acute diarrhea. Based on these studies, the estimates by the Centers for Disease Control and Prevention (CDC) suggest that 211 million episodes of acute gastroenteritis occur each year in the United States, resulting in over 900,000 hospitalizations and over 6000 deaths.[6] Although infectious diarrhea in the United States is often self-limited, the economic burden of GI infections still remains enormous.

Diarrheal illness accounts for 2 to 3.7 million doctor visits and 200,000 hospitalizations per year in children younger than 5 years of age in the United States.[7] The cost per diarrhea episode resulting in a physician visit in children younger than 5 years of age is estimated to be approximately $290. This extrapolates to a cost of over $2 billion per year for children younger than 5 years of age. In a study of claims data from a large insurance database from 1993 to 1996 for children younger than 5 years of age with diarrhea, an annual average rate of 35 hospitalizations and 943 outpatient visits per 10,000 children occurred.[8] Six deaths (0.08%) occurred during this period. The median payments (in constant 1998 dollars) for hospitalization decreased from $2528 in 1993 to $2101 in 1996. The median payment for outpatient visits was $47. The total payments for combined diarrhea-associated hospitalizations and outpatient visits averaged $7.1 million (in 1998 dollars) per year, with hospitalizations accounting for three-fourths of these payments. In addition, 50% of diarrheal illnesses lead to at least one full day of lost activity by patients or the parents of patients. This results in a total projected cost of diarrheal disease of $23 billion per year in the United States based on estimated medical costs and lost productivity.[9]

In addition, traveler's diarrhea interferes with planned activities or work in 30% of those affected, accounting for unknown but substantial direct and indirect lost dollars because of decreased productivity.[10]

CLINICAL PRESENTATION

In patients with GI illnesses, a careful history and physical examination are crucial in providing clues to the likely etiology. An organism-specific diagnosis is necessary for the appropriate management and treatment in moderate to severe cases. Unfortunately, the methods for diagnosis of diarrheal disease vary widely in clinical practice. One practice guideline recommends selective approaches to improving cost-effectiveness of stool cultures.[11] Fecal testing is recommended in patients with community-acquired diarrheal illnesses lasting for more than 1 day in patients with a recent use of antibiotics, day-care center attendance, hospitalization, or illness accompanied by fever, bloody stools, systemic illness, or dehydration. In hospitalized patients, fecal testing for standard bacterial pathogens (*Campylobacter, Salmonella, Shigella,* etc.) or ova and parasites is not recommended for diarrhea that occurs 3 days after the start of hospitalization owing to low yield, except in persons 65 years of age and older with comorbid disease, neutropenia, or human immunodeficiency virus (HIV) infection. Microscopic examination for fecal polymorphonuclear cells or a simple immunoassay for the neutrophil marker lactoferrin can further provide evidence of an inflammatory process and increase the yield of culture for invasive pathogens in patients presenting with fever or bloody stool.

For community-acquired or traveler's diarrhea, stool samples should be sent for culture of *Salmonella, Shigella, Campylobacter,* and *Escherichia coli* O157:H7.[11] A careful history may further point to specific etiologic agents. Bloody diarrhea may indicate enterohemorrhagic *E. coli.* Outbreaks should prompt consideration of *Staphylococcus aureus, Bacillus cereus, Clostridium perfringens, Vibrio, Salmonella, Campylobacter, Shigella,* or *E. coli* infection. Ingestion of inadequately cooked seafood should increase suspicions for infections with *Vibrio* or Norwalk-like viruses. Antibiotics predispose patients to cytotoxigenic *Clostridium difficile.* Travel to tropical areas increases the chances of developing enterotoxigenic *E. coli,* viral (Norwalk-like or rotaviral), and parasitic infections (*Giardia, Entamoeba, Strongyloides,* and *Cryptosporidium*).

For patients who develop diarrhea after 3 days of hospitalization, 15% to 20% of cases are due to *C. difficile.*[11] This suggests that in hospitalized patients, especially in those who are exposed to antimicrobial therapy or chemotherapy, the stool specimen should be tested for *C. difficile* toxin(s). In immunocompromised hosts, a wide range of viral, bacterial, and parasitic agents should be tested.

▶ TREATMENT: Diarrhea

▦ GENERAL APPROACHES TO TREATMENT

▦ REHYDRATION THERAPY

❷ Fluid replacement is the cornerstone of therapy for diarrhea regardless of etiology. Initial assessment of fluid loss is essential for rehydration, but an accurate baseline weight may not be available. Acute weight loss is the most reliable means of determining the extent of water loss. Clinical signs can be helpful in determining approximate deficits[12] (Table 111–1). Serum electrolyte concentrations should be measured. Physical assessment generally is more reliable in young children and infants than in adults.

Glucose-based oral rehydration therapy (ORT) reverses dehydration in nearly all patients with mild to moderate diarrhea.[12] Treatment failure is infrequent (3% to 6%).[13] Oral rehydration therapy offers the advantages of being inexpensive and noninvasive and does not require hospitalization for administration. In those who are able to take oral fluids, ORT is superior to administration of intravenous (IV) fluids. In addition, thirst drives ORT and provides a safeguard against overhydration. Glucose-based ORT generally does not decrease the duration of diarrhea or stool volume, but it does prevent dehydration, which is responsible for most diarrheal deaths. Weight loss of 9% to 10% is considered severe and requires IV fluid replacement with Ringer's lactate or normal saline. Intravenous therapy is also indicated in patients with uncontrolled vomiting, the presence of a paralytic ileus, stool output greater than 10 mL/kg per hour, shock, or loss of consciousness. Rapid IV rehydration is preferred over more prolonged deficit-replacement regimens for restoring extracellular fluids and electrolytes because it more effectively reestablishes gastrointestinal and renal perfusion.[14] Table 111–1 summarizes fluid-replacement guidelines for each dehydration category.

The necessary components of ORT solutions include glucose, sodium, potassium, chloride, and water[13,15] (Table 111–2). Oral rehydration therapy takes advantage of glucose-coupled sodium transport in the small bowel. Glucose enhances sodium and subsequently water transport across intestinal walls. Glucose concentrations greater than 5% may produce an osmotic diarrhea. Low-osmolarity ORT solutions (rice- or cereal-based) reduce the diarrhea stool number, volume, and frequency, as well as the duration of diarrhea and the ORT solution volume requirements when compared with isotonic high-glucose ORT solutions similar to the World Health Organization (WHO) formulation.[16] The efficacy of rice-based ORT solutions may be a result in part of their hypotonicity, which promotes intestinal water absorption.[17] Also, slow rice hydrolysis allows some rice (glucose) absorption to take place before hydrolysis occurs. Starch and simple proteins provide more cotransport molecules with a lower intraluminal osmotic load, thus increasing fluid and electrolyte uptake by enterocytes and reducing stool losses.[15] Therefore, a larger

TABLE 111–1. Clinical Assessment of Degree of Dehydration in Children Based on Percentage of Body Weight Loss*

Variable	Mild, 3%–5%	Moderate, 6%–9%	Severe, ≥10%
Blood pressure	Normal	Normal	Normal to reduced
Quality of pulses	Normal	Normal or slightly decreased	Moderately decreased
Heart rate	Normal	Increased	Increased (bradycardia in severe cases)
Skin turgor	Normal	Decreased	Decreased
Fontanelle	Normal	Sunken	Sunken
Mucous membranes	Slightly dry	Dry	Dry
Eyes	Normal	Sunken orbits/decreased tears	Deeply sunken orbits/decreased tears
Extremities	Warm, normal capillary refill	Delayed capillary refill	Cool, mottled
Mental status	Normal	Normal to listless	Normal to lethargic or comatose
Urine output	Slightly decreased	<1 mL/kg/h	<1 mL/kg/h
Thirst	Slightly increased	Moderately increased	Very thirsty or too lethargic to indicate
Fluid replacement	ORT 50 mL/kg over 2–4 h	ORT 100 mL/kg over 2–4 h	Ringer lactate 40 mL/kg in 15–30 min, then 20–40 mL/kg if skin turgor, alertness, and pulse have not returned to normal *or* Ringer lactate or NS 20 mL/kg, repeat if necessary, and then replace water and electrolyte deficits over 1–2 days
	Replace ongoing losses with low-sodium ORT (40–60 mEg/L Na$^+$) at 10 mL/kg per stool or emesis	Replace ongoing losses with low-sodium ORT (40–60 mEq/L Na$^+$) at 10 mL/kg per stool or emesis	Followed by ORT 100 mL/kg over 4 hours. Replace ongoing losses with low-sodium ORT (40–60 mEq/L Na$^+$) at 10 mL/kg per stool or emesis

*Percentages vary among authors for each dehydration category; hemodynamic and perfusion status is most important; when unsure of category, therapy for more severe category is recommended.
ORT, oval rehydration therapy
Adapted from refs. 10 and 15.

carbohydrate load can be given with rice solutions, resulting in a greater nutritional advantage. Amylase-resistant starch added to standard ORT solutions shortened the duration of diarrhea in cholera patients as compared with standard ORT solutions and rice-based ORT solutions.[18] Human breast milk, cow's milk, glycine, soy fiber formulas, and cereal preparations have been used successfully as rehydration substrates.[19,20]

Sodium content for oral replacement solutions should be between 50 and 90 mEq/L for initial rehydration. The American Academy of Pediatrics (AAP) recommends rehydration with a more electrolyte-concentrated rehydration phase and a subsequent maintenance phase using the more dilute solutions and larger volume[21] (see Table 111–1). In children with vomiting and diarrhea, ORT may be given as 5 mL

every 2 to 3 minutes in a teaspoon or oral syringe. Nasogastric administration of ORT is an alternative method of administration in a child with persistent vomiting.[12] Maintenance rehydration requires sodium concentrations between 40 and 60 mEq/L. ORT solutions with high sodium content may be alternated with water if a low-sodium fluid is not available. The maintenance phase should provide 100–150 mL/kg per day plus additional replacement for stool losses. Clear fluids, such as soda, apple juice, broth, and Gatorade, are hyperosmolar solutions that may draw free water into the gut lumen and cause hypernatremia. Use of these solutions should be avoided.

Early refeeding as tolerated is recommended.[22] The AAP guidelines recommend age-appropriate diet resumption as soon as dehydration is corrected.[21] Breast milk, lactose-free soy formula, and cow's

TABLE 111–2. Comparison of Common Solutions Used in Oral Rehydration and Maintenance

Product	Na (mEq/L)	K (mEq/L)	Base (mEq/L)	Carbohydrate (mmol/L)	Osmolality (mOsm/L)
Naturalyte (unlimited beverage)	45	20	48	140	265
Pediatric electrolyte (NutraMax)	45	20	30	140	250
Pedialyte (Ross)	45	20	30	140	250
Infalyte (formerly Ricelyte; Mead Johnson)	50	25	30	70	200
Rehydralyte (Ross)	75	20	30	140	310
WHO/UNICEF oral rehydration salts	90	20	30	111	310
Cola	2	0	13	700	750
Apple juice	5	32	0	690	730
Chicken broth	250	8	0	0	500
Sports beverage	20	3	3	255	330

Adapted from ref. 15.

milk–based formulas often can be continued.[12,22] Early initiation of feeding has shortened the course of diarrhea. In a study of severely malnourished children younger than 5 years of age with diarrhea, using a standardized protocol of slower oral rehydration, immediate feeding, and intensive management of complications resulted in a significant reduction of mortality as compared with standard therapy. Initially, easily digested foods, such as bananas, applesauce, and cereal, may be added. Foods high in fiber, sodium, and sugar should be avoided. Lactase deficiency may be exacerbated among known lactase-deficient patients and may persist up to 10 days.

After starting rehydration therapy, parents should be instructed to observe the child for a reversal of the signs of dehydration, increased stool consistency, and decreased stool frequency. If ORT is not improving the fluid status and the patient continues to produce frequent, large-volume watery stools, close supervision with medical support is justified.[22]

▣ ANTIMICROBIAL THERAPY

The indiscriminate use of antimicrobial therapy in GI infections produces increases in antimicrobial resistance, side effects of antimicrobial agents, and the threat of superinfections owing to eradication of normal flora. Increasing fluoroquinolone resistance in *Campylobacter* and multidrug resistance in *Salmonella* species worldwide reinforce the importance of local resistance patterns in making decisions about antimicrobial therapy.[23,24] Knowledge of the local patterns of susceptibility can guide the initial choice of antibiotic, but the appropriate choice ultimately depends on isolation of pathogens from recent clinical specimens. To decrease resistance, antibiotics should be prescribed judiciously in addition to adoption of prudent infection control measures.

◄3   Antibiotics are not essential in the treatment of most mild diarrheas, and empirical therapy for acute GI infections may result in courses of unnecessary antibiotics. However, appropriate antibiotic

TABLE 111–3. Recommendations for Antibiotic Therapy

Pathogen	First-Line Agents	Alternative Agents
Enterotoxigenic (Cholera-Like) Diarrhea		
Vibrio cholerae O1 or O139	Doxycycline 300 mg oral single dose; tetracycline 500 mg orally four times daily × 3 days; or trimethoprim-sulfamethoxazole DS tablet twice daily × 3 days; norfloxacin 400 mg orally twice daily × 3 days; or ciprofloxacin 500 mg orally twice daily × 3 days or 1 g orally single dose	Chloramphenicol 50 mg/kg IV every 6 hours, erythromycin 250–500 mg PO every 6–8 hours, and furazolidone
Enterotoxigenic *E. coli*	Norfloxacin 400 mg or ciprofloxacin 500 mg orally twice daily × 3 days	Trimethoprim-sulfamethoxazole DS tablet every 12 hours
C. difficile	Metronidazole 250 mg four times daily to 500 mg three times daily × 10 days	Vancomycin 125 mg orally four times daily × 10 days; bacitracin 20,000–25,000 units four times daily × 7–10 days
Invasive (Dysentery-Like) Diarrhea		
Shigella species[a]	Trimethoprim-sulfamethoxazole DS twice daily × 3–5 days	Ofloxacin 300 mg, norfloxacin 400 mg, or ciprofloxacin 500 mg twice daily × 3 days, or nalidixic acid 1 g/day ×5 days; azithromycin 500 mg orally × 1, then 250 mg orally daily × 4 days.
Salmonella		
Nontyphoidal[a]	Trimethoprim-sulfamethoxazole DS twice daily; ofloxacin 300 mg, norfloxacin 400 mg, or ciprofloxacin 500 mg twice daily × 5 days; or ceftriaxone 2 g IV daily or cefotaxime 2 g IV three times daily × 5 days	Azithromycin 1000 mg orally × 1 day, followed by 500 mg orally once daily × 6 days
Enteric fever	Ciprofloxacin 500 mg orally twice daily × 3–14 days (ofloxacin and perfloxacin equally efficacious)	Azithromycin 1000 mg orally × 1 day, followed by 500 mg daily × 5 days; or cefixime, cefotaxime, and cefuroxime; or chloramphenicol 500 mg four times daily orally or IV × 14 days
Campylobacter[a]	Erythromycin 500 mg orally twice daily × 5 days; azithromycin 1000 mg orally × 1 day, followed by 500 mg daily or clarithromycin 500 mg orally twice daily	Ciprofloxacin 500 mg or norfloxacin 400 mg orally twice daily × 5 days
Yersinia species[a]	A combination therapy with doxycycline, aminoglycosides, trimethoprim-sulfamethoxazole, or fluoroquinolones	
Traveler's Diarrhea		
Prophylaxis[a]	Norfloxacin 400 mg or ciprofloxacin 500 mg orally daily (in Asia, Africa, and South America); trimethoprim-sulfamethoxaxole DS tablet orally daily (in Mexico)	
Treatment	Norfloxacin 400 mg or ciprofloxacin 500 mg orally twice daily × 3 days, or trimethoprim-sulfamethoxazole DS tablet orally twice daily × 3 days (in Mexico), or azithromycin 500 mg orally once daily × 3 days (only in areas of high prevalence of quiniolone-resistant *Campylobacter* species, such as Thailand)	

[a]For high-risk patients only. See the preceding text for the high-risk patients in each infection.

therapy has been shown to shorten illness and reduce morbidity in some bacterial (cholera, enterotoxigenic *E. coli*, shigellosis, campylobacteriosis, yersiniosis) infections and can be lifesaving in invasive infections (*C. difficile*, salmonellosis). Antibiotic treatment also reduces the duration and shedding of organisms in infections with susceptible *Shigella* spp. and possibly in infection with susceptible *Campylobacter* spp.[25,26]

It is also important to note that outcomes of some bacterial diarrheal illnesses may be worsened by the use of antibiotics. Antibiotic treatment may prolong asymptomatic carriage of *Salmonella*.[27] In patients infected with *E. coli* O157, use of an antimicrobial agent may worsen the risk of hemolytic-uremic syndrome (HUS), which is defined by the triad of acute renal failure, thrombocytopenia, and microangiopathic hemolytic anemia, by increasing the production of shiga-like toxin.[28]

Table 111–3 summarizes antibiotic recommendations, and further details in the treatment of specific infections are discussed in appropriate sections.

ANTIMOTILITY AGENTS

Agents that inhibit peristalsis such as diphenoxylate and loperamide are contraindicated in most toxin-mediated diarrheal illnesses (enterohemorrhagic *E. coli*, pseudomembranous colitis, shigellosis). Slowing of fecal transit time is thought to result in extended toxin-associated damage. On the other hand, in traveler's diarrhea, a combination of appropriate antibiotics and loperamide controls symptoms within 10 hours.[29]

PREVENTION OF GASTROINTESTINAL INFECTIONS

Many diarrheal diseases can be prevented by following simple rules of personal hygiene and safe food preparation. Handwashing with soap is instrumental in preventing the spread of illness and should be emphasized for caregivers and persons with diarrheal illnesses. Safe food handling and preparation practices can decrease the incidence of certain types of enteric infections significantly. The public health measures of improved water supply and sanitation facilities and the quality control of commercial products are very important for the control of the majority of enteric infections.

Reporting suspected outbreaks and cases of notifiable illness to local health authorities is vital to allow measures to be taken to investigate threats of enteric infection arising from increasingly global and industrialized food supplies. The reporting of specific infectious diseases to the appropriate public health authorities is the cornerstone of public health surveillance, outbreak detection, and prevention and control efforts.

Vaccines also may be used to boost specific immune processes directed against the bacteria themselves or against adherence appendages, cytotoxins, or enterotoxins. Currently available vaccines for typhoid fever in the United States are the parenteral Vi capsular polysaccharide vaccine, the oral live-attenuated Ty21a vaccine, and the older heat-phenol-inactivated parenteral vaccine.[30] Only the older parenteral cholera vaccine is licensed for use in the United States, but it is not recommended owing to the low risk of cholera to the traveler and the limited efficacy of the vaccine.[31] New oral live and killed vaccines are licensed outside the United States and are used by some travelers. The rotavirus vaccine, although effective, has presented complications in the form of rare cases of intussusceptions; it is no longer marketed and thus is not recommended.[32]

PATIENT ASSESSMENT

Appropriate follow-up care of patients with acute diarrhea is based on successful restoration of fluid losses. The clinical signs and symptoms (see Table 111–1) that led to the diagnosis also can indicate adequate rehydration and should be assessed frequently. Because oral rehydration therapy is now preferred, routine laboratory testing often is unnecessary. Electrolytes should be measured in those receiving parenteral fluids, when oral replacement fails, or when signs of hypernatremia or hypokalemia are present. Follow-up stool samples to ensure complete evacuation of the infecting pathogen may be necessary only

in patients at high risk to initiate or contribute to a community outbreak. All patients should be monitored for complications associated with the infecting pathogen, resolution of the diarrhea, and adverse reactions to the pharmacologic agents used. One panel suggests prompt discharge of hospitalized children when rehydration is achieved, IV fluids have not been required, oral intake equals or exceeds losses, or adequate family education and medical follow-up are ensured. For most patients, discharge can occur in 16 to 24 hours.

BACTERIAL INFECTIONS

Bacterial agents are important causes of GI infections, and syndromes caused by these pathogens are better understood than viral gastroenteritis. For a simple generalization, the bacterial pathogens presented in this section are divided into either those which cause watery (enterotoxigenic) diarrhea or those which cause dysentery (invasive diarrhea). Watery diarrhea is usually self-limiting, whereas those who present with dysenteric symptoms, such as fever, tenesmus, and blood and/or pus in the stool, require close monitoring and intensive follow-up. Clinical signs and symptoms of these two broad categories are presented in the Table 111–4.

ENTEROTOXIGENIC (CHOLERA-LIKE) DIARRHEA

CHOLERA (*VIBRO CHOLERAE*)

Epidemiology

Cholera has been endemic in the Ganges delta, West Bengal, Bangladesh, and southern Asia (including Southeast Asia) since at least 1817.[33] A 1994 outbreak of a multidrug-resistant strain of cholera among Rwandan refugees resulted in more than 20,000 deaths. Cholera epidemics in 1991 and 1998 caused more than 1 million deaths in Latin America. As international travel has increased, the occurrence of cholera in the United States also has increased. Cholera has been reported in all major regions of the United States. However, the incidence, 1 case per 1 million persons, is extremely low.[34]

Vibrio cholerae O1 is the most common serogroup associated with epidemics and pandemics. Within this serogroup, there are two biotypes, classic and El Tor.[33] The six pandemics since 1817 presumably were caused by the classic biotype, and the seventh pandemic introduced the El Tor biotype. In 1992, a new serogroup, *V. cholerae* O139 Bengal, appeared in India and spread rapidly through Southeast

TABLE 111–4. Acute Infectious Diarrhea Clinical Syndromes: Watery vs. Dysenteric

	Watery	Dysenteric
Percentage of Patients	90	5–10
Stools		
Appearance	Watery	Bloody
Volume	Increased: ++/+++	Increased: +/++
Number per day	<10	>10
Reducing substances	0 to +++	0
pH	5.0–7.5	6.0–7.5
Occult blood	Negative	Positive
Fecal PMN cells	Absent or few	Many
Mechanisms	Toxins	Mucosal invasion
	Reduced absorption	
Complications		
Dehydration	Could be severe	Mild
Others	Acidosis, shock, electrolyte imbalance	Tenesmus, rectal prolapse, seizures
Etiology	Rotaviruses	*Shigella* spp.
	Enterotoxigenic *E. coli*	*Campylobacter* spp.
	V. cholerae	*S. enteritidis*

Adapted from Ref. 7.

Asia. *V. cholerae* O139 also has been isolated from food-production animals in the Netherlands. Four mechanisms for transmission have been proposed, including animal reservoirs, chronic carriers, asymptomatic or mild disease victims, and water reservoirs. A relatively large inoculum of 10^3 to 10^6 is required for infection if water is the vehicle and 10^2 to 10^4 if the vehicle is food. Approximately half the people infected with *V. cholerae* O1 are symptomatic, whereas only 1% to 5% of those infected with *V. cholerae* O139 manifest symptoms. The hallmark of cholera is the production of watery diarrhea, and severe dehydration may develop within a few hours, causing death within 24 hours. An estimated 25% to 50% of cases are fatal if left untreated. The prevention of cholera transmission depends on the provision of clean drinking water and public sanitation, which is difficult in impoverished developing countries.[33]

TREATMENT: Cholera

Regardless of the serotypes, the primary goal of therapy is restoration of fluid and electrolyte losses caused by watery diarrhea. ORT is the preferred method of rehydration, and several studies showed reduction in fluid requirements by 32% to 35% when rice-based instead of glucose-based ORT solutions are used (50–80 g rice instead of 20 g glucose per liter).[36] In patients who cannot tolerate ORT, IV Ringer's lactate solution can be used.[37] Normal saline is not recommended because it does not correct metabolic acidosis. After rehydration, maintenance fluid is given based on accurate recording of intake and output volumes.

Antibiotics shorten the duration of diarrhea, decrease fluid loss, and shorten the duration of the carrier state.[37] Table 111–3 provides recommendations on antibiotic selection. There appears to be substantial mobility in genetic elements encoding antibiotic resistance in *V. cholerae*, and the drug resistance patterns may change between outbreaks. For example, O139 strains isolated during 1992 and

Pathogenesis

V. cholerae is a gram-negative bacillus sharing similar characteristics with the family Enterobacteriaceae. Most pathology of cholera results from an enterotoxin (cholera toxin) produced by the bacteria.[33] Conditions that reduce gastric acidity, such as the use of antacids, histamine-receptor blockers, or proton pump inhibitors or infections with *Helicobacter pylori,* increase the risk for clinical disease. Cholera toxin stimulates adenylate cyclase, which increases intracellular cAMP and results in inhibition of sodium and chloride absorption by microvilli and promotes the secretion of chloride and water by crypt cells. The toxin likely acts along the entire intestinal tract, but most fluid loss occurs in the duodenum.[35] The net effect of the cholera toxin is isotonic fluid secretion (primarily in the small intestine) that exceeds the absorptive capacity of the intestinal tract (primarily the colon). This results in the production of watery diarrhea with electrolyte concentrations similar to that of plasma.

Clinical Presentation

The average incubation period for *V. cholerae* infection is 1 to 3 days.[35] The clinical presentation can vary from asymptomatic to life-threatening dehydration owing to watery diarrhea. The onset of diarrhea is abrupt and is followed rapidly or sometimes preceded by vomiting. Initial stools generally do not have the "rice water" appearance that is classically noted with cholera. Fever occurs in less than 5% of patients, and the physical examination correlates well with the severity of dehydration. In the most severe state, this disease can progress to death in 2 to 4 hours if not treated. In some cases, fluid accumulates within the intestinal lumen causing abdominal distension and ileus and may cause intravascular depletion without diarrhea. Patients may lose up to 1 liter of isotonic fluid every hour.

Laboratory abnormalities such as increased packed red blood cell volume and total protein, magnesium, and calcium levels are a result of hemoconcentration. Hypoglycemia, seizures, fever, and mental alterations are seen more often in children, perhaps as a reflection of the greater degree of dehydration and electrolyte losses observed with diarrhea in children.[33,35] Other complications include metabolic acidosis, prerenal azotemia, iatrogenic water intoxication from overrehydration, and aspiration pneumonia. Children, the elderly, and pregnant women are at an increased risk of complications due to cholera.

1993 showed a trend toward increased resistance to trimethoprim-sulfamethoxazole, but those isolated in India during 1996 and 1997 showed susceptibility to the same agent.[35] A single dose of doxycycline is the preferred agent, especially in endemic areas, although it has been associated with prolonged fecal excretion of bacteria. In children younger than 7 years of age, trimethoprim-sulfamethoxazole, erythromycin, and fuazolidone are preferred. In pregnant women, erythromycin or furazolidone can be used. In areas of high tetracycline resistance, fluoroquinolones such as ciprofloxacin are effective. Ciprofloxacin has been studied more extensively than other fluoroquinolones.[38]

The manufacture of the only licensed whole-cell cholera vaccine in the United States has been discontinued. Two vaccines are available in other countries.[35] These are oral vaccines; Dukoral consists of killed *V. cholerae* organisms and the cholera B subunit, and Orochol is an avirulent mutant of *V. cholerae* strain CVD103HgR.

Both vaccines are effective in field trials and volunteer studies, but their cost-effectiveness in endemic settings is uncertain. The WHO does not require vaccination for international travel to or from en-demic areas because the series of two injections is effective in only 50% of people and immunity wanes in 6 months or less. It is more cost-effective to provide counseling about avoiding risks.

ESCHERICHIA COLI

Epidemiology

E. coli is a gram-negative bacillus commonly found in the human GI tract. It is divided into five groups based on pathogenic features of diarrheal disease and toxin production: enterotoxigenic *E. coli* (ETEC), enteroinvasive *E. coli* (EIEC), enteropathogenic *E. coli* (EPEC), enteroadhesive *E. coli* (EAEC), and enterohemorrhagic *E. coli* (EHEC).[39] The most common group is ETEC; it accounts for about half of all cases of *E. coli* diarrhea and for more than 79,000 cases in the United States each year.[39,40] Enterotoxigenic *E. coli* is in-criminated as being the most common cause of traveler's diarrhea and a common cause of food- and water-associated outbreaks.[41] EAEC strains are also important causes of traveler's diarrhea in Mexico and North Africa. However, unlike ETEC, EAEC produces diarrhea more commonly in developing populations in association with per-sistent diarrhea ($\geq$14 days). EPEC infection is primarily a disease of children younger than 2 years of age in the developing world. The reason for the relative resistance of adults and older children is not known.

Recognized as a common and potentially deadly cause of in-fectious diarrhea, EHEC is believed to be the major etiologic factor responsible for the development of hemorrhagic colitis and HUS.[28] The CDC estimates the annual disease burden of *E. coli* O157:H7 in the Unites States to be more than 20,000 infections and as many as 250 deaths, but the failure of many clinical laboratories to screen for this organism greatly complicates any estimates. In the United States, serotype O157:H7 causes 50% to 80% of all EHEC infections, but in the southern hemisphere, such as Argentina, Australia, Chile, and South Africa, non-O157:H7 serotypes are often more important.[39] Transmission usually occurs via food and water, and outbreaks have been associated with undercooked ground beef.[28] Reports of EHEC enteritis continue to increase. EIEC strains are biochemically, genet-ically, and pathogenetically related closely to *Shigella* spp. and cause a disease similar to *Shigella*-like dysentery.

Pathogenesis

Enterotoxigenic *E. coli* are capable of producing two plasmid-mediated enterotoxins: heat-labile toxin (HLT) and heat-stable toxin (HST).[42] A cholera-like toxin, HLT has two subunits (A and B) that have similar antigenic properties and action on the gut mucosa. The net effect of this toxin on the mucosa is production of a cholera-like secretory diarrhea. HST is nonantigenic and has a low molecular weight. HST has a rapid onset of action and probably acts only on the small intestine.[43]

The mode of pathogenesis of the non-ETEC varieties is less well understood. The hallmark histopathologic lesion of EPEC infection is the effacing of microvilli and intimate adherence between the bac-terium and the epithelial cell membrane. EAEC adheres to intestinal mucosal Hep-2 cells, eliciting mucus production and bacterial biofilm layering. The final step in the pathogenesis of EAEC is cytotoxin elab-oration from the organism causing damage to intestinal cells. This can result in persistent diarrhea ($\geq$14 days). The pathogenicity of EHEC is related to the production of cytotoxins, commonly called *shiga-like toxins* because of their resemblance to the shiga toxin of *Shigella dysenteriae*.[44] EIEC invades the colonic epithelium.

Clinical Presentation

Nausea and watery stools, with or without abdominal cramping, are characteristic of the disease caused by ETEC.[39] Usually there is no blood or pus in the stool. Signs and symptoms are depend directly on the extent of fluid loss, which in most cases is subclinical. Most ETEC diarrhea is typically abrupt in onset and resolves within 24 to 48 hours without complication. The clinical features of EAEC diar-rhea are characterized as watery, mucoid, secretory diarrhea with low-grade fever and little or no vomiting. Common symptoms of EPEC infection include profuse watery diarrhea, vomiting, and low-grade fever.

Symptoms from EHEC infection can be severe, with as many as 11 to 12 bloody stools per day.[44,45] Cramping and severe abdominal pain are common. Nausea occurs in about two-thirds of patients, and vomiting occurs in less than a third. Symptoms usually last 1 week. The white blood cell (WBC) count is elevated and accompanied by a left shift, but patients often remain afebrile. Stool cultures should be performed when EHEC is suspected.[28] Death may occur rarely, usu-ally as a result of HUS.[37] EIEC infection presents most commonly as watery diarrhea, which can be indistinguishable from the secre-tory diarrhea seen with ETEC, but in a minority of cases, patients experience the dysentery syndrome, manifested as blood, mucus, and leukocytes in the stool with tenesmus and fever.

► TREATMENT: *E. coli* Diarrhea

The cornerstone of management of diarrheogenic *E. coli* infection is to prevent dehydration by correcting fluid and electrolyte imbal-ances. ORT is often lifesaving in infants and children.[39] Treatment of EHEC infection is primarily limited to supportive care, which may include dialysis, hemofiltration, transfusion of packed erythrocytes, platelet infusions, and other interventions as indicated clinically.[46] Se-vere disease may require renal transplant. Bismuth subsalicylate and loperamide are effective in decreasing the severity of ETEC diarrhea.

CLINICAL CONTROVERSY

Loperamide should not be used in patients with fever or dysentery because antimotility agents are contraindicated in the management of diarrhea due to EHEC. There is evidence that the use of such agents can increase the risk for develop-ment of HUS, possibly by delaying intestinal clearance of the organism and thereby increasing toxin absorption.

Although antimicrobial prophylaxis with doxycycline, trimethoprim-sulfamethoxazole, or a fluoroquinolone is effective in preventing ETEC diarrhea, the growing problem of antibiotic resistance and the possibility of adverse effects from antimicrobial agents deter recommendations of prophylaxis. Instead, experts recommend avoiding risk factors while traveling. In addition, if significant disease occurs, bismuth subsalicylate given four times daily may alleviate symptoms, and empirical antibiotics may shorten the duration of the disease.[47] Fluoroquinolones (e.g., ciprofloxacin, norfloxacin, and ofloxacin) are the most commonly recommended agents owing to increasing antimicrobial resistance among other drug classes. Vaccines that target colonization factor antigens are under development for ETEC infection.[48]

A number of antibiotics have been used to treat EPEC, but multiple-antibiotic resistance is common. The use of antibiotics remains controversial in EHEC infection.[49] Their use may be harmful owing to lysis of bacteria leading to increased release of toxin and alteration of normal intracolonic bacterial flora thereby increasing the systemic absorption of the toxin.

PSEUDOMEMBRANOUS COLITIS (*CLOSTRIDIUM DIFFICILE*)

Epidemiology

Pseudomembranous colitis (PMC) was first reported in 1893 and was associated with antibiotic therapy in 1955. Although described in the preantibiotic era, the incidence increasingly has been associated with antibiotic administration. *C. difficile* is thought to be the cause in 10% to 20% of patients experiencing antibiotic-associated diarrhea, 50% to 75% of those with antibiotic-associated colitis, and greater than 90% of those with antibiotic-associated pseudomembranous colits.[50] It is also the most common cause of nosocomial diarrhea, infecting 16% to 20% of inpatients, one-third of whom are symptomatic.[51]

The incidence of intestinal colonization is variable, ranging from 30% to 70% in infants to 3% to 5% in healthy adults.[50] The relationship between the colonized state and active disease is poorly understood. Many people are colonized with the bacteria yet do not go on to develop PMC. It occurs most often in high-risk groups, such as the elderly, debilitated patients, cancer patients, surgical patients, any patient receiving antibiotics, patients with nasogastric tubes, and patients who frequently use laxatives. PMC has been associated with use of broad-spectrum antimicrobials, including clindamycin, ampicillin, or third-generation cephalosporins.[50] Other agents that have been implicated, albeit at a lower incidence rate, include aminoglycosides, erythromycin, fluoroquinolones, trimethoprim-sulfmethoxazole, and surprisingly, vancomycin and metronidazole, two of the most commonly used antimicrobials for treatment of *C. difficile*.[52]

Pathogenesis

C. difficile is a gram-positive spore-forming anaerobic bacillus and causes a toxin-mediated disease. Once antibiotics disrupt normal colonic flora and colonization of *C. difficile* occurs, two toxins (A and B) are released to mediate diarrhea and colitis. Toxin A is the major pathogenic factor and has been characterized as an enterotoxin that causes intestinal fluid secretion, mucosal injury, and inflammation through actin disaggregation, intracellular calcium release, and damage to neurons. Toxin B is a nonenterotoxic cytotoxin that causes depolymerization of filamentous actin and mediates more potent damage to human colonic mucosa than toxin A. Initially, raised white and yellowish plaques form, and the surrounding mucosa may be inflamed. With progression of disease, these pseudomembranous plaques become enlarged and scatted over the colorectal mucosa.[53]

Clinical Presentation

C. difficile infection may cause a spectrum of disease from mild antibiotic-associated diarrhea to pseudomembranous entercolitis.[50] In colitis without pseudomenbrane formation, patients present with malaise, abdominal pain, nausea, anorexia, watery diarrhea, low-grade fever, and leukocytosis. PMC is characterized by more severe illness, with severe abdominal pain, perfuse diarrhea, high fever, marked leukocytosis, and classic pseudomembrane formation evident with sigmoidoscopic examination. Symptoms can start a few days after the start of antibiotic therapy or several weeks after antibiotics have been discontinued. The onset of illness is often abrupt.

C. difficile infection should be suspected in patients experiencing diarrhea with a recent history of antibiotic use (within the previous 2 months) or in those whose diarrhea began 72 hours after hospitalization. Diagnosis can be established by detection of toxin A or B, stool culture for *C. difficile,* or endoscopy. If the stool sample is negative, a second analysis is recommended because the testing sensitivity may be increased with repeat testing. Endoscopy should be reserved for situations where rapid diagnosis is needed, ileus is present, a stool is not available, or other colonic diseases are in the differential diagnosis.[54]

▶ TREATMENT: Pseudomembranous Colitis

Initial therapy should include discontinuation of the offending agent with a change to an alternative antibiotic if possible.[50] Fluid and electrolyte replacement therapy is necessary. Although diarrhea will resolve in 15% to 23% of patients without therapy, most patients will require antibiotics. Both vancomycin and metronidazole are effective, but metronidazole 250 mg orally four times daily is the drug of choice.[50] It is similar to vancomycin in time to resolution of diarrhea, incidence of side effects, and relapse rates. However, it is less expensive than vancomycin, and the concern for vancomycin resistance promotes metronidazole use.

Oral vancomycin 125 mg four times daily is second-line therapy. Its use is appropriate in the following situations: The patient has not responded to oral metronidazole; the organism is resistant to metronidazole; the patient is allergic or intolerant to metronidazole; treatment includes ethanol-containing solutions; the patient is either pregnant or younger than 10 years of age; the patient is critically ill because of *C. difficile* diarrhea or colitis (the duration of diarrhea is reduced

to 3 versus 4.6 days with metronidazole); and there is evidence suggesting that the diarrhea is caused by *S. aureus*.[50] Vancomcyin must be administered orally because IV vancomycin does not achieve gut lumen concentrations high enough for effective bacterial elimination.

Bacitracin is third-line treatment. In resolving symptoms, 80,000 units of bacitracin orally daily is as effective as vancomycin but is not as effective in eradicating the organism. Bacitracin's poor taste, which reduces patient adherence, limits its use.[54] Teicoplanin and fusidic acid have been effective in resolving symptoms and eradicating the organism.[54]

Relapse after antibiotic treatment occurs in about 20% to 25% of patients and does not appear to be influenced by the choice of initial therapy, dose of drug used, or duration of treatment.[50] Recurrences occur because of the persistence of the spore forms of *C. difficile* that are not killed by antibiotic therapy or reinfection by a new strain. Recurrences usually occur 3 to 21 days after antibiotics are stopped. Retreatment with metronidazole or vancomycin at the previous dose for 10 to 14 days generally is successful. The addition of rifampin to vancomycin also has been effective.[50]

CLINICAL CONTROVERSY

Some investigators have found prophylaxis with competing, nonpathogenic organisms such as *Lactobacillus* spp. or *Saccharomyces* spp. to be helpful in preventing relapse in small numbers of patients.[55,56] It is thought that these organisms help to restore the natural flora in the gut and make patients more resistant to colonization by *C. difficile*.

Vancomycin has been used in combination with anion-exchange resins dosed to avoid drug-resin binding, and this has been used successfully in a small number of cases.[54] Cholestyramine 4 g orally three to four times daily and colestipol 5 g orally twice daily have been used as alternatives to antibiotics in mild cases.

Drugs that inhibit peristalsis, such as diphenoxylate, are contraindicated in PMC.[50] Slowing of fecal transit time is thought to result in extended toxin-associated damage. Strict handwashing and contact precautions are imperative measures in preventing the spread of the organism. *C. difficile* can be cultured in rooms of infected individuals up to 40 days of after discharge.[51]

INVASIVE (DYSENTERY-LIKE) DIARRHEA

BACILLARY DYSENTERY (SHIGELLOSIS)

Epidemiology

The shigellae are gram-negative bacilli belonging to the family Enterobacteriaceae. Four species most often associated with disease are *Shigella dysenteriae* type I, *S. flexneri*, *S. boydii*, and *S. sonnei*.[57] The shigellae have worldwide distribution, with regional differences in prevalence of subgroups responsible for disease. For example, in the United States, the common causes of shigellosis are *S. sonnei* and *S. flexneri*. Cases caused by other shigellae are successfully acquired successfully during travel to developing countries. Because of overuse of antibiotics in human and animal feed, Southeast Asia and India have higher levels of resistance. Poor sanitation, poor personal hygiene, inadequate water supply, malnutrition, and increased population density are associated with an increased risk of *Shigella* gastroenteritis epidemics, even in developed countries.

Most cases result from fecal-oral transmission. A few well-documented food- and water-associated outbreaks have been reported. Peak incidence in the United States is in late summer. Estimates indicate that 450,000 cases of shigellosis occur in the United States and that 165 million cases occur in the world annually, resulting in over 1 million deaths worldwide each year.[57]

Shigellosis is primarily a disease of children, with the highest incidence between the ages of 6 months and 5 years. Infection among infants is uncommon, and only a third of all cases occur in adults.

Pathogenesis

Ingestion of as few as 10 to 200 viable organisms of the *Shigella* species causes disease in healthy adults, explaining the ease with which the disease is transmitted from person to person.[58] The bacteria multiply and spread within the submucosa of the small bowel, but they rarely extend beyond the mucosa. Penetration of the mucosa

is conferred genetically by large "invasion plasmids" and results in distortion of the crypts, death to intestinal epithelium causing focal ulceration, sloughing of mucosal cells, bloody mucoid exudate into the gut lumen, and submucosal accumulation of inflammatory cells with microabscess formation.[59] Microabscesses eventually may coalesce, forming larger abscesses. Infection frequently involves the entire colon. In addition to the virulence characteristics of invasiveness, *S. dysenteriae* type 1 and, to lesser degree, *S. flexneri* and *S. sonnei* produce a cytotoxin, or shiga toxin, the pathogenic role of which is unclear, although it is thought to damage endothelial cells of the lamina propria, resulting in microangiopathic changes that can progress to HUS.[60] Watery diarrhea commonly precedes the dysentery and may be a result of these toxins.

Clinical Presentation

Initial signs and symptoms include abdominal pain, cramping, and fever followed by frequent watery stools.[61] Within a few days, patients experience a decrease in fever, severe abdominal pain, and tenderness prior to the development of bloody diarrhea and other signs of dysentery (see Table 111–4). Stools are often greenish in color and contain leukocytes. Fluid and electrolyte losses may be significant, particularly in infants and elderly patients. In the early stages of the disease, stool cultures are positive. A rapid diagnostic test kit that uses DNA amplification by the polymerase chain reaction (PCR) is also available.

If left untreated, bacillary dysentery usually lasts about 1 week (range 1–30 days). Complications are unusual but may include severe dehydration, generalized seizures, septicemia, toxic megacolon, perforated colon, arthritis, protein-losing enteropathy, and HUS. Mortality is rare, but it may be more likely with *S. dysenteriae* type I. Less than 3% of persons who are infected with *S. flexneri* will later develop Reiter's syndrome, characterized by pains in the joints, irritation of the eyes, and painful urination. This can lead to chronic arthritis.[62]

▶ TREATMENT: Bacillary Dysentery (Shigellosis)

Shigelloisis is usually a self-limiting disease. Most patients recover in 4 to 7 days, although 10% may experience a recurrence. Oral fluid and electrolyte replacement is the foundation of treatment (dysentery is not generally associated with significant fluid loss). However, intravenous fluid replacement therapy may be necessary, especially in children and the elderly.

Owing to the self-limiting nature of the illness and rapid development of antimicrobial resistance on completion of therapy, antibiotic treatment is reserved for the elderly and infirmed, those who are immunocompromised, children in day-care centers, malnourished children, and health care workers. Antibiotics shorten

the period of fecal shedding and attenuate the clinical illness. The choice of agent depends on location (see Table 111–3). For infections acquired in the United States, the agent of choice is trimethoprim-sulfamethoxazole (only 4% resistance). For infections acquired outside the United States, the agents of choice are ciprofloxacin, norfloxacin, and azithromycin.[26]

Antimotility agents such as diphenoxylate are not recommended because they can worsen bacillary dysentery and could be involved in the development of toxic dilatation of the colon. Oral vaccines currently in development contain attenuated strains of *Shigella* and provide protection against shigellosis in human challenges.[63]

SALMONELLOSIS

Epidemiology

Salmonella species are gram-negative bacilli belonging to the family Enterobacteriaceae. As a result of DNA hybridization experiments, the classification and nomenclature of *Salmonella* spp. have been changing, causing much confusion.[64] Owing to a high degree of DNA similarity, all important *Salmonella* isolates have been classified into a single species, *S. choleraesuis,* with approximately 2500 different serotypes. Because various serotypes were known formally as species, it has been acceptable to refer to serotypes as species. For example *S. enterica* serotype Typhi is commonly referred to as *S. typhi.* Unfortunately, there is also a serotype Choleraesuis within *S. choleraesuis.* To decrease misunderstanding, a new name, *S. enterica,* was proposed to replace *S. choeraesuis,* and thus much of the current literature uses this name.

Specific *Salmonella* serotypes produce characteristic human disease. For example *S. enterica* serotypes Typhimurium or Enteritidis causes gastroenteritis, whereas serotypes Typhi or Paratyphi causes enteric fever. Clinical manifestations produced by *Salmonella* serotypes commonly include acute gastroenteritis (enterocolitis), bacteremia, extraintestinal localized infection, enteric fever (typhoid and paratyphoid fever), and a chronic carrier state.

In the United States, approximately 1.4 million cases of salmonellosis, 16,000 hospitalizations, and 600 deaths occur annually.[6] Salmonellosis is a disease primarily of infants, children, and adolescents. Children younger than 5 years of age account for about 25% of all diagnosed cases.[27] Conditions that may predispose to infection include those which decrease gastric acidity, antibiotic use, malnutrition, and immunodeficiency states. Contaminated food or water has been implicated in the majority of cases. Direct fecal-oral transmission occurs less frequently but is particularly important in children. Foods most often implicated in human salmonellosis are poultry, poultry products, beef, pork, and dairy products. Pets, particularly reptiles, are a common source of infection.

There is decreasing incidence in rates of salmonellosis in the United States. Foodborne outbreaks of enteric fever are rare, and a small number of cases often are associated with international travel, especially to developing countries. The most common *Salmonella* serotypes are Typhimurium and Enteritidis, accounting for approximately 50% of isolates from patients.[65] The overall downward trend in rates of salmonellosis is believed to be due to the improved food-handling practices and water treatment.

Pathogenesis

The incubation period, symptoms, and disease severity depend on the amount of organism ingested. The inoculum necessary for infection is estimated to less than 1000 organisms, and this infectious dose is lowered in patients with acholorhydria (gastric pH > 4.0). If the organisms survive the gastric acid barrier, mucosal invasion of the small intestine begins.[66] After penetration, microorganisms translocate to the intestinal lymphoid follicles and the draining mesenteric lymph nodes, in addition to the reticuloendothelial cells of the liver and spleen. Thereafter, the ability of organisms to survive and multiply within the mononuclear phagocytic cells of the lymphoid follicles, liver, and spleen plays an instrumental role in the pathogenesis. In the asymptomatic phase, the organisms are sequestered intracellularly. Once the critical number of organisms has been reached, bacteria are released into the bloodstream, and the symptoms of enteric fever are manifested. This dissemination of organisms via bloodstream also causes secondary infection in the liver, spleen, bone marrow, gallblad-

der, and Peyer's patches of the terminal ileum. After several weeks of infection, recruitment of mononuclear cells and lymphocytes induced by *Salmonella* is thought to be responsible for necrosis of Peyer patches and the abdominal pain observed in enteric fever.[66]

The mechanism by which nontyphoidal salmonellae cause enterocolitis is less well understood. Although a number of enterotoxins have been described in salmonellae, their role remains illusive.[67] Some salmonellae, such as *S. enterica* serotype Choleraesuis, which is the most invasive, are frequently associated with bacteremia and metastatic localization, whereas others seldom cause disease. Enterocolitis often is characterized by massive neutrophil infiltration into both the large and small bowel mucosa. The serotypes that are responsible for human illness cause intestinal epithelial cells to secrete interleukin 8 (IL-8), a potent neutrophil chemotactic factor. Degranulation and release of toxic substances by neutrophils may contribute to inflammation and result in tissue damage, fluid secretion, or leakage across the intestinal mucosa.

Clinical Presentation

Enterocolitis. Most patients experience symptoms within 72 hours of ingestion of contaminated food or water.[67] Patients often complain of nausea and vomiting followed by abdominal cramps, headache, fever, and diarrhea, although the actual presentation is quite variable. Some patients do not have increased stool frequency, whereas others have more than one stool per hour. Stools generally are loose and may be mucoid or bloody (dysentery-like) or both. Febrile episodes usually range between 100 and 102°F (37.7 and 38.8°C) but may be higher. Some evidence suggests that fever of 104°F (40°C) or higher is associated with shorter bacterial excretion.[68] Diarrhea and fever usually resolve spontaneously within 1 to 5 days but may last 2 weeks.

Stool cultures inevitably yield the causative organism if obtained early (i.e., in patients hospitalized less than 3 days).[52] Recovery of organisms continues to decrease with time so that by 3 to 4 weeks, only 5% to 15% of adult patients are passing *Salmonella*. Infants and children tend to pass bacteria for longer periods than adults. Some patients may continue to shed *Salmonella* for a year or longer. These "chronic carrier" states are rare for serotypes other than Typhi.[66]

Bacteremia. Salmonellae can produce bacteremia without classic enterocolitis or enteric fever. Bacteremia rarely occurs in older adults, but it can occur in up to 40% of infants.[69] It is also reported more frequently in persons with severe underlying illness or immunosuppression, including AIDS. The clinical syndrome is characterized by persistent bacteremia and prolonged intermittent fever with chills. Stool cultures frequently are negative. This clinical syndrome is most frequent with serotype Choleraesuis infections (50%). Leukocyte counts are often within the normal range.

Localized Infections. Localized infections develop in 5% to 10% patients with bacteremia.[67] Extraluminal infection or abscess formation or both can occur at any site. They may follow any of the other syndromes, or they may be the primary presentation. Metastatic infections involve bone, cysts, heart, kidney, liver, lungs, pericardium, spleen, and tumors. The clinical presentation usually is determined by the organ systems involved. Polymorphonuclear leukocyte counts often are elevated.

Enteric Fever (Typhoid and Paratyphoid). Enteric fever caused by serotype Typhi is called *typhoid fever.*[66] If caused by any other serotype, it is referred to as *paratyphoid fever.* The clinical presentations of typhoid fever and paratyphoid fever generally are indistinguishable, although paratyphoid fever tends to be less severe than typhoid fever. The incubation period can range from 10 to 14 days. The onset of symptoms is gradual. Nonspecific symptoms of fever, dull headache, malaise, anorexia, and myalgias are most common. Initially, fever tends to be remittent, but it progresses gradually over the first week to temperatures that are often sustained over 104°F (40°C). Other frequently encountered symptoms include chills, nausea, vomiting, cough, weakness, and sore throat. Symptoms subside slowly within 4 weeks.

Physical examination generally reveals an acutely ill patient. An erythematous maculopapular rash known as *rose spots* appears primarily on the abdomen in 15% to 50% of patients. The abdomen also may be tender, particularly in the lower quadrants. Hepatomegaly,

splenomegaly, or both also may be present in 50% of the cases, and cervical lymph nodes may be enlarged.

A normochromic anemia may develop rapidly without evidence of GI blood loss, although intestinal bleeding may be contributory. Leukopenia may be reflective of a relative decrease in polymorphonuclear leukocytes. WBC counts may range from 1200 to 20,000 cells/mm³. As many as one-third of the patients have elevated levels of the liver enzymes glutamic-oxaloacetic transaminase and alkaline phosphatase in serum. About 80% of patients have positive blood cultures. Bacteremia persists in about a third of cases for several weeks if not treated. Intestinal perforation, intestinal hemorrhage, thrombophlebitis, toxemia with circulatory collapse, encephalopathy, and pneumonia all contribute to a fatality rate of 1% to 2%. Without treatment, mortality may be 10%.[66]

▶ TREATMENT: Salmonellosis

▩ ENTEROCOLITIS

Fluid and electrolyte replacement is the primary mode of treatment. Most patients respond well to ORT (self-limited illness).[67] Antimotility drugs should be avoided because they increase the risk of mucosal invasion and complications. Antibiotic therapy is *not* indicated in healthy adults. Antibiotics have no effect on the duration of fever or diarrhea, and their frequent use increases the likelihood of resistance and the duration of fecal shedding. Antibiotics should be used in: (1) neonates or infants younger than 6 months of age because young children have an increased risk of complicated infection, (2) patients with primary or secondary immunodeficiency, such as AIDS or chemotherapy patients, (3) severely symptomatic patients with fever and bloody diarrhea, and (4) patients after splenectomy.[67] Susceptibility testing is recommended because many drug-resistant strains of *Salmonella* have emerged. Recommended antibiotics include the fluoroquinolones, trimethoprim-sulfamethoxazole, ampicillin, and third-generation cephalosporins. If susceptibility results are not available, a fluoroquinolone or third-generation cephalosporins should be instituted owing to resistance with trimethoprim-sulfamethoxazole and ampicillin. Azithromycin and aztreonam also have been studied and may be used as alternative agents.

▩ BACTEREMIA AND LOCALIZED INFECTIONS

Owing to increasing resistance, empirical therapy for life-threatening bacteremia or focal infections following nontyphoidal *Salmonella* infection should include both a third-generation cephalosporin (such as ceftriaxone 2 g IV daily) and a fluoroquinolone (ciprofloxacin 500 mg orally twice daily) until the susceptibilities are known.[69] The duration of antibiotic therapy is dictated by the site of infection. Bacteremia without endovascular infection should be treated for 7 to 14 days. In documented or suspected endovascular infection, 6 weeks of intravenous therapy with ampicillin or ceftriaxone is recommended. Chloramphenicol is no longer recommended in patients with endovascular infection owing to high rates of failure.

▩ ENTERIC FEVER (TYPHOID AND PARATYPHOID)

Antibiotic choice is dictated by susceptibility testing.[66] Fluoroquinolones are the drugs of choice for the treatment of enteric fever.[70]

A short course of 3 to 5 days is effective in uncomplicated enteric fever, but a minimum of 10 days is recommended in severe cases. In patients who are infected with fluoroquinolone-susceptible S. *enterica* serotype Typhi, the average time for defervescence is less than 4 days, and the cure rates exceed 96%, with fewer than 2% of treated patients having persistent fecal carriage or relapse. Unfortunately, fluoroquinolone resistance is increasing in some areas, and these strains are also often multidrug-resistant, limiting the choice of antibiotics. Among patients with fluoroquinolone-resistant S. *enterica* serotype Typhi infection, fluoroquinolones still can be used but at the maximal possible dose for a minimum of 10 to 14 days. These patients should be monitored carefully to determine whether they are excreting the organism in their feces. High-dose fluoroquinolone regimens have been successful in 90% to 95% of patients with multidrug-resistant infection.[71] However, the average time to defervescence is 7 days, and the rate of fecal carriage during convalescence can be as high as 20%.

The third-generation cephalosporins (e.g., ceftriaxone, cefixime, cefotaxime, and cefoperazole) and azithromycin are also effective drugs for typhoid. Chloramphenicol, amoxicillin, and trimethoprim-sulfamethoxazole remain appropriate for the treatment of typhoid fever in areas of the world where the bacterium is still fully susceptible to these drugs and where the fluoroquinolones are not available or affordable.[66] Although fluoroquinolones are not recommended in children, the pediatric use of ciprofloxacin in areas where multidrug-resistant S. *typhi* occurs is acceptable. In pregnant women, the β-lactam antibiotics are safe, and there are some case reports to support fluoroquinolone use.

Adults and children with severe enteric fever characterized by delirium, obtundation, stupor, coma, or shock benefit from prompt administration of dexamethasone 1 mg/kg every 6 hours for 24 to 48 hours.[72] Three vaccines against S. *typhi* are licensed in the United States: a heat-phenol-inactivated parenteral vaccine (Typhoid Vaccine, USP), an orally administered vaccine (Ty21a, Vivotif Berna), and a parenteral polysaccharide vaccine (ViCPS, Typhim Vi).[30] The efficacy of these vaccines ranges from 42% to 77%, and immunity persists for 3 to 5 years. The parenteral inactivated vaccine causes substantially more adverse reactions than the other two but provides more prolonged protection. The Ty21a and Vi vaccines are recommended for travelers to areas of endemic disease and those in high-risk groups, including household contacts of S. *typhi* carriers, laboratory technicians with repeated exposure, and sanitation workers in endemic areas. Since the Ty21a vaccine is a live, attenuated vaccine, it should not be administered to immunocompromised persons, patients taking antibiotics, or patients with gastroenteritis.

■ "CHRONIC CARRIERS" OF *SALMONELLA*

"Chronic carriers" of *Salmonella* usually have negative stool cultures at 12 weeks after the onset of illness, but some may have continued positive stool cultures at 6 to 12 months. Chronic fecal shedding of *Salmonella* has been associated with chronic biliary infection and cholelithiasis. To alleviate the chronic carrier state, the drug of choice is norfloxacin 400 mg orally twice daily for 28 days. In addition, amoxicillin and trimethoprime-sulfamethoxazole are effective in eradicating the bacteria in greater than 80% of cases after 6 weeks of therapy.[27] Chronic carriers should take preventative measures (i.e., antibiotics and hygiene) so that they do not serve as reservoirs of infection to the community.

CAMPYLOBACTERIOSIS

Epidemiology

The *Campylobacter* spp. are flagellated, curved, gram-negative rods that are thought to be one of the most common bacterial causes of diarrheal illnesses worldwide. Although there are 14 different species, *C. jejuni* is the species responsible for more than 99% of *Campylobacter*-associated gastroenteritis.[73] In the United States, the incidence of *Campylobacter* infection decreased 26% from 1996 to 1999. However, surveillance studies indicate that *Campylobacter* spp. remain the most commonly isolated enteric pathogen, detected two to seven times more frequently than *Salmonella* or *Shigella*.[74] Currently, the CDC estimates that 2.4 million persons are affected each year in the United States, involving almost 1% of the entire population.

In developed countries, the peak incidence of *Campylobacter* infections occurs in children younger than 1 year of age and young adults of 15 to 44 years of age. The incidence is also higher in males than in females, although the reason for this is unknown. Patients with AIDS are particularly susceptible; the incidence in AIDS patients is 40 times that of the general population.[73] Most reported cases occur during the summer months, beginning in May and peaking in August. In tropical developing countries, *Campylobacter* infections are common among children younger than 2 years of age, and asymptomatic infections of children and adults are more common than those seen in industrialized nations. This decrease in the case-to-infection ratio suggests that previous exposure confers immunity to the infecting strain.

The transmission of infection occurs primarily by ingestion of contaminated food or water. Although *Campylobacter* spp. have varied reservoirs, such as livestock, dogs, cats, and birds, the consumption of chicken has been shown to be the major vector of infections in industrialized nations.[75] Poultry products are nearly always contaminated with *Campylobacter* spp. during the slaughtering process, and it is estimated that 1 drop of chicken juice may contain 500 infectious organisms. Although public education emphasizes safe handling and cooking of chicken, it is easy to see how simple errors may result in human illness.

Pathogenesis

Campylobacter spp. are labile in acidic environments, much like *Salmonella*. Therefore, an inoculum of approximately 800 organisms is required to initiate infection. Conditions in the upper small intestine are favorable for multiplication. Flagella-mediated adherence and tissue invasion by bacteria have been demonstrated in the jejunum, ileum, and colon. Infection results in an acute inflammatory enteritis. *C. jejuni* can produce an enterotoxin or cytotoxin.[76] Both cytotoxins and enterotoxins may be produced in many strains. Symptom manifestation depends on immunity. Patients infected with *Campylobacter* develop specific IgG, IgM, and IgA antibodies in serum and IgA antibodies in intestinal secretions. Volunteer studies indicate that immunity does protect against illness.

Clinical Presentation

The average incubation period of *Campylobacter* is 2 to 4 days.[74] The most common presenting symptoms include diarrhea, abdominal pain, and fever. Nausea, vomiting, headache, myalgias, and malaise also may occur. Bowel movements may be numerous, bloody (dysentery-like), and foul smelling and range from loose to watery. Cramping and abdominal pain usually are relieved by defecation. In 75% of cases, leukocytes and red blood cells are detected in the stool samples. Peripheral leukocytosis also may be present. The disease usually is self-limited to about 1 week, but it may persist for several weeks in 10% to 20% of patients. The case-fatality rate is 0.05 per 1000 infections.

Complications, including pseudoappendicitis, pancreatitis, gastrointestinal hemorrhage, thrombophlebitis, abscess, septicemia, peritonitis, empyema, urinary tract infection, and cholecystitis, are uncommon but occur more frequently in those who are immunocompromised. *C. jejuni* has been associated with Guillain-Barré syndrome (GBS), but the relationship is not well understood.[77] *C. jejuni* infections are a common trigger of GBS, accounting for approximately 30% of GBS cases, but the risk of developing GBS after *C. jejuni* infection appears to be low (<1 case of GBS per 1000 *C. jejuni* infections). A reactive arthritis may develop several weeks after infection in persons with the HLA-B27 histocompatibility antigens.[62] Diagnosis is made by stool culture, but the bacteria sometimes are identifiable with Gram stain or carbol-fuchsin stain.

► TREATMENT: Campylobacteriosis

The primary treatment of campylobacteriosis is oral fluid and electrolyte replacement.[74] Most people recover from this self-limiting disease in 4 to 7 days. Antibiotics are *not* useful unless started within 4 days of the start of the illness because they do not shorten the duration or severity of diarrhea but only shorten the duration of bacterial excretion. However, antibiotics are warranted in patients who present with high fevers, severe bloody diarrhea, prolonged illnesses (>1 week), pregnancy, and immunocompromised states, including HIV infection (see Table 111–3).

C. jejuni is susceptible to a wide variety of antimicrobial agents. Fluoroquinolone resistance has increased to 10% to 13% in the United States (41% to 88% in Europe and Asia) in recent years and may be a result of the use of quinolone antibiotics in poultry feed and their frequent use overseas in treating enteric infections. Erythromycin is considered the drug of choice owing to its low cost, high efficacy, safety profile, and ease of administration. Newer macrolides such as clarithromycin and azithromycin are equally effective. Tetracycline, chloramphenicol, clindamycin, and aminoglycosides may be effective.[73] Antimotility agents such as loperamide are contraindicated because slowing fecal transit time may extend the duration of infection and increase toxin mucosal invasion.

YERSINIOSIS

Yersinia spp. are non-lactose-fermenting gram-negative coccobacilli that are widely distributed in nature. The genus *Yersinia* includes six species known to cause disease in humans. The best known species is *Y. pestis*, the causative agent of plague, which is usually spread by bites from infected animals, such as fleas, rodents, or cats. *Y. enterocolitica* and, to lesser extent, *Y. pseudotuberculosis* are most likely associated with intestinal infection, but overall, both are a relatively infrequent cause of diarrhea and abdominal pain. More than 50 serotypes of *Y. enterocolitica* exist; of these, serotypes 0:3, 0:8, and 0:9 are associated most frequently with enterocolitis.[78] Infections are reported commonly from northern Europe, and the peak incidence occurs during the winter months.

Children are most likely to experience illness with *Y. enterocolitica* infection.[79] Transmission of infection occurs frequently by ingestion of contaminated food or water. The organisms have been isolated from a variety of food sources, including pigs and raw goat and cow milk. Refrigeration does not deter the development of adherence and invasive virulence factors.

Y. enterocolitica invade the intestinal epithelium and penetrate the intestinal mucosa.[80] An inoculum of 10^9 organisms may be required for infection. Most strains produce an enterotoxin, but the role of toxin production in causing diarrhea is not well established. However, this infection causes mucosal ulcerations in the terminal ileum, necrotic lesions in Peyer's patches, and enlargement of mesenteric lymph nodes.

Clinical Presentation

These bacteria cause a wide spectrum of clinical syndromes.[79] Most patients with *Y. enterocolitica* infection present with enterocolitis that is mild and self-limiting. Symptoms include vomiting, abdominal pain, diarrhea, and fever; up to 60% of patients will have blood-streaked stools. Diarrhea resolves after 1 to 3 weeks, but bacteria excretion may continue for up to 3 months after diarrhea subsides. Most patients with this type of infection are younger than 5 years of age. In older children and adolescents, mesenteric adenitis and/or terminal ileitis with fever, right lower quadrant pain, and leukocytois are common. Mesenteric adenitis, which is difficult to distinguish from acute appendicitis, is also seen in patients infected with *Y. pseudotuberculosis*.

Approximately 10% to 30% of adult patients develop a reactive arthritis 1 to 2 weeks after recovery from enteritis. This arthritis, involving the knees, ankles, toes, fingers, and wrists, usually resolves in 1 to 4 months but may persist in about 10% of patients.[79] This complication is more common in persons with the HLA-B27 antigen.[62] Other postinfection complications include erythema nodosum, exudative pharyngitis, pneumonia, empyema, and lung abscess. Although rare, *Y. enterocolitica* bacteremia has been reported in patients with diabetes mellitus, severe anemia, hemochromatosis, cirrhosis, and malignancy. Other groups at risk include the elderly and those who received frequent red blood cell transfusions (iron overload).[81] These patients are at increased risk for hepatic or splenic abscesses, peritonitis, septic arthritis, osteomyelitis, wound infections, meningitis, and endocarditis.

▶ TREATMENT: Yersiniosis

Oral fluid and electrolyte replacement is an important initial approach. Owing to the self-limiting nature of the illness, antibiotics may not alter the time to resolution of the diarrhea or the rate of bacteriologic cure. Antibiotics should be used in high-risk patients who develop bacteremia (i.e., infants younger than 3 months of age and patients with cirrhosis or iron overload) or in patients with bone and joint infections.[79]

Drugs of choice are not yet identified. Fluoroquinolones alone or in combination with third-generation cephalosporins or aminoglycosides may be effective for *Yersinia* bacteremia or for those with bone and joint infections.[79] Other antibiotics effective in vitro are chloramphenicol, tetracyclines, and trimethoprim-sulfamethoxazole. Agents frequently resistant to *Yersinia* are penicillin G, ampicillin, and first-generation cephalosporins.

ACUTE VIRAL GASTROENTERITIS

Acute viral gastroenteritis was unknown until the 1970s. Viruses are now recognized as the leading cause of diarrhea in the world, although in many cases an exact pathogen cannot be determined. In Asia, Africa, and Latin America, viral gastroenteritis accounts for an estimated 3 to 5 billion cases and is associated with 5 to 10 million deaths.[82] Viruses that cause gastroenteritis include rotavirus, calicivirus, enteric adenovirus, and astrovirus. Other viruses, such as toroviruses, coronaviruses, picobirnaviruses, and pestiviruses, are being identified increasingly as causative agents of diarrhea.

ROTAVIRUSES

EPIDEMIOLOGY

Rotavirus is the most important cause of diarrhea worldwide, and 1 million people die annually from the infection. In the United States, approximately 3.5 million cases of diarrhea, 500,000 physician visits, 50,000 hospitalizations, and 20 deaths occur each year in children younger than 5 years of age. In developing countries, almost all children younger than 5 years of age are infected with rotaviruses.[83] The fecal-oral route is thought to be the most common mode of transmission. Although infection is seen most often in children aged 3 to 24 months, adults can be infected and may act as a reservoir for transmission. Serologic surveys show that nearly all children are infected by age 4 years. Rotavirus infection rates peak from November to May each year. In the first 5 years of life, four of five children in the United States will develop diarrhea from a rotavirus infection.

PATHOGENESIS

Rotaviruses are double-stranded wheel-shaped RNA viruses. These strains cause diarrhea by infecting the enterocyts of the villi in the small intestine. Changes to the villi include shortening of villus height, crypt hyperplasia, and mononuclear cell infiltration of the lamina propria. Diarrhea results from decreased absorption across intestinal mucosal surface.[84]

CLINICAL PRESENTATION

The rotavirus incubation period is less than 48 hours.[85] Clinical manifestations of rotavirus infections vary from asymptomatic (which is common in adults) to severe nausea, vomiting, and diarrhea with dehydration. The first infection tends to be the most severe. Symptoms are characterized initially by nausea and vomiting (67% to 90%). Fever occurs in about two-thirds of children. Diarrhea occurs in most patients and lasts from 1 to 9 days. Other signs and symptoms include respiratory symptoms, irritability, lethargy, pharyngeal erythema, rhinitis, red tympanic membranes, and palpable cervical lymph nodes. Dehydration and electrolyte disturbances occur more frequently in children.

Laboratory findings reflect the degree of vomiting, diarrhea, or both. Transient rises in liver enzymes may be seen in 60% of children hospitalized for rotavirus diarrhea. The WBC count is usually normal. Stools rarely contain blood or leukocytes. Rotavirus detection in stool samples is possible with an enzyme immunoassay and a latex agglutination assay, both of which are available commercially.

▶ TREATMENT: Rotavirus Infection

Oral fluid and electrolyte replacement is the cornerstone of treatment.[86] Oral *Lactobacillus* therapy may reduce the duration of diarrhea and of viral excretion. There is no role for antibiotics in acute infection. Bismuth subsalicylate, although shown to decrease the duration of diarrhea and stool output, is not recommended for routine use because of the self-limiting nature of the disease and the risk of bismuth subsalicylate overdose. Antimotility agents are not recommended because they have not been shown to decrease the duration or volume of diarrhea.

The first vaccine (RotaShield) to prevent rotavirus infection was licensed for use in the United States in 1998, but it was withdrawn from the market after 1.5 million doses were administered owing to an increased rate of idiopathic intussusception.[32] A number of rotavirus vaccines are under development, but the one that shows early promise is the rotavirus oral vaccine (Rotateq, Merck). This is a reassortant pentavalent vaccine with a backbone of bovine rotavirus and surface proteins of virus strains representing G types (G1–G4) and P1A. The preliminary results from the trial of 1946 healthy infants (aged 2 to 8 months) showed a level of protection of approximately 75%.[87]

NORWALK AND NORWALK-LIKE AGENTS

The human caliciviruses are assigned to two genera, Norwalk-like virus and Sapporo-like viruses, responsible for gastroenteritis. The Norwalk-like viruses cause illness in all age groups, whereas Sapporo-like viruses cause illness mainly in children.[88] Although the relative importance of these viruses as causes of GI infections is unknown, Norwalk-like viruses are important causes of outbreaks. The Norwalk virus was the first of these agents to be described in 1972 in Norwalk, Ohio. Other viruses that are morphorlogically indistinguishable from Norwalk virus and thus belong in this family were named according to the location of the outbreak of illness or contaminated source, such as Norwalk, Hawaii, Montgomery County, Ditchling, Cockle, Paramatta, Snow Mountain, and Marin County.

As with most viruses, the epidemiology of the Norwalk-like organism is not well understood. The disease commonly affects children and adults, but it is not often associated with disease in neonates and preschool children.[89] Outbreaks occur throughout the year and have been documented in families, health care systems, cruise ships, and college dormitories. Norwalk-like viruses are often spread from person to person. Other vectors of transmission include contaminated water supplies, fecal-oral spread, and food-borne outbreaks. Almost any food that has come in contact with contaminated water can serve as a vehicle for an outbreak. A major source of food-borne gastroenteritis is contamination of shellfish beds from raw sewage dumped into the water supply.

The pathophysiology of this disease is similar to that caused by the rotavirus. Human volunteer studies show histopathologic changes in the jejunum within 24 hours of viral challenge, and clinical manifestations appear within 48 hours.[88] Brush-border enzyme activity may be decreased, resulting in lactose intolerance, but it generally returns to preinfection levels within 2 weeks. The exact mechanisms of virus-induced vomiting or diarrhea are unknown. Virus shedding in the stool can occur over the first 24 to 48 hours after illness.

Norwalk-like viral gastroenteritis is characterized by sudden onset of abdominal cramps with nausea, vomiting, or both.[89] Although adults frequently experience nonbloody diarrhea, and children experience vomiting more often than diarrhea. Other complaints are myalgias, headache, and malaise, which are accompanied by fever in about 50% of patients. Signs and symptoms generally last 12 to 48 hours.[72]

The disease is generally self-limiting. Oral fluid and electrolyte replacement should be used, if necessary.[89] An oral Norwalk virus vaccine produced via expression of viral antigens in plants is under investigation, but the clinical availability of such a product is several years in the future.

ASTROVIRUSES

Astroviruses are being recognized increasingly as important causes of gastroenteritis. Astroviral illness is often reported in children younger than 3 years of age, but it also been described in adults and elderly.[90] Astroviruses have been detected in the stools of children, as well as in patients with immunodeficiency conditions such as HIV infection or bone marrow transplantation. Transmission is suspected to occur via the fecal-oral route. Outbreaks have been reported in schools, day-care settings, and pediatric wards. The pathogenesis of astroviral infection is believed to be similar to that noted for rotavirus. The clinical presentation consists of diarrhea, headache, malaise, nausea, and to lesser extent, vomiting. These symptoms appear to be similar to those observed with rotavirus but milder. The incubation period is estimated to be 3 to 4 days, and the disease is usually self-limiting within 5 days. Maintenance of adequate hydration and electrolyte balance is the only therapeutic issue. The duration of viral shedding may be as long as 35 days.[91]

ENTERIC ADENOVIRUS

Adenovirus is an icosahedral virus previously associated with respiratory, ocular, and genitourinary infections; however, serotypes 40 and 41 have been identified as GI pathogens. The peak incidence is in children younger than 2 years of age, and infections occur year-round. Transmission is primarily person to person and fecal-oral, and viral shedding from the gut may occur for extended periods. The incubation time is 8 to 10 days. Diarrhea and vomiting often last 1 to 2 weeks. Low-grade fever and respiratory symptoms are also common.[92] The diagnosis can be made by enzyme immunoassay that identifies serotypes.

TABLE 111–5. Agents Responsible for Acute Viral Gastroenteritis and Diarrhea

Virus	Peak Age of Onset	Time of Year	Duration	Mode of Transmission	Symptoms
Rotavirus	6 mo–2 yr	October to April	3–8 days	Fecal-oral, water, food	Vomiting, diarrhea, fever, abdominal pain, lactose intolerance
Enteric adenovirus	<2 yr	Year-round	7–9 days	Fecal-oral	Diarrhea, respiratory symptoms, vomiting, fever
Calicivirus	3 mo–6 yr	Peak in winter	4 days	Fecal-oral, water, shellfish	Vomiting, diarrhea
Astrovirus	<7 yr	Winter	1–4 days	Fecal-oral, water, shellfish	Vomiting, diarrhea, fever, abdominal pain
Pestivirus	<2 yr	NR	3 days	NR	Mild
Coronavirus-like particles	<2 yr	Fall and early winter	7 days	NR	Respiratory disease
Enterovirus	NR	NR	NR	NR	Mild diarrhea, secondary organ damage
Norwalk	>5 yr	Variable	12–24 h	Fecal-oral, food, aerosol	Nausea, vomiting, diarrhea, abdominal cramps, headache, fever, chills, myalgias

NR = not reported.
Compiled from refs. 85, 91, and 92.

OTHER POTENTIAL VIRAL PATHOGENS

Although less commonly associated with severe GI disease, pestivirus, torovirus, and coronavirus-like particles have been recovered from diarrheal stools. In HIV-infected patients, the presence of diarrhea is associated with virus in 35% of stool specimens. Astrovirus, picobirnavirus, calicivirus, and adenovirus appear to be the most commonly isolated viral pathogens.[92,93] Table 111–5 presents specific characteristics of these agents.

TRAVELER'S DIARRHEA

Traveler's diarrhea is identified by multiple names depending on where the disease occurs, but all describes the clinical syndrome manifested by malaise, anorexia, and abdominal cramps followed by the sudden onset of diarrhea that incapacitates many travelers.[25] In particular, an increased risk lies with North Americans and northern Europeans traveling to Latin America, southern Europe, Africa, and Asia. The highest risk is observed with patients with immunocompromised conditions, achlorhydria, or inflammatory bowel disease and people taking diuretics, digoxin, lithium, or insulin (because of the need for appropriate hydration). Overall, an estimated 20% to 50% of people traveling to high-risk areas will develop the illness.

◄5 The onset of symptoms usually occurs during the first 2 weeks of travel but can occur anytime during the visit or after returning home.[10] The severity of the syndrome is determined by the number of stools per day and the presence or absence of cramping, nausea, and vomiting. Traveler's diarrhea is rarely life-threatening and is caused by contaminated food or water. Foods at high risk for contamination include raw or undercooked meat and seafood and raw fruits and vegetables. Tap water, ice, and unpasteurized milk and dairy products may be associated with increased risk. The most common pathogens include ETEC (20% to 72%), *Shigella* (3% to 25%), *Campylobacter* (3% to 17%), *Salmonella* (3% to 7%), and viruses (0% to 30%).[10]

PROPHYLAXIS

◄6 Patient education in avoiding high-risk food and beverages may reduce the risk to less than 15%, even in endemic areas. Slogans such as "Peel it, boil it, cook it, or forget it" remind travelers to avoid contaminated food and to use water purification or reliable bottled beverages.[94] Bismuth subsalicylate 525 mg orally once to four times daily for up to 3 weeks is a commonly recommended prophylactic regimen. Bismuth subsalicylate may inhibit enterotoxin activity and prevent diarrhea. Although efficacy of prophylactic antibiotics have been documented, their uses are discouraged owing to the increased risk of selection of drug-resistant organisms, side effects of antibiotics (e.g., photosensitivity), and possible acquisition of more severe infections. Prophylactic antibiotics (see Table 111–3) are recommended only in high-risk individuals or in situations in which short-term illness could ruin the purpose of the trip.[25] Travelers to high-risk areas should pack a kit that includes a thermometer, loperamide, 3 days of antibiotics (see below), oral rehydration solution salts, and a water purification method.[94] No vaccines are currently marketed in United States, and those which are available and in development are ineffective.

► TREATMENT: Traveler's Diarrhea

Fluid and electrolyte replacement should be initiated at the onset of diarrhea. (ORT generally is not required in healthy individuals; flavored mineral water offers a good source of sodium and glucose.[10,25]) For symptom relief, loperamide (preferred because of its quicker onset and longer duration of relief relative to bismuth) should be taken (4 mg orally initially and then 2 mg with each subsequent loose stool to a maximum of 16 mg/day in patients without bloody diarrhea and discontinued if symptoms persist for over 48 hours). Other symptomatic therapy includes bismuth subsalicylate 525 mg every 30 minutes up to 8 doses. Antibiotics (see Table 111–3) are recommended in addition to loperamide in moderate or severe diarrhea with systemic symptoms. Currently, the drug of choice is a fluoroquinolone. In pregnant women and children younger than 16 years of age, a combination of trimethoprim-sulfamethoxazole and erythromycin has been suggested. Macrolides are the drugs of choices only in areas of high prevalence of *Campylobacter* species resistant to quinolones, such as Thailand.

FOOD POISONING

Food poisoning results from the ingestion of food containing pathogenic microorganisms, preformed toxins that were produced by microorganisms, or other toxic compounds. In the United States, food-borne disease causes approximately 76 million illnesses, 325,000 hospitalizations, and 5200 deaths each year.[6] Food-borne transmission may account for up to 35% of acute gastroenteritis cases caused by unknown agents. A number of bacteria can cause food poisoning (Table 111–6). Common bacterial (*Campylobacter, Salmonella, Shigella, E. coli, Yersinia, Vibrio*) and viral (Norwalk-like virus) causes of GI infections have been discussed in the preceding sections. Other common food-borne pathogens that cause gastroenteritis include *S. aureus, Bacillus cereus, C. perfringens,* and *C. botulinum.* Unfortunately, sporadic illness caused by these pathogens is not reportable through passive or active systems, and thus it is difficult to determine their disease burden.

Since food-borne disease can appear as sporadic cases or outbreaks, the diagnosis should be suspected whenever two or more people present with acute gastrointestinal or neurologic manifestations after sharing a meal within the previous 72 hours. Important clues about etiologic agents can be gathered from demographic information (age, gender, etc.), the clinical syndrome, incubation period, medical history, type of foods consumed, seasonality, and geographic location of the outbreak.

Staphylococcal food poisoning results from the ingestion of food contaminated by an enterotoxin produced by certain strains of *S. au-*reus growing within the food.[95] Enterotoxin production generally results from leaving foods at room temperature, allowing the staphylococci to grow. Symptoms are rapid in onset, generally occurring within 1 to 6 hours of ingestion of preformed toxin-containing foods. The condition is characterized by nausea and vomiting (75%), although abdominal cramps and diarrhea also may be present. Symptoms resolve in less than 12 hours. ORT should be provided in severe cases, but antibiotics are not indicated.

B. cereus causes two different types of clinical syndromes.[96] The first one is characterized by a short incubation period with vomiting, abdominal cramps, and to a lesser extent, diarrhea within 1 to 6 hours of ingestion of contaminated food. This syndrome is caused by a preformed heat-stable toxin. Similar to staphylococcal food poisoning, illnesses caused by *B. cereus* usually last less than 12 hours. The second syndrome has a longer incubation period (8–16 hours) and is caused by toxins produced in vivo after the ingestion of contaminated food. In this syndrome, patients experience diarrhea, abdominal cramps, and less frequently, vomiting. The heat-labile enterotoxin produced in this syndrome activates intestinal adenylate cyclase and causes intestinal fluid secretion. This illness usually resolves within 24 hours, but symptom durations of several days to weeks also have been observed.

Food-borne *C. perfringens* infection may present as two distinct syndromes.[97] Type A organisms are seen in Western nations and result in a 24-hour illness characterized by watery diarrhea and epigastric pain. Symptoms generally resolve within 24 hours. This enterotoxin-related syndrome damages the brush borders of epithelial cells at the

TABLE 111–6. Food Poisonings

Organism	Time to Symptoms (h)	Principal Foods	Peak Incidence (U.S.A)	Principal Mechanism of Pathophysiology	Duration	Treatment
Staphylococcus aureus	1–6	Salad, pastries, ham, poultry	Summer	Preformed toxins A–E (heat stable)	12 h	Supportive
Bacillus cereus	1–6	Meats, vegetables, fried rice	None	Preformed toxin	12 h	Supportive
	8–16			Toxin production (*in vivo*)	24 h	Supportive
Clostridium perfringens (type A)	6–24	Meats, poultry	Fall, winter, spring	Toxin production (*in vivo*)	24 h	Supportive
Vibrio parahemolyticus	16–72	Shellfish	Spring, summer, fall	Toxin production and tissue invasion	2–7 day	Supportive
Salmonella spp.	16–48	Beef, poultry, water, eggs, dairy products	Summer	Tissue invasion	2–7 day	Supportive
Shigella spp.	16–48	Salad, water	Summer	Tissue invasion	2–7 day	Supportive
EPEC	16–48	Water	None	Tissue invasion	2–7 day	Supportive
Campylobacter	16–48	Poultry, dairy products, clams, water	Spring, summer	Tissue invasion	2–7 day	Supportive
ETEC	16–72	Water	None	Toxin production (*in vivo*)	1–7 day	Supportive
Vibrio cholerae	16–72	Water		Toxin production (*in vivo*)	2–12 day	Supportive, antibiotics
Yersinia enterocolitica	16–48	Dairy products		Toxin production and/or tissue invasion	1–30 day	Supportive
Clostridium botulinum	12–72	Canned fruits, vegetables, meats, honey	None	Preformed toxins A, B, and E (children and adults)		Supportive (including mechanically assisted ventilation)
				Toxin production (*in vivo*) (infants)		Trivalent antitoxin

EPEC = enteropathogenic *E. coli*; ETEC = enterotoxigenic *E. coli*.

villus tips to cause a noninflammatory diarrhea. Type C organisms can be found in undercooked pork and occur in underdeveloped tropical regions. Type C organisms can produce a toxin-related syndrome called *enteritis necroticans,* which is a coagulative transmural necrosis of the intestinal wall. This syndrome can result in intestinal perforation leading to sepsis and mortality in approximately 40% of victims.

Food-borne botulism results from the ingestion of food contaminated with preformed toxins or toxin-producing spores from *C. botulinum. C. botulinum* poisoning is relatively rare; only 110 cases are reported per year in the United States. Botulism is almost always associated with improper preparation or storage of food. Seven distinct toxins (A to G) have been described. The toxins, which are produced by the bacteria and released on lysis, are the most potent biologic or chemical toxins known to humans. The toxin prevents the release of acetylcholine at the peripheral cholinergic nerve terminal. Toxin activity has prompted the use of minute locally injected doses to treat select spastic disorders, such as blepharospasm, hemifacial spasm, and certain dystonias.[98]

Food-borne botulism is suspected when patients present with acute GI symptoms concurrently or just prior to the onset of a symmetric descending paralysis without sensory or central nervous system involvement. Symptoms usually begin 18 to 24 hours after ingestion and progress over days to weeks. Other symptoms can include blurred vision, photophobia (90%), dysphagia (76%), generalized weakness (58%), nausea and vomiting (56%), and dysphonia (55%). Diagnosis is made by culturing *C. botulinum* from the stool. Guillain-Barré syndrome associated with *C. jejuni* infection has been a common differential diagnosis in patients who present with these symptoms. The difference lies in the onset of neurologic symptoms, which typically occur 1 to 3 weeks after the onset of *C. jejuni* infection, and the condition usually is manifested by an ascending paralysis in *C. jejuni*–associated Guillain-Barré syndrome.[77]

Treatment consists primarily of respiratory support and use of botulinum antitoxin.[99] Respiratory failure may occur prior to involvement of other upper muscle groups. If evaluation is performed within several hours of ingestion, gastric lavage or induction of vomiting is suggested. Cathartics and enemas also can be used to remove residual toxin from the bowel, but they are contraindicated in cases of ileus. Although the effectiveness of antitoxins is unknown, patients diagnosed with botulism should receive botulinum antitoxin. Botulinum antitoxin is a concentrated preparation of equine globulins obtained from horses immunized with toxins A, B, and E. Because trivalent antitoxin is equine in origin, patients should be tested for hypersensitivity before receiving the product intravenously. Other agents used experimentally as adjunctive therapy are guanidine, which antagonizes the effect of botulinum toxin at the neuromuscular junction, and 4-aminopyridine, which increases acetylcholine release.[100] Newer and more effective methods of treatment and prevention are under development, including a botulinum toxin vaccine consisting of nontoxic botulinum fragments. Prevention always should be stressed. Botulinum toxins are heat labile and readily destroyed by 10 minutes of boiling. All home-canned foods should be processed according to directions and boiled, not just warmed, prior to consumption.

In food-borne illnesses, the cornerstone of therapy remains supportive care. ORT is preferred in replenishing and maintaining fluid and electrolyte balance, and intravenous fluid therapy should be reserved for those who are severely ill and cannot tolerate oral therapy. Antiemetics and antiperistaltic agents offer symptomatic relief, but the latter should not be given in patients who present with high fever, bloody diarrhea, or fecal leukocytes. Antimicrobial therapy is not effective in the management of *S. aureus, C. perfringens*, or *B. cereus* food poisonings. In developed countries, many of the food-borne illness can be prevented with proper food selection, preparation, and storage. However, in developing countries, sanitation and clean water supply are larger concerns.

ABBREVIATIONS

AAP: American Academy of Pediatrics
AIDS: acquired immunodeficiency syndrome
CDC: Centers for Disease Control and Prevention
EAEC: enteroadhesive *E. coli*
EHEC: enterohemorrhagic *E. coli*
EIEC: enteroinvasive *E. coli*
EPEC: enteropathogenic *E. coli*
ETEC: enterotoxigenic *E. coli*
GBS: Guillain-Barré syndrome
HLT: heat-labile toxin
HST: heat-stable toxin
HUS: hemolytic-uremic syndrome
ORT: oral rehydration solution
WHO: World Health Organization

Review Questions and other resources can be found at *www.pharmacotherapyonline.com.*

REFERENCES

1. Kosek M, Bern C, Guerrant RL. The global burden of diarrheal disease, as estimated from studies published between 1992 and 2000. Bull WHO 2003;81:197–204.
2. Snyder JD, Merson MH. The magnitude of the global problem of acute diarrhoeal disease: A review of active surveillance data. Bull WHO 1982;60:604–613.
3. Bern C, Martines J, de Zoysa I, et al. The magnitude of the global problem of diarrhoeal disease: A ten-year update. Bull WHO 1992;70:705–714.
4. Lew JF, Glass RI, Gangarosa RE, et al. Diarrheal deaths in the United States, 1979 through 1987: A special problem for the elderly. JAMA 1991;265:3280–3284.
5. Ganarosa RE, Glass RI, Lew JF, et al. Hospitalizations involving gastroenteritis in the United States, 1985: The special burden of the disease among the elderly. Am J Epidemiol 1992;135:281–290.
6. Mead PS, Slutsker L, Dietz V, et al. Food-related illness and death in the United States. Emerg Infect Dis 1999;5:607–625.
7. American Academy of Pediatrics. Practice parameter: The management of acute gastroenteritis in young children. Pediatrics 1996;97:424–435.
8. Zimmerman CM, Bresee JS, Parashar UD, et al. Cost of diarrhea-associated hospitalizations and outpatient visits in an insured population of young children in the United States. Pediatr Infect Dis J 2001;20: 14–19.
9. Cheney CP, Wong RKH. Acute infectious diarrhea. Med Clin North Am 1993;77:1169–1196.
10. Passaro DJ, Parsonnet J. Advances in the prevention and management of traveler's diarrhea. Curr Clin Top Infect Dis 1998;18:217–236.
11. Guerrant RL, Van Gilder T, Steiner TS, et al. Practice guidelines for the management of infectious diarrhea. Clin Infect Dis 2001;32:331–350.
12. Armon K, Stephenson T, MacFaul R, et al. An evidence and consensus based guideline for acute diarrhoea management. Arch Dis Child 2001;85:132–142
13. Gavin N, Merrick N, Davidson B. Efficacy of glucose-based oral rehydration therapy. Pediatrics 1996;98:45–51.
14. Holliday MA, Friedman AL, Wassner SJ. Extracellular fluid restoration in dehydration: A critique of rapid versus slow. Pediatr Nephrol 1999;13:292–297.
15. Farthing MJG. Oral rehydration: An evolving solution. J Pediatr Gastroenterol Nutr 2002;34:S64–67.

16. Gore SM, Fontaine O, Pierce MF. Impact of rice-based oral rehydration solution on stool output and duration of diarrhoea: Meta-analysis of 13 clinical trials. BMJ 1992;304:287–291.

17. Molina S, Vettorazzi C, Peerson JM. Clinical trial of glucose-oral rehydration solution (ORS), rice dextrin-ORS, and rice flour-ORS for the management of children with acute diarrhea and mild or moderate dehydration. Pediatrics 1995;95:191–197.

18. Ramakrishna BS, Venkataraman S, Srinivasan P, et al. Amylase-resistant starch plus oral rehydration solution for cholera. New Engl J Med 2000;342:308–313.

19. Fayed IM, Hashem M, Hussein A, et al. Comparison of soy-based formulas with lactose and with sucrose in the treatment of acute diarrhea in infants. Arch Pediatr Adolesc Med 1999;153:675–680.

20. Faruque ASG, Mahalanabis D, Islam A, et al. Breast-feeding and oral rehydration at home during diarrhoea to prevent dehydration. Arch Dis Child 1992;67:1027–1029.

21. American Academy of Pediatrics. Practice parameter: The management of acute gastroenteritis in young children. Pediatrics 1996;97:424–435.

22. Sandhu BK. Rationale for early feeding in childhood gastroenteritis. J Pediatr Gastroenterol Nutr 2001;33:S13–16.

23. Hoge CW, Gambel JM, Srijan A, et al. Trends in antibiotic resistance among diarrheal pathogens isolated in Thailand over 15 years. Clin Infect Dis 1998;26:341–345.

24. Parry CM. Antimicrobial drug resistance in *Salmonella enterica*. Curr Opin Infect Dis 2003;16:467–72.

25. Khan WA, Seas C, Dhar U, et al. Treatment of shigellosis: V. Comparison of azithromycin and ciprofloxacin. A double-blind, randomized, controlled trial. Ann Intern Med 1997;126:697–703.

26. Mandal BK, Ellis ME, Dunbar EM, et al. Double-blind placebo-controlled trial of erythromycin in the treatment of clinical Campylobacter infection. J Antimicrob Chemother 1984;13:619–623.

27. Graham SM. Salmonellosis in children in developing and developed countries and population. Curr Opin Infect Dis 2002;15:507–512.

28. Carter AO, Borczyk AA, Carlson JAK, et al. A severe outbreak of *Escherichia coli* O157:H7–associated hemorrhagic colitis in a nursing home New Engl J Med. 1987;317:1496–1500.

29. Ramzan NN. Traveler's diarrhea. Gastroenterol Clin North Am 2001;30: 665–678.

30. Centers for Disease Control and Prevention. Typhoid immunization: Recommendations for the Immunization Practice Advisory Committee (ACIP). MMWR 1990;39:1–5.

31. Centers for Disease Control and Prevention. Cholera vaccine. MMWR 1990;37:617–678.

32. Centers for Disease Control and Prevention. Withdrawal of rotavirus vaccine recommendations. MMWR 1999;48:1007.

33. Faruque SM, Albert MJ, Mekalanos JJ. Epidemiology, genetics, and ecology of toxigenic *Vibrio cholerae*. Microbiol Mol Bio Rev 1998;64: 1301–1314.

34. Chang MH, Glynn MK, Groseclose SL. Endemic, notifiable bioterrorism-related diseases, United States, 1992–1999. Emerg Infect Dis 2003;9:556–564.

35. Sack DA, Sack RB, Nair GB, et al. Cholera. Lancet 2004;363:223–33.

36. Molla A, Sarker S, Hossain M, et al. Rice-power electrolyte solution as oral-therapy in diarrhea due to *Vibrio cholerae* and *Escherichia coli*. Lancet 1982;1:1317–1319

37. Banerjee S, LaMont JT. Treatment of gastrointestinal infections. Gastroenterology 2000;18(2 suppl 1):S48–67.

38. Khan WA, Bennish ML, Seas C, et al. Randomized, controlled comparison of single-dose ciprofloxacin and doxycycline for cholera caused by *Vibrio cholerae* 01 or 0139. Lancet 1996;348:296–300

39. Nataro JP, Kaper JB. Diarrheagenic *Escherichia coli*. Clin Microbiol Rev 1998;11:142–201.

40. Cantey JR. *Escherichia coli* diarrhea. Gastroenterol Clin North Am 1993;22:609–622.

41. Afghani B, Stutman HR. Toxin-related diarrheas. Pediatr Ann 1994;23: 549–555.

42. Sears CL, Kaper JB. Enteric bacterial toxins: mechanisms of action and linkage to intestinal secretion. Microbiol Rev 1996;60:167–215.

43. Brook MG, Bannister BA. Diarrhoea-causing *Escherichia coli*. Dig Dis 1993;11:288–297.

44. Slutsker L, Ries AA, Greene KD, et al. *Escherichia coli* O157:H7 diarrhea in the United States: Clinical and epidemiologic features. Ann Intern Med 1997;126:505–513.

45. Mead PS, Griffin PM. *Escherichia coli* O157:H7. Lancet 1998;352: 1207–1212.

46. Karch H, Bielaszewask M, Bitzan M, et al. Epidemiology and diagnosis of shiga toxin–producing *Escherichia coli* infections. Diagn Microbiol Infect Dis 1999;34:229–243.

47. Ericsson CD, DuPont HL, Mathewson JJ, et al. Treatment of traveler's diarrhea with sulfamethoxazole and trimethoprim and loperamide. JAMA 1990;263:257.

48. Katz DE, DeLorimier AJ, Wolf MK, et al. Oral immunization of adult volunteers with microencapsulated enterotoxigenic *Escherichia coli* (ETEC) CS6 antigen. Vaccine 2003;21:341–346.

49. Wong CS, Jelacic S, Habeeb RL, et al. The risk of the hemolytic-uremic syndrome after antibiotic treatment of *Escherichia coli* O157:H7 infections. New Engl J Med 2000;342:1930–1936.

50. Bartlett JG. Antibiotic-associated diarrhea. New Engl J Med 2002;346: 334–339.

51. McFarland LV, Mulligan ME, Kwok RY, et al. Nosocomial acquisition of *Clostridium difficile* infection. New Engl J Med 1989;320:204–210.

52. Rohner P, Pittet D, Pepey B, et al. Etiological agents of infectious diarrhea: Implications for requests for microbial culture. J Clin Microbiol 1997;35:1427–1432.

53. Hurley BW, Nguyen CC. The spectrum of pseudomembranous enterocolitis and antibiotic-associated diarrhea. Arch Intern Med 2002;162:2177–2184.

54. Feteky R. Guidelines for the diagnosis and management of *Clostridium difficile*–associated diarrhea and colitis. Am J Gastroenterol 1997;92: 739–750.

55. Elmer GW, Surawicz CM, McFarland LV. Biotherapeutic agents: A neglected modality for the treatment and prevention of selected intestinal and vaginal infections. JAMA 1996;275:870–876.

56. Vanderhoof JA, Young RJ. Use of probiotics in childhood gastrointestinal disorders. J Pediatr Gastroenterol Nutr 1998;27:323–331.

57. Kotloff KL, Winickoff B, Ivanoff JD, et al. Global burden of *Shigella* infections: Implications for vaccine development and implementation. Bull WHO 1999;77:651–656.

58. DuPont HL, Levine MM, Hornick RB, et al. Inoculum size in shigellosis and implications for expected mode of transmission. J Infect Dis 1989;159:1126–1128

59. Fernandez MI, Sansonetti PJ. *Shigella* interaction with intestinal epithelial cells determines the innate immune response in shigellosis. Int J Med Microbiol. 2003;293:55–67.

60. Keusch GT, Jacewicz M. The pathogenesis of shigella diarrhea: VI. Toxin and antitoxin in *Shigella flexneri* and *Shigella sonnei* infections in humans. J Infect Dis 1977;135:552–556.

61. Lopez EL, Prado-Jimenez V, O'Ryan-Gallardo M. Shigella and shiga toxin–producing *Escherichia coli* causing bloody diarrhea in Latin America. Infect Dis Clin North Am 2000;14:41–65

62. Hill Gaston JS, Lillicrap MS. Arthritis associated with enteric infection. Best Pract Res Clin Rheumatol. 2003;17:219–239.

63. Katz DE, Coster TS, Wolf MK, et al. Two studies evaluating the safety and immunogenicity of a live, attenuated *Shigella flexneri* 2a vaccine (SC602) and excretion of vaccine organisms in North American volunteers. Infect Immun 2004;72:923–930.

64. Brenner F, Villar R, Angulo F, et al. *Salmonella* nomenclature. J Clin Microbiol 2000;38:2465–2467.

65. Olsen SJ, Bishop R, Brenner FW, et al. The changing epidemiology of *Salmonella*: Trends in serotypes isolated from humans in the United States, 1987–1997. J Infect Dis 2001;183:753–761.

66. Parry CM, Hien TT, Dougan G, et al. Typhoid fever. New Engl J Med 2002;347:1770–1782.

67. Hohmann EL. Nontyphoidal salmonellosis. Clin Infect Dis 2001;32: 263–269.

68. El-Radhi AS, Rostila T, Vesikari T. Association of high fever and short bacterial excretion after salmonellosis. Arch Dis Child 1992;67:531–532.

69. Stutman HR. *Salmonella, Shigella,* and *Campylobacter:* Common bacterial causes of infectious diarrhea. Pediatr Ann 1994;23:538–543.

70. Hosek G, Leschinsky D, Irons S, Safranek TJ. Multidrug-resistant *Salmonella* serotype typhimurium—United States, 1996. JAMA 1997;277:1513.

71. Wain J, Hoa NT, Chinh NT, et al. Quinolone-resistant *Salmonella typhi* in Viet Nam: Molecular basis of resistance and clinical response to treatment. Clin Infect Dis 1997;25:1404–1410.

72. Hogan DE. The emergency department approach to diarrhea. Emerg Med Clin North Am 1996;14:673–694.

73. Allos BM, Blaser MJ. *Campylobacter jejuni* and the expanding spectrum of related infections. Clin Infect Dis 1995;20:1092–1101.

74. llos BM. *Campylobacter jejuni* infections: Update on emerging issues and trends. Clin Infect Dis 2001;32:1201–1206

75. Harris NV, Weiss NS, Nolan CM. The role of poultry and meats in the etiology of *Campylobacter jejunii* enteritis. Am J Public Health 1986;76:407–410

76. Wallis MR. The pathogenesis of *Campylobacter jejuni.* Br J Biomed Sci 1994;51:57–64.

77. Allos BM. Association between *Campylobacter* infection and Guillain-Barré syndrome. J Infect Dis 1997;(suppl 2):S125–128.

78. Hoogkamp-Korstanje JAA, de Koning J, Samsom JP. Incidence of human infection with *Yersinia enterocolitica* serotypes O3, O8, an dO9 and the use of indirect immunofluorescence in diagnosis. J Infect Dis 1986;153:138–141

79. Marks MI, Pai CH, LaFleur L, et al. *Yersinia enterocolitica* gastroenteritis: A prospective study of clinical, bacteriologic, and epidemiologic features. J Pediatr 1980;96:26–31.

80. San Joaquin VH. *Aeromonas, Yersinia,* and miscellaneous bacterial enteropathogens. Pediatr Ann 1994;23:544–548.

81. Haverly RM, Harrison CR, Dougherty TH. *Yersinia enterocolitica* bacteremia associated with red blood cell transfusion. Arch Pathol Lab Med 1996;120:499–500.

82. Wilhelmi I, Roman E, Sanchez-Fauquier A. Viruses causing gastroenteritis. Clin Microbiol Infect 2003;9:247–262.

83. Glass R, Kilgore P, Holman R, et al. The epidemiology of rotavirus diarrhea in the United States: Surveillance and estimates of disease burden. J Infect Dis 1996;174(suppl 1):S5–11.

84. Lundgren O, Svensson L. Pathogenesis of rotavirus diarrhea. Microb Infect 2001;3:1145–1156

85. Parashar UD, Holman RC, Clarke MJ, et al. Hospitalizations associated with rotavirus diarrhea in the United States, 1993 through 1995: Surveillance based on the new ICD-9-CM rotavirus-specific diagnostic code. J Infect Dis 1998;177:13–17

86. Centers for Disease Control and Prevention (CDC). Outbreak of severe rotavirus gastroenteritis among children—Jamaica, 2003. MMWR 2003;52:1103–1105.

87. Orellana C. Rotavirus vaccine shows promise. Lancet 2003;3:396

88. Koopmans M, von Bonsdorff CH, Vinje J, et al. Food-borne viruses. FEMS Microbiol Rev 2002;26:187–205

89. Bresee JS, Widdowson MA, Monroe SS, et al. Food-borne viral gastroenteritis: Challenges and opportunities. Clin Infect Dis 2002;35:748–753.

90. Oishi I, Yamazaki K, Kimoto T, et al. A large outbreak of acute gastroenteritis associated with astrovirus among students and teachers in Osaka, Japan. J Infect Dis 1994;170:439–443

91. Walter JE, Mitchell DK. Astrovirus infection in children. Curr Opin Infect Dis 2003;16:247–253.

92. Taterka JA, Cuff CF, Rubin DH. Viral gastrointestinal infections. Gastroenterol Clin North Am 1992;21:303–329.

93. Grohmann GS, Glass RI, Pereira HG, et al. Enteric viruses and diarrhea in HIV-infected patients. New Engl J Med 1993;329:14–20.

94. Centers for Disease Control and Prevention. Health Information for International Travel 1999–2000. Atlanta, Department of Health and Human Services (also *www.cdc.gov/travel/diarrhea.htm*).

95. Le Loir Y, Baron F, Gautier M. *Staphylococcus aureus* and food poisoning. Genet Mol Res 2003;2:63–76.

96. Terranova W, Blake PA. *Bacillus cereus* food poisoning. New Engl J Med 1978;298:143–144.

97. Hatheway CL. Toxigenic clostridia. Clin Microbiol Rev 1990;3:66–98.

98. Roblot P, Roblot F, Fauchere JL, et al. Retrospective study of 108 cases of botulism in Poitiers, France. J Med Microbiol 1994;40:379–384.

99. Shapiro RL, Hatheway C, Swerdlow DL. Botulism in the United States: A clinical and epidemiologic review. Ann Intern Med 1998;129:221–228.

100. Middlebrook JL. Protection strategies against botulinum toxin. Adv Exper Med Biol 1995;383:93–98.

112

INTRAABDOMINAL INFECTIONS

Joseph T. DiPiro and Thomas R. Howdieshell

Learning Objectives and other resources can be found at *www.pharmacotherapyonline.com.*

KEY CONCEPTS

❶ Most intraabdominal infections are "secondary" infections that are caused by a defect in the gastrointestinal tract that must be treated by surgical drainage, resection, and/or repair.

❷ Primary peritonitis generally is caused by a single organism (*Staphylococcus aureus* in patients undergoing chronic ambulatory peritoneal dialysis [CAPD] or *Escherichia coli* in patients with cirrhosis).

❸ Secondary intraabdominal infections usually are caused by a mixture of enteric gram-negative bacilli and anaerobes. This mix of organisms enhances the pathogenic potential of the bacteria.

❹ For peritonitis, early and aggressive intravenous fluid resuscitation and electrolyte replacement therapy are essential. A common cause of early death is hypovolemic shock caused by inadequate intravascular volume and tissue perfusion.

❺ Cultures of secondary intraabdominal infection sites generally are not useful for directing antimicrobial therapy. Treatment generally is initiated on a "presumptive" or empirical basis.

❻ Antimicrobial regimens for secondary intraabdominal infections should include coverage for enteric gram-negative bacilli and anaerobes. Antimicrobials that may be used for the treatment of secondary intraabdominal infections include (a) a β-lactam/β-lactamase inhibitor combination, (b) a carbapenem, (c) quinolone plus metronidazole, or an aminoglycoside plus clindamycin (or metronidazole).

❼ Treatment of primary peritonitis for CAPD patients should include an antistaphylococcal antimicrobial such as a first-generation cephalosporin or vancomycin (usually given by the intraperitoneal route).

❽ The duration of antimicrobial treatment should be for a total of 5 to 7 days for most intraabdominal infections.

❾ Patients treated for intraabdominal infections should be assessed for the occurrence of drug-related adverse effects, particularly hypersensitivity reactions (β-lactam antimicrobials), diarrhea (most agents), fungal infections (most agents), and nephrotoxicity (aminoglycosides).

Intraabdominal infections are those contained within the peritoneal cavity or retroperitoneal space. The peritoneal cavity extends from the undersurface of the diaphragm to the floor of the pelvis and contains the stomach, small bowel, large bowel, liver, gallbladder, and spleen. The duodenum, pancreas, kidneys, adrenal glands, great vessels (aorta and vena cava), and most mesenteric vascular structures reside in the retroperitoneum. Intraabdominal infections may be generalized or localized. They may be contained within visceral structures, such as the liver, gallbladder, spleen, pancreas, kidney, or female reproductive organs. Two general types of intraabdominal infection are discussed throughout this chapter: peritonitis and abscess. *Peritonitis* is defined as the acute inflammatory response of the peritoneal lining to microorganisms, chemicals, irradiation, or foreign-body injury. This chapter deals only with peritonitis of infectious origin.

An *abscess* is a purulent collection of fluid separated from surrounding tissue by a wall consisting of inflammatory cells and adjacent organs. It usually contains necrotic debris, bacteria, and inflammatory cells. These processes differ considerably in presentation and approach to treatment.

EPIDEMIOLOGY

Peritonitis may be classified as primary, secondary, or tertiary. Primary peritonitis, also called *spontaneous bacterial peritonitis,* is an infection of the peritoneal cavity without an evident source in the abdomen.[1,2] Bacteria may be transported from the bloodstream to the peritoneal cavity, where the inflammatory process begins. In secondary peritonitis, a focal disease process is evident within the abdomen. Secondary peritonitis may involve perforation of the gastrointestinal (GI) tract (possibly because of ulceration, ischemia, or obstruction), postoperative peritonitis, or posttraumatic peritonitis (blunt or penetrating trauma). Tertiary peritonitis occurs in critically ill patients and is infection that persists or recurs at least 48 hours after apparently adequate management of primary or secondary peritonitis.

❶ Primary peritonitis develops in up to 25% of patients with alcoholic cirrhosis.[3] Patients undergoing chronic ambulatory peritoneal dialysis (CAPD) average one episode of peritonitis every 2 years.[4] Epidemiologic data for secondary and tertiary intraabdominal infections are limited. Secondary peritonitis may be caused by perforation of a peptic ulcer; traumatic perforation of the stomach, small or large bowel, uterus, or urinary bladder; appendicitis; pancreatitis; diverticulitis; bowel infarction; inflammatory bowel disease, cholecystitis; operative contamination of the peritoneum; or diseases of the female genital tract such as septic abortion, postoperative uterine infection, endometritis, or salpingitis. Appendicitis is one of the most common causes of intraabdominal infection. In 1998, 278,000 appendectomies were performed in the United States for suspected appendicitis.[5]

ETIOLOGY

Primary peritonitis in adults occurs most commonly in association with alcoholic cirrhosis, especially in its end stage, or with ascites caused by postnecrotic cirrhosis, chronic active hepatitis, acute viral hepatitis, congestive heart failure, malignancy, systemic lupus erythematosus, or nephritic syndrome. It also may result from the use of a peritoneal catheter for dialysis or central nervous system ventriculoperitoneal shunting for hydrocephalus. Rarely, primary peritonitis occurs without apparent underlying disease.

Table 112–1 summarizes many of the potential causes of bacterial peritonitis. These include inflammatory processes of the GI tract or abdominal organs, bowel obstruction, vascular occlusions that may lead to gangrene of the intestines, and neoplasia that may cause intestinal perforation or obstruction. Other possible causes include those resulting from traumatic injuries or postoperative infections.

Abscesses are the result of chronic inflammation and may occur without preceding generalized peritonitis. They may be located within one of the spaces of the peritoneal cavity or within one of the visceral organs and may range from a few milliliters to a liter or more in volume. These collections often have a fibrinous capsule and may take from a few weeks to years to form.

The causes of intraabdominal abscess overlap those of peritonitis and, in fact, may occur sequentially or simultaneously. Appendicitis is the most frequent cause of abscess. Other potential causes of intraabdominal abscess include pancreatitis, diverticulitis, lesions of the biliary tract, genitourinary tract infections, perforating tumors in the abdomen, trauma, and leaking intestinal anastomoses. In addition, pelvic inflammatory disease in women may lead to tuboovarian abscess. For certain diseases, such as appendicitis and diverticulitis, abscesses occur more frequently than generalized peritonitis.

TABLE 112–1. Causes of Bacterial Peritonitis

Primary Bacterial Peritonitis
Peritoneal dialysis
Cirrhosis with ascites
Nephrotic syndrome
Secondary Bacterial Peritonitis
Miscellaneous causes
  Diverticulitis
  Appendicitis
  Inflammatory bowel diseases
  Salpingitis
  Biliary tract infections
  Necrotizing pancreatitis
Neoplasms
  Intestinal obstruction
  Perforation
Mechanical gastrointestinal problems
  Any cause of small bowel obstruction (adhesions, hernia)
Vascular causes
  Mesenteric arterial or venous occlusion (atrial fibrillation)
  Mesenteric ischemia without occlusion
Trauma
  Blunt abdominal trauma with rupture of intestine
  Penetrating abdominal trauma
Iatrogenic intestinal perforation (endoscopy)
Intraoperative events
Peritoneal contamination during abdominal operation
Leakage from gastrointestinal anastomosis

MICROFLORA OF THE GASTROINTESTINAL TRACT AND FEMALE GENITAL TRACT

A full appreciation of intraabdominal infection requires an understanding of the normal microflora within the GI tract. There are striking differences in bacterial species and concentrations of flora within the various segments of the GI tract (Table 112–2), and this bacterial environment usually determines the severity of infectious processes in the abdomen. Generally, the low gastric pH eradicates bacteria that enter the stomach. With achlorhydria, bacterial counts may rise to 10^5 to 10^7 organisms per milliliter. The normally low bacterial count also may increase by 1000- or 10,000-fold with gastric outlet obstruction, hemorrhage, gastric cancer, and in patients receiving histamine 2 (H_2)–receptor antagonists, proton pump inhibitors, or antacids.

TABLE 112–2. Usual Microflora of the Gastrointestinal Tract

Site	Commonly Found Bacteria	Approximate Concentration (Log No. Organisms/mL)	
		Aerobes	Anaerobes
Stomach[a]	Streptococcus, Lactobacillus	10–100	Rare
Biliary tract	Normally sterile (Escherichia coli, Klebsiella, or enterococci in some patients)	0	0
Proximal small bowel	Streptococcus (including enterococci), E. coli, Klebsiella, Lactobacillus, diphtheroids	100	Few
Distal ileum	E. coli, Klebsiella, Enterobacter, enterococci, Bacteroides fragilis, Clostridium, peptostreptococci	10^4–10^6	10^5–10^7
Colon	Bacteroides spp., peptostreptococci, Clostridium, E. coli, Klebsiella, enterococci, Enterobacter, and many others	10^5–10^8	10^9–10^{11}

[a]With achlorhydria, H_2-antagonist therapy, gastric cancer, or gastric outlet obstruction, bacterial counts may rise to 10^5/mL.

The biliary tract (gallbladder and bile ducts) is sterile in most healthy individuals, but in certain groups (age greater than 70 years, acute cholecystitis, jaundice, or common bile duct stones), it is likely to be colonized by aerobic gram-negative bacilli (particularly *Escherichia coli* and *Klebsiella* spp.) and enterococci.[6] Patients with biliary tract bacterial colonization are at greater risk of intraabdominal infection.

In the distal ileum, bacterial counts of aerobes and anaerobes are quite high. In the colon, there may be 400 to 500 different types of bacteria, with concentrations often reaching 10^{11} organisms per milliliter and anaerobic bacteria outnumbering aerobic bacteria by more than 1000 to 1. In fact, up to 50% of the dry mass of stool is bacteria. Fortunately, most colonic bacteria are not pathogens because they cannot survive in environments outside the colon. Perforation of the colon results in the release of large numbers of anaerobic and aerobic bacteria into the peritoneum. The colonic flora generally are consistent unless broad-spectrum antimicrobials have been used, in which case there are increases in *Candida* or gram-negative bacteria.

The lower female genital tract generally is colonized by a large number of aerobic and anaerobic bacteria. Anaerobes may number 10^9 organisms per milliliter and often include lactobacilli, eubacteria, clostridia, anaerobic streptococci, and less frequently, *Bacteroides fragilis.* Aerobic bacteria most often are streptococci and *Staphylococcus epidermidis,* and these may number 10^8 organisms per milliliter.

PATHOPHYSIOLOGY

Intraabdominal infection results from bacterial entry into the peritoneal or retroperitoneal spaces or from bacterial collections within intraabdominal organs. In primary peritonitis, bacteria may enter the abdomen via the bloodstream or the lymphatic system by transmigration through the bowel wall, through an indwelling peritoneal dialysis catheter, or via the fallopian tubes in females. Hematogenous bacterial spread (through the bloodstream) occurs more frequently with tuberculosis peritonitis or peritonitis associated with cirrhotic ascites. When peritonitis results from peritoneal dialysis, skin surface flora are introduced via the peritoneal catheter.[7] In secondary peritonitis, bacteria most often enter the peritoneum or retroperitoneum as a result of perforation of the GI or female genital tracts caused by diseases or traumatic injuries. Also, peritonitis or abscess may result from contamination of the peritoneum during a surgical procedure or following anastomotic leak.

The physiologic characteristics of the peritoneal cavity determine the nature of the response to infection or inflammation within it. The peritoneum is lined by a highly permeable serous membrane with a surface area approximately that of skin. The peritoneal cavity is lubricated with less than 100 mL of sterile, clear yellow fluid, normally with fewer than 300 cells/mm³, a specific gravity below 1.016, and protein content below 3 g/dL. These conditions change drastically with peritoneal infection or inflammation, as described below.

After bacteria are introduced into the peritoneal cavity, there is an immediate response to contain the insult. Humoral and cellular defenses respond first; then the omentum adheres to the affected area. A limited bacterial inoculum is handled rapidly by defense mechanisms, including complement activation. Under certain conditions, the bacterial insult is not contained, and bacteria disseminate throughout the peritoneal cavity, resulting in peritonitis. This is more likely to occur in the presence of a foreign body, hematoma, dead tissue, a large bacterial inoculum, continuing bacterial contamination, and contamination involving a mixture of synergistic organisms. Protein-calorie

malnutrition, antecedent steroid therapy, and diabetes mellitus also may contribute to the formation of an intraabdominal abscess.

When bacteria become dispersed throughout the peritoneum, the inflammatory process involves most of the peritoneal lining. There is an outpouring into the peritoneum of fluid containing leukocytes, fibrin, and other proteins that form exudates on the inflamed peritoneal surfaces and begin to form adhesions between peritoneal structures. This process, combined with a paralysis of the intestines (ileus), may result in confinement of the contamination to one or more locations within the peritoneum. Fluid also begins to collect in the bowel lumen and wall, and distension may result.

The fluid and protein shift into the abdomen (called *third-spacing*) may be so dramatic that circulating blood volume is decreased, which causes decreased cardiac output and hypovolemic shock. Accompanying fever, vomiting, or diarrhea may worsen the fluid imbalance. A reflex sympathetic response, manifested by sweating, tachycardia, and vasoconstriction, may be evident. With an inflamed peritoneum, bacteria and endotoxins are absorbed easily into the bloodstream (translocation), and this may result in septic shock. Other foreign substances present in the peritoneal cavity potentiate peritonitis. These adjuvants, notably feces, dead tissues, barium, mucus, bile, and blood, have detrimental effects on host defense mechanisms, particularly on bacterial phagocytosis.

Many of the manifestations of intraabdominal infections, particularly peritonitis, result from cytokine activity. Inflammatory cytokines, such as tumor necrosis factor α (TNF-α), interleukin 1 (IL-1), IL-6, IL-8, and interferon-γ (INF-γ), are produced by macrophages and neutrophils in response to bacteria and bacterial products or in response to tissue injury resulting from the surgical incision.[8] These cytokines produce wide-ranging effects on the endothelium of organs, particularly the liver, lungs, kidneys, and heart. With uncontrolled activation of these mediators, sepsis may result[9] (see Chap. 117).

Peritonitis may result in death because of the effects on major organ systems. Fluid shifts and endotoxin may result in hypovolemic and septic shock. Hypoalbuminemia may result from protein loss into the peritoneum exacerbating intravascular volume loss. Pulmonary function may be compromised by the inflamed peritoneum producing splinting (muscle rigidity caused by pain) that inhibits adequate diaphragmatic movement leading to atelectasis and pneumonia. Increased kung vascular permeability and resulting shunting of blood may induce onset of the respiratory distress syndrome and associated hypoxemia and hypercarbia. With fluid loss, hypotension, endotoxemia, and renal and hepatic perfusion may be compromised, and acute renal and hepatic failure are potential threats.

If peritoneal contamination is localized but bacterial elimination is incomplete, an abscess results. This collection of necrotic tissue, bacteria, and white blood cells (WBCs) may be at single or multiple sites and may be within one of the spaces of the peritoneal cavity or in one of the visceral organs. The location of the abscess often is related to the site of primary disease. For example, abscesses resulting from appendicitis tend to appear in the right lower quadrant or the pelvis; those resulting from diverticulitis tend to appear in the left lower quadrant or pelvis.

An abscess begins by the combined action of inflammatory cells (such as neutrophils), bacteria, fibrin, and other inflammatory mediators. Bacteria may release heparinases that cause local thrombosis and tissue necrosis or fibrinolysins, collagenases, or other enzymes that allow extension of the process into surrounding tissues. Neutrophils gathered in the abscess cavity die in 3 to 5 days, releasing lysosomal enzymes that liquefy the core of the abscess. A mature abscess may have a fibrinous capsule that isolates bacteria and the liquid core from antimicrobials and immunologic defenses.

Within the abscess, the oxygen tension is low, and anaerobic bacteria thrive, and thus the size of the abscess may increase because it is hypertonic, resulting in an additional influx of fluid. Hypertonicity promotes the formation of bacterial L forms, which are resistant to antimicrobial agents that disrupt cell walls. Abscess formation may continue and mature for long periods of time and may not be readily evident to either patient or physician. In some instances, the abscess may resolve spontaneously, and infrequently, it may erode into adjacent organs or rupture and cause diffuse peritonitis. If the abscess erodes through the skin, it may result in an enterocutaneous fistula, connecting bowel to skin, or in a draining sinus tract.

MICROBIOLOGY OF INTRAABDOMINAL INFECTION

Primary bacterial peritonitis often is caused by a single organism. In children, the pathogen is usually *Streptococcus pneumoniae* or a group A *Streptococcus*.[4] When peritonitis occurs in association with cirrhotic ascites, *Escherichia coli* is isolated most frequently. Other potential pathogens are: *Hemophilus pneumoniae, Klebsiella, Pseudomonas,* anaerobes, and *S. pneumoniae*.[10] Occasionally, primary peritonitis may be caused by *Mycobacterium tuberculosis*. Peritonitis in patients undergoing peritoneal dialysis is caused most often by common skin organisms, such as *S. epidermidis, Staphylococcus aureus,* streptococci, and diphtheroids. Occasionally, aerobic gram-negative bacilli may cause infections, particularly in patients undergoing dialysis during hospitalization. Mortality from primary peritonitis caused by gram-negative bacteria is much greater than that from gram-positive bacteria.[11]

Because of the diverse bacteria present in the GI tract, secondary intraabdominal infections often are polymicrobial.[13] The mean number of different bacterial species isolated from infected intraabdominal sites ranged from 2.9 to 3.7, including an average of 1.3 to 1.6 aerobes and 1.7 to 2.1 anaerobes.[14,15] With proper anaerobic specimen collection, anaerobic organisms are isolated in most patients. In one report of patients with gangrenous and perforated appendicitis, an average of 10.2 different organisms was isolated from each patient, including 2.7 aerobes and 7.5 anaerobes.[16] Purely aerobic or anaerobic infections are uncommon, as are infections caused by fungi. The frequencies with which specific bacteria were isolated from patients with peritonitis are given in Table 112–3.[17] *E. coli, Streptococcus* spp., and *Bacteroides* spp. were isolated most often from the infection site, as well as from blood cultures. In patients diagnosed with severe infections, the pattern of bacterial isolates may change and

TABLE 112–3. Pathogens Isolated from Patients with Secondary Peritonitis

Gram-Negative Bacteria	
E. coli	32–61%
Enterobacter	8–26%
Klebsiella	6–26%
Proteus	4–23%
Gram-Positive Bacteria	
Enterococci	18–24%
Streptococci	6–55%
Staphylococci	6–16%
Anaerobic Bacteria	
Bacteroides	25–80%
Clostridium	5–18%
Fungi	2–5%

Adapted from ref. 2.

commonly includes *Candida,* enterococci, Enterobacteriaceae, and *S. epidermidis.*

Visceral abscesses differ in character from the typical intraabdominal abscess. Hepatic abscesses may be polymicrobial (involving *E. coli* and anaerobes) or occasionally may be caused by amoeba. Pancreatic abscesses are often polymicrobial, involving enteric bacteria that ascend through the biliary system. Splenic abscesses usually result from hematogenous dissemination of bacteria, such as *S. aureus,* streptococci, and occasionally, *Salmonella* or anaerobic organisms. Pelvic inflammatory disease is associated initially with *Neisseria gonorrhoeae* or *Chlamydia trachomatis.* However, tuboovarian abscesses usually are polymicrobial, having a mix of gram-positive and gram-negative aerobes and anaerobes.

BACTERIAL SYNERGISM

The size of the bacterial inoculum and the number and types of bacterial species present in intraabdominal infections influence patient outcome. The combination of aerobic and anaerobic organisms appears to increase the severity of infection greatly. In animal studies, combinations of aerobic and anaerobic bacteria were much more lethal than infections caused by aerobes or anaerobes alone.

Facultative bacteria may provide an environment conducive to the growth of anaerobic bacteria.[13] Although many bacteria isolated in mixed infections are nonpathogenic by themselves, their presence may be essential for the pathogenicity of the bacterial mixture.[3] The role of facultative bacteria in mixed infections can include (1) promotion of an appropriate environment for anaerobic growth through oxygen consumption, (2) production of nutrients necessary for anaerobes, and (3) production of extracellular enzymes that promote tissue invasion by anaerobes.

Rat models of intraabdominal infection demonstrate that uncontrolled infection with an implanted mix of aerobes and anaerobes leads to a two-stage infectious process. There is an early peritonitis phase with a high mortality rate and isolation of *E. coli* from blood and a late abscess formation phase in all survivors with isolation of anaerobes such as *B. fragilis* and *Fusobacterium varium.* These experiments and others support the concept that aerobic enteric organisms and anaerobes are pathogens in intraabdominal infection. Aerobic bacteria, particularly *E. coli,* appear responsible for the early mortality from peritonitis, whereas anaerobic bacteria are major pathogens in abscesses, with *B. fragilis* predominating.[18]

Enterococcus can be isolated from many intraabdominal infections in humans, but its role as a pathogen is not clear.[19] Enterococcal infection occurs more commonly in postoperative peritonitis, in the presence of specific risk factors indicating failure of the host's defenses (immunocompromised patients), or with the use of broad-spectrum antibiotics.[20,21]

CLINICAL PRESENTATION

Intraabdominal infections have a wide spectrum of clinical features often depending on the specific disease process, the location and magnitude of bacterial contamination, and concurrent host factors. Peritonitis usually is recognized easily, but intraabdominal abscess often may continue for considerable periods of time, either going unrecognized or being attributed to an unrelated disease process. Patients with primary and secondary peritonitis present quite differently (Table 112–4).

Primary peritonitis can develop over a period of days to weeks and usually is a more indolent process than secondary peritonitis. The

TABLE 112–4. Clinical Presentation of Peritonitis

Primary Peritonitis

General

The patient may not be in acute distress, particularly with peritoneal dialysis.

Signs and Symptoms

The patient may complain of nausea, vomiting (sometimes with diarrhea), and abdominal tenderness.

Temperature may be only mildly elevated or not elevated in patients undergoing peritoneal dialysis.

Bowel sounds are hypoactive.

The cirrhotic patient may have worsening encephalopathy.

Cloudy dialysate fluid with peritoneal dialysis.

Laboratory Tests

The patient's WBC count may be only mildly elevated.

Ascitic fluid usually contains greater than 300 leukocytes/mm^3, and bacteria may be evident on Gram stain of a centrifuged specimen.

In 60% to 80% of patients with cirrhotic ascites, the Gram stain is negative.

Other Diagnostic Tests

Culture of peritoneal dialysate or ascitic fluid should be positive.

Secondary Peritonitis

Signs and Symptoms

Generalized abdominal pain.

Tachypnea.

Tachycardia.

Nausea and vomiting.

Temperature normal initially then increasing to 100 to 102°F (37.7 to 38.8°C) within the first few hours and may continue to rise for the next several hours.

Hypotension and shock if volume is not restored.

Decreased urine output due to dehydration.

Physical Examination

Voluntary abdominal guarding changing to involuntary guarding and a "board-like abdomen."

Abdominal tenderness and distension.

Faint bowel sounds that cease over time.

Laboratory Tests

Leukocytosis (15,000–20,000 WBC/mm^3, with neutrophils predominating and an elevated percentage of immature neutrophils (bands).

Elevated hematocrit and blood urea nitrogen because of dehydration.

Patient progresses from early alkalosis because of hyperventilation and vomiting to acidosis and lactic acidemia.

Other Diagnostic Tests

Abdominal radiographs may be useful because free air in the abdomen (indicating intestinal perforation) or distension of the small or large bowel is often evident.

---

first sign of peritonitis may be a cloudy dialysate in patients undergoing peritoneal dialysis or worsening encephalopathy in a cirrhotic patient.

The patient with generalized bacterial peritonitis presents most often in acute distress. The patient lies still, usually on his or her back, possibly with hips slightly flexed. Any movement of the patient, including rocking the bed or breathing, worsens the generalized abdominal pain.

If peritonitis continues untreated, the patient may experience hypovolemic shock from third-space fluid loss into the peritoneum, bowel wall, and lumen. This may be accompanied by sepsis because the inflamed peritoneum absorbs bacteria and toxins into mesenteric blood vessels and lymph nodes, initiating production of inflammatory

cytokines. Hypovolemic shock is the major factor contributing to mortality in the early stage of peritonitis.

Intraabdominal abscess may pose a difficult diagnostic challenge because the symptoms are neither specific nor dramatic. The patient may complain of abdominal pain or discomfort, but these symptoms are not reliable. Fever usually is present; often it is low grade, but it may be high, with a spiking pattern. The patient may have a paralytic ileus and abdominal distension. The abdominal examination is unreliable; tenderness and pain may be present, and a mass may be palpated.

Peritonitis may result from an abscess that ruptures, spreading bacteria and toxins throughout the peritoneum. In other patients, the entry of bacterial toxins into the systemic circulation from the abscess may lead to sepsis and progressive multisystem organ failure (e.g., renal, hepatic, pulmonary, or cardiovascular).

Laboratory studies generally are not helpful in the diagnosis of intraabdominal abscess, although most patients will have leukocytosis. Some patients may have positive blood cultures, whereas others, particularly diabetics, may have hyperglycemia. The finding of *Bacteroides* or any two enteric bacteria in the bloodstream is often indicative of an intraabdominal infectious process.

Radiographic methods are used to make the diagnosis of an intraabdominal abscess. Plain radiographs may show air-fluid levels or a shift of normal intraabdominal contents by the abscess mass. GI contrast studies also may demonstrate this displacement of abdominal structures. Both these modalities provide indirect evidence of abscess presence but are not generally helpful in precisely locating the abscess.

Ultrasound is a frequent first diagnostic method used when an intraabdominal abscess is suspected. The procedure may be done at the bedside, which is particularly helpful in the patient in the intensive care unit. In some patients, particularly the obese, it is technically difficult to perform and interpret the examination.[22]

Computed tomographic (CT) scan is used frequently to evaluate the abdomen for the presence of an abscess and is the imaging modality of greatest value. An oral radiocontrast agent should be given to allow differentiation of the abscess from the bowel. Intravenous radiocontrast material will be taken up preferentially in the wall of the abscess, creating a unique radiographic appearance, so-called rim enhancement.

Magnetic resonance imaging (MRI) is used infrequently to locate an intraabdominal abscess, particularly in the retroperitoneum, but this modality offers no significant advantage when compared with CT scan.

Radioactive isotope imaging with ^{67}Ga citrate-, ^{99m}Tc-, or ^{111}In-labeled leukocytes also may be used.[23] These studies require long preparation and image acquisition and are not used routinely unless CT scanning fails to demonstrate a suspected abscess.

Intraabdominal infection caused by disease processes at specific sites often produces characteristic manifestations that are helpful in diagnosis. For example, a patient with diverticulitis may exhibit stabbing left lower quadrant abdominal pain and constipation. Fever and leukocytosis frequently are present, and a tender mass sometimes is palpable. With appendicitis, the findings may be inconsistent, but many patients have a sudden onset of periumbilical or epigastric pain that usually is colicky and later shifts to the right lower quadrant. The location of pain may vary because the appendix can be in many locations (e.g., retrocecal or pelvic) in the abdomen. A mass may be palpable on abdominal, pelvic, or rectal examination. The patient's temperature generally is mildly elevated early and then increases. If perforation and peritonitis occur, findings would include diffuse abdominal pain, rigidity, and sustained fever. More frequently, however, appendiceal perforation results in a local abscess.

▶ TREATMENT: Intraabdominal Infections

▓ DESIRED OUTCOME

The primary goals of treatment are correction of the intraabdominal disease processes or injuries that have caused infection and the drainage of collections of purulent material (abscesses). A secondary objective is to achieve a resolution of infection without major organ system complications (pulmonary, hepatic, cardiovascular, or renal failure) or adverse drug effects. Ideally, the patient should be discharged from the hospital with full function for self-care and routine daily activities.

▓ GENERAL APPROACH TO TREATMENT

The treatment of intraabdominal infection most often requires the coordinated use of three major modalities: (1) prompt drainage, (2) support of vital functions, and (3) appropriate antimicrobial therapy to treat infection not eradicated by surgery.

Antimicrobials are an important adjunct to drainage procedures in the treatment of secondary intraabdominal infections; however, the use of antimicrobial agents without surgical intervention usually is inadequate. For most cases of primary peritonitis, drainage procedures may not be required, and antimicrobial agents become the mainstay of therapy.

◀ In the early phase of serious intraabdominal infections, attention should be given to the maintenance of organ system functions. With generalized peritonitis, large volumes of intravenous (IV) fluids are required to restore vascular volume, to improve cardiovascular function, and to maintain adequate tissue perfusion and oxygenation. Adequate urine output should be maintained to ensure adequate resuscitation and proper renal function. Respiratory function can be assisted by a variety of methods, including oxygen therapy, pulmonary physiotherapy, and ventilatory support in severely ill patients. Often the critically ill patient with intraabdominal infection will require intensive care management, particularly if there is cardiovascular or respiratory instability. Also, isolation procedures may be required if the infectious process poses a threat to other hospitalized patients.

An additional important component of therapy is nutrition. Intraabdominal infections often directly involve the GI tract or disrupt its function (paralytic ileus). The return of GI motility may take days, weeks, and occasionally, months. In the interim, enteral or parenteral nutrition as indicated facilitates improved immune function and wound healing to ensure recovery.

▓ NONPHARMACOLOGIC TREATMENT

▓ DRAINAGE PROCEDURES

Primary peritonitis is treated with antimicrobials and rarely requires drainage. Secondary peritonitis requires surgical correction of the underlying pathology. The drainage of the purulent material is the critical component of management of an intraabdominal abscess. Without adequate drainage of the abscess, antimicrobial therapy and fluid resuscitation can be expected to fail.

Secondary peritonitis is treated surgically. At the time of laparotomy, attempts are made to correct the cause of the peritonitis. This may include patching a perforated ulcer with omentum, resection of a segment of perforated colon, or excision of a portion of gangrenous small intestine. The goal of all these procedures is to repair or remove the inflamed or gangrenous viscus and to prevent further bacterial contamination. The presence of active inflammation increases the difficulty of the surgical procedure. This results in a higher morbidity and mortality rate than if the same procedures were performed in an elective setting without inflammation.

The presence of active inflammation may make it technically impossible to perform the ultimate surgical procedure. In this situation attempts are made to provide drainage of the infected or gangrenous structures. If an intraabdominal abscess, separate from any intraabdominal organ, is discovered during an exploratory laparotomy, it may be débrided, excised, or drained. If the intraabdominal abscess involves an abdominal structure, then a resection of part or all of that organ may be required. An example of this situation is an abscess associated with diverticular disease of the colon. Management may include drainage of the abscess and resection of the involved colon. All foreign material, necrotic tissue, feces, blood, or pus should be removed from the operative field, and the peritoneum should be copiously irrigated with 0.9% sodium chloride to decrease the concentrations of bacteria or other noxious substances.

After an abscess is located, it must be drained. This may be performed surgically or using percutaneous, image-guided techniques.[24,25] Typically, image-guided techniques are done using ultrasound or CT scanning. The management of an intraabdominal abscess with percutaneous catheter drainage may be sufficient to resolve the infection. Some patients may require a subsequent procedure to treat the underlying gastrointestinal conditions; however, a significant advantage is obtained by first draining the abscess percutaneously. This allows the surgical procedure to be performed on a patient who is no longer suffering the systemic manifestations of uncontrolled infection.

A number of drainage techniques have been described using endoscopy and laparoscopy.[26,27] These minimal-access techniques may offer advantages when compared with traditional surgery but probably will be used less often than radiologically assisted percutaneous drainage techniques.

The most valuable microbiologic information may be obtained at the time of percutaneous or operative abscess drainage. If pus or fluid is found that is believed to be infected, it is best to aspirate 2 to 3 mL into a syringe, remove any air, and tightly cap the syringe. The specimen should be taken promptly to the microbiology laboratory, where a Gram stain should be performed immediately and cultures prepared for identification of aerobic and anaerobic bacteria. If no fluid is available for collection, culture swab devices may be applied to the infected area; however, anaerobic organisms often are not isolated from swabs.

▓ FLUID THERAPY

◀ Aggressive fluid repletion and management are required for successful treatment of intraabdominal infections. Fluid therapy is instituted for the purposes of achieving or maintaining proper intravascular volume to ensure adequate cardiac output, tissue perfusion, and correction of acidosis. Loss of fluid through vomiting, diarrhea, or a nasogastric suction contributes to dehydration. Intravascular volume can be assessed by blood pressure and heart rate but more accurately

TABLE 112–5. Likely Intraabdominal Pathogens

Type of Infection	Aerobes	Anaerobes
Primary Bacterial Peritonitis		
Children (spontaneous)	Pneumococci, group A *Streptococcus*	—
Cirrhosis	*E. coli, Klebsiella,* pneumococci (many others)	—
Peritoneal dialysis	*Staphylococcus, Streptococcus*	—
Secondary Bacterial Peritonitis		
Gastroduodenal	*Streptococcus, E. coli*	—
Biliary tract	*E. coli, Klebsiella,* enterococci	*Clostridium* or *Bacteroides* (infrequent)
Small or large bowel	*E. coli, Klebsiella* spp., *Proteus* spp.	*Bacteroides fragilis* and other *Bacteroides, Clostridium*
Appendicitis	*E. coli, Pseudomonas*	*Bacteroides* spp.
Abscesses	*E. coli, Klebsiella,* enterococci	*B. fragilis* and other *Bacteroides, Clostridium,* anaerobic cocci
Liver	*E. coli, Klebsiella,* enterococci staphylococci, amoeba	*Bacteroides* (infrequent)
Spleen	*Staphylococcus, Streptococcus*	

y measurement of central venous pressure, pulmonary capillary wedge pressure, or urinary output. When a contracted vascular volume is accompanied by hemorrhage, the initial hematocrit may be normal, but if there is no associated hemorrhage, the hematocrit usually is elevated as an indication of hemoconcentration. Urine output should be monitored continuously in severely ill patients by use of a urinary bladder catheter, quantitated hourly, and should equal or exceed 0.5 mL/kg of body weight per hour.

In patients with peritonitis, hypovolemia often is accompanied by acidosis, so a reasonable IV fluid would be lactated Ringer's solution, which contains the bicarbonate precursor lactate, as well as sodium, chloride, potassium, and calcium. In the initial hour of treatment, large volumes of solution may be required to restore intravascular volume. Hours thereafter, fluids may be required at a rate of 1 L/h. Maintenance fluids should be instituted (after intravascular volume is restored) with 0.9% sodium chloride and potassium chloride (20 mEq/L) or 5% dextrose and 0.45% sodium chloride with potassium chloride (20 mEq/L). The administration rate should be based on estimated daily fluid loss through urine and nasogastric suction, including 0.5 to 1.0 L for insensible fluid loss. Potassium would not be included routinely if the patient is hyperkalemic or has renal insufficiency.

In patients with significant blood loss, blood transfusion may be indicated. This is generally in the form of packed red blood cells. The criteria for blood transfusion are controversial, but a hematocrit of 25% generally is accepted. In the individual patient, the decision is often determined by the overall clinical status and the ability of the patient to compensate for the reduction in oxygen-carrying capacity associated with an acute anemia. Additional blood component therapy with fresh frozen plasma or platelets is also based on the needs of the individual patient. Aggressive fluid therapy often must be continued in the postoperative period because fluid will continue to sequester in the peritoneal cavity, bowel wall, and lumen.

PHARMACOLOGIC TREATMENT

ANTIMICROBIAL THERAPY

The goals of antimicrobial therapy are (1) to control bacteremia and prevent the establishment of metastatic foci of infection, (2) to reduce

suppurative complications after bacterial contamination, and (3) to prevent local spread of existing infection. After suppuration has occurred (e.g., an abscess has formed), a cure by antibiotic therapy alone is very difficult to achieve; antimicrobials may serve to improve the results with surgery.

An empirical antimicrobial regimen should be started as soon as the presence of intraabdominal infection is suspected. Therefore, antibiotics usually are initiated before identification of the infecting organisms is complete. Therapy must be initiated based on the likely pathogens. Predominant pathogens, as discussed in the preceding section, vary depending on the site of intraabdominal infection and the underlying disease process. Table 112–5 lists the likely pathogens against which antimicrobial agents should be directed.

Antimicrobial Experience

Many studies have been conducted evaluating or comparing the effectiveness of antimicrobials for the treatment of intraabdominal infections. Substantial differences in patient outcomes from treatment with a variety of agents generally have not been demonstrated.

Important findings from the last 20 years of clinical trials regarding selection of antimicrobials for intraabdominal infections are

- Antimicrobial regimens should cover a broad spectrum of aerobic and anaerobic bacteria from the gastrointestinal tract.
- Single-agent regimens (such as antianaerobic cephalosporins, extended-spectrum penicillins with β-lactamase inhibitors, or carbapenems) are as effective as combinations of aminoglycosides with antianaerobic agents. This is also true for antimicrobial treatment of acute bacterial contamination from penetrating abdominal trauma.[28,29]
- Clindamycin and metronidazole appear to be equivalent in efficacy when combined with agents effective against aerobic gram-negative bacilli (gentamicin or aztreonam).
- For most patients, antimicrobial treatment can be completed orally with amoxicillin-clavulanate or the combination of ciprofloxacin and metronidazole.
- Five to seven days of antimicrobial treatment is sufficient for most intraabdominal infections of mild to moderate severity.

Intraabdominal infection presents in many different ways and with a wide spectrum of severity. The regimen employed and duration of treatment depend on the specific clinical circumstances (i.e., the nature of the underlying disease process and the condition of the patient). Compromised patients require more aggressive therapies than do otherwise healthy patients who experience the same intraabdominal infection.

Recommendations

⑥ For most intraabdominal infections, the antimicrobial regimen should be effective against both aerobic and anaerobic bacteria.[30] Although it is impossible to provide antimicrobial activity against every possible pathogen, agents with activity against enteric gram-negative bacilli such as *E. coli* and *Klebsiella* and anaerobes such as *B. fragilis* and *Clostridia* spp. should be administered. If most of the organisms can be eliminated through drainage or antimicrobials, the synergistic effect may be removed, and the patient's defenses may be able to eradicate the remaining infection.

Table 112–6 presents the recommended agents for treatment of community-acquired and complicated intraabdominal infections from the Infectious Diseases Society of America and the Surgical Infection Society.[30–32] These recommendations were formulated using an evidence-based approach. Most community-acquired infections are "mild to moderate," whereas health care–associated infections tend to be more severe and difficult to treat. Table 112–7 presents guidelines for treatment and alternative regimens for specific situations. These are general guidelines; there are many factors that cannot be incorporated into such a table.

Most patients with severe intraabdominal infection, generalized peritonitis, or sepsis should be placed on a β-lactam/β-lactamase inhibitor combination or carbapenem such as imipenem, ertapenem, or meropenem. Combinations of an aminoglycoside with an antianaerobic agent, such as clindamycin or metronidazole, may be used, but some authorities consider such combinations to be obsolete.[1,30] Gentamicin is the aminoglycoside of choice based on its lower cost. Other aminoglycosides, such as tobramycin, amikacin, and netilmicin, have

no advantage in intraabdominal infection and generally are not drugs of first choice. Aztreonam may be used as an alternative to an aminoglycoside to avoid potential nephrotoxicity.

The dosage for aminoglycosides should be determined initially based on the patient's weight and renal function. Dosage adjustment should be performed by applying pharmacokinetic principles and by using peak and trough serum drug levels. Because enteric gram-negative bacilli usually are very susceptible to aminoglycosides and the aminoglycosides are well distributed into peritoneal fluid,[33,34] high serum aminoglycoside concentrations generally are not required. Unless relatively resistant bacteria are suspected, a gentamicin or tobramycin peak concentration of 5–6 mcg/mL usually is effective. To achieve these serum concentrations, gentamicin or tobramycin dosage may range from 1–3 mg/kg per dose given as often as every 6 hours or as infrequently as every 48 hours if the patient has renal failure. Because aminoglycosides have concentration-dependent killing and a relatively long postantibiotic effect for aerobic gram-negative bacilli, once-daily administration (5–7 mg/kg) is a reasonable alternative and appears to be equivalent to multiple daily dosing.

When used for intraabdominal infection, aminoglycosides should be combined with agents that are effective against the majority of *B. fragilis*. Clindamycin or metronidazole is the agent of first choice, but others, such as antianaerobic cephalosporins (e.g., cefoxitin, cefotetan, or ceftizoxime), piperacillin, mezlocillin, and combinations of extended-spectrum penicillins with β-lactamase inhibitors, would be suitable alternatives. Clindamycin should be administered intravenously in a dosage of 600 or 900 mg every 8 hours. Patients receiving multiple broad-spectrum antimicrobial agents who are immunocompromised should receive an oral antifungal agent (nystatin) for prevention of fungal overgrowth in the mouth and GI tract. The benefits of systemic antifungal prophylaxis (with fluconazole) have not been established for intraabdominal infection and should not be used routinely.

With intraabdominal contamination from the upper GI tract (perforation of a peptic ulcer or biliary tract disease), *B. fragilis* is an uncommon pathogen, and other agents therefore may be substituted for clindamycin or metronidazole. Alternatives include ampicillin, penicillin, or first-generation cephalosporins.

CLINICAL CONTROVERSY

Enterococci often are isolated from intraabdominal infections, and many antimicrobials are ineffective against enterococci (such as cephalosporins and fluoroquinolones). Regimens without activity against enterococci (gentamicin with clindamycin or cephalosporins) generally are effective in treating intraabdominal infections; however, there are numerous reports of enterococcal superinfection in immunocompromised patients, particularly after broad-spectrum antimicrobial use. The Infectious Disease Society of America guidelines state that "Routine coverage against enterococcus is not necessary for patients with community-acquired intraabdominal infections. Antimicrobial therapy for enterococci [e.g., ampicillin, penicillin, or vancomcyin] should be given when enterococci are recovered from patients with health-care associated infections."

The failure of host defenses may be a critical factor in the pathogenicity of enterococci. In immunocompromised patients or patients with valvular heart disease or a prosthetic heart valve, there is justification to provide specific antimicrobial activity against enterococci. Ampicillin or other penicillins that are active against

TABLE 112–6. Recommended Agents for the Treatment of Community-Acquired Complicated Intraabdominal Infections

Agents Recommended for Mild to Moderate Infections	Agents Recommended for High-Severity Infections
β-Lactam/β-Lactamase Inhibitor Combinations	
Ampicillin-sulbactam	Piperacillin-tazobactam
Ticarcillin-clavulanate	
Carbapenems	
Ertapenem	Imipenem/cilistatin
	Meropenem
Combination Regimens	
Cefazolin or cefuroxime plus metronidazole	Third- or fourth-generation cephalosporins (cefotaxime, ceftriaxone, ceftizoxime, ceftazidime, cefepime) plus metronidazole
Ciprofloxacin, levofloxacin, moxifloxacin, or gatifloxacin in combination with metronidazole	Ciprofloxacin in combination with metronidazole
	Aztreonam plus metronidazole

From refs. 30, 31, and 32.

TABLE 112–7. Guidelines for Initial Antimicrobial Agents for Intraabdominal Infections

	Primary Agents	Alternatives
Primary Bacterial Peritonitis		
Cirrhosis	Cefotaxime	1. Add clindamycin or metronidazole if anaerobes are suspected 2. Other third-generation cephalosporins, extended-spectrum penicillins, aztreonam, and imipenem as alternatives 3. Aminoglycoside with antipseudomonal penicillin
Peritoneal dialysis	Regimen based on organism isolated 1. Staphylococcus: penicillinase-resistant penicillin or first-generation cephalosporin 2. *Streptococcus:* penicillin G 3. Aerobic gram-negative bacilli: cefotaxime, ceftazidime, or aminoglycoside plus an antipseudomonal penicillin 4. *Pseudomonas aeruginosa:* aminoglycoside plus antipseudomonal penicillin or ceftazidime	1. Alternative for resistant staphylococci is vancomycin 2. Alternative for Streptococcus is a first-generation cephalosporin 3. Alternatives for gram-negative bacilli are other third-generation cephalosporins, aztreonam, and extended-spectrum penicillins with β-lactamase inhibitors
Secondary Bacterial Peritonitis		
Perforated peptic ulcer	First-generation cephalosporins	1. Antianaerobic cephalosporins[a] 2. Possibly add aminoglycoside if patient condition is poor 3. Aminoglycoside with clindamycin or metronidazole; add ampicillin if patient is immunocompromised or if biliary tract origin of infection
Other	Imipenem/cilistatin, meropenem, ertapenem, or extended-spectrum penicillins with β-lactamase inhibitor	1. Ciprofloxacin with metronidazole 2. Aztreonam with clindamycin or metronidazole 3. Antianaerobic cephalosporins.[a]
Abscess		
General	Imipenem/cilastatin, meropenem, ertapenem, or extended-spectrum penicillins with β-lactamase inhibitor	1. Aztreonam with clindamycin or metronidazole 2. Ciprofloxacin with metronidazole 3. Aminoglycoside with clindamycin or metronidazole;
Liver	As above but add a first-generation cephalosporin	Use metronidazole if amoebic liver abscess is suspected
Spleen	Aminoglycoside plus penicillinase-resistant penicillin	Alternatives for penicillinase-resistant penicillin are first-generation cephalosporins or vancomycin
Appendicitis		
Normal or inflamed	Antianaerobic cephalosporins[a] (discontinued immediately postoperation)	1. Ampicillin-sulbactam
Gangrenous or perforated	Imipenem/cilastatin, meropenem, ertapenem, antianaerobic cephalosporins or extended-spectrum penicillins with β-lactamase inhibitor	1. Aztreonam with clindamycin or metronidazole 2. Ciprofloxacin with metronidazole 3. Aminoglycoside with clindamycin or metronidazole
Acute Cholecystitis	First-generation cephalosporin	Aminoglycoside plus ampicillin if severe infection
Cholangitis	Aminoglycoside with ampicillin with or without clindamycin or metronidazole	Use vancomycin instead of ampicillin if patient is allergic to penicillin
Acute Contamination from Abdominal Trauma	Antianaerobic cephalosporins[a] or ampicillin-sulbactam	1. A carbapenem 2. Ciprofloxacin plus metronidazole
Pelvic Inflammatory Disease	Cefotetan or cefoxitin with doxycycline	1. Clindamycin with gentamicin 2. Ampicillin-sulbactam with doxycycline 3. Ciprofloxacin with doxycycline and metronidazole

[a]Cefoxitin, cefotetan, and ceftizoxime.

enterococci (e.g., penicillin, piperacillin, and mezlocillin) should be used in patients at high risk, patients with persistent or recurrent intraabdominal infection, or patients who are immunosuppressed, such as after organ transplantation. Ampicillin remains the drug of choice for this indication because it is most active in vitro against enterococcus and is relatively inexpensive. Vancomycin is active against most enterococci; however, resistance is increasing, and this agent should be reserved for established infections when first-line therapies cannot be used.

With peritonitis that occurs from CAPD, the antimicrobial regimen used should be tailored to the isolated organism. The

selection of a specific agent or combination should be based on culture and susceptibility data. If microbiologic data are unavailable, empirical therapy with a first-generation cephalosporin plus an aminoglycoside is recommended. In less severe infections, a first-generation cephalosporin alone given intraperitoneally may suffice. Infection with staphylococci may be treated with a penicillinase-resistant penicillin (e.g., methicillin, nafcillin, or oxacillin), first-generation cephalosporins, or vancomycin if the patient is allergic to penicillin or the isolate is resistant to methicillin. For streptococcal infections, penicillin or ampicillin would be preferable to penicillinase-resistant penicillins. Most aerobic gram-negative bacilli may be treated effectively with an aminoglycoside. For infections caused by *P. aeruginosa,* an antipseudomonal penicillin (e.g., ticarcillin, piperacillin, mezlocillin, or azlocillin) or ceftazidime may be added.

Patients with peritonitis who are undergoing CAPD may receive parenteral as well as intraperitoneal antimicrobial agents. Intraperitoneal antimicrobial agents alone often are sufficient unless severe infection is present. A number of agents may be instilled through peritoneal catheters. Recommended concentrations of antimicrobial agents for intraperitoneal irrigation solutions are 8 mg/L for gentamicin and tobramycin, 1–3 mg/L for clindamycin, 50,000 units/L for penicillin G, 125 mg/L for cephalosporins, 100–150 mg/L for ticarcillin or carbenicillin, 50 mg/L for ampicillin, 100 mg/L for methicillin, 30 mg/L for vancomycin, and 3 mg/L for amphotericin B.[35]

The usual duration of therapy for peritonitis associated with CAPD is 10 to 14 days, but up to 3 weeks of therapy may be required. Antimicrobial therapy should be continued until dialysate fluid is clear, cultures are negative for 2 to 3 days, and the patient is asymptomatic. When parenteral agents are administered, the initial dose would be the same as that for patients with normal renal function, whereas subsequent doses should be much less or given less frequently for renally excreted agents and should account for possible loss through peritoneal dialysis. Serum concentrations should be performed for aminoglycosides and vancomycin. Some studies have demonstrated that for patients with spontaneous bacterial peritonitis associated with cirrhotic ascites, treatment duration may be as short as 5 days when ascitic fluid polymorphonuclear cell counts are used to guide treatment.[36,37]

After acute bacterial contamination, such as with abdominal trauma where GI contents spill into the peritoneum, combination antimicrobial regimens are not required. If the patient is seen soon after injury (within 2 hours) and surgical measures are instituted promptly, antianaerobic cephalosporins (such as cefoxitin or cefotetan) or extended-spectrum penicillins are effective in preventing most infectious complications. Antimicrobials should be administered as soon as possible after injury.

For appendicitis, the antimicrobial regimen used should depend on the appearance of the appendix at the time of operation, which may be normal, inflamed, gangrenous, or perforated. Because the condition of the appendix is unknown preoperatively, it is advisable to begin antimicrobial agents before the appendectomy is performed. Reasonable regimens would be antianaerobic cephalosporins or, if the patient is seriously ill, a carbapenem or β-lactam/β-lactamase inhibitor combination. If, at operation, the appendix is normal or inflamed, postoperative antimicrobials are not be required. If the appendix is gangrenous or perforated, a treatment course of 5 to 7 days with the agents listed in Table 112–7 is appropriate.

❽ The necessary duration of treatment for intraabdominal infections is not clearly defined. Acute intraabdominal contamination, such as after a traumatic injury, may be treated with a very short course (24 hours).[38] For established infections (i.e., peritonitis or intraabdominal abscess), an antimicrobial course limited to 5 to 7 days is justified. This allows eradication of bacteria remaining in the peritoneum after a surgical procedure that may enter the peritoneum through healing suture lines. Under certain conditions, therapy for longer than 7 days would be justified, e.g., if the patient remains febrile or is in poor general condition, when relatively resistant bacteria are isolated, or when a focus of infection in the abdomen may still be present. For some abscesses, such as pyogenic liver abscess, antimicrobials may be required for a month or longer.

Intraperitoneal irrigation of antimicrobial agents for treatment of intraabdominal infection has been studied often with conflicting results.[39] Intraoperative antimicrobial irrigation does not improve patient outcomes in comparison with copious intraoperative irrigation with normal saline. Possibly the most important aspect of peritoneal irrigation is the dilutional effect on bacteria and adjuvants that promotes infection (intestinal contents and hemoglobin). Most systemically administered antimicrobials easily cross the peritoneal membrane so that peritoneal fluid concentrations are similar to serum.[33,40] Confined areas, such as an abscess, can be expected to attain much lower antimicrobial concentrations.

EVALUATION OF THERAPEUTIC OUTCOMES

Whichever antimicrobial regimen is chosen, the patient should be reassessed continually to determine the success or failure of therapies. The clinician should recognize that there are many reasons for poor patient outcome with intraabdominal infection; improper antimicrobial administration is only one. The patient may be immunocompromised, which decreases the likelihood of successful outcome with any regimen. It is impossible for antimicrobials to compensate for a nonfunctioning immune system. There may be surgical reasons for poor patient outcome. Failure to identify all intraabdominal foci of infection or leaks from a GI anastomosis may cause continued intraabdominal infection. Even when intraabdominal infection is controlled, accompanying organ system failure, most often renal or respiratory, may lead to patient demise.

The outcome from intraabdominal infection is not determined solely by what transpires in the abdomen. Unsatisfactory outcomes in patients with intraabdominal infections may result from complications that arise in other organ systems. A complication commonly associated with mortality after intraabdominal infection is pneumonia.[41] A high APACHE (Acute Physiology and Chronic Health Evaluation) II score, low serum albumin concentration, and high New York Heart Association cardiac function status were significantly and in-

dependently associated with increased mortality from intraabdominal infection.[42]

❾ Once antimicrobials are initiated and the other important therapies described earlier are used, most patients should show improvement within 2 to 3 days. Usually, temperature will return to near normal, vital signs should stabilize, and the patient should not appear in distress, with the exception of recognized discomfort and pain from incisions, drains, and nasogastric tube. At 24 to 48 hours, aerobic bacterial culture results should return. If a suspected pathogen is not sensitive to the antimicrobial agents being given, the regimen should be changed if the patient has not shown sufficient improvement. If the isolated pathogen is extremely sensitive to one antimicrobial and the patient is progressing well, concurrent antimicrobial therapy often may be discontinued.

CLINICAL CONTROVERSY

❺ Although some investigators suggest that routine culturing of patients with community-acquired intraabdominal infections contributes little to their management,[43] other investigators suggest that antimicrobial therapy should be based on susceptibility of the bacteria collected from the operative site because this has been shown to correlate with clinical outcome.[44]

With anaerobic culturing techniques and the slow growth of these organisms, anaerobes often are not identified until 4 to 7 days after culture, and sensitivity information is difficult to obtain. For this reason, there are usually few data with which to alter the antianaerobic component of the antimicrobial regimen. A report indicating that anaerobes were not isolated should not be the sole justification for discontinuing antianaerobic drugs because anaerobic bacteria that were present in the infectious process may not have been transported properly to the microbiology laboratory, or other problems may have led to cell death in vitro.

Reasons for antimicrobial failure may not always be apparent. Even when antimicrobial susceptibility tests indicate that an organism is susceptible in vitro to the antimicrobial agent, therapeutic failures may occur. Possibly there is poor penetration of the antimicrobial agent into the focus of infection, or bacterial resistance may develop after initiation of antimicrobial therapy. Also, it is possible that an antimicrobial regimen may encourage the development of infection by organisms not susceptible to the regimen being used. Superinfection in patients being treated for intraabdominal infection can be caused by *Candida;* however, enterococci or opportunistic gram-negative bacilli such as *Pseudomonas* or *Serratia* may be involved.

Treatment regimens for intraabdominal infection can be judged as successful if the patient recovers from the infection without recurrent peritonitis or intraabdominal abscess and without the need for additional antimicrobials. A regimen can be considered unsuccessful if a significant adverse drug reaction occurs, reoperation or percutaneous drainage is necessary, or patient improvement is delayed beyond 1 or 2 weeks.

ABBREVIATIONS

APACHE: Acute Physiology and Chronic Health Evaluation
CAPD: chronic ambulatory peritoneal dialysis
CT: computed tomography
IL: interleukin
INF: interferon
TNF: tumor necrosis factor

Review Questions and other resources can be found at *www.pharmacotherapyonline.com.*

REFERENCES

1. Whittmann DH, Schein M, Condon RE. Management of secondary peritonitis. Ann Surg 1996;224:10–18.
2. Marshall JC, Innes M. Intensive care unit management of intraabdominal infection. Crit Care Med 2003;31:2228–2237.
3. Johnson CC, Baldessarre J, Levinson ME. Peritonitis: Update on pathophysiology, clinical manifestations, and management. Clin Infect Dis 1997;24:1035–1047.
4. Vas S, Oreopoulos DG. Infections in patients undergoing peritoneal dialysis. Infect Dis Clin North Am 2001;15:743–774.
5. Hall MJ, Popovic JR. 1998 Summary: National Hospital Discharge Survey, Number 316. Washington, National Center for Health Statistics, 2000.
6. Toloza EM, Wilson SE. Cholecystitis and cholangitis. In: Fry DE, ed. Surgical Infections. Boston, Little, Brown, 1995:254–263.
7. Keene WF, Alexander SR, Bailie GR, et al. Peritoneal dialysis—Related peritonitis treatment recommendations: 1996 update. Perit Dial Int 1996;16:557–573.
8. Schein M, Wittman DH, Holzheimer R, et al. Hypothesis: Compartmentalization of cytokines in intraabdominal infection. Surgery 1996;119:694–700.
9. Riche FC, Cholley BP, Panis YH, et al. Inflammatory cytokine response in patients with septic shock secondary to generalized peritonitis. Crit Care Med 2000;28:433–437.
10. Johnson DH, Cuhna BA. Infections in cirrhosis. Infect Dis Clin North Am. 2001;15:363–371.
11. Troidle L, Gordon-Brennan N, Kliger A, Finkelstein F. Differing outcomes of gram-positive and gram-negative peritonitis. Am J Kidney Dis 1998;32:623–628.
12. McClean KL, Shhehan GJ, Harding GKM. Intraabdominal infection: A review. Clin Infect Dis 1994;19:100–116.
13. Brook I, Frazier EH. Microbiology subphrenic abscesses: A 14-year experience. Am Surg 1999;65:1049–1053.
14. Brook I, Frazier EH. Aerobic and anaerobic microbiology of retroperitoneal abscesses. Clin Infect Dis 1998;26:938–941.
15. Bennion RS, Baron EJ, Thompson JE, et al. The bacteriology of gangrenous and perforated appendicitis—Revisited. Ann Surg 1990;211:165–171.
16. Sawyer RG, Rosenlof LK, Adams RB, et al. Peritonitis into the 1990s: Changing pathogens and changing strategies in the critically ill. Am Surg 1992;58:82–87.
17. Onderdonk AB, Bartlett JG, Louie T, et al. Microbial synergy in experimental intraabdominal abscess. Infect Immun 1997;13:22–26.
18. Montravers P, Andremont A, Massias L, Carbon C. Investigation of the potential role of *Streptococcus faecalis* in the pathophysiology of experimental peritonitis. J Infect Dis 1994;169:821–830.
19. Burnett RJ, Haverstock DC, Dellinger EP, et al. Definition of the role of enterococcus in intraabdominal infection: Analysis of a prospective randomized trial. Surgery 1995;118:721–723.
20. Donskey CJ, Chowdhry TK, Hecker MT, et al. Effect of antibiotic therapy on the density of vancomcyin-resistant enterococci in the stool of colonized patients. Ann Surg 2000;343:1925–1932.
21. Sitges-Serra A, Lopez MJ, Girvent M, et al. Postoperative enterococcal infection after treatment of complicated intraabdominal sepsis. Br J Surg 2002;89:361–367.
22. Gazelle GS, Mueller PR. Abdominal abscess: Imaging and intervention. Radiol Clin North Am 1994;32:913–932.
23. Datz FL. Abdominal abscess detection: Gallium-, ^{111}In-, and ^{99m}Tc-labeled leukocytes, and polyclonal and monoclonal antibodies. Semin Nucl Med 1996;26:51–64.
24. Montgomery RS, Wilson SE. Intraabdominal abscesses: Image-guided diagnosis and therapy. Clin Infect Dis 1996;23:28–36.
25. Shuler FW, Newman CN, Angood PB, et al. Nonoperative management for intraabdominal abscesses. Am Surg 1996;62:218–222.
26. Robles PJ, Lancaster B. Laparoscopic drainage of right subphrenic abscess: Report of one case. J Laparoendosc Surg 1996;6:55–60.
27. Kim HB, Gregor MB, Boley SJ, Kleinhaus S. Digitally assisted laparoscopic drainage of multiple intraabdominal abscesses. J Laparoendosc Surg 1993;3:477–479.
28. Hooker KD, DiPiro JT, Wynn JJ. Aminoglycoside combinations versus single β-lactams for penetrating abdominal trauma: A meta analysis. J Trauma 1991;31:1155–1160.
29. Solomkin JS, Dellinger EP, Christou NV, et al. Results of a multicenter trial comparing imipenem/cilastatin to tobramycin/clindamycin for intraabdominal infections. Ann Surg 1990;212:581–591.
30. Solomkin JS, Mazuski JE, Baron EJ, et al. Guidelines for the selection of anti-infective agents for complicated intraabdominal infections. Clin Infect Dis 2003;37:997–1005.
31. Mazuski JE, Sawyer RG, Nathens AB, et al. The Surgical Infection Society guidelines on antimicrobial therapy for intraabdominal infections: an executive summary. Surg Infect 2002;3:161–174.
32. Mazuski JE, Sawyer RG, Nathens AB, et al. The Surgical Infection Society guidelines on antimicrobial therapy for intraabdominal infections: evidence for recommendations. Surg Infect 2002;3:175–234.
33. Serour F, Dan M, Gorea A, et al. Penetration of aminoglycosides into human peritoneal tissue. Chemotherapy 1990;36:251–253.
34. Hodgman T, Dasta JK, Armstrong DK, et al. Tobramycin disposition into ascitic fluid. Clin Pharmacol 1984;3:203–205.

35. Levison ME, Pontzer RE. Peritonitis and other intraabdominal infections. In: Mardell GL, Douglas RG, Bennett JE, eds. Principles and Practice of Infectious Diseases. New York, Wiley, 1985:488.

36. Fong T, Akriviadis ES, Runyon BA, et al. Polymorphonuclear cell count response and duration of antibiotic therapy in spontaneous bacterial peritonitis. Hepatology 1989;9:423–426.

37. Runyon BA, McHutchison JG, Antillon MR, et al. Short-course versus long-course antibiotic treatment of spontaneous bacterial peritonitis. Gastroenterology 1991;100:1737–1742.

38. Bozorgzadeh A, Pizzi WF, Barie PS, et al. The duration of antibiotic administration in predicting abdominal trauma. Am J Surg 1999;172:125–135.

39. Schein M, Gecelter G, Freinkel W, et al. Peritoneal lavage in abdominal sepsis: A controlled clinical study. Arch Surg 1990;125:1132–1135.

40. Wittman DH, Schassan HH. Penetration of eight β-lactam antibiotics into peritoneal fluid. Arch Surg 1983;118:205–213.

41. Mustard RA, Bohnen JMA, Rosati C, Schouten D. Pneumonia complicating abdominal sepsis. Arch Surg 1991;126:170–175.

42. Christou NV, Barie PS, Dellinger EP, et al. Surgical infection society intraabdominal infection study. Arch Surg 1993;128:193–199.

43. Dougherty SH. Antimicrobial culture and susceptibility testing has little value for routine management of secondary bacterial peritonitis. Clin Infect Dis 1997;25(suppl 2):S258–261.

44. Nathens AB. Relevance and utility of peritoneal cultures in patients with peritonitis. Surg Infect (Larchmt) 2001;2:153–160.

113

PARASITIC DISEASES

JV Anandan

Learning Objectives and other resources can be found at *www.pharmacotherapyonline.com*.

KEY CONCEPTS

1 Parasites normally inflict some degree of injury to the host, the extent of which depends on such factors as parasite load, nutritional status, and immunologic competence of the host.

2 The primary reasons for deaths due to malaria are failure to take chemoprophylaxis, inappropriate chemoprophylaxis, delay in seeking medical care, and misdiagnosis.

3 In adults (including pregnant women), the chemoprophylaxis for all species of plasmodia is chloroquine phosphate 300 mg (base) once weekly beginning 1 week prior to departure and continuing for 4 weeks after leaving an endemic area.

4 In an uncomplicated attack of malaria (for all plasmodia except chloroquine-resistant *Plasmodium falciparum*), the recommended regimen is chloroquine 600 mg (base) initially, followed by 300 mg (base) 6 hours later, and then 300 mg (base) daily for 2 days.

5 Because falciparum malaria is associated with serious complications including pulmonary edema, hypoglycemia, jaundice, renal failure, confusion, delirium, seizures, coma, and death, careful monitoring of fluid status and hemodynamic parameters is mandatory.

6 Intestinal amebiasis is diagnosed by demonstrating *Entamoeba histolytica* cysts or trophozoites (may contain ingested erythrocytes) in fresh stool or from a specimen obtained by sigmoidoscopy. Three stool samples obtained 24 hours apart will produce a 60% to 90% yield for *E. histolytica*.

7 All symptomatic adults and children older than 8 years of age with giardiasis should be treated with metronidazole 250 mg three times daily for 7 days.

8 In the adult, both the cutaneous and mucocutaneous forms of leishmaniasis (*Leishmania braziliensis* and *L. mexicana*) are treated with stibogluconate. An alternative drug for the visceral form is amphotericin B.

9 In chronic trypanosomiasis (Chagas' disease), patients present with cardiomyopathy and heart failure.

10 The agents used commonly for the treatment of enterobiasis include pyrantel pamoate, mebendazole, or albendazole.

11 The resistance of lice to permethrin is increasing, and 0.5% malathion is an effective alternative.

Parasitic diseases are receiving increasing attention from clinicians in the United States because of the high frequency of travel, deployment of personnel for humanitarian and military missions (e.g., Peace Corps volunteers), inflow of immigrants from a wider geographic distribution, and the presence of immunosuppressed populations (e.g., AIDS and transplant patients). Migrant farm workers who work and live in substandard hygienic conditions, the large and growing Central and South American immigrant population, and other poorly screened immigrants from Asia represent significant sources of parasitic infections in the United States.[1–9] Clinicians need to have a heightened awareness for parasitic diseases and how to treat them. Clinical signs and symptoms, together with the patient's travel history, should be used with other diagnostic aids in the identification of parasitic diseases. Parasitic infections caused by pathogenic protozoa or helminths affect more than 3 billion people worldwide and impose tremendous health and economic burdens on developing countries.[9]

This chapter discusses the major parasitic diseases, including protozoan diseases (amebiasis, malaria), helminthic infections (ascariasis, enterobiasis), and ectoparasitic infestations (head and body lice). Emphasis is placed on diseases seen more frequently in the

United States. World distribution of parasites depends on the presence of suitable hosts, habitats, and environmental conditions.[9] A human parasite that does not use an intermediate host is likely to be found in any inhabited region of the world as long as the environmental conditions are suitable. *Ascaris* (round worm) and *Trichuris* (whip worm) require carelessness of habits for transfer and require time outside the body, where they are exposed to heat and dryness, to reach the infective stage. The distribution of the hookworm is more limited because the free-living forms are unprotected by resistant shells or cysts. African trypanosomiasis never occurs outside the range of the tsetse fly, malaria never occurs beyond the range of the infective *Anopheles* mosquito, and schistosomiasis never occurs in the absence of a specific water snail. The prevalence of clonorchiasis (Chinese liver fluke) is an example of the impact of both environmental and geographic factors. Clonorchiasis requires the simultaneous presence of not only humans, specific snail species, and certain fish but also unsanitary conditions that make the eggs accessible to the snails, an association of the snail and fish, and the established local habit of eating raw fish. The ability of some parasites to infect hosts other than humans may perpetuate an infection even when human habits preclude the possibility of more than occasional access to the human body. In North America, the broad tapeworm (*Diphyllobothrium latus*) would perish if it were not that dogs and other carnivores, such as the brown bear, serve as reservoir hosts.

HOST-PARASITE RELATIONSHIP

Symbiosis is the association of two species for the purpose of obtaining food for either one or the other. *Parasitism* is a symbiotic relationship in which one species, the host, is injured through the activities of the other. Through evolution, parasites have made specific morphologic adaptations. Adaptation to the host has taken a number of forms: loss of locomotor organelles in the protozoan *Sporozoa*, partial and complete lack of digestive systems in the trematodes and cestodes, respectively, elaboration of proteolytic enzymes to penetrate the host intestinal mucosa by *Entamoeba histolytica*, the cercariae of the blood fluke that penetrate the skin of the host by elaborate enzymes, and finally, the ability to infect an intermediate host to increase reproductive capacity, as seen among the cestodes and trematodes.[9]

Parasites normally inflict some degree of injury to the host, the extent of which depends on such factors as parasite load, nutritional status, and immunologic competence of the host. *Entamoeba coli* is considered commensal because it subsists on the bacterial flora of the gut and does not cause any harm to the host. Unlike *Entamoeba coli, Fasciolopsis buski,* the giant intestinal fluke, can produce severe local damage to the intestinal wall. *Ascaris,* the roundworm, can perforate the bowel wall, cause intestinal obstruction, and invade the appendix and bile duct. Malarial parasites destroy red cells by multiplying inside them. *Diphyllobothrium latum,* or the broad fish tapeworm, removes vitamin B_{12} from the gastrointestinal tract (GI) tract, resulting in megaloblastic anemia.[9]

PROTOZOAN DISEASES

MALARIA

Malaria represents the most devastating disease in terms of human suffering and economics. It affects the largest number of people (between 300 and 500 million new infections are reported annually) in the world, with more than 2 million deaths worldwide.[10,11] In the United States, deaths from malaria are preventable. The primary reasons for deaths are failure to take chemoprophylaxis, inappropriate chemoprophylaxis, delay in seeking medical care, and misdiagnosis.[4,5,10,11]

EPIDEMIOLOGY

The exact geographic distribution of the various species is not well documented; however, it is reported that *Plasmodium vivax* is more prevalent in India, Pakistan, Bangladesh, Sri Lanka, and Central America, whereas *P. falciparum* is predominant in Africa, Haiti, Dominican Republic, the Amazon region of South America, and New Guinea. Both *P. falciparum* and *P. vivax* are prevalent in all of Southeast Asia, South America, Middle East, North Africa, Ethiopia, Somalia, and Sudan.[10–13] Most of the infections with *P. ovale* occur in Africa, and the distribution of *P. malariae* is considered worldwide.

In the United States, most cases of malaria are reported in immigrants from endemic areas and in American travelers. Blood transfusion also has been cited as a cause of malarial infection.[12] The transmission of malaria from recent immigrants from endemic areas is a real threat because of the presence of a number of mosquito vectors—*Anopheles quadrimaculatatus* and *A. punctipennis*—in the United States.[14]

ETIOLOGY

Malaria is transmitted by the bite of an infected *Anopheles* mosquito that introduces the sporozoites (tissue parasites) of the plasmodia (*P. falciparum, P. vivax, P. malariae,* and *P. ovale*) into the bloodstream. The asexual reproduction stage develops in humans, whereas the sexual stage occurs in the mosquito.[9,12] The sporozoites invade parenchymal hepatocytes, multiply in stages referred to as *exoerythrocytic stages,* and become hepatic vegetative forms or schizonts. Schizonts rupture to release daughter cells, or merozoites, that then infect erythrocytes.

P. falciparum and *P. malariae* remain in the primary exoerythrocytic stage in the liver for about 4 weeks before invading erythrocytes, whereas *P. vivax* and *P. ovale* can exist in the liver in the latent exoerythrocytic form for extended periods, and therefore, infected subjects can experience relapses. The merozoites that invade the erythrocytes develop sequentially into ring forms, trophozoites, schizonts, and finally, merozoites, which can invade other erythrocytes or can develop into gametocytes, which undergo the sexual stage in the *Anopheles* vector. Erythrocytic forms never reinvade the liver without developing into sporozoites in the vector, and therefore, malaria infections from transfusion never result in the exoerythrocytic, or "liver," form.[9,12] *P. falciparum* can result in high levels of parasitemia because of its ability to invade erythrocytes of all ages, unlike *P. vivax* and *P. ovale,* which only invade young cells.[12]

PATHOLOGY

The erythrocytic phase causes extensive hemolysis, which results in anemia and splenomegaly. The most serious complications usually

---

TABLE 113–1. Clinical Presentation of Malaria

Initial Presentation
Nonspecific fever, chills, rigors, diaphoresis, malaise, vomiting[12]
Orthostatic hypotension
Electrolyte abnormalities

Erythrocytic Phase
Prodrome: Headache, anorexia, malaise, fatigue, myalgias
Nonspecific complaints such as abdominal pain, diarrhea, chest pain, and arthralgias
Paroxysm: High fever, chills, and rigor[9–12]
Cold phase: Severe pallor, cyanosis of the lips and nail bed, and cutis anserina ("goose flesh")[9–12]
Hot phase: Fever between 40.5°C (104.9°F) and 41°C (105.8°F).
Sweating phase:
  Follows hot phase by 2–6 hours
  Fever resolves
  Marked fatigue and drowsiness, warm, dry skin, tachycardia, cough, severe headache, nausea, vomiting, abdominal pain, diarrhea, and delirium
  Lactic acidosis and hypoglycemia (with falciparum malaria)[12,15]
Anemia
Splenomegaly

***P. falciparum* Infections**
Hypoglycemia, acute renal failure, pulmonary edema, severe anemia, thrombocytopenia, high-output heart failure, cerebral congestion, seizures and coma, and adult respiratory syndrome[15–21]

are associated with *P. falciparum* infections.[15–21] Infants and children younger than 5 years of age and nonimmune women who are pregnant are at high risk for severe complications from falciparum malaria.[15–19] The complications associated with falciparum malaria are primarily a result of the high parasitemia and the ability of the parasites to sequester in capillaries and postcapillary vessels of organs such as the brain and the kidney. It has been postulated that tissue hypoxia from anemia, together with *P. falciparum*–parasitized red blood cell adherence to endothelial cells in capillaries, contributes to extensive vascular disease and severe metabolic effects.[12,15] *P. malariae*

is implicated in immune-mediated glomerulonephritis and nephrotic syndrome[12,18] (Table 113–1).

To ensure a positive diagnosis, blood smears should be obtained every 12 to 24 hours for 3 consecutive days.[9,12,15] The presence of parasites in the blood 3 to 5 days after initiation of therapy suggests drug resistance. Recent advances for detecting malaria parasite have included DNA or RNA probes by polymerase chain reaction (PCR) and a rapid dipstick test (PARASIGHT F, Becton-Dickinson, Cockeysville, MD).[9,12,22,23] The dipstick is reported to have a sensitivity of 88% and a specificity of 97%, which is comparable with microscopy.[22]

▶ TREATMENT: Malaria

■ DESIRED OUTCOME

The primary goal in the management of malaria is the rapid diagnosis of the *Plasmodia* spp. by blood smears (repeated every 12 hours for 3 days) so as to initiate timely antimalarial therapy to eradicate the infection within 48 to 72 hours and to avoid complications such as hypoglycemia, pulmonary edema, and renal failure that are responsible for increased mortality in malaria.

■ PHARMACOLOGIC THERAPY

In adults (including pregnant women), the chemoprophylaxis for all species of *Plasmodium* is chloroquine phosphate 300 mg (base) once weekly beginning 1 week prior to departure and continued for 4 weeks after leaving an endemic area.[10,12,13,23,27] The pediatric dose of chloroquine phosphate is 5 mg (base) per kilogram of body weight (maximum 300 mg). When visiting or leaving an area endemic for *P. vivax* or *P. ovale*, primaquine phosphate (Primaquine) 15 mg (base) daily for 14 days beginning the last 2 weeks of chloroquine prophylaxis should be added to the regimen. The pediatric dose of primaquine is 0.3 mg (base) per kilogram of body weight per day for 14 days. The pediatric doses of chloroquine can be calculated based on body weight, and the tablets can be pulverized and placed in gelatin capsules. Parents can be instructed to suspend the dose in food, simple syrup, chocolate milk, or drink.[10,15]

In areas where chloroquine-resistant *P. falciparum* strains exist, travelers should receive mefloquine (Lariam) for prophylaxis. The adult dose of mefloquine is 250 mg once weekly beginning 1 week prior to departure and continuing for the full period of exposure, followed by 250 mg for 4 weeks after last exposure.[23–30] The pediatric dose of mefloquine for prophylaxis is

Body Weight (kg)	Dose
15–19 kg	5 mg/kg
15–19 kg	1/4 tablet
20–30 kg	1/2 tablet
31–45 kg	3/4 tablet
>45 kg	1 tablet

In travelers who are at immediate risk for drug-resistant falciparum malaria, a loading dose of mefloquine may be considered. Mefloquine is administered at 250 mg daily for 3 days before travel, followed by 250 mg once weekly while in the endemic area and

continued for 4 weeks after last exposure.[24,26] Some patients may experience neuropsychiatric reactions from this regimen and may need to be monitored closely.[12,24]

An alternative regimen for prophylaxis in chloroquine-resistant areas for those who cannot tolerate mefloquine is to take doxycycline 100 mg daily starting 1 to 2 days prior to departure, during the exposure period, and continuing for 4 weeks after leaving the endemic area.[12,24] Children older than 8 years of age should receive 2 mg/kg per day (up to 100 mg) of doxycycline. Doxycycline is contraindicated in children younger than 8 years of age, in pregnant women, and during breast-feeding.[13,24]

Another alternative regimen for chemoprophylaxis is the combination of atovaquone and proguanil (Malarone): 1 tablet daily beginning 1 to 2 days prior to travel and continuing for the duration of stay and 1 week after leaving the area.[13,14] Daily primaquine 15 mg (base) also has been recommended for prophylaxis for both *P. vivax* and *P. falciparum* malaria.[30]

In an uncomplicated attack of malaria (for all plasmodia except chloroquine-resistant *P. falciparum*), the recommended regimen is chloroquine 600 mg (base) initially, followed by 300 mg (base) 6 hours later, and then 300 mg (base) daily for 2 days. In severe illness or when oral therapy is not tolerated or parenteral quinine is not available, quinidine gluconate 10 mg/kg as a loading dose (maximum 600 mg) in 250 mL normal saline should be administered slowly over 1 to 2 hours, followed by continuous infusion of 0.02 mg/kg per minute until oral therapy can be started.[23,24] In patients who have received either quinine or mefloquine, the loading dose of quinidine should be omitted. Oral quinine (300 mg every 8 hours) should follow the intravenous dose of quinidine to complete 3 days for all infections, except for *P. falciparum* acquired in Thailand, in which case a full 7-day course should be given.[23,24] The pediatric dose of intravenous quinidine gluconate is the same as the dose for adults.[24] The pediatric dose of quinine is 25 mg/kg per day in three divided doses for 3 or 7 days.[24]

In *P. falciparum* (chloroquine-resistant) infections, a dose of 750 mg mefloquine followed by 500 mg 12 hours later is recommended. The pediatric dose of mefloquine is 15 mg/kg (<45 kg) followed by 10 mg/kg 8 to 12 hours later.[24] Intravenous quinidine gluconate followed by oral quinine should be administered for severe illness, as already indicated.[12,24] A second drug needs to be administered in chloroquine-resistant *P. falciparum*, and this second drug should follow the oral quinidine regimen: either a single dose of three tablets of pyrimethamine-sulfadoxine (Fansidar) on the last day of intravenous quinidine or clindamycin 900 mg three times daily for 3 to 5 days.[23,24] An alternative oral treatment for chloroquine-resistant *P. falciparum* infection in adults, especially in those with a history of seizures or psychiatric disorders, is the combination of atovaquone 250 mg and proguanil 100 mg (Malarone) (4 tablets daily for 3 days).[13,23,24] The intravenous quinidine regimen requires close monitoring of the electrocardiogram and other vital signs (e.g., hypotension and hypoglycemia).[15,23,24] Because falciparum malaria is associated with serious complications, including pulmonary edema, hypoglycemia, jaundice, renal failure, confusion, delirium, seizures, coma, and death, careful monitoring of fluid status and hemodynamic parameters is mandatory.[15–21,23] Exchange transfusion that may be required in patients with *P. falciparum* malaria in whom parasitemia is 5% to 15% remain a questionable modality.[20] Either peritoneal or hemodialysis may be indicated in renal failure.[23]

EVALUATION OF THERAPEUTIC OUTCOMES

When advising potential travelers on prophylaxis for malaria, be aware of the incidence of chloroquine-resistant *P. falciparum* malaria and the countries where this is prevalent.[11,13,23,24,29] Detailed recommendations for prevention of malaria may be obtained by checking the World Wide Web (e.g., www.cdc.gov/travel/ or www2.cdc.gov/mmwr/)[34,41] or by calling the Centers for Disease Control and Prevention (CDC) (see Appendix 113–1). A number of newer drugs are under active study and include the water-soluble artesunate and the oil-soluble artemether (Lumefantrine, also known as benflumetol) and combinations of this with other agents and the recently approval combination atovaquone and proguanil (Malarone) in the United States.[10,13,23,36–40] Halofantrine (Halfan) has poor bioavailability, prolongs the QTc interval at the recommended doses, and has been reported to have therapeutic failures.[24]

Acute *P. falciparum* malaria resistant to chloroquine should be treated with intravenous quinidine. These patients should have a central venous catheter to follow fluid status, and the electrocardiogram should be monitored closely. Hypoglycemia that is associated with *P. falciparum* should be checked and corrected with dextrose infusions.[15] Quinidine infusion should be slowed temporarily or stopped if there is a QT interval of greater than 0.6 second, an increase in the QRS complex to greater than 50%, or hypotension unresponsive to fluid challenge results. The suggested quinidine levels should be maintained at 3–7 mg/L.[15,23] Blood smears should be checked every 12 hours until parasitemia is less than 1%. Resolution of fever should take place between 36 and 48 hours after initiation of the intravenous quinidine therapy, and the blood should be clear of parasites in 5 days.[15,23] If parenteral therapy is required for more than 48 hours, it is suggested that the dose of quinidine be lowered by half.[24]

Travelers to endemic areas for malaria should be advised to remain in well-screened areas, to wear clothes that cover most of the body, and to sleep in mosquito nets.[4,41] It is prudent to carry the insect repellent DEET (*N,N*-diethylmetatoluamide) or other insect sprays containing DEET for use in mosquito-infested areas.[41] Readers are urged to check publications from the CDC for the list of countries where chloroquine-resistant *P. falciparum* exist.[24,34]

AMEBIASIS

EPIDEMIOLOGY AND ETIOLOGY

Because of its worldwide distribution and serious gastrointestinal manifestations, amebiasis is one of the most important parasitic diseases of humans.[9,42–45] The major causative organism in amebiasis is *Entamoeba histolytica*, which inhabits the colon and must be differentiated from the *E. dispar*, which is associated with an asymptomatic carrier state and is considered nonpathogenic. Although *E. histolytica* and *E. dispar* are indistinguishable morphologically, recent research

Malarial infection does not produce immunity in patients, and active research has been initiated to develop a malaria vaccine.[23,31–3] A vaccine that blocks the entry of sporozoites into the liver cells will prevent malaria at this stage. However, immunity to sporozoites does not protect the host against parasites in the erythrocytic cycle.[33] Infective sporozoites of *P. falciparum* are covered by a polypeptide circumsporozoite protein.[35] Isolation and identification of the gene encoding for this circumsporozoite protein have led to the development of a monoclonal antibody by recombinant DNA technology *P. falciparum* sporozoite vaccine is now under investigation.[33,35]

using monoclonal antibodies has been able to separate the two.[44,4] Invasive amebiasis is almost exclusively the result of *E. histolytica* infection. Approximately 50 million cases of invasive disease result each year worldwide, leading to an excess of 100,000 deaths.[43,44] In the United States, the incidence of amebiasis is estimated at about 4% in the general population.[45] The highest incidence is found in institutionalized mentally retarded patients, sexually active homosexuals patients with acquired immune deficiency syndrome (AIDS), the Native American population, and new immigrants from endemic areas (e.g., Mexico, India, West and South Africa, and portions of Central and South America).[44–49]

PATHOLOGY

E. histolytica invades mucosal cells of colonic epithelium, producing the classic flask-shaped ulcer in the submucosa.[42,44,45] The trophozoite has a cytolethal effect on cells through a toxin. If the trophozoite gets into the portal circulation, it will be carried to the liver, where it produces abscess and periportal fibrosis.[46,47,50–51] Amebic ulceration can affect the perineum and genitalia, and abscesses may occur in the lung and brain.[42,43,45,52]

CLINICAL PRESENTATION

The most frequent clinical manifestations of the disease are gastrointestinal (Table 113–2).

Liver abscesses that are located in the right lobe can spread to the lungs and pleura.[42–45] Pericardial infection, although rare, may be associated with extension of the amebic abscess from the left lobe of the liver. Erosion of liver abscesses also present as peritonitis.[42,47,50,5]

Review of the patient's history and recent travel cannot be overemphasized. Intestinal amebiasis is diagnosed by demonstrating *E. histolytica* cysts or trophozoites (may contain ingested erythrocytes) in fresh stool or from a specimen obtained by

TABLE 113–2. Most Common Manifestations of Amebiasis

Intestinal Disease

Vague abdominal discomfort, malaise to severe abdominal cramps, flatulence, bloody diarrhea (heme-positive in 100% of cases) with mucus[42–45]

Eosinophilia is usually absent, although mild leukocytosis is not unusual[42]

Amebic Liver Abscess

High fever, significant leukocytosis with left shift, elevated alkaline phosphatase, and liver tenderness on palpation[42,44,45]

Right upper quadrant pain, hepatomegaly, and liver tenderness, with referred pain to the left or right shoulder

Erosion of liver abscesses also present as peritonitis[42,47,50,51]

sigmoidoscopy. Three stool samples obtained 24 hours apart will produce a 60% to 90% yield for *E. histolytica*. Microscopy may not differentiate between the pathogenic *E. histolytica* and the nonpathogenic *E. dispar* in stools. Sensitive techniques are available to detect *E. histolytica* in stool, including antigen detection and PCR.[43–45,51] Endoscopy with scraping or biopsy may provide more definitive diagnosis where stool examinations do not provide adequate evidence.[45]

When amebic liver abscess is suspected from initial physical examination and history, confirmatory diagnostic procedures will include serology and liver scans (using isotopes by ultrasound or computed tomography) or magnetic resonance imaging.[42,45] Leukocytosis ($>10,000/mm^3$) and an elevated alkaline phosphatase concentration ($>75\%$) are common findings. In rare instances, needle aspiration of the hepatic abscess may be attempted using ultrasound guidance.[45,50]

▶ TREATMENT: Amebiasis

■ DESIRED OUTCOME

In amebiasis, the goals of therapy are initially to eradicate the parasite by use of specific amebicides and then to render supportive therapy.

■ TREATMENT REGIMENS

A number of different regimens have been suggested depending on the category of amebiasis: asymptomatic cyst passers, intestinal amebiasis, and amebic liver abscess.[42–45] Electrolyte replacement and nutritional support are essential adjunctive treatment modalities. Large hepatic abscess or amebic pericarditis may require needle aspiration, percutaneous catheter drainage, or rarely, surgery before drug therapy.[42,44,45] Most regimens require a combination of drugs administered concurrently or sequentially.[24,45]

A careful history should be taken when one of the differential diagnoses is ulcerative colitis because corticosteroid administration has the potential to unmask amebiasis and produce toxic megacolon.[45] All patients diagnosed as having inflammatory bowel disease should have their stools examined carefully and serologic testing done for amebiasis to avoid the serious consequence that results from the administration of corticosteroids.

■ PHARMACOLOGIC THERAPY

Metronidazole (Flagyl), tetracycline, dehydroemetine, and chloroquine (Aralen) are tissue-acting agents, whereas iodoquinol (Yodoxin), diloxanide furoate (Furamide), and paromomycin (Humatin) are luminal amebicides. A systemic agent may be so well absorbed that only small amounts of the drug stay in the bowel, which might prove ineffective as a luminal agent.[24,42,45,53,54] A luminal-acting agent, on the other hand, may be too poorly absorbed to be effective in the tissue. In the asymptomatic cyst passer, it is necessary to eradicate the causative agent from the lumen to prevent intestinal amebiasis or the development of amebic liver abscess. Drug effectiveness must be monitored by stool examination, i.e., from one to three negative specimens from 1 to 3 months after treatment.

Asymptomatic cyst passers and patients with mild intestinal amebiasis should receive one of the following luminal agents: paromomycin 25–30 mg/kg per day three times daily for 7 days, iodoquinol 650 mg three times daily for 20 days, or diloxanide furoate 500 mg three times daily for 10 days. These regimens have cure rates of between 84% and 96%.[45] Diloxanide furoate is only available from Ponorama Compounding Pharmacy [6744 Balboa Blvd., Van Nuys, CA 91406; (800)-247-9767].[24] The pediatric dose for paromomycin is the same as in adults, whereas the dose of iodoquinol is 30–40 mg/kg per day in three doses for 20 days, and the dose of diloxanide furoate is 20 mg/kg per day in three doses for 10 days.[24] Paromomycin is the preferred luminal agent in pregnant patients.[24,45]

Patients with severe intestinal disease or liver abscess should receive metronidazole 750 mg three times daily for 10 days, followed by a course of one of the luminal agents indicated earlier.[24,42–45] An alternative regimen of metronidazole 2.4 g/day for 2 days has been suggested to treat intestinal amebiasis.[45] In the pediatric patient, the dose of oral metronidazole is 50 mg/kg per day in divided doses to be followed by a luminal agent.[24] Patients who are too ill to take oral metronidazole should receive the drug in equivalent doses by the intravenous route.[42,45]

EVALUATION OF THERAPEUTIC OUTCOMES

Follow-up in patients with amebiasis should include repeat stool examination, serology, colonoscopy (in colitis), or computed tomography (CT; in liver abscess) between days 5 and 7, at the end of the course of therapy, and a month after the end of therapy.[42] Most patients with either intestinal amebiasis or colitis will respond in 3 to 5 days with amelioration of symptoms. Patients with liver abscesses may take from 7 to 10 days to respond; patients not responding during this period may require aspiration of abscesses or exploratory laparotomy. Serial liver scans have demonstrated healing of liver abscesses over 4 to 8 months after adequate therapy.[42]

SANITATION AND PREVENTIVE MEASURES

Travelers and tourists visiting an epidemic area should avoid local tap water, ice, salads, and unpeeled fruits. Water can be disinfected by the use of iodine (tincture of iodine or commercial sources: Potable Aqua tablet, Wisconsin Pharmacal, or Globaline, Wallace & Ternain) or a strong chlorine (laundry bleach) solution, but boiled water is probably the safest. An alternative or additional measure may be to carry a portable water purifier (Safewater, Durango, CO; *www.outgear.com*). Because food handlers in Asia and Latin America may be a source of amebiasis, travelers should avoid eating at food stalls and open markets.

GIARDIASIS

EPIDEMIOLOGY AND ETIOLOGY

Giardia lamblia (also known as *G. intestinalis* or *G. duodenalis*), an enteric protozoan, is the most common intestinal parasite responsible for diarrheal syndromes throughout the world.[55–69] *Giardia* is the most frequently identified intestinal parasite in the United States, with a prevalence rate of 16% in some areas. *G. lamblia* has been identified as the first enteric pathogen seen in children in developing countries, with prevalence rates between 15% and 30%.[57]

There are two stages in the life cycle of *G. lamblia*: the trophozoite and the cyst. *G. lamblia*, which is found in the small intestine, the gallbladder, and biliary drainage, is a pear-shaped trophozoite with four pairs of flagella. Two nuclei lie in the area of the sucking disk, giving the protozoan a characteristic facelike image.

The distribution of giardiasis is worldwide. Children seem to be affected more frequently than adults. Children in day-care centers may infect parents and other family members.[67] In less developed countries, fecal contamination of the environment and lack of potable water, education, and housing continue to be risk factors for giardiasis among children.

PATHOLOGY

Giardiasis results from ingestion of *G. lamblia* cysts in fecally contaminated water or food. The protozoan excysts under the stimulus of low gastric pH to release the trophozoite.[56] Colonization and multiplication of the trophozoite lead to mucosal invasion, localized edema, and flattening of the villi, resulting in malabsorption states in the host.[57–69]

Lactose intolerance precipitated by giardiasis can persist even after eradication of the protozoan. Achlorhydria, hypogammaglobu-

TABLE 113–3. Clinical Presentation of Giardiasis

Acute Onset
Diarrhea, cramplike abdominal pain, bloating, and flatulence[55–68]
Malaise, anorexia, nausea, and belching[60]
Chronic
Diarrhea: Foul-smelling, copious, light-colored, fatty stools; weight loss
Periods of diarrhea alternating with constipation
Steatorrhea, vitamin B_{12} and fat-soluble vitamin deficiencies[60–62]

linemia, or deficiency in secretory immunoglobulin A (IgA) are predispositions for giardiasis[55,57–69] (Table 113–3).

Diagnosis of giardiasis is made by examination of fresh stool or a preserved specimen during the acute diarrheal phase. Fresh stool specimens may show the trophozoites, whereas preserved specimen usually yield the cysts. If both the stool examination and string test prove unsuccessful, it may be necessary to attempt duodenal aspiration and biopsy to confirm the diagnosis; this may be more important in AIDS patients and in patients with hypogammaglobulinemia.[42,45] Most clinicians would advocate a clinical trial of the standard therapy before undertaking invasive diagnostic tests.[56,57] An indirect fluorescent antibody (IFA) test that uses a monoclonal antibody to a protein in *Giardia* cysts is available commercially for the detection of the *Giardia* antigen (Meridan Diagnostics, Cincinnati, OH).[66,67]

▶ TREATMENT: Giardiasis

▦ DESIRED OUTCOME

To reduce morbidity and to avoid complications in patients identified with prolonged diarrhea and malabsorption and who have a recent history of travel to an endemic area, rapid identification by ova and parasite (O&P) examination or by antigen detection test should be used to institute appropriate therapy.

▦ PHARMACOLOGIC THERAPY

 All symptomatic adults and children older than 8 years of age should be treated with metronidazole 250 mg three times daily

for 7 days. The alternative drugs include furazolidone 100 mg four times or paromomycin 25–30 mg/kg per day in divided doses daily for 1 week.[24,55–68] Paromomycin 25–30 mg/kg per day in three doses for 7 days or bacitracin or bacitracin zinc may be safe agents in pregnancy.[24,55,56] The pediatric dose for metronidazole is 15 mg/kg per day three times daily for 5 to 7 days.[24] Furazolidone suspension 6 mg/kg per day in four doses for 7 to 10 days and nitazoxanide (Alinia) suspension (a recently approved agent) 100–200 mg every 12 hours for 3 days are alternative drugs for children.[24,63] Quinacrine which was the drug of choice in giardiasis, has been discontinued by the manufacturer but is obtained in the United States from a Specialized Pharmacy (see Appendix 113–1). Albendazole 400 mg daily for 5 days has been cited to produce cure rates of 97% and as being equivalent to metronidazole in children. However, other investigators have disputed the efficacy of this agent.[56]

EVALUATION OF THERAPEUTIC OUTCOMES

Patients with symptomatic giardiasis, positive stool samples, or the detection of *Giardia* antigen by IFA or enzyme-linked immunosorbent assay (ELISA) should be treated with metronidazole for 7 days. Metronidazole produces cure rates of between 85% and 95%.[56–67] Diarrhea will stop within a few days, although in some patients it may take 1 to 2 weeks. Cyst excretion will cease within days; however, intestinal dysfunction (manifested as increased transit time) and radiologic changes (irregular thickening of the folds in the upper small intestine) may take a few months to resolve.[67] Patients who fail initial therapy with metronidazole should receive a second course of therapy. Pregnant patients can receive paromomycin 25–30 mg/kg per day in divided doses for 7 days. Metronidazole has been used in the second and third trimesters of pregnancy.[66,57]

Giardiasis can be prevented by good personal hygiene and by caution in food and drink consumption. Preventive measures are similar to those discussed under amebiasis (see "Sanitation and Preventive Measures").

LEISHMANIASIS

EPIDEMIOLOGY AND ETIOLOGY

This disease is caused by a protozoan belonging to the genus *Leishmania*. The three variations of the disease are visceral leishmaniasis (*kala*-azar, "black fever," or Assam fever), cutaneous leishmaniasis, and mucocutaneous leishmaniasis.[64–67] The visceral form is caused predominantly by *L. donovani*, whereas the other two forms are caused

y other species. Leishmaniasis is a complex disease, but space con-
traints do not justify an extended discussion here; interested readers
re urged to consult other sources.[64,67,68]

Leishmania exist in two forms: as a flagellated extracellular para-
te in the sandfly vector (Phlebotomus in the Indian subcontinent and
utzomyia and Psychodopygus in North and South America, Africa,
r the Middle East) and an aflagellar amastigote (intracellular form)
1 the host.[67,68] The major reservoirs for Leishmania, depending on
eographic location, are dogs, foxes, squirrels, and rodents. The sand-
ies ingest the parasite when they feed on the reservoir animals. After
metamorphosis in the gut of the sandfly, the parasite is transferred to
the human host when the infected sandfly takes a blood meal. Cu-
neous leishmaniasis seen most frequently in the United States is
aused by either L. braziliensis or L. mexicana, which are endemic to
outh Mexico and Central America.[67,68]

The disease can range from cutaneous ulcers to the mucocuta-
eous form affecting the nose, oral cavity, and pharynx. The highest
ncidence usually is seen in the summer months, especially in sub-
ects working near forested areas. Visceral leishmaniasis may be ac-

---

TABLE 113–4. Clinical Manifestation of Leishmaniasis

Visceral: Early
Papule that may ulcerate
Asymptomatic period (dissemination of the amastigote to organs:
  spleen, liver, bone marrow, and lymphatic tissue)
Visceral: Late (3–8 Months)[65,67]
Fever, chills, malaise, weight loss, abdominal distension, and
  hepatosplenomegaly[65,67]
Persisting raised ulcer
Cutaneous and Mucocutaneous
Mutilation of nose, soft palate, and trachea (L. braziliensis)

---

quired from transfusion of contaminated blood and accidental needle
stick injuries.[64,67] Patients with advanced-stage acquired immunodeficiency syndrome (AIDS) are reported to be highly susceptible to
leishmaniasis[67] (Table 113–4).

Demonstration of amastigote in tissue or bone marrow confirms
the diagnosis of leishmaniasis.[64–67]

▶ TREATMENT: Leishmaniasis

DESIRED OUTCOME

he major goal is to eradicate the amastigote in the tissue and to
ninimize the ensuing complications of leishmaniasis.

PHARMACOLOGIC THERAPY

All three forms of leishmaniasis are treated with stibogluconate sodium (antimony sodium gluconate-pentavalent anti-
nony, Pentostam), which is obtained from the CDC. In adults, both

the cutaneous and mucocutaneous forms (L. braziliensis and L. mexicana) are treated with stibogluconate 20 mg/kg per day for 20 to
28 days.[24] The drug may be administered by either the intravenous or
intramuscular route. Therapy for all forms of leishmaniasis may be
repeated.[24] An alternative drug for the visceral form is amphotericin
B (Fungizone) or liposomal amphotericin B (AmBisome). Liposomal
amphotericin B is also recommended for mucocutaneous and cutaneous forms.[24,70–73] Pediatric patients receive the same dose as adults
(see Appendix 113–1 for side effects of the drugs). Pentavalent antimony therapy combined with interferon-γ or liposomal amphotericin
may be alternatives in refractory leishmaniasis.[24] Other combination
therapies and alternative agents for the various forms of leishmaniasis
are discussed in detail by a number of authors.[64,72,73]

VALUATION OF THERAPEUTIC OUTCOMES

he presence of dead amastigotes in tissue and bone marrow, resolu-
ion of anemia and leukopenia, and disappearance of splenomegaly
nd hepatomegaly may be used as monitoring parameters for the dis-
ase. Travelers to endemic areas should use insect repellents and sleep
n fine-mesh netting to avoid exposure to the sandfly.[67,68] No effective
hemoprophylaxis against leishmaniasis is available.

AMERICAN TRYPANOSOMIASIS

TIOLOGY

wo distinct forms of the genus Trypanosoma occur in humans.
One is associated with African trypanosomiasis (sleeping sickness)
nd the other with American trypanosomiasis (Chagas' disease).[74–76]
. brucei gambiense and T. brucei rhodesiense are the causative or-
anisms for African trypanosomiasis. In Chagas' disease, the trypo-
mastigote is found in the bloodstream, and an ovoid, unflagellated
ntracellular form is found in cardiac and other tissues.[74,75]

T. cruzi is the agent that causes American trypanosomiasis.
American trypanosomiasis is transmitted by a number of species of a
eduviid bug (Triatoma infestans, Rhodrium prolixus) that live in wall
racks of houses in rural areas of North, Central, and South America.

The reduviid bug is infected by sucking blood from animals (e.g.,
opossums, dogs, and cats) or humans infected with circulating trypo-
mastigotes (Table 113–5).

In chronic disease, patients present with cardiomyopathy and
heart failure. Electrocardiograms are usually abnormal, demonstrating extrasystoles, first-degree heart block, right bundle-branch
block, and other serious conduction disturbances.[75,78] Degeneration

---

TABLE 113–5. Clinical Presentation of South American Trypanosomiasis

Acute
Unilateral orbital edema ("Romana's sign")[74,76]
Granuloma or "chagoma"
Fever, hepatosplenomegaly, and lymphadenopathy
Chronic
Cardiac: Cardiomyopathy and heart failure
ECG: First-degree heart block, right bundle-branch block, and
  arrhythmias[75,78]
Gastrointestinal: Enlargement of esophagus and colon ("mega"
  syndrome)[74,76,77]
Central nervous system: Meningoencephalitis, strokes, seizures, and
  focal paralysis[74,76,79–81]

of the autonomic ganglia in the smooth muscle of the esophagus and colon leads to uncoordinated peristalsis. The end result has been reported to be "megasyndromes" of affected organs.[74,76,77] Penetration of central nervous system results in meningoencephalitis, strokes, seizures, and focal paralysis.[74,76,79–81]

A history to verify the possible exposure to *T. cruzi* should be an important initial diagnostic work-up. Recovery of *T. cruzi* is defini-tive, but this is not always possible, especially in chronic disease. Positive serologic tests using indirect hemagglutination tests, ELISA (Chagas EIA, Abbott Labs), and a complement fixation (CF) test are diagnostic.[74] The CDC has used PCR to diagnosis *T. cruzi*.[82] Specimens may be sent to the CDC for testing. False-positive reactions are seen, especially in those exposed to leishmaniasis, syphilis, or malaria.[74]

▶ TREATMENT: American Trypanosomiasis

■ DESIRED OUTCOME

The primary goal of drug therapy in trypanosomiasis is to reduce the duration and severity of the illness and possibly to decrease mortality.

■ PHARMACOLOGIC THERAPY

The drugs that have been used to treat *T. cruzi* infections include ni-furtimox (Lampit, Bayer 2502) and benznidazole (Rochagan).[24,83,84] However, it has been suggested that benznidazole and related compounds may not be safe treatment for *T. cruzi*.[84] Oral nifurtimox is available from the CDC, whereas benznidazole is only available in Brazil. The adult dose of nifurtimox is 8–10 mg/kg per day in divided doses for 120 days. Because pediatric patients tolerate the drug better than adults, the dose for children aged 1 to 10 years is 15–20 mg/kg per day, and for children aged 11 to 16 years it is 12.5–15 mg/kg per day in divided doses.[24] Symptomatic treatment for heart failure includes digitalis and diuretics; the gastrointestinal complications, however, may require surgical revisions and reconstruction.[76]

EVALUATION OF THERAPEUTIC OUTCOMES

American trypanosomiasis (Chagas' disease), which is endemic in all Latin American countries, can be transmitted congenitally, by blood transfusion, and by organ transplantation.[74,76] Treatment with nifur-timox of the acute phase (i.e., fever, malaise, edema of face, generalized lymphadenopathy, and hepatosplenomegaly) produces between 50% and 75% cure rates.[74,76] Treatment of chronic infection with nifurtimox is not recommended. It is essential to identify *T. cruzi*–infected patients by serology and to monitor the cardiovascular status of these patients by electrocardiogram periodically. The congestive failure of cardiomyopathic Chagas' disease is treated the same way as cardiomyopathies from other causes.[75,76]

HELMINTHIC DISEASES

Most intestinal helminthic infections may not be associated with clearly defined manifestation of disease, but they can cause significant pathology.[85–94] One factor that determines the pathogenicity of helminths is their population density. Light infections may be fairly well tolerated, whereas high populations of intestinal helminths can result in predictable disease presentations. In the United States, these infections are seen most frequently in recent immigrants from Southeast Asia, the Caribbean, Mexico, and Central America.[1,3,9] There is a higher incidence of helminthic infections in the southern states. Other populations that have a high risk of infestation include institutionalized patients (both young and elderly), preschool children in day-care centers, residents of Indian reservations, and homosexual individuals. Certain conditions and drugs (fever, corticosteroids, and anesthesia) can cause atypical localization of worms.[93,94] Immunocompromised hosts can be overwhelmed by some helminthic infections, such as strongyloidiasis.[94]

NEMATODES

HOOKWORM DISEASE

This is an infection of the small intestine caused by either *Ancylostoma duodenale* or *Necator americanus*. *N. americanus* is found in the southeastern United States, where the temperature and humidity provide the proper environment. *Ancylostoma* is seen rarely in the United States.

The life cycles of both species of hookworm are similar. The adult worms live in the small intestine attached to the mucosa. The females liberate eggs, which are eliminated in the feces and develop into larvae. Infective larva enter the host in contaminated food or water or penetrate the skin, where a papular eruption with localized edema and erythema can result.

In the small intestine, where the adult worm lives attached to the mucosa, injury is usually caused by mechanical and lytic destruction of tissue. The loss of blood can lead to anemia and hypoproteinemia.[89–91]

Stool should be examined for eggs and the rhabditiform larvae. Eosinophilia (30% to 60%) is present in patients with chronic infection.

▶ TREATMENT: Hookworm Disease

Mebendazole (Vermox), an oral synthetic benzimidazole, is the agent of first choice. It is also effective against ascariasis, enterobiasis, and trichuriasis.[24,25,95,96] The adult dose for treatment of hookworm infestation is 100 mg twice daily for 3 days. Pediatric patients older than 2 years of age should receive the same dose as adults.[24]

ASCARIASIS

Ascariasis is caused by the giant roundworm *Ascaris lumbricoides*. Female worms range from 20 to 35 cm in length. The worm is found worldwide but more commonly in areas where sanitation is poor. In the United States, endemic areas include southeastern parts of the Appalachian range and the Gulf Coast states. Approximately 4 million people in the United States have ascariasis.[85]

Clinical Manifestations

During migration of the larvae through the lungs, patients can present with pneumonitis, fever, cough, eosinophilia, and pulmonary infiltrates.[9,85,93] Other symptoms of ascariasis include abdominal discomfort, abdominal obstruction, vomiting, and appendicitis.[86–88,93] Diagnosis is made by demonstrating the characteristic egg in the stool.

▶ TREATMENT: Ascariasis

In both adults and pediatric patients older than 2 years of age, the treatment for ascariasis is mebendazole (Vermox) 100 mg twice daily for 3 days. An alternative drug for ascariasis is pyrantel pamoate (Antiminth).[24,98]

ENTEROBIASIS

Enterobiasis, or pinworm infection, is caused by *Enterobius vermicularis*. The pinworm is a small, threadlike, spindle-shaped worm about cm in length. It is the most widely distributed helminthic infection in the world. There are estimated to be 42 million cases in the United States.[85,99] The majority of those infected are children.

There are no significant pathologic changes with the infection. The most common problem is cutaneous irritation in the perianal region, made by the migrating females or the presence of eggs. The intense pruritus and scratching can cause dermatitis and secondary bacterial infections. In children, the itching can cause loss of sleep and restlessness.

The most effective method of diagnosing pinworm infections is by the use of perianal swab using adhesive Scotch tape. The Scotch tape, which is applied to the perianal region with a tongue depressor, is examined microscopically for eggs.[9,85,99]

▶ TREATMENT: Enterobiasis

Helminthic drugs are used to eradicate or reduce the parasitic load in patients. The common agents for treatment include pyrantel pamoate, mebendazole, or albendazole (Zentel). The dose of pyrantel pamoate is 11 mg/kg (maximum 1 g) as a single dose that can be repeated in 2 weeks. The dose of mebendazole for adults and children older than 2 years of age is 100 mg as a single dose; this may be repeated in 2 weeks.[24,98] The dose of albendazole for adults and children older than 2 years of age is 400 mg, and this dose should be repeated in 2 weeks.[98] Following treatment, all bedding and underclothes should be sterilized by steaming or washing in the hot water cycle of a regular washing machine; this will eradicate the eggs. Bathroom rugs and toilet accessories also should be cleaned in a similar way.

EVALUATION OF THERAPEUTIC OUTCOME: NEMATODES

Morbidity and disease with intestinal nematodes are related to the intensity of infection or worm burden; subjects with transient exposure have less severe disease. The major adverse effects of intestinal nematodes are malnutrition, fatigue, and diminished work capacity. Treatment with antihelmintic agents results in complete eradication and significant change in the well-being of patients. Unlike other nematodes, strongyloidiasis can perpetuate itself by autoinfection, and under immunosuppression, the filariform can invade various organs (e.g., lungs, central nervous system, and the like) to produce disseminated infection that can be fatal.[9,85,94]

ECTOPARASITES

A parasite that lives on the outside the body of the host is called an *ectoparasite*. Approximately 6 to 12 million people become infested with pediculosis yearly in the United States.[108] Pediculosis usually is associated with poor personal hygiene, and infections are passed from person to person through social and sexual contact. The three types of human lice belong to two genera: *Pediculus,* including the head and body lice, and *Phthirus,* with only one species, the crab louse.[9,100–105] The human louse is detectable to the human naked eye and measures approximately 2 to 3 mm in length.

LICE

The two species that belong to this group include *Pediculus humanus capitis* (head louse) and *P. humanus corporis* (body louse). Female lice deposit eggs on the hair. The eggs (or nits) remain firmly attached to the hair, and in about 10 days, the lice hatch to form nymphs, which mature in 2 weeks. Using both their piercing mouth parts and a pumping device, the larvae and adults feed on the blood of the host. The body louse and head louse are essentially identical, although they live on different parts of the body. Unlike the head louse, which lives on the hair, the body louse is more frequently found on clothing of the infected host.

Pubic or crab lice are found on the hairs around the genitals, although they can occur in other areas of the body (e.g., eyelashes, beards, and axillae). Patients usually complain of severe pruritus from papular lesions produced by the bite of the louse. Hypersensitivity to foreign material injected by the lice can produce macular swellings and occasionally can lead to secondary bacterial infections.[101]

▶ TREATMENT: Lice

The goal of therapy is to eradicate the causative organisms and provide symptomatic relief to patients. The agent of choice for all three infections (body, head, and crab lice) is 1% permethrin (Nix).[100–109] Permethrin is a derivative of the flowers of the plant *Chrysanthemum cinerariifolium*. The term *pyrethrin* is usually applied to several esters of chrysanthemic acid and pyrethric acid. Permethrin has both pediculicidal and ovicidal activity against *P. humanus* var. *capitis*. The cure rate is reported to be in the range of 90% to 97%.[106–109] Individuals who have a history of ragweed or chrysanthemum allergy should use this compound with caution. The side effects reported with permethrin products include itching, burning, stinging, and tingling.[109] Permethrin 1% is applied to the scalp after the hair has been dried following a shampooing. The scalp should be saturated with permethrin liquid, and a towel should be wrapped around the scalp to allow the application to stay on for 10 minutes. The hair then should be rinsed off. A cream rinse of permethrin 1% (Nix-Creme Rinse) is also available. To ensure complete eradication, especially of newly hatched lice, ◀ it may be necessary to repeat the application.[104] Recent reports have suggested increasing lice resistance to permethrin 1%.[105–109] An alternative preparation for lice is 0.5% malathion (Ovide), which is very effective.[24,105] To ensure complete eradication of lice infestation, the malathion application should be left on the scalp for about 90 minutes.[109] For the relief of pruritus, a soothing lotion of calamine liniment or lotion with 0.1% menthol may be used. Other members of the family or sexual partners also should be treated. All bedding and clothes should be sterilized by boiling or washing in the hot water cycle of the washing machine to avoid reinfections. Seams of clothes should be examined to verify that all organisms are eradicated. An ocular lubricant (e.g., Lacri-Lube S.O.P.) applied twice daily may be used to remove crab louse infection of the eyelids.

SCABIES

Scabies is caused by the itch mite *Sarcoptes scabiei*, which affects both humans and animals. Mange in domestic animals is caused by the same organism. Infection usually affects the interdigital and popliteal folds, axillary folds, the umbilicus, and the scrotum.[100,102,110]

CLINICAL PRESENTATION

Patients will complain of severe itching and an inability to sleep and may have excoriations in the interdigital web spaces, wrists, elbows, buttocks, groin, and scalp. Excoriations may lead to secondary bacterial infections. The diagnosis is made by looking for burrows formed by the mite and taking skin scrapings, which will demonstrate the mite on a wet mount.

▶ TREATMENT: Scabies

Because these infections cause a great deal of discomfort and distress to patients and families, the goals of therapy are to eradicate the infestations rapidly, to institute symptomatic treatment, and to provide counseling and reassurance. The treatment of choice is permethrin 5% (Elimite) cream.[24,100,102,110] To initiate the treatment, the skin should be scrubbed thoroughly in a warm soapy bath using a soft brush to remove all scabs. The lotion is then applied to the whole body, avoiding the face, mucous membranes, and eyes. The application should be left on for 8 to 14 hours before bathing.[24] A single application eradicates 97% of scabies in subjects.[110] All close contacts should be checked and treated appropriately.

Other agents used to treat scabies are Crotamiton 10% (Eurax) and oral ivermectin (Stromectal) 200 mcg/kg once.[24,100,110] These should be used in patients who have hypersensitivity to permethrin preparations. Topical corticosteroids and antihistamines may be used to decrease pruritus.

Permethrin (1% to 5 %) for pediculosis and scabies is the preferred agent and remains the safest agent, especially in infants and children.[100,102] One application of permethrin is consistently effective in eradicating more than 90% of all infections. However, pruritus may persist for 2 to 4 weeks because of the remnants of mite parts in the skin.

Review Questions and other resources can be found at *www.pharmacotherapyonline.com*.

REFERENCES

1. Freedman DO, Woodall J. Emerging infectious diseases and the risk to the traveler. Med Clin North Am 1999;83:865–883.
2. Bechtel GA. Parasitic infections among migrant farm families. J Community Nurs 1998;15:1–7.
3. Walker PF, Jaranson J. Refuge and immigrant health care. Med Clin North Am 1999;83:1103–1120.
4. Dardick K. Educating travelers about malaria:dealing with resistance and patient noncompliance. Cleveland Clin J Med 2000;69:469–479.
5. Malaria Surveillance—United States, 2000. MMWR 2002;51(SS-5): 9–23.
6. Beigel Y, Greenberg Z, Ostfeld I. Letting the patient off the hook. N Engl J Med 2000;342:1658–1661.
7. Dorsey G, Gandhi M, Oyugi JH, Rosenthal PJ. Difficulties in the prevention, diagnosis and treatment of imported malaria. Arch Intern Med 2000;160:2505–2510.
8. Sinha A, Grace C, Alston WK, et al. African trypanosomiasis in two travelers from the United States. Clin Infect Dis 1999;29:840–844.
9. Markell EK, John DT, Krotoski WA. Markell and Voge's Medical Parasitology, 8th ed. Philadelphia, Saunders, 1999.
10. Magill AJ. The prevention of malaria. Prim Care Clin Off Pract 2002;29:815–842.
11. Malaria deaths following inappropriate malaria chemoprophylaxis—United States, 2001. MMWR 2001;50:597–599.
12. Krogstad DJ. Plasmodium species (Malaria). In: Mandell GL, Dolin R, Bennett JE, eds. Principles and Practice of Infectious Diseases, 5th ed. New York, Churchill-Livingstone, 2000:2817–2831.
13. Kain KC, Shanks GD, Keystone JS. Malaria chemoprophylaxis in the age of drug resistance: I. Currently recommended drug regimens. Clin Infect Dis 2001;33:226–234.
14. Local transmission of *Plasmodium vivax* malaria—Virginia, 2002. MMWR 2002;51:921–923.

15. Murphy GS, Oldfield EC III. Falciparum malaria. Infect Dis Clin North Am 1996;10:747–775.

16. Newton CRJC, Warrell DA. Neurological manifestations of falciparum malaria. Ann Neurol 1998;43:695–702.

17. Blum PG, Stephens D. Severe falciparum malaria in five soldiers from East Timor: A case series and literature review. Anaesth Intensive Care 2001;29:426–434.

18. Eiam-Ong S. Malarial nephropathy. Semin Nephrol 2003;23:21–33.

19. Murphy SC, Breman JG. Gaps in childhood malaria burden in Africa: Cerebral malaria, neurological sequelae, anemia, respiratory distress, hypoglycemia, and complications of pregnancy. Am J Trop Med Hyg 2001;64:57–67.

20. Riddle MS, Jackson JL, Sanders JW, Blazes DL. Exchange transfusion as an adjunct therapy in severe *Plasmodium falciparum* malaria: A meta-analysis. Clin Infect Dis 2002;34:1192–1198.

21. Taylor WRJ, White NJ. Malaria and the lung. Clin Chest Med 2002;23: 457–468.

22. Humar A, Ohrt C, Kain KC, et al. PARASIGHT F test compared with the polymerase chain reaction and microscopy for the diagnosis of *Plasmodium falciparum* malaria in travelers. Am J Trop Med Hyg 1997;56: 44–48.

23. White NJ. Malaria. In: Cook GC and Zumla A, eds. Manson's Tropical Diseases, 21st ed. London, Saunders, 2003:1205–1295.

24. Anonymous. Drugs for parasitic infections. In: Handbook of Antimicrobial Therapy, 16th ed. New Rochelle, NY, Medical Letter, Inc. 2002:120–143.

25. Tracey JW, Webster LT Jr. Drugs used in the chemotherapy of protozoal infections: Malaria. In: Hardman JG, Limbird LE, Gilman AG, eds. The Pharmacological Basis of Therapeutics, 10th ed. New York, McGraw-Hill, 2001:1069–1095.

26. Schlagenhauf P. Mefloquine for malaria chemoprophylaxis 1992–1998: A review. J Travel Med 1999;6:122–133.

27. Taylor TE, Strickland GT. Infections of the blood and reticuloendothelial system: Malaria. In: Hunter's Tropical Medicine and Emerging Infectious Diseases, 8th ed. Philadelphia, Saunders, 2000:614–643.

28. Alecrim WD, Espinosa FEM, Alecrim MGC. *Plasmodium falciparum* infection in the pregnant patient. Infect Dis Clin North Am 2000;14:83–95.

29. Shanks GD, Kain KC, Keystone JS. Malaria chemoprophylaxis in the age of drug resistance: II. Drugs that may be available in the future. Clin Infect Dis 2001;33:381–385.

30. Schwartz E, Regev-Yochay G. Primaquine as prophylaxis for malaria for nonimmune travelers: A comparison with mefloquine and doxycycline. Clin Infect Dis 1999;29:1502–1506.

31. Hoffman SL, Subramanian GM, Collins FH, Venter JC. *Plasmodium,* human and *Anopheles* genomics and malaria. Nature 2002;415:702–709.

32. Whitty CJM, Rowland M, Sanderson F, Mutabingwa TK. Malaria. Br Med J 2002;325:1221–1224.

33. Moore SA, Surgery EG, Cadwgan AM. Malaria vaccines: Where are we and where are we going? Lancet Infect Dis 2002;2:737–743.

34. Angus BJ. Malaria on the World Wide Web. Clin Infect Dis 2001;33:651–661.

35. Carvalho LJ, Daniel-Ribeiro CT, Goto H. Malaria vaccine: Candidate antigens, mechanisms, constraints and prospects. Scand J Immunol 2002;56:327–343.

36. Newton P, Suputtamongkol Y, White NJ, et al. Antimalarial bioavailability and disposition of artesunate in acute falciparum malaria. Antimicrob Agents Chemother 2000;44:972–977.

37. Ezzet F, van Vugt M, Nosten F, et al. Pharmacokinetics and pharmacodynamics of lumefantrine (Benflumetol) in acute falciparum malaria. Antimicrob Agents Chemother 2000;44:697–704.

38. Looareesuwan S, Wilairatana P, Royce C, et al. A randomized, double-blind, comparative trial of a new oral combination of artemether and benflumetol (CGP 56697) with mefloquine in the treatment of acute *Plasmodium falciparum* malaria in Thailand. Am J Trop Med Hyg 1999;60:238–243.

39. Looareesuwan S, Chulay JD, Canfield CJ, Hutchinson DBA, for the Malarone clinical trials study group. Malarone (atovaquone and proguanil hydrochloride): Review of its clinical development for treatment of malaria. Am J Trop Med Hyg 1999;60:533–541.

40. Looareesuwan S, Wilairatana P, Hutchinson DBA, et al. Efficacy and safety of atovaquone/proguanil compared with mefloquine for treatment of acute *Plasmodium falciparum* malaria in Thailand. Am J Trop Med Hyg 1999;60:526–532.

41. Fradin MS, Day JF. Comparative efficacy of insect repellents against mosquito bites. N Engl J Med 2002;347:13–18.

42. Jackson TFHG, Gathiram V. Intestinal and genital infections: Amebiasis. In: Strickland GT, ed. Tropical Medicine and Emerging Infections, 8th ed. Philadelphia, Saunders, 2000:577–588.

43. Haque R, Huston CD, Hughes M, et al. Amebiasis. N Engl J Med 2003;348:1565–1573.

44. Petr WA, Singh U. Diagnosis and management of amebiasis. Clin Infect Dis 1999;29:1117–1125.

45. Ravdin J. *Entamoeba histolytica* (amebiasis). In: Mandell GL, Dolin R, Bennett JA, eds. Principles and Practice of Infectious Diseases, 5th ed. New York, Churchill-Livingstone, 2000:2798–2810.

46. Hughes MA, Petri WA Jr. Amebic liver abscess. Infect Dis Clin North Am 2000;14:565–581.

47. Hoffner R, Kilaghbian T, Esekogwa VI, Henderson SO. Common presentations of amebic liver abscess. Ann Emerg Med 1999;34:351–355.

48. Antony S, Lopez-Po P. Genital amebiasis: Historical perspective of an unusual disease presentation. Urology 1999;54:952–955.

49. Yoshikawa I, Murata I, Yano K, et al. Asymptomatic amebic colitis in a homosexual man. Am J Gastroenterol 1999;94:2306–2308.

50. Akgun Y, Tacyildiz I, Celik Y. Amebic liver abscess: Changing trends over 20 years. World J Surg 1999;23:102–106.

51. Katz DE, Taylor DN. Parasitic infections of the gastrointestinal tract. Gastroenterol Clin North Am 2001;30:797–815.

52. Lyche KD, Jensen WA. Pleuropulmonary amebiasis. Semin Respir Infect 1997;12:106–112.

53. Tracy JW, Webster LT Jr. Drugs used in the chemotherapy of protozoal infections (continued). In: Hardman JG, Limbird LE, Molinoff PB, Gilman AG, eds. The Pharmacological Basis of Therapeutics, 10th ed. New York, McGraw-Hill, 2001:1097–1120.

54. Rosenthal PJ, Goldsmith R. Antiprotozoal drugs. In: Katzung BG, ed. Basic and Clinical Pharmacology, 8th ed. New York, McGraw-Hill, 2001:882–902.

55. Wright SG. Giardiasis. In: Strickland GT, ed. Tropical Medicine and Emerging Infectious Diseases, 8th ed. Philadelphia, Saunders, 2000: 589–593.

56. Gardner TB, Hill DR. Treatment of giardiasis. Clin Microbiol Rev 2001;14:14–128.

57. Hill DR. *Giardia lamblia*. In: Mandell GL, Dolin R, Bennett JE, eds. Principles and Practice of Infectious Diseases, 5th ed. New York, Churchill-Livingstone, 2000:2888–2894.

58. Ortega YR, Adam RD. Giardia: Overview and update. Clin Infect Dis 1997;25:545–550.

59. Heregi G, Cleary TG. Giardia. Pediatr Rev 1997;18:243–247.

60. Thielman NM, Guerrant RL. Persistent diarrhea in the returned traveler. Infect Dis Clin North Am 1998;12:489–501.

61. Bai JC. Malabsorption syndromes. Digestion 1998;59:530–546.

62. Carroccio A, Montalto G, Notarbartolo A, et al. Secondary impairment of pancreatic function as a cause of severe malabsorption in intestinal giardiasis: A case report. Am J Trop Med Hyg 1997;56:599–602.

63. Nitazoxanide (Alina): A new antiprotozoal agent. Med Lett 2003;45: 29–31.

64. Herwaldt B. Leishmaniasis. Lancet 1999;354:1191–1199.

65. Davidson RN. Visceral leishmaniasis in clinical practice. J Infect 1999;39:112–116.

66. Salman SM, Rubeiz NG, Kibbi A. Cutaneous leishmaniasis: Clinical features and diagnosis. Clin Dermatol 1999;17:291–296.

67. Pearson RD, De Queiroz Souża A, Jeronimo SMB. Leishmania species: Visceral (kala-azar), cutaneous, and mucosal leishmaniasis. In: Mandell GL, Bennett JE, Dolin R, eds. Principles and Practice of Infectious Diseases, 5th ed. New York, Churchill-Livingstone, 2000:2831–2845.

68. Magill AJ. Leishmaniasis. In: Strickland GT, ed. Hunter's Tropical Medicine and Emerging Infectious Diseases, 8th ed. Philadelphia, Saunders, 2000:665–687.

69. Sundar S, Jha TK, Berman J. Oral miltefosine for Indian visceral leishmaniasis. N Engl J Med 2002;347:1739–1746.

70. Sundar S, Agrawal NK, Murray HW, et al. Short-course, low-dose amphotericin-B lipid complex therapy for visceral leishmaniasis unresponsive to antimony. Ann Intern Med 1997;127:133–137.

71. Meyerhoff A. U.S. Food and Drug Administration approval of AmBisome (liposomal amphotericin B) for treatment of visceral leishmaniasis. Clin Infect Dis 1999;28:42–48.

72. Davidson RN. Practical guide for the treatment of leishmaniasis. Drugs 1998;56:1009–1018.

73. Moskowitz PF, Kurban AK. Treatment of cutaneous leishmaniasis: Retrospectives and advances for the 21st century. Clin Dermatol 1999;17:305–315.

74. Magill AJ, Reed SG. American trypanosomiasis. In: Strickland GT, ed. Hunter's Tropical Medicine and Emerging Infectious Diseases, 8th ed. Philadelphia, Saunders, 2000:653–664.

75. Rassi A Jr, Rassi A, Little WC. Chagas' heart disease. Clin Cardiol 2000;23:883–889.

76. Kirchhoff LV. Trypanosoma species (American trypanosomiasis, Chagas' disease): Biology of trypanosomes. In: Mandell GL, Bennett JE, Dolin R, eds. Principles and Practice of Infectious Diseases, 5th ed. New York, Churchill-Livingstone, 2000:2845–2853.

77. de Oliveira RB, Troncon LEA, Dantas RO, Meneghelli UG. Gastrointestinal manifestations of Chagas' disease. Am J Gastroenterol 1998;93:884–889.

78. Chagas' disease after organ transplantation—United States 2001. MMWR 2002;51:210–212.

79. Carod-Artal FJ, Vargas AP, Melo M, Horan TA. American trypanosomiasis (Chagas' disease): An unrecognized cause of stroke. J Neurol Neurosurg Psychiatry 2003;74:516–518.

80. Silva N, O'Bryan L, Masur H, et al. Trypanosoma cruzi meningoencephalitis in HIV-infected patients. J Acquir Immune Defic Syndr 1999;20:342–349.

81. Sartori AM, Shikansai-Yasuda NVA, Lopes MH. Follow-up of 18 patients with human immunodeficiency virus infection and chronic Chagas'disease, with reactivation of Chagas's disease causing cardiac disease in three patients. Clin Infect Dis 1998;26:177–179.

82. Herwaldt BL, Grijalva MJ, Newsome AL, et al. Use of polymerase chain reaction to diagnose the fifth reported US case of autochthonous transmission of Trypanosoma cruzi, in Tennessee, 1998. J Infect Dis 2000;181:395–399.

83. Estani SS, Segura EL, Ruiz AM, et al. Efficacy of chemotherapy with benznidazole in children in the indeterminate phase of Chagas' disease. Am J Trop Med Hyg 1998;39:526–529.

84. Lauria-Pires L, Braga MS, Vexenat AC, et al. Progressive chronic Chagas's heart disease after treatment with anti-Trypanosoma cruzi nitroderivatives. Am J Trop Med Hyg 2000;63:111–118.

85. Mahmoud AA. Intestinal nematodes (roundworms). In: Mandell GL, Bennett JE, Dolin R, eds. Principles and Practice of Infectious Diseases, 5th ed. New York, Churchill-Livingstone, 2000:2938–2943.

86. Ferreyra NP, Cerri GG. Ascariasis of the alimentary tract, liver, pancreas and biliary system: Its diagnosis by ultrasonography. Heptogastroenterology 1998;45:932–937.

87. Goenka MK, Chowdhury A, Das K. Appendicular ascariasis: Colonoscopic management. Gastrointest Endosc 1999;50:435–436.

88. Javid G, Wani N, Gulzar GM, et al. Gallbladder ascariasis: Presentation and management. Br J Surg 1999;86:1526–1527.

89. Brooker S, Peshu N, Warn PA, et al. The epidemiology of hookworm infection and its contribution to anaemia among preschool children in the Kenya Coast. Trans R Soc Trop Med Hyg 1999;93:240–246.

90. Olsen A, Magnussen P, Ouma JH, Andreassen J, Friis H. The contribution of hookworm and other parasitic infections to haemoglobin and iron status among children and adults in Western Kenya. Trans R Soc Trop Med Hyg 1998;92:643–649.

91. Stoltzfus RJ, Chwaya HM, Tielsch JM, et al. Epidemiology of iron deficiency anemia in Zanzibari school children: The importance of hookworms. Am J Clin Nutr 1997;65:153–159.

92. De Silva NR, Guyatt HL, Bundy DA. Morbidity and mortality due to ascaris-induced intestinal obstruction. Trans R Soc Trop Med Hyg 1997;91:31–36.

93. Bundy DAP, De Silva N. Intestinal nematodes that migrate through lungs (ascariasis). In: Strickland GT, ed. Hunter's Tropical Medicine and Emerging Infectious Diseases, 8th ed. Philadelphia, Saunders, 2000:726–730.

94. Gilman RH. Intestinal nematodes that migrate through skin and lung: Strongyloides infections. In: Strickland GT, ed. Hunter's Tropical Medicine and Emerging Infectious Diseases, 8th ed. Philadelphia, Saunders, 2000:736–740.

95. Albonico M, Stoltzfus RJ, Savioli L, et al. Controlled evaluation of two school-based anthelminthic chemotherapy regimens on the intensity of intestinal helminth infections. Int J Epidemiol 1999;28:591–596.

96. Bennett A, Guyatt H. Reducing intestinal nematode infection: Efficacy of albendazole and mebendazole. Parasitol Today 2000;16:71–74.

97. de Silva NR, Sirisena JLGJ, Gunasekera DPS, et al. Effect of mebendazole therapy during pregnancy on birth outcome. Lancet 1999;353:1145–1149.

98. Goldsmith RS. Clinical pharmacology of the anthelmintic drugs. In: Katzung BG, ed. Basic and Clinical Pharmacology, 8th ed. New York, McGraw-Hill, 2001:903–922.

99. Bundy DA, Cooper E. Nematodes limited to the intestinal tract (Enterobius vermicularis, Trichuris trichiura and Capillaria philippinensis). In: Strickland GT, ed. Hunter's Tropical Medicine and Emerging Infectious Diseases, 8th ed. Philadelphia, Saunders, 2000:719–726.

100. Chosidow O. Scabies and pediculosis. Lancet 2000;355:819–826.

101. Mathieu ME, Wilson BB. Lice (pediculosis). In: Mandell GL, Bennett JR, Dolin R, eds. Principles and Practice of Infectious Diseases, 5th ed. New York, Churchill-Livingstone, 2000:2972–2974.

102. Parish LC, Witkowski JA. The saga of ectoparasitosis: Scabies and pediculosis. Int J Dermatol 1999;8:432–433.

103. Roberts RJ. Head lice. New Engl J Med 2002;346:1645–1650.

104. Mazurek CM, Lee NP. How to manage head lice. West J Med 2000;172: 342–345.

105. Yoon KS, Gao J-R, Taplin D, et al. Permethrin-resistant human head lice, Pediculus capitis, and their treatment. Arch Dermatol 2003;139:994–1000.

106. Meinking TL, Entzel P, Porcelein SL, et al. Comparative efficacy of treatments for Pediculus capitis infections. Arch Dermatol 2001;137: 287–292.

107. Meinking TL, Clineschmidt CM, Chen C, et al. An observer blinded study of 10% permethrin crème rinse with and without adjunctive combing in patients with head lice. J Pediatr 2002;141:665–670.

108. Meinking TL, Serrano L, Hard B, et al. Comparative in vitro pediculicidal efficacy of treatments in a resistant head lice population in the United States. Arch Dermatol 2002;138:220–224.

109. Jones KN, English III JC. Review of common therapeutic options in the United States for the treatment of pediculosis capitis. Clin Infect Dis 2003;36:1355–1361.

110. Wendel K, Rompalo A. Scabies and pediculosis pubis. Clin Infect Dis 2002;35(suppl 2):S146–151.

Drug	Indications	Side Effects	Comments	References
Albendazole 200 mg tablet (zentel)	Giardiasis Ascariasis Neurocysticercosis	GI: Abdominal pain, nausea, diarrhea, increase in liver function enzymes	Not recommended in children <2 years old	9, 24, 94, 96, 98
Atovaquone 250 mg *plus* Proguanil 100 mg (Malarone)[a]	Prevention and treatment of *P. falciparum* malaria	Abdominal pain, nausea, vomiting and headache		13, 23, 24, 25, 39–40
Chloroquine phosphate (Aralen, Nivaquine) 250- and 500-mg tablets; 50 mg/mL (as HCl); 5-mL ampule	Malaria	GI: Nausea, vomiting, diarrhea CNS: Dizziness, headache, blurring of vision, confusion, fatigue Derm.: Pruritus	Administer oral dose after meals IV route: Recommend ECG monitoring *Contraindication:* Patients with psoriasis or porphyria	10, 13, 15, 23, 24, 27, 28
Diloxanide furoate[b] (Furamide) 500-mg tablet	Amebiasis	GI: Nausea, flatulence Derm.: Pruritus		9, 24, 42, 44, 45, 53, 54
Furazolidone (Furoxone) 100-mg tablet Suspension: 50 mg/5 mL	Giardiasis Alternative to metronidazole	GI: Nausea, vomiting Hypersensitivity: Hypotension, fever, arthralgia, uticaria Other: Headache	Disulfiram-like reaction with alcohol; avoid in G6PD[c] deficiency; may cause hemolysis; chances color of urine to brown	9, 24, 42, 45, 53, 54
Halofantrine (Halfan) 250-mg tablet	*P. falciparum* malaria	GI: Abdominal pain, diarrhea Card.: Prolongation of QT interval	Should *not* be taken with fatty meals. *Contraindication:* Preexisting conduction defects.	23, 24, 27
Iodoquinol (Yodoxin) 210-mg tablet	Amebiasis	GI: Abdominal pain, diarrhea Derm.: Rash	May interfere with thyroid function test *Contraindication:* Patients with iodine intolerance	24, 42–45, 53, 54
Ivermectin (Stromectal) 6-mg tablet	Strongyloidiasis Pediculosis	Dizziness, somnolence, tremor, vertigo, pruritus, abdominal pain	Should be taken with a full glass of water	24, 98, 100, 101, 109, 110
Mebendazole (Vermox) 100-mg chewable tablet	Ascariasis, trichuriasis, hookworm, pinworm,	GI: Abdominal pain, diarrhea CNS: Headache, dizziness Other: Pyrexia, neutropenia	Drug should be taken with meals *Contraindication:* Pregnancy *Drug interaction:* Can increase serum levels of theophylline	9, 24, 85, 93, 98
Mefloquine (Lariam) 250-mg tablet	*P. falciparum* malaria	Incidence 17% GI: Nausea, vomiting, abdominal pain, diarrhea Card.: Sinus bradycardia CNS: vertigo, dizziness, confusion, hallucinations, psychosis, convulsions Derm.: Itching, skin rash	Patients given doses in excess of 12 mg/kg should be monitored carefully because the side effects are dose-related	10–13, 15, 23, 24, 25, 26
Metronidazole (Flagyl) Oral: 250-mg, 500-mg tablets	Amebiasis Giardiasis	GI: Nausea, anorexia, vomiting, diarrhea, abdominal cramping, glossitis, metallic taste CNS: Dizziness, vertigo, headache, paresthesias	Avoid alcohol; alcohol ingestion will cause the disulfiram reaction: abdominal distress, vomiting, hypotension *Contraindication:* First trimester of pregnancy	9, 24, 54–59

(continued)

Drug	Indications	Side Effects	Comments	References
Nifurtimox[d] (Lampit, Bayer 2502)	South American trypanosomiasis	GI: Anorexia, nausea CNS: Peripheral neuritis, psychosis Hemat: Hemolysis in G6PD[c] deficiency patients	Monitor pulmonary function and hematologic parameters	24, 74, 76
Nitazoxanide (Alinia)100 mg/5 mL suspension	Cryptosporidiosis Giardiasis	Abdominal pain, diarrhea, vomiting, and headache	Rarely may produce yellow sclerae	59, 63
Primaquine phosphate 26.3-mg tablet	Malaria (P. vivax) (P. ovale)	GI: Nausea, abdominal pain CNS: Mental depression	In G6PD deficiency can cause hemolysis	9, 10–13, 23, 24, 25
Pyrantel pamoate (Antiminth) 50-mg/mL suspension	Pinworm Hookworm	GI: Anorexia, nausea, abdominal cramps, diarrhea CNS: Headache, dizziness		9, 24, 9, 99
Pyrimethamine (Daraprim) 25-mg tablet	Malaria (see pyrimethamine-sulfadoxime)	GI: Abdominal pain, vomiting, glossitis Hemat.: Megaloblastic anemia, hemolytic anemia	Recommended that folinic acid 1–5 mg/day be concurrently administered; can cause hemolysis in patients with G6PD[c] deficiency	9, 24, 25
Pyrimethamine 25 mg plus sulfadoxime 500 mg (Fansidar)	P. falciparium–resistant malaria	For pyrimethamine, see above GI: Nausea, abdominal pain, stomatitis Hemat.: Agranulocytosis, aplastic anemia, leukopenia	Combination has been reported recently to cause the Stevens-Johnson syndrome; patients should be advised to call their physician/ pharmacist if a skin rash or other reactions are seen	9, 10–13, 23, 24, 25
Quinacrine 100 mg[e]	Giardiasis	GI: Nausea, anorexia, vomiting Headache, toxic psychosis, hepatitis, and aplastic anemia	Avoid in pregnancy, psychosis and psoriasis	9, 23, 24, 25, 56, 57
Quinidine gluconate 500 mg base/mL; 10 mL	Acute malaria	GI: Nausea, vomiting, diarrhea Card.: Hypotension, widening of QRS and QT on ECG, heart block	Administration of IV quinidine requires close monitoring; should normally monitor ECG and all vital signs	9, 12, 15, 23, 24
Quinine sulfate 325-mg and 650-mg tablets	Acute malaria	Cinchonism: Flushing, dizziness, nausea, vomiting, diarrhea (levels over 10 mcg/mL) Card.: Hypotension, widening of QRS complex Hemat.: Hemolysis, leukopenia, thrombocytopenia	When drug is administered IV, it should be administered by slow infusion (600 mg over 8 h); close monitoring of vitals and ECG *Avoid use:* IM administration	9, 23–25, 27
Sodium stibogluconate (Pentostam)[f]	Leishmaniasis	GI: Nausea, vomiting, abdominal pain, pancreatitis, increase LFTs Musculoskel: Myalgia, fatigue Card.: T-wave inversion, bradycardia Hemat.: Leukopenia, thrombocytopenia pancreatitis	Highly toxic, requires careful monitoring of vitals and ECG; caution in patients with liver or cardiac problems	24, 64, 65, 67, 68

[a]Atovaquone 62.5 mg/proguanil 25 mg (Malarone), pediatric dosage strength.

[b]Investigational drugs obtained from Ponorama Compounding Pharmacy, 6744 Balboa Blvd, Van Nuys CA 91406. (800) 247-9767.

[c]G6PD-glucose-6-phosphate dehydrogenase.

[d]Investigational drug obtained from the Centers for Disease Control and Prevention, Parasitic Disease Service, Atlanta, GA 30333. (707) 488-7760 (business hours: 8:00 A.M. to 4:30 P.M. EST), (404) 639-2888 (night, weekends, or holidays, for emergency calls only).

[e]Available from Ponorama Compounding Pharmacy.

[f]Investigational drug obtained from Centers for Disease Control.

114

URINARY TRACT INFECTIONS AND PROSTATITIS

Elizabeth A. Coyle and Randall A. Prince

Learning Objectives and other resources can be found at *www.pharmacotherapyonline.com.*

KEY CONCEPTS

◀ Urinary tract infections are classified as uncomplicated and complicated. *Uncomplicated* refers to an infection in an otherwise healthy female who lacks structural or functional abnormalities of the urinary tract. Most often complicated infections are associated with a predisposing lesion of the urinary tract; however, the term may be used to refer to all other infections, except for those in the otherwise healthy adult female.

◀ Eighty-five percent of uncomplicated urinary tract infections are caused by *Escherichia coli,* and the remainder are caused primarily by *Staphylococcus saprophyticus, Proteus* spp., and *Klebsiella* spp. Complicated infections are more frequently associated with gram-negative organisms and *Enterococcus faecalis.*

◀ Symptoms of lower urinary tract infections include dysuria, urgency, frequency, nocturia, and suprapubic heaviness, whereas upper urinary tract infections involve more systemic symptoms such as fever, nausea, vomiting, and flank pain.

◀ Significant bacteriuria traditionally has been defined as bacterial counts of greater than 100,000 (10^5)/mL of urine. Many clinicians, however, have challenged this as too general a statement. Indeed, significant bacteriuria in patients with symptoms of a urinary tract infection may be defined as greater than 10^2 organisms per milliliter.

◀ The goals of treatment of urinary tract infections are to prevent or treat systemic consequences of infections, eradicate the invading organism(s), and prevent the recurrence of infection.

◀ Uncomplicated urinary tract infections can be managed most effectively with short-course (3 days) therapy with either trimethoprim-sulfamethoxazole or a fluoroquinolone. Complicated infections require longer treatment periods (2 weeks) usually with one of these agents.

◀ In choosing appropriate antibiotic therapy, practitioners need to be cognizant of antibiotic resistance patterns, particularly to *E. coli.* Recently, trimethoprim-sulfamethoxazole has demonstrated diminished activity against *E. coli* in some areas of the country, with reported resistance up to 20%.

◀ Acute bacterial prostatitis can be managed with many agents that have activity against the causative organism. Chronic prostatitis requires an agent that is not only active against the causative organism but also concentrates in the prostatic secretions. Therapy with trimethoprim-sulfamethoxazole or a fluoroquinolone is preferred for 4 to 6 weeks.

Infections of the urinary tract represent a wide variety of syndromes, including urethritis, cystitis, prostatitis, and pyelonephritis. Urinary tract infections (UTIs) are one of the most commonly occurring bacterial infections and account for 8 million patient visits annually.[1–3] Approximately one in three females will have had a urinary tract infection by age 24.[4] Infections in men occur much less frequently until the age of 65, at which point the incidence rates in men and women are similar.

A UTI is defined as the presence of microorganisms in the urinary tract that cannot be accounted for by contamination. The organisms present have the potential to invade the tissues of the urinary tract and adjacent structures. Infection may be limited to the growth of bacteria in the urine, which frequently may not produce symptoms. A UTI can present as several syndromes associated with an inflammatory response to microbial invasion and can range from asymptomatic bacteriuria to pyelonephritis with bacteremia or sepsis.

UTIs are be classified by several methods. Typically, they have been described by anatomic site of involvement. Lower tract infections include cystitis (bladder), urethritis (urethra), prostatitis (prostate gland), and epididymitis. Pyelonephritis is an infection involving the kidneys and represents upper tract infection.

◀ Also, UTIs are designated as uncomplicated or complicated. Uncomplicated infections occur in individuals who lack structural or functional abnormalities of the urinary tract that interfere with the normal flow of urine or voiding mechanism. These infections occur in females of childbearing age (15 to 45 years) who are otherwise normal, healthy individuals. Infections in males generally are not classified as uncomplicated because these infections are rare and most often represent a structural or neurologic abnormality.

Complicated UTIs are the result of a predisposing lesion of the urinary tract, such as a congenital abnormality or distortion of the urinary tract, a stone, indwelling catheter, prostatic hypertrophy, obstruction, or neurologic deficit that interferes with the normal flow of urine and urinary tract defenses. Complicated infections occur in both genders and frequently involve the upper and lower urinary tract.

TABLE 114–1. Diagnostic Criteria for Significant Bacteriuria

$\geq 10^2$ CFU coliforms/mL or $\geq 10^5$ CFU noncoliforms/mL in a
  symptomatic female
$\geq 10^3$ CFU bacteria/mL in a symptomatic male
$\geq 10^5$ CFU bacteria/mL in asymptomatic individuals on two consecutive
  specimens
Any growth of bacteria on suprapubic catheterization in a symptomatic
  patient
$\geq 10^2$ CFU bacteria/mL in a catheterized patient

Recurrent UTIs are characterized by multiple symptomatic infections with asymptomatic periods occurring between each episode. Either reinfection or relapse causes these infections. Reinfections are caused by a different organism than originally isolated and account for the majority of recurrent UTIs. Relapse is the development of repeated infections with the same initial organism and usually indicates a persistent infectious source.

Asymptomatic bacteriuria is a common finding, particularly among those 65 years of age and older, when there is significant bacteriuria ($>10^5$ bacteria/mL of urine) in the absence of symptoms. Symptomatic abacteriuria or acute urethral syndrome consists of symptoms of frequency and dysuria in the absence of significant bacteriuria. This syndrome is commonly associated with *Chlamydia* infections.

Significant bacteriuria is a term used to distinguish the presence of microorganisms that represent true infection versus contamination of the urine as it passes through the distal urethra prior to collection. Historically, bacterial counts equal to or greater than 100,000 organisms/mL of urine in a "clean catch" specimen were judged to indicate true infection.[5] Counts of less than 100,000, however, may represent true infection in certain situations, e.g., with concurrent antibacterial drug administration, rapid urine flow, low urinary pH, or upper tract obstruction.[6] Table 114–1 lists the clinical definitions of significant bacteriuria, which are dependent on the clinical setting and the method of specimen collection.[5] These criteria allow for more appropriate specificity and sensitivity in documenting infection under differing clinical circumstances.

EPIDEMIOLOGY

The prevalence of UTIs varies with age and gender. In newborns and infants up to 6 months of age, the prevalence of bacteriuria is about 1% and is more common in boys. Most of these infections are associated with structural or functional abnormalities of the urinary tract and have been correlated with the lack of circumcision.[7] Between the ages of 1 and 5 years, UTIs occur more frequently in females. The prevalence of bacteriuria in females and males of this age group is 4.5% and 0.5%, respectively.[8] Infections occurring in preschool boys usually are associated with congenital abnormalities of the urinary tract. These infections are difficult to recognize because of the age of the patient, but they often are symptomatic. In addition, it is believed that the majority of renal damage associated with UTI develops at this age.[8]

Through grade school and before puberty, the prevalence of UTI is about 1%, with 5% of females reported to have significant bacteriuria prior to leaving high school. This percentage increases dramatically to 1% to 4% after puberty in nonpregnant females primarily as a result of sexual activity. Approximately one in five women will suffer a symptomatic UTI at some point in their lives. Many women have recurrent infections, with a significant proportion of these women having a history of childhood infections. In contrast, the prevalence of bacteriuria in adult men is very low ($<0.1\%$).[9]

In the elderly, the ratio of bacteriuria in women and men is dramatically altered and is approximately equal in persons over the age of 65.[10] The overall incidence of UTI increases substantially in this population, with the majority of infections being asymptomatic. The rate of infection increases further for elderly persons who are residing in nursing homes, particularly those who are hospitalized frequently. The increase is probably the result of a number of factors, including obstruction from prostatic hypertrophy in males, poor bladder emptying as a result of prolapse in females, fecal incontinence in demented patients, neuromuscular disease, including strokes, and increased urinary instrumentation (catheterization).

ETIOLOGY

The bacteria causing UTIs usually originate from bowel flora of the host. Although virtually every organism is associated with UTIs, certain organisms predominate as a result of specific virulence factors. The most common cause of uncomplicated UTIs is *Escherichia coli*, which accounts for 85% of community-acquired infections. Additional causative organisms in uncomplicated infections include *Staphylococcus saprophyticus* (5% to 15%), *Klebsiella pneumoniae*, *Proteus* spp., *Pseudomonas aeruginosa*, and *Enterococcus* spp. (5% to 10%). Because *S. epidermidis* is frequently isolated from the urinary tract, it should be considered initially a contaminant. Repeat cultures should be performed to help confirm the organism as a real pathogen.

Organisms isolated from individuals with complicated infections are more varied and generally are more resistant than those found in uncomplicated infections. *E. coli* is a frequently isolated pathogen, but it accounts for less than 50% of infections. Other frequently isolated organisms include *Proteus* spp., *K. pneumoniae*, *Enterobacter* spp., *P. aeruginosa*, staphylococci, and enterococci. Enterococci represent the second most frequently isolated organisms in hospitalized patients.[11] In part, this finding may be related to the extensive use of third-generation cephalosporin antibiotics, which are not active against the enterococci. Vancomycin resistant *E. faecalis* and *S. faecium* (VRE) have become more widespread, especially in patients with long-term hospitalizations or underlying malignancies. VRE is a major therapeutic and infection control issue.[11,12]

Staphylococus aureus infections may arise from the urinary tract, but they are more commonly a result of bacteremia producing metastatic abscesses in the kidney. *Candida* spp. are common causes of UTI in the critically ill and chronically catheterized patient.

Most UTIs are caused by a single organism; however, in patients with stones, indwelling urinary catheters, or chronic renal abscesses, multiple organisms may be isolated. Depending on the clinical situation, the recovery of multiple organisms may represent contamination, and a repeat evaluation should be done.

PATHOPHYSIOLOGY

ROUTE OF INFECTION

In general, organisms gain entry into the urinary tract via three possible routes: the ascending, hematogenous (descending), and lymphatic pathways. The female urethra usually is colonized by bacteria believed o originate from the fecal flora. The short length of the female urethra and its proximity to the perirectal area make colonization of the urethra likely. Other factors that promote urethral colonization include the use of spermicides and diaphragms as methods of contraception.[2,3] Although there is evidence in females that bladder infections follow colonization of the urethra, the mode of ascent of the microorganisms is not completely understood. Massage of the female urethra and sexual intercourse allow bacteria to reach the bladder.[13] Once bacteria have reached the bladder, the organisms quickly multiply and can ascend the ureters to the kidneys. This sequence of events is more likely to occur if vesicoureteral reflux (reflux of urine into the ureters and kidneys while voiding) is present. The fact that UTIs are more common in females than in males because of the anatomic differences in location and length of the urethra tends to support the ascending route of infections as the primary acquisition route.

Infection of the kidney by hematogenous spread of microorganisms usually occurs as the result of dissemination of organisms from a distant primary infection in the body. Infections via the descending route are uncommon and involve a relatively small number of invasive pathogens. Bacteremia caused by *S. aureus* may produce renal abscesses. Additional organisms include *Candida* spp., *Mycobacterium tuberculosis, Salmonella* spp., and enterococci. Of particular interest, it is difficult to produce experimental pyelonephritis by intravenously administering common gram-negative organisms such as *E. coli* and *P. aeruginosa.* Overall, less than 5% of documented UTIs result from hematogenous spread of microorganisms.

There appears to be little evidence supporting a significant role for renal lymphatics in the pathogenesis of UTIs. There are lymphatic communications between the bowel and kidney, as well as between the bladder and kidney. There is no evidence, however, that microorganisms are transferred to the kidney via this route.

After bacteria reach the urinary tract, three factors determine the development of infection: the size of the inoculum, the virulence of the microorganism, and the competency of the natural host defense mechanisms. Most UTIs reflect a failure in host defense mechanisms.

HOST DEFENSE MECHANISMS

The normal urinary tract generally is resistant to invasion by bacteria and is efficient in rapidly eliminating microorganisms that reach the bladder. The urine under normal circumstances is capable of inhibiting and killing microorganisms. The factors thought to be responsible include a low pH, extremes in osmolality, high urea concentration, and high organic acid concentration. Bacterial growth is further inhibited in males by the addition of prostatic secretions.[14,15]

The introduction of bacteria into the bladder stimulates micturition, with increased diuresis and efficient emptying of the bladder. These factors are critical in preventing the initiation and maintenance of bladder infections. Patients who are unable to void urine completely are at greater risk of developing UTIs and frequently have recurrent infections. Also, patients with even small residual amounts of urine in their bladder respond less favorably to treatment than patients who are able to empty their bladders completely.[16]

An important virulence factor of bacteria is their ability to adhere to urinary epithelial cells, resulting in colonization of the urinary tract, bladder infections, and pyelonephritis. Various factors that act as antiadherence mechanisms are present in the bladder, preventing bacterial colonization and infection. The epithelial cells of the bladder are coated with a urinary mucus or slime called *glycosaminoglycan.* This thin layer of surface mucopolysaccharide is hydrophilic and strongly negatively charged. When bound to the uroepithelium, it attracts water molecules and forms a layer between the bladder and urine. The antiadherence characteristics of the glycosaminoglycan layer are nonspecific, and when the layer is removed by dilute acid solutions, rapid bacterial adherence results.[17]

In addition, the Tamm-Horsfall protein is a glycoprotein produced by the ascending limb of Henle and distal tubule that is secreted into the urine and contains mannose residues. These mannose residues bind *E. coli* that contain small surface projecting organellae on their surfaces called *pili* or *fimbriae.* Type 1 fimbriae are mannose-sensitive, and this interaction prevents the bacteria from binding to similar receptors present on the mucosal surface of the bladder. Other factors that possibly prevent adherence of bacteria include immunoglobulins (Ig) G and A. Investigators have documented both systemic and local kidney Ig synthesis in upper tract infections. The role of Igs in preventing bladder infection is less clear. Patients with reduced urinary levels of secretory IgA are, however, at increased risk of infections of the urinary tract.[14]

After bacteria actually have invaded the bladder mucosa, an inflammatory response is stimulated with the mobilization of polymorphonuclear leukocytes (PMNs) and resulting phagocytosis. PMNs are primarily responsible for limiting the tissue invasion and controlling the spread of infection in the bladder and kidney. They do not play a role in preventing bladder colonization or infections and actually contribute to renal tissue damage.

Other host factors that may play a role in the prevention of UTIs are the presence of *Lactobacillus* in the vaginal flora and circulating estrogen levels. In premenopausal women, circulating estrogen supports the vaginal tract growth of lactobacilli, which produce lactic acid to help maintain a low vaginal pH, thereby preventing *E. coli* vaginal colonization. Spermicide use, β-lactam antimicrobials use, lower estrogen levels, intercourse with a new partner, and douching can lead to decreases in lactobacilli colonization.[18,19]

BACTERIAL VIRULENCE FACTORS

Pathogenic organisms have differing degrees of pathogenicity (virulence), which play a role in the development and severity of infection. Bacteria that adhere to the epithelium of the urinary tract are associated with colonization and infection. The mechanism of adhesion of gram-negative bacteria, particularly *E. coli,* is related to bacterial fimbriae that are rigid hairlike appendages of the cell wall.[20] These fimbriae adhere to specific glycolipid components on epithelial cells. The most common type of fimbriae is type 1, which binds to mannose residues present in glycoproteins. Glycosaminoglycan and Tamm-Horsfall protein are rich in mannose residues that readily trap those organisms which contain type 1 fimbriae, which are then washed out of the bladder.[21] Other fimbriae are mannose-resistant and are associated more frequently with pyelonephritis, such as P fimbriae, which bind avidly to specific glycolipid receptors on uroepithelial cells. These bacteria are resistant to washout or removal by glycosaminoglycan and are able to multiply and invade tissue, especially the kidney. In addition, PMNs, as well as secretory IgA antibodies, contain receptors for type 1 fimbriae, which facilitates phagocytosis, but they lack receptors for P fimbriae.

Other virulence factors include the production of hemolysin and aerobactin.[20] Hemolysin is a cytotoxic protein produced by bacteria that lyses a wide range of cells, including erythrocytes, PMNs, and monocytes. *E. coli* and other gram-negative bacteria require iron for aerobic metabolism and multiplication. Aerobactin facilitates the binding and uptake of iron by *E. coli;* however, the significance of this property in the pathogenesis of UTIs remains unknown.

PREDISPOSING FACTORS TO INFECTION

The normal urinary tract typically is resistant to infection and colonization by pathogenic bacteria. In patients with underlying structural abnormalities of the urinary tract, the typical host defenses previously discussed usually are lacking. There are several known abnormalities of the urinary tract system that interfere with its natural defense mechanisms, the most important of which is obstruction. Obstruction can inhibit the normal flow of urine, disrupting the natural flushing and voiding effect in removing bacteria from the bladder and resulting in incomplete emptying. Common conditions that result in residual urine volumes include prostatic hypertrophy, urethral strictures, calculi, tumors, bladder diverticula, and drugs such as anticholinergic agents. Additional causes of incomplete bladder emptying include neurologic malfunctions associated with stroke, diabetes, spinal cord injuries, tabes dorsalis, and other neuropathies.

Vesicoureteral reflux represents a condition in which urine is forced up the ureters to the kidneys. Urinary reflux is associated not only with an increased incidence of UTIs and pyelonephritis but also with renal damage.[22] Reflux may be the result of a congenital abnormality or, more commonly, bladder overdistension from obstruction.

Other risk factors include urinary catheterization, mechanical instrumentation, pregnancy, and the use of spermicides and diaphragms.

CLINICAL PRESENTATION

The presenting signs and symptoms of UTIs in adults are recognized easily (Table 114–2). Women frequently will report gross hematuria. Systemic symptoms, including fever, typically are absent in this setting. Unfortunately, large numbers of patients with significant bacteriuria are asymptomatic. These patients may be normal, healthy patients, elderly patients, children, pregnant patients, and patients with indwelling catheters. It is important to note that attempts at differentiating upper tract from lower tract infections on the basis of symptoms alone are not reliable.

Elderly patients frequently do not experience specific urinary symptoms, but they will present with altered mental status, change in eating habits, or gastrointestinal symptoms. In addition, patients with indwelling catheters or neurologic disorders commonly will not have lower tract symptoms, whereas flank pain and fever may be recognized. Many of the aforementioned patients, however, frequently will develop upper tract infections with bacteremia and no or minimal urinary tract symptoms.

Symptoms alone are unreliable for the diagnosis of bacterial UTIs. The key to the diagnosis of UTI is the ability to demonstrate

TABLE 114–2. Clinical Presentation of Urinary Tract Infections in Adults

Signs and Symptoms
Lower UTI: Dysuria, urgency, frequency, nocturia, suprapubic heaviness
Gross hematuria
Upper UTI: Flank pain, fever, nausea, vomiting, malaise
Physical Examination
Upper UTI: Costovertebral tenderness
Laboratory Tests
Bacteriuria
Pyuria (white blood cell count >10/mm³)
Nitrite-positive urine (with nitrite reducers)
Leukocyte esterase–positive urine
Antibody-coated bacteria (upper UTI)

significant numbers of microorganisms in an appropriate urine specimen to distinguish contamination from infection. The type and extent of laboratory examination required depend on the clinical situation.

URINE COLLECTION

Examination of the urine is the cornerstone of laboratory evaluation for UTIs. There are three acceptable methods of urine collection. The first is the *midstream clean-catch method.* After cleaning the urethral opening area in both men and women, 20 to 30 mL of urine is voided and discarded. The next part of the urine flow is collected and should be processed immediately (refrigerated as soon as possible). Specimens that are allowed to sit at room temperature for several hours may result in falsely elevated bacterial counts. The midstream clean catch is the preferred method for the routine collection of urine for culture. When a routine urine specimen cannot be collected or contamination occurs, alternative collection techniques must be used.

The two acceptable alternative methods include catheterization and suprapubic bladder aspiration. Catheterization may be necessary for patients who are uncooperative or who are unable to void urine. If catheterization is performed carefully with aseptic technique, the method yields reliable results. Note, however, that introduction of bacteria into the bladder may result, and the procedure is associated with infection in 1% to 2% of patients. Suprapubic bladder aspiration involves inserting a needle directly into the bladder and aspirating the urine. This procedure bypasses the contaminating organisms present in the urethra, and any bacteria found using this technique generally are considered to represent significant bacteriuria. Suprapubic aspiration is a safe and painless procedure that is most useful in newborns, infants, paraplegics, seriously ill patients, and others in whom infection is suspected and routine procedures have provided confusing or equivocal results.

BACTERIAL COUNT

The diagnosis of UTI is based on the isolation of significant numbers of bacteria from a urine specimen. Microscopic examination of a urine sample is an easy-to-perform and reliable method for the presumptive diagnosis of bacteriuria. The examination may be performed by preparing a Gram stain of unspun or centrifuged urine. The presence of at least one organism per oil-immersion field in a properly collected uncentrifuged specimen correlates well with more than 100,000 bacteria/mL of urine. For detecting smaller numbers of organisms, a centrifuged specimen is more sensitive. Such examinations detect more than 10^5 bacteria/mL with a sensitivity of greater than 90% and a specificity of greater than 70%.[23] Counts of less than 30,000/mL, however, usually are not recognized reliably by these methods.[24]

PYURIA, HEMATURIA, AND PROTEINURIA

Microscopic examination of the urine for leukocytes is also used to determine the presence of pyuria. The presence of pyuria in a symptomatic patient correlates with significant bacteriuria.[25] Pyuria is defined as a white blood cell (WBC) count of greater than 10 WBCs/mm³ of urine. A count of 5 to 10 WBCs/mm³ is accepted as the upper limit of normal. It should be emphasized that pyuria is nonspecific and signifies only the presence of inflammation and not necessarily infection. Thus patients with pyuria may or may not have infection. Sterile pyuria has long been associated with urinary tuberculosis, as well as chlamydial and fungal urinary infections.

Hematuria, microscopic or gross, is frequently present in patients with UTI but is nonspecific. Hematuria may indicate the presence of other disorders, such as renal calculi, tumors, or glomerulonephritis. Proteinuria is found commonly in the presence of infection.

CHEMISTRY

Several biochemical tests have been developed for screening urine for the presence of bacteria. A common dipstick test detects the presence of nitrite in the urine, which is formed by bacteria that reduce nitrate normally present in the urine. False-positive tests are uncommon. False-negative tests are more common and frequently are caused by the presence of gram-positive organisms or *P. aeruginosa* that do not reduce nitrate.[26] Other causes of false tests include low urinary pH, frequent voiding, and dilute urine.

The leukocyte esterase (LE) dipstick test is a rapid screening test for detecting the presence of pyuria. Leukocytes esterase is found in primary neutrophil granules and indicates the presence of WBCs. The LE test is a sensitive and highly specific test for detecting more than 10 WBCs/mm^3 of urine. When the LE test is used with the nitrite test, the range of reported sensitivity and specificity is 45.5% to 100% and 60% to 98%, respectively, for the detection of bacteriuria.[27,28] These tests can be useful in the outpatient evaluation of uncomplicated UTIs. However, urine culture is still the "gold standard" test in determining the presence of UTIs.

CULTURE

The most reliable method of diagnosing UTI is by quantitative urine culture. Urine in the bladder is normally sterile, making it statistically possible to differentiate contamination of the urine from infection by quantifying the number of bacteria present in a urine sample. This criterion is based on a properly collected midstream clean-catch urine specimen. Patients with infection usually have greater than 10^5 bacteria/mL of urine. It should be emphasized that as many as one-third of women with symptomatic infection have less than 10^5 bacteria/mL. A significant portion of patients with UTIs, either symptomatic or asymptomatic, also have less than 10^5 bacteria/mL of urine.

Several laboratory methods are used to quantify bacteria present in the urine. The most accurate method is the pour-plate technique. This method is unsuitable for a high-volume laboratory because it is expensive and time-consuming. The streak-plate method is an alternative that involves using a calibrated-loop technique to streak a fixed amount of urine on an agar plate. This method is used most commonly in diagnostic laboratories because it is simple to perform and less costly.

After identification and quantification are complete, the next step is to determine the susceptibility of the organism. There are several methods by which bacterial susceptibility testing may be performed. Knowledge of bacterial susceptibility and achievable urine concentration of the antibiotics puts the clinician in a better position to select an appropriate agent for treatment.

INFECTION SITE

Several methods have been evaluated to determine the location of infection within the urinary system and differentiate upper tract from lower tract involvement. The most direct method is a ureteral catheterization procedure, as described by Stamey and colleagues.[29] The method involves the passage of a catheter into the bladder and then into each ureter, where quantitative cultures are obtained. History and physical examination were of little value in predicting the site of infection. Although this method provides direct quantitative evidence for UTI, it is invasive, technically difficult, and expensive. The Fairley bladder washout technique is a modification of the Stamey procedure that involves Foley catheterization only.[30] After the catheter is passed into the bladder, bladder samples are obtained, and the bladder is washed out, with culture samples taken at 10, 20, and 30 minutes. The procedure shows that up to 50% of patients have renal involvement regardless of signs and symptoms. Other investigators found 10% to 20% of tests to be equivocal.[31]

Noninvasive methods of localization may be more acceptable for routine use; however, they have limited clinical value. Patients with pyelonephritis can have abnormalities in urinary concentrating ability. The use of concentrating ability for localization of UTIs, however, is associated with high false-positive and false-negative responses and is not useful clinically.[26] The antibody-coated bacteria (ACB) test is an immunofluorescent method that detects bacteria coated with Ig in freshly voided urine, indicating upper urinary tract infection. The sensitivity and specificity of this test to localize the site of infection are reported to average 88% and 76%, respectively.[31] Because of the high incidence of false-positive and false-negative results, ACB testing is not used routinely in the management of UTIs.

Virtually all patients with uncomplicated lower tract infections can be cured with a short course of antibiotic therapy, and this assumption sometimes can be used to distinguish patients with lower and upper tract infections. Patients who do not respond or who relapse do so because of upper tract involvement. It is rarely necessary to localize the site of infection to direct the clinical management of such patients.

▶ TREATMENT: Urinary Tract Infections

■ DESIRED OUTCOME

5 The goals of UTI treatments are (1) to prevent or to treat systemic consequences of infection, (2) to eradicate the invading organism(s), and (3) to prevent the recurrence of infection.

■ MANAGEMENT

The management of a patient with a UTI includes initial evaluation, selection of an antibacterial agent and duration of therapy, and follow-up evaluation. The initial selection of an antimicrobial agent for the treatment of UTI is based primarily on the severity of the presenting signs and symptoms, the site of infection, and whether the infection is determined to be uncomplicated or complicated. Other considerations include antibiotic susceptibility, side-effect potential, cost, and the comparative inconvenience of different therapies.

Various pharmacologic factors may affect the action of antibacterial agents. Certainly the ability of the agent to achieve appropriate concentrations in the urine is of utmost importance. Factors that affect the rate and extent of excretion through the kidney include the patient's glomerular filtration rate and whether or not the agent is actively secreted. Filtration depends on the molecular size and degree of protein binding of the agent. Agents such as sulfonamides, tetracyclines, and aminoglycosides enter the urine via filtration. As the glomerular filtration rate is reduced, the amount of drug that enters the urine is reduced.

Most β-lactam agents and quinolones are filtered and are actively secreted into the urine. For this reason, these agents achieve high urinary concentrations despite unfavorable protein-binding characteristics or the presence of renal dysfunction.

The ability to eradicate bacteria from the urine is related directly to the sensitivity of the microorganism and the achievable concentrations of the antimicrobial agent in the urine. Unfortunately, most susceptibility testing is directed at achievable concentrations in the blood. There is a poor correlation between achievable blood levels of antimicrobial agents and the eradication of bacteria from the urine.[32] In the treatment of lower tract infections, plasma concentrations of antibacterial agents may not be important, but achieving appropriate plasma concentrations appears critical in patients with bacteremia and renal abscesses.

A number of nonspecific therapies have been advocated in the treatment and prevention of UTIs. Fluid hydration has been used to produce rapid dilution of bacteria and removal of infected urine by increased voiding. A critical factor appears to be the amount of residual volume remaining after voiding. As little as 10 mL of residual urine can alter the eradication of infection significantly.[16] Paradoxically, increased diuresis also may promote susceptibility to infection by diluting the normal antibacterial properties of the urine. Often in clinical practice the concentrations of antimicrobial agents in the urine are so high that dilution has little effect on efficacy.

The antibacterial activity of the urine is related to the low pH, which is the result of high concentrations of various organic acids. Large volumes of cranberry juice increase the antibacterial activity of the urine and prevent the development of UTIs.[2,23] Apparently, the cranberry juice content of fructose and other unknown substances (condensed tannins) acts to interfere with adherence mechanisms of some pathogens, thereby preventing infection. Acidification of the urine by cranberry juice does not appear to play a significant role. The use of other agents (ascorbic acid) to acidify the urine to hinder bacterial growth does not achieve significant acidification. Therefore, attempts to acidify urine with systemic agents are not recommended. *Lactobacillus* probiotics also may aid in the prevention of female UTIs by the vaginal pH, thereby decreasing *E. coli* colonization.[19] In postmenopausal women, estrogen replacement may be of help in the prevention of recurrent UTIs. After 1 month of topical estrogen replacement, decreases in vaginal *Lactobacillus*, as well as decreases in and pH and *E. coli* colonization, have been found.[18]

Urinary analgesics such as phenazopyridine hydrochloride are used frequently by many clinicians.[2] If the pain or dysuria present in a UTI is a consequence of infection, then urinary analgesics have little clinical role because most patients' symptoms respond quite rapidly to appropriate antibacterial therapy. Urinary analgesics also may mask signs and symptoms of UTIs not responding to antimicrobial therapy.

PHARMACOLOGIC THERAPY

Ideally, the antimicrobial agent chosen should be well tolerated, well absorbed, achieve high urinary concentrations, and have a spectrum of activity limited to the known or suspected pathogen(s). Table 114–3 lists the most common agents used in the treatment of UTIs along with comments concerning their general use. Table 114–4 presents an overview of various therapeutic options for outpatient therapy of UTI. Table 114–5 describes empirical treatment regimens for selected clinical situations.

The therapeutic management of UTIs is best accomplished by first categorizing the type of infection: acute uncomplicated cysti-

tis, symptomatic bacteriuria, asymptomatic bacteriuria, complicated UTIs, recurrent infections, or prostatitis. In choosing the appropriate antibiotic therapy, it is important to be aware of the increasing resistance of *E. coli* and other pathogens to many antimicrobials. Resistance to *E. coli* is as high as 30% for amoxicillin and cephalosporins.[34,35] Overall, trimethoprim-sulfamethoxazole remains susceptible, although resistance as high as 22% has been reported in various places.[35–39] However, resistant infections still may be treated successfully with trimethoprim-sulfamethoxazole, most likely owing to its high urinary concentrations. Current or recent antibiotic exposure is the most significant risk factor associated with *E. coli* resistance.[36–38] Antibiotic therapy should be determined based on the geographic resistance patterns of the prescriber, as well as the patient's recent history of antibiotic exposure.

ACUTE UNCOMPLICATED CYSTITIS

Acute uncomplicated cystitis is the most common form of UTI. These infections typically occur in women of childbearing age and often are related to sexual activity. Although the presence of dysuria, frequency, urgency, and suprapubic discomfort frequently is associated with lower tract infection, a significant number of patients have upper tract involvement as well.[40] Because these infections are predominantly caused by *E. coli*, antimicrobial therapy initially should be directed against this organism. Other common causes include *S. saprophyticus* and, occasionally, *K. pneumoniae* and *Proteus mirabilis*. Because the causative organisms and their susceptibility generally are known, many clinicians advocate a cost-effective approach to management. This approach includes a urinalysis and initiation of empirical therapy without a urine culture[40] (Fig. 114–1).

The goal of treatment for uncomplicated cystitis is to eradicate the causative organism and to reduce the incidence of recurrence caused by relapse or reinfection. The ability to reduce the chance of recurrence depends on the agent's efficacy in eradicating the uropathogenic bacteria from the vaginal and gastrointestinal reservoir. In the past, conventional therapy consisted of an effective oral antibiotic administered for 7 to 14 days. It is now apparent, however, that acute cystitis is a superficial mucosal infection that can be eradicated with much shorter courses of therapy. Advantages of short-course therapy include increased compliance, fewer side effects, decreased cost, and less potential for the development of resistance.

CLINICAL CONTROVERSY

Single-dose therapy is used frequently, although it can be associated with lower cure rates and increased reoccurrence compared with longer therapies.[1,32,44] Clinicians should not assume that all antimicrobial agents are effective as single-dose therapies. Data suggest that trimethoprim-sulfamethoxazole or the fluoroquinolones are most efficacious as single-dose therapies. Fosfomycin once daily also has been used, although other therapies appear superior.[1,45] The efficacy of these agents probably is related to observations that *E. coli* causing community-acquired UTIs are increasingly resistant to ampicillin, amoxicillin, and sulfonamides. In addition, oral β-lactam antibiotics are eliminated more rapidly and do not achieve high renal tissue concentrations compared with trimethoprim-sulfamethoxazole and are less successful in eradicating uropathogens from the vaginal and gastrointestinal reservoirs.

TABLE 114–3. Commonly Used Antimicrobial Agents in the Treatment of Urinary Tract Infections

Agent	Comments
Oral Therapy	
Sulfonamides	These agents generally have been replaced by more agents due to resistance.
Trimethoprim-sulfamethoxazole (TMP-SMX)	This combination is highly effective against most aerobic enteric bacteria except *Pseudomonas aeruginosa*. High urinary tract tissue levels and urine levels are achieved, which may be important in complicated infection treatment. Also effective as prophylaxis for recurrent infections.
Penicillins	
Ampicillin	Ampicillin is the standard penicillin that has broad-spectrum activity. Increasing *Escherichia coli* resistance
Amoxicillin–clavulanic acid	has limited amoxicillin use in acute cystitis. Drug of choice for enterococci sensitive to penicillin.
Carbenicillin indanyl	Amoxicillin-clavulanate is preferred for resistance problems. Carbenicillin indanyl is only indicated for the treatment of urinary tract infections.
Cephalosporins	There are no major advantages of these agents over other agents in the treatment of UTIs, and they are
Cephalexin	more expensive. They may be useful in cases of resistance to amoxicillin and
Cephradine	trimethoprim-sulfamethoxazole. These agents are not active against enterococci.
Cefaclor	
Cefadroxil	
Cefuroxime	
Cefixime	
Cefzil	
Cefpodoxime	
Tetracyclines	These agents have been effective for initial episodes of urinary tract infections; however, resistance
Tetracycline	develops rapidly, and their use is limited. These agents also lead to candidal overgrowth. They are useful
Doxycycline	primarily for chlamydial infections.
Minocycline	
Fluoroquinolones	The newer quinolones have a greater spectrum of activity, including *P. aeruginosa*. These agents are
Ciprofloxacin	effective for pyelonephritis and prostatitis. Avoid in pregnancy and children. Moxifloxacin should not be
Norfloxacin	used owing to inadequate urinary concentrations.
Levofloxacin	
Nitrofurantoin	This agent is effective as both a therapeutic and prophylactic agent in patients with recurrent UTIs. Main advantage is the lack of resistance even after long courses of therapy. Adverse effects may limit use (GI intolerance, neuropathies, pulmonary reactions).
Azithromycin	Single-dose therapy for chlamydial infections.
Methanamine hippurate–mandalate	These agents are reserved for prophylactic therapy or suppressive use between episodes of infection.
Fosfomycin	Single-dose therapy for uncomplicated infections.
Parenteral Therapy	
Aminoglycosides	Gentamicin and tobramycin are equally effective; gentamicin is less expensive. Tobramycin has better
Gentamicin	pseudomonal activity, which may be important in serious systemic infections. Amikacin generally is
Tobramycin	reserved for multiresistant bacteria.
Amikacin	
Netilmicin	
Penicillins	These agents generally are equally effective for susceptible bacteria. The extended-spectrum penicillins are
Ampicillin	more active against *P. aeruginosa* and enterococci and often are preferred over cephalosporins. They are
Ampicillin-sulbactam	very useful in renally impaired patients or when an aminoglycoside is to be avoided.
Ticarcillin-clavulanate	
Piperacillin	
Piperacillin-tazobactam	
Cephalosporins, first-, second-, and third-generation	Second- and third-generation cephalosporins have a broad spectrum of activity against gram-negative bacteria but are not active against enterococci and have limited activity against *P. aeruginosa*. Ceftazidime and cefepime are active against *P. aeruginosa*. They are useful for nosocomial infections and urosepsis due to susceptible pathogens.
Carbapenems	These agents have broad spectrum of activity, including gram-positive, gram-negative, and anaerobic
Imipenem-cilastatin	bacteria.
Meropenem	Imipenem and meropenem are active against *P. aeruginosa* and enterococci, but ertapenem is not. All may
Ertapenem	be associated with candidal superinfections.
Aztreonam	A monobactam that is only active against gram-negative bacteria, including some strains of *P. aeruginosa*. Generally useful for nosocomial infections when aminoglycosides are to be avoided and in penicillin-sensitive patients.
Quinolones	These agents have broad-spectrum activity against both gram-negative and gram-positive bacteria. They
Ciprofloxacin	provide urine and high-tissue concentrations and are actively secreted in reduced renal function.
Levofloxacin	
Gatifloxacin	

TABLE 114–4. Overview of Outpatient Antimicrobial Therapy for Lower Tract Infections in Adults

Indications	Antibiotic	Dose[a]	Interval	Duration
Lower tract Infections		2 DS tablets	Single dose	1 day
Uncomplicated	Trimethoprim-sulfamethoxazole	1 DS tablet	Twice a day	3 days
	Ciprofloxacin	250 mg	Twice a day	3 days
	Norfloxacin	400 mg	Twice a day	3 days
	Gatifloxacin	200–400 mg	Once a day	3 days
	Levofloxacin	250 mg	Once a day	3 days
	Lomefloxacin	400 mg	Once a day	3 days
	Enoxacin	200 mg	Once a day	3 days
	Amoxicillin	6 × 500 mg	Single dose	1 day
		500 mg	Twice a day	3 days
	Amoxicillin-clavulanate	500 mg	Every 8 hours	3 days
	Trimethoprim	100 mg	Twice a day	3 days
	Nitrofurantoin	100 mg	Every 6 hours	3 days
	Fosfomycin	3 g	Single dose	1 day
Complicated	Trimethoprim-sulfamethoxazole	1 DS tablet	Twice a day	7–10 days
	Trimethoprim	100 mg	Twice a day	7–10 days
	Norfloxacin	400 mg	Twice a day	7–10 days
	Ciprofloxacin	250–500 mg	Twice a day	7–10 days
	Gatifloxacin	400 mg	Once a day	7–10 days
	Moxifloxacin (PO only)	400 mg	Once a day	7–10 days
	Lomefloxacin	400 mg	Once a day	7–10 days
	Levofloxacin	250 mg	Once a day	7–10 days
	Amoxicillin-clavulanate	500 mg	Every 8 hours	7–10 days
Recurrent Infections	Nitrofurantion	50 mg	Once a day	6 months
	Trimethoprim	100 mg	Once a day	6 months
	Trimethoprim-sulfamethoxazole	1/2 ss tablet	Once a day	6 months
Acute urethral syndrome	Trimethoprim-sulfamethoxazole	1 DS	Twice a day	3 days
Failure of TMP-SMX	Azithromycin	1 g	Single dose	
	Doxycycline	100 mg	Twice a day	7 days
Acute pyelonephritis	Trimethoprim-sulfamethoxazole	1 DS tablet	Twice a day	14 days
	Ciprofloxacin	500 mg	Twice a day	14 days
	Gatifloxacin	400 mg	Once a day	14 days
	Norfloxacin	400 mg	Twice a day	14 days
	Levofloxacin	250 mg	Once a day	14 days
	Lomefloxacin	400 mg	Once a day	14 days
	Enoxacin	400 mg	Twice a day	14 days
	Amoxicillin-clavulanate	500 mg	Every 8 hours	14 days

[a]Dosing intervals for normal renal function.

[6] Three-day courses of trimethoprim-sulfamethoxazole or a fluoroquinolone (e.g., ciprofloxacin, levofloxacin, norfloxacin, or gatifloxacin) are superior to single-dose therapies.[41,42] The fluoroquinolone moxifloxacin is not recommended for use in UTIs owing to the inadequate urinary concentrations.[43] The use of amoxicillin and sulfonamides is not recommended because of the high incidence of resistant *E. coli*. For most adult females, short-course therapy is the treatment of choice for uncomplicated lower UTIs. Short-course therapy is inappropriate for patients who have had previous infections caused by resistant bacteria, for male patients, and for patients with complicated UTIs. If symptoms do not respond or recur, a urine culture should be obtained and conventional therapy with a suitable agent instituted.[1,3,46–48]

SYMPTOMATIC ABACTERIURIA

Symptomatic abacteriuria or acute urethral syndrome represents a clinical syndrome in which females present with dysuria and pyuria, but the urine culture reveals less than 10⁵ bacteria/mL of urine. Acute urethral syndrome is estimated to account for more than half the complaints of dysuria seen in the community today. These women most likely are infected with small numbers of coliform bacteria, including *E. coli*, *Staphylococcus* spp., or *Chlamydia trachomatis*. Additional causes include *Neisseria gonorrhoeae*, *Gardnerella vaginalis*, and *Ureaplasma urealyticum*.

Most patients presenting with pyuria will, in fact, have infection that requires treatment. Single-dose or short-course therapy with trimethoprim-sulfamethoxazole has been used effectively, and prolonged courses of therapy are not necessary for most patients. If single-dose or short-course therapy is ineffective, a culture should be obtained. If the patient reports recent sexual activity, therapy for *C. trachomatis* should be considered. Chlamydial treatment should consist of 1-g azithromycin or doxycycline 100 mg twice daily for 7 days. Often, concomitant treatment of all sexual partners is required to cure chlamydial infections and prevent reacquisition (see Chap. 115).

ASYMPTOMATIC BACTERIURIA

Asymptomatic bacteriuria represents patients who, in the absence of urinary symptoms, are found to have two consecutive urine cultures

TABLE 114–5. Empirical Treatment of Urinary Tract Infections and Prostatitis

Diagnosis	Pathogens	Treatment	Comments
Acute uncomplicated cystitis	E. coli S. saprophyticus	1. Trimethoprim-sulfamethoxazole × 3 days 2. Quinolone × 3 days	Short-course therapy more effective than single dose
Pregnancy	As above	1. Amoxicillin-clavulanate × 7 days 2. Cephalosporin × 7 days 3. Trimethoprim-sulfamethoxazole × 7 days	Avoid trimethoprim-sulfamethoxazole during third trimester
Acute pyelonephritis Uncomplicated	E. coli	1. Trimethoprim-sulfamethoxazole × 14 days 2. Quinolone × 14 days	Can be managed as outpatient
Complicated	E. coli Proteus mirabilis K. pneumoniae Pseudomonas aeruginosa E. fecalis	1. Quinolone × 14 days 2. Extended-spectrum penicillin Plus aminoglycoside	Severity of illness will determine duration of IV therapy. Culture results should direct therapy Oral therapy may complete 14 days of therapy
Prostatitis	E. coli K. pneumoniae Proteus spp P. aeruginosa	1. Trimethoprim-sulfamethoxazole × 4–6 weeks 2. Quinolone × 4–6 weeks	Acute prostatitis may require IV therapy initially Chronic prostatitis may require longer treatment periods or surgery

with more than 10^5 organisms/mL of the same organism. Most patients with asymptomatic bacteriuria are elderly and female. Pregnant women are another group of patients that frequently presents with asymptomatic bacteriuria. Although this group of patients typically responds to treatment, relapse and reinfection are very common, and chronic asymptomatic bacteriuria is difficult to eradicate.

The management of asymptomatic bacteriuria depends on the age of the patient and whether or not the patient is pregnant. In children, because of a greater risk of developing renal scarring and long-standing renal damage, treatment should consist of conventional courses of therapy as that for symptomatic infection. The greatest risk of renal damage occurs during the first 5 years of life.[49] In the nonpregnant female, therapy is controversial; however, treatment has little effect on the natural course of infections. Two groups characterize asymptomatic bacteriuria in the elderly: those with persistent bacteriuria and those with intermittent bacteriuria.

CLINICAL CONTROVERSY

Most clinicians feel that asymptomatic bacteriuria in the elderly is a benign disease that does not warrant treatment. Most data indicate that the patient without urinary tract obstruction is not destined to develop progressive renal damage. Investigators who have demonstrated an association between bacteriuria and decreased survival, however, have questioned this approach. In this setting, there is no apparent urgency in initiating therapy, so two cultures should be obtained to confirm the presence of bacteriuria. Treating ambulatory, nonhospitalized elderly women is effective in eliminating bacteria for at least 6 months and may protect against the development of symptomatic bacteriuria; however, only 50% of patients remained free of bacteria after 1 year.[50]

Several studies in hospitalized elderly subjects, however, have not found antimicrobial therapy to be efficacious.[51,52] A number of questions remain unanswered, e.g., the effect of eradication of bacteri-

uria on life expectancy, the cost-effectiveness and risk-benefit ratio of therapy, and the effect on morbidity. Certainly, with the information available and the high adverse reaction rate in the elderly, vigorous treatment and screening programs cannot be advocated.

◼ COMPLICATED URINARY TRACT INFECTIONS

◼ Acute Pyelonephritis

The presentation of high-grade fever ($>38.3°$C, or $100.9°$F) and severe flank pain should be treated as acute pyelonephritis, warranting aggressive management. Severely ill patients with pyelonephritis should be hospitalized and intravenous antimicrobials administered initially (Table 114–5). However, milder cases may be managed with orally administered antibiotics in an outpatient setting. Symptoms of nausea, vomiting, and dehydration may require hospitalization.

At the time of presentation, a Gram stain of the urine should be performed, along with a urinalysis, culture, and sensitivity tests. The Gram stain should indicate the morphology of the infecting organism(s) and help to direct the selection of an appropriate antibiotic. However, the precise identity and susceptibility of the infecting organism(s) will be unknown initially, warranting empirical therapy. The goals of treatment include the achievement of therapeutic concentrations of an antimicrobial agent in the bloodstream and urinary tract to which the invading organism is susceptible and sufficient therapy to eradicate residual infection in the tissues of the urinary tract.

In the mildly to moderately symptomatic patient in whom oral therapy is considered, an effective agent should be administered for at least a 2-week period, although use of highly active agents for 7 to 10 days may be sufficient.[1,53] Oral antibiotics that are highly active against the probable pathogens and that are sufficiently bioavailable are preferred. Although the sulfonamides and ampicillin or amoxicillin have been the primary choices for the treatment of gram-negative bacillary infections, they are no longer considered reliable agents for UTIs.[32] Reports of increasing resistance to E. coli have tempered their

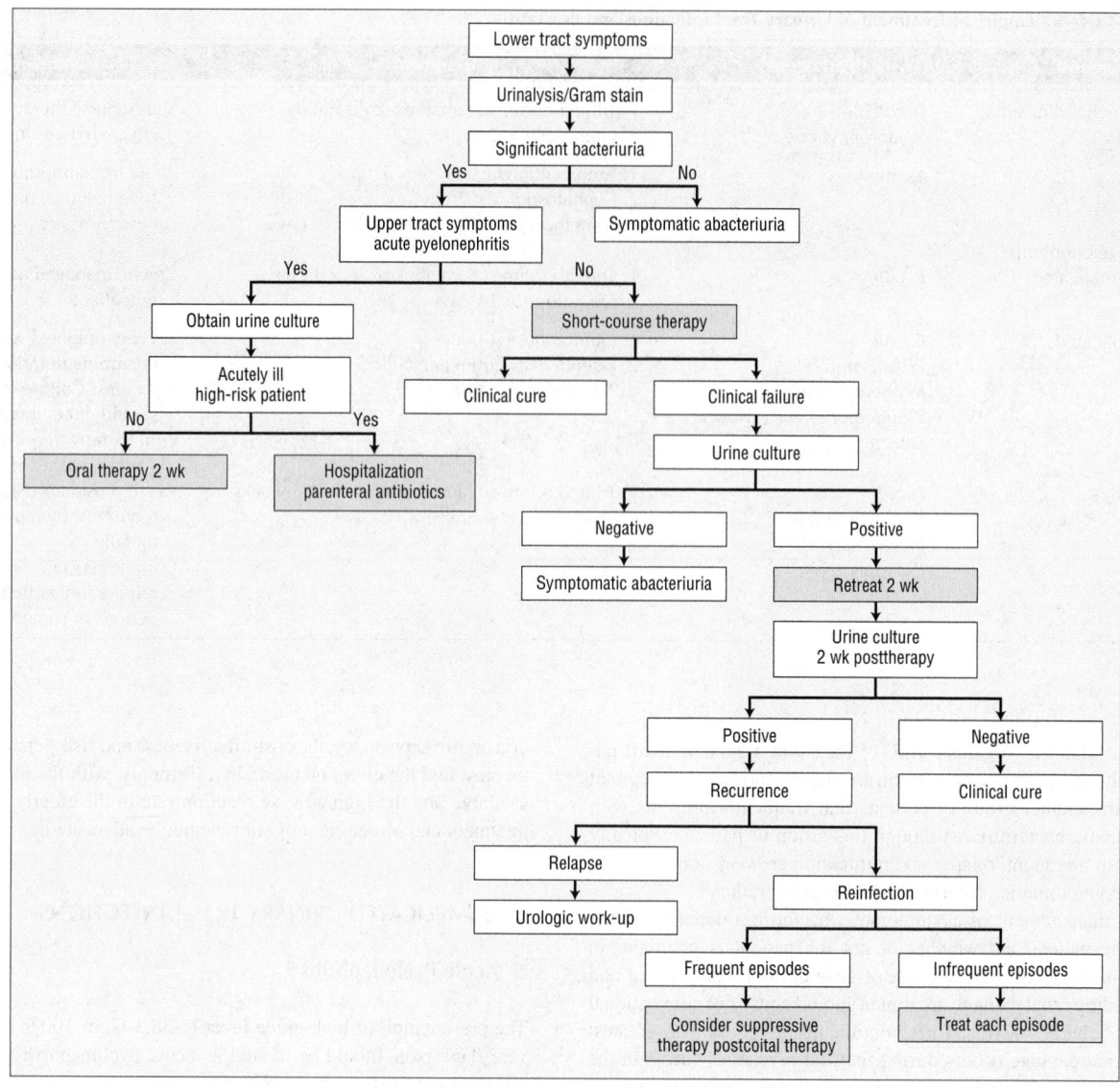

FIGURE 114–1. Management of UTIs in females.

use. In addition, treatment with trimethoprim-sulfamethoxazole (one double-strength tablet twice daily) for 2 weeks was superior to ampicillin, despite the organism being susceptible to both agents.[54] Agents such as trimethoprim-sulfamethoxazole and the fluoroquinolones are the agents of choice. If a Gram stain reveals gram-positive cocci, *S. faecalis* should be considered and treatment directed against this potential pathogen (ampicillin). Close follow-up of outpatient treatment is mandatory to ensure success.

In the seriously ill patient, parenteral therapy should be administered initially. Therapy should provide a broad spectrum of coverage and should be directed toward bacteremia or sepsis, if present. A number of antibiotic regimens have been used as empirical therapy, including an intravenous fluoroquinolone, an aminoglycoside with or without ampicillin, and extended-spectrum cephalosporins with or without an aminoglycoside.[1] Other options include aztreonam, the β-lactamase inhibitor combinations (e.g., ampicillin-sulbactam, ticarcillin-clavulanate, and piperacillin-tazobactam), carbapenems (e.g., imipenem, meropenem, or ertapenem), or intravenous trimethoprim-sulfamethoxazole. If the patient has been hospitalized within the past 6 months, has a urinary catheter, or is a nursing

home resident, the possibility of *P. aeruginosa* and enterococci, as well as multiply resistant organisms, should be considered. In this setting, ceftazidime, ticarcillin-clavulanate, piperacillin, aztreonam, meropenem, or imipenem in combination with an aminoglycoside is recommended. Ertapenem should not be used in this case owing to its inactivity against enterococci and *P. aeruginosa*.[55] The rationale for combination therapy is that in experimental animals, 3 days of aminoglycoside combination therapy followed by nonaminoglycoside single-agent therapy for 7 days resulted in a 100% cure rate.[56] If the patient responds to initial combination therapy, the aminoglycoside may be discontinued after 3 days. Although the aminoglycoside therapy is stopped, renal tissue concentrations of the aminoglycoside will persist for days. Based on sensitivity data, the patient then can be maintained or switched to a less expensive single agent, and ultimately, an appropriate oral agent may be used.

Effective therapy should stabilize the patient within 12 to 24 hours. A significant reduction in urine bacterial concentrations should occur in 48 hours. If bacteriologic response has not occurred, an alternative agent should be considered based on susceptibility testing. If the patient fails to respond clinically within 3 to 4 days or

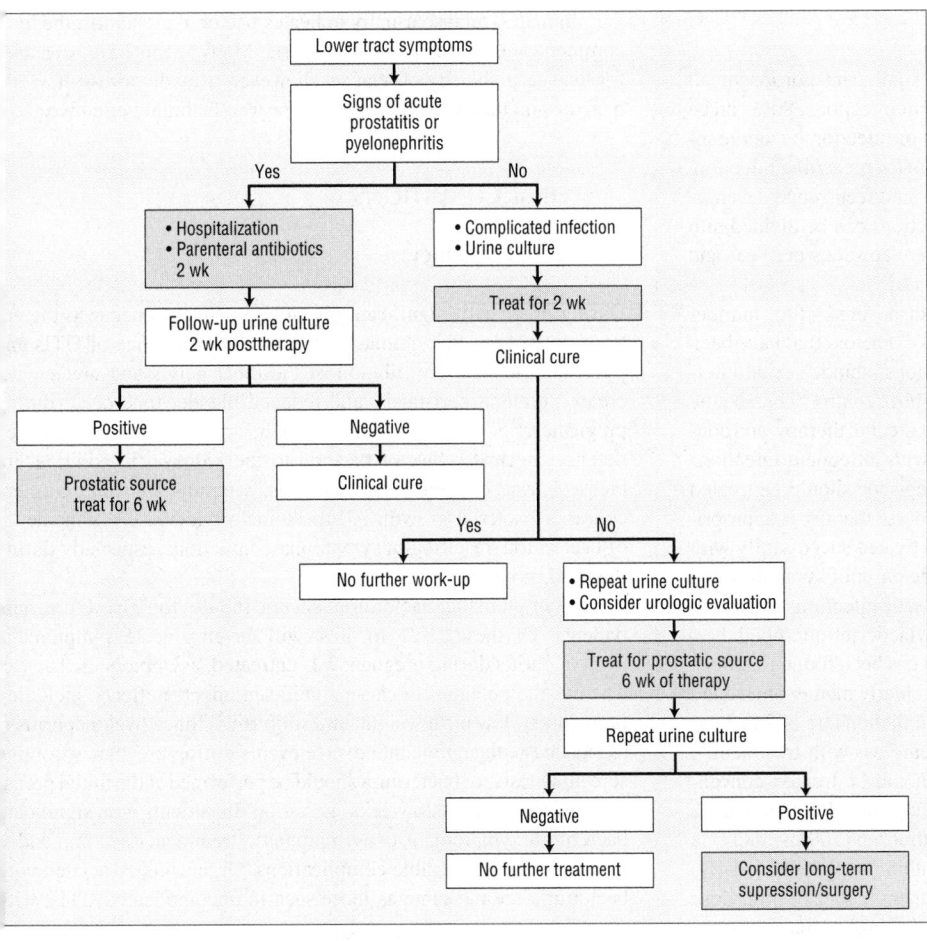

FIGURE 114–2. Management of UTIs in male.

has persistently positive blood or urine cultures, further investigation is needed to exclude bacterial resistance, possible obstruction, papillary necrosis, intrarenal or perinephric abscess, or some other disease process. Usually by the third day of therapy the patient is afebrile and significantly less symptomatic. In general, after the patient has been afebrile for 24 hours, parenteral therapy may be discontinued, and oral therapy instituted to complete a 2-week course. Follow-up urine cultures should be obtained 2 weeks after completion of therapy to ensure a satisfactory response and detect possible relapse.

Urinary Tract Infections in Males

The management of UTIs in males is distinctly different and often more difficult than in females. Infections in male patients are considered to be complicated because endogenous bacteria in the presence of functional or structural abnormalities that disrupt the normal defense mechanisms of the urinary tract cause them. The incidence of infections in males younger than 60 years of age is much less than the incidence in females. During the adult years, the occurrence of infection can be related directly to some manipulation of the urinary tract. The most common causes are instrumentation of the urinary tract, catheterization, and renal and urinary stones. Uncomplicated infections are rare, but they may occur in young males as a result of homosexual activity, lack of circumcision, and having sex with partners who are colonized with uropathogenic bacteria. As the patient ages, the most common cause of infection is related to bladder outlet

obstruction because of prostatic hypertrophy. In addition, the prostate gland may become infected and provide a nidus for recurrent infection in males.

The conventional view is that therapy in males requires prolonged treatment (Fig. 114–2). A urine culture should be obtained before treatment because the cause of infection in men is not as predictable as in women. Single-dose or short-course therapy is not recommended in this setting. Considerably fewer data are available comparing various antimicrobial agents in males as compared with females. If gram-negative bacteria are presumed, trimethoprim-sulfamethoxazole or the quinolone antimicrobials should be considered because these agents achieve high renal tissue, urine, and prostatic concentrations.[15]

Initial therapy should be for 10 to 14 days. Factors associated with treatment success are isolation of a single organism, the absence of significant obstruction or anatomic abnormalities, a normally functioning urinary tract, and the absence of prostatic involvement. Parenteral therapy may be required in certain situations, such as in severely ill patients, in the presence of acute prostatitis or epididymitis, and in patients who cannot tolerate oral medications. A comparison of 2-week versus 6-week therapy in males with recurrent infections who were given trimethoprim-sulfamethoxazole had cure rates of 29% and 62%, respectively.[57] Other investigators advocate longer treatment periods in males as well.[58] Follow-up cultures at 4 to 6 weeks after treatment are important in males to ensure bacteriologic cure. Many patients require longer periods of treatment and possible alterations in antibiotics depending on culture and sensitivity results and clinical response.

Recurrent Infections

Recurrent episodes of UTI account for a significant portion of all UTIs. Of the patients suffering from recurrent infections, 80% can be considered reinfections, i.e., the recurrence of infection by an organism different from the organism isolated from the preceding infection. These patients most commonly are female, and recurrence develops in about 20% of them with cystitis. Reinfections can be divided into two groups: those with less than two or three episodes per year and those who develop more frequent infections.

Management strategies depend on predisposing factors, number of episodes per year, and patient's preference. Factors that have been associated commonly with recurrent infections include sexual intercourse and diaphragm or spermicide use for birth control. Therapeutic options include self-administered therapy, postcoital therapy, and continuous low-dose prophylaxis. In patients with infrequent infections (less than three infections per year), each episode should be treated as a separately occurring infection. Short-course therapy is appropriate in this setting. Many women have been treated successfully with self-administered short-course therapy at the onset of symptoms.[59]

In patients with more frequent symptomatic infections and no apparent precipitating event, long-term prophylactic antimicrobial therapy may be instituted. Prophylactic therapy has been found to reduce the frequency of symptomatic infections in elderly men, women, and children. In women, most studies show a reinfection rate of 2 to 3 per patient-year reduced to 0.1 to 0.2 per patient-year with treatment.[60] Before prophylaxis is initiated, patients should be treated conventionally with an appropriate agent. Trimethoprim-sulfamethoxazole (one-half of a single-strength tablet), trimethoprim (100 mg daily), a fluoroquinolone (one tablet), and nitrofurantoin (50 or 100 mg daily) all reduce the rate of reinfection as single-agent therapy.[13] Full-dose therapy with these agents is unnecessary, and single daily doses can be used. Therapy generally is prescribed for a period of 6 months, during which time urine cultures are followed monthly. If symptomatic episodes develop, the patient should receive a full course of therapy with an effective agent and should be restarted on prophylactic therapy.

In women who experience symptomatic reinfections in association with sexual activity, voiding after intercourse may help to prevent infection. Also, single-dose prophylactic therapy with trimethoprim-sulfamethoxazole taken after intercourse has been found to reduce the incidence of recurrent infection significantly.[61]

In postmenopausal women with recurrent infections, the lack of estrogen results in changes in the bacterial flora of the vagina, resulting in increased colonization with uropathogenic *E. coli*. Topically administered estrogen cream is reported to reduce the incidence of infections in this population.[47]

The remaining 20% of recurrent UTIs are relapses, i.e., persistence of infection with the same organism after therapy for an isolated UTI. The recurrence of symptomatic or asymptomatic bacteriuria after therapy usually indicates that the patient has renal involvement, a structural abnormality of the urinary tract, or chronic bacterial prostatitis. In the absence of structural abnormalities, relapse often is related to renal infection and requires a long duration of treatment. Women who relapse after short-course therapy should receive a 2-week course of therapy. In patients who relapse after 2 weeks of therapy, therapy should be continued for another 2 to 4 weeks. If relapse occurs after 6 weeks of therapy, urologic evaluation should be performed, and any obstructive lesion should be corrected. If this is not possible, therapy for 6 months or longer may be considered. Asymptomatic adults who have no evidence of urinary obstruction should not receive long-term therapy.

In males, relapse usually indicates bacterial prostatitis, the most common cause of persistent bacteriuria. Many agents have been used for long-term therapy of relapses; however, trimethoprim-sulfamethoxazole and the fluoroquinolones appear to be highly effective.

SPECIAL CONDITIONS

UTIs in Pregnancy

During pregnancy, significant physiologic changes occur to the entire urinary tract that dramatically alter the prevalence of UTIs and pyelonephritis. Severe dilation of the renal pelvis and ureters, decreased ureteral peristalsis, and reduced bladder tone occur during pregnancy.[62,63] These changes result in urinary stasis and reduced defenses against reflux of bacteria to the kidneys. In addition, increased urine content of amino acids, vitamins, and nutrients encourages bacterial growth. All these factors increase the incidence of bacteriuria, resulting in symptomatic infections, especially during the third trimester.

Asymptomatic bacteriuria occurs in 4% to 7% of pregnant patients. Of these, 20% to 40% will develop acute symptomatic pyelonephritis during pregnancy. If untreated, asymptomatic bacteriuria has the potential to cause significant adverse effects, including prematurity, low birth weight, and stillbirth.[64] Since pyelonephritis is associated with significant adverse events during pregnancy, routine screening tests for bacteriuria should be performed at the initial prenatal visit and again at 28 weeks' gestation. In patients with significant bacteriuria, symptomatic or asymptomatic, treatment is recommended in order to avoid possible complications. Organisms associated with bacteriuria are the same as those seen in uncomplicated UTIs, with *E. coli* isolated most frequently.

Therapy should consist of an agent administered for 7 days that has a relatively low adverse-effect potential and is safe for the mother and baby. The administration of a sulfonamide, amoxicillin, amoxicillin-clavulanate, cephalexin, or nitrofurantoin is effective in 70% to 80% of patients. Tetracyclines should be avoided because of teratogenic effects, and sulfonamides should not be administered during the third trimester because of the possible development of kernicterus and hyperbilirubinemia. In addition, the available fluoroquinolones should not be given because of their potential to inhibit cartilage and bone development in the newborn. A follow-up urine culture 1 to 2 weeks after completing therapy and then monthly until gestation is complete is recommended.

Catheterized Patients

The use of an indwelling catheter frequently is associated with infection of the urinary tract and represents the most common cause of hospital-acquired infection. The incidence of catheter-associated infection is related to a variety of factors, including method and duration of catheterization, the catheter system (open or closed), the care of the system, the susceptibility of the patient, and the technique of the health care personnel inserting the catheter. The incidence of infection from a single catheterization in a healthy ambulatory patient is 1%.[65]

Bacteria may enter the bladder in a number of ways. During the catheterization, bacteria may be introduced directly into the bladder from the urethra. Once the catheter is in place, bacteria may pass up the lumen of the catheter via the movement of air bubbles, by motility of the bacteria, or by capillary action. In addition, bacteria may reach the bladder from around the exudative sheath that surrounds the catheter in the urethra. Cleaning the periurethral area thoroughly and applying an antiseptic (povidone-iodine) can minimize infection occurring during insertion of the catheter. The use of closed drainage systems has reduced significantly the ability of bacteria to pass up the lumen of the catheter and cause infection. A bacterium passing around the catheter sheath in the urethra is probably the most important pathway for infection. Avoiding manipulation of the catheter and trauma to the urethra and urethral meatus can minimize this path of acquisition.

Patients with indwelling catheters acquire UTIs at a rate of 5% per day. [65] The closed systems are capable of preventing bacteriuria in most patients for up to 10 days with appropriate care. After 30 days of catheterization, however, there is a 78% to 95% incidence of bacteriuria despite use of a closed system.[65] Unfortunately, UTI symptoms in catheterized patient are not clearly defined. Fever, peripheral leukocytosis, and urinary signs and symptoms may be of little predictive value.[66] When bacteriuria occurs in the asymptomatic, short-term catheterized patient (<30 days), the use of systemic antibiotics should be withheld and the catheter removed as soon as possible. If the patient becomes symptomatic, the catheter should be removed and treatment as described for complicated infections started. The optimal duration of therapy is not known. In the long-term catheterized patient (>30 days), bacteriuria is inevitable.[65] The administration of systemic antibiotics active against the infecting organism will sterilize the urine; however, reinfection occurs rapidly in more than 50% of patients. In addition, recolonization of the urine is with resistant organisms. Symptomatic patients must be treated because they are at risk of developing pyelonephritis and bacteremia. Bacteria have been found to adhere to the catheter and to produce a biofilm consisting of bacterial glycocalyces, Tamm-Horsfall protein, as wellas apatite and struvite salts, that act to protect the bacteria from antibiotics.[67] Recatheterization with a new, sterile unit should be performed in those symptomatic patients if the existing catheter has been in place for more than 2 weeks.

Various methods have been proposed to prevent the development of bacteriuria and infection in the patient with an indwelling catheter (see Table 114–5). The success of these methods depends on the type of catheter and the length of time it is in place. The use of constant bladder irrigation with antiseptic or antibacterial solutions has been investigated and found to reduce the incidence of infection in those with open drainage systems, but this approach has no advantage in those with closed systems. The use of prophylactic systemic antibiotics in patients with short-term catheterization reduces the incidence of infection over the first 4 to 7 days.[68] In long-term catheterized patients, however, antibiotics only postpone the development of bacteriuria and lead to the emergence of resistant organisms.

PROSTATITIS

Bacterial prostatitis is an inflammation of the prostate gland and surrounding tissue as a result of infection. It is classified as either acute or chronic. By definition, pathogenic bacteria and significant inflammatory cells must be present in prostatic secretions and urine to make the diagnosis of bacterial prostatitis. Prostatitis occurs rarely in young males, but it is commonly associated with recurrent infections in persons older than 30 years of age. As many as 50% of all males develop some form of prostatitis at some period in their life.[69] The acute form typically is an acute infectious disease characterized by a sudden onset of fever, tenderness, and urinary and constitutional symptoms. Chronic prostatitis presents with few symptoms related to the prostate but rather symptoms of urinating difficulty, low back pain, perineal pressure, or a combination of these. It represents a recurring infection with the same organism that results from incomplete eradication of bacteria from the prostate gland.

PATHOGENESIS AND ETIOLOGY

The exact mechanism of bacterial infection of the prostate is not well understood. The possible routes of infection are the same as those for UTIs. Reflux of infected urine into the prostate gland is thought to play an important role in causing infection. Intraprostatic reflux of urine occurs commonly and results in direct inoculation of infected urine into the prostate.[70] In addition, intraprostatic reflux of sterile urine can result in a chemical prostatitis and may be the cause of nonbacterial prostatitis. Sexual intercourse may contribute to infection of the prostate gland because prostatic secretions from men with chronic prostatitis and vaginal cultures from their sexual partners grew identical organisms. Other known causes of bacterial prostatitis include indwelling urethral and condom catheterization, urethral instrumentation, and transurethral prostatectomy in patients with infected urine.

A number of physiologic factors are believed to contribute to the development of prostatitis. Functional abnormalities found in bacterial prostatitis include altered prostate secretory functions. Prostatic fluid obtained from normal males contains prostatic antibacterial factor (PAF). This heat-stable, low-molecular-weight cation is a zinc-complexed polypeptide that is bactericidal to most urinary tract pathogens.[71] The antibacterial activity of PAF is related directly to the zinc content of prostatic fluid. Prostate fluid zinc levels and PAF activity also appear diminished in patients with prostatitis, as well as in the elderly.[70] Whether these changes are a cause or effect of prostatitis remains to be determined.

The pH of prostatic secretions in patients with prostatitis also has been reported to be altered.[72] Normal prostatic secretions have a pH in the range of 6.6 to 7.6. With increasing age, the pH tends to become more alkaline. In patients with inflammation of the prostate, prostatic secretions may have an alkaline pH in the range of 7 to 9. These changes suggest a generalized secretory dysfunction of the prostate that not only can affect the pathogenesis of prostatitis but also can influence the mode of therapy.

Gram-negative enteric organisms are the most frequent pathogens in acute bacterial prostatitis.[70] E. coli is the predominant organism, occurring in 75% of cases. Other gram-negative organisms frequently isolated include K. pneumoniae, P. mirabilis, and less frequently, P. aeruginosa, Enterobacter spp., and Serratia spp. Occasionally, cases of gonococcal and staphylococcal prostatitis occur, but they are infrequent.

E. coli most commonly causes chronic bacterial prostatitis, with other gram-negative organisms isolated less frequently. The importance of gram-positive organisms in chronic bacterial prostatitis remains controversial. S. epidermidis, S. aureus, and diphtheroids have been isolated in some studies.

CLINICAL PRESENTATION

Acute bacterial prostatitis presents as other acute infections (Table 114–6). Massage of the prostate will express a purulent discharge that will readily grow the pathogenic organism. Prostatic massage is contraindicated in acute bacterial prostatitis, however, because of the

TABLE 114–6. Clinical Presentation of Bacterial Prostatitis

Signs and Symptoms

Acute bacterial prostatitis: High fever, chills, malaise, myalgia, localized pain (perineal, rectal, sacrococcygeal), frequency, urgency, dysuria, nocturia, and retention

Chronic bacterial prostatitis: Voiding difficulties (frequency, urgency, dysuria), low back pain, and perineal and suprapubic discomfort

Physical Examination

Acute bacterial prostatitis: Swollen, tender, tense, or indurated gland

Chronic bacterial prostatitis: Boggy, indurated (enlarged) prostate in most patients

Laboratory Tests

Bacteriuria

Bacteria in expressed prostatic secretions

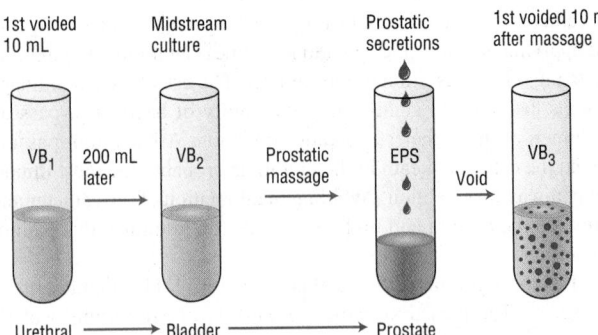

FIGURE 114–3. Segmented cultures of the lower tract in men.

risk of inducing bacteremia and associated local pain. The diagnosis of acute bacterial prostatitis can be made from the patient's clinical presentation and the presence of significant bacteriuria. As with other UTIs, the infecting organism can be isolated from a midstream specimen.

In contrast, chronic bacterial prostatitis is more difficult to diagnose and treat. Chronic bacterial prostatitis typically is characterized by recurrent UTIs with the same pathogen and is the most common cause of recurrent UTI in males. The patient's clinical presentation can vary widely (see Table 114–6). Many adults, however, are asymptomatic.

Because physical examination of the prostate is often normal, urinary tract localization studies are critical to the diagnosis of chronic bacterial prostatitis. The method of quantitative localization culture, as described by Meares and Stamey,[73] remains the diagnostic standard

(Fig. 114–3). The method compares the bacterial growth in sequential urine and prostatic fluid cultures obtained during micturition. The first 10 mL of voided urine is collected (voiding bladder 1, or VB1) and constitutes urethral urine. After approximately 200 mL of urine has been voided, a 10-mL midstream sample is collected (VB2). This specimen represents bladder urine. After the patient voids, the prostate is massaged, and expressed prostatic secretions (EPS) are collected. After prostatic massage, the patient voids again, and 10 mL of urine is collected (VB3).

The diagnosis of bacterial prostatitis is made when the number of bacteria in EPS is 10 times that of the urethral sample (VB1) and midstream sample (VB2). If no EPS is available, the urine sample following massage (VB3) should contain a bacterial count 10-fold greater than that of VB1 or VB2. If significant bacteriuria is present, ampicillin, cephalexin, or nitrofurantoin should be given for 2 to 3 days to sterilize the urine prior to performing the localization study.

▶ TREATMENT: Prostatitis

8 The goals in the management of bacterial prostatitis are, in general, the same as those for UTIs. Acute bacterial prostatitis responds well to appropriate antimicrobial therapy that is directed at the most commonly isolated organisms. Prostatic penetration of antimicrobials occurs because the acute inflammatory reaction alters the cellular membrane barrier between the bloodstream and the prostate. Most patients can be managed with oral antimicrobial agents, such as trimethoprim-sulfamethoxazole and the fluoroquinolones (e.g., ciprofloxacin, levofloxacin, and gatifloxacin) (see Table 114–5). Other effective agents in this setting include cephalosporins, and β-lactam/β-lactamase combinations. Although intravenous therapy is rarely necessary for total treatment, intravenous to oral sequential therapy with trimethoprim-sulfamethoxazole or the fluoroquinolones is appropriate. The conversion to an oral antibiotic can be considered after the patient is afebrile for 48 hours or after 3 to 5 days of intravenous therapy. The total course of antibiotic therapy should be 4 weeks in order to reduce the risk of development of chronic prostatitis. Therapy may be prolonged with chronic prostatitis (6 to 12 weeks). Long-term suppressive therapy also may be initiated for recurrent infections, such as three times weekly ciprofloxacin, trimethoprim-sulfamethoxazole regular-strength tablet daily, or nitrofurantoin 100 mg daily.[15]

Chronic bacterial prostatitis often presents a more vexing situation because cures are obtained rarely. In the past, it was recognized that despite high serum concentrations of antibacterial drugs in excess of the minimal inhibitory concentrations (MICs) of the infecting or-

ganisms, bacteria persisted in prostatic fluid. Most likely the failure to eradicate sensitive bacteria was caused by the inability of antibiotics to reach sufficient concentrations in the prostatic fluid and cross the prostatic epithelium.

Several factors that determine antibiotic diffusion into prostatic secretions were delineated from the canine model. Lipid solubility is a major determinant in the ability of drugs to diffuse from plasma across epithelial membranes. The degree of ionization in plasma also affects the diffusion of drugs. Only un-ionized molecules can cross the lipid barrier of prostatic cells, and the drug's pK_a directly determines the fraction of unchanged drug.

The pH gradient across the membrane has an influence on tissue penetration as well. A pH gradient of at least 1 pH unit between separate compartments allows for ion trapping. As the un-ionized drug crosses the epithelial barrier into prostatic fluid, it becomes ionized, allowing less drug to diffuse back across the lipid barrier. In early studies with the canine model, the prostatic pH was reported to be acidic (6.4).[70] More recent studies in humans, however, have reported that the pH of prostatic secretions from an inflamed prostate is actually basic (8.1 to 8.3).[70]

The choice of antibiotics in chronic bacterial prostatitis should include agents that are capable of reaching therapeutic concentrations in the prostatic fluid and whch possess the spectrum of activity to be effective. Agents that achieve therapeutic prostatic concentrations include trimethoprim and the fluoroquinolones. Sulfamethoxazole penetrates poorly and probably contributes very little to trimethoprim.

The fluoroquinolones appear to provide the best therapeutic options in the management of chronic bacterial prostatitis. Trimethoprim-sulfamethoxazole is also effective. Therapy should be continued for 4 to 6 weeks initially. Longer treatment periods may be necessary in some cases. If therapy fails with these regimens, chronic suppressive therapy may be used or surgery considered.

PHARMACOECONOMIC CONSIDERATIONS

The cost-effective management of UTIs requires knowledge of its pathogenesis and causative organisms associated with the various clinical syndromes described in this chapter. The costs associated with managing a UTI include direct costs, such a laboratory tests, medication, and health care visits. The indirect costs include lost work time and general quality-of-life issues such as disease or therapy adverse effects.

Direct costs are those associated with diagnosis, treatment, and follow-up. Reported percentages for these costs in cystitis are physician consultation 23%, laboratory costs 64%, and pharmaceuticals 13%.[74] The cost of pharmaceuticals varies according to the agents used and the duration of therapy. When trimethoprim-sulfamethoxazole and amoxicillin have been compared, trimethoprim-sulfamethoxazole results in a higher cure rate, lower relapse, fewer symptoms, and lower costs.[75] The fluoroquinolones also have been found to be highly effective agents but generally are more expensive. The outcome and total cost depend on whether therapy is empirical or definitive (based on a culture diagnosis for acute infection).

ABBREVIATIONS

ACB: antibody-coated bacteria
EPS: expressed prostatic secretions
LE: leukocyte esterase
PAF: prostatic antibacterial factor
PMN: polymorphonuclear leukocyte
UTI: urinary tract infection
WBC: white blood cell

Review Questions and other resources can be found at *www.pharmacotherapyonline.com.*

REFERENCES

1. Warren JW, Abrutyn E, Hebel JR, et al. Guidelines for antimicrobial treatment of uncomplicated acute bacterial cystitis and acute pyelonephritis. Clin Infect Dis 1999;29:745–758.
2. Fihn SD. Acute uncomplicated urinary tract infection in women. N Engl J Med 2003;349:259–266.
3. Bacheller CD, Bernstein JM. Urinary tract infections. Med Clin North Am 1997;81:719–729.
4. Foxman B. Epidemiology of urinary tract infections: Incidence, morbidity, and economic considerations. Am J Med 2002;113(suppl 1A):5–13S.
5. Johnson CC. Definitions, classification, and clinical presentation of urinary tract infections. Med Clin North Am 1991;75:241–252.
6. Platt R. Quantitative definition of bacteriuria. Am J Med 1983;75:44–52.
7. Stull TL, LiPuma JJ. Epidemiology and natural history of urinary tract infections in children. Med Clin North Am 1991;75:287–298.
8. Smellie JM. Reflections of thirty years of treating children with urinary tract infections. J Urol 1991;146:665–668.
9. Sobel JD, Kaye D. Urinary tract infections. In: Mandell GL, Bennett JE, Dolin R, eds. Principles and Practice of Infectious Diseases, 5th ed. New York, Churchill-Livingstone, 2000:773–800.
10. Baldassarre JS, Kaye D. Special problems in urinary tract infections in the elderly. Med Clin North Am 1991;75:375–390.
11. Gordon KA, Jones RN, et al. Susceptibility patterns of orally administered antimicrobials among urinary tract infections pathogens from hospitalized patients in North America: Comparison report to Europe and Latin America. Results from the SENTRY Antimicrobial Surveillance Program (2000). Diagn Microbiol Infect Dis 2003;45:295–301.
12. Wong AH, Wnzel RP, Edmond MB. Epidemiology of bacteriuria caused by vancomycin-resistant enterococci: A retrospective study. Am J Infect Control 2000;28:277–281.
13. Nicolle LE, Harding GKM, Preiksaitis J, et al. The association of urinary tract infection with sexual intercourse. J Infect Dis 1982;146:579–583.
14. Stamey TA, Fair WR, Timothy MM, et al. Antibacterial nature of prostatic fluid. Nature 1968;218:444–447.
15. Lipsky BA. Prostatitis and urinary tract infection in men: What's new; what's true? Am J Med 1999;106:327–334.
16. Shand DG, Nimmon CC, O'Grady F, et al. Relation between residual urine volume and response to treatment of urinary infection. Lancet 1970;1:1305–1306.
17. Parsons CL, Schrom SH, Hanno P, et al. Bladder surface mucin: Examination of possible mechanisms for its antibacterial effect. Invest Urol 1978;6:196–200.
18. Raz R, Stamm WE. A controlled trial of intravaginal estriol in postmenopausal women with recurrent urinary tract infections. N Engl J Med 1993;329:753–756.
19. Gupta K, Stapleton AE, Hooton TM, et al. Inverse association of H_2O_2-producing lactobacilli and vaginal *Escherichia coli* colonization in women with recurrent urinary tract infections. J Infect Dis 1998;178:446–450.
20. Sobel JD. Bacterial etiologic agents in the pathogenesis of urinary tract infections. Med Clin North Am 1991;75:253–273.
21. Orskov I, Ferencz A, Orskov F. Tamm-Horsfall protein or uromucoid is the normal urinary slime that traps type-1 fimbriated *Escherichia coli.* Lancet 1980;1:887.
22. Measley RE, Levison ME. Host defense mechanisms in the pathogenesis of urinary tract infection. Med Clin North Am 1991;75:275–286.
23. Jenkins RD, Fenn JP, Matsen JM. Review of urine microscopy for bacteriuria. JAMA 1986;255:3397–3403.
24. Pezzlo M. Detection of urinary tract infections by rapid methods. Clin Microbiol Rev 1988;2:268–280.
25. Stamm WE. Measurement of pyuria and its relation to bacteriuria. Am J Med 1983;75(suppl 1):53–58.
26. Pappas PG. Laboratory in the diagnosis and management of urinary tract infections. Med Clin North Am 1991;75:313–325.
27. Pels RJ, Bor DH, Woolhandler S, et al. Dipstick urinalysis screening of asymptomatic adults for urinary tract disorders. JAMA 1989;262:1221–1224.
28. VanNostrand JD, Junkins AD, Bartholdi RK. Poor predictive ability of urinalysis and microscopic examination to detect urinary tract infection. Am J Clin Pathol 2000;113:709–713.
29. Stamey TA, Govan DE, Palmer JM. The localization and treatment of urinary tract infections: The role of bactericidal urine levels as opposed to serum levels. Medicine 1965;44:1–36.
30. Fairley KF, Bond AG, Brown RB, et al. Simple test to determine the site of urinary tract infection. Lancet 1967;2:427–428.
31. Thomas VC, Forland M. Antibody-coated bacteria in urinary tract infection. Kidney Int 1982;21:1–7.
32. Stamey TA, Fair WR, Timothy MM, et al. Serum versus urinary antimicrobial concentrations in cure of urinary tract infections. N Engl J Med 1974;291:1159–1163.
33. Avorn J, Monane M, Gurwitz JH, et al. Reduction of bacteriuria and pyuria after ingestion of cranberry juice. JAMA 1994;271:751–754.
34. Barrett SP, Savage MA, Rebec MP, et al. Antibiotic sensitivity of bacteria associated with community acquired UTI in Britain. J Antimicrob Chemother 1999;44:359–365.

35. Kahlmeter G. The ECO-SENS Project: A prospective, multinational, multicenter, epidemiological survey of the prevalence and antimicrobial susceptibility of urinary tract pathogens-interim report. J Antimicrob Chemother 2000;46(suppl S1):15–22.

36. Steinke DT, Seaton RA, Phillips G, et al. Factors associated with trimethoprim-resistant bacteria isolated from urine samples. J Antimicrob Chemother 1999;43:841–843.

37. Goettsch W, VanPelt W, Naglekerke N, et al. Increasing resistance to fluoroquinolones in *Escherichia coli* from urinary tract infections in the Netherlands. J Antimicrob Chemother 2000;46:223–228.

38. Gupta K, Hooton TM, and Stamm WE. Increasing antimicrobial resistance and the management of uncomplicated community-acquired urinary tract infections. Ann Intern Med 2001;135:41–50.

39. Gupta K, Sahm DF, Mayfield D, Stamm WE. Antimicrobial resistance among uropathogens that cause community-acquired urinary tract infections in women: A nationwide analysis. Clin Infect Dis. 2001;33:89–94.

40. Johnson JR, Stamm WE. Urinary tract infection in women: Diagnosis and treatment. Ann Intern Med 1989;11:906–917.

41. Stamm WE, Hooton TM. Management of urinary tract infections in adults. N Engl J Med 1993;329:1328–1334.

42. Cox CE, Marbury TC, Pittman WG, et al. A randomized, double-blind, multicenter comparison of gatifloxacin versus ciprofloxacin in the treatment of complicated urinary tract infection and pyelonephritis. Clin Ther 2002;24:223–236.

43. Stass H, Kubitza D. Pharmacokinetics and elimination of moxifloxacin after oral and intravenous administration in man. J Antimicrob Chemother 1999;43(suppl B):83–90.

44. Naber KG. Treatment options for acute uncomplicated cystitis in adults. J Antimicrob Chemother 2000;46(suppl S1):23–27.

45. Stein GE. Comparison of single-dose fosfomycin and a 7-day course of nitrofurantoin in female patients with uncomplicated urinary tract infections. Clin Ther 1999;21:1864–1872.

46. Irvani A, Klimberg I, Briefer C, et al. A trial comparing low-dose, short-course ciprofloxacin and standard 7-day therapy with co-trimoxazole or nitrofurantoin in the treatment of uncomplicated urinary tract infections. J Antimicrob Chemother 1999;43(suppl A):67–75.

47. McCarty JM, Richard G, Huck W, et al. A randomized trial of short-course ciprofloxacin, ofloxacin, or trimethoprim-sulfamethoxazole for treatment of acute urinary tract infections in women. Am J Med 1999;106:292–299.

48. Tice AD. Short course therapy of acute cystitis: A brief review of therapeutic strategies. J Antimicrob Chemother 1999;43(suppl A):85–93.

49. Sherbotie JR, Cornfield D. Management of urinary tract infections in children. Med Clin North Am 1991;75:327–338.

50. Boscia JA, Kobasa WD, Knight RA, et al. Therapy versus no therapy for bacteriuria in elderly ambulatory nonhospitalized women. JAMA 1987;257:1067–1071.

51. Nicolle LE. Urinary tract infection in long-term-care facility residents. Clin Infect Dis 2000;31:757–761.

52. Nicolle LE, Bjornson J, Harding GKM, et al. Bacteriuria in elderly institutionalized men. N Engl J Med 1983;309:1420–1425.

53. Melekos MD, Naber KG. Complicated urinary tract infections. Int J Antimicrob Agents 2000;15:247–256.

54. Norrby SR. Short-term treatment of uncomplicated lower urinary tract infections in women. Rev Infect Dis 1990;12:458–467.

55. Curran MP, Simpson D, Perry CM. Ertapenem, a review of its use in the management of bacterial infections. Drugs 2003;63:1855–1878.

56. Bergeron MG, Beauchamp D, Poirier A, et al. Continuous vs intermittent administration of antimicrobial agents: Tissue penetration and efficacy in vivo. Rev Infect Dis 1985;3:84–97.

57. Gleckman R, Crowley M, Natsios GA. Therapy of recurrent invasive urinary tract infection in men. N Engl J Med 1979;301:878–880.

58. Lipsky GA. Urinary tract infections in men: Epidemiology, pathophysiology, diagnosis, and treatment. Ann Intern Med 1989;110:138–150.

59. Wong ES, McKevitt M, Running K, et al. Management of recurrent urinary tract infections with patient-administered single-dose therapy. Ann Intern Med 1985;102:302–307.

60. Hooton TM. Recurrent urinary tract infection in women. Int J Antimicrob Agents 2001;17:259–268.

61. Stapleton A, Latham RH, Johnson C, et al. Post-coital antimicrobial prophylaxis for recurrent urinary tract infection. JAMA 1990;264:703–706.

62. Andriole VT, Patterson TF. Epidemiology, natural history, and management of urinary tract infection in pregnancy. Med Clin North Am 1991;75:359–373.

63. Christensen B. Which antibiotics are appropriate for treating bacteriuria in pregnancy. J Antimicrob Chemother 2000;46(suppl S1):29–34.

64. McDermott S, Dagiuse V, Mann H, et al. Perinatal reis for mortality and mental retardation associated with maternal urinary tract infections. J Fam Pract 2001;50:433–437.

65. Warren JW. The catheter and urinary tract infection. Med Clin North Am 1991;75:481–493.

66. Tambyah PA, Maki DG. Catheter-associated urinary tract infection is rarely symptomatic. Arch Intern Med 2000;160:678–682.

67. Ohkawa M, Sugata T, Sawaki M, et al. Bacterial and crystal adherence to the surfaces of indwelling urethral catheters. J Urol 1990;143:717–721.

68. Stamm WE. Catheter-associated urinary tract infection: Epidemiology, pathogenesis, and prevention. Am J Med 1991;91(suppl 3):65s–71s.

69. Schaefer AJ. Urinary tract infection in men: State of the art. Infection 1994;22(suppl 1):S19–S21.

70. Meares EM. Prostatitis. Med Clin North Am 1991;75:405–424.

71. Fair WR, Couch J, Wehner M. Prostatic antibacterial factor: Identity and significance. Urology 1976;7:169–177.

72. Pfau A, Perlberg S, Shapiro A. The pH of prostatic fluid in health and disease: Implications of treatment in chronic bacterial prostatitis. J Urol 1978;119:384–387.

73. Meares EM, Stamey TA. Bacteriologic localization patterns in bacterial prostatitis and urethritis. Invest Urol 1968;5:492–518.

74. Patton JP, Nash DB, Abrutyn E. Urinary tract infection: Economic considerations. Med Clin North Am 1991;75:495–513.

75. MacDonald TM, Collins D, McGilchrist MM, et al. The utilization and economic evaluation of antibiotics prescribed in primary care. J Antimicrob Chemother 1995;35:191–204.

115

SEXUALLY TRANSMITTED DISEASES

Leroy C. Knodel

Learning Objectives and other resources can be found at *www.pharmacotherapyonline.com.*

KEY CONCEPTS

◀1 All recommended treatment regimens for gonorrhea also include antibiotic therapy directed against *Chlamydia* because of the high prevalence of coexisting *Chlamydia* infections in patients diagnosed with gonorrhea.

◀2 Parenteral penicillin is the treatment of choice for all syphilis infections. For patients who are penicillin-allergic, few well-studied alternative agents are available, and all are oral medications that require 2 to 4 weeks of therapy to be effective. Patient compliance and thus efficacy are a concern when alternative regimens must be used.

◀3 *Chlamydia* genital tract infections represent the most frequently reported communicable disease in the United States. In females, these infections are frequently asymptomatic or minimally symptomatic and, if left untreated, are associated with the development of pelvic inflammatory disease and attendant complications such as ectopic pregnancy and infertility. As a result, all sexually active females, females aged 20 to 25 years, and sexually active

women with multiple sexual partners should be screened annually for this infection.

◀4 Oral acyclovir, famciclovir, and valacyclovir are effective in reducing viral shedding, duration of symptoms, and time to healing of first-episode genital herpes infections, with maximal benefits seen when therapy is initiated at the earliest stages of infection. Depending on the severity of recurrent infections, which generally tend to be of shorter duration and produce less severe symptoms, symptomatic benefits may not be as obvious.

◀5 Metronidazole and tinidazole are the only agents currently approved in the United States to treat trichomoniasis. Although a single 2-g dose of either agent is widely used for compliance and other reasons, the alternative 7-day metronidazole regimen may be a better choice if sexual partners of treated individuals cannot be treated concurrently.

The spectrum of sexually transmitted diseases (STDs) has broadened from the classic venereal diseases—gonorrhea, syphilis, chancroid, lymphogranuloma venereum, and granuloma inguinale—to include a variety of pathogens known to be spread by sexual contact (Table 115–1). Because of the large number of infected individuals, the diversity of clinical manifestations, the changing drug-susceptibility patterns of some pathogens, and the high frequency of multiple STDs occurring simultaneously in infected individuals, the diagnosis and management of patients with STDs are much more complex today than they were even a decade ago.[1–4]

Despite a higher reported incidence of most major STDs in men, the complications of STDs generally are more frequent and severe in women. In particular, serious effects on maternal and infant health during pregnancy are well documented. Damage to reproductive organs, increased risk of cancer, complications associated with pregnancy, and transmission of disease to the fetus or newborn are associated with several STDs. As a result of the physiologic, psychosocial, and economic consequences of STDs, and because of the increasing prevalence of some viral STDs, such as human immunodeficiency virus (HIV) and genital herpes, for which curative therapy is not available, there is continuing research into STDs and the primary prevention of these diseases.[2–5]

With the exception of HIV infection, which is reviewed in detail in Chap. 123, the most frequently occurring STDs in the United States are discussed in this chapter. For other less common STDs, only

recommended treatment regimens are presented. The most current information on the epidemiology, diagnosis, and treatment of STDs provided by the Centers for Disease Control and Prevention (CDC) can be obtained at the CDC Web site on the Internet (*www.cdc.gov/*).

Numerous interrelated factors contribute to the epidemic nature of STDs. Sociocultural, demographic, and economic factors, together with patterns of sexual behavior, host susceptibility to infection, changing properties of the causative pathogens, disease transmission by asymptomatic individuals, and environmental factors, are important determinants of the frequency and distribution of STDs in the United States and worldwide.

Age is one of the most important demographic determinants of STD incidence. Overall, two-thirds of STD cases each year occur in persons in their teens and twenties, the peak years of sexual activity. With increasing age, the incidence of most STDs decreases exponentially. In sexually active teenagers, STD rates are highest in the youngest, suggesting that physiologic differences may contribute to increased susceptibility.[2–5]

Age-specific rates of STDs are higher in men than in women; however, reported rates may not represent true gender differences but rather may reflect greater ease of detection in men. In recent years, the ratio of male-to-female cases for most STDs has declined, possibly reflecting improvements in the diagnosis of STDs in asymptomatic women or changes in female sexual behavior following the availability of improved methods of contraception. Although some racial disparity

TABLE 115–1. Sexually Transmitted Diseases

Disease	Associated Pathogens
Bacterial	
Gonorrhea	*Neisseria gonorrhoeae*
Syphilis	*Treponema pallidum*
Chancroid	*Hemophilus ducreyi*
Granuloma inguinale	*Calymmatobacterium granulomatis*
Enteric disease	*Salmonella* spp., *Shigella* spp., *Campylobacter fetus*
Campylobacter infection	*Campylobacter jejuni*
Bacterial vaginosis	*Gardnerella vaginalis, Mycoplasma hominis, Bacteroides* spp., *Mobiluncus* spp.
Group B streptococcal infections	Group B *Streptococcus*
Chlamydial	
Nongonococcal urethritis	*Chlamydia trachomatis*
Lymphogranuloma venereum	*Chlamydia trachomatis*, type L
Viral	
Acquired immune-deficiency syndrome (AIDS)	Human immunodeficiency virus
Herpes genitalis	Herpes simplex virus, types I and II
Viral hepatitis	Hepatitis A, B, C, and D viruses
Condylomata acuminata	Human papillomavirus
Molluscum contagiosum	Poxvirus
Cytomegalovirus infection	Cytomegalovirus
Mycoplasmal	
Nongonococcal urethritis	*Ureaplasma urealyticum*
Protozoal	
Trichomoniasis	*Trichomonas vaginalis*
Amebiasis	*Entamoeba histolytica*
Giardiasis	*Giardia lamblia*
Fungal	
Vaginal candidiasis	*Candida albicans*
Parasitic	
Scabies	*Sarcoptes scabiei*
Pediculosis pubis	*Phthirus pubis*
Enterobiasis	*Enterobius vermicularis*

exists for rates of STD infection, it is possible that this is a reflection of socioeconomic differences.[2–5]

The single greatest risk factor for contracting STDs is the number of sexual partners. As the number of sexual partners increases, the risk of being exposed to someone infected with an STD increases. Sexual preference also plays a major role in the transmission of STDs. For all major STDs, rates are disproportionately greater in men who have sex with men (MSM) than in heterosexuals. Also, a number of less common STDs, including several caused by enteric protozoans and bacterial pathogens, occur primarily in MSM. The major risk factors for MSM appear to be related to the greater number of sexual partners and the practice of unprotected anal-genital, oral-genital, and oral-anal intercourse. In addition, prostitution and illicit drug use are associated with a higher incidence of most STDs.[1–4]

Some of the most serious sequelae of STDs are associated with congenital or perinatal infections. Most neonatal infections are acquired at birth, after infant passage through an infected cervix or vagina. Neonatal *Chlamydia trachomatis, Neisseria gonorrhoeae,* and herpes simplex virus (HSV) infections are associated with this type of spread. For pregnant women with syphilis, infection is usu-

ally transmitted transplacentally, producing a congenital infection. Depending on the organism, neonatal infections can manifest in a variety of ways, produce significant morbidity, and in some cases result in infant death.[1–4]

Other than complete abstinence, the most effective way to prevent STD transmission is by maintaining a mutually monogamous sexual relationship between uninfected partners. Short of this, use of barrier contraceptive methods, such as the male and female condoms, diaphragm, cervical cap, vaginal sponges, and vaginal spermicides alone or in combination, provides varying degrees of protection from a number of STDs. When used correctly and consistently, male latex condoms with or without spermicide are more effective than natural skin condoms in protecting against STD transmission, including HIV, gonorrhea, chlamydia, HSV, and hepatitis B. When lubrication is desired with latex condoms, water-based products, such as K-Y Jelly, are recommended because oil-based agents (e.g., petroleum jelly) can weaken latex condoms and reduce their effectiveness. The female condom is a lubricated polyurethane sheath with a diaphragm-like ring on each end that can be used as a protective device for women with male sexual partners who do not desire to use a condom. Limited data suggest that the female condom blocks penetration of viruses, including HIV; for nonviral STDs, the female condom provides STD protection similar to the male condom.[1,3,5,6] At one time, use of nonoxynol-9, a vaginal spermicide with cytolytic activity, was advocated to reduce the transmissibility of several STDs. This was based in large part on in vitro and animal data. However, recent data suggest that nonoxynol-9 does not reduce significantly the risk of transmission of common STDs but actually may increase the risk of HIV transmission in frequent users. Frequent use of nonoxynol-9 damages vaginal, cervical, and rectal epithelium, leading to increased transmissibility of HIV and possibly other STDs. Some evidence exists that diaphragms may protect against cervical gonorrheal, chlamydial, and trichomonal infections.[1,6–8]

The varied spectrum of clinical syndromes produced by common STDs is determined not only by the etiologic pathogen(s) but also by differences in male and female anatomy and reproductive physiology. For a number of STDs, the signs and symptoms overlap sufficiently to prevent accurate diagnosis without microbiologic confirmation. Frequently, symptoms are minimal or absent despite the presence of infection. Table 115–2 lists common clinical syndromes associated with STDs.[1–3]

GONORRHEA

EPIDEMIOLOGY AND ETIOLOGY

Neisseria gonorrhoeae is a gram-negative diplococcus estimated to cause up to 600,000 infections per year in the United States.[1] Of even greater concern are the substantial number of infections that remain undiagnosed and unreported.[1,9] Humans are the only known natural host of this intracellular parasite. Because of its rapid incubation period and the large number of infected individuals with asymptomatic disease, gonorrhea is difficult to control.[1,10–15]

The risk of a female acquiring a cervical infection after a single episode of vaginal intercourse with an infected male is approximately 50% to 60%, and the risk increases with multiple exposures.[10] While the risk of disease transmission from an infected female to an uninfected male is less, it still is as high as 20% to 30% following a single act of coitus. No data are available on the risk of transmission after other types of sexual contact.[10–12]

TABLE 115–2. Selected Syndromes Associated with Common Sexually Transmitted Pathogens

Syndrome	Commonly Implicated Pathogens	Common Clinical Manifestations[a]
Urethritis	*Chlamydia trachomatis*, herpes simplex virus, *Neisseria gonorrhoeae*, *Trichomonas vaginalis*, *Ureaplasma urealyticum*	Urethral discharge, dysuria
Epididymitis	*C. trachomatis*, *N. gonorrhoeae*	Scrotal pain, inguinal pain, flank pain, urethral discharge
Cervicitis/vulvovaginitis	*C. trachomatis*, *Gardnerella vaginalis*, herpes simplex virus, human papillomavirus, *N. gonorrhoeae*, *T. vaginalis*	Abnormal vaginal discharge, vulvar itching/irritation, dysuria, dyspareunia
Genital ulcers (painful)	*Hemophilus ducreyi*, herpes simplex virus	Usually multiple vesicular/pustular (herpes) or papular/pustular (*H. ducreyi*) lesions that may coalesce; painful, tender lymphadenopathy[b]
Genital ulcers (painless)	*Treponema pallidum*	Usually single papular lesion
Genital/anal warts	Human papillomavirus	Multiple lesions ranging in size from small papular warts to large exophytic condylomas
Pharyngitis	*C. trachomatis* (?), herpes simplex virus, *N. gonorrhoeae*	Symptoms of acute pharyngitis, cervical lymphadenopathy, fever[c]
Proctitis	*C. trachomatis*, herpes simplex virus *N. gonorrhoeae*, *T. pallidum*	Constipation, anorectal discomfort, tenesmus, mucopurulent rectal discharge
Salpingitis	*C. trachomatis*, *N. gonorrhoeae*	Lower abdominal pain, purulent cervical or vaginal discharge, adnexal swelling, fever[d]

[a]For some syndromes, clinical manifestations may be minimal or absent.
[b]Recurrent herpes infection may manifest as a single lesion.
[c]Most cases of pharyngeal gonococcal infection are asymptomatic.
[d]Salpingitis increases the risk of subsequent ectopic pregnancy and infertility.

PATHOPHYSIOLOGY

On contact with a mucosal surface lined by columnar, cuboidal, or noncornified squamous epithelial cells, the gonococci attach to cell membranes by means of surface pili and are then pinocytosed. The virulence of the organism is mediated primarily by the presence of pili and other outer membrane proteins. After mucosal damage is established, polymorphonuclear leukocytes (PMNs) invade the tissue, submucosal abscesses form, and purulent exudates are secreted.[10,11]

CLINICAL PRESENTATION

Individuals infected with gonorrhea can be symptomatic or asymptomatic, have complicated or uncomplicated infections, and have infections involving several anatomic sites. Interestingly, most of the symptomatic patients who are not treated become asymptomatic within 6 months, with only a few becoming asymptomatic carriers of the disease.[10–12] The most common clinical features of gonococcal infections are presented in Table 115-3.

TABLE 115–3. Presentation of Gonorrhea Infections

	Males	Females
General	Incubation period 1–14 days Symptom onset in 2–8 days	Incubation period 1–14 days Symptom onset in 10 days
Site of infection	Most common—urethra Others—rectum (usually due to rectal intercourse in MSM), oropharynx, eye	Most common—endocervical canal Others—urethra, rectum (usually due to perineal contamination), oropharynx, eye
Symptoms	May be asymptomatic or minimally symptomatic Urethral infection—dysuria and urinary frequency Anorectal infection—asymptomatic to severe rectal pain Pharyngeal infection—asymptomatic to mild pharyngitis	May be asymptomatic or minimally symptomatic Endocervical infection—usually asymptomatic or mildly symptomatic Urethral infection—dysuria, urinary frequency Anorectal and pharyngeal infection— symptoms same as for men
Signs	Purulent urethral or rectal discharge can be scant to profuse Anorectal—pruritus, mucopurulent discharge, bleeding	Abnormal vaginal discharge or uterine bleeding; purulent urethral or rectal discharge can be scant to profuse
Complications	Rare (epididymitis, prostatitis, inguinal lymphadenopathy, urethral stricture) Disseminated gonorrhea	Pelvic inflammatory disease disease and associated complications (i.e., ectopic pregnancy, infertility) Disseminated gonorrhea (three times more common than in men)

Complications associated with untreated gonorrhea appear more pronounced in women, likely a result of a high percentage who experience signs and symptoms that are nonspecific and minimally symptomatic. As a result, many women do not seek treatment until after the development of serious complications, such as pelvic inflammatory disease (PID). Approximately 15% of women with gonorrhea develop PID. Left untreated, PID can be an indirect cause of infertility and ectopic pregnancies. In 0.5% to 3.0% of patients with gonorrhea, the gonococci invade the bloodstream and produce disseminated disease. Disseminated gonorrhea infection (DGI) is three times more common in women than in men. The usual clinical manifestations of DGI are tender necrotic skin lesions, tenosynovitis, and monarticular arthritis.[1,10–13]

DIAGNOSIS

Diagnosis of gonococcal infections can be made by Gram-stained smears, culture, or methods based on the detection of cellular components of the gonococcus (e.g., enzymes, antigens, DNA, or lipopolysaccharide) in clinical specimens. Various stains have been used to identify gonococci microscopically, with the Gram stain the most widely used in clinical practice. Gram-stained smears are positive for gonococci when gram-negative diplococci of typical kidney bean morphology are identified within PMNs.[1,10–13] In the presence of equivocal smears (extracellular gonococcal forms that can be nonpathogenic, commensal *Neisseria,* or gram-negative diplococci of atypical morphology), culture is mandatory. In urethral smears from men with symptomatic urethritis, the smear is highly sensitive and specific, and culture is considered optional. Gram-stained smears are specific but insensitive for endocervical, rectal, cutaneous, and asymptomatic male urethral infections. In these situations, culture is the most reliable means of diagnosis. Because of the presence of non-pathogenic *Neisseria* in the pharynx, the Gram stain is not useful in the diagnosis of pharyngeal infection.[1,10,11,14]

Culture is considered the most reliable means of diagnosing gonococcal infections. Anatomic sites to be cultured depend on the individual's sexual preferences and body areas exposed. In women, because the urethra and other sites are rarely the sole locus of infection, cervical cultures produce the highest yield and frequently are performed in conjunction with rectal cultures. Urethral cultures are recommended in women who have had hysterectomies and heterosexual men. In MSM, anorectal cultures generally produce the highest yields, and pharyngeal and urethral cultures are considered optional.[1,10–14]

Because technical constraints and cost preclude the use of culture techniques in most office settings and clinics, alternative methods of diagnosis have been developed, including enzyme immunoassay, DNA probe techniques, and nucleic acid amplification techniques employing polymerase chain reaction (PCR) and ligase chain reaction (LCR). With the exception of Gram stain for symptomatic gonococcal urethritis, these tests offer increased sensitivity and/or specificity over both Gram stain and culture.[10] Additionally, many of these tests can provide a more rapid means of diagnosis than culture. Of particular clinical importance is the high sensitivity of DNA probe and PCR methods for detecting *N. gonorrhoeae* either in first-void urine samples of infected individuals or from vaginal swabs of infected women, and the extension of this technology to concurrently test for *Chlamydia trachomatis* in a single specimen.[1,14,17]

▶ TREATMENT: Gonorrhea

N. gonorrhoeae are susceptible to a variety of antibiotics. The development of chromosomally mediated and plasmid-mediated resistance has resulted, however, in an increasing number of isolates resistant to former first-line antibiotics such as penicillin, ampicillin, amoxicillin, and tetracycline.[1,10–13,18,19]

◀ All gonorrhea treatment regimens recommended by the CDC consist of various oral or parenteral cephalosporins and fluoroquinolones given as a single dose[1] (Table 115–4). These regimens have documented efficacy in the treatment of urethral, cervical, rectal, and pharyngeal infections. Coexisting chlamydial infection, which is documented in up to 50% of women and 20% of men with gonorrhea, constitutes the major cause of postgonococcal urethritis, cervicitis, and salpingitis in patients treated for gonorrhea.[1,15,16] As a result, concomitant treatment with doxycycline or azithromycin is recommended in all patients treated for gonorrhea. While none of the single-dose regimens recommended for gonorrhea in the CDC guidelines is effective against chlamydia, azithromycin (2 g) as a single dose is highly effective in eradicating both gonorrhea and chlamydia.

CLINICAL CONTROVERSY

Some clinicians advocate that a single 2-g dose of azithromycin should be the treatment of choice for gonorrhea because it is also effective in eradicating concomitant chalmydia infection. However, azithromycin therapy is associated with a greater incidence of gastrointestinal side effects and is much more expensive than other recommended first-line therapies.

Ceftriaxone, the only parenteral agent included in CDC recommended first-line agents for the treatment of gonorrhea, is administered intramuscularly (IM) as a single 125-mg dose, and in comparison with recommended oral antibiotics, it is an expensive alternative.[1,14–19]

Although oral therapy offers a promising alternative to the expense and pain associated with parenteral therapy, it may not be preferred for all cases of gonorrhea. Of the regimens of choice, only ceftriaxone is effective in eradicating both gonorrhea and incubating syphilis. Because the overall incidence of concomitant infection with both gonorrhea and syphilis appears low in most areas, selection of ceftriaxone based on this criterion should be considered only in areas in which the incidence of syphilis infection is high.[1,13,18,19] Resistance to the broad-spectrum cephalosporins recommended for the treatment of gonorrhea has not been reported. However, because of the increasing prevalence of high-level resistance to fluoroquinolones in some parts of the United States (i.e., Hawaii and California) and the world, these agents are no longer recommended for treating infections acquired in these locations. Similarly, fluoroquinolones are no longer recommended as first-line therapy in MSM due to data indicating increasing resistance in this population.[1,19] Ofloxacin is useful in eradicating both *N. gonorrhoeae* and *C. trachomatis;* however, different dosage regimens are required for each pathogen, and it is unknown whether the lower, multiple-dose daily regimen used in chlamydial infections is effective in eradicating gonorrheal infections.[1,18,19] Spectinomycin is still the preferred alternative for patients unable to tolerate the recommended cephalosporin or fluoroquinolone regimens. Although some resistance to spectinomycin is reported, its limited use appears to have prevented widespread resistance from developing.

TABLE 115–4. Treatment of Gonorrhea

Type of Infection	Recommended Regimens[a]	Alternative Regimens[b]
Uncomplicated infections of the cervix, urethra, and rectum in adults[c,d]	Ceftriaxone 125 mg IM once[e]; or ciprofloxacin 500 mg PO once[e]; or cefixime 400 mg PO once[f]; or ofloxacin 400 mg PO once[e] *plus* A treatment regimen for presumptive *C. trachomatis* coinfection (see Table 115–5)	Spectinomycin 2 g IM once; or ceftizoxime 500 mg IM once; or cefotaxime 500 mg IM once; or cefotetan 1 g IM once; or cefoxitin 2 g IM once with probenecid 1 g PO once; or lomefloxacin 400 mg PO once; or enoxacin 400 mg PO once; or norfloxacin 800 mg PO once *plus* A treatment regimen for presumptive *C. trachomatis* coinfection (see Table 115–5)
Gonococcal infections in pregnancy	Ceftriaxone 125 mg IM once[g,h] *plus* A recommended treatment regimen for presumptive *C. trachomatis* infection during pregnancy[h] (see Table 115–5)	Spectinomycin 2 g IM once *plus* a recommended treatment regimen for presumptive *C. trachomatis* infection during pregnancy[h] (see Table 115–5)
Disseminated gonococcal infection in adults (>45 kg)[h,i,j,k]	Ceftriaxone 1 g IM or IV every 24 hours[l]	Ceftizoxime 1 g IV every 8 hours[l] *or* Cefotaxime 1 g IV every 8 hours[l]
Uncomplicated infections of the cervix, urethra, and rectum in children (<45 kg)	Ceftriaxone 125 mg IM once[m]	Spectinomycin 40 mg/kg IM once (not to exceed 2 g)
Gonococcal conjunctivitis in adults	Ceftriaxone 1 g IM once[n]	
Ophthalmia neonatorum	Ceftriaxone 25–50 mg/kg IV or IM once (not to exceed 125 mg)	
Infants born to mothers with gonococcal infection (prophylaxis)	Ceftriaxone 25–50 mg/kg IV or IM once (not to exceed 125 mg)	

[a]Recommendations are those of the CDC.

[b]A number of other antimicrobials have demonstrated efficacy in treating uncomplicated gonorrhea but are not included in the CDC guidelines.

[c]Treatment failures are usually due to reinfection and necessitate patient education and sex-partner referral; additional treatment regimens for gonorrhea and chlamydia infections should be administered. Epididymitis should be treated for 10 days (see Table 115–8).

[d]Patients allergic to β-lactams should receive a quinolone. Persons unable to tolerate a β-lactam (penicillin or cephalosporin) or a quinolone should receive spectinomycin.

[e]Also recommended for the treatment of uncomplicated infections of the pharynx in combination with a treatment regimen for presumptive *C. trachomatis* infection; fluoroquinolones are *not* recommended for treating infections in MSM or infections acquired in Hawaii, California, or other parts of the world where high-level resistance to fluoroquinolones is reported.

[f]In July, 2002, Wyeth Pharmaceutical discontinued manufacturing cefixime; at the time of publication, there were no generic manufacturers of cefixime.

[g]Another recommended IM or PO cephalosporin also may be used.

[h]The fluoroquinolones, doxycycline, and erythromycin ethylsuccinate are contraindicated during pregnancy.

[i]Patients treated with one of the recommended regimens should be treated with doxycycline or azithromycin for possible coexistent chlamydial infection.

[j]Patients with gonococcal meningitis should be treated for 10 to 14 days and those with endocarditis for at least 4 weeks with ceftriaxone 1–2 g IV every 12 hours.

[k]All treatment regimens should be continued for 24–48 hours after improvement begins; at this time therapy can be switched to one of the following oral regimens to complete a 7-day course of treatment: cefixime 400 mg PO 2 times daily, or ciprofloxacin 500 mg PO 2 times daily, or ofloxacin 400 mg PO 2 time daily.

[l]All regimens should be continued for 24–48 hours after improvement begins; at this time therapy can be switched to one of the following oral regimens to complete a 7-day course of treatment: cefixime 400 mg PO 2 times daily or ciprofloxacin 500 mg PO 2 times daily or ofloxacin 400 mg PO 2 times daily.

[m]Patients with bacteremia or arthritis should receive ceftriaxone 50 mg/kg (maximum 1 g) IM or IV once daily for 7 days.

[n]The eye should be lavaged one time with saline solution.

Unlike ceftriaxone and the fluoroquinolones, spectinomycin has only limited efficacy in treating pharyngeal infections.

Pregnant women infected with *N. gonorrhoeae* should be treated with either a cephalosporin or spectinomycin because fluoroquinolones are contraindicated. For the treatment of presumed or diagnosed concurrent *C. trachomatis* infection, erythromycin and amoxicillin are the preferred treatments.[1,10,11,18,19]

Ceftriaxone is the recommended therapy for DGI, gonococcal meningitis, endocarditis, and any type of gonococcal infection in children. Although oral antibiotic regimens have not been studied adequately in children who weigh less than 45 kg, oral cefixime may provide a more patient acceptable alternative (*Note:* As of July 2002, Wyeth Pharmaceuticals discontinued manufacturing cefixime, and at the time of publication, there were no generic manufacturers of cefixime.) In cases of DGI, patients should be hospitalized and treated initially with one of the recommended parenteral antibiotics (see

Table 115–4). Although marked improvement is usually noted within 48 hours of initiating therapy, treatment should be continued as an outpatient with one of the recommended oral antibiotics to complete at least 7 days of antibiotic therapy.[1,18,19] Children and pregnant or lactating women should not receive fluoroquinolones because of the concern for bone and joint disorders. In MSM with DGI, ceftriaxone is preferred because of its efficacy in treating coexisting rectal, pharyngeal, and urethral infections.[1,10,18]

Gonococcal ophthalmia is highly contagious in adults and neonates and requires IM ceftriaxone therapy. Single-dose therapy is adequate for gonococcal conjunctivitis, although some physicians recommend continuing therapy until cultures are negative at 48 to 72 hours. Topical antibiotics are not sufficiently effective when used alone for ocular infections and are not necessary with appropriate systemic therapy. Infants with either type of ophthalmologic infection should be evaluated for signs of DGI.[1,10,18–20]

Treatment of gonorrhea during pregnancy is essential to prevent ophthalmia neonatorum. Gonococcal infection in newborns results primarily from passage through an infected birth canal, but it also can be transmitted in utero. Ophthalmia neonatorum is the most common ophthalmic infection in newborns (1.6% to 12%), although membranes of the vagina, pharynx, or rectum also can become colonized. Conjunctival involvement usually develops within 7 days of delivery and is characterized by intense, bilateral conjunctival inflammation with chemosis. If not treated promptly, corneal ulceration and blindness can develop. Because the law in most states requires neonatal prophylaxis with topical ocular antimicrobials, gonococcal ophthalmia neonatorum is rare in the United States. The American Academy of Pediatrics recommends that either silver nitrate (1%), tetracycline (1%), or erythromycin (0.5%) be instilled in each conjunctival sac immediately postpartum. Infants born to infected mothers should receive an IM or intravenous (IV) injection of ceftriaxone 25–50 mg/kg (not to exceed 125 mg); topical therapy is not necessary in such cases.[1,10–13,18,19]

EVALUATION OF THERAPEUTIC OUTCOMES

Although some clinicians recommend obtaining follow-up cultures at least 3 days after treatment, combination gonorrhea and chlamydial therapy rarely results in treatment failures, and routine follow-up of patients treated with a regimen included in the CDC guidelines is not recommended. Persistence of symptoms following any treatment requires culture of the site(s) of gonorrheal infection, as well as susceptibility testing if gonococci are isolated. In most cases, the presence of gonococci indicates reinfection rather than treatment failure and reflects the need for improved patient education and sex partner referral. Persistence of symptoms also can be caused by other infectious causes, such as *C. trachomatis*.[1,18,19]

SYPHILIS

EPIDEMIOLOGY AND ETIOLOGY

Although syphilis was the fifth most frequently reported communicable disease in the United States in 2001, the incidence of this disease has declined by almost 80% since 1990.[9] In addition to being highly contagious, syphilis is of major concern because, if left untreated, it can progress to a chronic systemic disease that can be fatal or seriously disabling.[22–25]

Syphilis usually is acquired by sexual contact with infected mucous membranes or cutaneous lesions, although on rare occasions it can be acquired by nonsexual personal contact, accidental inoculation, or blood transfusion. The causative organism of syphilis is *Treponema pallidum,* a spirochete. The risk of acquiring syphilis from an infected individual after a single sexual encounter is approximately 50% to 60%. After sexual contact, the organism penetrates the intact mucous membrane or a break in the cornified epithelium, and spirochetemia occurs.[24,25]

Evidence of a strong association between syphilis and HIV infection has been noted. Although complex and incompletely understood, it appears that syphilis, similar to other sexually transmitted genital ulcer diseases, can increase the risk of acquiring HIV in exposed individuals. Also, immunologic defects in HIV-infected individuals can modify the serologic response to syphilis. In particular, the possibility of delayed seroreactivity, markedly elevated serologic titers, and increased false-positive results could complicate the diagnosis, as well as assessment of treatment efficacy, in HIV-positive individuals infected with syphilis. Furthermore, anecdotal evidence suggests that compromised immune function may result in an accelerated progression of syphilis, particularly to neurosyphilis, requiring more aggressive antibiotic therapy in comparison with an immunocompetent host. As a result of this association, the CDC recommends that all patients diagnosed with syphilis be tested for HIV infection.[1,22–24]

CLINICAL PRESENTATION

The clinical presentation of syphilis is varied, with progression through multiple stages possible in untreated or inadequately treated patients (Table 115–5).

PRIMARY SYPHILIS

The primary stage, characterized by the appearance of a chancre on cutaneous or mucocutaneous tissue exposed to the organism, is highly infectious. Even without treatment, chancres persist only for 1 to 8 weeks before healing spontaneously. Because syphilitic chancres can be confused with other infectious etiologies, appropriate diagnostic testing is important.[22–24]

SECONDARY SYPHILIS

The secondary stage of syphilis is characterized by a variety of mucocutaneous eruptions resulting from widespread hematogenous and lymphatic spread of *T. pallidum*. Skin lesions can be either generalized or localized to a small portion of the body and, with the exception of follicular lesions, are nonpruritic. Generalized lymphadenopathy also is seen in the majority of patients, as are nonspecific symptoms such as mild and transitory malaise, fever, pharyngitis, headache, anorexia, and arthralgia. If untreated, secondary syphilis disappears in 4 to 10 weeks; however, lesions may recur at any time within 4 years.[12,22–24]

LATENT SYPHILIS

By definition, persons with a positive serologic test for syphilis but with no other evidence of disease have latent syphilis. Latent syphilis is further divided into early and late latency. During early latency, the patient is considered potentially infectious because of the 25% risk of spontaneous mucocutaneous relapse. The U.S. Public Health Service defines early latency as 1 year from the onset of infection, although other investigators propose a longer interval, such as 2 to 4 years. With the exception of pregnancy in which the mother may pass the disease to the fetus, late latency is considered noninfectious, although the patient remains a host.[1,22–24]

Most untreated patients with late latent syphilis have no further sequelae; however, approximately 25% to 30% progress either to neurosyphilis or to late syphilis with clinical manifestations other than neurosyphilis. Treatment of all patients with latent syphilis is essential because there is no way to predict which patients will have progression of their disease.[22–24]

TERTIARY SYPHILIS AND NEUROSYPHILIS

If left untreated, syphilis can slowly produce an inflammatory reaction in virtually any organ in the body. Manifestations of this disease

TABLE 115–5. Presentation of Syphilis Infections

General	
Primary	Incubation period 10–90 days (mean 21 days)
Secondary	Develops 2–8 weeks after initial infection in untreated or inadequately treated individuals
Latent	Develops 4–10 weeks after secondary stage in untreated or inadequately treated individuals
Tertiary	Develops in approximately 30% of untreated or inadequately treated individuals 10–30 years after initial infection
Site of Infection	
Primary	External genitalia, perianal region, mouth, and throat
Secondary	Multisystem involvement secondary to hematogenous and lymphatic spread
Latent	Potentially multisystem involvement (dormant)
Tertiary	CNS, heart, eyes, bones, and joints
Signs and Symptoms	
Primary	Single, painless, indurated lesion (chancre) that erodes, ulcerates, and eventually heals (typical); regional lymphadenopathy is common; multiple, painful, purulent lesions possible but uncommon
Secondary	Pruritic or nonpruritic rash, mucocutaneous lesions, flulike symptoms, lymphadenopathy
Latent	Asymptomatic
Tertiary	Cardiovascular syphilis (aoritits or aortic insufficiency), neurosyphilis (meningitis, general paresis, dementia, tabes dorsalis, eighth cranial nerve deafness, blindness), gummatous lesions involving any organ or tissue

progression were referred to previously as *tertiary syphilis*.[24] These clinical manifestations now are differentiated into two subgroups based on the presence or absence of central nervous system (CNS) involvement: neurosyphilis or tertiary syphilis (i.e., gumma and cardiovascular syphilis).[1,22–24]

Currently, the term *neurosyphilis* encompasses any patient with cerebrospinal fluid (CSF) abnormalities consistent with CNS infection.[1,24] Approximately 40% of patients with primary or secondary syphilis exhibit such abnormalities, although most remain asymptomatic. Persistence of CSF abnormalities into late latency is associated with a greater risk of progression to symptomatic neurosyphilis. Although data are conflicting, some investigators suggest that HIV-infected patients are at greater risk of developing symptomatic neurosyphilis than patients with intact immune systems.[1,22,25]

Rarely seen, the most common manifestations of disease progression from late latency are benign gumma formation and cardiovascular syphilis. The gumma, a nonspecific granulomatous lesion, is the classic lesion of late syphilis and develops in 50% of patients with disease progression. These chronic, destructive lesions characteristically infiltrate the skin, bone, soft tissue, and liver but can be found in any organ or tissue. Gummas of critical organs, such as the heart or brain, can be fatal.[1,24–28]

CONGENITAL SYPHILIS

In pregnant women with syphilis, *T. pallidum* can cross the placenta at any time during pregnancy. The risk of fetal infection is greatest in pregnant women with primary and secondary syphilis and declines in pregnant women with late disease. Transmission of syphilis during pregnancy occurs primarily transplacentally and can result in fetal death, prematurity, or congenital syphilis. Symptoms can be seen during the first months of life (early congenital syphilis) or later in childhood or adolescence (late congenital syphilis). Manifestations of early congenital syphilis resemble those of secondary syphilis, whereas those of late congenital syphilis correspond to the tertiary stage in adults.[22–25]

DIAGNOSIS

Because *T. pallidum* is difficult to culture in vitro, diagnosis is based primarily on microscopic examination of serous material from a suspected syphilitic lesion or on results from serologic testing. In primary syphilis, diagnosis is established by the presence of *T. pallidum* on dark-field microscopic examination of material from cutaneous lesions and enlarged lymph nodes in patients with secondary syphilis. In incubating syphilis, confirmation frequently is by dark-field microscopic examination because serologic tests can be unreactive early in the disease. Another method of direct microscopic examination, the direct fluorescent-antibody test (DFA-TP), which uses monoclonal or polyclonal antibodies specific for *T. pallidum*, has greater specificity and sensitivity than does dark-field examination, and does not require the immediate examination of fresh specimens.[12,24–28]

Serologic tests are the mainstay in the diagnosis of syphilis and traditionally are categorized as nontreponemal or treponemal. Common nontreponemal tests include the Venereal Disease Research Laboratory (VDRL) slide test, rapid plasma reagin (RPR) card test, unheated serum reagin (USR) test, and the tuluidine red unheated serum test (TRUST). Nontreponemal tests, which are inexpensive and easily performed, rely on the detection of treponemal antibodies directed against an alcoholic solution of cardiolipin, lecithin, and cholesterol contained in these tests. A positive nontreponemal test can indicate the presence of any stage of syphilis or congenital syphilis, although incubating syphilis and very early primary syphilis produce a negative reaction; however, because they are nonspecific tests, false-positive reactions occur, making them inappropriate to confirm the diagnosis alone. Transiently false-positive results can be seen in patients with acute febrile illnesses, after immunizations, and during pregnancy. Chronic false-positive results are commonly associated with heroin addiction, aging, chronic infections, autoimmune diseases, and malignant disease. In some cases, false-positive reactions are familial and are related to abnormal serum globulin levels.[23–28]

Nontreponemal tests are used primarily as screening tests; however, because *T. pallidum* antibody titers also can be quantitated by testing serial dilutions of the patient's serum for reactivity, they are useful in following the progression of the disease, recovery after therapy, and possible reinfection. Because antibody titers vary to some extent between tests, it is important that sequential serologic testing be performed using the same method each time. In patients treated successfully for primary and secondary syphilis, nontreponemal tests almost always will return to seronegativity. If these tests are going to return to negative in patients with early latent syphilis, they will do so within the first 4 years after adequate therapy; patients with disease of longer duration usually remain seropositive for life. In addition to their use in serologic testing, nontreponemal tests often are used on CSF to diagnose neurosyphilis.[23–28]

In some patients with secondary syphilis, a prozone phenomenon occurs that produces a negative VDRL test despite the presence of high reaginic antibody titers. This is corrected by diluting the patient's serum prior to testing.[26,27] For HIV-positive individuals with syphilis, the reactivity of nontreponemal tests can vary depending on the stage of the HIV infection. In the early stages, reaginic titers higher than in non–HIV-infected patients have been seen, resulting in the prozone phenomenon. During the later stages of HIV infection, however, when immune function deteriorates to a greater extent, serologic responses can be reduced or delayed. As a result, the diagnosis of syphilis in HIV-infected individuals can be more difficult.[1,24–28]

In diagnosing all stages of syphilis, treponemal tests are more sensitive than nontreponemal tests. Because these tests are technically more demanding and are more expensive, they are used primarily as confirmatory rather than as screening tests. The fluorescent treponemal antibody absorption (FTA-ABS) test is the most frequently used treponemal test. The FTA-ABS test uses the *T. pallidum* antigen to detect specific antibodies to treponemal organisms. The FTA-ABS test becomes positive earlier than nontreponemal tests in primary syphilis. After adequate antibiotic therapy for any stage of syphilis, the FTA-ABS test usually remains reactive for life and therefore is not useful in assessing serologic response to therapy, relapse, or reinfection. In suspected neurosyphilis when the CSF is negative with nontreponemal tests, FTA-ABS testing of the CSF is sometimes recommended. While less specific than the VDRL test for CSF involvement, the FTA-ABS test appears to be highly sensitive. Other serologic tests that are specific for the treponemal antibody are the *T. pallidum* hemagglutination assay (TPHA), microhemagglutination assay for antibodies to *T. pallidum* (MHA-TP), and the *T. pallidum* particle agglutination assay (TPPA). Recently, several enzyme immunoassays for *T. pallidum* have become available and are gaining wide use as confirmatory tests. PCR-based tests also are being investigated, particularly in situations in which serologic testing has poor sensitivity and specificity (e.g., congenital syphilis, early primary syphilis, and neurosyphilis). Additionally, multiplex PCR tests that can identify the presence of *T. pallidum,* herpes simplex virus type 1 (HSV-1) and HSV-2, and *Hemophilus ducreyi* from genital ulcer specimens are under study.[23,24,26–28]

▶ TREATMENT: Syphilis

Table 115–6 presents the CDC's treatment recommendations.[1] Parenteral penicillin G is the treatment of choice for all stages of syphilis. Because *T. pallidum* multiplies slowly, single doses of short- or intermediate-acting penicillins do not provide the prolonged, low-level exposure to penicillin required for eradication of the treponeme. As a result, benzathine penicillin G is the only penicillin effective for single-dose therapy.[1,12,22–25,29]

The recommended treatment for syphilis of less than 1 year's duration is benzathine penicillin G 2.4 million units as a single dose. Although the relapse rate for this regimen is less than 3%, some investigators advocate that 2.4 million units be administered once a week for 2 consecutive weeks. In patients with syphilis of greater than 1 year's duration and normal CSF examination, benzathine penicillin G is administered weekly for three successive doses. Although not specifically recommended by the CDC, this three-dose regimen is used by some experts to treat HIV-infected patients with syphilis of less than 1 year's duration based on data suggesting a greater risk of treatment failure with single-dose therapy.[1,24,25,29]

CLINICAL CONTROVERSY

Some experts even prefer to treat all patients with syphilis of less than 1 year's duration with the three-dose regimen because single-dose therapy is not consistently effective in eradicating treponemes from the CSF; this is of primary concern in patients with undiagnosed CSF involvement, such as HIV-infected individuals.

Patients with abnormal CSF findings should be treated as having neurosyphilis. Preferred regimens for neurosyphilis provide treatment over 10 to 14 days with parenteral penicillin G administered every 4 hours. Benzathine penicillin G alone in standard weekly doses and procaine penicillin G in doses under 2.4 million units do not consistently provide treponemicidal levels in the CSF and have resulted in treatment failures.[1,24,25,29] Because *T. pallidum* resistance to penicillin has not emerged, the primary need for alternative drugs in treating syphilis is for penicillin-allergic patients.[1,24,25,29]

Alternative regimens recommended for penicillin-allergic patients are doxycycline 100 mg orally twice daily or tetracycline 500 mg orally four times daily for 2 to 4 weeks depending on the duration of syphilis infection. Although erythromycin 500 mg orally four times daily was recommended in the past as an alternative regimen in nonpregnant, penicillin-allergic patients, evidence suggests that it is not as effective as other recommended regimens.[1,24,25,29]

Alternative treatment regimens should be used only in cases of documented penicillin allergy, and given concerns regarding patient compliance with these regimens, follow-up serologic testing is of particular importance.[1,23,24]

Other antibiotics used successfully in treating syphilis include various β-lactam antibiotics; however, none offers significant advantages over benzathine penicillin G. Even though ceftriaxone is considered effective in eradicating incubating syphilis when given as a single 125-mg dose, higher doses and more frequent administration (e.g., 1000 mg daily for 8 to 10 days) appear necessary for more advanced syphilis, and treatment failures are reported in HIV-infected patients. Preliminary data indicate that azithromycin 2 g as a single dose produces good results in patients with early syphilis.[1,24,25,29]

For pregnant patients, penicillin is the treatment of choice at the dosage recommended for that particular stage of syphilis. To ensure treatment success and prevent transmission to the fetus, some experts advocate an additional IM dose of benzathine penicillin G 2.4 million units 1 week after completion of the recommended regimen. In women allergic to penicillin, safe and effective alternatives are not available; therefore, skin testing should be performed to confirm a penicillin

TABLE 115–6. Drug Therapy and Follow-up of Syphilis

Stage/Type of Syphilis	Recommended Regimens[a]	Follow-Up Serology
Primary, secondary, or latent syphilis of less than 1 year's duration (early latent syphilis)	Benzathine penicillin G 2.4 million units IM in a single dose[b]	Quantitative nontreponemal tests at 6 and 12 months for primary and secondary syphilis; at 6, 12, and 24 months for early latent syphilis[c]
Latent syphilis of more than 1 year's duration (late latent syphilis) or syphilis of unknown duration	Benzathine penicillin G 2.4 million units IM once a week for 3 successive weeks (7.2 million units total)	Quantitative nontreponemal tests at 6, 12, and 24 months[d]
Neurosyphilis	Aqueous crystalline penicillin G 18–24 million units IV (3–4 million units every 4 hours or by continuous infusion) for 10–14 days[e] *or* Aqueous procaine penicillin G 2.4 million units IM daily plus probenecid 500 mg PO four times daily, both for 10–14 days[e]	CSF[f] examination every 6 months until the cell count is normal; if it has not decreased at 6 months or is not normal by 2 years, retreatment should be considered
Congenital syphilis	Aqueous crystalline penicillin G 50,000 units/kg IV every 12 hours during the first 7 days of life and every 8 hours thereafter for a total of 10 days *or* Procaine penicillin G 50,000 units/kg IM daily for 10 days	Quantitative nontreponemal tests every 2–3 months until nonreactive or titers have decreased 4-fold
Penicillin-allergic patients[g]		
Primary, secondary, or early latent syphilis	Doxycycline 100 mg PO two times daily for 2 weeks[h,i] *or* Tetracycline 500 mg PO four times daily for 2 weeks[h,i]	Same as for non–penicillin-allergic patients
Latent syphilis of more than 1 year's duration (late latent syphilis) or syphilis of unknown duration	Doxycycline 100 mg PO two times a day for 4 weeks[i] *or* Tetracycline 500 mg PO four times daily for 4 weeks[i]	Same as for non–penicillin-allergic patients

[a]Recommendations are those of the CDC.
[b]Some experts recommend multiple doses of benzathine penicillin G or other supplemental antibiotics in addition to benzathine penicillin G in HIV-infected patients with primary or secondary syphilis; HIV-infected patients with early latent syphilis should be treated with the recommended regimen for latent syphilis of more than 1 year's duration.
[c]More frequent follow-up (i.e., 3, 6, 9, 12, and 24 months) recommended for HIV-infected patients.
[d]More frequent follow-up (i.e., 6, 12, 18, and 24 months) recommended for HIV-infected patients.
[e]Some experts administer benzathine penicillin G 2.4 million units IM once per week for up to 3 weeks after completion of the neurosyphilis regimens to provide a total duration of therapy comparable to that used for late syphilis in the absence of neurosyphilis.
[f]CSF = cerebrospinal fluid.
[g]For nonpregnant patients; pregnant patients should be treated with penicillin after desensitization.
[h]Although less effective than either the doxycycline or tetracycline regimen, erythromycin 500 mg PO 4 times daily can be considered as an alternative regimen for nonpregnant patients.
[i]Pregnant patients allergic to penicillin should be desensitized and treated with penicillin.

allergy. It is recommended that women with positive skin tests undergo penicillin desensitization and receive the appropriate treatment regimen for their stage of disease.[1,24,25]

Most patients treated for primary and secondary syphilis experience the Jarisch-Herxheimer reaction after treatment. This benign, self-limiting reaction is characterized by flulike symptoms, such as transient headache, fever, chills, malaise, arthralgia, myalgia, tachypnea, peripheral vasodilation, and aggravation of syphilitic lesions. The exact mechanism of the reaction is unknown, although proposed etiologies, including immunologic mechanisms and release of endotoxin or other toxic treponemal products, are not substantiated. The Jarisch-Herxheimer reaction is independent of the drug and dose used and should not be confused with penicillin allergy. It usually begins within 2 to 4 hours of initiating therapy, peaks at 8 hours, and is complete within 12 to 24 hours. Most reactions can be managed symptomatically with analgesics, antipyretics, and rest. Steroids and antihistamines have been administered prior to initiation of syphilitic therapy but are of limited value.[1,23–25]

EVALUATION OF THERAPEUTIC OUTCOMES

Table 115–6 lists the CDC recommendations for serologic follow-up of patients treated for syphilis.[1] Quantitative nontreponemal tests should be performed at 6 and 12 months in all patients treated for primary and secondary syphilis and at 6, 12, and 24 months for early and late latent disease. The CDC recommends more frequent monitoring of HIV-infected individuals (i.e., 3, 6, 9, 12, and 24 months after therapy). In general, the time to reach seronegativity is proportional to the duration of the disease. Table 115–6 also includes specific testing recommendations for other stages of syphilis. Despite adequate therapy, some patients may remain seropositive based on nontreponemal test results. In these cases, stabilization of low antibody titers is indicative of adequate therapy. For women treated during pregnancy, monthly quantitative nontreponemal tests are recommended in those at high risk of reinfection.[1,23–25]

CHLAMYDIA TRACHOMATIS

EPIDEMIOLOGY AND ETIOLOGY

Based on CDC data, the number of reported cases of *Chlamydia* infection, the most frequently reported infectious disease in the United States, has more than doubled in the past 10 years.[1,7] Similar to other STDs, gross underreporting is believed to exist partly because of the large number of individuals who are treated presumptively without confirmatory microbiologic testing and partly because of the large number of individuals with asymptomatic infections. Chlamydial infections represent the most common cause of nongonococcal urethritis (NGU), accounting for as much as 50% of such infections.[30,31]

PATHOPHYSIOLOGY

C. trachomatis is an obligate intracellular parasite that shares properties of both viruses and bacteria. Like viruses, chlamydiae require cellular material from host cells for replication; however, unlike viruses, chlamydiae maintain their cellular identity throughout development. Although *C. trachomatis* lacks a cell wall peptidoglycan, its major outer membrane is similar to gram-negative bacteria. At least 18 serovars (subspecies) of *C. trachomatis* exist, of which only the lymphogranuloma venereum strains produce potentially invasive infections. The remaining serovars are involved primarily with superficial infection of epithelial cells.[31–33]

The risk of transmissibility of *Chlamydia* after exposure is unknown but is believed to be less than that following exposure to *N. gonorrhoeae*.[31–33] Coinfection with *Chlamydia* occurs in a substantial number of individuals with gonorrhea. All individuals diagnosed with *N. gonorrhoeae* should be assumed also to have *C. trachomatis* present.[1,15,16,34] Of major concern are data indicating that chlamydial infections are associated with up to a fivefold increased risk of acquiring HIV infection.[33] In addition to genital infections, ocular infections in adults owing to autoinoculation and infants owing to vaginal delivery through an infected birth canal are reported. Pharyngeal and rectal infections can develop secondary to orogenital or receptive anal intercourse, respectively, with an infected individual.[1,30–34]

CLINICAL PRESENTATION

In comparison with gonorrhea, chlamydial genital tract infections are more frequently asymptomatic, and when present, symptoms tend to be less noticeable. Urethral discharge usually is less profuse and more mucoid or watery than the urethral discharge associated with gonorrhea.[30–34] Table 115–7 summarizes the usual clinical presentation of chlamydial infections.

Similar to gonorrhea, chlamydia may be transmitted to an infant during contact with infected cervicovaginal secretions. Nearly two-thirds of infants acquire chlamydial infection after endocervical exposure, with the primary morbidity associated with seeding of the infant's eyes, nasopharynx, rectum, or vagina. In exposed infants, neonatal conjunctivitis develops in as many as 50%, and pneumonia develops in up to 16%. Inclusion conjunctivitis in newborns is usually self-limited, but it can result in scarring and micropannus of the cornea. Interstitial pneumonitis occurring secondary to carriage in the nasopharynx typically is mild, but it can be severe and require hospitalization.[1,30–34]

DIAGNOSIS

Because of the high rate of asymptomatic disease and the high prevalence of chlamydial infection in sexually active adolescent females, females aged 20 to 25 years, and sexually active women with multiple sex partners, the CDC recommends routine annual screening in these individuals. Laboratory confirmation of chlamydial infection is important because of the relative lack of specificity of symptoms when present.[1,32]

TABLE 115–7. Presentation of *Chlamydia* Infections

	Males	Females
General	Incubation period—35 days	Incubation period—7–35 days
	Symptom onset—7–21 days	Usual symptom onset—7–21 days
Site of infection	Most common—urethra	Most common—endocervical canal
	Others—rectum (receptive anal intercourse), oropharynx, eye	Others—urethra, rectum (usually due to perineal contamination), oropharynx, eye
Symptoms	Over 50% of urethral and rectal infections are asymptomatic	Over 66% of cervical infections are asymptomatic
	Urethral infection—mild dysuria, discharge	Urethral infection—usually subclinical; dysuria and frequency uncommon
	Pharyngeal infection—asymptomatic to mild pharyngitis	Rectal and pharyngeal infection—symptoms same as for men
Signs	Scant to profuse, mucoid to purulent urethral or rectal discharge	Abnormal vaginal discharge or uterine bleeding, purulent urethral or rectal discharge can be scant to profuse
	Rectal infection—pain, discharge, bleeding	
Complications	Epididymitis, Reiter's syndrome (rare)	Pelvic inflammatory disease and associated complications (i.e., ectopic pregnancy, infertility)
		Reiter's syndrome (rare)

Cell culture is the reference standard against which all other diagnostic tests are measured. Because chlamydiae are obligate intracellular parasites, specimens for culture must be obtained from endocervical (women) or urethral (men) epithelial cell scrapings rather than from urine or urethral discharges. Although tissue culture techniques have close to 100% specificity, the sensitivity is reported to be as low as 70% in part because of problems of improper specimen collection, transport, or processing. Because of the technical demands, expense, and length of time until results are available (3 to 7 days), culture is not used widely for diagnostic purposes today. However, culture remains the diagnostic standard in medicolegal cases such as sexual assault and child abuse because of its high specificity and ability to detect only viable organisms.[14,32,34,37–39]

Serologic tests are of limited value in diagnosing genital chlamydial infections because false-positive results may be obtained from previously infected individuals owing to persistence of chlamydial antibodies for prolonged periods.[14,32,34,37–39]

Tests that detect chlamydial antigens and nucleic acid provide more rapid results, are technically less demanding to perform, are less costly, and in some situations have greater sensitivity than culture. Commonly used nonculture tests for detection of *C. trachomatis* are the enzyme immunoassay (EIA), DNA hybridization probe, and the direct fluorescent monoclonal antibody (DFA) test. In comparison with culture, these tests have reduced sensitivities and slightly reduced specificities overall. Although the DFA test can be conducted in a short period of time, its sensitivity is highly dependent on skilled personnel in preparing the specimen for viewing under a fluorescent microscope and in interpreting the results. This test is used frequently as a confirmatory test for positive results seen with other nonculture tests.[14,32,34,37–39]

Most commercially available tests used to detect *C. trachomatis* use EIA techniques that detect chlamydial lipopolysaccharide (LPS) antigen. Some EIA methods, however, are not specific for *C. trachomatis*, and false-positive results are reported with other *Chlamydia* species, as well as with some gram-negative bacteria. The sensitivity and specificity of the test are generally lower when urine specimens are used.[14,32,34,37–40]

Rapid office tests that employ EIA technology for diagnosing chlamydial infections are widely available, and most provide results in 30 minutes. These tests generally are much less sensitive and specific than laboratory-performed EIA, and they are subject to a high false-positive rate because of the cross-reactivity of LPS from other microorganisms. As a result, a positive rapid office test should only be considered presumptive, and test results should be confirmed by a laboratory-based method.[14,38–40]

The greatest advances in the detection of chlamydial infection involved the development of various nucleic acid detection methods. Similar to EIA, the DNA hybridization probe test is easy to perform, and a large number of samples can be processed at the same time. Overall, the sensitivity and specificity of the DNA probe tests are greater than with EIA.[14,38–40]

Of all the advances in the diagnosis of *C. trachomatis* infections, the development of DNA amplification tests that can detect small amounts of chlamydial DNA such as PCR and LCR has been the most important. These tests are highly sensitive and specific for detecting infection in both urogenital specimens and urine. Use of self-collected vaginal specimens (swabs or tampons) or first-void urine samples offers greater patient acceptability, particularly when used to screen asymptomatic individuals. A further advantage of tests that can screen urine for the presence of infection is that up to 30% of women are reported to have urethral infection only, which would be missed using a test on endocervical samples. Because of their ability to detect as little as a single gene copy in a specimen, nucleic acid residues that persist following successful antibiotic therapy of a chlamydial infection can result in a false-positive test for several weeks following eradication of the organism.[14,32–41]

▶ TREATMENT: Chlamydia

A number of antimicrobials, including tetracyclines, macrolides, azithromycin, and some fluoroquinolones, display good in vitro and in vivo activity against *C. trachomatis*. In most clinical trials, cure rates exceeding 90% are reported for these agents. All these antimicrobials also appear to have good efficacy against *Ureaplasma urealyticum*, the second most common cause of NGU.[30–33]

Azithromycin 1 g orally as a single dose and doxycycline 100 mg orally twice daily for 7 days are the regimens of choice for the treatment of uncomplicated chlamydial infections[1] (Table 115–8). Because of its prolonged serum and tissue half-life, azithromycin is the only single-dose therapy that is effective in treating *C. trachomatis*. Of the fluoroquinolones, ofloxacin and levofloxacin are included in the CDC recommendations, but neither appears to offer an advantage over other first-line or alternative therapies. Although ciprofloxacin and some other fluoroquinolones have activity against *C. trachomatis* and *U. urealyticum*, high dosages have not consistently eradicated chlamydial infections.[1,34–37,41,42]

For pregnant women with chlamydial urogenital infections, treatment can reduce the risk of pregnancy complications and transmission to the newborn significantly. Because the use of tetracyclines and fluoroquinolones is contraindicated during pregnancy, erythromycin base and amoxicillin are the recommended drug treatments (see Table 115–8). Some clinicians prefer amoxicillin to erythromycin because of better patient tolerability and, as a result, improved patient compliance. Patients intolerant of the recommended erythromycin dosage can be treated with half the daily dose for 14 days instead of 7 days. Recommended alternatives to erythromycin base are erythromycin ethylsuccinate and azithromycin. Like erythromycin, azithromycin is in pregnancy category B and probably is an acceptable agent for use during pregnancy.[1,34–37,41,42]

CLINICAL CONTROVERSY

Although not recommended as first-line therapy in pregnant patients with chlamydial infections because of limited data on its safety, azithromycin is the only agent with documented efficacy in a single dose.

It is recommended that posttreatment cultures be obtained for pregnant patients treated for chlamydial infections to ensure eradication of the infection.[1,35–37]

C. trachomatis transmission during perinatal exposure can result in infections of the eye, oropharynx, lungs, urogenital tract, and rectum of the neonate or infant. Despite their efficacy in preventing gonococcal ophthalmia, topical erythromycin ointment (0.5%), tetracycline ointment (1%), and silver nitrate solution (1%) appear less effective in preventing chlamydial ophthalmia. Additionally, topical therapy has no effect on nasal carriage or colonization of other parts of the infant's body, so the potential for other infections, including

TABLE 115–8. Treatment of Chlamydial Infections

Infection	Recommended Regimens[a]	Alternative Regimen
Uncomplicated urethral, endocervical, or rectal infection in adults	Azithromycin 1 g PO once, or doxycycline 100 mg PO 2 times daily for 7 days	Ofloxacin 300 mg PO 2 times daily for 7 days, or levofloxacin 500 mg PO once daily for 7 days, or erythromycin base 500 mg PO 4 times daily for 7 days, or erythromycin ethyl succinate 800 mg PO 4 times daily for 7 days
Urogenital infections during pregnancy	Erythromycin base 500 mg PO 4 times daily for 7 days, or amoxicillin 500 mg PO 3 times daily for 7 days	Erythromycin base 250 mg PO 4 times daily for 14 days, or erythromycin ethyl succinate 800 mg PO 4 times daily for 7 days (or 400 mg PO 4 times daily for 14 days), or azithromycin 1 g PO as a single dose[b]
Conjunctivitis of the newborn or pneumonia in infants	Erythromycin base 50 mg/kg/day PO in 4 divided doses for 14 days[c]	

[a]Recommendations are those of the CDC.
[b]Data are insufficient to recommend routine use of azithromycin in pregnant women at this time.
[c]Topical therapy alone is inadequate and is unnecessary when systemic therapy is administered.

pneumonia, still remains. Because of the high percentage of treatment failures, topical therapy is not recommended to treat ophthalmia caused by *C. trachomatis*. Instead, an oral erythromycin regimen is recommended.[1,31–33]

EVALUATION OF THERAPEUTIC OUTCOMES

Treatment of chlamydial infections with the recommended regimens is highly effective; therefore, posttreatment laboratory testing is not recommended routinely unless symptoms persist or there are other specific concerns (e.g., pregnancy). Posttreatment tests should not be performed for at least 3 weeks following completion of therapy.[1] When posttreatment tests are positive, they usually represent noncompliance, failure to treat sexual partners, or laboratory error rather than inadequate therapy or resistance to therapy. Infants with pneumonitis should receive follow-up testing because erythromycin is only 80% effective, and a second course of therapy may be necessary.[1,30–34,36]

GENITAL HERPES

EPIDEMIOLOGY AND ETIOLOGY

Genital herpes infections represent the most common cause of genital ulceration seen in the United States. More than 50 million Americans have genital herpes, and this number is increasing by at least 500,000 each year.[1,7,43–48] Because of its morbidity, recurrent nature, and potential for complications, as well as its ability to be transmitted asymptomatically, genital herpes is of major public health importance.[45–54] Similar to syphilis and other STDs, the presence of genital herpes lesions is associated with an increased risk of acquiring HIV following exposure.[1,47]

PATHOPHYSIOLOGY

Herpes comes from the Greek word meaning "to creep" and is used to describe two distinct but antigenically related serotypes of herpes simplex virus. Herpes simplex virus type 1 (HSV-1) is associated most commonly with oropharyngeal disease, and herpes simplex virus type 2 (HSV-2) is associated most closely with genital disease; however, each virus is capable of causing clinically indistinguishable infection in both anatomic areas.[46,47,50,54]

Humans are the sole known reservoir for HSV. Infection is transmitted via inoculation of virus from infected secretions onto mucosal surfaces (e.g., urethra, oropharynx, cervix, and conjunctivae) or through abraded skin. Evidence that the virus survives for a limited time on environmental surfaces suggests the possibility of fomitic transfer as a nonvenereal route of transmission.[46,48–50]

The cycle of HSV infection occurs in five stages: primary mucocutaneous infection, infection of the ganglia, establishment of latency, reactivation, and recurrent infection. After viral inoculation, HSV infection is associated with cytoplasmic granulation, ballooning degeneration of cells, and production of mononucleated giant cells. Initially, the cellular response is predominantly polymorphonuclear, followed by a lymphocytic response. Replication occurs with viral spread to contiguous cells and peripheral sensory nerves. Latency then is established in sensory or autonomic nerve root ganglia. Latency appears to be lifelong, interrupted only by reactivation of the viral infection. It is unclear what factors are important in maintaining latency, but immune responses and emotional and physical stresses appear important in reactivating latent virus.[46,48]

CLINICAL PRESENTATION

The signs and symptoms of genital herpes infection are influenced by many factors, including previous exposure to HSV, viral type, and host factors such as age and site of infection. Because a high percentage of initial and recurrent infections are asymptomatic, and because viral shedding can occur in the absence of apparent lesions or symptoms, identification and education of individuals with genital herpes are essential in controlling its transmission.[46,53,55] A summary of the clinical presentation of genital herpes is provided in Table 115–9.

TABLE 115–9. Presentation of Genital Herpes Infections

General	Incubation period 2–14 days (mean - 4 days)
	Can be caused by either HSV-1 or HSV-2
Classification of Infection	
First-episode primary	Initial genital infection in individuals lacking antibody to either HSV-1 or HSV-2
First-episode nonprimary	Initial genital infection in individuals with clinical or serologic evidence of prior HSV (usually HSV-1) infection
Recurrent	Appearance of genital lesions at some time following healing of first-episode infection
Signs and Symptoms	
First-episode infections	Most primary infections are asymptomatic or minimally symptomatic
	Multiple painful pustular or ulcerative lesions on external genitalia developing over a period of 7–10 days; lesions heal in 2–4 weeks (mean 21 days)
	Flulike symptoms (e.g., fever, headache, malaise) during first fews after appearance of lesions
	Others—local itching, pain or discomfort; vaginal or urethral discharge, tender inguinal adenopathy, paresthesias, urinary retention
	Severity of symptoms greater in females than in males
	Symptoms are less severe (e.g., fewer lesions, more rapid lesion healing, fewer or milder systemic symptoms) with nonprimary infections
	Symptoms more severe and prolonged in the immunocompromised
	On average viral shedding lasts approximately 11–12 days for primary infections and 7 days for nonprimary infections
Recurrent	Prodrome seen in approximately 50% of patients prior to appearance of recurrent lesions; mild burning, itching, or tingling are typical prodromal symptoms
	Compared to primary infections, recurrent infections associated with (1) fewer lesions that are more localized, (2) shorter duration of active infection (lesions heal within 7 days), and (3) milder symptoms
	Severity of symptoms greater in females than in males
	Symptoms more severe and prolonged in the immunocompromised
	On average viral shedding lasts approximately 4 days
Therapeutic implications of HSV-1 versus HSV-2 genital infection	Primary infections due to HSV-1 and HSV-2 virtually indistinguishable
	Recurrence rate is greater following primary infection with HSV-2
	Recurrent infections with HSV-2 tend to be more severe
Complications	Secondary infection of lesions; extragenital infection due to autoinoculation; disseminated infection (primarily in immuncompromised patients); meningitis or encephalitis; neonatal transmission

COMPLICATIONS

Complications from genital herpes infections result from both genital spread and autoinoculation of the virus and occur most commonly with primary first episodes. Lesions at extragenital sites, such as the eye, rectum, pharynx, and fingers, are not uncommon. CNS involvement is seen occasionally and may take several forms, including an aseptic meningitis, transverse myelitis, or sacral radiculopathy syndrome.[47,50,51,54]

A major concern is the effect of genital herpes on neonates exposed during pregnancy. Neonatal herpes is associated with a high mortality and significant morbidity. It is transmitted to the newborn primarily through exposure to HSV in the birth canal but, in rare cases, also is transmitted transplacentally. The risk of transmission during birth appears much greater for first-episode primary infections than for recurrent infections. Neonatal herpes infection has a case-fatality rate of approximately 50%, with a large proportion of surviving infants experiencing significant morbidity, including permanent neurologic damage.[49–51]

DIAGNOSIS

Confirmation of a genital herpes infection can be made only with laboratory testing. Tissue culture is the most specific (100%) and sensitive method (80% to 90%) of confirming the diagnosis of first-episode genital herpes; however, culture is relatively insensitive in detecting HSV in ulcers in the latter stages of healing and in recurrent infections, as a result, in part, of reduced viral load. Viral culture is expensive and time-consuming, and improper collection or transport of specimens can result in false-negative results. In most situations, HSV isolation on tissue culture takes 48 to 96 hours. Following isolation, it is recommended that typing of the virus be performed because of prognostic implications (HSV-1 is associated with a lower rate of asymptomatic and symptomatic recurrence).[54–57] In instances in which rapid detection is necessary, such as an impending birth, other detection methods may be more useful. Amplified culture techniques that combine cell culture for 24 hours and subsequent staining for HSV antigen have sensitivities and specificities only slightly less than those of culture.[47,49,50,52–57]

Several serologic tests capable of distinguishing HSV-1 and HSV-2 antibodies have been marketed recently. These tests detect antibodies to type-specific HSV-1 and HSV-2 proteins gG-1 and gG-2, respectively. While antibody formation begins immediately following a primary herpes infection, complete seroconversion (i.e., complete antibody development) may take several months. Until the full expression of all antigenic determinants of HSV-1 and HSV-2 occurs, these tests are not useful in differentiating HSV-1 and HSV-2 infection[48,53,54,57] Older antibody detection tests, some of which are still marketed, are unable to distinguish between HSV-1 and HSV-2 owing to the considerable cross-reactivity between the two serotypes. Given the high prevalence of HSV-1 antibody in the adult population, accurate interpretation of positive results is not possible.[46,54]

In recent years, PCR assays that detect HSV DNA and can differentiate HSV-1 and HSV-2 infections have become increasingly available. These assays are more sensitive than culture and are considered the diagnostic test of choice for suspected CNS infections (i.e., HSV encephalitis and HSV meningitis). Although PCR assays are not used widely in diagnosing genital ulcer disease at this time, some data suggest that they also may prove useful in diagnosing asymptomatic viral shedding.[52,55–57]

While the diagnosis of genital herpes can be confirmed only by laboratory tests, less stringent diagnostic criteria (e.g., characteristic physical findings or clinical history) frequently are used in clinical practice. A presumptive diagnosis of genital herpes commonly is made based on the presence of dark-field-negative, vesicular, or ulcerative genital lesions. A prior history of similar lesions or recent sexual contact with an individual with similar lesions also is useful in making the diagnosis. Other STDs, including chancroid, lymphogranuloma venereum, and granuloma inguinale, and causes such as trauma, allergic reactions, and bacterial or fungal infections are considered in the differential diagnosis.[48,55–57]

▶ TREATMENT: Genital Herpes

The most achievable goals in the management of genital herpes are to relieve symptoms and to shorten the clinical course, to prevent complications and recurrences, and to decrease disease transmission. Although research has focused primarily on the treatment of active infection and suppression of recurrences, increasing emphasis is being placed on various approaches, including immunotherapy that might provide protection from disease transmission or possibly eliminate established latency.[47,48,55]

Palliative and supportive measures are the cornerstone of therapy for patients with genital herpes. Pain and discomfort usually respond to warm saline baths or the use of analgesics, antipyretics, or antipruritics; good genital hygiene can prevent the development of bacterial superinfection.

❹ Specific chemotherapeutic approaches to treating genital herpes include antiviral compounds, topical surfactants, photodynamic dyes, immune modulators, vaccines, and interferons. Few of these have undergone extensive evaluation, however, and only the antiviral agents have demonstrated any consistent clinical efficacy. The most recent CDC recommendations for the treatment of genital herpes include the antiviral agents acyclovir, valacyclovir, and famciclovir[1] (Table 115–10). The overall efficacy of these agents in treating genital HSV infection appears comparable, although once-daily valacyclovir and famciclovir regimens may have greater patient acceptability.[1,42–51,58]

◼ FIRST-EPISODE INFECTIONS

Oral formulations of acyclovir, famciclovir, and valacyclovir have demonstrated efficacy in reducing viral shedding, duration of symptoms, and time to healing of first-episode genital herpes infections, with maximal benefits seen when therapy is initiated at the earliest stages of infection.[1,44–48,58–61] Table 115–10 lists the recommended acyclovir, famciclovir, and valacyclovir oral regimens for first-episode infections. In immunocompromised patients or those with severe symptoms or complications necessitating hospitalization, parenteral acyclovir may be beneficial; however, the IV regimen has been associated with renal, gastrointestinal, bone marrow, and CNS toxicity, particularly in patients with renal dysfunction receiving high doses. No antiviral regimen is known to prevent latency or alter the subsequent frequency and severity of recurrences in humans.[1,42–51,61–64]

◼ RECURRENT INFECTIONS

CLINICAL CONTROVERSY

The role of antiviral agents in the treatment of most recurrent genital herpes episodes is controversial. Because signs and symptoms of recurrent infections generally are milder and of shorter duration than those of first-episode infections in immunocompetent hosts, demonstration of clinically important therapeutic benefits is difficult.

There are two approaches to management of recurrent episodes: episodic or chronic suppressive therapy.[1,47,50,51,55,56,61–64] Episodic therapy is initiated early during the course of the recurrence, preferably at the onset of prodromal symptoms, but no more than 24 hours after the appearance of lesions. In most patients, appreciable effects on symptomatology are not seen. Patients with prolonged episodes of recurrent infection or severe symptomatology are most likely to benefit from episodic therapy. Table 115–10 lists the recommended acyclovir, famciclovir, and valacyclovir suppressive regimens. Because of the relative mildness and brevity of recurrent infections, parenteral administration of acyclovir usually is not justifiable.[32,47,51,55,56]

Cost and the potential for adverse effects preclude available antiviral agents from being recommended routinely for use as suppressive therapy in all patients with recurrent genital herpes. Patients with frequent (greater than six per year) and physically or psychologically distressing recurrences, however, are candidates for suppressive therapy.[1,55,56,61–64]

Continuous therapy with recommended antivirals reduces the frequency and severity of recurrences in 70% to 90% of patients experiencing frequent recurrences. Asymptomatic viral shedding is markedly reduced in patients receiving suppressive therapy; however, the extent to which this decreases disease transmission to sexual partners remains to be determined. Despite antiviral suppressive therapy, low-level virus shedding still occurs. Since the frequency of recurrences tends to diminish over time, periodic "drug holidays" are advocated to assess changes in the underlying recurrence rate and determine if continued suppressive therapy is warranted.[1,55,56,61–64]

Resistant HSV isolates have been identified in some patients experiencing breakthrough recurrences while taking acyclovir. Although there is concern about the development of resistant strains

TABLE 115–10. Treatment of Genital Herpes

Type of Infection	Recommended Regimens[a,b]	Alternative Regimen
First clinical episode of genital herpes[c]	Acyclovir 400 mg PO 3 times daily for 7–10 days, *or* Acyclovir 200 mg PO 5 times daily for 7–10 days, *or* Famciclovir 250 mg PO 3 times daily for 7–10 days, *or* Valacyclovir 1 g PO 2 times daily for 7–10 days	Acyclovir 5–10 mg/kg IV every 8 hours for 2–7 days until clinical improvement occurs, followed by oral therapy to complete at least 10 days of total therapy[d]
First clinical episode of herpes proctitis or oral infection including stomatitis or pharyngitis	Acyclovir 400 mg PO 5 times daily for 7–10 days[e]	Acyclovir 5–10 mg/kg IV every 8 hours for 2–7 days until clinical improvement occurs, followed by oral therapy to complete at least 10 days of total therapy[d]
Recurrent infection Episodic therapy	Acyclovir 400 mg PO 3 times daily for 5 days,[f] *or* Acyclovir 800 mg PO 2 times daily for 5 days,[f] *or* Famciclovir 125 mg PO 2 times daily for 5 days,[f] *or* Valacyclovir 500 mg PO 2 times daily for 3–5 days,[f] *or* Valacyclovir 1 g PO once daily for 5 days[f] Acyclovir 400 mg PO twice daily,[g] *or*	
Suppressive therapy	Famciclovir 250 mg PO 2 times daily, *or* Valacyclovir 500 mg or 1000 mg PO once daily[h]	

[a]Recommendations are those of the CDC.
[b]HIV-infected patients may require more aggressive therapy.
[c]Primary or nonprimary first episode.
[d]Only for patients with severe symptoms or complications that necessitate hospitalization.
[e]Recommendations based on studies utilizing this dosage regimen rather than the lower dosage regimens recommended for first clinical episodes of genital herpes. It is not clear whether lower dosage regimens would have comparable efficacy. Famciclovir and valacyclovir are probably also effective for proctitis and oral infection, but clinical experience is limited.
[f]Requires initiation of therapy within 24 hours of lesion onset or during the prodrome that precedes some outbreaks.
[g]Indicated only for patients with frequent and/or severe recurrences; although safety and efficacy are documented in patients receiving acyclovir daily therapy for as long as 6 years and valacyclovir and famciclovir therapy for 1 year, it is recommended that therapy be discontinued periodically (e.g., once a year) to reassess the need for continued suppressive therapy.
[h]Valacyclovir 500 mg appears less effective than valacyclovir 1000 mg in patients with approximately 10 recurrences per year.

with suppressive therapy, clinical trials have found no evidence of cumulative toxicity or significant resistance in patients treated continuously with the recommended antivirals.[44,46,47,50,56,58,60,61]

■ SELECTED POPULATIONS

Immunocompromised patients are at greatest risk for severe and recurrent HSV infections. Acyclovir, valacyclovir, and famciclovir have been used to prevent reactivation of infection in patients seropositive for HSV who undergo transplantation procedures or induction chemotherapy for acute leukemia. Immunocompromised individuals, such as patients with AIDS, who fail treatment or prophylaxis with recommended antiviral doses frequently demonstrate improved response with higher doses. If resistance is suspected or confirmed with recommended first-line antivirals, foscarnet is usually effective. However, its use is associated with a greater risk of serious

adverse effects.[45,51,52,56] Lesional application of an extemporaneous compounded cidofovir gel or trifluridine ophthalmic solution appears to offer some benefits also.[1,43]

The safety of acyclovir, famciclovir, and valacyclovir during pregnancy is not established, although considerable experience with acyclovir in pregnant patients has produced no evidence of teratogenic effects. Because of the high maternal and infant morbidity associated with first-episode primary genital infections or severe recurrent infections at or near term, many clinicians advocate the use of systemic acyclovir as the standard of care in such cases; however, the effectiveness of such therapy is unknown. The use of acyclovir to suppress recurrent episodes near term is more controversial primarily because of the lack of data demonstrating significant benefits in this situation.[32,50,55,56,59–61]

With the increasing prevalence of genital herpes worldwide, the potential exists for widespread use and misuse of acyclovir, valacyclovir, and famciclovir, resulting in development of resistant HSV isolates. In vitro resistance to these three agents usually is mediated by alterations in viral thymidine kinase; most resistant isolates are either thymidine kinase–deficient or have altered thymidine kinase. The incidence and clinical implications of HSV resistance require further study particularly with respect to immunocompromised hosts, in whom resistance may develop with greater frequency and be of greater clinical importance. Unlike acyclovir, valacyclovir, and famciclovir, foscarnet does not require the presence of thymidine kinase to be effective.[47,50,52,55,56]

Numerous agents for the prophylaxis and treatment of genital herpes infections are being studied. Neither topical nor systemic interferons have demonstrated consistent beneficial effects in genital HSV infections; however, a reduction in pain and time of healing of lesions has been reported with an interferon preparation incorporated into a gel containing nonoxynol-9. Other treatments under investigation include cidofovir and immune modulators such as im-

iquimod and resiquimod.[47,53,56] Agents that can eliminate ganglionic latency and prevent recurrent HSV infections are not expected to be available in the near future. Development of vaccines capable of protecting against HSV infection has proved challenging given the relative lack of protection offered by humoral and cell-mediated immunity in preventing naturally occurring recurrent infections. Safety concerns with live attenuated virus vaccines resulted in research focused primarily on recombinant protein vaccines that have exhibited relatively poor immunogenicity. In recent years, investigations using replication-defective HSV mutants that are not pathogenic, as well as DNA vaccines that foster host cell uptake of foreign DNA that encode for an antigenic viral protein, have shown some promise in animal models. Use of heterologous vaccines (bacillus Calmette-Guérin and influenza vaccines) to stimulate the immune system in patients with recurrent genital herpes has proved of no significant benefit.[47,55,62-6]

EVALUATION OF THERAPEUTIC OUTCOMES

Available antiviral compounds are of greatest benefit in patients experiencing first-episode primary infections, immunocompromised patients, and patients with frequent or severe recurrent infections. Antivirals, however, are palliative and not curative, and patients receiving these agents should be monitored closely for adverse drug effects. CDC guidelines suggest that discontinuation of suppressive therapy after 1 year should be considered to assess for possible changes in the patient's intrinsic pattern of recurrence. In many patients, decreases in recurrence rates and the severity of symptoms occur over time. However, some clinicians prefer to continue suppressive therapy indefinitely because it significantly reduces asymptomatic viral shedding, a potential benefit in reducing the risk of disease transmission to uninfected sexual partners.[1,47,48,61]

TRICHOMONIASIS

EPIDEMIOLOGY AND ETIOLOGY

Trichomonas vaginalis, a flagellated, motile protozoan is responsible for 3 to 5 million cases of trichomoniasis annually in the United States.[65-68] Humans are host to two other *Trichomonas* species, *T. tenax* and *T. hominis,* but *T. vaginalis* is the only species thought to be pathogenic. Although infection by nonsexual contact is reported, it is rare. Contamination of inanimate objects and spread of infection via communal bathing or contact with infected bath or toilet articles is possible because *T. vaginalis* can survive for several hours on moist surfaces.[65-73] Neonatal infections also represent another possible nonvenereal route of disease transmission.[67-71,73,74]

Coinfection with other STDs is not unusual in patients diagnosed with trichomoniasis. Women infected with *T. vaginalis* are three times more likely to have gonorrhea than those who do not have trichomoniasis; approximately 20% of men with gonococcal urethritis also have trichomoniasis.[67,68] In patients treated appropriately for genital *C. trachomatis* or *U. urealyticum* infection, persistent urethritis can result from coexisting trichomonal infection.[1,70,71] Although not well documented, it is proposed that the inflammatory response produced by trichomoniasis may increased the risk of acquiring HIV.[66,68,74]

PATHOPHYSIOLOGY

Trichomonads typically can be isolated from the vagina, urethra, and paraurethral ducts and glands in the majority of infected women.

Infrequently, they are recovered from the endocervix. Extragenital sites are epidemiologically important because infection can persist and result in reinfection of the vagina if local therapy alone is used.[68,71,72] This may account for the higher relapse rates reported for local versus systemic therapy.[71,72,75] After attachment to the vaginal or urethral mucosa, trichomonads usually elicit an inflammatory response that manifests as a discharge containing large numbers of PMNs.[68-72]

CLINICAL PRESENTATION

Trichomonal infections are reported more commonly in women than in men. In part this may be due to the smaller number of organisms found in the male urethra making detection more difficult, greater disease transmission rates from males to females, and the nature of male infections, which have a high spontaneous cure rate even in the absence of treatment.[66,67,70-72] The typical clinical presentation of trichomoniasis in males and females is presented in Table 115-11.

DIAGNOSIS

T. vaginalis produces nonspecific symptoms also consistent with bacterial vaginosis; as a result, laboratory diagnosis is required. Because *T. vaginalis* requires a pH range of 4.9 to 7.5 for survival, a vaginal discharge pH of greater than 5.0 usually indicates the presence of either *T. vaginalis* or *Gardnerella vaginalis,* a common cause of bacterial vaginosis. The simplest and most reliable means of diagnosis is a wet-mount examination of the vaginal discharge.[67,70-72] Trichomoniasis is confirmed if characteristic pear-shaped, flagellating organisms are observed. The wet mount is only about 75% to 80% sensitive in detecting the presence of trichomonads, with lower sensitivities reported in men and in women with low-grade, subacute, or chronic infections.[68-70,72]

Although the presence of trichomonads may be reported on a Papanicolaou (Pap) smear, the sensitivity of this cytologic technique is less than for wet mount and also is associated with a number of false-positive results. Stained smears of cervical specimens have been used in diagnosis, but they are less sensitive and more time-consuming than the wet mount and therefore are not recommended. Culture techniques for trichomonads are highly specific and more sensitive than the wet mount, but they are not useful in rapid diagnosis because up to 48 hours or longer is necessary for growth. Cultures may be

TABLE 115–11. Presentation of Trichomonas Infections

	Males	Females
General	Incubation period 3–28 days Organism may be detectable within 48 hours after exposure to infected partner	Incubation period 3–28 days
Site of infection	Most common—urethra Others—rectum (usually due to rectal intercourse in MSM), oropharynx, eye	Most common—endocervical canal Others—urethra, rectum (usually due to perineal contamination), oropharynx, eye
Symptoms	May be asymptomatic (more common in males than females) or minimally symptomatic Urethral discharge (clear to mucopurulent) Dysuria, prurius	May be asymptomatic or minimally symptomatic Scant to copious, typically malodorous vaginal discharge (50–75%) and pruritus (worse during menses) Dysuria, dyspareunia
Signs	Urethral discharge	Vaginal discharge Vaginal pH 4.5–6 Inflammation/erythema of vulva, vagina, and/or cervix Urethritis
Complications	Epididymitis and chronic prostatitis (uncommon) Male infertility (decreased sperm motility and viability)	Pelvic inflammatory disease and associated complications (i.e., ectopic pregnancy, infertility) Premature labor, premature rupture of membranes, and low-birth-weight infants (risk of neonatal infections is low) Cervical neoplasia

necessary, however, to confirm the diagnosis in the absence of a positive wet mount or to determine antimicrobial susceptibility in intractable cases.[1,67–72]

Newer diagnostic tests such as monoclonal antibody or DNA probe techniques, as well as PCR tests that can detect small amounts of trichomonal DNA, have been developed. These tests are highly sensitive and specific for detecting infection in both urogenital specimens and urine. Such tests could replace more traditional diagnostic tests in the future.[66,68,71,72]

In males, demonstration of trichomonads in urethral specimens or urine sediment by wet mount is difficult, and diagnosis depends largely on culture. Specimens from males should be taken prior to first voiding because the small number of trichomonads in males may be reduced by micturition.[70–72]

▶ TREATMENT: Trichomoniasis

Recommended treatment regimens for *T. vaginalis* have changed little over the past 20 years. Metronidazole is the only antimicrobial agent available in the United States that is consistently effective in treating these infections. In only a few cases have *T. vaginalis* isolates been resistant to standard metronidazole doses. In these instances, longer courses of therapy or doses higher than those recommended routinely as initial therapy usually produce a cure.[1,67,68,70–76]

Table 115–12 provides treatment recommendations for *Trichomonas* infections.[1] The standard therapy for trichomoniasis is metronidazole 2 g orally as a single dose; cure rates are comparable with the recommended alternative regimen of 500 mg twice daily for 7 days. When sexual partners are treated simultaneously, cure rates greater than 95% are reported. If sexual partners are not treated concurrently, cure rates are somewhat lower. In limited clinical testing, single metronidazole doses of less than 1.5 g are associated with high failure rates.[1,65,67,68,70–77]

Advantages of single-dose therapy over the multidose alternative regimen include better patient compliance, lower total dose, lower cost, and shorter exposure of the patient's gastrointestinal and urogenital anaerobic bacterial flora to the drug. As a result of the latter, the likelihood of developing pseudomembranous colitis or symptomatic candidal vulvovaginitis is decreased.[68,69,71,76,77] Because high doses of metronidazole have mutagenic effects in bacteria and oncogenic effects in mice, a reduced time of exposure in humans may be beneficial. There is no conclusive evidence for either of these effects in humans after short-term therapy with recommended doses.[69,71,75,76] Gastrointestinal complaints (e.g., anorexia, nausea, vomiting, and diarrhea) are more common with the single 2-g dose, occurring in 5% to 10% of treated patients. Some patients also complain of a bitter metallic taste in the mouth. Patients intolerant of the single 2-g dose because of gastrointestinal adverse effects usually tolerate the multidose regimen.[68–73,74,76]

To achieve maximal cure rates and prevent relapse with the single 2-g dose of metronidazole, simultaneous treatment of infected sexual partners is necessary. In women treated with the alternative 7-day course, however, relapse rates are not appreciably different regardless of whether or not sexual partners are treated. It is speculated that in men, spontaneous resolution of trichomonal infection or a reduction in the number of trichomonads below the inoculum necessary to transmit disease may occur during the 7 days of a female's therapy. In patients who fail to respond to an initial course of metronidazole therapy, a second course of therapy with metronidazole 500 mg twice daily for 7 days is recommended. Patients refractory to a second course of treatment usually respond to a regimen using higher

TABLE 115–12. Treatment of Trichomoniasis

Type	Recommended Regimen[a]	Alternative Regimen
Symptomatic and asymptomatic infections	Metronidazole 2 g PO in a single dose[b]	Metronidazole 500 mg PO 2 times daily for 7 days[c]
Treatment in pregnancy	Metronidazole 2 g PO in a single dose[d]	
Neonatal infections[e]	Metronidazole 10–30 mg/kg daily for 5–8 days	

Note: Tinidazole was approved by the FDA in 2004 for the treatment of trichomonasis. The recommended dosage is 2 g PO in a single dose.

[a]Recommendations are those of the CDC.

[b]Treatment failures should be treated with metronidazole 500 mg PO 2 times daily for 7 days. Persistent failures should be managed in consultation with an expert. Metronidazole 2 g PO daily for 3–5 days has been effective in patients infected with *T. vaginalis* strains mildly resistant to metronidazole, but experience is limited; higher doses also have been used.

[c]Metronidazole labeling approved by the FDA does not include this regimen. Dosage regimens for treatment of trichomoniasis included in the product labeling are the single 2 g dose; 250 mg 3 times daily for 7 days; and 375 mg 2 times daily for 7 days. The 250 mg and 375 mg dosage regimens are currently not included in the CDC recommendations.

[d]Metronidazole is contraindicated in the first trimester of pregnancy. While the CDC recommends a single 2 g dose for treatment during pregnancy, a 7-day regimen is preferred by some since it produces lower peak serum drug concentrations.

[e]Only infants with symptomatic trichomoniasis or with urogenital trichomonal colonization that persists beyond the fourth week of life.

dosages of metronidazole (i.e., 2 to 4 grams daily for 3 to 14 days). Good response rates also are reported for metronidazole 2 to 3 g orally plus either a single 500-mg tablet administered intravaginally or intravaginal metronidazole gel (0.75%) for 7 to 14 days.[65,67,68,70–77] Topical vaginal therapy alone is associated with low cure rates because infections involving the urethra or periurethral glands are unaffected and can serve as source of reinfection.[67] Use of intravenous metronidazole may be warranted for rare cases of intolerance to oral medication or infections resistant to high-dose oral metronidazole. Sexual partners of all patients who require retreatment also should be treated or retreated because the majority of apparent treatment failures appear to be due to reinfection or noncompliance.[65,67,68,70–77]

Concerns regarding the use of metronidazole in women who are pregnant or breast-feeding have been raised. Because metronidazole is secreted in breast milk, it is recommended that breast-feeding be interrupted for 12 to 24 hours after maternal ingestion of a single 2-g dose.[1,70,74–77] Although metronidazole is contraindicated during the first trimester of pregnancy based on Food and Drug Administration (FDA)–approved labeling, and although some experts recommend avoiding its use throughout pregnancy, other experts advocate its use during any stage of pregnancy because of the potential adverse pregnancy outcomes associated with trichomoniasis.[1,74,75] Metronidazole easily crosses the placenta, and fetal blood levels are comparable with maternal levels. However, a clear association between terato-genic effects and maternal ingestion during pregnancy has not been shown.[1,68–70,74–76] No consensus exists on whether or how to treat trichomonas infections in pregnant women.

Various local therapies for trichomoniasis have been proposed, particularly for pregnant patients. Clotrimazole vaginal suppositories, 100 mg at bedtime for 1 to 2 weeks, relieve symptoms in many women and produce cure rates of 50% or greater.[68,72–74,76] An alternative therapy is gentle douching with either a diluted solution of vinegar or a 1% zinc sulfate solution until symptoms improve and then less frequently thereafter. This therapy generally provides some symptomatic improvement but few cures. Although once recommended, povidone-iodine douches should be avoided during pregnancy because of the risk of fetal thyroid suppression.[70,71,74,75]

Several 5-nitroimidazole antibiotics related to metronidazole (e.g., tinidazole, nimorazole, ornidazole, and carnidazole) are being investigated worldwide for the treatment of trichomoniasis. Unfortunately, none of these agents differs significantly from metronidazole in terms of efficacy or toxicity against metronidazole-susceptible strains of *T. vaginalis*. Tinidazole is reported to have produced cures in some metronidazole-resistant infections, but overall, cross-resistance between metronidazole and other 5-nitroimidazoles is high.[69–71,74,77] *Note:* Since this chapter was prepared, tinidazole was approved by the FDA for the treatment of trichomoniasis. The recommended dosage is 2 g orally as a single dose.

EVALUATION OF THERAPEUTIC OUTCOMES

Follow-up is considered unnecessary in patients who become asymptomatic after treatment with metronidazole. When patients remain symptomatic, it is important to determine if reinfection has occurred. In these cases, a repeat course of therapy, as well as identification and treatment or retreatment of infected sexual partners, is recommended. In situations in which reinfection can be excluded, a relative resistance to metronidazole should be assumed, and an alternative multidose metronidazole regimen should be prescribed. Culture and sensitivity are warranted for infections unresponsive to alternative metronidazole regimens.

HUMAN PAPILLOMAVIRUS AND OTHER STDs

Several STDs other than those just discussed occur with varying frequency in the United States and throughout the world. While an in-depth discussion of these diseases is beyond the scope of this chapter, Table 115–13 lists recommended treatment regimens.[1] Of notable

TABLE 115–13. Treatment Regimens for Miscellaneous Sexually Transmitted Diseases

Infection	Recommended Regimen[a]	Alternative Regimen
Chancroid (*Haemophilus ducreyi*)	Azithromycin 1 g PO in a single dose, or Ceftriaxone 250 mg IM in a single dose, or Ciprofloxacin 500 mg PO 2 times daily for 3 days,[b] or Erythromycin base 500 mg PO 4 times daily for 7 days	
Lymphogranuloma venereum	Doxycycline 100 mg PO 2 times daily for 21 days	Erythromycin base 500 mg PO 4 times daily for 21 days
Human Papillomavirus Infection: 　External genital warts	*Provider-Administered Therapies:* Cryotherapy (e.g., liquid nitrogen or cryoprobe), or Podophyllin 10–25% in compound tincture of benzoin applied to lesions; repeat weekly if necessary,[c,d] or Trichloroacetic acid (TCA) 80–90% or bichloroacetic acid (BCA) 80–90% applied to warts; repeat weekly if necessary, or Surgical removal (tangential scissor excision, tangential shave excision, curettage, or electrosurgery) *Patient-Applied Therapies:* Podofilox 0.5% solution or gel applied 2 times daily for 3 days, followed by 4 days of no therapy; cycle is repeated as necessary for a total of 4 cycles,[d] or Imiquimod 5% cream applied at bedtime 3 times weekly for up to 16 weeks[d]	Intralesional interferon or laser surgery
Human Papillomavirus Infection: 　Vaginal, urethral meatus, and anal warts	Cryotherapy with liquid nitrogen, or TCA or BCA 80–90% as for external HPV warts; repeat weekly as necessary (*not* for urethral meatus warts) or Podophyllin 10–25% in compound tincture of benzoin applied at weekly intervals (*not* for vaginal or anal warts),[d] or Surgical removal (*not* for vaginal or urethral meatus warts)	

[a]Recommendations are those of the CDC.
[b]Ciprofloxacin is contraindicated for pregnant and lactating women and for persons aged <18 years.
[c]Some experts recommended washing podophyllin off after 1–4 hours to minimize local irritation.
[d]Safety during pregnancy is not established.

importance among these other STDs, however, is genital human papillomavirus (HPV) infection, the most common viral STD in the United States. More than 80 HPV types have been characterized by genomic makeup, with approximately 30 types associated with genital tract lesions.[78–81] Of these, types 6 and 11 are associated most commonly with the development of low-grade dysplasia manifested as exophytic genital warts. In most individuals, genital infection with HPV is subclinical, and patients with visible acuminate warts represent less than 1% of all infected individuals. When present, genital warts can be large and multifocal, producing variable degrees of discomfort. Based on HPV DNA detection methods, most warts will regress spontaneously within 1 to 2 years of their initial appearance. However, reinfection is common in young, sexually active populations.[1,80,81]

Infection with several HPV types, particularly HPV-16, HPV-18, and HPV-45, is considered the major risk factor for the development of cervical neoplasia, the second most common cancer in women worldwide. While epidemiologic, virologic, and clinical data strongly support this association, HPV infection alone is insufficient to cause cervical cancer development because only a small percentage of infected women develop the disease. It appears that the interplay of host immune defenses, genetic factors, and infection with HPV types containing a more aggressive variant all contribute to the risk of developing cervical neoplasia.[78–81]

The Pap smear is the most cost-effective and frequently used diagnostic test for HPV. It can detect abnormal cytology in patients with clinical manifestations and those with subclinical disease (i.e., no overt condylomata) but not latent HPV infection. Visual inspection of genital surfaces under magnification can assist in making the diagnosis. Various tests for detecting HPV DNA, although not used routinely, also are available.[78–81]

No consensus exists on the best approach to treating patients with genital HPV infection, particularly because most cases appear to be transient with spontaneous regression of lesions. A number of treatments are recommended (see Table 115–13), but none is clearly superior to the others. Treatment generally is directed toward patients with manifestations of genital warts, with the goal of removing or destroying these lesions and grossly infected surrounding tissue. Because such treatment neither stops viral expression in surrounding tissue nor eliminates viral latency, recurrence of lesions is not uncommon.[78–81]

The development of a vaccine against HPV is a major focus of research related to genital HPV infections. An important consideration in vaccine development is the need to incorporate viral particles from multiple HPV types because there is limited cross-protection between the different HPV types known to cause genital infections. Current research emphasis is on the development of polyvalent vaccines that would offer protection against the most common types of HPV, as well as those types known to be associated with cervical cancer. Additionally, therapeutic vaccines aimed at either suppressing replicating virus or reversing neoplastic transformation in infected individuals are being evaluated.[78,81]

CONCLUSION

More than 20 different diseases have been identified for which sexual transmission is epidemiologically important. For most STDs, curative drug therapies are available; however, therapeutic approaches to viral STDs, such as genital herpes, provide only palliation and suppression of symptoms. Technologic advances in laboratory medicine have resulted in improved and more rapid diagnostic capabilities for many STDs. These advances are of particular importance for individuals with undiagnosed, asymptomatic disease who comprise a vast reservoir for continued disease transmission. Sexually active persons can reduce their risk of transmitting or acquiring an STD by avoidance of unsafe sexual practices, maintaining a mutually monogamous sexual relationship, or proper use of physical barriers during intercourse. In the future, vaccines providing protection from common STDs may have a significant effect on reducing the incidence of these infections.

ABBREVIATIONS

CDC: Centers for Disease Control and Prevention
CSF: cerebrospinal fluid
DFA: direct fluorescent monoclonal antibody
DFA-TP: direct fluorescent-antibody test
DGI: disseminated gonorrhea infection
EIA: enzyme immunoassay
FDA: Food and Drug Administration
FTA-ABS: flourescent treponemal antibody absorption
HIV: human immunodeficiency virus
HPV: human papillomavirus
HSV: herpes simplex virus
HSV-1: herpes simplex virus type 1
HSV-2: herpes simplex virus type 2
LCR: ligase chain reaction
MHA-TP: microhemagglutination assay for antibodies to
   T. pallidum
MSM: men who have sex with men
NGU: nongonococcal urethritis
Pap: Papanicolaou
PCR: polymerase chain reaction
PID: pelvic inflammatory disease
RPR: rapid plasma reagin
STD: sexually transmitted disease
TPHA: *T. pallidum* hemagglutination assay
TPPA: *T. pallidum* particle agglutination assay
TRUST: tuluidine red unheated serum test
USR: unheated serum reagin
VDRL: Veneral Disease Research Laboratory

Review Questions and other resources can be found at *www.pharmacotherapyonline.com*.

REFERENCES

1. Anonymous. Sexually transmitted diseases treatment guidelines 2002. MMWR 2002;51(RR-6):1–82.
2. Holmes KK, Handsfield HH. Sexually transmitted diseases: Overview and clinical approach. In: Braunwald E, Fauci AS, Kasper DL, et al, eds. Harrison's Principles of Internal Medicine, 15th ed. New York, McGraw-Hill, 2001:839–848.
3. Braverman PK. Sexually transmitted diseases in adolescents. Med Clin North Am 2000;84:869–889.
4. Handsfield HH. Sex, science, and society: A look at sexually transmitted diseases. Postgrad Med 1997;101:268–273, 277–278.
5. Rietmeijer CA, McMillan A. Some aspects of the prevention of sexually transmissible infections. In: McMillan A, Young H, Ogilvie MM, Scott GR, eds. Clinical Practice in Sexually Transmissible Infections. London, Saunders, 2002:11–28.
6. Gilliam ML, Derman RJ. Barrier methods of contraception. Obstet Gynecol Clin North Am 2000;27:841–858.
7. Roddy RE, Zekeng L, Ryan KA, et al. Effect of nonoxynol-9 gel on urogenital gonorrhea and chlamydial infection: A randomized, controlled trial. JAMA 2002;287:1117–1122.
8. Stone A. Microbicides: A new approach to preventing HIV and other sexually transmitted infections. Nat Rev Drug Discov 2002;1:977–985.
9. Anonymous. Summary of notifiable diseases, United States, 2001. MMWR 2001;50(53):1–136.
10. Ram S, Rice PA. Gonococcal infections. In: Braunwald E, Fauci AS, Kasper DL, et al, eds. Harrison's Principles of Internal Medicine, 15th ed. New York, McGraw-Hill, 2001:931–937.
11. Sparling PF, Handsfield HH. *Neisseria gonorrhoeae.* In: Mandell GL, Bennett JE, Dolin R, eds. Principles and Practice of Infectious Diseases, 5th ed. New York, Churchill-Livingstone, 2000:2242–2257.
12. Emmert DH, Kirchner JT. Sexually transmitted diseases in women: Gonorrhea and syphilis. Postgrad Med 2000;107:181–197.
13. Marrazzo JM. Infections due to *Neisseria.* In: Federman DD, Dale DC, eds. WebMD Scientific American Medicine (Internet). New York, WebMD Corporation, 2004; available at *http://online.statref.com/document.aspx?fxid=48&docid=1019.*
14. Anonymous. Screening tests to detect *Chlamydia trachomatis* and *Nesisseria gonorrhoeae* infections—2002. MMWR 2002;51(RR-15):1–39.
15. Lyss SB, Kamb ML, Peterman TA, et al. *Chlamydia trachomatis* among patients infected with and treated for *Neisseria gonorrhoeae* in sexually transmitted disease clinics in the United States. Ann Intern Med 2003;139:178–185.
16. Dicker LW, Mosure DJ, Berman SM, et al. Gonorrhea prevalence and coinfection with chlamydia in women in the United States, 2000. Sex Transm Dis 2003;30:472–476.
17. Koumans EH, Johnson RE, Knapp JS, St Louis ME. Laboratory testing for *Neisseria gonorrhoeae* by recently introduced nonculture tests: A performance review with clinical and public health considerations. Clin Infect Dis 1998;27:1171–1180.
18. Fox KK, Cohen MS. Gonococcal, chlamydial, and mycoplasma urethritis. In: Cohen J, Powderly WG, Berkley SF, et al, eds. Infectious Diseases, 2d ed. St Louis, Mosby, 2003:795–805.
19. Young H, McMillan A. Gonorrhea. In: McMillan A, Young H, Ogilvie MM, Scott GR, eds. Clinical Practice in Sexually Transmissible Infections. London, Saunders, 2002:313–356.
20. Smith J, Finn A. Antimicrobial prophylaxis. Arch Dis Child 1999;80:388–392.
21. Singh AE, Romanowski B. Syphilis: Review with emphasis on clinical, epidemiologic, and some biologic features. Clin Microbiol Rev 1999;12:187–209.
22. Golden MR, Marra CM, Holmes KK. Update on syphilis: Resurgence of an old problem. JAMA 2003;290:1510–1514.
23. Lukehart SA. Syphilis. In: Braunwald E, Fauci AS, Kasper DL, et al, eds. Harrison's Principles of Internal Medicine, 15th ed. New York, McGraw-Hill, 2001:1044–1052.
24. Young H, McMillan A. Syphilis and the endemic treponematoses. In: McMillan A, Young H, Ogilvie MM, Scott GR, eds. Clinical Practice in Sexually Transmissible Infections. London, W.B. Saunders, 2002:395–456.
25. Kinghorn GR. Syphilis. In: Cohen J, Powderly WG, Berkley SF, et al, eds. Infectious Diseases, 2d ed. St Louis, Mosby, 2003:807–816.
26. Birnbaum NR, Goldschmidt RH, Buffett WO. Resolving the common clinical dilemmas of syphilis. Am Fam Phys 1999;59:2233–2240, 2245–2246.

7. Wicher K, Horowitz HW, Wicher V. Laboratory methods of diagnosis of syphilis for the beginning of the third millennium. Microbes Infect 1999;1:1035–1049.

8. Clyne B, Jerrard DA. Syphilis testing. J Emerg Med 2000;18:361–367.

9. Pao D, Goh BT, Bingham JS. Management issues in syphilis. Drugs 2002;61:1447–1461.

0. Kirchner JT, Emmert DH. Sexually transmitted diseases in women: *Chlamydia trachomatis* and herpes simplex infections. Postgrad Med 2000:107:55–58, 61–65.

1. Jones RB, Batteiger BE. *Chlamydia trachomatis* (trachoma, perinatal infections, lymphogranuloma venereum, and other genital infections). In: Mandell GL, Bennett JE, Dolin R, eds. Principles and Practice of Infectious Diseases, 5th ed. New York, Churchill-Livingstone, 2000: 1989–2004.

2. Stamm WE. Chlamydial infections. In: Braunwald E, Fauci AS, Kasper DL, et al, eds. Harrison's Principles of Internal Medicine, 15th ed. New York, McGraw-Hill, 2001:1075–1081.

3. Fox KK, Cohen MS. Gonococcal, chlamydial and *Mycoplasma* urethritis. In: Cohen J, Powderly WG, Berkley SF, et al, eds. Infectious Diseases, 2d ed. St Louis, Mosby, 2003:795–805.

4. McMillan A, Ballard RC. Non-specific genital tract infection and chlamydial infection, including lymphogranuloma venereum. In: McMillan A, Young H, Ogilvie MM, Scott GR, eds. Clinical Practice in Sexually Transmissible Infections. London, Saunders, 2002:281–312.

5. Morton RS, Kinghorn GR. Genitourinary chlamydial infection: A reappraisal and hypothesis. Int J STD AIDS 1999;10:765–775.

6. Anonymous. National guideline for the management of *Chlamydia trachomatis* genital tract infection. Sex Transm Infect 1999;75(suppl 1): 4–8S.

7. Peipert JF. Genital chlamydial infections. N Engl J Med 2003;349: 2424–2430.

8. Hollblad-Fadiman K, Goldman SM. American College of Preventive Medicine practice policy statement: Screening for *Chlamydia trachomatis*. Am J Prev Med 2003;24:287–292.

9. Ostergaard L. Microbiological aspects of the diagnosis of *Chlamydia trachomatis*. Best Pract Res Clin Obstet Gynaecol 2002;16:789–799.

0. Watson EJ, Templeton A, Russell I, et al. The accuracy and efficacy of screening tests for *Chlamydia trachomatis*: A systematic review. J Med Microbiol 2002;51:1021–1031.

1. Guaschino S, Ricci G. How, and how efficiently, can we treat *Chlamydia trachomatis* infections in women? Best Pract Res Clin Obstet Gynaecol 2002:16:875–888.

2. Anonymous. Drugs for sexually transmitted infections. Med Lett Drugs Ther 1999;41:85–90.

3. McMillan A, Ogilvie MM. Herpes simplex virus infection. In: McMillan A, Young H, Ogilvie MM, Scott GR, eds. Clinical Practice in Sexually Transmissible Infections. London, Saunders, 2002:107–144.

4. Corey L. Herpes simplex virus. In: Mandell GL, Bennett JE, Dolin R, eds. Principles and Practice of Infectious Diseases, 5th ed. New York, Churchill-Livingstone, 2000:1564–1580.

5. Marques AR, Straus SE. Herpes simplex type 2 infections: An update. Dis Month 2000;46:325–359.

6. Sacks SL. Improving the management of genital herpes. Hosp Pract (Off Ed) 1999;34:41–49.

7. Goade D. Genital herpes. In: Cohen J, Powderly WG, Berkley SF, et al, eds. Infectious Diseases, 2d ed. St Louis, Mosby, 2003:817–826.

8. Corey L. Herpes simplex viruses. In: Braunwald E, Fauci AS, Kasper DL, et al, eds. Harrison's Principles of Internal Medicine, 15th ed. New York, McGraw-Hill, 2001:1100–1106.

9. Dwyer DE, Cunningham AL. Herpes simplex and varicella-zoster virus infections. Med J Aust 2002;177:267–273.

0. Whitley RJ, Roizman B. Herpes simplex virus infections. Lancet 2001; 357:1513–1518.

1. Simmons A. Clinical manifestations and treatment considerations of herpes simplex virus infection. J Infect Dis 2002;186(suppl 1):S71–77.

2. Ashley RL, Wald A. Genital herpes: Review of the epidemic and potential use of type-specific serology. Clin Microbiol Rev 1999;12:1–8.

53. Leung DT, Sacks SL. Current recommendations for the treatment of genital herpes. Drugs 2000;60:1329–1352.

54. Geers TA, Isada CM. Update on antiviral therapy for genital herpes infection. Cleve Clin J Med 2000;67:567–573.

55. Wald A, Ashley-Morrow R. Serological testing for herpes simplex virus (HSV)-1 and HSV-2 infection. Clin Infect Dis 2002;35(suppl 2): S173–182.

56. Wald A. Testing for genital herpes: How, who, and why. Curr Clin Top Infect Dis 2002;22:166–180.

57. Scoular A. Using the evidence base on genital herpes: Optimising the use of diagnostic tests and information provision. Sex Transm Infect 2002;78:160–165.

58. Patel R. Progress in meeting today's demands in genital herpes: An overview of current management. J Infect Dis 2002;186(suppl 1):S47–56.

59. Scott LL. Prevention of perinatal herpes: prophylactic antiviral therapy? Clin Obstet Gynecol 1999;42:134–148.

60. Corey L. Challenges in genital herpes simplex virus management. J Infect Dis 2002;186(suppl 1):S29–33.

61. Mills J, Mindel A. Genital herpes simplex infections: Some therapeutic dilemmas. Sex Transm Dis 2003;30:232–233.

62. Krause PR, Straus SE. Herpesvirus vaccines: Development, controversies, and applications. Infect Dis Clin North Am 1999;13:61–81.

63. Snoeck R, De Clercq E. New treatments for genital herpes. Curr Opin Infect Dis 2002;15:49–55.

64. Miller RL, Tomai MA, Harrison CJ, Bernstein DI. Immunomodulation as a treatment strategy for genital herpes: Review of the evidence. Int Immunopharmacol 2002;2:443–451.

65. Weller PF. Protozoal intestinal infections and trichomoniasis. In: Braunwald E, Fauci AS, Kasper DL, et al, eds. Harrison's Principles of Internal Medicine, 15th ed. New York, McGraw-Hill, 2001:1227–1230.

66. Soper D. Trichomoniasis: Under control or undercontrolled? Am J Obstet Gynecol 2004;190:281–290.

67. Sobel JD. Vaginitis, vulvitis, cervicitis and cutaneous vulval lesions. In: Cohen J, Powderly WG, Berkley SF, et al, eds. Infectious Diseases, 2d ed. St Louis, Mosby, 2003:683–691.

68. McMillan A. Vaginal infections and vulvodynia. In: McMillan A, Young H, Ogilvie MM, Scott GR, eds. Clinical Practice in Sexually Transmissible Infections. London, Saunders, 2002:473–516.

69. Rein MF. *Trichomonas vaginalis*. In: Mandell GL, Bennett JE, Dolin R, eds. Principles and Practice of Infectious Diseases, 5th ed. New York, Churchill-Livingstone, 2000:2894–2898.

70. Petrin D, Delgaty K, Bhattt R, Garber G. Clinical and microbiological aspects of *Trichomonas vaginalis*. Clin Microbiol Rev 1998;11:300–317.

71. Schwebke JR. Update on trichomoniasis. Sex Transm Infect 2002;78: 378–379.

72. Carr PL, Felsenstein D, Friedman RH. Evaluation and management of vaginitis. J Gen Intern Med 1998;13:335–346.

73. Faro S. Vaginitis: Differential Diagnosis and Management. Boca Raton, FL, Parthenon Publishing, 2004:67–92.

74. Cleveland A. Vaginitis: Finding the cause prevents treatment failure. Cleve Clin J Med 2000;67:634, 637–642, 645–646.

75. Sobel JD. Vaginitis. N Engl J Med 1997;337:1896–1903.

76. Forna F, Gulmezoglu AM. Interventions for treating trichomoniasis in women. Cochrane Database Syst Rev 2003(3).

77. Spence MR, Harwell TS, Davies MC, Smith JL. The minimum single oral metronidazole dose for treating trichomoniasis: A randomized, blinded study. Obstet Gynecol 1997;89:699–703.

78. Carr J, Gyorfi T. Human papillomavirus: Epidemiology, transmission, and pathogenesis. Clin Lab Med 2000;20:235–255.

79. Gunter J. Genital and perianal warts: New treatment opportunities for human papillomavirus infection. Am J Obstet Gynecol 2003;189(suppl 3): S3–11.

80. Eiley DJ, Douglas J, Beutner K, et al. External genital warts: Diagnosis, treatment, and prevention. Clin Infect Dis 2002;35(suppl 2): S210–224.

81. Zanotii KM, Belinson J. Update on the diagnosis and treatment of human papillomavirus infection. Cleve Clin J Med 2002;69:948–961.

116

BONE AND JOINT INFECTIONS

Edward P. Armstrong and Leslie L. Barton

Learning Objectives and other resources can be found at *www.pharmacotherapyonline.com.*

KEY CONCEPTS

❶ The most common cause of osteomyelitis (particularly that acquired by hematogenous spread) and infectious arthritis is *Staphylococcus aureus*.

❷ Culture and susceptibility information are essential as a guide for antimicrobial treatment of osteomyelitis and infectious arthritis.

❸ Joint aspiration and examination of synovial fluid are extremely important to evaluate the possibility of infectious arthritis.

❹ The most important treatment modality of acute osteomyelitis is the administration of appropriate antibiotics in adequate doses for a sufficient length of time.

❺ Antibiotics generally are given in high doses so that adequate antimicrobial concentrations are reached within infected bone and joints.

❻ The standard duration of antimicrobial treatment for osteomyelitis is 4 to 6 weeks.

❼ Oral antimicrobial therapy may be used for osteomyelitis to complete a parenteral regimen in children who have had a good clinical response to intravenous antibiotics and in adults without diabetes mellitus or peripheral vascular disease when the organism is susceptible to the oral antimicrobial, a suitable oral agent is available, and compliance is ensured.

❽ The three most important therapeutic maneuvers in the management of infectious arthritis are appropriate antibiotics, joint drainage, and joint rest.

Bone and joint infections are comprised of two disease processes known, respectively, as *osteomyelitis* and *septic,* or *infectious, arthritis.* As such, they are unique and separate infectious entities with different signs and symptoms and infecting organisms. Despite advances in therapy, however, these infections continue to cause significant morbidity from residual damage and chronic recurring infections. Emphasis on initiating antibiotic therapy as soon as possible is important in reducing long-term complications.

EPIDEMIOLOGY

Osteomyelitis generally is an uncommon disease. One classic publication reported that 247 patients had osteomyelitis in a prominent American teaching hospital during a 4-year period.[1] Acute osteomyelitis has an estimated annual incidence of 0.1 per 1000 children.[2] Osteomyelitis caused by contiguous spread, including postoperative, direct puncture, and that associated with adjacent soft tissue infections, comprises 47% of infections. Hematogenous osteomyelitis comprises 19% of infections, and osteomyelitis occurring in patients with significant peripheral vascular disease comprises 34% of infections. A review of osteomyelitis cases based on duration of disease shows that acute disease constitutes 56% of patients and that chronic osteomyelitis, defined as having a previous hospitalization for the same infection, constitutes 44% of patients.

Infectious or septic arthritis is an inflammatory reaction within the joint space. Distinct from osteomyelitis, septic arthritis is a more common disease and is known to be one of the most common causes of new cases of arthritis. One study identified 1158 cases of septic arthritis in a 4-year period.[3] Another hospital study reported 64 children with septic arthritis during a 6-year time frame.[4] A study from The Netherlands estimated the incidence of bacterial arthritis to be 5.7 cases per year per 100,000 inhabitants.[5]

ETIOLOGY

OSTEOMYELITIS

The most common method of classifying osteomyelitis is based on the route in which the infecting organism reaches the bone. Infection that results from spread through the bloodstream is termed *hematogenous osteomyelitis.* When the organism reaches the bone from an adjoining soft tissue infection, it is termed *contiguous osteomyelitis.* Osteomyelitis that results from direct inoculation, such as from trauma, puncture wounds, or surgery, generally is also classified under the contiguous osteomyelitis category. Patients with peripheral vascular disease are at risk for the development of osteomyelitis, and these patients often are separated into a third distinct category because of their unique management features.

Osteomyelitis also may be classified based on the duration of the disease. Acute osteomyelitis describes infections of recent onset, usually several days to 1 week, whereas chronic infections are those of a longer duration. Some authors describe chronic infections as those with symptoms for more than 1 month before therapy, whereas other authors define chronic infections as relapse of an initial infection. Yet a third system sometimes used to classify osteomyelitis is based on the anatomic location of the infection (medullary or superficial) and the physiologic status of the patient (otherwise healthy, systemic immunologic compromise, local immunologic compromise).[6,7] This classification system may be useful when comparing patients among different studies and attempting to categorize the severity of infection.

INFECTIOUS ARTHRITIS

Infectious arthritis may occur from many different types of microorganisms. Most infecting organisms are known to produce an infection in a single joint, termed *monarticular infections;* however, infections also may involve two or more joints.[8] As with osteomyelitis, joint infections also may be classified according to the mechanisms by which the infecting organism reaches the joint. Infectious arthritis may result from the spread of an adjacent bone infection, direct contamination of the joint space, or hematogenous dissemination. Hematogenous spread of the disease comprises the majority of infections; spread from osteomyelitis and direct inoculation is much less frequent.[9] Infectious arthritis occurs most commonly in patients older than age 16; 24% of cases occur in children 15 years of age or younger.[10]

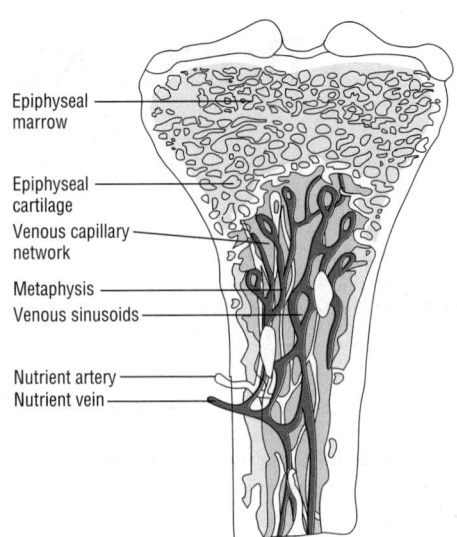

FIGURE 116–1. Cross-section of normal bone.

PATHOPHYSIOLOGY

HEMATOGENOUS OSTEOMYELITIS

Hematogenous osteomyelitis is described classically as a disease of children because most cases occur in patients younger than 16 years of age.[7] Table 116–1 summarizes the primary characteristics of osteomyelitis. Less commonly, these infections occur in adults. One exception, vertebral osteomyelitis, involves the vertebrae and occurs most frequently in patients older than 50 years of age.

Unique features of the anatomy and physiology of some bones appear to predispose them to become infected.[11] The vascular structure within the long bones appears to predispose the bone for hematogenous infections to begin within the metaphyses (Fig. 116–1). The nutrient arteries of the long bones divide within the medullary canal of the bone into small arterioles. These end in hairpin turns near the growth plate and flow into veins, of much wider diameter, that drain the medullary cavity.[1] An infection in hematogenous disease is initiated within the bend of the arterioles. There is considerable slowing of blood flow passing through the hairpin turns within the arterioles and then into the wider venous structures. This sludging of blood flow allows bacteria present within the bloodstream to settle and initiate an inflammatory response. In addition to these structural

features, there also appears to be less active phagocytosis within the metaphysis. After the bacteria settle in the bone, avascular necrosis may occur from occlusion of the nutrient vessels and release of bacterial enzymes.

In addition to these anatomic and functional features, there is some evidence that trauma is associated with developing an infection in specific bones. Children who develop hematogenous osteomyelitis may report some type of trauma as an etiologic event. Animal data also indicate that traumatized bone is more likely to become infected than normal bone.

Once the infection is initiated, exudate begins to form within the bone, which produces increased pressure. The age of the patient largely determines the next stage in the pathophysiology. In children older than 12 to 18 months, the infection that started in the metaphysis of a long bone is prevented from spreading into the joint because of the growth plate; however, the exudate often expands laterally through the thin outer cortex of the bone and raises the loose periosteum. The periosteum is thick and not easily broken, and the resulting pus usually remains subperiosteal. If there is significant periosteal damage, a soft-tissue abscess may develop. Impairment of blood flow to the outer portion of the cortical bone may occur, producing dead bone that separates from healthy bone, termed *sequestra*. The elevated periosteum remains viable because its blood supply, derived from the

TABLE 116–1. Types of Osteomyelitis, Age Distribution, Common Sites, and Risk Factors

Type of Osteomyelitis	Typical Age (yr)	Site(s) Involved	Risk Factors
Hematogenous	Less than 1	Long bones and joints	Prematurity, umbilical catheter or venous cutdown, respiratory distress syndrome, perinatal asphyxia
	1–20	Long bones (femur, tibia, humerus)	Infection (pharyngitis, cellulitis, respiratory infections), trauma, sickle cell disease, puncture wounds to feet
	Older than 50	Vertebrae	Diabetes mellitus, blunt trauma to spine, urinary tract infection
Contiguous	Older than 50	Femur, tibia, mandible	Hip fractures, open fractures
Vascular insufficiency	Older than 50	Feet, toes	Diabetes mellitus, peripheral vascular disease, pressure sores

overlying muscle, is unaffected. The raised periosteum will continue to produce bone; however, this new bone is now separated from the cortex because the periosteum has been raised from the infection. This new bone is termed *involucrum.*

In adults, the periosteum is tightly bound, and the cortex is thick. These anatomic features generally cause the infections to remain intramedullary. As expected, subperiosteal abscess formations are less common in this population. The infection may spread to adjacent bone structures through the Haversian and Volkmann canals. Chronic osteomyelitis is more likely to occur if large segments of bone become avascular and necrotic.

Neonatal patients also have unique characteristics. In these patients, there are blood vessels that spread through the cortex of the metaphyses and up into the epiphyses. This enables an infection that started within the metaphyseal area to spread easily to involve the epiphyses and then into the joint. Therefore, in infants, not only can the infection spread to involve the periosteum and the shaft as in children, but the infection also can spread to involve the joint.

Hematogenous osteomyelitis also is known to have a predilection for certain bones. The specific bones most likely to be involved also depend on the age of the patient. Children most commonly develop infections within the femur, tibia, humerus, and fibula.[12] Vertebral infections are more common in patients older than 50 years of age. Neonatal infections commonly involve multiple bones.

◀ The bacteriology of hematogenous osteomyelitis is unique compared with osteomyelitis caused by other routes of infection. A single organism is responsible for the vast majority of hematogenous infections. *Staphylococcus aureus* is isolated most frequently with hematogenous infections in children. In immunocompetent children who have been fully vaccinated with the *Hemophilus influenzae* type b vaccine, this is now an uncommon pathogen causing bone and joint infections.[13] However, neonatal osteomyelitis has a wider spectrum of infecting organisms.[14] The three most common etiologic agents are *S. aureus,* group B *Streptococcus,* and *Escherichia coli.* The infections from *S. aureus* and *E. coli* have been linked to complications occurring during pregnancy or delivery, and they are involved most frequently in multiple-bone infections.

Vertebral osteomyelitis has several unique features. Vertebral osteomyelitis occurs most commonly in adults 50 to 60 years of age. The lumbar and thoracic regions are the locations of most infections. Hematogenous infections are most likely to develop in the vascular areas near the subchondral plate region of the vertebral body. Staphylococci cause approximately 60% of these infections; however, gram-negative organisms now play a significant role. It is presumed that these gram-negative organisms, particularly *E. coli,* most likely originate within the urinary tract. *E. coli* vertebral infections have been associated with urinary tract infections, positive urine cultures, and bacteremias. *Mycobacterium tuberculosis* also is known to cause infections in the spine. Skin and respiratory tract infections are other foci of infections known to lead to vertebral infections.

A unique category of osteomyelitis patients consists of individuals with a history of intravenous drug abuse. More than 50% of the osteomyelitis infections in this group of patients are found in the vertebral column. Less than 20% of infections are located in either the sternoarticular or pelvic girdle. Infections are much less frequent within the extremities. An unusual feature of osteomyelitis in the intravenous drug-abusing population is the spectrum of organisms. Gram-negative organisms are responsible for 88% of infections. *Pseudomonas aeruginosa,* either singly or in combination with other organisms, is cultured in 78% of all infections. *Klebsiella, Enterobacter,* and *Serratia* also may be found but less commonly.

In addition, staphylococcal and streptococcal organisms may be cultured.

Patients with sickle cell anemia and related hemoglobinopathies have a much higher rate of infection with *Salmonella* as compared with other populations. *Salmonella* spp. are responsible for two-thirds of the infections in these patients. Bowel infarctions from the sickle cell disease may facilitate salmonellae entry into the bloodstream from the colon and spread hematogenously to the bone. Osteomyelitis in patients with sickle cell disease may occur in any bone, but it is observed to be most common in the medullary cavity of long or tubular bones. Because of the difficulty in separating bone pain during a sickle cell crisis from that of an infection, osteomyelitis may be relatively advanced in these patients when the diagnosis is made. Although salmonellae are cultured most frequently, staphylococci and other gram-negative organisms also may be isolated.

CONTIGUOUS-SPREAD OSTEOMYELITIS

This category of osteomyelitis includes infections caused by direct entrance of organisms from a source outside the body or progressive spread of an infection from tissue adjacent to the bone. Penetrating wounds (e.g., trauma), open fractures, and various invasive orthopedic procedures may result in direct inoculation of organisms into the bone. Infections also may occur secondary to pressure ulcers.[15] More than 80% of cases of postoperative osteomyelitis are known to occur following open reductions of fractures. Specifically, these infections occur most commonly after internal fixation of a hip fracture or femoral or tibial shaft fracture.

Osteomyelitis secondary to an adjoining soft tissue infection comprises another very important group of contiguous infections and most often involves the fingers and toes. Less commonly, infections may spread from infected teeth to involve the mandible or occur secondary to sinus infections by spreading through the mucosal lining of the sinuses into the vascular system surrounding the bone.

In contrast to hematogenous osteomyelitis, which occurs most commonly in children, contiguous-spread osteomyelitis occurs most commonly in patients older than age 50. Most likely this is so because important predisposing factors, such as hip fractures, are more common in this age group.

Contiguous-spread disease has several important differences compared with hematogenous osteomyelitis. Although *S. aureus* is still the most common organism isolated, infections with multiple organisms, including gram-negative bacilli, occur frequently. *P. aeruginosa, Proteus, Streptococcus, E. coli, S. epidermidis,* and anaerobes all may be isolated. One important exception to this wide range of organisms is puncture wounds of the feet. There is a strong correlation between puncture wounds of the feet and gram-negative osteomyelitis (often classified as *osteochondritis*), especially infections caused by *P. aeruginosa.*[16]

Patients with osteomyelitis in association with severe vascular insufficiency are extremely difficult to manage.[17,18] As anticipated, most of these patients have diabetes mellitus or severe atherosclerosis, and they develop their infections from contiguous-spread mechanisms. Generally, these patients are between the ages of 50 and 70 years when they develop osteomyelitis. Frequently, patients with vascular disease develop osteomyelitis in their toes and fingers, and there is usually an adjacent area of infection, such as cellulitis or dermal ulcers.

Another important characteristic of osteomyelitis in association with vascular insufficiency is the spectrum of infecting organisms.

Infections in these patients almost always include multiple organisms. The mixed-flora infections often include *Staphylococcus* and *Streptococcus* or the combination of *Staphylococcus, Streptococcus,* and Enterobacteriaceae. Enterococci and anaerobic organisms also may be seen.

Anaerobic organisms also play a role in osteomyelitis. When anaerobes are grown from cultures, they usually are found in association with other organisms, including aerobic bacteria. The two most common predisposing factors in patients who have anaerobic osteomyelitis are previous fractures and diabetes mellitus. The anaerobic infections in association with diabetes mellitus almost always occur within the feet. *Bacteroides fragilis* and *B. melaninogenicus* comprise the majority of anaerobic isolates.

INFECTIOUS ARTHRITIS

Distinct from osteomyelitis, infectious arthritis usually is acquired by hematogenous spread.[8] The synovial tissue is highly vascular and does not have a basement membrane, so organisms in the blood can easily reach the synovial fluid. Table 116–2 summarizes the characteristics of acute infectious arthritis. Some organisms, such as *Neisseria gonorrhoeae,* are especially likely to infect a joint during bacteremia. In addition, organisms also may gain access to the joint from a deep-penetrating wound, an intraarticular steroid injection, arthroscopy, prosthetic joint surgery, and contiguous osteomyelitis expansion into the joint.[3]

The risk factors associated with adult infectious arthritis (more than one factor may be present) are systemic corticosteroid use, preexisting arthritis, arthrocentesis, distant infection, diabetes mellitus, trauma, and other diseases.

Trauma also appears to be a risk factor in facilitating microorganism entry into the synovial space. One study found that 35% of patients with infectious arthritis had preexisting joint disease.[10] Unlike children, adults often have significant systemic diseases that predispose them to infectious arthritis, such as diabetes mellitus, immunosuppressive states (cancer, liver disease), or preexisting arthritis. Intravenous drug abusers also are prone to develop septic arthritis. Arthritis, joint trauma, and surgery are other important risk factors because chronic inflammation or trauma makes the joint more susceptible to infection.[19] In addition, rheumatoid arthritis patients may be prone to

bacterial infection because of an inherent phagocytic defect, as well as concomitant corticosteroid therapy. Hormonal factors appear to play a role in *N. gonorrhoeae* infectious arthritis. Women are more prone to develop disseminated gonococcal infections than men. The second and third trimesters of pregnancy and during menstruation appear to be the times of greatest risk for developing gonococcal bacteremia.

After bacteria gain access to the joint, the organisms begin to multiply and produce a persistent purulent effusion within the joint. If this joint effusion is present beyond 7 days, chronic, and sometimes irreversible, damage may occur. Purulent effusions may promote cartilage destruction by increasing leukocyte enzyme activity. In conjunction with the development of the effusion, almost all patients will develop a hot, swollen, painful joint. The proteolytic enzymes within the effusion and pressure necrosis may lead to cartilage and bone damage.

◀ *S. aureus,* the single most common infecting organism, is found in 48% of cases of nongonococcal bacterial arthritis. Streptococcal infections account for 18% of cases, and gram-negative organisms are less common.[10] Overall, *E. coli* is the most common of the gram-negative organisms; however, *P. aeruginosa* is the most frequent organism in intravenous drug abusers. Neonates may have infectious arthritis because of a broad range of organisms, with *S. aureus, Streptococcus,* and gram-negative organisms being most common. *S. aureus* and *Streptococcus* are the most common pathogens in children younger than 5 years of age. If the child has not been fully vaccinated or is immunocompromised, *H. influenzae* type b may be seen. Within the adult population, *S. aureus* is responsible for the vast majority of nongonococcal infections. The most common cause of bacterial arthritis in adults 18 to 30 years of age is *N. gonorrhoeae,* which are the most common infections in women.[20] Patients with a terminal complement deficiency (C5–C9) are at increased risk of disseminated infections with *Neisseria* spp. Although less common, nonbacterial causes of osteomyelitis and septic arthritis include fungi and viruses.[21]

CLINICAL PRESENTATION

The clinical presentation of acute hematogenous osteomyelitis is summarized in Table 116–3. Although neonatal hematogenous

TABLE 116–2. Characteristics of Acute Infectious Arthritis

Feature	Finding
Peak incidence	Children younger than 16 years
	Adults older than 50 years
Clinical findings	Fever of 38–40°C in children; painful swollen joint in the absence of trauma
	Physical exam: Effusion, restriction of joint motion, tenderness, and warmth of joint
Most commonly affected joints	Knee, hip, ankle, elbow, wrist, and shoulder
Laboratory findings:	
Erythrocyte sedimentation rate	Elevated in 90% of cases
White blood cell count	Elevated in 30–60% of cases
Left shift	Seen in two-thirds of patients
Blood culture	Positive in 40% of cases
Needle aspiration of joint	Gram-stain diagnostic in 30–50% of cases. Synovial fluid cultures are positive in 60–80% of cases. Synovial fluid differential reveals 90% polymorphonuclear leukocytes. Synovial fluid glucose decreased relative to serum glucose. Lactic acid levels elevated in nongonococcal infectious arthritis but not in gonococcal infectious arthritis

ABLE 116–3. Clinical Presentation of Hematogenous steomyelitis

gns and Symptoms

gnificant tenderness of the affected area, pain, swelling, fever, chills, decreased motion, and malaise

aboratory Tests

evated erythrocyte sedimentation rate, C-reactive protein, and white blood cell count

0% of patients will have positive blood cultures

iagnostic Studies

one changes observed on radiographs 10–14 days after the onset of infection. Technetium and gallium scans positive as early as 1 day after the onset of infection

---

steomyelitis may spread rapidly to involve the joint, often there are w systemic symptoms present. A joint effusion is present in 60% to 0% of neonatal infections. Decreased limb motion and edema over e affected area may be the only signs from which to make a diagno- s. Pyogenic vertebral osteomyelitis produces nonspecific symptoms, ch as severe back pain, fever or night sweats, and weight loss. The ain typically is present at rest and increases in severity with move- ent. Neurologic symptoms may occur if the infection extends and ompresses the spinal cord. With contiguous-spread osteomyelitis ere is often an area of localized tenderness, warmth, edema, and rythema over the infected site. Patients with significant vascular in- ufficiency usually have local symptoms, such as pain, swelling, and dness. Less commonly, patients with vascular disease also may have fever and elevated white blood cell (WBC) count. The presentation f osteomyelitis from surgery or trauma depends on the precipitating ause. If the infection follows surgery or bone trauma, the symptoms sually are noted within 1 month. The most frequent symptom is sim- ly pain in the area of infection. Less commonly, patients also may evelop a fever and elevated WBC count.

Patients with nongonococcal bacterial arthritis almost always resent with a fever, and 50% of patients have an elevated WBC ount (see Table 116–2). The average initial synovial WBC count 100,000 cells/mm^3 or greater in nongonococcal bacterial disease. he most frequent initial sign of disseminated gonococcal infections a migratory polyarthralgia. In addition, two-thirds of patients also omplain of fever, dermatitis, and tenosynovitis (inflammation of the endon sheath).

Nongonococcal bacterial arthritis almost always involves only single joint. The knee is the most commonly involved joint, but fections also may occur in the shoulder, wrist, hip, ankle, interpha- angeal joints, and elbow joints. Usually, the initial focus of infection at acted as the source for bacterial or microbial entrance can be iden- fied. Common routes for bacterial entrance include infections of the espiratory tract, skin, and urinary tract. Blood cultures are important these patients because they may be positive in 50% of patients.

Another type of infectious arthritis occurs following prosthetic oint surgery. With these infections, the erythrocyte sedimentation rate sually is elevated, although a leukocytosis often is absent. Infections at result from postoperative contamination usually become apparent ithin 1 year of surgery.

RADIOLOGIC AND LABORATORY TESTS

he evaluation of a patient who potentially may have osteomyelitis as several unusual aspects. Radiographs of the involved area should e obtained; however, bone changes characteristic of osteomyelitis

are not seen for at least 10 to 14 days after the onset of the infection.[22] Radiologists may note soft tissue swelling before any bone changes become obvious. Bone lesions do not appear on roentgenogram films until 10 days after infection because more than 50% of the bone matrix must be removed before the lesions can be detected. As an aide to improve the diagnosis, bone scanning is used commonly.[23]

Despite the seriousness of osteomyelitis, often there are few laboratory abnormalities. The erythrocyte sedimentation rate (ESR), C-reactive protein, and WBC count may be the only laboratory abnormalities.[12] The degree of abnormality of these laboratory find- ings does not correlate with the disease outcome; however, they are useful for monitoring therapy. C-reactive protein may be elevated be- cause of the presence of inflammation, and it may be substituted for the ESR. C-reactive protein is generally the more sensitive and spe- cific marker of response to therapy and often increases and decreases before the ESR.

When a clinical assessment of osteomyelitis is suspected, it is important to establish a bacteriologic diagnosis by culture of the in- fected bone. Accurate culture information is especially important as a guide for treatment of osteomyelitis. Bone aspiration is valuable in de- termining an accurate bacteriologic diagnosis.[24] In addition, perform- ing a bone aspiration determines whether or not there is an abscess present. If an abscess is located, the pus is cultured, and a Gram stain is performed. If an abscess is found, the fluid needs to be drained and cultured. Aspirates of subperiosteal pus or metaphyseal fluid yield a pathogen in 70% of cases. Cultures should be done for both aerobic and anaerobic bacteria. A Gram stain of the aspirate may be useful in initiating empirical antibiotic therapy. This allows a more appropriate choice of antibiotics from the first day of therapy rather than waiting several days while culture results are pending.

If a specimen is obtained from a previously undrained or un- opened wound abscess, the pathogen usually can be identified. In chronic osteomyelitis, however, identification may be more difficult. Open wounds and draining sinuses frequently are contaminated with other organisms and thus provide inaccurate culture information.[25] Therefore, because of the inaccuracies with sinus tract cultures, they cannot be relied on to reflect the pathogen. Cultures of loculated pus aspirates in the area of orthopedic devices removed from infected bone can be trusted, however, to identify the infecting organism. The preferable time to obtain culture material in a patient with a chronic draining sinus is at the time of open surgical débridement.

In addition to performing cultures from the involved bone, it also is important to obtain cultures from any site believed to be the source of a bacteremia. Blood cultures should be obtained. Approximately 50% of patients with hematogenous osteomyelitis will have positive blood cultures.

When evaluating the possibility of a patient having infectious arthritis, immediate joint aspiration with subsequent analysis of the synovial fluid is extremely important. The presence of purulent fluid usually indicates the presence of a septic joint. The synovial fluid WBC count is usually 50,000–200,000 cells/mm^3 when an in- fection is present. Approximately half the patients with an infected joint have a low synovial glucose level, usually less than 40 mg/dL. Gram stains of joint fluid demonstrate bacteria in 50% of patients with septic arthritis; however, such stains may be positive in only 25% of patients with gonococcal arthritis infections. Synovial fluid cultures usually are positive in patients with nongonococcal infections. Both blood and joint fluid should be cultured aerobically and anaerobically in a patient suspected of having an infected joint. Blood cultures are positive in one-half of patients with nongonococcal infections but in only 20% of those with gonococcal infections. Pharyngeal, rec- tal, cervical, or urethral smears and cultures, as well as cultures of cutaneous lesions, should be performed if a disseminated gonococcal infection is considered. As with osteomyelitis, most patients will have an elevated C-reactive protein concentration and ESR. Radiographs of infected joints often reveal distension of the joint capsule with soft

tissue swelling in the adjacent space. Magnetic resonance imaging may be helpful in identifying an infected hip. In patients who have developed an infected prosthetic joint, loosening of the prosthesis may be seen radiographically.

▶ TREATMENT: Bone and Joint Infections

DESIRED OUTCOME

The goals of treatment are resolution of the infection and prevention of long-term sequelae. The ultimate outcome of osteomyelitis depends on the acute or chronic nature of the disease and how rapidly appropriate therapy is initiated. Patients with acute osteomyelitis have the best prognosis. Cure rates exceeding 80% may be expected for patients with acute osteomyelitis who have surgery as indicated and received injectable antibiotics for 4 to 6 weeks.[26] In contrast, patients with chronic osteomyelitis have a much poorer prognosis.[27] Dead bone and other necrotic material from the infection act as a bacterial reservoir and make the infection very difficult to eliminate. Adequate surgical débridement to remove all the dead bone and necrotic material, combined with prolonged administration of antibiotics, provides the best chance to obtain a cure.[28] The inability to remove all the dead bone may allow residual infection and require suppressive antibiotics to control the infection.

In comparison, many patients who develop infectious arthritis recover with no long-term sequelae. Gonococcal arthritis usually resolves rapidly with antibiotics; however, patients with staphylococcal arthritis have a higher incidence of joint damage. Individuals at greatest risk for long-term sequelae are those who have symptoms present for more than 7 days before starting therapy and those with infections occurring within the hip joint and infections caused by gram-negative organisms. Common long-term residual effects following infectious arthritis are limited joint motion and persistent pain. Shortening of the affected extremity is another well-known complication. More than half the children who subsequently developed residual joint damage were believed normal at the time of hospital discharge.

GENERAL APPROACH TO TREATMENT

❹ Following completion of the steps needed to determine the infecting organism, the most important treatment modality of acute osteomyelitis is the administration of appropriate antibiotics in adequate doses for a sufficient length of time. It is important to stress that early antibiotic therapy may mitigate the need for surgery.[29] A delay in treatment may allow bone necrosis to occur and make eradication of the infection much more difficult. In these patients, recurrent exacerbations of the infection may result if all necrotic tissue is not removed surgically and all microorganisms eliminated. Adjunctive treatment with hyperbaric oxygen or antibiotic-impregnated implants during surgery also has been used.[30-32]

If a patient with hematogenous osteomyelitis does not respond by having a decrease in fever, local swelling, redness, and pain following the initiation of adequate antibiotic therapy, the patient should undergo surgical débridement of the infected area. It is important to emphasize the priority of starting antibiotics immediately after the cultures have been obtained. No treatment failures have been reported when injectable antibiotics were started within 48 hours of the onset of symptoms in children with osteomyelitis.

PHARMACOLOGIC THERAPY

ANTIBIOTIC BONE CONCENTRATION

❺ Antibiotics used in the management of acute osteomyelitis generally are given in high doses (adjusted for weight, renal function, hepatic function, or both) so that adequate antimicrobial concentrations are reached within the infected bone and joint. Between 8 and 12 g/day of a penicillinase-resistant penicillin (nafcillin or oxacillin), ampicillin, or cephalosporin or a similar large dose of another parenteral antibiotic is used in the initial management of adults with osteomyelitis. These dosing recommendations, however, are empirical; the relationship between a specific dose of a given antibiotic and its resulting concentration within the infected bone is largely unknown.[33] Semisynthetic penicillins, cephalosporins, clindamycin, and the aminoglycosides can be detected in bone homogenates soon after their administration.

DURATION OF ANTIBIOTIC THERAPY

❻ The specific duration of antibiotic therapy needed in the management of osteomyelitis is usually 4 to 6 weeks.[34] Failures approaching 20% have been observed in children treated with injectable antibiotics for 3 weeks or less. Thus, with the data indicating a minimum of 3 weeks of antibiotic therapy, the standard treatment for osteomyelitis has been parenteral antibiotics for 4 to 6 weeks.[35-37] Although these data were determined in children, this duration-of-therapy recommendation is also used in adults. A trial assessing ceftriaxone 2 g intravenously once daily for at least 6 weeks for S. aureus osteomyelitis achieved a cure rate of 77%.[38] The failures in this study were in patients with infected necrotic bone or infected hardware (wires, plates, screws, and rods) that could not be removed.

A modification of this recommendation has been used in some patients. Children receiving an appropriate oral antibiotic regimen and adults receiving an oral fluoroquinolone antibiotic, such as ciprofloxacin, for a duration of 6 weeks have been treated successfully. Monitoring the patient's clinical signs and symptoms and the C-reactive protein level or ESR is an important parameter to assess therapy. If signs or symptoms are still present at 6 weeks, therapy should be extended. In contrast, children who have had a puncture wound of the foot resulting in P. aeruginosa osteochondritis and who have had surgical débridement of infected material may be treated with parenteral antibiotics for 10 days.[39]

ORAL ANTIBIOTIC THERAPY

❼ One of the most significant changes in the management of osteomyelitis is the use of oral antibiotics to complete therapy.[40] Criteria for the use of oral outpatient antibiotic therapy for osteomyelitis are

- Confirmed osteomyelitis
- Clinical response to parenteral antibiotics

Suitable oral agent available

Compliance ensured

Suitable candidates are children with good clinical response to intravenous therapy and adults without diabetes mellitus or peripheral vascular disease.

Two primary populations have benefited from oral treatment. Children responding to initial parenteral therapy may be excellent candidates to receive follow-up oral therapy with an agent such as dicloxacillin, cephalexin, or amoxicillin depending on their culture and sensitivity results.[41] Although more controversial, the other population to benefit from oral therapy is adults with an infecting organism sensitive to a fluoroquinolone.[42] These two populations now no longer routinely require expensive and complicated courses of long-term parenteral antibiotics.

The use of oral antibiotics is well studied in children. Several studies documenting the effectiveness of oral therapy used injectable antibiotics initially and then switched to oral antibiotics when there was a decrease in the signs of inflammation and the ESR or when the patient was afebrile for 3 days.[41] If pus was obtained on the initial needle aspirate, or if a reduction in fever, local swelling, and tenderness did not occur despite adequate rest, immobilization, and intensive antibiotic therapy, the patients underwent surgical drainage.

The patients enrolled in oral antibiotic trials generally had disease of recent onset, identification of a specific infecting organism, enforced compliance, and surgery as indicated. In patients who meet these criteria, oral antibiotics appear to offer a great advantage in the treatment of osteomyelitis. Patients not meeting these criteria are more likely to develop chronic osteomyelitis with resulting recurrent exacerbations of the infection if oral therapy is attempted. One trial found no treatment failures in children with acute S. aureus osteomyelitis who were treated with either 150 mg/kg per day of cephradine or 40 mg/kg per day of clindamycin that was started initially intravenously and was converted to oral therapy within 4 days.[43]

Ciprofloxacin is effective in the treatment of osteomyelitis caused by gram-negative strains, such as E. cloacae and S. marcescens.[44] Many strains of streptococci are relatively resistant. Its activity against gram-negative bacilli allows patients to be treated orally and avoids the potential toxic complications of 4 to 6 weeks of aminoglycoside therapy. Ciprofloxacin and other fluoroquinolones also have demonstrated effectiveness in the treatment of chronic osteomyelitis along with adequate surgical débridement.[45,46] Another benefit with this agent is that it may be administered on an every-12-hour schedule. An important limitation of this antibiotic class, however, is that fluoroquinolones should not be used in children younger than 16 to 18 years of age or in pregnant women because of the potential to cause cartilage damage. Other limitations of ciprofloxacin are that it has poor coverage against anaerobic organisms and staphylococci and that P. aeruginosa may develop resistance.[47] Newer fluoroquinolones have additional gram-positive activity; however, additional well-controlled clinical trials are needed to determine most appropriately their role in the treatment of osteomyelitis.[48,49]

CLINICAL CONTROVERSY

Some clinicians believe that oral fluoroquinolones should be preferred treatments for osteomyelitis, whereas others believe that there have been inadequate studies to date to determine their comparative clinical effectiveness.

Concern has been raised about staphylococci resistance to fluoroquinolones. Methicillin-resistant S. aureus infections do not respond well to ciprofloxacin; however, resistance also may be troublesome for methicillin-sensitive strains. It is now recommended that when ciprofloxacin is to be used to treat osteomyelitis with mixed etiologies that include S. aureus, ciprofloxacin should be combined with an antistaphylococcal drug such as dicloxacillin, cephalexin, or clindamycin.

ANTIBIOTIC SELECTION

A critical component in the management of osteomyelitis is the selection of appropriate antibiotics. Empirical therapy must be selected on the basis of the most likely infecting organism while the results of culture and sensitivity data are pending. Table 116–4 summarizes empirical therapy recommendations. Dosages expressed in terms of milligrams per kilograms per day generally are given in divided doses every 6 to 8 hours (three to four times a day).

Because S. aureus, streptococci, and E. coli are the most common infecting organisms in newborns, an intravenous dosage of 150 mg/kg per day (given in four divided doses) of oxacillin or nafcillin plus cefotaxime 150 mg/kg per day (given in three to four divided doses) is appropriate. For children 5 years of age or younger, S. aureus and streptococci are the most common infecting organisms. Appropriate therapy in this age group is nafcillin or oxacillin 150 mg/kg per day intravenously or cefazolin 100 mg/kg per day. If the patient is immunocompromised or has not been fully vaccinated, empirical therapy is needed to also cover H. influenzae type b. In this setting, intravenous cefuroxime 150 mg/kg per day is appropriate empirical therapy. For children older than 5 years, S. aureus is the most likely infecting organism, and either nafcillin 150–200 mg/kg per day intravenously or cefazolin 100 mg/kg per day intravenously is recommended. If patients are allergic to penicillins or cephalosporins or are infected with methicillin-resistant S. aureus, vancomycin, clindamycin, or linezolid may be used.[50] Children with culture-negative osteomyelitis can be managed as presumed staphylococcal disease with excellent long-term results.[51] Children with osteomyelitis usually can be treated successfully with 4 weeks of parenteral therapy or parenteral followed by oral therapy.

CLINICAL CONTROVERSY

Some clinicians believe that empirical therapy of osteomyelitis and septic arthritis in a child younger than 5 years of age no longer requires H. influenzae type b coverage, whereas others are concerned about children not being fully vaccinated and desire to use an antibiotic with activity against this organism.

An oral regimen may be an alternative to the previous recommendation in many cases of osteomyelitis in children. Children who have undergone surgery, if needed, and have had a good clinical response to intravenous therapy may be candidates for the alternate oral antibiotic regimen. Parenteral antibiotic therapy should be initiated and continued until there has been a resolution in the erythema, swelling, and tenderness and until the patient is afebrile. Dicloxacillin, cloxacillin, and cephalexin (100 mg/kg per day) are effective oral agents. Patients should be monitored with periodic WBC counts, C-reactive protein (or ESR) determinations, and radiographic findings. When oral antibiotics are used, the total duration of oral and injectable therapy is usually at least 4 to 6 weeks. As stated previously, because of the risk of cartilage damage, fluoroquinolones should not be used in children. Hematogenous osteomyelitis in adults is caused most frequently by S. aureus and thus is treated appropriately with 8–12 g/day

TABLE 116–4. Empirical Treatment of Osteomyelitis

Patient Subtype	Likely Infecting Organism	Antibiotic[a]
Newborn	S. aureus, streptococci, E. coli	Nafcillin or oxacillin 50–150 mg/kg/day IV plus cefotaxime 100–200 mg/kg/day IV
Children 5 years of age or younger	1. If vaccinated for H. influenzae type b: S. aureus or streptococci	1. Nafcillin 150 mg/kg/day IV or cefazolin 100 mg/kg/day IV
	2. If not vaccinated against H. influenzae type b	2. Cefuroxime 150 mg/kg/day IV
Children older than 5 years of age	S. aureus	Nafcillin 150 mg/kg/day IV or cefazolin 100 mg/kg/day IV
Adults	S. aureus	Nafcillin 2 g IV every 4 hours or cefazolin 2 g IV every 8 hours
Intravenous drug abusers	Pseudomonas	Ciprofloxacin 750 mg PO twice daily or ceftazidime 2 g IV every 8 hours plus tobramycin 5 mg/kg/day IV
Postoperative or posttrauma patients	Gram-positive and gram-negative organisms	Nafcillin 2 g IV every 4 hours plus ceftazidime 2 g IV every 8 hours or ticarcillin-clavulanate 3.1 g IV every 4 hours
Patients with vascular insufficiency	Gram-positive and gram-negative organisms	Nafcillin 2 g IV every 4 hours or cefazolin 2 g IV every 8 hours plus ceftazidime 2 g IV every 8 hours
	If anaerobes suspected	Cefotetan 2 g IV every 12 hours or clindamycin 900 mg IV every 8 hours plus ceftazidime 2 g IV every 8 hours

[a]Dosage should be adjusted for some agents in patients with renal and/or hepatic dysfunction.

of a penicillinase-resistant penicillin such as nafcillin. A similar dose of a first-generation cephalosporin (e.g., cefazolin), clindamycin 2.4 g/day, or vancomycin 2 g/day (with normal renal function) may be used in individuals allergic to penicillin; however, if the infection is located within the vertebrae, E. coli must be considered, and thus, depending on the culture and sensitivity data, a switch to a cephalosporin may be needed.[52] After institution of appropriate antibiotic therapy, the antimicrobial agent should be continued for at least 4 to 6 weeks total (parenteral plus oral).

Special Populations

Osteomyelitis in a patient with a hemoglobinopathy, such as sickle cell anemia, is commonly caused by either *Salmonella* or *S. aureus*. Thus empirical antibiotics of first choice are ceftriaxone or cefotaxime. Alternatives are chloramphenicol and ciprofloxacin (in adults).

Bone infections in patients with a history of intravenous drug abuse require coverage for gram-negative organisms; therefore, empirical treatment with ceftazidime 2 g intravenously every 8 hours plus an aminoglycoside is indicated. If compliance can be ensured, these patients are excellent candidates to receive oral ciprofloxacin 750 mg twice daily. Antibiotic therapy in these patients should be continued for at least 4 to 6 weeks.

As discussed previously, several microorganisms can cause bone infections that occur after surgery or from contiguous spread of an adjacent soft tissue infection. *S. aureus* is the single most common organism, but multiple organisms may be involved. To provide the required broad-spectrum coverage, nafcillin 2 g intravenously every 4 hours plus ceftazidime 2 g intravenously every 8 hours should be used as initial therapy. An alternative single agent is ticarcillin–clavulanate potassium 3.1 g intravenously every 4 hours; however, there is less experience with this agent. Other broad-spectrum alternatives may be cefepime and imipenem. The antibiotic regimen may require modification after culture and sensitivity information is

evaluated. Based on the culture and sensitivity data, ciprofloxacin may be an appropriate oral alternative for these patients. Frequently, the antibiotics must be continued for 6 weeks to obtain a cure, and surgery often is required to remove any infected or devitalized tissue.

Patients with established vascular insufficiency who subsequently develop osteomyelitis are extremely difficult to manage.[6] Impaired blood flow to the extremities impedes the healing process, possibly requiring vascular bypass surgery.[53] Infections in these patients involve a wide range of organisms, including *S. aureus, Streptococcus,* anaerobes, and gram-negative organisms. Broad-spectrum therapy with a penicillinase-resistant penicillin in combination with ceftazidime is the preferred initial therapy. If anaerobes are suspected, an antianaerobic cephalosporin (e.g., cefoxitin) or clindamycin plus ceftazidime may be substituted. Ampicillin may need to be added to the regimen to provide coverage against enterococci. Despite aggressive antibiotic therapy along with surgical débridement, these patients continue to have very low cure rates. Amputation of the involved area may be required to obtain a cure of the infection.[54]

Home Antibiotic Therapy

Because the management of bone and joint infections frequently requires prolonged parenteral antibiotics, newer antibiotic regimens are being evaluated.[55] Administration of antibiotics in the home environment and the use of antibiotics with extended elimination half-lives are being studied.[56] Although acute osteomyelitis is one of the more common infectious diseases that may be treated with home intravenous antibiotics, not all patients are acceptable candidates for home administration.[57] Patients must be screened to include only those who are receiving a stable treatment program, those who are interested and are motivated in participating, and those who have good venous access, as well as those who have support from family members or neighbors and have home facilities for storage and refrigeration.[58]

Patients with adequate vascular access may be able to use a peripheral intravenous catheter; however, a central intravenous catheter may be required if venous access difficulties occur. Certain exclusion criteria also must be considered. Complications of other preexisting diseases, such as diabetic retinopathy, intention tremor, disabling inflammation or degenerative joint disease, coagulopathies, or various neurologic disorders may prevent individuals from receiving home antibiotics. A history of alcoholism or of intravenous drug abuse also are important exclusion criteria. Patients who are fluent in only a foreign language and patients who are illiterate or hard of hearing may have to be excluded if a qualified guardian is unavailable. In addition to meeting these initial screening criteria, patients must complete a thorough training program successfully before hospital discharge. Aseptic technique, proper catheter care, and correct administration techniques must be documented. Once a patient is receiving therapy in the home environment, continued monitoring of their antimicrobial therapy is important. It is vital to ensure compliance with the antimicrobial regimen.

In addition, the specific antibiotic regimen characteristics must be considered when evaluating a patient for home antibiotics.[59] Some important features are microbiologic culture and sensitivity data, the number of required daily antimicrobial doses, antibiotic stability data, and requirements for unique monitoring for the specific antimicrobial regimen, such as serum creatinine and peak and trough concentration measurements with aminoglycosides. Although an organism may be sensitive to several antimicrobial agents, one antibiotic may provide practical benefits over other agents. Patients who have an infecting organism that is sensitive to one of the longer-acting (less frequently dosed) cephalosporins and is resistant to less expensive agents (cefazolin) may benefit from the newer antibiotics. It is important, however, to monitor for the development of resistant strains and superinfections.

Infectious Arthritis

The three most important therapeutic maneuvers in the management of infectious arthritis are appropriate antibiotics, joint drainage, and joint rest.[60] Smears of the synovial fluid may be useful to select appropriate antibiotic therapy initially.[61] If bacteria are not observed on the Gram stain in a patient who has a purulent joint effusion, antibiotics still should be initiated because of the high risk of an infection being present.[62] A delay in initiating antibiotics significantly increases the likelihood for long-term complications.

The specific antibiotic selected depends on the most likely infecting organism. In infants younger than 1 month of age, the infecting organisms vary widely, and empirical therapy thus must provide broad-spectrum coverage. A penicillinase-resistant penicillin such as nafcillin or oxacillin plus an aminoglycoside is appropriate. Children younger than 5 years of age who have been immunized for *H. influenzae* type b should receive nafcillin, oxacillin, or cefazolin.

In children older than 5 years of age and in adults, initial therapy with a penicillinase-resistant penicillin is appropriate to provide the necessary coverage against *S. aureus*. Therapy should be changed to clindamycin, vancomycin, or linezolid if the *S. aureus* is resistant to methicillin. Preliminary data indicate that children with infectious arthritis may be converted to oral therapy after initial intravenous therapy.[63,64] As with osteomyelitis, intravenous drug abusers require coverage for *P. aeruginosa,* and therefore, combination therapy with an aminoglycoside is needed. The antibiotics selected usually are administered parenterally. Antibiotics administered by this route achieve sufficient concentrations within the synovial fluid, and thus intraarticular antibiotic injections are unnecessary. Although studies to define clearly the appropriate length of therapy have not been conducted, 2 to 3 weeks of antibiotic therapy generally is adequate in nongonococcal infections. Joint fluid cultures usually are no longer positive after 7 days of antibiotics.

Disseminated gonococcal infections often respond quickly to antibiotics.[65] Ceftriaxone 1 g/day for 7 to 10 days is the treatment of choice. After culture and sensitivity results are available and the organism is determined to be sensitive, therapy can be switched on the fourth day to oral amoxicillin or to doxycycline or tetracycline to complete the 7- to 10-day course. Clinical resolution of signs and symptoms usually is rapid.

Closed-needle aspiration is recommended for all infected joints except the hip. Joint drainage may be repeated daily for 5 to 7 days until effusions no longer reaccumulate. Open drainage is required in hip infections because closed-needle aspiration is difficult and inadequate. During the initial phase of the infection, weight bearing, such as walking, on the joint should be avoided. Passive range-of-motion exercises should be initiated when the pain begins to subside in order to maintain joint mobility.[66] Approximately one-third of patients with bacterial arthritis have a poor joint outcome, such as severe functional deterioration.[67] Poor joint outcomes are associated with older patients, those with preexisting joint disease, and patients with an infected joint containing synthetic material. Treatment guidelines have been shown to be useful with septic arthritis of the hip.[68]

PHARMACOECONOMIC CONSIDERATIONS

Cost and outcome issues are important in osteomyelitis and infectious arthritis. If long-term sequelae develop, such as impaired joint motion or draining sinus tracts, or if amputation is required, patient quality of life may be significantly diminished. Cost and quality-of-life issues have clearly played a major role in evaluating other treatment alternatives (oral therapy or home antibiotic treatment) rather than requiring patients to remain hospitalized to receive 4 to 6 weeks of parenteral antibiotics.[69] One study compared a series of decision analytic models to provide estimates of the costs and outcomes of different regimens.[70] Another study used a Markov model to compare different treatments in non–insulin-dependent diabetes mellitus patients who had foot infections and suspected osteomyelitis.[71] This study found that a 10-week course of culture-guided oral antibiotics after surgical débridement may be as effective as and less costly than other treatment approaches, such as immediate amputation.

EVALUATION OF THERAPEUTIC OUTCOMES

Patients with bone and joint infections must be monitored closely. Table 116–5 summarizes a pharmaceutical care monitoring protocol. An assessment of a therapy's success or failure is based on the patient's clinical findings and laboratory values. The clinical signs of inflammation, such as swelling, tenderness, pain, redness, and fever, should resolve with appropriate therapy. Initially, the clinical signs are assessed daily until improvement and then periodically thereafter. Elevations in WBC count also should decline gradually. The ESR usually is determined weekly. Elevations in the C-reactive protein or ESR may not return to normal for several weeks of therapy. The WBC count usually is obtained once or twice per week until it returns to the normal range. If by the end of the 4- to 6-week antibiotic course the clinical findings of osteomyelitis are no longer present and the C-reactive protein or ESR is within normal limits, the patient may be considered a clinical cure. Patients may relapse, however, after

TABLE 116–5. Monitoring Protocol

Parameter	Frequency	Notes
Culture and sensitivity	At initiation of treatment	
White blood cell count	1 time/week until within normal range	
C-reactive protein or erythrocyte sedimentation rate	Weekly	May not decrease to normal range until several weeks of therapy
Clinical signs of inflammation (redness, pain, swelling, tenderness, fever)	Daily during initiation of therapy	
Compliance of outpatient therapy	Reinforce before starting oral therapy and with each health care visit	Compliance is critical if treatment is to be successful

initially appearing to be cured. No relapse for 1 year generally is considered a complete cure.

If a patient fails to resolve the clinical signs and symptoms of inflammation after appropriate empirical antibiotics, surgical débridement may be needed. In addition, the patient may have a resistant infecting organism or an atypical infecting organism that may require a modification of the antibiotic therapy. It is especially important to note the infecting organism and its sensitivity pattern. Follow-up cultures at subsequent débridements may be useful to assess the antibiotic therapy.

Despite apparently adequate surgery and antibiotics, some patients may fail therapy and have recurrent relapses in their infection. This scenario is more common in the population with chronic osteomyelitis. These patients may require long-term oral antibiotics in order to keep the infection under control.

ABBREVIATIONS

ESR: erythrocyte sedimentation rate
WBC: white blood cell count

Review Questions and other resources can be found at *www.pharmacotherapyonline.com.*

REFERENCES

1. Waldvogel FA, Medoff G, Swartz MN. Osteomyelitis: A review of clinical features, therapeutic considerations and unusual aspects. N Engl J Med 1970;282:198–206, 260–266, 316–322.
2. Dahl LB, Hoyland AL, Dramsdahl H, Kaaresen PI. Acute osteomyelitis in children: A population-based retrospective study 1965 to 1994. Scand J Infect Dis 1998;30:573–577.
3. Atkins BL, Bowler CJW. The diagnosis of large joint sepsis. J Hosp Infect 1998;40:263–274.
4. Luhmann JD, Luhmann SJ. Etiology of septic arthritis in children: An update for the 1990s. Pediatr Emerg Care 1999;15:40–42.
5. Kaandorp CJ, Dinant HJ, van de Laar MA, et al. Incidence and sources of native and prosthetic joint infections: A community based prospective survey. Ann Rheum Dis 1997;56:470–475.
6. Mader JT, Mohan D, Calhoun JH. A practical guide to the diagnosis and management of bone and joint infections. Drugs 1997;54:253–264.
7. Mader JT, Shirtliff M, Calhoun JH. Staging and staging application in osteomyelitis. Clin Infect Dis 1997;25:1303–1309.
8. Perry CR. Septic arthritis. Am J Orthop 1999;28:168–178.
9. Stimmler MM. Infectious arthritis: Tailoring initial treatment to clinical findings. Postgrad Med 1996;99:127–139.
10. Weston VC, Jones AC, Bradbury N, et al. Clinical features and outcomes of septic arthritis in a single UK Health District 1982–1991. Ann Rheum Dis 1999;58:214–219.
11. Lew DP, Waldvogel FA. Osteomyelitis. N Engl J Med 1997;336:999–1007.
12. Trobs R, Moritz R, Buhligen U, et al. Changing pattern of osteomyelitis in infants and children. Pediatr Surg Int 1999;15:363–372.
13. Lundy DW, Kehl DK. Increasing prevalence of *Kingella kingae* in osteoarticular infections in young children. J Pediatr Orthop 1998;18:262–267.
14. Barton LL, Villar RG, Rice SA. Neonatal group B streptococcal vertebral osteomyelitis. Pediatrics 1996;98:459–461.
15. Hirshberg J, Rees RS, Marchant B, Dean S. Osteomyelitis related to pressure ulcers: the cost of neglect. Adv Skin Wound Care 2000;13:25–29.
16. Puffingarger WR, Gruel CR, Herndon WA, Sullivan JA. Osteomyelitis of the calcaneus in children. J Pediatr Orthop 1996;16:224–230.
17. Eneroth M, Larsson J, Apelqvist J. Deep foot infections in patients with diabetes and foot ulcer: An entity with different characteristics, treatments, and prognosis. J Diabetes Complications 1999;13:254–263.
18. Tice AD. Outpatient parenteral antimicrobial therapy for osteomyelitis. Infect Dis Clin North Am 1998;12:903–919.
19. Gupta MN, Sturrock RD, Field M. A prospective 2-year study of 75 patients with adult-onset septic arthritis. Rheumatology 2001;40:24–30.
20. Cucurull E, Expinoza LR. Gonococcal arthritis. Rheum Dis Clin North Am 1998;24:305–322.
21. Perez-Gomez A, Prieto A, Torresano M, et al. Role of the new azoles in the treatment of fungal osteoarticular infections. Semin Arthritis Rheum 1998;27:226–244.
22. Song KM, Sloboda JF. Acute hematogenous osteomyelitis in children. J Am Acad Orthop Surg 2001;9:166–175.
23. Sutter CW, Shelton DK. Three-phase bone scan in osteomyelitis and other musculoskeletal disorders. Am Fam Phys 1996;54:1639–1647.
24. Khatri G, Wagner DK, Sohnle PG. Effect of bone biopsy in guiding antimicrobial therapy for osteomyelitis complicating open wounds. Am J Med Sci 2001;321:367–371.
25. Zuluaga AF, Galvis W, Jaimes F, Vesga O. Lack of microbiological concordance between bone and non-bone specimens in chronic osteomyelitis: An observational study. BMC Infect Dis 2002;2:8–17.
26. Ezra E, Cohen N, Segev E, et al. Primary subacute epiphyseal osteomyelitis: Role of conservative treatment. J Pediatr Orthop 2002;22:333–337.
27. Ray PS, Simonis RB. Management of acute and chronic osteomyelitis. Hosp Med 2002;63:401–407.
28. Reinehr T, Burk G, Michel E, Andler W. Chronic osteomyelitis in childhood: is surgery always indicated? Infection 2000;28:282–286.

9. Hamdy RC, Lawton L, Carey T, et al. Subacute hematogenous osteomyelitis: Are biopsy and surgery always indicated? J Pediatr Orthop 1996;16:220–223.

0. Wang J, Li F, Calhoun JH, Mader JT. The role and effectiveness of adjunctive hyperbaric oxygen therapy in the management of musculskeletal disorders. J Postgrad Med 2002;48:226–231.

1. Gitelis S, Brebach GT. The treatment of chronic osteomyelitis with a biodegradable antibiotic-impregnated implant. J Orthop Surg 2002;10:53–60.

2. Strauss MB, Bryant B. Hyperbaric oxygen. Orthopedics 2002;25:303–310.

3. Xue IB, Davey PG, Phillips G. Variation in postantibiotic effect of clindamycin against clinical isolates of *Staphylococcus aureus* and implications for dosing of patients with osteomyelitis. Antimicrob Agents Chemother 1996;40:1403–1407.

4. Mader JT, Shirtliff ME, Bergquist SC, Calhoun J. Antimicrobial treatment of chronic osteomyelitis. Clin Orthop Res 1999;360:47–65.

5. Le Saux N, Howard A, Barrowman NJ, et al. Shorter courses of parenteral antibiotic therapy do not appear to influence response rates for children with acute hematogenous osteomyelitis: A systematic review. BMC Infect Dis 2002;2:16–24.

6. Vinod MB, Matussek J, Curtis N, et al. Duration of antibiotics in children with osteomyelitis and septic arthritis. J Paediat Child Health 2002;38:363–367.

7. Jaberi FM, Shahcheraghi GH, Ahadzadeh M. Short-term intravenous antibiotic treatment of acute hematogenous bone and joint infection in children: A prospective, randomized trial. J Pediatr Orthop 2002;22:317–320.

8. Guglielmo BJ, Luber AD, Paletta D, Jacobs RA. Ceftriaxone therapy for staphylococcal osteomyelitis: A review. Clin Infect Dis 2000;30:205–207.

9. Bradley JS, Nelson JD. 2002–2003 Nelson's Pocket Book of Pediatric Antimicrobial Therapy, 15th ed. Philadelphia, Lippincott Williams & Wilkins, 2002:24.

0. Karwowska A, Davies HD, Jadavji T. Epidemiology and outcome of osteomyelitis in the era of sequential intravenous-oral therapy. Pediatr Infect Dis J 1998;17:1021–1026.

1. Peltola H, Unkila-Kallio L, Kallio MJT. Simplified treatment of acute staphylococcal osteomyelitis of childhood. Pediatrics 1997;99:846–850.

2. Greenberg RN, Newman MT, Shariaty S, Pectol RW. Ciprofloxacin, lomefloxacin, or levofloxacin as treatment for chronic osteomyelitis. Antimicrob Agents Chemother 2000;44:164–166.

3. Peltola H, Unkila-Kallio L, Kallio MJT, Finnish Study Group. Simplified treatment of acute staphylococcal osteomyelitis of childhood. Pediatrics 1997;99:846–850.

4. Lew DP, Waldvogel FA. Use of quinolones in osteomyelitis and infected orthopaedic prosthesis. Drugs 1999;58(suppl 2):85–91.

5. Rissing JP. Antimicrobial therapy for chronic osteomyelitis in adults: Role of the quinolones. Clin Infect Dis 1997;25:1327–1333.

6. Galanakis N, Giamarellou H, Moussas T, Dounis E. Chronic osteomyelitis caused by multi-resistant gram-negative bacteria: Evaluation of treatment with newer quinolones after prolonged follow-up. J Antimicrob Chemother 1997;39:241–246.

7. Greenberg RN, Newman MT, Shariaty S, Pectol RW. Ciprofloxacin, lomefloxacin, or levofloxacin as treatment for chronic osteomyelitis. Antimicrob Agents Chemother 2000;44:164–166.

8. Stengel D, Bauwens K, Sehouli J, et al. Systematic review and meta-analysis of antibiotic therapy for bone and joint infections. Lancet Infect Dis 2001;1:175–188.

49. Lew DP, Waldvogel FA. Use of quinolones in osteomyelitis and infected orthopaedic prosthesis. Drugs 1999;58(suppl 2):85–91.

50. Till M, Wixson RL, Pertel PE. Linezolid treatment for osteomyelitis due to vancomycin-resistant *Enterococcus faecium*. Clin Infect Dis 2002;34:1412–1414.

51. Floyed RL, Steele RW. Culture-negative osteomyelitis. Pediatr Infect Dis J 2003;22:731–735.

52. Sapico FL. Microbiology and antimicrobial therapy of spinal infections. Orthop Clin North Am 1996;27:9–13.

53. Hill SL, Holtzman GI, Buse R. The effects of peripheral vascular disease with osteomyelitis in the diabetic foot. Am J Surg 1999;177:282–286.

54. Eneroth M, Larsson J, Apelqvist J. Deep foot infections in patients with diabetes and foot ulcer: An entity with different characteristics, treatments, and prognosis. J Diabetes Complications 1999;13:254–263.

55. Tice A. The use of outpatient parenteral antimicrobial therapy in the management of osteomyelitis: Data from the outpatient parenteral antimicrobial therapy outcomes registries. Chemotherapy 2001;47(suppl 1):5–16.

56. Williams DN, Rehm SJ, Tice AD, et al. Practice guidelines for community-based parenteral anti-infective therapy. Clin Infect Dis 1997;25:787–801.

57. Tice AD. Outpatient antimicrobial therapy for osteomyelitis. Infect Dis Clin North Am 1998;12:903–919.

58. Gomez M, Maraqa N, Alvarez A, Rathore M. Complications of outpatient parenteral antimicrobial therapy in childhood. Pediatr Infect Dis J 2001;20:541–543.

59. Tice AD, Hoaglund PA, Shoultz DA. Outcomes of osteomyelitis among patients treated with outpatient parenteral antimicrobial therapy. Am J Med 2003;114:723–728.

60. Cimmino MA. Recognition and management of bacterial arthritis. Drugs 1997;54:50–60.

61. Carreno PL. Septic arthritis. Best Pract Res Clin Rheumatol 1999;13:37–58.

62. Lyon RM, Evanich JD. Culture-negative septic arthritis in children. J Pediatr Orthop 1999;19:655–659.

63. Newton PO, Ballock RT, Bradley JS. Oral antibiotic therapy of bacterial arthritis. Pediatr Infect J 1999;18:1102–1103.

64. Kim HKW, Alman B, Cole WG. A shortened course of parenteral antibiotic therapy in the management of acute septic arthritis of the hip. J Pediatr Orthop 2000;20:44–47.

65. Angulo JM, Espinoza LR. Gonococcal arthritis. Compr Ther 1999;25:155–162.

66. Boustred AM, Singer M, Hudson DA, Bolitho GE. Septic arthritis of the metacarpophalangeal and interphalangeal joints of the hand. Ann Plast Surg 1999;42:623–629.

67. Kaandorp CJE, Krijnen P, Bernelot Moens HJ, et al. The outcome of bacterial arthritis. Arthritis Rheum 1997;40:884–892.

68. Kocher MS, Mandiga R, Murphy JM, et al. A clinical practice guideline for treatment of septic arthritis in children: Efficacy in improving process of care and effect on outcome of septic arthritis of the hip. J Bone Joint Surg 2003;85A:994–999.

69. Bernard L, El-Hajj PB, Lotthe A, et al. Outpatient parenteral antimicrobial therapy (OPAT) for the treatment of osteomyelitis: Evaluation of efficacy, tolerance and cost. J Clin Pharmacol Ther 2001;26:445–451.

70. Tavakoli M, Davey P, Clift BA, Davies HT. Diagnosis and management of osteomyelitis: Decision analytic and pharmacoeconomic considerations. Pharmacoeconomics 1999;16:627–647.

71. Eckman MH, Greenfield S, Mackey WC, et al. Foot infections in diabetic patients: Decision and cost-effectiveness. JAMA 1995;273:712–720.

117

SEPSIS AND SEPTIC SHOCK

S. Lena Kang-Birken and Joseph T. DiPiro

Learning Objectives and other resources can be found at *www.pharmacotherapyonline.com.*

KEY CONCEPTS

◀1 The spectrum of microorganisms associated with sepsis has changed from predominantly gram-negative bacteria in the late 1970s and 1980s to gram-positive bacteria as the major pathogens since 1987.

◀2 The rate of fungal infections has increased more than 200% from 1979 to 2000, and despite the recent addition of several potent antifungal agents, mortality ranges from 41% to 71%.

◀3 Sepsis represents a complex pathophysiology characterized by the activation of multiple overlapping and interacting cascades leading to systemic inflammation, a procoagulant state, and decreased fibrinolysis.

◀4 Mortality rates with sepsis are higher for patients with preexisting disease, intensive care unit care, and multiple-organ failure.

◀5 Timely diagnosis and identification of the pathogen are critical to successful management of the septic patient.

◀6 Prompt, aggressive initiation of broad-spectrum parenteral antibiotic therapy is required owing to high incidence of complications and mortality.

◀7 Significant fluid leaks from the vasculature occur with sepsis, and administration of large volumes of crystalloid solution such as normal saline is required.

◀8 Early goal-directed therapy of sepsis consisting of hemodynamic monitoring with a central venous catheter, volume resuscitation, inotropic therapy, and red blood cell transfusions demonstrated a significant clinical outcome benefit with a 16% absolute reduction in 28-day mortality.

◀9 Recombinant human activated protein C, which has both anti-inflammatory and anticoagulant properties, was associated with a 6.1% reduction in 28-day all-cause mortality in comparison with placebo.

Sepsis represents a significant burden to the national health care system. In 2000, sepsis affected approximately 660,000 people, an increase of 8.7% per year since 1979.[1] Over half the patients were admitted to the intensive care unit (ICU) with a mean length of stay of 15.7 days.[2] The total number of deaths increased from 21.9 per 100,000 population in 1979 to 43.9 per 100,000 populations in 2000.[1] With the annual cost of approximately $16.7 billion, there remains a vital need for clinicians to comprehend the pathophysiology and to appreciate the management options available for acutely ill patients with sepsis or septic shock.[2]

DEFINITIONS

In 1992, a joint committee of the American College of Chest Physicians and the Society of Critical Care Medicine standardized the terminology related to sepsis for several reasons: (1) widespread confusion with the use of these terms, (2) the need to provide a flexible classification scheme for patient identification, (3) identification of an earlier therapeutic intervention, and (4) standardization of research protocols.[3]

The criteria for the new terms provide specific physiologic variables that can be used to categorize a patient as having bacteremia, systemic inflammatory response syndrome (SIRS), sepsis, severe sepsis, septic shock, or multiple-organ-dysfunction syndrome (MODS),

suggesting an important continuum of progressive physiologic decline (Table 117–1). Introduction of the term *systemic inflammatory response syndrome* (SIRS) reflects the knowledge that a physiologically similar systemic inflammatory response can be seen even in the absence of identifiable infection[4,5] (Fig. 117–1). It is important to note that progression from sepsis to MODS can occur in the absence of an intervening period of septic shock.

At the most recent consensus conference, the definitions were revised to include additional criteria for the diagnosis of SIRS and sepsis.[6] A new staging system was developed to facilitate a more accurate staging of sepsis disease and the associated risks and prognosis. However, extensive testing and further refinement are needed before clinical application.

INFECTION SITES AND PATHOGENS

The leading primary sites of microbiologically documented infections that led to sepsis were the respiratory tract (40%), urinary tract (18%), and intraabdominal space (14%).[7] While almost any microorganism can be associated with sepsis and septic shock, the most common etiologic pathogens are gram-positive bacteria, followed by gram-negative bacteria and fungi. Certain viruses and rickettsiae may produce a similar syndrome.

TABLE 117–1. Definitions Related to Sepsis

Condition	Definition
Bacteremia (fungemia)	Presence of viable bacteria (fungi) in the bloodstream.
Infection	Inflammatory response to invasion of normally sterile host tissue by the microorganisms.
Systemic inflammatory response syndrome (SIRS)	Systemic inflammatory response to a variety of clinical insults which can be infection, but can be noninfectious etiology. The response is manifested by two or more of the following conditions: T > 38°C (100.4°F) or < 36°C (96.8°F); HR > 90 beats/min; RR > 20 breaths/min or Pa_{CO_2} < 32 torr; WBC > 12,000 cells/mm^3, < 4,000 cells/mm^3, or > 10% immature (band) forms.
Sepsis	The SIRS secondary to infection.
Severe sepsis	Sepsis associated with organ dysfunction, hypoperfusion, or hypotension. Hypoperfusion and perfusion abnormalities may include, but are not limited to, lactic acidosis, oliguria, or acute alteration in mental status.
Septic shock	Sepsis with hypotension, despite fluid resuscitation, along with the presence of perfusion abnormalities. Patients who are on inotropic or vasopressor agents may not be hypotensive at the time perfusion abnormalities are measured.
Multiple-organ dysfunction syndrome (MODS)	Presence of altered organ function requiring intervention to maintain homeostasis.
Compensatory anti-inflammatory response syndrome (CARS)	Compensatory physiologic response to systemic inflammatory response syndrome that is considered secondary to the actions of anti-inflammatory cytokine mediators.

HR = heart rate; RR = respiratory rate; T = temperature.
From ref. 3–6.

GRAM-POSITIVE BACTERIAL SEPSIS

Since 1987, gram-positive organisms are the predominant pathogens in sepsis and septic shock, accounting for approximately 50% of all cases.[1] The causes are *Staphylococcus aureus*, *Streptococcus pneumoniae*, coagulase-negative staphylococci, and enterococci. *Streptococcus* pyogenes and viridans streptococci are less commonly involved.[7,8]

S. pneumoniae sepsis is associated with an overall mortality rate of over 25%. Factors related to a higher mortality include shock, respiratory insufficiency, preexisting renal failure, and the presence of a rapidly fatal underlying disease. *Staphylococcus epidermidis* is related most often to infected intravascular devices, such as artificial heart valves and stents and the use of intravenous and intraarterial catheters. The rates of nosocomial enterococcal bacteremia and associated sepsis are also increasing. Enterococci are isolated most commonly in blood cultures following a prolonged hospitalization and treatment with broad-spectrum cephalosporins.

GRAM-NEGATIVE BACTERIAL SEPSIS

A greater proportion of patients with gram-negative bacteremia develop clinical sepsis, and gram-negative bacteria are also more likely to produce septic shock in comparison with gram-positive organisms (50% versus 25%, respectively).[9]

Escherichia coli is the most commonly isolated pathogen in sepsis.[7-9] Other common gram-negative pathogens include *Klebsiella* spp., *Serratia* spp., *Enterobacter* spp., and *Proteus* spp. *Pseudomonas aeruginosa*, although not considered a predominant endogenous flora, is found widely in the environment and is the most frequent cause of sepsis fatality. These commensal organisms generally are not aggressive pathogens because normal host flora inhibit the overgrowth. However, when immunity breaks down, these organisms extend beyond normal sites and often progress from colonization to illness. With the administration of antimicrobial agents having broad spectra of activity, the protective microflora presumably are removed, thus allowing overgrowth of more virulent species. Additionally, the integrity of the gastrointestinal mucosa as a mechanical barrier is critical. The infectious implications of trauma, penetrating wounds, small surface ulcerations, mechanical obstructions, and ischemic necrosis of the bowel carry a high risk of subsequent gram-negative infection that often progresses to sepsis.

Gram-negative sepsis results in a higher mortality rate compared with sepsis from any other groups of organisms.[10-12] The major factor

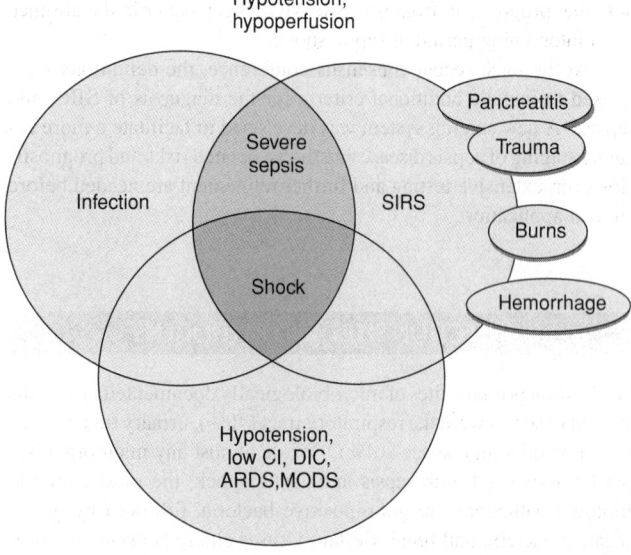

FIGURE 117–1. Relationship of infection, systemic inflammatory response syndrome (SIRS), sepsis, severe sepsis, and septic shock.

associated with the outcome of gram-negative sepsis appears to be the severity of any underlying condition. Patients with rapidly fatal conditions, such as acute leukemia, aplastic anemia, and more than 70% body surface area burn injury, have a significantly worse prognosis than do those patients with nonfatal underlying conditions, such as diabetes mellitus or chronic renal insufficiency.[1,2,9]

ANAEROBIC AND MISCELLANEOUS BACTERIAL SEPSIS

Anaerobes usually are considered low-risk organisms for the development of sepsis. If present, anaerobes often are found together with other pathogenic bacteria that are found commonly in sepsis. Epidemiology reports suggested that polymicrobial infections accounted for 5% to 39% of sepsis.[1,7] Mortality rates associated with polymicrobial infections are similar to sepsis caused by a single organism. Although some clinicians believe that the particular combination of organisms present in polymicrobial sepsis may provide clues to the source of infection, no clear source for the infection can be identified in up to 25% of cases. Other less common pathogens include meningococci, gonococci, rickettsiae, chlamydiae, and spirochetes.[10]

FUNGAL SEPSIS

The rate of fungal infections increased more than 200% from 1979 to 2000.[1] *Candida* spp. are common causes of fungal sepsis in hospitalized patients. While *C. albicans* remains the most dominant species, non-*albicans Candida* species, particularly *C. glabrata, C. parapsilosis, C. tropicalis,* and *C. krusei,* have emerged gradually from 24% in the 1980s to 46% between 1997 and 2000.[11,12] Other fungi identified as causes of sepsis include *Cryptococcus, Coccidioides, Fusarium,* and *Aspergillus.* Risk factors for fungal infection include abdominal surgery, poorly controlled diabetes mellitus, prolonged granulocytopenia, broad-spectrum antibiotic treatment, corticosteroid treatment, prolonged hospitalization, central venous catheter, total parenteral nutrition, hematologic malignancy, and chronic indwelling bladder (Foley) catheter.

Mortality ranges from 41% to 71% in patients with fungemia.[13] Hematologic diseases, neutropenia, and a higher number of positive blood cultures were associated with poor outcome irrespective of patient's gender, age, or days of antifungal drug treatment.

VIRAL SEPSIS

Viremia is common to many viral illnesses, but it does not usually lead to the development of clinical sepsis. Hypotension and disseminated intravascular coagulation (DIC) may occur with unusual viruses, such as Ebola virus and Lassa fever virus, and may be seen occasionally with influenza A, arbovirus, and possibly severe measles.[10]

PATHOPHYSIOLOGY

The pathophysiologic sequelae resulting from the interaction between the invading pathogen and the human host are diverse, complex, and incompletely understood.[14] Definitive relationships between infection and progression to septic shock have been difficult to demonstrate. Furthermore, clinical and histopathologic changes attributed to infection may be similar to those of coexisting conditions. Finally, observations from work with animal models of sepsis are difficult to apply to humans because of potential marked differences in responses.

CELLULAR COMPONENTS FOR INITIATING THE INFLAMMATORY PROCESS

The pathophysiologic focus of gram-negative sepsis has been on the lipopolysaccharide component of the bacterial cell wall. Commonly referred to as *endotoxin,* this substance is unique to the outer membrane of the gram-negative cell wall and generally is released with bacterial lysis. Lipid A, the innermost region of the lipopolysaccharide, is highly immunoreactive and is considered responsible for most of the toxic effects observed with gram-negative sepsis. Although lipid A may affect tissues directly, its predominant effect is to activate macrophages and trigger inflammatory cascades critical in the progression to sepsis and septic shock.[14,15] The endotoxin forms a complex with a protein called a *lipopolysaccharide-binding protein* that then engages the specific CD14 receptor on the surface of a macrophage. Subsequently, cytokine mediators are activated and released.

In gram-positive sepsis, peptidoglycan appears to exhibit proinflammatory activity. Peptidoglycan comprises up to 40% of gram-positive cell mass and is exposed on the cell wall surface. Although it competes with lipid A for similar binding sites on CD14, the potency of peptidoglycan is less than that of endotoxin.[14]

PRO- AND ANTI-INFLAMMATORY MEDIATORS

Sepsis involves activation of inflammatory pathways, and a complex interaction between proinflammatory and anti-inflammatory mediators plays a major role in the pathogenesis of sepsis. The key proinflammatory mediators include tumor necrosis factor-α (TNF-α), interleukin 1β (IL-1β), and interleukin 6 (IL-6), which are released by activated macrophages. Other mediators that may be important for the pathogenesis of sepsis include interleukin 8 (IL-8), platelet-activating factor (PAF), leukotrienes, and thromboxane A_2.[14,16,17] The significant anti-inflammatory mediators include IL-1 receptor antagonist (IL-1ra), IL-4, and IL-10.[15,17,18] These anti-inflammatory cytokines inhibit the production of the proinflammatory cytokines and downregulate some inflammatory cells.

TNF-α is considered the primary mediator of sepsis.[14–17] The TNF-α level is highly elevated very early in the inflammatory response in most patients with sepsis. In meningococcemia, increased morbidity and mortality are associated with high plasma concentrations of TNF-α. TNF-α release leads to activation of other cytokines (IL-1β and IL-6) associated with cellular damage. In addition, TNF-α stimulates the release of cyclooxygenase-derived arachidonic acid metabolites (thromboxane A_2 and prostaglandins) that contribute to vascular endothelial damage. TNF-α also causes endothelial cells to express adhesion molecules, facilitating influx of granulocytes.

The net effect of a given mediator can vary depending on the state of activation of the target cell, the presence of other mediators near the target cell, and the ability of the target cell to release mediators that can augment or inhibit the primary mediator. When the balance in the localized response is lost, the patient becomes systemically ill. As Fig. 117–2 illustrates, when there is a systemic spillover of excessive proinflammatory mediators, the patient presents with SIRS

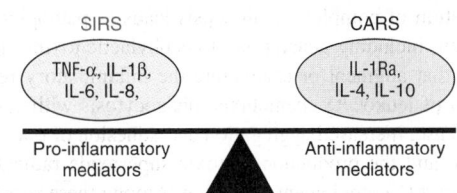

FIGURE 117–2. The balance between pro- and anti-inflammatory mediators.

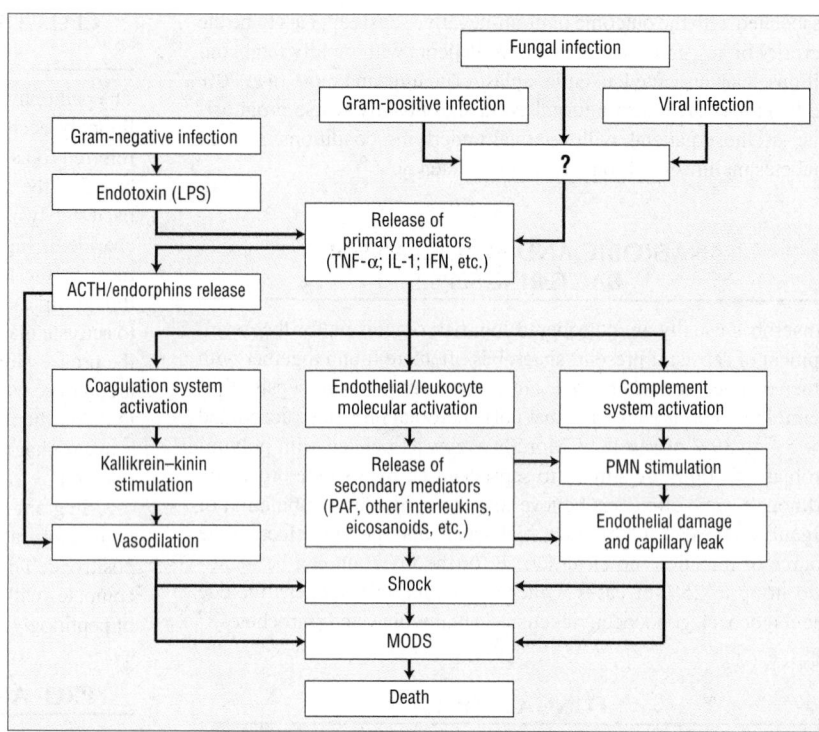

FIGURE 117–3. Cascades of sepsis. ACTH = adrenocorticotropic hormone.

and possibly MODS. Shortly after this initial phase, counterregulatory pathways become activated, and there is a systemic spillover of excessive anti-inflammatory mediators, representing a compensatory anti-inflammatory response syndrome (CARS). The balance between pro- and anti-inflammatory mechanisms determines the degree of inflammation, ranging from local antibacterial activity to systemic tissue toxicity or organ failure[7,14,17]

CASCADE OF SEPSIS

The cascade leading to the development of sepsis is complex and multifactorial, involving various mediators and cell lines[16,17,19] (Fig. 117–3). Through the actions of the mediators, a variety of cells become activated, initiating detrimental cascades. Initially, macrophages become activated and produce inflammatory cytokines. These cytokines then influence a wide range of cells, including endothelial cells, lymphocytes, hepatocytes, neutrophils, and platelets. Endothelial cells that respond to and produce a variety of cytokines mediate a primary mechanism of injury with sepsis. When injured, endothelial cells allow circulating cells such as granulocytes and plasma constituents to enter inflamed tissues, which may result in organ damage.

The microcirculation is affected by sepsis-induced inflammation.[20] The arterioles become less responsive to either vasoconstrictors or vasodilators. The capillaries are less perfused, and there is neutrophil infiltration and protein leakage into the venules. Pulmonary dysfunction may result from the destructive mechanisms of neutrophils that are attracted to lung tissue through the action mainly of IL-8.

Activation of complement in sepsis leads to pathophysiologic consequences including generation of anaphylactic toxins and other substances that augment or exaggerate the inflammatory response. Stimulation of leukocyte chemotaxis, phagocytosis with lysosomal enzyme release, increased aggregation and adhesion of platelets and neutrophils, and the production of toxic superoxide radicals is attributed in part to complement activation. Among these responses is the release of histamine from mast cells and the resulting increase in capillary permeability and the "third spacing" of fluid in interstitial spaces.

The inflammatory process in sepsis is also directly linked to the coagulation system. Proinflammatory mechanisms that promote sepsis are also procoagulant and antifibrinolytic, whereas fibrinolytic mechanisms may be anti-inflammatory. A key endogenous substance involved in the inflammation of sepsis is activated protein C, which enhances fibrinolysis and inhibits inflammation. Levels of protein C are reduced in patients with sepsis.[21]

PREDICTIVE MARKERS OF SEPSIS PROGRESSION

Correlation between the plasma levels of endotoxin and cytokines and the progression of sepsis has been evaluated.[22–26] While the TNF-α levels may be increased in patients with a variety of diseases and in many healthy people, there is a correlation of TNF-α levels with the severity of sepsis. High TNF-α levels are found in patients with septic shock. In contrast, IL-1 levels have been inconsistently associated with sepsis.[24] IL-6 may be a more consistent predictor of sepsis because it remains elevated for a longer period of time than does TNF-α and it appears to be related to sepsis severity and mortality.[23,25] Circulating concentrations of IL-8 also have been related to the severity of sepsis and mortality.[26] Although the plasma endotoxin concentration does not correlate with the development of gram-negative sepsis or outcome from infection, decreased antiendotoxin core immunoglobulin G concentrations are associated with increased mortality in patients with sepsis syndrome.[27]

COMPLICATIONS

Shock is the most ominous complication associated with sepsis, and mortality occurs in approximately half the patients with septic shock. Severe hypotension appears to be caused in part by the release of vasoactive peptides such as bradykinin and serotonin and by endothelial cell damage leading to the extravasation of fluids into interstitial spaces. Septic shock is associated with several complications, including DIC, acute respiratory distress syndrome (ARDS), and MODS.

DISSEMINATED INTRAVASCULAR COAGULATION (DIC)

Sepsis remains the most common cause of DIC. The incidence of DIC increases as the severity of sepsis increases. In sepsis alone, the incidence was 16%, in comparison with 38% in septic shock.[28] DIC occurs in up to 50% of patients with gram-negative sepsis, but it is also common in patients with gram-positive sepsis.

DIC begins with the activation and production of the proinflammatory cytokines such as TNF, IL-1, and IL-6, which appear to be the principal mediators, along with endotoxin, of endothelial injury, activation of the coagulation cascade, and inhibition of fibrinolysis. The combination of excessive fibrin formation, inhibited fibrin removal from a depressed fibrinolytic system, and endothelial injury results in microvascular thrombosis and DIC.[28]

Complications of DIC vary and depend on the target organ affected and the severity of the coagulopathy. DIC may produce acute renal failure, hemorrhagic necrosis of the gastrointestinal mucosa, liver failure, acute pancreatitis, ARDS, and pulmonary failure. Furthermore, since the procoagulant state appears to be the key in the pathogenesis of MODS, coagulation dysfunction and MODS often coexist in sepsis.

ACUTE RESPIRATORY DISTRESS SYNDROME (ARDS)

Pulmonary dysfunction usually precedes dysfunction in other organs, and it may even initiate the development of SIRS with resulting MODS. In sepsis caused by *S. aureus,* pulmonary involvement was reported in 82% of the patients.[29] Overall mortality rate ranges from 19% to 90% depending on the causative microorganism.[29,30]

Activated neutrophils and platelets adhere to the pulmonary capillary endothelium, initiating multiple inflammatory cascades with a release a variety of toxic substances. There is diffuse pulmonary endothelial cell injury, increased capillary permeability, and alveolar epithelial cell injury.[31] Consequently, interstitial pulmonary edema occurs and gradually progresses to alveolar flooding and collapse. The end result is loss of functional alveolar volume, impaired pulmonary compliance, and profound hypoxemia.[32]

HEMODYNAMIC EFFECTS

The hallmark of the hemodynamic effect of sepsis is the hyperdynamic state characterized by high cardiac output and an abnormally low systemic vascular resistance (SVR).[33] TNF-α and endotoxin directly depress cardiovascular function. Endotoxin depresses left ventricular function independent of changes in left ventricular volume or vascular resistance.

Persistent hypotension raises concern for the balance of oxygen delivery to the tissues (Do$_2$) and oxygen consumption by the tissues (Vo$_2$).[31] Sepsis results in a distributive shock characterized by inappropriately increased blood flow to selected tissues at the expense of other tissues that is independent of specific tissue oxygen needs. This perfusion defect is accentuated by an increased precapillary atrioventricular (AV) shunt. If perfusion decreases, oxygen extraction increases, and the AV oxygen gradient widens. Cellular Do$_2$ is decreased, but Vo$_2$ remains unaffected. When increased oxygen demand

occurs without increased blood flow, the increased Vo$_2$ is compensated by increased oxygen extraction. If perfusion decreases sufficiently in the face of high metabolic demands, then the reserve Do$_2$ can be exceeded, and tissue ischemia results. Significant tissue ischemia leads to organ dysfunction and failure. Therefore, systemic Do$_2$ relative to Vo$_2$ should be optimized by increasing oxygen delivery or decreasing oxygen consumption in a hypermetabolic patient.

ACUTE RENAL FAILURE

Renal dysfunction such as acute oliguric or anuric renal failure occurs in approximately one-quarter of the patients, and in the event of severe sepsis and MODS, renal dysfunction is potentially lethal, with a mortality of 50% to 90%.[2,31] Without normal urine output, fluid overload in the extravascular space, including the lungs, develops, leading to impairment of pulmonary gas exchange and severe hypoxemia. Consequently, compromised oxygen delivery would exacerbate peripheral ischemia and organ damage. Adequate renal perfusion and a trial of loop diuretics should be initiated promptly in oliguric or anuric patients with MODS. In addition, renal replacement therapy such as continuous hemofiltration should be used to facilitate volume and electrolytes.[31]

CLINICAL PRESENTATION

Table 117–2 lists some of the common clinical features of sepsis, although a number of these findings are not limited to infectious processes. The initial clinical presentation can be referred to as signs and symptoms of early sepsis, and they typically include fever, chills, and change in mental status. Hypothermia may occur with a systemic infection, and this is often associated with a poor prognosis.[10] In patients with sepsis caused by gram-negative bacilli, hyperventilation may occur even before fever and chills, and it may lead to respiratory alkalosis as the earliest metabolic change.

Progression of uncontrolled sepsis leads to clinical evidence of organ system dysfunction, as represented by the signs and symptoms attributed to late sepsis. With the exception of rapidly progressing cases, as in meningococcemia and *P. aeruginosa* or *Aeromonas* infection, the onset of shock is slow and usually follows a period of several hours of hemodynamic instability. Oliguria often follows hypotension. Increased glycolysis with impaired clearance of the resulting lactate by the liver and kidneys and tissue hypoxia because of hypoperfusion result in elevated lactate levels, contributing to metabolic

TABLE 117–2. Signs and Symptoms Associated with Sepsis

Early Sepsis	Late Sepsis
Fever or hypothermia	Lactic acidosis
Rigors, chills	Oliguria
Tachycardia	Leukopenia
Tachypnea	DIC
Nausea, vomiting	Myocardial depression
Hyperglycemia	Pulmonary edema
Myalgias	Hypotension (shock)
Lethargy, malaise	Hypoglycemia
Proteinuria	Azotemia
Hypoxia	Thrombocytopenia
Leukocytosis	ARDS
Hyperbilirubinemia	Gastrointestinal hemorrhage
	Coma

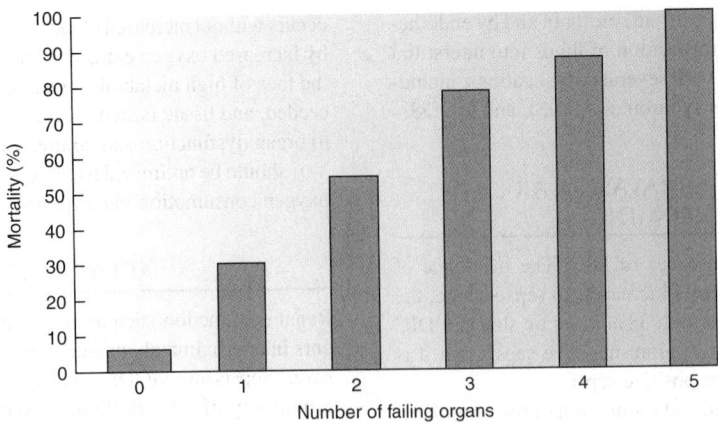

FIGURE 117–4. Mortality related to the number of failing organs.

acidosis. Altered glucose metabolism, including impaired gluconeo-genesis and excessive insulin release, is evidenced by either hyper-glycemia or hypoglycemia. The distinction between early and late sepsis is arbitrary, and it is recognized that sepsis represents a spectrum of clinical findings.

PROGNOSIS

 As the patient progresses from SIRS to sepsis to severe sepsis to septic shock, mortality increases in a stepwise fashion. Mortality

rates are higher for patients with advanced age; preexisting disease, including chronic obstructive pulmonary disease (COPD), neoplasm, and human immunodeficiency virus (HIV) disease; ICU care; and more organ failure. Mortality increased with age from 10% in children to 38.4% in those ≥85 years.[2] ICU admission was required in 51.1% of the patients with severe sepsis, and of those patients, mortality was reported in 34.1%.[2] Mortality from severe sepsis and MODS is most closely related to the number of dysfunctioning organs. As the number of failing organs increased from two to five, mortality increased from 54% to 100%[31] (Fig. 117–4). Duration of organ dysfunction also may affect the overall mortality rate.

▶ TREATMENT: Sepsis and Septic Shock

The primary goals of therapy for patients with sepsis include (1) timely diagnosis and identification of pathogen, (2) rapid elimination of the source of infection medically and/or surgically, (3) early initiation of aggressive antimicrobial therapy, (4) interruption of pathogenic sequence leading to septic shock, and (5) avoidance of organ failure. Supportive care such as stress ulcer prophylaxis and nutritional support is important to prevent complications during the stay in the ICU.

■ DIAGNOSIS AND IDENTIFICATION OF PATHOGEN

⬛ The presence of clinical features suggesting sepsis should prompt further evaluation of the patient. In addition to obtaining a careful history of any underlying conditions and recent travel, injury, animal exposure, infection, or use of antibiotics, a complete physical examination should be performed to determine the source of the infection.

A collection of specimens should be sent for culture prior to initiating any antimicrobial therapy. Generally, at least two sets of blood samples should be obtained for aerobic and anaerobic culture, as well as the samples of urine and sputum. A lumbar puncture is indicated in case of mental alteration, severe headache, or a seizure, assuming that no focal cranial lesions have been identified by computed tomographic (CT) scan. Further tests may be indicated to assess any systemic organ dysfunction owing to severe sepsis. The laboratory tests should include hemoglobin, white blood cell count with differential, platelet count, complete chemistry profile, coagulation parameters, serum lactate concentration, and arterial blood gases.[34]

■ ELIMINATION OF SOURCE OF INFECTION

After the source of infection is identified, prompt efforts to remove or eliminate the source should be initiated. With an infected intravascular catheter, the catheter should be removed and cultured. Urinary tract catheters should be removed if association with sepsis is suspected. Suspicion of soft tissue (cellulitis or wound infection) or bone involvement should lead to aggressive débridement of the affected area. Evidence of an abscess or sepsis associated with any intraabdominal pathology should prompt surgical intervention.

■ ANTIMICROBIAL THERAPY

⬛ Aggressive, early antimicrobial therapy is critical in the management of septic patients because of high incidence of complications and mortality. Because of the inherent problems associated with timely identification of the infecting organism or organisms, empirical antimicrobial regimens usually are started initially. Selection of empirical regimen should be based on the suspected site of infection, the most likely pathogens, acquisition of the organism from the community or hospital, the patient's immune status, and the antibiotic susceptibility and resistance profile for the institution. All patients should be treated initially with parenteral antibiotics for optimal drug concentrations. Empirical therapy for an immunocompromised patient should consist of antimicrobial combinations likely to be

TABLE 117–3. Empirical Antimicrobial Regimens in Sepsis

Infection (Site or Type)	Antimicrobial Regimen	
	Community-Acquired	*Hospital-Acquired*
Urinary tract	Ciprofloxacin *or* levofloxacin	Piperacillin *or* ceftazidime, ceftriaxone *or* ciprofloxacin, levofloxacin } ± gentamicin
Respiratory tract	Newer fluoroquinolone[a] *or* ceftriaxone + clarithromycin-azithromycin	Piperacillin, ticarcillin *or* ceftazidime, cefipime } + gentamicin or ciprofloxacin
Intra-abdominal	β-Lactamase inhibitor combo[b] *or* ciprofloxacin + metronidazole	Piperacillin-tazobactam *or* meropenem
Skin/soft tissue	Nafcillin *or* cefazolin	Ceftriaxone +/− vancomycin
Catheter-related		Vancomycin
Unknown		Piperacillin *or* ceftazidime-cefipime *or* meropenem } +gentamicin +/− vancomycin

[a]Levofloxacin, gatifloxacin, moxifloxacin, gemifloxacin.
[b]Ampicillin–sulbactam, ticarcillin–clavulanic acid.

synergistic. Once the pathogen and its susceptibility pattern are known, antimicrobial regimen should be modified accordingly.

SELECTION OF ANTIMICROBIAL AGENTS

In a study evaluating 904 patients with microbiologically confirmed severe sepsis or septic shock, appropriate initial antimicrobial therapy was an important determinant of survival.[7] The 28-day mortality was 24% in patients who received appropriate initial antimicrobial treatment versus 39% in those who received inappropriate initial treatment.

Table 117–3 lists antimicrobial regimens that can be used empirically based on the possible source of infection. In the nonneutropenic patient with an urinary tract infection, a third-generation cephalosporin, fluoroquinolone, or extended-spectrum penicillin, each with or without an aminoglycoside, should be considered.[35] *S. pneumoniae* is the most common cause of community-acquired pneumonia, and it accounts for approximately 60% of all deaths. The rising incidence of penicillin-resistant *S. pneumoniae* requires empirical use of newer "respiratory" fluoroquinolones. Newer fluoroquinolones, such as levofloxacin, gatifloxacin, moxifloxacin, and gemifloxacin, can be used as monotherapy because they offer excellent coverage against penicillin-resistant pneumococci and aerobic gram-negative bacteria, as well as atypical pathogens, including *Legionella pneumophila, Mycoplasma pneumoniae,* and *Chlamydia pneumoniae*.[36,37] Newer macrolides, such as clarithromycin and azithromycin, are very effective against atypical pathogens and better tolerated than erythromycin.

In nosocomial pneumonia, enteric gram-negative bacteria such as *Enterobacter* and *Klebsiella* spp., and *P. aeruginosa* are the major pathogens in addition to *S. aureus*. If *P. aeruginosa* infection is suspected, a dual regimen of antipseudomonal penicillin or third- or fourth-generation cephalosporin and an aminoglycoside is recommended because of the high mortality rate associated with *Pseudomonas* infection.[35] When an aminoglycoside is undesirable, an antipseudomonal fluoroquinolone such as ciprofloxacin or levofloxacin can be used instead. In case of methicillin-resistant *S. aureus*, vancomycin should be initiated. However, worldwide emergence of glycopeptide intermediately resistant *S. aureus* and vancomycin-resistant enterococci has led to development of alternative antimicrobial agents such as teicoplanin, quinupristin-dalfopristin, and linezolid.[38–40]

Secondary peritonitis as a consequence of perforation of the gastrointestinal tract usually is polymicrobial, involving enteric aerobes and anaerobes, and as many as five organisms are isolated per patient. In addition to surgical intervention, broad-spectrum antibiotics such as β-lactamase inhibitor combination agents (piperacillin-tazobactam or ticarcillin-clavulanate) are appropriate in intraabdominal infections.[41] Imipenem or meropenem may be indicated if resistance patterns prohibit the use of other, less expensive therapies.[42,43] Currently, most clinicians prefer meropenem to imipenem because it offers similar activity as imipenem with less propensity to cause seizures. In a multicenter study, meropenem was efficacious and safe when compared with a combination regimen of cefuroxime and gentamicin for the treatment of sepsis syndrome in patients who were 65 years of age or older.[42] Metronidazole is preferred over clindamycin against anaerobes because approximately 20% of *Bacteroides* spp. are resistant to clindamycin.[44]

In soft tissue infection caused by group A *Streptococcus,* streptococcal toxic shock syndrome may occur. Although penicillin and cefazolin are efficacious, experimental models of group A streptococcal infection show clindamycin to be more effective than penicillin.[35]

In addition to selecting the most appropriate antimicrobial agents, a clinician must ensure effective antibiotic usage, such as proper dosing, interval administration, optimal duration of treatment, monitoring of drug levels when appropriate, and avoidance of unwanted drug interactions. Lack of adherence to these requirements may lead to suboptimal or excessive tissue concentrations that may promote antibiotic resistance, toxicity, and inadequate efficacy despite appropriate antibiotic selection.

THERAPEUTIC CONSIDERATIONS WITH AMINOGLYCOSIDES

In vitro, tobramycin appears somewhat more active (based on concentrations achievable in serum relative to usual minimum inhibitory concentration) than gentamicin against *P. aeruginosa*. Gentamicin, however, appears more active than tobramycin against *Serratia* spp. Overall, amikacin exhibits most potent in vitro activity against the *Klebsiella-Enterobacter-Serratia* group. In addition, amikacin is less susceptible than gentamicin and tobramycin to plasmid-mediated enzyme inactivation, and it should be reserved as an alternative in situations of suspected or established resistance to gentamicin and tobramycin.

CLINICAL CONTROVERSY

Although aminoglycosides traditionally have been administered in divided doses, there has been increasing acceptance of administering aminoglycosides in a single daily dose of 4 to 7 mg/kg for gentamicin and tobramycin and 10 to 15 mg/kg for amikacin.[45-47] A single daily dose maximizes the well-defined, concentration-dependent killing activity of aminoglycosides, as well as the prolonged postantibiotic effect against gram-negative bacterial pathogens. Furthermore, nephrotoxicity is reduced significantly. With a single daily dose, there is a prolonged drug-free period during which the reported saturable or rate-limiting uptake of aminoglycosides into proximal renal tubular cells can be completed. Because of insufficient clinical data, single daily dose administration should not be used in pediatric patients, burn victims, pregnant patients, patients with preexisting or progressive renal dysfunction, or patients requiring aminoglycosides for synergy against gram-positive pathogens.

ANTIFUNGAL THERAPY

Candida species are associated most frequently with fungal infections, and the resulting candidemia frequently is associated with sepsis syndrome and a high mortality rate.[11,12,48] Treatment of invasive candidiasis involves amphotericin B–based preparations, the azole antifungal agents, the echinocandin antifungal agents, or combination therapy with fluconazole plus amphotericin B. The choice depends on the clinical status of the patient, the fungal species and its susceptibility, the relative drug toxicity, the presence of organ dysfunction that would affect drug clearance, and the patient's prior exposure to antifungal agents. In general, suspected systemic mycotic infection leading to sepsis is treated frequently with parenteral amphotericin B empirically, especially if the patient is clinically unstable, because of its greater activity against *Candida* species and non-*albicans* species including *C. glabrata* and *C. krusei*.[48]

Fluconazole is less toxic and easier to administer than amphotericin B. However, fluconazole resistance among *C. albicans* has been well described among HIV-infected individuals and is increasing in immunocompetent adults.[48] *C. glabrata* often has reduced susceptibility to fluconazole. Itraconazole exhibits a similar activity profile to fluconazole and is well known to be active against mucosal forms of candidiasis. However, formal clinical trials using intravenous

itraconazole are not available for invasive candidiasis. Voriconazole appears to be active against *Candida* species, including fluconazole-resistant isolates. A recently completed worldwide study will aid in analyzing voriconazole for the indication of treatment of serious invasive, fluconzole-resistant *Candida* infections including *C. krusei*.[48]

CLINICAL CONTROVERSY

Three new lipid formulations of amphotericin (amphotericin B lipid complex, amphotericin B cholesteryl sulfate, and liposomal amphotericin B) offer several advantages over amphotericin B deoxycholate.[49] They are less nephrotoxic, allow increased daily doses, have high tissue concentrations in the reticuloendothelial organs such as lungs, liver, and spleen, and have decreased infusion-associated side effects. However, superior clinical efficacy over the conventional amphotericin B or between the lipid formulations has not established clearly in comparative clinical trials. Higher cost and the lack of overall benefit of using a lipid formulation have led to placing the lipid-associated preparations as primarily for patients who are intolerant of or have an infection refractory to the deoxycholate preparation.[50] However, recent data reported an association of amphotericin B–induced nephrotoxicty with increased mortality, up to 6.6-fold, suggesting the use of a lipid formulation initially for patients at high risk of being intolerant.[48,51]

Caspofungin, the first echinocandin antifungal agent, appears to be potent against all *Candida* spp., including *C. glabrata*, *C. krusei*, and *C. lusitaniae* and *Aspergillus* spp. Intravenous caspofungin was reported to be equally effective but better tolerated than amphotericin B deoxycholate for invasive candidiasis.[52]

ANTIVIRAL THERAPY

When sepsis is caused by a systemic viral infection, parenteral antivirals such as acyclovir, ganciclovir, foscarnet, or ribavirin are used, depending on the suspected or documented viral pathogen. Aerosol administration of ribavirin may be indicated in serious illness secondary to respiratory syncytial virus.

DURATION OF THERAPY

The average duration of antimicrobial therapy in the normal host with sepsis is 10 to 14 days.[7,48] However, the duration may vary depending on the site of the infection, as well as the overall response to therapy. After the patient is stable hemodynamically, has been afebrile for 48 to 72 hours, has a normalizing white blood cell (WBC) count, and is able to take oral medications, then a step-down from parenteral to oral antibiotics can be considered for the remaining duration of therapy. Treatment may continue considerably longer if the infection is persistent. In a neutropenic patient, therapy usually is continued until the patient is no longer neutropenic and has been afebrile for at least 72 hours.

HEMODYNAMIC SUPPORT

A high cardiac output and a low systemic vascular resistance characterize septic shock. Patients may have hypotension as a result of low systemic vascular resistance and abnormal distribution of blood flow in the microcirculation, resulting in compromised tissue perfusion. Because approximately half of patients with septic shock die of MOSF, they should be monitored carefully, and aggressive hemodynamic support should be initiated.

Hemodynamics change rapidly in sepsis, and noninvasive evaluation may give inaccurate assessment of filling pressures and cardiac output, requiring a right-sided heart catheter in an intensive care unit.[53] Hemodynamic support can be divided into three main categories: fluid therapy, vasopressor therapy, and inotropic therapy.

FLUID THERAPY

Septic patients have enormous fluid requirements as a result of peripheral vasodilation and capillary leakage.[53] Rapid fluid resuscitation is the best initial therapeutic intervention for the treatment of hypotension in sepsis. The goal of fluid therapy is to maximize cardiac output by increasing the left ventricular preload, which ultimately will restore tissue perfusion.[53] Fluid administration should be titrated to clinical end points such as heart rate, urine output, blood pressure, and mental status. An increased serum lactate level, a byproduct of cellular anaerobic metabolism, should normalize as the tissue perfusion improves.

Isotonic crystalloids, such as 0.9% sodium chloride (normal saline) or lactated Ringer's solution, are used commonly for fluid resuscitation. A patient in septic shock typically requires up to 10 L of crystalloid solution during the first 24-hour period. These solutions distribute into the extracellular compartment. Approximately 25% of the infused volume of crystalloid remains in the intravascular space, whereas the balance distributes to extravascular spaces. Although this could impair diffusion of oxygen to tissues, clinical impact is unproven.

The most commonly used colloids are 5% albumin, naturally occurring plasma protein, and 6% hetastarch, a synthetic colloid formulation. These solutions offer more rapid restoration of intravascular volume because they produce greater intravascular volume expansion per quantity of volume infused. Colloids produce less peripheral edema than crystalloid, but there is no significant clinical impact. The use of colloid solutions and blood products may be particularly important if there is significant blood loss associated with sepsis or if the patient had severe preexisting anemia.

The major complications with fluid resuscitation are pulmonary and systemic edema. Aggressive volume expansion may cause an increase in pulmonary capillary pressure leading to an increase in lung water and associated hypoxemia. Currently available studies and reports suggest that there is no significant difference in the incidence of pulmonary edema between the crystalloid and colloid solutions. A meta-analysis of clinical studies comparing crystalloid and colloid resuscitation indicated no clinical outcome differences.[54]

Although crystalloid solutions require two to four times more volume than colloids, they are generally recommended for fluid resuscitation owing to the lower cost. However, colloids may be preferred, especially when the serum albumin concentration is less than 2.0 g/dL.

VASOPRESSOR AND INOTROPIC THERAPY

When fluid resuscitation alone provides inadequate arterial pressure and organ perfusion, vasopressors and inotropic agents should be initiated. Inotropic agents such as dopamine and dobutamine have been effective in improving cardiac output. Vasopressors should be considered when a systolic blood pressure is less than 90 mm Hg or mean arterial pressure (MAP) is lower than 60 to 65 mm Hg after adequate left ventricular preload and inotrope therapy. Although inotropes and vasopressors are effective in life-threatening hypotension and in improving cardiac index, there are significant complications, such as tachycardia and myocardial ischemia and infarction, as a result of the change in myocardial oxygen consumption in patients with coexisting coronary disease. Thus a catecholamine infusion should be titrated gradually to restore MAP without impairing stroke volume.

Agents commonly considered for vasopressor or inotropic support include dopamine, dobutamine, norepinephrine, phenylephrine, and epinephrine[55,56] (Table 117–4). Dopamine, an α- and β-adrenergic agent with dopaminergic activity, appears to increase MAP effectively in patients who remain hypotensive with reduced cardiac function after aggressive fluid resuscitation. Thus it is often the initial choice in sepsis because of combined vasopressor and inotropic effects. While low-dose dopamine (1 to 5 mcg/kg per minute) is effective in maintaining renal perfusion, higher doses (>5 mcg/kg per minute) exhibit α and β activity and are used frequently to support blood pressure and to improve cardiac function such as an increase in cardiac index (CI).

Dobutamine is a β-adrenergic inotropic agent that many clinicians consider to be the preferred drug for improvement of cardiac output and oxygen delivery, particularly in early sepsis before significant peripheral vasodilation has occurred. Doses of 2 to 20 mcg/kg per minute increases the CI, ranging from 20% to 66%. However, heart rate often increases significantly.[53] Dobutamine should be considered in severely septic patients with adequate filling pressures and blood pressure but low CI.

Norepinephrine is a potent α-adrenergic agent with less pronounced β-adrenergic activity, and it can be useful in septic shock when the clinician desires potent vasoconstriction of peripheral vascular beds. Doses of 0.01 to 3 mcg/kg per minute can reliably increase blood pressure with little change in heart rate or cardiac index. Norepinephrine is a more potent agent than dopamine in refractory septic shock. Despite the earlier concern of decreased renal blood flow associated with norepinephrine, data in humans and animals demonstrate a

TABLE 117–4. Receptor Activity of Cardiovascular Agents Commonly Used in Septic Shock

Agent	α_1	α_2	β_1	β_2	Dopaminergic
Dopamine	++/+++	?	++++	++	++++
Dobutamine	+	+	++++	++	0
Norepinephrine	+++	+++	+++	++	0
Phenylephrine	++/+++	+	?	0	0
Epinephrine	++++	++++	++++	+++	0

$\alpha_1 = \alpha_1$-adrenergic receptor; $\alpha_2 = \alpha_2$-adrenergic receptor; $\beta_1 = \beta_1$-adrenergic receptor; $\beta_2 = \beta_2$-adrenergic receptor; 0 = no activity; ++++ = maximal activity; ? = unknown activity.

norepinephrine-induced renal blood flow as well as urine and cardiac output.[55–57]

Phenylephrine, a selective α_1-agonist, has a rapid onset, short duration, and primary vascular effects, making it an attractive agent in the management of hypotension associated with septic shock. The limited available information suggests that it can increase blood pressure in fluid-resuscitated patients, and it does not appear to impair cardiac or renal function. Phenylephrine appears useful when tachycardia limits the use of other vasopressors.

Epinephrine, a nonspecific α- and β-adrenergic agonist, is capable of increasing CI and producing significant peripheral vasoconstriction in doses of 0.1 to 0.5 mcg/kg per minute. However, because of its undesirable effects, including a propensity to increase lactate level and to impair blood flow to the splanchnic system, it should be reserved for patients who fail to respond to traditional therapies for increasing or maintaining blood pressure.

During hypotension, endogenous vasopressin levels increase and maintain arterial blood pressure by vasoconstriction. However, there is a vasopressin deficiency in septic shock. Low doses of vasopressin (0.01 to 0.04 units/min) have been demonstrated to produce a significant rise in MAP in septic shock, leading to the discontinuation of other vasopressors.[55,58] While it may be beneficial to patients requiring high-dose vasopressors, routine use is not currently recommended owing to a lack of large, randomized, prospective clinical trials.[55,57]

In summary, for the septic patient with clinical signs of shock and significant hypotension unresponsive to aggressive fluid therapy, dopamine is the preferred agent for increasing the blood pressure. If dopamine does not produce the desired hemodynamic response, norepinephrine can be used. Epinephrine should be considered for refractory hypotension. Dopamine and epinephrine are more likely to induce or exacerbate tachycardia than norepinephrine and phenylephrine. In a septic patient with low CI after adequate fluid therapy and an adequate MAP, dobutamine is the first-line agent. Alternatively, dopamine in moderate doses (5 to 10 mcg/kg per minute) also can be used as an initial agent because of its selective effect on increasing cardiac output with its minimal effect on the systemic vascular resistance.

■ EARLY GOAL-DIRECTED THERAPY

8 A trial evaluated the timing of the goal-directed therapy involving adjustments of cardiac preload, afterload, and contractility to balance oxygen delivery with demand prior to admission to the intensive care unit. The mortality rate was 30% in the group receiving early goal-directed therapy including a placement of central venous catheter, more fluid than with traditional therapy, dobutamine therapy to a maximum of 20 mcg/kg per minute, and red blood cell transfusions during the first 6 hours. In comparison, the mortality rate was 46.5% in the traditional therapy group consisting of fluid resuscitation followed by vasopressor therapy if required.[59] Increased oxygen delivery from the red blood cell transfusions in the early goal-directed therapy group appeared to be the primary difference between the two groups.

■ ADJUNCTIVE THERAPIES

ARDS and hypoxia are common in septic patients, even in septic patients without pulmonary infection. Oxygen therapy is indicated to maintain oxygen saturation greater than 90%, and with progressive pulmonary insufficiency, the patient may require assisted ventilation.

The management of patients with ARDS is primarily supportive. Uncontrolled reports suggest that intravenous methylprednisolone in doses of 75 to 250 mg every 6 hours may improve survival in severely ill patients with refractory late ARDS.[60,61] Ketoconazole reduced the progression to ARDS and increased survival in a small study of septic surgical patients, possibly as a result of its inhibitory effects on alveolar macrophage production of leukotriene B_4 and thromboxane A_2.[62]

Nitric oxide (NO), a potent endogenous vasodilator, improved arterial oxygenation and reduced pulmonary artery pressures in patients with ARDS. However, it is also associated with hypotension, as well as being a mediator of sepsis-induced refractoriness to the vasopressor effects of catecholamines.[63] Additional work is needed to define any role for NO and ketoconazole in the management of sepsis.

Hyperglycemia frequently is associated with sepsis, and it is usually quite refractory to exogenous insulin. Intensive insulin therapy, maintaining blood glucose level at 80 to 110 mg/dL resulted in lower morbidity and mortality among critically ill patients in comparison with those with blood glucose levels of 180 to 200 mg/dL.[64] Insulin therapy also reduced the rate of death from multiple-organ failure among patients with sepsis, regardless of presence of diabetes prior to sepsis.

The corticosteroids have been the subject of much controversy in the management of septic patients.[65,66] Corticosteroids suppress the activation of polymorphonuclear leukocytes, complement activation, release of TNF, and activation of the coagulation system involved in the cascades of sepsis. A recent study demonstrated a decrease in mortality (absolute reduction of 10%) with lower doses of hydrocortisone and fludrocortisone in patients with adrenal insufficiency requiring high-dose or increasing vasopressor therapy within the first 8 hours of septic shock.[67] There was no benefit for those patients without adrenal insufficiency. In summary, routine use of corticosteroids in patients with sepsis or septic shock is not recommended until further study.

Heparin therapy for DIC is discouraged by most clinicians because there is no evidence that heparin prolongs the survival of patients despite its effect on the hypercoagulable condition found in DIC.[68] Hemorrhage is best managed by the replacement of clotting factors, platelets, and packed red blood cells.

Patients with severe sepsis are susceptible to progressive malnutrition secondary to the hypermetabolism associated with severe illness and injury.[69] Hence early enteral nutrition is recommended in patients with severe sepsis and septic shock to meet the increased energy and protein requirements. Protein requirements are increased to 1.5 to 2.5 g/kg per day, and increased amounts of branched-chain amino acids may be beneficial in septic patients.[70] Nonprotein caloric requirements range from 25 to 40 kcal/kg per day, and overfeeding of carbohydrates should be avoided to reduce the ventilatory requirements of the patient. The use of increased amounts of lipid to meet nonprotein caloric needs while reducing carbohydrate administration may be useful in this setting.

■ IMMUNOTHERAPY

A number of strategies have been used to reverse or control the inflammatory process initiated during sepsis[71] (Table 117–5). Despite the initial enthusiasm in immunotherapeutic interventions for sepsis,

TABLE 117-5. Summary of Selected Clinical Trials for Sepsis

Experimental Agent	Comments
HA-1A (antilipid A MAb)	No overall benefit; favorable trend in meningococcemia (preliminary report)
E5 (antilipid A MAb)	No overall benefit; improved organ dysfunction in some subgroups
Interleukin 1 receptor antagonist	No overall benefit
Platelet-activating factor inhibitors	No overall benefit; favorable trend in gram-negative sepsis
Bradykinin antagonists	No overall benefit; favorable trend in gram-negative sepsis
Anti-TNF MAb	No overall benefit; some evidence of improvement in subgroups of shock patients
TNF receptor: immunoglobulin constructs	Phase II: p75 receptor worsened outcome ($p < .01$); p55 receptor no overall benefit in phase III despite favorable trends in phase II
L-N-Monomethylarginine	No overall benefit, preliminary report

overall results generally have been disappointing with the exception of recombinant human activated protein C (Drotrecogin-alfa).

Recombinant human activated protein C, the first anti-inflammatory agent to be approved for sepsis, promotes fibrinolysis and associated anti-inflammatory mechanisms. The Recombinant Human Activated Protein C Worldwide Evaluation in Severe Sepsis (PROWESS) trial studied the effects of 96 hours of continuous infusion of recombinant activated protein C.[21] All-cause mortality at 28 days was reduced significantly from 30.8% with placebo to 24.7% in those receiving activated protein C.

The debate regarding certain aspects of the study design, patient selection, and safety continues.[72,73] A higher incidence of serious bleeding occurred during the 28-day period in the activated protein C group (3.5%) than in the placebo group (2.0%).[21] Despite the controversy, activated protein C appears to have a significant role in the treatment of septic shock. Subgroup analysis of the four stratified Acute Physiology and Chronic Health Evaluation (APACHE) II and recent cost-benefit analysis studies suggests the patients with APACHE II scores greater than 25 are the optimal candidates for activated protein C therapy.[21,74,75]

ABBREVIATIONS

APACHE: Acute Physiology and Chronic Health Evaluation
ARDS: acute respiratory distress syndrome
CARS: compensatory anti-inflammatory response syndrome
CI: cardias index
DIC: disseminated intravascular coagulation
Do$_2$: oxygen delivery to tissues
ICU: intensive care unit
IL: interleukin
MAP: mean arterial pressure
MODS: multiple organ dysfunction syndrome
NO: nitric oxide
PAF: platelet-activating factor
SIRS: systemic inflammatory response syndrome
SVR: systemic vascular resistance
TNF: tumor necrosis factor
Vo$_2$: tissue oxygen utilization
WBC: white blood cell

Review Questions and other resources can be found at *www.pharmacotherapyonline.com.*

REFERENCES

1. Martin GS, Mannino DM, Eaton S, Moss M. The epidemiology of sepsis in the United States from 1979 through 2000. N Engl J Med 2003;348:1546–1554.
2. Angus DC, Linde-Zwirble WT, Lidicker J, et al. Epidemiology of severe sepsis in the United States: Analysis of incidence, outcome, and associated costs of care. Crit Care Med 2001;29:1303–1310.
3. American College of Chest Physicians/Society of Critical Care Medicine Consensus Conference. Definitions for sepsis and organ failure and guidelines for the use of innovative therapies in sepsis. Crit Care Med 1992;20:864–874.
4. Fry DE. Sepsis syndrome. Am Surg 2000;66:126–132.
5. Nystrom PO. The systemic inflammatory response syndrome: Definitions and aetiology. J Antimicrob Chemother 1998;41(suppl A):1–7.
6. Levy MM, Fink MP, Marshall JC, et al. 2001 SCCM/ESICM/ACCP/ATS/SIS International Sepsis Definitions Conference. Crit Care Med 2003;31:1250–1256.
7. Harbarth S, Garbino J, Pugin J, et al. Inappropriate initial therapy and its effect on survival in a clinical trial of immunomodulating therapy for severe sepsis. Am J Med 2003;115:529–535.
8. Garnacho-Montero J, Garcia-Garmendia JL, Barrero-Almodovar A, et al. Impact of adequate empirical antibiotic therapy on the outcome of patients admitted to the intensive care unit with sepsis. Crit Care Med 2003;31:2742–2751.
9. Lazaron V. Gram-negative sepsis and the sepsis syndrome. Urol Clin North Am 1999;26:687–699.
10. Young LS. Sepsis syndrome. In: Mandell GL, Bennett JE, Dolin R, eds. Principles and Practice of Infectious Diseases, 5th ed. New York, Churchill-Livingstone, 2000;806–819.
11. Pfaller MA, Diekema DJ, Jones RN, et al. Trends in antifungal susceptibility of Candida spp. isolated from pediatric and adult patients with bloodstream infection: SENTRY Antimicrobial Surveillance Program, 1997–2000. J Clin Microbiol 2002;40:852–856.
12. Bodey GP, Mardani M, Hanna HA, et al. The epidemiology of Candida glabrata and Candida albicans fungemia in immunocompromised patients with cancer. Am J Med 2002;112:380–385.
13. Costa SF, Marinho I, Araujo EA, et al. Nosocomial fungaemia: A 2-year prospective study. J Hosp Infect 2000;45:69–72.
14. Bone RC, Grodzin CJ, Balk RJ. Sepsis: A new hypothesis for the pathogenesis of the diseases process. Chest 1997;112:235–243.
15. Marie C, Muret J, Fitting C, et al. Interleukin-1 receptor antagonist production during infectious and noninfectious systemic inflammatory response syndrome. Crit Care Med 2000;28:2277–2282.
16. Kim PK, Deutschman CS. Inflammatory responses and mediators. Surg Clin North Am 2000;80:885–894.
17. Van der Poll T, van Deventer SJH. Cytokines and anticytokines in the pathogenesis of sepsis. Infect Dis Clinic North Am 1999;13:413–426.
18. Van der Poll T, Malefyt RW, Coyle SM, Lowry SF. Antiinflammatory cytokine responses during clinical sepsis and experimental endotoxemia: Sequential measurements of plasma soluble interleukin (IL)–1 receptor type II, IL-10, IL-13. J Infect Dis 1997;175:118–122.
19. Hardaway RM. A review of septic shock. Am Surg 2000;66:22–29.
20. Lush CW, Kvietys PR. Microvascular dysfunction in sepsis. Microcirculation 2000;7:83–101.
21. Bernard GR, Vincent JL, Laterre PF, et al. Efficacy and safety of recombinant human activated protein C for severe sepsis. N Engl J Med 2001;344:699–709.

22. Damas P, Canivet J, De Groote D, et al. Sepsis and serum cytokine concentrations. Crit Care Med 1997;25:405–412.

23. Damas P, Ledoux D, Nys M, et al. Cytokine serum level during sepsis in human IL-6 as a marker of severity. Ann Surg 1992;215:356–362.

24. Damas P, Reuter A, Gysen P, et al. Tumor necrosis factor and interleukin-1 serum levels during severe sepsis in humans. Crit Care Med 1989;17:975–978.

25. Steinmetz HT, Herbertz A, Bertram M, Diehl V. Increase in interleukin-6 serum level preceding fever in granulocytopenia and correlation with death from sepsis. J Infect Dis 1995;171:225–228.

26. Marty C, Misset B, Tamion F, et al. Circulating interleukin-8 concentrations in patients with multiple organ failure of septic and nonseptic origin. Crit Care Med 1994;22:673–679.

27. Strutz F, Heller G, Krasemann K, et al. Relationship of antibodies to endotoxin core to mortality in medical patients with sepsis syndrome. Intensive Care Med 1999;25:435–444.

28. Nimah M, Brill RJ. Coagulation dysfunction in sepsis and multiple organ failure. Crit Care Med 2003;19:441–458.

29. Caksen H, Ozturk MK, Uzum K, et al. Pulmonary complications in patients with staphylococcal sepsis. Pediatr Int 2000;42:268–271.

30. Martin MA, Silverman HJ. Gram-negative sepsis and the adult respiratory distress syndrome. Clin Infect Dis 1992;14:1213–1228.

31. Awad SS. State-of-the-art therapy for severe sepsis and multisystem organ failure. Am J Surg 2003;186:23–30S.

32. Hirrela E. Advances in the management of acute respiratory distress syndrome. Arch Surg 2000;135:126–134.

33. Bunnell E, Parrillo JE. Cardiac dysfunction during septic shock. Clin Chest Med 1996;17:237–248.

34. Dellinger RP. Current therapy for sepsis. Infect Dis Clin North Am 1999;13:495–509.

35. Simon D, Trenholme G. Antibiotic selection for patients with septic shock. Crit Care Clin 2000;16:215–231.

36. Kays MB, Conklin M. Comparative in vitro activity and pharmacodynamics of five fluoroquinolones against clinical isolates of *Streptococcus pneumoniae*. Pharmacotherapy 2000;20:1310–1317.

37. Blondeau JM. A review of the comparative in-vitro activities of 12 antimicrobial agents, with a focus on five new "respiratory quinolones." J Antimicrob Chemother 1999;43(suppl B):1–11.

38. Wood MJ. Chemotherapy for gram-positive nosocomial sepsis. J Chemother 1999;11:446–452.

39. Harding I, MacGowan AP, White LO, et al. Teicoplanin therapy for *Staphylococcus aureus* septicaemia: Relationship between predose serum concentrations and outcome. J Antimicrob Chemother 2000;45:835–841.

40. Chien JW, Kucia ML, Salata RA. Use of linezolid, an oxazolidinone, in the treatment of multidrug-resistant gram-positive bacterial infections. Clin Infect Dis 2000;30:146–151.

41. Solomkin JS, Mazuski JE, Baron EJ, et al. Guidelines for the selection of anti-infective agents for complicated intra-abdominal infections. Clin Infect Dis 2003;37:997–1005.

42. Jaspers CA, Kieft H, Speelberg B, et al. Meropenem versus cefuroxime plus gentamicin for treatment of serious infections in elderly patients. Antimicrob Agents Chemother 1998;42;1233–1238.

43. Bradley JS, Garau J, Lode H, et al. Carbapenems in clinical practice: A guide to their use in serious infection. Int J Antimicrob Agents 1999;11:93–100.

44. Dalmau D, Cayouette M, Lamothe F, et al. Clindamycin resistance in *Bacteroides fragilis* group: Association with hospital-acquired infection. Clin Infect Dis 1997:24:874–877.

45. Hatala R, Dinh T, Cook DJ. Single daily dosing of aminoglycosides in immunocompromised adults: A systemic review. Clin Infect Dis 1997;24:810–815.

46. Chuck SK, Raber SR, Rodvold KA, Areff D. National survey of extended-interval aminoglycoside dosing. Clin Infect Dis 2000;30:433–439.

47. Wallace AW, Jones M, Bertino JS. Evaluation of four once-daily aminoglycoside dosing nomograms. Pharmacotherapy 2002;22:1077–1083.

48. Pappas PG, Rex JH, Sobel JD, et al. Guidelines for treatment of candidiasis. Infectious Diseases Society of America. Clin Infect Dis 2004;38:161–189.

49. Robinson RF, Nahata MC. A comparative review of conventional and lipid formulations of amphotericin B. J Clin Pharmacol Ther 1999;24:249–257.

50. Cagnoni PJ, Walsh TJ, Prendergast MM, et al. Pharmacoeconomic analysis of liposomal amphotericin B versus conventional amphotericin B in the empirical treatment of persistently febrile neutropenic patients. J Clin Oncol 2000;18:2476–2483.

51. DW, Su L, Yu DT, et al. Mortality and costs of acute renal failure associated with amphotericin-B therapy. Clin Infect Dis 2001;32:686–693.

52. Mora-Duarte J, Betts R, Rotstein R, et al. Comparison of caspofungin and amphotericin B for invasive candidiasis. N Engl J Med 2002;347:2020–2029.

53. Practice parameters for hemodynamic support of sepsis in adult patients in sepsis. Task force of the American College of Critical Care Medicine, Society of Critical Care Medicine. Crit Care Med 1999;27:639–660.

54. Choi PTL, Yip G, Quinonez LG, et al. Crystalloids versus colloids in fluid resuscitation: systemic review. Crit Care Med 1999;27:200–210.

55. Dellinger RP. Cardiovascular management of septic shock. Crit Care Med 2003;31:946–955.

56. Rendl-Wenzel EM, Armbruster C, Edelmann G, et al. The effects of norepinephrine on hemodynamics and renal function in severe septic shock states. Intensiv Care Med 1993;19:151–154.

57. Russell JA. Vasopressin in septic shock: Clinical equipoise mandates a time for restraint. Crit Care Med 2003;31:2707–2708.

58. Klinzing S, Simon M, Reinhart K, et al. High-dose vasopressin is not superior to norepinephrine in septic shock. Crit Care Med 2003;31:2646–2650.

59. Rivers E, Nguyen B, Havstad S, et al. Early goal-directed therapy in the treatment of severe sepsis and septic shock. N Engl J Med 2001;345:1368–1377.

60. Hooper RG, Kearl RA. Established adult respiratory distress syndrome successfully treated with corticosteroids. South Med J 1996;89:449–451.

61. Biffl WL, Moore FA, Moore EE, et al. Are corticosteroids salvage therapy for refractory acute respiratory distress syndrome? Am J Surg 1995;170:591–596.

62. Yu M, Tomasa G. A double-blind, prospective, randomized trial for ketoconazole, a thromboxane synthetase inhibitor, in the prophylaxis of the adult respiratory distress syndrome. Crit Care Med 1993;21:1635–1642.

63. Rossaint R, Falke KJ, Lopez F, et al. Inhaled nitric oxide for the adult respiratory distress syndrome. New Engl J Med 1993;328:339–405.

64. Van Den Berghe G, Wouters P, Weekers F, et al. Intensive insulin therapy in critically ill patients. N Engl J Med 2001;345:1359–1367.

65. Sessler CN. Steroids for septic shock back from the dead? (Con). Chest 2003;123:482–489S.

66. Balk RA. Steroids for septic shock back from the dead? (Pro). Chest 2003;123:490–499S.

67. Annane D, Sebille V, Charpentier C, et al. Effects of treatment with low-dose hydrocortisone and fludrocortisone on mortality in patients with septic shock. JAMA 2002;288:862–871.

68. Staudinger T, Locker GJ, Frass M. Management of acquired coagulation disorders in emergency and intensive-care medicine. Semin Thromb Hemost 1996;22:93–104.

69. DeWitt RC, Kudsk KA. The gut's role in metabolism, mucosal barrier function, and gut immunology. Infect Dis Clin North Am 1999;13:465–481.

70. Garcia-de-Lorenzo A, Ortiz-Leyba C, Planas M, et al. Parenteral administration of different amounts of branch-chain amino acids in septic patients: Clinical and metabolic aspects. Crit Care Med 1997;25:418–424.

71. Nasraway SA. The problems and challenges of immunotherapy in sepsis. Chest 2003;123:451–459S.

72. Bernard GR. Drotrecogin alfa (activated) recombinant human activated

protein C for the treatment of severe sepsis. Crit Care Med 2003;31: S85–93.

73. Eichacker RQ, Natanson C. Recombinant human activated protein C in sepsis: Inconsistent trial results, an unclear mechanism of action, and safety concerns resulted in labeling restrictions and the need for phase IV trials. Crit Care Med 2003:31:S94–96.

74. Manns BJ, Lee H, Doig CJ, et al. An economic evaluation of activated protein C treatment for severe sepsis. N Engl J Med 2002;347: 993–1000.

75. Angus DC, Linde-Zwirble WT, Clermont G, et al. Cost-effectiveness of drotrecogin alfa (activated) in the treatment of severe sepsis. Crit Care Med 2003;31:1–11.

118

SUPERFICIAL FUNGAL INFECTIONS

Thomas E. R. Brown and Thomas W. F. Chin

Learning Objectives and other resources can be found at *www.pharmacotherapyonline.com.*

KEY CONCEPTS

1. Vulvovaginal candidiasis (VVC) can be classified as uncomplicated or complicated. This classification is useful in determining appropriate pharmacotherapy.

2. *Candida albicans* is the major pathogen responsible for VVC. The number of cases of non-*albicans* species appears to be increasing.

3. Signs and symptoms of VVC are not pathogonmonic, and reliable diagnosis must be made with laboratory tests.

4. *Candida albicans* is the predominant species causing all forms of mucosal candidiasis. A number of host and exogenous factors have been identified as important risk factors predisposing an individual to the development of mucosal candidiasis. In oropharyngeal and esophageal candidiasis, the key risk factor is impaired host immune system.

5. A topical agent is the first choice for treating oropharyngeal candidiasis, whereas systemic therapy may be used in patients not responding to an adequate trial of topical treatment or unable to tolerate topical agents and in those at high risk for systemic candidiasis. Fluconazole and intraconazole solution are the most effective azole agents.

6. In esophageal candidiasis, topical agents are not of proven benefit; fluconazole or intraconazole solution is the first choice.

7. It is important that patients with human immunodeficiency virus (HIV) infection be on concurrent optimal antiretroviral therapy, which is important for the prevention of recurrent and refractory candidiasis.

8. Primary or secondary prophylaxis of fungal infection is not recommended routinely for HIV-infected patients; use of secondary prophylaxis should be individualized for each patient.

9. Topical agents are first-line agents for fungal skin infections. Exceptions are for the treatment of extensive or severe infection or those of tinea capitis or onychomycosis. Oral therapy is preferred in such situations.

10. Oral agents, in particular terbinafine and itraconazole, are first-line treatment for toenail and fingernail onychomycosis.

Superficial mycoses are among the most common infections in the world and the second most common vaginal infections in North America. Mucocutaneous candidiasis may occur in three forms, oropharyngeal, esophageal, and vulvovaginal disease, with oropharyngeal and vulvovaginal disease being the most common forms. These infections were reported in humans as far back as 1839. Over the last 15 to 20 years, the occurrence rates of some fungal infections have increased dramatically. The prevalence of fungal skin infections varies throughout different parts of the world from the most common causes of skin infections in the tropics to relatively rare disorders in the United States. This chapter reviews the pharmacotherapy of vulvovaginal candidiasis, oropharyngeal and esophageal candidiasis, and common dermatophyte infections.

VULVOVAGINAL CANDIDIASIS

1. *Vulvovaginal candidiasis* (VVC) refers to infections in individuals with or without symptoms who have positive vaginal cultures for *Candida*. Depending on episodic frequency, VVC can be classified as either sporadic or recurrent.[1] This classification is essential to understanding the pathophysiology, as well as the pharmacother-

apy, of VVC. Furthermore, VVC may be defined as *uncomplicated,* which refers to sporadic infections that are susceptible to all forms of antifungal therapy regardless of the duration of treatment, or *complicated,* in which consideration of factors affecting the host, microorganism, and pharmacotherapy all have an essential role in successful treatment.[1] Complicated VVC includes recurrent VVC, severe disease, non-*albicans* candidiasis, and abnormal host factors, including diabetes mellitus, immunosuppression, and pregnancy.[1]

EPIDEMIOLOGY

Minimal information on the incidence and prevalence of VVC exists. Health care workers are not required to report cases of VVC; therefore, estimates are derived from self-reported histories. Epidemiologic data are limited because VVC usually is diagnosed without microscopy and/or cultures, and antifungal nonprescription preparations are available for self-treatment.[1] By 25 years of age, approximately 50% of college women will have had at least one episode of VVC.[1] It is rare before menarche and increases dramatically around 20 years of age, with the peak incidence between 30 and 40 years of age. It is associated with the initial act of sexual intercourse. As many as 75% of women experience one bout of symptomatic VVC in their lifetime.

Bewteen 40% and 50% of women who experience one episode of VVC experience a second episode, and 5% experience recurrent VVC.[2,3] Black women appear to be at higher risk of developing VVC as compared with whites (62.8% versus 55%, respectively).[4] The incidence after menopause remains unknown.

PATHOPHYSIOLOGY

Candida albicans is the major pathogen responsible for VVC, accounting for 80% to 92% of symptomatic episodes. The remainder are caused by non-*albicans* species, with *C. glabrata* dominating.[5] The number of cases of non-*albicans* candidiasis appears to be increasing, possibly related to the use of nonprescription vaginal antifungal preparations and short-course therapy and/or the increased use of long-term maintenance therapy in preventing recurrent infections.[1]

Candida species can act as commensal members of the vaginal flora. Asymptomatic colonization with *Candida* has been found in 10% to 20% of reproductive-aged women.[5,6] *Candida* organisms are dimorphic; blastospores are believed to be responsible for colonization (transmission and spread), whereas germinated *Candida* forms are associated with tissue invasion and symptomatic infections.[7] To colonize the vagina, *Candida* must be able to attach to the mucosa. The attachment process is complex. Not only are candidal surface structures important for attachment, but appropriate receptors for attachment must be present in the epithelial tissue. Not all women have the same range of receptors, which may explain variation in colonization.[6] Changes in the host's vaginal environment or response are necessary to induce a symptomatic infection. Unfortunately, in most cases of symptomatic VVC, no precipitating factor can be identified.[7]

RISK FACTORS

Several factors predispose a woman to VVC. Vulvovaginal candidiasis is not considered to be a sexually transmitted disease, although sexual factors may be important. There is a dramatic increase in the frequency of VVC when women become sexually active. In addition, oral-genital contact may increase the risk.[1] However, current guidelines do not recommend the treatment of asymptomatic partners.[5] Contraceptive agents, including the diaphragm with spermicide, the contraceptive sponge, and the intrauterine device, increase the risk of VVC. Oral contraceptive users demonstrated increased risk of

TABLE 118–1. Clinical Presentation of Vulvovaginal Candidiasis

General Symptoms	Often involves both the vulva and the vagina Intense vulvar itching, soreness, irritation, burning on urination, and dyspareunia
Signs	Erythema, fissuring, curdy "cheese"-like discharge, satellite lesions, edema
Laboratory tests	Vaginal pH—normal, saline and 10% KOH microscopy—blastospores or pseudohyphae
Other diagnostic tests	*Candida* cultures not recommended unless classic signs and symptoms with normal vaginal pH and microscopy is inconclusive or recurrence is suspected

candidiasis; however, these reports were with the higher-dose oral contraceptive pills, and the risk may not be as great with the lower estrogen-dose oral contraceptives.[8]

Antibiotic use may increase the risk of VVC, but it is only significant in a small number of women. The mechanism by which antibiotics can increase the risk of VVC is unknown; colonization, however, is a prerequisite.[1] Diet (excess refined carbohydrate), douching, and tight-fitting clothing often are listed as important risk factors; however, no association has been established between these factors and increased risk of VVC.[1]

CLINICAL PRESENTATION

The clinical presentation of VVC is given in Table 118–1.[1] These signs and symptoms are not pathognomonic, and a reliable diagnosis cannot be made without laboratory tests. Self-diagnosis has a sensitivity of 35% and a specificity of 89% and a positive predictive value of 62%.[4] More than 50% of women who had self-diagnosed VVC did not have yeast as the causative agent.[9] Diagnosis should be based on both clinical presentation and investigations, including vaginal pH, saline microscopy, and 10% potassium hydroxide (KOH) microscopy. The vaginal pH remains normal in VVC, and microscopic investigations should detect blastospores or pseudohyphae. *Candida* cultures usually are not required in the diagnosis of uncomplicated VVC; however, they are recommended when an individual presents with classic signs and symptoms of VVC, has a normal vaginal pH, but microscopy is inconclusive or recurrence is suspected.[5]

▶ TREATMENT: Vulvovaginal Candidiasis

GOALS OF THERAPY

The goal of therapy is complete resolution of symptoms in patients who have symptomatic VVC. Test of cure is not necessary if symptoms resolve.[5] Antimycotic agents used in the treatment of VVC do not meet the definition of being fungicidal agents because of their slower killing rate. At the end of therapy, the number of viable organisms drops below the detectable range. However, by 6 weeks after a course of therapy, 25% to 40% of women will have positive yeast cultures and remain asymptomatic.[1] Asymptomatic colonization with *Candida* does not require therapy.

GENERAL APPROACHES TO TREATMENT

The approach to therapy is to remove or improve any predisposing factors if they can be identified. A pharmacologic agent should have limited local and systemic side effects, a high cure rate, and easy administration. Additionally, it would be advantageous to use a therapy that is able to resolve symptoms within 24 hours, that has broad antimycotic activity (to cover increasing rates on non-*albicans Candida*), that prevents recurrence, and that can be used over a shortened period of time such as 1 to 3 days.

Avoid harsh soaps and perfumes that may cause or worsen vulvar irritation. Keep the genital area clean and dry by avoiding constrictive clothing and frequent or prolonged exposure to hot tub use.[3] Cool baths may soothe the skin.[3] Daily ingestion of 240 mL yogurt containing *Lactobacillus acidophilus* decreased colonization and symptomatic infections of VVC in women with recurrent infections.[10]

PHARMACOLOGIC TREATMENTS

UNCOMPLICATED VULVOVAGINAL CANDIDIASIS

Cure rates for uncomplicated VVC are between 80% and 95% with topical or oral azoles and between 70% and 90% with nystatin preparations. Table 118–2 lists available topical and oral preparations for the treatment of uncomplicated VVC. There are many topical nonprescription preparations for the treatment of VVC. No significant differences in in vitro activity or clinical efficacy exist between the topical azole agents.[1,3,5] The selection of a topical azole should be based primarily on an individual patient's preference as to product formulation. Some topical products may cause vaginal burning, stinging, or irritation; on the other hand, the vehicle used in topical creams or gels can provide initial symptomatic relief.[1] Of note, though, most topical preparations can decrease the efficacy of latex condoms or diaphragms.

Oral azoles have been used in the treatment of VVC. Patients' prefer oral therapy because of its convenience.[11] Oral and topical therapy are therapeutically equivalent.[1] In the treatment of uncomplicated VVC, the duration of therapy is not critical. Cure rates with different lengths of treatment have not demonstrated that one therapy is significantly better.[12,13] Shorter-duration therapies (e.g., clotrimazole 1-day therapy) consist of higher concentrations of azoles that maintain the local therapeutic effect for up to 72 hours and allow for resolution of signs and symptoms.[14] A review of 14 trials that examined 1-day treatments showed less than 7% difference in short-term cure rates or improvement between any two treatments in any two studies and no significant differences in short- or long-term clinical cure rates among 1-day regimens.[12]

If the vulva is significantly irritated, topical application of a low-potency corticosteroid may be beneficial.[1,3,5] Anecdotal evidence suggests that high-potency corticosteroids may exacerbate the burning sensation initially.[1] Table 118–2 lists the therapeutic options for the treatment of uncomplicated VVC.

COMPLICATED VULVOVAGINAL CANDIDIASIS

Complicated VVC occurs in patients who are immunocompromised or have uncontrolled diabetes mellitus.[1] The main approach to the treatment of these individuals is to increase the length of therapy. Current recommendations are to lengthen therapy to 10 to 14 days regardless of the route of administration.[16] Therapeutic options include those listed in Table 118–2; however, regimens should be continued for 10 to 14 days. In a study of patients experiencing severe infections, better outcomes were achieved with 7-day topical azole therapy compared with single-dose fluconazole.[16] Length of therapy also should be extended in infections caused by non-*albicans* species. Most of these organisms have higher minimum inhibitory concentrations (MICs) to the azoles compared with *C. albicans*. They are still susceptible to the azoles but require a longer duration of treatment.[1]

VVC during pregnancy also may be considered complicated because consideration of host factors such as hormonal changes that

TABLE 118–2. Treatment for Uncomplicated Vulvovaginal Candidiasis

Active Ingredient	Preparation	Regimen
Over the Counter/Topical Vaginal Products		
Butoconazole	2% cream	1 applicator × 3 days
Clotrimazole	1% cream	1 applicator or
	100-mg tablet	1 100 mg tablet × 7 days
	2% cream	1 applicator or
	200-mg tablet	1 200 mg tablet × 3 days
	10% cream	1 applicator or
	500-mg tablet	1 500 mg tablet × 1 day
Miconazole[a]	2% cream	1 applicator or
	100-mg suppository	1 100 mg suppository × 7 days
	200-mg suppository	1 200 mg suppository × 3 days
	1200-mg ovule	1 ovule × 1 day
Ticonazole	6.5% cream	1 applicator or
	300-mg ovule	1 ovule × 1 day
Prescription/Topical		
Econazole	150-mg tablet	1 tablet × 3 days
Fenticonazole	2% cream	1 applicator × 7 days
Nystatin	100,000-unit tablet	1 tablet × 14 days
Terconazole	0.4% cream	1 applicator × 7 days
	0.8% cream	1 applicator or
	80-mg suppository	1 suppository × 3 days
Oral Products		
Ketoconazole	200 mg	1 tablet twice daily × 5 days
Itraconazole	200 mg	1 tablet twice daily × 1 day
Fluconazole	150 mg	1 tablet × 1 day

[a]The U.S. Food and Drug Administration warns of possible increase in anticoagulant effects of warfarin with concomitant use.

can affect normal flora are essential in selecting therapeutic regimens. Topical agents are considered to be safe throughout pregnancy. Nystatin topical cream used for treating VVC was the regimen of choice in the first trimester, but recent guidelines recommend the use of topical azoles and that 10 to 14 days of treatment may be necessary.[5] Oral agents are contraindicated in pregnancy because of the concern for fetal complications. However, a prospective assessment of pregnancy outcomes in 226 women exposed to fluconazole in the first trimester did not indicate increased risk of congenital abnormalities or other adverse outcomes.[17] The median dose of fluconazole was 200 mg, with 46.5% of the cohort receiving a single dose of fluconazole 150 mg.

RECURRENT VULVOVAGINAL CANDIDIASIS

Recurrent vulvovaginal candidiasis (RVVC) is defined as having more than four episodes of VVC within a 12-month period.[1,5] Fewer than 5% of women develop RVVC, and its pathogenesis is poorly understood. A proper diagnosis should be obtained to rule out other infections or nonmycotic contact dermatitis. Most of the therapies are empirical and not based on proper randomized, controlled trials.[5] Treatments include induction therapy, which should be administered for a minimum of 14 days or until clinical remission and negative cultures have been obtained.[1] Table 118–2 lists the medications used for induction therapy. Induction therapy should be followed by a

maintenance regimen that is used for 6 months. The following are recommended maintenance regimens:

Clotrimazole 500 mg vaginally once weekly for 6 months
Fluconazole 100 mg once weekly for 6 months
Ketoconazole 100 mg daily for 6 months
Itraconazole 400 mg once monthly for 6 months

Fifty percent of women may experience a relapse after maintenance therapy is discontinued.[5] A relapse may be treated as an individual episode if relapses are infrequent. However, if the relapses establish a repetitive pattern, then induction and maintenance regimens are indicated.[1]

ANTIFUNGAL RESISTANT VULVOVAGINAL CANDIDIASIS

Resistance to azole antifungals should be considered in individuals who have persistently positive yeast cultures and fail to respond to therapy despite adherence to prescribed regimens.[1] These infections can be treated with boric acid or 5-flucytosine.[18,19] Boric acid is administered as a 600-mg intravaginal capsule daily for 14 days of induction therapy, followed by a maintenance regimen of one capsule intravaginally twice weekly. Boric acid is toxic if administered orally. 5-Flucytosine cream is administered vaginally, 1000 mg inserted nightly for 7 days.

PHARMACOECONOMIC CONSIDERATIONS

There is little information on the pharmacoeconomics associated with VVC. One study examined the direct costs, including medical expenses (medications and clinic charges) and nonmedical expenses (costs of travel and time required in obtaining treatment) of VVC. Indirect costs (output loss through disability and premature death) were excluded from their estimates. The estimated total cost for all episodes of VVC in the United States in 1995 was $1.8 billion. The costs were higher in black women compared with white women ($34 versus $16 per capita cost, respectively). This difference is largely a result of the higher incidence of VVC among black women and because black women tend to seek medical advice rather than relying on self-diagnosis and treatment.[4]

EVALUATION OF THERAPEUTIC OUTCOMES

Treatment of VVC will be considered to have positive outcomes if the symptoms of VVC are resolved within 24 to 48 hours and no adverse medication events are experienced. Self-assessment of symptom relief is appropriate for most cases of VVC. If symptoms remain unresolved or recur, then further testing and treatment may be required.

OROPHARYNGEAL AND ESOPHAGEAL CANDIDIASIS

Oropharyngeal candidiasis (OPC) refers to an infection of the oral mucosa, and it is usually referred to informally as *thrush. Candida* is the predominant fungi responsible for the majority of oral fungal infections, and *C. albicans* is the principal species causing the infection, commonly referred to as *candidiasis* (the proper but less commonly used term being *candidosis*). The infection may extend into the esophagus, causing esophageal candidiasis.

EPIDEMIOLOGY AND MICROBIOLOGY

Candida can be isolated from the oral cavity in 30% to 60% of healthy adults but usually in low numbers and with no evidence of infection.[20,21] This is referred to as *asymptomatic colonization. C. albicans* is the predominant colonizing *Candida* species (70% to 80%), but any of the non-*albicans Candida* species may be seen.[20,21] Colonization rates are influenced by the severity and nature of the underlying medical illness and the duration of hospitalization, as well as age (highest in infants younger than 18 months of age and in adults over age 60 years). A variety of host and exogenous factors (Table 118–3) can lead to the transformation of asymptomatic colonization to symptomatic disease such as oropharyngeal and esophageal candidiasis. *C. albicans* is the most common species causing all forms of mucosal candidiasis in humans. Although OPC usually is linked synonymously with *C. albicans* infection, a number of other *Candida* species also can be pathogenic. These include *C. glabrata, C. tropicalis, C. krusei, C. guilliermondi, C. parapsilosis,* and others.[20,22,23] *C. krusei,* although relatively uncommon, generally is recovered from mucosal surfaces of neutropenic patients with hematologic malignancies.[24] Another species, *C. dubliniesis,* has been identified in both human immunodeficiency virus (HIV)–infected and noninfected patients.[23,24] There has been a noteworthy increase in the frequency of infections caused by the non-*albicans* species, which accounted for approximately 17% of *Candida* infections by the early 1990s.[22] In patients with cancer, almost half (46%) of all *Candida* infections are caused by non-*albicans* species.[25]

The incidence of OPC has increased significantly over the past 15 to 20 years. OPC is the most common opportunistic infection in patients with HIV disease, and it may be the first clinical manifestation of the HIV infection in the majority of untreated patients. Reported prevalence rates of OPC in the HIV-positive population vary from 12% to 96%.[22] However, up to 90% of untreated advanced HIV-infected patients likely have developed at least one episode of OPC at some stage during the progressive course of their disease.[22,23] The incidence

TABLE 118–3. Risk Factors for Development of Oropharyngeal and/or Esophageal Candidiasis

Local Factors	Potential Mechanisms
Use of steroids and antibiotics	Suppression of cellular immunity and inhibition of phagocytosis by steroids, including chronic use of inhaled and topical steroids. Alteration of endogenous oral flora by broad-spectrum antibiotics, especially when used with steroids, creates a milieu for proliferation of *Candida* due to reduced environmental and nutritional competition.
Dentures	Enhanced adherence of *Candida* to acrylic material of dentures, reduced saliva flow under surfaces of denture fittings, improperly fitted dentures, or poor oral hygiene; these provide a milieu conducive to survival of microorganisms.
Xerostomia caused by drugs (e.g., tricyclic antidepressants, phenothiazine) and chemotherapy, radiotherapy to head-neck and various diseases, e.g., Sjögren's syndrome, HIV, cancer of head-neck, bone marrow transplant recipients	Reduced dilutional and cleansing effect due to low secretion rate and low pH in saliva. Saliva and mucosa secretions have defense factors, such as lactoferrin, sialoperoxidase, lysozyme, histidine-rich polypeptide, secretory IgA antibodies, specific anti-*Candida* antibodies which help prevent adhesion and overgrowth of *Candida*.
Smoking Disruption of oral mucosa due to chemotherapy and radiotherapy, ulcers, endotracheal intubation trauma, and burns	Oral mucositis induced by radiation and breaks in physical barrier of oral epithelium, which is protective against invasion by microorganisms; altered rate of mucosa regeneration by cancer chemotherapy, which increases vulnerability to infection.

Systemic Factors	Potential Mechanisms
Drugs (cytotoxic agents, corticosteroids, immunosuppressants after organ transplant), omeprazole, environmental chemicals (benzene, pesticides)	Reduced immunity due to drug-induced neutropenia or cell-mediated immunity. Potent inhibition of gastric acid by proton pump inhibitors (PPI) can facilitate growth of *Candida*; PPI also may inhibit cytotoxic effect of lymphocytes and reduce salivary secretion.
Neonates or elderly	Immature immune system of neonates who usually acquire infection during birth to a mother with vaginal candidiasis or from exposure to infected bottle nipples or to skin of adult care giver. Elderly—Unclear if this is the direct effect of age per se or contribution from dentures or underlying comorbidity.
HIV infection/AIDS	Depletion of CD4 T-lymphocytes especially below 200–300 cells/mm^3; anti-*Candida* protective mechanism of T-lymphocytes at a mucosal level is unclear but may be due to altered cytokines, especially gamma-interferon which inhibit transformation of *Candida* blastocondia to the more invasive hyphal phase.
Diabetes	Higher than normal numbers of *C. albicans* cultured from saliva of daibetic patients. May be related to the elevated glucose levels and reduced chemotactic factor in saliva, altered neutrophil function, and reduced saliva volume and flow.
Malignancies (e.g., leukemia, head-neck cancer)	Use of intensive radiotherapy and chemotherapy can disrupt oral mucosa and also cause xerostomia; also prolonged use of broad-spectrum antibiotics in neutropenic patients can alter the normal oral flora. Because of the prolonged neutropenia, the principal immune defect, seen especially in leukemic patients, the initial oropharyngeal candidiasis can become systemic or invasive.
Nutritional deficiencies (e.g., iron, folate, vitamins B$_1$, B$_2$, B$_6$, B$_{12}$, and C)	May be related to dietary restriction or GI absorption problems. Deficiencies may serve to enhance the pathogenic potential of the candida inhabitants, alter host defense mechanisms, or change epithelial barrier integrity.

From refs. 2, 4, 5, and 8.

of OPC increases as the level of immunity (CD4 lymphocyte cell count) decreases, and OPC occurs in approximately 60% of those with a CD4 cell count of less than 100 to 200 cells/mm^3, 50% to 60% of whom will experience frequent recurrences. In non-HIV diseases, such as cancer, the incidence of OPC varies depending on the type of malignant neoplastic disease, level of immune suppression, and type and duration of treatment. OPC is reported in up to one-third of leukemic patients.[21]

After the oropharynx, the esophagus is the most common site of gastrointestinal candidiasis. The prevalence of esophageal candidiasis has increased mainly because of acquired immune-deficiency syndrome (AIDS), as well as the increased numbers of other severely immunocompromised patients.[24] Esophageal candidiasis is the first opportunistic infection in 3% to 10% of HIV-infected patients and is the second most common AIDS-defining disease after *Pneumocystis jiroveci* pneumonia.[25] The mean incidence of esophageal candidiasis among HIV-infected patients ranges from 15% to 20%.[25] The incidence of esophageal candidiasis in non–HIV-infected immunocompromised patients is not well established. *C. albicans* is also the most common cause of esophageal candidiasis, accounting for approximately 80% of cases, with the rest being caused by non-*albicans* species.[24,25]

The epidemiology of mucosal candidiasis has been affected by two factors. The widespread use of the azoles has led to a decline in the prevalence of mucosal candidiasis while leading to the emergence of refractory infections that have become difficult to treat. The introduction of highly active antiretroviral therapy (HAART) appears to have resulted in a significant decline in the incidence of OPC and esophageal candidiasis from over 30% to under 7%.[22,23]

PATHOPHYSIOLOGY

Significant differences exist in the virulence among *Candida* species. Although host and yeast virulence factors responsible for the pathogenesis of esophageal candidiasis are not as well known as for OPC, it is likely that they apply in both diseases. One virulence factor is the ability of the organism to adapt and survive in response to changes in the host environment.[24] The genes required for virulence are regulated in response to the environmental signals (i.e., temperature, pH, osmotic pressure, and iron and calcium ion concentrations). The ability of *C. albicans* to undergo reversible morphologic transition between the budding pseudohyphal and the more invasive hyphal growth forms is also a determinant of virulence, and genes are recognized to play a role.[24] Other virulence factors include adhesive ability of *C. albicans* to epithelial cells and proteins and ability to invade host cells by means of phospholipase and proteinase enzymes.[24]

The presence of *Candida* usually stimulates antibody formation and cell-mediated immunity in most healthy adults without causing any signs or symptoms of infection. Effective antifungal host-defense mechanisms in the oral cavity play an important role in maintaining the colonizing organisms in low numbers for years in the absence of inflammation. The changeover of the role of *Candida* from commensal to pathogenic in the human host usually occurs when host defenses are impaired, such as the T-lymphocyte–mediated immune system and neutrophils. In HIV disease, oral carriage of yeasts and risk of mucosal invasion increase with progressive decline in CD4 cells. Cytokines, especially interferon-γ, inhibit transformation of *Candida* blastoconidia to the more invasive hyphal phase.[20] Neutropenic patients are at highest risk of developing candidiasis, which underscores

the importance of neutrophils in host defense against *Candida*. Several host and exogenous factors contribute to the ability of *Candida* to cause infection (see Table 118–3). Oropharyngeal candidiasis is considered one of the earliest indicators of HIV infection and is a relatively reliable indirect marker of disease progression.[22] Several studies show that OPC, regardless of CD4 cell count, predicts the development of AIDS-related illnesses.[22,25]

Although OPC usually is not a life-threatening infection, i may predispose patients to develop more invasive disease, including esophageal candidiasis.[25] The combined presence of OPC and esophageal symptoms is both specific and sensitive in predicting esophageal disease. The presence of OPC or esophageal candidiasis usually suggests a reduced CD4 cell count and/or elevated HIV load and may be predictive of the progression and prognosis of HIV infection. The incidence of OPC increases, especially when the CD4 cell counts fall to between 500 and 200 cells/mm³.[26] Esophageal candidiasis can be as common or even more common than OPC in patients with more advanced HIV infection. It occurs more commonly later in the natural history of AIDS and almost invariably at a lower CD4 count (range 10–105 cells/mm³).[24] In more than half of HIV-infected patients, HIV infection evolves into AIDS as early as 1 to 3 years after the appearance of oral *Candida* lesions if the HIV infection remains inadequately controlled. Thus OPC has become one of the criteria frequently used in staging systems for HIV infection. For example, the Centers for Disease Control and Prevention (CDC) classifies OPC as indicative of symptomatic HIV infection but does not similarly classify it as AIDS.[25]

RISK FACTORS

 Local and systemic factors, as well as characteristics of the organism itself, can increase the susceptibility of an individual

TABLE 118–4. Clinical Presentation of Oropharyngeal and Esophageal

Oropharyngeal Candidiasis	Esophageal Candidiasis
General The clinical features can be quite diverse (see Table 118–5)	**General** This usually occurs as an extension of OPC. However, the esophagus can be the only site involved. The distal two-thirds, rather than the proximal one-third, is the most common site.
Symptoms Symptoms are diverse and range from none to sore, painful mouth, burning tongue, metallic taste, and dysphagia and odynophagia with involvement of hypopharynx.	**Symptoms** Typically the symptoms are dysphagia, odynophagia, and retrosternal chest pain but may be asymptomatic in some patients. Although rare, epigastric pain may be the dominant symptom.
Signs Signs are variable and may include diffuse erythema and white patches on the surfaces of buccal mucosa, throat, tongue, or gums. Constitutional signs are absent.	**Signs** Constitutional signs, including fever, occasionally occur. Physical findings may range from a few to numerous white or beige plaques of variable size. Plaques may be hyperemic or edematous, with ulceration in more severe cases. Most advanced cases may occur with increased mucosal friability and narrowing of lumen. Uncommon complications include perforation and aortic–esophageal fistula formation.
Laboratory Tests Scraping of an active lesion for microscopic examination can help confirm the diagnosis (presence of psuedohyphae and budding yeast) but is usually not necessary. Cultures are also not necessary since isolation of *Candida* does not distinguish between colonization and true infection. Cultures may be taken in patients responding poorly to therapy to determine the infecting species and to predict likely drug resistance.	**Laboratory Tests** The best test is upper GI endoscopy (more useful than barium swallow); helps exclude other causes of esophagitis (e.g., viral, aphthous ulcers). Diagnosis is confirmed by the histologic presence of *Candida* in biopsy lesions taken during endoscopy. Cultures to look for drug-resistant *Candida* are warranted in patients who require endoscopy.

From refs. 1, 4, 5, and 7.

TABLE 118–5. Clinical Classification of Oropharyngeal Candidiasis

Types	Population at Risk	Clinical Signs and Appearance
Pseudomembranous (thrush)	Neonates, patients with HIV or cancer, debilitated elderly, patients on broad-spectrum antibiotics or steroid inhalers, patients with dry mouth from various causes, smokers	Classic "cottage cheese" appearance, yellowish-white, soft plaques (or milk-curds) overlying areas of erythema on the buccal mucosa, tongue, gums and throat; plaques are easily removed by vigorous rubbing but may leave red or bleeding sites when removed; lesions on the tongue dorsum gives it a bald depapillated appearance.
Erythematous (acute atrophic)	Patients with HIV, patients on broad-spectrum antibiotics or steroid inhalers	Sensitive and painful erythematous mucosa with few, if any, white plaques; lesions are generally on dorsal surface of tongue or hard palate, occasionally on soft palate, but any part of mucosa can be involved; appear as flat red patches on the palate or atrophic patches on tongue dorsum with loss of papillae.
Hyperplastic (candidal leukoplakia)	Smokers; uncommon in patients with HIV	Thick white and adherent keratotic plaques commonly seen on the buccal mucosa and lateral border of tongue; may also see on lips and bottom of mouth; plaques cannot be easily scraped off or only partially removed. This condition is distinct from oral hairy leukoplakia, and it may progress to severe dysplasia or malignancy.
Angular cheilitis	Patients with HIV, denture wearers	Painful red, ulcerative, cracking or fissuring lesion at one or both corners of the mouth due to inflammatory reaction; usually lesions are small and rather punctate, but occasionally may extend in a linear fashion from the angles onto the facial skin.
Denture stomatis (chronic atrophic)	Denture wearers who tend to be elderly and have poor oral hygiene	Red, flat lesions on mucosa beneath the denture and extends to right up to the denture border; more commonly located beneath a maxillary denture, although can be encountered beneath a mandibular denture.

From refs. 1, 2, 7, and 8.

to *Candida* infections[21,23,24,27] (see Table 118–3). Endocrine disorders besides diabetes mellitus, such as hypothyroidism, hypoparathyroidism, and hypoadrenalism, also can predispose patients to *Candida* overgrowth. Patients with primary immune deficiencies such as lymphocytic abnormalities, phagocytic dysfunction, IgA deficiency, viral-induced immune paralysis, and severe congenital immunodeficiencies are also at risk for oropharyngeal candidiasis as well as disseminated candidiasis. Oral mucosal disease, such as lichen planus, can be pre-existent causes of candidiasis. Smoking has been suggested as a predisposing risk factor. In many cases, multiple concurrent predisposing factors to candidiasis may exist; e.g., xerostomia with mucositis and a break in the epithelial surface or immunosuppression, such as might occur in a leukemic patient receiving radiation and chemotherapy. The severity and extent of *Candida* infections increase with the number and severity of predisposing risk factors.

CLINICAL PRESENTATION AND DIAGNOSIS

The clinical signs and symptoms of OPC and the locations of the lesions can be quite diverse[20,23,24,26] (Table 118–4). Oropharyngeal candidiasis can manifest in several major forms[20,21,26,27] (Table 118–5). A presumptive diagnosis of OPC usually is made by the characteristic appearance on the oral mucosa, with resolution of signs and symptoms after antifungal therapy. Pseudomembranous candidiasis, commonly known as *oral thrush,* is the classic and most common form seen in immunosuppressed and immunocompetent hosts. Erythematous and hyperplastic candidiasis and angular cheilitis occur less commonly in the HIV-infected population. Complaints of dysphagia and/or odynophagia in the presence of OPC, along with a therapeutic trial of antifungal, can provide a reliable presumptive diagnosis of esophageal candidiasis. If antifungal therapy does not lead to resolution, more invasive tests can be undertaken.

▶ TREATMENT: Oropharyngeal Candidiasis

■ DESIRED OUTCOMES

The primary desired outcome in the management of OPC is a clinical cure, i.e., elimination of clinical signs and symptoms. Even when the patient is relatively asymptomatic, it is important to treat the initial episode of OPC to avoid progression to more extensive disease. In the most severe cases, the patient's quality of life may be impaired, and this may result in decreased fluid and food intake. Lack of appropriate treatment of OPC may lead to more extensive oral disease, especially in patients who are immunocompromised. The most serious complication of untreated OPC is extension of the in-

fection to esophageal candidiasis. Because esophageal candidiasis is more debilitating, the patient's quality of life is more affected. It is important to initiate appropriate antifungal therapy for both OPC and esophageal candidiasis. Preventing or minimizing the number of future recurrences of both types of candidiasis is an equally important outcome. The approach depends largely on the underlying predisposing conditions. Mycologic cure is not a necessary treatment outcome because it may not be feasible or realistic given that *Candida* species exist commonly as part of the normal mouth flora.

Minimizing toxicities and drug-drug interactions of systemic antifungal agents, as well as maximizing adherence by ensuring that the patient understands directions to take the medication appropriately, is an important secondary outcome of therapy.

GENERAL APPROACH TO TREATMENT

The management of *Candida* infections should be individualized for each patient, taking into consideration the underlying immune status, other concurrent mucosal and medical diseases, concomitant medications, and exogenous infectious sources. If possible, it is desirable to minimize all predisposing factors, such as administration of corticosteroids, chemotherapeutic agents, and antimicrobials, as well as instituting proper oral hygiene and resolving concurrent conditions such as denture stomatitis. Selection of an appropriate antifungal agent for treatment of candidiasis requires consideration of several factors, including the patient's drug adherence, adequate saliva for dissolution of solid topical medications, risk of caries from sucrose- or dextrose-containing preparations, potential drug interactions, co-existing medication conditions (e.g., liver disease may affect certain systemic drugs), location and severity of the infection, and the need for long-term maintenance therapy. Another factor that could affect drug selection is overuse of fluconazole leading to the emergence of fluconazole-resistant species of *C. albicans,* and in some cases to all azoles, and other intrinsically more resistant species such as *C. krusei, C. glabrata,* and *C. tropicalis.*

5   Topical therapies should be the first choice for localized infections. The efficacy of antifungal agents for OPC varies in different patient populations. Until the polyene antifungal agents became available in the 1950s, gentian violet, an aniline dye, was used commonly to treat oropharyngeal candidiasis.[21] Problems with gentian violet include fungal resistance, skin irritation, and especially the unaesthetic staining of the oral mucosa. Topical agents, such as nystatin and clotrimazole, have been the standard of treatment for uncomplicated OPC and generally are effective for treatment in otherwise healthy adults and infants with no underlying immunodeficiencies. Topical agents are available in an assortment of formulations, including oral rinses (suspension), troches, powder, vaginal tablets, and creams. The two most common types of formulations currently used are the suspension and troches (Table 118–6).

Topical agents require frequent applications because of the short contact time with the oral mucosa; the ideal contact time is 20 to 30 minutes. Sufficient saliva is needed to dissolve clotrimazole troches, and this may be problematic for patients with xerostomia. Also, the rough surface of the tablet may become irritating to the oral soft tissue. Troches also contain dextrose, which has cariogenic potential. Nystatin suspension may be a better choice for patients with xerostomia, but it is difficult to maintain adequate contact time with the oral mucosa. Some patients complain of the unpleasant taste of nystatin, which may cause nausea and vomiting, and this is problematic in cancer patients experiencing chemotherapy-induced nausea. The high sucrose content of nystatin suspension is cariogenic in dentate patients, and it should be used with caution in diabetic patients. Topical creams, such as clotrimazole, ketoconazole, miconazole, and nystatin (usually mixed with a steroid), are more appropriate for application three times dialy to the corners of the mouth in treating angular cheilitis.[27]

Systemic therapy is necessary in patients with OPC that is refractory to topical treatment, those who cannot tolerate topical agents, and those at high risk for disseminated systemic or invasive candidiasis. Effective treatment of esophageal candidiasis generally requires the use of systemic antifungal agents. However, these agents have the disadvantage of producing more side effects (see Table 118–6) and drug-drug interactions (see Chap. 119). Flucoanzole is generally well tolerated, and its absorption is unaffected by food or gastric acidity. Ketoconazole requires gastric acidity for absorption,

TABLE 118–6. Therapeutic Options for Mucosal Candidiasis

Antifungal	Preparation	Use[a]	Treatment Dosage/Duration	Common/Significant Side Effects
Clotrimazole	10-mg troche	OC	Hold 1 trouche in mouth for 15–20 minutes for slow dissolution 4–5 times daily for 7–14 days	Altered taste, mild nausea, vomiting
Nystatin	100,000 units/mL suspension	OC	5-mL swish and swallow four times daily for 7–14 days	Mild nausea, vomiting, diarrhea
Fluconazole	100-mg tablets	OC	100–200 mg daily for 7–14 days	GI upset; hepatitis not common
		EC	100–400 mg daily for 14–21 days	
Itraconazole	10 mg/mL solution[b] 100-mg capsule	OC	100-200 mg (solution) or 200 mg (tablets) daily for 7–14 days	GI upset; not common: hepatotoxicity, CHF, pulmonary edema with long-term use[e]
		EC	200-mg for 14–21 days	
Ketoconazole	200-mg tablets[c]	OC	200 mg daily for 7–14 days	Most common are nausea, vomiting, abdominal pain, itching, headache; endocrine effects; hepatotoxicity with long-term use—elevated ALT/AST in 2–10%; severe (hepatitis, liver failure) 1:10,000 to 1:2,000.[2]
		EC	400 mg daily for 14–21 days	
Amphotericin B	100 mg/mL suspension[d] 50-mg injection	RC	1–5 mL swish and swallow 4–5 times daily for 7–14 days	Oral: Nausea, vomiting, diarrhea with higher dose.
		EC	0.3–0.6 mg/kg/day or 10–20 mg IV infusion for 10–14 days or up to 21 days	IV: Fever, chills, sweats, electrolyte disturbance, bone marrow suppression

[a]OC = oropharyngeal candidiasis; EC = esophageal candidiasis; RC = refractory candidiasis.
[b]Solution is preferred over capsule; solution taken on empty stomach, capsules taken with food ± acidic beverage.
[c]Best taken with acidic beverage, e.g., Coke.
[d]Suspension is not marketed; can be prepared extemporaneously by pharmacy.[23]
[e]See discussion under onychomycosis.

which may be problematic in AIDS patients with achlorhydria, and hence it is best given with an acidic beverage. Itraconazole capsules also suffer from the same absorption problem. In contrast, itraconazole solution is well absorbed, best in a fasting state; in addition, the solution provides the benefit of both topical effects to the oral mucosa and systemic effects and is beneficial to patients with mucositis or swallowing problems. Whenever possible, it is generally beneficial to limit the use of systemic azole agents to prevent unnecessary drug exposure and to minimize the potential for occurrence of drug-resistant candidiasis, particularly from fluconazole resistance.

Antifungal agents generally are less efficacious in patients with HIV infection than in patients with cancer, and the time to response is also more prolonged.[25] In addition, treatment in HIV-infected patients usually produces a transient clinical response by lowering the quantity of organisms in the affected area without completely eradicating the yeast. The relapse rates are also higher in the HIV-infected patients than in other patient populations. As HIV infection progresses, and if antiretroviral treatment is suboptimal, patients usually experience more frequent recurrences of OPC, as well as esophageal candidiasis. In patients with HIV disease, it is equally important for them to be receiving HAART because this would provide the best prophylaxis against recolonization and recurrence of symptoms.[26]

◼ OROPHARYNGEAL CANDIDIASIS—HIV-INFECTED PATIENTS

It is appropriate to initiate therapy with topical agents for initial or recurrent episodes of OPC, provided that clinical symptoms are not severe and that there is minimal risk of esophageal involvement.[22,26] Clinical responses with the resolution of signs and symptoms generally occur within 5 to 7 days of starting treatment.[22] Clotrimazole appears to be the most effective topical agent and demonstrates comparable clinical response rates with both fluconazole and itraconazole.[20,22,23,25] However, the mycologic cure rates generally are significantly lower and the 4-week relapse rates tend to be higher for clotrimazole as compared with the systemic triazoles.[25] This may be of limited clinical significance in patients receiving effective HAART owing to their decreased susceptibility to opportunistic infection. Nystatin suspension, although still used frequently, appears to be the least effective agent and is associated with frequent treatment failures and early relapses, especially in patients with advanced HIV disease or neutropenia.[20–22,25]

Systemic oral azoles should be reserved for use in the more severe episodes of OPC unresponsive to topical agents or in patients with concurrent esophageal involvement.[20,22,25] Although clinical response in more than 80% of patients can be obtained with 50 to 200 mg/day of fluconazole, response occurs within 10 days with the 50-mg daily dose compared to within 5 days for 100- to 200-mg daily doses even for the most intractable forms of OPC.[20] The lower dose potentially may contribute to selection of resistance. Itraconazole oral solution with an improved absorption profile compared with the capsule formulation is comparable with fluconazole with respect to clinical and mycologic response and relapse rates.[23,25] A 14-day treatment course of itraconazole seems to be more effective than a 7-day course—the shorter course is associated with lower rates of mycologic cure and higher relapse rates. Itraconazole solution can be used as first-line therapy for OPC, and it may be used for cases not responding to fluconazole.[22,25,28] In clinical practice, fluconazole usually is the systemic azole agent of choice because of its favorable absorption, safety, and drug-interaction profiles.

◼ OROPHARYNGEAL CANDIDIASIS—NON–HIV-INFECTED PATIENTS

This patient population includes patients with hematologic malignancy (e.g., leukemias) or blood and marrow transplant (BMT) with a long duration of neutropenia and chronic graft-versus-host disease, patients with solid tumors, patients with solid-organ transplants who are receiving immunosuppressive therapy, and patients with diabetes mellitus; as well as patients on prolonged courses of antibiotics or corticosteroids and the debilitated elderly. Factors to consider in deciding whether to use topical or systemic antifungal therapy include the severity and extent of mucosal involvement (oropharyngeal versus esophageal), predisposing risk factors, and risk for dissemination. Patients who develop neutropenia (e.g., leukemic and BMT patients) are usually at high risk for disseminated and invasive fungal disease, and treatment of oral candidiasis is more aggressive. Patients with cell-mediated immune deficits but normal or near-normal granulocyte function and number (e.g., solid tumors, solid-organ transplants, or diabetic patients) are at low risk for dissemination of infection.

Specific antifungal therapy may be unnecessary for asymptomatic patients at relatively low risk for disseminated candidiasis, such as those who are not granulocytopenic or who are expected to have a short duration of granulocytopenia.[29] Many of these infections will clear spontaneously after recovery of the granulocytes or discontinuation of antibiotic and/or immunosuppressive therapy. However, antifungal therapy usually is required for patients who have persistent infection or significant symptoms, usually pain, or who are granulocytopenic with a relatively high risk of fungal dissemination.[29] Topical agents first may be given a therapeutic trial depending on the severity of infection and degree of immunosuppression. Although both nystatin and clotrimazole can be effective in treating OPC, nystatin suspension does not effectively reduce the incidence of either oropharyngeal or systemic *Candida* infections in immunocompromised patients receiving chemotherapy or radiation; its use often is associated with treatment failures and early relapses.[21,29,30] Clotrimazole appears to more effective in reducing colonization and treating acute episodes in cancer patients who are immunocompromised.

Systemic azole agents are used for treating OPC in patients who have failed or who are unable to take topical therapy.[21,28,29] The preceding discussion on the relative efficacy of fluconazole, itraconazole, and ketoconazole in HIV-infected patients may be extrapolated to the non–HIV-infected population. Fluconazole 100 to 200 mg daily is used more commonly because of more extensive experience with its use, and it is more effective and has a more favorable absorption and side-effect profile compared with ketoconazole.[23,25] If the oral route is not feasible for reasons such as severe chemotherapy-induced mucositis, fluconazole may be administered intravenously. In patients unresponsive to azoles, intravenous amphotericin B in relatively low doses of 0.1–0.3 mg/kg per day may be tried.[29] Because of the higher risk for dissemination in patients who are severely neutropenic ($<0.1 \times 10^9$ neutrophils/L) or clinically unstable (hypotensive, febrile), some clinicians may prefer to initiate therapy with intravenous amphotericin B at 0.6 mg/kg per day, with therapy continued until the neutropenia has resolved.[29]

Topical therapy with clotrimazole or nystatin for 7 days is usually adequate for treating mucocutaneous candidiasis in most solid-organ transplant patients.[31] Use of topical therapy will reduce the number of systemic drugs that these patients receive and hence minimize the risk of drug-drug interactions. Failure to respond to topical agents warrants the use of fluconazole. Low-dose amphotericin B 5–10 mg daily for 7 to 10 days is reserved for the unusual cases of treatment failure.

Patients who develop OPC because of prolonged antibiotic use or aerosolized corticosteroids use usually can be managed successfully by discontinuation of the offending agent, and the infection usually will resolve. If there is a strong desire to treat because of discomfort or need to hasten symptom resolution or an inability to stop the offending agent, therapy with a topical agent, either clotrimazole or nystatin, is effective in most cases. The advantage of systemic azoles is the convenience of less frequent dosing. Symptoms usually improve in 3 to 4 days. Infants should be given smaller amounts more frequently (e.g., nystatin 100,000 units every 2 to 3 hours) to ensure better contact time. For denture-related OPC, the patient should be instructed on proper daily oral hygiene. Dentures should be disinfected every night by soaking in antiseptic solution, such as chlorhexidine gluconate 0.12% to 0.25%.[27,32]

ESOPHAGEAL CANDIDIASIS—HIV-INFECTED PATIENTS

6 Treatment of esophageal candidiasis has not been as well studied as OPC. Because of the significant morbidity of esophageal candidiasis and the absence of evidence supporting the value of topical antifungals, treatment requires systemic antifungal agents.[20,23] Fluconazole is superior to ketoconazole with respect to endoscopic cure and clinical response and usually produces a more rapid onset of action and resolution of symptoms.[25] Fluconazole is more effective than oral itraconazole capsules but is as effective as itraconazole solution.[20,25] Patients who fail to respond to fluconazole should be treated with itraconazole solution. The use of fluconazole solution may be an effective alternative, although no comparative trials have been conducted.

In more advanced esophageal disease, oral azoles may be ineffective. Until recently, intravenous amphotericin B deoxycholate has been the alternative for patients with endoscopically proven disease who have failed fluconazole or itraconazole therapy.[22,24] Moderate disease may be treated adequately with low- to moderate-dose amphotericin B for 10 days, although higher doses may be necessary for patients with AIDS or advanced disease.[24,28] Voriconzole, a new triazole antifungal available in both oral and intravenous preparations, produces comparable clinical response to fluconazole.[37] Voriconazole has been associated with more side effects and multiple pharmacokinetic drug interactions.[24,38]

CLINICAL CONTROVERSY

Caspofungin, the first approved drug from a new class of antifungals, the echinocandins, has been demonstrated in three clinical trials to produce comparable clinical response to fluconazole and amphotericin B for esophageal candidiasis.[33–35] The incidence of adverse events of caspo-

fungin is comparable with that of intravenous fluconazole and significantly less than that of amphotericin B.[36] Caspofungin is neither a significant substrate nor an inhibitor of the cytochrome P450 enzymes or P-glycoprotein, and there are fewer drug-drug interactions.[24,36] However caspofungin is available only as an intravenous formulation and is more expensive than fluconazole and amphotericin B deoxycholate. Caspofungin thus is an appropriate alternative for patients who have failed on oral azoles and are intolerant of amphotericin B or have preexisting renal impairment.

ESOPHAGEAL CANDIDIASIS—NON–HIV-INFECTED PATIENTS

As in the case of HIV-infected patients, treatment of esophageal candidiasis requires systemic therapy. Patients may be started on fluconazole 100–200 mg/day for 2 to 3 weeks.[28] However, higher fluconazole doses (up to 400 mg/day) have been suggested for patients with severe symptoms or those who are neutropenic.[29] Itraconazole solution is an effective alternative for those not responding adequately to fluconazole. If the symptoms worsen or fail to respond, intravenous amphotericin B 0.6 mg/kg per day may be used. Intravenous amphotericin B may be considered for initial therapy in neutropenic patients who present with severe symptoms or who are at high risk for dissemination of *Candida,* such as those receiving other aggressive immunosuppressive therapy (e.g., corticosteroids, total-body irradiation, or antithymocyte globulin) and who have documented evidence of esophageal candidiasis or who have failed an initial empirical trial of oral nonabsorbable agents or systemic azoles.[29] Amphotericin B should be continued until at least the neutropenia resolves. For patients whose symptoms have resolved and who are afebrile and clinically stable, amphotericin B should be discontinued, and the patients should be monitored closely for infection recurrence. In high-risk patients, particularly those with persistent fever and neutropenia, the potential presence of clinically occult, diffuse gastrointestinal or disseminated candidiasis should be considered. With the availability of caspofungin and voriconazole, additional alternatives are present for patients who are intolerant of amphotericin B deoxycholate or who have preexisting renal impairment.[24,36,38]

ANTIFUNGAL PROPHYLAXIS

7 Ensuring that the HIV-infected patient is receiving appropriate antiretroviral therapy to enhance the immune system is perhaps the most important measure in preventing future episodes of mucosal candidiasis (oropharyngeal, esophageal, and vulvovaginal).[22,23] Initial success of treatment often is followed by symptomatic recurrences, especially in patients with advanced HIV disease. Current evidence only supports the efficacy of fluconazole in preventing recurrences or new infections of OPC; there is insufficient evidence to support prophylactic efficacy of the other antifungals.[39] However, the indications for antifungal prophylaxis and the best long-term management strategy still have not been well established. Although fluconazole is effective in reducing the risk for mucosal candidiasis in patients with advanced HIV disease, it does not provide complete protection, and breakthrough infections still may occur.[20,23] The reduced risk of recurrence of OPC also has not been demonstrated to improve survival. In addition, continuous long-term exposure to fluconazole has been associated with emergence of resistance and **8** refractory disease.[22,23] Thus recent guidelines from the U.S.

Public Health Service and the Infectious Diseases Society of America, as well as other experts in the area, do not recommend routine primary prophylaxis for OPC.[40] The rationale includes effectiveness of therapy for acute episodes of OPC, low incidence of serious invasive fungal disease, low mortality associated with mucosal candidiasis, the potential development of resistant candidiasis, the possibility of drug interactions, and the prohibitive long-term cost of prophylaxis. For the same reasons, chronic suppressive therapy (i.e., secondary prophylaxis of recurrent OPC) is also not recommended routinely, but rather clinicians should treat each acute episode as it occurs.[22,23,40]

The decision to use secondary prophylaxis should be individualized for each patient. Some clinicians may recommend secondary prophylaxis to HIV-infected patients with multiple recurrent episodes of symptomatic OPC or when the disease is sufficiently severe and affecting the quality of life or in those who are at risk of developing esophageal candidiasis or who have advanced AIDS (e.g., CD4 cell counts below 50 cells/mm^3).[22,23,40] Patients with a history of documented esophageal candidiasis may be candidates for chronic suppressive therapy if they are experiencing disabling recurrent infections, especially if associated with malnutrition.[24,40] Fluconazole 100 mg daily is the preferred agent for OPC and esophageal candidiasis. Once-weekly fluconazole (200 mg) is also effective for preventing OPC recurrences in those with less advanced AIDS.[23,41] Itraconazole solution 100 mg daily may be an alternative, although it has not been evaluated in controlled trials.[23]

Patients with malignant neoplastic diseases who are receiving irradiation, cytotoxic, and/or immunosuppressive therapy are at high risk for fungal infections in addition to bacterial and viral infections. The value of antifungal prophylaxis in these patients needs to be considered in the broader context of not only reducing colonization and the risk of superficial candidiasis but also, more important, reducing the risk for invasive candidiasis and improving survival. Management of these infections is discussed in detail in Chap. 120.

ANTIFUNGAL-REFRACTORY ORAL MUCOSAL CANDIDIASIS

Treatment of refractory or recurrent oral mucosal candidiasis (i.e., defined as clinically unresponsive to appropriate antifungal regimen) is frequently unsatisfactory, and clinical response is usually short-lived, with rapid and periodic recurrences. The key risk factors for occurrence of refractory candidiasis are advanced stage of AIDS with low CD4 cell counts (<50 cells/mm^3) and repeated or prolonged courses of various systemic antifungal agents, in particular

systemic azoles.[20,22–24] Although not necessarily the case, emergence of fluconazole-resistant *C. albicans* or selection for more resistant *Candida* species may be associated with frequent or prolonged use of fluconazole.[22,24] An important initial management strategy is to assess and optimize the antiretroviral therapy of the patient with refractory OPC to help improve the immune function. In fact, the incidence of fluconazole-refractory OPC, previously reported to be 5% or less in advanced HIV disease, is expected to be lower with the use of effective HAART.[22,23] It is important to identify potentially correctable causes of clinical failures of mucosal candidiasis, such as poor drug adherence, reduced drug absorption associated with hypochlorhydria, and drug-drug interactions.[22,23]

There have been few controlled studies that assess the effectiveness of antifungals. Doubling of the fluconazole dosage to 400 or 800 mg/day may be effective in some patients with infection caused by *Candida* of intermediate resistance, although the response may be only transient.[20] Fluconazole oral suspension may be beneficial in some patients because of increased salivary concentrations obtained when the suspension is taken with the swish-and-swallow technique.[20] Itraconazole oral suspension is effective in 55% to 70% of patients; however, the benefit is short-lived if chronic suppressive therapy is not maintained, and there is a high likelihood of the development of itraconazole resistance.[20] Amphotericin B oral suspension is limited primarily to use in azole-refractory patients.[22,28] It has broad spectrum activity against many fungal species and low likelihood of *Candida* resistance. There are limited data and experience on its use in immunosuppressed patients, and results from small studies have yielded mixed results, with clinical efficacy of 50% to 75% and a high relapse rate.[22,42] It is no longer available commercially in the United States, but it may be prepared extemporaneously by the pharmacy.[42] Patients with severe disease unresponsive to other agents require intravenous amphotericin B 0.4–0.6 mg/kg per day for 7 to 10 days to achieve clinical response; higher dose or longer treatment duration may be needed in more severe disease.[20,23,24] After response, suppressive therapy with amphotericin B is required to increase disease-free intervals. Patients who fail to respond to amphotericin B and require more than 1 mg/kg per day may be candidates for liposomal amphotericin B preparations because of renal and/or bone marrow toxicities, although at a markedly higher cost. Flucytosine usually is not used as monotherapy because of rapid development of resistance but may be used in combination with an azole or amphotericin B.[20,23] Newer antifungal agents, such as caspofungin and voriconazole, as discussed earlier, may be considered when current agents have failed or produce serious adverse effects.[24,36,38] Investigational agents for future use include micafungin and anidulafungin (both echinocandins), posaconazole, and ravuconazole.[24]

EVALUATION OF THERAPEUTIC OUTCOMES

Efficacy end points for oropharyngeal and esophageal candidiasis include rapid relief of symptoms and prevention of complications without early relapse after completion of the course of therapy. Sterilization of the oral cavity is not a feasible end point because mycologic eradication is rarely achievable, especially in HIV-positive patients. Symptomatic relief of presenting signs and symptoms generally occurs within 2 to 3 days of starting therapy, with complete resolution by 7 to 10 days. Patients should be advised about the time course and told to return for reassessment when signs and symptoms recur. It is usually unnecessary for the patient to be reassessed soon after finishing the treatment course. However, HIV patients should be questioned and examined for the occurrence of mucosa candidiasis as part

of their regular follow-up. The frequency of monitoring may be more often in neutropenic patients because of concern for dissemination of candidiasis. During the period of neutropenia, temperature should be monitored daily, as well as signs of dissemination. Hospitalized patients who are receiving intravenous amphotericin B also require daily monitoring by the pharmacist.

Efficacy of the antifungal agent is partly influenced by patient adherence to the medication regimen. Patients must be counseled on proper administration and dosing, in particular for topical agents[27,43] (Table 118–7). The likelihood of drug-related problems pertaining to drug toxicity and drug interactions depends on which antifungal agent is used. Safety end points include monitoring for occurrence of the relevant drug side effects and drug interactions.

TABLE 118–7. Patient Counseling Tips for Managing Oropharyngeal Candidiasis[8,24]

1. Clean the oral cavity prior to administering the topical antifungal agent. Daily fluoride rinses may help reduce the risk of caries when using an agent containing sucrose or dextrose.
2. Use the topical antifungal agent after meals as saliva flow and mouth movements can reduce the contact time.
3. Troches should be slowly dissolved in mouth, not chewed or swallowed whole, over 15 to 30 minutes and the saliva swallowed.
4. Suspension should be swished around the mouth in the oral cavity to cover all areas for as long as possible, ideally at least 1 minute, then gargled and swallowed.
5. Remove dentures while medication is being applied to the oral tissues.
6. Use a suspension instead of a troche if xerostomia is present; if a troche is preferred, the patient should rinse or drink water prior to dosing. For xerostomia, suggest nonpharmacologic measures for symptomatic relief, e.g., ice chips, sugarless gum or hard candy, citrus beverages.
7. Dentures should be removed and disinfected overnight using an antiseptic solution, e.g., chlorhexidine 0.12–0.2%. Disinfect oral tissues in addition to dental prosthesis.
8. Complete treatment course even though symptomatic improvement may occur in 48–72 hours.
9. Maintain good oral hygiene. Brush teeth daily (twice daily) and floss, rinse mouth or brush teeth after eating sweets.
10. Stop smoking; avoid alcohol.

From refs. 8 and 24.

MYCOTIC INFECTIONS OF THE SKIN, HAIR, AND NAILS

Superficial mycotic infections of the skin are referred to as *dermatophytoses*. They are common infections that usually are caused by dermatophytes classified by genera: *Trichophyton, Epidermophyton,* or *Microsporum*.[44] Dermatophytes have the ability to penetrate keratinous structures of the body. These infections affect both male and female genders and all races. Reservoirs of mycotic infections include humans, animals, and soil.[44] Individuals may develop an infection if they come in contact with a reservoir in addition to having a conducive environment for mycotic growth (i.e., moist conditions).[45] Risk factors for the development of an infection include prolonged exposure to sweaty clothes, failure to bathe regularly, many skin folds, sedentariness, and confinement to bed.[45]

Mycotic infections of the skin have a classic appearance that consists of a central clearing surrounded by an advancing red, scaly, elevated border.[45] Infections of the nail can appear chalky and dull yellow or white and become brittle and crumbly.

Diagnosis usually is based on patient history, as well as the physical examination.[46] Diagnostic tests include direct microscopic examination of a specimen after the addition of potassium hydroxide (KOH) or fungal cultures. The KOH test is quick, inexpensive, and easy to perform, whereas cultures are more expensive and take longer to obtain results. Diagnostic tests are recommended when systemic therapy is likely to be prescribed.[46]

❾ A general approach to treatment of superficial mycotic infections includes keeping the infected area dry and clean and limiting exposure to the infected reservoir. Topical agents generally are considered to be first-line therapy for infections of the skin. Oral therapy is preferred when the infection is extensive or severe or when treating tinea capitis or onychomycosis.[47–49] Table 118–8 lists spe-

cific treatments for each mycotic infection. Superficial mycotic infections are categorized by the pattern and site of infection.[44] The most commonly occurring infections in North America are detailed below.

TINEA PEDIS

Tinea pedis is the most common dermatophytoses (affecting approximately 70% of adults). It is better known as "athletes foot" and occurs in hot weather, with exposure to surface reservoirs (locker room floors), and with use of occlusive footwear.[45] Treatment with topical therapy for 2 to 4 weeks often is adequate for mild infections; however, severe infections or involvement of the nails requires oral therapy[45] (see Table 118–8). Recurrence of infection occurs in up to 70% of individuals. Prolonged treatment with either topical or systemic therapy may be required.[46,47]

TINEA MANUUM

Tinea manuum usually involves the palmar surface of the hands, is unilateral, and may involve the feet. Treatment of this infection is similar to tinea pedis (see Table 118–8). Emollients that contain lactic acid also may be useful.[45]

TINEA CRURIS

Tinea cruris is an infection of the proximal thighs and buttocks.[48] It is referred to as "jock itch" and is more common in males. The scrotum and penis often are spared from infection. Treatment with topical therapy is recommended and should continue for 1 to 2 weeks after symptom resolution. Severe infections may require oral therapy (see Table 118–8). Relief of pruritus and burning may be facilitated by the use of short-term (2 to 3 days) topical steroids (2.5% hydrocortisone).[45]

TINEA CORPORIS

Tinea corporis is an infection the glabrous skin of the trunk and extremities.[48] Therapy is similar to that for tinea pedis, tinea manuum, and tinea cruris (see Table 118–8).

TINEA CAPITIS

Tinea capitis is a mycotic infection involving the scalp, hair follicles, and adjacent skin[49,50] that primarily affects children. Treatment should consist of oral therapy, as well as the cleaning of combs and brushes, which may be contaminated[2] (see Table 118–8). Daily shampooing is recommended for removal of scales. Some children and adults may be asymptomatic carriers, thereby facilitating spread of the infection.[49] Family members who culture positive for tinea tonsurans should be treated with an antifungal shampoo (e.g., ketoconazole, selenium sulfide, or povidone-iodine).[49]

TINEA BARBAE

Tinea barbae affects the hairs and follicles of beards and mustaches.[49] Treatment is similar to that for tinea capitis (see Table 118–8). Removal of the beard or mustache is recommended.[45]

PITYRIASIS VERSICOLOR

Hyperpigmented and hypopigmented scaly patches characterize pityriasis versicolor. These patches are found on the trunk and

TABLE 118–8. Treatment of Mycoses of the Skin, Hair, and Nails

	Topical[a,b]	Oral[c]
Tinea pedis	Butenafine, daily	Fluconazole 150 mg 1 × per wk 1–4 wks
Tinea manuum	Ciclopirox, twice daily	Ketoconazole 200 mg daily × 4 wks
Tinea cruris	Clotrimazole, twice daily	Itraconazole 200–400 mg/day × 1 wk
Tinea coporis	Econazole, daily	Terbinafine 250 mg/d × 2 wks
	Haloprogen, twice daily	
	Ketoconazole cream, daily	
	Miconazole, twice daily	
	Naftifine cream, daily; gel, twice daily	
	Oxiconazole, twice daily	
	Sulconazole, twice daily	
	Terbinafine, twice daily	
	Tolnaftate, twice daily	
	Triacetin cream, solution, three times daily	
	Undecylenic acid, various preparations apply as directed	
Tinea capitis	Shampoo only in conjunction with oral therapy or for treatment	Terbinafine 250 mg/d 4–8 wks
Tinea barbae	of asymptomatic carriers	Ketoconazole 200 mg daily × 4 wks
	Ketaconazole 2 × per wk × 4 wks	Itraconazole 100–200 mg/day × 4–6 wks
	Selenium sulfide daily × 2 wks	Griseofulvin 500 mg/day × 4–6 wks
Pityriasis versicolor	Clotrimazole, twice daily	Ketoconazole 400 mg × 1
	Econazole, daily	Fluconazole 400 mg × 1
	Halprogin, twice daily	Itraconazole 200 mg daily × 3–7 days
	Ketoconazole, daily	
	Miconazole, twice daily	
	Oxiconazole cream only, twice daily	
	Sulconazole, twice daily	
	Terbinafine, twice daily	
	Tolnaftate, three times daily	
Onychomycosis	Ciclopirax nail lacquer apply solution at night for up to 48 wks	Terbinafine 250 mg/d × 6 wks (finger), 12 wks (toe)
Fingernail		Itraconazole[a] 200 mg twice daily × 1 wk per
Toenail		month for 2 months (finger), for 3 months (toe),
		or 200 mg daily for 2 months (finger), for
		3 months (toe)
		Fluconazole 150–300 mg once weekly ×
		3–6 months (finger), × 6–9 months (toe)

[a]Other products are available, including combination products.
[b]Length of therapy depends on mycotic sensitivity and severity of infection.
[c]Only capsule formulation studied; give with food for increased absorption.

extremities.[51] It is more common in adults and in areas with tropical ambient temperatures. Topical treatment usually is adequate unless there is extensive involvement, recurrent infections, or failure of topical therapy[51] (see Table 118–8).

ONYCHOMYCOSIS (TINEA UNGUIUM)

Onychomycosis is a fungal infection of the nail apparatus, and it is a common condition that accounts for up to 50% of all nail problems.[52] Onychomycosis more commonly affects the toenails, approximately 80% of cases, than the fingernails.[2] The dermatophyte *Trichophyton rubrum* is responsible for over 90% of onychomycosis.[52–54] Less common fungi causing onychomycosis are the yeasts (mainly *C. albicans*) and nondermatophyte molds.[52,54] There are four major clinical presentations of onychomycosis, of which the distal subungal is the most common type. In distal subungual infection, the nail plate, nail bed, and matrix areas are all affected.[52,53] The worst case of onychomycosis is progression of the infection to total dystrophic onychomycosis, characterized by almost complete destruction of the nail plate.[52,53] The prevalence of onychomycosis is higher with increasing age (especially above age 40 years), familial history, smoking, peripheral vascular disease, diabetes mellitus, and HIV disease.[52] It

is important to differentiate onychomycosis from other causes of nail abnormalities so that the patient receives appropriate therapy and is not subjected to prolonged treatment with unnecessary drugs. Besides clinical history and physical examination, proper diagnosis of onychomycosis may include direct microscopy of nail scrapings to look for fungal hyphae, fungal cultures, and histology.[52,55] Onychomycosis merits proper treatment because it can exert a negative impact on quality of life (cosmetic and psychosocial reasons, pain, discomfort, and decreased ambulation); it can lead to complications such as cellulitis or reduced mobility, which further compromises peripheral circulation in those with diabetes or peripheral vascular disease; and infected nails can serve as a source for transmission of fungi to other areas of the body, as well as to other people, such as close household contacts or in communal bathing places.[53,55,56] The primary end point of treatment is eradication of the organism, with secondary end points being clinical cure or improvement.[53] Successful eradication of the fungus does not always result in normalization of the nails because they may have been dystrophic prior to infection.

Systemic therapy is the preferred route of treating onychomycosis. Terbinafine and itraconazole (capsule), the current first-line agents for treatment, have yielded higher efficacy rates using shorter treatment periods (generally 3 months or shorter) for toenail and fingernail onychomycosis compared with the traditional agents (i.e., griseofulvin and ketoconazole). Terbinafine, an allylamine, exerts fungicidal activity and demonstrates the greatest in vitro activity against dermatophytes compared with the other oral antifungals; it has good activity against nondermatophyte molds and only marginal activity against *Candida*.[57] Itraconazole, generally considered fungistatic, has a broader antifungal spectrum and is very active against dermatophytes, nondermatophytes, and *Candida*.[57] Itraconazole can be administered as a daily regimen or as an intermittent regimen given daily for 1 week once monthly (pulse dosing). Both agents have lipophilic and keratinophilic properties, which explain their excellent penetration (appearing in the nail plate within days of treatment initiation) and accumulation in the nails, achieving concentrations far exceeding the MIC of most dermatophytes.[54,57] Both drugs are slowly eliminated from the nail, with mean half-lives of approximately 88 and 80 days for terbinafine and itraconazole (daily dosing), respectively; the nail half-life of itraconazole is shorter with pulse dosing.[54] Thus effective drug concentrations persist in nails for 30 to 36 weeks after completion of treatment with terbinafine and for at least 24 weeks with itraconazole.[54,57] This explains in part the long-term protection against relapses after the end of treatment.

Toenail onychomycoses usually are more difficult to treat than fingernail onychomycoses and require longer duration of treatment. Treatment of toenail onychomycosis requires a 12-week course, whereas a 6-week course generally is adequate for fingernail onychomycosis with either drug.[53,55] Itraconazole pulse therapy is the preferred method over continuous dosing for fingernail infections, and it consists of twice-daily dosing for a 1-week cycle per month for 2 consecutive months (i.e., two pulses); although not approved by the Food and Drug Administration (FDA), three to four pulses are effective for toenail infections; otherwise, half the dose is taken daily for 3 to 4 months[53,55,57] (see Table 118–8). In addition to lower drug cost, potential advantages of itraconazole pulse therapy compared with continuous therapy include a lower risk of adverse drug effects and improved patient adherence. Pulse dosing is as effective as continuous dosing.[55,59] Terbinafine pulse therapy also may be effective, although data are insufficient to currently recommend this method of administration.[55,57]

Direct comparative trials generally have shown that terbinafine is more effective than itraconazole either by continuous or pulse dosing. Mycologic and clinical cure rates for terbinafine ranged from 73% to 80% and from 69% to 76%, respectively; for itraconazole, the respective cure rates ranged from 38% to 63% and from 32% to 61%.[58,59] Three systematic reviews of the literature also reported that continuous terbinafine therapy is more effective than continuous or pulse itraconazole therapy.[59–61] In addition, a pharmacoeconomic analysis of oral and topical (ciclopirox) therapies showed that from a managed-care perspective, terbinafine was the most cost-effective therapy in terms of highest success rate, lowest relapse rate, and highest number of disease-free days for both fingernail and toenail infections.[62]

Both terbinafine and itraconazole generally are well tolerated. The more common adverse effects reported with terbinafine are gastrointestinal (e.g., diarrhea, dyspepsia, nausea, and abdominal pain), dermatologic (e.g., rash, urticaria, and pruritus), and headache; less common adverse effects include taste disturbances, fatigue, inability to concentrate, and asymptomatic liver enzyme abnormalities.[56,57] Although uncommon, severe adverse effects have been reported with terbinafine, including erythema multiforme, Stevens-Johnson syndrome and toxic epidermal necrolysis, neutropenia, lupus erythematosus, psoriasis, hair loss, and hepatotoxicity.[56,57,61,63] Although the incidence of severe hepatotoxicity is considered rare, the FDA issued a Public Health Advisory in 2001 regarding the association of terbinafine tablets with 16 possible cases of liver failure, including 2 liver transplants and 11 deaths.[64] Terbinafine thus is not recommended for patients with chronic or active liver disease, although hepatotoxicity may occur in patients with no preexisting liver disease or serious underlying medical condition. Prior to initiating terbinafine treatment, it is recommended to obtain appropriate nail specimens for laboratory testing to confirm the diagnosis of onychomycosis. Liver function parameters (serum transaminases) should be assessed prior to and periodically during treatment with terbinafine.

The common adverse effects of itraconazole are similar to those of terbinafine, such as gastrointestinal disturbance, dermatologic disorders, and headache; less common adverse effects include dizziness, fatigue, fever, decreased libido, and asymptomatic liver enzyme abnormalities (1% to 5% with continuous dosing and about 2% with pulse dosing).[56,57,65] Although still considered rare, 24 serious cases of liver failure, including transplantation and death, have been reported with the use of itraconazole, resulting in a recent FDA Public Health Advisory warning.[64] Some of these patients did not have preexisting liver disease or serious underlying medical conditions, and some developed within the first week of treatment. It has been suggested to avoid itraconazole in patients with elevated liver enzymes or active liver disease or in those who have experienced other drug-induced liver toxicity. Liver function parameters (serum transaminases) should be assessed prior to and periodically during treatment. However, some experts have suggested that frequent monitoring is not as necessary if pulse therapy is used because symptomatic hepatotoxicity has not been reported with pulse therapy.[65] In addition, there is an FDA warning on the risk of developing congestive heart failure (CHF) associated with the use of itraconazole, possibly related to its potential negative inotropic effect.[64,66] Therefore, itraconazole should not be used in patients with evidence of ventricular dysfunction, such as CHF. Symptomatic assessment for the development of CHF also should be included as part of therapy monitoring. Before a patient is subjected to several months of itraconazole treatment, it is important to confirm the diagnosis of onychomycosis.

In contrast to the azoles, terbinafine does not inhibit the cytochrome P450 3A4 isoenzymes, but it is a potent inhibitor of the CYP 2D6 isoenzymes, which are responsible for metabolism of tricyclic antidepressants and other psychotropic drugs.[54] The most significant drug interactions with terbinafine are decreased clearance of 33% by cimetidine and increased clearance of 100% by rifampin.[54,56] Other drug interactions of variable clinical significance include cyclosporine, caffeine, theophylline, and terfenadine.[54,56] A case was reported of nortriptyline toxicity when given concomitantly with terbinafine.[56] Itraconazole and its major metabolite can inhibit the CYP 3A4 isoenzymes and result in numerous clinically significant drug interactions.[54,56] (Refer to Chap. 119 for specific examples.)

Fluconazole is also active against dermatophytes, *Candida*, and some nondermatophytes.[55,56] Fluconazole does not have current FDA indication for treatment of onychomycosis. Limited studies showed that fluconazole pulse regimens produced mycologic cure rates from 51% to 87%.[56] The most effective dose and treatment duration have not been clearly established, with dosages ranging from 150 to 450 mg once weekly for 3 to 9 months (see Table 118–8). One study showed that a 9-month regimen of 450 mg once weekly was superior to 3- and 6-month durations.[67] In direct comparative studies, fluconazole was less effective than terbinafine or itraconazole.[68,69] Advantages of fluconazole include a relatively good safety profile, few drug interactions, and infrequent dosing.

These three oral antifungal agents have superseded the use of griseofulvin and ketoconazole as treatments of choice for onychomycosis.[53,55] Griseofulvin has a narrow antifungal spectrum, low clinical efficacy, especially for toenail infections, high relapse rates, and the need for prolonged treatment duration (up to 12 to 18 months for toenails). Use of ketoconazole is also associated with high relapse rates, and the prolonged treatment duration carries an increased risk of hepatotoxicity.

A number of topical antifungal products are available, and they provide variable success rates. Topical treatment requires regular applications for prolonged periods and strict patient adherence, which can be problematic. The most recently approved topical agent is a nail lacquer—ciclopirox 8% (Penlac)—for the treatment of mild to moderate onychomycosis caused by *Tricophyton rubrum* that does not involve the lunula.[70] Ciclopirox, a hydroxypyridine, has a broad spectrum of antifungal activity. Initial improvement may take as long as 6 months to occur. However, complete cure is reported in less than 10% of treated patients, with only about 60% of responders still remaining disease-free at 12 weeks after stopping treatment. Most experts consider topical therapy a feasible alternative when the infection is superficial involving the nail plate and limited to a few nails and to a partial area of the nail plate (owing to difficulty of applying treatment to the margin of the nail) or in the very early stages of a distal subungual type of infection when it is still confined to the distal edge of the nail.[53,54]

Recurrence rates of infection range from 20% to 30%, which could be either a relapse (original infection not completely cured) or reinfection (new infection after achieving a cure of the original).[53,54,56] Factors associated with poor response to systemic therapy include a compromised immune system (AIDS), reduced blood flow (diabetes, peripheral vascular disease, vasculitis, connective tissue disease, congestive heart failure), coexisting nail disease (psoriasis), nail factors (slow growth, thick nails, severe disease), drug-resistant organisms because of extensive prior drug exposure, and reduced bioavailability (absorption problems, poor compliance, drug interactions).[53,54,71] To help to improve treatment outcomes and reduce recurrence, patients should be counseled on the importance of proper foot hygiene, e.g., wearing breathable footwear and 100% cotton socks with frequent changes, keeping the nails short and clean, keeping the feet dry, protecting the feet in shared bathing areas, treating tinea pedis, and controlling other predisposing medical conditions.[56] The combined use of topical and systemic therapy has been proposed as a potential approach to help improve cure rates or shorten treatment duration, but randomized, controlled trials are needed to evaluate this approach.[53,71] Physical interventions such as surgical or chemical nail avulsion are used primarily as adjunct therapy in patients with total dystrophic onychomycosis, in whom there is severe onycholysis and extensive nail thickening or longitudinal spikes; response to oral therapy may be improved with partial nail avulsion in these patients.[55,71]

ABBREVIATIONS

BMT: bone marrow transplant
CHF: congestive heart failure
HAART: highly active antiretroviral therapy
HIV: human immunodeficiency virus
KOH: potassium hydroxide
OPC: oropharyngeal candidiasis
RVVC: recurrent vulvovagninal candidiasis
VVC: vulvovagninal candidiasis

Review Questions and other resources can be found at *www.pharmacotherapyonline.com.*

REFERENCES

1. Sobel JD, Faro S, Force R, et al. Vulvovaginal candidiasis: Epidemiologic, diagnostic and therapeutic considerations. Am J Obstet Gynecol 1998;178:203–211.
2. Hurley R. Recurrent *Candida* infection. Clin Obstet Gynecol 1981;8:209–213.
3. Haefner HK. Current evaluation and management of vulvovaginitis. Clin Obstet Gynecol 1999;42:184–195.
4. Foxman B, Barlow R, D'arcy H, et al. *Candida* vaginitis self-reported incidence and associated costs. Sex Transm Dis 2000;27:230–235.
5. Clinical Effectiveness Group. National guideline for the management of vulvovaginal candidiasis. Sex Transm Infect 1999;75(suppl 1):S19–20.
6. Larsen B. Vaginal flora in health and disease. Clin Obstet Gynecol 1993;36:107–121.
7. Sobel JD. Clinical vulvovaginitis. Clin Obstet Gynecol 1993;36:153–165.
8. Barbone F, Austin H, Louv WC, Alexander WJ. A follow-up study of the methods of contraception, sexual activity, and rates of trichomoniasis, candidiasis, and bacterial vaginosis. Am J Obstet Gynecol 1990;163:510–514.
9. Ferris DG, Dekle C, Litaker MS. Women's use of over-the-counter antifungal pharmaceutical products for gynecologic symptoms. J Fam Pract 1996;42:595–600.
10. Hilton E, Isenberg HD, Alperstein P, et al. Ingestion of yogurt containing *Lactobacillus acidophilus* as prophylaxis for candidal vaginitis. Ann Intern Med 1992;116:353–357.
11. Tooley PJ. Patient and doctor preferences in the treatment of vaginal candidiasis. Practitioner 1985;229:655–662.
12. Edelman DA, Grant S. One-day therapy for vaginal candidiasis a review. J Reprod Med 1999;44:543–547.
13. Perry CM, Whittington R, McTavish D. Fluconazole: An update of its antimicrobial activity, pharmacokinetic properties, and therapeutic use in vaginal candidiasis. Drugs 1995;49:984–1006.
14. Mendling W, Plempel M. Vaginal secretion levels after 6 days, 3 days and 1 day of treatment with 100-, 200-, 500-mg vaginal tablets of clotrimazole and their therapeutic efficacy. Chemotherapy 1982;28(suppl 1):43–47.
15. Kaplan B, Royburt M, Rabinerson D, Neri A. Once-daily fluocinonide-bifonazole combination for the treatment of vulvar itching and vulvovaginal candidiasis: Preliminary study. Clin Exp Obstet Gynecol 1996;23:173–176.
16. Sobel JD, Brooker JD, Stein GE, et al. Single oral dose of fluconazole compared with conventional clotrimazole topical therapy of candida vaginitis. Am J Obstet Gynecol 1995;172:1263–1268.
17. Mastroiacovo P, Mazzone T, Botto L, et al. Prospective assessment of pregnancy outcomes after first-trimester exposure to fluconazole. Am J Obstet Gynecol 1996;175:1645–1650.
18. Horowitz BJ. Topical flucytosine therapy for chronic recurrent *Candida tropicalis* infections. J Reprod Med 1986;31:821–824.
19. Sobel JD, Chaim W. Treatment of *Torulopsis glabrata* vaginitis: Retrospective review of boric acid therapy. Clin Infect Dis 1996;22:336–340.
20. Vasquez JA, Sobel JD. Mucosal candidiasis. Infect Dis Clin North Am 2002;16:793–820.
21. Epstein JB, Polsky B. Oropharyngeal candidiasis: A review of its clinical spectrum and current therapies. Clin Ther 1998;20:40–57.
22. Powderly WG, Mayer KH, Perfect JR. Diagnosis and treatment of oropharyngeal candiasis in patients infected with HIV: A critical reassessment. AIDS Res Hum Retroviruses 1999;15:1405–1412.
23. Fichtenbaum CJ, Aberg JA. Candidiasis and HIV. In: HIV Insite Knowledge Base Chapter, November 2002; available at *http://hivinsite.ucsf.edu.*
24. Vasquez JA. Invasive oesophageal candidiasis: Current and developing treatment options. Drugs 2003;63:971–989.
25. Darouiche RO. Oropharyngeal and esophageal candidiasis in immunocompromised patients: Treatment issues. Clin Infect Dis 1998;26:259–274.
26. Powderly WG, Gallant JE, Ghannoum MA, et al. Oropharyngeal candidiasis in patients with HIV: Suggested guidelines for therapy. AIDS Res Hum Retroviruses 1999;15:1619–1623.

27. Akpan A, Morgan R. Oral candidiasis. Postgrad Med J 2002;78:455–459.

28. Rex JH, Walsh TJ, Sobel JD, et al. Practice guidelines for the treatment of candidiasis. Clin Infect Dis 2000;30:663–678.

29. Freifeld AG, Walsh TJ, Pizzo PA. Clinical approaches to infections in the compromised host. In: Hoffman R, Benz EJ Jr, Shattil SJ, et al, eds. Hematology: Basic Principles and Practice, 3d ed. New York, Churchill-Livingstone, 2000.

30. Gotzsche PC, Johansen HK. Nystatin prophylaxis and treatment in severely immunodepressed patients. Cochrane Database Syst Rev 2003;1.

31. Anonymous. International conference for the development of a consensus on the management and prevention of severe candidal infections. Clin Infect Dis 1997;25:43–59.

32. Anonymous. Oropharyngeal candidiasis; available at *www.doctorfungus.org/mycoses/human/candidia;* accessed October 2003.

33. Villanueva A, Arathoon EG, Gotuzzo E, et al. A randomized double-blind study of caspofungin versus amphotericin for the treatment of candidal esophagitis. Clin Infect Dis 2001;33:1529–1535.

34. Arathoon EG, Gotuzzo E, Noriega LM, et al. Randomized, double-blind, multicenter study of caspofungin versus amphotericin B for treatment of oropharyngeal and esophageal candidiasis. Antimicrob Agents Chemother 2002;46:451–457.

35. Villanueva A, Gotuzzo E, Arathoon EG, et al. A randomized double-blind study of caspofungin versus fluconazole for the treatment of esophageal candidiasis. Am J Med 2002;113:294–299.

36. Deresinski SC, Stevens DA. Caspofungin. Clin Infect Dis 2003;36:1445–1457.

37. Ally R, Schurmann D, Kreisel W, et al. A randomized, double-blind, double-dummy, multicenter trial of voriconazole and fluconazole in the treatment of esophageal candidiasis in immunocompromised patients. Clin Infect Dis 2001;33:1447–1454.

38. Johnson LB, Kauffman CA. Voriconazole: A new triazole antifungal agent. Clin Infect Dis 2003;36:630–637.

39. Patton LL, Bonito AJ, Shugars DA. A systematic review of the effectiveness of antifungal drugs for the prevention and treatment of oropharyngeal candidiasis in HIV-positive patients. Oral Surg Oral Med Oral Pathol Oral Radiol Endod 2001;92:170–179.

40. USPHS/IDSA Prevention of Opportunistic Infections Working Group. 1999 USPHS/IDSA guidelines for the prevention of opportunistic infections in persons infected with human immunodeficiency virus. Clin Infect Dis 2000;30:S29–65.

41. Havlir DV, Dube MP, McCutchan JA, et al. Prophylaxis with weekly versus daily fluconazole for fungal infections in patients with AIDS. Clin Infect Dis 1998;27:1369–1375.

42. Grim SA, Smith KM, Romanelli F, Ofotokun I. Treatment of azole-resistant oropharygeal candidiasis with topical amphotericin B. Ann Pharmacother 2002;36:1383–1386.

43. Glick M, Siegel MA. Viral and fungal infections of the oral cavity in immunocompetent patients. Infect Dis Clin North Am 1999;13:817–831.

44. Nowak MA, Brodell RT. Rapid diagnosis of superficial fungal infections. Postgrad Med 1999;2:179–180.

45. Goldstein AO, Smith KM, Ives TJ, Goldstein B. Mycotic infections effective management of conditions involving the skin, hair, and nails. Geriatrics 2000;55:40–52.

46. Drake LA, Dinehart SM, Farmer ER, et al. Guidelines of care for superficial mycotic infections of the skin: Tinea corporis, tinea cruris, tinea faciei, tinea manuum, and tinea pedis. J Am Acad Dermatol 1996;34:282–286.

47. Gupta AK, Chow M, Daniel CR, Aly R. Treatments of tinea pedis. Dermatol Clin 2003;21:431–462.

48. Gupta AK, Chaudhry M Elewski B. Tinea corporis, tinea cruris, tinea nigra, and piedra. Dermatol Clin 2003;21:395–400.

49. Drake LA, Dinehart SM, Farmer ER, et al. Guidelines of care for superficial mycotic infections of the skin: Tinea capitis and tinea barbae. J Am Acad Dermatol 1996;34:290–294.

50. Higgins EM, Fuller LC, Smith CH. Guidelines for the management of tinea capitis. Br J Dermatol 2000;143:53–58.

51. Gupta AK, Batra R, Bluhm R, Faergemann J. Pityriasis versicolor. Dermatol Clin 2003;21:413–429.

52. Faergemann J, Baran R. Epidemiology, clinical presentation and diagnosis of onychomycosis. Br J Dermatol 2003;149(suppl 5):1–4.

53. Roberts DT, Taylor WD, Boyle J. Guidelines for treatment of onychomycosis. Br J Dermatol 2003;148:402–410.

54. Debruyne D, Coquerel A. Pharmacokinetics of antifungal agents in onychomycoses. Clin Pharmacokinet 2001;40:441–472.

55. Rodgers P, Bassler M. Treating onychomycosis. Am Fam Phys 2001;63:663–672, 677–678.

56. Gupta AK, Shear NH. A risk-benefit assessment of the newer oral antifungal agents used to treat onychomycosis. Drug Saf 2000;22:33–52.

57. Jain S, Sehgal VN. Itraconazole versus terbinafine in the management of onychomycosis: an overview. J Dermatol Treat 2003;14:30–42.

58. Evans EGV, Sigurgeisson B, for the LION Study Group. Double-blind, randomized study of continuous terbinafine compared with intermittent itraconazole in the treatment of toenail onychomycosis. Br Med J 1999;318:1031–1035.

59. Crawford F, Young P, Godfrey C, et al. Oral treatments for toenail onychomycosis: A systematic review. Arch Dermatol 2002;138:811–816.

60. Haugh M, Helou S, Boissel JP, Cribier BJ. Terbinafine in fungal infections of the nails: A meta-analysis of randomized clinical trials. Br J Dermatol 2002;147:118–121.

61. Cribier BJ, Paul C. Long-term efficacy of antifungals in toenail onychomycosis: a critical review. Br J Dermatol 2001;145:446–452.

62. Casciano J, Amaya K, Doyle J, et al. Economic analysis of oral and topical therapies for onychomycosis of the toenails and fingernails. Managed Care 2003;12:47–54.

63. Chambers WM, Millar A, Jain S, Burroughs AK. Terbinafine-induced hepatic dysfunction. Eur J Gastroenterol Hepatol 2001;13:1115–1118.

64. FDA Talk Paper. FDA issues health advisory regarding the safety of Sporanox products and Lamisil tablets to treat finger nail infections, May 2001, T01-22; available at *www.fda.gov/cder/ drug/advisory/sporanox-lamisil/advisory.htm.*

65. Gupta AK, Chwetzoff, Del Rosso J, Baran R. Hepatic safety of itraconazole. J Cutan Med Surg 2002;6:210–213.

66. Ahmad SR, Singer SJ, Leissa BG. Congestive heart failure associated with itraconazole. Lancet 2001;357:1766–1767.

67. Ling MR, Swinyer LJ, Jarratt MT, et al. Once-weekly fluconazole (450 mg) for 4, 6, or 9 months of treatment for distal subungual onychomycosis of the toenail. J Am Acad Dermatol 1998;38:S95–102.

68. Havu V, Heikkila H, Kuokkanen K, et al. A double-blind, randomized study to compare the efficacy and safety of terbinafine (Lamisil) with fluconazole (Diflucan) in the treatment of onychomycosis. Br J Dermatol 2000;142:97–102.

69. Arca E, Tastan HB, Akar A, et al. An open, randomized, comparative study of oral fluconazole, itraconazole and terbinafine therapy in onychomycosis. J Dermatol Treat 2002;13:3–9.

70. Ciclopirox (Penlac) nail lacquer for onychomycosis. Med Lett 2000;42:51–52.

71. Hay RJ. The future of onychomycosis therapy may involve a combination of approaches. Br J Dermatol 2001;145(supp 60):3–8.

119

INVASIVE FUNGAL INFECTIONS

Peggy L. Carver

Learning Objectives and other resources can be found at *www.pharmacotherapyonline.com*.

KEY CONCEPTS

◀1 Systemic mycoses may be caused by pathogenic fungi and include histoplasmosis, coccidioidomycosis, cryptococcosis, blastomycosis, paracoccidioidmycosis, and sporotrichosis, or infections by opportunistic fungi such as *Candida albicans, Aspergillus* spp., *Trichosporon, C. glabrata, Fusarium, Alternaria,* and *Mucor.*

◀2 The diagnosis of fungal infection generally is accomplished by careful evaluation of clinical symptoms, results of serologic tests, and histopathologic examination and culture of clinical specimens.

◀3 Histoplasmosis is caused by *Histoplasma capsulatum* and is endemic in parts of the central United States along the Ohio and Mississippi River valleys. Although most patients experience asymptomatic infection, some may experience chronic, disseminated disease.

◀4 Asymptomatic patients with histoplasmosis are not treated, although non-AIDS patients with evident disease are treated with either oral ketoconazole or intravenous amphotericin B; AIDS patients are treated with amphotericin B and then receive lifelong suppression.

◀5 Blastomycosis is caused by *Blastomyces dermatitidis* and generally is an asymptomatic, self-limited disease; however, reactivation can lead to chronic disease. Although treatment for self-limited disease is controversial, patients with chronic pulmonary disease or extrapulmonary disease

should be treated with ketoconazole, and those with central nervous system (CNS), progressive, or life-threatening disease should receive amphotericin B.

◀6 Coccidioidomycosis is caused by *Coccidioides immitis* and is endemic in some parts of the southwestern United States. It may cause nonspecific symptoms, acute pneumonia, or chronic pulmonary or disseminated disease. Primary pulmonary disease (unless severe) frequently is not treated, whereas extrapulmonary disease is treated with amphotericin B, and meningitis is treated with fluconazole.

◀7 Cryptococcosis is caused by *Cryptococcus neoformans* and occurs primarily in immunocompromised patients. Patients with acute meningitis are treated with amphotericin B with flucytosine. Patients infected with HIV require long-term suppressive therapy with fluconazole or itraconazole.

◀8 A variety of *Candida* spp. (including *C. albicans, C. glabrata, C. tropicalis,* and *C. krusei*) may cause diseases such as mucocutaneous, oral, esophageal, vaginal, and hematogenous candidiasis, as well as candiduria.

◀9 Aspergillosis may be caused by a variety of *Aspergillus* spp. that may cause superficial infections, pneumonia, allergic bronchopulmonary aspergillosis, or invasive infection. Treatment with amphotericin B or voriconazole generally is instituted but often is not successful.

For many years, fungal infections were classified as either superficial "nuisance diseases," such as athlete's foot or vulvovaginal candidiasis, or as relatively rare infections confined primarily to endemic areas of the country. When invasive fungal infections were encountered, amphotericin B was the only consistently effective, systemically active agent available for the treatment of systemic mycoses. ◀1 Advances in medical technology, including organ and bone marrow transplantation, cytotoxic chemotherapy, the widespread use of indwelling intravenous (IV) catheters, and the increased use of potent broad-spectrum antimicrobial agents all have contributed to the dramatic increase in the incidence of fungal infections worldwide.

Fungal infections have emerged as a major cause of death among cancer patients and transplant recipients.[1–4] In addition, patients with acquired immune-deficiency syndrome (AIDS) experience substantially more frequent and severe forms of cryptococcosis, histoplasmosis, coccidioidomycosis, and mucocutaneous (esophageal, oral, and vulvovaginal) candidiasis.

Problems remain in the diagnosis, prevention, and treatment of fungal infections. Unlike the available diagnostic techniques for most bacterial pathogens, there remains a host of unresolved issues regarding standardization of susceptibility testing methods, in vitro and in vivo models of infection, the utility of monitoring antifungal plasma concentrations, and the development and identification of resistant pathogens.[1,5–7] The Infectious Diseases Society of America published guidelines for the treatment of many commonly encountered fungal infections. These guidelines provide summaries of the literature and a consensus of expert opinions regarding the treatment of these difficult infections.[7]

MYCOLOGY

Fungi are eucaryotic organisms with a defined nucleus enclosed by a nuclear membrane; a cytoplasmic membrane containing lipids,

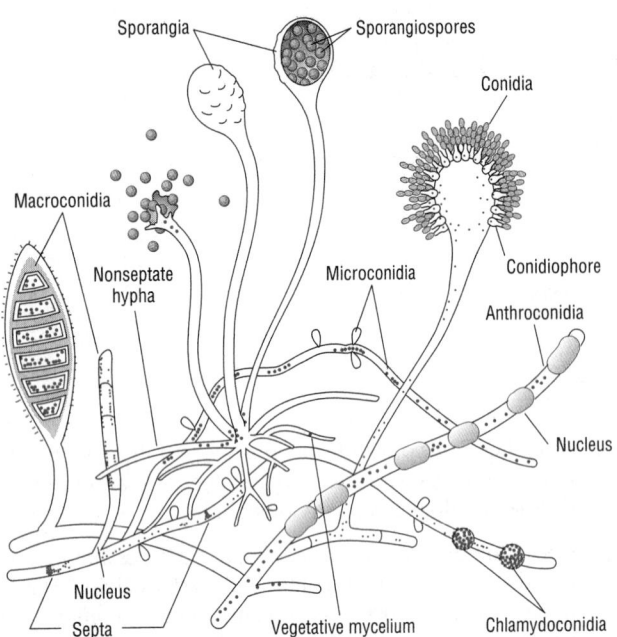

FIGURE 119–1. Forms of molds. The tubelike hyphae form their basic structure. Examples of spores and conidia and of the structures that bear them are shown. *(From Ryan KJ. Pathogenic fungi, in Sherris JC (ed): Medical Microbiology, 2d ed. New York, Elsevier, 1990:630, with permission.)*

cross walls) (Fig. 119–1). On agar media, molds grow outward from the point of inoculation by extension of the tips of filaments and then branch repeatedly, interweaving to form fuzzy, matted growths called *mycelia.* Yeasts are oval or spherically shaped unicellular forms that generally produce pasty or mucoid colonies on agar medium similar to those observed with bacterial cultures. Yeasts have rigid cell walls and reproduce by budding, a process in which daughter cells arise from pinching off a portion of the parent cell.

Fungi reproduce by forming spores asexually via mitosis to produce motile sporangiospores or nonmotile conidia (singular, conidium), or they reproduce sexually through meiosis to produce ascospores, basidiospores, oospores, or zygospores. Although terms such as *spore* and *conidia* should no longer be used interchangeably, some newer literature and much of the older medical literature continue to confuse these terms.

Many pathogenic fungi, termed *dimorphic fungi,* exist as either a yeast or a mold, depending on pathogen, site of growth (in the host or in the laboratory setting), and temperature. Usually yeasts are the parasitic form that invades human or animal host tissue, whereas molds are the free-living form found in the environment. For example, *Histoplasma capsulatum* exists as a yeast in humans and as a mold in the laboratory.[1,8]

SUSCEPTIBILITY TESTING OF ANTIFUNGAL AGENTS

Most laboratories do not routinely perform susceptibility tests on fungal isolates, but standardized methods for performing these tests are being developed and are now available for testing selected yeasts. To date, reference broth macrodilution and microdilution methods have been established for *Candida* and *Cryptococcus* spp., whereas broth the microdilution method has been standardized for filamentous fungi. Additionally, minimal inhibitory concentration (MIC) reference ranges for American Type Culture Collection (ATCC) quality control strains have been established against various antifungal agents, as well as interpretive breakpoints for fluconazole, itraconazole, and flucytosine against *Candida* spp[5] (Table 119–1). For further detail, refer to the section outlining treatment of *Candida* infections. Reliable and convincing interpretive breakpoints are not yet available for amphotericin B. The National Committee for Clinical Laboratory Standards (NCCLS) M27-A methodology does not reliably identify

glycoproteins, and sterols, mitochondria, Golgi apparatus, and ribosomes bound to endoplasmic reticulum; and a cytoskeleton with microtubules, microfilaments, and intermediate filaments. Fungi have rigid cell walls composed of chitin, cellulose, or both that stain with Gomori methenamine silver or periodic acid–Schiff reagent. Most fungi, except *Candida,* are too weakly gram-positive to be seen well on Gram's stain. *Cryptococcus neoformans* has a polysaccharide capsule surrounding the cell wall.[7]

Morphologically, pathogenic fungi can be grouped as either filamentous molds or unicellular yeasts. *Molds* grow as multicellular branching, threadlike filaments (hyphae) that are either septate (divided by transverse walls) or coenocytic (multinucleate without

TABLE 119–1. General Patterns of Susceptibility and Interpretive Breakpoints of *Candida Species*[a]

	Patterns of Susceptibility			
Candida Species	*Fluconazole*	*Itraconazole*	*Flucytosine*	*Amphotericin B*
C. albicans	S	S	S	S
C. tropicalis	S	S	S	S
C. parapsilosis	S	S	S	S
C. glabrata	S-DD to R[b]	S-DD to R[c]	S	S-I[d]
C. krusei	R	S-DD to R[c]	I-R	S-I[d]
C. lusitaniae	S	S	S	S to R[e]
Interpretive Breakpoints				
Sensitive	≤8	≤0.125	≤4	NA
S-DD or I	S-DD: 16–32	S-DD: 0.25–0.5	I: 8–16	NA
R	>32	>0.5	>16	NA

[a]Except for amphotericin B, interpretations are based on the use of a broth sensitivity test.
[b]Approximately 15% of *C. glabrata* isolates are resistant to fluconazole.
[c]Approximately 46% of *C. glabrata* isolates and 31% of *C. krusei* isolates are resistant to itraconazole.
[d]A significant proportion of *C. glabrata* and *C. krusei* isolates have reduced susceptibility to amphotericin B.
[e]Although frank resistance to amphotericin B is not observed in all isolates, it is well described for isolates of *C. lusitaniae.*
S = susceptible; S-DD = susceptible-dose dependent (see text); I = intermediate; R = resistant.
Adapted from refs. 5, and 9.

amphotericin B–resistant isolates; variations of the methodology using different media appear to enhance detection of resistant isolates.[5,9] It is important that the breakpoints be used following testing with the standardized, reproducible laboratory methodology (NCCLS 27-A) used to develop the test and that they be interpreted in the context of the delivered dose of the antifungal agent.

Because in vitro correlations with in vivo outcomes in patients are not yet known, the role of routine susceptibility testing is unknown at this time. Several concerns need to be considered as the use of MIC breakpoints is incorporated into the clinical practice setting: First, MICs are not actual physical measurements; rather, they provide estimates of drug activity. Since the MICs obtained can span greater than three twofold dilutions for the same isolate despite meticulous technique, MICs must be interpreted with caution. Second, host factors contribute greatly to clinical outcome. The same isolate in an immunocompetent patient may not result in the same outcome as in an immunocompromised patient. Thus, in vitro susceptibility does *not* necessarily equate with in vivo clinical success, and in vitro resistance may *not* always correlate with treatment failure. Susceptibility testing occasionally is indicated, e.g., in a patient with prolonged fungemia with a presumed susceptible isolate. Because of wide interlaboratory variability in test results, isolates should be tested at specialty laboratories that routinely perform these specialized tests. Susceptibility testing is most helpful in dealing with infections caused by non-*albicans* species of *Candida*.[5,9]

RESISTANCE TO ANTIFUNGAL AGENTS

It is important to distinguish between clinical resistance and microbial resistance. *Clinical resistance* refers to failure of an antifungal agent in the treatment of a fungal infection that arises from factors other than microbial resistance, such as failure of the antifungal agent to reach the site of infection or inability of a patient's immune system to eradicate a fungus whose growth is retarded by an antifungal agent.[10]

Microbial resistance can refer to *primary* or *secondary* resistance, as determined by in vitro susceptibility testing using standardized methodology. NCCLS resistance breakpoints are based on data relating treatment outcomes and fungal MICs and indicate the MIC at which clinical responses demonstrate a marked decline.[10] However, they do not serve as absolute predictors of therapeutic success or failure.

Primary, or *intrinsic, resistance* refers to resistance recorded prior to drug exposure in vitro or in vivo. *Secondary*, or *acquired resistance* develops on exposure to an antifungal agent and can be either reversible, owing to transient adaptation, or acquired as a result of one or more genetic alterations. The clinical consequences of antifungal resistance can be observed in treatment failures and in changes in the prevalences of *Candida* spp. causing disease. The evidence for the emergence of antifungal-resistant yeasts in patients other than those with HIV infection is confounded by the lack of standardized susceptibility testing methods and definitions of resistance. Large-scale surveys of yeasts from blood cultures, tested by standardized methodology, do not yet suggest that antifungal resistance is a significant or growing therapeutic problem.[10]

It is possible for a patient to respond clinically to treatment with an antifungal agent despite resistance to that agent in vitro because the patient's own immune system may eradicate the infection, or the agent may reach the site of infection in high concentrations.[10] Resistance to azole antifungal agents has been studied intensively partly because of the increased number of fluconazole-resistant *Candida* strains isolated from AIDS patients. Resistance may be acquired (i.e., transferred from other organisms or developed during therapy as a result of exposure to the antifungal agent) or intrinsic (innate lack of susceptibility of the antifungal agent to a pathogen). This issue has been reviewed extensively.[2,3,10]

The most exhaustive and definitive accounts of antifungal resistance have been described in *Candida* spp., in particular *Candida albicans* and, to a lesser extent, *C. glabrata*, *C. tropicalis*, and *C. krusei*, as well as in a few *Cryptococcus neoformans* isolates.[11–13] There are four different mechanisms that result in azole resistance: (1) mutations or upregulation of *ERG11*, (2) expression of multidrug efflux transport pumps that decrease antifungal drug accumulation within the fungal cell, (3) alteration of the structure or concentration of antifungal drug target proteins, and (4) alteration of membrane sterol proteins (Fig. 119–2). It is beyond the scope of this chapter to provide a complete discussion of the biochemical mechanisms of fungal resistance. Interested readers are referred to several excellent reviews concerning this topic.[10–13] Efflux pumps have been identified in *C. albicans, C. glabrata, C. tropicalis,* and *C. dubliniensis* and appear to be the most common mechanism of resistance encountered in clinical isolates. It is interesting to note that some of these mechanisms (efflux pumps in particular) appear to be reversible when selective pressure of antifungal agents is withdrawn.

Even though ketoconazole was used widely for the treatment of mucocutaneous candidiasis, resistant strains appeared very rarely. In patients with the uncommon syndrome of chronic mucocutaneous candidiasis, however, the chronic use of ketoconazole was associated with the emergence of ketoconazole-resistant *C. albicans*. Resistance likely developed in this specific population of patients because of two factors: the chronic use of ketoconazole and the inability of patients with this syndrome to eradicate the organism by normal host defense mechanisms. Fluconazole-resistant *C. albicans* have been noted almost entirely in AIDS patients and usually only after CD4 counts are less than 50 cells/mm^3 and after fluconazole was used chronically for repeated episodes of thrush over months to years. It appears that resistance develops in a stepwise progression in patients who have repeated episodes of thrush with one or several persisting strains of *C. albicans*. In vitro susceptibility testing shows a progressive decrease in susceptibility to fluconazole, and this has been correlated with clinical failure. This type of resistance has not yet become a problem in hospitalized patients treated with short courses of fluconazole or in patients in whom fluconazole has been used for prophylaxis.[14,15]

In the last few years, among hospitalized patients, there is increasing evidence for a shift toward isolation of other resistant species, such as *C. glabrata* and *C. krusei,* that have moderate or high-level resistance to fluconazole. This phenomenon has been especially common among patients in whom fluconazole has been used extensively.[2,3]

Resistance has not been described widely with itraconazole. This may be partly related to the fact that the drug has been used primarily for the treatment of endemic mycoses and not candidiasis. Even in patients never treated with itraconazole, however, *C. albicans* strains that are resistant to fluconazole also show decreased susceptibility to itraconazole.

The most commonly reported mechanisms of azole resistance among *C. albicans* isolates include reduced permeability of the fungal cell membrane to azoles, alteration in the target fungal enzymes (cytochrome P450) resulting in decreased binding of the azole to the target site, and overproduction of the fungal cytochrome P450 enzymes.[14,15] Studies also suggest the presence of efflux pumps capable of actively pumping azoles from the target pathogen, thereby conferring multidrug resistance to azole antifungals.[14,15]

C. glabrata is intrinsically more resistant than *C. albicans* to ketoconazole. Several strains of *C. glabrata* have been well characterized in terms of the mechanism of ketoconazole resistance.

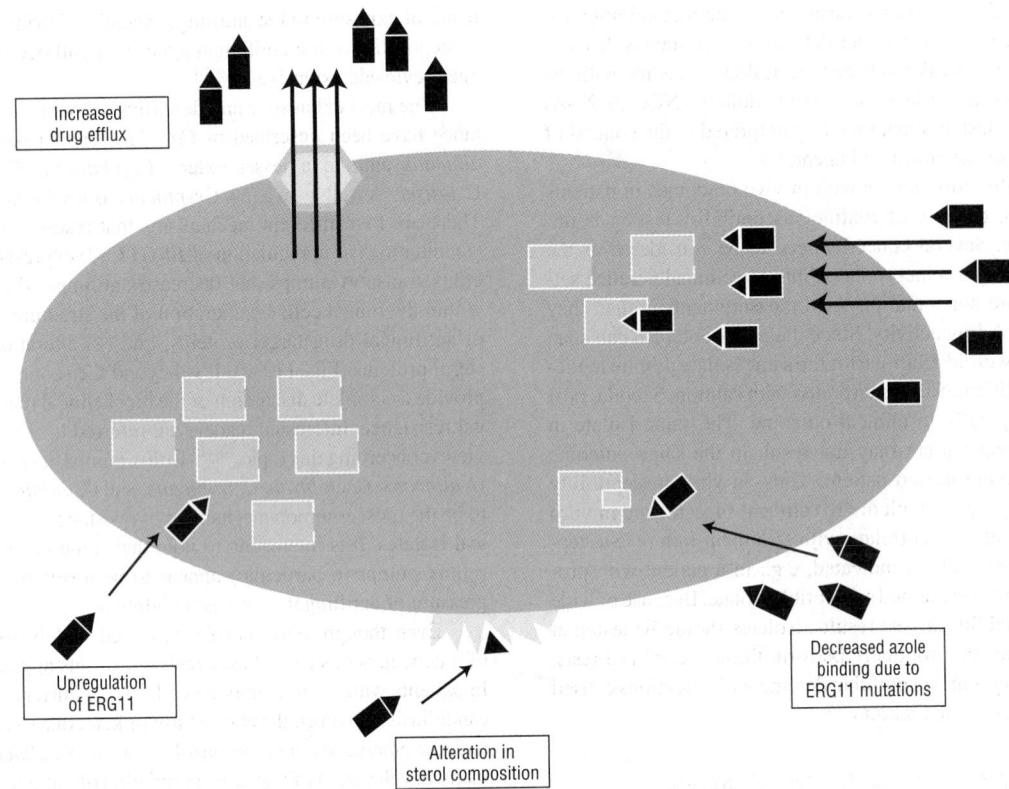

FIGURE 119–2. Resistance mechanisms of antifungal agents.

Decreased permeability to azoles has been described, but other strains show enhanced activity of the P450 cell membrane enzymes as well. *C. krusei* is inherently resistant to fluconazole, but it appears to be more susceptible to the other azoles. Decreased uptake of fluconazole into the fungal cell has been noted for several *C. krusei* strains.[14,15]

While rare, in vitro intrinsic resistance to amphotericin B is described, mainly in *C. lusitaniae*, *C. guillermondii*, and some molds (*Fusarium* spp., and *Pseudallescheria boydii*).[13] However, it is important to keep in mind that the current in vitro M27-A methodology discriminates poorly between rates of susceptibility of *Candida* spp. to amphotericin B. Although the rate of apparent resistance to amphotericin B appears to be quite low, breakthrough bacteremias in patients treated with amphotericin B have been observed. *C. glabrata*, *C. guilliermondii*, *C. krusei*, and *C. lusitaniae* appear to have a higher propensity than other *Candida* spp. to develop resistance to amphotericin B; this point should be kept in mind when treating patients with infections caused by one of these pathogens.[10] Since polyenes target ergosterol in the membranes of fungal cells, it is not surprising that amphotericin B–resistant strains of *Candida* generally have a marked decrease in ergosterol content compared with amphotericin B–susceptible strains. Resistant isolates of *Cryptococcus neoformans* have been reported to have a mutation in the C8 isomerization step of ergosterol synthesis.[13]

PATHOGENESIS AND EPIDEMIOLOGY

Systemic mycoses caused by primary or pathogenic fungi include histoplasmosis, coccidioidomycosis, cryptococcosis, blastomycosis, paracoccidioidomycosis, and sporotrichosis. Primary pathogens can cause disease in both healthy and immunocompromised individuals, although disease generally is more severe or disseminated in the immunocompromised host. In contrast, mycoses caused by opportunistic fungi such as *C. albicans*, *Aspergillus* spp., *Trichosporon*, *Torulopsis* (*Candida*) *glabrata*, *Fusarium*, *Alternaria*, and *Mucor* generally are found only in the immunocompromised host.[1]

Most fungal infections are acquired as a result of accidental inhalation of airborne conidia. For example, *H. capsulatum* is found in soil contaminated by bat, chicken, or starling excreta, and *C. neoformans* is associated with pigeon droppings. Although some fungi, including *C. albicans*, *C. neoformans*, and *Aspergillus* spp., are ubiquitous pathogens with worldwide distribution, other fungi have regional distributions associated with specific geographic environments.[1]

Systemic fungal infections are a major cause of morbidity and mortality in the immunocompromised patient. Fungal infections account for 20% to 30% of fatal infections in patients with acute leukemia, 10% to 15% of fatal infections in patients with lymphoma, and 5% of fatal infections in patients with solid tumors. The frequency of fungal infections among transplant recipients ranges from 0% to 20% for kidney and bone marrow transplant recipients to 10% to 35% for heart transplant recipients and 30% to 40% for liver transplant recipients.[4]

Approximately 2% to 4% of all hospitalized patients develop a nosocomial infection. Of these, bacteria comprise the most common etiologic agent.[1] Fungi, however, are becoming increasingly significant nosocomial pathogens. Fungi account for 10% of all bloodstream isolates. *Candida* spp. (primarily *C. albicans*) are the fourth most commonly isolated bloodstream isolate and account for 78% of all nosocomial fungal infections.[8,16]

Nosocomially acquired fungal infections may arise from either exogenous or endogenous flora. Endogenous flora may include normal commensals of the skin, gastrointestinal (GI), genitourinary, or respiratory tract. *C. albicans* is found as a normal commensal of the GI tract in 20% to 30% of humans.[8]

A complex interplay of host and pathogen factors influences the acquisition and development of fungal infections. Intact skin or mucosal surfaces serve as primary barriers to infection. Desiccation, epithelial cell turnover, fatty acid content, and low pH of the skin are believed to be important factors in host resistance. Bacterial flora of the skin and mucous membranes compete with fungi for growth. Alterations in the balance of normal flora caused by the use of antibiotics or alterations in nutritional status can allow the proliferation of fungi such as *Candida*, increasing the likelihood of systemic invasion and infection.[1]

The growth of fungi within tissues is restrained by a number of mechanisms. For example, serum has fungistatic activity against *Candida* in part because of transferrins, the human iron-binding proteins that deprive microbes of the iron needed for synthesis of respiratory enzymes. Serum also contains globulins, which cause a nonimmunologic clumping of *Candida*, facilitating their elimination by inflammatory cells.[1,8]

Tissue reaction in the presence of fungi varies with fungal species, site of proliferation, and duration of infection. Phagocyto-sis by neutrophils and macrophages is the earliest mechanism that prevents the establishment of fungi. Consequently, patients with decreased neutrophil counts or decreased neutrophil function are at higher risk of infections, particularly infections caused by *Candida* and *Aspergillus* spp. Some mycoses are characterized by a low-grade inflammatory response that does not eliminate the fungi. Fungal cells sometimes can persist within macrophages without being killed, perhaps because of resistance to the effects of lysosomal enzymes.[1]

DIAGNOSIS

The diagnosis of invasive fungal infections generally is accomplished by careful evaluation of clinical symptoms, results of serologic tests, and histopathologic examination and culture of clinical specimens. Skin tests generally are not useful diagnostically because they do not distinguish between active and past infection. They remain useful as screening tools and in epidemiologic studies to determine endemic areas. It is beyond the scope of this chapter to discuss the relative merits of each of the immunologic tests used in the diagnosis of invasive fungal infections. Interested readers, however, are referred to several excellent reviews concerning this topic.[17]

▶ TREATMENT: Invasive Mycoses

Strategies for the prevention or treatment of invasive mycoses can be classified broadly as prophylaxis, early empirical therapy, empirical therapy, and secondary prophylaxis or suppression.[1] In patients undergoing cytotoxic chemotherapy, antifungal therapy is directed primarily at the prevention or treatment of infections caused by *Candida* and *Aspergillus*. Prophylactic therapy with topical, oral, or intravenous antifungal agents is administered prior to and throughout periods of granulocytopenia (absolute neutrophil count < 1000/L). The potential benefits of prophylactic therapy must be weighed against the potential risks inherent in each regimen. Perfect[18] suggests that each clinician consider at least six criteria before justifying antifungal prophylaxis: (1) safety, (2) efficacy, (3) cost, (4) consequence, (5) prevalence, and (6) resistance.

Early empirical therapy is the administration of systemic antifungal agents at the onset of fever and neutropenia. Empirical therapy with systemic antifungal agents is administered to granulocytopenic patients with persistent or recurrent fever despite the administration of appropriate antimicrobial therapy.

Secondary prophylaxis (or suppressive therapy) is the administration of systemic antifungal agents (generally prior to and throughout the period of granulocytopenia) to prevent relapse of a documented invasive fungal infection that was treated during a previous episode of granulocytopenia.

Although these treatment classifications also have been applied to the treatment of fungal infections in AIDS, patients with AIDS rarely acquire systemic infections caused by *Candida* or *Aspergillus* spp. unless they become granulocytopenic because of disease or drugs. The use of antifungal prophylaxis is much less widely studied in this population, although studies suggest that early antifungal prophylaxis decreases the incidence of invasive cryptococcal disease.[19] Suppressive therapy generally is necessary following acute therapy for histoplasmosis, coccidioidomycosis, and cryptococcosis because of the high rates of relapse when antifungal therapy is discontinued.

▮ PROPHYLAXIS OF FUNGAL INFECTION IN THE HIV-INFECTED PATIENT

The use of antifungal prophylaxis to prevent fungal infections in HIV-infected patients has been assessed. Fluconazole prevented cryptococcosis and local *Candida* infections, including esophagitis, in HIV-infected patients, but overall mortality was not improved.[14] Because of the high costs of long-term prophylaxis, improved therapeutic regimens available for treating cryptococcal meningitis, and increasing reports of fluconazole resistance among *Candida* isolates from AIDS patients, many clinicians prefer not to use fluconazole prophylaxis in AIDS patients. For some patients with very low CD4 counts, however, some clinicians feel that it is cost-effective to use fluconazole prophylaxis to prevent cryptococcosis.[14]

HISTOPLASMOSIS

In humans, histoplasmosis is caused by inhalation of dust-borne microconidia of the dimorphic fungus *Histoplasma capsulatum*. Although there exist two dimorphic varieties of *H. capsulatum*, the small-celled (2–5 microns) form (var. *capsulatum*) occurs globally, whereas the large-celled (8–15 microns) form (var. *duboisii*) is confined to the African continent and Madagascar. In tissues stained by conventional techniques, *H. capsulatum* appears as an oval or round, narrow-pore, budding, unencapsulated yeast.[20]

EPIDEMIOLOGY

Although histoplasmosis is found worldwide, certain areas of North and Latin America are recognized as endemic areas; in the United States, most disease is localized along the Ohio and Mississippi River valleys, where more than 90% of residents may be affected. Precise reasons for this endemic distribution pattern are unknown but are thought to include moderate climate, humidity, and soil characteristics. *H. capsulatum* is found in nitrogen-enriched soils, particularly those heavily contaminated by avian or bat guano, which accelerates sporulation. Blackbird or pigeon roosts, chicken coops, and sites frequented by bats, such as caves, attics, or old buildings, serve as "microfoci" of infections. Although birds are not infected because of their high body temperature, bats (mammals) may be infected and can pass yeast forms in their feces, allowing the spread of *H. capsulatum* to new habitats. Air currents carry the spores for great distances, exposing individuals who were unaware of contact with the contaminated site.[20–22]

PATHOPHYSIOLOGY

At ambient temperatures, *H. capsulatum* grows as a mold. The mycelial phase consists of septate branching hyphae with terminal micro- and macroconidia that range in size from 2 to 14 microns in diameter. When soil is disturbed, these conidia become aerosolized and reach the bronchioles or alveoli.[20]

Animal studies demonstrate that within 2 to 3 days after reaching lung tissue, the conidia germinate, releasing yeast forms that begin multiplying by binary fission. During the next 9 to 15 days, organisms are ingested but not destroyed by large numbers of macrophages that are recruited to the infected site, resulting in small infiltrates. Infected macrophages migrate to the mediastinal lymph nodes and other sites within the mononuclear phagocyte system, particularly the spleen and liver. At this time, the onset of specific T-cell immunity in the non-immune host activates the macrophages, rendering them capable of fungicidal activity. Tissue granulomas form, many of which develop central caseation and necrosis over the next 2 to 4 months. Over a period of several years, these foci become encapsulated and calcified, often with viable yeast trapped within the necrotic tissue.[20,23]

Cellular immunity, as measured by histoplasmin skin-test reactivity, wanes in the absence of occasional reexposure. Although exposure to heavy inocula may overcome these immune mechanisms, resulting in severe disease, reinfection occurs frequently in endemic areas. In the immune individual, the reactions of acquired immunity begin 24 to 48 hours after the appearance of yeast forms, resulting in milder forms of illness and little proliferation of organisms. Although viable organisms may be found within granulomas years after initial infection, the organisms appear to have little ability to proliferate within the fibrous capsules, except in immunocompromised patients.[20,23]

CLINICAL PRESENTATION[14,17,19,20,22,23]

GENERAL

The outcome of infection with *H. capsulatum* depends on a complex interplay of host, pathogen, and environmental factors. Host factors include the degree of immunosuppression and the presence of immunity (from prior infection). Environmental factors include inoculum size, exposure within an enclosed area, and duration of exposure. Hematogenous dissemination from the lungs to other tissues probably occurs in all infected individuals during the first 2 weeks of infection before specific immunity has developed but is nonprogressive in most cases, which leads to the development of calcified granulomas of the liver and/or spleen. Progressive pulmonary infection is common in patients with underlying centrilobular emphysema.

A number of acute and chronic manifestations of histoplasmosis appear to result from unusual inflammatory or fibrotic responses to the pathogen, including pericarditis and rheumatologic syndromes during the first year after exposure, with chronic mediastinal inflammation or fibrosis, broncholithiasis, and enlarging parenchymal granulomas later in the course of disease.

ACUTE PULMONARY HISTOPLASMOSIS

In the vast majority of patients, low-inoculum exposure to *H. capsulatum* results in mild or asymptomatic pulmonary histoplasmosis. The course of disease generally is benign, and symptoms usually abate within a few weeks of onset. Patients exposed to a higher inoculum during an acute primary infection or reinfection may experience an acute, self-limited illness with flulike pulmonary symptoms, including fever, chills, headache, myalgia, and a nonproductive cough. Patients with diffuse pulmonary histoplasmosis may have diffuse radiographic involvement, become hypoxic, and require ventilatory support. A small percentage of patients present with arthritis, erythema nodosum, pericarditis, or mediastinal granuloma.

CHRONIC PULMONARY HISTOPLASMOSIS

Chronic pulmonary histoplasmosis generally presents as an opportunistic infection imposed on a preexisting structural abnormality, such as lesions resulting from emphysema. Patients demonstrate chronic pulmonary symptoms and apical lung lesions that progress with inflammation, calcified granulomas, and fibrosis. Patients with early, noncavitary disease often recover without treatment. Progression of disease over a period of years, seen in 25% to 30% of patients, is associated with cavitation, bronchopleural fistulas, extension to the other lung, pulmonary insufficiency, and often death.

DISSEMINATED HISTOPLASMOSIS

In patients exposed to a large inoculum and in immunocompromised hosts, successful containment of the organism within macrophages may not occur, resulting in a progressive illness characterized by yeast-filled phagocytic cells and an inability to produce granulomas. This disease, termed *disseminated histoplasmosis,* is characterized by persistent parasitization of macrophages. The clinical severity of the diverse forms of disseminated histoplasmosis (Table 119–2) generally parallels the degree of macrophage parasitization observed.

Acute (infantile) disseminated histoplasmosis is characterized by massive involvement of the mononuclear phagocyte system by yeast-engorged macrophages. Classically, this severe type of infection is seen in infants and young children and (rarely) in adults with Hodgkin's disease or other lymphoproliferative disorders. In infants or children, acute disseminated histoplasmosis is characterized by unrelenting fever, anemia, leukopenia or thrombocytopenia, enlargement of the liver, spleen, and visceral lymph nodes, and GI symptoms, particularly nausea, vomiting, and diarrhea. The chest roentgenogram often demonstrates remnants of the initiating acute pulmonary lesion. Untreated disease is uniformly fatal in 1 to 2 months. A less severe "subacute" form of the disease, which occurs in both infants and immunocompetent adults, is characterized by focal destructive lesions in various organs, weight loss, weakness, fever, and malaise. Untreated disease generally is fatal in approximately 10 months.

TABLE 119–2. Clinical Manifestations and Therapy of Histoplasmosis

Type of Disease and Common Clinical Manifestations	Approximate Frequency (%)[a]	Therapy/Comments
Nonimmunosuppressed Host		
Acute pulmonary histoplasmosis		
Asymptomatic or mild disease	50–99	*Asymptomatic, mild, or symptoms <4 weeks:* No therapy generally required
		Symptoms >4 weeks: Itraconazole 200 mg once daily × 6–12 weeks[b]
Self-limited disease	1–50	*Self-limited disease:* Amphotericin B[c] 0.3–0.5 mg/kg/day × 2–4 weeks (total dose 500 mg) or ketoconazole 400 mg orally daily × 3–6 months may be beneficial in patients with severe hypoxia following inhalation of large inocula
		Antifungal therapy generally not useful for arthritis or pericarditis; NSAIDs[d] or corticosteroids may be useful in some cases
Mediastinal granulomas	1–50	Most lesions resolve spontaneously; surgery or antifungal therapy with amphotericin B 40–50 mg/day × 2–3 weeks or itraconazole 400 mg/day orally × 6–12 months may be beneficial in some severe cases; mild to moderate disease may be treated with itraconazole for 6–12 months
Severe diffuse pulmonary disease		Amphotericin B 0.7 mg/kg/day, for a total dose of ≤35 mg/kg (or 3 mg/kg/day of one of the lipid preparations) + prednisone 60 mg daily tapered over 2 weeks,[e] followed by itraconazole 200 mg twice daily for 6–12 weeks; in patients who do not require hospitalization, itraconazole 200 mg once or twice daily for 6–12 weeks can be used
Inflammatory/fibrotic disease	0.02	*Fibrosing mediastinitis:* The benefit of antifungal therapy (itraconazole 200 mg twice daily × 3 months) is controversial but should be considered, especially in patients with elevated ESR[f] or CF[g] titers ≥1:32; surgery may be of benefit if disease is detected early; late disease may not respond to therapy
		Sarcoid-like: NSAIDs or corticosteroids may be of benefit for some patients
		Pericarditis: Severe disease: corticosteroids 1 mg/kg/day or pericardial drainage procedure
Chronic pulmonary histoplasmosis	0.05	Antifungal therapy generally recommended for all patients to halt further lung destruction and reduce mortality
		Mild–moderate disease: Itraconazole 200–400 mg PO daily × 6–24 months is the treatment of choice
		Itraconazole and ketoconazole (200–800 mg/day orally for 1 year) are effective in 74% to 86% of cases, but relapses are common; fluconazole 200–400 mg daily is less effective (64%) than ketoconazole or itraconazole, and relapses are seen in 29% of responders
		Severe disease: Amphotericin B 0.7 mg/kg/day for a minimum total dose of 35 mg/kg is effective in 59% to 100% of cases and should be used in patients who require hospitalization or are unable to take itraconazole due to drug interactions, allergies, failure to absorb drug, or failure to improve clinically after a minimum of 12 weeks of itraconazole therapy
Immunosuppressed Host		
Disseminated histoplasmosis	0.02–0.05	*Disseminated histoplasmosis:* Untreated mortality 83% to 93%; relapse 5% to 23% in non-AIDS patients; therapy is recommended for all patients
Acute (Infantile)		*Nonimmunosuppressed patients:* Ketoconazole 400 mg/day orally × 6–12 months or amphotericin B 35 mg/kg IV
Subacute		*Immunosuppressed patients: (non-AIDS) or endocarditis or CNS disease:* Amphotericin B >35 mg/kg × 3 months followed by fluconazole or itraconazole 200 mg orally twice daily × 12 months
Progressive histoplasmosis (immunocompetent patients and immunosuppressed patients without AIDS)		*Life-threatening disease:* Amphotericin B 0.7–1 mg/kg/day IV for a total dosage of 35 mg/kg over 2–4 months; once the patient is afebrile, able to take oral medications, and no longer requires blood pressure or ventilatory support, therapy can be changed to itraconazole 200 mg orally twice daily for 6–18 months
		Non-life-threatening disease: Itraconazole 200–400 mg orally daily for 6–18 months; fluconazole therapy 400–800 mg daily) should be reserved for patients intolerant to itraconazole, and the development of resistance may lead to relapses
Progressive disease of AIDS	25–50[h]	Amphotericin B 15–30 mg/kg (1–2 g over 4–10 weeks)[i] or itraconazole 200 mg 3 times daily for 3 days then twice daily for 12 weeks, followed by lifelong suppressive therapy with itraconazole 200–400 mg orally daily; a study is in progress to determine whether itraconazole therapy can be discontinued after one year if CD4+ counts are >150 cells/mm³

[a] As a percentage of all patients presenting with histoplasmosis.
[b] Itraconazole plasma concentrations should be measured during the second week of therapy to ensure that detectable concentrations have been achieved. If the concentration is below 1 mcg/mL, the dose may be insufficient or drug interactions may be impairing absorption or accelerating metabolism, requiring a change in dosage. If plasma concentrations are greater than 10 mcg/mL, the dosage may be reduced.
[c] Desoxycholate amphotericin B.
[d] NSAIDs = nonsteroidal anti-inflammatory drugs.
[e] Effectiveness of corticosteroids is controversial.
[f] ESR = erythrocyte sedimention rate.
[g] CF = complement fixation.
[h] As a percentage of AIDS patients presenting with histoplasmosis as the initial manifestation of their disease.
[i] Liposomal amphotericin B (Ambisome) may be more appropriate for disseminated disease.
Compiled from refs. 20, 22, and 23.

Most adults with disseminated histoplasmosis demonstrate a mild, chronic form of the disease. Untreated patients often are ill for 10 to 20 years, demonstrating long asymptomatic periods interrupted by relapses of clinical illness characterized primarily by weight loss, weakness, and fatigue. Chronic disseminated histoplasmosis can be seen in patients with lymphoreticular neoplasms (Hodgkin's disease) and patients undergoing immunosuppressant chemotherapy for organ transplantation or for rheumatic diseases. Although CNS involvement occurs in 10% to 20% of patients with severe underlying immunosuppressive conditions, focal organ involvement is uncommon. The disease is characterized by the development of focal granulomatous lesions, often with bone marrow involvement resulting in thrombocytopenia, anemia, and leukemia. Fever, hepatosplenomegaly, and GI ulceration are common.

HISTOPLASMOSIS IN HIV-INFECTED PATIENTS

Adult patients with AIDS demonstrate an acute form of disseminated disease that resembles the syndrome seen in infants and children. Progressive disseminated histoplasmosis (PDH) can occur as the direct result of initial infection or because of the reactivation of dormant foci. In endemic areas, 50% of AIDS patients demonstrate PDH as the first manifestation of their disease. Progressive disseminated histoplasmosis is characterized by fever (75% of patients), weight loss, chills, night sweats, enlargement of the spleen, liver, or lymph nodes, and anemia. Pulmonary symptoms occur in only one-third of patients and do not always correlate with the presence of infiltrates on chest roentgenogram. A clinical syndrome resembling septicemia is seen in approximately 25% to 50% of patients.

DIAGNOSIS

Detection of single, yeastlike cells 2 to 5 microns in diameter with narrow-based budding by direct examination or by histologic study of blood smears or tissues should raise strong suspicion of infection with *H. capsulatum* because colonization does not occur as with *Aspergillus* or *Candida* infection. Identification of mycelial isolates from clinical cultures can be made by conversion of the mycelium to the yeast form (requires 3 to 6 weeks) or via a rapid (2-hour)

and 100% sensitive DNA probe that recognizes ribosomal DNA. In patients with suspected disseminated or chronic cavitary histoplasmosis, two to three blood, sputum, and bone marrow cultures and stains should be obtained using the lysis centrifugation technique, and the cultures should be held for 14 to 21 days for optimal yield of *H. capsulatum*. In patients with acute self-limited histoplasmosis, extensive testing to verify the diagnosis may not be necessary.

In most patients, serologic evidence remains the primary method in the diagnosis of histoplasmosis. Results obtained from commercially available complement fixation (CF), immunodiffusion (ID), and latex agglutination (LA) antibody tests are used alone or in combination. In general, the use of histoplasmin skin tests is of little value except in epidemiologic studies because histoplasmin reactivity waxes in the absence of occasional reexposure. In addition, histoplasmin skin testing may result in a false increase in the CF titer for mycelial antigen (CF-M) to *H. capsulatum*. A fourfold rise in the CF titer is usually indicative of recent infection, although some patients with severe disease or profound immunosuppression may demonstrate a weaker antibody response.

Because the ID test is not as sensitive as CF, it should be used to assess the importance of weakly reactive results obtained by CF rather than as a screening procedure. Radioimmunoassay (RIA), which measures immunoglobulin M (IgM) and IgG antibodies against a histoplasmin extract, is the most sensitive test, but it may show a large number of false-positive reactions in patients living in an endemic area.

In the AIDS patient with PDH, the diagnosis is best established by bone marrow biopsy and culture, which yield positive cultures in more than 90% of patients, although blood cultures and histopathologic examination and culture of pulmonary tissue, sputum, skin, and lymph nodes also may be helpful. Detection of *H. capsulatum* polysaccharide antigen (HPA) in urine, blood, or cerebrospinal fluid (CSF) by enzyme-linked immunosorbent assay (ELISA) or by modified radioimmunoassay assay offer promising new techniques for the rapid diagnosis of histoplasmosis. The HPA (RIA) levels also have been used successfully to monitor the course of therapy and to detect relapses in patients with AIDS, and the clearance of antigen from serum and urine correlates with clinical efficacy during maintenance therapy with itraconazole. Unfortunately, these tests are not yet available for clinical use.

▶ TREATMENT: Histoplasmosis

■ NON–HIV-INFECTED PATIENT

Table 119–2 summarizes the recommended therapy for the treatment of histoplasmosis. In general, asymptomatic or mildly ill patients and patients with sarcoid-like disease do not benefit from antifungal therapy. In the vast majority of patients, low-inoculum exposure to *H. capsulatum* results in *mild* or *asymptomatic* pulmonary histoplasmosis. The course of disease generally is benign, and symptoms usually abate within a few weeks of onset. Therapy may be helpful in symptomatic patients whose conditions have not improved during the first month of infection. Fever persisting more than 3 weeks may indicate that the patient is developing progressive disseminated disease, which may be aborted by antifungal therapy. Whether antifungal therapy hastens recovery or prevents complications is unknown because it has never been studied in prospective trials.

Patients with mild, self-limited disease, chronic disseminated disease, or chronic pulmonary histoplasmosis who have no underlying immunosuppression usually can be treated with either oral

ketoconazole or IV amphotericin B. The goals of therapy are resolution of clinical abnormalities, prevention of relapse, and eradication of infection whenever possible, although chronic suppression of infection may be adequate in immunosuppressed patients, including those with HIV disease.[22,23]

Patients with arthritis, erythema nodosum, pericarditis, or mediastinal granuloma may require the addition of a 2-week course of corticosteroids to their therapy.[20]

■ HIV-INFECTED PATIENT

In AIDS patients, intensive 12-week primary antifungal therapy (induction and consolidation therapy) is followed by lifelong suppressive (maintenance) therapy with itraconazole. Amphotericin B dosages of 50 mg/day (up to 1 mg/kg per day) should be administered intravenously to a cumulative dose of 15 to 35 mg/kg (1 to 2 g) in patients who require hospitalization. Amphotericin B can be replaced with itraconazole 200 mg orally twice daily when the patient no longer requires hospitalization or intravenous therapy to complete a 12-week total course of induction therapy. In patients who do not require hospitalization, itraconazole therapy for 12 weeks may be used.

Fluconazole 800 mg/day orally as induction, followed by 400 mg/day, was effective in 88% of patients, but relapses occurred in approximately one-third of patients, and in vitro resistance developed in approximately 50% of patients who relapsed.

In regions experiencing high rates of histoplasmosis (>5 cases/100 patient-years), itraconazole 200 mg/day is recommended as prophylactic therapy in HIV-infected patients. Fluconazole is not an acceptable alternative because of its inferior activity against *H. capsulatum* and its lower efficacy for the treatment of histoplasmosis.[22]

EVALUATION OF THERAPEUTIC OUTCOMES

Response to therapy should be measured by resolution of radiologic, serologic, and microbiologic parameters and by improvement in signs and symptoms of infection. Although investigators are limited by the lack of standardized criteria to quantify the extent of infection, degree of immunosuppression, or treatment response, response rates (based on resolution or improvement in presenting signs and symptoms) of greater than 80% have been reported in case series in AIDS patients receiving varied dosages of amphotericin B. Rapid responses are reported, with the resolution of symptoms in 25% and 75% of patients by days 3 and 7 of therapy, respectively.

After the initial course of therapy for histoplasmosis is complete, lifelong suppressive therapy with oral azoles or amphotericin B (1–1.5 mg/kg weekly or biweekly) is recommended because of the frequent recurrence of infection.[25] Relapse rates in AIDS patients not receiving maintenance therapy range from 50% to 90%.[22]

Antigen testing may be useful for monitoring therapy in patients with disseminated histoplasmosis. Antigen concentrations decrease with therapy and increase with relapse. Some investigators recommend that treatment should continue until antigen concentrations revert to negative or less than 4 units. If treatment is discontinued before antigen concentrations in serum and urine revert to negative, patients should be followed closely for relapse, and antigen levels should be monitored every 3 to 6 months until they become negative.[22]

BLASTOMYCOSIS

North American blastomycosis is a systemic fungal infection caused by *Blastomyces dermatitidis*, a dimorphic fungus that infects primarily the lungs. Patients, however, may present with a variety of pulmonary and extrapulmonary clinical manifestations. Pulmonary disease may be acute or chronic and can mimic infection with tuberculosis, pyogenic bacteria, other fungi, or malignancy. Blastomycosis can disseminate to virtually every other body organ, and approximately 40% of patients with blastomycosis present with skin, bone and joint, or genitourinary tract involvement without any evidence of pulmonary disease.[24]

Pulmonary infection probably occurs by inhalation of conidia, which convert to the yeast form in the lung. A vigorous inflammatory response ensues, with neutrophilic recruitment to the lungs followed by the development of cell-mediated immunity and the formation of noncaseating granulomas.

EPIDEMIOLOGY

Blastomycosis was renamed *North American blastomycosis* in 1942, when Conant and Howell named a similar fungus endemic to South America, *Blastomyces braziliensis*, and the disease it caused *South American blastomycosis*. Although the disease is now recognized to be endemic to the southeastern and south central states of the United States (especially those bordering on the Mississippi and Ohio River basins) and the midwestern states and Canadian provinces bordering on the Great Lakes, numerous cases of North American blastomycosis have been diagnosed in Africa, northern parts of South America, India, and Europe. Endemic areas have been defined primarily by analysis of sporadic cases and epidemics or clusters of disease because the lack of a dependable skin or laboratory test makes wide-scale epidemiologic testing to determine the incidence of infection unfeasible at present.[23,25] Although initial review of sporadic cases suggested that males with outdoor occupations that exposed them to soil were at greatest risk for blastomycosis, more recent data suggest that there is no sex, age, or occupational predilection for blastomycosis.[23,24]

Although *B. dermatitidis* generally is considered to be a soil inhabitant, attempts to isolate the organism in nature frequently have been unsuccessful. *B. dermatitidis* has been isolated from soil containing decayed vegetation, decomposed wood, and pigeon manure, frequently in association with warm, moist soil of wooded areas that is rich in organic debris.[23,24]

PATHOPHYSIOLOGY AND CLINICAL PRESENTATION[16,17,23,24]

GENERAL

Colonization does not occur with *Blastomyces*. *Acute pulmonary blastomycosis* generally is an asymptomatic or self-limited disease characterized by fever, shaking chills, and productive, purulent cough, with or without hemoptysis, in immunocompetent individuals. The clinical presentation may be difficult to differentiate from other respiratory infections, including bacterial pneumonia, on the basis of clinical symptoms alone.

Sporadic (nonepidemic) pulmonary blastomycosis may present as a more chronic or subacute disease, with low-grade fever, night sweats, weight loss, and productive cough that resembles tuberculosis rather than bacterial pneumonia. *Chronic pulmonary blastomycosis* is characterized by fever, malaise, weight loss, night sweats, chest pain, and productive cough. Patients often are thought to have tuberculosis and frequently have evidence of disseminated disease that may appear 1 to 3 years after the primary pneumonia has resolved. Reactivation of disease may occur in the lungs or as the focus of new infection in other organs.

In approximately 40% of patients, dissemination is not accompanied by reactivation of pulmonary disease. The most common sites for disseminated disease include the skin and bony skeleton, although less commonly the prostate, oropharyngeal mucosa, and abdominal viscera are involved. CNS disease, while exceedingly uncommon, is associated with the highest mortality rate.

LABORATORY AND DIAGNOSTIC TESTS

The simplest and most successful method of diagnosing blastomycosis is by direct microscopic visualization of the large, multinucleated yeast with single, broad-based buds in sputum or other respiratory specimens following digestion of cells and debris with 10% potassium hydroxide. Histopathologic examination of tissue biopsies and culture of secretions also should be used to identify *B. dermatitidis,* although it may require up to 30 days to isolate and identify a small inoculum.

No reliable skin test exists to determine the incidence and prevalence of disease in endemic populations, and reliable serologic diagnosis of blastomycosis has long been hampered by the lack of specific and standardized reagents. Serologic response does not always correlate with clinical improvement, although some investigators have noted that a decline in the number of precipitins or CF titers may offer evidence of a favorable prognosis in patients with established disease.

Acute pulmonary blastomycosis generally is an asymptomatic or self-limited disease characterized by fever, shaking chills, and productive, purulent cough, with or without hemoptysis, in immunocompetent individuals. The clinical presentation may be difficult to differentiate from other respiratory infections, including bacterial pneumonia, on the basis of clinical symptoms alone. Sporadic (nonepidemic) cases of pulmonary blastomycosis may present as a more chronic or subacute disease with low-grade fever, night sweats, weight loss, and productive cough that resembles tuberculosis rather than bacterial pneumonia.

▶ TREATMENT: Blastomycosis

▦ NON–HIV-INFECTED PATIENT

◀5   In patients with mild pulmonary blastomycosis, the clinical presentation of the patient, the immune competence of the patient, and the toxicity of the antifungal agents are the main determinants of whether or not to administer antifungal therapy. All immunocompromised patients and patients with progressive pulmonary disease or with extrapulmonary disease should be treated (Table 119–3). In the

case of disease limited to the lungs, cure may have occurred before the diagnosis is made and without treatment. Regardless of whether or not the patient receives treatment, however, he or she must be followed carefully for many years for evidence of reactivation or progressive disease.[23,24]

Some authors recommend ketoconazole therapy for the treatment of self-limited pulmonary disease, with the hope of preventing late extrapulmonary disease; however, data supporting the efficacy of these regimens are lacking.[23,24] Itraconazole 200 to 400 mg/day

TABLE 119–3. Therapy of Blastomycosis

Type of Disease	Preferred Treatment	Comments
Pulmonary[a]		
Life-threatening	Amphotericin B[b] IV 0.7–1 mg/kg/day IV (total dose 1.5–2.5 g)	Patients may be initiated on amphotericin B and changed to oral itraconazole 200–400 mg orally daily once patient is clinically stabilized and a minimum dose of 500 mg of amphotericin B has been administered
Mild to moderate	Itraconazole 200 mg orally twice daily × ≥6 months[c]	*Alternative therapy:* Ketoconazole 400–800 mg orally daily × ≥6 months or fluconazole 400–800 mg orally daily × ≥6 months[d]
		In patients intolerant of azoles or in whom disease progresses during azole therapy: Amphotericin B 0.5–0.7 mg/kg/day IV (total dose 1.5–2.5 g)
Disseminated or Extrapulmonary		
CNS	Amphotericin B 0.7–1 mg/kg/day IV (total dose 1.5–2.5 g)	For patients unable to tolerate a full course of amphotericin B, consider lipid formulations of amphotericin B or fluconazole ≥ 800 mg orally daily
Non-CNS		
Life-threatening	Amphotericin B 0.7–1 mg/kg/day IV (total dose 1.5–2.5 g)	Patients may be initiated on amphotericin B and changed to oral itraconazole 200–400 mg orally daily once stabilized
Mild to moderate	Itraconazole 200–400 mg orally daily × ≥6 months	Ketoconazole 400–800 mg orally daily or fluconazole 400–800 mg orally daily × ≥6 months
		In patients intolerant of azoles or in whom disease progresses during azole therapy: Amphotericin B 0.5–0.7 mg/kg/day IV (total dose 1.5–2.5 g)
		Bone disease: Therapy with azoles should be continued for 12 months
Immunocompromised Host (Including Patients with AIDS, Transplants, or Receiving Chronic Glucocorticoid Therapy)		
Acute disease	Amphotericin B 0.7–1 mg/kg/day IV (total dose 1.5–2.5 g)	Patients without CNS infection may be switched to itraconazole once clinically stabilized and a minimum dose of 1 g of amphotericin B has been administered; long-term suppressive therapy with an azole is advised
Suppressive therapy	Itraconazole 200–400 mg orally daily	For patients with CNS disease or those intolerant of itraconazole, consider fluconazole 800 mg orally daily

[a]Some patients with acute pulmonary infection may have a spontaneous cure. Patients with progressive pulmonary disease should be treated.
[b]Desoxycholate amphotericin B.
[c]In patients not responding to 400 mg, dosage should be increased by 200 mg increments every 4 weeks to a maximum of 800 mg daily.
[d]Therapy with ketoconazole is associated with relapses, and fluconazole therapy achieves a lower response rate than itraconazole.
CNS = central nervous system.
Compiled from refs. 23, and 24.

demonstrated 90% efficacy as a first-line agent in the treatment of non-life-threatening non-CNS blastomycosis, and for compliant patients who completed at least 2 months of therapy, a success rate of 95% was noted. No therapeutic advantage was noted with the higher (400 mg) dosage as compared with patients treated with 200 mg.

All patients with disseminated blastomycosis, as well as those with extrapulmonary disease, require therapy. Ketoconazole 400 mg/day orally for 6 months cures more than 80% of patients with chronic pulmonary and nonmeningeal disseminated blastomycosis. Amphotericin B is more efficacious but more toxic and therefore is reserved for noncompliant patients and patients with overwhelming or life-threatening disease, CNS infection, and treatment failures. Cumulative amphotericin B dosages of more than 1 g have resulted in cure without relapse in 70% to 91% of patients with blastomycosis. Relapse rates depend on the total dosage of amphotericin B administered.[23,24] Patients with genitourinary tract disease should be treated initially with 600–800 mg/day of ketoconazole because of the low concentrations of drug achieved in the urine and prostate tissue.

Patients should be monitored carefully for signs of clinical failure, and those who fail or are unable to tolerate itraconazole therapy or who develop CNS disease should be treated with amphotericin B for a total cumulative dose of 1.5 to 2.5 g.[23,24]

Lipid preparations of amphotericin B are effective in animal models of blastomycosis, but they have not been evaluated adequately in humans. Limited clinical experience suggests that these preparations may provide an alternative for patients unable to experience standard therapy with amphotericin B because of toxicity. Surgery has only a limited role in the treatment of blastomycosis.

HIV-INFECTED PATIENT

For unclear reasons, blastomycosis is an uncommon opportunistic disease among immunocompromised individuals, including AIDS patients; however, blastomycosis may occur as a late (CD4 lymphocytes < 200 cells/mm^3) and frequently fatal complication of HIV infection. In this population, overwhelming disseminated disease with frequent involvement of the CNS is common.[23] Following induction therapy with amphotericin B (total cumulative dose of 1 g), HIV-infected patients should receive chronic suppressive therapy with an oral azole antifungal. Despite its higher cost, itraconazole has become the drug of choice for non-life-threatening histoplasmosis (mild to moderate disease) in HIV-infected patients.[24]

COCCIDIOIDOMYCOSIS

EPIDEMIOLOGY

Coccidioidomycosis is caused by infection with *Coccidioides immitis,* a dimorphic fungus found in the southwestern and western United States, as well as in parts of Mexico and South America. In North America, the endemic regions encompass the semiarid areas of the southwestern United States from California to Texas known as the Lower Sonoran Zone, where there is scant annual rainfall, hot summers, and sandy, alkaline soil. *C. immitis* grows in the soil as a mold, and mycelia proliferate during the rainy season. During the dry season, resistant arthroconidia form and become airborne when the soil is disturbed.

Although generally considered to be a regional disease, coccidioidomycosis has increased in importance in recent years because of the increased tourism and population in endemic areas, the increased use of immunosuppressive therapy in transplantation and oncology, and the AIDS epidemic. Although there is no racial, hormonal, or immunologic predisposition for acquiring primary disease, these factors affect the risk of subsequent dissemination of disease[25] (Table 119–4).

PATHOPHYSIOLOGY

When individuals come in contact with contaminated soil during ranching, dust storms, or proximity to construction sites or archaeologic excavations, arthroconidia are inhaled into the respiratory tree, where they transform into spherules, which reproduce by cleavage of the cytoplasm to produce endospores. The endospores are released when the spherules reach maturity. Similar to histoplasmosis, an acute inflammatory response in the tissue leads to infiltration of mononuclear cells, ultimately resulting in granuloma formation.[25]

CLINICAL PRESENTATION OF COCCIDIODOMYCOSIS[13,23–26]

Coccidioidomycosis encompasses a spectrum of illnesses ranging from primary uncomplicated respiratory tract infection that resolves spontaneously to progressive pulmonary or disseminated infection. Initial or primary infection with *C. immitis* almost always involves the lungs. Although approximately one-third of the population in endemic areas is infected, the average incidence of symptomatic disease is only approximately 0.43%.

SIGNS AND SYMPTOMS

In *asymptomatic disease* (60% of patients), patients have nonspecific symptoms that are often indistinguishable from ordinary upper respiratory infections, including fever, cough, headache, sore throat, myalgias, and fatigue. A fine, diffuse rash may appear during the first few days of the illness. Primary pneumonia may be the first manifestation of disease, characterized by a productive cough that may be blood-streaked, as well as single or multiple soft or dense homogeneous hilar or basal infiltrates on chest roentgenogram. Chronic, persistent pneumonia or persistent pulmonary coccidioidomycosis (primary disease lasting more than 6 weeks) is complicated by hemoptysis, pulmonary scarring, and the formation of cavities or bronchopleural fistulas.

Necrosis of pulmonary tissue with drainage and cavity formation occurs commonly. Most parenchymal cavities close spontaneously or form dense nodular scar tissue that may become superinfected

TABLE 119–4. Risk Factors for Severe, Disseminated Infection with Coccidioidomycosis

Race (Filipinos > African-Americans > Native Americans > Hispanics > Asians)

Pregnancy (especially when infection is acquired or reactivated in the second or third trimester)

Compromised cellular immune system, including
  AIDS patients
  Patients receiving
    Corticosteroids
    Immunosuppressive agents
    Chemotherapy

Male gender

Neonates

Patients with B or AB blood types

From ref. 25.

with bacteria or spherules of *C. immitis*. These patients often have persistent cough, fevers, and weight loss.

Valley fever occurs in approximately 25% of patients and is characterized by erythema nodosum and erythema multiforme of the upper trunk and extremities in association with diffuse joint aches or fever. More commonly, a diffuse, mild erythroderma or maculopapular rash is observed. Patients may have pleuritic chest pain and peripheral eosinophilia.

Disseminated disease occurs in less than 1% of infected patients. The most common sites for dissemination are the skin, lymph nodes, bone, and meninges, although the spleen, liver, kidney, and adrenal gland also may be involved. Occasionally, miliary coccidioidomycosis occurs, with rapid, widespread dissemination, often in concert with positive blood cultures for *C. immitis*. Patients with AIDS frequently present with miliary disease. Coccidioidomycosis in AIDS patients appears to be caused by reactivation of disease in most patients.

CNS infection occurs in approximately 16% of patients with disseminated coccidioidomycosis. Patients may present with meningeal disease without previous symptoms of primary pulmonary infection, although disease usually occurs within 6 months of the primary infection. The signs and symptoms are often subtle and nonspecific, including headache, weakness, changes in mental status (lethargy and confusion), neck stiffness, low-grade fever, weight loss, and occasionally, hydrocephalus. Space-occupying lesions are rare, and the main areas of involvement are the basilar meninges.

DIAGNOSIS

LABORATORY TESTS

Recovery of *C. immitis* from infected tissues or secretions for direct examination and culture provides an accurate and rapid method of diagnosis. Direct microscopic examination and histopathologic studies of infected tissues will reveal the large, mature endosporulating spherules. Young spherules without endospores may be confused, however, with other fungi. Silver stains of body fluids or tissue biopsies are also helpful.

With chronic, persistent pneumonia, *C. immitis* often can be cultured from the sputum for a period of several years. Chest radiographs usually demonstrate apical fibronodular lesions or slowly progressive cavitation. With CNS infection, analysis of the CSF generally reveals a lymphocytic pleocytosis with elevated protein and a decreased glucose concentration. Although serum usually is positive for coccidioidal CF antibodies, the coccidioidal skin test is often negative.

OTHER DIAGNOSTIC TESTS

Most patients develop a positive skin test within 3 weeks of the onset of symptoms. Baseline evaluation of skin test reactivity and serology is essential in order to assess cell-mediated immunity. Patients who develop early positive skin-test reactivity or whose coccidioidin skin-test reactivity turns from negative to positive during therapy have an improved prognosis compared with patients whose skin-test reactivity develops later or does not change during therapy. Patients with disseminated coccidioidomycosis whose skin tests are persistently negative are more likely to require prolonged therapy, and they are more likely to relapse after completion of therapy.

Antibody production can be used to follow the course of disease because most patients produce antibodies in response to infection with *C. immitis*. Early infection is characterized by the development of the IgM antibody, which peaks within 2 to 3 weeks of infection and then declines rapidly. The IgM antibody can be detected by either tube precipitin or immunodiffusion techniques.

The IgG antibody levels rise between 4 and 12 weeks after infection and decrease slowly over months to years, and IgG can be detected in many body fluids, including serum, CSF, and pleural fluid, by CF and ID techniques. Higher titers (>1:16 or 1:32) occur more frequently with severe disease. Titers can be followed serially to evaluate the efficacy of antifungal therapy.

Radiographic features tend to be quite variable; hilar adenopathy with alveolar infiltrates, tissue excavation of an infiltrate (resulting in a thin-walled cavity), or small pleural effusions are all seen commonly. With chronic persistent pneumonia, chest radiographs usually demonstrate apical fibronodular lesions or slowly progressive cavitation.

▶ TREATMENT: Coccidioidomycosis

▓ GENERAL GUIDELINES

Therapy for coccidioidomycosis is difficult, and the results are unpredictable. Guidelines are available for treatment of this disease; however, optimal treatment for many forms of this disease still generates debate.[25] The efficacy of antifungal therapy for coccidioidomycosis is often less certain than that for other fungal etiologies, such as blastomycosis, histoplasmosis, or cryptococcus, even when in vitro susceptibilities and the sites of infections are similar. The refractoriness of coccidioidomycosis may relate to the ability of *C. immitis* spherules to release hundreds of endospores, maximally challenging host defenses.[25,26] Fortunately, only approximately 5% of infected patients require therapy.[26]

▓ SPECIFIC AGENTS USED FOR THE TREATMENT OF COCCIDIOIDOMYCOSIS

Specific antifungals (and their usual dosages) for the treatment of coccidioidomycosis include intravenous amphotericin B (0.5 to 0.7 mg/

kg per day), ketoconazole (400 mg/day orally), intravenous or oral fluconazole (usually 400 to 800 mg/day, although dosages as high as 1200 mg/day have been used without complications), and itraconazole (200 to 300 mg orally twice daily as either capsules or solution).[25,26] If itraconazole is used, measurement of serum concentrations may be helpful to ascertain whether oral bioavailability is adequate.

Amphotericin B generally is preferred as initial therapy in patients with rapidly progressive disease, whereas azoles generally are preferred in patients with subacute or chronic presentations. The lipid formulations of amphotericin B have not been studied extensively in coccidioidal infection but may offer a means of giving more drug with less toxicity. Fluconazole probably is the most frequently used medicine given its tolerability, although high relapse rates have been reported in some studies. Relapse rates with itraconazole therapy may be lower than with fluconazole.[25,26]

▓ PRIMARY RESPIRATORY INFECTION

Although most patients with symptomatic primary pulmonary disease recover without therapy, management should include follow-up visits for 1 to 2 years to document resolution of disease or to identify as early as possible evidence of pulmonary or extrapulmonary complications.

CLINICAL CONTROVERSY

Because of the lack of prospective, controlled trials, there is continued disagreement among experts in endemic areas whether patients with coccidioidomycosis should be treated and, if so, which ones and for how long. The excellent tolerability of oral azoles has lowered the threshold for deciding to treat primary infection, and some clinicians treat all primary infections. Rationale for treating a primary self-limiting infection include the ability to lessen the morbidity associated with the acute infection and the possible ability to reduce the development of more serious complications. However, there is currently no evidence that treatment of the primary infection accomplishes either of these goals.[26]

Patients with a large inoculum, severe infection, or concurrent risk factors (e.g., HIV infection, organ transplant, pregnancy, or high doses of corticosteroids) probably should be treated, particularly those with high CF titers, in whom incipient or occult dissemination is likely. Because some racial or ethnic populations have a higher risk of dissemination, some clinicians advocate their inclusion in the high-risk group. Common indicators used to judge the severity of infection include weight loss (>10%), intense night sweats persisting more than 3 weeks, infiltrates involving more than one-half of one lung or portions of both lungs, prominent or persistent hilar adenopathy, CF antibody titers of greater than 1:16, failure to develop dermal sensitivity to coccidial antigens, inability to work, or symptoms that persist for more than 2 months.[25,26]

Commonly prescribed therapies include currently available oral azole antifungals at their recommended doses for courses of therapy ranging from 3 to 6 months.[25,26] In patients with diffuse pneumonia with bilateral reticulonodular or miliary infiltrates, therapy usually is initiated with amphotericin B; several weeks of therapy generally are required to produce clear evidence of improvement. Consolidation therapy with oral azoles can be considered at that time. The total duration of therapy should be at least 1 year, and in patients with underlying immunodeficiency, oral azole therapy should be continued as secondary prophylaxis.

INFECTIONS OF THE PULMONARY CAVITY

Many pulmonary infections that are caused by *C. immitis* are benign in their course and do not require intervention. In the absence of controlled clinical trials, evidence of the benefit of antifungal therapy is lacking, and asymptomatic infections generally are left untreated. Symptomatic patients may benefit from oral azole therapy, although recurrence of symptoms may be seen in some patients once therapy is discontinued. Surgical resection of localized cavities provides resolution of the problem in patients in whom the risks of surgery are not too high.[25,26]

EXTRAPULMONARY (DISSEMINATED) DISEASE

NONMENINGEAL DISEASE

Almost all patients with disease located outside the lungs should receive antifungal therapy; therapy usually is initiated with 400 mg.day of an oral azole. Amphotericin B is an alternative therapy and may be necessary in patients with worsening lesions or with disease in particularly critical locations such as the vertebral column. Approximately 50% to 75% of patients treated with amphotericin B for nonmeningeal disease achieve a sustained remission, and therapy usually is curative in patients with infections localized strictly to skin and soft tissues without extensive abscess formation or tissue damage. The efficacy of local injection into joints or the peritoneum, as well as intraarticular or intradermal administration, remains poorly studied. Amphotericin B appears to be most efficacious when cell-mediated immunity is intact (as evidenced by a positive coccidioidin or spherulin skin test or low CF antibody titer). Controlled trials that document these clinical impressions are lacking, however.[25,26]

MENINGEAL DISEASE

Fluconazole has become the drug of choice for the treatment of coccidioidal meningitis.[14,15] A minimum dose of 400 mg/day orally leads to a clinical response in most patients and obviates the need for intrathecal amphotericin B. Some clinicians will initiate therapy with 800 or 1000 mg/day, and itraconazole dosages of 400–600 mg/day are comparably effective. It is also clear, however, that fluconazole only leads to remission rather than cure of the infections; thus suppressive therapy must be continued for life. Ketoconazole cannot be recommended routinely for the treatment of coccidioidal meningitis because of its poor CNS penetration following oral administration. Patients who do not respond to fluconazole or itraconazole therapy are candidates for intrathecal amphotericin B therapy with or without continuation of azole therapy. The intrathecal dose of amphotericin B ranges from 0.01–1.5 mg given at intervals ranging from daily to weekly. Therapy is initiated with a low dosage and is titrated upward as patient tolerance develops.[14,15,25,26]

CRYPTOCOCCOSIS

EPIDEMIOLOGY

Cryptococcosis is a noncontagious, systemic mycotic infection caused by the ubiquitous encapsulated soil yeast *Cryptococcus neoformans,* which is found in soil, particularly in pigeon droppings, although disease occurs throughout the world, even in areas where pigeons are absent. Infection is acquired by inhalation of the organism. The incidence of cryptococcosis has risen dramatically in recent years, reflecting the increased numbers of immunocompromised patients, including those with malignancies, diabetes mellitus, chronic renal failure, and organ transplants and those receiving immunosuppressive agents. The AIDS epidemic also has contributed to the increased numbers of patients; cryptococcosis is the fourth most common infectious complication of AIDS and the second most common fungal pathogen.[27]

Although *C. neoformans* produces no toxins and evokes only a minimal inflammatory response in tissue, the polysaccharide capsule appears to allow the organism to resist phagocytosis by the host. The capsular polysaccharide of *C. neoformans* appears to comprise the major virulence factor for this pathogen. Four serotypes of *C. neoformans* (A through D) have been identified; they vary in their polysaccharide content, virulence, geographic foci, and response to antifungal therapy. Serotypes A and D are commonly associated with pigeon droppings and other environmental sites and generally require shorter therapy than do infections caused by serotypes B or C, which have been found only in infected humans and animals. Serotypes B and C appear more resistant to antifungal agents in vitro. Patients with AIDS are almost always infected with serotypes A and D, even in areas endemic for serotypes B and C. There is no particular geographic area of endemic focus for *C. neoformans.*

Cell-mediated immunity appears to play a major role in host defense against infection with *C. neoformans;* 29% to 55% of patients with cryptococcal meningitis have a predisposing condition. Many patients with disseminated cryptococcosis demonstrate defects in cell-mediated immunity. The predilection of *C. neoformans* for the CNS appears to be caused by the lack of immunoglobulins and complement and the excellent growth medium afforded by CSF.[27]

Disease may remain localized in the lungs or may disseminate to other tissues, particularly the CNS, although the skin also can be affected. Hematogenous spread generally occurs in the immunocompromised host, although it also has been seen in individuals with intact immune systems. Cryptococcemia is the most common symptomatic extraneural infection associated with *C. neoformans.* Cryptococcemia can be documented in 5% to 22% of non-AIDS patients, and CNS involvement of *C. neoformans* can be found in 18% to 50% of AIDS patients. Cryptococcal disease is present in 7.5% to 10% of AIDS patients. Therefore, patients with evidence of extraneural cryptococcosis should be evaluated for CNS disease.

CLINICAL PRESENTATION OF CRYPTOCOCCOSIS[13,27,28]

Primary cryptococcosis in humans almost always occurs in the lungs, although the pulmonary focus usually produces a subclinical infection. Symptomatic infections usually are manifested by cough, rales, and shortness of breath that generally resolve spontaneously. In non-AIDS patients, the symptoms of cryptococcal meningitis are nonspecific. Headache, fever, nausea, vomiting, mental status changes, and neck stiffness generally are observed. Less common symptoms include visual disturbances (photophobia and blurred vision), papilledema, seizures, and aphasia. In AIDS patients, fever and headache are common, but meningismus and photophobia are much less common than in non-AIDS patients. Approximately 10% to 12% of AIDS patients have asymptomatic disease, similar to the rate observed in non-AIDS patients.[28]

LABORATORY TESTS

With cryptococcal meningitis, the CSF opening pressure generally is elevated. There is a CSF pleocytosis (usually lymphocytes), leukocytosis, a decreased glucose concentration, and an elevated CSF protein concentration. There is also a positive cryptococcal antigen (detected by latex agglutination). The test is rapid, specific, and extremely sensitive, but false-negative results can occur. False-positive tests can result from cross-reactivity with rheumatoid factor and *Trichosporon beigelli. C. neoformans* can be detected in approximately 60% of patients by india ink smear of CSF, and it can be cultured in more than 96% of patients. Occasionally, large volumes of CSF are required to confirm the diagnosis.

The CSF parameters in patients with AIDS are similar to those seen in non-AIDS patients, with the exception of a decreased inflammatory response to the pathogen, resulting in a strikingly low number of leukocytes in CSF and extraordinarily high cryptococcal antigen titers.

► TREATMENT: Cryptococcosis

The choice of treatment for disease caused by *C. neoformans* depends on both the anatomic sites of involvement and the host's immune status.

NONIMMUNOCOMPROMISED PATIENTS

For asymptomatic immunocompetent hosts with isolated pulmonary disease and no evidence of CNS disease, careful observation may be warranted; in the case of symptomatic infection, fluconazole or amphotericin B is warranted (Table 119–5). In individuals with non-CNS cryptococcemia, a positive serum cryptococcal antigen titer (>1:8), cutaneous infection, a positive urine culture, or prostatic disease, the clinician must decide whether to follow the regimen for isolated pulmonary disease or the more aggressive regimen for patients with CNS (disseminated) disease.[19]

Prior to the introduction of amphotericin B, cryptococcal meningitis was an almost uniformly fatal disease; approximately 86% of patients died within 1 year. The use of large (1 to 1.5 mg/kg) daily doses of amphotericin B resulted in cure rates of approximately 64%. When amphotericin B is combined with flucytosine, a smaller dose of amphotericin B can be employed because of the in vitro and in vivo synergy between the two antifungal agents. Resistance develops to flucytosine in up to 30% of patients treated with flucytosine alone, limiting its usefulness as monotherapy.[28,29] Combination therapy with amphotericin B and flucytosine will sterilize the CSF within 2 weeks of treatment in 60% to 90% of patients, and most immunocompetent patients will be treated successfully with 6 weeks of combination therapy.[27] However, because of the need for prolonged IV therapy and the potential for renal and hematologic toxicity with this regimen, alternative regimens have been advocated. Despite a lack of clinically controlled trials in this population, amphotericin B induction therapy for 2 weeks, followed by consolidation therapy with fluconazole for an additional 8 to 10 weeks, is frequently recommended based on data extrapolated from studies conducted in HIV-infected patients. Suppressive therapy with fluconazole 200 mg/day for 6 to 12 months after the completion of induction and consolidation therapy is optional.[19,29–31]

Pilot studies evaluating combination therapy with fluconazole plus flucytosine as initial therapy yielded unsatisfactory results, and this approach is discouraged even in "low risk" patients. Ketoconazole has been used successfully in the treatment of cutaneous cryptococcosis, but it is not useful in the treatment of CNS disease, probably because of its poor penetration into the CNS.[19]

Despite low CSF concentrations of amphotericin B (2% to 3% of those observed in plasma), the use of intrathecal amphotericin B is not recommended for the treatment of cryptococcal meningitis except in very ill patients or in patients with recurrent or progressive disease despite aggressive therapy with IV amphotericin B. The dosage of amphotericin B employed is usually 0.5 mg administered via the lumbar, cisternal, or intraventricular (via an Ommaya reservoir) route two or three times weekly. Side effects of intrathecal amphotericin B include arachnoiditis and paresthesias. Intrathecal

TABLE 119–5. Therapy of Cryptococcocosis[a,b]

Type of Disease and Common Clinical Manifestations	Therapy/Comments
Nonimmunocompromised Host	Comparative trials for amphotericin B[c] versus azoles not available
Isolated pulmonary disease (without evidence of CNS infection)	*Asymptomatic disease:* Durg therapy generally not required; observe carefully or fluconazole 400 mg orally daily × 3–6 months
	Mild to moderate symptoms: Fluconazole 200–400 mg orally daily × 3–6 months;
	Severe disease or inability to take azoles: Amphotericin B 0.4–0.7 mg/kg/day (total dose of 1–2 g)
Cryptococcemia with positive serum antigen titer (>1:8), cutaneous infection, a positive urine culture, or prostatic disease	Clinician must decide whether to follow the pulmonary therapeutic regimen or the CNS (disseminated) regimen
Recurrent or progressive disease not responsive to amphotericin B	Amphotericin B[d] IV 0.5–0.75 mg/kg/day ± IT amphotericin B 0.5 mg 2–3 times weekly
Isolated pulmonary disease (without evidence of CNS infection)	*Mild to moderate symptoms or asymptomatic with a positive pulmonary specimen:* Fluconazole 200–400 mg orally daily × lifelong *or* Itraconazole 200–400 mg orally daily × lifelong *or* Fluconazole 400 mg orally daily + flucytosine 100–150 mg/kg/day orally × 10 weeks *Severe disease:* Amphotericin B until symptoms are controlled, followed by fluconazole
CNS disease	
Acute (induction/consolidation therapy) (follow all regimens with suppressive therapy)	Amphotericin B[d] IV 0.7–1 mg/kg/day + flucytosine 100 mg/kg/day orally × ≥2 weeks, then fluconazole 400 mg orally daily × ≥8 weeks[e] *or* Amphotericin B[d] IV 0.7–1 mg/kg/day + flucytosine 100 mg/kg/day orally × 6–10 weeks[e] *or* Amphotericin B[d] IV 0.7–1 mg/kg/day × 6–10 weeks[e] *or* Fluconazole 400–800 mg orally daily × 10–12 weeks *or* Itraconazole 400–800 mg orally daily × 10–12 weeks *or* Fluconazole 400–800 mg orally daily + flucytosine 100–150 mg/kg/day orally × 6 weeks[e] *or* Lipid formulation of amphotericin B IV 3–6 mg/kg/day × 6–10 weeks *Note:* Induction therapy with azoles alone is discouraged.
CNS disease	Amphotericin B[d] IV 0.7–1 mg/kg/day + flucytosine 100 mg/kg/day orally × 2 weeks, followed by fluconazole 400 mg orally daily for a minimum of 10 weeks (in patients intolerant to fluconazole, substitute itraconazole 200–400 mg orally daily) *or* Amphotericin B[d] IV 0.7–1 mg/kg/day + 5-FC 100 mg/kg/day orally × 6–10 weeks *or* Amphotericin B[d] IV 0.7–1 mg/kg/day × 10 weeks *Refractory disease:* Intrathecal or intraventricular amphotericin B
Immunocompromised Patients	
Non-CNS pulmonary and extrapulmonary disease	Same as nonimmunocompromised patients with CNS disease
CNS disease	Amphotericin B[d] IV 0.7–1 mg/kg/day × 2 weeks, followed by fluconazole 400–800 mg orally daily 8–10 weeks, followed by fluconazole 200 mg orally daily × 6–12 months (in patients intolerant to fluconazole, substitute itraconazole 200–400 mg orally daily) *Refractory disease:* Intrathecal or intraventricular amphotericin B
HIV-Infected Patients	
Suppressive/maintenance therapy	Fluconazole 200–400 mg orally daily × lifelong *or* Itraconazole 200 mg orally twice daily × lifelong *or* Amphotericin B IV 1 mg/kg 1–3 times weekly × lifelong

[a]When more than one therapy is listed, they are listed in order of preference.
[b]See text for definitions of induction, consolidation, suppressive/maintenance therapy, and prophylactic therapy.
[c]Deoxycholate amphotericin B.
[d]In patients with significant renal disease, lipid formulations of amphotericin B can be substituted for deoxycholate amphotericin B during the induction.
[e]Or until CSF cultures are negative
IV = intravenous; IT = intrathecal; CNS = central nervous system.
Compiled from refs. 27–31.

amphotericin B therapy should be administered in combination with IV amphotericin B.[31]

IMMUNOCOMPROMISED PATIENTS

Immunocompromised hosts with isolated pulmonary and extrapulmonary disease without CNS disease should be treated similarly to nonimmunocompromised patients with CNS disease. Immunocompromised patients with CNS infection require more prolonged therapy; treatment regimens are based on those used in the HIV-infected population and follow induction and consolidation therapy with 6 to 12 months of suppressive therapy with fluconazole.[19]

HIV-INFECTED PATIENTS

There are no controlled clinical trials evaluating the therapy of isolated pulmonary infection; thus the specific treatment of choice is unclear. However, because these patients are at high risk for disseminated infection, antifungal therapy is warranted in all patients. Lifelong therapy with fluconazole is recommended; in patients for whom fluconazole is not an option, itraconazole can be used.

Fluconazole is beneficial for both acute and chronic maintenance therapy for cryptococcal meningitis. Amphotericin B 0.4–0.5 mg/kg IV daily was compared with oral fluconazole 200 mg/day. Although the overall 10-week mortality was the same in both groups, the time until the CSF culture became negative was longer and there were more deaths in the first 2 weeks of therapy in the fluconazole group.[30] In later trials,[31] amphotericin B 0.7 mg/kg IV daily for 2 weeks (with or without oral flucytosine 100 mg/kg per day), followed by consolidation therapy with either itraconazole 400 mg/day orally or fluconazole 400 mg/day orally, led to markedly improved outcomes in comparison with earlier regimens. This study confirmed the benefit of early high-dose (0.7 mg/kg per day) amphotericin B use, the utility of flucytosine added to amphotericin B for induction therapy, and the slight superiority of fluconazole over itraconazole for consolidation therapy.

Amphotericin B combined with flucytosine is the initial treatment of choice. In patients who cannot tolerate flucytosine, amphotericin B alone is an acceptable alternative. After the initially successful 2-week induction period, consolidation therapy with fluconazole can be administered for 8 weeks or until CSF cultures are negative. In patients in whom fluconazole cannot be given, itraconazole is an acceptable, albeit less effective, alternative. Combination therapy with fluconazole plus flucytosine is effective; however, it is recommended as an alternative to the preceding therapies because of its potential for toxicity. Lipid

formulations of amphotericin B are effective, but the optimal dosage is unknown.[19]

In HIV-infected patients with elevated intracranial pressure at the initiation of antifungal therapy, lumbar drainage should remove enough CSF to reduce the opening pressure by 50%. Patients initially should undergo daily lumbar punctures to maintain CSF opening pressure in the normal range. When the CSF pressure is normal for several days, the procedure can be suspended. Adjunctive steroid treatment is not recommended because therapy has resulted in mixed results and its impact on outcome is unclear. Similarly, neither mannitol nor acetazolamide therapy provides any clear benefit in the management of elevated intracranial pressure.[19]

SUPPRESSIVE (MAINTENANCE) THERAPY FOR CRYPTOCOCCAL MENINGITIS IN THE HIV-INFECTED PATIENT

Relapse of *C. neoformans* meningitis occurs in approximately 50% of AIDS patients after completion of primary therapy. Persistence of asymptomatic urinary *C. neoformans* has been documented in a high percentage of AIDS patients despite seemingly adequate courses of therapy for primary meningeal disease. The prostate appears to act as a sequestered reservoir of infection in these patients, resulting in systemic relapse. Fluconazole is recommended for chronic suppressive therapy of cryptococcal meningitis in AIDS patients. The AIDS Clinical Trials Group's (ACTG) 026 study demonstrated that oral fluconazole 200 mg/day was superior to IV administration of amphotericin B 1 mg/kg weekly in preventing relapse. In addition, the fluconazole-treated group showed a lower incidence of adverse drug reactions and bacterial infections.[31] Randomized comparative trials also demonstrated the superiority of fluconazole versus itraconazole as maintenance therapy. Thus itraconazole should be reserved for patients intolerant to fluconazole. Ketoconazole is not effective as maintenance therapy.

Although some preliminary studies suggest lower relapse rates of opportunistic infections when patients have been treated successfully with potent antiretroviral therapy, until proven otherwise, maintenance therapy for cryptococcal meningitis should be continued for life. For selected patients who have responded very well to highly active antiretroviral therapy (HAART), the clinician may consider discontinuation of maintenance therapy following 12 to 18 months of successful suppression of HIV viral replication. A prospective, randomized trial confirmed that discontinuation of secondary prophylaxis is safe in patients after adequate treatment for cryptococcal meningitis who had CD4 cell increases of greater than 100 cells/mm^3 and an HIV viral load of fewer than 50 copies/mL for more than 3 months.[19,29–32]

EVALUATION OF THERAPEUTIC OUTCOMES

Once the CNS is involved, the usual course is weeks to months of progressive deterioration, with 80% of untreated patients dying within the first year. The prognosis of cryptococcal meningitis depends largely on the underlying predisposing factors of the host. Although cryptococcal antigen is positive in 90% of patients with cryptococcal meningitis, fewer than half the patients with cryptococcal meningitis develop antibody to capsular polysaccharide. Those who produce antibody have a slightly improved prognosis. In contrast, the presence of headache is a favorable symptom presumably because it leads to

an earlier diagnosis. A favorable outcome is also associated with a normal mental status on diagnosis and a CSF white blood cell (WBC) count of less than 20 cells/mm^3. A poor outcome is predicted, however, by the presence of one or more underlying diseases (including hematopoietic disorders and AIDS), corticosteroid or immunosuppressive therapy, pretreatment serum cryptococcal antigen titers of 1:32, and posttherapy serum antigen titers of 1:8. In non-AIDS patients, the cryptococcal antigen titer can be followed during therapy to assess response to antifungal therapy. In AIDS patients, decreasing titers are not necessarily predictive of success, and titers rarely become negative at the completion of therapy.[14,15]

CANDIDA INFECTIONS

Candida spp. are yeasts that exist primarily as small (4–6 microns), unicellular, thin-walled, ovoid cells that reproduce by budding. On agar medium, they form smooth, white, creamy colonies resembling staphylococci. Although there are more than 150 species of *Candida*, eight species—*C. albicans, C. tropicalis, C. parapsilosis, C. krusei, C. stellatoidea, C. guilliermondi, C. lusitaniae,* and *C. glabrata*—are regarded as clinically important pathogens in human disease.[8,16] Yeast forms, hyphae, and pseudohyphae may be found in clinical specimens.

PATHOPHYSIOLOGY

C. albicans is a normal commensal of the skin, female genital tract, and entire GI tract of humans. Therefore, the mere presence of hyphae or pseudohyphae in a clinical specimen is insufficient for the diagnosis of invasive disease. The majority of infections with *C. albicans* are acquired endogenously, although human-to-human transmission also can occur. Oral candidiasis in the newborn probably is acquired during passage through the birth canal, and balanitis in the uncircumcised male may be acquired through contact with a female with vaginal candidiasis.[8] Although the term *fungemia* refers to the presence of fungi in the blood, the most commonly isolated organism is *C. albicans*. Candidiasis may cause mucocutaneous or systemic infection, including endocarditis, peritonitis, arthritis, and infection of the CNS. (Mucocutaneous infections caused by *Candida* are discussed in further detail in Chap.118.)

The role of an intact integument is crucial in the prevention of mucocutaneous or hematogenous candidiasis. After *Candida* invades the dermis or enters the bloodstream, polymorphonuclear leukocytes (PMNs) play a major role in the defense of the patient because PMNs are capable of damaging pseudohyphae and can phagocytize and kill blastoconidia.[8] In addition to neutrophils, lymphocytes, monocytes, macrophages, complement, and eosinophils play a role in the prevention of infection. Adherence of *C. albicans* is important in the pathogenesis of oral candidiasis and subsequent colonization of the GI tract. Because evidence suggests that the GI tract is often the portal of entry for *Candida* in disseminated disease, factors that alter the adherence of *Candida* are crucial in the development of local and systemic infection. *C. tropicalis* adheres to intravascular catheters at a higher rate than *C. albicans,* a factor that may help to account for the increased incidence of systemic infections caused by this pathogen.

HEMATOGENOUS CANDIDIASIS

EPIDEMIOLOGY

The incidence of fungal infections caused by *Candida* spp. has increased substantially in the past two decades, and *Candida* infections currently constitute a significant cause of morbidity and mortality among severely ill patients. *Candida* spp. now constitute the fourth most common cause of bloodstream infections (BSIs) for patients hospitalized in ICUs in the United States, following coagulase-negative staphylococci, *Staphylococcus aureus,* and enterococci. The Centers for Disease Control and Prevention's (CDC) National Nosocomial Infection Survey implicated fungi as the cause of 8% of nosocomial infections. Although *C. albicans* accounted for 53% of *Candida* spp.,[15] non-*albicans* species of *Candida*, including *C. glabrata, C. tropicalis, C. krusei,* and *C. parapsilosis,* are increasingly frequent causes of invasive candidal infections.[34–36] *C. lusitaniae* infections are a

cause of breakthrough fungemia in cancer patients; *C. parapsilosis* has emerged as the second most common pathogen, following *C. albicans,* in neonatal ICU patients; and fungemia caused by *C. glabrata* is observed more commonly in adults whose age is greater than 65 years.[34,37] The change in species is of concern clinically because certain pathogens, such as *C. krusei* and *C. glabrata,* are intrinsically more resistant to commonly used triazole drugs.

PATHOPHYSIOLOGY

Candida generally is acquired via the GI tract, although organisms also may enter the bloodstream via indwelling IV catheters. Immunosuppressed patients, including those with lymphoreticular or hematologic malignancies, diabetes, and immunodeficiency diseases and those receiving immunosuppressive therapy with high-dose corticosteroids, immunosuppressants, antineoplastic agents, or broad-spectrum antimicrobial agents, are at high risk for invasive fungal infections. However, a number of prospective, randomized, controlled trials have validated the efficacy of antifungal prophylaxis and the use of antifungal agents for the treatment of persistently febrile patients with neutropenia who do not respond to antibiotics.[8,14,15,38] These efforts have resulted in a reduction in the frequency of bloodstream infections caused by *Candida* spp. and systemic candidiasis in patients with neutropenia. In fact, most bloodstream infections caused by *Candida* spp. now occur in patients who have been hospitalized in ICUs, especially adult and neonatal ICUs. Retrospective studies have identified a number of risk factors for candidal bloodstream infections in ICU patients, most of which have been verified in multiple studies, although some remain controversial[39] (Table 119-6). Major risk factors include the use of central venous catheters, total parenteral nutrition, receipt of multiple antibiotics, extensive surgery and burns, renal failure and hemodialysis, mechanical ventilation, and prior fungal colonization. Patients who have undergone surgery (particularly surgery of the GI tract) are increasingly susceptible to disseminated candidal infections.[39,40]

CLINICAL PRESENTATION OF HEMATOGENOUS CANDIDIASIS[8,13,16]

Dissemination of *C. albicans* can result in infection in single or multiple organs, particularly the kidney, brain, myocardium, skin, eye, bone, and joints. In most patients, multiple micro- and macroabscesses are formed. Infection of the liver and spleen is becoming recognized as a particularly common and difficult-to-treat site of infection that

---

TABLE 119–6. Risk Factors for Invasive Candidiasis

Neutropenia
Lymphoreticular or hematologic malignancies
Diabetes
Immunodeficiency diseases
High-dose corticosteroids
Immunosuppressants
Antineoplastic agents
Central venous catheters
Total parenteral nutrition (TPN)
Receipt of multiple antibiotics
Extensive surgery (particularly surgery of the GI tract)
Burns
Renal failure and hemodialysis
Mechanical ventilation
Prior fungal colonization

Compiled from refs. 8, 14, 15, 39, and 40.

characteristically occurs in patients undergoing chemotherapy for acute leukemia or lymphoma.

DIAGNOSIS

SIGNS AND SYMPTOMS

Several distinct presentations of disseminated *C. albicans* have been recognized.[12]

1. Patients present with the acute onset of fever, tachycardia, tachypnea, and occasionally, chills or hypotension. The clinical presentation generally is indistinguishable from that seen with sepsis of bacterial origin.
2. Patients develop intermittent fevers and are ill only when febrile.
3. Patient manifests progressive deterioration of their condition with or without fever.
4. Hepatosplenic candidiasis often is manifested only as fever while the patient remains neutropenic (<1000 WBCs/mm^3).

LABORATORY TESTS

Patients with positive blood cultures for *C. tropicalis* should receive serious consideration as candidates for systemic antifungal therapy.

Although a variety of serologic tests have been proposed for the detection of *Candida* protein antigens, serum antibodies to *Candida*, and antibodies to cell wall components such as mannan, no test has demonstrated reliable accuracy in the clinical setting for the diagnosis of disseminated infection with *Candida*. Only 25% to 45% of neutropenic patients with disseminated candidiasis at autopsy had a positive blood culture with *C. albicans* prior to death. The interpretation of positive surveillance cultures of the skin, mouth, sputum, feces, or urine is hampered by their occurrence as commensal pathogens and in distinguishing colonization from invasive disease.

Until recently, a rapid presumptive identification of *C. albicans* could be made by incubation of the organism in serum; formation of a germ tube (the beginning of hyphae, which arise as perpendicular extensions from the yeast cell, with no constriction at their point of origin) within 1 to 2 hours offered a positive identification of *C. albicans*.[8] Unfortunately, *C. dubliniensis*, a new species of *Candida* that was identified recently as an important cause of mucosal colonization and infection in HIV-infected individuals, also can produce a germ tube. A negative germ tube test does not rule out the possibility of *C. albicans*, but further biochemical tests must be performed to differentiate between other non-*albicans* species.[8,33]

In patients with hepatosplenic candidiasis, as the WBC count increases to more than 1000 cells/mm^3, imaging studies can detect the presence of abscess or microabscesses in the liver and spleen, often found with acute suppurative and granulomatous reactions.

▶ TREATMENT: Hematogenous Candidiasis

Fraser and colleagues[39] documented the high rate of mortality in nonneutropenic patients with fungal blood cultures. Mortality was highest in patients with sustained positive blood cultures, those who did not receive antifungal therapy, and those infected with non-*albicans* strains of *Candida*. This study clearly documented the importance of early recognition and treatment of positive fungal blood cultures. However, despite increased awareness of the importance of treating patients with positive blood cultures, mortality associated with candidemia remains high (47% among adults versus 29% among children) in even nonneutropenic patients.[41,42]

Treatment of candidiasis should be guided by knowledge of the infecting species; the clinical status of the patient; when available, the antifungal susceptibility of the infecting isolate; and whether the patient has received antifungal therapy previously (Table 119–7). Therapy should be continued for 2 weeks after the last positive blood culture and resolution of signs and symptoms of infection. All patients should undergo an ophthalmologic examination to exclude the possibility of candidal endophthalmitis.[9] Amphotericin B may be switched to fluconazole (intravenous or oral) for the completion of therapy. Susceptibility testing of the infecting isolate is a useful adjunct to species identification during selection of a therapeutic approach because it can be used to identify isolates that are unlikely to respond to fluconazole or amphotericin B. However, this is not currently available at most institutions.

■ NONIMMUNOCOMPROMISED PATIENT

■ PROPHYLAXIS

In ICUs, the use of fluconazole for prophylaxis or empirical therapy has increased exponentially in the past decade. However, studies that

demonstrated benefit in the prevention of invasive candidal bloodstream infections did so either by using highly selective criteria or by studying patients in an unusually high-risk ICU setting, and the role of antifungal prophylaxis in the sugical ICU remains extremely controversial.[9,43,44]

■ EMPIRICAL THERAPY

Few data are available for assessing the role of fluconazole as empirical therapy for suspected fungemia or for isolates other than *C. albicans*. Because fluconazole has poor activity against *Aspergillus* spp. and some non-*albicans* strains of *Candida*, many clinicians advocate amphotericin B as the therapy of choice in patients with suspected fungemia. If therapy is given, its use should be limited to patients with (1) *Candida* colonization at multiple sites, (2) multiple other risk factors, and (3) the absence of any other uncorrected causes of fever.[9,45]

■ SPECIFIC THERAPY

Three large randomized studies in nonneutropenic patients have demonstrated that fluconazole at 400 mg/day and deoxycholate amphotericin B at 0.5–0.6 mg/kg per day are similarly effective; however, fewer adverse effects are observed with fluconazole therapy.[46,47] Similarly, caspofungin is at least as effective as amphotericin B 0.6–0.7 mg/kg per day in (mainly nonneutropenic) adult patients with candidemia with fewer drug-related adverse events. Although the use of combination therapy (high-dose fluconazole plus amphotericin B) was demonstrated recently to be superior to treatment with fluconazole alone, the routine use of combination therapy in this patient population is not yet recommended.[48,49] Neonates with disseminated

TABLE 119–7. Therapy of Invasive Candidiasis [5,9,41]

Type of Disease and Common Clinical Manifestations	Therapy/Comments
Prophylaxis of Candidemia	
Nonneutropenic patients[a]	Not recommended except for severely ill/high-risk patients in whom fluconazole IV/PO 400 mg daily should be used (see to text)
Neutropenic patients[a]	The optimal duration of therapy is unclear but at a minimum should include the period at risk for neutropenia: Fluconazole IV/PO 400 mg daily *or* itraconazole solution 2.5 mg/kg q12h PO *or* micafungin (unlicensed in U.S.) 50 mg (1 mg/kg in patients under 50 kg) intravenously daily
Solid-organ transplantation	
Liver transplantation	*Patients with two or more key risk factors[b]:* Amphotericin B IV 10–20 mg daily *or* lipoosmal amphotericin B (AmBisome) 1 mg/kg/day *or* fluconazole 400 mg orally daily
Empirical Antifungal Therapy (Unknown *Candida* Species)	
Suspected disseminated candidiasis in febrile nonneutropenic patients	None recommended; data are lacking defining subsets of patients who are appropriate for therapy (see text)
Febrile neutropenic patients with prolonged fever despite 4–6 days of empirical antibacterial therapy	*Treatment duration:* Until resolution of neutropenia Amphotericin B IV 0.5–0.7 mg/kg/day *or* liposomal amphotericin B (AmBisome) IV 3 mg/kg/day *or* itraconazole 200 mg IV q12h × 2 days, then 200 mg/day x 12 days, then 400 mg PO (solution) daily *or* voriconazole 6 mg/kg IV loading dose q12h x day, then 3 mg/kg q12h (restrict to allogeneic bone marrow transplant and relapsed leukemia patients) *or* fluconazole 400 mg/day IV/PO (restrict to patients with a low risk for invasive aspergillosis or azole-resistant strains of *Candida* in patients with no previous azole exposure or signs and symptoms suggesting aspergillosis)
Treatment of Candidemia and Acute Hematogenously Disseminated Candidiasis	
Nonimmunocompromised host[c]	*Treatment duration:* 2 weeks after the last positive blood culture and resolution of signs and symptoms of infection *Remove existing central venous catheters when feasible plus*
C. albicans, C. tropicalis, C. parapsilosis	Amphotericin B IV 0.6 mg/kg/day *or* fluconazole IV/PO 6 mg/kg/day *or* caspofungin 70 mg loading dose then 50 mg IV daily *or* amphotericin B IV 0.7 mg/kg/day plus fluconazole IV/PO 800 mg/day *Patients intolerant or refractory to other therapy[d]:* Amphotericin B lipid complex IV 5 mg/kg/day Liposomal amphotericin B IV 3–5 mg/kg/day Amphotericin B colloid dispersion IV 2–6 mg/kg/day
C. krusei	Amphotericin B IV ≥1 mg/kg/day *or* caspofungin 70 mg loading dose then 50 mg IV daily
C. lusitaniae	Fluconazole IV/PO 6 mg/kg/day
C. glabrata	Amphotericin B IV ≥0.7 mg/kg/day *or* fluconazole IV/PO 6–12 mg/kg/day (400–800 mg/day in a 70 kg patient) *or* Caspofungin 70 mg loading dose then 50 mg IV daily
Neutropenic host[e]	*Treatment duration:* Until resolution of neutropenia *Remove existing central venous catheters when feasible plus* Amphotericin B IV 0.7–1.0 mg/kg/day (total dosages 0.5–1 gram) *or Patients failing therapy with traditional amphotericin B:* Lipid formulation of amphotericin B IV 3–5 mg/kg/day
Chronic Disseminated Candidiasis (hepatosplenic candidiasis)	*Treatment duration:* Until calcification or resolution of lesions *Stable patients:* Fluconazole IV/PO 6 mg/kg/day *Acutely ill or refractory patients:* Amphotericin B IV 0.6–0.7 mg/kg/day
Urinary Candidiasis	*Asymptomatic disease:* Generally no therapy is required *Symptomatic or high-risk patients[f]:* Removal of urinary tract instruments, stents, and Foley catheters, +7–14 days therapy with fluconazole 200 mg orally daily *or* amphotericin B IV 0.3–1 mg/kg/day

[a]Patients at significant risk for invasive candidiasis include those receiving standard chemotherapy for acute myelogenous leukemia, allogeneic bone marrow transplants, or high-risk autologous bone marrow transplants. However, among these populations, chemotherapy or bone marrow transplant protocols do not all produce equivalent risk, and local experience should be used to determine the relevance of prophylaxis.

[b]Risk factors include retransplantation, creatinine of more than 2 mg/dL, choledochojejunostomy, intraoperative use of 40 units or more of blood products, fungal coonization detected within the first 3 days after transplantation.

[c]Therapy is generally the same for AIDS/non-AIDS patients except where indicated and should continued for 2 weeks after the last positive blood culture and resolution of signs and symptoms of infection. All patients should receive an ophthalmologic examination. Amphotericin B may be switched to fluconazole (intravenous or oral) for the completion of therapy. Susceptibility testing of the infecting isolate is a useful adjunct to species identification during selection of a therapeutic approach because it can be used to identify isolates that are unlikely to respond to fluconazole or amphotericin B. However, this is not currently available at most institutions.

[d]Often defined as failure of ≥500 mg amphotericin B, initial renal insufficiency (creatinine ≥2.5 mg/dL or creatinine clearance <25 mL/min), a significant increase in creatinine (to 2.5 mg/dL for adults or 1.5 mg/dL for children), or severe acute administration-related toxicity.

[e]Patients who are neutropenic at the time of developing candidemia should receive a recombinant cytokine (granulocyte colony-stimulating factor or granulocyte-monocyte colony-stimulating factor) that accelerates recovery from neutropenia.

[f]Patients at high risk for dissemination include neutropenic patients, low-birth-weight infants, patients with renal allografts, and patients who will undergo urologic manipulation.

IV = intravenous; PO = orally.

Compiled from refs. 5, 9, and 41.

candidiasis usually are treated with amphotericin B because of its low toxicity in this patient population and because of the lack of experience with other agents in this population.[9,41] Treatment should continue until 2 weeks following the last positive blood culture and resolution of signs and symptoms of infection.

CLINICAL CONTROVERSY

Because *C. glabrata* often has reduced susceptibility to both fluconazole and amphotericin B, optimal therapy is unclear. Larger doses of fluconazole (800 mg/day in a 70-kg patient) have been used in less critically ill patients or amphotericin B (≥0.7 mg/kg per day). However, recent observational studies demonstrated no difference in mortality in nonneutropenic patients administered fluconazole versus amphotericin B for bloodstream infections caused by *C. glabrata*.[41] The potential utility of caspofungin has not been assessed.[9,41]

C. krusei infections should be treated with large doses of amphotericin B (≥1 mg/kg per day) or with caspofungin (70-mg IV loading dose, followed by 50 mg/day IV).[9] *C. tropicalis*, and *C. parapsilosis* may be treated with either amphotericin B at 0.6 mg/kg per day or fluconazole at 6 mg/kg per day. Amphotericin B resistance remains relatively rare despite over 45 years of clinical use, although it has been reported in *C. lusitaniae* (now *Clavispora lusitaniae*) and *C. guilliermondii*. *C. rugosa* often is considered to be "polyene tolerant," and these isolates are believed to be selected owing to the wide use of amphotericin B.

Among the lipid-associated formulations of amphotericin B, only liposomal amphotericin B (AmBisome) and amphotericin B lipid complex (Abelcet) have been approved for use in proven cases of candidiasis; however, patients with invasive candidiasis also have been treated successfully with amphotericin B colloid dispersion (Amphotec or Amphocil). The lipid-associated formulations are less toxic but as effective as amphotericin B deoxycholate.

CLINICAL CONTROVERSY

Owing to the higher cost and paucity of randomized trials showing the efficacy of lipid-associated formulations of amphotericin B against proven invasive candidiasis, many clinicians limit their first-line use for the treatment of these infections to individuals who are intolerant to, at high risk of intolerance to, or refractory to amphotericin B deoxycholate. However, the data demonstrating up to a 6.6-fold increase in mortality in patients with amphotericin B–induced nephrotoxicity have convinced other clinicians that high-risk patients (e.g., residence in an ICU care or intermediate care unit at the time of initiation of amphoterin B therapy) warrant first-line therapy with these agents.

▮ IMMUNOCOMPROMISED PATIENTS

In immunocompromised patients, the presence of candidemia is associated with evidence of disseminated disease in more than 70% of patients and with a 70% to 80% fatality rate. Therapy should include removal of the catheter and administration of systemic antifungal therapy.[9] The optimal agent, dose, and duration of therapy are unclear, and patients must be monitored carefully with serial blood cultures and careful physical examinations, particularly of the retina. Patients who are neutropenic at the time of developing candidemia should receive a recombinant cytokine (granulocyte colony-stimulating factor or granulocyte-monocyte colony-stimulating factor) that accelerates recovery from neutropenia.[9]

▮ PROPHYLAXIS

Recognition of the role of the GI tract in invasive *Candida* infections has led to efforts to decrease infections by prophylactic administration of topical or systemically absorbed antifungal agents in immunocompromised patients. The use of systemically absorbable agents such as azole antifungal agents appears to decrease the risk of invasive fungal infections.[9,50,51]

A randomized, double-blind, placebo-controlled trial in mostly allogeneic marrow recipients has shown that fluconazole, given at 400 mg/day from the start of the conditioning regimen until day 75, can reduce the frequency of invasive *Candida* infections and decrease mortality at day 110.[51] Moreover, 8 years after completion of the study, there was persistent protection against invasive candidiasis and *Candida*-related death and a decreased frequency of severe, gut-related graft-versus-host disease (GVHD). There also was an overall survival benefit of 17% in fluconazole-treated patients; this benefit in survival was independent of the underlying condition and the occurrence of relapses.[52] In less risk-selected patients with hematologic malignancies who were undergoing remission-induction chemotherapy, both fluconazole (400 mg/day) and itraconazole cyclodextrin (2.5 mg/kg orally twice daily) have been shown to be effective in preventing systemic infection and death caused by *Candida* spp.[53,54]

▮ EMPIRICAL THERAPY

Many clinicians advocate early institution of empirical IV amphotericin B in patients with neutropenia and persistent (>5–7 days) fever. However, the potential toxicities (particularly nephrotoxicity) of this agent preclude its routine use in all patients. Suggested criteria for the empirical use of amphotericin B include (1) fever of 5 to 7 days' duration that is unresponsive to antibacterial agents, (2) neutropenia of more than 7 days' duration, (3) no other obvious cause for fever, (4) progressive debilitation, (5) chronic adrenal corticosteroid therapy, and (6) indwelling intravascular catheters. In patients who fail therapy with amphotericin B, lipid formulations of amphotericin B may be used (3–5 mg/kg per day).

Itraconazole and fluconazole have demonstrated efficacy equivalent to that of deoxycholate amphotericin B in patients with hematologic malignancy (not treated with allogeneic hematopoietic stem cell transplantation).[55,56] However, since fluconazole is not active against filamentous fungi, its use in patients at high risk for these pathogens should be avoided. If used, the intravenous formulation of itraconazole should be used because the bioavailability of the oral formulations (including the solution) is unreliable.[45,57] Recently, voriconazole was compared with liposomal amphotericin B in a large randomized, multicenter trial of empirical antifungal therapy in febrile neutropenic patients.[58] The results of this study showed comparable composite success rates; however, voriconazole did not fulfill the protocol-defined criteria for noninferiority (a difference in success rates between voriconazole and amphotericin B of no more than 10 percentage points) to liposomal amphotericin. Voriconazole was superior in reducing documented breakthrough infections, infusion-related toxicity, and nephrotoxicity. However, patients who received voriconazole had more frequent episodes of transient visual disturbances and hallucinations.[58]

SPECIFIC THERAPY

Amphotericin B and the azoles have roles in the treatment of hematogenous candidiasis, and the choice of therapy is guided by weighing the greater activity of amphotericin B for some non-*albicans* species (e.g., *C. krusei*) against the lower toxicity and ease of administration of fluconazole.[9]

Most clinicians recommend amphotericin B in total dosages of 0.5–1 g administered over approximately 1 to 2 weeks in patients with *Candida* endophthalmitis and in all neutropenic patients with candidemia.[8,16,45] Longer courses of therapy may be needed in some patients.[16] Observational studies suggest that fluconazole and amphotericin B are similarly effective for the treatment of *C. albicans* bloodstream infections in the neutropenic patient; controlled data, however, are lacking. In patients with uncomplicated *C. albicans* fungemia who have not received systemic prophylaxis with antifungal azoles, therapy with fluconazole 400–800 mg/day IV may be considered.[59] However, in patients who have undergone allogeneic hematopoietic stem cell transplantation, the role of fluconazole is becoming more limited because of its widespread use for antifungal prophylaxis. In this setting, particularly if the patient has been treated previously with an azole antifungal agent, the possibility of microbiologic resistance must be considered.[9] Infections with fluconazole-resistant *Candida* spp., including *C. glabrata*, *C. krusei*, and fluconazole-resistant *C. albicans*, are more likely. Susceptibility testing can be useful in dealing with infections caused by non-*albicans* species of *Candida*.

In patients intolerant to amphotericin B or fluconazole, one of the lipid formulations may be used. In a randomized trial, amphotericin B lipid complex (ABLC) was found to be equivalent to 0.6–1 mg/kg per day of amphotericin B, and open-label therapy with amphotericin B colloid dispersion (ABCD) has been successful.

CANDIDURIA

Within the urinary tract, most common lesions are either *Candida* cystitis or hematogenously disseminated renal abscesses. *Candida* cystitis often follows catheterization or therapy with broad-spectrum antimicrobial agents. The diagnosis of *Candida* cystitis may be problematic because of the frequent presence of *Candida* pseudohyphae and yeast cells in urine specimens secondary to urethral colonization. The usefulness of urine colony counts or antibody coating techniques is questionable. The recovery of 10,000 organisms or visualization of both yeast and pseudohyphae from fresh midstream urine or from bladder urine obtained by single catheterization (not indwelling) is suggestive of genitourinary candidiasis.[8] In most patients, the infection is asymptomatic and clears spontaneously without specific antifungal therapy.

Initial therapy of candidal cystitis should focus on removal of urinary catheters whenever possible. Changing the catheter will eliminate candiduria in only 20% of patients, whereas discontinuation will eradicate *Candida* in 40% of patients. Asymptomatic candiduria rarely requires therapy. Therapy should be used in symptomatic patients and in neutropenic patients, as well as in patients with renal allografts and those who will undergo urologic manipulation, because of the risk of dissemination.[60,61]

Fluconazole 200 mg/day for 14 days hastens the time to a negative urine culture as compared with placebo treatment, but 2 weeks after the end of therapy, the frequency of a negative urine culture remains the same with both treatments.[61] Short courses of therapy are not recommended; treatment should include removal of catheters and stents whenever possible plus 7 to 14 days of therapy. Bladder irrigation with amphotericin B (50 mg in 500 mL sterile water instilled twice daily into the bladder via a three-way catheter) is only transiently effective. Minimal quantities (<3%) of amphotericin B are absorbed systemically from the bladder.[21,61]

ROLE OF CATHETER REMOVAL

Although it is common practice in today's standard of care to place indwelling catheters in patients for the administration of medications and parenteral nutrition (TPN), catheter-related infections are a common complication. These foreign bodies (especially triple-lumen catheters) double as entry ports for normal skin flora or other nosocomial pathogens, and they provide a readily available site for the binding of pathogens via microbiotic biofilms. Their subsequent role as a source of bloodstream infections is facilitated by frequent use, TPN, and the potential for contamination of catheters by medical staff who are colonized with *Candida* spp.

Most consensus recommendations urge that, if feasible, initial nonmedical management should include removal of all existing tunneled central venous catheters (CVCs) and implantable devices, particularly in patients with fungemia caused by *C. parapsilosis,* which is very frequently associated with catheters.[9,62] Arguments against the removal of all catheters in patients with candidemia include the prominent role of the gut as a source for disseminated candidiasis, the significant cost and potential for complications, and the problems that can be encountered in patients with difficult vascular access.[63] However, in an individual patient it is often difficult to determine the relative contribution of gut versus catheter as the primary source of fungemia.[62] The evidence for this recommendation is weakest in cancer patients with severe neutropenia and mucositis (e.g., acute leukemia, stem cell transplant), in whom candidemia is almost always primarily of gut origin, and removal of CVCs is least likely to have an impact on mortality.[64] Nucci and Anaissie[59] have proposed that CVCs be removed in nonneutropenic patients without a short life expectancy who have one of the following criteria: (1) otherwise unexplained hemodynamic instability, (2) lack of clinical improvement of resolution of candidemia after more than 72 hours of an optimal dose of an appropriate antifungal agent, (3) established or at high risk for endocarditis or septic thrombophlebitis, or (4) a pocket infection or cellulitis. In patients with more than one CVC, they recommend removal if one tunneled or implanted CVC is the likely source of infection and the patient meets the preceding criteria.[59]

ASPERGILLOSIS

EPIDEMIOLOGY

Aspergillus is an ubiquitous mold that grows well on a variety of substrates, including soil, water, decaying vegetation, moldy hay or straw, and organic debris. Although more than 300 species of

Aspergillus have been characterized, three species are most commonly pathogenic: *A. fumigatus, A. flavus,* and *A. niger.* The varying degrees of pathogenicity of each species depend on their relative geographic prevalence, conidial size and shape, thermotolerance, and production of mycotoxins. For example, transport of *A. fumigatus* conidia into the lungs is facilitated by their smaller diameter in comparison with *A. flavus* and *A. niger.*

The term *aspergillosis* may be broadly defined as a spectrum of diseases attributed to allergy, colonization, or tissue invasion caused by members of the fungal genus *Aspergillus.* A single satisfactory classification system for these disease entities is difficult because different populations of patients may develop the same type of infection. For example, osteomyelitis may result from local trauma or hematogenous dissemination in an immunocompromised host. Colonization in normal hosts can lead to allergic diseases ranging from asthma to allergic bronchopulmonary aspergillosis or, rarely, invasive disease.[65]

PATHOPHYSIOLOGY

Aspergillosis generally is acquired by inhalation of airborne conidia that are small enough (2.5–3 microns) to reach alveoli or the paranasal sinuses. Each conidiophore releases 10^4 conidia that remain suspended for long periods and are viable for months in dry locations. Although some authors advocate monitoring of hospital air for *Aspergillus* conidia, guidelines for interpreting results do not exist. The use of high-efficiency particulate air (HEPA) filters in operating rooms and laminar flow rooms and removal of immunocompromised patients from hospital renovation sites may be helpful in preventing infection in this population. Although the fate of *Aspergillus* conidia in the GI tract has not been closely studied, limited evidence suggests that this route may provide an important portal of entry for disseminated infections in humans.[66]

SUPERFICIAL INFECTION

Superficial or locally invasive infections of the ear, skin, or appendages often can be managed with topical antifungal therapy. Skin infections in patients with burn wounds, although uncommon, may progress to deep-tissue invasion despite the use of topical or parenteral antifungal agents. Risk factors for deep infection include extensive thermal injuries, malnutrition, cirrhosis, and previous infection with *Pseudomonas aeruginosa.*[66]

ALLERGIC BRONCHOPULMONARY ASPERGILLOSIS

Allergic manifestations of *Aspergillus* range in severity from mild asthma to allergic bronchopulmonary aspergillosis (BPA). BPA, which is almost always caused by *A. fumigatus,* is characterized by severe asthma with wheezing, fever, malaise, weight loss, chest pain, and a cough productive of blood-streaked sputum. Following recurrent episodes of severe asthma, the disease usually progresses to fibrosis and bronchiectasis with granuloma formation. When *Aspergillus* conidia become trapped in the viscous mucus of asthmatic patients, BPA develops. The fungus grows, releasing toxins and antigens. The resulting host sensitization results in a variety of immune reactions. Early in the course of disease, an IgE-mediated (type I) immune reaction results in bronchospasm, eosinophilia, and immediate skin reactivity. The ensuing fibrosis and pulmonary infiltrates appear to be mediated by circulating or precipitating antibody

complexes of IgG antibody, followed by granuloma formation and mononuclear infiltration because of a type IV delayed hypersensitivity reaction. Therapy is aimed at minimizing the quantity of antigenic material released in the tracheobronchial tree. Management of acute asthma attacks minimizes trapping of *Aspergillus* by bronchial secretions, and administration of parenteral corticosteroids clears lung infiltrates.[66,67] Antifungal therapy generally is not indicated in the management of allergic manifestations of aspergillosis, although some patients have demonstrated a decrease in their corticosteroid dose following therapy with itraconazole. A recent double-blind, randomized, placebo-controlled trial showed that itraconazole 200 mg twice daily for 16 weeks resulted in significant differences in the amelioration of disease, as measured by the reduction in corticosteroid dose and improvement in exercise tolerance and pulmonary function.[65]

ASPERGILLOMA

In the nonimmunocompromised host, *Aspergillus* infections of the sinuses most commonly occur as saprophytic colonization (aspergillomas or "fungus balls") of previously abnormal sinus tissue. An aspergilloma is composed of intertwined *Aspergillus* hyphae matted together with fibrin, mucus, and cellular debris. Infection usually is localized in the maxillary sinus and rarely is associated with local invasion of adjacent bone or brain tissue. Sinus aspergillosis also can present as allergic sinusitis with nasal drainage of brownish mucous plugs. Therapy with corticosteroids and surgery generally is successful. In the immunocompromised host, subacute, chronic, or fulminant invasive disease can be seen, and a combination of antifungal and surgical therapy generally is required.[66-69]

Pulmonary aspergillomas are fungus balls arising in preexisting cavities because of tuberculosis, histoplasmosis, lung tumors, or radiation fibrosis, although occasionally no previous pulmonary disease is present. The diagnosis of aspergilloma generally is made on the basis of chest radiographs, on which aspergillomas appear as a solid rounded mass, sometimes mobile, of water density within a spherical or ovoid cavity and separated from the wall of the cavity by an airspace of variable size and shape. Patients generally experience chest pain, dyspnea, and sputum production. Hemoptysis is observed in 50% to 80% of patients probably because of ulceration of the epithelial lining of the cavity with formation of granulation tissue, and hemoptysis is the cause of death in up to 26% of patients with aspergilloma. A poor prognosis is associated with increasing size or number of aspergillomas, immunosuppression (including corticosteroids), increasing *Aspergillus*-specific titers, underlying sarcoidosis, and HIV infection. Although *Aspergillus* can be cultured in only 50% to 60% of patients, precipitating antibodies are positive in virtually 100% of patients.

Invasive disease occurs rarely, and therapy therefore is controversial. There are no controlled clinical trials with which to guide therapy, and recommendations for treatment have been generated from uncontrolled trials and case reports.[69] Concern regarding the risk of severe hemorrhage has led some clinicians to use aggressive surgical excision of aspergillomas or pulmonary resection in patients with hemoptysis. Complications, including bronchopulmonary fistulas, hemorrhage, empyema, and persistent airspace problems, have led to the recommendation that surgical intervention be reserved for patients with severe (>500 mL/24 h) hemoptysis, however. Bronchial artery embolization (BAE) has been used to occlude the vessel that supplies the bleeding site in patients experiencing hemoptysis. Unfortunately, BAE generally is unsuccessful or only temporarily effective. Collateral circulation eventually develops, supplying blood flow to the affected area, and hemoptysis often recurs; consequently, reembolization is often unsuccessful. BAE should be used as a temporizing procedure in a patient with life-threatening disease who might respond to more definitive therapy if hemoptysis is stabilized. Mild to moderate hemoptysis should be managed conservatively. Although IV amphotericin B generally is not useful in eradicating aspergillomas, inhaled or intracavitary instillation of amphotericin B has been employed successfully in a limited number of patients. Itraconazole has been efficacious in uncontrolled studies; however, the dose and duration of therapy have not been standardized. Hemoptysis generally ceases when the aspergilloma is eradicated.[66,67,69]

INVASIVE ASPERGILLOSIS

Although exposure to *Aspergillus* conidia is nearly universal, impaired host defenses are required for the development of invasive disease. Phagocytes (neutrophils, monocytes, and macrophages) rather than antibodies or lymphocytes constitute the primary host defense system against invasive disease with aspergillosis. Macrophages prevent germination of conidia and also eradicate conidia, providing the first line of defense against invasive disease. Administration of corticosteroids appears to impair the killing of conidia by macrophages and to impair mobilization of neutrophils. Neutrophils halt hyphal growth and dissemination and kill mycelia, constituting a second line of defense. Prolonged neutropenia appears to be the most important predisposing factor to the development of invasive aspergillosis, accounting for the high frequency of disease in patients with acute leukemia. Complement provides a source of chemotactic factor and facilitates neutrophil damage to hyphae and monocyte killing of conidia. Complement is not necessary for the attachment or ingestion of conidia by human alveolar macrophages.[66,67,70]

Until recently, aspergillosis was an uncommon fungal infection in patients with AIDS. AIDS patients may be at less risk for aspergillosis than other fungal infections because the primary cellular defect in AIDS patients is in the T-lymphocytes, whereas neutrophils and macrophages constitute the primary lines of defense to infection with aspergillosis. Until recently, aspergillosis was reported as a late complication of disease in AIDS patients with additional risk factors for aspergillosis, such as corticosteroid use, neutropenia, previous *Pneumocystis carinii* or cytomegalovirus pneumonia, marijuana smoking, or the use of broad-spectrum antibiotics. However, approximately 50% of patients with aspergillosis have no classic risk factors. The majority of these patients had CD4 counts of fewer than 50 cells/mm^3. Although some patients diagnosed early in their infection responded to treatment, most patients do not respond to therapy with amphotericin B 0.5 mg/kg per day or itraconazole 200–600 mg/day.[71]

Invasive disease with *Aspergillus* can arise de novo or from any of the allergic or colonizing forms of aspergillosis. Predisposing factors to the development of invasive aspergillosis include glucocorticoid therapy, particularly following chronic administration or with higher dosages (30–200 mg/day of prednisone), cytotoxic agents, and recent or concurrent therapy with broad-spectrum antimicrobial agents. Patients with chronic hepatitis, alcoholism, diabetes mellitus, chronic granulomatous disease, leukopenia (<1000 cells/mm^3), leukemia (particularly acute lymphocytic or myelogenous leukemia), lymphoma, and acute rejection of an organ transplant are also at a higher risk of invasive disease. Although rare, invasive aspergillosis has been reported in apparently normal hosts.[66,67]

CLINICAL PRESENTATION [66–69]

The lung is the most common site of invasive disease. In the immunocompromised host, aspergillosis is characterized by vascular invasion leading to thrombosis, infarction, necrosis of tissue, and dissemination to other tissues and organs in the body. Survival beyond 2 or 3 weeks is uncommon. If bone marrow function returns, cavitation of the pulmonary lesion generally occurs, and the spread of infection may be halted. The progressive nature of the disease and its refractoriness to therapy are, in part, caused by the organism's rapid growth and its tendency to invade blood vessels.

Signs and Symptoms

Patients often present with classic signs and symptoms of acute pulmonary embolus: pleuritic chest pain, fever, hemoptysis, and friction rubs. The CNS, liver, spleen, heart, GI tract, pericardium, and other body sites are involved in a substantial minority of cases. In neutropenic patients with *Aspergillus* pneumonia, hyphae invade the walls of bronchi and surrounding parenchyma, resulting in an acute necrotizing, pyogenic pneumonitis. As a result, patients often present with classic signs and symptoms of acute pulmonary embolus: pleuritic chest pain, fever, hemoptysis, and friction rubs.

DIAGNOSIS

The diagnosis of aspergillosis is complicated by the presence of *Aspergillus* as a normal commensal in the human GI tract and respiratory secretions, and establishment of a definitive diagnosis of disease is difficult. Though suggestive of infection, the presence of hyphae in a smear or biopsy specimen is not diagnostic. Demonstration of *Aspergillus* by repeated culture and microscopic examination of tissue provides the most firm diagnosis. The appearance of *Aspergillus* in tissues varies with increasing host resistance from the normal vegetative hyphae found with necrotic tissue and exudate in the alveoli of immunocompromised hosts to the compact, tangled filaments ("granules") observed in fungal balls. Identification of *Aspergillus* generally is based on the appearance of 2- to 4-micron-wide septate hyphae that are dichotomously branched at 45-degree angles. Sporulation is observed rarely in tissue.[17] Although growth on Sabouraud dextrose or brain-heart infusion agar may be used for primary culture, bronchoscopy or bronchoalveolar lavage cultures are positive in only 40% of histopathologically identified specimens. Blood, CSF, and bone marrow cultures are rarely positive for *Aspergillus*.

Many clinicians treat positive respiratory cultures of *Aspergillus* as a common contaminant and argue that a minimum of two to three positive cultures is necessary before antifungal therapy is indicated. Any positive culture, however, may be indicative of true infection in the immunocompromised host, and the positive predictive value may be as high as 80% to 90% in patients with leukemia or bone marrow transplants.

Diagnostic Tests

A rapid test to detect galactomannan antigen in blood was approved recently in the United States. Late findings on radiographic studies include wedge-shaped pleural-based infiltrates or cavities on chest radiographs. Findings on computed tomographic (CT) scans include the halo sign (an area of low attenuation surrounding a nodular lung lesion) initially (caused by edema or bleeding surrounding an ischemic area) and, later, the crescent sign (an air crescent near the periphery of a lung nodule caused by contraction of infarcted tissue). CT abnormalities are best documented in neutropenic marrow transplant recipients and commonly precede plain chest radiograph abnormalities.

▶ TREATMENT: Invasive Aspergillosis

Therapy for invasive aspergillosis is far from optimal at this time in part because of the difficulties in establishing a diagnosis and in part because of a lack of truly effective antifungal agents. Administration of amphotericin B appears to decrease mortality from more than 90% to approximately 45%. These data, however, are difficult to interpret because many patients were diagnosed postmortem, or amphotericin B therapy was not administered until the patient had very advanced disease. Mortality from pulmonary aspergillosis in bone marrow transplant recipients exceeds 94% regardless of therapy.[66] Although early diagnosis and administration of antifungal therapy may result in higher response rates, correction of underlying immune deficits (in particular, return of neutrophil counts) is of paramount importance in eradication of infection.[68,69]

Until the diagnosis of aspergillosis can be determined more rapidly and definitively, empirical therapy must be instituted when invasive disease is suspected. In patients at highest risk for invasive disease (acute leukemia and bone marrow transplant recipients), the most important predisposing factors include prolonged severe neutropenia (<100 cells/mm^3 for more than 1 week), graft rejection, chronic administration of corticosteroids, and tissue damage from preexisting infection. In these patients, antifungal therapy should be instituted in any of these conditions: (1) persistent fever or progressive sinusitis unresponsive to antimicrobial therapy, (2) an eschar over the nose, sinuses, or palate, (3) the presence of characteristic radiographic findings, including wedge-shaped infarcts, nodular densities, and new cavitary lesions, or (4) any clinical manifestation suggestive of orbital or cavernous sinus disease or an acute vascular event associated with fever. Isolation of *Aspergillus* spp. from nasal or respiratory tract secretions should be considered confirmatory evidence in any of the previously mentioned clinical settings.[66,67]

NON–HIV-INFECTED PATIENT

PROPHYLAXIS

Unfortunately, effective chemoprophylaxis against infections by *Aspergillus* spp. has not been demonstrated thus far.[9] Apart from studies that compare prophylaxis with itraconazole or current investigational agents with prophylaxis with fluconazole, clinical trials are under way that investigate preventive approaches in patients with allogeneic hematopoietic stem cell transplantation during phases of aggressive immunosuppression for chronic graft-versus-host disease.

SPECIFIC THERAPY

Intravenous therapy with amphotericin B remains the preferred therapy, at least initially, in acutely ill patients. Because *Aspergillus* is only moderately susceptible to amphotericin B, full doses (1–1.5 mg/kg per day) generally are recommended, with response measured by defervescence and radiographic clearing. To treat microfoci, therapy should be continued after resolution of clinical and radiographic abnormalities until cultures (if they can be obtained) are negative, and reversible underlying predispositions have abated. Clinical response rather than any arbitrary total dose should guide duration of therapy. The optimal dosage or duration of amphotericin B therapy for the treatment of invasive disease is unknown and depends on the extent of disease, the response to therapy, and the patient's underlying

disease(s) and immune status. Unfortunately, the response rate averages only 37% (range 14% to 83%), and the response to therapy is largely related to the extent of aspergillosis at the time of diagnosis and host factors such as resolution of neutropenia and the return of neutrophil function, lessening immunosuppression, and the return of graft function from a bone marrow or organ transplant.

Lipid formulations of amphotericin B may be indicated in patients with impaired renal function and in those who develop nephrotoxicity while receiving deoxycholate amphotericin B. The lipid-based formulations may be preferred as initial therapy in patients with marginal renal function or in patients receiving other nephrotoxic drugs. Although these preparations appear less toxic than standard preparations, only limited data regarding their relative efficacy for invasive aspergillosis are available at this time because the studies with the lipid preparations have been open label or with historical conventional amphotericin B controls.[71–73]

Even though older azole antifungal agents (miconazole and ketoconazole) possess poor in vitro activity against *Aspergillus* spp., newer triazoles demonstrate improved activity both in vitro and in animal models of infection.[75] Itraconazole (100–500 mg/day for 11 to 192 days) shows therapeutic benefit in patients with pulmonary, skeletal, and pericardial aspergillosis, particularly in patients who are less immunocompromised.[65–69] The wide range of dosages, durations of therapy, and degrees of immunosuppression in these trials makes selection of an appropriate regimen difficult. Jennings and Hardin[67] reviewed the role of itraconazole for aspergillosis and recommended that itraconazole be reserved as a second-line agent for patients intolerant or not responding to high-dose amphotericin B. If itraconazole is used, a loading dose of 200 mg three times daily for 2 to 3 days should be employed, followed by itraconazole 200 mg twice daily for a minimum of 6 months. Although early studies employing relatively low dosages (50–100 mg/day) of fluconazole demonstrated some activity against less invasive forms of aspergillosis, including chronic pulmonary disease and aspergillomas, data regarding the use of higher dosages (>100 mg/day) in patients with invasive disease are not available. Oral itraconazole is an alternative for patients who can take oral medication, are likely to be adherent, can be demonstrated (by serum level monitoring) to absorb the drug, and are unlikely to experience interactions with other medications and as follow-up therapy in patients who respond to initial IV therapy.[69]

Caspofungin was approved by the Food and Drug Administration (FDA) for use as salvage therapy in patients who are intolerant or who fail therapy with one of the amphotericin B formulations.[57,76] Caspofungin has in vitro activity against *Aspergillus* spp. and is indicated for the treatment of invasive aspergillosis in patients who are refractory to or intolerant of other therapies such as conventional amphotericin B, lipid formulations of amphotericin B, and/or itraconazole. Caspofungin has not yet been studied for first-line therapy for patients with aspergillosis. Because of the high risk of mortality from invasive aspergillosis even following treatment with standard therapy such as amphotericin B or itraconazole, caspofungin may offer a new mechanism for salvage therapy for patients with this disease.

A large, randomized, multicenter trial that compared voriconazole with liposomal amphotericin B for empirical antifungal therapy showed comparable composite success rates; however, voriconazole did not fulfill the protocol-defined criteria for noninferiority to liposomal amphotericin. Voriconazole was superior in reducing documented breakthrough infections, infusion-related toxicity, and nephrotoxicity. However, patients who received voriconazole had more frequent episodes of transient visual disturbances and hallucinations.[58,75] A recent randomized trial, which compared voriconazole with amphotericin B (followed by other licensed antifungal therapy) for primary therapy of aspergillosis, noted better responses, improved survival, and fewer severe side effects with voriconazole.[58]

The use of adjuvant therapies, such as granulocyte transfusions or recombinant colony-stimulating factors, remains controversial, and controlled trials are lacking at this time. Although some authors advocate combination therapy with azoles, flucytosine, or rifampin plus amphotericin B, controlled clinical studies verifying the efficacy of these combination therapies are lacking.

SECONDARY PROPHYLAXIS

The use of prophylactic antifungal therapy to prevent primary infection or reactivation of aspergillosis during subsequent courses of chemotherapy is controversial.[22,67] Studies assessing the utility of IV administration of amphotericin B in low doses (0.1 mg/kg per day) as prophylactic therapy or with higher dosages (0.5–0.6 mg/kg per day) as empirical therapy for invasive fungal infections in patients with granulocytopenia have not included sufficient numbers of patients to enable detection of differences in the number of *Aspergillus* infections.[67] The prophylactic use of intranasal

amphotericin B aerosol sprays (5 or 10 mg/day in three divided doses) appeared beneficial in small studies in human and animal models. A larger randomized trial found, however, that amphotericin B sprays reduced colonization of the nasal mucosal without any reduction in the frequency of invasive pulmonary infections with aspergillosis. Because failure of amphotericin B sprays may be a result of the ability of small airborne conidia to access the alveolar spaces directly and to establish infection, use of aerosolized forms of amphotericin B capable of reaching the alveolar spaces may be required.[67]

In granulocytopenic patients who recover from an episode of invasive aspergillosis, the risk of relapse of aspergillosis during subsequent courses of chemotherapy is greater than 50%. Secondary prophylaxis of aspergillosis with empirical administration of high-dose amphotericin B decreases the risk of relapse. Amphotericin B 1 mg/kg per day is started 24 to 48 hours prior to the start of chemotherapy and continued throughout the period of granulocytopenia. Some investigators recommend the addition of flucytosine (dosed to achieve peak serum concentrations of 30–60 mcg/mL) to the amphotericin B regimen. Although the use of itraconazole (alone or in combination with amphotericin B or flucytosine) may be beneficial in this patient population, little is known regarding its efficacy in this setting. If itraconazole is administered, serum levels should be monitored to assess absorption because poor absorption of drug has been documented in this patient population.[76]

EMERGING PATHOGENS

The increased frequency of fungal pathogens that were once rare is gaining attention from the medical community. Permissive environmental conditions, selective antifungal pressure, and increased numbers of immunosuppressed patients have led to increased numbers of infections caused by filamentous fungi such as *Scedosporium* or *Fusarium* spp. Unfortunately, the early presentation of *Fusarium* and *Scedosporidium* infections often mimics that of aspergillosis. On histopathology, *Scedosporidium* resembles *Aspergillus* spp. with dichotomously branching, septate hyphae and has a tendency for invasion of vascular structures.[77] These pathogens often demonstrate intrinsic resistance to amphotericin B and are associated with high mortality rates.[83,89] For example, mortality due to *Scedosporidium prolificans*, previously known as *S. inflatum*, exceeds 85%; *S. apiospermum* (the asexual state of *Pseudallescheria boydii*), was uniformly fatal in 23 solid-organ transplant recipients with disseminated disease.[77] However, in vitro data suggest that *S. prolificans* is more sensitive to voriconazole than to amphotericin B or itraconazole. Voriconazole recently received FDA approval for the treatment of serious fungal infections caused by *S. apiospermum* and *Fusarium* spp., including *F. solani*, in patients intolerant of or refractory to other therapy.[79]

ANTIFUNGAL THERAPY

The antifungal armamentarium for the treatment of invasive fungal infections includes (1) inhibitors of the fungal cell membrane, such as polyenes (e.g., amphotericin B) and azole antifungals, (2) inhibitors of DNA (5-flucytosine), and more recently, (3) inhibitors of cell wall biosynthesis such as the recently approved agent caspofungin.[14,15]

Antifungal therapy generally uses one or more of these agents depending on the severity of infection and the patients' immune status. Rarely are the agents used in combination. Often therapy is initiated

with an intravenous agent such as amphotericin B, and therapy is changed to an oral (azole) regimen as the patient's clinical status improves and oral therapy is tolerated. The most widely used combination therapy consists of flucytosine plus amphotericin B. The role of combination therapy is unclear at this time; controlled trials are lacking, and the possibility of therapeutic antagonism when using azoles in combination with amphotericin B remains debated. Controlled trials are needed to define the role of azoles plus amphotericin B and azoles or amphotericin B plus caspofungin.

AMPHOTERICIN B

Amphotericin B remains the therapy of choice for many systemic fungal infections despite a lack of controlled clinical trials documenting the optimal dosage, duration of therapy, or relative efficacy of this agent in comparison with newer azole antifungal agents such as ketoconazole, itraconazole, and fluconazole. During pregnancy, amphotericin B remains the treatment of choice for most fungal infections because azole antifungals are teratogenic.[21,80]

The side effects of amphotericin B generally are categorized as acute (infusion related) or long term. Gallis and Drew[21] recently reviewed the side effects and clinical uses of amphotericin B.

LIPID FORMULATIONS OF AMPHOTERICIN B

The use of deoxycholate amphotericin B frequently is associated with the development of induced nephrotoxicity. In an attempt to decrease the incidence of nephrotoxicity, three lipid formulations of amphotericin B have been developed and approved for use in humans: amphotericin B lipid complex (ABLC, Abelcet; Enzon Pharmaceuticals), amphotericin B colloidal dispersion (ABCD, Amphotec; Intermune Pharmaceuticals), and liposomal amphotericin B (AmBisome; Gilead Pharmaceuticals). In these preparations, amphotericin B is incorporated into the phospholipid bilayer membrane rather than in the enclosed aqueous phase.

The various lipid formulations of amphotericin B exhibit markedly different pharmacokinetics; however, the clinical implications of these differences remain unclear.[72] Although larger doses of these preparations are required to achieve similar pharmacologic effects as the deoxycholate form of amphotericin B, the toxicity appears to be much lower.[80] Although the FDA-approved dosages of these agents are 5 mg/kg per day (amphotericin B lipid complex), 3–6 mg/kg per day (amphotericin B colloid dispersion), and 3–5 mg/kg per day (liposomal amphotericin B), the agents appear generally equipotent. The optimal dose of these compounds for serious *Candida* infections is unknown; however, dosages of 3–5 mg/kg per day appear reasonable. The relative efficacy of these agents is unknown; whether differences in pharmacokinetic features result in different outcomes in the treatment of specific types of infections (e.g., CNS infections) is unclear.[9,72]

Lipid formulations of amphotericin B are indicated for patients intolerant of, refractory to, or at high risk of being intolerant to conventional antifungal therapy.[9,72,81] Intolerance generally is defined as initial renal insufficiency (creatinine > 2.5 mg/ dL or creatinine clearance < 25 mL/min), a significant increase in creatinine (to 2.5 mg/dL for adults or 1.5 mg/dL for children), or severe acute administration-related toxicity, whereas refractory infections are defined as therapeutic failure of more than 500 mg amphotericin B.

Only ABLC and liposomal amphotericin B have been approved for use in proven candidiasis. Both in vivo and clinical studies indicate that these compounds are less toxic but as effective as amphotericin B when used in appropriate dosages. Nevertheless, their higher cost and the paucity of randomized trials in proven invasive candidiasis limit their front-line use in these infections.[81]

CLINICAL CONTROVERSY

Should lipid formulations of amphotericin B be used rather than the traditonal deoxycholate formulation? Many clinicians feel that lipid formulations have shown clear superiority in the treatment of aspergillosis and histoplasmosis and are "at least as good" as deoxycholate amphotericin B for the treatment of *Candida*, cryptococcosis, and febrile neutropenia. However, they lack FDA approval for these infections except (in some cases) as salvage therapy.[81]

FLUCYTOSINE

Flucytosine (also known as 5-flucytosine or 5-FC) is a fluorinated pyrimidine analogue that is highly water-soluble. Patients with creatinine clearances of less than 40 mL/min should receive 100–150 mg/kg daily in four divided doses. The dosage should be reduced by 50% in patients with a creatinine clearance of 25–50 mL/min and by 75% in patients with a clearance of 13–25 mL/min. Peak serum concentrations (2 hours after an oral dose) should be monitored in all patients (particularly those with a creatinine clearance of less than 10 mL/min) to maintain peak serum concentrations of more than 100 mg/L.[28,29]

Flucytosine generally is associated with very few side effects in patients with normal renal, GI, and hematologic function, although rash, GI discomfort, diarrhea (5% to 10%), and reversible elevations in hepatic enzymes are observed occasionally. In patients with renal dysfunction or concomitant amphotericin B therapy, leukopenia, thrombocytopenia, and (rarely) enterocolitis may occur. Although studies have suggested that little or no conversion of flucytosine to fluorouracil occurs in vitro, serum concentrations of greater than 1000 ng/mL (therapeutic for the treatment of malignancies) have been

documented in some patients. Investigators have theorized that flucytosine may be secreted into the GI tract, deaminated by intestinal bacteria, and reabsorbed as 5-fluorouracil.[28,29]

Flucytosine is used in combination with amphotericin B or fluconazole in the treatment of cryptococcosis or (less commonly) candidiasis. The rapid development of resistance to flucytosine, however, precludes its use as single-agent therapy. Mechanisms for drug resistance may include loss of deaminase and decreased permeability to the drug.[28,29]

ECHINOCANDINS

The echinoocandins are a new class of antifungal agents that act as concentration-dependent, noncompetitive inhibitors of the formation of $\beta(1,3)$-D-glucan synthase, an essential component of the cell wall of susceptible filamentous fungi that is absent in mammalian cells. Caspofungin is the first of this class of agents approved in the United States; clinical trials are currently evaluating several other agents from this class, including micafungin (FK463) and anidulafungin (VER-002).[76]

CASPOFUNGIN

Caspofungin is metabolized by hydrolysis and *N*-acetylation, and excretion of the drug and its metabolites in humans is 35% of the dose in feces and 41% of the dose in urine. Renal clearance of caspofungin is low, and total clearance of the drug is 12 mL/min. Therefore, no dosage adjustment is necessary for patients with renal insufficiency. Becasue caspofungin is not dialyzable, supplementary dosing is not required following hemodialysis.[76]

Adverse effects of caspofungin include histamine release resulting in rash, facial swelling, and itchiness. In clinical trials, concomitant use of cyclosporine and caspofungin resulted in elevated liver function tests two to three times the upper limit of normal. Therefore, it is generally not recommended to use these two drugs in combination. Additionally, when caspofungin was administered concurrently with tacrolimus, tacrolimus levels were reduced by 20% compared with when the healthy volunteers received tacrolimus alone. The mechanism for these interactions is not yet known. Caspofungin is not a cytochrome P450 inducer of enzyme 3A4 and is considered a poor substrate of P450 enzymes. Overall, caspofungin was found to show no cytochrome P450 inhibition in clinical studies and did not interact when administered concomitantly with amphotericin B, itraconazole, or mycophenolate.[76]

The recommended dose for an adult patient is a 70-mg loading dose administered on day 1 of therapy, followed by subsequent doses of 50 mg once daily. Duration of treatment should be based on the severity of the patient's underlying disease, recovery from immunosuppression, and clinical response. Caspofungin should be administered slowly via intravenous infusion over 1 hour.[76]

AZOLE ANTIFUNGAL AGENTS

The introduction of the azole antifungal agents has rapidly expanded the armamentarium of agents useful in the treatment of systemic fungal infections.[11] Adverse effects of azoles include GI disturbances (primarily nausea, vomiting, epigastric pain, and diarrhea), which appear to be more common in patients receiving ketoconazole and the solution formulation of itraconazole. Although cyclodextrin is not absorbed following oral administration, use of the intravenous formulation of itraconazole is limited to 2 weeks because of concerns for potential nephrotoxicity secondary to accumulation of the cyclodextrin vehicle.[14,15,82] Fluconazole is well tolerated; intestinal complaints are the most frequently reported, followed by headaches and rash. Unlike ketoconazole, fluconazole does not inhibit testicular or adrenal steroidogenesis in healthy volunteers or hospitalized patients. Reversible alopecia occurs not infrequently and usually appears after several months of treatment with higher doses of fluconazole. Azoles are potentially teratogenic and should be avoided in pregnant women.[14,15,82]

ITRACONAZOLE

Itraconazole is triazole antifungal with a broad spectrum of antifungal activity. Despite its marked structural similarity to ketoconazole, itraconazole differs in several important respects. Itraconazole appears to have greater specificity against fungal versus mammalian cytochrome P450, resulting in greater potency and a decrease in P450-mediated side effects. In addition, itraconazole possesses excellent in vitro activity against *Aspergillus* and *Sporothrix* spp.

Like ketoconazole, the capsule formulation of itraconazole depends on the availability of low gastric pH for dissolution and absorption. Administration with food appears to enhance significantly the bioavailability of itraconazole capsules, whereas it decreases the bioavailability of the oral solution. Because itraconazole exhibits pH-dependent dissolution and absorption, absorption of the capsule formulation is impaired in patients receiving antacids or H_2-receptor antagonists and in patients with achlorhydria.[82] Plasma concentrations of itraconazole following a single oral dose (capsules) in HIV-infected patients are approximately 50% lower than concentrations observed in healthy volunteers. The capsule formulation of itraconazole exhibits unpredictable oral bioavailability, particularly in subjects with hypochlorhydria and in patients with enteropathy caused by mucositis or graft-versus-host gut disease. Recently, oral suspension and IV formulations of itraconazole became available; both use cyclodextrin as a solubilizing vehicle to increase the solubility of the drug. The oral bioavailability of the solution is unaffected by alterations in gastric pH or in patients with enteropathy.[8,9,82]

FLUCONAZOLE

Fluconazole is a triazole antifungal agent with markedly different pharmacologic features than previously marketed azole antifungals. The small molecular weight, low protein binding, and increased water solubility of fluconazole result in rapid, essentially complete absorption of drug following oral administration. Since fluconazole is excreted primarily (>80%) as unchanged drug in the urine, dosage adjustments are necessary in patients with renal dysfunction.

VORICONAZOLE

The most common side effect of voriconazole is a reversible disturbance of vision (photopsia), which occurs in approximately 30% of patients but rarely leads to discontinuation of the drug. Symptoms tend to occur during the first week of therapy and decrease or disappear despite of continued therapy. Patients experience altered color discrimination, blurred vision, the appearance of bright spots and wavy lines, and photophobia. Patients should be cautioned that driving may be hazardous because of the risk of visual disturbances. The visual effects are associated with changes in electroretinogram tracings, which revert to normal when treatment with the drug is stopped; no permanent damage to the retina has been demonstrated.[75]

DRUG INTERACTIONS WITH AZOLE ANTIFUNGAL AGENTS

Drug interactions with azole antifungals generally can be placed into three broad categories: (1) decreases in azole bioavailability because of chelation or secondary to increases in gastric pH, (2) interactions with other cytochrome P450–metabolized drugs, and (3) interactions caused by inhibition of *p*-glycoprotein. Drug interactions in the latter two categories may result in increases or decreases in the azole antifungal, in the interacting drug, or in both drugs.[14,15]

The interaction of azole antifungal agents with other cytochromes P450–metabolized drugs is well recognized. The azoles appear to be metabolized almost entirely via the cytochrome P450 3A4 subfamily. As expected, they interact with other drugs metabolized partly or wholly via this enzyme pathway. In addition, fluconazole and voriconazole use the cytochrome P450 2C19 pathway. Numerous clinically significant interactions have been documented with azole antifungals and a variety of other drugs. In most cases, the azole interferes with the metabolism of the other cytochrome P450–metabolized drug.[14,15]

The interaction between ketoconazole and cyclosporine has been exploited in order to reduce drug costs associated with administration of cyclosporine following organ transplantation. Relative to ketoconazole and itraconazole, fluconazole appears to be intermediate in its ability to inhibit human cytochromes P450. The magnitude of fluconazole-induced inhibition of cyclosporine metabolism appears, however, to depend on the dosage of fluconazole.

Predictably, drugs such as rifampin, rifabutin, isoniazid, phenytoin, and carbamazepine, which are known to induce the activity of cytochromes P450, result in increased metabolism of the azole antifungals and may result in therapeutic failures. Increased dosages of azole antifungals may be required in patients receiving these combinations of drugs.[14,15]

Itraconazole is an inhibitor of intestinal *p*-glycoprotein. Significant increases in digoxin (a *p*-glycoprotein substrate) have been observed in patients receiving both agents concurrently. Interactions with other substrates of *p*-glycoprotein would be expected to occur.

COMBINATION ANTIFUNGAL THERAPY

Based on extensive experience in the management of bacterial and, more recently, retroviral infections, the use of combination agents for synergistic or additive effects is now common practice. However, studies supporting the use of combinations of antifungal agents have produced less definitive results. In vitro and animal data have produced conflicting results, and human studies are lacking. Thus there are as yet no firm recommendations regarding the use of such combinations in humans. A recent study comparing the use of high-dose fluconazole alone or in combination with amphotericin B in nonimmunocompromised patients with candidemia demonstrated no antagonism and a trend toward improved success and more rapid clearance of *Candida* from the bloodstream.[49]

PLASMA CONCENTRATION MONITORING OF ANTIFUNGAL AGENTS

Routine monitoring of plasma concentrations of antifungal agents to assess efficacy or toxicity of these agents generally is not available. Correlations between plasma concentrations of antifungal agents and therapeutic outcomes have been poorly studied. Under certain circumstances, serum or plasma concentration monitoring is warranted, e.g., in patients susceptible to flucytosine toxicity or to document adequate oral absorption of ketoconazole or itraconazole in cases of suspected treatment failure, concern about compliance or absorption, or when drug interactions that might reduce the solubility or accelerate the metabolism of azoles are suspected. Although "therapeutic" levels have not been defined, some investigators recommend maintenance of serum concentrations of itraconazole (2 to 4 hours after administration) of 1 mcg/mL, measured by bioassay.[6,22] Among AIDS patients, those receiving a dosage of 200 mg once or twice daily achieved median plasma concentrations of 3 or 6 mcg/mL, respectively.[22]

ABBREVIATIONS

AIDS: acquired immunodeficiency syndrome
ACTG: AIDS Clinical Trials Groups
ATCC: American Type Culture Collection
ABCD: amphotericin B colloid dispersion
ABLC: amphotericin B lipid complex
ABC: ATP-binding cassette
BAE: bronchial artery embolization
BPA: bronchopulmonary aspergillosis
CDC: Centers for Disease Control and Prevention
CNS: central nervous system
CVC: central venous catheter
CSF: cerebrospinal fluid
CF-M: CF titer for mycelial antigen
CF: complement fixation
ELISA: enzyme-linked immunosorbent assay
GI: gastrointestinal
GVHD: graft-versus-host disease
HPA: *H. capsulatum* polysaccharide antigen
HEPA: high-efficiency particulate air
HAART: highly active antiretroviral therapy
ID: immunodiffusion
IgM: immunoglobulin M
ICUs: intensive care units
IV: intravenous
LA: latex agglutination
MF: major facilitators
PMN: polymorphonuclear leukocytes
PDH: progressive disseminated histoplasmosis
RIA: radioimmunoassay
TPN: total parenteral nutrition
WBC: white blood cell

Review Questions and other resources can be found at *www.pharmacotherapyonline.com.*

REFERENCES

1. Bennett JE. Introduction to mycoses. In: Mandell GL, Bennett JE, Dolin R, eds. Principles and Practice of Infectious Diseases, 5th ed. Philadelphia, Churchill Livingstone, 2000:2654–2656.
2. Pfaller MA, Jones RN, Messer SA, et al. National surveillance of nosocomial blood stream infection due to *Candida* albicans: Frequency of occurrence and antifungal susceptibility in the SCOPE program. Diagn Microbiol Infect Dis 1998;31:327–332.
3. Pfaller MA, Jones RN, Doern GV, et al. International surveillance of blood stream infections due to *Candida* species in the European SENTRY Program: Species distribution and antifungal susceptibility including the investigational triazole and echinocandin agents. SENTRY Participant Group (Europe). Diagn Microbiol Infect Dis 1999;35:19–25.
4. Singh N. Invasive mycoses in organ transplant recipients: Controversies in prophylaxis and management. J Antimicrob Chemother 2000;45:749–755.
5. National Committee for Clinical Laboratory Standards (NCCLS). Reference method for broth dilution antifungal susceptibility testing of yeasts: Approved Standard. NCCLS Document M27-A. Wayne, PA, NCCLS, 1997.
6. Summers KK, Hardin TC, Gore SJ, Graybill JR. Therapeutic drug monitoring of systemic antifungal therapy. J Antimicrob Chemother 1997;40:753–764.
7. Sobel JD. Practice guidelines for the treatment of fungal infections. Clin Infect Dis 2000;30:652.
8. Bennett JE. Pathogenic fungi. In: Sherris JC, ed. Medical Microbiology, 2d ed. New York, Elsevier, 1991:440.
9. Pappas PG, Rex JH, Walsh TJ, et al. Guidelines for treatment of candidiasis. Clin Infect Dis 2004;38:161–189.
10. Sanglard D, Odds FC. Resistance of *Candida* species to antifungal agents: molecular mechanisms and clinical consequences. Lancet Infect Dis 2002;2:73185.
11. White TC, Marr KA, Bowden RA. Clinical, cellular, and molecular factors that contribute to antifungal drug resistance. Clin Microbiol Rev 1998;11:382–402.
12. Lupetti A, Danesi R, Campa M, et al. Molecular basis of resistance to azole antifungals. Trends Mol Med 2002;8:76–81.
13. Bille J. Mechanisms and clinical significance of antifungal resistance. Int J Antimicrob Agents. 2000;16:331–333.
14. Kauffman CA, Carver PL. Antifungal agents in the 1990s: Current status and future developments. Drugs 1997;53:539–549.
15. Kauffman CA, Carver PL. Use of azoles for systemic antifungal therapy. Adv Pharmacol 1997;39:143–189.
16. Edwards JE. *Candida* species. In: Mandell GL, Bennett JE, Dolin R, eds. Principles and Practice of Infectious Diseases, 5th ed. New York, Churchill-Livingstone, 2000:2656–2671.
17. Kaufman L. Laboratory methods for the diagnosis and confirmation of systemic mycoses. Clin Infect Dis 1992;14(suppl 1):S23–29.
18. Perfect JR. Antifungal prophylaxis: To prevent or not. Am J Med 1993;94:233–234.
19. Saag MS, Graybill RJ, Larsen RA, et al. Practice guidelines for the management of cryptococcal disease. Clin Infect Dis 2000;30:710–718.
20. Deepe GS. Histoplasma capsulatum. In: Mandell GL, Bennett JE, Dolin R, eds. Principles and Practice of Infectious Diseases, 5th ed. New York, Churchill-Livingstone, 2000:2718–2733.
21. Gallis HA, Drew RH, Pickard WW. Amphotericin B: 30 years of clinical experience. Rev Infect Dis 1990;12:308–329.
22. Wheat J, Sarosi G, McKinsey D, et al. Practice guidelines for the management of patients with histoplasmosis. Clin Infect Dis 2000;30:688–695.
23. Wheat LJ, Kauffman CA. Histoplasmosis. Infect Dis Clin North Am 2003;17(1):1–19.
24. O'Shaughnessy EM, Shea YM, Witebsky FG. Laboratory diagnosis of invasive mycoses. Infect Dis Clin North Am 2003;17(1):135–158.
25. Galgiani JN, Ampel NM, Catanzaro A, et al. Practice guidelines for the treatment of coccidioidomycoses. Clin Infect Dis 2000;30:658–661.
26. Chiller TM, Galgiani JN, Stevens DA. Coccidioidomycosis. Infect Dis Clin North Am 2003;17:41–57.
27. Bennett JE, Dismukes WE, Duma RJ, et al. A comparison of amphotericin B alone and combined with flucytosine in the treatment of cryptococcal meningitis. N Engl J Med 1979;301:126–131.
28. Francis P, Walsh TJ. Evolving role of flucytosine in immunocompromised patients: New insights into safety, pharmacokinetics, and antifungal therapy. Clin Infect Dis 1992;15:1003–1018.
29. Powderly WG, Saag MS, Cloud GA, et al. A controlled trial of fluconazole or amphotericin B to prevent relapse of cryptococcal meningitis in patients with the acquired immunodeficiency syndrome. N Engl J Med 1992;326:793–798.
30. Saag MS, Powderly WG, Cloud GA, et al. Comparison of amphotericin B with fluconazole in the treatment of acute AIDS-associated cryptococcal meningitis: The NIAID Mycoses Study Group and the AIDS Clinical Trials Group. N Engl J Med 1992;326:83–89.

31. van der Horst CM, Saag MS, Cloud GA, et al. Treatment of cryptococcal meningitis associated with the acquired immunodeficiency syndrome. N Engl J Med 1997;37:15–21.

32. Vibhagool A, Sungkanuparph S, Mootsikapun P, et al. Discontinuation of secondary prophylaxis for cryptococcal meningitis in human immunodeficiency virus-infected patients treated with highly active antiretroviral therapy: A prospective, multicenter, randomized study. Clin Infect Dis 2003; 36:1329–1331.

33. Sullivan DJ, Westerneng TJ, Haynes KA, et al. *Candida dubliniensis* sp. *nov:* Phenotyping and molecular characterization of a novel species associated with oral candidosis in HIV-infected individuals. Microbiology 1995;141;1507–1521.

34. Minari A, Hachem R, Raad I. *Candida lusitaniae:* A cause of breakthrough fungemia in cancer patients. Clin Infect Dis 2001;32:186–190.

35. Pfaller MA, Jones RN, Doern GV, et al. International surveillance of bloodstream infections due to *Candida* species: Frequency of occurrence and antifungal susceptibilities of isolates collected in 1997 in the United States, Canada, and South America for the SENTRY program. J Clin Microbiol 1998;36:1886–1889.

36. Winston DJ, Chandrasekar PH, Lazarus HM, et al. Fluconazole prophylaxis of fungal infections in patients with acute leukemia: Results of a randomized placebo-controlled, double-blind, multicenter trial. Ann Intern Med 1993;118:495–503.

37. Rangel-Frausto MS, Wiblin T, Blumberg HM, et al. National Epidemiology of Mycoses Survey (NEMIS): Variations in rates of blood stream infections due to *Candida* species in seven surgical intensive care units and six neonatal intensive care units. Clin Infect Dis 1999;29: 253–258.

38. Edmond MB, Wallace SE, McClish DK, et al. Nosocomial bloodstream infections in United States hospitals: A three-year analysis. Clin Infect Dis 1999;29:239–244.

39. Fraser VJ, Jones M, Dunkel J, et al. Candidemia in a tertiary care hospital: Epidemiology, risk factors, and predictors of mortality. Clin Infect Dis 1992;15:414–421.

40. Wey SB, Mori M, Pfaller MA, et al. Risk factors for hospital-acquired candidemia: A matched case-control study. Arch Intern Med 1989;149: 2349–2353.

41. Pappas, PG, Rex JH, Lee J, et al. A prospective observational study of candidemia: Epidemiology, therapy, and influences on mortality in hospitalized adult and pediatric patients. Clin Infect Dis 2003;37:634–643.

42. Wey SB, Mori M, Pfaller MA, et al. Hospital acquired candidemia: The attributable mortality and excess length of stay. Arch Intern Med 1988; 148:2642–2645.

43. Eggimann P, Francioli P, Bille J, et al. Fluconazole prophylaxis prevents intraabdominal candidiasis in high-risk surgical patients. Crit Care Med 1999;27:1066–1072.

44. Rocco TR, Reinert SE, Simms H. Effect of fluconazole administration in critically ill patients. Arch Surg 2000;135:160–165.

45. Edwards DE. International conference for the development of a consensus on the management and prevention of severe candidal infections. Clin Infect Dis 1997;25:43–59.

46. Rex JH, Bennett JE, Sugar AM, et al. A randomized trial comparing fluconazole with amphotericin B for the treatment of candidemia in patients without neutropenia. N Engl J Med 1994;331:1325–1330.

47. Phillips P, Shafran S, Garber G, et al. Multicenter randomized trial of fluconazole versus amphotericin B for treatment of candidemia in nonneutropenic patients: Canadian candidemia study group. Eur J Clin Micro Infect Dis 1997;16:337–345.

48. Mora-Duarte J, Betts R, Rotstein C, et al. Comparison of caspofungin and amphotericin B for invasive candidiasis. N Engl J Med 2002;347: 2020–2029.

49. Rex JH, Pappas PG, Karchmer AW, et al. A randomized and blinded multicenter trial of high-dose fluconazole plus placebo versus fluconazole plus amphotericin B as therapy for candidemia and its consequences in nonneutropenic subjects. Clin Infect Dis 2003;36:1221–1228.

50. Goodman JL, Winston DJ, Greenfield RA, et al. A controlled trial of fluconazole to prevent fungal infections in patients undergoing bone marrow transplantation. N Engl J Med 1992;326:845–851.

51. Slavin MA, Osborne B, Adams R, et al. Efficacy and safety of fluconazole prophylaxis for fungal infections after marrow transplantation: A prospective, randomized, double-blind study. J Infect Dis 1995;171:1545–1552.

52. Marr KA, Seidel K, Slavin MA, et al. Prolonged fluconazole prophylaxis is associated with persistent protection against candidiasis-related death in allogeneic marrow transplant recipients: Long-term follow-up of a randomized, placebo-controlled trial. Blood 2000;96:2055–2061.

53. Menichetti F, Del Favero A, Martino P, et al. Itraconazole oral solution as prophylaxis for fungal infections in neutropenic patients with hematologic malignancies: A randomized, placebo-controlled, double-blind, multicenter trial. GIMEMA Infection Program. Gruppo Italiano Malattie Ematologiche dell' Adulto. Clin Infect Dis 1999;28:250–255.

54. Rotstein C, Bow EJ, Laverdiere M, et al. Randomized placebo-controlled trial of fluconazole prophylaxis for neutropenic cancer patients: Benefit based on purpose and intensity of cytotoxic therapy. Clin Infect Dis 1999;28:331–340.

55. Boogaerts M, Winston DJ, Bow EJ, et al. Intravenous and oral itraconazole versus intravenous amphotericin B as empirical antifungal therapy for persistent fever in neutropenic patients with cancer who are receiving broad-spectrum antibacterial therapy. Ann Intern Med 2001;135:412–422.

56. Winston DJ, Hathorn JW, Schuster MG, et al. A multicenter, randomized trial of fluconazole versus amphotericin B for empiric antifungal therapy of febrile neutropenic patients with cancer. Am J Med 2000;108:282–289.

57. Pfaller MA. Nosocomial candidiasis: Emerging species, reservoirs, and modes of transmission. Clin Infect Dis 1996;22(suppl 2):S89–94.

58. Walsh TJ, Pappas P, Winston DJ, et al. Voriconazole compared with liposomal amphotericin B for empirical antifungal therapy in patients with neutropenia and persistent fever. N Engl J Med 2002;346:225–234.

59. Anaissie EJ, Darouiche RO, Abi-Said D, et al. Management of invasive candidal infections: Results of a prospective, randomized, multicenter study of fluconazole versus amphotericin B and review of the literature. Clin Infect Dis 1996;23:964–972.

60. Kauffman CA, Vazquez JA, Sobel JD, et al. Prospective multicenter surveillance study of funguria in hospitalized patients. Clin Infect Dis 2000;30:14–18.

61. Sobel JD, Kauffman CA, McKinsey D, et al. Candiduria: A randomized, double-blind study of treatment with fluconazole and placebo. Clin Infect Dis 2000;30:19–24.

62. Anaissie EJ, Rex JH, Uzun O, Vartivarian S. Predictors of adverse outcome in cancer patients with candidemia. Am J Med 1998;104:238–245.

63. Nucci M, Anaissie E. Should vascular catheters be removed from all patients with candidemia? An evidence-based review. Clin Infect Dis 2002;34:591–599.

64. Nguyen MH, Peacock JE Jr, Tanner DC, et al. Therapeutic approaches in patients with candidemia:evaluation in a multicenter, prospective, observational study. Arch Intern Med 1995;155:2429–2435.

65. Stevens DA, Schwartz HJ, Lee JT, et al. A randomized trial of itraconazole in allergic bronchopulmonary aspergillosis. N Engl J Med 2000;342:756–762.

66. Steinbach WJ, Stevens DA. Review of newer antifungal and immunomodulatory strategies for invasive aspergillosis. Clin Infect Dis 2003; 37(suppl 3):S157–187.

67. Jennings TS, Hardin TC. Treatment of aspergillosis with itraconazole. Ann Pharmacother 1993;27:1206–1211.

68. Harari S. Current strategies in the treatment of invasive *Aspergillus* infections in immunocompromised patients. Drugs 1999;58:621–631.

69. Stevens DA, Kan VL, Judson MA, et al. Practice guidelines for diseases caused by *Aspergillus*. Clin Infect Dis 2000;30:696–709.

70. Lin SJ, Schranz J, Teutsch SM. Aspergillus case fatality rate: Systematic review of the literature. Clin Infect Dis 2001;32:358–366.

71. Holding KJ, Dworkin MS, Wan PCT, et al. Aspergillosis among people infected with human immunodeficiency virus: Incidence and survival. Clin Infect Dis 2000;31:1253–1257.

72. Wong-Beringer A, Jacobs RA, Guglielmo BJ. Lipid formulations of amphotericin B: Clinical efficacy and toxicities. Clin Infect Dis 1998;27: 603–618.

73. Ellis M, Spence D, de Pauw B, et al. An EORTC international multicenter randomized trial (EORTC no. 19923) comparing two dosages of liposomal

amphotericin B for treatment of invasive aspergillosis. Clin Infect Dis 1998;27:1406–1412.

74. Wingard JR, White ML, Anaissie E, et al. A randomized, double-blind, comparative trial evaluating the safety of liposomal amphotericin B versus amphotericin B lipid complex in the empirical treatment of febrile neutropenia. Clin Infect Dis 2000;31:1155–1163.

75. Johnson LB, Kauffman CA. Voriconazole: A new triazole antifungal agent. Clin Infect Dis 2003;36:630–637.

76. Pacetti SA, Gelone SP. Caspofungin acetate for treatment of invasive fungal infections. Ann Pharmacother 2003;37:90–98.

77. Castiglioni B, Sutton DA, Rinaldi MG, et al. Pseudallescheria boydii (anamorph *Scedosporium apispermum*) infection in solid organ transplant recipients in a tertiary medical center and review of the literature. Medicine 2002;81:333–348.

78. Boutati EI, Anaissie EJ. Fusarium, a significant emerging pathogen in patients with hematologic malignancy: Ten years' experience at a cancer center and implications for management. Blood 1997;90:999–1008.

79. Pfizer. Vfend (voriconazole) package insert. New York, 2002.

80. King CT, Rogers PD, Cleary JD, et al. Antifungal therapy during pregnancy. Clin Infect Dis 1998;27:1151–1160.

81. Ostrosky-Zeichner L, Marr KA, Rex JH, Cohen SH. Amphotericin B: Time for a new "gold standard." Clin Infect Dis 2003;37:415–425.

82. Stevens DA. Itraconazole in cyclodextrin solution. Pharmacotherapy 1999;19:603–611.

120

INFECTIONS IN IMMUNOCOMPROMISED PATIENTS

Douglas N. Fish and S. Diane Goodwin

Learning Objectives and other resources can be found at *www.pharmacotherapyonline.com.*

KEY CONCEPTS

❶ An *immunocompromised host* is a patient with defects in host defenses that predispose to infection. Risk factors include neutropenia, immune system defects (from disease or immunosuppressive drug therapy), compromise of natural host defenses, environmental contamination, and changes in normal flora of the host.

❷ Immunocompromised patients are at high risk for a variety of bacterial, fungal, viral, and protozoal infections. Bacterial infections caused by gram-positive cocci (staphylococci and streptococci) occur most frequently, followed by gram-negative bacterial infections caused by Enterobacteriaceae and *Pseudomonas aeruginosa.* Fungal infections caused by *Candida* and *Aspergillus,* as well as certain viral infections (herpes simplex virus, cytomegalovirus), are also important causes of morbidity and mortality.

❸ Risk of infection in neutropenic patients is associated with both the severity and duration of neutropenia. Patients with severe neutropenia (absolute neutrophil count [ANC] <500 cells/mm³) for greater than 7 to 10 days are considered to be at high risk of infection.

❹ Fever (single oral temperature of 38.3°C [101°F] or greater or a temperature of 38°C [100.4°F] or greater for 1 hour or more) is the most important clinical finding in neutropenic patients and usually is the stimulus for further diagnostic work-up and initiation of antimicrobial treatment. Infection should be considered as the cause of fever until proved otherwise. Usual signs and symptoms of infection may be altered or absent in neutropenic patients. Appropriate empirical broad-spectrum antimicrobial therapy must be instituted rapidly to prevent excessive morbidity and mortality.

❺ Empirical antimicrobial regimens for neutropenic infections should take into account patients' individual risk factors, as well as institutional infection and susceptibility patterns. The significant morbidity and mortality associated with gram-negative infections require that initial empirical regimens for treatment of febrile neutropenia have good activity against *Pseudomonas aeruginosa* and Enterobacteriaceae. Inpatient parenteral regimens most commonly recommended for initial treatment include monotherapy with an antipseudomonal cephalosporin or carbapenem or a combination regimen consisting of an antipseudomonal cephalosporin or carbapenem plus an aminoglycoside. Low-risk patients may be treated successfully with oral antibiotics (ciprofloxacin plus amoxicillin-clavulanate), with the treatment setting determined by the patient's clinical status.

❻ Neutropenic patients who remain febrile after 3 to 5 days of initial antimicrobial therapy should be reevaluated to determine whether treatment modifications are necessary. Common regimen modifications include the addition of vancomycin (if not already present) and antifungal therapy (amphotericin B or fluconazole). Therapy should be directed at causative organisms, if identified, but broad-spectrum regimens should be maintained during neutropenia.

❼ The optimal duration of therapy for febrile neutropenia is controversial. The decision to discontinue antimicrobials is based on resolution of neutropenia, defervescence, culture results, and clinical stability of the patient.

❽ Prophylactic antimicrobials are administered to cancer patients expected to experience prolonged neutropenia, as well as to both hematopoietic stem cell and solid-organ transplant recipients. Prophylactic regimens may include antibacterial, antifungal, antiviral, or antiprotozoal agents, or a combination of these, selected according to risk of infection with specific pathogens. Optimal prophylactic regimens should take into account individual patient risk for infection and institutional infection and susceptibility patterns.

❾ Patients undergoing hematopoietic stem cell transplantation are at an extremely high risk of infection because of prolonged neutropenia following intensive chemotherapy with or without irradiation, whereas solid-organ transplant recipients are at high risk because of prolonged administration of immunosuppressive drugs. Fungal *(Aspergillus)* and viral (cytomegalovirus) infections are particularly troublesome in these populations, and prophylactic regimens directed against these pathogens are used commonly. When documented, these infections must be treated aggressively in order to optimize patient outcomes. Nevertheless, mortality rates are often very high despite appropriate and aggressive antimicrobial therapy.

◀⑩ Immunocompromised patients must be assessed continuously for evidence of infection and response to antimicrobial therapy. Because a large number of antimicrobials potentially may be used, the occurrence of drug-related adverse effects also must be assessed carefully. Efforts should be directed at designing cost-effective treatment strategies that promote optimal patient outcomes.

An immunocompromised host is a patient with intrinsic or acquired defects in host defenses that predispose to infection. Advances in modern medicine are creating more immunocompromised hosts than ever before. Historically, many of these patients died from their underlying diseases. Dramatic improvements in survival have been achieved by more aggressive therapy of underlying diseases and improved supportive care. Because aggressive therapy often renders patients profoundly immunosuppressed for long periods, however, opportunistic infections remain important causes of morbidity and mortality. This chapter focuses on risk factors for infection, common pathogens and infection sites, and prevention and management of suspected or documented infections in cancer patients (including hematopoietic stem cell transplant [HSCT] patients) and solid-organ transplant recipients. Chapter 123 discusses infectious complications associated with human immunodeficiency virus (HIV) infection.

RISK FACTORS FOR INFECTION/EPIDEMIOLOGY

NEUTROPENIA

◀①◀②◀③ Neutropenia is an abnormally reduced number of neutrophils circulating in peripheral blood. Although exact definitions of neutropenia often vary, an absolute neutrophil count (ANC) of fewer than 1000 cells/mm³ indicates a reduction sufficient to predispose patients to infection.[1] The ANC is the sum of the absolute numbers of both mature neutrophils (polymorphonuclear cells [PMNs], also called *polys* or *segs*) and immature neutrophils (*bands*). The absolute number of PMNs and bands is determined by dividing the percentage of these cells (obtained from the white blood cell [WBC] differential) by 100 and then multiplying the quotient obtained by the total number of WBCs.

The degree or severity of neutropenia, rate of neutrophil decline, and duration of neutropenia are important risk factors for infection.[1–6] All neutropenic patients are considered to be at risk for infection, but those with an ANC of fewer than 500 cells/mm³ are at greater risk than those with ANCs of 500 to 1000 cells/mm³. Most treatment guidelines use an ANC of fewer than 500 cells/mm³ as the critical value in making therapeutic decisions regarding the management of suspected or documented infections.[1,3–6] Risk of infection and death are greatest among patients with fewer than 100 neutrophils/mm³.[2] In patients with chemotherapy-induced neutropenia, the risk of infection is increased according to the rapidity of ANC decline. Infection risk also increases as the duration of neutropenia increases; patients with severe neutropenia of more than 7 to 10 days' duration are considered to be at especially high risk for serious infections.[3] The duration of chemotherapy-induced neutropenia varies considerably among subsets of cancer patients according to the specific chemotherapeutic agents used and the intensity of treatment. Patients undergoing hematopoietic stem cell transplantation (HSCT) may have no detectable granulocytes in peripheral blood for up to 3 to 4 weeks and are at particular risk for severe infections with a variety of pathogens.[7]

Bacteria and fungi commonly cause infections in neutropenic patients. Gram-positive cocci (*Staphylococcus aureus*, *S. epidermidis*, streptococci, and enterococci) have emerged as the most common cause of acute bacterial infections among neutropenic patients. Gram-negative bacilli (*Escherichia coli*, *Klebsiella pneumoniae*, *Pseudomonas aeruginosa*) traditionally were the most common causes of bacterial infection and remain frequent pathogens, although now they are not as common as gram-positive bacteria.[4,5,8] However, gram-negative infections are associated with significant morbidity and mortality. Patients who are neutropenic for extended periods of time and who receive broad-spectrum antibiotics are at risk for fungal infection, usually due to *Candida* or *Aspergillus* spp.[4] Viral infections, although not as common as bacterial and fungal infections, also may cause severe infection in the neutropenic patient.[6,9] Successful treatment of infections in neutropenic patients depends on resolution of neutropenia.[1–4,6]

Although not readily quantifiable, abnormalities may exist in granulocyte function, as well as in cell numbers. Defects in phagocyte function may be caused by underlying disease (e.g., leukemia) or its treatment (e.g., corticosteroids, antineoplastic agents, and radiation).[3,10,11]

IMMUNE SYSTEM DEFECTS

In addition to neutropenia, defects in T-lymphocyte and macrophage function (cell-mediated immunity) and B-cell function (humoral immunity) or both predispose patients to infection. Cellular immune dysfunction is the result of underlying disease or immunosuppressive drug therapy; these defects result in a reduced ability of the host to defend against intracellular pathogens. Patients with Hodgkin's disease and transplant patients receiving immunosuppressive drugs such as cyclosporine, tacrolimus, sirolimus, mycophenolate, corticosteroids, antineoplastic agents, or azathioprine are at risk for a variety of bacterial, fungal, viral, and protozoal infections (Table 120–1). While some of these pathogens are associated with asymptomatic or mild disease in normal hosts, they can cause disseminated, life-threatening infections in immunocompromised hosts.

Underlying disease frequently causes defects in humoral immune function. Patients with multiple myeloma and chronic lymphocytic leukemia have progressive hypogammaglobulinemia that results in defective humoral immunity. Splenectomy performed as a part of the staging process for Hodgkin's disease places patients at risk for infectious complications. Disease states with humoral immune dysfunction predispose the patient to serious, life-threatening infection with encapsulated organisms such as *Streptococcus pneumoniae*, *Hemophilus influenzae*, and *Neisseria meningitidis*.

DESTRUCTION OF PROTECTIVE BARRIERS

Loss of protective barriers is a major factor predisposing immunocompromised patients to infection. Damage to skin and mucous membranes by surgery, venipuncture, intravenous (IV) and urinary catheters, radiation, and chemotherapy disrupts natural host defense systems, leaving patients at high risk for infection. Chemotherapy-induced mucositis may erode mucous membranes of the oropharynx and gastrointestinal (GI) tract and establish a portal for subsequent infection by bacteria, herpes simplex virus, and *Candida*.[12] Medical and surgical procedures, such as transplant surgery, indwelling IV

TABLE 120–1. Risk Factors and Common Pathogens in Immunocompromised Patients

Risk Factor	Patient Conditions	Common Pathogens
Neutropenia	Acute leukemia Chemotherapy	Bacteria: *Staphylococcus aureus, Staphylococcus epidermidis, Escherichia coli, Klebsiella pneumoniae, Pseudomonas aeruginosa,* streptococci, enterococci Fungi: *Candida, Aspergillus, Zygomycetes* Viruses: Herpes simplex
Impaired cell-mediated immunity	Lymphoma Immunosuppressive therapy (steroids, cyclosporine, chemotherapy)	Bacteria: *Listeria, Nocardia, Legionella,* Mycobacteria Fungi: *Cryptococcus neoformans, Candida, Aspergillus, Histoplasma capsulatum* Viruses: Cytomegalovirus, varicella-zoster, herpes simplex Protozoal: *Pneumocystis jiroveci*
Impaired humoral immunity	Multiple myeloma Chronic lymphocytic leukemia Splenectomy Immunosuppressive therapy (steroids, chemotherapy)	Bacteria: *S. pneumoniae, H. influenzae, N. meningitidis*
Loss of protective barriers		
Skin	Venipuncture, bone marrow aspiration, urinary catheterization, vascular access devices, radiation, biopsies	Bacteria: *S. aureus, S. epidermidis, Bacillus* spp., *Corynebacterium jeikeium* Fungi: *Candida*
Mucous membranes	Respiratory support equipment, endoscopy, chemotherapy, radiation	Bacteria: *S. aureus, S. epidermidis,* streptococci Enterobacteriaceae, *P. aeruginosa, Bacteroides* spp. Fungi: *Candida* Viruses: Herpes simplex
Surgery	Solid organ transplantation	Bacteria: *S. aureus, S. epidermidis,* Enterobacteriaceae, *P. aeruginosa, Bacteroides* spp. Fungi: *Candida* Viruses: Herpes simplex
Alteration of normal microbial flora	Antimicrobial therapy Chemotherapy Hospital environment	Bacteria: Enterobacteriaceae, *P. aeruginosa, Legionella, S. aureus, S. epidermidis* Fungi: *Candida, Aspergillus*
Blood products, donor organs	Bone marrow transplantation Solid organ transplantation	Fungi: *Candida* Viruses: Cytomegalovirus, Epstein-Barr virus, hepatitis B, hepatitis C Protozoal: *Toxoplasma gondii*

Compiled from refs. 1, 3, 5, 6, 8, 10, 16, 17, 20, 22, 23, and 26.

catheter placement, bone marrow aspiration, biopsies, and endoscopy, further damage the integument and predispose patients to infection. Infections resulting from disruption of protective barriers usually are a result of skin flora, such as *S. aureus, S. epidermidis,* and various streptococci.[1,6,10,12]

ENVIRONMENTAL CONTAMINATION/ALTERATION OF MICROBIAL FLORA

Infections in immunocompromised patients are caused by organisms either colonizing the host or acquired from the environment. Microorganisms may be transferred easily from patient to patient on the hands of hospital personnel unless strict infection control guidelines are followed. Contaminated equipment, such as nebulizers or ventilators, and contaminated water supplies have been responsible for outbreaks of *P. aeruginosa* and *Legionella pneumophila* infections, respectively. Foods, such as fruits and green leafy vegetables, which are often colonized with gram-negative bacteria and fungi, are also sources of microbial contamination in immunocompromised hosts.[3,13]

Most infections in cancer patients are caused by organisms colonizing body sites, such as the skin, oropharynx, and GI tract.[12,13] About 80% of infecting bacterial pathogens are from the patient's endogenous flora.[14] The GI tract is the most common site from which infections in immunocompromised hosts originate. Periodontitis,

pharyngitis, esophagitis, colitis, perirectal cellulitis, and bacteremias are caused predominantly by normal flora of the gut; bloodstream infections are thought to arise from microbial translocation across injured GI mucosa.[12,13] Normal flora may be significantly disrupted and altered; oropharyngeal flora rapidly change to primarily gram-negative bacilli in hospitalized patients. Many cancer patients already may be colonized with gram-negative bacilli on admission as a result of frequent hospitalizations and clinic visits. In hospitalized cancer patients, 50% of infections, however, are caused by colonizing organisms acquired after admission.[14]

Although hospitalization and severity of illness are risk factors for colonization by gram-negative bacilli, administration of broad-spectrum antimicrobial agents has the greatest impact on flora of immunocompromised hosts. Use of these agents disrupts the delicate balance of GI tract flora and predisposes patients to infection with more virulent pathogens. Antineoplastic drugs (e.g., cyclophosphamide, doxorubicin, and fluorouracil) and acid-suppressive therapy (e.g., H_2-receptor antagonists, proton pump inhibitors, and antacids) also may result in changes in GI flora and possibly predispose patients to infection.[15]

Numerous factors, such as underlying disease, immunosuppressive drug therapy, and antimicrobial administration, determine the immunocompromised host's risk of developing infection. Several risk factors are present concomitantly in many patients (see Table 120–1).

ETIOLOGY OF INFECTIONS IN NEUTROPENIC CANCER PATIENTS

Infection remains a significant cause of morbidity and mortality in neutropenic cancer patients. More than 50% of febrile neutropenic patients have an established or occult infection.[1,6] Patients with profound neutropenia are at greatest risk for systemic infection, with at least 20% of these individuals developing bacteremia. Areas of impaired or damaged host defenses, such as the oropharynx, lungs, skin, sinuses, and GI tract, are common sites of infection. These local infections may progress to cause systemic infection and bacteremia.[12] Febrile episodes in neutropenic cancer patients can be attributed to microbiologically documented infection in only about 30% of cases, about one-half of which are due to bacteremia. Further, infections can be documented clinically in another 30% to 40% of patients, with the remaining 30% of patients manifesting infection only by fever.[3,10]

Table 120–1 lists organisms commonly infecting immunocompromised patients. About 60% of bacteremic episodes in cancer patients are the result of gram-positive organisms as compared with less than 30% of episodes documented during the 1970s and 1980s.[1,4,5] This shift is attributed to the frequent use of indwelling IV catheters and broad-spectrum antibiotics with excellent gram-negative activity but relatively poor gram-positive coverage, higher rates of mucositis caused by aggressive cancer treatments, and prophylaxis with trimethoprim-sulfamethoxazole or quinolones.[4,5,8,10,13] S. aureus and coagulase-negative staphylococci (especially S. epidermidis) are the most common organisms, but Bacillus spp. and Corynebacterium jeikeium are also important pathogens.[1,6,10] Data from the United States Centers for Disease Control and Prevention's (CDC) National Nosocomial Infection Surveillance System (NNIS) indicate increasing rates of methicillin-resistant staphylococcal infections in the hospital setting,[16] and resistance also is being observed in community-acquired staphylococcal infections. Viridans streptococci, which may be resistant to β-lactams, also have emerged as important pathogens, particularly in patients with chemotherapy-induced mucositis of the oropharynx.[5,10,17] Enterococci, including vancomycin-resistant strains, also may be problematic in many institutions.[4,8] Bacteremia caused by vancomycin-resistant enterococci (VRE) in neutropenic patients is associated with a mortality rate exceeding 70%.[5]

Overall, gram-positive infections do not always cause immediately life-threatening infections and are associated with somewhat lower mortality rates as compared with gram-negative infections.[1,10] However, gram-positive infections may cause severe complications, such as disseminated intravascular coagulation (DIC) and acute respiratory distress syndrome (ARDS). Methicillin-resistant S. aureus infections are associated with increased morbidity and mortality and hospital costs compared with susceptible organisms.[18] Thus prevention and timely diagnosis and treatment of gram-positive infections are clearly of great importance in the management of neutropenic cancer patients.

Gram-negative infections remain important causes of morbidity and mortality in immunocompromised cancer patients, but the relative frequency of infection owing to specific pathogens has been shifting among gram-negative infections. Escherichia coli and Klebsiella spp. remain the most common isolates at many centers. Strains of Klebsiella spp. producing plasmid-mediated extended-spectrum β-lactamases that hydrolyze extended-spectrum cephalosporins have emerged and are cause for concern.[1] The frequency of infections resulting from other gram-negative organisms, such as Enterobacter, Serratia, and Citrobacter, has been increasing.[8] Enterobacter spp.

are important causes of bacteremias; the use of broad-spectrum antibiotics, particularly third-generation cephalosporins, is thought to have played a major role in this trend. Infections owing to Enterobacter, Serratia, and Citrobacter may be difficult to treat because of the ease of β-lactamase induction and the more frequent development of resistance to multiple antibiotics.[3,8,10]

P. aeruginosa has long been an important pathogen in cancer patients. P. aeruginosa infection rates are decreasing in patients with solid tumors but not in patients with hematologic malignancies.[4,19,20] Infections caused by P. aeruginosa are associated with significant morbidity and mortality in neutropenic patients, with mortality rates of 33% to 75% reported.[10] The frequency of infection caused by difficult-to-treat organisms such as Stenotrophomonas maltophilia and Burkholderia cepacia appears to be increasing at many centers, probably because of selective pressures of broad-spectrum antimicrobial use.[5,10] Although the GI tract is a common site of bacterial infection, severe infections caused by anaerobic organisms are relatively infrequent. Anaerobes are found most frequently in mixed infections, such as perirectal cellulitis and mucositis-associated oropharyngeal infections.[10]

In addition to bacterial infections, neutropenic cancer patients are at risk for invasive fungal infections. Patients with extended periods of profound neutropenia who have been receiving broad-spectrum antibiotics, corticosteroids, or both are at the highest risk for invasive fungal infection. Up to one-third of febrile neutropenic patients who fail to respond to a week of broad-spectrum antibiotic therapy will have a systemic fungal infection.[1] A large international autopsy study revealed that up to 40% of patients with hematologic malignancies had deep fungal infections, many of which were undiagnosed prior to the time of death. Approximately 65% of these infections were the result of Candida spp., and another 30% were caused by Aspergillus spp.[21]

C. albicans is the most common fungal pathogen in neutropenic cancer patients.[5,22] Other species of Candida, such as C. tropicalis, C. parapsilosis, and C. krusei, are being isolated with increasing frequency. An increase also has been noted in infections caused by C. glabrata, Trichosporon spp., Fusarium spp., and Curvularia.[22–24] Because candidal species are normal flora, alteration of body host defenses is an important risk factor for the development of these infections. Oral thrush is the most common clinical manifestation of fungal infection. Mucous membranes damaged from chemotherapy and radiation serve as areas of candidal surface colonization and subsequent entry into the bloodstream; disease may then disseminate throughout the body. Organs such as the liver, spleen, kidney, and lungs are commonly involved in disseminated disease.[11,21,23] Hepatosplenic candidiasis, also known as chronic disseminated candidiasis, is an important infection in patients with hematologic malignancies.[3,25] Diagnosis of candidal infections is difficult and often requires invasive tissue sampling.[7] Overall mortality attributed to candidal infections in patients with invasive candidiasis is as high as 38%.[5]

Invasive infections caused by Aspergillus spp. are a very serious complication of neutropenia, with mortality approaching 80% in patients with prolonged neutropenia and/or patients undergoing allogeneic HSCT.[5] Infections resulting from Aspergillus spp. (including A. fumigatus, A. terreus, A. flavus, and A. niger) usually are acquired via inhalation of airborne spores. After colonizing the lungs, Aspergillus invades the lung parenchyma and pulmonary vessels, resulting in hemorrhage, pulmonary infarcts, and a high mortality rate. Invasive pulmonary disease is the dominant manifestation of infection in patients with neutropenia. However, Aspergillus spp.

also may cause other infections in neutropenic patients, including sinusitis, cutaneous infection, and disseminated disease involving multiple organs, including the central nervous system (CNS).[26] Prolonged neutropenia is the primary risk factor for invasive pulmonary aspergillosis in neutropenic patients with acute leukemia; use of corticosteroids also may predispose patients to disease.[26] Invasive aspergillosis should be suspected in neutropenic cancer patients colonized with *Aspergillus* (in sputum and/or nasal cultures) who remain persistently febrile despite a week or more of broad-spectrum antibiotic therapy.[1,26]

Chemotherapy-induced mucous membrane damage may predispose neutropenic cancer patients to the reactivation of herpes simplex virus (HSV), manifesting as gingivostomatitis or recurrent genital infections. Untreated oropharyngeal HSV infections may spread to involve the esophagus and often coexist with candidal infections. Clinical disease resulting from HSV occurs most often in patients with serologic evidence (e.g., serum antibodies to HSV) of prior infection. Both HSV-seropositive HSCT patients and HSV-seropositive leukemics receiving intensive chemotherapy are at high risk for recurrent HSV disease during periods of immunosuppression.[7]

Pneumocystis jiroveci and *Toxoplasma gondii* are the most common parasitic pathogens in immunocompromised cancer patients. Patients with hematologic malignancies (i.e., acute lymphocytic leukemia, lymphoma, and Hodgkin's disease) and those receiving high-dose corticosteroids as part of chemotherapy regimens are at the greatest risk of infection.[7] Routine use of trimethoprim-sulfamethoxazole prophylaxis, however, has reduced the incidence of these infections substantially.[1,27]

Because the majority of infecting organisms in cancer patients are from the host's own flora, some centers have employed routine surveillance cultures in an attempt to prospectively identify causes of fever and suspected infection. In a typical surveillance culture program, cultures of the nose, mouth, axillae, and perirectal area are performed twice weekly, and culture results are correlated with the clinical status of the patient. Because these cultures are costly and of low diagnostic yield, the utility of surveillance culture programs is felt to be limited. Surveillance cultures are, however, useful as research tools and in certain clinical situations; these situations include patients with prolonged profound neutropenia and in institutions with high rates of antimicrobial resistance or that have problems with virulent pathogens such as *P. aeruginosa* or *A. flavus*. Surveillance cultures should be limited to the anterior nares for detecting colonization with methicillin-resistant *S. aureus, Aspergillus,* and penicillin-resistant pneumococci and to the rectum for detecting *P. aeruginosa,* multiple-antibiotic-resistant gram-negative rods, and VRE.[1,10]

Knowledge of infection rates and local susceptibility patterns is essential for guiding optimal management of febrile neutropenia. These parameters must be monitored closely because the spectrum of infectious complications is related to multiple factors, including cancer chemotherapy regimens and antimicrobial therapy used for treatment and prophylaxis.

CLINICAL PRESENTATION

◀ The most important clinical finding in the neutropenic cancer patient is the presence of fever. Because of the potential for significant morbidity and mortality associated with infection in these patients, fever should be considered to be the result of infection until proved otherwise. At the appearance of fever, the patient should be evaluated carefully for other signs and symptoms of infection (see below).

CLINICAL PRESENTATION OF FEBRILE NEUTROPENIA[1,3,4,6,10]

GENERAL

- Because neutropenic cancer patients are at high risk for serious infections, frequent (at least daily), careful clinical assessments must be performed to search for possible evidence of infection.
- Physical assessment should include examination of all common sites of infection, including mouth/pharynx, nose and sinuses, respiratory tract, gastrointestinal tract, urinary tract, skin, soft tissues, perineum, and intravascular catheter insertion sites.

SYMPTOMS

- Usual signs and symptoms of infection may be absent or altered in neutropenic patients owing to low numbers of leukocytes and an inability to mount an inflammatory response (e.g., no infiltrate on chest x-ray, urinary tract infection without pyuria).
- Pain may be present at the infection site(s).

SIGNS

- Fever in this setting is defined as a single oral temperature of 38.3°C (101°F) or greater in the absence of other causes or a temperature 38°C (100.4°F) or greater for 1 hour or more. Other causes of fever unrelated to infection in this patient population include reactions to blood products, chemotherapeutic agents (and other drugs, including biologics), cell lysis, and the underlying malignancy.
- Usual signs of infection may be absent or altered; patients with bacteremia commonly exhibit no signs of infection other than fever.

LABORATORY TESTS

- Neutropenia (ANC ≤ 1000 cells/mm³)
- Blood cultures (two or more sets, including vascular access devices) for bacteria and fungi; cultures of other suspected infection sites (infection can be documented microbiologically in only about 30% of cases, about one-half of which are due to bacteremia).
- Other cultures should be obtained as indicated clinically according to the presence of signs or symptoms.
- Recent surveillance cultures (nasal, rectal) should be reviewed, if available.
- Complete blood count and blood chemistries should be obtained frequently to monitor neutropenia, plan supportive care, guide drug dosing, and assess patient's overall status.

OTHER DIAGNOSTIC TESTS

- Chest x-ray
- Aspiration, biopsy of skin lesions
- Other diagnostic tests as indicated clinically on the basis of physical examination and other assessments

▶ TREATMENT: Infections in Cancer Patients

■ FEBRILE EPISODES IN NEUTROPENIC CANCER PATIENTS

◀ ◀ The goals of antimicrobial therapy in neutropenic patients (including HSCT recipients) are (1) to protect the neutropenic patient from early death caused by undiagnosed infection, (2) to prevent breakthrough bacterial, fungal, viral, and protozoal infections during periods of neutropenia, and (3) to treat established infections effectively, all aimed at reducing patient morbidity and mortality and allowing for administration of optimal neoplastic therapy. All these goals must be achieved at the lowest possible toxicity and cost.

■ APPROACH TO TREATMENT

Guidelines for management of febrile episodes and documented infections in neutropenic patients are presented in Fig. 120–1 (from the Infectious Diseases Society of America [IDSA], revised in 2002).[1] Although many controversies remain regarding optimal management of these patients, the IDSA guidelines and those of other expert panels, such as the National Comprehensive Cancer Network (NCCN), offer an evidence-based consensus approach to the management of febrile neutropenia.

Because fever in the neutropenic cancer patient is considered the result of infection until proved otherwise, high-dose broad-spectrum bactericidal, usually parenteral, empirical antibiotic therapy should be initiated at the onset of fever or at the first signs or symptoms of infection. Withholding antibiotic therapy until isolation of an organism results in unacceptably high mortality rates. At least 50% of febrile neutropenic cancer patients have an established or occult infection, and at least 20% of profoundly neutropenic patients (ANC < 100 cells/mm^3) experience bacteremia.[1,6] In immunocompromised patients, undiagnosed infection can disseminate rapidly and result in death if left untreated or if treated improperly. Failure to initiate appropriate antibiotic therapy for *P. aeruginosa* bacteremia at the onset of fever in neutropenic cancer patients resulted in mortality rates of 15% and 70% within 12 and 48 hours, respectively.[19] Empirical antibiotic therapy is 70% to 90% effective at reducing early morbidity and mortality.[10] Therapy must be appropriate, however, and initiated promptly. Antimicrobial therapy also should be initiated promptly in afebrile cancer patients with signs and symptoms of infection.

When designing optimal empirical antibiotic regimens, clinicians must consider infection patterns and antimicrobial susceptibility trends in their respective institutions. Also, patient factors, such as risk for infection, drug allergies and concomitant nephrotoxins, and previous antimicrobial exposure (including prophylaxis), must be considered.[6] The first step in choosing empirical antimicrobial therapy is to determine the patient's risk of infection, which will help to guide the route and setting for therapy administration. Patients with neutropenia can be divided into low-, moderate-, and high-risk groups based on the projected duration of neutropenia and other risk factors for serious infection[5,28] (Table 120–2). Patients with neutropenia of short duration (≤7 days) are considered to be at relatively low risk of severe infection. Patients with neutropenia lasting 7 to 14 days are considered to be at moderate risk for severe infection. High-risk patients are those with neutropenia for 14 or more days; these patients are at increased risk for severe infection from bacteria, as well as from fungi, viruses, and parasites. Oral empirical antimicrobial therapy may be appropriate for low-risk patients. The patient's overall clinical condition and other risk factors for infection determine whether this oral therapy is administered on an inpatient or outpatient basis. If therapy is administered on an outpatient basis, the patient must be compliant with treatment and have prompt access to medical care around the clock, should his or her condition worsen. Patients considered at moderate risk of infection should receive at least the first few days of therapy administered parenterally in the hospital

TABLE 120–2. Risk-Based Therapy for Febrile Patients with Neutropenia

Risk Group	Patient Characteristics	Treatment Strategies
High risk	*Neutropenia:* Severe (ANC < 100/mm^3) and/or prolonged (≥14 days) *Malignancy/treatment:* Hematologic malignancy or allogeneic HSCT *Comorbidities:* Substantial comorbidity; poor performance status *Clinical status:* Clinical or hemodynamic instability (e.g., shock) and/or complex infection (e.g., pneumonia, bacteremia) *Response to initial therapy:* Slow response	*Therapy/setting:* Broad-spectrum, parenteral (IV) therapy, hospital-based for duration of febrile neutropenia
Moderate risk	*Neutropenia:* Moderate duration (7–14 days) *Malignancy/treatment:* Solid tumor treated with autologous HSCT *Comorbidities:* Minimal medical comorbidity *Clinical status:* Clinically stable *Response to initial therapy:* Favorable (e.g., early defervescence)	*Therapy/setting:* Initial parenteral, hospital-based therapy, followed by early discharge on a parenteral or oral regimen (sequential)
Low risk	*Neutropenia:* Short duration (≤7 days) *Malignancy/treatment:* Solid tumor treated with conventional chemotherapy *Comorbidities:* None *Clinical status:* Clinically stable at onset of fever; no identified focus of infection, or simple infection (e.g., UTI)	*Therapy/setting:* Broad-spectrum outpatient therapy (parenteral, sequential, or oral) for the entire episode

Adapted from refs. 1, 5, 6, and 28–33.

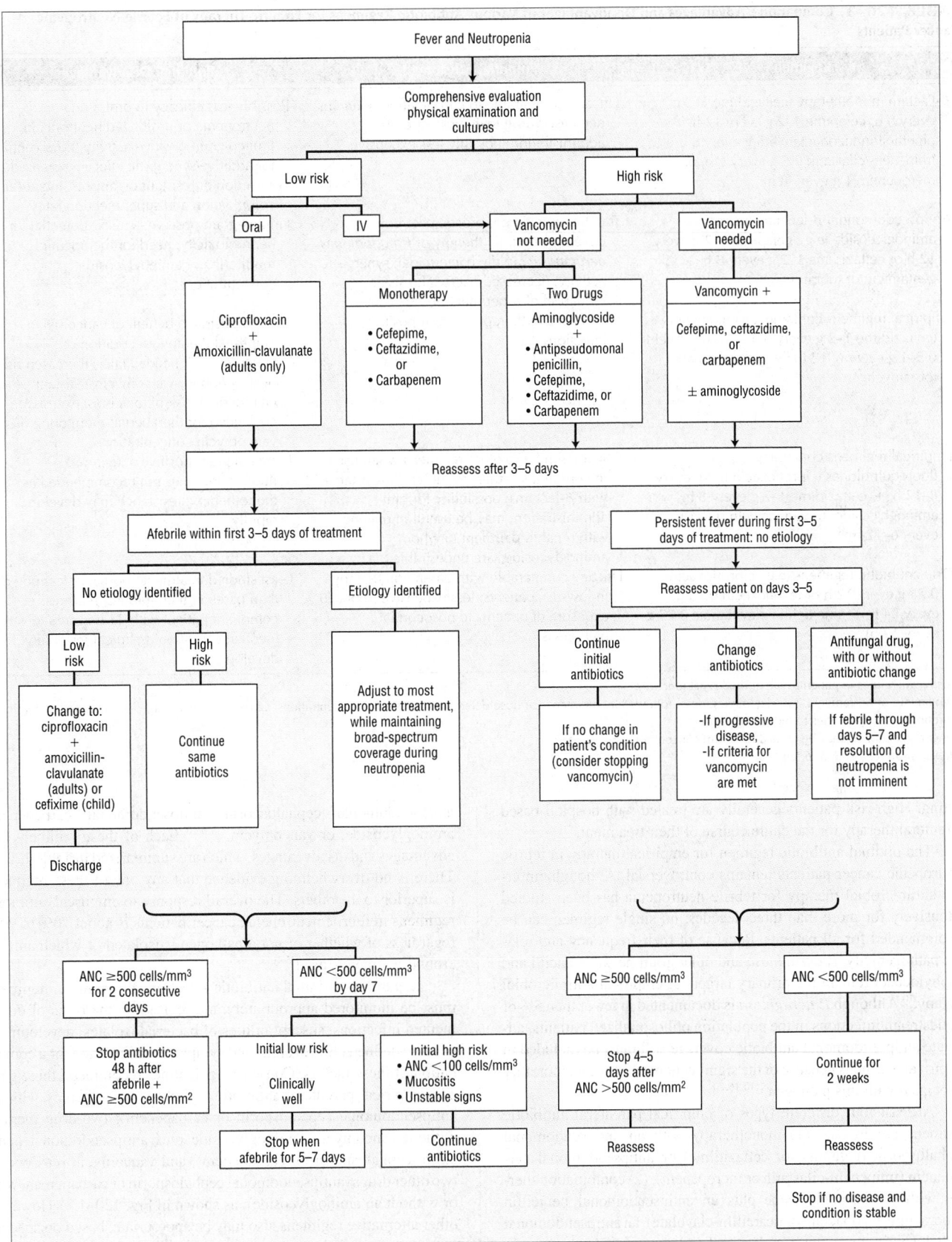

FIGURE 120–1. Management of febrile episodes in neutropenic cancer patients. ANC = absolute neutrophil count; carbapenem = imipenem-cilastatin, meropenem. *(Adapted from Ref. 2.)*

TABLE 120–3. Comparative Advantages and Disadvantages of Various Antibiotic Regimens for Empiric Therapy of Febrile Neutropenic Cancer Patients

Regimen	Potential Advantages	Potential Disadvantages
β-Lactam monotherapy (ceftazidime 1–2 g every 8 h, cefepime 1–2 g every 12 h, piperacillin/tazobactam 4.5 g every 6 h, imipenem/cilastatin 0.5 g every 6 h, or meropenem 1 g every 8 h)[a]	Efficacy comparable to combination regimens; decreased drug toxicities; ease of administration; possibly less expensive	Possibly less efficacy in profound neutropenia or prolonged neutropenia; limited gram-positive activity; no potential for additive/synergistic effects; increased selection of resistant organisms; increased colonization and superinfection rates
Antipseudomonal β-lactam plus aminoglycoside (e.g., cefepime 1–2 g every 12 h or ceftazidime 1–2 g every 8 h + gentamicin or tobramycin)[a,b]	Traditional regimen, broad-spectrum coverage; optimal therapy of Pseudomonas aeruginosa; rapidly bactericidal; synergistic activity; decreased bacterial resistance; reduction of superinfections	Limited gram-positive activity; potential for nephrotoxicity; need for therapeutic monitoring of aminoglycoside concentrations
Empirical regimens containing vancomycin (ceftazidime 1–2 g every 8 h + vancomycin 0.5–1 g every 6–12 h)[a] ± gentamicin or tobramycin[b]	Early effective therapy of gram-positive infections	No demonstrated benefit of vancomycin empirical therapy vs. addition of vancomycin if needed later; increased risk of selection for vancomycin-resistant enterococci; risk of toxicities; excessive cost; need for therapeutic monitoring of vancomycin concentrations
Empirical regimens containing fluoroquinolones (ciprofloxacin 0.4 g every 8–12 h + ceftazidime 1–2 g every 8 h, aminoglycoside, or vancomycin 0.5–1 g every 6–12 h)[a]	Efficacy similar to other regimens when used in combination therapy; no cross-resistance with β-lactams; possibility for oral administration; may be useful in patients with renal impairment in whom aminoglycosides are undesirable	Marginal gram-positive activity; fluoroquinolones not recommended as monotherapy; resistance may develop rapidly
Oral antibiotic regimens (e.g., ciprofloxacin 0.75 g every 12 h or levofloxacin 0.75 g every 24 h + amoxicillin-clavulanate 0.75 g every 12 h)	Efficacy comparable with parenteral therapy in low-risk patients; less expensive; reduced exposure of patients to nosocomial pathogens	Least studied treatment approach; less potent than parenteral antibiotics; requires compliant patient with 24 h access to medical care should clinical instability develop

[a]Dosing guidelines in patients with normal renal function.
[b]Gentamicin or tobramycin 2 mg/kg loading dose, followed by maintenance dose determined by serum concentrations. Choice of specific agent determined according to institutional susceptibilities to individual drugs.
[c]Vancomycin dosing may be guided by serum concentrations.
Adapted from refs. 1, 3, 5, 6, and 10.

setting. High-risk patients generally are treated with hospital-based parenteral therapy for the entire course of their treatment.

The optimal antibiotic regimen for empirical therapy in febrile neutropenic cancer patients remains controversial. Although empirical antimicrobial therapy for febrile neutropenia has been studied extensively for more than three decades, no single regimen can be recommended for all patients. Because of their frequency and relative pathogenicity, P. aeruginosa and other gram-negative bacilli and staphylococci remain the primary targets of empirical antimicrobial therapy.[10] Although P. aeruginosa is documented in fewer than 5% of bloodstream infections in the population of hospitalized patients, adequate antipseudomonal antibiotic coverage still must be included in empirical regimens because of the significant morbidity and mortality associated with this pathogen.[1,10,16,20]

At least four different types of empirical parenteral antibiotic regimens are in use: (1) monotherapy with an antipseudomonal cephalosporin (cefepime or ceftazidime) or antipseudomonal carbapenem (imipenem-cilastatin or meropenem), (2) combination therapy with an aminoglycoside plus an antipseudomonal penicillin (piperacillin-tazobactam or ticarcillin-clavulate), an antipseudomonal cephalosporin, or an antipseudomonal carbapenem, (3) vancomycin plus an antipseudomonal cephalosporin or antipseudomonal carbapenem, with or without an aminoglycoside, and (4) a fluoroquinolone (ciprofloxacin or levofloxacin) in combination with an

antipseudomonal cephalosporin, antipseudomonal carbapenem, aminoglycoside, or vancomycin.[1,3,6,10] Each of these regimens has advantages and disadvantages, which are summarized in Table 120–3. There is no overwhelming evidence that any one of these regimens is superior to the others. The overall response to empirical antibiotic regimens in febrile neutropenic cancer patients is about 70% to 90% regardless of whether or not a pathogen is isolated or which antimicrobial regimen is used.[5,10]

Regardless of initial antibiotic selection, all empirical regimens must be monitored appropriately and revised on the basis of documented infections, susceptibilities of bacterial isolates, development of more defined clinical signs and symptoms of infection, or a combination of these factors. Consensus guidelines recommend three general empirical parenteral antibiotic regimens (monotherapy with an antipseudomonal cephalosporin or carbapenem): two-drug therapy without vancomycin (aminoglycoside plus antipseudomonal penicillin, cephalosporin, or carbapenem), and vancomycin plus one to two other drugs (antipseudomonal cephalosporin or carbapenem, with or without an aminoglycoside), as shown in Fig. 120–1.[1,6] However, other alternative regimens also may be appropriate, based on specific patient characteristics.

Prompt initiation of broad-spectrum empirical antibiotic therapy is essential to prevent early morbidity and mortality in febrile neutropenic patients with cancer. Choice of empirical regimens should take into account the patient's risk of infection and clinical status, as well as patterns of hospital infections and susceptibility.

β-LACTAM MONOTHERAPY

Several β-lactam antibiotics in current use have been evaluated as monotherapy for the management of febrile episodes in neutropenic cancer patients, including antipseudomonal cephalosporins (ceftazidime and cefepime), antipseudomonal penicillins (ticarcillin–clavulanic acid and piperacillin-tazobactam), and antipseudomonal carbapenems (imipenem-cilastatin and meropenem).[1,3,6,10] An early landmark study compared ceftazidime monotherapy with a three-drug combination (cephalothin, gentamicin, and carbenicillin) in 550 episodes of fever and neutropenia.[34] Ceftazidime monotherapy was as effective as combination therapy in initial empirical management (first 72 hours); 78% of febrile patients with undocumented infections were managed successfully with one antibiotic, and no morbidity or mortality resulted from adding other antimicrobial agents only when indicated clinically. Similar favorable results were reported with cefepime and the antipseudomonal carbapenems.[1,35–38] A meta-analysis of 29 randomized clinical trials involving almost 4800 patients revealed that monotherapy with an antipseudomonal cephalosporin or carbapenem is at least as effective as aminoglycoside-containing combination regimens in the empirical treatment of febrile neutropenia.[39] These results were confirmed in a second meta-analysis of 46 clinical trials involving more than 7600 patients that revealed no significant differences between monotherapy and combination therapy (β-lactam/aminoglycoside) in rates of survival, treatment response, and bacterial/fungal superinfections but a higher rate of adverse events in patients receiving combination therapy.[40]

The use of monotherapy has several potential advantages and disadvantages (see Table 120–3). Perhaps the most common concerns are those regarding the selection of resistant strains of organisms, such as *P. aeruginosa, Enterobacter* spp., and *Serratia* spp., through extended-spectrum β-lactamases and type 1 β-lactamases, especially with ceftazidime.[1,6,41] Activity against gram-positive organisms, such as coagulase-negative staphylococci, methicillin-resistant *S. aureus,* enterococci (including vancomycin-resistant enterococci), penicillin-resistant *S. pneumoniae,* and some strains of viridans streptococci is poor with some single β-lactams, but cefepime and antipseudomonal carbapenems have good activity against viridans streptococci and pneumococci.[1] Although ceftazidime has been studied widely and used in the treatment of febrile neutropenia, newer agents may be more optimal owing to ceftazidime's susceptibility to β-lactamase induction and lower activity against gram-positive organisms.[1] For example, higher clinical response rates are achieved with meropenem than with ceftazidime.[42]

As with all empirical antibiotic regimens, patients receiving monotherapy should be monitored closely for treatment failure, secondary infections, and the development of resistance. Use of monotherapy may not be appropriate in institutions with high rates of gram-positive infections or infections caused by gram-negative pathogens such as *P. aeruginosa* and *Enterobacter* spp. Imipenem-cilastatin and meropenem, however, are less susceptible to inducible β-lactamases and often may be used effectively in these institutions. Overall, similar efficacy has been observed with monotherapy with antipseudomonal β-lactams and aminoglycoside combination therapy in the treatment of *P. aeruginosa* infections.[20]

AMINOGLYCOSIDE PLUS ANTIPSEUDOMONAL β-LACTAM

Regimens consisting of an aminoglycoside plus an antipseudomonal penicillin, antipseudomonal cephalosporin, or antipseudomonal carbapenem traditionally have been the most commonly used regimens for empirical treatment of febrile neutropenia, although many such regimens may lack adequate gram-positive activity[14] (see Table 120–3). This relative lack of activity remains a concern because of the increasing frequency of gram-positive infections. The choice of aminoglycoside and β-lactam for inclusion in empirical regimens should be based on institutional epidemiology and antimicrobial susceptibility patterns. If *P. aeruginosa* is a common institutional pathogen, use of empirical tobramycin or amikacin may be strongly considered because they are generally more active than gentamicin against this organism. However, gentamicin is still an appropriate choice in many institutions based on known susceptibility patterns in those locations. Similar efficacy is observed with an antipseudomonal penicillin, antipseudomonal cephalosporin, or antipseudomonal carbapenem in combination with an aminoglycoside.[1]

Combinations of broad-spectrum β-lactams and aminoglycosides often provide synergistic activity against bacteria commonly infecting neutropenic patients. The exact role of synergy in the outcome of febrile neutropenic patients treated with empirical antibiotic therapy, however, remains somewhat controversial, particularly in light of the efficacy of single-drug regimens. Nevertheless, synergistic combinations of antibiotics appear to be beneficial in patients with persistent, profound neutropenia. Moreover, administration of antipseudomonal β-lactams in combination with an aminoglycoside may result in a lower rate of drug resistance.[5]

Aminoglycoside toxicity may be a concern in patients receiving these regimens who are already receiving other nephrotoxic drugs, such as cisplatin and cyclosporine. Administration of aminoglycosides in large single daily doses (once-daily dosing) may be as effective, less costly, and no more toxic than conventional dosing methods.[43] A review of randomized, prospective trials in febrile neutropenia failed to find significant differences in either efficacy or toxicity between once-daily dosing and traditional dosing of aminoglycosides.[43] Although once-daily aminoglycoside dosing regimens appear to be safe and effective in these patients, there are not yet sufficient data to recommend once-daily dosing for routine use in this population.[5]

EMPIRICAL REGIMENS CONTAINING VANCOMYCIN

There has been considerable debate over the inclusion of vancomycin in initial empirical therapy of febrile neutropenic cancer patients. This controversy continues because of the increasing incidence of gram-positive infections in this population. One approach is to include vancomycin in the initial empirical antibiotic regimen, thereby providing early effective treatment of possible gram-positive infections. Decreased mortality from penicillin-resistant viridans streptococcal infections has been observed when vancomycin was included in initial therapy.[1,5] A second approach is to withhold vancomycin from initial empirical regimens, later adding the drug if gram-positive organisms are isolated from cultures or if there is no response to initial therapy. Support for both these approaches can be found in the medical literature.[1,6,10,44] Prospective studies indicate that there is no advantage to adding vancomycin to initial empirical regimens routinely if vancomcyin can be added later as needed.[14,44,45] In addition to increased costs of therapy, there is overwhelming evidence that the selection of vancomycin-resistant enterococci (VRE) is associated with excessive vancomycin use.[46]

Inclusion of vancomycin in initial empirical regimens may be more appropriate today because of higher rates of methicillin-resistant staphylococcal infections, as well as aggressive chemotherapy regimens causing significant mucosal damage that increases the risk for streptococcal infections. Vancomycin is recommended for inclusion in initial empirical regimens in patients at high risk of gram-positive infection, particularly due to methicillin-resistant *S. aureus* and coagulase-negative staphylococci (including those with evidence of infection of central venous catheters and other indwelling lines), high risk of viridans streptococcal infection due to severe mucositis, or pneumonitis in hospitals with high rates of methicillin-resistant staphylococcal infections.[1,3,6,10,17,46] Rates of β-lactam resistance among viridians streptococci are in the range of 18% to 29%.[6] Empirical vancomycin use also may be justified in institutions employing empirical or prophylactic antibiotic regimens without good activity against streptococci (e.g., ciprofloxacin) and in patients known to be colonized with methicillin-resistant staphylococci or β-lactam–resistant pneumococci. In patients with preliminary culture results indicating gram-positive infection, empirical vancomycin is appropriate while the susceptibility results are pending. Lastly, empirical use of vancomycin may be recommended in patients with hypotension or other evidence of cardiovascular impairment without an identified pathogen.[6,17,46] If empirical vancomycin therapy is initiated and no evidence of gram-positive infection is found after 24 to 48 hours, the drug should be discontinued.[1,5,6] Continuing vancomycin when not warranted results in higher costs, more toxicities, and greater risk of development of VRE.[44]

Vancomycin plus carbapenem regimens may have advantages over vancomcyin plus cephalosporin regimens because of lower rates of carbapenem resistance to gram-negative bacilli.[1] Newer antimicrobial agents such as quinupristin-dalfopristin and linezolid should be reserved for documented infections caused by multiresistant gram-positive pathogens such as VRE; the role of these drugs in the routine treatment of fever in neutropenic patients is undetermined, and linezolid is associated with myelosuppression.[1,6]

CLINICAL CONTROVERSY

Inclusion of vancomycin into empirical antimicrobial regimens for febrile neutropenia remains controversial. Vancomycin should be included in initial regimens for patients with evidence of gram-positive infections or at high risk for these infections, as determined by patient characteristics and institutional infection and susceptibility patterns.

FLUOROQUINOLONES AS A COMPONENT OF EMPIRICAL REGIMENS

Because the fluoroquinolone antibiotics have broad-spectrum activity (particularly against gram-negative pathogens), rapid bactericidal activity, and favorable pharmacokinetic and toxicity profiles, these agents have been investigated as empirical therapy in febrile neutropenic cancer patients. Ciprofloxacin is the preferred quinolone for use in this clinical setting because of its relatively better activity against *P. aeruginosa*. Response rates of quinolone-containing combination regimens are comparable with those obtained with the other regimens described previously.[1,5,47,48] Ciprofloxacin is not rec-

ommended for monotherapy, however, because of its relatively poor activity against gram-positive pathogens, particularly streptococci, and variable response rates in clinical studies.[1] Quinolones should not be used as empirical therapy in patients who have received quinolones as infection prophylaxis because of the risk of drug resistance.[1,6,10] Rates of fluoroquinolone resistance are increasing, and streptococcal treatment failures are a concern.[49] Although fluoroquinolones are not generally considered first-line empirical therapy, they may be useful as one component of combination regimens in patients with allergies or other contraindications to first-line agents.

ORAL ANTIBIOTIC THERAPY FOR MANAGEMENT OF FEBRILE NEUTROPENIA

An individual patient's risk of severe infection (influenced by degree/duration of neutropenia and other patient variables) determines appropriate antibiotic therapy and setting for administration (see Table 120–2 for patient characteristics and levels of infection risk in patients with neutropenia).[1,5,6,28] Risk stratification is based on several parameters, including duration and extent of neutropenia, type of cancer and its management (including history of HSCT), clinical status, comorbidities, and response to empirical antimicrobial therapy.[28] Because of the excellent spectrum of activity and favorable pharmacokinetics of relatively newer oral antibiotics, particularly the fluoroquinolones, oral antibiotics may have a role in the management of selected patients. In patients at low risk for severe bacterial infection, empirical therapy with broad-spectrum oral antibiotic agents achieves similar patient outcomes as parenteral antibiotics, with response rates of 77% to 95%.[5,29,30] The availability of oral antibiotics with broad spectra of activity has made possible the treatment of febrile neutropenia in low-risk patients completely in the outpatient setting. Patients with solid tumors undergoing conventional chemotherapy with an expected duration of neutropenia of less than 7 to 10 days and who are clinically stable may be appropriate candidates for oral antibiotic therapy administered on an outpatient basis.[5,28–31] Fluoroquinolones, either as monotherapy or in combination with amoxicillin-clavulanate (or clindamycin for penicillin-allergic patients) for enhanced gram-positive coverage, have been studied most commonly for outpatient therapy in low-risk patients. IDSA and NCCN guidelines recommend oral antibiotic therapy with ciprofloxacin plus amoxicillin-clavulanate in clinically stable low-risk adults (particularly those with recovering neutrophils) with no focus of bacterial infection and no signs of infection other than fever.[1,6] Oral cephalosporins such as cefixime also may be suitable for outpatient treatment.[1] Careful patient selection obviously is required for such management strategies; important patient characteristics include a history of medication compliance, good caregiver support, and close proximity to medical care in the event of failure to respond to outpatient antibiotic therapy. Benefits of oral therapy on an outpatient basis include increased convenience and quality of life for patients and caregivers and reduced exposure to multidrug-resistant institutional pathogens.[5] Outpatient therapy of low-risk patients is now common practice in many institutions.

In patients at moderate risk for severe bacterial infection, oral antibiotics may place a role in step-down therapy. Carefully selected neutropenic patients may be switched safely from broad-spectrum parenteral therapy to oral antibiotic regimens (e.g., ciprofloxacin plus amoxicillin-clavulanate) with response rates comparable to patients remaining on IV therapy.[10,28,32] Patient selection criteria generally include defervescence within 72 hours of initiation of parenteral therapy, hemodynamic stability, absence of positive cultures or a discernible site of infection, and ability to take oral medications. Many of these patients are able to complete their course of therapy at home.[1,10,28,32]

Changing parenteral antimicrobials to oral regimens in carefully selected patients is now relatively common practice and allows for less expensive hospitalizations and earlier patient discharges.

ANTIMICROBIAL THERAPY AFTER INITIATION OF EMPIRICAL THERAPY

After initiation of empirical antimicrobial therapy, judicious assessment of febrile neutropenic cancer patients is mandatory to evaluate response, clinical status, laboratory data, and potential need for therapy adjustments. After the administration of 72 hours or more of empirical antimicrobial therapy, the clinical status and culture results of febrile neutropenic patients should be reevaluated to determine whether or not therapeutic modifications are necessary. Additions or modifications to the initial antimicrobial regimen likely will be required in patients with ANCs of fewer than 500 cells/mm³ for greater than a week. Modifications of antimicrobial therapy should be based on clinical and laboratory data; antibiotic therapy should be optimized based on culture results. However, during periods of neutropenia, patients generally should continue to receive broad-spectrum therapy because of the risk of secondary infections or breakthrough bacteremias when antimicrobial coverage is too narrow.[1,5,10]

In patients who become afebrile after 3 to 5 days of therapy with no infection identified, it is generally optimal to continue antibiotic therapy until neutropenia has resolved (ANC ≥ 500 cells/mm³). Some clinicians elect to switch therapy from IV antibiotics to an oral regimen of ciprofloxacin plus amoxicillin-clavulanate after 2 days of IV therapy in low- to moderate-risk patients who become afebrile and have no evidence of infection. This approach may facilitate earlier hospital discharge. In high-risk patients, the parenteral antibiotic regimen should be continued for 7 days or more.[1,6] However, in afebrile patients with prolonged neutropenia but no signs or symptoms of infection, consideration can be given to discontinuing antibiotic therapy, provided patients can be observed carefully and have ready access to medical care.

The optimal management of patients who remain febrile in the absence of microbiologic or clinical documentation of infection remains highly controversial. The median time to defervescence of febrile neutropenic cancer patients receiving empirical antibiotic therapy is 5 to 7 days.[50] Persistently febrile patients should be evaluated carefully, but modifications generally are not made to initial antimicrobial regimens within the first 5 days of therapy unless there is evidence of clinical deterioration[1,5,6,14] (see Fig. 120–1). It important to note that the persistence of fever does not necessarily mean failure of a given antimicrobial regimen. This is particularly true if patients are otherwise clinically stable. Fever after 3 or more days of antibiotic therapy can be due to a number of causes, including nonbacterial infection, resistant bacterial infection or infection slow to respond to therapy, emergence of a secondary infection, inadequate drug concentrations, drug fever, cell wall–deficient bacteremia, and fever at an avascular site (e.g., catheter infection or abscess).[1,5] Patients with documented infection who are receiving appropriate antimicrobial therapy (based on in vitro susceptibility tests) often will remain febrile until resolution of neutropenia occurs.

Need for modification of antimicrobial therapy should be evaluated in neutropenic cancer patients who remain febrile despite 3 to 5 days of antibiotic therapy. The same antibiotic regimen can be continued in febrile but stable patients, especially if neutropenia is expected to resolve within a week. The antibiotic regimen may require modification in patients experiencing toxicities, as well as in patients

with evidence of progressive disease or documentation of an organism not covered by the initial regimen. When a causative organism is identified, specific therapy directed at the organism should be included; however, patients should continue to receive broad-spectrum therapy while they remain neutropenic.[1,3,5,10] Need for the addition of vancomycin should be considered as warranted by clinical and laboratory findings; however, if vancomycin was a component of the initial empirical regimen and the patient is still febrile after 3 days of therapy, discontinuation of vancomycin should be considered to reduce the risk of resistance.

INITIATION OF ANTIFUNGAL THERAPY

Neutropenic patients who remain febrile despite 5 or more days of broad-spectrum antibiotic therapy are candidates for antifungal therapy. A high percentage of febrile patients who die during prolonged neutropenia have evidence of invasive fungal infection on autopsy, even though many had no evidence of fungal disease before death.[21] Persistence of fever or development of a new fever during broad-spectrum antibiotic therapy may indicate the presence of a fungal infection most commonly due to *Candida* and *Aspergillus* spp. in approximately 33% of patients.[10] Blood cultures are positive in fewer than 50% of neutropenic patients with invasive fungal infections.[10] The lack of rapid, sensitive diagnostic tests for fungi and the high morbidity and mortality associated with waiting for isolation of fungal organisms justify the empirical addition of antifungal therapy in this clinical setting.[10] Therefore, empirical antifungal therapy should be initiated after 5 to 7 days of broad-spectrum antibiotic therapy at adequate doses to treat undiagnosed fungal infection and prevent fungal superinfection in high-risk febrile neutropenic patients.[22]

The optimal empirical antifungal regimen is not known presently. Empirical coverage for both *Candida* spp. and *Aspergillus* should be considered because these organisms are responsible for more than 90% of fungal infections in neutropenic cancer patients.[7] *Aspergillus* is particularly common in patients with hematologic malignancies and in patients undergoing HSCT; therefore, amphotericin B usually is preferred in these patients.[10,21] In the setting of febrile neutropenia, lipid-associated amphotericin B products are similar in efficacy to conventional amphotericin B while causing fewer toxicities.[51,52] However, the relative lack of experience with these products and significantly higher cost in comparison with conventional amphotericin B make their role in the empirical therapy of febrile neutropenia uncertain at this time.[1,10,51,52] Amphotericin B lipid-associated drugs may be appropriate in patients with preexisting renal dysfunction, renal dysfunction or infusion-related toxicities from conventional amphotericin B therapy, and in patients experiencing treatment failure of suspected/documented fungal infections on conventional amphotericin B therapy.[1,12]

The azole compounds fluconazole and itraconazole are used in the management of febrile neutropenia. Despite the high rate of amphotericin B toxicities, concerns regarding the emergence of azole-resistant fungi have prevented these agents from replacing amphotericin B as the "gold standard" in persistently febrile neutropenic patients. However, fluconazole can be a useful alternative to amphotericin B for empirical antifungal use in hospitals in which *Aspergillus* infections and infections due to *C. krusei* and drug-resistant *C. glabrata* are not common.[1] If fluconazole is used as antifungal prophylaxis in cancer patients, it should not be included in empirical antifungal regimens. Itraconazole has similar efficacy as amphotericin B, with fewer toxicities, and availability in both parenteral and oral forms provides a platform for step-down therapy if

TABLE 120–4. Infectious Complications after Bone Marrow and Solid Organ Transplantation: Syndromes of Disease and Treatment Guidelines

Pathogen	Syndromes of Disease	Treatment
Bacterial		
Gram-negative aerobic bacilli (Enterobacteriaceae, *Pseudomonas aeruginosa, Hemophilus influenzae*)	Blood, urinary tract, pulmonary, abdomen	*Empiric:* Ceftazidime 1–2 g every 8 h + Aminoglycoside,[a,b] cefepime 1–2 g every 12 h + aminoglycoside;[a,b] piperacillin-tazobactam 3.375–4.5 g every 4–6 h; imipenem-cilastatin 0.25–0.5 g every 6 h ± aminoglycoside[a,b] *Definitive:* According to culture and sensitivity results
Gram-positive cocci (*Staphylococcus aureus, S. epidermidis, Streptococcus pneumoniae, E. faecalis*)	Skin, blood, urinary tract, pulmonary, abdomen	*Empiric:* Nafcillin 1–2 g every 4–6 h; vancomycin 0.5–1 g every 6–12 h[c] *Definitive:* According to culture and sensitivity results
Legionella spp.	Pulmonary	Erythromycin 0.5–1 g every 6 h
Listeria monocytogenes	Central nervous system	Ampicillin 1–2 g every 4–6 h with gentamicin;[a] TMP-SMX 4 mg/kg every 12 h[d]
Nocardia spp.	Skin, pulmonary, central nervous system	Sulfadiazine 1 g every 4–6 h; TMP/SMX 4 mg/kg every 12 h[d]
Fungal		
Candida spp.	Blood, urinary tract, mucous membranes, skin	Clotrimazole 10 mg five times daily; nystatin 100,000 U every 6 h; ketoconazole 200 mg daily; fluconazole 100–400 mg daily; itraconazole 200–400 mg daily; amphotericin B 0.5–0.7 mg/kg/day ± 5-flucytosine 100–150 mg/kg/day divided every 6 h
Aspergillus spp.	Skin, pulmonary, central nervous system	Amphotericin B 1 mg/kg/day ± 5-flucytosine; itraconazole 200–400 mg daily; lipid-associated amphotericin B 4–5 mg/kg daily;[e] caspofungin 50 mg daily[e]; voriconizole 4 mg/kg every 12 h[e]
Cryptococcus neoformans	Skin, pulmonary, central nervous system	Amphotericin 0.5 mg/kg/day ± 5-flucytosine; fluconazole 400 mg daily
Zygomycetes (Mucor)	Rhinocerebral disease	Amphotericin B 1 mg/kg/day; lipid-associated amphotericin B 4–5 mg/kg daily[e]
Viral		
Herpes simplex virus	Skin, central nervous system, mucous membranes, pulmonary	Acyclovir 5–10 mg/kg every 8 h; foscarnet 60 mg/kg every 8 h
Cytomegalovirus	Pulmonary, blood, urinary tract, GI tract	Ganciclovir 5 mg/kg every 12 h; foscarnet 60 mg/kg every 8 h; hyperimmune globulins 100–500 mg/kg every 1–2 wk
Varicella-zoster virus	Skin, disseminated disease	Acyclovir 10 mg/kg every 8 h; foscarnet 60 mg/kg every 8 h
Epstein-Barr virus	Lymphoproliferative disease	No effective treatment
Papoviruses (BK, JC)	Skin, central nervous system	No effective treatment
Protozoal/parasitic		
Pneumocystis jiroveci	Pulmonary	TMP-SMX 15–20 mg/kg/day divided every 6 h[d]; atovaquone 750 mg every 12 h; pentamidine 4 mg/kg daily; dapsone 100 mg daily + TMP 15–20 mg/kg/day divided every 6 h; clindamycin 450–600 mg every 6 h + primaquine 15 mg daily
Toxoplasma gondii	Central nervous system	Pyrimethamine 50–100 mg daily + sulfadiazine 1 g every 4–6 h[f]; pyrimethamine 50–100 mg daily + clindamycin 450–600 mg every 6 h[f]
Strongyloides stercoralis	Pulmonary, central nervous system	Thiabendazole 25 mg/kg every 12 h (max 3 g/day)

[a]Gentamicin or tobramycin 2 mg/kg loading dose, followed by maintenance dose determined by serum concentrations. Choice of specific agent determined according to institutional susceptibilities to individual drugs.
[b]For penicillin-allergic adults, use ciprofloxacin 0.4 g every 8–12 h plus an aminoglycoside.
[c]Vancomycin dosing may be guided by serum concentrations.
[d]Based on the trimethoprim component of the combination.
[e]For use in cases refractory to amphotericin B or itraconazole.
[f]Folinic acid (5–10 mg/day) often recommended in conjunction with pyrimethamine-containing regimens for prevention of bone marrow toxicity.
TMP-SMX = trimethoprim-sulfamethoxazole

dicated clinically.[53] Use of voriconazole should be limited to allogeneic HSCT patients and patients with relapsed leukemia, and the ole of caspofungin in the setting of neutropenic fever remains to be etermined.[22,54]

As with antibiotic therapy, the optimal duration of antifungal herapy remains controversial. Most clinicians agree that antifungal herapy can be discontinued when neutropenia has resolved in clincally stable patients with no evidence of fungal infection. In neuropenic patients, antifungal therapy generally should be continued or at least 2 weeks in the absence of signs and symptoms of acive fungal disease, but many experts advocate continuing therapy ntil resolution of the neutropenia.[5,22] In neutropenic patients with locumented fungal disease, antifungal therapy should be directed at he causative organism, and therapy should be continued for at least weeks and clinical and culture data indicate resolution of the inection. In addition to fungal infections, other causes of persistent ever of unknown origin include resistant bacterial infection, tissue lecrosis as a result of underlying tumor, nonbacterial and nonfungal nfection (e.g., viral, mycobacterial, or parasitic), and drug or blood product administration. Treatment recommendations for specific fungal infections can be found in Table 120–4.

INITIATION OF ANTIVIRAL THERAPY

Febrile neutropenic patients with vesicular or ulcerative skin or mucosal lesions should be evaluated carefully for infection due to herpes simplex virus (HSV) or varicella-zoster virus (VZV). Mucosal lesions rom viral infections provide a portal of entry for bacteria and fungi luring periods of immunosuppression. If viral infection is presumed or documented, neutropenic patients should receive aggressive antivial therapy to aid healing of primary lesions and prevent disseminated lisease. Acyclovir traditionally has been used in this population. However, the newer antivirals valacyclovir and famciclovir have better oral absorption and more convenient dosing schedules. Routine use of aniviral agents in the management of patients without mucosal lesions or other evidence of viral infection generally is not recommended.[1] Treatment recommendations for viral infections are located in Table 120–4.

MANAGEMENT OF CATHETER INFECTIONS

Cancer patients are at high risk for the development of catheter-related infections, most often owing to coagulase-negative staphylococci or *S. aureus*.[1,5] Strategies for prevention and management of catheter-related infections are outlined in the practice guidelines published jointly by the IDSA in conjunction with other professional organizations.[55,56]

DURATION OF ANTIMICROBIAL THERAPY

The optimal duration of antimicrobial therapy in the neutropenic cancer patient remains controversial. Decisions regarding discontinuation of empirical antimicrobial therapy often are more difficult and complex than those regarding initiation of therapy (see Fig. 120–1). One point on which experts agree, however, is that the most important determinant of the total duration of antibiotic therapy is the patient's ANC.[1,3,4,6,10] If the ANC is 500 cells/mm³ or greater for 2 consecutive days, if the patient is afebrile and clinically stable

for 48 to 72 hours or more, and if no pathogen has been isolated, then antibiotics may be discontinued. Some clinicians advocate that patients with ANCs of fewer than 500 cells/mm³ be maintained on antibiotic therapy until resolution of neutropenia, even if afebrile. However, prolonged antibiotic use has been associated with superinfections resulting from resistant bacteria and fungi and increases the risk of antibiotic-related toxicities.[10] If low-risk patients are stable clinically but the ANC is still fewer than 500 cells/mm³, antibiotics may be discontinued after a total of 5 to 7 afebrile days. Patients, however, who experience profound neutropenia (ANC < 100 cells/mm³), have mucosal lesions, or have unstable vital signs or other risk factors should continue to receive antibiotics until the ANC has increased to 500 cells/mm³ or greater or the patient is stable clinically.

Patients who are persistently neutropenic and febrile but who are stable clinically with no active site of infection often may be discontinued successfully from antimicrobial therapy after 2 weeks or more. These patients, however, must be monitored carefully because reinstitution of antibiotics may be necessary.[1,10] An alternative approach is to place these patients on antimicrobial prophylaxis, as discussed below. Patients with documented infections should receive antimicrobial therapy until the infecting organism is eradicated and signs and symptoms of infection have resolved (at least 10 to 14 days of therapy).

Consensus guidelines provide useful information regarding the management of febrile episodes in cancer patients with neutropenia.[1,6] However, therapy (including initial empirical regimens, modifications, and duration of treatment) must be individualized based on individual patient parameters and response to therapy.

CLINICAL CONTROVERSY

A key controversy in the management of febrile neutropenia in cancer patients is the optimal time to stop empirical antimicrobial therapy in patients who remain persistently febrile. Patients' individual risk of severe infection (determined by extent and duration of neutropenia, as well as other risk factors) helps to guide treatment decisions in this setting.

COLONY-STIMULATING FACTORS

Because resolution of neutropenia is the most important determinant of patient outcome from both febrile episodes and documented infections, numerous studies have evaluated hematopoietic colony-stimulating factors (CSFs) (sargramostim, granulocyte-macrophage colony-stimulating factor, and filgrastim, granulocyte colony-stimulating factor) as adjunct therapy to antimicrobial treatment of febrile neutropenic cancer patients.[57] These studies consistently found that the use of CSFs reduces the total duration and severity of chemotherapy-related neutropenia. However, these studies failed to demonstrate consistent benefits of CSFs compared with placebo related to important outcome variables, such as overall survival and disease-free survival, but use of CSFs did result in fewer hospitalizations.[57,58] An expert panel of the American Society of Clinical Oncology (ASCO) has concluded that there is no clear support for the routine use of CSFs in uncomplicated fever and neutropenia.[57] The ASCO panel reported that the use of CSFs may be useful in patients with ANC of 500 cells/mm³ or fewer, uncontrolled primary disease, pneumonia, invasive fungal infections, multiorgan dysfunction, sepsis syndrome, hypotension, or other factors likely to cause rapid clinical deterioration, but the panel emphasized that even under these severe circumstances, the benefits of CSF therapy were not substantiated.[57] Clinical judgment must be exercised in determining which patients likely may benefit from judicious use of these expensive agents. Patients with prolonged neutropenia and documented infections who are not responding to appropriate antimicrobial therapy may benefit from treatment with CSFs.[57] Primary prophylaxis with CSFs may be warranted in patients with preexisting neutropenia or other risk factors for severe infection, especially when the risk of febrile neutropenia is 40% or greater.[57]

The direct transfusion of neutrophils also has been studied for the treatment of febrile neutropenia or opportunistic infections. Routine use of neutrophil transfusions is not supported, but use should be considered in profoundly neutropenic patients with documented infections in whom causative organisms cannot be eradicated with appropriate antimicrobial therapy in combination with CSFs.[1,6] At present, the use of neutrophil transfusions is considered experimental and is not recommended for routine management of febrile neutropenic patients.[59]

PROPHYLAXIS OF INFECTIONS IN NEUTROPENIC CANCER PATIENTS

Owing to the potential morbidity and mortality of infections in neutropenic cancer patients, measures have been taken to prevent these complications through a number of environmental modifications and prophylactic antimicrobial regimens. The goal of antimicrobial prophylaxis in cancer patients is to decrease the number and severity of systemic infections during prolonged periods of neutropenia. Decisions regarding prophylactic antimicrobials must be made with the realization of associated issues, such as resistance concerns.

GENERAL MEASURES

Because approximately 50% of pathogens infecting neutropenic cancer patients are acquired in the hospital, reducing acquisition of infectious organisms from the environment is a basic component in controlling nosocomial infection rates.[13,14] Neutropenic patients should be placed in reverse isolation (isolation to protect patients from contracting infections after exposure to others) with strict adherence to infection control guidelines by hospital personnel.[7] Proper, meticulous hand washing by hospital personnel is a simple yet very effective infection control measure.

To reduce the risk of infection caused by airborne pathogens, such as *Aspergillus* spp., laminar airflow rooms are in use at some cancer centers performing HSCTs. Laminar airflow rooms work by directing filtered air away from the patient, thus minimizing the risk of infection from airborne or environmental pathogens. Laminar airflow rooms are expensive, however, and use of these protective environments does not improve overall survival in HSCT recipients.[7,14]

BACTERIAL INFECTIONS

Early attempts at pharmacologic reduction of flora colonizing the GI tract used combinations of nonabsorbable antibiotics, including gentamicin, nystatin, vancomycin, polymyxin B, and colistin. The goal is to preserve colonization resistance to reduce gut colonization with virulent pathogens, such as *P. aeruginosa*, and their translocation into the bloodstream. When anaerobic flora are preserved by selective gut decontamination to prevent colonization by potentially pathogenic gram-negative organisms, this is termed *colonization resistance*.[3] This

concept is based on studies conducted in immunosuppressed animal in which selective gut decontamination resulted in a lower number o infections and minimal colonization by potential pathogens.[14]

Although clinical trials have demonstrated that oral nonabsorbable antibiotics reduce infections successfully, these regimens are not recommended routinely for infection prophylaxis because o several problems, including unpalatability, high cost, and frequen adverse effects (e.g., nausea, vomiting, and diarrhea).[1,13,14] Use o nonabsorbable antibiotic regimens also has been associated with the development of resistance to aminoglycosides among gram-negative bacilli, rendering the aminoglycosides useless as treatment alternatives for ensuing infections.[1,13,14] Owing to concerns regarding development of resistance, prophylaxis with aminoglycosides and vancomycin should be avoided.[1]

The concept of combining selective intestinal decontamination with systemic antimicrobial prophylaxis has been employed using oral agents, particularly the fluoroquinolones.[14] Prospective clinical trials have shown that orally absorbed prophylactic antibiotics, including trimethoprim-sulfamethoxazole and fluoroquinolones, are more effective and better tolerated than nonabsorbable antibiotics.[1] Data from most placebo-controlled studies indicate that trimethoprim-sulfamethoxazole significantly reduces infection rates in cancer patients.[1] Although trimethoprim-sulfamethoxazole is also effective as prophylaxis against *P. jiroveci*, its lack of activity against *P. aeruginosa* is worrisome, particularly in institutions in which pseudomonal infections are frequent.[1] Other concerns with trimethoprim-sulfamethoxazole prophylaxis include selection of resistant organisms, predisposition to development of oral fungal infections, and delay in bone marrow recovery resulting in prolonged neutropenic episodes.[10,13,14]

Numerous studies have shown that oral fluoroquinolones (ciprofloxacin and ofloxacin) are more effective than placebo, nonabsorbable antibiotics, and trimethoprim-sulfamethoxazole in preventing gram-negative infections in neutropenic cancer patients.[60,61] Fluoroquinolone prophylaxis during periods of neutropenia decreases the incidence of fever and microbiologically documented gram-negative infections.[60–62] There are, however, several limitations to their use. In particular, quinolones may lack adequate gram-positive activity. As a result, combination of a quinolone with a second agent providing enhanced gram-positive activity (e.g., rifampin, penicillin, or a macrolide) may be required for effective prophylaxis.[63] Fluoroquinolone prophylaxis has been associated with the development of resistant gram-negative organisms.[60] Rates of quinolone-resistant gram-negative bacilli infections exceed 25% in some centers at which quinolones have been used for prophylaxis.[8] Use of fluoroquinolone prophylaxis precludes these agents from consideration for inclusion in empirical antibiotic regimens in febrile neutropenic patients. Moreover, patients experiencing breakthrough infection during fluoroquinolone prophylaxis should not be placed on a fluoroquinolone subsequently for empirical therapy.

The use of antibacterial prophylaxis remains controversial owing to a lack of consistent efficacy, potential for development of resistant bacteria, high cost, and lack of impact on patient survival.[1] Therefore, antibacterial prophylaxis is not recommended routinely for all neutropenic patients. Prophylaxis (with trimethoprim-sulfamethoxazole or quinolone-penicillin) generally is indicated for patients expected to be profoundly neutropenic for more than 1 week, such as HSCT patients.[1,7] Additional risk factors that may provide justification for prophylaxis include mucous membrane or skin lesions, presence of indwelling catheters, need for instrumentation, severe periodontal disease, or other risk factors.[1] Neutrophil recovery eliminates the need for continued prophylaxis, and recovery may be facilitated by use of

CSFs.[57] In contrast to their unclear role in the treatment of febrile neutropenia, CSFs have been formally recommended by the ASCO for prevention of febrile neutropenia in high-risk patients.[57] Such patients include those receiving chemotherapy regimens that produce a high rate of febrile neutropenia (>40% incidence) or patients with active tissue infection at the time of chemotherapy, history of febrile neutropenia with previous courses of chemotherapy, or underlying bone marrow compromise.[57]

FUNGAL INFECTIONS

Because neutropenic patients are at risk for mucocutaneous and invasive fungal infections that are difficult to diagnose and treat in this population, antifungal prophylaxis may be considered during high-risk periods at institutions where fungal infections in cancer patients are frequent.[64] The goal of antifungal prophylaxis is to prevent development of invasive fungal infections during periods of risk, thereby reducing morbidity and mortality. A meta-analysis of antifungal prophylaxis in 38 trials involving more than 7000 cancer patients reported a decrease in the use of parenteral antifungal therapy, superficial and invasive systemic fungal infections, and fungal infection–related mortality rate.[65] Antifungal prophylaxis resulted in decreased mortality in patients with prolonged neutropenia and HSCT but had no effect on rates of invasive *Aspergillus* infections.

Although the choice of antifungal prophylaxis agents remains controversial, fluconazole prophylaxis (400 mg/day) has been particularly well studied and reduces the incidence of both superficial and systemic fungal infections, as well as significantly decreases mortality from fungal infections in patients with leukemia and HSCT recipients.[63,66–68] However, the use of fluconazole prophylaxis has resulted in the emergence of infections caused by *C. krusei* and *C. glabrata*, pathogens that frequently are resistant to fluconazole and other azole-type antifungal agents.[64,69] Routine antifungal prophylaxis with oral fluconazole (400 mg/day) or itraconazole oral solution (2.5 mg/kg every 12 hours) therefore should be limited to patients undergoing allogeneic HSCT (usually administered from the day of HSCT until engraftment to prevent candidiasis).[7,22] Prophylaxis against fungal infection is beneficial in leukemic patients, and the choice of either fluconazole, itraconazole, or amphotericin B should be determined by the types of fungal isolates at individual institutions.[22,68] Recent data indicate that itraconazole may be more effective than fluconazole for long-term antifungal prophylaxis in allogeneic HSCT recipients; however, itraconazole use was associated with more frequent GI side effects.[70] After initiation, antifungal prophylaxis should be continued until resolution of neutropenia or the need for institution of antifungal therapy for suspected/documented infection.[22]

Antifungal prophylaxis does not decrease the incidence of invasive mold infections.[65] In addition to environmental precautions, strategies being investigated for *Aspergillus* prophylaxis in neutropenic patients include oral itraconazole, low (0.1–0.25 mg/kg per day) to moderate (0.5 mg/kg per day) doses of amphotericin B, intranasal and aerosolized amphotericin B, and lipid-associated amphotericin B products.[7] None of these interventions can be recommended routinely in clinical practice at this time.

OTHER INFECTIONS

The use of trimethoprim-sulfamethoxazole in cancer patients at risk for *P. jiroveci* pneumonia has reduced the incidence of this protozoal infection substantially.[27] Antiviral prophylaxis with acyclovir or newer agents (valacyclovir and famciclovir) is employed in most centers to reduce the risk of HSV reactivation in patients with acute leukemia undergoing intensive chemotherapy. Varicella vaccine provides good protection (90%) in leukemic children and also may be useful in seronegative adults, although the vaccine has been less well studied in this population.

When considering use of antimicrobial (antibacterial, antifungal, antiprotozoal, and antiviral) prophylaxis in neutropenic patients with cancer, the risks and benefits of the prophylaxis versus issues with development of resistance, toxicities, and other concerns must be weighed.

PHARMACOECONOMIC CONSIDERATIONS

As in all areas of modern health care, attention has been directed increasingly to providing cost-effective management of febrile neutropenia in cancer patients. Use of oral and/or outpatient antimicrobial therapy in low-risk patients is an effective, less costly alternative that is preferred by patients.[71] Potent oral antimicrobials facilitate the conversion from IV antibiotics to oral therapy when appropriate. Judicious use of antimicrobials, such as reserving lipid-associated amphotericin B products for patients intolerant to conventional amphotericin B, helps to contain costs. In the situation of febrile neutropenia in a cancer patient, one may be tempted to "throw the kitchen sink" at suspected/documented infections; however, following guidelines such as those published by the IDSA and NCCN helps to guide the most appropriate use of available antimicrobials. Future consequences of antimicrobial overuse, such as resistance and limited treatment options, must be considered when choosing antimicrobial therapy for any indication, including management of febrile neutropenia. Each institution should examine its own infection and susceptibility patterns and use this information to guide empirical treatment decisions while individualizing therapy for each patient.

EVALUATION OF THERAPEUTIC OUTCOMES

Close monitoring of febrile neutropenic patients, including both clinical and laboratory parameters, is essential for early detection and treatment of infectious complications. Three general therapeutic outcomes have been defined in the setting of febrile neutropenia: (1) success (survival during the febrile episode until resolution of neutropenia by judicious selection of empirical antimicrobial therapy), (2) success with modification (same as 1 but with additions/modifications to empirical therapy), and (3) failure (death during febrile neutropenia).[10] Because many of the drugs that may be used in this setting have significant toxicity potential (e.g., aminoglycosides and amphotericin B), careful attention must be paid to the prevention and management of drug-related adverse effects. Evaluations of the parameters in the "Clinical Presentation" box are appropriate to help monitor and guide therapy. In addition, the NCCN guidelines for febrile neutropenia provide comprehensive recommendations on clinical/laboratory monitoring parameters, including schedules.[6] The reader is referred to individual chapters within this book for more detailed discussions of monitoring parameters related to specific types of infections (e.g., pneumonia and urinary tract infections).

INFECTIONS IN PATIENTS UNDERGOING HEMATOPOIETIC STEM CELL TRANSPLANTATION (HSCT)

◀1 Infection remains a major barrier to successful HSCT. Numerous advances in HSCT have taken place over the past decade and have resulted in greatly improved patient outcomes. Recipients of HSCT are at enhanced risk of infection because of prolonged periods of neutropenia. In addition, patients receiving allogeneic or matched unrelated donor transplants have added immune system insults imposed by prolonged immunosuppressive drug therapy for the prevention and treatment of graft-versus-host disease (GVHD). Intensive pretransplant conditioning regimens (high-dose chemotherapy and total-body irradiation), as well as GVHD itself, often disrupt protective barriers, such as mucous membranes, skin, and the GI tract, placing patients at further risk of infection. Patients experiencing marrow graft failure have extended periods of profound neutropenia often resulting in death from infectious causes. The Food and Drug Administration (FDA) approved sargramostim for marrow graft failure in both autologous and allogeneic transplants.

ETIOLOGY AND CLINICAL PRESENTATION OF INFECTIONS

◀2 ◀10 The timing with which specific types of infections typically occur following HSCT is represented in Fig. 120–2. Although the figure illustrates the general time course for infections in all types of HSCT, the relative incidence and importance of specific pathogens vary greatly according to the specific type of HSCT performed. Patients receiving allogeneic transplants are at greatest risk of infection at all times after HSCT and are predisposed to earlier and more severe infections with opportunistic pathogens such as *Aspergillus*. The presence of GVHD also has an impact on the incidence and timing of various infections.

After the administration of intensive conditioning regimens to eliminate malignant cells and prevent rejection of donor marrow, patients may remain profoundly neutropenic for 3 to 4 weeks. During this preengraftment period, they are at risk for the same types of infectious complications noted in other granulocytopenic cancer patients (e.g., bacterial and fungal infections) and should be managed accordingly (see Table 120–1). Table 120–4 lists regimens for the treatment of specific infections.

Fungal infections, especially those caused by *Candida* and *Aspergillus* spp., are serious and often fatal complications associated with HSCT. Fungi remain a serious cause of infection, particularly in allogeneic HSCT recipients, for up to 1 to 2 years following transplantation and may occur in as many as 10% of patients.[72] Mortality rates associated with invasive aspergillosis infections may be as high as 90%.[73]

In addition to bacterial and fungal infections, HSCT recipients also are at risk for serious HSV infections manifesting as severe gingivostomatitis, esophagitis, genital lesions, and rarely, pneumonia during the first month after transplant. Clinical disease is more common in patients with serologic evidence (e.g., serum antibodies)

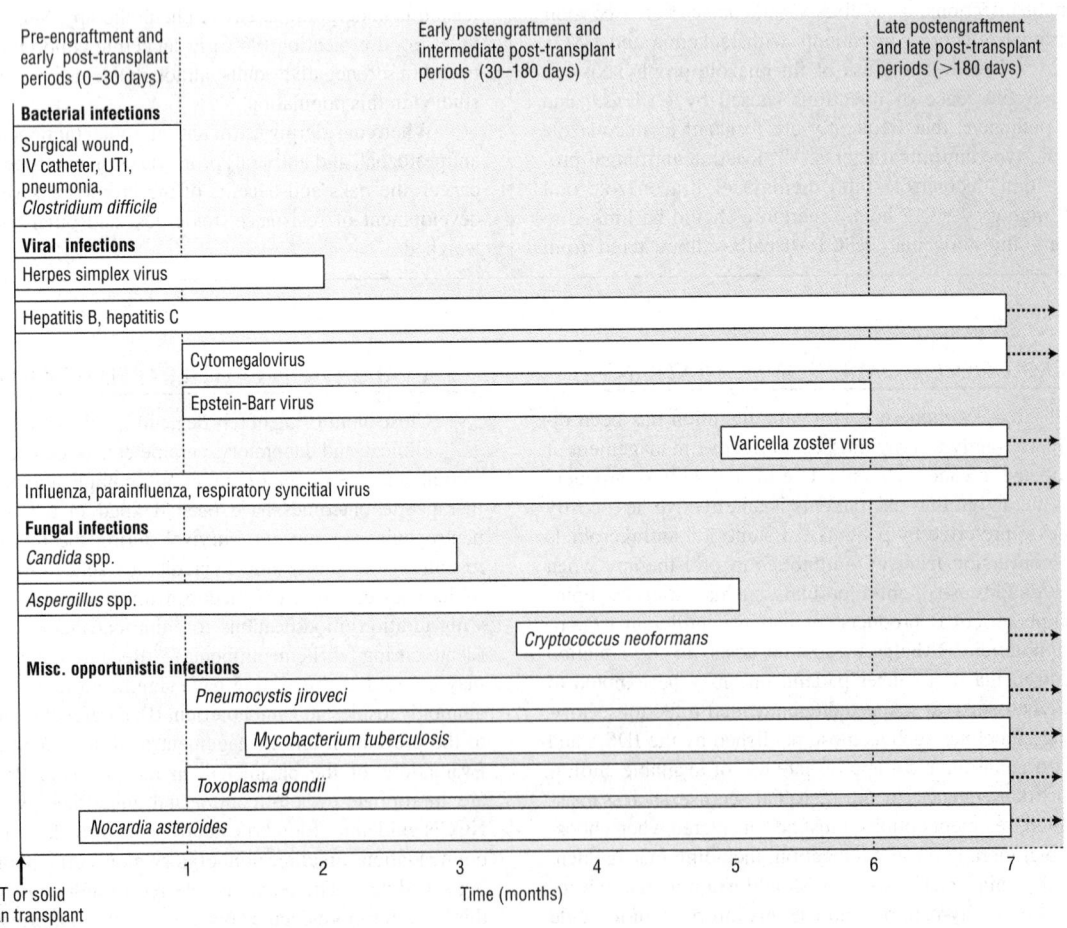

FIGURE 120–2. Timetable for the occurrence of infections in HSCT and solid organ-transplant patients. IV = intravenous; UTI = urinary tract infection.

of prior exposure and latent HSV infection pretransplant. Therefore, reactivation of latent disease during periods of immunosuppression is the most common etiology of HSV infection. Without prophylaxis, as many as 80% of HSV-seropositive patients experience mucocutaneous disease after intensive chemotherapy as compared with fewer than 25% of seronegative patients.[72,74] The HSV infections often coexist with candidal infection and mucositis secondary to chemotherapy, radiation, or both.[75] Acyclovir-resistant HSV infections also occur following HSCT but are not common.[72,76] Painful swallowing associated with these conditions often makes it difficult for patients to take oral medications and maintain adequate nutritional intake. Because of the considerable morbidity associated with reactivation of HSV after transplantation, the HSV serologic status of patients should be determined prior to transplant.

Recipients of HSCT remain at high risk for infection after bone marrow engraftment has occurred. Significant defects in neutrophil function and cell-mediated and humoral immunity, persisting for several months after transplantation, predispose patients to infectious complications. Acute and chronic GVHD also result in prolonged periods of immunosuppression and increased infection rates.

Bone marrow transplant patients are at high risk for cytomegalovirus (CMV) infections during the early postengraftment period. These range in severity from asymptomatic viral shedding (urine, throat, lungs) to life-threatening disseminated disease and interstitial pneumonia.[72,75]

As with HSV, patients seropositive for CMV before transplantation are at high risk for recurrent disease during periods of immunosuppression; about 70% of seropositive patients develop recurrent CMV disease after transplantation compared with only 3% of seronegative patients.[72,74,75] Other risk factors for CMV disease in HSCT patients include advanced age, human lymphocyte antigen (HLA) mismatch, total-body irradiation, multiagent conditioning regimens, and the presence of GVHD.[72] Patients without evidence of latent CMV infection (CMV seronegative) before transplantation may develop primary CMV disease after receiving bone marrow or blood products from CMV-seropositive donors. Although the typical onset of both primary and recurrent CMV infection is 1 to 2 months after transplantation, late-onset infections occurring more than 100 days after transplantation are increasing in frequency.[72,74,75,77] Patients receiving allogeneic transplants are at highest risk for CMV disease.[72,74,75]

The most serious clinical manifestation of CMV disease and the leading cause of infectious death in HSCT recipients is interstitial pneumonia (IP), which is associated with an 85% mortality rate if untreated.[72,74] This clinical syndrome manifests as fever, dyspnea, hypoxia, nonproductive cough, and diffuse pulmonary infiltrates. As many as 40% of allogeneic HSCT patients will develop IP; of these patients with IP, up to 40% of cases are the result of CMV.[72,74] IP also may result from other infectious (*P. jiroveci,* varicella-zoster virus) and noninfectious causes (pulmonary damage by radiation and chemotherapy).[72]

During the late postengraftment period (beginning about 100 days after transplantation), infections remain a major problem in patients suffering from chronic GVHD. Additional immunosuppressive therapy for the treatment of GVHD places these patients at added risk for infection. Infections common during the late postengraftment period include those caused by encapsulated bacteria, such as *S. pneumoniae* and *H. influenzae,* and viruses, including CMV and VZV.[72,74] Patients not undergoing allogeneic transplantation or suffering from chronic GVHD generally have few infections in this period.

Up to 50% of all patients surviving up to 10 months after transplantation develop an infection caused by VZV.[72] Infection with VZV is most common in patients receiving allogeneic transplants with acute or chronic GVHD.[72,74,75] Both primary (varicella) or recurrent disease (herpes zoster) usually present as skin lesions, most of which remain contained to local areas; however, 30% to 45% of these infections may disseminate to other cutaneous areas or body organs, causing mortality as high as 50%.[72,74,75]

▶ PROPHYLAXIS AND MANAGEMENT: Infections in Recipients of HSCT

8 **9** The goals of antimicrobial drug use in HSCT patients include (1) prevention of bacterial, fungal, viral, and protozoal infections during preengraftment and postengraftment periods and (2) effective treatment of established infections. The overall goal of prophylaxis and treatment of infection in HSCT patients is the prevention of infectious morbidity and mortality. These goals must be achieved at the lowest possible toxicity and cost. Prophylactic therapy should be specifically aimed at pathogens known to cause a high incidence of infection within the HSCT population, the specific institution, or both. In addition, prophylactic therapy should be limited to regimens proved to be effective through well-designed clinical trials.

Appropriate immunizations should be a primary consideration in the prevention of infections in HSCT recipients. Immunizations against common bacterial and viral pathogens are timed to avoid periods of severe immunosuppression following HSCT when the protective response to vaccination potentially would be decreased.[78] Current recommendations for immunization of HSCT patients include three doses each of diphtheria-pertussis-tetanus or diphtheria-tetanus, inactivated polio, conjugated *H. influenzae* type b, and hepatitis B vaccines at 12, 14, and 24 months after transplantation. The 23-valent pneumococcal vaccine should be administered at 12 and 24 months after HSCT, and the influenza vaccine should be administered prior to HSCT, resumed at least 6 months after transplantation, and continued for life. Family, close contacts, and health care providers of HSCT patients also should be vaccinated annually against influenza. Finally, the measles-mumps-rubella vaccine should be administered no sooner than 24 months after HSCT when the patient is considered to be immunocompetent. The varicella vaccine is contraindicated for administration to HSCT patients owing to the live-attenuated nature of the product and the risk of VZV infection.[78]

▇ BACTERIAL INFECTIONS

Prophylaxis of infections in HSCT patients is in many ways similar to that used in other neutropenic patients. Selective decontamination with oral antimicrobials is used commonly; considerations are the same as those discussed previously. Although some studies have shown decreased rates of bacteremia and other bacterial infections after HSCT, overall mortality rates were not reduced.[72,78] The routine use of prophylactic antibiotics in HSCT therefore is still controversial. Fluoroquinolones have become the most frequently used agents, often combined with another agent (e.g., macrolides or rifampin) for enhanced gram-positive activity.[72,74] These regimens usually are begun either within 72 hours of beginning the chemotherapy conditioning regimens or on the day of hematopoietic stem cell infusion and continued throughout the neutropenic period. Patients who become febrile while receiving prophylaxis should be managed according to general guidelines for febrile neutropenic patients.

The routine use of parenteral vancomycin for prophylactic therapy is not recommended. Prophylaxis with vancomycin has been studied because of the high incidence of gram-positive infections following transplantation. Vancomycin prophylaxis appears to decrease the overall incidence of gram-positive bacterial infections, number of days of empirical antimicrobial therapy, and cost of therapy.[72,78] However, important mortality benefits were not demonstrated consistently, and there are significant concerns regarding the selection of vancomycin-intermediate *S. aureus* and vancomycin-resistant enterococci. Prophylactic vancomycin use thus is not generally recommended except in institutions with high rates of infection with methicillin-resistant staphylococci among HSCT recipients.[74,78] There is currently no role for linezolid or quinupristin-dalfopristin except in documented infections caused by VRE.

Antibiotic prophylaxis against bacterial infection is recommended in the late postengraftment period (>100 days after transplantation) in certain high-risk patients, specifically allogeneic transplant recipients with chronic GVHD.[78] Antibiotics should be targeted against encapsulated bacteria such as *S. pneumoniae* and *H. influenzae* and should be selected based on local susceptibility patterns for these organisms. Patients receiving trimethoprim-sulfamethoxazole for prophylaxis of other opportunistic infections may be protected adequately and do not necessarily require an additional antibiotic.[72] Prophylaxis should be continued as long as the chronic GVHD is being actively treated.

▪ VIRAL INFECTIONS

Prophylaxis of recurrent HSV infection is recommended for all HSV-seropositive patients undergoing HSCT.[72,78] Approximately 0% to 10% of HSV-seropositive patients receiving acyclovir experienced viral shedding, clinical symptoms of viral reactivation, or both as compared with 60% to 80% of patients receiving placebo.[74] Acyclovir doses recommended for prophylaxis are 250 mg/m^2 (5 mg/kg) IV every 12 hours or 200 mg orally three times daily.[72,78] Intravenous therapy eventually will be necessary in most patients because of the development of severe mucositis from conditioning regimens. Oral acyclovir, however, is effective and considerably less expensive in patients who can take oral medications. Valacyclovir also has been used in doses of 500–1000 mg/day, but clinical experience is limited, and it is not currently recommended as first-line prophylaxis therapy.[78] Although the duration of antiviral prophylaxis differs between centers, acyclovir usually is begun at the time of the conditioning regimen and continued until bone marrow engraftment or until resolution of mucositis (approximately 30 days after HSCT).[78] Besides preventing recurrence of HSV disease, acyclovir prophylaxis also may reduce the incidence of CMV reactivation.[79] Patients developing active HSV or VZV infection should be treated with high-dose acyclovir (10 mg/kg IV every 8 hours).

Although high-dose oral acyclovir given for 6 months after transplantation also significantly reduces reactivation of VZV infections, routine use of long-term acyclovir is controversial and not generally recommended for this indication.[72,78] Patients who received HSCT within the previous 24 months or those beyond 24 months after HSCT who have chronic GVHD or are on immunosuppressive therapy should receive varicella-zoster immunoglobulin 625 units intramuscularly within 48 to 96 hours after close contact with persons with chickenpox or shingles for prevention of VZV-related disease.[78]

Acyclovir-resistant HSV has been reported occasionally in HSCT patients receiving acyclovir prophylaxis. Foscarnet is the drug of choice for treatment of acyclovir-resistant HSV. Foscarnet, however, has not been well studied for HSV prophylaxis.[72,74,78]

Prevention of CMV disease has been studied extensively in HSCT patients and is a well-accepted indication for prophylaxis because of the high associated infectious morbidity and mortality. If possible, CMV-seronegative patients should receive donor marrow and supportive blood products from seronegative donors only; however, CMV-seropositive patients are not at additional risk by receiving blood or marrow from seropositive donors.[72] Although acyclovir has relatively poor in vitro activity against CMV, a decrease in CMV infection and an improvement in overall survival were reported in HSV- and CMV-seropositive allogeneic HSCT recipients receiving IV acyclovir.[79]

CLINICAL CONTROVERSY

Although acyclovir is used commonly in many transplant centers for prophylaxis of CMV infection, this practice is somewhat controversial and is not universally recommended because of the intrinsically poor activity of acyclovir against CMV.[72]

Ganciclovir also has been well studied for prophylaxis because of its superior activity against CMV compared with acyclovir. Although administration of prophylactic ganciclovir to CMV-seropositive patients may decrease the occurrence of CMV disease significantly, studies found no clear survival benefit, and ganciclovir-related bone marrow suppression frequently was problematic. Ganciclovir prophylaxis therefore is only recommended routinely among allogeneic HSCT recipients for the first 100 days after transplantation.[72,78] The recommended dose of ganciclovir in these patients is 5 mg/kg IV every 12 hours for the first 5 to 7 days, followed by 5–6 mg/kg IV once daily five times per week until day 100 after HSCT.[78]

Perhaps a more appropriate role for ganciclovir is in early or preemptive therapy, in which ganciclovir is administered at first isolation of CMV from the blood or bronchoalveolar lavage (BAL) fluid. Detection of CMV may be accomplished through the use either of a monoclonal antibody–based test for viral antigens or by detection of viral DNA through polymerase chain reaction (PCR)–based tests. Preemptive therapy was evaluated in several studies and significantly reduced the occurrence of CMV disease (including CMV pneumonia), and it improved survival significantly up to 180 days after transplantation.[72] Because CMV viremia and BAL cultures are highly predictive of subsequent CMV disease, preemptive ganciclovir therapy should be considered for autologous HSCT recipients within the first 100 days after transplantation or in allogeneic HSCT recipients at any time point after transplantation.[72,78] The dose of ganciclovir for preemptive therapy is the same as that used for prophylaxis. Foscarnet may be used for either prophylaxis or preemptive therapy of CMV disease in patients intolerant of ganciclovir; the recommended foscarnet dose is 60 mg/kg IV every 12 hours for 7 days, followed by 90–120 mg/kg IV daily.[80] Oral valganciclovir 900 mg every 12 hours has not been well studied in the setting of HSCT and is not recommended routinely. CSFs are beneficial in this setting, providing benefits similar to those noted in neutropenic AIDS patients receiving ganciclovir therapy for CMV retinitis.

Pharmacologic prevention of CMV disease with either intravenous immunoglobulin (IVIG) or hyperimmune CMV-IVIG produced variable and inconclusive results.[74,81] The benefits of immunoglobulins for CMV prophylaxis in HSCT patients have not been demonstrated conclusively, and their use is not currently recommended.[72]

Ganciclovir is the drug of choice in the treatment of active CMV infection in HSCT patients (see Table 120–4). Foscarnet is effective in the treatment of severe CMV disease in AIDS patients and also may be of benefit for the treatment or prevention of infections in HSCT patients. Foscarnet may be used as an alternative to ganciclovir because of its relative lack of bone marrow toxicity. Foscarnet-related nephrotoxicity may be problematic, however, especially in the posttransplant period when patients may be receiving other nephrotoxic agents. Use of cidofovir also is limited by the risk of nephrotoxicity, and this agent has not been well studied in HSCT patients.

Numerous single-agent treatments, such as vidarabine, interferon, and ganciclovir, have been employed unsuccessfully as treatment for CMV pneumonitis. The combination of high-dose IVIG and ganciclovir, however, may decrease the mortality of this syndrome from 85% to only 30% to 50%.[72] Ganciclovir plus hyperimmune CMV-IVIG is also considered to be effective for the treatment of CMV disease, although this regimen has not been studied as extensively in the HSCT population in a controlled fashion. The potential for ganciclovir-associated bone marrow suppression prior to marrow engraftment and in patients who are just recovering from granulocytopenia remains a concern, especially in patients with unstable renal function. Ganciclovir plus CMV-IVIG is employed widely as the treatment regimen of choice for severe or life-threatening CMV disease. Ganciclovir plus IVIG also is used frequently, although CMV-IVIG is replacing IVIG in most institutions.[74,81]

FUNGAL INFECTIONS

Fluconazole prophylaxis is safe and efficacious for prevention of mucocutaneous and disseminated candidal infections in high-risk HSCT patients.[22,72,78,82] Patients specifically recommended for prophylaxis include all allogeneic transplant recipients and autologous recipients who are expected to have prolonged neutropenia, have received intensive conditioning regimens associated with extensive mucositis, or have recently received fludarabine.[72,78] Fluconazole 400 mg IV or orally given once daily is begun on the day of transplantation and continued until engraftment or resolution of neutropenia.[22,72,78] The variable activity of fluconazole against non-*albicans* species of *Candida* may be problematic in this population, as is lack of activity against

Aspergillus.[82] Prophylaxis with fluconazole (as well as itraconazole), although effectively reducing colonization and infection with yeasts, has not been demonstrated consistently to reduce overall mortality or invasive infections such as aspergillosis in HSCT recipients.[72,82,83] Low-dose amphotericin B (0.10–0.25 mg/kg per day) is used occasionally in institutions with high rates of *Aspergillus* infection after HSCT. Low-dose liposomal amphotericin B (1 mg/kg per day) also has been studied.[82,84] As with the azoles, amphotericin B prophylaxis has not been demonstrated clearly to provide benefits in either overall or infection-related mortality following HSCT.[13,22,74,83] Despite the controversies regarding absolute benefits of prophylaxis, fluconazole generally is recommended for most patients undergoing HSCT.[74,78,83] Low-dose amphotericin B prophylaxis should be reserved for institutions with high rates of infection owing to azole-resistant yeasts (e.g., *C. krusei*) or high rates of invasive disease such as aspergillosis.[74] Fluconazole and other azole antifungals may cause significant elevations in serum cyclosporine concentrations and predispose to cyclosporine toxicities; this interaction should be monitored closely in HSCT patients receiving these agents concurrently.[22]

PROTOZOAL INFECTIONS

Pulmonary infection with *P. jiroveci* is a relatively infrequent complication of HSCT. Mortality rates in this population, however, are approximately 60% and are especially high in patients with GVHD.[72,74,78] Prophylactic use of trimethoprim-sulfamethoxazole (one double-strength tablet three times per week or one single-strength tablet daily) is employed commonly in this setting. Toxoplasmosis is not a common infection in HSCT patients but is associated with mortality rates of approximately 70%.[85] Toxoplasmosis also should be prevented by trimethoprim-sulfamethoxazole prophylaxis.[72,78]

USE OF COLONY-STIMULATING FACTORS

Several studies have evaluated the use of filgrastim and sargramostim in HSCT patients in an effort to speed bone marrow recovery, to reduce the period of neutropenia, and to decrease infectious complications. Although the time to neutrophil recovery was consistently decreased, these studies failed to show significant differences in infection rates, transplant-related mortality, or overall survival. The use of CSFs appears to be safe, but their use in HSCT patients has not been formally recommended because of lack of clear benefits.[57]

EVALUATION OF THERAPEUTIC OUTCOMES

❿ Close monitoring of HSCT patients, including both clinical and laboratory data, is essential for early detection and treatment of infectious complications. In addition, because many of the drugs that may be used commonly in this setting have significant toxicity potential in HSCT patients (e.g., ganciclovir, amphotericin B, and trimethoprim-sulfamethoxazole), careful attention must be paid to the prevention and management of drug-related adverse effects. Monitoring parameters related to specific types of infections (e.g., pneumonia and urinary tract infections) should be applied as appropriate. The reader is referred to other chapters within this book for more specific information.

INFECTIONS IN SOLID-ORGAN TRANSPLANT RECIPIENTS

Since the introduction of cyclosporine in 1980, solid-organ transplantation has become an established mode of treatment for end-stage diseases of the kidney, liver, heart, lungs, and pancreas; small bowel transplantation is also now becoming more common. Both patient and allograft survival rates greatly exceed those of the past. Reasons for improved survival include continuous improvements in immunosuppressive drug therapy, candidate selection, and transplant surgery techniques and more experience in the management of complications (including infection) in these patients. Major hindrances to successful transplantation and extended long-term survival include problems with allograft dysfunction and rejection and infectious complications. Despite advances in diagnostic techniques and antimicrobial therapy, infection remains an important cause of morbidity and mortality.

RISK FACTORS

Many of the risk factors for infection discussed at the beginning of this chapter are present in solid-organ transplant patients (see Table 120–1). The most important risk factor in this population is the immunosuppressive drug therapy that patients receive for prevention and treatment of allograft rejection. Risk of infection depends on specific immunosuppressive drug regimens as well as on the intensity (dose) and duration of immunosuppression. Most opportunistic infections in transplant patients occur during the first 6 months after transplantation when the intensity and total cumulative doses of immunosuppressive therapy are very high.[84,86]

Current immunosuppressive regimens may have an impact on the pattern of infections after transplantation. Tacrolimus may be associated with lower rates of serious bacterial and viral infections than are seen with cyclosporine-based immunosuppressive regimens,[87] possibly because of a steroid-sparing effect of tacrolimus that enables patients to be maintained on greatly reduced doses of corticosteroids. Mycophenolate has been associated with higher rates of CMV disease and VZV infections compared with older azathioprine-based immunosuppressive regimens but conversely may have protective effects against *P. jiroveci* in patients undergoing renal transplantation.[86] Compared with mycophenolate-based regimens, sirolimus has been associated with significantly higher rates of surgical wound infections in renal transplant patients.[86] When evaluating published literature on infection patterns after solid-organ transplantation, one always must consider the organ being transplanted and the nature of the immunosuppressive drug regimens in use at reporting centers.

Immunosuppressive drugs, often in escalated doses, also are used to treat episodes of graft rejection. Drugs used to treat rejection include immunoglobulins directed against T cells (e.g., antithymocyte globulin [ATG]), murine monoclonal antibodies (muronomab), antibodies against interleukin 2 receptors (daclizumab and basiliximab), and high-dose IV or oral corticosteroids. Rejection episodes often occur during the posttransplant period when the overall cumulative dose or net state of immunosuppression is highest (2 to 4 months).[84] Therefore, patients already at risk for infection are placed at even higher risk if additional immunosuppressive therapy is needed to treat one or more episodes of graft rejection. Immunosuppressive drug therapy must be evaluated carefully when infections occur because, in many cases, immunosuppression may have to be reduced in order for the patient to survive the infectious episode; this is done at the expense of increased risk of graft rejection. Risk of increased infectious complications from immunosuppressive therapy used to treat rejection episodes is also determined, at least in part, by the specific therapy employed.[84,86]

ETIOLOGY

As with cancer patients, microorganisms infecting solid-organ transplant patients are present before transplantation or are acquired from exogenous sources. All transplant recipients are at risk for mucocutaneous candidiasis from species colonizing body sites. Invasive fungal infection is less common following kidney and pancreas transplantation (5% to 15%) but also may occur in 30% to 60% of heart, lung, liver, and small bowel transplant recipients; rates are high-

est following liver and small bowel transplantation and are associated with mortality rates of up to 60% to 70%.[73,84,88,89] Approximately 50% to 90% of all systemic fungal infections in transplant recipients are caused by *Candida* spp.[73,84,88,89] Abdominal surgery, especially the demanding operations required for liver and small bowel transplantation, predispose patients to serious fungal disease most likely as a consequence of entering an area highly colonized with *Candida* spp.[88] Lung and heart transplant recipients are particularly at risk for invasive aspergillosis; these infections may occur in up to 10% of patients.[88] Liver and lung transplant recipients are also at particularly high risk for serious gram-negative bacterial infections as a result of the technically difficult surgical procedures.[84]

Organisms present as latent tissue infections may reactivate and cause clinical disease after transplantation after the administration of immunosuppressive drug therapy. Disease resulting from infection reactivation has been noted with viral (HSV I and II, CMV, VZV, Epstein-Barr virus [EBV]), protozoal (*Toxoplasma gondii, P. jiroveci*), and mycobacterial (*Mycobacterium tuberculosis*) pathogens. Serologic or immunologic tests are performed prior to transplantation to assess the risk for infection because of reactivation and identify other subclinical infections (hepatitis B, *Legionella*). Many patients with reactivated disease have no clinical symptoms; often the only evidence of active infection is a rise in antibody titer from the pretransplant baseline, a positive culture, or histologic evidence. Reactivation of latent infection also may result in severe, life-threatening disease in immunosuppressed hosts.

Exogenous sources of infection in transplant patients include environmental contamination and transmission of microorganisms via transplanted organs and blood products. Environmental sources of infection are similar to those noted in other immunocompromised hosts, such as cancer patients. Airborne pathogens, especially fungi, such as *Aspergillus* and *C. neoformans,* may cause infections in transplant patients; this is thought to be a direct cause of increased *Aspergillus* infections among lung transplant patients.[84,88] Transplant patients are also at risk for common nosocomial infections and infections occurring as hospital outbreaks (*P. aeruginosa* and *Legionella*). Optimal prevention and management of nosocomial infections in transplant patients require knowledge of the current epidemiology of infections and susceptibility patterns in the institution.

Infections transmitted via donor organs or blood products are major causes of morbidity and mortality in transplant patients and may include HSV, *T. gondii,* and hepatitis B and C. The most important infections transmitted from the donor, however, are caused by CMV. These infections may cause serious disease (e.g., pneumonia, hepatitis, hematologic disorders, and chorioretinitis), as well as predisposing patients to other opportunistic infections and contributing to allograft dysfunction.[84] In contrast to reactivation disease, transplant patients contracting primary CMV disease are at increased risk for serious, life-threatening infections.[84,90,91] The most important source of primary CMV infection in transplant patients is the donor organ. Efforts are made to avoid transplanting organs from CMV-seropositive donors into CMV-seronegative recipients because of the potentially severe consequences. With the relative scarcity of suitable organs and the rapidity with which transplant decisions often must be made, however, this is not always possible. The consequences of transplanting an organ from a CMV-seropositive donor into an already CMV-seropositive recipient are less clear. Evidence exists that CMV reinfection (as well as reactivation) syndromes may occur in these patients.[84,86] Organs from donors seropositive for *T. gondii* or HSV generally are not withheld from seronegative patients. Organs from known HIV-infected donors, however, are not used for transplantation. Asymptomatic

HIV-seropositive individuals with a CD4 + lymphocyte count of greater than 400 cells/mm^3 may be considered for liver, heart, or lung transplantation without prohibitively high risk of acceleration of HIV disease.[91,92] However, this practice is not widespread because of the shortage of donor organs. The impact of protease inhibitors and highly active antiretroviral therapy (HAART) on long-term outcome of HIV-infected patients following transplantation is not known precisely but is felt to have improved the overall feasibility of transplanting these individuals.[92]

In addition to transmission from donor organs, primary CMV disease also may be transmitted from seropositive blood products, although this is a much less common mode of transmission. Risk of such transmission increases with the administration of large numbers of blood products.

Table 120–4 contains information on microbiology, clinical presentation, and treatment of infections in HSCT and solid-organ transplant recipients. Although opportunistic viral, fungal, and protozoal infections may occur commonly, bacterial infections remain the most frequent infectious complications after transplantation in all allograft recipients.

TIMING OF INFECTIONS AFTER TRANSPLANTATION

Although risk of infection with specific pathogens varies with the type of transplant, the time course of infections is similar in all transplant recipients. The overall risk of infection is greatest during the first 6 months after transplantation when the greatest number of risk factors are present. Both daily and cumulative doses of immunosuppressive drugs are at high levels, and additional agents may be necessary for the treatment of acute rejection episodes.[84,86]

As with HSCT, the overall time course for infections can be divided into three general periods after transplantation (see Fig. 120–2). During the early posttransplant period (within the first month after transplantation), patients are at risk for infections already present and brought forward from the pretransplant period (e.g., hepatitis B); postoperative infections, such as surgical wound and catheter infections; infection resulting from colonized donor organs (pneumonia following lung transplant); and reactivation of HSV.[84,86] In the intermediate posttransplant period (2 to 6 months after transplant), risk is highest for viral infections, including CMV, EBV, and hepatitis B and C. The combination of these "immunomodulating" viruses plus sustained immunosuppressive therapy leads to a high risk for opportunistic infections with pathogens such as *P. jiroveci, Aspergillus,* and *Nocardia asteroides.*[84,86,88] In the late posttransplant period (>6 months after transplant), the patient is at risk for persistent infections (particularly viral) from earlier posttransplant periods, reactivation of VZV and *C. neoformans,* and routine infections affecting the general population.[84] In addition, patients who have required additional immunosuppression therapy for acute or chronic rejection are at continued high risk for opportunistic infections *(Aspergillus and P. jiroveci).*[84,86,88] Although Fig. 120–2 illustrates infection patterns common to all solid-organ transplants, the relative incidence and importance of a particular pathogen will vary according to the type of transplant.

TYPES OF INFECTIONS AND CLINICAL PRESENTATION

Transplant patients are at risk for infections occurring at a variety of sites, including skin, surgical wound, urinary tract, lungs, blood, abdomen, and CNS; however, most infections occur at or near the site of the transplanted organ. For example, heart transplant and heart and lung transplant recipients most often are infected within the lungs or thoracic cavity. Urinary tract infections remain an important cause of morbidity in renal transplant patients, especially in the early posttransplant period. Administration of prophylactic antibiotics, such as trimethoprim-sulfamethoxazole, to these patients has, however, reduced the incidence and severity of urinary tract infections.[84,86] Serious, life-threatening bacterial and fungal infections originating from the abdomen and GI tract are most common after liver transplantation and are related to variables such as length of surgery and surgical procedures performed. Risk of bacteremia, usually originating from the gut, is highest in liver transplant patients. Renal transplant recipients are at the lowest risk of infections and infectious deaths, whereas patients receiving heart, lung, and liver transplants are at the highest risk of infection-related morbidity and mortality.[84,86,88]

CLINICAL PRESENTATION OF INFECTIONS IN SOLID-ORGAN TRANSPLANT PATIENTS

GENERAL

- Because transplant patients are at high risk for serious infections, frequent (at least daily), careful clinical assessments must be performed to search for possible evidence of infection.
- Clinical presentation of infection is variable and depends on the type and site of infection, type of transplant, time after transplantation, immune status of the host, and dose and duration of immunosuppressive therapy.
- Primary viral disease usually is more symptomatic and severe than disease caused by reactivation.
- Physical assessment should include examination of all common sites of infection, including mouth/pharynx, nose and sinuses, respiratory tract, GI tract, urinary tract, skin, soft tissues, perineum, and intravascular catheter insertion sites.

SYMPTOMS

- Usual signs and symptoms of infection may be absent or altered in patients receiving intensive immunosuppressive regimens owing to an inability to mount a typical inflammatory response (e.g., no infiltrate on chest x-ray, urinary tract infection without pyuria).
- Pain may be present at infection site(s).

SIGNS

- Fever is the single most important clinical sign indicating the presence of infection. Other causes of fever unrelated to infection in this patient population include reactions to blood products, drugs, embolic events, and ischemic injury.
- Usual signs of infection may be absent or altered.
- Signs of allograft dysfunction may be related to infection. Distinguishing fever as a result of allograft rejection versus infection often is very difficult and frequently requires allograft biopsy.

LABORATORY TESTS

- Blood cultures (two or more sets, including vascular access devices) for bacteria and fungi; cultures of other suspected or potential infection sites (urine, lungs, etc.).
- Other cultures should be obtained as clinically indicated according to the presence of signs or symptoms.
- Complete blood count and chemistries should be obtained frequently to monitor allograft function, plan supportive care, guide drug dosing, and assess patient's overall status.
- Surveillance cultures for CMV and HSV may be useful during first 3 months after transplantation for early detection of infection.

OTHER DIAGNOSTIC TESTS

- Chest x-ray
- Aspiration, biopsy of skin lesions
- Other diagnostic tests as indicated clinically on the basis of physical examination and other assessments

In contrast to febrile neutropenic patients, the threshold for initiating empirical antimicrobial therapy is higher in febrile transplant patients. As seen in Table 120–4, appropriate therapy for the large numbers of pathogens that may cause infections in transplant patients varies greatly from organism to organism. Therefore, careful attempts at definitive diagnosis of suspected infections must be made. If comprehensive work-up reveals no source of infection, careful observation of the febrile transplant patient (rather than empirical therapy) is a common practice. Surveillance cultures may be useful during the first 3 months for detecting CMV and HSV infections.[84,88,90,91] Management and monitoring of documented infections, such as urinary tract infections, pneumonias, and intraabdominal infections, are similar to that in other types of patients.

PREVENTION OF INFECTION IN SOLID ORGAN TRANSPLANTATION

The goals of antimicrobial drug use in solid-organ transplant recipients include (1) prevention of infectious complications in the immediate postoperative period, (2) prevention of late infectious complications associated with prolonged periods of immunosuppression, and (3) effective treatment of established infections in order to prevent graft dysfunction and rejection and decrease patient morbidity and mortality. All these goals must be achieved at the lowest possible toxicity and cost.

Prevention of infection in the transplant patient can be accomplished in a number of ways. First, risk of environmental contamination should be minimized.[93] Patients should be protected from institutional infectious outbreaks. Transplant patients should receive the pneumococcal vaccine once and the influenza vaccine yearly; however, their immunologic responses to these vaccines may be blunted by immunosuppressive therapy.[84]

Because the most important source of primary CMV disease is an infected donor organ, CMV-seronegative patients should not receive organs or blood products from seropositive donors if possible. A number of pharmacologic strategies also have been studied in an attempt to prevent CMV infection. Prophylactic ganciclovir (administered either as 5 mg/kg IV every 12 hours or as oral valganciclovir in doses ranging from 900 mg once daily to 1000 mg three times daily) is effective in reducing the incidence of both primary and reac-

tivated CMV disease in solid-organ transplantation.[80,84,86,90,91] Ganciclovir prophylaxis also may reduce reactivation of CMV disease significantly in seropositive patients receiving ALG or muronomab for treatment of acute rejection.[86,91] High-dose oral acyclovir effectively reduces the incidence of CMV infection and disease following renal transplantation.[94] However, acyclovir is less efficacious in high-risk renal transplant patients (donor positive, recipient negative for CMV serum antibodies) and other nonrenal transplant types.[84,86,91,95] Preemptive ganciclovir (initiated following actual isolation of CMV from blood, urine, BAL fluid, or other site) is more effective than acyclovir in the prevention of both primary and reactivation disease in liver transplant recipients. Preemptive ganciclovir effectively prevents CMV disease in other types of solid-organ transplants as well.[90,91] Ganciclovir-related bone marrow suppression is not as problematic in solid-organ transplant recipients as in HSCT patients; most studies report the drug as being reasonably well tolerated.[84,91,95]

Whether prophylaxis or preemptive therapy is the best approach to prevention of CMV disease is still controversial.[84,90,91] Prophylaxis is effective and easy to administer without the need for careful discrimination among suitable patients. However, universal prophylaxis results in unnecessary exposure of low-risk individuals to adverse effects of drugs, and there are concerns that prolonged exposure may increase the risk of viral resistance to drugs.[90,91,95] Preemptive therapy is effective and results in exposure of fewer patients to drugs. However, this strategy requires the availability and routine use of sensitive and specific diagnostic tests in order to identify high-risk individuals at an early stage of CMV infection. Although currently available PCR-based methods make this latter consideration less of an issue, PCR testing is not available at all centers. Prophylactic therapy should be used primarily in patients at highest risk of disease (i.e., seronegative patients receiving organs from seropositive donors), whereas other lower-risk patients should receive only preemptive therapy.[84,90,91] These recommendations are not universally accepted or practiced, however.

A number of studies also have demonstrated the value of CMV hyperimmune globulin (CMV-IVIG) in decreasing the incidence and severity of CMV disease following kidney, heart, lung, and liver transplantation.[84,90] Although prophylaxis with CMV-IVIG has been strongly recommended for CMV-seronegative transplant recipients receiving organs from seropositive donors, the benefits of CMV-IVIG relative to other therapies (e.g., prophylactic or preemptive ganciclovir) are not well known, and available studies are sometimes conflicting in their results. Whether or not the combination of CMV-IVIG plus ganciclovir offers advantages over the use of either agent alone, either for primary prophylaxis or for treatment of established CMV disease, is also unclear in solid-organ transplantation.[84,90]

Although the use of prophylactic acyclovir in HSV-seropositive patients undergoing HSCT is well accepted, prophylaxis in solid-organ transplant recipients remains controversial. Reactivation disease caused by HSV occurs in approximately 25% of HSV-seropositive patients who are not receiving prophylaxis.[84] Oral or genital mucocutaneous disease is the most common presentation, but HSV pneumonitis also is seen occasionally and is associated with a mortality rate of approximately 75%.[84] Acyclovir is being used at some centers because of the high incidence of clinical HSV infection, including pneumonias, after transplantation.

Prophylactic antimicrobial agents are of benefit to transplant patients in certain clinical situations. Antibiotic prophylaxis, with agents such as cefazolin begun perioperatively and continued for less than 24 hours is considered to reduce wound infection rates effectively following renal transplantation.[84,93] Although the benefits of erioperative prophylaxis have not been well demonstrated in other ypes of transplantation procedures, surgical prophylaxis usually is onsidered mandatory in liver, heart, and lung transplant patients be-ause of the high risk of perioperative bacterial infections.[84,93] Pul-nonary infections are particularly common in lung and heart-lung ransplant recipients, and these infections often are caused by bacteria olonizing the airways prior to transplantation. Perioperative an-ibiotics for lung and heart-lung procedures therefore often are elected based on pretransplant sputum cultures.[84,93] In addition, osttransplant antibiotic prophylaxis is effective in decreasing the umber of bacterial infections in renal transplant patients. Prophy-actic trimethoprim-sulfamethoxazole traditionally has been used be-ause it is inexpensive and well tolerated; other antibiotics, such as he fluoroquinolones, have been evaluated.[84] Administration of oral ow-dose trimethoprim-sulfamethoxazole (one double-strength tablet laily) for 6 to 12 months for prevention of *P. jiroveci* infection follow-ng heart and lung transplantation is common, although the efficacy nd optimal duration are still somewhat controversial.[84,96] Selective owel decontamination with nonabsorbable antibiotics in combina-ion with a low-bacterial diet (no fresh fruits and vegetables) effec-ively reduces oropharyngeal and GI colonization with gram-negative erobes and *Candida* in liver transplant patients. However, selec-ive bowel contamination is less efficacious when administered for period of less than 1 week prior to transplantation.[93] Since liver ransplantation usually is performed without advance notice as or-ans become emergently available, the practice of selective bowel lecontamination remains controversial and is not recommended outinely.[84,93]

Because immunosuppressed transplant recipients are at risk for mucocutaneous fungal infections, prophylactic oral or topical antifun-gal agents may be indicated in these patients. Liver transplant patients re clearly at high risk for invasive fungal infections and should re-eive prophylaxis with fluconazole (400 mg/day).[22,84,88,97] It also has een suggested that lung and heart-lung transplant recipients receive igh-dose fluconazole prophylaxis, although data for this recommen-lation are lacking.[22,88] Cyclosporine concentrations should be mon-tored closely in transplant patients receiving fluconazole and other zole antifungal agents.

Transplant patients, especially heart and heart-lung recipients, without serologic evidence of prior exposure to *T. gondii* who receive organs from seropositive donors are at high risk for toxoplasmosis.[84] Many of these patients will be receiving trimethoprim-sulfametho-xazole for prophylaxis of *P. jiroveci* infection; this agent also will provide effective prophylaxis against *T. gondii,* as well as against *V. asteroides.* Although prophylaxis is not given routinely at all centers, this therapy may be justified in high-risk patients because of the delays in diagnosis and serious infections associated with oxoplasmosis.[84]

The use of prophylactic isoniazid therapy for transplant patients with evidence of exposure to *M. tuberculosis* (those with a positive ourified protein derivative skin test) remains controversial. Risk of re-activation and development of clinical tuberculosis is enhanced with oosttransplant immunosuppression. Some clinicians believe, how-ever, that the risk of isoniazid-induced hepatotoxicity, especially in liver transplant recipients, in whom the rate of hepatotoxicity has been reported as high as 40%, outweighs the benefits of treatment. High-risk patients who may be considered for isoniazid prophylaxis include those with a positive skin test, those with previously diagnosed tuber-culosis who may not have been treated adequately, patients in close contact with individuals with active pulmonary disease, and patients with abnormal chest radiographs consistent with old tuberculosis who have not received prior prophylaxis.[84]

EVALUATION OF THERAPEUTIC OUTCOMES

Close monitoring of transplant recipients, including both clinical and laboratory data, is essential for early detection and treatment of po-tentially severe opportunistic infections.

ABBREVIATIONS

ANC: absolute neutrophil count
ARDS: acute respiratory distress syndrome
ASCO: American Society for Clinical Oncology
ATG: antithymocyte globulin
BAL: bronchoalveolar lavage
CDC: U.S. Centers for Disease Control and Prevention
CSF: colony-stimulating factor
DIC: disseminated intravascualr coagulation
EORTC: European Organization for the Research and Treatment of Cancer
GVHD: graft versus host disease
HAART: highly active anti-retroviral therapy
HLA: human leukocyte antigen
HSCT: hematopoietic stem cell transplantation
IDSA: Infectious Diseases Society of America
IP: interstitial pneumonia
MRSA: methicillin-resistant *Staphylococcus aureus*
NCCN: National Comprehensive Cancer Network
NNIS: National Nosocomial Infection Surveillance
PMN: polymorphonuclear leukocyte
VRE: vancomycin-resistant enterococci

Review Questions and other resources can be found at *www.pharmacotherapyonline.com.*

REFERENCES

1. Hughes WT, Armstrong D, Bodey GP, et al. 2002 guidelines for the use of antimicrobial agents in neutropenic patients with cancer. Clin Infect Dis 2002;34:730–751.
2. Bodey GP, Buckley M, Sathe YS, Freireich EJ. Quantitative relation-ships between circulating leukocytes and infection in patients with acute leukemia. Ann Intern Med 1966;64:328–340.
3. Pizzo PA. Management of fever in patients with cancer and treatment-induced neutropenia. N Engl J Med 1993;328:1323–1332.
4. Pizzo PA. Current concepts: Fever in immunocompromised patients. New Engl J Med 1999;341:893–900.
5. Donowitz GR, Maki DG, Crnich CJ, et al. Infections in the neutropenic patient: New views of an old problem. Hematology (Am Soc Hematol Educ Program) 2001:113–139.
6. National Comprehensive Cancer Network. Fever and neutropenia. Pract Guidelines Oncol 2002;1.
7. Sullivan KM, Dykewicz CA, Longworth DL, et al. Preventing opportunis-tic infections after hematopoietic stem cell transplantation: The Centers for Disease Control and Prevention, Infectious Diseases Society of America, and American Society for Blood and Marrow Transplantation practice guidelines and beyond. Hematology (Am Soc Hematol Educ Program) 2001:392–421.
8. Jones RN. Contemporary antimicrobial susceptibility patterns of bacterial pathogens commonly associated with febrile patients with neutropenia. Clin Infect Dis 1999;29:495–502.
9. Hicks KL, Chemaly RF, Kontoyiannis DP. Common community respi-ratory viruses in patients with cancer: More than just "common colds." Cancer 2003;97:2576–2587.

10. Giamarellou H, Antoniadou A. Infectious complications of febrile leukopenia. Infect Dis Clin North Am 2001;15:457–482.

11. Safdar A. Managing opportunistic infections against the odds of neutropenia. Abstr Hematol Oncol 2003;6:20–26.

12. O'Brien SN, Blijlevens NMA, Mahfouz TH, Anaissie EJ. Infections in patients with hematological cancer: Recent developments. Hematology (Am Soc Hematol Educ Program) 2003:438–472.

13. Hathorn JW. Critical appraisal of antimicrobials for prevention of infections in immunocompromised hosts. Hematol Oncol Clin North Am 1993; 7:1051–1099.

14. Viscoli C, Castagnola E. Planned progressive antimicrobial therapy in neutropenic patients. Br J Haematol 1998;102:879–888.

15. Bonten MJ, Gaillard CA, van der Geest S, et al. The role of intragastric acidity and stress ulcus prophylaxis on colonization and infection in mechanically ventilated ICU patients: A stratified, randomized, double-blind study of sucralfate versus antacids. Am J Respir Crit Care Med 1995; 152:1825–1834.

16. Centers for Disease Control and Prevention. National Nosocomial Infections Surveillance (NNIS) System Report: Data summary from January 1990–May 1999, issued June 1999. Am J Infect Control 1999;27: 520–532.

17. Tunkel AR, Sepkowitz KA. Infections caused by viridans streptococci in patients with neutropenia. Clin Infect Dis 2002;34:1524–1529.

18. Engemann JJ, Carmeli Y, Cosgrove SE, et al. Adverse clinical and economic outcomes attributable to methicillin resistance among patients with *Staphylococcus aureus* surgical site infection. Clin Infect Dis 2003;36:592–598.

19. Bodey GP, Jadeja L, Elting L. *Pseudomonas* bacteremia: Retrospective analysis of 410 episodes. Arch Intern Med 1985;145:1621–1629.

20. Chatzinikolaou I, Abi-Said D, Bodey, GP, et al. Recent experience with *Pseudomonas aeruginosa* bacteremia in patients with cancer: Retrospective analysis of 245 episodes. Arch Intern Med 2000;160:501–509.

21. Bodey GP, Bueltmann B, Duguid W, et al. Fungal infections in cancer patients: An international autopsy survey. Eur J Clin Microbiol Infect Dis 1992;11:99–109.

22. Pappas PG, Rex JH, Sobel JD, et al. Guidelines for treatment of candidiasis. Clin Infect Dis 2004;38:161–189.

23. Segal BH, Bow EJ, Menichetti F. Fungal infections in nontransplant patients with hematologic malignancies. Infect Dis Clin North Am 2002;16: 935–964.

24. Groll AH, Walsh TJ. Uncommon opportunistic fungi: New nosocomial threats. Clin Microbiol Infect 2001;7(suppl 2):8–24.

25. Walsh TJ, Whitcomb PO, Revankar SG, Pizzo PA. Successful treatment of hepatosplenic candidiasis through repeated cycles of chemotherapy and neutropenia. Cancer 1995;76:2357–2362.

26. Stevens DA, Kan VL, Judson MA, et al. Practice guidelines for diseases caused by *Aspergillus*. Clin Infect Dis 2000;30:696–709.

27. Hughes WT, Rivera GK, Schell MJ, et al. Successful intermittent chemoprophylaxis for *Pneumocystis jiroveci* pneumonitis. N Engl J Med 1987; 316:1627–1632.

28. Rolston KV. New trends in patient management: Risk-based therapy for febrile patients with neutropenia. Clin Infect Dis 1999;29:515–521.

29. Freifeld A, Marchigiani D, Walsh T, et al. A double-blind comparison of empirical oral and intravenous antibiotic therapy for low-risk febrile patients with neutropenia during cancer chemotherapy. N Engl J Med 1999;341:305–311.

30. Kern WV, Cometta A, DeBock R, et al. Oral versus intravenous empirical antimicrobial therapy for fever in patients with granulocytopenia who are receiving cancer chemotherapy. N Engl J Med 1999;341:312–318.

31. Escalante CP, Rubenstein EB, Rolston KV. Outpatient antibiotic therapy for febrile episodes in low-risk neutropenic patients with cancer. Cancer Invest 1997;15:237–242.

32. Shenep JL, Flynn PM, Baker DK, et al. Oral cefixime is similar to continued intravenous antibiotics in the empirical treatment of febrile neutropenic children with cancer. Clin Infect Dis 2001;32:36–43.

33. Giamarellou H, Bassaris HP, Petrikkos G, et al. Monotherapy with intravenous followed by oral high-dose ciprofloxacin versus combination therapy with ceftazidime plus amikacin as initial empirical therapy for granu-locytopenic patients with fever. Antimicrob Agents Chemother 2000;44: 3264–3271.

34. Pizzo PA, Hathorn JW, Hiemenz J, et al. A randomized trial comparing ceftazidime alone with combination antibiotic therapy in cancer patients with fever and neutropenia. N Engl J Med 1986;315:552–558.

35. Engervall P, Kalin M, Dornbusch K, Bjorkholm M. Cefepime as empirical monotherapy in febrile patients with hematological malignancies and neutropenia: A randomized, single-center phase II trial. J Chemother 1999;11:278–286.

36. Rolston KV, Berkey P, Bodey GP, et al. A comparison of imipenem to ceftazidime with or without amikacin as empirical therapy in febrile neutropenic patients. Arch Intern Med 1992;152:283–291.

37. Cometta A, Calandra T, Gaya H, et al. Monotherapy with meropenem versus combination therapy with ceftazidime plus amikacin as empirical therapy for fever in granulocytopenic patients with cancer. Antimicrob Agents Chemother 1996;40:1108–1115.

38. Fish DN, Singletary TJ. Meropenem: A new carbapenem antibiotic. Pharmacotherapy 1997;17:644–669.

39. Furno P, Bucaneve G, Del Favero A. Monotherapy or aminoglycoside-containing combinations for empirical antibiotic treatment of febrile neutropenic patients: A meta-analysis. Lancet Infect Dis 2002;2:231–242.

40. Paul M, Soares-Weiser K, Grozinsky S, Leibovici L. Beta-lactam versus beta-lactam-aminoglycoside combination therapy in cancer patients with neutropaenia. Cochrane Database Syst Rev 2003;3:CD003038.

41. Johnson MP, Ramphal R. β-Lactam-resistant *Enterobacter* bacteremia in febrile neutropenic patients receiving monotherapy. J Infect Dis 1990; 162:981–983.

42. Vandercam B, Gerain J, Humblet Y, et al. Meropenem versus ceftazidime as empirical monotherapy for febrile neutropenic cancer patients. Ann Hematol 2000;79:152–157.

43. Hatala R, Dinh TT, Cook DJ. Single daily dosing of aminoglycosides in immunocompromised adults: A systematic review. Clin Infect Dis 1997; 24:810–815.

44. Feld R. Vancomycin as part of initial empirical antibiotic therapy for febrile neutropenia in patients with cancer: Pros and cons. Clin Infect Dis 1999;29:503–507.

45. Cometta A, Kern WV, De Bock R, et al. Vancomycin versus placebo for treating persistent fever in patients with neutropenic cancer receiving piperacillin-tazobactam monotherapy. Clin Infect Dis 2003;37: 382–289.

46. Centers for Disease Control and Prevention. Recommendations for preventing the spread of vancomycin resistance: Recommendations of the Hospital Infection Control Practices Advisory Committee (HICPAC). MMWR 1995(Sept 22);44(No. RR-12):1–13.

47. Antabli BA, Bross P, Siegel RS, et al. Empirical antimicrobial therapy of febrile neutropenic patients undergoing haematopoietic stem cell transplantation. Int J Antimicrob Agents 1999;13:127–130.

48. Peacock JE Jr, Herrington DA, Wade JC, et al. Ciprofloxacin plus piperacillin compared with tobramycin plus piperacillin as empirical therapy in febrile neutropenia patients: A randomized, double-blind trial. Ann Intern Med 2002;137:77–87.

49. Scheld WM. Maintaining fluoroquinolone class efficacy: Review of influencing factors. Emerg Infect Dis, 2003; available from *//www.cdc.gov/ncidod/EID/vol9no1/02-0277.htm.*

50. Elting LS, Rubenstein EB, Rolston K, et al. Time to clinical response: An outcome of antibiotic therapy of febrile neutropenia with implications for quality and cost of care. J Clin Oncol 2000;18:3699–3706.

51. White MH, Anaissie EJ, Kusne S, et al. Amphotericin B colloidal dispersion vs amphotericin B as therapy for invasive aspergillosis. Clin Infect Dis 1997;24:635–642.

52. Walsh TJ, Finberg RW, Arndt C, et al. Liposomal amphotericin B for empirical therapy in patients with persistent fever and neutropenia. N Engl J Med 1999;340:764–771.

53. Boogaerts M, Winston DJ, Bow EJ, et al. Intravenous and oral itraconazole versus intravenous amphotericin B deoxycholate as empirical antifungal therapy for persistent fever in neutropenic patients with cancer who are receiving broad-spectrum antibacterial therapy: A randomized, controlled trial. Ann Intern Med 2001;135:412–422.

54. Walsh TJ, Pappas P, Winston DJ, et al. Voriconazole compared with liposomal amphotericin B for empirical antifungal therapy in patients with neutropenia and persistent fever. N Engl J Med 2002;346:225–234.

55. O'Grady NP, Alexander M, Dellinger P, et al. Guidelines for the prevention of intravascular catheter-related infections. Clin Infect Dis 2002;35:1281–1307.

56. Mermel LA, Farr BM, Sherertz RJ, et al. Guidelines for the management of intravascular catheter-related infections. Clin Infect Dis 2001;32:1249–1272.

57. Ozer H, Armitage JO, Bennett CL, et al. 2000 update of recommendations for the use of hematopoietic colony-stimulating factors: Evidence-based, clinical practice guidelines. J Clin Oncol 2000;18:3558–3585.

58. Clark OA, Lyman G, Castro AA, et al. Colony-stimulating factors for chemotherapy-induced febrile neutropenia. Cochrane Database Syst Rev 2003;3:CD003039.

59. Hubel K, Dale DC, Engert A, Liles WC. Current status of granulocyte (neutrophil) transfusion therapy for infectious diseases. J Infect Dis 2001;183:321–328.

60. Cruciani M, Rampazzo R, Malena M, et al. Prophylaxis with fluoroquinolones for bacterial infections in neutropenic patients: A meta-analysis. Clin Infect Dis 1996;23:795–805.

61. Kern W, Kurrle E. Ofloxacin versus trimethoprim-sulfamethoxazole for prevention of infection in patients with acute leukemia and granulocytopenia. Infection 1991;19:73–80.

62. Engels EA, Lau J, Barza M. Efficacy of quinolone prophylaxis in neutropenic cancer patients: A meta-analysis. J Clin Oncol 1998;16:1179–1187.

63. Munoz L, Martino R, Subira M, et al. Intensified prophylaxis of febrile neutropenia with ofloxacin plus rifampin during severe short-duration neutropenia in patients with lymphoma. Leuk Lymphoma 1999;34:585–589.

64. Cornely OA, Ullmann AJ, Karthaus M. Evidence-based assessment of primary antifungal prophylaxis in patients with hematologic malignancies. Blood 2003;101:3365–3372.

65. Bow EJ, Laverdiere M, Lussier N, et al. Antifungal prophylaxis for severely neutropenic chemotherapy recipients: A meta-analysis of randomized-controlled clinical trials. Cancer 2002;94:3230–3246.

66. Goodman JL, Winston DJ, Greenfield RA, et al. A controlled trial of fluconazole to prevent fungal infections in patients undergoing bone marrow transplantation. N Engl J Med 1992;326:845–851.

67. Slavin MA, Osborne B, Adams R, et al. Efficacy and safety of fluconazole prophylaxis for fungal infections after marrow transplantation: A prospective, randomized, double-blind study. J Infect Dis 1995;171:1545–1552.

68. Rotstein C, Bow EJ, Laverdiere M, et al. Randomized placebo-controlled trial of fluconazole prophylaxis for neutropenic cancer patients: Benefit based on purpose and intensity of cytotoxic therapy. Clin Infect Dis 1999;28:331–340.

69. Wingard JR, Merz WG, Rinaldi MG, et al. Increase in *Candida krusei* infection among patients with bone marrow transplantation and neutropenia treated prophylactically with fluconazole. N Engl J Med 1991;325:1274–1277.

70. Winston DJ, Maziarz RT, Chandrasekar PH, et al. Intravenous and oral itraconazole versus intravenous and oral fluconazole for long-term antifungal prophylaxis in allogeneic hematopoietic stem-cell transplant recipients: A multicenter, randomized trial. Ann Intern Med 2003;138:705–713.

71. de Lalla F. Antibiotic treatment of febrile episodes in neutropenic cancer patients: Clinical and economic considerations. Drugs 1997;53:789–804.

72. Leather HL, Wingard JR. Infections following hematopoietic stem cell transplantation. Infect Dis Clin North Am 2001;15:483–520.

73. Lin S-J, Schranz J, Teutsch SM. Aspergillosis case-fatality rate: Systematic review of the literature. Clin Infect Dis 2001;32:358–366.

74. Momin F, Chandrasekar PH. Antimicrobial prophylaxis in bone marrow transplantation. Ann Intern Med 1995;123:205–215.

75. Ketterer N, Espinouse D, Chomarat M, et al. Infections following peripheral blood progenitor cell transplantation for lymphoproliferative malignancies: Etiology and potential risk factors. Am J Med 1999;106:191–197.

76. Darville JM, Ley BE, Roome AP, et al. Acyclovir-resistant herpes simplex virus infections in a bone marrow transplant transplant population. Bone Marrow Tranplant 1998;22:587–589.

77. Nguyen Q, Champlin R, Giralt S, et al. Late cytomegalovirus pneumonia in adult allogeneic blood and marrow transplant recipients. Clin Infect Dis 1999;28:618–623.

78. Centers for Disease Control and Prevention. Guidelines for preventing opportunistic infections among hematopoietic stem cell transplant recipients: Recommendations of CDC, the Infectious Diseases Society of America, and the American Society of Blood and Marrow Transplantation. MMWR 2000;49(RR-10):1–110.

79. Meyers JD, Reed EC, Shepp DH, et al. Acyclovir for prevention of cytomegalovirus infection and disease after allogeneic marrow transplantation. N Engl J Med 1988;318:70–75.

80. Razonable RR, Paya CV. Valganciclovir for the prevention and treatment of cytomegalovirus disease in immunocompromised hosts. Expert Rev Anti-Infect Ther 2004;2:27–42.

81. Barnes RA. Immunotherapy and immunoprophylaxis in bone marrow transplantation. J Hosp Infect 1995;30(suppl):223–231.

82. Marr KA. Antifungal prophylaxis in hematopoitec stem cell transplant recipients. Curr Opin Infect Dis 2001;14:423–426.

83. Gubbins PO, Bowman JL, Penzak SR. Antifungal prophylaxis to prevent invasive mycoses among bone marrow transplantation patients. Pharmacotherapy 1998;18:549–564.

84. Simon DM, Levin S. Infectious complications of solid organ transplantations. Infect Dis Clin North Am 2001;15:521–549.

85. Mele A, Paterson PJ, Prentice HG, et al: Toxoplasmosis in bone marrow transplantation: A report of two cases and systematic review of the literature. Bone Marrow Transplant 2002;29:691–698.

86. Varon NF, Alangaden GJ. Emerging trends in infections among renal transplant recipients. Expert Rev Anti-Infect Ther 2004;2:95–109.

87. The U.S. Multicenter FK506 Liver Study Group. A comparison of tacrolimus (FK506) and cyclosporine for immunosuppression in liver transplantation. N Engl J Med 1994;331:1110–1115.

88. Singh N. Fungal infections in the recipients of solid organ transplantation. Infect Dis Clin North Am 2003;17:113–134.

89. Montoya JG, Giraldo LF, Efron B, et al: Infectious complications among 620 consecutive heart transplant recipients at Stanford University Medical Center. Clin Infect Dis 2001;33:629–640.

90. Kletzmayr J, Kreuzwieser E, Klauser R. New developments in the management of cytomegalovirus infection and disease after renal transplantation. Curr Opin Urol 2001;11:153–158.

91. Singh N. Preemptive therapy versus universal prophylaxis with ganciclovir for cytomegalovirus in solid organ transplant recipients. Clin Infect Dis 2001;32:742–751.

92. Roland ME, Adey D, Carlson LL, Terrault NA. Kidney and liver transplantation in HIV-infected patients: Case presentations and review. AIDS Patient Care Stds 2003;17:501–507.

93. Soave R. Prophylaxis strategies for solid-organ transplantation. Clin Infect Dis 2001;33(suppl 1):S26–31.

94. Singh N, Yu VL, Mieles L, et al. High-dose acyclovir compared with short-course preemptive ganciclovir therapy to prevent cytomegalovirus disease in liver transplant recipients. Ann Intern Med 1994;120:375–381.

95. Van der Bij W, Speich R. Management of cytomegalovirus infection and disease after solid-organ transplantation. Clin Infect Dis 2001;33(suppl 1):S33–S37.

96. Fishman JA. Prevention of infection caused by *Pneumocystis jiroveci* in transplant recipients. Clin Infect Dis 2001;33:1397–1405.

97. Paya CV. Prevention of fungal and hepatitis viral infections in liver transplantation. Clin Infect Dis 2001;33(suppl 1):S47–52.

121

ANTIMICROBIAL PROPHYLAXIS IN SURGERY

Salmaan Kanji and John W. Devlin

Learning Objectives and other resources can be found at *www.pharmacotherapyonline.com.*

KEY CONCEPTS

◀① *Prophylactic* antibiotic therapy differs from *presumptive* and *therapeutic* antibiotic therapy in that the latter two involve treatment regimens for documented or presumed infections, whereas the goal of prophylactic therapy is to prevent infections in high-risk patients or procedures.

◀② The risk of a surgical site infection (SSI) is determined from both the type of surgery and patient-specific risk factors; however, most commonly used classification systems only account for procedure-related risk factors.

◀③ Timing of antimicrobial prophylaxis is of paramount importance. Antibiotics should be administered 1 hour before the surgery to ensure adequate drug levels at the surgical site prior to the initial incision.

◀④ Antimicrobial agents with short half-lives (e.g., cefazolin) may need to be redosed intraoperatively during long (>3 hours) procedures.

◀⑤ One must consider the type of surgery, intrinsic patient risk factors, the most commonly identified pathogenic organisms, institutional antimicrobial resistance patterns, and cost when choosing an antimicrobial agent for prophylaxis.

◀⑥ Single-dose prophylaxis is appropriate for many types of surgery. First-generation cephalosporins (e.g., cefazolin) are the mainstay for prophylaxis in most surgical procedures because of their spectrum of activity, safety, and cost.

◀⑦ Vancomycin as a prophylactic agent should be limited to cases in which there is a documented history of life-threatening β-lactam hypersensitivity or where the incidence of infections with organisms resistant to cefazolin (e.g., methicillin resistant *Staphylococcus aureus* [MRSA]) is high enough to justify use.

According to the National Center for Health Statistics, approximately 46 million surgical procedures are performed annually in the United States, the majority of which are done in an outpatient setting.[1] Infection is the most common complication of surgery.[2] Surgical-site infections (SSIs) occur in about 3% to 6% of patients and prolong hospitalization by an average of 7 days at a direct annual cost of $5 to $10 billion.[3,4] SSIs are the third (14% to 16%) most frequent cause of nosocomial infections among hospitalized patients and the primary (40%) cause of nosocomial infection in surgical patients.[3] The prophylactic administration of antibiotics decreases the risk of infection after many surgical procedures and represents an important component of care for this population.

Antibiotics administered prior to the contamination of previously sterile tissues or fluids are deemed *prophylactic* antibiotics. The goal of therapy is to *prevent* an infection from developing. While eradication of distal (preexisting, unrelated to surgery) infections lowers the risk for subsequent postoperative infections, it does not, per se, constitute a prophylactic regimen. In fact, surgical prophylaxis often is prescribed concurrently under these circumstances because of important antimicrobial spectrum- and timing-related concerns. Both SSIs and infections not directly related to the surgical site are termed *nosocomial* (e.g., urinary tract infections, pneumonia, etc.). Prevention of these hospital-acquired infections is a major goal of antibiotic prophylaxis.

◀① *Presumptive* antibiotic therapy is administered when an infection is suspected but not yet proven. Clinical scenarios where presumptive therapy is employed commonly include acute cholecystitis, open compound fractures, and acute appendicitis of less than

24 hours' duration. In these situations, if signs of perforation or infection are absent during surgery, then routine prophylactic rather than presumptive therapy is warranted. An operative finding of a gangrenous gallbladder or a perforated appendix, however, is suggestive of an established infectious process, and thus a *therapeutic* antibiotic regimen would be required.[3]

According to the Center for Disease Control and Prevention's (CDC) National Nosocomial Infections Surveillance System (NNIS),[3] SSIs can be categorized as either incisional (e.g., cellulitis of the incision site) or organ/space (e.g., meningitis) (Fig. 121–1). Incisional SSIs are further subcategorized into superficial (involving only the skin or subcutaneous tissue) and deep (fascial and muscle layers) infections. Organ/space SSIs can involve any anatomic area other than the incision site. For example, a patient who develops bacterial peritonitis after bowel surgery would have an organ/space SSI. By definition, SSIs must occur within 30 days of surgery. If a prosthetic implant is involved, however, a deep incisional or organ/space SSI still can be reported up to 1 year from the date of surgery. Although microbiologic testing of surgical drainage material or sites may help to guide care, the specificity of a negative culture is poor and generally does not rule out an SSI.[3]

SSI RISK FACTORS

◀② SSI incidence depends on both procedure- and patient-related factors. Traditionally, the risk for SSIs has been stratified by surgical procedure in a classification system developed by the National

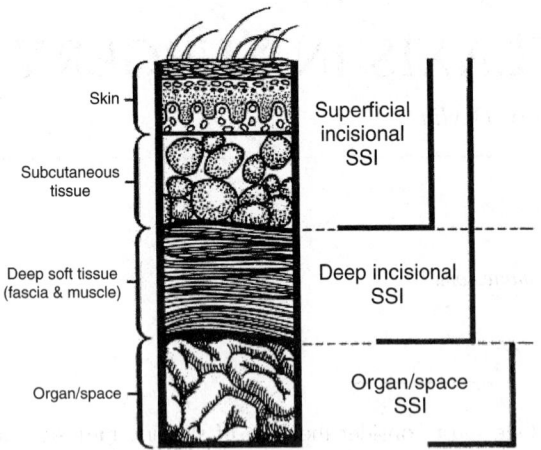

FIGURE 121–1. Cross section of abdominal wall depicting CDC classifications of SSIs. *(From ref. 3).*

TABLE 121–2. Patient and Operation Characteristics that May Influence the Risk of SSI

Patient	Operation
Age	Duration of surgical scrub
Nutritional status	Preoperative skin preparation
Diabetes	Preoperative shaving
Smoking	Duration of operation
Obesity	Antimicrobial prophylaxis
Coexisting infections at distal body sites	Operating room ventilation
Colonization with resistant microorganisms	Sterilization of instruments
Altered immune response	Implantation of prosthetic materials
Length of preoperative stay	Surgical drains
	Surgical technique

Adapted from ref. 3.

Research Council (NRC)[5] (Table 121–1). The NRC classification system proposes that the risk of an SSI depends on the microbiology of the surgical site, the presence of a preexisting infection, the likelihood of contaminating previously sterile tissue during surgery, and events during and after surgery.[5,6] A patient's NRC procedure classification is the primary determinant of whether antibiotic prophylaxis is warranted. It should be emphasized, however, that because a patient's NRC wound classification is influenced by surgical findings (e.g., gangrenous gallbladder) and perioperative events (e.g., major technique breaks), that categorization generally occurs intraoperatively.[7]

INHERENT PATIENT RISK

The NRC classification system does not account for the influence of underlying patient risk factors for SSI development, instead categorizing the risks for SSIs simply based on a specific surgical procedure. Disease states and conditions known to increase SSI risk are presented in Table 121–2. Preexisting distal infections increase SSI rates and should be resolved prior to surgery whenever possible. Diabetic patients have an increased risk of SSIs, especially those with uncon-

trolled perioperative blood sugars.[8] Preoperative smoking has been identified as an independent risk factor for SSI because of the deleterious effects of nicotine on wound healing. Preoperative immunosuppression, including corticosteroid use, also may increase infection risk. Malnutrition is a well-described risk factor for postoperative complications, including SSI, impaired wound and colonic anastomosis healing, and prolonged hospital stay. While enteral feeding in the perioperative period can reduce bacterial translocation by maintaining the integrity of the intestinal mucosa, nutritional supplementation has not been shown to decrease the incidence of infection.[9]

CLINICAL CONTROVERSY

Several recent studies have investigated the role of specialized enteral formulas fortified with a variety of immunomodulating micronutrients thought to enhance the immune response and gut function after trauma or surgery. While many clinicians are exploring the role of supplements such as glutamine, arginine, omega-3 fatty acids, and nucleotides, no study to date has shown a significant reduction in postoperative infection rates using these formulations.

TABLE 121–1. NRC[a] Wound Classification, Risk of SSI[b], and Indication for Antibiotics

Classification	SWI Rate (%) Preoperative Antibiotics	SWI Rate (%) No Preoperative Antibiotics	Criteria	Antibiotics
Clean	5.1	0.8	No acute inflammation or transection of gastrointestinal, oropharyngeal, genitourinary, biliary, or respiratory tracts. Elective case, no technique break	Not indicated unless high-risk procedure[c]
Clean-contaminated	10.1	1.3	Controlled opening of aforementioned tracts with minimal spillage/minor technique break. Clean procedures performed emergently or with major technique breaks.	Prophylactic antibiotics indicated
Contaminated	21.9	10.2	Acute, nonpurulent inflammation present. Major spillage/technique break during clean-contaminated procedure	Prophylactic antibiotics indicated
Dirty	N/A	N/A	Obvious preexisting infection present (abscess, pus, or necrotic tissue present)	Therapeutic antibiotics required

[a]NRC = National Research Council.
[b]SSI = surgical-site infection.
[c]High-risk procedures include implantation of prosthetic materials and other procedures where surgical-site infection is associated with high morbidity (see text).
Adapted from refs. 5 and 11.

TABLE 121–3. Surgical Site Infection Incidence (%) Stratified by National Research Council Wound Classification and SENIC Risk Factors[a]

No. of SENIC Risk Factors	Clean	Clean-Contaminated	Contaminated	Dirty
0	1.1	0.6	N/A	N/A
1	3.9	2.8	4.5	6.7
2	8.4	8.4	8.3	10.9
3	15.8	17.7	11.0	18.8
4	N/A	N/A	23.9	27.4

[a]The Study on the Efficacy of Nosocomial Infection Control (SENIC) risk factors include abdominal operation, operations lasting >2 hours, contaminated or dirty procedures by National Research Council (NRC) classification, and more than three underlying medical diagnoses.
Adapted from ref. 13.

Colonization of the nares with *Staphylococcus aureus* is a well-described SSI risk factor.[3] Two small prospective trials suggest that eradication of nasal *S. aureus* with mupirocin significantly reduces the incidence of SSI when compared with historical controls in patients undergoing both cardiac and upper gastrointestinal surgery. Larger prospective trials, however, are needed before this therapy can be advocated routinely. Other factors shown to increase the risk of SSI include age, length of preoperative hospital stay, and obesity.[3]

IDENTIFYING SSI RISK

Two large epidemiologic studies have objectively quantified SSI risk based on specific patient- and procedure-related factors. The Study on the Efficacy of Nosocomial Infection Control (SENIC) analyzed more than 100,000 surgery cases to identify and validate risk factors for SSI.[10] Abdominal operations, operations lasting longer than 2 hours, contaminated or "dirty" procedures (as per NRC classification), and more than three underlying medical diagnoses each were associated with an increased incidence of SSI. When NRC classification was stratified by number of SENIC risk factors present, SSI incidence varied by as much as a factor of 15 within the same NRC operative category[11] (Table 121–3).

The NNIS, in a subsequent analysis of more than 84,000 surgical cases, attempted to simplify and refine the SENIC system by quantifying intrinsic patient risk using the American Society of Anesthesiologists' (ASA) preoperative assessment score[12,13] (Table 121–4). An ASA score of 3 or greater was found to be a strong predictor for the development of an SSI. Other factors associated with increased SSI incidence include contaminated or "dirty" operations (NRC criteria) and surgical procedures lasting longer than average. Similar to the SENIC study, the SSI rate was linked to the number of risk factors present and varied considerably within NRC class.

Although evidence-based recommendations for antimicrobial prophylaxis during surgery are best established using the results of

randomized clinical trials, many studies have small sample sizes and do not stratify patients according to overall SSI risk. Future studies, particularly those involving clean procedures, should be stratified by SSI risk so that the subset of high-risk patients who might benefit the most from prophylaxis is clearly established.

BACTERIOLOGY

The most important consideration when choosing antibiotic prophylaxis is the bacteriology of the surgical site. Organisms involved in an SSI are acquired one of two ways: endogenously (from the patient's own normal flora) and exogenously (from contamination during the surgical procedure). Based on the type and anatomic location of the procedure and the NRC classification (see Table 121–1), resident flora can be predicted, and appropriate antibiotic choices can be made. According to NNIS data, *S. aureus*, coagulase-negative staphylococci, enterococci, *Escherichia coli*, and *Pseudomonas aeruginosa* are the pathogens most commonly isolated[3] (Table 121–5). With the widespread use of broad-spectrum antibiotics, however, *Candida* spp. and methicillin-resistant *S. aureus* are becoming more prevalent.[9]

Factors affecting the ability of an organism to induce an SSI depend on organism count, organism virulence, and host immunocompetency. Organisms in the commensal flora generally are not pathogenic. These organisms often serve the host as a form of protection against invasive organisms that otherwise would colonize the surgical site. Opportunistic organisms usually are kept in check by normal flora and rarely are problematic unless they are found in large numbers. Loss of this normal flora through the use of broad-spectrum antibiotics can destabilize this homeostasis, thus allowing pathogenic bacteria to proliferate and infection to occur.[14]

If translocated to a normally sterile tissue site or fluid during a surgical procedure, normal flora can become pathogenic. For example, *S. aureus* or *S. epidermidis* may be translocated from the surface of the skin to deeper tissues or *E. coli* from the colon to the peritoneal cavity, bloodstream, or urinary tract. Studies in animals and healthy volunteers have shown bacterial virulence to be an important determinant in the development of secondary infections.[15,16] Animal models of infection have demonstrated that while more than 1 million *S. aureus* per square centimeter or gram of tissue are required to produce infection, less than 100,000 *Streptococcus pyogenes* per square centimeter or gram of tissue would be required at the same site.[16,17]

Impaired host defense reduces the number of bacteria required to establish an infection. A breach of normal host defenses through surgical intervention (e.g., insertion of a prosthetic device) may

TABLE 121–4. American Society of Anesthesiologists Physical Status Classification

Class	Description
1	Normal healthy patient
2	Mild systemic disease
3	Severe systemic disease that is not incapacitating
4	Incapacitating systemic disease that is a constant threat to life
5	Not expected to survive 24 hours with or without operation

From ref. 15.

TABLE 121–5. Major Pathogens in Surgical Wound Infections

Pathogen	Percent of Infections[a]
Staphylococcus aureus	20
Coagulase-negative staphylococci	14
Enterococci	12
Escherichia coli	8
Pseudomonas aeruginosa	8
Enterobacter spp.	7
Proteus mirabilis	3
Klebsiella pneumoniae	3
Other *Streptococcus* spp.	3
Candida albicans	3
Group D streptococci	2
Other gram-positive aerobes	2
Bacteroides fragilis	2

[a]Data reported by the NNIS from 1990–1996, adapted from ref. 5.

enable organisms to cause infection. In addition, the loss of specific immune factors, such as complement activation, tissue-derived inhibitors (e.g., proinflammatory cytokines), cell-mediated response (e.g., T-cell function), and granulocytic or phagocytic function (e.g., neutrophils or macrophages) can greatly increase the risk for SSI development.[18] Vascular occlusive states related to the surgical procedure or those occurring from hypovolemic shock can greatly affect blood flow to the surgical site, thus diminishing host defense mechanisms against microbial invasion. Traumatized tissue, hematomas, and the presence of foreign material also lead to more infections. When a foreign body is introduced during a surgical procedure, fewer than 100 bacterial colony-forming units (CFUs) are required to cause an SSI.[19] Studies examining *S. aureus*–contaminated wound infections on the skin of healthy volunteers demonstrate a 10,000-fold reduction in the number of organisms required to establish a wound infection if sutures are not present.[15]

ANTIMICROBIAL RESISTANCE

Colonization of the host with antibiotic-resistant hospital flora prior to or during surgery may lead to an SSI that is unresponsive to routine antibiotic therapy. Epidemiologic studies demonstrate that the most common cause for nosocomially acquired multiresistant organisms is transmission from hospital personnel.[20] Patients treated with broad-spectrum antibiotic therapy also are at increased risk of colonization with hospital flora.

With cephalosporins established as first-line agents for prophylaxis over the past decade, organisms resistant to cephalosporins represent the majority of pathogens causing SSIs. The CDC has reported an alarming increase in the incidence of vancomycin-resistant enterococci (VRE) infections, particularly those with *E. faecium*.[3] Risk factors for VRE colonization include severe concomitant diseases, immunosuppression, admission to the intensive care unit, previous intraabdominal or cardiothoracic surgery, placement of indwelling catheters, and prolonged courses of antimicrobials, particularily vancomycin.[21] In an effort to control the spread of VRE, the CDC has published recommendations that include strict criteria for the use of vancomycin as surgical prophylaxis.[22] The guidelines suggest vancomycin substitution for cefazolin as SSI prophylaxis only when there is a high suspicion of methicillin-resistant *S. aureus* or in patients who have a documented history of a life-threatening allergy to penicillins or cephalosporins. Other limitations to vancomycin use, besides the risk of inducing resistant organisms, include its narrow spectrum of activity, its poor penetration into some tissues, and the potential for infusion-related reactions. The emergence of *S. aureus* displaying intermediate resistance (minimum inhibitory concentration [MIC] $\geq$ 8 mcg/mL) further underscores the need to limit routine use of vancomycin for prophylaxis.[23]

Although cefazolin remains a mainstay in cardiovascular SSI prophylaxis, its failure has been reported in cases involving methicillin-sensitive *S. aureus* (MSSA). In a comparison trial between cefamandole and cefazolin, significantly more failures were attributed to cefazolin, even though the primary pathogen was MSSA.[24] A similar trial comparing cefazolin and cefuroxime, however, did not show any difference in SSI incidence between the two regimens.[25] It has been proposed that the β-lactamase expressed by some MSSA is capable of hydrolyzing cefazolin more readily than cefuroxime or cefamandole. Although this trend is disturbing, the overall incidence of cefazolin failure remains low, and cefazolin remains the drug of choice for SSI prophylaxis in cardiovascular surgery.

The increase in frequency of fungal infections in surgical patients has drawn concern. In hospitalized patients, the incidence of nosocomial *Candida* infections has approximately doubled from 1991 to 1996.[26] Overzealous use of broad-spectrum antibiotics is the most likely cause for this increase. A study in patients undergoing cardiovascular surgery identified sex (female), length of stay in the intensive care unit, and duration of central venous catheterization as risk factors for postoperative *Candida* infections.[27] While presurgical *Candida* colonization is associated with a higher risk of fungal SSIs, the routine preoperative use of prophylactic antifungal agents is not being advocated at this time.[26,28]

SCHEDULING ANTIBIOTIC ADMINISTRATION

The following principles must be considered when providing antimicrobial surgical prophylaxis: (1) The agents should be delivered to the surgical site prior to the initial incision, and (2) bactericidal antibiotic concentrations should be maintained at the surgical site throughout the surgical procedure. While animal and human models have demonstrated the efficacy of a single dose of an antibiotic administered just prior to bacterial contamination, long operations often require intraoperative doses of antibiotics to maintain adequate concentrations at the surgical site for the duration of the surgery.[2] Antibiotics should be administered with anesthesia just prior to the initial incision. Administration of antibiotics too early may result in concentrations below the MIC toward the end of the operation, and administration too late leaves the patient unprotected at the time of the initial incision. In a study examining the timing of antibiotics in 2847 patients receiving prophylaxis, Classen and colleagues[29] evaluated patients who received prophylaxis early (2 to 24 hours before surgery), preoperative prophylaxis (0 to 2 hours prior to surgery), perioperative prophylaxis (up to 3 hours after first incision), and postoperative prophylaxis (>3 hours after the first incision). The risk of infection was lowest (0.6%) for those patients who received preoperative prophylaxis, moderate (1.4%) for those who received perioperative antibiotics, and greatest for those who received postoperative antibiotics (3.3%) or preoperative antibiotics too early (3.8%). These results indicate that the risk for an SSI increases dramatically with each hour that elapses from the initial incision to the time when antibiotics are administered eventually. For these reasons, prophylactic antibiotics should not be prescribed to be given "on call to the OR," which can occur 2 or more hours prior to the initial incision, nor should concurrent therapeutic antibiotics be relied on to provide adequate protection. In both situations, the chance for improperly timed doses is high.

Despite the importance of appropriately timed prophylactic antibiotic therapy, few patients receive antibiotics at the optimal time in relation to surgery. Potential barriers include antibiotics ordered after the patient has arrived in the operating room, delayed antibiotic preparation or delivery, and the use of antibiotics that require long infusion times. One study assessed the timing of prophylactic antibiotics in 100 patients and found that only 26% of patients received an antibiotic dose within 2 hours of the initial surgical incision.[30]

Although most studies comparing single versus multiple doses of prophylactic antibiotics have failed to show a benefit of multi-dose regimens, the duration of operations in these studies may not be as long as that which is frequently observed in clinical practice. Proponents of administering a second antibiotic dose during lengthy operations suggest that the risk for SSI is just as great at the end of surgery, during wound closing, as it is during the initial incision.[31] One study in patients undergoing clean-contaminated operations suggests that procedures longer than 3 hours require a second intraoperative dose of cefazolin or the substitution of cefazolin with a longer-acting antimicrobial agent.[32] A second study of patients undergoing elective colorectal surgery suggests that low serum antimicrobial concentrations at the time of surgical closure is the strongest predictor of postoperative SSI.[33] Studies in patients undergoing cardiac surgery also have demonstrated a higher infection rate among patients with undetectable antibiotic serum concentrations at the conclusion of the procedure.[34]

One strategy to ensure appropriate redosing of prophylactic antibiotics during long operations is to employ a visual or auditory reminder system. One hospital has published its experience with such a system and found that an automated reminder improved compliance and reduced SSIs. However, even with the reminder system, intraoperative redosing was done in only 68% of eligible patients.[35] Another strategy currently being evaluated is the role of continuous infusions of cefazolin. One pilot study has found this a feasible way to ensure adequate serum concentrations of antibiotic during prolonged surgeries.[36] Further trials are required before such an intervention can be recommended.

Underlying disease states that may affect antibiotic metabolism and/or elimination should be considered when developing a prophylactic regimen. For example, patients with thermal burn and spinal cord injuries eliminate certain classes of antibiotics, primarily the aminoglycosides and β-lactams, at unusually high rates compared with controls.[37] Individuals undergoing cardiac bypass may have altered antibiotic disposition related to increased volume of distribution and reduced total-body clearance and thus require special dosing consideration.[38]

ANTIMICROBIAL CHOICE

5 The choice of prophylactic antibiotic depends on the type of surgical procedure, the most frequent pathogens seen with this procedure, the safety and efficacy profile of the antimicrobial agent, the current literature evidence to support its use, and cost. Although most SSIs involve the patient's normal flora, antimicrobial selection also must take into account the susceptibility patterns of nosocomial pathogens within each institution. Typically, gram-positive coverage should be included in the choice of surgical prophylaxis because organisms such as S. aureus and S. epidermidis are encountered commonly as skin flora. The decision to broaden antibiotic prophylaxis to agents with gram-negative and anaerobic spectra of activity depends on both the surgical site (e.g., upper respiratory tract, gastrointestinal tract, genitourinary tract, etc.) and whether the operation will transect a hollow viscous or mucous membrane that may contain resident flora.[3]

Although antimicrobial prophylaxis may be administered through a variety of routes (e.g., oral, topical, intramuscular, etc.), the parenteral route is favored because of the reliability by which adequate tissue concentrations may be acheived.[39] Cephalosporins are the most commonly prescribed agents for surgical prophylaxis because of their broad antimicrobial spectrum, their favorable pharmacokinetic profile, their low incidence of adverse side effects, and low cost. First-generation cephalosporins, such as cefazolin, are the preferred choice for surgical prophylaxis, particularly for clean surgical procedures.[3,7,14] In cases where broader gram-negative and anaerobic coverage is desired, antianaerobic cephalosporins, such as cefoxitin or cefotetan, are appropriate choices. Although third-generation cephalosporins (e.g., ceftriaxone) have been advocated for prophylaxis because of their increased gram-negative coverage and

prolonged half-lives, their inferior gram-positive and anaerobic activity, in addition to their high cost, has discouraged the widespread use of these agents.[3,7,14]

Allergic reactions are the most common side effects associated with cephalosporin use. These can range from minor skin manifestations at the site of infusion to rash, pruritus, and on rare occasions anaphylaxis (<0.02%). The structural similarity between penicillins and cephalosporins (each containing a β-lactam ring) has led to considerable confusion about the cross-allergenicity between these two classes of drugs. Twenty percent of the general population is labeled "penicillin allergic," yet studies suggest that of these patients, only 10% to 20% will have positive results in a penicillin skin test.[40] The rate of cross-reactivity is approximately 2%, but since only 20% of all "penicillin allergic" patients are truly penicillin-allergic, the true incidence of cross-reactivity is likely less than 1%. Routine penicillin skin testing is not cost-effective.[40] In summary, the administration of cephalosporins is both safe and cost-effective for many patients who are labeled "penicillin allergic," and they may be used in patients who have not experienced an immediate or type I penicillin allergy.

Vancomycin may be considered for prophylactic therapy in surgical procedures involving implantation of a prosthetic device in which the rate of MRSA is high.[22] If the risk of MRSA is low and a β-lactam hypersensitivity exists, clindamycin can be used for many procedures instead of cefazolin in order to limit vancomycin use. Infusion-related side effects, such as thrombophlebitis and hypotension, particularly with vancomycin, usually can be controlled by adequate dilution and slower administration rates.[41]

Pseudomembranous colitis secondary to cephalosporins is uncommon and generally easily treated with a short course of oral metronidazole. Although infrequent, bleeding abnormalities related to cephalosporin use have been reported.[42] The primary hematologic effect appears to be an inhibition of vitamin K–dependent clotting factors that results in a prolongation of the prothrombin time. The mechanism for this effect, most commonly seen with cefotetan, is related to the methylthiotetrazole side chain of the β-lactam molecule. Patients at greatest risk for this hypoprothrombinemic effect have received a prolonged course of these agents and have underlying risk factors for vitamin K deficiency, such as malnutrition.[43]

Since inappropriate prophylactic antibiotic use not only can induce antibiotic resistance but also can negatively affect an institution's antibiotic budget, initiatives to curtail inappropriate antibiotic use have become the focus of many drug use evaluation efforts. Potential sources of inappropriate antibiotic prophylaxis include the use of broad-spectrum antimicrobials when a narrow-spectrum agent is warranted, extending prophylaxis for durations beyond that recommended in published guidelines, and using expensive antibiotics when equivalent, cheaper agents are available. The most effective tools to ensure appropriate prophylactic antibiotic prescribing are knowledge of one's institutional postoperative infection rate for each type of surgical procedure and the bacterial epidemiology patterns for each surgical population. Individualized institutional guidelines that take into account best literature evidence, institution-based antibiotic susceptibility data, and surgeon preference are also important tools to rationalize antibiotic prophylaxis use.[44]

RECOMMENDATIONS FOR SPECIFIC TYPES OF SURGERY

Guidelines for surgical prophylaxis usually are structured according to the affected tissues during an operation. While many different surgical procedures may be performed at any one anatomical site, this method of categorization is still optimal because the factors related to the success of a prophylactic regimen such as the endogenous flora that is expected and the pharmacokinetics, pharmacodynamics, and spectrum of selected antimicrobials generally are constant for a particular surgical site (see section on antimicrobial choice). The choice of antimicrobial prophylaxis is always best evaluated using the results of properly conducted clinical trials. In the absence of studies specific to the procedure in question, extrapolation from data on regimens for different procedures in the same anatomic site in question usually can be made. Subsequent modifications to each prophylactic regimen should be based on intraoperative findings or events.

While a comprehensive review of the surgical prophylaxis literature is beyond the scope of this chapter, there are important factors that should be reviewed for each type/site of surgery. Specific recommendations are summarized in Table 121–6. The reader is also referred to recently published guidelines and review articles.[3,7,14,39,45]

GASTROINTESTINAL SURGERY

Gastrointestinal surgery can be categorized according to surgical site and infectious risk. Gastroduodenal surgery and hepatobiliary surgery generally are considered to be clean or clean-contaminated surgeries with SSI rates generally less than 5%. Colorectal surgery, including appendectomies, is considered contaminated owing to the large quantities and polymicrobial nature of bacterial flora within the colon. SSI rates for these types of surgeries generally range from 15% to 30%. Emergent abdominal surgery involving bowel perforation or peritonitis is considered a dirty surgical procedure, associated with more than a 30% risk of SSI, and should be treated with *therapeutic* rather than *prophylactic* antibiotics.[3]

GASTRODUODENAL SURGERY

Insignificant numbers of bacteria usually are found in the stomach and duodenum because of their acidity. The rate of SSIs in gastroduodenal

TABLE 121–6. Most Likely Pathogens and Specific Recommendations for Surgical Prophylaxis

Type of Operation	Likely Pathogens	Recommended Prophylaxis Regimen[a]	Comments
Gastroduodenal	Enteric gram-negative bacilli, gram-positive cocci, oral anaerobes	Cefazolin 1 g × 1 (see text for recommendations for percutaneous endoscopic gastrostomy)	High-risk patients only (obstruction, hemorrhage, malignancy, acid suppression therapy, morbid obesity)
Biliary tract	Enteric gram-negative bacilli, anaerobes	Cefazolin 1 g × 1 for high-risk patients Laparoscopic: None	High-risk patients only (acute cholecystitis, common duct stones, previous biliary surgery, jaundice, age >60, obesity, diabetes mellitus)
Colorectal	Enteric gram-negative bacilli, anaerobes	PO: Neomycin 1 g + erythromycin base 1 g at 1 P.M., 2 P.M., and 11 P.M. 1 day preop plus mechanical bowel prep. IV: Cefoxitin or cefotetan 1 g × 1	Benefits of oral plus IV is controversial except for colostomy reversal and rectal resection
Appendectomy	Enteric gram-negative bacilli, anaerobes	Cefoxitin or cefotetan 1 g × 1	A second intraoperative dose of cefoxitin may be required if procedure lasts longer than 3 hours
Urologic	E. coli	Cefazolin 1 g × 1	Generally not recommended in patients with sterile pre-op urine cultures
Cesarean section	Enteric gram-negative bacilli, anaerobes, group B streptococci, enterococci	Cefazolin 2 g × 1	Give after cord is clamped
Hysterectomy	Enteric gram-negative bacilli, anaerobes, group B streptococci, enterococci	Vaginal: Cefazolin 1 g × 1 Abdominal: Cefotetan 1 g × 1 or Cefazolin 1 g × 1	Antibiotic prophylaxis should not exceed 24 hours
Head and neck	S. aureus, streptococci oral anaerobes	Cefazolin 2 g or clindamycin 600 mg at induction and q8h × 2 more doses	Addition of gentamicin to clindiamycin is controversial
Cardiothoracic	S. aureus, S. epidermidis, Corynebacterium, enteric gram-negative bacilli	Cefazolin 1 g q8h × 48h	Second-generation cephalosporins also have been advocated In areas with high prevalence of S. aureus resistance, vancomycin should be considered
Vascular	S. aureus, S. epidermidis, enteric gram-negative bacilli	Cefazolin 1 g at induction and q8h × 2 more doses	Abdominal and lower extremities have the highest infection rates
Orthopedic	S. aureus, S. epidermidis	Joint replacement: Cefazolin 1 g × 1 preop, then q8h × 2 more doses Hip fracture repair: Same as above except continue for 48 hours	Open fractures assumed contaminated with gram-negative bacilli; aminoglycosides often used—see text
Neurosurgery	S. aureus, S. epidermidis	CSF shunt procedures: Cefazolin 1 g × 1 or ceftriaxone 2 g × 1 Craniotomy: Cefazolin 1 g × 1 or cefotaxime 1 g × 1 or trimethoprim-sulfamethoxazole (160/800) IV × 1	No agents have been shown better than cefazolin in randomized control comparative trials.

[a]One-time doses are optimally infused at induction of anesthesia except as noted. Repeat doses may be required for long procedures. See text for references.

surgery generally is low, and thus procedures in this region can be classified as clean procedures. The risk for an SSI in this population increases with any condition that can lead to bacterial overgrowth, such as obstruction, hemorrhage, malignancy, or increasing the pH of gastroduodenal secretions with concomitant acid suppression therapy. Antimicrobial prophylaxis is of clinical benefit only in this high-risk population. In most cases, a single dose of intravenous cefazolin will provide adequate prophylaxis.[45] For patients with a β-lactam allergy, oral ciprofloxacin is as efficacious as parenteral cefuroxime as prophylactic therapy for gastroduodenal surgery.[46] Antimicrobial prophylaxis is only indicated in esophageal surgery in the presence of obstruction. Postoperative *therapeutic* antibiotics may be indicated if perforation is detected during surgery, depending on whether an established infection is present.

The use of antibiotic prophylaxis for percutaneous endoscopic gastrostomy (PEG) is controversial. Although postoperative peristomal infection can occur in up to 30% of patients, clinical trials with cefazolin given 30 minutes preoperatively in this population are conflicting. A pharmacoeconomic study using a meta-analysis of available studies to determine efficacy suggested that antibiotic prophylaxis cost was effective for patients undergoing PEG placements.[47,48]

HEPATOBILIARY SURGERY

Although bile is normally sterile, and the SSI rate after biliary surgery is low, antibiotic prophylaxis has been proved to be of benefit in this population. Bile contamination (bactobilia) can increase the frequency of SSIs and is present in many patients (e.g., acute cholecystitis, biliary obstruction, and advanced age).[45] In general, however, the correlation between bactobilia in surgical specimens and the subsequent pathogens implicated in an SSI is poor. The most frequently encountered organisms include *E. coli*, *Klebsiella* spp., and enterococci. *Pseudomonas* is an uncommon finding in the absence of cholangitis. Trials comparing first-, second-, and third-generation cephalosporins have not demonstrated benefit over single-dose cefazolin prophylaxis even in high-risk patients (e.g., age greater than 60 years, previous biliary surgery, acute cholecystitis, jaundice, obesity, diabetes, and common bile duct stones).[49] Ciprofloxacin and levofloxacin are effective alternatives for β-lactam-allergic patients undergoing open cholecystectomy.[50,51] In fact, orally administered levofloxacin appears to provide similar intraoperative gallbladder tissue concentrations.[51] For low-risk patients undergoing elective laparoscopic cholecystectomy, antibiotic prophylaxis is not of benefit and is not recommended.[52] The risk for SSIs in cirrhotic patients undergoing transjugular intrahepatic portosystemic shunt (TIPS) surgery may be reduced with a single prophylactic dose of ceftriaxone[53] but not with single doses of shorter-acting cephalosporins.[54] Antibiotic prophylaxis is not currently recommended prior to endoscopic retrograde cholangiopancreatography (ERCP).[55]

While surgeons may use *presumptive* antibiotic therapy for patients with acute cholecystitis or cholangitis and defer surgery until the patient is afebrile in an effort to decrease the risk of subsequent infections, this practice is controversial. Detection of an active infection during surgery (e.g., gangrenous gallbladder, suppurative cholangitis) is an indication for a course of postoperative *therapeutic* antibiotics. In either case, antibiotics with additional antianaerobic activity (e.g., cefoxitin or cefotetan) are indicated.[56]

COLORECTAL SURGERY

In the absence of adequate prophylactic therapy, the risk for SSI after colorectal surgery is large because of the significant bacterial

counts in fecal material present in the colon (frequently exceeds 10^9 per gram). Anaerobes and gram-negative aerobes predominate, although gram-positive aerobes also may play an important role. Reducing this bacteria load with a thorough bowel preparation regimen (4 L polyethylene glycol solution or 90 ml sodium phosphate solution administered orally the day before surgery) is controversial, even though 99% in a recent survey of surgeons routinely use mechanical preparation.[57] Risk factors for SSIs include age greater than 60 years, hypoalbuminemia, poor preoperative bowel preparation, corticosteroid therapy, malignancy, and operations lasting longer than 3.5 hours.[7]

CLINICAL CONTROVERSY

A recent randomized trial of 380 patients undergoing elective colorectal surgery suggests that SSIs are not reduced by preoperative mechanical bowel preparation.[58] This has been confirmed by a recent meta-analysis that shows that mechanical bowel preparation does not reduce the risk of anastamotic leakage or other complications, including postoperative infection.[59] Despite this new evidence, mechanical bowel preparations continue to be a standard of practice prior to elective bowel surgery.

Antimicrobial prophylaxis reduced mortality from 11.2% to 4.5% in a pooled analysis of trials comparing antimicrobial prophylaxis with no prophylaxis for colon surgery.[60] Effective antibiotic prophylaxis reduces the risk for an SSI even further. Several oral regimens designed to reduce bacterial counts in the colon have been studied.[61] The combination of 1 g neomycin and 1 g erythromycin base given orally 19, 18, and 9 hours preoperatively is the most commonly used regimen in the United States.[61] Neomycin, while poorly absorbed, provides intralumenal concentrations that are high enough to effectively kill most gram-negative aerobes. Oral erythromycin, although partially absorbed, still produces concentrations in the colon that are sufficient to suppress common anaerobes. If surgery is postponed, the antibiotics must be readministered to maintain efficacy. Optimally, the bowel preparation regimen should be completed prior to starting the oral antibiotic regimen. This is of particular concern because most procedures are now performed electively on a "same-day surgery" basis. In this case, the bowel preparation regimen is self-administered by the patient at home on the day prior to hospital admission, and thus compliance cannot be monitored carefully.

Patients who cannot take oral medications should receive parenteral antibiotics. Cefoxitin or cefotetan is used most commonly, but a number of other second-generation and some third-generation cephalosporins are also effective.[62] The role of metronidazole in combination with cephalosporin therapy is unclear. Currently, only retrospective evidence suggests that the addition of metronidazole to a cephalosporin or extended-spectrum penicillin may provide additional benefit.[63] Until this can be confirmed in prospective studies, metronidazole should be reserved for combination therapy with cephalosporins with poor anaerobic coverage (e.g., cefazolin). At this time, there is not enough evidence to recommend the addition of metronidazole to cephalosporins with anaerobic activity (e.g., cefotaxime, cefoxitin, and ceftriaxone). For β-lactam-allergic patients, perioperative doses of gentamicin and metronidazole have been used.[64] It is controversial whether the addition of preoperative parenteral antibiotics to the standard preoperative oral antibiotic regimen described earlier will decrease SSI rates lower than oral prophylaxis alone; however, combination therapy is superior to parenteral therapy alone.[65] Postoperative antibiotics generally are unnecessary in the absence of any untoward events or findings during surgery. Intravenous antibiotics are required for colostomy reversal and rectal resection because enterally administered antibiotics will not reach the distal segment that is to be reanastomosed or resected.[66]

APPENDECTOMY

Suspected appendicitis is a frequent cause for abdominal surgery. Numerous antibiotic regimens, all with activity against gram-positive and gram-negative aerobes and anaerobic pathogens, have been studied and found to be effective in reducing SSI incidence. A cephalosporin with antianaerobic activity, such as cefoxitin or cefotetan, is recommended as first-line therapy; however, a comparative trial of cefoxitin and cefotetan suggests that cefotetan may be superior, possibly because of its longer duration of action.[67] In the case of β-lactam allergy, metronidazole in combination with gentamicin is also an effective regimen. Broad-spectrum antibiotics covering nosocomial pathogens (e.g., *Pseudomonas*) do not further reduce SSI risk[68] and instead may increase the cost of therapy and promote bacterial resistance. While single-dose therapy with cefotetan is adequate, prophylaxis with cefoxitin may require intraoperative dosing if the procedure extends beyond 3 hours in duration. Established intraabdominal infections (e.g., gangrenous or perforated appendix) require an appropriate course of postoperative *therapeutic* antibiotics. Laparoscopic appendectomy produces lower postoperative infection rates that open appendectomy; however, antimicrobial prophylaxis was used in all patients in these studies, and thus the role for prophylaxis in this population remains unstudied.[69]

UROLOGIC PROCEDURES

Preoperative bacteriuria is the most important risk factor for development of an SSI after urologic surgery. All patients should have a preoperative urinalysis and should receive *therapeutic* antibiotics if bacteriuria is detected. Patients with sterile urine preoperativey are at low risk for developing an SSI, and the benefit of *prophylactic* antibiotics in this setting is controversial.[70] Reviews suggest that antibiotic prophylaxis is warranted in high-risk patients (e.g., prolonged indwelling catheterizaton, positive urine cultures, and neutropenia) undergoing transurethral, perineal, or suprapubic resection of the prostate, resection of bladder tumors, or cystoscopy.[70] The exact incidence of SSIs in this population is obscured, however, by the frequent use of postoperative urinary catheters and the subsequent risk of bacteriuria. *E. coli* is the most frequently encountered organism. Routine use of broad-spectrum antibiotics such as third-generation cephalosporins and fluoroquinolones has not been demonstrated to decrease SSI rates more than cefazolin, and thus such regimens are not recommended. One comparative trial determined that a single dose of oral ciprofloxacin was as effective as intravenous cefazolin and suggests that this may be a cheaper and easier alternative for outpatient urologic surgery.[71] Regimens longer than a single dose do not improve outcome. Urologic procedures requiring an abdominal approach, such as a nephrectomy or cystectomy, require antibiotic prophylaxis similar to that which would be used for a clean-contaminated abdominal procedure.[70]

CESAREAN SECTION

Cesarean section is the most frequently performed surgical procedure in the United States.[7] Prophylactic antibiotics are given to avoid endometritis, the most commonly occurring SSI. In the past, antibiotics were recommended for only high-risk patients, including those with premature membrane rupture or those not receiving prenatal care. Several large trials, as well as a meta-analysis, have shown bene-

fit in administering prophylactic antibiotics to all women undergoing emergent cesarean section regardless of their underlying risk factors.[72] Cefazolin remains the drug of choice despite a wide spectrum of potential pathogens, and a single 2-g dose appears to be superior to single or multiple 1-g doses.[73] Providing a broader spectrum of coverage with cefoxitin (for anaerobes) or piperacillin (for *Pseudomonas* or enterococci), does not lower postoperative infection rates further. For patients with a β-lactam allergy, preoperative metronidazole is an acceptable alternative.[72]

During a cesarean section, unlike other surgical procedures, antibiotics should be administered *after* the initial incision is made and after the umbilical cord is clamped. This will minimize infant drug exposure and thus potentially decrease the incidence of neonatal sepsis. Longer durations of prophylactic therapy have not been shown to result in lower infection rates.[74]

HYSTERECTOMY

The most important factor affecting the incidence of SSI after hysterectomy is the type of procedure that was performed. Vaginal hysterectomies are associated with a high rate of postoperative infection when performed without the benefit of prophylactic antibiotics because of the polymicrobial flora normally present at the operative site.[75] As with cesarean sections, cefazolin is the drug of choice for vaginal hysterectomies despite the wide spectrum of possible pathogens.[75] Single-dose therapy should be adequate, but most reports use a 24-hour regimen. The American College of Obstetricians and Gynecologists (ACOG) recommends the use of a first-, second-, or third-generation cephalosporin.[76] For patients with a β-lactam allergy, a single preoperative dose of doxycycline also is effective.[75]

Prophylactic antibiotics are recommended for abdominal hysterectomy despite the lack of bacterial contamination from the vaginal flora. Both cefazolin and antianaerobic cephalosporins (e.g., cefoxitin and cefotetan) have been studied extensively. Single-dose cefotetan is superior to single-dose cefazolin,[78] and the investigators suggest that cefotetan should be the drug of choice for abdominal hysterectomies. However, other authors suggest that either agent is appropriate, provided that 24 hours of antimicrobial coverage is not exceeded.[7] ACOG guidelines suggest that first-, second-, or third-generation cephalosporins can be used for prophylaxis.[76] Metronidazole is also effective and may be used if patients are allergic to β-lactam antibiotics.[75] Antibiotic prophylaxis may not be required in laparoscopic gynecologic surgery or tubal microsurgery.[79] Similar to other surgical procedures, perioperative events and findings may require the use of *therapeutic* antibiotics after surgery.

HEAD AND NECK SURGERY

Use of prophylactic antibiotics during head and neck surgery depends on the procedure type. Clean procedures (as per NRC definition), such as parotidectomy or simple tooth extraction, are associated with a very low incidence of SSI. Head and neck procedures involving an incision through a mucosal layer carry with them a higher risk for SSI. The normal flora of the mouth is polymicrobial; both anaerobes and gram-positive aerobes predominate. While typical doses of cefazolin usually are ineffective for anaerobic infections, a 2-g dose produces concentrations high enough to inhibit these organisms. A pharmacokinetic study suggested that a single dose of clindamycin is adequate for prophylaxis in maxillofacial surgery unless the procedure lasts longer than 4 hours, when a second dose should be administered intraoperatively.[80] A combination of clindamycin plus gentamicin also has been described but was found to offer no advantage over clindamycin alone.[81] For most head and neck cancer resection surgeries, including free-flap reconstruction, 24 hours of clindamycin is appropriate, and there is no additional benefit in extending therapy beyond 24 hours.[82] Topical therapy with clindamycin, amoxicillin-clavulanate, and ticarcillin-clavulanate has been described in small trials, but the exact role for topical antibiotics has yet to be defined.[83] Antimicrobial prophylaxis is not indicated for endoscopic sinus surgery without nasal packing.[39]

CARDIOTHORACIC SURGERY

Although cardiac surgery generally is considered a clean procedure, antibiotic prophylaxis has been demonstrated to lower SSI incidence. The substantial morbidity related to an SSI in this population, coupled with the routine implementation of prosthetic devices, further justifies the routine use of prophylaxis.[84] Patients who develop SSIs after coronary artery bypass graft (CABG) surgery have a mortality rate of 22% at 1 year compared with 0.6% for those who do not develop an SSI.[85] Risk factors for developing an SSI after cardiac surgery include obesity, renal insufficiency, connective tissue disease, reexploration for bleeding, and poorly timed administration of antibiotics.[84] Skin flora pathogens predominate; gram-negative organisms are rare.

Cefazolin has been studied extensively and is considered the drug of choice.[25] Although several studies and a meta-analysis have been published that advocate the use of second-generation cephalosporins (e.g., cefuroxime) rather than cefazolin, various methodologic flaws in these studies have limited the extrapolation of these results to practice. Cefazolin is as effective as cefuroxime in a large randomized trial of 702 patients undergoing open heart surgery and thus remains the standard of care.[86] Both patient weight and timing of cefazolin administration relative to surgery must be considered when developing a dosing strategy. Patients weighing more than 80 kg should receive 2 g cefazolin rather than 1 g. Doses should be administered no earlier than 60 minutes before the first incision and no later than at the beginning of induction.[84] Extending therapy beyond 48 hours does not lower SSI rates further.[87] Single-dose cefazolin therapy, in fact, may be sufficient.[88]

Routine vancomycin administration is potentially justified in hospitals having a high incidence of MRSA or when sternal wounds are to be explored surgically for possible mediastinitis. However, a recent large comparative trial enrolling almost 900 patients in a single center with a high prevalence of MRSA infections found that both cefazolin and vancomycin had similar efficacy in preventing SSI in patients undergoing cardiac surgery that required sternotomy.[89] Mediastinitis constitutes a failure of a prior prophylactic regimen. Continued postoperative vancomycin should be guided by culture and sensitivity data.[40] Subsequent antibiotic therapy is guided by intraoperative findings.

Pulmonary resection is associated with significant SSI risk, and prophylactic antibiotics have an established role in preventing postoperative infectious morbidity. Pleuropulmonary infections are much more common than wound infections, and pathogenic organisms likely migrate from the oral cavity or pharynx.[90] First-generation cephalosporins are inadequate; 48 hours of cefuroxime is preferred. A regimen of ampicillin-sulbactam is superior to first-generation cephalosporins, but further studies are required before this agent can be recommended as first-line prophylactic therapy.[91]

VASCULAR SURGERY

Vascular surgery, like cardiac surgery, generally is considered a clean surgery by NRC criteria. Although vascular graft infections occur infrequently (3% to 5%), the associated morbidity and mortality are extensive because treatment often requires surgical graft removal along with *therapeutic* antibiotic therapy.[92] Prophylactic antibiotics are of benefit, particularly for procedures involving the abdominal aorta and the lower extremities. Cefazolin is regarded as the drug of choice.[93] Twenty-four hours of prophylaxis with cefazolin is adequate; longer courses may lead to bacterial resistance.[94] For patients with β-lactam allergy, 24 hours of oral ciprofloxacin also has been shown to be effective.[92]

ORTHOPEDIC SURGERY

Most orthopedic surgery is clean by definition, and thus prophylactic antibiotics generally are indicated only when prosthetic materials (e.g., pins, plates, and artificial joints) are implanted.[19] A late-occurring infectious complication in this surgical population can result in substantial morbidity and may lead to prosthesis failure and subsequent removal. Staphylococci are the most frequently encountered pathogens; gram-negative aerobes are infrequent. Similar to many other surgical sites, cefazolin use is supported by substantial literature evidence and therefore is the prophylactic agent of choice. Vancomycin, although effective, is not recommended for routine use unless a patient has a documented history of a serious allergy to β-lactams or the propensity for MRSA infections at a particular institution necessitates its use. The current recommended duration of prophylaxis for joint replacement and hip fracture surgery is 24 hours.[7] Antibiotic-impregnated cement and beads have been used to lower SSI rates, but conclusive data regarding their efficacy are lacking.[19]

Patients suffering open (compound) fractures are particularly susceptible to infection because bacterial contamination almost always has occurred already. The use of antibiotics is *presumptive* under these circumstances. Cefazolin is often combined with an aminoglycoside in this setting, but controlled trials are lacking.[95] A clinical trial comparing clindamycin and cloxacillin suggests that clindamycin is superior and may be appropriate as monotherapy for Gustillo type I and II open fractures but not for type III fractures, where added gram-negative activity is recommended.[96] Duration of antibiotic therapy is highly variable and depends on surgical findings during débridement, results of intraoperative cultures, and clinical status. A prospective trial comparing short (<24 hours) and long (>24 hours) courses of antimicrobial prophylaxis for severe trauma suggests that longer courses of antibiotics do not offer additional benefit and may be associated with the development of resistant infections.[97] However, established joint infections and osteomyelitis require an extended course of *therapeutic* antibiotics.

NEUROSURGERY

Definitive recommendations on the role of antibiotic prophylaxis in neurosurgery cannot yet be made at this time.[98] While the rates of SSI after these generally clean operations are low, the morbidity and mortality of SSI, should it occur, are high. Procedures involving cerebrospinal fluid (CSF) shunt placement should be considered separately because this involves placement of a foreign body and is associated with higher infection rates. When choosing an antibiotic, one must consider not only the spectrum of activity but also the penetration of the agent into the site of action (CSF). A meta-analysis suggested that single doses of cefazolin or, where required, vancomycin appear to lower SSI risk after craniotomy.[99] The largest prospective, randomized trial to date of 826 patients undergoing clean neurosurgical procedures suggested that a single dose of ceftizoxime was as effective as a combination regimen of single-dose vancomycin and gentamicin. The authors also report that ceftizoxime was better tolerated and more consistently achieved adequate CSF levels to inhibit the most common organisms.[100] A more recent study of 780 patients undergoing neurosurgical procedures that included shunt surgery reported that single doses of cefotaxime and trimethoprim-sulfamethoxazole are equally effective in preventing SSIs.[101] Studies performed on procedures involving a shunt have been small in size and do not consistently show lower infection rates with antibiotic prophylaxis, although the results of two meta-analyses suggest that they may.[102,103] Since no trials have shown superiority of any one agent, single doses of cefazolin appear to be an acceptable choice.[99]

SSIs associated with spinal surgery are rare but devastating when they occur. The use of antimcrobial prophylaxis in this setting therefore is warranted and recommended by a meta-analysis.[104] Large randomized, controlled trials are lacking, but cefazolin is the antibiotic recommended most commonly. Cefazolin penetration into both intervertebral disks and CSF may not be adequate, and a combination of cefuroxime and gentamicin may be better. There is a paucity of clinical trials comparing these two regimens.[105]

MINIMALLY INVASIVE AND LAPAROSCOPIC SURGERY

Laparoscopic surgeries are being performed more frequently for a variety of different operations, including gynecologic, orthopedic, and biliary surgeries. This minimally invasive technique is associated with smaller wounds, fewer infectious complications, less of an inflammatory response, and therefore a better-preserved immune response to infection when compared with the open surgical approach.[106] The role of antimicrobial prophylaxis in this setting depends on the type of surgery performed and preexisting risk factors for infection. Unfortunately, there are few large prospective, placebo-controlled trials to determine in which patients and surgeries antimicrobial prophylaxis is warranted.

In addition to the recommendations for previously mentioned laparoscopic procedures, there is a variety of levels of evidence for prophylaxis in other laparoscopic and endoscopic procedures. Patients undergoing endoscopic retrograde cholaniopancreatography (ERCP) do not need antimicrobial prophylaxis unless biliary obstruction is evident. In these situations, a single 1-g dose of cefazolin will suffice.[107] The role of antimicrobial prophylaxis for transurethral resection of the prostate (TURP) is better established. A third-generation cephalosporin such as ceftriaxone (or cotrimoxazole for severely β-lactam-allergic patients) can be recommended as single-dose prophylaxis, especially for patients with nonsterile urine preoperatively or indwelling catheters.[107] The insertion of peritoneal dialysis catheters by laparoscopic technique is associated with significantly lower rates of postoperative infection. With SSI rates of less than 5%, prophylactic antimicrobial therapy may not be warranted, but this has not been studied in a large enough placebo-controlled trial. If the decision to provide antimicrobial prophylaxis is made, a single dose of cefazolin will suffice.[107]

NONPHARMACOLOGIC INTERVENTIONS

Besides antimicrobial strategies and aseptic technique, other strategies have been investigated in different types of surgeries to reduce postoperative infections. The most commonly cited and practiced interventions include maintenance of normothermia intraoperatively,

provision of supplemental oxygen in the perioperative period, and aggressive perioperative glucose control.

Core body temperature can fall by 1 to 1.5°C intraoperatively in patients under general anesthesia. Intraoperative hypothermia has been associated with impaired immune function, decreased blood flow to the surgical site, decreased tissue oxygen tension, and an increased risk of SSI. Efforts to maintain intraoperative normothermia should be exercised and may include the use of warming blankets and intravenous fluid warmers to mainatain core body temperature above 36°C. One prospective trial of 200 patients undergoing colorectal surgery found that maintenance of normothermia reduced postoperative infection rates along with other morbidity parameters, including length of stay.[108]

Low oxygen tension in the tissues that make up the surgical site increases the risk of bacterial colonization and subsequent SSI by decreasing the efficiency of neutrophil activity. Administration of high concentrations of oxygen (80% via ventilator or 12 L/min via a nonrebreather mask) reduced postoperative infection rates significantly in a multicenter randomized trial of 500 patients undergoing colorectal surgery.[109]

Diabetes and poor glucose control are well-known risk factors for SSI. The increased risk of infection is thought to be due to both macrovascular (vasculopathy and venoocclusive disease) and microvascular (subtle immunologic deficiencies, including neutrophil dysfunction and reduced complement and antibody activity) complications. Aggressive control of perioperative blood glucose decreases the incidence of SSI in diabetics undergoing cardiac surgery and is currently being evaluated in other types of surgery and in nondiabetic patients.[110]

CLINICAL CONTROVERSY

Although interventions to maintain normothermia intraoperatively, provide supplemental oxygen in the perioperative period, and aggressively control perioperative glucose show a significant reduction in SSI, they cannot be generalized to all types of surgeries. However, given the simplicity and low cost of these interventions, many clinicians are considering the applicability of such measures outside the studied population. At this time, pending further research, these interventions can only be recommended for routine use in the type of patient or surgery for which it was studied.

PHARMACOECONOMIC AND SAFETY IMPLICATIONS

It is paramount to consider the cost implications of pharmacotherapy guidelines that affect a large number of patients. While investigators have incorporated basic financial analysis into the results of antibiotic prophylaxis comparative trials,[40,44,47,85] robust pharmacoeconomic studies of various regimens of antimicrobial prophylaxis in surgery are lacking. Most of these studies are cost-minimization studies because only drug acquisition costs are considered. Studies that incorporate all relevant drug and treatment costs in relation to pertinent patient outcomes such as incidence of SSIs, hospital length of stay, and antibiotic related adverse events are needed.

The recommendations and literature reviewed in this chapter show that SSIs are preventable with appropriately chosen and timed prophylactic therapy in combination with meticulous aseptic technique and a variety of nonantimicrobial methods. Despite this, infection is the most common complication postoperatively. For this

TABLE 121–7. Strategies for Implementing an Institutional Program to Ensure the Appropriate Use of Antimicrobial Prophylaxis in Surgery

1. Educate

Develop an educational program that enforces the importance and rationale of timely antimicrobial prophylaxis.

Make this educational program available to all health care practitioners involved in the patient's care.

2. Standardize the Ordering Process

Establish a protocol (e.g., a preprinted order sheet) that standardizes antibiotic choice according to current published evidence, formulary availability, institutional resistance patterns, and cost.

3. Standardize the Delivery and Administration Process

Employ as system that ensures that antibiotics are prepared and delivered to the holding area in a timely fashion.

Standardize the administration time to less than 1 hour preoperatively.

Designate responsibility and accountability for antibiotic administration.

Provide visible reminders to prescribe/administer prophylactic antibiotics (e.g., checklists).

Develop a system to remind surgeons/nurses to readminister antibiotics intraoperatively during long procedures.

4. Provide Feedback

Follow up with regular reports of compliance and infection rates.

---

reason, many institutions, including the Joint Commission on Accreditation of Healthcare Organizations (JCAHO), have mandated a formalized approach to improving patient safety and reducing SSIs. Standardized institutional guidelines can effectively ensure appropriate prophylactic antimicrial therapy and ultimately reduce SSIs at individual institutions. Strategies to implement such a program are outlined in Table 121–7.

EVALUATION OF THERAPEUTIC OUTCOMES

When evaluating the outcome of surgical antibiotic prophylaxis, it is important to differentiate any potential SSI from other postoperative infection or complication. While fever and leukocytosis are common in the immediate postoperative period, they typically resolve with prompt ambulation, timely removal of invasive devices, prevention and/or resolution of atelectasis through optimal respiratory care, and effective analgesia. It is also important to remember that the emergence of distal infections, such as pneumonia, does not constitute a failure of surgical prophylaxis. Prophylaxis should be as short as possible because prolonged prophylactic regimens may contribute to the selection of resistant organisms and may make any infection more difficult to treat.

Surgical-site appearance is the most important determinant of the presence of an infection. Drainage of pus from the incision accompanied by redness, warmth, and pain or tenderness is highly suggestive of an SSI. By definition, any surgical site that requires incision and drainage by the surgeon is considered infected regardless of appearance. Failure to heal and wound dehiscence also are seen commonly with SSIs, although surgical technique and nutritional status may be important contributing factors.

The presentation of signs and symptoms consistent with an SSI in relation to previous surgery is an important consideration when evaluating therapeutic outcomes after surgical prophylaxis. Many SSIs will not be evident during acute hospitalization. In fact, SSIs may not become evident until up to 30 days later or, in the case of prosthe-

sis implantation, up to 1 year later. Thus the true incidence of SSI can only be determined by completing comprehensive postdischarge surveillance. All studies investigating the efficacy of surgical prophylaxis must include adequate postdischarge follow-up in order to be able to thoroughly assess the success of any prophylactic regimen.

ABBREVIATIONS

ACOG: American College of Obstetricians and Gynecologists
ASA: American Society of Anesthesiologists
CABG: coronary artery bypass graft
CDC: Centers for Disease Control and Prevention
CFU: colony-forming units
CSF: cerebrospinal fluid
ERCP: endoscopic retrograde cholangiopancreatography
JCAHO: Joint Commission on Accreditation of Healthcare Organizations
MIC: minimum inhibitory concentration
MRSA: methicillin-resistant *S. aureus*
MSSA: methicillin-sensitive *S. aureus*
NNIS: National Nosocomial Infections Surveillance System
NRC: National Research Council
PEG: percutaneous endoscopic gastrostomy
SENIC: Study on the Efficacy of Nosocomial Infection Control
SSI: surgical-site infection
TIPS: transjugular intrahepatic portosystemic shunt
TURP: transurethral resection of the prostate
VRE: vancomycin-resistant enterococci

Review Questions and other resources can be found at *www.pharmacotherapyonline.com*

REFERENCES

1. Mitka M. Preventing surgical infection is more important than ever. JAMA 2000;283:44–45.
2. de Lalla F. Antimicrobial chemotherapy in the control of surgical infectious complications. J Chemother 1999;11:440–445.
3. Mangram AJ, Horan TC, Pearson ML, et al. Guideline for prevention of surgical site infection, 1999. Centers for Disease Control and Prevention (CDC) Hospital Infection Control Practices Advisory Committee. Am J Infect Control 1999;27:97–132.
4. Polk HC, Christmas AB. Prophylactic antibiotics in surgery and surgical wound infections. Am Surg 2000;66:105–111.
5. National Academy of Sciences, National Research Council. Postoperative wound infections: The influence of ultraviolet irradiation of the operating room and of various other factors. Ann Surg 1964;160:32–135.
6. Cruse PJE, Foord R. A five-year prospective study of 23,649 surgical wounds. Arch Surg 1973;107:206–210.
7. ASHP Commission on Therapeutics. ASHP therapeutic guidelines on antimicrobial prophylaxis in surgery. In: Deffenbaugh J, ed. Best Practices for Health System Pharmacy. Bethesda, MD, ASHP, 1999:349–396.
8. Furnary AP, Zerr KJ, Grunkemeier GL, Starr A. Continuous intravenous insulin infusion reduces the incidence of deep sternal wound infection in diabetic patients after cardiac surgical procedures. Ann Thorac Surg 1999;67:352–360.
9. Dionigi R, Rovera F, Dionigi G, et al. Risk factors in surgery. J Chemother 2001;13: 6–11.
10. Haley RW, Culver DH, Morgan WM, et al. Identifying patients at high risk of surgical wound infection: A simple multivariate index of patient susceptibility and wound contamination. Am J Epidemiol 1985;121:206–215.

11. Weigelt JA, Dryer D, Haley RW. The necessity and efficiency of wound surveillance after discharge. Arch Surg 1992;127:77–82.

12. Culver DH, Horan TC, Gaynes RP, et al. Surgical wound infection rates by wound class, operative procedure, and patient risk index. Am J Med 1991;91(suppl 3B):152–157S.

13. Owens WD, Felts JA, Spitznagel EL. ASA physical status classifications: A study of consistency of ratings. Anesthesiology 1978;49:239–243.

14. Gyssens IC. Preventing postoperative infections: current treatment recommendations. Drugs 1999;57:175–185.

15. Elek SD, Conen PE. The virulence of *Staphylococcus pyogenes* for man: A study of the problems of wound infection. Br J Exp Pathol 1958; 38:573–586.

16. Burke JF. Identification of the sources of staphylococci contaminating the surgical wound during operation. Ann Surg 1963;158:898–904.

17. Kaiser AB, Kernodle DS, Parker RA. Low-inoculum model of surgical wound infection. J Infect Dis 1992;166:393–399.

18. Esposito S. Immune system and surgical site infection. J Chemother 2001;13:12–16.

19. De Lalla F. Antibiotic prophylaxis in orthopedic prosthetic surgery. J Chemother 2001;13:48–53.

20. Schaberg D. Major trends in the microbial etiology of nosocomial infection. Am J Med 1991;91(suppl 3B):72–75S.

21. Murray BE. Vancomycin-resistant enterococcal infections. N Engl J Med 2000;342:710–721.

22. Hospital Infection Control Practices Advisory Committee. Recommendations for preventing the spread of vancomycin resistance. MMWR 1995;44:1–13.

23. Centers for Disease Control and Prevention. Interim guidelines for prevention and control of *Staphylococcus aureus* infection associated with reduced susceptibility to vancomycin. MMWR 1997;46:626–635.

24. Kaiser AB, Petracek MR, Lea JW IV, et al. Efficacy of cefazolin, cefamandole, and gentamicin as prophylactic agents in cardiac surgery. Ann Surg 1987;206:791–797.

25. Ariano RE, Zhanel GG. Antimicrobial prophylaxis in coronary bypass surgery: A critical appraisal. DICP 1991;25:478–484.

26. Munoz P, Burrillo A, Bouza E. Criteria used when initiating antifungal therapy against *Candida* spp. in the intensive care unit. Int J Antimicrob Agents 2000;15:83–90.

27. Tran LT, Auger P, Marchand R, et al. Epidemiological study of *Candida* spp. colonization in cardiovascular surgical patients. Mycoses 1997; 40:169–173.

28. Pittet D, Monod M, Suter PM, et al. *Candida* colonization and subsequent infections in critically ill surgical patients. Ann Surg 1994;220:751–758.

29. Classen DC, Evans RS, Pestotnik SL, et al. The timing of prophylactic administration of antibiotics and the risk of surgical wound infection. N Engl J Med 1992;326:281–286.

30. Collier PE, Rudolph M, Ruckert D, et al. Are preoperative antibiotics administered preoperatively? Am J Med Qual 1998;13:94–97.

31. Esposito S. Is single-dose antibiotic prophylaxis sufficient for any surgical procedure? J Chemother 1999;11:556–564.

32. Scher KS. Studies on the duration of antibiotic administration for surgical prophylaxis. Am Surg 1997;63:59–62.

33. Zelenitzky SA, Ariano RE, Harding GKM, et al. Antibiotic pharmacodynamics in surgical prophylaxis: an association between intraoperative antibiotic concentrations and efficacy. Antimicrob Agents Chemother 2002;46:3026–3030.

34. Goldman DA, Hopkins CC, Karchmer AW. Cephalothin prophylaxis in cardiac valve surgery: A prospective, double-blind comparison of two-day and six-day regimen. J Thorac Cardiovasc Surg 1977;73:470–479.

35. Zanetti G, Flanagan HL Jr, Cohn LH, et al. Improvement of intraoperative antibiotic prophylaxis in prolonged cardiac surgery by automated alerts in the operating room. Infect Control Hosp Epidemiol 2003;24:7–9.

36. Waltrip T, Lewis R, Young V, et al. A pilot study to determine the feasibility of continuous cefazolin infusion. Surg Infect 2002;3:5–9.

37. Weinbren MJ. Pharmacokinetics of antibiotics in burn patients. J Antimicrob Chemother 1999;44:319–327.

38. Lewis DR, Longman RJ, Wisheart JD, et al. The pharmacokineics of a single dose of gentamicing (4 mg/kg) as prophylaxis in cardiac surgery requiring cardiopulmonary bypass. Cardiovasc Surg 1999;7:398–401.

39. Weed HG. Antimicrobial prophylaxis in the surgical patient. Med Clin North Am 2003;27:59–75.

40. Salkind AR, Cuddy PG, Foxworth JW. The rational clinical examination. Is this patient allergic to penicillin? An evidence-based analysis of the likelihood of penicillin allergy. JAMA 2001;285:2498–2505.

41. Hadaway L, Chamallas SN. Vancomycin: N perspectives on an old drug. J Infus Nurs 2003;26:278–284.

42. Sattler FR, Weitekamp MR, Ballard JO. Potential for bleeding with the new beta lactam antibiotics. Ann Intern Med 1986;105:924–931.

43. Williams KJ, Bax RP, Brown H, Machin SJ. Antibiotic treatment and associated prolonged prothrombin time. J Clin Pathol 1991;44:738–741.

44. Frighetto L, Marra CA, Stiver HG, et al. Economic impact of standardized orders for antimicrobial prophylaxis program. Ann Pharmacother 2000;34:154–160.

45. Bratzler DW, Houck PM. Antimicrobial prophylaxis for surgery: An advisory statement from the National Surgical Infection Prevention Project. Clin Infect Dis 2004;38:1706–1715.

46. McArdle CS, Morran CG, Anderson JR, et al. Oral ciprofloxacin as prophylaxis in gastroduodenal surgery. J Hosp Infect 1995;30: 211–216.

47. Kulling D, Sonnenberg A, Fried M, Bauerfeind P. Cost analysis of antibiotic prophylaxis for PEG. Gastrointest Endosc 2000;51:152–156.

48. Sharma VK, Howden CW. Meta-analysis of randomized, controlled trials of antibiotic prophylaxis before percutaneous endoscopic gastrostomy. Am J Gastroenterol 2000;95:3133–3136.

49. Jewesson PJ, Stiver G, Wai A, et al. Double-blind comparison of cefazolin and ceftizoxime for prophylaxis against infections following elective biliary tract surgery. Antimicrob Agents Chemother 1996;40:70–74.

50. Agrawal CS, Sehgal R, Singh RK, Gupta AK. Antibiotic prophylaxis in elective cholecystectomy: A randomized, double-blinded study comparing ciprofloxacin and cefuroxime. Ind J Physiol Pharmacol 1999;43: 501–504.

51. Swoboda S, Oberdorfer K, Klee F, et al. Tissue and serum concentrations of levofloxacin 500 mg administered intravenously or orally for antibiotic prophylaxis in biliary surgery. J Antimicrob Chemother 2003;51:459–462.

52. Koc M, Zulfikaroglu B, Kece C, et al. A prospective, randomized study of prophlactic antibiotics in elective laparoscopic cholecystectomy. Surg Endosc 2003;17:1716–1718.

53. Gulberg V, Deibert P, Ochs A, et al. Prevention of infectious complications after transjugular intrahepatic portosystemic shunt in cirrhotic patients with a single dose of ceftriaxone. Hepatogastroenterology 1999;46:1126–1130.

54. Deibert P, Schwartz S, Olschewski M, et al. Risk factors and prevention of early infection after implantation or revision of transjugular intrahepatic portosystemic shunts: Results of a randomized study. Dig Dis Sci 1998;43:1708–1713.

55. Harris A, Chan AC, Torres-Viera C, et al. Meta-analysis of antibiotic prophylaxis in endoscopic retrograde cholaniopancreatography (ERCP). Endoscopy 1999;31:718–724.

56. Sheen-Chen SM, Chen WJ, Eng HL, et al. Bacteriology and antimicrobial choice in hepatolithiasis. Am J Infect Control 2000;28:298–301.

57. Zmora O, Wexner SD, Hajjar L, et al. Trend in preparation for colorectal surgery: Survey of the members of the American Society of Colon and Rectal Surgeons. Am Surg 2003;69:150–154.

58. Zmora O, Mahajna A, Bar-Zakai B, et al. Colon and rectal surgery without mechanical bowel preparation: A randomized, prospective trial. Ann Surg 2003;237:363–367.

59. Guenaga KF, Matos D, Castro AA, et al. Mechanical bowel preparation for elective colorectal surgery. Cochrane Database Syst Rev 2003; 2:CD001544.

60. Baum ML, Anish DS, Chalmers TC, et al. A survey of clinical trials of antibiotic prophylaxis in colon surgery: Evidence against further use of no-treatment controls. N Engl J Med 1981;305:795–799.

61. Solla JA, Rothenberger DA. Preoperative bowel preparation: A survey of colon and rectal surgeons. Dis Colon Rectum 1990;33:154–159.

62. Jewesson P, Chow A, Wai A, et al. A double-blind, randomized study of three antimicrobial regimens in the prevention of infections after colorectal surgery. Diagn Microbiol Infect Dis 1997;29:155–165.

63. Mittelkötter U. Antimicrobial prophylaxis for abdominal surgery: Is there a need for metronidazole? J Chemother 2001;13:27–34.

64. McDonald PJ, Karran SJ. A comparison of intravenous cefoxitin and a combination of gentamicin and metronidazole as prophylaxis in colorectal surgery. Dis Colon Rectum 1983;26:661–664.

65. Lewis RT. Oral versus systemic antibiotic prophylaxis in elective colon surgery: A randomized study and meta-analysis send a message from the 1990s. Can J Surg 2002;45:173–180.

66. Ghorra SG, Rzeczycki TP, Natarajan R, Pricolo VE. Colostomy closure: Impact of preoperative risk factors on morbidity. Am Surg 1999;65:266–269.

67. Liberman MA, Greason KL, Frame S, Ragland JJ. Single-dose cefotetan or cefoxitin versus multiple-dose cefoxitin as prophylaxis in patients undergoing appendectomy for acute nonperforated appendicitis. J Am Coll Surg 1995;180:77–80.

68. Colliza S, Rossi S. Antibiotic prophylaxis and treatment of surgical abdominal sepsis. J Chemother 2001;13:193–201.

69. Chung RS, Rowland DY, Li P, Diaz J. A meta-analysis of randomized, controlled trials of laparoscopic versus conventional appendectomy. Am J Surg 1999;177:250–256.

70. Olson ES, Cookson BD. Do antimicrobials have a role in preventing septicaemia following instrumentation of the urinary tract? J Hosp Infect 2000;45:85–97.

71. Christiano AP, Hollowell CM, Kim H, et al. Double-blind, randomized comparison of single-dose ciprofloxacin versus intravenous cefazolin in patients undergoing outpatient endourologic surgery. Urology 2000;55:182–185.

72. Smaill F, Hofmeyr GJ. Antibiotic prophylaxis for cesarean section. Cochrane Database Syst Rev 2000;2:CD000933.

73. Rouzi AA, Khalifa F, Ba'aqeel H, et al. The routine use of cefazolin in cesarean section. Int J Gynaecol Obstet 2000;69:107–112.

74. Hopkins L, Smaill F. Antibiotic prophylaxis regimens and drugs for cesarean section. Cochrane Database Syst Rev 2000;2:CD001136.

75. Guaschino S, De Santo D, De Seta F. New perspectives in antibiotic prophylaxis for obstetric and gynaecological surgery. J Hosp Infect 2002;50(suppl A):S13–16.

76. American College of Obstetricians and Gynecologists. Antibiotics and gynecologic infections. Int J Gynaecol Obstet 1997;58:333–340.

77. Hemsell DL, Johnson ER, Hemsell PG, et al. Cefazolin is inferior to cefotetan as single dose prophylaxis for women undergoing elective total abdominal hysterectomy. Clin Infect Dis 1995;20:677–684.

79. Sturlese E, Retto G, Pulia A, et al. Benefits of antibiotic prophylaxis in laparoscopic gynaecological surgery. Clin Exp Obstet Gynecol 1999;26:217–218.

80. Meuller SC, Henkel KO, Neumann J, et al. Perioperative antibiotic prophylaxis in maxillofacial surgery: Penetration of clindamycin into various tissues. J Craniomaxillofac Surg 1999;27:172–176.

81. Johnson JT, Yu VL, Myers EN, Wagner RL. An assessment of the need for gram-negative bacterial coverage in antibiotic prophylaxis for oncological head and neck surgery. J Infect Dis 1987;155:331–333.

82. Carroll WR, Rosenstiel D, Fix JR, et al. Three-dose vs extended-course clindamycin prophylaxis for free-flap reconstruction of the head and neck. Arch Otolaryngol Head Neck Surg 2003;129:771–774.

83. Grandis JR, Vickers RM, Rihs JD, et al. Efficacy of topical amoxicillin plus clavulanate-ticarcillin plus clavulanate and clindamycin in contaminated head and neck surgery: Effect of antibiotic spectra and duration of therapy. J Infect Dis 1994;170:729–732.

84. Roy MC. Surgical-site infections after coronary artery bypass graft surgery: Discriminating site-specific risk factors to improve prevention efforts. Infect Control Hosp Epidemiol 1998;19:229–233.

85. Hollenbeak CS, Murphy DM, Koenig S, et al. The clinical and economic impact of deep chest surgical site infections following coronary artery bypass graft surgery. Chest 2000;118:397–402.

86. Curtis JJ, Boley TM, Walls JT, et al. Randomized, prospective comparison of first- and second-generation cephalosporins as infection prophylaxis for cardiac surgery. Am J Surg 1993;166:734–737.

87. Harbath S, Samore MH, Lichtenberg D, Carmeli Y. Prolonged antibiotic prophylaxis after cardiovascular surgery and its effect on surgical site infections and antimicrobial resistance. Circulation 2000;101:2916–2921.

88. Bucknell SJ, Mohajeri M, Low J, et al. Singe-versus multiple-dose antibiotics prophylaxis for cardiac surgery. Aust NZ J Surg 2000;70:409–411.

89. Finkelstein R, Rabino G, Masiah T, et al. Vancomycin versus cefazolin prophylaxis for cardiac surgery in the setting of a high prevalence of methicillin-resistant staphylococcal infections. J Thorac Cardiovasc Surg 2002;123:326–332.

90. Sok M, Dragas AZ, Erzen J, et al. Sources of pathogens causing pleuropulmonary infections after lung cancer resection. Eur J Cardiothorac Surg 2002;22:23–27.

91. Boldt J, Piper S, Uphus D, et al. Preoperative microbiologic screening and antibiotic prophylaxis in pulmonary resection operations. Ann Thorac Surg 1999;68:208–211.

92. Pratesi C, Russo D, Dorigo W, et al. Antibiotic prophylaxis in clean surgery: Vascular surgery. J Chemother 2001;13:123–128.

93. Marroni M, Cao P, Fiorio M, et al. Prospective, randomized, double-blind trial comparing teicoplanin and cefazolin as antibotic prophylaxis in prosthetic vascular surgery. Eur J Clin Microbiol Infect Dis 1999;18:175–178.

94. Terpstra S, Noorkhoek GT, Voesten HG, et al. Rapid emergence of resistant coagulase-negative staphylococci on the skin after antibiotic prophylaxis. J Hosp Infect 1999;43:195–202.

95. Gillespie WJ, Walenkamp G. Antibiotic prophylaxis for surgery for proximal femoral and other closed long bone fractures. Cochrane Database Syst Rev 2001;1:CD000244.

96. Vasenius J, Tulikoura I, Vainionpaa S, Rokkanen P. Clindamycin versus cloxacillin in the treatment of 240 open fractures: A randomized, prospective study. Ann Chir Gynaecol 1998;87:224–228.

97. Velmahos GC, Toutouzas KG, Sarkisyan G, et al. Severe trauma is not an excuse for prolonged antibiotic prophylaxis. Arch Surg 2002;137:537–541.

98. Hosein IK, Hill DW, Hatfield RH. Controversies in the prevention of neurosurgical infection. J Hosp Infect 1999;43:5–11.

99. Barker FG. Efficacy of prophylactic antibiotics for craniotomy: A meta-analysis. Neurosurgery 1994;35:484–492.

100. Pons VG, Denlinger SL, Guglielmo BJ, et al. Ceftizoxime versus vancomycin and gentamicin in neurosurgical prophylaxis: A randomized, prospective, blinded clinical trial. Neurosurg 1993;33:416–422.

101. Whitby M, Johnson BC, Atkinson RL, Stuart G. The comparative efficacy of intravenous cefotaxime and trimethoprim-sulfamethoxazole in preventing infection after neurosurgery: A prospective, randomized study. Brisbane Neurosurgical Infection Group. Br J Neurosurg 2000;14:13–18.

102. Haines SJ, Walters BC. Antibiotic prophylaxis for cerebrospinal fluid shunts: A meta-analysis. Neurosurgery 1994;34:87–93.

103. Langley JM, Leblanc JC, Drake J, Milner R. Efficacy of antimicrobial prophylaxis in placement of cerebrospinal fluid shunts: Meta-analysis. Clin Infect Dis 1993;17:98–103.

104. Barker FG. Efficacy of prophylactic antibiotic therapy in spinal surgery: A meta-analysis. Neurosurgery 2002;51:391–400.

105. Riley LH 3d. Prophylactic antibiotics for spine surgery: Description of a regimen and its rationale. J South Orthop Assoc 1998;7:212–217.

106. Balague Ponz C, Trias M. Laparoscopic surgery and surgical infection. J Chemother 2001;13:17–22.

107. Wilson APR. Antibiotic prophylaxis in endoscopic and minimally invasive surgery. J Chemother 2001;13:102–107.

108. Kurz A, Sessler DI, Lenhardt R. Perioperative normothermia to reduce the incidence of surgical-wound infection and shorten hospitalization. Study of Wound Infection and Temperature Group. N Engl J Med 1996;334:1209–1215.

109. Greif R, Akca O, Horn EP, et al. Supplemental perioperative oxygen to reduce the incidence of surgical-wound infection. Outcomes Research Group. N Engl J Med 2000;342:161–167.

110. Furnary AP, Zerr KJ, Grunkemeier GL, et al. Continuous intravenous insulin infusion reduces the incidence of deep sternal wound infection in diabetic patients after cardiac surgical procedures. Ann Thorac Surg 1999;67:352–360.

111. Olson M, O'Connor M, Schwartz ML. Surgical wound infection: A 5-year prospective study of 20,193 wounds at the Minneapolis VA Medical Center. Ann Surg 1984;199:253–259.

122

VACCINES, TOXOIDS, AND OTHER IMMUNOBIOLOGICS

Mary S. Hayney

Learning Objectives and other resources can be found at *www.pharmacotherapyonline.com*.

Vaccines have become modern medical miracles along with bypass surgery and the CAT scan, but with this difference—vaccines have saved more lives and prevented more deaths than any other modern medical intervention since the chlorination of water and the pasteurization of milk.

Richard M. Krause,
"The Jordan Report: Accelerated Development of
Vaccines 1996," NIAID/NIH

Immunization is defined as rendering a person protected from an infectious agent. Immunity to an infectious agent can be acquired by exposure to the disease, by the transfer of antibodies from mother to fetus, through the administration of immune globulin, and from vaccination. Immunization is the process of introducing an antigen into the body to induce protection against the infectious agent without causing disease. An antigen is a substance that induces an immune response. The antibody produced by the humoral arm of the immune system is usually the response that is measured as evidence of successful vaccination. However, increasing evidence exists that the cellular immune response, which is much more difficult to measure, is also a very important aspect of vaccine response.

This chapter introduces the reader to three groups of agents: vaccines, toxoids, and immune sera (together known as *immunobiologics*). These groups are defined, and related agents are dealt with concurrently to illustrate total immunotherapy. Obscure agents and agents with a limited scope of use, such as agents for bioterrorism, are not included in the interest of brevity.

PRODUCTS TO PRODUCE IMMUNIZATION

Vaccines and toxoids are separate and distinct products. Both types of products, however, act to induce active immunity, i.e., immunity generated by a natural immunologic response to an antigen. Viral vaccines can be live attenuated or killed. Killed viral vaccines may consist of whole or split viral particles, specific viral fragments (subunits), or virus-like particles. Bacterial vaccines generally are killed whole bacteria or specific bacterial antigens or conjugates. Live attenuated vaccines induce an immunologic response more consistent with that occurring with natural infection. Because the organisms in live attenuated vaccines undergo limited replication in the vaccinated individual after administration, they may confer lifelong immunity with one dose (as does a primary natural infection). Multiple doses of killed vaccines usually are needed to induce long-lasting, effective immunity. Often, additional doses at varying time intervals (booster doses) are required to maintain immunity. The booster doses of such vaccines elicit memory responses from the B cells that produce immunoglobulin G (IgG). The immune system has developed an array of antibodies to the antigen already, and on restimulation with a booster dose, the B cells that produce the most specific antibodies against the antigen are activated. This restimulation allows the most active antibodies against the antigen to be selected and maintained in the "immunologic memory." Thus the booster dose results in a rapid, intense antibody response that is long-lasting. Killed vaccines also can differ in immunity potential depending on their composition. For example, polysaccharide vaccines tend to be poorly immunogenic in infants, whereas conjugated vaccines of the same antigen tend to be highly immunogenic (e.g., pneumococcal polysaccharide vaccine versus pneumococcal conjugated vaccine). A T-cell–independent immune response is made to polysaccharide antigens that stimulate B cells directly.[1] There is no maturation or booster response with a T-cell–independent immune response, and children younger than 2 years of age cannot make this type of response. Protein-polysaccharide conjugate vaccines stimulate T cells and promote interactions between T cells and B cells when producing the protective immune responses consisting of immunologic memory and high-affinity IgG.

Toxoids are inactivated bacterial toxins that generally are combined with aluminum salts to enhance their antigenicity by prolonging antigen absorption and exposure. These adjuvants also increase local tissue irritation when injected. Toxoids stimulate the production of antibodies against the bacterial toxins rather than the infecting bacterial pathogens.

Immune sera are sterile solutions containing antibody derived from human (immunoglobulin) or equine (horse antitoxin) sources. Immunoglobulins are derived from donor pools of blood plasma and are processed using cold ethanol fractionation in order to inactivate known potential pathogens. Antitoxins are made by immunizing animals with an antigen and then harvesting the antibodies (antitoxins) made against the antigens. These sera are indicated for induction of passive immunity (temporary immunity to infection as a result of the administration of antibodies not produced by the host). Human immune sera is preferred because of its lower incidence of serum sickness and other allergic reactions as compared with equine derived sera (see the section "Other Immunobiologics" below).

In addition to the active component in an immunobiologic, other active and inert ingredients are often present. Suspending agents, such as water, saline, or complex fluids containing proteins (such as albumin) or antigens, are used as the vehicle for the immunobiologic agent. Preservatives, stabilizers, and antibiotics often are added to help maintain sterility. Immunized individuals may respond with allergic reactions not to the immunobiologic agent itself but to the other components of the pharmaceutical preparation. Different manufacturers of the same immunobiologic may have different active and inert ingredients or different quantities of these ingredients in their products.

The use of combination vaccines can decrease the number of injections required at a single visit. The childhood immunization schedule has become increasingly complex with up to seven injections in a single immunization visit. Licensed combination vaccines should be used whenever any of their components are indicated.[2]

Certain vaccines manufactured by various companies are considered interchangeable. Hepatitis A and hepatitis B vaccines are considered interchangeable. It is preferable to use diphtheria-tetanus-acellular pertussis (DTaP) vaccine from the same manufacturer to complete the entire primary series. However, immunization should not be delayed if the particular type of vaccine administered for the initial doses cannot be ascertained easily. Finally, all licensed *Hemophilus influenzae* type b conjugate vaccines are considered interchangeable for the primary series of three doses of vaccine.[3]

In general, vaccines and toxoids must be kept refrigerated because breaking the "cold chain" may result in loss of potency. Certain vaccines, such as measles-mumps-rubella (MMR), also may be frozen. Immune sera generally should be kept refrigerated and not frozen except for lyophilized intravenous human immunoglobulin (IVIG), which can be stored at room temperature. Certain vaccines, such as yellow fever, live attenuated influenza, and varicella, are sensitive to increased temperature. While some vaccines may be stored below 0°C (32°F), toxoids in general tend to aggregate on freezing, leading to increased adverse local effects. On the other hand, some vaccines, when stored under incorrect conditions, may not be easily distinguished from potent vaccines.

FACTORS AFFECTING RESPONSE TO IMMUNIZATION

Various factors are known to affect response to vaccines and toxoids. Viability of the antigen is an important factor (live attenuated versus killed), as discussed previously. Total dose is also important because there seems to exist a threshold dose above which no further increase in antibody titer is seen. The use of split doses or multiple reduced doses of a vaccine (such as those used in patients with allergies to some immunobiologic component as both a desensitization and an immunization program), however, may result in inadequate protection. In such instances, serologic testing should be performed to ascertain whether or not protection to the antigen had been attained. The interval between immunization doses, the number of doses given, or both may change immune response to an agent. For hepatitis B vaccine nonresponders, a significant proportion of individuals will mount a vaccine response when given additional doses of vaccine.[4] Alternatively, additional doses of influenza vaccine are minimally effective in immunocompetent elderly individuals, individuals with human immunodeficiency virus (HIV) infections, or patients with cancer.[5,6] Generally, intervals longer than those recommended between vaccine doses do not reduce immune response.[3]

The route and site of administration of the immunobiologic also are important. This is best illustrated by the hepatitis B vaccine, which elicits a satisfactory antibody response when given in the deltoid muscle but not consistently when administered in the gluteal area.[7] Injections should be administered in a site where there is little likelihood of site damage. Immunobiologics containing adjuvants should be given into muscle mass because they can cause irritation when given subcutaneously or intradermally.

Host factors also influence vaccine response. Immunodeficiency, increasing age, underlying disease, and genetic background have been associated with poor response rates.[8–11]

VACCINE ADMINISTRATION

Subcutaneous injections should be administered into the thigh of infants and in the upper arm area of older children and adults. A $5/8$-in, 25-gauge needle should be used, being careful not to administer the dose intradermally or intramuscularly. For intramuscular (IM) injection, the anterolateral aspect of the upper thigh (infants and toddlers) or the deltoid muscle of the upper arm (children and adults) should be used. When giving an IM injection to an adult, at least a 1-in needle should be used for persons weighing less than 90 kg and a 1.5-in needle for persons weighing more than 90 kg to ensure injection in the muscle.[7] The buttock should not be used because of the potential for inadequate immunologic response and because of the potential risk of injury to the sciatic nerve. When the buttock must be used (as for large doses of immunoglobulin), only the upper outer quadrant should be used, with the needle being inserted anteriorly. Intradermal injections should be administered on the volar surface of the forearm, except for human diploid cell (rabies) vaccine (HDCV), which should be given into the deltoid area to reduce reactions. A $3/8$- to $3/4$-in, 25- or 27-gauge needle should be used, with care being taken to not inject the immunobiologic substance into the subcutaneous tissue.

For orally administered vaccines, the general recommendation is to readminister the vaccine at the same visit if the vaccine is regurgitated within 5 to 10 minutes of administration. If the second dose is not retained, that dose should not be counted, and the vaccine should be readministered at the next visit.

The live attenuated influenza vaccine is administered intranasally. A specially designed sprayer is inserted just inside the nostril, and the dose is squirted by depressing the plunger of the sprayer. The clip is removed from the plunger so that the second half of the dose can be administered into the other nostril. The vaccinated individual should breathe normally. There is no need to repeat the dose if the individual sneezes during or shortly after administration.[12]

Questions often arise concerning the simultaneous administration of vaccines. In general, inactivated and live attenuated vaccines can be administered simultaneously at separate sites. If two or more killed antigens cannot be administered simultaneously, they may be administered without regard to spacing between doses. Killed and live antigens may be administered simultaneously or, if they cannot be administered simultaneously, at any interval between doses, with the exception of cholera (killed) and yellow fever (live) vaccine, which should be given at least 3 weeks apart. If live vaccines are not administered simultaneously, their administration should be separated by at least 4 weeks. Live viral vaccines may interfere with purified protein derivative (PPD) response; thus tuberculin testing should be postponed 4 to 6 weeks after live virus vaccine administration.

The simultaneous administration of immunoglobulin and live attenuated vaccines may inhibit host antibody response because of impairment of viral replication. A dose relationship between administration of immunoglobulin and inhibition of immune response to a vaccine exists (Table 122–1). Whole blood and other blood products containing antibodies may interfere with the response to the MMR and varicella vaccines. For rubella-seronegative women who are immediately postpartum and have received a blood product in the last trimester or anti-RhoD immunoglobulin (IG) at the time of delivery, vaccination with MMR should be done immediately, with rubella antibody testing at least 3 months later to determine vaccine response. In any patient, if vaccination with MMR or varicella is followed by emergency immunoglobulin administration, the vaccine can be repeated or seroconversion to the viral antigens can be confirmed after sufficient time has elapsed (see Table 122–1). Immunoglobulin does not interfere with the response to oral vaccines or yellow fever vaccine.[3]

TABLE 122–1. Suggested Intervals Between Administration of Antibody-Containing Products for Different Indications and Measles-Containing Vaccine and Varicella Vaccine[a]

Product/Indication	Dose, Including mg Immunoglobulin G (IgG)/kg of Body Weight[a]	Recommended Interval before Measles or Varicella (months)
Respiratory syncytial virus immune globulin (IG)[b]	15 mg/kg intramuscularly (IM)	None
Tetanus IG	250 units (10 mg IgG/kg) IM	3
Hepatitis A IG		
Contact prophylaxis	0.02 mL/kg (3.3 mg IgG/kg) IM	3
International travel	0.06 mL/kg (10 mg IgG/kg) IM	3
Hepatitis B IG	0.05 mL/kg (10 mg IgG/kg) IM	3
Rabies IG	20 IU/kg (22 mg IgG/kg) IM	4
Varicella IG	125 units/10 kg (20–40 mg IgG/kg) IM	5
Measles prophylaxis IG		
Standard (i.e., nonimmunocompromised) contact	0.25 mL/kg (40 mg IgG/kg) IM	5
Immunocompromised contact	0.50 mL/kg (80 mg IgG/kg) IM	6
Blood transfusion		
Red blood cells (RBCs), washed	10 mL/kg negligible IgG/kg	None
RBCs, adenine-saline added	10 mL/kg (10 mg IgG/kg) IV	3
Packed RBCs (hematocrit 65%)[c]	10 mL/kg (60 mg IgG/kg) IV	6
Whole blood (hematocrit 35%–50%)[c]	10 mL/kg (80–100 mg IgG/kg) IV	6
Plasma/platelet products	10 mL/kg (160 mg IgG/kg) IV	7
Cytomegalovirus intravenous immune globulin (IVIG)	150 mg/kg maximum	6
Respiratory syncytial virus prophylaxis IVIG	750 mg/kg	9
IVIG		
Replacement therapy for immune deficiencies[d]	300–400 mg/kg IV[d]	8
Immune thrombocytopenic purpura	400 mg/kg IV	8
	1000 mg/kg IV	10
Kawasaki disease	2 g/kg IV	11

[a]This table is not intended for determining the correct indications and dosages for using antibody-containing products. Unvaccinated persons might not be fully protected against measles during the entire recommended interval, and additional doses of Immune globulin or measles vaccine might be indicated after measles exposure. Concentrations of measles antibody in an immune globulin preparation can vary by manufacturer's lot. Rates of antibody clearance after receipt of an immune globulin preparation might vary also. Recommended intervals are extrapolated from an estimated half-life of 30 days for passively acquired antibody and an observed interference with the immune response to measles vaccine for 5 months after a dose of 80 mg IgG/kg. [Source: Mason W, Takahashi M, Schneider T. Persisting passively acquired measles antibody following gamma globulin therapy for Kawasaki disease and response to live virus vaccination (abstract 311). Presented at the 32nd meeting of the Interscience Conference on Antimicrobial Agents and Chemotherapy, Los Angeles, California, October 1992.]
[b]Contains antibody only to respiratory syncytial virus.
[c]Assumes a serum IgG concentration of 16 mg/mL.
[d]Measles and varicella vaccination is recommended for children with asymptomatic or mildly symptomatic human immunodeficiency virus (HIV) infection but is contraindicated for persons with severe immunosuppression from HIV or any other immunosuppressive disorder.
From MMWR 2002;53(2).

Simultaneous administration of killed vaccines along with immunoglobulins is not contraindicated. Different sites are recommended, however, for killed vaccine and immunoglobulin administration. It is not recommended to increase the dose or number of vaccines used in this circumstance.

IMMUNIZATION OF SPECIAL POPULATIONS

NEONATES, INFANTS, AND PREGNANT WOMEN

The age of the recipient is another important determining factor in vaccine and toxoid response. In the first few months of life, maternal antibodies acquired via transplacental transfer during the third trimester of gestation protect an infant. However, the maternal antibody also inhibits the immune response to live vaccines because the circulating antibodies neutralize the vaccine before the infant has the opportunity to mount an immune response. For this reason, live vaccines are not administered until maternal antibody has waned, generally by age 12 months.[3]

Premature infants should be vaccinated at the same chronologic age using the same schedule and precautions as full-term infants. The full recommended doses of vaccines should be used, regardless of age or birth weight. Hepatitis B vaccine should be administered if the infant weighs 2000 g, or it should be held until the infant is 2 months of age. Breast-fed infants should be vaccinated according to standard pediatric schedules.

Most vaccines are pregnancy category C. As with most drugs, this category assignment is not because there is a known risk to the fetus but rather because of lack of information. No birth defect has ever been attributed to vaccine exposure.[3] For example, no cases of congenital rubella syndrome from inadvertent administration of rubella vaccine to a pregnant woman have ever been reported. Despite this, vaccination of pregnant women generally is deferred until after delivery because of concern over potential risk to the fetus.

Universal influenza immunization is recommended for women who will be pregnant during influenza season. Tetanus-diphtheria (Td) vaccine is recommended for pregnant women who have not received a Td booster in the past 10 years. Although live vaccines generally are avoided because of the theoretical risk of transmission of the vaccine organism to the fetus, inactivated vaccines may be administered to pregnant women when the benefits outweigh the risks.[3] Hepatitis B, hepatitis A, meningococcal, inactivated polio, and pneumococcal polysaccharide vaccines should be administered to pregnant women who are at risk for contracting these infections.[13]

IMMUNOCOMPROMISED HOSTS

Vaccination in compromised hosts (e.g., those with chronic disease, such as diabetes, connective tissue disease, or alcoholics or those with cancer or HIV disease) must be individualized based on the disease state and its treatment. The Centers for Disease Control and Prevention (CDC) has classified persons with immunocompromised conditions into three groups[14]:

1. Persons with a condition that causes limited immune deficiency (e.g., renal disease, diabetes, liver disease, and asplenia)
2. Individuals who are severely immunocompromised but not as a result of HIV infection (e.g., congenital immunodeficiency, drug- or radiation-induced disease, hematologic disease, or solid tumor)
3. Persons with HIV infection

Patients with chronic pulmonary, renal, hepatic, or metabolic disease who are not receiving immunosuppressants may receive both live attenuated and killed vaccines and toxoids to induce active immunity. These patients often need higher doses of vaccines or more frequent dosing to induce immunity. Generally, immunization should be considered early in the course of the disease in an attempt to induce immunity at a point when the disease is less severe.

Patients with active malignant disease may receive killed vaccines or toxoids but should not be given live vaccines. The MMR vaccine is not contraindicated for close contacts, however. Live virus vaccines may be administered to persons with leukemia who have not received chemotherapy for at least 3 months. Vaccines should be timed to avoid coinciding with the start of chemotherapy or radiation therapy. Annual influenza vaccine should be administered 2 weeks prior to chemotherapy or between cycles.[6] If vaccines cannot be given at least 2 weeks or more before the start of these therapies, immunization should be postponed until 3 months after the therapy has been completed. Passive immunization with immunoglobulin may be used in place of active immunization regardless of the history of immunization.

Glucocorticoids may cause suppressed responses to vaccines. For the purposes of immunization, the immunosuppressing dose of corticosteroids is prednisone 20 mg or more daily or 2 mg/kg daily, or an equivalent dose of another steroid, for at least 2 weeks. Patients receiving long-term alternate-day steroid therapy with short-acting agents, administration of maintenance physiologic doses of steroids (such as 5–10 mg/day of prednisone) via topical, aerosol, intraarticular, bursal, or tendon steroid injections require no special consideration for immunization. If patients have been receiving high-dose corticosteroids or have had a course lasting longer than 2 weeks, then at least 1 month should pass before immunization with live virus vaccines.[3]

The patient with HIV infection requires special consideration. Responses to live and killed antigens generally are suboptimal and decrease as the disease progresses because HIV produces defects in cell-mediated immunity and humoral immunity.

For children up to age 16 years with HIV infection, immunization following the standard schedules is recommended for hepatitis B, DTaP, pneumococcal conjugate vaccine (PCV7), *H. influenzae* type b (Hib), inactivated polio vaccine (IPV), and annual influenza. Two doses of MMR vaccine should be administered at least 1 month apart as soon as possible after the first birthday. MMR should be administered only to children who have no evidence or moderate evidence of immunosuppression. Two doses of varicella vaccine separated by 3 months are recommended only in children with no evidence of immunosuppression.[15] Children with HIV infection are at high risk for invasive pneumococcal disease, so children aged 24 to 59 months who did not receive the primary series as infants also should receive two doses of PCV7 separated by at least 2 months. These children also should receive pneumococcal polysaccharide vaccine (PPV23). Other killed vaccines may be used without concern for increased risk. Live typhoid vaccine should be avoided. Yellow fever vaccine may be used if absolutely necessary, but it may pose a theoretical risk of encephalitis.[16]

TRANSPLANT PATIENTS

SOLID-ORGAN TRANSPLANT PATIENTS

Organ transplantation has become a routine treatment for end-stage organ disease of many causes. Although the number of organ transplants performed is severely limited by the availability of donor organs, survival of transplant recipients is increasing. Solid-organ transplant patients remain on immunosuppressive regimens for the rest of their lives. These immunosuppressive regimens result in a higher risk of infection and also decrease the protection conferred by immunization.[17]

Whenever possible, transplant patients should be immunized prior to transplantation. Live vaccines generally are not given after transplantation. Posttransplantation diphtheria, tetanus, pneumococcal, and influenza vaccine responses are unpredictable. Decreased immune response has been documented following hepatitis B vaccine.[18–23]

HEMATOPOIETIC STEM CELL TRANSPLANT PATIENTS

Reimmunization of hematopoietic stem cell transplant (HSCT) patients is necessary because antibody concentrations wane rapidly. Annual influenza immunization may begin as soon as 6 months following successful engraftment. Reimmunization with diphtheria-tetanus-pertussis (DTaP) vaccine if age 7 or younger, *H. influenzae* type b, inactivated polio, hepatitis B, and pneumococcal polysaccharide vaccines should begin approximately 12 months following HSCT. MMR can be administered at 24 months. Varicella, meningococcal, and pneumococcal conjugate vaccines are not recommended. Immunization of household contacts and health care workers is also necessary.[24]

CONTRAINDICATIONS AND PRECAUTIONS

There are very few contraindications to the use of vaccines except those outlined earlier. These contraindications include a history of anaphylactic reactions to the vaccine or a component of the vaccine or an unexplained encephalopathy occurring within 7 days of a dose of pertussis vaccine. Immunosuppression and pregnancy are temporary contraindications to live vaccines. An interval of time must elapse based on the dose of immunoglobulin before a live vaccine can be administered (see Table 122–1). Precautions for DTaP administration include hypotonic hyporesponsive episode, fever of 40.5°C (104.9°F) or greater, crying lasting more than 3 hours within 48 hours of a previous dose, and seizures with or without fever within 3 days after a dose.[3] Generally, mild to moderate local reactions, mild acute illnesses, concurrent antibiotic use, prematurity, family history of adverse events, diarrhea, and breast-feeding are not contraindications to immunization.

OBTAINING AN IMMUNIZATION HISTORY

An immunization history should be obtained from every patient, regardless of the reason for the health care visit. Ideally, any history provided by the patient from memory should be verified by reviewing the patient's personal written immunization record or a database that contains the complete immunization history. State-based immunization registries are being developed to improve immunization coverage by allowing health care providers access to records at any contact with the health care system. Registries are aimed primarily at facilitation childhood immunization records.[25] If an official written record is not available, patient characteristics (e.g., military service, travel history, and occupation) may provide clues as to the immunization history. Serologic testing for immunity against certain diseases can provide specific information, but it is employed routinely for only a few selected diseases (e.g., measles, rubella, hepatitis A and B, and varicella) and selected circumstances (e.g., employment in a health care facility). If a written record does not exist, one should be generated at the time of initiation of immunization. Patients without a written record should be considered susceptible and an immunization program started and completed unless a serious adverse reaction occurs. As a general rule, the risks associated with overimmunization are minimal relative to the risks associated with contracting vaccine-preventable diseases.[3]

VACCINE DELIVERY

Shortfalls in vaccine coverage targets exist in both the adult and pediatric populations.[26] Among children, those of preschool age historically have been the most neglected. Entry into public school is contingent on receipt of certain required immunizations, resulting in vaccine coverage rates above 97% in children 6 years of age and older. The lack of a similar enforcement mechanism in younger patients, however, has contributed to exceptionally low immunization rates (<50%), particularly in children younger than 2 years of age. From 1989 to 1991, the United States experienced a national measles epidemic largely caused by inadequately immunized preschool-aged children. Additionally, other segments of the population (i.e., adolescents and senior citizens) have been identified as needing better vaccine coverage.[26,27]

According to the CDC, every health care visit, regardless of its purpose, should be viewed as an opportunity to review a patient's immunization status and to administer needed vaccines. Immunization is perhaps the most cost-effective medical practice available. Each visit should encompass assessment of individuals' vaccine needs, administration of indicated agents, and documentation of immunization histories. The outcome measurement of what percentage of patients in a particular practice site is completely immunized is extremely important because the benefits of optimal vaccine use extend beyond the individual patient to the public as a whole.

NATIONAL VACCINE INJURY COMPENSATION ACT

The National Child Vaccine Injury Act of 1986 was passed by the U.S. Congress in response to reports of vaccine side effects and liability concerns of vaccine manufacturers and health care providers. With vaccine safety being questioned and manufacturers ceasing the development and marketing of vaccines, the National Vaccine Injury Compensation Program was instituted to offer a no-fault alternative means to compensate victims for injury owing to vaccination. The program offers liability protection to manufacturers and an efficient means of recovering damages for individuals potentially injured by vaccines. Compensation for vaccine-related injuries is outlined in the Vaccine Injury Table.[28] The act also instituted mandatory record keeping by health care providers in the permanent medical record. Specifically, the manufacturer and lot number of the vaccine, date of administration, and name, address, and title of the person giving the vaccine must be recorded. Additionally, the act mandates that health care providers report to their local health department or to the Food and Drug Administration (FDA) any occurrence of adverse reactions.

Health care providers must report all events requiring medical attention within 30 days of vaccination to the Vaccine Adverse Event Reporting System (VAERS), which serves as a central depot for vaccine-related adverse effects. Only a temporal association between the adverse event and vaccine administration needs to be made. No adverse event rates can be determined because only the number of adverse events reported is known; the number of vaccines administered is not known. This database can be used to determine changes in adverse-event frequencies, to evaluate risk factors for adverse events, and to find rare adverse events.[29] VAERS report forms can be obtained by calling 1-800-822-7967, or reports can be made online at *www.vaers.com.*

USE OF VACCINES AND TOXOIDS

Appendices 122–1 and 122–2 show the recommended schedules for routine immunization of children and adults. Many states require children to be fully immunized prior to entering elementary school; however, optimal protection is achieved by immunizing at the recommended ages, which requires special attention to children younger than 2 years of age. Adults and adolescents also require vaccination and often are unaware of this need. Adults should receive routine tetanus-diphtheria boosters and be immune to measles, mumps, rubella, and varicella by either immunization or history of infection. Certain individuals with conditions or lifestyles that put them at high risk for vaccine-preventable diseases also should be immunized as described in the text that follows and outlined in the immunization schedules in the appendices.

TOXOIDS

DIPHTHERIA TOXOID ADSORBED AND DIPHTHERIA ANTITOXIN

Diphtheria is an acute illness caused by the toxin released by a *Corynebacterium diphtheriae* infection. The toxin inhibits cellular protein synthesis, with membranes forming on mucosal surfaces. Systemic toxemia can result in myocarditis, neuritis, and thrombocytopenia. Membrane formation can cause respiratory obstruction, and significant toxin absorption can lead to severe illness and death.

Diphtheria toxoid adsorbed is a sterile suspension of modified toxins of *C. diphtheriae* that induces immunity against the exotoxin of this organism. Two strengths of diphtheria toxoid are available in the United States: the pediatric strength (D) and the adult strength (d), which contains less antigen because of the higher rate of adverse effects seen when the pediatric strength is used in adult patients.[30] The widespread use of diphtheria toxoid essentially has eliminated diphtheria from the United States.

Primary immunization with diphtheria toxoid (D) is indicated for children older than 6 weeks of age. The usual dose is 0.5 mL IM at rotating sites. Generally, the toxoid is given in combination with tetanus toxoid and acellular pertussis vaccine (as DTaP or in combination with hepatitis B surface antigen and IPV as well) at 2, 4, and 6 months of age. Additional doses are given at 15 to 18 months of age and again at 4 to 6 years of age.[30,31] Completing the primary diphtheria toxoid immunization series usually induces immunity of at least 10 years' duration in 90% of persons. Booster doses should be given every 10 years.

If primary immunization is given to an immunosuppressed patient, an additional dose of diphtheria toxoid should be administered 1 month following the return to normal immune status. Diphtheria toxoid may be administered to persons with mild febrile illnesses and with other live or killed vaccines.[30]

For unimmunized adults, a complete three-dose series of diphtheria toxoid should be administered, with the first two doses given at least 4 weeks apart and the third dose given 6 to 12 months after the second. The combined preparation diphtheria-tetanus (Td) is recommended in adults because it contains less diphtheria toxoid than the pediatric dose and is associated with fewer reactions to the diphtheria component. It also includes the recommended tetanus toxoid, but it omits the pertussis component, which is not used in patients older than 7 years of age. All adults should receive booster doses of Td every 10 years. Adverse effects of diphtheria toxoid include mild to moderate tenderness, erythema, and induration at the injection site. Systemic reactions occur very rarely.[30]

Diphtheria antitoxin is a sterile antitoxin derived from hyperimmunized horses and is indicated for immediate use in patients with diphtheria. Diphtheria antitoxin is used in addition to antibiotics. Antibiotics have no effect on the diphtheria toxin but must be used to control transmission of the organism. Sensitivity testing by performing an intradermal or scratch test and a conjunctival test should be done before administration. Desensitization should be performed prior to administration of diphtheria antitoxin in anyone with a positive hypersensitivity test. The diphtheria antitoxin is given IM or IV in a dosage related to the site and size of the diphtheric membrane, severity of illness, and duration of illness. The dose is the same for adults and children. The usual dose of diphtheria antitoxin is 20,000–40,000 units for pharyngeal disease, 40,000–60,000 units for nasopharyngeal lesions, and 80,000–120,000 units for extensive disease of 3 days or more. When given IV, the dose should be diluted 1:20 in 0.9% saline or dextrose 5% in water and infused at 1 mL/min after being warmed to 32 to 34°C (89.6 to 93.2°F).[30]

Adverse reactions to diphtheria antitoxin include anaphylactic reactions in 7% of patients, serum sickness occurring 12 days postadministration, or both. Serum sickness may be accelerated (7 to 12 days) in persons previously sensitized. Fortunately, the widespread use of diphtheria toxoid has greatly reduced the incidence of the disease and thus the use of diphtheria antitoxin.

TETANUS TOXOID, TETANUS TOXOID ADSORBED, AND TETANUS IMMUNOGLOBULIN

Tetanus is a severe acute illness caused by the exotoxin of *Clostridium tetani*. Sustained muscle contractions are characteristic of tetanus. Tetanus toxin interferes with neurotransmitters that promote muscle relaxation leading to continuous muscle spasms. Death can be due to the tetanus toxin itself or secondary to a complication such as aspiration pneumonia, dysregulation of the autonomic nervous system, or pulmonary embolism.

TABLE 122–2. Tetanus Prophylaxis

	Clean, Minor		All Other	
Vaccination history	Td	TIG	Td	TIG
Unknown or fewer than three doses	Yes	No	Yes	Yes
Three or more doses	No[a]	No	No[b]	No

[a]Yes if more than 10 years since last dose.
[b]Yes if more than 5 years since last dose.

Tetanus toxoid and tetanus toxoid adsorbed (adsorbed onto aluminum hydroxide, phosphate, or potassium sulfate to increase antigenicity) are sterile suspensions of the toxoid derived from *C. tetani*. Both toxoids are used to promote active immunity against tetanus; however, tetanus toxoid adsorbed is the preferred agent because it elicits a greater immune response and is associated with fewer adverse reactions.

Although a single dose of tetanus toxoid in a nonimmunized individual does not produce sufficient antibody response, a series of three 0.5-mL doses results in protection for 90% of vaccinees. Primary vaccination provides protection for at least 10 years. Additional doses of tetanus toxoid (combined with diphtheria toxoid, i.e., Td) are recommended as part of traumatic wound management if a patient has not received a dose of tetanus toxoid within the preceding 5 years. For minor or clean wounds, no dose is given. Table 112–2 summarizes these recommendations. Tetanus immunoglobulin (TIG) also should be given to individuals who have received fewer than three doses of tetanus toxoid and have more serious wounds. It can be administered with tetanus toxoid, provided that separate syringes and separate injection sites are used.[31]

In children, primary immunization against tetanus usually is offered in conjunction with diphtheria and pertussis vaccination (using DTaP or a combination vaccine that includes hepatitis B and polio vaccines as well). A 0.5-mL dose is recommended at 2, 4, 6, and 15 to 18 months of age, but the first dose can be administered as early as 6 weeks of age.[31] In children 7 years old and older and in adults who have not been immunized previously, a series of three 0.5-mL doses of Td are administered IM initially. The first two doses are given 1 to 2 months apart, and the third dose is recommended at 6 to 12 months after the second dose. Boosters are recommended every 10 years, and unless there is contraindication to diphtheria toxoid, Td should be used. Tetanus toxoid may be given simultaneously with other killed and live vaccines, and if indicated, it may be given to immunosuppressed patients.

Adverse reactions to tetanus toxoid include mild to moderate local reactions at the injection site, such as warmth, erythema, and induration. Rarely, fever, malaise, aches and pains, or neurologic disorders have been reported. In general, major local reactions occur within 2 to 8 hours of administration to patients with high serum tetanus antitoxin levels. This type of reaction is indicative of high preexisting antibody concentrations, and additional doses of toxoid should not be given any sooner than 10 years. Local reactions do not limit the use of the toxoid for further dosing. Although safety during pregnancy has not been definitely established, tetanus toxoid has been administered to pregnant women for the prevention of neonatal tetanus. Generally, waiting until the second trimester is suggested.

TIG is a sterile, concentrated, nonpyrogenic solution of immunoglobulins prepared from hyperimmunized humans. It is used to provide passive immunity to tetanus following the occurrence of traumatic wounds in nonimmunized or suboptimally immunized persons (see Table 122–2). A dose of 250–500 units IM should be administered. When administered with tetanus toxoid, separate sites for administration should be used. Also, TIG is used for the treatment of tetanus. In this setting, a single dose of 3000–6000 units IM is administered.

Adverse effects of TIG include pain, tenderness, erythema, and muscle stiffness at the injection site, which may persist for several hours. Systemic reactions occur rarely. IV administration has been associated with severe adverse reactions and is not recommended.

VACCINES

H. INFLUENZAE TYPE B VACCINES

Before 1995, *H. influenzae* type b (Hib) was responsible for thousands of cases of serious illnesses (e.g., meningitis, epiglottitis, pneumonia, sepsis, and septic arthritis). The incidence of Hib disease has declined more than 99% since introduction of the conjugate vaccines based on the organism's capsular substance, polyribosyl ribitol phosphate (PRP).[32]

The Hib vaccines in use are conjugate products consisting either of a polysaccharide or oligosaccharide of PRP covalently linked to a protein carrier. The protein carrier is important because it provides for T-lymphocyte–dependent immunologic response, whereas earlier Hib vaccines that consisted of only unconjugated PRP elicited a response that was T-cell-independent. T-cell involvement in the response provides for (1) a greater antibody response regardless of the age of the patient receiving the vaccine, (2) immunologic response at an earlier age (including infants), and (3) a booster effect on subsequent exposure to the Hib capsule, whether through revaccination or natural exposure. The protein carrier is not considered a vaccine and should not be substituted for immunization against tetanus, diphtheria, or *Neisseria meningitidis*.

The Hib conjugate vaccines are stable at 2 to 8°C (35.6 to 46.4°F) and should not be frozen. They are indicated for routine use in all infants and children younger than 5 years of age. Additionally, these three products differ in their immunogenicity and schedule of administration (Table 122–3). The primary series of Hib vaccination consists of a 0.5-mL IM dose at ages 2, 4, and 6 months if HbOC (HibTITER) or PRP-T (ActHIB) is used. If PRP-OMP is being used, the primary series consists of doses given at 2 and 4 months of age. A combination vaccine containing hepatitis B and Hib conjugate vaccines can be used for the primary series to decrease the number of injections needed for infant immunization.[33] The series should not be initiated in an infant younger than 6 weeks of age. Although use of one product for the entire primary series is desirable, adequate protection is achieved even when different products are used during the initial doses. Following the primary series, a booster dose is recommended at age 12 to 15 months. Any of the Hib conjugate vaccines are suitable for the booster dose regardless of which conjugate was used for the

primary series of doses.[3,32] Additionally, the DTaP-Hib combination can be used for this booster dose.

Schedules become more complex for infants who do not begin their Hib immunization at the recommended age or who have fallen behind in the immunization schedule. For infants 7 to 11 months of age who have not been vaccinated, three doses of HbOC, PRP-OMP, or PRP-T should be given: two doses spaced 4 weeks apart and then a booster dose at age 12 to 15 months (but at least 8 weeks since dose two). For unvaccinated children ages 12 to 14 months, two doses should be given, with an interval of 2 months between them. In a child older than 15 months, a single dose of any of the four conjugate vaccines is indicated.[33] The American Academy of Pediatrics has made recommendations for children with lapsed immunization. For infants 7 to 11 months who have received one or two doses of Hib vaccine, one dose of vaccine with a booster dose give at least 8 weeks later at age 12 to 15 months should be given. For children 12 to 14 months who received two doses, a single dose is indicated. If the child received only one dose before 12 months of age, two additional doses separated by 8 weeks should be given. A single dose of vaccine is needed for a child who is 15 to 59 months of age and who has received any incomplete schedule.[34]

Vaccines for Hib are recommended for routine use only for patients up through 59 months of age; beyond this age, most individuals will have natural immunity to Hib infection. Patients with certain underlying conditions (e.g., HIV infection, IgG_2 subclass deficiency, sickle cell disease, splenectomy, and bone marrow transplants and those receiving chemotherapy for malignancies) are at higher-than-normal risk for Hib infection, and use of at least one dose of vaccine in these patients should be considered, although efficacy data are lacking in most of these situations.[14,35]

Adverse reactions to the Hib vaccine are uncommon. Erythema and induration at the injection site occur in approximately 25% of children and resolve within 24 hours. Fever, diarrhea, and vomiting are reported occasionally. Fever of greater than 38°C (100.4°F) is reported in 2.4% of children.

HEPATITIS VACCINES

Information on vaccination for viral hepatitis can be found in Chap. 40.

INFLUENZA VIRUS VACCINE

Influenza is respiratory illness that is characterized by abrupt onset of fever, myalgia, headache, severe malaise, cough, sore throat, and rhinitis. The illness typically resolves in several days but can exacerbate a chronic medical condition or lead to secondary bacterial pneumonia. Influenza activity each winter results in increased numbers of physician visits, hospitalizations, and deaths.

The Advisory Committee on Immunization Practices (ACIP) makes yearly recommendations concerning the use and composition of influenza virus vaccine. These are published in *Morbidity and Mortality Weekly Report* annually. The reader should refer to these annual guidelines as a supplemental update to this chapter.

Influenza is classified as type A or B, with influenza A further subtyped based on hemagglutinin (H) and neuraminidase (N) surface antigens. Influenza A causes significant disease in humans, and the virus is subject to mutation by a phenomenon known as *antigenic drift and shift,* resulting in the development of different influenza strains. Previous exposure to or vaccination against one strain does not confer protection against other strains. Influenza B, also a significant cause of

TABLE 122–3. *H. influenzae* **Type b Conjugate Vaccine Products**

Vaccine	Trade Name	Protein Carrier
HbOC	HibTITER (Wyeth Vaccines)	Mutant diphtheria toxin protein
PRP-T	ActHIB (Aventis Pasteur)	Tetanus toxoid
PRP-OMP	PedvaxHIB (Merck)	*Neisseria meningitides* serogroup B outer membrane protein

The polysaccharide is polyribosyl-ribitol-phosphate (PRP).

human disease, is less likely to mutate. The antigenic composition of influenza vaccine is determined from year to year by the predominant circulating strains worldwide and generally changes on a yearly basis.

Influenza vaccines are available as inactivated trivalent split or subunit vaccine or as a live attenuated vaccine administered intranasally. Though both types of influenza vaccine probably are equally effective in protection from infection,[36] they are indicated for distinct populations and should not be considered interchangeable.

The inactivated influenza vaccine preparations generally contain 45 mcg antigen in 15-mcg trivalent units per 0.5 mL and are administered by IM injection. Split-virus vaccine must be used for children from 6 months to 12 years of age. Children 6 to 35 months old receive 0.25 mL of split-virus vaccine. Two doses of vaccine administered at least 1 month apart are necessary for all children younger than 9 years of age who are receiving the vaccine for the first time. Split-virus vaccine is less reactogenic than whole-virus vaccine, particularly in children. Whole- or split-virus vaccine can be administered to individuals older than 12 years of age. However, whole-virus vaccines are not available in the United States.[5]

The live attenuated influenza vaccine (LAIV) is derived from a master influenza vaccine strain that has been adapted to grow at 25°C most efficiently. The hemagglutinin and neuraminidase antigens specific to the circulating strains are inserted into the master strain. LAIV is administered by spraying into each nostril of the vaccine recipient. The vaccine virus undergoes limited replication in the upper respiratory tract, inducing a local and systemic response. LAIV is indicated for healthy individuals aged 5 to 49 years. It should not be used in individuals who are at high risk of complications from influenza infection. Two doses separated by at least 6 weeks are needed for children aged 5 to 8 years who are receiving it for the first season. LAIV is packaged in a prefilled sprayer that must be frozen until use.[36–39]

Response to influenza vaccine generally is measured in terms of antibody response and, more important, efficacy. The elderly and individuals with chronic diseases are less likely to develop antibody levels that are considered protective and may remain susceptible to influenza infection. However, vaccination confers protection from secondary complications and reduces the risk of hospitalization or pneumonia by 50% to 60% and death by 80%. Influenza vaccine is cost-effective in nursing home populations, in the elderly who live in the community, and in healthy working adults.[39–41]

Annual influenza vaccination is strongly recommended for individuals over the age of 6 months with chronic medical conditions that make them at increased risk for the complications of influenza. Annual influenza vaccination should be given to (1) all individuals 50 years of age and older, (2) residents of nursing homes, (3) adults and children with chronic cardiovascular or pulmonary diseases including asthma, (4) adults and children with chronic metabolic disease, renal dysfunction, hemoglobinopathies, or immunosuppression (including immunosuppression from medications or HIV), (5) children and teenagers receiving chronic aspirin therapy, and (6) pregnant women. Children younger than 2 years of age have a risk of hospitalization equivalent to other individuals with high-risk conditions, and immunization of children aged 6 to 23 months is recommended. The inactivated influenza vaccine has not been studied in infants younger than 6 months. Immunization of their household contacts and out-of-home caregivers may decrease the risk of influenza infection in these young infants. In addition, the influenza vaccination should be recommended for the following groups that can transmit influenza to high-risk groups: (1) health care workers in both inpatient and outpatient settings, (2) employees of residential care facilities for high-risk patients, and (3) household members (including children)

of persons in high-risk groups. Finally, influenza vaccination should be offered to anyone wishing to avoid influenza infection.[5] The optimal time period for influenza vaccination administration is October through mid-November. However, the vaccine can be administered to unvaccinated individuals in high-risk groups throughout the influenza season, which typically lasts until April. Administration of influenza vaccines is contraindicated in persons with known anaphylactic reaction to eggs or another component of the vaccine. Adults with acute febrile illness should be vaccinated when their symptoms have subsided. Vaccination need not be delayed in individuals with minor illness with or without fever.

Antiviral prophylaxis should be considered in individuals for whom the vaccine is contraindicated or for unvaccinated high-risk individuals as a bridge until a response to the vaccine has been mounted, usually about 2 weeks. Both amantadine and rimantadine are highly effective in preventing influenza A infection. Rimantadine is much better tolerated in the nursing home population.[42] The neuraminidase inhibitors zanamivir and oseltamivir are effective for infection prophylaxis, although only oseltamivir is approved for influenza prevention.[43,44]

Adverse reactions to the vaccine include local tenderness and low-grade fever in 3% to 5% of vaccinees beginning 6 to 12 hours postimmunization and lasting 1 to 2 days. Treatment with salicylates or acetaminophen is recommended. A slight increase in the risk of Guillain-Barré syndrome may follow in the weeks after influenza vaccination. The risk is estimated to be one case of Guillain-Barré syndrome per million doses of influenza vaccine administered.[45] Runny nose is the most commonly reported adverse reaction in both adults and children following administration of LAIV. Adults complained of headache and sore throat more frequently after receiving LAIV than after placebo. Children experienced higher rates of fever, vomiting, abdominal pain, and myalgias with vaccine than placebo. An increase in asthma and reactive airways disease was noted in a study of children aged 12 to 59 months. Therefore, the vaccine should not be used for children younger than 5 years old.[46]

MEASLES VACCINE

Measles (rubeola) is a highly contagious viral illness that is characterized by rash and high fever. Complications of measles infections include severe diarrhea, otitis media, pneumonia, and encephalitis. Measles results in 1 to 2 deaths per 1000 cases, with the death rate being much higher in developing countries. With widespread vaccination, measles is on the verge of eradication in the Americas.[47]

The measles vaccine is a live attenuated viral vaccine that produces a subclinical, noncommunicable infection. Approximately 95% of vaccine recipients seroconvert after a single dose, and most are protected for life.[48] Most persons failing to respond to the initial dose of measles vaccine will seroconvert following a second dose, and this forms the basis for the two-dose vaccine strategy that was implemented in the United States in 1989.

The measles vaccine is administered subcutaneously as a 0.5-mL dose in the arm (or in the thigh if the patient is younger than 15 months of age). The vaccine is administered routinely for primary immunization to persons 12 to 15 months of age, usually as the MMR vaccine. The measles vaccine is not administered earlier than 12 months (except in certain outbreak circumstances) because persisting maternal antibody that was acquired transplacentally late in gestation can neutralize the vaccine virus before the vaccinated person can mount an immune response. A second dose of MMR is recommended when children are aged 4 to 6 years.[33] The second dose of vaccine results in seroconversion in 95% of those individuals who were first-dose nonresponders.[49]

Measles-containing vaccine should not be given to pregnant women or immunosuppressed patients. The one exception is HIV-infected patients, who are at very high risk for severe complications if they develop measles.[3] Persons with HIV infection who have never had measles or have never been vaccinated against it should be given measles-containing vaccine unless there is evidence of severe immunosuppression. The second dose should be given 1 month later rather than waiting for entry to school.

Recent administration of immunoglobulin interferes with measles vaccine response, so the recommended interval between the immunoglobulin and vaccine is determined by the dose of immunoglobulin[3] (see Table 122–1). The administration of other live vaccines not administered on the same day should be delayed for at least 30 days following measles or MMR vaccine. Live measles vaccine may suppress a positive tuberculin skin test for up to 6 weeks postadministration.[3] Historically, persons with a history of anaphylactic reaction to egg protein were considered to be at high risk for serious reactions to measles vaccine, a product derived from chick embryo fibroblasts. However, the risk of measles vaccination to egg-allergic patients has been shown to be exceedingly low. Therefore, individuals in need of measles vaccine should receive it regardless of a history of egg allergy.[48] A history of serious neomycin hypersensitivity remains a contraindication to measles vaccine use because each 0.5-mL dose contains 25 mcg neomycin. Finally, mild febrile illness and upper respiratory tract infections are not contraindications to vaccination.[48]

Measles vaccination is indicated in all persons born after 1956 or in those who lack documentation of wild virus infection either by history or antibody titers. Persons who received killed measles vaccine alone, who were given live vaccine within 3 months of receiving killed vaccine, or who received a vaccine of unknown type between 1963 and 1967 should be revaccinated. Revaccination should be considered for students entering college because of outbreaks on college campuses. It is also important to vaccinate health care workers who have no documentation of vaccination and who were born in 1957 or later because of the possibility of becoming infected by patients and transmitting the disease to their patients.[50] If two doses are needed (the person has never been vaccinated), the doses should be given at least 1 month apart. Following vaccination, antibodies may be detected within 2 to 3 weeks in patients 12 months of age or older.

For postexposure prophylaxis, the vaccine is effective if given within 72 hours of exposure. In addition, immunoglobulin may be administered at a dose of 0.25 mg/kg IM (maximum dose 15 mL) if given within 6 days of exposure. In infants, postexposure vaccination may be given as early as 6 months of age, but it should be repeated at 12 to 15 months of age.

The measles vaccine has an excellent safety record. The most common side effect following vaccination is fever, which occurs in 5% to 15% of vaccinees. Transient generalized rash may occur in about 5% of vaccine recipients. These reactions generally appear 5 to 12 days postvaccination and last 2 to 5 days. Other adverse effects, such as headache, cough, sore throat, eye pain, malaise, and transient thrombocytopenia, occur less frequently. Local reactions at the injection site, while rare, may occur in subjects who have been vaccinated previously with killed vaccine. No association between MMR vaccination and the development of autism has been made following extensive study.[51–53] Febrile seizures occur rarely, and there is no association between MMR vaccination and the development of a subsequent seizure disorder.[54]

MENINGOCOCCAL POLYSACCHARIDE VACCINE

N. meningitidis is a leading cause of meningitis and sepsis in children and young adults in the United States. The vast majority of cases are sporadic, although the frequency of outbreaks, most often involving serogroup C, is increasing.

A quadrivalent vaccine containing capsular polysaccharides for serotypes A, C, Y, and W-135 has been available since the early 1970s. Although serogroup B causes approximately one-third of all cases, it has not been incorporated into the vaccine because group B polysaccharide is not immunogenic. The meningococcal polysaccharide vaccine is indicated in high-risk populations, such as those exposed to the disease, those in the midst of uncontrolled outbreaks, travelers to an area with epidemic or hyperendemic meningococcal disease, or individuals who have terminal complement component deficiencies or asplenia.

College freshmen, particularly those living in dormitories or residence halls, are at modestly increased risk of invasive meningococcal disease as compared with the rest of the population in this age group.[55,56] The Advisory Committee on Immunization Practices recommends that health care providers inform students and parents about the increased risk and that a safe, effective vaccine is available. The meningococcal polysaccharide vaccine should be made easily available for college freshmen wishing to decrease their risk for meningococcal disease.

Meningococcal polysaccharide vaccine is administered subcutaneously as a single 0.5-mL dose. Vaccinees should be older than 2 years of age because of the difficulty younger patients have responding to polysaccharide antigens. Younger children may produce sufficient antibody levels against serogroup A, however, if given two doses 3 months apart. Antibody levels thought to be protective are attained within 10 to 14 days. Revaccination may be considered in 2 to 3 years in high-risk children who are younger than 4 years of age on initial vaccination because of rapid antibody decline. Older children and adults who remain at high risk should be revaccinated after 3 to 5 years. The vaccine shows documented effectiveness in preventing meningococcal disease in 85% to 95% of recipients for serotypes A and C.[56] Efficacy of the vaccine for serotypes Y and W-135 is presumed but not documented. Adverse effects of meningococcal polysaccharide vaccine include fever and erythema at the injection site lasting 1 to 2 days.

MUMPS VACCINE

Mumps is a viral illness that classically causes bilateral parotitis 16 to 18 days after exposure. Fever, headache, malaise, myalgia, and anorexia may precede the parotitis. Serious complications are rare, although more common in adults. The mumps vaccine is a lyophilized live attenuated vaccine prepared from chick embryo cultures. Each 0.5-mL dose of the vaccine also contains 25 mcg neomycin. The vaccine is available alone or in combinations with measles and rubella vaccines.

The mumps vaccine is used to produce active immunity while producing a subclinical, noncommunicable infection. A single dose induces antibody formation in 97% of children older than 12 months of age and 93% of adults. Clinical efficacy ranges from 75% to 95%. The duration of immunity following vaccination is unknown, but data collected in the 30 years of use indicate that the efficacy persists.[48]

The vaccine usually is given in combination with measles and rubella vaccines (as MMR) and is administered as a 0.5-mL subcutaneous injection in the upper arm. Dosing recommendations coincide with those for measles vaccine, with the first dose being administered at age 12 to 15 months and the second dose prior to entry into elementary school. If the vaccine is given before 12 months of age, revaccination is necessary and should be given after reaching 1 year of age. The vaccine is also indicated in previously unvaccinated adults born in 1957 or later, in those who have been vaccinated previously with killed mumps vaccine (an older product no longer available), and in those with an uncertain history of wild virus infection. Postexposure vaccination is of no benefit.[48]

Mumps vaccine should not be given to pregnant women or immunosuppressed patients. Additionally, conception should be avoided for 28 days following vaccination.[57] Anaphylactic reactions to mumps-containing vaccines are very rare and generally not associated with hypersensitivity to eggs. Therefore, egg allergy is not a contraindication to vaccination. The effect of immunoglobulin preparations on mumps vaccine response is unknown, but the response to measles and rubella is compromised if administered after immunoglobulins. The recommended interval between the immunoglobulin and vaccine is determined by the dose of immunoglobulin[3] (see Table 122–1). Finally, the vaccine should not be given to individuals with anaphylactic reactions to neomycin.

Serious adverse reactions to the vaccine are reported rarely. Parotitis, rash, pruritus, and purpura occur rarely. Local reactions, including soreness, burning, and stinging, may occur at the injection site.

PERTUSSIS VACCINE

Pertussis is caused by a bacterial infection with *Bordetella pertussis*. The illness is characterized by paroxysms of coughing to expel thick mucous. In the early part of this century, pertussis was a common childhood infection and was a significant cause of childhood mortality. In recent years, the incidence of disease has been increasing in all age groups. Although infants and young children remain at highest risk for infections and its complications, investigators recently determined that older adults also are at increased risk of complications from pertussis.[58]

Acellular pertussis vaccines contain selective components of the *B. pertussis* organism. All acellular vaccines contain pertussis toxin (PT), and some contain one or more additional bacterial components (e.g., filamentous hemagglutinin [FHA], pertactin [a 69-kDa outer membrane protein], and fimbriae types 2 and 3). Acellular pertussis vaccine is recommended for all doses of the pertussis schedule at 2, 4, 6, and 15 to 18 months of age. A fifth dose of pertussis vaccine is given to children 4 to 6 years of age.[33,59] Pertussis vaccine is administered in combination with diphtheria and tetanus (DTaP). Although the pertussis vaccine is not recommended for individuals 7 years of age and older, booster doses for adolescents and adults may be incorporated into future recommendations because members of these groups are important reservoirs of infection.

Local administration site reactions occur relatively commonly. Systemic reactions, such as moderate fever, occur in 3% to 5% of vaccinees. Very rarely, high fever, febrile seizures, persistent crying spells, and hypotonic hyporesponsive episodes occur following vaccination. Allergy to a vaccine component and encephalopathy without known cause within 7 days of a pertussis vaccine are contraindications to future doses of vaccine. Efficacy of the vaccine is estimated to be about 80%.[59]

PNEUMOCOCCAL VACCINES

S. pneumoniae is a common pathogen with a range of manifestations including asymptomatic upper respiratory tract colonization,

sinusitis, acute otitis media, pharyngitis, pneumonia, meningitis, and bacteremia. Rates of invasive infections are highest in children under 2 years of age (approximately 200 per 100,000 population). The incidence increases again to 61 per 100,000 population in the elderly. In between the two age extremes, the incidence of invasive disease is about 24 per 100,000 population. Invasive pneumococcal infections cause approximately 40,000 deaths annually. Most of the deaths occur in the elderly or in those with underlying medical conditions. Approximately half the deaths could be vaccine-preventable. Two pneumococcal vaccine preparations, 23-valent pneumococcal polysaccharide vaccine (PPV23) and heptavalent pneumococcal conjugate vaccine (PCV7), are available. The vaccines have different indications and are not interchangeable.

PNEUMOCOCCAL POLYSACCHARIDE VACCINE

Pneumococcal polysaccharide vaccine (Pneumovax 23 and Pnu-Immune 23) is a mixture of highly purified capsular polysaccharides from 23 of the most prevalent or invasive types of *S. pneumoniae* seen in the United States. Serotypes included are 1, 2, 3, 4, 5, 6B, 7F, 8, 9N, 9V, 10A, 12F, 14, 15B, 17F, 18C, 19A, 20, 22F, 23F, and 33F. These 23 types represent 85% to 90% of all blood isolates and 85% of pneumococcal isolates from other generally sterile sites seen in the United States. The vaccine is administered intramuscularly or subcutaneously as a single 0.5-mL dose. Each 0.5-mL dose of vaccine contains 25 mcg of each polysaccharide type dissolved in isotonic saline solution (for a total of 575 mcg polysaccharide) and 0.25% phenol as preservative. Significant cross-reactivity with other pneumococcal capsular antigens not represented in the vaccine does not occur.[60]

PPV23 is recommended for the following immunocompetent persons[60]:

- Persons 65 years of age or older (If an individual received vaccine more than 5 years earlier and was younger than age 65 at the time of administration, revaccination should be given.)
- Persons aged 2 to 64 years with a chronic illness
- Persons aged 2 to 64 years with functional or anatomic asplenia (When splenectomy is planned, PPV23 should be given at least 2 weeks prior to surgery. A single revaccination is recommended at 5 years in subjects older than 10 years of age and at 3 years in subjects younger than 10 years of age.)
- Persons aged 2 to 64 years of age living in environments where the risk of invasive pneumococcal disease or its complications is increased (This does not include day-care center employees and children.)

PPV23 is recommended for immunocompromised persons 2 years of age or older with (1) HIV infection, (2) leukemia, (3) lymphoma, (4) Hodgkin's disease, (5) multiple myeloma, (6) generalized malignancy, (7) chronic renal failure or nephrotic syndrome, (8) patients receiving immunosuppressive therapy including corticosteroids, and (9) organ and bone marrow transplant recipients. A single revaccination should be given if 5 years or more have passed since receipt of the first dose in subjects older than 10 years of age. In subjects 10 years of age or younger, revaccination should be given 3 years after the previous dose.

PPV23 induces type-specific antibodies (T-cell-independent mechanisms) with a twofold rise within 2 to 3 weeks in 80% of young healthy adults. No correlation of antibody levels and protection has been determined. Antibody levels to these strains remain elevated for at least 5 years. In certain individuals, these levels decline within 10 years. Children may be protected for only 3 to 5 years. Elderly individuals and patients with chronic disease may have lower antibody levels produced with the vaccine. Children younger than 2 years of age do not respond adequately to the vaccine.

A number of other groups, including immunocompromised patients (e.g., leukemia, lymphoma, and multiple myeloma), dialysis patients, and acquired immunodeficiency syndrome (AIDS) patients, have reduced antibody production with the vaccine. Asymptomatic HIV-infected patients respond sufficiently to the vaccine. Patients with Hodgkin's disease respond to the vaccine better before splenectomy, chemotherapy, or radiation therapy.

PPV23 vaccine efficacy has been debated in the literature. Although prelicensure trials in young, healthy gold miners in South Africa showed a reduction in nonbacteremic disease rates, in the postmarketing period, randomized clinical trials performed in elderly persons with chronic disease did not confirm these findings.[60] A large study of elderly individuals demonstrated a decreased risk of pneumonia caused by *S. pneumoniae* in vaccinated individuals but showed no change in the risk of community-acquired pneumonia even though most community-acquired pneumonias are caused by *S. pneumoniae*.[61] For invasive disease, reduction rates of 56% to 81% have been shown with the vaccine. A meta-analysis of nine randomized, controlled trials concluded that the vaccine was efficacious in reducing the frequency of bacteremic pneumococcal disease among adults in low-risk groups. Cost-effectiveness also has been shown.[60]

While the safety of PPV23 during the first trimester of pregnancy has not been evaluated, no adverse effects have been seen in newborns whose mothers received the vaccine during pregnancy.[60]

PPV23 safety is well documented. Local reactions occur frequently within the first 48 hours and generally are mild. Local erythema and induration (30%), local discomfort (40%), and local swelling (3%) are the side effects observed most commonly. Revaccination has been associated with self-limited injection-site reactions more commonly than after the first dose.[62] Rarely, severe systemic reactions can occur, and they consist of weakness, myalgia, headache, photophobia, chills, and fever. Guillain-Barré syndrome has not been reported. In patients with HIV infection, pneumococcal vaccine may cause a transient increase in viral replication, but the importance of this is unknown.

PNEUMOCOCCAL CONJUGATE POLYSACCHARIDE VACCINE

Because of the lack of immune responsiveness in children younger than 2 years of age when exposed to polysaccharide vaccines, manufacturers have been developing conjugate vaccines to offer children protection from certain strains of *S. pneumoniae*. Formation of serotype conjugates to ensure stability and immunogenicity of each strain is complex and difficult. Thus work has progressed slowly.

Currently, a heptavalent vaccine (Prevnar) is available for use in children. This vaccine contains the conjugated capsular polysaccharides of serotypes 4, 6B, 9V, 14, 18C, 19F, and 23F, which cause approximately 80% of pediatric pneumococcal bacteremias in the United States.[63] The vaccine elicits a primary T-cell–dependent antibody response with the first dose and an immunologic memory effect after four doses.

PCV7 is administered as a 0.5-mL IM injection at 2, 4, and 6 months of age and between 12 and 15 months of age. PCV7 also should be used in older children aged 24 to 59 months who are at high risk. Children with sickle cell disease or splenic dysfunction, HIV infection, immunocompromising conditions, or chronic illnesses should be immunized. PPV23 can be used in conjunction with

PCV7. PPV23 should be administered after 2 years of age and at least 2 months after the last dose of PCV7.

The vaccine was 100% effective in preventing invasive disease by vaccine serotypes.[64] In clinical use, the vaccine is associated with a dramatic decline in invasive disease not only in vaccinees but also in adults. A 35% decline in the rate of disease caused by penicillin-resistant isolates also has been noted.[65]

The vaccine series generally is well tolerated. Injection-site reactions and fever were the most commonly reported adverse effects.[63]

POLIOVIRUS VACCINES

Poliomyelitis is a contagious viral infection that usually causes asymptomatic infection but in its serious form causes acute flaccid paralysis. Poliovirus is spread via the fecal-oral route. The virus replicates in the upper respiratory tract, gastrointestinal tract, and local lymphatics. The vast majority of polio infections are subclinical and asymptomatic. Indigenous polio has been absent from the United States since 1979, and the last case in the Americas was reported in 1991. Global eradication efforts are entering the final stages, and the eradication of polio should be accomplished in the next few years.

An inactivated trivalent vaccine developed by Jonas Salk was licensed for use in 1955. In 1987, an enhanced-potency inactivated polio vaccine (IPV) was introduced, and it has replaced the original inactivated vaccine. A live attenuated oral polio vaccine (OPV) was developed by Albert Sabin in 1962. OPV was the primary immunizing agent for poliovirus infection. Widespread OPV use is responsible for eradication of wild-type polio in most of the world. However, with no poliovirus circulation in the United States for years, IPV is the recommended vaccine for the primary series and booster dose for children. OPV will continue to be used in the areas of the world that have circulating poliovirus. The CDC maintains a stockpile of OPV to be used only in case of an outbreak.[66]

The IPV series is administered routinely to children at ages 2, 4, and 6 to 18 months, and 4 to 6 years. Protective antibodies to all three serotypes develop in 90% to 100% of children after two doses of vaccine. After three doses, 99% to 100% develop protective immunity, and the fourth dose results in long-term immunity.[66]

Primary poliomyelitis immunization is recommended for all children up to age 18. Primary immunization of adults over the age of 18 is not recommended routinely because a high level of immunity already exists in this age group and the risk of exposure in developed countries is exceedingly small. Unimmunized adults who are at increased risk for exposure because of travel, residence, or occupation should, however, receive IPV series. Incompletely immunized adults or children should complete the series of IPV regardless of the interval since initiation of primary immunization. Adults do not need a booster dose routinely unless there is an increased risk of exposure (travel), in which case a single dose of IPV can be given.[66]

Allergies to any component of IPV, including streptomycin, polymyxin B, and neomycin, are contraindications to vaccine use. There are no serious side effects attributable to IPV, and the only other contraindication is pregnancy, in which case IPV should be given only if there is a clear need, such as women who will be traveling or living in an area with endemic or epidemic poliovirus. IPV is recommended for immunodeficient individuals and their household contacts. Although the response may be lower, some protection against infection may be conferred.[66]

The routine use of OPV in the United States has been discontinued because OPV is rarely associated with vaccine-associated paralytic poliomyelitis (VAPP) in vaccinees (1 in 6.2 million doses) or contacts (1 in 7.6 million doses). Individuals with primary immune deficiency are at increased risk for this adverse reaction,[67] and for this reason, OPV is not recommended for persons who are immunodeficient or for normal individuals who reside in a household with an immunocompromised person. The use of OPV is reserved for polio outbreak control.[66]

RABIES VACCINE

Human diploid cell vaccine (HDCV), rabies vaccine adsorbed (RVA), and purified chick embryo cell culture rabies vaccine (PCEC) are killed vaccines used for preexposure and postexposure rabies virus prophylaxis. Transmission of rabies can occur via percutaneous, permucosal, or airborne exposure to the rabies virus. Circumstances favoring such transmission include animal bites or attacks and contamination of scratches, cuts, abrasions, or mucous membranes with saliva or other infectious material (brain tissue). Unprovoked attacks and daytime attacks by nocturnal animals are considered highly suspect. Common wild animal transmitters include skunks, coyotes, foxes, and raccoons. Almost 60% of human rabies deaths in the United States since 1980 were associated with bat contact. Canine rabies is very common in many foreign countries (most of Asia, Africa, and Latin America). Rodents, rabbits, and hares are infected rarely. There have been a few reports of a person-to-person transmission.[68,69]

Preexposure indications for using HDCV, RVA, or PCEC include persons whose vocation or avocation place them at high risk for rabies exposure, e.g., veterinarians, animal handlers, laboratory workers in rabies research laboratories, and field personnel (trappers, hunters, cave explorers). Travelers who will be in a country or area of a country where there is a constant threat of rabies, whose stay is likely to extend beyond 1 month, and who may not have readily available medical services (e.g., Peace Corps workers and missionaries) also should be considered for preexposure prophylaxis.[69] Rabies immunization of immunocompromised individuals should be postponed until the immunosuppression has resolved, or activities should be modified to minimize the potential exposure to rabies. If the vaccine is used in immunocompromised persons, it should be given by the IM route only, and antibody titers should be checked postimmunization. Pregnancy is not a contraindication if the risk of rabies is great. A rabies immunization series should be completed with the same product because no data exist on interchangeability of products.

All three vaccine preparations may be administered for preexposure prophylaxis as a three-dose series of 1 mL IM on days 0 and 7 and once between days 21 and 28. Alternatively, HDCV can be administered intradermally in a dose of 0.1 mL using the same schedule. HDCV must be given using the specific intradermal dosage form and syringe. Lower rabies antibody concentrations have been observed in individuals immunized using the intradermal route while taking malaria prophylaxis concurrently. The IM route is recommended in this situation.[69]

Individuals with ongoing risk of exposure—either continuous risk (e.g., research laboratory staff or those involved in rabies biologics production) or individuals with frequent exposures (e.g., those involved with rabies diagnosis, spelunkers, veterinarians, animal control workers, and wildlife workers in rabies-enzootic areas) should undergo serologic testing every 6 months and 2 years, respectively, to monitor rabies antibody concentrations. An IM or intradermal booster dose is recommended if the complete virus neutralization is below 1:5 serum dilution by the rapid fluorescent focus inhibition test.

Preexposure prophylaxis does not eliminate the need for postexposure therapy. Persons previously immunized with HDCV, RVA,

or PCEC or those who have received postexposure prophylaxis previously should receive two 1-mL IM doses of HDCV, RVA, or PCEC on postexposure days 0 and 3. Rabies immunoglobulin should not be given to this group.

Postexposure prophylaxis should be given after percutaneous or permucosal exposure to saliva or other infectious material from a high-risk source. Each case needs to be considered individually. Consideration needs to be given to the geographic area, species of animal, circumstances of the incident, and type of exposure. Local or state health departments should be contacted for assistance. Thorough cleansing of the wound with soap and water followed by irrigation with a virucidal agent such as povidone-iodine solution is an extremely important part of the management of rabies-prone wounds. Individuals who have not been immunized previously should receive the recommended regimen of rabies immunoglobulin (see rabies immunoglobulin section) and five doses of HDCV, RVA, or PCEC 1 mL IM on days 0, 3, 7, 14, and 28 after exposure.[69] The intradermal route should not be used for postexposure prophylaxis.

Intramuscular vaccine should be given in the deltoid muscle in adults and in the anterolateral thigh in children. The gluteal region should not be used. The lateral aspect of the deltoid should be used for intradermal injection of HDCV when used for preexposure prophylaxis

Adverse reactions to HDCV, RVA, and PCEC are less common and less serious with the currently available vaccines compared with previously used preparations. Injection-site reactions, including pain, erythema, swelling, and itching, are reported frequently. Another 5% to 40% of vaccinees may have headache, nausea, abdominal pain, muscle aches, dizziness, or a combination of these. Systemic allergic reactions ranging from hives to anaphylaxis occur in a very small number of subjects. Given the lack of alternative therapy and that rabies infection is almost always fatal, persons exposed to rabies who do have adverse reactions should continue the vaccine series in a setting with medical support services. In persons receiving booster doses of HDCV, an immune-complex-like disease has been seen 2 to 21 days later in as many as 6% of vaccinees.[69]

RABIES IMMUNOGLOBULIN

Human rabies immunoglobulin is used in conjunction with rabies vaccine as part of postexposure rabies management for previously unvaccinated individuals. The product is derived from plasma obtained from donors who have been hyperimmunized with rabies vaccine and have high titers of circulating antibody.

In persons who have not been immunized against rabies previously, rabies immunoglobulin is given simultaneously with rabies HDCV, RVA, or PCEC to provide optimal coverage in the interval before immune response to the vaccine occurs. The efficacy of this regimen has been clearly demonstrated. In situations in which a vaccine has been used alone, mortality rates of 50% to 60% have been observed. Mortality after the combination vaccine and rabies immunoglobulin regimens is an exceedingly rare event; however, failures have been reported when the wound was not infiltrated with rabies immunoglobulin.[70]

Rabies immunoglobulin does not interfere with vaccine-induced antibody formation. Its use is not recommended beyond 8 days after initiation of the vaccine series nor in persons previously immunized to rabies.

Human rabies immunoglobulin is administered in a dose of 20 IU/kg (0.133 mL/kg). If anatomically feasible, the entire dose should be infiltrated around the wound(s). Any remaining volume should be administered intramuscularly at a site distant from the rabies vaccination site. This product should never be administered by the intravenous route. Because other antibodies in the rabies immunoglobulin may interfere with the response to live-virus vaccines (MMR and varicella), it is recommended that these immunizations be delayed for 3 months.[3]

Side effects are rare but may include local soreness at the wound or IM injection site and mild temperature elevations. Caution is advised when administering this product to persons with known systemic allergies to immunoglobulin or thimerosal. Pregnancy is not a contraindication for its use.

RUBELLA VACCINE

An erythematous rash, lymphadenopathy, arthralgia, and low-grade fever characterize rubella (German measles). As many as 20% to 50% of rubella infections are asymptomatic.[71] The most important consequence of rubella infection occurs during pregnancy, particularly during the first trimester. Congenital rubella syndrome is associated with auditory, ophthalmic, cardiac, and neurologic defects. Rubella infection during pregnancy also can result in miscarriage or stillbirth. The primary goal of rubella immunization is to prevent congenital rubella syndrome.

Rubella vaccine contains lyophilized live attenuated rubella virus grown in human diploid cell culture. The vaccine is available alone or in combination with measles or mumps vaccine or both. Each 0.5-mL dose also contains 25 mcg neomycin.

Rubella vaccine induces antibodies that are protective against wild-virus infection. Following a single 0.5-mL subcutaneous dose, 98% of children 1 year of age or older become rubella antibody–positive within 2 to 6 weeks.[72] The duration of immunity has not been established. A second dose is recommended, however, at the same time measles vaccine is administered (as a second dose of MMR). The vaccine is indicated for children older than 1 year of age. Although individuals born before 1957 are assumed to be immune to rubella, this is not sufficient for women who could become pregnant. Therefore, all women of childbearing potential should have documentation of receiving at least one dose of a rubella-containing vaccine or laboratory evidence of immunity.[71] Recent administration of immunoglobulin interferes with rubella vaccine response for at least 3 months and depends on the dose of immunoglobulin that is administered.[3,48,71] Table 122–1 can be used as a guide for the recommended interval. The vaccine should not be given to immunosuppressed individuals, although MMR vaccine should be administered to young children with HIV infection without severe immunosuppression as soon as possible after their first birthday.[48] The vaccine should not be given to individuals who have experienced anaphylactic reactions to neomycin.[48]

Adverse effects of the rubella virus vaccine tend to increase with the age of the recipient. Symptoms are similar to wild-virus infection and include lymphadenopathy, rash, urticaria, fever, malaise, sore throat, headache, myalgias, and paresthesias of the extremities. These occur 7 to 12 days after vaccination and last 1 to 5 days. Joint symptoms occur more often in susceptible postpubertal females. Arthralgia occurs in 25% of such vaccinees, and 10% will have arthritis-like symptoms. These symptoms usually begin 1 to 3 weeks after vaccination and persist for 1 day to 3 weeks. A very small excess risk of chronic arthropathy exists.[73] The vaccine may cause suppression of tuberculin skin tests for up to 6 weeks after vaccination. While the vaccine virus may be excreted in nose and throat secretions, it is not contagious.

Although the rubella vaccine has never been associated with congenital rubella syndrome, its use during pregnancy is contraindicated. However, routine pregnancy testing prior to vaccination is not recommended. Women should be counseled not to become pregnant for 4 weeks following vaccination.[57] Termination of pregnancy is not indicated in women who are accidentally given the vaccine or who become pregnant during the month after vaccination.

VARICELLA VACCINE

Varicella is a highly contagious disease caused by varicella-zoster virus. The clinical illness is characterized by the appearance of successive waves of pruritic vesicles that rapidly crust over. Malaise and fever are common and last for 2 to 3 days. The virus remains dormant in the dorsal ganglia and reactivates as herpes zoster, also known as *shingles*. Although the exact stimulus for reactivation is unknown, a decrease in varicella-specific cell-mediated immunity associated with age or immunosuppression appears to be necessary but not sufficient for reactivation.

Live attenuated varicella vaccine contains the Oka-Merck strain of varicella virus, which was attenuated by propagation through several different cell culture lines. Varicella vaccine is a lyophilized product that must be kept frozen and protected from light. Once reconstituted, it must be administered subcutaneously within 30 minutes. Each 0.5-mL dose contains a minimum of 1350 plaque-forming units of virus, as well as 12.5 mg of hydrolyzed gelatin and trace amounts of neomycin, fetal bovine serum, and residual components from cell culture.[15]

The varicella vaccine is safe and immunogenic in healthy children and adults. A single dose results in seroconversion in greater than 94% of healthy children, and over 90% have persisting antibodies 1 year later. Studies in normal, healthy adults have shown lower seroconversion rates (as low as 80%) following a single dose, but this increases to 95% when a two-dose regimen is used. In clinical studies, varicella vaccine has been 70% to more than 95% effective in preventing chickenpox. Vaccinated individuals who develop chickenpox typically experience milder disease, with less fever and fewer skin lesions, many of which do not vesiculate. Similarly, vaccinated individuals who develop breakthrough infections transmit the varicella virus to others at a lower rate.[74]

The duration of protection provided by varicella vaccine is unknown but is believed to be long lasting. Potential self-boosting of vaccinated individuals as the latent vaccine virus reactivates in those with the lowest varicella antibody titer is one possibility by which lifelong immunity may be conferred.[75] Additionally, children who are immunized against varicella and then exposed to wild-virus experience an immunologic boost.[75] As varicella vaccine use becomes more widespread, the circulation of wild virus can be expected to diminish, and the opportunity for immunologic boosting because of natural exposure also will decline. It is not known whether booster doses will be needed under these circumstances or if reactivation of latent vaccine virus will be sufficient to confer long-term protection. Long-term studies assessing the duration of protection and the advisability of booster doses are ongoing.

The varicella vaccine is recommended for all children at 12 to 18 months of age. It is also recommended for patients above this age if they have not already had chickenpox. Individuals who are 12 months to 12 years of age require one dose. Persons 13 years of age and older should receive two doses, separated by 4 to 8 weeks.[74] Varicella vaccine can be used for postexposure prophylaxis. The vaccine is effective in the prevention or modification of varicella infection when given within 3 days and possibly 5 days of exposure.[76] Because the varicella vaccine is a live vaccine, it is contraindicated in pregnant or immunocompromised individuals. An exception is that children with asymptomatic or mildly symptomatic HIV infection should receive two doses of varicella vaccine 3 months apart. Also, children with humoral immune deficiencies may be immunized.[15] Varicella vaccination is contraindicated in individuals with a history of anaphylactic reaction to any component of the vaccine. Persons who have received blood, plasma, or immunoglobulin products in recent past should not receive varicella vaccine because of concern that passively acquired antibody will interfere with response to the vaccine. The recommended time interval between antibody-containing products and varicella vaccine depends on the dose of immune globulin (see Table 122–1). Although no adverse events associated with salicylate use after vaccination have been reported, salicylates should be avoided for 6 weeks after vaccination because of the association of salicylate use and Reye's syndrome following varicella infection.[74]

The varicella vaccine has an excellent safety record. Pain, local swelling, and erythema at the injection site occur in up to 32% of patients and fever in 10% to 15%. A varicella-like rash occurs in approximately 4% of vaccinees, accompanied by few, if any, systemic symptoms. The rash may be localized at the injection site or generalized. Lesions are usually few in number (2 to 10) and often papular rather than vesicular. Transmission of vaccine virus to susceptible close contacts has occurred, but it is very rare and is believed to occur only when the vaccinee develops a rash. Because the risk of vaccine virus transmission is very low and primary infection can be very severe, vaccination of household contacts of immunocompromised patients is recommended to prevent introduction of varicella into the household.[15,74]

Acquisition of either wild virus or the vaccine strain of varicella renders an individual susceptible to zoster (shingles) at a later date because of reactivation of latent virus. Data indicate that following varicella vaccination, zoster occurs less frequently than following natural infection.[15] In fact, the varicella vaccine is being investigated as a means to boost cellular immunity in the elderly to prevent shingles.[77]

VARICELLA-ZOSTER IMMUNOGLOBULIN

Varicella-zoster immunoglobulin (VZIg) is used for passive immunization of susceptible immunodeficient patients exposed to varicella infection. VZIg is prepared from plasma found in routine screening of normal volunteer blood donors to contain high titers of varicella antibody. On average, VZIg contains 10 to 20 times more varicella antibody than immunoglobulin.[74]

Postexposure prophylaxis with VZIg is indicated for the following susceptible individuals: (1) children with primary or acquired immunodeficiency, with neoplastic disease, or who require immunosuppressive therapy, (2) neonates whose mothers develop varicella within 5 days before or 2 days after delivery, (3) preterm infants (<28 weeks' gestation or who weigh <1000 g) who are exposed to varicella while hospitalized, (4) susceptible pregnant women, and (5) immunosuppressed adults and adolescents. Because healthy adults and adolescents who develop varicella are at increased risk for severe disease, complications, and death, VZIg could be considered in this population, with disease modification rather than prevention being the goal. If varicella is prevented, vaccination should be offered at a later date. Exposure to varicella is defined as direct indoor contact for more than 1 hour with an infectious person. A negative history of clinical disease is not a reliable indicator of varicella susceptibility. Most people with a negative clinical history will have detectable antibody on laboratory testing. Caution is warranted when interpreting a low positive result in an immunosuppressed patient who has received blood products or immunoglobulin because the circulating antibody may be acquired passively.

The clinical efficacy of VZIg can be measured by the rate at which it prevents infection, modifies disease, or prevents subclinical disease. Following household exposure, 30% to 50% of immunocompromised children who receive VZIg will develop disease. Neonates receiving VZIg exposed in utero will develop infection at about the same rate as neonates who did not receive VZIg, but the complication rate is substantially reduced among the infants treated with VZIg.[74]

For maximum effectiveness, VZIg must be given within 48 hours and not more than 96 hours following exposure. Because this agent may only attenuate infection, patients who receive VZIg still may have a period of communicability, and VZIg may prolong the incubation period to 28 days. Exact duration of antibody protection is not known but is assumed to be at least one half-life of the immunoglobulin or approximately 3 weeks.

VZIg is distributed by the American Red Cross Services. Contact with the distribution centers must be made within 72 hours of exposure, and specific criteria must be met in order for the product to be released.

Administration of VZIg is by the IM route (never intravenously) at doses of 125 units/10 kg of body weight up to 625 units (five vials) for patients weighing more than 40 kg. The dose for newborn infants is 125 units. VZIg may be indicated for individuals with bleeding diatheses, in whom IM injection generally should be avoided; the benefits of VZIg likely may outweigh the risks in many cases. Common adverse events include injection-site reactions.

OTHER IMMUNOBIOLOGICS

IMMUNOGLOBULIN

Immunoglobulin is available as both intramuscular (IMIG) and intravenous preparations (IVIG). The IMIG preparation, or the Cohn fraction II, is prepared from pooled plasma of several thousand donors by cold ethanol fractionation. It typically contains greater than 95% IgG and trace amounts of IgM, IgA, and other plasma proteins. Because Ig is harvested from a large donor pool, it contains a wide spectrum of IgG antibodies to the pathogens prevalent in the area from which the donors were obtained. In the fractionation process, high-molecular-weight IgG aggregates are formed, which can activate complement in the absence of antigen and precipitate anaphylactoid reactions. For this reason, IMIG is unsuitable for IV administration. IMIG typically contains 15% to 18% protein and not less than 90% IgG. A number of IVIG preparations are available commercially in the United States. Generally, these preparations contain greater than 90% IgG monomers and trace to small amounts of IgA. These products are available as lyophilized powders or solutions.

When administered either IV or IM, immunoglobulin distributes in approximately 5% of the body weight of the recipient. The plasma half-life of immunoglobulin ranges from 18 to 32 days. This range of half-life probably is attributable to the variation in the half-life of IgG subclasses. Peak serum concentrations occur immediately with IVIG, whereas IMIG produces peak concentrations within 2 days. After the initial period of equilibration, circulating IgG levels are superimposable between IV and IM equivalent dosages. No dosage adjustment is necessary in patients with renal or hepatic insufficiency, or both, or dialysis patients or geriatric patients.

Immunoglobulin is indicated in a wide variety of circumstances to provide passive immunity to individuals.[78] The indications for IMIG differ from those for IVIG. IMIG is indicated for providing

TABLE 122–4. Indications and Dosage of Intramuscular Immune Globulin in Infectious Diseases

Primary immunodeficiency states	1.2 mL/kg IM then 0.6 mL/kg every 2–4 weeks
Hepatitis A exposure	0.02 mL/kg IM within 2 weeks
Hepatitis A prophylaxis	0.02 mL/kg IM for exposure <3 months' duration
	0.06 mL/kg IM for exposure up to 5 months' duration
Hepatitis B exposure	0.06 mL/kg (HBIG preferred in known exposures)
Measles exposure	0.25 mL/kg (maximum dose 15 mL) as soon as possible
	0.5 mL/kg (maximum dose 15 mL) as soon as possible for immunocompromised individuals
Varicella exposure	0.6–1.2 mL/kg as soon as possible when VZIG not available

passive immunity in hepatitis A infections, hepatitis B exposures (however, HBIg is significantly more effective), measles, varicella, and primary immunodeficiency diseases. Although IMIG is indicated for the treatment of primary immunodeficiency, IVIG is better tolerated and more effective. IMIG is not indicated for prevention of rubella, mumps, or poliomyelitis. Table 122–4 lists the suggested dosages for IMIG for the prevention or attenuation of various infectious diseases.

There are many approved indications, as well as off-label uses, for IVIG. The therapeutic dose of IVIG is set empirically at 2 g/kg. Often this dose is given in five daily doses of 400 mg/kg each, but it may be preferable to divide the total dose into two daily doses of 1 g/kg if the patient can tolerate the volume of the infusion.[78,79]

- *Primary immunodeficiency states.* In primary immunodeficiency states, monthly doses of between 100 and 800 mg/kg are administered, with the average dose being 200–400 mg/kg. The immunodeficiency states for which IVIG is indicated include both antibody deficiencies and combined immune deficiencies. Significant reactions can occur in patients with low intrinsic levels of IgA given IVIG with greater amounts of IgA. An IVIG product with very low amounts of IgA should be used for these patients. IVIG is indicated for some patients with HIV infection; however, the data to support its use are better in the pediatric population.[16] With the advent of new antiretroviral agents and combination therapies, the usefulness of IVIG may be even more limited.

- *Immune thrombocytopenic purpura.* For the treatment of hemorrhage associated with immune (or idiopathic) thrombocytopenic purpura (ITP), doses of 1 g/kg daily for 2 to 3 days plus high-dose methylprednisolone are indicated. $Rh_o(D)$ immunoglobulin may be used in Rh-positive individuals as an alternative to IVIG (see next section). Adults tend to respond less well to IVIG than do children. IVIG is acceptable for treatment of both chronic and acute ITP, and IVIG has been used in ITP associated with pregnancy without adverse effects on the fetus. Corticosteroids remain the drugs of choice for adult ITP.[80] In thrombotic thrombocytopenia purpura, IVIG is reported to be effective in patients who do not respond to plasmapheresis. Other platelet disorders in which IVIG may be useful include neonatal immune thrombocytopenia, perinatal autoimmune thrombocytopenia,

drug-induced thrombocytopenia, thrombocytopenia secondary to infection, and transfusion-refractory thrombocytopenia; however, the data to support these uses are minimal.[78–80]

- *Chronic lymphocytic leukemia (CLL).* IVIG is used as a prophylactic measure in CLL patients who have had a serious bacterial infection. Doses of 400 mg/kg every 3 to 4 weeks are used.

- *Kawasaki disease (mucocutaneous lymph node syndrome).* This disease, which generally occurs in children, carries the hallmark of development of coronary artery abnormalities. Generally, it is recommended by the American Academy of Pediatrics that if the strict criteria for Kawasaki disease are met, an IVIG dose of 400 mg/kg per day for 4 consecutive days be used or, preferably, 2 g/kg as a single dose. The dose should be administered within 10 days of disease onset. Aspirin therapy also should be initiated.[81]

- *Bone marrow transplant.* IVIG is approved for reducing graft-versus-host disease and infections in patients over the age of 20 years. Patients receive 500 mg/kg 7 and 2 days before transplantation and weekly up to 3 months after. At 100 days posttransplant, patients receive a monthly dose of IVIG for 1 year. Following this regimen, infection (e.g., cytomegalovirus, fungal, bacterial, and interstitial pneumonia) decreased from 51% to 34% in bone marrow transplant patients. IVIG is not indicated in patients younger than 20 years of age.

- *Varicella-zoster.* Another approved indication for IVIG is in the prophylaxis of varicella-zoster if VZIg is not available.

A number of other proposed uses of IVIG can be identified. It is important to note that these are off-label uses but generally may be accepted in the medical community for routine treatment.[78] These uses include

- *Neonatal sepsis.* Neonatal sepsis can cause significant morbidity within 24 hours of birth. While group B *Streptococcus* and *Escherichia coli* remain the primary infecting organisms, other bacteria and fungi may be associated with sepsis. IVIG appears to be effective in neonates older than 34 weeks' gestational age or who weigh less than 1500 g. Routine use is not recommended; however, IVIG may be useful in neonates with recurrent infections.

- *Guillain-Barré syndrome.* IVIG is effective and is considered an alternative to plasmapheresis.[82]

- *Autoimmune diseases.* IVIG may be effective in self-limited immunoregulatory diseases but less effective in chronic diseases such as systemic lupus erythematosus. Overall, there is little evidence that IVIG is useful in the management of autoimmune diseases, except for patients with severe active disease who have not responded to or tolerated other interventions.[83]

- *Intractable epilepsy.* In patients who have confirmed IgG deficiency, IVIG may be useful. For certain syndromes, such as West or Lennox-Gastaut syndrome, IVIG may be considered.[78]

- *Chronic inflammatory demyelinating polyneuropathy.* Although steroids are the first-line therapy, IVIG may be used in patients who fail steroids or do not tolerate steroids.[79]

- *Cytomegalovirus (CMV) infection.* The use of CMV-IVIG is recommended instead of the use of IVIG.

Adverse effects of immunoglobulin vary with the route of administration. Following IMIG, pain, tenderness, and muscle stiffness persisting for hours or days are common. Repeat courses may cause sensitization with resulting allergic reactions. With IVIG, adverse effects occur in fewer than 1% of immunocompetent patients and in fewer than 10% of others. Chills, fever, nausea, and vomiting often are related to the rate of the infusion. Infusion should be given at a rate of 0.01–0.02 mL/kg per minute for 30 minutes and then, if no reactions occur, increased to 0.02–0.04 mL/kg per minute. Although infusion-rate recommendations vary slightly depending on the preparation, the guidelines presented can be followed for the various IV preparations.

Most adverse reactions are mild and transient. Arthralgia, myalgia, fever, pruritus, nausea, vomiting, chest tightness, palpitations, diaphoresis, dizziness, pallor, and respiratory distress have been reported. Rarely, aseptic meningitis has occurred from a few hours to 2 days after high-dose infusion. The syndrome resolves within days without sequelae. Also, acute renal failure has been reported primarily in individuals with underlying renal dysfunction, diabetes, sepsis, volume depletion, other nephrotoxic drugs, or age greater than 65 years. To minimize the risk, ensure adequate hydration prior to infusion, and choose an IVIG product that does not contain high sucrose concentrations for individuals at high risk.[84]

Immunoglobulin products are derived from human blood. Precautions such as donor screening and fractionation procedures and solvent-detergent treatment during the manufacturing process render the IVIG products free of HIV and hepatitis B and C viruses. Although no manufacturing process can guarantee that there is no viral contamination, the potential infection risk from immunoglobulin preparations is very small.[85]

RH$_O$(D) IMMUNOGLOBULIN

Second only to the ABO blood group system, Rhesus antigen D [Rh$_o$(D)] is an important antigen in human blood. The Rh$_o$(D) locus encodes this antigen, but this locus is absent in approximately 15% of the population. These individuals are Rh$_o$(D)-negative and have the potential to mount an antibody response to erythrocytes with the Rh$_o$(D) present. Rh$_o$(D) incompatibility during pregnancy can lead to sensitization of the mother. The maternal antibodies developed following normal fetal leakage of erythrocytes to the mother can cause hemolytic disease of the newborn during subsequent pregnancies.

Rh$_o$(D) immunoglobulin (RDIg) is a sterile solution of immunoglobulins prepared from human sera with high titers of Rh$_o$(D) antibody. RDIg suppresses the antibody response and formation of anti-Rh$_o$(D) in Rh$_o$(D)-negative women exposed to Rh$_o$(D)-positive blood. Administration of RDIg prevents hemolytic disease of the newborn in subsequent pregnancies with a Rh$_o$(D)-positive fetus. When administered within 72 hours of delivery of a full-term infant, RDIg reduces active antibody formation from 12% to 1% to 2%. The reduction in antibody formation is lower when RDIg is given beyond 72 hours postpartum. Smaller doses of RDIg are used after abortion, miscarriage, amniocentesis, or abdominal trauma. In addition, RDIg is also used in the case of a premenopausal woman who is Rh$_o$(D)-negative and who has inadvertently received Rh$_o$(D)-positive blood or blood products.

The dosage of RDIg varies with the indication. A standard dose of 300 mcg is given within 72 hours of a term delivery. Occasionally, where the fetus is known to be Rh$_o$(D)-positive, a 300-mcg dose is given at 28 weeks' gestation and within 72 hours after delivery. For postpregnancy termination occurring up to 13 weeks' gestation, one microdose (50 mcg) vial is given within 72 hours. For pregnancy termination after 13 weeks, one standard dose (300 mcg) is given within 72 hours. In other circumstances, such as in abdominal trauma, amniocentesis, or transfusion accidents, the dosage (number of standard dose vials) is based on the estimated packed red blood cell volume of

the fetal/maternal hemorrhage divided by 15. RDIg is administered intramuscularly only.

When considering RDIg for use, one must be certain of the mother's Rh$_o$(D) antigen status; RDIg should not be given to individuals positive for this antigen or to those with anti-Rh$_o$(D) antibodies. Occasionally, a large fetal bleed of Rh$_o$(D)-positive blood may make cross-matching of the mother difficult. In these cases, RDIg should be given only if previous tests have shown the mother to be Rh$_o$(D)-negative with no anti-Rh$_o$(D) antibody.

Adverse reactions to RDIg include injection-site tenderness and fever. Rh$_o$(D) does not interfere with response to rubella vaccine. Rubella-seronegative women should be immunized at hospital discharge even if they received RDIg postpartum.

CYTOMEGALOVIRUS IMMUNOGLOBULIN

CMV intravenous immunoglobulin (CMV-IVIG) contains IgG antibodies obtained from healthy persons with high titers of antibodies to CMV.

Attenuation of primary CMV disease associated with solid-organ transplantation in seronegative recipients of seropositive organs is the indication for CMV-IVIG. It is dosed using a tapering schedule. Dosage is 150 mg/kg preoperatively or within 72 hours postoperatively; 100 mg/kg at 2, 4, 6, and 8 weeks; and 50 mg/kg at weeks 12 and 16. These doses are for all ages. The use of CMV-IVIG has resulted in a significant decrease in CMV-related syndromes. Further studies are needed to determine the efficacy of CMV-IVIG in bone marrow transplantation. CMV-IVIG has been effective in some studies but ineffective in others.

Adverse effects of CMV-IVIG are seen in fewer than 5% of recipients and include flushing, chills, muscle cramps, back pain, chest tightness, fever, nausea, vomiting, hypotension, and tachycardia. These adverse events may be related to the infusion rate and can be managed by temporarily discontinuing the infusion. The infusion may be restarted at a decreased rate. Anaphylaxis occurs rarely and should be considered if hypotension develops during the infusion. Because CMV-IVIG contains other antibodies, live-virus vaccines should be withheld until 3 months after CMV-IVIG administration.

VACCINES FOR TRAVEL

The use of a few vaccines is reserved for individuals who travel to areas of the world where these vaccine-preventable infections are common. Immunization is only a part of travel medicine. Recommendations for the use of hepatitis A and hepatitis B vaccines can be found in Chap. 40. Meningococcal polysaccharide vaccine is recommended for seasonal travel in sub-Saharan Africa, and the use of this vaccine was described earlier in this chapter.

The CDC publishes annual editions of *Health Information for International Travel* (commonly referred to as the "Yellow Book"). The information contained in the book can be viewed and used at *www.cdc.gov/travel*. Additionally, this Web site offers information on disease outbreaks and updates of interest to the international traveler and to health care providers caring for international travelers.

JAPANESE ENCEPHALITIS VIRUS VACCINE

Japanese encephalitis is an arboviral infection spread by mosquitoes in Asia and Oceania. Infection leads to encephalitis in 1 in 20 to 1 in 1000 cases. However, the encephalitis is fatal in about 25% of cases, and neurologic sequelae are manifest in about 30% of cases. Transmission s seasonal, with the highest times of transmission occurring in the summer and early fall. Although the risk for the most travelers is quite low, the risk for individuals depends on the season, rural location, and duration of travel.[86] The Japanese encephalitis virus vaccine is recommended for U.S. expatriates residing in areas where Japanese encephalitis is endemic or epidemic. The vaccine is not recommended routinely for travelers to Asia.

Monovalent inactivated Japanese encephalitis virus vaccine has been available commercially in the United States since 1992. Three doses are needed to provide protective concentrations of neutralizing antibodies. The vaccine series produced higher antibody concentrations when administered in a 0-, 7-, and 30-day schedule rather that in a 0-, 7-, and 14-day regimen, but all subjects mounted a protective response regardless of regimen. Duration of antibody protection is unknown. Protective titers have been reported for up to 3 years after primary immunization. Additionally, single booster doses given 1 year after primary immunization have resulted in substantial rises in antibody titers. The Japanese encephalitis vaccine is administered to individuals at least 3 years of age as 1 mL given subcutaneously on days 0, 7, and 30. The 0-, 7-, and 14-day schedule can be used if time is a constraint. In addition, a 0- and 7-day schedule can be used if absolutely necessary, and it will provide protection for 80% of persons. The last dose should be administered at least 10 days before traveling to observe for adverse reactions. For children ages 1 to 3 years, 0.5 mL of vaccine is administered subcutaneously using the schedules already noted. No data are available for infants. Booster doses are recommended every 36 months, with 1-mL booster doses being given to children 3 years of age or older even if they received 0.5 mL as the initial dose. Pregnant women who travel to an epidemic or endemic area should be vaccinated. No data are available for immunocompromised patients.

Adverse reactions include pain and tenderness at the injection site (20%) and systemic side effects such as fever, headache, malaise, rash, chills, dizziness, myalgia, nausea, vomiting, and abdominal pain in 10%.[86] In addition, there are sporadic reports of hypersensitivity reactions to the vaccine. The manifestations of this type of reaction include urticaria, angioedema, and respiratory distress. These reactions have generally occurred after a median of 12 hours after the first dose of vaccine, with 88% of reactions occurring within 3 days. After a second dose, these hypersensitivity reactions may occur 3 to 14 days after injection.

TYPHOID VACCINE

Typhoid fever is an illness caused by infection with *Salmonella typhi*. Typhoid is spread via the fecal-oral route. Clinical illness in its severe form is characterized by gradually rising fever that reaches 39 to 41°C (102.2 to 105.8°F) and persists for up to 2 weeks. Headaches, abdominal discomfort, malaise, myalgia, and anorexia usually are present. Older children and adults usually have constipation, whereas diarrhea is common in infants. Complications include intestinal perforation and hemorrhage. Between 2% and 5% of patients become chronic gallbladder carriers of *S. typhi*.

Although rare in developed countries, typhoid is common in Africa, Asia, Central America, and South America. Travelers to these areas should be advised that careful selection of food and beverages is the most effective means of preventing infection but should be offered immunization if the itinerary puts the travelers at high risk for typhoid.

Three typhoid vaccines are available in the United States. The oral typhoid vaccine is a live attenuated preparation that is given as a four-dose series with one capsule administered every other day. The capsules should be taken on an empty stomach with cool or lukewarm liquid. The series should be completed 1 week prior to travel and should not be used in anyone younger than 6 years of age. The oral vaccine should not be administered during a course of antibiotics. The injectable typhoid vaccine (ViCPS) is a polysaccharide vaccine given as a single intramuscular dose at least 2 weeks before travel. This polysaccharide vaccine should not be given to children younger than 2 years of age. Another injectable typhoid vaccine is also available (Typhoid Vaccine USP). It is a heat-phenol–inactivated bacterial vaccine. This vaccine can be used in adults and children as young as 6 months of age. The vaccine series consists of two doses at least 4 weeks apart. This inactivated typhoid vaccine should be used only when the other two preparations cannot be used because Typhoid Vaccine USP is associated with significantly more adverse effects and is no more effective.[87]

Booster doses of all three vaccine preparations are recommended if continued or repeated exposure is expected. The entire four-dose oral vaccine series should be repeated every 5 years. The ViCPS preparation requires revaccination every 2 years, whereas the Typhoid Vaccine USP should be readministered every 3 years. A single dose is required even if more than 3 years have elapsed since the primary series.

Because the oral vaccine is a live attenuated preparation, its use in the immunocompromised should be avoided. Both parenteral vaccines can be administered to immunocompromised persons because they are inactivated. None of the vaccines should be given to febrile individuals. Pregnancy is not an absolute contraindication to use of any of the vaccines, but the benefits versus the risks must be weighed.[87]

The oral typhoid vaccine is well tolerated, with rare reports of gastrointestinal discomfort, fever, headache, or rash. Local injection-site reactions are the most commonly reported adverse event following the injectable typhoid vaccine (ViCPS). Systemic symptoms, such as fever, flulike symptoms, gastrointestinal discomfort, tremor, or neck pain, are reported occasionally. Most vaccinees will report injection-site reactions after the injectable Typhoid Vaccine USP. Malaise, headache, muscle aches, and fever also may occur. Very rarely, serious adverse events, such as chest paint, hypotension, and shock, have been reported.

YELLOW FEVER VACCINE

Yellow fever is caused by a virus transmitted via *Aedes* mosquito bites. Yellow fever is endemic in areas of South America and Africa. Symptoms of infection include fever, prostration, headache, photophobia, myalgias, arthralgias, anorexia, and vomiting. Management consists solely of supportive care. The fatality rate is approximately 20%.

Live attenuated yellow fever virus vaccine is recommended for persons who will be traveling to or living in areas where yellow fever infection occurs and is required for entry into certain countries.[88] The reconstituted vaccine is thermolabile, and unused portions must be discarded 1 hour after reconstitution.

The recommended dose is 0.5 mL subcutaneously given once, with similar booster doses recommended every 10 years. The vaccine, however, has been shown to be highly immunogenic, with antibodies persisting for at least 35 years and perhaps for life.

Mild side effects consisting of headache, myalgias, and low-grade fever 1 to 2 weeks after vaccination occur in fewer than 10% of vaccinees; treatment should be symptomatic. Immediate hypersensitivity reactions are rare and occur primarily in persons who have anaphylactic reactions to eggs or other substances. Neurotropic disease following yellow fever immunization is very rare (23 reported cases to date). Infants are likely more susceptible to neurotropic disease, and use of the yellow fever vaccine in infants younger than 9 months of age should be avoided.[88]

Yellow fever vaccine–associated viscerotropic syndrome occurs in a clinical spectrum from moderate illness with focal organ dysfunction to severe disease with multiple-organ-system failure and death. Yellow fever vaccine virus has been isolated from clinical samples collected from individuals with viscertropic syndrome. The viscertropic syndrome is more likely to occur with the first dose of vaccine than in individuals who have been vaccinated previously.

On theoretical grounds, the vaccine should be avoided during pregnancy unless travel to a high-risk area is imperative. It may be given to breast-feeding mothers. The vaccine may be used in immunocompromised patients if the risk of infection in an endemic area outweighs the potential vaccine risk. Additionally, it should not be given to infants younger than 4 months of age and, in general, should be used only if a child is 9 months of age or older. Children 4 to 9 months of age must be considered on an individual basis. Individuals 65 years of age and older appear to be at higher risk for serious vaccine-related adverse effects.[89] Decisions about travel to yellow fever endemic areas and vaccine use must be considered carefully given the seriousness of yellow fever infection.[88] It is contraindicated in persons with a history of an anaphylactic reaction to eggs. Where the history is in question, intradermal testing consisting of 0.02-mL doses of vaccine and normal saline control applied to the volar surface of the forearm should be done. The demonstration of an erythematous, urticarial wheal and negative control constitutes a positive response and contraindicates vaccination. This intradermal testing may be sufficient to produce antibodies, but serologic testing should be done to confirm this.

Yellow fever vaccine may be administered simultaneously with all other vaccines except cholera; a 3-week interval between vaccines is recommended. Simultaneous administration of immunoglobulin does not interfere with the immune response to this agent.

VACCINE INFORMATION RESOURCES

The field of vaccinology is developing ever more rapidly, with numerous changes being made in recommendations for vaccine use each year. Keeping up to date with the current recommendations can be a challenge. The childhood and adolescent immunization schedule is updated each January. Recommendations for the use of influenza vaccine are issued annually. Updates to the adult immunization schedule are made periodically. Health care providers involved in primary care and immunization delivery must keep themselves abreast of these changes in a systematic way. Reading electronic newsletters and browsing reliable Web sites are efficient methods of obtaining information (Table 122–5). Although several excellent, reliable, and timely Web sites exist, hundreds of sites with misleading and incorrect information also exist. Many of these sites are targeted at parents.

Vaccines are the only class of medications to which nearly every patient is exposed. Knowledge of these agents is critical in providing pharmaceutical care. Dramatic progress in public health has been made through the appropriate use of immunization. Additional improvements in quality of life and mortality can be made through continued increases in vaccination coverage with careful attention to this aspect of care by all health care providers.

TABLE 122–5. Web Resources for Vaccine Information

Recommended Internet Sites for Vaccine Information

www.cdc.gov/nip	National Immunization Program
www.cdc.gov/ncidod/ diseases/hepatitis	Center for Disease Control and Prevention's National Center for Infectious Diseases Viral Hepatitis
www.immunize.org	Immunization Action Coalition
www.vaccines.org	Allied Vaccine Group
www.nfid.org/NCAI/	National Coalition for Adult Immunization
www.cdc.gov/mmwr/	Morbidity and Mortality Weekly Report
www.hrsa.gov/osp/vicp/	Vaccine Injury Compensation Program
www.vaers.org	Vaccine Adverse Event Reporting System
www.iom.edu/	Institute of Medicine of the National Academies
www.immunizationinfo.org/	National Network for Immunization Information

Recommended Electronic Newsletters

www.immunize.org/express	The Immunization Action Coalition's newsletter
www.cdc.gov/mmwr/	Morbidity and Mortality Weekly Report

ABBREVIATIONS

ACIP: Advisory Committee on Immunization Practices
CDC: Centers for Disease Control and Prevention
CMV-IVIG: cytomegalovirus intravenous immunoglobulin
DTaP: diphtheria-tetanus-acellular pertussis vaccine
HBIg: hepatitis B immune globulin
HDCV: human diploid cell vaccine (rabies)
Hib: *Hemophilus influenzae* type b
HSCT: hematopoietic stem cell transplant
IMIG: intramuscular immunoglobulin
IPV: inactivated polio vaccine
ITP: immune thrombocytopenic purpura
IVIG: intravenous immunoglobulin
LAIV: live attenuated influenza vaccine
MMR: measles-mumps-rubella vaccine
OPV: oral polio vaccine
PCEC: purified chick embryo cell culture rabies vaccine
PCV: pneumococcal conjugate vaccine
PPD: purified protein derivative
PPV: pneumococcal polysaccharide vaccine
PRP: polyribosyl ribitolphosphate
PT: pertussis toxin
RDIg: Rho(D) immune globulin
RVA: rabies vaccine absorbed
Td: tetanus diphtheria
TIG: tetanus immune globulin
VAERS: Vaccine Adverse Event Reporting System
VAPP: vaccine-associated paralytic poliomyelitis
VZIG: varicella immune globulin

Review Questions and other resources can be found at *www.pharmacotherapyonline.com.*

REFERENCES

1. Ada G. Vaccines and vaccination. N Engl J Med 2001;345:1042–1053.
2. Centers for Disease Control and Prevention. Combination vaccines for childhood immunization. MMWR1999;48:1–15.

3. Centers for Disease Control and Prevention. General recommendations on immunization: Recommendations of the Advisory Committee on Immunization Practices (ACIP) and the American Academy of Family Physicians (AAFP). MMWR 2002;51:1–35.

4. Poland GA. Hepatitis B immunization in health care workers: Dealing with vaccine nonresponse. Am J Prev Med 1998;15:73–77.

5. Centers for Disease Control and Prevention. Prevention and control of influenza: Recommendations of the Advisory Committee on Immunization Practices (ACIP). MMWR 2004;53:1–40.

6. Arrowood JR, Hayney MS. Immunization recommendations for adults with cancer. Ann Pharmacother 2002;36:1219–1229.

7. Poland GA, Borrud A, Jacobson RM, et al. Determination of deltoid fat pad thickness: Implications for needle length in adult immunization. JAMA 1997;277:1709–1711.

8. Alimonos K, Nafziger AN, Murray J, Bertino JS Jr. Prediction of response to hepatitis B vaccine in health care workers: Whose titers of antibody to hepatitis B surface antigen should be determined after a three-dose series, and what are the implications in terms of cost-effectiveness? Clin Infect Dis 1998;26:566–571.

9. Dorrell L, Hassan I, Marshall S, et al. Clinical and serological responses to an inactivated influenza vaccine in adults with HIV infection, diabetes, obstructive airways disease, elderly adults and healthy volunteers. Int J STD AIDS 1997;8:776–779.

10. Pirofski LA, Casadevall A. Use of licensed vaccines for active immunization of the immunocompromised host. Clin Microbiol Rev 1998;11:1–26.

11. Hayney MS. Pharmacogenomics and infectious diseases: Impact on drug response and applications to disease management. Am J Health Syst Pharm 2002;59:1626–1631.

12. MedImmune Vaccines I. Influenza virus vaccine live, intranasal FluMist 2003–2004 Formula. Package Insert 2003:1–19.

13. Centers for Disease Control and Prevention. Guidelines for Vaccinating Pregnant Women from the Recommendations of the Advisory Committee on Immunization Practices (ACIP). Washington, U.S. Department of Health and Human Services, 1998:1–11 (updated October 2003).

14. Centers for Disease Control and Prevention. Recommendations of the Advisory Committee on Immunization Practices (ACIP): Use of vaccines and immune globulins for persons with altered immunocompetence. MMWR 1993;42:1–18.

15. Centers for Disease Control and Prevention. Prevention of varicella: Updated recommendations of the Advisory Committee on Immunization Practices (ACIP). MMWR 1999;48:1–5.

16. Centers for Disease Control and Prevention. Guidelines for preventing opportunistic infections among HIV-infected persons—2002. MMWR 2002;51:1–52.

17. Stark K, Gunther M, Schonfeld C, et al. Immunisations in solid-organ transplant recipients. Lancet 2002;359:957–965.

18. Huzly D, Neifer S, Reinke P, et al. Routine immunizations in adult renal transplant recipients. Transplantation 1997;63:839–845.

19. Dengler TJ, Strnad N, Buhring I, et al. Differential immune response to influenza and pneumococcal vaccination in immunosuppressed patients after heart transplantation. Transplantation 1998;66:1340–1347.

20. Burroughs M, Moscona A. Immunization of pediatric solid organ transplant candidates and recipients. Clin Infect Dis 2000;30:857–869.

21. Edvardsson VO, Flynn JT, Deforest A, et al. Effective immunization against influenza in pediatric renal transplant recipients. Clin Transplant 1996;10:556–560.

22. Fuchshuber A, Kuhnemund O, Keuth B, et al. Pneumococcal vaccine in children and young adults with chronic renal disease. Neph Dial Transplant 1996;11:468–473.

23. Loinaz C, de Juanes JR, Gonzalez EM, et al. Hepatitis B vaccination results in 140 liver transplant recipients. Hepato-Gastroenterology 1997;44:235–238.

24. Centers for Disease Control and Prevention. Guidelines for preventing opportunistic infections among hematopoietic stem cell transplant recipients: Recommendations of CDC, the Infectious Disease Society of America, and the American Society of Blood and Bone Marrow Transplantation. MMWR 2000;49. No. RR-10:52–53 and 97–118.

25. Centers for Disease Control and Prevention. Development of community- and state-based immunization registries: CDC response to a report from the National Vaccine Advisory Committee. MMWR 2001;50:1–17.

26. U.S. Department of Health and Human Services. Healthy People 2010: Understanding and Improving Health. Washington, US Government Printing Office, 2000:62.

27. Centers for Disease Control and Prevention. Immunization of adolescents: Recommendations of the Advisory Committee on Immunization Practices, the American Academy of Pediatrics, the American Academy of Family Physicians, and the American Medical Association. MMWR 1996;45:1–19.

28. US Department of Health and Human Services. National Vaccine Injury Compensation Program. Available at *www.hrsa.gov/osp/vicp/;* accessed January 27, 2004.

29. Chen RT, DeStefano F, Pless R, et al. Challenges and controversies in immunization safety. Infect Dis Clin North Am 2001;15:21–39, viii.

30. American Academy of Pediatrics. Diphtheria. In: Pickering LK, Peter G, Baker CJ, et al, eds. 2000 Red Book: Report of the Committee on Infectious Diseases. Elk Grove Village, IL, American Academy of Pediatrics, 2000:230–234.

31. American Academy of Pediatrics. Tetanus. In: Pickering LK, Peter G, Baker CJ, et al, eds. 2000 Red Book: Report of the Committee on Infectious Diseases. Elk Grove Village, IL, American Academy of Pediatrics, 2000:563–569.

32. Centers for Disease Control and Prevention. Progress toward elimination of *Haemophilus influenzae* type b invasive disease among infants and children—United States, 1998–2000. MMWR 2002;51:234–237.

33. Centers for Disease Control and Prevention. Recommended childhood and adolescent immunization schedule—United States, 2005. MMWR 2005;53:Q1–Q3.

34. American Academy of Pediatrics. *Haemophilus influenzae* infections. In: Pickering LK, Peter G, Baker CJ, et al, eds. 2000 Red Book: Report of the Committee on Infectious Diseases. Elk Grove Village, IL, American Academy of Pediatrics, 2000:262–272.

35. Centers for Disease Control and Prevention. Update on adult immunization: Recommendations of the Immunization Practices Advisory Committee (ACIP). MMWR 1991;40:1–94.

36. Treanor JJ, Kotloff K, Betts RF, et al. Evaluation of trivalent, live, cold-adapted (CAIV-T) and inactivated (TIV) influenza vaccines in prevention of virus infection and illness following challenge of adults with wild-type influenza A (H1N1), A (H3N2), and B viruses. Vaccine 1999;18:899–906.

37. Belshe RB, Mendelman PM, Treanor J, et al. The efficacy of live attenuated, cold-adapted, trivalent, intranasal influenzavirus vaccine in children. N Engl J Med 1998;338:1405–1412.

38. Belshe RB, Gruber WC, Mendelman PM, et al. Efficacy of vaccination with live attenuated, cold-adapted, trivalent, intranasal influenza virus vaccine against a variant (A/Sydney) not contained in the vaccine. J Pediatr 2000;136:168–175.

39. Nichol KL, Mendelman PM, Mallon KP, et al. Effectiveness of live, attenuated intranasal influenza virus vaccine in healthy, working adults: A randomized, controlled trial. JAMA 1999;282:137–144.

40. Nichol KL, Lind A, Margolis KL, et al. The effectiveness of vaccination against influenza in healthy, working adults (see comments). N Engl J Med 1995;333:889–893.

41. Nichol KL, Nordin J, Mullooly J, et al. Influenza vaccination and reduction in hospitalizations for cardiac disease and stroke among the elderly. N Engl J Med 2003;348:1322–1332.

42. Keyser LA, Karl M, Nafziger AN, Bertino JS Jr. Comparison of central nervous system adverse effects of amantadine and rimantadine used as sequential prophylaxis of influenza A in elderly nursing home patients. Arch Intern Med 2000;160:1485–1488.

43. Monto AS, Robinson DP, Herlocher ML, et al. Zanamivir in the prevention of influenza among healthy adults: A randomized controlled trial. JAMA 1999;282:31–35.

44. Hayden FG, Atmar RL, Schilling M, et al. Use of the selective oral neuraminidase inhibitor oseltamivir to prevent influenza. New Engl J Med 1999;341:1336–1343.

45. Lasky T, Terracciano GJ, Magder L, et al. The Guillain-Barré syndrome and the 1992–1993 and 1993–1994 influenza vaccines. N Engl J Med 1998;339:1797–1802.

46. Centers for Disease Control and Prevention. Using live, attenuated influenza vaccine for prevention and control of influenza: Supplemental recommendations of the Advisory Committee on Immunization Practices (ACIP). MMWR 2003;52:1–8.

47. Centers for Disease Control and Prevention. Absence of transmission of d9 measles virus: Region of the Americas, November 2002–March003. MMWR 2003;52:228–229.

48. Centers for Disease Control and Prevention. Measles, mumps, and rubella: Vaccine use and strategies for elimination of measles, rubella, and congenital rubella syndrome and control of mumps. Recommendations of the Advisory Committee on Immunization Practices (ACIP). MMWR 1998; 47:1–57.

49. Poland GA, Jacobson RM, Thampy AM, et al. Measles reimmunization in children seronegative after initial immunization. JAMA 1997;277: 1156–1158.

50. Centers for Disease Control and Prevention. Immunization of health-care workers. MMWR 1997;46:1–42.

51. Madsen KM, Hviid A, Vestergaard M, et al. A population-based study of measles, mumps, and rubella vaccination and autism. N Engl J Med 2002;347:1477–1482.

52. Makela A, Nuorti JP, Peltola H. Neurologic disorders after measles-mumps-rubella vaccination. Pediatrics 2002;110:957–963.

53. Institute of Medicine. Immunization safety review: Measles-mumps-rubella vaccine and autism. In: Stratton K, Gable A, Shetty P, McCormick M, eds. Washington, National Academy Press, 2001:1–69.

54. Institute of Medicine. Measles and mumps vaccines. In: Stratton K, Howe C, Johnston R, eds. Adverse Events Associated with Childhood Vaccines: Evidence Bearing on Causality. Washington, National Academy Press, 1994:118–186.

55. Bruce MG, Rosenstein NE, Capparella JM, et al. Risk factors for meningococcal disease in college students. JAMA 2001;286:688–693.

56. Centers for Disease Control and Prevention. Prevention and control of meningococcal disease and meningococcal disease and college students: Recommendations of the Advisory Committee on Immunization Practices (ACIP). MMWR 2000;49:1–20.

57. Centers for Disease Control and Prevention. Revised ACIP recommendation for avoiding pregnancy after receiving a rubella-containing vaccine. MMWR 2001;50:1117.

58. De Serres G, Shadmani R, Duval B, et al. Morbidity of pertussis in adolescents and adults. J Infect Dis 2000;182:174–179.

59. Centers for Disease Control and Prevention. Pertussis vaccination: Use of acellular pertussis vaccines among infants and young children. Recommendations of the Advisory Committee on Immunization Practices (ACIP). MMWR 1997;46:1–25.

60. Centers for Disease Control and Prevention. Prevention of pneumococcal disease: Recommendations of the Advisory Committee on Immunization Practices (ACIP). MMWR 1997;46:1–24.

61. Jackson LA, Neuzil KM, Yu O, et al. Effectiveness of pneumococcal polysaccharide vaccine in older adults. N Engl J Med 2003;348: 1747–1755.

62. Jackson LA, Benson P, Sneller VP, et al. Safety of revaccination with pneumococcal polysaccharide vaccine. JAMA 1999;281:243–248.

63. Centers for Disease Control and Prevention. Preventing pneumococcal disease among infants and young children: Recommendations of the Advisory Committee on Immunization Practices (ACIP). MMWR 2000;49: 1–35.

64. Black S, Shinefield H, Fireman B, et al. Efficacy, safety and immunogenicity of heptavalent pneumococcal conjugate vaccine in children. Northern California Kaiser Permanente Vaccine Study Center Group. Pediatr Infect Dis J 2000;19:187–195.

65. Whitney CG, Farley MM, Hadler J, et al. Decline in invasive pneumococcal disease after the introduction of protein-polysaccharide conjugate vaccine. N Engl J Med 2003;348:1737–1746.

66. Centers for Disease Control and Prevention. Poliomyelitis prevention in the United States: Updated recommendations of the Advisory Committee on Immunization Practices (ACIP). MMWR 2000;49:1–22.

67. Centers for Disease Control and Prevention. Prolonged poliovirus excretion in an immunodeficient person with vaccine-associated paralytic poliomyelitis. MMWR 1997;46:641–643.

68. Centers for Disease Control and Prevention. Compendium of animal rabies prevention and control, 2003. National Association of State Public Health Veterinariuans, Inc. (NASPHV). MMWR 2003;52:1–6.

69. Centers for Disease Control and Prevention. Human rabies prevention—United States, 1999: Recommendations of the Advisory Committee on Immunization Practices (ACIP). MMWR 1999;48:1–21.

70. Wilde H, Sirikawin S, Sabcharoen A, et al. Failure of postexposure treatment of rabies in children. Clin Infect Dis 1996;22:228–232.

71. Centers for Disease Control and Prevention. Control and prevention of rubella: Evaluation and management of suspected outbreaks, rubella in pregnant women, and surveillance for congenital rubella syndrome. MMWR 2001;50:1–23.

72. King GE, Markowitz LE, Heath J, et al. Antibody response to measles-mumps-rubella vaccine of children with mild illness at the time of vaccination. JAMA 1996;275:704–707.

73. Tingle AJ, Mitchell LA, Grace M, et al. Randomised, double-blind, placebo-controlled study on adverse effects of rubella immunisation in seronegative women. Lancet 1997;349:1277–1281.

74. Centers for Disease Control and Prevention. Prevention of varicella: Recommendations of the Advisory Committee on Immunization Practices (ACIP). MMWR 1996;45:1–36.

75. Krause PR, Klinman DM. Varicella vaccination: Evidence for frequent reactivation of the vaccine strain in healthy children. Nature Med 2000;6:451–454.

76. Watson B, Seward J, Yang A, et al. Postexposure effectiveness of varicella vaccine. Pediatrics 2000;105:84–88.

77. Raeder CK, Hayney MS. Immunology of varicella immunization in the elderly. Ann Pharmacother 2000;34:228–234.

78. Ratko TA, Burnett DA, Foulke GE, et al. Recommendations for off-label use of intravenously administered immunoglobulin preparations. University Hospital Consortium Expert Panel for off-label use of polyvalent intravenously administered immunoglobulin preparations. JAMA 1995;273:1865–1870.

79. Chen C, Danekas LH, Ratko TA, et al. A multicenter drug use surveillance of intravenous immunoglobulin utilization in US academic health centers. Ann Pharmacother 2000;34:295–299.

80. Cines DB, Blanchette VS. Immune thrombocytopenic purpura. N Engl J Med 2002;346:995–1008.

81. American Academy of Pediatrics. Kawasaki disease. In: Pickering LK, Peter G, Baker CJ, et al, eds. 2000 Red Book: Report of the Committee on Infectious Diseases. Elk Grove Village, IL, American Academy of Pediatrics, 2000:360–363.

82. Kieseier BC, Hartung HP. Therapeutic strategies in the Guillain-Barré syndrome. Semin Neurol 2003;23:159–168.

83. Kazatchkine MD, Kaveri SV. Immunomodulation of autoimmune and inflammatory diseases with intravenous immune globulin. N Engl J Med 2001;345:747–755.

84. Centers for Disease Control and Prevention. Renal insufficiency and failure associated with immune globulin intravenous therapy—United States, 1985–1998. MMWR 1999;48:581–521.

85. Chapel HM. Safety and availability of immunoglobulin replacement therapy in relation to potentially transmissable agents. IUIS Committee on Primary Immunodeficiency Disease. International Union of Immunological Societies. Clin Exp Immunol 1999;118:29–34.

86. Centers for Disease Control and Prevention. Inactivated Japanese encephalitis virus vaccine: Recommendations of the Advisory Committee on Immunization Practices (ACIP). MMWR 1993;42:1–15.

87. Centers for Disease Control and Prevention. Typhoid immunization: Recommendations of the Advisory Committee on Immunization Practices (ACIP). MMWR 1994;43:1–7.

88. Centers for Disease Control and Prevention. Yellow fever vaccine: Recommendations of the Advisory Committee on Immunization Practices (ACIP). MMWR 2002;51:1–11.

89. Martin M, Weld LH, Tsai TF, et al. Advanced age a risk factor for illness temporally associated with yellow fever vaccination. Emerg Infect Dis 2001;7:945–951.

2004 Childhood Immunization Schedule

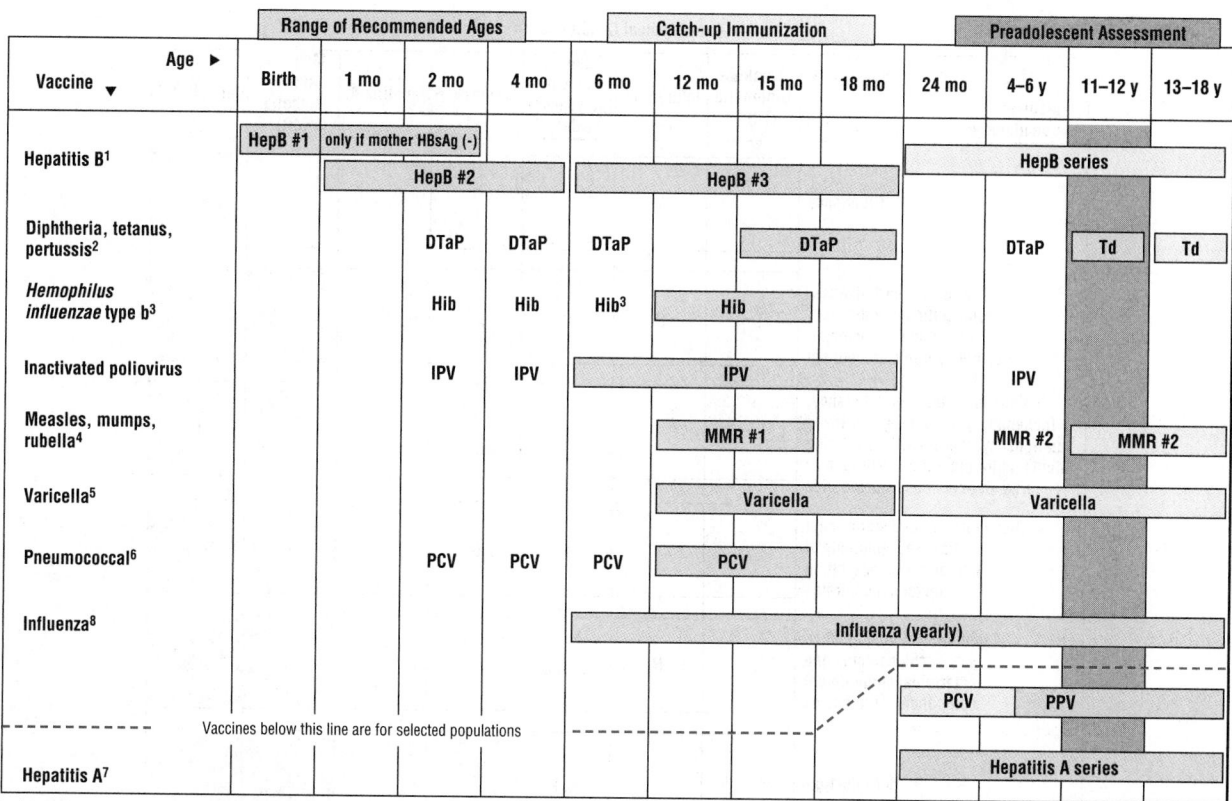

Vaccine	Age ▶	Birth	1 mo	2 mo	4 mo	6 mo	12 mo	15 mo	18 mo	24 mo	4–6 y	11–12 y	13–18 y
				Range of Recommended Ages			**Catch-up Immunization**				**Preadolescent Assessment**		
Hepatitis B¹		HepB #1	only if mother HBsAg (-)								HepB series		
				HepB #2			HepB #3						
Diphtheria, tetanus, pertussis²				DTaP	DTaP	DTaP		DTaP			DTaP	Td	Td
Hemophilus influenzae type b³				Hib	Hib	Hib³	Hib						
Inactivated poliovirus				IPV	IPV		IPV				IPV		
Measles, mumps, rubella⁴							MMR #1				MMR #2	MMR #2	
Varicella⁵							Varicella				Varicella		
Pneumococcal⁶				PCV	PCV	PCV	PCV						
Influenza⁸							Influenza (yearly)						
											PCV	PPV	
		Vaccines below this line are for selected populations											
Hepatitis A⁷											Hepatitis A series		

This schedule indicates the recommended ages for routine administration of currently licensed childhood vaccines, as of December 1, 2003, for children through age 18 years. Any dose not given at the recommended age should be given at any subsequent visit when indicated and feasible. ☐ Indicates age groups that warrant special effort to administer those vaccines not previously given. Additional vaccines may be licensed and recommended during the year. Licensed combination vaccines may be used whenever any components of the combination are indicated and the vaccine's other components are not contraindicated. Providers should consult the manufacturers' package inserts for detailed recommendations. Clinically significant adverse events that follow immunization should be reported to the Vaccine Adverse Event Reporting System (VAERS). Guidance about how to obtain and complete a VAERS form can be found on the Internet: *http:www.vaers.org/* or by calling 1-800-822-7967.

1. Hepatitis B (HepB) vaccine. All infants should receive the first dose of hepatitis B vaccine soon after birth and before hospital discharge; the first dose may also be given by age 2 months if the infant's mother is hepatitis B surface antigen (HBsAg) negative. Only monovalent HepB can be used for the birth dose. Monovalent or combination vaccine containing HepB may be used to complete the series. Four doses of vaccine may be administered when a birth dose is given. The second dose should be given at least 4 weeks after the first dose, except for combination vaccines, which cannot be administered before age 6 weeks. The third dose should be given at least 16 weeks after the first dose and at least 8 weeks after the second dose. The last dose in the vaccination series (third or fourth dose) should not be administered before age 24 weeks.

Infants born to HBsAg-positive mothers should receive HepB and 0.5 mL of Hepatitis B Immune Globulin (HBIG) within 12 hours of birth at separate sites. The second dose is recommended at age 1 to 2 months. The last dose in the immunization series should not be administered before age 24 weeks. These infants should be tested for HBsAg and antibody to HBsAg (anti-HBs) at age 9 to 15 months.

Infants born to mothers whose HBsAg status is unknown should receive the first dose of the HepB series within 12 hours of birth. Maternal blood should be drawn as soon as possible to determine the mother's HBsAg status; if the HBsAg test is positive, the infant should receive HBIG as soon as possible (no later than age 1 week). The second dose is recommended at age 1 or 2 months. The last dose in the immunization series should not be administered before age 24 weeks.

2. Diphtheria and tetanus toxoids and acellular pertussis (DTaP) vaccine. The fourth dose of DTaP may be administered as early as age 12 months, provided 6 months have elapsed since the third dose and the child is unlikely to return at age 15 to 18 months. The final dose in the series should be given at age ≥4 years. **Tetanus and diphtheria toxoids (Td)** is recommended at age 11 to 12 years if at least 5 years have elapsed since the last dose of tetanus and diphtheria toxoid–containing vaccine. Subsequent outline Td boosters are recommended every 10 years.

3. Haemophilus influenzae type b (Hib) conjugate vaccine. Three Hib conjugate vaccines are licensed for infant use. If PRP-OMP (PedvaxHIB or ComVax [Merck]) is administered at ages 2 and 4 months, a dose at age 6 months is not required. DTaP/Hib combination products should not be used for primary immunization in infants at ages 2, 4, or 6 months but can be used as boosters following any Hib vaccine. The final dose in the series should be given at age ≥12 months.

4. Measles, mumps, and rubella vaccine (MMR). The second dose of MMR is recommended routinely at age 4 to 6 years but may be administered during any visit, provided at least 4 weeks have elapsed since the first dose and both doses are administered beginning at or after age 12 months. Those who have not previously received the second dose should complete the schedule by the 11- to 12-year-old visit.

5. Varicella vaccine. Varicella vaccine is recommended at any visit at or after age 12 months for susceptible children (i.e., those who lack a reliable history of chickenpox). Susceptible persons age ≥13 years should receive 2 doses, given at least 4 weeks apart.

6. Pneumococcal vaccine. The heptavalent **pneumococcal conjugate vaccine (PCV)** is recommended for all children age 2 to 23 months. It is also recommended for certain children age 24 to 59 months. The final dose in the series should be given at age ≥12 months. **Pneumococcal polysaccharide vaccine (PPV)** is recommended in addition to PCV for certain high-risk groups. See *MMWR* 2000;49(RR-9):1–38.

7. Hepatitis A vaccine. Hepatitis A vaccine is recommended for children and adolescents in selected states and regions and for certain high-risk groups; consult your local public health authority. Children and adolescents in these states, regions, and high-risk groups who have not been immunized against hepatitis A can begin the hepatitis A immunization series during any visit. The 2 doses in the series should be administered at least 6 months apart. See *MMWR* 1999;48(RR-12):1–37.

8. Influenza vaccine. Influenza vaccine is recommended annually for children age ≥6 months with certain risk factors (including but not limited to children with asthma, cardiac disease, sickle cell disease, human immunodeficiency virus infection, and diabetes; and household members of persons in high-risk groups [see *MMWR* 2003;52(RR):1–36]) and can be administered to all others wishing to obtain immunity. In addition, healthy children age 6 to 23 months are encouraged to receive influenza vaccine if feasible, because children in this age group are at substantially increased risk of influenza-related hospitalizations. For healthy persons age 5 to 49 years, the intranasally administered live-attenuated influenza vaccine (LAIV) is an acceptable alternative to the intramuscular trivalent inactivated influenza vaccine (TIV). See *MMWR* 2003;52(RR-13):1–8. Children receiving TIV should be administered a dosage appropriate for their age (0.25 mL if age 6 to 35 months or 0.5 mL if age ≥3 years). Children age ≤8 years who are receiving influenza vaccine for the first time should receive 2 doses (separated by at least 4 weeks for TIV and at least 6 weeks for LAIV).

Adapted from material approved by the Advisory Committee on Immunization Practices (www.cdc.gov/nip/acip), the American Academy of Pediatrics (www.aap.org), and the American Academy of Family Physicians (www.aafp.org).

2004 Adult Immunization Schedule

by Medical Conditions

Medical Conditions ▼ / Vaccine ▶	Tetanus-Diphtheria (Td)*,1	Influenza2	Pneumo-coccal (polysacch-aride)3,4	Hepatitis B*,5	Hepatitis A6	Measles, Mumps, Rubella (MMR)*,7	Varicella*,8
Pregnancy		A					
Diabetes, heart disease, chronic pulmonary disease, chronic liver disease, including chronic alcoholism		B	C		D		
Congenital Immunodeficiency, leukemia, lymphoma, generalized malignancy, therapy with alkylating agents, antimetabolites, radiation or large amounts of corticosteroids			E				F
Renal failure / end stage renal disease, recipients of hemodialysis or clotting factor concentrates			E	G			
Asplenia including elective splenectomy and terminal complement component deficiencies		H	E, I, J				
HIV infection			E, K			L	

Legend:
- For all persons in this group
- Catch-up on childhood vaccinations
- For persons with medical / exposure indications
- Contraindicated

Special Notes for Medical Conditions

A. For women, vaccinate if pregnancy will be during influenza season. For women with chronic deseases/conditions, vaccinate at any time during the pregnancy.

B. Although chronic liver disease and alcoholism are not indicator conditions for influenza vaccination, give 1 dose annually if the patient is ≥ 50 years, has other indications for influenza vaccine, or if the patient requests vaccination.

C. Asthma is an indicator condition for influenza but not for pneumococcal vaccination.

D. For all persons with chronic liver disease.

E. For persons <65 years, revaccinate once after 5 years or more have elapsed since initial vaccination.

F. Persons with impaired humoral immunity but intact cellular immunity may be vaccinated. *MMWR* 1999;48 (RR-06): 1–5.

G. Hemodialysis patients: Use special formulation of vaccine (40 ug/mL) or two 1 mL 20 ug doses given at one site. Vaccinate early in the course of renal disease. Assess antibody titers to hep B surface antigen (anti-HBs) levels annually. Administer additional doses if anti-HBs levels decline to <10 milliinternational units (mIU)/ mL.

H. There are no data specifically on risk of severe or complicated influenza infections among persons with asplenia. However, influenza is a risk factor for secondary bacterial infections that may cause severe disease in asplenics.

I. Administer meningococcal vaccine and consider Hib vaccine.

J. Elective splenectomy: vaccinate at least 2 weeks before surgery.

K. Vaccinate as close to diagnosis as possible when CD4 cell counts are highest.

L. Withhold MMR or other measles containing vaccines from HIV-infected persons with evidence of severe immunosuppression. *MMWR* 1998;47 (RR-8):21–22; *MMWR* 2002;51 (RR-02): 22–24.

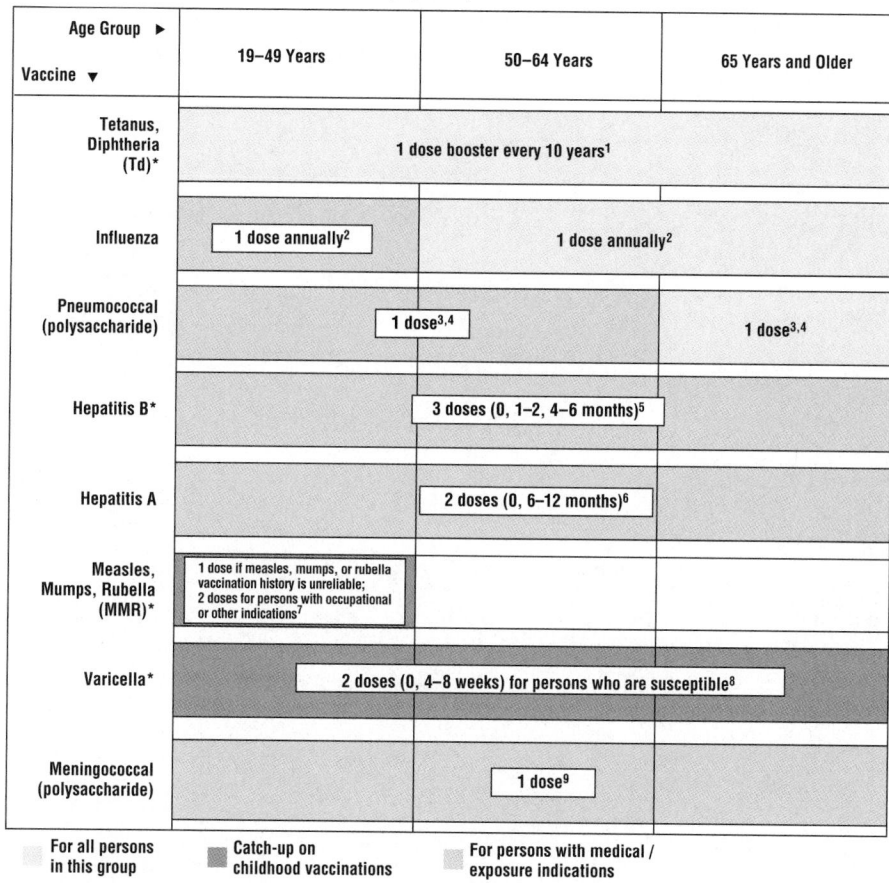

by Age Group

Age Group ▶ Vaccine ▼	19–49 Years	50–64 Years	65 Years and Older
Tetanus, Diphtheria (Td)*	1 dose booster every 10 years[1]		
Influenza	1 dose annually[2]	1 dose annually[2]	
Pneumococcal (polysaccharide)	1 dose[3,4]		1 dose[3,4]
Hepatitis B*	3 doses (0, 1–2, 4–6 months)[5]		
Hepatitis A	2 doses (0, 6–12 months)[6]		
Measles, Mumps, Rubella (MMR)*	1 dose if measles, mumps, or rubella vaccination history is unreliable; 2 doses for persons with occupational or other indications[7]		
Varicella*	2 doses (0, 4–8 weeks) for persons who are susceptible[8]		
Meningococcal (polysaccharide)	1 dose[9]		

☐ For all persons in this group   ■ Catch-up on childhood vaccinations   ▧ For persons with medical / exposure indications

*Covered by the Vaccine Injury Compensation Program.

This schedule indicates the recommended age groups for routine administration of currently licensed vaccines for persons 19 years of age and older. Licensed combination vaccines may be used whenever any components of the combination are indicated and the vaccine's other components are not contraindicated. Providers should consult the manufacturers' package inserts for detailed recommendations.

Report all clinically significant post-vaccination reactions to the Vaccine Adverse Event Reporting System (VAERS). Reporting forms and instructions on filing a VAERS report are available by calling 800-822-7967 or from the VAERS website at www.vaers.org.

For additional information about the vaccines listed above and contraindications for immunization, visit the National Immunization Program Website at www.cdc.gov/nip/ or call the National Immunization Hotline at 800-232-2522 (English) or 800-232-0233 (Spanish).

1. **Tetanus and diphtheria (Td)**—Adults including pregnant women with uncertain histories of a complete primary vaccination series should receive a primary series of Td. A primary series for adults is 3 doses: the first 2 doses given at least 4 weeks apart and the 3rd dose, 6–12 months after the second. Administer 1 dose if the person had received the primary series and the last vaccination was 10 years ago or longer. Consult *MMWR* 1991; 40 (RR-10): 1–21 for administering Td as prophylaxis in wound management. The ACP Task Force on Adult Immunization supports a second option for Td use in adults: a single Td booster at age 50 years for persons who have completed the full pediatric series, including the teenage/young adult booster. *Guide for Adult Immunization*. 3rd ed. ACP 1994: 20.

2. **Influenza vaccination**—Medical indications: chronic disorders of the cardiovascular or pulmonary systems including asthma; chronic metabolic diseases including diabetes mellitus, renal dysfunction, hemoglobinopathies, or immunosuppression (including immunosuppression caused by medications or by human immunodeficiency virus [HIV]), requiring regular medical follow-up or hospitalization during the preceding year; women who will be pregnant during the influenza season. Occupational indications: health-care workers. Other indications: residents of nursing homes and other long-term care facilities; persons likely to transmit influenza to persons at high-risk (in-home care givers to persons with medical indications, household contacts and out-of-home caregivers of children birth to 23 months of age, or children with asthma or other indicator conditions for influenza vaccination, household members and care givers of elderly and adults with high-risk conditions); and anyone who wishes to be vaccinated. For healthy persons aged 5–49 years without high risk conditions, either the inactivated vaccine or the intranasally administered influenza vaccine (Flumist) may be given. *MMWR* 2003;52 (RR-8):1–36;*MMWR* 2003;53 (RR-13): 1–8.

3. **Pneumococcal polysaccharide vaccination**—Medical indications: chronic disorders of the pulmonary system (excluding asthma), cardiovascular diseases, diabetes mellitus, chronic liver diseases including liver disease as a result of alcohol abuse (e.g., cirrhosis), chronic renal failure or nephrotic syndrome, functional or anatomic asplenia (e.g., sickle cell disease or splenectomy), immunosuppressive conditions (e.g., congenital immunodeficiency, HIV infection, leukemia, lymphoma, multiple myeloma, Hodgkins disease, generalized malignancy, organ or bone marrow transplantation), chemotherapy with alkylating agents, anti-metabolites, or long-term systemic corticosteroids. Geographic/other indications: Alaskan Natives and certain American Indian populations. Other indications: residents of nursing homes and other long-term care facilities. *MMWR* 1997;46 (RR-8):1–24.

4. **Revaccination with pneumococcal polysaccharide vaccine**—One time revaccination after 5 years for persons with chronic renal failure or nephrotic syndrome, functional or anatomic asplenia (e.g., sickle cell disease or splenectomy), immunosuppressive conditions (e.g., congenital immunodeficiency, HIV infection, leukemia, lymphoma, multiple myeloma, Hodgkin's disease, generalized malignancy, organ or bone marrow transplantation), chemotherapy with alkylating agents, anti-metabolites, or long-term systemic corticosteroids. For persons 65 and older, one-time revaccination if they were vaccinated 5 or more years previously and were aged less than 65 years at the time of primary vaccination. *MMWR* 1997;46 (RR-8):1–24.

5. **Hepatitis B vaccination**—Medical indications: hemodialysis patients, patients who receive clotting-factor concentrates. Occupational indications: health-care workers and public-safety workers who have exposure to blood in the workplace, persons in training in schools of medicine, dentistry, nursing, laboratory technology, and other allied health professions. Behavioral indications: injecting drug users, persons with more than one sex partner in the previous 6 months, persons with a recently acquired sexually transmitted disease (STD), all clients in STD clinics, men who have sex with men. Other indications: household contacts and sex partners of persons with chronic HBV infection, clients and staff of institutions for the developmentally disabled, international travelers who will be in countries with high or intermediate prevalence of chronic HBV infection for more than 6 months, inmates of correctional facilities. *MMWR* 1991;40 (RR-13):1–19.

6. **Hepatitis A vaccination**—For the combined HepA-HepB vaccine use 3 doses at 0, 1, 6 months. Medical indications: persons with clotting-factor disorders or chronic liver disease. Behavioral indications: men who have sex with men, users of injecting and noninjecting illegal drugs. Occupational indications: persons working with HAV-infected primates or with HAV in a research laboratory setting. Other indications: persons traveling to or working in countries that have high or intermediate endemicity of hepatitis A. *MMWR* 1999;48 (RR-12):1–37.

7. **Measles, Mumps, Rubella vaccination (MMR)**—Measles component: Adults born before 1957 may be considered immune to measles. Adults born in or after 1957 should receive at least one dose of MMR unless they have a medical contraindication, documentation of at least one dose or other acceptable evidence of immunity. A second dose of MMR is recommended for adults who:

- are recently exposed to measles or in an outbreak setting
- were previously vaccinated with killed measles vaccine
- were vaccinated with an unknown vaccine between 1963 and 1967
- are students in post-secondary educational institutions
- work in health care facilities
- plan to travel internationally

Mumps component: 1 dose of MMR should be adequate for protection. Rubella component: Give 1 dose of MMR to women whose rubella vaccination history is unreliable and counsel women to avoid becoming pregnant for 4 weeks after vaccination. For women of child-bearing age, regardless of birth year, routinely determine rubella immunity and counsel women regarding congenital rubella syndrome. Do not vaccinate pregnant women or those planning to become pregnant in the next 4 weeks. If pregnant and susceptible, vaccinate as early in postpartum period as possible. *MMWR* 1998;47 (RR-8): 1–57; *MMWR* 2001;50:1117.

8. **Varicella vaccination**—Recommended for all persons who do not have reliable clinical history of varicella infection, or serological evidence of varicella zoster virus (VZV) infection who may be at high risk for exposure or transmission. This includes, health-care workers and family contacts of immunocompromised persons, those who live or work in environments where transmission is likely (e.g., teachers of young children, day care employees, and residents and staff members in institutional settings), persons who live or work in environments where VZV transmission can occur (e.g., college students, inmates and staff members of correctional institutions, and military personnel), adolescents and adults living in households with children,women who are not pregnant but who may become pregnant in the future, international travelers who are not immune to infection. Note: Greater than 95% of U.S. born adults are immune to VZV. Do not vaccinate pregnant women or those planning to become pregnant in the next 4 weeks. If pregnant and susceptible, vaccinate as early in postpartum period as possible. *MMWR* 1996; 45 (RR-11): 1–36;*MMWR* 1999;48 (RR-6):1–5.

9. **Meningococcal vaccine (quadrivalent polysaccharide for serogroups A, C, Y, and W-135)**—Consider vaccination for persons with medical indications: adults with terminal complement component deficiencies, with anatomic or functional asplenia. Other indications: travelers to countries in which disease is hyperendemic or epidemic ("meningitis belt" of sub-Saharan Africa, Mecca, Saudi Arabia for Hajj). Revaccination at 3–5 years may be indicated for persons at high risk for infection (e.g., persons residing in areas in which disease is epidemic). Counsel college freshmen, especially those who live in dormitories, regarding meningococcal disease and the vaccine so that they can make an educated decision about receiving the vaccination. *MMWR* 2000;49 (RR-7): 1–20. Note: The AAFP recommends that colleges should take the lead in providing education on meningococcal infection and vaccination and offer it to those who are interested. Physicians need not initiate discussion of the meningococcal quadravalent polysaccharide vaccine as part of routine medical care.

Adapted from material approved by the Advisory Committee on Immunization Practices (ACIP), and accepted by the American College of Obstetricians and Gynecologists (ACOG) and the American Academy of Family Physicians (AAFP)

123

HUMAN IMMUNODEFICIENCY VIRUS INFECTION

Courtney V. Fletcher and Thomas N. Kakuda

Learning Objectives and other resources can be found at *www.pharmacotherapyonline.com.*

KEY CONCEPTS

❶ Infection with human immunodeficiency virus (HIV) occurs through three primary modes: sexual, parenteral, and perinatal. Sexual intercourse, primarily receptive anal and vaginal intercourse, is the most common method for transmission

❷ Once HIV enters the human body, the outer glycoprotein (gp160) expressed on the virus allows HIV to bind to CD4 receptors, proteins present on the surfaces of T-helper lymphocytes, monocytes, macrophages, dendritic cells, and brain microglia. The gp120 subunit of gp160 has high affinity for CD4 receptors and is responsible for the initial binding of the virus to the cell

❸ The goal of antiretroviral therapy is to achieve maximum suppression of HIV replication, interpreted to be a plasma viral load less than the lower limit of quantitation. Another equally important outcome is an increase in CD4 lymphocytes because this determines the risk for developing opportunistic infections.

❹ The use of potent combination antiretroviral therapy to suppress HIV replication to below the levels of detection of sensitive plasma HIV RNA assays limits the potential for selection of antiretroviral-resistant HIV variants, the major factor limiting the ability of antiretroviral drugs to inhibit virus replication and delay disease progression. Therefore, maximum achievable suppression of HIV replication should be the goal of therapy.

❺ The clinical use of antiretroviral agents is complicated by significant drug-drug interactions. Some interactions are beneficial and used purposely; others may be harmful, leading to inadequate drug concentrations. Clinicians involved in the pharmacotherapy of HIV infection must maintain a current knowledge of drug interactions for these reasons.

❻ Current recommendations for treating HIV infection advocate a minimum of three antiretroviral agents. The typical regimen consists of two nucleoside analogues with either a protease inhibitor (often pharmacologically enhanced with ritonavir) or a nonnucleoside.

❼ General principles for the management of opportunistic infections include prospective immunologic monitoring, primary prophylaxis, treatment, and secondary prophylaxis.

❽ Treatment of *Pneumocystis carinii* pneumonia with agents such as trimethoprim-sulfamethoxazole (or cotrimoxazole) or parenteral pentamidine is associated with a 60% to 100% response rate. Trimethoprim-sulfamethoxazole is the regimen of choice for the treatment and prophylaxis of PCP patients with and without HIV because it is less toxic.

❾ The combination of pyrimethamine and sulfadiazine is the most effective regimen for acute therapy of acquired immune deficiency syndrome (AIDS)–related CNS toxoplasmosis. Therapy with this combination should be continued for at least 3 weeks, but 6 weeks of treatment is recommended for more severely ill patients.

❿ Amphotericin B is more effective than fluconazole for treatment of cryptococcal meningitis because of its lower rates of early death and disease progression. Most patients with cryptococcal meningitis probably should receive amphotericin B in an intravenous dose of at least 0.5 mg/kg per day for a minimum of 2 weeks as acute therapy.

⓫ Treatment regimens for *Mycobacterium avium* complex infection should contain at least two antimycobacterial agents. Every regimen should contain either clarithromycin or azithromycin plus a second agent such as ethambutol.

⓬ Acyclovir is the drug of choice for treatment of herpes simplex virus (HSV) infection. Recurrent HSV disease often can be managed with low-dose suppressive oral acyclovir therapy.

The acquired immune deficiency syndrome (AIDS) was first recognized by the medical community as a distinct clinical entity in 1981. This syndrome was described initially in a cohort of young homosexual men with profound immunologic deficits, *Pneumocystis carinii* pneumonia (PCP), and Kaposi's sarcoma. A retrovirus, human immunodeficiency virus type 1 (HIV-1) is the major cause of AIDS.[1,2] A second retrovirus, HIV-2, also has been recognized to cause AIDS, although it is far less prevalent than HIV-1. These retroviruses are transmitted primarily by sexual contact and by contact with contaminated blood or blood products. Several risk behaviors for the acquisition of HIV infection have been identified, most notably the practice of anorectal intercourse and the sharing of blood-contaminated needles by injection-drug users. Transmission of HIV between heterosexuals and from childbearing women to their offspring is an increasing problem worldwide. Global statistics on the prevalence and incidence of this disease remain grim, and all treatments to date have been unsuccessful in eradicating HIV. However, potent combinations of antiretroviral agents, also known as *highly active antiretroviral therapy* (HAART), have been able to suppress HIV replication, delay the onset of AIDS, and prolong patient survival.[3] Unfortunately, this success is tempered by the long-term toxicities that may arise from using these agents.[4] The purpose of this chapter is to provide a discussion of the epidemiology and manifestations of HIV disease, therapeutic strategies directed at inhibiting the virus, and management of HIV-associated opportunistic infections.

THE HUMAN IMMUNODEFICIENCY VIRUS

EPIDEMIOLOGY

Persons infected with HIV and AIDS cases in the United States conform to the Centers for Disease Control and Prevention (CDC) surveillance case definition (Table 123–1) and are reported by health care providers to a public health department.[5] The cumulative number of reported AIDS cases in the United States at the end of December 2001 was 816,149; 467,910 (more than half) have already died. The number of individuals living with HIV infection or AIDS in the United States at the end of December 2001 was 181,976 and 344,178, respectively. Reported cases in men outnumbered women by approximately 6 to 1. Compared with their distribution in the overall population, African-American and Hispanic populations are disproportionately affected by AIDS, representing 42% and 20% of AIDS cases, respectively.[6] The estimated prevalence of HIV in the United States is 850,000 to 950,000 individuals. Each year the CDC estimates that 40,000 new cases of HIV infection occur in the United States, with approximately 70% of individuals diagnosed. Only half are linked to

appropriate prevention, care, and treatment services. Women account for a growing proportion of those newly infected.[7] Men who have sex with men (MSM) account for most cases. The increase in unprotected sex and recent outbreaks of syphilis among this population are growing concerns in the United States.[8] HIV infection, however, is a worldwide epidemic. The World Health Organization (WHO) estimates that 34 to 46 million adults and children are infected with HIV worldwide—primarily in sub-Saharan Africa (25 to 28.2 million) and Southeast Asia (4.6 to 8.2 million). Children younger than 15 years of age account for 2.5 million infections worldwide. Approximately 5 million additional infections occur each year, mainly (95%) in developing countries. Most of these infections will be acquired through heterosexual transmission.[9]

ETIOLOGY

HIV is a member of the lentivirinae (*lenti,* meaning "slow") subfamily of retroviruses. Lentiviruses are characterized by their indolent infectious cycle. There are two related but distinct types of HIV, HIV-1 and HIV-2. HIV-2, found mostly in western Africa, consists of six distinct phylogenetic lineages designated as subtypes (clades) A through F. HIV-1 also can be categorized based on phylogeny. Three groups of HIV-1 are currently recognized: M (main), N (new or non-M, non-O), and O (outlier). The nine subtypes of HIV-1 group M are identified as A through D, F through H, and J and K. Mixtures of subtypes are referred to as *circulating recombinant forms.*[10] HIV-1 subtype B is primarily responsible for the epidemic in North America and western Europe.

The origin of HIV is of considerable interest. The accumulated evidence suggests that HIV in humans was the result of a cross-species transmission (zoonosis) from primates infected with simian immunodeficiency virus (SIV). Phylogenetic and geographic relationships suggest that HIV-2 arose from SIV that infects sooty mangabeys. The

TABLE 123–1. Centers for Disease Control and Prevention 1993 Revised Classification System for HIV Infection in Adults and AIDS Surveillance Case Definition

CD4+ T-Cell Categories (Absolute Number and Percentage)	(A) Asymptomatic, Acute (Primary) HIV or PGL	(B) Symptomatic, not (A) or (C) Conditions	(C) AIDS-Indicator Conditions
≥500/mcL or ≥29%	A1	B1	C1
200–499/mcL or 14–28%	A2	B2	C2
<200/mcL or <14%	A3	B3	C3

AIDS-Indicator Conditions

Candidiasis of bronchi, trachea, or lungs	Lymphoma, Burkitt's
Candidiasis, esophageal	Lymphoma, immunoblastic
Cervical cancer, invasive	Lymphoma, primary, or brain
Coccidioidomycosis, disseminated or extrapulmonary	*Mycobacterium avium* complex or *M. kansasii,* disseminated or extrapulmonary
Cryptococcosis, extrapulmonary	*Mycobacterium tuberculosis,* any site (pulmonary or extrapulmonary)
Cryptosporidiosis, chronic intestinal (duration >1 month)	*Mycobacterium,* other species or unidentified species, disseminated or extrapulmonary
Cytomegalovirus disease (other than liver, spleen or nodes)	*Pneumocystis carinii* pneumonia
Cytomegalovirus retinitis (with loss of vision)	Pneumonia, recurrent
Encephalopathy, HIV-related	Progressive multifocal leukoencephalopathy
Herpes simplex: chronic ulcer(s) (duration >1 month); or bronchitis, pneumonitis, or esophagitis	*Salmonella* septicemia, recurrent
Histoplasmosis, disseminated or extrapulmonary	Toxoplasmosis of brain
Isosporiasis, chronic intestinal (duration >1 month)	Wasting syndrome due to HIV
Kaposi's sarcoma	

PCL = persistent generalized lymphadenopathy.

origin of HIV-1 is less clear, but similarities exist between SIVcpz, a virus that infects chimpanzees (*Pan troglodytes troglodytes*), and HIV-1. Cultural practices such as the preparation and eating of bush-meat or keeping chimpanzees as pets may have allowed the virus to jump from primate to humans. The earliest known human infection with HIV has been traced to central Africa in 1959. Modern transportation, promiscuity, and drug abuse have caused the rapid spread of the virus within the United States and throughout the world.[11] This chapter will focus on HIV-1 because this is the predominant strain likely to be encountered in the Western world.

DETECTION OF HIV AND SURROGATE MARKERS OF DISEASE PROGRESSION

When HIV-1 infection is suspected, whether owing to symptoms or high-risk behavior, it should be confirmed by laboratory methods. The most common method is an enzyme-linked immunosorbent assay (ELISA), which detects antibodies against HIV-1. The ELISA test is both highly sensitive (>99%) and highly specific (>99%), but false-positive results can occur in multiparous women; recent recipients of hepatitis B, HIV, influenza, or rabies vaccine; patients with multiple blood transfusion, liver disease, and renal failure; or those on chronic hemodialysis. False-negative results may occur if the patient is newly infected and the test is performed before antibody production is adequate. The minimum time to develop antibodies is 3 to 4 weeks from initial exposure, with greater than 95% of individuals developing antibodies after 6 months. Convenient methods for obtaining an ELISA sample have been developed, including an oral collection device (OraSure), an over-the-counter home fingerstick blood-collection test system (Home Access), and a urine test (Calpyte). Positive ELISAs are repeated in duplicate, and if one or both tests are reactive, a confirmatory test is performed for final diagnosis. Western blot is the most commonly used confirmatory test, although an indirect immunofluorescence assay is also available. A reactive ELISA test and a positive confirmatory test indicate an established HIV infection. If the confirmatory test is indeterminate, the dilemma can be resolved by retesting the individual after 30 days or performing a viral load assay if the patient is at high risk or symptomatic.[12]

Once diagnosed, HIV disease is monitored primarily by two surrogate markers, viral load and CD4 cell count. The viral load test quantifies the degree of viremia by measuring the amount of viral RNA (HIV RNA) in the plasma. There are several methods for determining HIV RNA, including reverse transcriptase–coupled polymerase chain reaction (RT-PCR), branched-chain DNA (bDNA), transcription-mediated amplification, and nucleic acid sequence–based assay. RT-PCR and bDNA are used more widely than the other techniques. Irrespective of the method used, viral load is reported as the number of viral RNA copies per milliliter. Each assay has its own lower limit of sensitivity to viral subtypes, and results can vary from one assay method to the other; therefore, it is recommended that the same assay method be used consistently within patients. Reductions in viral load often are reported in base 10 logarithm. For example, if a patient presents initially with a viral load of 100,000 copies/mL (10^5 copies/mL) and subsequently has a viral load of 10,000 copies/mL (10^4 copies/mL), the decrease in viral load is 1 $\log_{10}$. In general, a clinical response is considered sufficient if the response is greater than 0.5 $\log_{10}$. Viral load assays have greater than 99% specificity and can be used to detect most strains of HIV. More important, viral load can be used as a prognostic factor to monitor disease progression and the effects of treatment.[12]

Because HIV attacks and destroys cells bearing the CD4 receptor, the number of CD4 lymphocytes in the blood is a surrogate marker of disease progression. The normal adult CD4 lymphocyte count ranges from 500 to 1600 cells/mcL, or 40% to 70% of all lymphocytes. CD4 counts in children are age-dependent, with younger children having higher CD4 counts. Depletion of CD4 cells has been associated with the development of opportunistic infections and other AIDS malignancies.[13]

TRANSMISSION OF HIV

Infection with HIV occurs through three primary modes: sexual, parenteral, and perinatal. Sexual intercourse, primarily receptive anal and vaginal intercourse, is the most common method for transmission.[6] HIV can be found in semen and cervical secretions, and exposure to either of these infected body fluids may transmit the virus. No sexual act between individuals can be considered absolutely safe. The probability of HIV transmission from receptive anorectal intercourse is 0.1% to 3% per sexual contact; for receptive vaginal intercourse, the risk is approximately 0.1% to 0.2%.[14] In general, the probability of infection is increased when the index partner is in an advanced stage of disease. Persons at highest risk for heterosexual transmission include those with ulcerative sexually transmitted diseases, individuals with multiple sex partners, and sexual partners of injection-drug users. Risk of transmission is elevated when women experience vaginal bleeding during intercourse. Individuals with genital ulcers such as from syphilis, chancroid, or herpes are at a fourfold greater risk of contracting HIV. Gonorrhea, chlamydia, and trichomoniasis increase the risk two- to threefold. Sexual partners of circumcised males are less likely to acquire HIV infection when compared with sex partners of uncircumcised males, suggesting that the absence of the foreskin has a protective effect for the partner. Infections also can occur from artificial insemination with infected semen. The risk of acquiring HIV infection from oral intercourse is less well established. Casual contact with AIDS patients or persons with HIV infection is not a significant risk factor for HIV transmission. Prevention of sexual transmission in adults has been focused primarily on encouraging the use of condoms, reducing high-risk behavior (anal intercourse and promiscuity), and the treatment of sexually transmitted diseases. A combined approach has been advocated for successful prevention. Abstinence is encouraged among adolescents. Future interventions under development such as HIV vaccines and topical vaginal microbicides may further limit the spread of sexually transmitted HIV.

Parenteral transmission of HIV broadly encompasses infections owing to contaminated blood exposure such as from needlesticks, intravenous injection with used needles, receipt of blood products, or organ transplants. The use of contaminated needles or other injection-related paraphernalia by drug abusers has been the main cause of parenteral transmissions and currently accounts for a quarter of AIDS cases reported in the United States. Cases in which receipt of infected blood transfusion, blood components, or organ transplant was involved currently portray less than 1% of reports.[6] This low incidence is attributable to blood- and organ-donor screening and viral inactivation procedures for many clotting factors. These preventative measures have reduced the estimated risk for receiving tainted blood or blood products to 1 in 493,000.[15] Health care workers have a small but definite occupational risk of contracting HIV through accidental injury. Most cases of occupationally acquired HIV have been the result of a percutaneous needle stick injury. Studies indicate that the risk of HIV infection following this route is approximately 0.3%. Significant risk factors for seroconversion include deep injury, injury with a device visibly contaminated with blood, and exposure from a source who later died of AIDS. Guidelines for health care and public safety workers have been developed to minimize the hazard of occupational exposure.[16]

Perinatal infection, or vertical transmission, is the most common cause of pediatric HIV infection. Most infections occur during or near to the time of birth, and therefore, treatment of the infected mother is important. The risk of mother-to-child transmission is approximately 25% in the absence of breast-feeding and antiretroviral therapy. Factors that increase the likelihood of vertical transmission include prolonged rupture of membranes, chorioamnionitis, genital infections during pregnancy, preterm delivery, vaginal delivery, birth weight below 2500 g, illicit drug use during pregnancy, and a high maternal viral load.[17] Breast-feeding also can transmit HIV. The estimated frequency of breast milk transmission in one study was 16.2%, with the majority of infections developing within the first 6 months. Formula feeding prevented 44% of infections and was associated with a higher HIV-free survival rate after 2 years.[18] In countries where safe and available alternatives to breast-feeding exist, HIV-infected mothers are strongly recommended not to breast-feed.

PATHOGENESIS

The life cycle of HIV (Fig. 123–1) is complicated but necessary to understand because the current strategies employed in the treatment of HIV target various points in this cycle. Once HIV enters the human body, the outer glycoprotein (gp160) expressed on the virus allows HIV to bind to CD4 (cluster designation 4) receptors, proteins present on the surface of T-helper lymphocytes, monocytes, macrophages, dendritic cells, and brain microglia. The glycoprotein consists of two subunits, gp120 and gp41. The gp120 subunit has high affinity for CD4 receptors and is responsible for the initial binding of the virus to the cell. Once initial binding occurs, the intimate association of HIV with the cell is further enhanced by chemokine coreceptors. The two major chemokine receptors used by HIV are CCR5 and CXCR4. HIV that preferentially use CCR5, R5 viruses, are macrophage-tropic and non-syncytium-inducing. The R5 virus is typically implicated in most cases of sexually transmitted HIV. The X4 virus preferentially uses CXCR4 as a coreceptor and is T-cell-tropic—this virus is often predominant in the later stage of disease and is syncytium-inducing. Clinical isolates may contain a mixture of R5 and X4 viruses, and some viral strains, designated R5X4, may be dual-tropic (i.e., can use both coreceptors). Genetic defects in the expression of chemokine receptors appear to protect some individuals from developing AIDS despite their being exposed to the virus.[19] Attachment of HIV to the cell promotes fusion and internalization (adsorption) of the virus—a process mediated by the gp41 subunit.

After internalization, the virus is uncoated in preparation for replication. The genetic material of HIV is positive-sense single-strand RNA (ssRNA); the virus must transcribe this RNA into DNA to optimally replicate in human cells (transcription normally occurs from DNA to RNA—HIV works backward, hence the name *retrovirus*). To do so, HIV is equipped with a unique enzyme, RNA-dependent DNA polymerase (reverse transcriptase). Reverse transcriptase first synthesizes a complementary strand of DNA using the viral RNA as a template. The RNA portion of this DNA-RNA hybrid is then partially removed by ribonuclease H (RNase H), allowing reverse transcriptase to complete the synthesis of a double-stranded DNA (dsDNA) molecule. Unfortunately, the fidelity of reverse transcriptase is poor,

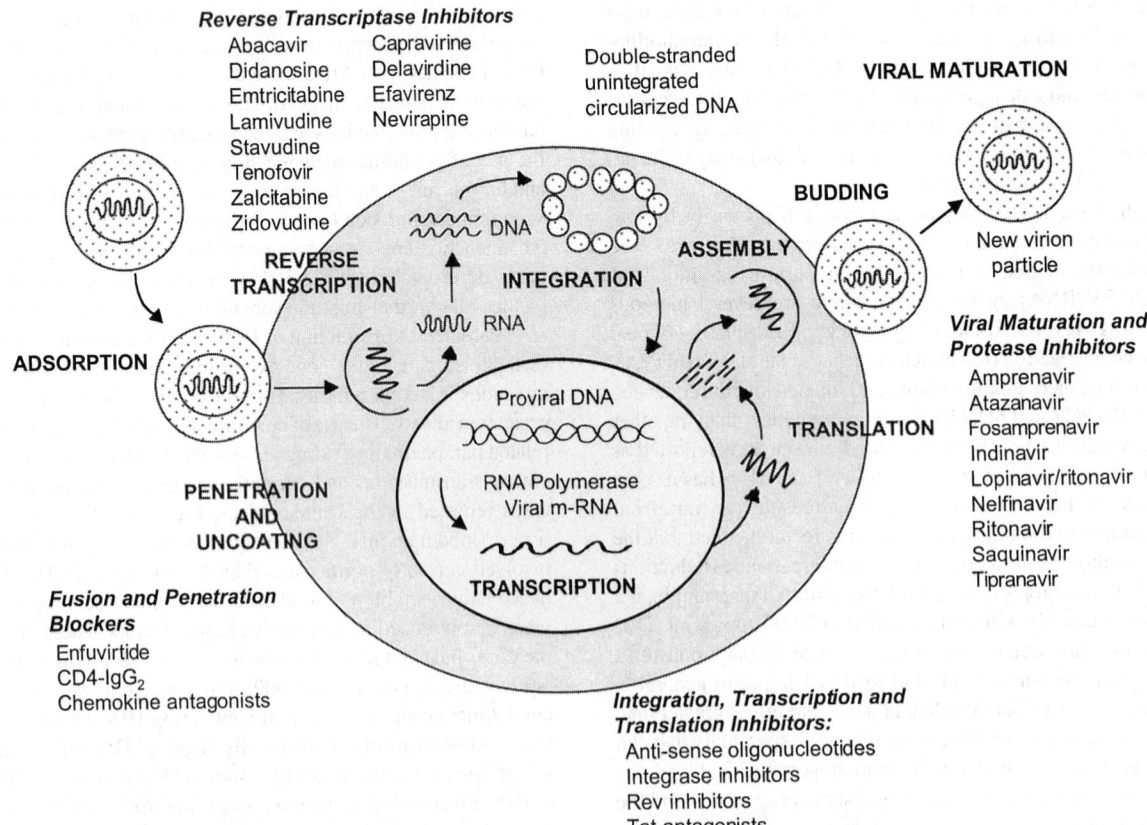

FIGURE 123–1. Life cycle of HIV with potential targets where replication may be interrupted and known or putative antiretroviral agents. *(Reprinted with permission, © Courtney V. Fletcher, 2004.)*

and many mistakes are made during the process. These errors in the final DNA product contribute to the rapid mutation of the virus and allow drug resistance to evolve. Following reverse transcription, the final dsDNA product migrates into the nucleus and is integrated into the host cell chromosome by integrase, another enzyme unique to HIV.

The integration of HIV into the host chromosome is troublesome for several reasons. First, HIV can establish a chronic and persistent infection, particularly in long-lived cells of the immune system such as memory T-lymphocytes.[20] Second, integration is random, thus making it difficult to target and extract integrated HIV. Last, random integration of HIV may cause cellular abnormalities and induce apoptosis.

Activation of the infected cell by antigens, cytokines, or other factors stimulates the cell to produce nuclear factor κB (NF-κB), an enhancer-binding protein. NF-κB normally regulates the expression of T-lymphocyte genes involved in growth but also can inadvertently activate replication of HIV. When HIV replication is induced, the host DNA polymerase transcribes the integrated proviral DNA into messenger RNA (mRNA) with subsequent translation of the mRNA into viral proteins. At first, transcription and translation are done at a low level, yielding various regulatory HIV proteins such as Tat, Nef, and Rev. The Tat protein is a potent amplifier of HIV gene expression; it binds to a specific RNA sequence of HIV that initiates and stabilizes transcription elongation. There is no evident function for Nef, although it appears to downregulate class I molecules and protect infected cells from cytotoxic T-lymphocytes.[21] Deletion of the *Nef* gene has been noted in HIV strains that have infected a cohort of long-term nonprogressors.[22] The Rev protein regulates posttranscriptional activity and, like Tat, is essential for HIV replication. Rev essentially shifts synthesis of HIV regulatory proteins to structural proteins (e.g., gp120) by inhibiting viral mRNA splicing and exporting the mRNA outside the nucleus.[21]

Assembly of new virion particles occurs in a stepwise manner beginning with the coalescence of HIV proteins beneath the host cell lipid bilayer. The nucleocapsid subsequently is formed with viral ssRNA and other components packaged inside. Once packaged, the virion then buds through the plasma membrane, acquiring the characteristics of the host lipid bilayer. After the virus buds, the maturation process begins. Within the virion, HIV protease begins cleaving a large precursor polypeptide into functional proteins that are necessary to produce a complete virus. Without this enzyme, the virion is immature and unable to adequately infect cells.[23]

HIV-1 exhibits a very high turnover rate, with an estimated 10 billion new viruses produced each day. More than 99% of these viruses are produced in newly infected cells. Ultimately, most infected cells will be destroyed from a number of mechanisms, including cell lysis by newly budding virions, cytotoxic T-lymphocyte–induced cell killing, syncytia formation, or apoptosis. Syncytia formation occurs when viral proteins expressed on the surface of the infected cell act as ligands for receptors expressed on uninfected cells. Uninfected cells clump onto the infected cell and fuse into a giant multinucleated cell. The syncytium-inducing X4 virus phenotype may develop later in disease and is associated with more rapid disease progression. Destruction of the CD4 cells leads to compromised immune function and consequently AIDS.

CLINICAL PRESENTATION

Clinical presentation of primary HIV infection may vary, but patients often have an acute retroviral syndrome or mononucleosis-like illness[24,25] (Table 123–2). Symptoms often last 2 weeks, and hospi-

TABLE 123–2. Clinical Presentation of Primary HIV Infection in Adults

Symptoms

Fever, sore throat, fatigue, weight loss, and myalgia

40% to 80% of patients will also exhibit a morbilliform or maculopapular rash usually involving the trunk

Diarrhea, nausea, and vomiting

Lymphadenopathy, night sweats

Aseptic meningitis (fever, headache, photophobia, and stiff neck) may be present in a quarter of presenting cases

Other

High viral load (exceeding 50,000 copies/mL in the adult or 500,000 copies/mL in the child)

Persistent decrease in CD4 lymphocytes

talization may be required for 15% of patients.[24] Primary infection is often associated with a high viral load and development of an immune response that for a period of time suppresses, but does not eliminate, viral replication. During this period, HIV is trapped by follicular dendritic cells in lymphoid tissue and replicates in the germinal center. The amount of HIV RNA in plasma falls substantially at this point, and symptoms resolve gradually. This decline coincides with the development of an immune response to HIV. The clinically latent period, however, is not virologically latent because HIV replication and immune system deterioration are ongoing. A persistent decrease in CD4 cells is the most measurable aspect of this immune system destruction.[20] Plasma viral load, on the other hand, will appear to have stabilized at a particular level or "set point." The set point that is established correlates directly with progression to AIDS and morbidity. The Multicenter AIDS Cohort Study (MACS) measured viral load in 181 HIV-positive men and followed them for as long as 11 years. Only 8% of patients with viral loads of less than 4530 copies/mL progressed to AIDS within 5 years, whereas the 5-year progression rate for those with initial viral loads above 36,270 copies/mL was 62%. The mortality rates within 5 years were 5% and 49%, respectively. Those with viral loads between 4531 and 13,020 progressed to AIDS at a rate of 26%, with a mortality rate of 10%, and those with viral loads from 13,021 to 36,270 progressed to AIDS at a rate of 49%, with a mortality rate of 25%. Clearly, a higher level of viremia at the onset is associated with poorer prognosis.[26]

Most children born with HIV are asymptomatic. On physical examination, children often present with unexplained physical signs such as lymphadenopathy, hepatomegaly, splenomegaly, failure to thrive, weight loss or unexplained low birth weight (in prenatally exposed infants), and fever of unknown origin. Laboratory findings include anemia, hypergammaglobulinemia (primarily IgA and IgM), altered mononuclear cell function, and altered T-cell subset ratios.[27] Of note, the normal range for CD4 cell counts in young children is much different from that in adults (Table 123–3). Bacterial infections, including *Streptococcus pneumoniae, Salmonella* spp., and *Mycobacterium tuberculosis,* may be more prevalent in children with AIDS than in adults with the disease. Kaposi's sarcoma is rare in children. Children with HIV infection may develop lymphocytic interstitial pneumonitis without evidence of *Pneumocystis carinii* or other pathogens on lung biopsy. Some children present with progressive, unexplained neurologic deterioration, including late-onset seizures, loss of developmental milestones, cessation of brain growth, and diffuse, unexplained encephalopathy. A history of recurrent or persistent bacterial, fungal, or viral infections, which may be chronic and initially subclinical or slowly progressive, has been observed. Included in this group are children with recurrent bacterial sepsis, meningitis,

TABLE 123–3. Centers for Disease Control and Prevention 1994 Revised Classification System for HIV Infection in Children Younger than 13 Years of Age

Immunologic Categories	12 Months Cells/mcL (%)[a]	1–5 Years Cells/mcL (%)*	6–12 Years Cells/mcL (%)*
1. No evidence of suppression	≥1500 (≥25%)	≥1000 (≥25%)	≥500 (≥25%)
2. Evidence of moderate suppression	750–1499 (15%–24%)	500–999 (15%–24%)	200–499 (15%–24%)
3. Severe suppression	<750 (<15%)	<500 (<15%)	<200 (<15%)

Immunologic Categories	N: No Signs/Symptoms	A: Mild Signs/Symptoms	B: Moderate Signs/Symptoms	C: Severe Signs/Symptoms
1. No evidence of suppression	N1	A1	B1	C1
2. Evidence of moderate suppression	N2	A2	B2	C2
3. Severe suppression	N3	A3	B3	C3

*Percentage of total lymphocytes.

and chronic otitis media and children with chronic oral candidiasis and presumed disseminated histoplasmosis. The current CDC pediatric AIDS surveillance definition (see Table 123–3) excludes children with congenital or perinatally acquired cytomegalovirus or other iden-

tified causes of congenital immunodeficiency.[28] Management of the HIV-infected child involves similar principles as the adult: antiretroviral therapy, treatment and prophylaxis of opportunistic infections, and supportive care.[29]

▶ TREATMENT: Human Immunodeficiency Virus Infection

▦ DESIRED OUTCOME

◀3 The goal of antiretroviral therapy is to achieve maximum suppression of HIV replication. This is commonly interpreted to be a plasma viral load less than the lower limit of quantitation (i.e., undetectable). Long-term response to therapy (i.e., durability) is determined by the viral load nadir achieved.[30,31] Another equally important outcome is an increase in CD4 lymphocytes because this determines the risk for developing opportunistic infections.[32] Occasionally, patients may respond virologically or immunologically without the other—the reasons for this discordance are unclear. The ultimate goal of antiretroviral therapy, however, is decreased morbidity and mortality.

▦ GENERAL APPROACH TO TREATMENT

In mid-1997, the National Institutes of Health Office of AIDS Research convened a panel to define the scientific principles that might serve as a guide for the clinical use of antiretroviral agents.[33] The 11 principles presented below are an amalgamation of knowledge of the life cycle of HIV, the consequences of HIV replication, clinical trials of antiretroviral agents, and scientific opinion.

1. Ongoing HIV replication leads to immune system damage and progression to AIDS. HIV infection is always harmful, and true long-term survival free of clinically significant immune dysfunction is unusual.
2. Plasma HIV RNA levels indicate the magnitude of HIV replication and its associated rate of CD4 cell destruction, whereas CD4 cell counts indicate the extent of HIV-induced immune damage already suffered. Regular, periodic measurement of plasma HIV RNA levels and CD4 cell counts is necessary to determine the risk of disease progression in an HIV-infected individual and to determine when to initiate or modify antiretroviral treatment regimens.

3. Because rates of disease progression differ among individuals, treatment decisions should be individualized by level of risk indicated by plasma HIV RNA levels and CD4 cell counts.
◀4 4. The use of potent combination antiretroviral therapy to suppress HIV replication to below the levels of detection of sensitive plasma HIV RNA assays limits the potential for selection of antiretroviral-resistant HIV variants, the major factor limiting the ability of antiretroviral drugs to inhibit virus replication and delay disease progression. Therefore, maximum achievable suppression of HIV replication should be the goal of therapy.
5. The most effective means to accomplish durable suppression of HIV replication is the simultaneous initiation of combinations of effective anti-HIV drugs with which the patient has not been treated previously and that are not cross-resistant with antiretroviral agents with which the patient has been treated previously.
6. Each of the antiretroviral drugs used in combination therapy regimens always should be used according to optimal schedules and dosages.
7. The available effective antiretroviral drugs are limited in number and mechanism of action, and cross-resistance between specific drugs has been documented. Therefore, any change in antiretroviral therapy increases future therapeutic constraints.
8. Women should receive optimal antiretroviral therapy regardless of pregnancy status.
9. The same principles of antiretroviral therapy apply to both HIV-infected children and adults, although the treatment of HIV-infected children involves unique pharmacologic, virologic, and immunologic considerations.
10. Persons with acute primary HIV infections should be treated with combination antiretroviral therapy to suppress virus replication to levels below the limit of detection of sensitive plasma HIV RNA assays.

TABLE 123–4. Treatment of HIV Infection: Antiretroviral Regimens Recommended in Antiretroviral-Naive Persons

Nonnucleoside Reverse Transcriptase Inhibitor (NNRTI)–Based Regimens

Preferred	Efavirenz *plus* lamivudine *plus* zidovudine (or tenofovir DF or stavudine) except for pregnant women or women with pregnancy potential
Alternatives	Efavirenz *plus* emtricitabine *plus* zidovudine (or tenofovir DF or stavudine) except for pregnant women or women with pregnancy potential
	or
	Efavirenz *plus* (lamivudine or emtricitabine) *plus* didanosine except for pregnant women or women with pregnancy potential
	or
	Nevirapine *plus* (lamivudine or emtricitabine) *plus* zidovudine (or stavudine or didanosine)

Protease Inhibitor (PI)–Based Regimens

Preferred	Lopinavir/ritonavir *plus* lamivudine *plus* zidovudine (or stavudine)
Alternatives	Amprenavir/ritonavir *plus* lamivudine (or emtricitabine) *plus* zidovudine (or stavudine)
	Atazanavir *plus* lamivudine (or emtricitabine) *plus* zidovudine (or stavudine)
	Indinavir-ritonavir *plus* lamivudine (or emtricitabine) *plus* zidovudine (or stavudine)
	Lopinavir-ritonavir *plus* emtricitabine *plus* zidovudine (or stavudine)
	Nelfinavir *plus* lamivudine (or emtricitabine) *plus* zidovudine (or stavudine)
	Saquinavir-ritonavir *plus* lamivudine (or emtricitabine) *plus* zidovudine (or stavudine)

Triple Nucleoside Reverse Transcriptase Inhibitor–Based Regimen

(Only as an alternative to NNRTI- or PI-based regimens when these cannot be used as preferred therapy)

Abacavir *plus* lamivudine *plus* zidovudine

Abacavir *plus* lamivudine *plus* stavudine

NRTI = nucleoside reverse transcriptase inhibitor; NNRTI = nonnucleoside reverse transcriptase inhibitor; PI = protease inhibitor.

From Panel on Clinical Practice for Treatment of HIV Infection. Guidelines for the use of antiretroviral agents in HIV-infected adults and adolescents. November 3, 2003, http://AIDSinfo.NIH.gov; accessed, January 5, 2004.

11. HIV-infected persons, even those with viral loads below detectable limits, should be considered infectious and should be counseled to avoid sexual and drug-use behaviors that are associated with transmission or acquisition of HIV and other infectious pathogens.

The extent to which these principles will stand the test of time is unknown; new information on the pathogenesis of HIV accrues constantly. The field of antiretroviral therapy is also evolving rapidly. Twenty antiretroviral agents are now approved by the Food and Drug Administration (FDA), and more are certain to come. Health care professionals involved in care of the HIV-infected person always must consult the most current literature with respect to the principles and strategies for therapy. At this time, a particularly excellent source for information on treatment guidelines can be found at: *www.AIDSinfo.NIH.gov.* With these caveats, Table 123–4 presents the state of the art for treatment of the HIV-infected individual as of November 2003. Treatment is recommended for all HIV-infected persons with symptomatic disease, CD4 lymphocyte counts below 350 cells/mcL, or plasma HIV RNA greater than 55,000 copies/mL regardless of the CD4 count.[34]

PHARMACOLOGIC THERAPY

Conceptually, there are three primary methods of therapeutic intervention against HIV: inhibition of viral replication, vaccination to stimulate a more effective immune response, and restoration of the immune system with immunomodulators. Several approaches for an

HIV vaccine are in development, including whole killed virus, subunit and peptide vaccination, recombinant live vector, and naked DNA delivery. While clinical studies of vaccines have been done, at this point, optimal vaccine strategies are still being explored. Genetic variability in HIV and a nascent understanding the role of the immune system in suppressing viral replication are significant barriers to the development of an effective HIV vaccine with long-lasting and protective immunity.[35] Among immunomodulators, interleukin 2 (aldesleukin or IL-2) appears to be the most promising. Several methods of dosing and administration have been attempted—the most common is subcutaneous administration for 5 consecutive days in 2-month cycles. The main benefit of IL-2 is increased CD4 cells; unfortunately, it is also associated with significant toxicities. Studies to assess clinical end points are underway.[36]

ANTIRETROVIRAL AGENTS

Inhibiting viral replication with combinations of potent antiretroviral agents has been the most clinically successful strategy. Thus far there are three primary groups of drugs used: entry inhibition, reverse transcriptase inhibitors, and protease inhibitors (Table 123–5). Reverse transcriptase inhibitors are of two types, those which are chemical derivatives of purine- and pyrimidine-based nucleosides and nucleotides (nucleoside/nucleotide reverse transcriptase inhibitors [NRTIs]) and those which are not (nonnucleoside reverse transcriptase inhibitors [NNRTIs]). NRTIs include thymidine analogues such as stavudine (d4T) and zidovudine (AZT or ZDV); cytosine analogues such as emtricitabine (FTC), lamivudine (3TC), and zalcitabine (ddC); the inosine derivative didanosine (ddI); and the guanosine analogue abacavir sulfate (ABC). Tenofovir disoproxil

TABLE 123–5. Pharmacologic Parameters of Antiretroviral Compounds

Drug	In Vitro Susceptibility (mcM IC$_{50}$ range)	F (%)	V$_d$ (L/kg)	t$_{1/2}$ (h)	CL/F (L/h)	Adult Dose[a] (doses/day)	Plasma C$_{max}$/C$_{min}$ (mcM)	Ratio Fetal-Maternal Conc.	Ratio CSF-Plasma Conc.
Nucleoside Reverse Transcriptase Inhibitors									
Abacavir	0.07–5.8	83	0.86	1.5	49.8	300 mg (2)	10.7/0.04	?	0.3
Didanosine	0.01–10	40	0.83	1.4	26.9	200 mg (2) 400 mg (1)	4/0.02	0.3–0.5	0.22
Emtricitabine	0.0013–0.64	93	3	10	21	200 mg (1)	7.3/0.04	?	?
Lamivudine	0.002–15	86	1.3	5	23.1	150 mg (2) 300 mg (1)	7.5/0.22	>0.7	0.12
Stavudine	0.009–4	86	0.53	1.4	34	40 mg (2)	4/0.004	>0.7	0.02
Tenofovir	0.04–8.5	40	1.2	17	35.7	300 mg (1)	1.13/0.2[g]	?	?
Zalcitabine	0.03–0.5	85	0.53	2	12	0.75 mg (3)	0.05/0.001	0.3–0.5	0.2
Zidovudine	0.01–0.048	64	1.6	1.1	112	200 mg (3) 300 mg (2)	2/0.2	>0.7	0.6
Nonnucleoside Reverse Transcriptase Inhibitors									
Delavirdine	0.05–0.1[c]	85	0.48[b]	5.8	4	400 mg (3)	35/14	?	0.004
Efavirenz	0.0017–0.025[c]	43	10.2[b]	48	10.3	600 mg (1)	12.9/5.6	?	0.007
Nevirapine	0.010–0.1	50	1.21	25	2.6	200 mg (2)[d]	5.5/3.0	1	0.45
Protease Inhibitors									
Amprenavir	0.012–0.41	?	6.1[b]	9	64.9	1200 mg (2)	10.7/0.56	?	0.02
Atazanavir	0.002–0.005	68	3.6[b]	7	25.2	400 mg (1)	3.26/0.17	?	0.0021–0.0226
Indinavir	0.025–0.1[c]	60	1.2[b]	1.5	43	800 mg (3)	13/0.25	?	0.07
Lopinavir[e]	0.004–0.027	?	0.74[b]	5.5	6.5	400 mg (2)	15.4/8.8	?	?
Nelfinavir	0.009–0.06	?	2[b]	2.6	37.4	750 mg (3) 1250 mg (2)	5.6/0.7	?	IND
Ritonavir	0.0038–0.154	60	0.41[b]	3–5	8.8	600 mg (2)[d]	16/5	?	IND
Saquinavir[f]	0.001–0.03	12	10	3	80	1200 mg (3)	0.4/0.15	?	IND

[a]Dose adjustment may be required for weight, renal or hepatic disease, and drug interactions.
[b]V$_d$/F.
[c]Range given is for IC$_{90}$ or IC$_{95}$.
[d]Initial dose escalation recommended to minimize side effects.
[e]Available as coformulation 4:1 lopinavir to ritonavir.
[f]Soft-gel formulation.
[g]Using PMPA molecular weight, not prodrug.
IND = indeterminate with standard analytical techniques; F = bioavailability; V$_d$ = distribution volume; t$_{1/2}$ = elimination half-life; CL = total-body clearance; C$_{max}$ = maximum plasma concentration; C$_{min}$ = minimum plasma concentration; CSF = cerebrospinal fluid; IC$_{50-90}$ = concentration required to produce 50% or 90% inhibition of HIV strains in vitro.

fumarate (TDF or PMPA) is an adenosine-derived nucleotide reverse transcriptase inhibitor. Several nucleoside analogues in various stages of development include alovudine (FLT), dOTC, and β-L-d4FC. As a class, the NRTIs require phosphorylation to the 5′-triphosphate moiety to be active. Intracellular phosphorylation occurs by cytoplasmic or mitochondrial kinases and phosphotransferases. Following prodrug activation, the 5′-triphosphate moiety acts in two ways: (1) It competes with endogenous deoxynucleotides for reverse transcriptase, and (2) it prematurely terminates DNA elongation owing to the modified 3′-hydroxyl group.[37] Hydroxyurea, a ribonucleotide reductase inhibitor, depletes intracellular deoxynucleotides and has been used in combination with NRTIs. Presumably, the reduction of endogenous triphosphates by hydroxyurea shifts the competition for reverse transcriptase in favor of the exogenous triphosphate (i.e., NRTI). In doing so, however, hydroxyurea may accentuate adverse effects such as pancreatitis from didanosine and peripheral neuropathy from stavudine-didanosine combinations.[38] Mycophenolic acid, an inosine monophosphate dehydrogenase inhibitor, can cause similar shifts in endogenous nucleotide pools. Although NRTIs are specific for HIV reverse transcriptase, their adverse effects in part may be owing to some inhibition of human DNA polymerases, particularly mitochondrial DNA polymerase γ.[39]

NNRTIs are a chemically heterogeneous group of agents that bind noncompetitively to reverse transcriptase close to the catalytic site. Unlike NRTIs, NNRTIs do not require intracellular activation, do not compete against endogenous deoxynucleotides, and do not have strong antiviral activity against HIV-2. Available NNRTIs include efavirenz, delavirdine, and nevirapine.[40] Capravirine and calanolide A are two agents in clinical development under this class.

The protease inhibitors (PIs) are a potent class of antiretrovirals that includes amprenavir, atazanavir, fosamprenavir, indinavir, lopinavir, nelfinavir, ritonavir, and saquinavir. Tipranavir is an investigational PI at the time of this writing. The pharmacology, safety, and efficacy of these drugs are reviewed elsewhere.[41] Briefly, PIs block the maturation process, thereby resulting in the production of immature, noninfectious virions.[23]

Enfuvirtide (T-20, or pentafuside) is the only entry inhibitor available at this time. An inhibitor of fusion, enfuvirtide is a synthetic 36-amino-acid peptide derived from the second heptad repeat (HR2) domain of gp41. It prevents fusion of HIV with the target cell by binding to the first heptad repeat (HR1) domain of gp41, thereby interfering with the "zipping" process of HR1 and HR2. Because of the peptide nature of enfuvirtide, oral delivery is impossible, and subcutaneous injection is the preferred route of administration.[42] A derivative of enfuvirtide designated T-1249 is currently under investigation—this too must be administered by subcutaneous injection.

Novel antiviral agents are currently in development and exploit other areas of HIV replication. Entry can be aborted by chemokine receptor antagonists and integrase, which represents another HIV-specific enzyme that can be targeted for inhibition. Drugs that block the assembly of HIV are also in development.[43]

DRUG INTERACTIONS

5 The clinical use of antiretroviral agents is complicated by the significant drug-drug interactions that can occur with many of these agents. Some interactions are beneficial and used purposely; others may be harmful, leading to inadequate drug concentrations. Clinicians involved in the pharmacotherapy of HIV must maintain a current knowledge of drug interactions for these reasons. The Internet provides a useful resource for updated information on antiretroviral drug interaction—recommended Web sites can be found in the ref. 44. In general, amprenavir, efavirenz, nevirapine, and tipranavir are inducers of drug metabolism, whereas delavirdine and the PIs inhibit drug metabolism.[44] Ritonavir is a potent inhibitor of cytochrome P450 3A–mediated metabolism and is now used primarily as a pharmacokinetic enhancer of other PIs. Lopinavir is coformulated with ritonavir (LPV/r) for this reason.[45] NRTIs also may have interactions among themselves. Zidovudine and stavudine, for example, are phosphorylated by the same kinases; antagonism occurs between these two drugs both in vitro and in vivo; thus the two should never be given together.[46] Complicating matters is the drug interaction potential of antituberculosis agents, particularly rifamycins. Rifampin is contraindicated with most PIs because drug concentrations of the PIs are reduced substantially. If patients require simultaneous treatment for both HIV and tuberculosis, a regimen consisting of efavirenz, ritonavir, or saquinavir-ritonavir should be considered.[47] The herbal product Saint John's wort (*Hypericum perforatum*) is a potent inducer of metabolism and is contraindicated with PIs and NNRTIs. Among health volunteers, St. John's wort decreased indinavir area under the curve on average 57%.[48]

PIVOTAL DEVELOPMENTS IN TREATMENT STRATEGIES

The pharmacotherapy of HIV infection has changed rapidly over the years as newer agents have become available and treatment paradigms have evolved. Highlights of the development of antiretroviral therapeutics are

- The demonstration that zidovudine monotherapy confers a survival benefit in persons who have AIDS.[49]
- The demonstration that combination regimens of two NRTIs (e.g., zidovudine and didanosine or zalcitabine) are superior to zidovudine monotherapy in immunologic and virologic parameters, particularly in patients with no previous antiretroviral therapy, and confer a superior survival benefit (ACTG 175).[50]
- The use of triple therapy with combinations of two NRTIs with NNRTIs or PIs, which has been clearly associated with a reduced incidence of opportunistic infections and improved survival.[3]

6 Current recommendations for treating HIV infection advocate a minimum of three antiretroviral agents. The typical regimen consists of two nucleoside analogues with either a PI (often pharmacologically enhanced with ritonavir) or an NNRTI, e.g., tenofovir, emtricitabine, lopinavir-ritonavir and zidovudine, lamivudine, efavirenz, respectively. Other combinations may include triple nucleoside analogues, dual PIs (two PIs both at active doses), dual boosted

PIs (two PIs pharmacologically enhanced with ritonavir), or a PI with a NNRTI. The initial choice in drugs is critical to long-term success, and factors such as adherence, efficacy (virologic and immunologic), durability, which drugs to start with and what to change to (i.e., sequencing), and tolerability are paramount to success.[34] Brief comments on these factors follow.

The simplest definition of adherence is the patient's ability to take medication as directed. Antiretroviral therapy is complex and long term, and the risk for virologic failure increases as adherence decreases. Patients with greater than 95% adherence on a PI regimen had better virologic and immunologic outcomes and a lower hospitalization rate than those with adherence below this threshold.[51] As clinicians, it is important to communicate to the patient the importance of proper medication taking with specific education aimed at understanding the disease process, monitoring, and goals of therapy. An individual's "readiness" to take medications should be clearly established before any treatment is initiated.[34] Caregivers, friends, and/or family members should be included in this process because social and psychological support are among the most important factors that influence adherence in this patient population.[52]

Several clinical trials have demonstrated the virologic and immunologic efficacy of antiretrovirals—the results are summarized succinctly elsewhere.[53–55] Unfortunately, only a few have been large, randomized, comparative (head-to-head) trials. Nevertheless, these trials provide insight on the subtle differences in efficacy among antiretrovirals. Superior virologic efficacy was seen with lopinavir-ritonavir 400/100 mg twice daily compared with nelfinavir 750 mg three times daily in antiretroviral-naive patients concomitantly treated with 40 mg twice daily of stavudine and lamivudine 150 mg twice daily. This double-blind, randomized, placebo-controlled trial involving 637 patients resulted in 75% of patients treated with lopinavir-ritonavir achieving viral loads of less than 400 copies/mL versus 63% of nelfinavir-treated patients after 48 weeks. The mean increases in CD4 cell counts were similar for both agents, 195 cells/mcL with nelfinavir and 207 cells/mcL with lopinavir-ritonavir. Overall tolerability was similar between the two agents.[56] Significantly more patients achieved viral suppression after 48 weeks with the NNRTI efavirenz given in combination with zidovudine-lamivudine when compared with a regimen of indinavir-zidovudine-lamivudine or indinavir-efavirenz in a multicenter, randomized, open-label study involving 432 patients. Both zidovudine and lamivudine were dosed twice daily, 300 and 150 mg, respectively. The administered dose for efavirenz was 600 mg once daily and that for indinavir was 800 mg every 8 hours. For the indinavir-efavirenz arm, efavirenz was given 600 mg once daily with indinavir 1000 mg every 8 hours to account for the drug interaction. The proportion of patients achieving HIV RNA of less than 400 copies/mL was 70% for those receiving treatment with efavirenz-zidovudine-lamivudine and 53% and 48% for indinavir-efavirenz and indinavir-zidovudine-lamivudine, respectively; mean increases in CD4 cell counts were 201, 180, and 185 cells/mcL, respectively.[57]

The durability and sequencing of a regimen are equally important as its efficacy. Since the advent of HAART, patients have been living longer with improved quality of life. The consequence of this is that patients will have to rely on their treatment for years to come, not months. Data on the long-term durability of HAART are scarce. The initiation of antiretroviral therapy in a treatment-naive person must come with consideration for what agents will be available should the first regimen fail. Antiretroviral resistance testing is a useful tool in this regard. There are two types of resistance tests: phenotype and genotype. A phenotype test determines the concentration of antiretroviral necessary to inhibit 50% of viral replication

(IC_{50}) in a recombinant viral assay. Results usually are expressed as a fold-change in susceptibility compared with wild-type virus. While an increase in the fold-change suggests reduced susceptibility to that antiretroviral, resistance is never absolute, and partial susceptibility may remain. Alternatively, drug levels may be increased to overcome reduced susceptibility—this strategy is currently under evaluation. Genotyping assesses the codon changes in gp41, reverse transcriptase, or protease in the patient and compares it to the wild-type sequence. Mutations, when present, are listed by the wild-type amino acid followed by the position in the genetic sequence of the protein or enzyme and end with the mutation found in the patient. For example, a common mutation caused by lamivudine and emtricitabine is the M184V mutation—a substitution of valine (V) for methionine (M) at the 184 position of reverse transcriptase. Interpretation of genotypes is complex, and the reader is encouraged to consult the most recent guidelines on HIV resistance testing.[58]

As with any medication, adverse effects occur with antiretroviral agents that may limit the patient's ability to tolerate medication. Several important adverse effects have been recognized with the currently available antiretrovirals. These include mitochondrial toxicity with NRTIs, rash with NNRTIs, and metabolic perturbations with PIs. A discussion on the specific presentation and management of these adverse effects is beyond the scope of this chapter but can be found elsewhere.[4,39,59–61]

TREATMENT IN SPECIAL POPULATIONS

PREGNANCY

Treatment recommendations have been made to address the specific requirements for HIV-infected pregnant women and the prevention of vertical transmission.[62] Therapy is warranted particularly in light of the dramatic reduction in transmission seen with zidovudine monotherapy (ACTG protocol 076). ACTG protocol 076 randomized 477 HIV-infected pregnant women (14 to 34 weeks' gestation) to either zidovudine or placebo. The zidovudine regimen consisted of antepartum zidovudine (100 mg five times daily) plus a continuous infusion of zidovudine during labor (2 mg/kg intravenously over 1 hour followed by 1 mg/kg per hour), and zidovudine for the newborn (2 mg/kg orally every 6 hours for 6 weeks). The HIV transmission rate was

25.5% among those who received placebo but was 8.3% when the mothers and their babies received zidovudine. This difference corresponds to a two-thirds reduction in the risk of maternal-to-infant HIV transmission. Adverse reactions associated with zidovudine therapy in the study were minimal: Hemoglobin concentrations were significantly lower at birth in infants whose mothers received zidovudine, but this difference disappeared by 12 weeks of age; there was no difference in minor or major structural abnormalities in the two groups.[63]

CLINICAL CONTROVERSY

Unfortunately, little is known about the use of other antiretrovirals in pregnant women and the effect these drugs may have on the developing fetus. PI use among 89 pregnant women appeared generally safe to both mother and baby in a retrospective multicenter survey.[66] In general, pregnant women should be treated similarly as nonpregnant adults; if possible, zidovudine should be used for both mother and infant.[62]

An abbreviated course of zidovudine (i.e., given during labor or in the first 48 hours of life) also can reduce transmission substantially and may be easier for the patient to take.[64] Alternatively, single-dose nevirapine given to the mother during labor and to the baby within 3 days of birth also can reduce transmission of HIV.[65]

POSTEXPOSURE PROPHYLAXIS

Protection of health care workers from accidental exposure to HIV is an important concern. The CDC has issued guidelines governing treatment for occupational HIV exposure. Postexposure prophylaxis (PEP) with a triple-drug regimen consisting of two NRTIs and a PI is recommended for percutaneous blood exposure involving significant risk (large volume of blood or blood from patients with advanced AIDS). Two NRTIs may be offered to the health care worker with lower risk of exposure, such as those involving the mucous membrane or skin. Treatment is not necessary if the source of exposure is urine or saliva. The optimal duration of treatment is unknown, but at least 4 weeks of therapy is advocated. Treatment ideally should be initiated within 1 to 2 hours of exposure.[16] Guidelines also have been developed for postcoital and postinjection-drug-use prophylaxis.[67]

EVALUATION OF THERAPEUTIC OUTCOMES

Following the initiation of therapy, patients usually are monitored at 3-month intervals with immunologic (CD4 count), virologic (HIV RNA), and clinical assessments. There are two general indications to change therapy: significant toxicity or treatment failure. Each of the available antiretroviral agents has its own set of drug-limiting adverse reactions[4]; fortunately, alternatives with nonoverlapping adverse effects are available. For example, the patient who experiences significant peripheral neuropathy on the combination of didanosine and stavudine could be changed to a combination of zidovudine and lamivudine. Specific criteria to indicate treatment failure have not been established through controlled clinical trials. As a general guide, the following events should prompt consideration for changing therapy:

1. Less than 1 $\log_{10}$ reduction in HIV RNA 1 month after the initiation of therapy or a failure to achieve maximal suppression of HIV replication within 4 to 6 months

2. A persistent decline in the CD4 cell count or a return to pretreatment value or an increase in HIV RNA of 0.3 to 0.5 $\log_{10}$ copies per milliliter from nadir

3. Clinical disease progression, usually the development of a new opportunistic infection

THERAPEUTIC FAILURE

Therapeutic failure in HIV therapy may be the result of nonadherence to medication, development of drug resistance, intolerance to one or more medications, adverse drug-drug interactions, or pharmacokinetic-pharmacodynamic variability. Few clinical data are available to indicate what alternative strategies should be employed for patients who fail their initial regimen. Moreover, the data that are available are confounded by the heterogeneity in the patients and their infecting viruses, which makes the results difficult to interpret. In general, patients failing their first regimen should be treated with a drug representing a new class (e.g., if the patient was treated initially with a PI, the PI can be switched to an NNRTI). The guiding principles (numbers 5 and 7) recommend changing to at least two new antiretroviral drugs that are not cross-resistant with agents the patient has received previously. Table 123–4 presents some examples of alternative regimens. Virologic resistance testing may help to guide the health care provider in selecting appropriate agents.[58] In addition to an alternative antiretroviral regimen, other investigational strategies suggested for therapeutic failure include drug holidays, structured or strategic treatment interruptions (STIs), and structured intermittent therapy (SIT). While there are subtle differences between these strategies, the overall premise is similar—stop all antiretrovirals and allow the patient time off medication. Undoubtedly, any strategy that discontinues antiretroviral therapy will allow viral replication to occur with subsequent declines in CD4 lymphocytes. Reinitiation of therapy then is intended to reestablish control of the disease. There remain numerous uncertainties about these discontinuation strategies, including how long the patient can remain off medications, how often this cycle can be done, and most important, the ability of the strategy to reduce morbidity and mortality, as has conventional HAART. Prospective studies are necessary to answer these questions.

INFECTIOUS COMPLICATIONS OF AIDS

The consequence of uncontrolled HIV replication is a steady decline in CD4 cells. Ironically, these are the cells that coordinate the immune system—the system designed to prevent infections from occurring in the first place. HIV is an insidious disease in that persons infected often present with opportunistic infections (OIs), a consequence of the weakened immune system rather than HIV per se. Most OIs are caused by organisms that are common in the environment and often represent the reactivation of quiescent infections. The development of certain OIs is related directly or indirectly to the level of CD4 lymphocytes and can be predicted with some degree of accuracy[16] (Fig. 123–2). Until the immunosuppression induced by HIV can be prevented, the prevention and management of OIs will remain an essential component of the comprehensive care of HIV-infected individuals.

Surveillance data indicate that the incidence of certain OIs in HIV-infected persons in the United States continues to change. The three major OIs—*Pneumocystis carinii* pneumonia (PCP), *Mycobacterium avium* complex (MAC) disease, and cytomegalovirus (CMV) retinitis—all have decreased in incidence.[3,68] Potent antiretroviral regimens and prophylactic strategies for OIs are major factors associated with these decreases. Nevertheless, opportunistic diseases continue to be complications of HIV disease and occur at low CD4 lymphocyte counts. For example, the risk of an OI was almost sixfold higher in persons receiving HAART with a baseline CD4 count of fewer than 50 cells/mcL compared with more than 200 cells/mcL.[69]

The spectrum of infectious diseases observed in HIV-infected individuals and recommended first-line regimens for treatment are shown in Table 123–6, and recommended therapies for primary prophylaxis are shown in Table 123–7. An exhaustive review of all OIs associated with HIV infection is beyond the scope of this chapter. The major OIs include: PCP, candidal esophagitis (discussed elsewhere in this text), central nervous system toxoplasmosis, cryptococcosis, mycobacterial disease, and herpes group virus infections. The following discussion will emphasize these pathogens and will provide an overview of the epidemiology, diagnosis, clinical manifestations, and results of treatment for these infections. Readers desiring more specific information, either for the diseases or agents mentioned, will need to consult additional references.

PNEUMOCYSTIS CARINII

P. carinii pneumonia (PCP) is the most common life-threatening opportunistic infection in patients with AIDS. Early in the AIDS epidemic, approximately 60% of patients with AIDS had PCP as their AIDS-defining event, and 80% experienced PCP at some point during their lifetime.[70] The advent of effective prophylaxis for PCP has decreased the relative incidence of PCP. However, PCP prophylaxis has not eliminated the disease because of persons unaware of their HIV infection, breakthrough PCP in those receiving prophylaxis, and variable compliance with prophylaxis. The taxonomy of the organism is unclear, having been classified as both protozoan and fungal, but genomic sequences suggests that *P. carinii* is a fungus.[71] Exposure to *P. carinii* is widespread because 80% of the population has developed serum antibodies by age 2 or 3 years.[72] The organism appears to reside without consequence in the human unless the host becomes immunologically compromised; immunosuppression allows the organism to multiply, giving rise to clinical disease.

PCP in patients with AIDS differs in clinical presentation from that in patients with other immunosuppressive conditions, such as malignant neoplasms. In AIDS patients, the presentation is often more subacute. Characteristic symptoms include fever and dyspnea; clinical signs are tachypnea with or without rales or rhonchi, and a nonproductive or mildly productive cough. Chest radiographs may show florid or subtle infiltrates or occasionally be normal. Infiltrates are usually interstitial and bilateral, however. Arterial blood gases may show minimal hypoxia (PaO$_2$ 80 to 95 mm Hg), but in more advanced disease they may be markedly abnormal. The onset of PCP is often insidious, occurring over a period of weeks, although more fulminant presentations can occur. The diagnosis of PCP is sually made by identification of the organism in induced sputum or in specimens obtained from bronchoalveolar lavage. Less commonly, transbronchial biopsy is used for diagnosis.

Untreated PCP has a mortality of nearly 100%. Treatment with agents such as trimethoprim-sulfamethoxazole (or cotrimoxazole) or parenteral pentamidine is associated with a 60% to 100% response rate. Both agents appear to be equally efficacious, but trimethoprim-sulfamethoxazole was less toxic. Trimethoprim-sulfamethoxazole is the regimen of choice for treatment and prophylaxis of PCP in patients with and without HIV.[73,74]

Trimethoprim-sulfamethoxazole, when used for the treatment of PCP, usually is given in doses of 15 to 20 mg/kg per day (based on

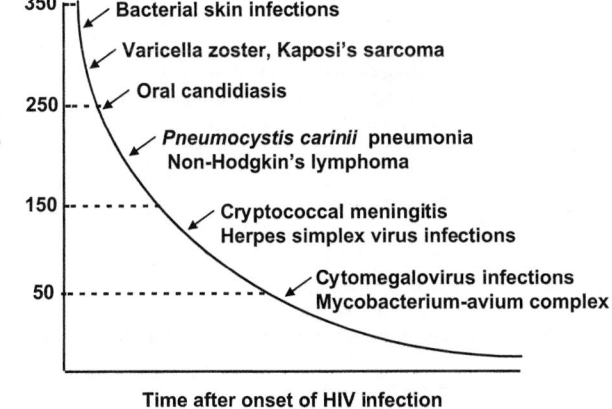

FIGURE 123–2. Natural history of opportunistic infections associated with HIV infection. *(Reprinted with permission, © Courtney V. Fletcher, 1995.)*

TABLE 123–6. Therapies for Common Opportunistic Pathogens in HIV-Infected Individuals

Clinical Disease	Selected Initial Therapies for Acute Infection in Adults	Common Drug- or Dose-Limiting Adverse Reactions
Fungi		
Candidiasis, oral	Fluconazole 200 mg orally single dose or 100 mg orally for 5 days	Taste, patient acceptance
	or	
	Nystatin 500,000 units oral swish 4–6 times daily for 7–10 days	
	or	
	Clotrimazole 10 mg (1 troche) orally 5 times daily for 7–10 days	
Candidiasis, esophageal	Fluconazole 200 mg orally or intravenously on the first day then 100 mg/d for 10–14 days	Elevated liver function tests, hepatotoxicity, nausea and vomiting
	or	Elevated liver function tests, hepatotoxicity, rash, nausea and vomiting
	Ketoconazole 400 mg/d orally for 10–14 days	
Pneumocystis carinii pneumonia	Trimethoprim-sulfamethoxazole intravenously or orally 12–20 mg/kg/day as TMP component in 3–4 divided doses for 21 days[a]	Skin rash, fever, leukopenia Thrombocytopenia
	or	
	Pentamidine intravenously 3–4 mg/kg/day for 21 days[a]	Azotemia, hypoglycemia, hyperglycemia
	Mild episodes	
	Atovaquone suspension 750 mg (5 mL) orally twice daily with meals for 21 days[a]	Rash, elevated liver enzymes, diarrhea
Cryptococcal meningitis	Amphotericin B 0.5–1.0 mg/kg/day intravenously for a minimum of 2 weeks *with* or *without* flucytosine 100–150 mg/kg/day orally in 4 divided doses *followed by*	Nephrotoxicity, hypokalemia, anemia, fever, chills Bone marrow suppression Elevated liver enzymes Same as above
	Fluconazole 100 to 200 mg/day, orally[a]	
Histoplasmosis	Amphotericin B 0.5–1 mg/kg/day intravenously for 6–8 weeks[a]	Same as above
	or	
	Itraconazole 200–400 mg/day orally for 3 months[a]	Elevated liver function tests, hepatotoxicity, nausea and vomiting, hypertension
Coccidioidomycosis	Amphotericin B 0.5–1 mg/kg/day intravenously for ≥6–8 weeks[a]	Same as above
Protozoa		
Toxoplasmic encephalitis	Pyrimethamine 200 mg orally once then 50–100 mg/day	Bone marrow suppression
	plus	
	Sulfadiazine 1–1.5 g orally four times daily	Allergy, rash, drug fever
	and	
	Folinic acid 10–20 mg orally daily for a minimum of 28 days[a]	
Isosporiasis	Trimethoprim and sulfamethoxazole 1–2 double-strength tablets (160 mg trimethoprim and 800 mg sulfamethoxazole) orally twice daily for 2–4 weeks	Same as above
Bacteria		
Organisms associated with T-cell defects:		
Mycobacterium avium complex	Clarithromycin 500 mg orally twice daily, *plus* ethambutol 15 mg/kg/day orally to a maximum of 1000 mg/day, *and*	Gastrointestinal intolerance Optic neuritis, peripheral neuritis
	Rifabutin 300 mg/day[a]	Rash, gastrointestinal intolerance Neutropenia, discolored urine, uveitis
Salmonella enterocolitis or bacteremia	Ciprofloxacin 500–750 mg orally twice daily for 14 days	Gastrointestinal intolerance
	or	
	Trimethoprim (160 mg)–sulfamethoxazole (800 mg) 1 tablet orally twice daily for 14 days	Same as above
Organisms associated with B-cell defects:		
Campylobacter enterocolitis	Ciprofloxacin 500 mg orally twice daily for 7 days	Same as above
	or	
	Erythromycin 250–500 mg orally four times daily for 7 days	Gastrointestinal intolerance, colitis ototoxicity
Shigella enterocolitis	Ciprofloxacin 500 mg orally twice daily for 5 days	Same as above

(continued)

TABLE 123–6. (*Continued*)

Clinical Disease	Selected Initial Therapies for Acute Infection in Adults	Common Drug- or Dose-Limiting Adverse Reactions
Viruses		
Mucocutaneous herpes simplex	Acyclovir 1–2 g/day orally in 3–5 divided doses for 7–10 days	Gastrointestinal intolerance
	or	
	Valacyclovir 500 mg orally every 12 hours for 7–10 days	Gastrointestinal intolerance
	or	
	Famciclovir 500 mg orally every 12 hours for 7–10 days	Headache, gastrointestinal intolerance
Varicella-zoster	Acyclovir 30 mg/kg/day intravenously in 3 divided doses *or* 4 g/day orally for 7–10 days	Obstructive nephropathy, CNS symptomatology
	or	
	Valacyclovir, 1 g orally every 8 hours for 7–10 days	Gastrointestinal intolerance
	or	
	Famciclovir 500 mg orally every 8 hours for 7–10 days	
Cytomegalovirus	Ganciclovir 7.5–10 mg/kg/day in 2–3 divided doses intravenously for 14 days[a]	Neutropenia, thrombocytopenia
	or	
	Foscarnet 180 mg/kg/day in 2 or 3 divided doses intravenously for 14 days[a]	Nephrotoxicity, hypohypercalcemia, hypohyperphosphatemia, anemia
Cytomegalovirus retinitis	Ganciclovir intraocular implant	

[a]Maintenance therapy is recommended.

the trimethoprim component) as three to four divided doses. Doses of 12 to 15 mg/kg per day may be as effective and perhaps reduce the incidence of toxicity. Trimethoprim-sulfamethoxazole usually is initiated by the intravenous route, although oral therapy (since oral absorption is high) may suffice in mildly ill and reliable patients or to complete a course of therapy after a response has been achieved with intravenous administration. If oral therapy is used, it may be prudent to document absorption with serum concentrations of trimethoprim or sulfamethoxazole because gastrointestinal disturbances or a malabsorption syndrome is known to alter drug absorption in patients with AIDS. Target concentrations for trimethoprim are between 5 and 8 mcg/mL.

For treatment of HIV-associated PCP, pentamidine isethionate is administered intravenously usually in doses of 4 mg/kg per day, although a pilot study has reported successful treatment with 3 mg/kg per day.[75,76] Aerosolized pentamidine should not be used for treatment of PCP because comparative studies with intravenous pentamidine indicate that aerosolized treatment is associated with a slower clinical response and higher rates of therapeutic failure and PCP relapse.[76,77]

The efficacy of trimethoprim-sulfamethoxazole or pentamidine for treatment of an initial episode of PCP in HIV-infected individuals is similar, with published response rates between 60% to 80%. While comparative studies between the two regimens are few, one prospective, randomized trial found that oxygenation improved more quickly and survival was better in those who received trimethoprim-sulfamethoxazole.[78]

CLINICAL CONTROVERSY

The optimal length of therapy for treatment of PCP with either agent is not known, but 21 days is commonly recommended. Clinical improvement in patients with AIDS is often slower than in non-AIDS patients. One study demonstrated improvement in chest radiograph or gallium scan in only two-thirds of patients at the end of treatment.[79] Thus the lack of prompt clinical improvement is not necessarily an indication of no response. In fact, patients frequently may worsen before they

improve. However, continued worsening after 4 days or lack of improvement after 7 to 10 days is an indication for a change in therapy regardless which agent was started initially. There are no data regarding the utility of concurrent therapy with both trimethoprim-sulfamethoxazole and pentamidine, and this approach is not recommended

Adverse reactions to both trimethoprim-sulfamethoxazole and pentamidine are common and range between 20% to 85% in this setting. The more common adverse reactions seen with trimethoprim-sulfamethoxazole are rash, fever, leukopenia, elevated serum transaminases, and thrombocytopenia. Mild rashes should be watched closely for progression to more severe reactions but are not an absolute contraindication to continuing therapy. The incidence of these adverse reactions is higher in HIV-infected individuals than in those not infected with HIV.[80] For pentamidine, side effects include hypotension, tachycardia, nausea, vomiting, severe hypoglycemia or hyperglycemia, pancreatitis, irreversible diabetes mellitus, elevated serum transaminases, nephrotoxicity, leukopenia, and cardiac arrhythmias. Some of these reactions appear to be infusion-rate-related (e.g., hypotension and tachycardia) and can be minimized by infusing pentamidine over 1 hour or more. The overall incidence of adverse reactions to pentamidine appears to be similar between individuals infected with HIV and those not infected. Dosage modification or pharmacokinetic monitoring can reduce somewhat the toxicity of both pentamidine and trimethoprim-sulfamethoxazole.[79] Dose reduction of pentamidine from 4 to 3 mg/kg per day appears to be successful in minimizing further rises in serum creatinine. Maintenance of serum trimethoprim concentrations between 5 and 8 mcg/mL may help to prevent severe myelosuppression.

The early addition of adjunctive corticosteroid therapy to anti-PCP regimens decreases the risk of respiratory failure and improves survival in patients with AIDS and moderate to severe PCP (PaO$_2 \leq$ 70 mm Hg or A–a gradient $\geq$ 35 mm Hg).[81,82] The adverse effects associated with corticosteroid therapy in these patients were minimal, primarily an increased incidence of herpetic lesions, although some

TABLE 123–7. Therapies for Prophylaxis of First Episode Opportunistic Diseases in Adults and Adolescents

Pathogen	Indication	First Choice
I. Standard of Care		
Pneumocystis carinii	CD4 + count <200/mcL *or* oropharyngeal candidiasis	Trimethoprim-sulfamethoxazole, 1 double-strength tablet orally once daily or 1 single-strength tablet orally once daily
Mycobacterium tuberculosis		
Isoniazid-sensitive	TST reaction ≥5 mm *or* prior positive TST result without treatment *or* contact with case of active tuberculosis	Isoniazid 300 mg orally plus pyridoxine, 50 mg orally once daily for qmo *or* isoniazid 900 mg orally plus pyridoxine 50 mg orally twice weekly × 12 mo 5
Isoniazid-resistant	Same as isoniazid-sensitive; high probability of exposure to isoniazid-resistant tuberculosis	Rifampin 600 mg orally once daily plus pyrazinamide 200 mg/kg orally once daily for 2 mo
Toxoplasma gondii	IgG antibody to *Toxoplasma* and CD4 + count <100/mcL	Trimethoprim-sulfamethoxazole 1 double-strength tablet orally once daily
Mycobacterium avium complex	CD4 + count <50/mcL	Azithromycin, 1200 mg orally once weekly or clarithromycin, 500 mg orally twice daily
Varicella zoster virus (VZV)	Significant exposure to chickenpox or shingles for patients who have no history of either condition or, if available, negative antibody to VZV	Varicella zoster immune globulin (VZIG), 5 vials (1.25 mL each) intramuscularly administered ideally within 48 h of exposure but ≤96 h
II. Usually Recommended		
Streptococcus pneumoniae	CD4 count of ≥200 cells/mcL	23-valent polysaccharide vaccine, 0.5 mL intramuscularly
Hepatitis B virus	All susceptible (antihepatitis B core antigen negative) patients	Hepatitis B vaccine, 3 doses
Influenza virus	All patients (annually, before influenza season)	Inactivated trivalent influenza virus vaccine: 0.5 mL intramuscularly
Hepatitis A virus	All susceptible (anti-HAV-negative) patients at increased risk for hepatitis A infection (e.g., illegal drug users, men who have sex with men, hemophiliacs) or patients with chronic liver disease Including chronic hepatitis B or C	Hepatitis A vaccine: 2 doses
III. Indicated for Use Only in Selected Circumstances		
Bacteria	Neutropenia	Granulocyte-colony-stimulating factor (G-CSF), 5–10 mcg/kg subcutaneously once daily for 2–4 weeks; or granulocyte-macrophage colony-stimulating factor (GM-CSF), 250 mcg/m^2 subcutaneously for 2–4 weeks
Cryptococcus neoformans	CD4 + count <50/mcL	Fluconazole, 100–200 mg orally once daily
Histoplasma capsulatum	CD4 + count < 100/mcL, endemic Geographic area	Itraconazole capsule, 200 mg orally once daily
Cytomegalovirus	CD4 + count < 50/μL and CMV antibody positivity	Oral ganciclovir, 1 g po three times daily

From Centers for Disease Control and Prevention. Guidelines for Preventing Opportunistic Infections Among HIV-Infected Persons—2002 Recommendations of the USPHS/IDSA. MMWR 2002;51:1–52.

concerns exist about the potential for reactivation of tuberculosis. The optimal dose and duration of corticosteroid therapy have not been identified. The regimen currently recommended is 40 mg prednisone orally twice daily during days 1 through 5, 40 mg once daily on days 6 through 10, and 20 mg once daily on days 11 through 21 or for the duration of therapy.[83] Methylprednisolone at 75% of the prednisone dose can be used if parenteral therapy is necessary. In general, adjunctive corticosteroid therapy should be initiated when antipneumocystis therapy is started because the data supporting the use of corticosteroids are based on initiation within the first 24 to 72 hours of the start of antipneumocystis therapy.

HIV-infected individuals who have had PCP are at high risk for recurrent PCP if no prophylactic measures are taken. Even though the treatment of PCP is becoming increasingly successful, the mortality rate from first-episode PCP is still between 5% and 20%, and therapy frequently is complicated by adverse reactions. Prevention of PCP is clearly a preferable strategy to treatment. The relative risk of PCP in 1665 HIV-infected participants who did not have AIDS was 4.9 in those with CD4 lymphocyte counts of fewer than 200 cells/mcL.[84] Currently in the United States, PCP prophylaxis is recommended for all HIV-infected individuals who have already had previous PCP. Prophylaxis is also recommended for any HIV-infected person who has a CD4 lymphocyte count of fewer than 200 cells/mcL or in whom the CD4 cells are less than 20% of total lymphocytes or who has oropharyngeal candidiasis.[16]

Trimethoprim-sulfamethoxazole is the preferred therapy for both primary and secondary prophylaxis of PCP in adults and adolescents. Trimethoprim-sulfamethoxazole is the most effective and least expensive agent for prophylaxis; it also appears to confer cross-protection against toxoplasmosis and many bacterial infections. The recommended dose in adults and adolescents is one double-strength tablet daily, although other regimens, such as one double-strength tablet thrice weekly or one single-strength tablet daily and gradual dose escalation using liquid trimethoprim-sulfamethoxazole, have been used in an attempt to reduce the incidence of adverse reactions and improve compliance. Alternative prophylactic regimens if trimethoprim-sulfamethoxazole cannot be tolerated include dapsone, dapsone plus pyrimethamine and leucovorin, aerosolized pentamidine, and atovaquone.[85]

Trimethoprim-sulfamethoxazole is also the recommended drug of choice for PCP prophylaxis in children. As described previously, the normal range for CD4 lymphocytes is very different for children than for adults. Both the absolute CD4 count and CD4 cells as a percentage of the total should be determined. A CD4 percentage of less than 25% is an indication of immunosuppression. The utility of trimethoprim-sulfamethoxazole for prophylaxis is well established for children not HIV-infected receiving myelosuppressive therapy.[86] The trimethoprim-sulfamethoxazole regimen recommended (although other acceptable alternatives exist) is 150 mg/m^2 per day of trimethoprim and 750 mg/m^2 per day of sulfamethoxazole given in divided doses twice daily three times weekly on consecutive days (e.g., Monday, Tuesday, and Wednesday). The total daily dose of trimethoprim-sulfamethoxazole in children should not exceed 320 mg trimethoprim and 1600 mg sulfamethoxazole. PCP prophylaxis in HIV-exposed/infected children is strongly recommended as follows: (1) all HIV-exposed infants beginning between 4 to 6 weeks of age and continuing to 12 months of age if infection status is unknown, (2) all HIV-infected infants beginning at 4 to 6 weeks of age and continuing to 12 months of age, and (3) all HIV-infected children older than 1 year of age with severe immunosuppression.[68]

TOXOPLASMA GONDII

The seroprevalence of *T. gondii* in HIV-infected individuals from major urban areas of the United States varies from 10% to 45%. The parasite is passed to humans from raw or undercooked meat and contact with feces from infected cats. *T. gondii* can infect any organ of the body and cause an acute infection; it has a predilection for the brain and the eye. Once an individual is infected, the organism can replicate, forming tissue cysts that persist for the life of the host. Many individuals will not have symptoms of disease. Immunosuppression, however, allows the release of tachyzoites from tissue cysts that produce a necrotic foci of infection, most often in the brain. In the patient with AIDS, *T. gondii* is an important opportunistic pathogen that is responsible for most focal intracerebral lesions.[87]

The clinical signs and symptoms of toxoplasmosis are associated most frequently with involvement of the CNS and less commonly the lungs and eyes, although any organ can be affected. Clinical presentation often includes: fever, headache, seizures (in approximately 10% to 25% of patients), focal neurologic abnormalities (in approximately 60% to 90%), and mental status changes. Brain biopsy is required to make a definitive diagnosis of toxoplasmic encephalitis, although presumptive diagnosis is made commonly in *T. gondii*–seropositive patients with typical CNS lesions. Characteristic radiographic abnormalities found by computed tomographic (CT) scan or magnetic resonance imaging (MRI) also have been useful in the diagnosis of CNS toxoplasmosis.

The initial treatment of CNS toxoplasmosis is usually empirical. Brain biopsy in patients with AIDS may be complicated by

potential morbidity, location of the lesion(s), or thrombocytopenia. Anti-*Toxoplasma* therapy usually is initiated in patients with AIDS who are seropositive for *Toxoplasma* and have clinical symptoms suspicious for toxoplasmosis and characteristic findings on neuroradiographic studies (multiple ring-enhancing lesions). In this setting, brain biopsy usually is not undertaken unless the patient fails to respond clinically or radiologically to 10 to 14 days of therapy or deteriorates clinically. Brain biopsy is an initial consideration in the *T. gondii*–seronegative patient or in patients with atypical lesions.

The combination of pyrimethamine and sulfadiazine is considered the most effective regimen for acute therapy of AIDS-related CNS toxoplasmosis.[88] This regimen works synergistically by sequentially inhibiting two steps in folic acid synthesis of the proliferative form of *T. gondii*. There is no widespread agreement on the optimal doses of pyrimethamine and sulfadiazine. Pyrimethamine loading doses of 75 mg orally on the first day, followed by 25 mg/day thereafter, have been used commonly. The erratic concentrations of pyrimethamine found in patients with AIDS and toxoplasmic encephalitis at lower doses (25 mg/day) have prompted some investigators to use larger doses.[89] Loading doses of 100 to 200 mg followed by daily oral doses of 1 to 1.5 mg/kg per day (50 to 100 mg/day) have been recommended.[90] The usual dose of sulfadiazine is 1 to 1.5 g every 6 hours (4 to 8 g/day). Folinic acid, in doses of 10–20 mg/day (although doses as high as 50 mg/day have been used), usually is added to the combination to reduce the pyrimethamine-induced bone marrow toxicity. Acute therapy with this combination should be continued for at least 3 weeks, but 6 weeks of treatment is recommended for more severely ill patients. Response rates (combined partial and complete) of approximately 85% have been observed following a minimum of 4 weeks of therapy. Adverse reactions, primarily bone marrow suppression associated with pyrimethamine and sulfadiazine hypersensitivity reactions, may limit therapy in as many as 40% of AIDS patients.[89] A regimen of pyrimethamine (50 mg/day) plus clindamycin (2400 mg/day) for 6 weeks, followed by reduced-dose maintenance therapy, was less effective (disease progression risk 1.8 times higher) than pyrimethamine-sulfadiazine.[88] The combination of pyrimethamine plus clindamycin does appear to be less toxic than pyrimethamine plus sulfadiazine. Other investigational alternative regimens include trimethoprim-sulfamethoxazole and pyrimethamine and leucovorin plus either clarithromycin, azithromycin, atovaquone, or dapsone.

The discontinuation of pyrimethamine-sulfadiazine after successful initial therapy may be considered in persons who have a sustained CD4 cell count of greater than 200 cells/mcL for at least 6 months and have completed initial therapy and are asymptomatic.[68] A regimen of sulfadiazine 500 to 1000 mg orally 4 times daily plus pyrimethamine 25 to 50 mg orally and leucovorin 10 to 25 mg orally once daily is recommended for maintenance therapy. Pyrimethamine plus clindamycin also can be considered for maintenance therapy, but this regimen may be associated with a higher relapse rate. A further advantage to the combination of pyrimethamine plus sulfadiazine is that an additional agent for prophylaxis of PCP is unnecessary, which is not the case with the pyrimethamine plus clindamycin combination.[91]

Only limited information about primary prophylaxis of *T. gondii* in the HIV-infected person is available from carefully controlled prospective studies. Primary prophylaxis is recommended, but in HIV-infected persons who have immunoglobulin G antibody to *T. gondii* and a CD4 cell count of fewer than 100 cells/mcL, the preferred regimen is trimethoprim-sulfamethoxazole one double-strength tablet orally once daily.[68]

CRYPTOCOCCUS NEOFORMANS

Infection with *C. neoformans* is now uncommon in the HAART era and occurs primarily in those with limited access to health care.[92] Infections probably are contracted originally through inhalation, and the respiratory tract is believed to be the first infected site. The usual clinical presentation of cryptococcal infection is meningitis, although pneumonia and disseminated disease also occur. The clinical features of cryptococcal meningitis may be subtle, nonspecific, and not localize to the CNS.[93] Fever, headache, and malaise are the most frequent symptoms. Meningeal features, mental status changes, and other focal neurologic signs occur only in a minority of patients. The diagnosis of cryptococcal meningitis always should be considered when HIV-infected individuals with advanced disease or low CD4 lymphocyte counts present with nonspecific symptoms or pulmonary or CNS findings.

Methods for diagnosis of cryptococcal infection includes serum and cerebrospinal fluid (CSF) testing for cryptococcal antigen and fungal cultures. Detection of cryptococcal antigen in serum and CSF is the most sensitive and specific test; an antigen titer of greater than 1:8 should be regarded as evidence for infection. Identification of *C. neoformans* on india ink examination of the CSF or from culture also may be used to confirm the diagnosis when antigen is unavailable. Factors suggestive of a poor prognosis in patients with cryptococcal meningitis include alteration in mental status, CSF antigen greater than 1:1024, a low CSF leukocyte count, and age younger than 35 years.

10 The goals of therapy for cryptococcal meningitis in patients with AIDS are to induce a remission and maintain a high quality of life. The standard therapeutic approach has been amphotericin B for both acute and maintenance therapy, although the introduction of azole compounds has changed the therapeutic approach for clinically stable patients. The largest controlled clinical trial of amphotericin B (mean daily dose ≈ 0.4 mg/kg) plus flucytosine versus fluconazole for cryptococcal meningitis in 194 patients with AIDS found that treatment was successful in 40% of the amphotericin recipients and in 34% of fluconazole recipients.[94] The death rate in the first 2 weeks of treatment was 18% in the fluconazole arm and 14% in the amphotericin arm. The death rate after 2 weeks was 4% and 6%, respectively, in the fluconazole and amphotericin groups. The median time to sterilization of CSF cultures was 42 days in amphotericin B recipients and 64 days in those who received fluconazole. These data suggest that while fluconazole is effective for treatment of cryptococcal meningitis, amphotericin B is more effective because of its lower rates of early death and disease progression. Most patients with cryptococcal meningitis probably should receive amphotericin B in an intravenous dose of at least 0.5 mg/kg per day for a minimum of 2 weeks as acute therapy. Flucytosine in doses of 100 to 150 mg/kg per day can be considered for combination with amphotericin B; serum concentrations should be monitored and peak levels kept below 100 mcg/mL to minimize hematologic adverse reactions. The addition of flucytosine to an amphotericin B regimen of 0.7 mg/kg per day for 2 weeks significantly improved mortality, clinical course, or CSF culture status at 2 weeks.[95]

Once the acute treatment of cryptococcal meningitis is completed, maintenance therapy is necessary to prevent relapse. Placebo-controlled trials of 100 to 200 mg/day fluconazole, as well as controlled trials versus 1 mg/kg per week of amphotericin B, have been conducted to prevent recurrence of cryptococcal disease in patients who completed acute therapy.[96,97] Compared with patients receiving amphotericin B maintenance therapy, the probability of remaining relapse-free at 1 year was higher for fluconazole recipients (97% versus 78%), and the rate of serious drug toxicity was lower (7% versus 31%). Fluconazole is superior to either placebo, amphotericin, or itraconazole for maintenance therapy and is the drug of choice to prevent relapse of cryptococcal meningitis.

In addition to treatment strategies, investigations are underway to determine whether fungal infections can be prevented. Results of a controlled trial of fluconazole (200 mg/day) versus clotrimazole troches (10 mg five times daily) suggest that after a median follow-up of 35 months, fluconazole recipients had a significant benefit in terms of reduced rate of invasive fungal infection (primarily cryptococcosis) and esophageal candidiasis.[98] The benefit of fluconazole therapy was greater for patients with fewer than 50 CD4 cells/mcL. The 2-year cumulative risk of cryptococcosis was 1.6% in the fluconazole group and 9.9% in the clotrimazole group ($p = 0.02$) in contrast to risks of 0.8% and 4.3%, respectively, in patients with higher CD4 counts. There was, however, no survival difference between the two groups. Despite fluconazole therapy, 10.6% of recipients developed proved or presumed candidiasis, raising the possibility of emergence of resistance to fluconazole. Drug-resistant candidiasis caused by *Candida albicans* and *C. krusei* has been observed in patients infected with HIV who are receiving fluconazole. The central question of whether the benefit of fluconazole and other agents for prophylaxis of fungal infections outweighs the risks, including resistance, remains to be clearly delineated. Presently, routine antifungal prophylaxis of cryptococcosis is not recommended.

MYCOBACTERIUM INFECTIONS

M. tuberculosis infection is a well-recognized and treatable complication of HIV infection and AIDS.[47] A discussion of the clinical presentation and treatment is found elsewhere in this book (Chap. 110).

Infections with non-tuberculous mycobacterial organisms, especially *M. avium* complex (MAC), were recognized early in the AIDS epidemic. Disseminated MAC is now uncommon, occurring in 1% to 3% of HIV-infected individuals. The major risk factor for MAC is advanced immunosuppression; the mean CD4 lymphocyte count in patients with disseminated MAC is usually fewer than 50 cells/mcL, and infection is rare in individuals with more than 100 cells/mcL. The organism is a common water and soil saprophyte; the routes of acquisition in patients with AIDS are thought to be gastrointestinal and/or respiratory. In patients with advanced HIV disease, MAC causes a widely disseminated infection. Local colonization also can occur and precede disseminated disease, although cultures of sputum or the gastrointestinal tract have a poor predictive value for subsequent disseminated MAC. The clinical syndrome associated with MAC includes high spiking fevers, diarrhea, night sweats, malaise, weight loss, anemia, and neutropenia. Persistent diarrhea and abdominal pain, a malabsorption syndrome, and extrahepatic biliary obstruction are manifestations associated with MAC gastrointestinal infection. Diagnosis of MAC infection usually is based on culture of the organisms from the blood, although biopsies of the liver, bone marrow, and lymph nodes are also highly sensitive and specific. Diagnosis of disseminated MAC in advanced HIV disease suggests a poor long-term prognosis without therapy.

Unfortunately, MAC is resistant to the standard drugs used for tuberculosis, such as isoniazid and pyrazinamide. Multiple agents such as rifampin, rifabutin (ansamycin), clofazimine, imipenem, amikacin, ethambutol, ciprofloxacin, clarithromycin, and azithromycin have varying degrees of in vitro anti-MAC activity.[99] Controversy formerly existed as to whether treatment for MAC is beneficial, but data indicate that an aggressive therapeutic approach decreases symptoms and prolongs survival. The largest randomized comparison of MAC treatment regimens evaluated clarithromycin with either ethambutol (C + E), rifabutin (C + R), or both (C + E + R) in 160 HIV-infected persons with MAC bacteremia. The proportion of subjects with a complete microbiologic response at week 12 was 40% in the C + E group, 42% in the C + R group, and 51% in the C + E + R group (no statistical differences). Relapse while receiving C + R (24%) was significantly higher than the other two arms (6% to 7%).[100]

There are several important issues regarding therapy of MAC, most notably who to treat, which drugs to use and for how long, and how to assess response to therapy. First, treatment regimens should contain at least two antimycobacterial agents. Second, every regimen should contain either clarithromycin or azithromycin because both have excellent activity against MAC. Of these agents, clarithromycin (500 mg twice daily) is the preferred agent for MAC treatment based on greater clinical experience and data that indicate that clarithromycin and ethambutol versus azithromycin and ethambutol produced a more rapid resolution of MAC bacteremia.[101] For the second agent, numerous choices are available, although ethambutol (15 mg/kg per day) is preferred by many experts. Many clinicians would add a third and some a fourth drug to this regimen. Among the alternatives available for the third drug, only rifabutin (300 mg/day) adds a significant microbiologic benefit. Clofazimine appears to be associated with an increase in mortality when used for therapy of MAC and should not be used.[102] Clinical responses usually occur within 2 to 8 weeks of the start of therapy. If a clinical and microbiologic response is observed, therapy should continue for the duration of the patient's life. The recommended regimen for secondary prophylaxis is clarithromycin 500 mg orally twice daily plus ethambutol 15 mg/kg orally once daily with or without rifabutin 300 mg orally once daily.

Disseminated MAC infection contributes significantly to morbidity and mortality in the HIV-infected person, therapy is not uniformly successful, and a high-risk population can be identified. Therefore, a strong basis for prophylaxis of MAC exists. Clarithromycin and azithromycin both reduce the risk of disseminated MAC. In a double-blind, placebo-controlled study, 682 persons with AIDS and CD4 lymphocyte counts of fewer than 100 cells/mcL were randomized to receive clarithromycin 500 mg twice daily or placebo.[103] MAC bacteremia developed nearly three times as often in placebo recipients as in clarithromycin recipients. There were 19 (6%) breakthrough MAC infections in the clarithromycin group versus 53 (16%) in the placebo arm (p <0.001). Clarithromycin-resistant strains of MAC were detected in some patients. During about 10 months of follow-up, 32% of the patients who received clarithromycin died compared with 41% (p = 0.026) in the placebo group. Azithromycin also has been shown to have a protective benefit against MAC infection. A three-arm trial evaluated azithromycin (1200 mg weekly), rifabutin (300 mg/day), and the combination in 693 HIV-infected persons with fewer than 100 CD4 cells/mcL.[104] The incidence of disseminated MAC infection at 1 year was 7.6% for azithromycin, 15.3% for rifabutin, and 2.6% for the combination. MAC isolates resistant to azithromycin were found in 11% of the patients who failed azithromycin prophylaxis. Dose-limiting adverse reactions, primarily gastrointestinal, were more common in the azithromycin plus rifabutin group. There was no difference in survival among the three regimens.

MAC prophylaxis is now strongly recommended for all HIV-infected adults and adolescents with CD4 counts of fewer than 50 cells/mcL.[16] The first-line choices are either azithromycin (1200 mg once weekly) or clarithromycin (500 mg twice daily); rifabutin is an alternative. Persons considered for prophylaxis should be evaluated to be sure that they do not have active disease owing to MAC or *M. tuberculosis*.

HERPESVIRUS INFECTIONS

HERPES SIMPLEX VIRUS

Herpes simplex viruses (HSV) types 1 and 2 cause significant morbidity in patients with AIDS. Seropositivity for HSV is widespread among adults with AIDS, and clinical disease usually is the result of reactivation of latent virus. The manifestations of HSV disease observed in persons with AIDS include orolabial, genital, and anorectal mucocutaneous disease; esophagitis; and less commonly, encephalitis. Ulcerative HSV lesions present for longer than 1 month in an individual with laboratory evidence for HIV infection or no other apparent cause for immunodeficiency are considered an AIDS-defining condition.

Anorectal lesions are common clinically evident HSV disease causing morbidity in homosexual men with AIDS and likely reflect the common risk factors for acquisition (sexual contact) of both HSV and HIV. Chronic perianal HSV lesions were among the first opportunistic infections associated with AIDS.[105] Symptoms include pain, itching, and painful defecation. The clinical presentation of anal, orolabial, and genital herpes in the patient with AIDS is similar to that in other immunosuppressed individuals. The severity of the episode can range from mild to severely destructive. The severity of mucocutaneous HSV disease increases with progressive immunosuppression. Other HSV manifestations, such as encephalitis, are rare in the patient with AIDS but are life-threatening. Differentiation from other CNS infections such as those caused by *C. neoformans* or *T. gondii* is important, and prompt treatment is essential.

Acyclovir is the drug of choice for the treatment of HSV disease.

For mild to moderate mucocutaneous disease, oral acyclovir in doses of 200 mg five times daily or 400 mg three times daily are used, although regimens of 400 mg five times daily have been described occasionally as clinically necessary. Intravenous acyclovir (15 mg/kg per day) should be used in settings where absorption of oral drug is questionable or oral tolerance is unlikely (HSV esophagitis) or perhaps when severe mucocutaneous disease is present. Treatment of mucocutaneous disease should be continued until all lesions have crusted. Intravenous acyclovir (30 mg/kg per day) also should be used for viscerally disseminated disease and for HSV encephalitis. Famciclovir and the oral prodrug of acyclovir, valacyclovir, are alternatives to oral acyclovir.

Recurrent HSV disease is common in many patients with AIDS following discontinuation of therapy. These individuals often can be managed with low-dose suppressive oral acyclovir therapy, as have other immunosuppressed patients at risk for frequently recurring HSV diseases.[106] Regimens commonly used include acyclovir 200 mg four times daily, 400 mg twice daily, and 800 mg once daily.

Acyclovir-resistant HSV has been isolated from patients with AIDS.[107] The primary mechanism of resistance appears to be a deficiency in viral thymidine kinase. Strategies that have been employed for management of severe acyclovir-resistant HSV infections include increasing the dose of acyclovir, discontinuing acyclovir, and use of an alternative antiviral agent. Vidarabine and foscarnet, because they do not require phosphorylation by thymidine kinase, are examples of potential alternative agents.[108,109] A randomized comparison of foscarnet and vidarabine indicated that foscarnet is more effective and associated with fewer adverse reactions than vidarabine.[110]

VARICELLA-ZOSTER VIRUS

Most adults with AIDS have been infected previously with varicella-zoster virus (VZV) and thus are not susceptible to primary infection (chickenpox) but may develop recurrent infection (zoster). The prevalence of zoster in HIV-infected individuals appears higher than in other age-matched immunocompetent persons and seems to reliably herald the loss of cell-mediated immunity and progression to AIDS.[111]

Zoster usually begins as radicular pain followed by localized erythematous rash and characteristic vesicles. Zoster usually remains confined to a limited number of dermatomes, but complications such as widespread cutaneous involvement and disseminated visceral zoster may occur. As in the treatment of HSV infections, acyclovir is the drug of choice for VZV infections. While an oral acyclovir regimen of 4 g/day is effective for the treatment of zoster in immunocompetent adults, the drug has not been fully evaluated in immunocompromised patients such as those with AIDS.[112] For practical reasons, oral acyclovir, famciclovir, or valacyclovir is often used for localized zoster. However, careful monitoring for signs of progression of zoster is essential. AIDS patients with disseminated cutaneous or visceral zoster should receive treatment with intravenous acyclovir in doses of 30 mg/kg per day for at least 7 days or until all lesions are crusted. Acyclovir-resistant VZV infections have been reported in patients with AIDS.[113]

CYTOMEGALOVIRUS

Cytomegalovirus (CMV) is the most common life-threatening viral infection in patients with AIDS. As with infection with other herpes group viruses, infection with CMV is ubiquitous; seropositivity among homosexual men with AIDS approaches 100%.[114] There are numerous manifestations of CMV infection, including retinitis, esophagitis, hepatitis, gastrointestinal involvement, and less commonly, radiculopathy, encephalitis, and pneumonitis. CMV end-organ disease occurs in up to 44.9% of AIDS patients, particularly when their CD4 count is below 50 cells/mcL. The incidence, however, has decreased in the era of HAART.[115]

CMV retinitis, the most commonly recognized CMV disease associated with AIDS, usually is associated with a painless progressive loss of vision. Patients initially may complain of blurry vision, loss of visual acuity, or "floaters." CMV retinitis usually begins unilaterally, but bilateral involvement may occur. Untreated, CMV retinitis invariably leads to blindness. The diagnosis of CMV retinitis is made by funduscopic examination and identification of characteristic findings. Lesions characteristic of CMV retinitis include a fluffy white perivascular exudate frequently associated with hemorrhage. Early diagnosis and treatment are crucial to prevent further visual deterioration.

The first approved agent of treatment for CMV diseases was ganciclovir. Structurally, ganciclovir differs from acyclovir only by a single hydroxyl side chain, but it is 30 to 50 times more active in vitro against CMV. The use of ganciclovir therapy traditionally has been divided into two phases, induction and maintenance, because high relapse rates are found after discontinuation of the drug following successful completion of a 2- to 3-week course of initial therapy. Induction regimens with ganciclovir are typically 7.5–10 mg/kg per day intravenously in two or three equally divided doses for 14 days or longer if there is a slow clinical response. Maintenance therapy is usually 5 to 6 mg/kg once daily, although doses of 10 mg/kg have been used 5 to 7 days per week for an indefinite period of time. Initial response rates for retinal CMV disease range from 60% to 90%.[116] Unfortunately, even with intravenous maintenance therapy, relapse of CMV retinitis is common and occurs at a median of approximately 55 to 80 days. Valganciclovir, an orally administered prodrug of ganciclovir, also can be used for induction therapy. A randomized trial of valganciclovir [900 mg twice daily for 3 weeks (induction), followed by 900 mg once daily for 1 week (maintenance)] versus intravenous ganciclovir [5 mg/kg twice daily (induction), followed by 5 mg/kg

once daily (maintenance)] resulted in a faster median time to progression of retinitis for the group assigned to intravenous ganciclovir (125 days) compared with the group assigned to oral valganciclovir (160 days).[117]

Neutropenia and thrombocytopenia are the most common drug- or dose-limiting adverse reactions associated with use of intravenous ganciclovir. Up to 50% of patients with AIDS receiving ganciclovir (alone) may need a dose reduction or interruption of therapy as a result of hematologic toxicity. Filgrastim (granulocyte-CSF), erythropoietin, or sargramostim (granulocyte-monocyte-CSF) offers some potential amelioration of the adverse hematologic effects of ganciclovir. Intravitreal administration also has been used as salvage therapy in an attempt to circumvent these adverse reactions.[118] Sustained-release intraocular ganciclovir implants represent another strategy developed not only to overcome systemic toxicity but also to avoid the need for intravitreal injections. One-hundred and seventy three patients representing 222 eyes were randomized to receive either ganciclovir implant 1 mcg/h (75 eyes), 2 mcg/h (71 eyes), or intravenous ganciclovir (76 eyes). Median progression to CMV retinitis was similar in the 1 and 2 mcg/h implant groups, 221 days and 191 days, respectively, but median time to progression in the patients treated with intravenous ganciclovir was 71 days ($p < 0.001$). Intravenous ganciclovir was associated with an almost threefold risk of progression compared with ganciclovir implants.[119] Ganciclovir implants, however, do not protect patients from CMV occurring elsewhere, including the initially uninvolved eye. Intravenous ganciclovir cuts the risk of CMV retinitis in the initially uninvolved eye by half. Extraocular involvement of CMV did not occur in patients receiving intravenous ganciclovir compared with 10.3% of patients who received an implant only. Therefore, patients having an implant also should receive systemic therapy, such as oral ganciclovir.

Foscarnet is a pyrophosphate analogue with both anti-HIV and anti-CMV activity. Controlled trials to evaluate immediate versus delayed foscarnet therapy of CMV retinitis in HIV-infected individuals found immediate foscarnet therapy more effective than delayed therapy in preventing progression of CMV disease.[120] Furthermore, prolonged survival and an anti-HIV effect (as assessed by a decline in HIV or p24 antigen) were observed.[121] An unblinded, randomized trial comparing ganciclovir with foscarnet therapy of CMV retinitis was conducted in 234 patients with AIDS.[122] Both drugs were administered in standard 14-day induction regimens, followed by maintenance therapy. Ganciclovir and foscarnet were equally effective in delaying the progression of CMV disease. The median time to progression of retinitis was 56 days in the ganciclovir groups and 59 days in the foscarnet group. There was a difference, however, in survival between these two groups. Median survival was 8.5 months for ganciclovir recipients, whereas it was 12.6 months for those who received foscarnet. The explanation for this survival difference is unknown. It is conceivable that the difference in mortality was due to the anti-HIV effect of foscarnet. Adverse reactions that necessitated a switch in therapy were more common among the foscarnet recipients. The choice of therapy for CMV retinitis is largely dictated by the adverse-reaction profiles of the two agents, convenience, concomitant medications being taken by the patient, and underlying disease states.

While foscarnet appears less likely to cause neutropenia than ganciclovir, it has a variety of potential adverse effects. The most common side effects are renal insufficiency and metabolic disturbances (both increases and decreases) in calcium and phosphorus. Other adverse reactions include anemia, thrombocytopenia, infusion-site reactions, nausea and vomiting, penile ulcerations, and seizures. Hydration reduces the incidence of serum creatinine elevations from 66% in a nonhydrated control group to 13% in hydrated individuals.[123] Foscarnet, like ganciclovir, is currently administered in two phases, induction and maintenance. Induction doses are 180 mg/kg per day intravenously in two or three divided doses for 14 days, followed by maintenance therapy in doses of 90 to 120 mg/kg intravenously once daily; foscarnet doses must be adjusted in individuals with renal insufficiency.

Other approaches to the treatment of CMV disease include the combination of ganciclovir and foscarnet and cidofovir. In patients who have relapsed CMV retinitis, the ganciclovir-foscarnet combination was compared with retreatment with either drug alone.[124] The median times to retinitis progression were foscarnet 1.3 months, ganciclovir 2.0 months, and ganciclovir-foscarnet 4.3 months. Adverse events among the three groups were similar. However, the combined use of ganciclovir-foscarnet had the greatest negative impact on quality of life most likely because of the time-intensive and complex administration requirements. Cidofovir is a nucleotide analogue shown to delay the progression of CMV retinitis. In a study of 64 patients with AIDS and previously untreated CMV retinitis, the median time to progression was 21 days in the deferred-therapy group versus 64 days in those who received low-dose cidofovir.[125] While cidofovir has certain advantages over ganciclovir and foscarnet, including a less frequent dosing schedule, the drug is nephrotoxic and can cause irreversible damage to the proximal renal tubules. Cidofovir must be given with aggressive intravenous hydration and concomitant probenecid, although these efforts only reduce, not prevent, nephrotoxicity. Also concerning is the finding that cidofovir did not show a significant effect on CMV viremia at the 3-week assessment point in the trial previously mentioned; this finding is in contrast to ganciclovir or foscarnet, which both suppress CMV viremia.

CMV infection of the gastrointestinal tract can involve sites ranging from the esophagus and stomach to the colon and rectum. In one series of AIDS patients with gastrointestinal tract infection, the colon was the most common site of infection, followed by the stomach or esophagus.[126] CMV colitis may be characterized by abdominal pain, fever, weight loss, and diarrhea, symptoms quite common among patients with HIV disease even in the absence of CMV infection. Characteristic symptoms of CMV esophagitis are dysphagia and substernal chest pain. Barium contrast studies may demonstrate abnormalities but will not distinguish among other etiologic agents, such as *Candida* and HSV, both of which are more common. The definitive diagnosis of CMV gastrointestinal infection requires endoscopy and biopsy with histologic identification of CMV inclusions or in situ antigen detection.

The therapy of CMV gastrointestinal disease has been more controversial. Few randomized, controlled trials have been conducted. A small randomized comparison of ganciclovir and foscarnet for AIDS-associated gastrointestinal disease found both therapies to be equally effective.[127] Judged by endoscopy, 83% of foscarnet recipients and 85% of ganciclovir recipients showed a response. Survival, however, was poor at less than 40 weeks for both groups. Although patients were not randomized to receive maintenance therapy or not, it is interesting that there was no difference in the time to progression of disease between those who did and those who did not. Symptomatic CMV gastrointestinal disease warrants treatment, and it appears that ganciclovir and foscarnet are equivalent. The role of maintenance therapy is less clear.

Various strategies have been evaluated to determine whether CMV disease in HIV-infected individuals can be prevented. A randomized, double-blind, placebo-controlled study of oral ganciclovir (1000 mg every 8 hours) in CMV-seropositive patients with AIDS found that oral ganciclovir significantly reduced the incidence of CMV disease.[128] CMV disease occurred in 26% of placebo recipients versus 14% of ganciclovir recipients ($p < 0.001$). However, there was no difference in survival between the two groups; the 1-year

mortality rate was 26% for placebo recipients versus 21% for ganciclovir recipients. A study of oral ganciclovir for prevention in patients with a slightly higher CD4 lymphocyte count did not find any protective benefit. Currently, prophylaxis with oral ganciclovir may be considered in HIV-infected adults and adolescents who have a CD4 cell count of fewer than 50 cells/mcL and are CMV antibody–positive, but it is not a recommended standard of care.

DISCONTINUATION OF PROPHYLAXIS FOR OPPORTUNISTIC INFECTIONS

The ability of HAART regimens to restore the CD4 cell count to levels rarely associated with the development of OIs provides a basis for the discontinuation of primary and secondary prophylaxis for certain patients. The current recommendations are found in ref. 68; select examples are as follows.[68] For PCP, primary prophylaxis can be discontinued in patients receiving and responding to HAART who have a CD4 cell count of more than 200 cells/mcL sustained for 3 months or more. Prophylaxis should be reinstated if the CD4 count drops to fewer than 200 cells/mcL. These same criteria apply for both the discontinuation and the reinitiation of secondary prophylaxis of PCP. Primary prophylaxis for MAC disease can be discontinued in patients who have had CD4 counts of more than 100 cells/mcL for a period of 3 months. Prophylaxis should be restarted if the CD4 count returns to fewer than 50 to 100 cells/mcL. Secondary prophylaxis for MAC can be considered for discontinuation in persons who have had a CD4 count sustained above 100 cells/mcL for at least 6 months and have completed 12 months of MAC therapy and are asymptomatic for MAC. Maintenance therapy (secondary prophylaxis) for CMV retinitis can be discontinued in patients whose CD4 cells have increased to more than 100 to 150 cells/mcL for 6 months or more and who have no evidence of active disease. Additional considerations should include the anatomic location of the CMV lesion (sight-threatening or not), adequate vision in the other eye, and the availability of regular eye examinations. Readers are advised that data continue to emerge on the safety of stopping primary and secondary prophylaxis, as well as criteria for when to restart secondary prophylaxis, and the most current guidelines always should be consulted.

CONCLUSION

Irrefutable progress has been made in the management of HIV: Disease progression can be delayed, survival can be prolonged, and the risk of maternal-to-fetal HIV transmission can be reduced. Twenty antiretroviral agents are now available for clinical use, and additional compounds are likely to follow. However, therapy is still suboptimal in that complete suppression of viral replication has not been achieved. There remain significant deficits in our understanding of the virologic and immunologic processes associated with HIV infection and the clinical pharmacology of anti-HIV compounds. Critical issues include the need for simpler and more potent regimens, emergence of drug-resistant viral isolates, and the inexorably progressive nature of HIV infection in some patients despite antiretroviral therapy. There is a clear need for more selective and potent inhibitors of HIV. The medical management of opportunistic infections associated with HIV disease also has changed dramatically since the recognition of AIDS early in the 1980s and has improved survival. The approach to PCP is most illustrative. The transition from an era marked by treatment of only established disease to one where primary and secondary prophylaxis based on CD4 lymphocyte count are standards of care reflects both progress in understanding the risk factors for OIs and in pharmacologic therapy. Collectively, three important lessons have been learned from the treatment of HIV and associated OIs: the need for prospective immunologic and virologic monitoring and early recognition of HIV infection, the use of potent combinations of antiretroviral agents to maximally inhibit viral replication and restore immune function, and primary and secondary prophylaxis of OIs. Emphasis on these principles, coupled with carefully controlled investigations of novel agents and therapeutic strategies, will continue to offer definite benefit and improve the quality of life for HIV-infected individuals and yield an advantage over this pernicious virus that causes AIDS.

ACKNOWLEDGMENTS

Grant support: RO1 AI33835, UO1 AI41089, and UO1 AI38858, from the National Institute of Allergy and Infectious Disease.

ABBREVIATIONS

ACTG: AIDS Clinical Trail Group
AIDS: acquired immune deficiency syndrome
bDNA: branched DNA
CD: cluster designation
CDC: Centers for Disease Control and Prevention
CMV: cytomegalovirus
CSF: cerebrospinal fluid
dsDNA: double-stranded DNA
ELISA: enzyme-linked immunosorbent assay
gp: glycoprotein
HAART: highy active antirertoviral therapy
HIV: human immunodeficiency virus
HSV: herpes simplex virus
IC_{50}: concentration of antiretroviral agent necessary to inhibit 50% of viral replication
MAC: *Mycobacterium avium* complex
MSM: men who have sex with men
NNRTI: nonnucleoside reverse transcriptase inhibitor
NRTI: nucleoside/nucleotide reverse transcriptase inhibitor
OI: opportunistic infection
PCP: *Pneumocystis carinii* pneumonia
PEP: postexposure prophylaxis
PI: protease inhibitor
SIV: simian immunodeficiency virus
SIT: structured intermittent therapy
ssRNA: single-stranded RNA
STI: structured or strategic treatment interruptions
WHO: World Health Organization
VZV: varicella-zoster virus

Review Questions and other resources can be found at *www.pharmacotherapyonline.com.*

REFERENCES

1. Barre-Sinoussi F, Chermann J, Rey F, et al. Isolation of a T-lymphotropic retrovirus from a patient at risk for acquired immunodeficiency syndrome (AIDS). Science 1983;220:868–871.
2. Gallo R, Salahuddin S, Popovic M, et al. Frequent detection and isolation of cytopathic retroviruses (HTLV-III) from patients with AIDS and at risk for AIDS. Science 1984;224:500–503.
3. Palella FJ Jr, Delaney KM, Moorman AC, et al. Declining morbidity and mortality among patients with advanced human immunodeficiency virus infection. N Engl J Med 1998;338:853–860.
4. Carr A. Toxicity of antiretroviral therapy and implications for drug development. Nature Rev Drug Discov 2003;2:624–634.
5. Centers for Disease Control and Prevention. Guidelines for national human immunodeficiency virus case surveillance, including monitoring for human immunodeficiency virus infection and acquired immunodeficiency syndrome. MMWR 1999;48:1–31.
6. Nakashima AK, Fleming PL. HIV/AIDS surveillance in the United States, 1981–2001. J Acquir Immune Defic Syndr 2003;32:68–85.
7. Centers for Disease Control and Prevention. HIV Prevention Strategic Plan Through 2005 (*www.cdc.gov/hiv/pubs/prev-strat-plan.pdf*).
8. Chen SY, Gibson S, Katz MH, et al. Continuing increases in sexual risk behavior and sexually transmitted diseases among men who have sex with men: San Francisco, California, 1999–2001. Am J Public Health 2002;92:1387–1388.
9. UNAIDS. AIDS Epidemic Update: 2003: Joint United Nations Programme on HIV/AIDS (UNAIDS) and World Health Organization, Geneva, WHO, 2003.
10. Robertson DL, Anderson JP, Bradac JA, et al. HIV-1 nomenclature proposal. Science 2000;288:55–56.
11. Hahn BH, Shaw GM, De Cock KM, Sharp PM. AIDS as a zoonosis: Scientific and public health implications. Science 2000;287:607–614.
12. Mylonakis E, Paliou M, Lally M, et al. Laboratory testing for infection with the human immunodeficiency virus: Established and novel approaches. Am J Med 2000;109:568–576.
13. Kovacs JA, Masur H. Prophylaxis against opportunistic infections in patients with human immunodeficiency virus infection. N Engl J Med 2000;342:1416–1429.
14. Mastro TD, de Vincenzi I. Probabilities of sexual HIV-1 transmission. AIDS 1996;10(suppl A):S75–82.
15. Schreiber GB, Busch MP, Kleinman SH. The risk of transfusion-transmitted viral infections. N Engl J Med 1996;26:1685–1690.
16. Centers for Disease Control and Prevention. Updated U.S. Public Health Service guidelines for the management of occupational exposures to HBV, HCV, and HIV and recommendations for postexposure prophylaxis. MMWR 2001;50:1–52.
17. Van Dyke RB, Korber BT, Popek E, et al. The Ariel project: A prospective cohort study of maternal-child transmission of human immunodeficiency virus type 1 in the era of maternal antiviral therapy. J Infect Dis 1999;179:319–328.
18. Nduati R, John G, Mbori-Ngacha D, et al. Effect of breastfeeding and formula feeding on transmission of HIV-1. JAMA 2000;283:1167–1174.
19. Dean M, Carrington M, Winkler C, et al. Genetic restriction of HIV-1 infection and progression to AIDS by a deletion allele of the *CKR5* structural gene. Science 1996;273:1856–1862.
20. Pierson T, McArthur J, Siliciano RF. Reservoirs for HIV-1: Mechanisms for viral persistence in the presence of antiviral immune responses and antiretroviral therapy. Annu Rev Immunol 2000;18:665–708.
21. Frankel AD, Young JAT. HIV-1: Fifteen proteins and an RNA. Annu Rev Biochem 1998;67:1–25.
22. Learmont JC, Geczy AF, Mills J, et al. Immunologic and virologic status after 14 to 18 years of infection with an attenuated strain of HIV-1: A report from the Sydney Blood Bank Cohort. N Engl J Med 1999;340:1715–1722.
23. Kohl NE, Emini EA, Schleif WA, et al. Active human immunodeficiency virus protease is required for viral infectivity. Proc Natl Acad Sci USA 1988;85:4686–4690.
24. Schacker T, Collier AC, Hughes J, et al. Clinical and epidemiologic features of primary HIV infection. Ann Intern Med 1996;125:257–264.
25. Kahn JO, Walker BD. Acute human immunodeficiency virus type 1 infection. New Engl J Med 1998;339:33–39.
26. Mellors JW, Rinaldo CR Jr, Gupta P, et al. Prognosis in HIV-1 infection predicted by the quantity of virus in plasma. Science 1996;272:1167–1170.
27. Love JT Jr, Shearer WT. Prevention, diagnosis, and treatment of pediatric HIV infection. Comp Ther 1996;22:719–726.

28. Centers for Disease Control and Prevention. 1994 revised classification system for human immunodeficiency virus infection in children less than 13 years of age. MMWR 1994;43:1–10.

29. The Working Group on Antiretroviral Therapy and Medical Management of HIV-Infected Children. Guidelines for the use of antiretroviral agents in pediatric HIV infection (*www.AIDSinfo.NIH.gov*).

30. Kempf DJ, Rode RA, Xu Y, et al. The duration of viral suppression during protease inhibitor therapy for HIV-1 infection is predicted by plasma HIV-1 RNA at the nadir. AIDS 1998;12:F9–14.

31. Raboud JM, Montaner JS, Conway B, et al. Suppression of plasma viral load below 20 copies/mL is required to achieve a long-term response to therapy. AIDS 1998;12:1619–1624.

32. Masur H, Kaplan JE, Holmes KK. Guidelines for the prevention of opportunistic infections in persons infected with human immunodeficiency virus: Recommendations of the U.S. Public Health Service and the Infectious Diseases Society of America. Ann Intern Med 2002;137:435–478.

33. NIH Panel to Define Principles of Therapy of HIV Infection. Report of the NIH panel to define principles of therapy of HIV infection, 1997 (www.hivatis.org).

34. US Department of Health and Human Services Panel on Clinical Practices for the Treatment of HIV Infection. Guidelines for the use of antiretroviral agents in HIV-infected adults and adolescents, 2003 (*www.AIDSinfo.nih.gov*).

35. Tramont EC, Johnston MI. Progress in the development of an HIV vaccine. Expert Opin Emerg Drugs 2003;8:37–45.

36. Piscitelli SC, Bhat N, Pau A. A risk-benefit assessment of interleukin-2 as an adjunct to antiviral therapy in HIV infection. Drug Saf 2000;22:19–31.

37. Stein DS, Moore KH. Phosphorylation of nucleoside analog antiretrovirals: A review for clinicians. Pharmacotherapy 2001;21:11–34.

38. Lisziewicz J, Foli A, Wainberg M, Lori F. Hydroxyurea in the treatment of HIV infection: Clinical efficacy and safety concerns. Drug Saf 2003;26:605–624.

39. Kakuda TN. Pharmacology of nucleoside and nucleotide reverse transcriptase inhibitor-induced mitochondrial toxicity. Clin Ther 2000;22:685–708.

40. Moyle G. The emerging roles of non-nucleoside reverse transcriptase inhibitors in antiretroviral therapy. Drugs 2001;61:19–26.

41. Eron JJ Jr. HIV-1 protease inhibitors. Clin Infect Dis 2000;30(suppl 2):S160–170.

42. Fletcher CV. Enfuvirtide, a new drug for HIV infection. Lancet 2003;361:1577–1578.

43. Condra JH, Miller MD, Hazuda DJ, Emini EA. Potential new therapies for the treatment of HIV-1 infection. Annu Rev Med 2002;53:541–555.

44. de Maat MM, Ekhart GC, Huitema AD, et al. Drug interactions between antiretroviral drugs and comedicated agents. Clin Pharmacokinet 2003;42:223–282.

45. Becker SL. The role of pharmacological enhancement in protease inhibitor-based highly active antiretroviral therapy. Exp Opin Invest Drugs 2003;12:401–412.

46. Havlir DV, Tierney C, Friedland GH, et al. In vivo antagonism with zidovudine plus stavudine combination therapy. J Infect Dis 2000;182:321–325.

47. Blumberg H, Burman W, Chaisson R, et al. American Thoracic Society/Centers for Disease Control and Prevention/Infectious Diseases Society of America: Treatment of tuberculosis. Am J Respir Crit Care Med 2003;167:603–662.

48. Piscitelli SC, Burstein AH, Chaitt D, et al. Indinavir concentrations and St John's wort. Lancet 2000;355:547–548.

49. Fischl MA, Richman DD, Grieco MH, et al. The efficacy of azidothymidine (AZT) in the treatment of patients with AIDS and AIDS-related complex. N Engl J Med 1987;317:185–191.

50. Hammer SM, Katzenstein DA, Hughes MD, et al. A trial comparing nucleoside monotherapy with combination therapy in HIV-infected adults with CD4 cell counts from 200 to 500 per cubic millimeter. N Engl J Med 1996;335:1081–1090.

51. Paterson DL, Swindells S, Mohr J, et al. Adherence to protease inhibitor therapy and outcomes in patients with HIV infection. Ann Intern Med 2000;133:21–30.

52. Singh N, Berman SM, Swindells S, et al. Adherence to human immunodeficiency virus-infected patients to antiretroviral therapy. J Infect Dis 1999;29:824–830.

53. Spooner KM, Lane HC, Masur H. Antiretroviral therapy: reference guide to major clinical trials in patients infected with human immunodeficiency virus. Clin Infect Dis 1995;20:1145–1151.

54. Spooner KM, Lane HC, Masur H. Guide to major clinical trials of antiretroviral therapy administered to patients infected with human immunodeficiency virus. Clin Infect Dis 1996;23:15–27.

55. Tavel JA, Miller KD, Masur H. Guide to major clinical trials of antiretroviral therapy in human immunodeficiency virus-infected patients: protease inhibitors, non-nucleoside reverse transcriptase inhibitors, and nucleotide reverse transcriptase inhibitors. Clin Infect Dis 1999;28:643–676.

56. Walmsley S, Bernstein B, King M, et al. Lopinavir-ritonavir versus nelfinavir for the initial treatment of HIV infection. N Eng J Med 2002;346:2039–2046.

57. Staszewski S, Morales-Ramirez J, Tashima KT, et al. Efavirenz plus zidovudine and lamivudine, efavirenz plus indinavir, and indinavir plus zidovudine and lamivudine in the treatment of HIV-1 infection in adults. N Engl J Med 1999;341:1865–1873.

58. Hirsch MS, Brun-Vezinet F, Clotet B, et al. Antiretroviral drug resistance testing in adults infected with human immunodeficiency virus type 1: 2003 Recommendations of an International AIDS Society—USA Panel. Clin Infect Dis 2003;37:113–128.

59. Gangar M, Arias G, O'Brien JG, Kemper CA. Frequency of cutaneous reactions on rechallenge with nevirapine and delavirdine. Ann Pharmacother 2003;34:839–842.

60. Schambelan M, Benson CA, Carr A, et al. Management of metabolic complications associated with antiretroviral therapy for HIV-1 infection: Recommendations of an International AIDS Society—USA Panel. J Acquir Immune Defic Syndr 2002;31:257–275.

61. Dube MP, Stein JH, Aberg JA, et al. Guidelines for the evaluation and management of dyslipidemia in human immunodeficiency virus (HIV)–infected adults receiving antiretroviral therapy: Recommendations of the HIV Medicine Association of the Infectious Disease Society of America and the Adult AIDS Clinical Trials Group. Clin Infect Dis 2003;37:613–627.

62. Public Health Services Task Force. Recommendations for the use of antiretroviral drugs in pregnant HIV-1 infected women for maternal health and interventions to reduce perinatal HIV-1 transmission in the United States, 2003 (*www.AIDSinfo.NIH.gov*).

63. Connor EM, Sperling RS, Gelber R, et al. Reduction in maternal-infant transmission of human immunodeficiency virus type 1 with zidovudine treatment. N Engl J Med 1994;331:1173–1180.

64. Wade NA, Birkhead GS, Warren BL, et al. Abbreviated regimens of zidovudine prophylaxis and perinatal transmission of the human immunodeficiency virus. N Engl J Med 1998;339:1409–1414.

65. Guay LA, Musoke P, Fleming T, et al. Intrapartum and neonatal single-dose nevirapine compared with zidovudine for prevention of mother-to-child transmission of HIV-1 in Kampala, Uganda: HIVNET 012 randomised trial. Lancet 1999;354:795–802.

66. Morris AB, Cu-Uvin S, Harwell JI, et al. Multicenter review of protease inhibitors in 89 pregnancies. J Acquir Immune Defic Syndr 2000;25:306–311.

67. Centers for Disease Control and Prevention. Management of possible sexual, injecting-drug-use, or other nonoccupational exposure to HIV, including considerations related to antiretroviral therapy. MMWR 1998;47:1–15.

68. Centers for Disease Control and Prevention. Guidelines for preventing opportunistic infections among HIV-infected persons—2002 recommendations of the U.S. Public Health Service and the Infectious Diseases Society of America. MMWR 2002;51:1–52.

69. Ledergerber B, Egger M, Erard V, et al. AIDS-related opportunistic illnesses occurring after initiation of potent antiretroviral therapy. JAMA 2000;282:2220–26.

70. Centers for Disease Control and Prevention. AIDS Weekly Surveillance Report. Atlanta, CDC, 1989.

71. Davey RJ, Masur H. Recent advances in the diagnosis, treatment, and prevention of *Pneumocystis carinii* pneumonia. Antimicrob Agents Chemother 1990;34:499–504.

72. Santamauro J, Stover D. *Pneumocystis carinii* pneumonia. Med Clin North Am 1997;81:299–318.

73. Hughes W, Feldman S, Chaudary S, et al. Comparison of pentamidine isethionate and trimethoprim-sulfamethoxazole in the treatment of *Pneumocystis carinii* pnemonia. J Pediatr 1978;92:285–291.

74. Masur H. Prevention and treatment of *Pneumocystis* pneumonia. N Eng J Med 1992;327:1853–60.

75. Conte J, Chernoff D, Feigal D, et al. Intravenous or inhaled pentamidine for treating *Pneumocystis carinii* pneumonia in AIDS. Ann Intern Med 1990;113:203–209.

76. Conte J Jr, Hollander H, Golden J, et al. Inhaled pentamidine or reduced dose intravenous pentamidine for *Pneumocystis carinii* pneumonia: A pilot study. Ann Intern Med 1987;107:495–498.

77. Soo Hoo G, Mohsenifar Z, Meyer R. Inhaled or intravenous pentamidine therapy for *Pneumocystis carinii* pneumonia. Ann Intern Med 1990;113: 195–202.

78. Sattler F, Cowan R, Nielsen D, et al. Trimethorprim-sulfamethoxazole compared with pentamidine for treatment of *Pneumocystis carinii* pneumonia in the acquired immunodeficiency syndrome. Ann Intern Med 1988;109:280–287.

79. Wharton J, Coleman D, Wofsy C, et al. Trimethorprim-sulfamethoxazole or pentamidine for *Pneumocystis carinii* pneumonia in the acquired immunodeficiency syndrome. Ann Intern Med 1986;105:37–44.

80. Wofsy C. Use of trimethoprim-sulfamethoxazole in the treatment of *Pneumocystis carinii* pneumonitis in patients with acquired immunodeficiency syndrome. Rev Infect Dis 1987;9(suppl 2):S184–194.

81. Bozzette S, Sattler F, Chiu J, et al. A controlled trial of early adjunctive treatment with coricosteriods for *Pneumocystis carinii* pneumonia in the acquired immunodeficiency syndrome. N Engl J Med 1990;323: 1451–1457.

82. Gagnon S, Boota A, Fischl M, et al. Corticosteriods as adjunctive therapy for severe *Pneumocystis carinii* pneumonia in the acquired immunodeficiency syndrome. N Engl J Med 1990;323:1444–1450.

83. The National Institutes of Health–University of California Expert Panel for Corticosteriods as Adjunctive Therapy for *Pneumocystis carinii* Pneumonia. Consensus statement on the use of corticosteriods as adjunctive therapy for *Pneumocystis* pneumonia in the acquired immunodeficiency syndrome. N Engl J Med 1990;323:1500–1504.

84. Phair J, Munoz A, Detels R, et al. The risk of *Pneumocystis carinii* pneumonia among men infected with human immunodeficiency virus type 1. N Engl J Med 1990;322:161–165.

85. Bozzette S, Finkelstein D, Spector S, et al. A randomized trial of three antipneumocystis agents in patients with advanced human immunodeficiency virus infection. NIAID AIDS Clinical Trials Group. N Engl J Med 1995;332:693–699.

86. Hughes W, Kuhn S, Chaudhary S, et al. Successful chemoprophylaxis for *Pneumocystis carinii* pneumonitis. N Engl J Med 1977;297: 1419–1426.

87. Tuazon C. Toxoplasmosis in AIDS patients. J Antimicrob Chemother 1989;23(suppl A):77–82.

88. Katlama C, Wit S, O'Doherty E, et al. Pyrimethamine-clindamycin vs pyrimethamine-sulfadiazine as acute and long-term therapy for toxoplasmic encephalitis in patients with AIDS. Clin Infect Dis 1996;22:268–275.

89. Weiss L, Harris C, Berger M, et al. Pyrimethamine concentrations in serum and cerebrospinal fluid during treatment of acute *Toxoplasma* encephalitis in patients with AIDS. J Infect Dis 1988;157:580–583.

90. Wong S, Remington J. Toxoplasmosis in the Setting of AIDS. Baltimore, Williams & Wilkins; 1994.

91. Herald A, Flepp M, Chave J-P, et al. Treatment for cerebral toxoplasmosis protects against *Pneumocystis carinii* pneumonia in patients with AIDS. Ann Intern Med 1991;115:760–763.

92. Mirza SA, Phelan M, Rimland D, et al. The changing epidemiology of cryptococcosis: An update from population-based active surveillance in 2 large metropolitan areas, 1992–2000. Clin Infect Dis 2003;36:789–794.

93. Chuck S, Sande M. Infections with *Cryptococcus neoformans* in the acquired immunodeficiency syndrome. N Engl J Med 1989;321: 794–799.

94. Saag M, Powderly W, Cloud G, et al. Comparison of amphotericin B with fluconzale in the treatment of acute AIDS-associated cryptococcal meningitis. N Engl J Med 1992;326:83–89.

95. van der Horst C, Saag M, Cloud G, et al. Treatment of cryptococcal meningitis associated with the acquired immunodeficiency syndrome. National Institute of Allergy and Infectious Diseases Mycoses Study Group and AIDS Clinical Trials Group. N Engl J Med 1997;337: 15–21.

96. Bozzette S, Larsen R, Chiu J, et al. A placebo-controlled trial of maintenance therapy with fluconazole after treatment of cryptococcal meningitis in the acquired immunodeficiency syndrome. N Engl J Med 1991; 324:580–584.

97. Powderly W, Saag M, Cloud G, et al. A controlled trial of fluconazole or amphotericin B to prevent relapse of cryptococcal meningitis in patients with the acquired immunodeficiency syndrome. N Engl J Med 1992; 326:793–798.

98. Powderly W, Finkelstein D, Feinberg J, et al. A randomized trial comparing fluconazole with clotrimazole troches for the prevention of fungal infections in patients with advanced human immunodeficiency virus infection. N Engl J Med 1995;332:700–705.

99. Peloquin C. *Mycobacterium avium* complex infection: Pharmacokinetic and pharmacodynamic considerations that may improve clinical outcomes. Clin Pharmacokinet 1997;32:132–144.

100. Benson CA, Williams PL, Currier JS, et al. A prospective, randomized trial examining the efficacy and safety of clarithromycin in combination with ethambutol, rifabutin, or both for the treatment of disseminated *Mycobacterium avium* complex disease in persons with acquired immunodeficiency syndrome. Clin Infect Dis 2003;37:1234–1243.

101. Ward T, Rimland D, Kauffman C, et al. Randomized, open-label trial of azithromycin plus ethambutol vs clarithromycin plus ethambutol as therapy for *Mycobacterium avium* complex bacteremia in patients with human immunodeficiency virus infection. Clin Infect Dis 1998;27: 1278–1285.

102. Lundgren J, Masur H. New approaches to managing opportunistic infections. AIDS 1999;13:S227–234.

103. Pierce M, Crampton S, Henry D, et al. A randomized trial of clarithromycin as prophylaxis against disseminated *Mycobacterium avium* complex infections in patients with advanced acquired immunodeficiency syndrome. N Engl J Med 1996;335:383–391.

104. Havlir D, Dube M, Sattler F, et al. Prophylaxis against disseminated *Mycobacterium avium* complex with weekly azithromycin, daily rifabutin, or both. N Engl J Med 1996;335:392–398.

105. Siegel F, Lopez C, Hammer B, et al. Severe acquired immunodeficiency in male homosexuals, manifested by chronic perianal ulcerative herpes simplex lesions. N Engl J Med 1981;305:1439–1444.

106. Wade J, Newton B, Flournoy N, et al. Oral acyclovir for prevention of herpes simplex virus reactivation after marrow transplantation. Ann Intern Med 1984;100:823–828.

107. Erlich K, Mills J, Chatis P, et al. Acyclovir-resistant herpes simples virus infections in patients with the acquired immunodeficiency syndrome. N Engl J Med 1989;320:293–296.

108. Erlich K, Jacobson M, Koehler J, et al. Foscarnet therapy for severe acyclovir-resistant herpes simples virus type-2 infections in patients with the acquired immunodeficiency syndrome. Ann Intern Med 1989;110:710–713.

109. Fletcher CV, Englund JA, Bean B, et al. Continuous infusion high-dose acyclovir for serious herpesvirus infections. Antimicrob Agents Chemother 1989;33:1375–1378.

110. Safrin S, Crumpacker C, Chatis P, et al. A controlled trial comparing foscarnet with vidarabine for acyclovir-resistant mucocutaneous herpes simplex virus in the acquired immunodeficiency syndrome. N Engl J Med 1991;325:551–555.

111. Melbye M, Grossman R, Goedert J, et al. Risk of AIDS after herpes zoster. Lancet 1987;1:728–731.

112. Huff J, Bean B, Balfour H Jr, et al. Therapy of herpes zoster with oral acyclovir. Am J Med 1988;85(suppl 2A):84–89.

113. Jacobson M, Berger T, Fikrig S, et al. Acyclovir-resistant varicella-zoster virus infection after chronic oral acyclovir therapy in patients with the acquired immunodeficiency syndrome. Ann Intern Med 1990;112: 187–191.

114. Quinnan G, Masur H, Rook A, et al. Herpesvirus infections in the acquired immunodeficiency syndrome. JAMA 1984;252:72–77.

115. Kaplan JE, Hanson D, Dworkin MS, et al. Epidemiology of human immunodeficiency virus–associated opportunistic infections in the Unitted States in the era of highly active antiretroviral therapy. Clin Infect Dis 2000;30:S5–14.

116. Fletcher CV, Balfour HH Jr. Evaluation of ganciclovir for cytomegalovirus disease. Ann Pharmocother 1989;23:5–12.

117. Martin DF, Sierra-Madero J, Walmsley S, et al. A controlled trial of valganciclovir as induction therapy for cytomegalovirus retinitis. N Engl J Med 2002;346:1119–1126.

118. Smith C. Local therapy for cytomegalovirus retinitis. Ann Pharmacother 1998;32:248–255.

119. Musch D, Martin D, Gordon J, et al. Treatment of cytomegalovirus retinitis with a sustained-release ganciclovir implant. N Engl J Med 1997;337:83–90.

120. Palestine A, Polis M, de Smet M, et al. A randomized, controlled trial of foscarnet in the treatment of cytomegalovirus retinitis in patients with AIDS. Ann Intern Med 1991;115:665–673.

121. Polis M, de Smet M, Bard B, et al. Increased survival of a cohort of patients with acquired immunodeficiency syndrome and cytomegalovirus retinitis who received sodium phosphonoformate (foscarnet). Am J Med 1993;94:175–180.

122. Studies of the Ocular Complications of AIDS Research Group. Mortality in patients with the acquired immunodeficiency syndrome treated with either foscarnet or ganciclovir for cytomegalovirus retinitis. N Engl J Med 1992;326:213–220.

123. Deray G, Katlama C, Dohin E. Prevention of foscarnet nephrotoxicity. Ann Intern Med 1990;113:332.

124. Studies of Ocular Complications of AIDS Research Group in Collaboration with the AIDS Clinical Trial Group. Combination foscarnet and ganciclovir therapy vs monotherapy for the treatment of relapsed cytomegalovirus retinitis in patients with AIDS. Arch Ophthamol 1996; 114:23–33.

125. Studies of Ocular Complications of AIDS Research Group in Collaboration with the AIDS Clinical Trials Group. Parenteral cidofovir for cytomegalovirus retinitis in patients with AIDS: The HPMPC peripheral cytomegalovirus retinitis trial. Ann Intern Med 1997;126: 264–274.

126. Dietrich D, Chachoua A, LaFleur F, et al. Ganciclovir treatment of gastronintestinal infections caused by cytomegalovirus in patients with AIDS. Rev Infect Dis 1988;10(suppl 3):S532–537.

127. Blanshard C, Benhamou Y, Dohin E, et al. Treatment of AIDS-associated gastrointestinal xytomegalovirus infection with foscarnet and ganciclovir: A randomized comparison. J Infect Dis 1995;172:622–628.

128. Spector S, McKinley G, Lelezari J, et al. Oral ganciclovir for the prevention of cytomegalovirus disease in persons with AIDS. N Engl J Med 1996;334:1491–1497.

124

CANCER TREATMENT AND CHEMOTHERAPY

Carol McManus Balmer, Amy Wells Valley, and Andrea Iannucci

Learning Objectives and other resources can be found at *www.pharmacotherapyonline.com.*

KEY CONCEPTS

◀1 Carcinogenesis is a multi-step process that includes initiation, promotion, conversion, and progression. The growth of both normal and cancerous cells is genetically controlled by the balance or imbalance of oncogene, protooncogene, and tumor suppressor gene protein products. Multiple genetic mutations are required to convert normal cells to cancerous cells. Apoptosis and cellular senescence (aging) are normal mechanisms for cell death.

◀2 Tumor growth patterns can be described mathematically by the Gompertzian growth curve. Most of the life span of an individual's cancer takes place before the cancer is clinically evident. The growth curve illustrates concepts of exponential tumor grown, growth fraction, tumor burden, and doubling time.

◀3 Because patients with clinically evident metastatic cancer can rarely be cured, early detection is critical. Screening programs are designed to detect cancers in asymptomatic people who are at risk of a specific type of cancer. Knowing the early warning signs of cancer is also important in early detection, when cancers are most likely to be localized.

◀4 Treatment for cancer should not begin until the presence of cancer is confirmed by a tissue (i.e., histologic) diagnosis. Clinical cancer staging provides prognostic information, and in conjunction with the patient's treatment goals, guides the selection of cancer treatment. The goals of cancer treatment include cure, prolongation of life, and relief of symptoms. Surgery and radiation therapy provide the best chance of cure for patients with localized cancers, but systemic treatment methods are required for systemic cancers.

◀5 Adjuvant therapy is usually systemic therapy that is administered to treat any existing micrometastases remaining after treatment of localized disease. Because adjuvant therapy is given to patients with no clinical evidence of cancer, the benefit of the treatment cannot be proven for an individual patient, but only for patient populations. Treatment decisions are based largely on an assessment of the presence of risk factors in an individual patient and the patient's estimated risk for cancer recurrence. The effectiveness of adjuvant therapies is measured statistically, by the relative and absolute reduction in the risk of recurrence. In con-

trast, outcomes can be assessed for individual patients with metastatic disease with carefully defined response criteria. Response criteria are disease-specific and usually include complete response, partial response, stable disease, progression, and clinical benefit.

◀6 Cancer cells are genetically unstable, which results in tumor masses of heterogeneous cells, and makes the cancer a "moving target" for drug therapy. Existence of many different clones of cancer cells in most patients provides the rationale for use of cancer drugs in combination, and is the likely reason for failure of cancer drug therapy to cure most patients with advanced cancer.

◀7 Compromising dose intensity of cancer drug therapy by delaying or reducing doses can compromise outcomes of therapy. Dose regimen and method of administration of some anticancer drugs can greatly affect their efficacy and toxicity. Rescue agents, antidotes, or other chemoprotectants are available for a few cancer drugs, and can be used to minimize toxicity to normal cells. Understanding the pathophysiology of chemotherapy drug toxicities can lead to more effective prevention and treatment of these toxicities. Prospective dose modification of some cancer drugs is essential in patients with impaired renal or hepatic function, to reduce the risk of severe toxicities. Identification of genetic variations that affect drug activation and metabolism may permit the development of individualized drug therapy regimens that optimize effectiveness and minimize toxicity.

◀8 The immune system is a natural defense against cancer, and can be utilized to treat existing cancers.

◀9 Development of biologically targeted agents that exploit differences between cancerous and normal cells permits greater specificity for cancer cells with less damage to normal cells. Monoclonal antibodies in cancer treatment recognize an antigen that is expressed preferentially on cancer cells, and can be used to target drugs or radioisotopes to the antigen-expressing cells.

◀10 The growth of some breast and prostate cancers is fed by gonadal hormones. Elimination of the effects of the feeding hormone can result in regression of the cancer.

◀11 Tumors must develop new blood vessels in order to grow.

◀12 Myelosuppression, which creates risk of infection and bleeding, is the acute dose-limiting toxicity for most non-specific cancer drugs. The risk of infection in neutropenic patients is related to the depth and duration of neutropenia. The only reliable indicator of infection in neutropenic patients is fever. Unexplained fever in neutropenic patients requires prompt initiation of empiric antibiotic therapy. Colony-stimulating factors may reduce the risk of febrile neutropenia. Evidence-based clinical guidelines should direct the use of costly supportive care resources such as hematopoietic growth factors.

◀13 Fatigue in cancer patients is multifactorial and can greatly compromise quality of life. Correctable causes of fatigue such as anemia should be identified and addressed.

◀14 Long-term complications of cancer treatment, such as infertility, secondary malignancies, effects on physical or intellectual development, and major organ damage, can negatively affect health and quality of life for cancer survivors.

◀15 The risk of developing some cancers may be modified prospectively by changes in lifestyle, diet, exposure to known carcinogens, and by other interventions.

Cancer is a group of more than 100 different diseases, characterized by uncontrolled cellular growth, local tissue invasion, and distant metastases.[1] It is second only to cardiovascular disease as a cause of mortality in Americans. More than 1.3 million cases of cancer are diagnosed annually, and cancer claims an estimated 570,280 lives in the United States each year.[2] The estimated incidence of common cancers and cancer-related deaths is illustrated in Fig. 124–1. The four most common cancers are prostate, breast, lung, and colorectal cancer. The most common cause of cancer-related deaths in the United States is lung cancer, which accounts for about 160,000 deaths each year. These cancers are discussed in further detail in the chapters that follow.

The roles of health professionals in the management of cancer patients can be very diverse. Thorough knowledge of antineoplastic drug pharmacology and pharmacokinetics is essential to prevent and to manage many drug-induced toxicities. Supportive-care issues such as nutritional support, pain management, infection, and nausea and vomiting require application of both clinical and pharmacologic principles. Provision of drug information to other health professionals and to patients and their families is another critical role. Experienced

health professionals are able to fulfill these roles and to make valuable contributions to patient care in the oncology setting.

This chapter introduces the basic concepts of carcinogenesis, tumor growth, and cancer treatment, provides general information on the pharmacology and clinical use of the antineoplastic agents, and presents an overview of supportive care issues in the oncology patient.

ETIOLOGY OF CANCER

CARCINOGENESIS

◀1 The mechanism by which cancers occur is incompletely understood. A cancer, or neoplasm, is thought to develop from a cell in which the normal mechanisms for control of growth and proliferation are altered. Current evidence supports the concept of carcinogenesis as a multistage process that is genetically regulated (Fig. 124–2).[3–6] The first step in this process is *initiation*, which requires exposure of normal cells to carcinogenic substances. These carcinogens produce genetic damage that, if not repaired, results in irreversible cellular

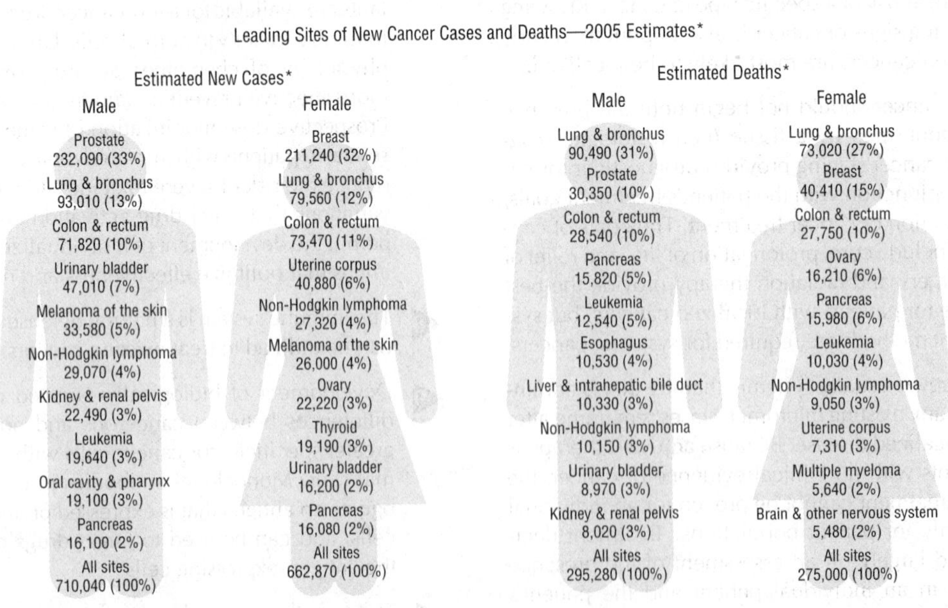

Leading Sites of New Cancer Cases and Deaths—2005 Estimates*

Estimated New Cases*

Male	Female
Prostate 232,090 (33%)	Breast 211,240 (32%)
Lung & bronchus 93,010 (13%)	Lung & bronchus 79,560 (12%)
Colon & rectum 71,820 (10%)	Colon & rectum 73,470 (11%)
Urinary bladder 47,010 (7%)	Uterine corpus 40,880 (6%)
Melanoma of the skin 33,580 (5%)	Non-Hodgkin lymphoma 27,320 (4%)
Non-Hodgkin lymphoma 29,070 (4%)	Melanoma of the skin 26,000 (4%)
Kidney & renal pelvis 22,490 (3%)	Ovary 22,220 (3%)
Leukemia 19,640 (3%)	Thyroid 19,190 (3%)
Oral cavity & pharynx 19,100 (3%)	Urinary bladder 16,200 (2%)
Pancreas 16,100 (2%)	Pancreas 16,080 (2%)
All sites 710,040 (100%)	All sites 662,870 (100%)

Estimated Deaths*

Male	Female
Lung & bronchus 90,490 (31%)	Lung & bronchus 73,020 (27%)
Prostate 30,350 (10%)	Breast 40,410 (15%)
Colon & rectum 28,540 (10%)	Colon & rectum 27,750 (10%)
Pancreas 15,820 (5%)	Ovary 16,210 (6%)
Leukemia 12,540 (5%)	Pancreas 15,980 (6%)
Esophagus 10,530 (4%)	Leukemia 10,030 (4%)
Liver & intrahepatic bile duct 10,330 (3%)	Non-Hodgkin lymphoma 9,050 (3%)
Non-Hodgkin lymphoma 10,150 (3%)	Uterine corpus 7,310 (3%)
Urinary bladder 8,970 (3%)	Multiple myeloma 5,640 (2%)
Kidney & renal pelvis 8,020 (3%)	Brain & other nervous system 5,480 (2%)
All sites 295,280 (100%)	All sites 275,000 (100%)

* Excludes basal and squamous cell skin cancers in situ carcinomas, except urinary bladder, American Cancer Society, Inc., Surveillance Research, 2005.

FIGURE 124–1. Estimated 2005 cancer incidences (*left*) and deaths (*right*) in the United States for males and females. (*Reproduced with permission from American Cancer Society.[2]*)

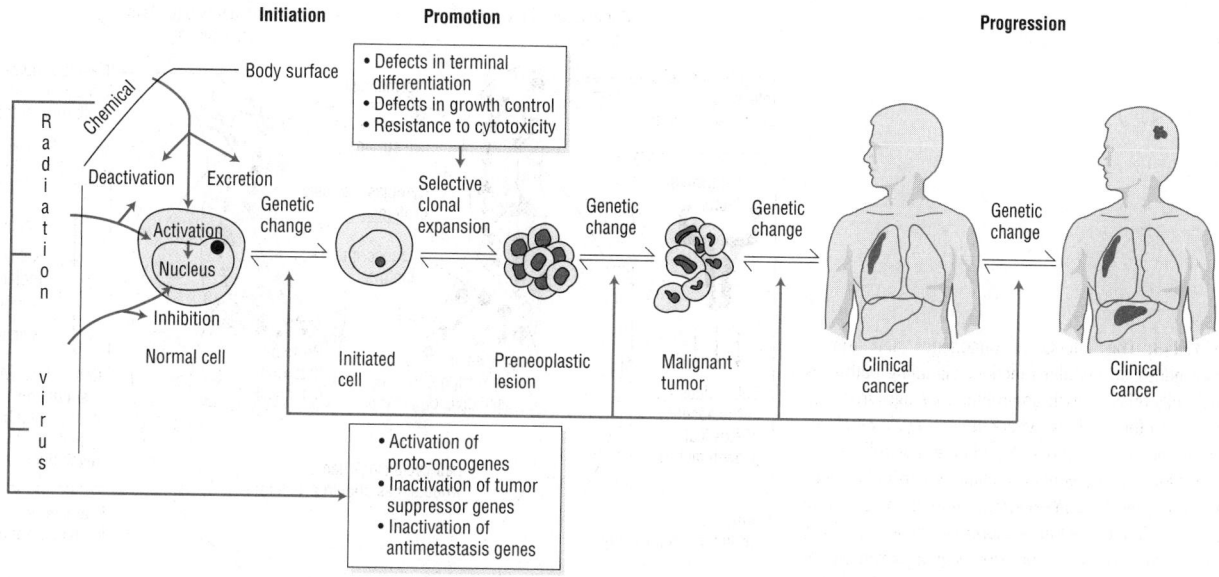

FIGURE 124–2. Multistage model of carcinogenesis. *(Adapted with permission from Weston et al.[5])*

mutations. This mutated cell has an altered response to its environment and a selective growth advantage, giving it the potential to develop into a clonal population of neoplastic cells. During the second phase, known as *promotion*, carcinogens or other factors alter the environment to favor growth of the mutated cell population over normal cells. The primary difference between initiation and promotion is that promotion is a reversible process. In fact, because it is reversible, the promotion phase may be the target of future chemoprevention strategies, including changes in lifestyle and diet. At some point, however, the mutated cell becomes cancerous (*conversion* or *transformation*). Depending on the type of cancer, 5 to 20 years may elapse between the carcinogenic phases and the development of a clinically detectable cancer. The final stage of neoplastic growth, called *progression*, involves further genetic changes leading to increased cell proliferation. The critical elements of this phase include tumor invasion into local tissues and the development of metastases.

Substances that may act as carcinogens or initiators include chemical, physical, and biologic agents.[5,6] Exposure to chemicals may occur by virtue of occupational and environmental means, as well as lifestyle habits. The association of aniline dye exposure and bladder cancer is one such example. Benzene is known to cause some leukemias. Some drugs and hormones used for therapeutic purposes are also classified as carcinogenic chemicals (Table 124–1). Physical agents that act as carcinogens include ionizing radiation and ultraviolet light. These types of radiation induce mutations by forming free radicals that damage DNA and other cellular components. Viruses are biologic agents that are associated with certain cancers. The Epstein-Barr virus is believed to be an important factor in the initiation of African Burkitt's lymphoma. Likewise, infection with hepatitis B virus is known to be a major cause of hepatocellular cancer. All the previously mentioned carcinogens, as well as age, gender, diet, growth factors, and chronic irritation, are among the factors considered to be promoters of carcinogenesis.

GENETIC BASIS OF CANCER

Cancer has been described as "a malady of genes, arising from genetic damage of diverse sorts and leading to distortions of either expression or biochemical function of genes."[7] In recent years, there has been marked progress in the understanding of the genetic changes that lead to the development of cancer, largely because of improvements in research techniques and new information generated as part of the human genome project.[3,5,6,8,9] There are two major classes of genes involved in carcinogenesis: oncogenes and tumor-suppressor genes. Figure 124–3 illustrates the effects of oncogenes and tumor-suppressor genes on normal cellular function. Oncogenes develop from normal genes, called protooncogenes, and may have important roles in all phases of carcinogenesis. Protooncogenes are present in all cells and are essential regulators of normal cellular functions, including the cell cycle. Genetic alteration of the protooncogene through point mutation, chromosomal rearrangement, or gene amplification

TABLE 124–1. Selected Drugs and Hormones Known to Cause Cancer in Humans

Drug or Hormone	Type of Cancer Caused
Alkylating agents (e.g., chlorambucil, mechlorethamine, melphalan, nitrosoureas)	Leukemia
Anabolic steroids	Liver
Analgesics containing phenacetin	Renal, urinary bladder
Anthracyclines (e.g., doxorubicin)	Leukemia
Antiestrogens (tamoxifen)	Endometrium
Coal tars (topical)	Skin
Estrogens	
Nonsteroidal (diethylstilbestrol)	Vagina/cervix, endometrium, breast, testes
Steroidal (estrogen replacement therapy, oral contraceptives)	Endometrium, breast, liver
Epipodophyllotoxins (etoposide, teniposide)	Leukemia
Immunosuppressive drugs (cyclosporine, azathioprine)	Lymphoma, skin
Oxazaphosphorines (cyclophosphamide, ifosfamide)	Urinary bladder, leukemia

Adapted from Compagni et al[4] and Cotran et al.[6]

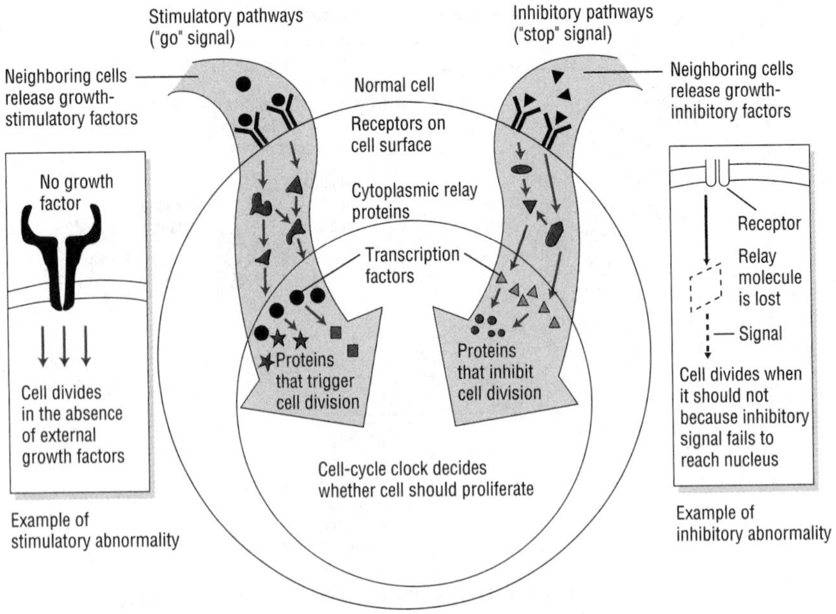

FIGURE 124–3. The effects of oncogenes and tumor-suppressor genes on cellular function. Signaling pathways in normal cells relay growth-controlling messages from the outer surface to the nucleus, where the cell-cycle clock receives these messages and decides whether the cell should divide. In cancer cells, genetic mutations can either activate oncogenes, resulting in excessive stimulation (too many "go" signals) or inactivate tumor-suppressor genes, resulting in loss of cell-cycle inhibition (no "stop" signals). Examples of abnormal stimulatory or inhibitory processes are provided in the boxes. *(Adapted with permission from Weinberg.[9])*

activates the oncogene. These genetic alterations may be caused by carcinogenic agents such as radiation, chemicals, or viruses (somatic mutations), or they may be inherited (germ-line mutations). Once activated, the oncogene produces either excessive amounts of the normal gene product or an abnormal gene product. The result is dysregulation of normal cell growth and proliferation, which imparts a distinct growth advantage to the cell and increases the probability of neoplastic transformation. An example is the *myc* family of oncogenes. The normal gene product of *myc* acts as a signal for cellular proliferation. As an oncogene, the gene product is overexpressed or amplified, resulting in excessive cellular proliferation. Table 124–2 lists examples of other oncogenes and their classification by mechanism.

In contrast, tumor-suppressor genes regulate and inhibit inappropriate cellular growth and proliferation.[3,6,8,9] Gene loss or mutation results in loss of control over normal cell growth (see Fig. 124–3). Two common examples of tumor-suppressor genes are the retinoblastoma and *p53* genes. Mutation of *p53* is one of the most common genetic changes associated with cancer, and is estimated to occur in half of all malignancies.[9] The normal gene product of *p53* is responsible for negative regulation of the cell cycle, allowing the cell cycle to halt for repairs, corrections, and responses to other external signals. Inactivation of *p53* removes this checkpoint, allowing mutations to occur. Mutation of *p53* has been linked to a variety of malignancies, including brain tumors (astrocytoma); carcinomas of the breast, colon, lung, cervix, and anus; and osteosarcoma. Another important function of *p53* may be modulation of cytotoxic drug effects. Loss of *p53* has been associated with antineoplastic drug resistance.

Another group of genes important in carcinogenesis is the DNA repair genes.[6] The normal function of these genes is to repair DNA that is damaged by environmental factors, or errors in DNA that occur during replication. If not corrected, these errors can result in mutations that activate oncogenes or inactivate tumor suppressor genes. As more mutations in the genome occur, the risk for malignant transformation increases. The DNA repair genes have been classified as tumor suppressor genes, because a loss in their function results in increased risk for carcinogenesis. Deficiencies in DNA repair genes have been discovered in familial colon cancer (hereditary nonpolyposis colon cancer) and breast cancer syndromes.

Oncogenes and tumor-suppressor genes provide the stimulatory and inhibitory signals that ultimately regulate the cell cycle.[9–11] These signals converge on a molecular system in the nucleus known as the cell cycle clock (see Fig. 124–3). The function of the clock in normal tissue is to integrate the signal input and to determine if the cell cycle should proceed. The clock is composed of a series of interacting proteins, the most important of which are cyclins and cyclin-dependent kinases (CDKs). Cyclins (especially cyclin D1) and CDKs promote entry into the cell cycle and are overexpressed in several cancers, including breast cancer. CDK inhibitors have been identified as important negative regulators of the cell cycle.

When the normal regulatory mechanisms for cellular growth fail, back-up defense systems may be activated. The secondary defenses include apoptosis (programmed cell death or suicide) and cellular senescence (aging). Apoptosis is a normal mechanism of cell death required for tissue homeostasis.[9–12] This process is regulated by oncogenes and tumor-suppressor genes and is also a mechanism of cellular death after exposure to cytotoxic agents. Overexpression of oncogenes responsible for apoptosis may produce an "immortal" cell, which has increased potential for malignancy. The *bcl-2* oncogene is an example. The most common chromosomal abnormality found in lymphoid malignancies is the t(14;18) translocation. The *bcl-2* protooncogene is normally located on chromosome 18. Translocation of this protooncogene to chromosome 14 in proximity to the immunoglobulin heavy chain gene leads to overexpression of *bcl-2*, which decreases apoptosis and confers a survival advantage to the cell. Studies show that *p53* is also a regulator of apoptosis. Loss of *p53* disrupts normal apoptotic pathways, imparting a survival advantage to the cell. Recent evidence also has revealed an important role for apoptosis as a mechanism of inherent resistance to chemotherapy.[12]

Cellular senescence is another important defense mechanism.[6,8–10] Laboratory studies demonstrate that once a cell population has undergone a preset number of doublings, growth stops and cells die. This is known as senescence, a process that is regulated by telomeres. Telomeres are the DNA segments or caps at the ends of chromosomes. They are responsible for protecting the end of the DNA from damage. With each replication, the length of the telomeres is shortened. After the telomeres are shortened to a critical

TABLE 124–2. Examples of Oncogenes and Tumor Suppressor Genes

Gene	Function	Associated Human Cancer
Oncogenes		
Genes for growth factors or their receptors		
EGFR or ERB-B1	Codes for epidermal growth factor (EGFR) receptor	Glioblastoma, breast cancer, squamous carcinoma
HER-2/neu or ERB-B2	Codes for a growth factor receptor	Breast, salivary gland, prostate, bladder and ovarian cancers
RET	Codes for a growth factor receptor	Thyroid cancer
Genes for cytoplasmic relays in stimulatory signaling pathways		
K-RAS	Code for guanine nucleotide-proteins with GTPase activity	Lung, ovarian, colon, pancreatic binding cancers
N-RAS		Neuroblastoma, acute leukemia
Genes for transcription factors that activate growth-promoting genes		
c-MYC		Leukemia and breast, colon, gastric, and lung cancers
N-MYC		Neuroblastoma, small cell lung cancer, and glioblastoma
Genes for cytoplasmic kinases		
BCR-ABL	Codes for a nonreceptor tyrosine kinase	Chronic myelogenous leukemia
Genes for other molecules		
BCL-2	Codes for a protein that blocks apoptosis	Indolent B-cell lymphomas
BCL-1 or PRAD1	Codes for cyclin D1, a cell cycle clock stimulator	Breast, head and neck cancers
MDM2	Protein antagonist of p53 tumor suppressor protein	Sarcomas
Tumor suppressor genes		
Genes for proteins in the cytoplasm		
APC	Step in a signaling pathway	Colon and gastric cancer
NF-1	Codes for a protein that inhibits the stimulatory Ras protein	Neurofibroma, leukemia, and pheochromocytoma
NF-2	Codes for a protein that inhibits the stimulatory Ras protein	Meningioma, ependymoma, and schwannoma
Genes for proteins in the nucleus		
MTS1	Codes for p16 protein, a cyclin-dependent kinase inhibitor	Involved in a wide range of cancers
RB1	Codes for the pRB protein, a master brake of the cell cycle	Retinoblastoma, osteosarcoma, and bladder, small cell lung, prostate and breast cancers
p53	Codes for the p53 protein, which can halt cell division and induce apoptosis	Involved in a wide range of cancers
Genes for protein whose cellular location is unclear		
BRCA1	DNA repair, transcriptional regulation	Breast and ovarian cancers
BRCA2	DNA repair	Breast cancer
VHL	Regulator of protein stability	Renal cell cancer
MSH2, MLH1, PMS1, PMS2, MSH6	DNA mismatch repair enzymes	Hereditary nonpolyposis colorectal cancer

Adapted from Liotta et al,[3] Cotran et al,[6] and Weinberg.[9]

length, senescence is triggered. In this way, telomeres tally and limit the number of cell doublings. In cancer cells, the function of telomeres is overcome by overexpression of an enzyme known as telomerase. Telomerase replaces the portion of the telomeres that is lost with each cell division, thereby avoiding senescence and permitting an infinite number of cell doublings. Telomerase is a target for antineoplastic drug development.

As information regarding the role of oncogenes and tumor-suppressor genes accumulated, it became evident that a single mutation is probably not sufficient to initiate cancer.[4–9] Scientists postulate that combinations of mutations are required for carcinogenesis and that each mutation is inherited by the next generation of cells

(Fig. 124–4). Thus, several detectable genetic mutations may be present in an established tumor. Early mutations are found in both premalignant lesions and in established tumors, whereas later mutations are found only in the established tumor. This theory of sequential genetic mutations resulting in cancer has been demonstrated in colon cancer and in brain tumors. In colon cancer, the initial genetic mutation is believed to be loss of the adenomatous polyposis coli gene, which results in formation of a small benign polyp. Oncogenic mutation of the *ras* gene is often the next step, leading to enlargement of the polyp. Loss of function of DNA mismatch repair enzymes may occur at many points in the progression of malignant transformation. Loss of the *p53* gene and another gene, believed to be the "deleted in

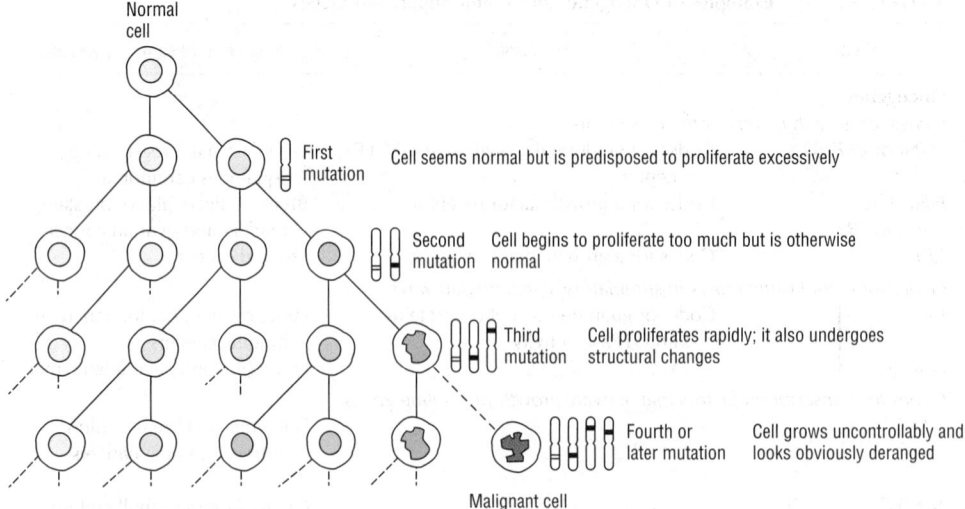

FIGURE 124–4. Emergence of a cancer cell from a normal cell is thought to occur through a process known as clonal evolution. First, one daughter cell inherits or acquires a cancer-promoting mutation and passes the defect to its progeny and all future generations. At some point, one of the descendants acquires a second mutation, and a later descendant acquires a third, and so on. Eventually, some cell accumulates enough mutations to cross the threshold to cancer. *(Reproduced with permission from Cotran et al.[6])*

colorectal cancer" gene, complete the transformation into a malignant lesion. Loss of *p53* is thought to be a late event in the development and progression of the malignancy.

Identification of genes and other proteins involved in carcinogenesis has several important clinical implications. In the future, they may be used in cancer screening to identify individuals at increased risk for cancer, and in cancer treatment to design new anticancer agents and gene therapies. Specific genetic abnormalities are so commonly associated with some types of cancers that the presence of that abnormality aids in the diagnosis of that cancer. If the presence of these genes (i.e., gene expression profile) can reliably predict the clinical course of a cancer or response to certain cancer therapies,

then genetic analysis may also become an important prognostic and treatment decision tool.[13]

PRINCIPLES OF TUMOR GROWTH

The study of tumor growth forms the foundation for many of the basic principles of modern cancer chemotherapy. The growth of most tumors is illustrated by the Gompertzian tumor growth curve (Fig. 124–5).[6,11,14] Gompertz was a German insurance actuary who described the relationship between age and expected death. This mathematical model also approximates tumor-cell proliferation. In the

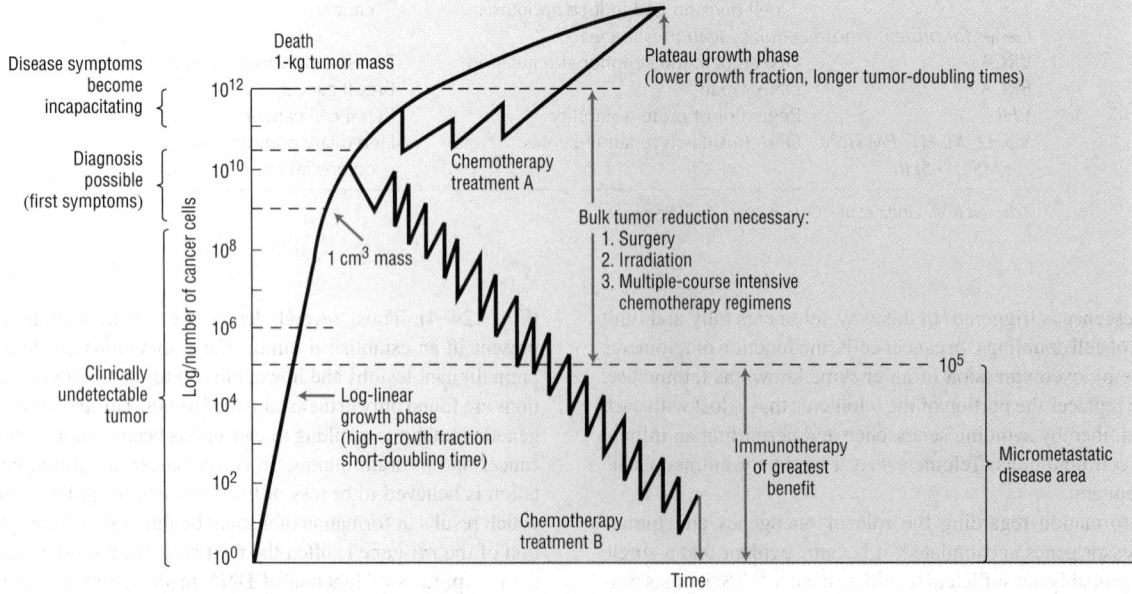

FIGURE 124–5. Gompertzian kinetics tumor-growth curve; relationship to symptoms, diagnosis, and various treatment regimens. *(Reproduced with permission from Buick.[14])*

early stages, tumor growth is exponential, which means that the tumor takes a constant amount of time to double its size. During this early phase, a large portion of the tumor cells is actively dividing. This population of cells is called the *growth fraction*. The doubling time, or time required for the tumor to double in size, is very short. Because most anticancer drugs have greater effect on rapidly dividing cells, tumors are most sensitive to the effects of chemotherapy when the tumor is small and the growth fraction is high. However, as the tumor grows, the doubling time is slowed.[11,14] The growth fraction is decreased, probably owing to the tumor outgrowing its blood and nutrient supply or the inability of blood and nutrients to diffuse throughout the tumor mass. Wide variability exists in measured doubling times for different cancers. The doubling time of most solid tumors is about 2 to 3 months. However, some tumors have doubling times of only days (e.g., aggressive lymphomas) and others have even longer doubling times (e.g., some salivary gland tumors).[6]

Figure 124–5 also illustrates the impact of tumor burden. It takes about 10^9 cancer cells (1-g mass, 1 cm in diameter) for a tumor to be clinically detectable by palpation or radiography. Such a tumor has undergone approximately 30 doublings in cell number. It only takes 10 additional doublings for this 1-g mass to reach 1 kg in size. A tumor possessing 10^{12} cancer cells (1-kg mass) is considered lethal. Thus a tumor is clinically undetectable for most of its life span. Tumor burden also impacts response to chemotherapy. The cell kill hypothesis states that a certain percentage of cancer cells (not a certain number of cells) will be killed with each course of chemotherapy. For example, if a tumor consists of 1,000 cancer cells and the chemotherapy regimen kills 90% of the cells, then 10% or 100 cancer cells would remain. The second chemotherapy course kills another 90% of cells, and again only 10% or 10 cells remain. According to this hypothesis, the tumor burden will never reach zero. Tumors consisting of less than 10^4 cells are believed to be small enough for elimination by host factors, including immunologic mechanisms, and these factors must be in place for a cure to be possible. The limitations of this theory are that it assumes all cancers are equally responsive and that drug resistance and metastases do not occur.[1,6,11,14]

INVASION AND METASTASIS

Metastasis is the spread of neoplastic cells from the primary tumor site to distant sites.[6,15] Despite advances in diagnostic techniques and screening for cancer, many patients have detectable metastatic disease at diagnosis. Once clinically evident distant metastases are present, cancers are seldom curable. Newly diagnosed cancer patients may also have microscopic cancer metastases. Although clinically undetectable, these small clusters of diseased cells must be present, because many patients subsequently relapse at distant sites despite removal of the primary tumor. Some patients with micrometastatic disease may be cured with systemic chemotherapy.

The two primary pathways of metastasis are hematogenous and lymphatic. Other, less-common modes of disease spread include dissemination via cerebrospinal fluid and transabdominal spread within the peritoneal cavity. Tumors are constantly shedding neoplastic cells into the systemic circulation or surrounding lymphatics. This process may begin early in the life of the tumor and often increases with time. The time course for metastasis depends largely on the biology of the tumor. Breast cancer, for example, tends to metastasize very early. Not all of the shed cancer cells, or "seeds," result in a metastatic lesion. The "seed" must first find the appropriate "soil," or an environment suitable for growth.[15] This process is illustrated in the diverse patterns

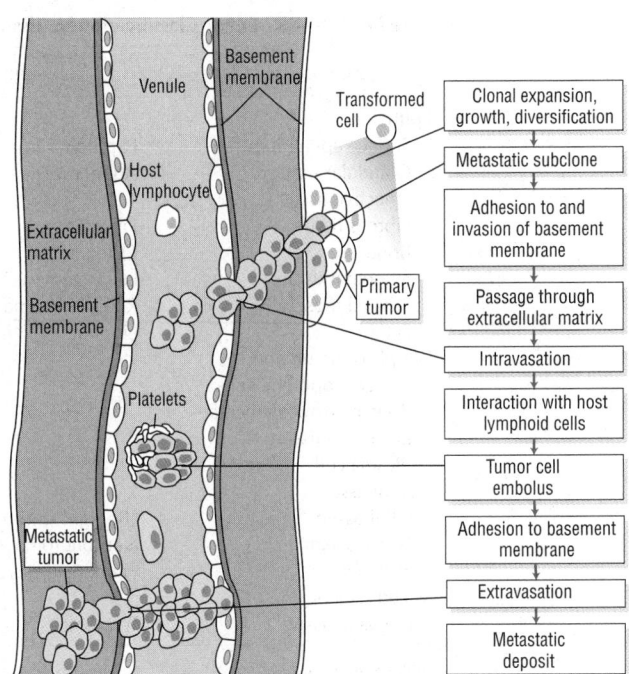

FIGURE 124–6. The process of developing a cancer metastasis. *(Reproduced with permission from Cotran et al.[6])*

of metastasis that are characteristic of individual types of cancer. An example is prostate cancer, which commonly metastasizes to bone, but rarely to the brain.

The process of invasion and metastasis involves several essential steps (Fig. 124–6). After neoplastic transformation, the malignant cells and surrounding host tissue secrete substances that stimulate the formation of new blood vessels to provide oxygen and nutrients. This process is known as *angiogenesis* or *neovascularization*.[16] Tumor cells must then detach from the primary mass and invade surrounding blood and lymph vessels. The tumor cells or cell aggregates detach and embolize through these vessels, but most do not survive circulation. The disseminated cells must then attach to the vascular endothelium. The cells may proliferate within the lumen of the vessel, but most commonly extravasate into the surrounding tissue. The local microenvironment may provide growth factors that can serve as "fertilizer" to potentiate the proliferation of the metastasis. At every step of the way, the potential metastatic cell must fight the host immune system. Last, the metastasis must again initiate angiogenesis to ensure continued growth and proliferation. Because angiogenesis has been recognized as a critical element in primary tumor growth as well as metastasis, it has become a target for development of new anticancer agents.

PATHOLOGY OF CANCER

TUMOR CHARACTERISTICS

Tumors may be either benign or malignant. Benign tumors are noncancerous growths that are often encapsulated, localized, and indolent. Cells of benign tumors resemble the cells from which they developed. These masses seldom metastasize, and once removed they rarely recur. In contrast, malignant tumors invade and destroy the surrounding tissue. The cells of malignant tumors are genetically unstable, and

TABLE 124–3. Tumor Classification by Tissue Type

Tissue of Origin	Benign	Malignant
Epithelial		
Surface epithelium	Papilloma	Carcinoma (squamous, epidermoid)
Glandular tissue	Adenoma	Adenocarcinoma
Connective tissue		
Fibrous tissue	Fibroma	Fibrosarcoma
Bone	Osteoma	Osteosarcoma
Smooth muscle	Leiomyoma	Leiomyosarcoma
Striated muscle	Rhabdomyoma	Rhabdomyosarcoma
Fat	Lipoma	Liposarcoma
Lymphoid tissue and		
hematopoietic cells		
Bone marrow elements		Leukemias
Lymphoid tissue		Hodgkin's and non-Hodgkin's lymphoma
Plasma cell		Multiple myeloma
Neural tissue		
Glial tissue	"Benign" gliomas	Glioblastoma multiforme, astrocytoma
Nerve sheath	Neurofibroma	Neurofibrosarcoma
Melanocytes	Pigmented nevus (mole)	Malignant melanoma
Mixed tumors		
Gonadal tissue	Teratoma	Teratocarcinoma

Adapted from Cotran.[6]

loss of normal cell architecture results in cells that are atypical of their tissue or cell of origin. These cells lose the ability to perform their usual functions. This loss of structure and function is defined as anaplasia. In contrast to benign tumors, malignant tumors tend to metastasize, and consequently recurrences are common after removal or destruction of the primary tumor.

TUMOR ORIGIN

Tumors may arise from any of four basic tissue types: epithelial tissue, connective tissue (i.e., muscle, bone, and cartilage), lymphoid tissue, and nerve tissue. Although some malignant cells are atypical of their cells of origin, the involved cells usually retain enough of their parent's traits to identify their origin. Benign tumors are named by adding the suffix -oma to the name of the cell type. Hence, adenomas are benign growths of glandular origin, or growths that exhibit a glandular pattern. Table 124–3 lists common tumor nomenclature by tissue type.[6]

Some cancers are preceded by cellular changes that are abnormal, but not yet malignant. Correction of these early changes could potentially prevent the occurrence of a cancer. Precancerous lesions may be described as consisting of either hyperplastic or dysplastic cells. Hyperplasia is an increase in the number of cells in a particular tissue or organ, which results in an increased size of the organ. It should not be confused with hypertrophy, which is an increase in the size of the individual cells. Hyperplasia occurs in response to a stimulus and reverses when the stimulus is removed. Dysplasia is defined as an abnormal change in the size, shape, or organization of cells or tissues. Hyperplasia and dysplasia may precede the appearance of a cancer by several months or years.

Malignant cells are divided into those of epithelial origin or the other tissue types. Carcinomas are malignant growths arising from epithelial cells. Malignant growths of muscle or connective tissue are called sarcomas. Therefore an adenocarcinoma is a malignant tumor arising from glandular tissue. Another term used frequently in the description of malignancy is *carcinoma in situ*. In this instance, the cancer is limited to the epithelial cells of origin; it has not yet invaded

the basement membrane. Carcinoma in situ is a preinvasive stage of malignancy, and most tumors have progressed well beyond this stage at diagnosis. Like all classification systems, there are exceptions to these rules. Malignancies of hematologic origin, such as leukemias and lymphomas, are classified separately. Leukemias and lymphomas are discussed in later chapters.

DIAGNOSIS AND STAGING

SCREENING

◀3 Because cancers are most curable with surgery or radiation before they have metastasized, early detection and treatment have obvious potential benefits. In addition, small tumors are more responsive to chemotherapy, as discussed previously. Early diagnosis is difficult for many cancers because they do not produce clinical signs or symptoms until they have become large or have metastasized. Cancer screening programs are designed to detect signs of cancer in people who have not yet developed symptoms from cancer. Lack of effective screening methods for some cancers and inaccessibility of some anatomic sites further complicate the process. Education of the public on the early warning signs of common cancers is extremely important for facilitating early detection. For some cancers, effective screening procedures do exist. The Papanicolaou (Pap) smear test, for example, is an effective tool to detect cervical cancer in its early stages. Self-examination of the breasts in women and of the testicles in men may lead to early diagnosis of cancers in these organs. The American Cancer Society has published guidelines for routine screening examinations (Table 124–4).[17]

DIAGNOSIS

◀4 The presenting signs and symptoms of cancer vary widely and depend on the type of cancer. The presentation in adults may include any of cancer's seven warning signs (Table 124–5), as well as pain or loss of appetite.[18] The warning signs of cancer in

TABLE 124–4. Screening Guidelines for Early Detection of Cancer in Asymptomatic People

Disease	Test or Procedure	Sex	Age (y)	Frequency
Breast cancer	Breast self-examination	F	20 and over	Monthly
	Clinical breast examination	F	20–39	Every 3 years
		40 and over	Every year	
	Mammography	F	40 and over	Every year[a]
Colon and rectal cancer	One of the following examination schedules should be followed:			
	Fecal occult blood test (FOBT) or fecal immunochemical test (FIT)	M and F	50 and over	Every year
	Flexible sigmoidoscopy	M and F	50 and over	Every 5 years
	Annual FOBT or FIT and flexible sigmoidoscopy[b]	M and F	50 and over	Every 5 years
	Colonoscopy	M and F	50 and over	Every 10 years
	Double contrast barium enema	M and F	50 and over	Every 5 years
Prostate cancer	Digital rectal exam and	M	50 and over	Every year[c]
	prostate-specific antigen (PSA) blood test	M	50 and over	Every year[c]
Cervical cancer	Pap test or liquid-based test	F	3 years after beginning vaginal intercourse	Every year[d] Every 2 years
Endometrial cancer	Information on risks and symptoms	F	Menopause	Once[e]
Cancer-related check-up	Health counseling and physical exam[f]	M and F 40 and over	20–40	Every 3 years Every year

[a]Women at increased risk (e.g., family history, genetic tendency, or past breast cancer) should talk with their physician about benefits and limitations of starting earlier, having additional tests, or more frequent examinations.
[b]Flexible sigmoidoscopy together with FOBT or FIT is preferable to either test alone, although annual FOBT/FIT alone and flexible sigmoidoscopy every 5 years without FOBT/FIT has some benefit. People at moderate to high risk for colorectal cancer should discuss a different testing schedule with their physician.
[c]Digital rectal examination and PSA testing should be offered annually to men with a life expectancy of at least 10 years. Men at high risk (e.g., African-American men and men with a strong family history) should begin testing at age 45. Information should be provided regarded benefits and limitations of prostate cancer screening.
[d]At or after age 30, women with three consecutive normal tests may be screened at less frequent intervals (every 2–3 years). Alternatively, HPV DNA testing and conventional or liquid-based testing could be performed every 3 years. Women at high risk (e.g., human immunodeficiency virus infection or weak immune system) may be screened more frequently. Women over the age of 70 years may stop screening if they have three normal tests in the last 10 years.
[e]Women with or at risk for hereditary nonpolyposis colon cancer should begin annual endometrial biopsy starting at age 35.
[f]To include examination for cancers of the mouth, thyroid, testicles, skin, lymph nodes, and ovaries, as well as health counseling about tobacco, sun exposure, diet and nutrition, risk factors, sexual practices, and environmental and occupational exposures. From The American Cancer Society.[17]

children are different, and reflect the types of tumors more common in this patient population (Table 124–6).[18] Even with increased public awareness, the fear of a cancer diagnosis can deter patients from seeking medical attention. The definitive diagnosis of cancer relies on the procurement of a sample of the tissue or cells suspected of malignancy and pathologic assessment of this sample. This sample can be obtained by numerous methods, including biopsy, exfoliative cytology, or fine-needle aspiration. A tissue diagnosis is essential, because many benign conditions can masquerade as cancer. Definitive treatment should not begin without a pathologic diagnosis.

TABLE 124–5. Cancer's Seven Warning Signs

Change in bowel or bladder habits
A sore that does not heal
Unusual bleeding or discharge
Thickening or lump in breast or elsewhere
Indigestion or difficulty in swallowing
Obvious change in wart or mole
Nagging cough or hoarseness
If YOU have a warning signal, see your doctor!

From American Cancer Society. Seven warning signs of cancer. Atlanta, American Cancer Society.

TABLE 124–6. Cancer's Warning Signs in Children

Continued, unexplained weight loss
Headaches with vomiting in the morning
Increased swelling or persistent pain in bones or joints
Lump or mass in abdomen, neck, or elsewhere
Development of a whitish appearance in the pupil of the eye
Recurrent fevers not caused by infections
Excessive bruising or bleeding
Noticeable paleness or prolonged tiredness

From American Cancer Society. Eight warning signs of cancer in children. Atlanta, American Cancer Society.

TABLE 124–7. TNM Staging Classification System for Colorectal Cancer

Primary tumor (T)

T_X Primary tumor cannot be assessed
T_0 No evidence of primary tumor
T_{is} Carcinoma in situ: intraepithelial or invasion of lamina propria
T_1 Tumor invades submucosa
T_2 Tumor invades muscularis propria
T_3 Tumor invades through the muscularis propria into the subserosa, or into nonperitonealized pericolic or perirectal tissues
T_4 Tumor perforates the visceral peritoneum, and/or directly invades other organs or structures

Regional lymph nodes (N)

N_X Regional lymph nodes cannot be assessed
N_0 No regional lymph node metastasis
N_1 Metastasis in one to three pericolic or perirectal lymph nodes
N_2 Metastasis in four or more pericolic or perirectal lymph nodes

Distant metastasis (M)

M_X Presence of distant metastasis cannot be assessed
M_0 No distant metastasis
M_1 Distant metastasis

Stage		Grouping		Dukes	Modified Astler-Collier
Stage 0	T_{is}	N_0	M_0		
Stage I	T_1	N_0	M_0	A	A
	T_2	N_0	M_0	A	B1
Stage IIA	T_3	N_0	M_0	B	B2
Stage IIB	T_4	N_0	M_0	B	B2, B3
Stage IIIA	T_{1-2}	N_1	M_0	C	C1–3
Stage IIIB	T_{3-4}	N_1	M_0	C	C1–3
Stage IIIC	Any T	N_2	M_0	C	C1–3
Stage IV	Any T	Any N	M_0	"D"	D

From Greene et al.[19]

STAGING

In addition to tissue diagnosis, tumors should be staged to determine the extent of disease before any definitive treatment is initiated.[18] The process is dictated by knowledge of the biology of the tumor and by the signs and symptoms elicited in the history and physical examination. Staging provides information on prognosis and guides treatment selection. After treatment is implemented, the staging work-up is usually repeated to evaluate the effectiveness of the treatment. Uniform staging criteria are imperative in clinical research aimed at evaluating cancer treatment regimens. Staging has been valuable in learning more about the biology of various tumor types. A staging work-up may involve x-rays, computed tomography scans, magnetic resonance imaging, ultrasounds, bone-marrow biopsies, bone scans, lumbar puncture, and a variety of laboratory tests, including appropriate tumor markers. Some cancers produce antigens or other substances that are characteristic of that particular cancer. These so-called tumor markers are often nonspecific and may be elevated in many different cancer types, or in patients with nonmalignant diseases. As a result, tumor markers are generally more useful for monitoring response and detecting recurrence than as diagnostic tools. Examples are the measure of human chorionic gonadotropin and

α-fetoprotein in patients with testicular cancer, or prostate-specific antigen in prostate cancer.[6]

The most commonly applied staging system for solid tumors is the TNM classification, where T = tumor, N = node, and M = metastases. A numerical value is assigned to each letter to indicate the size or extent of disease. The designated rating for tumor describes the size of the primary mass and ranges from T_1 to T_4. Carcinoma in situ is designated T_{is}. Nodes are described in terms of the extent and quality of nodal involvement (N_0 to N_3). Metastases are generally scored depending on their presence or absence (M_0 or M_1). To simplify the staging process, most cancers are classified according to the extent of disease by a numerical system involving stages I through IV. Stage I usually indicates localized tumor, stages II and III represent local and regional extension of disease, and stage IV denotes the presence of distant metastases. The assigned TNM rating translates into a particular stage classification. For example, $T_3N_1M_0$ describes a moderate- to large-sized primary mass, with regional lymph node involvement and no distant metastases, and for most cancers is stage III. The criteria for classifying disease extent are quite specific for each different type of cancer. For some tumors, alternative alphabetical systems (stage A, B, C, or D) are used in clinical practice. Table 124–7 provides an example of the staging system for colorectal cancer.[19]

▶ TREATMENT: Modalities of Cancer Treatment

Four primary modalities are employed in the approach to cancer treatment: surgery, radiation, chemotherapy, and biologic therapy.[20] The oldest of these is surgery, which plays a major role in the diagnosis and treatment of cancer. Surgery remains the treatment

of choice for most solid tumors diagnosed in the early stages. Radiation therapy was first used for cancer treatment in the late 1800s and remains a mainstay in the management of cancer. Although very effective for treating many types of cancer, surgery and radiation are local treatments. These modalities are likely to produce a cure in patients with truly localized disease. But because most patients with cancer have metastatic disease at diagnosis, localized therapies often fail to completely eliminate the cancer. In addition, systemic diseases such as leukemia cannot be treated with a localized modality. Chemotherapy (including hormonal therapy) accesses the systemic circulation and can theoretically treat the primary tumor and any metastatic disease. Biologic therapies are currently considered in the broader sense of "biologically directed" therapies. Immunotherapy, the earliest important form of biologic therapy, usually involves stimulating the host's immune system to fight the cancer. The agents used in immunotherapy are usually naturally occurring cytokines, which have been produced with recombinant DNA technology. Examples of agents used in immunotherapy include interferons (IFNs) and interleukins (ILs). Biologically directed therapies include monoclonal antibodies, other targeted therapies such as tyrosine kinase inhibitors or proteosome inhibitors, and tumor vaccines.

5 Many cancers appear to be eliminated by surgery or radiation. However, the high incidence of later recurrence implies that the primary tumor began to metastasize before it was removed. These early metastases are too small to detect with currently available diagnostic tests and are known as micrometastases. Adjuvant therapy is defined as the use of systemic agents to eradicate micrometastatic

disease following localized modalities such as surgery or radiation or both. The goal of systemic therapy given in this setting is to reduce subsequent recurrence rates and prolong long-term survival. Thus adjuvant therapy is given to patients with potentially curable malignancies who have no clinically detectable disease after surgery or radiation. Because adjuvant therapy is given at a time that the cancer is undetectable, its effectiveness cannot be measured by response rates; instead it is evaluated by recurrence rates and survival. The value of adjuvant therapy is best established in colorectal and breast cancers. Chemotherapy may also be given in the neoadjuvant or preoperative setting. The goals in this instance are to make other treatment modalities more effective by reducing tumor burden and to destroy micrometastases. For example, in head and neck cancer, neoadjuvant chemotherapy is employed in an attempt to shrink large tumors and to make them more amenable to later surgical resection, and possibly spare critical organs, such as the larynx.

The management of most types of cancer involves the use of combined modalities. Early stage breast cancer is a good example of the use of a combined-modality approach. The primary tumor is removed surgically, and radiation therapy is delivered to the remaining breast (after lumpectomy) or to the axilla (if there is marked lymph node involvement). Adjuvant chemotherapy and/or hormonal therapy is then administered to eradicate any micrometastatic disease.

► TREATMENT: Principles of Chemotherapy

PURPOSES OF CHEMOTHERAPY

4 The era of modern cancer chemotherapy was born in 1941, when Goodman and Gilman first administered nitrogen mustard to patients with lymphoma.[21] Since that time, numerous antineoplastic agents have been developed, and a variety of chemotherapy regimens have been investigated in every type of cancer. Table 124–8 lists tumors and their responsiveness to chemotherapy.[14,22] Cancer chemotherapy may be indicated as a primary, palliative, adjuvant, or neoadjuvant treatment modality. Treatment with cytotoxic drugs is the primary curative modality for a few diseases, including leukemias, lymphomas, choriocarcinomas, and testicular cancer. Most solid tumors are not curable with chemotherapy alone, either because of the biology of the tumor or because of advanced disease at presentation. Chemotherapy in this setting is often initiated for palliative purposes. It is often possible to decrease tumor size or to retard growth enough to reduce untoward symptoms caused by the tumor. Adjuvant and neoadjuvant chemotherapy are defined in the previous section.

RESPONSE CRITERIA

5 The response to chemotherapy and other treatment modalities may be described as a cure, complete response, partial response, stable disease, or progression.[22,23] These terms are used routinely in oncology to define the response to chemotherapy and other treatment modalities. A cure implies that the patient is entirely free of disease and has the same life expectancy as a cancer-free individual. Although there is no way to be absolutely certain that an individual patient is cured, a stable plateau in the survival curve after cancer treatment is taken as evidence of cure. For most cancers, the survival curves have plateaued by about 5 years. Thus 5 years of survival without

disease recurrence is often equated with a cure. However, there are some malignancies, such as breast cancer and melanoma for example, in which patients are still at significant risk for relapse after 5 years.

Complete response (CR) means complete disappearance of all cancer without evidence of new disease for at least 1 month after treatment. The terms "cure" and "CR" are not synonymous. Although an individual must have a CR to be cured, many individuals who achieve a CR will eventually relapse. A *partial response* (PR) is defined as a 50% or greater decrease in the tumor size or other objective disease markers, and no evidence of any new disease for at least 1 month. Overall objective response rates for a given treatment are determined by adding the CR and PR rates. Despite the small changes in tumor size, some patients may experience subjective improvement in the symptoms caused by their cancer. Although clinically important, this does not indicate an objective response. The term *clinical benefit response* was recently coined; it refers to patients who have clinical benefit as measured by decreases in pain or analgesic consumption, or improved quality of life or performance status. A patient whose tumor size neither grows nor shrinks by more than 25% has stable disease. Progression of disease is defined as a 25% increase in the tumor size or the development of any new lesions while receiving treatment. These response definitions are applicable to solid tumors, but diseases such as leukemias and multiple myeloma are not characterized by discrete, measurable masses. Responses in these diseases are measured by elimination of abnormal cells (e.g., return to normal hematology parameters and normal bone marrow in leukemia), return of tumor markers to normal levels (e.g., normal serum protein electrophoresis in multiple myeloma), disappearance of pleural or peritoneal effusions, or improved function of affected organs (e.g., improved renal function after obstructive uropathy). Cytogenetic markers and molecular techniques have an increasingly important role in determining whether all cancer has been truly eliminated. For example, in chronic myelogenous leukemia, the Philadelphia chromosome [a (9:22) chromosomal translocation resulting in the *bcr-abl* gene] can be detected

TABLE 124–8. The Role of Chemotherapy in the Treatment of Cancer

Chemotherapy used alone with curative intent

Acute lymphocytic leukemia	Acute nonlymphocytic (myelogenous) leukemia
Burkitt's lymphoma	Diffuse large cell lymphoma
Hodgkin's lymphoma	Testicular cancer
Choriocarcinoma (gestational trophoblastic neoplasm)	

Chemotherapy used as adjuvant therapy with curative intent

Breast cancer	Colorectal cancer
Ewing's sarcoma	Osteosarcoma
Wilms' tumor	Ovarian cancer

Chemotherapy used as neoadjuvant therapy

Anal carcinoma[a]	Bladder cancer
Breast cancer (locally advanced)[a]	Cervical cancer
Esophageal cancer	Head and neck cancers[a]
Osteosarcoma[a]	Rectal cancer
Soft tissue sarcoma[a]	

Chemotherapy used to palliate symptoms in advanced disease

Bladder cancer[a]	Brain tumors
Breast cancer[a]	Carcinoid tumors
Cervical cancer	Chronic lymphocytic leukemia
Chronic myelogenous leukemia[a]	Colorectal cancer
Endometrial cancer	Esophageal cancer
Gastric cancer	Head and neck cancers
Hairy cell leukemia[a]	Kaposi's sarcoma
Indolent lymphomas	Metastatic melanoma
Multiple myeloma[a]	Mycosis fungoides
Neuroblastoma[a]	Non-small-cell lung cancer
Osteosarcoma	Ovarian cancer[a]
Pancreatic cancer	Prostate cancer
Small cell lung cancer[a]	Soft tissue sarcoma

Chemotherapy has little or no effect on palliation

Hepatocellular cancer	Renal cell carcinoma
Thyroid cancer	

[a]Significant increase in survival is achieved.
Adapted from Cotran et al,[6] Buick,[14] and Haskell.[22]

by polymerase chain reaction techniques, even when no leukemia is evident in the bone marrow or bloodstream. Patients without evidence of the Philadelphia chromosome are classified as a complete cytogenetic response.

FACTORS AFFECTING RESPONSE TO CHEMOTHERAPY

◀6   These include tumor burden, tumor-cell heterogeneity, drug resistance, dose intensity, and patient-specific factors. The significance of tumor burden has been discussed earlier. Tumors consist of a heterogeneous population of cell types. Because of the genetic instability of cancer cells compared to normal cells, mutations commonly occur during cell division. Large tumors have undergone many cell divisions and express multiple cell mutations resulting in genetically varied cell populations.[6,14,22] In 1979, Goldie and Coldman proposed that these cytogenetic changes were not completely random and were highly associated with the development of the ability of tumors to resist drug action.[1,6,14] The probability of developing resistant cell populations increases as tumor size increases. It is believed that a small percentage of resistant cancer cells may survive initial chemotherapy. Resistant populations later proliferate and eventually become the dominant cell types. This explains the common pattern of an initial response to chemotherapy, followed by progressive tumor regrowth despite continuing the same treatment regimen.

Drug resistance may be either an acquired or inherited property of a neoplastic cell. Mechanisms of drug resistance include decreased activation of prodrugs, decreased uptake of drugs secondary to alterations in drug transport systems, changes in target enzymes, alterations in the cell's ability to repair drug-induced damage, increased drug inactivation, and decreased apoptosis.[6,12,14,20] One focus of research in this area is pleiotropic drug resistance or multidrug resistance.[14,20,24,25] When some cancer cells are exposed to increasing concentrations of a specific antineoplastic agent in vitro, they become resistant to that agent. Surprisingly, these same cells also become resistant to other structurally unrelated antineoplastic agents; that is, they are multidrug resistant. Cytotoxic agents derived from natural products, such as the anthracyclines, actinomycin D, mitomycin C, the vinca alkaloids, the epipodophyllotoxins, and the taxanes, produce multidrug resistance. The resistant cancer cells possess a membrane-associated protein known as P170 or P-glycoprotein, which appears to enhance the export of toxins, such as chemotherapy agents, out of the cell (Fig. 124–7). The gene that encodes for P-glycoprotein is known as the *mdr-1* gene. Expression of this gene is amplified in cells that are resistant to the natural products listed previously. P-glycoprotein is also found in high concentrations in tumors that are traditionally resistant to chemotherapy (e.g., renal cell and non-small-cell lung cancers) and thus may also be an important mechanism of intrinsic or inherited drug resistance. Several drugs have been investigated as possible inhibitors of this efflux pump, such as the calcium channel blockers, quinidine, cyclosporine, and the phenothiazines. Another

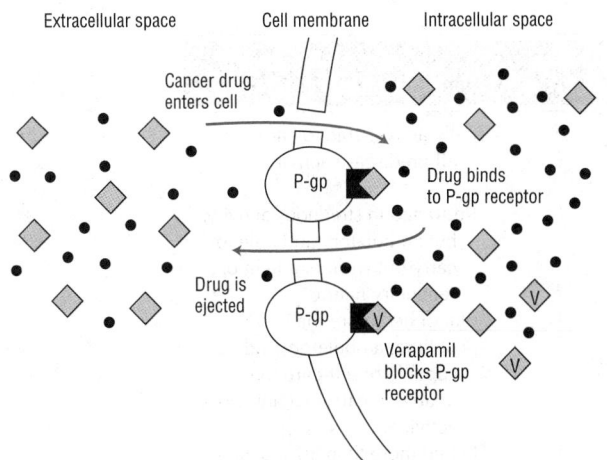

FIGURE 124–7. P-glycoprotein (P-gp) is a membrane-associated protein that acts as a drug efflux pump. Anticancer agents enter the cell, bind to the P-gp receptor, and are ejected. Some agents that modify multidrug resistance, like verapamil, block the P-gp receptor, allowing the anticancer agent to remain in the cell.

efflux pump, known as the multidrug resistance–associated protein, was also recently identified. Other potential mechanisms of drug resistance include inactivation of chemotherapy agents by glutathione metabolism, upregulation of target enzymes such as topoisomerases or dihydrofolate reductase, and decreased apoptosis after exposure to chemotherapy.[24] The last mechanism can be mediated by *bcl-2* oncogene overexpression or loss of the *p53* gene, as discussed in the oncogene section. The interplay between apoptosis and drug resistance is an area of intense research.[12]

The relationship between dose and response has been extensively explored in cancer chemotherapy. Dose is believed to be a critical factor in determining response for many types of cancers. Dose intensity is defined as the dose delivered to the patient over a specified period of time.[1,26,27] The three main variables that determine delivered dose intensity are the dose per course, the interval between doses, and the total cumulative dose. Dose density refers to shortening of the usual interval between doses (e.g., every 2 weeks instead of every 3 weeks) and is designed to maximize the drugs' effects on tumor growth kinetics. This strategy has been most extensively studied in breast cancer, with positive results in adjuvant therapy of patients with high-risk node-positive disease. The delivery of optimal dose intensity is often compromised by the toxicities of the oncologic drugs. Treatment cycles are commonly delayed because of inadequate recovery from drug toxicity, especially myelosuppression. Subsequent doses of chemotherapy are often reduced to prevent or reduce the severity of these toxicities. The impact of this issue on patient outcome has been proven in studies showing reduced rates of response and survival in individuals receiving less-than-optimal chemotherapy doses.[26] Understanding the pathophysiology of drug-induced toxicities has led to the development of more effective agents for prevention and management of these toxicities. The development of drug- and toxicity-specific chemoprotective agents has facilitated application of dose-intensity principles.[28] The colony-stimulating factors avert neutropenia and permit delivery of dose-intensive or dose-dense regimens that are usually dose-compromised by neutropenia. The issue of dose intensity is brought into a new light in the era of high-dose chemotherapy with autologous hematopoietic stem cell support. Although lethal myelosuppression is avoided by administering hematopoietic stem cells, other severe end-organ toxicities emerge as antineoplastic doses are increased.

Patient-specific factors create unpredictable variability in response to chemotherapy. The biology of cancer is strongly affected by host characteristics and genetics. The pathway of genetic mutations that resulted in malignancy can also affect response to therapy. For example, breast cancers that overexpress the *HER-2/neu* (*EGFR-2*) oncogene are often refractory to regimens like CMF (cyclophosphamide, methotrexate, and 5-fluorouracil), but sensitive to anthracycline-based regimens.[29] Likewise, patients with EGFR mutations that result in enhanced tyrosine kinase activity are more likely to respond to the tyrosine kinase inhibitor gefitinib.[30] Interindividual variations in drug absorption, disposition, elimination, or metabolism may lead to sub- or supratherapeutic levels of antineoplastic agents and their metabolites.[31,32] As a result, both drug efficacy and drug toxicity can be affected. Until recently, health professionals in oncology have focused on dose modification based on variation in body size, blood counts, and renal and hepatic function. Prospective dose modifications based on these parameters are still very important to optimize the effectiveness of therapy and minimize toxicity. But recently, more specific tools are becoming available, as we learn how to identify and apply differences in people's genetic make-up to their cancer drug therapy. The study of the role of inheritance in individual variation in drug response is known as *pharmacogenomics*. In oncology, several clinically relevant genetic polymorphisms, or variations, have been identified that can affect drug pharmacokinetics and pharmacodynamics. Examples include polymorphisms in genes responsible for production of the enzymes dihydropyrimidine dehydrogenase (responsible for 5-fluorouracil metabolism), thiopurine S-methyltransferase (responsible for thiopurine metabolism), and uridine diphosphate-glucuronosyltransferase 1A1 (responsible for irinotecan metabolism). Patients with deficiencies in these enzymes can experience significant and possibly life-threatening toxicity. Screening for these genetic abnormalities will permit individualization of regimens to avoid toxicity and maximize antitumor effects. Monitoring of antineoplastic drug concentrations may also improve the therapeutic index.[33] Pharmacokinetic and pharmacodynamic modeling is associated with improved responses and decreased toxicity in children with acute lymphoblastic leukemia.[34]

The presence of other disease states may also affect response to treatment by limiting treatment options. The overall functional status of a patient may be assessed using performance status scales, such as the Karnofsky and Eastern Cooperative Oncology Group scales (Table 124–9).[23] These scales can be used to predict patient tolerance of chemotherapy, as well as to assess the effects of chemotherapy on the patient's level of activity and quality of life. In many cancers, performance status at diagnosis is the most important prognostic indicator.

Today's oncology clinician has a wealth of information to consider when designing a treatment approach for an individual patient. Patient-specific factors (e.g., performance status, comorbidities, renal and hepatic function, and pharmacogenomics), tumor-specific factors (e.g., pathology, stage, and molecular profile), and treatment goals (e.g., palliation and cure) are all considered when determining the best treatment option.

COMBINATION CHEMOTHERAPY

Although single-agent therapy is sometimes employed, the more common approach to chemotherapy involves administration of multiple agents.[1,21,23] This approach is based on the Goldie-Coldman hypothesis, which addresses the issue of tumor cell heterogeneity and the inevitable development of drug resistance. Combination chemotherapy is employed to target as many types of cells in the tumor as possible.

TABLE 124–9. Performance Status Scales

Description: Karnofsky Scale	Karnofsky Scale (%)	Zubrod Scale (ECOG)	Description: ECOG Scale
No complaints; no evidence of disease	100	0	Fully active, able to carry on all predisease activity
Able to carry on normal activity; minor signs or symptoms of disease	90		
Normal activity with effort, some signs or symptoms of disease	80	1	Restricted in strenuous activity, but ambulatory and able to carry out work of a light or sedentary nature
Cares for self; unable to carry on normal activity or to do active work	70		
Requires occasional assistance but is able to care for most personal needs	60	2	Out of bed more than 50% of time; ambulatory and capable of self-care, but unable to carry out any work activities
Requires considerable assistance and frequent medical care	50		
Disabled; requires special care and assistance	40	3	In bed more than 50% of time; capable of only limited self-care
Severely disabled; hospitalization indicated, although death not imminent	30		
Very sick; hospitalization necessary; requires active supportive treatment	20	4	Bedridden; cannot carry out any self-care; completely disabled
Moribund; fatal processes progressing rapidly	10		
Dead	0		

ECOG, Eastern Cooperative Oncology Group.
Adapted from Haskell.[22]

Selection of agents for combination chemotherapy regimens involves consideration of drug-specific factors such as mechanism of action, antitumor activity, and toxicity profile. Drugs that possess minimally overlapping mechanisms of action and toxicities are combined, when possible. Myelosuppressive combinations are sometimes alternated with nonmyelosuppressive combinations to allow bone marrow recovery, while gaining additive antitumor effects. The selected agents should each have significant activity against the tumor that is to be treated. If a synergistic reaction is known to exist for two agents, they may be combined in various treatment regimens. Development of more specifically targeted agents may decrease the need for combining multiple agents.

CELL CYCLE

Both cancer cells and normal cells reproduce in a series of steps known as the cell cycle. Figure 124–8 depicts the cell cycle and the phases of activity for commonly used antineoplastic agents.[11,14] The first phase is mitosis (M). Mitosis lasts for approximately 30 to 60 minutes and during this phase, cell division occurs. After mitosis, the cell might enter a dormant phase (G_0), or might proceed to the first gap phase (G_1). G_0 is the largest variable in the cell cycle, and during this resting phase, the cell is not actively committed to cell division. Some stimulus results in the cell entering the first gap phase (G_1). During G_1, the cell prepares for DNA synthesis by manufacturing necessary enzymes. DNA synthesis (S) occurs next, and this phase lasts 10 to 20 hours. The percentage of cells in the S phase can be measured by flow cytometry and is an indicator of the rate of tumor-cell proliferation. Tumors with a high percentage of S-phase cells are aggressively growing. The synthesis phase is followed by a second gap or premitotic phase (G_2), lasting 2 to 10 hours. During this second gap, the cell prepares for mitosis by producing ribonucleic acid (RNA) and specialized proteins, as well as the mitotic spindle apparatus. The cycle then begins again with the M phase. Most normal human cells exist in the G_0 phase, and most cancer cells are not sensitive to the effects of chemotherapy when in this stage. The cell cycle is regulated by external mitogens, including cytokines, hormones, and growth factors. As mentioned earlier, some of the genes that regulate the cell cycle are known to be protooncogenes and tumor-suppressor genes.

All cancer cells do not proliferate faster than normal cells; some cancer cells reproduce more rapidly, and others are more indolent. Many anticancer drugs target rapidly-proliferating cells (both normal and cancerous cells), and these agents may act at selective or multiple sites of the cell cycle. Agents with major activity in a particular phase of the cell cycle are known as cell-cycle phase–specific agents. The antimetabolites exert their major effect during the S phase. Cell-cycle phase–specific agents may also be active to a lesser extent in other phases of the cycle. Cell-cycle phase–nonspecific agents are those with significant activity in multiple phases. The alkylating agents such as nitrogen mustard are examples. In many cases, the cytotoxic effects of a drug may result from interactions with other intracellular activities and are not related to specific cell-cycle events. Hormones are an example of this type of drug.

Knowledge of cell-cycle specificity has been applied to the scheduling of chemotherapy administration. By definition, phase-specific agents exert their major activity when cells are in a particular phase of the cell cycle. At any given time, the heterogeneous cell populations within a tumor are at various phases in the cell cycle. By giving phase-specific agents as a continuous infusion or in multiple repeated fractions, it is theoretically possible to target more cells as they progress into the drug-sensitive phase. Thus phase-specific

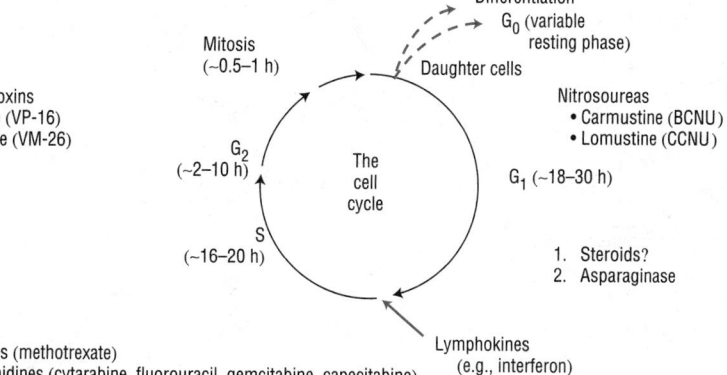

1. Vinca alkaloids
   • Vincristine, vinblastine, vinorelbine
2. Taxanes
   • Paclitaxel, docetaxel

1. Bleomycin
2. Podophyllotoxins
   • Etoposide (VP-16)
   • Teniposide (VM-26)

Differentiation
G_0 (variable resting phase)
Daughter cells

Mitosis (~0.5–1 h)

G_2 (~2–10 h)

The cell cycle

S (~16–20 h)

G_1 (~18–30 h)

Nitrosoureas
   • Carmustine (BCNU)
   • Lomustine (CCNU)

1. Steroids?
2. Asparaginase

Cell cycle phase–nonspecific agents
1. Classic alkylating agents (mechlorethamine, melphalan, busulfan, chlorambucil, cyclophosphamide, ifosfamide)
2. Anthracycline antibiotics (doxorubicin, daunorubicin, idarubicin)
3. Miscellaneous (dacarbazine, cisplatin, carboplatin)
4. Nitrosoureas (also G_0)
5. Mitomycin C
6. Dactinomycin

Antimetabolites
1. Antifolates (methotrexate)
2. Antipyrimidines (cytarabine, fluorouracil, gemcitabine, capecitabine)
3. Antipurines (mercaptopurine, thioguanine, fludarabine, chlorodeoxyadenosine)
4. Miscellaneous (hydroxyurea, procarbazine)
5. Steroids? (also G_1)

Lymphokines (e.g., interferon)

FIGURE 124–8. Cell cycle activity for anticancer drugs. Cell cycle phase-specific agents appear to be most active during a particular phase, but may also be active in another phase. Cell cycle phase-nonspecific agents may have greater activity in one phase than another, but not to the degree of cell cycle (phase)-specific agents. In many cases, it is likely that drug cytotoxicity involves multiple intracellular sites of action and may not be linked to specific cell-cycle events.

agents are also termed *schedule dependent*. In contrast, cell-cycle phase–nonspecific drugs are active in many phases, and consequently are not schedule dependent. The activity of this group of drugs is dependent on the magnitude of the dose, and these drugs are termed *dose dependent*.

MOLECULAR BIOLOGY

Because many antineoplastic agents interfere with the cellular synthesis of DNA, RNA, and proteins, it is important to review the basic principles of molecular biology.[3,35] Each normal human cell contains 46 chromosomes, which are composed of DNA (deoxyribonucleic acid; Fig. 124–9). DNA carries hereditary information in units called genes. A single chromosome can contain 20,000 or more genes. Genes code for specific proteins that regulate cellular activity and inherited traits (some of which affect carcinogenesis and cancer growth, as well as the efficacy and metabolism of anticancer drugs). The genetic information is encoded in DNA by precise sequencing of subunits known as nucleotides. Each nucleotide consists of a sugar (deoxyribose), phosphoric acid, and a base. Four bases exist in DNA: adenine, thymine, guanine, and cytosine. Adenine and guanine are purine-type bases; thymine and cytosine are pyrimidine-type bases (Fig. 124–10). These nucleotides are connected linearly to form a chain. Each DNA molecule is made up of two chains of nucleotides, which wind around each other to form a double helix (see Fig. 124–9). The two strands are held together by chemical bonding between the bases. The bonding process is very specific; adenine binds only with thymine, and guanine binds only with cytosine. This is known as complementary base pairing. RNA (ribonucleic acid) is important in the DNA-directed synthesis of proteins or enzymes. RNA differs from DNA in that it is composed of a single strand of nucleotides, the sugar is ribose, and the base uracil is substituted for thymine. There are three known

types of RNA: messenger RNA (mRNA), transfer RNA (tRNA), and ribosomal RNA (rRNA).

DNA SYNTHESIS

During the DNA synthesis phase, which takes place in the cell nucleus, the DNA unwinds and exposes its nucleotides. When DNA unwinds for replication or protein synthesis, only the portion of the molecule containing the needed nucleotides needs to be exposed. Rather than unwinding the entire strand, topoisomerase I and II enzymes cleave the DNA strands to facilitate unwinding of the section that is needed. The enzyme DNA polymerase matches free complementary nucleotides from the environment to the exposed nucleotides of the DNA (see Fig. 124–9). The newly created strands rewind, resulting in two complete double helices. The topoisomerase enzymes are also responsible for resealing the cleaved DNA strands.

PROTEIN SYNTHESIS

The synthesis of proteins is a more complex process (Fig. 124–11). Proteins consist of chains of amino acids in very specific sequences. As in DNA synthesis, the double helix must unwind. However, in protein synthesis, only the portion of the DNA molecule that codes for the desired protein is exposed. The enzyme RNA polymerase matches free complementary RNA nucleotides to the exposed DNA nucleotides, and the resultant chain of nucleotides is called mRNA. This process is called transcription. The mRNA travels to ribosomes in the cytoplasm, where protein synthesis occurs. Each three nucleotides of the mRNA chain compose a codon, whose sequence is specific for a particular amino acid. The codon is recognized by tRNA, which then carries the amino acid to the ribosome, where it is added to the growing peptide chain. This process is known as translation. The

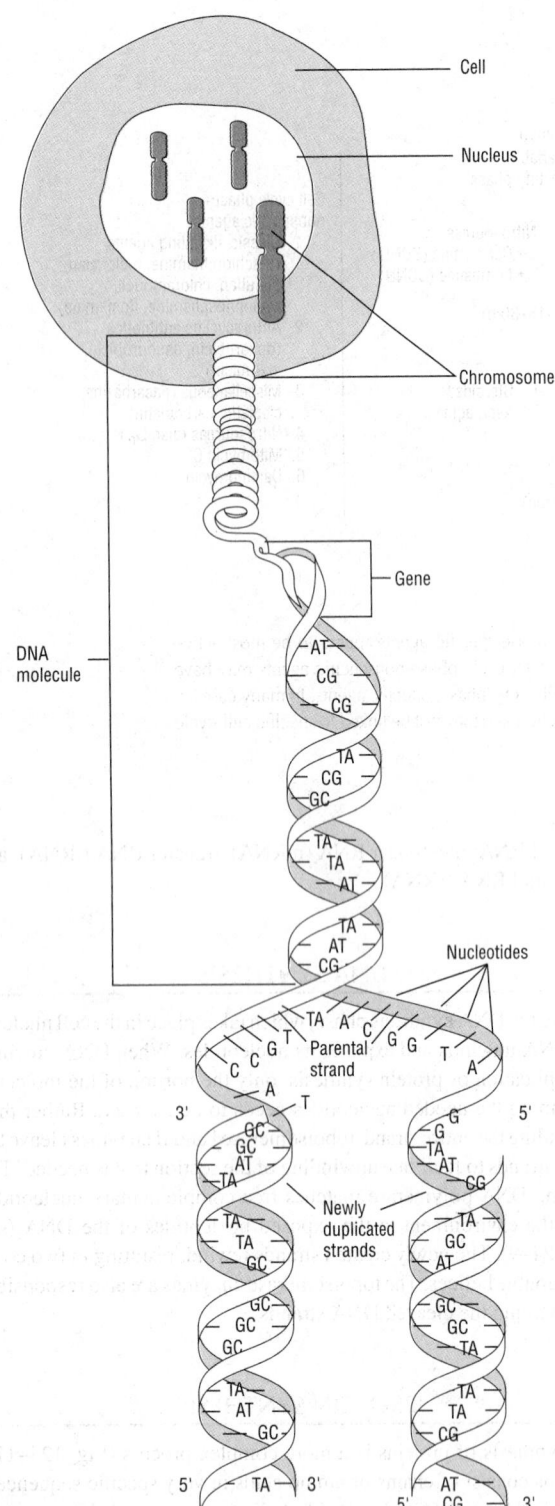

FIGURE 124–9. Structure and function of DNA. Within the cellular nucleus, tightly coiled strands of DNA are packaged in units called chromosomes. Working subunits of chromosomes are called genes. During DNA replication, the double-stranded DNA helix unwinds, exposing individual nucleotides. Complementary nucleotides are retrieved and assembled by DNA polymerases to form new strands of DNA.

Bases

Adenine (A)

Thymine (T)

Guanine (G)

Cytosine (C)

FIGURE 124–10. Structures of DNA constituents.

completed protein is then ready for its intended use as an enzyme or as a structural component.

CLINICAL PHARMACOLOGY OF ANTICANCER AGENTS

Agents used in cancer chemotherapy are commonly categorized by their mechanism of action or by their origin. The alkylating agents exert their effects on DNA and protein synthesis by binding to DNA and preventing the unwinding of the DNA molecule. The antimetabolites resemble naturally occurring nuclear structural components ("metabolites"), such as the nucleotide bases, or inhibit enzymes involved in the synthesis of DNA and proteins. Antitumor antibiotics gain their name from their source; they are fermentation products of *Streptomyces* species. Figure 124–12 shows the sites of action of common categories of antineoplastic agents. The following section addresses these and other classes of agents used in the treatment of cancer. The clinical uses, mechanisms, side effects, and practical patient management suggestions for commonly used agents in each class are detailed in the accompanying tables. Unless otherwise indicated, information included in the tables is derived from FDA-approved drug labeling for individual agents. Dose modifications of individual agents are summarized in Table 124–10.

ANTIMETABOLITES

FLUORINATED PYRIMIDINES

Fluorouracil

Fluorouracil (5-FU) is a fluorinated analog of the naturally occurring pyrimidine uracil, originally synthesized in the late 1950s (Table 124–11). It is a prodrug and must be metabolized to the nucleotide form, fluorodeoxyuridine monophosphate (FdUMP), to be active. In the presence of folates, FdUMP binds tightly to and interferes with

Nucleus
Cytoplasm
DNA
Gene
Nucleotides
mRNA
tRNA
AA
Chain of amino acids forms protein
AA AA AA AA
Ribosome
mRNA

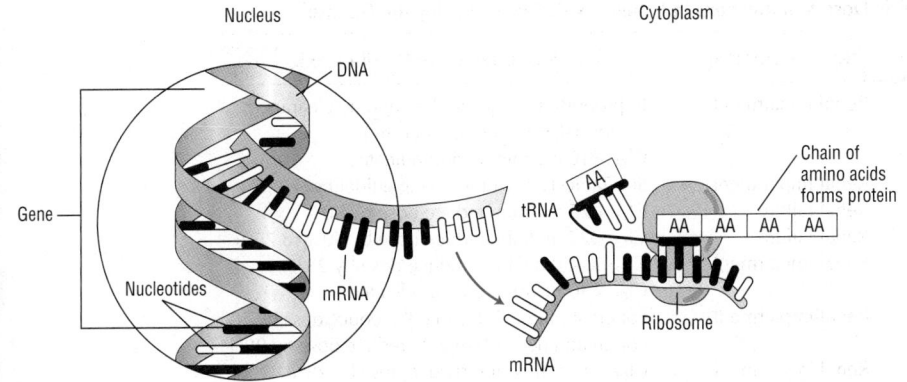

FIGURE 124–11. Protein synthesis. When a specific protein is needed, the portion of DNA responsible for that protein unwinds, exposing the necessary nucleotide sequence. Complementary nucleotides are assembled to form messenger RNA (mRNA), which travels to ribosomes in the cytoplasm. There, transfer RNA (tRNA) matches amino acids to the nucleotide sequence on the mRNA. The amino acids are assembled to form proteins.

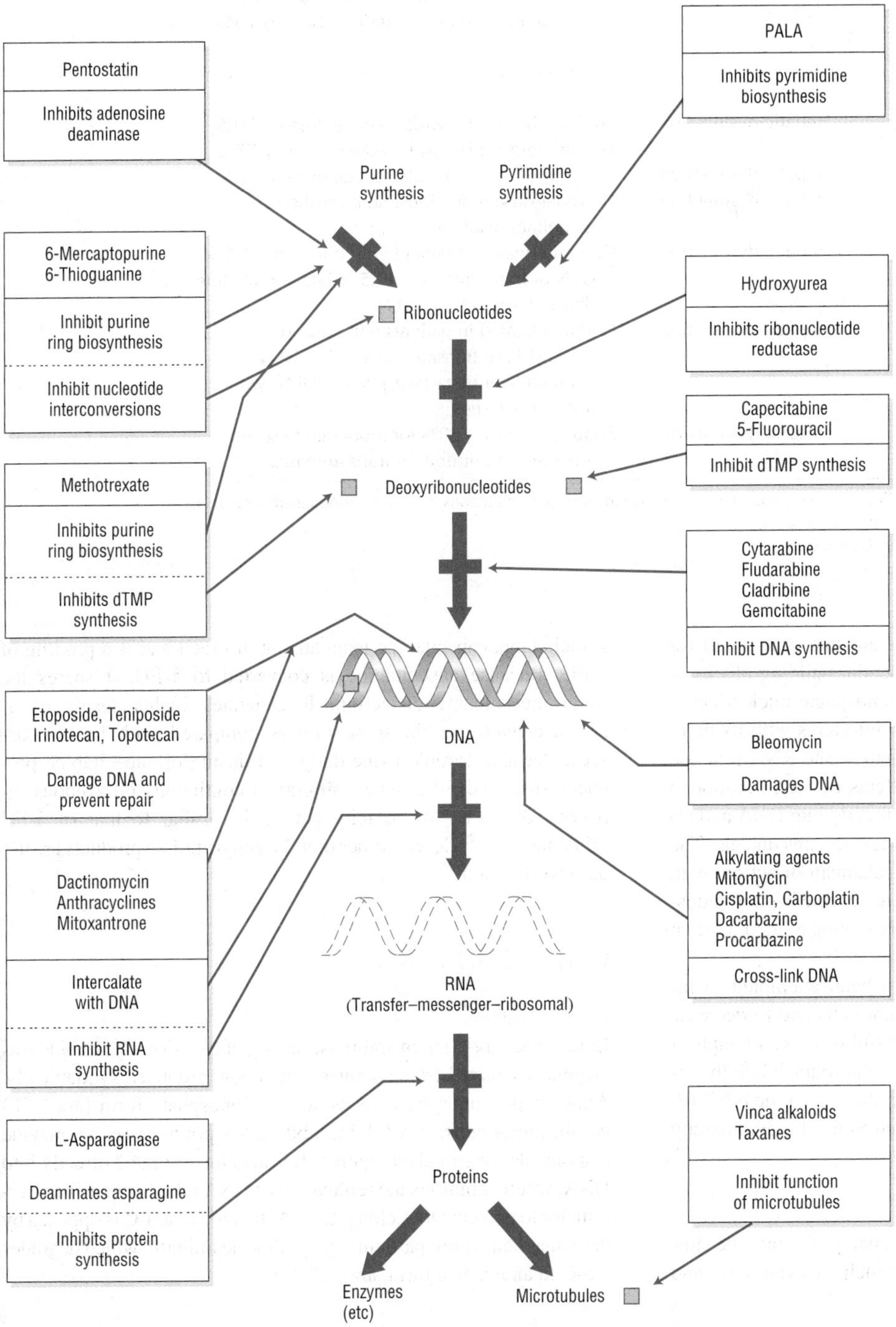

Pentostatin
Inhibits adenosine deaminase
6-Mercaptopurine
6-Thioguanine
Inhibit purine ring biosynthesis
Inhibit nucleotide interconversions
Methotrexate
Inhibits purine ring biosynthesis
Inhibits dTMP synthesis
Etoposide, Teniposide
Irinotecan, Topotecan
Damage DNA and prevent repair
Dactinomycin
Anthracyclines
Mitoxantrone
Intercalate with DNA
Inhibit RNA synthesis
L-Asparaginase
Deaminates asparagine
Inhibits protein synthesis
Purine synthesis
Pyrimidine synthesis
Ribonucleotides
Deoxyribonucleotides
DNA
RNA
(Transfer–messenger–ribosomal)
Proteins
Enzymes
(etc)
Microtubules
PALA
Inhibits pyrimidine biosynthesis
Hydroxyurea
Inhibits ribonucleotide reductase
Capecitabine
5-Fluorouracil
Inhibit dTMP synthesis
Cytarabine
Fludarabine
Cladribine
Gemcitabine
Inhibit DNA synthesis
Bleomycin
Damages DNA
Alkylating agents
Mitomycin
Cisplatin, Carboplatin
Dacarbazine
Procarbazine
Cross-link DNA
Vinca alkaloids
Taxanes
Inhibit function of microtubules

FIGURE 124–12. Mechanisms of action of commonly used antineoplastic agents. *(From Chabner BA, Ryan DP, Paz-Ares L, Garcia-Carbonero R, Calabresi P. Antineoplastic agents. In: Hardman JG, Limbird LE, Gilman AG, eds. Goodman & Gilman's The Pharmacologic Basis of Therapeutics, 10th ed. New York, McGraw-Hill, 2001: 1381.)*

TABLE 124–10. Empiric Dose Modifications in Patients with Renal and Hepatic Disease[a]

Agent	Organ Dysfunction	Suggested Dose Modification
Methotrexate, cisplatin	Renal impairment	In proportion to lowered creatinine clearance (normal = 60 mL/min per m^2) Cl$_{cr}$ <10 mL/min, contraindicated
Carboplatin	Renal impairment	See Table 124–14 for dosing guideline
Cyclophosphamide	Renal failure	Cl$_{cr}$ <25 mL/min; reduce dose by 50%
Bleomycin	Renal failure	Cl$_{cr}$ <25 mL/min; reduce dose by 50% to 75%
Capecitabine	Renal impairment	Cl$_{cr}$ 30–50 mL/min; reduce dose by 25% Cl$_{cr}$ <30 mL/min, contraindicated
Cytarabine (high dose: >1 g/m^2)	Renal impairment	For creatinine 1.5–1.9 mg/dL, reduce dose by 50% For creatinine >2.0 mg/dL, reduce dose by 95%
Topotecan	Renal impairment	Cl$_{cr}$ 20–39 mL/min; reduce dose by 25%
Cladribine Fludarabine	Renal impairment	In proportion to lowered creatinine clearance
Hydroxyurea, doxorubicin, daunorubicin, vincristine, vinblastine	Hepatic dysfunction	For bilirubin >1.5 mg/dL, reduce dose by 50% For bilirubin >3.0 mg/dL, reduce dose by 75%
Vinorelbine	Hepatic dysfunction	For bilirubin >2.0 mg/dL, reduce dose by 50% For bilirubin >3.0 mg/gL, reduce dose by 75%
Gemcitabine	Hepatic dysfunction	For bilirubin >1.6 mg/dL, reduce dose by 20%
Idarubicin, mitoxantrone	Hepatic dysfunction	Consider dose reductions; no published guidelines available
Docetaxel	Hepatic dysfunction	Contraindicated in patient with bilirubin >1.5 × ULN or transaminases >1.5 × ULN or alkaline phosphtases >2.5 × ULN
Irinotecan	Hepatic dysfunction	Contraindicated in patients with bilirubin >2 mg/dL, or transaminases >3 × ULN (without liver metastases), >5 × ULN (with liver metastases)
Paclitaxel	Hepatic dysfunction	Reduce dose by ≥50% for moderate to severe increases in bilirubin or transaminases

[a]Only approximate guidelines can be given. See text for explanations and limitations. Cl$_{cr}$, creatinine clearance; ULN, upper limit of normal laboratory values.
Adapted from ref. 1 and package inserts.

the function of thymidylate synthase. This enzyme is required for synthesis of thymidine, one of the four essential building blocks of DNA. Another metabolite of 5-FU, the triphosphate nucleotide, is incorporated into RNA as a false base, and interferes with its function. Interference with both thymidine formation and RNA function is important in producing the cytotoxic effects of 5-FU. Although 5-FU nucleotides can also be incorporated directly into DNA and affect its stability, the contribution to cell damage remains unclear. The method of administration influences the mechanism of action, with thymidylate synthesis inhibition playing a greater role in continuous-infusion regimens, and incorporation into RNA being more important for intermittent-bolus schedules.[36]

Several pharmacologic strategies have been attempted to increase the cytotoxicity of 5-FU against tumor cells and to decrease its toxicity to normal cells. The most successful of these attempts at biochemical modulation are combinations of fluorouracil and the reduced folate leucovorin. Folates increase the stability of the FdUMP-thymidylate synthase complex, thereby increasing the cytotoxicity and clinical usefulness of the drug.[36–40]

Oral Fluoropyrimidines

Capecitabine is an orally active pyrimidine analog. Despite the similarity of its name to cytidine derivatives such as cytarabine and gemcitabine, capecitabine is an analog of uracil and is a prodrug of 5-FU. Because capecitabine is converted to 5-FU, it shares the same mechanisms of action. It generates higher levels of 5-FU selectively within some tumors compared with healthy tissues. Because chronic twice-daily oral dosing of capecitabine produces sustained 5-FU levels similar to continuous intravenous infusions of 5-FU, the toxicity pattern is similar to that of 5-FU infusions.[36,41–43] Several other oral fluoropyrimidine products are under investigation.[44]

CYTIDINE ANALOGS

Cytarabine

Cytarabine (ara-C) is an arabinose analog of cytosine. Cytarabine was originally isolated from sponges, but is now produced synthetically. Ara-C is phosphorylated to its active triphosphate form (ara-CTP) within tumor cells. Ara-CTP inhibits DNA polymerase, an enzyme responsible for strand elongation. It is also incorporated directly into DNA, where it inhibits the replication of DNA and acts as a chain terminator to prevent DNA elongation. Activation of ara-C is opposed by deaminase enzymes, particularly cytidine deaminase, which degrades ara-C to an inactive form, ara-U.[36,45,46]

TABLE 124–11. Antimetabolites

Agent/Major Uses	Class/Mechanism	Major Side Effects	Comments
Azacitidine [5-azacytidine, 5-AC, Ara C, Vidaza][a] MDS Sickle cell anemia; thalassemia	Pyrimidine [cytidine] nucleoside analog antimetabolite; induces differentiation in malignant cells; causes demethylation or hypomethylation of DNA; this can alter gene tanscription and expression, restoring normal function to tumor suppressor genes responsible for cell differentiation and growth	Myelosuppression; low emetogenic potential; constitutional symptoms (fatigue, weakness, fever, rigors); musculoskeletal symptoms (arthralgias, pain in limbs); pulmonary (cough, dyspnea)	Suspension for subcutaneous injection; approved for treatment of all MDS subtypes; onset of response usually requires 3–4 months; myelosuppression decreases with onset of response in MDS patients; drug toxicity may be difficult to distinguish from symptoms of MDS
Capecitabine (Xeloda)[b] Breast cancer; colorectal cancer; GI tract cancers	Similar to 5-fluorouracil: converted to 5-FU in three-step process; greater activation in tumor cells than in normal cells	Diarrhea may require fluid and electrolyte replacement; warn patients to stop drug if they experience an increase of 4–6 or more stools per day or nocturnal stools; hand-foot syndrome (palmar-plantar erythema): numbness, dysesthesia, tingling, swelling, redness, pain, sometimes blistering, ulceration in hands and feet; stop drug and restart at lower dose when resolved; topical emollients may be helpful; nausea common but mild; low risk of myelosuppression	Pharmacokinetics and toxicity mimic continuous-infusion 5-FU; drug interactions: Warfarin—(*major interaction*), results in increased anticoagulant effects, increased risk of bleeding; monitor coagulation parameters closely; phenytoin—may require phenytoin dose reduction; monitor phenytoin levels closely; leucovorin increases the activity and toxicity of capecitabine Dose adjustment for renal dysfunction: reduce dose by 25% for Cl_{cr} 30–50 mL/min; avoid with Cl_{cr} <30 mL/min
Cladribine [2-chlorodeoxyadenosine, 2-CDA, Leustatin][c] Hairy cell leukemia; CLL; NHL	Purine [adenosine] nucleoside antimetabolite; active triphosphate form can prevent elongation of DNA chain; also inhibits ribonucleotide reductase, depleting intracellular deoxynucleotides and impairing DNA synthesis	Myelosuppression; fever (onset by day 6, persisting for about 3 days); immunosuppressive; severe opportunistic infections occur; low emetogenic potential	Usually administered by continuous infusion for 7 days
Cytarabine (ara-C; cytosine arabinoside; Cytosar U)[d] ANLL; ALL; lymphomatous meningitis; NHL; MDS High-dose ara-C (HDAC) Liposomal cytarabine (Depocyt) for intrathecal use for lymphomatous meningitis	Antipyrimidine antimetabolite; inhibits DNA polymerase with inhibition of DNA strand elongation and replication; activated in tumor cells to triphosphate form; competes with conversion of cytidine to deoxycytidine nucleotides, further blocking polymerization of DNA; leads to production of short DNA strands; cell-cycle specific (S phase): acts only on proliferating cells	Myelosuppression; alopecia; moderate emetogen; worse with high dose (>1 g/m²) or IT administration; diarrhea; mucositis; flu-like syndrome with fever and arthralgias; rash often followed by desquamation on palms and soles *HDAC toxicities*: Cerebellar toxicity; direct neurotoxicity: ataxia, slurred speech, nystagmus; conjunctivitis (drug is excreted into tears and blocks corneal DNA synthesis)	HDAC infusions should be administered over 2–3 hours to decrease risk of CNS toxicity; use steroid eyedrops during treatment and for 48 hours posttreatment to prevent conjunctivitis with HDAC Increased HDAC neurotoxicity in patients with impaired renal function; dose reduction recommended; frequent neurologic exams; monitor creatinine; avoid concurrent administration of nephrotoxic drugs Rapid cell kill: may see tumor lysis syndrome with large tumor burden (WBC >100,000/mm³)
Fludarabine (FAMP; Fludara)[e] CLL; low-grade NHL; ANLL; Waldenstrom's macroglobulinemia	Inhibits ribonucleotide reductase via inhibition of DNA synthesis; inhibits DNA polymerase via inhibition of DNA repair	Myelosuppression, including decreased T cells; low emetogenic potential; diarrhea; rare CNS toxicity: somnolence, peripheral neuropathies, hearing loss that is dose related, may be severe with high cumulative doses; may induce altered mental status, seizures; pulmonary toxicity: interstitial pneumonitis	Risk of opportunistic infections associated with decreased T-cell function for several months after treatment (PCP, mycobacterial infections); prophylactic antibiotics for PCP and HSV should be considered, particularly when fludarabine is used in combination with corticosteroids Rapid cell kill: tumor lysis syndrome precautions needed; reduce dose with impaired renal function

(continued)

TABLE 124–11. (Continued)

Agent/Major Uses	Class/Mechanism	Major Side Effects	Comments
Fluorouracil (5-FU)[f] Breast cancer; colorectal cancer; gastric and pancreatic cancers; esophageal, head, and neck cancer; cervical cancer Radiosensitizer Cataract surgery	Fluorinated antipyrimidine analog of uracil; prodrug fluorodeoxyuridine monophosphate (FdUMP) is active form; thymidylate synthase (TS) inhibitor; interferes with RNA/DNA function; "false" pyrimidine; leucovorin enhances binding of FdUMP to TS; potentiates cytotoxicity as well as toxicity; cell-cycle specific: S phase	Mucositis and diarrhea resulting from damage to normally rapidly proliferating cells of GI tract (worse with continuous infusion, concurrent leucovorin regimens); mild emetogen; myelosuppression (worse with bolus administration); rash, hyperpigmentation, photosensitivity; hand-foot syndrome (palmar-plantar erythema) with continuous-infusion regimens; alopecia uncommon; ocular toxicity (excess tearing, itching, burning); myocardial ischemic symptoms (especially high-dose continuous infusions)	Various routes of administration: IV bolus or short or continuous infusion; dose, schedule, and inclusion of leucovorin affect toxicity pattern *Diarrhea can be severe and life threatening*; treat aggressively with antimotility agents; leucovorin can worsen 5-FU diarrhea; special caution in elderly females Deficiency of dihydropyrimidine dehydrogenase (DPD) correlates with increased toxicity; DPD required to metabolize 5-FU *Drug interaction with warfarin:* increased anticoagulant effect; monitor closely
Gemcitabine (Gemzar)[g] Pancreatic cancer; NSCLC; breast cancer; head and neck cancer; bladder cancer; testicular cancer; ovarian cancers, HD	Related to cytarabine, incorporated into DNA, inhibits DNA synthesis; ribonucleotide reductase inhibitor; interferes with DNA chain elongation	Myelosuppression; neutropenia, thrombocytopenia; may be more severe with infusions >1 hour; myelosuppression may necessitate dose reduction and/or delay in therapy; flu-like syndrome: fever, myalgias; rash: typically erythematous, pruritic, starts 48–72 hours after dose; elevations in liver transaminases; low emetogenic potential; rare pulmonary toxicity: dyspnea, bronchospasm; radiation-recall reactions	Generally very well-tolerated; rash may respond to topical steroids, dose reduction; fevers may respond to acetaminophen Dose reduction recommended for patients with elevated total bilirubin (>1.5 mg/dL) Breast cancer indication is in combination with paclitaxel
Hydroxyurea (Hydrea)[c] CML; sickle cell disease; melanoma;[h] head and neck cancers;[h] ovarian cancer;[h] cervical cancer	Inhibits ribonucleotide reductase; inhibits DNA synthesis (does not interfere with RNA or protein synthesis)	Myelosuppression; low emetogenic potential; rash, pruritus, skin hyperpigmentation; hyperuricemia may occur with rapid cytoreduction; secondary leukemias may occur with long-term use	Drug is degraded by moisture; keep capsules in a tightly sealed container with a desiccant
6-Mercaptopurine (Purinethol; 6-MP)[c] ALL	Antipurine antimetabolite; purine analog; inhibits DNA, RNA, protein synthesis; metabolized by xanthine oxidase	Myelosuppression: mild; anorexia, low emetogenic potential; dry skin rash, photosensitivity; hepatotoxicity: jaundice and hyperbilirubinemia occur after 1–2 months of therapy and may be dose-limiting	Drug interactions: allopurinol increases the toxicity of 6-MP by interfering with metabolism: *75% dose reduction* of 6-MP is required if used with allopurinol; 6-MP reduces anticoagulant effects of warfarin; concurrent use of 6-MP with other hepatotoxic drugs increases the risk of hepatotoxicity
Methotrexate [MTX] ALL CNS leukemia [IT] Breast cancer NHL Osteosarcoma Head and neck cancer Bladder cancer Rheumatoid arthritis	**Folic acid antagonist;** inhibits dihydrofolate reductase (DHFR); blocks reduction of folate to tetrahydrofolate; inhibits *de novo* purine synthesis; results in arrest of DNA, RNA, and protein synthesis Leucovorin provides reduced folate to bypass the metabolic block.	Myelosuppression: can be prevented with leucovorin rescue Mucositis: can be prevented with leucovorin Renal dysfunction: (high dose regimens) caused by precipitation of drug in renal tubules; hydration (3 L/m²/day) and alkalinization of urine (to	Avoid drugs that decrease renal excretion of cisplatin, salicylates, sulfas, probenecid, penicillins Methotrexate distributes readily into third space fluids (ascites, pleural effusions), prolonging exposure and increasing toxicity. May be contraindication for use.

TABLE 124–11. (Continued)

Agent/Major Uses	Class/Mechanism	Major Side Effects	Comments
SLE and other autoimmune disorders Ectopic pregnancy		increase drug solubility; keep urine pH >7) minimize nephrotoxicity. Reduce dose for renal dysfunction; avoid use in severe renal impairment Emetogenic potential generally low, but higher emetogenicity with high-dose therapy CNS toxicity: malaise, dizziness; may be more severe with IT administration (nausea, vomiting, seizures, headache) Hepatotoxicity: cirrhosis/portal fibrosis (more common with chronic administration) Photosensitivity	**Monitor methotrexate levels with high-dose administration** Toxicities (mucositis, BM suppression) correlate with MTX levels >1 μM (1×10^{-6}M) for >48 hours. High-dose regimens must include leucovorin (LCV) rescue to prevent irreversible BM toxicity. LCV continued until MTX level <0.1 μM to 0.01 μM. Use preservative-free preparations for IT and high-dose administration.
Pemetrexed [Allmeta] Mesothelioma NSCLC	Multitargeted antifolate; disrupts folate-dependent processes essential for cell reproduction. Inhibits thymidylate synthase, dihydrofolate reductase [DHFR], and glycinamide ribonucleotide formyltransferase [GARFT], all involved in synthesis of thymidine and purine nucleotides.	Myelosuppression: increased in patients with elevated cystathioneine or homocysteine concentrations. Folic acid and vitamin B_{12} supplementation decrease myelosuppression by decreasing elevated cystathionine and homocysteine levels. Stomatitis, pharyngitis Rash, desquamation. Premedicate with dexamethasone 4 mg twice daily the day before, day of, and day after administration.	Approved for use in combination with cisplatin Renally eliminated. No dose changes require creatinine clearance ≥45 mL/min. Not recommended in patients with lower creatinine clearances. Avoid short-acting NSAIDs [eg ibuprofen] for before and after pemetrexed administration. Avoid longer acting NSAIDs for 5 days prior to and 2 days after pemetrexed administration. Supplementation with folic acid [400 mcg daily starting 1 week before first dose; continued days after last dose] and vitamin B_{12} [1000 mcg IM during week prior to first dose and even cycles thereafter] is required during administration to reduce toxicity. Leucovorin rescue is indicated for Grade 4 toxicities.

[a]From Silverman et al.[49]
[b]From Pizzorno et al,[36] Schuller et al,[41] Reigner et al,[42] Wagstaff et al,[43] and Cunningham et al.[44]
[c]From Pizzorno et al.[36]
[d]From Pizzorno et al,[36] Johnson,[45] and Smith et al.[46]
[e]From Pizzorno et al,[36] Rossi et al,[50] and Plosker et al.[51]
[f]From Pizzorno et al,[36] 5-Fluorouracil,[37] Sobrero et al,[38] Rich et al,[39] and Sloan et al.[40]
[g]From Pizzorno et al,[36] Johnson,[45] Venook et al,[47] and Friedlander et al.[48]
[h]Although an FDA-approved indication, the drug is no longer used for this disease.
ANLL, acute nonleukocytic leukemia; ALL, acute lymphocytic leukemia; BM, bone marrow; Cl$_{cr}$, creatinine clearance; CLL, chronic lymphocytic leukemia; CML, chronic myelogenous leukemia; DNA, deoxyribonucleic acid; HD, Hodgkin's disease; HSV, herpes simplex virus; IT, intrathecal; MDS, myelodysplastic syndrome; NHL, non-Hodgkin's lymphoma; NSCLC, non-small-cell lung cancer; PCP, *Pneumocystis carinii* pneumonia; RNA, ribonucleic acid; WBC, white blood cells.

Cytidine deaminase levels are very low in the CNS. Cytotoxic concentrations are maintained in the CNS for several hours after CNS administration of traditional cytarabine formulations, and for more than 2 weeks following CNS administration of depot formulated cytarabine.

The toxicity of cytarabine is dose dependent. The most characteristic toxicity of high-dose ara-C (HDAC; >1 g/m² per dose) regimens is a cerebellar syndrome of dysarthria, nystagmus, and ataxia. Risk of CNS toxicity is strongly correlated with advanced age and renal dysfunction. Renal insufficiency permits accumulation of high levels of ara-CTP, which is believed to be neurotoxic. Hepatic dysfunction, high cumulative doses, and bolus dosing may also increase the risks of neurotoxicity.[36,45,46]

Gemcitabine

Gemcitabine is a fluorine-substituted deoxycytidine analog related structurally to cytarabine (see Table 124–11). Its activation and mechanism of action are similar to those of cytarabine. Gemcitabine is incorporated into DNA, where it inhibits DNA polymerase activity. It also inhibits ribonucleotide reductase. Compared with cytarabine, gemcitabine achieves intracellular concentrations about 20 times higher than does ara-C, secondary to increased penetration of cell membranes, and greater affinity for the activating enzyme deoxycytidine kinase. Gemcitabine that is incorporated into DNA has a prolonged intracellular half-life. Its stereoconfiguration causes another normal base pair to be added next to the fraudulent gemcitabine base pair in the DNA strand. This "masked chain termination" protects the gemcitabine from excision and elimination.[36,45,47,48]

Azacytidine

Azacytidine was approved in 2004 for the treatment of patients with myelodysplastic syndrome, a disorder of hematopoietic cell maturation that can progress to acute leukemia. Azacytidine, a cytidine nucleoside analog, causes hypomethylation of DNA. Hypomethylation may normalize the function of genes that control cell differentiation and proliferation, promoting normal cell maturation.[49]

PURINES AND PURINE ANTIMETABOLITES

6-Mercaptopurine and 6-Thioguanine

Some of the oldest and newest anticancer agents are synthetic analogs of the naturally occurring purines guanine and adenine (see Table 124–11). 6-Mercaptopurine (6-MP) was the first purine analog to be used in cancer chemotherapy. Thioguanine (6-TG) is the two-amino analog of 6-MP. Both drugs are rapidly converted to ribonucleotides that inhibit purine biosynthesis. They also undergo purine interconversion reactions needed to supply purine precursors for synthesis of nucleic acids. Clinical cross-resistance is generally observed.[36]

6-MP depends on xanthine oxidase for an initial oxidation step. Its metabolism is markedly decreased by concomitant administration of the xanthine oxidase inhibitor allopurinol, and serious toxicity may result. Oral 6-MP doses must be reduced when allopurinol is administered together with 6-MP.[36]

Fludarabine Monophosphate

Fludarabine monophosphate (FAMP) is an analog of the purine adenine. Like cytarabine, fludarabine interferes with DNA polymerase, causing chain termination. Unlike ara-C, fludarabine is also incorporated into RNA, resulting in inhibited transcription. The usual dose-limiting toxicity is myelosuppression. Fludarabine is also immunosuppressive, with associated opportunistic infections.[36,50,51]

Cladribine

Cladribine (2-chlorodeoxyadenosine; 2-CDA) is a purine nucleoside analog that is resistant to inactivation by adenosine deaminase. The triphosphate form of this agent is incorporated into DNA, resulting in inhibition of DNA synthesis and early chain termination. Cladribine's antitumor activity is unusual for an antimetabolite in that it affects both actively dividing and resting cancer cells. Like fludarabine, cladribine possesses immunosuppressive effects that place patients at risk for serious opportunistic infections.[36,45]

ANTIFOLATES

Folate vitamins are essential cofactors in DNA synthesis. They carry one-carbon groups in transfer reactions that are required for purine and thymidylic acid synthesis, and in turn for formation of DNA and for cell division. Natural folates circulating in the blood have a single glutamic acid group, but within cells they are converted to polyglutamates, which are more efficient cofactors and which are preferentially retained inside the cells.[52]

Dietary folates must be chemically reduced to their tetrahydro forms, with four hydrogens on the pteridine ring, to be active. The enzyme responsible for this reduction is dihydrofolate reductase (DHFR), a key enzyme whose actions are inhibited by methotrexate and other antifolates. The result of this inhibition is depletion of intracellular pools of reduced folates (tetrahydrofolates) essential for thymidylate and purine synthesis. Lack of either thymidine or purines prevents synthesis of DNA. The DHFR-mediated effects of antifolate drugs on normal and probably also on cancerous cells may be neutralized by supplying reduced folates exogenously. The reduced folate used clinically for "rescue" is leucovorin (folinic acid), which bypasses the metabolic block induced by DHFR inhibitors.[52]

Methotrexate

The folic acid analog methotrexate (MTX) is the best understood of all drugs in the broad category of antimetabolites (see Table 124–11). It has been in clinical use for about 50 years. Like physiologic folates, methotrexate is transported intracellularly by an active transport system. In high doses, passive diffusion may overcome tumor cell resistance caused by saturated active transport systems. Resistance to the antifolates can also be caused by increased production of DHFR. Other potential causes of resistance are slow rates of thymidylate synthesis, decreased affinity of DHFR for methotrexate, and lack of polyglutamation within tumor cells. Polyglutamated forms of folates are better retained within cells. Malignant cells may achieve greater MTX polyglutamate levels than normal cells, which may in part explain the selective effects of MTX on malignant versus normal cells.[52]

Accurate and readily available assays for serum MTX levels have made therapeutic drug monitoring of MTX a valuable clinical tool. The threshold for cytotoxic effects of MTX is approximately 5×10^{-8} M. Toxicity and efficacy are related not only to peak concentrations, but more importantly, to time that concentrations remain above this threshold level. For MTX doses requiring leucovorin rescue (generally doses greater than 100 mg/m^2), leucovorin must be administered until levels fall below 5×10^{-8} M. Therapeutic drug monitoring is also an effective means of increasing the likelihood of therapeutic success, by individualizing doses based on target parameters.[52]

Pemetrexed

Pemetrexed is a multitargeted antifolate that inhibits at least three biosynthetic pathways in thymidine and purine synthesis (see Table 124–11). In addition to inhibition of DHFR, it also inhibits thymidine synthase and glycinamide ribonucleotide formyltransferase, decreasing the risk of development of drug resistance. Supplementation of folic acid and vitamin B$_{12}$ is required to decrease myelosuppression.[52,53]

MICROTUBULE-TARGETING DRUGS

VINCA ALKALOIDS

Vincristine, vinblastine, and vinorelbine are natural alkaloids derived from the periwinkle (vinca) plant. They act as mitotic inhibitors, or "spindle poisons." Although the alkaloids are very similar structurally, they have different activities and patterns of toxicity (Table 124–12).

Vinca alkaloids bind to tubulin, the structural protein that polymerizes to form microtubules. These are the hollow tubes that make up the mitotic spindle and that are also important in nerve conduction and neurotransmission. Vinca alkaloids disrupt the normal balance between polymerization and depolymerization of microtubules, inhibiting assembly of microtubules and disrupting microtubule dynamics. This interferes with formation of the mitotic spindle and

TABLE 124–12. Antimicrotubule Agents

Agent/Major Uses	Mechanism	Adverse Effects	Comments
Taxanes			
Docetaxel (Taxotere)[a] Breast cancer; NSCLC; prostate cancer; ovarian cancer; SCLC; bladder cancer; gastric cancer; head and neck cancers; melanoma; soft tissue sarcomas	Similar to paclitaxel, promotes microtubule assembly; inhibits depolymerization of tubulin; inhibits cell division	Myelosuppression; fluid retention syndrome: edema, weight gain, pleural effusions, ascites; typically occurs when cumulative dose exceeds 400 mg/m^2; alopecia; rash: forearms, hands; nail disorders: onycholysis, banding, hypo- or hyperpigmentation; mild peripheral neuropathy; mildly emetogen; hypersensitivity reactions	Dexamethasone 8 mg orally twice daily for 3 days (starting 1 day prior to docetaxel) is recommended to lower risk of fluid retention syndrome; shorter dexamethasone regimens used for weekly docetaxel dosing Requires dose reduction for liver dysfunction (elevated total bilirubin, elevated transaminases and/or alkaline phosphatase) Prepare and administer using glass or non-PVC IV bags and tubing
Paclitaxel (Taxol)[c] Ovarian cancer; breast cancer; KS; NSCLC; SCLC; esophageal and head and neck cancers; testicular cancer; bladder cancer; cervical and endometrial cancers	Induces polymerization of microtubules, stabilizing the microtubules to make them nonfunctional; derived from the Pacific yew tree (*Taxus brevifolia*)	Myelosuppression may be dose-limiting; hypersensitivity reactions (preventable with appropriate premedications); peripheral neuropathy: paresthesias may be cumulative, dose-related; myalgias/arthralgias typically occur 3–5 days after administration and persist for 3–5 days; mucositis: more common with high doses; mildly emetogen: cardiac: asymptomatic bradycardia most common; ventricular arrhythmias, third-degree heart block, and MI rarely reported; alopecia: total body	Premedicate patients to prevent hypersensitivity reactions: dexamethasone 20 mg IV **or** orally 12 hours and 6 hours prior to paclitaxel, and diphenhydramine 50 mg IV 30 minutes prior to paclitaxel, and ranitidine 50 mg IV or cimetidine 300 mg IV 30 minutes prior to paclitaxel Reduce dose in patients with elevated total bilirubin (>1.5 mg/dL) and/or elevated transaminases (guidelines not well established) Neurotoxicity may be severe enough to require discontinuation; treat myalgias/arthralgias with NSAIDs, narcotic analgesics In paclitaxel-cisplatin combination regimens, give paclitaxel first to decrease neutropenia
Nitrogen-mustard type alkylating agent			
Estramustine (Emcyt)[b] Prostate cancer	Structurally is a combined estrogen and alkylating agent, but functions mainly as an antimicrotubule agent; interferes with microtubule associated proteins (MAPs)	Nausea and vomiting (may be dose-limiting); diarrhea; cardiovascular: lowers arterial circulation; ischemic heart disease patients with CHF may develop increased symptoms of heart failure; thromboembolic events; gynecomastia, nipple tenderness; increased liver function tests	Patients with pre-existing heart disease, cerebrovascular disease, and hypertension should be closely monitored during treatment; most cardiovascular complications occur within the first 2 months to 1 year of treatment; low-dose warfarin (1–2 mg/day) is commonly used to decrease risk of thromboembolic events, but its value is not proven Doses should be taken on an empty stomach (1 hour before or 2 hours after a meal); avoid concurrent administration with dairy products or calcium compounds; refrigerate
Vinca alkaloids			
Vinblastine (Velban)[b] Testicular cancer; NHL; HD; KS; bladder cancer; breast cancer; NSCLC; melanoma; prostate cancer; renal cell carcinoma	Antimicrotubule agent/vinca alkaloid; derived from the periwinkle plant; disrupts formation of microtubules	Myelosuppression may be dose-limiting; mucositis; mildly emetogen; neurotoxicity: less common than with vincristine; myalgias; SIADH (rarely); vesicant: extravasation injury	Treat extravasation injury with warm soaks, and injection of hyaluronidase Reduce dose by 50% for total bilirubin 1.5–3 mg/dL; by 75% for total bilirubin >3 mg/dL

(continued)

TABLE 124–12. (Continued)

Agent/Major Uses	Mechanism	Adverse Effects	Comments
Vincristine (VCR, Oncovin)[b] ALL; HD; NHL; multiple myeloma; breast cancer; SCLC; KS; brain tumors; soft tissue sarcomas; osteosarcomas; neuroblastoma; Wilms' tumor	Antimicrotubule agent/vinca alkaloid; derived from the periwinkle plant; disrupts formation of microtubules	Peripheral neuropathy: primary dose-limiting toxicity; motor, sensory, autonomic, and cranial nerves may all be affected (paresthesias, ileus, urinary retention, facial palsies); may be irreversible; mild emetogen; SIADH; vesicant: extravasation injury	*Prevent ileus:* treat constipation aggressively; doses range from 1–1.4 mg/m^2 (max); doses are traditionally capped at 2 mg to minimize neurotoxicity, but capping is controversial Reduce dose by 50% for total bilirubin 1.5–3 mg/dL; by 75% for total bilirubin >3 mg/dL; treat extravasation injury with warm soaks, and injection of hyaluronidase *LETHAL* if administered intrathecally!
Vinorelbine (Navelbine)[b] NSCLC; breast cancer; HD; cervical cancer; ovarian cancer; prostate cancer	Antimicrotubule agent/synthetic vinca alkaloid; disrupts formation of microtubules	Myelosuppression (neutropenia); neurotoxicity: peripheral neuropathy (less common than with vincristine); constipation; low back pain; mild emetogen; vesciant: causes painful phlebitis with administration; alopecia is uncommon	Eliminated primarily by metabolism and biliary excretion: follow package insert for dose adjustments Drug interaction with phenytoin: decreases phenytoin levels; drug interaction with erythromycin (may inhibit vinorelbine metabolism): increased risk of vinorelbine toxicity

[a]From Rowinsky et al,[54] Hainsworth et al,[55] and Krieger et al.[56]
[b]From Kitamura et al.[36]
[c]From Rowinsky et al[54] and Krieger et al.[56]

All, acute lymphocytic leukemia; CHF, congestive heart failure; HD, Hodgkin's disease; KS, Kaposi's sarcoma; MI, myocardial infarction; NHL, non-Hodgkin's lymphoma; NSAID, nonsteroidal anti-inflammatory drug; NSCLC, non-small-cell lung cancer; PVC, polyvinyl chloride; SIADH, syndrome of inappropriate secretion of antidiuretic hormone; SCLC, small cell lung cancer.

causes cells to accumulate in mitosis. They also disturb a variety of microtubule-related processes in cells, and induce apoptosis. Resistance to the vinca alkaloids develops primarily from P-glycoprotein–mediated multidrug resistance, which decreases drug accumulation and retention within tumor cells.[54]

TAXANES

Paclitaxel and docetaxel are taxane plant alkaloids with antimitotic activity (see Table 124–12). Paclitaxel was isolated from the bark of the Pacific yew tree, *Taxus brevifolia*, but is now produced semisynthetically from the needles of the European yew, *Taxus baccata*. Docetaxel is a semisynthetic taxoid extracted from 10-deacetyl baccatin III, a noncytotoxic precursor found in the renewable needle biomass of yew plants.[54]

Paclitaxel and docetaxel both act by binding to tubulin, but unlike the vincas do not interfere with tubulin assembly. Instead, the taxanes promote microtubule assembly and interfere with microtubule disassembly. They induce tubulin polymerization, resulting in formation of inappropriately stable, nonfunctional microtubules. The stability of the microtubles damages cells, because the dynamics of microtubule-dependent structures required for mitosis and other cellular functions are disrupted. Taxanes also have some nonmitotic actions that can promote cancer cell death, such as inhibition of angiogenesis. Resistance to the antitumor effects of the taxanes is attributable to alterations in tubulin or tubulin binding sites, or to P-glycoprotein–mediated multidrug resistance. Although paclitaxel and docetaxel have very similar mechanisms of action, cross-resistance between the two agents is incomplete.[54–56]

ESTRAMUSTINE

Estramustine is an unusual drug in that it structurally combines the alkylating agent nor-nitrogen mustard with the hormone estradiol. It was designed with the intent that the estradiol portion of the molecule would facilitate uptake of the alkylating agent into hormone-sensitive prostate cancer cells. Despite the inclusion of an alkylator, estramustine does not function in vivo as an alkylating agent. Estrogens are released after its administration and are responsible for much of the toxicity of estramustine, but are not believed to contribute to its cytotoxic effect. In the mid-1980s, estramustine was redefined as an antimicrotubule agent. It binds covalently to microtubule-associated proteins that are part of the structural support for microtubules. The binding causes the separation of microtubule-associated proteins from the microtubules, inhibiting microtubule assembly and eventually causing their disassembly.[57]

TOPOISOMERASE INHIBITORS

Topoisomerases are essential enzymes involved in maintaining DNA topologic structure during replication and transcription. DNA topoisomerase enzymes relieve torsional strain during DNA unwinding by producing strand breaks. They cleave DNA strands and form intermediates with the strands, producing a gap through which DNA strands can pass, then reseal the strand breaks. Topoisomerase I produces single-strand breaks; topoisomerase II produces double-strand breaks.[58] Several important anticancer agents target topoisomerase enzymes: anthracyclines, camptothecins, and the epipodophyllotoxins (Table 124–13).

TABLE 124–13. Topoisomerase-Active Agents

Agent/Major Uses	Mechanism	Adverse Effects	Comments
Topoisomerase I inhibitors **Irinotecan** (CPT-11; Camptosar)[a] Colon cancer; NSCLC; SCLC; cervical and ovarian cancers; gastric cancer; pancreatic cancer	Topoisomerase I inhibitor; inhibits DNA binding activity of topoisomerase I, resulting in multiple DNA single-strand breaks; ultimately interferes with DNA synthesis	Diarrhea: acute (cramping, flushing, vomiting, diaphoresis within 1 hour of completion; related to cholinergic effects) and delayed (>12 hours after administration; usually after the second or third dose); may be severe; moderately high emetogenic potential; myelosuppression: neutropenia; alopecia; fatigue; increased liver function tests; pulmonary toxicity: diffuse infiltrates, fever, dyspnea	Acute diarrhea is best treated or prevented with atropine; delayed diarrhea managed with antimotility agents (loperamide 4 mg at first sign of diarrhea then 2 mg every 2 hours until no diarrhea for 12 hours); octreotide is not usually effective; ensure that patients have a supply of antimotility agents to take with the first symptoms of diarrhea; ensure fluid and electrolyte replacement in patients with severe diarrhea Dose should be reduced in patients with elevated total bilirubin, no specific guidelines available Drug administration sequence affects pharmacokinetics and tolerability of irinotecan in 5-FU + irinotecan regimens
Topotecan (Hycamtin)[b] Ovarian cancer; SCLC; MDS	Topoisomerase I inhibitor; inhibits DNA binding activity of topoisomerase I, resulting in multiple DNA single-strand breaks; ultimately interferes with DNA synthesis	Myelosuppression (neutropenia); mucositis (dose-related; worse with continuous infusion); very low to low emetogenic potential; diarrhea (mild); reversible elevations in transaminases	Dose adjustments may be necessary for Cl_{cr} <60 mL/min
Topoisomerase II inhibitors **Daunorubicin** (Daunomycin, Dauno, Cerubidine)[c] Liposomal daunorubicin (DaunoXome) ANLL; ALL; KS (liposomal)	Antitumor antibiotic; topoisomerase II inhibitor; DNA intercalator; free-radical formation (thought to be related to cardiac toxicity and tissue injury)	Myelosuppression (dose-related); mucositis (worse with continuous infusion); moderate emetogenic potential; alopecia; vesicant: severe extravasation injury; cardiac toxicities: *acute*—not related to cumulative dose; arrhythmias, pericarditis; *chronic*—cumulative injury to myocardium (total dose >550 mg/m^2; lower total cumulative doses cause damage to myocardium in children (e.g., 350 mg/m^2)	Apply ice to areas of extravasation to lessen extent of injury Dose reduction required for total bilirubin >1.5 mg/dL (50% of full dose) and >3 mg/dL (25% of full dose) May discolor urine (red-orange) Liposomal form: decreased risk of cardiac and vesicant toxicity
Doxorubicin (Adriamycin, Adria, Doxo, hydroxydaunorubicin)[c] Liposomal doxorubicin (Doxil) Breast cancer; osteosarcoma and soft tissue sarcomas; NHL; HD; ALL; ANLL; bladder cancer; ovarian cancer; thyroid cancer; Wilms' tumor; neuroblastoma; SCLC; KS (liposomal); gastric cancer; multiple myeloma; NSCLC; endometrial cancer	Antitumor antibiotic; topoisomerase II inhibitor; DNA intercalator; free-radical formation (thought to be related to cardiac toxicity and tissue injury)	Myelosuppression; mucositis: worse with continuous infusion; moderate emetogenic potential: may cause acute and delayed (by 24–48 hours) emesis; vesicant: severe extravasation injury; cardiac toxicities: *acute*—not related to cumulative dose; arrhythmias, pericarditis; *chronic*—cumulative injury to myocardium (total dose >550 mg/m^2); lower total cumulative doses cause damage to myocardium in children (e.g. 350 mg/m^2); radiation recall reactions	Apply ice to areas of extravasation to lessen extent of injury; dose reduction required for total bilirubin >1.5 mg/dL (50% of full dose) and >3 mg/dL (25% of full dose) May discolor urine (red-orange) Dexrazoxane (Zinecard), a cardioprotectant, decreases risk of cardiotoxicity; approved for use in breast cancer patients with >300 mg/m^2 doxorubicin; concerns over possible tumor protection limit its use Liposomal form: decreased risk of cardiac and vesicant toxicities

(continued)

TABLE 124–13. (Continued)

Agent/Major Uses	Mechanism	Adverse Effects	Comments
Epirubicin (Ellence)[e] Breast cancer; gastric cancer	Antitumor antibiotic (see daunorubicin and doxorubicin)	Myelosuppression; mucositis: worse with continuous infusion; moderately emetogenic: may cause acute and delayed (by 24–48 hours) emesis; vesicant: severe extravasation injury; cardiotoxicity (similar to other anthracyclines); may be less cardiotoxic than doxorubicin; controversy about equivalent doses; cardiac toxicity associated with cumulative doses >900 mg/m^2	Apply ice to areas of extravasation to lessen extent of injury; dose reduction required for total bilirubin >1.5 mg/dL (50% of full dose) and >3 mg/dL (25% of full dose) May discolor urine (red-orange)
Etoposide (VP-16; Vepesid), Etoposide phosphate (Etopophos)[d] Testicular cancer; SCLC; NSCLC; ANLL; KS; HD; NHL; BMT preparative chemotherapy; gastric cancer	Plant alkaloid, epipodophyllotoxin; inhibits DNA binding activity of topoisomerase II, resulting in multiple DNA double-strand breaks	Myelosuppression; moderately emetogenic: may be worse with oral and high-dose regimens; alopecia; mucositis; hypotension: infusion rate–related; etoposide phosphate can be given IV push without hypotension risk; hypersensitivity reactions: especially common in children	Requires large volumes of fluid for IV administration due to limited solubility (max concentration 0.4 mg/mL); if hypotension occurs, stop infusion until BP stable, then resume at decreased rate Available orally in liquid-filled gelatin capsules; approximately 50% bioavailability, but absorption is variable and greater at lower oral doses
Idarubicin (Idamycin)[e] ANLL; oral preparation investigational	Antitumor antibiotic (similar to daunorubicin and doxorubicin, but more potent); topoisomerase II inhibition; DNA intercalation; free-radical formation	Myelosuppression; mucositis; moderately emetogenic; vesicant: extravasation; alopecia; cardiac toxicities: *acute* and *chronic*, as with daunorubicin and doxorubicin (total cumulative dose not well established; >150 mg/m^2 reported to be associated with decreased LVEF	Apply ice to areas of extravasation to lessen extent of injury Dose reduction required for total bilirubin >1.5 mg/dL (50% of full dose) and >3 mg/dL (25% of full dose) May discolor urine red-orange Produces cumulative cardiotoxicity with other anthracyclines
Mitoxantrone (Novantrone)[f] ANLL; prostate cancer; NHL; HD; breast cancer Multiple sclerosis	Anthracenedione (not an anthracycline); topoisomerase II inhibitor; DNA intercalator; low potential compared with anthracyclines for formation of free radicals	Myelosuppression; low emetogenic potential; mucositis; alopecia; less cardiotoxic than the anthracyclines	Not a vesicant (may cause vein irritation, but not associated with severe tissue injury like anthracyclines) May discolor urine blue-green

[a]From Rubin et al,[58] Kellner et al,[60] Ulukan et al,[61] Vanhoefer et al,[62] Raymond et al,[63] and Falcome et al.[64]
[b]From Rubin et al[58] and Kellner et al.[60]
[c]From Rubin et al[58] and Danesi et al.[65]
[d]From Rubin et al[58] and Hande.[59]
[e]From Rubin et al[58] and Danesi et al.[65]
[f]From Rubin et al.[58]
ALL, acute lymphocytic leukemia; ANLL, acute nonlymphocytic leukemia; BMT, bone marrow transplantation; BP, blood pressure; Cl$_{Cr}$, creatinine clearance; HD, Hodgkin's disease; KS, Kaposi's sarcoma; LVEF, left ventricular ejection fraction; MDS, myelodysplastic syndrome; NHL, non-Hodgkin's lymphoma; NSCLC, non-small-cell lung cancer; SCLC small cell lung cancer.

ETOPOSIDE AND TENIPOSIDE

Etoposide and teniposide are semisynthetic podophyllotoxin derivatives (see Table 124–13). Podophyllin is extracted from the mayapple or mandrake plant. Like the vinca alkaloids, podophyllin itself binds to tubulin and interferes with microtubule formation. Unlike the parent compound, however, etoposide and teniposide damage tumor cells by causing strand breakage through inhibiting topoisomerase II.[58,59] Resistance may be caused by differences in topoisomerase II levels, by increased cell ability to repair strand breaks, or by increased levels of P-glycoproteins. Etoposide and teniposide are usually clinically cross-resistant. They are cell-cycle phase–specific and arrest cells in the S or early G$_2$ phase. As a result, activity is much greater when they are administered in divided doses over several days, rather than in large single doses.[58,59]

CAMPTOTHECIN DERIVATIVES

Camptothecin, a plant alkaloid derived from *Camptotheca acuminata*, is a potent inhibitor of DNA topoisomerase I. Clinical trials failed to show expected antitumor activity, and the drug produced severe, unpredictable toxicity. The camptothecin analogs irinotecan and topotecan were synthesized to reduce toxicity and improve therapeutic effects. Both irinotecan and topotecan, through its active metabolite SN-38, poison the actions of the topoisomerase I enzymes. Topoisomerase I enzymes stabilize DNA single-strand breaks and inhibit strand resealing (see Table 124–13).[58,60–64]

ANTHRACENE DERIVATIVES

The most widely used and best understood anthracene derivative is doxorubicin, also commonly known by its earliest trade name, Adriamycin or "Adria." Other members of the anthracene group include daunorubicin (daunomycin), idarubicin, epirubicin, and mitoxantrone (see Table 124–13). All of these agents except mitoxantrone are anthracyclines and share a common, four-membered anthracene ring complex with an attached aglycone or sugar portion. The ring complex is a chromophore and accounts for the intense colors of these compounds. Doxorubicin differs from its parent compound daunorubicin by the addition of a hydroxyl group on the attached sugar, and it is sometimes referred to as hydroxydaunorubicin. A hydroxyl group on epirubicin is in the *epi* conformation compared with doxorubicin (epidoxorubicin), and idarubicin is demethoxydaunorubicin. Mitoxantrone is an anthracenedione rather than an anthracycline, and has no sugar group attached to the three-membered anthracene ring complex.[58,65]

Doxorubicin, Daunorubicin, Idarubicin, and Epirubicin

Anthracyclines have been classified as antitumor antibiotics, but it is more accurate to refer to them as intercalating topoisomerase inhibitors (see Table 124–13). Intercalating agents are compounds that insert or stack between base pairs of DNA. Although it is well established that the planar groups of the anthracene ring complex do intercalate with DNA, causing structural changes that interfere with DNA and RNA synthesis, this is not their primary mechanism of cytotoxicity. The anthracyclines are primarily topoisomerase II poisons, producing double-strand DNA breaks.[58,65]

The anthracyclines also undergo electron reductions to reactive compounds that can damage DNA and cell membranes. Free radicals formed from reduction of the anthracyclines first donate electrons to oxygen to make superoxide, which can react with itself to make hydrogen peroxide. Cleavage of hydrogen peroxide produces the highly reactive and destructive hydroxyl radical. This last step requires iron, and the anthracyclines are potent iron binders. Iron-anthracycline complexes can bind to DNA and react rapidly with hydrogen peroxide to produce the hydroxyl radicals that actually cleave DNA. Human cells have natural defenses against oxygen radical damage, in the form of enzymes that can convert the radicals to less reactive compounds, or that can repair DNA damage. Differences in distribution of these defensive enzymes may account for characteristic sites of toxicities of the anthracyclines. For example, cardiac muscle has low levels of defensive enzymes and high levels of enzymes that activate anthracyclines. Oxygen free-radical formation is firmly established as a cause of cardiac damage and extravasation injury, but is not a major mechanism of tumor-cell killing. Resistance to the anthracyclines is usually secondary to P-glycoprotein–dependent multidrug resistance, causing the anthracyclines to be actively pumped out of tumor cells. Altered topoisomerase II activity may also be clinically important.[58,65]

Mitoxantrone

The anthracenedione mitoxantrone was synthesized in an attempt to develop agents with comparable antitumor activity to doxorubicin, but with an improved safety profile (see Table 124–13). Like the anthracyclines, mitoxantrone is an intercalating topoisomerase II inhibitor,

but its potential for free-radical formation is much less than that of the anthracyclines. Perhaps because of the decreased tendency for free-radical formation, the risks of cardiac toxicity and ulceration after extravasation, although still present, are markedly reduced.[57,65]

ALKYLATING AGENTS

The alkylating agents are among the oldest and most useful of antineoplastic drugs. Their clinical use evolved from the observation of bone marrow suppression and lymph node shrinkage in soldiers exposed to sulfur mustard gas warfare during World War I. In an effort to develop similar agents that might be useful in treating cancerous overgrowths of lymphoid tissues, less reactive derivatives were synthesized. Their effectiveness as anticancer agents was confirmed by clinical trials in the middle 1940s.[66]

All of the alkylating agents work through the covalent bonding of highly reactive alkyl groups or substituted alkyl groups with nucleophilic groups of proteins and nucleic acids. Some alkylating agents react directly with biologic molecules; others form an intermediate compound that reacts with the targets. The most common binding site for alkylating agents is the seven-nitrogen group of guanine. These covalent interactions result in cross-linking between two DNA strands or between two bases in the same strand of DNA. Reactions between DNA and RNA and between drug and proteins may also occur, but the main insult that results in cell death is inhibition of DNA replication, because the interlinked strands do not separate as required. Because the alkylating agents can damage DNA during any phase of the cell cycle, they are not cell-cycle–phase specific. However, their greatest effect is seen in rapidly dividing cells.

As a class, alkylators are cytotoxic, mutagenic, teratogenic, carcinogenic, and myelosuppressive. Resistance to these agents can occur from increased DNA repair capabilities, from decreased entry into or accelerated exit from cells, from increased inactivation of the agents inside cells, or from lack of cellular mechanisms to result in cell death following DNA damage. They react with water and are inactivated by hydrolysis, making spontaneous degradation an important component of their elimination.[67]

CYCLOPHOSPHAMIDE AND IFOSFAMIDE

Cyclophosphamide and ifosfamide are nitrogen mustard derivatives, and are widely used alkylating agents (Table 124–14). They are closely related in structure, clinical use, and toxicity. Neither agent is active in its parent form and must be activated by mixed hepatic oxidase enzymes. The active metabolite of cyclophosphamide is phosphoramide mustard. Another metabolite, 4-hydroxycyclophosphamide is cytotoxic, but is not an alkylating agent. Ifosfamide is hepatically activated to ifosfamide mustard. Acrolein, a metabolite of both cyclophosphamide and ifosfamide, has little antitumor activity, but is responsible for some of their toxicity.[67,68]

NITROSOUREAS

The nitrosoureas are alkylating agents characterized by lipophilicity and ability to cross the blood-brain barrier. Carmustine or bischloroethylnitrosourea (BCNU) and lomustine (CCNU) are commercially available. BCNU is available as an intravenous preparation and as a drug-impregnated biodegradable wafer (Gliadel) for direct application to residual tumor tissue following surgical resection of brain tumors. The nitrosoureas decompose to reactive alkylating metabolites and to isocyanate compounds that have several effects on reproducing cells (see Table 124–14).[67]

TABLE 124–14. Alkylating Agents

Agent/Major Uses	Class/Mechanism	Major Side Effects	Comments
Busulfan (Myleran tablets, Busulfex injection)[a] CML; BMT preparative regimens	DNA-DNA and DNA-protein cross-links; inhibition of DNA replication; selective cytotoxicity for myeloid cells; crosses blood-brain barrier	Myelosuppression; skin hyperpigmentation; pulmonary fibrosis; low emetogenic potential (in standard doses); endocrine: gynecomastia, adrenal insufficiency; *high- and BMT-dose toxicities:* seizures (generalized tonic-clonic); hepatic veno-occlusive disease; highly emetogenic in BMT doses	Bone marrow recovery may be delayed (3–6 weeks); pulmonary fibrosis associated with >3 years exposure, prior chest radiation; seizure prophylaxis (phenytoin 300 mg/day with BMT doses) Pharmacokinetic monitoring is required with IV busulfan, preferably in an experienced BMT setting *IV and oral preparations are not interchangeable;* put tablets in gelatin capsules for easier administration with high-dose administration
Carboplatin (Paraplatin)[b] Ovarian cancer; NSCLC; SCLC; head and neck cancer; testicular cancer; bladder cancer; breast cancer	Platinum agent; forms inter- and instrastrand DNA cross-links; inhibition of DNA synthesis	Myelosuppression: thrombocytopenia, neutropenia, anemia; moderately emetogenic; risk of hypersensitivity reactions, frequently delayed, after 5+ doses; may necessitate discontinuation of carboplatin; frequently results in cross-hypersensitivity to cisplatin	Reduce dose for Cl_{cr} <60 mL/min; platelet recovery may be delayed (4–5 weeks) Calvert formula for dose modifications: Dose (mg) = target AUC × (CL_{cr} + 25); Cl_{cr} calculated using Cockcroft-Gault equation; note that the calculated dose is *total dose, not dose per m^2 body surface area*
Carmustine (BCNU, *bischloro-nitrosourea;* BiCNU)[a] Brain tumors; myeloma; NHL; HD; BMT preparative regimens; melanoma; also available in wafer form for implantation into brain tumor cavities after resection (Gliadel)	Nitrosourea; cross-links DNA strands; inhibits DNA replication; highly lipophilic: penetrates CNS	Myelosuppression (may be delayed, nadir at 3–4 weeks); highly emetogenic; cumulative nephrotoxicity; pulmonary fibrosis; facial flushing during infusion	Bone marrow recovery may require 6–8 weeks postadministration; not a vesicant; vein irritation and facial flushing may be related to alcohol vehicle Prepare in glass bottles or non-PVC bags and non-PVC (such as nitroglycerin-designated) tubing to avoid adsorption of drug to PVC plastics
Chlorambucil (Leukeran)[a] CLL; NHL; HD Available only as 2-mg tablets	Nitrogen mustard derivative; forms interstrand DNA cross-links; selective cytotoxicity for lymphocytes	Myelosuppression (dose-limiting); increased liver function tests; skin rash; low emetogenic potential; menstrual irregularities; pulmonary toxicity: interstitial pneumonitis/fibrosis; carcinogenic: risk of secondary malignancies; causes infertility and sterility; teratogenic	Should be taken on an empty stomach; food decreases absorption May be dosed in low daily-dosing regimens or in higher dose, "pulse" or intermittent dosing schedules administered biweekly or monthly; *note: pulse dosing may require patients to take several tablets (e.g., 10–20 tablets) per dose*
Cisplatin (CDDP; *cis-diaminodicholoro-platinum;* Platinol)[c] Ovarian cancer; bladder cancer; testicular cancer; cervical cancer; NSCLC; SCLC; esophageal and head and neck cancers; NHL; sarcomas; melanoma; endometrial cancer; gastric cancer Radiosensitizer	Platinum agent; forms inter- and intrastrand DNA cross-links; inhibition of DNA synthesis; aquated species is cytotoxic	*Nephrotoxic!* Direct toxicity to renal tubules; severe and prolonged potassium and magnesium wasting; highly emetogenic (acute and/or delayed onset); neurotoxicity: peripheral neuropathy that is cumulative and dose-related in stocking-glove pattern; may be reversible; ototoxicity: may cause permanent hearing loss; may require dose reduction or drug discontinuation; anemia with chronic dosing; may respond to epoetin; generally not myelosuppressive; doses should not exceed 100 mg/m^2 (maximum single dose *and* per-cycle dose); inactivated by contact with aluminum needles	*Hydration required!* 1–2 liters of 0.9% sodium chloride minimum pre- and post cisplatin administration; ensure good urine output (>100 mL/hour); potassium chloride and magnesium sulfate in IV fluid to replace losses; with or without mannitol 12.5–50 g to increase urine flow; dose reductions with CL_{cr} <60 mL/min; carboplatin may be an alternative agent for patients with impaired renal function; aggressive antiemetics required pretreatment and for 3–5 days after to prevent delayed nausea/vomiting Amifostine chemoprotective agent; may reduce cisplatin renal toxicity; little impact on neurotoxicity or myelosuppression; adds to nausea and causes hypotension; limited evidence of efficacy of vitamin E for prevention of neurotoxicity

TABLE 124–14. (Continued)

Agent/Major Uses	Class/Mechanism	Major Side Effects	Comments
Cyclophosphamide (Cytoxan)[d] Breast cancer; NHL; ALL; ANLL; CLL; ovarian cancer; myeloma; retinoblastoma; neuroblastoma; HD; NSCLC; SCLC; endometrial cancer; soft-tissue sarcomas; BMT-preparative (high-dose); bladder cancer SLE; autoimmune disorders	Alkylating agent; nitrogen mustard derivative; cross-links DNA-DNA or DNA-protein; inhibits DNA synthesis; activated by hepatic microsomal (CYP450) mixed function oxidases; acrolein metabolite (no antitumor activity) associated with hemorrhagic cystitis	Hemorrhagic cystitis Moderately emetogenic: worse with high doses; nausea may be delayed 12–24 hours; myelosuppression; alopecia; SIADH, typically with high doses (>2 g/m^2); secondary malignancies (bladder cancers, acute leukemia); infertility, sterility	Hydration needed to prevent hemorrhagic cystitis (oral/IV ~3 L/day × 72h); mesna may be required with high-dose regimens (see ifosfamide) Instruct patients to take oral tablets in the morning to allow for elimination of toxic metabolite; absorbed through skin: *avoid spills* Drug interactions: CYP450 inducers (e.g., barbiturates) may increase formation of toxic metabolites; CYP450 inhibitors (e.g., cimetidine) may increase myelosuppression
Dacarbazine (DTIC; *d*imethyl*t*riazeno-*i*midazole-*c*arboxamide)[a] Melanoma; HD; soft-tissue sarcomas; brain tumors	Exact mechanism unclear; alkylation most likely mechanism, but does not cause DNA cross-linking; also appears to inhibit DNA, RNA, and protein synthesis; activated by hepatic microsomal mixed function oxidases (CYP450 enzymes)	Myelosuppression; highly emetogenic; flu-like syndrome: fever, myalgia, malaise (may last for several days after dacarbazine administration); facial flushing; photosensitivity: use caution with sun exposure	Not a vesicant, but may cause burning pain at injection site Light-sensitive: dispense in lightproof bags; pink color indicates decomposition
Ifosfamide (Ifex)[d] Testicular cancer; soft-tissue sarcomas; NHL; NSCLC; cervical cancer; head and neck cancers	Alkylating agent; cross-links DNA strands; activated in the liver by microsomal (CYP450) mixed function oxidases	Hemorrhagic cystitis: *always* given with mesna and hydration; nephrotoxicity: renal tubular acidosis; potassium, magnesium, and phosphate wasting, especially in high-dose regimens; myelosuppression; CNS effects: somnolence, confusion, disorientation, cerebellar symptoms that are dose-related; moderately emetogenic; alopecia	3–4 L/day fluid for hydration; potassium, magnesium, and phosphate may be required to replace losses Mesna dose is typically 60–100% of ifosfamide dose (1:1 for continuous infusion ifosfamide); ifosfamide and mesna are physically compatible and may be delivered in same IV bag CNS toxicity and nausea and vomiting may be more severe with rapid infusion; case reports suggest methylene blue may be effective treatment for CNS toxicity
Mechlorethamine (nitrogen mustard; H$_2$N; Mustargen)[a] HD; NHL; Mycosis fungoides (topical)	Bifunctional alkylating agent (two reactive groups); forms inter-and intrastrand DNA cross-links; inhibits DNA, RNA, and protein synthesis	Myelosuppression; highly emetogenic: rapid onset, within 1–2 hours of dose; vesicant: extravasation injury; secondary malignancies; sterility and infertility	Antidote for extravasation: sodium thiosulfate; very short stability in aqueous solutions, about 1 hour Used as topical solution or in compounded ointments for mycosis fungoides
Oxaliplatin (Eloxatin)[d] Colorectal cancer; ovarian cancer; gastric cancer	Platinum agent (see cisplatin, carboplatin)	Peripheral neuropathy >50% patients: *acute form:* <14 days, rapid onset, reversible, exacerbated by cold, affects hands, feet, perioral area, and throat; *persistent form:* onset >14 days, mainly hands and feet; may affect proprioception; may be permanent; pharyngolaryngeal dysesthesias in 1–2%; nausea, vomiting: moderately emetogenic; abdominal pain, diarrhea; anaphylaxis risk	Renally eliminated; reduce dose in patients with impaired renal function Glutathione, magnesium, and calcium supplementation being evaluated for prevention of neuropathies Avoid exposure to cold
Procarbazine (Matulane)[a] HD; brain tumors; NSCLC Only available orally	Exact mechanism unclear; alkylation most likely mechanism of action; also appears to inhibit DNA, RNA, and protein synthesis; activated by hepatic microsomal mixed function oxidases (CYP450 enzymes); good CNS penetration	Myelosuppression: thrombocytopenia, neutropenia (may be prolonged 4–6 weeks); low emetogenic potential may be more severe initially; diarrhea; neurotoxicity: paresthesias, neuropathy; flu-like syndrome; infertility and sterility; secondary malignancies	Administered as a single, daily dose on an empty stomach Monoamine oxidase inhibitors: drug-food interactions with tyramine-rich foods such as red wines, dark beers, aged cheeses, yogurt; may precipitate hypertensive crisis; drug interactions: tricyclic antidepressants and SSRIs, sympathomimetics; disulfiram-like reaction with alcohol

(continued)

TABLE 124–14. (Continued)

Agent/Major Uses	Class/Mechanism	Major Side Effects	Comments
Temozolomide (Temodar)[f] Brain tumors; brain metastases; melanoma	Similar to dacarbazine; same reactive metabolite as dacarbazine (MTIC); does not require liver for activation; well absorbed orally; achieves therapeutic levels in CNS	Headache and fatigue; moderately emetogenic; myelosuppression: neutropenia, thrombocytopenia; myalgias, back pain; diplopia; lymphopenia, especially in chronic dosing	Crosses blood-brain barrier in therapeutic concentrations Administer on an empty stomach; capsules should not be opened or chewed Drug interaction: valproic acid may decease clearance of temozolomide slightly PCP prophylaxis should be considered for patients who develop lymphopenia
Thiotepa (thiethylene thiophosphoramide; ThioTEPA)[a] Breast cancer; bladder cancer (instillation); BMT preparation	Trifunctional alkylating agent; active metabolite TEPA; crosses blood-brain barrier	Myelosuppression (dose-limiting); nausea and vomiting: severe at high doses for BMT preparation; mucositis; pruritus and dermatitis	Very old drug, now most commonly used as preparative regimen for stem cell transplants

[a]From Bast et al.[66]
[b]From Bast et al,[66] Su et al,[70] and Guminski et al.[71]
[c]From Bast et al,[66] Su et al,[70] Guminski et al.[71] O'Dwyer et al.[72]
[d]From Bast et al,[66] Colvin.[67]
[e]From Bast et al,[66] Su et al,[70] and Pace et al.[73]
[f]From Bast et al,[66] Boddy et al,[68] and Stupp et al.[69]
ALL, acute lymphocytic leukemia; ANLL, acute nonlymphocytic leukemia; AUC, area under the curve; BMT, bone marrow transplantation; Cl$_{cr}$, creatinine clearance; CLL, chronic lymphocytic leukemia; CML, chronic myelogenous leukemia; CNS, central nervous system; CYP450, cytochrome P450 isoenzyme; HD, Hodgkin's disease; NHL, non-Hodgkin's lymphoma; NSCLC, non-small-cell lung cancer; PCP, *Pneumocystis carinii* pneumonia; PVC, polyvinyl chloride; SCLC, small cell lung cancer; SIADH, syndrome of inappropriate secretion of antidiuretic hormone; SLE, systemic lupus erythematosus; SSRI, selective serotonin reuptake inhibitor; TEPA, thiethylene phosphoramide.

NONCLASSIC ALKYLATING AGENTS

Several other cytotoxic agents appear to act as alkylators, although their structures do not include the classic alkylating groups. They are capable of binding covalently to cellular components and include procarbazine, dacarbazine, temozolamide, the heavy metal compounds, and some antitumor antibiotics (see Table 124–14).[67]

Dacarbazine and Temozolomide

Dacarbazine, or dimethyl triazeno-imidazole-carboxamide (DTIC), and temozolomide (dihydro methyl oxoimidazo tetrazino carboxamide) are nonclassic alkylating agents (see Table 124–14). Both compounds undergo demethylation to the same active intermediate (monomethyl triazeno imidazole carboxamide [MTIC]) that interrupts DNA replication by causing methylation of guanine. Unlike dacarbazine, temozolomide does not require the liver for activation, and is chemically degraded to MTIC at physiologic pH. Both drugs inhibit DNA, RNA, and protein synthesis.[67,69,70]

Important pharmacokinetic differences exist between the two drugs. Dacarbazine is poorly absorbed, and must be administered by intravenous infusion. Temozolomide is rapidly absorbed after oral administration, and is approximately 100% bioavailable when given on a completely empty stomach. Darcarbazine penetrates the CNS poorly, but temozolomide readily crosses the blood-brain barrier, achieving therapeutically active concentrations in cerebrospinal fluid and brain tumor tissues.[67,69,70]

HEAVY METAL COMPOUNDS

CISPLATIN, CARBOPLATIN, AND OXALIPLATIN

The platinum derivatives, cisplatin, carboplatin, and oxaliplatin are anticancer agents with remarkable usefulness in cancer treatment (see Table 124–14). Recognition of cisplatin's cytotoxic activity was the result of a serendipitous observation that bacterial growth in culture was altered when an electric current was delivered to the media through platinum electrodes. The growth change was noted to be similar to that produced by alkylating agents and radiation. It was found that a platinum-chloride complex, now known as cisplatin, generated by the current was responsible for the changes. Carboplatin is a structural analog of cisplatin in which the chloride groups of the parent compound are replaced by a carboxycyclobutane moiety. It shares a similar spectrum of clinical activity with cisplatin, and cross-resistance is common. Oxaliplatin is an organoplatinum compound in which the platinum is complexed with an oxalate ligand as the leaving group and to diaminocyclohexane. Its spectrum of activity differs substantially from the other platinum compounds, and includes notable activity against colorectal cancers.[67,71]

The cytotoxicity of the platinum derivatives depends on platinum binding to DNA and the formation of intrastrand cross-links or adducts between neighboring guanines. These intrastrand links cause a major bending of the DNA. They may cause cellular damage by distorting the normal DNA conformation and preventing bases that are normally paired from lining up with each other. Interstrand cross-links also occur.[67,71]

The cytotoxic form of cisplatin is the aquated species, in which hydroxyl groups or water molecules replace the two chloride groups. This reaction occurs readily in low concentrations of chloride, such as the concentrations present within cells, and produces a positively charged compound that can react with DNA. The aquated species is responsible for both the efficacy and toxicity of cisplatin. Carboplatin also undergoes aquation, but at a slower rate. Oxaliplatin becomes active when the oxalate ligand is displaced in physiologic solutions.[67,71]

Resistance to the therapeutic effects of platinum compounds may occur through several mechanisms. The ability to repair platinum-induced DNA damage may be increased, or the agents may be inactivated by increased levels of intracellular glutathione, metallothioneins, or other thiol-containing proteins. Altered uptake into cells may also affect sensitivity to platinum compounds.[67,71,72]

Cisplatin is a highly toxic antineoplastic agent, with potential for producing serious nephrotoxicity, ototoxicity, peripheral neuropathy, emesis, and anemia. The significant efficacy of cisplatin against many tumor types makes it a valuable agent despite these toxicities, most of which can be prevented or managed with aggressive supportive care measures.[67,72,73] In contrast, carboplatin administration is limited by hematologic toxicity. Patients with compromised renal function require dose reductions to limit myelosuppressive toxicity. The most widely used dosage schema, the Calvert formula (see Table 124–14), uses a target area under the curve and renal function parameters to estimate the carboplatin dose.[67,71] Carboplatin's potential to cause renal damage, peripheral neuropathy, ototoxicity, and nausea and vomiting is much less than that of comparable cisplatin doses.[67] Oxaliplatin is not nephrotoxic, ototoxic, or highly emetogenic, but produces peripheral neuropathies and unique cold-induced neuropathies.[74] All of the platinum derivatives have significant potential to cause hypersensitivity reactions, including anaphylaxis.

MISCELLANEOUS AGENTS

BLEOMYCIN

Bleomycin or "bleo" is an antitumor antibiotic (Table 124–15). It is a mixture of peptides from fungal *Streptomyces* species, and as such its strength is expressed in units of drug activity. One unit is roughly equal to 1 mg of polypeptide protein. The predominant peptide is bleomycin A2, which makes up approximately 70% of the commercial product. Bleomycin's cytotoxicity is secondary to DNA strand breakage, or scission, which it produces via free-radical formation. Cytotoxicity depends on binding of an iron-bleomycin complex to DNA. The bleomycin-iron complex then reduces molecular oxygen to free oxygen radicals that cause primarily single-strand breaks in DNA. Bleomycin has greatest effect on cells in the G_2 phase of the cell cycle and in mitosis.[75]

Bleomycin is inactivated within cells by the enzyme aminohydrolase. This enzyme is widely distributed, but is present in only low concentrations in the skin and the lungs, explaining the predominant toxicities of bleomycin to those sites. The presence of hydrolase enzymes in tumor cells is the primary mechanism of resistance to bleomycin. Cells can also become resistant by repairing the DNA breaks produced by bleomycin.[75]

HYDROXYUREA

Hydroxyurea is a unique drug that inhibits ribonucleotide reductase, the enzyme required to convert ribonucleotides into the deoxyribonucleotide forms required for both DNA synthesis and repair (see Table 124–15). Cells accumulate in the S phase because DNA synthesis is inhibited, and only abnormally short DNA strands are produced.[36]

L-ASPARAGINASE

L-Asparaginase is unique among cytotoxic drugs in its unusual mechanism of action, patterns of toxicity, and source (see Table 124–15). It is an enzyme produced by *Escherichia coli* and other bacteria.

L-Asparagine is a nonessential amino acid that can be synthesized by most mammalian cells, except for those of certain lymphoid human malignancies, which lack or have very low levels of the synthetase enzyme required for L-asparagine formation. L-Asparagine is degraded by the enzyme L-asparaginase, which depletes existing supplies and inhibits protein synthesis. Increased L-asparagine synthetase activity within tumor cells causes resistance to L-asparaginase treatment.[76]

ARSENIC TRIOXIDE

Arsenic is an organic element and a well-known poison that is an effective treatment for acute promyelocytic leukemia (see Table 124–15).[77] As an antineoplastic, arsenic trioxide acts as a differentiating agent, inducing the growth progression of cancerous cells into mature, more normal cells. It also induces programmed cell death or apoptosis.

MITOMYCIN C

Mitomycin C is a natural product sometimes classified as an antitumor antibiotic (see Table 124–15).[67,78] It has functional similarities to nitrogen mustard compounds and may function as an alkylating agent, although its toxicity pattern differs from conventional alkylators.

IMMUNE THERAPIES

◀8 An intact immune system is believed to play an important role in the control of cancer growth, as evidenced by the high incidence of cancers in immunosuppressed patients such as solid organ transplant recipients or those with human immunodeficiency virus infections. There are also rare but well documented spontaneous remissions of immunologically-linked cancers, particularly melanoma and renal cell carcinoma. Immune therapies attempt to harness the immune system to treat cancer (Table 124–16).[79–81]

INTERFERONS

The interferons (IFNs) are a family of proteins produced by nucleated cells and by recombinant DNA technology, with antiviral, antiproliferative, and immunoregulatory activities. They are classified as α, β, or γ interferons based on antigenic, biologic, and pharmacologic properties. Many subtypes of IFN α are known. IFN α-2a and IFN α-2b, approved for anticancer indications, are very similar single-species recombinant products.

The mechanisms of IFN α's antitumor action are complex. IFN increases the activity of cytotoxic cells within the immune system, but direct antiproliferative effects also play a role. IFNs prolong the cell cycle, which results in cytostasis, an increase in cell size, and apoptosis. They can inhibit new blood vessel formation in tumors and can increase the expression of antigens on tumor cell surfaces, making the cancerous cells more easily recognized by the cells of the immune system. They also inhibit or block certain oncogenes that can direct the unregulated cell growth that is characteristic of cancerous cells. Alterations in gene expression may change the levels of receptors for other cytokines, or the concentration of regulatory proteins on immune cells, or may activate enzymes that alter cellular growth and function.[79,80]

INTERLEUKIN-2 (ALDESLEUKIN)

Interleukin-2 (aldesleukin; IL-2) is a lymphokine produced by recombinant DNA technology that promotes B- and T-cell proliferation and differentiation and initiates a cytokine cascade with multiple interacting immunologic effects. The IL-2 receptor is expressed in increased amounts on activated T cells and mediates most of the effects of IL-2. Antitumor effects depend on proliferation of

TABLE 124–15. Miscellaneous Agents

Agent/Major Uses	Class/Mechanism	Major Side Effects	Comments
Arsenic trioxide (Trisenox)[a] APL	Differentiating agent; exact mechanism unclear; causes morphologic changes and DNA fragmentation characteristic of apoptosis	Retinoic acid syndrome: pulmonary infiltrates, respiratory distress, and hypotension; cardiovascular: tachycardia, edema, QT prolongation, chest pain, hypotension; low to moderate emetogenic potential; electrolyte abnormalities: hypokalemia or hyperkalemia, hypomagnesemia, hyperglycemia; rash; light-headedness or vasomotor symptoms; fatigue; musculoskeletal pain	Retinoic acid syndrome must be treated promptly with corticosteroids; weight gain secondary to fluid retention may be dose limiting
Asparaginase (L-asparaginase, Elspar) **Pegaspargase** (Oncospar)[b] ALL	Antitumor enzyme, hydrolyzes L-asparagine in bloodstream, depriving tumor cells of the essential amino acid; results in inhibition of protein, DNA, and RNA synthesis and cell proliferation; derived from *Escherichia coli*	Hypersensitivity reactions (fever, hypotension, rash, dyspnea in 25%), much lower risk with polyethylene glycol form; low emetogenic potential; pancreatitis; decreased synthesis of proteins, clotting factors; CNS: lethargy	Skin test prior to administration; anaphylaxis precautions; Pegaspargase complexed with polyethylene glycol to decrease immunogenicity and prolong duration of action (dose every 2 weeks vs. 2–5 times/week); more costly, may be difficult to obtain Monitor clotting function
Bleomycin (Bleo, Blenoxane)[c] NHL, HD; testicular cancer; squamous cell cancers of the head and neck, cervix, skin, penis, or vulva; malignant pleural effusions; KS	Antitumor antibiotic, causes single- and double-strand DNA scission (free-radical mediated); inhibition of protein, DNA, and RNA synthesis	Anaphylaxis and hypersensitivity reactions; fever and flu-like symptoms; mucositis; pulmonary fibrosis secondary to oxygen free-radical formation; low emetogenic potential; alopecia; not myelosuppressive	Test dose (1 unit) is recommended, but controversial: premedicate for subsequent doses with acetaminophen Dose reduction for CL_{cr} <60 mL/min Pulmonary toxicity associated with: single doses >30 units, cumulative dose >400 units, bolus administration; risk factors: age >70, pre-existing pulmonary disease, prior chest radiation, exposure to high oxygen concentrations
Mitomycin C (Mutamycin)[d] Gastric cancer, breast cancer; bladder cancer (instillation); esophageal cancer; cervical cancer; colorectal cancer; NSCLC	Antitumor antibiotic activated to an alkylating agent; cross-links DNA; inhibits DNA and RNA synthesis; superoxide free radicals may produce DNA strand breaks	Myelosuppression: may be delayed and prolonged (up to 8 weeks); mucositis; moderately emetogenic; extravasation: severe vesicant; pulmonary toxicity: pneumonitis, fibrosis (worse with concurrent vincristine or vinblastine); hemolytic anemia and uremic syndrome	Apply ice or cold packs to site for extravasation; tissue damage may be delayed for 3–4 months after extravasation Sometimes administered intra-arterially, but systemic side effects may still occur

[a]From Kurtzberg et al.[76]
[b]From Laxo et al. [75]
[c]From Andre et al.[74]
[d]From Bast et al,[66] Soignet et al.[77]

ALL, acute lymphocytic leukemia; APL, acute promyelocytic leukemia; CL_{cr}, creatinine clearance; CNS, central nervous system; HD, Hodgkin's disease; KS, Kaposi's sarcoma; NHL, non-Hodgkin's lymphoma; NSCLC, non-small-cell lung cancer.

cytotoxic immune cells that can recognize and destroy tumor cells without damaging normal cells. Some of these cytotoxic cells are natural killer cells, lymphokine-activated killer cells, and tumor-infiltrating lymphocytes.[81]

The toxicity of IL-2 is related to dose, route, and duration of therapy, but in general, IL-2 is toxic therapy that requires vigorous supportive care. The most common dose-limiting toxicities are hypotension, fluid retention, and renal dysfunction. IL-2 decreases peripheral vascular resistance, producing peripheral vasodilation, tachycardia, and hypotension. A characteristic vascular- or capillary-leak syndrome produces fluid retention, which in turn can cause respiratory compromise. These toxicities require administration of vasopressors in most patients, judicious use of fluid support and diuretics, and supplemental oxygen. Patients with underlying cardiovascular or renal abnormalities are more susceptible to these adverse effects, making careful patient selection important.[81] Most patients treated with IL-2 in full doses experience thrombocytopenia, anemia, eosinophilia, reversible cholestasis, and skin erythema with burning and pruritus, and some have neuropsychiatric changes, hypothyroidism, and bacterial infections.[82–85] In general, the

TABLE 124–16. Immune Therapies

Agent/Major Uses	Mechanism	Adverse Effects	Comments
Interferon alfa (interferon α-2b; Intron A and Interferon α-2a; Roferon-A, IFN)[a] KS; CML; melanoma; hairy cell leukemia; renal cell carcinoma; NHL; multiple myeloma Hepatitis B and C; condyloma acuminata	Stimulates the immune system against tumor cells; direct and indirect cytotoxic activity; increases expression of tumor-associated antigens	Flu-like syndrome: fever, malaise, chills, headaches; fatigue: often dose-limiting; anorexia and altered taste; increased liver function tests (transient); myelosuppression: mild leukopenia, thrombocytopenia; depression; vivid dreams or nightmares	Patients should be advised to administer interferon in the evening to reduce excessive daytime sedation; premedication and scheduled dosing with acetaminophen or an NSAID may alleviate flu-like symptoms Flu-like symptoms typically subside with chronic use; no tolerance to fatigue, may necessitate dose reduction; antidepressants valuable for depressive symptoms Polyethylene glycol interferon forms have sustained duration of effect
Aldesleukin (interleukin-2, IL-2; Proleukin)[b] Renal cell cancer; melanoma	Stimulates growth, differentiation, and proliferation of activated T cells; generates lymphokine-activated killer cell activity and other killer cells; stimulates the immune system against tumor cells	Flu-like syndrome: fevers, chills, malaise; vascular or capillary leak syndrome: hypotension, pulmonary and peripheral edema; GI: moderately emetogenic, diarrhea; nephrotoxicity: partially due to hypotension or decreased renal perfusion; myelosuppression: thrombocytopenia, leukopenia, generally transient; cardiac: arrhythmias, reflex tachycardia; skin rash, flushing, itching, peeling, dryness; CNS: somnolence, confusion; bacterial infections common, especially staphylococcal	Addition of dopamine in "renal" doses (1–5 mcg/kg per minute) may help maintain good renal blood flow and blood pressure Pulmonary edema can be managed with cautious use of diuretics; short courses of albumin may also be beneficial Patients with history of cardiac arrhythmias may require cardiac monitoring during IL-2 administration Itching may respond to treatment with antihistamines (hydroxyzine or diphenhydramine); emollient skin creams or occlusive agents are effective for dry, peeling skin; avoid corticosteroids: may counteract the antitumor effects of IL-2.

[a]From Bradner[78] and Border.[79]
[b]From Kirkwood et al.[80]
CML, chronic myelogenous leukemia; CNS, central nervous system; KS, Kaposi's sarcoma; NHL, non-Hodgkin's lymphoma; NSAID, nonsteroidal anti-inflammatory drug.

toxicities from IL-2 therapy reverse quickly once therapy is stopped, and can be managed or prevented by careful prospective monitoring and pharmacologic supportive care.[81]

BIOLOGICALLY DIRECTED THERAPIES

Most anticancer drugs are relatively indiscriminant cellular poisons. Although a few, such as methotrexate, capecitabine, L-asparaginase, and the immune therapies demonstrate some degree of selectivity for malignant cells, the selectivity is incomplete, and dose-limiting damage to normal cells also occurs. Recently anticancer research has focused on development of anticancer agents that target malignant cells more specifically, or the biochemical processes that control cancerous cell growth.

DENILEUKIN DIFTITOX

Denileukin diftitox (Ontak) is a recombinant fusion protein that combines the active sections of both IL-2 and diphtheria toxin. Unconjugated diphtheria toxin is much too toxic to administer to humans. As

the "payload" of the fusion protein, however, its cytotoxic effects are directed toward cells that express the high-affinity form of the IL-2 receptor, such as cancer cells of some patients with cutaneous T-cell lymphoma. Once denileukin diftitox interacts with the IL-2 receptors, the toxin inhibits protein synthesis in the cancer cells and causes cell death.[66]

Although denileukin diftitox is directed therapy, its targeting of cells that express high-affinity IL-2 receptors is not specific; that is, these receptors are expressed on cells other than cancer cells. Denileukin diftitox produces acute hypersensitivity reactions, flu-like symptoms, sometimes with prominent diarrhea, and vascular-leak syndrome. It differs from the vascular-leak syndrome produced by high-dose IL-2 in that it occurs in fewer patients, is delayed in onset, is usually self-limited, and does not consistently recur on retreatment.[81]

ENDOCRINE THERAPIES

Perhaps the earliest successful approach to target the growth processes of cancerous cells was the use of endocrine therapies. Endocrine manipulation is an option for management of cancers from tissues whose growth is under gonadal hormonal control, especially breast, prostate, and endometrial cancers. These cancers may regress if the "feeding" hormone is eliminated or antagonized. Major organ system toxicity is uncommon from hormonal treatment, making it the least toxic of systemic anticancer therapies. Increasingly specific agents such as the selective estrogen receptor modulators (SERMs) and aromatase inhibitors have increased the utility of

hormonal therapies in the treatment of cancer. Individual agents are described in Table 124–17.[86–93]

Corticosteroid hormones are also useful anticancer agents because of their lymphotoxic effects. Their primary use is in management of hematologic malignancies, especially lymphomas, lymphocytic leukemias, and multiple myeloma. In addition to their cytotoxic effects, corticosteroids have many other applications in

TABLE 124–17. Endocrine Agents Commonly Used in Cancer Treatment

Agent/Major Uses	Class/Mechanism	Major Side Effects	Comments
Antiandrogens			
Bicalutamide (Casodex)[a] Prostate cancer	Nonsteroidal antiandrogen; androgen receptor antagonist; inhibits testosterone and dihydrotestosterone uptake and binding in prostate cells	Hot flashes; gynecomastia, breast tenderness; decreased libido; hepatotoxicity, elevated transaminases; diarrhea	Monitor serum transaminases Drug interactions: may displace warfarin from protein binding sites, increasing anticoagulant effects Often used in combination with an LHRH agonist at initiation of therapy to prevent symptoms of tumor flare
Flutamide (Eulexin)[a] Prostate cancer	Nonsteroidal antiandrogen; androgen receptor antagonist; inhibits testosterone and dihydrotestosterone uptake and binding in prostate cells	Hot flashes; gynecomastia, breast tenderness, nipple pain; decreased libido; diarrhea; low emetogenic potential; mild transient elevations in liver transaminases	Use with caution in G6PD deficiency: may lead to methemoglobinemia Monitor serum transaminases Drug interactions: substrate of CYP450 1A2, CYP450 3A4; inhibits CYP450 1A2; may lead to increased warfarin anticoagulant effects Often used in combination with LHRH agonist at initiation of therapy to prevent symptoms of tumor flare
Nilutamide (Nilandron)[a] Prostate cancer	Nonsteroidal antiandrogen; androgen receptor antagonist; inhibits testosterone and dihydrotestosterone uptake and binding in prostate cells	Pulmonary: dyspnea; may cause interstitial pneumonitis (dyspnea on exertion, chest pain, fever) symptom onset in the first 3 months; hot flashes; gynecomastia; low emetogenic potential; testicular atrophy, decreased libido; hepatic toxicity: elevated transaminases; rare fatal hepatitis; visual disturbances: delayed adaptation to darkness, photophobia, cataracts; isolated cases of aplastic anemia reported; disulfiram-like reaction with alcohol	Visual disturbances (impaired adaptation to darkness) may reverse with dose reduction; monitor serum transaminases; obtain chest x-ray if patient reports dyspnea; evidence of interstitial pneumonitis necessitates discontinuation of treatment Often used in combination with an LHRH agonist at initiation of therapy to prevent symptoms of tumor flare
Antiestrogens			
Aminoglutethimide (Cytadren)[b] Breast cancer; prostate cancer	Nonsteroidal aromatase inhibitor; inhibits conversion of cholesterol to delta-5-pregnenolone; results in decreased synthesis of corticosteroid hormones (glucocorticoids, estrogens, and androgens); also blocks conversion of androgens to estrogens	Adrenocorticoid suppression and insufficiency; skin rash, typically within the first week, usually self-limiting, disappears after 5–8 days, but may require discontinuation of therapy; lethargy, somnolence, dizziness; mild nausea, anorexia; leukopenia and agranulocytosis have been rarely reported	Mineralocorticoid (fludrocortisone) and glucocorticoid (e.g., hydrocortisone 20–30 mg/day) replacement therapy may be required in as many as 50% of patients Salvage therapy for breast cancer and prostate cancer
Anastrazole (Arimidex)[c] Breast cancer	Selective, nonsteroidal aromatase inhibitor; inhibits conversion of androgens to estrogens	Hot flashes; vasodilation, peripheral edema; weakness; arthralgias; elevated transaminases; hyperlipidemia; thrombosis less common than with tamoxifen	Should not be used concurrently with tamoxifen; not indicated for premenopausal women or women with ER-negative tumors; used in postmenopausal women because peripheral conversion of adrenal androgens to estrogens is the primary source of estrogen; not used in premenopausal women because it does not interfere with production of ovarian estrogens

TABLE 124–17. (Continued)

Agent/Major Uses	Class/Mechanism	Major Side Effects	Comments
Exemestane (Aromasin)[c] Breast cancer	Irreversible steroidal aromatase inactivator; prevents conversion of androgens to estrogens by inhibiting the aromatase enzyme	Hot flashes; fatigue; depression, anxiety, insomnia; mild nausea, anorexia; edema; dyspnea; elevated transaminases	Not indicated for premenopausal women Drug interactions: CYP450 3A4 substrate, but no significant interactions yet reported; St. John's wort may decrease exemestane levels Food interactions: plasma levels increase when taken with a fatty meal; recommended to be taken after a meal
Fulvestrant (Faslodex)[d] Breast cancer	Antiestrogen; estrogen receptor antagonist; downregulates estrogen receptor protein in human breast cancer cells; no estrogen agonist properties	Hot flashes; low emetogenic potential; diarrhea, constipation, abdominal pain; headache; back pain and myalgia; pharyngitis; dizziness; insomnia; depression	Available in prefilled syringes for IM injection once a month IM injection should be administered into buttocks; should not be used in patients with thrombocytopenia or on anticoagulant therapy Not indicated for premenopausal or women with ER-negative tumors
Letrozole (Femara)[e] Breast cancer	Selective, nonsteroidal aromatase inhibitor; inhibits conversion of androgens	Hot flashes; arthralgias, myalgias; headache; fatigue; low emetogenic potential; dyspnea, cough; breast pain; hyperlipidemia; elevated transaminases	Not indicated for premenopausal women; emerging evidence supports the use of letrozole for 5 years following completion of 5 years of adjuvant tamoxifen to further prolong survival in postmenopausal women Drug interactions: substrate of CYP450 2A6 and 3A4; inhibits CYP450 2A6 and C19; potential for interactions with inhibitors or inducers of these enzymes as well as other substrates, but specific drug interactions have not been identified
Megestrol acetate (Megace)[f] Breast cancer; endometrial cancer; cancer cachexia and anorexia; prostate cancer	Synthetic progestin with antiestrogen properties; interferes with normal estrogen cycle; may also have direct effects on the endometrium	Fluid retention and edema; weight gain; hot flashes; vaginal bleeding and spotting, amenorrhea and menstrual irregularities; decreased libido; breast tenderness; adrenal corticoid suppression and adrenal insufficiency; hepatotoxicity; thrombosis; photosensitivity	Suspension is compatible with water, apple juice, and orange juice High doses required for appetite stimulation
Tamoxifen (Nolvadex)[e] Breast cancer	Nonsteroidal estrogen receptor antagonist; competitively binds to estrogen receptors on estrogen-dependent breast cells	Hot flashes; fluid retention; weight loss; mood swings, depression; bone pain, tumor pain; thrombosis; vaginal bleeding and spotting, vaginal discharge, menstrual irregularities, decreased libido; endometrial and uterine cancer; low emetogenic potential; hyperlipidemia; decreased visual acuity, retinopathy, corneal changes, cataracts; rash, photosensitivity; hepatotoxicity, elevated transaminases; thrombocytopenia	Breast cancer treatment or adjuvant therapy in ER-positive patients; preventive therapy in women at high risk for breast cancer Monitor patients closely for endometrial hyperplasia or cancer; monitor serum transaminases CYP450 substrate (CYP450 2A6, 2B6, 2C8/9, 2D6, 2E1, 3A4) and inhibitor (CYP450 3A4, 2B6, 2C8/9); significantly increases anticoagulant effects of warfarin
Toremifene (Fareston)[e] Breast cancer; endometrial cancer; desmoid tumors	Nonsteroidal antiestrogen; estrogen receptor antagonist	Hot flashes; vaginal discharge or bleeding; low emetogenic potential; diaphoresis; thromboembolism; dizziness; hypercalcemia; dry eyes, visual acuity changes	Hypercalcemia and tumor flare have been reported during the first weeks of treatment Drug interactions: substrate of CYP450 1A2, 3A4; enzyme inhibitors may increase toremifene blood levels; toremifene can increase anticoagulant effects of warfarin; anticonvulsants can decrease toremifene blood levels

(continued)

TABLE 124–17. (Continued)

Agent/Major Uses	Class/Mechanism	Major Side Effects	Comments
LHRH Agonists			
Goserelin (Zoladex)[g] Prostate cancer; breast cancer	LHRH agonist; initially stimulates steroidogenesis by increasing levels of LH and FSH, but ultimately inhibits gonadotropin secretion with continuous administration by negative feedback mechanism; results in decreased testosterone and estrogen levels	Testicular atrophy, decreased libido, impotence; gynecomastia, breast tenderness; hot flashes; low emetogenic potential; depression, confusion; angina, CHF; thrombosis; elevated liver function tests; injection site reactions or abscess; hyperlipidemia; decreased bone density	Antiandrogens are coadministered during initial therapy to decrease symptoms of tumor flare (bone pain, urinary tract obstruction, or spinal cord compression) associated with the initial increase in serum testosterone levels Administered as a subcutaneous injection of implanted pellets every 1–3 months
Leuprolide (Lupron, Lupron Depot, Eligard)[g] Prostate cancer; breast cancer	LHRH agonist; initially stimulates steroidogenesis by increasing levels of LH and FSH, but ultimately inhibits gonadotropin secretion with continuous administration by negative feedback mechanism; ultimately results in decreased testosterone and estrogen levels	Testicular atrophy, decreased libido, impotence; gynecomastia, breast tenderness; hot flashes; low emetogenic potential; depression, confusion; angina, CHF, thrombosis; elevated liver function tests; pain at injection site; hyperlipidemia; decreased bone density	Antiandrogens are coadministered during initial therapy to decrease symptoms of tumor flare (bone pain, urinary tract obstruction, or spinal cord compression) associated with the initial increase in serum testosterone levels Administered as IM injection every 1–4 months
LHRH Antagonists			
Abarelix (Plenaxis)[h] Prostate cancer	GnRH antagonist; directly competes with GnRH receptors in pituitary, suppressing LH and FSH production, and reducing testosterone secretion by testes	*Life-threatening hypersensitivity reactions, sometimes severe and immediate, limit use:* urticaria, hypotension, syncope; reactions may occur after any dose; risk increases with cumulative dosing; hot flashes; breast enlargement or pain; can prolong QT interval	No initial surge in testosterone production, therefore no risk of tumor flare Observe patients for allergic reactions for at least 30 minutes after each dose Patients must sign consent before drug administration to confirm understanding of risks and benefits; risks limit use to men who require androgen suppression, cannot risk tumor flare, and refuse orchiectomy

[a]From Jordan.[86]
[b]From Plosker et al.[84]
[c]From Anonymous.[85]
[d]From Schally et al.[88]
[e]From Anonymous[82] and Witzig et al.[83]
[f]From Osborne et al.[87]
[g]From Plosker et al[84] and Jordan.[86]
[h]From Budzar et al.[89]
CBC, complete blood cell count; CHF, congestive heart failure; CYP450, cytochrome P450 isoenzyme; G6PD, glucose-6-phosphate dehydrogenase; ER, estrogen receptor; FSH, follicle-stimulating hormone; GnRH, gonadotropin-releasing hormone; IM, intramuscular; LH, luteinizing hormone; LHRH, luteinizing-hormone releasing hormone.

supportive care of cancer patients. Corticosteroids have diverse toxicities in chronic or high-dose use, but are generally well tolerated in the short-term therapies usually used in cancer patient care.[94]

RETINOIDS

Vitamin A and its metabolites, collectively referred to as the retinoids, play important roles in numerous biologic processes, including normal cellular differentiation. Because cancerous growth is characterized by abnormal cellular differentiation, retinoids are proving to have important therapeutic roles in the treatment and perhaps in the prevention of cancers. Tretinoin (all-*trans*-retinoic acid) is a naturally occurring derivative of vitamin A (retinol). Other retinoids indicated for treatment of cancers include alitretinoin (9-*cis*-retinoic acid), available in gel form for topical management of Kaposi's sarcoma lesions and bexarotene (Targretin) gel or capsules for treatment of cutaneous T-cell lymphoma (Table 124–18).[95,96]

Retinoids are classed as morphogens, small molecules released from one type of cells that can affect the growth and differentiation of neighboring cells. Their normal roles in the human body are to induce differentiation of some cells, stop the differentiation of others, and both suppress and induce apoptosis in different cell types. Their diverse actions come from the diversity of their receptors. The two classes of retinoid receptors are retinoid X receptors (RXRs) and retinoic acid receptors (RARs), each with α, β, and γ subclasses. RXRs are versatile; they bind to RARs and to other nuclear receptors such as thyroid hormone receptors. Once activated, the receptors act as transcription factors that in turn regulate the expression of genes that control cellular growth and differentiation.[95]

Tretinoin binds primarily to the RAR-α receptors. Alitretinoin is considered a panagonist; that is, it binds to all known retinoid receptors, producing diverse regulatory effects. Bexarotene is synthetic and is classed as a rexinoid. It is the first RXR-selective retinoid agonist. The exact mechanism of action of alitretinoin and bexarotene as anticancer agents is unknown.[95,96]

TABLE 124–18. Biologically-Directed Therapies

Agent/Major Uses	Class/Mechanism	Major Side Effects	Comments
Molecular targets			
Bexarotene (Targretin)[a] Cutaneous T-cell lymphoma	Retinoid analog that may activate retinoid receptors	Peripheral edema; insomnia, headache; fever, chills; lipid abnormalities, increased triglycerides, cholesterol, reduced high-density lipoproteins; hypothyroidism (reduced thyroxine, thyroid-stimulating hormone); diarrhea; low emetogenic potential; leukopenia and anemia; dry skin; increased liver function tests; pancreatitis	Drug interactions: metabolized by CYP450 3A4, may interact with drugs that inhibit or induce this enzyme May cause hypoglycemia in patients receiving insulin, sulfonylureas, or metformin; contraindicated in pregnant women Limit vitamin A supplements
Bortezomib (PA-341, Velcade)[b] Multiple myeloma; prostate cancer	Boronic acid dipeptide that reversibly inhibits the proteosome; proteosomes are enzyme complexes in cells that degrade proteins that regulate cell-cycle progression; actions are mediated through inhibition of the degradation of NF-κB	Fatigue or malaise; nausea, diarrhea, anorexia, constipation, vomiting; low to moderate GI effects; myelosuppression, especially thrombocytopenia; hyponatremia, hypokalemia; peripheral neuropathy may be dose-limiting, cumulative, and dose-related, but reversible; fever	First proteosome inhibitor; administered as rapid IV bolus twice weekly for 2 weeks in 21-day cycle Increased risk of severe neuropathy in patients with pre-existing neuropathy
Gefitinib (Iressa)[c] NSCLC	EGFR tyrosine kinase inhibitor; inhibits signal transduction pathways essential for tumor cell proliferation, differentiation, angiogenesis, and metastasis	Pulmonary toxicity: interstitial lung disease (ILD), symptoms of cough, dyspnea, and fever (~1% overall incidence, but 1/3 of cases have been fatal); diarrhea; skin reactions: acne-like rash, dry skin, may require interruption of treatment; low emetogenic potential; hepatotoxicity; eye pain	Therapy should be interrupted if patients develop symptoms of ILD and drug should be discontinued if ILD is confirmed Patients with symptoms of eye pain should be evaluated for aberrant eyelash growth Drug interactions: metabolized by CYP450 3A4, gefitinib effects may be decreased by CYP450 3A4 inducers (e.g., rifampin, phenytoin) and increased by CYP450 3A4 inhibitors (e.g., ketoconazole, voriconazole); major interaction with warfarin leading to increased anticoagulant effects and increased bleeding risk; histamine-2 blockers may decrease gefitinib levels
Imatinib mesylate (Gleevec, STI 571)[d] CML (adults and pediatrics); GIST; Ph + ALL	Tyrosine kinase inhibitor; relatively specific for the tyrosine kinase coded for by the *bcr-abl* translocation in CML patients	Moderate emetogenic potential: take with meals and a full glass of water; edema: periorbital edema is characteristic; pleural effusions, ascites, or pulmonary edema also occur; rash; diarrhea; neutropenia, thrombocytopenia (sometimes difficult to distinguish from CML-induced cytopenias); increased liver function tests	Metabolized primarily by CYP450 3A4; competitive inhibitor of CYP450 3A4, 2C9, and 2D6, so beware of drug interactions; may increase warfarin effects Dose reductions should be considered for liver dysfunction and myelosuppression per manufacturer recommendations Usual dose: 400 mg orally per day; cost ~$2,400 per month
Tretinoin (All-*trans*-retinoic acid [ATRA], Vesenoid)[e] APL	Vitamin A derivative (retinoid); induces differentiation, maturation of immature promyelocytic cells	Headache is most common side effect; severe headache may be sign of pseudotumor cerebri (intracranial hypertension); "ATRA syndrome": pulmonary symptoms (dyspnea, respiratory distress, fever, pleural effusions); low emetogenic potential; dry skin and mucous membranes, mucositis; bone pain; transient elevations in transaminases, bilirubin	Headaches are usually manageable with mild analgesics; ATRA syndrome treated with corticosteroid administration (initiate when WBC ≥10,000) and/or holding ATRA until symptoms resolve; bone pain typically responds to mild analgesics; teratogenic: contraindicated in pregnancy; female patients should be educated about proper contraceptive measures Give daily dose orally in two divided doses; round to nearest 10 mg (available only as 10 mg capsules)

(continued)

TABLE 124–18. (Continued)

Agent/Major Uses	Class/Mechanism	Major Side Effects	Comments
Monoclonal antibodies			
Alemtuzumab (Campath)[f] B-cell CLL	Anti-CD52 monoclonal antibody, results in antibody-dependent lysis of CD52+ B and T lymphocytes	Myelosuppression and immunosuppression; infection; infusion-related nausea and vomiting; fever; hypotension; rash; headache; fatigue	Patients should be started on antiviral and PCP prophylaxis during and 6 months posttreatment; some evidence suggests that subcutaneous administration may be associated with less acute toxicity
Bevacizumab (Avastin)[g] Colorectal cancer; renal cell carcinoma	Recombinant humanized MoAB; binds to vascular endothelial growth factor to prevent it from binding to its receptors; this inhibits new vessel formation (angiogenesis)	Most serious adverse effect (2% incidence, idiosyncratic) is GI bleeding or perforation, sometimes with intra-abdominal abscess formation; impaired wound healing; hypertension; proteinuria; rare severe pulmonary hemorrhage	Presenting symptoms of GI bleeding or perforation: abdominal pain, nausea, vomiting, and constipation; risk not correlated with duration of therapy; treat hypertension with standard antihypertensives; avoid within 28 days after major surgery; suspend treatment before elective surgery
Cetuximab (Erbitux)[h] Colorectal cancer	Recombinant human/mouse MoAB that binds to the EGFR and inhibits the binding of EGFR and other growth factors; EGFR is overexpressed in some solid tumors such as colorectal cancer; cetuximab inhibits cell cycle progression; induces apoptosis; may enhance the effects of some chemotherapy agents and radiation	Acne-like rash in most patients, sometimes severe, on face and upper torso, onset in 1–3 weeks, may improve with continued treatment, reversible; paronychial cracking in fingers or toes, may take several months to heal; asthenia; abdominal pain, nausea, constipation, diarrhea; infusion and hypersensitivity reactions	Acne-like rash is poorly responsive to standard acne treatments; dose reductions may be required; skin rash may correlate with response; premedicate with antihistamine; medical resources for the treatment of severe infusion reactions should be available; reduce infusion rate for mild to moderate infusion reactions, discontinue infusion for severe toxicity
Gemtuzumab ozogamicin (Mylotarg)[i] CD33+ ANLL	Humanized anti-CD33 antibody linked to calicheamicin, a potent toxin; binding to the CD33 receptor results in internalization of the antibody-antigen complex; calicheamicin is then released intracellularly and exerts cytotoxicity by causing DNA double-strand breaks, resulting in cell death	Infusion reactions: fevers, chills, nausea, vomiting, hypotension, dyspnea; myelosuppression may be severe and prolonged; tumor lysis syndrome: WBCs should be reduced to <30,000/mm^3 prior to administration if possible, to decrease risk; increased liver function tests and bilirubin, hepatic veno-occlusive disease	Premedicate with acetaminophen 1000 mg and diphenhydramine 50 mg; requires 4–8 hours of observation postinfusion; light-sensitive Requires preparation in darkened hood and light protective bag for administration
Ibrotumomab tiuxetan (Zevalin)[j] NHL (low-grade CD20+)	Anti-CD20 MoAB linked to radioactive yttrium (Y^{90}); murine version of the rituximab antibody; monoclonal antibody to CD20 (a B-lymphocyte surface antigen)–positive cells; binds complement and increases antibody dependent cellular cytotoxicity; radioactive linkage delivers radiation dose directly to tumor cells to decrease damage to normal cells	Must consider toxicities of rituximab also, since always given in combination; hematologic toxicity very delayed in onset, occurring 7 ± 9 *weeks* after drug administration with 2–4 weeks for recovery; infusion reactions: asthenia, nausea, chills, fever; tumor pain	Rituximab administered prior to ibritumomab to decrease circulating B-cells, improves targeting of the radiation (see rituximab); imaging dose of ibritumomab chelated to indium-111 to map the expected distribution of the radioisotope is administered ~1 week prior to treatment dose; repeated treatment not usually required
Rituximab (Rituxan)[k] Low-grade NHL; CLL; intermediate-grade NHL Idiopathic thrombocytopenic purpura; rheumatoid arthritis	Monoclonal antibody that reacts with CD20 (a B-lymphocyte surface antigen)–positive cells; binds complement and increases antibody dependent cellular cytotoxicity	Hypersensitivity reactions, infusion rate–related; infusion-related side effects: flushing, chills, fever, rigors, hypotension; bronchospasm, dyspnea, angioedema; tumor lysis syndrome, especially with large tumor burden (e.g., CLL with a high WBC); low emetogenic potential; thrombocytopenia; myalgias; tachycardia	Infusion-related reactions may be severe; increase rate of infusion gradually (e.g., start at 25–50 mg/min increasing by 25–50 mg/min at 30-minute intervals; maximum infusion rate = 400 mg/h); premedicate with 650–1000 mg acetaminophen, 50 mg diphenhydramine with or without dexamethasone; use meperidine 25 mg IV as needed for rigors; consider hospitalization for first dose

TABLE 124–18. (Continued)

Agent/Major Uses	Class/Mechanism	Major Side Effects	Comments
Tositumomab (Bexxar)[l] NHL (low-grade CD20+)	Anti-CD20 MoAB linked to radioactive iodine (^{131}I); monoclonal antibody to CD20 (a B-lymphocyte surface antigen)–positive cells; binds complement and increases antibody dependent cellular cytotoxicity; radioactive linkage delivers radiation dose directly to tumor cells, resulting in additional cytotoxicity	Cytopenias (especially thrombocytopenia and neutropenia): severe and prolonged; late onset 4–7 weeks after treatment, persisting >3 months; nausea, vomiting, abdominal pain (within days), diarrhea (within days to weeks after infusion); infusion reactions: fever, rigors, chills, sweating, hypotension, dyspnea, bronchospasm; anaphylaxis may occur; premedicate; hypothyroidism: all patients must receive thyroid-blocking agents; asthenia, myalgias, arthralgias; cough; rash	Radiopharmaceutical, to be prepared and administered only by personnel trained in radiopharmaceuticals; premedicate with acetaminophen and antihistamines; slow infusion rate or interrupt infusion for infusion reactions; medications for treatment of hypersensitivity reactions should be available for immediate use; avoid in pregnant females; may cause hypothyroidism in fetus; two-step administration; MoAB and low radioisotope dose is followed after 1–2 weeks by MoAB and therapeutic radioisotope dose; renally excreted; impaired renal function may increase exposure to radioactive components; patients must be trained in precautions to decrease radiation exposure to family, friends, and general public
Trastuzumab (Herceptin)[m] Breast cancer; prostate cancer; pancreatic cancer; lung cancer; ovarian cancer	MoAB directed against *HER2* receptors, overexpressed in some breast cancer patients and related to epidermal growth factor	Cardiac toxicity: congestive cardiomyopathy, usually reversible with medical management; infusion reactions	Do not administer with anthracyclines; best response seen in patients highly positive for *HER2* overexpression

[a]From McCarty et al[91] and McKeage et al.[92]
[b]From Peng et al[99] and Croom et al.[100]
[c]From Anonymous,[93] Heinrich et al,[97] and Druker.[98]
[d]From Anonymous,[93] McKay et al,[94] Sporn et al,[95] and Duvic et al.[96]
[e]From McCarty et al.[91]
[f]From Ekmekcioglu et al[81] and Giaccone et al.[102]
[g]From Richardson et al,[103] Mitchell,[104] and Harris.[105]
[h]From Harris,[105] Frampton et al,[106] and Miller et al.[107]
[i]From Ekmekcioglu et al,[81] Hurwitz et al,[108] and Anonymous.[109]
[j]From Reynolds et al[110] and Saltz et al.[111]
[k]From Ekmekcioglu et al[81] and Giles et al.[112]
[l]From Ekmekcioglu et al[81] and Larson et al.[113]
[m]From Ekmekcioglu et al,[81] Vogel et al,[114] and Perez et al.[115]
ANLL, acute nonlymphocytic leukemia; APL, acute promyelocytic leukemia; CLL, chronic lymphocytic leukemia; CML, chronic myelogenous leukemia; EGFR, epidermal growth factor receptor; GIST, gastrointestinal stromal tumor; MoAB, monoclonal antibody; NF-κB, nuclear factor-κB; Ph+ ALL, Philadelphia chromosome–positive acute lymphocytic leukemia; PCP, *Pneumocystis carinii* pneumonia; WBC, white blood cell.

TYROSINE KINASE INHIBITORS

Imatinib

Imatinib mesylate was the first tyrosine kinase inhibitor to be approved for treatment of cancer (see Table 124–18). It inhibits deregulated *bcr-abl* tyrosine kinase, the molecular abnormality in patients with chronic myelogenous leukemia that results from the characteristic "Philadelphia chromosome" translocation. The deregulated tyrosine kinase constantly drives leukemic cell proliferation. Imatinib inhibits cell proliferation and induces apoptosis in the Philadelphia chromosome–positive cells. It is relatively, but not completely, selective for these cells.[97–100]

Gefitinib

Gefitinib is a selective inhibitor of epidermal growth factor receptor [EGFR] tyrosine kinase (see Table 124–18). EGFR is a cell surface receptor expressed or overexpressed in many solid tumors. When ligand binds to the EGFR receptor, tyrosine kinase activity initiates a cascade of signaling events within the cancer cells that stimulates their proliferation and promotes their survival. Gefitinib inhibits EGFR ac-

tivity by competing with adenosine triphosphate for its binding site on the EGFR tyrosine kinase. This blocks the tyrosine kinase cascade of downstream signaling, and ultimately interferes with the proliferation and growth of cancer cells. It is orally administered and well tolerated, most commonly producing diarrhea and mild skin rashes.[97,101,102]

PROTEOSOME INHIBITORS

Proteosomes are protein complexes within cells that are responsible for degrading and eliminating cellular proteins. Some of the proteins that are degraded by proteosomes are proteins that regulate critical functions for successful cancer growth, such as regulation of the cell cycle, transcription factors, apoptosis, angiogenesis, and cell adhesion.[103,104] One proteosome inhibitor, bortezomib, is commercially available (see Table 124–18). Bortezomib has very specific affinity for the catalytic portion of the proteosome. It can induce apoptosis in cancer cells indirectly. Although many actions may contribute to its effects, one pathway of action is well established. Bortezomib interferes with degradation of the inhibitory partner protein of a transcription factor, nuclear factor-κB [NF-κB]. NF-κB induces transcription of genes that block cell death pathways and promote cell proliferation, but in order for it to do so, NF-κB must be released from its inhibitory partner protein in the cytoplasm and move to the nucleus. When NF-κB's partner protein fails to degrade, through the actions of bortezomib, NF-κB is held in the cytoplasm and prevented from transcribing the genes that promote cancer growth. Bortezomib is approved for the treatment of patients with multiple myeloma.[103,104]

MONOCLONAL ANTIBODIES

The monoclonal antibodies have become established agents in the treatment of cancer. Monoclonal antibodies (MoABs) consist of immunoglobulin sequences that are known to recognize a specific antigen or protein on the surface of cells. There are several mechanisms by which monoclonal antibodies may induce death of cancer cells. Direct mechanisms include induction of apoptosis, blockade of growth factor receptors, or induction of anti-idiotype antibodies. Important indirect mechanisms include antibody-dependent cellular toxicity and complement-mediated cellular toxicity.[66,105] Antibodies may also be carriers for cytotoxic drugs or toxins (i.e., immunoconjugates) that are targeted by the antibody directly to the antigen-bearing cancer cells. Once the antibody binds to its cellular surface receptor, the complex can be internalized, and the toxic "payload" liberated into the cytoplasm to cause cell damage. MoABs can also serve as carriers for radioisotopes. Delivery of radiation therapy in this manner is called radioimmunotherapy. Drug and toxin conjugates kill only the targeted cell, but radiation delivered via MoAB is less narrowly targeted. Depending on the penetration of the radioisotope through tissue, the radiation can also damage nearby cells that do not express the targeted antigen.[66,105] Table 124–18 summarizes the characteristics and clinical uses of monoclonal antibodies.[82–85,106–115]

Several limitations affect the success and specificity of treatment with MoABs. Although monoclonal antibodies are designed to be specific to a particular target antigen, that target antigen may also be expressed on normal tissues to some degree, decreasing their selectivity. Thus toxicity often occurs when the monoclonal antibodies bind to normal cells, or are recognized by the immune system. All of the monoclonal antibodies are also associated with some degree of infusion-related reactions. The severity of these reactions can range from mild (e.g., fever, chills, nausea, and rash) to severe, life-threatening anaphylaxis with cardiopulmonary collapse. Many patients also experience chest or back pain during the infusion. Patients with circulating tumor cells in the bloodstream are at highest risk for more severe reactions. For these reasons, patients must be monitored closely during drug infusion. The reactions tend to be more severe with the initial infusion, and subside with subsequent treatment. Most agents require premedication with antihistamines and acetaminophen. Recommended infusion rates are usually lower for the initial dose, with incremental increases as tolerated by the patient. For patients experiencing signs or symptoms of infusion-related reactions, the infusion should be interrupted and prompt treatment with antihistamines, corticosteroids, and other supportive measures should be initiated. Pulmonary toxicity may occur as part of the infusion-related reaction or may occur as a distinct entity.[66,82–86,105–115]

ANGIOGENESIS INHIBITORS

Angiogenesis refers to the development of new capillaries to increase vascular supply of tissue. Although angiogenesis is a normal function, and is essential to wound healing, reproduction, and growth, it is also central to the successful growth of tumor masses. Tumors need blood supply to grow. Interference with their ability to

develop new blood vessels by means of antiangiogenic drugs can limit or prevent tumor growth.[107]

There are many potential means of interfering with angiogenesis. Examples are targeting vascular growth factors, or the production and control of the endothelial cells that make up the vessel linings. Most antiangiogenic drugs are cytostatic rather than truly cytotoxic, since they prevent new vessel growth and thus cause growth delay of the tumors. Some vascular targeting agents, however, can destroy existing blood vessels. These could be cytotoxic.[107,116]

Bevacizumab is a humanized monoclonal antibody directed against vascular endothelial growth factor (VEGF), a growth factor that regulates proliferation and permeability of blood vessels (see Table 124–18). VEGF acts through two receptors. Bevacizumab inhibits the signaling process for new blood vessels by binding VEGF ligand to prevent it from interacting with its receptors. It was approved in 2004 for treatment of patients with colorectal cancer.[107–109]

THALIDOMIDE

Thalidomide, the infamous drug that caused severe limb deformities (phocomelia or "seal limbs") when used by pregnant women as an over-the-counter sedative in the 1960s, is approved for treatment of leprosy and has orphan drug status for multiple myeloma. It also has documented clinical activity in several other types of cancer. Thalidomide is a glutamic acid derivative, and is broadly classed as an immunomodulatory agent. It has many potential mechanisms of action as an anticancer agent. It is an angiogenesis inhibitor, interfering with the growth of new blood vessels needed for tumor growth. This action is also linked to its teratogenic effects. Other possible mechanisms include: direct inhibition of cancer cells, free-radical oxidative damage to DNA, interfering with adhesion of cancer cells, inhibiting tumor necrosis factor-α production, or altering secretion of cytokines that affect the growth of cancer cells. Great care must be taken to prevent thalidomide's use during pregnancy.[107,116,117]

GENERAL SUPPORTIVE CARE ISSUES

The treatment of cancer with most antineoplastic drugs is complicated by the risk of multiple serious toxicities, many of which are life threatening. Drug-specific toxicities, such as doxorubicin-induced cardiotoxicity and bleomycin-related pulmonary toxicity, were summarized in the previous section (see Tables 124–11 through 124–18). Several adverse effects are common to many antineoplastic agents. These include nausea and vomiting, myelosuppression, mucositis, alopecia, infertility, and carcinogenesis. Nutritional support and pain management are also important supportive care issues, although malnutrition and pain are not usually direct results of drug toxicity. The management of chemotherapy-induced nausea and vomiting and the basic principles of nutritional support and pain management are discussed in detail in other sections of this text.

Because many antineoplastic drugs affect DNA synthesis, any cell with a high turnover rate will be more sensitive to the toxic effects of chemotherapy. Cancer cells do not necessarily proliferate faster than normal cells. Normal tissues that consist of rapidly proliferating cells are targets for the toxicities of many anticancer drugs.[14] The bone marrow, intestinal mucosa, and hair follicles are such tissue sites where drug effects are manifested.

MYELOSUPPRESSION

 Although not seen with all antineoplastic agents, myelosuppression is the most common dose-limiting side effect of cytotoxic agents. Bone marrow suppression does not usually occur immediately after chemotherapy administration. Blood components that have already been produced must be consumed before the effect is evident. White blood cells (WBCs), especially neutrophil precursors, are most significantly affected because of their rapid proliferation and short life-span (6 to 12 hours). Platelets (5- to 10-day life-span) are also affected, but to a much less degree than neutrophils. Erythrocytes, with a 120-day life-span, are affected the least. Usual nadirs, or lowest blood cell counts, occur at 10 to 14 days following chemotherapy administration, with recovery by 3 to 4 weeks. There are some exceptions to this general rule. The nitrosoureas and mitomycin C exhibit a delayed pattern of nadir (4 to 6 weeks) and recovery (6 to 8 weeks). Planned courses of chemotherapy may have to be delayed while waiting for the granulocyte count to return to normal. For a patient to safely receive another cycle of myelosuppressive chemotherapy, a WBC count $\geq 3,000/mm^3$ or an absolute neutrophil count (ANC) of $\geq 1,500/mm^3$ and a platelet count of $\geq 100,000/mm^3$ are usually required.

Myelotoxicity is a desired therapeutic effect in leukemia patients during induction chemotherapy. However, myelosuppression is an undesirable side effect during chemotherapy for other malignancies. If significant myelosuppression has occurred with prior courses of chemotherapy, the doses of the offending agent(s) in subsequent courses may be reduced. The magnitude of dose reduction is dictated by the degree of myelosuppression incurred and the incidence and severity of infection or bleeding. Empiric dosage reductions may be made for the first chemotherapy treatment if the patient has a low baseline WBC or platelet count, has diminished bone marrow reserve, has impaired drug-elimination capabilities, or is to receive a combination of several drugs that cause myelosuppression. Patients who have received multiple prior courses of other myelotoxic chemotherapy regimens or extensive radiation therapy, especially to the pelvis, may have a decreased bone marrow reserve. They are more sensitive to the myelosuppressive effects of chemotherapy, and normal doses may produce profound marrow toxicity. The pharmacokinetic profile of a myelosuppressive agent is also important in determining the appropriate dose. For example, the anthracyclines produce bone marrow suppression as an acute dose-limiting toxicity, and these agents depend on biliary excretion as their primary route of elimination. A patient with biliary obstruction may have compromised elimination of anthracyclines and is at increased risk for severe bone marrow suppression. Although dosage reduction can prevent myelotoxicity, it may also compromise antitumor response for some tumors (e.g., breast cancer or lymphoma). For such tumors, empiric use of hematopoietic growth factors provides an alternative to dose reduction in patients at high risk for toxicity.

NEUTROPENIA

When the ANC falls below $500/mm^3$, infection risk increases.[118-120] The ANC may be calculated by multiplying the percentage of neutrophils (segmented plus banded neutrophils) by the total WBC count. The risk of infection is also directly proportional to the duration of neutropenia. Other risk factors for infection include alteration in the integrity of physical defense barriers and the functional integrity of WBCs. The patient's underlying cancer, as well as treatment with cytotoxic drugs and radiation, can affect neutrophil function. The diagnosis of infection in the neutropenic patient is complicated by the lack of WBCs. Usual signs and symptoms of infection, such as pus, abscesses, and infiltrates on chest x-ray, depend on the presence of WBCs. The only reliable indication of infection in these patients is fever. Definitive culture results may take days, and a septic neutropenic cancer patient can die within hours if not treated. Therefore the basic approach to the manage-

ment of the febrile neutropenic cancer patient is prompt initiation of empiric antibiotics. The antibiotics are chosen based on reliable coverage of the most likely organisms, antibiotic sensitivities at the institution, the patient's signs and symptoms (if present), side-effect profiles, and cost.[120] The most common source of infection in these patients is self-infection with body flora, which includes both gram-positive and gram-negative bacteria. Although bacteria cause most early infections, fungi become important pathogens as the course of neutropenia is prolonged. Traditionally, all febrile neutropenic cancer patients have received intravenous antibiotics in the hospital setting until full recovery of neutrophils. However, it is possible to identify patients at low risk for infectious complications who are candidates for alternative treatment strategies, including early discharge from the hospital and outpatient oral or intravenous antibiotics.[120,121] Specific treatment of infections in immunocompromised hosts is discussed elsewhere in this text.

Numerous methods have been explored to prevent infections in cancer patients.[120,122] Colony-stimulating factors (CSFs) are commonly employed for this purpose.[122-124] These hormones are naturally occurring proteins that are essential for the normal growth and maturation of blood cell components (Fig. 124–13). The CSFs have the ability to enhance the production and also the function of their target cells. Two agents, G-CSF (granulocyte colony-stimulating factor) and GM-CSF (granulocyte-macrophage colony-stimulating factor) are commercially available in the United States. G-CSF (filgrastim) specifically stimulates the production of neutrophilic granulocytes. GM-CSF (sargramostim) promotes the proliferation of granulocytes (neutrophils and eosinophils) and monocytes/macrophages. Although GM-CSF stimulates megakaryocytes, no consistent effect on platelet production has been observed in clinical trials. Both agents initially enhance demargination and mobilization of mature cells from the marrow and then provide constant stimulation of stem cell progenitors. Colony-stimulating factors are produced by recombinant DNA technology, and several host cells are used to produce CSFs, including bacteria (*Escherichia coli*), yeast, and mammalian cells (Chinese hamster ovary cells) (Table 124–19). Products derived from yeast or mammalian sources are glycosylated to varying degrees, as are naturally occurring CSFs, whereas those derived from *E. coli* are nonglycosylated. This difference does not result in any clinically significant effects on neutrophil production. Pegfilgrastim is a long-acting CSF, created by addition of a polyethylene glycol molecule to G-CSF. Clinical trials have demonstrated that a single dose of pegfilgrastim provides equivalent effects to 10 to 11 days of daily G-CSF, with similar side-effect profiles.

The CSFs reduce the incidence, magnitude, and duration of neutropenia when used as preventive therapy following a variety of myelosuppressive chemotherapy regimens.[122-124] These effects have been accompanied by a modest decrease in febrile days, fewer infections, and fewer days on antibiotics. In some studies, use of CSFs also resulted in a decrease in the incidence of mucositis. Growth factors have also permitted the administration of subsequent chemotherapy courses on schedule, resulting in enhanced dose intensity. However, the increased dose intensity provided by the CSFs has not yet been found to translate into improved tumor response or survival. Because of lack of impact on response rates and survival, decisions regarding appropriate use of growth factors are based on weighing proven clinical benefits against economic considerations. The American Society of Clinical Oncology has developed evidence-based clinical practice guidelines to promote appropriate use of the CSFs.[123-124]

Growth factors may be used in either the primary or secondary prophylaxis of neutropenia. Primary prophylaxis refers to the use of CSFs to prevent neutropenia with the first cycle of chemotherapy. This strategy is only clinically and economically appropriate for

FIGURE 124–13. Sites of action of hematopoietic growth factors in the differentiation and maturation of marrow cell lines. A self-sustaining pool of marrow stem cells differentiates under the influence of specific hematopoietic growth factors to form a variety of hematopoietic and lymphopoietic cells. Stem cell factor (SCF), FTL-3 ligand (FL), interleukin-3 (IL-3), and granulocyte/macrophage colony-stimulating factor (GM-CSF), together with cell–cell interactions in the marrow, stimulate stem cells to form a series of burst-forming units (BFU) and colony-forming units (CFU): CFU-GEMM, CFU-GM, CFU-Meg, BFU-E, and CFU-E (GEMM, granulocyte, erythrocyte, monocyte, and megakaryocytes; GM, granulocyte and macrophage; Meg, megakaryocyte; E, erythrocyte). After considerable proliferation, further differentiation is stimulated by synergistic interactions with growth factors for each of the major cell lines—granulocyte colony-stimulating factor (G-CSF), monocyte/macrophage-stimulating factor (M-CSF), thrombopoietin, and erythropoietin. Each of these factors also influences the proliferation, maturation, and, in some cases, the function of the derivative cell line. *(Adapted from Hillman RS. Hematopoietic agents: Growth factors, minerals and vitamins. In: Hardman JG, Limbird LE, Gilman AG, eds. Goodman & Gilman's The Pharmacologic Basis of Therapeutics, 10th ed. New York, McGraw-Hill, 2001:1489.)*

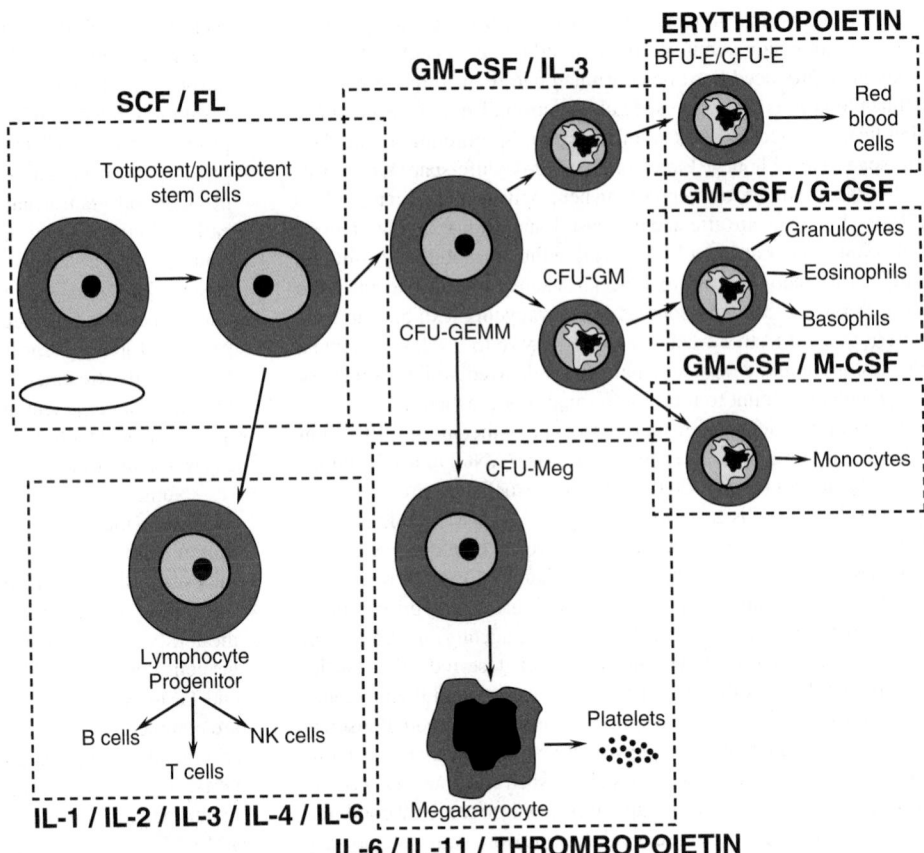

patients who are receiving a chemotherapy regimen associated with febrile neutropenia in more than 40% of patients.[124] Models to predict the likelihood of developing neutropenia after chemotherapy are under development, and if validated, may serve to identify patients most likely to benefit from primary prophylaxis.[125] Secondary prophylaxis refers to the use of growth factors to prevent recurrent neutropenia in patients who experienced neutropenia with the prior cycle of chemotherapy. Because this method of using CSFs has not been demonstrated to improve disease-free or overall survival, it is recommended that secondary prophylaxis be reserved for patients with curable malignancies where dose should not be compromised.[124]

Although both G-CSF and GM-CSF are used clinically to prevent febrile neutropenia after administration of standard doses of chemotherapy, only G-CSF is FDA-approved for this indication. One exception is in the induction treatment of acute myelogenous leukemia, in which both G-CSF and GM-CSF have been demonstrated to reduce the duration of neutropenia, often accompanied by modest decreases in hospitalization and infectious complications. Benefits

have been most clearly documented in patients older than age 55 years. Similar data are available for G-CSF in the treatment of patients with acute lymphoblastic leukemia. These beneficial effects, however, have not resulted in improved response rates or overall survival.[124]

Only a few studies have addressed the role of CSFs in the treatment of established neutropenia.[123,124] These studies suggest no or only minimal clinical benefit from use of CSFs. At this time, the CSFs should not be routinely employed in patients with established neutropenia, regardless of the presence of fever. Both CSFs have also proven effective in acceleration of hematopoietic engraftment and in treatment of graft failure following hematopoietic stem cell transplantation. Other uses for the CSFs include peripheral blood stem cell mobilization, neutropenia in patients with acquired immune deficiency syndrome, myelodysplastic syndromes, congenital neutropenia, and aplastic anemia. Growth factors should not be used in patients receiving concomitant chemotherapy and radiotherapy, especially if the radiation involves the mediastinum. These patients appear to experience more significant thrombocytopenia when administered CSFs.

TABLE 124–19. Granulocyte Colony-Stimulating Factor (G-CSF) and Granulocyte-Macrophage Colony-Stimulating Factor (GM-CSF) Products and Sources

CSF	Generic Name	Brand Name	Manufacturer	Recombinant DNA Source
G-CSF	Filgrastim	Neupogen	Amgen	*Escherichia coli*
	Pegfilgrastim	Neulasta	Amgen	
	Lenograstim	Granocyte[a]	Chugai/Rhone Poulenc	Chinese hamster ovary cells
GM-CSF	Sargramostim	Leukine	Berlex	*Saccharomyces cerevisiae* (yeast)
	Molgramostim	Leucomax[a]	Novartis/Schering-Plough	*E. coli*

[a]Not approved by the FDA; available outside the U.S.

At currently recommended doses, the CSFs are well tolerated. Side effects are more commonly seen with GM-CSF and may be related to the drug's ability to enhance binding of neutrophils to endothelial cells or to activation of monocytes/macrophages, which may stimulate the release of cytokines such as IL-1 and tumor necrosis factor.[122] The most common toxicity of the CSFs is bone pain (20% to 25% of patients), which can be treated with acetaminophen or nonsteroidal anti-inflammatory drugs. Bone pain was the most significant toxicity seen in clinical trials with G-CSF. Other side effects of G-CSF include an increase in lactate dehydrogenase, alkaline phosphatase, and uric acid levels. Additional toxicities of GM-CSF include constitutional symptoms, such as low-grade fever, myalgias, arthralgias, lethargy, and mild headache. GM-CSF may also produce an elevation in liver transaminases. At higher doses of GM-CSF, pleural and pericardial effusions, capillary-leak syndrome, and thrombus formation may occur. A first-dose reaction described after GM-CSF administration has been reported more commonly with the *E. coli*–derived product (molgramostim), which is not commercially available in the United States. This reaction is more common after intravenous infusion and consists of dyspnea, facial flushing, hypotension, hypoxia, and tachycardia. Both G-CSF and GM-CSF may produce mild erythema at subcutaneous injection sites, as well as a generalized maculopapular rash with either subcutaneous or intravenous administration.

For prophylaxis of chemotherapy-induced neutropenia, CSF therapy should not begin sooner than 24 hours after the last dose of chemotherapy and should be continued until the ANC exceeds a safe level following the expected chemotherapy nadir. In the setting of bone marrow transplantation, CSFs should not begin sooner than 24 hours after the last dose of chemotherapy or 12 hours after the last radiotherapy treatment. The recommended starting dose of G-CSF is 5 mcg/kg per day in all settings except for peripheral blood stem cell mobilization, where doses of 10 mcg/kg per day are usually used. For pegfilgrastim, a single dose of 6 mg administered 24 hours after chemotherapy is used. The recommended dose of yeast-derived GM-CSF is 250 mcg/m^2 per day. Pharmacokinetic data favor subcutaneous injection as the most effective route. However, in patients in whom subcutaneous injections are not feasible (e.g., where there is anasarca), G-CSF and GM-CSF may be given intravenously. Pegfilgrastim should not be given intravenously. Because of the high cost associated with CSF use, alternative dosing regimens have been explored. These regimens attempt to decrease the total amount of CSF used by either delaying the start of CSFs (e.g., to day 3 after chemotherapy), decreasing the dose (e.g., to 3 mcg/kg per day of G-CSF), or decreasing the duration of CSF therapy. Specifically, the posttreatment target ANC of 10,000/mm^3 recommended by product information is often reduced to an ANC of greater than 2,000 or 5,000/mm^3 in clinical practice. Standardized doses of 300 mcg or 480 mcg of G-CSF and 500 mcg of GM-CSF, based on product vial sizes, are often used to minimize waste. For patients receiving pegfilgrastim, it is important that additional CSF not be administered for the 10 days following administration, as additional benefit is not realized.

THROMBOCYTOPENIA

Chemotherapy-induced thrombocytopenia puts the patient at risk for significant bleeding. To date, platelet transfusions remain the mainstay of management.[126] At most centers, platelet transfusion is indicated for patients with a platelet count of <10,000/mm^3, or for patients with lesser degrees of thrombocytopenia with signs or symptoms of hemorrhage. Patients with thrombocytopenia who must undergo a surgical procedure are also appropriate candidates for transfusion. For patients with nonmyeloid malignancies who experienced significant

thrombocytopenia with a prior cycle of chemotherapy, oprelvekin (IL-11) may be considered as secondary prophylaxis. When used after chemotherapy regimens associated with a high risk of thrombocytopenia, oprelvekin decreased the need for platelet transfusions, as well as the numbers of platelets required for transfusion.[127] Unfortunately, oprelvekin is associated with some significant adverse effects, mostly related to fluid retention (e.g., edema, dilutional anemia, dyspnea, and pleural effusions). Cardiac toxicity, especially tachycardia, and atrial fibrillation and flutter have also been observed. Prophylactic oprelvekin is also significantly more expensive than platelet transfusions.[128] Considering the modest clinical benefit, the adverse effects, and the high cost, oprelvekin use should be reserved for patients at high risk for severe thrombocytopenia from chemotherapy where dose reduction is known to compromise disease response. Other CSFs such as interleukins-1, -3, and -6, have also been studied, but significant impact on platelet counts with an acceptable adverse-effect profile has not been demonstrated. The discovery and development of thrombopoietin, a megakaryocyte-stimulating factor, may represent the most significant factor in the future of thrombocytopenia treatment.

ANEMIA

Anemia is a common hematologic complication of cancer chemotherapy.[129] The incidence of anemia depends on several factors, including the type and duration of therapy, and the type and stage of the underlying malignancy. For example, cisplatin and carboplatin are more commonly associated with anemia than many other chemotherapeutic agents. Multiple conditions are known to cause anemia in cancer patients, including chronic gastrointestinal blood loss, nutrient deficiency (e.g., iron and folate), chemotherapy and radiation therapy, bone marrow invasion by the tumor, hemolysis, renal dysfunction, and anemia of chronic disease. Of all the signs and symptoms of anemia, fatigue is most common in cancer patients.[129,130] In fact, fatigue is the most commonly reported symptom overall in patients undergoing chemotherapy. The presence of fatigue is correlated with the severity of anemia; treatment of anemia results in improvement in fatigue and quality of life. Anemia is only one of many possible causes of fatigue in patients with cancer. Other common causes of fatigue include insomnia, depression, unrelieved pain, and the underlying malignancy.

Previously, the only option for the treatment of chemotherapy-related anemia was red blood cell transfusions. This intervention is still the mainstay of acute management, but the availability of the recombinant human erythropoietic products—epoetin alfa and darbepoetin alfa—has provided another therapeutic tool.[129] Several studies have documented the efficacy of these agents in the anemia associated with chemotherapy. Both epoetin alfa and darbepoetin alfa increase hemoglobin and hematocrit, decrease transfusion requirements, and improve quality of life. Several early indicators of response have been derived, including an increase in hemoglobin of 0.5 to 1 g/dL above baseline, a decline in ferritin, or an increase in the absolute reticulocyte count after 2 to 4 weeks of therapy. These surrogate end points can be used to identify nonresponders early, so that therapy may be modified or discontinued, as indicated. Serum erythropoietin levels have minimal utility in predicting response or monitoring therapy.

Clinical practice guidelines to guide the appropriate use of erythropoietic agents have been developed (Fig. 124–14).[131] The first step is to evaluate the underlying cause of the anemia and initiate specific therapy as indicated. For example, patients with iron deficiency anemia should receive iron supplementation. Patients with chronic bleeding or hemolysis should not receive erythropoietic therapy, as

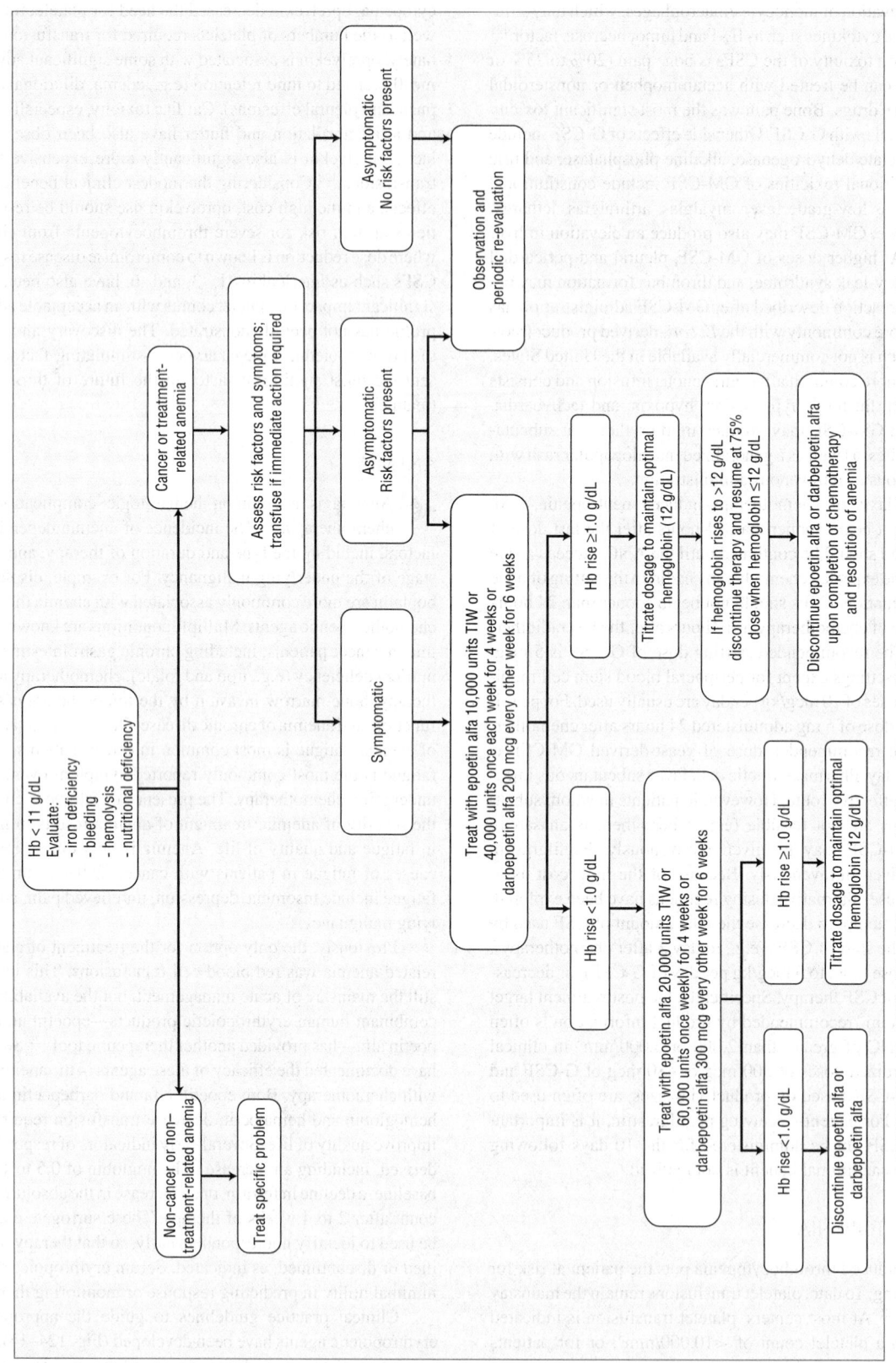

FIGURE 124-14. 2004 National Comprehensive Cancer Network clinical practice guidelines for cancer and treatment-related anemia.

this does not target the underlying cause of their anemia. Epoetin alfa and darbepoetin alfa should be considered for chemotherapy- or cancer-related anemia only after otherwise treated causes of anemia have been ruled out. These patients can be started on either epoetin alfa at a dose of 10,000 units three times a week or 40,000 units once each week, or darbepoetin alfa at a dose of 200 mcg every other week. After 4 to 6 weeks, the hemoglobin should be reassessed. In patients who do not achieve at least a 1-g/dL rise in hemoglobin, the dose should be increased as shown in Fig. 124–14. Treatment should be discontinued in patients who do not respond after 4 to 6 weeks at the higher dose. Iron deficiency should be ruled out as a cause of treatment failure prior to discontinuing therapy. Erythropoietic therapy should also be discontinued in patients who complete planned chemotherapy or in those who have resolution of their anemia (hemoglobin level 12 to 13 g/dL).

MUCOSITIS

The gastrointestinal mucosa is composed of epithelial cells with a high mitotic index and rapid turnover rate, making it a common site of chemotherapy-induced toxicity.[132,133] The subsequent inflammation, or mucositis, can lead to painful ulcerations, local infection, and inability to eat, drink, or swallow. Disruption of the GI mucosal barrier may also provide an avenue for systemic microbial invasion. The time course for development and resolution of mucositis often parallels that of neutropenia. Agents most commonly associated with mucositis include 5-FU, doxorubicin, and methotrexate. Currently, the most effective means of preventing mucositis is through good oral hygiene. Patients at high risk for this toxicity (those with poor dentition, high-dose chemotherapy, or radiation therapy involving the oropharynx) should be evaluated by a dentist prior to chemotherapy and should be instructed to rinse their mouths frequently with baking soda and salt water or plain saline rinses during and between courses of chemotherapy. Clinical practice guidelines for the prevention and treatment of cancer therapy-induced mucositis have recently been published.[134] The benefit of chlorhexidine rinses over saline rinses is unclear. In patients undergoing radiation therapy to the head and neck region, chlorhexidine rinses have detrimental effects on the oral mucosa. For patients receiving 5-FU treatment, the use of ice (oral cryotherapy) may decrease the risk for mucositis by decreasing drug delivery to the oral mucosa. A better understanding of the pathobiology of mucositis has resulted in identification of promising new agents to better prevent mucositis. The keratinocyte growth factors palifermin and repifermin are in clinical trials for prevention of chemotherapy-induced mucositis, and one of these agents (i.e., palifermin) was approved by the FDA in December 2004 for use in patients receiving high-dose chemoradiotherapy prior to hematopoietic stem cell transplantation.

After mucositis has developed, treatment is mainly supportive, including use of topical or systemic analgesics and oral hygiene (including the rinses described).[132,134] Viscous lidocaine, diphenhydramine liquid, and dyclonine are topical anesthetics commonly employed. Severe cases of mucositis may lead to dehydration and require intravenous hydration. Local infections caused by *Candida* species and reactivation of herpes simplex viruses are common in these patients. Suspicious lesions should be cultured, and appropriate antifungal and/or antiviral treatment should then be instituted. Antifungal therapy may be delivered topically for mild infections (thrush) using clotrimazole troches or nystatin oral suspension. For more severe oral or esophageal fungal infections, systemic treatment with oral fluconazole or intravenous amphotericin B is indicated.

Mucosal damage can occur at any point along the entire length of the GI tract. In the lower portion of the GI tract, this damage is usually manifested as diarrhea (mild to life-threatening in nature) and abdominal pain. Support with intravenous fluids and electrolyte supplementation should be initiated promptly in severe cases. After infectious causes have been ruled out, diarrhea can safely be treated with antispasmodics such as Lomotil or loperamide. The somatostatin analog octreotide has also been used successfully to treat severe cases of chemotherapy-induced diarrhea. The specific treatment of early and late diarrhea from irinotecan is summarized in Table 124–13.

ALOPECIA

Although not a life-threatening side effect of chemotherapy, the toxicity that many patients find most distressing is alopecia. Alopecia from chemotherapy is usually temporary, and the degree of hair loss varies widely.[135] Loss of hair is not limited to the scalp; any area of the body may be affected. Patients receiving a taxane as part of their chemotherapy regimen are especially prone to total body alopecia. Hair loss usually begins 1 to 2 weeks after chemotherapy, and regrowth may begin before the chemotherapy courses are completed. Cryotherapy (local application of ice) and scalp tourniquets have both been investigated as methods of preventing alopecia. Both techniques produce vasoconstriction, resulting in decreased exposure of hair follicles to the chemotherapy agents. These techniques are not uniformly effective and are contraindicated in patients with cancers that may metastasize to the scalp, such as leukemia and lymphoma.

EXTRAVASATION

Vesicants are antineoplastic agents that may cause severe tissue damage if they escape from the vasculature.[136,137] These agents include the anthracyclines, actinomycin D, the vinca alkaloids, mitomycin C, nitrogen mustard, and the taxanes. The anthracyclines are the most notorious agents, and the most extensively investigated. The tissue damage may result in prolonged pain, tissue sloughing, infection, and loss of mobility. Prompt initiation of the appropriate interventions is important to minimize morbidity. Unfortunately, most information on extravasation management is anecdotal; few controlled clinical studies have been conducted to determine optimal intervention strategies. Therefore prevention has become the focus of extravasation management. The most important method of prevention is good administration technique,[136] but even then, extravasations may occur. The vein selected for administration should be on the distal portion of the arm. The large veins of the forearm are desirable because if a drug does extravasate, there is adequate soft-tissue coverage to protect crucial structures like nerves and tendons, and joint function is not put at risk. Peripherally administered vesicants should be given slowly via intravenous injection (IV push) through the side arm of a running IV. The person administering the vesicant should verify needle stability and adequate blood return after each 1 to 2 mL of drug is injected. Vesicants should not be administered by intravenous infusion unless the patient has a central venous catheter. For extravasation of vesicants, one of the most important interventions is the application of ice packs to the affected area. One exception to this rule is the vinca alkaloids, which are better managed with application of heat. Only a few antidotes to vesicant agents are employed clinically. Sodium thiosulfate is used to neutralize nitrogen mustard extravasations, and hyaluronidase (if available) can improve the outcome after extravasation of vinca alkaloids, etoposide, and taxanes. Topical application of dimethyl sulfoxide may be an effective method for managing anthracycline and mitomycin C extravasations.[137]

INFERTILITY

Advances in the treatment of some cancers, such as Hodgkin's disease and testicular cancer, have produced long-term survivors and the opportunity to examine the late consequences of chemotherapy administration. Infertility and secondary cancers have emerged as important late effects. The gonadal toxicities of chemotherapy have not received much attention in the past because they are not life threatening. High rates of fertility deficits and sexual dysfunction have been noted for both men and women.[138,139] In men the antitumor drugs have been shown to produce severe oligospermia or azoospermia as well as infertility. Serum testosterone levels are only rarely altered. The recovery of spermatogenesis after completion of chemotherapy is unpredictable. Men receiving combination chemotherapy appear to sustain more long-lasting adverse effects on fertility than men receiving single-agent therapy. Age, total dose, duration of therapy, and type of drug are other important variables. In women, toxic effects on the ovaries result clinically in amenorrhea, vaginal epithelial atrophy, and menopausal symptoms. These effects are related to dose and age. Younger patients are more resistant to the effects on the ovaries. As with men, the recovery of fertility is unpredictable, but women younger then 25 years of age appear to have the best outcomes. The effects of the alkylating agents on fertility have been extensively studied. This group of drugs exerts profound and consistently detrimental effects on reproductive function. Less is known about commonly used agents such as doxorubicin, taxanes, and platinum compounds. Patients with potentially curable tumors who desire to have children in the future should be informed about the risk for infertility and sperm or oocyte banking options.

SECONDARY MALIGNANCIES

Secondary cancers induced by chemotherapy and radiation are a serious long-term complication.[140] Although many types of solid tumors have been reported as chemotherapy-induced malignancies, acute nonlymphocytic leukemia (ANLL) or myelodysplastic syndrome is the most common secondary cancer. ANLL or myelodysplastic syndrome has been reported following successful treatment of Hodgkin's lymphoma, acute leukemias, non-Hodgkin's lymphomas, multiple myeloma, breast cancer, and advanced ovarian cancer. For curable cancers, the relatively small risk for occurrence of secondary malignancies is far outweighed by the benefits of survival in large numbers of patients. However, for cancers such as ovarian cancer, the risk of leukemia is not offset by improved survival in chemotherapy recipients. The issue of secondary malignancies is of particular concern in patients receiving adjuvant chemotherapy. As with the late complication of infertility, the antineoplastic agents primarily associated with secondary cancers are the alkylating agents. Etoposide, teniposide, and the anthracyclines have also been linked to secondary leukemias. Solid tumors as secondary malignancies occur more commonly after treatment with radiation than with chemotherapy.

SAFETY AND HANDLING ISSUES

As discussed previously, the cytotoxic drugs used to treat cancer are carcinogenic, mutagenic, and teratogenic. Consequently, these drugs should be handled with care to avoid inadvertent exposure of health care professionals.[141] All pharmacies should have written procedures for handling these drugs safely, and all personnel should be oriented to these procedures. The most common avenue of exposure is via inhalation of aerosolized drug. Individuals preparing chemotherapy should work in a class II biologic safety cabinet and wear gowns and powder-free disposable latex gloves. The gowns should be made of lint-free, low-permeability fabric with a solid front, long sleeves, and tight-fitting elastic cuffs. Negative-pressure techniques should be employed in drug preparation to minimize aerosolization. Health care workers administering these agents should take similar precautions to avoid exposure. Kits for cleaning up chemotherapy spills should be located in all areas of the institution in which chemotherapy is handled. Cytotoxic waste should be disposed of properly, and patients should be informed of proper methods of disposing of potentially contaminated body excreta and cytotoxic waste.

CANCER PREVENTION

Since many cancers are difficult to treat, especially in the advanced stages, cancer prevention has become an intense focus of cancer research. For some cancers, effective pharmacologic means of cancer prevention have been identified, such as tamoxifen for breast cancer prevention. Specific chemoprevention strategies will be discussed in disease-specific cancer chapters of this text. There are also general strategies known to prevent or reduce the risk of many malignancies, including modification of nutritional factors, increased physical activity, and reductions in exposure to known carcinogens, such as tobacco and the sun.

NUTRITION AND PHYSICAL ACTIVITY

The relationship between diet and cancer is the subject of intense investigation. There is evidence that suggests that up to one-third of cancer deaths in the United States are attributable to dietary factors.[17] Although controversy exists over the true role of diet in carcinogenesis, some general recommendations have been developed by the American Cancer Society (Table 124–20).[17] There is strong evidence that increased consumption of fruits and vegetables lowers the risk for many cancers, especially those of the gastrointestinal and respiratory tracts. Consumption of a high-fat diet appears to increase the risk for breast, colorectal, and prostate cancers. The average American consumes 36% to 38% of daily calories as fat. A decrease in fat intake to less than 30% of daily calories may decrease the risk for developing cancer, as well as heart disease. Obese individuals have increased risk of several cancers, including colorectal, breast, biliary, and uterine cancers. The inverse relationship between dietary fiber and colon cancer has received much attention. The American diet is typically low in fiber (11 g/day). High fiber intake (20 to 30 g/day) may decrease the risk of colon cancer. A high alcohol intake has been shown to increase the risk for many upper aerodigestive tract malignancies, especially in smokers.

Obesity and inactivity are also an important determinant of cancer risk. Increased physical activity is known to decrease the risk for breast, colon, endometrial, and prostate cancers.[17] Recommendations to increase physical activity and maintain a healthful weight are included in the American Cancer Society Cancer Prevention Guidelines.

TOBACCO

Cigarette smoking remains the most preventable cause of premature death in the United States. More than 400,000 deaths per year and 30% of all cancers in the United States are due to smoking.[142] For many types of cancer, the underlying etiology is unknown. One notable exception is lung cancer; cigarette smoking is the major cause of this disease. More than 90% of all cases of lung cancer are diagnosed in smokers. Tobacco smoking also increases the relative risk for development of many other types of cancer, including cancers of

TABLE 124–20. American Cancer Society Guidelines on Nutrition and Physical Activity for Cancer Prevention

Recommendations for individuals

1. *Eat a variety of healthful foods, with an emphasis on plant sources.*
   - Eat five or more servings of a variety of vegetables and fruits each day.
   - Choose whole grains in preference to processed (refined) grains and sugars.
   - Limit consumption of red meats, especially high-fat and processed meats.
   - Choose foods that help maintain a healthful weight.
2. *Adopt a physically active lifestyle.*
   - Adults should engage in at least moderate activity for 30 minutes or more on five or more days of the week; 45 minutes or more of moderate to vigorous activity on five or more days per week may further enhance reductions in risk of breast and colon cancer.
3. *Maintain a healthful weight throughout life.*
   - Balance caloric intake with physical activity.
   - Lose weight if currently overweight or obese.
4. *If you drink alcoholic beverages, limit consumption.*

Recommendations for community action

Public, private, and community organizations should work to create social and physical environments that support the adoption and maintenance of healthy nutrition and physical activity behaviors.
- Increase access to healthful foods in schools, worksites, and communities.
- Provide safe, enjoyable, and accessible environments for physical activity in schools and for transportation and recreation in communities.

From American Cancer Society.[17]

---

the mouth, pharynx, larynx, esophagus, and bladder. Passive inhalation of exhaled tobacco by-products and cigarette smoke represents a significant risk factor for lung cancer in the nonsmoking population. Smokeless tobacco has been connected to the development of oral cancers. Abstinence from chewing and smoking tobacco is believed to be a major factor in the prevention of these malignancies.

SUN EXPOSURE

The association between sun exposure and skin neoplasms is also well established. The incidence of both nonmelanomatous skin cancer and melanoma has steadily increased in past decades, paralleling the increase in recreational sun exposure.[143] During this same time period, protection from ultraviolet light exposure normally provided by the ozone layer has been compromised. Fair-skinned individuals who sunburn easily are particularly at high risk. Melanoma and skin cancers can be largely prevented by minimizing exposure to the sun and by applying strong sunscreens and sunblocks to sun-exposed areas (SPF-15 or greater).

ABBREVIATIONS

ANC: absolute neutrophil count
ANLL: acute nonlymphocytic leukemia
ara-C: cytarabine
ara-CTP: active triphosphate form of cytarabine
BCNU: carmustine
CCNU: lomustine
2-CDA: cladribine (2-chlorodeoxyadenosine)
CDK: cyclin-dependent kinase
CMF: cyclophosphamide, methotrexate, and 5-fluorouracil
CR: complete response
CSF: colony-stimulating factor
DHFR: dihydrofolate reductase
DNA: deoxyribonucleic acid
EGFR: epidermal growth factor receptor
FAMP: fludarabine monophosphate

FdUMP: fluorodeoxyuridine monophosphate
5-FU: fluorouracil
G_0: dormant phase of the cell cycle
G_1: first gap phase of the cell cycle
G_2: second gap or premitotic phase of the cell cycle
G-CSF: granulocyte colony-stimulating factor
GM-CSF: granulocyte-macrophage colony-stimulating factor
HDAC: high-dose ara-C
IFN: interferon
IL: interleukin
M: mitosis
MoAB: monoclonal antibody
6-MP: 6-mercaptopurine
mRNA: messenger RNA
MTIC: monomethyl triazeno imidazole carboxamide
MTX: methotrexate
NF-κB: nuclear factor-κB
PR: partial response
RAR: retinoic acid receptor
RNA: ribonucleic acid
rRNA: ribosomal RNA
RXR: retinoid X receptor
S: DNA synthesis phase of the cell cycle
6-TG: thioguanine
tRNA: transfer RNA
VEGF: vascular endothelial growth factor
WBC: white blood cell

Review Questions and other resources can be found at *www.pharmacotherapyonline.com.*

REFERENCES

1. Kaufman D, Chabner BA. Clinical strategies for cancer treatment: The role of drugs. In: Chabner BA, Longo DL, eds. Cancer Chemotherapy and Biotherapy: Principles and Practice. Philadelphia, Lippincott-Raven, 1996:1–16.

2. American Cancer Society. Cancer facts and figures—2005. Atlanta, American Cancer Society, 2005.

3. Liotta LA, Liu ET. Essentials of molecular biology: Genomics and cancer. In: DeVita VT, Hellman S, Rosenberg SA, eds. Cancer: Principles and Practice of Oncology, 6th ed. Philadelphia, Lippincott Williams & Wilkins, 2000:17–30.

4. Compagni A, Christofori G. Recent advances in research on multistage tumorigenesis. Br J Cancer 2000;83:1–5.

5. Weston A, Harris CC. Chemical carcinogenesis. In: Kufe DW, Pollock RE, Weichselbaum RR, et al, eds. Cancer Medicine, 6th ed. Hamilton, Ontario, BC Decker, 2003:267–278.

6. Cotran RS, Kumar V, Collins T: Neoplasia. In: Cotran RS, Kumar V, Collins T, eds. Robbins' Pathologic Basis of Disease, 6th ed. Philadelphia, WB Saunders, 1999:260–328.

7. Bishop JM. The molecular genetics of cancer. Science 1987;235: 305–311.

8. Gibbs WW. Untangling the roots of cancer. Sci Am 2003;289:56–65.

9. Weinberg RA. How cancer arises. Sci Am 1996;275:62–70.

10. Lundberg AS, Weinberg RA. Control of the cell cycle and apoptosis. Eur J Cancer 1999;35:531–539.

11. Dang C, Gilweski TA, Sarbone A, Norton L. Chemotherapy: cytokinetics. In: Kufe DW, Pollock RE, Weichselbaum RR, et al, eds. Cancer Medicine, 6th ed. Hamilton, Ontario, BC Decker, 2003:645–668.

12. Johnstone RW, Ruefli AA, Lowe SW. Apoptosis: a link between cancer genetics and chemotherapy. Cell 2002;108:153–164.

13. Marx J. DNA arrays reveal cancer in its many forms. Science 2000;289: 1670–1672.

14. Buick RN. Cellular basis of chemotherapy. In: Dorr RT, Von Hoff DD, eds. Cancer Chemotherapy Handbook, 2nd ed. New York, Elsevier, 1994: 3–14.

15. Stetler-Stevenson WG, Kleiner DE Jr. Molecular biology of cancer: Invasion and metastasis. In: DeVita VT, Hellman S, Rosenberg SA, eds. Cancer: Principles and Practice of Oncology, 6th ed. Philadelphia, Lippincott Williams & Wilkins, 2000:123–136.

16. Folkman J, Kalluri R. Tumor angiogenesis. In: Kufe DW, Pollock RE, Weichselbaum RR, et al, eds. Cancer Medicine, 6th ed. Hamilton, Ontario, BC Decker, 2003:161–194.

17. American Cancer Society. Cancer Prevention and Early Detection Facts and Figures 2004. Atlanta, American Cancer Society, 2004.

18. American Cancer Society. Warning signs of cancer. Atlanta, American Cancer Society.

19. Greene FL, Page DL, Fleming ID, et al, eds. AJCC Cancer Staging Manual, 6th ed. New York, Springer-Verlag, 2002:113–119.

20. Yaeger TE, Brady LW. Basis for major current therapies for cancer. In: Lenhard RE, Osteen RT, Gansler T, eds. Clinical Oncology. Atlanta, American Cancer Society, 2001:159–230.

21. Calabresi P, Chabner BA. Chemotherapy of neoplastic diseases. In: Hardman JG, Limbird LE, Molinoff PB, et al, eds: Goodman & Gilman's The Pharmacologic Basis of Therapeutics, 10th ed. New York, McGraw-Hill, 2001:1381–1388.

22. Haskell CM. Principles of cancer chemotherapy. In: Haskell CM, ed. Cancer Treatment, 5th ed. Philadelphia, WB Saunders, 2001:62–86.

23. Balmer CB, Finley RS. Principles of cancer treatment. In: Finley RS, Balmer C, eds. Concepts in Oncology Therapeutics, 2nd ed. Bethesda MD, Amer Soc Health-System Pharmacists, 1998:15–32.

24. Safa AR. Multidrug resistance. In: Schilsky RL, Milano GA, Ratain MJ, eds. Principles of Antineoplastic Drug Development and Pharmacology. New York, Marcel Dekker, 1996:457–486.

25. Tan B, Piwnica-Worms D, Ratner L. Multidrug resistance transporters and modulation. Curr Opin Oncol 2000;12:450–458.

26. Hryniuk WM. Dose intensity. In: Schilsky RL, Milano GA, Ratain MJ, eds. Principles of Antineoplastic Drug Development and Pharmacology. New York, Marcel Dekker, 1996:263–280.

27. Piccart MJ, Biganzoli L, Di Leo A. The impact of chemotherapy dose density and dose intensity on breast cancer outcome: what have we learned? Eur J Cancer 2000; 36(Suppl 1):S4–S10.

28. Links M, Lewis C. Chemoprotectants: A review of their clinical pharmacology and therapeutic efficacy. Drugs 1999;57:293–308.

29. Ravdin P. The use of HER2 testing in the management of breast cancer. Semin Oncol 2000;27(5 Suppl 9):33–42.

30. Lynch TJ, Bell DW, Sordella R, et al. Activating mutations in the epidermal growth factor receptor underlying responsiveness of non-small-cell lung cancer to gefitinib. N Engl J Med 2004;350:2129–2139.

31. Weinshilboum R. Inheritance and drug response. N Engl J Med 2003;348: 529–537.

32. Evans WE, McLeod HL. Pharmacogenomics—drug disposition, drug targets, and side effects. N Engl J Med 2003;348:538–549.

33. Collins JM. Pharmacokinetics and clinical monitoring. In: Chabner BA, Longo DL, eds. Cancer Chemotherapy and Biotherapy: Principles and Practice. Philadelphia, Lippincott-Raven, 1996:17–29.

34. Burke GA, Estlin EJ, Lowis SP. The role of pharmacokinetic and pharmacodynamic studies in the planning of protocols for the treatment of childhood cancer. Cancer Treat Rev 1999;25:13–27.

35. Ross J. Structure and function of the gene. In: Abeloff MD, Armitage JO, Lichter AS, Niederhuber JE, eds. Clinical Oncology, 2nd ed. Philadelphia, Churchill Livingstone, 2000:3–9.

36. Pizzorno G, Diasio RB, Cheng Y-C. Pyrimidines and purine antimetabolites. In: Kufe DW, Pollock RE, Weichselbaum RR, et al, eds. Cancer Medicine, 6th ed. Hamilton, Ontario, BC Decker, 2003:739–757.

37. 5-Fluorouracil: Forty-plus and still ticking. A review of its preclinical and clinical development. Invest New Drugs 2000;18:299–313.

38. Sobrero AF, Aschele C, Bertino JR. Fluorouracil in colorectal cancer—A tale of two drugs: Implications for biochemical modulation. J Clin Oncol 1997;15:368–381.

39. Rich TA, Shepard RC, Mosley ST. Four decades of continuing innovation with fluorouracil: current and future approaches to fluorouracil chemoradiation therapy. J Clin Oncol 2004;22:2214–2232.

40. Sloan JA, Goldberg RM, Sargent DJ, et al. Women experience greater toxicity with fluorouracil-based chemotherapy for colorectal cancer. J Clin Oncol 2002;20:1491–1498.

41. Schuller J, Cassidy J, Dumont E, et al. Preferential activation of capecitabine in tumor following oral administration to colorectal cancer patients. Cancer Chemother Pharmacol 2000;45:291–297.

42. Reigner B, Blesch K, Weidekamm E. Clinical pharmacokinetics of capecitabine. Clin Pharmacokinet 2001;40:85–104.

43. Wagstaff AJ, Ibbotson T, Goa KL. Capecitabine: a review of its pharmacology and therapeutic efficacy in the management of advanced breast cancer. Drugs 2003;63:217–236.

44. Cunningham D, Coleman R. New options for outpatient chemotherapy—the role of oral fluoropyrimidines. Cancer Treatment Reviews 2001;27: 211–220.

45. Johnson SA. Clinical pharmacokinetics of nucleoside analogues: focus on haematological malignancies. Clin Pharmacokinet 2000;39:5–26.

46. Smith GA, Damon LE, Rugo HS, et al. High-dose cytarabine dose modification reduces the incidence of neurotoxicity in patients with renal insufficiency. J Clin Oncol 1997;15:833–839.

47. Venook AP, Egorin MJ, Rosner GL, et al. Phase I and pharmacokinetic trial of gemcitabine in patients with hepatic or renal dysfunction: cancer and leukemia group B 9565. J Clin Oncol 2000;18:2780–2787.

48. Friedlander PA, Bansa R, Schwartz L, et al. Gemcitabine-related radiation recall preferentially involves internal tissue and organs. Cancer 2004; 100:1793–1799.

49. Silverman LR, Demakos EP, Peterson BL, et al. Randomized controlled trial of azacytidine in patients with the myelodysplastic syndrome: a study of the Cancer and Leukemia Group B. J Clin Oncol 2002;20: 2429–2440.

50. Rossi JF, Van Hoof A, De Boeck K, et al. Efficacy and safety of oral fludarabine phosphate in previously untreated patients with chronic lymphocytic leukemia. J Clin Oncol 2004;22:1260–1267.

51. Plosker GL, Figgitt DP. Oral fludarabine. Drugs 2003;63:2317–2323.

52. Kamen BA, Cole PD, Bertino JR. Folate antagonists. In: Kufe DW, Pollock RE, Weichselbaum RR, et al, eds. Cancer Medicine, 6th ed. Hamilton, Ontario, BC Decker, 2003:727–738.

53. Curtin NJ, Hughes AN. Pemetrexed disodium, a novel antifolate with multiple targets. Lancet Oncol 2001;2:298–306.

54. Rowinsky E. Microtubule-targeting natural products. In: Kufe DW,

Pollock RE, Weichselbaum RR, et al, eds. Cancer Medicine, 6th ed. Hamilton, Ontario, BC Decker, 2003:791–810.

55. Hainsworth JD, Burris HA III, Yardley DA, et al. Weekly docetaxel in the treatment of elderly patients with advanced breast cancer: a Minnie Pearl Cancer Research Network phase II trial. J Clin Oncol 2001;19: 3500–3505.

56. Krieger JA, Stanford BL, Ballard EE, Rabinowitz I. Implementation and results of a test dose program with taxanes. Cancer J 2002;8:337–341.

57. Kitamura T, Nishimatsu H, Tomita K, et al: Estramustine combination chemotherapy and low-dose monotherapy in advanced prostate cancer. Expert Rev Anticancer Ther 2002;2:59–71.

58. Rubin EH, Hait WN. Anthracyclines and DNA intercalators/epipodo-phyllotoxins/camptothecins/DNA topoisomerases. In: Kufe DW, Pollock RE, Weichselbaum RR, et al, eds. Cancer Medicine, 6th ed. Hamilton, Ontario, BC Decker, 2003:781–790.

59. Hande KR. Etoposide: four decades of development of a topoisomerase II inhibitor. Eur J Cancer 1998;34:1514–1521.

60. Kellner U, Sehested M, Jensen PB, et al: Culprit and victim—DNA topoisomerase II. Lancet Oncol 2002;3:235–242.

61. Ulukan H, Swaan PW. Camptothecins: a review of their chemotherapeutic potential. Drugs 2002;62:2039–2057.

62. Vanhoefer U, Harstrick A, Achterrath W, et al. Irinotecan in the treatment of colorectal cancer: clinical overview. J Clin Oncol 2001;19: 1501–1518.

63. Raymond E, Boige V, Faivre S, et al. Dosage adjustment and pharma-cokinetic profile of irinotecan in cancer patients with hepatic dysfunction. J Clin Oncol 2002;20:4303–4312.

64. Falcome A, Di Paolo A, Masi G, et al. Sequence effect of irinotecan and fluorouracil treatment on pharmacokinetics and toxicity in chemotherapy-naive metastatic colorectal cancer patients. J Clin Oncol 2001;19:3456–3462.

65. Danesi R, Fogli S, Gennari A, et al. Pharmacokinetic—pharmacodynamic relationships of the anthracycline anticancer drugs. Clin Pharmacokinet 2002;41:431–444.

66. Bast RC Jr, Kousparou CA, Epenetos AA, et al. Monoclonal serotherapy. In: Kufe DW, Pollock RE, Weichselbaum RR, et al, eds. Cancer Medicine, 6th ed. Hamilton, Ontario, BC Decker, 2003:881–898.

67. Colvin M. Alkylating agents and platinum antitumor compounds. In: Kufe DW, Pollock RE, Weichselbaum RR, et al, eds. Cancer Medicine, 6th ed. Hamilton, Ontario, BC Decker, 2003:759–779.

68. Boddy AV, Yule SM. Metabolism and pharmacokinetics of oxazaphosphorines. Clin Pharmacokinet 2000;38:291–304.

69. Stupp R, Gander M, Leyvraz S, Newlands E. Current and future developments in the use of temozolomide for the treatment of brain tumors. Lancet Oncol 2001;2:552–560.

70. Su YB, Sohn S, Krown SE, et al. Selective CD4+ lymphopenia in melanoma patients treated with temozolomide: a toxicity with therapeutic implications. J Clin Oncol 2004;22:610–616.

71. Guminski AD, Harnett PR, deFazio A. Scientists and clinicians test their metal—back to the future with platinum compounds. Lancet Oncol 2002;3:312–318.

72. O'Dwyer PJ, Stevenson JP, Johnson SW. Clinical pharmacokinetics and administration of established platinum drugs. Drugs 2000;59(Suppl 4): 19–27.

73. Pace A, Savarese A, Picardo M, et al. Neuroprotective effect of vitamin E supplementation in patients treated with cisplatin chemotherapy. J Clin Oncol 2003;21:927–931.

74. Andre T, Boni C, Mounedji-Boudiaf L, et al. Oxaliplatin, fluorouracil, and leucovorin as adjuvant treatment for colon cancer. N Engl J Med 2004;350:2343–2351.

75. Laxo JS. Bleomycin. Cancer Chemother Biol Response Modif 1999;18: 39–45.

76. Kurtzberg J, Yousem D, Beauchamp N Jr. Asparaginase. In: Kufe DW, Pollock RE, Weichselbaum RR, et al, eds. Cancer Medicine, 6th ed. Hamilton, Ontario, BC Decker, 2003:823–830.

77. Soignet SL, Frankel SR, Douer D, et al. United States multicenter study of arsenic trioxide in relapsed acute promyelocytic leukemia. J Clin Oncol 2001;19;3852–3860.

78. Bradner WT. Mitomycin C: a clinical update. Cancer Treat Rev 2001; 27:35–50.

79. Borden EC. Interferons. In: Kufe DW, Pollock RE, Weichselbaum RR, et al, eds. Cancer Medicine, 6th ed. Hamilton, Ontario, BC Decker, 2003: 831–841.

80. Kirkwood JM, Bender C, Agarwala S, et al. Mechanisms and management of toxicities associated with high-dose interferon alfa-2b therapy. J Clin Oncol 2002;20:3703–3718.

81. Ekmekcioglu S, Grimm EA. Cytokines: biology and applications in cancer medicine. In: Kufe DW, Pollock RE, Weichselbaum RR, et al, eds. Cancer Medicine, 6th ed. Hamilton, Ontario, BC Decker, 2003: 843–851.

82. Anonymous. Ibritumomab tiuxetan [Zevalin] for non-Hodgkin's lymphoma. Med Lett 2002;44:101–102.

83. Witzig TE, Flinn IW, Gordon LI, et al. Treatment with ibritumomab tiuxetan radioimmunotherapy in patients with rituximab-refractory follicular non-Hodgkin's lymphoma. J Clin Oncol 2002;20:3262–3269.

84. Plosker GL, Figgitt DP. Rituximab: a review of its use in non-Hodgkin's lymphoma and chronic lymphocytic leukemia. Drugs 2004;63:803–843.

85. Anonymous. Iodine-131 tositumomab [Bexxar] for treatment of lymphoma. Med Lett 2003;45:86–87.

86. Jordan VC. Estrogens and antiestrogens. In: Kufe DW, Pollock RE, Weichselbaum RR, et al, eds. Cancer Medicine, 6th ed. Hamilton, Ontario, BC Decker, 2003:939–946.

87. Osborne CK, Zhao H, Fuqua SAW. Selective estrogen receptor modulators: structure, function, and clinical use. J Clin Oncol 2000;18: 3172–3186.

88. Schally AV, Comaru-Schally AM. Hypothalamic and other peptide hormones. In: Kufe DW, Pollock RE, Weichselbaum RR, et al, eds. Cancer Medicine, 6th ed. Hamilton, Ontario, BC Decker, 2003:911–926.

89. Buzdar AU, Harvey HA. Aromatase inhibitors. In: Kufe DW, Pollock RE, Weichselbaum RR, et al, eds. Cancer Medicine, 6th ed. Hamilton, Ontario, BC Decker, 2003:947–959.

90. Denmeade SR, Isaacs JT. Androgen deprivation strategies in the treatment of advanced prostate cancer. In: Kufe DW, Pollock RE, Weichselbaum RR, et al, eds. Cancer Medicine, 6th ed. Hamilton, Ontario, BC Decker, 2003:967–979.

91. McCarty KS Jr, Nichols M, McCarty DS Sr. Progestins. In: Kufe DW, Pollock RE, Weichselbaum RR, et al, eds. Cancer Medicine, 6th ed. Hamilton, Ontario, BC Decker, 2003:961–966.

92. McKeage K, Curran MP, Plosker GL. Fulvestrant: a review of its use in hormone receptor-positive metastatic breast cancer in postmenopausal women with disease progression following antiestrogen therapy. Drugs 2004;64:633–648.

93. Anonymous. Abarelix [Plenaxis] for advanced prostate cancer. Med Lett 2004;46:22–23.

94. McKay LI, Cidlowski JA. Corticosteroids. In: Kufe DW, Pollock RE, Weichselbaum RR, et al, eds. Cancer Medicine, 6th ed. Hamilton, Ontario, BC Decker, 2003:927–938.

95. Sporn MB, Lippman SM. Chemoprevention of cancer. In: Kufe DW, Pollock RE, Weichselbaum RR, et al, eds. Cancer Medicine, 6th ed. Hamilton, Ontario, BC Decker, 2003:414–422.

96. Duvic M, Hymes K, Heald P, et al. Bexarotene is effective and safe for treatment of refractory advanced-state cutaneous T-cell lymphoma: multinational phase II-III trial results. J Clin Oncol 2001;19: 2456–2471.

97. Heinrich MC, Blanke CD, Corless CL, Druker BJ. Small-molecule inhibitors of protein kinases in the treatment of human cancer. In: Kufe DW, Pollock RE, Weichselbaum RR, et al, eds. Cancer Medicine, 6th ed. Hamilton, Ontario, BC Decker, 2003:811–821.

98. Druker BJ. Imatinib as a paradigm of targeted therapies. J Clin Oncol 2003;21(Suppl):239s–245s.

99. Peng B, Hayes M, Resta D, et al. Pharmacokinetics and pharmacodynamics of imatinib in a phase I trial with chronic myeloid leukemia patients. J Clin Oncol 2004;22:935–942.

100. Croom KF, Perry CM. Imatinib mesylate in the treatment of gastrointestinal stromal tumors. Drugs 2003;63:513–522.

101. Culy CR, Faulds D. Gefitinib. Drugs 2002;62:2237–2248.

102. Giaccone G, Herbst RS, Manegold C, et al. Gefitinib in combination with gemcitabine and cisplatin in advanced non-small-cell lung cancer: a phase III trial—INTACT 1. J Clin Oncol 2004;22:777–784.

103. Richardson PG, Barlogie B, Berenson J. A phase 2 study of bortezomib in relapsed, refractory myeloma. N Engl J Med 2003;348:2609–2617.

104. Mitchell BS. The proteosome—an emerging therapeutic target in cancer. N Engl J Med 2003;348:2597–2598.

105. Harris M. Monoclonal antibodies as therapeutic agents for cancer. Lancet Oncol 2004;5:292–302.

106. Frampton JE, Wagstaff AJ. Alemtuzumab. Drugs 2003;63:1229–1243.

107. Miller KD, Sweeney CJ, Sledge GW Jr. Redefining the target: chemotherapeutics as antiangiogenics. J Clin Oncol 2001;19:1195–1206.

108. Hurwitz H, Fehrenbacher L, Novotny W, et al. Bevacizumab plus irinotecan, fluorouracil, and leucovorin for metastatic colorectal cancer. N Engl J Med 2004;350:2335–2342.

109. Anonymous. Two new drugs for colon cancer. Med Lett 2004;46:46–48.

110. Reynolds NA, Wagstaff AJ. Cetuximab in the treatment of metastatic colon cancer. Drugs 2004;64:109–118.

111. Saltz LB, Meropol NJ, Loehrer PJ Sr, et al. Phase II trial of cetuximab in patients with refractory colorectal cancer that expresses the epidermal growth factor receptor. J Clin Oncol 2004;22:1201–1208.

112. Giles F, Estey E, O'Brian S. Gemtuzumab ozogamicin in the treatment of acute myeloid leukemia. Cancer 2004;98:2095–2104.

113. Larson RA, Boogaerts M, Estey E, et al. Antibody-targeted chemotherapy of older patients with acute myeloid leukemia in first relapse using Mylotarg [gemtuzumab ozogamicin]. Leukemia 2002;16:1627–1636.

114. Vogel CL, Cobleigh MA, Tripathy D, et al. Efficacy and safety of trastuzumab as a single agent in first-line treatment of HER2-overexpressing metastatic breast cancer. J Clin Oncol 2002;20:719–726.

115. Perez EA, Rodeheffer R. Clinical cardiac tolerability of trastuzumab. J Clin Oncol 2004;22:322–329.

116. Fine HA, Figg WD, Jaeckle K, et al. Phase II trial of the antiangiogenic agent thalidomide in patients with recurrent high-grade gliomas. J Clin Oncol 2000;18;708–715.

117. Weber D, Rankin K, Gavino M, Delasalle K, Alexanian R. Thalidomide alone or with dexamethasone for previously untreated multiple myeloma. J Clin Oncol 2003;21:16–19.

118. DePauw BE, Donelly JP. Infections in the immunocompromised host: General principles. In: Mandell GP, Bennett JE, Dolin R, eds. Principles and Practice of Infectious Disease, 5th ed. Philadelphia, Churchill Livingstone, 2000:3079–3090.

119. Pizzo PA. Empirical therapy and prevention of infection in the immunocompromised host. In: Mandell GP, Bennett JE, Dolin R, eds. Principles and Practice of Infectious Disease, 5th ed. Philadelphia, Churchill Livingstone, 2000:3102–3112.

120. Hughes WT, Armstrong D, Bodey GP, et al. 2002 Guidelines for the use of antimicrobial agents in neutropenic patients with cancer. Clin Infect Dis 2002;34:730–751.

121. Rolston KV, Talcott JA. Ambulatory antimicrobial therapy for hematologic malignancies. Oncology (Huntingt) 2000;14:17–22.

122. Nemunaitis J. A comparative review of the colony-stimulating factors. Drugs 1997;54:709–729.

123. ASCO Ad Hoc Colony-Stimulating Factor Guideline Expert Panel. American Society of Clinical Oncology recommendations for the use of hematopoietic colony-stimulating factors: Evidence-based, clinical practice guidelines. J Clin Oncol 1994;12:2471–2508.

124. ASCO Ad Hoc Colony-Stimulating Factor Guideline Expert Panel. 2000 Update of recommendations for the use of hematopoietic colony-stimulating factors: Evidence-based, clinical practice guidelines. J Clin Oncol 2000;3558–3585.

125. Crawford J, Dale DC, Lyman GH. Chemotherapy-induced neutropenia: Risks, consequences, and new directions for its management. Cancer 2004;100:228–237.

126. Schiffer CA, Anderson KC, Bennett CL, et al. Platelet transfusion for patients with cancer: Clinical practice guidelines of the American Society of Clinical Oncology. J Clin Oncol 2001;19:1519–1538.

127. Demetri GD. Pharmacologic treatment options in patients with thrombocytopenia. Semin Hematol 2000;37(2 Suppl 4):11–18.

128. Cantor SB, Elting LS, Hudson DV, et al. Pharmacoeconomic analysis of oprelvekin (recombinant human interleukin-11) for secondary prophylaxis of thrombocytopenia in solid tumor patients receiving chemotherapy. Cancer 2003;97:3099–3106.

129. Johnston E, Crawford J. The hematologic support of the cancer patient. In: Berger A, Portenoy RK, Weissman DE, eds. Principles and Practice of Supportive Oncology, 2nd ed. Philadelphia, Lippincott-Raven, 2002: 549–555.

130. Cella D. The effects of anemia and anemia treatment on the quality of life of people with cancer. Oncology (Huntingt) 2002;16(9 Suppl 10): 125–132.

131. Rizzo JD, Lichtin AE, Woolf SH, et al. Use of epoetin in patients with cancer: Evidence-based clinical practice guidelines of the American Society of Clinical Oncology and the American Society of Hematology. Blood 2002;100:2303–2320.

132. Berger AM, Kilroy TJ. Oral Complications. In: DeVita VT Jr., Hellman S, Rosenberg SA, eds. Cancer: Principles and Practice of Oncology, 6th ed. Philadelphia, Lippincott Williams & Wilkins, 2001:2881–2893.

133. Sonis ST, Elting LS, Keefe D, et al. Perspectives on cancer therapy-induced mucosal injury. Cancer 2004;100(suppl 9):1995–2025.

134. Rubenstein EB, Peterson DE, Schubert M, et al. Clinical practice guidelines for the prevention and treatment of cancer therapy-induced oral and gastrointestinal mucosa. Cancer 2004;100(suppl 9):2026–2046.

135. Siepp CA. Hair loss. In: DeVita VT Jr, Hellman S, Rosenberg SA, eds. Cancer: Principles and Practice of Oncology, 6th ed. Philadelphia, Lippincott Williams & Wilkins, 2001:2922–2923.

136. Albanell J, Baselga J. Systemic therapy emergencies. Semin Oncol 2000; 27:347–361.

137. Dorr RT. Pharmacologic management of vesicant chemotherapy extravasations. In: Dorr RT, Von Hoff DD, eds. Cancer Chemotherapy Handbook, 2nd ed. Stamford, Appleton & Lange, 1994;109–118.

138. Howell S, Shalet S. Gonadal damage from chemotherapy and radiotherapy. Endocrin Metab Clin North Am 1998;27:927–943.

139. Lenz KL, Valley AW. Infertility after chemotherapy: A review of the risks and strategies for prevention. J Oncol Pharm Pract 1996;2:75–100.

140. Green DM, D'Angio GJD. Second malignant neoplasms. In: Albeoff MD, Armitage JO, Lichter AS, Niederhuber JE, eds. Clinical Oncology, 2nd ed. Philadelphia, Churchill Livingstone, 2000:1082–1100.

141. ASHP technical assistance bulletin on handling cytotoxic and hazardous drugs. Am J Hosp Pharm 1990;47:1033–1049.

142. Bergen AW, Caporaso N. Cigarette smoking. J Natl Cancer Inst 1999; 91: 1365–1375.

143. Gilchriest BA, Eller MS, Geller AC, Yaar M. The pathogenesis of melanoma induced by ultraviolet radiation. N Engl J Med 1999;340: 1341–1348.

125
BREAST CANCER

Celeste Lindley and Laura Boehnke Michaud

Learning Objectives and other resources can be found at *www.pharmacotherapyonline.com.*

KEY CONCEPTS

◀1 Breast cancer is most commonly diagnosed in early stages, when it is a highly curable malignancy.

◀2 Local therapy of early stage breast cancer consists of modified radical mastectomy or lumpectomy plus external beam radiation therapy. The surgical approach to the ipsilateral axilla may consist of a full level I/II axillary lymph node dissection or a lymph node mapping procedure with sentinel lymph node biopsy.

◀3 Adjuvant endocrine therapy reduces the rates of relapse and death in patients with hormone-receptor positive early breast cancer tumors. Adjuvant chemotherapy reduces the rates of relapse and death in all patients with early stage breast cancer.

◀4 The choice of chemotherapy regimen, dose, schedule and duration of therapy, and the choice of endocrine therapy are controversial and rapidly changing as results from ongoing randomized clinical trials are reported.

◀5 Neoadjuvant chemotherapy is appropriate for patients with locally advanced or inflammatory breast cancer, followed by local therapy and further adjuvant systemic therapy.

◀6 Initial therapy of metastatic breast cancer in women with hormone receptor–positive tumors should consist of hormonal therapy.

◀7 Women with metastatic breast cancer who have hormone receptor–positive tumors and respond to an initial hormonal manipulation will usually respond to a second hormonal manipulation.

◀8 Approximately 40% of women with metastatic breast cancer will respond to chemotherapy regimens; doxorubicin- and taxane-containing regimens are the most active.

◀9 The goal of adjuvant chemotherapy is curative, while the goal of chemotherapy in the metastatic setting is palliative.

◀10 Although controversial, the benefits of annual screening mammography in women younger than 50 years of age are apparent and a large number of national and international studies demonstrate a 20% to 40% reduction in breast cancer mortality from annual or biannual screening mammography in women aged 50 to 70 years.

Breast cancer is the most common site of cancer and is second only to lung cancer as a cause of cancer death in American women. It is estimated that 211,240 new cases of breast cancer will be diagnosed and that 40,410 women will die of breast cancer in 2005.[1] Whites account for the largest portion of estimated cases (82%) and deaths (80%). In addition to invasive breast cancers, it is estimated that 58,490 cases of in situ cancer will be diagnosed among women in the United States in 2005.

Female breast cancer incidence rates vary considerably across racial and ethnic groups. The average annual age-adjusted incidence rate from 1997 to 2001 was 141.7 cases per 100,000 among white females, 119.9 among blacks, 96.8 among Asian-Americans/Pacific Islanders, 89.6 in Hispanics, and 54.2 in American Indians/Alaska Natives.[2] Probable reasons for the higher incidence rates in whites than other racial and ethnic groups include genetic, reproductive, and lifestyle factors.[3] Female breast cancer incidence rates increased for all women combined from 1980 to 2001, although the rate of increase slowed in the 1990s. The temporal trends in incidence are shown by race and ethnicity in Fig. 125–1. Incidence rates continued to increase in white women (0.4% per year, 1987–2001), but have stabilized in black women since 1992. In other racial and ethnic groups, rates increased from 1992 through 2001 in Asian-Americans/Pacific

Islanders (1.7% per year) and Hispanics (0.7% per year), but decreased among American Indians/Alaska Natives (3.7% per year).[2]

◀11 Most breast cancers diagnosed are small tumors (≤2 cm) and disease is localized in all racial and ethnic groups. However, blacks and other minority women have proportionally more cases of disease diagnosed at more advanced stages compared with white women. This is thought to reflect access to and use of screening mammography and timely treatment. The incidence of ductal carcinoma in situ (DCIS) increased rapidly between the early and late 1980s, stabilized between the late 1980s and early 1990s, and increased rapidly thereafter. The rapid increases in DCIS are largely attributed to increased use of screening mammography, because most cases of DCIS manifest solely as clustered microcalcifications seen on mammography.[3]

Figure 125–1 shows trends in female breast cancer mortality rate by race and ethnicity. From 1997 to 2001, the average breast cancer death rate was highest in blacks (35.4 cases per 100,000 women), followed by whites (26.4), Hispanics (17.3), American Indians/Alaska Natives (13.6), and Asian-Americans/Pacific Islanders (12.6).[2] The death rate is higher among blacks than white women despite the lower incidence. Breast cancer death rates decreased by 2.6% per year among white women and by 1.2% per year since 1992 among

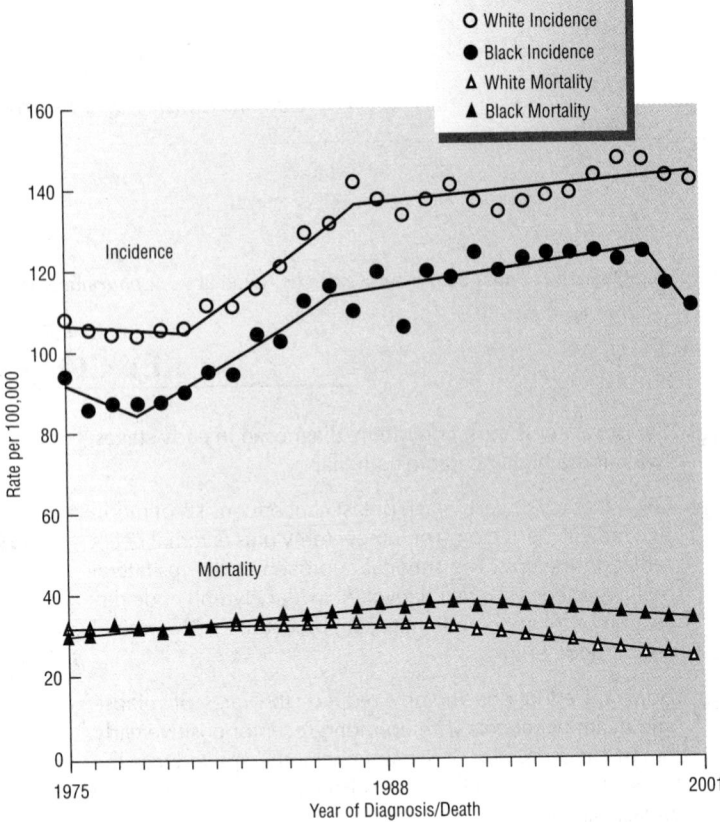

FIGURE 125–1. Breast cancer incidence and mortality rates by race, 1975–2001. (From Ries et al.[2])

black women. These declines in breast cancer mortality have been attributed to changes in screening practices and effectiveness of adjuvant systemic therapy following primary local regional therapy. The disparity between white and black women can be explained by differences in timely diagnosis through mammography screening and unequal access to prompt, high-quality treatment.[3]

EPIDEMIOLOGY AND ETIOLOGY

The two variables most strongly associated with the occurrence of breast cancer are gender and age. Although one commonly thinks of breast cancer as a disease confined to women, about 1,690 cases of male breast cancer were projected to be diagnosed in the United States in 2005.[1] Although male gender had been considered a poor prognostic factor in some investigations, it is now believed that higher mortality rates in men are attributable to more advanced disease at the time of diagnosis. When stage and other known prognostic factors are controlled for, men do not fare any differently from their female counterparts. Similarly, treatment of male breast cancer is no different from treatment of breast cancer in females.

The incidence of breast cancer increases with advancing age. Perhaps the most frequently quoted breast cancer statistic is that one in seven women will develop breast cancer during their lifetime. It should be emphasized that this is a cumulative lifetime risk of developing the disease from birth to age 110, and that the estimates are weighted by the probability of surviving through each decade of life.[4] Women older than 90 years of age contribute very little to the overall risk statistic because their numbers are so small. The "one in seven women" figure is often misinterpreted by women who assume that it

translates into one in seven women being diagnosed with breast cancer each year. Feuer and colleagues developed a more useful method of presenting the risk data based on age intervals.[4] As Table 125–1 demonstrates, the risk of a woman developing breast cancer before the age of 40 years is about 1 in 250. It is apparent from this table that although the cumulative probability of developing breast cancer increases with increasing age, more than half of the risk occurs after age 60 years.

An understanding of the relationship between age and the incidence of breast cancer is particularly relevant when one discusses "risk factors" or factors other than age that increase a woman's probability of developing breast cancer. The relative risk (RR) of developing breast cancer for an individual woman in a defined risk group is usually multiplied by the probability of a woman developing breast cancer during her lifetime, and this figure is taken as the cumulative lifetime risk of that individual developing breast cancer. However, the

TABLE 125–1. Risk of Developing Breast Cancer in SEER Areas, Women, All Races 1998–2000

Age Interval (y)	Probability (%) of Developing Invasive Breast Cancer During the Interval
30–40	0.40 or 1 in 250
40–50	1.45 or 1 in 69
50–60	2.78 or 1 in 36
60–70	3.81 or 1 in 26
From birth to death	13.51 or 1 in 7

From Ries LAG, Eisner MP, Kosary CL, eds. SEER Cancer Statistics Review: 1975–2001. Bethesda. MD, http://seer.cancer.gov/csr/1975–2001/, 2004.

risk of developing breast cancer is age dependent. Therefore a more meaningful way to counsel patients regarding their risk of developing breast cancer based on the presence of a known risk factor incorporates an age-specific incidence rate, not cumulative lifetime risk. For example, if a 40-year-old woman with a strong family history of breast cancer is thought to have a relative risk ratio of 2.0, her risk of developing breast cancer by the age of 50 is only 2.9% (2 × 1.45) not 27.02% (2 × 13.51) (see Table 125–1). It is also important to note that recognized risk factors are not additive in a simple mathematical sense and that the observed cumulative lifetime risk associated with nongenetic risk factors has rarely exceeded 30% (1 in 3) in any study, regardless of the number and significance of individual risk factors. Finally, it should be emphasized that more than 60% of women with breast cancer have no identifiable major risk factor, indicating that the search for the etiology of this disease is largely incomplete.

A number of calculators are available on the internet to estimate a patient's risk of developing breast cancer. The National Cancer Institute (NCI) has an online version of the Breast Cancer Risk Assessment Tool that is considered the most authoritative and accurate standard (http://brca.nci.nih.gov/brc/q1.htm). This tool used the original Gail Model, named after the author of a number of publications that described the scientific basis for risk calculations and applied it to data from the Breast Cancer Detection and Demonstration Project, a mammography screening project conducted in the 1970s. The Breast Cancer Risk Assessment Tool was designed for health professionals to project a women's individualized risk for invasive breast cancer over a 5-year period and over her lifetime.

ENDOCRINE FACTORS

A number of endocrine factors have been linked to the incidence of breast cancer.[5,6] Many of these relate to the total duration of menstrual life. Early menarche, generally defined as menstruation beginning before age 12, has been shown by a number of investigators to increase the cumulative lifetime risk of breast cancer development compared to menarche at age 16 or greater. Conversely, early age of natural menopause has been shown to result in a reduction of risk. Similarly, investigators have reported that bilateral oophorectomy prior to age 35 reduces the relative risk of developing breast cancer.

Nulliparity and a late age at first birth (≥30 years) have been reported to increase the lifetime risk of developing breast cancer twofold. Women who have their first child after the age of 35 have a slightly higher risk than a nulliparous woman. It has been suggested that the period between the onset of menses and the age of first pregnancy provides a "window of initiation" for the development of breast cancer. This is a time when an unbalanced hormonal environment reacts with the abundant and highly responsive breast tissue. Investigators have postulated that international differences in age of menarche, age at menopause, and childbearing may account for a substantial part of the international differences in the incidence of breast cancer. In underdeveloped countries where the incidence of breast cancer is low compared to the United States, a late onset of menarche is the rule, and frequently there is a decreased interval between puberty and first pregnancy, followed by several pregnancies and early menopause.

Many studies have evaluated the relationship between exogenous hormones and development of breast cancer. Postmenopausal estrogen replacement therapy has been the subject of several recent meta-analyses, with conflicting results.[7,8] The recently reported NCI-sponsored Women's Health Initiative study randomized 80,000 women to take postmenopausal estrogen replacement therapy combined with progesterone or a placebo.[9] This study reported an increased risk of breast cancer (38 vs. 30 cases per 10,000 person years [RR = 1.26]) when women taking combined estrogen/progesterone for an average of 5.2 years were compared to those receiving placebo. The increase in risk was observed in year three in women who had previously used menopausal hormones, but not until year four in women with no previous use. Women who had a hysterectomy, and therefore did not require progestin therapy to decrease risk of endometrial carcinoma, did not have an increased or decreased risk of breast cancer as compared to women receiving placebo. Thus long-term use of hormone replacement therapy and concurrent use of progestins appear to contribute to breast cancer risk.

The use of postmenopausal estrogen replacement therapy in women with a history of breast cancer is generally considered contraindicated. Because of the association of estrogen and risk of breast cancer, many clinicians believe that patients with a strong family history or other risk factors for breast cancer should not receive postmenopausal estrogen replacement therapy. This dogma has recently been challenged in the medical literature. Proponents of estrogen replacement therapy in patients with successfully treated operable breast cancer often state that the possible benefits of replacement therapy in terms of prevention of chronic conditions outweigh an unknown but potential increased risk of breast cancer development. However, a recent report from the Women's Health Initiative showed no reduction in the risk of coronary heart disease in women randomized to receive hormone replacement therapy.[10] Women who are considering estrogen replacement therapy should carefully consider the risks versus benefits (see Chap. 80 for a detailed discussion of hormone replacement therapy).

There are more than 20 epidemiologic studies of the potential carcinogenic effect of oral contraceptives, most of which have not shown a relationship between use of birth control pills and breast cancer incidence. But results are conflicting and assessment of the studies necessitates consideration of the particular oral contraceptive products involved, daily and cumulative doses of the hormones administered, and the latency for development of breast cancer. A review and meta-analysis suggest that the risk of breast cancer is not increased in women who had ever received oral contraceptive drugs. However, women who were current oral contraceptive users did show a small but significant increase in the relative risk of breast cancer (RR = 1.24).[11] It should be pointed out that early use of oral contraceptives may be associated with early menarche and may result in late age of first birth, both of which are recognized risk factors for breast cancer. Reassuring data that oral contraceptives do not increase breast cancer risk later in life have recently been published.[12,13] Although it is not entirely possible to rule out a promotional effect of oral contraceptives on breast cancer development in young patients, most experts believe that the safety and benefits of low-dose oral contraceptives currently outweigh the potential risks and that changes in the prescribing practice for the use of oral contraceptives are not warranted. Oral contraceptives are known to reduce the risk of ovarian cancer by about 40% and the risk of endometrial cancer by about 60%.

GENETIC FACTORS

Both personal and family histories influence a woman's risk of developing breast cancer. A past medical history for breast cancer is associated with about a fivefold increased risk of contralateral breast cancer. Cancer of the uterus and ovary has also been associated with an increased risk of the development of breast cancer. Breast cancer is observed as part of cancer family syndromes in association with other tumors. Only 5% of breast cancer patients are thought to have a pedigree consistent with hereditary breast cancer.

A topic that bears some discussion because of its prevalence in the general population is the relationship of fibrocystic breast disease to the development of invasive breast cancer. As many as 85% of American women have "lumpy breasts" and may have a clinical diagnosis of fibrocystic breast disease or benign breast disease. The relative risk of breast cancer in patients with a history of fibrocystic breast disease has ranged from 1.5 to 2.0 in reported studies. But fibrocystic disease involves a heterogeneous group of pathologic changes associated with various degrees of breast cancer risk. Thus a clinical diagnosis of fibrocystic or benign breast disease has little practical significance for counseling patients regarding individual risk of breast cancer. Benign breast conditions are classified as nonproliferative or proliferative. On the basis of a review of more than 10,000 breast biopsies,[14] women with proliferative disease were found to have a relative risk of 1.9, and the subcategory of women with atypical hyperplasia had a relative risk of 4.4. Nonproliferative benign breast disease was not associated with an excess risk of breast cancer. About 80% of the reviewed biopsies were found to have nonproliferative benign breast disease, and of those demonstrating proliferation, only 3.6% were "atypical." These data suggest that benign breast disease or fibrocystic disease is most often not associated with proliferation, and that women with benign breast disease or fibrocystic disease are not at an increased risk for developing breast cancer. However, it must be noted that "lumpy breasts" may lead to a delay in diagnosis of breast cancer because of inability of the patient or physician to detect a true malignant lesion.

It has been recognized for some time that a family history of breast cancer is associated rather strongly with a woman's own risk for developing the disease. Empirical estimates of the risks associated with particular patterns of family history of breast cancer indicate the following:[15]

1. Having any first-degree relative with breast cancer increases a woman's risk of breast cancer 1.5- to 3-fold, depending on age.
2. The higher relative risk is associated with breast cancer with onset younger than age 45 years in one or more first-degree relatives.
3. Having multiple first-degree relatives affected has been inconsistently associated with elevated risks.
4. Having a second-degree relative affected increases a woman's risk of developing breast cancer by approximately 50% (RR = 1.5).
5. Affected family members on the maternal side and the paternal side contribute similarly to the risk.

Although certain patterns of family history are associated with substantial elevations in the risk of breast cancer, these high-risk patterns occur infrequently in the general population (Table 125–2). The percentage of all breast cancers in the population that can be attributed to family history range between 6% and 12%.[15] Thus it appears that genetically transmitted susceptibility contributes to their etiology of breast cancer in a sizable minority of patients.

In the early 1990s, pedigree analysis of 23 high-risk families for breast and ovarian cancer provided evidence for a rare autosomal dominant allele.[16,17] From these families, a gene on the long arm of chromosome 17 (17q21) was identified as abnormal in a large percentage of these hereditary breast and ovarian cancer patients. Isolation of the *BRCA1* gene was initially reported in 1994. A second

TABLE 125–2. Established and Probable Risk Factors for Breast Cancer

Risk Factor	Comparison Category	Risk Category	Typical Relative Risk
Family history of breast cancer	No first-degree relatives affected	Mother affected before the age of 60 y	2.0
		Mother affected after the age of 60 y	1.4
		Two first-degree relatives affected	4–6
		Breast cancer in one or more second-degree relatives	1.36
		Ovarian cancer in one or more first-degree relatives	1.59
Age at menarche	16 y	11 y	1.3
Age at birth of first child	Before 20 y	20–24 y	1.3
		25–29 y	1.6
		≥30 y	1.9
Age at menopause	45–54 y	After 55 y	1.5
		Before 45 y	0.7
		Oophrectomy before 35 y	0.4
Benign breast disease	No biopsy or aspiration	Proliferation only	1.5
		Atypical hyperplasia	3.5
		Lobular carcinoma *in situ*	7.2
Obesity	10th percentile	90th percentile	
		Age, 30–49 y	0.8
		Age ≥50 y	1.2
Oral contraceptive use	Never used	Ever used	1.0
		≥4 y before first pregnancy	1.7
Postmenopausal estrogen replacement	Never used	Current use all ages	1.4
		15 + y	1.3
		Past use	1.0
Alcohol use	Nondrinker	1 drink/day	1.10
		2 drinks/day	1.25
		3 drinks/day	1.50

Adapted from Colditz GA, Stampfer MJ, Willett WC. Prospective study of estrogen replacement therapy and risk of breast cancer in postmenopausal women. JAMA 1990;264:2648–2653.

breast cancer gene, called *BRCA2*, has been mapped to chromosome 13. From these data, a woman with a strong family history of breast or ovarian cancer, or both, who carries a germline mutation of *BRCA1* faces roughly an 85% lifetime risk of breast cancer and a 60% risk of ovarian cancer. Carriers of the *BRCA2* mutation have similar risks for breast cancer, but much lower risks for ovarian cancer.

It has been reported that Jewish people of Eastern European decent (Ashkenazi Jews) have an unusually high (2.5%) carrier rate of germline mutations in *BRCA1* and *BRCA2* as compared to the rest of the U.S. population. A recent study that examined 1,008 Ashkenazi Jewish women with breast cancer in the New York area found that by age 80, a woman with a mutation in either gene had an 82% risk of developing breast cancer, compared to an average woman's risk of about 13%.[18] Risks were 20% by age 40 and 55% by age 60. Lifetime risks for ovarian cancer were 54% for women with *BRCA1* mutations and 23% for those with *BRCA2* mutations. Surprisingly, half of the patients with BRCA mutations had no breast or ovarian cancer among mothers, sisters, grandmothers, or aunts, which raised the question of the importance of family history and whether all Ashkenazi Jewish women should undergo genetic testing.[18] The results of this study are in contrast with an earlier reported study of similar design in which Ashkenazi Jewish families were reported to have lifetime risks of 50% and 16% for breast and ovarian cancer, respectively.[19]

The question of who should receive screening for BRCA is unresolved. The probability of being a carrier of the gene is related to ethnicity and family history. Important factors in family history include the number of affected and unaffected family members, the age at which cancer is diagnosed, and the presence of ovarian cancer. It is currently estimated that the risk of a *BRCA1* mutation increases 20-fold if breast and ovarian cancer occur concurrently in one or more family members. However, as pointed out in the recent study in Ashkenazi Jewish women, the importance of family history appears to diminish as family size decreases.

To date, there are no clear recommendations for carriers of *BRCA1* and *BRCA2* from high-risk families. Bilateral total mastectomy does reduce the risk of breast cancer occurrence; however, both breast and ovarian cancer have been reported in patients who have had prophylactic removal of these organs. In BRCA carriers who do not opt for surgical prophylaxis, mammography every 6 months is recommended. Because no effective screening for ovarian cancer exists, most experts recommend bilateral oophorectomy at completion of childbearing and estrogen replacement therapy until the age of 50 years. Estrogen replacement therapy provides approximately one-third of physiologic estrogen concentrations, and although controversial, some experts suggest that the benefits in terms of prevention of chronic diseases outweigh the risk of cancer. The benefit of tamoxifen for chemoprevention in BRCA carriers is not clear.[20] In the recently reported New York study in women who were BRCA gene mutation carriers, women who exercised and maintained a healthy weight during adolescence had a later onset of breast cancer compared with inactive or overweight women. Of many potential risk modifiers examined, including smoking, alcohol, exposure to radiation and pesticides, and reproductive behavior, the only other factor to influence risk was that women who had at least one pregnancy also had later cancer onset.[18]

Isolation and cloning of *BRCA1* and *BRCA2* should ultimately lead to a greater understanding of the biology of malignant transformation of mammary epithelium, and to major advances in diagnostics and therapeutics benefiting all breast cancer patients. It is hoped that an improved basic understanding of the molecular mechanisms involved in breast cancer development and the discovery of novel approaches

to reverse or prevent these processes will ultimately lead to the ability to cure this extremely common and often fatal disease.

ENVIRONMENTAL AND LIFESTYLE FACTORS

The observation that breast cancer incidence rates vary 10-fold between countries suggests that environmental factors play an important role in the etiology of breast cancer. Perhaps the most compelling evidence is derived from studies of Asian women who migrated from Japan to the San Francisco Bay area. Although the incidence of breast cancer in Asian women is quite low (about 97 cases per 100,000 women), the incidence of breast cancer in Asian women who were born in the United States, or who migrated from Asia to the United States, gradually increases to equal that of the white population in the same area.

Diet is an obvious environmental factor, and possible relationships between fat or cholesterol intake and steroid hormone metabolism have led to an emphasis on dietary fat as a possible etiologic agent. International studies demonstrate a positive correlation between age-adjusted cancer mortality rate and national per capita fat intake. The correlation is stronger in postmenopausal than in premenopausal women. Studies in laboratory animals provide further evidence of a relationship between dietary fat intake and breast cancer. Despite these compelling indirect data, case control and prospective studies performed in the United States have not clearly demonstrated an association between dietary fat and breast cancer risk. In fact, the relative risk of developing breast cancer among the women with the highest quintile of total fat intake was 0.85 as compared to women in the lowest quintile. However, the difference in fat intake among women at these two extremes was only 25%.[21] The results of this study show that women who reduce fat intake in the context of the usual American diet are not likely to reduce their breast cancer risk. The possible benefits of lowering fat intake to levels substantially below 30% of caloric intake will need to be tested in randomized trials.

Additional investigated dietary factors include micronutrients and food-derived heterocyclic amines. Many of the studies that have examined the relative risk for breast cancer for high fat intake have also examined the association between breast cancer and intake of fiber, β-carotene, and vitamins C, E, and A. The relationship between vitamin A and breast cancer risk is unclear. In contrast, most studies support some benefit from β-carotene, vitamin C, and/or dietary fiber. Experimental and epidemiologic evidence suggests an association between breast cancer and the Western diet, which typically includes a large amount of cooked meats and fat, as well as a high caloric intake. One group of compounds that may play a role in human breast cancer is the heterocyclic amines found commonly in cooked beef, fish, and chicken. At least 19 heterocyclic amines with mutagenic activity have been identified in grilled, broiled, and fried meat and fish. Among these heterocyclic amines, 10 were examined for long-term carcinogenicity and all proved to be positive.[22] Experimental studies examining the interaction between heterocyclic amines and other dietary factors with respect to mammary carcinogenesis are warranted.

Both body weight and height are associated with breast cancer. Indices of obesity are related to breast cancer risks in a complex way that differs by age and menopausal status. Most studies of premenopausal women show either no relationship with body weight, or slightly declining breast cancer risks with increasing body weight. One plausible biologic mechanism to explain this phenomenon is reduced ovarian activity in obese women. Most studies in postmenopausal women, however, show increasing breast cancer risks with increasing body weight. In addition to obesity, the distribution of body fat also may play an independent role in breast cancer. Upper body (central or abdominal) adiposity increases the risk of breast cancer independent of overall obesity. This association may be related to the excess levels of free-circulating estrogen resulting from the conversion of androstenedione to estradiol in peripheral adipose tissue, in conjunction with suppressed levels of circulating sex hormone binding globulin in women with central adiposity.[23]

Exercise may provide modest protection against breast cancer, but the relationship is complex. Strenuous physical activity can delay menarche, and thereby decrease risk. Moderate levels of physical activity in premenopausal women are associated with anovulatory cycles, which also are associated with decreased risk. The reduction in breast cancer seen in postmenopausal women who exercise might be mediated through weight control,[24–26] although some studies have not shown an influence of body mass index on the relationship between physical activity and breast cancer risk.[27,28] At least one case-control study failed to show a protective role of physical activity in women of any age group.[29] Overall, excess body weight appears to result in a slightly increased risk of breast cancer, and those that do develop breast cancer are more likely to be estrogen receptor–positive. Although controlled weight loss probably leads to an overall healthier condition, the data to support a direct link between weight loss and breast cancer risk reduction do not exist. Research in this area is relatively recent; further progress is dependent on the development of accurate measurements of physical activity, past and present.

Reports of more than 50 epidemiologic investigations of the relationship between alcohol and breast cancer have appeared in the literature. A recent meta-analysis[30] of these studies indicates both a modest positive association between alcohol and breast cancer and a dose-response relationship. Data suggest that risk increases with consumption of alcohol in general, regardless of the beverage type. Several factors, including age, weight, and estrogen use, have been shown to modify this relation in some studies. The mechanism of the alcohol-breast cancer hypothesis may include increased levels of estradiol or other reproductive steroid hormones; altered hepatic metabolism of carcinogens; production of cytotoxic protein products; diminished immunologic surveillance; impaired DNA repair; or possibly an influencing effect of alcohol on cell membrane integrity and/or metabolism of intracellular substrates.[30] In addition, animal studies have yielded mixed results regarding the influence of alcohol on the incidence of breast cancer. Although a causal relationship between alcohol consumption and breast cancer has not been proven in a prospective trial, the weight of the evidence suggests that a relationship, direct or indirect, may exist.

Radiation is associated with an increased risk of breast cancer in survivors of the atomic bomb, in patients given radiation for postpartum mastitis, in women receiving multiple fluoroscopic exams during therapy for tuberculosis, and in patients who receive mediastinal radiation for malignancies. Interestingly, this risk appears to be confined to exposure to radiation prior to the age of 40, which again suggests that a "window of initiation" for breast cancer occurs at a relatively early age. Exposure to diagnostic x-rays including annual screening mammography does not impart a sufficient dose of radiation for clinical concern. A critical reassessment of benefits versus risks from screening mammography found recently that for a woman beginning annual screening mammography at age 50 years and continuing to age 75 years, the benefit exceeds the radiation risk by a factor of 100. Even for a woman who begins annual screening at age 35 years and continues until age 75 years, the benefit of reduced mortality is projected to exceed the radiation risk by a factor of more than 25.[31]

Cigarette smoking and augmentation mammoplasty do not appear to increase the risk of breast cancer. Blood pressure medications, reserpine, and other drugs that increase prolactin levels have not been shown to increase the risk of breast cancer. Caffeine also has no predisposing effect on breast cancer, but may play a role in exacerbation of benign breast disease. The role of environmental carcinogens has not been systematically evaluated.

CLINICAL PRESENTATION

A painless lump is the initial sign in more than 90% of women with breast cancer. The typical malignant mass is solitary, unilateral, solid, hard, irregular, and nonmobile. In approximately 10% of cases, stabbing or aching pain is the first symptom. Less commonly, nipple discharge, retraction, or dimpling may herald the onset of the disease. In more advanced cases, prominent skin edema, redness, warmth, and induration of the underlying tissue may be observed.

The breast is a complex organ composed of skin, subcutaneous tissue, fatty tissue, and branching ductal and glandular structures. Various diseases that affect these structures can produce a palpable mass. In addition, the physiologic changes associated with the menstrual cycle can cause abnormalities of the breast that produce a three-dimensional mass. The most common causes of breast masses in young women are fibroadenoma, fibrocystic disease, carcinoma, and fat necrosis.

About 80% of women first detect some breast abnormalities themselves, underscoring the importance of breast self-examination. In the United States, it is increasingly common for breast cancer to be detected during routine screening mammography in asymptomatic women. It is widely accepted that the smaller the mass, the higher the likelihood of cure, and the more conservative the treatment options offered to the patient. Thus as the number of breast cancer cases found by screening mammography increases, overall survival of breast cancer patients is expected to improve.

Breast cancer that is confined to a localized breast lesion is often referred to as *early, primary, localized,* or *curable.* Unfortunately, as is discussed shortly, breast cancer cells often spread by contiguity, lymph channels, and through the blood to distant sites. As discussed in subsequent sections, this often occurs early in the breast cancer growth, and deposits of tumor cells form in distant sites that cannot be detected with current diagnostic methods and equipment (micrometastases). When breast cancer cells can be detected clinically or radiologically in sites distant from the breast, the disease is referred to as *advanced* or *metastatic* breast cancer. Tissues most commonly involved with metastases are lymph nodes (other than axillary or internal mammary), skin, bone, liver, lungs, and brain. Symptoms of bone pain, difficulty breathing, abdominal enlargement, jaundice, and mental status changes may herald the clinical presentation of metastatic breast cancer. About 10% of women have signs and symptoms of distant metastases when they first seek treatment. In virtually all of them, a breast mass has been present for several months to years. In addition, about one-half of all patients who initially are treated for localized disease develop signs and symptoms of metastatic breast cancer, most commonly 3 to 5 years following local potentially curative therapy with surgery, radiation, and systemic adjuvant therapy.

DIAGNOSIS

Initial work-up for a woman presenting with a lesion or symptoms suggestive of breast cancer should include a careful history, physical examination of the breast, three-dimensional mammography, and possibly other breast imaging techniques such as ultrasound. Most (80% to 85%) breast cancers can be visualized on a mammogram as a mass, a cluster of calcifications, or a combination of both. The detection of a mass smaller than 2 mm is considered ideal, but it is difficult in practice to detect tumors smaller than 5 mm. Large, noncalcified masses may be difficult to detect in the dense glandular breast, which is common in premenopausal women. The threshold for the detection of a cancer is variable and depends on the radiographic abnormality, the fat:glandular tissue ratio of the breast, the technical quality of the examination, and the diligence and expertise of the radiologist.

Interpretations of mammography obtained either for screening or to evaluate a new breast mass generally fall into one of three categories: (1) the radiologist notes nothing suspicious for malignancy; (2) something of concern is seen and follow-up or further testing is advised; or (3) something clearly suspicious is present and a biopsy is indicated. A detailed discussion of abnormal mammogram radiographic findings and their significance is beyond the scope of this chapter, although excellent references are available.[32,33] It should be noted, however, that well-circumscribed x-ray masses are benign in 98% of cases; such lesions may not require a biopsy, but may be followed radiographically at 6-month intervals. Masses interpreted as "suspicious and a biopsy should be performed" have a 20% to 30% probability of malignancy. Masses interpreted as "highly suspicious radiographically" are malignant in 75% to 90% of cases. The overall probability of malignancy when a biopsy is performed on a nonpalpable mammographic abnormality ranges from 20% to 35%.

Breast biopsy is indicated for a mammographic abnormality that suggests malignancy or for a palpable mass on physical examination. Biopsy can be accomplished percutaneously in most circumstances, making excisional biopsy unnecessary. Excisional biopsy indicates the complete removal of the abnormal tissue. Excisional biopsy is performed with either a local or general anesthetic, and is usually done as an outpatient operative procedure. Needle biopsies have included both core-needle biopsy (which removes a core of tissue) and fine-needle aspiration (which removes cells from the suspicious site). These procedures are associated with minimal discomfort and anxiety, few complications, and no disfigurement, and could represent significant cost savings when compared to conventional surgical excisional biopsy. The accuracy of fine-needle aspiration is quite good in experienced hands, but its limitations include false-negatives, specimens with insufficient material for diagnosis, and the inability to distinguish invasive from in situ cancer. In the United States, stereotactic core needle biopsy is the most common initial biopsy method for mammographically detected, nonpalpable abnormalities. Core needle biopsy offers a more definitive histologic diagnosis, avoids inadequate samples, and can distinguish invasive from in situ breast cancer. It should be pointed out that biopsy is used only to establish the diagnosis. Following confirmation of malignancy, subsequent surgical procedures are performed to assure complete removal of the abnormal tissue.[5]

STAGING AND PROGNOSIS

Few malignant diseases illustrate the importance of stage (anatomic extent of disease) at the time of diagnosis and overall survival more clearly than breast cancer. Stage is defined on the basis of the primary tumor size (T_{1-4}), presence and extent of lymph node involvement (N_{1-3}), and presence or absence of distant metastases (M_{0-1}) (Table 125–3 and Fig. 125–2). Although many possible combinations of T and N are possible within a given stage, simplistically, stage 0

TABLE 125–3. TNM Stage Grouping for Breast Cancer

Stage Grouping			
0	T_{is}	N_0	M_0
I	T_1*	N_0	M_0
IIA	T_0	N_1	M_0
	T_1*	N_1	M_0
	T_2	N_0	M_0
IIB	T_2	N_1	M_0
	T_3	N_0	M_0
IIIA	T_0	N_2	M_0
	T_1*	N_2	M_0
	T_2	N_2	M_0
	T_3	N_1	M_0
	T_3	N_2	M_0
IIIB	T_4	N_0	M_0
	T_4	N_1	M_0
	T_4	N_2	M_0
IIIC	Any T	N_3	M_0
IV	Any T	Any N	M_1

*T_1 includes T_1mic

Adapted with permission of the American Joint Committee on Cancer (AJCC), Chicago, IL. The original source for this material is the AJCC Cancer Staging Manual, Sixth Edition (2002) published by Springer-Verlag New York, www.springer-ny.com.

represents carcinoma in situ (T_{is}) or disease that has not invaded the basement membrane. Stage I represents small primary tumor without lymph node involvement, and the majority of stage II disease involves regional lymph nodes. Stages I and II are often referred to as *early breast cancer*. It is in these early stages that the disease is curable. Stage III, also referred to as *locally advanced disease,* usually represents a large tumor with extensive nodal involvement in which either node or tumor is fixed to the chest wall. Stage IV disease is characterized by the presence of metastases to organs distant from the primary tumor and is often referred to as *advanced or metastatic disease* as described earlier. Most cancer today presents in early stages where the prognosis is favorable (Table 125–4).

The American Joint Committee for Cancer (AJCC) recently published new staging criteria for breast cancer which were officially implemented in January 2003.[34] Tumor staging systems are periodically updated to incorporate new diagnostic and therapeutic advances that affect risk of disease recurrence and survival. Major changes included in the 2003 staging system from the 1988 version included size-based discrimination between micrometastases and isolated tumor cells, classification of lymph node status by number of involved axillary lymph nodes, and new classification for metastases to the infraclavicular, internal mammary, and supraclavicular lymph nodes. A new substage, IIIC, was also designated. The net effect of changes in the staging system appears to be a shifting of the population in each stage toward more advanced stages or substages. A recent report compared survival in 1,350 breast cancer patients according to the 1988 and 2003 staging system.[35] In this report, adoption of the 2003 AJCC staging system for breast cancer improved stage-specific overall survival by as much as 15%. This improvement in stage-specific overall survival applied across every disease stage except stage IV. It is important to note that comparison among patients staged with the different staging systems will likely result in the appearance of an improvement in treatment efficacy. However, this would be an inaccurate assessment because, for example, women staged as stage IIA based on the 1988 staging system would likely be considered to have a more advanced stage (i.e., IIB based on the 2003 staging system), and thus a worse prognosis.

Tumor (T)

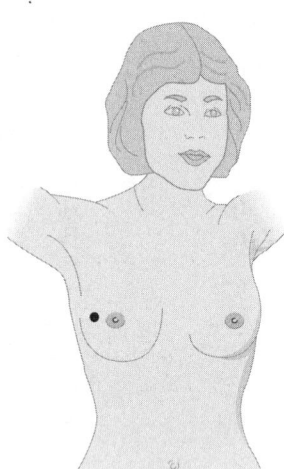

T_0	No evidence of tumor
T_{is}	Carcinoma in situ or Paget's disease of nipple with no tumor
T_1	≤ 2 cm
	T_1 mic ≤ 0.1 cm
	$T_{1a} > 0.1$ cm–0.5 cm
	$T_{1b} > 0.5$ cm–1 cm
	$T_{1c} > 1$ cm–2 cm
T_2	> 2 cm–5 cm
T_3	> 5 cm
T_4	Any size; direct extension to chest wall (excluding pectoral muscle); skin infiltration; peau d' orange; satellite nodules
	T_{4a} Extension to chest wall
	T_{4b} Edema or ulceration of skin or presence of satellite nodules
	T_{4c} Both T_{4a} and T_{4b}
	T_{4d} Inflammatory carcinoma

Nodes (N)

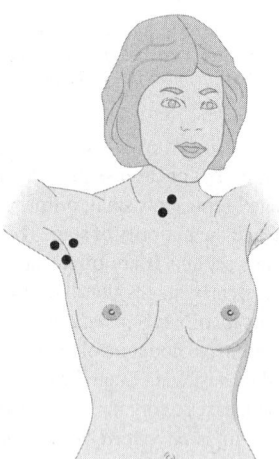

N_X	Regional lymph nodes cannot be assessed (e.g., previously removed)
N_0	No regional lymph node metastasis
N_1	Metastasis in movable ipsilateral axillary lymph node(s)
N_2	Metastases in ipsilateral axillary lymph nodes fixed or matted, or in clinically apparent ipsilateral internal mammary nodes in the absence of clinically evident axillary lymph node metastasis
	N_{2a} Metastasis in ipsilateral axillary lymph nodes fixed to one another (matted) or to other structures
	N_{2b} Metastasis only in clinically apparent ipsilateral internal mammary nodes and in the absence of clinically evident axillary lymph node metastasis
N_3	Metastasis in ipsilateral infraclavicular lymph node(s), or in clinically apparent ipsilateral internal mammary lymph node(s) and in the presence of clinically evident axillary lymph node metastasis; or metastasis in ipsilateral supraclavicular lymph node(s) with or without axillary or internal mammary lymph node involvement
	N_{3a} Metastasis in ipsilateral infraclavicular lymph node(s) and axillary lymph node(s)
	N_{3b} Metastasis in ipsilateral internal mammary lymph node(s) and axillary lymph node(s)
	N_{3c} Metastasis in ipsilateral supraclavicular lymph node(s)

Metastasis (M)

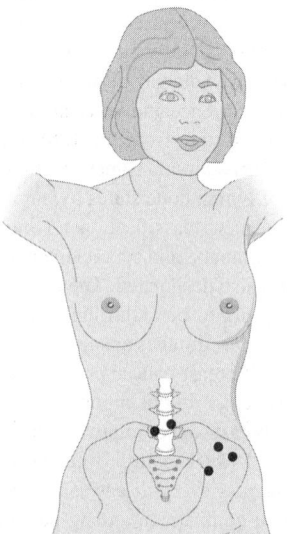

M_0	No distant metastases
M_1	Distant metastasis, including metastasis to ipsilateral supraclavicular lymph node(s)

FIGURE 125–2. TNM staging system for breast cancer. (Adapted from Singletary SE et al. Revision of the American Joint Committee on Cancer Staging System for Breast Cancer. J Clin Oncol 2002;20:3628–3636.)

TABLE 125–4. Estimated Stage at Presentation and 5-Year Disease-Free Survival (DFS): Breast Cancer

	Percentage of Total Cases	5-Year DFS[a] (%)
Stage I	40	70–90
Stage II	40	50–70
Stage III	15	20–30
Stage IV	5	0–10[b]

[a]With current conventional local and systemic therapy.
[b]Patients in stage IV are rarely free of disease; however, 10% to 20% of these patients may survive with minimal disease for 5 to 10 years.

PATHOLOGY

The pathologic evaluation of breast lesions serves to establish the histologic diagnosis and to confirm the presence or absence of other factors believed to influence prognosis. These prognostic factors include the presence of necrosis, lymphatic or vascular invasion, nuclear grade, hormone receptor status, proliferative index, amount of aneuploidy, presence or absence of oncogenes, presence or absence of mutations in the tumor suppressor *p53* gene, and perhaps presence or absence of elevated growth factor levels, as well as enzymes (cathepsin D), proteins, and angiogenesis factors.

INVASIVE CARCINOMA

Invasive breast cancers are a histologically heterogeneous group of lesions. Most breast carcinomas are adenocarcinomas and are classified on the basis of their microscopic appearance as either ductal or lobular, corresponding to the ducts and lobules of the normal breast. The various histologic types of breast cancer have different prognoses, but it is unknown whether their response to therapy differs, because patients in therapeutic trials are not typically stratified according to histologic type. The five most common types of invasive breast cancer are briefly described.

Invasive or *infiltrating ductal carcinoma* is the most common histology. The other histologic patterns can occur alone or with infiltrating ductal carcinoma. These tumors are generally referred to as infiltrating ductal carcinoma "not otherwise specified," and account for about 75% of all invasive breast cancers. These tumors commonly spread to the axillary lymph nodes and their prognosis is poorer than for other histologic types (specifically tubular, medullary, and mucinous/colloid). *Infiltrating lobular carcinoma* accounts for 5% to 10% of breast tumors. Typical presentation is an area of ill-defined thickening in the breast, in contrast to a prominent lump characteristic of infiltrating ductal carcinoma. A greater proportion of infiltrating lobular carcinomas are multicentric tumors, either in the same or opposite breast, as compared with infiltrating ductal carcinoma. Overall, infiltrating lobular carcinoma and infiltrating ductal carcinoma have similar likelihoods of axillary node involvement and prognosis, yet the sites of metastases tend to differ. Ductal carcinoma more frequently metastasizes to the bone or to the liver, lung, or brain, whereas lobular carcinoma more commonly metastasizes to meningeal and serosal surfaces and other unusual sites.

The three most common special types of invasive cancer are *tubular, medullary,* and *mucinous. Medullary carcinoma* is a well-defined lesion with a characteristic microscopic appearance that includes a well-circumscribed border, intense infiltration with small lymphocytes, and other factors. It accounts for 5% to 7% of all breast carcinomas and is believed to have a better prognosis than infiltrat-

ing ductal carcinoma. *Mucinous (or colloid) carcinoma* constitutes approximately 3% of all breast carcinomas and is characterized by the abundant accumulation of extracellular mucin around clusters of tumor cells. It is slow growing and can be bulky. When the tumor is predominantly mucinous, the prognosis tends to be more favorable. *Tubular carcinoma* accounts for approximately 2% of all breast cancers and is a type of carcinoma in which tubule formation is conspicuous on pathology. Axillary metastases are uncommon and the prognosis is considerably better than for infiltrating ductal carcinomas. Histologies rarely reported include adenocystic carcinoma, carcinosarcomas, and papillary carcinoma. In some pathology reports, infiltrating ductal carcinoma may include small areas containing these special tumor types.

Special situations seen clinically and histologically include Paget's disease of the breast and inflammatory breast cancer. Paget's disease of the breast occurs in 1% to 4% of all patients with breast cancer. Clinically, the patient presents with a relatively long history of eczematous changes in the nipple with itching, burning, oozing, bleeding, or some combination of these. The nipple changes are associated with an underlying carcinoma in the breast that is usually palpable. The histology of the tumor type is either ductal carcinoma in situ (DCIS) or invasive ductal carcinoma. Prognosis is related to the histologic type of the associated tumor.

Inflammatory breast cancer is characterized clinically by prominent skin, edema, redness and warmth, visible erysipeloid margin, and induration of the underlying tissue. Biopsies of the involved skin reveal cancer cells in the dermal lymphatics. Inflammatory breast cancer typically has a very rapid onset and although it may look somewhat similar to a neglected mass, its presentation with rapid onset and progression of local symptoms distinguishes it from other cases of locally advanced disease. Prognosis of patients with inflammatory breast cancer is poor, even if the disease is apparently localized.

NONINVASIVE CARCINOMA

As with invasive carcinoma, the noninvasive lesions may be divided broadly into ductal and lobular categories. Evidence supports that the development of malignancy is a multistep process and that invasive breast cancer has a preinvasive phase. During the carcinoma in situ phase, normal epithelial cells undergo genetic alterations that result in malignant transformation. Transformed epithelial cells proliferate and pile up within lobules or ducts, but lack the required genetic alterations that enable the cells to penetrate the basement membrane. Therefore carcinoma in situ is diagnosed when malignant transformation of cells has occurred, but the basement membrane is intact by light microscopy.

The widespread use of screening mammography and subsequent biopsy coupled with recognition of noninvasive breast carcinoma by pathologists has resulted in a significant increase in the diagnosis of in situ breast cancer during the past decade. Its incidence has risen from 1% to 5% in the early 1970s to 28% in the late 1980s; between 1988 and 1996, the incidence of in situ cancer rose steadily at a rate of 6% per year.[2] The natural history of these disorders is not well described in the literature, and thus the debate continues regarding carcinoma in situ: Is carcinoma in situ preinvasive cancer or simply a marker of unstable epithelium that represents an increased risk for the development of subsequent aggressive cancer? Although a detailed discussion of the biology and appropriate management of noninvasive breast cancer is beyond the scope of this chapter, some of the more salient characteristics of DCIS and lobular carcinoma in situ (LCIS) are described below and the reader is referred to a number of excellent reviews for a more comprehensive discussion.[36,37]

DCIS is seen more frequently than LCIS at a ratio of about 6 to 3:1. Most DCIS cases diagnosed currently are small nonpalpable lesions, unlike its presentation as a palpable mass in more than half of cases in years prior to mammography. Most cases of DCIS today are found by biopsies performed for clustered microcalcifications seen on screening mammography. There are five distinct histologic patterns of DCIS: comedo, cribriform, micropapillary, papillary, and solid. The biologic characteristics are consistent with its role as a direct precursor to invasive carcinoma, which appears to develop in most, but not all, cases if left untreated within 10 years of diagnosis. The peak incidence of DCIS is 51 to 59 years, which closely parallels that of invasive carcinoma.

Treatment of DCIS depends on its presentation, size, and pathology. The patient and physician have the following options: (1) excision with negative margins, preferably 1 to 2 cm; (2) excision followed by breast irradiation; and (3) traditional total mastectomy with reconstruction. It is important to note, however, that in all cases, carcinoma in situ is treated as cancer. Mastectomy had been the standard treatment of DCIS for several decades. The combined data from 1,061 women who underwent mastectomy for DCIS, reported in 14 published studies, with follow-up ranging from 2 years to more than 15 years, show an overall local recurrence rate of only 0.75% and an overall cancer mortality rate of less than 1%. Breast conservation, that is, wide local excision followed by irradiation of breast tissue, may be an effective alternative to mastectomy. The recently completed National Surgical Adjuvant Breast and Bowel Project (NSABP) B17 trial randomized 808 women with DCIS to receive lumpectomy alone or lumpectomy with radiation.[38] The results of this trial demonstrated an advantage for radiation plus lumpectomy in terms of fewer local recurrences. Although radiation following lumpectomy does not appear to change the survival of patients with DCIS, it significantly reduces the incidence of local recurrences and enhances the breast preservation rate in these women. The EORTC Trial which was identical in design reported very similar results, which supports lumpectomy followed by radiation in women with DCIS.[39] However, if more than one area of the breast is involved with DCIS, a mastectomy is the preferred option. It has also been suggested that breast conservation may not be appropriate for younger women whose lifetime risk of breast cancer is high given a diagnosis of DCIS. Axillary dissection is generally not indicated. There is currently no proven benefit for the use of cytotoxic chemotherapy in patients who receive local therapy for DCIS. The value of tamoxifen in patients with DCIS is controversial. The NSABP B-24 trial, which randomized 1,804 women with DCIS to lumpectomy plus radiation plus either tamoxifen or placebo, showed a benefit of tamoxifen in reduction in ipsilateral invasive breast cancer (44% reduction, $p = 0.03$).[40] However, the UK/AN2 trial which was similar in design failed to show a benefit of tamoxifen in reduction in ipsilateral invasive breast cancer in women with DCIS.[41] Most experts would agree that there is little evidence to support the routine use of tamoxifen in this patient population. However, there may be subgroups of patients with DCIS, such as hormone receptor–positive patients, who may benefit from the addition of tamoxifen to lumpectomy plus radiation. In fact, tamoxifen use in patients with DCIS that is hormone receptor–positive was recommended by the International Expert Consensus on Primary Therapy of Early Breast Cancer in their recently published update.[42] Follow-up of women who have been treated for DCIS should be as comprehensive as that of a woman with invasive carcinoma to facilitate early detection of any subsequent malignancy.

LCIS is a microscopic diagnosis, not a gross abnormality. Therefore it is always nonpalpable and it is virtually impossible to make the diagnosis of LCIS by clinical examination. Unlike DCIS, LCIS does not demonstrate calcifications on mammography, and in fact is not associated with mammographic abnormalities. LCIS is most frequently diagnosed in biopsy specimens that were obtained because of symptoms or mammography findings consistent with benign lesions. Multicentricity is common (>30%) with LCIS, and the opposite breast is affected in up to 50% of patients. It is unclear whether LCIS proceeds to invasive carcinoma or serves as a marker for a high probability of invasive carcinoma developing elsewhere in the breast. Thus the management of LCIS is very controversial. Some experts favor a program of breast examination, periodic physician examination, and mammography as management of LCIS. In selected patients who are particularly anxious about the development of cancer, bilateral total mastectomies and prompt reconstruction represent a reasonable approach. Radiation and systemic chemotherapy has no role in the management of LCIS. Patients with LCIS were included in the Tamoxifen Chemoprevention Trial and thus patients with LCIS should be offered tamoxifen as a preventive strategy.

PROGNOSTIC FACTORS

The natural history of breast cancer varies between patients, with some having an extremely aggressive disease that progresses rapidly, whereas others follow a more indolent course. The ability to predict which patients have a better disease prognosis is extremely important in designing treatment recommendations to maximize quantity and quality of life. A number of potential pathologic prognostic and predictive factors have been identified. Prognostic factors are measurements available at diagnosis or time of surgery, that in the absence of adjuvant therapy are associated with recurrence rate, death rate, or other clinical outcome. Predictive factors are measurements available at diagnosis that are associated with the response to a specific therapy. Prognostic and predictive factors fall into three categories: patient characteristics that are independent of the disease such as age; disease characteristics such as tumor size or histologic type; and biomarkers that are measurable parameters in tissues, cells, or fluids, such as hormone receptor status.

The median age for the diagnosis of breast cancer is between the ages of 60 and 65 years.[2] Younger women, particularly women younger than 35 years of age, have a more aggressive form of the disease, and elderly women, particularly those older than 70 years of age with breast cancer, frequently have hormone receptor protein in their malignant tissue, suggesting a more indolent tumor pattern and a higher likelihood of response to hormonal therapy. Race appears to be prognostic but not predictive. Black breast cancer patients are generally younger and often have larger tumors at diagnosis, and a smaller percentage have hormone receptors in their tumor tissue. These factors contribute to a poorer prognosis. It should be emphasized that for both age and race, in cases of similar clinical presentation, adjuvant treatment confers similar benefits to black and white women.

Tumor size and the presence and number of involved axillary lymph nodes are established primary factors in assessing the risk for breast cancer recurrence and subsequent metastatic disease. Table 125–5 shows the 5-year relapse rate according to size of the primary tumor and axillary node involvement from results of three investigations.[43–45] These data clearly demonstrate that the major factor that influences the likelihood of recurrence is the presence of positive axillary nodes. But regardless of axillary node studies, the size of the primary tumor remains an independent prognostic factor for disease recurrence. In axillary node–negative patients, a tumor size of less than 2 cm is associated with a very favorable prognosis. However, there does not appear to be a large difference between prognosis in patients with large (>5 cm) tumors and negative nodes, as

TABLE 125–5. Five-Year Relapse Rate (%) Based on Size of Primary Tumor and Axillary Nodal Status

Axillary Status	Size of Primary Tumor (cm)		
	<2	2–5	>5
Axillary nodes negative			
Fisher et al[43]	12	24	27
Nemoto et al[44]	13	19	25
Valagussa et al[45]	8	24	19
Axillary nodes positive			
Fisher et al[43]	50	60	79
Nemoto et al[44]	39	50	65
Valagussa et al[45]	37	64	74

compared to patients with 2- to 5-cm tumors and negative nodes. Thus the size of the primary tumor in patients with negative axillary lymph nodes may not provide as much information regarding prognosis as in node-positive patients.

The number of affected nodes is directly related to disease recurrence. The recently revised staging system for breast cancer differs from the 1988 version in that it recognizes the absolute number of positive nodes as a prognostic factor, with N_1 representing one to three positive nodes, N_2 representing four to nine positive nodes, and N_3 representing ten or more positive nodes in its pathologic staging system.[44] In addition, metastases to ipsilateral internal mammary and supraclavicular nodes are noted as N_2 and N_3, respectively (if detected macroscopically, but N_1 if detected only by microscopy), compared to axillary lymph node metastases alone, which are designated N_1. Although determination of the number of involved axillary nodes by hematoxylin and eosin staining is still the preferred technique, identifiers have been added to indicate the use of sentinel lymph node dissection and use of immunohistochemical and molecular techniques (microscopic vs. macroscopic) to determine presence of metastases.

Aside from the tumor-node-metastasis (TNM) stage of the disease, hormone receptor studies have received the most attention in the characterization of primary breast cancer. Hormone receptors are used clinically as indicators of prognosis and to predict response to hormone therapy. Hormone receptors are cytoplasmic proteins that transmit signals to the nucleus of the cell for growth and proliferation. The hormone receptors clinically useful in discussions of breast cancer include the estrogen receptor (ER) and the progesterone receptor (PR). The presence of these proteins in the primary tumor (or less often metastases) is routinely measured by enzyme-linked immunochemical assays and radioassays (enzyme-linked immunosorbent assay). Concentrations of hormone receptors less than 3 femtomoles (fmol) per milligram of cytosol protein are considered negative, 3 to 10 fmol/mg of cytosol protein are intermediate, and concentrations of hormone receptors greater than 10 fmol/mg of cytosol protein are positive. The level (i.e., quantitative) of hormone receptor and the methodology used to assess hormone receptors are important for predictive ability. Although the estrogen receptor has received the most attention to date, more recent data suggest that the presence of the progesterone receptor protein is required for the functional effects of the estrogen receptor protein to occur. This is evidenced by studies that have reported that response to hormonal manipulation and prognosis are highly correlated with the presence of both positive estrogen receptor protein and positive progesterone receptor protein. Hormone receptors are most valuable in predicting response to hormone therapy. About 70% to 80% of patients who are ER-positive and PR-positive will respond to hormonal manipulation. ER-negative patients rarely

respond to hormonal manipulation. The response rate in patients who are ER-negative and PR-positive is somewhere in between.

About 50% to 70% of patients with primary or metastatic breast cancer have hormone receptor–positive tumors. The median level and frequency of hormone receptor–positive tumors are higher in postmenopausal patients as compared to premenopausal patients. That difference is the primary reason for the different recommendations for adjuvant and metastatic treatment of breast cancer between premenopausal and postmenopausal patients that are discussed in later sections of this chapter. Many experts suggest that breast cancer in postmenopausal women is substantively different than that occurring in premenopausal women. Breast cancer is predominantly a disease of the elderly. When it occurs in younger patients, the course of the disease is more aggressive. Hormone receptor positivity, more common in postmenopausal women, is associated with a superior response to hormone therapy and a longer disease-free interval between primary and subsequent metastatic disease, and overall a more favorable prognosis. The presence of hormone receptors in tumors is associated with a favorable disease-free interval and perhaps an overall survival difference of 5% to 10% (as compared to hormone receptor–negative patients).

The rate of tumor cell proliferation also has prognostic significance in breast cancer recurrence. Rate of cell proliferation can be determined with either the tritiated thymidine-labeling index or DNA flow cytometry, which determines the percentage of tumor cells actively dividing (S-phase fraction). Both techniques have shown that patients with rapidly proliferating tumors have a decreased disease-free survival as compared to patients with slowly proliferating tumors.[46] Flow cytometry can also detect abnormal DNA content, or aneuploidy, in breast cancer cells. Although there are conflicting reports regarding the clinical significance of ploidy status, some studies report that patients with aneuploid tumors have significantly shorter relapse-free survival times than do patients with diploid tumors.[46] Newer methods of determining proliferative rate include the use of monoclonal antibodies to antigens in proliferating cells, such as Ki-67. As an example, in one report of 371 node-negative breast cancer women with a high Ki-67 labeling index, they had a 20-fold greater mortality rate than those with a labeling index of $\leq 10\%$.[47]

Nuclear grade and tumor (histologic) differentiation are known, independent prognostic indicators. Several histologic grading systems have been developed and shown to have prognostic value in the evaluation of breast cancer. Fisher and associates[47] have shown a 5-year survival of 93% for patients with good nuclear grade, compared to 79% for patients with poor nuclear grade. However, lack of concordance between pathologists' grading results has thwarted the use of this prognostic indicator in clinical trials.

A number of additional potential prognostic factors have been identified in the past 5 years. These include overexpression of the *erbB-2* (or *HER-2/neu*) oncogene, cathepsin D, angiogenic growth factors, mutations in the tumor suppressor *p53* gene, and others.[48] Many of the new potential prognostic factors have been shown to be strongly correlated with established risk factors. For example, many ER-positive tumors are also *HER-2*–negative and cathepsin D–negative, which makes it difficult to discern the relative importance of potential prognostic factors. Identification of these numerous factors and correlations between these and known prognostic factors that affect clinical outcome is of interest because each correlation allows basic mechanistic insights into disease processes. Practically, they allow prediction of probable clinical outcomes that can guide therapeutic decision making. Several of these new prognostic factors, specifically the *HER-2* oncogene overexpression and *p53* mutations, have shown early promise as predictors of efficacy of adjuvant chemotherapy.

The *HER-2/neu* gene is located on 17q21 and is transcribed into a 4.5-kd mRNA, which is translated into a 185-kd glycoprotein. The HER-2/neu protein is expressed at low levels in the epithelial cells of normal breast tissue. *HER-2/neu* is a member of the erbB (or HER) growth factor receptor family and its overexpression is associated with transmission of growth signals that control aspects of normal cell growth and division. Preclinical and clinical studies indicate that *HER-2* overexpression may have prognostic and predictive value. In some studies, *HER-2/neu* gene amplification and protein overexpression, measured by fluorescence in situ hybridization (FISH) and immunohistochemistry (IHC), respectively, correlates with factors associated with a poor prognosis. However, not all studies have found this association. A number of reports have found that *HER-2/neu* amplification and overexpression are significant independent predictors of shorter disease-free survival and reduced overall survival in node-positive breast cancer.[49,50] The relationship between *HER-2/neu* amplification and overexpression in node-negative patients has also been reported to confer less favorable outcomes in some, but not all, studies. The data regarding the predictive value of *HER-2/neu* and response to hormonal and chemotherapy is similarly conflicted. However, most experts would agree that women whose tumors overexpress *HER-2/neu* appear to be relatively resistant to alkylating agent–based adjuvant therapy, and they might derive greater benefit from an anthracycline-based adjuvant therapy regimen.[51] It is important to note that the strength of the evidence to support anthracycline-based adjuvant regimens in women with *HER-2/neu*–overexpressing tumors is not considered adequate to warrant a recommendation by most consensus groups. Although some evidence supports that *HER-2/neu* overexpression is associated with relative resistance to adjuvant endocrine therapy, particularly tamoxifen, data are conflicting. *HER-2/neu* overexpression more likely represents a negative prognostic factor in hormone receptor–positive women. Hormone receptor–positive women who are also *HER-2/neu* positive should receive adjuvant hormonal therapy. Clearly, *HER-2/neu* positively predicts response to trastuzumab therapy, which is a monoclonal antibody directed against the *HER-2/neu* receptor. Currently, the use of trastuzumab is indicated for treatment of metastatic breast cancer in patients who have tumors that overexpress *HER-2/neu*. However, trials in the adjuvant setting are ongoing. A final controversy surrounds the testing method employed to determine *HER-2/neu* status. Although there are many methods, *HER-2/neu* gene amplification measured by FISH and overexpression of the HER-2/neu protein product measured by IHC are the most commonly used methods. Discordant FISH and IHC assays are most commonly the result of false-positive results in patients with a 2+ screen by IHC testing, which suggests that overexpression of *HER-2/neu* in these cases should be confirmed by FISH.[52]

Although there is a growing understanding of the prognostic significance of individual factors, it is not clear how to practically use multiple prognostic factors in concert. The development of decision-making systems for clinical applications will require improvements in the areas of (1) standardization of methodologies and interlaboratory quality control for prognostic factor determinations, (2) definition of a limited set of prognostic markers that are independently predictive, and (3) staging systems that integrate this information. The National Institutes of Health (NIH) convened an expert panel to develop a consensus statement on adjuvant therapy for breast cancer.[53] One question addressed by the Consensus Development Panel was which factors should be used to select systemic adjuvant therapy. The panel identified age, tumor size, axillary node status, histologic tumor type, standardized pathologic grade, and hormone receptor status as the only currently accepted prognostic and predictive factors. In addition, the updated International Expert Consensus on the Primary Therapy of Early Breast Cancer concluded that ER and PR expression of the primary tumor cells are the only tumor-related markers with clear predictive value for treatment response that has unequivocal clinical utility regarding adjuvant therapy.[42] This central importance of the steroid hormone receptors emphasizes the absolute necessity to measure ER and PR, report results in a standardized quantitative manner (e.g., percentage of cells stained), and use quality-assured procedures in experienced laboratories. The predictive utility of *HER-2* overexpression, cell proliferation markers, and the interaction of these factors with steroid hormone receptor expression await confirmation. The prognostic usefulness of features such as expression of the components of uPA and PAI-1,[54,55] deregulated expression of cyclin E,[56,57] and presence of tumor cells in bone marrow and in circulating blood is not clear.[58–60]

▶ TREATMENT: Early Breast Cancer

▤ EARLY BREAST CANCER

▤ LOCAL-REGIONAL THERAPY

Most patients presenting with breast cancer today have either an in situ tumor, a small tumor with negative lymph nodes (stage I), or a small stage II cancer. Surgery alone can cure most, if not all, patients with in situ cancers and approximately half of all patients with stage II cancers. The choice of surgical procedures has changed drastically over the past 50 years. This in part is a result of changes in our understanding of the biology of breast cancer, and is due in part to a series of well-conducted trials performed over this time period.

The Halstedian theory and concept of tumor growth, formulated at the end of the nineteenth century, held that breast cancer was a local-regional disease that spread to involve larger contiguous areas of the breast, chest wall, and adjacent lymph nodes. This hypothesis gave rise to emphasis throughout most of the twentieth century on the Halsted radical mastectomy, the hallmark of an approach maintaining that cure of early disease could best be achieved with expansive, meticulously performed surgical procedures. The *radical mastectomy* involves removal of the breast and both major and minor pectoralis muscles. The axillary nodes on the same side (ipsilateral) as the breast lesion are also removed. Substantial morbidity is associated with this procedure. Muscle resection decreases strength and range of motion, and removal of axillary lymph nodes can produce edema of the arm and resected breast area. This procedure was often followed by external beam radiation therapy to the involved area.

During the 1960s, it was recognized that breast cancer is often microscopically disseminated at the time of initial diagnosis. The evolutionary concept that breast cancer is not only a local, but also a systemic, disease has resulted in major changes in local and systemic therapy. In 1980, the Commission on Cancer of the American College of Surgeons reported that there had been an apparent gradual shift from a radical to modified radical mastectomy since December of 1972.[61] The modified radical mastectomy, also termed *total mastectomy with axillary lymph node dissection,* is not as precisely defined or standardized as the radical mastectomy. The pectoralis minor muscle may be excised, divided, or left intact, and more importantly, there may be variation in the extent of axillary lymph node dissection, ranging from sampling to full dissection. It was recognized during this time period that a major factor in prognosis was involvement of axillary lymph nodes rather than the type of initial surgical procedure performed.

Results of a large trial conducted in the United States by the NSABP repudiated the Halsted theory and supported the alternative systemic hypothesis. NSABP B-04, randomized nearly 2,000 women among three treatment regimens: radical mastectomy, simple mastectomy with local-regional irradiation, and simple mastectomy and removal of nodes if they later became clinically positive.[62] Forty percent of patients who underwent the radical mastectomy had pathologically positive lymph nodes; thus it can be assumed that 40% of patients in the other two groups had positive axillary nodes that were not removed. Despite the disparity in local-regional treatment, no significant difference in treatment failure, distant metastases, or overall survival was observed through more than 25 years of follow-up.

Based on the results of that trial, the NSABP instituted a second trial (B-06) in which patients with stage I or stage II breast cancer with a tumor size 4 cm or less were treated with either modified radical mastectomy or lumpectomy with or without radiation therapy.[63] Lumpectomy followed by radiation resulted in a 5-year survival of 85% compared to 76% for modified radical mastectomy; the 20-year results were consistent with the earlier results. This study also found that radiation therapy reduced the probability of local tumor recurrence by about 30% in patients treated with lumpectomy. The local failure rate of modified radical mastectomy was 8.1% compared to 7.2% for lumpectomy alone and 1.1% for lumpectomy and radiation therapy. Neither the rate of development of distant metastases nor contralateral breast cancer was different in the treatment groups.

The NIH Consensus Conference on the Treatment of Early Stage Breast Cancer addressed the roles of modified radical mastectomy versus breast conservation and concluded that primary therapy for breast cancer stages I and II should be *breast conservation*.[53] Breast conservation consists of lumpectomy, also referred to as segmental mastectomy or partial mastectomy, and is defined as excision of the primary tumor and adjacent breast tissue, followed by radiation therapy to reduce the risk of local recurrence. Removal of level I/II axillary lymph nodes is recommended for completeness of staging and prognostic information. The reason given for favoring breast conservation therapy is that it achieved similar results to more extensive surgical procedures, and had cosmetically superior results.

Most patients with breast cancer can be treated by lumpectomy and radiation therapy. Several factors should be considered in selecting patients for breast conservation therapy. Multiple sites of cancer within the breast and the inability to attain negative pathologic margins on the excised breast specimen are predictive for an increased risk of recurrence with breast-conserving therapy and are indications for mastectomy. Some pre-existing collagen vascular diseases (e.g., scleroderma and systemic lupus erythematosus) are a contraindication for the use of breast-conserving radiation and surgery. Although local recurrence following breast-conservation therapy is not associated with increased mortality, it is distressing to the patient and requires surgical removal of the breast. In addition, reconstructive therapy is often not feasible in a breast that has previously received irradiation. Another major consideration in selecting patients for breast-conserving therapy is the expected cosmetic result. Although the size of the tumor is not an important consideration for breast cancer recurrence, the relationship of the size of the tumor to the total breast volume is

an important cosmetic consideration. If the volume of the tissue removed is large in a woman with small breasts, better results can often be obtained with mastectomy and reconstruction. Despite the desire of the patient and the willingness of the surgeon to avoid mastectomy, in some circumstances a lumpectomy will approximate so closely a mastectomy that both the patient and the physician will agree that preservation of a very limited amount of breast tissue would not justify the inconvenience of radiation therapy. Another approach to therapy for these patients would be primary systemic therapy to potentially shrink the tumor and minimize surgery (see section on adjuvant systemic therapy for further details). Aside from the probability of local recurrence and the ability to achieve a satisfactory cosmetic result, consideration must be given to the availability of an external beam radiation facility and the patient's willingness to comply with the prescribed course of radiotherapy. In most instances, external beam radiation therapy used in conjunction with breast-conserving procedures involves 4 to 6 weeks of radiation therapy directed to the breast tissue (a total of 5,000 cGy administered in 200-cGy doses daily to eradicate residual disease). Complications associated with radiation therapy to the breast are minor and include reddening and erythema of the breast tissue and subsequent shrinkage of total breast mass beyond that predicted on the basis of breast tissue removal. Some clinical situations also require postmastectomy radiation therapy as well (see section on locally advanced breast cancer).

Simple or *total mastectomy* involves removal of the entire breast without dissection of the underlying muscle or axillary nodes. The major disadvantage of this procedure is that axillary nodal status is not determined, and therefore important prognostic information may be lost. This procedure is used in patients with carcinoma in situ, in whom there is a 1% incidence of axillary node involvement, or in cases of local recurrence following breast-conservation therapy. While axillary lymph node dissection with histopathologic study of the axillary specimen was the gold standard for detecting axillary nodal involvement and determining the number of lymph nodes containing tumor, the importance of stage I/II axillary dissection is being challenged. Although highly accurate, its morbidity is significant, with an acute complication rate as high as 20% to 30% and rates of chronic lymphedema also on the order of 20% to 30%.[64,65]

A new procedure involving lymphatic mapping and sentinel lymph node biopsy is becoming more acceptable at many academic centers across the United States.[66] This procedure was first utilized in melanoma, but has been adapted for use with breast tumors.[67] The sentinel lymph node is the first lymph node that drains a cancer. Injection of a vital blue dye around the primary breast tumor results in identification of the sentinel lymph node in the majority of patients, and the status of this lymph node may predict the status of the remaining nodes in the nodal basin. In more recent series, the use of a radiolabeled colloid alone or in addition to the blue dye is generally associated with a higher rate of identification of the sentinel lymph node, but this is a controversial topic and may be related to experience of the surgeon or other factors. Regardless of the mapping technique and patient populations studied, a sentinel lymph node can be identified in 90% of patients, and can accurately predict the status of the remaining axillary nodes in 95% of patients.[67] Contraindications to this procedure are patients with clinically apparent lymph node involvement, tumors >5 cm in size or locally advanced, neoadjuvant chemotherapy, multicentric cancers, prior axillary surgery, and/or a large biopsy cavity. Patients who are pregnant or lactating are also not eligible for this procedure. Another issue that is raised is the experience and mastery of the procedure by the surgical team. It has been shown that an individual surgeon must perform approximately

20-60 procedures to attain competency.[68,69] At present the long-term outcome of patients undergoing this procedure alone (without completion axillary dissection) are not available. Ongoing clinical trials will hopefully answer these questions, but this is a very controversial subject with much debate amongst even the most highly regarded breast surgeons. Thus, simple mastectomy may be a reasonable alternative for women who wish to avoid the inconvenience of radiation therapy and preserve their option for breast reconstruction in the future, understanding the lack of long-term data with sentinel lymph node biopsy alone.

The NSABP B-04 and B-06 trials are widely credited with the finding that breast conservation is an appropriate primary therapy for most women with stages I and II disease, and is preferable because it provides survival rates equivalent to those of modified radical mastectomy. But these trials were also important for the valuable information they provided regarding the natural history of the disease and the identification of pathologic prognostic factors associated with early cancer spread. The preponderance of information available regarding selecting women most likely to benefit from systemic adjuvant therapy was derived from pathologic evaluation of tissues archived from these trials. It is hoped that further investigation into less extensive surgery (now focused on the axilla) will continue to provide valuable information for the future.

SYSTEMIC ADJUVANT THERAPY

3 *Systemic adjuvant therapy* is defined as the administration of systemic therapy following definitive local therapy (surgery, radiation, or a combination of these) when there is no evidence of metastatic disease, but a high likelihood of disease recurrence. The concept of breast cancer being a systemic disease and the rationale of adjuvant chemotherapy was based on a series of laboratory and clinical investigations conducted during the 1960s and 1970s that were directed primarily toward achieving a better understanding of tumor metastases. Table 125–6 illustrates the laboratory findings, clinical ab-

TABLE 125–6. Laboratory Findings, Clinical Observations, and Biologic Hypothesis of Breast Cancer as a Systemic Disease and the Value of Adjuvant Chemotherapy

- By the time cancer becomes clinically detectable, it is advanced (about 30 doublings) and has had ample opportunity to establish distant micrometastases.
- There is no orderly pattern of tumor cell dissemination, and the bloodstream is of considerable importance in tumor spread.
- Operable breast cancer is often a systemic disease and variations in local-regional therapy have not substantially affected survival. Only by control of distant disease can there be an improvement in the outcome of breast cancer patients.
- Likelihood of disease recurrence is related to size of tumor mass and axillary node involvement at diagnosis.
- Recurrence of breast cancer following local-regional therapy is most commonly at sites distant from the breast.
- Tumor growth fraction is inversely related to tumor population site. Therefore, optimal kinetic conditions to achieve cure with chemotherapy exist in the setting of micrometastatic disease.
- Efficacy of chemotherapy is dose dependent and optimal doses of combination chemotherapy can be more safely and effectively administered in the adjuvant setting as opposed to the setting of advanced disease.

normalities, and biologic hypothesis that lead to recognition of breast cancer as a systemic disease and documented the value of adjuvant chemotherapy. The very earliest adjuvant trials in breast cancer consisted of perioperative administration of alkylating agents with the intent of eradicating micrometastases that were disseminated at the time of surgical excision of the tumor. Many collaborative research groups have conducted stepwise series of studies designed to identify appropriate candidates for systemic adjuvant therapy, as well as optimal regimens and duration of systemic adjuvant therapy. Several hundred randomized clinical trials evaluating various systemic adjuvant modalities have been reported. Most published results confirm that chemotherapy, hormonal therapy, or both, result in improved disease-free survival (DFS) and/or overall survival (OS) for all treated patients, or more commonly for patients in specific prognostic subgroups (e.g., nodal involvement, menopausal status, hormonal receptor status, growth fraction, or nuclear grade). The huge amount of data generated by these trials has resulted in a great deal of controversy, with different conclusions being reached by various experts.

A number of factors make interpretation of results of systemic adjuvant therapy trials difficult. These include differences in the patient populations studied, the variation in natural history of breast cancer, the absence of information regarding pathologic prognostic factors in many studies, and differences in treatment approach and methods of analysis. It is important to remember that the goal of systemic adjuvant therapy is cure. Therefore patients in these studies must be followed for long periods of time before results can be determined. In addition, because most patients with early breast cancer (50% to 90%) in the various trials are cured with local-regional therapy alone, large numbers of patients are required to show a statistically significant difference that can be attributed to systemic adjuvant therapy. For these reasons, combined analysis, or meta-analysis, of all breast cancer trials has been conducted, and until recently was the most frequently referred to information regarding systemic adjuvant therapy. This effort, organized by the Early Breast Cancer Trialists' Collaborative Group, is based on a worldwide collaboration involving 133 randomized trials conducted between 1957 and 1985.[70] The results of the Early Breast Cancer Trialists' Collaborative Group meta-analyses were published in 1988, 1992, and 1998. Many important questions regarding the optimal way to administer adjuvant chemotherapy[70,71] and hormonal therapy,[70–73] and the degree of benefit in terms of DFS or OS to clinically relevant subsets of patients have been answered by these meta-analyses. Simply stated, the results of the meta-analyses support the use of adjuvant hormonal therapy in all patients with positive hormone-receptor status, and this finding is reflected in the 2000 NIH Consensus Development Conference Statement[53] that adjuvant hormonal therapy should be recommended to women whose tumors contain hormone receptor protein regardless of age, menopausal status, involvement of axillary lymph nodes, or tumor size. The results of these meta-analyses also support a benefit of adjuvant chemotherapy, again reflected in the 2000 NIH Consensus Development Conference Statement that it is accepted practice to offer cytotoxic chemotherapy to most women with lymph node metastases or with primary breast cancers larger than 1 cm in diameter (both node-negative and node-positive).[53]

It is important to understand the relative and absolute magnitude of the benefit associated with adjuvant systemic therapy in breast cancer. Table 125–7 shows the proportional reduction in the annual odds of recurrence and death by age for adjuvant polychemotherapy and adjuvant tamoxifen given for 5 years in women with tumors that are positive for hormone receptors based on the results of these meta-analyses. Throughout these reports, the results are presented as they

TABLE 125–7. Ten-Year Results of the Overview Analysis

| Age | Tamoxifen | | Polychemotherapy | |
| | Reduction in Annual Odds | | Reduction in Annual Odds | |
	Recurrence (%)	Death (%)	Recurrence (%)	Death (%)
All patients	47 ± 3	26 ± 4	24 ± 2	15 ± 2
<40	54 ± 13	52 ± 17	37 ± 7	27 ± 5
40–49	41 ± 10	22 ± 13	34 ± 5	27 ± 5
50–59	37 ± 6	11 ± 8	22 ± 4	14 ± 4
60–69	54 ± 5	33 ± 6	18 ± 4	8 ± 4
≥70	54 ± 13	34 ± 13	NS	NS

NS, not significant.
From Paridaens et al[111] and Mauras et al.[112]

are in Table 125–7, as proportional benefits that compare the effects of two groups, in this case, chemotherapy or hormonal therapy versus no chemotherapy or hormonal therapy. A proportional reduction of 25% might equivalently be described as an odds ratio or hazard ratio of 0.75, an odds reduction of 25%, or a 25% reduction in the death rate. For a given proportional reduction in death rate, the absolute improvement in 10-year survival will depend on the risk of death with no treatment, which for breast cancer is known to vary based on prognostic factors that include patient characteristics, disease characteristics and biomarkers identified earlier in this chapter. Table 125–8 shows the number of deaths avoided per 100 patients treated in several hypothetical subsets of patients with different estimated 10-year survivals without adjuvant therapy, as a function of different estimates of treatment benefit shown as the proportional reductions in mortality if they did receive adjuvant therapy. Approximately 15 of every 100 patients benefited at 10 years from adjuvant therapy when a 30% proportional reduction in mortality is observed in the highest-risk subgroups (50% death rate with no adjuvant therapy). In contrast, the same 30% proportional reduction in mortality translated into a benefit for 3 of 100 patients in the lowest-risk subset (10% death rate with no adjuvant therapy). Thus the absolute benefit of adjuvant therapy depends on both the proportional reduction in mortality and the risk of disease recurrence, with the greatest benefit observed in the highest-risk treatment groups given a fixed proportional reduction in mortality. Table 125–9 further demonstrates this by using data from the meta-analysis to show the absolute benefits of adjuvant chemotherapy in terms of age and nodal status. In the highest-risk group, node-positive women younger than 50 years of age, only 41.4% were alive at 10 years with no polychemotherapy as compared with 53.8% with polychemotherapy,

which translates into an absolute survival benefit of 12.4%. However, in the node-negative group, patients less than 50 years old where survival with no polychemotherapy was highest (i.e., 71.9%), the addition of polychemotherapy produced an absolute benefit of only 5.7%. It should be pointed out that all of these differences in survival are highly statistically significant and form the basis of the 2000 NIH Consensus Development Group recommendation that it is accepted medical practice to offer cytotoxic chemotherapy to most women with early-stage breast cancer.[53] However, the absolute benefit in node-positive women age 50 to 69 years is quite small (2.3%), and depending on other disease characteristics and comorbid conditions, patients may elect not to pursue treatment. Although a 2% absolute reduction in death attributable to polychemotherapy may appear small, at least two investigators have reported that most patients with breast cancer would accept severe toxicity from treatment to achieve as little as a 1% to 5% improvement in survival.[74,75]

Several international and national groups have developed guidelines for treatment of early-stage breast cancer based on specific patient and disease characteristics and the results of these meta-analyses. In March 2003, an international group of researchers met in St. Gallen, Switzerland for the Eighth International Conference of Adjuvant Therapy of Primary Breast Cancer.[76] At the conclusion of the conference, a consensus panel of experts reviewed and modified its previous guidelines and recommendations for selection of adjuvant systemic therapies in specific patient populations outside of the framework of clinical trials (Table 125–10). Criteria used to construct Table 125–10 included risk of relapse, predicted response, results of treatment from randomized clinical trials, and patient preferences concerning risks and benefits of effective therapy. Patient populations are categorized into groups based on risk of relapse. The panel defined node-negative, minimal/low-risk as patients with all of the following: ER/PR-positive tumors with all of the following characteristics: pathologic tumor size ≤2 cm, grade 1, and age ≥35 years. Average-risk node-negative patients have at least one of the following: pathologic tumor size >2 cm, grade 2 or 3, or age <35 years. Patients with average-risk, node-negative tumors are further classified into endocrine responsive or nonresponsive disease, based on the presence or absence of hormone receptors, respectively. Node-positive patients are by definition at high risk of relapse.

The National Comprehensive Cancer Network (NCCN) has also developed practice guidelines for the treatment of breast cancer. Figure 125–3 illustrates the NCCN 2004 guidelines for adjuvant treatment of stages I to IIIA breast cancer following total mastectomy or lumpectomy. These more recent guidelines reflect the increasing trend toward the use of chemotherapy in postmenopausal (age >50 years)

TABLE 125–8. Absolute Reduction in Mortality at 10 Years per 100 Patients Treated

| Estimated 10-year Death Rate With No Therapy | Hypothetical Proportional Reduction in Mortality Due to Treatment | | | | |
	50%	40%	30%	20%	10%
50% (5-cm tumor, negative nodes)	25	20	15	10	5
30% (average tumor diameter, negative nodes)	15	12	9	6	3
10% (≤1-cm tumor, negative nodes)	5	4	3	2	1

TABLE 125–9. Absolute Benefits of Adjuvant Chemotherapy by Age and Nodal Status

	With Polychemotherapy (%)	With No Polychemotherapy (%)	Absolute Benefit (%)
Disease-free survival			
Age <50 y			
Node-negative	68.3	58.0	10.3
Node-positive	47.6	32.2	15.4
Age 50–69 y			
Node-negative	65.6	59.9	5.7
Node-positive	43.4	39.0	5.4
Overall survival			
Age <50 y			
Node-negative	77.6	71.9	5.7
Node-positive	53.8	41.4	12.4
Age 50–69 y			
Node-negative	71.2	64.8	6.4
Node-positive	48.6	46.3	2.3

TABLE 125–10. Adjuvant Treatment for Patients with Node-Negative and Node-Positive Breast Cancer

Node-Negative		
Patient Group	*Minimal Risk*	*Average Risk*
Premenopausal, endocrine-responsive	Tamoxifen or none	• GnRH analog[a] + tamoxifen[b] ± chemotherapy[c,d] or • Chemotherapy → tamoxifen[b] (± GnRH analog[a]) or • Tamoxifen or • GnRH analog[a,e]
Premenopausal, endocrine-nonresponsive	Not applicable	• Chemotherapy
Postmenopausal, endocrine-responsive	Tamoxifen[d,f] or none	• Tamoxifen,[f] or • Chemotherapy[c] → tamoxifen[b,e]
Postmenopausal, endocrine-nonresponsive	Not applicable	• Chemotherapy

Node-Positive	
Patient Group	*Treatments*
Premenopausal, endocrine-responsive	• Chemotherapy → tamoxifen[b] (± GnRH analog[a]) or • GnRH analog + tamoxifen[b] (± chemotherapy[c])
Premenopausal, endocrine-nonresponsive	• Chemotherapy
Postmenopausal, endocrine-responsive	• Chemotherapy[c] → tamoxifen[b,e] or • Tamoxifen[e]
Postmenopausal, endocrine-nonresponsive	• Chemotherapy

[a]Or ovarian ablation.
[b]Tamoxifen therapy should not be started until after chemotherapy is finished.
[c]The addition of chemotherapy is considered an acceptable option based on evidence from clinical trials. Considerations about a low relative risk of relapse, age, toxic effects, socioeconomic implications, and information on patient preference might justify the use of endocrine therapy alone.
[d]Indicates treatments sill being tested in randomized clinical trials.
[e]In the presence of chemotherapy, adding tamoxifen to ovarian suppression may improve outcome. Use of a GnRH analog alone has been shown to be as effective as chemotherapy and is an option if tamoxifen is not indicated.
[f]In women in whom tamoxifen is not acceptable (contraindicated or not tolerated), then an aromatase inhibitor (data are limited to anastrozole) may be used.
GnRH, gonadotropin-releasing hormone (goserelin is most extensively studied).

SYSTEMIC ADJUVANT TREATMENT

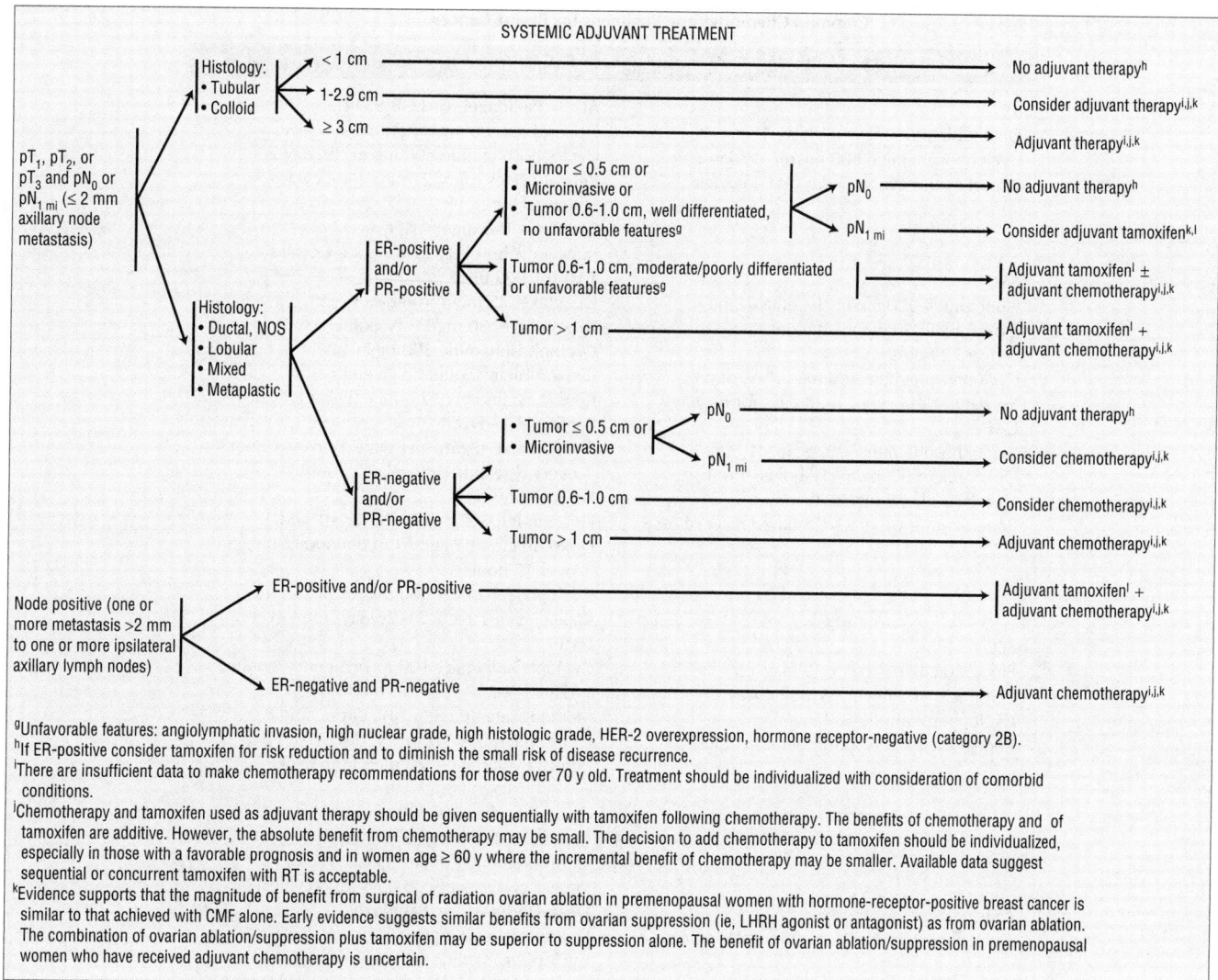

^{g}Unfavorable features: angiolymphatic invasion, high nuclear grade, high histologic grade, HER-2 overexpression, hormone receptor-negative (category 2B).
^{h}If ER-positive consider tamoxifen for risk reduction and to diminish the small risk of disease recurrence.
^{i}There are insufficient data to make chemotherapy recommendations for those over 70 y old. Treatment should be individualized with consideration of comorbid conditions.
^{j}Chemotherapy and tamoxifen used as adjuvant therapy should be given sequentially with tamoxifen following chemotherapy. The benefits of chemotherapy and of tamoxifen are additive. However, the absolute benefit from chemotherapy may be small. The decision to add chemotherapy to tamoxifen should be individualized, especially in those with a favorable prognosis and in women age ≥ 60 y where the incremental benefit of chemotherapy may be smaller. Available data suggest sequential or concurrent tamoxifen with RT is acceptable.
^{k}Evidence supports that the magnitude of benefit from surgical of radiation ovarian ablation in premenopausal women with hormone-receptor-positive breast cancer is similar to that achieved with CMF alone. Early evidence suggests similar benefits from ovarian suppression (ie, LHRH agonist or antagonist) as from ovarian ablation. The combination of ovarian ablation/suppression plus tamoxifen may be superior to suppression alone. The benefit of ovarian ablation/suppression in premenopausal women who have received adjuvant chemotherapy is uncertain.

FIGURE 125–3. National Comprehensive Cancer Network 2004 treatment guidelines for invasive breast cancer. (*Reproduced with permission from NCCN.*)

patients, as well as the well-established premenopausal (age <50 years) patient group, hormonal therapy in all hormone receptor–positive women regardless of age or menopausal status, and the combination of both chemotherapy and hormonal therapy.[77] These guidelines differ from the St. Gallen expert consensus guidelines in the recommendation of chemotherapy for women with node-negative tumors 0.6 to 1 cm in size. If the characteristics of these tumors are unfavorable (angiolymphatic invasion, high nuclear or histologic grade, *HER-2* overexpression, or hormone receptor–negative), then chemotherapy is recommended with or without hormonal therapy, depending on hormone-receptor status.

Intensive research efforts are directed toward identifying those characteristics of the primary tumor (pathologic prognostic factors) that may predict for a higher or lower likelihood of metastases and death in node-negative patients. Although a multitude of prognostic factors are being investigated, no single factor or combination of factors sufficiently identifies those at risk of metastases or is sufficiently standardized to be reproducibly applicable to all patients. For a more in-depth discussion of the issues and controversies regarding adjuvant therapy of breast cancer, the reader is referred to two excellent references.[78,79]

In contrast to adjuvant systemic therapy, the use of preoperative systemic therapy is gaining favor in both early-stage and locally-advanced breast cancers. This approach to therapy, referred to as *neoadjuvant* or *primary systemic therapy*, most often consists of chemotherapy, but in special circumstances may also include hormonal therapy (e.g., in inoperable patients with significant comorbidities). The advantages of preoperative systemic therapy include: (1) decrease in the size of the tumor to minimize surgery; and (2) to determine response to chemotherapy/hormone therapy in vivo (an important prognostic indicator). In a pivotal study conducted by the NSABP (B18), preoperative chemotherapy was compared to traditional chemotherapy given after surgery (same chemotherapy and same number of cycles).[80] While no difference was found in DFS or OS between these two groups, rates of breast-conserving surgery were higher in the group receiving preoperative chemotherapy (67.8% vs. 59.8%).[81] This study also identified a small subset of patients (13%) who had a pathologically complete response (pCR; no tumor left at surgery) after chemotherapy. These patients went on to have a significantly better DFS compared with patients that did not achieve a pCR ($p < 0.0001$).[81] While this approach to therapy is generally reserved for patients with inoperable tumors (locally advanced),

TABLE 125–11. Common Chemotherapy Regimens for Breast Cancer

Adjuvant Chemotherapy Regimens	
AC	**AC → Paclitaxel (CALGB 9344)**
Doxorubicin 60 mg/m^2 IV, day 1	Doxorubicin 60 mg/m^2 IV, day 1
Cyclophosphamide 600 mg/m^2 IV, day 1	Cyclophosphamide 600 mg/m^2 IV, day 1
Repeat cycles every 21 days for 4 cycles[a]	Repeat cycles every 21 days for 4 cycles
	Followed by:
	Paclitaxel 175 mg/m^2 IV over 3 hours
	Repeat cycles every 21 days for 4 cycles[b]
FAC[w]	**TAC (BCIRG 001)**
Fluorouracil 500 mg/m^2 IV, days 1 and 4	Docetaxel 75 mg/m^2 IV, day 1
Doxorubicin 50 mg/m^2 IV continuous infusion over 72 hours[w]	Doxorubicin 50 mg/m^2 IV bolus, day 1
	Cyclophosphamide 500 mg/m^2 IV, day 1
Cyclophosphamide 500 mg/m^2 IV, day 1	(Doxorubicin should be given first)
Repeat cycles every 21–28 days for 6 cycles[c]	Repeat cycles every 21–28 days for 6 cycles[d]
CAF	**Paclitaxel → FAC[w]**
Cyclophosphamide 600 mg/m^2 IV, day 1	Paclitaxel 80 mg/m^2 per week IV over 1 hour every week for 12 weeks
Doxorubicin 60 mg/m^2 IV bolus, day 1	Followed by:
Fluorouracil 600 mg/m^2 IV, day 1	Fluorouracil 500 mg/m^2 IV, days 1 and 4
Repeat cycles every 21–28 days for 6 cycles[e]	Doxorubicin 50 mg/m^2 IV continuous infusion over 72 hours
	Cyclophosphamide 500 mg/m^2 IV, day 1
	Repeat cycles every 21–28 days for 4 cycles[n]
FEC	**CMF**
Fluorouracil 500 mg/m^2 IV, day 1	Cyclophosphamide 100 mg/m^2 per day orally, days 1–14
Epirubicin 100 mg/m^2 IV bolus, day 1	Methotrexate 40 mg/m^2 IV, days 1 and 8
Cyclophosphamide 500 mg/m^2 IV, day 1	Fluorouracil 600 mg/m^2 IV, days 1 and 8
Repeat cycle every 21 days for 6 cycles[g]	Repeat cycles every 28 days for 6 cycles[h]
	or
	Cyclophosphamide 600 mg/m^2 IV, day 1
	Methotrexate 40 mg/m^2 IV, day 1
	Fluorouracil 600 mg/m^2 IV, days 1 and 8
	Repeat cycles every 28 days for 6 cycles[i]
CEF	**Dose-Dense AC → Paclitaxel**
Cyclophosphamide 75 mg/m^2 orally on days 1–14	Doxorubicin 60 mg/m^2 IV bolus, day 1
Epirubicin 60 mg/m^2 IV, days 1 and 8	Cyclophosphamide 600 mg/m^2 IV, day 1
Fluorouracil 600 mg/m^2 IV, days 1 and 8	Repeat cycles every 14 days for 4 cycles (must be given with growth factor support)
Repeat cycles every 21 days for 6 cycles (requires prophylactic antibiotics or growth factor support)[j]	Followed by:
	Paclitaxel 175 mg/m^2 IV over 3 hours
	Repeat cycles every 14 days for 4 cycles (must be given with growth factor support)[k]

Metastatic Single-Agent Chemotherapy	
Paclitaxel	**Vinorelbine**
Paclitaxel 175 mg/m^2 IV over 3 hours	Vinorelbine 30 mg/m^2 IV, days 1 and 8
Repeat cycles every 21 days[l]	Repeat cycles every 21 days
or	or
Paclitaxel 80 mg/m^2 per week IV over 1 hour	Vinorelbine 25–30 mg/m^2 per week IV
Repeat dose every 7 days[m]	Repeat cycles every 7 days (adjust dose based on absolute neutrophil count; see product information)[n]
Docetaxel	**Gemcitabine**
Docetaxel 60–100 mg/m^2 IV over 1 hour	Gemcitabine 600–1000 mg/m^2 per week IV, days 1, 8, and 15
Repeat cycles every 21 days[o]	Repeat cycles every 28 days (may need to hold day-15 dose based on blood counts)[q]
or	
Docetaxel 30–35 mg/m^2 per week IV over 30 minutes	
Repeat dose every 7 days[p]	
Capecitabine	**Liposomal doxorubicin**
Capecitabine 2,000–2,500 mg/m^2 per day orally, divided twice daily for 14 days	Liposomal doxorubicin 30–50 mg/m^2 IV over 90 minutes
Repeat cycles every 21 days[q,r]	Repeat cycles every 21–28 days[s]

TABLE 125–11. (Continued)

Metastatic Combination Chemotherapy Regimens	
Docetaxel + capecitabine Docetaxel 75 mg/m² IV over 1 hour, day 1 Capecitabine 2000–2500 mg/m² per day orally divided twice daily for 14 days Repeat cycles every 21 days[t] **Epirubicin + docetaxel[x]** Epirubicin 70–90 mg/m² IV bolus Followed by: Docetaxel 70–90 mg/m² IV over 1 hour Repeat cycles every 21 days[v]	**Doxorubicin + docetaxel[x]** Doxorubicin 50 mg/m² IV bolus, day 1 Followed by: Docetaxel 75 mg/m² IV over 1 hour, day 1 Repeat cycles every 21 days[u]

[a]From Fisher B, et al. J Clin Oncol 1990;8:1483.

[b]From Henderson CI, et al. J Clin Oncol 2003;21:976.

[c]From Buzdar AU, et al. In: Salmon S, ed. Adjuvant Therapy of Cancer, VIII. Philadelphia, Lippincott-Raven, 1997: 93–100.

[d]From Martin et al.[84]

[e]From Wood WC, et al. N Engl J Med 1994;330:1253.

[f]From Green et al.[88]

[g]French Adjuvant Study Group. J Clin Oncol 2001;19:602.

[h]From Bonadonna G, et al. N Engl J Med 1976;294:405.

[i]From Fisher B, et al. N Engl J Med 1989;32:473.

[k]From Citron et al.[87]

[l]From Taxol (paclitaxel) product information. Bristol-Myers Squibb, April 2003.

[m]From Perez EA, et al. Clin Oncol 2001;19:4216.

[n]From Zelek L. Cancer 2001;92:2267.

[o]From Taxotere (docetaxel) product information. Aventis Pharmaceuticals Inc., April 2003.

[p]From Hainsworth JD, et al. J Clin Oncol 1998;16:2164.

[q]From Carmichael J, et al. J Clin Oncol 1995;13:2731.

[p]From Xeloda product information.[122]

[r]From Michaud et al.[123]

[s]From Ranson MR, et al. J Clin Oncol 1997;15:3185.

[t]From O'Shaughnessy et al.[127]

[u]From Nabholtz JM, et al. J Clin Oncol 2003;21:968.

[v]From Levin MN, et al. J Clin Oncol 1998;16:2651.

[w]FAC may also be given with bolus doxorubicin administration, and the fluorouracil dose is then given on days 1 and 8.

[x]Paclitaxel may also be given concurrently with doxorubicin **or** epirubicin as a combination regimen. Pharmacokinetic interactions make these regimens more difficult to give.

early-stage breast cancer patients who meet the criteria for breast-conserving therapy except for the size of the tumor may be considered for preoperative systemic therapy in order to decrease the size of the tumor, allowing for less radical surgery and better cosmetic results.

Adjuvant Chemotherapy

Cytotoxic drugs that have been used alone and in combination as adjuvant therapy in breast cancer include doxorubicin, epirubicin, cyclophosphamide, methotrexate, fluorouracil, paclitaxel, docetaxel, melphalan, prednisone, vinorelbine, and vincristine. The most common combination chemotherapy regimens employed in the adjuvant and metastatic setting are listed in Table 125–11.

The basic principle of adjuvant therapy for any cancer type is that the regimen with the highest response rate in advanced disease should be the optimal regimen for use in the adjuvant setting. However, results from individual clinical trials investigating specific regimens in the adjuvant setting are required to be able to identify the benefits and risks to a specific patient population. Early administration of effective combination chemotherapy at a time when the tumor burden is low should increase the likelihood of cure and minimize the emergence of drug-resistant tumor cell clones. Anthracyclines (doxorubicin and epirubicin) have historically been referred to as the most active class of chemotherapy agents in the treatment of metastatic breast cancer. This has led to the assumption that anthracycline-containing regimens are associated with a higher cure rate than non–anthracycline-containing regimens when used in the adjuvant setting. The meta-analysis of polychemotherapy (discussed previously) investigated this question, presenting indirect evidence from 11 trials that compared an anthracycline-containing regimen with a cyclophosphamide, methotrexate, fluorouracil (CMF)–type regimen and demonstrating a significant advantage for the anthracycline regimens.[72] In this meta-analysis, anthracycline-containing regimens were modestly superior in reducing recurrence and death compared to regimens without anthracyclines. A 12% ± 4% reduction in annual odds of recurrence and an 11% ± 5% reduction in annual odds of death were reported in the 1998 update, and this translated into an absolute difference in overall mortality at 5 years of 3%.[72]

The taxanes (paclitaxel and docetaxel) are a newer class of agents that rival the anthracyclines in their activity in metastatic breast cancer, becoming (arguably) the most active class of chemotherapy for this disease. Since these agents are relatively new, adjuvant studies including them have not yet been incorporated into the overview meta-analysis. However, results from a few clinical trials have been reported and are reaching substantial follow-up to provide meaningful information. All trials have enrolled node-positive patients only, and all

TABLE 125–12. Adjuvant Taxane-Containing Regimens from Clinical Trials

	CALGB 9344 n = 3,170	NSABP B28 n = 3,060	BCIRG 001 n = 1,491
Median follow-up	69 months	67 months	55 months
Treatment arms	AC → Pac[a] vs AC	AC → Pac[a] vs AC	TAC vs FAC
Disease-free survival			
Reduction in risk of recurrence	17%	17%	28%
Hazard ratio	0.83	0.83	0.72
95% Confidence interval	0.73–0.94	0.73–0.95	0.59–0.88
p Value	0.0013	0.008	0.001
Overall survival			
Reduction in risk of death	26%	18%	30%
Hazard ratio	0.74	0.82	0.70
95% Confidence interval	(0.60–0.92)	(0.71–0.95)	(0.53–0.91)
p Value	0.0065	0.0061	0.008

AC, doxorubicin, cyclophosphamide; BCIRG, Breast Cancer International Research Group; CALGB, Cancer and Leukemia Group B; FAC, fluorouracil, doxorubicin, cyclophosphamide; NSABP, National Surgical Adjuvant Breast and Bowel Project; Pac, paclitaxel; TAC, docetaxel, doxorubicin, cyclophosphamide.

[a]The dose of paclitaxel differs in these two studies. The CALGB study used the dosing and schedule listed in Table 125–11. The NSABP study administered a higher dose of paclitaxel, at 225 mg/m^2 IV over 3 hours, every 21 days, for 4 cycles.

but one has been published in abstract form only (Table 125–12).[82–84] Two studies have incorporated four cycles of paclitaxel into the adjuvant regimen sequentially after four cycles of AC.[82,83] These two studies compared this new regimen to the standard regimen of four cycles of AC. Results from these studies indicate a modest but statistically significant advantage in DFS with the addition of paclitaxel (see Table 125–12). However, the increase in OS in one of these studies has not yet reached statistical significance. In earlier trials with anthracycline-containing regimens (meta-analysis), differences in survival were not seen until 7 to 10 years of follow-up were completed. Therefore this trial may require longer follow-up in order to demonstrate a difference in OS. Nonetheless, advantages in DFS and OS in one trial are sufficient for many clinicians to justify use of this regimen in the adjuvant setting.

Investigating the concurrent use of a taxane with an anthracycline has also been investigated in node-positive breast cancer patients. The Breast Cancer International Research Group (BCIRG) randomized node-positive breast cancer patients to receive six cycles of the standard fluorouracil, doxorubicin, and cyclophosphamide (FAC) regimen or six cycles of the paclitaxel, doxorubicin, and cyclophosphamide (TAC) regimen. Substantial increases in DFS and OS were found with the taxane regimen in this study, substantiating the role of the taxanes in the adjuvant setting for node-positive patients.[84] Because these studies were limited to node-positive patients, the benefits in node-negative patients are unknown.

CLINICAL CONTROVERSY

While the incorporation of the taxanes into many different regimens, both sequentially and concurrently, has lead to a shift in therapy for node-positive breast cancer patients, the use of taxane-containing regimens in node-negative patients remains controversial. The use of an anthracycline-containing regimen has been established for both node-negative and node-positive breast cancer patients.

However, there is no apparent biological reason why node-negative disease should respond differently to the taxanes than node-

positive disease. The only difference may be that the absolute benefit for this patient population may be smaller, and may not be large enough to warrant a change from the standard of care. Further follow-up from these trials will continue to address this issue.

No validated predictive factors exist for response to chemotherapy. However, HER-2/neu status and ER-negativity may be useful predictors of response, depending on the outcome of several ongoing clinical trials. Retrospective studies have suggested that the benefit with the anthracycline-containing regimens over CMF-like regimens may be limited to those tumors that overexpress HER2/neu. However, this is based on retrospective data and should be viewed with skepticism. The use of trastuzumab, a monoclonal antibody directed against the HER2/neu receptor (see section on metastatic breast cancer), is currently being investigated for use in the adjuvant setting with chemotherapy.

CLINICAL CONTROVERSY

The addition of trastuzumab to chemotherapy has resulted in a survival advantage for metastatic breast cancer patients with HER2-overexpressing/amplified tumors compared with chemotherapy alone. However, the use of trastuzumab-chemotherapy combinations in the adjuvant setting has yet to be substantiated. These patients tend to have a poor prognosis with chemotherapy alone and may benefit from additional therapy. However, there are not yet data to demonstrate additional benefit with this combination compared with chemotherapy alone.

These trials are still ongoing and preliminary efficacy data are not yet available. ER-status has also been looked at for predictability. Several clinical trials have attempted to correlate ER-negative status with better response to adjuvant chemotherapy. These results are inconsistent and current practice does not recommend tailoring chemotherapy based on ER-status. Further investigation into both of these markers may provide evidence to suggest otherwise, but until those data are available, current practice does not incorporate these into decisions regarding adjuvant chemotherapy.

Although the optimal duration of adjuvant chemotherapy administration is unknown, it appears to be on the order of 12 to 24 weeks and may depend on the regimen being used. Chemotherapy is usually initiated within 3 weeks of surgical removal of the primary tumor. "Dose intensity" and "dose density" appear to be critical factors in achieving optimal outcomes in adjuvant breast cancer therapy. *Dose intensity* is defined as the amount of drug administered per unit of time and is typically reported in milligrams per square meter of body surface area per week (mg/m^2 per week). Increasing dose, decreasing time, or both can increase dose intensity. *Dose density* is equivalent to the concept of increasing dose intensity, but not by increasing the amount of drug given, as occurs with dose escalation, but instead by decreasing the time between treatment cycles. The issue of dose intensity first received wide attention in 1981, when the Milan group reported a retrospective analysis of their original CMF adjuvant study, suggesting that only those patients who received at least 85% of their planned CMF dose benefited significantly from adjuvant therapy, whereas those receiving less than 65% of the planned dose had the same disease-free survival and overall survival as the group of control patients treated by surgery alone.[85] More recent studies that have escalated the dose of cyclophosphamide or doxorubicin in standard anthracycline-containing regimens reported that this intervention offers no therapeutic advantage and is associated with greater toxicity. A study by the Cancer and Leukemia Group B (CALGB) that is often discussed assigned 1,572 women to three treatment groups given different doses and schedules of CAF.[86] The high-dose arm had twice the dose intensity and twice the drug dose as the low-dose arm (basically representing what we now consider "standard dose" CAF). The moderate-dose arm had two-thirds the dose intensity as the high-dose arm, but the same total drug dose. At a median follow-up of 9 years, DFS and OS for patients on the moderate- and high-dose arms were superior to those for the patients in the low-dose arm. There was no difference in DFS or OS between the moderate- and the high-dose arms. Therefore it would appear that reducing the dose for standard treatment regimens should be avoided, unless necessitated by severe toxicity. But increasing doses beyond those contained in standard treatment regimens does not appear to be beneficial. In a more recent study conducted by the CALGB, the dose of doxorubicin was escalated (60 mg/m^2, 75 mg/m^2, or 90 mg/m^2) in combination with cyclophosphamide at a fixed dose of 600 mg/m^2.[82] No benefits were seen with the higher dose levels in this trial. Therefore it appears that there is a threshold for dosing adjuvant chemotherapy under which there may be a lack of benefit. *Dose intensity* above that threshold does not appear to add benefit and imparts additional toxicity.

A recent study investigating the idea of *dose density* has now been reported. The CALGB conducted yet another study looking not only at dose density, but also at the question of using sequential versus combination chemotherapy regimens. Using a 2×2 factorial design, investigators randomized node-positive breast cancer patients after surgery to compare sequential versus concurrent chemotherapy, and standard dose versus dose density.[87] The arms of the study were as follows: (1) sequential doxorubicin (A) for four cycles, followed by paclitaxel (P) for four cycles, followed by cyclophosphamide (C) for four cycles, with all cycles given every 3 weeks; (2) sequential A for four cycles, followed by P for four cycles, followed by C for four cycles, with all cycles given every 2 weeks with filgrastim; (3) concurrent AC for four cycles, followed by P for four cycles, with all cycles given every 3 weeks; and (4) concurrent AC for four cycles, followed by P for four cycles, with all cycles given every 2 weeks with filgrastim. After a median follow-up of 36 months, the patients receiving every-2-week chemotherapy had a significantly prolonged DFS (at 3 years 85% vs. 81%; RR = 0.74, $p = 0.01$) and OS (92% vs. 90%; RR = 0.69, $p = 0.013$) compared with every 3-week chemotherapy.[87] The use of sequential versus concurrent chemotherapy did not show a benefit for one over the other in terms of DFS or OS. Due to the statistical design of this trial, it does not indicate which of the four regimens tested is the best one to use. It does, however, indicate a benefit with more frequent dosing, at least with the drugs, doses, and combinations used here. Patients in the concurrent every-2-week group (group 4) had significantly more regimen-related toxicity, including a very high rate of red blood cell transfusions for anemia (13% of cycles).[87] Red blood cell transfusions are rarely required with most other standard adjuvant chemotherapy regimens used for breast cancer. Previous data with paclitaxel given weekly versus every 3 weeks indicates that this drug is more effective when given weekly in the neoadjuvant setting.[88] Therefore some have speculated that the different paclitaxel schedule is the primary reason for the success with this approach to therapy. All of this information leaves many clinicians wondering whether it is prudent, based on the available evidence, to incorporate this regimen into standard of care. Hopefully, as other clinical trials investigate this and other questions, clinicians will be better equipped to choose the optimal adjuvant chemotherapy regimen for their patients. Until that time this approach to therapy is certainly an option for some patients, recognizing the additive toxicity.

A major focus in clinical investigation was the use of more high-dose chemotherapy regimens as adjuvant therapy. Because bone marrow suppression is the dose-limiting toxicity for most chemotherapeutic agents, high-dose chemotherapy regimens followed by colony-stimulating factors or reinfusion of autologous hematopoietic stem cells have been developed. Trials to define the specific usefulness of high-dose regimens, as well as autologous hematopoietic stem cell transplantation in conjunction with dose-intense regimens, were justified given the positive response rates seen in the metastatic breast cancer setting and the very poor prognosis associated with disease that involves 4 to 9, and particularly 10 or more, axillary lymph nodes. Several cooperative groups have conducted trials of high-dose chemotherapy versus conventional adjuvant therapy. None of the trials have shown a significant difference in DFS or OS. Based on available evidence, this approach to therapy is not worth the added toxicity.

The short-term toxic effects of chemotherapy used in the adjuvant setting are generally well tolerated. Although a number of investigators have demonstrated a reduction in quality of life, most patients are able to maintain a reasonable level of function and emotional and social well being during treatment.[89] In general, supportive therapy of the patient receiving systemic adjuvant chemotherapy has improved in the past decade. Increased attention to the impact of symptoms on quality of life may account for some of this improvement. In addition, serotonin-antagonist antiemetics have become available to assist in managing chemotherapy-induced nausea and vomiting, and colony-stimulating factors are often helpful in preventing febrile neutropenia, particularly in elderly patients or patients receiving high-dose and dose-dense chemotherapy regimens. However, a number of side effects are common with the regimens employed and patients should be appropriately counseled regarding the likelihood of alopecia, weight gain, and fatigue. Patients who are menstruating will often experience a cessation of menses that may or may not return. Along with cessation of menses are accompanying signs and symptoms of menopause. Deep vein thrombosis has been reported in women receiving combination chemotherapy regimens.[90] A recent study estimated that 1 to 10 of 10,000 patients treated for 6 months with cyclophosphamide-based regimens might be expected to have leukemia within 10 years of diagnosis of breast cancer.[91]

Cardiomyopathy induced by doxorubicin occurs less than 1% of the time in women whose total dose of doxorubicin is less than 320 mg/m^2.[92] It should be noted that epirubicin in the adjuvant setting is given at a dose of 100 to 120 mg/m^2.[93] At this dose epirubicin has an equal chance of causing cardiomyopathy as standard doxorubicin doses when both agents are given as bolus or short infusions. Taxanes are often associated with hypersensitivity reactions, peripheral neuropathy and/or myalgias and arthralgias for a few days following the infusion.

Before we leave the topic of adjuvant chemotherapy in stage I and II breast cancer, it is important to note that the magnitude of survival benefit for chemotherapy appears to be small, with an absolute reduction in mortality of only 5% at 10 years for patients with negative axillary lymph nodes and 10% for patients with positive axillary lymph nodes. In addition, there is currently no means to identify patients who will attain this survival benefit. However, two investigators report that most patients with breast cancer would accept severe toxicity from treatment to achieve as little as a 1% to 5% improvement in survival.[74,75] Therefore in the absence of the ability to predict who will benefit, it is likely that most patients with stage I and stage II breast cancer will choose an adjuvant chemotherapy treatment. The optimal chemotherapy regimen for use in the adjuvant setting has yet to be identified and depends on many patient and tumor characteristics. All of the regimens previously mentioned are appropriate in the settings in which they were discussed.

Adjuvant Endocrine Therapy

4 Hormonal therapies that have been studied in the treatment of primary or early breast cancer include tamoxifen, oophorectomy, ovarian irradiation, luteinizing hormone-releasing hormone (LHRH) agonists, anastrozole, letrozole, and exemestane.

Tamoxifen was traditionally the gold standard adjuvant hormonal therapy and has been used in the adjuvant setting for three decades. Tamoxifen is antiestrogenic in breast cancer cells, but it appears to have estrogenic properties in other tissues and organs.[94,95] Newer information confirms that tamoxifen and other similar drugs have many estrogenic and antiestrogenic effects that depend on the tissue and the gene in question, and they are more appropriately called selective estrogen receptor modulators (SERMs). Women receiving adjuvant tamoxifen therapy have a reduction in recurrence and mortality compared to women not receiving adjuvant tamoxifen therapy.[71] This observation, coupled with evidence of tamoxifen's tolerability including beneficial estrogenic effects on the lipid profile and bone density, led to tamoxifen being the hormonal agent of choice, at least until evidence with the antiaromatase agents became available in postmenopausal women. Premenopausal patients may derive equivalent benefit from ovarian ablation via surgery or administration of LHRH agonists.[73]

The optimal dose of tamoxifen is unclear. The Early Breast Cancer Trialists' Group showed that more is not necessarily better for response rates.[71] Lower doses of tamoxifen may be effective, but no clinical trials have addressed this question. Therefore the current recommended dose for tamoxifen in both the adjuvant, as well as the metastatic and preventative settings, is 20 mg/day. Because tamoxifen has a long biologic half-life, it can be administered as a single daily dose. Adjuvant tamoxifen therapy is generally initiated shortly after surgery or as soon as pathology results are known and the decision to administer tamoxifen as adjuvant therapy is made. An interesting theory with some laboratory and clinical support held that tamoxifen antagonized the beneficial effect of chemotherapy in women aged 50 years or younger. Chemotherapy acts by inhibiting DNA synthesis, resulting in death of tumor cells, whereas tamoxifen is believed to have a static effect on tumor cell growth. The growth inhibitory effect of tamoxifen may therefore diminish the cytotoxic effect of chemotherapy, resulting in subsequent recurrence of disease in women who received the two agents concurrently. A phase III intergroup trial conducted investigating this question was reported in 2002.[96] Investigators randomized patients to receive chemotherapy for six cycles with concurrent tamoxifen, followed by continued tamoxifen for a total of 5 years, or chemotherapy with sequential tamoxifen for 5 years. After a median follow-up of 8.5 years, the administration of sequential tamoxifen resulted in an estimated DFS advantage of 18% (hazard ratio [HR] = 1.18) compared to the concurrent use of tamoxifen with chemotherapy.[96] Therefore the administration of tamoxifen should be limited to administration after completion of chemotherapy.

The optimal duration of tamoxifen therapy in the adjuvant setting is currently defined as 5 years. Studies examining prolonged administration (e.g., 10 years) have failed to demonstrate any advantage and may in fact be associated with a slightly worse survival.[97]

The best information regarding the side effects of tamoxifen come from the National Surgical Adjuvant Breast and Bowel Project (NSABP), Breast Cancer Prevention Trial (P1).[98] This trial randomized 13,388 women at increased risk for breast cancer, 35 years of age or older, to placebo (n = 6,707) or 20 mg/day of tamoxifen (n = 6,681) for 5 years. Although the primary finding of this study was that tamoxifen reduced the risk of invasive breast cancer by 49%, this study also provides an excellent opportunity to objectively quantitate side effects associated with tamoxifen, due to its placebo control. Information was collected with regard to the occurrence of hot flashes, vaginal discharge, irregular menses, fluid retention, nausea, skin changes, diarrhea, and weight gain or loss. The self-administered depression scale and a global quality of life and a sexual function scale were administered at each follow-up visit. The only symptomatic differences noted between the placebo and tamoxifen group were related to hot flashes and vaginal discharge, both of which occurred more often in the latter group. There were no notable differences between the two groups relative to any of the findings obtained from the various self-reporting instruments. Tamoxifen administration did not alter the average annual rate of ischemic heart disease, but a reduction in hip radius and spine fractures was observed. Of note, the rates of stroke, pulmonary embolism, and deep vein thrombosis were elevated in the tamoxifen group (stroke, RR = 1.59; pulmonary embolism, RR = 3.01; and deep vein thrombosis, RR = 1.60). These events occurred more frequently in women age 50 years or older. The rate of endometrial cancer was increased in the tamoxifen group (RR = 2.53), and this increased risk occurred predominantly in women age 50 years or older. The increased risk of endometrial carcinoma is similar in magnitude to that associated with postmenopausal estrogen replacement therapy and is likely a consequence of an estrogenic effect of tamoxifen on the endometrium. Some experts argue that this risk is acceptable because the endometrial cancer induced by tamoxifen is low-stage, low-grade, and easily treated with surgery or other means and does not pose a life-threatening risk to women. There is also an increased risk of uterine sarcomas (a more aggressive form of endometrial cancer) with tamoxifen use, but this risk appears to be lower than the more common endometrial cancers identified in the NSABP P-1 study.[99] Currently, routine endometrial biopsy is not recommended for women receiving tamoxifen therapy. However, gynecologic exams and education regarding the importance of immediately reporting vaginal bleeding to primary physicians for further evaluation are important counseling points to women receiving tamoxifen therapy. In the NSABP-P1 trial, no increase in liver, colon, rectal, ovarian, or other tumors was observed in the tamoxifen group as compared to the group who received placebo.

Toremifene is a recently marketed antiestrogen whose primary advantage is a lower estrogenic:antiestrogenic ratio as compared to tamoxifen (based on laboratory data).[100] Toremifene (60 mg orally daily) has been found to have efficacy similar to that of tamoxifen in metastatic disease and a generally similar side-effect profile.[101] Currently, toremifene is indicated as an alternative to tamoxifen in patients with metastatic breast cancer, but studies are ongoing that evaluate its safety and efficacy in the adjuvant setting.

In premenopausal women, the use of LHRH-agonists or other means of ovarian ablation have been shown to provide benefit in the adjuvant setting.[73] The use of goserelin (an LHRH-agonist), alone or with tamoxifen, has been compared with standard chemotherapy (CMF) for six cycles. As a single agent, goserelin appears to provide similar benefit compared with CMF for six cycles for node-positive, ER-positive, premenopausal breast cancer patients.[102] In another trial, the combination of goserelin and tamoxifen was compared with CMF for 6 cycles.[103] After a median follow-up of 6 years, this trial demonstrated a significant advantage over endocrine therapy in terms of DFS. Both of these trials require longer follow-up to determine the long-term consequences of this type of therapy. Similar comparative evidence is not available with anthracycline-containing regimens, although a clinical trial designed to answer this question was stopped due to slow accrual. However, ongoing studies are underway to look at this question. There are no data comparing an LHRH-agonist to tamoxifen alone in the adjuvant setting. Therefore optimal endocrine therapy is not known for these women. Also, based on retrospective reviews, premenopausal women who cease to menstruate with chemotherapy may have a better survival compared to women who continue to menstruate.[104] Therefore the role of an LHRH-agonist after chemotherapy in women who continue to menstruate is also being investigated.

In postmenopausal women, recently reported evidence supporting the use of aromatase inhibitors in the adjuvant setting is intriguing and may usurp the role of tamoxifen. Three different approaches to therapy have been undertaken with these new agents: (1) direct comparison with tamoxifen for adjuvant hormonal therapy, (2) sequential use after 5 years of adjuvant tamoxifen therapy, and (3) sequential use after 2 to 3 years of adjuvant tamoxifen. In the former setting, anastrozole was compared with tamoxifen or the combination in postmenopausal women with hormone-receptor positive, early-stage breast cancer (ATAC trial). In the most recent preliminary analysis of this study, after a median of 47 months of follow-up, anastrozole continues to produce superior DFS (86.9% vs. 84.5%; HR = 0.86; $p = 0.03$) compared with tamoxifen alone.[105] The combination of anastrozole and tamoxifen resulted in similar outcomes as tamoxifen alone, imparting no benefit for patients in that arm of the study. These data are very controversial due to the preliminary nature of the results and the lack of long-term safety information with the aromatase inhibitors. Concerns surrounding loss of bone density and an increased risk of osteoporosis are evident from the preliminary data.[105] However, the overall impact on quality of life and survival has yet to be determined, but successful coadministration of bisphosphonates with the aromatase inhibitors has been accomplished in many patients in the metastatic setting.

The other approach to adjuvant hormonal therapy advances looks at the sequential use of newer agents after the optimal 5 years of tamoxifen or only 2 to 3 years of tamoxifen. Five additional years of letrozole, in a highly publicized study reported in the *New England*

Journal of Medicine, was compared with placebo in postmenopausal breast cancer patients who had completed 5 years of tamoxifen therapy.[106] After a median follow-up of 2.4 years, letrozole was associated with superior estimated 4-year DFS compared with placebo in this setting (93% vs. 87%; $p < 0.001$). While these results were preliminary, patients were unblinded and allowed to crossover to the active arm of therapy. Therefore effects on survival will never be ascertained. However, further follow-up will be completed with regard to safety and DFS in those patients randomized to letrozole from the beginning of the trial. Based on the results of this study, letrozole received FDA approval in November 2004 for extended adjuvant therapy (i.e., after 5 years of tamoxifen therapy). In another recent trial, patients who had completed 2 to 3 years of adjuvant tamoxifen therapy were randomized to continue tamoxifen or crossover to exemestane for the remainder of the 5 years. After a median follow-up of 30.6 months, DFS was substantially longer with exemestane compared with continuation of tamoxifen (91.5% vs. 86.8%; HR = 0.68, $p = 0.00005$).[107] Concerns regarding long-term safety also arise with this study, with data indicating a possible increase in cardiovascular disease, osteoporosis, and visual disturbances with exemestane compared with tamoxifen.

CLINICAL CONTROVERSY

The optimal use of antiaromatase agents in the adjuvant setting for postmenopausal women with hormone-receptor positive tumors is controversial. Multiple studies have recently been published with results indicating a benefit to regimens that include an aromatase inhibitor as initial therapy or after tamoxifen. However, many questions remain as to the optimal drug, dose, sequence, and duration of therapy for these newer agents.

Tamoxifen, as mentioned previously, has been utilized in the adjuvant setting for nearly 30 years and has a very well defined safety and efficacy profile in this setting. It is difficult to change the entire way early breast cancer is treated based on the results of single studies, albeit very large, well designed studies. Nonetheless, these data should be discussed with breast cancer patients who are postmenopausal and have tumors that are hormone-receptor positive.

LOCALLY ADVANCED BREAST CANCER (STAGE III)

Locally advanced cancer breast cancer generally refers to breast carcinomas with significant primary tumor and nodal disease, but in which distant metastases cannot be documented. A wide variety of clinical scenarios can be seen within this group of patients, including neglected tumors that have spread locally, to inflammatory breast cancers that are a unique entity. Inflammatory breast cancer is associated with similar clinical findings compared to other neglected, locally advanced breast tumors (e.g., erythema representing skin involvement). The distinction between the two diagnoses lies in the rapidity of onset of symptoms. Many locally advanced breast cancers are diagnosed in patients that have had symptoms for months to years and have neglected to seek medical attention. While these women have a poor prognosis due to the delay in diagnosis, they are not classified as inflammatory breast cancer. The hallmark of inflammatory breast cancers is the rapid onset of symptoms within weeks to months, including erythema of the skin with or without a detectable underlying breast mass. These patients are often inappropriately treated for cellulitis with antibiotics for several weeks to months. Due to the aggressive nature of this disease, a delay in diagnosis may be fatal for some of these women.

The natural history of locally advanced breast cancer suggested that even when local-regional control was accomplished, systemic relapse and death from breast cancer eventually occurred in most patients.[108] This led to interest in the use of neoadjuvant or primary chemotherapy in locally advanced breast cancer, as discussed previously. This approach to therapy renders inoperable tumors resectable, and can increase rates of breast-conserving therapy. Theoretical advantages also include potential benefits related to early initiation of systemic therapy, delivery of drugs through an intact vasculature, in vivo assessment of response to therapy, and the opportunity to study the biologic effects of the systemic treatment. However, this approach to therapy also results in a loss of standard, well-validated pathologic prognostic markers, such as initial tumor size and the number of axillary lymph nodes involved. Also, as discussed earlier, OS with adjuvant compared with neoadjuvant chemotherapy is similar, making either approach reasonable for a patient with operable breast cancer. For patients with inoperable breast cancer, including inflammatory breast cancer, the initial approach to therapy should be chemotherapy with the goal of achieving resectability.

After neoadjuvant chemotherapy, most tumors respond with more than a 50% decrease in tumor size; about 70% of patients experience downstaging. Chemotherapy regimens used in this setting are similar to those used in the adjuvant setting. Supporting evidence for each individual regimen differs, but most of the available data support the use of anthracycline-containing regimens, incorporation of the taxanes in some manner, and other approaches to improve dose-density or dose-intensity. For more detailed information regarding the specific regimen-related information, the reader is referred to a recently published review.[108] Neoadjuvant endocrine therapy may be an option for patients who have unresectable, hormone receptor–positive tumors who are unable to receive chemotherapy (e.g., multiple comorbid conditions). In terms of local therapy, this usually follows chemotherapy and the extent of surgery will be determined by response to chemotherapy, the wishes of the patient, and the cosmetic results likely to be achieved. However, many patients may be able to have breast-conserving surgery if an acceptable response to chemotherapy is achieved. Adjuvant radiation therapy should be administered to all locally advanced breast cancer patients to minimize local recurrences, regardless of the type of surgery utilized for that individual patient (e.g., mastectomy or segmental mastectomy). Inoperable tumors that are unresponsive to systemic chemotherapy may require radiation therapy for local management and may or may not be eligible for surgical resection after that radiation. These patients are not commonly seen, but have a very poor prognosis. For most patients in this category, cure is still the primary goal of therapy and can be achieved in a large number of patients when all treatment modalities are employed.

METASTATIC BREAST CANCER (STAGE IV)

The goal of therapy with early and locally advanced breast cancer is to cure the disease. But breast cancer is currently incurable after it has advanced beyond local-regional disease. The goal of treatment of metastatic breast cancer is to improve symptoms and quality of life and extended survival. Thus it is important to choose therapy with good activity while minimizing toxicities. Treatment of metastatic breast cancer with either cytotoxic or endocrine therapy often results in regression of disease and improvements in quality of life. In patients who respond to therapy, duration of survival is also increased. The choice of therapy for metastatic disease is based on the site of disease involvement and presence or absence of certain characteristics. For example, patients who experience a long DFS following local-regional therapy, or have disease that is primarily located in the bone or soft tissue will likely respond to endocrine therapy. The most important factor predicting response to endocrine therapy is the presence of estrogen and progesterone receptors in the primary tumor tissue. Fifty to sixty percent of ER-positive patients and 75% to 80% of ER- and PR-positive patients will respond to hormonal therapy, while those with ER- and PR-negative tumors have a less than 10% response rate. Thus the largest factor determining choice of endocrine versus cytotoxic chemotherapy is the presence of hormone receptors in the primary breast tumor. Site of disease is also important in that numerous studies have shown that endocrine therapy is more likely to be effective in patients with bone and soft tissue metastases. Patients with asymptomatic visceral involvement (e.g., liver or lung) may be candidates for hormonal therapy, depending on the clinical circumstance (generally hormones work more slowly than chemotherapy). Patients with symptomatic visceral and/or central nervous system involvement generally have more rapidly growing cancer that requires chemotherapy. Endocrine therapy is the treatment of choice for patients who are hormone receptor–positive and exhibit the first sign of metastatic disease in soft tissue, bone, or pleura, owing to the equal probability of response to hormonal compared to chemotherapy, and the lower toxicity profile of endocrine therapy.

Patients who respond to initial endocrine therapy often respond to a second (or even third) hormonal manipulation. Response rate is lower and duration of response is shorter with second (and third) hormonal manipulations. Patients are sequentially treated with endocrine therapy until their tumors cease to respond, at which time cytotoxic chemotherapy can be given. Combinations of different hormonal therapies or chemotherapy plus hormones are not employed in the setting of metastatic breast cancer, secondary to lack of increased efficacy and evidence of increased toxicity. Women with hormone receptor–negative tumors, with rapidly progressive or symptomatic lung, liver, or bone marrow involvement, or those having progressed on initial endocrine therapy are usually treated initially with cytotoxic chemotherapy. Patients with tumors that have *HER2* overexpression or amplification should be considered for treatment with trastuzumab alone or with chemotherapy.

ENDOCRINE THERAPY

The pharmacologic goals of endocrine therapy for breast cancer are to either decrease circulating levels of estrogen and/or prevent the effects of estrogen at the breast cancer cell (targeted therapy) through blocking the hormone receptors or downregulating the presence of those receptors. Achievement of the first goal depends on the menopausal status of the patient, but achievement of the second goal is independent of menopausal status. Many endocrine therapies are available to target either goal of therapy, and combination studies have also been conducted, attempting to combine differing mechanisms of action and improve outcomes. Unfortunately, combinations have not demonstrated any efficacy benefits, but have increased toxicity. Therefore combinations of endocrine agents for breast cancer are not recommended outside the context of a clinical trial. The concept of sequencing these agents is now becoming popular in the adjuvant setting and may play a role in the metastatic setting when a patient

TABLE 125–13. Endocrine Therapies Used for Metastatic Breast Cancer

Class	Drug	Dose	Side Effects
Aromatase inhibitors			
Nonsteroidal	Anastrozole	1 mg orally daily	Hot flashes, arthralgias,
	Letrozole	2.5 mg orally daily	myalgias, headaches,
Steroidal	Exemestane	25 mg orally daily	diarrhea, mild nausea
Antiestrogens			
SERMs	Tamoxifen	20 mg orally daily	Hot flashes, vaginal
	Toremifene	60 mg orally daily	discharge, mild
			nausea,
			thromboembolism,
			endometrial cancer
SERDs	Fulvestrant	250 mg IM every 28 days	Hot flashes, injection
			site reactions,
			possibly
			thromboembolism.
LHRH analogs	Goserelin	3.6 mg SC every 28 days	Hot flashes,
	Leuprolide	7.5 mg IM every 28 days	amenorrhea,
	Triptorelin	3.75 mg IM every 28 days	menopausal
			symptoms, injection
			site reactions
Progestins	Megestrol acetate	40 mg orally four for a day	Weight gain, hot
	Medroxyprogesterone	400–1000 mg IM every week	flashes, vaginal
			bleeding, edema,
			thromboembolism
Androgens	Fluoxymesterone	10 mg orally twice a day	Deepening voice,
			alopecia, hirsutism,
			facial/truncal acne,
			fluid retention,
			menstrual
			irregularities,
			cholestatic jaundice
Estrogens	Diethylstilbestrol	5 mg orally three for a day	Nausea/vomiting, fluid
	Ethinyl estradiol	1 mg orally three for a day	retention, anorexia,
	Conjugated estrogens	2.5 mg orally three for a day	thromboembolism,
			hepatic dysfunction

SERM, selective estrogen receptor modulator; SERD, selective estrogen receptor downregulator; LHRH, luteinizing hormone-releasing hormone.

is progressing on one agent after gaining significant benefit. These patients are often treated with a series of endocrine agents, often over several years, before chemotherapy is considered.

Until recently, there was little evidence that the response or survival benefit from one endocrine therapy was clearly superior to that achieved with other therapies. Antiestrogens, progestins, aminoglutethimide, estrogens, and androgens, as well as surgical procedures including oophorectomy, adrenalectomy, and hypophysectomy were equivalent in many randomized trials in patients with metastatic breast cancer. Due to the equality in efficacy, the choice of a particular endocrine therapy was based primarily on toxicity (Table 125–13). Based on these criteria, tamoxifen was the preferred initial agent when metastases are present. An exception to this occurs when the patient is receiving adjuvant tamoxifen at the time or within 1 year of occurrence of metastatic disease. In these cases, other agents are generally employed.

Over the past decade, new information has been published regarding the use of a new generation of aromatase inhibitors. These data have changed the way we treat metastatic breast cancer, as well as early-stage breast cancer (as was noted previously). In postmenopausal and castrated women, the main source of estrogen is derived from the peripheral conversion of androstenedione, produced by the adrenal gland, into estrone and estradiol. This conversion requires

the enzyme aromatase. Aromatase also catalyzes the conversion of androgens to estrogens in the ovary in premenopausal women and in extraglandular tissue, including the breast itself, in postmenopausal women. Therefore aromatase inhibitors effectively reduce the level of circulating estrogens, as well as estrogens in the target organ. Aminoglutethimide was the prototype aromatase inhibitor, but was a nonspecific, weak enzyme inhibitor associated with a many toxicities. Many analogues and derivatives of aminoglutethimide have been tested over the years to try and improve on the efficacy:toxicity ratio of this agent. Third-generation aromatase inhibitors are now available, including anastrozole, letrozole, and exemestane. These agents have far greater selectivity and higher potency for the aromatase enzyme than aminoglutethimide. A major advantage of these newer compounds is their reduced toxicity profile, which consists mainly of nausea, hot flashes, arthralgias/myalgias, and mild fatigue. Anastrozole and letrozole are nonsteroidal compounds that exhibit reversible, competitive inhibition of aromatase. These are triazole compounds and have no intrinsic hormonal activity in and of themselves. Exemestane is a steroidal compound and binds irreversibly to aromatase, forming a covalent bond. While this mechanism may appear to be superior to the reversible binding seen with the nonsteroidal agents, there is no clinical evidence that this drug produces superior results over the other agents in this class. Exemestane does possess some androgenic properties that are evident at very high doses, generally much higher than what is used clinically.

The new inhibitors have been compared with megestrol acetate as second-line therapy in postmenopausal women with positive or unknown hormone receptor status who have progressed while on tamoxifen therapy. While response rates with these agents have not been significantly better with the newer agents, time to progression and OS have been significantly better with at least two of the three aromatase inhibitors (anastrozole and exemestane).[109] Rates of clinical benefit (objective response + stabilization of disease for 24 weeks) are also improved with the new aromatase inhibitors. Clinical benefit, a category of response used in metastatic breast cancer clinical trials, is a clinically relevant end point, due to its similar OS compared to tumors that exhibit an objective response.[110] Tolerability is also improved with the aromatase inhibitors compared with megestrol acetate. Toxicity patterns showed more nausea, vomiting, and hot flashes with the aromatase inhibitor and more weight gain and fluid retention with megestrol acetate. All three agents are approved for second-line therapy of advanced breast cancer in postmenopausal women, moving megestrol acetate to third-line therapy.

Both anastrozole and letrozole are also approved for first-line therapy for advanced breast cancer in postmenopausal women. Large trials have compared these agents to tamoxifen and found similar response rates and a longer median time to progression for patients receiving the selective aromatase inhibitor.[109] A consistent finding in these trials was a lower incidence of thromboembolic events and vaginal bleeding in patients who received selective aromatase inhibitors, which, together with the advantage in terms of time to progression, led to the conclusion that the new aromatase inhibitors are superior to tamoxifen as first-line therapy for advanced breast cancer in postmenopausal women. Phase III data with exemestane as first-line therapy compared with tamoxifen are expected in late 2004. A small, randomized phase II trial comparing exemestane to tamoxifen in this setting has demonstrated an advantage with exemestane over tamoxifen in terms of response rates and time to progression.[111] However, this study is not large enough to draw conclusions from, and we await the results of the larger, phase III study to help guide decisions in this setting. Use of a steroidal aromatase inhibitor (exemestane) after a patient progresses on a nonsteroidal inhibitor (anastrozole or letrozole) may provide some benefit and is a common practice based on small clinical trials investigating this sequential approach to therapy.[109] The opposite sequence has also shown some benefit. Therefore patients may receive two aromatase inhibitors (first-line and second-line, sequentially), especially in patients who progress while on adjuvant tamoxifen therapy.

As mentioned several times so far, the aromatase inhibitors are only appropriately used in women who are postmenopausal. Pre- or perimenopausal women, whose ovaries are functioning, are not appropriate candidates for these therapies, at least based on the available evidence. Use of the aromatase inhibitors in addition to ovarian ablation (e.g., oophorectomy or LHRH-agonists) is currently being investigated. Also, the use of aromatase inhibitors in men with advanced breast cancer should be avoided. Available evidence suggests that use of these agents in men increases circulating levels of testosterone, which may negate the therapeutic effects of the drug.[112]

Antiestrogens bind to estrogen receptors, preventing receptor-mediated gene transcription and are therefore used to block the effect of estrogen on the end target. This class of agents is now subdivided into two pharmacologic categories, SERMs and pure antiestrogens. SERMs include tamoxifen and toremifene and demonstrate tissue-specific activity, both estrogenic and antiestrogenic, as described previously. The agonistic activity is thought to be responsible for many of the adverse reactions seen with these agents, including the increased risk of endometrial cancer. Research into how to minimize this agonistic activity has lead to the production of pure estrogen receptor antagonists that lack estrogen agonist activity. Pure antiestrogens are a new class of agents that are also referred to as selective estrogen receptor downregulators (SERDs). These molecules bind to the ER, inhibiting estrogen binding, but cause a degradation of the drug-ER complex, decreasing the amount of ER on the tumor cell surface. There is currently only one pure antiestrogen commercially available in the United States, fulvestrant.

Tamoxifen is generally considered to be the antiestrogen of choice in both premenopausal and postmenopausal women with metastatic breast cancer who have tumors that are hormone receptor–positive. Tamoxifen is usually administered in 20 mg once-daily doses. There is no advantage for higher doses of tamoxifen. Moreover, long-term administration of very high doses of tamoxifen (e.g., 12 months of 60 to 100 mg/m^2 twice daily) is associated with decreased visual acuity and retinopathy.

A dose schedule of tamoxifen 20 mg/day reaches a steady-state concentration after about 4 months of therapy. The half-life of tamoxifen during chronic dosing is 7 days. Serum tamoxifen concentrations can be detected 6 weeks after discontinuation of therapy. Thus the maximum beneficial effects of tamoxifen are not observed for at least 2 months following initiation of therapy, and it is unlikely that symptoms of metastatic disease will return if patients miss several doses. The toxicities of tamoxifen are described in the section on adjuvant endocrine therapy. The only additional toxicity that one might expect to find in the setting of metastatic breast cancer (specifically bone metastases) is a tumor flare or hypercalcemia, which occurs in approximately 5% of patients following the initiation of any SERM therapy and is not an indication to discontinue SERM therapy. It is generally accepted that this is a positive indication that the patient will respond to endocrine therapy. As was mentioned previously, toremifene is another commercially available SERM for the treatment of breast cancer. It exhibits similar efficacy and tolerability compared with tamoxifen in the metastatic setting and is given at a dose of 60 mg daily. The same issues apply to toremifene as were discussed with tamoxifen. Cross-resistance to toremifene has been demonstrated in patients with tamoxifen-refractory disease.[113] Therefore at the current time, toremifene appears to be an alternative to tamoxifen in postmenopausal patients with positive or unknown hormone receptor status with metastatic breast cancer. Raloxifene, another SERM, received approval in December 1997 for prevention of osteoporosis in postmenopausal women. Currently, available data with raloxifene as a treatment for breast cancer are not encouraging (very low response rates, no clinical benefit). The use of this agent for breast cancer treatment should be discouraged. Investigation into the use of raloxifene for prevention of breast cancer in women at high risk is currently underway (see section on prevention and screening).

Fulvestrant is a new agent approved for the second-line therapy of postmenopausal metastatic breast cancer patients who have tumors that are hormone receptor–positive. It is given as an intramuscular injection every 28 days and is marketed as a single injection of 5 mL or two injections of 2.5 mL each.[114] Studies examining the role of fulvestrant in the treatment of metastatic breast cancer have compared this agent to anastrozole. Due to the nature of anastrozole's mechanism of action, only postmenopausal women were eligible for these trials. There is no biologic reason why fulvestrant should not produce similar outcomes in premenopausal women, but no data exist to confirm the safety or efficacy in premenopausal women. In the comparative trials with fulvestrant and anastrozole, similar efficacy and safety were demonstrated with both agents when given after patients progressed on tamoxifen therapy.[115,116] Adverse events related to fulvestrant include injection site reactions, hot flashes, asthenia, and headaches. The dose of fulvestrant is 250 mg given intramuscularly every 28 days. This agent is covered by Medicare and is a good option for patients who are unable to take an oral medication.

Another goal of antitumor treatment is to reduce estrogen production in premenopausal women with surgery, irradiation, or medication. No difference has been found in two randomized trials of the overall response rate between tamoxifen and oophorectomy in premenopausal women. However, the secondary response rate to oophorectomy after tamoxifen treatment was somewhat higher than the response to tamoxifen after primary oophorectomy (33% vs. 11%).[117] Some experts interpret this as suggesting that tamoxifen does not completely antagonize available estrogen, particularly in premenopausal women. Ovarian ablation (surgically or chemically) is still commonly used in some parts of the United States and is considered by many specialists to be the endocrine therapy of choice in premenopausal women. The mortality rate with surgical oophorectomy is low, usually less than 2% to 3% in appropriately selected patients. Irradiation of the ovaries was a means of castration many years ago, but was associated with multiple complications and is no longer performed for these purposes. Chemical castration with LHRH analogs is increasingly used in lieu of oophorectomy in premenopausal women.

Medical castration with LHRH analogs has been used in premenopausal metastatic breast cancer patients and induces remission in about one-third of unselected cases. The mechanism of action of LHRH analogs in breast cancer is thought to result from downregulation of LHRH receptors in the pituitary. Decreased levels of luteinizing hormone subsequently lead to a decrease in estrogen to castrated levels. Thus the effect of LHRH analogs on circulating estrogen levels in premenopausal breast cancer simulates oophorectomy. The three agents available in the United States are leuprolide, goserelin, and triptorelin, but only goserelin is approved for the treatment of metastatic breast cancer. These agents are administered as an injection every 4 weeks (all products have extended formulations, lasting 3 to 4 months) and are associated with minimal side effects including amenorrhea, hot flashes, and occasional nausea (see Table 125–13). A recent meta-analysis was reported on combined tamoxifen and LHRH agonists versus LHRH agonists alone in premenopausal patients with metastatic breast cancer.[118] With a median follow-up of 6.8 years, there was a significant survival benefit and progression-free survival benefit in favor of the combined treatment. The overall response rate was significantly higher on combined endocrine treatment. However, this analysis did not compare tamoxifen alone to the combination of an LHRH agonist with tamoxifen. Therefore if an LHRH agonist is used as first-line therapy for metastatic breast cancer, it should be used in combination with tamoxifen. If tamoxifen is used as first-line therapy for metastatic breast cancer, then there are no data supporting adding an LHRH agonist to this setting. This is a very controversial topic that may be answered through clinical trials in the next few years, but currently it is up to the individual clinician and patient to decide. LHRH agonists may also produce a flare response due to an initial surge in LH and estrogen production for the first 2 to 4 weeks. This flare response is similar to that seen with tamoxifen and patients should be monitored for increasing pain and/or hypercalcemia during the initiation period.

Progestins such as megestrol acetate and medroxyprogesterone acetate have been compared with tamoxifen in randomized trials and have been found to yield equal response rates. Although there were no direct comparisons of these two forms of progestational therapy, they appear to be equally effective. Medroxyprogesterone acetate is more frequently used in Europe, and megestrol acetate is more frequently used in the United States. Based on efficacy and tolerability, these agents are generally reserved as third-line therapy after patients have received an aromatase inhibitor and a SERM (tamoxifen or toremifene). The most common dose used for megestrol acetate is 160 mg/day; the most common side effect is weight gain, occurring in 20% to 50% of patients. Patients experiencing weight gain may have fluid retention, but fluid retention is not totally responsible for total weight gain. In cachectic cancer patients, the weight gain may be desirable, but this is not uniformly true of all patients with metastatic breast cancer. Additional side effects associated with progestins include vaginal bleeding in 5% to 10% of patients either while patients are taking the progestational agent or when it is discontinued, and somewhat less than a 10% incidence of hot flashes. Thromboembolic complications are also significant with these agents.

High-dose estrogens and androgens are rarely used today because these agents are more toxic than the other hormonal agents discussed thus far. About one-third of patients placed on high-dose estrogens will discontinue them because of side effects, the most important of which are thromboembolic events, vomiting, and fluid retention. Less common side effects include areolar hyperpigmentation, breast tenderness and engorgement, vaginal discharge, incontinence, hot flashes, and phlebitis. All the effective androgens cause masculinizing effects, including hirsutism and acne, in more than 50% of patients. In addition to their toxicities, the mechanism by which these agents exert a therapeutic effect in breast cancer is unknown. About 20% response rates were reported in clinical trials conducted in the 1960s and 1970s in unselected groups of breast cancer patients. Given the recent availability of the aromatase inhibitors, use of androgens and estrogens has become rare.

CYTOTOXIC THERAPY

Cytotoxic chemotherapy is eventually required in most patients with metastatic breast cancer. Patients with hormone receptor–negative tumors require chemotherapy as initial therapy of symptomatic metastases. Patients who initially respond to hormonal manipulations eventually cease to respond and go on to require chemotherapy. Combination chemotherapy results in an objective response in about 40% of patients previously unexposed to chemotherapy. Most patients have partial responses, and complete disappearance of disease occurs in fewer than 10% of patients treated. The median duration of response is 5 to 12 months, but some patients will have an excellent response to an initial course of chemotherapy and may live 5 to 10 years or longer without evidence of disease. In general, median survival of patients after treatment with commonly used drug combinations for metastatic breast cancer is 14 to 33 months. The median time to response has ranged from 2 to 3 months in most studies, but this period depends in large part on the site of measurable disease. The median time to appearance of response is between 3 and 6 weeks in patients whose disease is primarily in the skin and lymph nodes, 6 to 9 weeks for patients with metastatic lung involvement, 15 weeks with hepatic involvement, and nearly 18 weeks in patients with bone involvement. Thus it is often the case that an immediate response to therapy is not apparent, and in general, once a chemotherapy regimen has been initiated, it is continued until there is unequivocal evidence of progressive disease.

There are no well-defined clinical characteristics or established tests to identify patients likely to benefit from chemotherapy. Factors associated with an increased probability of response that have been identified include a good performance status, a limited number (one to two) of disease sites, and patients who respond to chemotherapy or hormonal therapy with a long disease-free interval. Patients who have progressive disease during chemotherapy have a lower probability of response to a different type of chemotherapy. However, this is not necessarily true for patients who are given chemotherapy after some interval during which they have received no chemotherapy. Patients who do not respond to endocrine therapy are as likely to respond to chemotherapy as patients who are treated with chemotherapy as their initial treatment modality. Age, menopausal status, and receptor status have not been associated with favorable or unfavorable response to chemotherapy.

A number of chemotherapeutic agents have demonstrated activity in the treatment of breast cancer, including doxorubicin, epirubicin, paclitaxel, docetaxel, capecitabine, fluorouracil, cyclophosphamide, methotrexate, vinblastine, vinorelbine, gemcitabine, mitoxantrone, mitomycin-C, thiotepa, and melphalan. The most active classes of chemotherapy in metastatic breast cancer are the anthracyclines and the taxanes, producing response rates as high as 50% to 60% in patients who have not received prior chemotherapy for metastatic disease.[119] Paclitaxel was approved by the FDA in 1994 for single-agent treatment of metastatic breast cancer for patients who had relapsed following therapy with a doxorubicin-containing regimen. The FDA-recommended dose of paclitaxel is 175 mg/m^2 every 21 days, which is considerably higher than the dose used for treatment of ovarian cancer, the other disease for which paclitaxel has obtained FDA approval for use. Studies investigating the optimal dose and schedule of paclitaxel indicate higher response rates and less toxicity with weekly administration versus every-3-week administration.[88] The most useful weekly dose in the metastatic setting appears to be 80 mg/m^2 per week with no breaks in therapy. With this approach, the toxicity profile of paclitaxel changes with less myelosuppression and delayed onset of peripheral neuropathy, but slightly more fluid retention and skin and nail changes. Also, at such low doses, the incidence of hypersensitivity reactions is slightly less, requiring fewer premedications. However, the incidence of hypersensitivity reactions remains approximately 3%, even with all available preventive measures. Docetaxel has also demonstrated high single-agent activity against metastatic breast cancer. The FDA approved it in 1995 for treatment of metastatic breast cancer for patients with relapse following therapy with doxorubicin-containing regimens. The approved dose is 60 to 100 mg/m^2 administered every 3 weeks. Impressive overall response rates of 54% to 68% were reported in four studies of docetaxel 100 mg/m^2 as first-line chemotherapy. A randomized study comparing doses of 60 mg/m^2, 75 mg/m^2, and 100 mg/m^2 was recently published, demonstrating a dose-response relationship with regard to response rates only.[120] Time to progression and overall survival were similar between all three dose levels. Therefore dose remains important for symptomatic patients who require a rapid response to therapy. In asymptomatic patients requiring docetaxel chemotherapy, lower doses may be appropriate. Myelosuppression is the major dose-limiting toxicity of docetaxel. Nonhematologic toxicities include fatigue, mucosal toxicity, mild to moderate nausea and vomiting, diarrhea, and neurosensory complaints. Results from a single randomized trial appear to indicate that docetaxel is associated with less neuropathy, myalgia, and hypersensitivity than paclitaxel given every 3 weeks; but febrile neutropenia, fluid retention, and skin reactions appear to occur more frequently with the newer taxane.[121] The median cumulative docetaxel dose to the onset of fluid retention is 400 mg/m^2 in nonpremedicated patients. Recent data demonstrate that the prophylactic use of dexamethasone 8 mg orally, twice a day for 3 days, starting 24 hours before the docetaxel infusion can significantly delay the onset and reduce the severity of fluid retention, as well as decrease the incidence and severity of hypersensitivity reactions, nausea, and skin rashes.

Capecitabine is a novel agent approved in the mid-1990s with significant activity in metastatic breast cancer patients who have progressed on an anthracycline-containing regimen as well as a taxane regimen. This agent is a prodrug for fluorouracil with somewhat targeted activity towards malignant cells. The parent compound undergoes a three-step enzymatic conversion to become fluorouracil at the target cell. The third and final step in this conversion is more likely to occur in malignant cells than normal cells due to the presence of higher levels of the responsible enzyme in malignant tissues. In patients who have been exposed to an anthracycline and a taxane, capecitabine produces response rates of about 25%, which is impressive compared to other tested chemotherapy agents.[122] The dose-limiting side effects with this agent are unique and include palmar-plantar erythrodysesthesia (hand-foot syndrome), diarrhea, and mucositis. Very little myelosuppression or nausea is experienced with this agent, but monitoring patients for these adverse events is still warranted. Capecitabine is an oral chemotherapy agent that is given twice a day for 14 days, followed by 1 week of rest in a 21-day cycle. The approved dose of capecitabine is 2,500 mg/m^2 per day divided twice daily as indicated above. In retrospective studies, this dose appears to be poorly tolerated and dose reductions are required in nearly all patients.[123,124] Therefore, many clinicians prefer to start at 2,000 mg/m^2 per day in a similar schedule, especially in light of the goals of therapy for metastatic breast cancer. The retrospective analyses appear to indicate no loss of efficacy with this approach, but randomized controlled trials looking at different doses of capecitabine have not yet been completed.

Vinorelbine, a microtubule interactive agent, has also shown impressive response rates in metastatic breast cancer.[125] Vinorelbine was approved by the FDA in 1994 for the treatment of non-small-cell lung cancer. It is not approved for breast cancer, but response rates to weekly IV doses of 30 mg/m^2 of vinorelbine range from 30% to 50%, with an overall 5% complete response rate in the phase I and phase II studies in patients with advanced breast cancer. As has been observed with paclitaxel and docetaxel, patients with less prior treatment have a higher response rate than those who are more heavily pretreated. Importantly, paclitaxel, docetaxel, and vinorelbine do not appear to be cross-resistant with anthracyclines, which are arguably considered first-line in treatment of metastatic breast cancer.

Gemcitabine is another agent that is used quite frequently in patients who have received the aforementioned chemotherapy regimens, who still have a good performance status and may benefit from additional chemotherapy. This is a nucleotide analogue that inhibits DNA synthesis. Response rates ranging from 13% to 42% have been reported in a number of phase II trials.[125] In patients who have been exposed to an anthracycline and a taxane, gemcitabine appears to provide similar benefit to capecitabine. However, the studies with gemcitabine are much smaller than with capecitabine. Nonetheless, gemcitabine is utilized for the treatment of metastatic breast cancer and many ongoing trials are further investigating where this agent may fit into therapy. The dose of gemcitabine varies depending on the extent of prior therapy and bone marrow reserve, but generally ranges from 800 to 1,250 mg/m^2 given IV on days 1, 8, and 15 every 28 days. The day 15 dose is often omitted due to myelosuppression. This agent appears to affect platelets more frequently than other chemotherapy previously mentioned, and close monitoring is required for patients receiving this agent. Other common adverse events include a flu-like syndrome with fever, chills, myalgias and arthralgias, and mild nausea.

Combination chemotherapy regimens are associated with higher response rates than are single-agent therapies in the treatment of metastatic breast cancer, but the higher response rates have not usually translated into significant differences in time to progression and OS. The use of sequential single-agent chemotherapies versus the combination regimens has been widely debated for metastatic breast cancer.

CLINICAL CONTROVERSY

The benefits of combination chemotherapy regimens for metastatic breast cancer over sequential single agents have not been clearly defined. There are a few trials that have compared combination regimens to single agent chemotherapy, with higher response rates seen with the combination. However, these trials fail to include an arm with the same agents given sequentially. Therefore it is not clear whether sequential single agents or combination regimens are optimal in this setting.

One trial investigating the combination of doxorubicin with paclitaxel versus each single agent with crossover to the other agent upon progression set out to help answer the question of which is more effective.[126] While response rates were higher with the combination regimen, time to progression and OS were similar between all arms of the study. This was more than likely due to the fact that most patients who progressed on their first single agent, went on to receive the second-line single agent, thereby negating any potential survival benefits seen with improved response rates. In another study comparing single-agent docetaxel to the combination of docetaxel with capecitabine, the combination arm produced higher response rates, time to progression, and OS compared with the single agent.[127] However, only 15% of patients in the docetaxel alone arm received capecitabine after progression. Therefore this study does not answer the question of whether combination therapy is better than sequential single-agent therapy. It is widely accepted that combination regimens do impart greater toxicity. In the palliative metastatic setting, using the least toxic approach is preferred when efficacy is considered equal. In clinical practice, patients who require a rapid response to chemotherapy (e.g., those with symptomatic bulky metastases) often receive combination therapy despite the added toxicity. This decision is complex and should be made on an individual patient basis.

Because most patients are given adjuvant chemotherapy, regimens chosen for first-line use in the metastatic setting are often different from those used in the adjuvant setting. If a patient's cancer recurs within 1 year of finishing adjuvant chemotherapy, those chemotherapy agents are not considered effective for treatment of her metastatic disease. However, if the patient recurs more than 1 year after the end of her adjuvant chemotherapy, the same agents may also be helpful in the metastatic setting.

BIOLOGIC THERAPY

Trastuzumab is a humanized monoclonal antibody that binds with a specific epitope of the HER-2/neu protein. The parent antibody (monoclonal antibody, 4D5) induces a specific biologic response through activation of *HER-2/neu*; this response includes autophosphorylation of the tyrosine kinase internal domain leading to inhibition of cellular growth, decreased malignant potential, and possibly reversal of resistance to certain chemotherapies and possibly endocrine therapy. Single-agent treatment with trastuzumab has a response rate of 15% to 20% and a clinical benefit rate of nearly 40% of patients with *HER-2/neu*–overexpressing cancers.[128] Moreover, the results of a large randomized trial demonstrated that trastuzumab is at least

additive, and perhaps has synergistic activity with other chemotherapeutic agents.[129] In this pivotal trial comparing chemotherapy in combination with trastuzumab versus chemotherapy alone, the addition of trastuzumab increased response rates, time to progression, and overall survival when compared to chemotherapy alone. Patients in this trial who were anthracycline naïve were treated with an anthracycline (mostly doxorubicin, some epirubicin) plus cyclophosphamide, and patients who had received an adjuvant anthracycline regimen were treated with paclitaxel. During this trial, it became apparent that patients receiving the anthracycline-trastuzumab combination had a very high incidence of cardiotoxicity (27%), leading to discontinuation of this arm of the study and a black box warning regarding this contraindication in the product information for trastuzumab. Many investigators are attempting to circumvent this toxicity while giving these two classes of agents together (e.g., liposomal doxorubicin or continuous-infusion doxorubicin). However, until further information regarding the safety of these approaches becomes available, this combination should not be given outside the context of a clinical trial. Many other chemotherapy agents have successfully been administered with trastuzumab. Only one other phase III trial has been published comparing chemotherapy alone versus chemotherapy plus trastuzumab. Extra and colleagues compared docetaxel alone versus docetaxel with trastuzumab in patients with previously untreated *HER2/neu*-positive metastatic breast cancer.[130] This trial demonstrated significant advantages to the combination in terms of response rates, time to progression, and OS.

Other chemotherapy agents that have been evaluated in several phase II trials include vinorelbine, gemcitabine, capecitabine, and the platinum agents (cisplatin and carboplatin). In phase II trials vinorelbine in combination with trastuzumab has shown very high response rates even in heavily pretreated patients.[131] This combination is now in phase III clinical trials to investigate whether this combination may be better than a taxane-trastuzumab combination as front-line therapy for metastatic breast cancer. In another phase III trial, the triplet combination of paclitaxel, carboplatin, and trastuzumab was compared with paclitaxel and trastuzumab as a dual therapy.[132] This study demonstrated superior response rates and time to progression with the triplet regimen versus the doublet regimen. However, toxicities with the addition of carboplatin were significantly greater in terms of myelosuppression and nausea. This is important information to keep in mind when making treatment decisions for metastatic breast cancer patients, recalling the importance of palliation of symptoms in this setting.

These studies suggest that trastuzumab is reasonably well tolerated. The most common adverse effects are infusion-related, primarily fever and chills, and occur in about 40% of patients during the initial infusion. These effects generally are mild to moderate and last approximately 1 to 2 hours after the infusion is started. Other infusion-related reactions include nausea, vomiting, pain at tumor sites, rigors, headaches, dizziness, dyspnea, hypotension, rash, and asthenia, which are much less common.[133] These reactions are also usually mild to moderate and rarely require discontinuation of therapy. Acetaminophen and diphenhydramine may be given and/or the infusion rate reduced to help alleviate the symptoms related to these reactions. If infusion-related symptoms occur, subsequent doses should be infused over 90 minutes. Infusion over 30 minutes is appropriate if symptoms subside. A more severe reaction consisting of severe hypersensitivity and/or pulmonary reactions have been reported, but are rare. It is important to educate patients regarding the pulmonary reactions, as these may occur up to 24 hours after the infusion and can be fatal if not promptly treated. Again, this is a rare occurrence, but patient education is paramount to ensure a successful outcome.

Trastuzumab may increase the incidence of infection, diarrhea, and/or other adverse events when given with chemotherapy. However, most of these increases are not clinically significant for the individual patient.

One exception to this statement is the cardiotoxicity seen with this agent both in combination and as a single agent. As mentioned previously, when given with an anthracycline the rates of heart failure are unacceptably high, but even when given as a single agent there is about a 5% incidence of heart failure. Fortunately, the heart failure seen with trastuzumab is somewhat reversible with pharmacologic management and some patients have continued therapy with trastuzumab after their left ventricular ejection fraction has returned to normal. There are no systematic guidelines for cardiac monitoring with this agent. However, close monitoring for clinical signs and symptoms of heart failure is important in order to intervene with appropriate cardiac treatments.

Trastuzumab is administered as an initial loading dose of 4 mg/kg; this is followed by a 2-mg/kg dose administered weekly. One small, phase II study has demonstrated successful administration of trastuzumab on a 3-week schedule with a 8-mg/kg loading dose followed 3 weeks later with a 6-mg/kg maintenance dose given every 3 weeks.[134] This method of administration is more convenient than weekly administration, but comparative data with this dose and schedule versus the standard dose and schedule are not available at this time. When patients progress on therapy with trastuzumab, many clinicians will continue the trastuzumab and change the chemotherapy regimen. This approach to management is not systematically addressed in the literature, but is a very important question to answer. It is hoped that in the near future there will be a clinical trial to answer this question. Until that time, continuing trastuzumab and changing chemotherapy appears to be a reasonable approach to managing metastatic breast cancer patients.

Although trastuzumab is currently indicated only for the treatment of metastatic breast cancer, several cooperative groups are evaluating its safety and efficacy in women with HER-2/neu-overexpressing breast cancer in the adjuvant and neoadjuvant settings. It should be noted that only 20% to 30% of patients with metastatic breast cancer overexpress HER-2/neu, and commercially available IHC tests that are reported back as 2+ for HER-2/neu are often negative by the more sensitive and specific FISH technique. To date, there is no benefit associated with the administration of trastuzumab to the subset of patients who are HER-2/neu–negative, and a very questionable benefit associated with administration of trastuzumab to women who are 2+ for HER-2/neu by IHC staining alone. The patients who benefit most from trastuzumab therapy include those whose tumors express HER2 protein at the 3+ level and/or demonstrate gene amplification by FISH testing.

■ RADIATION THERAPY

Radiation is an important modality in the treatment of symptomatic metastatic disease. The most common indication for the treatment with radiation therapy is painful bone metastases or other localized sites of disease refractory to systemic therapy. Radiation therapy gives significant pain relief to approximately 90% of patients who are treated for painful bone metastases. Radiation is also an important modality in the palliative treatment of metastatic brain lesions and spinal cord lesions, which respond poorly to systemic therapy, as well as eye or orbit lesions and other sites where significant accumulation of tumor cells occurs. Skin and/or lymph node metastases confined to the chest wall area may also be treated with radiation therapy for palliation (e.g., open wounds or painful lesions).

PREVENTION AND EARLY DETECTION

Current efforts at breast cancer prevention are directed toward the identification and removal of risk factors. Unfortunately, a number of risk factors associated with development of breast cancer, such as family history of breast cancer or personal history of breast or other gynecologic malignancies, cannot be modified. Isolation and cloning of breast cancer susceptibility genes now allows screening of women with histories suggestive of "breast cancer families" and identification of appropriate candidates for prophylactic bilateral mastectomy. There are currently no absolute indications for prophylactic bilateral mastectomy. This surgery is considered for women at very high risk for the development of breast cancer, particularly if the women's breasts are difficult to evaluate by both physical examination and mammography, and they have persistent disabling fears that they will be diagnosed with the disease.

In the past 10 years, there has been increasing interest in chemoprevention of breast cancer. This includes interventions directed at inhibiting neoplastic development through pharmacologic measures. Two important classes of agents being studied for breast cancer chemoprevention are the retinoids and SERMs. Retinoids (all vitamin A and its isomer derivatives and synthetic analogs) are biologic regulators of orderly epithelial cell development, and are therefore potentially ideal agents for controlling abnormal epithelial proliferation that occurs in carcinogenesis. While only preclinical data are available suggesting a benefit with these types of therapies, clinical trials are needed to further investigate the role of the retinoids in prevention of breast cancer.

The agent that is currently receiving the most attention as a chemoprevention agent for breast cancer is tamoxifen. As previously described, tamoxifen is useful as an adjunct after treatment of primary breast cancer. In randomized trials of tamoxifen as an adjuvant treatment for breast cancer, women who received tamoxifen were also found to have a reduced incidence of contralateral primary breast carcinomas.[71] The NSABP, in a large, randomized placebo-controlled study, demonstrated significant reductions in risk of invasive and noninvasive breast cancers with 5 years of tamoxifen therapy (20 mg/day).[98] While this study is controversial, other studies have also been reported around the world investigating the role of tamoxifen in chemoprevention. A recent meta-analysis of these trials is available and indicates a consistent benefit in reducing the incidence of ER-positive breast cancers (48%).[135] Tamoxifen has been repeatedly shown to be a relatively safe drug with an acceptable toxicity profile when used to treat patients with breast cancer. However, its estrogenic effects on the uterus and the coagulation system increase the risk of serious adverse effects that may be critical for patients taking this agent in the prevention setting. Toxicities associated with tamoxifen were further described in the section on adjuvant endocrine therapy. Therefore any decision to use tamoxifen for chemoprevention should not be made lightly, and all the information regarding the individual woman's risk of breast cancer, the potential benefits of tamoxifen, and the potential serious adverse events associated with tamoxifen,

TABLE 125–14. Guidelines for Early Detection of Breast Cancer

	American Cancer Society[136]	U.S. Preventive Services Task Force[137]	National Cancer Institute[138]
BSE	Age ≥20: risk/benefit discussion	All ages: ±	NR
CBS	Age 20–30: every 3 years	All ages: ± (recommended with mammogram)	All ages: every year
	Age ≥40: every year		
Mammogram	Age ≥40: interval not designated	Age ≥40: every 1–2 years (± CBE)	Age 40–49: every 1–2 years
			Age ≥50: every 1–2 years

BSE, breast self-examination; CBE, clinical breast examination; NR, not recommended; ±, insufficient data to recommend for or against.

should all be discussed at length with every patient considering this agent.

Although raloxifene was shown to reduce the risk of invasive breast cancer by a similar percentage (in clinical trials in which it was evaluated for osteoporosis), the use of raloxifene should be reserved for its approved indication, which is to prevent bone loss in postmenopausal women. The ongoing Study of Tamoxifen and Raloxifene trial directly compares the efficacy and safety of tamoxifen and raloxifene in the chemoprevention of breast cancer. Use of raloxifene for this indication should await the results of this trial. At the present time, the use of tamoxifen or raloxifene with other medications, such as hormone replacement therapy, and tamoxifen and raloxifene in combination or sequentially, has not been adequately studied. However, an increased risk of thromboembolic complications may be seen with these combinations, possibly causing more harm than good. A similar reduction in the incidence of contralateral primary breast cancers was demonstrated with anastrozole in the adjuvant ATAC study (discussed previously), leading to the premise that aromatase inhibitors may also play a role in chemoprevention of breast cancer.[105] No data are yet available investigating these agents in the setting of prevention, but clinical trials are planned.

The rationale for early detection of breast cancer is based on the clear relationship between stage of breast cancer at diagnosis and the probability for cure. Thus if all breast cancer could be detected at a very early stage of the disease (i.e., small primary tumor and negative lymph nodes), then more patients with the disease could be cured. Screening guidelines for early detection of breast cancer have been put forward by the American Cancer Society, the U.S. Preventive Services Task Force, and the National Cancer Institute (Table 125–14).[136–138] These all include recommendations for women at average risk, with some general statements regarding screening for high-risk women as well.

Currently, the American Cancer Society recommends that all women over the age of 20 years be informed of the benefits and limitations of breast self-examinations (BSE).[136] There are several studies that have attempted to investigate the benefits of BSE. These trials were primarily conducted prior to the age of mammographic screening and demonstrated an inferential benefit in diagnosis of earlier stages of breast cancer. One more recent trial, the Shanghai trial, appeared to indicate no benefit, but a higher rate of biopsies in women who were taught BSE compared with women who were not taught BSE.[139] The investigators from this trial caution that this was a study of BSE instruction and not BSE performance. Compliance and competency with the BSE were not guaranteed nor looked at in this trial. Due to the lack of direct evidence to support or refute a benefit with BSE, the ACS has taken the stance that it is not recommended, but women of all ages should be instructed and encouraged to be aware

of their breasts in order to recognize any changes and promptly report these to a health professional.[136] The U.S. Preventive Services Task Force and the NCI came to similar conclusions.[137,138]

Recommendations for breast examination by a health care professional (clinical breast examination) vary among the three available screening guidelines. The rate of breast cancer detection using clinical breast examination (CBE) alone is low, with even lower rates in younger women and women with higher body weight.[136] Randomized clinical trials have inconsistent results and often looked at use of this screening tool in conjunction with mammograms. The American Cancer Society recommends CBE in conjunction with mammography for women aged 40 and older.[136] For younger patients it is recommended as part of a periodic health examination every 3 years, but this recommendation is based on weak evidence. The NCI recommends CBE for women 40 and older in conjunction with mammography every 1 to 2 years.[138] The U.S. Preventive Services Task Force guidelines for screening state that there is insufficient evidence to recommend for or against CBE alone.[137] Nonetheless, with most yearly visits for gynecologic examination (e.g., pelvic exam and Pap smears), the health professional usually performs a breast exam as part of that evaluation.

Clearly, the largest area of controversy in screening recommendations for breast cancer surrounds annual mammography. Most, if not all, guidelines recommend annual mammography for women 50 years of age and older. Nearly 75% of all breast cancer occurs in women 50 years of age or older, and it has been conclusively demonstrated that regular use of screening mammography can reduce mortality from breast cancer by 20% to 40% in this age group. Controversy regarding the use of screening mammography is largely confined to women younger than 50 years of age. After many years of debate, the three available guidelines discussed here recommend mammograms in this age group of women every 1 to 2 years.[136–138] Controversy lies in the nuances of these data. Clearly the benefits in terms of mortality with screening a younger population are numerically smaller. Nonetheless, there is a reduction in mortality with screening mammograms in women ages 40 to 49. There are also many other debates within this controversial area and the reader is referred to these references for further details.[136–138] Other radiologic methods of breast imaging are also being investigated (e.g., digital mammography and magnetic resonance imaging [MRI]). Recommendations for women with a high risk of breast cancer are not fully established.

It should also be noted here that the risks associated with screening mammography are present and should be discussed with each patient so they are able to make an informed decision regarding these procedures. The risks involved with screening mammograms include false-negative results, false-positive results, overdiagnosis (true-positives that will not become clinically significant), and radiation risk. The rate of false-negative results with the current technology is about 20%, which is why CBE is an important adjunct to screening for many women. While the specificity of mammography is quite high (90%), the majority of abnormal exams are false-positives, leading to additional biopsies and psychological distress. The issue of overdiagnosis refers primarily to the growth in detection of DCIS from screening mammography. The biological significance of these tumors is unknown, as only a portion of them would become invasive if left in place. So the question remains, are we treating women who do not require treatment? Experts in the field continue to debate this issue. Radiation exposure also has been discussed in the context of screening mammography, but the small doses of radiation exposure with mammograms (2 to 4 mGy per standard two-view exam) appears to be overshadowed by other benefits in terms of reduction in mortality due to early cancer detection.[138]

Significant advances in the safety and efficacy of screening mammography have occurred during the past two decades. These advances have enabled superior visualization of breast and breast tissue with a concurrent reduction in the dose of radiation that is delivered. About 10% of all palpable masses are not detected by mammography. This is most commonly observed in premenopausal women, and may be directly related to the increased density of breast tissue in this estrogen-rich environment.

Although the safety and efficacy of screening mammography in terms of image quality and dosimetry are very acceptable, the American College of Radiology (ACR) has recognized for some years the need for greater quality control in mammography. A voluntary accreditation program developed by this organization and adopted by various state and federal agencies has greatly improved the overall quality of mammography in the majority of facilities in this country. Many of the details of the accreditation process have recently been adopted for use by governmental agencies, culminating in the Mammography Quality Standards of 1992. This act, which essentially codifies the ACR program, assures that all mammographic facilities will now be required to achieve a common high standard of quality assurance. Responsibility for operation of the act has been given to the FDA. As of October 1, 1994, all facilities that offer mammography must be FDA-certified to remain open. Passage of this landmark legislation, as well as provision of appropriate levels of funding to conduct this program, represents an important contribution to the health of women.

EVALUATION OF THERAPEUTIC OUTCOMES

The desired therapeutic outcome of adjuvant therapy of breast cancer differs significantly from that of metastatic disease. Adjuvant therapy—chemotherapy, hormonal therapy, or both—is administered with curative intent. The rationale for adjuvant therapy is that breast cancer, even when diagnosed in early stages when clinical evidence of distant spread is not apparent, is a systemic disease that spreads early to distant sites. Adjuvant therapy is intended to eradicate these micrometastases and thus cure the patient of breast cancer. Therefore the overall goal of adjuvant therapy is to cure the disease, which is something that cannot be fully evaluated for years following initial diagnosis and treatment. In addition, because there is no clinical evidence of disease at the time adjuvant therapy is started, assessment of disease response is not possible. Instead, a predetermined number of cycles of adjuvant therapy and/or years of hormonal therapy are administered. Adjuvant chemotherapy is often associated with significant toxicity. Maintaining dose intensity has been demonstrated to be important in the cure of disease, and therefore optimizing supportive care measures such as antiemetics and growth factors is highly

recommended. The goals of therapy with neoadjuvant chemotherapy are slightly different. These goals focus on earlier end points of tumor response in order to minimize surgery, determine prognosis, and potentially conserve the breast tissue for a better cosmetic result. The other outcomes discussed with adjuvant therapy also apply to this scenario as well, in terms of improving survival and decreasing recurrences compared to no systemic therapy.

Palliation is the therapeutic outcome in treatment of metastatic breast cancer. In general, the least toxic therapies are used initially, with increasingly aggressive therapies applied in a sequential fashion and in a manner that does not significantly compromise the quality of the patient's life. Tumor response to a particular treatment regimen may be measured by clinical chemistry such as liver enzyme elevation in a patient with hepatic metastases, or imaging techniques such as bone scans or chest x-rays. However, assessment of the patient's clinical status and symptom control is often adequate to evaluate response to the therapy administered. In the patient with metastatic breast cancer, it is common to initiate hormonal therapy or chemotherapy and continue administration until signs and symptoms of disease progress or new signs and symptoms present. Optimizing quality of life is the therapeutic end point in the treatment of patients with metastatic breast cancer. A number of valid and reliable tools are available for objective assessment of quality of life in patients with breast cancer.

CONCLUSIONS

Breast cancer is the most commonly occurring cancer in women in the United States, and is second only to lung cancer as the most common cancer cause of death. The etiology of breast cancer is unknown, but a number of factors that increase a woman's chances of developing the disease have been identified. These risk factors, as well as information regarding the biology of the disease, suggest that a complex interplay between hormones, genetic factors, and environmental and lifestyle influences all contribute to the etiology of this disease. The recent identification of the *BRCA1* and *BRCA2* genes, tumor-suppressor genes important in the development of inherited and perhaps sporadic breast and ovarian cancer, holds promise in identifying patients at high risk, as well as improving our basic understanding of the causes of breast and ovarian cancer.

Most breast cancers are diagnosed in early stages before the disease has disseminated to sites distant from the breast. Treatment consists of local management, as well as systemic adjuvant therapy with chemotherapy, hormonal therapy, or a combination of these. Breast-conservation therapy, which consists of complete removal of the tumor (lumpectomy), combined with breast irradiation and axillary lymph node sampling, is currently the preferred method of treatment for most patients with localized breast cancer. Patients who are not candidates for breast conservation or who do not choose this local therapy will generally receive the modified radical mastectomy.

It is apparent from clinical and laboratory experiments and observation that the spread of breast cancer via the bloodstream occurs early in the course of the disease. This results in patients relapsing with systemic metastatic disease following local curative therapy. The likelihood of later development of metastatic disease is related to the size of the primary tumor, presence of lymph node involvement and number of nodes affected, and a number of additional pathologic prognostic factors, which include proliferative capacity, nuclear grade, hormone receptor status, and presence or absence of oncogenes and other protein products. Systemic adjuvant therapy is commonly administered to patients with localized breast cancer following surgical procedures to diminish the risk of or delay disease recurrence. The NIH and other groups have developed guidelines for adjuvant systemic therapy for early-stage breast cancer based on expert consensus, and these treatment recommendations continue to evolve as new data become available.

Advanced breast cancer includes locally advanced breast cancer (stage III) and metastatic breast cancer (stage IV). Treatment of stage III breast cancer generally consists of a combination of surgery, radiation, and chemotherapy administered in an aggressive approach. Although response rates and survival have improved, there is still much progress to be made in stage III breast cancer. Metastatic breast cancer is usually incurable. The only exception to this is that some promising long-term response rates have been observed in a subset of patients with metastatic disease who have a complete or near complete response to conventional chemotherapy. Unfortunately, this represents a small number of the total population of patients with metastatic breast cancer. Metastatic breast cancer is treated with endocrine therapy or chemotherapy. Patients who are hormone receptor–positive will generally receive initial endocrine therapy followed by combination chemotherapy when endocrine therapy fails. Patients who are hormone receptor–negative or who have symptomatic disease involving the liver, lung, or central nervous system will generally receive chemotherapy as first-line therapy of metastatic disease. Chemotherapy will result in an objective response in about 50% to 60% of patients previously unexposed to chemotherapy. Most patients have partial response, and complete disappearance of disease occurs in fewer than 20% of patients treated. Median duration of response is 5 to 12 months; although some patients will have an excellent response to an initial course of chemotherapy and may live 5 to 10 years without evidence of disease. In general, survival of patients after treatment with commonly used drug combinations for metastatic breast cancer is a median of 14 to 33 months. The response rate to second- and third-line combination chemotherapy varies from 20% to 40%, depending on the previous chemotherapy regimens the patient has received. The availability of capecitabine, vinorelbine, and gemcitabine offers the promise of more successful second- and third-line treatments for metastatic breast cancer in the future. Development of novel targeted agents (e.g., trastuzumab) has also changed the outlook for patients whose tumors overexpress *HER2/neu*.

Current efforts at breast cancer prevention are directed toward the identification and removal of risk factors. In addition, two classes of agents, the retinoids and SERMs, are being evaluated for their ability to prevent breast cancer. Any statement regarding the value of these modalities awaits the results of ongoing clinical trials. Early detection of breast cancer remains important for decreasing breast cancer mortality. The rationale for early detection of breast cancer is based on the clear relationship between stage of breast cancer at diagnosis and the probability of a cure. The American Cancer Society, the U.S. Preventive Services Task Force, and the National Cancer Institute have developed screening guidelines for early detection of breast cancer. While these guidelines differ in their nuances, the overall benefits of screening mammography are apparent in their recommendations. However, the debate continues as to the absolute benefits and risks of these procedures.

Intensive research efforts are ongoing in all aspects of breast cancer etiology, detection, prevention, and treatment. Thanks to the thousands of patients who volunteered for these clinical trials, a substantial reduction in mortality has been seen in selected patient subsets. It is hoped that the information obtained in the next decade will result in the knowledge required to significantly reduce mortality from breast cancer for all women. Only through these continued efforts and participation of patient volunteers will advances be made in the management of this disease.

ABBREVIATIONS

ACR: American College of Radiology
AJCC: American Joint Committee for Cancer
BCIRG: Breast Cancer International Research Group
BSE: breast self-examination
CALGB: Cancer and Leukemia Group B
CBE: clinical breast examination
CMF: cyclophosphamide, methotrexate, fluorouracil (regimen)
DCIS: ductal carcinoma in situ
DFS: disease-free survival
ER: estrogen receptor
FAC: fluorouracil, doxorubicin, and cyclophosphamide (regimen)
FISH: fluorescence in situ hybridization
IHC: immunohistochemistry
LCIS: lobular carcinoma in situ
LHRH: luteinizing hormone-releasing hormone
NCCN: National Comprehensive Cancer Network
NCI: National Cancer Institute
NIH: National Institutes of Health
NSABP: National Surgical Adjuvant Breast and Bowel Project
OS: overall survival
pCR: pathologically complete response
PR: progesterone receptor
RR: relative risk
SERD: selective estrogen receptor downregulator
SERM: selective estrogen receptor modulators
TAC: paclitaxel, doxorubicin, and cyclophosphamide (regimen)
TNM: tumor-node-metastasis staging system

Review Questions and other resources can be found at *www.pharmacotherapyonline.com*.

REFERENCES

1. Jemal A, Murray T, Ward E, et al. Cancer statistics, 2005. CA Cancer J Clin 2005;55:10–30.
2. Ries LAG, Eisner MP, Kosary CL, et al. SEER Cancer Statistics Review, 1975–2001. Bethesda, MD, National Cancer Institute, 2004.
3. Ghafoor A, Jenial A, Ward E, et al. Trends in breast cancer by race and ethnicity. CA Cancer J Clin 2003;53:342–355.
4. Feuer EJ, Wun LM, Boring CC, et al. The lifetime risk of developing breast cancer. J Natl Cancer Inst 1993;85:892–897.
5. Clemons M, Goss P. Estrogen and the risk of breast cancer. N Engl J Med 2001;344:276–285.
6. Kelsey JL, Gammon MD, John EM. Reproductive factors and breast cancer. Epidemiol Rev 1993;15:36.
7. Dupont WD, Page DL. Menopausal estrogen replacement therapy and breast cancer. Arch Intern Med 1991;151:67–72.
8. Steinberg KK, Thacker SB, Smith SJ, et al. A meta-analysis of the effect of estrogen replacement therapy on the risk of breast cancer. JAMA 1991;265:1985–1990.
9. Risks and benefits of estrogen and progestin in healthy postmenopausal women: Principal results from the Women's Health Initiative randomized controlled trial. JAMA 2002;288:321.
10. Manson JE, Hsia J, Johnson KC, et al. Estrogen plus progestin and the risk of coronary heart disease. N Engl J Med 2003;349:523–534.
11. Breast cancer and hormonal contraceptives: Collaborative reanalysis of individual data on 53,297 women with breast cancer and 100,239 women

without breast cancer from 54 epidemiological studies. Collaborative Group on Hormonal Factors in Breast Cancer. Lancet 1996;347:1713.

12. Hankinson SE, Colditz GA, Manson JE, et al. A prospective study of oral contraceptive use and risk of breast cancer. Cancer Causes Control 1997;8:65.

13. Marchbanks PA, McDonald JA, Wilson HG, et al. Oral contraceptives and the risk of breast cancer. N Engl J Med 2002;346:2025.

14. Dupont WD. Risk factors for breast cancer in women with proliferative breast disease. N Engl J Med 1985;312:146–151.

15. Familial breast cancer: Collaborative reanalysis of individual data from 52 epidemiological studies including 58,209 women with breast cancer and 101,986 women without the disease. Lancet 2001;358:1389.

16. Thompson WD. Genetic epidemiology of breast cancer. Cancer 1994;74:279–287.

17. Weber BL, Abel JK, Brody LC, et al. Familial breast cancer. Cancer 1994;74:1013–1020.

18. King MC, Marks JH, Mandell JB. Breast and ovarian cancer risks due to inherited mutations in BRCA1 and BRCA2. Science 2003;302:643–646.

19. Struewing JP, Hartge P, Wacholder S, et al. The risk of cancer associated with specific mutations of BRCA1 and BRCA2 among Ashkenazi Jews. N Engl J Med 1997;336:1401–1408.

20. Robson M. Tamoxifen for primary breast cancer prevention in BRCA heterozygotes. Eur J Cancer 2002;38:S18–S19.

21. Howe GR, Friedenreich CM, Jain M, Miller AB. A cohort study of fat intake and risk of breast cancer. J Natl Cancer Inst 1991;83:336–340.

22. Nagao M, Ushijima T, Wakabayashi K, et al. Dietary carcinogens and mammary carcinogenesis. Cancer 1994;74:1063–1069.

23. Schapira DV, Kumar NB, Lyman GH. Obesity, body fat distribution and sex hormones in breast cancer patients. Cancer 1991;67:2215–2218.

24. Romieu I, Berlin JA, Colditz G. Oral contraceptives and breast cancer: Review and meta-analysis. Cancer 1990;66:2253–2263.

25. Thune I, Brenn T, Lund E, Gaard M. Physical activity and the risk of breast cancer. N Engl J Med 1997;336:1269.

26. Brinton LA, Bernstein L, Colditz GA. Summary of the workshop: Workshop on physical activity and breast cancer, November 13–14, 1997. Cancer 1998;83:595.

27. Friedenreich CM, Bryant HE, Courneya KS. Case-control study of lifetime physical activity and breast cancer risk. Am J Epidemiol 2001;154:336.

28. Yang D, Bernstein L, Wu AH. Physical activity and breast cancer risk among Asian-American women in Los Angeles: A case-control study. Cancer 2003;97:2565.

29. Lee IM, Cook NR, Rexrode KM, Buring JE. Lifetime physical activity and risk of breast cancer. Br J Cancer 2001;85:962.

30. Longnecker MP. Alcohol consumption in relation to risk of breast cancer. Cancer Causes Control 1994;5:73–82.

31. Feig SA, Ehrlich SM. Estimation of radiation risk from screening mammography: Recent trends and comparison with expected benefits. Radiology 1990;174:639–647.

32. McKenna RJ. The abnormal mammogram radiographic findings, diagnostic optional, pathology, and stage of cancer diagnosis. Cancer 1994;79:244–255.

33. Baines CJ, Miller AB, Kopans DB. Canadian national breast screening study: Assessment of technical quality by external review. Am J Radiol 1990;155:743–747.

34. Singletary SE, Allred C, Ashley P, et al. Revision of the American Joint Committee on Cancer staging system for breast cancer. J Clin Oncol 2002;20:3628–3636.

35. Woodward WA, Strom EA, Tucker SL, et al. Changes in the 2003 American Joint Committee on Cancer Staging for Breast Cancer dramatically affect stage-specific survival. J Clin Oncol 2003;21:3244–3248.

36. Frykberg ER, Bland KI. Overview of the biology and management of ductal carcinoma in situ of the breast. Cancer 1994;74:350–361.

37. Frykberg ER, Ames FC, Bland KI. Current concepts for management of early (in situ and occult invasive) breast carcinoma. In: Bland KI, Copeland EM, eds. The Breast: Comprehensive Management of Benign and Malignant Diseases. Philadelphia, WB Saunders, 1991:731–751.

38. Fisher B, Constantio J, Redmond C, et al. Lumpectomy compared with lumpectomy and radiation therapy for the treatment of intraductal breast cancer. N Engl J Med 1993;328:1581–1586.

39. Julien JP, Bijker N, Fentiman IS, et al. Radiotherapy in breast-conserving treatment for ductal carcinoma in situ: First results of the EORTC randomized phase III trial 10853. EORTC Breast Cancer Cooperative Group and EORTC Radiotherapy Group. Lancet 2000;355:528–533.

40. Fisher B, Dignam J, Wolmark N, et al. Tamoxifen in treatment of intraductal breast cancer: National surgical adjuvant breast and bowel project B-24 randomised controlled trial. Lancet 1999;353:1993–2000.

41. Houghton J, George WD, Cuzick J, et al. Radiotherapy and tamoxifen in women with completely excised ductal carcinoma in situ of the breast in the UK, Australia, and New Zealand: Randomised controlled trial. Lancet 2003;362:95–102.

42. Goldhirsch A, Wood WC, Gelber RD, et al. Meeting highlights: Updated international expert consensus on the primary therapy of early breast cancer. J Clin Oncol 2003;21:3357–3365.

43. Fisher B, Slack NH, Bross IDJ. Cancer of the breast: Size of neoplasm and prognosis. Cancer 1969;24:1071–1080.

44. Nemoto T, Vana T, Bedwani RN, et al. Management and survival of female breast cancer. Cancer 1980;45:2917–2924.

45. Valagussa P, Bonadonna G, Veronesi U. Patterns of relapse and survival in operable breast carcinoma with positive and negative axillary nodes. Tumori 1978;64:241–258.

46. Hedley DW, Clark GM, Cornelisse CJ, et al. Consensus review of the clinical utility of DNA cytometry in carcinoma of the breast. Cytometry 1993;14:482–485.

47. Fisher B, Redmond C, Fisher E, et al. Relative worth of estrogen or progesterone receptor and pathologic characteristics of differentiation as indicators of prognosis in node-negative breast and Bowel Project Protocol B-06. J Clin Oncol 1988;6:1076–1087.

48. Hayes DF. Measurement of prognostic factors in breast cancer. UpToDate 2003.

49. Tandon AK, Clark GM, Chamness GC, et al. Her-2/neu oncogene protein and prognosis in breast cancer. J Clin Oncol 1989;7:1120.

50. Gusterson BA, Gelber RD, Goldhirsch A, et al. Prognostic importance of c-erbB-2 expression in breast cancer. International (Ludwig) Breast Cancer Study Group. J Clin Oncol 1992;10:1049.

51. Yamauchi H, Hayes DF. Her-2/neu (c-erbB-2) and predicting response to therapy in breast cancer. UpToDate 2004.

52. Perez EA, Roche PC, Jenkins RB, et al. HER2 testing in patients with breast cancer: Poor correlation between weak positivity by immunohistochemistry and gene amplification by fluorescence in situ hybridization. Mayo Clin Proc 2002;77:148.

53. NIH Consensus Development Conference Statement. Adjuvant therapy for breast cancer 2000, November 1–3:1–23. www.nih.gov website. Accessed February 28, 2001.

54. Harbeck N, Kates RE, Look MP, et al. Enhanced benefit from adjuvant chemotherapy in breast cancer patients classified high-risk according to urokinase-type plasminogen activator (uPA) and plasminogen activator inhibitor type 1 (n=3424). Cancer Res 2002;62:4617–4622.

55. Look MP, van Putten WL, Duffy MJ, et al. Pooled analysis of prognostic impact of urokinase-type plasminogen activator and its inhibitor PAI-1 in 8377 breast cancer patients. J Natl Cancer Inst 2002;94:116–128.

56. Keyomarsi K, Tucker SL, Buchholz TA, et al. Cyclin E and survival in patients with breast cancer. N Engl J Med 2002;347:1566–1575.

57. Keyomarsi K, Tucker SL, Bedrosian I. Cyclin E is a more powerful predictor of breast cancer outcome than proliferation. Nat Med 2003;9:152.

58. Hayes DF. Markers of increased risk for failure of adjuvant therapies. Breast 2003;12:S14 (suppl 1, abstr S37).

59. Braun S, Pantel K, Muller P, et al. Cytokeratin-positive cells in the bone marrow and survival of patients with stage I, II, or III breast cancer. N Engl J Med 2000;342:525–533.

60. Piccart MJ. New data on chemotherapy in the adjuvant setting. Breast 2003;12:S4 (suppl 1, abstr S5).

61. Nemoto T, Vana J, Bedwani RN, et al. Management and survival of female breast cancer: Results of a national survey by the American College of Surgeons. Cancer 1980;45:2917–2924.

62. Fisher B, Jeong JH, Anderson S, et al. Twenty-five-year follow-up of a randomized trial comparing radical mastectomy, total mastectomy, and total mastectomy followed by irradiation. N Engl J Med 2002;347:567–575.

63. Fisher B, Anderson S, Bryant J, et al. Twenty-year follow-up of a randomized trial comparing total mastectomy, lumpectomy and lumpectomy plus irradiation for the treatment of invasive breast cancer. N Engl J Med 2002;347:1233–1241.

64. Ivens D, Hoe AL, Podd TJ, et al. Assessment of morbidity from complete axillary dissection. Br J Cancer 1992;66:136–138.

65. Keramopoulos A, Tsionou C, Minaretzis D, et al. Arm morbidity following treatment of breast cancer with total axillary dissection: A multivariated approach. Oncology 1993;50:445–449.

66. Hsueh EC, Hansen N, Giuliano A. Intraoperative lymphatic mapping and sentinel lymph node dissection in breast cancer. CA Cancer J Clin 2000;50:279–291.

67. Morrow M, Harris JR. Local management of invasive breast cancer. In: Diseases of the Breast, 2nd ed. Lippincott Philadelphia, Williams & Wilkins, 2000:515–560.

68. Cox CE, Haddad F, Cox JM, et al. Lymphatic mapping in the treatment of breast cancer. Oncology 1998;12:1283.

69. Morton DL. Intraoperative lymphatic mapping and sentinel lymphadenectomy: community standard care of clinical investigation? Cancer 1997;3:341.

70. Early Breast Cancer Trialists' Collaborative Group T. Systemic treatment of early breast cancer by hormonal, cytotoxic, or immune therapy: 133 randomized trials involving 31,000 recurrences and 24,000 deaths among 75,000 women. Lancet 1992;339:1–15.

71. Early Breast Cancer Trialists' Collaborative Group. Tamoxifen for early breast cancer: An overview of the randomized trials. Lancet 1998;351:1451–1467.

72. Early Breast Cancer Trialists' Collaborative Group. Polychemotherapy for early breast cancer: An overview of the randomized trials. Lancet 1998;352:930–942.

73. Early Breast Cancer Trialists' Collaborative Group. Ovarian ablation for early breast cancer: An overview of the randomized trials. Cochrane Database Sys Rev 2000 CD000485 Up to Date™ 2005.

74. Ravdin PM, Siminoff IA, Harvey JA. Survey of breast cancer patients concerning their knowledge and expectations of adjuvant therapy. J Clin Oncol 1998;16:515–521.

75. Lindley C, Vasa S, Sawyer WT, Winer EP. Quality of life and preferences for treatment following systemic adjuvant therapy for early stage breast cancer. J Clin Oncol 1998;16:380–387.

76. Goldhirsch A, Wood WC, Gelber RD, et al. Meeting highlights: Updated international expert consensus on the primary therapy of early breast cancer. J Clin Oncol 2003;21:3357–3365.

77. NCCN Clinical Practice Guidelines in Oncology: Breast cancer: v.1.2004; www.nccn.org.

78. McCarthy NJ. Update on adjuvant chemotherapy for early breast cancer. Oncology 2000;14:1267–1288.

79. Thomas E, Hortobagyi GN. New paradigms in adjuvant systemic therapy of breast cancer. Endocr Relat Cancer 2003;10:75–89.

80. Fisher B, Brown A, Mamounas E, et al. Effect of preoperative chemotherapy on local-regional disease in women with operable breast cancer: Findings from National Surgical Adjuvant Breast and Bowel Project B-18. J Clin Oncol 1997;15:2483–2893.

81. Fisher B, Bryant J, Wolmark N, et al. Effect of preoperative chemotherapy on the outcome of women with operable breast cancer. J Clin Oncol 1998;16:2672–2685.

82. Henderson IC, Berry DA, Demetri GD, et al. Improved outcomes from adding sequential paclitaxel but not from escalating doxorubicin dose in an adjuvant chemotherapy regimen for patients with node-positive primary breast cancer. J Clin Oncol 2003;21:976–983.

83. Mamounas EP, Bryant J, Lembersky BC, et al. Paclitaxel (T) following doxorubicin/cyclophosphamide (AC) as adjuvant chemotherapy for node-positive breast cancer: results from NSABP B-28 (Meeting abstract). Proc Am Soc Clin Oncol 2003;A12.

84. Martin M, Pienkowski T, Mackey J, et al. TAC improves disease free survival and overall survival over FAC in node positive early breast cancer patients, BCIRG 001: 55 months follow-up (Meeting abstract). San Antonio Breast Cancer Symposium 2003;A43.

85. Bonadonna G, Valagussa P, Moliterni A, et al. Adjuvant cyclophosphamide, methotrexate, and fluorouracil in node-positive breast cancer: The results of 20 years of follow-up. N Engl J Med 1995;332:901–906.

86. Wood WC, Budman DR, Korzun AH, et al. Dose and dose intensity of adjuvant chemotherapy for stage II, node-positive breast carcinoma. N Engl J Med 1994;18:1253–1259.

87. Citron ML, Berry DA, Cirrincione C, et al. Randomized trial of dose-dense versus conventionally scheduled and sequential versus concurrent combination chemotherapy as postoperative adjuvant treatment of node-positive primary breast cancer: First report of Intergroup Trial C9741/Cancer and Leukemia Group B Trial 9741. J Clin Oncol 2003;21:1431–1439.

88. Green MC, Buzdar AU, Smith T, et al. Weekly (wkly) paclitaxel (P) followed by FAC as primary systemic chemotherapy (PSC) of operable breast cancer improves pathologic complete remission (pCR) rates when compared to every 3-week (Q 3 wk) P therapy (tx) followed by FAC—final results of a prospective phase III randomized trial (Meeting abstract). Proc Am Soc Clin Oncol 2002;A135.

89. Winer EP. Quality-of-life research in patients with breast cancer. Cancer 1994;74:410–415.

90. Levine MN, Gent M, Hirsh J, et al. The thrombogenic effect of anticancer drug therapy in women with stage II breast cancer. N Engl J Med 1988;318:404–407.

91. Smith RE, Bryant J, DeCillis A, et al. Acute myeloid leukemia and myelodysplastic syndrome after doxorubicin-cyclophosphamide adjuvant therapy for operable breast cancer: the National Surgical Adjuvant Breast and Bowel Project experience. J Clin Oncol 2003;21:1195–1204.

92. Henderson IC, Sloss JL, Jaffe N, et al. Serial studies of cardiac function in patients receiving adriamycin. Cancer Treat Rep 1978;62:923–929.

93. Ellence (epirubicin) product information. Pharmacia and Upjohn Co., April 2003.

94. Love RR, Mazess RB, Barden HS, et al. Effects of tamoxifen on bone mineral density in postmenopausal women with breast cancer. N Engl J Med 1992;326:852–856.

95. Love RR, Wiebe DA, Newcomb PA, et al. Effects of tamoxifen on cardiovascular risk factors in postmenopausal women. Ann Intern Med 1992;115:860–864.

96. Albain KS, Green SJ, Ravdin PM, et al. Adjuvant chemohormonal therapy for primary breast cancer should be sequential instead of concurrent: Initial results from intergroup trial 0100 (SWOG-8814) (Meeting abstract). Proc Am Soc Clin Oncol 2002;A143.

97. Fisher B, Dignam J, Bryant J, et al. Five versus more than five years of tamoxifen for lymph node-negative breast cancer: updated findings from the National Surgical Adjuvant Breast and Bowel Project B-14 randomized trial. J Natl Cancer Inst 2001;93:684–690.

98. Fisher B, Costantino JP, Wickerham DL, et al. Tamoxifen for prevention of breast cancer: Report of the national surgical adjuvant breast and bowel project P-1 study. J Natl Cancer Inst 1998;90:1371–1388.

99. Nolvadex (tamoxifen) product information. AstraZeneca Pharmaceuticals LP, June 2003.

100. Fareston (toremifene) product information. Shire US Inc., May 2003.

101. Hayes DF, Van Zyl JA, Hacking A, et al. Randomized comparison of tamoxifen and two separate doses of toremifene in postmenopausal patients with metastatic breast cancer. J Clin Oncol 1995;13:2556–2566.

102. Jonat W, Kaufmann M, Sauerbrei W, et al. Goserelin versus cyclophosphamide, methotrexate and fluorouracil as adjuvant therapy is premenopausal patients with node-positive breast cancer: The Zoladex Early Breast Cancer Research Association Study. J Clin Oncol 2002;20:4628–4635.

103. Jakesz R, Hausmaninger H, Kubista E, et al. Randomized adjuvant trial of tamoxifen and goserelin versus cyclophosphamide, methotrexate, and fluorouracil: Evidence for the superiority of treatment with endocrine blockade in premenopausal patients with hormone-responsive breast cancer—Austrian Breast and Colorectal Cancer Study Group Trial 5. J Clin Oncol 2002;20:4621–4627.

104. Laurentiis MD, Martignetti A, Isernia G, et al. Amenorrhea induced by adjuvant chemotherapy in breast cancer patients strongly correlates with a better survival: a long follow-up study (Meeting abstract). Proc Am Soc Clin Oncol 1998;A519.

105. The ATAC Trialists' Group. Anastrozole alone or in combination with tamoxifen versus tamoxifen alone for adjuvant treatment of postmenopausal women with early-stage breast cancer: Results of the ATAC trial efficacy and safety update analyses. Cancer 2003;98:1802–1810.

106. Goss PE, Ingle JN, Martino S, et al. A randomized trial of letrozole in postmenopausal women after five years of tamoxifen therapy for early-stage breast cancer. N Engl J Med 2003;349:1793–1802.

107. Coombes C, Hall E, Gibson LJ, et al. A randomized trial of exemestane after two to three years of tamoxifen therapy in postmenopausal women with primary breast cancer. N Engl J Med 2004;350:1081–1092.

108. Giordano SH. Update on locally advanced breast cancer. Oncologist 2003;8:521–530.

109. Assikis VJ, Buzdar AU. Recent advances in aromatase inhibitor therapy for breast cancer. Semin Oncol 2002;29(3 Suppl 11):120–128.

110. Robertson J, Lee D. Static disease of long duration (greater than 24 weeks) is a important remission criterion in breast cancer patients treated with the aromatase inhibitor "Arimadex" (anastrozole) (Meeting abstract). Breast Cancer Res Treat 1997;46:214.

111. Paridaens R, Dirix LY, Beex L, et al. Exemestane in active and well tolerated as first-line hormonal therapy of metastatic breast cancer patients: Results of a randomized phase II trial (Meeting abstract). Proc Am Soc Clin Oncol 2000;A316.

112. Mauras N, O'Brien KO, Klein KO. Estrogen suppression in males: metabolic effects. J Clin Endocrinol Metab 2000;85:2370–2377.

113. Stenbygaard LE, Herrstedt J, Thomsen JF, et al. Toremifene and tamoxifen in advanced breast cancer—a double-blind cross-over trial. Breast Cancer Res Treat 1993;25:57–63.

114. Faslodex (Fulvestrant) product information. AstraZeneca Pharmaceuticals LP, December 2003.

115. Osborne CK, Pippen J, Jones SE, et al. Double-blind, randomized trial comparing the efficacy and tolerability of fulvestrant versus anastrozole in postmenopausal women with advanced breast cancer progressing on prior endocrine therapy: Results of a North American Trial. J Clin Oncol 2002;20:3386–3395.

116. Howell A, Robertson JFR, Albano JQ, et al. Fulvestrant, formerly ICI 182,780, is as effective as anastrozole in postmenopausal women with advanced breast cancer progressing after prior endocrine treatment. J Clin Oncol 2002;20:3396–3403.

117. Ingle JN, Krook JE, Green SJ, et al. Randomized trial of bilateral oophorectomy versus tamoxifen in premenopausal women with metastatic breast cancer. J Clin Oncol 1986;4:178–185.

118. Klijn JGM, Blamey RW, Boccardo F, et al. Combined tamoxifen and luteinizing hormone-releasing hormone (LHRH) agonist versus LHRH agonist alone in premenopausal advanced breast cancer: A meta-analysis of four randomized trials. J Clin Oncol 2001;19:343–353.

119. Michaud LB, Valero V, Hortobagyi G. Risks and benefits of taxanes in breast and ovarian cancer. Drug Saf 2000;23:401–428.

120. Mouridsen H, Harvey V, Semiglazov V, et al. Phase III trial of docetaxel 100 versus 75 versus 60 mg/m2 as second line chemotherapy in advanced breast cancer (Meeting abstract). San Antonio Breast Cancer Symposium 2002;A327.

121. Jones S, Erban J, Overmoyer B, et al. Randomized trial comparing docetaxel and paclitaxel in patients with metastatic breast cancer (Meeting abstract). San Antonio Breast Cancer Symposium 2003;A10.

122. Xeloda (Capecitabine) product information. Roche Pharmaceuticals April 2003.

123. Michaud LB, Gauthier AM, Wojdylo JR, et al. Improved therapeutic index with lower dose capecitabine in metastatic breast cancer (MBC) patients (Pts) (Meeting abstract). Proc Am Soc Clin Oncol 2000;A402.

124. O'Shaughnessy J, Blum J. A retrospective evaluation of the impact of dose reduction in patients treated with Xeloda (Capecitabine) (Meeting abstract). Proc Am Soc Clin Oncol 2000;A400.

125. Esteva FJ, Valero V, Pusztai L, et al. Chemotherapy of metastatic breast cancer: What to expect in 2001 and beyond. Oncologist 2001;6:133–146.

126. Sledge GW, Neuberg D, Bernardo P, et al. Phase III trial of doxorubicin, paclitaxel, and the combination of doxorubicin and paclitaxel as front-line chemotherapy for metastatic breast cancer: An Intergroup Trial (E1193). J Clin Oncol 2003;21:588–592.

127. O'Shaughnessy J, Miles D, Vukelja S, et al. Superior survival with capecitabine plus docetaxel combination therapy in anthracycline-pretreated patients with advanced breast cancer: phase III trial results. J Clin Oncol 2002;20:2812–2823.

128. Cobleigh MA, Vogel CL, Tripathy D, et al. Multinational study of the efficacy and safety of humanized anti-HER2 monoclonal antibody in women who have HER2-overexpressing metastatic breast cancer that progressed after chemotherapy for metastatic disease. J Clin Oncol 1999;17:2639–2648.

129. Slamon DJ, Leyland-Jones B, Shak S, et al. Use of chemotherapy plus a monoclonal antibody against HER2 for metastatic breast cancer that overexpresses HER2. N Engl J Med 2001;344:783–792.

130. Extra JM, Cognetti F, Chan S, et al. First-line trastuzumab (Herceptin) plus docetaxel versus docetaxel alone in women with HER2-positive metastatic breast cancer (MBC): Results from a randomized phase II trial (M77001) (Meeting abstract). San Antonio Breast Cancer Symposium 2003;A217.

131. Burstein HJ, Harris LN, Marcom PK, et al. Trastuzumab and vinorelbine as first-line therapy for HER2-overexpressing metastatic breast cancer: multicenter phase II trial with clinical outcomes, analysis of serum tumor markers as predictive factors, and cardiac surveillance algorithm. J Clin Oncol 2003;21:2889–2895.

132. Robert N, Leyland-Jones B, Asmar L, et al. Phase III comparative study of trastuzumab and paclitaxel with and without caraboplatin in patients with HER2/neu positive advanced breast cancer (Meeting abstract). San Antonio Breast Cancer Symposium 2002;A35.

133. Treish I, Schwartz R, Lindley C. Pharmacology and therapeutic use of trastuzumab in breast cancer. Am J Health Syst Pharm 2000;57:2063–2076.

134. Leyland-Jones B, Gelmon K, Ayoub JP, et al. Pharmacokinetics, safety and efficacy of trastuzumab administered every three weeks in combination with paclitaxel. J Clin Oncol 2003;21:3965–3971.

135. Cuzick J, Powles T, Veronesi U, et al. Overview of the main outcomes in breast cancer prevention trials. Lancet 2003;361:296–300.

136. Smith RA, Saslow D, Sawyer KA, et al. American Cancer Society guidelines for breast cancer screening: Update 2003. CA Cancer J Clin 2003;54:141–169.

137. U.S. Preventive Services Task Force. Breast cancer screening. February 2002, www.ahcpr.gov/clinic/uspstf/uspsbrca.htm.

138. National Cancer Institute. Breast cancer screening recommendations. www.cancer.gov/cancerinfo/pdq/screening/breast/healthprofessional.

139. Thomas DB, Gao DL, Self SG, et al. Randomized trial of breast self-examination in Shanghai: Methodology and preliminary results. J Natl Cancer Inst 1997;89:355–365.

126

LUNG CANCER

Rebecca S. Finley and Jeannine S. McCune

Learning Objectives and other resources can be found at *www.pharmacotherapyonline.com*.

KEY CONCEPTS

1 Lung cancer is the leading cause of cancer deaths in both men and women in the United States. The overall 5-year survival rate for all types of lung cancer is approximately 15%.

2 Cigarette smoking is responsible for about 83% of all lung cancers. Smoking cessation should be encouraged, particularly in those receiving curative treatment (i.e., stage I to IIIA non-small cell lung cancer and limited stage small cell lung cancer).

3 Non-small cell lung cancer (NSCLC) is diagnosed in the majority (80%) of lung cancer patients. NSCLC typically has a slower growth rate and doubling time than small cell lung cancer (SCLC).

4 Many lung cancers go undetected until they are advanced because individuals who have a long history of cigarette smoking are unlikely to notice the early symptoms of cough or dyspnea. It is often symptoms associated with large tumors or metastatic disease that prompt medical attention.

5 Surgery has had an established role in curing early-stage NSCLC, but SCLC rapidly metastasizes and thus surgery has a minimal role in its management. Radiotherapy has a role in the management of both diseases, particularly for management of symptomatic metastatic disease. Chemotherapy has had an established role in the management of SCLC for over 25 years. For NSCLC patients, chemotherapy for stage IV NSCLC is preferred over best supportive care, and data continue to be positive for the role of chemotherapy in earlier stages of NSCLC.

6 The most appropriate treatment for NSCLC is determined by the size and location of the tumor, extent of lymph node spread, presence or absence of metastatic sites, and condition of the patient. Surgery is the treatment of choice for early-stage NSCLC (stage I or II); some patients may benefit from postoperative chemotherapy and/or radiation. For patients with locally advanced NSCLC (stage III), chemotherapy with or without radiation followed by surgery improves survival over radiation followed by surgery. Doublet chemotherapy including cisplatin or carboplatin and another active drug (e.g., vinorelbine, paclitaxel, docetaxel, or gemcitabine) is recommended for patients with unresectable stage III or stage IV disease.

7 Because SCLC has the propensity to disseminate early on in the disease, surgery is not usually indicated. SCLC is radiosensitive, and radiotherapy is used in combination with chemotherapy in patients with limited disease. Prophylactic cranial irradiation is used in select patients to reduce the risk of CNS metastases. Combination chemotherapy will prolong the survival of most patients with SCLC. Patients with limited disease are more likely to have a complete response to chemotherapy and longer survival than those who have extensive disease at the time of diagnosis. The most widely used chemotherapy regimens for SCLC include cisplatin or carboplatin plus etoposide. Despite very high response rates to chemotherapy, most patients with SCLC eventually have disease progression and die from this disease.

Lung cancer is a major cause of morbidity and mortality that has reached epidemic proportions in many industrialized countries and is the most frequently fatal malignancy in the world. The American Cancer Society estimates that the age-adjusted incidence of lung cancer will be 90 and 54 per 100,000 for men and women, respectively, in the United States during 2005, which represents nearly 175,000 new cases during this year. Approximately 163,510 deaths will be attributed to this malignancy.[1] Despite major advances in the understanding and management of lung cancer, the overall 5-year survival rate for all types of lung cancer remains a dismal 15%, although evidence suggests that the death rate from lung cancer in the U.S. has declined slightly in recent years.[1,2] This is in contrast to many developing countries where the death rate from lung cancer is increasing. These differences are attributed to changes in smoking habits (de-

creasing in the U.S. and increasing in developing countries), the tar content of cigarettes, and to a lesser extent, availability of treatment. Although the overall 5-year survival rate for lung cancer is low, it may be curable with surgical resection if detected in the early stages, and many patients experience significant survival and symptom-relief benefits from systemic chemotherapy or radiation.

1 Lung cancer is estimated to account for 13% of all newly diagnosed cancers in adults.[1] It remains the leading cause of cancer death in both adult men and women.[1] The incidence and death rate due to lung cancer are declining more rapidly in men than women, which reflects the patterns of tobacco use. In 1987, for the first time, lung cancer surpassed breast cancer as the primary cause of cancer death among American women.[1] Because the risk of lung cancer increases with the duration and extent of tobacco exposure, it is not surprising that the incidence of lung cancer increases with age; the peak age of diagnosis is between 55 and 65 years. Among patients 40 years of age and older, the likelihood that a solitary pulmonary nodule seen on chest x-ray is a carcinoma is high and this probability increases proportionately with age. Patients with lung cancer may undergo surgery, chemotherapy, radiation, or multimodality therapy, depending on the histologic type of the tumor, its size and location, and the presence of metastases at diagnosis. Two leading oncology groups representing leading clinicians in the U.S. have published clinical practice guidelines for the treatment of lung cancer. The National Comprehensive Cancer Network (NCCN) has developed evidence-based guidelines that provide recommendations regarding the screening, staging, and treatment of both SCLC and NSCLC.[3,4] The American Society of Clinical Oncology (ASCO) first published evidence-based guidelines regarding the staging and treatment of NSCLC in 1997, which were subsequently updated in 2003.[5]

ETIOLOGY

Lung carcinomas arise from normal bronchial epithelial cells that have acquired multiple genetic lesions and are capable of expressing a variety of phenotypes.[6] The natural history of lung cancer begins with exposure of these normal cells to carcinogens, which cause chronic inflammation eventually leading to the genetic and cytologic changes that progress to carcinoma. Activation of protooncogenes, inhibition or mutation of tumor-suppressor genes, and production of autocrine growth factors also contribute to cellular proliferation and malignant transformation.[6] Under normal circumstances, cell surface peptidases produced by epithelial cells degrade and regulate these growth factors, but these enzymes are expressed at low or undetectable levels by most lung cancer cells, thus facilitating uncontrolled growth.[7] Although individual lung carcinomas may have multiple molecular abnormalities, some specific changes have been associated with the various types of lung cancer. For example, p53 mutations have been observed in about 90% of small cell lung cancers, but in only about 50% of non-small cell lung cancers, and this type of mutation appears to be more frequent in the squamous cell and large cell subtypes of non-small cell

lung cancers than in adenocarcinomas.[8,9] Evidence is accumulating that such molecular changes not only influence the transformation from normal to malignant cell, but also may have an impact on the progression of the disease and its response to therapy, and therefore strongly influence the patient's prognosis (Table 126–1). In particular, the overexpression of epidermal growth factor receptor (EGFR) on the surface of NSCLC cells has become an important target for new treatment strategies discussed later in the chapter. As in many other malignant diseases, further elucidation of the molecular profile of lung cancer has led to improved preventive, diagnostic, prognostic, and therapeutic strategies.

Numerous studies have established the relationship between tobacco exposure and lung cancer. The American Cancer Society estimates that cigarette smoking is responsible for about 83% of all lung cancer cases, and studies have established a dose-response relationship between the number of cigarettes smoked, the number of years an individual has smoked, the tar and nicotine content of cigarettes, and the development of lung cancer.[2] Likewise, smokers with obstructive airway disease or chronic bronchitis have a three- to fivefold greater risk of developing lung cancer than do smokers with normal pulmonary function.[16] Mattson and associates estimated that a 35-year-old man who smokes 25 cigarettes per day or more has a 13% risk of dying of lung cancer before age 75.[17] The increased rate of lung cancer deaths among women has also been attributed to increased smoking.[1] Cessation of smoking is associated with a gradual decrease in the risk, but a long period of time (more than 6 years) is necessary before an appreciable decline of the risk occurs. Antismoking campaigns, increased tobacco taxes, and smoke-free areas in many public areas and businesses, along with societal pressures have been somewhat successful in reducing the number of adult Americans who smoke. However, the high number of lung cancers in ex-smokers emphasizes the need to prevent individuals from ever starting to smoke. Passive exposure to cigarette smoke is believed to contribute to the increased risk of lung cancer in nonsmokers living with smokers. Other carcinogens also increase the risk of lung cancer and may act synergistically with cigarette smoking.[2] Occupational or environmental exposure to asbestos, chloromethyl ethers, various heavy metals, polycyclic aromatic hydrocarbons, and radon has also

TABLE 126–1. Examples of Relationship of Molecular Changes in Lung Cancer to Clinical Outcomes

Molecular Changes	Impact on Clinical Outcome	Reference
Microsatellite alterations	Reduced survival	Sekido et al[6]
Overexpression of BCL2	Decreased response to chemotherapy and radiation therapy	Sekido et al[6]
Expression of gastrin-releasing peptide and other bombesin-like peptides (SCLC)	Promote tumor growth	Sekido et al[6]
Overexpression of MYC (SCLC)	Reduced survival	Sekido et al[6]
Overexpression of HER2/neu (NSCLC)	Shorter survival, multidrug resistance	Tsai et al[10]
High hepatocyte growth factor levels (NSCLC)	Poor outcome	Siedfried et al[11]
K-ras mutations (NSCLC)	Poor prognosis	Rosell et al,[12] Huncharek et al[13]
Absent Rb expression (NSCLC)	Poor prognosis	Sekido et al[6]
E-cadherin expression (NSCLC)	Increased lymph node metastases; poor survival	Sulzer et al[14]
Decreased alpha3 integrin expression (NSCLC)	Poor prognosis	Adachi et al[15]

NSCLC, non-small cell lung cancer; SCLC, small cell lung cancer.

been associated with the development of lung cancer.[2] In addition, the incidence of lung cancer is higher in urban than in rural areas, and air pollution has been implicated as a possible causative agent.

Data from observational studies suggest that intake of β-carotene and carotene (vitamin A) is inversely associated with lung cancer risk.[18] The first prospective randomized chemoprevention trial with antioxidants in a large, well-nourished population was reported in 1994.[19] In that trial, more than 29,000 middle-aged male smokers were randomized to receive dietary supplementation with β-carotene, α-tocopherol, or both for 6 years. Interestingly, the trial failed to detect any significant protective effect of either vitamin, and surprisingly, significantly more new cases of lung cancer developed in the group treated with β-carotene. Other prospective trials have also failed to demonstrate beneficial effects of carotenoids, vitamin C, or vitamin E against lung cancer. Conversely, several other trials and case-control studies show a significant difference in relative risk related to intake of one of these antioxidants.[2,18] Additional studies are necessary to define the role of antioxidants in lung cancer prevention.

HISTOLOGIC CLASSIFICATION

The World Health Organization lung cancer classification is accepted worldwide (Table 126–2).[20] Four major cell types of carcinomas (squamous cell, adenocarcinoma, large cell, and small cell carcinomas) account for more than 90% of all lung tumors. Histologic confirmation of cell type is usually made by light microscopy and is essential in treatment planning because of differences in the natural histories, clinical features, and response to therapy of the various types. As noted earlier, several additional biologic and cytogenetic characteristics (e.g., secretion of peptide hormones, autocrine growth factor receptors, specific mutations, or chromosomal deletions of lung tumors) are currently being evaluated for their prognostic significance. In terms of management strategy and overall prognosis, adenocarcinoma, squamous cell, and large cell carcinomas are frequently grouped together and referred to as non-small cell lung cancer (NSCLC).

Although once the most common type of NSCLC, squamous cell (or epidermoid) carcinoma now accounts for less than 30% of all lung cancers, and is distinguished histologically by evidence of squamous differentiation. This tumor tends to be central in origin, arising from metaplastic bronchial epithelium, and frequently extends into the bronchial lumen, resulting in obstruction. Squamous cell carcinomas (along with small cell lung cancers [SCLC]) have a much higher incidence among smokers and among males and appear to have a strong dose-response relationship to tobacco exposure.[2,21] Although they can grow rapidly, most squamous cell carcinomas tend to be slow growing and confined to the lungs (especially early in the disease course). Such tumors may eventually metastasize to the hilar and mediastinal lymph nodes, liver, adrenal glands, kidneys, bone, and gastrointestinal tract.

Adenocarcinoma is now the most common type of lung cancer in the United States, accounting for about 40% of cases. This is partly a result of the increased incidence of lung cancer in women, who tend to have more adenocarcinomas than epidermoid cancers. Interestingly, it does not have a dose-response relationship to tobacco exposure. These tumors are usually located in the peripheral sections of the lung and are distinguished pathologically by a glandular or papillary pattern and mucin production.[2] The presentation and natural history of adenocarcinomas are quite variable. These tumors can present as a single nodule, multifocal nodules, or rapidly progressing, bilateral, diffuse processes. They are likely to metastasize at an early stage (often before the diagnosis of the primary tumor) and spread widely to distant sites including the contralateral lung, liver, bone, adrenal glands, kidneys, and central nervous system. As a result, adenocarcinoma has a worse prognosis than squamous cell carcinoma.

Large cell carcinomas are anaplastic tumors that show no evidence of differentiation. These tumors account for only about 15% of all lung cancers.[2] These tumors tend to be large and bulky tumors arising in the periphery of the lung, to have a propensity to metastasize in a pattern quite similar to adenocarcinomas, and to be associated with a similar poor prognosis.

Small cell carcinomas account for about 20% of all lung tumors. Almost all cases are associated with a history of smoking. They are distinguished by a proliferation of neoplastic cells with round to oval nuclei. These tumors tend to arise in the central portion of the lung, but may also be found in the lung periphery. SCLC is a very aggressive and rapidly growing tumor with approximately 60% to 70% of patients initially presenting with disseminated disease outside of the hemithorax.[21] These tumors commonly express neuroendocrine differentiation that may account for some of the paraneoplastic syndromes frequently associated with this disease. SCLC secretes gastrin-releasing peptide that acts as an autocrine growth factor. Secretion of other peptide hormones, cytogenetic abnormalities, and amplification and increased expression of oncogenes are also common. This disease has a propensity to metastasize to the lymph nodes, opposite lung, liver, adrenal glands and other endocrine organs, bone, bone marrow, and central nervous system.

Lung tumors frequently exhibit more than one histology, and it is now evident that all types of lung cancer share a common pluripotent stem cell. Studies of lung cancer cells have also shown that cell lines may spontaneously change phenotype, which may explain the mixed histology. Occasionally, patients can also have multiple lung nodules arising in different lobes or the contralateral lung. This is referred to as *synchronous tumors,* and the nodules may be of similar or different cell types. This usually worsens the patient's overall prognosis.

TABLE 126–2. World Health Organization Classification of Lung Cancer

I. Benign
II. Dysplasia and carcinoma in situ
III. Malignant
   A. Squamous cell carcinoma (epidermoid)
   B. Small cell carcinoma
     1. Oat cell
     2. Intermediate cell
     3. Combined oat cell
   C. Adenocarcinoma
     1. Acinar
     2. Papillary
     3. Bronchoalveolar
     4. Mucus secreting
   D. Large cell carcinoma
     1. Giant cell
     2. Clear cell

From Sobin.[20]

CLINICAL PRESENTATION

Location and extent of the tumor determine the presenting signs and symptoms. If the lesion is in the central portion of the bronchial tree, it is likely to cause symptoms at an earlier stage than will a lesion in the periphery of the lung, which may remain asymptomatic until the lesion is quite large or has spread to other areas. The most common initial signs and symptoms include cough, dyspnea, chest pain, sputum production, and hemoptysis. Unfortunately, many patients with lung cancer also have chronic pulmonary and/or cardiovascular diseases (usually related to smoking), and such symptoms may go unnoticed or be attributed to the concomitant disease. Many patients also exhibit systemic symptoms such as anorexia, weight loss, and fatigue that are suggestive of a malignancy.[2,21] Patients can also have other signs and symptoms at the time of diagnosis or at any point during its recurrence or progression. Disseminated disease also may be responsible for extrapulmonary signs and symptoms such as neurologic deficits resulting from central nervous system metastases, bone pain or pathologic fractures secondary to bone metastases, or liver dysfunction resulting from tumor involvement in the liver.

CLINICAL PRESENTATION OF LUNG CANCER

LOCAL SIGNS AND SYMPTOMS ASSOCIATED WITH PRIMARY TUMOR OR REGIONAL SPREAD WITHIN THE THORAX

Cough
Hemoptysis
Dyspnea
Rust-streaked or purulent sputum
Chest, shoulder, or arm pain
Wheeze and stridor
Superior vena caval obstruction
Pleural effusion or pneumonitis
Dysphagia (secondary to esophageal compression)
Hoarseness (secondary to laryngeal nerve paralysis)
Horner's syndrome
Phrenic nerve paralysis
Pericardial effusion/tamponade
Tracheal obstruction

EXTRAPULMONARY SIGNS AND SYMPTOMS ASSOCIATED WITH METASTATIC INVOLVEMENT

Bone pain and/or pathologic fractures
Liver dysfunction
Neurologic deficits
Spinal cord compression

PARANEOPLASTIC SYNDROMES

Weight loss
Cushing's syndrome
Hypercalcemia
Syndrome of inappropriate secretion of antidiuretic hormone (SIADH)
Pulmonary hypertrophic osteoarthropathy
Clubbing
Anemia
Eaton-Lambert myasthenic syndrome

Paraneoplastic syndromes are signs and symptoms that occur at sites away from the primary tumor or its metastases and are not associated with direct tumor involvement. They may be caused by the production of biologically active substances (e.g., peptide hormones) or antibodies, or by other undefined mechanisms. Paraneoplastic syndromes occur more frequently with lung cancer than with any other tumor. These syndromes may be the first signs of a tumor and may prompt the search for an underlying malignancy. Paraneoplastic syndromes that commonly occur in association with lung cancers include cachexia, hypercalcemia, syndrome of inappropriate secretion of antidiuretic hormone, and Cushing's syndrome.[2,21]

SCREENING

At the time of initial diagnosis, many patients with lung cancer have advanced disease, and unfortunately the prognosis for these patients is poor. In tumor types such as breast and colon cancers, early detection has contributed to a substantial improvement in overall survival rates, and over the past 30 years numerous trials have evaluated the impact of using various techniques in the early detection of lung cancer. In particular, large screening studies have been conducted in high-risk populations (e.g., men older than age 40 who smoke).[22–24] Chest x-rays and sputum cytology are the most commonly used screening techniques in these older studies. Although several of these studies have reported that lung cancers may be detected at an earlier stage, actual mortality rates were not affected.[23,24] Other investigations have also documented that chest x-rays are not sensitive enough to detect very small (<2 cm) lung tumors, which might account for the lack of impact of this screening technique.[25,26] Furthermore, chest x-rays and sputum cytology may be associated with false-positive results in these high-risk individuals, leading to unnecessary and costly work-ups and anxiety. A recent reanalysis of one of the earlier screening trials that used different methods to remove or control potential bias indicated that early detection may improve survival because more tumors are diagnosed while they are still able to be surgically resected.[22,27] However, the American Cancer Society does not currently recommend screening for early detection of lung cancer.

Over the years, since these early screening studies, diagnostic technologies have improved and have been evaluated in screening studies. In several uncontrolled trials, low-dose spiral or helical computed tomography (CT) has detected lung tumors at sizes significantly smaller than with conventional chest x-rays (approximately 1.5 cm vs. 2 to 3 cm).[26,28,29] Controlled trials that assess the impact on survival and mortality of spiral CT versus conventional methods of lung cancer detection are underway, but until they are completed, it should not be assumed that detection at this smaller size will change outcomes, because many lung tumors are known to develop micrometastases while the primary tumors are quite small.[30] Although evidence shows that conventional sputum cytology as an early detection tool does not lead to improvement in lung cancer outcomes, several serum and sputum biomarkers of malignant transformation are under evaluation in high-risk populations. However, none have been identified as having sufficient sensitivity and specificity to reliably screen for early lung cancer.

DIAGNOSIS

Once signs and symptoms of lung cancer have been recognized, chest x-rays, CT scans, and positron emission tomography (PET) scans are the most valuable diagnostic tests. Chest x-ray is the primary method of lung cancer detection, and may also be useful in measuring tumor size, establishing gross lymph node enlargement, and aiding in detection of other tumor-related findings, such as pleural effusion, lobar collapse, and metastatic bone involvement of ribs, spine, and shoulders. CT is helpful in all of the foregoing, as well as in evaluation of parenchymal lung abnormalities, detection of masses only suspected on the chest x-ray, and assessment of mediastinal and hilar lymph nodes. PET scans, however, are reportedly more accurate than CT scans in distinguishing malignant from benign lesions, detecting mediastinal lymph node metastases, and identifying metastatic spread.[31–33] Most recently, the use of integrated CT-PET technology has been reported to improve the diagnostic accuracy in the staging of NSCLC over either CT or PET technology alone.[33]

Clinical characteristics of a lung nodule may also help to differentiate benign from malignant nodules and thus determine when invasive diagnostic tests are warranted. For example, benign lesions usually have sharp borders, whereas malignant lesions usually have irregular or radiating borders.

When there is clinical and radiologic evidence of a tumor, pathologic confirmation must be established. This may be accomplished by examination of sputum cytology and/or tumor biopsy by fiberoptic bronchoscopy, percutaneous needle biopsy, or open-lung biopsy. All patients must also have a thorough history and physical examination with emphasis on detecting signs and symptoms of the primary tumor, regional spread of the tumor, distant metastases, and paraneoplastic syndromes. The physical examination also aids in determining whether or not a patient may be able to withstand aggressive surgery or chemotherapy.

Unfortunately, by the time the tumor is diagnosed, dissemination has already occurred in many patients. Determination of the extent (or stage) of the tumor involvement is important because it will aid in the selection of treatment, and estimation of the probability of cure and survival, as well as facilitating comparison of the individual patient to large-scale clinical trials.

STAGING

NON-SMALL CELL LUNG CANCER

The American Joint Committee on Cancer[34] has established a TNM staging classification for lung cancer based on the primary tumor size and extent (T), regional lymph node involvement (N), and presence or absence of distant metastases (M). Table 126–3 outlines this staging system. For comparison of various therapeutic modalities, a simpler stage grouping system is also used in which stage I refers to tumors confined to the lung without lymphatic spread; stage II refers to large tumors with ipsilateral peribronchial or hilar lymph node involvement; stage III includes other lymph node and regional involvement; and stage IV includes any tumor with distant metastases.[34]

The primary tumor is assessed with chest x-rays and fiberoptic bronchoscopy, whereas lymphatic spread is usually assessed by mediastinoscopy, gallium-67 citrate scanning, and CT and/or PET scans.[2] If the history and physical examination or other routine clinical studies (e.g., complete blood cell count and liver function tests) suggest the possibility of metastatic disease, then special scans (e.g., bone, brain, or liver) or biopsies (e.g., bone marrow or liver) may be necessary for staging.[2]

SMALL CELL LUNG CANCER

A two-stage classification established by the Veterans Administration Lung Cancer Study Group is widely used in the United States to stage SCLC.[21] Limited disease is classified as disease confined to one hemithorax and to the regional lymph nodes. All other disease is classified as extensive. Approximately 70% of patients initially present

TABLE 126–3. Tumor (T), Node (N), Metastasis (M) Staging for Lung Cancer

T_x	Positive malignant cell; no lesion seen
T_1	≤3 cm surrounded by lung or visceral pleura
T_2	>3 cm or involvement of main bronchus 2 cm or more distal to the carina, or invasion of visceral pleura, or associated atelectasis or obstructive pneumonitis extending to hilar region
T_3	Direct invasion of chest wall, diaphragm, mediastinal pleura, or parietal pericardium; or tumor in main bronchus less than 2 cm distal to the carina; or associated atelectasis or obstructive pneumonitis of the entire lung
T_4	Invasion of mediastinum, heart, great vessel, trachea, esophagus, vertebral body, or carina; or tumor with a malignant pleural effusion
N_0	No regional lymph node involvement
N_1	Metastasis in ipsilateral peribronchial and/or ipsilateral hilar lymph node(s), including direct extension
N_2	Metastasis in ipsilateral mediastinal and/or subcarinal lymph node(s)
N_3	Metastasis in contralateral mediastinal, contralateral hilar, ipsilateral or contralateral scalene, or supraclavicular lymph node(s)
M_0	No distant metastases
M_1	Distant metastases

Stage Groupings			
Stage IA	T_1	N_0	M_0
Stage IB	T_2	N_0	M_0
Stage IIA	T_1	N_1	M_0
Stage IIB	T_2	N_1	M_0
	T_3	N_0	M_0
Stage IIIA	T_1–T_3	N_2	M_0
	T_3	N_1	M_0
Stage IIIB	Any T	N_3	M_0
	T_4	Any N	M_0
Stage IV	Any T	Any N	M_1

From AJCC.[34]

with extensive disease. Because of this high frequency of disseminated disease at diagnosis (bone 38%; liver 22% to 28%; bone marrow 17% to 23%; central nervous system [CNS] 8% to 14%), a comprehensive past medical history and physical examination are necessary. Any suspicious signs or symptoms detected during the physical examination should be carefully investigated. In addition, it is necessary to obtain laboratory tests (i.e., complete blood cell count with differential, platelet count, serum electrolytes, liver function tests, calcium, lactate dehydrogenase [LDH], blood urea nitrogen, and serum creatinine), chest CT, bone scan, and brain imaging.[3] The need for a bone marrow biopsy is controversial;[35] recent NCCN guidelines recommend a bone marrow aspirate for those who have limited stage disease, but not for those with extensive stage disease.[3] Pulmonary function tests, electrocardiogram, and cardiac function tests should be conducted if clinically indicated, especially if chest radiotherapy is being considered.[3]

▶ TREATMENT: Lung Cancer

■ NON-SMALL CELL LUNG CANCER

◄5 ◄6   Surgery, radiation therapy, and systemic therapy using nonspecific cytotoxic chemotherapy or targeted therapies are all used in the management of NSCLC. Currently, only surgery, and to a lesser extent radiation therapy, offer an opportunity for long-

term survival in a significant percentage of patients, although only about 30% of unselected patients have localized disease (stage I or II) that is amenable to local therapy.[2] Curative therapy in this disease is determined by the anatomic stage of the disease (it must be localized with no evidence of distant metastases) and the ability of the patient to tolerate aggressive therapy. If left untreated, most patients with NSCLC die within 1 year of diagnosis.

Radiation therapy (radiotherapy) is used in a variety of settings for the treatment of NSCLC. Thoracic radiotherapy may be administered with curative intent for treatment of small localized tumors in some patients. Radiotherapy is most commonly administered postsurgically (adjuvant therapy) for prevention of local disease recurrence, as well as in advanced disease for the palliation of tumor-related symptoms (i.e., control of pain from bone metastases, hemoptysis, or obstructive symptoms).

Historically, NCSLC has been considered less responsive to conventional cytotoxic chemotherapy than many other types of cancer including leukemias, lymphomas, breast cancer, and even SCLC. Until recently, the use of chemotherapy was considered controversial. However, studies have consistently shown that although chemotherapy is not curative, patients with advanced stage NSCLC who respond to chemotherapy are more likely to have a survival benefit and reduced symptoms as compared to patients who do not respond to chemotherapy.[2] Combination chemotherapy regimens that include newer active agents are demonstrating higher response rates and longer median survival durations than ever before. In addition, as discussed below, chemotherapy now appears to have a role in the management of early stage disease in combination with surgery and radiation. The use of chemotherapy in the management of NSCLC is most extensively discussed in the section on stage IV disease (advanced NSCLC).

STAGE I AND IIA NON-SMALL CELL LUNG CANCER

5 **6** Surgical resection (pneumonectomy or lobectomy) is the treatment of choice for NSCLC patients with clinical stage I and II (disease that by all evidence is stage I or II prior to surgical resection and examination of lymph nodes) disease. Overall, more than 50% of patients with stage I and 35% of patients with stage II disease who undergo complete surgical resection survive 5 years without disease recurrence.[36] The most important prognostic factors for patients undergoing surgical resection are the size of the tumor, the presence or absence of lymph node involvement, and residual tumor in the surgical margins.[4] The addition of spiral CT and PET scanning of the chest to the initial preoperative staging plan have markedly improved the accuracy of clinical staging. However, mediastinal lymph node sampling via mediastinoscopy or dissection at the time of surgery is important to confirm the presence or absence of lymph node involvement. If mediastinal lymph nodes are found to be involved at the time of surgery, a complete lymph node dissection should be done.

The size of the tumor is of prognostic importance in stage I and stage II disease, with tumors <2 cm having the best long-term survival rates. Typically, removal of the involved lobe of the lung (e.g., lobectomy) is the recommended surgical procedure for stage IA tumors, but there is some evidence that pneumonectomy may reduce the rate of local recurrences for patients with larger size stage IB tumors.[36,37]

Stage II (T_1N_1) disease has a poorer prognosis, with a 5-year survival rate after complete surgical resection of approximately 40%.[2] Pneumonectomy, or removal of the entire lung (versus lobectomy), is the recommended surgical procedure for stage II disease with lymph node involvement ($T_{1-3}N_1$). Despite complete resection (no apparent residual disease remaining), as many as 50% of patients with stage II disease develop recurrent disease and die within 2 years.[2] It is therefore postulated that many of these patients may benefit from postoperative radiotherapy to improve local control, as well as from chemotherapy to decrease the risk of undiagnosed systemic micrometastasis.[36] Although some trials have reported benefit from postoperative adjuvant radiation in patients with stage I or II disease, others have not

shown benefit and several have reported adverse outcomes associated with radiation.[38–40] Therefore adjuvant thoracic radiotherapy is recommended postoperatively when surgical margins indicate that there is residual disease.[4,40] The goal of radiotherapy in this setting is curative, by eliminating the residual disease and reducing the risk of local disease recurrence. Because micrometastases are known to develop while lung tumors are quite small, the use of systemic postoperative chemotherapy has been extensively evaluated. Cisplatin-based systemic chemotherapy with or without radiation therapy is recommended for patients with positive surgical margins, when there is documented involvement of the ipsilateral mediastinal or subcarinal lymph nodes, and in patients with primary tumors >3 cm.[4] Although many clinical trials evaluating adjuvant chemotherapy following surgical resection have not demonstrated a clear-cut benefit, a recent report by the International Adjuvant Lung Cancer Trial Collaborative Group reported a 17% improvement in disease-free survival and a 14% improvement in overall survival for patients receiving cisplatin-based adjuvant therapy versus those receiving no adjuvant therapy.[41] This trial included 1867 patients with stages I, II, and III NSCLC who received cisplatin in combination with either etoposide, vinblastine, vinorelbine, or vindesine without radiation therapy.

CLINICAL CONTROVERSY

The use of adjuvant chemotherapy in patients with stage I or IIA NSCLC is controversial. The recent report by the International Adjuvant Lung Cancer Collaborative Group shows that adjuvant chemotherapy results in a modest improvement in disease-free and overall survival. It is not clear, however, whether this modest improvement is worth the cost and side effects associated with chemotherapy.

Radiotherapy alone (without chemotherapy or surgery) is the treatment of choice for stage I and II patients who refuse surgery or who are considered high surgical risks because of concomitant illness or restrictive pulmonary reserve.[2] It is also used when the tumor is unresectable because of fixation to a major blood vessel, the trachea, or the esophagus. Of those patients, the 2- and 5-year survival rates appear to be highest for patients whose tumors would otherwise be considered resectable.

STAGE IIB, IIIA, AND IIIB NON-SMALL CELL LUNG CANCER

6 Management of locally advanced NSCLC stage IIB, IIIA ($T_{1-3}N_2$, T_3N_1), and IIIB tumors is more controversial. Although many of these tumors are resectable or potentially resectable, the prognosis is poor, with 5-year survival rates ranging from 10% to 30%, depending on tumor size and lymph node involvement.[2] Both postoperative adjuvant and preoperative neoadjuvant chemotherapy and/or radiation therapy have been extensively evaluated in an effort to improve the overall survival rate. Adjuvant or neoadjuvant thoracic radiotherapy is used to reduce the risk of local disease recurrence. However, when given without chemotherapy, it does not impact overall survival rates because many of these patients develop systemic (distant) metastases.[2] The use of radiotherapy alone or postoperatively (without chemotherapy) in stage III disease should be reserved for those patients with a poor performance status who are at high risk for significant chemotherapy-induced toxicity.

For patients with surgically resectable, locally advanced stage IIB, IIIA, and more advanced IIIB (any T N_3 or T_4 any N) disease, neoadjuvant (before surgery) chemotherapy with or without concurrent radiotherapy, followed by surgery, improves local and regional control and overall survival when compared to preoperative radiation followed by surgery.[4,40] As in earlier-stage disease, cisplatin-based two-drug combinations are generally recommended for preoperative chemotherapy regimens. Cisplatin plus etoposide or cisplatin plus vinorelbine or another vinca alkaloid have been the most widely studied cisplatin-based two-drug regimens in adjuvant and neoadjuvant trials, but newer combinations such as cisplatin and paclitaxel or cisplatin and docetaxel have demonstrated improved outcomes in patients with advanced NSCLC, and may be used in these earlier stages. Preoperative chemotherapy may also increase the likelihood that an advanced local tumor may be completely resected at the time of surgery.[2] Alternatively, depending on the tumor location and size and the extent of lymph node involvement, NCCN guidelines also indicate that initial surgery followed by postoperative RT and/or cisplatin-based chemotherapy is also an acceptable treatment plan.[4] Large phase III trials continue to evaluate various combinations of neoadjuvant chemotherapy with or without radiotherapy versus initial surgery followed by adjuvant therapy. Accurate disease staging, consistent eligibility criteria, and multidisciplinary communication are essential to the success of these trials in elucidating the role of future neoadjuvant therapy in locally advanced NSCLC. Stage IV disease with systemic metastasis is, by definition, not surgically resectable for cure, and is therefore classified as nonresectable.

CLINICAL CONTROVERSY

Management of locally advanced (stage IIB, IIIA, and IIIB) NSCLC is controversial. Both postoperative adjuvant and preoperative neoadjuvant chemotherapy, with or without concurrent radiotherapy, have been used.

STAGE IV METASTATIC OR RECURRENT AND UNRESECTABLE STAGE III NON-SMALL CELL LUNG CANCER

Although surgery and radiation therapies have been the mainstay of treatment options for patients with localized or regional disease, about 70% of NSCLC patients present with advanced, poor-prognosis stage III and IV disease at the time of diagnosis. The majority of these advanced tumors are not surgically resectable due to disseminated (multiple sites) metastatic disease or metastatic sites that are not amenable to surgery. Patients with single metastatic sites may undergo surgical resection of both the primary tumor in the lung and the metastatic site.[4] Patients who have recurrent disease following surgical resection are usually not candidates for further surgical interventions and are managed similarly to those who present with stage IV disease. Although chemotherapy (single-agent and combination regimens) has been used for treatment of NSCLC for more than three decades, the overall survival benefits were not clearly established until just a few years ago. Beneficial effects of chemotherapy have been recognized both due to the discovery of new more active drugs, more optimal use of drugs, and improvement in the design of clinical trials.[2] Several studies have compared chemotherapy to the best supportive care and have shown a consistently better outcome for chemotherapy.[2,42-44] In 1995, the Non-small Cell Lung Cancer Collaborative Group reported the results of a large meta-analysis encompassing over 25 years of clinical trials of chemotherapy in the management of NSCLC.[45] This meta-analysis included data for 9387 patients from 52 randomized clinical trials that compared chemotherapy alone versus best supportive care and chemotherapy plus radiotherapy or surgery versus either single-treatment modality. Best supportive care generally consisted of symptom management with palliative radiotherapy, corticosteroids, pain management, and antibiotics as required. The results of this meta-analysis and other evidence suggest that chemotherapy, when combined with either surgery and/or radiotherapy, improves survival for patients with advanced stage NSCLC by 2 to 4 months, and increases the 1-year survival rate by 10% to 20%.[38,45] Cisplatin-containing chemotherapy regimens appear to be superior to older non–cisplatin-containing regimens, and regimens containing alkylating agents generally produced inferior outcomes. The roles of individual chemotherapy agents or regimens were not compared in this particular meta-analysis and require further evaluation.[45]

Both the NCCN and ASCO guidelines recommend the use of platinum-based (cisplatin or carboplatin) chemotherapy for unresectable NSCLC.[4,5] Duration of treatment with combination chemotherapy plus radiotherapy for advanced-stage NSCLC should be a minimum of two cycles to a maximum of eight cycles in most cases.[4,5]

Over the past 30 years, thousands of clinical trials have evaluated chemotherapy for the treatment of advanced NSCLC. The results have often been inconsistent or even conflicting. Direct comparison of study results between clinical trials is difficult and requires critical assessment of the study design, inclusion criteria (performance status, history of prior weight loss, and staging criteria), exclusion criteria, and assessment methodology. An excellent example is the importance of enrollment criteria for stage III locally advanced disease. Subset analysis is particularly important for stage III disease, because IIIA includes locally advanced disease, while stage IIIB includes more bulky regional disease with an overall poorer prognosis. Also, whether or not pathologic documentation of stage IIIA (N_2) disease was required in the trial is important because, if it was not, then some stage II (N_1) patients with a better prognosis may have been erroneously enrolled. Poorly defined stage III patient enrollment, with or without documented N_2 disease, may have contributed to the wide ranges reported in long-term survival rates and response rates between study arms in many of the early clinical trials.

Standardized response criteria are also important for the comparison of clinical trial results. The standard definition of a complete response (CR) is the complete disappearance of all evidence of the tumor as verified by two scans at least 4 weeks apart, whereas a partial response (PR) is defined as a reduction in measurable tumor mass of more than 50% for ≥ 4 weeks. Because many lung tumors do not have definite margins and are difficult to measure, the term *objective response* (OR) has been used to describe disease in which there has been a definite decrease in the size of the lesion without the appearance of any new lesions.[2] Tumor response to chemotherapy is generally evaluated at the end of the second or third cycle and at the end of every second cycle thereafter. Patients with stable disease, with OR, or with measurable decrease in tumor size (CR or PR) should continue with the same chemotherapy regimen, although several trials have found that prolonged administration of chemotherapy does not appear to improve survival, but may be associated with increased toxicity.[46-48] Although the ASCO and NCCN guidelines recommend a maximum of eight and six cycles of chemotherapy, respectively, other experts recommend that the number of cycles be limited to three or four cycles in patients with advanced disease.[4,5,38] The chemotherapy regimen should always be discontinued for documented progressive disease, and an alternative regimen or investigational protocol should be considered.

Several prognostic factors have important implications in terms of response and survival for NSCLC patients selected to receive chemotherapy. These factors include the patient's current performance status, percentage of weight loss from baseline, and extent of disease (stage).[2] Among these factors, an initial favorable performance status (Eastern Cooperative Oncology Group [ECOG] performance status of 0 to 2) appears to be the most consistent factor predicting a better response and improved survival after chemotherapy. There is little evidence to support the usefulness of chemotherapy in persons with an ECOG performance status of ≥3 (Karnofsky performance status of less than 50%).[2] Patients with an unfavorable prognosis (poor performance status, elevated LDH, weight loss >5%, and/or significant concomitant diseases) should receive supportive care and palliative radiation when necessary.

Phase II and phase III randomized trials with subset selection and disease documentation are ongoing to evaluate the efficacy of various combinations of chemotherapy, radiation, and surgery. Clinicians must refrain from extrapolating the results from early clinical trials into their general daily practice and should continue, whenever possible, to refer patients to carefully designed randomized trials to define the optimal therapy for the various subsets of NSCLC.

Chemotherapy for stage IV NSCLC is not curative, despite significant advances in available treatment options. But improved response rates, a modest increase in survival, and decreased toxicity profiles observed with many of the newer chemotherapy agents and combination regimens have led most experts to agree that most patients with stage IV disease should receive at least one chemotherapy regimen.[4,5]

The cost-effectiveness ratio for the use of chemotherapy versus best supportive care in advanced stages III and IV NSCLC has also been evaluated. Jaakimainen and colleagues demonstrated a modest increase in survival, improved symptom management, and decreased medical costs for patients receiving chemotherapy versus those receiving best supportive care.[49] The potentially high costs of chemotherapy, especially with the newer agents, are generally offset by the use of outpatient oncology clinics for drug administration and by the decreased costs incurred from best supportive care for symptom management and hospitalization (often prolonged). Cost calculations for cisplatin plus one of the new agents given in a combination regimen for advanced stage NSCLC is less than $20,000 per life-year gained, which is in the range of other widely accepted interventions.[50]

SINGLE-AGENT CHEMOTHERAPY

Single-agent chemotherapy has generally demonstrated objective response rates of 5% to 25% with no significant effect on overall survival. When responses do occur with single-agent chemotherapy, the duration of the response is usually brief (2 to 4 months) and complete responses are rare.[2] Among the most active single agents in NSCLC are cisplatin, carboplatin, docetaxel, etoposide, gemcitabine, ifosfamide, irinotecan, mitomycin, paclitaxel, topotecan, vinblastine, vinorelbine, and the EGFR tyrosine kinase inhibitors, gefitinib and erlotinib. Numerous other investigational agents, including marimastat, a matrix metalloproteinase inhibitor (cytostatic agent); tirapazamine, a cytotoxic that targets hypoxic cells; and other EGFR inhibitors are currently undergoing evaluation as single agents and in combination therapy in phase II and phase III clinical trials.

COMBINATION CHEMOTHERAPY

Combinations of two or more chemotherapy agents have been used in the management of NSCLC since the late 1960s. Response rates for combination chemotherapy regimens generally have been better than single-agent therapy, but improvement in overall survival rates has not been consistently observed.[51,52] Active combination chemotherapy regimens that have consistently reported response rates exceeding 30% have used various combinations of cisplatin, carboplatin, gemcitabine, ifosfamide, or mitomycin, and vinblastine, vindesine, or vinorelbine (Table 126–4). Evidence suggests that cisplatin dose may have an impact on tumor response, and the most widely recommended first-line regimens now include either cisplatin or carboplatin in combination with one other active agent.

For a number of years, the combination of cisplatin (60 to 100 mg/m^2 on day 1) and etoposide (80 to 120 mg/m^2 on days 1, 2, and 3 of the treatment cycle) given every 21 to 28 days was regarded as the most active regimen in the treatment of advanced NSCLC.[2] Newer chemotherapeutic agents in several distinct classes have shown single-agent activity of greater than 20% in NSCLC. The plant alkaloids (vinorelbine), taxanes (antimicrotubule agents; paclitaxel and docetaxel), antimetabolites (gemcitabine), and topoisomerase I inhibitors (topotecan and irinotecan) have being extensively studied in various combinations with platinum compounds (cisplatin or carboplatin). In 2000, the first trial documenting a superior response rate to cisplatin and etoposide was reported with the combination of cisplatin and paclitaxel.[53] Other trials have subsequently reported similar survival and adverse event outcomes with other platinum-based two-drug combinations.[54–56] Whereas earlier studies of chemotherapy focused primarily on response rates, newer studies focus on disease-free survival and overall survival, time to disease progression, quality of life, toxicity (short- and long-term), and cost effectiveness. These outcome measures are felt to provide more insight regarding the meaningful impact of the therapy on patients' lives. Results from many recently published trials combining these new chemotherapy agents with platinum-based regimens suggest improved 1-year survival rates in advanced NSCLC of 30% to 40% vs. 15% to 25% with the older cisplatin-based combination regimens (see Table 126–4).

Addition of a third drug to these two-drug combinations has not appeared to provide benefit and in some cases has been associated with increased toxicity.[64,65]

Vinorelbine is a semisynthetic vinca alkaloid. Single-agent activity has been demonstrated in advanced NSCLC, with response rates of up to 33%, median survivals of 40 weeks, and 1-year survival rates of 24% to 30%.[59] The combination of vinorelbine plus cisplatin has demonstrated superior efficacy to either agent alone, and to vindesine plus cisplatin in randomized phase III trials.[59,66]

The taxanes, paclitaxel and docetaxel, are antimicrotubular agents that bind to the microtubules and promote and stabilize microtubular assembly, resulting in the inhibition of mitosis and cell death. Paclitaxel as a single agent and in combination regimens has been evaluated in patients with advanced NSCLC with positive results. Regimens have included paclitaxel administered by 1-hour, 3-hour, and 24-hour continuous infusion schedules at low doses (175 mg/m^2) and high doses (250 mg/m^2) with granulocyte colony-stimulating factor (G-CSF) support.

In a study conducted by ECOG, 574 evaluable patients were randomized to receive either cisplatin plus paclitaxel 175 mg/m^2 given as a 24-hour continuous infusion; cisplatin plus paclitaxel 250 mg/m^2 given as a 24-hour continuous infusion with G-CSF support; or the standard regimen of cisplatin plus etoposide.[53] Survival for patients who received paclitaxel was significantly longer than those receiving etoposide. Although no difference in survival was observed between the low- and high-dose paclitaxel arms (median of 9.9 months; 1-year survival rate of 39%), the high-dose arm resulted in significantly greater toxicity (myalgia, peripheral neuropathy, and possibly

TABLE 126–4. Combination Regimens Using Newer Agents for Non-Small Cell Lung Cancer

Reference	Evaluable/Total Patients and Stage	Regimen	Overall Response Rates (%)	Median Survival Duration	Median 1-Year Survival (%)	Time to Disease Progression
Paclitaxel + cisplatin versus etoposide + cisplatin						
Bonomi et al[53]	574/599 IIIB 109 IV 465	Etoposide 100 mg/m² IV days 1,2, and 3; cisplatin 75 mg/m² IV day 1; cycle: every 21 days	12%	7.6 mo	31.8%	2.8 mo
		Paclitaxel 250 mg/m² over 24 hours IV day 1; cisplatin 75 mg/m² IV day 2; filgrastim 5 mcg/kg SC from day 3 until ANC ≥10,000/mm³; cycle: every 21 days	27.7%	10 mo	40.3%	5 mo
		Paclitaxel 135 mg/m² over 24 hours IV day 1; cisplatin 75 mg/m² IV day 2; cycle: every 21 days	25.3%	9.5 mo	37.4%	4.4 mo
Cisplatin (C) + paclitaxel (P) or gemcitabine (G) or docetaxel (D) versus carboplatin (Cb) + paclitaxel						
ECOG trial 1594, phase III Schiller et al[57]	1155/1,207 (1083 PS 0–1) (63 PS 2) 98 IIIB 968 IV	CP (reference arm for trial); cisplatin 75 mg/m² IV day 1; paclitaxel 175 mg/m² over 24 hours IV day 1; cycle: every 21 days	21%	7.8 mo	31%	3.4 mo
		GC; gemcitabine 1000 mg/m² IV days 1, 8, 15; cisplatin 100 mg/m² IV day 1; cycle: every 28 days	22%	8.1 mo	36%	4.2 mo[a]
		DC; docetaxel 75 mg/m² IV day 1; cisplatin 75 mg/m² IV day 1; cycle: every 21 days	17%	7.4 mo	31%	3.7 mo
		PCb; paclitaxel 225 mg/m² over 3 hours IV day 1; carboplatin AUC 6 IV day 1; cycle: every 21 days	17%	8.1 mo	34%	3.1 mo
Paclitaxel + carboplatin versus vinorelbine (V) + cisplatin						
SWOG Phase III Kelly et al[58]	408/444 chemo-naïve (PS 0–1); 12% IIIB; n = 207 11% III B; n = 201	Pcb; paclitaxel 225 mg/m² over 3 hours IV day 1; carboplatin AUC 6 IV day 1; cycle: every 21 days	PR 27%	8.0 mo	36%	NR
		VC; vinorelbine 25 mg/m² IV weekly; cisplatin 100 mg/m² IV day 1; cycle: every 28 days	PR 27%	8.0 mo	33%	NR
Cisplatin (C) + vinorelbine or vindesine (Vind) versus vinorelbine						
LeChavalier et al[59]	192/206 chemo-naïve (PS ≤2) 23 IIIA 58 IIIB 102 IV	VC; vinorelbine 30 mg/m² IV weekly; cisplatin 120 mg/m² days 1 and 29, then every 6 weeks	30%	9.2 mo[a]	35%[a]	NR
	183/200 21 IIIA 49 IIIB 109 IV	Vind/C; vindesine 3 mg/m² every week for 6 wk then every 2 weeks thereafter; cisplatin 120 mg/m² days 1 and 29, then every 6 weeks	19%	7.4 mo	27%	NR
	199/206 20 IIIA 65 IIIB 97 IV	V; vinorelbine 30 mg/m² weekly	14%	7.2 mo	30%	NR
Cisplatin + gemcitabine or etoposide						
Abratt et al[60]	50/53 chemo-naïve; (PS 0 = 1, 1 = 34, 2 = 18) 14 IIIA 19 IIIB 20 IV	GC; gemcitabine 1000 mg/m² IV weekly on days 1, 8, 15; cisplatin 100 mg/m² IV day 15; cycle: every 28 days	52% (CR 4%) (PR 48%)	13 mo	61%	NR
Cardenal et al[61]	135/135 chemo-naïve (PS 0–1) 67 IIIB 68 IV	GC; gemicitabine 1250 mg/m² IV weekly on days 1 and 8; cisplatin 100 mg/m² IV day 1; cycle: every 21 days	40.6%[a] (p = .02)	8.7 mo	NR	TDP 8.7 mo[a] (p = .01)
		EC; etoposide 100 mg/m² IV days 1, 2, 3; cisplatin 100 mg/m² IV day 1; cycle: every 21 days	21.9%	7.2 mo	NR	7.2 mo
Irinotecan + cisplatin						
DeVore et al[62]	52 chemo-naïve (PS 0 = 12, 1 = 32, 2 = 8) 11 IIIB 44 IV	IC; irinotecan 60 mg/m² IV days 1, 8, 15; required ≤40 mg/m² in 60% of patients; cisplatin 80 mg/m² IV day 1; cycle: every 28 days	28.8%	9.9 mo	37%	NR
Masuda et al[63]	378/398 chemo-naïve; (PS 0–1, 93%; PS 2, 7%) 37% IIIB 63% IV	IC; irinotecan 60 mg/m² IV days 1, 8, 15; cisplatin 80 mg/m² IV day 1; cycle: every 28 days	43%	50.3 wk	47.5%	
		C/Vind; cisplatin 80 mg/m² IV day 1; vindesine 3 mg/m² IV days 1, 8, 15; cycle: every 28 days	31%	47.7 wk	37.9%	
		I (CPT-11); irinotecan 100 mg/m² IV days 1, 8, 15	21%	46.1 wk	40.7%	

[a]Statistically significant difference.

ANC, absolute neutrophil count; CR, complete response; NR, not reported; PR, partial response; PS, performance status; TDP, time to disease progression.

cardiac toxicity) and was more costly, whereas the lower-dose paclitaxel regimen (without filgrastim) had a higher incidence of grade 4 granulocytopenia. The median duration of survival in the cisplatin plus etoposide group was 7.6 months (1-year survival rate 32%).

Other studies have evaluated paclitaxel given for shorter durations of infusion. In a phase II trial, 53 patients with stage IIIB or IV NSCLC were treated with paclitaxel (135 to 215 mg/m^2) via 24-hour continuous infusion plus carboplatin dosed to an area under the curve (AUC) of 7.5 on day 2 and given every 3 weeks.[67] Severe myelosuppression was observed, with moderate-to-severe neutropenia in 57% of patients after the first cycle, which led to the addition of G-CSF for the second and subsequent cycles. Significant thrombocytopenia and anemia were also reported in 47% and 33% of patients, respectively. Despite initially high response rates of 62% and an encouraging 1-year survival rate of 54%, the 2-year and 3-year survival rates remain poor at 15% and 4%, respectively. A subsequent trial by Langer and colleagues[68] compared a 1-hour versus a 24-hour infusion of paclitaxel plus carboplatin. The 1-hour regimen was associated with an increased rate of peripheral neuropathy and minimal myelosuppression, but the response rate decreased to 27%. The shorter (<3 hours) infusions of paclitaxel are easily administered in the outpatient oncology setting and rarely require G-CSF support, which makes them more convenient and acceptable to patients than the 24-hour infusions. The results of ongoing cooperative trials in advanced NSCLC will clarify the most appropriate infusion schedule and the role of paclitaxel in combination with platinum compounds and the other newer agents.

Docetaxel is an active semisynthetic taxoid, without the schedule-dependent efficacy and somewhat different toxicity issues than those associated with paclitaxel administration. Most of the early docetaxel clinical trials used dosages of 60, 75, or 100 mg/m^2 infused intravenously over 1 hour every 3 weeks. Initial phase II single-agent docetaxel studies reported response rates from 25% to 38%, median survivals of 9 months, and a 1-year survival rate of about 38% in chemotherapy-naive patients with advanced NSCLC.[2,69] Docetaxel 75 mg/m^2 every 3 weeks in combination with cisplatin is indicated in previously untreated patients with unresectable NSCLC and also as a second-line single agent (100 mg/m^2 every 3 weeks) against previously platinum-treated NSCLC with response rates of 15% to 21%, median survival of 7 months, and 1-year survival of 25%.[2,69,70]

Docetaxel received FDA approval in 1999 for the treatment of advanced stage IIIB and stage IV metastatic NSCLC after failure of a platinum-based chemotherapy regimen. Approval was granted based on the preliminary analysis of data from two randomized trials. The first trial compared docetaxel to best supportive care in 204 patients previously treated with platinum. The initial dose of docetaxel of 100 mg/m^2 (D 100) IV over 1 hour every 3 weeks was decreased to 75 mg/m^2 (D 75) after an interim study analysis reported a greater risk of severe neutropenia with the higher dose. The D 75 dose level was active and reported a significant advantage to best supportive care in terms of time-to-disease progression (10.6 weeks vs. 6.7 weeks), median survival (7.5 months vs. 4.6 months; $p = 0.047$), and 1-year survival (37% vs. 11%; $p = 0.003$).[71]

Docetaxel has been successfully administered to chemotherapy-naïve patients in combination with either cisplatin or carboplatin. Docetaxel 75 mg/m^2 plus cisplatin (75 to 100 mg/m^2) infused on day 1 every 3 weeks is active and well tolerated, with neutropenia being the dose-limiting toxicity.[69] Based on phase II data, this combination was included as one of the four arms in the randomized phase III ECOG 1594 trial (see discussion of this trial in the gemcitabine section).[57] The addition of filgrastim allowed a greater dose intensity in one phase II docetaxel plus cisplatin trial, resulting in a higher initial response rate and a slightly increased median survival. The

combination of docetaxel (65 to 80 mg/m^2) plus carboplatin (AUC 5 to 6) administered every 3 weeks is also active.[69] Decreasing the carboplatin AUC to 5 while maintaining a higher docetaxel dose intensity appears to maintain efficacy and to cause less neutropenia, and is thus being further investigated. However, the results of these encouraging studies must be confirmed in larger phase III trials. Numerous phase II and III multi-institutional and cooperative group trials are ongoing to evaluate the efficacy and toxicity of docetaxel with carboplatin, cisplatin, vinorelbine, gemcitabine, irinotecan, and thoracic radiation therapy.

Gemcitabine is a nucleoside analog (antimetabolite) that is phosphorylated intracellularly by deoxycytidine kinase. It has an increased membrane permeability and affinity for deoxycytidine kinase, yielding higher intracellular concentrations of the active metabolite and prolonged inhibition of DNA, as compared to its structurally related predecessor cytarabine. Phase I and II trials of gemcitabine have demonstrated antitumor activity against a variety of solid tumors, including lung, breast, ovarian, and pancreatic cancers. The overall toxicity profile for single-agent gemcitabine is modest. Gemcitabine was approved in the United States in 1998 for use in first-line combination therapy with cisplatin for the treatment of nonresectable, locally advanced or metastatic NSCLC. This indication for gemcitabine was based on data presented from 657 patients who participated in two randomized clinical trials with cisplatin. In one trial, gemcitabine 1000 mg/m^2 IV on days 1, 8, and 15 plus cisplatin 100 mg/m^2 IV on day 1 every 28 days was compared to single-agent cisplatin.[72] The second registration trial compared gemcitabine 1250 mg/m^2 IV on days 1 and 8 plus cisplatin 100 mg/m^2 IV on day 1 every 21 days, to cisplatin 100 mg/m^2 IV on day 1 plus etoposide 100 mg/m^2 IV on days 1, 2, and 3[61] (see Table 126–4). In both studies, the objective response rates (26% vs. 10% and 33% vs. 14%, respectively), median survival (9 months vs. 7.6 months and 8.7 months vs. 7 months, respectively), and time to disease progression was significantly better for the gemcitabine plus cisplatin combinations.

An Eastern Cooperative Oncology Group (ECOG 1594) trial randomized patients with advanced NSCLC to three platinum-containing regimens (cisplatin plus either gemcitabine [GC] or docetaxel [DC] vs. paclitaxel plus carboplatin [PCb]) to the standard reference arm of cisplatin plus paclitaxel (CP).[57] Of the 1207 patients enrolled from October 1996 through May 1999, 1155 were eligible for data analysis. Enrollment included patients with stage IIIB with a poorer prognosis, which included a pleural or pericardial effusion (disease not responsive to radiotherapy), and patients with stage IV NSCLC. Patients were stratified by performance status and baseline weight loss. Patients with performance status 0 to 2 were initially eligible for the trial, but an interim analysis revealed that patients with a performance status of 2 experienced increased toxicity with the cisplatin-containing regimens, and the study was subsequently limited to patients with performance status 0 and 1 only. There were no significant differences between the paclitaxel plus cisplatin control arm and the other three regimens in response rate, median survival, or 1-year survival (see Table 127–4). However, the GC regimen resulted in a modest 1 month advantage in time to disease progression ($p = .002$).

As expected, different toxicity patterns were reported for the four regimens. The PCb regimen was the most well-tolerated regimen, but it also had the lowest response rate and time to disease progression. The GC regimen had a higher incidence of severe thrombocytopenia and moderate to severe renal dysfunction, but the lowest incidence of severe neutropenia and febrile neutropenia. Moderate nausea was a problem for all of the cisplatin-containing regimens and was the greatest in the GC regimen with the higher dosage of cisplatin (100 mg/m^2 vs. 75 mg/m^2). Overall, the results of the four regimens were quite similar in this trial, and no clear advantage for one regimen over another was evident.[57] The high proportion of patients with stage IV disease in this trial is probably responsible for the disappointingly low overall response rates and median survival. In the community setting, the PCb regimen may be slightly easier to administer and monitor. Both the GC and DC regimens warrant further investigation in advanced NSCLC with varying dosages and infusion schedules to evaluate efficacy and improve toxicity. Altering the gemcitabine dose and schedule to days 1 and 8 only, eliminating the day 15 dose, has successfully improved the toxicity profile in other gemcitabine-containing regimens.

Irinotecan is a water-soluble analog of camptothecin, which is a potent inhibitor of topoisomerase I, the nuclear enzyme responsible for maintaining DNA topologic structure. Inhibition of topoisomerase I stabilizes single-strand DNA breaks and prevents religation (resealing), resulting in DNA dysfunction and apoptosis. Single-agent irinotecan studies reported initial response rates of up to 35% in chemotherapy-naïve advanced-stage NSCLC patients.[2,4] Unfortunately, response rates were low for previously treated patients with refractory disease. Combination chemotherapy with irinotecan plus cisplatin yielded response rates of 40% to 54% in patients with chemotherapy-naïve advanced-stage NSCLC. The irinotecan-cisplatin combination produced modest improvements in 1-year survival rates of 35% to 47%.[62,63,73] Irinotecan plus cisplatin is currently being evaluated worldwide in numerous combination regimens combined with gemcitabine, docetaxel, and/or vinorelbine.

Preclinical data indicate that radiotherapy increases the proportion of cells in the S phase, which may enhance the efficacy of topoisomerase I inhibitors. Thus trials evaluating irinotecan as a single agent in combination chemotherapy regimens plus radiotherapy have been undertaken. A phase I/II trial of bimodality therapy for locally advanced NSCLC with single-agent irinotecan 60 mg/m^2 weekly for 6 weeks, plus concurrent thoracic radiotherapy to the tumor site and regional lymph nodes resulted in an objective response rate of 77%.[74] The combined modality therapy resulted in dose-limiting esophagitis, severe pneumonitis, and diarrhea. The combination initially appears to be promising, and a phase II continuation trial with irinotecan decreased to 45 mg/m^2 weekly plus concurrent radiotherapy will provide further toxicity evaluation and survival data for the regimen.

Recognition that many NSCLCs overexpress the EGFR has led to the evaluation of several EGFR inhibitors in the management of NSCLC. In 2003, gefitinib, an orally active EGFR inhibitor, was approved by the FDA as a single agent for patients with advanced NSCLC whose disease progressed despite a platinum plus docetaxel regimen. Gefitinib is a small molecule that blocks the intracellular tyrosine kinase portion of the EGFR. Signals initiated by cell surface membrane EGFRs are vital in the proliferation and survival of cancer cells. Because the EGFR is frequently overexpressed in NSCLC cells, it is a logical target in the treatment of this disease. Early clinical trials demonstrated that gefitinib was well tolerated and demonstrated antitumor responses in 12% to 18% of patients who had previously progressed following other chemotherapy for NSCLC.[75,76] About 40% of patients in that trial experienced relief of symptoms associated with the disease. Presently the use of gefitinib is controversial because of its low response rates and the data regarding its effects on survival.

CLINICAL CONTROVERSY

The approval of the orally active EGFR inhibitor gefitinib provides clinicians with a drug with a novel mechanism of action. However, its use is controversial because of its low response rate and its lack of survival benefit.

Two large randomized phase III studies, however, failed to demonstrate improved response rates or survival when gefitinib was added to chemotherapy as compared to chemotherapy alone.[77,78] Further analyses of these two phase III trials showed that responses were more common in women, patients who had never smoked, and in patients with bronchoalveolar carcinomas or adenocarcinomas with bronchoalveoloar features. However, the response rate was low, even in patients with these favorable prognostic factors. In addition, the intensity of immunohistochemical staining of the tumor for EGFR also did not correlate with the likelihood of a response. It has been recently reported that tumors with heterozygous mutations within the tyrosine kinase portion of the EGFR are more likely to respond to gefitinib.[79] These mutations appear to activate growth factor signaling due to enhanced stabilization between the tyrosine kinase and adenosine triphosphate or its competitive inhibitor, gefitinib. Prospective evaluation of this molecular marker of gefitinib response may assist clinicians in selecting patients who are most likely to respond to this targeted therapy.

In November 2004, a second orally active EGFR inhibitor, erlotinib (Tarceva), was approved by the FDA as a single agent for patients with locally advanced or metastatic NSCLC after failure of at least one prior chemotherapy regimen. Its approval was based on an international, multicenter, randomized, double-blind phase III trial in 731 patients with locally advanced or metastatic (stage IIIB or IV) NSCLC who had failed at least one prior chemotherapy regimen.[80] Patients were randomized to receive either erlotinib 150 mg or placebo orally once daily. Patients in the erlotinib group had a significantly higher objective response rate (8.9% vs. 0.9%, $p < .001$) and longer median progression-free and overall survival (9.9 wk vs. 7.9 wk, $p < .001$ and 6.7 mo vs. 4.7 mo [hazard ratio = 0.73], $p < .001$, respectively) than those in the placebo group. Patients in the erlotinib group also had significantly improved symptom control, as measured as time to deterioration of cough, dyspnea, and pain. Erlotinib, like gefitinib, showed no benefit when added to conventional platinum-based chemotherapy.

Although there are no head-to-head comparisons of erlotinib and gefitinib, review of the available evidence suggests that erlotinib is more active than gefitinib. Erlotinib has been shown to significantly prolong survival in a large randomized controlled trial, whereas gefitinib failed to show a significant survival benefit in the ISEL (Iressa Survival Evaluation in Lung cancer) trial.[81]

RADIATION THERAPY FOR ADVANCED NON-SMALL CELL LUNG CANCER

Palliative radiotherapy with chemotherapy may be used in selected patients to control local and systemic disease and to reduce disease-related symptoms. Brain metastases are also commonly treated with radiotherapy; in the case of a solitary brain lesion, surgical resection may be used.

When thoracic radiotherapy is used with curative intent, high total-dose fractions (≥ 60 Gy) are required because of the correlation between dose and local control of NSCLC. These higher dosages of radiotherapy frequently result in severe esophagitis, pneumonitis, and pulmonary toxicity in the surrounding normal tissues. Improved radiotherapy delivery techniques, such as multiple daily radiation fractions (hyperfractionated radiotherapy) and three dimensional treatment planning, allow delivery of greater dosage fractions specifically to the tumor site while decreasing the toxicity to surrounding normal tissues, as compared to standard radiotherapy. However, concurrent radiotherapy plus chemotherapy with radiosensitizing agents, such as cisplatin, paclitaxel, and gemcitabine, further complicate the risks for severe toxicity, often necessitating dose reductions in one or both treatment modalities.[82] Numerous randomized combined modality trials have been initiated to evaluate the optimal delivery method, schedule, and dosages for radiotherapy in concert with cisplatin and the newer chemotherapy agents.

EVALUATION OF THERAPEUTIC OUTCOMES

Following initial therapy for NSCLC, patients must be monitored for evidence of disease recurrence. For patients who have undergone surgical resection with or without chemotherapy and/or radiation, a physical examination and chest x-ray are recommended every 3 to 4 months for the first 2 years, then every 6 months for 3 years, and then annually; and a low-dose spiral chest CT scan is recommended annually to monitor for evidence of locoregional recurrence. Suspicious symptoms or physical findings (e.g., bone pain, visual abnormalities or headache, or elevated liver function tests) should prompt an evaluation to rule out distant metastases.[4]

For patients with advanced disease receiving chemotherapy, diagnostic tests used in initial staging should be repeated after the second cycle to evaluate for response to determine if further therapy is warranted.

▶ TREATMENT: Small Cell Lung Cancer

◀5 ◀7 The use of aggressive combination chemotherapy regimens in SCLC results in four- to fivefold increases in median survival. Without treatment, survival is generally less than 5 to 7 weeks for patients with metastatic disease (extensive-disease SCLC) and less than 12 weeks for patients with regional disease (limited-disease SCLC). With treatment, median survival rates for extensive- and limited-disease are 8 to 13 months and 14 to 20 months, respectively.[3]

Prognostic factors used to determine the appropriate therapy for SCLC patients include the stage of disease (i.e., limited stage vs. extensive stage) and performance status (e.g., an ECOG performance status of 0, or ability to carry out all normal activity without restriction). Patients who initially present with limited disease and are treated with aggressive chemotherapy regimens demonstrate a significantly longer median survival than do patients presenting with extensive disease treated with the same regimens.[21] Patients with a better performance status at the time of initial diagnosis also have an improved prognosis.[21] Patients with normal pretreatment serum LDH are more likely to have limited disease, higher complete response rates, and longer median survivals.[21] Females appear to have a better prognosis than do males, as do patients younger than age 60 to 70 years. Weight loss and serum neuron-specific enolase, a biologic marker, have also been suggested as relevant prognostic factors.[83]

■ SURGERY AND RADIATION THERAPY

Because SCLC has the propensity to disseminate early on in the disease, surgery is indicated only for the rare patient with small, isolated lesions.[3]

◀7 SCLC is considered very radiosensitive. Radiotherapy is used in combination with chemotherapy to treat limited-stage disease or used alone for management of symptomatic metastases. The rationale for combined modality therapy is based on the premise that the addition of radiotherapy to chemotherapy will better control bulky disease within the chest primary tumor site.[21] In most randomized trials, combined modality therapy has only modestly improved disease-free survival and 2-year survival over that achieved with chemotherapy alone. The optimal dose and scheduling of thoracic radiotherapy (once-daily vs. twice-daily) plus chemotherapy have not been fully defined by large-scale randomized clinical trials. However, it appears that thoracic radiotherapy given concurrently with cycle one of chemotherapy versus later cycles, or alternating with chemotherapy, are more likely to produce favorable responses than when radiotherapy is administered following chemotherapy.[21,84] Unfortunately, many studies of combined-modality therapy have been associated with increased morbidity when compared to chemotherapy alone or radiotherapy after chemotherapy. Patients who receive twice-daily radiotherapy experience a greater incidence of severe esophagitis, and those who receive radiotherapy combined with radiosensitizing drugs (e.g., doxorubicin) have a higher incidence of radiation esophagitis and pneumonitis. Factors that are associated with a higher risk for severe radiation pneumonitis include performance status of 1, female gender, and forced expiratory volume of the lungs in 1 second <2 L.[85] Interestingly, chemotherapy regimen, radiotherapy dose, and field size were not predictors of severe radiation pneumonitis. Combined-modality clinical trials currently underway are evaluating various dosages, schedules, and new techniques such as three-dimensional radiotherapy, in combination with a variety of chemotherapeutic agents in an attempt to maximize tumor control with an acceptable degree of toxicity.

For SCLC patients, radiotherapy is utilized to prevent and treat brain metastases. Brain metastases are present at the time of diagnosis in 10% of SCLC patients. The cumulative incidence of brain metastasis rises to 50% in patients alive at 2 years.[21,86] The role of prophylactic cranial irradiation (PCI) is based on the theory that eradication of microscopic or subclinical brain metastases would prevent or delay the onset of brain metastases. Based on the potential toxicity of PCI and an unconfirmed survival advantage, the role of PCI has been a point of controversy for many years.[21,87] However, the Prophylactic Cranial Irradiation Overview Collaborative Group recently published meta-analysis results from seven SCLC trials enrolling patients from 1985 onward. The analysis included data from 987 patients with SCLC in complete remission after initial therapy, and compared overall survival with the addition of PCI to an observation group. The pooled relative risk of death in the patients receiving PCI compared to the observation group was 0.84, which corresponded to a modest 5.4% absolute increase in overall survival at 3 years (15.3% alive in the observation group vs. 20.7% alive in the PCI group; $p = .01$).[87] In addition, PCI increased the rate of disease-free survival and decreased the incidence of brain metastases with a trend toward greater benefit with earlier delivery of PCI. Based on this analysis, in patients without significant cognitive impairment or cerebral atrophy, PCI is recommended in those with limited disease in complete response, and should be considered in those with extensive disease in complete response.[3] PCI is also not recommended in patients with advanced age or poor performance status.[3] Doses ranging from 24 Gy in 8 fractions to 36 Gy in 18 fractions are recommended.[3]

For patients with symptomatic brain metastases, therapeutic dosages of cranial irradiation usually control the CNS disease.

Dexamethasone (to decrease intracranial pressure) and anticonvulsants are routinely administered to patients with brain metastases for symptomatic control and seizure prevention, respectively. Combination chemotherapy should also be administered, with administration occurring after whole-brain irradiation in those patients with symptomatic brain metastases.[3]

CHEMOTHERAPY

A number of cytotoxic agents have demonstrated significant single-agent activity in chemotherapy-naïve patients with limited- and extensive-disease SCLC, but the activity in recurrent or refractory SCLC is modest. Among the more commonly used chemotherapy agents in the United States are cisplatin, carboplatin, etoposide (intravenous and oral regimens), topotecan, paclitaxel, docetaxel, and gemcitabine.

Combination chemotherapy is clearly superior to single-agent therapy.[88] Despite the apparent benefit of combination chemotherapy, the higher incidence of acute toxicity, neutropenic fever, and toxic death in the palliative (metastatic disease, noncurable) treatment setting must be considered.

In the United States, the most frequently used regimens in newly diagnosed patients are: PE (or EP): cisplatin (P) + etoposide (E); EC (CE): etoposide (E) + carboplatin (C); and CP: irinotecan (CPT-11; C) + cisplatin (P).[3,89] Overall response rates (80% to 90% vs. 60% to 80%) and survival durations (12 to 20 months vs. 7 to 11 months) are generally superior for patients with limited disease versus those with extensive disease. According to the NCCN guidelines, chemotherapy with concurrent radiation is recommended for patients with limited-disease SCLC and good performance status (a category 1 recommendation, which indicates uniform consensus based on high-level evidence).[3] The same recommendation was made for patients with limited-disease SCLC with poor performance status, although the grade of evidence was lower (category 2A, which indicates uniform consensus based on lower-level evidence including clinical experience).[3] The 2-year disease-free survival rate for patients with limited disease at diagnosis is 15% to 40%.[3] In comparison, very few patients with extensive disease at diagnosis are alive at 2 years without disease.[3]

The optimal choice of combination chemotherapy regimen and scheduling is not clear. A meta-analysis of 19 randomized trials (4054 evaluable patients) compared cisplatin-based to non–cisplatin-based chemotherapy regimens.[90] Of these 19 trials, 10 trials randomized patients to cisplatin plus etoposide (PE) versus a regimen without either drug (e.g., CAV or cyclophosphamide + doxorubicin + vincristine), and 9 trials compared PE to a regimen without cisplatin, but that may have included etoposide. Both the overall and subset analysis concluded that cisplatin-containing regimens had a higher response rate, improved overall survival, lower incidence of life-threatening myelosuppression, and no increased risk of treatment-related mortality versus the non–cisplatin-containing regimens.

Carboplatin is often substituted for cisplatin in numerous SCLC regimens and has been shown to have similar efficacy with somewhat less toxicity, particularly for patients with pre-existing renal dysfunction or severe neuropathy.[21] In a randomized comparison of carboplatin and etoposide (CE) versus PE in patients with SCLC, the overall survival was 11.8 months for the CE group and 12.5 months for the PE group.[93] Based on these data, PE or CE have become the most commonly used regimens to treat SCLC in the United States.

ALTERNATING CROSS-RESISTANT CHEMOTHERAPY

Because the duration of response is usually brief (less than 1 year) for patients achieving a complete response, drug-resistant cells are often responsible for treatment failure. The Goldie-Coldman theory predicts that cycling of two active, non–cross-resistant chemotherapy regimens may overcome this problem.[94] At least two phase III clinical trials have used alternating, non–cross-resistant regimens in the management of SCLC, and most have failed to demonstrate substantial benefits.[91,92] Four cycles of PE has equivalent efficacy to six cycles of CAV and CAV alternating with PE with no significant difference in response rate or median survival.[91,92] Toxicity differed between the arms, with the PE regimen causing more severe nausea and vomiting, and the CAV regimen more frequent severe myelosuppression, neurotoxicity, and cardiac toxicity.

DOSE INTENSITY AND DOSE DENSITY

Experimental animal and human tumor data suggest that the amount of drug administered over a unit of time (i.e., mg/m^2 per week) may be critical to the degree of tumor cell kill.[95] The importance of dose-intensity has been evaluated in many types of human cancer, particularly those like SCLC, which are initially responsive to chemotherapy, but are not usually curable with conventional therapies. Randomized trials comparing dose-intensive (high-dose) CAE (cyclophosphamide, doxorubicin, and etoposide), CAV (cyclophosphamide, doxorubicin, and vincristine), PE, CEEP (cyclophosphamide, 4'-epidoxorubicin, etoposide, and cisplatin), and cyclophosphamide plus vincristine, versus standard-dose regimens have failed to demonstrate significant differences in overall survival.[96,97] Furthermore, a meta-analysis of 60 clinical trials failed to show a consistent relationship between dose intensity and survival for most SCLC chemotherapy regimens.[98] Although a significant difference in survival was observed in limited-stage SCLC patients receiving two dosage levels of cisplatin, cyclophosphamide, doxorubicin, and etoposide,[99] some researchers suggest that this study compared insufficient to sufficient doses of chemotherapy.[96]

Dose intensity can be increased by shortening the interval between cycles (i.e., dose density). The data with dose-dense chemotherapy regimens is conflicting, with findings of both no survival difference[100–102] and improved survival with dose-dense regimens.[103,104]

The incidence and severity of toxicities such as granulocytopenia, febrile neutropenia, mucositis, and weight loss are significantly higher in patients who receive dose-intensive treatment regimens. Currently, dose-intensive chemotherapy regimens should not be considered as standard oncology practice and should be reserved for clinical trials, in patients with limited-disease stage SCLC, and for the evaluation of newer agents.

ALTERNATIVE COMBINATION CHEMOTHERAPY REGIMENS

The addition of other active chemotherapy agents in patients who have relapsed following PE have provided minimal improvement in survival. The addition of ifosfamide improved survival, but also toxicity.[105,106] The addition of paclitaxel to PE resulted in similar overall survival,[107,108] while adding paclitaxel to CE increased overall survival only in limited-disease SCLC patients.[109] The addition of paclitaxel to PE increases myelosuppression and grade 3 and 4 neurotoxicity, diarrhea, and asthenia.[107]

Combination chemotherapy regimens that include irinotecan have shown promise in both chemotherapy-naive and previously treated limited-disease stage and extensive-disease stage SCLC.[89] The Japanese Clinical Oncology Group compared CP (irinotecan [CPT-11] 60 mg/m^2 IV on days 1, 8, and 15 combined with cisplatin 60 mg/m^2 IV day 1 given every 4 weeks for four cycles) versus EP (etoposide and cisplatin given every 3 weeks for four cycles) in 154 patients with extensive-disease stage SCLC.[89] Study enrollment was halted after the interim analysis results showed a statistically significant difference in median survival and 1-year survival in the CP arm. CP was well tolerated, with significantly less moderate to severe neutropenia (66% vs. 92%) and thrombocytopenia (5% vs. 18%) versus the EP arm, respectively. As expected, moderate to severe diarrhea was reported in 16% of patients receiving irinotecan. It should be noted, however, that the difference in overall survival, while statistically significant, represents only a modest improvement. Additional studies are ongoing to evaluate combinations of irinotecan with various conventional and newer agents.

MAINTENANCE CHEMOTHERAPY

Maintenance chemotherapy after induction appears to offer minimal benefit, although study design flaws have been noted in the available trials.[110] Since 1980, over 13 randomized clinical trials have evaluated the benefit of maintenance chemotherapy. Most trials, however, were conducted with older induction chemotherapy regimens (i.e., CAV) and not with PE or CE. It is possible that there is a subset of patients, perhaps those with particularly chemotherapy-sensitive

disease treated with moderately intensive chemotherapy, who may benefit from a maintenance program. In unselected patients, treatment programs that extend beyond four cycles of chemotherapy have not demonstrated an advantage in survival and may be associated with reduced quality of life.[3,21] Maintenance with the targeted therapy marimastat, a matrix metalloproteinase inhibitor, did not improve progression-free or overall survival, but diminished quality of life in limited- and extensive-disease SCLC.[111] Similarly, inhibition of c-kit tyrosine kinase by imatinib does not appear to be an effective agent for monotherapy for SCLC, based on preclinical xenograft models.[112]

CHEMOTHERAPY FOR RELAPSED DISEASE

After disease recurrence, the median survival is about 4 months.[3] Unfortunately, when disease recurs, it is usually less sensitive to chemotherapy. The agent of choice for second-line chemotherapy is often based on the time span between completion of the induction chemotherapy regimen and relapse.[3] Ifosfamide, paclitaxel, docetaxel, and gemcitabine are options for those with a good performance status (i.e., performance status 0 to 2) who relapse <3 months after induction chemotherapy was completed.[3] In those who relapse between 3 and 6 months after PE or CE, options include topotecan, irinotecan, CAV (cyclophosphamide, doxorubicin, and vincristine), gemcitabine, paclitaxel, docetaxel, oral etoposide, methotrexate, or vinorelbine. Topotecan administered as a second-line agent in patients with drug-resistant tumors produced objective responses and decreased symptoms in 25% to 38% of patients.[113,114] The original chemotherapy regimen is used for those who have a long duration of disease control (i.e., >6 months between induction chemotherapy and relapse).[3]

EVALUATION OF THERAPEUTIC OUTCOMES

Restaging to determine the efficacy of induction therapy is done after two to three cycles of treatment. At this point, therapy is continued for patients with a complete or partial response or stable disease, and discontinued or changed to a non–cross-resistant regimen in patients demonstrating evidence of progressive disease. The induction chemotherapy regimen is administered for four to six cycles if the SCLC disease is responsive. In those with a complete response, PCI is offered as discussed above. After recovery from initial therapy, follow-up visits should occur every 3 months for years 1, 2, and 3, then every 6 months for years 4 and 5, then annually for patients with either a partial or complete response.[3]

COMPLICATIONS AND SUPPORTIVE CARE

Patients with lung cancer frequently have numerous concurrent medical problems. Such problems may be related to invasion of the primary tumor and its metastases, paraneoplastic syndromes (see clinical presentation, above), chemotherapy and radiotherapy toxicity, or concomitant disease states (e.g., cardiac disease, renal dysfunction, chronic obstructive pulmonary disease, asthma, or diabetes). Depression is also common and sometimes persistent in patients with SCLC and NSCLC and should be treated. Identification, diagnosis, and treatment of the patient as a whole may improve the patient's overall quality of life and tolerance to cancer treatments.

The chemotherapy regimens used in the management of lung cancer are intensive and are associated with a wide variety of toxic

effects. Nausea and vomiting may be severe. Cisplatin-containing regimens require the use of aggressive acute and delayed antiemetic regimens containing a serotonin antagonist plus dexamethasone. Patients experiencing protracted nausea and vomiting may require intravenous hydration and nutritional support. Myelosuppression is often the dose-limiting toxicity associated with chemotherapy. Granulocytopenia places patients at a high risk for serious infections. Other toxic effects associated with these chemotherapy regimens include mucositis, nephrotoxicity, peripheral neuropathies, and ototoxicity.

Patients receiving radiation therapy may experience complications including severe esophagitis, fatigue, radiation pneumonitis, and cardiac toxicity. These toxicities are usually more common and severe when radiation is combined with chemotherapy. The patient's baseline performance status and the degree of pulmonary dysfunction (e.g., chronic obstructive pulmonary disease from years of tobacco use) must be considered in the decision of radiation dosage and fractionation.

It is readily apparent that many lung cancer patients receive complex pharmacologic regimens that may include chemotherapeutic agents, antiemetics, antibiotics, analgesics, anticoagulants, bronchodilators, corticosteroids, anticonvulsants, and cardiovascular agents. Such regimens necessitate intensive therapeutic monitoring in order to avoid drug-related and radiotherapy-related toxic effects and to optimize therapeutic outcome for individual patients.

ABBREVIATIONS

ASCO: American Society of Clinical Oncology
AUC: area under the curve

CNS: central nervous system
CR: complete response
CT: computed tomography
ECOG: Eastern Cooperative Oncology Group
EGFR: epidermal growth factor receptor
G-CSF: granulocyte colony-stimulating factor
LDH: lactate dehydrogenase
NCCN: National Comprehensive Cancer Network
NSCLC: non-small cell lung cancer
OR: objective response
PCI: prophylactic cranial irradiation
PET: positron emission tomography
PR: partial response
SCLC: small cell lung cancer

Review Questions and other resources can be found at *www.pharmacotherapyonline.com.*

REFERENCES

1. Jemal A, Murray T, Word E, et al. Cancer statistics, 2005. CA Cancer J Clin 2005;55:10–30.
2. Ginsberg RJ, Vokes EE, Rosenzweig K. Non-small cell lung cancer. In: DeVita VT, Hellman S, Rosenberg SA, eds. Cancer. Principles and Practice of Oncology, 6th ed. Philadelphia, Lippincott Williams & Wilkins, 2001:925–983.
3. NCCN Clinical Practice Guidelines for small cell lung cancer [website]. January 7, 2004. Available at: *http://www.nccn.org/professionals/ physician_gls/PDF/sclc.pdf.* Accessed June 7, 2004.
4. NCCN Clinical Practice Guidelines for non-small cell lung cancer [website]. February 9, 2004. Available at: *http://www.nccn.org/ professionals/physician_gls/PDF/nscl.pdf.* Accessed June 2004.
5. Pfister DG, Johnson DH, Azzoli CG, et al. American Society of Clinical Oncology treatment of unresectable non-small-cell lung cancer guideline: Update 2003. J Clin Oncol 2004;22:330–353.
6. Sekido Y, Fong KM, Minna JM. Molecular biology of lung cancer. In: DeVita VT, Hellman S, Rosenberg SA, eds. Cancer. Principles and Practice of Oncology, 6th ed. Philadelphia, Lippincott Williams & Wilkins, 2001:917–925.
7. Miller YE, Franklin WA. Molecular events in lung carcinogenesis. Hematol Oncol Clin North Am 1997;11:215–234.
8. Bennett WP, Hussein SP, Vahakangas KH, et al. Molecular epidemiology of human cancer risk: Gene-environment interactions and p53 mutations spectrum in human lung cancer. J Pathol 1999;187:8–18.
9. Tammemagi MC, McLaughlin JR, Bull SB. Meta-analysis of p53 tumor-suppressor gene alternations and clinicopathological features in resected lung cancers. Cancer Epidemiol Biomarkers Prev 1999;8:625–634.
10. Tsai CM, Chang KT, Wu LH, et al. Correlations between intrinsic chemoresistance and HER-2/neu gene expression, p53 gene mutations, and cell proliferation characteristics in non-small cell lung cancer cell lines. Cancer Res 1996;56:206–209.
11. Siegfried JM, Weissfeld LA, Singh-Kaw P, et al. Association of immunoreactive hepatocyte growth factor with poor survival in resectable non-small cell lung cancer. Cancer Res 1997;57:433–439.
12. Rosell R, Li S, Skacel Z, et al. Prognostic impact of mutated *K-ras* gene in surgically resected non-small cell lung cancer patients. Oncogene 1993;8:2407–2412.
13. Huncharek M, Muscat J, Geschwind JF. *K-ras* oncogene mutation as a prognostic marker in non-small cell lung cancer: A combined analysis of 881 cases. Carcinogenesis 1999;20:1507–1510.
14. Sulzer MA, Leers MP, van Noord JA, et al. Reduced E-cadherin expression is associated with increased lymph node metastasis and unfavorable prognosis in non-small cell lung cancer. Am J Res Crit Care Med 1998;157:1319–1323.
15. Adachi M, Taki T, Huang C, et al. Reduced integrin alpha-3 expression

as a factor of poor prognosis in patients with adenocarcinoma of the lung. J Clin Oncol 1998;16:1060–1067.
16. Islam SS, Schottenfeld D. Declining FEV_1 and chronic productive cough in cigarette smokers: A 25-year prospective study of lung cancer incidence in Tecumseh, Michigan. Cancer Epidemiol Biomarkers Prev 1994; 3:289–298.
17. Mattson ME, Pollack ES, Cullen JW. What are the odds that smoking will kill you? Am J Public Health 1987;77:425–431.
18. Menkes MS, Comstock GW, Vulleumier JP, et al. Serum beta-carotene, vitamin A and E, selenium and the risk of lung cancer. N Engl J Med 1986; 315:1250–1254.
19. The Alpha-Tocopherol, Beta Carotene Cancer Prevention Study Group. The effect of vitamin E and beta carotene on the incidence of lung cancer and other cancers in male smokers. N Engl J Med 1994;330:1029–1035.
20. Sobin LH. The World Health Organization's histological classification of lung tumors: A comparison of the first and second editions. Cancer Detect Prev 1982;5:391–406.
21. Murren J, Glatstein E, Pass HI. Small cell lung cancer. In: DeVita VT, Hellman S, Rosenberg SA, eds. Cancer: Principles and Practice of Oncology, 6th ed. Philadelphia, Lippincott Williams & Wilkins, 2001: 983–1018.
22. Fontana RS, Sanderson DR, Woolner LB, et al. Lung cancer screening: The Mayo program. J Occup Med 1986;28:746–750.
23. Melamed MR, Flehinger BJ, Zaman MB, et al. Screening for early lung cancer. Results of the Memorial Sloan-Kettering study in New York. Chest 1984;86:44–53.
24. Tockman MS. Survival and mortality from lung cancer in a screened population. The Johns Hopkins study. Chest 1986;89(Suppl):324S–325S.
25. Quekel GBA, Kessels AGH, Goei R, et al. Miss rate of lung cancer: On the chest radiograph in clinical practice. Chest 1999;115:720–724.
26. Sone S, Li F, Yang ZG, et al. Results of three-year mass screening program for lung cancer: Cancer using mobile low-dose spiral computed tomography scanner. Br J Cancer 2001;84:25–32.
27. Strauss GM. The Mayo Lung Cohort: A regression analysis focusing on lung cancer incidence and mortality. J Clin Oncol 2002;20:1973–1983.
28. Ohmatsu H, Kakinuma R, Kaneko M, et al. Successful lung cancer screening with low-dose helical CT in addition to chest x-ray and sputum cytology: The comparison of two screening periods with or without helical CT. Radiology 2000;217(Suppl):242 (Abstract).
29. Swensen SJ, Jett JR, Sloan JA, et al. Screening for lung cancer with low-dose spiral computed tomography. Am J Resp Crit Care Med 2002; 165:508–513.
30. Patz EF, Rossi S, Harpole DH, et al. Correlation of tumor size and survival in patients with 1A non-small cell lung cancer. Chest 2000;117: 1568–1571.
31. Saunders CA, Dussek JE, O'Doherty MJ, et al. Evaluation of fluorine-18-fluorodeoxy-glucose whole-body positron emission tomography imaging in the staging of lung cancer. Ann Thorac Surg 1999;67:790–797.
32. Kalff V, Hicks RJ, ManManus MP, et al. Clinical impact of (18)F fluorodeoxyglucose positron emission tomography in patients with non-small cell lung cancer: A prospective study. J Clin Oncol 2001;19: 111–118.
33. Lardinois D, Weder W, Hany TF, et al. Staging of non-small cell lung cancer with integrated positron-emission tomography and computed tomography. N Engl J Med 2003;348:2500–2507.
34. American Joint Committee on Cancer (AJCC). Manual for Staging of Cancer, 4th ed. Philadelphia, Lippincott, 1997:127–137.
35. Argiris A, Murren JR. Staging and clinical prognostic factors for small-cell lung cancer. Cancer J 2001;7:437–447.
36. Deslauriers J, Grégoire J. Surgical therapy for early non-small cell lung cancer. Chest 2000;177(Suppl 4):104S–109S.
37. Martini N, Bains MS, Burt ME, et al. Incidence of local recurrence and second primary tumors in resected stage I lung cancer. J Thorac Cardiovasc Surg 1995;109:120–129.
38. Spira A, Ettinger DS. Multidisciplinary management of lung cancer. N Engl J Med 2004;350:379–392.
39. PORT Meta-analysis Trialists Group. Postoperative radiotherapy in non-small-cell lung cancer: Systematic review and meta-analysis of

individual patient data from nine randomized controlled trials. Lancet 1998;352:257–263.

40. The Lung Cancer Study Group. Effects of postoperative mediastinal radiation on completely resected stage II and III epidermoid cancer of the lung. N Engl J Med 1986;315:1377–1381.

41. The International Adjuvant Lung Cancer Trial Collaborative Group. Cisplatin-based adjuvant chemotherapy in patients with completely resected non-small-cell lung cancer. N Engl J Med 2004;350:351–360.

42. Cormesir Y, Bergeron D, LaForge J, et al. Benefits of polychemotherapy in advanced non-small-cell bronchogenic carcinoma. Cancer 1982; 50:845–849.

43. Rapp E, Pater J, Willan A, et al. Chemotherapy can prolong survival in patients with advanced non-small cell lung cancer: Report of a Canadian multicenter randomized trial. J Clin Oncol 1988;6:633–641.

44. Cartei G, Cartei F, Cantone A, et al. Cisplatin-cyclophosphamide-mitomycin combination chemotherapy with supportive care versus supportive care alone for treatment of metastatic nonsmall-cell lung cancer. J Natl Cancer Inst 1993;85:794–800.

45. Non-small Cell Lung Cancer Collaborative Group. Chemotherapy in non-small cell lung cancer: A meta-analysis using updated data on individual patients from 52 randomized clinical trials. BMJ 1995;311: 899–909.

46. Smith IE, O'Brien ME, Talbot DC, et al. Duration of the chemotherapy in advanced non-small-cell lung cancer: A randomized trial of three versus six courses of mitomycin, vinblastine, and cisplatin. J Clin Oncol 2001; 19:1336–1343.

47. Depierre A, Quoix E, Mercier M, et al. Maintenance chemotherapy in advanced non-small cell lung cancer (NSCLC): A randomized study of vinorelbine (V) versus observation (OB) in patients (pts) responding to induction therapy. Proc Am Soc Clin Oncol 2001;20:309a (Abstract).

48. Socinski MA, Schell MJ, Peterman A, et al. Phase III trial comparing a defined duration of therapy versus continuous therapy followed by second-line therapy in advanced-stage IIIB/IV non-small-cell lung cancer. J Clin Oncol 2002;20:1335–1343.

49. Jaakimainen L, Goodwin J, Pater J, et al. Counting the costs of chemotherapy in a National Cancer Institute of Canada randomized trial in non-small cell lung cancer. J Clin Oncol 1990;8:1301–1309.

50. Evans WK, Will BP, Berthelot JM, et al. The cost of managing lung cancer in Canada. Oncology 1995;9:147–153.

51. Marino P, Preatoni A, Cantoni A, et al. Single-agent chemotherapy versus combination chemotherapy in advanced non-small cell lung cancer: A quality and meta-analysis study. Lung Cancer 1995;13:1–12.

52. Lilenbaum RC, Langenberg P, Dickersin K. Single agent versus combination chemotherapy in patients with advanced nonsmall cell lung carcinoma. Cancer 1998;82:116–126.

53. Bonomi P, Kim K, Fairclough D, et al. Comparison of survival and quality of life in advanced non-small-cell lung cancer patients treated with two dose levels of paclitaxel combined with cisplatin versus etoposide with cisplatin: results of an Eastern Cooperative Oncology Group trial. J Clin Oncol 2000;18:623–631.

54. Schiller JH, Harrington D, Belani CP, et al. Comparison of four chemotherapy regimens for advanced non-small-cell lung cancer. N Engl J Med 2002;346:92–98.

55. Kosmidis P, Mylonakis N, Nicolaides C, et al. Paclitaxel plus carboplatin versus gemcitabine plus paclitaxel in advanced non-small-cell lung cancer: A phase III randomized trial. J Clin Oncol 2002;20:3578–3585.

56. Kelly K, Crowley J, Bunn PA. Randomized phase III trial of paclitaxel plus carboplatin versus vinorelbine plus cisplatin in the treatment of patients with non-small-cell lung cancer: A Southwest Oncology Group trial. J Clin Oncol 2001;19:3210–3218.

57. Schiller JH, Harrington D, Belani C, et al. Comparison of four chemotherapy regimens for adverse non-small-cell lung cancer. N Engl J Med 2002; 346:92–98.

58. Kelly K, Crowley J, Bunn RB, et al. A randomized phase III trial of paclitaxel plus carboplatin (PC) versus vinorelbine plus cisplatin (VC) in untreated advanced non-small cell lung cancer (NSCLC): A Southwest Oncology Group (SWOG) trial. Proc Am Soc Clin Oncol 1999;18: A-1777 (Abstract).

59. LeChevalier T, Brisgand D, Douillard J, et al. Randomized study of vinorelbine and cisplatin versus vindesine and cisplatin versus vinorelbine alone in advanced non-small-cell lung cancer: Results of a European multicenter trial including 612 patients. J Clin Oncol 1994;12:360–367.

60. Abratt RP, Bezwoda WR, Falkson G, et al. Efficacy and safety profile of gemcitabine in nonsmall cell lung cancer: A phase II study. J Clin Oncol 1994;12:1535–1540.

61. Cardenal F, Lopez-Cabrerizo MP, Anton A, et al. Randomized phase III study of gemcitabine-cisplatin versus etoposide-cisplatin in the treatment of locally advanced or metastatic non-small-cell lung cancer. J Clin Oncol 1999;17:12–18.

62. DeVore RF, Johnson DH, Crawford J, et al. Phase II study of irinotecan plus cisplatin in patients with advanced non-small-cell lung cancer. J Clin Oncol 1999;17:2710–2720.

63. Masuda N, Fukoka M, Negro S, et al. Randomized trial comparing cisplatin (CDDP) and irinotecan (CPT-11) versus CDDP and vindesine (VDS) versus CPT-11 alone in advanced nonsmall cell lung cancer (NSCLC), a multicenter phase III study. Proc Am Soc Clin Oncol 1999; 18:1774 (Abstract).

64. Kelly K, Mikhaeel-Kamel N, Pan Z, et al. A phase I/II trial of paclitaxel, carboplatin, and gemcitabine in untreated patients with advanced non-small cell lung cancer. Clin Cancer Res 2000;6:3474–3479.

65. Frasci G, Panza N, Comella P, et al. Cisplatin, gemcitabine, and paclitaxel in locally advanced or metastatic non-small-cell lung cancer: A phase I-II study. J Clin Oncol 1999;17:2316–2325.

66. Wozniak AJ, Crowley JJ, Balcerzak SP, et al. Randomized trial comparing cisplatin with cisplatin plus vinorelbine in the treatment of advanced non-small cell lung cancer: A Southwestern Oncology Group study. J Clin Oncol 1998;16:459–465.

67. Langer C, Leighton J, Comis RL, et al. Paclitaxel and carboplatin in combination in the treatment of advanced non-small-cell-lung cancer: A phase II toxicity, response, and survival analysis. J Clin Oncol 1995; 13:1860–1870.

68. Langer CJ, Rosvold E, Millenson M, et al. Paclitaxel by 1- or 24-hour infusion combined with carboplatin in advanced non-small cell lung cancer (NSCLC): A comparative analysis. Proc Am Soc Clin Oncol 1997;16: A-1625 (Abstract).

69. Belani CP. Paclitaxel and docetaxel combination in non-small cell lung cancer. Chest 2000;17:144S–151S.

70. Gandara DR, Vokes E, Green M, et al. Docetaxel (Taxotere) in platinum-treated non-small cell lung cancer (NSCLC): Confirmation of prolonged survival in a multicenter trial. Proc Am Soc Clin Oncol 1997;16:A-1632 (Abstract).

71. Shepherd FA, Dancey J, Ramlau R. Prospective randomized trial of docetaxel versus best supportive care in patients with non-small cell lung cancer previously treated with platinum-based chemotherapy. J Clin Oncol 2000;18:2095–2103.

72. Fossella FV, Lippman SM, Shin DM, et al. Maximum-tolerated dose defined for single-agent gemcitabine: A phase I dose-escalation study in chemotherapy-naive patients with advanced non-small cell lung cancer. J Clin Oncol 1997;15:310–316.

73. Masuda N, Fukuoka M, Fujita A, et al. A phase II trial of combination CPT-11 and cisplatin for advanced non-small cell lung cancer. CPT-11 Lung Cancer Study Group. Br J Cancer 1998;78:251–256.

74. Takeda K, Negoro S, Kudoh S, et al. Phase I/II study of weekly irinotecan and concurrent radiation therapy for locally advanced non-small cell lung cancer. Br J Cancer 1999;79:1462–1467.

75. Fukuoka M, Yano S, Giaccone G, et al. Multi-institutional randomized phase II trial of gefitinib for previously treated patients with advanced non-small-cell lung cancer. J Clin Oncol 2003;21:2237–2246.

76. Kris MG, Natale RB, Herbst RS, et al. Efficacy of gefitinib, an inhibitor of the epidermal growth factor receptor tyrosine kinase, in symptomatic patients with non-small cell lung cancer: A randomized trial. JAMA 2003; 290:2149–2158.

77. Herbst RS, Giaccone G, Schiller JH, et al. Gefitinib in combination with paclitaxel and carboplatin in advanced non-small-cell lung cancer: A phase III trial–INTACT 2. J Clin Oncol 2004;22:785–794.

78. Giaccone G, Herbst RS, Manegold C, et al. Gefitinib in combination

with gemcitabine and cisplatin in advanced non-small-cell lung cancer: A phase III trial–INTACT 1. J Clin Oncol 2004;22:777–784.

79. Lynch TJ, Bell DW, Sordella R, et al. Activating mutations in the epidermal growth factor receptor underlying responsiveness of non-small-cell lung cancer to gefitinib. N Engl J Med 2004;350:2129–2139.

80. Shepherd FA, Pereira J, Ciuleanu TE, et al. A randomized placebo-controlled trial of erlotinib in patients with advanced non-small cell lung cancer following failure of 1st or 2nd line chemotherapy. Proc Am Soc Clin Oncol 2004;22:6225(Abstract).

81. Gefitinib (Iressa) lung cancer ISEL trial shows no overall survival advantage in a highly refractory population [press release 2004 Dec 17]. Available from http://www.astrazeneca-us.com/.

82. Johnson DH. Locally advanced unresectable non-small cell lung cancer: New treatment strategies. Chest 2000;117:123S–125S.

83. Bremnes RM, Sundstrom S, Aasebo U, et al. The value of prognostic factors in small cell lung cancer: Results from a randomised multicenter study with minimum 5 year follow-up. Lung Cancer 2003;39:303–313.

84. Turrisi AT 3rd, Kim K, Blum R, et al. Twice-daily compared with once-daily thoracic radiotherapy in limited small-cell lung cancer treated concurrently with cisplatin and etoposide. N Engl J Med 1999;340:265–271.

85. Robnett TJ, Machtay M, Vines EF, et al. Factors predicting severe radiation pneumonitis in patients receiving definitive chemoradiation for lung cancer. Int J Radiat Oncol Biol Phys 2000;48:89–94.

86. Arriagada R, Le Chevalier T, Borie F, et al. Prophylactic cranial irradiation for patients with small-cell lung cancer in complete remission. J Natl Cancer Inst 1995;87:183–190.

87. Auperin A, Arriagada R, Pignon JP, et al. Prophylactic cranial irradiation for patients with small-cell lung cancer in complete remission. Prophylactic Cranial Irradiation Overview Collaborative Group. N Engl J Med 1999;341:476–484.

88. Aisner J, Alberto P, Bitran J, et al. Role of chemotherapy in small cell lung cancer: a consensus report of the International Association for the Study of Lung Cancer workshop. Cancer Treat Rep 1983;67:37–43.

89. Noda K, Nishiwaki Y, Kawahara M, et al. Irinotecan plus cisplatin compared with etoposide plus cisplatin for extensive small-cell lung cancer. N Engl J Med 2002;346:85–91.

90. Pujol JL, Carestia L, Daures JP. Is there a case for cisplatin in the treatment of small-cell lung cancer? A meta-analysis of randomized trials of a cisplatin-containing regimen versus a regimen without this alkylating agent. Br J Cancer 2000;83:8–15.

91. Roth BJ, Johnson DH, Einhorn LH, et al. Randomized study of cyclophosphamide, doxorubicin, and vincristine versus etoposide and cisplatin versus alternation of these two regimens in extensive small-cell lung cancer: A phase III trial of the Southeastern Cancer Study Group. J Clin Oncol 1992;10:282–291.

92. Fukuoka M, Furuse K, Saijo N, et al. Randomized trial of cyclophosphamide, doxorubicin, and vincristine versus cisplatin and etoposide versus alternation of these regimens in small-cell lung cancer. J Natl Cancer Inst 1991;83:855–861.

93. Skarlos DV, Samantas E, Kosmidis P, et al. Randomized comparison of etoposide-cisplatin vs. etoposide-carboplatin and irradiation in small-cell lung cancer. A Hellenic Co-operative Oncology Group study. Ann Oncol 1994;5:601–607.

94. Goldie JH, Coldman AJ, Gudauskas GA. Rationale for the use of alternating non-cross–resistant chemotherapy. Cancer Treat Rep 1982;66:439–449.

95. Hryniuk W, Bush H. The importance of dose intensity in chemotherapy of metastatic breast cancer. J Clin Oncol 1984;2:1281–1288.

96. Galani E, Ellis PA, Harper PG. Small-cell lung cancer, high growth rate, high response rate to chemotherapy: Ideal for high-dose chemotherapy? J Clin Oncol 2002;20:3941–3943.

97. Johnson DH, Carbone DP. Increased dose-intensity in small-cell lung cancer: A failed strategy? J Clin Oncol 1999;17:2297–2299.

98. Klasa RJ, Murray N, Coldman AJ. Dose-intensity meta-analysis of chemotherapy regimens in small-cell carcinoma of the lung. J Clin Oncol 1991;9:499–508.

99. Arriagada R, Le Chevalier T, Pignon JP, et al. Initial chemotherapeutic doses and survival in patients with limited small-cell lung cancer. N Engl J Med 1993;329:1848–1852.

100. Sculier JP, Paesmans M, Lecomte J, et al. A three-arm phase III randomised trial assessing, in patients with extensive-disease small-cell lung cancer, accelerated chemotherapy with support of haematological growth factor or oral antibiotics. Br J Cancer 2001;85:1444–1451.

101. Ardizzoni A, Tjan-Heijnen VC, Postmus PE, et al. Standard versus intensified chemotherapy with granulocyte colony-stimulating factor support in small-cell lung cancer: A prospective European Organization for Research and Treatment of Cancer-Lung Cancer Group Phase III Trial-08923. J Clin Oncol 2002;20:3947–3955.

102. Murray N, Livingston RB, Shepherd FA, et al. Randomized study of CODE versus alternating CAV/EP for extensive-stage small-cell lung cancer: An Intergroup Study of the National Cancer Institute of Canada Clinical Trials Group and the Southwest Oncology Group. J Clin Oncol 1999;17:2300–2308.

103. Steward WP, von Pawel J, Gatzemeier U, et al. Effects of granulocyte-macrophage colony-stimulating factor and dose intensification of V-ICE chemotherapy in small-cell lung cancer: A prospective randomized study of 300 patients. J Clin Oncol 1998;16:642–650.

104. Thatcher N, Girling DJ, Hopwood P, et al. Improving survival without reducing quality of life in small-cell lung cancer patients by increasing the dose-intensity of chemotherapy with granulocyte colony-stimulating factor support: Results of a British Medical Research Council Multicenter Randomized Trial. Medical Research Council Lung Cancer Working Party. J Clin Oncol 2000;18:395–404.

105. Loehrer PJ Sr. The role of ifosfamide in small cell lung cancer. Semin Oncol 1996;23(3 Suppl 7):40–44.

106. Miyamoto H, Nakabayashi T, Isobe H, et al. A phase III comparison of etoposide/cisplatin with or without added ifosfamide in small-cell lung cancer. Oncology 1992;49:431–435.

107. Mavroudis D, Papadakis E, Veslemes M, et al. A multicenter randomized clinical trial comparing paclitaxel-cisplatin-etoposide versus cisplatin-etoposide as first-line treatment in patients with small-cell lung cancer. Ann Oncol 2001;12:463–470.

108. Niell HB, Herndon JE, Miller AA, et al. Randomized phase III Integroup trial (CALGB 9732) of etoposide (VP-16) and cisplatin (DDP) with or without paclitaxel (TAX) in patients with extensive stage small cell lung cancer [abstract]. Proc ASCO 2002;21:293a.

109. Reck M, von Pawel J, Macha HN, et al. Randomized phase III trial of paclitaxel, etoposide, and carboplatin versus carboplatin, etoposide, and vincristine in patients with small-cell lung cancer. J Natl Cancer Inst 2003;95:1118–1127.

110. Sculier JP, Joss RA, Schefer H, et al. Should maintenance chemotherapy be used to treat small cell lung cancer? Eur J Cancer 1998;34:1148–1155.

111. Shepherd FA, Giaccone G, Seymour L, et al. Prospective, randomized, double-blind, placebo-controlled trial of marimastat after response to first-line chemotherapy in patients with small-cell lung cancer: A trial of the National Cancer Institute of Canada-Clinical Trials Group and the European Organization for Research and Treatment of Cancer. J Clin Oncol 2002;20:4434–4439.

112. Wolff NC, Randle DE, Egorin MJ, et al. Imatinib mesylate efficiently achieves therapeutic intratumor concentrations in vivo but has limited activity in a xenograft model of small cell lung cancer. Clin Cancer Res 2004;10:3528–3534.

113. Ardizzoni A, Hansen H, Dombernowsky P, et al. Topotecan, a new active drug in the second-line treatment of small-cell lung cancer: A phase II study in patients with refractory and sensitive disease. The European Organization for Research and Treatment of Cancer Early Clinical Studies Group and New Drug Development Office, and the Lung Cancer Cooperative Group. J Clin Oncol 1997;15:2090–2096.

114. Perez-Soler R, Glisson BS, Lee JS, et al. Treatment of patients with small-cell lung cancer refractory to etoposide and cisplatin with the topoisomerase I poison topotecan. J Clin Oncol 1996;14:2785–2790.

127

COLORECTAL CANCER

Patrick J. Medina and Lisa E. Davis

Learning Objectives and other resources can be found at *www.pharmacotherapyonline.com.*

KEY CONCEPTS

◀1 Maintaining a diet with high-fiber and low fat intake has not been proved to reduce colorectal cancer risk, but is beneficial for reducing risk of other chronic diseases.

◀2 In certain patient populations, the risk of colon cancer may be reduced by the use of aspirin and other nonsteroidal anti-inflammatory drugs, hormone replacement therapy, and calcium supplementation.

◀3 Effective colorectal cancer screening programs incorporate annual fecal occult blood testing in combination with regular examination of the entire colon starting at age 50 for average-risk individuals. Colorectal adenomas can progress to cancer and should be removed.

◀4 The stage of colorectal cancer upon diagnosis—determined by depth of bowel invasion, lymph node involvement, and presence of metastases—is the most important prognostic factor for disease recurrence and survival.

◀5 The goal for stage I, II, and III colon cancer is cure; surgery should be offered to all eligible patients for this purpose. Adjuvant chemotherapy, consisting of 6 months of fluorouracil plus leucovorin, significantly reduces the risk of cancer recurrence and overall mortality compared to observation alone in patients with stage III disease.

◀6 Adjuvant therapy consisting of fluorouracil-based chemosensitized radiation therapy should be offered to patients with stage II or III cancer of the rectum. Adjuvant fluorouracil chemotherapy plus radiation decreases risk of local and distant disease recurrence as compared to observation alone.

◀7 Chemotherapy is palliative for metastatic disease. Fluorouracil-based chemotherapy regimens combined with leucovorin, administered in a variety of schedules, provide a modest improvement in survival and can be highly beneficial in reducing patient symptoms.

◀8 Triple-drug therapy consisting of fluorouracil and leucovorin with oxaliplatin or irinotecan improves survival compared to fluorouracil plus leucovorin alone, and is considered as standard first-line therapy for metastatic disease. Bevacizumab, in combination with fluorouracil-based chemotherapy, is also indicated for initial treatment of metastatic colorectal cancer. Patients may benefit from more than one regimen during the treatment of their disease.

◀9 Capecitabine is an acceptable alternative to intravenous fluorouracil for metastatic colorectal cancer, as it provides similar efficacy and its oral dosing may offer greater patient convenience. The role of capecitabine as a replacement for intravenous fluorouracil in combination regimens is under investigation.

◀10 Individuals whose disease progresses during or is refractory to irinotecan may benefit from cetuximab, either alone or combined with continuing irinotecan. Their tumor should be epidermal growth factor receptor–positive.

Colorectal cancer involves the colon, rectum, and the anal canal. It is one of the three most common cancers occurring in adult men and women in the United States, and accounts for approximately one in nine cancer diagnoses. In 2005, an estimated 145,290 new cases will be diagnosed, of which 104,950 will involve the colon and 40,340 the rectum.[1]

For both adult men and women, colorectal cancer is the third leading cause of cancer-related deaths in the United States. An estimated 56,290 deaths will occur during 2005.[1] Overall, the mortality and incidence associated with colorectal cancer has decreased during the past 30 years. Mortality rates associated with colorectal cancer in the United States are comparable to those of other industrialized areas around the world.[2]

Multiple factors are associated with the development of colorectal cancer, including acquired and inherited genetic susceptibility, environmental elements, and lifestyle choices. Overall, about 37% of affected individuals undergo a surgical procedure alone intended for cure. An additional 37% of individuals can potentially be cured by undergoing surgery followed by radiation therapy (XRT), chemotherapy, or both. Curability is influenced primarily by extent of tumor invasion into adjacent tissues or organs and presence of metastatic disease. Five-year survival rates are close to 91% and 88% for persons with early stages of colon and rectal cancer, respectively.[3] After the tumor has spread regionally to adjacent lymph nodes or tissues, five-year survival rates drop to 69% for colon cancer and to 63% for cancer of the rectum. Five-year survival for individuals with metastatic disease is about 9%.

Treatment modalities for colorectal cancer include surgery, XRT, chemotherapy, immunotherapy, and new targeted molecular therapies. Surgery is the most important and definitive procedure associated with cure; radiation therapy can be used to improve curability following surgical resection and to reduce symptoms and complications associated with advanced disease. Chemotherapy is used in adjuvant treatment regimens as well as in treatment for advanced stages of disease. Much progress has been made in the treatment of advanced disease, in the ability to identify candidates for potentially curative surgical procedures, and the availability of active drug regimens that can improve patients' survival.

EPIDEMIOLOGY

Incidence rates worldwide vary by as much as 20-fold. The highest incidence rates occur in highly industrialized areas such as North America, Northern and Western Europe, Australia, and New Zealand. The lowest incidence rates are seen in India and in less-developed areas such as South America and rural Africa.[4] Rates have increased substantially, however, in previously lower-risk countries such as Japan and China, as well as among persons migrating from low-risk areas to the United States. Within one or two generations, the incidence rates among migrating groups approximate those of the new host country, suggesting that environmental and dietary factors may influence a late stage in colorectal carcinogenesis. However, colorectal cancers are known to develop more frequently in certain families and genetic predisposition to this disease is also well-recognized.

The incidence of colon cancer is greatest among males, who have an age-adjusted incidence rate of 44.3 per 100,000, as compared to females for whom the rate is 34.8 per 100,000.[3] Cancer of the rectum occurs less frequently; the incidence rate is 19.1 and 11.6 per 100,000 for males and females, respectively. Cancer of the colon and rectum is the third most frequent malignancy among U.S. men and white and African-American women, but is second next to breast cancer for Hispanic, American Indian/Alaskan Native, and Asian/Pacific Islander women. The overall incidence of colon and rectal cancers in the United States has declined since 1992 at an average rate of 0.7% per year; this rate of decrease is beginning to level off.[3] This decline is attributable primarily to decreasing rates among white males and females, although rates in African-American males and females have also declined but more slowly.

Although it is difficult to compare trends because of large year-to-year variations in colorectal cancer incidence rates in minority population groups, downward trends in colorectal cancer incidence appear to be greater for whites, African-Americans, Asian/Pacific Islanders, and American Indian/Alaskan Native Americans than for Hispanics. Trends for incidence and mortality rates among white and African-American males and females in the United States can be compared in Fig. 127–1.

The median age at diagnosis is about 72 years.[3] Fewer than 5% of affected persons are younger than age 44 years. An individual's risk, however, increases with increasing age. Seventy percent of cases develop in adults older than 65 years of age. The stage of disease at presentation is similar among different ethnic groups, although the tendency to present with later-stage disease is slightly higher for African-Americans.

About 10% of all cancer deaths are a result of cancer of the colon or rectum. It is estimated that 56,290 individuals will die of colorectal cancer in the United States in 2005, despite a decline in overall combined mortality for both colon and rectal cancer observed during the last 20 years. For women, the decline in colorectal cancer mortality rates has been evident since 1950, whereas death rates among men did not start to decline until the late 1970s.[3] These trends in mortality rates are similar to those observed in other countries. Overall mortality rates remain higher among African-American males and females, and the rates of decline are lower as compared to those for white males and females. Colorectal cancer mortality rates are lower for Hispanics, American Indians/Alaskan Natives, and Asian/Pacific Islanders than for whites or African-Americans. Factors contributing to the overall

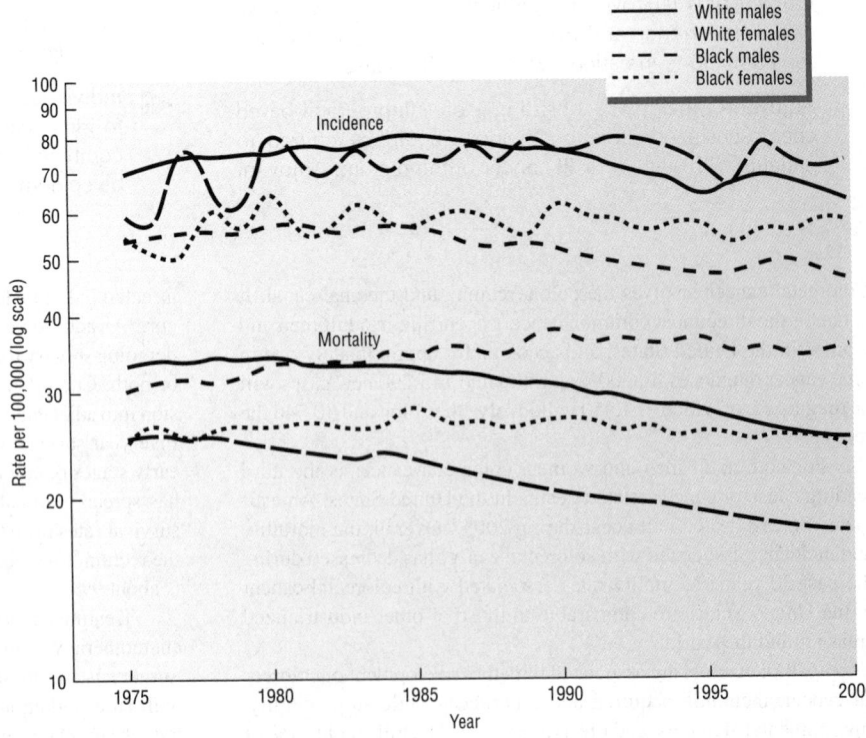

FIGURE 127–1. SEER incidence and mortality rates for invasive colon and rectum cancer, 1975–2000, age-adjusted and age-specific. Rates are per 100,000 and age-adjusted to the 2000 U.S. standard population. (From Ries et al.[3])

decline in colorectal cancer mortality likely include decreasing incidence rates, screening programs with early polyp removal, and more effective and better-tolerated treatments.

ETIOLOGY AND RISK FACTORS

Numerous studies suggest that the development of colorectal cancer can be caused or promoted by dietary or environmental factors that affect the bowel, lifestyle choices, and certain comorbid conditions, in addition to physical and genetic susceptibilities.

DIETARY INTAKE AND NUTRIENTS

◁ Epidemiologic studies of worldwide incidence of colorectal cancer suggest that economic development and dietary habits strongly influence its development. Although findings based on epidemiologic data are subject to potential biases, as well as inconsistencies in how dietary factors are categorized and measured, numerous studies have attempted to ascertain the true contribution of dietary habits as independent risk factors for colon cancer development.

FIBER

◁ Dietary fiber is the part of ingested plant material that is not processed by normal human digestive enzymes. Fibers are frequently classified as either water soluble (pectins, gums, and mucilages) or insoluble (celluloses, hemicellulose, and lignins). The insoluble fibers have been most consistently associated with reduced cancer risk. Foods that are high in fiber include vegetables, fruit, grains, and cereals. Postulated protective effects of dietary fiber include dilution or reduced absorption of carcinogens in the bowel, reduced fecal pH, reduced bowel transit time, alterations in bile acid metabolism, or increased production of short-chain fatty acids.[5] The protective effects of fiber may also reflect an associated concomitant reduction in dietary fat intake associated with high-fiber diets. The degree of colorectal cancer risk reduction associated with increased consumption of vegetables and fruit is variable but generally modest. Conflicting data exist as to whether one category of dietary fiber is superior to another.

In a meta-analysis of six case-control studies of vegetable consumption and colon cancer risk, a combined odds ratio of 0.48 was observed between the highest and lowest quintiles of consumption.[6] Two large prospective studies have also demonstrated an inverse relationship between fiber intake and colon cancer. The Prostate, Lung, Colorectal, and Ovarian Cancer Screening Trial found that participants in the highest quintile of dietary fiber intake had a 27% lower risk of adenoma than those in the lowest quintile.[7] The inverse association was strongest for fiber from grains and cereals and from fruits. A European trial has reported similar results with a 25% risk reduction in the incidence of colorectal cancer for the highest versus lowest quintile of intake.[8] In contrast, data from a prospective, cohort study of dietary factors and risk of colorectal adenomas in men and women using data from the Health Professionals Follow-Up Study and from the Nurse's Health Study found no association between fiber intake and risk of colorectal adenoma or cancer in over 120,000 participants, although a weak inverse association existed between dietary fiber and colorectal cancer with respect to participants with low folate consumption.[9] Thus the evidence that increased dietary fiber consumption reduces colorectal cancer risk is suggestive, but not conclusive, and the amount, type, and duration of fiber intake may determine who benefits.

FAT

◁ Epidemiologic studies suggest that a relationship exists between dietary fat intake and colorectal cancer risk, although this has not been consistently seen.[6] This may have resulted from the use of dietary evaluations that focused on the quantity, origin, or type (saturated, monounsaturated, and polyunsaturated) of fat rather than specific fatty acids ingested. The association between red meat consumption and colorectal cancer is strongest, possibly a result of the heterocyclic amines formed during cooking or the presence of specific fatty acids in red meat such as arachidonic acid.

The role of dietary fat in cancer development may be a result of its influence on fecal bile acid concentrations. The release of bile acids is stimulated following ingestion of dietary fat. These acids are then converted by colonic flora to secondary bile acids, which are associated with bowel mucosal irritation and cell proliferation responses and may promote tumor growth.[10]

Therefore while data indicate that animal meat and saturated fat intake and processing appear to be associated with an increased risk of colorectal cancer, the magnitude of this risk has not been determined.

CALCIUM AND MICRONUTRIENTS

◁ The role of calcium intake on colorectal cancer risk has been investigated in cohort, case-control, and randomized studies. The risk of colon cancer was shown in two prospective cohort studies to be inversely related to calcium intake. The decrease in risk was limited to distal colon cancer with no change seen in the incidence of proximal cancers. Calcium's protective effect may be related to a reduction in mucosal cell proliferation rates or through its binding to bile salts in the intestine. High levels of dietary folate, a key constituent of vegetables, are also associated with decreased colorectal cancer and adenoma risk.[5] Folate availability influences DNA methylation, which is an important process in maintaining normal bowel mucosa. Evidence exists that an adequate dietary folate intake may be enough to lower the risk of colon cancer, and exceeding normal intake may not add any protective effects. Additional micronutrient deficiencies that have been demonstrated through several studies to increase colorectal cancer risk include selenium, vitamin C, vitamin D, vitamin E, and β-carotene; however, the benefit of dietary supplementation does not appear to be substantial.[10]

LIFESTYLE FACTORS

NONSTEROIDAL ANTI-INFLAMMATORY DRUG AND ASPIRIN USE

◁ Several lifestyle factors are known to affect colorectal cancer risk (Table 127–1). Studies have consistently demonstrated that regular (at least two doses per week) nonsteroidal anti-inflammatory drug (NSAID) and aspirin use is associated with a reduced risk of colorectal cancer.[5] In the Nurse's Health Study, a decreased risk of colorectal cancer was seen in women who took aspirin regularly for at least 10 consecutive years, with the greatest reduction occurring with an intake of four to six tablets per week.[11] This benefit has also been seen with NSAID users. A population-based study of individuals who had taken NSAIDs for at least 48 months of the previous 5 years demonstrated a relative risk of colorectal cancer one-half that of nonusers.[12] Additional studies support these findings that regular aspirin or NSAID use may decrease the risk of colorectal cancer by as much as 50%. The potential mechanisms by which these agents exert their protective effects appear to be linked primarily to their inhibition

TABLE 127–1. Lifestyle Factors Associated with Colorectal Cancer Risk

Factor	Comments
Aspirin and non-aspirin NSAID use	Regular use associated with risk reduction, perhaps as much as 50%
Postmenopausal hormone use	Exogenous hormone intake decreases risk 19%–34%
Alcohol intake	Heavy use increases colorectal risk two- to threefold
Physical inactivity and obesity	Elevated BMI and physical inactivity associated with increased risk
Tobacco use	Use of tobacco products estimated to contribute to up to 12% of colorectal cancer deaths annually
Diabetes	Hyperinsulinemia may promote colorectal cancer development
Western diet	High fat, red meat consumption, and low fiber intake possibly associated with increased risk

BMI, body mass index; NSAID, nonsteroidal anti-inflammatory drug.
From Potter.[5]

of cyclooxygenase-2 (COX-2) and free radical formation. COX-2 overexpression is seen in precancerous and cancerous lesions in the colon and is associated with a decrease in colon cancer cell apoptosis, as well as enhanced production of angiogenesis-promoting factors.[13] Inhibition of COX by NSAIDs, aspirin, and coxibs restores apoptosis and decreases expression of proangiogenic factors.

EXOGENOUS HORMONE USE

Exogenous hormone use, particularly postmenopausal hormone replacement therapy, is associated with a significant reduction in colorectal cancer risk in most studies.[5,14] A meta-analysis of 18 epidemiologic studies of postmenopausal hormone replacement therapy showed a 20% reduction in risk of colon cancer, and a 19% reduction in risk of rectal cancer, in women who received hormone replacement therapy as compared to women who never used hormone replacement therapy.[14] The risk is reduced in postmenopausal women receiving both estrogen only and combined estrogen and progestin therapy, and persists for approximately 10 years after therapy is discontinued. Risk reduction appears greatest among women who are currently receiving hormone replacement therapy. However, prospective data on exogenous hormone use and colon cancer risk are conflicting. The Women's Health Initiative showed that colorectal cancer rates were reduced by 37% with combined estrogen/progestin use, whereas the Heart and Estrogen/Progestin Replacement Study Follow-up study demonstrated no significant decrease in risk.[14,15] Furthermore, although invasive colorectal cancer occurred less frequently with estrogen/progestin use in the Women's Health Initiative, colorectal cancers were diagnosed at a much later stage in women who took hormones as compared to placebo.[16]

Several mechanisms for a protective effect of estrogens on the bowel have been identified.[5,14] Declining estrogen levels associated with aging are associated with estrogen receptor hypermethylation, resulting in reduced expression of the estrogen receptor gene and dysregulated colonic mucosal cell growth. In addition, estrogen use may reduce serum levels of insulin-like growth factor-1, an important mitogen that influences cell-cycle progression in certain cells.

OBESITY AND PHYSICAL INACTIVITY

Physical inactivity and elevated body mass index (BMI), independent of level of physical activity, are associated with an elevated risk of colon adenoma, colon cancer, and rectal cancer.[10] Individuals with a total higher level of activity throughout life have the lowest risk. Hypotheses for these relationships include the observation that physical activity stimulates bowel peristalsis, resulting in decreased bowel transit time, and the possibility that exercise-induced alterations in body glucose, insulin levels, and perhaps other hormones may reduce tumor cell growth.[5]

The risk of colon cancer may be increased as much as twofold in men who are in the highest quintile of body size. The evidence linking elevated BMI with increased colon cancer risk is less consistent for women, although, the Iowa Women's Health Study showed that cancer risk was 40% higher in women who were in the highest quintile of BMI as compared to the cancer risk of women in the lowest quintile.[5] The relationship between obesity and colorectal cancer among women may diminish with age. Premenopausal obese women appear to be at the greatest risk, while postmenopausal obese women do not have an elevated risk of colon cancer. In a prospective cohort study, obesity (BMI ≥ 30 kg/m^2) was associated with a 75% higher risk of colon cancer among women who were premenopausal at baseline; no association was found between BMI and colon cancer risk in postmenopausal women.[17] Type 2 diabetes mellitus, independent of body mass size and physical activity level, is also associated with an increased risk of colorectal cancer in women. Data from the Nurse's Health Study suggest that colon cancer risk may be increased by 49% in diabetic women as compared to nondiabetic women.[18] These and other findings support a role for hyperinsulinemia as a possible link between obesity, sedentary lifestyle, and diabetes mellitus and colon cancer.

ALCOHOL AND TOBACCO USE

High alcohol consumption increases the risk of rectal and colon cancer, perhaps as much as two- to threefold, although some studies have found no significant increase in risk.[6,10] The evidence is strongest in men, but alcohol consumption is generally greater in men than in women. The impact of alcohol consumption and colon cancer may be greatest when folate intake is low, possibly resulting from the antifolate properties of alcohol. Smoking tobacco products, including cigarettes, cigars, and pipes, may contribute to as much as 12% of all colorectal cancer deaths.[19] The cancer-promoting effects of alcohol and tobacco may be through generation of carcinogens or their direct toxic effects on bowel tissue.

CLINICAL RISK FACTORS

CHRONIC INFLAMMATORY DISEASES

Chronic ulcerative colitis, particularly when it involves the entire large intestine, predisposes individuals to colorectal cancer at a rate that is 4- to 20-fold greater than average.[20] The risk is even greater for young individuals and increases for all affected individuals with increasing extent of bowel involvement and disease duration. The cumulative risk of colorectal cancer is low early in life, and increases by 0.5% to 1% each year for 8 to 10 years after diagnosis.[20] Although a precise causative link has not been established, chronic underlying inflammation may be a significant predisposing factor. The progressive dysplastic changes that bowel mucosa undergo are similar to those observed in adenomatous polyps. Similarly, patients with Crohn's disease are also at increased risk, although the relative risk is slightly lower than that of patients with ulcerative colitis. This difference may be related to the decreased length of bowel affected by the chronic inflammatory process in individuals with Crohn's disease. Overall, persons diagnosed with either disease constitute about 1% to 2% of all new cases of colorectal cancer each year.

GENETIC SUSCEPTIBILITY

HEREDITARY

There are three specific patterns in which colon cancer is generally observed: sporadic, inherited, and familial.[21] While the majority of cases of colon cancer are sporadic in nature, as many as 10% of cases are thought to be hereditary. The two most common forms of hereditary colon cancer are familial adenomatous polyposis (FAP) and hereditary nonpolyposis colorectal cancer (HNPCC). Each of these results from a specific germline mutation.[21] FAP is a rare autosomal dominant trait that is caused by inactivating mutations of the adenomatous polyposis coli (*APC*) gene and accounts for 0.5% to 1% of all colorectal cancers. The disease is manifested by hundreds to thousands of tiny sessile adenomatous polyps that carpet the colon and rectum, typically arising during adolescence.[5] Symptoms generally present between the ages of 25 and 35 years, at which time cancer is already present in about half of patients. The risk of developing colorectal cancer for individuals with untreated FAP is virtually 100%; most will develop colorectal cancer by their fourth decade of life. Several variants of FAP exist and are associated with different extracolonic manifestations.[5]

HNPCC, also referred to as Lynch syndrome I or II, is an autosomal dominant inherited syndrome that accounts for 1% to 5% of colon cancer cases.[5] A mutation in one of the DNA mismatch-repair (MMR) genes, most commonly *MLH1* or *MSH2*, is responsible for HNPCC.[21] In contrast to FAP, adenomatous polyps are not a primary manifestation of the HNPCC. Polyps that do form tend to be located primarily in the proximal colon. The average age of these patients is between 40 and 44 years. Because the clinical presentation of HNPCC is difficult to distinguish from "sporadic" forms of colorectal cancer, the diagnosis of HNPCC can be confirmed by the presence of germline mutations in a family of genes responsible for DNA MMR. Criteria for diagnosis of HNPCC have been established.[21] Testing for *MLH1/MSH2* mutations is generally reserved for those individuals who meet these strict criteria. Carriers of a germline mutation have an 80% to 85% risk of developing colorectal cancer over their lifetime.[22]

Familial colon cancer represents the least understood pattern of colorectal cancer. Up to 25% of patients who develop colorectal cancer will have a family history of colorectal cancer. In these families, the frequency of colorectal cancer is too high to be considered sporadic, but the pattern is not consistent with an inherited syndrome. First-degree relatives of patients diagnosed with colorectal cancer have an increased risk of the disease that is at least two to four times that of persons in the general population without a family history.[23]

ENZYME POLYMORPHISMS

Increasing evidence suggests that certain high-prevalence genetic polymorphisms, such as *N*-acetyltransferases (NAT1 and NAT2), certain cytochrome (CYP450) isoenzymes, methylenetetrahydrofolate reductase (MTHFR) enzymes, and hemochromatosis gene mutations may confer genetic susceptibility to colorectal cancer.[5] Individuals with certain variations in NAT1, NAT2, and CYP450 1A2 enzyme genotypes may be particularly susceptible to carcinogenic effects of a high dietary intake of meat or tobacco smoke. Variants of MTHFR may influence the association of colorectal cancer risk with dietary folate or vitamin B_{12} intake. Mutations in the hemochromatosis gene are associated with increased colon cancer risk with increasing age and total iron intake.

SUMMARY OF RISK FACTORS

In summary, the true association between most dietary factors and risk of colon cancer is unclear. The protective effects of fiber, calcium, and a diet low in fat are not completely known at this time. Lifestyle factors such as NSAID use and hormone replacement use appear to decrease the risk of colorectal cancer, but questions remain about how to best use these agents. Obesity and alcohol use appear to increase risk of colon cancer, but their association is not well defined. Genetic and clinical risk factors such as inflammatory bowel disease are well known risks for colon cancer.

PATHOPHYSIOLOGY

ANATOMY AND BOWEL FUNCTION

The large intestine consists of the cecum; ascending, transverse, descending, and sigmoid colon; and the rectum (Fig. 127–2). In adults, it extends approximately 1.5 m and has a diameter ranging from 8 cm in the cecum to 2 cm in the sigmoid colon. The function of the large intestine is to receive 500 to 2000 mL of ileal contents per day. Absorption of fluid and solutes occurs in the right colon or the segments proximal to the middle of the transverse colon, with movement and storage of fecal material in the left colon and distal segments of the colon. Mucus secretion from goblet cells into the intestinal lumen lubricates the mucosal surface and facilitates movement of the dehydrated feces. It also serves to protect the luminal wall from bacteria and colonic irritants such as bile acids.

Four major tissue layers, from the lumen outward, form the large intestine: the mucosa, submucosa, muscularis externa, and serosa (Fig. 127–3). Embedded in the submucosa and muscularis externa is a rich lymphatic capillary system. Lymphatic channels do not extend into the mucosa. The muscularis externa consists of circular smooth

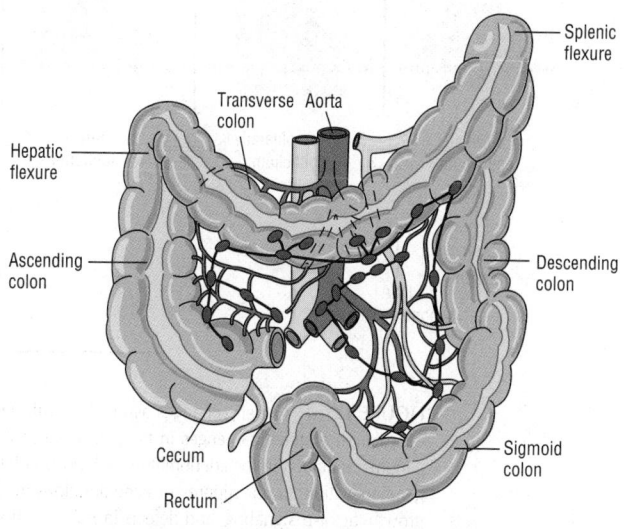

FIGURE 127–2. Colon and rectum anatomy.

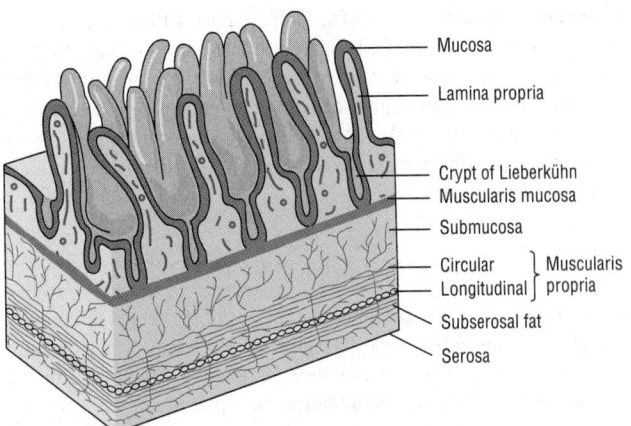

FIGURE 127–3. Cross-section of bowel wall.

muscle and three outer longitudinal smooth muscle bands. Contraction of these muscle groups moves colonic material toward the anal canal. The outermost layer of the colon, the serosa, secretes a fluid that allows the colon to slide easily over nearby structures within the peritoneum. The serosa covers only the anterior and lateral aspects of the upper third of the rectum. The lower third lies completely extraperitoneal and is surrounded by fibrofatty tissue as well as adjacent organs and structures.

The surface epithelium of the colonic mucosa undergoes continual renewal, and complete replacement of epithelial cells occurs every 4 to 8 days. Cell replication normally takes place within the lower third of crypts, the tubular glands located within the intestinal mucosa. The cells then mature and differentiate to either goblet or absorptive cells as they migrate toward the bowel lumen. The total number of epithelial cells remains relatively constant as the number of cells migrating from the crypts is balanced by the rate of exfoliation of cells from the mucosal surface. This two-phase process is critical to the malignant transformation of the epithelial cells. The number of dysplastic and hyperplastic aberrant crypt foci increases with increasing age; as the mass of abnormal cells accumulates at the top of the crypt and starts to protrude into the stream of fecal matter, their contact with fecal mutagens can lead to further cell mutations and eventual adenoma formation.[5]

COLORECTAL TUMORIGENESIS

The development of a colorectal neoplasm is a multi-step process of several genetic and phenotypic alterations of normal bowel epithelium structure and function, leading to unregulated cell growth, proliferation, and tumor development. Since the majority of colorectal cancers develop sporadically, with no inherited or familial disposition, efforts have been directed toward identifying these alterations and learning whether detection of such changes may lead to improved cancer detection and/or treatment outcomes.

A genetic model has been proposed for colorectal tumorigenesis that describes a process of transformation from adenoma to carcinoma. However, at least three separate additional molecular pathways to developing colorectal cancer have been identified.[5] These include a pathway for HNPCC, an ulcerative colitis–dysplasia-carcinoma sequence, and a pathway involving loss of function of the estrogen receptor gene through hypermethylation. Some of the molecular processes are common to more than one pathway.

Figure 127–4 is an overview of the adenoma-carcinoma model. The adenoma-carcinoma sequence of tumor development reflects an accumulation of mutations within colonic epithelium which confer a selective growth advantage to the affected cells. Key elements of this process include hyperproliferation of epithelial cells to form a small benign neoplasm or adenoma in conjunction with cellular gene mutations.[24,25] These mutations occur early and frequently in sporadic cases of both adenomas and colorectal cancer. Somatic mutations

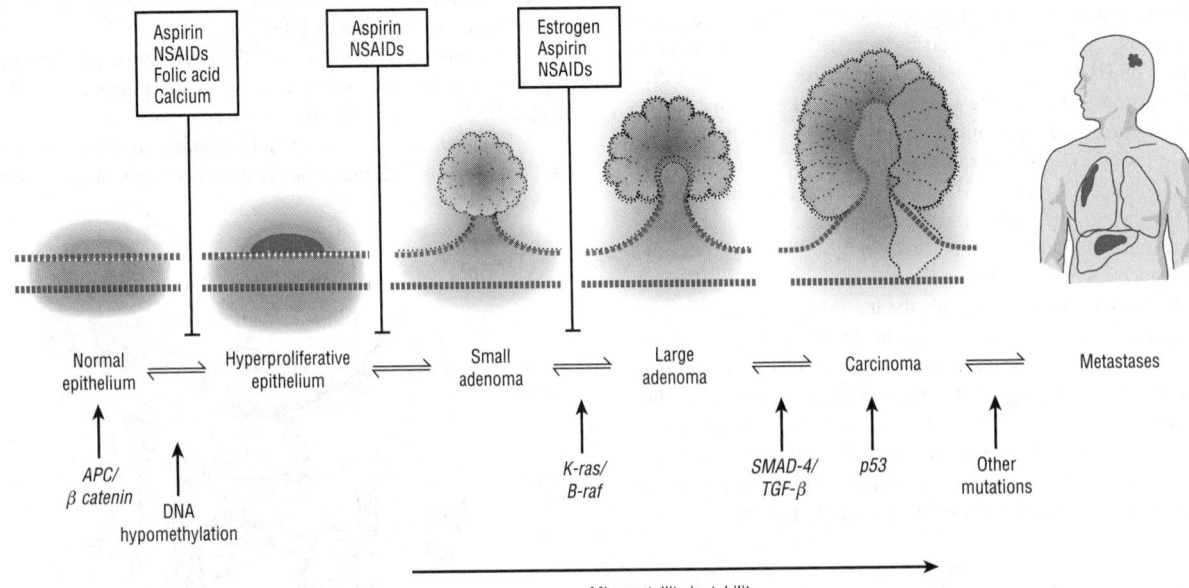

FIGURE 127–4. Genetic changes associated with the adenoma-carcinoma sequence in colorectal cancer. The accumulation of genetic changes in the pathogenesis of colorectal cancer includes DNA hypomethylation across the genome, mutation in the adenomatous polyposis coli (APC) gene or abnormalities in β catenin; k-Ras or B-raf oncogene activation; tumor suppressor gene deletions in chromosome 18q (SMAD-4 mutations) and disruption of tumor growth factor-β signaling; and defects in p53 function. Shown also are points of possible chemopreventive activity by various agents. (From Midgley et al,[24] Robbins et al,[25] Arends,[26] and Jänne et al.[30])

TABLE 127–2. Genetic Mutations Associated with Colorectal Cancer

Type of Mutation	Genes	Associated Disease
Germline	APC	Familial adenomatous polyposis (FAP)
	DNA mismatch-repair	Hereditary nonpolyposis colorectal cancer (HNPCC)
Somatic	Oncogenes:	Sporadic colorectal cancer
	ras	
	B-raf	
	myc	
	src	
	erbB2[a]	
	Tumor suppressor genes:	
	p53	
	SMAD-4	
	APC	
	DNA mismatch-repair genes:	
	MSH2	
	MLH1	
	PMS1	
	PMS2	
	MSH6	
	MSH3	
Genetic polymorphism	APC	Familial colon cancer in Ashkenazi Jewish individuals

[a]Controversial.
APC, adenomatous polyposis coli.
Modified with permission from Calvert et al.[21]

must occur in at least four or five genes to produce the malignant transformation.[21]

Genetic changes include activating mutations of oncogenes, inactivating mutations of tumor suppressor genes, and defects in DNA MMR genes. Specific genetic mutations that cause colorectal cancer are listed in Table 127–2. Activating mutations of *ras* protooncogenes, primarily involving the K-*ras* and N-*ras* genes, occur frequently in colorectal cancer.[22,23] The *ras* family of genes is responsible for encoding proteins involved in transmission of extracellular growth signals to the nucleus. Activation of *ras* leads to a constitutive activity of the protein, resulting in continuous stimulus of cell proliferation and other activities that promote carcinogenesis.[21]

Tumor suppressor genes are normal cellular genes that are capable of transforming normal cells to cancerous cells through their deletion or inactivation. One of the earliest genetic changes in colorectal tumorigenesis involves the mutation or loss of the *APC* gene, a tumor suppressor gene localized on the long arm of chromosome 5q21. The *APC* gene encodes for a protein that binds to α- and β-catenin, which belong to a family of proteins associated with intracellular adhesion.[25] β-Catenin binds to the cytoplasmic domain of E-cadherin, an important molecule responsible for cell-cell adhesion. These activities, among others, are believed to be involved in regulation of cell shape and cell-to-cell communication, and may affect cell-cycle regulation or apoptosis. β-Catenin alterations may also lead to abnormal epithelial proliferation and differentiation of cells. Inactivation of the *APC* gene is the single gene defect responsible for FAP,

and is frequently an early event in the development of sporadic colorectal cancer cases.[21] A specific *APC* mutation, I1307K, is a factor in the development of familial colon cancer in individuals of Ashkenazi Jewish ancestry.[21]

Mutational inactivation of two additional important tumor suppressor genes, *p53*, located on chromosome 17p, and the *DPC-4* (deleted in pancreatic cancer) gene, located on chromosome 18q, occur later during the adenoma-carcinoma sequence.[24–26] Normal *p53* gene expression is important for G_1 cell-cycle arrest to facilitate DNA repair during replication, and to induce apoptosis, an irreversible cell process resulting in cell death. Inactivation of *p53* occurs in up to 75% of sporadic colorectal cancers.[21]

Previously, the *DCC* (deleted in colorectal carcinoma) gene was thought to be the tumor suppressor gene involved in 18q deletions. The protein encoded by the normal *DCC* gene is believed to share similar structural features to certain types of cell adhesion molecules, and as such may interact with various proteins to control cell-cell or cell-matrix interactions and cellular proliferation. Mutations of *DCC* are found in approximately 50% of advanced adenomas.[21] The *DPC-4* gene, also referred to as *SMAD-4*, is located adjacent to the *DCC* gene, and has become identified as an important component involved in the transforming growth factor-β (TGF-β) signaling pathway.[26] The frequency of *SMAD-4* mutations in colorectal cancer is reported to be from 6% to 30%.[26]

A distinct group of genetic traits has also been identified for individuals with HNPCC, but occur in sporadic cases of colorectal cancer, as well. Replication errors occur frequently and represent widespread alterations in the length of a series of repeated nucleotides, or microsatellites, within tumor DNA.[24] Mutations of those genes that appear to recognize and regulate DNA mismatch-repair errors, or MMR genes, contribute to microsatellite instability and colorectal tumorigenesis.[25] Failure to repair DNA mismatches results in microsatellite instability, which accelerates further gene mutations, leading to oncogene activation or tumor suppressor gene inactivation. Tumor progression may then be facilitated through a link between DNA repair defects and mutations of critical growth regulatory genes. Inactivation of a receptor for type II transforming growth factor-β, a protein that has antiproliferative effects on colonic epithelial cell growth, has been demonstrated in cells with replication errors.[27]

Several additional genes and protein receptors are believed important in colorectal tumorigenesis, although their roles have not been completely determined. COX-2, which is induced in colorectal cancer cells, influences apoptosis and other cellular functions. The peroxisome proliferator activated receptor gene, a nuclear receptor that serves as a transcription factor, may interact with the COX pathway and affect tumorigenesis.[21] The protooncogene c-*erb*-B is activated in a high percentage of human tumors, including colorectal cancer, and encodes for expression of epidermal growth factor receptor (EGFR), a transmembrane glycoprotein involved in signaling pathways that affect cell growth, differentiation, proliferation, and angiogenesis. These mechanisms are potentially important because of the availability of pharmacologic agents that can influence these processes and affect cell growth.

HISTOLOGY

Adenocarcinomas account for more than 90% of tumors of the large intestine.[28] Other histologic types such as mucinous adenocarcinoma, signet-ring adenocarcinoma, carcinoid simplex, and carcinoid tumors occur less frequently. Adenocarcinomas are assigned one of three tumor grade designations based on the degree of cellular differentiation, the degree to which the tumor resembles the structure, and function of its cell of origin. The most differentiated adenocarcinomas, or grade I tumors, generally resemble adenomas, whereas grade III tumors are considered "high grade," the most undifferentiated, and have frequently lost the characteristics of mature normal cells. Poorly differentiated tumors are associated with a worse prognosis than those that are better differentiated.[28]

Mucinous adenocarcinomas possess the same basic structure as adenocarcinomas, but differ in that they secrete an abundant quantity of extracellular mucus. They account for only about 10% of colorectal carcinomas but tend to be frequent in patients with HNPCC and patients with coexisting ulcerative colitis.[28] Signet-ring adenocarcinomas have a characteristic appearance because of the displacement of the nucleus to one side by large vacuoles of intracellular mucin. Patients tend to present with a more advanced stage of disease and have a highly invasive tumor. Both mucinous and signet-ring adenocarcinoma histologies confer a poor prognosis.

PREVENTION AND SCREENING

Cancer prevention efforts can be considered as either primary or secondary. Primary prevention strategies are aimed at preventing the development of colorectal cancer in a population at risk. Secondary prevention approaches are undertaken to prevent malignancy in a population that has already manifested an initial disease process. The basis for primary prevention depends on identification of risk factors followed by eradication or alteration of their effects on carcinogenesis. Primary prevention also includes lifestyle and diet modification.[29,30] Several primary preventive measures have undergone or are currently undergoing study; Table 127–3 lists some of the most promising strategies.

HIGH-FIBER LOW-FAT DIET

Although early studies suggest that a substantial increase in daily dietary fiber and/or decrease in dietary fat intake might significantly, reduce colorectal cancer risk results from recent randomized trials are inconsistent. The role of a diet high in fiber, or the use of fiber supplementation, as a prevention strategy requires further investigation.

CHEMOPREVENTION

The most widely studied agents for the chemoprevention of colorectal cancer are aspirin and the NSAIDs. Although COX-2 expression is not elevated in normal colonic epithelium, up to 40% of colorectal adenomas and 90% of sporadic colon carcinomas have elevated levels of COX-2.[13,33] COX-2 appears to play a role in polyp formation and COX-2 inhibition suppresses polyp growth. In contrast, COX-1 levels remain normal in both normal and malignant tissue. In randomized studies of individuals with FAP, sulindac and celecoxib, a selective COX-2 inhibitor, have been shown to reduce the size and number of adenomatous polyps.[13,29] In 1999, the FDA approved the use of celecoxib to reduce the number of adenomatous colorectal polyps in FAP, as an adjunct to usual care. This approval was based primarily on results from a trial of 77 patients with FAP who received celecoxib, 400 mg orally twice daily, or placebo, for 6 months. Celecoxib administration resulted in a statistically significant reduction in mean polyp number (28% vs. 4.5%) and polyp burden (30.7% vs. 4.9%) compared to placebo.[33] The efficacy of celecoxib has not been compared to that of other agents. In addition, its effects are likely to be transient, because patients receiving sulindac were noted to experience an increase in size and number of polyps within 3 months after the sulindac was discontinued.[30] The use of aspirin as both a primary and secondary chemopreventive agent has also been studied. In a prospective, randomized trial, low-dose (81 mg/day) but not high-dose (325 mg/day) aspirin was shown to decrease the incidence of adenoma formation by 19% in patients with a previous history of at least one adenoma.[34] A similar benefit was seen in patients with a history of colorectal cancer.

The Calcium Polyp Prevention Study evaluated the effect of calcium carbonate supplementation on risk of recurrence of colorectal adenomas. Calcium supplementation was associated with a moderate reduction in risk of recurrent colorectal adenomas.[35] In a separate randomized study, calcium supplementation was associated with a reduced risk of adenoma recurrence as compared to placebo, but only in individuals with a serum vitamin D level above 29.1 ng/mL.[36]

TABLE 127–3. Prevention Strategies for Colorectal Cancer

Prevention Strategy	Proposed Mechanism of Protective Effect
High-fiber diet supplementation[a]	Decreases fecal bile acids; decreases bowel tansit time; direct binding to fecal mutagens; dilution of fecal material
Dietary fat reduction[a]	Decreases fecal bile acids; reduces consumption of heterocyclic amines and other carcinogens that are produced through meat preparation and processing techniques
Nonsteroidal anti-inflammatory agents	Inhibit COX-2; induce apoptosis via 15-LOX-1
Folic acid	Increases levels of intracellular folate
Calcium	Direct binding to bile and fatty acids; inhibits epithelial cell proliferation
Estrogens	Decrease synthesis of secondary bile acids; decrease production of IGF-1; direct antiproliferative effects on colorectal epithelium
Ursodeoxycholic acid	Modulates bile acid composition; inhibits cell proliferation
Aminosalicylates[b]	Inhibit cellular proliferation and induce apoptosis
Eflornithine	Inhibits cellular proliferation through alterations in polyamine metabolism
Oltipraz	Detoxifies activated carcinogens via glutathione S transferase inhibition

[a]To date, findings from randomized trials have failed to demonstrate a protective effect of low-fat high-fiber fruit and vegetable dietary intake in reducing risk of recurrence of colorectal adenomas or colorectal cancer.
[b]In individuals with pre-existing ulcerative colitis or inflammatory bowel disease.
COX-2, cyclooxygenase-2; 15-LOX-1, 15-lipoxygenase-1; IGF-1, insulin-like growth factor 1.
From Jänne et al,[30] Redaeli et al,[31] and Steele.[32]

Additional prospective studies have not shown a significant decrease in adenoma recurrence at 3 years. Although calcium intake appears to be inversely related to colon cancer, its role as a chemoprevention agent is still under investigation.

Additional intervention trials of various micronutrients, including selenium and folic acid, and other chemopreventive agents have been completed or are ongoing.[29,30] Because of their different mechanisms of action and sites of influence on the process of colorectal carcinogenesis, certain populations of individuals may benefit most from selected agents.

SURGICAL RESECTION

Surgical resection remains an option to prevent colon cancer in individuals at extremely high risk for its development. Despite the potential for NSAIDs to reduce adenoma development and to induce adenoma regression in individuals with FAP, their effects are incomplete and therefore inadequate to replace surgical resection as an important means of cancer prevention for these high-risk individuals. Individuals with FAP who are found to have polyposis on lower endoscopy screening examinations should undergo total proctocolectomy and ileal pouch–anal anastomosis or total abdominal colectomy with an ileorectal anastomosis.[37] Because of the high incidence of metachronous cancers (25% to 40%) in patients with HNPCC, prophylactic total colectomy with an ileorectal anastomosis is recommended for those individuals.[37] Colonoscopic polypectomy, removal of polyps detected during screening colonoscopy, is considered the standard of care for all individuals to prevent the progression of premalignant adenomatous polyps to adenocarcinomas.

SCREENING

Based on the recognized incidence of colorectal cancer, identification of high-risk individuals, and the high rate of curability associated with localized lesions, screening recommendations for early detection of colorectal cancer have been established.[38] This section reviews available screening techniques for colon cancer.

DIGITAL RECTAL EXAMINATION

The digital rectal examination has been a traditional part of the annual physical examination in patients older than 40 years of age and accounts for the detection of about 10% of all colorectal cancers that are within 7 to 10 cm of the anus. By itself, the digital rectal

examination is not an effective screening tool; it should be performed at the same time as other screening examinations.[38]

FECAL OCCULT BLOOD TESTING

The use of fecal occult blood tests (FOBT) annually or biannually have resulted in an increased number of asymptomatic individuals diagnosed with early stages of disease. Results from three randomized, controlled trials with a combined enrollment of over 250,000 patients have demonstrated that repeated FOBTs reduce colorectal cancer mortality by 15% to 33%.[39] Two main methods are available to detect occult blood in the feces: guaiac dye or derivative, and immunochemical methods. The Hemoccult II is the most commonly used FOBT in the U.S. This is a guaiac-based test that detects pseudoperoxidase activity in hemoglobin when hemoglobin comes in contact with a guaiac-impregnated paper. When a solution containing hydrogen peroxide is poured over the paper a blue color appears if the test is positive. The testing process is complex and requires specific patient counseling to avoid inaccurate results (Table 127–4). The Hemoccult Sensa, another guaiac-based test, is preferred by some organizations, as it may have increased sensitivity and specificity compared to the Hemoccult II. Clinical guidelines have been developed for performing and interpreting results of FOBT.[39] The limitations associated with fecal occult blood screening remain an issue of active concern. Many early-stage tumors do not bleed, and therefore the false-negative rates are about 70% for cancer and 90% for polyps. However, these concerns are addressed somewhat through continued serial screening with FOBT. In addition, about 1% to 5% of randomly selected individuals will have a positive test result and about 2% to 17% of those individuals will be found to have colorectal cancer.[39] False-positive results can prove to be very expensive and inconvenient for a patient because of the follow-up tests required to confirm a positive result. Nevertheless, studies evaluating the effects of FOBT as a screening modality have established that their annual use reduces colorectal cancer mortality by up to 33%.[39]

Newer tests such immunochemical assays were developed to reduce the rate of false-positive results associated with the guaiac based tests. Immunochemical tests (InSure, and others) use antibodies to detect the globin protein portion of human hemoglobin. These tests have the advantage of improved specificity and sensitivity.[40] A potential increase in patient compliance is expected since these tests do not react with dietary factors or medications. To date these tests have not found widespread use in the United States because of commercial and technical reasons, although they, along with guaiac based tests, can be recommended in screening protocols.

TABLE 127–4. Patient Counseling Points Prior to Hemoccult II Testing

To avoid false-positives:
1. Dietary restrictions
   - Avoid rare red meat and vegetables with peroxidase activity (turnips, broccoli, cauliflower, and radishes) for 3 days prior to testing
2. Medical restrictions
   - Avoid iron products, rectal administration of medications and digital rectal exams for 3 days prior to testing
   - Avoid nonsteroidal anti-inflammatory drugs for up to 7 days prior to testing

To avoid false-negatives:
- Avoid vitamin C for 3 days prior to testing
- Avoid testing dehydrated samples (rehydrating of samples is not recommended)

Procedure for Hemoccult II Testing:
Patient applies two separate samples of three different stools to six test card windows

FLEXIBLE SIGMOIDOSCOPY

Sigmoidoscopy is useful for examining the lower 35% to 60% of the bowel, depending on the instrument, and thus increases the detection rate by approximately two- to threefold.[39] A 60-cm flexible sigmoidoscope can be used to reach the splenic flexure in order to detect 50% to 60% of cancers, but it requires more operator training, is associated with increased risk, and is not tolerated as well as the 35-cm instrument. The combination of sigmoidoscopy plus FOBT improves sensitivity for lesions that will be missed by sigmoidoscopy alone, but not nonbleeding lesions such as polyps. Findings from the Kaiser-Permanente Medical Care Program show that screening sigmoidoscopy could effectively reduce mortality from colorectal cancer by 60%.[41] These data, however, have yet to be validated through randomized trials.

TOTAL COLONIC EXAMINATION

Total colonic examination can be accomplished with colonoscopy or double-contrast barium enema. A colonoscope facilitates examination of the whole bowel to the cecum in the majority of patients, and allows for simultaneous removal of premalignant lesions. Although it allows for greater visualization of the colon, colonoscopy involves greater risk and inconvenience to patients. However, it is the preferred screening method based on its superior ability to detect lesions in the proximal colon as compared to sigmoidoscopy.[38] This may become increasingly important, as the proportion of tumors occurring in the proximal or right (cecum, ascending, and transverse colon) side of the colon has increased over the past 30 years, with fewer occurring in the rectum and distal or left (descending and sigmoid colon) side. It remains controversial whether this observation reflects a change in the biology of the disease or the nature of screening techniques. The majority of lesions, however, still occur in the distal colon.

A double-contrast barium enema (DCBE) produces an image of the entire colon in most examinations, and the retained barium outlines small polyps and mucosal lesions. This approach is the least expensive method of examining the entire colon, but is considered inferior to colonoscopy for detecting polyps and colorectal cancer.[38] In addition, a supplemental colonoscopy is required if suspicious lesions are identified. Because of these limitations, the combination of DCBE with flexible sigmoidoscopy is used to increase the sensitivity for detecting a colorectal malignancy versus DCBE alone, and is generally reserved for use when a colonoscopy is not feasible.

NOVEL SCREENING STRATEGIES

Molecular screening strategies include the analysis of stool samples for presence of oncogenes, tumor suppressor genes, or mutant DNA MMR genes in cells that are shed from premalignant polyps or adenocarcinomas in the bowel.[40] Although available tests have reliable sensitivity and specificity, the cost and complexity associated with their analysis make them unlikely screening tools for the general population at present. Genetic testing is an important cancer-screening approach for family members of individuals diagnosed with FAP or HNPCC, and is appropriate for selected individuals, but should only be offered in conjunction with genetic counseling.

Computed tomography (CT) colonography (virtual colonoscopy) is an imaging procedure that creates two- or three-dimensional images of the colon by combining multiple helical CT scans. Initial tests are promising, though patients still require bowel cleansing and colonoscopy to remove detected lesions.[40]

SCREENING SUMMARY

Table 127–5 outlines the current American Cancer Society guidelines for screening and surveillance for early detection of colorectal polyps and cancer. Men and women who are 50 years of age and are at average risk (their only risk factor is age >50 years) should be screened with annual FOBT with examination of the colon every 5 to 10 years, depending on the type of test used.[42] Although several methods for examining the colon are available, there is no evidence that one test should be chosen over another.[39] More rigorous (usually starting at an earlier age) screening recommendations are recommended for moderate-to high-risk individuals.

DIAGNOSIS

SIGNS AND SYMPTOMS

The signs and symptoms associated with colorectal cancer can be extremely varied, subtle, and nonspecific. Patients with early-stage colorectal cancer are often asymptomatic and lesions are usually found as a result of screening studies. Any change in bowel habits (e.g., constipation, diarrhea, or alteration in size or shape of stool), vague abdominal discomfort, abdominal pain, or distention may all be warning signs of a malignant process. Obstructive symptoms and changes in bowel habits frequently develop with tumors located in the transverse and descending colon. Bleeding may be acute or chronic and most commonly appears as bright red blood mixed with stool. Iron deficiency anemia, presenting as weakness and occasionally high-output congestive heart failure, frequently develops as a result of chronic occult blood loss.

PRESENTATION OF COLORECTAL CANCER

GENERAL
Patient symptoms are usually nonspecific and can vary drastically among patients.

SYMPTOMS
- Change in bowel habits (generally an increase in frequency) or rectal bleeding.
- Constipation, depending on the location of the tumor.
- Nausea, vomiting, and abdominal discomfort.
- Fatigue may be present if anemia is severe.

SIGNS
- Blood in the stool is the most common sign.
- Hepatomegaly and jaundice in advanced disease.
- Leg edema as a consequence of lymph node involvement, thrombophlebitis, fistula formation, weight loss, and pain in the lower back or radiating down the legs are indicative of widespread disease.

LABORATORY TESTS
- Positive guaiac stool test and anemia (iron deficiency) from blood loss
- Elevated carcinoembryonic antigen (most patients)
- Elevated liver enzymes may be present with metastatic disease.

About 20% of patients with colorectal cancer present with metastatic disease.[3] Metastatic spread occurs as a result of direct tumor invasion of adjacent tissues or by lymphatic or hematogenous spread. The venous drainage of the colon and rectum influences the

TABLE 127–5. American Cancer Society Guidelines for Screening and Surveillance for Early Detection of Colorectal Polyps and Cancer

Risk Category	Recommendation[a]	Age to Begin (Years)	Interval
Average risk	FOBT *or*	50	Annually
	Flexible sigmoidoscopy *or*	50	Every 5 years
	FOBT plus flexible sigmoidoscopy[b] *or*	50	Annual FOBT with flexible sigmoidoscopy every 5 years
	DCBE *or*	50	Every 5 years
	Colonoscopy	50	Every 10 years
Increased risk			
People with single, small (<1 cm) or multiple adenomatous polyps of any size	Colonoscopy[c]	3–6 years after initial polypectomy	If exam is normal, screening as for average risk person
People with large (≥1 cm) or multiple adenomatous polyps, or adenomas with high-grade dysplasia or villous change	Colonoscopy[c]	Within 3 years after initial polypectomy	If normal, repeat in 3 years; if still normal, screening as per average risk
Personal history of curative-intent resection of colorectal cancer	Colonoscopy[c]	Within 1 year after resection	If normal, repeat in 3 years; if still normal, repeat every 5 years
Colorectal cancer or adenomatous polyps in first-degree relative younger than 60 years or in two or more first-degree relatives at any ages	Colonoscopy[c]	Age 40 or 10 years before the youngest case in family, whichever is earlier	Every 5–10 years
High risk			
Family history of familial adenomatous polyposis (FAP)	Early surveillance with endoscopy, and counseling to consider genetic testing	Puberty	If genetic test positive, colectomy is indicated
Family history of hereditary nonpolyposis colon cancer (HNPCC)	Colonoscopy and counseling to consider genetic testing	Age 21	If genetic test positive, or if the patient has not had genetic testing, every 1–2 years until age 40, then annually
Inflammatory bowel disease; chronic ulcerative colitis; Crohn's disease	Colonoscoy biopsies for dysplasia	8 years after the start of pancolitis or 12–15 years after the start of left-sided colitis	Every 1–2 years

[a]Digital rectal examination should be done at the time of each sigmoidoscopy, colonoscopy, or DCBE.
[b]FOBT together with flexible sigmoidoscopy is preferred over FOBT or flexible sigmoidoscopy alone.
[c]If colonoscopy is not available or feasible, DCBE alone or together with flexible sigmoidoscopy are acceptable alternatives.
DCBE, double-contrast barium enema; FOBT, fecal occult blood testing.
Modified with permission from Smith et al.[42]

pattern of metastases most commonly seen. The most common site of metastasis is the liver, often the only site of metastatic disease in 40% of patients, followed by the lungs and then bones, specifically the sacrum, coccyx, pelvis, and lumbar vertebrae. Liver metastases are present in 5% to 10% of patients at presentation.

WORK-UP

When a patient is suspected of having colorectal carcinoma, a careful history and physical examination should be performed. The patient history should include a past medical history and family history, especially noting the presence of inflammatory bowel disease, colorectal cancer, polyps, and cancers of the breast, ovary, and endometrium. A complete physical examination includes careful abdominal examination for the presence of masses or ascites, a rectal examination, and an assessment for possible hepatomegaly and lymphadenopathy. In all women, a breast and pelvic examination is recommended, especially in women with a history of breast, ovarian, or endometrial

cancer. Table 127–6 summarizes the recommended tests for pretreatment evaluation of patients with potentially curable colorectal cancer.

An unexplained anemia in an older patient requires surveillance of the entire large bowel, especially the right colon. Red blood cell indices (e.g., hemoglobin, hematocrit, mean corpuscular volume, and reticulocyte count) and a work-up of iron status (e.g., serum ferritin, serum iron, and total iron-binding capacity) may be useful to confirm acute or chronic blood loss and/or iron-deficiency anemia. An evaluation of the entire large bowel is undertaken with either colonoscopy or sigmoidoscopy and a double-contrast barium enema. A barium enema may be preferred in situations in which a partially obstructing lesion prohibits passage of the endoscope; however, it should be avoided if complete obstruction or perforation of the bowel is suspected. A characteristic finding indicative of colon cancer seen on barium enema is an apple core–shaped lesion with tumor involving the circumference of the bowel. When possible, the endoscope is used to collect tissue for a histologic evaluation and provide a preliminary diagnosis following the procedure.

TABLE 127–6. Recommended Pretreatment Evaluation for Patients with Potentially Curable Colorectal Cancer

- Personal medical history and family history of colorectal polyps, cancer, or other malignancies
- Physical examination, including evaluation for lymphadenopathy, hepatomegaly, and ascites; women should have appropriate evaluations to rule out breast, ovarian, or endometrial cancers
- Complete blood count, liver chemistries, and serum carcinoembryonic antigen
- Total colonic evaluation with colonoscopy or flexible sigmoidoscopy with double-contrast barium enema
- Chest x-ray
- Chest/abdominal/pelvic computed tomography scan
- Additional studies as indicated

From Skibber et al.[28]

Baseline laboratory tests should be obtained and include a complete blood cell (CBC) count, platelet count, prothrombin time, activated partial thromboplastin time, and liver and renal function tests. Abnormal liver function tests may suggest liver involvement with tumor. However, patients with metastatic disease to the liver may have normal liver function tests, and abnormal liver function tests are not always indicative of metastatic disease.

Additional laboratory tests include a baseline carcinoembryonic antigen (CEA) level. CEA belongs to a group of cell-surface glycoproteins termed "oncofetal proteins," which are expressed during embryonic development and re-expressed on the cell surfaces of many carcinomas, particularly those of the gastrointestinal tract. The concentration of CEA can be measured in the blood and can therefore potentially serve as a marker for colorectal cancer. However, not all colorectal cancers produce CEA, and elevated concentrations are even more frequent in patients with metastatic disease. It is important to recognize, however, several concomitant disease states that can elevate CEA: alcoholic and chronic hepatitis, diverticulitis, renal failure, cholelithiasis, fibrocystic breast disease, smoking, and other carcinomas.[44] Most commercially available assays list a normal range of less than 3 ng/mL and 5 ng/mL for nonsmokers and smokers, respectively. Although CEA measurement is too insensitive and nonspecific to be used as a screening test for early-stage colorectal cancer, it is useful for monitoring colorectal cancer response to treatment, particularly if the pretreatment concentration is elevated. The CEA test also has preoperative prognostic implications because it has been shown to correlate with the size and degree of differentiation of the carcinoma. Elevated preoperative CEA levels correlate with a poor survival and may predict likelihood of recurrence, regardless of tumor stage at diagnosis. After a potentially curative resection, CEA levels should return to normal within 4 to 6 weeks.[44] Persistently elevated CEA levels may indicate residual disease, while elevations after normalization may indicate relapsed disease.

Radiographic imaging studies evaluate the extent of disease involvement. A chest x-ray should be performed to rule out the presence of metastatic spread to the lungs. A CT scan of the abdomen and pelvis is often performed to evaluate hepatic and retroperitoneal involvement and occult abdominal and pelvic disease, and to determine the depth of tumor penetration into the bowel wall and/or invasion to adjacent organs. Detection of lymph node involvement with either study is limited by the difficulty of distinguishing inflammatory or reactive lymph nodes from those infiltrated with tumor. Because CT scans may not adequately detect peritoneal seeding, small distant lymph node metastasis, or liver metastasis in colon cancer, an occasional patient may need to undergo a laparotomy, spiral CT, MRI, or positron emission tomography (PET) scan in order to confirm metastatic disease. PET imaging is also useful to discriminate between benign and malignant disease by detecting tumor-related metabolic alterations in affected tissues.[45] PET scans are commonly used for the detection of recurrent colorectal cancer in patients with rising CEA levels and inconclusive findings on standard imaging studies.

Intrarectal or transrectal ultrasonography is a technique that is becoming more widely available for the evaluation of patients with rectal cancer. It is useful for detecting the depth of tumor penetration, and like pelvic CT scans, is fair to good in determining lymph node involvement. Cystoscopy or IV pyelography studies are rarely indicated except for very large rectal tumors found on examination, if the patient exhibits symptoms, or if a CT scan suggests bladder involvement. Intraluminal and hepatic MRI studies may also provide useful information.

Immunodetection of tumors using tumor-directed antibodies is receiving greater recognition as an imaging technique for the early detection and imaging of colorectal cancers. Several tumor-associated proteins have been identified within or on the surface membrane of colorectal malignant cells to which monoclonal antibodies have been targeted. Of these, TAG-72 and CEA have undergone the greatest amount of study.[46] Radiolabeled monoclonal antibodies directed against these antigens have been used in clinical studies for both external immunoscintigraphy as well as intraoperative localization of tumor. OncoScint, an indium-111–labeled monoclonal antibody targeted to the TAG-72 antigen is an FDA-approved diagnostic imaging agent available for determining the location and extent of extrahepatic disease in patients with colorectal cancer. The CEA scan is a Tc-99m–labeled anti-CEA antibody for the assessment of recurrent colorectal carcinoma. The use of these tests is generally reserved for those patients who have completed standard diagnostic imaging tests, but may still require additional information regarding the extent of disease. They may also play an important role in identifying metastatic or recurrent disease in individuals with rising CEA levels and negative standard radiographic studies.

STAGING

The purpose of the staging examinations is to precisely describe the malignancy at a point in its natural history that assists in developing patient treatment options and determining their overall prognosis. Traditionally, the Dukes classification, originally published in 1932, was used in the staging of colorectal cancers.[28] Since its original publication, it has undergone several modifications; a modified Astler-Coller (MAC) version is now used more extensively. However, because multiple staging systems exist and have been used for various clinical trials, the literature is often difficult to evaluate. Therefore, in an effort to standardize the staging system for colorectal cancer, the American Joint Committee on Cancer (AJCC) and the International Union Against Cancer (IUAC) jointly agreed to use and recommend the TNM classification system. This classification takes three aspects of cancer growth—T (tumor size), N (lymph node involvement), and M (presence or absence of metastases) into account. The TNM classification also allows for various subdivisions within each of the three categories, which is then used for determining the disease stage.[20] Table 127–7 is a summary of staging using the TNM system. Table 127–8 shows the stage assignment based on TNM classifications. Figure 127–5 is a representation of the relationship between the MAC and AJCC/IUAC staging systems.

TABLE 127–7. TNM Staging Definitions for Colorectal Cancer

Criteria	Classification	Definition
Primary tumor (T)	T_X	Primary tumor cannot be assessed
	T_0	No evidence of primary tumor
	T_{is}	Carcinoma in situ: intraepithelial or invasion of the lamina propria[a]
	T_1	Tumor invades submucosa
	T_2	Tumor invades muscularis propria
	T_3	Tumor invades through the muscularis propria into the subserosa, or into the nonperitonealized pericolic or perirectal tissues
	T_4	Tumor directly invades other organs or structures and/or perforates the visceral peritoneum[b,c]
Regional lymph nodes (N)	N_X	Regional nodes cannot be assessed
	N_0	No regional lymph node metastasis
	N_1	Metastasis in one to three regional lymph nodes
	N_2	Metastasis in four or more regional lymph nodes
Distant metastasis (M)	M_X	Distant metastasis cannot be assessed
	M_0	No distant metastasis
	M_1	Distant metastasis

[a]Tis includes cancer cells confined within the glandular basement membrane (intraepithelial) or lamina propria (intramucosal) with no extension through the muscularis mucosae into the submucosa.
[b]Direct invasion in T_4 includes invasion of other segments of the colorectum by way of the serosa; for example, invasion of the sigmoid colon by a carcinoma of the cecum.
[c]Tumor that is adherent to other organs or structures macroscopically is classified T_4. However, if no tumor is present in the adhesion microscopically, the classification should be pT_3. The V and L substaging should be used to identify the presence or absence of vascular or lymphatic invasion.
Used with the permission of the American Joint Committee on Cancer (AJCC), from AJCC Cancer Staging Manual.[47]

PROGNOSIS

The stage of colorectal cancer upon diagnosis is the most important independent prognostic factor for survival and disease recurrence. Table 127–9 compares the stage of disease upon presentation and relative survival rates for individuals with colon and rectum cancer. Additional clinical and pathologic variables may affect the prognosis of patients with colorectal cancer. Consideration of these factors plays an important role in determining optimal strategies for treatment as well as appropriate follow-up. Clinical factors present at time of diagnosis that are associated with a poor prognosis and decreased survival include bowel obstruction or perforation, rectal bleeding, high preoperative CEA level, distant metastases, and location of the primary tumor in the rectum or rectosigmoid area.[28,44]

Pathologic variables associated with a negative influence on prognosis include increasing depth of muscular invasion; presence of venous, lymphatic, or perineural invasion; increasing number of involved lymph nodes; presence of peritumoral lymphoid reaction; mucinous or signet-ring histology; high proliferation indices; tumor aneuploidy; and presence of certain molecular markers (18q/DCC mutation or loss, microsatellite stability, elevated thymidylate synthase [TS] expression, and p53 mutation or loss).[28,48]

Allelic loss of chromosome 18q, which is located on the DCC gene, is predictive of mortality, independent of tumor differentiation, vascular invasion, and TNM stage. Five-year survival rates decrease by 39% and 14% in patients with allelic loss of chromosome 18q and stage II or III colorectal cancer, respectively.[49] Tumors that overexpress TS, which is responsible for converting deoxyuridine monophosphate to deoxythymidine monophosphate, an

TABLE 127–8. Colon Cancer Stage by TNM Classification

Stage	T	N	M	Dukes[a]	MAC[a]
0	T_{is}	N_0	M_0	—	—
I	T_1	N_0	M_0	A	A
	T_2	N_0	M_0	A	B1
IIA	T_3	N_0	M_0	B	B2
IIB	T_4	N_0	M_0	B	B3
IIIA	T_1–T_2	N_1	M_0	C	C1
IIIB	T_3–T_4	N_1	M_0	C	C2/C3
IIIC	Any T	N_2	M_0	C	C1/C2/C3
IV	Any T	Any N	M_1	—	D

[a]Dukes B is a composite of better ($T_3 N_0 M_0$) and worse ($T_4 N_0 M_0$) prognostic groups, as is Dukes C (any T $N_1 M_0$ and any T $N_2 M_0$). MAC is the modified Astler-Coller classification.
Used with the permission of the American Joint Committee on Cancer (AJCC), from AJCC Cancer Staging Manual.[47]

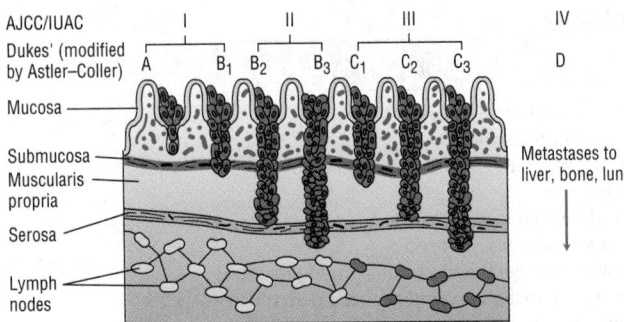

FIGURE 127–5. Staging systems for colorectal cancer.

TABLE 127–9. Colon and Rectal Cancer Disease Stage and Survival Rates (SEER Data, 1995–2000)

Tumor Stage at Diagnosis	Stage Distribution (%)[a]		5-Year Relative Survival (%)	
	Colon	*Rectum*	*Colon*	*Rectum*
Localized	36	44	91.1	87.7
Regional	39	34	69.0	62.7
Distant	21	15	10.1	8.2
All stages	—	—	63.0	64.3

[a]Approximately 4% and 6% of cancers of the colon and rectum, respectively, were unstaged.
From Ries et al.[3]

essential step for DNA synthesis, are less sensitive to fluorouracil chemotherapy. Patients whose colon cancers have higher levels of TS appear to have a significantly worse overall 5-year survival than patients whose cancers have a low level of TS.[28,48] The importance of elevated TS and type of therapeutic interventions is unclear. Theoretically, patients with high levels of TS may benefit from a non–fluorouracil containing chemotherapy regimen, although a large cooperative group trial failed to identify any subgroup of patients that failed to benefit from fluorouracil plus leucovorin therapy based on tumor TS levels.

Similarly, tumors that overexpress mutant *p53* demonstrate a high degree of resistance to radiation, fluorouracil, and certain other chemotherapeutic agents and are associated with a poorer prognosis.[48] In contrast, colorectal cancers that demonstrate low frequency microsatellite instability or microsatellite stability appear to be associated with a more favorable outcome and may respond better to fluorouracil.[50] Tumors that have a high rate of proliferation are generally associated with a poor prognosis. Ki-67 is expressed in cells actively engaged in the cell cycle and has also been used as a measure of colon cancer proliferation. Interestingly, for unknown reasons, high levels of Ki-67 were associated with an increase in overall survival in patients with early-stage colon cancer. A large number of additional molecular factors including K-*ras* mutations, lack of p27 expression, and *bcl*-2 and EGFR overexpression appear to have prognostic significance but have been studied less sufficiently to date.[48] Evaluation of these factors may provide important clues as to which patients will benefit most from more aggressive therapy, individuals who may not require systemic chemotherapy, and new therapeutic targets for the treatment of colorectal cancer.

▶ TREATMENT: Colorectal Cancer

■ DESIRED OUTCOME

Treatment goals for cancer of the colon or rectum are based on the stage of disease at presentation. Stages I, II, and III disease are considered potentially curable, and as such, are managed ideally with the intent of eradicating known and micrometastatic sites of tumor to achieve remission and avoid disease recurrence. Because stage IV disease is generally not curable, treatments are offered to reduce symptoms, avoid disease-related complications, and prolong survival. Treatment strategies for individuals who manifest premalignant forms of the disease (e.g., adenomatous polyps) should be undertaken to prevent polyp progression and transformation to malignancy.

■ GENERAL APPROACH TO TREATMENT

Although advanced age is not an absolute contraindication for relatively aggressive therapies, a consideration of the age of the patient, concomitant disease states, lifestyle factors, and the patient's preferences are incorporated into the treatment planning process. Special or emergent conditions, such as bowel perforation, spinal cord compression, and severe pain, anemia, or other symptomatic problems, need to be addressed acutely, after which time a more long-term disease-specific plan can be developed. The treatment approaches for colorectal cancer reflect two primary treatment goals: curative therapy for localized disease, and palliative therapy for metastatic cancer.

For patients for whom treatment intent is curative, surgical resection of the primary tumor is the most important component of therapy.[28] Depending on the extent of disease and whether the tumor originated in the colon or rectum, further adjuvant chemotherapy or chemotherapy plus XRT may be appropriate. With few exceptions, surgery is used infrequently for metastatic disease. In this setting, systemic chemotherapy is the mainstay of treatment; XRT may also be useful for disease palliation of localized symptoms or when chemotherapy is no longer effective. Patients with metastatic disease who are asymptomatic may benefit from initiation of therapy and treatment should not be withheld until they develop symptoms.

■ OPERABLE DISEASE

■ SURGERY

Individuals with operable—stages I, II, and III—colorectal cancer should undergo a complete surgical resection of the primary tumor mass with a regional lymphadenectomy as a curative approach for their disease.[28] The surgical approach for colon cancer generally involves a complete resection of the tumor with an appropriate margin of tumor-free bowel and a regional lymphadenectomy. A total colectomy is rarely needed in colon cancer, but may be indicated for selected patients with FAP or chronic ulcerative colitis.

Surgery for rectal cancer depends on the region of tumor involvement. A low anterior resection is the procedure of choice in patients with lesions in the middle to upper rectum.[51] Patients with lesions in the lower portion of the rectum may require an abdominoperineal resection if either the amount of unaffected bowel is insufficient for a resection far enough away from the tumor, or too close to areas that cannot permit an anastomosis. Newer surgical techniques have been developed in an attempt to retain function of the rectal sphincter and still achieve complete tumor resection. Individuals who are not candidates for sphincter-sparing resections or have extensive local spread of tumor will require an abdominoperineal resection. This involves removal of the distal sigmoid, rectosigmoid, rectum, and anus with the establishment of a permanent sigmoid colostomy. Less than one-third of patients will require a permanent colostomy for rectal cancer.[51] Other complications that occur frequently with surgery for rectal cancer include urinary retention, incontinence, impotence, and locoregional recurrence.

Overall, surgery for colorectal cancer is associated with a morbidity and mortality rate of 8% to 15% and 1% to 2%, respectively, depending on the type and extent of procedure.[28,51] Common complications associated with colorectal surgery include infection, anastomotic leakage, obstruction, adhesion formation, and malabsorption syndromes.

ADJUVANT THERAPY FOR COLON CANCER

Adjuvant therapy in colorectal cancer is administered to selected individuals after complete tumor resection in an attempt to eliminate residual local or micrometastatic disease, thereby decreasing tumor relapse and improving patient survival. Since greater than 90% of patients with stage I colon or rectal cancer are cured by surgical resection alone, adjuvant therapy is not indicated.[28] The role of adjuvant chemotherapy for stage II colon cancer is less clear. Certain patients with stage II colon cancer are at a higher risk for recurrence, although adjuvant chemotherapy for all patients with stage II disease has not been shown to be superior to surgery alone. Although there is no lymph node involvement, these tumors can penetrate through the muscle wall, into surrounding structures, or through the visceral peritoneum. Consequently, an intermediate risk of relapse still exists because of the invasive nature of stage II disease.

Results of studies that have attempted to determine whether patients with stage II disease benefit from adjuvant therapy are conflicting. Most trials that suggest adjuvant therapy improves survival for stage II disease frequently enroll individuals with a high risk of relapse and do not include an untreated control group. Therefore at present, various tumor molecular genetic factors (e.g., chromosome 18q deletion, tumor ploidy, mutations of protooncogenes or tumor-suppressor genes, tumor TS expression, and tumor microsatellite instability) are being studied in an effort to identify subsets of patients with stage II disease who have an increased risk of relapse. Patients with stage II colon cancer should be enrolled in carefully controlled clinical trials to assess the impact of newer agents and whether molecular genetic factors can be used in this group of patients to predict risk of recurrence.

Adjuvant chemotherapy is standard therapy for patients with stage III colon cancer. The presence of lymph node involvement with tumor places patients with stage III colon cancer at high risk for relapse, and the risk of death within 5 years of surgical resection alone is as high as 70%.[28] In this population of patients, adjuvant chemotherapy significantly decreases risk of cancer recurrence and death and is considered standard of care.

Adjuvant XRT plus chemotherapy is considered standard treatment for patients with stage II/III rectal cancer.[51] Tumors arising in the rectum are technically more difficult to resect with wide circumferential margins, and lead to local recurrences more frequently than that seen with colon cancers. Therefore XRT is an important aspect of adjuvant therapy for rectal cancer to reduce risk of local tumor recurrence.

Adjuvant Radiation Therapy

There is currently no definitive role for adjuvant XRT in colon cancer because most recurrences are extrapelvic and occur in the abdomen.[28] Although local recurrence and debilitating pelvic pain are uncommon, a subset of patients with T_3 or T_4 tumors located in the cecum, hepatic and splenic flexures, and sigmoid are at increased risk of local recurrence and may benefit from postoperative XRT and chemotherapy. Early trials using effective doses of whole abdominal XRT were limited by considerable toxicity.[51] However, results from studies combining abdominal XRT plus fluorouracil are promising. To date, postoperative local XRT may reduce the risk of local recurrence and improve survival compared to adjuvant chemotherapy alone, but should only be considered for select patients with colon cancer.[28]

In patients undergoing surgery for rectal cancer, XRT is used to reduce risk of local tumor recurrence. Radiation therapy is given prior to or following surgery and can be delivered using a variety of dosing regimens, administration schedules, and techniques.[51] Accumulating data suggest that preoperative XRT may be used to reduce the initial size of the tumor to such an extent that the tumor could be reclassified to a lower stage, or "downstaged," and therefore rendered more resectable. This might then lead to improved patient survival or result in the need for a less extensive surgical procedure. Preoperative XRT is also administered to reduce the amount of tumor seeding that can occur during surgery; however, this approach is more likely to affect a greater area than is necessary.[51] Postoperative administration of XRT may more adequately treat a defined area, but is associated with more toxicity because of a greater amount of bowel being present in the treatment field.

Adverse effects associated with XRT in colorectal cancer can be acute or chronic. Acute effects primarily include hematologic depression, dysuria, diarrhea, abdominal cramping, and proctitis. Chronic symptoms that sometimes persist for months following discontinuation of XRT may involve persistent diarrhea, proctitis or enteritis, small bowel obstruction, perineal tenderness, and impaired wound healing.

Adjuvant Chemotherapy

For more than 40 years, fluorouracil has been the most widely used chemotherapeutic agent for the adjuvant treatment of colorectal cancer, both as a single agent and in combination with other agents. Newer agents such as irinotecan, capecitabine, and oxaliplatin are currently being studied in combination chemotherapy regimens for the adjuvant treatment of colon cancer. Investigational chemotherapy agents, biologic therapies that target the underlying tumor biology, and new administration methods are also being developed.

Figure 127–6 depicts the National Comprehensive Cancer Network (NCCN) Practice Guidelines for adjuvant therapy of colon cancer.

Single Agents. Early results of adjuvant chemotherapy in colon cancer were disappointing and failed to improve results associated with surgery alone. Based on their activity for metastatic colon cancer, fluorouracil and floxuridine were investigated as single-agent

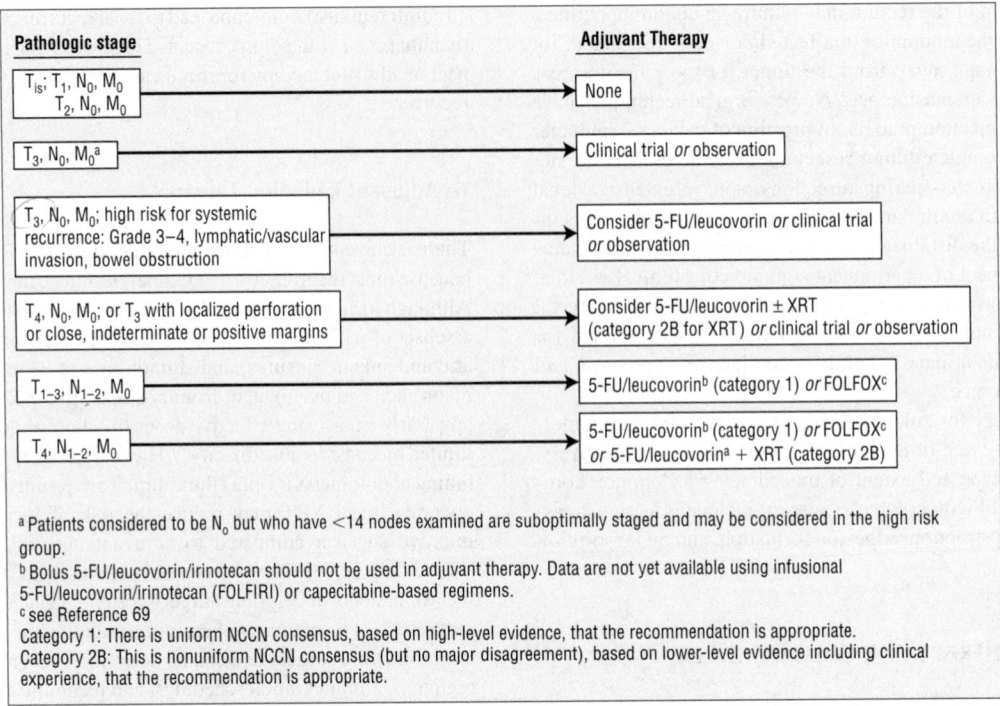

FIGURE 127–6. National Comprehensive Cancer Network practice guidelines for adjuvant therapy of colon cancer. *Adapted with permission from the NCCN 2.2004 Colon Cancer and Rectal Cancer Guidelines, the Complete Library of NCCN Clinical Practice Guidelines in Oncology [CD-ROM]. Jenkintown, Pennsylvania: © National Comprehensive Cancer Network, June 2004. To view the most recent and complete version of the guideline, go online to www.nccn.org.*

chemotherapy agents for use after surgery. In 1988, a meta-analysis of fluorouracil-based adjuvant therapy was published that evaluated phase III trials that compared adjuvant fluorouracil to surgery alone.[52] A small, statistically insignificant improvement in survival was noted with fluorouracil-based regimens. These findings questioned the value of the standard use of IV bolus fluorouracil alone as adjuvant therapy for colon cancer, but results from recent studies suggest that protracted or continuous IV fluorouracil infusion treatment schedules are effective as adjuvant therapy.[53]

Clinical studies comparing efficacy of bolus and continuous infusion schedules generally favor continuous infusion of fluorouracil. This is consistent with evidence that suggests that the duration of infusion may be an important determinant of the biologic activity of fluorouracil, particularly because of its short plasma half-life and S-phase specificity for optimal TS inhibition. Continuous IV infusions also permit increased fluorouracil dose intensity, which may account for the higher response rates observed with prolonged infusions of fluorouracil. However, because of the more costly and cumbersome nature of continuous IV infusions, fluorouracil has most commonly been administered as an IV bolus injection in the United States. Unlike continuous IV infusion where fluorouracil can be given alone, IV bolus regimens only include fluorouracil in combination with at least one other agent.

Clinically significant differences in toxicity also differ based on the dose, route, and schedule of fluorouracil administration. Leukopenia is the primary dose-limiting toxicity of IV bolus fluorouracil, although diarrhea, stomatitis, and nausea and vomiting can also occur.[54] The incidence and severity of stomatitis can be significantly reduced with the use of oral cryotherapy. In this approach, the patient is required to chew and hold ice chips in the mouth during the period between 5 minutes prior to and 30 minutes following the bolus

injection of fluorouracil. The basis for the protective effects of this procedure is based on the premise that local vasoconstriction caused by the ice chips temporarily reduces blood flow to the oral mucosa, thereby reducing drug exposure to the oral mucosa.

Although continuous IV infusion fluorouracil is generally well tolerated, dose-limiting toxicities can be substantial. A distinct toxicity, palmar-plantar erythrodysesthesia ("hand-foot syndrome"), and stomatitis occur most frequently with this route of administration.[28,54] Hand-foot syndrome occurs in 24% to 40% of patients receiving extended continuous IV infusions and is characterized by painful swelling and erythroderma of the soles of the feet, palms of the hands, and distal fingers. This type of skin toxicity is fully reversible upon interruption of therapy or dose reduction and is not life-threatening; however, it can be significant and acutely disabling. The incidence of stomatitis, diarrhea, and hematologic toxicity is not substantial at standard doses, but increases with increasing doses of fluorouracil. No significant difference is noted in the incidence of mucositis, diarrhea, nausea and vomiting, or alopecia between continuous and bolus IV fluorouracil administration.[28,54]

An additional determinant of fluorouracil toxicity, regardless of the method of administration, is related to its catabolism and pharmacogenomic factors. Dihydropyrimidine dehydrogenase (DPD) is the main enzyme responsible for the catabolism of fluorouracil to inactive metabolites. A pharmacogenetic disorder has been identified in cancer patients in which they have a complete or near-complete deficiency of this enzyme, resulting in severe toxicity, including death, after the administration of fluorouracil. Molecular studies have suggested there is a relationship between allelic variants in the *DPYD* gene (the gene that encodes DPD) and a deficiency in DPD activity.[55] About 3% of patients may be genotypically heterozygous for a mutant DPYD allele, although differences between sex and races are unknown at this time.

TABLE 127–10. Examples of Combination Fluorouracil Plus Leucovorin Treatment Regimens for Colorectal Cancer

Regimen	Fluorouracil	Leucovorin	Frequency
Roswell Park regimen[60]	600 mg/m^2 per day IV, day 1	500 mg/m^2 per day IV over 2 hours	Repeat weekly for 6 out of 8 weeks
Mayo Clinic regimen[61]	425 mg/m^2 per day IV, days 1–5	20 mg/m^2 per day IV, days 1–5	Repeat every 4–5 weeks
de Gramont regimen[62]	400 mg/m^2 per day IV bolus, followed by 600 mg/m^2 CIV over 22 hours, days 1 and 2 for 2 consecutive days	200 mg/m^2 per day IV over 2 hours days 1 and 2	Repeat every 2 weeks
Modified Machover regimen[63]	370–400 mg/m^2 per day IV, days 1–5	200 mg/m^2 per day IV, days 1–5	Repeat every 4–5 weeks

CIV, continuous intravenous infusion.

Combination Regimens

FLUOROURACIL PLUS LEVAMISOLE

In 1990, the National Institutes of Health Consensus Development Conference recommended that the use of fluorouracil and levamisole be considered standard therapy for patients with surgically treated stage III colon cancer. Levamisole is a synthetic, oral anthelmintic drug with immunomodulatory properties and minimal, generally reversible toxicities that include metallic taste, arthralgias, central nervous system toxicities (mood changes, sleep disorders, or cerebellar ataxia), rare myelosuppression, and hepatic toxicity.

In a study sponsored by the Mayo Clinic and the North Central Cancer Treatment Group (NCCTG), surgery alone was compared with postoperative levamisole and postoperative levamisole plus fluorouracil in patients with surgically treated stage II and stage III colorectal cancer.[56] Fluorouracil, 450 mg/m^2 per day, was administered by IV bolus injection for 5 consecutive days, starting within 21 to 35 days following surgery. Starting 1 month later, patients received fluorouracil, 450 mg/m^2, as a single IV bolus injection each week for 48 weeks. Levamisole was administered 50 mg orally every 8 hours for 3 consecutive days. Each 3-day cycle was repeated every 2 weeks and continued for 1 year. Although the combination of levamisole and fluorouracil significantly reduced recurrence rates, it did not confer a statistically significant survival advantage. However, a small but significant survival benefit for patients with stage III disease was identified through subset analysis of the data. Results of a larger Intergroup trial, first published in 1990 and later updated in 1995 after a median follow-up of 6.5 years, demonstrated that the combination of fluorouracil plus levamisole following surgical resection in patients with stage III colon cancer reduced the recurrence rate by 40% and the death rate by 33%.[57] Levamisole alone provided no significant reduction in either recurrence or deaths.

FLUOROURACIL PLUS LEUCOVORIN

The nature of the pharmacology of fluorouracil provides several opportunities to increase its antitumor activity, the most common of which is accomplished by using concomitant leucovorin. The addition of leucovorin increases the binding affinity of the active fluorouracil metabolite to TS, thus enhancing its cytotoxic activity. The combination of fluorouracil plus leucovorin has undergone extensive study in the adjuvant setting, based on the observation that fluorouracil plus leucovorin substantially improves response rates compared to fluorouracil alone for metastatic disease. Since the mid-1980s, several large randomized trials have evaluated the efficacy of fluorouracil plus leucovorin as adjuvant therapy for patients with stage II or III

colon cancer. In each of the studies, rates of recurrence and survival improved substantially for patients receiving fluorouracil plus "high dose" (200 to 500 mg/m^2 per day) or "low dose" (20 to 25 mg/m^2 per day) leucovorin compared to surgery alone.[58] The International Multicentre Pooled Analysis of Colon Cancer Trials (IMPACT) analyzed pooled data from three ongoing trials comparing surgery alone to adjuvant fluorouracil (370 to 400 mg/m^2 per day) plus high-dose leucovorin (200 mg/m^2 per day) given daily for 5 consecutive days, repeated every 28 days for 6 cycles (6 months).[59] The recurrence and death rates were reduced by 35% and 22%, respectively. These studies were initiated when a surgery-alone control group was appropriate for stage III colon cancer, before the results were available from the fluorouracil plus levamisole adjuvant trial.

Fluorouracil and leucovorin can be administered in a variety of treatment schedules, but none has proven superior with regard to overall patient survival. Table 127–10 lists examples of some of these regimens. In the U.S., the most common regimens include the Roswell Park regimen[60] and the Mayo Clinic regimen,[61] while in Europe, treatments such as the de Gramont regimen[62] favor a continuous intravenous schedule of fluorouracil. The weekly fluorouracil plus high-dose leucovorin (Roswell Park) and the daily fluorouracil plus low-dose leucovorin (Mayo Clinic) regimens were compared in a 4-arm U.S. Intergroup trial (INT-0089), that randomized patients with high-risk stage II and stage III colon cancer to either regimen, fluorouracil plus levamisole, or a combination of fluorouracil, leucovorin, and levamisole.[64] The standard fluorouracil plus levamisole regimen was administered over 12 months and the leucovorin-containing regimens were given for 6 cycles over a time period of 6 to 8 months. Overall survival (OS) was the primary end point with disease-free survival (DFS) as a secondary end point. For patients with stage II and III disease, the only significant difference was between fluorouracil plus levamisole versus fluorouracil plus leucovorin plus levamisole in terms of 5-year DFS (56% vs. 60%) and 5-year OS (63% vs. 67%). The high-dose leucovorin regimen was not superior to the low-dose leucovorin regimen, and the 3-drug combination was not superior to fluorouracil plus leucovorin alone. In addition, 6 months of adjuvant therapy with fluorouracil plus leucovorin was as effective as 12 months of fluorouracil plus levamisole.

An analysis of the treatment-related toxicities in the INT-0089 trial reveals several important differences (Table 127–11).[58] Grade 3 or worse toxicities, consisting of diarrhea, leukopenia, and stomatitis, usually occurred during the first month of therapy. Toxicities were most prevalent in the low-dose leucovorin arms with or without levamisole. The incidence of granulocytopenia and stomatitis were more commonly observed with low-dose leucovorin, while diarrhea occurred more frequently in the high-dose leucovorin arm. In a preliminary analysis of toxicity based on patient age, the risk of stomatitis and leukopenia appears greater in patients older than 70 years and in women.

TABLE 127–11. Treatment Toxicities in Intergroup Trial 0089

Toxicity	Percentage of Grade III Toxicity or Worse			
	5-FU/LD-LV	5-FU/HD-LV	5-FU/LEV	5-FU/LV/LEV
Leukopenia	11.9	2.8	9	14.9
Neutropenia	24.1	3.9	18.8	35.1
Stomatitis	18.2	1.4	3.6	22.6
Diarrhea	21.1	30	11.4	17.9

5-FU, fluorouracil; HD-LV, high-dose leucovorin; LD-LV, low-dose leucovorin; LEV = levamisole.
Reproduced with permission from Macdonald.[58]

Other large trials have consistently shown 6 months of fluorouracil plus leucovorin to be at least equivalent to 12-month regimens containing levamisole.[65,66] In the National Surgical Adjuvant Breast and Bowel Project (NSABP) C-04 trial, patients with stage II and III colon cancer were randomized to one of three study arms consisting of weekly fluorouracil plus high-dose (HD) leucovorin for 6 months, fluorouracil plus levamisole for 12 months, or the combination of fluorouracil plus HD-leucovorin and levamisole.[65] The fluorouracil and leucovorin were administered for 6 months; the levamisole was continued for a total of 12 months. In a pairwise comparison between fluorouracil plus HD-leucovorin versus fluorouracil plus levamisole, there was a significant prolongation in 5-year DFS (65% vs. 60%) and a trend toward improved 5-year OS (74% vs. 70%; $p = 0.07$) with HD-leucovorin. No difference was seen in DFS or OS between fluorouracil plus HD-leucovorin and fluorouracil plus HD-leucovorin plus levamisole.

Continuous IV infusion fluorouracil also does not improve efficacy in the adjuvant treatment setting.[53,67] In a comparison of a 12-week protracted venous infusion (PVI) of fluorouracil versus the Mayo Clinic regimen for 6 months, OS was similar, but the PVI fluorouracil was associated with less toxicity.[53] Thus a 6-month regimen of fluorouracil plus leucovorin is the standard chemotherapy for patients with stage III colon cancer. Levamisole is no longer a required component of adjuvant chemotherapy regimens for colon cancer. Also, no standard exists for the best schedule of fluorouracil and leucovorin administration. Although there are no significant differences in efficacy between the Roswell Park and the Mayo Clinic regimen, toxicities can be different. With the exception of diarrhea, the Roswell Park regimen weekly HD-leucovorin regimen may be less toxic and is preferred by many practitioners. Although efficacy of HD- and LD-leucovorin with each of the regimens is similar, the costs of leucovorin doses ranging from 20 to 500 mg/m^2 are significantly different, and compliance issues regarding daily or weekly drug administration should be considered. Therefore the toxicity profiles of these regimens, overall treatment costs, and patient compliance issues should be considered to help determine the optimal adjuvant chemotherapy regimen for an individual patient.

The impact of adjuvant therapy on patients with stage II colon cancer is currently unknown. Most adjuvant trials have been conducted in mixed patient populations that included both stage II and stage III patients. Subset analyses of these trials, done in an attempt to identify the benefit of adjuvant therapy in stage II colon cancer, have produced conflicting results.[28] High-risk individuals (e.g., greater depth of muscle invasion, venous or lymphatic invasion, chromosome 18q allelic loss, tumor aneuploidy, mucinous or signet-ring histology, poor tumor differentiation, or mutant $p53$ gene overexpression) probably benefit from adjuvant therapy. These individuals should be offered adjuvant chemotherapy, preferably in the setting of a randomized clinical trial, based on individual clinical, pathologic, and biologic prognostic factors. Despite the lack of a consensus regarding the use of adjuvant chemotherapy for individuals with high-risk stage II colon cancer, many practitioners offer this therapy to selected patients. Optimal dosing, administration schedule, and duration of therapy have yet to be determined, but most practitioners choose to apply the same treatment approach as for stage III colon cancer.

CLINICAL CONTROVERSY

There is a lack of agreement among clinicians as to whether patients with stage II colon cancer should receive adjuvant chemotherapy. Some believe all patients should receive some form of chemotherapy, while others only recommend treatment or clinical trials for high-risk individuals.

Investigational Approaches. Despite the significant reduction in cancer recurrence and increased survival afforded with fluorouracil-based adjuvant chemotherapy, the results obtained thus far indicate need for continued improvement. Several strategies are underway, including protracted fluorouracil infusion, oral fluorinated pyrimidines, irinotecan, oxaliplatin, and immunotherapy-based therapies.[58,68]

New chemotherapy agents and chemotherapy regimens are constantly being investigated in an attempt to improve on the response and safety of fluorouracil plus leucovorin in the adjuvant setting. Most attempts to improve the adjuvant therapy for colon cancer add a third active chemotherapy agent to existing fluorouracil/leucovorin regimens. Irinotecan and oxaliplatin, both active drugs in metastatic colon cancer, are currently being investigated in stage II and III colon cancer in regimens similar to those used in the metastatic setting.[68] In the MOSAIC trial, 2,246 patients with stage II or III colon cancer were randomized to receive fluorouracil plus leucovorin or FOLFOX4 postoperatively.[69] Results are promising; the addition of oxaliplatin resulted in a 23% risk reduction in disease recurrence and increased 3-year overall DFS (78.2% vs. 72.9%) compared to fluorouracil plus leucovorin alone. The addition of oxaliplatin did not substantially increase the toxicity of fluorouracil and leucovorin in the trial. These results will require longer follow-up prior to becoming standard of care in the adjuvant setting, although some practitioners are encouraged by these findings and have begun to incorporate oxaliplatin into adjuvant treatment regimens. Further modifications of the FOLFOX4 regimen may also improve tolerability. Capecitabine, an oral prodrug of fluorouracil, and other oral pyrimidines are also being evaluated in adjuvant studies as a replacement for fluorouracil in an attempt to improve the safety and ease of administration of the chemotherapy regimens.[68,70]

Portal Administration. Because the liver is the site of recurrence in about 40% of patients, infusion of chemotherapy via the portal vein provides an additional adjuvant treatment approach. The rationale for this is based on a belief that intraoperative manipulation of the tumor provides emboli of tumor that travel directly into the portal vein circulation, ultimately developing into hepatic micrometastasis.[28] Historically, fluorouracil has been the most common agent used for hepatic portal vein infusion. Because greater than 80% of a dose of fluorouracil administered systemically is metabolized by the liver, direct hepatic infusion of fluorouracil provides high local concentrations of the drug at the most common site of recurrence and minimizes systemic toxicity. Perioperative portal vein chemotherapy administration might then destroy cells before they can establish tumor growth.

An early trial evaluated the effect of a postoperative infusion of 1 g of fluorouracil infused via the portal vein daily for 7 days as compared to no further therapy following surgical resection in patients with stages I to III colorectal cancer. Heparin was also infused to reduce thrombosis.[71] Those patients who received fluorouracil and heparin experienced a significant benefit in the reduction of hepatic metastasis and a dramatic improvement in survival. Results from a trial of 1,158 patients with stages I to III colon cancer, who were randomized to receive either a continuous infusion of fluorouracil 600 mg/m^2 per day for 7 days with heparin via the portal vein, or no therapy following surgical resection, showed a modest but statistically significant improvement in DFS (68% vs. 60%) and OS (76% vs. 71%) in the chemotherapy group.[72]

Results of other trials evaluating postoperative portal vein infusions and fluorouracil or other agents are mixed. A meta-analysis of 4,000 patients in 10 randomized trials of portal vein infusion suggests a small (about 4%) improvement in 5-year OS with portal vein infusion.[73] However, these authors acknowledge that the flaws in some study designs and inadequate data to date require additional evidence from large randomized trials to determine whether this approach improves patient outcome. At this time, therefore, the value of portal vein infusion of fluorouracil for colon cancer remains unproven.

Biologic Therapy. Edrecolomab (17-1A monoclonal antibody) has been studied alone and in combination with fluorouracil following curative surgery for stage III colorectal cancer. It is administered as a 500-mg IV infusion given postoperatively that is followed by four monthly infusions of 100 mg. Edrecolomab's mechanism of action and common toxicities are described in Table 127–12. Compared to observation alone, antibody treatment with edrecolomab resulted in a 23% reduction in cancer recurrence and a 32% reduction in overall mortality in 189 patients with stage III cancer of the colon or rectum.[74] A randomized trial of 2761 patients who were randomly assigned to fluorouracil plus leucovorin alone, in combination with edrecolomab, or edrecolomab alone showed that DFS was lower with edrecolomab, and the addition of edrecolomab to fluorouracil plus leucovorin did not improve survival.[75] The future role of edrecolomab in adjuvant therapy is unclear.

TABLE 127–12. Investigational Agents for the Treatment of Colorectal Cancer

Drug Name	Mechanism of Action	Common Adverse Reactions	Phase in Development
Oral Fluorinated Pyrimidines			
Uracil-Tegafur (UFT, Ftorafur)	Tegafur: oral prodrug of fluorouracil; converted to fluorouracil by thymidine/uridine phosphorylase in the liver Uracil: Substrate for dihydropyridimidine dehydrogenase (DPD); inhibits degradation of fluorouracil	Vomiting, stomatitis, diarrhea, skin rash, and neurotoxicity (dizziness, confusion, ataxia)	Phase II/III
Eniluracil (776C85, 5-ethynyluracil)	DPD inactivator: binds to enzyme first in a reversible manner and then irreversibly inactivates it; inhibits fluorouracil degradation	Lacks systemic toxicity when administered alone	Phase III
Raltitrexed (ZD1694, Tomudex)	Folate analog: acts as a potent and selective thymidylate synthase inhibitor	Myelosuppression, nausea, vomiting, diarrhea, anorexia, reversible elevation of liver enzymes	Phase II
Monoclonal Antibodies			
Edrecolomab (17-1A MoAb, Panorex)	Murine monoclonal antibody directed against a tumor-specific glycoprotein located on colorectal tumor cells; antitumor activity via antibody-dependent cellular cytotoxicity (ADCC)	Diarrhea, abdominal pain, nausea, vomiting, infusion-related reactions (fever, chills)	Phase III
Signal Pathway Inhibitors			
Erlotinib (OSI-774, Tarceva) and others	Epidermal growth factor receptor (EGFR) tyrosine kinase inhibitor; inhibits cell proliferation signal transduction pathway	Acneiform skin rash, diarrhea, headache, mucositis, hyperbilirubinemia, neutropenia, anemia	Phase I
Tumor Vaccines			
Tipifarnib (R115777, Zarnesta)	Farnesyl transferase inhibitor, blocks Ras-activated signal transduction pathway	Myelosuppression, rash, fatigue, neuropathy	Phase II/III
CEA Vac and others	Monoclonal antibody vaccine targeting carcinoembryonic antigen	None reported	Phase III
Onco Vax	Prepared from autologous tumor cells mixed with bacille Calmette-Guérin, an organism with antitumor activity	Flu-like symptoms	Phase III
Antisense Therapy			
Oblimersen (G3139, Genasense)	Oligonucleotide that targets *Bcl-2* mRNA and inhibits expression of *Bcl-2*, an antiapoptotic oncogene	Myelosuppression, hypotension, fatigue, elevation of serum transaminases, mild hyperglycemia, fever	Phase II/III

ADJUVANT CHEMOTHERAPY FOR RECTAL CANCER

6 Rectal cancer involves those tumors found below the peritoneal reflection in the most distal 15 cm of the large bowel, and as such is very distinct from colon cancer in that it has a propensity for both local and distant recurrence. The higher incidence of local failure and poorer overall prognosis associated with rectal cancer is due to anatomic limitations in excising adequate radial margins around the rectal tumor. Although an abdominoperitoneal surgical resection of the tumor and adjacent tissues results in a high probability of local control and long-term survival, the sequelae, including need for a permanent colostomy and high incidence of sexual and genitourinary dysfunction, has led to investigation of approaches that use multimodal therapies which preserve the integrity of the anal sphincter. In addition, because treatment with surgery, XRT, or systemic chemotherapy at the time of the recurrence is often suboptimal, adjuvant therapy after tumor resection is an important aspect of treatment of the primary tumor. The effectiveness of postoperative XRT and fluorouracil-based chemotherapy for stage II or III rectal cancer is well established. Although T_1 tumors with a favorable histology may be treated successfully with local excision alone, adjuvant XRT plus chemotherapy should be offered for larger lesions. Similar to adjuvant therapy for colon cancer, fluorouracil provides the basis for chemotherapy regimens for rectal cancer. The XRT decreases the rate of local pelvic recurrences, whereas the fluorouracil decreases the risk of distant tumor recurrence and enhances the effectiveness of the XRT. The optimal delivery schedule for these two therapies is the subject of ongoing investigation, but many trials have demonstrated improved local control and survival for patients who receive a combination of postoperative XRT and chemotherapy as compared to surgery alone. In 1990, based on results from the Gastrointestinal Tumor Study Group (GITSG) and the Mayo/NCCTG studies, the National Cancer Institute Consensus Conference recommended that standard postoperative adjuvant treatment for patients with stage II or III rectal tumors should consist of six cycles of fluorouracil-based chemotherapy with concurrent pelvic XRT.[76]

The GITSG trial was designed to evaluate adjuvant postoperative treatment for patients with stage II or III rectal cancer. Patients were randomized into one of four groups: (1) observation only (control); (2) XRT alone; (3) chemotherapy alone (fluorouracil and semustine) for 18 months; or (4) combination XRT and chemotherapy.[77] Despite protocol violations and a short median follow-up, the study finished earlier than anticipated because of the statistically significant results that favored the combined modality treatment. The patients receiving the combination therapy had a reduction in both local (11% vs. 24%) and distant (26% vs. 34%) recurrence rates as compared to the control group. Although not seen initially, a re-estimate of survival probabilities at a median follow-up of 94 months demonstrated that the combination treatment was associated with a 24% OS advantage over the control group.[78] As expected, combined modality therapy resulted in more severe hematologic toxicity, enteritis, and diarrhea than either chemotherapy or XRT alone.

The Mayo/NCCTG trial compared postoperative XRT alone, postoperative XRT with concurrent fluorouracil plus semustine chemotherapy, and pre- and postirradiation chemotherapy in a similar population of 204 patients with rectal cancer.[79] This was the first randomized trial in which one cycle of combination chemotherapy was given before and after XRT in addition to the administration of fluorouracil during XRT. The use of combined chemotherapy and XRT significantly affected local recurrence, relapse-free survival, and OS as compared to XRT alone.[51] Patients receiving combined therapy experienced an overall relative reduction of recurrence of 34% at

5 years as compared to the XRT-only group. A 36% improvement in DFS and 29% improvement in OS at 5 years were also observed in the combined group.

Acute complications such as severe hematologic toxicity (leukopenia and thrombocytopenia), enteritis, and diarrhea were commonly observed in the combined group. Hematologic toxicity was more noticeable during postirradiation chemotherapy, despite reduced doses. Although small bowel complications were uncommon, four deaths were reported as a result of complications as a consequence of small bowel obstruction, fistulas, septicemia resulting from perforation, and hemorrhage. There was a 6% incidence of primary cancers, equally divided between the XRT and combined groups. Because of the leukemogenic potential associated with semustine and results from prospective comparative trials that demonstrate that it does not contribute to overall treatment efficacy, semustine is no longer included in standard adjuvant treatment regimens. This regimen without semustine represents a popular adjuvant treatment regimen for rectal cancer.

Additional trials have sought to determine optimal combinations of concurrent radiation and fluorouracil. Based on preclinical studies that suggest continuous infusions of fluorouracil provide more effective radiosensitization than IV bolus injections, the Gastrointestinal Intergroup compared continuous IV fluorouracil infusion to intermittent bolus injections.[80] Six hundred sixty patients with stage II or III rectal cancer received either continuous infusion or IV bolus fluorouracil with postoperative pelvic XRT, in addition to pre- and postirradiation fluorouracil. At a median follow-up of 46 months, patients who received continuous infusion fluorouracil experienced a reduction in distant metastases and improved DFS and OS. The incidence of leukopenia (white blood cell count $<2000/mm^3$) was greater in the IV bolus fluorouracil group, whereas diarrhea was more frequent in the protracted infusion group. Many treatment centers now employ continuous-infusion fluorouracil throughout the 5- or 6-week schedule of postoperative XRT for rectal cancer. Despite evidence that leucovorin improves efficacy of fluorouracil in other treatment settings, it does not appear to improve efficacy of adjuvant treatment for rectal cancer.[81] Use of oral alternatives to fluorouracil that are also known to enhance radiation effects, such as capecitabine, are under investigation, with preliminary data suggesting the combination of capecitabine and XRT will be safe and effective.[82]

Preoperative (Neoadjuvant) Versus Postoperative Therapy

6 Interest in preoperative or neoadjuvant therapy has increased based on advances in imaging techniques to more accurately stage rectal tumors preoperatively and the success of combined XRT plus fluorouracil administered in the postoperative setting. Both pre- and postoperative XRT administered in conventional doses effectively decreases local recurrence rates for rectal cancer by up to 50% as compared to rates with surgery alone.[58] Preoperative XRT, by shrinking and thereby downstaging the tumor prior to surgical resection, improves sphincter preservation, but the primary concern with this approach is potential overtreatment with XRT. While this is a common treatment strategy in some European countries, the issue of pre- versus postoperative XRT is a subject of debate and investigation in the United States. Furthermore, the way that XRT and fluorouracil are delivered varies widely. Some practitioners deliver XRT as 45 to 55 Gy in small fractions of 1.8 to 2.0 Gy over a period of 5 to 6 weeks, whereas short, intensive courses deliver therapy in five fractions over a period of 1 week. Moreover, variability in surgical technique can also influence outcome.[83] Fluorouracil can be administered as IV bolus injections for 3 or 4 days during the first and last weeks of XRT or via a continuous IV infusion. Although concurrent XRT plus fluorouracil continuous infusion is theoretically more efficacious based on the results from postoperative chemoradiation trials, short intensive-course chemoradiation strategies are less expensive and more convenient for the patient. Preliminary results of NSABP Trial R-03 suggest that pre- and postoperative chemoradiation therapy are similarly safe and efficacious, but long-term survival and toxicity data will be needed to make a definitive conclusion.

Several trials that have compared preoperative therapy to surgery alone have failed to show a survival benefit with preoperative XRT; however, the Swedish Rectal Cancer Trial, a randomized trial of 1,168 patients with resectable rectal cancer who underwent a short course of intensive preoperative XRT followed by surgery within 1 week or surgery alone, was able to demonstrate improved local recurrence rates (11% vs. 27%) and 5-year survival for those patients who received XRT plus surgery versus surgery alone (58% vs. 48%).[84,85] These findings will need to be verified in future trials before this therapy can be considered the standard of care. Moreover, the short-course therapy is unlikely to sufficiently downstage the tumor because it will have only been completed 1 week prior to surgery. Whether fluorouracil can be safely incorporated into such a regimen will also require further evaluation.

Results from the GITSG, NSABP, and Intergroup trials indicate that survival benefits can be achieved with the addition of fluorouracil to postoperative XRT for resectable rectal cancer.[77–80] Adjuvant chemotherapy plus XRT decreases local tumor recurrence after surgery and increases the probability of sphincter preservation in patients with clinically resectable disease. Neoadjuvant therapy may provide similar benefits and additionally improve the rate of resectability in patients with locally advanced disease by downstaging the tumor, but regimens cannot be considered standard therapy at this time. The NCCN Practice Guidelines for rectal cancer indicate that postoperative fluorouracil-based chemotherapy plus XRT is considered appropriate adjuvant therapy for resectable T_2 or larger lesions.[86] Neoadjuvant fluorouracil chemoradiation followed by abdominoperineal or low anterior resection or surgery alone plus postoperative fluorouracil or fluorouracil plus XRT should be considered for locally unresectable tumors.

METASTATIC DISEASE

INITIAL THERAPY

Several advances have been made recently in developing efficacious treatment options for metastatic colorectal cancer. Whereas surgery and XRT are most often used to manage isolated sites of tumor, chemotherapy is most useful for patients with disseminated disease and is the primary treatment modality for unresectable metastatic colorectal cancer.

Surgery

Complete surgical resection of discrete hepatic, pulmonary, abdominal, or brain metastases in patients with colorectal cancer, if possible, may offer selected patients an opportunity to experience extended DFS. Patients who have from one to three small nodules isolated to the liver, lungs, or abdomen have the most favorable outcome. Up to 25% of patients will present with hepatic metastases at time of diagnosis, and 60% of patients with colorectal cancer will develop hepatic metastases sometime during the course of their disease.

Five-year survival for patients who undergo surgical resection of metastases isolated to the liver ranges from 20% to 39%, with a median survival duration of 28 to 40 months, and is associated with an operative mortality rate less than 5%.[87] These results are drastically greater than those in patients with unresectable metastatic colorectal cancer, in whom 5-year survival is uncommon and median survival is about 12 months. Patients with no significant general medical risk factors, fewer than four hepatic lesions, CEA levels less than 200 ng/mL, small tumor size, lack of extrahepatic tumor, and adequate surgical margins have the best opportunity for an improved long-term outcome. The primary site of tumor should also be completely resected. Ablative therapies that involve destroying the tumor through freezing and thawing (cryoablation), heat (radiofrequency), or alcohol injection may be useful for patients who have very small hepatic lesions and are unable to undergo liver resection surgery, but are less successful than surgical interventions.[87] Outcomes associated with resection of isolated pulmonary, abdominal, and brain metastases have been less studied; however, this approach is potentially curative and should be considered for patients with resectable disease who are appropriate surgical candidates.

Because approximately two-thirds of patients who undergo resection of hepatic metastases will have disease recurrence, adjuvant systemic and hepatic arterial infusion chemotherapy have been studied in an attempt to improve long-term outcomes. A randomized trial that compared 6 months of hepatic floxuridine and dexamethasone plus IV fluorouracil with leucovorin to IV fluorouracil with leucovorin alone following resection of hepatic metastases in 156 patients showed improved 2-year DFS (86% vs. 72%) and hepatic recurrence-free survival at 2 years (90% vs. 60%) with the combined therapy.[88] Many practitioners offer adjuvant chemotherapy to select patients following potentially curative hepatic resection, but further studies, especially those involving more active agents, are needed to determine an optimal treatment regimen.[89]

Radiation

Symptom reduction is the primary goal of XRT for patients with advanced or metastatic colorectal cancer.

Chemotherapy

Accepted initial chemotherapy regimens for metastatic cancer of the colon or rectum consist of oxaliplatin plus fluorouracil and leucovorin, irinotecan plus fluorouracil and leucovorin, bevacizumab plus a fluorouracil-based regimen, or fluorouracil plus leucovorin alone. Examples of treatment regimens for metastatic colorectal cancer are listed in Table 127–13. The site(s) of tumor involvement and history of prior chemotherapy help to define an appropriate management strategy. In general, treatment options are similar for metastatic cancer of the colon and rectum.

Currently, metastatic colorectal cancer is incurable and treatment goals are to reduce patient symptoms, improve quality of life, and extend survival. Two recent meta-analyses were performed to estimate the magnitude of benefit and harm associated with palliative chemotherapy for metastatic colorectal cancer. In a pooled analysis of randomized trials comparing chemotherapy to observation or supportive care alone, a total of nine trials that included 614 patients were evaluated.[102] All trials used fluorouracil-based chemotherapy, but three trials in which hepatic arterial or portal vein administration was used were also included. Several trials allowed delayed or

TABLE 127–13. Chemotherapeutic Regimens for Metastatic Colorectal Cancer

	Regimen	Major Dose-Limiting Toxicities
Initial therapy		
Pyrimidine only		
Weekly, high-dose leucovorin; Roswell Park regimen[61]	Fluorouracil 600 mg/m^2 IV + leucovorin 500 mg/m^2 IV weekly × 6 out of 8 weeks	Diarrhea, mucositis
Consecutive day, low-dose leucovorin; Mayo Clinic regimen[61]	Fluorouracil 425 mg/m^2 per day IV + leucovorin 20 mg/m^2 per day IV days 1–5, for 5 consecutive days, repeated every 4–5 weeks	Mucositis, neutropenia
Bolus plus infusional fluorouracil; (LV5FU2)[62]; de Gramont regimen	Leucovorin 200 mg/m^2 per day IV over 2 hours followed by fluorouracil 400 mg/m^2 per day IV bolus, then followed by fluorouracil 600 mg/m^2 per day continuous IV infusion over 22 hours, days 1 and 2 for 2 consecutive days; repeat every 2 weeks	Neutropenia, mucositis
Capecitabine[90]	1250 mg/m^2 orally twice daily for 14 days, repeated every 3 weeks	Diarrhea, hand-foot syndrome
Oxaliplatin plus fluorouracil plus leucovorin		
Oxaliplatin plus bimonthly infusional fluorouracil; FOLFOX4[91]	Oxaliplatin 85 mg/m^2 IV day 1 plus bolus fluorouracil 400 mg/m^2 IV plus leucovorin 200 mg/m^2 IV followed by fluorouracil 600 mg/m^2 IV in 22-hour infusion on days 1 and 2, every 2 weeks	Sensory neuropathy, neutropenia
High-dose oxaliplatin plus bimonthly infusional fluorouracil; FOLFOX7[92]	Oxaliplatin 130 mg/m^2 IV with leucovorin 400 mg/m^2 IV day 1, followed by fluorouracil 400 mg/m^2 IV bolus and 2400 mg/m^2 continuous IV infusion over 46 hours started on day 1, repeated every 2 weeks	Sensory neuropathy, diarrhea, myelosuppression
Irinotecan plus fluorouracil plus leucovorin		
Irinotecan plus bolus fluorouracil; IFL; Saltz regimen[93]	Irinotecan 125 mg/m^2 IV plus fluorouracil 500 mg/m^2 IV plus leucovorin 20 mg/m^2 IV weekly for 4 weeks out of 6 weeks	Diarrhea, neutropenia
Irinotecan plus infusional fluorouracil; FOLFIRI[94]	Irinotecan 180 mg/m^2 IV plus leucovorin 400 mg/m^2 IV plus bolus fluorouracil 400 mg/m^2 IV, followed by fluorouracil 2400 mg/m^2 continuous IV infusion over 46 hours on day 1, repeated every 2 weeks	Nausea, diarrhea, mucositis, neutropenia
Biweekly irinotecan plus infusional fluorouracil[95]	Irinotecan 180 mg/m^2 IV plus leucovorin 200 mg/m^2 plus fluorouracil 400 mg/m^2 IV, followed by fluorouracil 600 mg/m^2 continuous IV infusion over 22 hours, day 1, repeated every 2 weeks	Neutropenia, diarrhea
Weekly irinotecan plus infusional fluorouracil[95]	Irinotecan 80 mg/m^2 IV plus leucovorin 500 mg/m^2 IV plus fluorouracil 2300 mg/m^2 continuous IV infusion over 24 hours day 1, repeated weekly	Neutropenia, diarrhea
Bevacizumab		
Bevacizumab plus bolus IFL[96]	Irinotecan 125 mg/m^2 IV plus fluorouracil 500 mg/m^2 IV plus leucovorin 20 mg/m^2 IV weekly for 4 out of 6 weeks, with bevacizumab 5 mg/m^2 IV day 1, repeated every 2 weeks	Diarrhea, hypertension, asthenia, thrombosis, vomiting, proteinuria
Salvage therapy		
Irinotecan[a]		
Weekly irinotecan[93]	Irinotecan 125 mg/m^2 IV every week for 4 out of 6 weeks	Neutropenia, diarrhea
Every 3-weekly irinotecan[97]	Irinotecan 350 mg/m^2 IV every 3 weeks	Neutropenia, diarrhea
Oxaliplatin plus fluorouracil plus leucovorin[b]		
Oxaliplatin plus bimonthly infusional fluorouracil; FOLFOX4[91]	Oxaliplatin 85 mg/m^2 IV day 1 plus bolus fluorouracil 400 mg/m^2 IV plus leucovorin 200 mg/m^2 IV followed by fluorouracil 600 mg/m^2 IV in 22-hour infusion on days 1 and 2, every 2 weeks	Sensory neuropathy, neutropenia
High-dose oxaliplatin plus bimonthly infusional fluorouracil; FOLFOX7[92]	Oxaliplatin 130 mg/m^2 IV with leucovorin 400 mg/m^2 IV day 1, followed by fluorouracil 400 mg/m^2 IV bolus and 2400 mg/m^2 continuous IV infusion over 46 hours started on day 1, repeated every 2 weeks	Sensory neuropathy, diarrhea, myelosuppression
Cetuximab[c]		
Cetuximab plus irinotecan[98]	Continue irinotecan as previously dosed, plus cetuximab 400 mg/m^2 IV loading dose, then cetuximab 250 mg/m^2 IV weekly thereafter	Asthenia, diarrhea, nausea, acneiform rash, vomiting
Cetuximab[98]	Cetuximab 400 mg/m^2 IV loading dose, then cetuximab 250 mg/m^2 IV weekly thereafter	Acneform rash, asthenia, constipation, diarrhea
Fluorouracil		
Protracted continuous infusion[99]	Fluorouracil 250–300 mg/m^2 per day continuous IV infusion until disease progression	Mucositis, hand-foot syndrome
Investigational		
Xelox; CapOx[100]	Capecitabine 1000 mg/m^2 orally twice daily days 1–14 plus oxaliplatin 70 mg/m^2 IV days 1 and 8; repeat every 3 weeks	Diarrhea, sensory neuropathy
Xeliri; CapIri[100]	Capecitabine 1000 mg/m^2 orally twice daily days 1–14 plus irinotecan 100 mg/m^2 IV days 1 and 8; repeat every 3 weeks	Diarrhea, neutropenia
IROX[101]	Oxaliplatin 85 mg/m^2 IV plus irinotecan 200 mg/m^2 IV day 1, repeated every 3 weeks	Neutropenia, diarrhea, vomiting, sensory neuropathy

[a]If first-line therapy, fluorouracil plus leucovorin or oxaliplatin plus fluorouracil plus leucovorin.
[b]If first-line therapy, fluorouracil plus leucovorin or irinotecan plus fluorouracil plus leucovorin, or bevacizumab plus IFL.
[c]If irinotecan-refractory disease.

discretionary use of chemotherapy in patients assigned to observation or supportive care alone; 12% to 57% of control patients received at least one course of chemotherapy. Despite these discrepancies, chemotherapy was associated with a significant reduction in mortality at 1 (relative risk ratio 0.69) but not 2 years (relative risk ratio 0.93).

The second meta-analysis to determine the benefit of chemotherapy in metastatic disease analyzed individual patient data and summary statistics from 13 randomized trials that included 1,365 patients.[103] Eligible trials compared palliative chemotherapy given via any route of administration to supportive care alone or treatments not involving chemotherapy. Trials that allowed chemotherapy use in control patients were not excluded. In the analysis of seven trials in which individual patient data were available, palliative chemotherapy was shown to reduce risk of death by 35%, which translates to a prolongation of median survival by 3.7 months. The investigators were unable to determine the extent to which treatment resulted in significant toxicities or affected quality of life because of inadequate data. However, the results of both analyses suggest that palliative chemotherapy is beneficial and improves survival in metastatic colorectal cancer. Because many patients assigned to control arms eventually received chemotherapy, the magnitude of survival benefit associated with chemotherapy could be underestimated.

Fluorouracil continues to be incorporated into current first-line chemotherapy regimens used for metastatic colorectal cancer. When administered in bolus injection treatment schedules, fluorouracil is given most frequently with leucovorin, which improves response rates but has minimal impact on overall survival. The addition of irinotecan to fluorouracil plus leucovorin significantly improves response rates, progression-free survival, and median survival, without adversely affecting quality of life. Oxaliplatin in combination with fluorouracil and leucovorin has also shown improvements in median survival when compared to the combination of irinotecan plus fluorouracil and leucovorin in the initial treatment of metastatic colon cancer. The addition of bevacizumab to fluorouracil-based regimens improves efficacy compared to chemotherapy alone. Either of these three- or four-drug combinations may be considered as first-line therapy for metastatic colorectal cancer. Ongoing trials are evaluating the sequencing of these regimens, as well as comparing the efficacy of combinations of fluorouracil plus leucovorin, to investigational treatments with capecitabine, oral fluoropyrimidines and newer agents. Table 127–14 summarizes comparative outcome data from potentially useful chemotherapeutic treatments for metastatic colorectal cancer.

◀ ■ *Fluorouracil.*   Fluorouracil has been administered as a single agent by IV bolus injection but response rates are only 10% to 20%.[28,104] As such, IV bolus fluorouracil as a single agent is considered ineffective for metastatic colorectal cancer.

A variety of continuous IV infusion fluorouracil regimens have been developed to increase the duration of drug exposure during the S phase of the cell cycle and increase DNA-dependent cytotoxicity. Some of these schedules involve short (24- to 48-hour) weekly or biweekly or protracted continuous fluorouracil infusions for up to 12 weeks.[28] Doses of fluorouracil employed in 24 to 48 hour infusions generally range from 1000 to 2000 mg/m^2 per day. A regimen utilizing 300 mg/m^2 per day for 10 weeks is considered the maximally tolerated dose for protracted continuous infusion. Based on the assumption that a dose-response relationship exists for colorectal cancer, this approach is one of the most efficacious methods of dose intensification for fluorouracil. The maximum cumulative fluorouracil dose that can be administered via continuous IV infusion in a 28-day period is approximately 4000 to 7400 mg/m^2 as compared to 2,400 to 2,500 mg/m^2 with IV bolus fluorouracil.[105]

Despite differences in dose intensity among the different regimens, no clear survival advantages or trends are obvious for any particular regimen. However, in comparison to IV bolus fluorouracil, response rates with continuous infusion fluorouracil are approximately doubled. In a meta-analysis of six randomized trials evaluating 1219 patients with advanced colorectal cancer that compared efficacy of continuous infusion and bolus IV fluorouracil, a significantly higher tumor response rate (22% vs. 14%) was observed in patients receiving fluorouracil by continuous IV infusion.[106] Although continuous infusion fluorouracil was also associated with a significant OS benefit (overall hazard ratio 0.88), this effect is generally considered as marginal. Therefore, until future studies demonstrate a clinical benefit with continuous infusion fluorouracil with respect to the added expense and complications associated with venous access devices and portable infusion pumps, some clinicians continue to favor IV bolus schedules for initial therapy of metastatic disease. Increased acceptance and added clinical benefit with continuous infusion fluorouracil has been demonstrated when fluorouracil is administered with other agents and is becoming more commonplace in clinical practice.

◀ ■ *Fluorouracil Plus Leucovorin.*   Numerous studies have evaluated various doses and administration schedules of fluorouracil plus leucovorin in an attempt to improve treatment response rates and survival in metastatic colorectal cancer. Response rates of 14% to 58% have been observed with a variety of doses of fluorouracil in combination with leucovorin at doses ranging from 20 to 500 mg/m^2.[28] Leucovorin can be given by IV bolus, continuous infusion, and orally. The administration sequence and timing of leucovorin may be important factors in evaluating the efficacy of biochemical modulation with leucovorin. A schedule for administering leucovorin prior to fluorouracil is the most effective approach to enable the level of intracellular-reduced folates to accumulate prior to fluorouracil administration. However, the maximum tolerated dose of fluorouracil when given in combination with leucovorin is lower than that when given alone. In addition, a qualitative alteration of the toxicity pattern has been noted.

Despite significantly higher response rates and improved progression-free survival achieved with leucovorin-modulated fluorouracil regimens, their effect on OS is modest. The lack of any clear survival benefit detected in clinical trials might be explained by the generally short duration of tumor responses, the large number of patients who do not respond to treatment, or the effects of crossover administration of fluorouracil plus leucovorin in patients who fail single-agent fluorouracil. Phase III trials evaluating fluorouracil and leucovorin for metastatic colorectal cancer have been criticized because doses of fluorouracil used in control groups have been below the maximum-tolerated dose. As a result, the addition of leucovorin may appear to produce a greater antitumor effect when in fact it is being compared to a suboptimal dose of fluorouracil in the control group.

The most practical issue at present, however, is whether a weekly, biweekly, or monthly regimen of fluorouracil given as an IV bolus or continuous infusion with high- or low-dose leucovorin is most preferable. The most commonly used regimens for metastatic colorectal cancer in the U.S. have involved the Mayo Clinic regimen and the Roswell Park regimen (see Table 127–13). These regimens have been compared in randomized trials with conflicting results.

For a number of years the Mayo Clinic regimen has been the reference regimen in metastatic colon cancer. However, limitations with

TABLE 127–14. Comparative Outcomes from Selected Trials in Metastatic Colorectal Cancer

Trial	Number	Outcome Measures	Results
First-line			
Goldberg et al[101]	795	Primary: TTP; secondary: OS, RR time to treatment discontinuation	Median TTP: IFL vs. FOLFOX 6.9 vs. 8.7 mo (p = .0014). Median survival 15.0 mo with IFL vs. 19.5 mo with FOLFOX (p = .001). Response rate with FOLFOX (45%) higher compared to IFL (31%; p = .002) and IROX (35%, p = .03). TTP and OS with IROX (6.5 and 17.4 mo) no different from FOLFOX.
de Gramont et al[91]	420	Primary: PFS; secondary: RR, OS, tolerability, QOL	Median PFS: 9.0 vs. 6.2 mo (p = .0003); RR: 50.7 vs. 22.3% (p = .0001), oxaliplatin plus LV5FU2 vs. LF5FU2 alone; no oxaliplatin plus LV5FU2 vs. LV5FU2 alone difference in OS (16.2 vs. 14.7 mo) or QOL
Saltz et al[93]	683	Primary: PFS; secondary: RR, OS	Median PFS longer with IFL (7.0 mo) vs. FU/LV (4.3 mo; p = .004); PFS similar with irinotecan alone (4.2 mo) compared to FU/LV; RR higher with IFL vs. FU/LV (50 vs. 28%; p < .001); median survival longer with IFL (14.8 mo) vs. 12.6 mo with FU/LV (p = .04), which was similar to irinotecan (12.0 mo)
Douillard et al[95]	387	Primary: RR; secondary: TTP, response duration, TTF, OS, QOL	Significantly higher RR with infusional IFL vs. infusional FU/LV alone (35 vs 22%; p < .005) by ITT; TTP longer with IFL (6.7 vs. 4.4 mo; p < .001) and OS longer with IFL vs. infusional FU/LV alone (17.4 vs. 14.1 mo; p = .031)
Tournigand et al[94]	226	Test the best sequence of FOLFIRI vs. FOLFOX6; primary: second PFS; secondary: PFS, OS, RR, safety	Median survival 21.5 mo with FOLFIRI then FOLFOX6 vs. 20.6 mo with FOLFOX6 then FOLFIRI; median PFS also no different (14.2 vs. 10.9 mo), or RR or median PFS with first treatment: FOLFOX6 54% and 8.0 mo, vs. 56% and 8.5 mo with FOLFIRI
Hurwitz et al[96]	925	Primary: OS; secondary: PFS, RR, response duration, QOL	Bevacizumab plus IFL increased median survival (20.3 mo) vs. IFL alone (15.6 mo; p = .00003), PFS (10.6 vs. 6.24 mo; p < .00001), RR (45% vs. 35%; p = .0029), and duration of response (10.4 vs. 7.1 mo; p = .0014)
Twelves[90]	1,207	Primary: RR; secondary: TTP, OS, response duration	Tumor response to capecitabine greater than with FU/LV (25.7 vs. 16.7%; p < .0002), but no difference in median TTP (4.6 vs. 4.7 mo) or median survival (392 vs. 391 days)
Second-line			
Rougier et al[99]	267	Primary: OS; secondary: PFS, RR, symptom-free survival, adverse effects, QOL	Irinotecan improved median PFS (4.2 vs. 2.9 mo; p = .030) compared to infusion fluorouracil and 1-year survival (45% vs. 35%; p = .035) but not median OS (10.8 vs. 8.5 mo). Median pain-free survival was similar (p = .06; 10.3 vs. 8.5 mo) between irinotecan and fluorouracil, as was QOL
Cunningham et al[97]	279	Primary: OS; secondary; performance status, body weight, tumor-related symptoms, QOL	Compared to best supportive care, OS was improved with irinotecan (13.8% 1-year survival vs. 36.2%; p = .0001); survival without deterioration in performance status, weight loss greater than 5%, and pain-free survival were also improved with irinotecan
Cunningham et al[98]	329	Primary: RR; secondary: TTP, OS	Addition of cetuximab to continuing irinotecan associated with 22.9% response rate compared to 10.9% with cetuximab alone (p = .0074); median survival with cetuximab plus irinotecan similar to cetuximab alone (8.6 vs. 6.9 mo; p = 0.48), but TTP was longer with cetuximab plus irinotecan (4.1 vs. 1.5 mo; hazard ratio 0.54; 95% CI, 0.42–0.71)

FU5LV2, bolus plus infusional fluorouracil and leucovorin; FU/LV, fluorouracil plus leucovorin; IFL, irinotecan plus fluorouracil plus leucovorin; IROX, irinotecan plus oxaliplatin; ITT, intention to treat; OS, overall survival; PFS, progression-free survival; QOL, quality of life; RR, response rate; TTF, time to treatment failure; TTP, time to tumor progression.

this regimen are becoming more apparent. A trial comparing the Mayo Clinic regimen to either fluorouracil alone or fluorouracil (370 mg/m^2 per day for 5 days) with HD-dose leucovorin (200 mg/m^2 per day) found the Mayo Clinic regimen to be more effective, with a response rate of 42%, compared to response rates of 10% and 31% for fluorouracil alone or in combination with HD-leucovorin, respectively.[107] Although the LD-leucovorin regimen was more effective than the HD regimen, the difference in response could be attributed to the higher doses of fluorouracil that were administered in the Mayo Clinic regimen. Median survival, 12.7 months, was no different in either leucovorin-containing regimen. A subsequent collaborative trial

compared the Mayo Clinic regimen to the Roswell Park regimen in 372 patients with metastatic disease.[108] There were no differences in tumor response (35% vs. 31%), median survival (9.3 months vs. 10.7 months), or palliative responses. The LD-leucovorin regimen was, however, associated with significantly more leukopenia and stomatitis, whereas HD-leucovorin caused more diarrhea and a greater hospitalization requirement to manage toxicity. Similar modifications of leucovorin have been studied with the Roswell Park regimen. In a trial comparing high- (500 mg/m^2) and low-dose (20 mg/m^2) leucovorin plus weekly fluorouracil at equal doses (500 mg/m^2) in 291 patients with inoperable or metastatic colorectal cancer, there were no differences in median response duration, progression-free, or overall survival.[109] While the incidence of mucositis was similar for both groups (9.8% vs. 11.5%), grade 3 or 4 diarrhea was more common with high-dose leucovorin (27% vs. 16.1%).

Overall, response rates and survival outcomes with weekly and daily regimens of bolus fluorouracil plus LD- or HD-leucovorin appear comparable. Leucovorin doses greater than 20 mg/m² do not appear to increase overall survival, but rather add to the toxicity of either daily or weekly regimens of fluorouracil. Weekly (HD-leucovorin) treatment schedules are associated with a higher incidence of diarrhea, the primary dose-limiting toxicity, whereas mucositis and leukopenia are relatively infrequent.[110] Mucositis tends to be dose-limiting and leukopenia is more common with the daily (LD-leucovorin) treatment schedule.

The Mayo Clinic regimen has also been compared to bimonthly and weekly regimens of infusional fluorouracil. Higher response rates of 24% to 54% have been noted in bimonthly regimens of fluorouracil administered first as an IV bolus infusion followed by a 22-hour continuous infusion in combination with high-dose leucovorin administered over 2 hours.[110] However, the bimonthly combined IV bolus and continuous infusion fluorouracil schedule (de Gramont regimen) did not improve median survival compared to the Mayo Clinic schedule, although it was associated with a lower incidence of severe granulocytopenia, diarrhea, and mucositis.[62] High response rates (39% to 58%) have also been observed in previously untreated and treated patients receiving weekly fluorouracil as a continuous 24-hour infusion in combination with HD-leucovorin given over 2 to 24 hours. In a recent trial of untreated metastatic colorectal cancer, 497 patients were randomly assigned to receive the Mayo Clinic regimen of fluorouracil/leucovorin or fluorouracil 2600 mg/m² as a 24-hour continuous infusion alone or in combination with HD-leucovorin weekly.[111] Though median survival rates were not different between groups, progression-free survival was prolonged when weekly fluorouracil was administered with HD-leucovorin. Similar to other toxicity results, leukopenia and mucositis were more frequent in patients receiving bolus fluorouracil plus leucovorin (Mayo Clinic regimen), while patients receiving continuous infusion fluorouracil plus leucovorin experienced more diarrhea and hand-foot syndrome.

In summary, the Mayo Clinic regimen of fluorouracil plus low-dose leucovorin is still an acceptable regimen, although a weekly schedule of leucovorin plus fluorouracil (either bolus or continuous infusion) may be more convenient for the patient in terms of fewer scheduled clinic appointments, less interference with work schedules, and ease of dose adjustments based on toxicity. Bimonthly infusions of fluorouracil given over 2 days produce higher response rates when compared to daily regimens and are gaining in acceptability. However, the incorporation of newer agents into treatment regimens rather than continual adjustments of fluorouracil and leucovorin doses and administration schedules will most likely result in the greatest advances in drug therapy for metastatic colorectal cancer.

CLINICAL CONTROVERSY

The best way to administer fluorouracil has been debated by clinicians for years. Although higher response rates are seen with continuous infusions of fluorouracil, many argue that this benefit is not clinically meaningful.

◀ ■ *Irinotecan Plus Fluorouracil and Leucovorin.*   Based on irinotecan's activity against untreated and fluorouracil-resistant colorectal cancer, in addition to its unique mechanism of action, several investigations have been completed to determine whether the addition of irinotecan to fluorouracil plus leucovorin as initial therapy for metastatic disease could further improve survival. In a randomized trial of 387 previously untreated patients with advanced colorectal cancer, irinotecan plus fluorouracil and leucovorin was compared to fluorouracil plus leucovorin with regard to tumor response, survival, and quality of life[95] (see Table 127–14). The choice of one of two fluorouracil plus leucovorin regimens was left to the discretion of participating investigators. Patients randomized to fluorouracil plus leucovorin could receive weekly fluorouracil (2,600 mg/m²) as a 24-hour IV infusion plus leucovorin (500 mg/m²), or the de Gramont regimen of IV bolus and infusional fluorouracil. For the three-drug treatment, a weekly regimen of irinotecan (80 mg/m²) with a 24-hour infusion of fluorouracil (2300 mg/m²) plus leucovorin 500 mg/m², or an every 2-week regimen consisting of irinotecan (180 mg/m²) on day 1 with IV bolus fluorouracil (400 mg/m²) followed by a 22-hour IV infusion (600 mg/m²) plus leucovorin (200 mg/m² given on days 1 and 2) could be used. Tumor response, median time to disease progression, and OS were all greater in the irinotecan group. Diarrhea and neutropenia were the most common toxicities and were worse in the irinotecan-containing groups. Diarrhea was the most common reason for dose reduction or treatment discontinuation with the weekly regimens, and led to hospital admission for 32% of patients receiving irinotecan compared to 12% of patients who received only fluorouracil plus leucovorin. Neutropenia was the most common cause of dose reductions with the every-2-week regimens. Results from questionnaires indicated that a definite deterioration in quality of life developed consistently later in the irinotecan group.

A second randomized trial compared the addition of irinotecan (125 mg/m²) to weekly fluorouracil plus leucovorin (fluorouracil 500 mg/m² IV bolus plus leucovorin 20 mg/m² IV bolus, each given weekly for 4 weeks, repeated every 6 weeks) to the Mayo Clinic regimen and to irinotecan alone (125 mg/m² IV weekly for 4 weeks, repeated every 6 weeks) as first-line therapy in 683 patients with metastatic colorectal cancer.[93] The combination of irinotecan, fluorouracil, and leucovorin resulted in significantly increased tumor response rates and improved progression-free survival and OS as compared to fluorouracil plus leucovorin and irinotecan alone, respectively. The combined incidence of grade 3 or 4 diarrhea was 22.7% with the three-drug combination, compared to 13.2% with fluorouracil plus leucovorin and 31% with irinotecan alone. However, the incidence of grade 3 diarrhea was almost threefold greater with triple-drug therapy as compared to the two-drug regimen. Mid-cycle dose reductions caused by neutropenia, which were more common with the three-drug treatment, could potentially have lowered subsequent risk of grade 4 diarrhea. Mucositis was more frequent in the fluorouracil plus leucovorin group. Quality-of-life analyses did not indicate that the addition of irinotecan to fluorouracil plus leucovorin compromised quality of life. Based on these results, this became the most common administration schedule for irinotecan plus fluorouracil and leucovorin in the United States, although irinotecan-based regimens containing continuous infusions of fluorouracil (e.g., FOLFIRI) are preferred by many practitioners.

The most common adverse effects of irinotecan in these regimens are diarrhea, neutropenia, nausea and vomiting, asthenia, abdominal pain, and alopecia; diarrhea and neutropenia are dose limiting.[93,95] Two distinct patterns of diarrhea have been described. Early-onset diarrhea occurs during or within 2 to 6 hours after irinotecan administration and is characterized by lacrimation, diaphoresis, abdominal cramping, flushing, and/or diarrhea. These cholinergic symptoms, thought to be due to inhibition of acetylcholinesterase, respond to atropine 0.25 to 1 mg given intravenously or subcutaneously. Approximately 10% of patients experience the acute symptoms during or shortly following the irinotecan. More commonly, late-onset diarrhea appears, 1 to 12 days after irinotecan administration, and may last for 3 to 5 days.[28,112] Late-onset diarrhea may require hospitalization or discontinuation of therapy, and fatalities have been reported. The incidence of late-onset diarrhea has been as high as 39% in some studies, but is now much lower with aggressive antidiarrheal intervention.[28,112]

Aggressive intervention with high-dose loperamide therapy should consist of 4 mg taken at the first sign of soft or watery stools, followed by 2 mg orally every 2 hours until symptom free for 12 hours. This regimen can be modified to 4 mg every 4 hours taken during the night. Of note, a significant correlation has been identified between the severity of delayed diarrhea, irinotecan, and SN-38 (irinotecan's active metabolite) area under the concentration-versus-time curve, as well as pharmacogenetic abnormalities in the enzyme UDP-glucuronosyltransferase (UGT1A1), which is responsible for the glucuronidation of SN-38 to inactive metabolites. The UGT1A1 enzyme exists in polymorphic states, and reduced or deficient levels of this enzyme are observed in Gilbert's syndrome, a familial hyperbilirubinemia disorder, and correlate with irinotecan-induced diarrhea and neutropenia.[113]

Based on these studies, the addition of irinotecan to fluorouracil plus leucovorin (IFL) has been proved to increase survival when compared to fluorouracil plus leucovorin in the first-line treatment of metastatic colorectal cancer. These data support the current consensus that the three-drug treatment regimen be considered a first-line option for metastatic colorectal cancer. Accordingly, irinotecan received approval from the FDA in 2000 as first-line therapy for metastatic colorectal cancer in combination with fluorouracil and leucovorin. The use of fluorouracil plus leucovorin without irinotecan is appropriate as first-line therapy when a less-toxic regimen is desirable, especially for patients with a poor performance status.

8 ■ *Fluorouracil and Leucovorin Plus Oxaliplatin.* Oxaliplatin, a 1,2-diaminocyclohexane platinum carrier ligand with a mechanism of action similar to cisplatin, in combination with infusional fluorouracil plus leucovorin, is approved by the FDA for use in first-line and salvage regimens for metastatic colorectal cancer (see Table 127–13). Oxaliplatin differs from cisplatin in that the DNA damage induced by oxaliplatin may not be as easily recognized by the DNA MMR complex.[114] Thus oxaliplatin-induced DNA damage may play a particularly important role in colorectal cancers that are associated with defects in MMR genes, as are prevalent in HNPCC. Oxaliplatin's incorporation into fluorouracil-based regimens as first-line therapy for metastatic colorectal cancer is associated with higher response rates and improved progression-free survival and variable effects on OS. A comparison of the de Gramont regimen, with or without oxaliplatin 85 mg/m^2 as a 2-hour infusion on day 1 (FOLFOX4 regimen), was designed to evaluate progression-free survival as a primary end point in 420 previously untreated patients with metastatic disease.[103] Tumor response (50.7% vs. 22.3%) and progression-free survival (median, 9 months vs. 6.2 months) were improved with oxaliplatin compared to fluorouracil plus leucovorin alone; an observed improvement in OS did not reach statistical significance (median, 16.2 months vs. 14.7 months). Although the three-drug regimen was associated with higher frequencies of grade 3 and 4 toxicities, primarily neutropenia, diarrhea, and neurosensory toxicity, they did not significantly impair quality of life.

Intergroup Trial N9741, a comparison of oxaliplatin plus fluorouracil and leucovorin (FOLFOX4) to weekly irinotecan plus IV bolus fluorouracil and leucovorin (IFL), and a combination of irinotecan plus oxaliplatin (IROX) in 795 patients with previously untreated metastatic colorectal cancer showed superior efficacy with

FOLFOX4.[101] The IROX arm showed no advantage over either of the other two arms. Significant improvements in response rates, progression-free survival, and median survival were seen with FOLFOX4 compared to IFL (see Table 127–14).[101] The study design allowed patients who failed either regimen to crossover to irinotecan or oxaliplatin, depending on their initial treatment assignment. Sixty percent of patients who failed FOLFOX4 received salvage irinotecan, whereas 24% of IFL failures received salvage oxaliplatin. The impact that this crossover had on survival is unknown, but may have resulted in an improvement in survival for the FOLFOX4 arm. In addition, the method of fluorouracil administration, and its impact on study results, has been called into question. Patients on the IFL arm received weekly IV bolus fluorouracil, while FOLFOX4 administered fluorouracil as IV bolus followed by continuous infusion IV, which is known to increase response rates. Therefore it is not possible to compare the true contributions of oxaliplatin and irinotecan combined with fluorouracil plus leucovorin in this study. The deletion of fluorouracil (or any fluorinated pyrimidine) from a first-line regimen may be undesirable.

In a phase III cooperative group study, a simplified combined bolus and infusional fluorouracil regimen with irinotecan (FOLFIRI) was compared to oxaliplatin combined with the same fluorouracil plus leucovorin schedule (FOLFOX6) in previously untreated patients with advanced colorectal cancer to determine whether the sequence of administration of both regimens differed with regard to efficacy and toxicities.[94] Patients were randomized to receive initial treatment with FOLFIRI or FOLFOX6, and at disease progression the patients then received the alternate regimen. Both sequences resulted in similar response rates, progression-free survival, and median survival, but the toxicity profiles were different. As first-line therapy, the incidence of grade 3 or 4 mucositis, nausea and vomiting, neutropenia, thrombocytopenia, fatigue, and alopecia were significantly more common with FOLFIRI, and neurologic toxicities were more common with FOLFOX6. The comparative toxicities of FOLFOX6 and FOLFIRI[94] are consistent with those in the comparison between FOLFOX4 and IFL,[101] where neuropathy and neutropenia were more common with oxaliplatin, with diarrhea, nausea, vomiting, dehydration, and febrile neutropenia being more common with IFL.

The decreased toxicity profile may be a result of oxaliplatin's distinct toxicity profile as compared with other platinum drugs. Oxaliplatin has minimal renal toxicity, myelosuppression, and nausea and vomiting when compared to other platinum-based drugs. Oxaliplatin is associated with both acute and persistent neuropathies.[115] The acute neuropathies occur with 1 to 2 days of dosing and resolve within 2 weeks. The neuropathies usually occur peripherally, but may also occur in the jaw and tongue. A rare acute syndrome of pharyngolaryngeal dysesthesia (1% to 2% of patients) is characterized by subjective sensations of difficulty in swallowing and shortness of breath. Overall, acute neuropathies occur in approximately 90% of patients, and are precipitated or exacerbated by exposure to cold temperatures or cold objects. Therefore patients should be instructed to avoid cold drinks and use of ice, and to cover skin before exposure to cold or cold objects. Several prophylactic and treatment strategies have been studied with varying degrees of success. Carbamazepine, gabapentin, amifostine, and calcium and magnesium infusions have been used to both prevent and treat oxaliplatin-induced neuropathies. Persistent neuropathy is typically a cumulative adverse effect, occurring after 8 to 10 cycles, and is seen mostly in patients who are responding to therapy.[101] The neuropathy is characterized by paresthesias, dysesthesias, and hypoesthesias, but may also include deficits in proprioception that can interfere with daily activities (e.g., writing, buttoning, swallowing, and difficulty walking due to impaired proprioception), and occur in half of patients receiving oxaliplatin with infusional fluorouracil plus leucovorin, but usually resolve with dosage reductions or cessation of oxaliplatin therapy.[115]

CLINICAL CONTROVERSY

The results of N9741 have been debated between clinicians since their presentation. Whether an irinotecan-containing regimen (IFL or FOLFIRI) is still the standard of care for metastatic disease, or if it has been replaced by FOLFOX4 is an unanswered question. Most patients should receive irinotecan- and oxaliplatin-containing regimens at some point during treatment for their disease.

9 ◀ *Capecitabine.* Capecitabine (Xeloda) is an oral, tumor-activated and tumor-selective fluoropyrimidine carbamate. Capecitabine is converted to fluorouracil through a three-step activation process, the final step being activation by thymidine phosphorylase, which is present in greatest concentrations at the tumor site. These activation steps lead to an approximate threefold increase in tumor and 1.4-fold increase in hepatic fluorouracil levels. Capecitabine has been compared to fluorouracil plus leucovorin as first-line therapy for metastatic colorectal cancer in two randomized phase III trials. In a pooled analysis of 1,207 patients randomized to capecitabine (1,250 mg/m^2 orally twice daily for 14 days, repeated every 3 weeks) or the Mayo Clinic regimen, tumor response to capecitabine was superior to that with fluorouracil plus leucovorin (25.7% vs. 16.7%).[90] Time to tumor progression and median survival, however, were no different. Hand-foot syndrome was more common with capecitabine, whereas grade 3 or 4 neutropenia and stomatitis was more common with fluorouracil plus leucovorin. The convenience of oral administration and different toxicity profile makes capecitabine a potentially useful alternative to IV fluorouracil regimens in the setting of metastatic disease. However, since the IV treatment arm in these comparative studies could be considered more toxic than the weekly IV fluorouracil plus leucovorin treatment schedule, it is premature to conclude that capecitabine is as efficacious and less toxic than all parenteral fluorouracil-based regimens. There is increasing evidence that infusional fluorouracil is superior to bolus administration, and that oral capecitabine may mimic this method of fluorouracil administration. These data, along with capecitabine's ease of administration, and data that irinotecan and oxaliplatin appear to have a greater effect when combined with infusional fluorouracil has lead to capecitabine being evaluated as a replacement for infusional fluorouracil.

Both irinotecan and oxaliplatin have been combined with capecitabine and preliminary data suggest these combinations will be safe and effective in the initial treatment of metastatic colorectal cancer.[100,116] The current FDA-approved indication for capecitabine is for use in metastatic colon cancer when therapy with a fluoropyrimidine alone is desired. Replacement of fluorouracil/leucovorin with capecitabine in other regimens is not currently approved, although longer follow-up of completed trials may prove capecitabine a suitable replacement for infusional fluorouracil in combination with irinotecan or oxaliplatin.

8 ◀ *Biologic Therapy.* Bevacizumab (Avastin, rhu-MAb VEGF) is a recombinant, humanized monoclonal antibody that inhibits vascular endothelial growth factor (VEGF). Bevacizumab, in combination with intravenous fluorouracil-based chemotherapy, was approved by the FDA in 2004 for initial treatment of patients with metastatic colorectal cancer. This represents the third available combination regimen for first-line treatment. Results from two randomized trials show increased benefit compared to chemotherapy alone. In a phase II study, patients were randomized to one of three arms: fluorouracil plus leucovorin given as the Roswell Park regimen alone (control), or chemotherapy combined with bevacizumab 5 mg/kg or 10 mg/kg, with bevacizumab administered as an IV infusion every 2 weeks until disease progression.[117] Patients treated with bevacizumab 5 mg/kg responded significantly better than those treated with fluorouracil plus leucovorin alone, with a higher overall response rate (40% vs. 17%) and an increase in median survival (21.5 months vs. 13.8 months), respectively. Interestingly, for reasons unknown at this time, the 5-mg/kg group also had a better overall response than those who received bevacizumab 10 mg/kg.

A phase III trial of bevacizumab in combination with IFL as first-line therapy in patients with metastatic colorectal cancer has also been completed. Patients were randomized to receive IFL plus bevacizumab placebo or IFL plus bevacizumab 5 mg/kg every 2 weeks.[96] The addition of bevacizumab to IFL therapy resulted in an increase in median (15.6 vs. 20.3 months) and progression-free survival (6.24 vs. 10.6 months), as well as a higher response rate (34.7% vs. 44.9%) compared to IFL alone. The frequency of typical adverse effects associated with IFL chemotherapy was not increased with the addition of bevacizumab. Grade 3 hypertension was significantly increased in the bevacizumab group. The incidence of other safety concerns with bevacizumab, such as bleeding, thromboembolism, and proteinuria, were not increased in the bevacizumab group compared to placebo. The hypertension is easily managed with oral antihypertensive agents. The risk of gastrointestinal perforation was increased by the addition of bevacizumab to IFL, and patients complaining of abdominal pain associated with vomiting or constipation should be considered for this rare, but potentially fatal complication.

The results of this study show the relevance of angiogenesis as an important target for the treatment of metastatic colorectal cancer. Bevacizumab is currently being investigated in first-line and salvage treatment regimens in combination with other active agents, including oxaliplatin, capecitabine, and cetuximab. How the addition of bevacizumab to FOLFOX4 will compare to FOLFOX4 alone, or the other irinotecan-based combinations remains to be seen. Practitioners can select first-line treatment for metastatic colorectal cancer from among four currently approved treatments: oxaliplatin plus fluorouracil plus leucovorin; irinotecan plus fluorouracil plus leucovorin; bevacizumab plus fluorouracil-based chemotherapy; and capecitabine. Capecitabine may prove an appropriate substitute for intravenous fluorouracil in these combination regimens; fluorouracil plus leucovorin alone is also appropriate first-line treatment for those individuals for whom three-drug combination regimens are believed to be too toxic. Table 127–15 depicts current NCCN Practice Guidelines for treatment of advanced or metastatic colorectal cancer.

Investigational Approaches

Chemotherapy. Comparisons of fluorouracil-based regimens alone and in combination with other agents, including trimetrexate, raltitrexed, methotrexate, interferon-α, and N-(phosphonacetyl)-L-asparte (PALA), have also been investigated in previously untreated patients with metastatic colorectal cancer.[28] Trimetrexate, raltitrexed, and methotrexate improve response rates and have small effects on progression-free intervals with minimal or no effect on overall survival. The addition of interferon-α or PALA to fluorouracil plus leucovorin increases toxicities and does not improve overall efficacy.

CHEMOTHERAPY FOR ADVANCED OR METASTATIC DISEASE:[1]

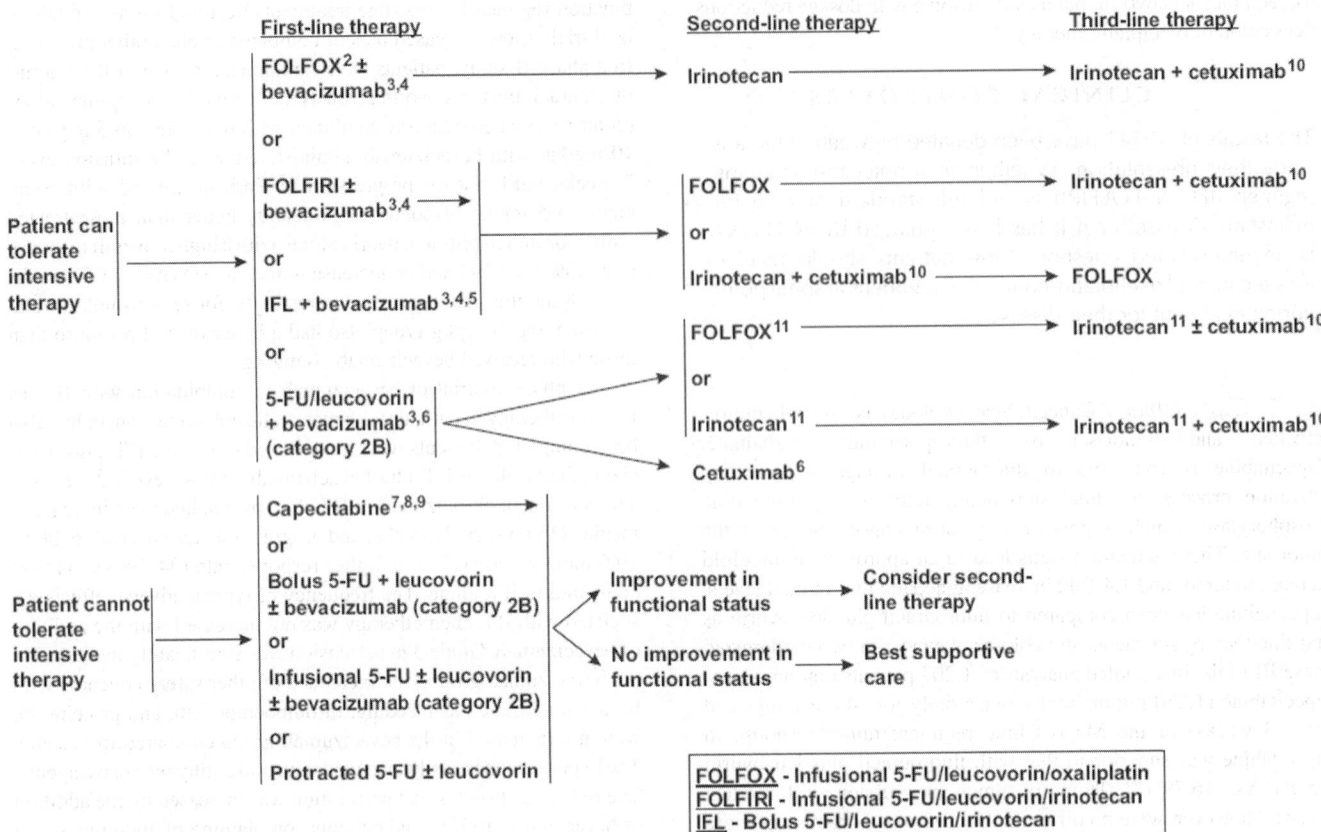

[1] For chemotherapy references, see Table 127-13.

[2] 5-FU/leucovorin/oxaliplatin has shown to be superior to bolus 5-FU/leucovorin/irinotecan as first-line therapy. Goldberg R, Sargent DJ, Morton RF, et al. A randomized controlled trial of fluorouracil plus leucovorin, irinotecan, and oxaliplatin combinations in patients with previously untreated metastatic colorectal cancer. J Clin Oncol 2004;22(1):23–30.

[3] Bevacizumab, used in combination with IV 5-FU based chemotherapy is approved for first-line therapy. Response data for bevacizumab/FOLFOX are not available. Elderly patients are at increased risk of stroke and other arterial events.

[4] There is no evidence of continuing bevacizumab as a single agent in the salvage setting.

[5] Bolus 5-FU/leucovorin/irinotecan (IFL) is an inferior regimen. If it is to be used, it would be in combination with bevacizumab.

[6] A treatment option for patients not able to tolerate oxaliplatin or irinotecan.

[7] There are no data to support the use of bevacizumab and capecitabine.

[8] Combination therapy with capecitabine cannot be recommended as standard therapy until data are available from phase III trials.

[9] Patients with diminished creatinine clearance may require dose modification of capecitabine.

[10] Cetuximab is indicated in combination with irinotecan-based therapy for patients refractory to irinotecan-based chemotherapy or as single agent therapy for patients intolerant to irinotecan.

[11] If patients are able to tolerate these agents.

FIGURE 127–7. National Comprehensive Cancer Network treatment guidelines for advanced or metastatic colon cancer. *(Adapted with permission from the NCCN v 4.2005 Colon Cancer Guidelines, the NCCN Clinical Practice Guidelines in Oncology, National Comprehensive Cancer Network www.nccn.org, accessed September 2005.)*

Pemetrexed, a multitargeted antifolate, and PTK787/ZK 222584, an oral tyrosine kinase VEGF receptor inhibitor, are among several agents that are in later phases of clinical trials.

■ *Hepatic Artery Infusion.* Although hepatic chemotherapy infusion for metastatic colorectal cancer remains an area of investigation, findings to date do not suggest superiority compared to systemic chemotherapy. The rationale for hepatic artery infusion (HAI) is based on the principle that normal liver hepatocytes and early micrometastases obtain their primary blood supply from the portal vein. In contrast, tumors in the liver are thought to receive most of their blood supply via the hepatic artery.[89] Therefore drug administration via the hepatic artery should result in delivery of high concentrations of drug

to the tumor cells with a much lower exposure to normal liver tissue. Also, for drugs that undergo a high first-pass extraction through the liver, systemic exposure and toxicity are minimized.

Because the liver is a common site of colorectal cancer metastasis, and the only site of metastatic involvement in up to one-third of patients, hepatic-directed therapies continue to be explored. Historically, floxuridine and fluorouracil have undergone the most study for hepatic artery infusion, particularly because of their high hepatic extraction rates, but newer active agents such as irinotecan and oxaliplatin have been studied as well. The observations seen with systemic therapy that continuous-infusion fluoropyrimidine provides greater response rates guide most strategies for HAI. Trials involving HAI have been conducted in patients with unresectable liver metastases and as adjuvant therapy following curative resection of isolated metastases.

The pharmacokinetic properties of floxuridine in particular provide for rapid systemic clearance and high liver drug extraction (94% to 99%).[28] Fluorouracil has a much lower extraction rate, but is also used frequently. Floxuridine is typically administered as a continuous 24-hour infusion at a dose of 0.1 to 0.3 mg/kg per day for a total of 14 days. This is in contrast to a comparable IV dose equal to 0.125 mg/kg per day. Heparin, in amounts up to 50,000 units per 50 mL of solution, is often added to the mixture in an attempt to decrease the incidence of arterial thromboses.

Regional HAI can be accomplished using a hepatic arterial port, a totally implantable pump, or a percutaneously placed catheter into the hepatic artery that is connected to an external pump. The volume of drug required to administer floxuridine can be contained within an implantable pump, whereas fluorouracil administration generally requires use of an external pump. Implanted infusion pumps are typically loaded with a 2-week volume of chemotherapy that is followed by an infusion of heparinized saline for 2 weeks.[89] Candidates are selected carefully based on documentation of hepatic-only disease, good performance status, and no significant comorbidities or liver anatomic variants.

Early trials of HAI revealed objective response rates ranging from 30% to 88%, many of which were observed in previously treated patients, as well as increased survival rates compared to historic controls. Because supportive care alone is no longer considered standard care for metastatic disease, when HAI was compared to systemic chemotherapy, most comparisons did not yield a survival benefit.[89] Furthermore, the majority of studies have allowed patients in the systemic therapy treatment groups to crossover to HAI upon tumor progression; therefore the impact of these treatments on survival is difficult to interpret.

In two randomized trials in which HAI floxuridine was compared to systemic fluorouracil plus leucovorin, and treatment crossover was not allowed, the European trial did not detect any treatment difference in progression-free or OS, whereas the CALGB trial showed improved time to hepatic progression (9.8 vs. 7.3 months) and median OS (22.7 vs. 19.8 months) with HAI.[89] However, both studies were affected by pump-related delays and complications, and the final analysis of the CALGB study has not been published.[89]

Given the significant improvements with systemic chemotherapy for metastatic disease achieved with systemic chemotherapy over the past several years, attention has been directed to HAI with non-fluoropyrimidines, including irinotecan, oxaliplatin, and biologic agents. Early studies have shown promising results, but whether this approach offers any advantage compared to systemic therapy will require significant further study. HAI has also been studied in alternating schedules with systemic fluoropyrimidines, but no survival advantages were observed.[89]

The primary limitations of HAI include development and/or progression of extrahepatic disease and treatment toxicities. Common toxicities include hepatobiliary toxicity and peptic ulceration, which can be life-threatening. Systemic chemotherapy-related side effects, such as myelosuppression, stomatitis, nausea, vomiting, or diarrhea, are uncommon.[89] Inflammation or ulceration of the stomach or duodenum can occur from inadvertent drug exposure to these areas. Patients who complain of persistent abdominal pain, diarrhea, or melena should have their HAI withheld and undergo endoscopic evaluation. The degree of hepatobiliary toxicity ranges from an elevation in hepatic enzymes resulting in a chemical hepatitis, to biliary sclerosis. Elevation of liver function enzymes or increased serum bilirubin levels occurred in approximately 42% of patients in the randomized trials.[89]

Progressive biliary sclerosis, usually associated with floxuridine, developed in 3% to 26% of patients in the randomized trials. Patients receiving HAI should have their liver enzymes and bilirubin monitored every 2 weeks during therapy, and guidelines are available for dose reductions or drug discontinuation.[89] Biliary sclerosis often resolves upon discontinuation of therapy within 2 to 4 weeks, although irreversible damage can occur. In an attempt to reduce inflammation and ischemia of bile ducts, dexamethasone is frequently added to HAI floxuridine, and appears to decrease the extent of liver function test abnormalities that occur in patients who experience hepatobiliary toxicity. Another approach is to alternate HAI floxuridine with hepatic arterial bolus fluorouracil, which does not cause hepatobiliary toxicity.

Gastritis and gastrointestinal or duodenal ulceration with risk of hemorrhage can also develop, which are reversible upon discontinuation of therapy. These effects are believed due to perfusion of chemotherapy into the stomach and duodenum via small vessels branching from the hepatic artery. These toxicities may be ameliorated by surgical ligation of the blood vessels supplying the stomach and duodenum, or H_2-antagonist therapy. Cholecystitis, which occurs in approximately one-third of patients, can be avoided through removal of the gallbladder at the time of catheter placement.[89]

Because of toxicities associated with HAI, most patients require some transient interruption of therapy, a decrease in dosage, or discontinuation of therapy. Furthermore, extrahepatic disease progression with HAI therapy alone remains a clinical problem. Although increased response rates and a trend toward improved survival have been reported, the costs and toxicities with this approach are significant. In a meta-analysis of actual costs (based on 1995 U.S. dollars) for HAI therapy, the average cost per patient was $25,208 and $29,562, for a patient in Palo Alto, California, and Paris, France, respectively.[89] In a comparison of costs with HAI floxuridine and systemic fluorouracil plus leucovorin, HAI was more cost effective than systemic chemotherapy. Therefore for the minority of patients who present with unresectable disease to the liver only, HAI may represent a reasonable therapeutic option, but it should not be considered standard therapy until the results of ongoing trials comparing HAI and systemic therapy, especially more effective regimens, become available.

SECOND-LINE THERAPY

Systemic chemotherapy represents the mainstay of therapy for patients whose disease progresses following initial treatment for metastatic disease. Figure 127–8 depicts an algorithm for treatment of refractory metastatic disease. Treatment options are based on type of and response to prior treatments, the site and extent of disease, and patient factors and treatment preferences.

Systemic Chemotherapy

Upon disease progression following standard initial therapy, appropriate treatment options may include oxaliplatin plus fluorouracil and leucovorin, irinotecan plus cetuximab, cetuximab, irinotecan, continuous-infusion fluorouracil, capecitabine plus irinotecan or oxaliplatin, capecitabine, intrahepatic therapy for selected patients, supportive care, or participation in a clinical trial. The choice of specific agents depends primarily on the type of prior therapy received. Since most patients will have received a combination of a pyrimidine with either irinotecan or oxaliplatin, second-line therapy with the alternate regimen should be considered; however, an optimal sequence for administration of both treatments has not been established.

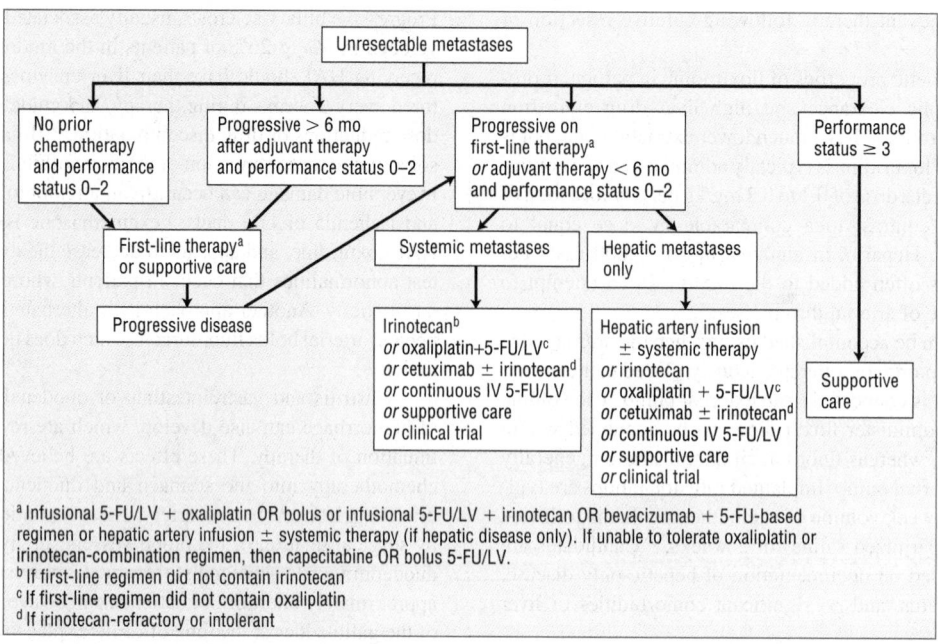

FIGURE 127–8. Algorithm for treatment of unresectable or refractory metastatic colorectal cancer.

■ *Irinotecan.* Two important trials have delineated an appropriate standard of care for patients who experience disease progression with fluorouracil therapy for metastatic colorectal cancer.[97,99] The results of these trials demonstrate a survival benefit associated with irinotecan, which was approved by the FDA in 1996, as second-line therapy for recurrent or progressive disease following fluorouracil. In phase II studies of previously treated patients with metastatic colorectal cancer, objective response rates of 13% to 27% have been observed.[97,99]

In a phase III trial of 189 patients with metastatic colorectal cancer that had progressed within 6 months of treatment with fluorouracil, irinotecan was compared to supportive care alone with regard to survival, quality of life, and other clinical variables.[97] Irinotecan was administered as 350 mg/m^2 IV every 3 weeks; the dose was reduced to 300 mg/m^2 for individuals who were 70 years of age or older, had a World Health Organization performance status of 2, or who had clinical risk factors for developing excessive treatment toxicity. Supportive care could include any symptomatic therapy with the exception of irinotecan or any other topoisomerase I inhibitor. With the exception of more patients with poor performance status being in the supportive care group, baseline patient characteristics were similar between groups. Median survival was 9.2 months with irinotecan, as compared to 6.5 months with supportive care alone. One-year survival was significantly greater with irinotecan (36.2% vs. 13.8%) and was not associated with significantly worse quality-of-life scores except for diarrhea. Clinical variables such as cognitive functioning, pain, dyspnea, and appetite loss were in favor of irinotecan therapy. The most common grade 3 or 4 side effects with irinotecan included leukopenia and neutropenia (22%), diarrhea (22%), nausea (14%), and vomiting (14%). Seventy-two percent of patients receiving irinotecan required hospital admission for adverse events, compared to 63% of supportive care patients. Thus irinotecan was associated with an improved survival and quality of life compared to supportive care alone, that appeared to balance treatment-related toxicities.

A comparison of irinotecan to continuous-infusion fluorouracil in a similar population of 267 patients allocated patients to irinotecan, 300 to 350 mg/m^2 IV every 3 weeks, or one of three continuous-infusion fluorouracil regimens: leucovorin 200 mg/m^2 IV over 2 hours followed by IV bolus fluorouracil (400 mg/m^2) and 22-hour

continuous-infusion fluorouracil (600 mg/m^2), given the first 2 days of every 2-week period; fluorouracil 250 to 300 mg/m^2 as prolonged continuous IV infusion until disease progression; or fluorouracil 2600 to 3000 mg/m^2 per day IV over 24 hours, with or without leucovorin (20 to 500 mg/m^2 IV), given weekly for 6 weeks, with a 2-week rest period between cycles.[99] Median follow-up after 15 months revealed a longer 1-year survival (45% vs. 32%) and median survival (10.8 months vs. 8.5 months) with irinotecan, as compared to fluorouracil. Sixty-nine percent of patients receiving irinotecan experienced at least one grade 3 or 4 toxicity, as compared to 54% of patients receiving fluorouracil. The most common toxicities with irinotecan were diarrhea, neutropenia, pain, vomiting, and asthenia, whereas pain, asthenia, diarrhea, and dermatologic toxicities were most common with fluorouracil. There was no difference in hospitalization requirement for adverse effects between treatments.

Based on the results of these trials, irinotecan should be considered standard second-line therapy for patients who have failed prior treatment with fluorouracil-based regimens. Either dosage regimen (irinotecan 125 mg/m^2 IV weekly for 4 weeks followed by a 2-week rest period or 300 to 350 mg/m^2 IV every 3 weeks) is acceptable. For the every 3-week regimen, initial administration of irinotecan at the lower dose should be considered for patients who have received significant prior pelvic or abdominal irradiation. Protracted continuous-infusion fluorouracil could be considered for those individuals with disease that no longer responds to bolus IV fluorouracil plus leucovorin or irinotecan.

■ *Oxaliplatin.* For patients who received primary treatment with irinotecan and fluorouracil, oxaliplatin plus fluorouracil and leucovorin should be considered. Despite the low activity of oxaliplatin alone against fluorouracil-refractory disease, when oxaliplatin has been administered in a bimonthly regimen with high-dose leucovorin and continuous fluorouracil infusion, a 20.6% response rate with a median survival in excess of 10 months has been observed.[118] The combination of oxaliplatin plus fluorouracil and leucovorin is also effective as salvage therapy after irinotecan plus fluorouracil and leucovorin triple therapy regimens that are standard for the initial treatment of metastatic colon cancer, with a response rate of about 20%.[119] Whereas irinotecan can be used effectively as a single agent in colorectal cancer, it should be noted that oxaliplatin does not have substantial activity alone, and should only be given in combination with a fluoropyrimidine. Patients with progressive disease who have received irinotecan and oxaliplatin-containing regimens and desire further treatment may benefit from therapy with cetuximab.

Biologic Therapy.

Cetuximab (IMC-C225, Erbitux) is a chimeric monoclonal antibody directed against an epidermal growth factor receptor (EGFR) that received FDA approval in 2004 for use in EGFR-expressing metastatic colorectal cancer. Cetuximab should be administered in combination with irinotecan, but can be used as a single agent in patients who cannot tolerate irinotecan-based chemotherapy.

In a phase II study, patients with EGFR-expressing metastatic colorectal cancer who had demonstrated clinical failure on an irinotecan-based regimen received open label cetuximab, 400 mg/m^2 IV as a loading dose, followed by weekly infusions of 250 mg/m^2 IV until disease progression.[120] Of 57 patients treated, 5 achieved a partial response, with a minor response or stable disease developing in 21 additional patients. The median survival was 6.4 months. The most common grade 3 or 4 adverse events were acne-like skin rash (18% grade 3) and adverse effects characterized as asthenia, lethargy, malaise, or fatigue (9% grade 3).

The combination of cetuximab plus irinotecan was also compared to cetuximab as a single agent in patients with EGFR-positive colorectal cancer that had progressed on irinotecan. Three hundred and twenty-nine patients were randomized in a 2:1 ratio to receive cetuximab plus continuation of the irinotecan or cetuximab alone.[98] The objective tumor response rates, 22.9% and 10.8% with cetuximab plus irinotecan and cetuximab alone, respectively, were very encouraging, and resulted in the endorsement of cetuximab by the FDA via accelerated approval. Median survival was 8.6 months for the combination and 6.9 months with monotherapy ($p = 0.48$). Time to disease progression was significantly longer with cetuximab plus irinotecan compared to cetuximab alone (4.1 vs. 1.5 months; hazard ratio 0.54), even among patients who also had oxaliplatin-refractory disease. The incidence of grade 3 or 4 adverse effects was as anticipated based on previous trials; asthenia and acne-like rash occurred most commonly with cetuximab alone, and in addition to typical irinotecan-related side effects (e.g., nausea, vomiting, and diarrhea) with combination treatment. Interestingly, there was no association between tumor response and intensity of EGFR-positive staining. Because patients who experienced disease progression on monotherapy were allowed to crossover to combination treatment, any difference in OS between the two groups would be difficult to ascertain.

Whether cetuximab adds benefit to oxaliplatin-based regimens or as part of initial therapy for metastatic colorectal cancer will depend on findings from ongoing studies. At present, there are no data that demonstrate increased survival or improvement in disease-related symptoms with cetuximab, but studies are attempting to address these end points. Nevertheless, cetuximab should be considered in patients with irinotecan- and oxaliplatin-refractory colorectal cancer. Immunohistochemical evidence of EGFR-positive staining should be obtained prior to initiating therapy.

Miscellaneous Salvage Chemotherapy.

Similar to initial treatment of metastatic colon cancer, capecitabine is being investigated as a replacement for infusional fluorouracil in salvage regimens in combination with irinotecan or oxaliplatin. Initial results from small trials suggest that this will be a safe and effective way to treat refractory disease.

Other agents used as salvage therapy include mitomycin C in combination with continuous-infusion fluorouracil, which produced a higher response rate (54% vs. 38%) and significantly longer median failure-free survival (7.9 months vs. 5.4 months) with no decrease in quality of life, as compared to fluorouracil alone.[121] Thus these agents may act synergistically with fluorouracil, particularly when it is administered as a continuous IV infusion, and these combinations deserve further study. Synergistic clinical activity between raltitrexed and fluorouracil has also been observed. Pilot studies of higher doses of single-agent raltitrexed and different treatment schedules of raltitrexed plus fluorouracil demonstrate modest activity as second-line therapy.

One interesting subject of debate is whether treatment could be suspended once disease stabilization occurs and restarted upon disease progression. In a small number of patients who achieved a partial response or disease stabilization with fluorouracil plus leucovorin, chemotherapy was discontinued and then restarted upon disease progression.[122] Reinstitution of therapy resulted in partial tumor response and disease stabilization in 18% and 53% of patients, respectively. While the efficacy of this approach requires confirmation from randomized trials, these preliminary data support the inclusion of fluorouracil in salvage treatment regimens with other agents. Finally, patients who fail standard treatment for metastatic colorectal cancer should be encouraged to participate in a clinical trial evaluating new treatment approaches for this incurable disease.

Hepatic-Directed Therapies.

Patients with hepatic-predominant disease whose disease progresses with systemic therapy may be candidates for HAI, chemoembolization, cryotherapy, or radiofrequency ablation. Percutaneous ethanol injection can be performed but is considered relatively ineffective against colorectal hepatic metastases.[123] Response rates to HAI therapy in patients who are refractory to fluorouracil-based therapy may be as high as 33%.[124] Although HAI has not been compared to IV irinotecan as second-line therapy, tumor response rates from historical data are similar. Future applications of HAI may include hepatic-targeted therapy with antiangiogenic factors, small molecules designed to interfere with molecular targets, or attenuated genetically modified viruses.

The largest experience with hepatic arterial chemoembolization has been seen in patients with metastatic carcinoid tumors or primary hepatocellular carcinomas. Most recently, small trials have been expanded to include hepatic metastases caused by colorectal cancer. Hepatic arterial chemoembolization delivers high concentrations of cytotoxic agents directly to the tumor and results in the embolization or devascularization of the liver, which blocks perfusion of the tumor and eliminates its blood supply. This procedure involves the instillation of a mixture that incorporates chemotherapeutic agents, radioactive contrast dye, and/or an embolic agent directly into the hepatic artery. Agents and doses most commonly studied include doxorubicin (40 to 60 mg), mitomycin (10 to 20 mg), and cisplatin (100 to 150 mg), which are usually dissolved in approximately 10 to 15 mL of a radiographic contrast dye.[125] Addition of an embolic agent to the mixture, such as a gelatin sponge (Gelfoam), polyvinyl alcohol particles, bovine collagen, or iodized poppy seed oil (Lipiodol and Ethiodol), results in either a temporary or permanent occlusion of the hepatic artery. Although about 80% of patients in one trial experienced a response, the number of patients with colorectal cancer who have undergone this procedure thus far is relatively low. In addition, patients still experience eventual disease progression. However, preliminary results from small series suggest that the high tumor responses may be associated with a survival benefit, and randomized trials comparing systemic therapy to hepatic chemoembolization for unresectable disease are ongoing.

Cryosurgery involves placement of a cryoprobe into the tumor, either percutaneously or intraoperatively, and then lowering the probe temperature to −100°C.[123] This is repeated in cycles, resulting in the formation of an ice ball; the ice crystal formation causes tumor destruction. Cryosurgery may be used alone or in conjunction with other localized procedures, such as radiofrequency ablation, which is becoming increasingly used for colorectal liver metastases. The technique involves placement of a chilled perfusion electrode needle into the tumor with subsequent application of alternating electrical current through the electrode, resulting in thermal coagulative necrosis of the tumor.[123] Laser interstitial thermal therapy represents an alternate method for causing tumor coagulative necrosis using a laser. Radiofrequency ablation is also being evaluated in conjunction with HAI, in an effort to reduce local recurrence of metastatic tumors. Procedure-related complications may include bleeding, coagulopathy, liver abscess, biliary stricture, and pleural effusion.[123] While these approaches represent potential treatment strategies for patients with unresectable, yet limited hepatic-only metastases, additional experience is needed to determine long-term outcomes. Furthermore, extrahepatic sites of disease continue to be a problem even for those individuals in whom the liver tumors can be eradicated. Thus far none of these approaches has become established as standard care.

NEW STRATEGIES AND AGENTS IN DEVELOPMENT

At present, fluorouracil plus leucovorin, bevacizumab, irinotecan, and oxaliplatin are the most frequently used chemotherapeutic agents for cancer of the colon and rectum. New chemotherapy agents have been studied in an attempt to further improve antitumor efficacy and reduce treatment toxicities. Oral fluorinated pyrimidines and TS inhibitors, such as fluorouracil prodrugs and inhibitors of fluorouracil catabolism, can prolong in vivo fluorouracil exposure and enhance antitumor effects without the use of continuous IV infusions. However, treatment with traditional chemotherapy agents, which target rapidly-dividing cells, kills both malignant and nonmalignant cells, and new cancer therapies are needed to improve therapeutic outcomes. In particular, targeted therapies aimed at the underlying cancer pathology are increasingly being developed and utilized in colorectal cancer treatment. A variety of agents targeted toward augmenting the host immune system response have undergone or are currently undergoing study for colorectal cancer, including monoclonal antibodies and tumor vaccines. Another potential strategy is regulating tumor growth through the inhibition of cell signal transduction processes, including farnesyl transferase inhibitors or targeting overexpressed growth factor receptors such as EGFR. Agents that can alter microenvironmental factors that support angiogenesis and tumor metastases may also be of benefit. Table 127–12 lists the mechanism of action, adverse effects, and phase of development for selected investigational agents for colorectal cancer.

In addition, observations that various tumor characteristics (e.g., TS expression), patient drug-metabolizing enzymes (e.g., DPD and plasma uracil:dihydrouracil ratio), and molecular markers (e.g., chromosome 18q allelic loss, microsatellite instability, and *p53* mutation or loss) may predict prognosis and response to certain therapies that lead to opportunities to select optimal first-line therapies for individual patients. Patients who are deficient in DPD experience severe and potentially life-threatening toxicities with conventional doses of fluorouracil. However, determination of DPD activity is relatively time-consuming and the techniques are not amenable to routine clinical practice. As an alternative, plasma ratio determinations of uracil and dihydrouracil, which are more easily obtainable, appear to identify individuals with DPD deficiency and who are therefore at risk of developing significant toxicities.[126] Of factors predictive for tumor sensitivity to fluorouracil, TS expression has been most studied.[28] Results from in vitro studies demonstrate that pretreatment intratumoral TS levels are inversely correlated to tumor response to fluorouracil. Whether increased tumor TS expression reflects a biologically more aggressive tumor or is directly related to fluorouracil resistance is unknown. Studies are underway to use this and other information to identify rational therapeutic approaches for select patients.

PHARMACOECONOMIC CONSIDERATIONS

The estimated costs of treating colorectal cancer in the United States alone exceeds 6.5 billion dollars per year.[127] The total cost for managing a patient with cancer of the colon is estimated to be approximately $45,000 to $61,000. Costs for patients with rectal cancer are approximately 15% higher because of the added expense of radiation therapy. These cost estimates are higher than estimated lifetime attributable costs for treating other common tumors such as cancer of the breast, prostate, and lung.[127] In addition, medical care costs vary, depending on the stage of disease. Medicare claims data reveal greater costs are incurred during the initial phase of care as compared to the terminal stage of disease. For all stages of disease, initial care accounted for approximately one-half of the long-term cancer-related cost, but the terminal phase of treatment also represents a high proportion of treatment costs.[31] Thus a long-term approach is needed to accurately estimate the cost of treating patients diagnosed with colorectal cancer. In addition, higher costs are noted for treating early-stage disease. The average total Medicare payments for treating stage II and IV colorectal cancer is $68,000 and $36,000, respectively.[128] This relates to higher continuing care costs for stage II patients such as adjuvant therapy and surveillance of patients not needed in patients with metastatic disease. The impact of changes in clinical practice on treatment costs, such as increased use of adjuvant therapy, changes in duration of hospital stay and outpatient delivery of health services, and incorporation of costly agents into standard treatment regimens, must also be continually considered.

An evaluation of the cost-effectiveness of adjuvant therapy for stage III colon cancer determined that 12 months of adjuvant therapy of fluorouracil plus levamisole resulted in 1.88 years of life-years gained for each treated patient, and a cost-effectiveness ratio of $2094 per life-year saved.[129] However, a more accurate estimate of cost-effectiveness of current adjuvant therapy will need to evaluate 6-month courses of fluorouracil plus leucovorin and consider patients with both stage III and high-risk stage II disease.

The cost-effectiveness of therapeutic regimens in the metastatic setting has also been calculated. The combination of both infusional and bolus irinotecan plus fluorouracil and leucovorin have been compared to fluorouracil plus leucovorin alone.[130] Results have varied depending on second-line therapies evaluated and have ranged from approximately $22,000 to $50,000 per life-year gained. In one trial the irinotecan group had an incremental cost of $8341 per patient. The relationships between costs associated with newer drugs on treatment outcomes, especially agents such as bevacizumab and cetuximab, will need to be considered, especially as they have become incorporated into standard care therapies.

Although several investigations have evaluated cost-effectiveness of various screening procedures, published data regarding costs associated with colorectal cancer prevention are not currently available. In a recent cost-effectiveness analysis, assuming a 75% compliance rate with the screening procedure, the incremental cost effectiveness of combined sigmoidoscopy and fecal occult blood testing compared with colonoscopy performed twice-lifetime (at the ages of 50 and 60) was approximately $330,000 and $42,000 per life-year gained, respectively.[131] The cost benefit for twice-lifetime colonoscopy remained when calculations were performed on compliance estimates ranging from 25% to 100%. In addition, a separate comparison of the cost-effectiveness of fecal occult blood testing, flexible sigmoidoscopy, and colonoscopy found colonoscopy to be the most cost-effective screening strategy when performed every 10 years. These evaluations are sensitive to the impact of uncertainty about actual compliance rates in different clinical practice settings, which must be considered in the interpretation of these data. Most accepted screening strategies, however, have cost-effectiveness ratios that are well below the accepted benchmark of $50,000 per life-year saved.[127] Overall, when compared to other commonly accepted screening modalities, colon cancer screening is cost-effective. The incremental cost for screening is $6600 per year of life saved, compared to breast cancer screening at $22,000 per year of life gained.

EVALUATION OF THERAPEUTIC OUTCOMES

The goal of monitoring is to evaluate whether the patient is receiving any benefit from the management of the disease or to detect recurrence. Similarly, follow-up examinations help to determine whether preventive interventions or screening studies effectively reduce an individual's risk for developing colorectal cancer or presenting with an advanced stage of disease. During treatment for active disease, patients should undergo monitoring for measurable tumor response, progression, or new metastases; these tests may include chest CT scans or x-rays, abdominal or pelvic CT scans or x-rays, depending on the site of disease being evaluated for response, and CEA measurements every 3 months if the CEA is or was previously elevated. In addition, a CBC should be obtained prior to each course of chemotherapy administration to ensure that hematologic indices are adequate. Baseline liver function tests and an assessment of renal function should be evaluated prior to and periodically during therapy. These tests and other selected serum chemistries should also be evaluated with the development of any new symptoms or significant change in disease status. Patients should be evaluated during every treatment visit for the presence of anticipated side effects, which generally include loose stools or diarrhea, nausea or vomiting, mouth sores, fatigue, and fever, as well as other side effects such as neuropathy and skin rash that are typically associated with oxaliplatin and cetuximab, respectively. Patients receiving bevacizumab should be evaluated for hypertension and proteinuria.

Symptoms of recurrence such as pain syndromes, changes in bowel habits, rectal or vaginal bleeding, pelvic masses, anorexia, and weight loss develop in fewer than 50% of patients. A greater percentage of recurrences are detected in asymptomatic patients because of increased serum CEA levels that lead to further examination. Although the value of CEA monitoring for asymptomatic disease recurrence is questioned by some because of the related expense and emotional stress associated with false-positive elevations, CEA monitoring plays an important role in postoperative follow-up studies for most individuals. A PET scan can be considered to identify localized

TABLE 127–15. NCCN Postoperative Surveillance Practice Guidelines for Colon and Rectal Cancer

- History and physical examination every 3 months for 2 years, then every 6 months for a total of 5 years
- CEA[a] every 3 months for 2 years, then every 6 months for years 2 to 5 for T_2 or greater lesions
- Colonoscopy[b] in 1 year, repeat in 1 year if abnormal or at least every 2 to 3 years if negative for polyps. If no preoperative colonoscopy was obtained due to obstructing lesion, then colonoscopy in 3 to 6 months

[a]If patient is a potential candidate for surgical resection of isolated metastases.
[b]All patients with colon cancer should be counseled for family history. Patients with suspected herediary nonpolyposis colon cancer (HNPCC), familial adenomatous polyposis (FAP), and attenuated FAP should be followed per the NCCN Colorectal Screening Guidelines.
Adapted with permission from the NCCN 2.2004 Colon Cancer and Rectal Cancer Guidelines, the Complete Library of NCCN Clinical Practice Guidelines in Oncology [CD-ROM]. Jenkintown, Pennsylvania: © National Comprehensive Cancer Network, June 2004. To view the most recent and complete version of the guideline, go online to www.nccn.org.

sites of metastatic disease in situations in which a rising CEA level suggests metastatic disease, but CT scans and other imaging studies are negative.

Patients who undergo curative surgical resection, with or without adjuvant therapy, require close follow-up based on the premise that early detection and treatment of recurrence could still render them cured. In addition, early treatment for asymptomatic metastatic colorectal cancer appears superior to delayed therapy. Specific practice guidelines for postoperative surveillance examinations have been developed by the NCCN (Table 127–15). Colorectal cancer surveillance guidelines published by the American Society of Clinical Oncology recommend against routinely monitoring liver function tests, CBC, fecal occult blood testing, CT scans, annual chest x-rays, or pelvic imaging in asymptomatic patients.[132]

Recent advances in the treatment for cancer of the colon and rectum now offer the potential to improve patient survival but for many patients, improved disease- and progression-free survival represent equally important therapeutic outcomes. Figure 127–7 depicts the NCCN Practice Guidelines for chemotherapy for advanced or metastatic colorectal cancer. Although treatment approaches for metastatic colorectal cancer have been historically assessed by their ability to produce a measurable objective tumor response, which is generally believed necessary for any treatment to improve survival, the effects of therapies on survival are clinically more meaningful than their ability to induce a tumor response. However, with the availability of multiple active treatments for metastatic disease, and the likelihood that patients will receive more than one during the course of their treatment, improvements in OS with new therapies will be increasingly difficult to determine.

In the absence of the ability of a specific treatment to demonstrate improved survival, important outcome measures should include the effects of the treatment on patient symptoms, daily activities and performance status, and other quality-of-life indicators, as well as progression-free survival and time to treatment failure. Because metastatic colorectal cancer is incurable, a specific decision regarding an individual patient's care will ultimately be required; this should be based on a careful assessment of the balance between risks associated with treatment (or lack thereof) and benefits of treatment. Effort should also be made to ensure that the costs of screening, diagnostic tests, treatments, and procedures for colorectal cancer are consistent with their value in improving patient outcomes.

ABBREVIATIONS

AJCC: American Joint Committee on Cancer
APC: adenomatous polyposis coli (gene)
BMI: body mass index
CBC: complete blood cell count
CEA: carcinoembryonic antigen
COX: cyclooxygenase
CT: computed tomography
CYP450: cytochrome P450 isoenzyme
DCBE: double-contrast barium enema
DCC: Deleted in colon cancer
DFS: disease-free survival
DPD: dihydropyrimidine dehydrogenase
EGFR: epidermal growth factor receptor
FAP: familial adenomatous polyposis
FOBT: fecal occult blood test
FOLFIRI: Fluorouracil, leucovorin, irinotecan
FOLFOX: Fluorouracil, leucovorin, oxaliplatin
5-FU: fluorouracil
FUDR: Floxuridine
GITSG: Gastrointestinal Tumor Study Group
HAI: hepatic artery infusion
HD: high-dose
HNPCC: hereditary nonpolyposis colorectal cancer
IFL: irinotecan plus fluorouracil plus leucovorin
IMPACT: International Multicentre Pooled Analysis of Colon
    Cancer Trials
IUAC: International Union Against Cancer
IGF-I: Insulin-like growth factor-I
LD: low-dose
LV: leucovorin
MAC: modified Astler-Coller (classification)
MMR: mismatch-repair (gene)
MTHFR: methylenetetrahydrofolate reductase
NAT: *N*-acetyltransferase
NCCN: National Comprehensive Cancer Network
NCCTG: North Central Cancer Treatment Group
NSABP: National Surgical Adjuvant Breast and Bowel Project
NSAID: nonsteroidal anti-inflammatory drug
OS: overall survival
PALA: N-(phosphonacetyl)-L-asparte
PET: positron emission tomography
PVI: protracted venous infusion
TGF-β: transforming growth factor-β
TS: Thymidylate synthase
UGT1A1: UDP-glucuronosyltransferase
VEGF: vascular endothelial growth factor
XRT: radiation therapy

Review Questions and other resources can be found at
www.pharmacotherapyonline.com.

REFERENCES

1. Jemal A, Murray T, Ward E, et al. Cancer statistics, 2005. CA Cancer J Clin 2005;55:10–30.
2. Bray F, Sankila R, Ferlay J, Parkin DM. Estimates of cancer incidence and mortality in Europe in 1995. Eur J Cancer 2002;38:99–166.
3. Ries LAG, Eisner MP, Kosary CL, et al, eds. SEER Cancer Statistics Review, 1975–2001, National Cancer Institute. Bethesda, MD, *http://seer.cancer.gov/csr/*1975_2001/, 2004.
4. Pisani P, Bray F, Parkin DM. Estimates of the world-wide prevalence of cancer for 25 sites in the adult population. Int J Cancer 2002;97:72–81.
5. Potter JD. Colorectal cancer: Molecules and populations. J Natl Cancer Inst 1999;91:916–932.
6. Trock B, Lanza E, Greenwald P. Dietary fiber, vegetables, and colon cancer: Critical review and meta-analyses of the epidemiologic evidence. J Natl Cancer Inst 1990;82:650–661.
7. Peters U, Sinha R, Chatterjee N, et al. Dietary fibre and colorectal adenoma in a colorectal cancer early detection programme. Lancet 2003;361:1491–1495.
8. Bingham SA, Day NE, Luben R, et al. Dietary fibre in food and protection against colorectal cancer in the European Prospective Investigation into Cancer and Nutrition (EPIC): An observational study. Lancet 2003;361:1496–1501.
9. Fuchs CS, Giovannucci EL, Colditz GA. Dietary fiber and the risk of colorectal cancer and adenoma in women. N Engl J Med 1999;340:169–176.
10. Giovannucci E. Modifiable risk factors for colon cancer. Gastroenterol Clin North Am 2002;31:925–943.
11. Giovannucci E, Egan KM, Hunter DJ, et al. Aspirin and the risk of colorectal cancer in women. N Engl J Med 1995;333:609–614.
12. Smalley W, Ray WA, Daugherty J, Griffin MR. Use of nonsteroidal anti-inflammatory drugs and incidence of colorectal cancer. Arch Intern Med 1999;159:161–166.
13. Thun MJ, Henley J, Patrono C. Nonsteroidal anti-inflammatory drugs as anticancer agents: Mechanistic, pharmacologic, and clinical issues. J Natl Cancer Inst 2002;94:252–266.
14. Grodstein F, Newcomb PA, Stampfer MJ. Postmenopausal hormone therapy and the risk of colorectal cancer: A review and meta-analysis. Am J Med 1999;106:574–582.
15. Nelson HD, Humphrey LL, Nygren P, et al. Postmenopausal hormone replacement therapy: scientific review. JAMA 2002;288:872–881.
16. Chlebowski RT, Wactawski-Wende J, Ritenbaugh C, et al. Estrogen plus progestin and colorectal cancer in postmenopausal women. N Engl J Med 2004;350:991–1004.
17. Terry PD, Miller AB, Rohan TE. Obesity and colorectal cancer risk in women. Gut 2002;51:191–194.
18. Hu FB, Manson JE, Liu S, et al. Prospective study of adult onset diabetes mellitus (Type 2) and risk of colorectal cancer in women. J Natl Cancer Inst 1999;91:542–547.
19. Chao A, Thun MJ, Jacobs EJ, et al. Cigarette smoking and colorectal cancer morality in the Cancer Prevention Study II. J Natl Cancer Inst 2000;92:1888–1896.
20. Munkholm P. Review article: The incidence and prevalence of colorectal cancer in inflammatory bowel. Aliment Pharmacol Ther 2003;18(Suppl 2):1–5.
21. Calvert PM, Frucht H. The genetics of colorectal cancer. Ann Intern Med 2003;137:603–612.
22. Lynch HT, Lynch J. Lynch syndrome: Genetics, natural history, genetic counseling, and prevention. J Clin Oncol 2000;18(Nov 1 suppl):19s–31s.
23. Fuchs CS, Giovannucci EL, Colditzs GA, et al. A prospective study of family history and the risk of colorectal cancer. N Engl J Med 1994;331:1669–1674.
24. Midgley R, Kerr D. Colorectal cancer. Lancet 1999;353:391–399.
25. Robbins DH, Ilkowitz SH. The molecular and genetic basis of colon cancer. Med Clin North Am 202;86:1467–1495.
26. Arends JW. Molecular interactions in the Vogelstein model of colorectal carcinoma. J Pathol 2000;190:412–416.
27. Markowitz S, Wang J, Myeroff L, et al. Inactivation of the type II TGF-β receptor in colon cancer cells with microsatellite instability. Science 1995;268:1336–1338.
28. Skibber JM, Minsky BD, Hoff PM. Cancer of the colon. In: DeVita VT, Hellman S, Rosenberg SA, eds. Cancer: Principles and Practice of Oncology, 6th ed. Philadelphia, Lippincott Williams & Wilkins, 2001:1216–1270.

29. Alberts DS, Slatery ML, Giovannucci E, et al. Primary prevention of colon cancer with dietary and micronutrient interventions. Cancer 1998;83:1734–1739.

30. Jänne PA, Mayer RJ. Chemoprevention of colorectal cancer. N Engl J Med 2000;342:1960–1968.

31. Redaelli A, Cranor CW, Okano GJ, Reese PR. Screening, prevention and socioeconomic costs associated with the treatment of colorectal cancer. Pharmacoeconomics 2003;21:1213–1238.

32. Steele VE. Current mechanistic approaches to the chemoprevention of cancer. J Biochem Mol Bio 2003;36:7–81.

33. Steinbach G, Lynch PM, Phillips RK, et al. The effect of celecoxib, a cyclooxygenase-2 inhibitor, in familial adenomatous polyposis. N Engl J Med 2000;342:1946–1952.

34. Baron JA, Cole BF, Sandler RS, et al. A randomized trial of aspirin to prevent colorectal adenomas. N Engl J Med 2003;348:891–899.

35. Baron JA, Beach M, Mandel JS, et al. Calcium supplements for the prevention of colorectal adenomas. N Engl J Med 1999;340: 101–107.

36. Grau MV, Baron JA, Sandler RS, et al. Vitamin D, calcium supplementation, and colorectal adenomas: Results of a randomized trial. J Natl Cancer Inst 2003;95:1765–1771.

37. Vasen HFA. Clinical diagnosis and management of hereditary colorectal cancer syndromes. J Clin Oncol 2000;18(Nov 1 suppl):81s–92s.

38. Smith RA, Cokkinides V, Eyre HJ. American Cancer Society guidelines for the early detection of cancer, CA Cancer J Clin 2003;53: 27–43.

39. Walsh JM, Terdiman JP. Colorectal cancer screening. JAMA 2003;289: 1288–1296.

40. Levin B, Brooks D, Smith RA, Stone A. Emerging technologies in screening for colorectal cancer. CA Cancer J Clin 2003;53:44–55.

41. Selby JV, Friedman GD, Quesenberry CP, Weiss NS. A case-control study of screening sigmoidoscopy and mortality from colorectal cancer. N Engl J Med 1992;326:653–657.

42. Smith RA, Cokkinides V, Eyre HJ. American Cancer Society guidelines for the early detection of cancer. CA Cancer J Clin 2003;53:27–43.

43. National Comprehensive Cancer Network. Colon Cancer. NCCN Clinical Practice Guidelines in Oncology v.2.2004, 04/30/2004, National Comprehensive Cancer Network, Inc., 2004.

44. 2000 Update of Recommendations for the Use of Tumor Markers in Breast and Colorectal Cancer: Clinical Practice Guidelines of the American Society of Clinical Oncology. J Clin Oncol 2001;19:1865–1878.

45. Akhurst T, Larson SM. Positron emission tomography imaging of colorectal cancer. Semin Oncol 1999;26:577–583.

46. Moffat FL, Gulec SA, Serafini AN, et al. A thousand points of light or just dim bulbs? Radiolabeled antibodies and colorectal cancer imaging. Cancer Invest 1999;17:322–334.

47. Colon and rectum. In: American Joint Commission on Cancer. AJCC Cancer Staging Manual. 6th ed. New York, Springer, 2002:113–124.

48. Compton C, Fenoglio-Preiser CM, Pettigrew N, Fielding LP. American Joint Committee on Cancer Prognostic Factors Consensus Conference Colorectal Working Group. Cancer 2000;88:1739–1757.

49. Ogunbiyi OA, Goodfellow PJ, Herfarth K, et al. Confirmation that chromosome 18q allelic loss in colon cancer is a prognostic indicator. J Clin Oncol 1998;16:427–433.

50. Ribic CM, Sargent DJ, Moore MJ, et al. Tumor microsatellite-instability status as a predictor of benefit from fluorouracil-based adjuvant chemotherapy for colon cancer. N Engl J Med 2003;349:247–257.

51. Skibber JM, Hoff PM, Minsky BD. Cancer of the rectum. In: DeVita VT, Hellman S, Rosenberg SA, eds. Cancer: Principles and Practice of Oncology, 6th ed. Philadelphia, Lippincott Williams & Wilkins, 2001: 1271–1318.

52. Buyse M, Zeleniuch-Jacquotte A, Chalmers TC. Adjuvant therapy of colorectal cancer—Why we still don't know. JAMA 1988;259: 3571–3578.

53. Saini A, Norman AR, Cunningham D, et al. Twelve weeks of protracted venous infusion of fluorouracil (5-FU) is as effective as 6 months of bolus 5-FU and folinic acid as adjuvant treatment in colorectal cancer. Br J Cancer 2003;88:1859–1865.

54. The Meta-Analysis Group in Cancer. Toxicity of fluorouracil in patients with advanced colorectal cancer: Effect of administration schedule and prognostic factors. J Clin Oncol 1998;16:3537–3541.

55. van Kuilenburg ABP, Haasjes J, Richel DJ, et al. Clinical implications of dihydropyrimidine dehydrogenase (DPD) deficiency in patients with severe 5-fluorouracil-associated toxicity: Identification of new mutations in the DPD gene. Clin Cancer Res 2000;6:4705–4712.

56. Laurie JA, Moertel CG, Fleming TR, et al. Surgical adjuvant therapy of large bowel carcinoma: An evaluation of levamisole and combination of levamisole and 5-fluorouracil. The North Central Cancer Treatment Group and the Mayo Clinic. J Clin Oncol 1989;7:1447–1456.

57. Moertel CG, Fleming TR, Macdonald JS, et al. Intergroup study of fluorouracil plus levamisole as adjuvant therapy for stage II/Dukes' B2 colon cancer. J Clin Oncol 1995;13:2936–2943.

58. Macdonald JS. Adjuvant therapy of colon cancer. CA Cancer J Clin 1999;49:202–219.

59. International Multicentre Pooled Analysis of Colon Cancer Trials (IMPACT) Investigators. Efficacy of adjuvant fluorouracil and folinic acid in colon cancer. Lancet 1995;345:939–944.

60. Wolmark N, Rockette H, Fisher B, et al. The benefit of leucovorin-modulated fluorouracil as postoperative adjuvant therapy for primary colon cancer: Results from National Surgical Adjuvant Breast and Bowel Project Protocol C-03. J Clin Oncol 1993;11:1879–1887.

61. O'Connell MJ, Mailliard J, Kahn MJ, et al. Controlled trial of fluorouracil and low-dose leucovorin given for 6 months as postoperative adjuvant therapy for colon cancer. J Clin Oncol 1997;15:246–250.

62. de Gramont A, Bosset JF, Milan C, et al. Randomized trial comparing monthly low-dose leucovorin and fluorouracil bolus with bimonthly high-dose leucovorin and fluorouracil bolus plus continuous infusion for advanced colorectal cancer: a French intergroup study. J Clin Oncol 1997;15:808–815.

63. Machover D, Goldschmidt E, Chollet P, et al. Treatment of advanced colorectal and gastric adenocarcinomas with 5-fluorouracil and high-dose folinic acid. J Clin Oncol 1986;4:685–696.

64. Haller DG, Catalano PJ, Macdonald JS, Mayer RJ. Fluorouracil (FU), leucovorin (LV) and levamisole (LEV) adjuvant therapy for colon cancer: Five-year final report of INT-0089. Proc Am Soc Clin Oncol 1998; 17:256a (Abstract).

65. Wolmark N, Rockette H, Mamounas E, et al. Clinical trial to assess the relative efficacy of fluorouracil and leucovorin, fluorouracil and levamisole, and fluorouracil, leucovorin, and levamisole in patients with Dukes' B and C carcinoma of the colon: Results from National Surgical Adjuvant Breast and Bowel Project C-04. J Clin Oncol 1999;17: 3553–3559.

66. O'Connell MJ, Laurie JA, Kahn M, et al. Prospectively randomized trial of postoperative adjuvant chemotherapy in patients with high-risk colon cancer. J Clin Oncol 1998;16:295–300.

67. Poplin E, Benedetti J, Estes N, et al. Phase III randomized trial of bolus 5-FU/leucovorin/levamisole versus 5-FU continuous infusion/levamisole as adjuvant therapy for high-risk colon cancer (SWOG 9415/INT-0153). Proc Am Soc Clin Onol 2000;19:240a (Abstract).

68. Kuebler JP, de Gramont A. Recent experience with oxaliplatin or irinotecan combined with 5-fluorouracil and leucovorin in the treatment of colorectal cancer. Semin Oncol 2003;30(4 Suppl 15):40–46.

69. Andre T, Boni C, Mounedji-Boudiaf L, et al. Oxaliplatin, fluorouracil, leucovorin as adjuvant treatment for colon cancer. N Engl J Med 2004; 350:2243–2351.

70. Scheithauer W, McKendrick J, Begbie S, et al. Oral capecitabine as an alternative to i.v. 5-fluorouracil-based adjuvant therapy for colon cancer: safety results of a randomized, phase III trial. Ann Oncol 2003;14: 1735–1743.

71. Taylor I, Machin D, Mullee M, et al. A randomized controlled trial of adjuvant portal vein cytotoxic perfusion in colorectal cancer. Br J Surg 1985;72:359–363.

72. Wolmark N, Rockette H, Petrelli N, et al. Long-term results of the efficacy of perioperative portal vein infusion of 5-FU for treatment of colon cancer: NSABP C-02. Proc Am Soc Clin Oncol 1994;13:194a (Abstract).

73. Liver Infusion Meta-analysis Group. Portal vein chemotherapy for colorectal cancer: A meta-analysis of 4000 patients in 10 studies. J Natl Cancer Inst 1997;89:497–505.

74. Riethmüller G, Holz E, Schlimok G, et al. Monoclonal antibody therapy of Dukes' C colorectal carcinoma: Seven-year outcome of a multicenter randomized trial. J Clin Oncol 1998;16:1788–1794.

75. Punt CJ, Nagy A, Douillard JY, et al. Edrecolomab alone or in combination with fluorouracil and folinic acid in the adjuvant treatment of stage III colon cancer: A randomised study. Lancet 2002;360:671–677.

76. National Institutes of Health Consensus Development Conference. Adjuvant therapy for patients with colon and rectal cancer. JAMA 1990;264:1444–1450.

77. Gastrointestinal Tumor Study Group. Prolongation of the disease-free interval in surgically treated rectal carcinoma. N Engl J Med 1985;312:1465–1472.

78. Douglass HO, Moertel CG, Mayer RJ, et al. Survival after postoperative combination treatment of rectal cancer. N Engl J Med 1986;315:1294–1295.

79. Krook JE, Moertel CG, Gunderson LL, et al. Effective surgical adjuvant therapy for high-risk rectal carcinoma. N Engl J Med 1991;324:709–715.

80. O'Connell MJ, Martenson JA, Wieand HS, et al. Improving adjuvant therapy for rectal cancer by combining protracted infusion fluorouracil with radiation therapy after curative surgery. N Engl J Med 1994;331:502–507.

81. Tepper JE, J O'Connell MJ, Niedzwiecki D, et al. Adjuvant therapy in rectal cancer: Analysis of stage, sex, and local control—Final report of Intergroup 0114. J Clin Oncol 2002;20:1744–1750.

82. Dunst J, Reese T, Sutter T, et al. Phase I trial evaluating the concurrent combination of radiotherapy and capecitabine in rectal cancer. J Clin Oncol 2002;20:3983–3991.

83. Kapiteijn E, Marijnen CAM, Nagtegall ID, et al. Preoperative radiotherapy combined with total mesorectal excision for resectable rectal cancer. N Engl J Med 2001;345:638–646.

84. Swedish Cancer Rectal Trial. Improved survival with preoperative radiotherapy in resectable rectal cancer. N Engl J Med 1997;336:980–987.

85. Swedish Cancer Rectal Trial. Correction to improved survival with preoperative radiotherapy in resectable rectal cancer. N Engl J Med 1997;336:1539.

86. National Comprehensive Cancer Network. Rectal Cancer. NCCN Clinical Practice Guidelines in Oncology v.2.2004, 04/30/2004, National Comprehensive Cancer Network, Inc., 2004.

87. Fong Y, Salo J. Surgical therapy of hepatic colorectal metastasis. Semin Oncol 1999;26:514–523.

88. Kemeny N, Huang Y, Cohen AM, et al. Hepatic arterial infusion of chemotherapy after resection of hepatic metastases from colorectal cancer. N Engl J Med 1999;341:2039–2048.

89. Cohen AD, Kemeny NE. An update on hepatic arterial infusion chemotherapy for colorectal cancer. Oncologist 2003;8:553–566.

90. Twelves C. Capecitabine as first-line treatment in colorectal cancer: Pooled data from two large, phase III trials. Eur J Cancer 2002;38(Suppl):15–20.

91. de Gramont A, Figer A, Seymour M, et al. Leucovorin and fluorouracil with or without oxaliplatin as first-line treatment in advanced colorectal cancer. J Clin Oncol 2000;18:2938–2947.

92. Maindrault-Gœbel, de Gramont A, Louvet C, et al. High-dose intensity oxaliplatin added to the simplified bimonthly leucovorin and 5-fluorouacil regimen as second-line therapy for metastatic colorectal cancer (FOLFOX7). Eur J Cancer 2001;37:1000–1005.

93. Saltz LB, Cox JV, Blanke C, et al. Irinotecan plus fluorouracil and leucovorin for metastatic colorectal cancer. N Engl J Med 2000;343:905–914.

94. Tournigand C, André T, Achille E, et al. FOLFIRI followed by FOLFOX6 or the reverse sequence in advanced colorectal cancer: A randomized GERCOR study. J Clin Oncol 2004;22:229–237.

95. Douillard JY, Cunningham D, Roth AD, et al. Irinotecan combined with fluorouracil compared with fluorouracil alone as first-line treatment for metastatic colorectal cancer: A multicentre randomized trial. Lancet 2000;355:1041–1047.

96. Hurwitz H, Fehrenbacher L, Novotny W, et al. Bevacizumab plus irinotecan, fluorouracil, and leucovorin for metastatic colorectal cancer. N Engl J Med 2004;350:2335–2342.

97. Cunningham D, Pyrhönen S, James RD, et al. Randomised trial of irinotecan plus supportive care versus supportive care alone after fluorouracil failure for patients with metastatic colorectal cancer. Lancet 1998;352:1413–1418.

98. Cunningham D, Humblet Y, Siena S, et al. Cetuximab monotherapy and cetuximab plus irinotecan in irinotecan-refractory metastatic colorectal cancer. N Engl J Med 2004;351:337–345.

99. Rougier P, Van Cutsem E, Bajetta E, et al. Randomised trial of irinotecan versus fluorouracil by continuous infusion after fluorouracil failure in patients with metastatic colorectal cancer. Lancet 1998;352:1407–1412.

100. Grothey A, Jordan K, Kellner O, et al. Randomized phase II trial of capecitabine plus irinotecan (CapIri) vs capecitabine plus oxaliplatin (CapOx) as first-line therapy of advanced colorectal cancer (ACRC). Proc Am Soc Clin Oncol 2003;22:255 (Abstract 1022).

101. Goldberg RM, Sargent DJ, Morton RF, et al. A randomized controlled trial of fluorouracil plus leucovorin, irinotecan, and oxaliplatin combinations in patients with previously untreated metastatic colorectal cancer. J Clin Oncol 2004;22:23–30.

102. Jonker DJ, Maroun JA, Kocha W. Survival benefit of chemotherapy in metastatic colorectal cancer: A meta-analysis of randomized controlled trials. Br J Cancer 2000;82:1789–1794.

103. Colorectal Cancer Collaborative Group. Palliative chemotherapy for advanced colorectal cancer: Systematic review and meta-analysis. BMJ 2000;321:531–535.

104. Sobrero AF, Aschele C, Bertino JR. Fluorouracil in colorectal cancer—A tale of two drugs: Implications for biochemical modulation. J Clin Oncol 1997;15:368–381.

105. Leichman CG. Prolonged infusion of fluorinated pyrimidines in gastrointestinal malignancies: A review of recent clinical trials. Cancer Invest 1994;12:166–175.

106. Meta-analysis Group In Cancer. Efficacy of intravenous continuous infusion of fluorouracil compared with bolus administration in advanced colorectal cancer. J Clin Oncol 1998;16:301–308.

107. Poon MA, O'Connell MJ, Wieand HS et al. Biochemical modulation of fluorouracil with leucovorin: confirmatory evidence of improved therapeutic efficacy in advanced colorectal cancer. J Clin Oncol 1991;9:1967–1972.

108. Buroker TR, O'Connell MJ, Wieand HS, et al. Randomized comparison of two schedules of fluorouracil and leucovorin in the treatment of advanced colorectal cancer. J Clin Oncol 1994;12:14–20.

109. Jüger E, Heike M, Bernhard H, et al. Weekly high-dose leucovorin versus low-dose leucovorin combined with fluorouracil in advanced colorectal cancer: Results of a randomized multicenter trial. J Clin Oncol 1996;14:2274–2279.

110. Machover D. A comprehensive review of 5-fluorouracil and leucovorin in patients with metastatic colorectal carcinoma. Cancer 1997;80:1179–1187.

111. Kohne C-H, Wils J, Lorenz M, et al. Randomized phase III study of high-dose fluorouracil given as a weekly 24-hour infusion with or without leucovorin versus bolus fluorouracil plus leucovorin in advanced colorectal cancer. J Clin Oncol 2003;21:3721–3728.

112. Cersosimo RJ. Irinotecan: A new antineoplastic agent for the management of colorectal cancer. Ann Pharmacother 1998;32:1324–1333.

113. Desai AA, Innocenti F, Ratain MJ. Pharmacogenomics: road to anticancer therapeutics in nirvana? Oncogene 2003;22:6621–6628.

114. Raymond E, Faivre S, Chaney S, et al. Cellular and molecular pharmacology of oxaliplatin. Mol Cancer Ther 2002;1:227–235.

115. Grothey A. Oxaliplatin-safety profile: neurotoxicity. Semin Oncol 2003;30(4 Suppl 15):5–13.

116. Patt YZ, Lin E, Leibman J, et al. Capecitabine plus irinotecan for chemotherapy naïve patients with metastatic colorectal cancer. Proc Am Soc Clin Oncol 2003;22:281 (Abstract 1130).

117. Kabbinavar F, Hurwitz HI, Fehrenbacher L, et al. Phase II, randomized trial comparing bevacizumab plus fluorouracil (FU)/leucovorin (LV) with FU/LV alone. J Clin Oncol 2003;21:60–65.

118. André T, Bensmaine MA, Louvet C, et al. Multicenter phase II study of bimonthly high-dose leucovorin, fluorouracil infusion, and oxaliplatin for metastatic colorectal cancer resistant to the same leucovorin and fluorouracil regimen. J Clin Oncol 1999;17:3560–3568.

119. Kouroussis C, Souglakos J, Mavroudis D, et al. Oxaliplatin with high-dose leucovorin and infusional 5-fluorouracil in irinotecan-pretreated patients with advanced colorectal cancer. Am J Clin Oncol 2002;25:627–631.

120. Saltz LB, Meropol NL, Loehrer PJ, et al. Phase II trial of cetuximab in patients with refractory colorectal cancer that expresses the epidermal growth factor receptor. J Clin Oncol 2004;22:1201–1208.

121. Ross P, Norman A, Cunningham D, et al. A prospective randomized trial of protracted venous infusion 5-fluorouracil with or without mitomycin C in advanced colorectal cancer. Ann Oncol 1997;8:995–1001.

122. Goldberg RM. Is repeated treatment with a fluorouracil-based regimen useful in colorectal cancer? Semin Oncol 1998;25(5 Suppl 11):21–28.

123. Dick EA, Taylor-Robinson SD, Thomas HC, Gedroyc WMW. Ablative therapy for liver tumors. Gut 2002;50:733–739.

124. Patt YZ, Hoque A, Lozano R, et al. Phase II trial of hepatic arterial infusion of fluorouracil and recombinant human interferon alfa-2b for liver metastases of colorectal cancer refractory to systemic fluorouracil and leucovorin. J Clin Oncol 1997;15:1432–1438.

125. Fraker DL, Soulen M. Regional therapy of hepatic metastases. Hematol Oncol Clin North Am 2002;16:947–967.

126. Gamelin E, Boisdron-Celle M, Guérin-Meyer V, et al. Correlation between uracil and dihydrouracil plasma ratio, fluorouracil (5-FU) pharmacokinetic parameters, and tolerance in patients with advanced colorectal cancer: A potential interest for predicting 5-FU toxicity and determining optimal 5-FU dosage. J Clin Oncol 1999;17:1105–1110.

127. Schrag D, Weeks J. Costs and cost-effectiveness of colorectal cancer prevention and therapy. Semin Oncol 1999;26:561–568.

128. Brown ML, Riley GF, Schussler N, Etizioni R. Estimating health care costs related to cancer treatment from SEER-medicare data. Med Care 2002;40(Suppl):IV104–IV117.

129. Brown ML, Nayfield SG, Shibley LM. Adjuvant therapy for stage III colon cancer: Economics returns to research and cost-effectiveness of treatment. J Natl Cancer Inst 1994;86:424–430.

130. Schmitt C, Blijham G, Jolain B, et al. Medical care consumption in a phase III trial comparing irinotecan with infusional 5-fluorouracil (5-FU) in patients with metastatic colorectal cancer after 5-FU failure. Anticancer Drugs 1999;10:617–623.

131. Vijan S, Hwang EW, Hofer TP, Hayward RA. Which colon cancer screening test? A comparison of costs, effectiveness, and compliance. Am J Med 2001;111:593–601.

132. Desch CE, Benson AB, Smith TJ, et al. Recommended colorectal cancer surveillance guidelines by the American Society of Clinical Oncology. J Clin Oncol 1999;17:1312–1321.

128
PROSTATE CANCER

Jill M. Kolesar

Learning Objectives and other resources can be found at *www.pharmacotherapyonline.com.*

KEY CONCEPTS

◀1 Prostate cancer is the most frequent cancer in U.S. men. African-American ancestry, family history, and increased age are the primary risk factors for prostate cancer.

◀2 Prostate-specific antigen is a useful marker for detecting prostate cancer at early stages, predicting outcome for localized disease, defining disease-free status, and monitoring response to androgen-deprivation therapy or chemotherapy for advanced-stage disease.

◀3 The prognosis for prostate cancer patients depends on the histologic grade, the tumor size, and disease stage. More than 85% of patients with stage A_1 disease but less than 1% of those with stage D_2 can be cured.

◀4 Androgen ablation with a luteinizing hormone–releasing hormone (LH-RH) agonist plus an antiandrogen should be used prior to radiation therapy for patients with locally advanced prostate cancer to improve outcomes over radiation therapy alone.

◀5 Androgen ablation therapy, with either orchiectomy, an LH-RH agonist alone or an LH-RH agonist plus an antiandrogen (combined hormonal blockade), can be used to provide palliation for patients with advanced (stage D_2) prostate cancer. The effects of androgen deprivation seem most pronounced in patients with minimal disease at diagnosis.

◀6 Antiandrogen withdrawal, for patients having progressive disease while receiving combined hormonal blockade with an LH-RH agonist plus an antiandrogen, can provide additional symptomatic relief. Mutations in the androgen receptor have been documented that cause antiandrogen compounds to act like receptor agonists.

◀7 Chemotherapy, with docetaxel and prednisone, improve survival in patients with hormone-refractory prostate cancer. Patients with hormone-refractory prostate cancer should be considered for entry into clinical trials investigating new therapies for prostate cancer.

◀1 Prostate cancer is the most frequent cancer among American men and represents the second leading cause of cancer-related deaths in all males.[1] In the United States alone, it is estimated that 232,090 new cases of prostatic carcinoma will be diagnosed and more than 30,350 men will die from this disease in 2005.[1] Although prostate cancer incidence increased during the late 1980s and early 1990s owing to widespread prostate-specific antigen (PSA) screening, deaths from prostate cancer have been continuously declining since 1995.[1]

Localized prostate cancer can be cured by surgery or radiation therapy, but advanced prostate cancer is not yet curable. Treatment for advanced prostate cancer can provide significant disease palliation for many patients for several years after diagnosis. The endocrine dependence of this tumor is well documented, and hormonal manipulation to decrease circulating androgens remains the basis for the treatment of advanced disease.

EPIDEMIOLOGY

◀1 Table 128–1 summarizes the possible factors associated with prostate cancer.[2,3] The only widely accepted risk factors for prostate cancer are age, race-ethnicity, and family history of prostate cancer.[3] The disease is rare under the age of 40, but the incidence sharply increases with each subsequent decade, most likely because the individual has had a lifetime exposure to testosterone, a known growth signal for the prostate.[3]

RACE AND ETHNICITY

The incidence of clinical prostate cancer varies across geographic regions. Scandinavian countries and the United States report the highest incidence of prostate cancer, while the disease is relatively rare in Japan and other Asian countries.[4] African-American men have the highest rate of prostate cancer in the world, and in the United States, prostate cancer mortality in African-Americans is more than twice that seen in Caucasian populations.[1] Hormonal, dietary, and genetic differences, as well as differences in access to health care may contribute to the altered susceptibility to prostate cancer in these populations.[3] Testosterone, commonly implicated in the pathogenesis of prostate cancer, is 15% higher in African-American men compared with Caucasian males. Activity of 5-α-reductase, the enzyme that converts testosterone to its more active form, dihydrotestosterone (DHT), in the prostate, is decreased in Japanese men compared with African-Americans and Caucasians.[3] In addition, genetic variations in the androgen receptor exist. Activation of the androgen receptor is inversely correlated with CAG repeat length. Shorter CAG repeat sequences have been found in African-Americans. Therefore the combination of increased testosterone and increased androgen receptor

TABLE 128–1. Risk Factors Associated with Prostate Cancer

Factor	Possible Relationship
Probable risk factors	
Age	More than 70% of cases are diagnosed in men greater than 65 years old
Race	African-Americans have higher incidence and death rate
Genetic	Familial prostate cancer inherited in an autosomal dominant manner
	Mutations in *p53*, *Rb*, E-cahedrin, α-catenin, androgen receptor, *KAI1*, microsatellite instability, loss of heterozygocity at 1, 2q, 12p, 15q, 16p, and 16q
	Candidate prostate cancer gene locus identified on chromosome 1
Possible risk factors	
Environmental	Clinical carcinoma incidence varies worldwide
	Latent carcinoma similar between regions
	Nationalized males adopt intermediate incidence rates between that of the United States and their native country
Occupational	Increased risk associated with cadmium exposure
Diet	Increased risk associated with high-meat and high-fat diets
	Decreased intake of 1,25-dihydroxyvitamin D, vitamin E, lycopene, and β-carotene increases risk
Hormonal	Does not occur in eunuchs
	Low incidence in cirrhotic patients
	Up to 80% are hormonally dependent
	African-Americans have 15% increased testosterone
	Japanese have decreased 5-α-reductase activities
	Polymorphic expression of the androgen receptor

Compiled from Carter et al,[2] Hsieh et al,[3] and Ross et al.[4]

activation may account for the increased risk of prostate cancer for African-American men.[3] The Asian diet generally is considered to be low in fat and high in fiber with a high concentration of phytoestrogens. Phytoestrogens, consisting of isoflavonoids, flavonoids, and lignans, are potential chemoprotectants.[5] Combining the protection from a low-fat diet with decreased DHT activity may explain the decreased risk of prostate cancer found in Asian men. A positive family history for prostate cancer is associated with a two- to threefold risk elevation. Three other factors, the age of the man at risk, the age of the affected relative, and the number of relatives diagnosed with prostate cancer, modify the magnitude of the excess risk. In general, younger age (<65) of the man at risk, younger age of affected relatives, and increased number of relatives with prostate cancer increase the risk of prostate cancer beyond two- to threefold.[3]

FAMILY HISTORY

Carter and colleagues[2] have demonstrated that familial clustering of prostate cancer can be explained by Mendelian inheritance of a rare autosomal dominant allele, which accounts for 9% of all prostate cancer and 45% of disease reported in men under the age of 55.[2] Genome-wide scans have identified potential prostate cancer susceptibility loci on chromosomes 1, 2q, 12p, 15q, 16p, and 16q; however,

none of these susceptibility loci have demonstrated linkage to currently known candidate genes.[6]

An alternative explanation for the familial clustering may be polymorphisms in genes important for prostate cancer function and development.[6] Candidate polymorphisms include a polymorphism in the androgen receptor, which has two different nucleotide repeat variants, the CAG or the GCC. The CAG repeat varies in repeat number from 11 to 31 repeats in healthy individuals, and the number of repeats is inversely proportional to the activity of the androgen receptor. Some studies have demonstrated that shorter CAG repeats are associated with increased prostate cancer risk. Another candidate polymorphism is SRD5A2, which is the gene that codes for 5-α-reductase, the enzyme that converts testosterone to the more active dihydrotestosterone. A variant in SRD5A2, the Ala49Thr, increases the activity and may increase prostate cancer risk.[6]

DIET

A number of epidemiologic studies support an association between high fat intake and risk of prostate cancer. A strong correlation between national per capita fat consumption and national prostate cancer mortality has been reported, and prospective case-control studies suggest that a high-fat diet doubles the risk of prostate cancer.

Other dietary factors implicated in prostate cancer include retinol, carotenoids, lycopene, and vitamin D consumption.[6,7] Retinol, or vitamin A, intake, especially in men older than 70, is correlated with an increased risk of prostate cancer, whereas intake of its precursor, β-carotene, has a protective or neutral effect. Lycopene, obtained primarily from tomatoes, decreases the risk of prostate cancer in small cohort studies. The antioxidant vitamin E also may decrease the risk of prostate cancer. Men who developed prostate cancer in one cohort study had lower levels of 1,25(OH)$_2$-vitamin D than matched controls, although a prospective study did not support this.[3] Clearly, dietary risk factors require further evaluation, but because fat and vitamins are modifiable risk factors, dietary intervention may be promising in prostate cancer prevention.

OTHER FACTORS

Benign prostatic hyperplasia (BPH) is one of the most common problems of elderly men, affecting more than 40% of men over the age of 70. BPH results in the urinary symptoms of hesitancy and frequency. Since prostate cancer affects a similar age group and often has similar presenting symptoms, the presence of BPH often complicates the diagnosis of prostate cancer, although it does not appear to increase the risk of developing prostate cancer.[3,6]

Smoking has not been associated with an increased risk of prostate cancer, but smokers with prostate cancer have an increased mortality resulting from the disease when compared with nonsmokers with prostate cancer (relative risk 1.5 to 2).[3,6] In addition, in a prospective cohort analysis, alcohol consumption was not associated with the development of prostate cancer.

ETIOLOGY

The growth and development of the prostate is under control of androgens and it is well known that men who undergo castration prior to puberty do not develop prostate cancer. The majority of risk factors for prostate cancer are factors that either increase or decrease testosterone exposure. Despite this, serum testosterone or DHT levels obtained at diagnosis are not directly associated with prostate cancer risk, suggesting a multifactorial cause of prostate cancer.[6]

PATHOPHYSIOLOGY

MOLECULAR GENETICS

As described in the epidemiology section, a familial association in prostate cancer has been recognized and generally is accepted to be genetically determined, although the precise genetic mutation of polymorphism has not been identified. In addition, a number of genes are mutated in sporadic cases of prostate cancer, although the relative contribution and interrelationship of these genes are still unknown.

E-cadherin gene inactivation via hypermethylation has been reported frequently in prostate cancer.[6] E-cadherin is a prognostic marker in prostate cancer, with aberrant E-cadherin expression associated with high-grade tumors and poor outcome in terms of disease progression and overall survival.[6] P-cadherin expression is absent in most prostate cancers, but in prostate cancers where P-cadherin is expressed, PSA is characteristically absent. The cadherin-catenin pathway may be inactivated by gene mutations or hypermethylation, and is thought to be an early event in prostate carcinogenesis.

In cells with DNA damage, *p53* is thought to function by halting cell-cycle progression, resulting in cell death via apoptotic pathways. The loss of functional *p53* may result in replication of damaged DNA and subsequently unregulated cell growth. Point mutations in *p53* thought to be caused by environmental toxins have been identified in 42% of prostate carcinomas. Mutations were present in stages B to D, although not in latent prostate carcinomas studied.[8] *Rb* mutations, also thought to be important in cell-cycle regulation, have been reported in prostate cancer patients.[6] Abnormal *p53* and *Rb,* as measured by immunohistochemistry, may be independent predictors of survival. In one study,[9] 15-year survival was 38% in patients with abnormal *p53* compared with 87% for those with normal *p53.* Aberrant *p53* also predicts radiation failure and is mutated in approximately 60% of metastatic bone marrow lesions.[10]

KAI1, or *Kang ai,* which is Chinese for anticancer, is an antimetastatic gene. The gene codes for a protein belonging to a family of leukocyte surface glycoproteins that function in cell-cell interactions and cell–extracellular matrix interactions and that is downregulated, without mutation, during the progression of prostate cancer.[11]

As of the most recent update, there are 374 different reported mutations in the androgen receptor gene.[12] Mutations in the androgen receptor gene appear to occur more frequently in advanced and hormone-refractory prostate cancer.[12] Mutated androgen receptors may be activated not only by testicular androgens, but also by several androgens, steroids, and nonsteroidal antiandrogens, promoting subsequent prostate cancer growth. Androgen receptor mutations are speculated to explain the antiandrogen withdrawal syndrome.[13]

An additional hormonal mechanism may be mutation in 5-α-reductase, the enzyme responsible for converting testosterone to active DHT. In one series, mutations were identified in 57% of prostate cancer patients.[14] While the function of the mutated enzyme has not been identified, it is hypothesized to be an activation, where increased amounts of DHT are formed. A significant number of latent prostatic carcinomas in Japanese men contain an inactivating mutation in the androgen receptor, whereas no such mutations were found in latent carcinomas of white American men.[15] It appears that the stage in which an androgen receptor mutation occurs (latent versus metastatic), as well as the functional significance of the mutation, can alter the clinical course of prostate cancer. Additional genetic analysis

has identified mutations in *H-ras* in less than 4% of American prostate carcinomas and up to 25% of Japanese carcinomas. Mutations in late-stage clinical carcinoma were identified in Ha-*ras;* however, latent prostate carcinoma had mutations in *K-ras,* possibly indicating a protective mutation.[3]

Although the molecular characterization of prostate cancer is evolving, this area of study represents a major advance in our understanding of disease pathology and may represent future avenues for diagnosis, staging, and treatment of prostate cancer.

PATHOLOGY

The normal prostate is composed of acinar secretory cells arranged in a radial shape and surrounded by a foundation of supporting tissue. The size, shape, or presence of acini is almost always altered in the gland that has been invaded by prostatic carcinoma. Adenocarcinoma, the major pathologic cell type, accounts for more than 95% of prostate cancer cases.[16] Much rarer tumor types include small cell neuroendocrine cancers, sarcomas, and transitional cell carcinomas.

Prostate cancer can be graded systematically according to the histologic appearance of the malignant cell and then grouped into well, moderately, or poorly differentiated grades.[17] Gland architecture is examined and then rated on a scale of 1 (well differentiated) to 5 (poorly differentiated). Two different specimens are examined, and the score for each specimen is added. Groupings for total Gleason score are 2 to 4 for well-differentiated, 5 or 6 for moderately-differentiated, and 7 to 10 for poorly differentiated tumors. Poorly differentiated tumors grow rapidly (poor prognosis), while well differentiated tumors grow slowly (better prognosis).

Metastatic spread can occur by local extension, lymphatic drainage, or hematogenous dissemination.[18] Lymph node metastases are more common in patients with large, undifferentiated tumors that invade the seminal vesicles. The pelvic and abdominal lymph node groups are the most common sites of lymph node involvement (Fig. 128–1). Skeletal metastases from hematogenous spread are the most common sites of distant spread. Typically, the bone lesions are osteoblastic or a combination of osteoblastic and osteolytic. The most common site of bone involvement is the lumbar spine. Other sites of bone involvement include the proximal femurs, pelvis, thoracic spine,

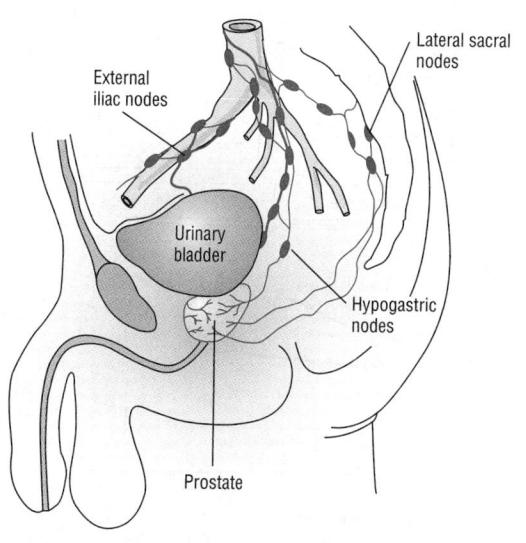

FIGURE 128–1. The prostate gland.

ribs, sternum, skull, and humerus. The lung, liver, brain, and adrenal glands are the most common sites of visceral involvement, although, these organs usually are not involved initially. About 25% to 35% of patients will have evidence of lymphangitic or nodular pulmonary infiltrates at autopsy. The prostate is a rare site for metastatic involvement from other solid tumors.

RATIONALE FOR HORMONAL MANAGEMENT

The prostate gland is a solid, rounded, heart-shaped organ positioned between the neck of the bladder and the urogenital diaphragm (see Fig. 128–1). The organ consists of single anterior, posterior, and median lobes and two lateral lobes. The posterior lobe is palpable by anterior rectal examination at 2 to 5 cm from the anal verge. Within the four morphologically defined areas of the prostate gland, 95% of the carcinomas arise from the glandular epithelium of the peripheral zone.[18] In contrast, BPH arises from the central or periurethral regions of the prostate gland.

Normal growth and differentiation of the prostate depends on the presence of androgens, specifically DHT.[19] The testes and the adrenal glands are the major sources of circulating androgens. Hormonal regulation of androgen synthesis is mediated through a series of biochemical interactions between the hypothalamus, pituitary, adrenal glands, and testes (Fig. 128–2). Luteinizing hormone–releasing hormone (LH-RH) released from the hypothalamus stimulates the release of luteinizing hormone (LH) and follicle-stimulating hormone (FSH) from the anterior pituitary gland. LH complexes with receptors on the Leydig cell testicular membrane and stimulates the production of testosterone and small amounts of estrogen. FSH acts on the Sertoli cells within the testes to promote the maturation of LH receptors and to produce an androgen-binding protein. Circulating testosterone and estradiol influence the synthesis of LH-RH, LH, and FSH by a negative feedback loop operating at the hypothalamic and pituitary level.[21]

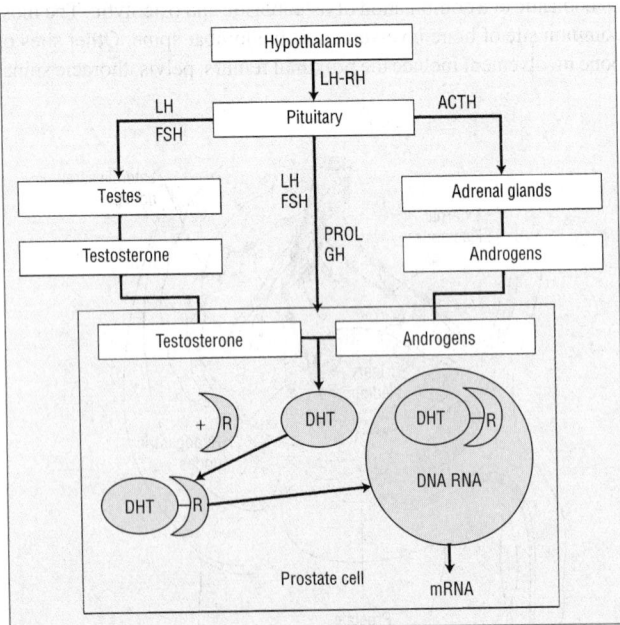

FIGURE 128–2. Hormonal regulation of the prostate gland. ACTH, adrenocorticotropic hormone; DHT, dihydrotestosterone; FSH, follicle-stimulating hormone; GH, growth hormone; LH, luteinizing hormone; LH-RH, luteinizing hormone–releasing hormone; PROL, prolactin; R, receptor.

TABLE 128–2. Hormonal Manipulations in Prostate Cancer

Androgen source ablation	Antiandrogens
Orchiectomy	Flutamide
Adrenalectomy	Bicalutamide
Hypophysectomy	Nilutamide
LH–RH or LH inhibition	Cyproterone acetate[b]
Estrogens	Progesterones
LH–RH agonists	5-α-Reductase inhibition
Progesterones[a]	Finasteride[b]
Cyproterone acetate[b]	
Androgen synthesis inhibition	
Aminoglutethimide	
Ketoconazole	
Progesterones[a]	

[a]Minor mechanisms of action.
[b]Investigational compounds or use.
LH, luteinizing hormone; LH–RH, luteinizing hormone–releasing hormone.

Prolactin, growth hormone, and estradiol appear to be important accessory regulators for prostatic tissue permeability, receptor binding, and testosterone synthesis.

Testosterone, the major androgenic hormone, accounts for 95% of the androgen concentration. The primary source of testosterone is the testes; however, 3% to 5% of the testosterone concentration is derived from direct adrenal cortical secretion of testosterone or C19 steroids such as androstenedione.[18,19]

Only 2% of total plasma testosterone is present in the physiologically active unbound state. The remaining testosterone is reversibly bound to a steroid hormone–binding globulin. The unbound testosterone or androgen precursors penetrate the prostatic cell by passive diffusion and are converted to DHT by 5-α-reductase.[18,19] DHT subsequently binds with a specific cytoplasmic receptor. This DHT-receptor complex is then transported to the nucleus of the cell, where transcription and ultimately translation of stored genetic material occur.[18,19]

Huggins and Hodges[20] observed that both normal and malignant prostatic tissue contains a high level of acid phosphatase, suggesting that prostatic malignancy represents an overgrowth of prostate tissue. They then demonstrated that a decrease in serum acid phosphatase along with symptomatic relief occurred in patients with metastatic prostate cancer treated with either estrogens or orchiectomy therapies known to reduce circulating androgens.[20] Androgen ablation is used in the treatment and palliation of advanced prostate cancer because prostatic epithelium undergoes atrophy when the normal physiologic effect of androgens is reduced.[8]

Hormonal manipulations to ablate or reduce circulating androgens can occur through several mechanisms[18,19] (Table 128–2). The organs responsible for androgen production can be removed surgically (orchiectomy, hypophysectomy, or adrenalectomy). Hormonal pathways that modulate prostatic growth can be interrupted at several steps (see Fig. 128–2). Interference with LH-RH or LH can reduce testosterone secretion by the testes (estrogens, LH-RH agonists, progestogens, and cyproterone acetate). Estrogen administration reduces androgens by directly inhibiting LH release, by acting directly on the prostate cell, or by decreasing free androgens by increasing steroid-binding globulin levels.[18,19]

Isolation of the naturally occurring hypothalamic decapeptide hormone luteinizing hormone–releasing hormone or LH-RH has provided another group of effective agents for advanced prostate cancer treatment.[20] The physiologic response to LH-RH depends on both the dose and the mode of administration. Intermittent pulsed LH-RH administration, which mimics the endogenous release pattern, causes sustained release of both LH and FSH, whereas high-dose or continuous intravenous administration of LH-RH inhibits gonadotropin release due to receptor downregulation.[21] Structural modification of the naturally occurring LH-RH and innovative delivery have produced a series of LH-RH agonists that cause a similar downregulation of pituitary receptors and a decrease in testosterone production.[21]

Androgen synthesis can be inhibited in the testes or in the adrenal gland. Aminoglutethimide inhibits the desmolase-enzyme complex in the adrenal gland, thereby preventing the conversion of cholesterol to pregnenolone. Pregnenolone is the precursor substrate for all adrenal-derived steroids, including androgens, glucocorticoids, and mineralocorticoids.[22] Ketoconazole, an imidazole antifungal agent, causes a dose-related reversible reduction in serum cortisol and testosterone concentration by inhibiting both adrenal and testicular steroidogenesis.[22,23] As a secondary mechanism to its antiandrogen action, megestrol acetate inhibits the synthesis of androgens. This inhibition appears to occur at the adrenal level, but circulating levels of testosterone also are reduced, suggesting that inhibition at the testicular level also may occur.[22]

Antiandrogens inhibit the formation of the DHT-receptor complex and thereby interfere with androgen-mediated action at the cellular level.[23] Megestrol acetate, a progestational agent, also is available and has antiandrogen actions.[22] Finally, the conversion of testosterone to DHT may be inhibited by 5-α-reductase inhibitors.[24]

CLINICAL PRESENTATION

Whereas prostatic carcinoma may be asymptomatic in patients with localized disease, most patients with signs and symptoms have advanced disease at presentation. In patients with locally invasive disease, the most common complaints arise from ureteral dysfunction or impingement. Patients complain of alterations in micturition manifested by urinary frequency, hesitancy, and dribbling.[16,17,25] New onset impotence or less firm penile erections in an elderly male may indicate prostate cancer.

Most commonly, patients with advanced disease present with back pain and stiffness due to osseous metastases.[25] Eventually, spinal cord lesions may lead to cord compression if not treated properly.[25] Rarely, pathologic fractures can occur. Lower extremity edema can occur as a result of lymphatic obstruction. Anemia and weight loss are nonspecific signs of advanced disease.

CLINICAL PRESENTATION OF PROSTATE CANCER[16,17,25]

LOCALIZED DISEASE
Asymptomatic

LOCALLY INVASIVE DISEASE
Ureteral dysfunction, frequency, hesitancy, and dribbling
Impotence

ADVANCED DISEASE
Back pain
Cord compression
Lower extremity edema
Pathologic fractures
Anemia
Weight loss

CHEMOPREVENTION

Considerable interest in preventing prostate cancer exists and several large chemoprevention trials are sponsored and ongoing by the National Cancer Institute. The first large chemoprevention trial in prostate cancer, the Prostate Cancer Prevention Trial (PCPT), began in 1993 and randomized 18,881 men older than 55 years with a low risk of prostate cancer (PSA = 3 ng/mL) to receive 5 mg finasteride daily (a 5-α-reductase inhibitor) or placebo to determine if inhibition of DHT synthesis in the prostate for a prolonged period (7 years) would lead to a decreased incidence of prostate cancer.[24] Finasteride is currently used in the treatment of BPH.

The results of the PCPT were recently published, and confirmed the efficacy of finasteride in reducing the rate of acute urinary retention, the need for surgery for symptomatic BPH, and a reduced risk of progression of BPH. In addition, finasteride demonstrated a 24.8% reduction in prostate cancer prevalence during the 7-year period. Another way of looking at these results is the number needed to treat to prevent one prostate cancer. With a prostate cancer incidence of 6.3% in the finasteride and 8.7% in the placebo arm, the absolute reduction is 2.4%, giving a number needed to treat to prevent one cancer of 41. However, tumors in the treated group had a higher Gleason score, suggesting more aggressive disease compared to the placebo group for all men in whom prostate cancer developed during the study period, and it is too early to evaluate survival end points. So, while we now know that finasteride reduces the risk of prostate cancer development, whether it improves survival is still open to question.[24]

CLINICAL CONTROVERSY

Prevention of prostate cancer with finasteride is controversial. In a recently completed trial comparing finasteride to placebo, those receiving finasteride had fewer prostate cancers, but those that developed were more aggressive. The effects of finasteride on survival are still unknown.

Therefore, the use of finasteride to prevent prostate cancer is currently under debate.[26] Because of its established benefit in treating BPH, the 20% to 30% of men over 50 with BPH may derive the additional benefit of prostate cancer prevention and should be offered treatment with finasteride. In the 70% to 80% of men without BPH, the benefits, side effects (primarily impotence), and risks of finasteride should be discussed prior to initiating therapy.

Selenium is a naturally occurring trace element that is an essential nutrient in the human diet. A large randomized clinical trial designed to examine skin cancer prevention first suggested that selenium has a beneficial effect in the prevention of prostate cancer.[27] The Alpha-Tocopherol Beta-Carotene Cancer Prevention Study conducted in Finland reported a 34% decrease in the incidence of prostate cancer in subjects receiving α-tocopherol (a form of vitamin E) compared with the placebo group. These results, in addition to previous data, prompted a second large-scale chemoprevention trial of prostate cancer. SELECT[28] is a phase III trial to determine whether selenium and/or vitamin E decreases the incidence of prostate cancer in healthy men. This trial, initiated by the National Cancer Institute in 2001 and with final results anticipated in 2013, is expected to shed more light on the role of these agents in the prevention of prostate cancer. Until results are available, supplementation with selenium or vitamin E for primary prevention of prostate cancer is not recommended.

SCREENING METHODS

Since prostate cancer is not curable in advanced stages, prevention efforts are under intensive evaluation. Early detection of potentially curable prostate cancers is the goal of prostate cancer screening. For cancer screening to be beneficial, it must reliably detect cancer at an early stage, when intervention would decrease mortality. Whether prostate cancer screening fits these criteria has generated considerable controversy.[29] Evidence from randomized clinical trials addressing whether screening reduces prostate cancer mortality may not be available for 10 to 15 years. In the interim, clinicians are faced with the dilemma of whether to screen or not to screen, as well as how best to treat early-stage prostate cancer.

DIGITAL RECTAL EXAMINATION

Digital rectal examination (DRE) has been recommended since the early 1900s for the detection of prostate cancer. The primary advantage of DRE is its specificity, reported at greater than 85%, for prostate cancer. Other advantages of DRE include low cost, safety, and ease of performance. However, DRE is relatively insensitive and is subject to interobserver variability. DRE as a single screening method has poor compliance and has had little effect on preventing metastatic prostate cancer in one large case-control study.[30]

PROSTATE-SPECIFIC ANTIGEN

PSA is a prostate-specific glycoprotein produced only in the cytoplasm of benign and malignant prostate cells.[31] PSA functions as a serine protease, which liquefies seminal fluid after ejaculation. In addition to its biologic activity, PSA also may enhance cellular growth by its ability to cleave insulin-like growth factor–binding proteins. Cleavage activates insulin-like growth factor (IGF), which can then bind to IGF receptors and stimulate growth in the prostate.[31]

Unlike acid phosphatase, PSA levels are not influenced by ambient conditions or subject to diurnal variation, but are influenced by sedentary conditions. Therefore it is recommended that all PSA measurements be made on sera collected from ambulatory patients. PSA levels not only rise with prostatic manipulation such as transrectal ultrasound (TRUS) and/or biopsy, but also remain above normal for several weeks thereafter. PSA has a serum half-life of 2 to 3 days.[31]

PSA is used widely for prostate cancer screening in the United States, with simplicity its major advantage and low specificity its primary limitation.[32] PSA may be elevated in men with acute urinary retention, acute prostatitis, and prostatic ischemia or infarction, as well as BPH, a nearly universal condition in men at risk for prostate cancer. PSA elevations between 4.1 and 10 ng/mL cannot distinguish between BPH and prostate cancer, limiting the utility of PSA alone for the early detection of prostate cancer. Additionally, only 38% to 48% of men with clinically significant prostate cancer have a serum PSA outside the reference range.[31]

Neither DRE nor PSA is sensitive or specific enough to be used alone as a screening test.[31] Although the relative predictability of DRE and PSA is similar, the tumors identified by each method are different. Catalona and associates[33] confirmed that the combination of a DRE plus PSA determination is a better method of detecting prostate cancer than DRE alone.

Efforts to increase PSA specificity include the use of free PSA measurements, age- and race-specific PSA levels, PSA density, and PSA velocity.[31,32]

CURRENT SCREENING RECOMMENDATIONS

The common approach to prostate cancer screening today involves offering PSA measurements beginning at age 50 to all men of normal risk with a 10-year or greater life expectancy.

CLINICAL CONTROVERSY

Prostate cancer screening is controversial. Increased screening has led to an increased incidence of early-stage prostate cancer for which the most appropriate management is still unknown. Prostate cancer screening has not been shown to improve survival. However, the American Cancer Society currently recommends that digital rectal examination and PSA be offered annually to men beginning at age 50 years with at least a 10-year life expectancy, and to younger men (45 years old) who are considered to be at high risk for prostate cancer development (strong familial predisposition or African-American).

Despite this common practice, the benefits of prostate cancer screening are unproven. PSA measurements can identify small, subclinical prostate cancers, where no intervention may be required. Detecting prostate cancer in those not needing therapy not only increases the cost of care through unnecessary screening and work-ups, but also increases the toxicity of therapy, by subjecting some patients to unnecessary therapy.[34] Currently, the American College of Physicians recommends that rather than screening all men for prostate cancer as a matter of routine, physicians should describe the potential benefits and known risks of screening, diagnosis, and treatment, listen to the patient's concerns, and then decide on an individual's screening method. In a randomized, controlled trial of an educational videotape describing the advantages and disadvantages of prostate cancer screening, patients who viewed the videotape had an increase of 78% ($p = .001$) in prostate cancer knowledge and a decrease of 18.5% ($p = .009$) in requests for screening over control patients.[35] The American Cancer Society (ACS) currently recommends that DRE and PSA be offered annually to men beginning at age 50 years with at least a 10-year life expectancy and to younger men (45 years old) who are considered to be at high risk for prostate cancer development (strong familial predisposition or African-American). The ACS defines an abnormal PSA value to be above 4 ng/mL. If both tests are normal, no further diagnostic action is required; however, if either is abnormal, further work-up by TRUS is indicated.

Two ongoing national randomized trials will provide important data to help resolve the prostate cancer screening controversies. The first is the Prostate, Lung, Colon, and Ovarian Trial, which is designed to test the efficacy of prostate cancer screening in 74,000 men aged 60 to 74.[31] The second is the Prostate Cancer Intervention Versus Observation Trial, which is a randomized study comparing radical prostatectomy with expectant management.[36] These trials, when complete, likely will provide key information regarding the costs and benefits of prostate cancer screening and the most appropriate early management.

DIAGNOSIS

Transperianal or transrectal prostate biopsy is necessary to confirm a prostate cancer diagnosis and to grade the tumor specimen. TRUS-guided biopsies of hypoechoic areas may help define extraprostatic extension.[37] For patients with visceral or lytic metastases, these lesions may be biopsied, because this presentation is common for one

TABLE 128–3. Diagnostic and Staging Work-Up for Prostate Cancer

Initial tests	Digital rectal examination (DRE)
	Prostate-specific antigen (PSA)
	Transrectal ultrasonography (TRUS) if either DRE is positive or PSA is elevated
	Biopsy
Staging tests	Gleason score on biopsy specimen
	Bone scan
	Complete blood count
	Liver function tests
	Serum phosphatases (acid/alkaline)
	Excretory urogram
	Chest x-ray
Additional staging tests (depends on tumor classification, PSA, and Gleason score)	Skeletal films
	Lymph node evaluation
	Pelvic computed tomography
	^{111}In-labeled capromab pendetide scan
	Bipedal lymphangiogram
	Transrectal magnetic resonance imaging

of the variant histologies (small cell neuroendocrine) that requires a treatment strategy different from that for adenocarcinomas.[37]

Table 128–3 summarizes the diagnostic staging work-up. When DRE is performed, prostatic carcinoma is classically characterized by a rock-hard nodule or mass in the gland, whereas the gland is smooth and rubbery in BPH.

STAGING

The information obtained from the diagnostic tests is used to stage the patient. There are two commonly recognized staging classification systems (Table 128–4). The formal international classification system (tumor, node, metastases; TNM), adopted by the International Union Against Cancer in 1974, was updated in 1992 in an effort to provide congruence with the classical American Urologic System (AUS) staging system for prostate cancer.[38] The AUS classification is the most commonly used staging system in the United States (see Table 128–4). Patients are assigned to stages A through D and corresponding subcategories based on size of the tumor (T), local or regional extension, presence of involved lymph node groups (N), and presence of metastases (M).[38] Some studies classify patients who have progressed after hormonal therapy as stage D_3.[38] Based on men diagnosed with prostate cancer at Walter Reed Army Medical Center from 1988 to 1998, including over 2042 prostate cancer diagnoses, localized prostate cancer (stage T_1 and T_2) was diagnosed more

TABLE 128–4. Staging and Classification Systems for Prostate Cancer

AUS[a] Stage (A–D)	AJC-UICC[b] Classification (TNM)
A (occult, nonpalpable)	$T_xN_xM_x$ (cannot be assessed)
	$T_0N_0M_0$ (nonpalpable)
A_1: Focal	T_0: Focal or diffuse
A_2: Diffuse	
B (confined to prostate)	$T_1N_0M_0$, $T_2N_0M_0$
B_1: Single nodule in one lobe, <1.5 cm	T_1 (Clinically inapparent tumor not palpable or visible by imaging)
	T_{1a}: Tumor incidental histologic finding in 5% or less of tissue resected
	T_{1b}: Tumor incidental histologic finding in 5% or more of tissue resected
	T_{1c}: Tumor identified by needle biopsy (e.g., because of elevated PSA)
B_2: Diffuse involvement of whole gland, >1.5 cm	T_2: (Tumor confined within the prostate[c])
	T_{2a}: Tumor involves half of a lobe or less
	T_{2b}: Tumor involves more than half a lobe, but not both lobes
	T_{2c}: Tumor involves both lobes
C (localized to periprostatic area)	$T_3N_0M_0$, $T_4N_0M_0$
C_1: No seminal vesicle involvement, <70 g	T_3: (Tumor extends through the prostatic capsule[d])
	T_{3a}: Unilateral extracapsular extension
	T_{3b}: Bilateral extracapsular extension
	T_{3c}: Tumor invades the seminal vesicle(s)
C_2: Seminal vesicle involvement, >70 g	T_4: (Tumor is fixed or invades adjacent structures other than the seminal vesicles)
	T_{4a}: Tumor invades any of bladder neck, external sphincter, or rectum
	T_{4b}: Tumor invades levator muscles and/or is fixed to the pelvic wall
D (metastatic disease)	Any T, N_{1-4}, M_0, or N_{0-4}, M_1
D_1: Pelvic lymph nodes or ureteral obstruction	N_1: Metastasis in a single lymph node, 2 cm or less in greatest dimension
D_2: Bone, distant lymph node, organ, or soft tissue metastases	N_2: Metastasis in single lymph node more than 2 cm but not more than 5 cm in greatest dimension; or multiple lymph node metastases, none more than 5 cm in greatest dimension
	N_3: Metastasis in lymph node more than 5 cm in greatest dimension
	M_{1a}: Nonregional lymph node(s)
	M_{1b}: Bone(s)
	M_{1c}: Other site(s)

[a]American Urologic System.
[b]American Joint Committee–International Union Against Cancer.
[c]Note: Tumor found in one or both lobes by needle biopsy, but not palpable or visible by imaging, is classified as T_{1c}.
[d]Note: Invasion into the prostatic apex or into (but not beyond) the prostatic capsule is not classified as T_3 but as T_2.
Reproduced with permission from Montie.[38]

frequently (89% vs. 68%), and advanced disease (stages T_3, T_4, and D) was diagnosed less frequently (11% vs. 32%) when comparing the 1998 to the 1988 incidence rates.

PROGNOSIS

3 The prognosis for patients with prostate cancer depends on the histologic grade, the tumor size, and the local extent of the primary tumor.[17] The most important prognostic criterion appears to be the histologic grade, because the degree of differentiation ultimately determines the stage of disease. Poorly differentiated tumors are highly associated with both regional lymph node involvement and distant metastases.[17] Other prognostic factors that are being explored include DNA content, cell proliferative activity, epidermal growth factor (EGF), transforming growth factor-α, EGF receptor, *erbB2* oncogene, *ras* oncogene, *RB1* tumor-suppressor gene, *p53* tumor-suppressor gene, and change in PSA.[39]

During 1992 to 1999, 5-year overall survival rates were estimated at 98% for whites and 93% for African-Americans.[1] For this same period, the survival rates for localized or regional disease (100%), and distant disease (33%) in white males were about the same as the survival rates for localized or regional disease (100%), and distant disease (26%) in African-American males.[1] A 6.3% decline in age-adjusted mortality has been documented for the period 1991 to 1995.[40] Ten-year cancer-specific survival is estimated as 95% for stage A_1, 80% for stages A_2 to B_2, 60% for stage C, 40% for stage D_1, and 10% for stage D_2.[41] It is estimated that more than 85% of patients with stage A_1 can be cured, whereas fewer than 1% of patients with stage D_2 will be cured.

▶ TREATMENT: Prostate Cancer

■ DESIRED OUTCOME

The desired outcome in early-stage prostate cancer is to minimize morbidity and mortality due to prostate cancer.[37] Unfortunately, the most appropriate therapy of early-stage prostate cancer is unknown.

CLINICAL CONTROVERSY

Treatment of localized prostate cancer is controversial. While early-stage disease is curable by surgery or radiation therapy, both modalities have significant morbidity and mortality and watchful waiting is an option for some patients.

Early-stage disease may be treated with surgery, radiation, or watchful waiting. While surgery and radiation are curative, they are associated with significant morbidity and mortality. Since the overall goal is to minimize morbidity and mortality associated with the disease, watchful waiting is appropriate in selected individuals. Advanced prostate cancer (stage D) is not currently curable, and treatment should focus on providing symptom relief and maintaining quality of life.[42]

■ GENERAL APPROACH TO TREATMENT

The initial treatment for prostate cancer depends primarily on the disease stage, the Gleason score, the presence of symptoms, and the life expectancy of the patient.[16,37] Figure 128–3 shows the National Comprehensive Cancer Network (NCCN) consensus-based practice guidelines for initial prostate cancer management.[37] All the treatment options were considered "category 2A" by the panel of experts that developed these guidelines; this means that the recommendations were uncontested and generally accepted by all panel members, but the recommendations were based on lower level evidence, including clinical experience.

Prostate cancer is usually initially diagnosed by PSA and DRE and confirmed by a biopsy, where the Gleason score is assigned. Asymptomatic patients with a low risk of recurrence, those with a T_1 or T_2, with a Gleason score of 2 through 6, and a PSA of <10 ng/mL may be managed by observation, radiation, or a radical prostatectomy. As patients with asymptomatic early-stage disease generally have an excellent 10-year survival, immediate morbidities of treatment must be balanced with the likelihood of dying from prostate cancer. In general, more aggressive treatments of early-stage prostate cancer are reserved for younger men, although patient preference is a major consideration in all treatment decisions. In a patient with a normal life expectancy of less than 10 years, observation and radiation therapy may be offered. In those with a normal life expectancy of 10 to 20 years, either observation, radiation (external beam or brachytherapy), or radical prostatectomy may be offered. Patients with a normal life expectancy of greater than 20 years are offered radiation therapy or a radical prostatectomy. Radical prostatectomy and radiation therapy generally are considered therapeutically equivalent for localized prostate cancer, although neither has been proved to be better than observation alone.[37,42,43] A prospective, randomized trial comparing the two treatments showed a cause-specific survival of 81.2% in the surgery group and 84.6% ($p = .024$) in the radiation group. Patients in the surgery group also had an increased incidence of incontinence and a poorer quality of life, suggesting that radiation therapy may be preferred.[44] Complications from radical prostatectomy include blood loss, stricture formation, incontinence, lymphocele, fistula formation, anesthetic risk, and impotence. Nerve-sparing radical prostatectomy can be performed in many patients; 50% to 80% regain sexual potency within the first year.[45] Acute complications from radiation therapy include cystitis, proctitis, hematuria, urinary retention, penoscrotal edema, and impotence (30% incidence).[16] Chronic complications include proctitis, diarrhea, cystitis, enteritis, impotence, urethral stricture, and incontinence.[16] Since radiation and prostatectomy have significant and immediate mortality when compared with observation alone, many patients may elect to postpone therapy until symptoms develop.

Individuals with T_{2b} and T_{2c} disease or a Gleason score of 7 or a PSA ranging from 10 to 20 ng/mL are considered at intermediate risk for prostate cancer recurrence.[37] Individuals with less than a 10-year expected survival may be offered observation, radiation therapy, or radical prostatectomy, and those with a greater than 10-year life expectancy may be offered either radical prostatectomy or radiation therapy.

4 The treatment of patients at high risk of recurrence (stages T_{3a} to T_{3b}, a Gleason score ranging from 8 to 10, or a PSA value >20 ng/mL) depends on life expectancy.[37] In those with a life expectancy of 5 years or less, either observation or hormonal therapy are options. For patients with this stage of disease and a life expectancy of greater than 5 years, a combination of radiation therapy and

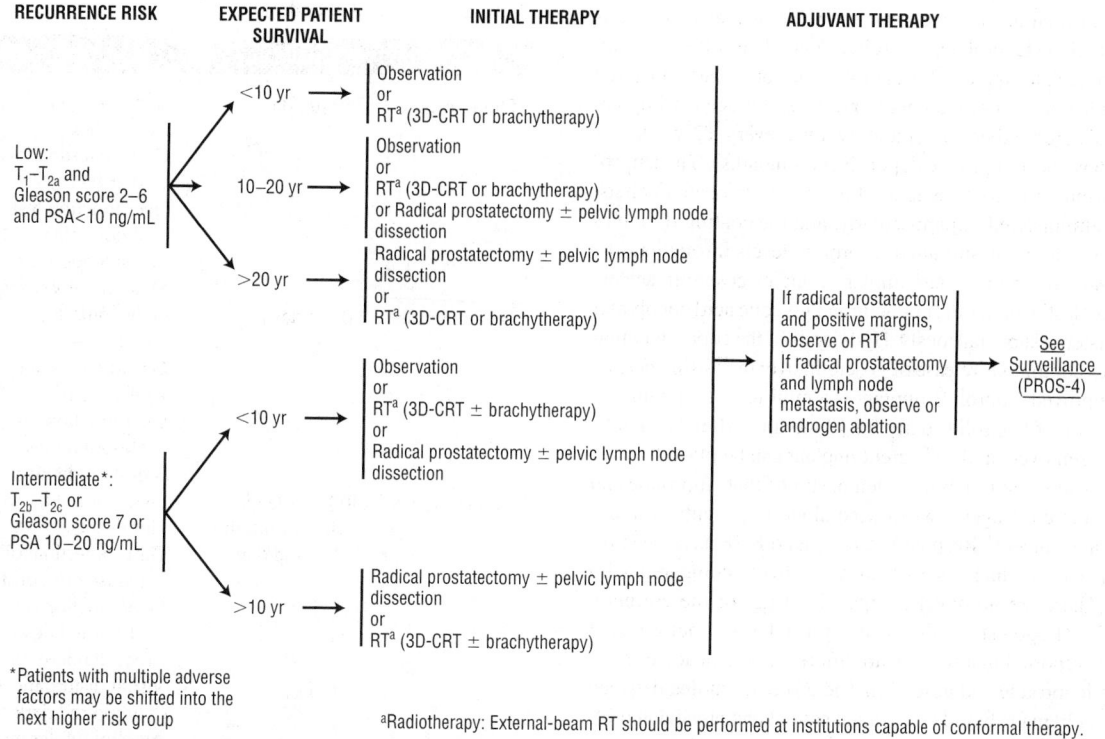

RECURRENCE RISK	EXPECTED PATIENT SURVIVAL	INITIAL THERAPY	ADJUVANT THERAPY

FIGURE 128–3. Initial management of T_1–T_{2c} prostate cancer. *(Reproduced from version 1.2002, January 7, 2002. © 2002 National Comprehensive Cancer Network, Inc. All rights reserved. These guidelines and this illustration may not be reproduced in any form without the express written permission of NCCN.)*

hormonal therapy is recommended, although select individuals with a low tumor volume may receive a radical prostatectomy in place of radiation therapy. A study supporting the combination of radiation therapy and hormonal therapy randomized over 400 subjects to receive goserelin, 3.6 mg every 4 weeks; and flutamide, 250 mg three times a day for 2 months before radiation therapy and during radiation therapy, or radiation therapy alone.[46] After 8 years of follow-up, androgen ablation was associated with an improvement in local control (42% vs. 30%), reduction in the incidence of distant metastases (34% vs. 45%), disease-free survival (33% vs. 21%), biochemical disease-free survival (PSA <1.5; 24% vs. 10%), and cause-specific mortality (23% vs. 31%). The authors performed an additional subset analysis, showing that the beneficial effect of short-term androgen ablation is most pronounced in patients with Gleason scores of 2 to 6, for whom there was a highly significant improvement in all end points, including survival (70% vs. 52%). Most clinicians continue the androgen ablation for a total of 2 to 3 years.[37,47]

Patients with T_{3c} and T_4 disease have a very high risk of recurrence and are not candidates for radical prostatectomy because of extensive local spread of disease.[37] Patients may be offered androgen ablation or a combination of radiation therapy and androgen ablation. Recent evidence suggests that androgen ablation should be instituted at diagnosis rather than waiting for symptomatic disease or progression to occur. In a randomized clinical trial enrolling 500 men with locally advanced prostate cancer who were randomized to either immediate initiation of androgen ablation with either orchiectomy or androgen ablation, or deferred hormonal therapy, individuals with immediate therapy had a median actuarial cause-specific survival duration of 7.5 years for immediate treatment and 5.8 years for deferred treatment.[48]

The major initial treatment modality for advanced prostate cancer (stage D_2) is androgen-ablative pharmacotherapy using either orchiectomy or LH-RH agonists, either alone or combined with antiandrogens.[37] Estrogens were once widely used; however, the primary estrogen, diethylstilbestrol (DES), was withdrawn from the U.S. market in 1997 due to increased cardiovascular risk. Secondary hormonal manipulations, cytotoxic chemotherapy, or supportive care is used for the patient who progresses after initial therapy.[22]

NONPHARMACOLOGIC THERAPY

ORCHIECTOMY

Bilateral orchiectomy, or removal of the testes, rapidly reduces circulating androgens to castrate levels (<50 ng/dL).[16] However, many patients are not surgical candidates owing to their advanced age, and other patients find this procedure psychologically unacceptable.[16] Orchiectomy is the preferred initial treatment in patients with impending spinal cord compression or ureteral obstruction.

PHARMACOLOGIC THERAPY

DRUG TREATMENTS OF FIRST CHOICE

LH-RH Agonists

Luteinizing hormone–releasing hormone (LH-RH) agonists are a reversible method of androgen ablation and are as effective as orchiectomy in treating prostate cancer.[49] Currently available LH-RH agonists include leuprolide, leuprolide depot, leuprolide implant, and goserelin acetate implant.[20] Leuprolide acetate is administered once daily, whereas leuprolide depot and goserelin acetate implant can be administered either once monthly, once every 12 weeks, or once every 16 weeks (leuprolide depot, every 4 months). The leuprolide depot formulation contains leuprolide acetate in coated pellets. The dose is administered intramuscularly, and the coating dissolves at different rates to allow sustained leuprolide levels throughout the dosing interval. Goserelin acetate implant contains goserelin acetate dispersed in a plastic matrix of D,L-lactic and glycolic acid copolymer and is administered subcutaneously. Hydrolysis of the copolymer material provides continuous release of goserelin over the dosing period. A recently approved leuprolide implant is a mini-osmotic pump that delivers 120 mcg of leuprolide daily for 12 months. After 12 months the implant is removed, and a different implant can be placed.

Several randomized trials have demonstrated that leuprolide and goserelin are effective agents when used alone in patients with advanced prostate cancer.[21] Response rates around 80% have been reported, with a lower incidence of adverse effects compared with estrogens.[21] There are no direct comparative trials of the currently available LH-RH agonists or the dosage formulations, but a recent meta-analysis reported that there is no difference in efficacy or toxicity between leuprolide and goserelin. Therefore the choice between the two is usually made based on cost and patient and physician preference for a dosing schedule.

The most common adverse effects reported with LH-RH agonist therapy include a disease flare-up during the first week of therapy, hot flashes, erectile impotence, decreased libido, and injection-site reactions.[21] The disease flare-up is thought to be caused by initial induction of LH and FSH by the LH-RH agonist, and manifests clinically as either increased bone pain or increased urinary symptoms.[21] This flare reaction usually resolves after 2 weeks and has a similar onset and duration pattern for the depot LH-RH products.[50,51]

LH-RH agonist monotherapy can be used as initial therapy, with similar response rates to orchiectomy and estrogen administration expected. There is a lower incidence of cardiovascular-related adverse effects associated with LH-RH therapy than with estrogen administration. Patients should be counseled to expect worsening symptoms during the first week of therapy, and caution should be exercised when initiating LH-RH agonist therapy in patients with widely metastatic disease involving the spinal cord or having the potential for ureteral obstruction because irreversible complications may occur.

Antiandrogens

Three antiandrogens, flutamide, bicalutamide,[33,72] and nilutamide,[32] are currently available (Table 128–5).

Antiandrogens have been used as monotherapy in previously untreated patients, but a recent meta-analysis determined that monotherapy with antiandrogens is less effective than LH-RH agonist therapy.[51] Efficacy of the antiandrogens was similar. Flutamide has a response rate of 50% to 87%,[22] bicalutamide has a response rate of 54% to 70%,[52,53] and nilutamide has a response rate of approximately 40%.[54] Objective responses are manifested as decreased bone pain, decreased prostate size, decreased PSA, and/or improved performance status. However, for advanced prostate cancer, all currently available antiandrogens are indicated only in combination with androgen-ablation therapy; flutamide and bicalutamide are indicated in combination with an LH-RH agonist, and nilutamide is indicated in combination with orchiectomy.[22]

TABLE 128–5. Antiandrogens

Antiandrogen	Usual Dose	Adverse Effects
Flutamide	750 mg/day	Gynecomastia Hot flushes Gastrointestinal disturbances (diarrhea) Liver function test abnormalities Breast tenderness Methemoglobinemia
Bicalutamide	50 mg/day	Gynecomastia Hot flushes Gastrointestinal disturbances (diarrhea) Liver function test abnormalities Breast tenderness
Nilutamide	300 mg/day for first month then 150 mg/day	Gynecomastia Hot flushes Gastrointestinal disturbances (nausea or constipation) Liver function test abnormalities Breast tenderness Visual disturbances (impaired dark adaptation) Alcohol intolerance Interstitial pneumonitis

The most common antiandrogen-related adverse effects are listed in Table 128–5. In the only randomized comparison of bicalutamide plus an LH-RH agonist versus flutamide plus an LH-RH agonist, diarrhea was more common in flutamide-treated patients.[55,56] Antiandrogens can reduce the symptoms from the flare phenomenon associated with LH-RH agonist therapy.

Combined Hormonal Blockade

Although up to 80% of patients with advanced prostate cancer will respond to initial hormonal manipulation, almost all patients will relapse within 2 to 4 years after initiating therapy.[16] Two mechanisms have been proposed to explain this tumor resistance.[57] The tumor could be heterogeneously composed of cells that are hormone-dependent and hormone-independent, or the tumor could be stimulated by extratesticular androgens that are converted intracellularly to DHT. The rationale for combination hormonal therapy is to interfere with multiple hormonal pathways to completely eliminate androgen action. In clinical trials, combination hormonal therapy, sometimes also referred to as *maximal androgen deprivation* or total androgen blockade, has been used. The combination of LH-RH agonists or orchiectomy with antiandrogens is the most extensively studied combined androgen-deprivation approach.

Labrie and colleagues[58] reported an initial study combining an LH-RH agonist with flutamide and subsequently have provided follow-up for 363 patients. Response rates, the main end point of these studies, have been greater than 90% in previously untreated patients.[58] However, response rates of less than 35% have been observed with this combination in patients previously treated with initial hormonal manipulation.

These studies, although quite encouraging, have been criticized for lack of a concurrent control arm and for using response rather than survival as the final end point. For these reasons, the National

Cancer Institute (NCI) sponsored a randomized, placebo-controlled, double-blind multicenter trial comparing leuprolide with leuprolide plus 250 mg flutamide orally three times a day in newly diagnosed patients with stage D prostate cancer.[58]

Both median progression-free survival (16.5 vs. 13.9 months) and median overall survival (35.6 vs. 28.3 months) were significantly longer in the 303 evaluable patients treated with leuprolide plus flutamide than in the 300 evaluable patients treated with leuprolide alone. The best response to combination therapy was observed in patients with minimal disease (no disease in ribs, long bones, or soft tissue other than lymph nodes) and a good performance status. An update of this trial has demonstrated that median survival was 61 months in the combination arm and 41 months in the leuprolide-alone arm in patients with minimal disease.[59] The addition of flutamide to leuprolide reduced the symptoms from the flare phenomenon associated with LH-RH agonist therapy. Patients in both groups experienced common adverse effects associated with LH-RH agonist treatment. Diarrhea was the only additional adverse effect attributable to flutamide administration. In a comparison of goserelin with goserelin and flutamide conducted in 589 patients with 10 years of follow-up, combined androgen blockade (CAB) showed no benefit over goserelin alone.[60]

Several other studies comparing CAB with conventional medical or surgical castration have been performed.[55,61–64] In studies with LH-RH agonists, the results have varied, with no consistent benefit demonstrated for CAB.

A recently completed NCI intergroup trial involving 1387 evaluable stage D_2 prostate cancer patients failed to show any significant survival benefits for the combination of orchiectomy plus flutamide over orchiectomy alone.[64] Like other studies of CAB, overall survival was longest in patients with minimal disease. Diarrhea, elevated liver function tests, and anemia were more common in those patients who received flutamide.

The most recent meta-analysis of 27 randomized trials in 8275 patients (4803 treated with flutamide, 1683 treated with nilutamide, and 1784 treated with cyproterone) comparing maximal androgen blockade with conventional medical or surgical castration showed a small survival benefit at 5 years for those treated with flutamide or nilutamide (27.6%) compared to those with castration alone (24.7%; $p = .0005$).[65]

In one of the few combination androgen-deprivation studies comparing two different antiandrogens (bicalutamide vs. flutamide), the time to treatment failure (the main study end point), time to progression (as defined by appearance of new or worsening bone or extraskeletal lesions), and time to death were equivalent, suggesting that the two treatments are equally effective.[66]

CLINICAL CONTROVERSY

The use of combined androgen blockade is controversial. Meta-analysis shows a small survival advantage when comparing combined androgen blockade to orchiectomy or LH-RH agonist alone. However, this modest benefit is achieved at significant financial cost and with additional toxicities.

Although some investigators now consider CAB to be the initial hormonal therapy of choice for newly diagnosed patients, the clinician is left to weigh the costs of combined therapy against potential benefits in light of conflicting results in the randomized trials[21] and the modest benefit seen in the meta-analysis.[65] For those trials that did show an advantage for CAB, whether these effects are specific to the testosterone-deprivation method (orchiectomy vs. leuprolide vs. goserelin), the antiandrogen, the duration of therapy, or patient

selection is not clear. Until further carefully designed studies that use survival, time to progression, quality of life, patient preference, and cost as end points are conducted, it is appropriate to use either LH-RH agonist monotherapy or CAB as initial therapy for metastatic prostate cancer. CAB may be most beneficial for improving survival in patients with minimal disease and for preventing tumor flare, particularly in those with advanced metastatic disease. All other patients may be started on LH-RH monotherapy, and an antiandrogen may be added after several months if androgen ablation is incomplete.

There is still considerable debate concerning when to start hormonal-deprivation therapy in patients with advanced prostate cancer.[67] The original recommendation to start therapy when symptoms appeared was based on the Veterans Administration Cooperative Urologic Research Group (VACURG) trials, in which no overall survival difference was demonstrated in patients who either started DES initially or crossed over to active treatment when symptoms appeared; the excess mortality was attributed to estrogen administration.[68] Because LH-RH agonists and antiandrogens are considered suitable alternatives with less cardiovascular toxicity, it is not clear whether delaying therapy is justified. Reanalysis of the original VACURG data[69] and recent combined androgen-deprivation trials[63,70] demonstrate a survival advantage for young, good-performance-status, minimal-disease patients treated initially with hormonal therapy, suggesting that early intervention before symptoms appear may be appropriate.[67] The issue of when best to start hormonal therapy is the subject of several clinical trials.[67]

CLINICAL CONTROVERSY

Older data, using DES, showed that initiation of hormonal therapy at symptom onset yielded equivalent survival to starting hormonal therapy at initial diagnosis. With equivalent survival, decreased costs, and decreased toxicity from DES, the standard of practice was to delay initiation of hormonal therapy until symptoms developed. The favorable toxicity profile of LH-RH agonists led to the re-evaluation of the starting time for therapy; current research shows that younger men with a good performance status may benefit from initiation of hormonal therapy at diagnosis, rather than waiting for symptoms to develop.

Estrogens

DES was once a mainstay of prostate cancer therapy. While very effective in androgen ablation, DES-treated patients experienced increased cardiovascular mortality.[68] LH-RH agonists, with equivalent efficacy and decreased cardiovascular toxicity, supplanted DES as a mainstay of therapy. Recent evidence suggesting that parenteral estrogen reduces or negates the adverse cardiovascular effects of estrogen has renewed interest in estrogen androgen ablation. Hedlund and colleagues compared monthly intramuscular injections of polyestradiol phosphate with total androgen blockade by orchiectomy or CAB in 915 men, showing no difference in survival or cardiovascular mortality.[50] Other available estrogenic substances, such as ethinyl estradiol, conjugated estrogens, chlorotrianisene, and polyestradiol phosphate, cost more than DES and have not been studied as extensively.

DRUG TREATMENTS OF SECOND CHOICE

Secondary or salvage therapies for patients who progress after their initial therapy depend on what was used for initial management[37]

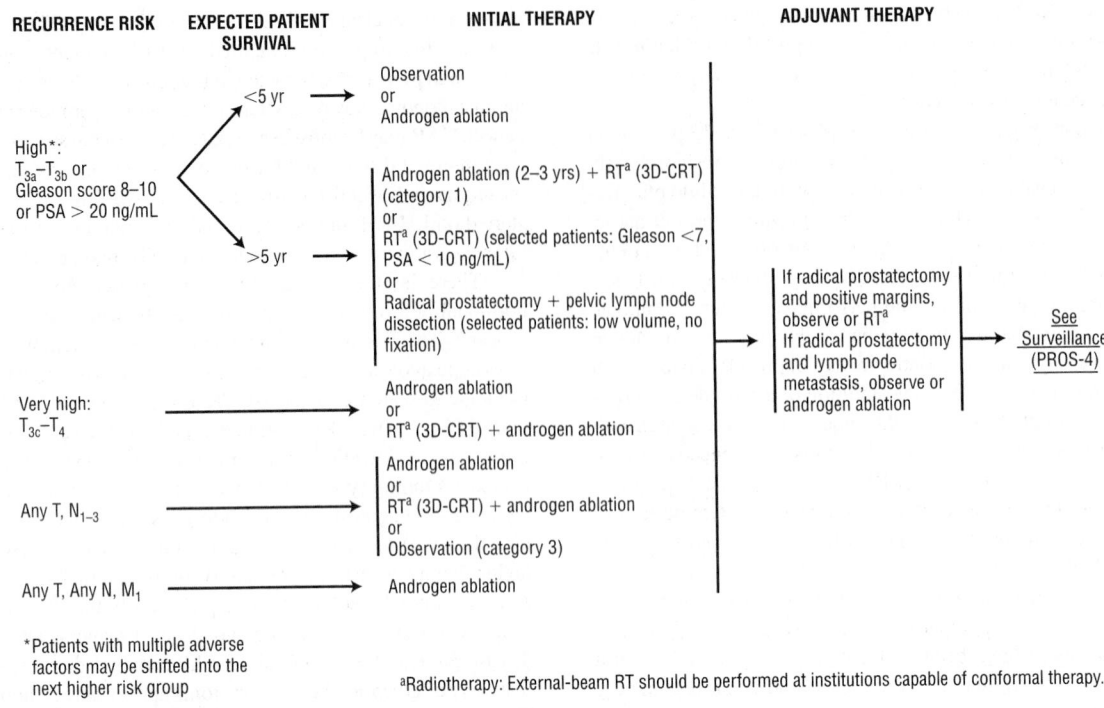

RECURRENCE RISK | EXPECTED PATIENT SURVIVAL | INITIAL THERAPY | ADJUVANT THERAPY

High*:
T_{3a}–T_{3b} or
Gleason score 8–10
or PSA > 20 ng/mL

<5 yr → Observation
or
Androgen ablation

>5 yr → Androgen ablation (2–3 yrs) + RT^a (3D-CRT) (category 1)
or
RT^a (3D-CRT) (selected patients: Gleason <7, PSA < 10 ng/mL)
or
Radical prostatectomy + pelvic lymph node dissection (selected patients: low volume, no fixation)

If radical prostatectomy and positive margins, observe or RT^a
If radical prostatectomy and lymph node metastasis, observe or androgen ablation → See Surveillance (PROS-4)

Very high:
T_{3c}–T_4 → Androgen ablation
or
RT^a (3D-CRT) + androgen ablation

Any T, N_{1-3} → Androgen ablation
or
RT^a (3D-CRT) + androgen ablation
or
Observation (category 3)

Any T, Any N, M_1 → Androgen ablation

*Patients with multiple adverse factors may be shifted into the next higher risk group

^{a}Radiotherapy: External-beam RT should be performed at institutions capable of conformal therapy.

Note: All recommendations are category 2A unless otherwise indicated.
Clinical Trials: NCCN believes that the best management of any cancer patient is in a clinical trial. Participation in clinical trials is especially encouraged.

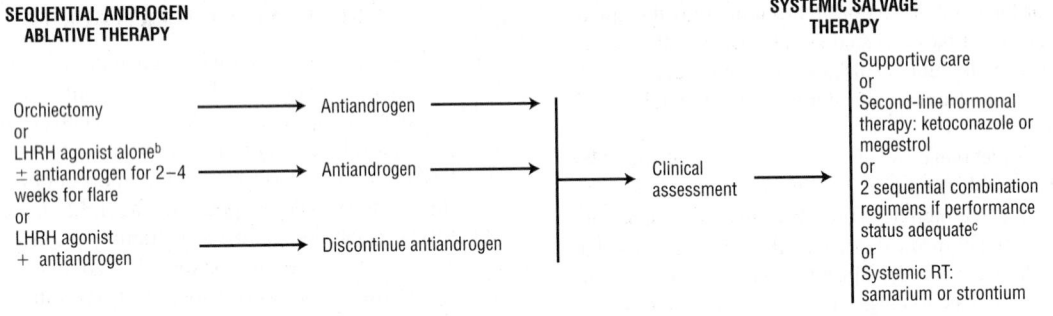

SEQUENTIAL ANDROGEN ABLATIVE THERAPY | SYSTEMIC SALVAGE THERAPY

Orchiectomy
or
LHRH agonist alone^b
± antiandrogen for 2–4 weeks for flare
or
LHRH agonist
+ antiandrogen

→ Antiandrogen →
→ Antiandrogen →
→ Discontinue antiandrogen

→ Clinical assessment →

Supportive care
or
Second-line hormonal therapy: ketoconazole or megestrol
or
2 sequential combination regimens if performance status adequate^c
or
Systemic RT: samarium or strontium

^{b}Check serum testosterone at 1 mo. If > 20 ng/dL, consider orchiectomy or adding antiandrogen.

^{c}Cytotoxic chemotherapy: Examples of regimens with documented activity in metastatic prostate cancer may include ketoconazole/doxorubicin, alternating with estramustine/vinblastine, estramustine/etoposide, mitoxantrone/prednisone, estramustine/paclitaxel, and docetaxel/estramustine.

Note: All recommendations are category 2A unless otherwise indicated.
Clinical Trials: NCCN believes that the best management of any cancer patient is in a clinical trial. Participation in clinical trials is especially encouraged.

FIGURE 128–4. Management of T_3–T_4 prostate cancer. *(Reproduced from version 1.2002, January 7, 2002. © 2002 National Comprehensive Cancer Network, Inc. All rights reserved. These guidelines and this illustration may not be reproduced in any form without the express written permission of NCCN.)*

(Fig. 128–4). For patients initially diagnosed with localized prostate cancer, radiotherapy can be used in the case of failed radical prostatectomy. Alternatively, androgen ablation can be used in patients who progress after either radiation therapy or radical prostatectomy.

Secondary hormonal manipulations, such as adding an antiandrogen to a patient who incompletely suppresses testosterone secretion with an LH-RH agonist, or withdrawing antiandrogens in a patient receiving combination therapy, or using agents that inhibit androgen synthesis, can be attempted in patients initially treated with one hormonal modality. Supportive care, chemotherapy, or local radiotherapy can be used in patients who have failed all forms of androgen-ablation manipulations because these patients are considered to have androgen-independent disease.

For patients who initially received an LH-RH agonist alone, castration testosterone levels should be documented. Patients with inadequate testosterone suppression (>20 ng/dL) can be treated by adding an antiandrogen or performing an orchiectomy. If castration testosterone levels have been achieved, the patient is considered to have androgen-independent disease, and palliative androgen-independent salvage therapy can be used.

◀**6**   If the patient initially received combined androgen blockade with an LH-RH agonist with an antiandrogen, then androgen withdrawal is the first salvage manipulation. Objective and subjective responses have been noted following the discontinuation of flutamide,[71] bicalutamide,[72] or nilutamide[73] in patients receiving these agents as part of combined androgen ablation with an LH-RH agonist. Mutations in the androgen receptor have been demonstrated that allow antiandrogens such as flutamide, bicalutamide, and nilutamide (or their metabolites) to become agonists and activate the androgen receptor.[74] Patient responses to androgen withdrawal manifest as significant PSA reductions and improved clinical symptoms. Androgen withdrawal responses lasting 3 to 14 months have been noted in up to 35% of patients, and predicting response seems to be most closely related to longer androgen exposure times.[13] Incomplete cross-resistance has been noted in some patients who received bicalutamide after they had progressed while receiving flutamide.[52] Adding an agent that blocks adrenal androgen synthesis, such as aminoglutethimide, at the time that androgens are withdrawn may produce a better response than androgen withdrawal alone.[74] Because of the potential for response immediately after antiandrogen withdrawal, a sufficient observation and assessment period (usually 4 to 6 weeks) is usually required before a patient can be enrolled on a clinical trial evaluating a new agent or therapy for advanced prostate cancer.

Androgen synthesis inhibitors, such as aminoglutethimide or ketoconazole, can provide symptomatic relief for a short time in approximately 50% of patients with progressive disease despite previous androgen-ablation therapy.[22] Adverse effects during aminoglutethimide therapy occur in approximately 50% of patients.[22] Central nervous system effects that include lethargy, ataxia, and dizziness are the major adverse reactions. A generalized morbilliform, pruritic rash has been reported in up to 30% of patients treated. The rash is usually self-limiting and resolves within 5 to 8 days with continued therapy. Adverse effects from ketoconazole include gastrointestinal intolerance, transient rises in liver and renal function tests, and hypoadrenalism.

After all hormonal manipulations are exhausted, the patient is considered to have androgen-independent disease. At this point, palliative supportive therapy is appropriate.[37,75] Palliation can be achieved by pain management, using radioisotopes such as strontium-89[76] or samarium-153 lexidronam[77] for bone-related pain, analgesics, corticosteroids, bisphosphonates,[78] or local radiotherapy.[37] Data are emerging that demonstrate that bisphosphonates such as pamidronate and zoledronic acid may prevent skeletal morbidity, such as pathologic fractures and spinal cord compression in men with hormone-refractory prostate cancer; however, other studies have shown no benefit. The early use of bisphosphonates has also been shown to prevent bone loss due to androgen deprivation therapy. The usual dose of pamidronate is 90 mg every month and the usual dose of zoledronic acid is 4 mg every 3 to 4 weeks. A trial of pamidronate or zoledronic acid can be initiated in prostate cancer patients with bone pain; if no benefit is observed, the drug may be discontinued.[79]

On May 19, 2004, docetaxel was approved for the treatment of metastatic prostate cancer. The approval was based on the TAX327 study, a randomized, multicenter global clinical trial enrolling over 1000 men with metastatic, hormone-refractory prostate cancer.[92,93] The study compared docetaxel 75 mg/m^2 every 3 weeks and prednisone 5 mg twice a day with docetaxel 35 mg/m^2 weekly five out of six weeks and prednisone 5 mg twice a day and mitoxantrone 75 ng/m^2 every 3 weeks and prednisone 5 mg twice a day. Docetaxel, in combination with prednisone, given every 3 weeks showed a survival advantage of approximately 2.5 months over the control group in the trial ($p = .009$). The most common adverse events reported were nausea, alopecia, and bone marrow suppression. In addition, fluid retention and peripheral neuropathy, known effects of docetaxel, were

also observed. Because this is the first chemotherapy regimen to show survival benefit in this setting, docetaxel and prednisone should be considered standard chemotherapy for hormone-refractory metastatic prostate cancer.

Androgen ablation is usually continued when chemotherapy is initiated.[37]

Docetaxel and prednisone have recently been shown to improve survival in hormone-refractory metastatic prostate cancer and should be considered standard therapy. Single agents with modest activity in prostate cancer include cyclophosphamide, estramustine, 5-fluorouracil, methotrexate, dacarbazine, mitoxantrone, doxorubicin, paclitaxel, gemcitabine, vinorelbine, and cisplatin.[80] If disease stabilization is included as a favorable response, response rates up to 46% have been reported.[80] Several trials have evaluated the various combination regimens containing the most active single agents.[80–82]

Both estramustine combined with vinblastine[81,83] and mitoxantrone combined with prednisone are active combination regimens for refractory prostate cancer.[84] Although estramustine as a single agent[81,89] produced similar response rates to other available chemotherapy agents, development of estramustine combinations (such as estramustine plus vinblastine or estramustine plus docetaxel) continued when its mechanism of action was discovered to involve microtubule proteins rather than alkylation.[82,83]

Estramustine and vinblastine combinations have been evaluated in several trials.[81,83] Response is manifested as objective tumor regression (partial response rate up to 50%), PSA declines, pain relief, and delay in bone scan progression. The toxicities of estramustine combined with vinblastine are nausea, gynecomastia, fatigue, and fluid retention. When vinblastine monotherapy was compared with estramustine plus vinblastine in a large phase III intergroup trial for men with metastatic androgen-independent prostate cancer, patients receiving the combination had improved time to progression and PSA improvement, although the difference in overall survival did not reach statistical significance.[86]

Mitoxantrone plus prednisone is another combination regimen that can palliate hormone-refractory prostate cancer.[84] One hundred and sixty-one patients with hormone-refractory prostate cancer with pain were randomized to receive either 10 mg/day prednisone alone, or this same prednisone dose with mitoxantrone. The primary end point was a palliative ("clinical benefit") response, as assessed by a pain scale and analgesic requirements. Quality of life was assessed with a series of linear analog health-assessment scales and the Prostate Cancer–Specific Quality of Life Instrument.

Palliative responses were noted in 29% of patients in the mitoxantrone plus prednisone group and 12% of patients in the prednisone-alone group. The duration of palliative response was greater and quality-of-life scores for pain, physical activity, constipation, and mood were better in patients who received mitoxantrone plus prednisone. Overall survival was the same in both groups. Patients treated with mitoxantrone plus prednisone experienced tolerable adverse effects, although five patients did develop some cardiac-related adverse effects. Mitoxantrone plus corticosteroids is approved by the FDA for hormone-refractory prostate cancer.

Other possible chemotherapeutic regimens suggested by the NCCN guidelines and clinical trials include ketoconazole plus doxorubicin, estramustine plus etoposide, or estramustine plus paclitaxel.[37]

Although it would seem rational that prostate cancer is a heterogeneous disease composed of cells sensitive to hormonal therapy, chemotherapy, both therapies, or neither therapy, attempts to combine endocrine therapy and chemotherapy to produce an additive effect have not produced significant response rates. When orchiectomy was compared with DES plus cyclophosphamide in a prospective, randomized trial in patients with stage D prostate cancer, the response rate, median survival, and time to progressive disease were similar between the two treatment groups.[87] Likewise, Osborne and colleagues[88] demonstrated a higher initial response rate for patients treated with hormonal therapy plus chemotherapy; however, overall median survival was similar. Furthermore, in a randomized trial involving 419 prostate cancer patients with bone metastases, subgroup analysis demonstrated that orchiectomy plus estramustine produced a longer time to progression compared with orchiectomy alone in patients less than 73 years old, although overall survival was similar.[87]

Fluoxymesterone has been used in some trials designed to test androgen-priming strategies to get the cells to cycle more rapidly and therefore be more susceptible to the effects of cytotoxic chemotherapy. However, the response rates have been inconsistent and spinal cord compression has occurred in some patients, so it appears that the risks of androgen priming outweigh the benefits.[88]

Cytotoxic chemotherapy for hormone-refractory prostate cancer may be offered to the patient as part of a clinical trial. To make the results of a clinical trial applicable to the majority of hormone-refractory prostate cancer patients, the patient populations need to be clearly defined with regard to disease extent and hormone sensitivity.[90] Likewise, responses should be quantified by accepted disease-regression measures. If surrogate markers, such as PSA changes, are used, the response needs to be described in terms of the percentage decline, the number of times the decline is documented, and the period during which the decline is maintained.[90,91] Quality-of-life end points are also appropriate outcome measures.

Many new drugs and new combinations are in development for prostate cancer management.[79] The first 38-patient trial of suramin demonstrated a 42-week median survival and significant PSA declines (greater than 75%).[94] Suramin also shows promise in combination with hydrocortisone. Other efforts include agents with novel anticancer targets and mechanisms (apoptosis inhibitors, growth factor inhibitors, and antimetastasis agents), targeted therapy (vaccines, monoclonal antibodies, or growth receptor antibodies), oncogene regulation (farnesyl transferase inhibitors), matrix metalloproteinase inhibitors, and gene therapy.[22]

PHARMACOECONOMIC CONSIDERATIONS

The main economic concerns for prostate cancer focus on prostate cancer screening for asymptomatic men, initial therapy of clinically localized disease, surgical vs. medical castration, and the use of combined hormonal blockade as treatment for advanced disease. Unfortunately, there is generally insufficient clinical evidence to determine the most appropriate therapy, making economic modeling essentially meaningless.

Prostate cancer screening remains highly controversial because the survival benefits and the associated costs are not well defined.[95] Krahn and colleagues[96] determined that annual screening of all eligible men would cost 45 million Canadian dollars, or 0.15% of total health care expenditures. Available cost-utility studies estimate that the cost per crude or quality-adjusted life-year gained from prostate cancer screening ranges from $3000 to $729,000.[95-98] Since the cost-effectiveness of prostate cancer screening cannot be determined until the benefits are documented, it is important to incorporate economic analysis into the large ongoing screening studies.

Treatment options for clinically localized prostate cancer include radiation therapy, surgery, or watchful waiting. There is currently no evidence to suggest which therapy is the most clinically effective, and treatment choice is often made by patient or physician preference. However, there are large economic differences in the therapies, with the cost of a radical prostatectomy $12,000 more expensive than watchful waiting, and radiation therapy $15,000 more expensive than watchful waiting.[99]

Surgical castration (by removal of the testes) and medical castration with LH-RH agonists yield similar clinical results, although the majority of patients prefer medical castration. In two economic analysis comparisons, the primary cost of the surgical castration was hospital length of stay and medical castration drug costs. Both analyses found that in patients surviving 18 to 24 months, a surgical castration was more cost effective.[100]

Table 128–6 lists the costs for the initial hormonal therapies for stage D_2 prostate cancer. Using a societal perspective and data from the original leuprolide plus flutamide versus leuprolide alone trial to calculate the incremental cost per life-year gained, Hillner and colleagues[97] concluded that CAB has an incremental cost-effectiveness of $25,300 per life-year gained, which is within current accepted benchmarks. The cost dropped to $13,700 per life-year gained in patients with minimal disease.

In a follow-up study, this same group used physician focus group estimates to generate quality-of-life factors and incorporated these factors into an economic model.[98] The incremental cost per quality-adjusted life-year gained seemed reasonable when data from the original CAB were used: $25,000 for patients with minimal disease and

TABLE 128–6. Comparative Costs of Hormonal Therapy for Advanced Prostate Cancer

Drug	Dose	Average Wholesale Price per Month of Therapy
Leuprolide depot	7.5 mg/mo	$566.85
Leuprolide depot	22.5 mg/12 wk	$1,700.63
Leuprolide depot	30 mg/16 wk	$2,267.50
Goserelin implant	3.6 mg every 28 days	$439.24
Goserelin implant	10.8 mg/12 wk	$1,317.74
Flutamide	750 mg/day	$315.70
Bicalutamide	50 mg/day	$319.74
Nilutamide	300 mg/day for first mo	$467.16
	then 150 mg/day	then $233.58

		Average Wholesale Price per 3 Months of Therapy
Combined androgen blockade		
Leuprolide depot 22.5 mg/12 wk		
+ flutamide	750 mg/day	$2,647.97
+ bicalutamide	50 mg/day	$2,659.85
+ nilutamide	150 mg/day	$2,401.37
		($2,634.95 1st month)
Goserelin depot 10.8 mg/12 wk		
+ flutamide	750 mg/day	$2,265.08
+ bicalutamide	50 mg/day	$2,270.96
+ nilutamide	150 mg/day	$2,018.48
		($2,252.06 1st month)

Compiled from Drug Topics, Annual Pharmacists' Reference (Redbook). Oradell, NJ, Medical Economics, 1998.

$18,000 for patients with severe disease. However, these incremental costs increased dramatically to $53,700 for patients with minimal disease and $41,000 for patients with severe disease when the same model was applied to survival data from a meta-analysis.

Because there is considerable debate about the value of using CAB for advanced prostate cancer, continued economic assessments of this therapy will be crucial to help policymakers and clinicians decide on the most appropriate therapy. It also will become very important to incorporate economic analyses into chemotherapy trials because these efforts move toward including clinical benefit response as a main end point.

EVALUATION OF THERAPEUTIC OUTCOMES

Monitoring of prostate cancer depends on the stage of the cancer.[37] When definitive, curative therapy is attempted, objective parameters to assess tumor response include assessment of the primary tumor size, evaluation of involved lymph nodes, and the response of tumor markers such as PSA to treatment. Following definitive therapy, the PSA level is checked every 6 months for the first 5 years, then annually. Local recurrence in the absence of a rising PSA may occur, so the DRE is also performed. In the metastatic setting, clinical benefit responses can be documented by evaluating performance status changes, weight changes, quality of life, and analgesic requirements, in addition to the PSA or DRE at 3-month intervals.

FUTURE DIRECTIONS

Prostate cancer occurs in older males and is curable when local disease is present. Efforts are underway to better define screening and early detection approaches and to determine how best to use PSA as a screening, diagnostic, and therapeutic monitoring test. Proper staging at initial patient presentation is essential because the therapy intensity will depend on the disease stage. Patients with localized prostate cancer can be managed effectively with surgery or radiation therapy. For patients with advanced disease, there are many treatment options. Androgen-ablative therapy is very effective for symptom palliation. Initial androgen-ablative measures include orchiectomy or an LH-RH agonist. CAB using an antiandrogen with either orchiectomy or an LH-RH agonist is used routinely despite equivocal studies and its cost. The effects of androgen ablation seem most pronounced in patients with minimal disease. Studies are still ongoing to define the best initial therapy, to determine when to start initial therapy, to identify which patient subpopulation might benefit best from a given treatment modality, and to identify which surrogate markers should be used to monitor disease activity.

Secondary therapies, including alternate hormonal therapies, antiandrogen withdrawal in a patient receiving CAB, chemotherapy, local radiotherapy, or supportive care can provide disease palliation. Continued efforts to develop new agents with novel mechanisms of action that prolong survival are ongoing. Further insight into the molecular basis for prostate cancer development may provide new therapeutic approaches.

ABBREVIATIONS

ACS: American Cancer Society
AUS: American Urologic System
BPH: benign prostatic hyperplasia

CAB: combined androgen blockade
DES: diethylstilbestrol
DHT: dihydrotestosterone
DRE: digital rectal examination
EGF: epidermal growth factor
FSH: follicle-stimulating hormone
IGF: insulin-like growth factor
LH: luteinizing hormone
LH-RH: luteinizing hormone–releasing hormone
NCCN: National Comprehensive Cancer Network
NCI: National Cancer Institute
PCPT: Prostate Cancer Prevention Trial
PSA: prostate-specific antigen
TRUS: transrectal ultrasound
VACURG: Veterans Administration Cooperative Urologic Research Group

Review Questions and other resources can be found at *www.pharmacotherapyonline.com.*

REFERENCES

1. Jemal A, Murray T, Ward E, et al. Cancer statistics, 2005. CA Cancer J Clin 2005;55:10–30.
2. Carter BS, Beaty TH, Steinberg GD, et al. Mendelian inheritance of familial prostate cancer. Proc Natl Acad Sci USA 1992;89:3367–3372.
3. Hsieh K, Albertsen PC. Populations at high risk for prostate cancer. Urol Clin North Am 2003;30:669–676.
4. Ross R, Coetzee GA, Reichardt J, et al. Does the racial-ethnic variation in prostate cancer have a hormonal basis? Cancer 1995;75:1778–1882.
5. Denis L, Morton MD, Griffiths K. Diet and its preventative role in prostate cancer. Eur Urol 1999;35:377–387.
6. Crawford ED. Epidemiology of prostate cancer. Urology 2003; 62(6 Suppl 1):3–12.
7. Norrish AE, Jackson RT, Sharpe SJ, Skeaff CM. Prostate cancer and dietary carotenoids. Am J Epidemiol 2000;15:124–127.
8. Visakorpi T. The molecular genetics of prostate cancer. Urology 2003; 62(5 Suppl 1):3–10.
9. Theodorescu D, Broder SR, Boyd JC, et al. p53, bcl-2 and retinoblastoma proteins as long-term prognostic markers in localized carcinoma of the prostate. J Urol 1997;158:131–137.
10. Rakozy C, Grignon DJ, Li Y, et al. p53 gene alteration in prostate cancer after radiation failure and their association with clinical outcome: A molecular and immunohistochemical analysis. Pathol Res Pract 1999;195:129–135.
11. Dong JT, Suzuki H, Pin SS, et al. Down-regulation of the KAI1 metastasis suppressor gene during the progression of human prostatic cancer infrequently involves gene mutation or allelic loss. Cancer Res 1996;56: 4387–4390.
12. Gottlieb B, Beitel LK, Lumbrosso R, et al. Update of the androgen receptor gene mutations database. Hum Mutat 1999;14:103–114.
13. Sommer A, Haendler B. Androgen receptor and prostate cancer: molecular aspects and gene expression profiling. Curr Opin Drug Discov Devel 2003;6:702–711.
14. Kelly WK, Slovin S, Scher HI. Steroid hormone withdrawal syndromes: Pathophysiology and clinical significance. Urol Clin North Am 1997;24:421–431.
15. Takahashi H, Furusato M, Allsbrook WC, et al. Prevalence of androgen receptor gene mutations in latent prostatic carcinomas from Japanese men. Cancer Res 1995;55:1621–1624.
16. Frydenberg M, Stricker PD, Kaye KW. Prostate cancer diagnosis and management. Lancet 1997;349:1681–1687.
17. Gleason DF. Histologic grade, clinical stage, and patient age in prostate cancer. Natl Cancer Inst Mongr 1988;7:15–18.

18. De Marzo AM. Meeker AK, Zha S, et al. Human prostate cancer precursors and pathobiology. Urology 2003;62(5 Suppl 1):55–62.

19. Culig Z. Role of the androgen receptor axis in prostate cancer. Urology 2003;62(5 Suppl 1):21–26.

20. Huggins C, Hodges CV. Studies on prostatic cancer: 1. The effect of castration, of estrogen, and of androgen injection on serum phosphatases in metastatic carcinoma of the prostate. Cancer Res 1941;1:293–297.

21. Marks LS. Luteinizing hormone-releasing hormone agonists in the treatment of men with prostate cancer: Timing, alternatives, and the 1-year implant. Urology 2003;62(6 Suppl 1):36–42.

22. Oh WK. Secondary hormonal therapies in the treatment of prostate cancer. Urology 2002;60(3 Suppl 1):87–92.

23. Anderson J. The role of antiandrogen monotherapy in the treatment of prostate cancer. BJU Int 2003;91:455–461.

24. Thompson IM, Goodman PJ, Tangen CM, et al. The influence of finasteride on the development of prostate cancer. N Engl J Med 2003;349:215–224.

25. Ung JO, Richie JP, Chen MH, et al. Evolution of the presentation and pathologic and biochemical outcomes after radical prostatectomy for patients with clinically localized prostate cancer diagnosed during the PSA era. Urology 2002;60:458–463.

26. Marberger M, Adolfsson J, Borkowski A, et al. The clinical implications of the prostate cancer prevention trial. BJU Int 2003;92:667–671.

27. Duffield-Lillico AJ, Slate EH, Reid ME, et al, and Nutritional Prevention of Cancer Study Group. Selenium supplementation and secondary prevention of nonmelanoma skin cancer in a randomized trial. J Natl Cancer Inst 2003;95:1477–1481.

28. Klein EA. Clinical models for testing chemopreventative agents in prostate cancer and overview of SELECT: The Selenium and Vitamin E Cancer Prevention Trial. Recent Results Cancer Res 2003;163:212–225.

29. Schmid HP, Prikler L, Semjonow A. Problems with prostate-specific antigen screening: A critical review. Recent Results Cancer Res 2003;163:226–231.

30. Galic J, Karner I, Cenan L, et al. Role of screening in detection of clinically localized prostate cancer. Coll Antropol 2003;27(Suppl 1):49–54.

31. Gohagan JK, Prorok PC, Kramer BS, et al. The prostate, lung, colorectal, and ovarian cancer screening trial of the National Cancer Institute. Cancer 1995;75:1869–1873.

32. Wilson SS, Crawford ED. Screening for prostate cancer: Current recommendations. Urol Clin North Am 2004;31:219–226.

33. Catalona WJ, Smith DS, Ratliff TL, et al. Measurement of prostate-specific antigen in serum as a screening test for prostate cancer. N Engl J Med 1991;324:1156–1161.

34. Ross KS, Carter HB, Pearson JD, Guess HA. Comparative efficacy of prostate specific antigen screening strategies for prostate cancer detection. JAMA 2000;284:1399–1405.

35. Volk R, Cass AR, Spann SJ. A randomized controlled trial of shared decision making for prostate cancer screening. Arch Fam Med 1999;8:333–340.

36. Wilt TJ, Brawer MK. Early intervention or expectant management for prostate cancer. The Prostate Cancer Intervention Versus Observation Trial (PIVOT): A randomized trial comparing radical prostatectomy with expectant management for the treatment of clinically localized prostate cancer. Semin Urol 1995;13:130–136.

37. Scherr D, Swindle PW, Scardino PT. National Comprehensive Cancer Network. National Comprehensive Cancer Network guidelines for the management of prostate cancer. Urology 2003;61(2 Suppl 1):14–24.

38. Montie JE. Staging of prostate cancer: Current TNM classification and future prospects for prognostic factors. Cancer 1995;75(Suppl):1814–1818.

39. Kumar-Sinha C, Rhodes DR, Yu J, Chinnaiyan AM. Prostate cancer biomarkers: a current perspective. Exp Rev Molec Diagn 2003;3:459–470.

40. Hoeksema M, Law C. Cancer mortality rates fall: A turning point for the nation. J Natl Cancer Inst 1996;88:1706–1707.

41. Scardino PT, Weaver R, Hudson MA. Early detection of prostate cancer. Hum Pathol 1992;23:211–222.

42. Schroder FH, de Vries SH, Bangma CH. Watchful waiting in prostate cancer: review and policy proposals. BJU Int 2003;92:851–859.

43. Scher HI. Prostate carcinoma: Defining therapeutic objectives and improving overall outcomes. Cancer 2003;97(3 Suppl):758–771.

44. Akakura A, Isaka S, Akimoto S, et al. Long-term results of a randomized trial for the treatment of stages B2 and C prostate cancer: Radical prostatectomy versus external beam radiation with a common endocrine therapy in both modalities. Urology 1999;54:313–318.

45. Walsh PC, Partin AW, Epstein JI. Cancer control and quality of life following anatomical radical retropubic prostatectomy: Results at 10 years. J Urol 1994;152:1831–1836.

46. Pilepich MV, Winter K, John MJ, et al. Phase III radiation therapy oncology group (RTOG) trial 86-10 of androgen deprivation adjuvant to definitive radiotherapy in locally advanced carcinoma of the prostate. Int J Radiat Oncol Biol Phys 2001;50:1243–1252.

47. Roach M. Hormonal therapy and radiotherapy for localized prostate cancer: Who, where and how long? J Urol 2003;170(6 Pt 2):S35–S40; discussion S40–1.

48. Medical Research Council Prostate Cancer Working Party Investigators Group. Immediate versus deferred treatment for advanced prostate cancer: Initial results of the Medical Research Council Trial. Br J Urol 1997;79:235–246.

49. Prostate Cancer Trialist's Collaborative Group. Maximum androgen blockade in advanced prostate cancer: An overview of the randomised trials. Lancet 2000;355:1491–1498.

50. Hedlund PO, Henriksson P. Parenteral estrogen versus total androgen blockade in the treatment of advanced prostate carcinoma: Effects of overall survival and cardiovascular mortality. Urology 2000;55:328–333.

51. Seidenfield J, Samson DJ, Hasselblad V, et al. Single therapy androgen suppression in men with advanced prostate cancer: A systematic review and meta analysis. Ann Intern Med 2000;132:566–577.

52. Scher H, Leibertz C, Kelly W, et al. Bicalutamide for advanced prostate cancer: The natural history versus treated history of disease. J Clin Oncol 1997;15:2928–2938.

53. Bales G, Chodak G. A controlled trial of bicalutamide versus castration in patients with advanced prostate cancer. Urology 1996;47:38–43.

54. Decensi A, Bocardo F, Guarneri D, et al. Monotherapy with nilutamide, a pure nonsteroidal antiandrogen, in untreated patients with metastatic carcinoma of the prostate. J Urol 1991;146:377–381.

55. Boccardo F, Rubagotti A, Barichello M, et al. Bicalutamide monotherapy versus flutamide plus gosrelin in prostate cancer patients: Results of an Italian Prostate Cancer Project study. J Clin Oncol 1999;17:2027–2038.

56. Schellhammer P, Sharifi R, Block N, et al. A controlled trial of bicalutamide versus flutamide, each in combination with luteinizing hormone-releasing hormone analogue therapy, in patients with advanced prostate cancer. Casodex Combination Study Group. Urology 1995;45:745–752.

57. Labrie F, Dupont A, Simard J, et al. Intracrinology: The basis for the rational design of endocrine therapy at all stages of prostate cancer. Eur Urol 1993;2:94–105.

58. Labrie F, Dupont A, Cusan L, et al. Combination therapy with flutamide and medical (LH-RH agonist) or surgical castration in advanced prostate cancer: 7-year clinical experience. J Steroid Biochem Mol Biol 1990;37:943–950.

59. Eisenberger M, Crawford ED, Blumenstein B, et al. National Cancer Institute Integroup Study 0036. Prognostic factors in stage D2 prostate cancer: Important implications for future trials: Results of a cooperative intergroup study (INT 0036). Semin Oncol 1994;21:613–619.

60. Tyrell CJ, Altwein JE, Klippel F, et al. Comparison of an LH-RH analogue with combined androgen blockade in advanced prostate cancer. Eur Urol 2000;37:205–211.

61. Iversen P, Rasmussen F, Klarskov P, Christensen IJ. Long-term results of Danish Prostatic Cancer Group Trial 86: Goserelin acetate plus flutamide versus orchiectomy in advanced prostate cancer. Cancer 1993;72:3851–3854.

62. Tyrell CJ, Altwein JE, Klippel F, et al. Multicenter randomized trial comparing Zoladex with Zoladex plus flutamide in the treatment of advanced prostate cancer: Survival update. International Prostate Cancer Study Group. Cancer 1993;72:3878–3879.

63. Denis LJ, Carnelro de Moura JL, Bono A, et al. Goserelin acetate and flutamide versus bilateral orchiectomy: A phase III EORTC trial (30853). EORTC GU Group and EORTC Data Center. Urology 1993;42:119–129.

64. Eisenberger MA, Blumenstein BA, Crawford ED, et al. Bilateral orchiectomy with or without flutamide for metastatic prostate cancer. N Engl J Med 1998;339:1036–1042.

65. Moul JW, Fowler JE Jr. Evolution of therapeutic approaches with luteinizing hormone-releasing hormone agonists in 2003. Urology 2003; 62(6 Suppl 1):20–28.

66. Schellhammer P, Sharifi R, Block N, et al. A controlled trial of bicalutamide versus flutamide, each in combination with luteinizing hormone-releasing hormone analogue therapy, in patients with advanced prostate carcinoma: Analysis of time to progression. Cancer 1996;78:2164–2169.

67. Mazeman E, Bertrand P. Early versus delayed hormonal therapy in advanced prostate cancer [Discussion 49]. Eur Urol 1996;30(Suppl 1):40–43.

68. The Veterans Administration Cooperative Urological Research Group. Carcinoma of the prostate: Treatment comparisons. J Urol 1967;98:516–522.

69. Byar DP, Corle DK. Hormone therapy for prostate cancer: Results of the Veterans Administration Cooperative Urologic Research Group studies. Natl Cancer Inst Monogr 1988;7:165–170.

70. Denis L, Murphy GP. Overview of phase III trials on combined androgen treatment in patients with metastatic prostate cancer. Cancer 1993; 72:3888–3895.

71. Scher HI, Kelly WK. Flutamide withdrawal syndrome: Its impact on clinical trials in hormone refractory prostate cancer. J Clin Oncol 1993;11:1566–1572.

72. Small E, Srinivas S. The androgen withdrawal syndrome: Experience in a large cohort of unselected patients with advanced prostate cancer. Cancer 1995;76:1428–1434.

73. Huan SD, Gerridzen RG, Yau JC, Stewart DJ. Antiandrogen withdrawal syndrome with nilutamide. Urology 1997;49:632–634.

74. Sartor O, Cooper M, Weinberger M, et al. Surprising activity of flutamide withdrawal, when combined with aminoglutethimide, in treatment of hormone-refractory prostate cancer. J Natl Cancer Inst 1994;86:222–227.

75. Esper PS, Pienta KJ. Supportive care in the patient with hormone refractory prostate cancer. Semin Urol Oncol 1997;15:56–64.

76. Crawford ED, Kozlowski JM, Debruyne FM, et al. The use of strontium 89 for palliation of pain from bone metastases associated with hormone-refractory prostate cancer. Urology 1994;44:481–485.

77. Resche I, Chatal JF, Pecking A, et al. A dose-controlled study of 153 Sm-ethylenediaminetetramethylenephosphonate (EDTMP) in the treatment of patients with painful bone metastases. Eur J Cancer 1997;33:1583–1591.

78. Posadas EM, Dahut WL, Gulley J. The emerging role of bisphosphonates in prostate cancer. Am J Ther 2004;11:60–73.

79. Moyer P. New treatment hope for prostate cancer. Lancet Oncol 2004;5:5.

80. Siu LL, Moore MJ. Other chemotherapy regimens including mitoxantrone and suramin. Semin Urol Oncol 1997;15:20–27.

81. Seidman AD, Scher HI, Petrylak D, et al. Estramustine and vinblastine: Use of prostate specific antigen as a clinical trial end point for hormone refractory prostatic cancer. J Urol 1992;147:931–934.

82. Hudes G. Estramustine-based chemotherapy. Semin Urol Oncol 1997;15:13–19.

83. Perry CM, McTavish D. Estramustine phosphate sodium: A review of its pharmacodynamic and pharmacokinetic properties, and therapeutic efficacy in prostate cancer. Drugs Aging 1995;7:49–74.

84. Tannock IF, Osoba D, Stockler MR, et al. Chemotherapy with mitoxantrone plus prednisone or prednisone alone for symptomatic hormone-resistant prostate cancer: A Canadian randomized trial with palliative end points. J Clin Oncol 1996;14:1756–1764.

85. Iversen P, Rasmussen F, Asmussen C, et al. Estramustine phosphate versus placebo as second line treatment after orchiectomy in patients with metastatic prostate cancer. DAPROCA study 9002. Danish Prostatic Cancer Group. J Urol 1997;157:929–934.

86. Hudes G, Einhorn L, Ross E, et al. Vinblastine versus vinblastine plus oral estramustine phosphate for patients with hormone refractory prostate cancer. J Clin Oncol 1999;17:3160–166.

87. Murphy GP, Beckley S, Brady MF, et al. Treatment of newly diagnosed metastatic prostate cancer patients with chemotherapy agents in combination with hormones versus hormones alone. Cancer 1983;51:1264–1272.

88. Osborne CK, Blumenstein B, Crawford ED, et al. Combined versus sequential chemo-endocrine therapy in advanced prostate cancer: Final results of a randomized southwest oncology group study. J Clin Oncol 1990;8:1675–1682.

89. Janknegt RA, Boon TA, van de Beek C, Grob P. Combined hormono/chemotherapy as primary treatment for metastatic prostate cancer: A randomized, multicenter study of orchiectomy alone versus orchiectomy plus estramustine phosphate. The Dutch Estracyt Study Group. Urology 1997;49:411–420.

90. Scher HI, Mazumdar M, Kelly WK. Clinical trials in relapsed prostate cancer: Defining the target. J Natl Cancer Inst 1996;88:1623–1634.

91. Kelly WK, Slovin S, Scher HI. Clinical use of posttherapy prostate-specific antigen changes in advanced prostate cancer. Semin Oncol 1996;23:8–14.

92. Petrylak DP, Macarthur R, O'Connor J, et al. Phase I/II studies of docetaxel combined with estramustine in men with hormone refractory prostate cancer. Semin Oncol 1999;26:28–33.

93. Eisenberger MA, DeWit R, Berry W, et al. A multicenter phase III comparison of docetaxel + prednisone and mitoxantvone + prednisone in patients with hormone-refractory prostate cancer. 2004 ASCO Annual Meeting Proceedings (Post-Meeting Edition). Vol. 22, (July 15 Supplement), 2004:2s (abstract no. 4).

94. Hussain M, Fisher EI, Petrylak DP, et al. Androgen deprivation and four courses of fixed-schedule suramin treatment in patients with newly diagnosed metastatic prostate cancer. J Clin Oncol 2000;18:1043–1049.

95. Benoit RM, Naslund MJ. The economics of prostate cancer screening. Oncology (Huntingt) 1997;11:1533–1543.

96. Krahn MD, Coombs AB, Levy IG. Current and projected annual direct costs of screening asymptomatic men for prostate cancer using prostate specific antigen. CMAJ 1999;160:49–57.

97. Hillner BE, McLeod DG, Crawford ED, Bennett CL. Estimating the cost-effectiveness of total androgen blockade with flutamide in M1 prostate cancer. Urology 1995;45:633–640.

98. Bennett CL, Matchar D, McCrory D, et al. Cost-effective models for flutamide for prostate carcinoma patients: Are they helpful to policy makers? Cancer 1996;77:1854–1861.

99. Turini M, Redaelli A, Gramegna P, Radice D. Quality of life and economic considerations in the management of prostate cancer. Pharmacoeconomics 2003;21:527–541.

100. Hummel S, Paisley S, Morgan A, et al. Clinical and cost-effectiveness of new and emerging technologies for early localised prostate cancer: A systematic review. Health Technol Assess 2003;7:iii, ix–x, 1–157.

129
LYMPHOMAS
Val R. Adams and Gary C. Yee

Learning Objectives and other resources can be found at *www.pharmacotherapyonline.com.*

KEY CONCEPTS

❶ The goal of treatment of patients with Hodgkin's lymphoma is cure, regardless of disease spread or prognostic factors.

❷ Most patients with early-stage Hodgkin's lymphoma should be treated with involved-field radiation and several cycles of combination chemotherapy.

❸ Combination chemotherapy with doxorubicin (Adriamycin), bleomycin, vinblastine, and dacarbazine (ABVD) is the primary treatment for patients with advanced-stage Hodgkin's lymphoma. Patients who attain a complete response do not require consolidative radiation therapy, but patients who only achieve a partial response may benefit from involved-field radiation.

❹ Many patients with Hodgkin's lymphoma will be refractory to initial therapy or will have a recurrence following a complete remission. Response to salvage therapy depends on the extent and site of recurrence, previous therapy, and duration of initial remission. High-dose chemotherapy and autologous hematopoietic stem cell transplantation should be considered in patients with refractory or relapsed disease.

❺ The current classification system for non-Hodgkin's lymphoma is the Revised European-American Classification of Lymphoid Neoplasms and World Health Organization (REAL-WHO) classification system, which is based on the principle that a classification is a list of specific disease entities defined by a combination of morphology, immunophenotype, genetic features, and clinical features.

❻ The Ann Arbor staging system correlates poorly with prognosis in non-Hodgkin's lymphoma. Several prognostic models have been developed to estimate prognosis in patients with non-Hodgkin's lymphoma. The International Prognostic Index (IPI) score is a well-established model for patients with aggressive non-Hodgkin's lymphomas. It is hoped that the Follicular Lymphoma International Prognostic Index (FLIPI) will become a useful model for patients with indolent lymphomas.

❼ The clinical behavior and degree of aggressiveness can be used to categorize non-Hodgkin's lymphoma into indolent and aggressive lymphomas. Patients with an indolent lymphoma usually have a relatively long survival, with or without aggressive chemotherapy. Although these lymphomas respond to a wide range of therapeutic approaches, few if any of these patients are cured of their disease. In contrast, aggressive lymphomas are rapidly growing tumors and patients have a short survival if appropriate therapy is not initiated. Many patients with aggressive lymphomas respond to intensive chemotherapy and some are cured of their disease.

❽ Patients with localized follicular lymphoma can be cured with radiation therapy alone. Advanced follicular lymphoma is not curable, and there are many treatment options, including watchful waiting, extended-field radiation therapy, single-agent alkylating agents, anthracycline-containing combination chemotherapy, purine analogues, interferon alfa, anti-CD20 monoclonal antibodies, and high-dose chemotherapy with hematopoietic stem cell rescue.

❾ Patients with localized aggressive lymphomas can be cured with several cycles of cyclophosphamide, hydroxydaunomycin (doxorubicin), vincristine (Oncovin), and prednisone (CHOP) chemotherapy and involved-field irradiation. Patients with bulky stage II, stage III, or stage IV aggressive lymphomas can be cured of their disease with CHOP chemotherapy. The addition of rituximab to CHOP (R-CHOP) is used by many centers in place of CHOP.

❿ Conventional-dose salvage therapy can induce responses in patients with aggressive lymphomas who relapse, but long-term survival and cure is uncommon. Some patients with aggressive lymphoma who relapse and respond to salvage therapy can be cured with high-dose chemotherapy and autologous hematopoietic stem cell transplantation.

Lymphomas are a heterogeneous group of malignancies that arise from malignant transformation of immune cells that reside predominantly in lymphoid tissues. They most commonly present as a solid tumor, but can sometimes present as circulating tumor cells in peripheral blood. The differing histology of lymphoma cells has led to classification of Hodgkin's lymphoma (Reed-Sternberg cells) or non-Hodgkin's lymphoma (B- or T-cell lymphocyte markers). Non-Hodgkin's lymphomas (NHLs) are further classified into distinct clinical entities, which are defined by a combination of morphology, immunophenotype, genetic features, and clinical features.

Chemotherapy is the mainstay of treatment in patients with lymphoma, especially those with widespread disease. Overall cure rates are high for many subtypes of lymphomas, even when patients present with advanced disease.

HODGKIN'S LYMPHOMA

Thomas Hodgkin first described the mysterious disease of the lymph system that bears his name in 1932. Hodgkin's disease is a form of lymphoma, the cause of which is still unknown, and is fatal in more than 90% of patients untreated for 2 to 3 years. Studies have demonstrated the orderly spread of this disease. The prognosis for patients with Hodgkin's lymphoma is primarily determined by stage, presence or absence of systemic symptoms, presence of absence of a large mass, and the use of appropriate therapy. When appropriate therapy is given, more than 75% of all newly diagnosed Hodgkin's lymphoma patients will be cured. This extraordinary success has not been without cost. The treatment programs are intense, technically demanding, and associated with considerable acute toxicity and long-term complications. The long-term effects, particularly secondary malignancies, account for a higher cumulative mortality than Hodgkin's lymphoma 15 to 20 years after treatment. Long-term toxicities with standard chemotherapy regimens have been more fully documented in recent years and are shaping future therapies.[1-4]

EPIDEMIOLOGY

It is estimated that nearly 7350 new cases of Hodgkin's lymphoma will be diagnosed in the United States in 2005, which represents less than 1% of all known cancers.[5] It is expected that there will be 1410 deaths associated with Hodgkin's lymphoma during this same time. This disease occurs slightly more frequently in males than in females. Once thought to be only a disease of the young, it is now recognized that Hodgkin's lymphoma exhibits a bimodal distribution in industrialized countries. The first peak occurs between the ages of 15 and 40 (usually 25 to 30) and again in those older than 55.[6] In recent years, the incidence has increased in younger patients and declined in those over 40, which may be due to more accurate diagnosis of lymphoid malignancies in this age group.[7] The 5- and 10-year overall survival for all stages according to the SEER database is 82% and 76%, respectively.[8] Death rates due to recurrent Hodgkin's lymphoma are less than those from other causes 15 years after treatment.[9]

ETIOLOGY

The etiology of Hodgkin's lymphoma is unknown. The cause of Hodgkin's lymphoma has been elusive for several reasons. Tissue taken from a Hodgkin's lymphoma mass reveals that only 1% to 2% of the cells are Reed-Sternberg cells (malignant), which has made it difficult to study.[2] Infection has been considered a potential cause of Hodgkin's lymphoma since the disease was first described. Viruses have emerged as the leading candidates for an infectious etiology. Studies have suggested an increased risk of Hodgkin's lymphoma in patients who have been infected with the Epstein-Barr virus (EBV). Reed-Sternberg cells (large, bilobate, multinuclear cells) are the malignant cells in Hodgkin's lymphoma, although they have also been found in mononucleosis patients. Consequently, the diagnosis of Hodgkin's lymphoma requires the presence of Reed-Sternberg cells and a history and physical examination consistent with the diagnosis of Hodgkin's lymphoma. Both serologic and molecular methods have linked EBV to Hodgkin's lymphoma, particularly in patients

over the age of 50 years.[6,10] Homosexual men infected with human immunodeficiency virus (HIV) are also at a slightly increased risk of developing Hodgkin's lymphoma. Occasional geographic clusters of cases further support the linkage between Hodgkin's lymphoma and an infectious agent. Genetic factors also predispose people to Hodgkin's lymphoma. The risk of Hodgkin's lymphoma is increased slightly in individuals with certain human leukocyte antigen types and in people with ataxia telangiectasia. The strongest evidence suggesting that genes are important in the etiology of Hodgkin's lymphoma comes from identical twin studies, which show that the unaffected identical twin has about a 100-fold increase in risk. Other environmental risk factors have been linked with Hodgkin's lymphoma, but only appear to play a minor role.[2,6,10,11]

PATHOPHYSIOLOGY

Hodgkin's lymphoma is a clonal malignant lymphoid disease of transformed lymphocytes. The malignant cell in Hodgkin's lymphoma is known as "Reed-Sternberg" after Dr. Carl Sternberg and Dr. Dorothy Reed who are credited with the first definitive microscopic description of Hodgkin's lymphoma in 1898 and 1902, respectively.[2] The origin of the Reed-Sternberg cell has eluded scientists because of the inability to isolate and analyze these cells to the necessary depth. A typical Hodgkin's lymphoma mass occurs in a lymph node and contains normal reactive and inflammatory cells, fibrosis, and a relatively small percentage (1% to 2%) of Reed-Sternberg cells. In recent years, new laboratory techniques have led to significant progress in identifying the origin of the Reed-Sternberg cell. Single-cell polymerase chain reaction (PCR) and DNA microarray analysis indicate that nearly all classic Hodgkin's lymphoma cases and all nodular lymphocyte-predominant Hodgkin's lymphomas have immunoglobulin gene rearrangements, which indicates a germinal center or postgerminal center B-cell origin (Table 129–1).[10,11] Interestingly, nearly all Reed-Sternberg cells fail to express B-cell specific cell surface proteins (CD19, CD20, CD79α). Current hypotheses about the transforming event and malignant process indicate that B-cell transcriptional processes are disrupted, which prevent B-cell surface marker expression and production of immunoglobulin mRNA. The normal cellular

TABLE 129–1. B-Cell Development and the Corresponding Neoplasm Derived at Each Stage

		B-Cells	Corresponding Neoplasm
Foreign antigen independent	Bone marrow	Stem cell	
		Pro-B-cell	
		Pre-B-cell	B-LBL/ALL
		Immature B-cell	
Foreign antigen dependent	Peripheral lymphoid tissue	Mature naïve B-cell	B-CLL, MCL
		Germinal center	BL, FL, LPHL, DLBCL, cHL
		Memory B-cell	MZL, B-CLL
Terminal differentiation		Plasma cell	Plasmacytoma/ myeloma

ALL, acute lymphocytic leukemia; BL, Burkitt lymphoma; B-CLL, B-cell chronic lymphocytic leukemia; B-LBL, B-cell lymphoblastic lymphoma; cHL, classic Hodgkin's lymphoma; DLBCL, diffuse large B-cell lymphoma; FL, follicular lymphoma; LPHL, lymphocyte-predominant Hodgkin's lymphoma; MCL, mantle cell lymphoma; MZL, marginal zone B-cell lymphoma.
Adapted from Harris et al.[42]

consequence of failure to express immunoglobulin is apoptosis, but due to alterations in the normal apoptotic pathways, cell survival and proliferation are favored. Reed-Sternberg cells have been shown to overexpress nuclear factor-κB, which is associated with cell proliferation and anti-apoptotic signals. Infections with viral and bacterial pathogens upregulate nuclear factor-κB and consequently are hypothesized to be involved with the etiology of Hodgkin's lymphoma.[10,11] This hypothesis is supported by the finding of EBV in many Hodgkin's lymphoma tumors, but it is important to note that not all tumors are associated with EBV.[12] As molecular techniques continue to improve, our understanding of the pathophysiology of Hodgkin's lymphoma will also improve.

The histopathologic classification of Hodgkin's lymphoma has undergone numerous changes over the last three decades. The current classification system used today is the WHO modification of the Revised European-American Classification of Lymphoid Neoplasms (Table 129–2).[13] This classification divides Hodgkin's lymphoma into two major groups: classical Hodgkin's lymphoma (cHL) and nodular lymphocyte-predominant Hodgkin's disease (NLPHD), which constitute approximately 95% and 5% of cases, respectively. Classical Hodgkin's lymphoma is further divided into four subtypes: nodular sclerosis, mixed cellularity, lymphocyte-depletion, and lymphocyte-rich. The subtypes in these classification systems are based on characteristics of the Reed-Sternberg cell, the surrounding cells, and connective tissue. Nodular sclerosis has features that make it distinct from the other three subtypes, which represent a continuum of background cellularity, with lymphocyte-predominance being the most cellular and lymphocyte-depletion being the least cellular. Nodular lymphocyte-predominant Hodgkin's lymphoma is separated because of its distinct immunophenotype: CD15$^-$, CD20$^+$, CD30$^-$, and CD45$^+$ (the opposite of classical Hodgkin's disease).[11] With the introduction of extensive staging, sophisticated megavolt radiotherapy, and effective combination chemotherapy, the true prognostic value of these subtypes is becoming less clear.

TABLE 129–2. WHO Classification of Lymphoid Malignancies

B Cell	T Cell	Hodgkin's Disease
Precursor B cell neoplasm	Precursor T cell neoplasm	Nodular lymphocyte-predominant Hodgkin's disease
Precursor B lymphoblastic leukemia/lymphoma (precursor B cell acute lymphoblastic leukemia)	**Precursor T lymphoblastic lymphoma/leukemia (precursor T cell acute lymphoblastic leukemia)**	
Mature (peripheral) B cell neoplasms	Mature (peripheral) T cell neoplasms	Classical Hodgkin's disease
B cell chronic lymphocytic leukemia/small lymphocytic lymphoma	T cell prolymphocytic leukemia	Nodular sclerosis Hodgkin's disease
B cell prolymphocytic leukemia	T cell granular lymphocytic leukemia	Lymphocyte-rich classical Hodgkin's disease
Lymphoplasmacytic lymphoma	Aggressive NK cell leukemia	Mixed-cellularity Hodgkin's disease
Splenic marginal zone B cell lymphoma ($\pm$ villous lymphocytes)	Adult T cell lymphoma/leukemia (HTLV-I+)	Lymphocyte-depletion Hodgkin's disease
Hairy cell leukemia	Extranodal NK/T cell lymphoma, nasal type	
	Enteropathy-type T cell lymphoma	
Plasma cell myeloma/plasmacytoma	Hepatosplenic $\gamma\delta$ T cell lymphoma	
Extranodal marginal zone B cell lymphoma of MALT type		
Mantle cell lymphoma	Subcutaneous panniculitis-like T cell lymphoma	
Follicular lymphoma	**Mycosis fungoides/Sézary syndrome**	
Nodal marginal zone B cell lymphoma ($\pm$ monocytoid B cells)	Anaplastic large cell lymphoma, primary cutaneous type	
Diffuse large B cell lymphoma	**Peripheral T cell lymphoma, not otherwise specified (NOS)**	
Burkitt's lymphoma/Burkitt cell leukemia	**Angioimmunoblastic T cell lymphoma**	
	Anaplastic large cell lymphoma, primary systemic type	

Bold type represents those malignancies that occur in at least 1% of patients.
HTLV, human T cell lymphotropic virus; MALT, mucosa-associated lymphoid tissue; NK, natural killer; WHO, World Health Organization.
Adapted from Harris et al.[42]

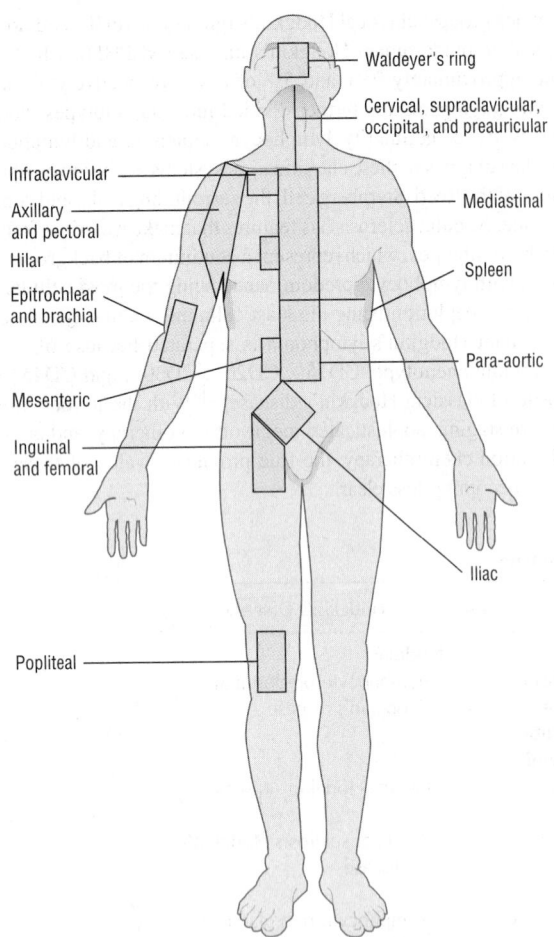

Waldeyer's ring

Cervical, supraclavicular,
occipital, and preauricular

Infraclavicular

Axillary
and pectoral

Hilar

Epitrochlear
and brachial

Mesenteric

Inguinal
and femoral

Mediastinal

Spleen

Para-aortic

Iliac

Popliteal

FIGURE 129–1. Representation of the anatomic regions used in the staging of Hodgkin's disease. (*Reproduced with permission from Rosenberg SA. Staging of Hodgkin's disease. Radiology 1966;87:146 [Letter].*)

CLINICAL PRESENTATION

Most patients with lymphoma present with some form of adenopathy that waxes and wanes for an average of 5 months before diagnosis. A painless, rubbery lymph node is discovered in and is localized to the cervical region. Adenopathy of the inguinal and axillary regions may be present at diagnosis but is less common, while involvement of Waldeyer's ring and the epitrochlear nodes rarely occurs (Fig. 129–1). Other common sites of nodal involvement include the mediastinal, hilar, and retroperitoneal regions. Up to 40% of patients with Hodgkin's lymphoma may also present with constitutional symptoms (B symptoms) including fever, drenching night sweats, and unexplained weight loss (>10% in the 6 months preceding diagnosis). Pruritus is also commonly noted in patients with Hodgkin's lymphoma, but its presence does not appear to have significant prognostic value.[2,6]

DIAGNOSIS, STAGING, AND PROGNOSTIC FACTORS

The diagnosis and pathologic classification of Hodgkin's lymphoma can only be made by review of a biopsy (preferably an excisional biopsy) of the enlarged node by an expert hematopathologist. Full evaluation of extent of disease, or staging, is necessary with Hodgkin's lymphoma. Staging determines appropriate treatment of the disease and provides useful information regarding prognosis. In addition, specific knowledge of the involved sites can be used to determine response. Presence of advanced stage, extensive B symptoms, and massive mediastinal involvement implies a poorer prognosis for a given patient.[2]

The Ann Arbor staging classification, which was developed at the 1970 Ann Arbor conference, has proven to be a good workable scheme. At the Cotswolds meeting in 1989, the Ann Arbor classification was modified to account for new diagnostic techniques (e.g., computed tomography [CT] and magnetic resonance imaging [MRI]), and the understanding that prognosis is associated with the bulk of the disease and the number of involved nodal sites (Table 129–3).[14] After careful staging, about one-half of patients have localized disease (stages I, II, and II_E) and the remainder has advanced disease (stages III or IV). About 10% to 15% present with metastatic disease (stage IV). It is important to note that Hodgkin's lymphoma appears to follow a predictable pattern of nodal spread that is not seen with the non-Hodgkin's lymphomas.

Diagnostic and staging procedures are based on recommendations made at the Ann Arbor and Cotswolds conferences and new scientific advances as outlined in the National Comprehensive Cancer Network (NCCN) guidelines.[15] In addition to a careful physical exam and routine laboratory tests, chest x-ray and CT scans of the chest, abdomen, and pelvis are routinely performed. Bone marrow biopsy is recommended in patients with more advanced stage disease. Staging can be based on clinical or pathologic findings. Clinical stage (CS) is based on all noninvasive procedures (history, physical exam, laboratory tests, and radiologic findings), while pathologic stage (PS) is based on the biopsy findings of strategic sites (muscle,

TABLE 129–3. The Cotswolds Staging Classification of Hodgkin's Disease

Stage I	Involvement of a single lymph node region or structure (I) or of a single extralymphatic organ or site (I_E)
Stage II	Involvement of two or more lymph node regions on the same side of the diaphragm (II) or localized involvement of an extralymphatic organ or site and of one or more lymph node regions on the same side of the diaphragm (II_E). The number of nodal regions involved should be indicated by a subscript (e.g., II_2)
Stage III	Involvement of lymph node regions on both sides of the diaphragm (III), which may also be accompanied by localized involvement of an extralymphatic organ or site (III_E) or by involvement of the spleen (IIIS) or both ($IIIS_E$). III_1: with or without splenic, hilar, celiac, or portal node involvement. III_2: with para-aortic, iliac, or mesenteric node involvement

Stage IV	Diffuse or disseminated involvement of one or more extralymphatic organs or tissues with or without associated lymph node enlargement
	A—No symptoms
	B—Fever, night sweats, weight loss (>10%)
	X—Bulky disease
	  >one-third the width of the mediastinum
	  >10 cm maximal dimension of nodal mass
	E—Involvement of extralymphatic tissue on one side of the diaphragm by limited direct extension from an adjacent, involved lymph node region
	S—Involvement of the spleen
	CS—Clinical stage
	PS—Pathologic stage

Adapted from Lister et al.[14]

TABLE 129–4. Prognostic Groups for Hodgkin's Lymphoma

	EORTC	GHLSG
Risk factors	A. Large mediastinal mass[a]	A. Large mediastinal mass[a]
	B. Age $\geq$50 years	B. Extranodal disease
	C. Elevated ESR[b]	C. Elevated ESR[b]
	D. $\geq$4 involved regions	D. $\geq$3 involved regions
Treatment groups		
Early-stage favorable	CS I–II supradiaphragmatic, no RF	CS I–II with no RF
Early-stage unfavorable	CS I–II supradiaphragmatic with $\geq$1 RF	CS I, CSIIA with $\geq$1 RF
		CS IIB with C/D but without A/B
		(see above)
Advanced-stage	CS III–IV	CS IIB with A/B (see above)
		CS III–IV

[a]Defined as a mediastinal mass larger than one-third of the greatest chest diameter on x-ray.
[b]Erythrocyte sedimentation rate ($\geq$50 without or $\geq$30 with B symptoms).
CS, clinical stage; EORTC, European Organization for Research and Treatment of Cancer; GHLSG, German Hodgkin's Lymphoma Study Group; RF, risk factor.
Adapted from Diehl et al.[11]

bone, skin, spleen, and abdominal nodes) with an invasive procedure such as a laparoscopy or laparotomy. Those patients with extranodal disease (muscle, skin, bone, of Waldeyer's ring) contiguous to involved nodes are classified with the subscript "E" in the Cotswolds staging system.[14]

Invasive staging procedures such as laparotomy and lymphangiogram are not usually performed during staging. These tests can detect occult disease in the abdomen, which would require systemic chemotherapy in addition to radiation for patients with early-stage supradiaphragmatic disease. Therefore these tests should only be considered for patients who will be treated with radiation alone if the results are negative. When the treatment plan includes systemic therapy, the use of these procedures does not impact treatment decisions or patient prognosis. Clinicians rarely order either procedure because the availability of lymphangiography is low and the complications of laparotomy are relatively high (about 5%).[11,16,17]

Analyses of early studies led to the identification of prognostic factors that could predict poor treatment outcomes of Hodgkin's lymphoma. Patient characteristics that have been determined as unfavorable prognostic factors include advanced stage, advanced age, male gender, presence of B symptoms, higher number of involved nodal regions, large mediastinal mass, extranodal disease, elevated erythrocyte sedimentation rate (ESR), presence of anemia, leukocytosis, lymphocytopenia, and low serum albumin.

Clinical trials performed by large cancer groups (e.g., European Organization for Research and Treatment of Cancer [EORTC] and German Hodgkin's Lymphoma Study Group [GHLSG]) have used combinations of these prognostic factors to stratify patients into early-stage favorable, early-stage unfavorable (intermediate) disease, or advanced disease (Table 129–4). Canadian and United States cooperative groups use similar criteria. In the NCCN guidelines, bulky disease, elevated ESR, and number of involved nodal sides are de-

fined as unfavorable features.[15] Although the exact criteria between groups or studies are not identical, stage, advanced age, bulky disease, and signs of systemic disease (B symptoms, elevated ESR, or extranodal disease) are of most prognostic significance.[11]

Some of these factors can also be used to predict prognosis in patients with advanced disease. The International Prognostic Factors Project uses seven factors to generate an International Prognostic Score (IPS), which can be used to predict progression-free and overall survival (Table 129–5).[18]

TABLE 129–5. The International Prognostic Factors Project Score for Advanced Hodgkin's Lymphoma

Risk factors
Serum albumin (<4 g/dL)
Hemoglobin (<10.5 g/dL)
Male gender
Stage IV disease
Age ($\geq$45 y)
White blood cell (WBC) count ($\geq$15,000/mm^3)
Lymphocytopenia (<600/mm^3 or <8% of WBC count)

Number of Factors	Freedom from Progression[a]	Overall Survival[a]
0	84 $\pm$ 4	89 $\pm$ 2
1	77 $\pm$ 3	90 $\pm$ 2
2	67 $\pm$ 2	81 $\pm$ 2
3	60 $\pm$ 3	78 $\pm$ 3
4	51 $\pm$ 4	61 $\pm$ 4
$\geq$5	42 $\pm$ 5	56 $\pm$ 5

[a]Percentage of patients at 5 years.
Adapted from Hasenclever et al.[18]

▶ TREATMENT: Hodgkin's Disease

The current goal in the treatment of Hodgkin's lymphoma is to maximize curability while minimizing short- and long-term treatment-related complications. According to the SEER database, the 5-year age-adjusted relative survival is greater than 80%.[8] The development of effective therapies for all stages of Hodgkin's lym-

phoma remains one of the most remarkable achievements in modern cancer care. The introduction of modern linear accelerators providing radiation beams in the range of <10 megaelectron volts, effective combination chemotherapy regimens, and new methods of combining these two modalities, have all contributed to high cure rates.

In general, most patients with early-stage Hodgkin's lymphoma are treated with combination chemotherapy and radiation. Patients with advanced-stage disease are usually treated with combination chemotherapy alone, although those with bulky disease receive radiation therapy to the site of bulky disease. Patients who do not achieve a complete remission may benefit from consolidative radiation. For the 15% to 20% of patients with refractory or recurrent disease, salvage therapy consists of multiagent chemotherapy with or without high-dose chemotherapy and autologous hematopoietic stem cell transplantation (HSCT), which can be curative. The following sections will review treatment of early-stage favorable disease, early-stage unfavorable disease (intermediate), advanced-stage disease, and salvage therapy.

For Hodgkin's lymphoma, surgery is not usually part of the therapeutic treatment regardless of stage. It is, however, important for diagnosis (excisional biopsy), and on some occasions, placement of a central line.[2]

Radiation is commonly an integral part of the treatment plan. Select patients with early-stage disease can receive radiation as the only treatment modality, while others will receive chemotherapy and radiation. Although radiation is a local therapy, many patients with advanced (widespread) disease will also receive radiation therapy to residual or bulky disease sites after chemotherapy. The major concern with radiation therapy is its long-term effects, such as cardiovascular disease and secondary malignancies, which commonly occur in the lung, breast, gastrointestinal tract, and connective tissue.[3,4] To avoid these toxicities, several studies have been completed and others are ongoing to maximize efficacy while minimizing the extent of radiation (radiation field) and the dose of radiation. The types of radiation fields used are shown in Fig. 129–2. Radiation to a single field that contains Hodgkin's lymphoma is called *involved-field radiation*; radiation to the involved field and a second uninvolved area is termed *extended-field radiation* or *subtotal nodal irradiation*; and radiation of all areas is called *total nodal irradiation*.[1,6] Specific therapies discussing radiation dose and field are discussed below with the pharmacologic therapy.

TREATMENT OF EARLY-STAGE FAVORABLE DISEASE

RADIATION THERAPY ALONE

Patients with stage IA or IIA disease and favorable prognostic factors can be successfully treated with radiation alone. Until recently, extended-field radiation has been considered to be the treatment of choice for stage IA and IIA disease. This treatment produces disease-free survival rates ranging from 65% to 85% and overall survival rates ranging from 75% to 93%.[2,6,11] If the decision is made to use radiation alone, extended-field radiation appears to be superior to involved-field radiation, based on a recent meta-analysis conducted by Specht and colleagues.[19] Results of that analysis showed that more extensive radiation reduces the risk of treatment failure at 10 years (31% vs. 43%), but does not improve 10-year overall survival (77% vs. 77.1%). When the intent is to use radiation alone, pathologic (i.e., surgical) staging is recommended to assure that the patient has limited-stage disease. Surgical staging consists of laparotomy and splenectomy, which has been associated with a morbidity and mortality rate of approximately 5%, primarily postoperative infection and sepsis.[2,6]

In an effort to avoid the long-term effects of extended-field radiation and risks of surgical staging, and improve treatment results, several studies have evaluated a combined modality approach that involves the use of short-duration chemotherapy and involved-field radiation.[11] Based on favorable results of these studies, most clinicians no longer treat patients with early-stage favorable disease with radiation alone.

CHEMOTHERAPY IN COMBINATION WITH RADIATION

Clinical trials comparing radiation alone to radiation plus chemotherapy have shown lower relapse rates in patients treated with combined modality therapy (radiation and chemotherapy), but no change in overall survival.[11,20] Current studies focus on questions such as the optimal number of chemotherapy cycles and the volume of radiation that must be used to obtain optimal patient outcomes. In patients with advanced-stage disease, a minimum of six cycles are usually given. However, results of recent studies suggest that as few as two to four cycles of chemotherapy is adequate.[11] Different combination chemotherapy regimens have been used in these studies, and it is not clear that any one regimen is superior to another. Other studies showed that extended-field radiation did not improve progression-free or overall survival as compared with involved-field irradiation, when radiation was combined with several cycles of chemotherapy.[11]

Based on these data, the current recommendation is to treat patients with early-stage favorable disease with two to four cycles of combination chemotherapy (i.e., ABVD; see below) and involved-field radiation.[15] With this approach, 5-year progression-free and overall survival rates of >90% can be achieved.

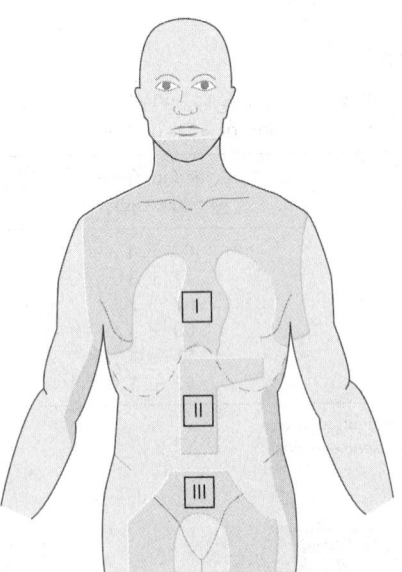

FIGURE 129–2. Radiation fields (shaded areas) commonly employed in Hodgkin's disease. I, mantle; II, para-aortic-splenic pedicle; III, pelvic; I + II, subtotal nodal irradiation; I + II + III, total nodal irradiation. (*Reproduced with permission from Eyre HI, Farver ML. Hodgkin's disease and non-Hodgkin's lymphoma. In: Holleb AI, Fink DJ, Murphy GP, eds. Textbook of Clinical Oncology. Atlanta, American Cancer Society, 1991:382.*)

TREATMENT OF EARLY-STAGE UNFAVORABLE DISEASE

Patients with early-stage disease who have certain features associated with a poor prognosis are defined as having unfavorable disease (see

Table 129–4). Because of the high relapse rate in patients with early-stage unfavorable disease treated with radiation alone, most clinicians currently favor combined modality therapy (combination chemotherapy and involved-field radiation) to reduce the relapse rate and avoid the toxicity associated with extended-field radiation and the mortality associated with surgical staging.[2,11]

CHEMOTHERAPY IN COMBINATION WITH RADIATION

Although randomized trials show that combined modality therapy reduces the relapse rate in patients with early-stage unfavorable disease, questions concerning the appropriate radiation volume, most effective chemotherapy regimen, and number of chemotherapy cycles remain.[11] In one recent trial (GHSG HD8), patients with early-stage unfavorable Hodgkin's lymphoma treated with chemotherapy and involved-field radiation had similar outcomes comes as those treated with the same chemotherapy regimen and extended-field radiation.[21]

Several ongoing trials compare different chemotherapy regimens or number of chemotherapy cycles.[11] A combination of doxorubicin (Adriamycin), bleomycin, vinblastine, and dacarbazine (ABVD) has become the standard regimen used to treat patients with early-stage unfavorable disease because of its established effectiveness in patients with advanced-stage disease and its favorable toxicity (both acute and chronic) profile (Table 129–6).[11] The use of a less toxic regimen, epirubicin, bleomycin, vinblastine, and prednisone (EBVP), which is effective in early-stage favorable disease, was found to be inferior to MOPP/ABV in patients with unfavorable disease. Other regimens that have been found to be effective include CVPP (see below) in combination with mantle irradiation.[2] A relatively new regimen, Stanford V, has generated a great amount of interest because in patients with bulky early-stage disease and advanced-stage disease, it has produced a 5-year overall survival of 96% and freedom from progression rate of 89%.[22] Finally, some trials are evaluating the number of chemotherapy cycles (4 vs. 6).

The current NCCN guidelines recommend four to six cycles of combination chemotherapy, followed by involved-field radiation (30 to 36 Gy).[15] ABVD is the most common regimen used, but other regimens can be used as an alternative to ABVD.

TREATMENT OF ADVANCED-STAGE DISEASE

Advanced-stage disease consists of stage III and IV disease. In some studies, stage IIB with a large mediastinal mass or extranodal disease is also considered advanced-stage disease (see Table 129–4). It is almost always widespread, which precludes the use of radiation alone as a therapeutic modality. Intensive combination chemotherapy is the mainstay of treatment, although some patients will benefit from consolidative radiation following chemotherapy.

CHEMOTHERAPY

One of the initial combination chemotherapy regimens introduced in the early 1960s that was shown to produce cures in advanced Hodgkin's disease was the MOPP (mechlorethamine, vincristine [Oncovin], procarbazine, and prednisone) regimen (see Table 129–6).[23] MOPP chemotherapy has been a mainstay of treatment for patients with stage III and IV advanced Hodgkin's disease. According

to the 20-year follow-up of the National Cancer Institute (NCI) trial, MOPP has produced complete remissions (disappearance of all measurable disease) in 84% of patients and has a 10-year cure rate of 54%. Forty-six percent of the original patients are still alive at a median of 14 years posttreatment (19% died due to other illness).[24] This is in contrast to the results of single-agent therapy, in which remissions occur less rapidly and are not as durable. Patients should receive two cycles of therapy beyond that required to produce a complete response; a minimum of six cycles should be administered. Maintenance therapy has not been shown to increase survival and may contribute to the long-term complications seen with therapy. The delivery of full or nearly full doses of chemotherapy is extremely important (e.g., dose intensity). Dose reduction within the various studies is probably the single most important factor explaining the differences in response rates between institutions administering seemingly similar regimens.[25] Dosage reductions based on toxicity may be made, but significant reductions can alter response and survival.[24]

Ever since MOPP therapy was created and the efficacy confirmed, researchers tried to modify the regimen in an attempt to improve efficacy and decrease toxicity.[25] Some MOPP variations include MVPP (vinblastine substituted for vincristine), CVPP (cyclophosphamide substituted for mechlorethamine), and ChlVPP (chlorambucil substituted for mechlorethamine, and vinblastine substituted for vincristine) were attractive alternatives to MOPP because they offered equal efficacy and differing or less severe toxicities. The various combination chemotherapy regimens appear to produce initial complete response rates in over 80% of the patients treated, and result in a 55% to 65% cure rate for advanced Hodgkin's lymphoma.

ABVD. The development of ABVD (doxorubicin [Adriamycin], bleomycin, vinblastine, and dacarbazine) by Bonnadonna and colleagues at the Milan Cancer Institute about a decade later represents the next important step in the evolution of therapy for Hodgkin's lymphoma (see Table 129–6). ABVD was initially shown to be effective in MOPP failures and was later compared directly to MOPP in advanced disease, where it produced an 82% complete response rate, as compared with a 67% complete response rate with MOPP. Improved failure-free survival was demonstrated with ABVD, but no significant differences in 5-year overall survival were noted.[26] Since ABVD is less toxic and provided similar or better outcomes than MOPP, it gradually replaced MOPP as the standard regimen for advanced-stage Hodgkin's lymphoma.

Alternating or Hybrid Regimens. In the early 1980s, the Goldie-Coldman hypothesis proposed that chemotherapy resistance was related to spontaneous mutation rates and the development of resistant clones. To test that hypothesis, researchers designed several clinical trials to evaluate the efficacy of alternating non–cross-resistant drug combinations in patients with Hodgkin's lymphoma.[27]

The initial approach investigators took was to alternate or combine the MOPP and ABVD regimens. When MOPP and ABVD (or ABV) are combined in a monthly cycle, it is referred to as a *hybrid* regimen. Besides a potential benefit in efficacy, a major potential benefit of alternating or hybrid regimens is decreased risk of long-term toxicities. In the alternating MOPP/ABVD regimen, the cumulative doses of procarbazine and mechlorethamine are reduced by 50% and the cumulative doxorubicin dose is reduced by 50%. In the hybrid regimen the cumulative doxorubicin dose is reduced by 33% and the cumulative bleomycin dose is reduced by 50%.

Several clinical trials have been performed to evaluate the efficacy of alternating or hybrid MOPP/ABVD regimens. The results of

TABLE 129–6. Combination Chemotherapy Regimens for Hodgkin's Lymphoma

Drug	Dosage (mg/m²)	Route	Days
MOPP			
Mechlorethamine	6	IV	1, 8
Vincristine	1.4	IV	1, 8
Procarbazine	100	Oral	1–14
Prednisone	40	Oral	1–14
Repeat every 21 days			
ABVD			
Adriamycin (doxorubicin)	25	IV	1, 15
Bleomycin	10	IV	1, 15
Vinblastine	6	IV	1, 15
Dacarbazine	375	IV	1, 15
Repeat every 28 days			
MOPP/ABVD			
Alternating months of MOPP and ABVD			
MOPP/ABV Hybrid			
Mechlorethamine	6	IV	1
Vincristine	1.4	IV	1
Procarbazine	100	Oral	1–7
Prednisone	40	Oral	1–14
Doxorubicin	35	IV	8
Bleomycin	10	IV	8
Vinblastine	6	IV	8
Repeat every 28 days			
Stanford V			
Doxorubicin	25	IV	Weeks 1, 3, 5, 7, 9, 11
Vinblastine	6	IV	Weeks 1, 3, 5, 7, 9, 11
Mechlorethamine	6	IV	Weeks 1, 5, 9
Etoposide	60	IV	Weeks 3, 7, 11
Vincristine	1.4[a]	IV	Weeks 2, 4, 6, 8, 10, 12
Bleomycin	5	IV	Weeks 2, 4, 6, 8
Prednisone	40	Oral	Every other day for
One course (12 weeks)			12 weeks; begin tapering at week 10
BEACOPP (baseline)			
Bleomycin	10	IV	8
Etoposide	100	IV	1–3
Adriamycin (doxorubicin)	25	IV	1
Cyclophosphamide	650	IV	1
Oncovin (vincristine)	1.4[a]	IV	8
Procarbazine	100	Oral	1–7
Prednisone	40	Oral	1–14
Repeat every 21 days			
BEACOPP (escalated)			
Bleomycin	10	IV	8
Etoposide	200	IV	1–3
Adriamycin (doxorubicin)	35	IV	1
Cyclophosphamide	1250	IV	1
Oncovin (vincristine)	1.4[a]	IV	8
Procarbazine	100	Oral	1–7
Prednisone	40	Oral	1–14
Granulocyte colony-stimulating factor		SC	8+
Repeat every 21 days			

[a]Vincristine dose capped at 2 mg.

these trials show that alternating and hybrid regimens are superior to MOPP but not to ABVD.[4,11,26] Another approach was to administer sequential cycles of MOPP and ABVD (MOPP → ABVD). Results of an intergroup trial showed sequential MOPP and ABVD to be inferior to the MOPP/ABV hybrid regimen in terms of response and survival.[28] In another randomized comparison of the MOPP/ABV hybrid regimen and ABVD, the complete remission rate, failure-free survival,

and overall survival were similar between the two regimens.[29] However, that trial was closed prematurely because of an increased number of treatment-related deaths and secondary malignancies in the patients who received the MOPP/ABV hybrid regimen.

In summary, alternating, hybrid, or sequential MOPP/ABVD (or MOPP/ABV) regimens have not been shown to be more effective than ABVD. ABVD has the advantage of less acute toxicity, no sterility, and a low risk of secondary acute myeloid leukemia/myelodysplastic syndrome. For these reasons, ABVD is the current standard for chemotherapy in advanced-stage Hodgkin's lymphoma.

■ *New Chemotherapy Regimens.* More recently, new regimens have been developed with increased dose-intensity or dose-density. Two relatively new regimens (BEACOPP and Stanford V) are variations of the above hybrid regimens that administer drugs with a shorter frequency or have escalated the dose of the most active agents. Since the majority of patients in the recent trials also received radiation therapy, results of these promising new trials are discussed in the next section.

■ *Summary.* In summary, the standard treatment of advanced-stage Hodgkin's lymphoma is six to eight cycles of ABVD chemotherapy. About 70% to 80% of patients will have a complete remission to ABVD chemotherapy, and about 60% to 70% will be cured of their disease. No further treatment is needed for patients attaining a complete remission. Patients achieving a partial remission should receive consolidative radiation to residual sites of disease (see below).

■ CHEMOTHERAPY IN COMBINATION WITH RADIATION

❸ The role of low-dose consolidative radiation when added to chemotherapy for the treatment of advanced-stage Hodgkin's disease is controversial.[11,30] The rationale for its use was based on the radiosensitivity of Hodgkin's lymphoma, a 20% to 40% relapse rate, and the tendency of Hodgkin's lymphoma to relapse at sites of initial involvement.[30] Many clinical trials were conducted to evaluate the benefit of additional radiation in patients who have a complete response to combination chemotherapy. The results of these studies were inconsistent, and a meta-analysis of 14 randomized trials showed a modest improvement in disease control at 10 years, but no difference in overall survival.[31] In a recently published study, patients with advanced disease were randomized to receive either involved-field radiation after MOPP/ABV hybrid chemotherapy or no further therapy.[32] Five-year event-free and overall survival were no different between patients who did not receive radiation and those who did (84% vs. 79% and 91% vs. 85%, respectively). However, in that study, patients who received radiation after a partial remission had 5-year event-free and overall survival that was similar to those in patients who achieved a complete remission to chemotherapy. These results suggest a role for consolidative radiation in patients who have a partial response after chemotherapy. Fewer secondary malignancies occurred in the group who did not receive radiation as compared to the radiation group (4% vs. 7.8%).

The Stanford V and BEACOPP regimens are relatively new regimens for advanced-stage Hodgkin's lymphoma (see Table 129–6). The Stanford V, a 7-drug regimen, was developed as a short-duration (12 weeks) regimen that maintained the dose-intensity of active agents, but reduced the cumulative doses of doxorubicin, bleomycin, and nitrogen mustard.[33] Developed by the German Hodgkin's Lymphoma Study Group, BEACOPP uses similar drugs as in the COPP/ABVD regimen (the same as MOPP/ABVD, with cyclophosphamide substituted for mechlorethamine), but rearranges the drugs in a shorter 3-week cycle.[11,34] Several different versions of BEACOPP have been developed: standard-dose BEACOPP (BEACOPP baseline), higher-dose BEACOPP (BEACOPP escalated), and dose-dense BEACOPP (BEACOPP-14). Granulocyte colony-stimulating factor (G-CSF) support is required for the BEACOPP escalated and BEACOPP-14 regimens. Most patients in these trials receiving these regimens have also received radiation therapy. Early studies with these regimens have reported 5-year overall survival rates of greater than 90%.[11,22,34] Few randomized clinical trials have evaluated these newer regimens. An intergroup trial is currently testing Stanford V versus ABVD in patients with advanced-stage Hodgkin's lymphoma. The German Hodgkin's Lymphoma Study Group recently reported the results of a prospective randomized trial comparing COPP/ABVD, standard BEACOPP, and increased-dose BEACOPP.[35] Freedom from treatment failure at 5 years was 69%, 76%, and 87% for COPP/ABVD, standard-dose BEACOPP, and increased-dose BEACOPP, respectively ($p < 0.001$ for comparison of increased-dose BEACOPP with the COPP/ABVD group and with the BEACOPP group). Five-year overall survival was 83%, 88%, and 91%, for COPP/ABVD, standard-dose BEACOPP, and increased-dose BEACOPP, respectively ($p = 0.002$ for comparison of COPP/ABVD vs. increased-dose BEACOPP). Despite filgrastim support, 90% of patients in the increased-dose BEACOPP group had grade IV leukopenia, as compared to 19% in patients in the COPP/ABVD arm and 37% in the standard-dose BEACOPP arm. However, the higher rate of acute toxicity did not translate into a difference in acute treatment-related fatalities (<2% for all three regimens). The increased-dose BEACOPP was also associated with a higher rate of secondary acute leukemias. Longer follow-up of this trial will be required to determine whether the survival gain with increased-dose BEACOPP is maintained and outweighs the increased risk of long-term toxicities such as secondary malignancies. The current German study group study compares eight courses of BEACOPP escalated to six courses of BEACOPP escalated and eight courses of BEACOPP-14.

CLINICAL CONTROVERSY

Some clinicians believe that Stanford V or increased-dose BEACOPP is superior to ABVD in the treatment of patients with advanced-stage Hodgkin's lymphoma. Increased-dose BEACOPP has been shown to be superior to COPP/ABVD, which is similar to MOPP/ABVD. Other clinicians believe that ABVD is still the treatment of choice because increased-dose BEACOPP has not been tested directly against it. They also express concern over the short- and long-term toxicity with increased-dose BEACOPP. This controversy will be answered with currently ongoing randomized studies and longer follow-up of the increased-dose BEACOPP trial.

■ SALVAGE CHEMOTHERAPY

❹ The goal of salvage therapy is cure regardless of the site(s) of recurrence or primary therapy. With the increasing use of chemotherapy with or without radiation, regardless of disease extent, the rate of primary refractory disease is decreasing. Patients who do not achieve a complete remission with the initial regimen are considered to have primary refractory disease. These patients have a poor prognosis when treated with salvage chemotherapy, and consequently are candidates for high-dose chemotherapy and HSCT.[35,36]

Patients who relapse after an initial complete response can be treated with the same regimen, a different potentially non–cross-resistant regimen, radiation, or high-dose chemotherapy and autologous HSCT (often preceded by conventional-dose chemotherapy). The response to salvage therapy depends on the extent and site of recurrence, previous therapy, and duration of initial remission. Patients who relapse after radiation therapy alone have a good chance of being cured with combination chemotherapy, although fewer patients are being treated with radiation alone. Other patient groups who have a favorable prognosis following salvage therapy include patients who experience a local recurrence in a nonirradiated location and those who relapse more than 1 year after completion of their initial chemotherapy. Patients who experience late relapses can be cured with retreatment with the same chemotherapy regimen, treatment with a different, potentially non–cross-resistant regimen, or high-dose chemotherapy and autologous HSCT. The NCI has reported on their long-term follow-up of MOPP-retreated patients. Patients with long initial remissions had a 45% disease-free survival rate at 10 years.[37]

Patients who have an early relapse (less than 1 year after treatment) generally respond poorly to standard-dose salvage chemotherapy, with cure occurring in less than 20% of patients. High-dose chemotherapy and autologous HSCT is more effective, but also produces a higher risk of treatment-related mortality. The choice of salvage treatment should therefore consider the patient's tolerance for a particular set of chemotherapeutic agents and treatment approach (standard-dose chemotherapy vs. high-dose chemotherapy and autologous HSCT).

HEMATOPOIETIC STEM CELL TRANSPLANTATION

High-dose therapy should be considered in patients that relapse within 12 months of initial remission and those who are refractory to first-line chemotherapy.[11,15,36] Although no one preparative regimen has been shown to be superior to another, most regimens do not include total body irradiation because of their potential pulmonary toxicity. Most patients are already at risk for pulmonary toxicity because they usually receive initial therapy containing one or more of the following: bleomycin, thoracic radiation, and nitrosoureas. High-dose chemotherapy with autologous HSCT produces long-term progression-free survival rates in patients with refractory and relapsed disease of 30% to 40% and 40% to 50%, respectively.[11,36] More details describing high-dose chemotherapy and HSCT for refractory or relapse chemotherapy can be found in Chap. 134.

LONG-TERM COMPLICATIONS

A variety of acute and chronic toxicities may occur as a result of treatment for Hodgkin's lymphoma. Long-term complications of radiation therapy, chemotherapy, and combined modality therapy have become more evident as the curability and long-term survival of Hodgkin's lymphoma patients has improved.[1,4] Gonadal dysfunction, secondary malignancies, and cardiac disease have become important considerations in the treatment of this malignancy. Almost all men and up to 50% of premenopausal women treated with six cycles of regimens containing alkylating agents will become sterile. This appears to be a dose-related phenomenon. For men, there does not appear to be a safe nonsterilizing dose of nitrogen mustard or chlorambucil, so if fertility is a major concern, ABVD may be the best alternative.[1,2]

Now that 10-, 15-, and 20-year survival data are available, evaluation of secondary malignancies can be made. Recent reports show that after treatment for Hodgkin's lymphoma, the relative risk for secondary cancers is increased.[1,2,4] Both solid tumors and hematologic malignancies (acute myelogenous leukemia/myelodysplastic syndrome and non-Hodgkin's lymphoma) have been observed. The increase in relative risk varies from about fourfold for solid tumors to over 100-fold for acute myelogenous leukemia. Radiation therapy is associated with the highest risk of developing a solid tumor (relative risk = 4.4).[4] The overall risk of developing acute leukemia (usually occurring in the first 10 years) ranges from 2% to 6%, but may be significantly higher in certain subsets of patients.[2] The relative risk is highest in patients who are treated initially with chemotherapy, either alone or combined with radiation.[4] Patients who receive MOPP or increased-dose BEACOPP therapy appear to have a higher risk of secondary acute leukemia as compared with ABVD; combined modality therapy further increases the risk of developing secondary leukemias.[4,11]

NON-HODGKIN'S LYMPHOMA

The non-Hodgkin's lymphomas (NHL) are a heterogeneous group of lymphoproliferative disorders that affect people from early childhood to late adulthood. Advances in molecular biology techniques and our understanding of the human immune system have led to major progress in understanding the pathogenesis and treatment of the lymphomas. NHLs are classified into distinct clinical entities that are defined by a combination of morphology, immunophenotype, genetic features, and clinical features. These differences influence the natural history and approach and response to treatment. The use of extensive combination chemotherapeutic regimens has resulted in dramatic improvements in survival and cure in patients with a disease that once was considered incurable. The 5-year survival rate for patients with NHL has increased from 47% to 59% over the past 20 years.[5,8] Further improvement in survival is anticipated with the continued expansion of our therapeutic armamentarium, including high-dose chemotherapy and biologic therapy.

EPIDEMIOLOGY AND ETIOLOGY

NHL is the fifth most common cause of newly diagnosed cancer in the United States and accounts for about 4% of all cancers. An estimated 56,390 new cases will be diagnosed in 2005, and it is estimated that 19,200 people will die from NHL during this same period.[5] Although the average age of patients at the time of diagnosis is about 65 years, NHL can occur at any age.[38] The incidence rate generally increases with age, and is higher in men than in women and in whites than in blacks.[8] The age-adjusted incidence rate of NHL has increased by more than 80% in the United States since the early 1970s, from about 11 cases per 100,000 in 1975 to more than 19 cases per 100,000 in the mid-1990s, with an average increase of about 3% to 4% per year.[8] The incidence of NHL appears to have stabilized or even declined since reaching its peak in 1994, but it is not clear whether this observation is a long-term trend. The increase in the incidence of NHL over the past three decades is second only to melanoma, and has been referred to as an epidemic of NHL. Although the increased incidence has been particularly noted among the elderly and patients with the acquired immunodeficiency syndrome (AIDS), much of this increase cannot be explained by known risk factors.

The etiology of NHL is unknown, although several genetic diseases, environmental agents, and infectious agents have been associated with the development of NHL.[38,39] An increased incidence of NHL is seen in many congenital and acquired immunodeficiency states, supporting the role of immune dysregulation in the etiology of NHL. Patients with congenital immunodeficiency disorders

(Wiskott-Aldrich syndrome, ataxia, or telangiectasia), acquired immunodeficiency disorders (AIDS, acquired hypogammaglobulinemia, or graft-versus-host disease), and chronic pharmacologic immunosuppression (solid organ transplantation) are predisposed to the development of NHL. Autoimmune diseases (Hashimoto's thyroiditis and Sjögren's syndrome) cause chronic inflammation in the mucosa-associated lymphoid tissue (MALT), which predisposes patients to subsequent lymphoid malignancies. Other autoimmune diseases such as systemic lupus erythematosus and rheumatoid arthritis have also been associated with the development of NHL, but the use of immunosuppressive agents in these diseases makes the pathologic cause less clear.

Certain infections have been associated with the development of lymphoma.[38–40] EBV was discovered in cell lines from tumors of patients with African (endemic) Burkitt's lymphoma, and EBV DNA is associated with 95% of endemic Burkitt's lymphoma. However, EBV is associated with sporadic Burkitt's lymphoma in about 30% of cases. EBV is also associated with posttransplant lymphoproliferative disorders and some lymphomas in patients with AIDS or congenital immunodeficiencies. The human T-cell lymphotropic virus type 1 (HTLV-1) was the first human retrovirus associated with a malignancy. Infection with HTLV-1, especially in early childhood, is strongly associated with an aggressive form of T-cell lymphoma, known as adult T-cell leukemia/lymphoma (ATL). HTLV-1 is endemic in southern Japan, Africa, and the Caribbean. In endemic areas, more than 50% of all NHL cases are ATL. A third virus associated with NHL is human herpes virus 8. This virus was originally isolated from Kaposi's sarcoma lesions in AIDS patients. Finally, gastric infection with *Helicobacter pylori*, a gram-negative bacteria that leads to chronic gastritis, is associated with gastric MALT lymphomas.

A number of physical agents have also been associated with the development of NHL.[38–40] Exposure to herbicides, particularly phenoxy herbicides, has been associated with the development of NHL. These observations may explain why workers in certain occupations, such as farmers, forestry workers, and agricultural workers, have been associated with a higher risk of NHL. Exposure to lawn care pesticides is also increasing in the general population. A higher risk of NHL has also been associated with exposure to other chemical solvents and dyes, exposure to radiation from nuclear explosions, and high intake of meats and dietary fats. Smoking or alcohol consumption has not been strongly associated with an increased risk of NHL.

GENETIC ABNORMALITIES

Chromosomal translocations have become a hallmark of many lymphoid malignancies.[41,42] The presence of these specific translocations can be helpful in the diagnosis and classification of lymphoid malignancies. The mechanisms leading to the translocations are unknown, but they usually involve the antigen receptor loci. In contrast to most myeloid and some lymphoid leukemias, NHL usually places a structurally intact cellular protooncogene under the regulatory influence of the highly expressed immunoglobulin or T-cell receptor genes, leading to effects on cell growth, cellular differentiation, or apoptosis. The most common chromosomal translocations involve t(8;14), t(14;18), and t(11;14); each translocation involves the immunoglobulin heavy-chain gene locus on chromosome 14 at 14q32. The translocation t(8;14) that involves c-*MYC*, a well-characterized oncogene clearly associated with malignancy, is implicated in nearly all cases of Burkitt's lymphoma. The translocation t(14;18) that involves *BCL*-2, one of several putative B-cell lymphoma–associated oncogenes, is found in about 90% of follicular B-cell lymphomas. The translocation t(11;14) that involves *BCL*-1, is found in most patients with mantle cell lymphoma. Another putative B-cell lymphoma–associated oncogene, *BCL*-6, is found in about a third of diffuse large B-cell lymphomas.

Although mutations in the *p53* tumor suppressor gene have been recognized in many human neoplasms, such mutations have not been consistently found in patients with lymphoma, which suggests that it may occur late in malignant evolution.

Detection of translocations, such as *BCL*-2 in follicular lymphomas, can be used clinically to monitor for minimal residual disease. In patients with follicular lymphoma who received monoclonal antibody–purged autologous bone marrow transplantation, those whose bone marrow was negative by PCR for the *BCL*-2 rearrangement after purging had significantly longer freedom from recurrence than those whose bone marrow remained PCR positive.[43]

PATHOLOGY AND CLASSIFICATION

NHLs are neoplasms derived from the monoclonal proliferation of malignant B or T lymphocytes and their precursors. About 85% of NHLs in the United States are of B-cell origin. Proliferation of malignant cells results in the replacement of the normal cells and architecture of lymph nodes or bone marrow with a relatively uniform population of lymphoid cells. The classification of NHLs has evolved over the last five decades, as advances in immunology and genetics have allowed scientists to recognize a number of previously unrecognized subtypes of NHLs (Table 129–7).[44] The current classification schemes characterize the NHLs according to the cell of origin (B-cell vs. T-cell), clinical features, and morphologic features. Additional immunohistochemical markers, cytogenetic features, and genotypic characteristics may also be help to further classify NHL into subtypes.

MORPHOLOGY

The macroscopic and microscopic appearance of the involved tissue remains one of the most important factors in the diagnosis and classification of NHLs. In the 1950s, Rappaport and coworkers proposed a morphologic classification of malignant lymphomas based on two features: (1) that the malignant cell would disrupt the nodal architecture in a *nodular* or *diffuse* manner, and (2) that lymphomas of histiocytic origin existed. The Rappaport classification gained rapid acceptance in the United States because of its precision, simplicity, and prognostic significance. Application of the system divided NHLs into those with large (i.e., incorrectly called "histiocytes") or small cells, with or without a nodular (i.e., follicular) growth pattern.

TABLE 129–7. Evolution in the Classification of Non-Hodgkin's Lymphomas

Time	Classification System	Basis for Classification
1950s–1960s	Rappaport	Morphology
1970s–1980s	Luke-Collins	Morphology and immunophenotype
1970s–1980s	Kiel	Morphology and immunophenotype
1980s–1990s	International Working Formulation	Morphology and clinical behavior
1990s	REAL	Disease entities
2001	WHO	Disease entities

REAL, Revised European-American Classification of Lymphoid Neoplasms developed by the International Lymphoma Study Group; WHO, World Health Organization.

IMMUNOLOGY

In the 1970s, it became apparent that NHLs were tumors of the immune system and were derived from B or T lymphocytes. The availability of techniques using antibodies to antigens on the surface of lymphoid cells (i.e., immunophenotyping) and cytochemical assays led to the following conclusions: (1) most NHLs were of B-cell origin; (2) all follicular or nodular lymphomas were of follicle center cell origin; and (3) most lymphomas previously classified as reticulum cell sarcoma or histiocytic lymphoma had the immunologic characteristics of transformed lymphocytes. Using this new information, a number of expert pathologists independently developed new classification schemes for NHL in the 1970s and 1980s.[44] The Kiel classification was based primarily on the work of Lennert and became widely used in Europe. In North America, the Luke-Collins classification scheme was used briefly, but was soon superceded by the International Working Formulation. Like the Rappaport classification, divisions within the International Working Formulation were based largely on cell size (large ["histiocytic"] versus small [lymphocytic]), cell shape (round vs. not round), and growth pattern (follicular [nodular] vs. diffuse). Both the Kiel and International Working Formulation classification schemes also considered the histologic grade of the tumor, but only the International Working Formulation considered actual survival curves of patients with the various subtypes of NHL. "Low-grade" indicated longer median survival (i.e., indolent) while "intermediate-grade" and "high-grade" indicated shorter median survival (i.e., aggressive). In the 1980s and early 1990s, the International Working Formulation became the most widely used classification scheme in North America, whereas the Kiel classification was widely used in Europe.[44] It was based on the premise that NHL was a single disease with a range of histologic grade and clinical aggressiveness.

NEW DISEASE ENTITIES

In the 1980s and early 1990s, rapid advances in immunology and genetics allowed scientists to recognize a number of previously unrecognized subtypes of NHLs. Cytogenetic and molecular genetic analyses identified the presence of many chromosomal translocations, oncogenes, and their gene products in patients with NHL (see the section on genetic abnormalities). In addition, diseases that would have been lumped together as "low grade" or "intermediate/high grade" in the International Working Formulation showed marked differences in survival, which prompted scientists to re-evaluate lymphoma classification schemes.

Information from these studies has allowed scientists to further classify B-cell lymphomas as malignant expansions of cells from either the germinal center, mantle zone, or marginal zone of normal lymph nodes (see Table 129–1).[42,45] Germinal centers are complex structures that form in spleen and lymph nodes in response to antigenic challenge. In addition to B cells, germinal centers contain antigen-presenting cells and helper T cells that cooperate in mediating the B-cell changes that result in a more potent secondary immune response. Malignant transformation often occurs or is initiated in germinal center B cells. Follicular, Burkitt's, and most large cell lymphomas are believed to be tumors of germinal center B cells. Three histologically distinct microenvironments have been described within the germinal center: a mantle zone surrounding interior dark and interior light zones. The mantle zone contains small resting B cells that have not been exposed to antigen ("naïve"). Tumors of cells from the mantle zone are usually clinically indolent and histologically low grade. Antigen-triggered activation of the densely packed

B cells of the dark zone causes cells to proliferate and causes genomic DNA to undergo somatic hypermutation. Surviving clones from within the dark zone then enter the light zone where proliferation slows and affinity selection occurs. During affinity selection, only cells with surface immunoglobulin receptors with high affinity for the antigen survive. Antigen-specific B cells generated in the germinal center reaction leave the follicle and reappear in the outer mantle zone, to form a marginal zone. Marginal zones are particularly prominent in mesenteric lymph nodes, Peyer's patches, and the spleen. These post–germinal center B cells include memory B cells of the marginal zone and plasma cells. Marginal cell B-cell lymphomas tend to be indolent and may be either extranodal or nodal; extranodal marginal cell B-cell lymphomas are also referred to as MALT lymphomas.

T-cell lymphomas can be classified on the basis of antigen expression as either precursor (thymic) or mature (peripheral) in origin. These classifications clinically translate to precursor lymphoblastic lymphomas or to a heterogeneous group of peripheral T-cell lymphomas. Tumors of natural killer or natural killer–like T cells are uncommon.

The International Lymphoma Study Group, an informal group of 19 hematopathologists from the United States, Europe, and Asia, adopted a new approach to lymphoma classification in 1993. Since it represented a revision of current or prior European and American lymphoma classifications, it was called the REAL. The REAL classification system is based on the principle that a classification is a list of "real" disease entities, which are defined by a combination of morphology, immunophenotype, genetic features, and clinical features.[46,47] The relative importance of each of these criteria for both definition and diagnosis differs among different diseases. Morphology is always important, and some diseases are primarily defined by morphology alone (e.g., follicular lymphoma), although immunophenotype can be helpful in difficult cases. Some diseases have a specific immunophenotype (e.g., mantle cell lymphoma or small lymphocytic lymphoma) that is virtually diagnostic of that disease. A specific genetic abnormality is important in some lymphomas—t(11;14) in mantle cell lymphoma, t(8;14) in Burkitt's lymphoma, and t(14;18) in follicular lymphoma—while other lymphomas lack specific genetic abnormalities (e.g., MALT lymphoma and diffuse large B-cell lymphoma). Finally, other lymphoma classes take into account clinical features (e.g., extranodal vs. nodal presentation in marginal zone lymphoma and peripheral T-cell lymphoma). A recent retrospective study of the REAL classification confirmed the clinical relevance of this approach.[48]

Since 1995, members of the European and American hematopathology societies have worked to develop a new WHO classification of hematologic malignancies. The final classification was published in 2001.[13] The WHO classification uses an updated version of the REAL classification and expands the principles of the REAL classification to the classification of myeloid and histiocytic malignancies.

The REAL-WHO classification categorizes lymphoid malignancies into three major categories: B-cell lymphomas, T-cell (and putative natural killer cell) lymphomas, and Hodgkin's lymphoma (see Table 129–2).[46,47] Within the B-cell and T-cell neoplasm category, there are two major categories: "precursor" neoplasms, which correspond to the earliest stages of differentiation (lymphoblastic), and "peripheral" neoplasms, which correspond to the more differentiated B- and T-cell stages. The REAL-WHO classification uses the term "grade" to refer to histologic parameters such as cell and nuclear size, density of chromatin, and proliferation fraction, and the term "aggressiveness" to denote clinical behavior of a tumor. This classification scheme includes both lymphomas and lymphoid leukemias, because there is no distinction between the solid and circulating forms of these diseases. The REAL-WHO classification includes several previously unrecognized types of lymphomas, including mantle cell lymphoma, monocytoid B-cell lymphoma, extranodal lymphoma of MALT, splenic marginal zone lymphoma, primary mediastinal large B-cell lymphoma, and a variety of T-cell lymphomas. New entities not specifically recognized in the International Working Formulation account for about 20% to 25% of the cases.

The REAL-WHO classification has broad clinical implications. The WHO Clinical Advisory Committee has agreed that clinical groupings of lymphoid neoplasms into prognostic categories are neither necessary nor desirable because such arbitrary groupings are of no practical value and may be misleading.[49] Treatment of a specific patient should be determined not by the broad prognostic group into which the patient's neoplasm falls, but by the specific type of neoplasm, with the addition of grade *within* the tumor type (if applicable), and clinical prognostic factors.

CLINICAL PRESENTATION

Patients with NHL present with a wide variety of symptoms, depending on the site of involvement and whether tumor involvement is nodal or extranodal.[38,40] Sites of involvement and dissemination of the malignant cells can sometimes be predicted based on the cell of origin and the fact that the tumor frequently disseminates to areas where the normal counterparts of the lymphoma cells are located. For example, B-cell lymphomas involve areas of the lymphoid system normally populated by B-lymphocytes, such as lymph nodes, spleen, and bone marrow. T-cell lymphomas commonly disseminate to various extranodal sites such as the skin and lungs. In contrast to Hodgkin's lymphoma, the bone marrow is commonly involved in NHL.

In general, patients may have either localized or generalized adenopathy, with the involved nodes being painless, rubbery, and discrete, and usually located in the cervical and supraclavicular regions as in Hodgkin's disease. The liver or spleen may be enlarged in patients with generalized adenopathy. Patients with mesenteric or gastrointestinal involvement may present with signs and symptoms of nausea, vomiting, obstruction, abdominal pain, a palpable abdominal mass, or gastrointestinal bleeding. Patients with bone marrow involvement may have symptoms related to anemia, neutropenia, or thrombocytopenia. NHL has a greater tendency to involve the testes, epitrochlear nodes, and Waldeyer's ring than Hodgkin's lymphoma. The incidence of solitary brain lymphoma is increasing, especially in patients with AIDS. Infrequently, patients with NHL may present with acute renal failure from retroperitoneal adenopathy causing ureteral obstruction, or from metabolic abnormalities such as hyperuricemia with uric acid nephropathy.

In contrast to Hodgkin's lymphoma, only about 20% of patients with NHL have the constitutional symptoms of fever, night sweats, and weight loss of greater than 10%.

DIAGNOSIS, STAGING, AND PROGNOSTIC FACTORS

As with Hodgkin's lymphoma, the diagnosis of NHL must be established by pathologic review of tissue obtained by biopsy. The preferred procedure is an excisional biopsy, in which the entire involved lymph node is removed for review by an experienced hematopathologist. This procedure should be done carefully to prevent distortional artifact of the architecture, which could lead to an inaccurate diagnosis. Needle biopsy of the node can sometimes provide adequate tissue for

pathologic diagnosis, if an excisional biopsy cannot be performed. When adenopathy is not present, diagnosis may be established by biopsy of cutaneous lesions, bone marrow biopsy and aspiration in patients with unexplained myelosuppression, liver biopsy in patients with hepatomegaly or elevated liver function transaminases, or biopsy of involved extranodal organs, such as bone, Waldeyer's ring, lung, and testis.

After the diagnosis is established, further work-up is required to determine the extent of involvement.[38,50] Clinical staging always begins with a thorough history and physical examination. Patients should be questioned about the presence or absence and extent of fever, night sweats, and weight loss. A detailed history of lymphadenopathy should also be obtained, including when and where the lymph nodes were first noted, and their rate of growth. A complete physical examination is performed to assess the extent of disease involvement, with special attention given to all nodal areas. All patients should have a complete blood count, serum chemistries including liver and renal profiles, a chest x-ray, and bone marrow aspiration and biopsy. The likelihood of bone marrow involvement varies among the different histologic types of lymphoma (Table 129–8). Lumbar puncture to evaluate the cerebrospinal fluid is recommended in patients who have histologic types of lymphoma that often spread to the central nervous system.

Imaging studies are usually important in the staging work-up.[38,50] CT scanning can identify both nodal and extranodal sites of disease, and has largely replaced lymphangiography for the evaluation of retroperitoneal lymphadenopathy. The abdominal and pelvic CT scan can identify mesenteric and retrocrural node involvement. CT scans can also detect tumor involvement of organs, including the kidneys, ovary, spleen, and liver. MRI is of limited usefulness in the staging of NHL. Gallium scans are sometimes used as part of the staging work-up. Other tests, such as liver-spleen scan, bone scan, upper gastrointestinal series, and intravenous pyelogram, are sometimes useful in patients with organ symptomatology or serum chemistry abnormalities.

Staging laparotomy was widely used in the late 1960s and 1970s as part of the staging work-up in patients with lymphoma, but it is rarely used today because of technical improvements in imaging studies and the morbidity and potential mortality associated with the procedure.

The Ann Arbor staging classification developed for the clinical staging of Hodgkin's lymphoma is also used to stage patients with NHL (see Table 129–3). After completion of the staging work-up, most patients will be found to have advanced disease (stages III and IV). The frequency of localized disease at the time of diagnosis varies depending on the histologic type of lymphoma (see Table 129–8). Stage is a more important prognostic factor in Hodgkin's lymphoma than in NHL.

The Ann Arbor system emphasizes the distribution of nodal disease sites because Hodgkin's lymphoma usually spreads through contiguous lymph nodes and does not involve extranodal sites. But NHL is a disease with tremendous heterogeneity that does not spread through contiguous lymph nodes, and that often involves extranodal sites. As a result of these clinical differences between Hodgkin's lymphoma and NHL, there is poor correlation between Ann Arbor stage and prognosis.

6 This lack of accuracy with the Ann Arbor staging system in NHL has lead to several international projects to develop prognostic models in the most common types of NHLs—diffuse large cell lymphomas and follicular lymphomas. The International Non-Hodgkin's Lymphoma Prognostic Factors Project was based on more than 2,000 patients with diffuse aggressive lymphomas treated with

TABLE 129–8. Patient Characteristics of the Common Histologic Types of Non-Hodgkin's Lymphoma

Histologic Type	% of Total	% Male	Median Age	% Stage I or II	% Marrow Positive	% IPI 0/1	% IPI 4/5
Small B-lymphocytic (B-CLL/B-SLL)	6.7	53	65	9	72	17	10
Mantle cell (MCL)	6	74	63	20	64	19	19
Follicular, all grades	22.1	42	59	33	42	39	6
Extranodal Marginal zone, B cell, MALT	7.6	48	60	67	14	38	5
Diffuse large B cell (DLBCL)	30.6	55	64	54	16	31	16
Primary mediastinal large B cell (PMBL)	2.4	34	37	66	3	44	9
Burkitt's	<1	89	31	62	33	44	22
Precursor T-lymphoblastic (T-LBL)	1.7	64	28	11	50	35	22
Peripheral T cell, all types	7	55	61	20	36	14	27
Anaplastic large T/null cell (ALCL)	2.4	69	34	51	13	50	19

IPI, International Prognostic Index; MALT, mucosa-associated lymphoid tissue.

an anthracycline-containing combination chemotherapy regimen in the United States, Europe, and Canada.[51] The Project identified five risk factors that correlated with low response to chemotherapy and poor survival: (1) age >60 years, (2) reduced performance status ≥ 2, (3) abnormal serum lactate dehydrogenase (LDH) levels, (4) two or more extranodal sites of disease, and (5) advanced tumor stage (Ann Arbor stages III or IV; Table 129–9). In patients ≤ 60 years old, three risk factors correlated with low response to chemotherapy and poor survival: (1) reduced performance status, (2) abnormal serum LDH levels, and (3) Ann Arbor stage. It is unclear whether the effect of

serum LDH level is related to a tumor or a host event. LDH likely measures cellular catabolism (the enzyme is released from injured cells), or the product of tumor burden and proliferation. Because each of the factors has approximately the same impact (e.g., relative risk) on prognosis, the number of adverse risk factors is summed to provide the IPI score. Patients could therefore have a score of 0 to 5. Table 129–9 shows the correlation between the IPI score and complete response rate and 5-year survival. For patients ≤ 60 years old, a simplified IPI score can be developed based on Ann Arbor stage, serum LDH, and performance status.

TABLE 129–9. Risk Factors and Survival According to the International Non-Hodgkin's Lymphoma Prognostic Factors Project

All Patients	Patients ≤ 60 Years of Age
Age >60 years of age	LDH > normal
LDH > normal	Performance status ≥ 2
Performance status ≥ 2	Ann Arbor stage III or IV
Ann Arbor stage III or IV	
Extranodal involvement ≥ 2 sites	

Risk Group	Number of Risk Factors	Complete Response Rate (%)	5-Year Survival Rate (%)
Patients of all ages			
Low	0, 1	87	73
Low–intermediate	2	67	51
High–intermediate	3	55	43
High	4, 5	44	26
Patients ≤ 60 years of age			
Low	0	92	83
Low–intermediate	1	78	69
High–intermediate	2	57	46
High	3	46	32

LDH, lactic dehydrogenase.
Adapted from the International Non-Hodgkin's Lymphoma Prognostic Factors Project.[51]

TABLE 129–10. Risk Factors and Survival According to the Follicular Lymphoma International Prognostic Index (FLIPI)

All patients
Age >60 years of age
Ann Arbor stage III or IV
Number of nodal sites >4
Abnormal lactate dehydrogenase level
Hemoglobin <12 g/dL

Risk Group (% of Patients)	Number of Risk Factors	5-Year Overall Survival (%)	10-Year Overall Survival (%)
Low (36)	0–1	91	71
Intermediate (37)	2	78	51
High (27)	≥3	53	36

Adapted from Solal-Celigny et al.[52]

Although the IPI is often used to predict prognosis in patients with other NHL subtypes, the IPI has several shortcomings when applied to patients with indolent lymphomas. Because only patients with diffuse aggressive lymphomas were used to develop the IPI system, some important prognostic factors may have been missed. Furthermore, the IPI system has limited discriminating power in follicular lymphoma because only about 10% of patients are categorized as high-risk in the IPI system. To address these concerns, several studies have attempted to develop a clinically useful prognostic model in patients with follicular lymphoma. However, none of these prognostic models has been validated or widely used. An international cooperative study was designed to develop a prognostic model similar to the IPI in patients with follicular lymphoma.

The results of that study, which was based on more than 4,000 patients with follicular lymphoma diagnosed between 1985 and 1992, was recently published.[52] Five factors were identified that correlated with poor survival: (1) age >60 years, (2) advanced tumor stage (Ann Arbor stages III or IV), (3) low hemoglobin level (<12 g/dL), (4) five or more nodal sites of disease, and (5) abnormal serum LDH level. Analogous to the IPI, the number of adverse risk factors is summed to provide the FLIPI. Three prognostic groups were identified: low-risk (0 to 1 factors), intermediate-risk (2 factors), and high-risk (≥3 factors). The new system appeared to have higher discriminating power among groups as compared with the IPI system. Table 129–10 shows the correlation between the FLIPI score and overall survival.

▶ TREATMENT: Non-Hodgkin's Lymphoma

GENERAL TREATMENT PRINCIPLES

The primary goals in the treatment of NHL are to relieve symptoms, cure the patient of their disease whenever possible, and minimize the risk of serious toxicities. The treatment strategy depends on many factors including patient age, concomitant disease, disease type, stage of disease, site of disease, and patient preference.

Historically, both the clinical behavior and degree of aggressiveness are often used to describe NHLs. The term *favorable* is used to describe indolent lymphomas because of their relatively slow growing behavior. Indolent lymphomas make up about 25% to 40% of all NHLs. Patients with an indolent lymphoma usually have a relatively long survival, with or without aggressive chemotherapy. Although these lymphomas respond to a wide range of therapeutic approaches, there is no evidence of a survival plateau, which indicates that patients are rarely cured of their disease. In contrast, aggressive lymphomas are termed *unfavorable* because of their rapid growth rate and short survival (measured in weeks to months), if appropriate therapy is not initiated. Aggressive lymphomas make up about 60% to 75% of all NHLs. Although these unfavorable lymphomas are generally more aggressive than indolent lymphomas, many patients with aggressive lymphomas who respond to chemotherapy can experience prolonged disease-free survival and some are cured of their disease. Therefore the terminology for the NHLs represents a paradox, where "favorable" is bad and "unfavorable" is good in terms of the likelihood for cure.

Therapeutic approaches to NHL include radiation therapy, chemotherapy, and biologic agents. The role of radiation therapy in the treatment of NHL differs from its role in the treatment of Hodgkin's disease. Although the disease is responsive to radiation therapy, only a small percentage of patients with NHL present with truly localized disease that can be treated with local or regional radiation therapy. Radiation therapy is used more commonly in advanced disease, primarily as a palliative measure to control local bulky disease.

Effective chemotherapy for NHL ranges from single-agent therapy in indolent lymphomas to aggressive, complex combination chemotherapy regimens in aggressive lymphomas. The most active agents used in the treatment of NHL include the alkylating agents (e.g., cyclophosphamide and chlorambucil), bleomycin, doxorubicin, purine analogues, etoposide, methotrexate, vincristine, and corticosteroids (e.g., prednisone and dexamethasone).

B-cell lymphomas have served as a model for immunotherapy with monoclonal antibodies for more than 20 years, beginning with the successful use of custom-made monoclonal antibodies targeted against the idiotype present on the patient's cancer cells.[53] These encouraging results led to the development of monoclonal antibodies against a more "generic" target, a molecule on the surface of B cells that would be present on tumor cells.[54] One potential target, the CD20 molecule, was present only on cells in the B-lymphocyte lineage. It is expressed on the surface of both normal and malignant B-cells, but not on other normal tissues. Rituximab (Rituxan) is a chimeric monoclonal antibody directed at the CD20 molecule.[55] Since rituximab was approved in November 1997 to treat relapsed or refractory indolent or follicular CD20[+] lymphomas, it has become one of the most widely used therapies for NHL. More recently, two radiolabeled monoclonal antibodies (i.e., radioimmunoconjugates) targeted against the CD20 antigen have been approved. With the availability of monoclonal antibodies and radioimmunoconjugates for the therapy of lymphoma, most patients with NHL will receive one or more biologic agents during the course of their disease.

Objective response to therapy for NHL should be defined according to the International Workshop to Standardize Response Criteria for Non-Hodgkin's Lymphoma.[56] Appropriate therapy for NHL depends on the patient's age, histologic type, stage of disease, site of disease, and IPI or FLIPI score (or presence of adverse prognostic factors). In general, treatment of lymphoma can be divided into that of limited disease and that of advanced disease. The limited disease group includes those patients with localized disease (Ann Arbor stages I and II). The advanced disease group is defined as all Ann Arbor stage III or IV patients, and also frequently includes Ann Arbor stage II patients with poor prognostic features (see Tables 129–9 and 129–10).[51,52]

The following section will discuss the clinical characteristics and therapy of the most common disease entities.

INDOLENT LYMPHOMAS

FOLLICULAR LYMPHOMAS

The combined group of follicular lymphomas makes up the second most common histologic type of NHL in the United States, comprising about 20% of all NHLs worldwide and up to 70% of indolent lymphomas reported in American and European clinical trials.[48,57] These lymphomas are classified as *follicular small cleaved cell, follicular mixed cell,* and *follicular large cell lymphoma* in the Working Formulation.[46] In the study that led to the development of the International Working Formulation, patients with follicular small cleaved cell and mixed cell lymphomas had significantly better survival than did those with follicular large cell lymphoma.[58] Therefore, follicular small cleaved cell and mixed cell lymphomas were considered as low-grade lymphomas, whereas follicular large cell lymphomas were considered to be intermediate-grade lymphomas. However, it is difficult to divide cases of follicular lymphoma into distinct subtypes because there is a continuous gradation in the number of large cells (i.e., centroblasts), and there are no uniform criteria for assignment of follicular lymphoma into the various subtypes. As a result, there is major disagreement, even among expert hematopathologists, on the subtype in many cases. In the International NHL Classification Project, the percentage of agreement for the various grades of the follicular lymphomas was only 61% to 73%.[48]

The WHO classification includes criteria for grading follicular lymphoma based on the number of centroblasts per high-power field (hpf): grade 1 (0 to 5 centroblasts/hpf), grade 2 (6 to 15 centroblasts/hpf), and grade 3 (>15 centroblasts/hpf).[13] The clinical behavior and treatment outcome of grades 1 and 2 follicular lymphoma are similar, and they are usually treated as indolent lymphomas. In contrast, grade 3 follicular lymphoma is synonymous with what is often referred to as follicular large cell lymphoma, and is usually treated as an aggressive lymphoma.

Follicular lymphomas tend to occur in older adults, with a slight female predominance (see Table 129–8). Most patients have advanced disease at diagnosis, but about 25% to 33% of patients have localized disease (clinical stage I or II) at diagnosis.[48] Extranodal disease, bulky disease, and B symptoms (constitutional symptoms) are uncommon features at diagnosis. Most patients with follicular lymphoma have the chromosomal translocation t(14;18) at the time of diagnosis.

The clinical course is generally indolent, with median survivals of 8 to 10 years. Most patients have dramatic responses to initial therapy, and their disease course is characterized by multiple relapses, with responses to salvage therapy becoming progressively shorter after every relapse, eventually leading to death from disease-related causes.[59] The natural history of follicular lymphoma shows a pattern of constant relapses over time (i.e., no evidence of a survival plateau), which suggests that patients are not cured of their disease. But the natural history of follicular lymphoma can be unpredictable. Spontaneous regression of objective disease has been noted in as many as 20% to 30% of patients.[59] There is also a high conversion rate of follicular lymphoma to a more aggressive histology over time that steadily increases after diagnosis and reaches 40% to 70% at 8 to 10 years.[59] At autopsy, 95% of patients with follicular lymphoma have some evidence of diffuse large B-cell lymphoma. Patients with transformed indolent lymphoma should be treated in the same way as an aggressive lymphoma.

Certain subsets of patients with follicular lymphoma have a much better or worse prognosis. Some studies suggest that the natural history of follicular large cell lymphoma (i.e., grade 3 follicular lymphoma) is similar to that of other aggressive lymphomas, and that treatment with intensive combination chemotherapy regimens may result in long-term disease-free survival, including a possible plateau in the survival curve.[57,60] The recent development of the FLIPI prognostic model should help clinicians to identify patients in different prognostic groups based on disease characteristics at the time of diagnosis.[52] Patients who are predicted to have a poor prognosis (i.e., high-risk) could then be offered aggressive or experimental therapy, while those who are predicted to have a good prognosis (i.e., low-risk) would be treated with standard therapy, therefore avoiding unnecessary toxicity.

Therapy of Localized Disease (Stages I and II)

Radiation therapy is the standard treatment for early-stage follicular lymphoma. Involved-field, extended-field, and total nodal irradiation have been used. Carefully staged patients with either stage I or contiguous stage II disease treated with radiation therapy alone can achieve disease-free survival rates of 40% to 50% and overall survival rates of 60% to 70% at 10 years.[57] Late relapses are uncommon; only 10% of patients who reached 10 years without relapse subsequently experienced a recurrence.

Chemotherapy is not usually given in most patients with localized follicular lymphoma, but it may be helpful in some patients with high-risk stage II disease (e.g., multiple sites of involvement or bulky disease).[61]

About 40% to 50% of patients with clinical stage I or II follicular lymphoma are cured of their disease with radiation therapy alone.[57] Most centers use radiation at a dose of 30 to 40 Gy to either involved (i.e., local) or regional fields, which would consist of irradiation to the involved nodal region plus one additional uninvolved region on each side of the involved nodes. Extended-field irradiation is not usually used because of the absence of a survival benefit and possible increased risk of secondary malignancies. In addition, previous use of extended-field irradiation compromises the ability of that patient to receive subsequent chemotherapy. The 2004 NCCN guidelines state that locoregional radiation therapy, chemotherapy followed by radiation therapy, or extended-field radiation therapy are appropriate options for patients with early-stage follicular lymphoma.[50]

Therapy of Advanced Disease (Stages III and IV)

The management of stage III and IV indolent lymphomas remains controversial, as standard therapeutic approaches have not been shown to be curative despite the high complete remission rates to initial therapy. Therapeutic options for these patients are diverse and include watchful waiting, radiation therapy, single-agent chemotherapy, combination chemotherapy, biologic therapy, and combined-modality therapy.[38,57,62] Although complete remission can be achieved in 50% to 80% of patients with various treatments, the median time to relapse is usually only 18 to 36 months. About 20% of patients who have a complete response remain in remission for longer than 10 years. After relapse, patients are re-treated and again high remission rates can be achieved (see below). Unfortunately, the response rates and duration of response both decrease with each re-treatment.

Two different initial treatment approaches exist and are described as conservative or aggressive. Patients treated with the conservative approach receive no initial therapy followed by single-agent chemotherapy or radiation therapy when treatment is needed. Candidates for the conservative approach are usually older, asymptomatic, and have minimal tumor burden. Patients with symptoms, extensive extranodal involvement, bulky disease, or impaired end-organ function at the time of diagnosis are not candidates for conservative treatment. With the aggressive approach, patients usually receive rituximab, combination chemotherapy, or both, early in the disease course. There are no convincing data to indicate that immediate aggressive therapy significantly improves survival as compared with conservative therapy. More than 80% of patients with stage III or IV follicular lymphoma are alive at 5 years, and the median survival is about 7 to 8 years.

CLINICAL CONTROVERSY

The management of advanced indolent lymphomas is controversial because none of the therapeutic approaches have been shown to be curative despite the high complete remission rates to initial therapy. Therapeutic options for these patients are diverse and include watchful waiting, radiation therapy, single-agent chemotherapy, combination chemotherapy, biologic therapy, and combined modality therapy. Although more intensive therapies have a higher complete response rate, they have not been shown to increase overall survival as compared with more conservative approaches.

At the time of relapse, many treatment options are available.[63] At the time of relapse, the following factors must be considered: age, symptomatic status of the patient, tumor burden, rate of regrowth (based on previous assessment of active disease sites), presence or absence of characteristics suggesting transformation or biologic progression, prior therapy, degree and duration of response to prior therapy, availability of clinical trials, and patient preferences.

No Initial Therapy.
Because there are no convincing data that standard treatment approaches have improved survival, some clinicians have adopted a "watch and wait" approach for asymptomatic patients in which therapy is delayed until the patient experiences systemic symptoms or disease progression such as rapidly progressive or bulky adenopathy, anemia, thrombocytopenia, or disease in threatening sites such as the orbit or spinal cord.[59] The median time until treatment is required is 3 to 5 years, and about 20% of patients do not require therapy for up to 10 years. The 10-year survival is 73%, which is not significantly different from patients who received therapy at the time of diagnosis. In a randomized study of asymptomatic patients

with indolent lymphomas (mostly follicular), patients who underwent watchful waiting had similar cause-specific and overall survival as compared with those who received immediate chlorambucil.[64] With a median length of follow-up of 16 years, about 17% of patients who were randomized to the watchful waiting group died of other causes without receiving chemotherapy and an additional 9% are alive and have not yet had chemotherapy. As described above, patients with follicular lymphoma who are followed without therapy sometimes have spontaneous regressions that can be complete, while the disease in other patients can convert to a more aggressive histology. If the watchful waiting approach is chosen, the patient should be evaluated at least every 2 months for the first year and quarterly thereafter, so that intervention can occur before serious problems occur.

Radiation.
Follicular lymphoma is sensitive to radiation therapy, and total lymphoid irradiation or whole body irradiation has been used to treat patients with advanced follicular lymphoma. Although the results with total lymphoid irradiation have been excellent in selected patients with limited stage III follicular lymphoma,[57] extensive radiation therapy is rarely used for patients with advanced follicular lymphoma requiring systemic therapy because of concerns regarding prolonged myelosuppression and difficulties in administering future treatments. Total lymphoid irradiation has been given in combination with chemotherapy, but studies have failed to show a survival advantage for combined modality treatment.[38,57] As a result, new high-dose chemotherapy regimens usually do not include the use of total lymphoid irradiation.

Chemotherapy.
Oral alkylating agents, given either alone or in combination, have been the mainstay of treatment for follicular lymphoma. More intensive chemotherapy has not been shown to improve patient outcome. In a randomized trial of oral chlorambucil (0.1 to 0.2 mg/kg per day), oral cyclophosphamide (1.5 to 2.5 mg/kg per day), or CVP (cyclophosphamide, vincristine, and prednisone) in patients with indolent lymphoma, no significant difference in overall survival or freedom from relapse between the three groups was observed.[59] In a more recently published randomized trial of single-agent cyclophosphamide (100 mg/m² per day) versus CHOP-B (cyclophosphamide, doxorubicin, vincristine, prednisone, and bleomycin), no significant difference in overall time to failure or overall survival was observed at 10 years.[65] The dosage of single-agent chlorambucil or cyclophosphamide is usually adjusted to maintain a platelet count above 100,000/mm³ and a white blood cell count above 3,000/mm³. Although single-agent alkylating agents have a high initial complete remission rate, the time required to achieve a complete response is slow (median time is 9 to 12 months). Complete responses occur more rapidly with combination chemotherapy, particularly with doxorubicin-containing regimens. Many clinicians will therefore give CHOP (cyclophosphamide, doxorubicin, vincristine, and prednisone) or CHOP-like chemotherapy when a rapid response is necessary. Table 129–11 shows the CHOP regimen that is widely used in the

TABLE 129–11. CHOP Regimen

Drug	Dose (mg/m²)	Route	Treatment Days
Cyclophosphamide	750	IV	1
Doxorubicin	50	IV	1
Vincristine	1.4	IV	1
Prednisone	100	Oral	1–5
One cycle is 21 days			

Note: Another name for doxorubicin is hydroxydaunomycin

treatment of NHL. In those who achieve a complete response, the duration of response is relatively short (about 2.5 years). There is no benefit of maintenance therapy. After the best response is achieved, many experts will discontinue therapy and observe.

Both single-agent alkylating agents and CVP are well tolerated by most patients. The advantages of oral chlorambucil are no hair loss, little or no nausea, and minimal myelosuppression. Because of its mild side-effect profile, oral chlorambucil is usually recommended for older patients who are minimally symptomatic or who have other comorbidities. There are some concerns with the risk of secondary acute leukemia in patients receiving continuous exposure to alkylating agents.

Purine Analogues. Several studies have reported encouraging results with two adenosine analogues, fludarabine phosphate and 2-chlorodeoxyadenosine (2-CdA; cladribine), in previously untreated and relapsed advanced follicular lymphoma. The mechanism of action for both drugs is not well understood, but both agents accumulate in lymphocytes and are resistant to adenosine deaminase. In patients with relapsed or refractory indolent lymphoma, single-agent fludarabine has an overall response rate of almost 50% and a complete response rate of 10% to 15%. Response rates are higher in previously untreated patients, with overall and complete response rates of 70% and almost 40%, respectively.[62] The median time to progression is less than 6 months for relapsed disease and more than 12 months for previously untreated patients. Although the response rates to 2-CdA in previously untreated patients is similar to those with fludarabine, the duration of response appears to be shorter with 2-CdA. Combination regimens that include one of these purine analogues are also being investigated.[62] Fludarabine and mitoxantrone (FN) and fludarabine, mitoxantrone, and dexamethasone (FND) are examples of fludarabine-containing regimens that have shown encouraging results in patients with indolent lymphoma.[66,67]

Purine analogues usually do not cause nausea and vomiting or hair loss, but they are associated with cumulative and prolonged myelosuppression and profound immunosuppression, which increases the risk of opportunistic infections such as fungal infections, *Pneumocystis carinii* pneumonia, and viral infections.

Interferon Alfa. Single-agent interferon alfa (IFN-α) is active in the treatment of follicular lymphoma, with objective response rates of 30% to 50% in patients with relapsed disease.[68] About 10% of patients have a complete response to IFN-α. Several randomized controlled trials have evaluated the potential benefit of adding IFN-α to combination chemotherapy. Based on the results of one of these trials, IFN-α-2b (Intron A) was granted FDA approval as initial treatment for patients with clinically aggressive follicular lymphoma and a large tumor burden, in combination with an anthracycline-containing regimen. Its approval was based on the Groupe d'Etude des Lymphomes Folliculaires trial, which compared CHVP (cyclophosphamide, doxorubicin, teniposide, and prednisone) to CHVP and IFN-α-2b.[69] CHVP was given monthly for six cycles, then every 2 months for six more cycles, whereas IFN-α-2b was given at a dose of 5 million units three times a week for 18 months. Patients who received concurrent IFN-α-2b had a significantly higher response rate (85% vs. 69%), which translated into significant differences in median progression-free interval (2.9 years vs. 1.5 years) and overall survival (not reached versus 5.6 years).

At least ten randomized controlled trials in the United States and Europe have evaluated the role of IFN-α either during induction, as maintenance therapy, or in both settings. The results of these trials have been inconsistent.[62,70] In a meta-analysis of more than 1,500 newly diagnosed patients from the various randomized trials, the efficacy of IFN-α depended on the intensity of the chemotherapy regimen and response to induction chemotherapy. The major conclusion of the meta-analysis was that IFN-α was probably beneficial in responsive patients (those who had a partial or complete response to induction chemotherapy) who were receiving more intensive chemotherapy (an anthracycline- or anthracene-containing regimen).

In the most recent randomized controlled trial, 571 patients with stage III or IV indolent NHLs (mostly follicular) were studied as part of a Southwest Oncology Group (SWOG) trial. Patients who responded to intensive chemotherapy that consisted of six to eight cycles of prednisone, methotrexate, doxorubicin, cyclophosphamide, and etoposide/mechlorethamine, vincristine, procarbazine, and prednisone (ProMACE/MOPP) or chemotherapy plus irradiation therapy were randomized to receive either consolidation IFN-α-2b (2 million units/m^2 given three times weekly SC) for 2 years or observation.[71] With a median follow-up of more than 6 years, no difference in progression-free or overall survival was observed.

The reasons for the divergent results cannot be easily explained.[70] Based on these negative results, the significant cost and toxicities associated with this agent, and the recent availability of other treatment options, most clinicians no longer use IFN-α in patients with indolent lymphomas.

Rituximab. The approval of rituximab is arguably the most important recent development in the treatment of NHL. Its initial approval was based on an open-label multicenter study that enrolled 166 patients with relapsed or recurrent indolent lymphoma.[72] Rituximab, given intravenously at a dose of 375 mg/m^2 weekly for 4 weeks, resulted in an overall response of 48% (complete response [CR]: 6%; partial response [PR]: 42%). Median time to progression for responders was 13.2 months and median duration of response was 11.6 months. Other studies of single-agent rituximab in patients with relapsed or refractory indolent NHL have reported overall response rates of 40% to 60% and complete response rates of 5% to 10%.[55,73] Investigators have evaluated different dosages and dosage schedules of single-agent rituximab, including higher dosages (up to 2 g/m^2), more frequent administration (three times per week), and more doses (weekly for 8 weeks). Although these alternative dosages or dosage schedules have been well tolerated (i.e., no dose-limiting toxicity was observed), they do not appear to increase the antitumor activity of rituximab.

Another advantage of rituximab is that it can be safely used as a retreatment option. About 40% of patients who relapsed after a response to rituximab have an objective response to re-treatment with rituximab.[74] Interestingly, patients who respond the second time usually have longer durations of remission than they did to the first course. Therefore, many clinicians will consider retreatment with rituximab for patients who have a sustained (i.e., more than 6 months) first remission and if their tumor has continued expression of CD20 antigen.

Based on the activity of rituximab in relapsed or refractory patients, it is increasingly being used as first-line therapy, either alone or in combination with chemotherapy.[55,73] When given as a single agent to patients with previously untreated indolent NHL, the overall response rate is 60% to 70% and the complete response rate is 20% to 30%. It is interesting to note that many of these patients remain in molecular remission (i.e., PCR-negative) at 12 months.[75] In patients who respond to the standard rituximab regimen (375 mg/m^2 weekly for 4 weeks), some studies have evaluated the role of maintenance rituximab, given at a dose of 375 mg/m^2 weekly for 4 weeks every 6 months, in an attempt to improve the initial therapeutic response and prolong duration of remission.[76] With continued maintenance therapy, the final response rate increased to 73%, with 37% complete responses. Median progression-free survival was 34 months. Based on these encouraging results, the role of maintenance rituximab is being investigated in a multicenter cooperative group randomized trial.

The rationale for the use of rituximab in combination with conventional agents is based on clinical activity of both agents/regimens, non–cross-resistant mechanisms of action, non-overlapping toxicities, and synergistic antitumor activity in vitro. Many clinical trials have evaluated the use of rituximab in combination with other chemotherapy agents.[55,73] In a phase II trial of six courses of rituximab and CHOP chemotherapy (R-CHOP), the overall and complete response rate in 40 patients with previously untreated or relapsed indolent lymphoma was 95% and 55%, respectively.[77] More than 70% of patients are progression-free after 4 years of follow-up. In an updated analysis, median time to progression was reached at 82 months. Rituximab and CHOP chemotherapy can be combined in many different ways. In the R-CHOP regimen developed by Czuczman and associates,[77] two doses of rituximab are given before the start of CHOP therapy, two more doses are given in the middle of the six cycles of CHOP, and two additional doses are given at the end of CHOP therapy. No significant additional toxicity was observed in patients who received R-CHOP. Similar overall and complete response rates have been reported with clinical trials of rituximab combined with other chemotherapy regimens.[55,73]

Most of the adverse effects of rituximab are infusion related, particularly after the first infusion, and consist of fever, chills, respiratory symptoms, fatigue, headache, pruritus, and angioedema.[55] Premedication with oral acetaminophen 650 mg and diphenhydramine 50 mg is usually given 30 minutes before rituximab infusion.

Radioimmunotherapy. The recent approval of the anti-CD20 radioimmunoconjugates ^{131}I-tositumomab (Bexxar) and ^{90}Y-ibritumomab tiuxetan (Zevalin) has provided clinicians with a novel treatment option for patients with indolent NHLs.[78,79] Both ^{131}I-tositumomab and ^{90}Y-ibritumomab tiuxetan are mouse antibodies linked to a radioisotope, either iodine 131 (^{131}I) or yttrium 90 (^{90}Y). Indolent lymphomas are known to be responsive to radiation therapy (i.e., radiosensitive), and the rationale of radioimmunotherapy is that the antibody will act as a "guided missile" to deliver its payload (i.e., radiation) to its target (i.e., lymphoma cells that express the CD20 antigen). The specificity of the monoclonal antibody allows delivery of the radiation selectively to the tumor (and adjacent normal tissues).

Radioimmunoconjugates have some advantages and disadvantages over unlabeled ("naked") monoclonal antibodies such as rituximab. Tumor cell kill following rituximab depends on binding of the antibody to the tumor cell and the host immune system. Therefore tumor cells that do not express the target antigen are not accessible to the antibody, or are resistant to immune-mediated attacks and may escape treatment. Radioimmunoconjugates, because of their ability to deliver radiation over a distance from a source, can not only kill tumor cells that are in contact with the antibody, but also adjacent tumor cells which may not have been in contact with the antibody or may not express the target antigen. This effect is sometimes referred to as the relevant bystander or "crossfire" effect. However, one disadvantage of radioimmunotherapy is that it can also damage adjacent normal tissues, such as bone marrow cells.

Both ^{131}I-tositumomab and ^{90}Y-ibritumomab tiuxetan have shown activity in relapsed and refractory patients with indolent or transformed lymphomas.[78,79] In patients who respond to radioimmunotherapy, the duration of remission can be more than several years. Based on these encouraging results, some clinicians are considering radioimmunotherapy earlier in the disease course, including patients with previously untreated disease. In a phase II study, patients with previously untreated follicular lymphoma were treated with six cycles of CHOP chemotherapy followed 4 to 8 weeks later by ^{131}I-tositumomab.[80] The overall response rate to the entire treatment regimen was 90%, including 67% complete remissions, and the 2-year progression-free survival is estimated to be 81%. A current multicenter cooperative group study (SWOG S0016) randomizes patients with advanced indolent lymphomas to either CHOP or rituximab (given concurrently, based on the Czuczman regimen[77]) or CHOP and ^{131}I-tositumomab (given sequentially).

Radioimmunotherapy is generally well tolerated. The major acute toxicities with both radioimmunoconjugates are infusion-related reactions and myelosuppression. ^{131}I-tositumomab can also cause thyroid dysfunction. The primary concern with radioimmunotherapy is the development of treatment-related myelodysplastic syndrome or acute myelogenous leukemia.[81]

The decision to use radioimmunotherapy must be made carefully because of the complexity, risks, and costs of the treatment regimen. Although oncologists usually select patients for therapy, the radioimmunotherapy regimen must be administered at a radiation oncology or nuclear medicine facility. Because of safety concerns related to delivery of radiation to bone marrow, candidates for radioimmunotherapy usually have limited bone marrow involvement and adequate absolute neutrophil and platelet counts.

Hematopoietic Stem Cell Transplantation. High-dose chemotherapy, followed by autologous or allogeneic HSCT, is another option for patients with relapsed follicular lymphoma.[63,82,83] In patients who are transplanted at the time of initial treatment failure, 5-year event-free survival is about 40% to 50%. Although the rate of recurrence is lower after allogeneic HSCT as compared with autologous HSCT, that benefit is offset by increased treatment-related mortality after allogeneic HSCT.[83] The presence of a survival plateau after allogeneic HSCT suggests that some patients may be cured of their disease. In a recently published randomized trial, patients with relapsed follicular lymphoma who received autologous HSCT had significantly longer progression-free and overall survival than those who received additional courses of combination chemotherapy.[84]

Based on these encouraging results, some studies have evaluated autologous HSCT as consolidation therapy after CHOP or CHOP-like chemotherapy in patients with poor-risk follicular lymphoma.[82] Several large randomized trials are ongoing, and the results of these trials should further define the role of autologous HSCT as first-line therapy of follicular lymphoma.

Rituximab is being evaluated in the setting of autologous HSCT.[73,85] It is given pretransplant as an in vivo purging agent prior to stem cell collection. In other studies, rituximab is given as post-transplant consolidation.

High-dose myeloablative transplants are usually reserved for younger patients without serious comorbidities, but nonmyeloablative allogeneic transplants may be an option for older patients who would not otherwise be eligible for autologous or allogeneic HSCT.

Investigational Therapies. As discussed above, the idiotype present on the patient's tumor cells serves as a potential target for immunotherapy. This idiotype can be used to manufacture a patient-specific vaccine.[53] Vaccines would potentially produce both humoral and cellular immune responses, and would also be longer acting than passive immunotherapy. Several vaccines are being evaluated in clinical trials.[39]

OTHER INDOLENT LYMPHOMAS

Marginal zone B-cell lymphomas, MALT (extranodal) and nodal types, are two of the new forms of NHL not previously recognized in the International Working Formulation.[86] Extranodal and nodal types of marginal zone B-cell lymphomas represent approximately 7.6% and 1.8% of new cases of NHLs.[48] Clinically, MALT lymphomas tend to be indolent. Most patients present with localized disease involving extranodal sites, which involves glandular epithelial tissues of various sites, such as the stomach, lungs, parotid gland, thyroid, and orbit (see Table 129–8). The stomach is the most frequent site and gastric MALT lymphomas are frequently associated with chronic gastritis and *Helicobacter pylori* infection. Because MALT lymphomas tend to remain localized for long periods, local treatment (surgery or local/regional radiation therapy) is effective and offers the opportunity for cure. Patients with gastric MALT lymphomas who are positive for *H. pylori* should be treated for their infection (e.g., antibiotics). Patients with disseminated MALT lymphoma should be treated with the same type of chemotherapy used in patients with follicular lymphoma.

AGGRESSIVE LYMPHOMAS

DIFFUSE LARGE B-CELL LYMPHOMA

Diffuse large B-cell lymphomas (DLBCLs) are the most common lymphoma in the International NHL Classification Project, accounting for about 30% of all NHLs.[48] Most DLBCLs are classified as *diffuse large cell cleaved, noncleaved,* or *immunoblastic* or *diffuse mixed cell* in the International Working Formulation.[46,87] DLBCLs are characterized by the presence of large cells, which are similar in size to or larger than tissue macrophages and usually more than twice the size of normal lymphocytes. The median age at the time of diagnosis is in the seventh decade, but DLBCL can affect individuals of all ages, from children to the elderly. Patients often present with a rapidly enlarging symptomatic mass, with B symptoms in about one-third of the cases.[38,88] About 30% to 40% of patients with DLBCL present with extranodal disease; common sites include the head and neck, gastrointestinal tract, skin, bone, testis, and CNS. DLBCL is the most common type of diffuse aggressive lymphoma, which share in common an aggressive clinical behavior that leads to death within weeks to months if the tumor is not treated. Diffuse aggressive lymphomas are also sensitive to many chemotherapeutic agents, and some patients treated with chemotherapy can be cured of their disease.

Several factors have been shown to correlate with response to chemotherapy and survival in patients with aggressive lymphoma. Since the IPI was originally developed based on patients with aggressive lymphoma, IPI score correlates with prognosis (see Table 129–9).[51] Although IPI is a clinically useful tool to estimate prognosis, the factors used to calculate the IPI score probably represent clinical surrogates for the biologic heterogeneity among DLBCLs, and many researchers are interested in determining the prognostic importance of certain phenotypic and molecular characteristics of DLBCLs. For example, markers of apoptosis, cell-cycle regulation, cell lineage, and cell proliferation are being evaluated as potentially clinically useful prognostic factors. Gene expression profiling with biochips may also correlate with survival. Using gene expression profiling, investigators identified three molecularly distinct forms of DLBCL based on gene expression patterns indicative of different stages of B-cell differentiation: germinal center B-cell-like, activated B-cell-like, and type 3.[89] The type 3 subgroup did not express either set of genes at a high level. The investigators used 17 genes to construct a model that correlated with overall survival after chemotherapy. In another study, investigators were able to develop a predictive model based on only six genes.[90] These results suggest that molecular classification of tumors on the basis of gene expression may allow identification of clinically significant subtypes of cancer.

Therapy of DLBCL is based on the Ann Arbor stage, IPI score, and other prognostic factors. About one-half of patients present with localized (stage I or II) disease. However, many patients present with large bulky masses (i.e., larger than 10 cm), and patients with bulky stage II disease are treated with the same approach as that used with those with advanced disease (stage III or IV).

Therapy of Localized Disease (Stages I and II)

Before 1980, radiation therapy was the primary treatment for patients with localized DLBCL. Five-year disease-free survival with radiation therapy alone was about 50% and 20% in patients with stage I and stage II disease, respectively.[38,87,88] Randomized trials in the 1980s showed that radiation therapy followed by chemotherapy resulted in significantly longer disease-free and overall survival as compared with radiation therapy alone. Other studies reported excellent results with a short course of chemotherapy (three cycles) followed by involved-field radiotherapy or six to eight cycles of CHOP chemotherapy, with or without consolidation radiotherapy. With either of these approaches, 5-year progression-free survival was >90% for patients with stage I disease and about 70% for patients with stage II disease.[38,87,88]

Since it was not clear which approach was more effective, the SWOG performed a randomized trial that compared three cycles of CHOP and involved-field radiotherapy or eight cycles of CHOP in patients with stage I and nonbulky stage II aggressive lymphoma.[91] Patients treated with three cycles of CHOP plus radiotherapy had significantly better 5-year progression-free (77% vs. 64%) and overall (82% vs. 72%) survival than patients treated with CHOP alone. The incidence of life-threatening toxicity was higher in patients who received CHOP alone. Based on the results of this trial, the current standard for therapy of most patients with localized nonbulky aggressive lymphoma is three to four cycles of CHOP followed by locoregional radiation therapy (30 to 40 Gy).[38,50,88] A stage-modified IPI score is sometimes used to identify patients with localized lymphoma who may have a poor prognosis. Patients with one or more of these poor prognostic factors (i.e., stage II, elevated LDH levels, age >60 years, or performance status ≥2) may benefit from more aggressive chemotherapy (six to eight cycles of CHOP) followed by locoregional radiation therapy. At some institutions, R-CHOP has replaced CHOP as standard therapy.

Therapy of Advanced Disease (Bulky Stage II and Stages III and IV)

It has been known since the late 1970s that intensive combination chemotherapy can cure some patients with disseminated DLBCL.[38,40,88] Initial studies with COP (same as CVP) produced a plateau on the survival curve of just 10%, with a median survival of less than 1 year. Based on the activity of single-agent doxorubicin, McKelvey and colleagues developed the CHOP regimen (see Table

129–11).[92] A few years later, a SWOG study showed that CHOP was more active than COP, and CHOP chemotherapy rapidly became the treatment of choice for patients with aggressive lymphomas.[93] Studies in larger numbers of patients showed that about 50% of patients had a complete remission to CHOP chemotherapy, and 50% to 75% of the patients who had a complete response (about one-third of all patients) experienced long-term disease-free survival and cure of their disease.

In an effort to improve these results, many investigators used several general approaches to develop second- and third-generation regimens in the 1980s and early 1990s.[40,88] The first approach was to add a nonmyelotoxic drug, most often bleomycin, to the three-week cycle (e.g., CHOP-Bleo or BACOP). The second approach was to add nonmyelosuppressive agents *between* cycles of CHOP or BACOP. One example of this strategy was the M-BACOD (methotrexate, bleomycin, doxorubicin, cyclophosphamide, vincristine, and dexamethasone) regimen, in which high-dose methotrexate with leucovorin rescue was administered on day 10. M-BACOD was later modified to m-BACOD, which included the same drugs but had a lower methotrexate dosage. Another variation on this strategy was to give semicontinuous or weekly therapy; relatively small doses of myelosuppressive agents are administered, alternating over a 12-week period with nonmyelosuppressive agents. An example of this strategy is MACOP-B (methotrexate with leucovorin rescue, doxorubicin, cyclophosphamide, vincristine, prednisone, and bleomycin). The third approach was to give as many drugs as possible, as flexibly as possible (e.g., ProMACE/MOPP). ProMACE/MOPP was later modified to ProMACE/CytaBOM (prednisone, doxorubicin, cyclophosphamide, and etoposide, followed by cytarabine, bleomycin, vincristine, and methotrexate with leucovorin rescue). Results of phase II trials suggested that these second- and third-generation regimens were more active than CHOP, with slightly higher complete response rates and improved disease-free survival rates.[38,40,88] However, they were also more difficult to administer, more toxic, and more expensive. Based on these results, oncologists generally adopted one of these second- or third-generation combination regimens as their standard regimen for patients with advanced aggressive lymphomas.

Many randomized studies have compared different combination regimens in patients with aggressive lymphoma.[38,40,88] Although the results of these studies show that no one regimen is clearly superior to another, they show the superiority of anthracycline-containing regimens over those that do not contain an anthracycline. In the largest and most widely quoted study, the SWOG initiated a randomized trial in 1986 that compared CHOP to three of the most commonly used third-generation regimens (m-BACOD, ProMACE/CytaBOM, and MACOP-B) in nearly 900 patients with bulky stage II, stage III, or stage IV aggressive lymphoma. At the time of the initial publication (median follow-up = 35 months), no differences in disease-free and overall survival were observed between the four groups.[94] Furthermore, no significant differences in disease-free or overall survival were observed in any subgroup of patients. The risk of treatment-related mortality, however, was higher in patients receiving one of the third-generation regimens. Extended follow-up of that trial shows that about 35% of patients who participated in that trial are probably cured of their disease, regardless of the initial combination chemotherapy regimen.[87] Interestingly, the overall survival is about 10% higher than the disease-free survival, which probably reflects the effectiveness of salvage high-dose chemotherapy with autologous HSCT (see below).

Based on the lack of survival benefit with the newer combination chemotherapy regimens, the less complicated and less expensive CHOP regimen should be considered as the treatment of choice for most patients with DLBCL and other aggressive lymphomas.

Unfortunately, the major conclusion from these studies is not that all of these regimens are extremely effective, but that all of these regimens are equally bad. Less than 50% of patients with DLBCL are currently cured of their disease with combination chemotherapy, and most patients who relapse after an initial response do so in the first 2 years. New treatment approaches are clearly needed.

The IPI score should be calculated for every patient with DLBCL and incorporated into treatment decisions for individual patients (see Table 129–9). Patients with a low IPI score should be treated with conventional CHOP (or R-CHOP) therapy. But patients with a high-intermediate or high-risk IPI score should be identified as candidates for more aggressive treatments. These include addition of rituximab to CHOP, dose-intense or dose-dense chemotherapy with growth factor support, or high-dose chemotherapy with autologous HSCT.

Based on the encouraging results of R-CHOP in indolent lymphomas, several studies have evaluated this combination in aggressive lymphomas.[55] In a multicenter pilot study of 33 patients with previously untreated CD20[+] aggressive NHL, the addition of rituximab to six cycles of CHOP chemotherapy produced a 94% objective response rate, with 61% of patients achieving a complete response.[95] Rituximab was given at a dosage of 375 mg/m^2 on day 1 of each cycle; cyclophosphamide, doxorubicin, and vincristine was given intravenously on day 3, and oral prednisone was given on days 3 to 7. In an updated analysis (62 months), progression-free and overall survival was 80% and 87%, respectively. In the 18 patients with an IPI score of ≥2, the overall response rate was 89% and complete response rate was 56%. No significant additional toxicity was noted. Based on these encouraging results, including the results of the GELA study in elderly patients (see below), many institutions currently recommend R-CHOP in all patients with aggressive lymphoma.[50]

Several studies have attempted to improve treatment results by increasing chemotherapy dose (i.e., dose-intensity), shortening the interval between chemotherapy cycles (i.e., dose-density), or both. Because of the increased risk of severe neutropenia, these approaches require growth factor support. Although results of these studies have not consistently shown improved survival, encouraging results from several recently published studies suggest that these approaches be evaluated in future randomized trials.[96,97]

Another approach in high-risk patients is to give high-dose chemotherapy with autologous HSCT as intensive consolidation in high-risk patients with DLBCL who achieve a remission with standard chemotherapy.[87] Several randomized controlled trials have been conducted in patients with aggressive NHLs, and the results of these trials have been critically reviewed recently by two independent panels of experts.[98,99] Based on a review of the available evidence, it was concluded that high-dose chemotherapy with autologous HSCT is effective in high-risk (i.e., high-intermediate/high-risk based on IPI score) patients who have a complete remission to conventional therapy (first complete remission in high-risk patients) and in untreated high-risk patients (high-dose sequential therapy in untreated high-risk patients).[99] There was inadequate evidence to make a treatment recommendation for the other possible clinical situations, such as in patients who do not respond to standard induction therapy (primary refractory disease) or in patients who have a partial remission to standard induction therapy (first partial remission after full-course induction therapy). Since those recommendations were published, another randomized study showed that high-dose chemotherapy with autologous HSCT improves event-free survival in patients with a lower IPI score (i.e., low, low-intermediate, or high-intermediate risk).[100]

Unfortunately, the available evidence has led to a discussion of when high-dose chemotherapy with autologous HSCT should be offered to high-risk patients with aggressive NHLs: early (i.e., when patients are in their first complete remission) or later (i.e., after patients have relapsed). To address this question, the various cooperative groups in the United States have agreed to conduct a randomized clinical trial of early versus delayed high-dose chemotherapy for patients with high-risk (high-intermediate or high-risk based on IPI score) DLBCL. In this trial, referred to as the North American High-Dose Therapy Trial, patients younger than 65 years old will receive five courses of CHOP chemotherapy. Patients who have a partial or complete response will then be randomized to receive either three more cycles of CHOP or one additional cycle of CHOP followed by high-dose chemotherapy with autologous HSCT. Patients on the standard CHOP treatment who relapse will then receive the same high-dose chemotherapy.

CLINICAL CONTROVERSY

Because of high relapse rate in patients who have a complete response to CHOP, some clinicians believe that high-dose chemotherapy with autologous HSCT should be given as consolidation therapy in high-risk patients with aggressive NHLs who have a complete remission to CHOP or R-CHOP chemotherapy. To address this question, the North American High-Dose Therapy Trial is a randomized clinical comparison of early versus delayed high-dose chemotherapy for patients with high-risk (high-intermediate or high-risk based on IPI score) diffuse large B-cell lymphoma. The results of this trial should determine when high-risk patients with aggressive lymphoma should receive high-dose chemotherapy with autologous HSCT.

In summary, all younger patients with bulky stage II, stage III, or stage IV disease should be treated with CHOP (or R-CHOP) or CHOP-like chemotherapy until a complete response is achieved (usually three to four cycles).[50] A rapid response to chemotherapy (i.e., a complete response achieved in the first three treatment cycles) is associated with a more durable remission compared with patients requiring longer treatment. Two or more cycles of chemotherapy should be given following attainment of a complete response (a total of six to eight cycles). The use of long-term maintenance therapy following a complete response has not been shown to improve survival. High-dose chemotherapy with autologous HSCT should be considered in high-risk patients who respond to standard chemotherapy. Patients should be enrolled in clinical trials of new treatment approaches whenever possible.

Therapy of Elderly Patients with Advanced Disease

More than one-half of patients with NHL are older than 60 years of age at diagnosis, and about one-third are over the age of 70 years. The International Non-Hodgkin's Lymphoma Prognostic Factors Project showed that patients older than 60 years of age had a significantly lower complete response rate and overall survival.[51] The reasons for the poorer outcome in elderly patients are not clear. Older patients do not tolerate intensive chemotherapy as well as younger patients, and some studies have reported that older patients have a higher risk of treatment-related mortality. As a result, many clinicians treat elderly patients with reduced-dose or less-aggressive chemotherapy regimens. In general, these less intensive regimens have used anthracyclines with less cardiotoxicity than doxorubicin, have substituted mitoxantrone for doxorubicin, or have used short-duration weekly therapy.[38,88]

Over the past few years, several nonrandomized and randomized trials have evaluated different treatment approaches in older patients with aggressive NHL.[38,88] The results of these studies suggest that carefully selected elderly patients with good performance status and without significant comorbidities may tolerate aggressive anthracycline-containing regimens as well as younger patients. These patients should be treated initially with full-dose CHOP or similar regimens; dosages can be reduced later if severe toxicity occurs. Hematopoietic growth factors may allow elderly patients to maintain dose intensity.

The combination of rituximab and CHOP (R-CHOP) has replaced CHOP as standard treatment for elderly patients with aggressive lymphoma, based on the results of the GELA study.[101] In that study of 399 elderly patients with DLBCL, patients who were randomized to receive R-CHOP had a significantly higher complete response rate (76% vs. 63%) and longer event-free and overall survival as compared with those who received CHOP. In an updated analysis of that trial, significant differences in 4-year event-free survival (51% vs. 29%) and overall survival (59% vs. 47%) were observed between the two treatment groups. Further analysis of that study showed that the treatment benefit was primarily observed in patients with tumors that overexpressed BCL-2 (BCL-2^+).[102] It is important to note that rituximab is given differently in the GELA study as compared with the Czuczman study in patients with indolent lymphomas. In the R-CHOP regimen developed by Czuczman and associates,[77] two doses of rituximab are given before the start of CHOP therapy; two more doses are given in the middle of the six cycles of CHOP; and two additional doses are given at the end of CHOP therapy. In the GELA study, rituximab is given on day 1 (the same day that cyclophosphamide, doxorubicin, and vincristine are administered) with each cycle of CHOP chemotherapy.

Salvage Therapy

Although many patients with aggressive NHL experience long-term survival and cure with intensive chemotherapy, nearly 50% of patients fail to achieve a complete remission, and of those patients who do achieve a complete remission, about 20% to 30% subsequently relapse. Therefore about 60% to 70% of all patients with aggressive NHL will require salvage therapy at some time during their disease course. Response to salvage therapy depends on the initial responsiveness of the tumor to chemotherapy. Patients who achieve an initial complete remission and then relapse generally have a better response to salvage therapy than those who are primarily or partially resistant to chemotherapy.

Many conventional-dose salvage chemotherapy regimens have been used in patients with relapsed or refractory NHL. Many patients who respond to salvage therapy (i.e., chemosensitive relapse) will then receive high-dose chemotherapy with autologous HSCT. In an effort to avoid cross-resistance, most salvage regimens incorporate drugs not used in the initial therapy. Some of the more commonly used salvage regimens include DHAP (dexamethasone, cytarabine, and cisplatin), ESHAP (etoposide, methylprednisolone, cytarabine, and cisplatin), and MINE (mesna, ifosfamide, mitoxantrone, and etoposide), and no one regimen appears to be clearly superior to any other regimen.[38,40,88,103] Rituximab is sometimes added to these salvage regimens. With these salvage regimens, about 25% to 35% of patients achieve a complete response, with a median duration of remission of

1 to 2 years. Only about 5% to 10% of patients will have long-term disease-free survival.

ICE (ifosfamide, carboplatin, and etoposide) chemotherapy is a newer regimen that has been used in patients with refractory disease. Some clinicians believe that ICE is better tolerated than older cisplatin-based regimens, particularly in older patients. The combination of ICE and rituximab (RICE) is currently being evaluated as a salvage regimen, and early results are encouraging.[104] Rituximab is given before the first dose of ICE and then weekly during the regimen.

To improve the cure rate, many studies have evaluated high-dose chemotherapy with autologous HSCT as intensive consolidation therapy in patients who respond to salvage therapy.[98,99] In the PARMA study, 215 patients with relapsed aggressive NHL who had a response to DHAP salvage therapy were randomized to receive either high-dose chemotherapy or continued DHAP therapy.[105] Patients who received high-dose chemotherapy had significantly longer 5-year disease-free survival (46% vs. 12%) and overall survival (53% vs. 32%) than those treated with conventional salvage therapy. Further analysis of that study showed that patients who relapsed within 12 months of their initial diagnosis were less likely to benefit from high-dose chemotherapy than patients who relapsed after 12 months. Based on a review of the available evidence, including the PARMA study, it was concluded that high-dose chemotherapy with autologous HSCT is effective in patients who relapse for the first time and have responded to salvage therapy (first chemotherapy-sensitive relapse).[98,99] Unfortunately, there was inadequate evidence to make a treatment recommendation for patients who relapse and have not responded to salvage therapy (chemotherapy-resistant relapse). Based on these studies, high-dose chemotherapy with autologous HSCT is considered to be the treatment of choice in younger patients with chemotherapy-sensitive relapse.[38,50,88,106] High-dose chemotherapy with autologous HSCT is not recommended in patients with untested or chemotherapy-refractory relapse.

Rituximab is being evaluated in the setting of autologous HSCT.[73,85] It is given pretransplant as an in vivo purging agent prior to stem cell collection. In one study of patients with aggressive lymphoma, two courses of rituximab (starting at day 42 and 6 months posttransplant) were given as posttransplant consolidation.[85]

OTHER AGGRESSIVE LYMPHOMAS

Mantle cell lymphoma (MCL) is one of the new disease entities previously unrecognized by other classification systems.[107] This histologic type was found in 6% of cases in the International Non-Hodgkin's Lymphoma Classification Project.[48] The chromosomal translocation t(11;14) occurs in most cases of MCL. MCL usually occurs in older adults, particularly in men, and most patients have advanced disease at the time of diagnosis (see Table 129–8).[107] Extranodal involvement is found in about 90% of cases. The course of the disease is moderately aggressive; the median overall survival is about 3 years, with no evidence of a survival plateau.

Patients with disseminated MCL are usually treated with the same intensive combination chemotherapy regimens that are used in diffuse aggressive lymphomas. Overall response rates to these regimens is about 80%, with about one-half of patients achieving a complete response.[107] Median progression-free and overall survival was 20 and 36 months, respectively. In patients who respond to initial therapy, interferon alfa may have a role as maintenance or consolidation therapy. Despite the high response rates, MCL is not considered curable with standard chemotherapy. Therefore younger patients who

have an initial response to chemotherapy often undergo autologous or allogeneic HSCT as consolidation therapy.[108] Because MCL usually expresses CD20, rituximab, either alone or combined with CHOP, has been used with some success in patients with newly diagnosed and relapsed MCL.[55,107] The NCCN Guidelines recommend that patients with advanced-stage MCL be treated initially with combination chemotherapy, either alone or combined with rituximab.[50]

Primary mediastinal large B-cell lymphoma (PMBL) is a distinct clinicopathologic entity, accounting for about 7% of all DLBCLs and 2.4% of all NHLs in the International NHL Classification Project.[48] This type of lymphoma tends to occur in younger patients (median age at presentation is 30 years old) and has a female predominance (see Table 129–8).[109] Patients present with a locally invasive mediastinal mass originating in the thymus, with frequent airway compromise and superior vena cava syndrome. Although the disease course is similar to that of other aggressive lymphomas, the biologic features of PMBL clearly differentiate PMBL from other types of DLBCL.[109] Patients with PMBL should be treated similarly to other patients with localized DLBCL.

NON-HODGKIN'S LYMPHOMA IN AIDS

The risk of NHL for patients with AIDS is increased about 150- to 250-fold as compared to the general population.[110] AIDS-related lymphoma arises as a consequence of long-term stimulation and proliferation of B lymphocytes from HIV and the reactivation of prior EBV infection due to HIV-induced immunosuppression.[38,40,111] AIDS-related lymphoma usually occurs late in the course of HIV infection and is the cause of death in about 15% of HIV-infected individuals. Although HIV infects T cells, more than 95% of AIDS-related lymphomas are B-cell neoplasms. About 60% of AIDS-related lymphomas are classified as Burkitt's (30%) or diffuse large B-cell type (30%).[111]

The clinical presentation is similar to that observed in other immunocompromised states. Most patients with AIDS-related lymphoma present with B (constitutional) symptoms and have advanced stage (III or IV) disease at the time of diagnosis.[38,40,111] Involvement of extranodal sites is common. The clinical course of AIDS-related lymphoma is aggressive; median survival is about 6 months and 2-year survival is only 10% to 20%. Factors associated with decreased survival include age greater than 35 years, history of injection drug use, CD4 cell count < 100/mm³, a history of AIDS prior to the diagnosis of lymphoma, stage III or IV disease, and elevated LDH levels.[111] The IPI has also been validated for use in patients with AIDS-related lymphoma.

The treatment of patients with AIDS-associated lymphomas is difficult because the immunocompromised state of these patients increases their risk of significant toxicity due to myelosuppressive therapy. Except for primary CNS lymphoma, AIDS-related lymphoma is never considered truly localized, and systemic chemotherapy is indicated. For patients with adequate immune function and without a history of an opportunistic infection, chemotherapy regimens similar to those used for aggressive lymphomas may be used.[38,40,111] However, many patients with AIDS-related lymphoma are treated with less intensive regimens because of the increased risk of treatment-related toxicity. In the era of highly active antiretroviral therapy (HAART), however, some clinicians believe that standard doses of chemotherapy can be safely administered to patients who achieve a virologic response to HAART.

The results of treatment with standard chemotherapy regimens, including CHOP, BACOD, and CDE (cyclophosphamide, doxorubicin, and etoposide), have been disappointing. The complete response rate with combination chemotherapy is about 40% to 50%, with a median survival of about 8 months. Newer approaches such as the dose-adjusted EPOCH (etoposide, prednisone, vincristine, cyclophosphamide, and doxorubicin) regimen developed at the National Cancer Institute appear promising.[112] At 53 months' median follow-up, disease-free and overall survival are 73% and 60%, respectively. Intrathecal chemotherapy should be administered to prevent CNS relapses. HAART and prophylactic antibiotics should be continued during chemotherapy.

EVALUATION OF THERAPEUTIC OUTCOMES

Hodgkin's and non-Hodgkin's lymphomas tend to respond well to radiation, chemotherapy, and biologic therapy. The goal of therapy for patients with Hodgkin's and aggressive non-Hodgkin's lymphoma is long-term survival and cure. The therapeutic goal in patients with indolent NHLs is less clear because of the indolent nature of the disease and the lack of convincing evidence showing that therapy prolongs survival. Therapeutic responses are evaluated based on physical exam, radiologic evidence, and other positive findings at baseline.[56] A complete response is defined as a normal physical exam, with normal lymph nodes and lymph node masses, and no evidence of disease in other sites. A classification of complete response "uncertain" is used when the patient has a normal physical exam and lymph nodes, shrinkage of >75% in lymph node masses, and a normal or indeterminate bone marrow biopsy. A partial response is defined as shrinkage of tumor in the lymph nodes or lymph node masses by ≥50%, or a completely normal exam except a positive bone marrow biopsy. Relapse or progression is defined as new nodes involved or an increase in nodal or spleen mass size.

Patients with Hodgkin's and aggressive non-Hodgkin's lymphoma are usually evaluated for response at the end of four cycles of therapy or at the end of treatment if less than four cycles of therapy are planned. If patients are treated with chemotherapy alone, two additional cycles of chemotherapy are given after the patient has achieved a complete remission. The rapidity of response to therapy in patients with indolent NHL depends on the choice of therapy. Responses occur slowly with therapy with oral alkylating agents, but occur much more rapidly with aggressive therapies such as combination chemotherapy with or without rituximab. If radiation alone is used, then a therapeutic evaluation should occur at the end of treatment.

CONCLUSIONS

Several decades ago, lymphomas were considered a fatal disease. Today most patients with Hodgkin's disease and many patients with aggressive NHLs can be cured with radiation therapy, chemotherapy, or a combination of radiation and chemotherapy. Our ability to achieve long-term survival and cure in these patients is the result of many factors, including development of accurate and reproducible classification systems; a more uniform approach to the staging of lymphoma; and advances in treatment strategies, especially the use of intensive combination chemotherapy. The routine use of hematopoietic growth factors allows oncologists to maintain dose intensity, which may be important for the treatment of aggressive lymphomas. The use of high-dose chemotherapy with autologous HSCT as intensive consolidation therapy for selected patients with aggressive NHL who respond to initial induction therapy, or as salvage therapy after relapse for patients with Hodgkin's lymphoma or aggressive NHL, has also contributed to increased cure rates.

New treatment approaches are needed, particularly for indolent NHLs. Although many new therapies have been developed recently for indolent lymphomas, there is no convincing evidence that any of these therapies have changed the natural history of the disease. One of the most exciting new therapies is biologic therapy with anti-CD20 monoclonal antibodies. The recent approval of radiolabeled anti-CD20 antibodies (i.e., radioimmunoconjugates) provides another therapeutic option for these patients. As these new biologic therapies become available, it will be important to better understand how to use these agents, either alone or combined with standard chemotherapy. Although about one-third of patients with aggressive lymphomas can be cured of their disease, most patients will relapse and eventually die of their disease. More effective induction chemotherapy regimens are needed for newly diagnosed patients, and more active salvage therapy is needed for patients with relapsed aggressive NHL.

The goal for the future is to develop treatment modalities to achieve cure in a larger number of patients. But the acute and chronic toxicities associated with treatment must also be considered, particularly in elderly patients and those with significant comorbidities. Consideration of long-term toxicities is of particular concern to patients with Hodgkin's lymphoma because of the high cure rate.

Finally, it is hoped that a better understanding of the pathogenesis of NHL through continued research in molecular biology and immunology will lead to the development of specific therapies aimed at molecular targets. In addition, gene expression profiling may also allow researchers to identify new clinically important subtypes of NHL, and to identify subgroups of patients who respond poorly to standard therapy.

ABBREVIATIONS

ABVD: doxorubicin (Adriamycin), bleomycin, vinblastine, and dacarbazine
AIDS: acquired immunodeficiency syndrome
ATL: adult T-cell leukemia/lymphoma
BACOP: bleomycin, cyclophosphamide, doxorubicin (hydroxydaunomycin), vincristine (Oncovin), and prednisone
BEACOPP: bleomycin, etoposide, doxorubicin (Adriamycin), cyclophosphamide, vincristine (Oncovin), procarbazine, and prednisone
2-CdA: cladribine
CDE: cyclophosphamide, doxorubicin, and etoposide
cHL: classical Hodgkin's lymphoma
ChlVPP: chlorambucil, vincristine (Oncovin), procarbazine, and prednisone
CHOP-B: cyclophosphamide, doxorubicin, vincristine, prednisone, and bleomycin
CHOP: cyclophosphamide, doxorubicin (hydroxydaunomycin), vincristine (Oncovin), and prednisone
CHVP: cyclophosphamide, doxorubicin (hydroxydaunomycin), teniposide, and prednisone
COPP: cyclophosphamide, vincristine (Oncovin), procarbazine, and prednisone

CR: complete response
CS: clinical stage
CT: computed tomography
CVP: cyclophosphamide, vincristine, and prednisone
CVPP: cyclophosphamide, vincristine (Oncovin), procarbazine, and prednisone
DHAP: dexamethasone, cytarabine, and cisplatin
DLBCL: diffuse large B-cell lymphoma
EBV: Epstein-Barr virus
EBVP: epirubicin, bleomycin, vinblastine, and prednisone
EORTC: European Organization for Research and Treatment of Cancer
EPOCH: etoposide, prednisone, vincristine, cyclophosphamide, and doxorubicin
ESHAP: etoposide, methylprednisolone, cytarabine, and cisplatin
ESR: erythrocyte sedimentation rate
FLIPI: Follicular Lymphoma International Prognostic Index
FND: fludarabine, mitoxantrone, and dexamethasone
FN: fludarabine and mitoxantrone
G-CSF: granulocyte colony-stimulating factor
GHLSG: German Hodgkin's Lymphoma Study Group
HAART: highly active antiretroviral therapy
HIV: human immunodeficiency virus
HPF: high-power field
HSCT: hematopoietic stem cell transplantation
HTLV-1: human T-cell lymphotropic virus type 1
ICE: ifosfamide, carboplatin, and etoposide
IFN-α: interferon alfa
IPI: International Prognostic Index
IPS: International Prognostic Score
LDH: lactate dehydrogenase
MACOP-B: methotrexate with leucovorin rescue, doxorubicin, cyclophosphamide, vincristine, prednisone, and bleomycin
MALT: mucosa-associated lymphoid tissue
M-BACOD: methotrexate, bleomycin, doxorubicin (Adriamycin), cyclophosphamide, vincristine (Oncovin), and dexamethasone
MCL: mantle cell lymphoma
MINE: mesna, ifosfamide, mitoxantrone, and etoposide
MOPP: mechlorethamine, vincristine (Oncovin), procarbazine, and prednisone
MRI: magnetic resonance imaging
MVPP: mechlorethamine, vinblastine, procarbazine, and prednisone
NCCN: National Comprehensive Cancer Network
NCI: National Cancer Institute
NHL: non-Hodgkin's lymphoma
NLPHD: nodular lymphocyte-predominant Hodgkin's disease
PCR: polymerase chain reaction
PMBL: primary mediastinal large B-cell lymphoma
PR: partial response
ProMACE/CytaBOM: prednisone, doxorubicin, cyclophosphamide, and etoposide, followed by cytarabine, bleomycin, vincristine, and methotrexate with leucovorin rescue
ProMACE/MOPP: prednisone, methotrexate, doxorubicin, cyclophosphamide, and etoposide/mechlorethamine, vincristine, procarbazine, and prednisone
PS: pathologic stage
R-CHOP: rituximab, cyclophosphamide hydroxydaunomycin, vincristine (Oncovin), and prednisone
REAL-WHO: Revised European-American Classification of Lymphoid Neoplasms and World Health Organization
RICE: rituximab, ifosfamide, carboplatin, and etoposide
SWOG: Southwest Oncology Group

Review Questions and other resources can be found at *www.pharmacotherapyonline.com.*

REFERENCES

1. Donaldson SS, Hancock SL, Hoppe RT. The Janeway lecture. Hodgkin's disease—finding the balance between cure and late effects. Cancer J Sci Am 1999;5:325–333.
2. Diehl V, Mauch P, Harris NL. Hodgkin's Disease. In: DeVita VT Jr, Hellman S, Rosenberg SA, eds. Cancer: Principles & Practice of Oncology, 6th ed. Philadelphia, Lippincott Williams & Wilkins, 2001:2339–2387.
3. Gustavsson A, Osterman B, Cavallin-Stahl E. A systematic overview of radiation therapy effects in Hodgkin's lymphoma. Acta Oncol 2003;42:589–604.
4. Linch DC, Gosden RG, Tulandi T, et al. Hodgkin's lymphoma: choice of therapy and late complications. Hematology (Am Soc Hematol Educ Program) 2000:205–221.
5. Jemal A, Murray T, Ward E, et al. Cancer statistics, 2004. CA Cancer J Clin 2005;55:10–30.
6. Kaufman D, Longo DL. Hodgkin's Disease. In: Abeloff MD, Armitage JO, Lichter AS, Niederhuber JE, eds. Clinical Oncology, 2nd ed. Philadelphia, Churchill Livingstone, 2000:2620–2657.
7. Glaser SL, Swartz WG. Time trends in Hodgkin's disease incidence. The role of diagnostic accuracy. Cancer 1990;66:2196–2204.
8. Ries L, Eisner M, Kosary C, et al. SEER cancer statistics review, 1975–2001. Bethesda, MD, National Cancer Institute, 2004.
9. Aleman BMP, van den Belt-Dusebout AW, Klokman WJ, et al. Long-term cause-specific mortality of patients treated for Hodgkin's disease. J Clin Oncol 2003;21:3431–3439.
10. Papadaki T, Stamatopoulos K. Hodgkin disease immunopathogenesis: long-standing questions, recent answers, further directions. Trends Immunol 2003;24:508–511.
11. Diehl V, Stein H, Hummel M, et al. Hodgkin's lymphoma: biology and treatment strategies for primary, refractory, and relapsed disease. Hematology (Am Soc Hematol Educ Program) 2003:225–247.
12. Jarrett RF, Krajewski AS, Angus B, et al. The Scotland and Newcastle epidemiological study of Hodgkin's disease: impact of histopathological review and EBV status on incidence estimates. J Clin Pathol 2003;56:811–816.
13. Jaffe ES, Harris NL, Stein H, Vardiman JW. World Health Organization Classification of Tumours: Pathology and Genetics of Tumours of the Haematopoietic and Lymphoid tissues. Lyon, France, IARC Press, 2001.
14. Lister TA, Crowther D, Sutcliffe SB, et al. Report of a committee convened to discuss the evaluation and staging of patients with Hodgkin's disease: Cotswolds meeting. J Clin Oncol 1989;7:1630–1636.
15. Hodgkin's Disease Guidelines. Practice Guidelines in Oncology: National Comprehensive Cancer Network, 2004.
16. Kaufman D, Longo DL. Hodgkin's Disease. In: Abeloff MD, Armitage JO, Lichter AS, Niederhuber JE, eds. Clinical Oncology, 2nd ed. Philadelphia, Churchill Livingstone, 2000:2620–2657.
17. Diehl V, Mauch P, Harris NL. Hodgkin's Disease. In: DeVita VT Jr, Hellman S, Rosenberg SA, eds. Cancer: Principles & Practice of Oncology, 6th ed. Philadelphia, Lippincott Williams & Wilkins, 2001:2339–2387.
18. Hasenclever D, Diehl V, Armitage JO, et al. A prognostic score for advanced Hodgkin's disease. N Engl J Med 1998;339:1506–1514.
19. Specht L, Gray RG, Clarke MJ, Peto R. Influence of more extensive radiotherapy and adjuvant chemotherapy on long-term outcome of early-stage Hodgkin's disease: a meta-analysis of 23 randomized trials involving 3,888 patients. International Hodgkin's Disease Collaborative Group. J Clin Oncol 1998;16:830–843.
20. Press OW, LeBlanc M, Lichter AS, et al. Phase III randomized intergroup trial of subtotal lymphoid irradiation versus doxorubicin, vinblastine, and subtotal lymphoid irradiation for stage IA to IIA Hodgkin's disease. J Clin Oncol 2001;19:4238–4244.

21. Engert A, Schiller P, Josting A, et al. Involved-field radiotherapy is equally effective and less toxic compared with extended-field radiotherapy after four cycles of chemotherapy in patients with early-stage unfavorable Hodgkin's lymphoma: results of the HD8 trial of the German Hodgkin's Lymphoma Study Group. J Clin Oncol 2003;21:3601–3608.

22. Horning SJ, Hoppe RT, Breslin S, et al. Stanford V and radiotherapy for locally extensive and advanced Hodgkin's disease: mature results of a prospective clinical trial. J Clin Oncol 2002;20:630–637.

23. DeVita VT Jr, Simon RM, Hubbard SM, et al. Curability of advanced Hodgkin's disease with chemotherapy. Long-term follow-up of MOPP-treated patients at the National Cancer Institute. Ann Intern Med 1980;92:587–595.

24. Longo DL, Young RC, Wesley M, et al. Twenty years of MOPP therapy for Hodgkin's disease. J Clin Oncol 1986;4:1295–306.

25. Longo DL. The use of chemotherapy in the treatment of Hodgkin's disease. Semin Oncol 1990;17:716–735.

26. Canellos GP, Anderson JR, Propert KJ, et al. Chemotherapy of advanced Hodgkin's disease with MOPP, ABVD, or MOPP alternating with ABVD. N Engl J Med 1992;327:1478–1484.

27. Goldie JH, Coldman AJ, Gudauskas GA. Rationale for the use of alternating non-cross-resistant chemotherapy. Cancer Treat Rep 1982;66:439–449.

28. Glick JH, Young ML, Harrington D, et al. MOPP/ABV hybrid chemotherapy for advanced Hodgkin's disease significantly improves failure-free and overall survival: the 8-year results of the intergroup trial. J Clin Oncol 1998;16:19–26.

29. Duggan DB, Petroni GR, Johnson JL, et al. Randomized comparison of ABVD and MOPP/ABV hybrid for the treatment of advanced Hodgkin's disease: report of an intergroup trial. J Clin Oncol 2003;21:607–614.

30. Prosnitz LR. Consolidative radiotherapy in the treatment of advanced Hodgkin's disease: is it dead? Int J Radiat Oncol Biol Phys 2003;56:605–608.

31. Loeffler M, Brosteanu O, Hasenclever D, et al. Meta-analysis of chemotherapy versus combined modality treatment trials in Hodgkin's disease. International Database on Hodgkin's Disease Overview Study Group. J Clin Oncol 1998;16:818–829.

32. Aleman BMP, Raemaekers JMM, Tirelli U, et al. Involved-field radiotherapy for advanced Hodgkin's lymphoma. N Engl J Med 2003;348:2396–2406.

33. Horning SJ, Williams J, Bartlett NL, et al. Assessment of the Stanford V regimen and consolidative radiotherapy for bulky and advanced Hodgkin's disease: Eastern Cooperative Oncology Group pilot study E1492. J Clin Oncol 2000;18:972–980.

34. Diehl V, Franklin J, Hasenclever D, et al. BEACOPP, a new dose-escalated and accelerated regimen, is at least as effective as COPP/ABVD in patients with advanced-stage Hodgkin's lymphoma: interim report from a trial of the German Hodgkin's Lymphoma Study Group. J Clin Oncol 1998;16:3810–3821.

35. Diehl V, Franklin J, Pfreundschuh M, et al. Standard and increased-dose BEACOPP chemotherapy compared with COPP-ABVD for advanced Hodgkin's disease. N Engl J Med 2003;348:2386–2395.

36. Bierman PJ, Nademanee A. Autologous and allogeneic hematopoietic cell transplantation for Hodgkin's disease. In: Blume KG, Forman SJ, Appelbaum FR, eds. Thomas' Hematopoietic Cell Transplantation. Malden, MA, Blackwell Science, 2004:1191–1206.

37. Longo DL, Duffey PL, Young RC, et al. Conventional-dose salvage combination chemotherapy in patients relapsing with Hodgkin's disease after combination chemotherapy: the low probability for cure. J Clin Oncol 1992;10:210–218.

38. Armitage JO, Mauch PM, Harris NL, Bierman P. Non-Hodgkin's lymphoma. In: DeVita VT, Hellman S, Rosenberg SA, eds. Cancer: Principles & Practice of Oncology, 6th ed. Philadelphia, Lippincott Williams & Wilkins, 2001:2256–2316.

39. Vose JM, Chiu BC-H, Cheson BD, et al. Update on epidemiology and therapeutics for non-Hodgkin's lymphoma. Hematology (Am Soc Hematol Educ Program) 2002:241–262.

40. Lister TA, Armitage JO. Non-Hodgkin's lymphoma. In: Abeloff MD, Armitage JO, Lichter AS, Niederhuber JE, eds. Clinical Oncology, 2nd ed. New York, Churchill Livingstone, 2000:2658–2719.

41. Macintyre E, Willerford D, Morris SW. Non-Hodgkin's lymphoma: molecular features of B cell lymphoma. In: Schechter GP, Berliner N, Telen MJ, eds. Hematology 2000, 2000:180–204.

42. Harris NL, Stein H, Coupland SE, et al. New approaches to lymphoma diagnosis. Hematology (Am Soc Hematol Educ Program) 2001:194–220.

43. Freeman AS, Neuberg D, Mauch P, et al. Long-term follow-up of autologous bone marrow transplantation in patients with relapsed follicular lymphoma. Blood 1999;94:3325–3333.

44. Trumper LH, Brittinger G, Diehl V, Harris NL. Non-Hodgkin's lymphoma: a history of classification and clinical observations. In: Mauch PM, Armitage JO, Coiffier B, et al, eds. Non-Hodgkin's Lymphomas. Philadelphia, Lippincott Williams & Wilkins, 2004:3–19.

45. Kuppers R, Klein U, Hansmann M-L, Rajewsky K. Cellular origins of human B-cell lymphomas. N Engl J Med 1999;341:1520–1529.

46. Harris NL, Jaffe ES, Stein H. A revised European-American classification of lymphoid neoplasms: a proposal from the International Lymphoma Study Group. Blood 1994;84:1361–1392.

47. Harris NL. Revised European-American and World Health Organization Classifications of Non-Hodgkin's Lymphoma. In: Mauch PM, Armitage JO, Coiffier B, et al, eds. Non-Hodgkin's Lymphoma. Philadelphia, Lippincott Williams & Wilkins, 2004:45–58.

48. The Non-Hodgkin's Lymphoma Classification Project. A clinical evaluation of the International Lymphoma Study Group classification of non-Hodgkin's lymphoma. Blood 1997;89:3909–3918.

49. Harris NL, Jaffe ES, Diebold J, et al. World Health Organization Classification of neoplastic diseases of the hematopoietic and lymphoid tissues: report of the Clinical Advisory Committee meeting—Airlie House, Virginia, November 1997. J Clin Oncol 1999;17:3835–3849.

50. Non-Hodgkin's Lymphoma Guidelines. Practice Guidelines in Oncology: National Comprehensive Cancer Network, 2004.

51. The International Non-Hodgkin's Lymphoma Prognostic Factors Project. A predictive model for aggressive non-Hodgkin's lymphoma. N Engl J Med 1993;329:987–994.

52. Solal-Celigny P, Roy P, Colombat P, et al. Follicular lymphoma international prognostic index. Blood 2004;104:1258–1265.

53. Levy R. Karnofsky lecture: immunotherapy of lymphoma. J Clin Oncol 1999;17:7–13.

54. Grillo-Lopez AJ, White CA, Varns C, et al. Overview of the clinical development of rituximab: first monoclonal antibody approved for treatment of lymphoma. Semin Oncol 1999;26(Suppl 14):66–73.

55. Plosker GL, Figgitt DP. Rituximab: a review of its use in non-Hodgkin's lymphoma and chronic lymphocytic leukemia. Drugs 2003;63:803–843.

56. Cheson BD, Horning SJ, Coiffier B, et al. Report of an international workshop to standardize response criteria for non-Hodgkin's lymphoma. J Clin Oncol 1999;17:1244–1253.

57. Freedman AS, Friedberg JW, Mauch PM, et al. Follicular lymphoma. In: Mauch PM, Armitage JO, Coiffier B, et al, eds. Non-Hodgkin's Lymphoma. Philadelphia, Lippincott Williams & Wilkins, 2004:367–388.

58. The Non-Hodgkin's Lymphoma Classification Project: National Cancer Institute sponsored study of classifications of non-Hodgkin's lymphomas. Summary and description of a working formulation for clinical usage. Cancer 1982;49:2112–2135.

59. Horning SJ. Natural history of and therapy for the indolent non-Hodgkin's lymphomas. Semin Oncol 1993;20(Suppl 5):75–88.

60. Rodriguez J, McLaughlin P, Hagenmeister FB, et al. Follicular large cell lymphoma: an aggressive lymphoma that often presents with favorable prognostic features. Blood 1999;93:2202–2207.

61. Seymour JF, Pro B, Fuller LM, et al. Long-term follow-up of a prospective study of combined modality therapy for stage I–II indolent non-Hodgkin's lymphoma. J Clin Oncol 2003;21:2115–2122.

62. Cheson BD. New therapeutic strategies for the treatment of indolent non-Hodgkin's lymphoma. In: Schechter GP, Hoffman R, Schrier S, eds. Hematology (Am Soc Hematol Educ Program), 1999:291–829.

63. Cabanillas F, Horning S, Kaminski M, Champlin R. Managing indolent lymphomas in relapse: working our way through a plethora of options. Hematology (Am Soc Hematol Educ Program) 2000:166–179.

64. Ardeshna KM, Smith P, Norton A, et al. Long-term effect of a watch and wait policy versus immediate systemic treatment for asymptomatic advanced-stage non-Hodgkin's lymphoma: a randomised controlled trial. Lancet 2003;362:516–522.

65. Peterson BA, Petroni GR, Frizzera G, et al. Prolonged single-agent versus combination chemotherapy in indolent follicular lymphomas: a study of the Cancer and Leukemia Group B. J Clin Oncol 2003;21:5–15.

66. McLaughlin P, Hagemeister F, Romaguera J, et al. Fludarabine, mitoxantrone, and dexamethasone: an effective new regimen for indolent lymphoma. J Clin Oncol 1996;14:1262–1268.

67. Velasquez WS, Lew D, Grogan TM, et al. Combination of fludarabine and mitoxantrone in untreated stages III and IV low-grade lymphoma: S9501. J Clin Oncol 2003;21:1996–2003.

68. Parkinson DR, Sznol M, Cheson BD. Biologic therapies for low-grade lymphomas. Semin Oncol 1993;20(Suppl 5):111–117.

69. Solal-Celigny P, Lepage E, Brousse N, et al. Doxorubicin-containing regimen with or without interferon alfa-2b for advanced follicular lymphoma: final analysis of survival and toxicity in the Groupe d'Etude des Lymphomes Folliculaires 86 Trial. J Clin Oncol 1998;16:2332–238.

70. Cheson BD. The curious case of the baffling biological. J Clin Oncol 2000;18:2007–2009.

71. Fisher RI, Dana BW, LeBlanc M, et al. Interferon alfa consolidation after intensive chemotherapy does not prolong the progression-free survival of patients with low-grade non-Hodgkin's lymphoma: results of the Southwest Oncology Group Randomized Phase III Study 8809. J Clin Oncol 2000;18:2010–2016.

72. McLaughlin P, Grillo-Lopez AJ, Link BK, et al. Rituximab chimeric anti-CD20 monoclonal antibody therapy for relapsed indolent lymphoma: half of patients respond to a four-dose treatment program. J Clin Oncol 1998;16:2825–2833.

73. Cohen Y, Solal-Celigny P, Polliack A. Rituximab therapy for follicular lymphoma: a comprehensive review of its efficacy as primary treatment, treatment for relapsed disease, re-treatment and maintenance. Haematologica 2003;88:811–823.

74. Davis TA, Grillo-Lopez AJ, White CA, et al. Rituximab anti-CD20 monoclonal antibody therapy in non-Hodgkin's lymphoma: safety and efficacy of re-treatment. J Clin Oncol 2000;18:3135–3143.

75. Colombat P, Salles G, Brousse N, et al. Rituximab (anti-CD20 monoclonal antibody) as single first-line therapy for patients with follicular lymphoma with a low tumor burden: clinical and molecular evaluation. Blood 2001;97:101–106.

76. Hainsworth JD, Litchy S, Burris HA, et al. Rituximab as first-line and maintenance therapy for patients with indolent non-Hodgkin's lymphoma. J Clin Oncol 2002;20:4261–4267.

77. Czuczman MS, Grillo-Lopez AJ, White CA, et al. Treatment of patients with low-grade B-cell lymphoma with the combination of chimeric anti-CD20 monoclonal antibody and CHOP chemotherapy. J Clin Oncol 1999;17:268–276.

78. Cheson BD. Radioimmunotherapy of non-Hodgkin lymphomas. Blood 2003;101:391–398.

79. Emmanouilldes C. Radioimmunotherapy for non-Hodgkin's lymphoma. Semin Oncol 2003;30:531–544.

80. Press OW, Unger JM, Braziel RM, et al. A phase 2 trial of CHOP chemotherapy followed by tositumomab/iodine I 131 tositumomab for previously untreated follicular non-Hodgkin lymphoma: Southwest Oncology Group Protocol S9911. Blood 2003;102:1606–1612.

81. Armitage JO, Carbone PP, Connors JM, et al. Treatment-related myelodysplasia and acute leukemia in non-Hodgkin's lymphoma patients. J Clin Oncol 2003;21:897–906.

82. Hunault-Berger M, Ifrah N, Solal-Celigny P, et al. Intensive therapies in follicular non-Hodgkin lymphomas. Blood 2002;100:1141–1152.

83. van Besien K, Loberiza FR, Bajorunaite R, et al. Comparison of autologous and allogeneic hematopoietic stem cell transplantation for follicular lymphoma. Blood 2003;102:3521–3529.

84. Schouten HC, Qian W, Kvaloy S, et al. High-dose therapy improves progression-free survival and survival in relapsed follicular non-Hodgkin's lymphoma: results from the randomized European CUP trial. J Clin Oncol 2003;21:3918–3927.

85. Horwitz SM, Negrin RS, Blume KG, et al. Rituximab as adjuvant to high-dose therapy and autologous hematopoietic cell transplantation for aggressive non-Hodgkin lymphoma. Blood 2004;103:777–783.

86. Cavalli F, Isaacson PG, Gascoyne RD, Zucca E. MALT lymphomas. Hematology (Am Soc Hematol Educ Program) 2001:241–258.

87. Fisher RI, Shah P. Current trends in large cell lymphoma. Leukemia 2003;17:1948–1960.

88. Armitage JO, Mauch PM, Harris NL, et al. Diffuse large B-cell lymphoma. In: Mauch PM, Armitage JO, Coiffier B, et al, eds. Non-Hodgkin's Lymphoma. Philadelphia, Lippincott Williams & Wilkins, 2004:427–453.

89. Rosenwald A, Wright G, Chan WC, et al. The use of molecular profiling to predict survival after chemotherapy for diffuse large-B-cell lymphoma. N Engl J Med 2002;346:1937–1947.

90. Lossos IS, Czerwinski DK, Alizadeh AA, et al. Prediction of survival in diffuse large-B-cell lymphoma based on the expression of six genes. N Engl J Med 2004;350:1828–1837.

91. Miller TP, Dahlberg S, Cassady JR, et al. Chemotherapy alone compared with chemotherapy plus radiotherapy for localized intermediate- and high-grade non-Hodgkin's lymphoma. N Engl J Med 1998;339:21–26.

92. McKelvey EM, Gottleib JA, Wilson HE, et al. Hydroxyldaunomycin (Adriamycin) combination chemotherapy in malignant lymphoma. Cancer 1976;38:1484–1493.

93. Jones SE, Grozea PN, Metz EN, et al. Superiority of Adriamycin containing combination chemotherapy in the treatment of diffuse lymphoma: a Southwest Oncology Group study. Cancer 1979;43:417–425.

94. Fisher RI, Gaynor ER, Dahlberg S, et al. Comparison of a standard regimen (CHOP) with three intensive chemotherapy regimens for advanced non-Hodgkin's lymphoma. N Engl J Med 1993;328:1002–1006.

95. Vose JM, Link BK, Grossbard ML, et al. Phase II study of rituximab in combination with CHOP chemotherapy in patients with previously untreated, aggressive non-Hodgkin's lymphoma. J Clin Oncol 2001;19:389–397.

96. Blayney DW, LeBlanc ML, Grogan T, et al. Dose-intense chemotherapy every 2 weeks with dose-intense cyclophosphamide, doxorubicin, vincristine, and prednisone may improve survival in intermediate- and high-grade lymphoma: a phase II study of the Southwest Oncology Group (SWOG 9349). J Clin Oncol 2003;21:2466–2473.

97. Coiffier B. Increasing chemotherapy intensity in aggressive lymphoma: a renewal? J Clin Oncol 2003;21:2457–2459.

98. Shipp MA, Abeloff MD, Antman KH, et al. International consensus conference on high-dose therapy with hematopoietic stem cell transplantation in aggressive non-Hodgkin's lymphomas: report of the jury. J Clin Oncol 1999;17:423–429.

99. Haln T, Wolff SN, Czuczman M, et al. The role of cytotoxic therapy with hematopoietic stem cell transplantation in the therapy of diffuse large cell B-cell non-Hodgkin's lymphoma: an evidence-based review. Biol Blood Marrow Transplant 2001;7:308–331.

100. Milpied N, Deconinck E, Gaillard F, et al. Initial treatment of aggressive lymphoma with high-dose chemotherapy and autologous stem-cell support. N Engl J Med 2004;350:1287–1295.

101. Coiffier B, Lepage E, Briere J, et al. CHOP chemotherapy plus rituximab compared with CHOP alone in elderly patients with diffuse large-B-cell lymphoma. N Engl J Med 2002;346:235–242.

102. Mounier N, Briere J, Gisselbrecht C, et al. Rituximab plus CHOP (R-CHOP) overcomes bcl-2-associated resistance to chemotherapy in elderly patients with diffuse large B-cell lymphoma (DLBCL). Blood 2003;101:4279–4284.

103. Rodriguez-Monge EJ, Cabanillas F. Long-term follow-up of platinum-based lymphoma salvage regimens. The M.D. Anderson Cancer Center experience. Hematol Oncol Clin North Am 1997;11:937–947.

104. Kewalramani T, Zelenetz AD, Nimer SD, et al. Rituximab and ICE as second-line therapy before autologous stem cell transplantation for relapsed or primary refractory diffuse large B-cell lymphoma. Blood 2004;103:3684–3688.

105. Philip T, Guglielmi C, Hagenbeek A, et al. Autologous bone marrow transplantation as compared with salvage chemotherapy in relapses of chemotherapy-sensitive non-Hodgkin's lymphoma. N Engl J Med 1995;333:1540–1545.

106. Lister TA. High-dose therapy for follicular lymphoma revisited: not if, but when? J Clin Oncol 2003;21:3894–3896.

107. Hiddemann W, Lenz G, Weisenburger DD, Dreyling MH. Mantle cell lymphoma. In: Mauch PM, Armitage JO, Coiffier B, et al, eds. Non-Hodgkin's Lymphoma. Philadelphia, Lippincott Williams & Wilkins, 2004:461–476.

108. Press OW. Treatment of mantle-cell lymphoma: stem-cell transplanta-tion, radioimmunotherapy, and management of mantle-cell lymphoma subsets. In: ASCO Education Book, 2002:407–415.

109. van Besien K, Kelta M, Bahaguna P. Primary mediastinal B-cell lymphoma: a review of pathology and management. J Clin Oncol 2001;19:1855–1864.

110. Goedert JJ. The epidemiology of acquired immunodeficiency syndrome malignancies. Semin Oncol 2000;27:390–401.

111. Levine AM, Said JW. Management of acquired immunodeficiency syndrome-related lymphoma. In: Mauch PM, Armitage JO, Coiffier B, et al, eds. Non-Hodgkin's Lymphoma. Philadelphia, Lippincott Williams & Wilkins, 2004:613–627.

112. Little RF, Pittaluga S, Grant N, et al. Highly effective treatment of acquired immunodeficiency syndrome-related lymphoma with dose-adjusted EPOCH: impact of antiretroviral therapy suspension and tumor biology. Blood 2003;101:4653–4659.

130
OVARIAN CANCER

William C. Zamboni, Laura L. Jung, and Margaret E. Tonda

Learning Objectives and other resources can be found at *www.pharmacotherapyonline.com.*

KEY CONCEPTS

❶ Patients with local disease have a 5-year survival rate greater than 90%, but most patients present with disseminated disease because symptoms are nonspecific and go unrecognized until late in the disease course. Patients with advanced disease have a 5-year survival rate of 10% to 30%.

❷ Ovarian cancer usually occurs in postmenopausal women in the sixth decade of life; the risk of developing ovarian cancer is increased in women with a family history involving two or more first-degree relatives.

❸ CA-125 is an antigen common to most nonmucinous epithelial ovarian carcinoma and is a useful marker for ovarian cancer; rising or falling CA-125 titers correlate with the disease extent.

❹ Ovarian cancer management is based on the histologic type, pathologic grade, and disease stage at initial presentation. In general, the treatment of patients with ovarian cancer involves surgical debulking at the time of staging laparotomy and primary or adjuvant chemotherapy.

❺ The beneficial effects of adjuvant chemotherapy in the treatment of local disease depend on the stage and disease subtype. Postoperative adjuvant chemotherapy is not required in stage IA or IB grade 1, whereas patients with stage IA or IB grade 2 or 3, and stage IC require adjuvant chemotherapy. All patients with stage II disease require adjuvant treatment. Paclitaxel plus carboplatin or cisplatin for three to six cycles is the current recommended adjuvant therapy for these patients.

❻ Survival of patients with advanced ovarian cancer is a function of stage at initial diagnosis and the amount of residual disease after surgical debulking. Patients with stage III disease treated with optimal debulking (<2 cm of residual tumor) have a 4-year survival rate of 30%, while patients with stage III or IV disease who have undergone suboptimal debulking (>2 cm of residual disease) have less than a 10% long-term survival rate.

❼ Current recommended treatment of advanced ovarian cancer (stage III or IV) is based on initial surgical debulking followed by paclitaxel plus carboplatin for six cycles.

❽ Approximately 20% to 50% of patients without evidence of disease on second-look laparotomy will relapse. In addition, patients who were initially sensitive to chemotherapy and whose response lasted the longest have the greatest likelihood of achieving a response to retreatment with the initial treatment regimen or treatment with salvage therapy.

❾ Patients with disease that was refractory to the initial platinum-containing chemotherapy or that recurs within 6 months after treatment (platinum-refractory) are unlikely to benefit from standard-dose platinum therapy. However, patients who relapse more than 6 months after the initial platinum-containing regimen (platinum-sensitive) have a response rate of 27% to 59% with a standard-dose second-line platinum regimen.

❿ The NCCN guidelines recommend retreatment with either paclitaxel or platinum, or the combination of paclitaxel and a platinum compound if disease recurs more than 6 months after the initial treatment with paclitaxel in combination with a platinum analog. Treatment options for patients with refractory disease or disease recurrence within 6 months after treatment include topotecan, altretamine, oral etoposide, liposomal doxorubicin, gemcitabine, tamoxifen, referral for a clinical trial, or supportive care therapy.

Ovarian cancer is the fifth most common noncutaneous malignancy diagnosed in women.[1] Overall, it is the fifth leading cause of cancer-related death and the most common death from gynecologic malignancy.[1] The incidence of ovarian cancer is highest in the United States, Europe, and Israel, and lowest in Japan and developing countries.[2] In the United States alone, it is estimated that 22,220 new cases of ovarian cancer will be diagnosed, and 16,210 women will die from this disease in 2005.[1] Based on Surveillance, Epidemiology, and End Results data collected from 1995 to 2000, 5-year survival

for all stages is nearly 50%, although it dramatically increases to over 90% in patients with localized disease.[1]

❶ Unfortunately, most patients have disseminated disease at diagnosis because symptoms are nonspecific and may not be recognized until late in the disease course.[4] Overall 5-year survival is slightly higher for white Americans (44%) as compared with African-Americans (38%). Survival for patients with localized disease is similar for white Americans and African-Americans (93%).[1] Surgery is an integral part of ovarian cancer management.[3] Chemotherapy, primarily the combination of a taxane plus a platinum analog, plays an important role for adjuvant therapy of localized and advanced disease.[3]

EPIDEMIOLOGY

Ovarian cancer usually occurs in postmenopausal white women during the sixth decade of life.[2] Only 5% to 10% of ovarian cancer is familial; the majority of ovarian cancer occurs sporadically. For women in the United States, the overall lifetime risk of developing ovarian cancer is 1.4% to 1.8%.[2] The most important risk factor appears to be family history of ovarian cancer. The lifetime risk for developing ovarian cancer markedly increases to 7% to 9% in women with a family history involving two or more first-degree relatives.[2] The risk for ovarian cancer is decreased to 0.6% in women who have had several pregnancies, especially in women who first became pregnant before age 25, and is increased to 3.4% in nulliparous women, suggesting that uninterrupted ovulation may be a contributing factor.[2] Prolonged oral contraceptive use or breast-feeding lowers the risk for developing ovarian cancer.[2] An increased risk has been associated with environmental exposure to asbestos or talc.[2]

GENETICS

Several hereditary ovarian cancer syndromes have been described, which include the development of breast and ovarian cancers or ovarian, endometrial, and nonpolyposis colon cancers.[2,3,5] These syndromes tend to occur at an earlier age than the usual development for each of the individual malignancies and account for about 5% of the total ovarian cancer incidence.[2,5] These syndromes may be linked to a number of genetic abnormalities that have been detected in patients with ovarian cancer.[6-8] The most common genetic alterations include mutations in *BRCA1* and *BRCA2*, but may also involve *p21*, *Her-2/Neu*, *p53*, *OVAC1*, *OVAC2*, and *Rb* gene function, and loss of heterozygosity on chromosomes 6, 9, 13q, 17, 18q, 19p, and 22q.

BRCA1 and *BRCA2* are tumor suppressor genes thought to be involved in one or more pathways of DNA damage recognition and repair. The *BRCA1* gene is located on chromosome 17q12-21 and the *BRCA2* gene is located on chromosome 13q12-13. Current risk estimates for the development of ovarian cancer in women with mutations in *BRCA1* are 26% to 85% by 70 years of age, whereas mutations in *BRCA2* appear to confer a lesser risk of developing this disease with an estimated risk of <10% by 70 years of age.[9,10] These estimates of ovarian cancer should to be interpreted with caution, as they are limited by selection bias of the study populations for families with large numbers of breast and ovarian cancers.

Patients with *BRCA1*-associated ovarian cancer are usually significantly younger than patients with *BRCA2* mutations, with a mean age of 54 years.[11] *BRCA1*-linked ovarian cancers are typically of serous histology, moderate to high grade, and advanced stage at diagnosis.[11] Identification of *BRCA1* mutations in patients may confer some survival benefit. Rubin and colleagues reported higher rates of overall survival in patients with ovarian cancer with *BRCA1* mutations than their matched controls not known to have hereditary cancer (77 months vs. 29 months, respectively).[8] In another study, patients with advanced-stage ovarian cancer with *BRCA1* mutations survived significantly longer than sporadic cases of ovarian cancer.[11] In this same study, patients with *BRCA1* or *BRCA2* mutations also had a significantly longer disease free interval (14 months vs. 7 months, respectively) compared to sporadic cases of ovarian cancer. Although it is unclear why *BRCA1* mutations may confer a survival advantage

in patients with ovarian cancer, one hypothesis suggests that these tumors may respond more favorably to chemotherapy. As *BRCA1* and *BRCA2* are thought to be involved in DNA damage or repair, their inactivation may result in an increased sensitivity of ovarian cancer cells to cytotoxic agents that act via induction of DNA damage.

Despite the progress made in understanding the genetic mechanisms and implications of ovarian cancer, much of this information is currently too premature to be clinically useful. Given current guidelines for the follow-up care of individuals at high genetic risk of ovarian cancer and the lack of clinically useful information, especially with BRCA mutations, additional clinical trials and research programs to further determine screening mechanisms for early detection, chemoprevention, and improved treatment are necessary.[9,10]

PATHOLOGY

Ovarian carcinomas can be separated into three major entities: epithelial carcinomas, germ cell tumors, and stromal carcinomas. Most ovarian tumors (85% to 90%) are derived from the epithelial surface of the ovary.[2] The classification of common epithelial tumors has been developed by the World Health Organization and the International Federation of Gynecology and Obstetrics.[12,20] The nomenclature takes into account cell type, location of the tumor, and the degree of the malignancy, ranging from benign tumors to tumors of low malignancy to invasive carcinomas. Low malignancy ("borderline malignancy") epithelial tumors have a much better prognosis compared to invasive carcinomas and are characterized by epithelial papillae with atypical cell clusters, cellular stratification, nuclear atypia and increased mitotic activity. Malignant tumors are characterized by an infiltrative destructive growth pattern with malignant cells growing in a disorganized manner and dissection into stromal planes. Invasive epithelial carcinomas are characterized by histologic type and grade (degree of cellular differentiation).

The histologic types of common epithelial tumors include serous, mucinous, endometrioid and clear cell.[3,13] Serous carcinoma is the most common type of epithelial ovarian cancer and accounts for more than 50% of cases. The peak age range is 45 to 65 years.[13] Typical serous carcinomas display complex papillary and solid patterns and qualify as high-grade carcinomas. Endometrioid carcinomas are seen in women 40 to 50 years of age and comprise about 10% to 15% of ovarian carcinomas, of which about 6% are surface epithelial neoplasms.[13] Endometrioid tumors are usually diagnosed as stage I disease and have a better prognosis than tumors with serous histology. Mucinous carcinomas occur in women between 40 and 70 years of age and account for about 12% of all ovarian cancers. The overall prognosis for mucinous carcinoma is better than for serous carcinoma because most patients present with stage 1 disease. Clear cell carcinoma comprises about 3% of ovarian epithelial neoplasms and about 8% to 10% of ovarian carcinomas in women, with a mean age of 57 years. Although clear cell carcinoma is the least common ovarian neoplasm, it is most commonly associated with paraneoplastic-related hypercalcemia.[13]

The true prognostic impact of histologic subtype and grade in patients with epithelial ovarian cancer remains to be determined. In early-stage ovarian cancer, clear cell histology is a poor prognostic factor, while mucinous and clear cell histologies are poor prognostic indicators in advanced-stage disease.[14,15]

Germ cell tumors of the ovary are very uncommon, occurring in about 2% to 3% of all ovarian cancers in Western countries with an increased incidence in black and Asian women.[20] These tumors are highly curable and affect primarily young women, with a peak age incidence in the early 20s. In contrast to epithelial tumors, approximately 60% to 70% of germ cell tumors are stage I at diagnosis. Serum markers (human β-chorionic gonadotropin [β-hCG] and α-fetoprotein [AFP]) are helpful in the diagnosis and management of these tumors.

Ovarian sex cord-stromal tumors account for about 5% of all ovarian cancers and tend to be diagnosed at stage I.[20] These tumors are associated with hormonal effects, such as precocious puberty, amenorrhea, and postmenopausal bleeding.

CLINICAL PRESENTATION

Patients with early ovarian cancer can present with nonspecific, vague abdominal symptoms such as nausea, discomfort, dyspepsia, flatulence, bloating, fullness, early satiety, and digestive disturbances.[3,4] These symptoms can easily be confused with symptoms that happen normally throughout the menstrual cycle. Late symptoms can include pain, abdominal distention, ascites, and abdominal or pelvic masses.[3,4] A palpable ovary in a postmenopausal woman should be promptly evaluated because functional cysts do not usually occur in this age group.[16]

CLINICAL PRESENTATION OF OVARIAN CANCER

GENERAL
The patient may not be in any acute distress and may complain of vague, nonspecific symptoms.

SYMPTOMS
The patient may complain of back pain, fatigue, bloating, constipation, abdominal pain, urinary urgency, nausea, or weight change.

SIGNS
Patients may have a palpable abdominal mass.
Patients may have lymphadenopathy.
Patients may have signs of ascites (abdominal distention, shifting, and dullness to percussion)

LABORATORY TESTS
CA-125 may be elevated.
Hepatic function abnormalities may suggest metastatic disease.
Abnormalities in renal function tests may suggest compression of the renal system by the tumor.

OTHER DIAGNOSTIC TESTS
Chest x-ray, cystoscopy, proctoscopy, MRI, and CT may indicate extent of disease and any possible metastases.

DIAGNOSIS

The diagnostic work-up for suspected ovarian cancer includes a careful physical examination including a thorough breast examination, a Pap smear, and a rectovaginal examination.[16,17] A detailed family history should be taken, especially noting the rate and pattern of relatives with malignancies.

A complete blood count, chemistry profile (including liver and renal function tests), and a CA-125 assay should be performed. CA-125 is an antigen common to most nonmucinous epithelial ovarian

cancers and is detected in the laboratory with a monoclonal antibody directed at this antigen.[18,19] CA-125 is a useful tumor marker because it is found in more than 80% of ovarian tumors and rising (or falling) titers correlate with disease extent.[18,19] Normal CA-125 values are less than 35 units/mL.[18,19]

Refractory disease is often associated with a CA-125 level that does not return to normal or that remains elevated after completion of chemotherapy.[18,19] A new elevation in the CA-125 level may be the first sign of relapse.[19]

Other diagnostic tests should include a chest x-ray, an intravenous pyelogram, cystoscopy, proctoscopy, and a barium enema. Depending on clinical evaluation, computed tomography (CT), magnetic resonance imaging (MRI), or ultrasound may be indicated. An upper GI series is indicated in patients with gastrointestinal symptoms or with bowel obstruction.

The approach to diagnosing an adnexal mass discovered on pelvic examination depends on several factors, including the patient's reproductive age, adnexal mass size, menopausal status, and symptoms.[20] Exploratory laparotomy is indicated in premenarchal women, women with masses greater than 8 cm, women with masses that increase or persist through several menstrual cycles or that are fixed to peritoneal surfaces, women with bilateral masses, or women with intra-abdominal pain or ascites.[20]

SCREENING

Ovarian cancer is an ideal malignancy for early screening efforts because more than 50% of cases are currently diagnosed with advanced disease.[1] However, for screening efforts to be successful, suitable sensitive, specific, cost-effective screening tests with an adequate positive predictive value must be available. Also, there must be a detectable preclinical phase, and the disease must be amenable to therapy.[21-23] Three screening tests have been used to detect ovarian cancer: bimanual rectovaginal pelvic examination, CA-125 determination, and transvaginal sonography (TVS).[23] Bimanual rectovaginal pelvic examination is inadequate for screening purposes because it lacks useful sensitivity and specificity.[21-23] CA-125 is elevated in only 50% of stage I cases and a significant number of women with benign ovarian disease have abnormal CA-125 values.[21-23] TVS is not specific enough to use as the sole screening modality.

The following screening guidelines were developed at a National Institutes of Health consensus conference.[24]

- All women should have a comprehensive family history taken that focuses on all the known ovarian cancer risk factors. Rectovaginal pelvic exam should be performed as part of ordinary medical care.

- For women without a family history of ovarian cancer or with a family history of ovarian cancer in one relative, routine screening with ultrasound or CA-125 is not recommended because current evidence does not support any benefit. Participation in ovarian cancer screening trials is appropriate.

- In women with a family history of ovarian cancer in two or more relatives, the risk for developing ovarian cancer is 7%. No conclusive data show that screening in these patients is beneficial. However, because this situation carries a 3% risk of having a hereditary ovarian cancer syndrome, these women should be counseled by a gynecologic oncologist or other qualified specialist regarding their individual risk.

- Women from families with hereditary ovarian cancer syndromes (i.e., Lynch II syndrome) have a 40% lifetime risk

TABLE 130–1. FIGO[a] Staging for Epithelial Ovarian Cancer

I: Confined to the ovaries
     IA: One ovary, no ascites, intact capsule
     IB: Both ovaries, no ascites, intact capsule
     IC: Ruptured capsule, capsular involvement, positive
           peritoneal washings, or malignant ascites
II: Ovarian tumor with pelvic extension
     IIA: Extension to uterus or tubes
     IIB: Extension to other pelvic organs (bladder, rectum, or vagina)
     IIC: Pelvic extension, plus findings for stage IC
III: Tumor involving the upper abdomen or lymph nodes
     IIIA: Microscopic seeding outside the true pelvis
     IIIB: Gross deposits ≤2 cm in diameter
     IIIC: Gross deposits >2 cm in diameter or nodal involvement
IV: Distant organ involvement, including or splenic liver parenchyma
     or pleural space

[a]International Federation of Gynecology and Obstetrics

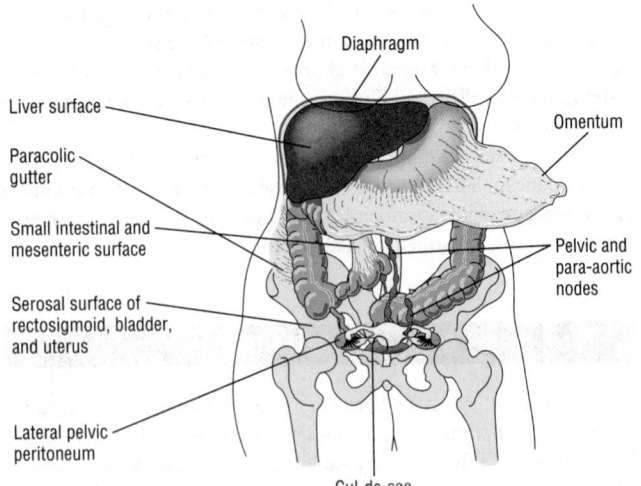

FIGURE 130–1. Staging laparotomy for ovarian cancer.

of developing ovarian cancer. Although no data indicate that screening will reduce mortality, annual rectovaginal pelvic examination, CA-125 determinations, and TVS are recommended in these women until age 35 or when childbearing is complete. Prophylactic bilateral oophorectomy should then be considered to reduce the overall risk.

With regard to possible ovarian cancer development, current recommendations for follow-up care for individuals with *BRCA1* and/or possibly *BRCA2* mutations include genetic counseling and annual or semiannual transvaginal ultrasound with color flow Doppler and serum CA-125 beginning at age 25 to 35 years.[17] There is not enough information to recommend for or against prophylactic oophorectomy or prophylactic use of oral contraceptives in *BRCA1* carriers. Participation in ongoing ovarian cancer screening trials should be encouraged.

STAGING

The stage of ovarian cancer depends on the extent of disease found at surgical exploration (Table 130–1). Epithelial ovarian cancer spreads by peritoneal surface shedding and lymphatic dissemination (Fig. 130–1).[16] A careful and accurate surgical staging laparotomy is necessary to properly stage the patient; it is therefore recommended that a gynecologic-oncologic surgeon do this procedure to prevent understaging.[25,26] Total abdominal hysterectomy, bilateral salpingo-oophorectomy, and partial omentectomy are performed.[16,17] A care-

ful examination of all serosal surfaces is done and biopsies of any grossly involved areas are taken. Ovarian capsule rupture, if present, is noted. Ascites and peritoneal washings are collected. Integral to the initial surgical staging procedure, the surgeon attempts to debulk as much gross tumor as possible because the amount of residual disease in patients with stage III ovarian cancer correlates with survival.[20]

PROGNOSIS

6 The prognosis for patients with epithelial ovarian cancer is related to disease stage, pathologic grade, and cell histology. Patients with well-differentiated stage IA or IB tumors have a 5-year survival rate of greater than 90% with no additional benefit derived from adjuvant therapy.[17,24] With adjuvant therapy, patients with any poorly differentiated stage I, stage IC, or stage II disease have an 80% 5-year survival rate.[17,27] Survival in patients with stage III disease is decreased compared to earlier stages, and is directly related to the size of residual tumors present after debulking surgery. Patients with implants less than 0.5 cm have a median survival of 40 months, those with implants 0.5 to 2 cm have a median survival of 18 months, and those with residual tumor greater than 2 cm have a median survival of 6 to 12 months.[28,29] The 5-year survival rate for stage IV patients is only 5% to 10%.[2] Patients with borderline ovarian cancer have an excellent prognosis, with a 5-year survival rate of 93% and a 10-year survival rate of 91%.[2]

▶ TREATMENT: Ovarian Cancer

4 Ovarian cancer management is based on the histologic type, pathologic grade, and the stage of disease at initial presentation (Fig. 130–2). In general, the treatment of patients with ovarian cancer initially involves surgical debulking at the time of staging laparotomy followed by adjuvant chemotherapy.[30]

However, the effect of debulking on outcome in patients with stage IV disease is unclear.[31] Second-line therapy is recommended if residual disease is found after adjuvant chemotherapy. Although response rates are high, many patients with ovarian cancer still die from their disease, so it is important to diagnose patients earlier, and

it is appropriate to enroll patients with any disease stage into clinical trials.

TREATMENT BY STAGE

EARLY-STAGE DISEASE (STAGES I AND II)

Approximately one-third of ovarian cancer patients present with localized disease (stage I or II) at initial diagnosis.[24] In patients with apparent early stage disease, comprehensive surgical staging is of utmost importance because approximately one-third of patients will have metastatic disease that is not apparent on gross total resection.[32]

◁ During laparotomy, the patient should undergo comprehensive staging, total abdominal hysterectomy, and bilateral salpingo-oophorectomy.[30] Women with stage IA, grade 1 ovarian tumors who wish to preserve ovarian and reproduction function can undergo a unilateral salpingo-oophorectomy without significant risk of decreased survival.[30,33] The beneficial effects of adjuvant chemotherapy in localized disease depend on the stage and the disease subtype.

◁ Postoperative adjuvant chemotherapy is not required in grade 1, stage IA or IB ovarian cancer, whereas patients with grade 2 or 3, stage IA or IB, and stage IC ovarian cancer benefit from adjuvant chemotherapy (see Fig. 130–2).[16,24,30] All patients with stage II disease should receive adjuvant treatment.[16,24,30] The role of adjuvant chemotherapy for patients with stage I disease is controversial. Recent data suggest that the outcome of patients with stage I disease who relapse following no adjuvant chemotherapy is similar to that of patients with stage III disease who relapse following chemotherapy.[34] For localized ovarian cancer (stage I or II), the recommended adjuvant regimen is paclitaxel plus cisplatin or carboplatin given for three to six cycles.[30]

ADVANCED DISEASE (STAGES III AND IV)

◁ The majority of women with ovarian cancer present with stage III or IV disease.[3] The approach to the treatment of advanced ovarian cancer is initial surgical debulking followed by adjuvant/consolidative paclitaxel plus cisplatin or carboplatin for six cycles[30] (see Fig. 130–2). Overall survival is a function of the initial disease stage (stage III vs. IV) and the amount of residual disease left after surgical debulking.

PRIMARY CYTOREDUCTIVE SURGERY

◁ The surgical removal of ovarian tumors should be as complete as possible to increase the likelihood of response to chemotherapy. The amount of residual disease after debulking is also a strong prognostic factor. Patients with stage III disease who have optimal debulking (<2 cm of residual tumor) have a 4-year survival rate of approximately 30%.[2] Patients with stage III or IV disease who have undergone suboptimal debulking (>2 cm of residual tumor) have less than a 10% chance of long-term survival.[28]

PRIMARY ADJUVANT CHEMOTHERAPY

TREATMENT REGIMENS

Systemic chemotherapy following optimal surgical debulking is the cornerstone of first-line treatment of advanced epithelial ovarian cancer. Although there have been only modest improvements in long-term survival, there have been significant improvements in 5-year survival of patients with advanced ovarian cancer. Table 130–2 summarizes the chemotherapeutic regimens used as the initial treatment of newly diagnosed ovarian cancer.

The combination of cyclophosphamide and cisplatin or carboplatin was once the first-line adjuvant therapy of choice in women with advanced-stage ovarian cancer.[29,35] However, paclitaxel alone, and in combination with platinum analogs, has shown significant

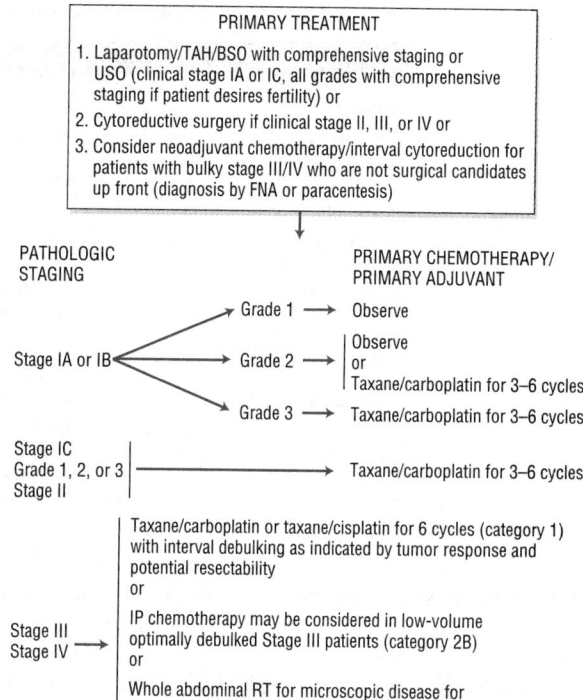

FIGURE 130–2. Initial management of epithelial ovarian cancer. All recommendations are category 2A unless otherwise indicated. BSO, bilateral salpingo-oophorectomy; TAH, total abdominal hysterectomy; USO, unilateral salpingo-oophorectomy. *Clear-cell pathology is considered high grade regardless of the stage. (Reproduced with permission from NCCN cancer practice guidelines in oncology, 2005. Copyrighted by the National Comprehensive Cancer Network. All rights reserved. These guidelines and illustrations may not be reproduced in any form without the express permission of the NCCN.)

activity in ovarian cancer.[36–38] McGuire and colleagues reported that the combination of paclitaxel 135 mg/m² over 24 hours and cisplatin 75 mg/m² achieved better response rates and survival outcomes than cyclophosphamide 750 mg/m² and cisplatin 75 mg/m² in patients with newly diagnosed, suboptimally debulked, stage III and IV ovarian cancer.[39] Survival improved significantly in the paclitaxel arm, with an increase in median progression-free survival (18 months vs. 13 months) and an overall survival (38 months vs. 24 months). Neutropenia, alopecia, and peripheral neuropathy were more severe in the paclitaxel/cisplatin group. Similar results have been reported in a large European-Canadian Phase III randomized trial study.[40]

Cisplatin and carboplatin have been used as single agents and in combination therapy in previously untreated ovarian cancer.[41] Combination chemotherapy regimens containing cisplatin achieved higher response rates and overall survival than regimens without cisplatin in patients with stage III or IV ovarian cancer.[17] A meta-analysis comparing treatment with platinum analogs, either as single agents or in combination regimens, reported a higher overall response rate and longer survival in the combination treatment group.

Single-agent carboplatin has been compared to platinum combination chemotherapy (paclitaxel plus carboplatin, or cyclophosphamide, doxorubicin, and cisplatin [CAP]) for first-line treatment of ovarian cancer in 2,074 patients with ovarian cancer, regardless of their stage at diagnosis.[42] No difference was found in overall survival after 51 months of follow-up between paclitaxel plus carboplatin and single-agent carboplatin or CAP. A small increase (1.2 months) in progression-free survival was noted in favor of paclitaxel plus carboplatin in comparison to either carboplatin or CAP. However, this

TABLE 130–2. Initial Chemotherapeutic Regimens of Epithelial Ovarian Cancer

Drug(s)	Dose(s)	Cycle Frequency
Cisplatin	100 mg/m² IV day 1	Every 28 days
Carboplatin	400–800 mg/m² IV day 1	Every 28–35 days
Cisplatin +	50–100 mg/m² IV day 1	Every 21–28 days
cyclophosphamide	500–1,000 mg/m² IV day 1	
Carboplatin +	200–300 mg/m² IV day 1	Every 28 days
cyclophosphamide	500–1,000 mg/m² IV day 1	
Cisplatin + doxorubicin +	50–60 mg/m² IV day 1	Every 28 days
cyclophosphamide	40–50 mg/m² IV day 1	
	500–750 mg/m² IV day 1	
Paclitaxel + cisplatin	135 mg/m² IV (24-h infusion) day 1	Every 21 days
	75 mg/m² IV day 1	
Paclitaxel + carboplatin	175 mg/m² IV (3-h infusion) day 1	Every 21 days
	Dosed to AUC 5–7.5 IV day 1	
Docetaxel + carboplatin	75 mg/m² IV day 1	Every 21 days
	Dosed to AUC 5 IV day 1	

AUC, area under the curve

increase in progression-free survival was associated with more alopecia, fever, and sensory neuropathy than single-agent carboplatin, and more sensory neuropathy than CAP.

Carboplatin has been used in place of cisplatin in combination therapy for patients with advanced ovarian cancer because of better tolerability, ease of administration, and apparent equivalent survival.[43–47] Several prospective, randomized phase III trials comparing carboplatin plus paclitaxel versus cisplatin plus paclitaxel in patients with advanced ovarian cancer have been conducted.[48–52] Results concluded that carboplatin plus paclitaxel is the preferred regimen because of equal efficacy and less toxicity. In the U.S. study (Gynecologic Oncology Group [GOG] 158), 840 previously untreated patients with optimally resected stage III disease (no residual tumor nodule >1 cm) were randomized to carboplatin (area under the curve [AUC] = 7.5) plus paclitaxel 175 mg/m² over 3 hours, or cisplatin 75 mg/m² plus paclitaxel 135 mg/m² over 24 hours administered every 21 days for 6 cycles.[48,49] The study was designed for equivalence with the primary end point being time to progression. Results demonstrated no difference in recurrence-free survival with median times of 19.4 months for the cisplatin arm versus 20.7 months for the carboplatin arm. More toxicity was observed in the cisplatin arm. The incidence of grade 4 leukopenia, grade 3 or 4 gastrointestinal toxicity, grade 1 to 4 fever, and grade 1 to 4 metabolic toxicity was higher for patients in the cisplatin arm, whereas patients in the carboplatin arm experienced more grade 3 or 4 thrombocytopenia and grade 1 or 2 pain. Neurotoxicity was similar between the two treatment arms, which may be related to the carboplatin dose (AUC = 7.5). These results suggest carboplatin plus paclitaxel is preferred over cisplatin plus paclitaxel because of equivalent efficacy, better tolerability, and ease of administration.

Docetaxel plus carboplatin may be emerging as the combination regimen of choice for first-line treatment of ovarian cancer. Preliminary results of the Scottish Randomized Trial in Ovarian Cancer (SCOTROC) Phase III trial comparing carboplatin (at an AUC of 5) in combination with docetaxel (75 mg/m² over 1 hour) or paclitaxel (175 mg/m² over 3 hours) administered every 21 days for 6 cycles as first-line chemotherapy for stages IC to IV epithelial ovarian cancer have been reported.[54] Although survival analyses are ongoing, the progression-free survival at 1 year, clinical response, and CA-125 responses were similar in the two treatment arms. The docetaxel-carboplatin regimen produced more myelotoxicity, edema, and hypersensitivity reactions than paclitaxel-carboplatin. However,

docetaxel-carboplatin was associated with significantly less neurotoxicity. The overall incidence of grade 3 and 4 toxicities was <10% in both arms. These preliminary results suggest that first-line treatment of ovarian cancer with docetaxel-carboplatin achieves similar response rates with significantly less neurotoxicity than treatment with paclitaxel-carboplatin.

The Progress in the Management of Gynecologic Cancer Conference recently published a consensus summary statement.[53] In that statement, carboplatin and paclitaxel (or carboplatin and docetaxel) was recommended as appropriate first-line chemotherapy for patients with advanced ovarian cancer. These recommendations are similar to those contained in the National Comprehensive Cancer Network (NCCN) guidelines. The 2005 NCCN guidelines list paclitaxel and carboplatin as the preferred regimen, although docetaxel and carboplatin is listed as an alternative regimen.

CLINICAL CONTROVERSY

Based on preliminary data of decreased neuropathy, some practitioners are treating patients newly diagnosed with ovarian cancer with docetaxel-carboplatin as first-line treatment. However, other practitioners are awaiting 5-year survival outcomes comparing paclitaxel-carboplatin to docetaxel-carboplatin to determine the preferred first-line treatment.

Dose Intensity

Dose intensity, or the amount of drug delivered over a specified time interval (expressed as mg/m² per week) may be an important factor in determining treatment outcomes with platinum-based regimens in patients with ovarian cancer.[84] However, a retrospective review of 45 randomized trials found no correlation between cisplatin dose and treatment outcome. A prospective randomized trial in patients with suboptimally debulked stage III (>1-cm residual masses) and any stage IV disease, randomized patients to receive cyclophosphamide 500 mg/m² IV plus either cisplatin 50 mg/m² IV or 100 mg/m² IV every 3 weeks.[55] Patients in the cisplatin 50 mg/m² group received eight cycles and patients in the cisplatin 100 mg/m² group received four cycles (same total cisplatin dose). Clinical and pathologic response rates, response duration, and survival were similar in both groups. Hematologic and gastrointestinal effects, febrile episodes, septic events, and renal toxicities were significantly more common and severe in the patients receiving the higher cisplatin dose. Similarly, Kaye and colleagues reported no survival difference in patients receiving six cycles of cyclophosphamide plus cisplatin 100 mg/m^2 IV or 50 mg/m^2 IV.[56] Neurotoxicity persisted in more patients in the high-dose arm (10 of 31), as compared to the low-dose arm (1 of 24). Likewise, dose-intensity analyses with carboplatin have demonstrated equivocal results.[57–59] Accumulating evidence seems to indicate that the dose-response curve for the platinum compounds levels off within the clinically useful dosage range.[57] However, it is not clear that providing higher cumulative platinum doses confers any survival advantage over the standard cisplatin 75 mg/m^2 IV dose.

Duration of Therapy

The duration of consolidative chemotherapy has been evaluated in several studies. In advanced ovarian cancer, the administration of five cycles of cyclophosphamide, cisplatin, and doxorubicin was equally effective and less toxic as compared to 10 cycles of chemotherapy.[60] Six to nine cycles of chemotherapy has become the standard approach and results in clinical response rates of approximately 60% to 70%, with 5-year survival rates of 10% to 20%. Because approximately 50% of patients with a confirmed pathologic response will ultimately relapse,[16] chemotherapy may be extended for two or three cycles beyond best response.[21]

The NCCN guidelines recommend three to six cycles of treatment for lower stage tumors and at least six cycles of treatment for patients with stage III or IV disease.[30] However, results of a recent randomized study showed that 12 months of maintenance paclitaxel significantly prolongs the duration of progression-free survival in patients with advanced ovarian cancer who attain a complete response to initial platinum and paclitaxel-based chemotherapy.[61]

Many questions still need to be answered about initial therapy for advanced stages of ovarian cancer. Ongoing clinical trials are addressing whether some of the paclitaxel-containing regimens are better than current regimens for early-stage disease. There are also several comparative trials for advanced-stage ovarian cancer. These studies include determining the optimal paclitaxel dose, schedule, and treatment duration, and determining whether dose intensification aided by growth factor support will achieve higher response rates and improve survival. The results of the SCOTROC trial may result in the combination of docetaxel and carboplatin becoming first-line therapy in newly diagnosed ovarian cancer.[54] In addition, low-dose weekly carboplatin-paclitaxel, new triplet combinations of carboplatin-paclitaxel with agents such as gemcitabine or topotecan, and sequential doublets such as cisplatin-topotecan followed by cisplatin-paclitaxel, are also under investigation.[61,62]

RECURRENT OR /REFRACTORY DISEASE

The choices for effective treatment of recurrent ovarian cancer are limited. In addition, approximately 20% to 50% of patients without evidence of residual disease on second-look laparotomy will relapse. Options include secondary cytoreductive surgery, salvage chemotherapy, hormonal therapy, radiotherapy, intraperitoneal chemotherapy, and high-dose chemotherapy with stem-cell support. Patients who respond to initial chemotherapy and whose response lasts the longest have the greatest likelihood of achieving a response to the same first-line regimen or to second-line treatment.[64] Also,

patients with recurrent or refractory disease after initial chemotherapy historically have a poor overall prognosis. Improved outcomes have been achieved in recurrent and refractory ovarian cancer with the use of high-dose chemotherapeutic agents such as cisplatin, carboplatin, and paclitaxel, and the use of combination regimens containing these agents. In addition, topotecan, pegylated liposomal doxorubicin, and gemcitabine have shown antitumor activity in patients with relapsed-refractory ovarian cancer.[64–72] Table 130–3 summarizes some of the chemotherapeutic regimens used in the treatment of recurrent or refractory ovarian cancer.

SECONDARY CYTOREDUCTIVE SURGERY AND INTERVAL SURGICAL DEBULKING

Operative re-exploration (or secondary laparotomy) was once an integral part of the management of advanced ovarian carcinoma. However, the role of secondary cytoreduction (or interval debulking) after consolidative chemotherapy is currently unclear. Several conflicting studies exist with regard to the survival advantages of secondary cytoreduction. A nonrandomized GOG study evaluated 112 International Federation of Gynecology and Obstetrics (FIGO) stage I or II ovarian cancer patients who first underwent initial surgical staging and then underwent a restaging operation following adjuvant therapy. The study reported that only 5% of the patients who were asymptomatic prior to surgery had disease confirmed by second-look laparotomy, as compared to half of the patients who were symptomatic prior to second-look laparotomy.[73] In patients with optimal (no residual tumor nodule >1 cm) stage III disease, preliminary results indicate second-look surgery does not influence the recurrence-free survival in this patient population. These data suggest that second-look laparotomy may not be warranted in asymptomatic patients with early-stage disease. In addition, the National Cancer Institute (NCI) consensus conference recommends that second-look operations should be performed only when the results will change management or as part of a clinical trial.[24]

Randomized trials of secondary surgical cytoreduction have reported conflicting results. In an older randomized trial, van der Burg and colleagues performed interval debulking surgery on 140 stage IIB to stage IV suboptimally debulked (>1 cm of residual disease) ovarian cancer patients after receiving three cycles of cisplatin plus cyclophosphamide.[74] Patients then received an additional three cycles of these same drugs after surgery. Patients randomized to the nonsurgical treatment arm received six cycles of chemotherapy. Interval debulking surgery significantly prolonged overall and progression-free survival and reduced the death risk by 33%. However, in a recently published study of 550 women with stage III or IV treated with maximal primary cytoreductive surgery and three cycles of paclitaxel and cisplatin, patients randomized to receive secondary cytoreductive surgery followed by three more cycles of chemotherapy had similar progression-free survival and overall survival as compared with those randomized to receive three more cycles of chemotherapy alone.[75]

The overall effect of interval debulking is influenced by several factors including initial response to chemotherapy, the amount of residual disease before and after second-look surgery, and the presence of microscopic residual disease. The results of recent trials suggest that secondary surgical cytoreduction does not prolong survival in patients who are treated with maximal primary cytoreductive surgery followed by appropriate postoperative chemotherapy.

CLINICAL CONTROVERSY

Some clinicians believe secondary cytoreduction improves survival in patients with ovarian cancer, while others do not. Factors that will affect the results of interval debulking are initial response to chemotherapy, amount of residual disease before and after secondary cytoreduction, and the presence of microscopic disease.

SALVAGE CHEMOTHERAPY

The NCCN guidelines for salvage therapy for recurrent or refractory disease include several treatment options (Fig. 130–3).[30] A useful guideline when treating a patient with refractory or relapsed disease is to administer a salvage regimen for two courses and then to evaluate for response.[64] If no response is observed, then an alternative salvage regimen may be selected. For topotecan or liposomal doxorubicin, evidence suggests continuation of treatment for four cycles and then re-evaluation for response.

Patients with prior low-stage, low-grade disease who have disease recurrence and who have never received chemotherapy should be treated as if they are newly diagnosed advanced-stage patients, undergoing surgical debulking and adjuvant chemotherapy with the combination of paclitaxel and a platinum agent. The NCCN guidelines suggest that tamoxifen is an appropriate therapy in patients with stage I or II ovarian cancer with a rising CA-125 as their only manifestation of disease progression.[30,76]

PLATINUM SENSITIVE VERSUS REFRACTORY DISEASE

The choice of retreatment with platinum-containing chemotherapy depends on the time frame in which the disease recurs.[3] Patients with advanced ovarian cancer that experience disease recurrence following initial chemotherapy are divided into two therapeutic groups. Patients who do not respond to the initial platinum-containing chemotherapy or who have recurrence within 6 months after discontinuing treatment are defined as *platinum-refractory*. These patients are unlikely to benefit from additional platinum or paclitaxel therapy and would be candidates for treatment with second-line salvage chemotherapy.[30] Patients who respond to the initial chemotherapy and relapse more than 6 months after discontinuation of chemotherapy are termed *platinum-sensitive*. These patients often benefit from secondary treatment with paclitaxel alone, a platinum agent alone, or paclitaxel in combination with a platinum analog.[77–83] Patients who had a long disease-free interval with a locally recurrent tumor might benefit from a second cytoreductive surgery.

Carboplatin has been used in the treatment of platinum-refractory ovarian cancer. Kavanagh and colleagues treated 33 platinum-refractory ovarian cancer patients with disease progression after taxane salvage therapy with carboplatin 300 mg/m[2] every 28 days.[84] These investigators noted a 21% partial response rate, a 39% stabilization rate, and a median response duration greater than 7 months. However, all responding patients had a platinum-free interval of at least 12 months.

Paclitaxel has also shown significant activity in platinum-refractory ovarian cancer.[37,85–90] At the approved dose of 175 mg/m[2] over 3 hours every 21 days, the response rate was 15% in patients with relapsed ovarian cancer.[85] Dose-intense paclitaxel regimens (250 mg/m[2] over 24 hours every 21 days plus filgrastim support) appear to produce higher objective response rates compared to conventional-dose regimens.[86–88] Altering infusion schedules of paclitaxel has been explored to maximize the cytotoxic activity of paclitaxel against ovarian cancer cells.[63] Weekly infusions may increase the dose intensity of paclitaxel while minimizing bone marrow suppression and other toxicities associated with paclitaxel administration.[63,89–90] Paclitaxel can be safely administered weekly at a dose of 80 mg/m[2] over 1 hour to heavily pretreated patients with advanced ovarian cancer, resulting in clinical response rates of approximately 30% in patients with relapsed ovarian cancer.[89–90] Ongoing and future clinical trials will help define the role of weekly paclitaxel in the treatment of patients with advanced ovarian cancer.

Docetaxel offers an alternative taxane treatment in patients with platinum-refractory ovarian cancer.[91–93] Preclinical studies show that docetaxel has more potent in vitro activity than does paclitaxel.[94] Docetaxel has produced overall response rates of 20% to 40% in patients with platinum-sensitive and platinum-refractory advanced

TABLE 130–3. Chemotherapeutic Regimens for Relapsed or Refractory Ovarian Cancer

Drug(s)	Dose(s)	Cycle Frequency
Gemcitabine	800–1,200 mg/m[2] IV days 1, 8, and 15	Every 28 days
Docetaxel	100 mg/m[2] IV day 1	Every 21 days
Pegylated-liposomal doxorubicin	40–50 mg/m[2] IV day 1	Every 28 days
Paclitaxel	80 mg/m[2] IV (1-h infusion) day 1	Every week
Paclitaxel	135–250[a] mg/m[2] IV[b] day 1	Every 21 days
Carboplatin	400–800 mg/m[2] IV day 1	Every 28–35 days
Paclitaxel	135 mg/m[2] IV (3-h infusion) day 1	Every 21 days
Cisplatin	75 mg/m[2] IV day 1	
Topotecan	1.5 mg/m[2] IV once daily for 5 days	Every 21 days
Tamoxifen	20 mg orally twice a day	Continuous
Etoposide	50 mg/m[2] orally once daily for 21 days	Every 28 days
Altretamine	260 mg/m[2] orally (total daily dose divided in four doses) for 14–21 days	Every 28 days

[a]Filgrastim used with 250 mg/m[2] dose.
[b]3-hour or 24-hour infusion.

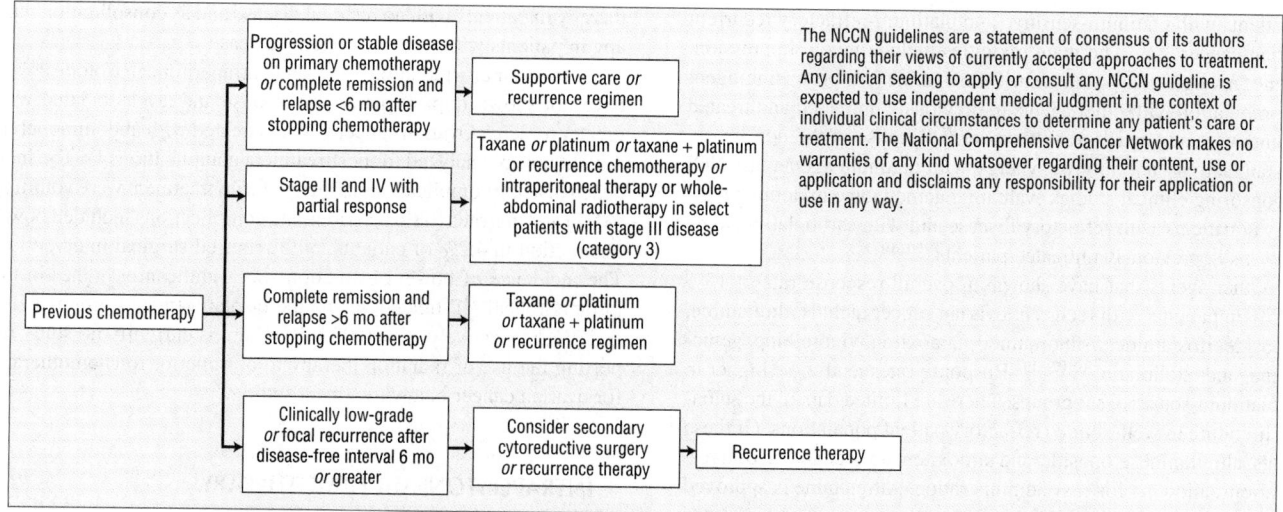

FIGURE 130–3. Management of recurrent/relapsed/progressive epithelial ovarian cancer. All recommendations are category 2A unless otherwise indicated. (Reproduced with permission from NCCN clinical practice guidelines in oncology, 2005. Copyrighted by the National Comprehensive Cancer Network. All rights reserved. These guidelines and illustrations may not be reproduced in any form without the express permission of the NCCN.)

ovarian cancer.[91–93] The response rates ranged from 17% to 20% in patients who were platinum-refractory, defined as a treatment-free interval of 0 to 4 months.[92] Neutropenia is the dose-limiting toxicity of docetaxel and fluid retention appears to be a cumulative toxicity, which can be managed with diuretics and steroids. Docetaxel is active in patients who have received prior platinum therapy, but it is important to assess the activity of docetaxel after paclitaxel failure, particularly because paclitaxel is considered a standard in front-line regimens. Further studies are also indicated to determine if docetaxel has a role as part of initial chemotherapy.

The combination of paclitaxel/platinum versus conventional platinum-based chemotherapy has been assessed in women with platinum-sensitive relapsed ovarian cancer.[95] A total of 802 patients were randomized between the two treatment groups and balanced for initial treatment with paclitaxel/platinum chemotherapy. Overall survival curves favored treatment with paclitaxel/platinum therapy with a hazard ratio of 0.82 ($p = 0.02$), corresponding to an absolute difference in 2-year survival of 7%. Progression-free survival curves also favored paclitaxel/platinum therapy, with a hazard ratio of 0.76 ($p = 0.0004$), corresponding to an absolute difference in 1-year progression-free survival of 10%.

CLINICAL CONTROVERSY

In patients with relapsed ovarian cancer that is platinum-sensitive, some clinicians believe patients should be immediately re-treated with a chemotherapy regimen including a platinum agent. Other clinicians believe the platinum-free interval for these patients should be extended by treating with a non-platinum regimen (i.e., topotecan) and reserving the platinum agent until the next relapse.

Regimens Not Containing Taxane or Platinum

As most patients will receive a taxane in combination with a platinum agent as initial therapy, there is a need for effective non–cross-resistant agents for use as second-line and salvage chemotherapy. In addition, the optimal chemotherapeutic agent or regimen in the treatment of platinum-refractory disease is currently unclear.

Topotecan, an analog of the plant alkaloid 20(S)-camptothecin, is active in patients with metastatic ovarian cancer and is non–cross-resistant with platinum-based chemotherapy.[65,66,96,97] Preclinical studies suggest that protracted schedules of administration using low doses of topotecan achieve the greatest antitumor response.[99] Topotecan has demonstrated efficacy in phase II trials as second-line and salvage therapy in patients who have relapsed after, or progressed during, platinum-based therapy.[65,66,96,97] A randomized phase III trial compared topotecan and paclitaxel in patients with advanced ovarian cancer who had failed one platinum-based regimen.[65] Patients were randomized to receive topotecan 1.5 mg/m² per day as a 30-minute infusion for 5 days repeated every 21 days or paclitaxel 175 mg/m² as a 3-hour infusion every 21 days. The overall response rate was 20.5% and 13.2% for the topotecan- and paclitaxel-treated groups, respectively. The median time to progression for topotecan-treated patients (32 weeks) was not significantly different than for paclitaxel-treated patients (20 weeks). Median survival was 61 weeks in the topotecan-treated group and 43 weeks in the paclitaxel-treated group. Topotecan was well tolerated with minimal nonhematologic toxicities.[65,66,96,97]

Pegylated liposomal doxorubicin is an emerging option for patients with recurrent ovarian cancer.[67–69] In an early phase II study, 35 patients with progressive disease after at least one platinum and paclitaxel–based regimen received pegylated liposomal doxorubicin 50 mg/m² every 3 weeks (with a dose reduction to 40 mg/m² in the event of grade 3 or 4 toxicities or a lengthening of the interval to 4 weeks);[67] the overall response rate was 25.7%. A large randomized phase III study was completed comparing pegylated liposomal doxorubicin 50 mg/m² every 4 weeks to topotecan 1.5 mg/m² per day for 5 days repeated every 21 days in patients who failed first-line platinum therapy.[69] A total of 474 patients were randomized, 239 to pegylated liposomal doxorubicin and 235 to topotecan. The overall confirmed response rate for the pegylated liposomal doxorubicin and topotecan groups were 20% and 17%, respectively. Overall survival tended to favor pegylated liposomal doxorubicin, with a median of 108 weeks versus 71.1 weeks for topotecan. Differences in toxicity were observed between the arms, with more hematologic toxicity occurring in the topotecan arm and more palmar-plantar erythrodysesthesia in the pegylated liposomal doxorubicin arm.

Gemcitabine, a novel pyrimidine antimetabolite, has achieved overall response rates of approximately 13% to 19% as a single agent in patients with platinum-sensitive and platinum-refractory recurrent ovarian cancer.[70-72] The main toxicities include myelosuppression, fatigue, myalgias, and skin rash. Gemcitabine is a promising agent in combination with other agents in previously untreated and treated patients with advanced ovarian cancer.[99] Because of the non–cross-resistant activity and in vivo synergy with platinum agents, the NCI is sponsoring clinical studies evaluating gemcitabine in doublet regimens in patients with refractory disease and with carboplatin/taxane regimens in previously untreated patients.[100,101]

Other agents that have shown an overall response rate of 15% to 25% in patients with recurrent ovarian cancer include altretamine, etoposide, ifosfamide, 5-fluorouracil, tamoxifen, vinorelbine, gemcitabine, and oxaliplatin.[76,102-107] Response rates tend to be higher in the platinum-sensitive subgroups. There are limited data in the scientific literature in well-defined refractory patient populations. Of these agents, altretamine, etoposide, and tamoxifen are available in oral formulations, allowing for easy administration. Altretamine is approved as single-agent therapy at doses of 260 mg/m^2 per day administered in four divided doses for 14 to 21 days given every 28 days.[103]

Much progress has been made in the treatment of refractory and relapsed ovarian cancer. However, because most patients will receive paclitaxel and platinum combinations as first-line adjuvant therapy, there is still a need to develop non–cross-resistant agents that are active in patients who have progressed on, or relapsed after, this combination regimen. Management of advanced ovarian cancer that is refractory to first-line therapy is not well defined. Selection of salvage regimens is based on the mechanisms of action and toxicity profiles of the particular agents. Additionally, there are a variety of innovative treatment options that may have a role in the treatment of patients with advanced ovarian cancer, including antitumor vaccines, gene therapy, and angiogenesis inhibitors. Therapies directed at reversing p53 gene–associated resistance are also being investigated.[108,109] There is also evidence suggesting the growth and proliferation of ovarian tumors depends on neovascularization, or angiogenesis.[110] Hence antiangiogenic agents may have a future role in the treatment of patients with advanced ovarian cancer.

RADIATION THERAPY

The use of radiation therapy in the treatment of ovarian cancer is controversial. The two forms of radiation therapy used in ovarian cancer are external beam whole-abdominal irradiation and intraperitoneal isotopes, such as ^{32}P. Radiation therapy has been used as adjuvant therapy in patients with no residual disease and as consolidation therapy in patients with minimal residual disease.

Abdominal irradiation[111,112] and intraperitoneal isotopes[113,114] have not shown improvements in response and are associated with greater toxicity. Ovarian cancer patients treated with abdominopelvic radiation were analyzed for posttreatment complications.[112] The incidence of acute complications associated with treatment were vomiting (61%) and diarrhea (68%). Serious late complications included bowel obstruction in 4.2% of patients; 64% required surgical intervention. The incidence of bowel obstruction was significantly higher in the intraperitoneal ^{32}P-treated versus the cisplatin-treated groups (11% and 2%, respectively; $p = 0.004$).[114] There is currently no study reporting the use of radiation therapy to be superior to chemotherapy for ovarian cancer in any treatment setting.

INTRAPERITONEAL CHEMOTHERAPY

Significant advances have occurred in understanding the advantages, limitations, and administration methods of intraperitoneal (IP) chemotherapy for ovarian cancer treatment.[115-117] Following initial treatment of advanced ovarian cancer, many patients who achieve a complete clinical response will have persistent disease or will develop recurrent disease. Overall, the proportion of patients achieving long-term survival is small. Ovarian cancer is an ideal disease for IP chemotherapy because the bulk of the disease remains in the peritoneal cavity.[115-117] The theoretical advantage of IP administration is to increase the dose intensity and total drug exposure directly to the tumor, while decreasing the systemic exposure and possible toxicity. With IP administration, cytotoxic agents are instilled directly into the peritoneal cavity in large volumes to allow these agents to reach all sites within the peritoneal cavity. Studies show potential value in IP administration for initial, consolidation, and salvage therapy. Data suggest that patients with small-volume tumors (<2 cm) are best suited for IP administration as initial therapy or as salvage therapy in relapsed disease. Therefore IP administration is a theoretically attractive approach, taking into account the biology of the disease, the anatomic characteristics of the peritoneal cavity, and the pharmacokinetic advantage of drugs administered intraperitoneally versus intravenously. Drugs that have been administered IP include cisplatin, carboplatin, cytarabine, etoposide, doxorubicin, mitoxantrone, paclitaxel, 5-fluorouracil, thiotepa, melphalan, methotrexate, and topotecan.[115-123] Table 130–4 summarizes IP chemotherapeutic regimens.

TABLE 130–4. Intraperitoneal (IP) Chemotherapeutic Regimens for Ovarian Cancer

Drug(s)	Dose(s)	Cycle Frequency
Topotecan	3 mg/m^2 (24-h infusion) day 1	Every 21 days
Cisplatin	50–100 mg/m^2 IP day 1	Every 21–28 days
Cisplatin Cyclophosphamide	100 mg/m^2 IP day 1 600 mg/m^2 IV day 1	Every 21 days
Etoposide Cisplatin Sodium thiosulfate	200–350 mg/m^2 IP day 1 100–200 mg/m^2 IP day 1 12–16 mg/m^2 IV day 1	Every 28 days
Cisplatin Cytarabine	100–150 mg/m^2 IP day 1 600–1,200 mg/m^2 IP day 1	Every 28 days
Paclitaxel	125 mg/m^2 IP day 1	Every 28 days
Mitoxantrone	20–30 mg/m^2 IP day 1	Every 28 days

Of particular interest are the agents that appear to be the most effective against ovarian cancer, which include the platinum analogs and paclitaxel. These agents appear to have a pharmacologic advantage when administered intraperitoneally. Peritoneal exposure of cisplatin or carboplatin after IP administration is approximately 10- to 20-fold greater than after systemic administration.[121] The exposure of the peritoneal cavity to paclitaxel after IP administration is approximately 30 times higher than plasma exposure.[122,123] Additionally, cytotoxic concentrations of paclitaxel may persist within the peritoneal cavity for 5 to 7 days after a single dose. Therefore weekly administration may result in continuous exposure of the peritoneal surface to the drug.[115]

■ FIRST-LINE INTRAPERITONEAL THERAPY

IP chemotherapy has been evaluated as treatment for newly diagnosed patients with advanced ovarian cancer. Multicenter, randomized trials using IP chemotherapy as first-line therapy have been conducted.[124–126] In a phase III trial, women with previously untreated stage III ovarian carcinoma with residual tumors of <2 cm were randomized to receive cyclophosphamide 600 mg/m^2 in combination with IP cisplatin 100 mg/m^2 or IV cisplatin 100 mg/m^2.[124] Median survival was significantly longer in the IP cisplatin-treated group (49 months) as compared to the IV cisplatin-treated group (41 months). In addition, moderate to severe tinnitus, hearing loss, and neuromuscular toxicities were significantly more frequent in the IV cisplatin-treated group. These data suggest that IP cisplatin is more effective and less toxic than IV cisplatin. However, further studies are needed to confirm the advantage of IP cisplatin over IV cisplatin.

A phase III trial examined a total of 462 eligible patients with small (<1 cm in maximal diameter), residual, advanced ovarian cancer who were randomized to receive two courses of either carboplatin (AUC = 9) followed by IV paclitaxel 135 mg/m^2 over 24 hours and IP cisplatin 100 mg/m^2 every 21 days for six cycles, or IV paclitaxel 135 mg/m^2 over 24 hours and IV cisplatin 75 mg/m^2 every 21 days for six cycles.[126] Progression-free survival was superior in the IP arm versus the IV arm (median 27.9 months vs. 22.2 months, respectively). Overall survival was 63.2 months in the IP arm versus 52.2 months in the IV arm. Although a significant improvement in progression-free survival was observed, toxicity was much greater in the experimental arm. Results from this study provide future direction for clinical studies in patients with small-volume disease.[30]

■ SALVAGE INTRAPERITONEAL THERAPY

Intraperitoneal therapy has also been evaluated as salvage therapy in patients with relapsed and refractory ovarian cancer in many phase I and II clinical trials.[115–117] Intraperitoneal cisplatin and carboplatin have achieved documented complete responses in relapsed patients initially treated with systemic platinum-containing regimens.[127,128] In the salvage setting, most of the IP experience has been with cisplatin, either alone or in combination. The primary toxicity associated with IP cisplatin was bone marrow suppression; neurotoxicity and nephrotoxicity have also been observed.[117] At doses greater than 125 mg/m^2, the dose-limiting toxicity of paclitaxel IP is abdominal pain.[123]

The impact of IP chemotherapy on survival in the salvage setting is limited because of the absence of randomized trials; however, there is some indirect evidence suggesting a positive influence.[117] Several studies have evaluated factors that influence the response to IP therapy.[115–117] A retrospective study evaluated the results of IP cisplatin with etoposide or cytarabine as salvage therapy.[127] Of patients

with microscopic disease at the time of IP therapy, 41% achieved a surgically-defined complete response, whereas only 29% of patients with macroscopic disease (largest residual tumor mass <0.5 cm in diameter) had a surgically-defined complete response. Patients whose largest residual tumor mass was greater than 1 cm had less than a 5% complete response rate. This is consistent with data showing a 1 to 2 cm depth of penetration of IP cisplatin into tumor or normal tissue.[129]

An objective response rate of less than 10% is anticipated for IP cisplatin in patients who fail to demonstrate at least a partial response to initial systemic cisplatin.[118] Thus IP cisplatin should not be used in cisplatin-refractory patients. In addition to platinum sensitivity and tumor size, extent of tumor spread must also be considered. IP therapy is most beneficial when the tumor is confined to the abdomen.[115–117] IP therapy is unlikely to have an advantage in patients with bulky disease because drug penetration into larger tumor nodules is limited. Additionally, patients best suited for IP administration should have limited IP adhesions with free fluid distribution.

Complications from IP therapy may be related to catheter function, infection, or bowel problems.[117,130] Mechanical obstruction to fluid inflow has been reported in approximately 5% of patients. Most commonly, this results from fibrin sheath formation around the catheter tip.[131] In some cases, peritoneal adhesions obstruct fluid entry into the abdominal cavity, causing uneven distribution of the chemotherapeutic agent. Infectious complications, such as superficial cellulitis around the catheter entry site, deep tissue infections, and peritonitis, are the most prevalent IP-related complications and are reported in approximately 10% of patients.[130,131] Bowel-related complications (approximately 3% incidence) include obstruction, ileus, and perforation. IP administration may also result in a false CA-125 elevation.[130]

Currently, IP chemotherapy outcomes for ovarian cancer treatment have been very encouraging, but additional well-designed comparative trials are needed to define the role of IP versus systemic chemotherapy. The NCCN guidelines consider IP therapy an investigational approach to ovarian cancer management.[30]

■ AUTOLOGOUS HEMATOPOIETIC STEM CELL TRANSPLANTATION

Ovarian cancer is initially very chemosensitive; however, drug resistance is a major issue. Increased drug exposure to chemotherapeutic agents is a likely way of overcoming resistance and of possibly increasing response rates and survival. The use of high-dose myeloablative chemotherapy followed by bone marrow or peripheral blood progenitor cell rescue has been used as salvage therapy in hematologic and solid tumor malignancies. The most common ablative regimens used in ovarian cancer contain platinum analogs (i.e., cisplatin or carboplatin), alkylating agents (i.e., melphalan, thiotepa, or cyclophosphamide), and/or etoposide.[132–134]

Shpall and associates evaluated the use of IP cisplatin and high-dose systemic cyclophosphamide and thiotepa followed by autologous bone marrow support in advanced ovarian cancer.[132] Of patients evaluated, 75% had pathologically documented partial response (i.e., >75% reduction in tumor mass). Legros and colleagues treated poor-prognosis ovarian cancer patients with either high-dose melphalan or high-dose carboplatin plus cyclophosphamide followed by autologous stem cell transplantation after receiving cisplatin induction therapy and second-look operations.[133] They reported an overall 60% 5-year survival rate and a 73% 5-year survival rate in patients with a pathologic complete response at second-look laparotomy. In patients with persistent or recurrent ovarian cancer treated with high-dose chemotherapy plus autologous stem cell transplantation, tumor bulk and chemosensitivity to prior regimens were the most important prognostic factors.[134] The use of high-dose chemotherapy in the setting of ovarian cancer has been reviewed.[135,136] The data demonstrate increased response rates with limited survival advantages.

Recently, Stiff and coworkers analyzed data from 421 women who were reported to the Autologous Blood and Marrow Transplant registry from 1989 to 1996.[137] This project was undertaken to assess the effectiveness of high-dose chemotherapy and autotransplantation. More than 80% of the patients analyzed had stage III or IV disease at diagnosis, and approximately 50% were in a clinically complete response before transplantation. Because of the limitations of this study, such as center-specific differences in selection of patients for transplant, varied timings of transplant, and varied high-dose chemotherapy regimens, the authors suggest data from this study can only be used to identify groups of patients that should or should not be studied further. The results indicate that patients with platinum-refractory disease have a 2.24 times higher mortality rate than do patients with platinum-sensitive disease. The probability of a 2-year survival after transplantation was 23% and 39% for patients with platinum-refractory and platinum-sensitive disease, respectively. The results from this study suggest better outcomes with autotransplantation than with conventional chemotherapy. However, there are inherent biases that must be considered because of the relatively small numbers of patients studied in this trial. Randomized trials are needed to fully understand the role of transplantation in patients with ovarian cancer.

A large, randomized phase III trial (GOG 164) comparing standard-dose chemotherapy to high-dose chemotherapy plus peripheral blood progenitor cell transplantation was recently closed in the United States because of slow accrual.[135] Currently, investigators in Europe are conducting randomized trials using high-dose chemotherapy and stem cell transplantation. Until the results from this and other ongoing trials are available, the role of bone marrow or peripheral blood progenitor cell transplantation in the initial and subsequent treatment of advanced refractory ovarian cancer is unclear and should be considered an investigational approach.

BORDERLINE OVARIAN CANCER

Borderline (low malignant potential) ovarian cancers account for approximately 15% of all epithelial ovarian cancers; the majority (75%) are stage I at the time of diagnosis.[138] These tumors must be recognized because their prognosis and treatment are clearly different from those of malignant invasive carcinomas. Trimble and Trimble reviewed 953 patients with a mean follow-up of 7 years and found a survival rate of 92% for advanced-stage tumors with the usual cause of death being benign disease complications (e.g., small-bowel obstruction) and therapy-related complications. Malignant transformation was rarely the cause of death. In one series, the 5-, 10-, 15-, and 20-year survival rates of patients with all stages of low malignant potential tumors were 97%, 95%, 92%, and 89%, respectively.[138]

In patients with stage I or II disease, no additional chemotherapy or radiation treatment is indicated for a completely resected tumor of low malignant potential.[139,140] In the presence of bilateral ovarian cystic neoplasms or a single ovary involvement, partial oophorectomy or a unilateral salpingo-oophorectomy can be performed if childbearing potential is to be maintained. When childbearing is not a consideration, a total abdominal hysterectomy and bilateral salpingo-oophorectomy is appropriate therapy because most clinicians favor removing the remaining ovarian tissue, which is at risk for recurrence of a borderline tumor or rarely developing invasive carcinoma.

Patients with advanced disease should undergo a total hysterectomy, bilateral salpingo-oophorectomy, omentectomy, node sampling, and aggressive cytoreductive surgery. However, there is little evidence that adjuvant chemotherapy or radiotherapy improves outcome.[138,140] There have been no controlled studies comparing postoperative treatment with no treatment.

NONEPITHELIAL OVARIAN CANCER

OVARIAN STROMAL TUMORS

Ovarian stromal tumors normally have an indolent natural history and rarely occur bilaterally. They are managed by unilateral salpingo-oophorectomy and usually do not require additional treatment.[16] Stage II stromal tumors require more extensive surgery owing to the lack of effective adjuvant therapy. Because this tumor is relatively rare, the role of chemotherapy is unclear.

OVARIAN GERM-CELL TUMORS

Ovarian-derived germ-cell tumors are rare and may have a mixed histology. Thus treatment should be directed toward the most malignant component of the tumor. Surgery alone has not been very effective, producing 2-year survival rates of 13% to 16%.[141] Combination chemotherapy has produced high cure rates and improved prognosis in patients with germ-cell tumors.

Endodermal sinus and dysgerminoma are two subtypes of germ-cell tumors. Endodermal sinus tumors are aggressive tumors that usually occur unilaterally. Without chemotherapy, most patients die from their disease; thus patients with all stages of disease should receive combination chemotherapy. The most common combination chemotherapeutic regimens used are vincristine, dactinomycin, and cyclophosphamide in combination, and cisplatin plus bleomycin in combination with vincristine or etoposide.[141] Dysgerminoma tumors have a high cure rate and are highly sensitive to radiation therapy; however, the sterility associated with abdominal irradiation has resulted in systemic chemotherapy becoming first-line therapy. The treatment of choice for newly diagnosed disease is a platinum-containing regimen.[141–143] The combination of bleomycin, etoposide, and cisplatin (BEP) demonstrated a 97% remission rate at 10 to 54 months in 35 patients with germ-cell tumors.[144] Also, two GOG trials demonstrated that 89 of 93 patients with stages I, II, and III disease and completely resected tumors were disease-free after three BEP cycles.[142–144] Patients with recurrent or refractory disease after cisplatin-based chemotherapy can be treated with radiation therapy.[141]

PHARMACOECONOMIC CONSIDERATIONS

The majority of economic analyses in ovarian cancer management have focused on the cost-effectiveness of paclitaxel combinations as initial treatment regimens because the combination of paclitaxel and cisplatin has increased the median survival of newly diagnosed patients with advanced-stage disease compared to the combination of cisplatin and cyclophosphamide.[39] In the United States, incremental costs per life-year gained $19,820 (inpatient) and $21,222 (outpatient),[146] and $19,603[146,147] have been calculated for patients treated with paclitaxel plus cisplatin compared to cyclophosphamide plus cisplatin. In comparison, the incremental costs per life-year gained of $20,355[148] and $32,213[149] have been reported for patients treated with paclitaxel plus cisplatin as compared to cyclophosphamide plus cisplatin in Canada. In addition, Messori and associates reported an $18,200 cost per quality-adjusted life-year gained.[146,147] The results of these studies suggest that the additional cost for the combination of paclitaxel and cisplatin compares favorably to costs for other medical interventions that are considered cost-effective. Cost considerations should be an important factor in the decision-making process of using a particular treatment strategy or deciding whether to pursue a new strategy in randomized trials.

EVALUATION OF THERAPEUTIC OUTCOMES

When applied mainly to clinical trials, complete response is defined as complete resolution of all disease and is further categorized either as a pathologic or a clinically complete response. A pathologic complete response is defined as no detectable disease on second-look laparotomy. A clinical complete response is defined as no detectable disease by radiologic imaging techniques. The National Institutes of Health consensus conference on ovarian cancer concluded that second-look laparotomy should be performed only in clinical trials.[24] Partial response is defined as a greater than 50% decrease in all measurable disease. Stable disease is defined as disease maintenance without progression. In addition, general definitions for response duration and survival apply to ovarian cancer. Disease-free survival is defined from the point of achieving a complete response to the time of disease recurrence. Recent studies have evaluated the percentage of CA-125 reduction as a surrogate marker for response.[150,151]

Localized ovarian cancer is highly curable by surgery, and if appropriate, chemotherapy. The goals of therapy should be to maintain the patient's quality of life and to preserve reproductive capabilities, if desired. Newly diagnosed advanced ovarian cancer is highly responsive to surgical debulking and subsequent consolidative chemotherapy; however, cure rates are much lower than with localized disease. The goals of therapy in advanced ovarian carcinoma are to cure the disease, to extend disease-free survival, and to prolong overall survival. Patients with recurrent or refractory disease are generally not curable and have a poor long-term prognosis. Thus the primary direction of therapy may be symptom management, quality-of-life maintenance, and minimization of treatment-related toxicity.[151]

FUTURE DIRECTIONS

Although the number of women in the United States dying from ovarian cancer continues to increase, substantial treatment progress has been made. However, there are still several therapeutic questions that need to be asked and problems that need to be solved. New approaches to the treatment of advanced primary as well as recurrent and refractory ovarian cancer, such as agents to overcome resistance, should be studied. The optimum adjuvant and consolidation treatment modalities should be determined. The results of the ongoing ICON5 trial may provide information on the most appropriate two- and three-agent combinations, and altering the sequence of chemotherapy regimens in the treatment of newly diagnosed ovarian cancer. However, these studies were initiated prior to the results of the SCOTROC trial, and

thus none of the treatment arms contain docetaxel. The role of IP chemotherapy in all stages of disease is unclear, as is the most appropriate salvage therapy. Answering these therapeutic questions and solving these therapeutic problems may prolong the long-term survival in patients with local and advanced ovarian cancer.

ABBREVIATIONS

AFP: α-fetoprotein
AUC: area under the curve
BEP: bleomycin, etoposide, and cisplatin
CAP: cyclophosphamide, doxorubicin, and cisplatin
CT: computed tomography
FIGO: International Federation of Gynecology and Obstetrics
GOG: Gynecologic Oncology Group
β-hCG: human β-chorionic gonadotropin
IP: intraperitoneal
MRI: magnetic resonance imaging
NCI: National Cancer Institute
NCCN: National Comprehensive Cancer Network
TVS: transvaginal sonography

Review Questions and other resources can be found at *www.pharmacotherapyonline.com.*

REFERENCES

1. Jemal A, Murray T, Ward E, et al. Cancer statistics, 2004. CA Cancer J Clin 2005;55:10–30.
2. Holschneider CH, Berek JS. Ovarian cancer: Epidemiology, biology, and prognostic factors. Semin Surg Oncol 2000;19:3–10.
3. Cannistra SA. Cancer of the ovary. NEJM 2004;351:2519–2529.
4. Goff BA, Mandel LS, Melancon CH, Muntz HG. Frequency of symptoms of ovarian cancer in women presenting to primary care clinics. JAMA 2004;291:2705–2712.
5. Lynch HT, Watson P, Lynch JF, et al. Hereditary ovarian cancer: Heterogeneity in age at onset. Cancer 1993;71(Suppl 2):573–581.
6. Lancaster JM, Wiseman RW. Recent advances in the molecular genetics of hereditary breast and ovarian cancer. Prog Clin Biol Res 1997;396:31–51.
7. Lynch HT, Casey MJ, Lynch J, et al. Genetics and ovarian carcinoma. Semin Oncol 1998;25:265–280.
8. Rubin SC, Benjamin I, Behbakht K. Clinical and pathological features in women with germ-line mutations of BRCA1. N Engl J Med 1996;335:1413–1416.
9. Eisinger F, Alby N, Bremond A, et al. Recommendations for medical management of hereditary breast and ovarian cancer: the French National Ad Hoc Committee. Ann Oncol 1998;9:939–950.
10. Burke W, Daly M, Garber J, et al. Recommendations for followup of individuals with an inherited predisposition to cancer, BRCA1 and BRCA2. Cancer genetics studies consortium. JAMA 1997;277:997–1003.
11. Boyd J, Sonoda Y, Federici MG, et al. Clinicopathologic features of BRCA-linked and sporadic ovarian cancer. JAMA 2000;283:2260–2265.
12. Scully RE. Tumors of the ovary and maldeveloped gonads, fallopian tube, and broad ligament. In: Young RH, Clement PB, eds. Atlas of Tumor Pathology, 3rd series. Washington, Armed Forces Institute of Pathology, 1996:27.
13. Seidman JD, Kuman RJ. Pathology of ovarian carcinoma. Hematol Oncol Clin North Am 2003;17:909–925.
14. Young RC, Walton LA, Ellenberg SS, et al. Adjuvant therapy in stage I and stage II epithelial ovarian cancer: results of two prospective randomized trials. N Engl J Med 1990;322:1021.

15. Omura GA, Brody MF, Homesly HD, et al. Long-term follow-up and prognostic factor analysis in advanced ovarian carcinomas: the Gynecologic Oncology Group experience. J Clin Oncol 1991;9:1138.

16. Ozols RF, Vermorken JB. Chemotherapy of advanced ovarian cancer: Current status and future directions. Semin Oncol 1997;24:S2-1–S2-9.

17. Hand R, Fremgen A, Chmiel JS, et al. Staging procedures, clinical management, and survival outcome for ovarian carcinoma. JAMA 1993;269:1119–1122.

18. Kenemans P, Yedema CA, Bon GG, von Mensdorff-Pouilly S. CA-125 in gynecologic oncology—A review. Eur J Obstet Gynecol Reprod Biol 1993;49:115–124.

19. Hempling RE. Tumor markers in epithelial ovarian cancer. Obstet Gynecol Clin North Am 1994;21:41–61.

20. Ozols RF, Schwartz PE, Eifel PJ. Ovarian cancer, fallopian tube carcinoma, and peritoneal carcinoma. In: Devita VT, Hellman S, Rosenberg SA, eds. Cancer: Principles and Practice of Oncology, 6th ed. Philadelphia, Lippincott Williams & Wilkins, 2001:1597–1632.

21. Mackey SE, Creasman WT. Ovarian cancer screening. J Clin Oncol 1995;13:783–793.

22. van Nagell JR, DePriest PD, Gallion HH, Pavlik EJ. Ovarian cancer screening. Cancer 1993;71:1523–1528.

23. Carlson KJ, Skates S, Singer DE. Screening for ovarian cancer. Ann Intern Med 1994;121:124–132.

24. NIH Consensus Conference. Ovarian cancer. Screening, treatment, and followup. NIH Consensus Development Panel on Ovarian Cancer [see comments]. JAMA 1995;273:491–497.

25. Nguyen HN, Averette HE, Hoskins W, et al. National survey of ovarian carcinoma. Part V. The impact of physician's specialty on patients' survival. Cancer 1993;72:3663–3670.

26. Boente MP, Yek K, Hogan VM, Ozols RF. Current status of staging laparotomy in colorectal and ovarian cancer. Cancer Treat Res 1996;82:337–357.

27. Kawai M, Kikkawa F, Hattori S, et al. Long-term followup of patients with epithelial carcinoma of the ovary. Int J Gynaecol Obstet 1994;44:259–266.

28. Louie KG, Ozols RF, Myers CE, et al. Long-term results of a cisplatin-containing combination chemotherapy regimen for the treatment of advanced ovarian carcinoma. J Clin Oncol 1986;4:1579–1585.

29. Omura GA, Brady MF, Homesley HD, et al. Long-term followup and prognostic factor analysis in advanced ovarian carcinoma: The Gynecologic Oncology Group experience. J Clin Oncol 1991;9:1138–1150.

30. Morgan RJ Jr, Alvarez RD, Armstrong DK, et al for the NCCN Cancer Panel. NCCN 2005 Ovarian Cancer Practice Guideline. www.NCCN.com [serial online]. Jan 2005.

31. Goodman HM, Harlow BL, Sheets EE, et al. The role of cytoreductive surgery in the management of stage IV epithelial ovarian carcinoma. Gynecol Oncol 1992;46:367–371.

32. Hoskins W, Rice L, Rubin S. Ovarian cancer surgical practice guidelines. Society of surgical oncology practice guidelines: Ovarian cancer. Oncology 1997;11:896–900, 903–904.

33. Miyazaki T, Tomoda Y, Ohta M, et al. Preservation of ovarian function and reproductive ability in patients with malignant ovarian tumors. Gynecol Oncol 1988;30:329–341.

34. Kolomainen DF, A'Hern R, Gore M. Can patients with relapsed previously untreated stage I epithelial ovarian cancer (EOC) be salvaged? J Clin Oncol 2003;21:3113–3118.

35. Neijt JP, ten Bokkel Huinink WW, van der Burg ME, et al. Randomized trial comparing two combination chemotherapy regimens (CHAP-5 v CP) in advanced ovarian carcinoma. J Clin Oncol 1987;5:1157–1168.

36. McGuire WP. Taxol: A new drug with significant activity as a salvage therapy in advanced epithelial ovarian carcinoma. Gynecol Oncol 1993;51:78–85.

37. Rowinsky EK, Donehower RC. Paclitaxel (Taxol) [published erratum appears in N Engl J Med 1995;333:75]. N Engl J Med 1995;332:1004–1014.

38. Kohler DR, Goldspiel BR. Paclitaxel (Taxol). Pharmacotherapy 1994;14:3–34.

39. McGuire WP, Hoskins WJ, Brady MF, et al. Cyclophosphamide and cisplatin compared with paclitaxel and cisplatin in patients with stage III and stage IV ovarian cancer. N Engl J Med 1996;334:1–6.

40. Piccart MJ, Bertelsen K, Stuart G, et al. Long-term follow-up confirms a survival advantage of the paclitaxel-cisplatin regimen over the cyclophosphamide-cisplatin combination in advanced ovarian cancer. Int J Gynecol Cancer 2003; 13(Suppl 2):144–148.

41. Taylor AE, Wiltshaw E, Gore ME, et al. Long-term followup of the first randomized study of cisplatin versus carboplatin for advanced epithelial ovarian cancer. J Clin Oncol 1994;12:2066–2070.

42. International Collaborative Ovarian Neoplasm Group. Paclitaxel plus carboplatin versus standard chemotherapy with either single-agent carboplatin or cyclophosphamide, doxorubicin and cisplatin in women with ovarian cancer: the ICON3 randomized trial. Lancet 2002;360:505–515.

43. Aabo K, Adams M, Adnitt P, et al. Chemotherapy in advanced ovarian cancer: Four systematic meta-analyses of individual patient data from 37 randomized trials. Br J Cancer 1998;78:1479–1487.

44. Go RS, Adjei AA. Review of the comparative pharmacology and clinical activity of cisplatin and carboplatin. J Clin Oncol 1999;17:409–422.

45. Alberts DS, Green S, Hannigan EV, et al. Improved therapeutic index of carboplatin plus cyclophosphamide versus cisplatin plus cyclophosphamide: Final report by the Southwest Oncology Group of a phase III randomized trial in stages III and IV ovarian cancer [published erratum appears in J Clin Oncol 1992;10:1505]. J Clin Oncol 1992;10:706–717.

46. Swenerton K, Jeffrey J, Stuart G, et al. Cisplatin-cyclophosphamide versus carboplatin-cyclophosphamide in advanced ovarian cancer: A randomized phase III study of the National Cancer Institute of Canada Clinical Trials Group. J Clin Oncol 1992;10:718–726.

47. Ozols RF. Carboplatin and paclitaxel in ovarian cancer. Semin Oncol 1995;22:78–83.

48. Bookman MA, Greer BE, Ozols RF. Optimal therapy of advanced ovarian cancer: carboplatin and paclitaxel vs. cisplatin and paclitaxel (GOG 158) and an update on GOG0 182-ICON5. Int J Gynecol Cancer 2003;136:735–740.

49. Ozols RF, Bundy BN, Green BE, et al. Phase III trial of carboplatin and paclitaxel compared with cisplatin and paclitaxel in patients with optimally resected stage III ovarian cancer: a Gynecologic Oncology Group Study. J Clin Oncol 2003;21:3194–3200.

50. du Bois A, Luck HJ, Meier W, et al. A randomized clinical trial of cisplatin/paclitaxel versus carboplatin/paclitaxel as first-line treatment of ovarian cancer. J Natl Cancer Inst 2003;3;95:1320–1329.

51. Neijt JP, Engelholm SA, Tuxen MK, et al. Exploratory phase III study of paclitaxel and cisplatin versus paclitaxel and carboplatin in advanced ovarian cancer. J Clin Oncol 2000;18:3084–3092.

52. Ozols RF. Paclitaxel (Taxol)/carboplatin combination chemotherapy in the treatment of advanced ovarian cancer. Semin Oncol 2000;27 (Suppl 7):3–7.

53. Cannistra SA, Bast RC, Berek JS, et al. Progress in the management of gynecologic cancer: consensus summary statement. J Clin Oncol 2003;21(May 15 suppl):129S–132S.

54. Vasey R. Preliminary results of the SCOTROC trial: A phase III comparison of paclitaxel-carboplatin (PC) and docetaxel-carboplatin (DC) as first-line chemotherapy for stage IC-IV epithelial ovarian cancer (EOC). Proc Am Soc Clin Oncol 2001;20:202a (Abstract).

55. McGuire WP, Hoskins WJ, Brady MF, et al. Assessment of dose-intensive therapy in suboptimally debulked ovarian cancer: A Gynecologic Oncology Group study. J Clin Oncol 1995;13:1589–1599.

56. Kaye SB, Paul J, Cassidy J, et al. Mature results of a randomized trial of two doses of cisplatin for the treatment of ovarian cancer. Scottish Gynecology Cancer Trials Group. J Clin Oncol 1996;14:2113–2119.

57. McGuire WP. How many more nails to seal the coffin of dose intensity? Ann Oncol 1997;8:311–313 (Editorial).

58. Jakobsen A, Bertelsen K, Andersen JE, et al. Dose-effect study of carboplatin in ovarian cancer: A Danish Ovarian Cancer Group study. J Clin Oncol 1997;15:193–198.

59. Gore M, Mainwaring P, Macfarlane V, et al. Randomized trial of dose-intensity with single-agent carboplatin in patients with epithelial ovarian cancer. J Clin Oncol 1998;16:2426–2434.

60. Hakes TB, Chalas E, Hoskins WJ, et al. Randomized prospective trial of 5 versus 10 cycles of cyclophosphamide, doxorubicin, and cisplatin in advanced ovarian carcinoma. Gynecol Oncol 1992;45:284–289.

61. Markman M, Lin PY, Wilczynski S, et al. Phase III randomized trial of 12 versus 3 months of maintenance paclitaxel in patients with advanced ovarian cancer after complete response to platinum and paclitaxel-based chemotherapy: a Southwest Oncology Group and Gynecologic Group trial. J Clin Oncol 2003;21:2460–2465.

62. Hansen SW, Anderson H, Boman K, et al. Gemcitabine, carboplatin and paclitaxel (GCP) as first-line treatment of ovarian cancer FIGO stages IIB-IV. Proc Am Soc Clin Oncol 1999;18:357a (Abstract).

63. Hoskins P, Eisenhauer E, Vergote I, et al. Phase II feasibility study of sequential couplets of Cisplatin/Topotecan followed by paclitaxel/cisplatin as primary treatment for advanced epithelial ovarian cancer: a National Cancer Institute of Canada Clinical Trials Group Study. J Clin Oncol 2000;18:4038–4044.

64. Dunton CJ. New options for the treatment of advanced ovarian cancer. Semin Oncol 1997;23:S5-2–S5-11.

65. ten Bokkel Huinink W, Gore M, Carmichael J, et al. Topotecan versus paclitaxel for the treatment of recurrent epithelial ovarian cancer. J Clin Oncol 1997;15:2183–2193.

66. Swisher EM, Mutch DG, Rader JS, et al. Topotecan in platinum- and paclitaxel-resistant ovarian cancer. Gynecol Oncol 1997;66:480–486.

67. Muggia FM, Hainsworth JD, Jeffers S, et al. Phase II study of liposomal doxorubicin in refractory ovarian cancer: Antitumor activity and toxicity modification by liposomal encapsulation. J Clin Oncol 1997;15:987–993.

68. Gordon AN, Cranai CO, Rose PG, et al. Phase II study of liposomal doxorubicin in platinum- and paclitaxel refractory epithelial ovarian cancer. J Clin Oncol 2000;18:3093–3100.

69. Gordon AN, Fleagle JT, Guthrie D, et al. Recurrent epithelial ovarian carcinoma: A randomized phase III trial of pegylated liposomal doxorubicin versus topotecan. J Clin Oncol 2001;19:3312–3322.

70. Lund B, Hansen P, Theilade K, et al. Phase II study of gemcitabine (2x, 2x-difluorodeoxycytidine in previously treated ovarian cancer patients. J Natl Cancer Inst 1994;6:1530–1533.

71. Shapiro JD, Millward MJ, Rischin D, et al. Activity of gemcitabine in patients with advanced ovarian cancer: Responses seen following platinum and paclitaxel. Gynecol Oncol 1996;63:89–93.

72. Friedlander M, Milward MJ, Bell D, et al. A phase II study of gemcitabine in platinum pre-treated patients with advanced epithelial ovarian cancer. Ann Oncol 1998;9:1343–1345.

73. Walton L, Ellenberg SS, Major F Jr, et al. Results of second-look laparotomy in patients with early stage ovarian carcinoma. Obstet Gynecol 1987;70:770–773.

74. van der Burg ME, van Lent M, Buyse M, et al. The effect of debulking surgery after induction chemotherapy on the prognosis in advanced epithelial ovarian cancer. Gynecological Cancer Cooperative Group of the European Organization for Research and Treatment of Cancer [see comments]. N Engl J Med 1995;332:629–634.

75. Rose PG, Nerenstone S, Brady MF, et al. Secondary surgical cytoreduction for advanced ovarian carcinoma. N Engl J Med 2004;351:2489–2497.

76. Hatch KD, Beecham JB, Blessing JA, Creasman WT. Responsiveness of patients with advanced ovarian carcinoma to tamoxifen. A Gynecologic Oncology Group study of second-line therapy in 105 patients. Cancer 1991;68:269–271.

77. Markman M, Rothman R, Hakes T, et al. Second-line platinum therapy in patients with ovarian cancer previously treated with cisplatin. J Clin Oncol 1991;9:389–393.

78. Seltzer V, Vogl S, Kaplan B. Recurrent ovarian carcinoma: retreatment utilizing combination chemotherapy including cis-diamminedichloroplatinum in patients previously responding to this agent. Gynecology 1989;21:167–176.

79. Rose PG, Fusco N, Fluellen L, et al. Second-line therapy with Paclitaxel and carboplatin following recurrent disease following first-line therapy with paclitaxel and platinum in ovarian or peritoneal carcinoma. J Clin Oncol 1998;16:1494–1497.

80. Gershenson DM, Kavanagh JJ, Copeland LJ, et al. Retreatment of patients with recurrent epithelial ovarian cancer with cisplatin-based chemotherapy. Obstet Gynecol 1989;73:798–802.

81. Parmar MK, Ledermann JA, Colombo N, et al. Paclitaxel plus platinum-based chemotherapy versus conventional platinum-based chemotherapy in women with relapsed ovarian cancer: the ICON4/AGO-OVAR-2.2 trial. Lancet 2003;21:2099–2106.

82. Zanotti KM, Belinson JL, Kennedy AW, et al. Treatment of relapsed carcinoma of the ovary with single-agent paclitaxel following exposure to paclitaxel and platinum employed as initial therapy. Gynecol Oncol 2000;79:211–215.

83. Markman M, Markman J, Webster K, et al. Duration of response to second-line, platinum-based chemotherapy for ovarian cancer: implications for patient management and clinical trial design. J Clin Oncol 2004;22:3120-3125.

84. Kavanagh J, Tresukosol D, Edwards C, et al. Carboplatin reinduction after taxane in patients with platinum-refractory epithelial ovarian cancer. J Clin Oncol 1995;13:1584–1588.

85. Eisenhauer EA, ten Bokkel Huinink WW, Swenerton KD, et al. European-Canadian randomized trial of paclitaxel in relapsed ovarian cancer: High-dose versus low-dose and long versus short infusion. J Clin Oncol 1994;12:2654–2666.

86. Kohn EC, Sarosy G, Bicher A, et al. Dose-intense Taxol: High response rate in patients with platinum-resistant recurrent ovarian cancer. J Natl Cancer Inst 1994;86:18–24.

87. Einzig AI. Review of phase II trials of Taxol (paclitaxel) in patients with advanced ovarian cancer. Ann Oncol 1994;5:S29–S32.

88. Omura G, Brady MF, Look KY, et al. Phase III trial of paclitaxel at two dose levels, the higher dose accompanied by filgrastim at two dose levels in platinum-pretreated epithelial ovarian cancer: an intergroup study. J Clin Oncol 2003;21:2843–2848.

89. Fennelly D, Aghajanian C, Schapiro F, et al. Phase I and pharmacologic study of paclitaxel administered weekly in patients with relapsed ovarian cancer. J Clin Oncol 1997;51:187.

90. Abu-Rustum NR, Aghajanian C, Barakat RR, et al. Salvage weekly paclitaxel in recurrent ovarian cancer. Semin Oncol 1997;24:S15-62–S15-67.

91. Kavanagh JJ, Kudelka AP, Gonzalez de Leon C, et al. Phase II study of docetaxel in patients with epithelial ovarian carcinoma refractory to platinum. Clin Cancer Research 1996;2:837–842.

92. Piccart MJ, Gore M, Ten Bokkel Huinink W, et al. Docetaxel: An active new drug for treatment of advanced epithelial ovarian cancer. J Natl Cancer Inst 1995;87:676–681.

93. Francis P, Schneider J, Hann L, et al. Phase II trial of docetaxel in patients with platinum-refractory advanced ovarian cancer. J Clin Oncol 1994;12:2301–2308.

94. Kellard LR, Abel G. Comparative in vitro cytotoxicity of Taxol and Taxotere against cisplatin-sensitive and resistant human ovarian carcinoma cell lines. Cancer Chemother Pharmacol 1992;30:444–450.

95. ICON and AGO Collaborators. Paclitaxel plus platinum-based chemotherapy versus conventional platinum-based chemotherapy in women with relapsed ovarian cancer: the ICON4/AGO-OVAR-2.2 trial. Lancet 2003;361:2099–2106.

96. Markman M. Topotecan: An important new drug in the management of ovarian cancer. Semin Oncol 1997;24:S5–S11.

97. Creemers GJ, Bolis G, Gore M, et al. Topotecan, an active drug in the second-line treatment of epithelial ovarian cancer: Results of a large European phase II study [see comments]. J Clin Oncol 1996;14:3056–3061.

98. Stewart CF, Zamboni WC, Crom WR, et al. Topoisomerase I interactive drugs in children with cancer. Invest New Drugs 1996;14:37–47.

99. Ozols RF. The role of gemcitabine in the treatment of ovarian cancer. Semin Oncol 2000;27:40–47.

100. Trimble EL. Innovative therapies for advanced ovarian cancer. Semin Oncol 2000;27:24–30.

101. Bergman AM, Ruiz van Haperen VWT, Veerman G, et al. Synergistic interaction between cisplatin and gemcitabine in vivo. Clin Cancer Res 1996;2:521–530.

102. Lee CR, Faulds D. Altretamine. A review of its pharmacodynamic and pharmacokinetic properties, and therapeutic potential in cancer chemotherapy. Drugs 1995;49:932–953.

103. Manetta A, MacNeill C, Lyter JA, et al. Hexamethylmelamine as a single second-line agent in ovarian cancer. Gynecol Oncol 1990;36:93–96.

104. Rose P, Blessing J, Mayer A, Homesley H. Prolonged oral etoposide as second-line therapy for platinum-resistant and platinum-sensitive ovarian carcinoma. A Gynecologic Oncology Group Study. J Clin Oncol 1998;16:405–410.

105. Gelmann EP. Tamoxifen for the treatment of malignancies other than breast and endometrial carcinoma. Semin Oncol 1997;24:S1-65–S1-70.

106. Bougnoux P, Dieras V, Petit T, et al. A multicenter phase II of oxaliplatin as a single agent in platinum and/or taxanes pretreated advanced ovarian cancer: Final results. Proc Am Soc Clin Oncol 1999;18:368 (Abstract).

107. Chollet P, Bensmaine MA, Brienza S, et al. Single agent activity of oxaliplatin in heavily advanced epithelial ovarian cancer. Ann Oncol 1996;7:1065–1070.

108. Gurnani M, Lipari P, Dell J, et al. Adenovirus-mediated p53 gene therapy has greater efficacy when combined with chemotherapy against human head and neck, ovarian, prostate, and breast cancer. Cancer Chemother Pharmacol 1996;44:143–151.

109. Song K, Cowan KH, Sinha BK. In vivo studies of adenovirus-mediated p53 gene therapy for cis-platinum-resistant human ovarian tumor xenografts. Oncol Res 1999;11:153–159.

110. Alvarez AA, Krigman HR, Whitaker RS, et al. The prognostic significance of angiogenesis in epithelial ovarian carcinoma. Clin Cancer Res 1999;5:587–591.

111. Chiara S, Conte P, Franzone P, et al. High-risk early-stage ovarian cancer. Randomized clinical trial comparing cisplatin plus cyclophosphamide versus whole abdominal radiotherapy. Am J Clin Oncol 1994;17:72–76.

112. Fyles AW, Dembo AJ, Bush RS, et al. Analysis of complications in patients treated with abdominopelvic radiation therapy for ovarian carcinoma. Int J Radiat Oncol Biol Phys 1992;22:847–851.

113. Soper JT, Berchuck A, Dodge R, Clarke-Pearson DL. Adjuvant therapy with intraperitoneal chromic phosphate (32P) in women with early ovarian carcinoma after comprehensive surgical staging. Obstet Gynecol 1992;79:993–997.

114. Vergotte IB, Vergote-De Vos LN, Abeler VM, et al. Randomized trial comparing cisplatin with radioactive phosphorus or whole-abdomen irradiation as adjuvant treatment of ovarian cancer. Cancer 1992;69:741–749.

115. Markman M. Intraperitoneal chemotherapy. Crit Rev Oncol Hematol 1999;31:239–246.

116. Vermorken JB. The role of intraperitoneal chemotherapy in epithelial ovarian cancer. Int J Gynecol Cancer 2000;10(Suppl 1):26–32.

117. Markman M. Intraperitoneal therapy of ovarian cancer. Semin Oncol 1998;25:356–360.

118. Plaxe SC, Christen RD, O'Quigley J, et al. Phase I and pharmacokinetic study of IP topotecan. Invest New Drugs 1998;16:147–153.

119. Feun LG, Blessing JA, Major FR, et al. A Phase II study of intraperitoneal cisplatin and thiotepa in residual ovarian carcinoma: A gynecologic oncology group study. Gynecol Oncol 1998;71:410–415.

120. Morgan RJ, Braly P, Leong L, et al. Phase II trial of combination intraperitoneal cisplatin and 5-fluorouracil in previously treated patients with advanced ovarian cancer: Long-term follow-up. Gynecol Oncol 2000;77:433–438.

121. Elferink F, van der Viigh WJF, Klein I, et al. Pharmacokinetics of carboplatin after intraperitoneal administration. Cancer Chemother Pharmacol 1988;21:57–60.

122. Markman M, Francis P, Rowinsky E, Hoskins W. Intraperitoneal paclitaxel: A possible role in the management of ovarian cancer? Semin Oncol 1995;22:84–87.

123. Markman M, Francis P, Rowinsky E, et al. Intraperitoneal Taxol (paclitaxel) in the management of ovarian cancer. Ann Oncol 1994;5:S55–S58.

124. Alberts DS, Liu PY, Hannigan EV, et al. Intraperitoneal cisplatin plus intravenous cyclophosphamide versus intravenous cisplatin plus intra-venous cyclophosphamide for stage III ovarian cancer. N Engl J Med 1996;335:1950–1955.

125. Kirmani S, Braly PS, McClay EF, et al. A comparison of intravenous versus intraperitoneal chemotherapy for the initial treatment of ovarian cancer. Gynecol Oncol 1994;54:338–344.

126. Markman M, Bundy B, Akberst DS, et al. Phase III trial of standard-dose of intravenous cisplatin plus paclitaxel versus moderately high-dose carboplatin followed by intravenous paclitaxel and intraperitoneal cisplatin in small-volume stage III ovarian carcinoma: An intergroup study of the Gynecologic Oncology Group, Southwestern Oncology Group and Eastern Cooperative Oncology Group. J Clin Oncol 2001;19:1001–1007.

127. Markman M, Reichman B, Hakes T, et al. Responses to second-line cisplatin-based intraperitoneal therapy in ovarian cancer: Influence of a prior response to intravenous cisplatin. J Clin Oncol 1991;9:1801–1805.

128. Piver MS, Recio FO, Baker TR, Driscoll D. Evaluation of survival after second-line intraperitoneal cisplatin-based chemotherapy for advanced ovarian cancer. Cancer 1994;73:1693–1698.

129. Los G, Mutsaers PH, Vijgh WJ. Direct diffusion of cis-diamminedichloroplatinum(II) in intraperitoneal rat tumors after intraperitoneal chemotherapy: A comparison with systemic chemotherapy. Cancer Res 1989;49:3380–3384.

130. Schneider JG. Intraperitoneal chemotherapy. Obstet Gynecol Clin North Am 1994;21:195–212.

131. Brandner P, Neis KJ. Use of an implantable catheter system for intraperitoneal chemotherapy in ovarian cancer. Artif Organs 1994;18:328–330.

132. Shpall EJ, Jones RB, Bearman S. High-dose therapy with autologous bone marrow transplantation for the treatment of solid tumors. Curr Opin Oncol 1994;6:135–138.

133. Legros M, Dauplat J, Fleury J, et al. High-dose chemotherapy with hematopoietic rescue in patients with stage III to IV ovarian cancer: Long-term results [see comments]. J Clin Oncol 1997;15:1302–1308.

134. Stiff PJ, Bayer R, Kerger C, et al. High-dose chemotherapy with autologous transplantation for persistent/relapsed ovarian cancer: A multivariate analysis of survival for 100 consecutively treated patients [see comments]. J Clin Oncol 1997;15:1309–1317.

135. McGuire WP. High-dose chemotherapeutic approaches to ovarian cancer. Semin Oncol 2000;27(Suppl 7):41–46.

136. Herrin VE, Thigpen JT. High-dose chemotherapy in ovarian carcinoma. Semin Oncol 1999;26:99–105.

137. Stiff PJ, Veum-Stone J, Lazarus HM, et al. High-dose chemotherapy and autologous stem cell transplantation for ovarian cancer: An autologous blood and marrow transplant registry report. Ann Intern Med 2000;133:504–515.

138. Trimble CL, Trimble EL. Management of epithelial ovarian tumors of low malignant potential. Gynecol Oncol 1994;55:S52–S61.

139. Leake JF. Tumors of low malignant potential. Curr Opin Obstet Gynecol 1992;4:81–85.

140. Trope C, Kaern J, Vergote IB, et al. Are borderline tumors of the ovary over-treated both surgically and systemically? A review of four prospective randomized trials including 253 patients with borderline tumors. Gynecol Oncol 1993;51:236–243.

141. Williams SD. Chemotherapy of ovarian germ cell tumors. Hematol Oncol Clin North Am 1991;5:1261–1269.

142. Segelov E, Campbell J, Ng M, et al. Cisplatin-based chemotherapy for ovarian germ cell malignancies: The Australian experience. J Clin Oncol 1994;12:378–384.

143. Williams S, Blessing JA, Liao SY, et al. Adjuvant therapy of ovarian germ cell tumors with cisplatin, etoposide, and bleomycin: A trial of the Gynecologic Oncology Group. J Clin Oncol 1994;12:701–706.

144. Gershenson DM. Update on malignant ovarian germ cell tumors. Cancer 1993;71:1581–1590.

145. McGuire W, Neugut AI, Arikian S, et al. Analysis of the cost-effectiveness of paclitaxel as alternative combination therapy for advanced ovarian cancer. J Clin Oncol 1997;15:640–645.

146. Messori A, Trippoli S, Becagli P, Tendi E. Pharmacoeconomic profile of paclitaxel as a first-line treatment for patients with advanced ovarian

carcinoma. A lifetime cost-effectiveness analysis. Cancer 1996;78:2366–2373.

147. Messori A, Cecchi M, Becagli P, Trippoli S. Pharmacoeconomic profile of paclitaxel as a first-line treatment for patients with advanced ovarian carcinoma. A lifetime cost-effectiveness analysis. Cancer 1997;79:2264–2266 (Letter).

148. Covens A, Boucher S, Roche K, et al. Is paclitaxel and cisplatin a cost-effective first-line therapy for advanced ovarian carcinoma? Cancer 1996;77:2086–2091.

149. Elit LM, Gafni A, Levine MN. Economic and policy implications of adopting paclitaxel as first-line therapy for advanced ovarian cancer: An Ontario perspective. J Clin Oncol 1997;15:632–639.

150. Rustin GJ, Nelstrop AE, McClean P, et al. Defining response of ovarian carcinoma to initial chemotherapy according to serum CA-125. J Clin Oncol 1996;14:1545–1551.

151. Montazeri A, McEwen J, Gillis CR. Quality of life in patients with ovarian cancer: Current state of research. Support Care Cancer 1996;4:169–179.

131
ACUTE LEUKEMIAS

Helen L. Leather and Betsy Bickert

Learning Objectives and other resources can be found at *www.pharmacotherapyonline.com.*

KEY CONCEPTS

1. Acute leukemias are the most common malignancies in children and the leading cause of cancer-related death in patients younger than age 35 years.

2. Despite the World Health Organization classification system for myeloid neoplasms, the French-American-British classification remains the most widely used.

3. To establish a definitive diagnosis of acute leukemia the following diagnostic components are required: bone marrow biopsy and aspirate (with >20% blasts), cytogenetics, and immunophenotyping.

4. There are several well-known risk factors that correlate with prognosis for ALL. Poor prognostic factors include high WBC counts at presentation, very young or very old age at presentation, delayed remission induction and presence of cytogenetic abnormalities (e.g., Ph+ chromosome).

5. Therapy of both ALL and AML are based on specific risk factors such as age or WBC count at time of diagnosis in ALL. For both ALL and AML, cytogenetic abnormalities provide significant information regarding risk stratification and identify subgroups that may benefit from novel molecularly targeted therapies.

6. There are several well-known poor prognostic factors for adult AML, and they include older age (>60 years), organ impairment, certain FAB subtypes (FAB M0, M5, M6, M7), presence of extramedullary disease, and presence of cytogenetic abnormalities (i.e., -5, -7, complex karyotype).

7. For children with ALL, induction therapy includes vincristine, a corticosteroid, and asparaginase, with or without an anthracycline. For adults with ALL, vincristine, prednisone, and an anthracycline are given, and asparaginase is sometimes added.

8. Because the high risk of central nervous system relapse in ALL, all patients require prophylactic therapy to prevent CNS disease. The choice for therapy includes a combination of the following: cranial irradiation and single-agent intrathecal chemotherapy, triple-drug intrathecal chemotherapy, or high-dose systemic chemotherapy that crosses the blood-brain barrier.

9. Patients with ALL frequently relapse after consolidation due to residual disease. Long-term maintenance therapy for 2 to 3 years is essential, and eradicates residual leukemia cells and prolongs the duration of remission. Maintenance therapy consists of pulse doses of vincristine, oral methotrexate, and oral mercaptopurine.

10. Colony-stimulating factors can be safely and effectively used with myelosuppressive chemotherapy for acute leukemias. The benefits can include reduced incidence of serious infections, reduced hospital stays, and fewer treatment delays, but do not include prolonged disease-free survival.

11. Therapy of AML usually includes induction therapy with an anthracycline and cytarabine. Post-remission therapy is required in all patients and can include either consolidation chemotherapy with or without maintenance therapy, or hematopoietic stem cell transplantation.

12. Treatment of acute promyelocytic leukemia consists of induction therapy, followed by consolidation and maintenance therapy. Induction includes tretinoin and an anthracycline; consolidation therapy consists of two to three cycles of anthracycline-based therapy; maintenance consists of pulse doses of tretinoin, mercaptopurine, and methotrexate for 2 years.

The leukemias are heterogeneous hematologic malignancies characterized by unregulated proliferation of the blood-forming cells of the bone marrow. These immature proliferating leukemia cells (blasts) physically "crowd out" or inhibit normal cellular maturation in bone marrow, resulting in anemia, neutropenia, and thrombocytopenia. Leukemic blasts may also infiltrate a variety of tissues such as lymph nodes, skin, liver, spleen, kidney, testes, and the central nervous system.

The term *leukemia* was coined by Virchow to describe the "white blood" of some patients that he saw under the microscope in 1845.[1] Historically, leukemia has been classified as acute or chronic based on differences in cell of origin and cell line maturation, clinical presentation, rapidity of progression of the untreated disease, and response to therapy. Four major leukemias are recognized: acute lymphocytic (or lymphoblastic) leukemia (ALL), acute myeloid leukemia (AML), chronic lymphocytic leukemia (CLL), and chronic myeloid leukemia (CML). Undifferentiated immature cells that proliferate autonomously characterize acute leukemias. Chronic leukemias also proliferate autonomously, but the cells are more differentiated and mature.[1] Untreated, the acute leukemias are rapidly progressive, resulting in death within 2 to 3 months.

EPIDEMIOLOGY

In 2005 it is estimated that 15,930 new cases of acute leukemias—11,960 cases of AML and 3970 cases of ALL—will be diagnosed in the United States, accounting for less than 2% of the total cancer incidence. The incidence has been relatively stable for two decades. An estimated 10,490 deaths per year, representing about 2% of all cancer deaths, are caused by acute leukemias. The acute leukemias are the leading cause of cancer-related deaths in persons younger than age 35, but an uncommon cause of cancer-related death after age 35 years.[1,2] Among adults, acute and chronic leukemias occur at equal rates. More than 90% of the cases of acute and chronic leukemia occur in adults. There are approximately 4.0 cases of AML and 1.4 cases of ALL per 100,000 individuals.[3] The median age at diagnosis of patients with AML is about 65 years, while the median age for ALL patients is about 10 years.[1-3] The incidence of AML rises with age from 1.8 per 100,000 in individuals younger than age 65 years to 17.7 per 100,000 in those 65 years or older.[3] Acute leukemia is slightly more common in males than in females. In the United States, acute leukemia is more common among whites than among African-Americans, American Indians, and Hispanic ethnicities.[1,3]

Despite the low incidence rate, the acute leukemias are the most common malignancy in persons younger than 15 years of age, constituting about 30% of all childhood malignancies.[3] In the United States, 9200 persons younger than 15 years of age are diagnosed with cancer each year; 2,200 of them have ALL.[4] AML accounts for about 20% of all childhood leukemias, and the chronic leukemias account for less than 5%.[3] Childhood ALL is 30% more common in males than females, peaks at 2 to 5 years of age, and is twice as likely to affect white children than African-American children.[3] The incidence of childhood AML is highest in the Hispanic population and occurs throughout childhood without any peak age period. Acute leukemia during the first year of life (infant leukemia) is twice as likely to be ALL as AML.[3]

Chemotherapy has dramatically improved the outlook of patients with acute leukemia. Over 85% of children and young adults with acute leukemia achieve an initial complete remission (CR) of their disease. Overall, 65% to 85% of adults achieve an initial CR.[1,4] For persons less than 20 years of age, the 5-year survival rate is 83% for ALL and 50% for AML.[3] The prognosis of adult acute leukemia is generally worse than that of childhood leukemia, with only 30% to 40% of patients becoming long-term survivors.[1,4]

ETIOLOGY

The exact cause of the acute leukemias is unknown. A multifactorial process involving genetics, environmental and socioeconomic factors, toxins, immunologic status, and viral exposures is likely. Table 131–1 summarizes the major factors that have been linked to acute leukemias. Infectious and genetic factors have the strongest associations to date.[1,5] In pediatric ALL, a number of environmental factors have been investigated as possible causes: exposure to ionizing radiation, toxic chemicals, herbicides and pesticides; maternal use of

TABLE 131–1. Clinical Conditions Associated with an Increased Frequency of Acute Leukemia

Drugs	**Chemical**
Alkylating agents	Benzene
Epidophyllotoxins	**Radiation**
Genetic conditions	Ionizing radiation
Down's syndrome	**Virus**
Bloom's syndrome	Epstein-Barr Virus
Fanconi's anemia	Human T-lymphocyte virus
Klinefelter's syndrome	(HTLV-1 and HTLV-2)
Ataxia telangiectasia	**Social habits**
Langerhans cell histiocytosis	Cigarette smoking
Shwachman's syndrome	Maternal marijuana use
Severe combined	Maternal ethanol use
immunodeficiency syndrome	
Kostmann's syndrome	
Neurofibromatosis type 1	
Familial monosomy 7	
Diamond-Blackfan anemia	

contraceptives, diethylstilbestrol, or cigarettes; parental exposure to drugs (amphetamines, diet pills, and mind-altering medications), diagnostic radiographs, alcohol consumption, or chemicals before and during pregnancy;[6] and chemical contamination of groundwater. A few studies have reported a possible link between electromagnetic fields of high-voltage power lines and the development of leukemia, but a recently published study could not confirm this association. In most patients who develop leukemia, a causative agent cannot be identified.

Risk factors associated with childhood AML include Hispanic ethnicity, prior exposure to alkylating agents or epipodophyllotoxins, and in utero exposure to ionizing radiation.[1] Maternal alcohol consumption, parental and child pesticide exposure, and parental benzene exposure are also potential risk factors for childhood AML.

PATHOPHYSIOLOGY

A basic understanding of normal hematopoiesis is needed before one can understand the pathogenesis of leukemia. The reader is referred to Chap. 98 for a detailed discussion of hematopoiesis. Normal hematopoiesis consists of multiple well-orchestrated steps of cellular development. A pool of pluripotent stem cells undergoes differentiation, proliferation, and maturation, to form the mature blood cells seen in the peripheral circulation. These pluripotent stem cells initially differentiate to form two distinct stem cell pools. The myeloid stem cell gives rise to six types of blood cells (erythrocytes, platelets, monocytes, basophils, neutrophils, and eosinophils), while the lymphoid stem cell differentiates to form circulating B and T lymphocytes. Leukemia may develop at any stage and within any cell line.

Two features are common to both AML and ALL: first, both arise from a single leukemic cell that expands and acquires additional mutations, culminating in a monoclonal population of leukemia cells. Second, there is a failure to maintain a relative balance between proliferation and differentiation, so that the cells do not differentiate past a particular stage of hematopoiesis. Cells (lymphoblasts or myeloblasts) then proliferate uncontrollably. Proliferation, differentiation, and apoptosis are under genetic control, and leukemia can occur when the balance between these processes is altered. New antileukemia drug therapies are being developed that are specifically targeted to the biologic processes involved in proliferation and differentiation.[4]

AML probably arises from a defect in the pluripotent stem cell or a more committed myeloid precursor, resulting in partial differentiation and proliferation of immature precursors of the myeloid blood-forming cells. In older patients, trilineage leukemic involvement is common, suggesting that the cell of origin is probably a stem or very early progenitor cell. In younger patients, a more differentiated progenitor becomes malignant, allowing maturation of some granulocytic and erythroid populations. These two forms of AML exhibit different patterns of resistance to chemotherapy, with resistance more evident in the older adults with AML. ALL is a disease characterized by proliferation of immature lymphoblasts. In this type of acute leukemia, the defect is probably at the level of the lymphopoietic stem cell or a very early lymphoid precursor.[1]

Leukemic cells have growth and/or survival advantages over normal cells, leading to a "crowding out" phenomenon in the bone marrow. This growth advantage is not caused by more rapid proliferation as compared with normal cells. Some studies suggest that it is caused by factors produced by leukemic cells that either inhibit normal cellular proliferation and differentiation, or reduce apoptosis as compared with normal blood cells.

The types of genetic alterations that lead to leukemia have only recently become evident. The genetic defects may include (1) activation of a normally suppressed gene (protooncogene) to create an oncogene that produces a protein product that signals increased proliferation; (2) loss of signals for the blood cell to differentiate; (3) loss of tumor suppressor genes that control normal proliferation; and (4) loss of signals for apoptosis. Most normal cells are programmed to die eventually through apoptosis, but the appropriate programmed signal is often interrupted in cancer cells, leading to continued survival, replication, and drug resistance. Signal transduction, RNA transcription, cell-cycle control factors, cell differentiation, and programmed cell death may all be affected.

One example of a genetic defect leading to acute leukemia is abnormal activation of the *ras* gene.[7] These genes produce G proteins (guanine nucleotide-binding proteins) that couple activation of outer cell membrane receptors to activation of signal transduction.

The abnormal activation of these signal transduction pathways can lead to increased cell proliferation. Point mutations in the *ras* gene lead to unregulated proliferation and differentiation. Defects in this gene are present in 25% to 44% of AML patients, and in 6% to 18% of ALL patients. Disruption of *ras* signaling also creates a useful target for therapeutic intervention. The investigational agents called farnesyl transferase inhibitors (such as tipifarnib [R115777, Zarnestra] or lonafarnib [Sarasar]) block an early part of the *ras* pathway, and are undergoing evaluation in various types of cancer, including leukemias.

LEUKEMIA CLASSIFICATION

The French-American-British (FAB) classification system identifies eight different subtypes of AML based on granulocytic differentiation and maturation (Table 131–2), and this system is used to determine prognosis and choice of therapy. However, it does not consider clinical characteristics, clonal cytogenetic abnormalities, immunophenotyping, or response to therapy. The World Health Organization (WHO) and the Society of Hematopathology have proposed a new classification system for myeloid neoplasms (Table 131–3).[8] This new classification system incorporates not only morphologic findings, but genetic, immunophenotypic, biologic, and clinical features. It has long been known that certain cytogenetic abnormalities have prognostic significance, but did not always correlate well with the FAB classification system.[9] In addition, this new classification attempts to formally incorporate the relationship between AML and myelodysplastic syndrome (MDS). A limitation of the WHO classification is that it does not account for some of the myeloid disorders of childhood. There are recommendations to expand the myelodysplastic/myeloproliferative disorders to include additional subclasses such as juvenile myelomonocytic leukemia and patients with Down's syndrome.[10]

Lymphoid leukemias are not addressed in the current WHO classification system. Markers on the cell surface or membrane of the lymphoblast can be used to classify ALL (Table 131–4). ALL may also be described by cytogenetic abnormalities. Chromosome alterations include numerical (hyperdiploidy and hypodiploidy), and structural

TABLE 131–2. Morphologic (FAB) Classification of Acute Myeloid Leukemia

		Frequency of FAB subtype[a]		
	Subtype	Adults (%)	Children <2 y (%)	Children >2 y (%)
M0	Acute myeloblastic leukemia, without maturation	5	Low	Low
M1	Acute myeloblastic leukemia with minimal maturation	15	17	25
M2	Acute myeloblastic with maturation	25		27
M3	Acute promyelocytic leukemia	10		5
M4	Acute myelomonocytic leukemia	25	30	26
M5a	Acute monoblastic leukemia, poorly differentiated	5	52	16
M5b	Acute monoblastic leukemia, well differentiated	5		
M6	Acute erythroleukemia	5		2
M7	Acute megakaryoblastic leukemia	10		5–7

[a]Percentages should be compared vertically and not horizontally.
FAB, French-American-British.

TABLE 131–3. World Health Organization Classification of Acute Myeloid Leukemia

Acute myeloid leukemia (AML) with recurrent genetic abnormalities
  AML with t(8;21)(q22;q22), (AML1/ETO)
  AML with abnormal bone marrow eosinophils and inv (16)(p13;q22) or t(16;16)(p13;q22),
    (CBFβ/MHY11)
  Acute promyelocytic leukemia with t(15;17)(q22;q12), (PML/RARα) and variants
  AML with 11q23 (MLL) abnormalities

Acute myeloid leukemia with multilineage dysplasia
  Following MDS or MDS/MPD disorder
  Without antecedent MDS or MDS/MPD, but with dysplasia in at least 50% of cells or two or more
    lineages

Acute myeloid leukemia and MDS, therapy related
  Alkylating agent/radiation-related type
  Topoisomerase II inhibitor-related type (some may be lymphoid)
  Others

Acute myeloid leukemia, not otherwise categorized
Classify as:
  Acute myeloid leukemia, minimally differentiated
  Acute myeloid leukemia without maturation
  Acute myeloid leukemia with maturation
  Acute myelomonocytic leukemia
  Acute monoblastic/acute monocytic leukemia
  Acute erythroid leukemia (erythroid/myeloid and pure erythroleukemia)
  Acute megakaryocytic leukemia
  Acute basophilic leukemia
  Acute panmyelosis with myelofibrosis
  Myeloid sarcoma

MDS, myelodysplastic syndrome; MLL, mixed lineage leukemia; MPD, myeloproliferative disease; PML, promyelocytic leukemia; RAR, retinoic acid receptor-α.
From Vardiman et al.[8]

abnormalities due to exchanges of genetic information within (inversing) or between (translocation) chromosomes.[11]

CLINICAL PRESENTATION

❸ Common signs and symptoms at presentation are described in the clinical presentation boxes. In addition to clinical presentation, laboratory and pathology evaluations are required for a definitive diagnosis of leukemia. The most important test is a bone marrow biopsy and aspirate, which is submitted to hematopathology for numerous evaluations. Cytochemical stains are helpful to determine if the acute leukemia is of myeloid or lymphoid lineage. Immunophenotyping involves the analysis of specific antigens, known as clusters of differentiation, often abbreviated "CD," present on the surface of hematopoietic cells. While no leukemia-specific antigens have been identified, the pattern of cell surface antigen expression reliably distinguishes between lymphoid and myeloid leukemia.[1] Common immunophenotypic markers seen in AML and ALL are listed in Table 131–5. Cytogenetic analysis of the marrow to determine the presence of nonrandom numerical and structural chromosomal abnormalities in leukemic cells is also helpful for diagnosis, establishing prognosis, and evaluating response to therapy.[9] Chromosome translocations can result in abnormal expression and/or function of cellular oncogenes. Unique translocations can identify specific subtypes of acute leukemia. For example, APL is characterized by a specific translocation between chromosomes 15 and 17: t(15;17). Recently, technically difficult cytogenetic analysis has been supplemented with fluorescent in situ hybridization (FISH) that allows for quick, sensitive analysis of samples that might be inadequate for karyotyping.[13,14] FISH is a process in which specific genes in an intact cell are visualized with fluorescent-labeled probes. Molecular tests may be used to identify products of specific translocations, such as promyelocytic leukemia–retinoic acid receptor-α (PML-RARα) in APL.

TABLE 131–4. Morphologic (FAB) Classification and Immunophenotype of Acute Lymphocytic Leukemia

Subtype	Cell of Origin	Frequency of FAB Subtype[a]	
		Adults (%)	Children (%)
L1	Early pre-B cell Pre-B cell B cell T cell	30	85
L2	Early pre-B cell Pre-B cell B cell T cell	60	14
L3	B cell	10	1

[a]Percentages should be compared vertically and not horizontally.
FAB, French-American-British.

TABLE 131–5. Common Immunophenotypes in Acute Leukemia

Leukemia	Common Immunophenotypes
Acute myeloid leukemia	CD13, CD15, CD33, CD14, CD64, and C-KIT
B-cell acute lymphoblastic leukemia	CD19, CD20, CD10, and CD22
T-cell acute lymphoblastic leukemia	CD2, CD3, CD4, CD5, and CD7

PRESENTATION OF ACUTE MYELOID LEUKEMIA[1,8,12]

GENERAL

Typically a 1- to 3-month history of vague symptoms such as tiredness, lack of exercise tolerance, chest pain, and "feeling unwell," but in no obvious distress.

SYMPTOMS

The patient may report weight loss, malaise, fatigue, and palpitations and dyspnea on exertion. They may also present with fever, chills, and rigors suggestive of infection; bruising (excessive vaginal bleeding, epistaxis, ecchymoses, and petechiae); gum hypertrophy (AML M4 and AML M5 subtypes); bone pain; seizures, headache, and diplopia.

SIGNS

Temperature may be elevated due to low neutrophil count; petechiae

LABORATORY TESTS

Complete blood cell count (with differential). Anemia is usually present and is normochromic and normocytic (without a compensatory increase in reticulocytes). Thrombocytopenia (severe, less than 50,000/mm^3 platelets) is present in approximately 50% of cases. Leukopenia/leukocytosis: approximately 20% of patients will present with an elevated white blood cell (WBC) count, 20% with a low WBC count, and the rest with normal counts. Even patients with elevated counts can be considered functionally neutropenic.

Uric acid is elevated in 50% of patients due to rapid cellular turnover (more common in patients presenting with elevated WBC counts).

Electrolytes: potassium and phosphate are usually elevated.

Coagulation: elevated prothrombin time, partial thromboplastin time, D-dimers; hypofibrinogenemia.

OTHER DIAGNOSTIC TESTS

Bone marrow biopsy and aspirate: send for morphologic examination, cytochemical staining, immunophenotyping, and cytogenetic (chromosome) analysis. At diagnosis the marrow is typically hypercellular, with normal erythropoiesis being replaced by leukemic blasts. To be diagnosed with AML, there needs to be more than 20% blasts.

For patients presenting with CNS signs, a diagnostic lumbar puncture should be performed. CNS involvement is common with AML M4 and M5 subtypes.

PRESENTATION OF ACUTE LYMPHOBLASTIC LEUKEMIA[1,8,12]

GENERAL

Typically a 1- to 3-month history of vague symptoms such as tiredness, lack of exercise tolerance, chest pain, and "feeling unwell," but in no obvious distress.

SYMPTOMS

The patient may report weight loss, malaise, fatigue, and palpitations and dyspnea on exertion. They may also present with fever, chills, and rigors suggestive of infection; bruising (excessive vaginal bleeding, epistaxis, ecchymoses, and petechiae); bone pain; seizures, headache, and diplopia.

SIGNS

Temperaure may be elevated due to low neutrophil count; petechiae; splenomegaly, hepatomegaly, and lymphadenopathy.

LABORATORY TESTS

Complete blood cell count (with differential). Anemia is usually present and is normochromic and normocytic (without a compensatory increase in reticulocytes). Thrombocytopenia (severe, less than 50,000/mm^3 platelets) is present in approximately 50% of cases. Leukopenia/leukocytosis: approximately 20% patients will present with an elevated white blood cell (WBC) count, 20% with a low WBC count, and the rest with normal counts. Even patients with elevated counts can be considered functionally neutropenic.

Uric acid is elevated in 50% of patients due to rapid cellular turnover (more common in patients presenting with elevated WBC counts).

Electrolytes: potassium and phosphate are usually elevated.

OTHER DIAGNOSTIC TESTS

Bone marrow biopsy and aspirate: send for morphologic examination, cytochemical staining, immunophenotyping, and cytogenetic (chromosome) analysis.

CNS involvement is common in all ALL patients, and is a common cause of relapse. All patients should have a screening lumbar puncture performed.

PROGNOSTIC FACTORS

Many clinical and laboratory features at diagnosis are associated with response to treatment, as measured by the CR rate, duration of remission, and long-term survival. Identification of these risk factors may allow the clinician to better understand the disease and to tailor treatment according to risk of disease recurrence. For example, if a patient has many clinical and laboratory features that are associated with a good response to chemotherapy ("good risk"), then the clinician may choose to give less intensive therapy to reduce the risk of long-term toxic effects. Conversely, if a patient is unlikely to respond well to therapy ("high risk" or "poor risk"), then the clinician may choose to give more intensive chemotherapy that might include hematopoietic stem cell transplantation (HSCT).

ACUTE LYMPHOBLASTIC LEUKEMIA

In both adults and children with ALL, recent studies have identified several risk factors that correlate with prognosis (Table 131–6). As most patients with ALL achieve a CR, these factors correlated with the risk of leukemic relapse rather than the risk of not achieving a CR.

Poor prognostic factors include high WBC count at presentation, very young or old age at presentation, delayed remission induction, and the presence of specific cytogenetic abnormalities.[15]

Several specific chromosomal translocations have been identified and are now being routinely used in risk assessment,

TABLE 131–6. Prognostic Factors in Acute Lymphoblastic Leukemia

	Risk for Leukemic Relapse	
Factor	Low	High
Morphology	L1	L2, L3
Immunologic phenotype	Early pre-B cell	Null cell, T cell, pre-B cell, B cell
WBC count at diagnosis	<10,000/mm^3	>50,000/mm^3
Platelets	>100,000/mm^3	<30,000/mm^3
Patient age	3–7 years	<1 year or >10 years
Cytogenetics	Normal karyotype	t(9;22); t(4;11); −7; +8
Myeloid markers	Absent	Present
CNS leukemia	Absent	Present
Node/liver/spleen enlargement	Absent	Massive
Mediastinal mass	Absent	Present
Time to remission	<4 weeks	>4 weeks

CNS, central nervous system; WBC, white blood cell.

and subsequently to direct therapy (Table 131–7). Adult patients generally have a worse prognosis than children due to disease biology and treatment tolerance. Adults typically have more cytogenetic abnormalities, particularly the presence of the Philadelphia chromosome (Ph$^+$) or t(9;22), which confer higher-risk disease. Other poor prognostic factors more common in adults include chemotherapy resistance, slower response to chemotherapy, high WBC at presentation, and a mediastinal mass or extramedullary involvement.

The National Cancer Institute developed an ALL risk stratification to create a standard for comparison in children[15] (Table 131–8). Therapy is initially selected based on this classification, but may be modified based on the presence or absence of cytogenetic abnormalities, slow response to induction treatment, or CNS involvement. In the adult population with ALL, age <35 years, good performance status, time to CR <4 weeks, timely clearance of blasts, and presenting WBC count of <30,000/mm^3 all qualify as "standard risk" factors.[5]

ACUTE MYELOID LEUKEMIA

◀5 ◀6 Several prognostic factors have been identified for adults with AML. The most important patient factor is age, with younger patients more likely to achieve a CR than older patients (older than age 60).[1,12] The lower CR rate in older patients appears to result from an increased frequency of fatal infectious and bleeding complications, as well as disease resistance to conventional chemotherapy.[12]

TABLE 131–8. National Cancer Institute Acute Lymphoblastic Leukemia Risk Stratification

Risk Group	Age (Years)	White Blood Cells (cells/mm^3)	Karyotype
Standard	1 to <10	<50,000	No t(9;22) or t(4;11)
High	1 to <10	≥50,000	
	<1 or ≥10	Any	
	Any	Any	t(9;22) or t(4;11)

From Wells et al.[16]

The duration of remission is also shorter in older patients compared to younger patients. Other patient-specific prognostic factors include concurrent infection and any major organ impairment.[12] FAB morphologic subtype may be a factor, with types M0, M5, M6, and M7 having the worst outcome.[1,12] Patients with extramedullary disease, CNS involvement, or underlying MDS have a worse prognosis.[1,12] Certain cytogenetic abnormalities are also known to worsen the response rate and survival of patients with AML (see Table 131–7).[1,9] In addition, patients who develop a "secondary" leukemia after treatment of another malignancy usually have a very poor response to antileukemic chemotherapy.[1]

Prognostic factors associated with pediatric AML have been reported but few have been shown to consistently predict treatment outcome. Historically, poor prognostic factors include an initial WBC count greater than 100,000/mm^3, FAB subtype M1 without Auer rods, certain chromosomal abnormalities (see Table 131–7), age <5 years, and having AML secondary to prior chemotherapy or radiation therapy. A recent report from the Children's Cancer Group identified both poor and favorable prognostic factors. Poor prognostic factors at diagnosis included male gender, platelet count ≤20,000/mm^3, hepatomegaly, MDS, FAB subtype M5, greater than 15% bone marrow blasts at day 14 of induction therapy, and trisomy 8.[16] Abnormal chromosome 16 was associated with a higher rate of CR.[16]

TREATMENT GOALS

The short-term goal of treatment for acute leukemia is to rapidly achieve a complete clinical and hematologic remission. In the absence of a CR, a rapid and fatal outcome is inevitable. Complete remission is defined as the disappearance of all clinical and bone marrow evidence (normal cellularity >20% with <5% blasts) of leukemia, with restoration of normal hematopoiesis (neutrophils ≥1,500/mm^3 and platelets >100,000/mm^3). Partial remission is a significant response

TABLE 131–7. Risk Category According to Cytogenetic Abnormalities Present

	Risk Category		
Disease	Good Risk	Intermediate Risk	High Risk
AML	t(8;21)(q22;q22); inv(16); t(15;17); t(9;11) trisomy 21	Normal karyotype; trisomy 8; 11q23; del(7q); del(9q); trisomy 22	Complex karyoptype; −5; −7; del(5q); inv(3p)
Probability of relapse	≤25%	50%	>70%
4-Year survival	≥70%	40–50%	≤20%
ALL	Hyperdiploidy; t(10;14); or 6q		t(9;22); t(8;14); t(4;11); t(1;9)

ALL, acute lymphoblastic leukemia; AML, acute myeloid leukemia.
From Hasle et al[10] and Thomas et al.[19]

to treatment, although evidence of residual disease in the bone marrow remains (5% to 25% blasts) and is considered a treatment failure requiring additional therapy. The definition of response for adult AML has recently been re-evaluated, and there is a proposal to change the definition of response to include not only CR, but also morphologic CR, CR with incomplete count recovery, cytogenetic CR, and molecular CR.[17,18]

After a CR is achieved, the goal is to maintain the patient in continuous CR. As discussed later, the occurrence of leukemic relapse in the bone marrow significantly reduces the likelihood of curing the disease. Most patients who will die from acute leukemia die within the first 6 years; the survival curve (percentage alive versus time) beyond the sixth year after therapy does not continue to decline as rapidly, and at this time patients can be considered "cured."[1]

▶ TREATMENT: Acute Lymphoblastic Leukemia

Successful treatment of ALL was first developed in children. Current regimens induce CR in 97% to 99% of children with ALL.[11] Cure rates in children have risen from less than 5% with treatments used in the 1960s to approximately 80% by 1995.[3] Although treatment results with adult ALL are worse than those with childhood ALL, recent use of aggressive chemotherapy in adult ALL has increased the CR rate to 60% to 85%. Long-term disease-free survival (DFS) in this population, however, remains low (between 30% and 40%) due to the higher proportion of adults presenting with poor-risk disease. CR rates and DFS vary according to a number of poor prognostic factors (see Tables 131–6 and 131–7), and certain types of ALL are associated with a very poor outcome. Ph+ ALL, characterized by the presence of the t(9;22) cytogenetic abnormality, has a dismal 5-year survival (10% adults; 25% children).[19] Although this specific type of ALL is treated essentially like all other ALL patients, patients with Ph+ ALL can benefit from the addition of a targeted molecular therapy, as discussed later.

Therapy for ALL has historically been divided into three phases: (1) remission induction; (2) consolidation therapy; and (3) maintenance therapy (Fig. 131–1). Central nervous system (CNS) prophylaxis is a mandatory component of any ALL treatment regimen and is administered longitudinally during the induction and consolidation phases. Recently more complex regimens have been explored. All patients still receive induction therapy to yield a CR. Post-remission therapy is needed to treat microscopic disease and may include intensive inpatient therapy (consolidation or intensification therapy) followed by less aggressive outpatient therapy (maintenance or continuation). Tables 131–9 and 131–10 illustrate representative treatment regimens for adult and pediatric ALL.[20–22]

REMISSION INDUCTION

The goal of remission induction is to rapidly induce a complete clinical and hematologic remission. The CR rate is 97% to 99%

in children treated with vincristine, dexamethasone or prednisone, and asparaginase or pegasparagase.[1] In children with high-risk ALL, daunorubicin is added to standard three-drug induction. Complete remission is achieved in 72% to 92% of adults with daunorubicin or doxorubicin, vincristine, and prednisone.[1,5] Since most adults are considered high-risk, adults usually receive more intensive remission induction regimens. However, the value of adding more drugs to the basic three- or four-drug induction regimen is unclear. Equally unclear is the value of higher doses of the standard combination of drugs for remission induction. Some studies suggest that high-dose methotrexate and cytarabine alternating with fractionated cyclophosphamide plus vincristine, doxorubicin, and dexamethasone (hyper-CVAD) may improve response and survival in adults with ALL.[23,24] However, this treatment may be associated with significant cerebellar toxicity.[25] Higher doses of cyclophosphamide may be indicated for patients with T-cell ALL.[5]

Some experts suggest that most treatment failures in childhood ALL result from inadequate initial reduction of the leukemic clone and the acquisition of drug resistance by residual lymphoblasts.[26] This is the basis upon which many trials have incorporated four-drug (or more) induction remission regimens and aggressive intensification or consolidation regimens in the management of higher-risk patients. Most treatment protocols add daunorubicin to induction for high-risk ALL, and some also add other agents, such as cyclophosphamide, methotrexate, cytarabine, and teniposide. The rate of clearance of blasts may be an important prognostic factor. Children with a slow rate of clearance of blasts from the bone marrow in the first 7 (high-risk) or 14 (standard-risk) days of therapy have an eventual outcome that is inferior to those with rapid clearance of blasts (see Table 131–8 for definitions of risk).[27] Additional therapy significantly improves outcome of children with a slow early response.[27] Historically, prednisone has been the primary glucocorticoid used in pediatric ALL regimens. Dexamethasone is now being used in some standard-risk protocols due to its longer duration of action and higher cerebrospinal fluid penetration compared to prednisone.[28] Dexamethasone, when used in place of prednisone during induction and maintenance, also improves event-free survival (EFS) and decreases the risk of CNS relapse.[28] However, dexamethasone increases side effects such as avascular necrosis, steroid myopathy, hyperglycemia, and infections.[28,29]

Ph+ ALL is associated with poor long-term outcomes, although the availability of imatinib mesylate, a molecularly targeted therapy, has prompted much research into the effect of this new drug on long-term survival rates. While responses may be seen with imatinib mesylate as monotherapy, this approach does not produce durable remissions.[30] Clinical trials are now exploring the addition of this targeted therapy to conventional chemotherapy, with encouraging early results. The combination of hyper-CVAD and imatinib appears to produce better outcomes compared to historical control data with hyper-CVAD alone, but additional studies and long-term follow-up are needed to conclusively determine if this

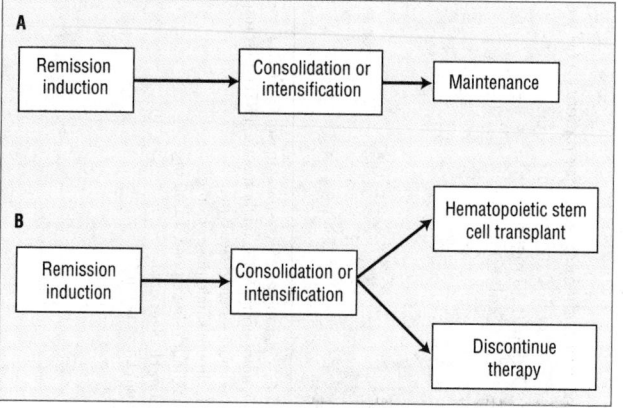

FIGURE 131–1. Treatment algorithm for (A) ALL and (B) AML.

TABLE 131–9. Representative Chemotherapy Regimens for Adult Acute Lymphoblastic Leukemia

Remission Induction		CNS Prophylaxis		Consolidation		Maintenance
Drug and Dose	Days	Prophylaxis	Days	Drug and Dose	Days	Drug, Dose, and Timing

German or Hoelzer Regimen (Adult)[d]

Remission Induction		CNS Prophylaxis		Consolidation		Maintenance
PRED (Oral) 60 mg/m²	1–28	Cranial irradiation		DEX (Oral) 10 mg/m²	1–28	MP (Oral) 60 mg/m² daily and
VCR (IV) 1.5 mg/m²[a]	1, 8, 15, 22	MTX (IT) 10 mg/m²[b]	31, 38, 45, 52	VCR (IV) 1.5 mg/m²[a]	1, 8, 15, 22	MTX (Oral/IV) 20 mg/m² weekly, weeks 10–18 and 29–130
DNR (IV) 25 mg/m²	1, 8, 15, 22			DOX (IV) 25 mg/m²	1, 8, 15, 22	
ASP (IV) 5,000 units/m²	1–14			CTX (IV) 650 mg/m²[c]	29	
CTX (IV) 650 mg/m²[c]	29, 43, 57			Ara-C (IV) 75 mg/m²	31–34, 38–41	
Ara-C (IV) 75 mg/m²	31–34, 38–41, 45–48, 52–55			TG (Oral) 60 mg/m²	29–42	
MP (Oral) 60 mg/m²	29–57					

CALGB 8811 (Adult)[e]

Course I		Course III		Course II: Early intensification		Course V
CTX (IV) 1,200 mg/m²	1	Cranial irradiation		MTX (IT) 15 mg	1	VCR (IV) 2 mg day 1 monthly
DNR (IV) 45 mg/m²	1, 2, 3	MTX (IT) 15 mg	1, 8, 15, 22, 29	CTX (IV) 1,000 mg/m²	1	PRED (Oral) 60 mg/m² days 1–5 monthly
VCR (IV) 2 mg	1, 8, 15, 22	MP (Oral) 60 mg/m²	1–70	MP (Oral) 60 mg/m²	1–14	MTX (Oral) 20 mg/m² days 1, 8, 15, 22 monthly
PRED (Oral) 60 mg/m²	1–21	MTX (Oral) 20 mg/m²	36, 43, 50, 57, 64	Ara-C (SC) 75 mg/m²	1–4, 8–11	MP (Oral) 60 mg/m² days 1–28 monthly
ASP (SC) 6,000 U/m²	5, 8, 11, 15, 18, 22			VCR (IV) 2 mg	15, 22	
				ASP (SC) 6,000 units/m²	15, 18, 22, 25	

Induction chemotherapy for patients ≥60 y old, use:

CTX (IV) 800 mg/m²	1
DNR (IV) 30 mg/m²	1–3
PRED (Oral) 60 mg/m²	1–7

Course IV: Late intensification

Drug and Dose	Days
DOX (IV) 30 mg/m²	1, 8, 15
VCR (IV) 2 mg	1, 8, 15
DEX (Oral) 10 mg/m²	1–14
CTX (IV) 1,000 mg/m²	29
TG (Oral) 60 mg/m²	29–42
Ara-C (SC) 75 mg/m²	29–32, 36–39

Ara-C, cytarabine; ASP, asparaginase; CALGB, Cancer and Leukemia Group B; CNS, central nervous system; CTX, cyclophosphamide; DEX, dexamethasone; DNR, daunorubicin; DOX, doxorubicin; IT, intrathecal; MP, mercaptopurine; MTX, methotrexate; PRED, prednisone; TG, thioguanine; VCR, vincristine.

[a]Maximum single dose, 2 mg.
[b]Maximum single dose, 15 mg.
[c]Maximum single dose, 1,000 mg.
[d]From Hoelzer et al.[20]
[e]From Larson et al.[21]

TABLE 131–10. Representative Chemotherapy Regimens for Pediatric Acute Lymphoblastic Leukemia

Induction (1 month)
Intrathecal cytarabine on day 0
Prednisone 40 mg/m^2 per day or dexamethasone 6 mg/m^2 per day orally for 28 days
Vincristine 1.5 mg/m^2 per dose (max 2 mg) IV weekly for 4 doses
Pegaspargase 2,500 units/m^2 per dose IM for 1 dose or asparaginase 6,000 units/m^2 per dose IM
    Mon, Weds, and Fri for 6 doses
Intrathecal methotrexate weekly for 2–4 doses

Consolidation (1 month)
Mercaptopurine 50–75 mg/m^2 per dose orally at bedtime for 28 days
Vincristine 1.5 mg/m^2 per dose (max 2 mg) IV on day 0
Intrathecal methotrexate weekly for 1–3 doses
Patients with CNS or testicular disease may receive radiation

Interim maintenance (1 or 2 cycles) (2 months)
Methotrexate 20 mg/m^2 per dose orally at bedtime weekly
Mercaptopurine 75 mg/m^2 per dose orally daily on days 0–49
Vincristine 1.5 mg/m^2 per dose (max 2 mg) IV on days 0 and 28
Dexamethasone 6 mg/m^2 per day orally on days 0–4 and 28–32

Delayed intensification (1 or 2 cycles) (2 months)
Dexamethasone 10 mg/m^2 per day orally on days 0–6 and 14–20
Vincristine 1.5 mg/m^2 per dose (max 2 mg) IV weekly for 3 doses
Pegaspargase 2,500 units/m^2 per dose IM for 1 dose
Doxorubicin 25 mg/m^2 per dose IV on days 0, 7, and 14
Cyclophosphamide 1,000 mg/m^2 per dose IV on day 28
Thioguanine 60 mg/m^2 per dose orally at bedtime on days 28–41
Cytarabine 75 mg/m^2 per dose SC or IV on days 28–31 and 35–38
Intrathecal methotrexate on days 0 and 28

Consolidation option #2 (3-week intervals for 6 courses on weeks 5–24)
Mercaptopurine 50 mg/m^2 per dose orally at bedtime
Prednisone 40 mg/m^2 per day for 7 days on weeks 8 and 17
Vincristine 1.5 mg/m^2 per dose (max 2 mg) IV on the first day of weeks 8, 9, 17, and 18
Methotrexate 200 mg/m^2 per dose IV + 800 mg/m^2 dose over 24 hours on day 1 of weeks 7, 10,
    13, 16, 19, and 22
Intrathecal methotrexate on weeks 5, 6, 9, 12, 15, and 18

Late intensification (weeks 25–52)
Methotrexate 20 mg/m^2 per dose IM weekly or 25 mg/m^2 per dose orally every 6 hours for 4 doses
    every other week
Mercaptopurine 75 mg/m^2 per dose orally at bedtime
Prednisone 40 mg/m^2 per day orally for 7 days on weeks 25 and 41
Vincristine 1.5 mg/m^2 per dose (max 2 mg) IV on the first day of weeks 25, 26, 41, and 42
Intrathecal methotrexate on day 1 of weeks 25, 33, 41, and 49

Maintenance (12-week cycles)
Methotrexate 20 mg/m^2 per dose orally at bedtime or IM weekly with dose escalation as tolerated
Mercaptopurine 75 mg/m^2 per dose orally at bedtime on days 0–83
Vincristine 1.5 mg/m^2 per dose (max 2 mg) IV on days 0, 28, and 56
Dexamethasone 6 mg/m^2 per day orally on days 0–4, 28–32, and 56–60
Intrathecal methotrexate on day 0

IM, intramuscularly; IV, intravenous.

strategy will become the new standard of care in this high-risk population.[19]

CENTRAL NERVOUS SYSTEM PROPHYLAXIS

8 CNS prophylaxis may overlap with or be incorporated into induction, consolidation, or maintenance. The rationale for CNS prophylaxis is based on two observations. First, many chemotherapeutic agents do not readily cross the blood-brain barrier. Second, results from early clinical trials of ALL showed that 50% to 75% of

patients with ALL and no CNS involvement at diagnosis experienced an extremely high rate of early isolated CNS relapse.[5] These observations indicate that the CNS is a potential sanctuary for leukemic cells and that undetectable leukemic cells are present in the CNS in many patients at the time of diagnosis. Detectable CNS involvement at the time of diagnosis is relatively uncommon (<10%) in ALL.[1] Factors that are associated with an increased risk of CNS involvement at diagnosis in children include a high initial WBC count, T-cell phenotype, mature B-cell phenotype, age ≤1 year, thrombocytopenia, lymphadenopathy, and hepatomegaly or splenomegaly. In adults, risk factors for CNS disease include mature B-cell ALL phenotype and a high proportion of cells in the S phase (indicator of cellular turnover).[5]

The goal of CNS prophylaxis is to eradicate undetectable leukemic cells from the CNS. Leukemic meningitis is more easily prevented than treated. Once CNS relapse has occurred, patients are at increased risk of bone marrow relapse and death from refractory leukemia. Initial trials in childhood ALL in the 1960s established craniospinal irradiation as the standard for prevention of CNS relapse.[11] However, this approach was associated with long-term sequelae including neuropsychological deficits, precocious puberty, osteoporosis, thyroid dysfunction, an increased incidence of brain tumors, short stature, and obesity. Subsequent trials have demonstrated that irradiation may be replaced by frequent administration of intrathecal chemotherapy in most children with ALL.[11]

The selection of a CNS prophylaxis regimen must consider efficacy, toxicity, and risk of CNS disease.

❽   Intrathecal chemotherapy, cranial irradiation, and high-dose intravenous methotrexate or cytarabine can be used to treat or prevent CNS disease. These treatment approaches have reduced CNS relapses to less than 2% among children.[1,11] Intrathecal therapy consists of methotrexate and cytarabine alone or in combination. When given together, hydrocortisone is commonly added to decrease the incidence of arachnoiditis. The doses of intrathecal chemotherapy used in pediatric ALL patients must be individualized based on age because of differences in the volume of cerebrospinal fluid at various ages. Due to the long-term sequelae associated with cranial or craniospinal irradiation, only children with CNS disease at diagnosis or who are in certain high-risk subsets receive this therapy in the United States.

CONSOLIDATION THERAPY

Consolidation (or intensification) therapy in ALL is started after a CR has been achieved, and refers to continued intensive chemotherapy in an attempt to eradicate clinically undetectable disease. Regimens usually incorporate either non–cross-resistant drugs that are different from the induction regimen, or more dose-intensive use of the same drugs.

Randomized trials show that consolidation therapy clearly improves patient outcome in children, but its benefit in adults is less clear.[1,11] The relative benefit of individual components of treatment regimens is difficult to demonstrate because of the overall complexity of therapy in ALL. The adult regimens listed in Table 131–9 offer two different approaches to consolidation with similar results. Consolidation therapy in the German regimen is similar to the remission induction regimen, but substitutes dexamethasone for prednisone (due to its better CNS penetration to prevent leukemic meningitis), doxorubicin for daunorubicin, and thioguanine for mercaptopurine.[31] Alternatively, the Cancer and Leukemia Group B (CALGB) trial uses a consolidation regimen far more complicated than the induction regimen. The latter includes different drugs and higher doses, at least for the cyclophosphamide dose.[21] The outcomes from these distinctly different approaches are similar. The German investigators found a median survival duration of 27.5 months and an estimated 5-year survival rate of 39%.[31] With a shorter follow-up time (median, 43 months), the CALBG study showed a median survival duration of 36 months and a 3-year survival rate of 39% for those 30 to 59 years old.[21] The results of these studies suggest that a consolidation phase in adult ALL therapy is necessary, although specific questions remain about drug selection, duration of therapy, dosing, and timing of administration.

In children, the intensity of consolidation therapy is based on the child's risk classification and rate of cytoreduction during induction.

Patients who respond slowly to induction therapy are at higher risk of relapse if they are not treated on more aggressive regimens. Various consolidation regimens have been studied with similar results. Two examples of consolidation regimens are presented in Table 131–10. One strategy is to include one or two delayed intensification phases separated by low-intensity interim maintenance cycles to maintain remission and to decrease cumulative toxicity. This strategy yields a 6-year EFS of 76% for a single delayed intensification and 83% for two cycles in intermediate-risk patients.[32] Current studies are testing similar regimens in standard-risk patients. The antimetabolite-based regimens may have a reduced risk of late toxicities, but the more intensive consolidation regimens appear to result in better survival for some patients, especially those with higher-risk disease.

Current studies are designed to continue the assessment of the intensity of consolidation needed for patients with different levels of risk and to determine whether methotrexate should be administered orally or intramuscularly due to compliance issues.

Children with Ph+ ALL or infants with t(4;11) mixed lineage leukemia (MLL), or children who only achieve a partial remission may be transplanted in first remission if a suitable donor is available.[1,33] In adults, the indications for transplantation are less clear,[1] but if the patient is not too old, and an allogeneic matched-sibling donor is available, many treatment centers would recommend allogeneic hematopoietic stem cell transplantation (alloHSCT) in first remission. Autologous hematopoietic stem cell transplantation (autoHSCT) has not been demonstrated to be superior to chemotherapy. The International Bone Marrow Transplant Registry (IBMTR) reports 44% DFS for matched unrelated donor (MUD) transplants. Haploidentical and cord blood transplants are being investigated since many patients do not have matched sibling donors available.

MAINTENANCE THERAPY

❾   Many adult ALL patients relapse shortly after completion of remission induction and consolidation therapy, presumably because of residual disease. Maintenance therapy allows long-term drug exposure to slowly dividing cells, allows the immune system time to eradicate leukemia cells, and promotes apoptosis (programmed cell death). The goal of maintenance therapy is therefore to further eradicate residual leukemic cells and prolong remission duration. Although maintenance therapy is clearly beneficial in childhood ALL, the possible benefit in adults has only recently been demonstrated. In some adult ALL trials that included induction and consolidation, but omitted maintenance, the DFS at 2 years was lower compared to trials that included maintenance.[1,34,35]

Maintenance therapy usually consists of mercaptopurine and methotrexate, at doses that produce relatively little myelosuppression, with intermittent "pulses" of vincristine and a steroid. Table 131–9 lists the typical doses for these agents in this phase. In an effort to determine the long-term outcome of the duration and intensity of maintenance therapy, the Childhood ALL Collaborative Group published findings from a large meta-analysis involving 12,000 randomized children from 42 trials initiated prior to 1987.[38] The analysis revealed that longer maintenance, pulses of vincristine and prednisone, and the inclusion of one or two intensive reinduction courses significantly reduced the total number of deaths or relapse. However, only intensive reinduction improved survival.

The optimal duration of maintenance therapy in adults is unknown, but most treatment programs continue maintenance therapy for 24 to 36 months. Based on the results of studies that show a trend toward an increase in late relapse (excluding isolated testicular relapse) among male children treated for 2 years versus 3 years, some centers treat female children for 2 years while males receive maintenance for 3 years. Decisions about maintenance therapy in adults are also based on the patient's subtype of ALL. Adults with common pre-B-cell ALL benefit from conventional maintenance therapy with methotrexate and mercaptopurine, while those with B-cell ALL or Ph+ ALL probably gain greater benefit from intensive induction and consolidation and little from maintenance.[5]

Interpatient variability in the pharmacokinetics of oral methotrexate and mercaptopurine may also be an important determinant of the effectiveness and toxicity of maintenance therapy. Patients who take their oral methotrexate and mercaptopurine on an evening versus a morning schedule appear to have a superior outcome.[36] To account for the interpatient variability, most pediatric protocols titrate the dose of either agent to maintain an absolute neutrophil count of 750 to 1,500/mm³. Some protocols circumvent bioavailability and poor compliance issues by administering methotrexate parenterally. The importance of these pharmacokinetic issues in adults is less well defined.

Genetic polymorphisms may affect drug metabolism, receptor expression, drug transportation, drug disposition, and pharmacologic response. These alterations may contribute to acute and chronic toxicity from ALL therapy as well as differences in treatment outcome. The most studied polymorphism involves thiopurine metabolism. Thiopurines are inactivated by S-methylation by cellular thiopurine methyltransferase (TPMT). About 10% of the population have intermediate TPMT activity due to heterozygous polymorphisms in the gene encoding for TPMT, and one in 300 has extremely low activity due to homozygous presence of this TMPT polymorphism.[37] Deficiency of TPMT activity results in excessive myelosuppression from mercaptopurine and thioguanine. Patients with low activity (homozygous mutant TPMT genotype) may require 85% to 90% dose reductions.[37] Prospective evaluation of TPMT status was complicated in the past, since many ALL patients receive transfusions prior to definitive diagnosis. TPMT status can now be determined directly by DNA-based testing, which may become a standard of care in the near future.

ACUTE LYMPHOBLASTIC LEUKEMIA IN INFANTS

ALL and AML in infants less than 1 year of age accounts for less than 5% of the reported acute leukemias in childhood, but they are associated with poor outcomes. EFS in infant ALL is 20% to 40%.[39] Sixty to seventy percent of infants with acute leukemia have a translocation that involves the MLL gene located at 11q23.[39] In infant ALL, the t(4;11) is most common and has been associated with an extremely poor outcome in the past, with only 10% to 20% EFS.[39] Other poor prognostic factors in infant ALL include age less than 6 months, a high WBC count, hepatosplenomegaly, and CNS disease. These factors are also closely associated with MLL translocations. Patients with infant ALL may have greater drug resistance to asparaginase and prednisone, but increased sensitivity to cytarabine.[39] Although the use of intensive regimens such as high-dose methotrexate and high-dose cytarabine have improved survival rates, unacceptably high mortality rates have also been observed with some regimens. Lack of pharmacokinetic data for chemotherapy in infants has contributed to toxicity from inappropriate dosing of doxorubicin and vincristine. To reduce neuropsychological complications, most protocols avoid cranial irradiation. The use of HSCT for infants with ALL remains controversial

due to a lack of donors, concerns over the long-term toxicity of total body irradiation, and excessive mortality in some series.

ACUTE LYMPHOBLASTIC LEUKEMIA IN THE ELDERLY

A considerable number of ALL cases occur in patients older than age 60 years, but no specific treatment recommendations can be made. The response to therapy and durability of response seem less than in younger adults or children. Older patients have a higher incidence of Ph+ ALL compared to younger patients, and a lower occurrence of T-cell ALL.[5,19] Based on data demonstrating excellent responses in CML, the addition of imatinib to conventional chemotherapy in Ph+ ALL patients is an increasingly common approach.[19] Whether this leads to any increase in EFS or overall survival (OS) remains to be seen. In general, older patients have a lower CR rate, and when achieved, the duration of remission is shorter than with younger patients.

TREATMENT OF RELAPSED ACUTE LYMPHOBLASTIC LEUKEMIA

The most common site for relapse is the bone marrow, although isolated relapses can occur in the CNS or testicles. Marrow relapse usually follows isolated CNS or testicular relapses. Therefore patients with isolated extramedullary relapses are treated with localized radiation (cranial or testicular) and aggressive systemic chemotherapy similar to that given to patients with a marrow relapse.[1]

Patients who have completed treatment and who have stayed in remission for longer periods are more likely to be reinduced into remission again. Patients with more favorable risk factors initially, and those who received less intensive initial treatments, are more likely to respond well to reinduction/salvage regimens.[33] In general, long-term survival after relapse is very poor, and aggressive therapies are used.

Matched sibling alloHSCT is the treatment of choice for all childhood ALL in second remission (CR2). Children who relapse more than 36 months after completion of initial therapy have reasonable outcomes with chemotherapy alone.[11] For patients with shorter initial remissions or who relapse on therapy (including most adults), alloHSCT performed while in CR2 is associated with longer DFS than chemotherapy (40% vs. 17%).[33] Patients who undergo HSCT are less likely to relapse, but are more likely to experience treatment-related morbidity and mortality. Recently published studies suggest that relapsed pediatric patients may have better 5-year DFS after alloHSCT in CR2 as compared to chemotherapy alone, regardless of duration of remission, WBC count at diagnosis, or number of agents used in initial induction.[40]

ROLE OF COLONY STIMULATING FACTORS IN ACUTE LYMPHOBLASTIC LEUKEMIA

The use of granulocyte colony-stimulating factor (G-CSF) in children and adults administered during, after, or between courses has been shown to shorten the duration of neutropenia by 2 to 10 days.[41–47] Standard-risk ALL therapy in children is not myelosuppressive and does not warrant the use of colony-stimulating factors (CSFs). It was initially thought that children with high-risk ALL may benefit from a CSF if treatment delays could be avoided. However, a recent trial in high-risk patients demonstrated that while there was a decrease in the median time to neutrophil recovery, this did not translate into any benefit in terms of episodes of febrile neutropenia, positive blood cultures, or serious infections.[46] Length of hospital stay and time to complete induction therapy were not significantly altered.[46] Similarly, there was no difference between filgrastim and placebo in hospitalization rate for fever and neutropenia, incidence of severe infection, or EFS.[46] Patients did have shorter hospital stays (average, 4 days) and fewer documented infections. A trial of filgrastim in high-risk pediatric ALL patients may be warranted in patients with treatment delays due to neutropenia if the patient's quality of life is not impaired by daily subcutaneous injections.

In the adult ALL population, one trial has demonstrated an improved CR rate, but this has not been confirmed in other large randomized studies.[47] No trial has shown improved EFS or OS in either the pediatric or adult populations. Several studies reported a decrease in the incidence of febrile neutropenia,[42,45] duration of hospitalization,[41,43,47] and duration of antibiotic use.[42]

Current American Society of Clinical Oncology (ASCO) guidelines recommend the initiation of CSFs after completion of the first few days of chemotherapy of either the initial induction or first remission course.[48] The British Society of Hematology has more recently published their recommendations for the use of CSFs in patients with hematologic malignancies, and recommend their use following intensive phases of treatment to decrease the severity of neutropenia.[49]

LATE EFFECTS OF ACUTE LYMPHOBLASTIC LEUKEMIA

Certain late effects associated with cranial or craniospinal irradiation and/or corticosteroids were discussed earlier. Some childhood ALL regimens that incorporate intensive use of topoisomerase II inhibitors (etoposide and teniposide) are associated with unacceptably high risks of development of secondary leukemia.[11] High cumulative doses of anthracyclines used in high-risk or relapsed patients can cause cardiomyopathy. Cranial irradiation has also been found to cause learning deficits, especially in patients less than 5 years of age at the time of treatment. Patients who received cranial radiation as children also have higher unemployment rates and lower marital rates among females two decades after diagnosis.[50]

▶ TREATMENT: Acute Myeloid Leukemia

AML accounts for most cases of acute leukemia in adults, and occurs with increasing frequency in elderly patients. It accounts for only 15% to 20% of the acute leukemias in children, but is responsible for 30% of leukemia-related mortality. With recent advances in chemotherapy and supportive care, 65% to 85% of all patients achieve CR and 20% to 40% become long-term survivors.[1,4] Overall, the median duration of remission is 1 to 2 years.[1,4] In patients older than age 60 years, the percentage of patients achieving a CR is lower (39% to 64%), and the median duration of remission is shorter than 1 year.[51] In contrast to ALL, effective therapies used in AML cause severe and often prolonged myelosuppression, with the exception of tretinoin. As a result, patients with AML, particularly patients older than age 60 years, are at greater risk for treatment-related fatal infectious and bleeding complications.

The 5-year survival in children with AML has increased from 17% in 1976 to 50% in 2000.[3] Children with Down's syndrome and AML receive less intense therapy and have EFS of 68% to 100%.[52] Treatment of AML, unlike that of ALL, usually only consists of induction and intensive post-remission therapy (see Fig. 131–1). CNS prophylaxis is not routinely given in adult AML (with the exception of some M4 and M5 leukemias), but is generally administered to pediatric patients. Table 131–11 presents several representative induction regimens for treatment of adult AML.[53–59]

REMISSION INDUCTION

As with ALL, the goal of remission induction for AML is to rapidly induce a CR. Compared to ALL, however, fewer patients with AML achieve CR. Since the CR rate in AML is related to the intensity of the remission induction regimen, the drugs used in AML are given at doses that uniformly cause severe marrow hypoplasia (except tretinoin). One reason for the lower CR rate in AML as compared to ALL is the inability to give optimal doses of chemotherapy because of marrow toxicity. With continued improvement of supportive care for patients undergoing chemotherapy, more intensive treatment regimens are being given in an effort to reduce the high rate of leukemic relapse and increase the proportion of long-term survivors. Most patients achieve a CR after one or two courses of chemotherapy. Patients who require additional chemotherapy to achieve a CR have been reported to have a poor prognosis, even if remission is ultimately achieved.[1]

The most active single agents in AML (non-M3) are the anthracycline antibiotics (daunorubicin, doxorubicin, and idarubicin), anthracenediones (mitoxantrone), and the antimetabolite cytarabine. The most common regimen ("7 + 3") combines daunorubicin administered as a short infusion of 45 to 60 mg/m² per day on days 1 to 3, along with cytarabine administered as a continuous 24-hour infusion of 100 mg/m² per day on days 1 to 7. The CR rate with the 7 + 3 regimen is 60% to 80% in younger adults. The remission rate decreases to 40% to 50% in patients older than age 60 years. OS rates with an anthracycline and cytarabine are 15% at 5 years.[60] Several trials have attempted to improve upon conventional 7 + 3 therapy, but have shown no improvement by (1) increasing cytarabine to 10 days, (2) shortening cytarabine to 5 days, (3) substituting doxorubicin for daunorubicin, (4) adding thioguanine, or (5) increasing cytarabine dosage to 200 mg/m² per day (given by continuous infusion).[4,12]

Other clinical trials have evaluated idarubicin or mitoxantrone as alternatives to daunorubicin in combination with standard continuous infusion cytarabine.[55,60–66] Preliminary data showed that idarubicin or mitoxantrone increased CR rates in adults younger than 60 years of age and increased survival durations.[55,62,66] Conversely, other trials in older adults showed no difference in CR rates or survival, but did report an increased number of patients achieving a CR with only one course of idarubicin plus cytarabine as compared to daunorubicin plus cytarabine.[60] In a review of long-term follow-up results from randomized trials evaluating idarubicin versus daunorubicin, only one trial maintained a significant difference favoring idarubicin. The effect of anthracycline choice on the CR rates in the elderly was studied by the Eastern Cooperative Oncology Group (ECOG).[64] Elderly AML patients were randomized to standard doses of cytarabine combined with either daunorubicin (45 mg/m² for 3 days), idarubicin

TABLE 131–11. Representative Chemotherapy Regimens for Adult AML

Induction therapy	
Yates/CALGB[54] ("7 + 3")	Daunorubicin 45 mg/m² IV daily on days 1 to 3
	Cytarabine 100 mg/m² CIV daily on days 1 to 7
Weirnik et al[55]	Idarubicin 13 mg/m² IV daily on days 1 to 3
	Cytarabine 100 mg/m² CIV daily on days 1 to 7
Weick et al[56]	Daunorubicin 45 mg/m² IV daily on days 1 to 3
	Cytarabine 2,000 mg/m² IV every 12 h × 12 doses on days 1 to 6
Mitus et al[57]	Cytarabine 100 mg/m² CIV daily on days 1 to 7
	Daunorubicin 45 mg/m² IV daily on days 1 to 3
	Cytarabine 2,000 mg/m² IV every 12 h × 6 doses on days 8 to 10
Bishop/ALSG[58]	Cytarabine 100 mg/m² CIV daily on days 1 to 7
("7 + 3 + 7")	Daunorubicin 50 mg/m² IV daily on days 1 to 3
	Etoposide 75 mg/m² IV daily on days 1 to 7
Bishop et al[59]	Cytarabine 3,000 mg/m² IV every 12 h on days 1, 3, 5, and 7
("HIDAC + 3 + 7")	Daunorubicin 50 mg/m² IV daily on days 1 to 3
	Etoposide 75 mg/m² IV daily on days 1 to 7
Post-remission chemotherapy[a]	
Mitus et al[57]	*Cycles 1 and 3*
	Cytarabine 200 mg/m² CIV daily on days 1 to 5
	Daunorubicin 60 mg/m² IV daily on days 1 and 2
	Cycle 2
	Cytarabine 2,000 mg/m² IV every 12 h × 6 doses on days 1 to 3
	Etoposide 100 mg/m² IV daily on days 4 and 5
Mayer et al[53]	Cytarabine 3,000 mg/m² IV every 12 h on days 1, 3, and 5
	(6 doses) × 1 to 4 cycles

[a]Number of postremission chemotherapy cycles is dependent on patient characteristics and inclusion of hematopoietic stem cell transplantation in treatment plan.
CIV, continuous intravenous infusion.

(12 mg/m² for 3 days), or mitoxantrone (12 mg/m² for 3 days). No difference in DFS, OS, or toxicity was seen between the three induction regimens.[64]

CLINICAL CONTROVERSY

Is there a superior anthracycline to use as part of the induction regimen for acute myeloid leukemia? Some clinicians believe that idarubicin is superior in attaining a complete remission following one cycle of induction compared to alternative anthracyclines or anthracenediones. Randomized trials in the elderly show similar remission rates with all anthracyclines and anthracenediones. Whether there is a difference in younger patients remains to be seen.

Thus the anthracycline of choice for a standard 7 + 3 regimen remains controversial, with many centers adopting idarubicin into the induction regimen in younger AML patients, and the choice in the elderly is based on individual clinician preference and institutional acquisition costs.

Other researchers have studied the impact of adding another agent, etoposide, to remission induction regimens for AML.[58] A comparison of standard 7 + 3 with or without etoposide on days 1 to 7 ("7 + 3 + 7") in newly diagnosed AML patients aged 15 to 70 years demonstrated no difference in CR rates or OS. A subset analysis of patients less than 55 years of age demonstrated a doubling of the duration of remission and OS in the etoposide-containing arm. The 7 + 3 + 7 regimen was more toxic in patients older than 55 years of age. A small trial in relapsed or refractory adults younger than 70 years of age also reported an increased duration of remission in patients receiving etoposide combined with high-dose cytarabine, as compared to high-dose cytarabine alone, thus confirming the activity of etoposide in the treatment of AML.[67]

Based on experimental tumor models that showed a steep dose-response curve for cytarabine, higher doses of cytarabine have also been evaluated as a means to enhance the outcome of remission induction therapy.[68] The addition of high-dose cytarabine on days 8 to 10 following conventional 7 + 3 therapy resulted in a CR rate of 89%, which is higher than that reported in the Southeastern Cancer Study Group or the CALGB trial (see Table 131–11).[57] In adults younger than 60 years of age, high-dose cytarabine (3,000 mg/m² every 12 hours on days 1, 3, 5, and 7) combined with daunorubicin and etoposide led to an improved duration of CR as compared with the same combination with standard-dose cytarabine, although the CR rate and OS were no different between the high-dose and standard-dose cytarabine groups.[59] The Southwest Oncology Group compared standard- and high-dose cytarabine (2,000 mg/m² every 12 hours for 12 doses), given in combination with daunorubicin.[56] High-dose cytarabine improved DFS, but did not significantly improve the CR rate or OS and was associated with more toxicity. A recent retrospective study conducted by the European Group for Blood and Marrow Transplantation showed that the cytarabine dose administered during induction and/or consolidation did not influence the outcome in patients who ultimately went on to receive allogeneic or autologous HSCT.[69] These data suggest that high doses of cytarabine during induction may not be needed in patients scheduled to receive a HSCT as post-remission therapy. In summary, the role of high-dose cytarabine during induction remains controversial. If used during induction, high-dose cytarabine is more appropriate in younger patients than in elderly patients because of poor tolerance by elderly patients.

The National Comprehensive Cancer Network (NCCN) has published guidelines for the treatment of AML.[70] The classic 7 + 3 regimen may be insufficient in adults younger than age 60 because the duration of remission is less than that reported in some studies that employed high-dose cytarabine in induction.[70] The NCCN committee recommends that adults younger than 60 years be treated with more aggressive chemotherapy with high-dose cytarabine with an anthracycline or anthracenedione. In patients older than age 60 years with good performance status, the conventional 7 + 3 regimen should be used or the patient should be enrolled in available clinical trials. The approach in patients with an antecedent hematologic disorder differs, and younger patients should be offered available clinical trials or proceed to alloHSCT (provided a suitable donor is available). Older patients (>60 years) with an antecedent hematologic disorder are usually offered best supportive care because of the dismal outcomes associated with conventional chemotherapy. All adult patients who present with CNS symptoms, and all AML M4 and AML M5 patients who are not symptomatic, should have a diagnostic lumbar puncture, and if it is positive, should be treated for disease. Methotrexate 12 to 15 mg, with or without cytarabine, should be administered intrathecally twice a week until clearance of leukemic blasts from the CSF, and then monthly for approximately 6 months.

The most effective induction regimens for children have included an anthracycline plus cytarabine, and either thioguanine or etoposide, yielding a remission rate of 75% to 85%.[71] Intensified therapy regimens, which include more antileukemic agents or compress the time in which the agents are delivered, have improved survival rates. In compressed or intensified treatment regimens, the second course of therapy is given 6 days after the first, without waiting for marrow recovery to occur. While there was an increased mortality rate associated with intensive versus standard timing in children with AML, the long-term EFS was significantly better in the intensive therapy group.[71]

Following induction therapy, patients should be evaluated for a response. A proportion of children will not enter into a CR, and will require additional chemotherapy called "reinduction." Typically a bone marrow biopsy is performed 7 to 10 days after the completion of chemotherapy (or day 14 from the start of chemotherapy), to document disease eradication. If there is persistent disease, a second course of therapy is administered. The second course may be identical to the initial induction regimen, or include high-dose cytarabine and asparaginase, or mitoxantrone and cytarabine. If the marrow is aplastic, a repeat marrow biopsy should be performed upon hematologic recovery to document a CR.

■ POST-REMISSION THERAPY

Although most adults with AML achieve a CR, the duration of remission is short (4 to 8 months) if no further treatment is given. Relapse is presumably a consequence of the presence of residual, but clinically undetectable, leukemic cells after remission induction therapy. The goal of intensive post-remission therapy is to eradicate these residual leukemic cells and to prevent the emergence of drug-resistant disease. The need for post-remission therapy is based on postmortem analysis and cell kinetic data suggesting that nearly 10^9 residual leukemic cells remain after effective remission induction therapy.[12] Strategies evaluated as post-remission therapy include (1) low-dose, prolonged maintenance therapy; (2) short-course intensive chemotherapy-alone regimens; and (3) high-dose chemotherapy with or without radiation therapy followed by allo- or autoHSCT.

■ CHEMOTHERAPY

In the treatment of AML, post-remission therapy is often referred to as consolidation or maintenance therapy. Results

of randomized trials in adults clearly show that post-remission therapy following remission induction therapy prolongs survival versus no therapy, although the exact duration of maintenance is controversial.[72,73] Trials have shown that a shorter duration of maintenance therapy is as effective as a longer duration of maintenance therapy. Alternatively, one to four courses of intensive chemotherapy can be administered over 6 months. An ECOG trial demonstrated that one course of more intensive chemotherapy, termed "consolidation therapy," increased EFS as compared to lower-dose maintenance therapy administered for 2 years, although alternative strategies might again be needed for the elderly due to toxicity.[74]

The intensity of post-remission therapy has been shown to be important. In a large CALGB trial, all patients received standard 7 + 3 induction, and once a CR was achieved, were randomized to receive one of three cytarabine-based consolidation regimens: 100 mg/m^2 per day or 400 mg/m^2 per day as a continuous 24-hour infusion, or 3,000 mg/m^2 every 12 hours on days 1, 3, and 5.[53] For adults younger than 60 years, the probability of remaining in CR after 4 years was significantly higher in patients who received high-dose cytarabine (25% vs. 29% vs. 44%, respectively).[53] Elderly patients had lower response rates in all arms and did not benefit from the administration of higher doses of cytarabine, probably because they were unable to tolerate the high-dose regimen. Dose-limiting neurotoxicity in the high-dose arm was greater in elderly patients.[53] Table 131–11 lists other approaches to intensive chemotherapy consolidation.

It is not clear whether the same agents (cytarabine and an anthracycline) given for remission induction should be used for post-remission therapy in higher doses, or whether different agents altogether should be given. If leukemic relapse is caused by a resistant cell line, then the use of different agents that are non–cross-resistant with drugs used in induction would appear to be beneficial.

High-dose cytarabine appears to be a key part of post-remission therapy, particularly if not used in induction therapy. However, many questions remain, such as the optimal dose (g/m^2), number of doses per cycle, and number of cycles of high-dose cytarabine. The only generally accepted practice is that induction alone is insufficient and that some form of post-remission therapy prolongs survival. The NCCN guidelines recommend four cycles of high-dose cytarabine for adults younger than 60 years of age and with good cytogenetics.[70] If a patient is older than age 60 years, standard-dose cytarabine with or without anthracycline, a dose-reduced high-dose cytarabine regimen (1 to 1.5 g/m^2 per day for four to six doses), or enrollment in a clinical trial is recommended. Patients with poor-risk cytogenetics, underlying MDS, or secondary AML should be referred for either a matched sibling or MUD alloHSCT.[70]

CLINICAL CONTROVERSY

What is the best dose of cytarabine to use for consolidation, how many doses and how many cycles should be administered? The optimal dose of high-dose cytarabine to administer, the number of doses per cycle, and the number of cycles to give remains unknown. What is known is that post-remission therapy is necessary to prevent relapse and that regimens containing high-dose cytarabine appear to be a key part of post-remission therapy.

Children with a matched sibling donor should proceed to alloHSCT once in remission. Children with no suitable stem cell donor should receive consolidation chemotherapy, with which survival results are similar to those seen with autoHSCT.[75]

ALLOGENEIC HEMATOPOIETIC STEM CELL TRANSPLANTATION

AlloHSCT represents the most aggressive approach to post-remission therapy in the management of AML. Much controversy surrounds this treatment approach, specifically the appropriateness, timing, treatment design, and donor selection.

The antileukemic activity of alloHSCT is based on the administration of pretransplant high-dose chemotherapy (or chemoradiotherapy) and the development of a posttransplant immune-based antileukemic response. The immune-based response, referred to as a graft-versus-leukemia (GVL) effect, often accompanies the graft-versus-host disease (GVHD) reaction. The immune-based benefit of alloHSCT has been demonstrated through the observation of consistently lower relapse rates with alloHSCT as compared to autologous or syngeneic HSCT. This potential benefit of alloHSCT can be offset by the risk of posttransplant complications such as GVHD, veno-occlusive disease, graft failure, and infections.

AlloHSCT was first evaluated as a treatment modality for AML in refractory patients, but because of initial success in small numbers of patients, it has also been evaluated as intensive post-remission therapy in AML patients in first or subsequent remission. Nonrandomized trials of human leukocyte antigen (HLA)-identical sibling alloHSCT performed in AML patients in first CR report 5-year survival rates of 45% to 60% with relapse rates of 10% to 20%.[76,77] Transplant-related mortality following sibling alloHSCT is 20% to 30% in most series. As clinicians have gained more experience in this intensive form of therapy and been provided with more effective immunosuppressive and antibiotic regimens, transplant-related mortality rates have decreased and survival rates have increased. Bone marrow registry data indicate that long-term survival rates in AML patients who receive a matched sibling alloHSCT while in first remission have increased from about 45% in the early 1980s to about 60% in the mid-1990s.[1,4]

Table 131–12 presents the results of randomized comparisons of alloHSCT to autoHSCT or intensive consolidation chemotherapy alone.[78-81] AlloHSCT from an HLA-matched sibling donor in AML patients in first CR results in long-term DFS in 43% to 55% of patients. Although the results vary, some of the studies show longer DFS and lower relapse rates with alloHSCT in AML in first CR as compared to chemotherapy-alone post-remission regimens.[82]

AlloHSCT is still generally restricted to patients younger than 60 years of age, which limits the number of patients eligible for treatment of a disease that primarily affects older adults. One new approach, termed nonmyeloablative stem cell transplant (NST), uses less toxic nonmyeloablative preparative regimens and is now being evaluated in AML patients, particularly older patients or those with comorbid illnesses that would limit their eligibility for conventional alloHSCT. NST is designed to provide enough immunosuppression in the preparative regimen to allow for engraftment of donor cells, and depends heavily on the development of a GVL effect as a means to treat and prevent relapse of AML. Initial results of NST in AML patients indicate that the procedure is well tolerated in a wide age range of patients, and that it is associated with low rates of regimen-related toxicity.[83,84] Evaluations in larger numbers of patients are necessary to determine the comparative impact of NST on GVHD, DFS, and OS. Because only 30% of patients will have an HLA-matched sibling donor, alloHSCT is further restricted as a treatment alternative for AML patients. MUD transplantation using a phenotypically HLA-matched donor identified from bone marrow registries is considered as a treatment alternative for young adults and pediatric AML patients. This approach is associated with long-term DFS rates of 30% to 40%, which are slightly lower than in AML patients undergoing HLA-matched sibling alloHSCT because of a higher risk of treatment-related mortality with the procedure.[85,86]

AUTOLOGOUS HEMATOPOIETIC STEM CELL TRANSPLANTATION

Compared to alloHSCT, autoHSCT has the advantage of a lower risk of posttransplant complications because of lack of immunosuppression and GVHD, and more broad applicability because of a lack of donor limitations and fewer age restrictions. While the preparative regimen still provides antileukemic activity, autoHSCT is associated with higher incidences of relapse because of a lack of a GVL effect and potential tumor contamination with autologous stem cells. DFS following autoHSCT for AML in first CR ranges from 40% to 60%, with treatment-related mortality of 5% to 15% and relapse rates of 30% to 50%.[74,78-81,87-89] Long-term response rates decrease proportionally as autoHSCT is employed in second or subsequent CR.

Controversies in autoHSCT include the optimal timing of therapy, the amount of consolidation therapy needed, the dose of stem cells needed, and the impact of posttransplant therapy.[89] Table 131–12 compares autoHSCT versus other post-remission therapies; they are discussed below.

TABLE 131–12. Comparative Trials of Allogeneic HSCT (AlloHSCT) or Autologous HSCT (AutoHSCT) or Chemotherapy (Chemo) Alone as Post-Remission Therapy for AML in First Complete Remission

	Disease-Free Survival at 4 Years (%)			Overall Survival at 4 Years (%)		
	AlloHSCT	AutoHSCT	Chemo	AlloHSCT	AutoHSCT	Chemo
Zittoun et al[78] (EORTC-GIMEMA)	55%[a]	48%[b]	30%	59%	56%	46%
Harousseau et al[79] (GOELAM)	44%	44%	40%	53%	50%	54%
Cassileth et al[80] (Intergroup)	43%	35%	35%	46%	43%	52%[c]
Burnett et al[81] (UK MRC)	47%	50%	40–58%	53%	52%	46–52%

[a]$p = 0.01$.
[b]$p = 0.05$.
[c]$p = 0.02$.

◼ COMPARISONS OF POST-REMISSION THERAPY OPTIONS

Several randomized trials in AML patients in first CR have compared outcomes following alloHSCT, autoHSCT, and/or intensive consolidation chemotherapy (see Table 131–12).[78–81] In most trials, eligible patients based on age and donor availability received an alloHSCT and the remaining patients were randomized between autoHSCT and chemotherapy alone. The EORTC-GIMEMA trial observed a DFS advantage and reduced relapse risk for alloHSCT or autoHSCT as compared to chemotherapy alone, but no differences in OS.[78] Survival rates were comparable because of a higher relapse rate in the chemotherapy group as compared to a higher treatment-related mortality rate in the alloHSCT group. This is the only trial that has demonstrated superior 4-year DFS with transplantation versus chemotherapy. Interestingly, the response rates in the conventional chemotherapy arm in this trial were lower than those reported in other studies, and this may account for the benefit. Several other trials have showed no difference in DFS or OS between autoHSCT, alloHSCT, and conventional chemotherapy.[79–81] In aggregate, these trials show that either autoHSCT or alloHSCT can reduce the risk of relapse, although this has not translated into a survival benefit. One of the trial design issues that may explain this lack of survival benefit was the low percentage of patients who progressed to transplantation when randomized, thus diluting the effect of transplantation. The effect of stem cell source on DFS and OS is controversial. Several comparative trials of bone marrow versus peripheral blood have been completed, with only two demonstrating a survival advantage for recipients of peripheral blood.[90,91]

5 Most transplant centers base their decision to transplant on cytogenetic risk category.[4] Patients with poor-risk cytogenetics do poorly with conventional chemotherapy or autoHSCT (DFS <15%), and therefore alloHSCT is the treatment of choice in this population. Patients with good-risk cytogenetics should not proceed to transplant in first CR, as their outcomes with conventional chemotherapy remain very good, and alloHSCT should be reserved in case of relapse. The optimal treatment of choice in patients with intermediate-risk cytogenetics is not clear and is based on clinician preference. Many centers consider a relapse probability of 40% to 50% sufficiently high enough to warrant the risk of transplant-related mortality.

According to the NCCN guidelines, the decision to proceed to HSCT depends on cytogenetics.[70] If the patient has a good-risk cytogenetic profile and is younger than age 60 years, then high-dose cytarabine for four cycles or one cycle of high-dose cytarabine–based therapy followed by autoHSCT is preferred over alloHSCT. If the patient has a poor-risk cytogenetic profile and is younger than age 60 years, then alloHSCT transplant should be considered early after remission induction. Patients with intermediate-risk cytogenetics should be entered into a clinical trial, but if a clinical trial is not available, either a matched sibling alloHSCT or an autoHSCT should be considered. AutoHSCT can be used if a hematologic and cytogenetic remission is achieved. For patients older than age 60 years, the NCCN guidelines do not favor HSCT and recommend either enrollment into a clinical trial, or consideration of conventional high-dose cytarabine. In recent years clinicians increasingly consider autoHSCT as a treatment option, and for selected patients older than 60 years of age, NST is being used more frequently.[83,84] For the AML patient who relapses early after induction therapy, if a sibling or matched related donor is available, then alloHSCT is the primary reinduction therapy because conventional chemotherapy offers little help. If the relapse occurs late, then HSCT can be used as post-remission consolidation after conventional induction therapy.[70]

◼ ACUTE MYELOID LEUKEMIA IN INFANTS

Infant AML is usually myelomonoblastic or monoblastic in morphology. Poor prognostic factors include t(1;22), high WBC count, and CNS disease. Neonates with Down's syndrome may develop transient clonal megakaryoblastic myeloproliferative syndrome that usually spontaneously resolves without treatment within a few months.[53] Infants with AML receive the same therapy as children of other ages, with the dosing per kilogram and not per squared meter.

◼ ACUTE MYELOID LEUKEMIA IN THE ELDERLY

As the median age at diagnosis is in the range of 65 to 70 years, AML is a disease of the elderly. Unfortunately, long-term DFS is lower in older patients, ranging from 5% to 15%, as compared to 40% in younger patients.[92,93] In patients older than age 55 years, a review of ECOG studies reported the median duration of survival to be 6 to 9 months, as compared to 11 months in patients younger than age 55 years. The actual response and survival rates may be even lower, as many elderly patients with AML are not included in clinical trials because of a lack of eligibility and poor performance status.[51]

Elderly patients with AML have a poor outcome as a result of the frequent presence of unfavorable prognostic factors, including poor-risk cytogenetic features, preceding myelodysplasia, and a higher incidence of inherent drug resistance.[4] Greater than 70% of de novo AML patients older than age 55 years will express the multidrug resistance (MDR1) phenotype associated with chemotherapy resistance, including resistance to the leukemia-active anthracyclines and etoposide.[94] Older patients with AML may also have poor outcome because of the inability to withstand aggressive therapy as a result of poor organ function, poor performance status, or existing comorbidities. Although older patients with AML may be able to tolerate aggressive induction therapy, intensive post-remission therapy is often too toxic, thus increasing the likelihood of patient relapse.[95] Older AML patients have also been reported to have an impaired capacity to recover from intensive therapy as a consequence of leukemic involvement of earlier hematopoietic cells.[51]

The potential therapeutic strategies in elderly AML patients include (1) no chemotherapy (i.e., best supportive care or palliative care therapy), (2) attenuated chemotherapy, or (3) standard-dose chemotherapy.[4] The palliative approach is most appropriate in patients with slowly progressive leukemia ("smoldering leukemia"). The difficulty lies in the ability to reliably identify these patients at diagnosis. While initially accepted in older patients, palliative care approaches in older patients with AML with moderate to good performance status and organ function are now considered inappropriate. An ECOG/CALGB study prospectively randomized patients to either a conventional chemotherapy arm or to an observation arm in which patients could receive modest doses of chemotherapy for symptom palliation. Survival was twice as long in the chemotherapy group. The quality of life of each group was similar, with each spending approximately 50% of the study time in the hospital.[96] Chemotherapy may prolong survival without significantly decreasing the quality of life for elderly patients. Thus chemotherapy is a viable treatment option for elderly patients, although the best chemotherapy regimen and overall treatment approach is controversial. One approach is to attenuate the dose of chemotherapy, preferably using oral agents where possible, or lower doses of intravenous agents. Agents used in this strategy include oral etoposide, low-dose subcutaneous cytarabine, and other oral agents such as thioguanine and idarubicin (oral idarubicin is not currently commercially available in the U.S.). Complete remission rates of 32% to 35% have been reported with low-dose subcutaneous cytarabine.[97]

Another approach is to use standard induction regimens that would be used in younger adults. With standard 7 + 3 induction therapy, the complete response rate in older AML patients ranges from 39% to 48%, compared with 65% to 73% in adults <60 years. Half of the remaining patients are likely to die during induction therapy from infection or other complications, and the other half often has refractory disease.[95] More elderly patients than younger patients will require two courses of induction therapy to achieve a remission. In an effort to improve response rates, some trials have attempted to determine the best anthracycline and the appropriate dose. Unlike younger patients, comparative data in elderly patients do not suggest any efficacy or toxicity advantages of idarubicin or mitoxantrone over daunorubicin for AML induction therapy.[64,98] Results of early uncontrolled trials reported high morbidity and mortality rates during induction in elderly AML patients who received aggressive doses of daunorubicin (>45 mg/m² per day for 3 days). More recent trials, however, suggest that older AML patients can safely withstand higher doses of daunorubicin (60 to 90 mg/m² per day), which may be a result of enhancements in supportive care.[96,99] Unlike younger patients, older patients with AML do not experience added benefit when etoposide is incorporated into an anthracycline and cytarabine–containing regimen, nor do they appear to benefit when etoposide is substituted for cytarabine in induction.[58,100]

Post-remission strategies in elderly AML patients are less well defined.[4] Even though high-dose cytarabine has become a standard component of post-remission therapy in younger patients, it has not been shown to be beneficial in the elderly. In the elderly, attenuated-dose cytarabine during induction decreases remission and survival rates while decreasing treatment-related mortality rates, which raises the concern that attenuated-dose cytarabine during post-remission therapy may cause similar outcome. In the CALGB trial comparing post-remission cytarabine doses, there was less benefit of higher doses of cytarabine (3,000 mg/m²) in patients older than age 60 years as compared to younger patients.[53] Serious toxicities, particularly neurotoxicity, were more frequent in the elderly, and these toxicities limited the ability to deliver the planned four courses of therapy. A recent ECOG review of lower doses of cytarabine (1,500 mg/m² for 6 to 12 doses) in older AML patients were well tolerated, with a treatment-related mortality rate of only 2% and median survival at 2 years of 30%.[99] Based on these data, some clinicians question the need for doses of cytarabine as high as 3,000 mg/m² and suggest that attenuated high-dose regimens (such as 1,500 mg/m²) may be sufficient and beneficial. The appropriate number of cycles of post-remission consolidation therapy is unknown and currently under investigation in a randomized ECOG trial.

While maintenance therapy is considered inferior to intensive consolidation chemotherapy in younger patients, its role in older patients with AML is still undefined. Some studies suggest that maintenance therapy following consolidation prolongs DFS but not OS as compared to no maintenance therapy.[92,101] Since older patients may not be able to tolerate more aggressive post-remission strategies such as HSCT, maintenance therapy may play an important role in improving outcomes.

More novel approaches to post-remission therapy targeted at immune modulation have been evaluated in elderly patients with AML. Early results with interleukin-2 (IL-2) as a means to enhance immune-mediated prevention of relapse have been promising.[102] The CALGB is currently conducting a randomized trial in the elderly comparing 90 days of post-remission low-dose, subcutaneous IL-2 versus observation. FLT-3 ligand is another immunomodulatory cytokine that enhances recovery and activity of hematopoietic and dendritic cells and is currently under investigation as post-remission therapy in elderly AML patients.

NST is another therapeutic option in elderly patients with AML and MDS. Two small studies suggest this is a feasible option, with actuarial OS and EFS rates of 44% to 69% and 37% to 56%, respectively.[83,84] The advantage of this approach is less intensive chemotherapy with less toxicity, and the immune system providing the ongoing antileukemia effect via GVHD/GVL mechanisms (see Chap. 134).

■ TREATMENT OF RELAPSED OR REFRACTORY ACUTE MYELOID LEUKEMIA

The most common cause of treatment failure in AML patients receiving chemotherapy alone or undergoing HSCT is relapse. In addition, a substantial number of patients, especially elderly patients, experience refractory disease as defined by the inability to achieve a CR after two courses of induction therapy. In most cases, the preferred method of treatment for relapse or refractory disease is HSCT. Prolonged DFS is observed in 30% to 40% of patients receiving allo- or autoHSCT in first relapse or second CR.[103,104] Unfortunately, only a small percentage of relapsed or refractory adult patients will be eligible for HSCT, particularly alloHSCT, because of age and donor restrictions. The role of NST is being evaluated as previously discussed.

The timing of HSCT to treat relapse is controversial. Some studies suggest that outcome of HLA-matched, related alloHSCT performed at the time of early first relapse is comparable to that observed when the procedure is performed in second CR.[103] The difficulty in this approach is identifying a patient in "early relapse," as often the patient will present in a florid relapse. While performing the alloHSCT in first relapse eliminates the need for and toxicity of salvage chemotherapy, the feasibility of this approach can be limited by the logistics required to prepare and to activate a donor. A comparison conducted by the IBMTR demonstrated the superiority of alloHSCT over chemotherapy for treatment of relapse occurring 1 to 2 years following induction.[105] Prolonged leukemia-free survival occurred in at least twofold more alloHSCT recipients as compared to patients receiving chemotherapy. In the treatment of refractory disease, alloHSCT is superior to autoHSCT in adults younger than age 55 years.[106,107]

Patients who relapse following alloHSCT have a poor outcome, with a median survival of about 3 to 4 months.[1] In this scenario, treatment options depend on performance status, clinical condition, and the time since alloHSCT. Patients relapsing less than 100 days following alloHSCT are unlikely to respond to current strategies, and salvage attempts are often associated with a high treatment-related mortality. For patients relapsing more than 1 year after alloHSCT, second alloHSCT may be an alternative in selected young adults, but the likelihood of prolonged survival is generally less than 10% with a second transplant.[1] Other strategies being investigated for AML relapsing after alloHSCT include immune manipulation to stimulate a GVL effect through donor lymphocyte infusions, and premature discontinuation of cyclosporine and other immunosuppressants.

AutoHSCT is an option at the time of first relapse if cells have been previously collected and stored during first remission. If such cells were not collected, then it is necessary to achieve a second CR in order to proceed to autoHSCT. Prolonged DFS of 30% and 20% are reported when autoHSCT is performed in second and third CR, respectively.[108] The advantages of autoHSCT are the lack of donor limitations and fewer age-based restrictions; the disadvantage is the need to achieve a CR, which requires exposure to more cytotoxic chemotherapy. If patients relapse following autoHSCT, alloHSCT from a related or unrelated donor is preferred in selected younger patients. NST or other investigational therapies can be considered for older patients who relapse after autoHSCT.

If patients with relapsed or refractory disease are not candidates for HSCT, until recently the primary mode of treatment was salvage chemotherapy. The ability to achieve a second CR with salvage chemotherapy is related to the duration of the first remission. About 50% to 60% of patients who relapse greater than 2 years after induction therapy will achieve a second CR, often with the same induction regimen.[109] If the patient relapses 1 to 2 years after induction therapy, the second CR rate decreases to 40%, and only 10% to 20% of patients who relapse within 6 to 12 months following induction are able to achieve a second CR with alternate salvage chemotherapy regimens. Long-term survival at 3 years ranges from zero in patients who relapse early to 20% to 25% in those who experience a prolonged duration of initial remission. Based on these data, a risk-adapted approach should be taken when considering treatment options. The most commonly used salvage regimens are high-dose cytarabine–based regimens with doses of 2,000 to 3,000 mg/m^2 every 12 hours for 8 to 12 doses. High-dose cytarabine schedules that use once-daily doses or alternate-day doses have also been used in an attempt to minimize toxicity.[1,109] Cytarabine has been administered alone or in combination with various agents, including etoposide, fludarabine, topotecan, and an anthracycline, as treatment of relapsed or refractory AML. Response rates to such salvage regimens range from 30% to 50%, but are often short-lived. Patients who received high-dose cytarabine during induction may be less likely to benefit from such a regimen for treatment of relapse, and thus require alternate salvage strategies. Patients with a remission duration of greater than a year appear to benefit most from high-dose cytarabine regimens.[109]

About 70% of relapsed or refractory AML express the MDR1 phenotype, which confers a high degree of chemotherapy resistance because of its encoding and overexpression of P-glycoprotein. P-glycoprotein is a membrane protein capable of removing certain antineoplastics from the intracellular to extracellular space. Antagonists of P-glycoprotein, such as cyclosporine or the cyclosporine analog valspodar (formerly PSC 833), have been investigated as a strategy to overcome resistance in these patients.[110–113] In addition to inhibiting P-glycoprotein, cyclosporine may also affect the disposition of agents such as anthracyclines, and thus increase the exposure to cytotoxic agents. Valspodar is 10-fold more effective in inhibiting P-glycoprotein than cyclosporine and lacks cyclosporine's renal toxicity. Unfortunately, randomized trials in previously untreated or relapsed/refractory patients have shown no advantages and more regimen-related deaths in patients older than age 60 years receiving the MDR modulator.[112,113] Other MDR inhibitors with limited interference with hepatic metabolism are currently under investigation.

Monoclonal antibodies have been the subject of recent investigations in the treatment of relapsed or refractory AML, and have the ability to deliver targeted therapy to the malignant cell. Gemtuzumab ozogamicin is an anti-CD33 antibody complexed to the antitumor antibiotic calicheamicin. Since CD33 is expressed in 90% of leukemic blasts, this anti-CD33–directed product provides targeted cell kill to leukemic cells. Patients with AML in first untreated relapse treated with gemtuzumab (9 mg/m^2 for two doses separated by 14 days) attained a CR in 16% of patients, with a further 13% of patients having normalization of blood counts with the exception of persistent platelet counts <100,000/mm^3.[114,115] Toxicity can be problematic with gemtuzumab. Common adverse effects include infusion-related reactions (fever and chills), prolonged neutropenia and thrombocytopenia, and transient elevations in hepatic enzymes. A more serious adverse event associated with gemtuzumab therapy is veno-occlusive disease. It was initially thought that this only occurred in patients receiving gemtuzumab following HSCT, but has now been described in several patients who were never exposed to HSCT. Close monitoring of a patient's weight should occur, as well as monitoring of liver function tests, particularly bilirubin. Because gemtuzumab lacks specific dose-limiting organ toxicities, it is also being investigated in combination with other chemotherapy agents.[116] Gemtuzumab therapy in pediatric patients has been limited by the incidence of veno-occlusive disease of the liver when given prior to HSCT. Other antibodies under investigation in salvage regimens and high-dose preparative regimens for AML include radiolabeled anti-CD45 agents and HuM195, a humanized mouse monoclonal antibody targeted against the CD33 antigen.

Numerous classes of new agents are being investigated as alternate treatment approaches for relapsed or refractory AML, including the ubiquitin-proteasome pathway inhibitors (bortezomib), new novel nucleoside analogues (troxacitabine),[117] hypomethylating agents (decitabine and 5-azacytidine),[118] histone deacetylase inhibitors (phenylbutyrate),[119] and angiogenesis modulators (bevacizumab and thalidomide).[120] Arsenic trioxide, which is effective in the treatment of APL, is also under investigation for treatment of AML via its modulation of apoptotic and chromatin remodeling pathways.[121] Imatinib mesylate, the tyrosine kinase inhibitor exhibiting efficacy in the treatment of CML, also inhibits AML cell lines and is currently undergoing clinical trials in AML.[122]

In children with AML, the duration of first remission predicts remission rates following relapse. The BFM group reported that patients who relapse within 1.5 years of initial diagnosis have a 5-year survival of 10%, versus 40% for those who relapse later than 1.5 years after initial diagnosis.[123] In children with relapsed or refractory AML, a regimen of mitoxantrone 12 mg/m^2 per day for 4 days starting on the third day of treatment and cytarabine 1,000 mg/m^2 per dose every 12 hours for eight doses can achieve a second CR rate of 76% with only a 3% mortality rate.[124] However, the 2-year OS rate was only 24%. Patients were eligible to receive intensification with high-dose cytarabine and etoposide at the investigator's discretion, and this arm was closed due to a toxic death rate of 10%. Currently, most pediatric patients in second CR receive alloHSCT if a suitable donor is available.

LATE EFFECTS OF THERAPY FOR ACUTE MYELOID LEUKEMIA

Due to the intense therapy received by children with AML, they are at risk for a variety of long-term sequelae. A recent study reported that more than 50% of survivors have growth abnormalities.[125] Other findings include neurocognitive deficits, transfusion-associated hepatitis, endocrine disorders, cataracts, and cardiomyopathy (median cumulative anthracycline dose 335 mg/m^2). The 20-year cumulative risk for a second malignancy is estimated to be 1.8%.

▶ TREATMENT: Acute Promyelocytic Leukemia

APL is a subclass of AML (FAB M3) that accounts for 10% of all cases, and is the most curable leukemia of all AML subtypes. Most patients are diagnosed between the age of 15 and 60 years. Five-year DFS rates of 70% to 80% are reported with APL.[18] APL has historically been diagnosed by the distinctive cytoplasmic granules seen on light microscopy. There are two variants: hypergranular (most common), and microgranular. APL is clinically unique from the other subclasses because of the common occurrence of severe coagulopathy (characterized by disseminated intravascular coagulation) at diagnosis and during induction therapy. In APL, differentiation and maturation arrest are caused by alterations in the retinoic acid receptor because of the translocation of chromosomes 15 and 17. The discovery of t(15;17) now provides a cytogenetic marker of the disease and is a prognostic marker in favor of response to differentiation therapy with tretinoin (commonly referred to as all-trans retinoic acid).[126] This translocation leads to a fusion protein of the promyelocytic leukemia (PML) gene on chromosome 15 and the retinoic acid receptor-α (RARα) on chromosome 17.[126]

Historically, treatment of APL involved combination chemotherapy regimens used in the treatment of other subclasses of AML. Such standard regimens produced CR rates of 50% to 60%, but were associated with a high treatment-related mortality rate caused by hemorrhagic complications. The introduction of molecularly targeted therapy with tretinoin allows for high CR rates with a significant reduction in life-threatening bleeding complications.

INDUCTION THERAPY

Tretinoin, an oral vitamin A analog, is usually given orally in a dose of 45 mg/m^2 per day, as a single dose or divided into two doses, given after a meal. Tretinoin-based regimens achieve CR rates as high as 95% in APL patients within 1 to 3 months. Tretinoin does not cross the blood-brain barrier; therefore leukemic meningitis should be treated with conventional intrathecal chemotherapy.

While being devoid of myelosuppressive effects, tretinoin therapy is associated with headache, skin and mucous membrane reactions, bone pain, nausea, and the retinoic acid syndrome. When tretinoin is started, rapid onset of differentiation of promyelocytes occurs, which can lead to leukocytosis and/or retinoic acid syndrome. The retinoic acid syndrome (fever, respiratory distress, interstitial pulmonary infiltrates, pleural effusions, and weight gain) is now referred to as the APL differentiation syndrome or APL hyperleukocytosis syndrome, because it has been associated with other treatment modalities in the management of APL. Among tretinoin-treated patients, this syndrome has been fatal in 5% to 29% of cases. A combination of chemotherapy with tretinoin induction decreases the incidence of retinoic acid syndrome, and rapid initiation of dexamethasone 10 mg (0.2 mg/kg per dose in children) twice daily for 3 days upon development of symptoms decreases associated mortality.

A number of clinical trials have evaluated optimum treatment regimens for APL since the discovery of tretinoin.[127–135] These trials have demonstrated that tretinoin induction therapy, followed by consolidation chemotherapy, produced similar CR rates but decreased relapse and increased EFS and OS as compared to chemotherapy alone for induction and consolidation.[127,128] However, a significant proportion of patients receiving tretinoin in that study relapsed by 4 years,

and 25% of patients experienced the retinoic acid syndrome.[127] In an effort to extend the duration of remission and decrease tretinoin-associated toxicity, other trials have evaluated the outcome of sequential and concurrent administration of tretinoin with chemotherapy during induction therapy. The UK MRC trial compared concurrent administration of tretinoin with chemotherapy to sequential tretinoin during induction (given 5 days before anthracycline-based induction chemotherapy) with the hope of reducing coagulopathy-related complications.[129] Concurrent administration was superior in terms of CR rates, early death, and EFS and OS at 3 years. The French study demonstrated similar CR rates with concurrent or sequential tretinoin and standard induction chemotherapy, but noted a better DFS and EFS at 2 years in the concurrent administration group (suggesting a synergistic or additive effect for the combination).[130] Based on these data, the current recommendations for induction therapy for newly diagnosed APL patients include tretinoin 45 mg/m^2 per day until a CR is achieved, in addition to an anthracycline (either daunorubicin 50 to 60 mg/m^2 per dose for 3 days, or idarubicin 12 mg/m^2 per dose every other day for four doses).[18] Similar CR rates are observed with daunorubicin or idarubicin. APL cells appear to be more sensitive to anthracyclines, perhaps due to decreased P-glycoprotein expression.

It is important to note that chemotherapy regimens used in combination with tretinoin differ from standard AML regimens, primarily due to the lack of a cytarabine backbone. Several studies have evaluated the role of cytarabine in induction regimens for APL. The addition of cytarabine has not improved the CR rate.[131] At some centers, children routinely receive both cytarabine and an anthracycline (usually the previously discussed 7 + 3 regimen) in combination with tretinoin.

POST-REMISSION THERAPY

Consolidation chemotherapy must also be administered to patients with APL due to the high relapse rate. Consolidation therapy usually consists of an anthracycline-based regimen. Recent studies suggest that there is a limited role for high-dose cytarabine in consolidation phases.[132] Current recommendations reserve high-dose cytarabine regimens for patients who remain polymerase chain reaction–positive after consolidation with an anthracycline-containing regimen.[18]

Unlike other subtypes of AML, the role of maintenance therapy is well defined in APL. Before the advent of tretinoin, nonrandomized trials supported a benefit of continuous low-dose methotrexate and mercaptopurine in prevention of relapse of APL.[133] Larger prospective trials have demonstrated decreased relapse rates in patients who received maintenance therapy (either tretinoin or combination chemotherapy),[18,127,132] and some trials have demonstrated increased EFS and OS.[130] In a study that compared maintenance with tretinoin, tretinoin plus chemotherapy, and chemotherapy or observation, observation was associated with the highest relapse rate and tretinoin plus chemotherapy with the lowest relapse rate.[130] Current recommendations for maintenance therapy in adult APL patients includes tretinoin 45 mg/m^2 per day for 15 days every 3 months, in addition to mercaptopurine 100 mg/m^2 orally daily and methotrexate 10 mg/m^2 per week, for 2 years in all patients.[18]

RELAPSED ACUTE PROMYELOCYTIC LEUKEMIA

Relapsed APL can also be effectively treated with tretinoin therapy in a large number of cases. Patients relapsing after tretinoin-based therapy are able to achieve second CR with tretinoin-based reinduction.[127] For patients resistant to induction or reinduction with tretinoin-based regimens, alternative strategies include arsenic trioxide, and allo- or autoHSCT. Outcomes with autoHSCT depend on the disease status of the patient at the time of transplant. AutoHSCT in CR2 (versus first CR) is associated with a lower OS, leukemia-free survival, and increased treatment-related mortality. Based on the sensitive nature of patients to chemotherapy, autoHSCT in first CR is currently not warranted, but offers an excellent option for polymerase chain reaction PML-RAR α–negative patients in CR2. AlloHSCT should not be offered to patients in first CR, as the mortality associated with alloHSCT outweighs the risks of conventional chemotherapy. In CR2, it is an appropriate choice as consolidation after reinduction with either arsenic trioxide or tretinoin.[136]

Arsenic trioxide has induced clinical remissions in relapsed APL through its induction of apoptosis and differentiation.[137–139] The recommended dose is 0.15 mg/kg per day IV until bone marrow remission, not to exceed 60 doses, followed by consolidation beginning 3 to 6 weeks after completion of induction at the same dose for a total of 25 doses over a period up to 5 weeks. Arsenic trioxide therapy is associated with two specific toxicities. First, it has been shown to cause the APL hyperleukocytosis syndrome, similar to that seen with tretinoin. Management is similar: corticosteroids at first signs of pulmonary distress or a rapidly rising WBC count. The second toxicity is a prolongation of the QTc interval.[140] It is therefore important to obtain a baseline 12-lead electrocardiogram (ECG) prior to starting therapy with arsenic trioxide, and correct any electrolyte abnormalities including potassium, calcium, and magnesium. Other medications known to prolong the QTc interval should be discontinued, if possible, during arsenic trioxide therapy. The QTc interval should not exceed 500 msec at baseline, and if it increases to >500 msec during therapy, the patient should be re-evaluated. Do not reintroduce the arsenic trioxide until the QTc is <460 msec. Following induction of a second CR with arsenic trioxide in relapsed patients, post-remission therapy with combination arsenic trioxide and chemotherapy can result in molecular remissions and improved DFS, as compared to chemotherapy or arsenic trioxide alone following remission.[139] Additional investigations are underway to evaluate the role of arsenic trioxide in multidrug post-remission regimens. Other drugs that are undergoing evaluation for efficacy in APL include gemtuzumab ozogamicin and Am 80.

PATIENT MONITORING

Detection of residual PML-RARα transcripts in the bone marrow at the end of consolidation therapy is strongly associated with subsequent hematologic relapse. Achievement of PML-RAR α–negative status is associated with a higher probability of cure. The use of this molecular technique allows the clinician to assess response to therapy and also detect relapse earlier, which might prevent the development of overt disease recurrence and is associated with improved outcome compared with delaying treatment until overt morphologic relapse.[18] Most experts recommend that APL patients should be routinely evaluated for continuous remission status. Suggested follow-up includes polymerase chain reaction for PML-RARα every 3 to 6 months for 2 years, and then every 6 months for 2 years.[18]

USE OF COLONY-STIMULATING FACTORS IN ACUTE MYELOID LEUKEMIA

In AML, colony-stimulating factors (CSFs) have been evaluated as a means to enhance chemotherapy cytotoxicity, shorten the duration of neutropenia, and reduce the incidence and severity of infection following induction and consolidation chemotherapy. Most studies showed limited benefit with the use of CSFs as "priming" agents administered during induction therapy in an effort to recruit leukemia cells into the cycle to enhance susceptibility to cell-cycle–specific chemotherapy agents, leading to increased cell kill. However, the positive results of a recently published study with filgrastim as a priming agent in AML patients has renewed interest in this principle.[141] While the response rates between the groups were no different, those patients in CR after induction chemotherapy receiving filgrastim had higher DFS. There was no effect on OS. Subgroup analysis did show improved OS and DFS for patients with standard-risk AML receiving filgrastim. Use of CSFs during chemotherapy administration is discouraged outside the setting of a clinical trial.

CLINICAL CONTROVERSY

Colony-stimulating factors were investigated a decade ago as "priming agents" to recruit cells into the cycle, so theoretically there was a greater leukemia cell kill. Most studies were negative and showed no incremental increases in CR rates. Recent data suggesting that there is improved disease-free survival has renewed interest in this principle.

Both filgrastim and sargramostim are approved by the FDA to treat neutropenia after antileukemia therapy. The original package inserts listed myeloid malignancies as contraindications to the use of filgrastim or sargramostim. Myeloid blast cells have receptors for G-CSF and GM-CSF, and there was initial concern that the use of these factors would stimulate regrowth of the myeloid leukemia. Although subsequent studies have not shown this not to be true, many pediatric clinicians do not initiate filgrastim until an initial remission is achieved.

A number of randomized trials, primarily in elderly patients, consistently demonstrate reduction in neutropenia when filgrastim or sargramostim is administered following AML induction chemotherapy.[64,142–150] While neutropenia can be reduced from 2 to 12 days depending on the trial, results vary in terms of improvements in infectious morbidity and mortality, resource utilization, and disease response rates (Table 131–13). Comparison of outcomes between trials is difficult because of differences in study design and patient populations. The use of CSFs in elderly AML patients has received particular attention because complications related to prolonged neutropenia, particularly infection, are one of the major causes of failure to achieve remission. In one large trial in elderly AML patients, administration of sargramostim following induction and consolidation therapy significantly reduced infection rates and increased OS.[64] But another randomized trial evaluating Escherichia coli–derived sargramostim during and after chemotherapy has shown a negative impact of CSF therapy by reporting an unexplained decreased CR rate in the sargramostim arm.[148]

As a result of these trials, the ASCO Guidelines for the Use of Hematopoietic Colony-Stimulating Factors only recommends the use of CSFs after initial induction therapy if the benefits of decreased hospitalization outweigh the CSF cost.[48] Patients older than age 55 years appear to derive the greatest benefit, and use is appropriate in

TABLE 131–13. Colony-Stimulating Factors Following Induction Therapy for Acute Myeloid Leukemia

Reference	Drug	Enhanced Neutrophil Recovery	Other Benefits Related to Colony-Stimulating Factor Therapy
Godwin et al[142]	Filgrastim	Yes	Fewer days of fever and antibiotics
Heil et al[143]	Filgrastim	Yes	Decreased duration of hospitalization
Dombert et al[144]	Filgrastim	Yes	Increased complete remission rate
Rowe et al[64]	Filgrastim	Yes	Decreased incidence of infection and increased survival
Usuki et al[150]	Filgrastim	Yes	None
Stone et al[145]	Sargramostim (*E. coli*)	Yes	None
Witz et al[146]	Sargramostim (*E. coli*)	Yes	Increased disease-free survival
Zittoun et al[147]	Sargramostim (*E. coli*)	No	Decreased complete remission rate
Lowenberg et al[148]	Sargramostim (*E. coli*)	Yes	None

this population where more rapid marrow recovery might decrease the duration of hospitalization.[48] Routine use in younger patients remains controversial. More recently, the British Society of Hematology has published guidelines on the use of CSFs in hematologic malignancies, which are in agreement with the ASCO guidelines. Both groups note that following consolidation therapy, there is a more profound shortening of the duration of neutropenia and a reduction in the use of antibiotic therapy.[49] Further pharmacoeconomic data are required in this setting, but the body of evidence supports their use following consolidation therapy in adults. Other controversial issues surrounding CSF use in AML include which CSF to use, what dose, which day to start after chemotherapy, how long to continue, and should the marrow be examined for leukemia prior to starting a CSF. The use of growth factors can also interfere with the interpretation of the day 14 bone marrow examination.

SUPPORTIVE CARE

The most common and significant toxic effect of antileukemic agents is marrow suppression. With the exception of prednisone (and dexamethasone), tretinoin, asparaginase, and vincristine, antineoplastic agents used to treat acute leukemia cause myelosuppression. During AML remission induction and post-remission therapy, daily monitoring of the complete blood count and the absolute neutrophil count is necessary to determine when red cell and platelet transfusions are needed and when neutropenia is achieved. Less frequent monitoring than daily may be sufficient during ALL induction. Marrow hypoplasia from the myelosuppressive regimens usually reaches its lowest point (nadir) after 1 to 2 weeks of therapy and lasts for another 1 to 2 weeks. During this period of hypoplasia, infectious and bleeding complications are major causes of death in leukemic patients. As typical signs and symptoms of infection may be absent in the neutropenic host, frequent monitoring of vital signs (especially fever) and daily physical examination are important.[151] Infection control strategies often include routine hand washing; dietary restrictions,; reverse isolation and laminar-air flow rooms; fungal, *Pneumocystis*, and bacterial prophylaxis; and the empiric use of broad-spectrum antibiotics when fever occurs (see Chap. 120).[151] The NCCN guidelines, in contrast to those of many institutions, do not recommend prophylactic antimicrobials or gut decontamination during induction or consolidation unless there is a documented recurrent problem at the institution.[70]

In children, prophylactic antibiotics have not proven useful and have resulted in increased resistance. Pediatric ALL patients on standard induction regimens, which generally are minimally myelosuppressive, often have recovered blood counts earlier and do not require very aggressive measures. However, they do require close monitoring of vital signs and blood counts until their counts recover. Pediatric AML patients are usually admitted for at least 1 month during induction and again for consolidation. Regardless of therapy, children with AML have a 10% to 20% induction mortality rate due to infection and bleeding complications.[52] The incidence of viridans streptococci has increased with the intensity of therapy and is most associated with high-dose cytarabine. These infections can lead to meningitis or delayed acute respiratory distress syndrome.

Pneumocystis carinii prophylaxis (usually trimethoprim-sulfamethoxazole) is begun in all adults and children with ALL by the end of induction and continues until 6 months after therapy is discontinued.

Acute leukemia patients, particularly those with an initial elevated WBC count, are at risk for tumor lysis syndrome. Preventive measures include allopurinol or rasburicase, and adequate hydration (with or without sodium bicarbonate) prior to and during chemotherapy to prevent the development of urate nephropathy from rapid destruction of white blood cells. In adults, 300 mg of allopurinol once daily, started 1 to 2 days prior to chemotherapy, is usually adequate. Children should receive 10 mg/kg per day of allopurinol in three divided doses. Rasburicase, a recombinant urate-oxidase enzyme produced by genetic modification of *Saccharomyces cerevisiae*, catalyzes the enzymatic oxidation of uric acid into the inactive soluble metabolite, allantoin. In children, rasburicase 0.15 to 0.2 mg/kg per day more rapidly reduces uric acid levels in patients with aggressive malignancies compared to allopurinol, and reduces the need for dialysis.[152–154] There are limited data supporting the use of this product in adults, although existing data suggest similar efficacy to that of the pediatric population.[152] Because of the expense, this product is usually limited to patients with ALL who have a high WBC count or bulky extramedullary disease, high-grade lymphoma, or patients with AML with a high presenting WBC. Most institutions also include an elevated uric acid as part of the criteria for use. Due to the rapid onset of action of rasburicase, many institutions also limit the use to a single dose and allow repeat doses when the criteria for use are met again. Rasburicase is contraindicated in patients with glucose-6-phosphate dehydrogenase deficiency.

Tumor lysis syndrome may lead not only to hyperuricemia, but also to hyperkalemia, hyperphosphatemia, and hypocalcemia.

Hematologic support consists primarily of platelet and packed red blood cell transfusions. Platelet transfusions are often given for peripheral counts below 5000 to 10,000/mm³ or clinical signs of bleeding. Transfusions of packed red cells may also be indicated for a hematocrit under 25%, profound fatigue, shortness of breath, tachycardia, or chest pain. APL can release procoagulants that can cause disseminated intravascular coagulation, necessitating close monitoring and replacement of coagulation factors with cryoprecipitate. Because of the gastrointestinal toxic effects of chemotherapy, parenteral nutrition may be required. Patients are frequently receiving infusions of antibiotics, fluids, hyperalimentation, and blood products simultaneously. To provide the total support needed for these patients, a multiple-lumen central venous access device such as a Hickman catheter may be placed at the start of therapy.

EVALUATION OF THERAPEUTIC OUTCOMES

Appropriate development of a pharmaceutical care plan for the acute leukemia patient begins with establishing the diagnosis and prognosis for the patient. Long-term therapeutic goals for the patient may include long-term DFS, although palliative care is a possibility in some patients. The desired short-term outcome is the establishment of remission. The return of hematologic values to normal and a repeat bone marrow biopsy that demonstrates no evidence of disease serve as documentation that remission has been achieved. Monitoring guidelines for induction or consolidation are similar (Table 131–14). After the appropriate post-remission therapy has been completed, the patient may return monthly for 1 year and then every 3 months, to check hematologic values. If no evidence of disease exists after 5 years from the diagnosis and the patient has been in continuous CR, the patient is considered cured.

Intense monitoring of fevers, hematologic and chemistry laboratory values, microbiology reports, and the patient's physical condition are necessary to identify infection, risk of bleeds, and tumor lysis syndrome early. A coagulation-screening panel will identify patients with ongoing disseminated intravascular coagulation, a particular risk with APL.

During therapy, the pharmacist can be an important provider of patient education. Patients should receive information regarding acute and chronic toxicities of the chemotherapy being administered, as well as possible treatments for those toxicities. The pharmacist can also be an important resource for information regarding antibiotics, antiemetics, nutritional support, CSFs, and other supportive care issues.

Pharmacists need to be involved in checking drug doses and any dose modifications for organ dysfunction or prior toxicity. Pharmacists are often in the best position to recognize the potential for

TABLE 131–14. Acute Myeloid Leukemia Assessment and Monitoring

Baseline Work-Up	Monitoring During Therapy	Post-Remission Monitoring
History and physical examination	Daily physical examination	Routine physical examination at clinic visit
CBC with differential, platelets	CBC with differential, platelets	CBC with differential, platelets
Serum chemistries (creatinine, bilirubin, AST, ALT to assess organ function)	Serum chemistries (including uric acid, K^+, PO_4^{3-}, Scr during tumor lysis syndrome risk period[a])	Bone marrow biopsy and aspirate at set intervals to evaluate ongoing remission
Coagulation (PT, PTT, D-dimers, fibrinogen)	Coagulation (PT, PTT, D-dimers, fibrinogen [if APL])	
Bone marrow biopsy and aspirate with cytogenetics	Bone marrow biopsy and aspirate 7–10 days after end of chemotherapy (with cytogenetics if initially abnormal)	
Immunophenotyping and cytochemistry	Temperature curve (initiate antibiotics when febrile)	
Human leukocyte antigen (HLA) typing	Lumbar puncture (with intrathecal chemotherapy) if initial lumbar puncture was positive for leukemia	
Cardiac work-up (MUGA or echocardiogram; ECG)		
Intravascular access		
Lumbar puncture (if symptomatic or AML M4 or M5)		
Chest x-ray		
Height and weight		

[a]Risk for tumor lysis syndrome during induction therapy only.
ALT, alanine aminotransferase; APL, acute promyelocytic leukemia; AST, aspartate aminotransferase; CBC, complete blood cell count; ECG, electrocardiogram; MUGA, multiple gated acquisition (blood pool scan); PT, prothrombin time; PTT, partial thromboplastin time; Scr, serum creatinine.

medication errors and drug interaction and to help avoid them. Similarly, pharmacists are often able to identify the possibility that patient problems are secondary to drug treatments.

Numerous late sequelae from leukemia therapy have been recognized and should be included in the monitoring plan after therapy is completed. The long-term consequences of HSCT are discussed in Chap. 134.

ABBREVIATIONS

ALL: acute lymphocytic (or lymphoblastic) leukemia
alloHSCT: allogeneic hematopoietic stem cell transplantation
AML: acute myeloid leukemia
APL: acute promyelocytic leukemia
ASCO: American Society of Clinical Oncology
autoHSCT: autologous hematopoietic stem cell transplantation
CALGB: Cancer and Leukemia Group B
CLL: chronic lymphocytic leukemia
CML: chronic myeloid leukemia
CR: complete remission
CR2: second remission
CSF: colony-stimulating factor
DFS: disease-free survival
ECG: electrocardiograph
ECOG: Eastern Cooperative Oncology Group
EFS: event-free survival
FAB: French–American–British classification system
FISH: fluorescent in situ hybridization
G-CSF: granulocyte colony-stimulating factor
GM-CSF: granulocyte macrophage-colony stimulating factor
GVHD: graft-versus-host disease
GVL: graft-versus-leukemia (effect)
HLA: human leukocyte antigen
HSCT: hematopoietic stem cell transplantation
hyper-CVAD: high-dose methotrexate and cytarabine alternating
    with fractionated cyclophosphamide plus vincristine,
    doxorubicin, and dexamethasone
IBMTR: International Bone Marrow Transplant Registry
IL-2: interleukin-2
MDS: myelodysplastic syndrome
MLL: mixed lineage leukemia
MUD: matched unrelated donor
NCCN: National Comprehensive Cancer Network
NST: nonmyeloablative stem cell transplant
OS: overall survival
Ph$^+$: Philadelphia chromosome
PML: promyelocytic leukemia (gene)
RARα: retinoic acid receptor-α
TPMT: thiopurine methyltransferase
WBC: white blood cell
WHO: World Health Organization

Review Questions and other resources can be found at
www.pharmacotherapyonline.com.

REFERENCES

1. Scheinberg DA, Maslak P, Weiss M. Acute leukemias. In: DeVita VT, Hellman S, Rosenberg SA, eds. Cancer: Principles and Practice of Oncology, 6th ed. Philadelphia, Lippincott Williams & Wilkins, 2001:2404–2433.

2. Jemal A, Murray T, Word E, et al. Cancer statistics, 2005. CA Cancer J Clin 2005;55:10–30.

3. Ries LAG, Eisner MP, Kosary CL, et al. SEER Cancer Statistics Review, 1975–2001, National Cancer Institute, Bethesda, MD, http://seer.cancer.gov/csr/1975_2001/,2004.

4. Stone RM, O'Donnell MR, Sekeres MA. Acute myeloid leukemia. Hematology (Am Soc Hematol Edouc Program) 2004:98–117.

5. Faderl S, Jeha S, Kantarjian HM. The biology and therapy of adult acute lymphoblastic leukemia. Cancer 2003;98:1337–1354.

6. Wen W, Shu XO, Potter JD, et al. Parental medication use and risk of childhood acute lymphoblastic leukemia. Cancer 2002;95:1786–1794.

7. Beaupre DM, Kurzrock R. RAS and leukemia: from basic mechanisms to gene-directed therapy. J Clin Oncol 1999;17:1071–1079.

8. Vardiman JW, Harris NL, Brunning RD. The World Health Organization (WHO) classification of the myeloid neoplasms. Blood 2002;100:2292–2302.

9. Byrd JC, Mrozek K, Dodge RK, et al. Pretreatment cytogenetic abnormalities are predictive of induction success, cumulative incidence of relapse, and OS in adult patients with de novo acute myeloid leukemia: results from Cancer and Leukemia Group B (CALGB 8461). Blood 2002;100:4325–4336.

10. Hasle H, Niemeyer CM, Chessells JM, et al. A pediatric approach to the WHO classification of myelodysplastic and myeloproliferative disease. Leukemia 2003;17:277–282.

11. Pui CH, Evans WE. Acute lymphoblastic leukemia. N Engl J Med 1998;339:605–615.

12. Schiffer CA. Acute myeloid leukemia in adults. In: Holland JF, Frei E, Bast RC, et al, eds. Cancer Medicine, 4th ed. Philadelphia, Williams & Wilkins, 1997:2617–2649.

13. Rubnitz JE, Camitta BM, Mahmoud H, et al. Childhood acute lymphoblastic leukemia with the MLL-ENL fusion and t(11;19)(q23;p13.3) translocation. J Clin Oncol 1999;17:191–196.

14. Brockman SR, Paternoster SF, Ketterling RP, Dewald GW. New highly sensitive fluorescence in situ hybridization method to detect PML/RARA fusion in acute promyelocytic leukemia. Cancer Genet Cytogenet 2003;145:144–151.

15. Smith M, Arthur D, Camitta B, et al. Uniform approach to risk classification and treatment assignment for children with acute lymphoblastic leukemia. J Clin Oncol 1996;14:18–24.

16. Wells RJ, Arthur DC, Srivastava A, et al. Prognostic variables in newly diagnosed children and adolescents with acute myeloid leukemia: Children's Cancer Group Study 213. Leukemia 2002;16:601–607.

17. Cheson B, Bennett JM, Kopecky KJ, et al. Revised recommendations of the International Working Group for diagnosis, standardization or response criteria, treatment outcomes, and reporting standards for therapeutic trials in acute myeloid leukemia. J Clin Oncol 2003;21:4642–4649.

18. Lowenberg B, Griffin JD, Tallman MS. Acute myeloid leukemia and acute promyelocytic leukemia. Hematology (Am Soc Hematol Educ Program) 2003:82–101.

19. Thomas DA, Faderl S, Cortes J, et al. Treatment of Philadelphia chromosome-positive acute lymphoblastic leukemia with Hyper-CVAD and imatinib mesylate. Blood 2004;103:4396–4407.

20. Hoelzer D, Ludwig WD, Thiel E, et al. Improved outcome in adult B-cell acute lymphoblastic leukemia. Blood 1996;87:495–508.

21. Larson RA, Dodge RK, Burns CP, et al. A five-drug remission induction regimen with intensive consolidation for adults with acute lymphoblastic leukemia: Cancer and Leuekmia Group B Study 8811. Blood 1995;85:2025–2037.

22. Lee EJ, Petroni GR, Schiffer CA, et al. Brief-duration high-intensity chemotherapy for patients with small noncleaved-cell lymphoma or FAB L3 acute lymphoblastic leukemia: results of cancer and leukemia group B study 9251. J Clin Oncol 2001;19:4014–4022.

23. Thomas DA, Cortes J, O'Brien S, et al. Hyper-CVAD program in Burkitt's-type adult acute lymphoblastic leukemia. J Clin Oncol 1999;17:2461–2470.

24. Kantarjian HM, O'Brien S, Smith TL, et al. Results of treatment with hyper-CVAD, a dose-intensive regimen, in adult acute lymphocytic leukemia. J Clin Oncol 2000;18:547–561.

25. Koh LP, Lim LC. Cerebellar toxicity following hyperCVAD regimen for acute lymphoblastic leukemia. Br J Haematol 1999;104:644–645.

26. Rivera GK, Raimondi SC, Hancock ML, et al. Improved outcome in childhood acute lymphoblastic leukaemia with reinforced early treatment and rotational combination chemotherapy. Lancet 1991;337:61–66.

27. Nachman J, Sather HN, Gaynon PS, et al. Augmented Berlin-Frankfurt-Munster therapy abrogates the adverse prognostic significance of slow early response to induction chemotherapy for children and adolescents with acute lymphoblastic leukemia and unfavorable presenting features: a report from the Children's Cancer Group. J Clin Oncol 1997;15: 2222–2230.

28. Gaynon PS, Carrel AL. Glucocorticoid therapy in childhood acute lymphoblastic leukemia. Adv Exp Med Biol 1999;457:593–605.

29. Ravindranath Y. Recent advances in pediatric acute lymphoblastic and myeloid leukemia. Curr Opin Oncol 2003;15:23–35.

30. Ottmann OG, Druker BJ, Sawyers CL, et al. A phase 2 study of imatinib in patients with relapsed or refractory Philadelphia chromosome-positive acute lymphoid leukemias. Blood 2002;100:1965–1971.

31. Hoelzer D, Thiel E, Löffler H, et al. Prognostic factors in a multicenter study for treatment of acute lymphoblastic leukemia in adults. Blood 1988;71:123–131.

32. Lange BJ, Bostrom BC, Cherlow JM, et al. Double-delayed intensification improves EFS for children with intermediate-risk acute lymphoblastic leukemia: a report from the Children's Cancer Group. Blood 2002; 99:825–833.

33. Popat U, Carrum G, Heslop HE. Haemopoietic stem cell transplantation for acute lymphoblastic leukaemia. Cancer Treat Rev 2003;29: 3–10.

34. Cassileth PA, Andersen JW, Bennett JM, et al. Adult acute lymphocytic leukemia: The Eastern Cooperative Oncology Group experience. Leukemia 1992;6(Suppl 2):178–181.

35. Dekker AW, van't Veer MB, Sizoo W, et al. Intensive postremission chemotherapy without maintenance therapy in adults with acute lymphoblastic leukemia. Dutch Hemato-Oncology Research Group. J Clin Oncol 1997;15:476–482.

36. Schmiegelow K, Glomstein A, Kristinsson J, et al. Impact of morning versus evening schedule for oral methotrexate and 6-mercaptopurine on relapse risk for children with acute lymphoblastic leukemia. Nordic Society for Pediatric Hematology and Oncology (NOPHO). J Pediatr Hematol Oncol 1997;2:102–109.

37. Wall AM, Rubnitz JE. Pharmacogenomic effects on therapy for acute lymphoblastic leukemia in children. Pharmacogenomics J 2003;3: 128–135.

38. Richards S, Gray R, Peto R, et al. Duration and intensity of maintenance chemotherapy in acute leukemia: Overview of 42 trials involving 12,000 randomised children. Childhood ALL Collaborative Group. Lancet 1996;347:1783–1788.

39. Biondi A, Cimino G, Pieters R, et al. Biological and therapeutic aspects of infant leukemia. Blood 2000;96:24–33.

40. Boulad F, Steinherz P, Reyes B, et al. Allogeneic bone marrow transplantation versus chemotherapy for the treatment of childhood acute lymphoblastic leukemia in second remission: A single institution study. J Clin Oncol 1999;17:197–207.

41. Pui CH, Boyett JM, Hughes WT, et al. Human granulocyte CSF after induction chemotherapy in children with acute lymphoblastic leukemia. N Engl J Med 1997;336:1781–1787.

42. Welte K, Reiter A, Mempel K, et al. A randomized phase-III study of the efficacy of granulocyte colony-stimulating factor in children with high-risk acute lymphoblastic leukemia. Berlin-Frankfurt-Munster Study Group. Blood 1996;87:3143–3150.

43. Clarke V, Dunstan FD, Webb DK. Granulocyte colony-stimulating factor ameliorates toxicity of intensification chemotherapy for acute lymphoblastic leukemia. Med Pediatr Oncol 1999;32:331–335.

44. Ottmann OG, Hoelzer D, Gracien E, et al. Concomitant granulocyte colony-stimulating factor and induction chemoradiotherapy in adult acute lymphoblastic leukemia: a randomized phase III trial. Blood 1995;86:444–450.

45. Geissler K, Koller E, Hubmann E, et al. Granulocyte colony-stimulating factor as an adjunct to induction chemotherapy for adult acute lymphoblastic leukemia—a randomized Phase-III study. Blood 1997;90: 590–596.

46. Heath JA, Steinherz PG, Altman A, et al. Human granulocyte colony-stimulating factor in children with high-risk acute lymphoblastic leukemia: a Children's Cancer Group Study. J Clin Oncol 2003;21: 1612–1617.

47. Larson RA, Dodge RK, Linker CA, et al. A randomized controlled trial of filgrastim during remission induction and consolidation chemotherapy for adults with acute lymphoblastic leukemia: CALGB Study 9111. Blood 1998;92:1556–1564.

48. Ozer H, Armitage JO, Bennett CL, et al. 2000 Update of recommendations for the use of hematopoietic colony-stimulating factors: evidence-based, clinical practice guidelines. American Society of Clinical Oncology Growth Factor Expert Panel. J Clin Oncol 2000;18:3558–3585.

49. Pagliuca A, Carrington PA, Pettengell R, et al. Guidelines on the use of colony-stimulating factors in haematological malignancies. Br J Haematol 2003;123:22–33.

50. Pui CH, Cheng C, Leung W, et al. Extended follow-up of long-term survivors of childhood acute lymphoblastic leukemia. N Engl J Med 2003; 349:640–649.

51. Hiddemann W, Kern W, Schoch C, et al. Management of acute myeloid leukemia in elderly patients. J Clin Oncol 1999;17:3569–3576.

52. Langmuir PB, Aplenc R, Lange BJ. Acute myeloid leukaemia in children. Best Pract Res Clin Hematol 2001;14:77–93.

53. Mayer RJ, Davis RB, Schiffer CA, et al. Intensive postremission chemotherapy in adults with acute myeloid leukemia. Cancer and Leukemia Group B. N Engl J Med 1994;331:896–903.

54. Yates J, Gildewell O, Wiernik P, et al. Cytosine arabinoside with daunorubicin or adriamycin for therapy of acute myelocytic leukemia: a CALGB study. Blood 1982;60:454–462.

55. Weirnik PH, Banks PLC, Case DC Jr, et al. Cytarabine plus idarubicin or daunorubicin as induction and consolidation therapy for previously untreated adult patients with acute myeloid leukemia. Blood 1992;79: 313–319.

56. Weick JK, Kopecky KJ, Appelbaum FR, et al. A randomized investigation of high-dose versus standard-dose cytosine arabinoside with daunorubicin in patients with previously untreated acute myeloid leukemia: a Southwest Oncology Group study. Blood 1996;88: 2841–2851.

57. Mitus AJ, Miller KB, Schenkein DP, et al. Improved survival for patients with acute myelogenous leukemia. J Clin Oncol 1995;13:560–569.

58. Bishop JF, Lowenthal RM, Joshua D, et al. Etoposide in acute nonlymphocytic leukemia. Australian Leukemia Study Group. Blood 1990;75: 27–32.

59. Bishop JF, Matthews JP, Young GA, et al. A randomized study of high-dose cytarabine in induction in acute myeloid leukemia. Blood 1996; 87:1710–1717.

60. Bennett JM, Young ML, Andersen JW, et al. Long-term survival in acute myeloid leukemia: the Eastern Cooperative Oncology Group experience. Cancer 1997;80(11 Suppl):2205–2209.

61. Mandelli F, Petti MC, Ardia A, et al. A randomised clinical trial comparing idarubicin and cytarabine to daunorubicin and cytarabine in the treatment of acute non-lymphoid leukemia: A multicentric study from the Italian Co-operative Group GIMEMA. Eur J Cancer 1991;27:750–755.

62. Berman E, Heller G, Santorsa J, et al. Results of a randomized trial comparing idarubicin and cytosine arabinoside with daunorubicin and cytosine arabinoside in adult patients with newly diagnosed acute myelogenous leukemia. Blood 1991;77:1666–1674.

63. Berman E, Wiernik P, Vogler R, et al. Long-term follow-up of three randomized trials comparing idarubicin and daunorubicin as induction therapies for patients with untreated acute myeloid leukemia. Cancer 1997;80(11 Suppl):2181–2185.

64. Rowe JM, Neuberg D, Friedenberg W, et al. A phase 3 study of three induction regimens and of priming with GM-CSF in older adults with

acute myeloid leukemia: a trial by the Eastern Cooperative Oncology Group. Blood 2004;103:479–485.

65. Arlin Z, Case DC Jr, Moore J, et al. Randomized multicenter trial of cytosine arabinoside with mitoxantrone or daunorubicin in previously untreated adult patients with acute nonlymphocytic leukemia (ANLL). Leukemia 1990;4:177–183.

66. Vogler WR, Velez-Garcia E, Weiner RS, et al. A phase III trial comparing idarubicin and daunorubicinin combination with cytarabine in acute myelogenous leukemia: a Southeast Cancer Study Group Study. J Clin Oncol 1992;10:1103–1111.

67. Vogler WR, McCarley DL, Stagg M, et al. A Phase III trial of high-dose cytosine arabinoside with or without etoposide in relapsed and refractory acute myelogenous leukemia. A Southwast Cancer Study Group trial. Leukemia 1994;8:1847–1853.

68. Plunkett W, Iacoboni S, Keating MJ. Cellular pharmacology and optimal therapy concentrations of 1-β-D-arabinofuranosylcytosine 51-triphosphate in leukemic blasts during treatment of refractory leukemia with high-dose 1-β-D-arabinofuranosylcytosine. Scand J Haematol 1986;44:51–59.

69. Cahn JY, Labopin M, Sierra J, et al. No impact of high-dose cytarabine on the outcome of patients transplanted for acute myeloblastic leukaemia in first remission. Acute Leukaemia Working Party of the European Group for Blood and Marrow Transplant (EBMT). Br J Haematol 2000;110:308–314.

70. National Comprehensive Cancer Network Clinical Practice Guidelines in Oncology. Acute Myeloid Leukemia. Version 1.2004. http://www.nccn.com/physician´gls/f´guidelines.html. Accessed 12/3/03.

71. Gregory J, Arceci R. Acute myeloid leukemia in children: a review of risk factors and recent trials. Cancer Invest 2002;20:1027–1037.

72. Buchner T, Urbanitz D, Hiddemann W, et al. Intensified induction and consolidation with and without maintenance chemotherapy for acute myeloid leukemia (AML): two multicenter studies of the German AML Cooperative Group. J Clin Oncol 1985;3:1583–1589.

73. Cassileth PA, Harrington DP, Hines JD, et al. Maintenance chemotherapy prolongs remission duration in adult acute nonlymphocytic leukemia. J Clin Oncol 1988;6:583–587.

74. Cassileth PA, Lynch E, Hines JD, et al. Varying intensity of postremission therapy in acute myeloid leukemia. Blood 1992;79:1924–1930.

75. Woods WG, Neudorf S, Gold S, et al. A comparison of allogeneic bone marrow transplantation, autologous bone marrow transplantation, and aggressive chemotherapy in children with acute myeloid leukemia in remission. Blood 2001;97:56–62.

76. Clift RA, Buckner CD, Appelbaum FR, et al. Allogeneic bone marrow transplantation in patients with acute myeloid leukemia in first remission. A randomized trial of two irradiation regimens. Blood 1990;76:1867–1871.

77. Geller RB, Saral R, Pianadosi S, et al. Allogeneic bone marrow transplantation after high-dose busulfan and cyclophosphamide in patients with acute nonlymphocytic leukemia. Blood 1989;73:2209–2218.

78. Zittoun RA, Mandelli F, Willemze R, et al. Autologous or allogeneic bone marrow transplantation compared with intensive chemotherapy in acute myelogenous leukemia in first remission. European Organization for Research and Treatment of Cancer (EORTC) and the Gruppo Italiano Malattie Ematologiche Maligne dell'Adulto (GIMEMA) Leukemia Cooperative Groups. N Engl J Med 1995;332:217–223.

79. Harrousseau JL, Cahn JY, Pignon B, et al. Comparison of autologous bone marrow transplantation and intensive chemotherapy as postremission therapy in adult acute myeloid leukemia. The Groupe Ouest Est Leucemies Aigues Myeloblastiques (GOELAM). Blood 1997;90:2978–2986.

80. Cassileth PA, Harrington DP, Appelbaum FR, et al. Chemotherapy compared with autologous or allogeneic bone marrow transplantation in the management of acute leukemia in first remission. N Engl J Med 1998;339:1649–1656.

81. Burnett AK, Wheatley K, Goldstone AH, et al. The value of allogeneic bone marrow transplant in patients with acute myeloid leukemia at differing risk of relapse: results of the UK MRC AML 10 trial. Br J Haematol 2002;118:385–400.

82. Reiffers J. HLA-identical sibling hematopoietic stem cell transplantation for acute myeloid leukemia. In: Atkinson K, ed. Clinical Bone Marrow and Stem Cell Transplantation, 2nd ed. New York, Cambridge University Press, 2000:433–445.

83. Taussig DC, Davies AJ, Cavenagh JD, et al. Durable remissions of myelodysplastic syndrome and acute myeloid leukemia after reduced-intensity allografting. J Clin Oncol 2003;21:3060–3065.

84. Wong R, Giralt S, Martin T, et al. Reduced-intensity conditioning for unrelated donor hematopoietic stem cell transplantation as treatment for myeloid malignancies in patients older than 55 years. Blood 2003;102:3052–3059.

85. Anasetti C. Transplantation of hematopoietic stem cells from alternate donors in acute myelogenous leukemia. Leukemia 2000;14:502–504.

86. Bertz H, Potthoff K, Finke J. Allogeneic stem-cell transplantation from related and unrelated donors in older patients with myeloid leukemia. J Clin Oncol 2003;21:1480–1484.

87. Archimbaud E, Thomas X, Michallet M, et al. Prospective genetically randomized comparison between intensive post-induction chemotherapy and bone marrow transplantation in adults with newly diagnosed acute myeloid leukemia. J Clin Oncol 1994;12:262–267.

88. Schiller GJ, Nimer SD, Territo MC, et al. Bone marrow transplantation versus high-dose cytarabine-based consolidation chemotherapy for acute myelogenous leukemia in first remission. J Clin Oncol 1992;10:41–46.

89. Linker CA. Autologous stem cell transplantation for acute myeloid leukemia. Bone Marrow Transplant 2003;31:731–738.

90. Bensinger WI, Martin PJ, Storer B, et al. Transplantation of bone marrow as compared with peripheral blood cells from HLA-identical relatives in patients with hematologic cancers. N Engl J Med 2001;344:175–181.

91. Couban S, Simpson D, Barnett MJ, et al. A randomized multicenter comparison of bone marrow and peripheral blood in recipients of matched sibling allogeneic transplants for myeloid malignancies. Blood 2002;100:1525–1531.

92. Lowenberg B, Sucieu S, Archimbaud E, et al. Mitoxantrone versus daunorubicin in induction and consolidation therapy: The value of low-dose cytarabine for maintenance of remission, and an assessment of prognostic factors in acute myeloid leukemia in the elderly: Final report of the Leukemia Organization for the Research and Treatment of Cancer and the Dutch-Belgium Hemato-Oncology Cooperative Hovon Group randomized phase III study AML-9. J Clin Oncol 1998;16:872–881.

93. Stone RM. Therapy of older adults with AML: CALGB studies. In: Hiddeman W, Buchner T, Wormann B, et al, eds. Acute Leukemias VIII: Prognostic Factors and Treatment Strategies. Berlin, Springer-Verlag, 1999.

94. Leith CP, Kopecky KJ, Godwin J, et al. Acute myeloid leukemia in the elderly: Assessment of multidrug resistance (MDR) and cytogenetics distinguishes biologic subgroups with remarkably distinct responses to standard chemotherapy: A Southwest Oncology Group study. Blood 1997;89:3323–3329.

95. Rowe JM. Treatment of acute myelogenous leukemia in older adults. Leukemia 2000;14:480–487.

96. Löwenberg B, Zittoun R, Kerkhofs H, et al. On the value of intensive remission-induction chemotherapy in elderly patients of 65 + years with acute myeloid leukemia: a randomized phase III study of the European Organization for Research and Treatment of Cancer Leukemia Group. J Clin Oncol 1989;7:1268–1274.

97. Cheson BD, Simon R. Low-dose ara-C in acute nonlymphocytic leukemia and myelodysplastic syndromes: a review of 20 years' experience. Semin Oncol 1987;14:126–133.

98. AML Collaborative Group. A systematic collaborative review of randomized trials comparing idarubicin with daunorubicin (or other anthracyclines) as induction therapy for acute myeloid leukemia. Br J Haematol 1998;103:100–109.

99. Rowe JM, Andersen JW, Mazza JJ, et al. Randomized placebo-controlled phase III study of granulocyte-macrophage colony stimulating factor in adult patients (>55–70 years) with acute myelogenous leukemia: A study of the Eastern Cooperative Oncology Group (E1490). Blood 1995;86:457–462.

100. Anderson JE, Kopecky KJ, Willman CL, et al. Outcome after induction chemotherapy for older patients with acute myeloid leukemia is not improved with mitoxantrone and etoposide compared to cytarabine and daunorubicin: a Southwest Oncology Group study. Blood 2002;100: 3869–3876.

101. Buchner T, Urbanitz D, Hiddeman W, et al. Intensified induction and consolidation with or without maintenance chemotherapy for acute myeloid leukemia (AML): Two multicenter studies of the German AML Cooperative Group. J Clin Oncol 1985;3:1583–1589.

102. Hellstrand K, Mellqvist U, Wallhut E, et al. Histamine and interleukin-2 in acute myelogenous leukemia. Leuk Lymphoma 1997;27:429–438.

103. Clift RA, Buckner CD, Appelbaum FR, et al. Allogeneic marrow transplantation during untreated first relapse of acute myeloid leukemia. J Clin Oncol 1992;10:1723–1729.

104. Petersen FB, Lynch MH, Clift RA, et al. Autologous marrow transplantation for patients with acute myeloid leukemia in untreated first relapse or in second complete remission. J Clin Oncol 1993;11:1353–1360.

105. Gale RP, Horowitz MM, Rees JKH, et al. Chemotherapy versus transplants for acute myelogenous leukemia in second remission. Leukemia 1996;10:13–19.

106. Forman SJ, Schmidt GM, Nademanne AP, et al. Allogeneic bone marrow transplantation as therapy for primary induction failure for patients with acute leukemia. J Clin Oncol 1991;9:1570–1574.

107. Biggs JC, Horowitz MM, Gale RP, et al. Bone marrow transplants may cure patients with acute leukemia never achieving remission with chemotherapy. Blood 1992;80:1090–1093.

108. Chopra R, Goldstone AH, McMillan AK, et al. Successful treatment of acute myeloid leukemia beyond first remission with autologous bone marrow transplantation using busulfan/cyclophosphamide and unpurged marrow: The British autograft group experience. J Clin Oncol 1991; 9:1840–1847.

109. Tallman MS, Mocharnuk RS. Acute myeloid leukemia: Review of Current Treatment Strategies. In: Medscape: Hematology-Oncology Clinical Management, Vol. 4: Acute Myeloid Leukemia. 2002:1–20.

110. List AF, Kopecky KJ, Willman CL, et al. Benefit of cyclosporine modulation of drug resistance in patients with poor-risk acute myeloid leukemia: A Southwest Oncology Group study. Blood 2001;98:3212–3220.

111. Gorin NC, Estey E, Jones RJ, et al. New developments in the therapy of acute myelocytic leukemia. Hematology (Am Soc Hematol Educ Program) 2000:69–89.

112. Greenberg P, Advani R, Tallman M, et al. Treatment of refractory/relapsed AML with PSC833 plus mitoxantrone, etoposide, cytarabine (PBSC-MEC) vs MEC: Randomized phase III trial (E2995). Blood 1999; 94(Suppl 1):383a.

113. Baer MR, George SL, Dodge RK. Phase 3 study of the multidrug resistance modulator PSC-833 in previously untreated patients 60 years of age and older with acute myeloid leukemia: Cancer and Leukemia Group B Study 9720. Blood 2002;100:1224–1232.

114. Sievers EL, Larson RA, Stadtmauer EA, et al. Efficacy and safety of gemtuzumab ozogamicin in patients with CD-33 positive acute myeloid leukemia in first relapse. J Clin Oncol 2001;19:3244–3254.

115. Giles F, Estey E, O'Brien S. Gemtuzumab ozogamicin in the treatment of acute myeloid leukemia. Cancer 2003;98:2095–2104.

116. Giles FJ. Novel agents for the therapy of acute leukemia. Curr Opinion Oncol 2002;14:3–9.

117. Giles FJ, Garcia-Manero G, Cortes JE, et al. Phase II study of troxacitabine, a novel dioxolane nucleoside analog, in patients with refractory leukemia. J Clin Oncol 2002;20:656–664.

118. Issa J, Garcia-Manero G, Giles FJ, et al. Phase I study of low-dose prolonged exposure schedules of the hypomethylating agent 5-aza-2'-deoxycytidine (decitabine) in hematopoietic malignancies. Blood 2004; 103:1635–1640.

119. Warrell RP, He LZ, Richon V, et al. Therapeutic targeting of transcription in acute promyelocytic leukemia by use of an inhibitor of histone deacetylase. J Natl Cancer Inst 1998;90:1621–1625.

120. Moehler TM, Ho AD, Goldschmidt H, Barlogie B. Angiogenesis in hematologic malignancies. Crit Rev Oncol Hematol 2003;45:227–244.

121. Perkins C, Kim CN, Fang G, et al. Arsenic induces apoptosis of multidrug-resistant human myeloid leukemia cells that express bcr-abl or overexpress MDR, MRP, Bcl-2 or Bcl-x(L). Blood 2000;95:1014–1022.

122. Cortes J, Giles F, O'Brien S, et al. Results of imatinib mesylate therapy in patients with refractory or recurrent acute myeloid leukemia, high-risk myelodysplastic syndrome, and myeloproliferative disorders. Cancer 2003;97:2760–2766.

123. Stahnke K, Boos J, Bender-Gotze C, et al. Duration of first remission predicts remission rates and long-term survival in children with relapsed acute myelogenous leukemia. Leukemia 1998;12:1534–1538.

124. Wells RJ, Adams MT, Alonzo TA, et al. Mitoxantrone and cytarabine induction, high-dose cytarabine, and etoposide intensification for pediatric patients with relapsed or refractory acute myeloid leukemia: Children's Cancer Group Study 2951. J Clin Oncol 2003;21:2940–2947.

125. Leung W, Hudson MM, Strickland DK, et al. Late effects of treatment in survivors of childhood acute myeloid leukemia. J Clin Oncol 2000;18:3273–3279.

126. Warrell RP, de Thè H, Wang Z, Degos L. Acute promyelocytic leukemia. N Engl J Med 1993;329:177–189.

127. Fenaux P, Chevret S, Guerci A, et al. Long-term follow-up confirms the benefit of all-trans-retinoic acid in acute promyelocytic leukemia. European APL group. Leukemia 2000;14:1371–1377.

128. Tallman MS, Andersen JW, Schiffer CA, et al, All-trans-retinoic acid in acute promyelocytic leukemia. N Engl J Med 1997;337:1021–1028.

129. Burnett AK, Goldstone AH, Gray RG, et al. All-trans-retinoic acid given concurrently with induction chemotherapy improves the outcomes of APL: Results of the UK MRC ATRA trial. Blood 1997;90(Suppl 1):1474.

130. Fenaux P, Chastang C, Chevret S, et al. A randomized comparison of all-trans-retinoic acid (ATRA) followed by chemotherapy and ATRA plus chemotherapy and the role of maintenance therapy in newly diagnosed acute promyelocytic leukemia. Blood 1999;94:1192–1200.

131. Avvisati G, Petti M, Lo Coco F, et al. Induction therapy with idarubicin alone significantly influences EFS duration in patients with newly diagnosed hypergranular acute promyelocytic leukemia: final results of the GIMEMA randomized study LAP 0389 with 7 years of minimal follow-up. Blood 2000;100:3141–3146.

132. Sanz M, Martin G, Raynon C, et al. A modified AIDA protocol with anthracycline-based consolidation results in high antileukemic efficacy and reduced toxicity in newly diagnosed PML-RARα-positive acute promyelocytic leukemia. PETHEMA group. Blood 1999;94:3015–3021.

133. Kantarjian H, Keating M, Walters RS, et al. Role of maintenance chemotherapy in acute promyelocytic leukemia. Cancer 1987;59:1258–1263.

134. Tallman MS, Andersen JW, Schiffer CA, et al. All-trans retinoic acid in acute promyelocytic leukemia: long term outcome and prognostic factor analysis from the North American Intergroup protocol. Blood 2002;100:4298–4302.

135. Sanz MA, Vellenga E, Rayon C, et al. All-trans retinoic acid and anthracycline monochemotherapy for the treatment of elderly patients with acute promyelocytic leukemia. Blood 2004;104:3490–3493.

136. Nabhan C, Mehta J, Tallman M. The role of bone marrow transplantation in acute promyelocytic leukemia. Bone Marrow Transplant 2001;28: 219–226.

137. Niu C, Yan H, Yu T, et al. Studies of treatment of acute promyelocytic leukemia with arsenic trioxide: remission induction, follow-up, and molecular monitoring in 11 newly diagnosed and 47 relapsed acute promyelocytic leukemia patients. Blood 1999;94:3315–3324.

138. Soignet S, Maslak P, Wang Z, et al. Complete remission after treatment of acute promyelocytic leukemia with arsenic trioxide. N Engl J Med 1998; 339:1341–1348.

139. Solignet S, Frankel S, Douer D, et al. United States multicenter study of arsenic trioxide in relapsed acute promyelocytic leukemia. J Clin Oncol 2001;19:3852–3860.

140. Barbey JT, Pezzullo JC, Soignet SL. Effect of arsenic trioxide on QT interval in patients with advanced malignancies. J Clin Oncol 2003; 21:3609–3615.

141. Lowenberg B, van Putten W, Theobald M, et al. Effect of priming with granulocyte colony-stimulating factor on the outcome of chemotherapy for acute myeloid leukemia. N Engl J Med 2003;349:743–752.

142. Godwin JE, Kopecky KJ, Head DR, et al. A double-blind placebo-controlled trial of granulocyte colony-stimulating factor in elderly patients with previously untreated acute myeloid leukemia: A Southwest Oncology Group Study (9031). Blood 1998;91:3607–3615.

143. Heil G, Hoelzer D, Sanz MA, et al. A randomized, double-blind, placebo-controlled, phase III study of filgrastim in remission induction and consolidation therapy for adults with de novo acute myeloid leukemia. The International Acute Myeloid Leukemia Study Group. Blood 1997;90:4710–4718.

144. Dombert H, Chastang C, Fenaux P, et al. A controlled study of recombinant human granulocyte colony-stimulating factor in elderly patients after treatment for acute myelogenous leukemia. AML Cooperative Study Group. N Engl J Med 1995;332:1678–1683.

145. Stone RM, Berg DT, George SL, et al. Granulocyte-macrophage colony-stimulating factor after initial chemotherapy for elderly patients with primary acute myelogenous leukemia. N Engl J Med 1995;332:1671–1677.

146. Witz F, Sadoun A, Perrin MC, et al. A placebo-controlled study of recombinant human granulocyte-macrophage colony-stimulating factor administered during and after induction treatment for de novo acute myelogenous leukemia in elderly patients. Groupe Ouest Est Leucemies Aigues Myeloblastiques (GOELAM). Blood 1998;91:2722–2730.

147. Zittoun R, Suciu S, Mandelli F, et al. Granulocyte-macrophage colony-stimulating factor associated with induction treatment of acute myelogenous leukemia: A randomized trial by the European Organization for Research and Treatment of Cancer Leukemia Cooperative Group. J Clin Oncol 1996;14:2150–2159.

148. Lowenberg B, Boogaerts MA, Daenen SM, et al. Value of different modalities of granulocyte-macrophage colony-stimulating factor applied during or after induction therapy of acute myeloid leukemia. J Clin Oncol 1997;15:3496–3506.

149. Bennett CL, Stinson TJ, Laver JH, et al. Cost analyses of adjunct colony stimulating factors for acute leukemia: Can they improve clinical decision making? Leuk Lymphoma 2000;37:65–70.

150. Usuki K, Urabe A, Masaoka T, et al. Efficacy of granulocyte colony-stimulating factor in the treatment of acute myelogenous leukaemia: a multicentre randomized study. Br J Haematol 2002;116:103–112.

151. Hughes WT, Armstrong D, Bodey GP, et al. 2002 guidelines for the use of antimicrobial agents in neutropenic patients with cancer. Clin Infect Dis 2002;34:730–751.

152. Pui CH, Jeha S, Irwin D, Camitta B, et al. Recombinant urate oxidase (rasburicase) in the prevention and treatment of malignancy-associated hyperuricemia in pediatric and adult patients: results of a compassionate-use trial. Leukemia 2001;15:1505–1509.

153. Pui CH, Mahmoud HH, Wiley JM, et al. Recombinant urate oxidase for the prophylaxis or treatment of hyperuricemia in patients with leukemia or lymphoma. J Clin Oncol 2001;19:697–704.

154. Bosly A, Sonet A, Pinkerton CR, et al. Rasburicase (recombinant urate oxidase) for the management of hyperuricemia in patients with cancer: report of an international compassionate use study. Cancer 2003;98:1048–1054.

132

CHRONIC LEUKEMIAS

Timothy R. McGuire and Steven Z. Pavletic

Learning Objectives and other resources can be found at *www.pharmacotherapyonline.com.*

KEY CONCEPTS

◀1 Chronic myelogenous leukemia (CML) patients who have a cytogenetic response have an improved survival.

◀2 Interferon alfa is generally not being used in newly diagnosed CML patients.

◀3 Imatinib has revolutionized the management of CML, and the majority of newly diagnosed patients will receive imatinib for at least a year, with patients who achieve a complete cytogenetic response continuing therapy indefinitely.

◀4 Allogeneic hematopoietic stem cell transplantation (HSCT) is the only modality currently available that is known to cure CML, and it is increasingly used in patients who have failed imatinib therapy.

◀5 The management of chronic lymphocytic leukemia (CLL) is highly variable and may include delaying therapy in asymptomatic older patients, well-tolerated single-agent chemotherapy in symptomatic older patients, and more aggressive therapy in younger patients.

◀6 Fludarabine is now being used as first-line therapy in younger patients, either alone or combined with cyclophosphamide or monoclonal antibodies (rituximab).

◀7 Alemtuzamab is generally used to produce a response in patients who have failed fludarabine therapy.

◀8 Nonmyeloablative HSCT may have an important role in CLL, with reports of high rates of complete remission, although it is not clear whether these patients are cured of their disease.

Chronic leukemia includes at least four disease types: chronic myelogenous leukemia (CML), chronic lymphocytic leukemia (CLL), prolymphocytic leukemia, and hairy cell leukemia. It differs from acute leukemia in that its clinical course is indolent. Most patients with chronic leukemia survive for several years after their initial diagnosis, even without treatment. Conversely, most patients with acute leukemia die of their disease within weeks to months after diagnosis if not treated. Because CML and CLL occur more frequently and represent approximately 40% of all cases of newly diagnosed leukemias occurring in the United States during 2005, this chapter focuses on these two cancers.[1]

CHRONIC MYELOGENOUS LEUKEMIA

CML is one of a group of hematologic cancers known as myeloproliferative disorders and results from the malignant transformation of a pluripotent stem cell. This malignant transformation leads to the clonal proliferation and accumulation of both progenitor and mature myeloid cells.[2,3] The clinical course of CML has three phases: it begins with an indolent chronic phase in which signs and symptoms can be controlled with well-tolerated low-intensity chemotherapy; next is a transition phase known as the accelerated phase, in which low-intensity chemotherapy no longer controls the white blood cell (WBC) count; and, finally, there is a terminal phase, also known as a blast crisis, which is similar to acute leukemia and leads to rapid clinical deterioration and death of the patient.

EPIDEMIOLOGY AND ETIOLOGY

It is estimated that approximately 4600 new cases of CML will be diagnosed in the United States in 2005, representing nearly 15% of all leukemias.[1] CML is predominantly a neoplasm of middle-aged adults, with a median age at diagnosis of approximately 50 years of age.[3] Although ionizing radiation and heavy occupational exposure to benzene are known to be associated with CML, it is rare for a newly diagnosed patient to give a history of exposure to a known risk factor. There is a 20- to 25-fold increase in the incidence of all leukemias in atomic bomb survivors. The risk of leukemia is highest in those who were exposed at a young age, with more CML cases than acute lymphoblastic leukemia cases.[4] CML can also occur after radiotherapy for ankylosing spondylitis, and it may be one of the secondary malignancies that can occur after cancer treatment with chemotherapy.[5] There are no known oncogenic viruses associated with CML.

PATHOPHYSIOLOGY

MOLECULAR BIOLOGY

CML was first described in 1845, but the extensive research into the genetic and molecular aspects of the disease began with the discovery of the Philadelphia chromosome (Ph) in 1960 by Nowell and Hungerford. Research in the 1980s identified the molecular changes that occur as a result of the Ph. An oncogenic protein resulting from the Ph was identified and implicated in the pathophysiology of CML.[6]

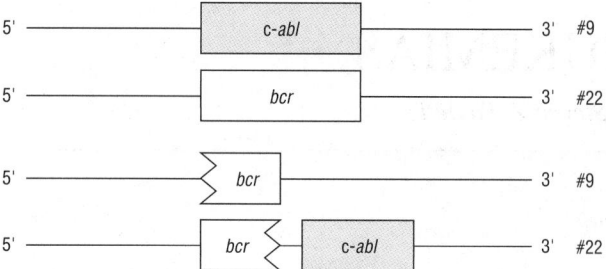

FIGURE 132–1. Diagram of the chromosomal translocation that results in the Philadelphia chromosome. This abnormality is encountered in 90% to 95% of patients who have chronic myelogenous leukemia. (From Fishleder AK. Oncogenes and cancer: clinical applications. Cleve Clin J Med 1990;57:721–726.)

Ph was the first karyotypic abnormality specifically implicated in the pathogenesis of cancer; its discovery has resulted in extensive research into the molecular biology of CML.[3,6] This chromosomal abnormality is characteristic of CML and is present in 90% to 95% of patients with a presumptive diagnosis of the disease. It can also occur in as many as 20% of adults and 5% of children with acute lymphoblastic leukemia, and in as many as 5% of adults and children with acute myelogenous leukemia.[3]

Ph, identified as a shortened long arm of chromosome 22, is found in granulocyte and erythrocyte progenitors, macrophages, megakaryocytes, and some lymphocytes.[3] This anomaly is the consequence of breaks in chromosomes 9 and 22, resulting in a transposition that relocates the 3′ end of *abl*, the Abelson protooncogene, from its normal site on chromosome 9 at band 34 to the 5′ end of the breakpoint cluster region (*bcr*) on chromosome 22 at band 11.[3] This reciprocal translocation is usually symbolized as t(9;22)(q34;q11) and results in the formation of the hybrid *bcr-abl* fusion gene (Fig. 132–1). Through this chromosomal translocation, the *abl* protooncogene is able to escape the normal genetic controls on its expression and is activated into a functional oncogene, directing the transcription of an 8.5-kilobase mRNA molecule that is translated into a 210-kilodalton protein. This protein, known as p210BCR-ABL, is unique and has higher tyrosine phosphokinase activity than the 145-kilodalton protein translated by the mRNA of the normal *abl* gene. The higher kinase activity of p210BCR-ABL is essential in the development of CML because the phosphorylation of tyrosine residues on growth factor receptors are believed to serve as an important intracellular signal in cell proliferation and programmed cell death. This stimulation of cell proliferation and inhibition of apoptosis leads to accumulation of the malignant clone. The p210BCR-ABL protein has also been shown to transform hematopoietic cells in vitro and to induce a CML-like myeloproliferative disorder in mice after infection of their bone marrow with a retrovirus that encodes the p210BCR-ABL.[7]

NATURAL HISTORY

It is generally accepted that CML begins with the malignant transformation of a single cell and therefore is considered a clonal disease. This alteration gives the transformed progenitor cell an inheritable selective growth advantage, leading to the proliferation of a neoplastic, monoclonal population of pluripotent stem cells.[8] The Ph can be found in both myeloid and lymphoid cells, which suggests that the transformed cell of CML is a pluripotent stem cell.[3,6] Granulocytosis, usually present in CML, results from the increased growth rate of the transformed clone and disruption of normal hematopoi-

etic cell maturation. Disrupted maturation leads to additional divisions by CML progenitor cells before reaching a nonproliferative stage; the resulting number of circulating granulocytes may be many times higher than normal. Later in the clinical course of CML, cytopenias may occur in association with fibrotic changes in the bone marrow.[3]

In the chronic phase, therapeutic intervention can effectively control the expansion of the CML clone and normalize the white blood cell count. As CML progresses, the malignant clone becomes more genetically unstable, and chromosomal abnormalities other than Ph may occur. Clinical evidence of the accelerated phase of CML begins to emerge as the patient's WBC count becomes increasingly difficult to manage. The rate of progression of CML is variable, and the blastic phase can sometimes erupt without any apparent accelerated phase. The relative mass of the chronic phase cell populations, genetic predetermination, and differences in either genetic stability or proliferative state of the leukemic cells are possible explanations for this variability in disease progression.[3,6] The final stage of CML, known as the acute phase or blastic phase, is marked by the presence of rapidly proliferating blast cells that have lost their ability to differentiate into nonproliferating cells.[3,6] The proliferative advantage of blast cells over normal hematopoietic cells is much greater than that of chronic phase leukemic cells. CML in blastic phase is relatively resistant to treatment. The poor response to chemotherapy is not exclusively a result of drug resistance; it also results from the high proliferative rate of blastic phase CML and the replacement of malignant cells eliminated by chemotherapy.[3,8] The increased proliferative rate of blastic phase CML is the consequence of a number of factors, such as the high levels of cytokines produced by CML cells and loss of tumor suppressor genes such as *p53*.[3,6] Several cytokines have been identified as potentially important in CML, including hematopoietic growth factors and vascular endothelial cell growth factor.[6,9]

bcr-abl AS A THERAPEUTIC TARGET

The *bcr-abl* fusion gene produces a mutant tyrosine kinase that is involved in both the increased proliferation of the CML clone, and in the reduction in FAS-mediated apoptosis. The characterization of the adenosine triphosphate (ATP) binding site on the tyrosine kinase has led to a new class of inhibitors. The first of these inhibitors, imatinib mesylate (Gleevec), was approved in 2001 for patients in chronic phase who had failed interferon alfa (IFN-α), and in accelerated phase or blast crisis. It obtained additional FDA approval in 2002 for first-line treatment in newly diagnosed CML. The clinical results associated with imatinib have changed the way CML is treated, and will be discussed in more detail under the treatment section of this chapter.[10,11]

CLINICAL PRESENTATION AND PROGNOSIS

The diagnosis of CML is usually made during the chronic phase following an abnormal complete blood cell count. The blood sample is occasionally obtained during a routine physical examination, but is usually obtained after the patient presents with symptoms such as weight loss, fatigue, malaise, night sweats, and fever. Splenomegaly and hepatomegaly are found in 30% to 40% of patients. Typical laboratory findings of the peripheral blood during the chronic phase include leukocytosis, thrombocytosis, basophilia, and low leukocyte alkaline phosphatase. In one series of newly diagnosed CML patients, the most common feature of the peripheral blood was a highly elevated WBC count (>100,000/mm^3) occurring in about 70% of patients.[3,12]

Important poor prognostic factors include older age, splenomegaly, high platelet count, and a high percentage of blasts at diagnosis. Although these factors have prognostic importance, they often fail to predict the risk for disease progression in an individual patient. Despite their limitations, these clinical features have been used to develop a widely used prognostic scoring system called the Sokal system. Using these disease and patient characteristics, clinicians can categorize patients into one of three risk groups: low-risk (median survival of about 6 years), intermediate-risk (median survival of about 4 years), and high-risk (median survival of about 2 years).[3]

Methylation of the *abl* gene and shortening of telomere length have been investigated for their ability to predict disease progression.[13,14] The *abl* gene may have an inhibitory effect on the *bcr-abl* oncogene, and methylation of *abl* reverses that inhibitory effect, leading to progression to blast crisis.[13] Telomere shortening has also been shown to reduce the time to the accelerated phase.[14] While neither methylation of *abl* or telomere shortening are standard clinical assays, these and other molecular markers may be used in the future to predict prognosis and guide therapy selection.

The accelerated phase is clinically the least distinct of the three phases of CML and may be difficult to recognize in some patients. Hematologic signs and symptoms reflect a progression in myeloproliferative acceleration and the approach of fatal blast crisis. Physical symptoms of acceleration include a resurgence of splenic enlargement, unexplained fever, and persistent bone pain. WBC counts and other signs and symptoms begin to be increasingly difficult to control with low-dose chemotherapy.

The clinical course of CML terminates in blastic phase, in which patients have peripheral blood and bone marrow findings very similar to those of acute leukemia. The blastic phase is of myeloid lineage in about two-thirds of patients and of lymphoid lineage in the other third of patients. Blastic phase is confirmed by the presence of greater than 30% blasts in the bone marrow or peripheral blood.[3] The median survival for patients in blastic phase is 4 to 6 months, with most treatment options providing modest or no survival advantage.

▶ TREATMENT: Chronic Myelogenous Leukemia

◀ Cure of CML can be achieved only by eradication of the malignant clone (i.e., Ph-positive cells). Treatment response can be defined in several different ways, depending on the tests used to measure response (Fig. 132–2). *Hematologic* response is defined as the normalization of peripheral blood counts. Although hematologic response is the easiest type of response to measure, this type of response is not associated with changes in the percentage of cells positive for the Ph. *Cytogenetic* responses evaluate the percentage of cells positive for Ph, with *complete* cytogenetic remission defined as the elimination of Ph from bone marrow, and *major* cytogenetic response defined as fewer than 35% Ph-positive cells in the bone marrow. Patients who have a cytogenetic response have an improved survival compared to those who fail to achieve a response. Conventional cytotoxic chemotherapy can be used in chronic-phase CML to attain a hematologic remission. However, low-dose chemotherapy used in chronic phase does not produce cytogenetic responses and has little or no effect on median survival. Interferon, imatinib, and hematopoietic stem cell transplantation (HSCT) can produce cytogenetic responses that are associated with longer median survivals. However, even complete cytogenetic response does not define cure.

More sensitive measures of residual disease are being used to identify the group of patients likely to be cured of their disease. *Molecular* remissions are determined by polymerase chain reaction (PCR), which is several logs more sensitive than methods used to measure cytogenetic remissions. Although bone marrow aspirates are the conventional method of determining cytogenetic response, the use of PCR in peripheral blood to measure *bcr* gene rearrangements is increasingly being used to monitor disease because of the ease of obtaining blood compared to bone marrow.[15] To date, only allogeneic HSCT (alloHSCT) has been shown to consistently eliminate the Ph-positive malignant clone. Fig. 132–2 illustrates the residual disease that remains after various types of responses and the response rates obtained with the common therapies for CML. Table 132–1 shows the effect of various treatment modalities on survival in chronic-phase CML.[16]

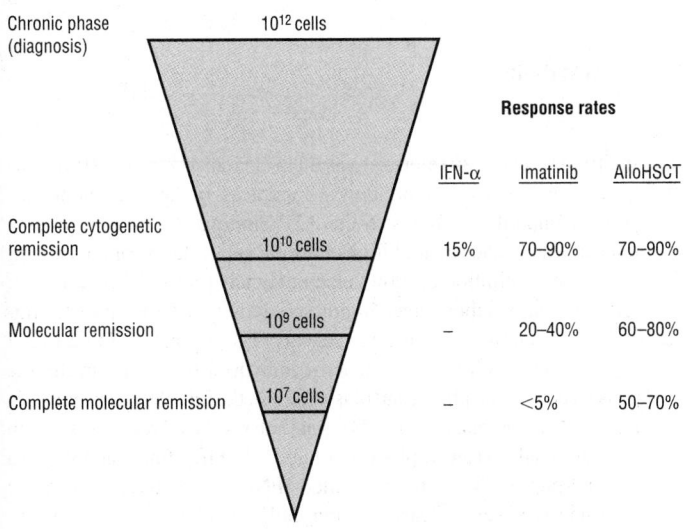

	Response rates		
	IFN-α	Imatinib	AlloHSCT
Chronic phase (diagnosis) — 10^{12} cells			
Complete cytogenetic remission — 10^{10} cells	15%	70–90%	70–90%
Molecular remission — 10^9 cells	–	20–40%	60–80%
Complete molecular remission — 10^7 cells	–	<5%	50–70%

FIGURE 132–2. Response rates, based on different measures of response, obtained with the common therapies for CML.

TABLE 132–1. Effect of Therapy on Survival in Patients with Early Chronic-Phase Chronic Myelogenous Leukemia

Therapy	5-Year Survival (%)	Median Survival (Months)
Busulfan	30–40	40–50
Hydroxyurea	40–50	50–60
IFN-α	50–70	60–80
IFN-α + cytarabine	60–80	NR
Allogeneic transplant		
Matched sibling	60–80	NR
Matched unrelated	50–70	NR
Imatinib	95[a]	NR

[a]Approximate 2-year survival.

IFN-α, interferon alfa; NR, not yet reached.

Adapted from Sawyers,[12] Hill et al,[16] Hehlmann et al,[17] Barrett,[33] and Melo et al.[48]

CONVENTIONAL CHEMOTHERAPY

Busulfan (Myleran) and hydroxyurea (Hydrea) can be used to reduce white cell count shortly after diagnosis. These agents can be taken orally, are inexpensive, have reasonable side-effect profiles, and are able to rapidly normalize elevated WBC counts in chronic-phase CML. Although both agents produce predictable declines in WBC count and hematologic remissions in 70% to 80% of chronic-phase CML patients, busulfan and hydroxyurea have very little effect on Ph-positive cells in bone marrow.[3] Based on results from a randomized study of nearly 500 CML patients by the German CML Study Group, which showed that hydroxyurea treatment provided a significant survival advantage over busulfan, hydroxyurea is the preferred conventional agent in newly diagnosed chronic-phase CML.[17]

Hydroxyurea inhibits the enzyme ribonucleotide reductase, leading to suppression of DNA synthesis, elimination of cells in the S phase of the cell cycle, and synchronization in the G_1 or pre-DNA synthesis phase.[18] The drug is usually administered daily and can be initiated at 40 to 50 mg/kg per day in divided doses until the WBC count falls below 10,000/mm^3. At that point, the dose can be decreased to a maintenance level of 20 mg/kg per day, but increasingly is tapered and stopped once imatinib therapy is started. Imatinib normalizes blood counts based on suppression of the malignant clone in the bone marrow, an effect not seen with hydroxyurea. Suppression of the malignant clone in the bone marrow is the desired therapeutic effect because of its impact on survival.[19]

INTERFERONS

Interferon was the first biologic therapy that showed important activity in cancer and was introduced into the market with a great deal of excitement. The interferons are a family of glycoproteins involved in many of the functional aspects of the hematopoietic system. Interferon alfa (IFN-α) and interferon beta (IFN-β) bind to the same cell-surface receptor on target cells, whereas interferon gamma (IFN-γ) binds to a separate receptor. Although all have been studied in the treatment of chronic-phase CML, IFN-α has been most extensively investigated in the management of CML and is FDA approved for this indication.[3] Two recombinant forms of IFN-α are presently marketed: IFN-α_{2a} (Roferon A) and IFN-α_{2b} (Intron A). In addition, two polyethylene glycol conjugated IFN products (PEG-IFN-α_{2b} and PEG-IFN-α_{2a}) are approved for the treatment of hepatitis C. Surprisingly, PEG-IFN-α_{2a} was found to be superior to conventional IFN-α in the treatment of hepatitis C, which gave hope that improved response might be seen in CML patients.[20] Unfortunately, a recent study reported that PEG-IFN-α_{2b} was not more effective and had a similar toxicity profile to the nonpegylated drug in CML patients.[21]

The exact mechanism of IFN-α activity in CML is unknown, but is complex with multiple effects on cellular function. Some of the proposed alterations include changes in gene transcription, substrate phosphorylation, antigen presentation, and apoptosis.[6,22]

❷ The past enthusiasm for the use of human IFN-α in the treatment of chronic-phase CML was based on the observation that 20% to 50% of patients achieve a cytogenetic response, which led to prolonged survival.[3,23] Because of its unique activity in CML, imatinib has generally replaced IFN-α for initial treatment in patients who are not candidates for alloHSCT. However, there are patients who have already achieved cytogenetic response on IFN-α and continue to receive the drug as maintenance therapy, and depending on the physician, may not be switched to imatinib. In addition, IFN-α may have a role in those patients who do not tolerate or respond to imatinib. However, if current trends continue, IFN-α usage will continue to decline in CML.[24] The lack of enthusiasm for the use of IFN-α in the treatment of CML is related in part to its significant toxicity profile. IFN-α produces both short-term constitutional toxicities and potentially dose-limiting long-term toxicities. The most predictable early toxicity is a flu-like syndrome characterized by fever, chills, myalgias, headache, and anorexia. These dose-dependent effects may be a result of IFN-α–induced leukocytosis and release of cytokines. This acute flu-like syndrome can be ameliorated by starting IFN-α dosing at 50% of the final dose during the first week, giving the drug at bedtime, and coadministering acetaminophen or indomethacin with each IFN-α dose. Reduction of initial WBC counts to around 10,000/mm^3 with hydroxyurea may also reduce these symptoms.[3] Despite these methods of ameliorating toxicity, the flu-like syndrome is an important source of morbidity, occasionally requiring termination of therapy. Cardiovascular toxicities (tachycardia and hypotension) are seen in about 15% of patients in the first few weeks. Long-term adverse effects include weight loss, alopecia, neurologic effects (paresthesias, cognitive impairment, and depression), and immune-mediated complications (hemolysis, thrombocytopenia, nephrotic syndrome, systemic lupus erythematosus, and hypothyroidism), which can be dose limiting in about 5% to 20% of patients.[3]

IMATINIB

Imatinib (previously referred to as STI571) inhibits the p210 tyrosine kinase, leading to differentiation and apoptosis of the CML clone. Imatinib competitively binds to the ATP-binding site on the tyrosine kinase, which leads to inhibition of the phosphorylation of kinase substrates and inhibition of growth factor signals for the CML clone.

❸ Imatinib demonstrated impressive activity in CML in early clinical trials and has changed the way CML is treated. Table 132–2 summarizes the clinical results of imatinib in CML patients in chronic phase, accelerated phase, and blast crisis. In the initial trials in chronic-phase CML and blast-crisis CML imatinib produced responses which are not usually seen in phase I studies.[10,11] Fifty-four patients with chronic-phase CML who had failed IFN-α were studied. Of those who had received at least 300 mg daily of imatinib, nearly 100% of patients achieved complete hematologic remission and 30% had

TABLE 132–2. Cytogenetic Response Rate Associated with Imatinib in Chronic Myelogenous Leukemia (CML)

Disease Status	Daily Dose (mg)	MCR (%)	CCR (%)	Median Follow-Up
Chronic-phase CML				
Newly diagnosed				
	400	87	79	18 months
	800	96	90	15 months
Prior treatment	400	60	41	18 months
Accelerated-phase CML				
	600	28	19	12 months
	400	16	11	
Blast-crisis CML				
	400–800	16	7.4	

CCR, complete cytogenetic response; MCR, major cytogenetic response.
Adapted from Kantarjian et al,[24] O'Brien et al,[25] Talpaz et al,[28] Sawyers et al,[29] and Kantarjian et al.[30]

a major cytogenetic remission. Hematologic responses were seen within 4 weeks, while major cytogenetic response occurred as early as 2 months and as late as 10 months after the start of treatment. A complete cytogenetic remission was obtained in seven patients (13%), and two of the seven patients had a molecular remission. The lack of a clear dose-limiting toxicity and the high response rates in these high-risk chronic-phase CML patients made imatinib unique among the various therapies for CML.[10] Imatinib has also been studied in patients with myeloid blast-crisis CML, and about 55% of patients have a response to imatinib, including 10% of patients who achieve a complete hematologic response.[11] Imatinib was well tolerated in patients with blast-crisis CML, although a higher rate of grade 3 and 4 neutropenia was reported in patients with advanced disease.

A phase II study of imatinib in chronic-phase CML patients who had failed IFN-α confirmed the initial results reported in phase I studies. Patients were dosed at 400 mg/day because the phase I studies suggested a suboptimal response at 300 mg/day or less. Nearly all patients attained a complete hematologic remission and 60% achieved a major cytogenetic response. Perhaps most importantly, a complete cytogenetic remission was obtained in about 40% of patients treated with imatinib.[24]

The most recently published study of imatinib was a phase III trial that compared IFN-α plus cytarabine to 400 mg daily of imatinib. This study, which is referred to as the International Randomized Study of Interferon versus STI571 (IRIS) trial, included over 1000 newly diagnosed CML patients. Patients who received imatinib had a significantly higher rate of complete hematologic remissions (95% vs. 55%), complete (74% vs. 8.5%), and major (85% vs. 22%) cytogenetic remissions, and a significantly lower percentage of patients who progressed to blast crisis in the imatinib group (96.7% vs. 91.5%).[25] The rate of response in the imatinib group was also more rapid, with most patients achieving complete hematologic responses in the first 6 weeks, and most complete cytogenetic responses occurring in the first 3 months of therapy. In a subsequent analysis of the IRIS data, Hughes and associates reported a higher molecular response in the imatinib-treated group (39%) compared to the IFN-α–treated group (2%) after 12 months of treatment.[26] In that study, molecular response was defined as a > 3-log decline in bcr-abl transcript expression. However, many experts believe that cure of CML requires a complete molecular remission, which requires at least an additional 2-log decline and loss of the bcr-abl signal (see Fig. 132–2). Complete molecular remissions occurred in only 3% of patients, which suggests that imatinib alone cannot cure most patients with CML. In addition to

superior activity, imatinib also was better tolerated, with less than 1% of patients intolerant to therapy, compared with about 25% in the IFN-α–treated group.

The role of molecular monitoring as a method to identify early relapse in imatinib-treated patients is unclear. Molecular monitoring would be helpful in patients on imatinib who have an initial molecular response, but who then have a gradual increase in the number of bcr-abl transcripts. If these patients were identified before they experienced a hematologic or cytogenetic relapse, clinicians could increase the imatinib dose or refer the patient for alloHSCT. However, the relationship between molecular and cytogenetic remission and the prognostic importance of molecular relapses are not clear. Therefore it is difficult at this time to integrate molecular relapse into clinical decision making.

In a recently published update of the IRIS trial, the complete cytogenetic remission rate in imatinib-treated patients is 79% at 24 months.[27] Nearly all patients in the IFN-α plus cytarabine group have crossed over to the imatinib arm due to better tolerability and higher activity.[25,27] Because of this high cross-over rate to the imatinib arm, it may not be possible to determine the relative survival benefit of imatinib when compared to IFN-α.

Imatinib was rapidly approved based on phase II studies. Because of its rapid approval and relatively recent entry into the market, the best way to use this drug continues to evolve. Imatinib is often dosed at 600 mg per day in accelerated-phase CML and 800 mg per day in blast-crisis CML. This practice is based in part on data from the phase I study in CML blast-crisis patients in whom the majority of patients who obtained a bone marrow response received doses above 600 mg per day.[11] In subsequent phase II studies that compared 400 mg to 600 mg of imatinib in patients with accelerated-phase CML[28] and blast crisis CML,[29] there was either a trend or a statistically significant improvement in response rate in patients on the 600-mg dose.

CLINICAL CONTROVERSY

Nearly all chronic-phase CML patients receive a course of 400 mg per day of imatinib. Because the phase I trials suggested that response in accelerated-phase and blast-crisis CML was dose related, high-dose regimens of 800 mg per day are being evaluated in chronic-phase CML. Early results suggest a more rapid and extensive response can be achieved, but at the cost of more toxicity and financial burden. If there are high rates of complete molecular remission and these remissions are durable with 800 mg per day of imatinib, initial dosing regimens may be changed.

An area of controversy in patients in chronic-phase CML involves the optimal dosing regimen for imatinib. While 400 mg per day of imatinib is the recommended dose in chronic-phase CML, results of some studies suggest that the use of doses higher than 400 mg per day can produce more rapid and more extensive responses. About a third of patients who had not achieved a cytogenetic response after 1 year on 400 mg per day of imatinib achieved a major cytogenetic response when the imatinib dose was increased to 800 mg per day.[19] In another study, Kantarjian and colleagues demonstrated in newly diagnosed patients the superior efficacy of 800 mg compared to 400 mg per day. Complete molecular responses after 18 months of therapy were uncommon at the 400-mg dose (7%), but occurred more commonly at 800 mg per day (28%).[30] However, higher imatinib doses are associated with greater toxicity, particularly grade 3 and 4 myelosuppression, and the cost of high-dose regimens may be prohibitive in some patients. Larger randomized studies that measure molecular responses and evaluate durability of response are required to determine if the higher activity of high-dose regimens is worth the increased toxicity and cost.

While the phase I studies of imatinib in CML were unable to determine a maximum tolerated dose, most serious toxicities occur in patients receiving 750 mg or more per day. While grade 3 or 4 myelosuppression only occurs in 5% to 10% of patients with chronic-phase CML, it occurs in 50% to 60% of patients in accelerated phase or blast crisis.[28,29] The myelosuppression often occurs during the first 2 to 4 weeks of starting the drug and is more common in patients with high blastic involvement of the bone marrow and in those with low hemoglobin counts.[31] The neutropenia associated with imatinib seems to be associated with fewer infectious complications compared to neutropenia from cytotoxic chemotherapy, which may be related to the absence of the mucositis usually associated with cancer chemotherapy. The myelosuppression associated with imatinib is believed to be related to its therapeutic effect against the CML clone since similar rates of bone marrow suppression are not seen in patients receiving imatinib for gastrointestinal stromal tumors.[32] Hematopoiesis in CML, particularly in accelerated phase and blast crisis, is so dependent on the CML clone that suppression of that clone can lead to myelosuppression.

Imatinib is also associated with some nonhematologic toxicities. Dose-related nausea and vomiting is the most common side effect and can be reduced by taking the drug with a meal. Edema and fluid retention are also dose related and most often manifests as periorbital edema. Rarely fluid retention can be severe, leading to pulmonary and cerebral edema. Risk factors for edema include female gender, age over 65, and a history of heart and kidney disease. About 20% to 40% of patients complain of musculoskeletal symptoms, which tend to occur during the first month of therapy and decline in severity over time. Drug rash can frequently occur but is usually mild. Severe rash, while uncommon, has been reported as an important cause for discontinuing therapy. Hepatotoxicity can occur, and the drug is usually stopped if liver function tests exceed five times normal. After the tests normalize, imatinib can be cautiously restarted at a reduced dose. The drug is then escalated upward to the prior dose if the liver function tests do not rise during 6 to 12 weeks of treatment at the reduced dose.[19]

Imatinib has several potentially clinically important drug interactions. Imatinib is metabolized by cytochrome P450 isoenzyme 3A4 (CYP3A4) and inducers of CYP3A4 metabolism may increase imatinib clearance. For example, a patient who was being treated with both imatinib and phenytoin had a suboptimal response and was found to have a 75% reduction in plasma imatinib concentrations as compared to patients not on phenytoin. The clinical significance of this interaction was confirmed by rapid disease response when phenytoin therapy was withdrawn.[10] Imatinib may increase levels of other drugs metabolized by CYP3A4. For example, there have been reports of increased blood levels of cyclosporine and simvastatin in the presence of imatinib.[19]

▨ HEMATOPOIETIC STEM CELL TRANSPLANTATION

◀4 Allogeneic hematopoietic stem cell transplantation (alloHSCT) is the only therapy proven to cure patients with CML, with many patients alive and disease-free more than 10 years after transplant.[3] A recent study from the International Bone Marrow Transplant Registry (IBMTR) reported a 5-year survival rate of 69% in patients undergoing matched sibling alloHSCT within the first year of diagnosis.[33] As stated previously, patients who undergo matched-sibling alloHSCT

within the first year of diagnosis have a better 5-year survival rate than those who undergo alloHSCT beyond 1 year of their diagnosis (70% to 80% vs. 50% to 60%).[33,34] The use of a targeted busulfan and cyclophosphamide preparative regimen may further improve survival following alloHSCT.[34] By adjusting busulfan doses based on plasma levels and eliminating total body irradiation, these investigators reported that the risk of leukemic relapse and transplant-related morbidity and mortality was reduced.

Unfortunately, fewer than 30% of patients eligible for alloHSCT will have a human leukocyte antigen (HLA)-matched sibling donor, and alternative donors must be considered. The most common alternative donor is an unrelated individual who is HLA matched. Results from several studies show that 50% to 70% of patients undergoing matched unrelated donor alloHSCT are alive at 3 to 5 years posttransplant.[33] The same predictors for good outcome in matched related alloHSCT, including undergoing transplantation within the first year after diagnosis and at a younger age at transplant, also apply to matched unrelated donor alloHSCT.[35–37] AlloHSCT from matched unrelated donors may be more sensitive to delay than matched sibling transplants.[37] Results from these studies and a decision analysis suggest that patients who are candidates for a matched unrelated donor alloHSCT should be transplanted within the first year of diagnosis to optimize outcomes.[38]

Because of the activity of imatinib, fewer transplants are being performed for CML. Data from the IBMTR showed that in 1998, over 600 transplants were performed for CML in 222 bone marrow transplant centers in North America. Transplants for CML accounted for 23% of the centers' total alloHSCT volume. In 2002, the same centers reported the number of transplants had declined to 268, accounting for only 9% of their alloHSCT volume.[39] As stated in the prior section, imatinib is likely to improve 5-year survival rates as compared to treatment with IFN-α.[25] However, neither IFN-α nor imatinib treatment is likely to cure patients, and no survival data exist comparing imatinib to alloHSCT.

CLINICAL CONTROVERSY

While the controversy of whether to use imatinib or alloHSCT as initial therapy is relevant to fewer than 30% of newly diagnosed CML patients, it is one of the major controversies in management of this disease. Current National Comprehensive Cancer Network (NCCN) guidelines demonstrate the imprecision of the decision-making process, suggesting that it is governed by the patient's preference. One reasonable approach is to evaluate hematologic remission at 3 months, and patients who have not had a complete remission and are eligible for transplant should have it offered. In patients receiving imatinib, cytogenetic responses should be evaluated every 3 months thereafter, and those who obtain a cytogenetic complete remission can be continued on imatinib, while those with incomplete cytogenetic responses at 9 to 12 months may consider transplantation. More sensitive measures of minimal residual disease (e.g., polymerase chain reaction) may allow further refinement of the decision making.

The controversy as to whether to use imatinib or alloHSCT is relevant only for those CML patients who are young enough to tolerate alloHSCT and who have a matched related or unrelated donor. With the median age of onset for CML being in the fifth or sixth decade of life and the high risk of mortality in patients over 50 years of age, at least half of CML patients will be excluded from alloHSCT based on age alone. Even when all the criteria are met (matched donor and younger age), 100-day mortality after alloHSCT exceeds 10%. This risk of early mortality associated with alloHSCT may be too high in the imatinib era, when most patients have elimination of the Ph without significant toxicity. The NCCN CML guidelines recommend that the use of transplantation or imatinib therapy should be a patient's decision, made after careful discussion of the benefits and risks of each therapy.[40] The clinical decision is further complicated by the observation that there is a well recognized window when transplant is optimally performed. Patients who are transplanted beyond the first year after diagnosis because they were initially started on imatinib and later had an inadequate response, are less likely to be cured of their disease.

Some studies suggest that the use of certain drugs in the initial management of CML may also affect the outcome of alloHSCT. For example, busulfan and IFN-α may have negative effects on alloHSCT.[3] Busulfan increases the risk of posttransplant complications and has been reported to reduce survival.[3] The effect of previous IFN-α use is more controversial. The most recent study reported that if IFN-α was discontinued at least 90 days before transplantation, no effect on survival posttransplant was observed.[41] The poorer outcomes in patients transplanted after busulfan therapy, and perhaps IFN-α therapy, is a cautionary experience that may have lessons for the use of imatinib in patients who are candidates for alloHSCT. Preliminary data suggest that patients previously treated with imatinib had significantly higher transplant-related mortality.[42] The results of this study, while provocative, must be confirmed in studies with larger numbers of patients. The effect of imatinib on transplant outcome remains an important unanswered question and is part of the clinical uncertainty associated with initial therapy in CML.

Given that most patients treated with imatinib achieve cytogenetic complete remission and are likely to be alive at 5 years, strategies to improve transplant outcomes are critical if its role is to be other than a salvage therapy. One method is the infusion of donor lymphocytes as a form of adoptive immunotherapy to induce a graft-versus-leukemia (GVL) effect. In relapsed CML, donor lymphocytes have been shown to induce durable responses, and these responses strongly correlate with the development of graft-versus-host disease (GVHD).[43] In addition to development of acute GVHD, tumor burden also predicts likelihood of response to donor lymphocyte infusion in relapsed CML. There was a 100% response to donor lymphocytes

when treating molecular relapse, 75% response in cytogenetic relapse, and 35% if patients relapsed in accelerated phase or blast crisis. The dose, timing, and method of administration of donor lymphocytes may also impact effectiveness. In one study, there was a significantly lower incidence of GVHD with escalating doses of donor lymphocyte infusion rather than single-dose donor lymphocytes, while maintaining a similar 70% to 90% complete cytogenetic remission rate.[44] This study suggests that the administration of donor lymphocytes in fractionated doses rather than a single large dose after recovery from tissue damage caused by the preparative regimen may induce a GVL effect while minimizing GVHD. In another study, Guglielmi and associates reported that the administration of lower cell doses decreased the risk of acute GVHD without compromising antitumor responses.[45] The optimal method of administering donor lymphocytes remains unclear, but these data suggest it may be possible to partially separate the GVL effect from GVHD.

Imatinib has been used in patients who relapsed after alloHSCT. Cytogenetic response rates exceeded 50%, but at the expense of acute GVHD and myelosuppression.[46] While more work needs to be done on imatinib salvage therapy after alloHSCT, this high response rate is promising.

The importance of detecting the *bcr-abl* fusion gene product in CML patients after alloHSCT was studied in 346 patients and 634 collected blood samples. A positive polymerase chain reaction (PCR) 3 months or 36 months after transplant did not predict for relapse, but a positive PCR at 6 or 12 months after transplant was highly predictive.[47] With this tool, it may be possible to identify patients who are at high risk for clinical relapse and to treat them with donor lymphocyte infusion or imatinib in an attempt to suppress or eradicate residual disease.

It is too early to define the role of nonmyeloablative transplants in CML, but early results suggest equivalent efficacy to myeloablative transplants. While early transplant-related mortality is low following nonmyeloablative transplantation, transplant-related mortality is nearly 20% at 1 year.[48] However, in a recently published study of 24 CML patients receiving nonmyeloablative transplants, the estimated 5-year disease-free survival was 85% with low transplant-related mortality.[49] The excellent results reported in this study will need to be confirmed by larger studies from experienced centers.

CHRONIC LYMPHOCYTIC LEUKEMIA

CLL is a lymphoproliferative disorder characterized by progressive accumulation of functionally incompetent clonal B lymphocytes. CLL is a common form of leukemia in the United States, but is rare in Japan and China. It is estimated that about 9730 new cases of CLL will be diagnosed in the United States in 2005.[1] Occasional family clusters have been recognized, and first-degree relatives of patients with CLL are at three times the risk of developing a lymphoid malignancy as compared to the general population. CLL is a disease of the elderly, with a median age of onset in the sixth decade of life, although about 10% of CLL occurs in patients who are younger than 50 years of age. Etiologic factors have not been identified in CLL, and there are no data supporting either radiation or viral oncogenesis.[3]

CLINICAL PRESENTATION

The diagnosis of CLL is often made incidentally during a routine blood draw or after the patient complains of various constitutional

symptoms such as fever or fatigue. These symptoms result from reduction in normal hematopoiesis and the production of dysfunctional lymphocytes.[3] Often an abnormal CBC is characterized by high numbers of mature-looking small lymphocytes. Lymphocytosis is nearly always present, and a bone marrow aspirate usually shows an infiltration of mature-appearing lymphocytes. The diagnosis is confirmed by analysis of the phenotypic characteristics of the peripheral blood lymphocytes. If there is a monoclonal B lymphocytosis, this is often sufficient to confirm the diagnosis. In about 60% of patients, there is lymphadenopathy, usually in the cervical, axillary, or inguinal areas. Intra-abdominal nodes may also be palpable, and about 50% of patients have spleen and liver enlargement. In addition to these relatively common presentations, lymphoid infiltrates can sometimes be detected at other anatomic sites, including skin, lung, gastrointestinal tract, and central nervous system.[3]

A number of laboratory abnormalities can be identified at the time of diagnosis. As stated above, lymphocytosis in the peripheral blood and lymphocytic infiltration of the bone marrow are usually seen at diagnosis. Anemia, thrombocytopenia, and neutropenia are frequently evident, either at the time of diagnosis or some time during the course of the disease. The underlying reason for these cytopenias is not clear, but they most likely result from infiltration of the bone marrow by malignant lymphocytes. Other potential causes of cytopenias include autoimmune consumption of red blood cells and platelets and excessive T-suppressor cell or diminished T-helper cell function.[3] Hypogammaglobulinemia is often present at diagnosis and develops in nearly all patients as the disease progresses. Unlike the Ph in CML, there is no single cytogenetic marker for CLL.

Although no single chromosomal rearrangement identifies CLL, more than 80% of patients with CLL have cytogenetic abnormalities. A number of the chromosomal rearrangements have been shown to correlate with prognosis.[3]

STAGING AND PROGNOSIS

There is a wide variability in survival times, with some patients dying within 3 years of diagnosis and others living two decades with CLL. The Rai staging system has helped to design appropriate management strategies for CLL. Prognosis depends on stage and tumor burden at diagnosis. The Rai staging system has been combined into a risk classification scheme: low-risk (stage 0), intermediate-risk (stages I and II), and high-risk (stages III and IV), with median survivals of greater than 10 years, 7 years, and 2 to 4 years, respectively.[3] The other common staging system is the Binet System, which is more commonly used in Europe. Table 132–3 summarizes the Rai staging system.

Despite the prognostic importance of staging, the disease course varies within each stage so that one patient may have an indolent course with long survival time, whereas another patient may have

TABLE 132–3. Rai Staging System for Chronic Lymphocytic Leukemia

Risk Class	Stage	Clinical Characteristics	% At Diagnosis	Median Survival (y)
Low	0	Lymphocytosis alone	60	>10
Intermediate	I–II	Lymphocytosis and lymphadenopathy or spleen or liver enlargement	20	6–8
High	III–IV	Lymphocytosis and anemia or thrombocytopenia	20	2–4

Adapted from Kantarjian et al.[3]

more aggressive disease and a relatively short survival time. Because staging systems, such as the Rai system, incompletely predict for subsets of patients who progress rapidly within each stage, numerous molecular markers are being investigated to identify patients who have poorer prognosis. One of the more promising markers is ZAP-70, an intracellular protein with tyrosine kinase activity. It is a surrogate measure for the unmutated variable region of the immunoglobulin heavy chain gene that is a strong predictor for rapid disease progression. Patients who have elevated ZAP-70 expression by flow cytometry have a poorer prognosis. The hope is that relatively easily measured molecular markers like ZAP-70 will allow the identification of patients who have poorer prognosis and may benefit from more aggressive treatment.[50]

▶ TREATMENT: Chronic Lymphocytic Leukemia

⑤ Since currently available treatments have not been shown to cure CLL, the primary goal of therapy is to improve quality of life.[3] Because molecular responses have been seen with newer therapies, it may be possible to cure CLL in a small subgroup of patients.[51] Since few if any patients are cured, it is not surprising that management of CLL patients is highly variable. Some clinicians delay drug therapy after diagnosis to obtain several weeks of baseline information on signs and symptoms of the disease.[3] The decision about whether drug therapy should be initiated after this baseline period is based on several parameters, including age of the patient, aggressiveness of the tumor, and symptoms. Treatment is often instituted for the following indications: signs and symptoms of progressive disease, worsening of blood dyscrasias, autoimmune complications, symptomatic splenomegaly, bulky lymph nodes, severe lymphocytosis ($>100,000$ to $200,000/mm^3$), and increased infectious complications.

Most stage 0 patients do not require treatment and are usually managed with close observation. In patients with stage I or II disease, management is controversial because the results of studies in this group of patients have not found a consistent survival benefit from drug therapy.[3] The use of cytotoxic chemotherapy in early-stage CLL is usually reserved for patients who have disease characteristics consistent with a more aggressive course, such as short lymphocyte doubling times and diffuse lymphocytic infiltrates in the bone marrow biopsy. In stage III and IV disease, treatment is required, with the goal of achieving a partial or complete remission. Median survival times for patients who achieve some form of remission exceed 4 years, whereas those who do not achieve remission have a median survival of less than 2 years.[3] Historically, drug therapy begins with

low-dose alkylating agents. Splenic radiation or splenectomy is often recommended in patients with stage III and IV disease to reduce symptoms and to improve autoimmune blood dyscrasias. The current treatment for patients requiring systemic therapy has shifted to fludarabine, unless the patient is elderly or has poor renal function.[51]

CYTOTOXIC CHEMOTHERAPY

The controversy surrounding CLL management with low-dose alkylating agents was evaluated in a meta-analysis.[52] The results of that analysis showed that delayed treatment did not have an adverse effect on 10-year survival. If only deaths caused by CLL were considered, there was a statistically significant improvement in survival when treatment was deferred. Chlorambucil continues to be widely used in elderly patients as initial treatment for CLL, but its use is based on a small number of studies.[3,53] The addition of prednisone to chlorambucil is likely to increase infectious risk with no advantage in the treatment of CLL. However, prednisone may have value in CLL-associated autoimmune blood dyscrasias.[54,55]

Cyclophosphamide produces a similar response rate as chlorambucil (30% to 40%) and can be used in patients who have difficulty tolerating chlorambucil or in whom response is not optimal. Some patients refractory to chlorambucil will respond to cyclophosphamide. Cyclophosphamide is less commonly used because of its risk of hemorrhagic cystitis and bladder cancer with prolonged treatment.[3]

The purine nucleoside analogs fludarabine, 2-chlorodeoxyadenosine (cladribine), and 2-deoxycoformycin (pentostatin), have an important role in the management of patients who have become resistant to chlorambucil, and as initial therapy for younger patients who can tolerate their immunosuppressive activity. Less data exist on the activity of pentostatin and cladribine in CLL than with fludarabine. There have been no randomized comparisons of the various purine nucleoside analogs, but the available data suggest that single-agent fludarabine and cladribine have similarly high activity in CLL.[56]

Fludarabine was initially studied in 369 CLL patients who were refractory to chlorambucil. In that study, fludarabine produced an overall response rate of 47% and a complete response rate of 32%.[57] Sorensen and associates reported a similar overall response rate of 32% in patients with refractory CLL who were treated with fludarabine.[58] The most durable responses occurred in patients with lower-stage disease. Patients who received prior alkylating therapy and did not respond to the purine nucleosides had a poor survival. Based on these encouraging response rates in patients with refractory disease, fludarabine is now being used in chemotherapy-naïve patients, resulting in overall response rates of about 60% to 80%.[59] One randomized study has compared fludarabine to chlorambucil in chemotherapy-naïve patients, and the results of that study showed a higher complete remission rate with fludarabine (20% vs. 5%) as compared with chlorambucil.[60] However, the higher complete remission rate did not translate into a significant difference in overall survival, and patients treated with fludarabine had a higher rate of severe neutropenia and infection. The study allowed chlorambucil failures to cross-over to the fludarabine arm, which may have reduced the ability to show a survival advantage in patients treated with fludarabine. Based on the higher complete remission rate and improved time to disease progression, this study helped to establish fludarabine as a front-line therapy for CLL.

Based on the single-agent activity of fludarabine, many fludarabine-based combination regimens have been evaluated in patients with CLL. The activity of fludarabine is potentiated by alkylating agents and monoclonal antibodies. These combinations have recently been shown to have superior activity to single-agent therapy. Table 132–4 gives the response rates reported with purine nucleosides alone and in combination with other therapies. Fludarabine combined with alkylating agents have produced complete response rates higher than those achieved with fludarabine alone. The combination produced complete response rates between 30% and 50%, as compared to 10% to 20% for single-agent fludarabine.[61–64] Complete remission rates are higher in previously untreated patients. As indicated by the study comparing chlorambucil to fludarabine, high complete remission rates do not necessarily lead to improved survival. However, an exciting finding from one of these studies was that 17% of patients achieved a molecular remission.[63] While pentostatin as a single agent has not been as active as fludarabine, it has promising activity when combined with alkylating agents. A trial studying pentostatin and cyclophosphamide combinations in previously treated patients reported a 17% complete remission rate.[65]

BIOLOGIC THERAPY

The most recent additions to therapy in CLL are the monoclonal antibodies directed against targets on lymphocytes.[66,67] Rituximab targets the CD20 molecule which is expressed on B lymphocytes. Alemtuzumab was approved in May 2001 for the treatment of patients with CLL who had failed fludarabine therapy. Alemtuzumab targets

TABLE 132–4. Treatment for Newly Diagnosed (i.e., Untreated) and Previously Treated Chronic Lymphocytic Leukemia

Treatment	Overall Response Rate	Complete Response Rate
Chlorambucil		
Untreated	37%	4%
Fludarabine alone		
Untreated	60–80%	20–30%
Previously treated	67%	13%
Fludarabine + cyclophosphamide		
Untreated	80–90%	30–50%
Previously treated	80%	15%
Rituximab alone		
Untreated	50–60%	10%
Previously treated	30–40%	0–3%
Fludarabine + rituximab		
Untreated	80–100%	30–50%
Previously treated	70–80%	20–30%
Alemtuzumab alone		
Untreated	80–90%	20–30%
Previously treated	30–50%	5–20%
Alemtuzumab + fludarabine[a]		
Previously treated (n = 6)	5 of 6	1 of 6

[a]Raw numbers, not percentages.
Adapted from Keating et al.[51]

the CD52 molecule, which is expressed on nearly all lymphocytes. The CD20 molecule is less densely expressed in CLL cells compared to the B lymphocytes in indolent non-Hodgkin's lymphoma, the approved indication for rituximab. Concentrations of soluble CD20 are also higher in the plasma of CLL patients, which may neutralize the antibody's activity. When rituximab was used as the sole therapy in CLL, higher doses than those used in indolent non-Hodgkin's lymphoma had to be given to overcome these biologic features of CLL. Three recent studies of standard doses of rituximab demonstrated high complete response rates when combined with fludarabine-containing chemotherapy (30% to 70%).[51,68,69]

Alemtuzumab has generally been used in CLL patients who are refractory to other available therapies. In this group of patients with refractory disease, the antibody produced an overall response rate of 30% to 40%, with a complete response rate of less than 10%. This level of response in refractory CLL is important, but is accompanied by a significant toxicity profile, including pancytopenia, infusion reactions, and opportunistic infections. An interesting finding with the combination of alemtuzumab and fludarabine is that patients resistant to each alone were sensitive to the combination.[70] This level of activity in refractory patients led to the evaluation of alemtuzumab earlier in therapy, alone or combined with purine nucleosides.[51,56] Results with the antibody alone in newly diagnosed patients were similar to those with fludarabine alone. The combination of fludarabine and alemtuzumab may be too toxic, with high rates of cytomegalovirus (CMV) infection from the resultant severe immunosuppression.

While alemtuzumab alone may not improve results in newly diagnosed patients, it may be an important therapy for refractory patients. There are also interesting data that suggest that alemtuzumab can clear minimal residual disease after patients have been treated with chemotherapy. O'Brien and colleagues demonstrated that 38% of patients with residual disease after chemotherapy could achieve a molecular remission with alemtuzumab, and some of these remissions appeared to be durable.[71] The major complication in this study was infectious, with relatively high rates of CMV and Epstein-Barr virus infections. Because of the risk of CMV reactivation and *Pneumocystis* infections, prophylaxis with trimethoprim-sulfamethoxazole and famciclovir or valaciclovir is recommended with the use of alemtuzumab.

HEMATOPOIETIC STEM CELL TRANSPLANTATION

There is a limited experience with the use of HSCT in CLL. Early mortality with autologous and allogeneic HSCT is approximately 10% and 40%, respectively. Those patients who achieve molecular remission as determined by PCR seem to have longer disease-free survival.[72] While autologous transplantation has lower transplant-related mortality than allogeneic transplantation, relapse rates are high and it is generally not a preferred therapy in CLL. While cure is currently not considered achievable in CLL, alloHSCT is the most likely method of producing molecular complete remissions by initiating a GVL effect.[73,74]

CLINICAL CONTROVERSY

CLL is currently not considered a curable disease. However, a GVL effect has been demonstrated for CLL which may produce a long-term complete remission and perhaps cure. Because most CLL patients are elderly, full-intensity alloHSCT causes high transplant-related mortality and is generally not used in CLL. Nonmyeloablative HSCT may be an important treatment in CLL if it is not too toxic and if the GVL effect is sufficiently potent to destroy often bulky tumor as well as minimal residual disease.

AlloHSCT for CLL is an area of growing interest. Although this modality of treatment may hold promise of cure, the advanced age of most CLL patients and high treatment-related mortality limit the applicability of alloHSCT. Older patients who are not candidates for alloHSCT may be candidates for nonmyeloablative alloHSCT.[3] A recent study reported a GVL effect in CLL patients treated with nonmyeloablative transplantation. This GVL effect may be potentiated by the treatment of patients with rituximab during the posttransplant course.[75]

EVALUATION OF THERAPEUTIC OUTCOMES

The goal of disease monitoring in CML, which measures hematologic, cytogenetic, and molecular response, is to identify patients who have optimally responded to an initial course of imatinib. A suboptimal response to imatinib—defined by no hematologic response at 3 months or no complete cytogenetic response at 12 months—can be helpful in patients who are eligible for alloHSCT. In patients who obtain a hematologic or cytogenetic response to imatinib, but who later relapse during imatinib treatment should also be considered for transplantation. Alternatively, the dose of imatinib may be increased in an attempt to induce response. The role of molecular responses in making therapeutic decisions is not clear, but increased levels of *bcr-abl* transcripts in patients who have had a molecular response should be considered in the decision to increase imatinib dose, or in eligible patients, perform alloHSCT.

CLL is considered an indolent disease that is incurable and the goal of therapy should be to increase the duration and quality of life. Except in those patients who are younger and have aggressive disease, aggressive therapy should be avoided. The benefits of aggressive therapy should be carefully weighed against the risks and costs in older patients with indolent disease. A reasonable strategy for these patients is to administer single-agent well-tolerated chemotherapy or no therapy at all in patients without symptoms. Younger patients with aggressive disease should receive more active therapies, such as combinations of fludarabine plus chemotherapy, fludarabine plus monoclonal antibodies, or nonmyeloablative transplantation. If the decision is made to use these aggressive therapies and to accept the risk of potentially life-threatening toxicities, the goal of therapy should be to achieve a durable complete remission.

TREATMENT SUMMARY

Several experts and groups, such as the NCCN, have published guidelines for the treatment of patients with chronic leukemia. For the past several decades, alloHSCT has been the only curative therapy for CML. Cytogenetic responses have been obtained with IFN-α, leading to an improved duration of survival. However, there are no convincing data to show that IFN-α can permanently eliminate the malignant CML clone, and its use is associated with many adverse effects. Imatinib has changed the management of CML. Most patients with chronic-phase CML receive imatinib as initial therapy at a dose of 400 mg per day, and attain a complete cytogenetic remission within the first year of therapy. It may be that imatinib can eliminate the malignant clone in a small subgroup of patients, particularly at higher doses, but longer follow-up will be required to determine the durability of these responses. NCCN guidelines indicate that patients who are candidates for alloHSCT and have a matched donor should receive alloHSCT if it is their preference. Based on recent trends in the number of transplants for CML, most clinicians and their patients prefer imatinib over alloHSCT. Patients who relapse after alloHSCT despite the development of acute GVHD should be placed on imatinib or possibly IFN-α. Patients undergoing alloHSCT who relapse or do not achieve remission and have not developed acute GVHD should be withdrawn from posttransplant immunosuppression to induce GVHD and GVL. If this is not successful, patients should receive donor lymphocyte infusion. Imatinib or IFN-α can be tried if donor lymphocyte infusion fails to produce a response.

Patients who are placed on imatinib at a dose of 400 mg per day as primary therapy and who do not achieve a hematologic remission 3 months after starting therapy may respond to an higher imatinib dose. Alternatively the patient should be evaluated for alloHSCT. Those patients on imatinib who achieve hematologic remission at 3 months should continue on imatinib, and cytogenetics should be evaluated every 3 to 6 months. Patients who have not achieved a complete cytogenetic remission at 1 year may respond to increased doses of imatinib or should be treated with alloHSCT if eligible. Patients in accelerated phase or blast crisis may respond to high doses of imatinib (600 to 800 mg/day), or in those with a matched related donor, alloHSCT can be offered. Unfortunately, responses in accelerated phase or blast crisis are usually not durable and patients usually die of their disease.

Because CLL is often an indolent disease that develops in older patients, an important goal is to optimize quality of life rather than to use aggressive, relatively toxic therapy. In younger patients, fludarabine with or without an alkylating agent is often given with the goal of obtaining complete remissions. However, in the older patient the use of chlorambucil may still be preferred to decrease the infectious risk associated with fludarabine. In younger patients or patients with more aggressive CLL, a combination of fludarabine and an alkylating agent or monoclonal antibody or alloHSCT may offer long-term disease-free survival.

ABBREVIATIONS

alloHSCT: allogeneic hematopoietic stem cell transplantation
ATP: adenosine triphosphate
CLL: chronic lymphocytic leukemia
CML: chronic myelogenous leukemia
CMV: cytomegalovirus
CYP 450: cytochrome P450 isoenzyme
GVHD: graft-versus-host disease
GVL: graft-versus-leukemia (effect)
HLA: human leukocyte antigen
HSCT: hematopoietic stem cell transplantation
IBMTR: International Bone Marrow Transplant Registry
IFN-α: interferon alfa
IFN-α_{2a}: interferon alfa$_{2a}$
IFN-α_{2b}: interferon alfa$_{2b}$
IFN-β: interferon beta
IFN-γ: interferon gamma
IRIS: International Randomized Study of Interferon (versus STI571 trial)
NCCN: National Comprehensive Cancer Network
PCR: polymerase chain reaction
PEG-IFN-α_{2a}: polyethylene glycol conjugated interferon alfa$_{2a}$
PEG-IFN-α_{2b}: polyethylene glycol conjugated interferon alfa$_{2b}$
Ph: Philadelphia chromosome
WBC: white blood cell

Review Questions and other resources can be found at *www.pharmacotherapyonline.com.*

REFERENCES

1. Jemal A, Murray T, Ward E, et al. Cancer statistics, 2004. CA Cancer J Clin 2005;55:10–30.
2. Goldman JM, Melo JV. Chronic myeloid leukemia—Advances in biology and new approaches to treatment. N Engl J Med 2003;349:1451–1464.
3. Kantarjian H, Faderl S, Talpaz M. Chronic leukemias. In: Devita VT, Hellman S, Rosenberg SA, eds. Cancer: Principles and Practice of Oncology, 6th ed. Philadelphia, Lippincott, 2001:2433–2447.
4. Butturini A, Gale RP. Age of onset and type of leukemia. Lancet 1989;2:789–791.
5. Waller CF, Fetscher S, Lange W. Treatment-related CML. Ann Hematol 1999;78:341–344.
6. Clarkson B, Strife A, Wisniewski D, et al. Chronic myelogenous leukemia as a paradigm of early cancer and possible curative strategies. Leukemia 2003;17:1211–1262.
7. Daley GQ, Van Etten RA, Baltimore D. Induction of chronic myelogenous leukemia in mice by the p210 bcr-abl gene of the Philadelphia chromosome. Science 1990;247:824–830.
8. Preisler H, Raza A. An overview of some studies of chronic myelogenous leukemia: Biological-clinical observations and viewing the disease as a chaotic system. Leuk Lymphoma 1993;11:145–150.
9. Srdan V, Kantarjian H, Manshouri T, et al. Prognostic significance of cellular vascular endothelial cell growth factor expression in chronic phase chronic myelogenous leukemia. Blood 2002;99:2265–2267.
10. Druker BJ, Talpaz M, Resta DJ, et al. Efficacy and safety of a specific inhibitor of the bcr-abl tyrosine kinase in chronic myelogenous leukemia. N Engl J Med 2001;344:1031–1037.
11. Druker BJ, Sawyers CL, Kantarjian H, et al. Activity of a specific inhibitor of the bcr-abl tyrosine kinase in the blast crisis of chronic myelogenous leukemia and acute lymphocytic leukemia with the Philadelphia chromosome. N Engl J Med 2001;344:1038–1042.
12. Sawyers CL. Chronic myelogenous leukemia. N Engl J Med 1999;340:1330–1340.
13. Asimakopoulos FA, Shteper PJ, Krichevsky S, et al. ABL methylation is a distinct molecular event associated with clonal evolution of chronic myelogenous leukemia. Blood 1999;94:2452–2460.
14. Boultwood J, Peniket A, Watkins et al. Telomere length shortening in chronic myelogenous leukemia is associated with reduced time to accelerated phase. Blood 2000;96:358–361.
15. Lowenberg B. Minimal residual disease in chronic myeloid leukemia. N Engl J Med 2003;349:1399–1401.
16. Hill JM, Meehan KR. Chronic myelogenous leukemia. Postgrad Med 1999;106:149–159.
17. Hehlmann R, Heimpel H, Hasford J, et al. Randomized comparison of busulfan and hydroxyurea in chronic myelogenous leukemia: Prolongation of survival by hydroxyurea. Blood 1993;82:398–407.
18. Kennedy BJ. The evolution of hydroxyurea therapy in chronic myelogenous leukemia. Semin Oncol 1992;19:21–26.
19. Deininger MW, O'Brien SG, Ford JM, Druker BJ. Practical management of patients with chronic myeloid leukemia receiving imatinib. J Clin Oncol 2003;21:1637–1647.
20. Zeuzem S, Feinman SV, Rasenack J, et al. Peginterferon alfa-2a in patients with chronic hepatitis C. N Engl J Med 2000;343:1666–1672.
21. Michallet M, Maloisel F, Delain M, et al. Pegylated recombinant interferon alpha-2b vs recombinant interferon alpha-2b for the initial treatment of chronic-phase chronic myelogenous leukemia: A phase III study. Leukemia 2004;18:309–315.
22. Guilhot F, Lacotte-Thierry L. Interferon-alpha: Mechanisms of action in chronic myelogenous leukemia in chronic phase. Hematol Cell Ther 1998;40:237–239.
23. Kantarjian HM, Smith TL, O'Brien SG, et al. Prolonged survival in chronic myelogenous leukemia after cytogenetic response to interferon-alpha therapy. Ann Intern Med 1995;122:254–261.
24. Kantarjian H, Sawyers C, Hochhaus A, et al. Hematologic and cytogenetic responses to imatinib mesylate in chronic myelogenous leukemia. N Engl J Med 2002;346:645–652.
25. O'Brien SG, Guilhot F, Larson RA, et al. Imatinib compared with interferon and low-dose cytarabine for newly diagnosed chronic-phase chronic myeloid leukemia. N Engl J Med 2003; 348:994–1004.
26. Hughes TP, Kaeda J, Branford S, et al. Frequency of major molecular responses to imatinib or interferon alfa plus cytarabine in newly diagnosed chronic myeloid leukemia. N Engl J Med 2003;349:1423–1432.
27. Cervantes F. Durability of responses to imatinib in newly diagnosed chronic-phase chronic myeloid leukemia: 24-month update from the IRIS study. Blood 2003;102:181a.
28. Talpaz M, Silver TR, Druker BJ, et al. Imatinib induces durable hematologic and cytogenetic responses in patients with accelerated phase chronic myeloid leukemia: Results of a phase 2 study. Blood 2002;99:1928–1937.
29. Sawyers CL, Hochhaus A, Feldman E, et al. Imatinib induces hematologic and cytogenetic responses in patients with chronic myeloid leukemia in myeloid blast crisis: Results of a phase II study. Blood 2002;99:3530–3539.
30. Kantarjian H, Talpaz M, O'Brien S, et al. High-dose imatinib mesylate therapy in newly diagnosed Philadelphia chromosome-positive chronic phase chronic myelogenous leukemia. Blood 2004;103:2873–2878.
31. Mauro MJ, O'Dwyer ME, Kurilik G, et al. Risk factors for myelosuppression in chronic phase CML patients treated with imatinib mesylate (STI571). Blood 2001;98:139a.

32. Demetri GD, von Mehren M, Blanke CD, et al. Efficacy and safety of imatinib mesylate in advanced gastrointestinal stromal tumors. N Engl J Med 2002;347:472–480.

33. Barrett J. Allogeneic stem cell transplantation for chronic myeloid leukemia. Semin Hematol 2003;40:59–71.

34. Radich JP, Gooley T, Bensinger W, et al. HLA-matched related hematopoietic cell transplantation for chronic-phase CML using a targeted busulfan and cyclophosphamide preparative regimen. Blood 2003;102:31–35.

35. Hansen J, Goolby TA, Martin PJ, et al. Bone marrow transplantation from unrelated donors for patients with chronic myelogenous leukemia. N Engl J Med 1998;338:962–968.

36. McGlave P, Shu XO, Wen W, et al. Unrelated donor marrow transplantation therapy for chronic myelogenous leukemia: 9 years' experience of the National Marrow Donor Program. Blood 2000;95:2219–2225.

37. Weisdorf DJ, Anasetti C, Antin JH, et al. Allogeneic bone marrow transplantation for chronic myelogenous leukemia: comparative analysis of unrelated versus matched sibling donor transplantation. Blood 2002;99:1971–1977.

38. Lee SJ, Kuntz KM, Horowitz MM, et al. Unrelated donor bone marrow transplantation for chronic myelogenous leukemia: A decision analysis. Ann Intern Med 1997;127:1080–1088.

39. Giralt S, Sobocinski K, Horowitz MH. Impact of imatinib therapy on the use of allogeneic hematopoietic stem cell transplantation for treatment of chronic myelogenous leukemia. Blood 2003;102:473a.

40. National Comprehensive Cancer Network Clinical Practice Guidelines in oncology. Chronic myelogenous leukemia. Version 2004. http://www.nccn.org.

41. Hehlmann R, Hochhaus A, Kolb HJ, et al. Interferon-α before allogeneic bone marrow transplantation in chronic myelogenous leukemia does not affect outcome adversely, provided it is discontinued at least 90 days before the procedure. Blood 1999;94:3668–3677.

42. Zander AR, Zabelina T, Renges H, et al. Pretreatment with Gleevec increases transplant-related mortality after allogeneic transplant. Blood 2003;102:468a.

43. Raiola AM, Lint MV, Valbonesi M, et al. Factors predicting response and graft-versus-host disease after donor lymphocyte infusions: A study on 593 infusions. Bone Marrow Transplant 2003;31:687–693.

44. Dazzi F, Szydlo M, Craddock C, et al. Comparison of single dose and escalating dose regimens of donor lymphocyte infusion for relapse after allografting for chronic myelogenous leukemia. Blood 2000;95:67–71.

45. Guglielmi C, Arcese W, Dazzi F, et al. Donor lymphocyte infusion for relapsed chronic myelogenous leukemia: prognostic relevance of the initial cell dose. Blood 2002;100:397–405.

46. Kantarjian HM, O'Brien S, Cortes JE, et al. Imatinib mesylate therapy for relapse after allogeneic stem cell transplantation for chronic myelogenous leukemia. Blood 2002;100:1590–1595.

47. Radich JP, Gehly G, Gooley T, et al. Polymerase chain reaction detection of the BCR-ABL fusion transcript after allogeneic bone marrow transplantation for chronic myelogenous leukemia: Results and implications in 346 patients. Blood 1995;85:2632–2638.

48. Melo JV, Hughes TP, Apperley JF. Chronic myelogenous leukemia. Hematology (Am Soc Hematol Educ Program) 2003:132–152.

49. Or R, Shapira MY, Resnick I, et al. Non-myeloablative stem cell transplantation for treatment of chronic myelogenous leukemia in first chronic phase. Blood 2003;101:441–445.

50. Shanaflet TD, Geyer SM, Kay NE. Prognosis at diagnosis: integrating molecular biologic insights into clinical practice for patients with chronic lymphocytic leukemia. Blood 2004;103:1202–1210.

51. Keating MJ, Chiorazzi N, Messmer B, et al. Biology and treatment of chronic lymphocytic leukemia. Hematology (Am Soc Hematol Educ Program) 2003:153–175.

52. CLL Trialists Collaborative Group. Chemotherapeutic options in chronic lymphocytic leukemia: A meta-analysis of the randomized trials. J Natl Cancer Inst 1999;91:861–868.

53. Manoharan A. Long-term remissions with weekly chlorambucil therapy in patients with intermediate risk chronic lymphocytic leukemia. Br J Hematol 2002;118:1192–1193.

54. Mauro FR, Foa R, Cerretti R, et al. Autoimmune hemolytic anemia in chronic lymphocytic leukemia: Clinical, therapeutic, and prognostic factors. Blood 2000;95:2736–2792.

55. Dighiero G, Binet JL. When and how to treat chronic lymphocytic leukemia. N Engl J Med 2000;343:799–801.

56. Johnson SA, Thomas W. Therapeutic potential of purine analogue combinations in the treatment of lymphoid malignancies. Hematol Oncol 2000;18:141–153.

57. Keating MJ, O'Brien S, Kantarjian H, et al. Nucleoside analogs in treatment of chronic lymphocytic leukemia. Leuk Lymphoma 1993;10:139–145.

58. Sorensen JM, Vena DA, Fallavollita, et al. Treatment of refractory chronic lymphocytic leukemia with fludarabine phosphate via the group C protocol mechanism of the National Cancer Institute: Five-year follow-up report. J Clin Oncol 1997;15:458–465.

59. Keating MJ, O'Brien S, Lerner S, et al. Long-term follow-up of patients with CLL receiving fludarabine regimens as initial therapy. Blood 1998;92:1165–1171.

60. Rai KR, Peterson BL, Appelbaum FR, et al. Fludarabine compared with chlorambucil as primary therapy for chronic lymphocytic leukemia. N Engl J Med 2000;343:1750–1757.

61. O'Brien SM, Kantarjian HM, Cortes J, et al. Results of the fludarabine and cyclophosphamide combination regimen in chronic lymphocytic leukemia. J Clin Oncol 2001;19:1414–1420.

62. Flinn IW, Byrd JC, Morrison C, et al. Fludarabine and cyclophosphamide with filgrastim support in patients with previously untreated indolent lymphoid malignancies. Blood 2000;96:71–75.

63. Bosch F, Ferrer A, Lopez-Guillermo A, et al. Fludarabine, cyclophosphamide, and mitoxantrone in the treatment of resistant or relapsed chronic lymphocytic leukemia. Br J Hematol 2002;119:976–984.

64. Schiavone EM, DeSimone M, Palmieri S, et al. Fludarabine plus cyclophosphamide for the treatment of advanced chronic lymphocytic leukemia. Eur J Hematol 2003;71:23–28.

65. Weiss MA, Maslak PG, Jurcic JG, et al. Pentostatin and cyclophosphamide: An effective new regimen in previously treated patients with chronic lymphocytic leukemia. J Clin Oncol 2003;21:1278–1284.

66. Lin TS, Lucas MS, Byrd JC. Rituximab in B-cell chronic lymphocytic leukemia. Semin Oncol 2003;30:483–492.

67. Moreton P, Hillmen P. Alemtuzumab therapy in B-cell lymphoproliferative disorders. Semin Oncol 2003;30:493–501.

68. Byrd JC, Peterson BL, Morrison VL, et al. Randomized phase 2 study of fludarabine with concurrent versus sequential treatment with rituximab in symptomatic, untreated patients with B-cell chronic lymphocytic leukemia: Results from Cancer and Leukemia Group B 9712. Blood 2003;101:6–14.

69. Schulz H, Klein SK, Rehnald U, et al. Phase 2 study of a combined immunochemotherapy using rituximab and fludarabine in patients with chronic lymphocytic leukemia. Blood 2002;100:3115–3120.

70. Kennedy B, Rawstron A, Carter C, et al. Campath-1H and fludarabine in combination are highly active in refractory chronic lymphocytic leukemia. Blood 2002;99:2245–2247.

71. O'Brien SM, Kantarjian HM, Thomas DA, et al. Alemtuzumab as treatment for residual disease after chemotherapy in patients with chronic lymphocytic leukemia. Cancer 2003;98:2657–2663.

72. Provan D, Bartlett-Pandite L, Zwicky C, et al. Eradication of PCR detectable chronic lymphocytic leukemia cells is associated with improved outcome after bone marrow transplantation. Blood 1996;88:2228–2235.

73. Pavletic ZS, Arrowsmith ER, Bierman PJ, et al. Outcome of allogeneic stem cell transplantation for B-cell CLL. Bone Marrow Transplant 2000;7:717–722.

74. Dreger P, Montserrat E. Autologous and allogeneic stem cell transplantation for chronic lymphocytic leukemia. Leukemia 2002;16:985–992.

75. Khouri IF, Lee MS, Saliba RM, et al. Non-myeloablative allogeneic stem cell transplantation for chronic lymphocytic leukemia: impact of rituximab on immunomodulation and survival. Exp Hematol 2004;32:28–35.

133

MELANOMA

Rowena N. Schwartz

Learning Objectives and other resources can be found at *www.pharmacotherapyonline.com.*

KEY CONCEPTS

❶ Cutaneous melanoma is becoming a common cancer, but it is a cancer that can be prevented and cured if detected early. Public education about screening and early detection is an effective strategy for controlling the increase in the incidence and the mortality associated with cutaneous melanoma.

❷ Surgical resection of early-stage melanoma is associated with complete response and cure.

❸ Patients with locally advanced disease should be evaluated for adjuvant therapy with interferon-α_{2b} or a clinical trial.

❹ The toxicities associated with interferon-α_{2b} therapy are significant and require patient education, close patient monitoring, and appropriate dose delay and/or reduction.

❺ Metastatic melanoma remains a clinical challenge. At this time, there is not a standard treatment approach for patients

with metastatic disease. Dacarbazine is still considered one of the most active agents and can be used as a single agent; the use of combination chemotherapy has not been shown to be superior to single-agent therapy with dacarbazine.

❻ High-dose aldesleukin (interleukin-2) is approved for the treatment of patients with metastatic melanoma. The toxicities with this regimen are high and close patient monitoring by an experienced health care team is essential during treatment. A small percentage of patients will experience a durable response.

❼ A number of melanoma tumor vaccines have been evaluated in clinical trials in metastatic melanoma and in the adjuvant setting. The role of specific melanoma vaccines has not been defined at this time.

The incidence and mortality rate of cutaneous melanoma have increased during the past several decades in the United States and in most Caucasian populations throughout the world. It is estimated that about 59,580 new cases of melanoma will be diagnosed in the United States in 2005, although projections may represent an underestimation, as many superficial and in situ melanomas are still thought to be underreported.[1] The increase in incidence has most affected industrialized countries. In the last decade of the twentieth century, the increase in incidence was still apparent, but there appears to be a decline in the rate of increase in certain subgroups (e.g., women in the United States). Analysts believe the increase in cutaneous melanoma over time is due to a cohort effect; it appears that those individuals born before 1950 show increased risk, whereas those born after 1950 show a stable or declining rate.[2] Worldwide, the incidence of melanoma varies dramatically. The incidence is approximately 0.2 to 35 per 100,000 among females in New Zealand, and as high as 40.5 per 100,000 among males in Australia.

Mortality for melanoma is the highest of all the skin cancers. It is estimated that about 8,000 individuals will die of melanoma in 2005.[1] The mortality rate from melanoma appears to have stabilized and possibly declined in recent years in Australia, the United States, and Europe. The stabilization of mortality rates appears to be in part due to efforts at both primary and secondary prevention of melanoma.

ETIOLOGY AND EPIDEMIOLOGY

The etiology of melanoma, like most other malignancies, is not fully understood. A number of host factors and environmental factors have

been identified, and it is likely that these factors alone or in combination increase the occurrence of cutaneous melanomas. These factors are listed in Table 133–1.

Genetic factors have been strongly linked to the development of melanoma, but appear to account for a small percentage of the overall incidence.[3] Familial atypical multiple mole syndrome (FAMMS) or hereditary dysplastic nevus syndrome (HDNS) is a hereditary disease characterized by a predisposition to develop dysplastic nevi and cutaneous melanoma. Approximately 8% to 10% of cases of melanoma are associated with family history or HDNS. The mode of inheritance is controversial and is believed to be polygenic. The p16^{INK4a} gene localized on the 9p21 locus is affected through germline mutations or deletions in approximately 50% of patients with familial melanoma. In individuals with dysplastic nevi and a family history of cutaneous melanoma, the cumulative lifetime incidence approaches 100%, whereas dysplastic nevi are thought to be precursors of 20% to 40% of sporadic melanoma.

Sunlight is one of the most important environmental factors in the pathogenesis of melanoma. Radiation in the ultraviolet B (UVB) range (280 to 320 nm) is thought to be a critical factor, although there is increasing concern that prolonged exposure to ultraviolet A (UVA) is also a risk factor for the development of melanoma. The use of UVB-blocking sunscreens may allow individuals to sustain more prolonged sun exposure without the ability to perceive erythema or pain, ultimately resulting in intense irradiation of the skin by UVA light.[4]

The incidence of melanoma has been associated with latitude and the intensity of solar exposure among susceptible populations. Skin characteristics are important in determining responses to

TABLE 133–1. Risk Factors for Melanoma

Host risk factors
  Adulthood (>15 years of age)
  History of cutaneous melanoma
  Dysplastic nevi
  Cutaneous melanoma in first-degree relative
  Immunodeficiency/immunosuppression
  High density of nevi
  High degree of freckling
  Sunburn easily/tan rarely
  Blonde or red hair
  Blue, green, or gray eyes
  Socioeconomic status (higher > lower)
  White (versus black) race
External risk factors
  Intense intermittent sun exposures
  History of sunburn
  More than four painful sunburns before the age of 15
  Outdoor leisure

ultraviolet radiation. Whites with fair hair (red and blond), light-colored eyes (blue and green), and high degrees of freckling who have a tendency to burn and rarely tan with exposure to sunlight are especially at risk. Nonmelanoma skin cancers, such as squamous cell and basal cell cancer, have long been shown to be directly related to the total sun exposure, and it was thought that melanoma was similarly related to lifetime exposure to the sun. Epidemiologic research has not been able to demonstrate such a relationship between cumulative exposure to sunlight and the occurrence of cutaneous melanoma. Studies have demonstrated a lower risk for the development of melanoma in outdoor workers when compared to indoor workers.[4] Intermittent overexposure to sunlight, blistering sunburns, and the time of life of exposure to the sun are now believed to be the more critical factors for development of cutaneous melanoma. Individuals who have a history of severe sunburns appear to have a higher risk of the development of melanoma than individuals who have had chronic sun exposure without a history of burning. The risk with sunlight and ultraviolet radiation seems to be greatest during childhood and adolescence. Intensive exposure to sunlight during infancy and early adolescence is more hazardous than exposure during adult life.

Immunocompromised patients are at increased risk for the development of cutaneous melanoma. Immunodeficiency includes those individuals with ataxia telangiectasia, chronic lymphocytic leukemia, Hodgkin's lymphoma, and immunosuppression following organ transplant. Acquired immunodeficiency syndrome also has been shown to increase the risk of developing cutaneous melanoma. Personal history of nonmelanoma or melanoma skin cancers is a risk factor for subsequent melanoma.

PATHOGENESIS

The pathogenesis of melanoma is not fully understood, but advances in the understanding of the immunology and molecular biology of melanoma provides a number of potential new avenues for the development of novel treatment strategies. Human melanocytes are dendritic pigmented cells that arise from the neural crest tissue during early fetal development and migrate by 4 to 6 weeks to a variety of sites within the body, such as the skin, uveal tract, meninges, and ectodermal mucosa. In the adult, most melanocytes are located at the epidermal-dermal junction of the skin and the choroid of the eye, but can be found in a variety of other tissues such as the meninges and the alimentary and respiratory tract. Primary melanoma can therefore arise in any area of the body with melanocytes. The skin is the most frequent site of melanoma; cutaneous melanoma constitutes 90% of all melanoma. Primary melanoma can also arise in the eye (ocular melanoma) and less frequently in the meninges, respiratory tract, and gallbladder.

Normal melanocytes arise from melanoblasts and undergo a series of differentiation events before reaching a final end-cell differentiation state. Normal melanocytes can be arrested in their differentiation process at any given state of maturation without loss of their proliferation capacity. Melanocytes adhere to the basement membrane of the epidermis, and despite a resting state maintain a lifelong proliferation potential. Melanocytes synthesize melanin to protect various tissues such as the skin from ultraviolet radiation (UVR)–induced damage, and reach the keratinocytes in the upper layers of the epidermis via dendrites. Tyrosinase is an essential enzyme used within the melanosomes to synthesize melanin.

There is a malignant transformation of skin melanocytes from preexisting nevocellular nevi in the development of melanoma. A series of distinct steps are involved in the development and progression of melanoma from melanocytes. The pathologic components of the progression in human melanoma appear to involve a series of morphologic stages: (1) an acquired or congenital melanocytic nevus, (2) melanocytic nevus with architectural atypia, (3) histologically dysplastic nevus with cytologic atypia and architectural atypia, (4) primary melanoma in the radial growth phase in which limited growth and radial expansion of the nevi may occur without metastatic competence (nontumorigenic melanoma), (5) primary melanoma in the vertical growth phase with or without in-transit metastases in which there appears to be uncontrolled proliferation and increased angiogenesis, (6) regional lymph node metastatic melanoma (lymphatic), and (7) distant metastatic melanoma (hematogenous).[5] Primary melanoma is characterized by radial growth and limited vertical thickness (less than 0.75 mm). Primary melanoma demonstrates little tendency to metastasize. Melanoma has a potential for metastasis formation with the onset of a vertical growth phase. Metastatic melanoma is seen with an increase in vertical thickness. Therefore the thickness of a primary melanoma is an important prognostic indicator, and is used in the staging classification of cutaneous melanoma. Individual melanomas can skip steps in this development. The progression from the melanocyte to the melanoma likely involves genetic aberrations.

Normal melanocytes require growth factors for proliferation, but melanoma cells are able to proliferate without growth factors.[6] Melanoma cells secrete a variety of growth autocrine and paracrine factors that facilitate proliferation. Additionally, with progression, melanoma cells increase production of certain growth factors and cytokines. Basic fibroblast growth factors (bFGFs) are thought to be an important mediator of growth stimulation and cell survival and act as a motility factor for melanoma cells. Additionally, bFGFs upregulate serine proteinases and metalloproteinases. Melanoma cells are strong producers of chemoattractive proteins such as interleukin-8. Vascular endothelial growth factor can be triggered in the vertical growth phase. Most of these changes occur between the radial growth phase and vertical growth phase of primarily melanoma, and metastatic cells often show highest productions of cytokines.

The types of products that have been isolated from melanoma include various growth factors, proteases, protease inhibitors, cell adhesion proteins, and host response modifiers. Melanoma cells express all major types of adhesion receptors including integrins and cadherins, and the expression of these receptors increases as melanoma progresses.

The understanding of the biology of melanoma has provided potential targets for drug therapy. Understanding of hematopoietic and dendritic cell growth factors has led to the clinical investigation of granulocyte macrophage-colony stimulating factor in melanoma as an adjunct to vaccine therapy, and it has demonstrated promising results in pilot studies[7] in the adjuvant treatment of melanoma. Identification of potential targets for therapy, such as bFGF, has led to the investigation of antisense oligonucleotides to block its role in modulating melanoma.

Immune factors appear to be involved in the progression of melanoma more often than in most other solid tumors. Spontaneous cancer regressions are rare, but are a well-documented phenomenon seen in melanoma. Focal regression in primary melanoma has also been reported. The regression of tumor appears to be associated with host immunity.

A number of different tumor antigens have been identified on melanoma cells by the use of monoclonal antibodies in both human and murine models. Melanoma-associated antigens (MAAs) have been identified in the cellular membrane and cytoplasm of melanoma cells. Ganglioside antigens have been of particular interest in the development of immunotherapy for melanoma. A large number of monoclonal antibodies to MAAs have been developed and are currently being used in clinical trials for the diagnosis and the therapy of melanoma.

The humoral and cellular responses of individuals with melanoma that express MAA have been described and provide the rationale for immunotherapy in the management of metastatic melanoma. Melanoma-directed antibodies have been isolated in the sera of patients with melanoma. The presence of antimelanoma antibodies in the sera of patients correlates with the clinical status of the patients, and the antibodies gradually disappear from the serum as the disease progresses. This phenomenon may be explained by the possible formation of anti-idiotype antibody directed against the antimelanoma antibody, an increase in the circulation of soluble tumor antigens that saturate all the antibody combining sites, increased levels of immunosuppression, or absorption of the antibodies on the tumor mass.

In recent years, interest has focused on the role of cell-mediated immune response in melanoma. Specific cell-mediated responses may play a role in tumor regression, but the role of specific cells such as cytotoxic T lymphocytes (CTLs) is not fully understood. Tumor-infiltrating lymphocytes (TILs) have been shown in vivo and in vitro to possess antitumor reactivity. TILs contain a large number of mature tumor-specific lymphocytes and have been a target for manipulation in immunotherapeutic approaches for melanoma.

Specific genetic alterations have been demonstrated in the pathogenesis of melanoma.[6] At least six genes with loci showing random deletions, rare translocations, and rare amplifications on chromosomes 1, 6, 7, 9, 10, and 11 have been identified in melanoma cells. Alterations in other genes located on other chromosomes may also contribute to the progression of melanoma. Alterations of chromosome 1 are seen in many forms of human cancer. The region of chromosome 1 that is involved in melanoma involves the tumor suppressor gene. The alterations seen in chromosome 6 potentially link melanoma and the major histocompatibility complex. The 9p21 locus is frequently affected in melanoma, and germline abnormalities are seen in approximately 50% of familial melanomas at this gene. In sporadic melanoma sporadic mutations are found in the *ras* gene; this mutation is seen more commonly in melanomas related to sun exposure. Genetic data suggest that familial melanoma is heterogenous

and likely due to several penetrant susceptibility genes acting alone or with multiple less-penetrant risk-factor modifier genes. *CDKN2A* and *DCK4* are highly penetrant susceptibility genes that have been identified. Variants of the *MC1R* (melanocortin-1 receptor) gene have also been associated with increased risk of melanoma. Additional deletions and mutations in *PEN/MMAC1* have been described in about 30% of cutaneous melanoma. The genetic influence to melanoma progression appears to involve a series of complex interactions. As these interactions are understood, the potential for gene therapy in melanoma expands.

HISTOLOGIC SUBTYPES OF MELANOMA

Cutaneous melanomas are categorized by growth patterns. The four histologic subtypes of cutaneous melanoma are distinctive in developmental phases and clinical features. The four major subtypes of cutaneous melanoma are superficial spreading melanoma, nodular melanoma, lentigo maligna melanoma, and acral lentiginous melanoma. There is no difference in the clinical outcome of the four subtypes if the comparison is controlled for depth of penetration. Any of the four subtypes of melanoma can occur as an amelanotic variant. Amelanotic melanomas appear to be devoid of clinically apparent pigmentation. Uveal melanoma is considered a separate disease from cutaneous melanoma.

Superficial spreading melanoma is the most common morphologic type of cutaneous melanoma and accounts for about 70% of all melanoma. The lesions usually arise from a preexisting nevus, known as a precursor lesion, and evolve slowly over 1 to 5 years. At some point, superficial spreading melanoma may progress to a more rapid growth phase. Early in lesion development the superficial spreading melanoma is flat, but as the lesion progresses, the surface becomes irregular and asymmetrical. The lesion enlarges when it enters into a rapid growth phase, and the edges appear notched or lacy. At times there are patches of regression within the lesion, signified by amelanotic areas. This subtype of melanoma is more common in women. The mean age of diagnosis of superficial spreading melanoma is 50 years, which is earlier than that noted for other subtypes. Superficial spreading melanoma usually occurs after puberty.

Nodular melanoma is the second most common growth pattern of melanoma and occurs in 15% to 30% of patients. Nodular melanoma is a pure vertical growth-phase disease. In nodular melanoma, a small expansive nodule in the papillary dermis invades the reticular dermis and subcutis. The radial growth phase is absent at all times. Nodular melanomas are more aggressive, and develop more rapidly than superficial spreading melanoma. Nodular melanomas are dark blue-black and often uniform in color with a shiny surface, although a small percentage of nodular melanomas are amelanotic and have a fleshy appearance. Nodular melanomas are raised and often symmetrical. They occur at any age, and are most common on the trunk, head, and neck. Nodular melanomas are more common in men.

Lentigo maligna melanoma represents a small percentage of melanomas and is unique from other histologic subtypes because it does not have the same propensity to metastasize. Lentigo maligna melanomas are generally large (>3 cm), flat, and tan-colored lesions with shades of brown and black. This subtype of melanoma occurs in an older age group, and is typically located on the chronically sun-exposed skin in older individuals. Lentigo maligna melanoma is uncommon before the age of 50, and may have been present for over 5 years. Lentigo maligna melanoma can be difficult to distinguish from solar lentigo.

Acral lentiginous melanoma presents as three distinct clinical subtypes: melanoma on the palms of the hands or soles of the feet, subungual melanoma, and mucosal melanoma. Most acral lentiginous melanomas are located on the soles of the feet and look like a large tan or brown stain. The lesions often have irregular convoluted borders. The initial macular component of palmar/plantar melanomas can be masked by the thickened stratum corneum at these sites. Many of these lesions look verrucous in appearance, making them difficult to distinguish from warts by the untrained eye. Suspicious lesions on the palms or soles of the feet should be evaluated. Acral lentiginous melanoma includes subungual melanoma, which arises in the nail matrix or nailbed. The most common presentation is a brown or black line in the great toe or the thumbnail. Mucosal melanoma is rare but can occur on any mucosal surface. Mucosal melanoma occurs most commonly in the oropharyngeal mucosa, followed by the anal/rectal mucosa, the genital mucosa, and the urinary mucosa. Unfortunately, mucosal melanoma often does not become clinically apparent until there is a large mass or the lesion bleeds. Acral lentiginous melanoma occurs in less than 10% of Caucasians with melanoma, but is the most common type of melanoma reported in blacks, Asians, and Hispanics.

Uveal melanoma is the most common primary intraocular malignancy seen in adults, but is an uncommon tumor. Unlike cutaneous melanoma, the frequency and mortality of uveal melanoma have remained steady. This melanoma arises from the pigmented epithelium of the choroid. Iris melanoma is a subset of uveal melanoma and tends to have a more benign course. The risk of metastasis varies with the histologic type and size of the tumor, as well as the location in the eye. Metastases occur most frequently in the liver, but have been documented in a variety of tissues.

CLINICAL PRESENTATION

The initial clinical presentation of melanoma is often a melanoma lesion. The lesion can be located anywhere on the body, but is most common on the lower extremities in women, and the back and trunk in men. The cardinal clinical feature of a cutaneous melanoma is a pigmented skin lesion that changes over a period of time. The clinical features used to describe or evaluate a questionable lesion are highlighted by the mnemonic "ABCD." Unlike benign pigmented lesions, the shape of a melanoma lesion is often (A) *asymmetric*. Benign lesions tend to have regular margins, whereas melanoma lesions often have irregular (B) *borders*. The (C) *color* of melanoma lesions are often variegated, ranging in color from tan to blue-black, and at times the lesion is intermingled with colors of red, purple, and white. The size or (D) *diameter* of a melanoma lesion is frequently 6 mm or greater when identified, whereas benign lesions are usually smaller. Early melanoma lesions may be diagnosed at a smaller size. Another warning sign of a potential melanoma is a change in preexisting nevi. Some clinicians use the ABCDE mnemonic for melanoma, adding (E) for *evolution* of a mole. Changes such as a sudden or continuous enlargement of a lesion, an elevation of a lesion, or any change in the skin surrounding a nevus, including redness or swelling are important clinical signs. Uncommonly, the sensation of the lesion may become itchy or tender and painful. Friability of the lesion resulting in bleeding or oozing is also a danger sign. Perhaps the most important warning sign of danger is the evolution in any characteristic of a lesion.

The clinical appearance of a melanoma depends on the histologic subtype and the stage of development of the lesion. It is usually possible to distinguish three variants of cutaneous melanoma including flat melanoma, nodular melanoma, and a flat melanoma with a nodular area. Flat melanoma usually corresponds to the histologic classification of superficial spreading melanoma.

The diagnosis of melanoma is complicated by a number of pigmented moles (melanocytic nevi) and nonmelanocytic lesions that resemble melanoma. Ordinary nevi, found on the skin of white adults, average between 10 and 40 lesions. These lesions are usually absent at birth and increase in number through adult life, and then gradually decline in number. They appear as tiny pinpoint macules and are usually uniform in color, but increase in size to a maximum of 4 to 6 mm. Nonmelanocytic pigmented lesions such as seborrheic keratoses, pigmented basal-cell carcinoma, and vascular lesions can also appear similar to a melanoma lesion.

Improved survival rates for melanoma have been attributed to treatment of lesions identified at an earlier stage of development. Efforts to improve survival rates are concentrated on the diagnosis and treatment of the primary lesion. The cost-effectiveness of massive screening for all adults by a physician has never been demonstrated. A number of agencies, such as the American Academy of Dermatology and the American Cancer Society, have sponsored free annual screenings. Routine examination of the skin by physicians is recommended for individuals at high risk. The entire cutaneous surface should be examined including the scalp.

Self-examination of the skin places the responsibilities of identification on the individual. Identification of early melanoma allows the opportunity to treat the lesions when they are thin and curable. Educational pamphlets describing the method of self-examination (Table 133–2) for the public are available through the American Cancer Society, the American Academy of Dermatology, and the Skin Cancer Foundation. If a newly discovered pigmented lesion is identified or if a preexisting pigmented lesion changes, the individual should be evaluated by a physician immediately.

A biopsy is critical in establishing the diagnosis of melanoma. The subsequent pathologic interpretation of the biopsy will determine the appropriate therapy and prognosis. An excisional biopsy with a margin of normal-appearing skin is recommended for a suspicious lesion, and should include a portion of underlying subcutaneous fat for microstaging. Although a biopsy is recommended for large lesions where an excisional biopsy is impractical, an incisional biopsy can be performed, but should include a core of full thickness of skin and subcutaneous tissue. When excisional biopsies are not appropriate, as with the face or palmar surface of the hands, a full-thickness incisional or punch biopsy is preferred to a shave biopsy.

Evaluation of any individual with a suspected melanoma includes a complete history and total body skin examination. The focus of the patient history is to identify potential risk factors. Risk-related

---

TABLE 133–2. Self-Examination of Suspicious Moles

1. Examine your body front and back in the mirror, and then right and left sides with arms raised.
2. Bend the elbows and look carefully at the forearms and upper arms and palms.
3. Look at the backs of the legs and feet. Look specifically in the spaces between toes and at the soles of the feet.
4. Examine the back of the neck and scalp with the help of a hand-held mirror; part hair (or use a blow dryer) to lift hair and give you a closer look.
5. Check the back and buttocks with a hand-held mirror.

Derived from publications of the American Academy of Dermatology.

TABLE 133–3. Clark Classification

Clark Level	Anatomic Landmark
N	Epidermis
I	Dermo-epidermal junction
II	Papillary dermis
III	Interface between papillar dermis and reticular dermis
IV	Reticular dermis and subcutaneous fat

questions include an assessment of family history of melanoma, personal history of skin cancer and/or nevus excisions, sun exposure, and phototype. Total dermatologic examination is necessary to determine melanoma risk factors (e.g., mole pattern, mole type, or freckling) and for staging. For patients with melanomas of 1 mm or more in thickness, a baseline chest x-ray and liver chemistries are generally recommended despite the fact that they are relatively insensitive at detecting clinically occult distant disease. Lactate dehydrogenase should be evaluated, as it has been correlated with prognosis. Elevated serum lactate dehydrogenase was one of the most predictive independent factors of decreased survival in published studies, even after accounting for site and number of metastases.[8] Any clinical indication of regional lymph node involvement should be confirmed with fine-needle aspiration or on biopsy of the enlarged lymph node. Additionally, any other signs or symptoms suggestive of metastatic disease should be completely evaluated.

There is a definite association between the size of a primary melanoma lesion and the likelihood of metastases. The prognostic factor originally used to determine survival was based on the cross-sectional profile of the primary tumor. The cross-sectional profile could be evaluated if the deepest invasive tumor cells lay above or below the sweat glands. This assessment was further clarified by Clark,[9] who described the relationship of depth of invasion of the cancer cells to the standard anatomic landmarks of the skin (Table 133–3). Clark's classification is a practical approach for patients with more superficial tumors, because tumors classified as Clark levels I through III seldom metastasize. That classification system has been criticized because of problems associated with practical measurements. Melanoma lesions that occur in the presence of lymphoid infiltration, fibrosis, or even the cells of preexisting nevi are difficult to assess with classic reference landmarks.

Breslow[10] replaced Clark's classification of reference landmarks with the use of thickness of the primary melanoma lesion. Tumor thickness is quantified to the nearest tenth of a millimeter with an ocular micrometer, measuring from the top of the granular layer of the overlying epidermis to the deepest contiguous invasive melanoma cell. The correlation between tumor thickness and probability of tumor metastases is strong, but does not include aspects such as tumor satellites, defined rather arbitrarily as skin involvement within 2 cm of the primary lesion, and vascular invasion. It was once thought that the presence of satellite nodule(s) had the same impact on prognosis as a high-risk primary lesion (tumor thickness >4 mm). It is now thought that patients with satellitosis have a worse prognosis than patients with thick primary lesions, and prognosis is more similar to that of patients with nodal metastases. There are a number of prognostic factors, in addition to tumor thickness and level of invasion, that are associated with the risk of developing metastatic disease.[11]

The American Joint Committee on Cancer (AJCC) developed a staging system for melanoma that divides patients with localized melanoma into four stages according to microstaging criteria of Breslow and Clark. In addition to consideration of the primary lesion, the AJCC staging system includes aspects of the tumor satellite, extent of lymph node involvement, and presence of metastatic disease. Recent analysis of several large databases worldwide has identified areas in which the AJCC staging system published in 1997 did not reflect the natural history of melanoma. Issues such as the appropriate cutoff values for primary tumor thickness, ulceration of the melanoma, and the satellite lesions of the primary tumor are important for determining the natural history of the disease in an individual, and should be considered when making decisions about therapy. The cutoff values initially proposed by Breslow for primary tumor thickness were initially used in the AJCC staging system, but it appears that cutoff depths of 1, 2, and 4 mm of thickness may better predict overall survival. Melanoma ulceration is associated with increased mitotic rate within a primary melanoma. The presence of ulceration of the primary lesion has been correlated with poorer survival for patients with very thin or thick lesions, but ulceration of the melanoma was not included in the 1997 AJCC staging system.

A revised staging system for cutaneous melanoma was approved by the AJCC.[12] Revisions of the new melanoma staging system include (1) melanoma thickness and ulceration for all tumors (except T_1 tumors); (2) the number of metastatic lymph nodes versus gross dimensions, and the delineation of clinically occult versus clinically apparent nodal metastases; (3) the site of distant metastases and the presence of elevated serum lactate dehydrogenase for metastatic disease; (4) upstaging of all patients with stage I, II, and III disease when a primary melanoma is ulcerated; and (5) a new convention for separating clinical and pathologic staging to include information obtained from intraoperative lymphatic mapping and sentinel node biopsy. Clinical staging includes microstaging of the primary melanoma and clinical and radiologic evaluation. It is used after the complete excision of the primary melanoma with clinical assessment for regional and distant metastasis. Pathologic staging includes the microstaging of the primary melanoma and pathologic information about the regional nodes after partial or complete lymphadenectomy. At this time it appears that patients with very limited disease (stage 0 or 1A disease) do not require pathologic evaluation of lymph nodes (Tables 133–4 and 133–5). It is important to look closely at the staging system used in clinical trials to appropriately interpret the results.

As with other solid tumors, the presence of regional lymph node involvement is a powerful predictor of tumor burden and patient outcome. In the past, the primary method to determine nodal status was by surgical resection and analysis of the lymph nodes via a regional lymph node dissection. In recent years, preoperative lymphoscintigraphy and intraoperative sentinel node mapping have become more widely used methods to identify the first or sentinel lymph node in the direct pathway of lymph drainage from the primary cutaneous melanoma. The rationale for lymphatic mapping and subsequent sentinel node biopsy is based on the observation that regions of the skin have patterns of lymphatic drainage to specific lymph nodes in the regional lymphatic basin. The sentinel lymph node is believed to be the first node in the lymphatic basin into which the primary melanoma drains. Unlike other solid tumors, melanoma appears to progress in an orderly nodal distribution. The evaluation of sentinel nodes has been used for detection of micrometastases in breast cancer and is gaining popularity in melanoma. Sentinel lymph node biopsy provides an avenue to perform a more thorough examination of a single sentinel node than is possible when examining multiple lymph nodes with a lymph node dissection, and may be most useful in melanomas located in ambiguous drainage sites such as the head and neck areas.

TABLE 133–4. Melanoma TNM Classification

T Classification	Thickness	Ulcerative Status
T_1	≤1 mm	A: without ulceration and level II/III
		B: with ulceration or level IV/V
T_2	1.01–2 mm	A: without ulceration
		B: with ulceration
T_3	2.01–4 mm	A: without ulceration
		B: with ulceration
T_4	>4 mm	A: without ulceration
		B: with ulceration

N Classification	No. of Metastatic Nodes	Nodal Metastatic Mass
N_1	1 node	A: micrometastasis
		B: macrometastasis
N_2	2–3 nodes	A: micrometastasis
		B: macrometastasis
		C: in-transit metastases/satellite(s) without metastatic nodes
N_3	4 or more metastatic lymph nodes, matted nodes, ulcerated melanoma, metastatic lymph nodes, or intransit metastatic or satellite lesions	

M Classification	Site	Serum Lactate Dehydrogenase
M_{1a}	Distant skin, subcutaneous, or nodal metastatic disease	Normal
M_{1b}	Lung metastases	Normal
M_{1c}	All other visceral metastases	Normal
	Any distant metastasis	Elevated

Micrometastases are diagnosed after sentinel or elective lymphadenectomy.
Macrometastases are defined as clinically detectable lymph node metastases confirmed by therapeutic lymphadenectomy or when any lymph node metastasis exhibits extracapsular extension.
Barch.[12]

Additionally, the detection of clinically undetectable disease in a lymph node basin that is not directly adjacent to the primary lesion may allow for the upstaging of patients who are initially believed to have node-negative disease. Currently, there is increasing interest in developing methods to improve the detection of occult micrometastases in biopsied lymph nodes with more sensitive reverse transcriptase polymerase chain reaction assays to detect the presence of tyrosinase messenger RNA. This may be a method for broad clinical use to detect occult melanoma cells in the blood of patients with small clinical lesions.[13]

TABLE 133–5. American Joint Committee on Cancer Tumor (T), Node (N), Metastasis (M) Stage Grouping for Cutaneous Melanoma

Pathologic Stage	T	N	M	Clinical Stage	T	N	M
0	T_{is}	N_0	M_0	0	T_{is}	N_0	M_0
IA	T_{1a}	N_0	M_0	IA	T_{1a}	N_0	M_0
IB	T_{1b}	N_0	M_0	IB	T_{1b}	N_0	M_0
	T_{2a}	N_0	M_0		T_{2a}	N_0	M_0
IIA	T_{2b}	N_0	M_0	IIA	T_{2b}	N_0	M_0
	T_{3a}	N_0	M_0		T_{3a}	N_0	M_0
IIB	T_{3b}	N_0	M_0	IIB	T_{3b}	N_0	M_0
	T_{4a}	N_0	M_0		T_{4a}	N_0	M_0
IIC	T_{4b}	N_0	M_0	IIC	T_{4b}	N_0	M_0
IIIA	T_{1-4a}	N_{1a}	M_0	IIIA	Any T_{1-4a}	N_{1b}	M_0
IIIB	T_{1-4a}	N_{1b}	M_0	IIIB	Any	N_{2b}	M_0
	T_{1-4a}	N_{2a}	M_0		T_{1-4a}		
IIIC	Any T	N_{2b}, N_{2c}	M_0	IIIC	Any T	N_{2c}	M_0
	Any T	N_3	M_0		Any T	N_3	M_0
IV	Any T	Any N	M_1	IV	Any T	Any N	M_1

The stage of the melanoma at time of diagnosis is one of the primary indicators of natural history of the disease; other factors have been shown to influence survival of primary melanoma. Factors such as tumor growth phase, mitotic rate, density of TILs infiltrating the tumor tissue, anatomic site of the primary tumor, gender and age, have all been demonstrated to have an impact on survival (Table 133–6). In addition, a number of additional prognostic factors have been identified for patients with advanced disease. The number of metastatic sites, disease involvement of the gastrointestinal tract, liver, pleura, or lung, or a Eastern Cooperative Oncology Group (ECOG) performance status of ≥ 1, male, and patients with prior immunotherapy have been associated with poor prognosis.

TABLE 133–6. Prognostic Factors for Cutaneous Melanoma

Tumor-related factors
  Tumor thickness
  Level of tumor invasion
  Anatomic site of primary tumor (increased survival in tumors of extremities versus axial, neck, head, and trunk tumors)
  Mitotic rate (correlated with decreased survival)
  Angiogenesis
  Occurrence of microsatellites
  Area of tumor regression
  Presence of tumor-infiltrating lymphocytes (correlated with increased survival)
Patient-related factors
  Age (decreased survival in patients >60 years of age)
  Gender (survival: female >male)

▶ TREATMENT: Melanoma

The treatment of a patient with cutaneous melanoma depends on the stage of the disease. Local disease is managed and often cured with surgical ablation. Regional disease is treated with surgical resection of the primary lesion, and depending on the risk of recurrence, possibly adjuvant therapy. The use of adjuvant therapy after surgical resection and the role of interferon-α as adjuvant therapy remain controversial. Treatment for disseminated melanoma remains a challenge. Although the literature provides numerous clinical trials of single-agent and combination chemotherapy, immunotherapy, and biotherapy regimens, there is not a single standard approach for management of the individual with metastatic melanoma.

SURGERY

Patients that present with a suspicious pigmented lesion should undergo a full thickness excisional biopsy, if possible. Sites in which excisional biopsy are inappropriate include the face, palm of the hand, sole of the foot, distal digit, and subungual lesions. A full thickness incisional or punch biopsy is preferred in these cases to provide microstaging and ultimately to determine therapy.

Cutaneous melanoma that is localized can often be cured with surgical excision. The extent of the excision margin is important in the prevention of local recurrence and ultimate survival. For melanoma in situ, excision of the lesion or biopsy site with 0.5 to 1 cm border of clinically normal skin and a layer of subcutaneous tissue is recommended at this time. Excision with a 1-cm margin of clinically normal skin and underlying subcutaneous tissue is recommended for invasive melanoma ≤ 1 mm thick.[14] This recommendation is a significant reduction from the previous recommendation of a 5-cm margin. The appropriate margin of excision for melanomas between 1 and 2 mm in thickness is controversial. A recent study suggests there is a greater risk of locoregional recurrence when melanomas that are at least 2 mm thick are excised with a 1-cm margin rather than a 2-cm margin.[15] Lesions that are 2 to 4 mm thick should be excised with a 2-cm margin. Primary tumors more than 4 mm thick require at least a 2-cm margin, but it is not clear if a larger margin is beneficial.[16]

Surgical management of lentigo maligna melanoma is problematic, as subclinical extension of atypical junctional melanocytic hyperplasia may extend beyond the visible margins; it is important to completely excise these lesions.

When isolated regional lymph nodes are detected via physical exam in the absence of distant disease, therapeutic lymphadenectomy is recommended. The extent of therapeutic lymph node dissection is often modified according to the anatomic area of the lymphadenopathy. The role of lymphadenectomy is not as established in situations in which the regional lymph nodes do not appear to be involved under clinical examination. Although a subgroup of patients with stage I melanoma will have microscopic metastatic disease in nonpalpable lymph nodes, prophylactic regional lymph node dissection has not been shown to prolong survival or decrease time to relapse in randomized clinical trials. Selective regional lymphadenectomy performed after scintigraphic and dye lymphographic identification of the affected sentinel draining lymph node(s) is becoming increasingly common. If the sentinel node is found to have micrometastatic melanoma, regional dissection of the involved nodal basin is performed. If lymphatic mapping with sentinel node biopsy is available, it should be considered in patients with melanomas that are over 1 mm thick or Clark level IV.

One of the most important aspects of the surgical management of cutaneous melanoma is the role of patient follow-up. Postsurgical follow-up of patients who have had a melanoma excised is essential to monitor for undetected metastatic disease and the development of a second primary cutaneous melanoma or second nonmelanoma primary malignancy. Scheduled screening in addition to routine surgical follow-up is required for any patient with a melanoma; the frequency and duration recommended depends on the stage of melanoma. The optimal duration of follow-up remains controversial. The majority of patients who are going to have recurrent disease will do so in the first 5 years following treatment, but late recurrences seen in patients over 10 years following surgery have been observed. The increased lifetime risk of developing a second primary melanoma supports lifetime dermatologic surveillance for all patients.

The role of curative surgery is limited to that of early-stage disease in cutaneous melanoma. The role of surgery beyond that of cure is less clear, although surgery may offer palliation for patients with isolated metastases. Resection of isolated lesions in the brain and the lungs may be appropriate in certain cases and should be evaluated based on individual patient criteria. Surgery can be an option in situations in which the lesion is accessible and when the lesion may cause problems if not removed. Melanoma in the gastrointestinal tract can lead to bowel obstruction, and appropriate resection or bypass may allow the patient significant relief of symptoms. Despite the lack of controlled clinical trials, the impact on palliative surgery should be evaluated in the context of a patient's comfort and quality of life. Surgery may be an appropriate option if the perceived outcome is to provide patient comfort. On the other hand, surgery may constitute a significant physical challenge or financial burden to a patient with a limited life expectancy. The clinical scenarios involving surgical resection should be fully evaluated in terms of overall quality of life.

The risk of relapse and death after the resection of a local or regional cutaneous melanoma is the primary determinant for the use of adjuvant therapy after primary resection. Adjuvant trials have focused on patients at intermediate or high risk of recurrence.

IMMUNOTHERAPY

Melanoma is considered one of the most immunogenic solid tumors; it appears to interact with and respond to the immune system of the host in which it arises. Spontaneous regressions of melanoma suggest the importance of the immune system in disease modulation. Lymphoid infiltration into the primary melanoma also suggests that immunomodulation may impact the biology of melanoma. Early work with nonspecific immunomodulators, such as levamisole and bacille Calmette-Guérin, in melanoma demonstrated that tumor regression could occur with these therapies, although many of these regressions were limited and short-lived. Coupled with the fact that melanoma is one of the tumors most resistant to other standard systemic treatment modalities used for cancer (i.e., radiation and chemotherapy), immunotherapy offers an avenue of treatment if surgery fails or is not an option. Although the complete response (CR) rate seen in those patients with melanoma treated with biotherapy is low, the durability of the responses can be significant. This has led to increasing research in the optimization of biotherapeutic approaches for patients with metastatic melanoma and for the establishment of biotherapy in the adjuvant setting.

INTERFERON

The *interferons* consist of a group of antigenically and genetically distinct species and subspecies; the interferons have differing immunomodulatory activity and are directly cytostatic and cytotoxic. A number of studies have evaluated various doses and schedules of recombinant interferon for the treatment of metastatic melanoma, but no standard strategy is recommended. Response rates in metastatic melanoma range from 10% to 30%, and overall response rates are approximately 15% for interferon-α. Unfortunately the optimal dose, treatment schedule, and treatment combination/regimens have not been established for the management of metastatic melanoma.

In initial clinical trials with interferon therapy for patients with metastatic cutaneous melanoma, response rates were highest in those patients with minimal disease. Additionally, responses were seen in all sites of disease, but were most frequent in subcutaneous, lymph node, and pulmonary metastases. Success of interferon in a setting with minimal disease has encouraged investigators to evaluate the benefit of interferon in patients after curative surgical resection who were at high risk for recurrent disease (bulky disease or regional lymph node involvement). Early trials of short-term and/or low-dose regimens of interferon-α did not demonstrate a survival benefit in the adjuvant setting. In an attempt to optimize response in the adjuvant setting, a strategy was developed to administer maximum tolerated doses of interferon-α for 1 month, followed by prolonged therapy of interferon-α at more tolerable doses for 48 weeks. The rationale for the induction phase was to provide peak levels of interferon sufficient to inhibit tumor growth and provide both antiangiogenesis and immunomodulatory effects while avoiding production of anti-interferon antibodies. A large, multicenter, cooperative group trial of interferon-α_{2b} versus observation was designed for patients with high-risk (stage IIB and III disease based on the 1997 AJCC staging criteria) melanoma following curative surgical resection. Interferon-α_{2b} was given intravenously as an induction therapy at maximum tolerated doses of 20 million international units/m^2 per dose 5 days per week for 4 weeks in an outpatient setting; treatment was continued for 48 weeks with subcutaneous interferon-α_{2b} 10 million international units/m^2 per dose three times per week at home. This therapy is now often referred to as high-dose interferon (HDI). Analysis of the 280 patients demonstrated a disease-free survival and an overall survival advantage with interferon-α treatment for patients with stage IIB and III disease following surgical resection.[17] With longer follow-up, however, the difference in overall survival is no longer significant.[18] The prolongation of overall survival was approximately 1 year, and the most significant reduction in melanoma recurrence was during the early treatment period. Subgroup analysis of this study indicated that patients with large primary tumors and node-negative disease ($T_4N_0M_0$) did not receive the same benefit from therapy, but the small number of patients in this group made it difficult to draw definite conclusions about the role of interferon treatment for adjuvant therapy in this subgroup. Whether the information from this trial should be extrapolated to patients with local recurrences, satellite lesions, or in-transit metastases is not known, and should be evaluated on an individual case basis.

Toxicities for the interferon therapy were common and severe in a majority of the patients at some point during therapy and necessitated dose reductions and/or delays during both the induction and maintenance phases of the study. Dose modifications were required for dose-limiting constitutional symptoms, hematologic toxicity, and hepatic toxicities, but 74% of the patients were able to complete the year of therapy in an outpatient setting.

The optimal dose of interferon in the adjuvant setting is not clear. A subsequent ECOG trial designed to evaluate the impact of lower doses of interferon (LDI; 3 million units per dose subcutaneous three times weekly) for 24 months compared to the high-dose regimen (HDI) described above versus observation did not demonstrate a survival advantage of HDI versus observation.[19] At a median follow-up of 52 months, the 5-year estimated relapse-free survival for HDI was 44%, LDI 40%, and observation 35%. HDI was shown to be statistically superior for relapse-free survival, prolonging the median time to relapse by 10 months compared to observation and LDI. With longer follow-up, however, the difference in relapse-free survival is no longer significant.[18] An overall survival benefit was not seen for HDI or LDI compared to observation, although the investigators speculated that this analysis of survival was affected by the number of patients in the observation arm that received interferon therapy after disease progression.[19]

The frequency and severity of toxicity seen with HDI in the adjuvant setting and the lack of overall survival benefit has raised several important questions: (1) Are the toxicities associated with HDI treatment worth the potential benefits for patients? (2) What are the mechanism(s) and best standard(s) of care for patients who experience interferon toxicity? (3) Is the regimen/schedule of interferon used in the initial positive trial (HDI) necessary to achieve the benefits seen in this study? Aggressive toxicity evaluation and individualized management is essential to help preserve quality of life in those individuals receiving interferon therapy.

One of the categories of toxicities seen with interferon-α therapy is actually a diverse group of side effects referred to as constitutional symptoms; this can include acute symptoms such as fever, chills, myalgia, and fatigue, and can encompass some of the more chronic toxicities such as fatigue, anorexia, and depression.[20] Acetaminophen may be used to prevent or minimize acute dose-related symptoms such as fever, myalgia, and chills. Opiates such as meperidine are often required when patients experience severe chills or rigors, most commonly during the initial month of the high-dose intravenous interferon-α induction phase. Nonsteroidal anti-inflammatory drugs (NSAIDs) have been used to manage interferon-related myalgia, but may have overlapping side effects with interferon, such as a decrease in renal blood flow and nausea. NSAIDs, like acetaminophen, may mask fevers that occur in those patients who experience neutropenia while on therapy. Fatigue is one of the most frequently observed dose-limiting toxicities seen with interferon therapy.[20] The mechanisms of interferon-induced fatigue are not fully understood at this time, and are often multifactorial in individual patients. Interferon-induced fatigue appears to be dose-related and may worsen with continued therapy. Pharmacologic (e.g., amantadine) and nonpharmacologic interventions (e.g., exercise, psychosocial techniques, distraction, energy management, and dietary modifications) are currently being evaluated to treat cancer-related fatigue and now interferon-related fatigue.[20,21] Anorexia was reported in approximately 70% of patients receiving adjuvant interferon therapy for melanoma and is thought to be mediated through direct effects on hypothalamic neurons, modification of normal hypothalamic neurotransmitters/neuropeptides, or effects from stimulation of other cytokines.[20,22] Depression is common and should be fully evaluated and treated based on patient-related symptoms.[20] Contributing factors such as interferon-induced hypothyroidism and/or concomitant interferon symptoms (e.g., nausea and fatigue) should be evaluated concurrently with depression symptoms to optimize treatment decisions. Taste alterations may contribute to anorexia. Investigational strategies for ameliorating interferon-induced anorexia include nutritional intervention, use of appetite stimulants such as megestrol acetate, and patient education. Glucocorticoids should not be used for appetite stimulation or as part of an antiemetic therapy, as they may adversely impact the immunomodulatory effects of the interferon. Other toxicities such as hematologic or hepatic toxicities require monitoring and appropriate dose modification.

Because of the associated toxicity and adverse effects seen with interferon-α therapy there has been worldwide concern about the usefulness of this intensive adjuvant therapy for melanoma despite the possible benefits in relapse-free and overall survival.[23] A subsequent report from the cooperative group study demonstrated a quality-of-life benefit with interferon therapy based on the quality-of-life-adjusted survival analysis.[24] This analysis calculates the quality-of-life-adjusted years gained as a result of interferon-α treatment or the clinical benefit of time without toxicities and without disease.

The role of interferon as adjuvant therapy is not clear at this time. The issue of patient side effects and cost needs to be carefully weighed against the disease-free survival benefit seen in those individuals with high risk of recurrence. As high-dose interferon remains the only therapy to demonstrate benefit in large comparative trials, it should be considered for patients with high-risk disease. According to the National Comprehensive Cancer Network (NCCN) Clinical Practice Guidelines for melanoma, interferon alfa is one of several options for select patients with high-risk disease.[25] Observation was also listed as an option. Individuals should be prescreened for potential problems associated with therapy; relative contraindications to high-dose interferon therapy include autoimmune diseases, immunosuppression, decompensated liver disease, severe neuropsychiatric diseases, or life-threatening infection.[20] Efforts continue to better define the optimal treatment regimen for high-dose interferon versus other strategies in well designed clinical trials.

CLINICAL CONTROVERSY

There is significant controversy regarding the role of interferon-α as adjuvant therapy in high-risk patients after surgical resection of melanoma. Assessment of patient risk factors, availability of clinical trials, and cost of therapy should be evaluated prior to initiation of therapy.

The role of interferon in advanced disease is even more unclear, especially for those patients who have recurred after treatment with adjuvant interferon therapy. Interferon-α has been used as a single agent in patients with metastatic disease who have not received adjuvant therapy, and in combination with chemotherapy and/or other biotherapy for metastatic melanoma. The challenges of combination therapy are that many of the toxicities seen with interferon can be exacerbated by concomitant chemotherapy (e.g., nausea, vomiting, and neutropenia). In an attempt to limit systemic toxicity and to potentiate local benefits, the regional administration has been evaluated in a variety of settings. Intralesional and perilesional application of interferon has been shown to have some efficacy in small lesions and appears to be well tolerated.[26]

INTERLEUKIN-2

Interleukin-2 (IL-2), a glycoprotein produced by activated lymphocytes, has been extensively studied in the management of metastatic melanoma. The precise mechanism of cytotoxicity of IL-2 is unknown; high concentrations of IL-2 have not been shown to have a direct antitumor effect on cancer cells in vitro. In vitro and in vivo, IL-2 stimulates the production and release of many secondary monocyte-derived and T-cell-derived cytokines, including IL-4, IL-5, IL-6, IL-8, tumor necrosis factor-α, granulocyte macrophage-colony stimulating factor, and interferon-γ, which may have direct or indirect antitumor activity. In addition, interleukin-2 appears to stimulate the cytotoxic activities of natural killer cells, monocytes, lymphokine-activated killer (LAK) cells, and cytotoxic T lymphocytes (CTLs). Although the clinical significance is not currently understood, preliminary studies have shown that several human melanoma cell lines express both α and β chains of the interleukin receptor that specifically bind to interleukin-2.

Based on preclinical studies that showed a dose-response relationship between recombinant IL-2 (aldesleukin) and tumor response, the initial clinical trials of aldesleukin in the treatment of patients with melanoma used relatively high doses of the drug as a single agent or in combination with LAK cells. The response rates seen in these trials ranged from 15% to 25%, and 2% to 5% of patients achieved complete responses, some of which were durable. Responses were seen at a number of metastatic sites such as lung, liver, bone, lymph nodes, and subcutaneous tissue. Based on the re-evaluation of early clinical trials,[27] recombinant IL-2 (aldesleukin) was approved by the FDA for treatment of metastatic melanoma. Overall, objective response rates were about 16%, but in some cases there were durable responses and responses seen in patients with large tumor burdens. The high aldesleukin doses used in the initial clinical trials and recommended in the labeling of the drug are associated with serious toxicities and may limit the practicality of therapy for individual patients and broad application in certain health care systems. At the high doses (600,000 international units/kg per dose every 8 hours for 14 doses maximum) approved for treatment of metastatic melanoma, cytokine-induced capillary leak syndrome is a common problem and may be accompanied by hypotension, visceral edema, dyspnea, tachycardia, and arrhythmias. Increased permeability of capillary walls allows for a fluid shift from the intravascular space into tissue. As the patient becomes intravascularly dehydrated, hypotension may occur, resulting in reflex tachycardia and arrhythmias. In addition, the decrease in blood volume may result in decreased renal blood flow and urine output, manifesting as an increase in blood urea nitrogen, serum creatinine, edema, and weight gain, and a decrease in urine output (input greater than output). Visceral edema can result in pulmonary congestion, pleural effusions, and edema. The management of patients receiving high-dose aldesleukin requires careful monitoring and a staff trained in aspects of critical care such as hypotension management. Although some institutions manage patients receiving high-dose aldesleukin in an intensive care unit, most patients can be managed on a designated oncology unit. Additional side effects seen with aldesleukin include constitutional symptoms, pruritus and eosinophilia, bone marrow suppression including thrombocytopenia, an increase in liver function tests, and nausea.[28]

CLINICAL CONTROVERSY

Although aldesleukin has been associated with long-term durable responses in a small subset of patients with metastatic melanoma, the toxicity profile, intensity of therapy, and cost has limited acceptance within the United States. Patients should be evaluated for treatment prior to initiation of therapy.

In an attempt to provide the benefit of aldesleukin therapy without the serious side effects, a number of studies have evaluated continuous-infusion aldesleukin therapy, and lower-dose aldesleukin alone or with chemotherapy and interferon therapy. Response rates have been promising, but survival has not been significantly affected. At this time, direct head-to-head comparisons of various dosing schedules and regimens are needed to determine the optimum approach to aldesleukin therapy in metastatic melanoma. The coadministration of LAK cells with aldesleukin does not appear to significantly improve clinical response. Although some studies have suggested improved response with coadministration of TILs with recombinant IL-2, the therapy is technically difficult and costly, and the overall clinical benefit has not been clearly demonstrated.

Histamine has been shown to inhibit the generation of reactive oxygen species by phagocytes and ultimately preserve natural killer cell and T-cell responsiveness to IL-2. Preclinical work led to a series of clinical trials evaluating the combination of aldesleukin and histamine dihydrochloride with the hope that the combination would increase the efficacy of aldesleukin in patients with metastatic melanoma. It was also hoped that lower doses of aldesleukin would allow for outpatient treatment for metastatic melanoma. In initial clinical trials, aldesleukin was administered subcutaneously with or without histamine dihydrochloride. A survival advantage was seen with the combination in a subset of patients, those patients with liver metastases.[29] Constitutional toxicities were common but less than those seen with high-dose aldesleukin; patients were able to maintain therapy at home. The addition of histamine dihydrochloride resulted in a significant toxicity secondary to the effects of the histamine, including vasodilation, cardiovascular effects, and injection-site reactions. Most toxicities were mild, except for headaches, and were managed symptomatically.[30]

One of the greatest challenges in the management of patients with metastatic melanoma with immunotherapy is to determine for an individual patient if the potential benefits of aldesleukin therapy outweigh the substantial risk. It is obvious from the reports of long-term responses (greater than 10 years) in some patients that the risk is certainly worth the benefit for those individuals. A number of parameters such as human leukocyte antigen (HLA) expression and pretreatment immunologic status have been evaluated as potential predictors to therapy. Unfortunately, at this time it is difficult to determine which individuals will respond to aldesleukin therapy, as no biologic or immunologic parameters have been found to correlate with response. The decision to treat an individual with high-dose aldesleukin should be based on an analysis of an individual patient's risk versus potential benefit. Patients with inadequate pulmonary function, cardiac function, renal insufficiency, active infection, or poor performance status are poor candidates for this therapy. Aldesleukin can be safely administered with a properly trained health care team, and is one of only two approved therapies for treatment of metastatic melanoma.

VACCINES

The rationale for vaccination as a therapeutic modality is based on the observation that tumor cells differ antigenically from normal cells, and the hope that vaccines might induce effective tumor-specific immune responses with fewer toxicities than conventional chemotherapy or other immunotherapies. Greater knowledge about tumor antigens and the mechanism of antigen presentation and immune response to antigens has led to the development of several vaccination strategies for the treatment of early and advanced melanoma. A number of these vaccine approaches are being evaluated in both metastatic disease and in the adjuvant setting (Table 133–7).[31,32]

Active immunization is one of the well-characterized strategies for immunotherapy of melanoma. Current melanoma vaccines upregulate the antibody response of CTLs to specific tumor antigens. Melanoma antigens are either tumor-associated antigens (TAAs) or melanoma-associated antigens (MAAs). TAAs are common to melanoma cells and other tumor cells, while MAAs are usually proteins or glycoproteins found predominantly in melanomas and less commonly in normal melanocytes. The use of TAAs or MAAs for melanoma vaccines can be difficult, as the expression of antigens in melanoma cells is often heterogeneous and may change in response to the patient's immune response. Unfortunately, MAAs and TAAs also tend to be weakly immunogenic, although immunogenicity can be increased by physical alterations.

Melanoma vaccines range from complex antigen mixtures to purified antigens. Complex vaccines are polyvalent and can stimulate an immune response to a number of tumor antigens and are less

TABLE 133–7. Melanoma Vaccines

Whole melanoma cells
　Autologous cells
　Allogeneic cells
　Haptenized cells
Melanoma cell lysates
　Viral oncolysates
　Shed melanoma cell supernatant
Defined antigen vaccines
　Gangliosides (GM2, GD2)
Anti-idiotype monoclonal antibodies
　Anti-GD3 gangliosides
Dendritic cell
Protein antigens
DNA vaccination
Recombinant viral vaccines

susceptible to antigenic modulation by the cancer cells. Single-antigen vaccines can be problematic if a single-resistant-antigen-negative tumor cell develops.

Melanoma vaccines can be prepared from a patient's own tumor (autologous preparations), and will therefore target antigens from that patient's melanoma cell. Autologous vaccines may involve modification of the tumor cells with a hapten to increase immunogenicity of the preparation. Allogeneic preparations do not require patient tissue to prepare the vaccine. Allogeneic preparations often include a number of cell lines to increase the content of immunogenic TAAs and MAAs.

Melanoma vaccines may also be prepared with tumor cell lysate. Lysate vaccines can be prepared from the whole cells or from the cellular elements most likely to contain the antigens important for the induction of protective immune responses. Material shed from the melanoma cells is believed to be rich in cell-surface antigens and has been used for preparation of a melanoma vaccine. Melacine is a lysate vaccine prepared from two human melanoma cell lines administered with an adjuvant immunostimulant monophosphoryl lipid A and purified mycobacterial cell-wall skeleton called DETOX.[33] Initial reports from uncontrolled clinical trials with Melacine have suggested a role in the treatment of patients with surgically resected and metastatic melanoma. It is thought that a subset of patients defined by HLA subtypes showed benefit, suggesting that this vaccine therapy may be a targeted approach for select patients. CancerVax is a polyvalent allogeneic whole-cell vaccine developed by Morton,[34] which is comprised of an irradiated live-cell preparation of three allogeneic melanoma cell lines selected for their high content of MAAs and TAAs. BCG is used as an adjuvant and the vaccine is administered intradermally. CancerVax is being evaluated for the postsurgical treatment of stage III melanoma and in stage IV disease after surgical resection.

An alternative approach to vaccine construction is to develop a vaccine from a single highly-specific antigen. Preparations currently in clinical trials include vaccines prepared from gangliosides, peptides such as MAGE or MART, and anti-idiotype monoclonal antibodies. Gangliosides G_{M2}, G_{D2}, G_{M3}, G_{D3}, and O-acetyl-G_{D3} are present on the surface of many melanoma cells, but G_{M2} is the most consistently expressed and immunogenic antigen. One vaccine composed of the ganglioside G_{M2} coupled with keyhole limpet hemocyanine is being evaluated in the adjuvant setting. The vaccines from a single antigen have the advantage that they can be prepared in a reproducible manner on a large scale. The problem with this approach is that it is unclear if targeting a single antigen or peptide on a melanoma will be sufficient to kill the tumor cell. As with other approaches for targeted therapy, there is a concern that cancer cells will develop strategies to circumvent the targeted treatment approach.

OTHER APPROACHES

Dendritic cells are potent antigen-presenting cells for the initiation of antigen-specific immune responses. Dendritic cells express high levels of major histocompatibility complex class I and class II molecules, which are essential in antigen presentations. Activation of T cells and recruitment of non–antigen specific effectors, such as natural killer cells and macrophages, result in a broad immune response. One strategy to use dendritic cells for inducing antitumor immune responses has been done with peptide-pulsed dendritic cells. Antimelanoma CTLs can be generated from healthy donors and patients with melanoma with dendritic cells pulsed with melanoma-derived peptides. A number of clinical trials are evaluating dendritic cell–based immunotherapy.[35]

Monoclonal antibodies have been used for the diagnosis and treatment of melanoma. Two strategies have been pursued: treatment

with a monoclonal antibody to activate the host immune system, and treatment with a conjugated monoclonal antibody (i.e., immunoconjugate). Monoclonal antibodies have been conjugated to cytotoxic agents, radioisotopes, and toxins such as ricin A. Trials of monoclonal antibodies were initially limited secondary to the production of the monoclonal antibody. A problem seen in current studies is the induction of neutralizing antibodies to the murine monoclonal antibodies. Chimeric, humanized, or pure human monoclonal antibodies against MAAs could potentially avoid the development of human antimouse antibody. A vaccine which is composed of three monoclonal anti-idiotype antibodies that include the internal image of several determinants of the MAA has been developed and looked at in clinical trials. One of the problems with this antibody is the inability to directly induce a cell-mediated antitumor effect; therefore adjuvants are now being used to increase the ability of the anti-idiotype antibodies to induce a greater immune response.

Gene therapy of human melanoma is still in its infancy, but suggests several exciting approaches to the management of metastatic melanoma. Several strategies for gene therapy are currently under investigation for the treatment of melanoma. One approach to gene therapy for melanoma is the modification of melanoma cells with the insertion of one or more cytokine genes, and then administering these altered allogeneic or autologous cells as a vaccine. Cytokine gene transduction has been accomplished with a number of cytokines including aldesleukin (IL-2), tumor necrosis factor-α, IL-4, and interferon. It is hoped that the insertion of cytokine genes into melanoma cells will significantly increase the cells' immunogenicity.

Genes can also be transferred in vitro into TILs associated with melanoma in an attempt to potentiate the cytotoxicity of these cells. Rosenberg and colleagues were the first to attempt to transduce the gene coding for resistance to neomycin into human TILs. This approach has since been used to transfer the tumor necrosis factor gene into TILs.

Thalidomide and thalidomide analogs are also being evaluated in the management of melanoma. Thalidomide, given as either a single agent or in combination with chemotherapy or cytokines, is being evaluated in a variety of studies. Thalidomide analogs are also being evaluated to try and avoid toxicities associated with the parent compound. The thalidomide analogs are grouped into two classes; the selective cytokine inhibitory drugs and the immunomodulatory derivatives. Both classes appear to have antiangiogenic and anti-inflammatory properties, but the selective cytokine inhibitory drugs are phosphodiesterase inhibitors. Immunomodulatory derivatives also have effects on T-cell stimulation and inhibition of tumor necrosis factor-α. Several of these agents are being evaluated in clinical trials in metastatic melanoma.

CHEMOTHERAPY

A number of cytotoxic agents have demonstrated in vitro activity to melanoma; only a few drugs have consistently shown a response rate greater than 10% in patients with melanoma. Since chemotherapy has rarely cured a patient with melanoma, the primary goal of chemotherapy is palliation.[36] The results of clinical trials are generally expressed in terms of response rates. The response rate usually includes the fraction of patients who experience a partial response plus those who experience a complete response. Partial response criteria vary but may require a 50% reduction of the tumor for a minimum of 1 month. A complete response would require total regression of all metastases for at least 1 month and is uncommon (<5%). It is essential to realize that these response rates do not reflect survival, and do not evaluate benefit to the patient. Response rates also do not represent the toxicities and the complications of therapy.

5 *Dacarbazine*, a cytotoxic drug thought to exert its antitumor effect through alkylation, is currently the most effective single agent for the treatment of melanoma. Dacarbazine remains the only FDA-approved chemotherapeutic agent for the treatment of metastatic melanoma in the United States. In prospective controlled clinical trials, response rates of 10% to 25% have been seen, with an average duration of response of 5 to 7 months. Complete responses are uncommon, with a dismal 2% of patients treated with single-agent dacarbazine sustaining long-term complete responses. There does not appear to be a survival benefit for dacarbazine relative to other treatments or supportive care. Early clinical trials demonstrate patients with skin, subcutaneous tissue, and lymph node involvement respond most frequently, whereas metastatic disease to the liver, bone, and central nervous system are often unresponsive. The optimum dose schedule of dacarbazine has never been determined; therefore single-dose regimens are often preferred for patient convenience. Common side effects of dacarbazine therapy include moderate myelosuppression, severe nausea and vomiting, and a flu-like syndrome after large doses. The nausea and vomiting can be prevented and managed with available antiemetics and is not a major complication. At this time, there is no known role of dacarbazine in the adjuvant setting.

Temozolomide is one of a series of imidazoletetrazine derivatives that was developed as a potential alternative to dacarbazine. Temozolomide is a prodrug of the active metabolite of dacarbazine. Dacarbazine requires hepatic transformation to its active intermediate, whereas at physiologic pH, temozolomide chemically degrades to the cytotoxic triazene monomethyl 5-triazeno imidazole carboxamide. Temozolomide is administered orally and appears to be less emetogenic than dacarbazine. Temozolomide appears to cross into the central nervous system, and therefore was initially thought to have benefit for patients with CNS metastases. In chemotherapy-naïve individuals with metastatic melanoma, response rates for temozolomide are similar to those seen with dacarbazine.

The *nitrosoureas* have also been shown to be active against melanoma. Nitrosoureas, such as carmustine and lomustine, have antitumor activity similar to dacarbazine, with reported response rates between 10% and 20%. Sites of responses are similar to those seen with dacarbazine. It was initially thought that there may be an added benefit to the use of the lipophilic nitrosoureas in a malignancy that can metastasize to the brain. Unfortunately, despite the ability of these agents to cross the blood-brain barrier, the commercially available nitrosoureas have not been shown to produce an increased response in melanoma in the central nervous system. Fotemustine, a nitrosourea available in Australia and some European countries, appears to cross the blood-brain barrier more rapidly than other nitrosoureas. Response rates of 30% have been reported in previously untreated patients, with response rates of 25% of patients who had cerebral metastases. Fotemustine is considered standard therapy in some countries.[37] The most common toxicity of the nitrosoureas is delayed myelosuppression, particularly thrombocytopenia. Leukopenia and thrombocytopenia may be seen as long as 3 to 5 weeks after drug administration, and may limit the inclusion of these agents to multidrug regimens.

Cisplatin and related compounds have also been evaluated in the management of metastatic melanoma. The effectiveness of platinum compounds as single agents is limited, with response rates reported to be less than 10%. The toxicities of cisplatin can be problematic, and include acute and delayed nausea and vomiting, renal toxicity, and neurotoxicity.

TABLE 133–8. Combination Chemotherapy Regimens for Metastatic Melanoma

Dartmouth regimen (CDBT): repeated every 3–4 weeks
Cisplatin 25 mg/m^2 IV daily × 3 (days 1, 2, and 3)
Dacarbazine 220 mg/m^2 IV daily × 3 (days 1, 2, and 3)
Carmustine 150 mg/m^2 IV daily × 1 (day 1)
Tamoxifen 10 mg orally twice a day
CVD
Cisplatin 20 mg/m^2 IV daily × 4 (days 2, 3, 4, 5)
Vinblastine 1.6 mg/m^2 IV daily × 5 (days 1, 2, 3, 4, 5)
Dacarbazine 800 mg/m^2 IV daily × 1 (day 1)

Taxanes have demonstrated encouraging results in initial trials of metastatic melanoma but require further evaluation to warrant the toxicities commonly seen.

COMBINATION CHEMOTHERAPY

In an attempt to extend the efficacy seen with single agents, a variety of combination chemotherapy regimens (Table 133-8) have been evaluated in small and large clinical trials; response rates reported are as high as 30% to 50% in single-institution phase II trials in patients with metastatic melanoma. The combination of dacarbazine with other chemotherapy, most commonly cisplatin, has been able to increase the response rates reported with dacarbazine alone, but the survival benefit has been minimal. Again, responses were often limited to metastases in soft tissue, lymph nodes, and the lung—the sites most likely to respond to single-agent dacarbazine therapy. The concern with combination chemotherapy is increased toxicity, and any reports of an increase in response rates should be weighed against the effect of toxicities on overall quality of life. The initial reports with CVD regimen (cisplatin, vinblastine, and dacarbazine) were exciting; reported response rates were greater than 50% and were seen with acceptable toxicities. Comparisons of this regimen to dacarbazine alone have been conflicting. Initial studies indicated an increase in response rate, response duration, and survival benefit with the combination regimen. Subsequent reports showed no difference in response rates or survival.

The Dartmouth regimen is a combination chemotherapy regimen that includes carmustine, dacarbazine, cisplatin, and tamoxifen. Initial reports from uncontrolled phase II trials of this combination have demonstrated high response rates of 20% to 50%, but few patients achieve long-term survival. The benefit of tamoxifen to this regimen has been controversial, but a controlled clinical trial from the National Cancer Institute of Canada demonstrates no benefit in response or survival from tamoxifen in this combination.[38] Careful analysis of the initial studies demonstrates that the criteria used to measure response were not consistent with standards used in large multicenter studies. Phase III trials have shown no benefit for the Dartmouth regimen as compared to single-agent dacarbazine.[39,40] Response rates were 15%, and median survival was about 7 months in both studies. Of concern, toxicities were higher with the combination study and included bone marrow suppression, nausea, vomiting, and fatigue.

ENDOCRINE THERAPY

The role of endocrine therapy in the management of melanoma has been debated over the last decade. Initial reports that described high-affinity cytoplasmic estrogen receptors in patients with metastatic melanoma caused some experts to speculate about the possibility that antiestrogens or other hormonal manipulation may be beneficial to modulate the biology of melanoma. Additionally, estrogens have been shown to suppress T-lymphocyte activity and to suppress or stimulate the activities of B lymphocytes, macrophages, and natural killer cells, supporting a hypothesis that estrogens may influence the immunologic mechanisms that appear to be important in melanoma.

Tamoxifen was shown to have a response and survival benefit in a randomized trial when combined with dacarbazine in patients with metastatic melanoma; this benefit was most pronounced in women. Well designed prospective randomized studies demonstrate that tamoxifen does not significantly enhance the antitumor effect of dacarbazine alone or of the combination of dacarbazine with cisplatin and carmustine. As discussed previously, subsequent trials have not been able to confirm the initial reported benefit of the antiestrogen when combined with chemotherapy, and tamoxifen is no longer routinely included in chemotherapy regimens.

BIOCHEMOTHERAPY

Low overall response rates and toxicity have limited the routine use of chemotherapy alone or immunotherapy alone in the management of metastatic disease. Over the past decade, the strategy of a combination of chemotherapy and cytokines, aldesleukin and/or interferon, often termed *biochemotherapy*, has been a major focus of investigation in the management of metastatic melanoma and more recently in the adjuvant setting. The primary rationale is to combine two therapies with some biological activity to increase overall activity, and perhaps response rates. Additionally, some preclinical trials suggest potential synergistic interactions between cytokines and some chemotherapy agents. As with other treatment strategies in melanoma, the results from initial trials suggested a higher response rate with biochemotherapy than those seen with either chemotherapy or biotherapy alone. Although several studies have suggested an increase in response rate with the addition of interferon to chemotherapy, results of most studies show that the addition of interferon does not increase the antitumor effect of dacarbazine, but does increase toxicity and cost. Similarly, the combination of aldesleukin to chemotherapy has not been consistently shown to increase response or survival. The most encouraging results have been seen with combination chemotherapy and combination biotherapy, but the results of phase III studies have not demonstrated a clear advantage of biochemotherapy as compared to chemotherapy alone.[41] Results to date suggest response rates similar to or slightly better than those seen with dacarbazine alone, with increased toxicity. Toxicities can be severe, and are consistent with the individual agents in the regimen.

One of the problems seen in most studies of biochemotherapy is the relatively short duration of response. Recurrence rates among patients who do respond to therapy are as high as 50% within 18 to 24 months. Strategies such as subcutaneous low-dose interleukin-2 are being investigated in an effort to prolong overall survival and time to progression in the patients who do respond to treatment. The initial response rates, durable complete remission, and activity in those patients in which HDI therapy has failed has stimulated interest in evaluating biochemotherapy in the adjuvant setting for patients with high-risk node-positive patients as compared to HDI.

LIMB PERFUSION AND LIMB INFUSION

Isolated limb perfusion (ILP)[42,43] is a surgical procedure of regional intravascular delivery of chemotherapy and/or biotherapy into an extremity with cutaneous melanoma. ILP is a method to escalate the dose of chemotherapeutic drugs in a specific region of the body while limiting the systemic toxicities of the agent. The majority of perfusions can be performed with drug exposures of less than 2%. The most significant side effect of ILP is regional toxicity; all of the skin, subcutaneous tissue, and tissue of the extremity receives the same dose and is subjected to the same perfusion conditions as the tumor located within the extremity. After regional perfusions, objective response rates have been reported to exceed 50% in treated limbs and overall response rates may be as high as 80%. The role of hyperthermia (39° to 40°C) with regional isolated perfusion is not clearly defined. Although most clinical trials have used melphalan, it is not known whether the combination of melphalan with other agents may improve results. Agents that have been combined with melphalan include actinomycin D, nitrogen mustard, thiotepa, and cisplatin. Recent work with the biologic response modifiers, such as tumor necrosis factor-α, have been encouraging. A simplified form of ILP, called isolated limb infusion (ILI), is a low-flow ILP performed under hypoxic conditions via small caliber arterial and venous catheters. It has been proposed that the hypoxia that develops during ILI may be beneficial with certain cytotoxic agents such as melphalan.

PREVENTION AND DETECTION

The results of early treatment emphasize the role for early detection and prevention. The American Academy of Dermatology recommends monthly self-examination of skin to serve as a mechanism of recognizing moles or marks on the skin that may be melanoma. Patients with a strong family history should have a clinical examination, and in some cases, screening photography to document size, shape, and location of moles.

Education and re-education about the importance of sun protection has the potential to help decrease the rising incidence of this disease. Historically, patients have been counseled that the risk of skin cancer can be limited by the use of sunscreens with a sun protection factor (SPF) of 15 or greater. It is important to include counseling about the appropriate use of sunscreens to optimize benefits from these products. One study noted that most consumers typically apply less sunscreen than is needed to establish the SPF number on the bottle; the actual SPF received is 20% to 50% of that number.[44,45] Sunscreens should be applied 15 to 30 minutes before going into the sun, and should be reapplied every 2 hours, after swimming, and after perspiring heavily.

Sunscreen lotions are more efficient in protecting against shorter ultraviolet wavelengths that lead to sunburns, than in protecting against the longer wavelengths in the UVA range which may lead to skin damage and skin cancers such as melanoma. It is not clear what the impact of the use of high potency sunscreens will have on the incidence of melanoma, as the lag time for melanoma is about two decades and the high potency sunscreens have only been popular for about 10 years.

It is important to educate the public that sunscreens should not be used to increase time in the sun. The slogan, "Slip! Slop! Slap!" (slip on a shirt, slop on the sunscreen, and slap on a hat), initially

TABLE 133–9. Sunscreens

Physical Blockers (Reflectants)	Chemical Absorbers
Zinc oxide	Ultraviolet B absorbers
Talc	Salicylates
Titanium dioxide	Chinnamates
Red petrolatum	Campho derivatives
	Aminobenzoates
	Ultraviolet A absorbers
	Benzopehnone-6
	Dibenzoylmethanes

developed for public health campaigns in Australia, provides a more comprehensive approach to sun protection. Sun avoidance, especially during the peak hours of the sun intensity (10 AM to 4 PM), use of protective clothing and head coverings, and staying in the shade when outdoors are important education concepts for those individuals who are in the sun for prolonged periods of time and/or who are at high risk of burning (Table 133–9).[46]

EVALUATION OF THERAPEUTIC OUTCOMES

The outcome of patients treated with melanoma depends on the stage of disease at presentation. The prognosis of patients with thin tumors (<1 mm in thickness) and localized disease is good, with long-term survival in more than 90% of patients. There is risk of regional nodal involvement with increasing tumor thickness, and therefore survival rates decrease in patients with nodal involvement. Long-term survival in patients with distant metastases is even lower. Therefore early diagnosis and appropriate treatment of early disease is essential. Patients with suspicious pigmented lesions should be evaluated and have the lesion excised whenever possible. Treatment is determined by patient factors and stage of disease.

There is no clear recommendation regarding appropriate follow-up of patients with melanoma. Clinical practice guidelines published by the NCCN provide some guidance for follow-up of patients with melanoma.[25] Intensive surveillance has the benefit of early detection of recurrent disease, which may lead to better options of surgical resection. Emphasis on evaluation of locoregional areas is important. For patients with in situ melanoma periodic skin examinations for life are recommended, although frequency is determined based on patient risk factors. For patients with stage IA disease, comprehensive history and physical examination is recommended every 3 to 12 months, again based on individual patient risk factors. Individuals with stage IB to III melanoma should have history and physical examination every 3 to 6 months for 3 years; then every 4 to 12 months for 2 years; and annually thereafter. Patients with stage IV disease who are disease-free after treatment should be followed as outlined for patients with stage III disease.

Local recurrence is associated with aggressive tumor biology and is frequently a manifestation of an aggressive primary tumor. If a local recurrence occurs after inadequate primary disease, the patient should undergo a work-up based on the lesion thickness of the original melanoma. Patients with nodal recurrence should be evaluated for lymph node metastases. Patients with systemic recurrence should be evaluated and treated in a fashion similar to those patients presenting with systemic disease.

ABBREVIATIONS

AJCC: American Joint Committee on Cancer
bFGFs: basic fibroblast growth factors
CR: complete response
CTL: cytotoxic T lymphocyte
ECOG: Eastern Cooperative Oncology Group
FAMMS: familial atypical multiple mole syndrome
HDI: high-dose interferon
HDNS: hereditary dysplastic nevus syndrome
HLA: human leukocyte antigen
IL-2: interleukin-2
ILI: isolated limb infusion
ILP: isolated limb perfusion
LAK: lymphokine-activated killer (cell)
LDI: low-dose interferon
MAA: melanoma-associated antigen
NSAID: nonsteroidalanti-inflammatory drug
SPF: sun protection factor
TAA: tumor-associated antigen
TIL: tumor-infiltrating lymphocyte
UVA: ultraviolet A
UVB: ultraviolet B

Review Questions and other resources can be found at *www.pharmacotherapyonline.com*.

REFERENCES

1. Jemal A, Murray T, Ward E, et al. Cancer statistics, 2005. CA Cancer J Clin 2005;55:10–30.
2. Berwick M, Weinstock MA. Epidemiology current trends. In: Balch CM, Houghton AN, Sober AJ, Soong S, eds. Cutaneous Melanoma. St. Louis, Quality Medical Publishing, 2003:15–23.
3. Tsao H, Haluska FG. Genetics of skin cancer. In: Sober AJ, Haluska F, eds. American Cancer Society Atlas of Clinical Oncology Skin Cancer. Hamilton, Ontario, Canada, BC Decker, 2001:16–30.
4. Gallagher RP, Elwood JM, Yang P. Is chronic sunlight exposure important in accounting for increases in melanoma incidence? Int J Cancer 1989; 44:813–815.
5. Dore JF, Carrel S. Biology of melanoma differentiation and progression. In: Lejeune FJ, Chaudhuri PK, Das Gupta K, eds. Malignant Melanoma: Medical and Surgical Management. New York, McGraw-Hill, 1994: 9–26.
6. Bogenrieder T, Elder DE, Herlyn M. Molecular and cellular biology. In: Balch CM, Houghton AN, Sober AJ, Soong S, eds. Cutaneous Melanoma. St. Louis, Quality Medical Publishing, 2003:15–23.
7. Spitler LE, Grossbard ML, Ernstoff ME, et al. Adjuvant therapy of stage III and IV malignant melanoma using granulocyte-macrophage colony-stimulating factor. J Clin Oncol 2000;18:1614–1620.
8. Balch CM, Soong SJ, Buzaid AC, et al. The new melanoma staging system and factors predicting melanoma survival. Clin Oncol Update 2002;5:3. 1–19.
9. Clark WH Jr. A classification of malignant melanoma in man correlated with histogenesis and biologic behavior. In: Montagna W, Hu F, eds. Advances in Biology of the Skin. The Pigmentary System. London, Pergamon, 1967:621–645.
10. Breslow A. Thickness, cross-sectional areas and depth of invasion in the prognosis of cutaneous melanoma. Ann Surg 1970;172:1902–1908.
11. Halpern AC, Schuchter LM. Prognostic models in melanoma. Semin Oncol 1997;24(Suppl 4):2–7.

12. Balch CM, Buzaid AC, Soong SJ, et al. Final version of the American Joint Committee on cancer staging system for cutaneous melanoma. J Clin Oncol 2001;19:3635–3648.

13. Hoon DS, Wang Y, Dale PS, et al. Detection of occult melanoma cells in blood with a multiple-marker polymerase chain reaction assay. J Clin Oncol 1995;13:2109–2116.

14. Balch CM, Urist MM, Karakousis CP, et al. Efficiency of 2-cm surgical margins for intermediate-thickness melanomas (1–4 mm): Results of a multi-institutional randomized surgical trial. Ann Surg 1993;218:262–269.

15. Meirion Thomas K, Newton-Bishop J, A'Hern R, Coombes G, et al. Excision margins in high-risk malignant melanoma. N Engl J Med 2004;350:757–766.

16. Mos ME, Balch CM, Cascinelli N, Edwards MJ. Excision of primary melanoma. In: Balch CM, Houghton AN, Sober AJ, Soong S, eds. Cutaneous Melanoma. St. Louis, Quality Medical Publishing, 2003:209–230.

17. Kirkwood JM, Straderman MH, Ernstoff MS, et al. Interferon alfa-2b adjuvant therapy of high-risk resected cutaneous melanoma: The Eastern cooperative oncology group trial EST 1684. J Clin Oncol 1996;14:7–17.

18. Kirkwood JM, Manola J, Ibrahim J, Sondak V, Ernstoff MS, Rao U. A pooled analysis of Eastern Cooperative Oncology Group and Intergroup trials of adjuvant high-dose interferon for melanoma. Clin Cancer Res 2004;10:1670–1677.

19. Kirkwood JM, Ibrahim JG, Sondak VK, et al. High- and low-dose interferon alfa-2b in high risk melanoma: first analysis of intergroup trial E1690/S9111/C9190. J Clin Oncol 2000;18:2444–2458.

20. Kirkwood JM, Bender C, Agarwala S, et al. Mechanisms and management of toxicities associated with high-dose interferon alfa-2b therapy. J Clin Oncol 2002;20:3703–3718.

21. Dalakas MC, Mock V, Hawkins MJ. Fatigue: Definitions, mechanisms, and paradigms for study. Semin Oncol 1998;25(Suppl 1):48–53.

22. Plata-Salaman CR. Cytokines and anorexia: A brief overview. Semin Oncol 1998;25(Suppl 1):64–72.

23. Moschos SJ, Kirkwood JM. Present status and future prospects for adjuvant therapy of melanoma: Time to build upon the foundation of high-dose interferon alfa-2b. J Clin Oncol 2004;22:11–14.

24. Cole BF, Gelber RD, Kirkwood JM, et al. A quality-of-life-adjusted survival analysis of interferon alfa-2b adjuvant treatment for high-risk resected cutaneous melanoma: An Eastern cooperative oncology group study (E1684). J Clin Oncol 1996;14:2666–2673.

25. Houghton A, Coit D, Bloomer W, Buzaid A, et al. NCCN melanoma practice guidelines. National Comprehensive Cancer Network. J NCCN 2004;2:46–60.

26. Von Wussow P, Bock B, Hartmann F, Deicher H. Intralesional interferon-alpha therapy in advanced malignant melanoma. Cancer 1988;61:1071–1074.

27. Atkins MB, Lotze MT, Dutcher JP, et al. High-dose recombinant interleukin-2 therapy for patients with metastatic melanoma: analysis of 270 patients between 1985 and 1993. J Clin Oncol 1999;17:2105–2116.

28. Schwartz RN, Stover L, Dutcher J. Managing toxicities of high-dose interleukin-2. Oncology 2002;16(Suppl 13):11–20.

29. Agarwala SS, Glaspy J, O'Day SJ, et al. Results from a randomized phase III study comparing combined treatment with histamine dihydrochloride plus interleukin-2 versus interleukin-2 alone in patients with malignant melanoma. J Clin Oncol 2001;20:125–133.

30. O'Day SJ, Agarwala SS, Naredi P, Kass CL, et al. Treatment with histamine dihydrochloride and interleukin-2 in patients with advanced metastatic malignant melanoma: a detailed safety analysis. Melanoma Res 2003;13:307–311.

31. Conforti AM, Ollila DW, Kelley MC, et al. Update on active specific immunotherapy with melanoma vaccines. J Surg Oncol 1997;66:55–64.

32. Wolchok JD, Weber JS, Houghton AN, Livingston PO. Melanoma vaccines. In: Balch CM, Houghton AN, Sober AJ, Soong S. Cutaneous Melanoma. St. Louis, Quality Medical Publishing, 2003:645–656.

33. Sosman JA, Unger JM, Liu P, et al. Significant impact of HLA class I alleles on outcome in T3N0 melanoma patients with Melacine: An allogeneic melanoma cell lysate vaccine. Prospective analysis of Southwest Oncology Group 9035. Proceedings of ASCO 2001:351 (Abstract).

34. Morton DL, Foshag LJ, Hoon DS, et al. Prolongation of survival in metastatic melanoma after active specific immunotherapy with a new polyvalent melanoma vaccine. Ann Surg 1992;216:463.

35. Mirev BR. Melanoma vaccines. Semin Oncol 2002;29:479–493.

36. Bajetta W, Del Vecchio M, Bernard-Marty C, Viteli M, et al. Metastatic melanoma: chemotherapy. Semin Oncol 2002;29:427–445.

37. Jacquillat C, Khayat D, Banzet P, et al. Final report of the French multicenter phase II study of the nitrosourea fotemustine in 153 evaluable patients with disseminated malignant melanoma including patients with cerebral metastases. Cancer 1990;66:1873–1878.

38. Rusthoven JJ, Quirt IC, Iscoe NA, et al. Randomized, double-blind, placebo-controlled trial comparing the response rates of carmustine, dacarbazine, and cisplatin with and without tamoxifen in patients with metastatic melanoma. National Cancer Institute of Canada clinical trials group. J Clin Oncol 1996;14:2083–2090.

39. Chapman PB, Einhorn L, Meyeres ML, et al. Phase III multicenter randomized trial of the Dartmouth regimen versus dacarbazine in patients with metastatic melanoma. J Clin Oncol 1999;17:2745.

40. Middleton MR, Lorigan P, Owen J, et al. A randomized phase III study comparing dacarbazine, BCNU, cisplatin and tamoxifen with dacarbazine and interferon in advanced melanoma. Br J Cancer 2000;82:1158.

41. Atkins MB, Lee S, Flaherty LE, et al. A prospective randomized phase III trial of concurrent biochemotherapy with cisplatin, vinblastine, dacarbazine, interleukin-2 and interferon alpha-2b versus CVD alone in patients with metastatic melanoma (E3695): An ECOG-coordinated intergroup trial. Proc Am Soc Clin Oncol 2003;22:708 (Abstract 2847).

42. Rossi CR, Foletto M, Pilati P, Mocellin S, Lise M. Isolated limb perfusion in locally advanced cutaneous melanoma. Semin Oncol 2002;29:400–409.

43. Kroon BBR. Regional isolation perfusion in melanoma of the limbs; accomplishments, unsolved problems, future. Eur J Surg Oncol 1998;14:101–110.

44. Westerdahl J, Olsson H, Masback A, et al. Is the use of sunscreens a risk factor for malignant melanoma? Melanoma Res 1995;5:59–65.

45. Stokes R, Diffey B: How well are sunscreen users protected? Photodermatol Photoimmunol Photomec 1997;13:186–188.

46. Marks R, Hill D. Prevention of skin cancer. In: Sober AJ, Haluska FG, eds. American Cancer Society Atlas of Clinical Oncology Skin Cancer. Hamilton, Ontario, Canada, BC Decker, 2001:325–339.

134

HEMATOPOIETIC STEM CELL TRANSPLANTATION

Janelle B. Perkins and Gary C. Yee

Learning Objectives and other resources can be found at *www.pharmacotherapyonline.com.*

KEY CONCEPTS

1. Hematopoietic stem cell transplantation (HSCT) is a process that involves intravenous infusion of hematopoietic stem cells from a donor into a recipient, following the administration of chemotherapy with or without radiation. The rationale is to increase tumor cell kill by increasing the dose of chemotherapy. Immune-mediated effects may also contribute to the tumor cell kill observed after allogeneic HSCT.

2. Hematopoietic stem cells used for transplantation can come from the recipient (autologous) or from a related or unrelated donor (allogeneic). If the related donor is a twin, the transplant is referred to as a syngeneic transplant.

3. Human leukocyte antigen (HLA) mismatching of allogeneic donor-recipient pairs at either class I or class II loci correlates with the risk of graft failure, graft-versus-host disease (GVHD), and survival. The ideal donor is one that is matched at HLA-A, -B, -C, and DRB1.

4. Hematopoietic stem cells are found in the bone marrow, peripheral blood, and umbilical cord blood. Because of the rarity and similarity to other cells, hematopoietic stem cells are difficult to isolate and measure. These stem cells express the CD34 antigen, and the number of $CD34^+$ cells has become a clinically useful measure of the number of hematopoietic stem cells.

5. Due to clinical and economic advantages, peripheral blood has replaced bone marrow as the source of hematopoietic stem cells in the autologous HSCT setting. Peripheral blood stem cells are increasingly used in allogeneic HSCT.

6. The purpose of the preparative (or conditioning) regimen in traditional myeloablative transplants is two-fold: (1) maximal tumor cell kill and (2) immunosuppression of the recipient to reduce the risk of graft rejection (allogeneic HSCT only).

7. Posttransplant immunotherapy is based on the graft-versus-tumor (GVT) effect caused by certain subsets of T cells responsible for eradication of malignant cells. Posttransplant immunotherapy includes the use of donor lymphocyte infusions, immunomodulatory cytokines, monoclonal antibodies, or antitumor vaccines.

8. Reduced intensity or nonmyeloablative transplants have been developed in order to reduce early posttranslant morbidity and mortality while maximizing the GVT effect of the allogeneic graft. The advantage to this approach is that many patients who would otherwise not be eligible for allogeneic HSCT can now be offered a potentially curative therapy.

9. Transplant-related mortality associated with allogeneic HSCT ranges from 10% to 80% depending mostly on age, donor, and disease status. Major causes of death include infection, organ toxicity, and GVHD. The most common cause of death post–autologous HSCT is disease relapse; transplant-related mortality is usually less than 5%, depending on the conditioning regimen, age, and disease status.

10. Treatment of acute GVHD is often unsuccessful and the resulting complications can be fatal. Patients undergoing allogeneic HSCT are given prophylactic immunosuppressive therapy which inhibits T-cell activation and/or proliferation. The most commonly used GVHD prophylaxis regimens are cyclosporine or tacrolimus and methotrexate.

11. Treatment of chronic GVHD consists of prednisone alone, or alternate-day prednisone and either daily or alternate-day cyclosporine. Tacrolimus can be substituted for cyclosporine.

1. Hematopoietic stem cell transplantation (HSCT) is a process that involves intravenous infusion of hematopoietic stem cells from a compatible donor into a recipient, usually following administration of high-dose chemotherapy. Hematopoietic stem cells can be derived from the bone marrow, peripheral blood, or umbilical cord blood. The rationale for HSCT in the treatment of malignant disease is based on studies that show that most anticancer drugs have a steep dose-response relationship and that bone marrow suppression limits the chemotherapy dosage that can be safely administered. Although standard-dose chemotherapy can prolong survival in many cancer patients, most patients are not cured of their disease (Fig. 134–1). The infusion of hematopoietic stem cells allows oncologists to administer very high chemotherapy doses (as much as 10-fold higher). If tumor cells that are resistant to standard doses are sensitive to higher doses

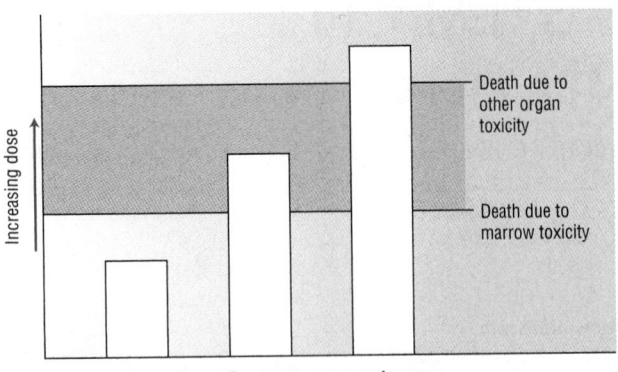

Window of opportunity for high-dose chemotherapy

FIGURE 134–1. Patients represented by the middle column are the best candidates for hematopoietic stem cell transplantation because this technique allows administration of chemotherapy or radiation in doses that would otherwise be intolerable due to severe myelosuppression.

of chemotherapy, then tumor cell kill will be greatly increased, and the likelihood of cure would be higher with HSCT. The chemotherapy dose cannot be escalated indefinitely, however, because of the risk of death caused by nonhematopoietic toxicity. The success and increasing use of nonmyeloablative transplants (NMT) shows that immune-mediated effects may also contribute to the tumor cell kill observed after allogeneic HSCT.

High-dose chemotherapy followed by HSCT has become an important treatment modality for a variety of malignant and nonmalignant diseases. Approximately 45,000 transplants are performed worldwide each year, primarily for malignant diseases.[1] About 40% of these transplants are performed in North America. The number of transplants has declined in recent years because of declining use for breast cancer (autologous) and chronic myelogenous leukemia (allogeneic).

Historically the most common type of donor was a genetically nonidentical individual such as a histocompatible sibling (referred to as allogeneic HSCT [alloHSCT]). But the number of autologous transplants—in which the patient serves as his or her own donor—has increased dramatically, and the number of autologous transplants (autoHSCT) performed (about 30,000) currently exceeds the number of alloHSCTs (about 15,000) performed each year.[1] Although this chapter focuses on the application of HSCT in the treatment of malignant disease, it is important to note that many nonmalignant diseases—including aplastic anemia, thalassemia, sickle cell anemia, immunodeficiency disorders, and other genetic disorders—are potentially curable with alloHSCT. Transplantation is also being investigated as a treatment modality in patients with life-threatening autoimmune diseases such as rheumatoid arthritis, systemic and multiple sclerosis, and systemic lupus erythematosus.

This chapter summarizes the procedures involved in HSCT, and current issues in the field of HSCT, as well as the application of HSCT in the treatment of malignant diseases. More detailed information on HSCT can be found in recently published reviews and books.[2–4] Information on HSCT can also be found on several Web sites (www.Bmtinfo.org, www.IBMTR.org, and www.Marrow.org).

DONORS AND HISTOCOMPATIBILITY TESTING

Different types of donors are used in HSCT. In *autologous* transplants, patients receive their own hematopoietic stem cells that were collected and stored before intensive cytotoxic therapy. In *syngeneic* transplants, an identical twin serves as the donor. In *allogeneic* transplants, the donor is genetically not identical to the recipient, but shares some common tissue antigens. Immunologic compatibility is evaluated with studies of cell surface antigens encoded by genes of the major histocompatibility complex (MHC), which is located on the sixth chromosome and is referred to as the HLA (human leukocyte antigen) complex.[5] The genes of the HLA system are clustered in three distinct regions designated as class I, class II, and class III. Class I and class II antigens function as major transplantation antigens, while products of class III genes play other important roles in the immune system. The major class I loci in humans are referred to as HLA-A, HLA-B, and HLA-C. There is one major class II locus (HLA-D); class II genes encode for the α and β polypeptide chains of the class II molecules. The designation of class II genes consists of three letters: the first (D) indicates the class, the second (M, O, P, Q, or R) the family, and the third (A or B) the chain (α and β, respectively). Class I and class II antigens differ in their tissue distribution, structure, and function. Class I antigens are expressed on virtually all nucleated cells and serve as the primary targets for cytotoxic T lymphocytes. In contrast, class II antigens are normally expressed only on macrophages, B lymphocytes, and activated T lymphocytes, and serve as the primary targets for helper T lymphocytes.

Historically, the most important HLA loci in alloHSCT were HLA-A, HLA-B, and HLA-D (or HLA-DR [D-related]). Typing for HLA-A, HLA-B, and HLA-DR has been traditionally performed by serologic typing with standard microcytotoxicity assays.[6] HLA types determined by this method are reported as the loci (A, B, or DR), followed by a number (e.g., HLA-A2). Typing for the HLA-D region also can be performed with cellular typing methods, such as the mixed lymphocyte reaction (MLR) or mixed lymphocyte culture (MLC). A "positive" MLR or MLC indicates incompatibility somewhere in the HLA-D region. Individuals who have a low degree of reactivity in the MLR or MLC (expressed as a low percentage of relative response), and who meet other selection criteria, could serve as donors. However, HSCT centers no longer use this method alone to determine HLA-D compatibility because studies show that MLR or MLC reactivity does not correlate significantly with the risk of acute graft-versus-host disease (GVHD) or graft failure.

Serologic methods detect *antigen* mismatches because they are based on the formation of alloantibodies against specific HLA antigens. However, any given HLA antigen can be encoded by a family of HLA alleles that differ by only a few amino acids. Over 100 alleles at HLA-A, 200 at HLA-B, and 50 at HLA-C have been identified in different human populations. The HLA class II DRB and DPB loci are extremely polymorphic, with over 200 DR alleles and over 75 DP alleles. Different alleles encoding the same antigen can be distinguished only by high-resolution (i.e., DNA-based) typing techniques such as polymerase chain reaction (PCR)-based techniques. As discussed later, these *allele* mismatches may have an adverse effect on patient outcome.

HLA mismatching at either class I and II loci correlates with the risk of graft failure, GVHD, and survival.[6] HLA *antigen* mismatches, particularly when they involve both class I and II antigens, are generally more important risk factors than *allele* mismatches. In an analysis of 1,876 patients who received matched unrelated donor (MUD) transplants under the auspices of the National Marrow Donor Program, high- or low-resolution mismatches at HLA-A, B, C, and DRB1 each had similar adverse effects on mortality.[7] Only HLA-A mismatches were associated with an increased risk of GVHD. However, among patients who received transplants from "6 antigen matched" (HLA-A, B, and DRB1 matched) donors, the number of allele mismatches correlated with the risk of grades III through IV acute GVHD and survival. The observation concerning the prognostic importance of HLA-C is particularly important, since this locus is omitted in most matching algorithms.

The most common donor for alloHSCT is an HLA-identical sibling. The odds that any one full sibling will match a patient are one in four. Only about 30% of Americans have an HLA-identical sibling. In an effort to offer alloHSCT to patients who lack an HLA-identical sibling donor, alternative donors are being used. Rarely, a parent can be HLA identical with his or her child. A relative can be a zero- (rare), one-, two-, or three-loci antigen mismatch (assuming testing for HLA-A, -B, and -DR antigens). It is estimated, however, that only an additional 10% of patients will have a closely HLA-matched related donor.

The most common type of alternative donor is an individual unrelated to the recipient who is fully or closely HLA matched. To facilitate identification of these donors, the National Marrow Donor Program (NMDP) was started in 1986 with initial funding from a U.S. Navy contract. To date, more than 5 million donors in the United States have been registered by the NMDP and the NMDP has facilitated more than 20,000 MUD transplants. About one-third of alloHSCTs performed worldwide are from unrelated donors. The NMDP currently requires that the selected donor and recipient are matched at HLA-A, -B, and -DRB1; low/intermediate resolution typing is required at HLA-A and -B, while high-resolution typing is required at DRB1. Since each patient has two phenotypes for each locus (one from each parent), matching is analyzed at six antigens (or alleles). Therefore, a "completely" matched (i.e., "6 of 6 match") unrelated donor is matched for HLA-A, -B, and -DR (or DRB1). A "closely" matched unrelated donor is usually incompatible at one HLA antigen. In addition to HLA-A, -B, and -DR (or DRB1), some NMDP transplant centers require additional testing for HLA-C (i.e., "8 of 8 match"). Based on the results of the recent study by Flomenberg and colleagues,[7] the NMDP plans to require HLA-C typing and high-resolution typing for all MUD transplants in the near future.

The ideal unrelated donor is an allele-matched donor at HLA-A, -B, -C, and DRB1 (i.e., "8 of 8 match"). However, given the extreme polymorphism of the HLA system, most patients who undergo matched unrelated donor HSCT will not have an allele-matched donor. Furthermore, the cost of conducting a search for an allele-matched donor would be prohibitive in most patients, and prolongation of the search process would increase the risk of relapse in patients with high-risk hematologic malignancies. The following guidelines should be used in unrelated donor selection: (1) assume that HLA-A, -B, -C, and DRB1 are equally important; (2) avoid antigen mismatches, if possible; (3) accept one allele mismatch over one antigen mismatch; and (4) minimize the number of allele mismatches.[8]

The likelihood of any one unrelated individual being a antigen-level match ranges from 1 in 100 to 1 in 1,000,000, depending on the prevalence of the patient's HLA type and ethnic background. With the current size of the NMDP registry, the matching likelihood is higher than 80% for Caucasians. Because most minorities are not as well represented in the program as whites, the likelihood of finding a donor for patients from certain ethnic groups is lower. Another limitation is the time needed to search for a potential donor. The average length of time from donor search to transplant is 3 to 4 months. Many patients with acute leukemia may relapse while waiting for completion of the search. Cost is also a concern, as the cost for donor search and marrow procurement ranges from $25,000 to $50,000. About two-thirds of MUD transplants are performed in patients with some form of leukemia, with chronic myelogenous leukemia (CML) being the most common diagnosis.

The clinical results of alloHSCT with alternative donors are encouraging. Although some patients who receive hematopoietic stem cells from an alternative donor are probably cured of their disease, the risk of transplant-related mortality is high. In a study of nearly 3,000 patients with chronic myelogenous leukemia treated with alloHSCT, transplant-related mortality was significantly higher after alternative donor transplants than after HLA-identical sibling transplants.[9] The difference in mortality was primarily related to a higher risk of graft failure and acute GVHD. Improved methods in HLA matching and supportive care have led to improved outcomes over the past few years.[6] Results of a recent study showed that patients with chronic myelogenous leukemia who received matched (6 of 6) unrelated donor transplants while in the early chronic phase (i.e., within 1 year from diagnosis) had similar disease-free survival as those who received matched sibling transplants.[9] When transplant was delayed beyond 1 to 2 years, however, outcome for the MUD transplants was worse than for those who received matched sibling transplants.

Allogeneic HSCT from a matched sibling or unrelated donor is not an option for some patients. In those cases, relatives who are partially HLA matched (i.e., mismatched) can serve as donors. About 10% of alloHSCTs are performed from related donors who are partially HLA matched. Although some patients who receive transplants from mismatched related donors experience long-term survival, the risks of graft failure and acute GVHD are higher than those for recipients of matched-sibling transplants.[10]

COLLECTION OF HEMATOPOIETIC STEM CELLS

Hematopoietic stem cells serve as "mother" cells for all blood cells including erythrocytes, leukocytes, and platelets (see Chap. 98).[11] Stem cells have varying degrees of "stemness"; true *pluripotent* stem cells are capable of replicating indefinitely and can give rise to stem and progenitor cells of *all* tissues. *Multipotent* stem cells, like the hematopoietic stem cell, have the capacity for self-renewal and can differentiate into more than one cell type in a particular tissue lineage. Because of their capacity for self-renewal, hematopoietic stem cells are capable of repopulating the marrow of the recipient.

Hematopoietic stem cells are rare cells, comprising less than 0.01% of all bone marrow cells. It is extremely difficult to isolate and measure stem cells quantitatively because of their rarity and their similarity in appearance to other cells. For these reasons, surrogate markers are used to measure the number of stem cells. Measurement of the number of cells expressing the CD34 antigen (CD34+ cells), as determined by flow cytometry, has become the standard method of measuring hematopoietic stem cell content.[12] CD34 is an antigen expressed on hematopoietic stem cells and other early progenitor cells.

Hematopoietic stem cells are found in the bone marrow, peripheral blood, and umbilical cord blood. Hematopoietic stem cells from the bone marrow are obtained by multiple aspirations from the anterior and posterior iliac crests while the donor is under general anesthesia. The procedure takes about an hour and yields 200 to 1,500 mL, depending on the size of the donor. The marrow is transferred into tissue culture medium containing preservative-free heparin. The pooled marrow is then passed through a series of stainless steel screens to break up aggregated particles, resulting essentially in a single-cell suspension. In alloHSCT, the marrow stem cells are given to the recipient within 12 to 24 hours after harvest. In autoHSCT, the marrow is frozen and stored until needed. After intravenous infusion, the marrow stem cells enter the systemic circulation and find their way to the bone marrow cavity, where they reseed and grow in the bone marrow microenvironment. Although the donor experiences local soreness for a few days, the procedure is usually well tolerated, with no delayed complications resulting from the marrow aspiration. The major risk of serving as a marrow donor is that of undergoing general anesthesia.

Hematopoietic stem cells in peripheral blood (peripheral blood progenitor cells [PBPCs] or stem cells [PBSCs]) are found in the mononuclear fraction of white blood cells (lymphocytes and monocytes) and are collected by a procedure called *leukapheresis (or apheresis)*. In this outpatient procedure, about 9 to 14 liters of blood are processed over several hours during each daily leukapheresis session. Most of the blood cells are returned to the donor, and each leukapheresis yields approximately 200 mL of cells.

The number of hematopoietic stem cells that circulate in peripheral blood is normally too low for this approach to be technically feasible. Without mobilization techniques, at least six leukaphereses are usually required to collect a sufficient number of PBSCs. Several methods have been used clinically to mobilize hematopoietic stem cells from the bone marrow into peripheral blood.[12-15] The first is to give chemotherapy, which can briefly increase the number of PBSCs as much as 100-fold. The second and most common method is to administer a recombinant hematopoietic growth factor such as granulocyte colony-stimulating factor (G-CSF; filgrastim) or granulocyte macrophage-colony stimulating factor (GM-CSF; sargramostim). Although both agents are FDA-approved for this indication, G-CSF is the most commonly used growth factor. Commonly used dosages are 5 to 16 mcg/kg per day for G-CSF and 250 mcg/m^2 per day for GM-CSF. The combination of chemotherapy followed by a hematopoietic growth factor increases the number of PBSCs to a greater extent than either method alone. This approach is more expensive and is associated with more adverse effects than a growth factor alone, but the number of leukaphereses is reduced, and the additional chemotherapy may further reduce the tumor burden before transplantation. With current mobilization techniques, most HSCT centers collect sufficient PBSCs with three or fewer leukaphereses. Figure 134-2 shows representative schemas for mobilization and collection of PBSCs.

Several studies show that the number of CD34$^+$ cells infused correlates significantly with the rate of neutrophil and platelet recovery after high-dose chemotherapy.[12-14] Rapid neutrophil recovery is usually observed in patients who receive at least 2 × 10^6 CD34$^+$ cells/kg (body weight of recipient). More rapid platelet recovery is observed when at least 5 × 10^6 CD34$^+$ cells/kg are transplanted as compared to lower cell doses. As a result, most transplant centers currently use 2 × 10^6 CD34$^+$ cells/kg as a minimum number to collect for autologous transplant, with 5 × 10^6 CD34$^+$ cells/kg as an optimal target. Some studies suggest that there are clinical and economic benefits associated with infusion of higher CD34$^+$ cell doses.[16,17] Although the difference in the *median* number of days to neutrophil or platelet recovery is usually no more than 1 to 2 days in patients who receive more than 5 × 10^6 CD34$^+$ cells/kg as compared to those who receive less than 5 × 10^6 CD34$^+$ cells/kg, fewer patients who receive more

than 5 × 10^6 CD34$^+$ cells/kg have delayed engraftment. This small effect may be important, because patients with delayed engraftment consume a disproportionate share of health care resources such as additional transfusions, hospital days, and drugs (e.g., antibiotics and growth factors).

The optimal regimen to mobilize PBSCs is not clear.[13-15] Results of some randomized studies show that G-CSF alone provides higher yields of CD34$^+$ cells as compared with GM-CSF alone.[15] Higher doses of G-CSF or twice-daily administration of G-CSF may also mobilize more CD34$^+$ cells. Many cytokines and other novel agents, given either alone or in combination with G-CSF, are being evaluated for use in mobilization regimens.[14,15]

CLINICAL CONTROVERSY

Multiple regimens exist for mobilization of peripheral blood stem cells. Most centers use G-CSF alone, but some centers use a combination of G-CSF and GM-CSF. The optimal dose of the hematopoietic growth factor is not known. Some centers use chemotherapy in combination with G-CSF or GM-CSF, depending on their disease status. The choice of a secondary mobilization strategy is also controversial.

In some otherwise-eligible transplant candidates, an optimal number of CD34$^+$ cells will not be obtained with standard mobilization methods. Risk factors associated with poor mobilization include the amount (greater than six cycles) and type of prior chemotherapy (alkylating agents) and prior radiation therapy.[13-15] Older age is also associated with poor mobilization in some studies. Several strategies have been evaluated to overcome the obstacle of poor mobilization: remobilization with the same or higher doses of the same hematopoietic growth factor, a combination of hematopoietic growth factors, or a combination of chemotherapy and a hematopoietic growth factor. Bone marrow harvest is also an option, but is often of limited value.

The use of peripheral blood instead of bone marrow as a source of hematopoietic stem cells offers several advantages. The most clinically important advantage is that patients who receive mobilized PBSCs experience more rapid hematopoietic engraftment.[18,19] Although engraftment of all lineages is more rapid when PBSCs are used, the most significant effect is observed with platelet recovery. Patients who receive mobilized PBSCs experience platelet recovery as much as 2 to 3 weeks earlier than those who receive bone marrow stem cells. Another advantage is that the donor does not experience the discomfort associated with marrow aspirations and is not exposed to the risk associated with general anesthesia. Also, PBSCs may be less likely to be contaminated with malignant cells compared with marrow stem cells. Finally, because PBSCs are collected from the mononuclear cell fraction, a fraction that also contains immunocompetent cells (e.g., natural killer cells and T lymphocytes), some investigators believe that infusion of PBSCs may represent a form of "adoptive immunotherapy." In this model, natural killer cells and lymphocytes targeted against tumor cells help to kill residual tumor cells.

Although studies have not reported a significant difference in disease-free survival between patients who receive mobilized PBSCs and those who receive bone marrow, the use of mobilized PBSCs is associated with other clinical and economic benefits. Patients who receive mobilized PBSCs require fewer platelet transfusions and are usually discharged earlier from the hospital.[18,19] In an economic analysis of a randomized controlled trial, Smith and colleagues reported that the total average cost of a PBSC transplant was $13,521 lower than that of bone marrow transplant (BMT) ($45,792 versus $59,314).[20] At transplant centers with intensive clinic support, patients are able

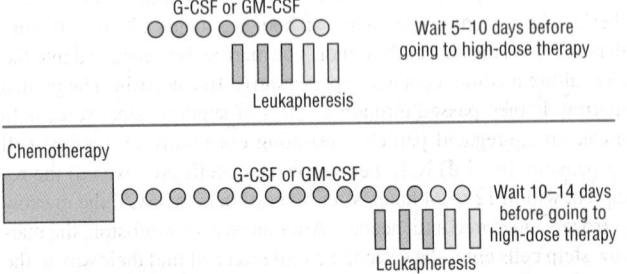

FIGURE 134–2. Schema for collection of PBPCs after hematopoietic growth factor administration (*top*) or after chemotherapy and hematopoietic growth factor administration (*bottom*). Symbols with gray shading represent procedures done only if adequate numbers of CD34$^+$ cells have not been collected.

to receive much of their posttransplant care as an outpatient, further reducing the cost of HSCT.[21] As a result of these clinical and economic advantages, peripheral blood has replaced bone marrow as the source of stem cells in the autologous setting.

Peripheral blood is increasingly being used as a source of hematopoietic stem cells in alloHSCT.[22,23] About 50% of the alloHSCTs performed currently come from PBSCs harvested from normal donors. This is despite early concerns that the increased numbers of T lymphocytes found in peripheral blood could increase the risk of GVHD. Concerns were also raised over the safety and ethics of administering G-CSF to normal individuals volunteering as donors. G-CSF is generally well-tolerated. Short-term effects are similar to those seen in cancer patients (e.g., bone pain, headache, fever, arthralgias, and malaise). Because the potential long-term effects related to G-CSF are unknown, careful follow-up of donors is recommended.

Randomized controlled trials show that patients who received allogeneic PBSC transplants from HLA-identical siblings experienced more rapid hematopoietic recovery and required fewer transfusions as compared to patients receiving BMT.[22,23] The difference in the rate of engraftment may be related to the threefold higher numbers of CD34[+] cells infused in recipients of PBSC transplants. Although most of these studies did not report an increased risk of acute GVHD or transplant-related mortality in patients receiving allogeneic PBSC transplants, a higher incidence of chronic GVHD was observed. In a meta-analysis of published reports, the risk of chronic GVHD was about 50% higher for patients who received allogeneic PBSC transplants as compared to those who received BMT.[24] Some studies have reported a correlation between the CD34[+] cell dose and the risk of chronic GVHD, which suggests that the higher CD34[+] cell dose may explain, in part, the increased risk of chronic GVHD.[25] Use of PBSCs from unrelated donors is also being investigated.[23] About 25% of the matched unrelated transplants coordinated by the NMDP use PBSCs.

In addition to bone marrow and peripheral blood, hematopoietic stem cells are also found in umbilical cord blood (UCB). UCB is an attractive source for several reasons. Because the stem cells are collected from placental blood, there is no risk to the mother or the baby. There is also very low risk of transmissible infectious diseases such as cytomegalovirus and Epstein-Barr virus. In addition, the cells are available immediately because the donor does not have to be located and harvested. Initially, UCB was obtained from siblings but now recipients of transplants from unrelated donors account for almost all patients who receive UCB transplants. It is estimated that more than 2,000 unrelated UCB transplants have been performed worldwide.[26]

Results of uncontrolled studies show that recipients of UCB transplantation have a lower risk of GVHD but a higher risk of graft failure as compared with recipients of BMT.[26] Recipients of UCB transplantation usually receive a CD34[+] cell dose more than 1 log lower than that given to recipients of BMT, and this difference in CD34[+] cell dose may explain the delayed engraftment in recipients of UCB transplantation. In one study, the number of infused CD34[+] cells correlated with the rate of engraftment, transplant-related mortality, and survival.[27] Although no randomized comparisons have been performed, a matched-pair analysis showed similar survival in children who underwent either unrelated UCB transplantation or BMT.[28]

A major limitation to UCB transplants is the limited volume of blood collected, usually 60 to 150 mL. Although the relatively low numbers of hematopoietic cells may be adequate for hematopoietic engraftment in children and small adults, it may not be adequate for larger recipients. Efforts to expand the number of hematopoietic stem cells include culturing them ex vivo with combinations of hematopoietic growth factors, or "pooling" several units of UCB for one recipient. Preliminary results with unrelated UCB transplants in adult recipients are encouraging,[26,29] but more experience is needed with adult recipients before this procedure can be recommended as a standard procedure in that population.

UCB represents an alternative source of hematopoietic stem cells in children and some adults who do not have a HLA-matched sibling donor.[26,29] As discussed above, UCB has some advantages over bone marrow stem cells. In addition, the time required to identify and obtain cells from an unrelated UCB donor is usually less than 1 month, which is significantly shorter than that required for an unrelated marrow donor. Therefore a UCB graft may be advantageous for patients who require an urgent transplant.

APPROACHES TO ERADICATE MALIGNANT CELLS

PRETRANSPLANT CHEMOTHERAPY OR CHEMORADIOTHERAPY

Nearly all patients who receive HSCT must be prepared (or "conditioned") before infusion of hematopoietic stem cells.[30] In patients with malignant disease, the goal of the preparative or conditioning regimen is to kill as many malignant cells as possible. Preparative regimens usually include commonly used anticancer drugs given at very high doses—doses that would be associated with severe and life-threatening bone marrow suppression if hematopoietic stem cells were not infused. In patients undergoing alloHSCT, another purpose of the preparative regimen is to suppress the immune system of the recipient so that the graft is not rejected.

In some preparative regimens, the only drug given is cyclophosphamide, a drug with both immunosuppressive and cytotoxic effects. Because of the inadequate antitumor activity of cyclophosphamide in some types of cancers, other drugs are often added. Examples of drugs that often are included in preparative regimens are cytarabine (ara-C), busulfan, thiotepa, etoposide (VP-16), carboplatin, cisplatin, carmustine (BCNU), melphalan, and ifosfamide.[30]

Total body irradiation (TBI) is also commonly used in pretransplant preparative regimens, particularly in patients with leukemia.[31] In patients with malignant disease, the rationale is to eradicate malignant cells located in areas inaccessible to the systemic circulation, and thus to the cytotoxic agents. TBI also has significant immunosuppressive activity. Historically, the standard TBI regimen involved the administration of a midline tissue dose of about 1000 cGy (1 cGy = 1 rad), which is more than twice the lethal dose of radiation for a normal person. Many centers currently give fractionated (split over several days, once or twice a day) rather than single-dose TBI to patients with malignant disease. The rationale for this approach is an improved therapeutic ratio—destruction of more leukemic cells and marrow stem cells while sparing other normal tissues. The acute toxicities of TBI consist of fever, nausea, vomiting, diarrhea, mucositis, and tender swelling of the parotid gland. Long-term complications of TBI-containing regimens include cataract formation, growth retardation, carcinogenesis, permanent reproductive sterility, and secondary malignancies.

LEUKEMIA

Most patients with leukemia undergoing alloHSCT receive either cyclophosphamide and TBI (CyTBI) or busulfan and cyclophosphamide (BuCy). When given with TBI, cyclophosphamide is usually given first, as two 60-mg/kg per day doses, followed by TBI. TBI can be given as a single dose or fractionated over several days. One variation of that regimen is to give hyperfractionated TBI first, followed by cyclophosphamide. In that regimen, which is primarily used in patients with acute lymphoblastic leukemia (ALL), 11 TBI doses of 120 cGy are given; doses are given three times a day on days –7 to –5 (day 0 is designated as the day of transplant), and twice a day on the last day (day –4). After TBI, two doses of cyclophosphamide are given intravenously once a day at a dosage of 60 mg/kg on days –3 and –2.

Because of the many acute and chronic toxicities of TBI, it would be advantageous to omit it from the preparative regimen. One widely used preparative regimen that does not include TBI is BuCy. In the original regimen (BuCy4), busulfan was given orally at a dosage of 1 mg/kg every 6 hours (4 mg/kg per day) for 16 doses on days –9 to –6, followed by four doses of cyclophosphamide, given intravenously once daily at a dosage of 50 mg/kg on days –5 to –2. In one widely used modification of that regimen (BuCy2), the total cyclophosphamide dosage is reduced from 200 (50 × 4) to 120 (60 × 2) mg/kg. Plasma busulfan concentrations are monitored at some centers because some studies suggest that systemic exposure may correlate with outcome,[32] and the use of a targeted busulfan and cyclophosphamide preparative regimen may improve patient outcome.[33] An intravenous form of busulfan is also available commercially (Busulfex), which reduces some of the interpatient variability in systemic exposure.[34] The use of intravenous busulfan may also reduce the risk of hepatic veno-occlusive disease. The dose of IV busulfan approved for pretransplant conditioning regimens is 0.8 mg/kg every 6 hours for 4 days. Once-a-day dosing regimens have also been developed, which may facilitate outpatient administration of intravenous busulfan.

Several prospective randomized studies have compared CyTBI to BuCy in patients with acute or chronic myelogenous leukemia undergoing alloHSCT.[35–37] The results of these studies show that BuCy has similar or greater antileukemic activity in patients with CML than CyTBI. But in patients with acute myelogenous leukemia (AML), some studies suggest that the CyTBI regimen was associated with slightly better disease-free survival rates than BuCy. However, none of the patients who were randomized to BuCy in these studies received busulfan doses adjusted on the basis of plasma concentrations. In children with ALL, a retrospective study showed higher survival in children who received CyTBI as a preparative regimen.[38] Long-term toxicities appear to be comparable between the two regimens.

Other drugs have been evaluated in addition to or instead of cyclophosphamide in the preparative regimen.[30,37] Examples include cytarabine or etoposide in combination with TBI. There are no convincing data to indicate that any of these regimens are superior to CyTBI or BuCy. The same preparative regimens are usually given to patients undergoing autoHSCT for leukemia.

LYMPHOMA

Based on experience in patients with leukemia, the initial regimen used in many patients with Hodgkin's and non-Hodgkin's lymphoma was CyTBI, particularly in alloHSCT. Most preparative regimens currently used in autoHSCT for lymphoma include an alkylating agent (either cyclophosphamide or melphalan), carmustine, and etoposide.[30,39] TBI is usually not included in the conditioning regimen because many patients with lymphoma have received prior radiotherapy. One widely used regimen in autoHSCT is the CBV regimen, which consists of cyclophosphamide, carmustine (BCNU), and etoposide (VP-16). In that original regimen, cyclophosphamide was given at a dosage of 1.5 g/m² on days –6 to –3, carmustine was given at a dosage of 300 mg/m² on day –6, and etoposide was given at a

dosage of 100 mg/m² every 12 hours for six doses on days –6 to –4. Some centers have modified the original CBV regimen by changing the dosage of some of the drugs or adding or substituting other drugs including cytosine arabinoside, etoposide, melphalan, lomustine, and thioguanine. Other widely used nitrosourea-based regimens are BEAC (BCNU, etoposide, ara-C, and cyclophosphamide) and BEAM (BCNU, etoposide, ara-C, and melphalan). No one preparative regimen has been shown to be clearly superior to other regimens in the treatment of lymphoma.

Although TBI is usually not included in the conditioning regimen, some form of radiation therapy is often given, depending on the type, location, and extent of disease. Instead of TBI, some patients receive localized radiation in high doses to areas of residual or bulky disease. Many patients with Hodgkin's lymphoma have received thoracic radiation as primary therapy for their disease, so TBI is usually avoided in patients with Hodgkin's lymphoma. Conversely, most patients with indolent non-Hodgkin's lymphoma receive TBI as part of their preparative regimen because of the known sensitivity of these tumors to low doses of radiation.[40]

One of the disadvantages of TBI is that it delivers as much radiation to normal organs as it does to tumor cells. The availability of anti-CD20 radiolabeled monoclonal antibodies offers the potential to deliver more radiation to tumor cells and less to normal organs. In these trials, ^{131}I-tositumomab was given, either alone or combined with high-dose cyclophosphamide and etoposide, with autoHSCT in patients with non-Hodgkin's lymphoma.[41,42] With this approach, very high radiation doses could be delivered to sites of disease. Preliminary results with this approach are encouraging.[43]

SOLID TUMORS

Most conditioning regimens in autoHSCT include at least one alkylating agent because of their steep dose-response curve and other favorable characteristics previously discussed.[30] Many regimens include more than one alkylating agent, based on preclinical studies that show that resistance to a specific alkylating agent does not impart cross-resistance to other alkylating agents. Other anticancer drugs that modulate the activity of alkylating agents in a synergistic manner, such as etoposide, are also attractive drugs to include in high-dose preparative regimens. The dose of nonalkylating agents with antitumor activity has also been escalated in patients with solid tumors based on tumor-specific activity. Examples include mitoxantrone, paclitaxel, and topotecan. It is not clear whether these regimens offer any clinical advantages over those that include only alkylating agents.

PURGING THE STEM CELL PRODUCT

One disadvantage of autoHSCT is that the stem cell product (graft) may be contaminated with malignant cells. Infusion of these malignant cells may contribute to tumor relapse. Many approaches have been developed to eliminate ("purge") the marrow of these tumor cells.[44] The most common approach is to add substances, such as chemicals or monoclonal antibodies, to the stem cell product while it is outside of the body (ex vivo) (Fig. 134–3). Because the substances are removed before infusion of the stem cells, nonhematopoietic tissues are not exposed to the substances and therefore are not damaged. However, these substances can remove or damage hematopoietic stem cells, which are essential for complete and rapid engraftment, and purging has been associated with a delay in marrow recovery. Ex vivo marrow purging is also performed in alloHSCT in an attempt to eliminate T lymphocytes believed to be responsible for acute GVHD (see

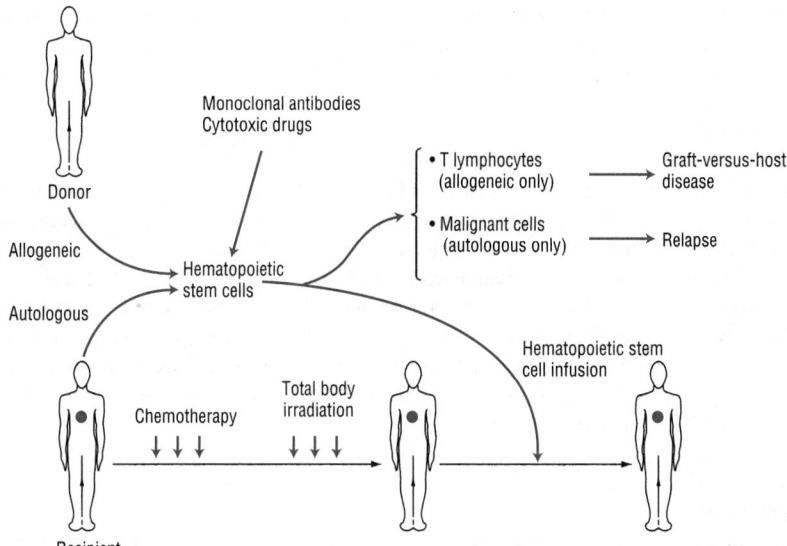

FIGURE 134–3. The use of ex vivo marrow purging to remove or destroy T cells (allogeneic only) or residual malignant cells (autologous only).

Fig. 134–3). Results with this approach are discussed below in the GVHD section.

One approach is to add one or more monoclonal antibodies that are directed against specific antigens present on the tumor cells, but which are absent on nearly all other cells.[42,45] Although this approach is theoretically attractive, it is limited because not all cells from patients with the same type of cancer will express a specific antigen. Furthermore, for some types of cancers, it has been difficult to identify antigens distinct from those present on normal hematopoietic stem cells. To date, this strategy has been used most commonly in patients with lymphoid malignancies, either ALL or non-Hodgkin's lymphoma.

Another method of ex vivo purging is to add chemicals or drugs to kill the tumor cells.[46] The advantage of this technique is that it can be used for a broader range of tumor types. However, chemical purging is not completely selective for tumor cells, and it is therefore important to add the precise amount of chemical or drug that kills sufficient numbers of tumor cells while sparing the largest number of hematopoietic stem cells. The chemical that is most commonly used for purging is 4-hydroperoxycyclophosphamide (4-HC, or perfosfamide), a congener of cyclophosphamide. A stable compound, 4-HC enters cells and is rapidly reduced to 4-hydroxycyclophosphamide, which serves as the precursor to the reactive phosphoramide mustard. The level of aldehyde dehydrogenase, the enzyme that inactivates 4-hydroxycyclophosphamide, appears to be highest in early hematopoietic progenitors and decreases as these cells differentiate. This observation may explain why 4-HC appears to have an acceptable therapeutic index. Other analogs of cyclophosphamide (e.g., mafosfamide) also are being investigated as chemical purging agents.

Another method to purge malignant cells is to identify, select, and concentrate hematopoietic stem cells, a process known as positive selection.[44] In this process, cells collected from marrow or peripheral blood are treated ex vivo with monoclonal antibodies against CD34. CD34+ cells are therefore separated from those that are CD34−, including most malignant cells. Although a randomized study showed that one of these techniques reduced the number of tumor cells by 1.6 to 6 (median 3.1) logs, no significant difference in disease-free or overall survival rate was observed.[47]

Although ex vivo purging has been extensively studied, there is a lack of convincing evidence that it improves transplant outcomes.

Since these techniques can be cumbersome and add cost to the transplant procedure, their use should be restricted to clinical trials.

Rituximab has been used pretransplant for in vivo purging of the stem cell graft prior to autoHSCT in patients with non-Hodgkin's lymphoma.[40,42] When used for in vivo purging, rituximab is usually given before each leukapheresis. Although the use of rituximab was effective in reducing the number of tumor cells in the stem cell graft, it is not clear whether this approach improves disease-free survival after autoHSCT.

POSTTRANSPLANT IMMUNOTHERAPY

The rationale for posttransplant immunotherapy is based on observations that certain subsets of T cells are responsible for the eradication of malignant cells. This is referred to as the graft-versus-leukemia (GVL) or graft-versus-tumor (GVT) effect. Evidence for GVL is based on retrospective studies that show that patients who developed graft-versus-host disease (GVHD) had a lower risk of leukemic relapse than those who did not develop GVHD.[48] But the overall survival rate was no different because of the increased non-relapse mortality associated with GVHD. Other anecdotal evidence supporting a T-cell mediated GVL effect was the increased risk of relapse found with T-cell-depleted transplants as compared to unmodified transplants, and the difference in relapse rates between recipients of syngeneic and HLA-identical sibling transplants.

DONOR LYMPHOCYTE INFUSIONS

Perhaps the most commonly used form of posttransplant immunotherapy is infusions of donor lymphocytes to treat disease relapse after alloHSCT.[49,50] Lymphocytes are collected from the same donor who provided hematopoietic stem cells. Most of the experiences with donor lymphocyte (or leukocyte) infusion (DLI) have been for patients with CML. More than 80% of patients who are in cytogenetic or molecular relapse respond to DLI. The response rate is slightly lower in chronic phase relapse, whereas the response rates in more advanced phases are about 15% to 30%. Although the time to response is delayed (median of 3 to 4 months), patients often have a durable molecular remission to DLI.

Response rates to DLI in patients with other myeloid malignancies, such as AML and myelodysplasia, are generally lower (25% to 30%) than those seen in CML.[49,51] This may be related to the rapid proliferation of acute leukemia versus the often prolonged time to response after DLI or to the lack of suitable target antigens on non-CML cells for recognition by donor cytotoxic T cells. Patients with AML are more likely to achieve a complete response to DLI post-HSCT if they have had a longer remission period after transplant and if they have had some GVHD after the DLI.[49,52] Administration of induction chemotherapy prior to DLI may improve the antitumor activity of DLI in patients with AML, but this has not been tested in a randomized study. DLI has been shown to have limited benefit in patients with relapsed ALL after transplant.

DLI appears to be effective in patients with multiple myeloma who relapse after alloHSCT, with reported response rates of 40% to 50% in patients relapsing after transplant.[49,51] Unfortunately, these responses tend to be transient and associated with the occurrence of GVHD. Anecdotal evidence suggests a graft-versus-lymphoma effect in patients with indolent non-Hodgkin's lymphoma and chronic lymphocytic leukemia (a disease entity that is closely related to the indolent non-Hodgkin's lymphomas).

The most serious complications of DLI are pancytopenia and GVHD. The cytopenias are generally transient and can be treated with hematopoietic growth factors. A small percentage of patients may have a more prolonged course of aplasia with associated risk of infection, bleeding, and anemia. Another infusion of donor stem cells may be beneficial in these patients. Acute GVHD (grade II or greater) occurs in 40% to 60% of those receiving DLI, and while the severity of GVHD has been correlated with GVL, complete responses have been seen in the absence of GVHD, suggesting that the effects can be separated. DLI is associated with 10% to 15% nonrelapse mortality at 1 year.

Because of the large potential of DLI as curative therapy for some patients with certain hematologic malignancies, investigators are evaluating strategies to separate the GVL effect from the GVH effect, thus making DLI more tolerable. Others are developing methods that would expand the efficacy of DLI to other malignancies. Some of these strategies include T-cell depletion from the stem cells followed by delayed T-cell add-back transplant for patients with evidence of residual disease around 3 months posttransplant; selective depletion

of CD8$^+$ cells from the DLI; in vivo or in vitro T-cell activation with interleukin-2; or infusion of T cells that are selected to recognize tumor-specific antigens.[49,51]

IMMUNOMODULATORY CYTOKINES

Another approach to induce a GVT effect in patients who relapse following HSCT is to administer a cytokine posttransplant with immunomodulatory activity, such as interleukin-2 (IL-2).[48,53,54] Some beneficial effects have been observed with the use of IL-2 with respect to effects on natural killer cells and other important antitumor immune responses. Toxicities have been tolerable in most patients but can be serious and life-threatening. Studies are necessary to define the role of these cytokines in prolonging relapse-free survival after HSCT.

MONOCLONAL ANTIBODIES

Rituximab is being evaluated as adjuvant therapy in patients with non-Hodgkin's lymphoma treated with autoHSCT.[42,55] The timing and number of doses of rituximab therapy varies. A recently published study by the Stanford program reported promising results with two 4-week courses starting at day 42 and 6 months posttransplant.[55] Neutropenia was observed in about 50% of the patients treated.

NONMYELOABLATIVE TRANSPLANTS

⑧ The newest approach to take advantage of the immunoreactivity between healthy donor T cells and host tumor cells is the use of nonmyeloablative transplants (NMT, "mini" transplants, or transplant "lite").[56–59] The number of NMTs has risen from about 500 in 1999 to more than 1,500 in 2002; the number of NMTs in 2002 represents about one-third of the allogeneic transplants registered with the International Bone Marrow Transplant Registry.[60] The rationale for NMT is based on the assumption that most of the antitumor activity associated with alloHSCT is the result of the donor T-cell–mediated GVT effect, and not the result of the myeloablative doses of chemotherapy or radiation (Fig. 134–4). If this assumption is correct, the major role of the preparative regimen is to suppress the host immune system, thus allowing engraftment of donor hematopoietic stem cells and donor

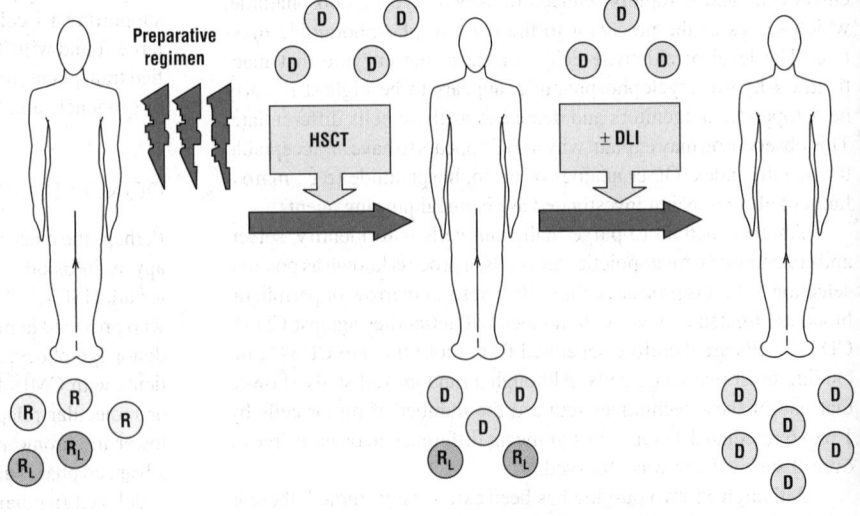

FIGURE 134–4. Schema for nonmyeloablative transplantation for hematologic malignancy. Recipients (R) receive a nonmyeloablative preparative regimen and an allogeneic hematopoietic stem cell transplant. Initially, mixed chimerism is present with the coexistence of donor (D) cells and recipient-derived normal and leukemia/lymphoma (R$_L$) cells. Donor-derived T cells mediate a graft-versus-host hematopoietic effect that eradicates residual recipient-derived normal and malignant hematopoietic cells. Donor lymphocyte infusions may be administered to enhance graft-versus-tumor effects. (Adapted from Champlin R, Khouri I, Anderlini P, et al. Nonmyeloablative preparative regimens for allogeneic hematopoietic transplantation: biology and current indications. Oncology 2003;17:94–100.)

T-cell cytotoxicity. To test this model in a clinical setting, regimens have been developed that include lower doses of drugs than those used in conventional transplants or other anticancer drugs that are immunosuppressive. A major advantage of this "reduced-intensity" approach is that potentially curative transplants can be offered to patients who would not typically be considered for alloHSCT because of their unacceptably high risk of transplant-related complications (e.g., increased age or those with moderately compromised organ function).

A number of preparative regimens have been developed for use in NMT, and these regimens vary in their cytotoxic (and thus myelosuppressive) and immunosuppressive activity.[56–59] Two general approaches have been used in the development of these regimens. The first consists of *reduced-intensity* regimens in which drugs with proven activity against the tumor are chosen. These regimens provide some immunosuppressive activity and are associated with some regimen-related toxicity. The second approach consists of *nonmyeloablative* regimens that have immunosuppressive conditioning regimens that are minimally myelosuppressive. Drugs that are often included in nonmyeloablative and reduced-intensity regimens include alkylating agents (busulfan, melphalan, or cyclophosphamide), purine analogs (fludarabine, pentostatin, or cladribine), and antithymocyte globulin. Low-dose (i.e., 200 cGy) TBI or alemtuzumab is included in some regimens.

DLIs are sometimes given posttransplant in NMT to convert mixed chimerism into full donor chimerism and to treat residual or progressive disease. Preliminary results show that DLI is effective and is associated with acceptable toxicity (mostly GVHD) in patients with early signs of disease persistence or progression after NMT.[61] Prophylactic DLI is being investigated at some centers to eradicate residual disease and reduce the risk of relapse.

Numerous clinical trials have reported the results of NMT from HLA-matched related or unrelated donors in relatively small cohorts of patients.[56–58] Follow-up is relatively short in most series. In the largest series, 253 patients received HLA-matched related NMT at one of several transplant centers that were part of an international consortium of transplant centers led by the Fred Hutchinson Cancer Research Center.[58,62] All patients had a hematologic malignancy. The source of hematopoietic stem cells was G-CSF–mobilized PBSCs. Median age was 54 years; the oldest patient was 73 years old. Median follow-up was 13 months. The first cohort of 58 patients was conditioned with TBI alone (2 Gy); 17% of these patients experienced nonfatal graft rejection. Fludarabine was then added to the conditioning regimen in the remaining patients, and the incidence of graft rejection decreased dramatically. A combination of cyclosporine and mycophenolate mofetil was given as GVHD prophylaxis. Most patients did not need platelet transfusions, and only about two-thirds required red blood cell transfusions. The majority of the transplant was done entirely in the ambulatory care setting. Typical side effects such as mucositis, diarrhea, and organ toxicities were absent. While the risk of infection in the first 100 days appeared to be lower than that seen with myeloablative alloHSCT, the risk of late viral and fungal infections persisted.[63,64] GVHD, although delayed compared to historical controls, was still a significant problem (discussed later).[65] Transplant-related mortality was only 5% at day 100. As compared with matched controls, patients who received NMT had significantly lower transplant-related mortality at day 100 and 1 year.[66] Follow-up is early, but remissions have been observed in virtually all disease categories, including molecular remissions. Disease remissions generally occurred slowly in 3 to 24 months, thus most likely making this form of therapy more beneficial in patients with chronic or indolent malignancies or those that can be effectively debulked prior to transplant.

Under a similar protocol, the same consortium of transplant centers treated 89 patients with HLA-matched unrelated NMT.[67] Both peripheral blood and marrow was used as a source of hematopoietic stem cells. Durable engraftment was observed in 85% of patients who received G-CSF–mobilized PBSCs, but only in 56% of marrow recipients. Transplant-related mortality was 11% at day 100. Patients who received PBSCs had improved progression-free and overall survival as compared with marrow recipients.

Antitumor responses have been observed with NMT in patients with renal cell carcinoma, melanoma, breast cancer, and other solid tumors.[59,68,69] In order to improve on the efficacy seen with NMT, some investigators are evaluating novel approaches to enhance allogeneic immune responses against tumor-associated antigens (if available) such as posttransplant vaccination.

NMTs are also being evaluated as salvage therapy in patients with a hematologic malignancy who do not respond to or have relapsed after autoHSCT,[70] and as intensive consolidation therapy in patients with multiple myeloma who are treated with autoHSCT.[71]

In summary, NMT from HLA-matched related or unrelated donors is a promising treatment modality for patients who are not candidates for myeloablative alloHSCT because of age or comorbidities. Myelosuppression is mild, and most patients do not develop severe neutropenia or thrombocytopenia. Because of the reduced intensity of the conditioning regimen, early transplant-related mortality is less than that seen with myeloablative alloHSCT. GVHD and infections, although occurring later after transplant, continue to be a significant cause of morbidity and mortality. Antitumor responses have been observed in hematologic malignancies and solid tumors.

TRANSPLANT-RELATED COMPLICATIONS

Although many patients with cancer who are treated with high-dose chemotherapy and autoHSCT or alloHSCT experience long-term survival and cure of their disease, this modality is associated with many serious and potentially life-threatening complications. In the early 1970s, early posttransplant mortality was extremely high, and most HSCT patients did not survive beyond 100 days. During those early years of alloHSCT, death was usually related to infection, GVHD, interstitial pneumonia, and leukemic relapse. Today, largely because of the availability of improved broad-spectrum antibiotics, immunosuppressive drugs, antiviral drugs, and hematopoietic growth factors, transplant-related mortality after alloHSCT with HLA-matched sibling donors has been reduced to less than 30% at most centers. Causes of death are usually related to transplant-related organ toxicity, GVHD, or immunosuppression. Until recently, alloHSCT was usually restricted to patients younger than 50 years old with an HLA-identical sibling donor. With advances in the prevention and treatment of transplant-related complications and the availability of NMT, alloHSCT is now being offered to patients older than 50 years of age. The risk of transplant-related mortality after high-dose chemotherapy with autoHSCT is less than 5% at many centers, depending on patient population and conditioning regimen. Mortality is lower with autologous transplants because of the lack of GVHD and associated complications of immunosuppression. Transplant-related mortality in autoHSCT is usually caused by regimen-related toxicity.

Table 134–1 lists the dose-limiting nonhematologic toxicity for several drugs that are commonly included in conditioning regimens.

TABLE 134–1. Dose-Limiting Nonhematologic Toxicities for Selected Chemotherapeutic Agents Included in Conditioning Regimens in Hematopoietic Stem Cell Transplantation

Drug	Conventional Dose[a] (mg/m^2)	ABMT[b] Dose (mg/m^2)	Dose-Limiting Toxicity
Busulfan (oral)	2	450	Hepatic
Carboplatin	400	2,000	Hepatic, renal
Carmustine	200	1,200	Pulmonary, hepatic
Cisplatin	100	200	Renal, peripheral neuropathy
Cyclophosphamide	1,000	7,500	Cardiomyopathy
Etoposide	300–600	2,400	Mucositis
Ifosfamide	5,000	18,000	Renal
Melphalan	40	225	Mucositis
Thiotepa	20–50	1125	Mucositis, CNS

[a]Doses are approximate and are for drugs as single agents. When combinations are used, doses may need to be decreased.
[b]ABMT, autologous bone marrow transplantation.
Modified from Eder JP, Elias A, Shea TC, et al. A phase I–II study of cyclophosphamide, thiotepa, and carboplatin with autologous bone marrow transplantation in solid tumor patients. J Clin Oncol 1990;8:1242.

These toxicities may be uncommon or rare with the administration of conventional doses of a specific drug. Toxicities seen with conventional doses can be expected to be more frequent and/or severe when these agents are given in high doses (e.g., mucositis, enteritis, nausea, vomiting, hematuria, etc). Several unusual and severe manifestations of regimen-related toxicities are discussed in detail below.

HEPATIC VENO-OCCLUSIVE DISEASE

Hepatic veno-occlusive disease (VOD), also known as sinusoidal-obstructive syndrome, occurs as a result of chemotherapy-induced damage and obliteration of the small intrahepatic central venules leading to necrosis of hepatocytes, portal hypertension, and hepatic failure.[72] Clinical signs of hepatic VOD include fluid retention leading to sudden weight gain and ascites, hepatomegaly (sometimes painful), and hyperbilirubinemia/jaundice usually occurring within the first 3 weeks after transplant. The incidence of hepatic VOD ranges from 5% to 20% in most series. Severe hepatic VOD is fatal in 50% to 75% of patients who develop it. Factors reported to increase the risk of hepatic VOD include the use of TBI-containing conditioning regimens and the presence of elevated liver function tests pretransplant. Pretransplant exposure to gemtuzumab ozogamicin (Mylotarg) has been implicated in the development of VOD.[73] The use of some drugs in the conditioning regimen, such as busulfan or carmustine, may also increase the risk of hepatic VOD. Busulfan concentrations have been correlated with the risk of hepatic VOD in some but not all studies.[32] Based on these studies, some HSCT centers adjust busulfan doses based on plasma concentrations. The use of IV busulfan reduces the interpatient variation in systemic exposure associated with the oral formulation, and has been associated with a reduced risk of hepatic VOD.[34]

Some studies suggest that prostaglandin E_1, unfractionated and low-molecular-weight heparin, or ursodiol may be partially effective in the prevention of hepatic VOD.[72] Prophylactic defibrotide may also be effective.[74] Treatment is generally supportive. Recombinant tissue plasminogen activator has been given to patients with severe hepatic VOD because of the possible role of the coagulation cascade in the pathogenesis of VOD. Responses have been reported but patients also experienced a higher risk of bleeding.[72] Defibrotide may also be beneficial in the treatment of VOD.[75]

PULMONARY COMPLICATIONS

Pulmonary complications following HSCT can be categorized as infectious and noninfectious (infectious complications are discussed in Chap. 120). Noninfectious complications are described as early (first 100 days posttransplant) and late (>100 days posttransplant). Patients receiving high-dose BCNU are also at risk for pulmonary fibrosis as a result of direct pulmonary tissue damage caused by this agent. Early complications include diffuse alveolar hemorrhage, engraftment syndrome, and idiopathic interstitial pneumonitis.[76] Diffuse alveolar hemorrhage (DAH) is characterized by dyspnea, hypoxia, dry cough, and fever. Chest x-ray usually shows diffuse infiltrates in an alveolar pattern. DAH is diagnosed by examination of bronchoalveolar lavage fluid, which reveals progressively bloodier fluid with each instilled aliquot, and by negative findings on microbiologic analysis. Although it can be life-threatening or fatal, prompt treatment with high doses of corticosteroids is sometimes beneficial.

Fever, erythrodermatous skin rash, and noncardiogenic pulmonary edema can occur during neutrophil recovery after HSCT. Because these clinical manifestations usually occur immediately before or at the time of neutrophil engraftment, this clinical entity has been referred to as "engraftment syndrome."[77] The incidence of engraftment syndrome is not known because of the lack of uniform diagnostic criteria, although some series report that about 10% of patients who receive autoHSCT develop this syndrome. Engraftment syndrome can progress to life-threatening respiratory failure with or without multiple organ failure. Corticosteroids are effective in some patients.

Idiopathic interstitial pneumonitis (IIP; also called idiopathic pneumonia syndrome) is defined as widespread alveolar injury in the absence of active lower respiratory tract infection following HSCT. Patients with idiopathic interstitial pneumonitis are clinically indistinguishable from those with interstitial pneumonitis related to infection. IIP is postulated to have a multifactorial etiology including toxic effects of myeloablative conditioning, immunologic cell-mediated injury, inflammatory cytokine-induced lung damage, and occult pulmonary infections. The risk is similar in recipients of autoHSCT or alloHSCT, but appears to be higher in patients who are conditioned with a TBI-containing regimen or who have acute GVHD. Mortality has been reported to be as high as 70% and treatment consists of supportive care only. The incidence of IIP may be lower after nonmyeloablative as compared to conventional preparative regimens.[78]

Late pulmonary complications cover a wide spectrum of disorders and include both obstructive and restrictive lung diseases. Included in these disorders are bronchiolitis obliterans with or without organizing pneumonia, diffuse alveolar damage, and lymphocytic interstitial pneumonia.[76,79,80] Therapy consists of steroids, which are about 50% effective; patients with mild-to-moderate airflow impairment appear to have the best response. Mortality from these disorders is about 40%.

GRAFT FAILURE

Initial engraftment after high-dose chemotherapy conditioning regimens usually occurs in the first 2 to 4 weeks posttransplant. Engraftment is evidenced by rising peripheral blood counts and the presence of hematopoietic precursor cells in the marrow. In alloHSCT, the presence of donor cells is confirmed with cytogenetic markers (i.e., chimerism). In most patients, engraftment is sustained with complete recovery of hematopoiesis.

Graft failure can occur after autologous, syngeneic, and allogeneic HSCT. It can be a result of an immunologic reaction between donor and host, infusion of insufficient numbers of hematopoietic stem cells, a viral infection, recurrence of primary hematologic malignancy, drug reaction (e.g., ganciclovir), or the development of a secondary myelodysplasia. Two syndromes have been observed: early graft failure occurs when the rate of hematopoietic recovery is delayed (primary graft failure or delayed engraftment), whereas late graft failure is characterized by a decline in the peripheral blood counts after initial engraftment (secondary graft failure). With widespread use of PBSCs and posttransplant growth factors, primary graft failure is rare after autologous and HLA-matched related alloHSCT. When graft failure occurs after alloHSCT and is characterized by the regrowth of immunocompetent host cells and a simultaneous loss of donor cells, it is referred to as graft rejection. Graft rejection occurs rarely after HLA-matched related alloHSCT. An increased risk of graft rejection has been observed in recipients of hematopoietic stem cells from HLA-mismatched related or unrelated donors, recipients of T-cell–depleted marrow, and patients with severe aplastic anemia.[6,9,10,81]

The long-term prognosis in patients with graft failure is poor. Despite supportive care, death may result from infection or bleeding. In some patients with an HLA-identical sibling donor, a second infusion of stem cells can be attempted. The most effective therapy for graft failure is G-CSF or GM-CSF. The 2000 American Society of Clinical Oncology guidelines recommend that patients with graft failure after HSCT be treated with GM-CSF 250 mcg/m^2 per day for 14 days followed by a 7-day break. Up to three such courses with dose escalation to 500 mcg/m^2 per day in the last course is advised.[82]

Hematopoietic growth factors are usually given posttransplant to accelerate engraftment, although some clinicians believe that posttransplant G-CSF or GM-CSF use is unnecessary due to the already rapid engraftment seen after mobilized PBSC transplants.[83] The usual dosage of GM-CSF is 250 mcg/m^2 per day. Many different dosages and schedules of G-CSF have been used after autoHSCT. Originally, G-CSF was given at a dose of 5 to 10 mcg/kg per day beginning on the day of or the day after infusion of stem cells and continued until neutrophil recovery to greater than an arbitrary number of neutrophils (500 to 1,000/mm^3). In one study of three different G-CSF dosages (5, 10, and 16 mcg/kg per day), there was no significant difference in the rate of hematopoietic recovery between the different dosages.[84] In another study, delayed initiation of G-CSF at a dosage of 5 mcg/kg per

day until day 5 posttransplant did not impair hematopoietic recovery after autologous PBSC transplantation.[85] Pegfilgrastim is currently being studied in the transplant setting.

Hematopoietic growth factors also accelerate the rate of hematopoietic recovery in patients undergoing alloHSCT. Although laboratory studies show that growth factors can modify T-cell and dendritic cell function, a meta-analysis of 18 studies, including 9 prospective randomized trials, showed no increased risk of acute GVHD when G-CSF or GM-CSF was used after alloHSCT.[86] However, a recently published retrospective study of patients with acute leukemia showed that G-CSF use after allogeneic BMT was significantly associated with an increased risk of acute GVHD and death.[87] It is interesting to note that no detrimental effects of G-CSF were noted in patients receiving allogeneic PBSC transplants.

None of the commercially available hematopoietic growth factors has a significant effect on platelet recovery. Results of studies with investigational platelet growth factors given posttransplant, such as thrombopoietin and interleukin-11, have been disappointing.[83] Platelet transfusions remain the standard of care in patients with thrombocytopenia below a given threshold (e.g., 10,000/mm^3) or who are having significant bleeding.

Anemia may also be problematic in the posttransplant setting, especially in patients receiving allogeneic transplants. The etiology is unclear and most likely multifactorial. Erythropoietin administration may be useful in reducing the need for red blood cell transfusions and may be given in regimens similar to those given for malignancy-associated anemia.[83]

GRAFT-VERSUS-HOST DISEASE

GVHD is caused by immunocompetent donor T cells reacting against antigens presented by antigen-presenting cells. In that setting, donor T cells recognize histocompatibility antigens of the host as genetically foreign, become activated, proliferate, and attack recipient tissue, thereby producing the clinical syndrome of GVHD.[88]

Two different clinical GVHD syndromes have been recognized, depending on the time of onset and clinical presentation.[89] While there is considerable overlap, acute GVHD occurs early, while chronic GVHD occurs late in the posttransplant course; acute GVHD is usually limited to the gastrointestinal tract, skin, and liver, while signs and symptoms of chronic GVHD resemble an autoimmune disorder and can affect many organ systems

Acute Graft-Versus-Host Disease

Acute GVHD usually becomes clinically evident during the first 100 days posttransplant and is characterized by selective epithelial damage of target organs by donor T cells.[89,90] The onset of acute GVHD is often delayed past day 100 following NMT.[65] The pathophysiology of acute GVHD has been described as a three-step process. In step 1, the high-dose preparative regimen leads to damage and activation of host tissues and the secretion of inflammatory cytokines such as interleukin-1 and tumor necrosis factor-α. In step 2, donor T cells are activated, and secretion of other cytokines by activated T cells results in the recruitment of other cell types (e.g., macrophages and natural killer cells) that also contribute to the pathology associated with GVHD. The third and final step is characterized by the generation of multiple cytotoxic effectors that contribute to target tissue injury. The term "cytokine storm" is sometimes used to describe the critical role of inflammatory cytokines in this process.

Based on this three-step model, three general approaches can be used to prevent GVHD in humans. The first is to reduce host tissue

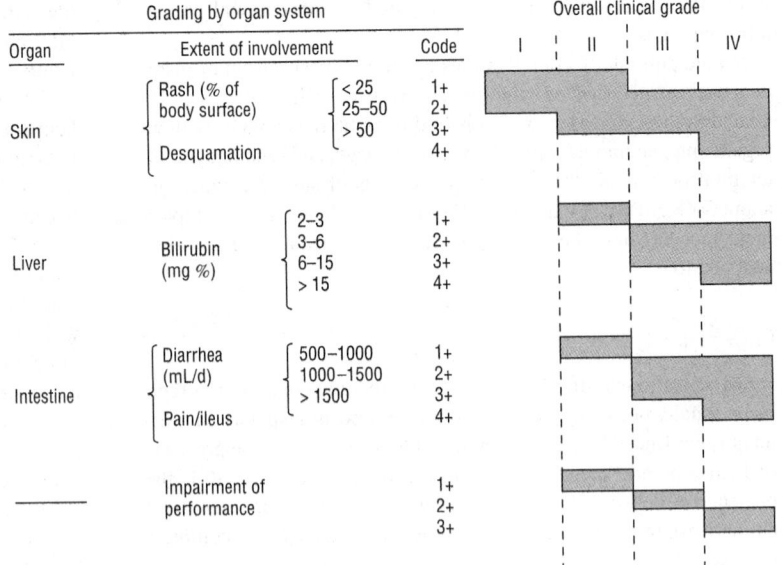

FIGURE 134–5. Clinical grading of acute GVHD. The left panel summarizes the grading by organ system; the right panel shows the overall clinical grade. With grade I, only the skin can be involved. With more extensive involvement of the skin or involvement of liver and intestinal tract and impairment of the clinical performance status, either alone or in any combination, the severity grade advances from II to IV.

damage with the use of reduced intensity or nonmyeloablative conditioning regimens. The second and most widely used approach is to modulate donor T cells by reducing T-cell numbers (T-cell depletion), inhibiting T-cell activation (most immunosuppressive agents), or inhibiting T-cell proliferation (antiproliferative agents). The third approach is to block inflammatory stimulation and effectors (e.g., tumor necrosis factor-α inhibitors).

The principal target organs for acute GVHD are the skin, liver, and gastrointestinal tract. Acute GVHD is classified into four grades, depending on the number of organs involved and the degree of involvement of each organ (Fig. 134–5). Grade I disease involves only the skin, while grades II through IV involve the skin and either the liver or gastrointestinal tract or both. The initial sign of acute GVHD is usually a generalized maculopapular rash that involves the face, ears, palms, soles, and upper trunk. The skin rash can spread to the rest of the body. Acute GVHD usually progresses to involve other organs. Gastrointestinal GVHD is manifested as diarrhea, but may progress to abdominal pain/cramping and ileus. GVHD of the upper intestinal tract has also been described presenting as nausea, vomiting, anorexia, and dyspepsia. The diagnosis of gastrointestinal GVHD must be made by mucosal biopsy. Hepatic GVHD is usually asymptomatic, consisting of hyperbilirubinemia and increases in serum aminotransferase and alkaline phosphatase levels. The diagnosis is usually made by biopsy, although many patients are not biopsied.

The overall incidence of moderate to severe (grades II to IV) GVHD ranges from 10% to more than 80% after alloHSCT. Mortality directly attributable to acute GVHD or its treatment occurs in 10% to 20% of patients. The incidence of GVHD is related to the degree of histocompatibility, number of T cells in the graft, donor and recipient age, and prophylactic regimen. In patients receiving PBSC grafts, CD34[+] cell dose and type of prophylactic regimen are also risk factors. The risk of acute GVHD is lower in recipients of NMT and UCB transplants as compared with myeloablative allogeneic transplants,[26,65] and is slightly higher in recipients of allogeneic PBSC transplants as compared with allogeneic BMT.[24] The most severe acute GVHD is observed in alloHSCT with non-HLA-identical related or unrelated donors. In these settings, the incidence of grades II to IV acute GVHD exceeds 50%, despite aggressive GVHD prophylaxis. The risk of acute GVHD is lower in

patients with a certain interleukin-10 genotype.[91] Interleukin-10 secreted by antigen-presenting cells promotes the development of immunologic tolerance and suppresses the production of inflammatory cytokines.

Multiorgan acute GVHD and the drugs given to prevent or treat it are associated with delayed immunologic recovery and increased susceptibility to infections. Infection is often the primary cause of death in patients with GVHD. Patients with GVHD on immunosuppressive therapy should receive prophylactic antiviral, antibacterial, and antifungal therapy.

Because treatment of established acute GVHD is often unsatisfactory, aggressive preventive measures are usually taken. The most common strategy used to prevent acute GVHD is to block the activation of T cells by administration of immunosuppressive agents.[89,90] Several immunosuppressive agents have been used, including methotrexate, cyclosporine, tacrolimus, mycophenolate mofetil, antithymocyte globulin, corticosteroids, and monoclonal antibodies directed at T cells. The pharmacology of these drugs is reviewed elsewhere.[92] Most GVHD prophylaxis regimens combine two or more immunosuppressive agents that affect different stages of T-cell activation. Another strategy is to remove or deplete most T cells from donor bone marrow ex vivo prior to transplant by physical separation (i.e., lectin agglutination) or by treatment with monoclonal antibodies directed at T cells (see Fig. 134–3).[81]

In alloHSCT with HLA-identical sibling donors, the combination of cyclosporine and either methotrexate or corticosteroids reduces the incidence of grades II to IV acute GVHD to 25% to 40%. Intravenous cyclosporine is usually started around day 0 at an initial dosage of 3 to 5 mg/kg per day, given in two divided doses. Dosages are adjusted based on trough cyclosporine concentrations. Patients are converted to oral cyclosporine when they can tolerate oral medications. Cyclosporine is given at full doses until about day 50 and in the absence of GVHD, is then gradually tapered and discontinued by day 180. Methotrexate is given intravenously on days 1, 3, 6, and 11 posttransplant. The methotrexate dosage is 10 mg/m^2, except for the first dose given on day 1 (15 mg/m^2). Some protocols omit the day 11 dose because of its myelosuppressive effects. When cyclosporine is given in combination with corticosteroids, methylprednisolone is usually started during the first 2 weeks posttransplant, given at full dosages for several weeks, and gradually tapered in the absence of GVHD. Although the efficacy of cyclosporine-methotrexate and cyclosporine-corticosteroids appears to be similar, the use of methotrexate may increase the risk of early graft failure, while corticosteroid administration has been associated with a higher incidence of infections. It is not clear whether three-drug regimens are more effective than two-drug regimens. In one prospective randomized study, the addition of methylprednisolone did not further increase the efficacy of the cyclosporine-methotrexate regimen.[93] Unexpectedly, patients who received the three-drug combination had a higher incidence of acute and chronic GVHD and infection than did those given cyclosporine and methotrexate.[94] In contrast, two other prospective randomized studies showed a benefit for the three-drug regimen versus a two-drug regimen.[95,96] It is not completely clear why the trials reached different conclusions, but the different schedules of methylprednisolone may have had some influence on the results. In the first trial, methylprednisolone was given from days 0 to 35 posttransplant. In contrast, methylprednisolone was not started in the other trials until after day 7 posttransplant. Some investigators speculate that early administration of methylprednisolone may have interfered with the antiproliferative effects of methotrexate on T cells.[93]

Tacrolimus, given either alone or combined with methotrexate or methylprednisolone, has also been studied as GVHD prophylaxis after alloHSCT.[89] Two large multicenter randomized trials compared cyclosporine and methotrexate with tacrolimus and methotrexate. One study was done in patients undergoing HLA-identical sibling alloHSCT,[97] while the other study was done in patients undergoing matched unrelated alloHSCT.[98] Both studies found the tacrolimus combination to be significantly superior to the cyclosporine combination in preventing grades II to IV acute GVHD. The incidence of renal impairment was higher in patients receiving tacrolimus, and more tacrolimus-treated patients in the HLA-sibling transplantation trial required hemodialysis. The incidence of hypertension was significantly higher in cyclosporine-treated patients in the HLA-matched sibling alloHSCT trial. No difference in the overall or relapse-free survival rate was reported in the two trials, although in the subgroup of patients with advanced disease in the HLA-sibling alloHSCT trial, cyclosporine-treated patients had significantly better overall and disease-free survival rates at 2 years as compared to those patients who received tacrolimus. The authors also explained that lowering the target blood levels to less than 20 ng/mL might reduce the renal toxicity of tacrolimus. Based on the results of these two studies, some transplant centers currently use tacrolimus and methotrexate as first-line acute GVHD prophylaxis.

Acute GVHD prophylaxis regimens used in NMT are usually similar to those used in myeloablative alloHSCT. Some centers, however, have developed novel prophylactic regimens specifically for patients undergoing NMT. An example of such a regimen is cyclosporine and mycophenolate mofetil,[58,62] which was developed based on preclinical studies.[99]

The role of ex vivo T-cell depletion from donor grafts is controversial (see Fig. 134–3).[81] Although the use of T-cell–depleted marrow can reduce the incidence and severity of acute GVHD, it is associated with an increased risk of graft failure, delayed immune reconstitution, leukemic relapse, cytomegalovirus reactivation, and Epstein-Barr virus–related lymphoproliferative disorders. As a result, this approach does not improve the survival rate in recipients of HLA-identical sibling donor marrow. These observations suggest that important cell populations are being eliminated in the depletion process. Various approaches are being investigated to selectively remove the T cells responsible for GVHD while leaving those cells that

mediate engraftment, antileukemic effect, and suppression of Epstein-Barr virus–transformed lymphocytes. Another approach is to infuse the T cells originally depleted from the graft later in the posttransplant period to prevent leukemic relapse.[100] Because of the higher risk of GVHD in alloHSCT with HLA-mismatched or matched unrelated donors, T-cell depletion is sometimes included as part of the GVHD prophylaxis regimen in that setting.

With HLA-mismatched or matched unrelated donors, the risk of moderate-to-severe (grades II to IV) acute GVHD is 50% or higher with conventional two-drug prophylaxis. Several approaches are used to reduce the risk of acute GVHD in this high-risk group of patients: three-drug GVHD prophylaxis, pretransplant administration of antithymocyte globulin, or ex vivo T-cell depletion of donor bone marrow (see Fig. 134–3). Encouraging results have been reported with the addition of novel immunosuppressive agents such as sirolimus to two-drug prophylaxis regimens.[101] The addition of rabbit antithymocyte globulin to the pretransplant conditioning regimen reduced the risk of acute GVHD, but increased the risk of lethal infections.[102] Uncontrolled studies suggest that ex vivo T-cell depletion significantly reduces the risk of early graft failure and acute GVHD, with apparent preservation of the GVL effect.[81]

If a patient develops grade II to IV acute GVHD, prophylactic agents are continued and high-dose corticosteroids, given as intravenously administered methylprednisolone, are started. The usual dosage is 2 mg/kg per day, given in two divided doses. The initial dosage is as high as 10 mg/kg per day in some protocols, although there is no convincing evidence that higher dosages are more effective. About 20% to 40% of patients with established acute GVHD respond to high-dose corticosteroids. If the patient responds, the corticosteroid dose is tapered gradually over several weeks, depending on response. In patients who experience a flare in their GVHD during the taper phase, therapy consists of increasing the steroid dose. GVHD-associated mortality is strongly correlated to response to initial treatment, and ranges from about 25% in patients who had a complete response to about 80% in those patients who had no response or progressive disease.

Several randomized trials have evaluated other agents combined with methylprednisolone.[89] In particular, the addition of anti-T-cell antibodies such as antithymocyte globulin or monoclonal antibodies to methylprednisolone has not been shown to improve patient outcome. Administration of enteric beclomethasone dipropionate capsules to systemic methylprednisolone is more effective than systemic methylprednisolone alone in the treatment of gastrointestinal acute GVHD.[103]

In patients who fail initial treatment with corticosteroids, salvage therapy with antithymocyte globulin, mycophenolate mofetil, thalidomide, sirolimus, or pentostatin has been given with some success.[89] In addition, a variety of humanized mononclonal antibodies or fusion proteins are being evaluated in the treatment of steroid-refractory acute GVHD: denileukin difitox (Ontak), daclizumab (Zenapax), infliximab (Remicade), and etanercept (Enbrel).[104–106]

Chronic Graft-Versus-Host Disease

Chronic GVHD usually occurs after day 100 and is the major determinant of late transplant-related morbidity and mortality.[89,90,107–109] The pathophysiology of chronic GVHD is poorly understood. Chronic GVHD is often considered an autoimmune disease because of its similarity to other autoimmune disorders.

The incidence of chronic GVHD in patients who survive more than 150 days ranges from 20% to 70%.[89,107] The risk of chronic GVHD increases with increasing donor and recipient age, and is higher in patients who receive transplants from HLA-nonidentical related or unrelated donors, patients who receive PBSC transplants, and patients who receive DLI. A meta-analysis reported that the risk of chronic GVHD is increased by about 50% in patients who receive allogeneic PBSC transplants as compared with BMT.[24] The risk of chronic GVHD is lower after UCB transplantation.[26] The incidence of chronic GVHD is increasing because of increasing use of alternative donors, PBSCs as the graft source, DLI for treatment of recurrence, and older recipient age. Previous acute GVHD increases the risk of chronic GVHD, but about 20% to 30% of patients who receive HLA-matched alloHSCT develop chronic GVHD with no history of acute GVHD (de novo). Unlike acute GVHD, prophylactic immunosuppression does not appear to reduce the incidence or severity of the chronic form of the disease.

The clinical manifestations of chronic GVHD can involve virtually all major organ systems.[89,107,109] The diagnosis of chronic GVHD requires at least one manifestation that is characteristic of chronic GVHD: lichenoid oral or vaginal findings, ocular sicca, skin dyspigmentation, scleroderma, bronchiolitis obliterans, and esophageal web formation.[107] The most common sites of involvement are the skin, mouth, liver, and eye. Since signs and symptoms are sometimes not noticeable for several months, many centers require their alloHSCT patients to undergo screening studies to detect early clinical chronic GVHD.

The most commonly used staging system is the limited/extensive classification proposed by the Seattle HSCT program.[89,107,109] In that system, chronic GVHD is classified as limited or extensive, depending on pathologic findings and the extent of systemic involvement. Limited chronic GVHD indicates localized skin involvement, mild hepatic dysfunction, or both. Most patients have extensive disease, with involvement of the skin, liver, eyes, mouth, esophagus, or other organs. Extensive disease is associated with a worse prognosis. The clinicopathologic findings of chronic GVHD are similar to those observed in various autoimmune diseases, with a marked increase in collagen deposition in the target organs. Several investigators have proposed improved staging systems based on larger numbers of patients and survival.[110]

If no functional impairment is present, patients with limited disease are not treated with systemic therapy. A variety of topical preparations may be used in patients with skin-only disease, such as clobetasol, tacrolimus, and pimecrolimus. Many patients with extensive chronic GVHD, if left untreated, will die of infections or become disabled. The long-term survival rate is worse in certain subgroups of patients, such as patients with extensive skin involvement, thrombocytopenia, progressive onset of chronic GVHD, and those who fail to respond to immunosuppressive therapy.

Initial treatment in patients with standard-risk chronic GVHD consists of prednisone (1 mg/kg per day) alone or alternate-day therapy with prednisone and cyclosporine (10 to 12 mg/kg per day in two divided doses).[90,107–109] Although many clinicians prefer alternate-day prednisone and cyclosporine, a recently published randomized trial showed no differences in response or survival between the two regimens in standard-risk patients.[111] Tacrolimus is substituted for cyclosporine at some centers. Patients with high-risk disease should be treated with alternate-day therapy with prednisone and cyclosporine or tacrolimus. The calcineurin inhibitor is given daily rather than on alternate days at some centers. Treatment is continued until signs and symptoms of the disease have resolved, usually over a period of several months. As chronic GVHD improves, immunosuppressive therapy is gradually tapered and finally discontinued provided there is no flare of GVHD. About 60% of standard-risk patients and 40% of high-risk patients treated for chronic GVHD

have all of their immunosuppressive therapy successfully discontinued. Patients who fail initial therapy have a very poor prognosis, and several therapies have been investigated with varying degrees of success: thalidomide, ultraviolet A irradiation after oral treatment with β-methoxypsoralen, extracorporeal photophoresis, tacrolimus, sirolimus, pentostatin, mycophenolate mofetil, hydroxychloroquine, and others.[89,107,109]

CLINICAL CONTROVERSY

The choice of initial treatment of chronic GVHD is controversial. Many clinicians will treat standard- and high-risk patients with alternate-day prednisone and either daily or alternate-day cyclosporine. However, a randomized trial showed no differences in response or survival between prednisone alone and alternate-day prednisone and cyclosporine in standard-risk patients. Other clinicians will substitute tacrolimus for cyclosporine. Several randomized trials are in progress, and the results of these trials should help to determine the optimal initial therapy for chronic GVHD.

Infection is the primary cause of death in patients with chronic GVHD, and antimicrobial prophylaxis is an important component of the care of patients being treated for chronic GVHD. Patients should receive oral trimethoprim-sulfamethoxazole, penicillin, and acyclovir to prevent those infections commonly seen in immunocompromised patients.[89,107,108] Some centers will also administer intravenous immunoglobulin to patients with low serum immunoglobulin G levels.

INFECTION

Patients undergoing high-dose chemotherapy with autoHSCT or alloHSCT are severely immunocompromised and therefore at high risk for bacterial, fungal, and viral infection. Management of these infections is discussed in detail in Chap. 120. Comprehensive guidelines for monitoring, prophylaxis, and treatment of infections in HSCT recipients are available at http://www.cdc.gov/mmwr/preview/mmwrhtml/rr4910a1.htm.

LATE COMPLICATIONS

With the success of HSCT, the number of long-term survivors has grown. Many survivors experience delayed complications of transplantation, especially those receiving alloHSCT, and primary care physicians will care for them.[112] Major late complications include restrictive and obstructive pulmonary disease; bone and joint disease; cataract formation; endocrine dysfunction, including sterility; impaired growth and development; infections; cardiovascular disease; and cirrhosis as a result of chronic hepatitis C infection and secondary malignancies.[113,114]

Physical recovery tends to occur earlier than psychological or work recovery.[115] Full recovery usually takes several years, and about two-thirds of patients do not have major limitations by 5 years.

CONCLUSIONS

Over the last few decades, HSCT has evolved from an idea into a well-established therapy used to treat thousands of patients with serious malignant and nonmalignant hematologic diseases. Transplantation is also being investigated as a treatment modality in patients with certain solid tumors or life-threatening autoimmune diseases. Because myelosuppression is the dose-limiting toxicity for many anticancer agents, HSCT allows the administration of higher and potentially more effective doses of chemotherapy. In patients who receive alloHSCT, cells in the graft can mediate a GVT effect.

Although HSCT is a potentially curative therapy, this modality is associated with many serious and potentially life-threatening complications. With improved supportive care and management of infection, transplant-related mortality after alloHSCT with HLA-matched sibling donors has been reduced over the last few years. Causes of death are usually related to transplant-related organ toxicity, GVHD, or immunosuppression. Until recently, alloHSCT was usually restricted to patients younger than 50 years old with an HLA-identical sibling donor. With the availability of NMT, alloHSCT is now being offered to patients who would not otherwise be candidates for alloHSCT because of age or comorbidities. The risk of transplant-related mortality after autoHSCT is very low, and is primarily related to regimen-related toxicity. Many long-term survivors of HSCT will experience delayed complications.

ABBREVIATIONS

ALL: acute lymphoblastic leukemia
alloHSCT: allogeneic hematopoietic stem cell transplantation
AML: acute myelogenous leukemia
autoHSCT: autogenous hematopoietic stem cell transplantation
BEAC: BCNU, etoposide, ara-C, and cyclophosphamide
BEAM: BCNU, etoposide, ara-C, and melphalan
BMT: bone marrow transplant
BuCy: busulfan and cyclophosphamide
CBV: cyclophosphamide, carmustine (BCNU), and etoposide (VP-16)
CML: chronic myelogenous leukemia
CyTBI: cyclophosphamide and total body irradiation
DAH: diffuse alveolar hemorrhage
DLI: donor lymphocyte infusion
G-CSF: granulocyte colony-stimulating factor
GM-CSF: granulocyte macrophage-colony stimulating factor
GVHD: graft-versus-host disease
GVL: graft-versus-leukemia (effect)
GVT: graft-versus-tumor (effect)
4-HC: 4-hydroperoxycyclophosphamide
HLA: human leukocyte antigen
HSCT: hematopoietic stem cell transplantation
IIP: idiopathic interstitial pneumonitis
IL-2: interleukin-2
MHC: major histocompatibility complex
MLC: mixed lymphocyte culture
MLR: mixed lymphocyte reaction
MUD: matched unrelated donor
NMDP: National Marrow Donor Program
NMT: nonmyeloablative transplant
PBPC: peripheral blood progenitor cell
PBSC: peripheral blood stem cell
PCR: polymerase chain reaction
TBI: total body irradiation
UCB: umbilical cord blood
VOD: (hepatic) veno-occlusive disease

Review Questions and other resources can be found at *www.pharmacotherapyonline.com*.

REFERENCES

1. Horowitz MM. Uses and growth of hematopoietic cell transplantation. In: Blume KG, Forman SJ, Appelbaum FR, eds. Thomas' Hematopoietic Cell Transplantation, 3rd ed. Malden, MA:, Blackwell Science, 2004: 9–15.
2. Armitage JO, Antman KH. High-Dose Cancer Therapy: Pharmacology, Hematopoietins, Stem Cells, 4th ed. Philadelphia, Lippincott Williams & Wilkins, 2000.
3. Blume KG, Forman SJ, Appelbaum FR. Thomas' Hematopoietic Cell Transplantation, 3rd ed. Malden, MA, Blackwell Science, 2004:???–???.
4. Appelbaum FR. The current status of hematopoietic cell transplantation. Annu Rev Med 2003;54:491–512.
5. Klein J, Sato A. The HLA system. N Engl J Med 2000;343:702–709.
6. Petersdorf EW. Hematopoietic cell transplantation from unrelated donors. In: Blume KG, Forman SJ, Appelbaum FR, eds. Thomas' Hematopoietic Cell Transplantation, 3rd ed. Malden, MA, Blackwell Science, 2004:1132–1149.
7. Flomenberg N, Baxter-Lowe LA, Confer D, et al. Impact of HLA class I and class II high resolution matching on outcomes of unrelated donor bone marrow transplantation: HLA-C mismatching is associated with a strong adverse effect on transplant outcome. Blood 2004;104:1923–1930.
8. Hurley CK, Lowe LB, Logan B, et al. National Marrow Donor Program HLA-matching guidelines for unrelated marrow transplants. Biol Blood Marrow Transplant 2003;9:610–615.
9. Weisdorf DJ, Anasetti C, Antin JH, et al. Allogeneic bone marrow transplantation for chronic myelogenous leukemia: comparative analysis of unrelated versus matched sibling donor transplantation. Blood 2002;99:1971–1977.
10. Anasetti C, Velardi A. Hematopoietic cell transplantation from HLA partially matched related donors. In: Blume KG, Forman SJ, Appelbaum FR, eds. Thomas' Hematopoietic Cell Transplantation, 3rd ed. Malden, MA, Blackwell Science, 2004:1116–1131.
11. Manz MG, Akashi K, Weissman IL. Biology of hematopoietic stem and progenitor cells. In: Blume KG, Forman SJ, Appelbaum FR, eds. Thomas' Hematopoietic Cell Transplantation, 3rd ed. Malden, MA, Blackwell Science, 2004:69–95.
12. Siena S, Schiavo R, Pedrazzoli P, Carlo-Stella C. Therapeutic relevance of $CD34^+$ cell dose in blood cell transplantation for cancer therapy. J Clin Oncol 2000;18:1360–1377.
13. Kessinger A, Sharp JG. The whys and hows of hematopoietic progenitor and stem cell mobilization. Bone Marrow Transplant 2003;31:319–329.
14. Fruehauf S, Seggewiss R. It's moving day: factors affecting peripheral blood stem cell mobilization and strategies for improvement. Br J Haematol 2003;122:360–375.
15. Ng-Cashin J, Shea T. Mobilization of autologous peripheral blood hematopoietic cells for support of high-dose cancer therapy. In: Blume KG, Forman SJ, Appelbaum FR, eds. Thomas' Hematopoietic Cell Transplantation, 3rd ed. Malden, MA, Blackwell Science, 2004:9–15.
16. Glaspy JA. Economic considerations in the use of peripheral blood progenitor cells to support high-dose chemotherapy. Bone Marrow Transplant 1999;23(Suppl 2):s21–s27.
17. Schulman KA, Birch R, Zhen B, et al. Effect of $CD34^+$ cell dose on resource utilization in patients after high-dose chemotherapy with peripheral blood stem cell support. J Clin Oncol 1999;17:1227–1233.
18. Beyer J, Schwella N, Zingsem J, et al. Hematopoietic rescue after high-dose chemotherapy using autologous peripheral blood progenitor cells or bone marrow: a randomized comparison. J Clin Oncol 1995;13:1328–1335.
19. Schmitz N, Linch DC, Dreger P, et al. Filgrastim-mobilized peripheral

blood progenitor cell transplantation: results of a randomized phase III trial in lymphoma patients. Lancet 1996;347:353–357.

20. Smith TJ, Hillner BE, Schmitz N, et al. Economic analysis of a randomized clinical trial to compare filgrastim-mobilized peripheral blood progenitor cell transplantation with autologous bone marrow transplantation in patients with Hodgkin's and non-Hodgkin's lymphoma. J Clin Oncol 1997;15:5–10.

21. Meisenberg BR, Ferran K, Hollenbach K, et al. Reduced charges and costs associated with outpatient autologous stem cell transplantation. Bone Marrow Transplant 1999;21:927–932.

22. Couban S, Barnett M. The source of cells for allografting. Biol Blood Marrow Transplant 2003;9:669–673.

23. Schmitz N. Peripheral blood hematopoietic cells for allogeneic transplantation. In: Blume KG, Forman SJ, Appelbaum FR, eds. Thomas' Hematopoietic Cell Transplantation, 3rd ed. Malden, MA, Blackwell Science, 2004:9–15.

24. Cutler C, Giri S, Jeyapalan S, et al. Acute and chronic graft-versus-host disease after allogeneic peripheral blood stem cell and bone marrow transplantation: A meta-analysis. J Clin Oncol 2001;19:3685–3691.

25. Heimfeld S. HLA-identical stem cell transplantation: is there an optimal CD34 cell dose? Bone Marrow Transplant 2003;31:839–845.

26. Grewal SS, Barker JN, Davies SM, Wagner JE. Unrelated donor hematopoietic cell transplantation: marrow or umbilical cord blood? Blood 2003;101:4233–4244.

27. Wagner JE, Barker JN, DeFor TE, et al. Transplantation of unrelated donor umbilical cord blood in 102 patients with malignant and non-malignant diseases: influence of CD34 cell dose and HLA disparity on treatment-related mortality and survival. Blood 2002;100:1611–1618.

28. Barker JN, Davies SM, DeFor TE, et al. Survival after transplantation of unrelated donor umbilical cord blood is comparable to that of human leukocyte antigen-matched-unrelated donor bone marrow: results of a matched-pair analysis. Blood 2001;97:2957–2961.

29. Koh L-P, Chao NJ. Umbilical cord blood transplantation in adults using myeloablative and nonmyeloablative preparative regimens. Biol Blood Marrow Transplant 2004;10:1–22.

30. Bensinger WI, Spielberger R. Preparative regimens and modification of regimen-related toxicities. In: Blume KG, Forman SJ, Appelbaum FR, eds. Thomas' Hematopoietic Cell Transplantation, 3rd ed. Malden, MA, Blackwell Science, 2004:158–177.

31. Shank B, Hoppe RT. Radiotherapeutic principles of hematopoietic cell transplantation. In: Blume KG, Forman SJ, Appelbaum FR, eds. Thomas' Hematopoietic Cell Transplantation, 3rd ed. Malden, MA, Blackwell Science, 2004:178–197.

32. McCune JS, Gibbs JP, Slattery JT. Plasma concentration monitoring of busulfan: does it improve outcome? Clin Pharmacokinet 2000;39:155–165.

33. Radich JP, Gooley T, Bensinger W, et al. HLA-matched related hematopoietic cell transplantation for chronic-phase CML using a targeted busulfan and cyclophosphamide preparative regimen. Blood 2003;102:31–35.

34. Kashyap A, Wingard J, Cagnoni P, et al. Intravenous versus oral busulfan as part of a busulfan/cyclophosphamide preparative regimen for allogeneic hematopoietic stem cell transplantation: decreased incidence of hepatic venoocclusive disease (HVOD), HVOD-related mortality, and overall 100-day mortality. Biol Blood Marrow Transplant 2002;8:493–500.

35. Socie G, Clift RA, Blaise D, et al. Busulfan plus cyclophosphamide compared with total-body irradiation plus cyclophosphamide before marrow transplantation for myeloid leukemia: long-term follow-up of 4 randomized studies. Blood 2001;98:3569–3574.

36. Ferry C, Socie G. Busulfan-cyclophosphamide versus total body irradiation-cyclophosphamide as preparative regimen before allogeneic hematopoietic stem cell transplantation for acute myeloid leukemia: what have we learned? Exp Hematol 2003;31:1182–1186.

37. Gupta V, Lazarus HM, Keating A. Myeloablative conditioning regimens for AML allografts: 30 years later. Bone Marrow Transplant 2003;32:969–978.

38. Davies SM, Ramsay NKC, Klein J, et al. Comparison of preparative regimens in transplants for children with acute lymphoblastic leukemia. J Clin Oncol 2000;18:340–347.

39. Mounier N, Gisselbrecht C. Conditioning regimens before transplantation in patients with aggressive non-Hodgkin's lymphoma. Ann Oncol 1998;9(Suppl 1):S15–S21.

40. Hunault-Berger M, Ifrah N, Solal-Celigny. Intensive therapies in follicular non-Hodgkin's lymphomas. Blood 2002;100:1141–51.

41. Press OW. Radioimmunotherapy for non-Hodgkin's lymphomas: a historical perspective. Semin Oncol 2003;30(Suppl 4):10–21.

42. Malek SN, Flinn IW. Incorporating monoclonal antibodies in blood and marrow transplantation. Semin Oncol 2003;30:520–530.

43. Gopal AK, Gooley TA, Maloney DG, et al. High-dose radioimmunotherapy versus conventional high-dose therapy and autologous hematopoietic stem cell transplantation for relapsed follicular non-Hodgkin's lymphoma: a multivariate cohort analysis. Blood 2003;102:2351–2357.

44. Roman-Unfer S, Cook B, Nieto Y, Shpall E. Negative and positive stem cell selection. In: Armitage JO, Antman KH, eds. High-Dose Cancer Therapy, 3rd ed. Philadelphia, Lippincott Williams & Wilkins, 2000:331–353.

45. Gribben JG. Antibody-mediated purging. In: Blume KG, Forman SJ, Appelbaum FR, eds. Thomas' Hematopoietic Cell Transplantation, 3rd ed. Malden, MA, Blackwell Science, 2004:244–253.

46. Colvin OM. Pharmacologic purging of bone marrow. In: Blume KG, Forman SJ, Appelbaum FR, eds. Thomas' Hematopoietic Cell Transplantation, 3rd ed. Malden, MA, Blackwell Science, 2004:254–257.

47. Stewart AK, Vescio R, Schiller G, et al. Purging of autologous peripheral-blood stem cells using CD34 selection does not improve overall or progression-free survival after high-dose chemotherapy for multiple myeloma: results of a multicenter randomized controlled trial. J Clin Oncol 2001;19:3771–3779.

48. Fefer A. Graft-versus-tumor responses. In: Blume KG, Forman SJ, Appelbaum FR, eds. Thomas' Hematopoietic Cell Transplantation, 3rd ed. Malden, MA, Blackwell Science, 2004:369–379.

49. Kolb HJ, Schmid C, Barrett AJ, Schendel DJ. Graft-versus-leukemia reactions in allogeneic chimeras. Blood 2004;103:767–776.

50. Mackinnon S. Who may benefit from donor leucocyte infusions after allogeneic stem cell transplantation? Br J Haematol 2000;110:12–17.

51. Collins RH. Management of relapse after allogeneic transplantation. In: Blume KG, Forman SJ, Appelbaum FR, eds. Thomas' Hematopoietic Cell Transplantation, 3rd ed. Malden, MA, Blackwell Science, 2004:1150–1163.

52. Levine JE, Braun T, Penza SL, et al. Prospective trial of chemotherapy and donor leukocyte infusions for relapse of advanced myeloid malignancies after allogeneic stem cell transplantation. J Clin Oncol 2002;20:405–412.

53. Stein AS, O'Donnell MR, Slovak ML, et al. Interleukin-2 after autologous stem cell transplantation for adult patients with acute myeloid leukemia in first complete remission. J Clin Oncol 2003;21:615–623.

54. Negrin RS. Prevention and therapy of relapse following autologous hematopoietic cell transplantation. In: Blume KG, Forman SJ, Appelbaum FR, eds. Thomas' Hematopoietic Cell Transplantation, 3rd ed. Malden, MA, Blackwell Science, 2004:1394–1405.

55. Horwitz SM, Negrin RS, Blume KG, et al. Rituximab as adjuvant to high-dose therapy and autologous hematopoietic cell transplantation for aggressive non-Hodgkin's lymphoma. Blood 2004;103:777–783.

56. Tabbara IA, Ingram RM. Nonmyeloablative therapy and allogeneic hematopoietic stem cell transplantation. Exp Hematol 2003;31:559–566.

57. Slavin S, Morecki S, Weiss L, et al. Nonmyeloablative stem cell transplantation: reduced-intensity conditioning for cancer immunotherapy—from bench to patient bedside. Semin Oncol 2004;31:4–21.

58. Sandmaier BM, Storb R. Nonmyeloablative therapy and hematopoietic cell transplantation for hematologic disorders. In: Blume KG, Forman SJ, Appelbaum FR, eds. Thomas' Hematopoietic Cell Transplantation, 3rd ed. Malden, MA, Blackwell Science, 2004:1165–1176.

59. Childs RW, Srinivasan R. Allogeneic hematopoietic cell transplantation for solid tumors. In: Blume KG, Forman SJ, Appelbaum FR, eds. Thomas' Hematopoietic Cell Transplantation, 3rd ed. Malden, MA, Blackwell Science, 2004:1177–1187.

60. Loberiza F. Report on the state of the art in blood and marrow transplantation—Part I of the IBMTR/ABMTR summary slides with guide. IBMTR/ABMTR Newsletter 2003;10:7–10.

61. Bethge A, Hegenbart U, Stuart MJ, et al. Adoptive immunotherapy with donor lymphocyte infusions after allogeneic hematopoietic cell transplantation following nonmyeloablative conditioning. Blood 2004; 103:790–795.

62. Mielcarek M, Storb R. Non-myeloablative hematopoietic cell transplantation as immunotherapy for hematologic malignances. Cancer Treat Rev 2003;29:283–290.

63. Junghanss C, Marr KA, Carter RA, et al. Incidence and outcome of bacterial and fungal infections following nonmyeloablative compared with myeloablative allogeneic hematopoietic stem cell transplantation: a matched control study. Biol Blood Marrow Transplant 2002;8:512–520.

64. Junghanss C, Boeckh M, Carter RA, et al. Incidence and outcome of cytomegalovirus infections following nonmyeloablative compared with myeloablative allogeneic stem cell transplantation: a matched control study. Blood 2002;99:1978–1985.

65. Mielcarek M, Martin PJ, Leisenring W, et al. Graft-versus host disease after nonmyeloablative versus conventional hematopoietic stem cell transplantation. Blood 2003;102:756–762.

66. Diaconescu R, Flowers CR, Storer B, et al. Morbidity and mortality with nonmyeloablative compared to myeloablative conditioning before hematopoietic cell transplantation from HLA matched related donors. Blood 2004;104:1550–1558.

67. Maris MB, Niederwieser D, Sandmaier BM, et al. HLA-Matched unrelated donor hematopoietic cell transplantation after nonmyeloablative conditioning for patients with hematologic malignancies. Blood 2003; 102:2021–2030.

68. Blaise D, Bay JO, Faucher C, et al. Reduced-intensity preparative regimen and allogeneic stem cell transplantation for advanced solid tumors. Blood 2004;103:435–441.

69. Ueno NT, Cheng YC, Rondon G, et al. Rapid induction of complete donor chimerism by the use of a reduced-intensity conditioning regimen composed of fludarabine and melphalan in allogeneic stem-cell transplantation for metastatic solid tumors. Blood 2003;102:3829–3836.

70. Fung HC, Cohen S, Rodriguez R, et al. Reduced-intensity allogeneic stem cell transplantation for patients whose prior autologous stem cell transplantation for hematologic malignancy failed. Biol Blood Marrow Transplant 2003;9:649–656.

71. Maloney DG, Molina AJ, Sagebi F, et al. Allografting with nonmyeloablative conditioning following cytoreductive autografts for the treatment of patients with multiple myeloma. Blood 2003;102:3447–3454.

72. Kumar S, DeLeve LD, Kamath PS, Tefferi A. Hepatic veno-occlusive disease (sinusoidal obstruction syndrome) after hematopoietic stem cell transplantation. Mayo Clin Proc 2003;78:589–598.

73. Wadleigh M, Richardson PG, Zahrieh D, et al. Prior gemtuzumab ozogamicin exposure significantly increases the risk of veno-occlusive disease in patients who undergo myeloablative allogeneic stem cell transplantation. Blood 2003;102:1578–1582.

74. Chalandon Y, Roosnek E, Mermillod B, et al. Prevention of veno-occlusive disease with defibrotide after allogeneic stem cell transplantation. Biol Blood Marrow Transplant 2004;10:347–354.

75. Richardson PG, Murakami C, Jin Z, et al. Multi-institutional use of defibrotide in 88 patients after stem cell transplantation with severe veno-occlusive disease and multisystem organ failure: response without significant toxicity in a high-risk population and factors predictive of outcome. Blood 2002;100:4337–4343.

76. Horak DA. Pulmonary complications after hematopoietic cell transplantation. In: Blume KG, Forman SJ, Appelbaum FR, eds. Thomas' Hematopoietic Cell Transplantation, 3rd ed. Malden, MA, Blackwell Science, 2004:873–882.

77. Spitzer TR. Engraftment syndrome following hematopoietic stem cell transplantation. Bone Marrow Transplant 2001;27:893–898.

78. Fukuda T, Hackman RC, Guthrie KA, et al. Risks and outcomes of idiopathic pneumonia syndrome after nonmyeloablative compared to conventional conditioning regimens for allogeneic hematopoietic stem cell transplantation. Blood 2003;102:2777–2785.

79. Palmas A, Tefferi A, Meyers JL, et al. Late-onset noninfectious pulmonary complications after allogeneic bone marrow transplantation. Br J Haematol 1998;100:680–687.

80. Dudek AZ, Mahaseth H, DeFor TE, Weisdorf DJ. Bronchiolitis obliterans in chronic graft-versus-host disease: analysis of risk factors and treatment outcomes. Biol Blood Marrow Transplant 2003;9:657–666.

81. Soiffer RJ. T-cell depletion to prevent graft-versus-host disease. In: Blume KG, Forman SJ, Appelbaum FR, eds. Thomas' Hematopoietic Cell Transplantation, 3rd ed. Malden, MA, Blackwell Science, 2004: 221–233.

82. Ozer H, Armitage JO, Bennett CL, et al. Update of recommendations for the use of hematopoietic colony stimulating factors: Evidence-based, clinical practice guidelines. J Clin Oncol 2000;18:3558–3585.

83. Finke J, Mertelsmann R. Recombinant growth factors after hematopoietic cell transplantation. In: Blume KG, Forman SJ, Appelbaum FR, eds. Thomas' Hematopoietic Cell Transplantation, 3rd ed. Malden, MA, Blackwell Science, 2004:613–623.

84. Bolwell B, Goomastic M, Dannley R, et al. G-CSF post-autologous progenitor cell transplantation: A randomized study of 5, 10, and 16 mcg/kg/ day. Bone Marrow Transplant 1997;19:215–219.

85. Bolwell B, Pohlman B, Andresen S, et al. Delayed G-CSF after autologous progenitor cell transplantation: prospective randomized trial. Bone Marrow Transplant 1998;21:369–373.

86. Ho VT, Mirza NQ, Junco DD, et al. The effect of hematopoietic growth factors on the risk of graft-versus-host disease after allogeneic hematopoietic stem cell transplantation: a meta-analysis. Bone Marrow Transplant 2003;32:771–775.

87. Ringden O, Labopin M, Gorin N-C, et al. Treatment with granulocyte colony-stimulating factor after allogeneic bone marrow transplantation for acute leukemia increases the risk of graft-versus-host disease and death: a study from the Acute Leukemia Working Party of the European Group for Blood and Marrow Transplantation. J Clin Oncol 2004; 22:416–423.

88. Ferrara JLM, Antin J. The pathophysiology of graft-versus-host disease. In: Blume KG, Forman SJ, Appelbaum FR, eds. Thomas' Hematopoietic Cell Transplantation, 3rd ed. Malden, MA, Blackwell Science, 2004:353–368.

89. Sullivan KM. Graft-versus-host disease. In: Blume KG, Forman SJ, Appelbaum FR, eds. Thomas' Hematopoietic Cell Transplantation, 3rd ed. Malden, MA, Blackwell Science, 2004:635–664.

90. Vogelsang GB, Lee L, Bensen-Kennedy DM. Pathogenesis and treatment of graft-versus-host disease after bone marrow transplant. Annu Rev Med 2003;54:29–52.

91. Lin M-T, Storer B, Martin PJ, et al. Relation of an interleukin-10 promoter polymorphism to graft-versus-host disease and survival after hematopoietic-cell transplantation. N Engl J Med 2003;349:2201–2210.

92. Chao NJ. Pharmacology and the use of immunosuppressive agents after hematopoietic cell transplantation. In: Blume KG, Forman SJ, Appelbaum FR, eds. Thomas' Hematopoietic Cell Transplantation, 3rd ed. Malden, MA, Blackwell Science, 2004:209–220.

93. Storb R, Pepe M, Anasetti C, et al. What role for prednisone in prevention of acute graft-versus-host disease in patients undergoing marrow transplants? Blood 1990;76:1337–1345.

94. Sayer HG, Longton G, Bowden R, et al. Increased risk of infection in marrow transplant patients receiving methylprednisolone for graft-versus-host disease prevention. Blood 1994;84:1328–1332.

95. Chao NJ, Schmidt GM, Niland JC, et al. Cyclosporine, methotrexate, and prednisone compared with cyclosporine and prednisone alone for the prophylaxis of acute graft-versus-host disease. N Engl J Med 1993; 329:1225–1230.

96. Ruutu T, Volin L, Parkkli T, et al. Cyclosporine, methotrexate, and methylprednisolone compared with cyclosporine and methotrexate for the prevention of graft-versus-host disease in bone marrow transplantation from HLA-identical sibling donor: A prospective randomized study. Blood 2000;96:2391–2398.

97. Ratanatharathorn V, Nash RA, Przepiorka D, et al. Phase III study comparing methotrexate and tacrolimus (Prograf, FK506) with methotrexate and cyclosporine for graft-versus-host disease prophylaxis after

HLA-identical sibling bone marrow transplantation. Blood 1998;92: 2303–2314.

98. Nash RA, Antin JH, Karanes C, et al. Phase 3 study comparing methotrexate and tacrolimus with methotrexate and cyclosporine for prophylaxis of acute graft-versus-host disease after marrow transplantation from unrelated donors. Blood 2000;96:2062–2068.

99. Yu C, Seidel K, Nash RA, et al. Synergism between mycophenolate mofetil and cyclosporine in preventing graft-versus-host disease among lethally irradiated dogs given DLA-identical unrelated marrow grafts. Blood 1998;91:2581–2587.

100. Elmaagacli AH, Peceny R, Steckel N, et al. Outcome of transplantation of highly purified peripheral blood CD34+ cells with T-cell add-back compared with unmanipulated bone marrow or peripheral blood stem cells from HLA-identical sibling donors in patients with first chronic phase chronic myeloid leukemia. Blood 2003;101:446–453.

101. Antin JH, Kim HT, Cutler C, et al. Sirolimus, tacrolimus, and low-dose methotrexate for graft-versus-host disease prophylaxis in mismatched related donor or unrelated donor transplantation. Blood 2003;102: 1601–1605.

102. Bacigalupo A, Lamparelli T, Bruzzi P, et al. Antithymocyte globulin for graft-versus-host disease prophylaxis in transplants from unrelated donors: 2 randomized studies from Gruppo Italiano Trapianti Midollo Osseo (GITMO). Blood 2001;98:2942–2947.

103. McDonald GB, Bouvier M, Hockenbery DM, et al. Oral beclomethasone dipropionate for treatment of intestinal graft-versus-host disease: a randomized, controlled trial. Gastroenterology 1998;115: 28–35.

104. Bruner RJ, Farag SS. Monoclonal antibodies for the prevention and treatment of graft-versus-host disease. Semin Oncol 2003;30:509–519.

105. Ho VT, Zahrieh D, Hochberg E, et al. Safety and efficacy of denileukin diftitox in patients with steroid-refractory acute graft-versus-host disease after allogeneic hematopoietic stem cell transplantation. Blood 2004;104:1224–1226.

106. Couriel D, Saliba R, Hicks K, et al. Tumor necrosis factor alpha blockade for the treatment of acute GVHD. Blood 2004;104:649–654.

107. Lee SJ, Vogelsang G, Flowers MED. Chronic graft-versus-host disease. Biol Blood Marrow Transplant 2003;9:215–233.

108. Bhushan V, Collins RH. Chronic graft-vs-host disease. JAMA 2003;290: 2599–2603.

109. Vogelsang GB. Chronic graft-versus-host disease. Br J Haematol 2004; 125:435–454.

110. Akpek G, Lee SJ, Flowers ME, et al. Performance of a new clinical grading system for chronic graft-versus-host disease: a multicenter study. Blood 2003;102:802–809.

111. Koc S, Leisenring W, Flowers MED, et al. Therapy for chronic graft-versus-host disease: a randomized trial comparing cyclosporine plus prednisone versus prednisone alone. Blood 2003;100:48–51.

112. Antin JH. Long-term care after hematopoietic-cell transplantation in adults. N Engl J Med 2002;347:36–42.

113. Socie G, Salooja N, Cohen A, et al. Nonmalignant late effects after allogeneic stem cell transplantation. Blood 2003;101:3373–3385.

114. Flowers MED, Deeg HJ. Delayed complications after hematopoietic cell transplantation. In: Blume KG, Forman SJ, Appelbaum FR, eds. Thomas' Hematopoietic Cell Transplantation, 3rd ed. Malden, MA, Blackwell Science, 2004:944–961.

115. Syrjala KL, Langer SL, Abrams JR, et al. Recovery and long-term function after hematopoietic cell transplantation for leukemia and lymphoma. JAMA 2004;291:2335–2343.

135

ASSESSMENT OF NUTRITION STATUS AND NUTRITION REQUIREMENTS

Katherine Hammond Chessman and Vanessa J. Kumpf

Learning Objectives and other resources can be found at *www.pharmacotherapyonline.com.*

KEY CONCEPTS

◀ Classification of nutrition status is often desired as a means to identify those who are nutritionally at risk or malnourished.

◀ Nutrition screening programs should identify those at risk for poor nutrition-related outcomes due to either over- or undernutrition.

◀ Nutrition assessment is the first step in formulating a patient-specific nutrition care plan for a patient who is found to be nutritionally at risk or malnourished.

◀ A nutrition-focused medical and dietary history and a nutrition-focused physical examination are key components of nutrition assessment and will reveal risk factors for and the likelihood of malnutrition and nutrient deficiencies.

◀ Appropriate anthropometric measurements are essential in a complete nutrition assessment and should be evaluated based on published standards.

◀ Biochemical (laboratory) tests are also essential for nutrition assessment, but must be interpreted in the context of the physical findings, medical history, and clinical status of the patient, as well as specific test limitations.

◀ Nutrient deficiencies involving micronutrients (e.g., vitamins or trace elements) or macronutrients (e.g., fat, protein, or carbohydrate) are possible, and a comprehensive nutrition assessment will identify the presence of these.

◀ When determining patient-specific nutrition requirements, goals should be established based on the patient's clinical condition and the need for maintenance or repletion in adults, as well as for continued growth and development in children.

◀ Drug-nutrient interactions can affect a patient's nutrition status as well as the response to or adverse effects seen with drug therapy and must be considered when evaluating a patient's nutrition care plan.

◀ An initial nutrition assessment and determination of nutrition requirements only defines an empirical starting point for a nutrition care plan. Close monitoring is required so that timely adjustments to the nutrition care plan can be made based on patient-specific responses to ensure appropriate nutrition-related outcomes.

Nutrition care is a vital component of quality patient care. This chapter reviews the current tools most commonly used for nutrition screening and accurate, relevant, and cost-effective nutrition assessment. Determination of patient-specific micro- and macronutrient requirements and potential drug-nutrient interactions are also discussed.

CLASSIFICATION OF NUTRITION DISEASE

◀ Undernutrition usually results from starvation (inadequate nutrient intake) or altered metabolism (inappropriate use of ingested nutrients). Pure starvation occurs when inadequate amounts of appropriate nutrients are available to support tissue repair or synthesis, and changes can be reversed by adequate feeding.[1] An alteration in nutrient metabolism exists when the cell has altered substrate demands

or use such as cachexia associated with inflammatory or neoplastic conditions. In such situations, enhancing nutritional intake may not be sufficient to meet the increased demand.[1] Regardless of the cause, undernutrition results in changes in subcellular, cellular, and/or organ function that expose the individual to increased risks of morbidity and mortality (see Chap. 136). In general, deficiency states can be categorized as those involving protein and calories or those involving single nutrients such as individual vitamins or trace elements. Depletion of individual nutrients leads to symptoms related to that nutrient's function. Protein-calorie malnutrition may be classified as marasmus, kwashiorkor, or mixed marasmus/kwashiorkor.

Marasmus is a chronic condition resulting from a prolonged deficiency in total intake and/or nutrient utilization. Somatic protein (skeletal muscle) and adipose tissue (subcutaneous fat) wasting occurs, but visceral protein production (e.g., albumin and transferrin) is preserved. Weight loss usually exceeds 10% of usual weight. When severe, cell-mediated immunity, measured by delayed cutaneous hypersensitivity (DCH), and muscle function are impaired. Patients with wasting diseases such as cancer commonly have marasmus and a prototypical starved, wasted appearance.

Kwashiorkor develops when there is adequate calorie but a relatively inadequate protein intake. These patients generally are well nourished but are extremely catabolic, usually secondary to trauma, infection, or burns. There is depletion of visceral (and to some degree somatic) protein pools with relative adipose tissue preservation, and hypoalbuminemia and edema are commonly seen. In the setting of severe metabolic stress and protein deprivation, kwashiorkor may develop rapidly and may result in impaired immune function.

Mixed marasmus/kwashiorkor is a form of severe protein-calorie malnutrition that develops in chronically ill, starved patients during periods of hypermetabolic stress. There is reduced visceral protein synthesis superimposed on wasting of somatic protein and energy (adipose tissue) stores. Immunocompetence is lowered, increasing the incidence of infection, and wound healing is compromised.

Obesity (overnutrition) is a major health care concern in the United States. Between 2000 and 2001, the prevalence of obesity in American adults (defined as a body mass index [BMI] of 30 kg/m^2 or greater) increased from 19.8% to 20.9%.[2] Additionally, approximately 15% of children and adolescents (ages 6 to 19 years) are obese (BMI at or above the 95th percentile for age[3] on the gender appropriate BMI-for-age growth chart published by the Centers for Disease Control National Center for Health Statistics [NCHS]).[4] Many more children are considered to be at-risk for obesity (BMI at or above the 85th percentile for age). Nutrition assessment allows identification of obese individuals or those at risk of becoming obese, and the numerous consequences of overnutrition, including type II diabetes mellitus, cardiovascular disease, and stroke (see Chap. 140).

NUTRITION SCREENING

Because a thorough nutrition assessment on every patient is not practical (or warranted), nutrition screening provides a systematic way of identifying individuals at risk for malnutrition. Risk factors for undernutrition include any disease state, complicating condition, treatment, or socioeconomic condition that may result in a decreased nutrient intake, altered metabolism, and/or malabsorption. Nutrition screening can be done in the home by the patient or home health care professional, in long-term care facilities, in ambulatory care clinics, or in the hospital. Various rating and classification systems have been proposed to assess nutrition risk and guide subsequent interventions.[5–7] Checklists are used in many clinical settings to quantify a person's food and alcohol consumption habits; ability to buy, prepare, and eat food; weight history; diagnoses; or medical/surgical procedures. Depending on the specific criteria evaluated, three to four risk factors may put a person at risk for malnutrition. Pediatric screening programs most often evaluate growth parameters against the NCHS growth charts[4] and medical conditions known to increase nutrition risk.[8] Hospital screening programs must also identify patients receiving specialized nutrition support, or enteral or parenteral nutrition prior to admission.

The Joint Commission on Accreditation of Healthcare Organizations hospital standards state: *"Based on the results of the nutrition screen and, when appropriate, nutrition assessment and re-assessment, the nutrition treatment plan is implemented for all patients determined to be at nutrition risk."*[9] For inpatients, a nutrition screening process should occur within an institution-designated period of time (usually 24 to 72 hours after admission). In the hospital setting, patients initially determined to be "not at risk" should be re-evaluated every 7 to 14 days to detect deterioration in nutrition status secondary to changes in food intake or clinical condition. By identifying at-risk individuals, nutrition screening can be a cost-effective way to help decrease complications and length of hospital stay.[10] Nutrition screening should also occur frequently in the outpatient setting, especially in young children and the elderly, to ensure that potential nutritional issues are addressed before they become significant problems.

NUTRITION ASSESSMENT

A comprehensive nutrition assessment is the first step in formulating a patient-specific nutrition care plan. Nutrition assessment has four major goals: (1) identification of the presence or risk of developing malnutrition, including disorders resulting from micro- or macronutrient deficiencies (undernutrition), obesity (overnutrition), or impaired metabolism, (2) determination of risk of malnutrition-associated complications, (3) establishment of estimated nutrition needs, and (4) establishment of baseline parameters against which to measure nutrition therapy outcomes.

A comprehensive nutrition assessment should include a nutrition-focused medical and dietary history, a physical examination including anthropometric measurements and laboratory measurements, and provides a basis for determining the patient's nutrition requirements and the optimal type and timing of nutrition intervention.

CLINICAL EVALUATION

Clinical evaluation with a nutrition-focused medical and dietary history and physical examination remains the oldest, simplest, and most widely used method of evaluating nutrition status. Clinical evaluation of nutrition status correlates well with objective evaluations (e.g., laboratory parameters and anthropometric measurements). The medical and dietary history components of the clinical evaluation will provide information about factors that predispose to malnutrition (e.g., prematurity, chronic diseases, gastrointestinal [GI] malfunction, and alcohol abuse). The clinician should direct the interview to elicit any history of weight loss, anorexia, vomiting, diarrhea, and decreased or unusual food intake (Table 135–1).

The nutrition-focused physical examination consists of an assessment of lean body mass (LBM) and the physical findings of vitamin deficiency, trace element deficiency, and essential fatty acid deficiency. The assessment should characterize the presence and degree of muscle wasting, edema, loss of subcutaneous fat, dermatitis, glossitis, cheilosis, and/or jaundice[11] (Table 135–2).

In the 1970s, an initial, comprehensive nutritional assessment required up to 3 days to complete and cost several thousand dollars. In the 1980s, the subjective global assessment (SGA), a streamlined, simplified, reproducible, cost-effective approach to nutrition assessment that took only 20 minutes to complete was introduced and is used extensively today. Five aspects of the medical and dietary history are used in the SGA: weight changes in the previous 6 months, dietary intake changes, GI symptoms, functional capacity, and disease states. Weight loss of less than 5% of usual body weight is considered a "small" loss, 5% to 10% loss is a "potentially significant loss," and more than a 10% loss is a "definitely significant loss." Dietary intake should be characterized as either normal or abnormal, and the length of time and degree of abnormal intake should be noted. The presence of GI symptoms (e.g., anorexia, nausea, vomiting, or diarrhea) on a daily basis for longer than 2 weeks is significant. Functional

TABLE 135–1. Pertinent Data from Nutrition-Focused Medical and Dietary History

Nutrition intake and dietary habits
  Anorexia or unusual or absent taste
  Dietary intake and special diets, including enteral or
    parenteral nutrition
  Formula or breast-feeding and age at initiation of solid foods
  Supplemental vitamin, mineral, or herbal intake
  Food allergies or intolerance
Underlying pathology with nutritional effects
  Chronic infections or inflammatory states
  Neoplastic diseases
  Endocrine disorders
  Chronic illness including pulmonary disease, cirrhosis, and
    renal failure
  Hypermetabolic states such as trauma, burns, and sepsis
  Digestive or absorptive disease, nausea, vomiting, or diarrhea
  Hyperlipidemia
  Prematurity
End-organ effects
  Weight change or failure to thrive
  Skin or hair changes
  Activity and energy level, exercise tolerance, and fatigue
  Obesity
  Gastrointestinal tract symptoms: diarrhea, vomiting, constipation
Miscellaneous
  Catabolic medications or therapies: corticosteroids,
    immunosuppressive agents, radiation, or chemotherapy
  Other medications: diuretics, laxatives, or anabolic steroids
  Genetic background: body habitus of parents, siblings, and family
  Alcohol or drug abuse

TABLE 135–2. Physical Findings Suggestive of Malnutrition

General appearance
  Edema (especially ankle and sacral)
  Cachexia or obesity
  Ascites
  Signs and symptoms of dehydration: poor skin turgor, sunken eyes,
    orthostasis, or dry mucous membranes
  Muscle wasting or loss of subcutaneous fat
  Obesity
Skin and mucous membranes
  Thin, shiny, or scaling skin
  Decubitus ulcers
  Ecchymoses or perifollicular petechiae
  Poorly healing of surgical or traumatic wounds
  Pallor or redness of gums or fissures at mouth edge
  Glossitis, stomatitis, or cheilosis
Musculoskeletal
  Retarded growth
  Bone pain or tenderness or epiphyseal swelling
  Muscle mass less than expected for habitus, genetic history, and
    level of exercise
Neurologic
  Ataxia, positive Romberg test, or decreased vibratory or
    position sense
  Nystagmus
  Convulsions or paralysis
  Encephalopathy
  Failure to meet age-appropriate developmental milestones
Hepatic
  Jaundice
  Hepatomegaly

capacity assesses the patient's energy level and whether the patient is active or bedridden. Finally, disease states present are assessed as to their impact on metabolic demands (i.e., no stress, low, moderate, or high stress). Four physical examination findings are rated as normal, mild, moderate, or severe: loss of subcutaneous fat (triceps and chest), muscle wasting (quadriceps and deltoids), edema (ankle and sacral), and ascites. The clinician then ranks the patient's nutritional status as adequately nourished, moderately malnourished, or severely malnourished.

ANTHROPOMETRIC MEASUREMENTS

⑤ Anthropometric measurements, gross measurements of body cell mass, are used to evaluate LBM and fat stores. The most common measurements are stature (height or length, depending on age), weight, head circumference (for children younger than 3 years of age), and measurements of limb size, such as skinfold thickness, midarm muscle circumference (MAMC), wrist circumference, and waist circumference. Bioelectrical impedance analysis (BIA) is also an anthropometric assessment tool. These parameters are used to compare an individual with normative standards for a population and as repeated measurements in an individual to monitor response to a nutrition care plan. In adults, nutrition-related changes in anthropometric measurements occur slowly; several weeks or more are usually required before detectable changes are noted. In infants and young children, however, changes may occur more quickly. Acute changes in anthropometric measurements, specifically weight and skinfold thickness, usually reflect changes in hydration status, and this must be considered when interpreting these parameters, particularly in hospitalized patients.

WEIGHT, STATURE, AND HEAD CIRCUMFERENCE

Body weight is a nonspecific measure of body cell mass, representing skeletal mass, body fat, and the energy-using component referred to as LBM. Change in weight over time, particularly in the absence of edema, ascites, and voluntary losses, is an important indicator of altered LBM. Interpretation of any actual body weight (ABW) measurement should take into consideration ideal weight-for-height, also referred to as ideal body weight (IBW) or LBM, usual body weight (UBW), fluid status, and age (Table 135–3). Dehydration will result in

TABLE 135–3. Evaluation of Actual Body Weight

Actual body weight (ABW) compared to ideal body weight (IBW)	
Undernutrition	
ABW <69% IBW	Severe malnutrition
ABW 70–79% IBW	Moderate malnutrition
ABW 80–90% IBW	Mild malnutrition
Normal	
ABW 90–120% IBW	Normal
Overnutrition	
ABW >120% IBW	Overweight
ABW ≥150% IBW	Obese
ABW ≥200% IBW	Morbidly obese

Actual body weight (ABW) compared to usual body weight (UBW)	
ABW 85–95% UBW	Mild malnutrition
ABW 75–84% UBW	Moderate malnutrition
ABW <74% UBW	Severe malnutrition

From McClave et al.[11]

TABLE 135–4. Ideal Body Weight Calculation and Assessment

Equations

Males: IBW (kg) = 50 kg + [2.3 × (inches over 5 feet)]

Females: IBW (kg) = 45.5 kg + [2.3 × (inches over 5 feet)]

Children (1–18 years): IBW (kg) = [(height in cm)^2 × 1.65]/1000

Adjusted body weight for obesity = [(ABW − IBW) × 0.25] + IBW

Examples

Male, weight 165 lb, height 6′2″	IBW = 50 kg + (2.3 × 14) = 82.2 kg
	ABW (75 kg) = 91% IBW
	Interpretation: normal
Female, weight 198 lb, height 5′6″	IBW = 45.5 kg + (2.3 × 6) = 59.3 kg
	ABW = 152% IBW
	Interpretation: obese
Child, weight 28.6 lb, height 3′2″	IBW = [(96.5)^2 × 1.65]/1,000 = 15.4 kg
	ABW = 84% IBW
	Interpretation: mild malnutrition

TABLE 135–5. Expected Growth Velocities in Children

Age	Weight (g/day)	Height (cm/month)
0–3 mo	24–35	2.8–3.4
3–6 mo	15–21	1.7–2.4
6–12 mo	10–13	1.3–1.6
1–3 y	5–9	0.6–1
4–6 y	5–6	0.5–0.6
7–10 y	7–11	0.4–0.5

Example of growth assessment:

Age: 2 months; weight: 3.9 kg; weight at 1 month of age, 3.1 kg; days since last wt: 30

Growth velocity = [(3.9 kg − 3.1 kg) × 1,000 g/kg]/30 days = 26.7 g/day

Interpretation: normal growth

From Centers for Disease Control.[4]

decreased ABW but not a loss in LBM. Once the patient is rehydrated, rechecking the weight is important to establish the baseline weight to use for nutrition evaluation. The presence of edema or ascites increases total body water (TBW), thus increasing ABW. Weights of patients with severe edema and ascites should not be used for nutrition assessment without taking the extra water weight into consideration. Subtle changes in fluid status that may affect ABW can be detected by monitoring the patient's daily fluid intake and output.

The IBW provides one population reference standard against which the ABW can be compared to detect both over- and undernutrition states. The IBW for a given height is the weight that correlates with maximum longevity. Numerous reference tables have been generated based on various population statistics. In clinical practice, mathematical equations based on gender and heights are used commonly to estimate IBW. Equations for adults (age 18 years and older) and children and examples of their use are given in Table 135–4.

Alternatively, IBW in children can be determined by identifying the weight that corresponds to the same growth percentile as the child's measured stature (length or height) on the appropriate NCHS growth chart.[4] For obese patients, an adjusted IBW should be used for nutrition-related calculations (see Table 135–4).

Change in weight over time can be calculated as the percentage of UBW, where percent change = (ABW/UBW) × 100 (see Table 135–3). Use of the UBW as a reference point provides a more accurate reflection of clinically and nutritionally significant weight changes. Determining a patient's UBW, however, depends on patient or family recall, which may be inaccurate. The use of UBW avoids the problems of normative tables, and it documents comparative changes in body weight. The change in weight also should be interpreted relative to time. In adults, unintentional weight loss of more than 10% in less than 6 months has been correlated with a poor clinical outcome.

The best indicator of adequate nutrition in a child is appropriate growth. At each medical encounter, weight, stature, and head circumference should be plotted on the appropriate NCHS gender- and age-based growth curve.[4] These charts were developed in 1977 from a large population of healthy, primarily Caucasian children and revised recently to better reflect the ethnic mix of the United States' population. Special growth charts are available for assessment of short- and long-term growth of premature infants[12] and children with Down syndrome.[13] For premature infants with corrected postnatal age of 40 weeks or more, the NCHS growth charts can be used; however, weight-for-age and length-for-age should be plotted according to corrected postnatal age until 2 years and 3.5 years of age, respectively.

Recommended intervals between measurements are weight, 7 days; length, 4 weeks; height, 8 weeks; and head circumference, 7 days in infants and 4 weeks in children up to 3 years of age.[14]

Growth velocity can be used to assess growth at intervals too close to plot accurately on a growth chart (Table 135–5). In newborns, average weight gain is 10 to 20 g/kg per day (20 to 30 g/day in term infants and 10 to 25 g/day in preterm infants).[15] Weight gain declines considerably after 2 to 3 months of age. Head growth (measured by head circumference), which is usually 0.5 cm/week during the first year of life, can be compromised during periods of critical illness or malnutrition. Sustained head growth, especially at a rate above expected, during these periods suggests hydrocephalus.

Growth failure or failure-to-thrive is defined as weight-for-age or weight-for-height (or length) below the 5th percentile or a falloff of two or more major percentiles (major percentiles are defined as 95th, 90th, 75th, 50th, 25th, 10th, and 5th). Weight-for-height evaluation is age-independent and helps differentiate the stunted child (chronic malnutrition) from the wasted child (acute malnutrition). Short stature, which is associated with many chronic diseases, is a manifestation of chronic undernutrition. Short stature in the absence of malnutrition suggests an endocrinopathy such as growth hormone deficiency, but may also be a normal variant.

BODY MASS INDEX

BMI, defined as body weight in kilograms divided by the square of the height in meters (kg/m^2), is another way to assess appropriateness of weight-for-height. BMI is more highly correlated with body fat than any other indicator using height and weight. It can be used to categorize both obesity and undernutrition in adults and children. Various tables listing BMI stratified by height and weight are available for quick reference.[16] A BMI greater than 25 kg/m^2 is considered overweight, 30 kg/m^2 or higher is obese, and a BMI less than 18.5 kg/m^2 is indicative of malnutrition. Suggested interpretation of BMI values is shown in Table 135–6.[17,18]

Although guidelines for BMI have not yet been universally accepted, in general, healthy weights are those associated with a reduction in disease risk. BMI values over 25 kg/m^2 are considered to be a risk factor for premature death and disability as a consequence of overweight and obesity (see Chap. 140). These health risks increase as the BMI increases. While BMI correlates strongly with total body fat, individual variation, especially in very muscular persons, may lead to erroneous classification of either obesity or malnutrition when BMI alone is used to assess nutrition status. As with other nutrition assessment parameters, BMI should be interpreted based on individual characteristics including gender and frame size. A major advantage of the revised NCHS growth charts for children was the addition of charts for assessment of BMI based on age and gender. It is hoped that

TABLE 135–6. Interpretation of Body Mass Index (BMI) Values

BMI (kg/m^2)	Nutrition Status
Adults	
<16	Severe malnutrition
16–17	Moderate malnutrition
17–18.5	Mild malnutrition
19–25	Healthy (19–34 years of age)
21–27	Healthy (over 35 years of age)
25–30	Overweight (19–34 years of age)
27.5–30	Overweight (over 35 years of age)
30–40	Moderate obesity
>40	Severe or morbid obesity
Children	
BMI-for-age <5th percentile	Underweight
BMI-for-age 5th–85th percentile	Healthy
BMI-for-age >85th percentile	At risk for overweight
BMI-for-age ≥95th percentile	Overweight
Example of BMI calculation and assessment	
Male, 40 y, wt 180 lb, ht 5′10″	BMI = 81.1/(1.78)^2 = 25.8 kg/m^2 Interpretation: healthy
Female, 25 y; wt 185 lb, ht 5′5″	BMI = 84.1/(1.65)^2 = 30.9 kg/m^2 Interpretation: moderately obese

From Meisler et al[17] and Himes et al.[18]

such charts will heighten parental and health care provider awareness of those children whose BMI and family history put them at risk for adult obesity and its associated risks.

CLINICAL CONTROVERSY

Historically, IBW has been used to evaluate an individual's nutrition status, specifically 1.5 times IBW has been designated as overweight. However, IBW is predicated on height, body frame size, and muscle mass. The use of IBW may lead to misclassification of nutrition status in some individuals. Body mass index is felt to be a better indicator of the level of adiposity in individuals and is becoming the standard for defining obesity. However, the BMI must also be interpreted carefully. While it is a convenient way to standardize over the normal range of height and weight seen in adults, it does not eliminate the need to consider gender and frame size.

SKINFOLD THICKNESS AND MIDARM MUSCLE CIRCUMFERENCE

Skinfold thickness measurement provides an estimate of subcutaneous fat, whereas MAMC estimates skeletal muscle mass. These simple, noninvasive anthropometric measurements are not used commonly in clinical practice, but are appropriate for both population analysis and individual long-term monitoring. Triceps skinfold thickness (TSF) is the most commonly used skinfold measurement, although reference standards also exist for subscapular and iliac sites. Over 50% of the body's fat is subcutaneous, and changes in subcutaneous fat usually reflect changes in total body fat. Careful technique in the use of pressure-regulated calipers is essential for reproducibility and reliability in measuring TSF. MAMC is a calculated value based on the measurement of the midarm circumference and TSF.

Individual anthropometric measurements should be interpreted cautiously because standards do not account for individual variations in bone size, large muscle mass, hydration status, or skin compressibil-

ity; reference standards do not account for obesity, ethnicity, illness, and increased age; and technique is critical and interobserver error may be as high as 30%. Furthermore, in adults these parameters are slow to change, often requiring weeks before significant alterations from baseline can be detected.

WAIST CIRCUMFERENCE

Waist circumference (WC) is used to assess abdominal fat content. Excess abdominal fat that is out of proportion to total body fat is considered an independent predictor of risk for obesity-related complications. Waist circumference is determined by measuring the distance around the smallest area below the rib cage and the top of the iliac crest. Interpretation varies with age. Men are considered at risk if the waist circumference is greater than 40 inches; women are at risk if the waist circumference is greater than 35 inches. These standards do not apply if the patient is less than 5 feet tall or has a BMI of 35 kg/m^2 or greater.

WAIST TO HIP RATIO

The waist:hip ratio has also been associated with undesirable health consequences. For most people, extra weight around the waist confers more of a health risk than extra weight around the hips and thighs. The waist:hip ratio is determined by dividing the waist circumference by the hip circumference. The hip circumference is determined by measuring the distance around the largest extension of the buttocks. For both men and women, a waist:hip ratio of 1 or greater is considered a risk factor for adverse health consequences. A ratio of less than 1 in men or 0.8 or less in women is considered "safe."

BIOELECTRICAL IMPEDANCE

Bioelectrical impedance (BIA) is a simple, noninvasive, and relatively inexpensive technique used to measure LBM.[19–21] The procedure is based on the fact that lean tissue has a higher electrical conductivity (less resistance) than fat, which is a poor current conductor because of its greater fluid and electrolyte content. By placing electrodes on the wrist and ankle and applying a very small electric current, impedance (resistance) to flow can be measured. Assessment of LBM, TBW, and water's distribution into compartments can be determined with BIA. Increased TBW decreases impedance; therefore, it is important to evaluate fluid status along with BIA measurements. Other potential limitations of BIA include variability with electrolyte imbalance, interference by large fat masses (obesity), and the lack of reference standards that reflect variations in individual body sizes and clinical conditions. While BIA equations have high validity when used in the population in which they were developed (mostly young, healthy adults), BIA equations are subject to errors that cannot be determined a priori unless they are validated in the specific population in which they are applied.[22–24]

BIOCHEMICAL ASSESSMENT OF LEAN BODY MASS

LBM includes skeletal muscle, somatic protein, and functional proteins such as circulating proteins and the visceral proteins. Biochemically, LBM can be assessed by measuring the serum visceral proteins, albumin (ALB), transferrin (TFN), and prealbumin (thyroxine-binding prealbumin or transthyretin). Other serum proteins, such as retinol-binding protein, fibronectin (an opsonic protein), and somatomedin-C (insulin-like growth factor-1), that have a very short half-life (less than 12 to 24 hours), have been suggested as

TABLE 135–7. Visceral Proteins Used for Assessment of Lean Body Mass

Serum Protein	Biosynthetic Site	Half-life (days)	Function	Factors Resulting in Increased Values	Factors Resulting in Decreased Values
Albumin	Hepatocyte	18–20	Maintains plasma oncotic pressure; transports small molecules	Dehydration, anabolic steroids, insulin, infection	Overhydration, edema, renal insufficiency, nephrotic syndrome, poor dietary intake, impaired digestion, burns, congestive heart failure, cirrhosis, thyroid/adrenal/pituitary hormones, trauma, sepsis
Transferrin	Hepatocyte	8	Binds Fe in plasma; transports Fe to bone	Fe deficiency, pregnancy, hypoxia, chronic blood loss, estrogens	Chronic infection, cirrhosis, burns, enteropathies, nephrotic syndrome, cortisone, testosterone
Prealbumin (transthyretin)	Hepatocyte	1–2	Binds T_3 and to a lesser extent T_4; carrier for retinol-binding protein	Renal dysfunction	Cirrhosis, hepatitis, stress, surgery, inflammation, hyperthyroidism, cystic fibrosis, renal dysfunction, zinc deficiency

Fe, iron; T_4, thyroxine; T_3, triiodothyronine.
From Spiekerman[27] and Erstad et al.[28]

indicators of nutrition status.[25] However, the clinical availability of these alternative tests is limited, and their relevance to nutrition status and the outcome of patients is debatable. Creatinine-height index has historically been used to assess LBM, but is seldom used today due to multiple concerns with its validity and a lack of evidence to support its usefulness in assessing muscle mass.[26]

VISCERAL PROTEINS

Measuring serum concentrations of the transport proteins synthesized by the liver can assess the visceral protein compartment. It is assumed that a low serum protein concentration in states of undernutrition reflects the hepatic protein synthetic mass, and therefore indirectly the functional protein mass of other organs such as heart, lung, kidney, and intestines. The visceral proteins with the greatest relevance for nutrition assessment are serum ALB, TFN, and prealbumin. Many factors other than nutrition may affect the serum concentration of these proteins, including age, abnormal renal (nephrotic syndrome) or GI tract (protein-losing enteropathy) losses, hydration status (dehydration results in hemoconcentration, overhydration in hemodilution), hepatic function (because this is the primary synthesis site), and metabolic stress (sepsis, trauma, surgery, and/or infection). Therefore visceral protein concentrations must be interpreted relative to the individual's overall clinical status (Table 135–7).[27–30]

ALB was one of the first identified biochemical markers of malnutrition and has long been used in population studies. ALB is a relatively insensitive index of early protein malnutrition because there is a large amount normally found in the body (4 to 5 g/kg of body weight), it is highly distributed in the extravascular compartment (60%), and it has a long half-life (18 to 20 days).[28] However, chronic protein deficiency in the setting of adequate nonprotein calorie intake leads to marked hypoalbuminemia because of a net ALB loss from the intravascular and extravascular compartments (kwashiorkor). Serum ALB concentrations also are affected by moderate-to-severe calorie deficiency; hepatic, renal, and GI disease; and infection, trauma, stress, and burns. In many cases, interpretation of serum ALB concentrations relative to nutrition status is difficult; however, a positive correlation between decreased serum ALB concentrations and poor clinical outcome has been demonstrated in a variety of settings. Additionally, serum ALB concentrations of 2.5 g/dL or less can be expected to exacerbate ascites and peripheral, pulmonary, and GI mucosal edema due to decreased colloid oncotic pressure.

TFN is a glycoprotein that binds and transports ferric iron to the liver and reticuloendothelial system for storage. As a surrogate marker of nutrition status, it is more likely to decrease in response to protein depletion before serum ALB concentrations decrease because it has a shorter biologic half-life (8 days), and there is less of it in the body (less than 100 mg/kg of body weight).[27] Serum TFN concentrations may be determined by direct measurement or can be estimated indirectly from measurement of total iron-binding capacity (TIBC), where $TFN = (TIBC \times 0.8) - 43$. Critical illness, hydration status, and iron stores affect the serum TFN concentration. In iron deficiency, hepatic TFN synthesis is increased, resulting in increased serum TFN concentrations unrelated to protein status.

Prealbumin is the transport protein for thyroxine and a carrier for retinol-binding protein. The body's content of prealbumin is low (10 mg/kg of body weight), and it has a very short biologic half-life (1 to 2 days).[27] Prealbumin may be reduced in as few as 3 days after calorie and protein intake is significantly decreased, or when hypercatabolism or severe metabolic stress (trauma or burns) is present. Because of its short half-life, it is most useful in monitoring the short-term, acute effects of nutrition support.[28] As with ALB and TFN, serum prealbumin concentrations are depressed in those with liver disease due to decreased hepatic synthesis. Increased serum prealbumin concentrations have been noted in patients with renal disease due to impaired renal excretion.

These serum visceral proteins are of greatest value in assessing uncomplicated semistarvation and recovery. During severe acute stress (trauma, burns, or sepsis), these proteins are relatively poor markers of nutrition status because their synthesis is downregulated as the liver increases the production of acute-phase reactants such as C-reactive protein, α_1-acid glycoprotein, and α_1-antitrypsin.

IMMUNE FUNCTION TESTS

The frequency of impaired immunocompetence and increased incidence of infection in malnourished patients suggests that certain immune function tests can be used as nutrition status markers. Nutrition affects immune status either directly, affecting primarily the lymphoid system, or indirectly by affecting cellular metabolism or organ systems that are involved with immune system regulation. Immune function tests used in nutrition assessment are the total lymphocyte count (TLC) and DCH reactions. Both tests are simple, readily available, and inexpensive. TLC reflects the number of circulating T and B lymphocytes. Tissues that generate T cells are very sensitive to malnutrition and undergo involution resulting in decreased T cell production[29] and eventually lymphopenia. TLC is calculated from a complete blood count with differential: TLC = (% lymphocytes × total number of white blood cells). Values of less than 1500 cells/mm[3] and 900 cells/mm[3] have been associated with moderate and severe nutrition depletion, respectively.[11]

DCH is commonly assessed using antigens to which the patient has been previously sensitized. The recall antigens used most frequently in nutrition assessment are mumps, *Candida albicans,* streptokinase-streptodornase, *Trichophyton,* coccidioidin, and purified protein derivative. Anergy is associated with severe malnutrition, and immune response may be restored with nutrition repletion. Other more sophisticated immune function tests have been used to evaluate nutrition status in research settings, including lymphocyte surface antigens (CD4 and CD8 counts, CD4:CD8 ratio), T-lymphocyte responsiveness, and serum interleukin concentrations. Many non–nutrition-related factors may affect immune function indicators. Non-nutrition factors that affect TLC include infection (e.g., human immunodeficiency virus/acquired immunodeficiency syndrome [HIV/AIDS], pertussis, viruses, and tuberculosis), immunosuppressive drugs (e.g., corticosteroids, cyclosporine, chemotherapy, and antilymphocyte globulin), and the presence of leukemia and lymphoma. DCH can be affected by a number of factors, including fever, viral illness, recent live virus vaccination, critical illness, irradiation, immunosuppressive drugs, diabetes mellitus, HIV/AIDS, cancer, and surgery. This lack of specificity currently limits the usefulness of these tests as nutrition status markers. There may be a role for these tests in monitoring response when a nutrition regimen includes immunotherapy.[30] Nutrients such as arginine, omega-3 fatty acids, and nucleic acids given in pharmacologic doses have been shown to improve immune function.[31–33] Monitoring the efficacy of a nutrition care plan that includes these potentially immunomodulating nutrients may need to include immune function assessment with these or other immune function indicators.

SPECIFIC NUTRIENT DEFICIENCIES

◁ A comprehensive nutrition assessment must include an evaluation of possible trace element, vitamin, and essential fatty acid deficiencies. Because of their key role in metabolic processes (as coenzymes and cofactors), a deficiency of any of these nutrients may result in altered metabolism and cell dysfunction, and may interfere with metabolic processes necessary for nutritional repletion. The evaluation of single-nutrient-deficiency states includes an accurate history to identify symptoms and risk factors that may indicate deficiency or predispose the patient to developing a deficiency state. A focused physical examination for signs of deficiencies and biochemical assessment to confirm a suspected diagnosis also should be done. Ideally, biochemical assessment would be based on the nutrient's function (e.g., metalloenzyme activity) rather than simply measuring the nutrient's serum concentration. Unfortunately, few practical methods to assess micronutrient function are available currently, and most assays measure serum concentrations of the individual nutrient.

TRACE ELEMENTS

Deficiency states have been described for the essential trace elements zinc, copper, manganese, selenium, chromium, iodine, fluoride, molybdenum, and iron. Each element is involved in a variety

of biologic functions and is necessary for normal metabolism, serving as a coenzyme and/or playing a role in hormonal metabolism or erythropoiesis. Other essential trace elements for which deficiency states have not been recognized include tin, nickel, vanadium, cobalt, gallium, aluminum, arsenic, boron, bromine, cadmium, germanium, and silicon. Toxicities can occur with excess intake of some trace elements. With the current public interest in alternative and complementary medicine, care should be taken to ask patients about their use of nutrition supplements and to assess for signs and symptoms of toxicities (overdose) as well as deficiencies (Table 135–8).

Zinc is a component of many enzymes and proteins and is involved in the regulation of gene expression. Zinc deficiency is characterized by several signs and symptoms, including a moist eczematous dermatitis most apparent in the nasolabial folds and around orifices (see Table 135–8).[34–36] Zinc deficiency occurs most frequently with abnormal GI losses, such as in Crohn's disease, malabsorptive states (e.g., short bowel syndrome), and extensive ostomy or fistula losses, or from prolonged inadequate intake, such as with zinc-free or inadequately zinc-supplemented parenteral nutrition. Zinc deficiency can be documented by the presence of low plasma zinc concentrations. However, plasma zinc concentration decreases in acute stress states such as trauma, surgery, burns, or sepsis and will generally remain depressed until the stress resolves. Also, because zinc is a normal contaminant of most blood collection tubes, special zinc-free collection tubes must be used for plasma assays. Hair zinc analysis by atomic absorption spectroscopy or neutron activation analysis may be a good indicator of zinc status in children.[37] Lymphocyte 5′-nucleotidase activity and leukocyte zinc content are better indicators of zinc status, but these assays are not widely available.

Copper is a component of enzymes involved in iron metabolism. Copper deficiency may present as hypochromic, microcytic anemia as well as leukopenia, neutropenia, skeletal demineralization, and hypercholesterolemia (see Table 135–8).[34,38] In severe cases, such as in Menkes' syndrome, copper deficiency is further manifested as hypothermia, hair and skin depigmentation, progressive mental deterioration, and growth retardation. Factors predisposing to copper deficiency include malabsorption states, protein-losing enteropathy, nephrotic syndrome, and copper-free parenteral nutrition.[33,34,38,39] Excess copper ingested or inadequate elimination on a chronic basis can result in liver cirrhosis (e.g., Wilson's disease). Copper deficiency is assessed most frequently on the basis of plasma copper or ceruloplasmin concentrations. As with zinc, serum copper concentrations may not accurately reflect total body copper status because serum concentrations may be altered by a variety of conditions and may remain normal even when hepatic stores are deficient (see Table 135–8). Copper function may be assessed by measuring activity of the cuproenzymes, erythrocyte superoxide dismutase activity, or cytochrome-C oxidase in platelets or leukocytes. Enzyme activity is decreased significantly in copper deficiency.[36,38] However, measurement of enzyme activity is method- and technique-sensitive and not available routinely.

Chromium is an important cofactor, along with insulin, in the maintenance of normal blood glucose concentrations. Chromium deficiency is characterized by glucose intolerance and impaired protein utilization. Patients with chromium deficiency also may have increased free fatty acid concentrations and a low respiratory quotient (RQ) (see Table 135–8). Chromium deficiency has only been identified in patients receiving long-term parenteral nutrition that provided inadequate chromium intake.[35,36,40,41] Plasma chromium concentrations do not accurately reflect total body chromium status, presumably because the biologically active form of chromium is an organic substance known as the *glucose tolerance factor.* Chromium toxicity

TABLE 135–8. Assessment of Trace Element Status

Trace Element	Signs of Deficiency	Signs of Toxicity	Factors Associated with Altered Plasma Concentrations
Chromium	Glucose intolerance, peripheral neuropathy, increased free fatty acid levels, low RQ, weight loss, increased LDL, glucosuria, impaired protein utilization	Industrial exposure: skin/nasal septal lesions, allergic dermatitis, increased incidence of lung cancer	Decreased: long-term inadequate intake Increased: renal failure
Copper	Neutropenia, leukopenia, hypochromic anemia, osteoporosis, hair and skin depigmentation, dermatitis, anorexia, diarrhea, mental deterioration, hypercholesterolemia	Wilson's disease: liver cirrhosis, diarrhea, vomiting, metallic taste	Decreased: high iron or vitamin C intake, corticosteroid use Increased: infection, rheumatoid arthritis, pregnancy, oral contraceptives, decreased biliary excretion
Iodine	Hypothyroid goiter, neuromuscular impairment, deaf-mutism, increased embryonic and postnatal mortality, cognitive impairment, impaired fertility, cretinism (severe cases)	Thyrotoxicosis: nodular goiter, weight loss, tachycardia, muscle weakness, warm skin	Decreased: long-term inadequate intake
Iron	Microcytic, hypochromic anemia, fatigue, weakness, pallor, glossitis, headache, dysphagia, fingernail changes, gastric atrophy, paresthesias	Liver cirrhosis, cardiomyopathy, pancreatic damage, skin pigmentation	Increased: blood transfusion Decreased: blood loss
Manganese	Nausea, vomiting, dermatitis, hair color changes, hypocholesterolemia, growth retardation, defective carbohydrate and protein metabolism	Parkinsonian-like symptoms, hyperirritability, hallucinations, libido disturbances, ataxia	Increased: decreased biliary excretion high iron or vitamin C intake
Molybdenum	Tachycardia, tachypnea, altered mental status, visual changes, headache, nausea, vomiting	Gout-like syndrome, increased urinary copper	Varies with assay used High iron or vitamin C intake
Selenium	Muscle weakness and pain, cardiomyopathy	Nausea, vomiting, hair and nail loss, tooth decay, skin lesions, irritability, fatigue, peripheral neuropathy	Decreased: malignancy, liver failure, pregnancy Increased: reticuloendothelial neoplasia
Zinc	Dermatitis, hypogeusia, alopecia, diarrhea, apathy, depression, growth retardation, impaired wound healing, immunosuppression	Acute: gastric distress, nausea, dizziness, death with large intravenous doses Chronic: immunosuppression, decreased HDL, copper deficiency	Decreased: infection, hypoalbuminemia, corticosteroids, pregnancy, burns, stress, inflammation Increased: tissue injury, hemolysis, contaminated collection tube

HDL, high-density-lipoprotein cholesterol; LDL, low-density-lipoprotein cholesterol; RQ, respiratory quotient.

is not a common clinical concern and has been reported only with contaminated drinking water or industrial exposure.

Manganese is important in the function of many enzymes, including arginase (amino acid metabolism), pyruvate carboxylase (carbohydrate metabolism), and superoxide dismutase (cholesterol metabolism; antioxidant), and in bone formation. Manganese deficiency has only been reported in association with the ingestion of chemically defined manganese-deficient oral diets.[34–36] Symptoms associated with manganese deficiency include nausea, vomiting, dermatitis, hair color changes, hypocholesterolemia, and growth retardation (see Table 135–8). Manganese toxicity is more concerning and has been described in several patients receiving long-term parenteral nutrition.[42–44]

Manganese appears to accumulate in brain tissue, especially in the setting of chronic cholestasis and short bowel syndrome. Clinical toxicity is evidenced primarily by extrapyramidal symptoms mimicking Parkinson's disease. Serum manganese concentrations do not correlate well with the clinical presentation, but magnetic resonance imaging (MRI) of the basal ganglia may show hyperintensity areas, especially in the globus pallidus. In most reported cases, discontinuation of manganese in the parenteral nutrition solution resulted in resolution of neurologic symptoms in 6 months with partial or total normalization of the MRI after 1 to 2 years. Other methods of evaluating man-

ganese status include measuring the manganese content of mononuclear blood cells[45] and the activity of manganese superoxide dismutase, a mitochondrial antioxidant enzyme.[46] While these methods are good indicators of manganese status, they are not widely available.

Selenium, as selenocysteine, is incorporated into glutathione peroxidase (antioxidant), iodothyronine deiodinase (thyroid hormone regulation), and selenoprotein P (vitamin C metabolism). Prematurity, acute illness, chronic GI losses, and long-term selenium-free parenteral nutrition are associated with low serum selenium concentrations and decreased glutathione peroxidase activity.[36,47–49] The clinical significance of reduced serum selenium concentrations is unclear. Selenium deficiency has been described in patients receiving long-term selenium-free parenteral nutrition. Muscle pain and weakness are the most frequently observed signs and symptoms (see Table 135–8), but severe biochemical deficiency is not always accompanied by these symptoms.[50] Fatal cardiomyopathy has been reported in several cases.

Selenium toxicity may occur when patients receive doses exceeding 200 mcg/kg per day for prolonged periods.[51] Selenium status may be assessed by measuring plasma selenium concentrations, which will reflect recent selenium intake. Decreased concentrations may indicate selenium deficiency, but reductions also have been observed in patients with malignancies, liver failure, and pregnancy. Assays that measure the activity of the selenium-containing enzyme glutathione peroxidase in erythrocytes or the plasma concentration of selenoprotein P may be more sensitive measurements of selenium status because they reflect chronic ingestion, but neither is widely available.[50]

Molybdenum is a cofactor for enzymes involved in catabolism of sulfur amino acids, purines, and pyrimidines (i.e., xanthine, aldehyde, and sulfite oxidases). Molybdenum deficiency is rare. One case of molybdenum deficiency has been reported in a patient receiving long-term home parenteral nutrition who presented with symptoms that included tachycardia, tachypnea, headache, night blindness, nausea, vomiting, central scotomas, lethargy, disorientation, and ultimately coma (see Table 135–8). Symptoms were reversed when molybdenum was added to the parenteral nutrition solution. Factors predisposing to molybdenum deficiency appear to be low birthweight,[52] excessive loss via the GI tract, such as with short bowel syndrome, and long-term inadequate intake, such as with molybdenum-free parenteral nutrition. Biochemical abnormalities expected in molybdenum deficiency include very low serum and urine uric acid concentrations (low xanthine oxidase activity) and low urine inorganic sulfate concentrations (low sulfate oxidase activity).[53]

Deficiency of iodine, a component of thyroid hormones, may result in goiter formation (see Chap. 73). However, not everyone with an iodine-deficient diet will develop a goiter. Thyroxine (T_4) and triiodothyronine (T_3) can be used to assess iodine status (see Table 135–8). Intravenous iodine supplements typically are not necessary except during long-term parenteral nutrition with minimal enteral intake. Iodine needs generally are met by cutaneous absorption of iodine from germicides (e.g., povidone-iodine) used in catheter care or consumption of iodized salt.[54,55] Use of povidone-iodine will likely decrease with the increased use of chlorhexidine for catheter care, and the need for iodine supplementation must be individualized. Iodine excess is rarely a clinical concern when thyroid function is normal.

Iron is an important component of hemoglobin, myoglobin, and cytochrome enzymes; therefore, it is important in oxygen transport, muscle iron storage, and cellular energy production. Patients with iron deficiency anemia generally present with fatigue, weakness, and pallor, but they also may have other symptoms[36,56] (see Chap. 99). Inadequate iron intake, malabsorption, and blood loss are the principal causes of iron deficiency anemia. Iron toxicity (overload) with possible organ damage can occur when chronic iron intake exceeds requirements. Iron deficiency is confirmed by assessment of body iron stores, as reflected indirectly by measurement of hemoglobin, serum iron, TIBC, and serum ferritin, or directly by marrow staining and liver biopsy.[56] Although the direct methods are the most accurate, they are invasive, and indirect measurements are used more commonly. However, indirect parameters may be altered by chronic illness independent of iron stores; thus concomitant illness must be considered in their interpretation.

VITAMINS

A thorough nutrition-focused history and physical examination is the most valuable means of screening patients for vitamin deficiency or toxicity (Table 135–9). It is uncommon to see a single vitamin deficiency; usually multiple vitamin deficiencies occur with general malnutrition. Single vitamin deficiencies do occur, however. Thiamine deficiency may result in lactic acidosis and encephalopathy,[57] whereas pernicious anemia due to vitamin B_{12} deficiency has been reported with increasing frequency, especially in the elderly. Recently, the incidence of vitamin D deficiency has increased in children. Laboratory assessment may be useful to confirm the clinical suspicion of a deficiency state. The first indication of a deficiency is usually a fall in circulating serum concentrations of the vitamin or its coenzyme.

Subsequently, there is a decrease in urinary excretion of the vitamin, which in turn is followed by diminished tissue concentrations of the vitamin. The most common measurements of vitamin status are assays of circulating amounts in plasma or serum. Assays of biochemical or metabolic function of the vitamin are more likely to reflect body stores than are serum concentrations. Most of these functional assays use erythrocyte or leukocyte extracts to determine apoenzyme activity, which is dependent on the vitamin coenzyme (see Table 135–9).

ESSENTIAL FATTY ACIDS

The body can synthesize most fatty acids except for linoleic acid (an omega-6 fatty acid) and linolenic acid (an omega-3 fatty acid). Therefore intake of approximately 2% to 4% of total calories as these fatty acids is essential to prevent deficiency. Essential fatty acid deficiency is rare in adults and children but can occur with prolonged use of lipid-free parenteral nutrition, with severe fat malabsorption, with very-low-fat enteral feeding formulations, or with severe malnutrition, especially in stressed patients.[58] In critically ill adults and older children with increased metabolic demands, essential fatty acid deficiency has been reported to occur within 1 week of starting lipid-free parenteral nutrition.[58,59] Newborns, especially those born prematurely, have limited fat stores; therefore, they may develop essential fatty acid deficiency more rapidly than adults. Biochemical essential fatty acid deficiency has been noted within 72 hours after birth in preterm infants receiving fat-free intravenous solutions.[60] Symptoms of essential fatty acid deficiency include dermatitis (dry, cracked, scaly skin), alopecia, impaired wound healing, growth failure, thrombocytopenia, and anemia.

Linoleic acid normally is converted to arachidonic acid (a tetraene fatty acid). If linoleic acid is unavailable, oleic acid will be substituted, which results in production of eicosatrienoic acid (a triene fatty acid) as the metabolic end product. Therefore essential fatty acid deficiency can be detected on the basis of decreased tetraene production and increased triene production. Normally, the ratio of trienes to tetraenes is less than 0.4; when this ratio becomes greater than 0.4, the diagnosis of essential fatty acid deficiency is established. Analysis of plasma fatty acids, however, is expensive and not widely available.

CARNITINE

Carnitine is a quaternary amine required for transport of long-chain fatty acids into the mitochondria for β-oxidation and energy production. Carnitine also binds acyl residues and helps in their elimination (detoxification), thereby decreasing the number conjugated with coenzyme A and increasing the ratio of free to acetylated coenzyme A. Carnitine is available from a wide variety of dietary sources (especially meats) and can be synthesized by the liver and kidneys from lysine and methionine. Hepatic synthesis is decreased in premature infants, and low plasma carnitine concentrations and/or overt carnitine deficiency have been documented in premature infants receiving parenteral nutrition or carnitine-free diets, as well as in those with inborn errors of metabolism.[61–64] Other predisposing factors for carnitine deficiency include chronic kidney or liver disease, vitamin C deficiency, chronic use of valproic acid and zidovudine, and a vegetarian diet.[63–65]

The clinical presentation of carnitine deficiency includes generalized skeletal muscle weakness, fatty liver, and fasting hypoglycemia. Carnitine status can be assessed by measurement of plasma, urine, or red blood cell total and free carnitine concentrations. Plasma and urine carnitine concentrations are most helpful in primary carnitine deficiency (an inborn error of metabolism). Plasma concentrations constitute less than 1% of the total body carnitine.[64,65]

TABLE 135–9. Assessment of Vitamin Status

Vitamin	Signs of Deficiency	Laboratory Assay	Comments
Water-soluble vitamins			
Thiamine (B$_1$)	Paresthesias, nystagmus, impaired memory, lactic acidosis, congestive heart failure, Wernicke-Korsakoff syndrome	Red blood transketolase activity	Increased need with hemodialysis, peritoneal dialysis, malabsorption
Riboflavin (B$_2$)	Mucositis, dermatitis, cheilosis, photophobia, corneal vascularization, lacrimation, decreased vision, impaired wound healing, normocytic anemia	Urinary riboflavin	
Pantothenic acid	Fatigue, malaise, headache, insomnia, vomiting, abdominal cramps	Serum pantothenic acid	
Niacin	Pellagra: dermatitis, dementia, glossitis, diarrhea, memory loss, headaches	Urinary niacin metabolites	Flushing and GI distress can be seen with supplements; increased need with hemo- and peritoneal dialysis, malabsorption
Pyridoxine (B$_6$)	Dermatitis, neuritis, convulsions, microcytic anemia	Plasma B$_6$	Sensory neuropathy (high supplement intake)
Folic acid	Megaloblastic anemia, diarrhea, glossitis	Serum folate	Decreased with increased cellular/tissue turnover (pregnancy, malignancy, hemolytic anemia); masks neurologic complications of vitamin B$_{12}$ deficiency; decreases risks of neural tube defects
Cobalamin (B$_{12}$)	Pernicious anemia, glossitis, spinal cord degeneration, peripheral neuropathy	Serum B$_{12}$	Decreased absorption in the elderly, distal ileal resection, loss of gastric intrinsic factor
Biotin	Dermatitis depression, lassitude, somnolence	Urinary biotin	
Ascorbic acid (C)	Enlargement and keratosis of hair follicles, impaired wound healing, anemia, lethargy, depression, bleeding, ecchymosis	Plasma ascorbic acid	GI disturbances, kidney stones, excess iron absorption with excess intake; smokers need 35 mg/day more than nonsmokers
Fat-soluble vitamins			
A	Dermatitis, night blindness, keratomalacia, xerophthalmia	Serum vitamin A	Teratogenic effects, liver toxicity with excessive intake; alcohol intake, liver disease, hyperlipidemia, and severe protein malnutrition increase susceptibility to adverse effects of high intake; β-carotene supplements recommended only for those at risk of deficiency (fat malabsorption)
D	Rickets, osteomalacia, muscle weakness	Plasma 25-hydroxy vitamin D	Elevated intake causes hypercalcemia; decreased in uremia, vitamin D at ages >60 y may be decreased in winter, fat malabsorption
E	Hemolysis	Serum vitamin E	Excess intake: hemorrhagic toxicity; anticoagulant effect should be monitored carefully if taking supplements
K	Bleeding	Prothrombin time	Anticoagulant therapy can be affected by supplements or diet

Acylcarnitine concentrations are more helpful in secondary causes of carnitine deficiency. When only total and free concentrations are available, the free is subtracted from the total to give the acylcarnitine concentration.

MUSCLE FUNCTION TESTS

A relatively new approach to nutrition assessment is to evaluate muscle function as an end-organ response. Hand-grip strength (forearm muscle dynamometry), respiratory muscle strength, and muscle re-

sponse to electrical stimulation have been used.[66] Hand-grip strength has been shown to correlate with patient outcome. Forearm muscle dynamometry is a relatively simple, noninvasive, and inexpensive procedure. Ulnar nerve stimulation causes measurable muscle contraction. In the setting of malnutrition, increased fatigue and a slowed muscle relaxation rate have been noted; these indices return to normal after refeeding. Both these parameters have the advantage of being indicators of tissue function rather than composition. Their utility in clinical practice is currently hampered by a lack of appropriate reference standards and limited data confirming their sensitivity and specificity as nutrition assessment tools.

OTHER NUTRITION ASSESSMENT TOOLS

Various methods to determine body composition have been used in the research setting. These methods generally are complex, require expensive technology, and at present are limited to research centers. One of the most promising for clinical practice is dual-energy x-ray absorptiometry (DEXA). This procedure is now available in many hospitals and clinics for measuring bone density. DEXA also can be used to quantify the mineral, fat, and LBM compartments. Ultrasound and infrared interactance can be used to measure subcutaneous fat. The latter uses an inexpensive and portable device, but these measurements have not been used extensively for nutrition assessment. MRI and computed tomography can measure subcutaneous, intra-abdominal, and regional fat distribution. Neutron activation is a means of measuring body nitrogen, calcium, sodium, chloride, and phosphorus. These measurements can then be used to calculate total body fat, bone, and protein. Isotope dilution methods determine TBW and underwater weighing determines density. In addition, these methods can be used to estimate LBM and body fat. Furthermore, LBM also can be estimated using total body electrical conductivity and by measuring the naturally occurring isotope ^{40}K.

ASSESSMENT OF NUTRIENT REQUIREMENTS

Nutrition requirements depend on an individual's clinical condition and the need for continued maintenance of adequate nutrition, or whether starvation or ongoing metabolic stress dictate a need for repletion. For obese patients, usual nutrition requirements may be altered due to the need for weight loss. In children, there is the added consideration of sustaining or re-establishing normal growth and development. Organ function (e.g., intestine, kidney, liver, and pancreas) may affect nutrient utilization.

Nutrient requirements vary with age, gender, size, disease state, clinical condition, nutrition status, and physical activity level. An estimate of nutrient requirements therefore must be made using guidelines interpreted in the context of these patient-specific factors. The recommended dietary allowances (RDAs) initially were intended to provide information to be used to prevent nutritional deficiencies in a healthy population of individuals,[67] but have often been used inappropriately to evaluate the diets of individuals. In the early 1990s, the Food and Nutrition Board began the task of revising the RDAs, and created a new family of nutrition reference values, the dietary reference intakes (DRIs) and seven nutrient groups.[68]

The four categories of the new DRIs are estimated average requirements (EARs), recommended dietary allowances (RDAs), adequate intakes (AIs), and tolerable upper intake level (UL). EARs can be used for planning recommended nutrient intake for groups, as they are defined as the amount of the nutrient that meets the needs of 50% of persons in a given group. The RDA is designated as nutrient intake that meets the needs of almost all persons in the designated group. The RDA is approximately two standard deviations above the EAR for nutrients for which the requirement is well defined, and 1.2 times the EAR for nutrients for which there is more variability. AIs are defined as the average intake of a designated group that appears to sustain a particular nutrition state, growth, or other functional indication of health. This category is reserved for nutrients for which no EAR or RDA has been determined. Finally the UL is the maximum nutrient intake that is unlikely to pose adverse affects in almost all persons in a designated group. DRIs have been established for six of the seven established nutrient groups: (1) calcium, phosphorus, magnesium, vitamin D, and fluoride;[69] (2) folate and other B vitamins;[70] (3) antioxidants (e.g., selenium and vitamins C and E);[71] (4) trace elements;[72] (5) macronutrients (e.g., protein, fat, carbohydrates, and fiber);[73] and (6) electrolytes and water.[74] Recommendations for group 7, which includes other food components (e.g., phytoestrogens), are still in development.

ENERGY REQUIREMENTS

The DRIs for macronutrients[73] recommend that adults consume 45% to 65% of their total calories from carbohydrates, 20% to 35% from fat, and 10% to 35% from protein. The recommendations for children are similar, except that infants and younger children need a higher proportion of fat (approximately 40% to 50% of total calories) in their diets. An RDA for total carbohydrates for adults and children of 130 g/day was set with the most recent revisions.[73]

CLINICAL CONTROVERSY

Clinicians have debated whether calorie requirements should be expressed in terms of total or nonprotein calories. Those that use nonprotein calories base the decision on the theory that protein should be used for synthesis, not energy production. Those that correctly use total calories know that in the presence of adequate calorie intake, protein is not necessarily prioritized solely for anabolism. Also, standard equations such as the HBEs used to estimate energy needs were derived from measurement of energy expenditure and thus estimate total calories. In fact, while daily protein intake is used primarily for synthesis, protein is constantly being metabolized to energy. Approximately 15% of the total caloric expenditure comes from the breakdown of protein and other nitrogen-containing molecules. Additionally, calorie goals should be consistent among enteral, parenteral, and oral routes, necessitating the use of total calories.

There are numerous published methods for determining an individual's total energy or calorie (kcal) requirement. The most commonly used methods to determine energy requirements use calories per kilogram of body weight (kcal/kg), equations that estimate energy expenditure, or indirect calorimetry. The simplest method to assess energy requirements is to use population estimates of calories required per kilogram of body weight. This method assumes standard values for the energy requirements associated with various disease states or clinical conditions, as well as the additional requirements for repletion of a malnourished individual. It does not take into consideration age- or gender-related differences in energy needs. Daily adult requirements determined by this method, using actual body weight or adjusted body weight in kilograms, generally are accepted to be:

Healthy, normal nutrition status: 20 to 25 kcal/kg per day
Malnourished or mildly metabolically stressed: 25 to 30 kcal/kg per day
Critically ill, hypermetabolic: 30 to 35 kcal/kg per day
Major burn injury (>50% total body surface area): 35 to 40 kcal/kg per day

Suggested calorie intakes for maintenance and normal growth of healthy infants and children are shown in Table 135–10.[73] For children, these maintenance energy requirements are approximately 150% of basal metabolic rate (BMR) with the additional calories

TABLE 135–10. Dietary Reference Intakes for Energy and Protein in Healthy Children

Age (Reference age/wt)	Estimated Energy Requirement (kcal/day) Male	Estimated Energy Requirement (kcal/day) Female	Protein RDA (g/kg/day)
0–6 mo (3 mo/6 kg)	570	520	1.52[a]
7–12 mo (9 mo/9 kg)	743	676	1.5
1–2 yr (24 mo/12 kg)	1046	992	
1–3 yr (24 mo/12 kg)			1.1
3–8 yr (6 y/20 kg)	1742	1642	
4–8 yr (6 y/20 kg)			0.95
9–13 yr (11 y/M: 36 kg; F: 37 kg)	2279	2071	0.95
14–18 yr (16 y/M: 61 kg; F: 54 kg)	3152	2368	0.85

F, female; M, male; RDA, recommended dietary allowance.
[a]Adequate intake.

TABLE 135–12. Stress Factors for Use in Children and Adults

Condition	Factor
No stress	
Confined to bed	1.2
Out of bed: normal activity	1.3
Mild stress	
Postoperative recovery: uncomplicated surgery	1
Trauma: mild (e.g., long bone fracture)	1.2
Moderate stress	
Sepsis (moderate)	1.3
Trauma: central nervous system (sedated)	1.3
Trauma: moderate to severe	1.5
Severe stress	
Sepsis (severe)	1.6
Trauma: central nervous system (severe)	Up to 2.0
Burns (proportionate to burned area)	Up to 2.0

needed to support activity and growth. Caloric requirements increase with fever, sepsis, major surgery, trauma, burns, and long-term growth failure, and in the presence of chronic conditions such as bronchopulmonary dysplasia, congenital heart disease, and cystic fibrosis. Caloric needs may decrease with obesity and neurologic disability (e.g., cerebral palsy). Clinical judgment and close monitoring are essential to ensure that the desired nutrition therapy outcomes are attained.

Various equations are used to estimate energy needs (Table 135–11). The Harris-Benedict equations, which were first published in 1919, remain one of the most popular means used to assess energy requirements in adults. They have the advantage of taking into consideration the patient's age, height, weight, gender, and clinical condition. The HBEs were derived from oxygen consumption

TABLE 135–11. Equations to Estimate Basal Energy Expenditure in Adults and Children

Harris-Benedict (kcal/day):
Males: BEE = 66 + [(13.7W(kg)] + [5H(cm)] − (6.8A)
Females: BEE = 655 + [(9.6W(kg)] + [1.8H(cm)] − (4.7A)
Modified Harris-Benedict (kcal/day) for adults >60 years of age:
Males: BEE = [(8.8W(kg)] + [1128H(m)] − 1071
Females: BEE = [(9.2W(kg)] + [637H(m)] − 302
Caldwell-Kennedy (kcal/day) for children <3 years of age:
BEE = 22 + (31W) + [1.2H(cm)]
Schofield (MJ/day) (to convert to kcal/day multiply by 239.2):
3–10 years of age
Males: BMR = (0.08W) + [0.55H(m)] + 1.74
Females: BMR = (0.07W) + [0.68H(m)] + 1.55
10–18 years of age
Males: BMR = (0.07W) + [0.57H(m)] + 2.16
Females: BMR = (0.04W) + [1.95H(m)] + 0.84
FAO/WHO/UNU (kcal/day):
3–10 years of age
Males: BMR = 22.7W + 495
Females: BMR = 22.5W + 499
10–18 years of age
Males: BMR = 17.5W + 651
Females: BMR = 12.2W + 746

A, age in years; BEE, basal energy expenditure; BMR, basal metabolic rate; FAO/WHO/UNU, Food and Agriculture Organization/World Health Organization/United Nations University; H, height in centimeters (cm) or meters (m), as indicated; MJ, megajoules; W, weight in kilograms.

measurements made on normally nourished individuals who were in a fasting and resting state. While these equations are commonly referred to as the basal energy expenditure (BEE) equations, they actually estimate resting energy expenditure (REE). This is the amount of energy expended by an awake individual to perform only basal functions such as breathing, circulating blood, and fasting metabolic processes. The original HBEs along with modifications for adults over age 60 years are shown in Table 135–11.

Because these equations approximate REE, their results must be modified by a factor that is most representative of the individual's clinical condition. For example, an individual who is confined to bed may require a calorie intake that is 20% above the REE, whereas a person who is suffering from a severe burn injury may require a 150% to 200% increase over the calculated REE. The metabolic response to stress in children appears to be similar to that seen in critically ill adults, and the "stress factors" used in adults shown in Table 135–12 can be used in children once the REE has been determined using one of the equations shown in Table 135–11.[75,76] Controversy exists over the accuracy and reliability of predicting energy expenditure based on these equations because clinical judgments will vary with each clinician.[77–79] Additionally, in validation studies in healthy subjects, these equations have been shown to overestimate REE by 5% to 15%.[79] It is also important to note that ABW (up to a BMI of 57 kg/m^2 in men and 40 kg/m^2 in women), not IBW, was used to generate the original data with these equations.[79]

The most accurate clinical tool for determining energy requirements is to measure them using indirect calorimetry, also referred to as metabolic gas monitoring.[80] Indirect calorimetry methodology is based on the fact that when substrates (carbohydrates, fat, and protein) are oxidized, oxygen (O_2) is consumed and carbon dioxide (CO_2) is produced in varying amounts depending on the substrate being oxidized. Indirect calorimetry is a noninvasive procedure in which oxygen consumption (Vo_2, mL/min) and carbon dioxide production (Vco_2, mL/min) are measured. Using the abbreviated Weir equation, REE (kcal/day) can be calculated as $(3.9Vo_2 + 1.1Vco_2) \times 1.44$.[80]

This measured energy expenditure represents the actual energy expended by the patient during the time period during which the measurements were taken. It is often extrapolated to a 24-hour period to approximate daily energy requirements. REE measurement reflects alterations in energy requirements due to disease or clinical condition, but does not include energy required for nutritional repletion of a malnourished individual or growth in a child. The energy intake required for these functions can be calculated as follows depending on nutrition goals: maintenance, 1 to 1.3 × REE; repletion or growth, 1.3 to 1.5 × REE; and depletion, less than 1 × REE.

The data obtained from indirect calorimetry also can be used to determine an RQ which reflects substrate oxidation, characterizes substrate use, and is calculated as V_{CO_2}/V_{O_2}. RQ values for nutrient substrates are fat, 0.7; carbohydrate, 1; protein, 0.8; and mixed substrate (fat, carbohydrate, and protein), 0.85. An RQ value of greater than 1 represents either lipogenesis or hyperventilation; an RQ value of less than 0.7 may indicate a ketogenic diet, fat gluconeogenesis, or ethanol oxidation. Values outside the 0.67 to 1.3 range should raise doubts as to the test's validity. Clinically the RQ is used to determine if a patient is being overfed, which is indicated by an RQ value greater than 1.

CLINICAL CONTROVERSY

The Harris-Benedict equations (HBEs) have been validated in many settings; however, depending on the "stress" factor chosen, may overestimate true needs in some populations. In patients with pulmonary artery catheters, energy needs can be determined using the Fick method assuming a respiratory quotient of 0.85, and using cardiac output and measurement of saturation of arterial and mixed venous blood. Indirect calorimetry can also be used to measure energy expenditure in an individual. All of these methods have advantages and disadvantages. Energy expenditure is not a fixed value that never changes. In critically ill patients particularly, energy expenditure can vary significantly from one period of time to the next, depending on other interventions (e.g., paralyzation, sedation, or analgesia), and the patient's clinical condition (e.g., sepsis, burns, or trauma). No one method has been shown to be superior to another. Estimates of energy needs derived from any of these techniques should be viewed as empiric estimates. The patient's response to these intakes should be carefully monitored.

There are limitations to the use of indirect calorimetry.[79,80] Not all institutions have metabolic carts available or personnel trained to use them. Calibration errors are common, and indirect calorimetry overestimates REE for patients with hyperventilation, metabolic acidosis, overfeeding, and air leaks anywhere in the system. Underestimates of REE are likely with hypoventilation, metabolic alkalosis, underfeeding, and gluconeogenesis. Mechanically ventilated patients are technically easier to study because the indirect calorimeter circuit can be plugged into the ventilator circuit. The patient must be at complete rest for 1 hour, must not receive bolus feedings either by feeding tube or orally for 4 hours, should have no changes in substrate delivery for 12 hours, must be on a fraction of inspired oxygen of less than 0.6, and the positive end-expiratory pressure must be less than 5 cm H_2O to ensure a steady-state reading. Unfortunately, most of the patients in whom indirect calorimetry would be desirable will not meet these requirements.

PROTEIN

Daily protein requirements are based on age, nutrition status, disease state, and clinical condition. The RDA for protein for children is shown in Table 135–10, and for individuals over 18 years of age the RDA is 0.8 g/kg per day, which is much less than most people typically consume.[73] In adults older than 60 years of age, protein needs are increased to 1 g/kg per day to help reduce the loss of LBM that occurs with aging, and up to 1.5 to 2 g/kg per day may be needed in states of metabolic stress such as infection, trauma, and surgery,

to prevent loss of LBM.[73,81] Protein requirements are also higher in pregnant and lactating women (1.1 g/kg per day).[73] In general, protein intake should be approximately 10% to 35% of total calories in the normal diet.

Protein metabolism depends on both kidney and liver function; therefore, protein requirements will be altered with decreased kidney or liver function (see Chap. 139). Critical illness (e.g., sepsis, burns, or trauma) will result in a hypercatabolic state in which there is increased protein synthesis and degradation. Consequently, protein requirements will be increased to 1.5 to 2 g/kg per day. In burn patients, protein requirements may be as high as 2.5 to 3 g/kg per day. Liver failure typically results in the need for protein restriction (0.5 g/kg per day) except if a hypercatabolic state is also present, in which case the requirement may be increased to 1.5 g/kg per day. Protein needs in renal failure are variable and affected by the various renal replacement therapies available. The application of these guidelines requires both clinical judgment and frequent monitoring of renal and liver function, serum chemistries, clinical condition, and nutrition outcomes (see Chap. 139).

Nitrogen is found only in protein and at a relatively constant ratio of 1 g nitrogen per 6.25 g protein. This ratio may vary somewhat for enteral and parenteral feeding formulations, depending on the biologic value of the protein source. Adequacy of protein intake can be assessed clinically by measuring urinary nitrogen excretion and comparing it with nitrogen intake—a nitrogen balance study. Nitrogen balance indirectly reflects an individual's protein use or protein catabolic rate, which increases in states associated with hypercatabolism.[82] As the stress level increases, the concomitant increase in protein catabolism results in an increase in urinary nitrogen excretion.[83] Usually the amount of urea nitrogen is measured in a 24-hour urine urea collection (24-h UUN). In healthy individuals, the quantity of UUN accounts for 80% to 90% of the total urine nitrogen (TUN) excreted. Nitrogen output (g/day) can be approximated as 24-h UUN + 4, where 4 is a factor representing usual skin, fecal, and respiratory nitrogen losses.[84] Alternatively, if available, TUN can be measured and may be more accurate, but it is generally more expensive.[88] If TUN is used, then the best estimate of nitrogen output is TUN × 1.05.[84] In patients with renal failure, in which case neither measured UUN nor TUN represents nitrogen generation, protein turnover can be approximated with equations based on urea kinetics that estimate the rate of urea production.[26]

FAT

The AI for men and women for fat is 1.6 and 1.1 g of α-linolenic acid daily, respectively, and for linoleic acid is 17 g/day for adult men and 12 g/day for adult women. Overall, fat should represent no more than 20% to 35% of total calories with the recommendation that saturated fatty acids, *trans* fatty acids, and dietary cholesterol intake be kept as low as possible while consuming a nutritionally adequate diet.[73] As mentioned previously, fat intake in children less than 2 years of age is critical for proper central nervous system growth and development; therefore, no fat restriction (e.g., skim milk) should be imposed until after the age of 2 years.

FIBER

Maintenance of normal bowel habits, lower blood pressure, and lower cholesterol serum concentrations have been attributed to adequate dietary fiber intake. Some evidence, although inconclusive, also suggests that fiber has a role in the prevention of colon cancer and promotion of weight control. Men and women 50 years of age and younger should ingest 38 g/day and 25 g/day, respectively, of total fiber. For men and women over the age of 50, the recommended intakes are 30 g/day and 21 g/day, respectively.[73] For children less than 16 years of age, the "age + 5" rule is often used. The recommended daily intake of fiber is calculated by adding 5 g to the child's age in years. For example, a 6-year-old child should ingest 11 g/day of dietary fiber.

FLUID

The daily fluid requirement for adults depends on many factors but is generally 30 to 35 mL/kg. It also can be estimated as 1 mL/kcal ingested or as 1500 mL/m^2 per 24 hours. Fluid requirements per kilogram are higher for children and even higher for preterm infants due to their higher percentage of TBW and BEE. Additionally, premature neonates have increased fluid requirements due to greater insensible losses and the kidney's inefficiency in concentrating urine. The Holliday-Segar method is a commonly employed, quick, and simple method for estimating minimum daily fluid needs of children that also can be applied to adults. Children who weigh less than 10 kg should receive at least 100 mL/kg per day. An additional 50 mL/kg per day should be provided for each kilogram of body weight between 11 and 20 kg, and 20 mL/kg per day for each kilogram above 20 kg. Thus maintenance fluid needs for a child weighing 8 kg would be 800 mL/day, whereas 1350 mL/day would be the projected need for a 17-kg child.

Factors that alter fluid needs for both adults and children are shown in Table 135–13. When determining daily fluid intake for an individual, all sources of fluid intake must be taken into consideration (e.g., fluid vehicles for intravenous medications and intravenous or feeding tube flushes). Monitoring of urine output and specific gravity as well as serum electrolytes and weight changes is used to assess fluid status. A urine output of at least 1 mL/kg per hour (in children) and approximately 50 mL/h (in adults) is considered adequate to ensure tissue perfusion. Urine output should be higher if large fluid volumes or high renal solute loads (e.g., parenteral nutrition or concentrated enteral feeding formulations) are being administered. Urine specific gravity depends on the kidney's concentrating and diluting capabilities. Concomitant diuretic therapy due to increased solute excretion will limit the usefulness of urine specific gravity as an index of fluid status.

TABLE 135–13. Factors that Alter Fluid Requirements

Increased Requirements	Decreased Requirements
Fever	Fluid overload
Radiant warmers	Cardiac failure
Diuretics	Decreased urinary output
Vomiting	Heat shields
Nasogastric suction	Relatively high humidity
Ostomy/fistula drainage	Humidified air via endotracheal tube
Diarrhea	Renal failure
Glycosuria	Hypoalbuminemia with starvation
Phototherapy	Syndrome of inappropriate secretion
Increased ambient temperatures	of antidiuretic hormone (SIADH)
Hyperventilation	
Prematurity	
Excessive sweating	
Increased metabolism	
(e.g., hyperthyroidism)	
Diabetes insipidus	

MICRONUTRIENTS

Requirements for micronutrients (e.g., electrolytes, trace elements, and vitamins) vary with age, gender, and the route by which the nutrient is ingested (Table 135–14).[69–72,74,85,86] The variability between oral and parenteral requirements is due to bioavailability considerations. Micronutrients poorly absorbed via the GI tract usually will be required in greater doses enterally than parenterally. However, many water-soluble micronutrients are excreted more rapidly via the kidneys when administered intravenously. In these situations, the intravenous dose will be greater than the oral dose. Other factors that affect micronutrient requirements include GI losses through diarrhea, vomiting, or high-output fistula; wound healing; and hypermetabolism/catabolism. Cutaneous micronutrient losses (e.g., zinc, copper, and selenium) also may be significant after major burn injury.[87,88] Sodium, potassium, magnesium, and phosphorus are particularly dependent on renal function, and in the setting of renal failure, intake will likely need to be restricted. Calcium needs, on the other hand, may be increased in these patients. Patients who are severely malnourished will have increased electrolyte requirements during early refeeding owing to preexisting deficiencies and/or rapid intracellular uptake with anabolism. Failure to provide adequate electrolytes during refeeding has resulted in death from the refeeding syndrome.[89]

DRUG-NUTRIENT INTERACTIONS

❾ Drug-induced nutrient deficiency, poor therapeutic response, enhanced drug toxicity, and failure to achieve desired nutrition outcomes can occur if either nutrition support or drug therapy is stopped due to adverse effects.[90–94] Patient outcomes may be enhanced when an effective screening method to identify significant drug-nutrient interactions is coupled with a patient counseling program.[9] An important part of the screening process is to recognize risk factors that influence drug-nutrient interactions. The potential for drug-nutrient interactions is greatest in pediatric and elderly individuals, those with poor nutrition status (obesity and marasmus), and those receiving multiple drug therapies.

Mineral and electrolyte serum concentrations may change due to drug therapy. For example, with diuretics, urine sodium, potassium, and magnesium wasting may occur, causing a reduction in their respective serum concentrations (see Chaps. 49 and 50). Serum electrolyte concentrations also may increase as a direct result of the drug's mechanism (e.g., potassium-sparing diuretics) or due to the drug's salt form. Corticosteroids and cyclosporine are known to cause hyperglycemia, whereas other drugs are prescribed to pharmacologically lower blood glucose concentrations, e.g., insulin and oral hypoglycemics (see Chap. 72).

Vitamin status also may be affected by drugs (Table 135–15). For example, sulfasalazine therapy has been noted to cause a decrease in folic acid, isoniazid therapy causes pyridoxine deficiency, and furosemide therapy may result in decreased thiamin concentrations. Furthermore, some drug therapy outcomes may be affected by vitamin intake. The ingestion of megadoses of folic acid may decrease methotrexate's therapeutic effect, whereas changes in an individual's usual vitamin K intake may cause variability in warfarin's anticoagulation effects.

Drug delivery vehicles also may contain nutrients. Most intravenous therapies (maintenance intravenous fluids, drugs, and electrolyte replacements) are delivered using either dextrose (e.g., dextrose 5% in water) or sodium (e.g., 0.9% normal saline) in the admixture. Lipid emulsion (10%) is used as the vehicle for the anesthetic

TABLE 135–14. Recommended Daily Electrolytes, Trace Elements, and Vitamins[a]

	Adult		Pediatric	
Nutrient	*Enteral*	*Parenteral*	*Enteral*	*Parenteral*
Electrolytes and minerals				
Acetate[b]	—	—	—	—
Calcium	1000–1200 mg	0–15 mEq	0–12 mo: 210–270 mg 1–3 y: 500 mg 4–8 y: 800 mg 9–18 y: 1300 mg	Premature: 2–4 mEq/kg Other: 2–3 mEq/kg
Chloride[b]	—	—	—	2–6 mEq/kg
Fluoride	3–4 mg	—	0–6 mo: 0.01 mg 7–12 mo: 0.5 mg 1–8 y: 0.7–1 mg 9–18 y: 2–3 mg	—
Magnesium	M: 400–420 mg F: 310–320 mg	10–20 mEq	0–6 mo: 30 mg 7–12 mo: 75 mg 1–3 y: 80 mg 4–8 y: 130 mg 9–13 y: 240 mg 14–18 y: 360–410 mg	0.25–1 mEq/kg
Phosphorus	700 mg	20–45 mmol	0–6 mo: 100 mg 7–12 mo: 275 mg 1–8 y: 460–500 mg 9–18 y: 1250 mg	Premature: 1.5–2 mmol/kg Others: 1–2 mmol/kg
Potassium[c,d]	4700 mg	60–100 mEq	0–6 mo: 400 mg 7–12 mo: 700 mg 1–8 y: 3000–3800 mg 9–18 y: 4500–4700 mg	2–5 mEq/kg
Sodium[c,d]	1200–1500 mg	60–100 mEq	0–6 mo: 120 mg 7–12 mo: 370 mg 1–8 y: 1000–1200 mg 9–18 y: 1500 mg	2–6 mEq/kg
Trace elements				
Chromium[e] (mcg)	M: 30–35 F: 20–25	10–15	0–6 mo: 0.2 7–12 mo: 5.5 1–8 y: 11–15 9–18 y: 21–35	0.14–0.2 mcg/kg (max 5 mcg)
Copper[f] (mcg)	900	0.5–1.5	0–12 mo: 200–220 1–8 y: 340–440 9–18 y: 700–890	20 mcg/kg (max 300 mcg)
Iodine[g] (mcg)	150	70–140	0–12 mo: 110–130 1–8 y: 90 9–18 y: 120–150	1 mcg/kg
Iron (mg)	M: 8 F (<50 y): 18 F (≥50 y): 8	Varies	0–6 mo: 0.27 7 mo–18 y: 7–11 F (14–18 y): 15	Varies
Manganese[f] (mg)	1.8–2.3	0.15–0.8	0–6 mo: 0.003 7–12 mo: 0.6 1–8 y: 1.2–1.5 9–18 y: 1.6–2.2	1 mcg/kg (max 50 mcg)
Molybdenum (mcg)	45	100–200	0–12 mo: 2–3 1–8 y: 17–22 9–18 y: 34–43	0.25 mcg/kg (max 5 mcg)
Selenium (mcg)	55	40–80	0–12 mo: 15–20 1–8 y: 20–30 9–18 y: 40–55	1.5–3 mcg/kg (max 30 mcg)
Zinc[h] (mg)	8–11	2.5–4	0–12 mo: 2–3 1–8 y: 5 9–18 y: 8–11	Premature: 300–400 mcg/kg Other: 50–250 mcg/kg
Vitamins				
Ascorbic acid (mg)	75–90	100	0–12 mo: 40–50 1–8 y: 15–25 9–18 y: 45–75	80
Biotin (mcg)	30	60	0–12 mo: 5–6 1–8 y: 8–12 9–18 y: 20–25	20

(continued)

TABLE 135–14. Continued

Nutrient	Adult		Pediatric	
	Enteral	*Parenteral*	*Enteral*	*Parenteral*
Choline (mg)	425–550	Not established	0–12 mo: 125–150 1–8 y: 200–250 9–18 y: 375–550	Not established
Cobalamin (mcg)	2.4	5	0–12 mo: 0.4–0.5 1–8 y: 0.9–1.2 9–18 y: 1.8–2.4	1
Folic acid (mcg)	400	400	0–12 mo: 65–80 1–8 y: 150–200 9–18y: 300–400	140
Niacin (mg NE)	14–16	40	0–12 mo: 2–4 1–8 y: 6–8 9–18 y: 12–16	17
Pantothenic acid (mg)	5	15	0–12 mo: 1.7–1.8 1–8 y: 2–3 9–18 y: 4–5	5
Pyridoxine (mg)	1.3–1.7	4	0–12 mo: 0.1–0.3 1–8 y: 0.5–0.6 9–18 y: 1–1.3	1
Riboflavin (mg)	1.1–1.3	3.6	0–12 mo: 0.3–0.4 1–8 y: 0.5–0.6 9–18 y: 0.9–1.3	1.4
Thiamin (mg)	1.1–1.2	3	0–12 mo: 0.2–0.3 1–8 y: 0.7–1 9–18 y: 2–3	1.2
Vitamin A (mcg RE)	700–900	600 (3300 IU)	0–12 mo: 400–500 1–8 y: 300–400 9–18 y: 600–900	700 (2300 IU)
Vitamin D (mcg)	≤50 y: 5 >50 y: 10 >70 y: 15	5 (200 IU)	All ages: 5 (200 IU)	5 (200 IU)
Vitamin E (mg TE) (α-tocopherol)	15	10 (10 IU)	0–12 mo: 4–5 1–8 y: 6–7 9–18 y: 11–15	7 (7 IU)
Vitamin K	90–120 mcg	0.7–2.5 mg	0–12 mo: 2–2.5 1–8 y: 30–55 9–18 y: 60–75	200 mcg

[a]Adapted from Food and Nutrition Board,[67] Food and Nutrition Information Center,[68] Food and Nutrition Board,[69] Food and Nutrition Board,[70] Food and Nutrition Board,[71] Jefferson,[90] Fuhr,[91] and Kirk.[92] Data represent either the RDA or the AI for each nutrient where established.

[b]As needed to maintain acid-base balance.

[c]Newborns and low-birth-weight or very-low-birth-weight infants or with concomitant disease (e.g., necrotizing enterocolitis) may have higher requirements. Intake in nonhealthy children must be individualized.

[d]No RDA or AI has been established.

[e]An additional 20 mcg of chromium per day is recommended in patients with intestinal losses.

[f]May accumulate in cholestasis.

[g]Long-term parenteral nutrition only; no topicals containing iodide or table salt are used.

[h]An additional 12.2 mg zinc/L of small bowel fluid lost and 17.1 mg zinc/kg of stool or ileostomy output is recommended; add an additional 2 mg zinc per day for acute catabolic stress.

[i]Higher doses (15 mcg) recommended in those over 70 years of age.

AI, adequate intakes; NE, niacin equivalents; PN, parenteral nutrition; RDA, recommended dietary allowances; RE, retinal equivalents; TE, tocopherol equivalent.

agent propofol and may contribute a large amount of calories when continuous propofol infusions are used. In these instances, nutrition support regimens must be adjusted to accommodate the calories and other nutrients delivered through other therapies.

PRACTICAL GUIDELINES FOR NUTRITION ASSESSMENT

◀10 The value of any given marker used for nutrition assessment is only as great as its ability to accurately identify the patient with malnutrition and to correlate with malnutrition-associated com-

plications. Most of the currently available markers of nutrition status were first used in epidemiologic studies to define large populations suffering from malnutrition caused by famine. The response of the various nutritional status markers to nutrition therapy and the correlation between improvement in these markers and decreased morbidity and mortality further support their validity. However, when applied to an individual, most of these markers lack specificity and sensitivity, which makes the development of a clinically useful, cost-effective approach to individual patient nutrition assessment challenging.

The importance of the nutrition-focused history and physical examination in both nutrition screening and nutrition assessment cannot be overemphasized. The least amount of objective data that can further

TABLE 135–15. Drug Effects on Vitamin Status

Drug	Effect
Antacids	Thiamin deficiency
Antibiotics	Vitamin K deficiency
Anticonvulsants	Vitamin D and folic acid malabsorption
Antineoplastics	Folic acid antagonism and malabsorption
Antipsychotics	Decreased riboflavin
Cathartics	Increased requirements for vitamins D, C, and B$_6$
Cholestyramine	Vitamins A, D, E, and K, β-carotene malabsorption
Colestipol	Vitamins A, D, E, and K, β-carotene malabsorption
Corticosteroids	Decreased vitamins A, D, and C
Diuretics (loop)	Thiamin deficiency
Histamine$_2$ antagonists	Vitamin B$_{12}$ deficiency
Isoniazid	Vitamin B$_6$ deficiency
Mineral oil	Vitamins A, D, E, and K malabsorption
Orlistat	Vitamins A, D, E, and K malabsorption
Pentamidine	Folic acid deficiency
Proton pump inhibitors	Vitamin B$_{12}$ deficiency

substantiate the clinical impression and provide a baseline for subsequent monitoring are those markers which show the best correlation with outcome: weight and serum albumin concentration. The cost-effectiveness of the addition of further biochemical parameters is yet to be determined. The assessment of other anthropometric measures is most useful in the setting of anticipated long-term nutrition support in which these measurements will serve as a longitudinal marker of an individual's response to the nutrition care plan.

Initially, nutrition requirements are determined on the basis of assumptions made about the patient's clinical condition and the nutrition needs associated with repletion or growth, if needed. Once a nutrition intervention has been initiated, periodic reassessment of nutrition status is critical to determine the accuracy of the initial estimate of nutrition requirements. Also, nutrition requirements are dynamic in the setting of acute or critical illness—as the patient's clinical status changes, so will protein and energy requirements, further emphasizing the need for continued reassessment.

Better markers of nutrition status and methods for determining patient-specific nutrition requirements are needed to allow further refinement of estimates of individual nutrition needs. Functional tests and simple, noninvasive tests for body composition analysis hold promise for the future. However, until better methods of assessment become available clinically and are demonstrated to be cost-effective, the currently available battery of tests will continue to be the mainstay of nutrition assessment.

Information in this chapter can be used to establish empiric goals for nutrition care. However, as with other forms of therapy, continuous monitoring and reassessment are required to determine if these goals are appropriate for an individual patient.

ABBREVIATIONS

ABW: actual body weight
AI: adequate intake
AIDS: acquired immunodeficiency syndrome
ALB: albumin
BEE: basal energy expenditure
BIA: bioelectrical impedance analysis

BMI: body mass index
BMR: basal metabolic rate
DCH: delayed cutaneous hypersensitivity
DEXA: dual-energy x-ray absorptiometry
DRI: dietary reference intake
EAR: estimated average requirement
HBE: Harris-Benedict equation
HIV: human immunodeficiency virus
IBW: ideal body weight
LBM: lean body mass
MAMC: midarm muscle circumference
NCHS: National Center for Health Statistics
RDA: recommended dietary allowance
REE: resting energy expenditure
RQ: respiratory quotient
SGA: subjective global assessment
T$_3$: triiodothyronine
T$_4$: thyroxine
TBW: total body water
TFN: transferrin
TIBC: total iron-binding capacity
TLC: total lymphocyte count
TSF: triceps skinfold thickness
TUN: total urine nitrogen
UBW: usual body weight
UL: tolerable upper intake level
UUN: urine urea nitrogen
Vco$_2$: carbon dioxide production
Vo$_2$: oxygen consumption

Review Questions and other resources can be found at *www.pharmacotherapyonline.com.*

REFERENCES

1. Kotler DP. Cachexia. Ann Intern Med 2000;133:622–634.
2. Mokdad AH, Ford ES, Bowman BA, et al. Prevalence of obesity, diabetes, and obesity-related health risk factors, 2001. JAMA 2003;299:76–79.
3. Ogden CL, Flegal KM, Carroll MD, Johnson CL. Prevalence and trends in overweight among US children and adolescents, 1999–2000. JAMA 2002;288:1728–1732.
4. Centers for Disease Control and Prevention, National Center for Health Statistics. CDC growth charts: United States, 2000. http://www.cdc.gov/growthcharts/. Accessed June 4, 2004.
5. American Academy of Family Physicians, American Dietetic Association, and National Council on the Aging, Inc. Nutrition Interventions Manual for Professionals Caring for Older Americans. Washington, Nutrition Screening Initiative, 1992. http://www.aafp.org/nsi/. Accessed June 4, 2004.
6. Council on Practice, Quality Management Committee. Identifying patients at risk: ADA's definitions for nutrition screening and nutrition assessment. J Am Diet Assoc 1994;94:838–839.
7. Kovacevich DS, Boney AR, Braunschweig CL, et al. Nutrition risk classification: A reproducible and valid tool for nurses. Nutr Clin Pract 1997;12:20–25.
8. A.S.P.E.N. Board of Directors. Definition of terms used in A.S.P.E.N. guidelines and standards. Nutr Clin Pract 1995;10:1–3.
9. Joint Commission on Accreditation of Healthcare Organizations. 2003 Hospital Accreditation Standards. Oakbrook Terrace, IL, Joint Commission Resources, 2003.
10. McClave SA, Mitoraj TE, Thielmeier KA, Greenburg RA. Differentiating subtypes (hypoalbuminemic versus marasmic) of protein-calorie malnutrition: incidence and clinical significance in a university hospital setting. JPEN J Parenter Enteral Nutr 1992;16:337–342.

11. Shopbell JM, Hopkins B, Shronts EP. Nutrition screening and assessment. In: Gottschlich MM, ed. The Science and Practice of Nutrition Support: A Case-Based Core Curriculum, America Society for Parenteral and Enteral Nutrition. Dubuque, IA, Kendall/Hunt, 2001:107–140.

12. Lair CS, Kennedy KA. Monitoring postnatal growth in the neonatal intensive care unit. Nutr Clin Pract 1997;12:124–129.

13. Cronk C, Crocker AC, Pueschel SM, et al. Growth charts for children with Down syndrome: 1 month to 18 years of age. Pediatrics 1988;81:102–110.

14. Klish WJ. Nutritional assessment. In: Wyllie R, Hyams JS, eds. Pediatric Gastrointestinal Disease: Pathophysiology, Diagnosis, Management. Philadelphia, Saunders, 1993:1090–1109.

15. Crouch JB. Anthropometric assessment. In: Groh-Wargo S, Thompson M, Cox JH, eds. Nutritional Care for High-Risk Newborns, rev. ed. Chicago, Precept Press, 1994:9–14.

16. Dickey RA, Baluska DG, Bray GW, et al. AACE/ACE Position Statement on the Prevention, Diagnosis, and Treatment of Obesity, 1998 revision. http://www.aace.com/clin/guidelines/obesityguide.pdf. Accessed June 4, 2004.

17. Meisler JG, St. Jeor S. Summary and recommendations from the American Health Foundation's expert panel on healthy weight. Am J Clin Nutr 1996;63(3 Suppl):474S–477S.

18. Himes JH, Dietz WH. Guidelines for overweight in adolescent preventive services: Recommendations from an expert committee. Am J Clin Nutr 1994;59:307–316.

19. Chumlea WC, Guo S. Bioelectrical impedance and body composition: Present status and future directions. Nutr Rev 1994;52:123–131.

20. Kyle UG, Pichard C. Dynamic assessment of fat-free mass during catabolism and recovery. Curr Opin Clin Nutr Metab Care 2000;3: 317–322.

21. Elia M, Ward LC. New techniques in nutritional assessment: Body composition methods. Proc Nutr Soc 1999;58:33–38.

22. Pichard C, Kyle UG, Janssens JP, et al. Body composition by x-ray absorptiometry and bio-electrical impedance in chronic respiratory insufficiency patients. Nutrition 1997;13:952–958.

23. Roubenoff R, Baumgartner RN, Harris TB, et al. Application of bioelectrical impedance analysis to elderly population. J Gerontol 1997;52A:M129–M136.

24. Kyle UG, Genton L, Mentha G, et al. Reliable bioelectrical impedance analysis estimate of fat-free mass in liver, lung, and heart transplant patients. JPEN J Parenter Enteral Nutr 2001;25:45–51.

25. Mattox TW, Brown RO, Boucher BA, et al. Use of fibronectin and somatomedin-C as markers of enteral nutrition support in traumatized patients using a modified amino acid formula. JPEN J Parenter Enteral Nutr 1988;12:592–596.

26. Russell MK, McAdams MP. Laboratory monitoring of nutritional status. In: Matarese LE, Gottschlich MM. Contemporary Nutrition Support Practice: A Clinical Guide. Philadelphia, Saunders, 1998:47–63.

27. Spiekerman AM. Proteins used in nutritional assessment. Clin Lab Med 1993;13:353–369.

28. Erstad BL, Campbell DJ, Rollins CJ, Rappaport WD. Albumin and prealbumin concentrations in patients receiving postoperative parenteral nutrition. Pharmacotherapy 1994;14:458–462.

29. Chandra RK, Sarchielli P. Nutritional status and immune response. Clin Lab Med 1993;13:455–461.

30. Alexander JW, Peck MD. Future prospects for adjunctive therapy: Pharmacologic and nutritional approaches to immune system modulation. Crit Care Med 1990;18:S159–S164.

31. Moore FA, Moore EE, Kudsk KA, et al. Clinical benefits of an immune-enhancing diet for early postinjury enteral feeding. J Trauma 1994;37:607–615.

32. Kudsk KA, Minard G, Croce MA, et al. A randomized trial of isonitrogenous enteral diets after severe trauma: An immune-enhancing diet reduces septic complications. Ann Surg 1996;224:531–543.

33. Barton RG. Immune-enhancing enteral formulas: Are they beneficial in critically ill patients. Nutr Clin Pract 1997;12:51–62.

34. Baumgartner TG. Trace elements in clinical nutrition. Nutr Clin Pract 1993;8:251–263.

35. Nielson FH. Other trace elements. In: Ziegler EE, Filer LJ, eds. Present Knowledge in Nutrition, 7th ed. Washington, ILSI Press, 1996:353–377.

36. Shenkin A. Micronutrients. In: Rombeau JL, Rolandelli RH, eds. Clinical Nutrition: Enteral and Tube Feeding, 3rd ed. Philadelphia, Saunders, 1997:96–111.

37. Weber CW, Nelson GW, Vasquez-de-Vaquera M, et al. Trace elements in the hair of healthy and malnourished children. J Trop Pediatr 1990;36: 230–234.

38. Tamura H, Hirose S, Watanabe O, et al. Anemia and neutropenia due to copper deficiency in enteral nutrition. JPEN J Parenter Enteral Nutr 1994;18:185–189.

39. Wasa M, Satani M, Tanano H, et al. Copper deficiency with pancytopenia during parenteral nutrition. JPEN J Parenter Enteral Nutr 1994;18:190–192.

40. Stoeker BJ. Chromium. In: Ziegler EE, Filer LJ, eds. Present Knowledge in Nutrition, 7th ed. Washington, ILSI Press,1996:344–352.

41. Verhage AH, Cheong WK, Jeejeebhoy KN. Neurologic symptoms due to possible chromium deficiency in long-term parenteral nutrition that closely mimic metronidazole-induced syndromes. JPEN J Parenter Enteral Nutr 1996;20:123–127.

42. Alves G, Thiebot J, Tracqui A, et al. Neurologic disorders due to brain manganese deposition in a jaundiced patient receiving long-term parenteral nutrition. JPEN J Parenter Enteral Nutr 1997;21:41–45.

43. Fell JME, Reynolds AP, Meadows N, et al. Manganese toxicity in children receiving long term parenteral nutrition. Lancet 1996;347:1218–1221.

44. Keen CL, Zidenbery-Cherr S, Lonnerdal B. Nutritional and toxicological aspects of manganese intake: An overview. In: Mertz W, Abernathy CO, Olin SS, eds. Risk Assessment of Essential Elements. Washington, ILSI Press, 1994:221–235.

45. Matasuda A, Kimura M, Takeda T, et al. Changes in manganese content of mononuclear blood cells in patients receiving total parenteral nutrition. Clin Chem 1994;40:829–832.

46. Malecki EA, Lo HC, Yang H, et al. Tissue manganese concentrations and antioxidant enzyme activities in rats given total parenteral nutrition with and without supplemental manganese. JPEN J Parenter Enteral Nutr 1995;19:222–226.

47. Abrams CK, Siram SM, Galsim C, et al. Selenium deficiency in long-term total parenteral nutrition. Nutr Clin Pract 1992;7:175–178.

48. Lockitch G, Jacobson B, Quigley G, et al. Selenium deficiency in low birth weight neonates: An unrecognized problem. J Pediatr 1989;114:865–870.

49. Rannem T, Ladefoged K, Hylander E, et al. The effect of selenium supplementation on skeletal and cardiac muscle in selenium-depleted patients. JPEN J Parenter Enteral Nutr 1995;19:351–355.

50. Rannem T, Persson-Moschos M, Huang W, et al. Selenoprotein P in patients on home parenteral nutrition. JPEN J Parenter Enteral Nutr 1996;20:287–291.

51. Levander OA, Burk PF. Selenium. In: Ziegler EE, Filer LJ, eds. Present Knowledge in Nutrition, 7th ed. Washington, ILSI Press, 1996:320–328.

52. Friel JK, MacDonald AC, Mercer CN, et al. Molybdenum requirements in low-birth-weight infants receiving parenteral and enteral nutrition. JPEN J Parenter Enteral Nutr 1999;23:155–159.

53. Sardesai VM. Molybdenum: An essential trace element. Nutr Clin Prac 1993;8:277–281.

54. Nicholalds GE. Iodine. In: Baumgartner TG, ed. Clinical Guide to Parenteral Micronutrition, 3d ed. Deerfield, IL, Fujisawa USA, 1997:361–374.

55. Moukarzel AA, Buchman AL, Salas JS, et al. Iodine supplementation in children receiving long-term parenteral nutrition. J Pediatr 1992;121:252–254.

56. Jordan NS. Hematology: Red and white blood cells. In: Traub SL, ed. Basic Skills in Interpreting Laboratory Data, 2d ed. Bethesda, MD, American Society of Health-System Pharmacists, 1996:297–320.

57. Centers for Disease Control and Prevention. Lactic acidosis traced to thiamin deficiency related to nationwide shortage of multivitamins for total parenteral nutrition—United States, 1997. JAMA 1997;278:109–111.

58. Adolph M, Hailer S, Echart J. Serum phospholipid fatty acids in severely injured patients on total parenteral nutrition with medium chain/long chain triglyceride emulsions. Ann Nutr Metab 1995;39:251–260.

59. Sacks GS, Brown RO, Collier P, Kudsk KA. Failure of tropical vegetable oils to prevent essential fatty acid deficiency in a critically ill patient receiving long-term parenteral nutrition. JPEN J Parenter Enteral Nutr 1994;18:274–277.

60. Foote KD, MacKinnon MJ, Innis SM. Effect of early introduction of formula versus fat-free parenteral nutrition on essential fatty acid status of preterm infants. Am J Clin Nutr 1991;54:93–97.

61. Tibboel D, Delemarre FMC, Przyrembel H, et al. Carnitine deficiency in surgical neonates receiving total parenteral nutrition. J Pediatr Surg 1990;25:418–421.

62. Borum PR. Carnitine in neonatal nutrition. J Child Neurol 1995;10(Suppl 2):S25–S31.

63. Broquist HP. Carnitine. In: Shils ME, Olson JA, Shike M, eds. Modern Nutrition in Health and Disease, 8th ed. Philadelphia, Lea & Febiger, 1994:459–465.

64. Scaglia F. Carnitine deficiencies. EMedicine.com, Inc., March 4, 2004. http://www.emedicine.com/ped/topic321.htm. Accessed June 4, 2004.

65. Borum PR. Carnitine. In: Baumgartner TG, ed. Clinical Guide to Parenteral Micronutrition, 3rd ed. Deerfield, IL, Fujisawa USA, 1997:629–641.

66. Cerra FB, Benitez MR, Blackburn GL, et al. Applied nutrition in ICU patients: A consensus statement of the American College of Chest Physicians. Chest 1997;111:769–778.

67. Food and Nutrition Board, National Research Council. Recommended Dietary Allowances, 10th ed. Washington, National Academy of Sciences, 1989.

68. Food and Nutrition Information Center. Dietary Reference Intakes (DRI) and Recommended Dietary Allowances (RDA). http://www.nal.usda.gov/fnic/etext/000105.html#q2. Accessed June 4, 2004.

69. Food and Nutrition Board, Institute of Medicine. Dietary Reference Intakes for Calcium, Phosphorus, Magnesium, Vitamin D, and Fluoride. Washington, National Academy Press, January 1, 1999. http://www.nap.edu/books/0309063507/html/index.html. Accessed June 4, 2004.

70. Food and Nutrition Board, Institute of Medicine. Dietary Reference Intakes for Thiamin, Riboflavin, Niacin, Vitamin B$_6$, Folate, Vitamin B$_{12}$, Pantothenic Acid, Biotin, and Choline. Washington, National Academy Press, January 1, 2000. http://www.nap.edu/books/0309065542/html/index.html. Accessed June 4, 2004.

71. Food and Nutrition Board, Institute of Medicine. Dietary Reference Intakes for Vitamin C, Vitamin E, Selenium, and Carotenoids. Washington, National Academy Press, January 1, 2000. http://www.nap.edu/books/0309069351/html/. Accessed June 4, 2004.

72. Food and Nutrition Board, Institute of Medicine. Dietary Reference Intakes for Vitamin A, Vitamin K, Arsenic, Boron, Chromium, Copper, Iodine, Iron, Manganese, Molybdenum, Nickel, Silicon, Vanadium, and Zinc. Washington, National Academy Press, January 9, 2001. http://www.nap.edu/books/0309072794/html/. Accessed June 4, 2004.

73. Food and Nutrition Board, Institute of Medicine. Dietary Reference Intakes for Energy, Carbohydrate, Fiber, Fat, Fatty Acids, Cholesterol, Protein, and Amino Acids. September 5, 2002. http://www.nap.edu/books/0309085373/html/. Accessed June 4, 2004.

74. Food and Nutrition Board, Institute of Medicine. Dietary Reference Intakes for Water, Potassium, Sodium, Chloride, and Sulfate. February 11, 2004. http://www.nap.edu/books/0309091691/html/. Accessed June 4, 2004.

75. Dimand RJ. Parenteral nutrition in the critically ill infant and child. In: Baker RD, Baker SS, Davis AM, eds. Pediatric Parenteral Nutrition. New York, Chapman & Hall, 1997:273–300.

76. Pollack MM. Nutritional support of children in the intensive care unit. In: Suskind RM, Lewinter-Suskind L, eds. Textbook of Pediatric Nutrition, 2d ed. New York, Raven Press, 1993:207–216.

77. Garrel DR, Jobin N, DeJonge LHM. Should we still use the Harris and Benedict equations? Nutr Clin Pract 1996;11:99–103.

78. Osborne BJ, Saba AK, Wood SJ, et al. Clinical comparison of three methods to determine resting energy expenditure. Nutr Clin Pract 1994;9:241–246.

79. Frankenfield D. Energy and macrosubstrate requirements. In: Gottschlich MM, ed. The Science and Practice of Nutrition Support: A Case-Based Core Curriculum, America Society for Parenteral and Enteral Nutrition. Dubuque, IA, Kendall/Hunt, 2001:31–52.

80. McClave SA, Snider HL. Use of indirect calorimetry in clinical nutrition. Nutr Clin Pract 1992;7:207–221.

81. McGee M, Binkley J, Jensen GL. Geriatric nutrition. In: Gottschlich MM, ed. The Science and Practice of Nutrition Support: A Case-Based Core Curriculum, America Society for Parenteral and Enteral Nutrition. Dubuque, IA, Kendall/Hunt, 2001:373–389.

82. Long CL, Lowry SR. Hormonal regulation of protein metabolism. JPEN J Parenter Enteral Nutr 1990;14:555–562.

83. Barton RG. Nutrition support in critical illness. Nutr Clin Pract 1994;9:127–139.

84. Velasco N, Long CL, Otto DA, et al. Comparison of three methods for the estimation of total nitrogen losses in hospitalized patients. JPEN J Parenter Enteral Nutr 1990;14:517–522.

85. Kleinman RE (ed). Committee on Nutrition, American Academy of Pediatrics. Pediatric Nutrition Handbook, 4th ed. Elk Grove Village, IL, American Academy of Pediatrics, 1998.

86. Greene HL, Hambidge KM, Schanler R, Tsang RC. Guidelines for the use of vitamins, trace elements, calcium, magnesium, and phosphorus in infants and children receiving total parenteral nutrition: Report of the Subcommittee on Pediatric Parenteral Nutrient Requirements from the Committee on Clinical Practice Issues of the American Society for Clinical Nutrition. Am J Clin Nutr 1988;48:1324–1342.

87. Berger MM, Cavadini C, Bart A, et al. Cutaneous copper and zinc losses in burns. Burns 1992;18:373–380.

88. Berger MM, Cavadini C, Bart A, et al. Selenium losses in 10 burned patients. Clin Nutr 1992;11:75–82.

89. Solomon SM, Kirby DF. The refeeding syndrome: A review. JPEN J Parenter Enteral Nutr 1990;14:90–97.

90. Jefferson JW. Drug and diet interactions: Avoiding therapeutic paralysis. J Clin Psychiatry 1998;59:31–39.

91. Fuhr U. Drug interactions with grapefruit juice: Extent, probable mechanism and clinical relevance. Drug Saf 1998;18:251–272.

92. Kirk JK. Significant drug-nutrient interactions. Am Fam Physician 1995;51:1175–1182.

93. Singh BN. Effects of food on clinical pharmacokinetics. Clin Pharmacokinet 1999;37:213–255.

94. Thomas JA, Burns RA. Important drug-nutrient interactions in the elderly. Drugs Aging 1998; 3:199–209.

136

PREVALENCE AND SIGNIFICANCE OF MALNUTRITION

Gordon Sacks and Pamela D. Reiter

Learning Objectives and other resources can be found at *www.pharmacotherapyonline.com.*

KEY CONCEPTS

◀1 Weight loss is a hallmark sign of malnutrition in the cancer patient and correlates with decreased survival for some cancer types.

◀2 Nutritional problems in human immunodeficiency virus/acquired immunodeficiency syndrome (HIV/AIDS) patients have shifted from complications of severe wasting to metabolic changes associated with subcutaneous fat atrophy, visceral fat accumulation, hypertriglyceridemia, and insulin resistance.

◀3 Immune function, growth, and survival can be improved in HIV-positive children with aggressive nutritional and antiviral therapy.

◀4 Enteral nutrition (EN) decreases septic complications when compared with parenteral nutrition (PN) in severely injured trauma patients.

◀5 EN and PN promote remission in the majority of patients with acute Crohn's disease.

◀6 Adults with less than 60 cm remaining of small bowel after massive surgery will require PN for months to years.

◀7 EN supplemented with immune-enhancing nutrients lowers metabolic and infectious complications in adult surgical patients.

◀8 Catch-up growth can be achieved more rapidly in infants with bronchopulmonary dysplasia if they receive a diet higher in protein, calcium, phosphorus, and zinc.

◀9 Optimizing nutritional status of pediatric solid organ transplant patients pre- and post-transplantation can improve outcomes and reduce morbidity.

◀10 Malnutrition is associated with increased utilization of health care resources and nutritional interventions can contribute to cost savings by lowering length of hospital stay and morbidity associated with malnutrition.

The term *malnutrition* has been used to characterize a broad range of altered nutritional states. *Overnutrition* is the term used to describe excess nutrient intake, whereas *undernutrition* is used to describe insufficient intake or substrate use. Both nutritional states can contribute to the poor outcome of many disease states. Unless specifically stated, this chapter will use the nomenclature of malnutrition as synonymous with undernutrition (refer to Chap. 140 for a discussion on overnutrition/obesity). In children, malnutrition can be defined by a variety of criteria. Stages (e.g., Waterlow stages) have been developed to define the severity of protein-energy malnutrition. Anthropometric evaluations, using established age-based growth curves, can define acute and chronic malnutrition using either Z scores or height and weight percentiles. In general, malnutrition in children is defined as growth that is below the fifth percentile for age or less than 90% to 95% of the median value for age. In this chapter, the prevalence of malnutrition as defined by a variety of nutrition assessment parameters is documented, and the significant impact of abnormalities in these nutrition assessment parameters on the morbidity and mortality of selected disease states is presented. Interventional strategies for the prevention and management of malnutrition and the economic consequences of malnutrition are also presented.

Although malnutrition occurs throughout the world, it is most prevalent in underdeveloped countries, where food supply, ignorance, poverty, overcrowding, and poor sanitation are contributing factors. The most susceptible individuals in developed and underdeveloped countries are infants (especially premature infants), pregnant or lactating women, and the elderly. Factors that contribute to malnutrition in developed countries include poor maternal nutrition before and during pregnancy, misconceptions about the use of certain foods, fad diets, maternal illiteracy, household poverty, and alcohol or drug abuse. The relationship between malnutrition and breast-feeding is time-dependent. While the benefit of breast-feeding during the first 6 months of life in reducing mortality and improving growth is well known, prolonged breast-feeding (beyond 6 months to 1 year) has been associated with a higher risk of malnutrition. However, this latter association may be due to lower use of complimentary foods within poor households, rather than breastfeeding per se.[1]

Malnutrition is associated most commonly with exacerbations of chronic disease and acute illness and thus is prevalent in the hospital setting. Recognition of the scope of the problem coincides with the systematic application of nutrition assessment techniques to hospitalized individuals in the last two decades. The prevalence of previously unrecognized malnutrition is 40% to 55% among adult patients from varying socioeconomic backgrounds hospitalized in a variety of institutions.[2] The prevalence of malnutrition has declined and there has been a heightened awareness of nutritional disease and better in-hospital nutrition management since the mid-1970s.[3] Worldwide, nearly 200 million children are moderately to severely underweight, and 70 million are severely malnourished.[4] Over one-half of global childhood deaths under 5 years of age can be attributed directly or indirectly to malnutrition.[5] Chronic malnutrition in children less than 2 years of age is an independent predictor of poor cognitive development lasting up to 11 years of age.[6] Severe malnutrition is both a medical and social disorder and successful management requires attention to both of these factors. Fortunately, the global trend indicates a modest but consistent decline in malnutrition-associated mortality in children less than 5 years of age.[7]

Because children have both limited body stores and high metabolic demands, they are at particular risk for developing malnutrition, especially during illness. While the majority of undernourished children are from underdeveloped countries, malnutrition is also seen in the United States and other industrial countries. In 1974, a publicly funded health and nutrition program known as the Pediatric Nutrition Surveillance System was established to generate data on the prevalence of malnutrition in children generally younger than 5 years of age. The most recent report published in 1998 revealed a reduction in the incidence of malnutrition.[8] The prevalence of shortness (height for age) in children younger than 24 months of age has declined from 10.5% in 1989 to 9.7% today, a value still more than twice the expected value. In older children (aged 2 to 5 years), the prevalence of shortness in 1989 of 7.5% was only slightly higher than expected and the prevalence has now fallen to 5.7%. Recent values for thinness, or weight for height, have also declined since 1989 and are currently at 3.1% in infants less than 24 months old and 1.9% in children aged 2 to 5 years old. These values are lower than the expected value of 5% and indicate that the prevalence of acute malnutrition in this population is low. Anemia, hematologic evidence of poor nutrition status, and/or iron deficiency was very high between 1980 and 1985 (20% to 30%), but has declined to 18.4% in those less than 24 months of age and 16.9% in those between 2 and 5 years of age.[8] Admittedly, the nutritional health of children in the United States has changed over the past decade. The focus on malnutrition has now been shifted to the prevention and treatment of childhood obesity, which has reached epidemic proportions (see Chap. 140).

Children with chronic disease and those in periods of rapid growth have the highest prevalence of malnutrition. Hendricks and colleagues described the change in prevalence of protein-energy malnutrition in hospitalized children over a 15-year period.[9] Overall prevalence was high, but significant reductions were detected in acute malnutrition (weight for height <90% of median) from 33.6% to 24.5%, and chronic malnutrition (weight for height <95% of median) from 46.8% in 1976 to 27.3% in the 1990s.

EFFECT ON ORGAN AND CELLULAR FUNCTION

The outcome of malnutrition is an inappropriate reduction in lean body mass resulting in alterations in the structure and/or function (Table 136–1) of essentially every organ. The clinical significance of the effect will depend on the specific anatomic structure or system and on the degree of malnutrition. For example, with mild malnutrition, loss of skeletal muscle mass may be apparent as weakness or a decreased level of physical activity. However, alterations in cardiac function usually are not apparent until severe malnutrition is present. Until recently, the effect of early malnutrition (fetal and neonatal) on organ and cellular function was only recognized in terms of short-term growth and development outcomes. Now we realize that "fetal programming" or "metabolic imprinting" is linked to adult health. Specifically, maternal body composition and dietary balance during pregnancy can influence the risk of adult-onset cardiac disease, type II diabetes, and obesity.[7,10,11]

There is also a well-established biochemical and clinical relationship between malnutrition and immune function. Alterations in the immune system (Table 136–2) represent an end-organ or functional response to malnutrition and may reflect a decline in lean body mass as well as a deficiency in specific nutrients such as zinc.[12] Clinically, this is manifested as an increased incidence of infection.

Malnourished patients have an increased likelihood of developing wound infections from altered immunity. Although wound healing

TABLE 136–1. **End-Organ Responses in Malnutrition**

Organ	Anatomic Responses	Physiologic Responses
Heart	Four-chamber dilation; atrophic degeneration with necrosis and fibrosis; myofibrillar disruption	QT prolongation, low voltage, bradycardia; decreased cardiac output, stroke volume, and contractility; preload intolerance; diminished responsiveness to drugs
Lung	Emphysematous changes; pulmonary infarcts; reduced bacterial clearance; muscle atrophy	Pneumonia; decreases in functional residual capacity, vital capacity, and maximum breathing capacity; depressed hypoxic/hypercarbic drives
Hematologic	Failure of stem-cell production; decreased PMN chemotaxis; decreased lymphocyte count with reduced helper T and increased suppressor T and killer cells; decreased blastogenesis to phytohemagglutinin	Anemia; anergy; decreased granuloma formation; impaired response to chemotherapy; increased infection rate
Renal system	Epithelial swelling; atrophy; mild cortical calcification; depressed erythropoietin synthesis	Reduced glomerular filtration rate and inability to handle sodium loads; polyuria; metabolic acidosis
Gastrointestinal system	Disproportionate mass loss; hypoplastic and atrophic changes; decrease in total mucosal height	Depressed enzymatic activity; shortened transit time; impaired motility; propensity for bacterial overgrowth; maldigestion and malabsorption
Liver	Mass loss; periportal fat accumulation	Decreased visceral protein synthesis; depressed microsomal activity; eventual hepatic insufficiency

PMN, polymorphonuclear leukocyte.
Reproduced with permission from Cerra FB (ed). Manual of Surgical Nutrition. St Louis, MO, CV Mosby, 1984:6.

TABLE 136–2. Immune Response Mechanisms in Malnutrition

Parameter	Observation in Malnutrition
Cell-mediated immune response	
Delayed cutaneous hypersensitivity	Decreased
Lymphocyte transformation	Decreased
Polymorphonuclear leukocyte response	
Phagocytosis	Normal or decreased
Metabolism	Decreased
Bactericidal capacity	Decreased
Chemotaxis	Decreased
Total lymphocyte count	Decreased
T cells	
CD4+	Decreased
CD8+	Decreased
Helper:suppressor ratio	Decreased
Humoral response	
Complement activity (CH50)	Decreased
Secretory Immunoglobulin A	Decreased
Serum complement	Decreased or normal
Serum immunoglobulins	Normal
Serum opsonization	Normal

occurs at the expense of other tissues, in the setting of protein-energy malnutrition, the rate at which wounds heal and the tensile strength of the wound are decreased.[9] Deficiency of arginine, copper, vitamin C, vitamin A, or zinc also may contribute to decreased wound healing (Table 136–3). Supplemental vitamin A can promote wound healing in animal models in the presence of deficiency,[13] and arginine has improved markers of wound healing (i.e., protein and hydroxyproline in the wound bed) in elderly healthy human volunteers.[14] Other nutrients, when ingested in excessive amounts, may impair wound healing. For example, excess vitamin E antagonizes the promotion of wound healing by vitamin A, and excess zinc will displace copper and interfere with lysyl oxidase (the enzyme necessary for collagen cross-link formation).[13]

DISEASE-SPECIFIC CONSEQUENCES

Malnutrition seldom exists as an isolated disease state, but rather is usually found in patients with other pre-existing illnesses. Often

TABLE 136–3. Nutritional Disorders and Wound Healing

Nutritional Disorder	Effect on Wound Healing
Arginine deficiency	Altered collagen formation
Copper deficiency	Impaired lysyl oxidase activity
Protein-energy malnutrition	Decreased wound strength because of reduced hydroxyproline content of wound; decreased rate of wound healing; increased incidence of wound infection
Vitamin C deficiency	Decreased fibroblast maturation with failure of collagen synthesis; decreased angiogenesis
Vitamin A deficiency	Decreased collagen accumulation; formation of abnormal collagen
Zinc deficiency	Impaired DNA and protein synthesis; impaired mitosis and cell proliferation

the primary disease or complications of the disease predispose an individual to the development of malnutrition. The primary factors that enhance the likelihood of developing malnutrition include decreased dietary intake (e.g., due to nausea, vomiting, or anorexia), malabsorption (e.g., due to short bowel syndrome, severe diarrhea, or high-output fistula), and altered metabolism (hypermetabolic and catabolic states due to sepsis, trauma, cancer, or AIDS). Malnutrition is also associated with major organ failure: renal, hepatic, cardiac, and pulmonary failure and multisystem organ failure (see Chap. 139).

CANCER

Patients with cancer have many factors that contribute to the likelihood of developing malnutrition (Table 136–4). The frequency is highest (>80%) in patients with gastric and pancreatic tumors, and lowest in patients with hematologic malignancies.[15] Weight loss, a sign of malnutrition, occurs in 30% to 80% of adult cancer patients. A significant relationship between weight loss and reduced survival has been demonstrated for some (lung, prostate, and colon cancer), but not all tumor types.[15] The degree of reduction in median survival is statistically significant for some cancers and ranges from 49% to 79%.

Malnutrition in children with cancer is common, and the prevalence is highest in those with Ewing's sarcoma (67%) and neuroblastoma (47%), and lowest in those with acute leukemias (6%) and non-Hodgkin's lymphomas (10% to 15%). While undernutrition has historically been an independent prognostic factor in the long-term outcome of children with certain cancers, not all researchers agree and it remains an area worthy of continued research.[16–18] Furthermore, due to advancements in cancer treatment strategies, the importance of nutritional status may diminish. The stage of disease progression and chemotherapy-related complications also has been associated with an increased prevalence.[19] Theoretically, early recognition and management of malnutrition in cancer patients may minimize the nutritional consequences, improve tumor response, reduce side effects of therapy, and improve survival. Cancer patients treated with bone marrow transplantation have shown improved tumor response and clinical outcome with parenteral nutrition (PN) compared with control groups not receiving PN.[20]

Improved nutrition status enhances survival and improves treatment tolerance in many but not all children.[19,21] Malnutrition in cancer patients due to simple starvation, characterized by normal metabolism but inadequate nutrient intake or malabsorption, appears to be responsive to nutrition intervention.[22] However, malnutrition due to cancer cachexia, characterized by altered nutrient use despite adequate supply, does not.[23,24]

CLINICAL CONTROVERSY

The intent of EN and PN should be to prevent or reverse protein-calorie malnutrition, and treatment of malnutrition due to cancer cachexia is controversial. Some clinicians believe nutrition support is warranted in terminally ill children if an improved quality of life can be attained.

AIDS

Generalized wasting and malnutrition were common characteristics of HIV/AIDS during the early years of this epidemic. The etiology and risk factors of AIDS-associated malnutrition are multifactorial (Table 136–5).[25–28] In many patients, weight loss and wasting were often the earliest symptoms along with opportunistic infection. The malnutrition was often progressive and led to death in

TABLE 136–4. Risk Factors for Malnutrition in Cancer Patients

Risk Factor	Nutrition Consequence
Primary disease	
Tumor type	Weight loss, anorexia, altered taste, altered metabolism
Complicating conditions	
Malabsorption	Impaired absorption of all or selected nutrients, diarrhea
Bowel obstruction	Nausea and vomiting, inability to ingest nutrients orally or by enteral nutrition
Infection	Increased energy expenditure and protein requirements, altered metabolism, anorexia, malabsorption
Psychological response	Anorexia, food aversion
Treatments	
Chemotherapy	Taste and appetite alterations, nausea and vomiting, mucositis, esophagitis, diarrhea, constipation
Surgery	
Radical resection of oropharyngeal region	Problems with chewing and swallowing
Esophageal reconstruction	Gastric stasis and hypochlorhydria secondary to vagotomy; diarrhea and steatorrhea
Gastrectomy	Dumping syndrome, malabsorption, lack of intrinsic factor, hypoglycemia
Intestinal resection	Malabsorption, renal oxalate stones, metabolic acidosis, diarrhea
Pancreatectomy	Malabsorption, diabetes mellitus
Radiation	
Head and neck	Stomatitis, dysgeusia, xerostomia
Abdomen and pelvis	Bowel obstruction, fistulae, radiation enteritis (diarrhea, protein-losing enteropathy, malabsorption)

some patients.[29,30] Poor nutrition status as indicated by weight loss and decreased serum prealbumin concentrations has been shown to be a predictor of survival in adult AIDS patients.[31,32] Furthermore, simultaneous micronutrient deficiencies such as vitamin A, vitamin B_{12}, zinc, and selenium have been significantly associated with HIV-related mortality, independent of CD4 counts <200 and changes in CD4 over time. When the individual effect of these micronutrient deficiencies was further delineated, selenium deficiency was the only independent predictor of HIV-related prognosis.[32] Recently, nutritional problems have shifted from the characteristic lethal wasting associated with opportunistic infections to a syndrome of subcutaneous fat atrophy, visceral fat accumulation, hypertriglyceridemia, and insulin resistance.[33] The etiology is unclear but may be related to new protease inhibitor therapy.[34] The implications of these metabolic and body compositional changes on outcome and development of comorbidities (i.e., atherosclerosis) are unclear at this time.

Most HIV-positive children will experience nutritional deficits and growth abnormalities.[26] Infants with perinatal-acquired AIDS have normal birthweights, but show signs of growth delay as early as 4 months.[35] Failure to thrive has been reported in up to 33% of HIV-infected children.[27] Impaired linear growth also appears to correlate with periods of rapid viral replication and lower CD4 T-lymphocyte counts during the first 18 months of life.[36,37] There is a direct relationship between these growth abnormalities and morbidity and mortality.[38] Fortunately, immune function, growth velocity, and survival can be improved markedly if aggressive nutritional therapy and antiviral therapy are initiated.[26,28,39]

The response to nutrition intervention in adults with AIDS has been variable. Supplemental dietary intake of selected micronutrients has been shown to have an impact on mortality in HIV-1 seropositive homosexual/bisexual men. High intakes of B-group vitamins (B_1, B_6, and niacin) and β-carotene were associated with improved survival, whereas an increased intake of zinc was associated with worse survival.[40] In a retrospective review of home PN in 22 AIDS patients with weight loss greater than 10% of usual body weight, 15 patients gained weight, 6 stabilized, and 2 continued to lose weight.[41] Lean body mass repletion in AIDS patients with weight loss and inadequate food intake has been reported when enteral nutrition was the sole source of nutrient intake.[42] Kotler and associates compared the effects of PN and an oral semi-elemental diet on body weight, body composition, survival, quality of life, and medical costs in AIDS outpatients with malabsorption syndromes.[43] At the end of 3 months, the PN group gained more weight and significantly more fat, but body cell mass measurements and survival did not differ between the groups. However, the group receiving an oral diet scored significantly better on a physical functioning subscale of quality of life. The

TABLE 136–5. Risk Factors for Malnutrition in AIDS

Risk Factor	Nutrition Consequence
General factors: decreased oral intake, malabsorption	Anorexia, poor diet, esophageal/oral lesions, emotional stress, HIV wasting syndrome, diarrhea, enteropathy, medication side effects
Opportunistic infections: bacterial (MAI, TB); viral (CMV, herpes); fungal (*Candida albicans*, cryptococcus); protozoal (*Pneumocystis carinii*, microsporidia, *Isospora belli*, cryptosporidia, *Giardia lamblia*)	Fever, hypermetabolism, anorexia, malabsorption
Malignancies: Kaposi's sarcoma, lymphoma	Anorexia, hypermetabolism, medication side effects
Medications: antibiotics, anticancer chemotherapy, antidepressants	Nausea, vomiting, diarrhea, anorexia, mucositis
Neuropsychiatric disorders: dementia, depression, anxiety, encephalopathy	Poor oral intake, anorexia, poor diet
Socioeconomic factors: IV drug abuse, low income	Poor oral intake, anorexia, poor diet

CMV, cytomegalovirus; MAI, *Mycobacterium avium-intercellulare*; TB, tuberculosis.

most dramatic differences were in medical costs, with a fourfold cost increase in patients receiving PN versus oral diet therapy.[43]

With earlier diagnosis and initiation of treatment for HIV-positive status prior to the onset of AIDS, the prevalence of malnutrition may decline. New treatment modalities for AIDS are also being developed that may affect the prevalence of malnutrition and the response to nutrition intervention in this patient population (see Chap. 123). For example, 12 weeks of recombinant human growth hormone treatment was evaluated in 178 HIV-infected patients with unintentional weight loss of $\geq 10\%$. In this double-blind, placebo-controlled, multicenter trial, growth hormone administration resulted in a mean increase of 3 kg of lean body mass with a decrease of about 1.7 kg of body fat. These changes in body composition were accompanied by an improvement in functional performance, reflected by treadmill work output.[44] However, concerns regarding the development of hyperglycemia and diabetes associated with long-term use of growth hormone have tempered its utilization. Other agents including thalidomide,[45] testosterone,[46] and nandrolone decanoate[47] have also shown promise in reversing cachexia associated with AIDS.

CRITICAL ILLNESS, TRAUMA, AND BURN INJURY

One of the characteristics of critical illness is hypermetabolism. Trauma, burn injury, and sepsis are all catalysts for the release of mediators that initiate and regulate the hypermetabolic response. The metabolic consequences of this response include altered carbohydrate metabolism, increased protein synthesis and degradation, and increased lipid oxidation, which ultimately result in loss of protein and lean body mass.[48] In a previously well-nourished individual, critical illness can result in the onset of kwashiorkor-like malnutrition within 5 to 7 days. In a previously malnourished individual, critical illness can precipitate severe mixed marasmus-kwashiorkor in 3 to 5 days. In a prospective study of 129 patients admitted to the intensive care unit (ICU), 43% were malnourished.[49] The malnourished patients had an increased length of stay in the ICU (a mean of 27 vs. 19 days) and a statistically significantly increased incidence of complications (55% vs. 40%) compared with well-nourished patients with a similar severity of illness.

◀4 The goal of nutrition support in critically ill patients is to prevent the development or worsening of malnutrition. Patient outcomes related to tissue repair and organ function may be improved through nutrition support in these patients.[48] Enteral nutrition (EN) initiated within 24 to 48 hours of injury may attenuate the hypermetabolic response.[50] Enteral nutrition also has been shown to result in fewer septic complications when compared with PN.[51] Two recent meta-analyses suggest that critically ill patients may derive the greatest benefit when enterally fed an immune-enhanced formula that contains pharmacologic doses of immune-modulating nutrients such as arginine, glutamine, nucleic acids, and omega-3 fatty acids.[52,53]

INFLAMMATORY BOWEL DISEASE

Malnutrition has been reported in 20% to 45% of patients with inflammatory bowel disease (IBD). Malabsorption, increased gastrointestinal losses, or poor oral intake are the predominant causes.[54] Decreased food intake may be due to pain, anorexia, or altered taste; malabsorption may be due to mucosal abnormalities, bacterial overgrowth, or diminished absorptive surface area after surgical resection of diseased bowel, and hypermetabolism may be a consequence of fever and infection.[55] Various nutrient abnormalities, such as anemia

and vitamin and trace mineral deficiencies, have been observed in IBD patients.[54] Growth failure occurs in 15% to 40% of prepubertal patients and is characterized by retarded skeletal maturation (which may be irreversible) and delayed development of secondary sex characteristics.[56] The nutrition consequences of ulcerative colitis tend to be less severe than those of Crohn's disease. Approximately 25% to 50% of patients with ulcerative colitis are hypoalbuminemic, and 2% to 20% experience growth failure.

◀5 Nutrition management of IBD may be achieved with enteral nutrition and/or PN.[57] Enteral is the preferred route except in patients with a high-output fistula or obstruction or if enteral feeding exacerbates pain. EN or PN is likely to facilitate remission in 60% to 80% of patients with acute Crohn's disease. However, the course of ulcerative colitis is not influenced by the use of nutrition support, although nutrition status may be maintained in an acute exacerbation.

CHRONIC INTESTINAL PSEUDO-OBSTRUCTION

Pseudo-obstruction, a hypomotility or dysmotility disorder of the gastrointestinal tract that is thought to be a neuromuscular disorder of the smooth muscle and/or its innervation, often presents with the symptoms of bowel obstruction. Prolonged dysmotility can result in malnutrition as well as growth failure in children.[58] Primary factors contributing to a risk of malnutrition are anorexia, nausea, vomiting, and obstruction, which may recur over years. Approximately 15% to 30% of patients with pseudo-obstruction require nutrition support with either PN or EN.[58]

SHORT BOWEL SYNDROME

Short bowel syndrome (SBS) is the result of the surgical resection of a large portion of the intestinal tract. The degree of nutrition impairment depends on the amount and location of excised bowel. Malabsorption is present to some extent immediately following surgery and may be permanent.[59] Bowel adaptation will occur over time (6 to 12 months), but may not result in restoration of the full absorptive capacity of the intestine. Intestinal adaptation occurs more frequently in children than in adults.[60] The minimal intestinal length required to achieve complete bowel adaptation in infants and children has been reported to vary from 10 cm to 57 cm.[61,62] Premature infants may have the best adaptive response to SBS owing to normal rapid intestinal growth during late gestation when the jejunum, ileum, and colon more than double in length.[63]

◀6 Adults who have 600 to 700 cm of ileum remaining after surgical resection (i.e., 100 to 200 cm of ileum resected) will require vitamin B_{12}, calcium, and magnesium supplementation. Massive resection of the small bowel leaving less than 60 cm in adults and less than 10 cm in children will result in severe malabsorption of all nutrients and these patients will require total or supplemental PN for months or years postoperatively.[60,64,65] Removal of the colon with the retention of <50 cm of jejunum and ileum may require that patients remain on PN for life.[64] One long-term study of 124 adults with nonmalignant SBS maintained on PN demonstrated that the presence of terminal ileum in continuity with the colon enhanced the probability of weaning from PN and survival.[66] In the absence of nutrition support, malnutrition is inevitable and can be life-threatening. For those children with extensive bowel loss or life-threatening complications from prolonged PN, innovative surgical procedures including bowel lengthening and transplantation can improve the gut's adaptive process and reduce the need for PN.[60,67,68]

SURGICAL PATIENTS

Malnourished patients tend to have a greater risk of postoperative morbidity and mortality than well-nourished patients. Several nutrition assessment parameters predict morbidity and mortality in surgical patients. In a classic study by Mullen and colleagues, the value of 16 nutritional and immunologic variables was examined and serum concentrations, of albumin and transferrin, as well as delayed cutaneous hypersensitivity reactions were found to be the most reliable predictors of outcome.[69] These factors have been confirmed by several authors to correlate with morbidity and mortality.[70,71] A retrospective study by Kudsk and colleagues[72] extended these findings by showing that operative site, in addition to the preoperative albumin concentration, was an independent risk factor in predicting clinical outcome: patients who underwent a colectomy and gastrectomy tolerated greater degrees of hypoalbuminemia than those patients who underwent esophagectomy or pancreatectomy. The complication rate was higher and resource utilization increased in patients who underwent pancreatic or esophageal surgery with serum albumin concentrations less than 3.25 g/dL. The Subjective Global Assessment (SGA), developed by Detsky and colleagues, is a clinical method that can aid in the recognition of undernutrition by evaluating a patient's nutritional status based on features of the medical history and physical examination.[73] In prospective studies, SGA has been shown to be very successful in predicting complications in surgical patients. One study demonstrated SGA to be a better predictor of postoperative infectious complications than serum albumin, serum transferrin, delayed hypersensitivity skin testing, anthropometry, creatinine-height index, and the prognostic nutritional index (PNI).[73] No studies have evaluated the effect of nutrition support on the PNI and the subsequent patient outcome. However, the use of preoperative PN in patients with malnutrition, particularly when associated with a low serum albumin concentration, has been demonstrated to reduce the incidence of major postoperative complications in several patient populations.[74] Parenteral nutrition administered solely after surgery was actually associated with an increased incidence of complications in approximately 10% of patients. Conflicting data were found in the multi-institutional VA Cooperative Study.[75] This prospective, randomized clinical trial in 395 malnourished patients evaluated the impact of perioperative PN on mortality and the rate of postoperative complications at 30 and 90 days. Differences in mortality at 30 and 90 days were not statistically significant, and there was no significant reduction in complication rate. The types of complications in the two groups were different. The PN group had a higher incidence of infectious complications and a lower incidence of noninfectious complications. The incidence of noninfectious complications was higher in those with the greatest degree of malnutrition (determined by calculation of a nutrition risk index using serum albumin concentration and weight). In the PN group, the highest incidence of infectious complications was in the borderline or mildly malnourished patients. The investigators concluded that perioperative PN did not result in an improved postoperative course except in patients who were severely malnourished preoperatively. In patients who were mildly to moderately malnourished, the incidence of infectious complications associated with the use of PN outweighed the benefits. As with critically ill patients, enteral feeding with immune-enhanced formulas in surgical patients appears to promote the best nutrition and clinical outcome with fewer metabolic and infectious complications.[76]

PEDIATRIC DISEASES

Regardless of the disease process, pediatric patients in general are at greater risk for nutrition disorders and develop the most severe con-

TABLE 136–6. Management Principles of Severe Pediatric Malnutrition

1. Recognize the physiologic effects of reductive adaptation. Every organ system has adapted to starvation and cannot tolerate aggressive reintroduction of nutrition.
2. Treat or prevent hypoglycemia, hypothermia, and dehydration (days 1–3). Initiate small, frequent feedings (every 2–3 hours) and provide only enough calories to meet basic metabolic demands.
3. Avoid a high-protein diet (days 1–3) secondary to liver incompetence.
4. Correct electrolyte imbalance (day 1 through week 6).
5. Assume the child has an infection and empirically treat with antibiotics (days 1–7).
6. Avoid cardiac failure secondary to aggressive rehydration. Parenteral rehydration should be avoided at all costs and only used if the child is in shock. Avoid diuretics during the first 1–5 days even if edema is evident.
7. Advance enteral feeding to recover lost weight and provide for "catch-up growth" (day 7 through week 26).
8. Correct micronutrient deficiencies with vitamins and minerals (without iron on days 1–7 and with iron on day 7 through week 6).
9. Correct emotional and social disorders.

sequences more frequently (Table 136–6). Nutrition deficiency in the young affects existing organs and cells, may impair normal development, and may result in permanent, irreversible damage. Pharmacologic and technologic advances in neonatal medicine have improved the survival of extremely premature infants (<750 g). However, the prevalence of neonatal diseases such as bronchopulmonary dysplasia and necrotizing enterocolitis also has increased, which may further complicate the infant's nutrition status (see Table 136–6).

BRONCHOPULMONARY DYSPLASIA

Bronchopulmonary dysplasia (BPD) or chronic lung disease is a clinical, pathologic, and radiographic disease of the newborn resulting from prolonged exposure to positive-pressure ventilation and elevated oxygen concentrations. Risk factors for developing BPD include extent of prematurity, nutrition status, and immunologic status. Characteristics of BPD include pulmonary edema and tissue destruction with subsequent repair, fibrosis, and inflammation. These infants also have an elevated metabolic rate and growth failure.

CLINICAL CONTROVERSY

Supplemental vitamin A is used in some neonatal treatment centers to reduce the risk of BPD and sepsis in preterm infants. However, concern over the risk of vitamin A toxicity (i.e., posthemorrhagic hydrocephalus or liver disease) and sequelae from repeated intramuscular injections of vitamin A prevent its widespread use.

Growth failure and altered body composition are common in infants with BPD when compared with their peers without BPD.[77,78] The persistence of this altered body composition can last into the first years of life.[78] Estimates of growth failure after hospital discharge range between 30% and 67%.[79] The origin of growth failure is multifactorial and has been associated with elevations in both resting and total energy expenditure, use of corticosteroids, intrauterine growth retardation, and feeding problems.[80,81] Given that pulmonary edema is common, fluid restriction is often necessary. This restriction further impedes provision of adequate calories and may contribute to poor growth.[80] Optimal oxygen therapy during the first year of life in infants with BPD can result in growth patterns similar to those seen in infants without BPD.[82] Growth failure during the first 2 years of life, early childhood, and beyond has been reported, but it appears that prematurity and sociodemographic factors rather than BPD per se are most predictive of future growth.[83,84] Catch-up growth can be attained faster when infants are fed higher intakes of protein, calcium, phosphorus, and zinc.[85] Vitamin A deficiency has been associated with BPD, but supplementation of vitamin A in all BPD patients is not universally endorsed. Benefits of vitamin A supplementation (i.e., a trend toward reduction in ventilatory support) must be considered with risks of repeated intramuscular injections.

NECROTIZING ENTEROCOLITIS

Necrotizing enterocolitis (NEC) is a complex disorder characterized by intestinal mucosal injury secondary to ischemia, bacterial overgrowth, and/or the presence of nutrients within the gut lumen. NEC typically occurs in the first 1 to 3 weeks of life and in premature infants (<38 weeks' gestational age) with inadequate immune function and an immature intestinal epithelial barrier.[86] Rapid advancement of EN has been linked to the development of NEC. The severe inflammation of the intestinal tract caused by mucosal injury results in malabsorption of nutrients. Total bowel rest is the treatment of choice; hence PN is required to prevent malnutrition. If NEC results in bowel perforation, necrosis, or stricture, surgery is required to resect the injured portion of the bowel. SBS may be a consequence if more than 70% of the bowel is resected, and long-term home PN will then be required. Additionally, infants with advanced disease who require surgery are at increased risk of growth failure. Fortunately, advances in surgical techniques have increased the survival rate of NEC over the past decade to between 60% and 80%, depending on the gestational age at the time of diagnosis.[87] If significant intestinal resection can be avoided, growth and nutrient absorption in these children may be normal.[61]

CYSTIC FIBROSIS

The predominant clinical findings of cystic fibrosis (CF) are related to altered pulmonary function and pancreatic exocrine function. Historically, growth retardation and failure to thrive have been classic features of CF. According to the National Cystic Fibrosis Patient Registry data, malnutrition (height for age or weight for age <5th percentile) was very prevalent in infants (47%), adolescents (34%), and children with newly diagnosed CF (44%).[88] Over the past decade, the nutritional status of children with CF has improved, largely due to the association of nutritional intervention with disease progression and clinical outcome. A recent longitudinal study confirmed that nutrition and lung function are codependent variables in CF.[89] Other factors that contribute to the nutrition disorders associated with CF include an increased energy expenditure, malabsorption, anorexia, gastroesophageal reflux, pharmacotherapy, glucosuria, and inadequate pulmonary toilet.[90,91] Increased energy requirements in CF patients are the result of the increased amount of work required to breathe and an elevated resting energy expenditure (REE) during pulmonary exacerbations. Recent data suggest that children with only mild to moderate lung disease may be spared from this rise in REE during an acute exacerbation.[92] It is also theorized that the genetic defect that causes CF affects metabolism, causing an increase in energy requirements. The physical pounding on the back of the patient while in a partially inverted position (i.e., pulmonary toilet) is designed to loosen the thickened bronchial secretions that impair breathing. It may be performed numerous times throughout the day and may result in an increase in energy expenditure. It also interferes with the feeding schedule, which needs to be designed to ensure that the stomach is empty or nearly empty before the pulmonary toilet process begins, to prevent pulmonary aspiration of stomach contents.

As life expectancy of patients with CF increases, the recognition of CF-associated diseases has also increased. CF-related diabetes mellitus is now a well-recognized problem and further complicates the nutritional management of those individuals.[93] Altered pancreatic function is common and over 90% of CF patients need pancreatic enzyme supplementation. Insufficiency of pancreatic enzyme secretion into the intestine reduces the absorption of fat and fat-soluble vitamins. Consequently, more than two-thirds of the CF centers in North America use a hydrolyzed (semi-elemental) enteral formula with low fat content for infants with CF. However, the nutrition benefits of this expensive hydrolyzed formula over a conventional cow's milk formula have been challenged. Several investigations do not support the use of a hydrolyzed formula as part of routine nutrition care.[94,95] Nutritional management typically focuses on the use of oral pancreatic enzymes (e.g., Viokase and Pancrease), supplemental fat-soluble vitamins, and a high-protein, high-calorie diet.[88] If nutrition status cannot be maintained with these measures, supplemental EN or PN may be indicated.

SOLID-ORGAN FAILURE IN CHILDHOOD

Malnutrition with growth impairment is a well-recognized complication of renal, hepatic, and cardiac failure in children. Evidence suggests that these factors increase the risk of morbidity and mortality. Mechanisms responsible for malnutrition include reduced energy intake, increased resting energy rates, and increased total energy expenditure.[96-99] Early clinical onset of organ failure can have profound effects on growth and development, especially in children with end-stage liver disease, in whom the liver is not able to perform intermediary metabolism. Among children diagnosed with hereditary renal disorders, 50% had marked growth retardation (mean age at observation = 10 years).[99] Prevalence of malnutrition in hospitalized children with cardiac disease varies with age and type of cardiac lesion. Seventy-nine percent of infants with heart disease had evidence of acute malnutrition, compared with less than 30% in all other age groups. The prevalence of chronic malnutrition was common in all age groups. An inverse relationship to age was observed with 82%, 84%, 61%, 58%, and 38% of infants, toddlers, preschool children, school-age children, and adolescents, respectively, being malnourished.[100] Children with complex cardiac disease or left-to-right intracardiac shunts had the highest prevalence of both acute and chronic malnutrition (38% to 80%). Catch-up growth in children with chronic renal failure, complex congenital heart lesions, and advanced cirrhosis can be attained with aggressive feeding regimens, including tube feedings.[97,101] Optimizing nutritional status during the pre- and post-transplant phase can improve outcomes and reduce morbidity.[102,103] After liver transplantation, catch-up growth can occur, but final height remains 0.5 to 1 standard deviation below normal.[104]

MANAGEMENT

The increased awareness of the prevalence and significance of untreated protein-calorie malnutrition has provided a strong incentive for a more rigorous evaluation of abnormalities of nutrition status and prompt initiation of nutrition support for malnourished patients.

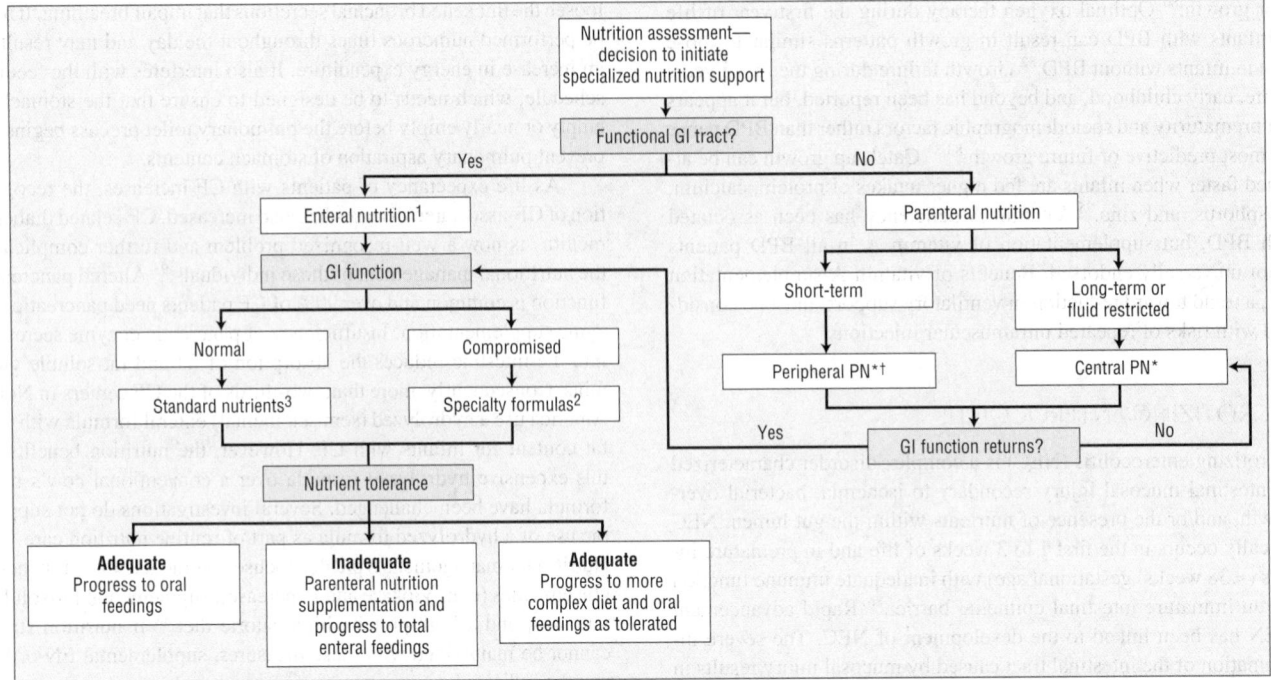

FIGURE 136–1. Routes to deliver nutrition support to adults: Clinical decision algorithm. *Formulation of enteral and parenteral solution should be made considering organ function (e.g., cardiac, renal, respiratory, or hepatic). †In selected patients, peripheral parenteral nutrition may be considered to provide partial or total nutrition support for up to 2 weeks in patients who cannot ingest or absorb oral or enteral-tube–delivered nutrients, or when central vein parenteral nutrition is not feasible. ¹Short-term: nasogastric, nasojejunal. Long-term: gastrostomy, jejunostomy. Feeding may be more appropriate distal to the pylorus if the patient has an increased risk of aspiration. ²Formulas should be tailored to patient GI tolerance and include elemental, low/high fat content, lactose-free, fiber-rich, and modular formulas. ³Polymeric, complete formulas are appropriate.

If nutrition assessment (see Chap. 135) reveals no malnutrition, then the patient should be counseled on appropriate maintenance goals for nutrition intake. If mild to moderate malnutrition is present, an anabolic feeding regimen should be initiated using oral supplements. If anorexia is a major contributing factor, enteral tube feeding may be indicated. Intact nutrients can be administered enterally when normal bowel function is present, but a specially designed formula that has a modified fat content, is lactose-free, contains fiber, and/or is calorie or protein enriched may be indicated if intestinal function is compromised (see Chap. 138). If malabsorption is a major contributing factor, tube feeding using a disease-specific formula, or alternatively, supplemental or total PN may be indicated. In the presence of severe malnutrition, an anabolic feeding regimen should be initiated either enterally or parenterally depending on intestinal function and malabsorption[105] (Fig. 136–1). Data from international studies show the median mortality rate secondary to severe malnutrition in children under 5 years of age is 25%. Since some institutions have reported a rate less than 5%, the treatment strategy that is employed appears to be critical. Therefore the World Health Organization has published guidelines for the management of severe malnutrition in children (see www.who.int/nut/manageme.pdf).

When bowel obstruction or SBS is present, PN is indicated. Equivocal data exist whether EN is absolutely contraindicated in hypoperfusion of the gut. The most recent recommendations advocate holding enteral nutrition when patients have; sustained hypotension (<70 mm Hg), a need for increasing doses of pressor agents to maintain the mean arterial pressure ≥70 mm Hg, increasing ventilatory support requirements, or worsening signs of GI intolerance to the enteral nutrition (i.e., sudden abdominal distention, abrupt increases in

nasogastric output, and sudden abdominal pain).[106] The anticipated duration of the need for parenteral support will dictate whether one uses the peripheral or central venous route of administration (see Chap. 137). Routine re-evaluation of the response to nutrition therapy and attainment of nutrition goals should be incorporated into the overall patient care plan.

PHARMACOECONOMIC CONSIDERATIONS

Malnourished patients have increased complications during their hospital course and an increased length of stay (LOS), and thereby incur increased health care costs.[3,107] Low serum albumin concentrations must also be interpreted in the context of the surgical site (esophagus vs. colon), since this has been shown to affect the complication rate, thereby influencing hospital and ICU LOS.[72] As disproportionate consumers of health care resources, malnourished patients rank among the top 10%.[108]

Although the evidence is strong that malnutrition is associated with increased health care costs, it has been more difficult to establish the cost-benefit or cost savings of nutrition intervention. Based on assumptions derived from the literature, Twomey and Patching[109] concluded that preoperative PN could be cost-saving in patients undergoing surgery for gastrointestinal cancer. A similar conclusion applied to a broader patient population is supported by a model that examines the financial implications of malnutrition and nutrition therapy.[108] This model takes into consideration the increased costs associated with an increased LOS, and morbidity and mortality caused by malnutrition, as well as the costs of identifying patients at risk for malnutrition, providing nutrition support, and managing the complications associated with the nutrition support. Tucker and Miguel confirmed the association between poor nutritional status and prolonged length of hospital stay, and also determined that when nutrition intervention occurred (oral, enteral, or parenteral nutrition), the average LOS was decreased by 2.1 days.[107]

Trauma patients are at an unusually high risk for developing malnutrition due to the hypermetabolic and hypercatabolic state associated with underlying injury. Although several clinical trials have compared the efficacy of EN versus PN, little data are available regarding the cost-effectiveness of these two routes of administration. Trice and colleagues[110] assessed the economic impact of the delivery of EN versus PN to trauma patients. Their evaluation of the data from nine prospective, randomized clinical trials revealed that postoperative PN was associated with an almost fourfold increased risk of infectious complications and 15-fold greater risk of catheter sepsis compared with EN. Estimated total costs thus were four- to 12.5-fold greater in patients receiving PN versus EN. Thus the decision to prescribe PN over EN should be evaluated carefully when considering nutrition support in trauma patients.

Economic savings also have been achieved when specialized nutrition support teams are involved with the provision of EN.[111] A benefit of $4.20 was realized for every $1 invested in nutrition support team management. Furthermore, management by the nutrition support team resulted in reductions in mortality rate, length of hospital stay, readmission rates, and complications, compared with management by a nonteam group. Thus intervention by specially trained health care practitioners, including pharmacists, can lower operating costs associated with nutrition intervention without compromising the quality of patient care.

EVALUATION OF THERAPEUTIC OUTCOMES

Although the cost-benefit analysis of nutrition intervention is weak, the issue that seems clear is that malnutrition is associated with significant morbidity and mortality in numerous disease states and clinical settings. Furthermore, it is likely that improved patient outcomes can be achieved by a systematic approach to identify the presence of risk factors for malnutrition, quantitate the degree of malnutrition, and initiate nutrition management.[112] The clinician's responsibilities in the management of nutrition disease include the following:

1. Assist in identifying patients at risk for malnutrition and/or candidates for nutrition intervention.
2. Assist in the design of patient-specific nutrition-support regimens.
3. Evaluate and manage all drug-nutrient interactions.
4. Evaluate laboratory data, especially parameters used to determine safety and efficacy of nutrition support.

ABBREVIATIONS

AIDS: acquired immunodeficiency syndrome
BPD: bronchopulmonary dysplasia
CF: cystic fibrosis
CLD: chronic lung disease
EN: enteral nutrition
HIV: human immunodeficiency virus
IBD: inflammatory bowel disease

LOS: length of stay
NEC: necrotizing enterocolitis
PNI: prognostic nutritional index
PN: parenteral nutrition
REE: resting energy expenditure
SBS: short bowel syndrome
SGA: Subjective Global Assessment

Review Questions and other resources can be found at *www.pharmacotherapyonline.com.*

REFERENCES

1. Fawzi WW, Herrera MG, Nestel P, et al. A longitudinal study of prolonged breastfeeding in relation to child undernutrition. Int J Epidemiol 1998;27:255–260.
2. Gallagher-Allred DR, Voss AC, Finn SC, et al. Malnutrition and clinical outcomes: The case for medical nutrition therapy. J Am Diet Assoc 1996;96:361–366.
3. Coats KG, Morgan SL, Bartolucci AA, Weinsier RL. Hospital-associated malnutrition: A re-evaluation 12 years later. J Am Diet Assoc 1993;93:27–33.
4. Iyengar GV, Nair PP. Global outlook on nutrition and the environment: Meeting challenges of the next millennium. Sci Total Environ 2000;249:331–346.
5. The state of the world's children 1998: A UNICEF report. Malnutrition: Causes, consequences, and solution. Nutr Rev 1998;56:115–123.
6. Mendez MA, Adair LS. Severity and timing of stunting in the first two years of life affect performance on cognitive tests in late childhood. J Nutr 1999;129:1555–1562.
7. Caballero B. Global patterns of child health: The role of nutrition. Ann Nutr Metab 2002;46(Suppl 1):3–7.
8. Centers for Disease Control And Prevention. Pediatric nutrition surveillance, 1997 full report. Atlanta, U.S. Department of Public Health and Human Services, Centers for Disease Control and Prevention, 1998.
9. Hendricks KM, Duggan C, Gallagher L, et al. Malnutrition in hospitalized pediatric patients. Arch Pediatr Adolesc Med 1995;149:1118–1122.
10. Sawaya Al, Martins P, Hoffman D, Roberts SB. The link between childhood undernutrition and risk of chronic diseases in adulthood: A case study of Brazil. Nutr Rev 2003;61(5 Pt 1):168–175.
11. Godfrey KM, Barker DJ. Fetal programming and adult health. Public Health Nutr 2001;4:611–624.
12. Prasad AS. Zinc: An overview. Nutrition 1995;11:93–99.
13. Albina JE. Nutrition and wound healing. JPEN J Parenter Enteral Nutr 1994;18:367–376.
14. Kirk SJ, Hurson M, Regan MC, et al. Arginine stimulates wound healing and immune function in elderly human beings. Surgery 1993;114:155–160.
15. Dewys WD, Begg C, Lavin PT, et al. Prognostic effect of weight loss prior to chemotherapy in cancer patients. Am J Med 1980;69:491–497.
16. Barr RD, Gibson B. Nutritional status and cancer in childhood. J Pediatr Hematol Oncol 2000;22:491–494.
17. Pedrosa F, Bonilla M, Liu A, et al. Effect of malnutrition at the time of diagnosis on the survival of children treated for cancer in El Salvador and Northern Brazil. J Pediatr Hematol Oncol 2000;22:502–505.
18. Lobato-Mendizabal E, Lopez-Martinez B, Ruiz-Arguelles GJ. A critical review of the prognostic value of the nutritional status at diagnosis in the outcome of therapy of children with acute lymphoblastic leukemia. Rev Invest Clin 2003;55:31–35.
19. Mauer AM, Burgess JB, Donaldson SS, et al. Special nutritional needs of children with malignancies: A review. JPEN J Parenter Enteral Nutr 1990;14:315–324.
20. Weisdorf SA, Lysne J, Wind D, et al. Positive effect of prophylactic total parenteral nutrition on long-term outcome of bone marrow transplantation. Transplantation 1987;43:833–838.

21. Holcomb GW, Ziegler MM. Nutrition and cancer in children. Surg Annu 1990;22:129–142.

22. Klein S, Simes J, Blackburn G. TPN and cancer clinical trials. Cancer 1986;58:1378–1386.

23. Brennan MF. Uncomplicated starvation versus cancer cachexia. Cancer Res 1977;37:2359–2364.

24. Kern KA, Norton JA. Cancer cachexia. JPEN J Parenter Enteral Nutr 1988;12:286–298.

25. Raiten DJ. Nutrition and HIV. Nutr Clin Pract 1991;6(3 Suppl):1S–94S.

26. Miller TL. Malnutrition: Metabolic changes in children, comparisons with adults. J Nutr 1996;126:2623S–2631S.

27. Winter H. Gastrointestinal tract function and malnutrition in HIV-infected children. J Nutr 1996;126:2620S–2622S.

28. Oleske JM, Rothpletz-Puglia PM, Winter H. Historical perspectives on the evolution in understanding the importance of nutritional care in pediatric HIV infection. J Nutr 1996;126:2616S–2619S.

29. ASPEN Board of Directors. Acquired immune deficiency syndrome. JPEN J Parenter Enteral Nutr 2002;26(Suppl):85SA–86SA.

30. Kotler D, Tierney A, Wang J, et al. Magnitude of body-cell-mass depletion and the timing of death from wasting in AIDS. Am J Clin Nutr 1989;50:444–447.

31. Guenter P, Muurahainen N, Simons G, et al. Relationships among nutritional status, disease progression, and survival in HIV infection. J Acquir Immune Defic Syndr 1993;6:1130–1138.

32. Baum MK, Shor-Posner G. Micronutrient status in relationship to mortality in HIV-1 disease. Nutr Rev 1998;56(1 Pt 2):S135–S139.

33. Kotler DP, Rosenbaum K, Wang J, et al. Studies of body composition and fat distribution in HIV-infected and control subjects. J Acquir Immune Defic Syndr Hum Retrovirol 1999;20:228–237.

34. Carr A, Semaras K, Chisholm DJ, et al. Pathogenesis of HIV-1 protease inhibitor-associated peripheral lipodystrophy, hyperlipidemia, and insulin resistance. Lancet 1998;351:1881–1883.

35. McKinney RE, Robertson JWR. Effect of human immunodeficiency virus infection on the growth of young children. J Pediatr 1993;123:579–582.

36. Pollack H, Glasberg H, Lee E, et al. Impaired early growth of infants perinatally infected with human immunodeficiency virus: Correlation with viral load. J Pediatr 1997;130:915–922.

37. Miller TL, Easley KA, Zhang W et al. Maternal and infant factors associated with failure to thrive in children with vertically transmitted human immunodeficiency virus-1 infection: The prospective, P2C2 human immunodeficiency virus multicenter study. Pediatrics 2001;108:1287–1296.

38. Brettler DB, Forsberg A, Bolivar E, et al. Growth failure as a prognostic indicator for progression to acquired immunodeficiency syndrome in children with hemophilia. J Pediatr 1990;117:584–588.

39. Beisel WR. Nutrition and immune function: Overview. J Nutr 1996;126:2611S–2615S.

40. Tang AM, Graham NMH, Saah AJ. Effects of micronutrient intake on survival in human immunodeficiency virus type 1 infection. Am J Epidemiol 1996;143:1244–1256.

41. Singer P, Rothkopf MM, Kvetan V, et al. Risks and benefits of home parenteral nutrition in the acquired immunodeficiency syndrome. JPEN J Parenter Enteral Nutr 1991;15:75–79.

42. Kotler DP, Tierney AR, Ferraro R, et al. Enteral alimentation and repletion of body cell mass in malnourished patients with acquired immunodeficiency syndrome. Am J Clin Nutr 1991;53:149–154.

43. Kotler DP, Fogleman L, Tierney AR. Comparison of total parenteral nutrition and an oral, semielemental diet on body composition, physical function, and nutrition-related costs in patients with malabsorption due to acquired immunodeficiency syndrome. JPEN J Parenter Enteral Nutr 1998;22:120–126.

44. Schambelan M, Mulligan K, Grunfeld C, et al. Recombinant human growth hormone in patients with HIV-associated wasting: A randomized, placebo-controlled trial. Ann Intern Med 1996;125:873–882.

45. Kaplan G, Thomas S, Fierer DS. Thalidomide for the treatment of AIDS-associated wasting. AIDS Res Hum Retroviruses 2000;16:1345–1355.

46. Grinspoon S, Corcoran C, Anderson E. Sustained anabolic effects of long-term androgen administration in men with AIDS-wasting. Clin Infect Dis 1999;28:634–636.

47. Miller K, Corcoran C, Armstrong C. Transdermal testosterone administration in women with acquired immunodeficiency syndrome wasting: A pilot study. J Clin Endocrinol Metab 1998;83:2717–2725.

48. Cerra FB, Benitez MR, Blackburn GL, et al. Applied nutrition in ICU patients: A consensus statement of the American College of Chest Physicians. Chest 1997;111:769–778.

49. Giner M, Laviano A, Meguid MM, Gleason JR. In 1995 a correlation between malnutrition and poor outcome in critically ill patients still exists. Nutrition 1996;12:23–29.

50. Chiarelli A, Enzi G, Casadei A, et al. Very early nutrition supplementation in burned patients. Am J Clin Nutr 1990;51:1035–1039.

51. Kudsk KA, Croce MA, Fabian TC, et al. Enteral versus parenteral feeding: Effects on septic morbidity after blunt and penetrating abdominal trauma. Ann Surg 1992;215:503–513.

52. Heys SD, Walker LG, Smith I, et al. Enteral nutritional supplementation with key nutrients in patients with critical illness and cancer: A meta-analysis of randomized controlled clinical trials. Ann Surg 1999;229:467–477.

53. Beale RJ, Bryg DJ, Bihari DJ. Immunonutrition in the critically ill: A systematic review of clinical outcome. Crit Care Med 1999;27:2799–2805.

54. Bowling TE. Inflammatory bowel disease. Eur J Gastroenterol Hepatol 1995;7:521–527.

55. Afonso JJ, Rombeau JL. Parenteral nutrition for patients with inflammatory bowel disease. In: Rombeau JL, Caldwell MD, eds. Clinical Nutrition: Parenteral Nutrition, 2nd ed. Philadelphia, Saunders, 1993:427–441.

56. Seidman EG, LeLeiko N, Ament M, et al. Nutritional issues in pediatric inflammatory bowel disease: Symposium report. J Pediatr Gastroenterol Nutr 1991;12:424–438.

57. ASPEN Board of Directors. Inflammatory bowel disease. JPEN J Parenter Enteral Nutr 2002;26(Suppl):73SA, 115SA–116SA.

58. Vargas JH, Sachs P, Ament ME. Chronic intestinal pseudo-obstruction syndrome in pediatrics: Results of a national survey by members of the North American Society for Pediatric Gastroenterology and Nutrition. J Pediatr Gastroenterol Nutr 1988;7:323–332.

59. Thompson JS. Management of the short bowel syndrome. Gastroenterol Clin North Am 1994;23:403–419.

60. Thompson JS, Langnas AN, Pinch LW, et al. Surgical approach to short-bowel syndrome: Experience in a population of 160 patients. Ann Surg 1995;222:600–607.

61. Wasa M, Takagi Y, Sando K, et al. Long-term outcome of short bowel syndrome in adult and pediatric patients. JPEN J Parenter Enteral Nutr 1999;23:S110–S112.

62. Kurkchubasche AG, Rowe MI, Smith SD. Adaptation in short-bowel syndrome: Reassessing old limits. J Pediatr Surg 1993;28:1069–1107.

63. Touloukian RJ, Walker Smith GJ. Normal intestinal length in preterm infants. J Pediatr Surg 1983;18:720–723.

64. Wilmore DW, Robinson MK. Short bowel syndrome. World J Surg 2000;24:1486–1492.

65. Jeejeebhoy KN. Short bowel syndrome: A nutritional and medical approach. CMAJ 2003;16:1297–1302.

66. Messing B, Crenn P, Beau P, et al. Long-term survival and parenteral nutrition dependence in adult patients with the short bowel syndrome. Gastroenterology 1999;117:1043–1050.

67. Figueroa-Colon R, Harris PR, Birdsong E, et al. Impact of intestinal lengthening on the nutritional outcome for children with short bowel syndrome. J Pediatr Surg 1996;31:912–916.

68. Langnas AN, Shaw BW, Antonson DL, et al. Preliminary experience with intestinal transplantation in infants and children. Pediatrics 1996;97:443–448.

69. Mullen JL, Gertner MH, Buzby GP, et al. Implications of malnutrition in the surgical patient. Arch Surg 1979;114:121–125.

70. Rudman D, Feller AB, Nagraj HS, et al. Relation of serum albumin concentration to death rate in nursing home men. JPEN J Parenter Enteral Nutr 1987;11:360–363.

71. Buzby GP, Mullen JL, Mathews DC, et al. Prognostic nutritional index in gastrointestinal surgery. Am J Surg 1980;139:160–166.

72. Kudsk KA, Tolley EA, DeWitt RC, et al. Preoperative albumin and surgical site identify surgical risk for major postoperative complications. JPEN J Parenter Enteral Nutr 2003;27:1–9.

73. Detsky AS, Baker JP, O'Rourke K, et al. Predicting nutrition-associated complications for residents undergoing gastrointestinal surgery. JPEN J Parenter Enteral Nutr 1987;11:440–446.

74. Klein S, Kinney J, Jeejeebhoy K, et al. Nutrition support in clinical practice: Review of published data and recommendations for future research directions. JPEN J Parenter Enteral Nutr 1997;21:133–156.

75. The Veterans Affairs Total Parenteral Nutrition Cooperative Study Group. Perioperative total parenteral nutrition. N Engl J Med 1991;325:525–532.

76. Sacks GS, Genton L, Kudsk KA. Controversy of immunonutrition for surgical, critical-illness patients. Curr Opin Crit Care 2003;9:300–305.

77. deRegnier RA, Guilbert TW, Mills MM, Georgieff MK. Growth failure and altered body composition are established by one month of age in infants with bronchopulmonary dysplasia. J Nutr 1996;126:168–175.

78. Huysman WA, de Ridder M, de Bruin NC, et al. Growth and body composition in preterm infants with bronchopulmonary dysplasia. Arch Dis Child Fetal Neonatal Ed 2003;88:F46–F51.

79. Johnson DB, Cheney C, Monsen ER. Nutrition and feeding in infants with bronchopulmonary dysplasia after initial hospital discharge: Risk factors for growth failure. J Am Diet Assoc 1998;98:649–656.

80. Atkinson SA. Special nutritional needs of infants for prevention of and recovery from bronchopulmonary dysplasia. J Nutr 2001;131:942S–946S.

81. Abrams SA. Chronic pulmonary insufficiency in children and its effects on growth and development. J Nutr 2001;131:938S–941S.

82. Chye JK, Gray PH. Rehospitalization and growth of infants with bronchopulmonary dysplasia: A matched control study. J Paediatr Child Health 1995;31:105–111.

83. Robertson CMT, Etches PC, Goldson E, Kyle JM. Eight-year school performance, neurodevelopmental, and growth outcome of neonates with bronchopulmonary dysplasia: A comparative study. Pediatrics 1992;89:365–372.

84. Vrienich LA, Bozynski MEA, Shyr Y, et al. The effect of bronchopulmonary dysplasia on growth at school age. Pediatrics 1995;95:855–859.

85. Brunton JA, Saigal S, Atkinson SA. Growth and body composition in infants with bronchopulmonary dysplasia up to 3 months corrected age: A randomized trial of high-energy nutrient-enriched formula fed after hospital discharge. J Pediatr 1998;133:340–345.

86. Neu J, Weiss MD. Necrotizing enterocolitis: Pathophysiology and prevention. JPEN J Parenter Enteral Nutr 1999;23:S13–S17.

87. Guthrie SO, Gordon PV, Thomas V, et al. Necrotizing enterocolitis among neonates in the United States. J Perinatol 2003;23:278–285.

88. Lai H, Kosorok MR, Sondel SA, et al. Growth status in children with cystic fibrosis based on the national Cystic Fibrosis Patient Registry data: Evaluation of various criteria used to identify malnutrition. J Pediatr 1998;132:478–485.

89. Steinkamp G, Wiedemann B. Relationship between nutritional status and lung function in cystic fibrosis: Cross sectional and longitudinal analyses from the German CF quality assurance (CFQA) project. Thorax 2002;57:596–601.

90. Ramsay BW, Farrell PM, Penchartz P, et al. Consensus report: Nutritional assessment and management of cystic fibrosis. Am J Clin Nutr 1992;55:108–116.

91. Pencharz PB, Durie PR. Pathogenesis of malnutrition in cystic fibrosis, and its treatment. Clin Nutr 2000;19:387–394.

92. Stallings VA, Fung EB, Hofley PM, Scanlin TF. Acute pulmonary exacerbation is not associated with increased energy expenditure in children with cystic fibrosis. J Pediatr 1998;132:493–499.

93. Wilson DC, Kalnins D, Stewart C, et al. Challenges in the dietary treatment of cystic fibrosis related diabetes mellitus. Clin Nutr 2000;19:87–93.

94. Erskine JM, Lingard CD, Sontage MK, Accurso FJ. Enteral nutrition for patients with cystic fibrosis: Comparison of a semi-elemental and non-elemental formula. J Pediatr 1998;132:265–269.

95. Ellis L, Kalnins D, Corey M, et al. Do infants with cystic fibrosis need a protein hydrolystate formula? A prospective, randomized, comparative study. J Pediatr 1998;132:270–276.

96. Haffner D, Weinfurth A, Manz F, et al. Long-term outcome of paediatric patients with hereditary tubular disorders. Nephron 1999;83:250–260.

97. Charlton CP, Buchanan E, Holden CE, et al. Intensive enteral feeding in advanced cirrhosis: Reversal of malnutrition without precipitation of hepatic encephalopathy. Arch Dis Child 1992;67:603–607.

98. Greer R, Lehnert M, Lewindon P, et al. Body composition and components of energy expenditure in children with end-stage liver disease. J Pediatr Gastroenterol Nutr 2003;36:358–363.

99. Leitch CA. Growth, nutrition and energy expenditure in pediatric heart failure. Prog Pediatr Cardiol 2000;11:195–202.

100. Cameron JW, Rosenthal A, Olson AD. Malnutrition in hospitalized children with congenital heart disease. Arch Pediatr Adolesc Med 1995;149:1098–1102.

101. Claris-Appiani A, Ardissino GL, Dacco V, et al. Catch-up growth in children with chronic renal failure treated with long-term enteral nutrition. JPEN J Parenter Enteral Nutr 1995;19:175–178.

102. Varan B, Tokel K, Yilmaz G. Malnutrition and growth failure in cyanotic and acyanotic congenital heart disease with and without pulmonary hypertension. Arch Dis Child 1999;81:49–52.

103. McDiarmid SV. Risk factors and outcomes after pediatric liver transplantation. Liver Transpl Surg 1996;2:44–45.

104. Sokal EM, Cleghorn G, Goulet O, et al. Liver and intestinal transplantation in children: Working group report of the first world congress of pediatric gastroenterology, hepatology and nutrition. J Pediatr Gastroenterol Nutr 2002;25:S159–S172.

105. ASPEN Board of Directors. Routes to deliver nutrition support to adults: Clinical decision algorithm. In: Clinical Pathways and Algorithms for Delivery of Parenteral and Enteral Nutrition Support in Adults. Silver Spring, MD, ASPEN, 1998:5.

106. McClave SA, Chang W-K. Feeding the hypotensive patient: Does enteral feeding precipitate or protect against ischemic bowel. Nutr Clin Pract 2003;18:279–284.

107. Tucker HN, Miguel SG. Cost containment through nutrition intervention (Review). Nutr Rev 1996;54:111–121.

108. Bernstein LH, Shaw-Stiffel TA, Schorow M, Brouillette R. Financial implications of malnutrition (review). Clin Lab Med 1993;13:491–507.

109. Twomey PL, Patching SC. Cost-effectiveness of nutritional support. JPEN J Parenter Enteral Nutr 1985;9:3–10.

110. Trice S, Melnik G, Page CP. Complications and costs of early postoperative parenteral versus enteral nutrition in trauma patients. Nutr Clin Pract 1997;12:114–119.

111. Hassell JT, Games AD, Shaffer B, Harkins LE. Nutrition support team management of enterally fed patients in a community hospital is cost-beneficial. J Am Diet Assoc 1994;94:993–998.

112. ASPEN Board of Directors. Rationale for adult nutrition support guidelines. JPEN J Parenter Enteral Nutr 2002;26(Suppl):9SA–21SA.

137
PARENTERAL NUTRITION

Todd W. Mattox and Pamela D. Reiter

Learning Objectives and other resources can be found at *www.pharmacotherapyonline.com.*

KEY CONCEPTS

1 Four steps to developing a successful nutrition plan include definition of nutrition goals, determination of nutrition requirements, determination of appropriate route of delivery of nutrients, and subsequent monitoring of the nutrition regimen to evaluate suitability of the regimen as a patient's clinical condition changes and to minimize or treat complications early.

2 The appropriate route of nutrition support depends on the functional condition of the patient's gastrointestinal (GI) tract, risk of aspiration, expected duration of nutrition therapy, and clinical condition.

3 Identifying the patient who is most likely to benefit from PN therapy includes consideration of the patient's age, nutrition status, expected duration of GI dysfunction, and potential risks of initiating therapy.

4 Parenteral nutrition (PN) solutions may be appropriately formulated for administration by peripheral or central venous access.

5 PN solutions may be infused continuously or intermittently.

6 Biochemical and clinical measurements considered necessary for effective monitoring of patients receiving PN include serum chemistries, vital signs, weight, total daily fluid intake and losses, and nutritional intake.

7 Non–catheter-related complications of PN therapy are minimized with application of age-appropriate nutrient dosing guidelines, frequent monitoring, and rational adjustments to the PN regimen when metabolic abnormalities occur.

8 Expenses associated with PN therapy may be minimized by using PN in appropriate patients, appropriate use of laboratory measurements associated with PN therapy, maximizing efficient purchasing practices for PN solutions and compounding supplies, streamlining compounding procedures, and minimizing PN waste.

Maintenance of adequate nutrition status during illness has been recognized for over 50 years as an integral part of the medical treatment plan for patients who are unable to use normal physiologic means of nourishment. Successful techniques for providing intravenous nutrition support were introduced to clinical practice in the early 1960s.[1] Metabolic complications associated with fluid overload and electrolyte imbalances stimulated the investigation of central venous access. The use of larger vessels permitted infusion of concentrated formulas, which decreased the fluid volume required and avoided the phlebitis that commonly occurred when hypertonic infusions were given peripherally.

By the late 1960s, Rhoads and Dudrick had documented continued growth and improvement in nutritional markers in humans with the use of central intravenous nutrition.[1] By the early 1970s, intravenous nutrition was used to sustain growth and development in premature infants.[2]

Further clinical experience and research fostered development of protocols that promoted better patient care and resulted in a decline in complications associated with parenteral nutrition (PN) therapy.[3] The scope of practice for nutrition support clinicians has broadened as a result of increasing knowledge regarding the metabolic consequences associated with acute injury and chronic disease states. The pharmacist's role in providing safe and effective nutrition-support care requires knowledge of the principles of patient selection, initial therapy design, preparation and dispensing of the nutritional formu-

lations, and outcome monitoring (Table 137–1).[4-7] However, the role of other health care professionals may be similar because of the evolving interdisciplinary approach to providing parenteral and enteral nutrition.[6-11] This chapter reviews indications for PN, components of PN formulations, routes of intravenous administration, practical aspects of regimen design, solution admixture, outcome monitoring, and management of complications for both adult and pediatric (neonates, infants, and children) patients.

DESIRED OUTCOMES

1 The overall objective of nutrition support therapy is to promote positive clinical outcomes of an illness or improve a patient's quality of life. Four fundamental steps are key to providing optimal care for patients who require nutrition support. They are definition of nutrition goals, determination of nutrient requirements for achievement of the nutrition goals, delivery of the required nutrients, and subsequent assessment of the nutrition regimen.[6-8]

A patient's nutrition goals can be established after a thorough nutritional assessment (see Chap. 135). Nutrient requirements and an appropriate route for delivery of the required nutrients can then be determined (see Chaps. 136 and 138). Goals of nutrition support include correction of the patient's caloric and nitrogen imbalances, fluid

TABLE 137–1. Scope of Practice for Nutrition Support Pharmacists

Assessment of the patient's nutrition care needs
- Determine nutrient requirements based on the patient's data.
- Prevent and/or identify nutrient–nutrient, drug–nutrient, drug–drug, and drug–disease/condition interactions.
- Assess suitability for specialized nutrition support.

Development of a nutrition care plan
- Define goals and objectives of specialized nutrition support therapy.
- Select the preferred route for administration of nutrition support therapy.
- Design patient-specific feeding formulations.

Implementation of the nutrition care plan
- Obtain or write prescriptions for feeding formulations.
- Be proficient with techniques of compounding feeding formulations.
- Perform or supervise the compounding and dispensing of parenteral feeding formulations.

Monitoring the patient response to the nutrition therapy
- Evaluate laboratory data to determine the patient's clinical, nutritional, and metabolic responses to specialized nutrition support.
- Prevent and/or identify nutrient–nutrient, drug–nutrient, drug–drug, and drug–disease/condition interactions.
- Evaluate continued need for specialized nutrition support.

Administrative management
- Participate in development of policy and procedures for patient care and operational aspects of specialized nutrition support.

Quality of care
- Develop and implement quality improvement activities directed at the process of nutritional and metabolic care.

Advancement of nutrition support pharmacy practice
- Contribute to the professional development of pharmacists and other health care professionals and to the education of patients through presentations, publications, and research.

From Holcombe et al.[4]

or electrolyte abnormalities, and any known vitamin or trace element abnormalities, without causing or worsening other metabolic complications. Specific caloric goals include (1) adequate energy intake to promote normal growth and development in neonates, infants, and children, (2) energy equilibrium and preservation of fat calorie stores in well-nourished adults, and (3) positive energy balance in malnourished patients with depleted endogenous fat stores. Obese patients with excess endogenous fat stores (>120% of ideal body weight) may require less caloric support than nonobese patients with the same clinical condition.[12] Specific nitrogen goals are positive nitrogen balance or nitrogen equilibrium and improvement in the serum concentration of visceral protein markers such as transferrin or prealbumin.

❷ The gastrointestinal (GI) tract is the optimal route for providing nutrients unless obstruction, severe pancreatitis, or other GI complications are present[13] (see Fig. 136–1). Other considerations that may have an impact on determination of an appropriate route for nutrition support include expected duration of nutrition therapy and risk of aspiration. Patients who have nonfunctional GI tracts or are otherwise not candidates for enteral nutrition (EN) may benefit from PN. Use of the intravenous route for nutrition support is also commonly referred to as total parenteral nutrition (TPN) or hyperalimentation. Routine monitoring is necessary to ensure that the nutrition regimen is suitable for a given patient as his or her clinical condition changes and to minimize or treat complications early.

INDICATIONS FOR NUTRITION SUPPORT

The association between malnutrition and development of complications and mortality has been well documented in adult and pediatric patients.[14–16] Although improvement in nutrition status as defined by various clinical nutrition markers has been reported in patients who received PN, the impact on clinical outcome has been difficult to demonstrate in many adult populations. Several investigations have reported a positive effect of PN on complications and mortality, whereas others have failed to demonstrate any difference.[14,15,17] Early studies have been criticized for defects in study design such as small sample sizes, inappropriate randomization, and inconsistent baseline nutrition status among the study group, which hindered demonstration of the effectiveness of PN therapy. The impact of PN on clinical outcome has been more successfully demonstrated in critically ill infants and children, particularly those with acquired or congenital GI tract anomalies.[2] Consensus guidelines for use of PN in adults and pediatric patients are based on clinical experience and investigations in specific patient populations[17–19] (Table 137–2). Unfortunately, conflicting data have resulted in a lack of consistency in published guidelines from different sources, which complicates identification of the patient who is most likely to benefit from PN. However, these published reports may serve as resources for development of institution-specific standards.

❸ The decision to initiate PN is based on the assessment that the patient cannot meet his or her nutritional requirements with use of the GI tract. This assessment must include an evaluation of the patient's nutrition status, clinical status, age, and potential risks of initiating therapy, such as infection and other metabolic abnormalities. The appropriate length of time to wait prior to starting PN therapy has not been well defined.[13]

CLINICAL CONTROVERSY

The most appropriate time to initiate PN in adults differs between various consensus reports because few data specifically address this issue. Hence some recommendations are evidence-based from findings extrapolated from clinical investigations of adult patients receiving PN or enteral nutrition, while others are based on meta-analysis review of PN use in adults.

However, adult PN therapy is not an emergent intervention and should not be initiated until the patient is hemodynamically stable.[13] In general, adults who are not candidates for EN should be considered candidates for PN after 7 to 14 days of suboptimal nutritional intake.[13] Guidelines for use in infants and children are primarily influenced by age. The younger the patient, the sooner PN should be considered.

CLINICAL CONTROVERSY

Although clinical data suggest that critically ill neonates will benefit from aggressive PN within the first 24 hours of life, some clinicians withhold PN therapy for 2 to 3 days after birth because of concerns for development of adverse effects associated with protein intolerance, such as hyperammonemia, azotemia, and metabolic acidosis.

However, the most appropriate time to initiate therapy is controversial. Early PN within the first 24 hours of life has been recommended.[19–21] Protein loss in extremely low-birth-weight infants can be twofold higher than in term infants, and frequently results in a negative nitrogen balance that cannot be corrected by

TABLE 137–2. Indications for Parenteral Nutrition (PN)

1. Inability to absorb nutrients via the gastrointestinal tract because of one or more of the following:
   a. Massive small bowel resection.
   Adults: Usually patients with <100 cm of small bowel distal to the ligament of Treitz without a colon, or <50 cm of small bowel without an intact colon.
   Pediatrics: PN should be initiated in all patients who undergo resection of any part of the small bowel significant enough to result in restriction of enteral intake.
   b. Intractable vomiting when adequate enteral intake is not expected for 7–14 days.
   c. *Severe diarrhea:*
   Intractable diarrhea of infancy: infants younger than 3 months who have persistent diarrhea for more than 2 weeks with three or more stool cultures negative for enteropathogens, who have failed a trial of enteral nutrition support.
   a. *Inflammatory bowel disease (Crohn's disease or ulcerative colitis):*
   PN may benefit patients with acute exacerbations of ulcerative colitis when surgery is being considered and when preservation of lean body mass and functional capacity with enteral nutrition is impossible. PN is indicated for children with Crohn's disease who have near-complete bowel obstruction, high-output fistulae, gastrointestinal bleeding, and progressive surgical resection resulting in short bowel syndrome.
   e. *Bowel obstruction:*
   Pseudo-obstruction: PN is indicated in patients with prolonged dysmotility of the gastrointestinal tract distal to the pylorus, or in patients who cannot grow and gain weight with enteral nutrition alone.
   f. *Gastrointestinal fistulae:* PN is indicated in patients in whom enteral intake must be restricted longer than 7 days.
2. *Cancer:* Antineoplastic therapy, radiation therapy, or hematopoietic stem cell transplantation.
   a. PN may benefit some severely malnourished cancer patients or those in whom gastrointestinal or other toxicities are anticipated to preclude adequate oral nutritional intake for a prolonged period of time.
   b. PN is not routinely indicated for well-nourished or mildly malnourished patients undergoing surgery, chemotherapy, or radiation treatment, and in whom adequate oral intake is anticipated.
   c. PN is unlikely to benefit patients with advanced cancer whose malignancy is documented as unresponsive to chemotherapy or radiation therapy. However, its use in carefully selected patients with good performance status, an estimated life expectancy >40–60 days, with strong social and financial support who have also failed trials of less invasive medical therapies may be appropriate.
3. *Pancreatitis:* It can be used in patients with moderate to severe pancreatitis when adequate enteral intake is not expected for 5–7 days. PN should be used when enteral feeding exacerbates abdominal pain, ascites, or fistula output in patients with pancreatitis and limited oral intake.
4. *Critical care:*
   a. PN should be used in those patients in whom enteral nutrition is contraindicated or is unlikely to provide adequate nutritional requirements within 5–10 days (e.g., major surgery, trauma, sepsis, traumatic brain injury, or cerebrovascular accident).
   b. Organ failure (liver, renal, or respiratory): PN should be used in patients with moderate to severe catabolism, with or without malnutrition, when enteral feeding is contraindicated.
   c. Burns: PN should be used in those patients in whom enteral nutrition is contraindicated or is unlikely to provide adequate nutritional requirements within 4–5 days.
5. *Perioperative PN:*
   a. Preoperative: For malnutrition when the gastrointestinal tract is not functional and surgery is not expected for at least 7 days.
   b. Postoperative: PN should be used in patients in whom enteral nutrition is contraindicated or is unlikely to provide adequate nutritional requirements within 7–10 days.
6. *Hyperemesis gravidarum:* When enteral tube feeding is not tolerated.
7. *Eating disorders:* PN should be considered for patients with anorexia nervosa and severe malnutrition who require nonvolitional feeding, but who cannot tolerate enteral support for physical or emotional reasons.
8. *Low-birth-weight (premature) infants:* PN is indicated within the first day of life in selected low-birth-weight infants such as those diagnosed with necrotizing enterocolitis or bronchopulmonary dysplasia, before enteral nutrition is initiated and as a supplement while enteral nutrition is being advanced.
9. *Inborn errors of metabolism:* PN use may be necessary in children who are unable to tolerate certain specialized formulas enterally because of disease-induced nausea and vomiting and poor palatability of the formulas.

From ASPEN Board of Directors.[13,18,19,110]

glucose as a sole nutrient. Additionally, decreased hyperglycemic events, improved growth, and other positive metabolic outcomes have been demonstrated with early aggressive PN in neonates.[22] However, many clinicians hesitate to initiate early PN due to concern of adverse effects associated with protein intolerance. Withholding PN for 2 to 3 days after birth, coupled with a slow advancement of substrate, only appears to contribute to the acute semistarvation and growth failure seen in many neonates.[21,23,24] Term infants who have failed EN support or have a dysfunctional GI tract will benefit from initiation of PN after 2 to 3 days of suboptimal nutritional intake.[19,20] Well-nourished children who are not candidates for EN should be considered candidates for PN after 5 to 7 days of suboptimal nutritional intake.[20,25] Children with preexisting malnutrition likely will require earlier intervention. Guidelines for older children are similar to those in adults.

COMPONENTS OF PARENTERAL NUTRITION

PN solutions should provide the optimal combination of macronutrients and micronutrients to meet the specific nutritional requirements of the patient. Macronutrients include water, protein, dextrose, and intravenous lipid emulsion. Micronutrients include vitamins, trace elements, and electrolytes. Both macronutrients and micronutrients are necessary for maintenance of normal metabolism. In general, macronutrients are used for energy (dextrose and fat) and as structural substrates (protein and fats). Micronutrients are required to support a variety of metabolic activities necessary for cellular homeostasis such as enzymatic reactions, fluid balance, and regulation of electrophysiologic processes. These components usually require individualized adjustments as the patient's clinical condition dictates changes in metabolic stress, organ function, fluid and electrolyte balance, and acid-base status.

AMINO ACIDS

Protein in PN solutions is provided in the form of crystalline amino acids (CAAs), which are used primarily for protein synthesis. When oxidized for energy, 1 g of protein yields 4 calories. However, including the caloric contribution from protein when calculating calories provided by the PN regimen is controversial.[26]

CLINICAL CONTROVERSY

While sufficient energy substrate should be provided to allow use of amino acids for protein synthesis rather than as an energy source, oxidation of amino acids for energy has been demonstrated in critically ill patients and is thought to occur because of metabolic derangements seen during severe metabolic stress. Hence some practice settings may differ in expressing calories provided by a PN regimen as total calories (protein, carbohydrate, and fat calories) or nonprotein calories (carbohydrate and fat calories).

Commercially available CAA solutions may be categorized as standard amino acid solutions or modified amino acid solutions. Standard CAA solutions are designed for use in patients with "normal" organ function and nutritional requirements (Table 137–3). Although standard CAA solutions differ in the proportion of specific amino acids, they contain a balanced profile of essential, semiessential, and nonessential L-amino acids. Despite these differences, similar effects on markers of protein use have been reported.[27] These products also differ in protein concentration, total nitrogen, and electrolyte content. Because the nitrogen concentration of dietary protein is approximately 16%, 6.25 (100 g protein/16 g nitrogen) is commonly accepted as the conversion figure for calculating the amount of nitrogen provided by CAA protein. Differences in nitrogen content per gram of amino acids among CAA products may affect calculation of nitrogen amounts infused when determining nitrogen balance.[27,28] The clinical significance of these differences in calculations of nitrogen balance for routine clinical use is not known.[28]

Electrolyte composition of standard CAA solutions varies from small, obligatory amounts, to the provision of maintenance requirements of most electrolytes for an adult. The contribution of electrolytes from CAA solutions must be considered when determining a patient's individual requirements. The availability of CAA in several different concentrations facilitates compounding of patient-specific PN regimens. Highly concentrated products (15% to 20%) are attractive for use in critically ill patients who typically require fluid restriction but have large protein needs. Modified amino acid solutions are designed for use in patients who have altered protein requirements such as those with hepatic encephalopathy, renal failure, and metabolic stress or trauma, as well as neonates and pediatric patients (see Table 137–3). These solutions tend to be more expensive than standard CAA solutions. The rationale for and clinical efficacy of modified amino acids in disease-specific PN regimens is controversial (see Chap. 139).

Several commercially available CAA solutions are designed to provide conditionally essential amino acids (CEAAs). CEAAs are considered nonessential during health because they are produced from other amino acids. However, under certain physiologic conditions such as prematurity or sepsis, these amino acids cannot be synthesized in sufficient quantities.[27] CAA solutions specifically designed for use in neonates and pediatric patients contain increased amounts of taurine, aspartic acid, and glutamic acid. Other CEAAs, such as cysteine, carnitine, and glutamine, are not available in commercial CAA solutions in pharmacologic amounts because they are relatively unstable or poorly soluble.[27]

PN solutions therefore may need to be modified by clinicians to provide supplemental amounts of CEAAs. Cysteine is a CEAA in preterm and term infants that may be added to PN solutions at the time of compounding. An additional benefit of including cysteine is that it enhances calcium and phosphate solubility in PN solutions by decreasing the solution's pH.[29] Carnitine is a quarternary amine required for transport of free fatty acids into the mitochondria for beta-oxidation and energy production.[30] Newborns are at risk for carnitine deficiency because of their immature synthetic and conservation mechanisms. Decreased plasma carnitine concentrations are associated with impaired lipid metabolism in patients receiving intravenous lipid emulsion (IVLE).[31]

Supplemental carnitine may be added to the PN solution at the time of compounding. However, routine addition to neonatal PN regimens is controversial because the effect of supplemental carnitine on clinical outcomes such as weight gain and lipid utilization is not clear.[31]

CLINICAL CONTROVERSY

Little evidence of sustained positive outcomes after carnitine supplementation exists. However, decreased plasma carnitine concentrations have been reported in neonates within 2 weeks of inadequate enteral intakes of carnitine-containing infant formula. Thus intravenous carnitine supplementation is generally reserved for patients receiving sole PN support for more than 2 weeks.

Glutamine is the most abundant free amino acid in the body and is an important intermediate for many metabolic processes. Glutamine is reported to have an important role in maintaining intestinal integrity, immune function, and protein synthesis during conditions of metabolic stress.[27,32] Investigations in humans and animals have reported positive effects on nutritional markers such as nitrogen balance, whereas others have reported significant improvement in other outcome markers such as decreased length of hospitalization, incidence of infections, and GI toxicities associated with chemotherapy or radiation.[33] However, the best adult candidate for response to glutamine therapy has not been clearly identified.[33] The clinical utility of glutamine in neonates is less clear.[34] The clinical use of glutamine is further complicated because there is no commercially available intravenous glutamine formulation. Currently available CAA solutions do not contain glutamine because of poor solubility and instability. Use of intravenous glutamine requires special manufacturing techniques not readily available in many institutional pharmacies.[35] Additional controlled trials are warranted to clearly justify risks and costs associated with extemporaneous compounding before routine use of intravenous glutamine can be recommended.[33,35] Dipeptide amino acids are a potential parenteral source for CEAAs that may provide a solution to the instability and solubility limitations. Dipeptides are synthesized by combining

TABLE 137-3. Macronutrient Components of Parenteral Nutrition Solutions

Nutritional Substrate	Intravenous Source	Commercial Product (Manufacturer)		Comments
Fluid	Sterile water for injection USP	Various manufacturers		
Nitrogen	Crystalline amino acids			
	Standard solutions	Aminosyn	(Abbott)	Contain a balanced profile of
		Aminosyn II	(Abbott)	essential, semiessential, and
		FreAmine III	(Braun)	nonessential L-amino acids
		Travasol	(Clintec)	
		Clinisol	(Clintec)	
		Novamine	(Clintec)	
		Prosol	(Clintec)	
	Disease-specific solutions			
	Hepatic encephalopathy	Aminosyn HF	(Abbott)	Amino acid profile includes higher
		Hepatasol	(Clintec)	concentrations of BCAA and lower
		Hepatamine	(Braun)	concentrations of AAA and methionine
	Renal failure	Aminosyn RF	(Abbott)	Amino acid profile includes higher
		RenAmine	(Clintec)	concentrations of EAA and
		Aminess	(Clintec)	histidine
		NephrAmine	(Braun)	
	Metabolic stress/trauma	Aminosyn HBC	(Abbott)	Amino acid profile provides standard
		BranchAmin[a]	(Clintec)	essential, semiessential and
		FreAmine HBC	(Braun)	nonessential amino acids with higher concentrations of BCAA
	Pediatrics	Aminosyn PF	(Abbott)	Amino acid profile includes standard
		Trophamine	(Braun)	essential, semiessential and
		Premasol	(Clintec)	nonessential amino acids with lower concentrations of methionine, phenylalanine, and glycine; these solutions also contain taurine, glutamate, and aspartate
	Conditional or essential amino acids[b]			
	Cysteine HCl		(Abbott, GensiaSicor)	
	L-Carnitine	Carnitor	(Sigma Tau)	
	L-Glutamine			Investigational
	Intravenous dipeptides			
	L-alanyl-L-glutamine			Investigational
	Glycyl-L-tyrosine			Investigational
	L-alanyl-L-tyrosine			Investigational
	N-acetyl-L-tyrosine			Used in Trophamine (Braun)
Energy				
Carbohydrate	Dextrose	Various manufacturers		
	Glycerol			Used in ProcalAmine (Braun)
	Xylitol			Investigational
Fat	Intravenous fat emulsion			
	LCT emulsions (oil source)	Liposyn II	(Abbott)	(Soybean/safflower)
		Liposyn III	(Abbott)	(Soybean)
		Intralipid	(Clintec)	(Soybean)
	LCT/MCT combination		Investigational	
	Short-chain fatty acids		Investigational	
	Omega-3 fatty acids		Investigational	

AAA, aromatic amino acids (includes phenylalanine and tyrosine); BCAA, branched-chain amino acids (leucine, isoleucine, and valine); EAA, essential amino acids (leucine, isoleucine, valine, phenylalanine, tryptophan, methionine, threonine, and lysine); LCT, long-chain triglycerides; MCT, medium-chain triglyceride.
[a]Used as a supplement to a standard amino acid solution to increase BCAA content.
[b]Used as a supplement to crystalline amino acid solutions.

two amino acids with a peptide bond. The resulting protein is more soluble and stable than the individual amino acids.[27] Intravenous dipeptide formulations would be advantageous clinically because they incorporate higher concentrations of some specific amino acids, as well as some low-solubility, low-stability amino acids that are omitted or present in small quantities in current CAA solu-

tions. In addition, use of dipeptides would allow formulation of CAA solutions with a higher nitrogen content. Further studies are needed to assess long-term safety and optimal combinations of amino acids in different disease states. Examples of commercially available CAA products and some investigational amino acids are listed in Table 137-3.

DEXTROSE

The primary energy source in PN solutions is carbohydrate, usually in the form of dextrose monohydrate. This nutritional substrate is available in a variety of concentrations ranging from 5% to 70%. When oxidized, each gram of hydrated dextrose provides 3.4 kcal. Dextrose is oxidized at a maximum rate of 4 to 7 mg/kg per minute in adults receiving intravenous dextrose infusions.[36] Premature infants have a higher rate of glucose oxidation because of their relatively large body proportion of metabolically active organs. Although the fetal nutrient delivery rate is approximately 5 to 6 mg/kg per minute, maximum glucose oxidation rates of 12 to 14 mg/kg per minute have been reported in very-low-birth-weight neonates and term infants.[19,22,37] However, an investigation of critically ill children from 1 to 11 years old reported glucose oxidation rates similar to those observed in adults.[38] The appropriate dose of intravenous dextrose depends on the patient's age and clinical condition. If the dextrose infusion rate exceeds the glucose oxidation rate, metabolically expensive pathways such as glycogen repletion and lipid synthesis will be favored, resulting in increased energy expenditure, increased oxygen consumption, and increased carbon dioxide production. Excessive dextrose infusion rates also may contribute to the development of hyperglycemia, excess carbon dioxide production, and increased biochemical markers for liver function associated with fatty infiltration of the liver.[38,39] Although infusion rates of up to 11 to 12 mg/kg per minute have been recommended for young children, the recommended dose of dextrose for routine clinical care rarely exceeds 5 mg/kg per minute in older critically ill children and adults.[25,35,36,38]

Insulin is essential to transport dextrose into many cells such as skeletal muscle for oxidation to yield energy. Because many clinical conditions associated with impaired insulin secretion or activity may complicate provision of PN, non-insulin-dependent sources of carbohydrate have been investigated (see Table 137–3). Of these nutrients, only glycerol is available commercially for clinical use in humans as a carbohydrate source for PN. Glycerol is a sugar alcohol that provides 4.3 kcal/g and is available as a 3% solution in combination with 3% amino acids and supplemental electrolytes (ProcalAmine, B. Braun). This product is nearly isotonic, so it may be infused peripherally. A major disadvantage of this formula is the dilute concentrations of amino acids and carbohydrate. Most adult patients require up to 3 to 4 L/day of ProcalAmine solution together with lipid emulsion as a caloric source to provide minimum energy requirements.[40] Intravenous glycerol use in catabolic adults is safe and effective, but similar data are not available for infants and children.[41]

LIPID EMULSION

IVLE is used as a concentrated source of calories and essential fatty acids. Commercially available IVLE products differ in source of triglycerides (soybean oil or a combination of soybean oil and safflower oil), fatty acid content, and commercially available concentrations (10%, 20%, and 30%; see Table 137–3). These products also contain egg phospholipids as an emulsifying agent and glycerol to make the emulsion isotonic. Although the caloric contribution of fat is 9 kcal/g, the caloric content of IVLE is 1.1 kcal/mL for 10% emulsion, 2 kcal/mL for 20% emulsion, and 3 kcal/mL for 30% emulsion because of the caloric contribution of the egg phospholipid and glycerol.[42] The sources of triglyceride in IVLEs differ in fatty acid composition. Soybean oil emulsions contain approximately 50% to 55% linoleic acid and 4% to 9% linolenic acid, whereas IVLEs that contain safflower oil are made of approximately 66% linoleic acid and 4% linolenic acid.[42] Linolenic acid, an omega-3 fatty acid,

and linoleic acid, an omega-6 fatty acid, are both polyunsaturated long-chain triglycerides (LCTs).[43] IVLE products also differ in phospholipid and triglyceride concentrations. Higher-concentrated IVLEs (20% and 30%) have a lower phospholipid:triglyceride ratio compared with 10% IVLE.[44] Because higher amounts of circulating phospholipids have been associated with impaired triglyceride clearance in neonates and infants, 20% IVLE is the preferred product for this population.[20,25,35,39,44,45]

Both types of IVLEs are effective in the treatment or prevention of essential fatty acid deficiency (EFAD). EFAD is the result of a biochemical deficiency of linoleic acid and arachidonic acid, which are considered essential in humans.[46] Although linolenic acid may be essential, all commercially available IVLEs contain soybean oil as a predominant source of linolenic acid. These fatty acids are important for a variety of functions such as cellular integrity, platelet function, postnatal brain development, and wound healing.[25,46] Normally, linoleic acid is converted to the tetraene arachidonic acid. When linoleic acid is not present in sufficient amounts, oleic acid is converted to the triene 5,8,11-eicosatrienoic acid, a fatty acid of lesser physiologic integrity, and EFAD occurs. EFAD may be prevented by providing 2% to 5% of total calories as linoleic acid. This may be achieved in most adult patients by giving approximately 100 g IVLE weekly.[47] Neonates and infants require a minimum of 0.5 to 1 g/kg daily.[20,25,39]

Plasma clearance of IVLE is directly related to gestational age of infants and appears to be influenced by the rate of infusion and the patient's clinical status.[25,44,45] The risk of developing hypertriglyceridemia lessens with longer infusion times.[35,39,45] Rapid IVLE infusions in neonates have been reported to contribute to pulmonary dysfunction such as decreased oxygenation.[39] Adverse pulmonary effects are thought to be caused by polyunsaturated fatty acid (PUFA)-driven prostaglandin production, which results in altered vascular tone. However, the association between IVFE and pulmonary dysfunction is not clear.[39] In addition, data in animals and humans also suggest that rapid infusion of long-chain fatty acid formulations may have a negative impact on immunocompetence by saturating the reticuloendothelial system.[43,45]

As a caloric source, use of IVLE may facilitate provision of adequate calories and minimize complications of nutrition therapy such as hyperglycemia, hepatotoxicity, or increased production of carbon dioxide.[43] Although the frequency of acute adverse effects is reported to be less than 1% with current formulations, patients receiving their first dose of IVLE should be monitored for dyspnea, chest tightness, palpitations, and chills. Headache, nausea, and fever also have been reported and may be associated with a rapid infusion rate. In general, the use of IVLE is contraindicated in patients with an impaired ability to clear lipid emulsion, such as patients with pathologic hyperlipidemia and hypertriglyceridemia associated with pancreatitis.[45] Finally, patients with a reported egg allergy should be evaluated carefully for the nature and severity of the reaction before deciding to initiate a lipid-based PN regimen.

Commercially available 10% and 20% IVLE products may be administered either by the central or peripheral route. They may be added directly to the PN solution as a total nutrient admixture (TNA) or 3-in-1 system (lipids, protein, glucose, and additives), or they may be piggybacked with the CAA-dextrose solution.[43] The more concentrated 30% IVLE is only approved for use in the preparation of TNA and is not intended for direct intravenous administration.

The negative effects of LCTs on immune function have stimulated a search for new sources of lipids.[43,48] Medium-chain triglycerides (MCTs) may offer several advantages, especially for critically ill patients. MCTs are hydrolyzed and cleared more rapidly than

LCTs, and they do not accumulate in the liver. In addition, MCTs do not require carnitine for entrance into mitochondria for oxidation. However, MCTs are not a source of essential fatty acids. Subsequent studies of intravenous MCT-LCT mixtures in a number of patients have demonstrated safety and efficacy comparable with standard LCT emulsions.[43,48] Several MCT-LCT products are available in Europe, although no intravenous MCT formulations are currently available commercially in the United States. Other intravenous lipid formulations currently being investigated contain omega-3 PUFAs.[43] Current IVLEs contain omega-6 PUFAs as linoleic acid and omega-3 PUFAs as linolenic acid. Omega-3 PUFAs are metabolized to cytokine mediators, which may be less inflammatory and immunosuppressive than those derived from omega-6 PUFAs. The effect of IVLE administration on immune function, as well as patient morbidity and mortality, is not clear.[39,49,50] However, investigations of enteral solutions with a higher concentration of omega-3 PUFAs have reported decreased infections and improvement in in vitro immunologic indices in critically ill patients.[51] Although IVLE products remain the most common source of parenteral lipids, a number of drugs have been introduced that contain lipid as either a vehicle for delivery or as a portion of the drug molecular formulation. Propofol, an intravenous anesthetic, is delivered in a soybean oil-in-water emulsion that is essentially the same as Intralipid 10%. This agent is used commonly for continuous sedation of ventilated patients and should be considered a potentially significant source of calories that may require adjustment of a patient's nutrition regimen.[52] The antifungal amphotericin B is available in several lipid-containing combinations such as liposomal and lipid complex formulations. The caloric contribution from these products when used in standard doses generally is small and is not relevant clinically.

VITAMINS

Vitamins are necessary for the maintenance of normal metabolism and cellular function. Fat-soluble vitamins (i.e., A, D, E, and K) are stored extensively in the body's fat tissue, whereas water-soluble vitamins are stored in limited amounts by the body. Maintenance guidelines for daily parenteral vitamin supplements have been established by the Nutrition Advisory Group of the American Medical Association (NAG-AMA) for adults, children, and infants.[53] The NAG-AMA identified 13 essential vitamins that include four fat-soluble vitamins and nine water-soluble vitamins. These guidelines are based on the recommended daily allowances (RDAs), which are designed to meet requirements of healthy people. Vitamin requirements for preterm infants and patients with metabolic stress or specific organ failures are controversial.[39,54–56] Revised NAG-AMA recommendations for parenteral vitamin requirements in infants and children reflect data reported in pediatric patients who received currently available formulations.[56] In general, the revised recommendations focused on changes for preterm infants requiring PN.

Several adult and pediatric parenteral multiple-vitamin products formulated to comply with the NAG-AMA guidelines are available commercially. Currently there are two commercially available parenteral vitamin products designed for use in pediatric patients. These parenteral multiple-vitamin formulations provide 13 essential vitamins, including vitamin K. MVI-Pediatric (Mayne Pharma) and Infuvite Pediatric (Baxter) are formulated to meet the revised NAG-AMA guidelines for infants weighing less than 1 kg to children up to 11 years old. However, there are no commercially available intravenous multivitamin products designed to specifically meet the unique requirements of premature infants, including higher vitamin A and lower

vitamin B_1, B_2, B_6, and B_{12} doses relative to recommendations for term infants and older children.

In the past, parenteral multiple-vitamin formulations for adults contained only 12 essential vitamins. Vitamin K was not included to minimize the risk of a drug-nutrient interaction in patients receiving anticoagulants, which antagonize vitamin K. However, in 2000, the Food and Drug Administration (FDA) mandated reformulation of adult parenteral multiple-vitamin products to include 150 mcg vitamin K in addition to higher doses of vitamins B_1, B_6, and C.[57] The NAG-AMA recommendation for vitamin K in adults is 2 to 4 mg weekly. However, other practitioners have recommended larger doses of 5 to 10 mg weekly. An investigation of patients receiving long-term IVLE-containing PN at home suggests that supplemental vitamin K may not be necessary to maintain normal prothrombin times and plasma vitamin K concentrations.[58] Vegetable oils such as soybean and safflower oils used in IVLEs are a natural source of phylloquinine (vitamin K_1). However, the vitamin K concentration depends on the type and concentration of vegetable oil in the IVLE.[57–59] Mean concentrations of 13.2 and 26.5 mcg/100 mL were reported for 10% and 20% Liposyn II (Abbott), which contains both soybean and safflower oil.[59] Mean concentrations of 30.9 and 67.5 mcg/100 mL were reported for 10% and 20% Intralipid (Kabivitrum), which contains only soybean oil. The bioavailability of vitamin K_1 from IVLEs is not known. Although hospitalized patients who received no additional vitamin K supplementation during short-term PN that included a low-vitamin K–containing IVLE experienced minimal effects on International Normalized Ratio, supplemental vitamin K may be given intramuscularly or subcutaneously or added to the PN solution if needed.[57,60] However, the role of supplemental vitamin K when using a vitamin K–containing multiple-vitamin product is not clear.

Vitamin requirements may be altered in malnutrition and other specific disease states or with certain drug therapies. Individual and combination products are available to provide additional or tailored supplementation, which may be necessary to prevent development of vitamin toxicities or deficiencies caused by altered metabolism or drug therapy.

TRACE ELEMENTS

Trace elements are minerals that are required in very small amounts for a variety of biochemical and physiologic functions. Many trace elements are an important part of metalloenzymes and also function as cofactors in a variety of regulatory metabolic pathways.[54,56] Although 17 trace elements have demonstrated biologic importance, clear deficiency syndromes in humans have been described only for iron, iodine, cobalt (as vitamin B_{12}), zinc, and copper.[56,61,62] The NAG-AMA recognized zinc, copper, and chromium as being essential for intravenous supplementation in patients receiving PN.[63] While a clear deficiency syndrome for manganese has not been reported in humans, the NAG-AMA considered manganese essential based on case reports of patients receiving PN with metabolic complications that corrected after manganese supplementation.[63] Reports of syndromes associated with selenium and molybdenum deficiency suggest that they also may be essential.[56,61,62] Recommendations for trace elements in pediatric patients receiving PN have been revised as well.[56]

Intravenous trace elements are available as single-mineral solutions and as multiple-mineral combinations with or without electrolytes. Most products provide the daily requirements for the trace minerals considered essential by the NAG-AMA (zinc, copper, chromium, and manganese), whereas some also include iodide,

TABLE 137–4. Fluid, Electrolyte, and Acid–Base Abnormalities

Problem	Possible Causes	Intervention
Hypovolemia	Gastrointestinal fluid losses, osmotic diuresis	Increase fluid intake
Hypervolemia	Renal failure, cardiac failure, excess fluid intake	Decrease fluid intake, diuretics
Hyponatremia	Gastrointestinal losses, fluid overload, diuretics	Varies with cause
Hypernatremia	Dehydration, net relative sodium excess	Increase fluid intake, decrease sodium intake
Hypokalemia	Gastrointestinal losses, diuretics, anabolism	Increase potassium intake
Hyperkalemia	Renal failure, potassium-sparing drug therapy, metabolic acidosis	Decrease potassium intake, correct metabolic acidosis
Hypophosphatemia	Phosphate-binding antacids, anabolism, phosphate-free dialysate	Discontinue phosphate binders, increase phosphorus intake
Hyperphosphatemia	Renal failure	Decrease phosphorus intake
Hypomagnesemia	Diarrhea, malabsorption, anabolism; magnesium-wasting drug therapy	Increase magnesium intake
Hypermagnesemia	Renal failure	Decrease magnesium intake
Hypocalcemia	Hypoalbuminemia, chronic renal failure	Calculate estimated serum calcium concentration corrected for hypoalbuminemia, or monitor serum ionized calcium concentrations to verify hypocalcemia, increase calcium intake if necessary
Hypercalcemia	Dehydration, malignancy	Decrease calcium intake, increase fluid intake
Metabolic acidosis	Diarrhea, high-output fistulae, renal failure	Treat underlying causes, increase acetate and decrease Cl in PN solution
Metabolic alkalosis	Gastric losses	Treat underlying cause, increase Cl and decrease acetate in PN solution

Adapted with permission from Teasley-Strausburg et al.[91]

molybdenum, or selenium. Combination products are available for pediatric patients that provide manganese, copper, chromium, zinc, and selenium.

Requirements for trace elements also change depending on the clinical condition of the patient. For example, higher doses of supplemental zinc likely are necessary in patients with high-output ostomies or diarrhea because the predominant route of excretion for zinc is via the GI tract. Manganese and copper are excreted through the biliary tract, whereas chromium, molybdenum, and selenium are excreted renally. Hence these trace elements should be restricted or withheld from PN solutions in patients with cholestatic liver disease and renal failure, respectively.

ELECTROLYTES

Electrolytes such as sodium, potassium, calcium, magnesium, phosphorus, chloride, and acetate are necessary components of PN for the maintenance of numerous cellular functions including acid-base balance and cellular growth. Electrolytes may be given to maintain normal serum concentrations or to correct deficits. Patients who have "normal" organ function and relatively normal serum concentrations of any electrolyte should receive normal maintenance doses of electrolytes on initiation of PN and daily thereafter (see Chap. 135). Requirements for specific electrolytes will vary according to the patient's age, disease state, organ function (see Chap. 139), previous and current drug therapy, nutrition status, and extrarenal losses (Table 137–4). Electrolytes are available commercially as single- and multiple-nutrient solutions. Multiple-electrolyte solutions are useful in stable patients with normal organ function who are receiving PN. Concentrated multiple-electrolyte solutions designed for addition to PN solutions generally contain only sodium, potassium, calcium, and magnesium. Phosphorus must be added as a separate additive. Further information regarding metabolism and requirements of vitamins, trace elements, and electrolytes is given elsewhere.[35]

DESIGNING A PARENTERAL NUTRITION REGIMEN

Several factors including venous access, fluid status of the patient, and macronutrient and micronutrient requirements are important considerations when designing the PN regimen for an individual patient. A patient's venous access and fluid status will determine how concentrated the PN solution may be compounded and hence will have an impact on the amount of nutrient that may be provided. PN solutions may be administered by central or peripheral venous access. The clinical condition of the patient will determine which route is most appropriate (Fig. 137–1).

ROUTES OF PARENTERAL NUTRITION ADMINISTRATION

PERIPHERAL ROUTE

Because of physical limitations of peripheral veins, peripheral parenteral nutrition (PPN) regimens usually are dilute solutions of amino acids, dextrose, and micronutrients. Although early PPN studies supported the use of amino acids alone as protein-sparing therapy, subsequent investigations have challenged this theory.[17,64] The rationale for protein-sparing PPN was based on the theory that the provision of dextrose in the setting of altered metabolism or stress would promote further increases in serum insulin concentrations and thereby hinder the use of endogenous fat stores and promote nitrogen catabolism. Protein-sparing PPN is used for patients with marginal nutrition status and inadequate oral intake who are not candidates for central catheter placement, and when the expected length of PN therapy is less than 1 week. However, investigations of adults receiving postoperative PN suggest that some patients who meet criteria for protein-sparing PPN may not benefit from PN support.[17]

The addition of IVLEs to PPN is referred to as the lipid system. The lipid system is designed for use in mild to moderately stressed

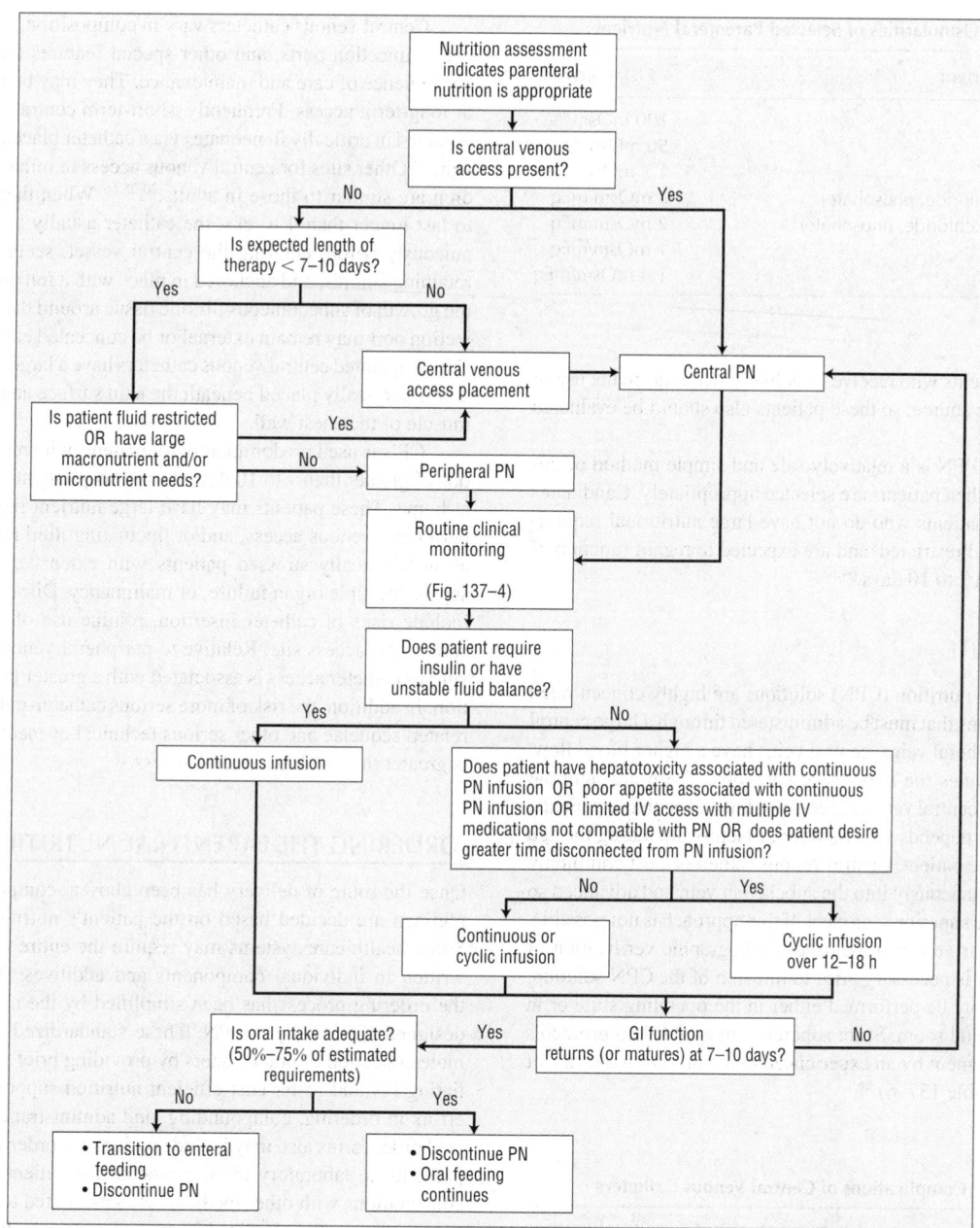

FIGURE 137–1. The route of PN and the infusion type depend on the patient's clinical status and the expected length of therapy.

patients in whom central access is unavailable or undesirable and function of the GI tract is expected to return within 7 to 10 days. The addition of IVLE increases caloric support to levels more consistent with PN regimens administered centrally. Advantages of PPN include a lower risk of infectious, metabolic, and technical complications that may occur with central vein catheterization. However, several other factors may complicate use of PPN in many patient populations. Patients who have received multiple courses of chemotherapy, malnourished patients, premature infants, elderly patients, and others with an illness of long duration who have already been subjected to multiple venous accesses for administration of fluids and medications are likely to have limited peripheral venous access. Use of PPN is also limited by relatively poor tolerance of peripheral veins to hypertonic solutions. Thrombophlebitis is a commonly reported complication in patients re-

ceiving PPN. Although the risk of developing phlebitis is greater with solution osmolarities greater than 600 to 900 mOsm/L, peripherally administered total nutrient admixtures with much higher osmolarities have been associated with low infusion-site complications in some centers.[64,65] Efforts to minimize development of phlebitis and/or infiltration sequelae in patients receiving PPN include addition of IVLEs to the regimen as a possible venous lumen protectant, subtherapeutic doses of heparin (0.5 to 1 unit/mL) to prevent thrombus formation, and/or small doses of hydrocortisone (5 mg/L) to minimize inflammation of the access site.[65] The osmolarity of a PN solution may be estimated by using the guidelines for osmolarities of selected PN components in Table 137–5. Because lower-osmolarity solutions are relatively dilute, much larger volumes of solution generally are required to meet nutritional requirements. Finally, patients with large

TABLE 137–5. Osmolarities of Selected Parenteral Nutrients

Nutrient	Osmolarity
Amino acid	100 mOsm/%
Dextrose	50 mOsm/%
Lipid emulsion	1.7 mOsm/%
Sodium (acetate, chloride, phosphate)	2 mOsm/mEq
Potassium (acetate, chloride, phosphate)	2 mOsm/mEq
Magnesium sulfate	1 mOsm/mEq
Calcium gluconate	1.4 mOsm/mEq

nutrition requirements who receive PPN likely will require the use of IVLEs as a caloric source, so these patients also should be evaluated for lipid tolerance.

In summary, PPN is a relatively safe and simple method of nutritional support when patients are selected appropriately. Candidates for PPN include patients who do not have large nutritional requirements, are not fluid restricted, and are expected to regain function of the GI tract within 7 to 10 days.[64,65]

CENTRAL ROUTE

Central parenteral nutrition (CPN) solutions are highly concentrated hypertonic solutions that must be administered through a large central vein. Unlike peripheral veins, central veins have a higher blood flow, which quickly dilutes the hypertonic solutions. There are multiple sites for obtaining central venous access in adult and pediatric patients. The choice of site depends on a number of factors, including the age and anatomy of the patient. Central venous catheters most commonly are inserted percutaneously into the subclavian vein and advanced so that the tip is at the superior vena cava. If this approach is not possible, the internal jugular vein may be used. Radiographic verification of correct placement is necessary prior to infusion of the CPN solution. Catheterization may be performed either in the operating suite or in the patient's hospital room. Strict adherence to established protocols and catheter placement by an experienced clinician lessen the risk of complications (Table 137–6).[66]

TABLE 137–6. Complications of Central Venous Catheters

Complication	Description
Arterial injury	Puncture of subclavian or carotid artery during catheter insertion
Pneumothorax	Perforation of the pleura or lung during insertion, which results in air collection in the pleural space
Air embolism	Introduction of air into the catheter, which subsequently enters the venous circulation
Catheter embolism	A portion of the catheter fragments and enters the venous circulation
Venous thrombosis	Formation of thrombosis inside the lumen of the catheter and/or inside the vessel around the catheter, which may result in catheter or vessel occlusion
Chylothorax	Injury to the thoracic duct during catheter insertion
Brachial plexus injury	Injury to the nerve during catheter insertion, or injury secondary to catheter malposition or extravasation of a hypertonic solution

Data from Grant.[66]

Central venous catheters vary in composition, lumen size, number of injection ports, and other special features that affect ease or convenience of care and maintenance. They may be placed for short- or long-term access. Frequently, short-term central venous access is obtained in critically ill neonates via a catheter placed in the umbilical vein.[20] Other sites for central venous access in infants and older children are similar to those in adults.[20,25,66] When therapy is expected to last longer than 4 weeks, the catheter usually is tunneled subcutaneously before entering the central vessel, secured initially with retaining sutures, and anchored in place with a felt cuff that promotes the growth of subcutaneous fibrotic tissue around the catheter. The injection port may remain external or be concealed entirely beneath the skin. Implanted central venous catheters have a larger port or reservoir that is surgically placed beneath the skin surface and anchored in the muscle of the chest wall.

CPN is used predominantly for patients who require PN for periods of greater than 7 to 10 days during hospitalization or indefinitely at home. These patients may have large nutrient requirements, poor peripheral venous access, and/or fluctuating fluid requirements such as metabolically stressed patients with extensive surgery, trauma, sepsis, multiple organ failure, or malignancy. Disadvantages of CPN include risks of catheter insertion, routine use of the catheter, and care of the access site. Relative to peripheral venous access, central venous catheter access is associated with a greater potential for infection. In addition, the risk of more serious catheter-induced trauma and related sequelae and other serious technical or mechanical problems is greater than with peripheral access.

ORDERING THE PARENTERAL NUTRITION REGIMEN

Once the route of delivery has been chosen, components of the PN regimen are decided based on the patient's nutritional assessment. Some health care systems may require the entire PN formula to be written in individual components and additives. More commonly, the ordering process has been simplified by the use of order forms designed specifically for PN. These standardized order forms promote education of practitioners by providing brief guidelines for initiating PN and foster cost-efficient nutrition support by minimizing errors in ordering, compounding, and administration.[67,68] Standardized order forms also may include options for ordering certain related procedures, laboratory tests, protocols for patient management, or consultations with other medical services related to the patient's nutrition support. Standardized forms and protocols should be reviewed and updated periodically to reflect changes in the practices and patient population of a practice setting and also advances in technology that may affect provision of nutrition support.

ADULT PARENTERAL NUTRITION SOLUTIONS

In general, there are two formats for ordering adult PN. The standard formula approach offers a variety of base formulas (CAA-dextrose combination) with a fixed nonprotein-calorie:nitrogen ratio (NPC:N). This format usually includes different formulas designed for mild to moderately stressed patients, renal failure patients, fluid-restricted patients, and liver failure patients. Because the NPC:N is fixed, the amount of nutrient delivered depends solely on the infusion rate. Other institutions may compound individualized formulas. This approach permits compounding of patient-specific solutions. Compounding of the PN solution is limited only by the concentrations of stock solutions and stability concerns. The amount of nutrient delivered depends on the daily volume of the PN solution infused and the nutrient concentrations in the PN solution. The total daily amount of PN solution may be prepared in multiple bags, or more cost-effectively in a single container.[35]

Traditionally, adult PN solutions have been ordered by expressing the final concentrations of each component in the solution. For example, CAA and dextrose are ordered commonly in final percentage, electrolytes in milliequivalents per liter, and other additives in amount (milliliters or units) per day. This inconsistency may promote confusion and misinterpretation of PN solution contents that may result in harm, especially when patients are transferred between health system environments. To ensure that PN labels in all health system environments clearly and accurately reflect the PN solution contents, guidelines for standardized adult PN labeling have been recommended.[35] In addition to including a variety of other information on the label such as dosing weight and route of administration, the guidelines suggest expressing PN ingredients in amounts per total volume, which minimizes the need for pharmaceutical calculations to determine the nutrient value of the admixture. Computer software for calculating PN solutions is widely available, and several programs have adapted the recommended labeling guidelines. However, because some institutions may continue to follow traditional ordering practices, the steps for pharmaceutical calculations of a PN base solution will be reviewed briefly (Fig. 137–2).

There are several guidelines or clinical rules of thumb that may help the pharmacist calculate a PN regimen after a patient's nutritional requirements have been decided. For example, adult patients receiving only PN therapy may need larger volumes of fluid to provide maintenance requirements and replace extrarenal losses. However, patients requiring other intravenous drug therapy may receive adequate fluid in their intravenous maintenance solution (e.g., 0.45% NaCl in 5% dextrose) and/or piggybacked medications. Depending on individual institutional practices, maximally concentrating the PN solution and using an inexpensive maintenance fluid to manage hydration may provide a cost-effective regimen that requires fewer adjustments. Another guideline that may be helpful in designing a PN regimen in which the CAA-dextrose base is infused separately from the IVLEs is to allow a volume of approximately 100 to 150 mL/L of base solution for electrolytes and other additives. PN regimens for patients who require very small amounts of additives, such as patients with renal failure, may be further concentrated.

PEDIATRIC PARENTERAL NUTRITION SOLUTIONS

Pediatric PN solutions are typically ordered using an individualized approach because clinical practice guidelines often recommend nutrient intakes based on the patient's weight. For that reason, many institutions use a PN order form that expresses daily nutrient amount based on kilogram weight. For example, protein and fat are ordered as grams per kilogram per day, dextrose as milligrams per kilogram per minute, and electrolytes as milliequivalents per kilogram per day. However, some institutions may order macronutrients by expressing the final concentration of each component in the solution. Current safe practice guidelines suggest that the pediatric PN label identify components as an "amount per day" with a secondary expression of components as "amount per kilogram per day."[35] Auxiliary labels may be needed when the format between PN ordering and PN labeling is different. Clinician awareness of institution-specific labeling practices is imperative to minimize the risk of misinterpreting orders and potentially causing patient harm. Calculations for determining a pediatric PN solution are reviewed to clarify fundamental concepts for ordering pediatric PN solutions (Fig. 137–3). Additional features of the pediatric PN label should include the dosing weight, adminis-

tration date and time, expiration date, infusion rate, and duration of infusion. Because infants and children generally receive daily maintenance fluid from the PN regimen, supplemental intravenous solutions are rarely needed. Pediatric PN may be provided as a 2-in-1 or TNA formulation. However, the TNA system is not recommended for use when compounding neonatal PN due to instability of lipid particles with higher calcium and phosphorus content.[35] The labeling guidelines for IVLE in children are similar to those in adults.

ADMINISTRATION TECHNIQUES

PN solutions should be administered with an infusion pump to ensure consistent and controlled delivery of the solution. The intravenous administration line may include an in-line filter at a point prior to connection to the catheter. A 0.22-micron filter is recommended for use with CAA-dextrose solutions to remove particulate matter, air, and any microorganisms that may be present in the solution from prior manipulations of the admixture or the administration line. Because the average size of IVLE particles is approximately 0.5 micron, IVLEs administered separately from the CAA-dextrose solution must be piggybacked into the PN line at a site beyond the in-line filter.[35] Routine use of in-line filters (>0.22 micron) with TNA solutions is controversial.[69,70] However, the FDA recommends use of a 1.2-micron filter, which may be effective in preventing catheter occlusion due to precipitates or lipid aggregates.[35] This filter size is also reported to remove *Candida albicans*.

INITIATING AND ADVANCING THE PARENTERAL NUTRITION INFUSION

ADULT PARENTERAL NUTRITION

The patient's nutrition status, current clinical status, history of glucose tolerance, and concentration of dextrose in the formula will dictate the infusion rate at which the adult PN solution should be initiated. Many institutions begin infusion of the goal PN slowly and increase the rate gradually over 12 to 24 hours to the desired rate. The infusion rate is likewise reduced in a stepwise fashion when the decision to end PN therapy is made. This approach should prevent development of hyperglycemia and rebound hypoglycemia, respectively. However, many patients should tolerate initiation of PN at the goal infusion rate. Stable patients with normal organ function and stable baseline serum glucose concentrations have demonstrated minimal effect on serum glucose concentrations when abruptly initiating or discontinuing PN therapy.[71–73] Tapered initiation and cessation has been recommended for patients receiving intermittent subcutaneous regular insulin, patients with severe renal or hepatic disease, patients with other disease states that may increase the risk for development of hypoglycemia, such as severe diabetes or pancreatic malignancy, and patients who are receiving concurrent drug therapy that may predispose to development of hypoglycemia or mask the cardiovascular symptoms of hypoglycemia (β-blockers).[71] Others have recommended routinely tapering the PN rate for all patients by decreasing the rate by 50% for 1 hour prior to discontinuation.[72]

Although the IVLE dose should not exceed 2.5 g/kg per day or 60% of total daily calories, lower doses of 1 g/kg per day not to exceed 30% of calories have been recommended to minimize negative effects associated with long-chain fatty acids.[35] Manufacturer's information recommends IVLE infusion over 4 to 8 hours for adults. However, infusion over 16 to 24 hours appears to be the best clinical strategy

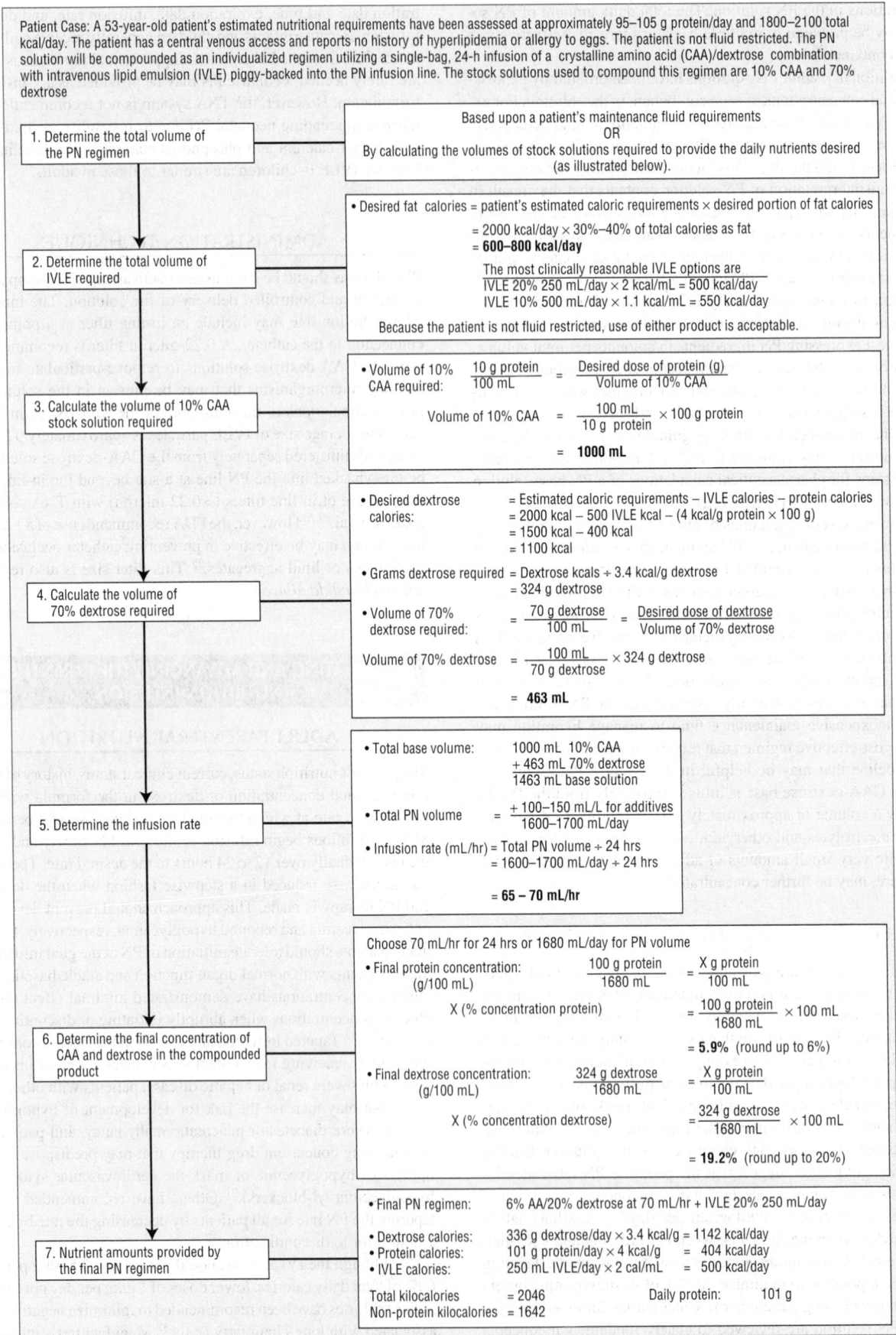

FIGURE 137–2. Calculation of a compounding plan for an adult PN regimen.

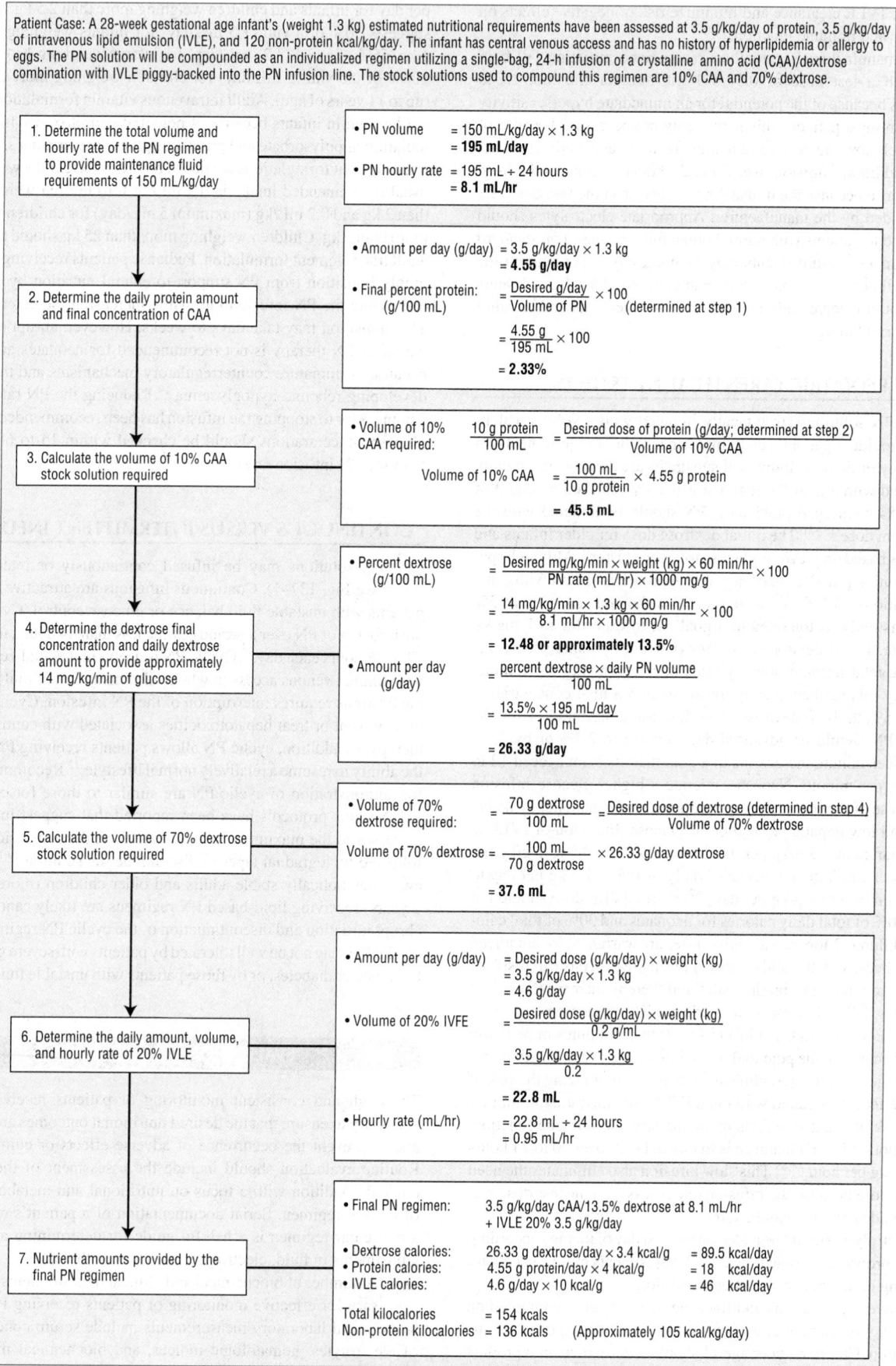

FIGURE 137–3. Calculation of a compounding plan for a pediatric PN regimen.

to promote IVLE clearance and minimize risk of negative effects on pulmonary and immune function.[44,45]

The manufacturer's guidelines recommend initiating IVLE in adults with a test dose of 0.5 to 1 mL/min for the first 15 to 30 minutes because of the potential for an immediate hypersensitivity reaction. In most patients, this is probably not necessary because of the relatively low incidence and benign nature of acute adverse reactions. In addition, infusion over 20 to 24 hours eliminates the need for a test dose because the infusion rate is less than the test-dose rate recommended by the manufacturer. Appropriate electrolytes should be provided to patients with normal organ function based on standard nutrient ranges.[35] Adjustments may be necessary depending on the patient's clinical condition. Adults and children older than 11 years of age should receive daily amounts of trace elements and an adult vitamin formulation.

PEDIATRIC PARENTERAL NUTRITION

Pediatric PN solutions are typically initiated with a volume calculated to provide a patient's daily maintenance fluid requirements on the first day of therapy. Individual substrates are then advanced daily as tolerated with a goal PN regimen generally achieved by day 3 of therapy. As mentioned previously, PN should be initiated with the goal protein dose.[19–21] The initial dextrose dose for older infants and children is based on previous glucose tolerance history. Although specific institution practices may vary, one approach is to start with (final concentration) 10% dextrose and advance the concentration in 5% increments daily as tolerated to a goal not to exceed 5 to 7 mg/kg per minute. Initial dextrose doses for premature infants should approximate fetal nutrient delivery rates of 5 to 6 mg/kg per minute. Frequently this mathematically translates into a final concentration range of 5% to 10% dextrose. The dextrose concentration for the neonatal PN should be advanced daily by 1% to 2.5% or by 2- to 4-mg/kg-per-minute increments to a goal that does not exceed 12 to 14 mg/kg per minute. Neonates tolerate a higher glucose infusion rate because of the relatively large proportion of metabolically active organs and low hepatic production of glucose. Initiation of IVLE is usually started at 0.5 g/kg per day in neonates and 0.5 to 1 g/kg per day in older children and increased daily by 0.5 to 1 g/kg per day to a maximum of 3 to 4 g/kg per day.[19,20,38] The IVLE dose should not exceed 60% of total daily calories for neonates and 30% of total calories for children. More conservative doses are warranted for jaundiced neonates because fatty acids released during hydrolysis can displace bilirubin from albumin-binding sites and thereby increase the risk of kernicterus.[16,38,39] The manufacturer's guidelines recommends initiating IVLE at 0.05 to 0.1 mL/min for 10 to 15 minutes in pediatric patients because of the potential for an immediate hypersensitivity reaction. In general, the best clinical strategy for minimizing the risk of adverse effects associated with rapid IVLE administration, minimizing the risk of negative effects on pulmonary and immune function, and promoting IVLE clearance is to infuse IVLE over 20 to 24 hours or 0.15 g/kg per hour.[44,45] This slow infusion also eliminates the need for a test dose because the infusion rate is less than the test-dose rate recommended by the manufacturer.

Electrolytes should be added on the first day of therapy according to age-appropriate nutrient ranges.[19,35] Adjustments may be necessary depending on the patient's clinical condition.

Intravenous vitamins and trace elements should be initiated on the first day of therapy and continued as a daily component of the PN solution. Children under age 11 should receive a vitamin product formulated for pediatric patients. Two multivitamin dosing schemas have been suggested for infants and children.[35] One method recommends 2 mL/kg per day for infants weighing less than 2.5 kg and 5 mL

per day for infants and children weighing more than 2.5 kg. The other suggests 30% of a vial (1.5 mL/day) for infants weighing less than 1 kg, 65% of a vial (3.25 mL/day) for infants weighing 1 to 3 kg, and 100% of the vial (5 mL/day) for children weighing more than 3 kg (up to 11 years of age). Adult intravenous vitamin formulations should not be used in infants because of potential neurotoxicity from accumulation of polysorbate and propylene glycol preservatives. Pediatric trace element formulations are dosed based on the child's weight. The usual recommended intake is 0.3 mL/kg for children weighing less than 3 kg and 0.2 mL/kg (maximum 5 mL/day) for children weighing more than 3 kg. Children weighing more than 25 kg should receive an adult trace element formulation. Pediatric patients receiving PN commonly transition from PN support to enteral nutrition by gradually decreasing the PN infusion rate while increasing the enteral intake. This transition may take days to weeks. However, abrupt discontinuation of PN therapy is not recommended for neonates and infants because of immature counterregulatory mechanisms and the risk for developing rebound hypoglycemia.[19] Reducing the PN rate for 1 to 2 hours prior to stopping the infusion has been recommended.[19] Blood glucose concentrations should be checked within 15 to 60 minutes after the PN infusion ends.

CONTINUOUS VERSUS INTERMITTENT INFUSIONS

PN solutions may be infused continuously or intermittently (see Fig. 137–1). Continuous infusions are attractive for use in patients with unstable fluid balance or glucose control. Cyclic PN is the infusion of PN over a period of time less than 24 hours, usually for 12 to 18 hours each day.[72] Cyclic PN is useful in hospitalized patients with limited venous access in whom administration of multiple other medications requires interruption of the PN infusion. Cyclic PN also may prevent or treat hepatotoxicities associated with continuous PN therapy. In addition, cyclic PN allows patients receiving PN at home the ability to resume a relatively normal lifestyle.[72] Recommendations for administration of cyclic PN are similar to those for continuous PN. Various protocols have been reported that suggest incremental increases to the maximum infusion rate for a desired period of time followed by a gradual taper to discontinue the solution.[19,71,72] However, metabolically stable adults and older children (more than age 2 years) receiving lipid-based PN regimens are likely candidates for abrupt initiation and discontinuation of the cyclic PN regimen.[19,71,73] Cyclic PN may not be well tolerated by patients with severe glucose intolerance or diabetes, or by those patients with unstable fluid balance.

EVALUATION OF OUTCOMES

Thorough and consistent monitoring of patients receiving PN is necessary to ensure that the desired nutritional outcomes are achieved and to prevent the occurrence of adverse effects or complications. Routine evaluation should include the assessment of the patient's clinical condition with a focus on nutritional and metabolic effects of the PN regimen. Serial documentation of a patient's response to a particular regimen is a helpful guide for determining appropriate adjustments in fluid, electrolyte, and nutrient therapies.

A number of biochemical and clinical measurements are necessary for effective monitoring of patients receiving PN. Important clinical laboratory measurements include serum concentrations of electrolytes, hematologic indices, and biochemical markers for renal function, liver function, and nutrition status. Other important clinical measurements include vital signs, weight, total fluid intake and losses, and nutritional intakes. Weekly height/length and head

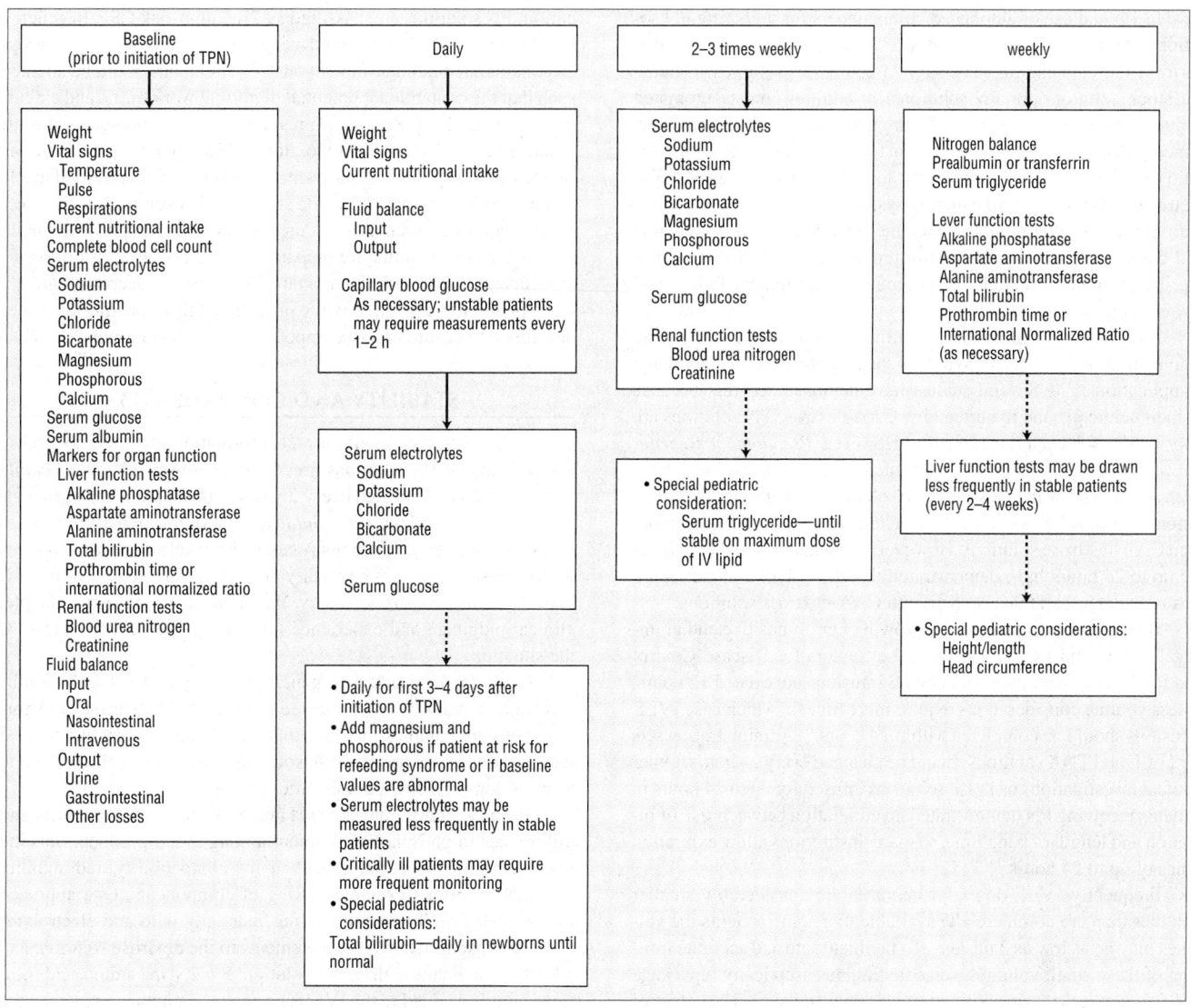

FIGURE 137–4. Monitoring strategy for patients receiving parenteral nutrition.

circumference measurements are helpful for monitoring nutritional changes in neonates. The frequency of clinical laboratory measurements usually depends on the stability of a patient's clinical condition and age. For example, frequency of blood laboratory measurements in neonates and infants tends to be more conservative due to their smaller circulating blood volumes, and in some cases, lack of central vascular access. Monitoring parameters considered important for patients receiving PN and the suggested frequency of measurement for each are outlined in Fig. 137–4. Appropriate assessment and evaluation of patient data can identify impending complications that may be avoided or treated early. Monitoring protocols should be developed and tailored for the patient population, medical practices, and resources of individual practice settings.

COMPOUNDING, STORAGE, AND INFECTION CONTROL

Several considerations are necessary when preparing and storing PN solutions. In general, the type of solution being prepared will dictate methods of compounding, storage, and infusion. Currently, the two most commonly used types of PN solutions are the CAA-dextrose combination with or without IVLEs piggybacked into the PN line, and TNAs. Use of TNA solutions offers several potential advantages, including reduced inventory (infusion pumps, tubing, and other related supplies), decreased time for compounding and administration, a potential decrease in manipulations of the infusion line (which should correspond with a decreased risk of catheter contamination), and ease of delivery and storage for patients receiving home PN.[74] Potential disadvantages include increased risk of infections, and stability and compatibility concerns. For example, the stability of TNA solutions may be less predictable compared with that of CAA-dextrose solutions, which make their use less desirable in specific patient populations such as neonates and infants.[35] In addition, the opaque solution that results after the addition of IVLEs makes detection of particulate matter difficult, and TNA solutions cannot be filtered with a bacteria-retentive 0.22-micron filter.[35] Methods for compounding PN solutions vary based on a health care system's patient population and medical practices and the number of PN solutions that need to be prepared. PN base solutions may be prepared by using gravity-driven transfer of CAA stock solutions to partially filled bags of concentrated dextrose stock solutions.[35,75] Other practice settings may use commercially prepared CAA-dextrose products that are separated within a single bag and then mixed prior to use.[35] Advances in compounding technology have facilitated use of automated compounders for preparing PN solutions. Automated compounders are computer-based systems that perform the calculations necessary to determine volumes of nutrient stock solutions for PN solutions. In addition, most automated compounder systems include software that communicates the determined calculations directly to a transfer pump device that delivers fluid from the source container to the final container by either a volumetric or gravimetric fluid pumping system.[75] Advantages associated with automated compounders include reduction in personnel time and compounding materials and improved accuracy of compounding. Disadvantages include the potential for equipment failure and power outages.

Assurance of solution sterility during compounding, storage, and administration is necessary to reduce the risk of infection and related complications.[76,77] Several studies have demonstrated that because of their acidic pH and hypertonicity, CAA-dextrose PN solutions are poor media for bacterial growth.[77] However, *Pseudomonas aeruginosa, Escherichia coli,* and fungi such as *Candida albicans* have been noted to grow in CAA-dextrose solutions.[77] In general, TNA solutions appear to support growth of bacteria less than IVLEs, but more than CAA-dextrose solutions. However, investigations of TNAs hung for up to 24 hours have demonstrated that the risk of contamination was no greater than that reported with CAA-dextrose solutions.[43,69]

Because IVLEs also support growth of gram-positive and gram-negative bacteria as well as fungi, the Centers for Disease Control and Prevention recommend that IVLE infusions not exceed 12 hours, unless volume considerations require more time, in which case IVLE infusions should be completed within 24 hours.[69] Administration sets for IVLE and TNA solutions should be changed every 24 hours. Other clinical investigations of IVLE solutions infused for up to 24 hours in patients receiving PN demonstrated no correlation between risk of infection and length of hang time, so many institutions allow expiration times of up to 24 hours.[78,79]

Frequently IVLE doses for neonates are considerably smaller volumes than are commercially available. For some patients the volumes may be as low as 2 mL/day. To facilitate safe and accurate infusion of these small volumes, some institutions aseptically repackage IVLE into plastic syringes for syringe pump infusion. The effect of this repackaging process on the risk of infection has not been studied in large well-designed trials. In addition, conflicting guidelines for use of other IVLE-containing medications such as propofol further confound application of Centers for Disease Control guidelines because these recommendations do not address the use of repackaged IVLE preparations.[69,80]

CLINICAL CONTROVERSY

The best delivery method for IVLE (manufacturer's bottle vs. repackaged syringe) and suggested interval of tubing change continue to be debated.

However, recent standards from the United States Pharmacopeia (USP) indicate administration of extemporaneously compounded lipid-based emulsions should be completed within 12 hours.[76]

The USP Chapter 797 details the procedures and requirements for compounding all sterile preparations including PN formulations.[76] These standards will apply to all health care settings in which sterile preparations are compounded and will be used by boards of pharmacy, the FDA, and accreditation organizations such as the Joint Commission on Accreditation of Healthcare Organizations. Compounded sterile preparations (CSP) are defined by risk level (high, medium, low) based on the probability of microbial, chemical, or physical contami-

nation. PN solutions are classified as a medium-risk CSP. In general, PN solutions should be prepared using aseptic technique under a properly maintained laminar flow hood.[69,76] The hood should be situated such that the contaminant potential of normal work traffic and air currents is minimized. Personnel must be trained adequately and must practice strict aseptic technique. Supervision by a pharmacist experienced in compounding intravenous solutions and knowledgeable about stability, compatibility, and storage of PN solutions is also necessary. Quality assurance procedures should be developed to maintain safe and accurate admixture preparation. The potential risk of sepsis associated with PN solution contamination can be decreased greatly when pharmacy-based admixture programs follow specific guidelines developed to ensure proper compounding of PN solutions.[76]

STABILITY AND COMPATIBILITY

Comprehensive sources of current information about compatibility and stability of PN solutions are *Trissel's Handbook on Injectable Drugs,* which is published every 2 years with supplements during alternating years, and the *King Guide to Parenteral Admixtures,* which is updated quarterly.[81,82] In many cases, the exact answer to a compatibility question may not be readily available, and a review of the primary literature may be necessary. When information is not available, clinical judgment and experience must be used carefully to resolve the situation.

CAA-dextrose solutions generally are stable for 1 to 2 months if refrigerated at 4°C and protected from light.[83] However, TNA formulations are complex mixtures that are inherently unstable. Several factors affect stability of TNA solutions, including pH, electrolyte charges, temperature, and time after compounding.[83]

Because of differences in pH among various CAA products and differences in phospholipid content among IVLE products, specific manufacturers should be consulted for compatibility and stability information prior to routine mixing of components. One approach to compounding TNA formulations manually is to add electrolytes (except phosphorus) and trace elements to the dextrose solution, and add phosphate salts to the CAA solution. Finally, the amino acid solution should be added to the IVLEs prior to or simultaneously with the dextrose solution. However, mixing components in this specific order and time sequence may not be possible with the use of automated compounders. The compounder's manufacturer should be consulted for the optimal mixing sequence to ensure safe compounding of TNA solutions.

The precipitation of calcium and phosphorus is a common interaction that is potentially life-threatening.[35,83] Factors that enhance the risk of precipitate formation include high concentrations of calcium and phosphorus salts, use of the chloride salt of calcium, decreased amino acid and dextrose concentrations, increased solution temperature, increased solution pH, use of an improper sequence when mixing calcium and phosphorus salts, and the presence of other additives including IVLEs.[35,82,83] Electrolyte stability in TNA solutions is difficult to assess because of poor visualization of a precipitate should one occur. PN solutions for neonates and infants tend to have a higher content of calcium and phosphorus as well as other divalent cations that limit the use of TNA formulations. Because of the relatively limited amount of published stability information, the use of a 2-in-1 formulation with separate administration of IVLEs is recommended for neonates and infants.[35] In general, alternative methods of delivering electrolytes or other medications should be pursued in any clinical situation in which compatibility information involving a TNA solution is lacking. Because the addition of bicarbonate to acidic PN solutions may result in the formation of carbon dioxide gas and insoluble calcium and magnesium carbonates, the use of sodium bicarbonate in PN solutions is not recommended.[35] Use of a bicarbonate precursor salt such as acetate usually is preferred.

Vitamins may be affected adversely by changes in solution pH, presence of other additives, storage time, solution temperature, and exposure to light.[83] Because of variable stabilities of individual vitamins, intravenous vitamin solutions should be added to the PN solution as near to the time of administration as is clinically feasible, and should not be in the PN solution longer than 24 hours.

Increased peroxide concentrations have been reported in dextrose–amino acid solutions after addition of intravenous multivitamins and/or exposure to air or light.[84,85] Increased peroxide production also has been reported in IVLEs after exposure to light.[86] Peroxide formation in dextrose–amino acid solutions depends on the concentration of intravenous multivitamins, amino acids, and dextrose, and the presence of IVLEs.[84] Peroxide production in IVLEs also depends on the intensity of light and is enhanced with phototherapy light in neonates.[86] Multiple in vitro experiments have reported negative effects of peroxides and associated metabolites on organ and immune function.[39,84–87] However, the clinical effects of PN containing peroxides are not clear.[39] Neonatal and infant PN regimens usually deliver a higher daily peroxide load when compared with those for adults.[84] To minimize the risk of negative metabolic effects from peroxide infusion, the use of light-protective PN bags and infusion tubing for neonatal and infant IVLE and PN solutions has been recommended.[84,85]

Many patients receiving PN at home or in a hospital also receive other intravenous medications. The compatibility of these medications and other intravenous solutions is an important concern in delivering safe and effective drug and nutritional therapy. Intravenous medications are infused most often as a separate admixture piggybacked in the PN line. However, some medications may be added directly to the PN solution and administered at the same rate as the PN infusion. Because of the potential for ineffective drug therapy or other complications associated with physiochemical incompatibility and stability of the PN solution, specific criteria should be considered before one adds a medication directly to the PN solution.[88] The dosage regimen should be stable for each 24-hour period and should have pharmacokinetic properties appropriate for continuous infusion. There should be documented chemical and physical compatibility of the medication with PN mixture components and other medications that may be piggybacked concomitantly into the PN line. Finally, the PN regimen should be infused continuously over 24 hours. Advantages of using PN admixtures as drug vehicles include consolidation of dosage units, improved pharmacotherapy for certain drugs, conservation of fluid in volume-restricted patients, fewer venous catheter violations, and decreased compounding and administration times.[88] However, a major disadvantage to the use of PN solutions as drug-delivery vehicles is the lack of compatibility and stability data in the PN solutions that are used commonly in clinical practice. Medications frequently added to PN solutions include albumin, regular insulin, and histamine₂-antagonists.[81,82,88]

COMPLICATIONS OF PARENTERAL NUTRITION

PN can be a safe and effective therapy when appropriate patients have been selected and the course of therapy is monitored and adjusted correctly. However, PN support is a complex therapy that is associated with numerous complications. These complications may be divided into four categories: mechanical or technical, infectious, metabolic, and nutritional.

MECHANICAL OR TECHNICAL COMPLICATIONS

Mechanical or technical complications include malfunctions in the system used for intravenous delivery of the solution. Examples of such malfunctions include infusion pump failure, problems with administration sets or tubing, and problems with the catheter. Catheter-related complications are potentially life-threatening.

Pneumothorax, catheter misdirection or migration into the wrong vein or improperly-positioned within the cardiac chambers, arterial puncture, bleeding, and hematoma formation may occur during surgical placement of the catheter. Many of these complications, in addition to venous thrombosis and air embolism, may occur after insertion as well. Catheters occasionally occlude or break during use. If these problems cannot be rectified easily, the catheter may need to be surgically replaced.[66]

INFECTIOUS COMPLICATIONS

Infectious complications can be a major hazard in patients receiving CPN. Often these patients are predisposed to infection as a result of compromised immunity and/or concomitant infection. Frequent use of broad-spectrum antibiotic therapy and malnutrition are also predisposing factors for development of infection. Infection rarely develops secondary to solution contamination.[69,77] However, strict adherence to specific protocols for preparation of PN solutions should minimize this occurrence.[76,77] A more common source of systemic infection is catheter-related infection. Catheter-related bloodstream infection is defined as the presence of bacterial or fungal growth from the catheter tip and peripheral blood cultures. Catheter infection or a colonized catheter is defined as microbial growth from the catheter tip or from a blood culture drawn from the catheter with no growth of the same organism in the peripheral blood culture.[69] Patients with catheter-related infections may exhibit signs of sepsis syndrome such as fever, chills, mental status changes, hypotension, or glucose intolerance. These infections occur when the catheter becomes colonized by direct microbial invasion of the skin at the insertion site or at the infusion site of the catheter. For example, colonization may occur after multiple manipulations of the line used for PN administration, which can occur when the PN line is used to administer other medications. Other examples include failure of in-line bacterial filters, poor placement technique, and poor care of the insertion site.[69]

When no other source of infection is apparent in symptomatic patients, the catheter should be evaluated as the potential source. Blood cultures are drawn from a peripheral site and from the central catheter. In many institutions the suspected catheter is removed, the tip is cultured quantitatively, and a new central catheter is inserted. If bacterial or fungal growth of the same organism occurs from the catheter tip and the peripheral blood culture, the exchanged catheter is removed, and another is placed in a different anatomic site. If bacterial or fungal growth occurs from the catheter tip or from a blood culture drawn from the catheter with no growth of the same organism in the peripheral culture, the catheter may be removed and replaced with another in the same anatomic location. However, because the clinical value of frequent central catheter replacement in patients with sepsis secondary to catheter-related infection is controversial, other treatment protocols have been suggested.[89]

METABOLIC AND NUTRITIONAL COMPLICATIONS

Metabolic complications associated with PN therapy are numerous, and if left untreated, may be potentially fatal. Common metabolic abnormalities related to substrate intolerance and fluid,

TABLE 137–7. Substrate Intolerance in Parenteral Nutrition

Complication	Possible Causes	Intervention
Hyperglycemia	Stress, infection, corticosteroids, pancreatitis, diabetes mellitus, peritoneal dialysis, excessive dextrose administration	Decrease dextrose load by decreasing infusion rate or dextrose concentration (may substitute fat calories); administer insulin
Hypoglycemia	Abrupt withdrawal of dextrose, insulin overdose	Increase dextrose intake; decrease exogenous insulin; taper infusion rate prior to discontinuing PN
Excess of carbon dioxide production	Excess dextrose intake	Decrease dextrose intake; balance calories from fat and dextrose
Hypertriglyceridemia	Stress, familial hyperlipidemia, pancreatitis; excess IVLE dose; rapid IVLE infusion rate	Decrease IVLE dose; decrease rate of IVLE infusion; discontinue IVLE if indicated
Abnormal liver function tests (elevated AST, alkaline phosphatase, and bilirubin)	Stress, infection, cancer, excess carbohydrate intake, excess caloric intake, essential fatty acid deficiency	Decrease dextrose load (substitute fat); decrease total calories; provide essential fatty acids; cycle PN infusion; transition to enteral nutrition regimen

AST, aspartate aminotransferase (SGOT); IVLE, intravenous lipid emulsion.
Adapted with permission from Teasley-Strausburg et al.[91]

electrolyte, and acid-base disorders are presented in Table 137–4 and Table 137–7 along with predisposing factors and general strategies for intervention. The etiology, mechanisms, and implications of individual metabolic abnormalities are multifactorial and have been summarized in multiple reviews.[20,25,35,39,45,47,52,72,90–92]

PN-associated hepatic dysfunction, as evidenced by elevations in serum liver function measurements such as total bilirubin, aspartate aminotransferase, alanine aminotransferase, and alkaline phosphatase is well documented.[92–94] No single etiology has been identified, although several risk factors have been reported. Risk factors for children include degree of prematurity, sepsis, hypoxia, lack of enteral nutrition, small bowel bacterial overgrowth, GI conditions requiring surgical intervention, duration of PN therapy, and long-term administration of excessive calories.[25,39,93–95] PN-associated hepatic dysfunction in infants is characterized clinically by a serum direct bilirubin concentration greater than 2 mg/dL.[95] Taurine deficiency has been proposed as an etiology of cholestasis in preterm infants and neonates.[25,95] Taurine is a CEAA not present in standard CAA solutions that is important in neonatal and infant bile metabolism. However, the effectiveness of PN regimens with CAA solutions containing supplemental taurine is unclear.[25,94,95] Risk factors for PN-associated hepatic dysfunction in adults include preexisting liver diseases, sepsis, preexisting malnutrition, large extent of bowel resection, duration of PN therapy, lack of enteral intake, and long-term administration of excessive calories.[92–94] PN-associated hepatic dysfunction in adults typically presents as steatosis and steatohepatosis on biopsy.[93,94] Clinically, PN-associated hepatic dysfunction is characterized by mild elevations in serum liver enzymes, usually less than three times the upper limit of normal, with peak enzyme levels usually occurring between 1 and 4 weeks after initiating PN.[93,94] In many cases, the liver abnormalities improve or resolve with manipulation of substrate intake or discontinuation of PN therapy. However, death from PN-associated liver failure in adults and pediatric patients receiving long-term home PN has been reported.[92]

Hypertriglyceridemia, defined as serum triglyceride concentrations of 400 to 500 mg/dL in adults and 150 to 200 mg/dL in preterm infants, neonates, and older pediatric patients, may occur in patients receiving IVLE-based PN. Risk factors include preexisting liver or pancreatic dysfunction, sepsis, multiple organ failure, degree of prematurity, rate of IVLE infusion, and dose.[37,44,45]

IVLE-associated hypertriglyceridemia generally is thought to be due to defective lipid clearance.[44] Premature infants and neonates have relatively slower lipid clearance compared with adults because of immature metabolic pathways, including decreased lipoprotein lipase activity.[37,44,45] Reducing the infusion rate or IVLE dose or withholding IVLE therapy should be considered when patients present with hypertriglyceridemia or lipemic serum.[44,45] Use of low-dose heparin to stimulate lipoprotein lipase activity has been suggested as a potential therapeutic intervention to treat IVLE-associated hypertriglyceridemia.[44,45] The role of carnitine for treatment of IVLE-associated hypertriglyceridemia is not clear.[44,45]

The refeeding syndrome (RS) is a nutritional complication reported in severely malnourished patients with significant weight loss who receive PN.[39,96] RS is associated primarily with hypophosphatemia, although hypokalemia, hypomagnesemia, and life-threatening cardiac dysfunction have been reported as well. The mechanism of the electrolyte abnormalities appears to be related to acute provision of macronutrient substrates that promote anabolism in an environment of depleted total body stores of phosphorus, potassium, and magnesium. Cardiac dysfunction is thought to occur because of an acute volume expansion that increases cardiac demand. Recommendations for initiating PN in adults at risk for RS include providing less than 50% of the calculated nonprotein caloric requirements initially. The dextrose dose should be initiated at approximately 150 to 200 g/day. Calories should be advanced over 3 to 4 days to the desired goal. Because the metabolic abnormalities described with RS appear to be related primarily to acute provision of large amounts of dextrose, the goal protein dose may be provided with the initial PN infusion.[96] Pediatric PN regimens are usually advanced over several days as a general practice for all patients. However, additional recommendations for minimizing the risk of refeeding syndrome in pediatric patients includes provision of additional phosphorus and potassium above standard nutrient requirements at the time PN is initiated.[39]

Other nutritional complications of PN therapy may develop over a prolonged course of therapy (weeks to months) as a result of inappropriate intake of a particular nutrient. Certain conditions, such as metabolic stress in a previously malnourished patient, may elicit symptoms of deficiency much earlier if a nutrient is not appropriately provided. For example, lactic acidosis and other life-threatening complications associated with severe thiamine deficiency have been reported in patients who received PN solutions without multivitamin supplementation.[97] At least maintenance doses of vitamins, trace elements, and essential fatty acids should be provided to all patients with normal age-related organ function receiving PN.

Patients receiving PN regimens without IVLEs for extended periods (weeks to months) are at risk for development of EFAD. Clinical signs of EFAD include hair loss, desquamative dermatitis, thrombocytopenia, and malabsorption and diarrhea resulting from changes in intestinal mucosa.[46,47] EFAD also may be diagnosed by evaluating plasma fatty acid profiles. A triene:tetraene ratio more than 0.4 is biochemical evidence for EFAD. These manifestations may occur 1 to 3 weeks after initiation of fat-free PN in adults and within 72 hours in premature infants.[37]

Metabolic bone disease is a complication usually reported in adults and children receiving long-term home PN.[92,98] This disorder in adults is characterized by osteomalacia with or without osteoporosis that may present without associated clinical, radiologic, or biochemical abnormalities. The diagnosis may not be made in premature infants until after the development of bone fractures or overt rickets. The etiology is poorly understood and likely multifactorial. Treatment options include pharmacologic intervention, calcium and vitamin D supplementation, and exercise. Others have recommended removal of vitamin D from the PN in patients with low serum parathyroid hormone and 1,25-hydroxyvitamin D concentrations.[92]

Clinical symptoms of trace element deficiencies, although rare, have been reported in patients receiving PN. More commonly, decreased serum trace element concentrations have been reported in a variety of patient populations. However, the clinical significance of decreased concentrations of many trace elements is not known because serum concentrations often do not correlate with total body stores.[61,62] Clinical signs and symptoms of trace element deficiencies have been reviewed elsewhere.[61]

Occasionally, patients may develop nutrient-induced toxicities, most commonly as a result of the accumulation of fat-soluble vitamins or trace elements due to either excessive intake or decreased excretion. Certain disease states (e.g., severe renal or hepatic failure) may necessitate reduction in vitamin and trace element intake.

Many trace elements are present in PN components as contaminants.[53,99,100] The content varies among components and manufacturers. Some investigations of patients with normal organ function receiving PN have reported concern with elevated serum concentrations of particular trace elements such as chromium and manganese.[61,99,100] Aluminum is a common contaminant of many sterile intravenous solutions including those used for compounding PN. Calcium and phosphorus solutions are among those components with higher levels of aluminum contamination.[101,102] Aluminum accumulation may occur during long-term PN therapy, especially in patients with renal insufficiency, and is associated with abnormal neurologic and hematologic function and metabolic bone disease in adults and premature infants.[98,101–104] Preterm infants are at higher risk of aluminum toxicities because they receive larger doses (micrograms per kilogram) from PN solutions than adults.[98,101–104] Preterm infants are also more likely to retain aluminum because of immature renal function. Although the maximum safe level of intravenous aluminum intake is not known, the FDA has defined parenteral doses of 4 to 5 mcg/kg per day as amounts associated with central nervous system and bone toxicity in patients with impaired renal function, including premature neonates.[102,103] Even lesser amounts may result in tissue accumulation but no documented toxicity.

Recent data suggest that the aluminum content of sterile solutions used for compounding PN has declined due to awareness of toxicity and improvements in industrial PN component preparation.[104] However, in 2004 the FDA implemented a restriction of aluminum content in large-volume PN stock solutions to a maximum of 25 mcg/L and require a statement of aluminum content on the label of small-volume PN solutions beginning in 2004.[103]

HOME PARENTERAL NUTRITION

Advances in technology for the delivery of intravenous solutions have allowed medically stable patients who require extended PN therapy to be maintained indefinitely on intravenous nutrition. An increasing concern for cost containment of health care services has fostered use of sophisticated infusion devices to provide PN at home. Numerous programs are now available outside the traditional health care setting to support patients with various long-term or permanent medical conditions. Standards have been developed to promote safe and effective care.[7] Home PN services may be coordinated and administered through a hospital, by a commercially operated corporation, or through a joint venture between the two.

Many factors are considered in selecting candidates for home PN therapy. Significant benefit must be expected from placing a patient into the program. Additionally, the patient and his or her caregiver must be willing to complete training successfully and assume numerous other responsibilities that are important for managing a new daily routine in the home. Other logistics such as funding, procurement of solutions and supplies, and clinical management and follow-up must be evaluated, resolved, and implemented for each patient in order to achieve the desired outcomes.[92,105]

Patients with Crohn's disease, ischemic bowel disease, severe GI motility disorders, extensive intestinal obstruction, and congenital bowel dysfunction have been maintained successfully with home PN.[105]

In the past, patients or their caregivers may have been trained to mix PN solutions in the home. Today patients commonly receive premixed PN solutions from the hospital or a commercial vendor. Intravenous vitamins or other additives may be added daily by the patient or caregiver, depending on the arrangement with the PN provider. The solution generally is administered through the night by infusion pump over 10 to 12 hours.[72] A cycled regimen allows the patient time away from the pump during daylight hours and provides many patients with the freedom to have a reasonably normal daily routine. Clinical management and follow-up are performed periodically according to the needs of the patient and the protocol of the care provider. A coordinated effort among several health care professionals, including physicians, pharmacists, nurses, social workers, and the patient and his or her caregiver, as well as the suppliers, is paramount to providing safe and effective management. Home PN affords some patients the potential for an ambulatory lifestyle while maintaining an intravenous feeding regimen that was previously only available in the hospital setting. For others, home PN may contribute to a better quality of life in the comfort of their home.

PHARMACOECONOMIC CONSIDERATIONS

Because numerous variables have an impact on the provision of PN support and the response to therapy, determining the true cost of PN is difficult.[106–108] In general, PN is an expensive intervention, and cost likely varies depending on the underlying indication for treatment and whether PN is provided at home or in an acute care

TABLE 137–8. Costs Associated with Parenteral Nutrition (PN) Therapy

Type of Cost	Description
Direct	
• PN solution	
Components	Dextrose, AA, IVLE, other additives
Preparation	Dependent on system used for compounding: solution transfer sets, bags, syringes, technician time, pharmacist time
Administration	Administration sets, solution filter, pump, nursing time
• Catheter placement and site management	Venous access device
	Central catheter: site of procedure (bedside vs. operating room), radiographic confirmation of placement, supplies used for site care
	Peripheral line: nursing time, supplies used for site care
• Monitoring	Routine laboratory and clinical measurements, changes in therapy to prevent complications or toxicities, nutrition support clinician time
• Complications	*Mechanical:* treatment of specific complication
	Infectious: cost of antibiotic therapy or venous access replacement
	Metabolic: increased clinical and laboratory measurements, possible waste of PN solution
Indirect	
• Morbidity	Quality-of-life expenses such as cost of patient discomfort, time lost from work or other activities as a result of PN therapy
• Mortality	Cost of premature death based, for example, on expected future wages

AA, amino acids; IVLE, intravenous lipid emulsion.

setting.[92,106–108] Expenses associated with PN therapy may be categorized as direct and indirect costs (Table 137–8).[108,109] Direct costs may be further categorized as fixed or variable costs. Fixed costs do not depend on the volume of patients receiving therapy. For example, an automatic compounder and the tubing sets required to transfer volumes of stock solutions to the administration bag would be considered fixed costs in many practice settings. These costs per patient tend to be highest in low-volume environments. Variable costs such as PN administration bags depend directly on the number of patients receiving PN. Other direct costs include ancillary services required by patients receiving PN and costs related to the management of nutritionally associated complications.

Benefits and other clinical effects of PN (i.e., length of stay and frequency of complications) in specific patient populations have been evaluated.[17,18,110] Few investigations have reported an economic assessment of the therapy. However, economic data from many of these reports would not necessarily reflect current costs. Indeed, the direct cost of PN solution components generally has declined over the past decade. Attempting to measure the cost or cost savings associated with reported benefits of PN therapy and other clinical effects based on results of controlled clinical trials is difficult.[106,107] Clinical outcomes measurements and hence economic outcomes are influenced by multiple factors, including experimental design, sample size, and specific health system practices. Several investigations used for determining costs and benefits of PN therapy have been criticized for such biases.[14,108]

While the results of economic analyses of PN remain controversial, similarities among several reports provide a basis for methods of limiting the costs of PN therapy. These include the following:

1. Use of PN only for appropriate patients as described by institution-specific criteria based on current consensus statements.[111] The costs and complications associated with EN have been demonstrated to be less than those associated with PN.[112,113]

2. Frequent evaluation of the need for routine laboratory measurements used for monitoring PN therapy. In general, the level of laboratory monitoring should decrease as a patient's clinical condition stabilizes (see Fig. 137–4).

3. Minimize the cost of PN by using efficient purchasing practices for PN solutions and compounding supplies through contract purchasing, streamlined compounding procedures, standardized administration times and 24-hour hang times to reduce waste, single-bag PN solutions, and optimized monitoring plans.

CONCLUSIONS

Appropriate patient selection, assessment, and monitoring are key to successful nutritional therapy and prevention of unnecessary complications or harm to the patient. Standardized order forms and monitoring protocols are useful tools to ensure appropriate administration and monitoring of PN therapy. Because pharmacists have been actively involved in the provision of PN at many levels, including direct patient care, education, and research, nutrition support has been recognized as a pharmacy practice specialty.[114] In addition, as the interdisciplinary approach to specialized nutrition support has evolved, standards of practice have been defined for pharmacists as well as other health care professionals who provide nutrition support care.[5,9–11] The future of PN therapy and the role of the nutrition-support clinician will be affected primarily by new insights from clinical research and economic challenges in the health care environment.

ABBREVIATIONS

CAA: crystalline amino acid
CEAA: conditionally essential amino acid
CPN: central parenteral nutrition
CSP: compounded sterile preparations
EFAD: essential fatty acid deficiency

EN: enteral nutrition
IVLE: intravenous lipid emulsion
LCT: long-chain triglyceride
MCT: medium-chain triglyceride
NAG-AMA: Nutrition Advisory Group of the American Medical
   Association
NPC:N: nonprotein-calorie:nitrogen ratio
PN: parenteral nutrition
PPN: peripheral parenteral nutrition
PUFA: polyunsaturated fatty acid
RDA: recommended daily allowance
RS: refeeding syndrome
TNA: total nutrient admixture
TPN: total parenteral nutrition
USP: United States Pharmacopeia

Review Questions and other resources can be found at
www.pharmacotherapyonline.com.

REFERENCES

1. Dudrick SJ. Early developments and clinical applications of total parenteral nutrition. JPEN J Parenter Enter Nutr 2003;27:291–299.
2. Schwenk WF. Specialized nutrition support: The pediatric perspective. JPEN J Parenter Enter Nutr 2003;27:160–167.
3. Wesley JR. Nutrition support teams: Past, present and future. Nutr Clin Pract 1995;10:219–228.
4. Holcombe BJ, Thorne DB, Strausburg KM, et al. Pharmacy practice insights: Analysis of the practice of nutrition support pharmacy specialists. Pharmacotherapy 1995;15:806–813.
5. American Society for Parenteral and Enteral Nutrition. Standards of practice for nutrition support pharmacists. Nutr Clin Pract 1999;14:275–281.
6. American Society for Parenteral and Enteral Nutrition. Standards for nutrition support: Hospitalized patients. Nutr Clin Pract 1995;10:208–219.
7. American Society for Parenteral and Enteral Nutrition. Standards for home nutrition support. Nutr Clin Pract 1999;14:151–162.
8. ASPEN Board of Directors. Standards for hospitalized pediatric patients. Nutr Clin Pract 1996;11:217–228.
9. ASPEN Board of Directors. Standards of practice for nutrition support dietitians. Nutr Clin Pract 2000;15:53–59.
10. ASPEN Board of Directors. Standards of practice for nutrition support nurses. Nutr Clin Pract 2001;16:56–62.
11. ASPEN and the Task Force on Standards for Nutrition Support Physicians. Standards of practice for nutrition support physicians. Nutr Clin Pract 2003;18:270–275.
12. Choban PS, Flancbaum L. Nourishing the obese patient. Clin Nutr 2000; 19:305–311.
13. ASPEN Board of Directors and The Clinical Guidelines Taskforce. Administration of specialized nutrition support. JPEN J Parenter Enter Nutr 2002;26:18SA–21SA.
14. Wolfe BM, Mathiesen KA. Clinical practice guidelines in nutrition support: Can they be based on randomized clinical trials? JPEN J Parenter Enter Nutr 1997;21:1–6.
15. ASPEN Board of Directors and The Clinical Guidelines Taskforce. Nutrition assessment-adults. JPEN J Parenter Enter Nutr 2002;26:9SA–12SA.
16. ASPEN Board of Directors and The Clinical Guidelines Taskforce. Nutrition Assessment-pediatrics. JPEN J Parenter Enter Nutr 2002;26:13SA–18SA.
17. Koretz RL, Lipman TO, Klein S. AGA technical review on parenteral nutrition. Gastroenterology 2001;121:970–1001.
18. ASPEN Board of Directors and The Clinical Guidelines Taskforce. Specific guidelines for disease-adults. JPEN J Parenter Enter Nutr 2002;26:61SA–96SA.
19. ASPEN Board of Directors and The Clinical Guidelines Taskforce. Administration of specialized nutrition support-issues unique to pediatrics. JPEN J Parenter Enter Nutr 2002;26:97SA–110SA.
20. Koo WWK, Cepeda EE. Parenteral nutrition in neonates. In Rombeau JL, Rolandelli RH, eds. Clinical Nutrition: Parenteral Nutrition, 3rd ed. Philadelphia, Saunders, 2001:463–475.
21. Thureen PJ, Hay WW. Early aggressive nutrition in preterm infants. Semin Neonatol 2001;6:403–415.
22. Thureen PJ. Early aggressive nutrition in the neonate. NeoReviews 1999;Sept:e45–e55.
23. Ziegler EE. Malnutrition in the premature infant. Acta Paediatr Scand Suppl 1991;374:58–66.
24. Clark RH, Wagner CL, Merritt RJ, et al. Nutrition in the neonatal intensive care unit: How do we reduce the incidence of extrauterine growth restriction? J Perinatol 2003;23:337–344.
25. Falcone RA, Warner BW. Pediatric parenteral nutrition. In Rombeau JL, Rolandelli RH, eds. Clinical Nutrition: Parenteral Nutrition, 3rd ed. Philadelphia, Saunders, 2001:476–496.
26. Miles JM, Klein JA. Should protein be included in caloric calculations for a TPN prescription? Point-counterpoint. Nutr Clin Pract 1996;11:204–206.
27. Furst P, Stehle P. Are intravenous amino acid solutions unbalanced? New Horizons 1994;2:215–223.
28. Miller SJ. The nitrogen balance revisited. Hosp Pharm 1990;25:61–65, 70.
29. Shatsky F, McFeely EJ, Takahashi D. A table for estimating calcium and phosphorus compatibility in parenteral nutrition formulas that contain trophamine plus cysteine. Hosp Pharm 1995;30:690–692, 793.
30. Scaglia F, Longo N. Primary and secondary alterations of neonatal carnitine metabolism. Semin Perinatol 1999;23:152–161.
31. Cairns PA, Stalker DJ. Carnitine supplementation of parenterally fed neonates (Cochrane Review). In The Cochrane Library, Issue 2, 2002. Oxford: Update Software.
32. Des Robert C, Le Bacquer O, Piloquet H, et al. Acute effects of intravenous glutamine supplementation on protein metabolism in very low birth weight infants: a stable isotope study. Pediatr Res 2002;51:87–93.
33. Buchman AL. Glutamine: Commercially essential or conditionally essential? A critical appraisal of the human data. Am J Clin Nutr 2001;74:25–32.
34. Tubman TR, Thompson SW. Glutamine supplementation for preventing morbidity in preterm infants. Cochrane Database Syst Rev 2000;2:CD001457.
35. Taskforce for the Revision of Safe Practices for Parenteral Nutrition. JPEN J Parenter Enter Nutr 2004;28:539–570.
36. Rosemarin DK, Wardlaw GM, Mirtallo JM. Hyperglycemia associated with high, continuous infusion rates of total parenteral nutrition dextrose. Nutr Clin Pract 1996;11:151–156.
37. Thureen PJ, Hay Jr WW. Intravenous nutrition and postnatal growth of the micropremie. Clin Perinatol 2000;27:197–219.
38. Sheridan RL, Yu YM, Prelack K, et al. Maximal parenteral glucose oxidation in hypermetabolic young children: A stable isotope study. JPEN J Parenter Enter Nutr 1998;22:212–216.
39. Shulman RJ, Phillips S. Parenteral nutrition in infants and children. J Pediatr Gastroenterol Nutr 2003;36:587–607.
40. Waxman K, Day AT, Stellin GP, et al. Safety and efficacy of glycerol and amino acids in combination with lipid emulsion for peripheral parenteral nutrition support. JPEN J Parenter Enter Nutr 1992;16:374–378.
41. Product information. ProcalAmine. Irvine, CA, B. Braun Medical, 1998.
42. Intravenous fat emulsions. In: Wickersham RM, Novak KK, managing eds. Drug Facts and Comparisons. St. Louis, Wolters Kluwer Health, 2003:109–110.
43. Driscoll DF, Adolph M, Bistrian BR. Lipid emulsions in parenteral nutrition. In Rombeau JL, Rolandelli RH, eds. Clinical Nutrition: Parenteral Nutrition, 3rd ed. Philadelphia, Saunders, 2001:35–59.
44. Putet G. Lipid metabolism of the micropremie. Clin Perinatol 2000;27:57–69.

45. Sacks GS, Mouser JF. Is IV lipid emulsion safe in patients with hyper-triglyceridemia? Nutr Clin Pract 1997;12:120–123.

46. Sardesai VM. The essential fatty acids. Nutr Clin Pract 1992;7:179–186.

47. Dickerson RN. Essential fatty acid deficiency: An "old" disorder that should not be forgotten. Hosp Pharm 1998;33:1435–1440.

48. Lai HS, Chen WJ. Effects of medium-chain and long-chain triacylglyc-erols in pediatric surgical patients. Nutrition 2000;16:401–406.

49. Battistella FD, Wildergren JT, Anderson JT, et al. A prospective, random-ized trial of intravenous fat emulsion administration in trauma victims requiring total parenteral nutrition. J Trauma 1997;43:52–58.

50. McCowen KC, Friel C, Sternberg J, et al. Hypocaloric total parenteral nutrition: Effectiveness in prevention of hyperglycemia and infectious complications. A randomized clinical trial. Crit Care Med 2000;28:3606–3611.

51. Heyland DK, Novak F, Drover JW, et al: Should immunonutrition become routine in critically ill patients? A systematic review of the evidence. JAMA 2001:286:944–953.

52. Roth MS, Martin AB, Katz JA. Nutritional implications of prolonged propofol use. Am J Health Syst Pharm 1997;54:694–695.

53. American Medical Association Department of Foods and Nutrition. Mul-tivitamin preparations for parenteral use: A statement by the nutritional advisory group. J Parenter Enter Nutr 1979;3:258–262.

54. Demling RH, DeBiasse MA. Micronutrients in critical illness. Crit Care Clin 1995;11:651–673.

55. Greer FR. Vitamin metabolism and requirements in the micropremie. Clin Perinatol 2000;27:95–118.

56. Green HL, Hambidge KM, Schanler R, Tsang RC. Guidelines for the use of vitamins, trace elements, calcium, magnesium, and phosphorus in infants and children receiving total parenteral nutrition: Report of the Subcommittee on Pediatric Parenteral Nutrient Requirements from the Committee on Clinical Practice Issues of the American Society for Clinical Nutrition. Am J Clin Nutr 1988;48:1324–1342.

57. Helphingstine CJ, Bistrian BR. New food and drug administration re-quirements for inclusion of vitamin K in adult parenteral multivitamins. J Parenter Enter Nutr 2003;27:220–224.

58. Chambrier C, Lellerq M, Saudin F, et al. Is vitamin K1 supplementation necessary in long-term parenteral nutrition? JPEN J Parenter Enter Nutr 1998;22:87–90.

59. Lennon C, Davidson KW, Sandowski JA, Mason JB. The vitamin K content of intravenous lipid emulsion. JPEN J Parenter Enter Nutr 1993;17:142–144.

60. Duerksen DR, Papineau N. Is routine vitamin K supplementation re-quired in hospitalized patients receiving parenteral nutrition? Nutr Clin Pract 2000;15:81–83.

61. Misra S, Kirby DF. Micronutrient and trace element monitoring in adult nutrition support. Nutr Clin Pract 2000;15:120–126.

62. Aggett PJ. Trace elements of the micropremie. Clin Perinatol 2000;27:119–129.

63. American Medical Association. Guidelines for essential trace element preparations for parenteral use: A statement by the Nutrition Advisory Group. JPEN J Parenter Enter Nutr 1979;3:263–267.

64. Miller SJ. Peripheral parenteral nutrition: Theory and practice. Hosp Pharm 1991;26:796–801.

65. Anderson ADG, Palmer D, MacFie J. Peripheral parenteral nutrition. Br J Surg 2003;90:1048–1054.

66. Grant JP. Vascular access for total parenteral nutrition: techniques and complications. In: Handbook of Total Parenteral Nutrition, 2nd ed. Philadelphia, Saunders, 1992:107–138.

67. Cerulli J, Malone M. Can changes to a total parenteral nutrition order form improve prescribing? Nutr Clin Pract 2000;15:143–151.

68. Peverini RL, Beach DS, Wan KW, Vyhmeister NR. Graphical user in-terface for a neonatal parenteral nutrition decision support system. Proc AMIA Symp 2000:650–654.

69. O'Grady NP, Alexander M, Dellinger EP, et al. Guidelines for the preven-tion of intravascular catheter-related infections. MMWR Morb Mortal Wkly Rep 2002;51(RR10):1–26.

70. Mirtallo JM. The complexity of mixing calcium and phosphate. Am J Hosp Pharm 1994;51:1535–1536.

71. Dickerson RN. How fast can I taper a TPN in a hospitalized patient? Hosp Pharm 1985;20:620–621.

72. Speerhas R, Wang J, Seidner D, Steiger E. Maintaining normal blood glucose concentrations with total parenteral nutrition: Is it necessary to taper total parenteral nutrition? Nutr Clin Pract 2003;18:414–416.

73. Krzyda EA, Andris DA, Whipple JK, et al. Glucose response to abrupt initiation and discontinuation of total parenteral nutrition. J Parenter Enter Nutr 1993;17:64–67.

74. Campos ACL, Paluzzi M, Meguid MM. Clinical use of total nutrient admixtures. Nutrition 1990;6:347–356.

75. American Society for Health-System Pharmacists. ASHP guidelines on the safe use of automated compounding devices for the preparation of parenteral nutrition admixtures. Am J Health Syst Pharm 2000;57:1343–1348.

76. USP General Information Chapter. Pharmaceutical Compounding: Ster-ile Preparations (797). USP 27/NF 22. Rockville, MD, United States Pharmacopeia Convention, 2003.

77. Thompson B, Robinson LA. Infection control of parenteral nutrition solutions. Nutr Clin Pract 1991;6:49–54.

78. Ebbert ML, Farraj M, Hwang LT. The incidence and clinical signifi-cance of intravenous fat emulsion contamination during infusion. JPEN J Parenter Enter Nutr 1987;11:42–45.

79. Fox M, Molesky M, Van Aerde JE, Muttitt S. Changing parenteral nutri-tion administration sets every 24 h versus every 48 h in newborn infants. Can J Gastroenterol 1999;13:147–151.

80. Sacks GS, Driscoll DF. Does lipid hang time make a difference? Time is of the essence. Nutr Clin Pract 2002;17:284–290.

81. Trissel LA. Handbook on Injectable Drugs, 12th ed. Bethesda, MD, American Society for Hospital Pharmacists, 2003.

82. King JC, Catania PN, ed. King Guide to Parenteral Admixtures. Napa, CA, King Guide Publications, 2003.

83. Trissel LA. Amino acid injection. In: Handbook on Injectable Drugs, 12th ed. Bethesda, MD, American Society for Hospital Pharmacists, 2003:45–90.

84. Laborie S, Lavoie JC, Pineault M, Chessex P. Contribution of mul-tivitamins, air and light in the generation of peroxides in adult and neonatal parenteral nutrition solutions. Ann Pharmacother 2000;34:440–445.

85. Laborie S, Lavoie JC, Pineault M, Chessex P. Protecting solutions of par-enteral nutrition from peroxidation. JPEN J Parenter Enter Nutr 1999;23:104–108.

86. Neuzil J, Darlow BA, Inder TE, et al. Oxidation of parenteral lipid emul-sion by ambient and phototherapy lights: Potential toxicity of routine parenteral feeding. J Pediatr 1995;126:785–790.

87. Helbock HJ, Ames BN. Use of intravenous lipids in neonates. J Pediatr 1995;126:747–748.

88. Driscoll DF, Baptista RJ, Mitrano FP, et al. Parenteral nutrient admixtures as drug vehicles: Theory and practice in the critical care setting. DICP 1991;25:276–283.

89. Mermel LA, Farr BM, Sherertz RJ, et al. Guidelines for the man-agement of intravascular catheter-related infections. Clin Infect Dis 2001;32:1249–1272.

90. McMahon MM. Management of parenteral nutrition in acutely ill patients with hyperglycemia. Nutr Clin Pract 2004;19:120–128.

91. Teasley-Strausburg KM, Shronts EP. Metabolic and gastrointestinal com-plications. In Teasley-Strausburg KM, ed. Nutrition Support Handbook: A Compendium of Products with Guidelines for Usage. Cincinnati, Harvey Whitney Books, 1992:295–303.

92. Howard L, Ashley C. Management of complications in patients receiving home parenteral nutrition. Gastroenterology 2003;124:1651–1661.

93. Briones ER, Iber FL. Liver and biliary tract changes and injury associated with total parenteral nutrition: Pathogenesis and prevention. J Am Coll Nutr 1995;14:219–228.

94. Quigley EMM, Marsh MN, Shaffer JL, Markin RS. Hepatobiliary complications of total parenteral nutrition. Gastroenterology 1993;104:286–301.

95. Btaiche IF, Khalidi N. Parenteral nutrition-associated liver complications in children. Pharmacotherapy 2002;22:188–211.

96. Brooks MJ, Melnik G. The refeeding syndrome: An approach to understanding its complications and preventing its occurrence. Pharmacotherapy 1995;15:713–726.

97. Centers for Disease Control. Lactic acidosis traced to thiamine deficiency related to nationwide shortage of multivitamins for total parenteral nutrition—United States, 1997. MMWR Morb Mortal Week Rep 1997;46:523–528.

98. Buchman AL, Moukarzel A. Metabolic bone disease associated with total parenteral nutrition. Clin Nutr 2000;19:217–231.

99. Mouser JF, Hak EB, Helms RA, et al. Chromium and zinc concentrations in pediatric patients receiving long-term parenteral nutrition. Am J Health Sys Pharm 1999;56:1950–1956.

100. Dickerson RN. Manganese intoxication and parenteral nutrition. Nutrition 2001;17:689–693.

101. Davis A, Spillane R, Zublena L. Aluminum: A problem trace metal in nutrition support. Nutr Clin Pract 1999;14:227–231.

102. Klein GL, Leichter AM, Heyman MB, and the Patient Care Committee of the North American Society for Pediatric Gastroenterology and Nutrition. Aluminum in large and small volume parenterals used in total parenteral nutrition: Response to the Food and Drug Administration notice proposed rule by the North American Society for Pediatric Gastroenterology and Nutrition. J Pediatr Gastroenterol Nutr 1998;27:457–460.

103. Food and Drug Administration. Aluminum in large and small volume parenterals used in total parenteral nutrition. Fed Regist 2000;65:4103–4111.

104. Advenier E, Landry C, Colomb V, et al. Aluminum contamination of parenteral nutrition and aluminum loading in children on long-term parenteral nutrition. J Pediatr Gastroenterol Nutr 2003;36:448–453.

105. DeLegge MH. Demographics of home parenteral nutrition. JPEN J Parenter Enter Nutr 2002;26:S60–S62.

106. Lipman TO. The cost of TPN: Is the price right? JPEN J Parenter Enter Nutr 1993;17:199–200.

107. Eisenberg JM, Glick HA, Buzby GP, et al. Does perioperative total parenteral nutrition reduce medical care costs? JPEN J Parenter Enter Nutr 1993;17:201–209.

108. Twomey PL, Patching SC. Cost effectiveness of nutritional support. JPEN J Parenter Enter Nutr 1985;9:3–10.

109. Eisenberg JM, Glick H, Hillman AL, et al. Measuring the economic impact of perioperative total parenteral nutrition: Principles and design. Am J Clin Nutr 1988;47:382–391.

110. ASPEN Board of Directors and The Clinical Guidelines Taskforce. Specific guidelines for disease-pediatrics. JPEN J Parenter Enter Nutr 2002;26:111SA–138SA.

111. Trujillo EB, Young LS, Chertow GM, et al. Metabolic and monetary costs of avoidable parenteral nutrition use. JPEN J Parenter Enter Nutr 1999;23:109–113.

112. Lipman TO. Grains or veins: Is enteral nutrition really better than parenteral nutrition? A look at the evidence. JPEN J Parenter Enter Nutr 1998;22:167–182.

113. Trice S, Melnik G, Page C. Complications and costs of early postoperative parenteral versus enteral nutrition in trauma patients. Nutr Clin Pract 1997;12:114–119.

114. Task Force on Specialty Recognition and Certification of Nutritional Support Pharmacists. Executive summary of petition requesting recognition of nutritional support pharmacy as a specialty. Am J Hosp Pharm 1991;48:1284.

138
ENTERAL NUTRITION

Vanessa J. Kumpf and Katherine Hammond Chessman

Learning Objectives and other resources can be found at *www.pharmacotherapyonline.com.*

KEY CONCEPTS

1 The gastrointestinal (GI) tract defends the host from toxins and antigens by both immunologic and nonimmunologic mechanisms, collectively referred to as the gut barrier function. Whenever possible, enteral nutrition (EN) is preferred over parenteral nutrition (PN) because it is as effective, may reduce metabolic and infectious complications, and is less expensive.

2 Candidates for EN are those who cannot or will not eat, those who exhibit a sufficiently functioning GI tract to allow adequate nutrient absorption, and in whom enteral access can be safely obtained.

3 The most common route for both short-term and long-term EN access is directly into the stomach. The method of delivery may be either continuously via an infusion pump, intermittently via a pump or gravity drip, or bolus administration.

4 Patients unable to tolerate feeding directly into the stomach due to impaired gastric motility or for those at high risk of aspiration, feeding tube tip placement into the duodenum or jejunum may be indicated. When feeding into the small bowel, the continuous method of delivery via an infusion pump is required in order to enhance tolerance.

5 Selection of the enteral feeding formulation depends on nutritional requirements, the patient's primary disease state and related complications, and nutrient digestibility and

absorption. A standard polymeric formulation will meet the needs of the majority of adult patients and children older than 10 years of age.

6 Measurement of gastric residual volumes can be used to monitor GI tolerance in patients receiving gastric feeding. Although not always reliable, excessive residual volumes may be associated with nausea, abdominal distention, and increased risk for aspiration.

7 Management of diarrhea in patients receiving EN should focus on identification and correction of the most likely cause(s). Tube feeding–related causes include too rapid delivery or advancement of formula, intolerance to the formula composition, and occasionally formula contamination.

8 Prior to administering medications through a feeding tube, the feeding tube tip location should be verified (stomach or small bowel) and the most suitable dosage form selected. Medications that should not be crushed and administered through a tube include enteric-coated or sustained-release capsules or tablets and sublingual or buccal tablets.

9 The coadministration of medications with EN can result in alterations in bioavailability and/or changes in the desired pharmacologic effects of several medications, including phenytoin, warfarin, selected antibiotics, antacids, and omeprazole.

Enteral nutrition (EN) is defined as the delivery of nutrients by tube or by mouth into the GI tract. This chapter focuses on nutrient delivery through a feeding tube rather than the oral ingestion of food. The terms EN and tube feeding are thus used interchangeably in this context. The goal of EN is to provide calories, macronutrients, and micronutrients to patients unable to achieve these requirements from an oral diet. Over the past 20 to 30 years, EN has replaced parenteral nutrition (PN) as the preferred method of specialized nutrition support in many patients at risk of malnutrition. Improvements in enteral access techniques and feeding formulations, and the recognition of methods to prevent and manage complications have resulted in an increased use of EN across all health care settings.

In this chapter, the principles and practices related to the successful use of EN support are described. Digestive and absorptive physiology is reviewed and the beneficial effects of EN are presented. The indications for EN, and descriptions of various enteral access and administration methods are also summarized. Characteristics of

commercially available enteral feeding formulations are presented, as well as initiation and monitoring guidelines to prevent and manage complications. Clinical therapeutic controversies are highlighted and discussed. In addition, issues of drug compatibility, drug-nutrient interactions, and drug administration via enteral feeding tubes are discussed. Finally, the effectiveness and pharmacoeconomics of EN in enhancing nutrition and disease outcome goals are reviewed.

GASTROINTESTINAL TRACT PHYSIOLOGY

DIGESTION AND ABSORPTION

Digestion and absorption are GI processes that generate the body's usable fuels.[1–3] Digestion consists of the stepwise conversion of a complex chemical and physical nutrient into a molecular form which is absorbable by the intestinal mucosa. Absorption from the GI tract

TABLE 138–1. Gastrointestinal Enzymes and Hormones

Enzyme/Hormone	Site of Secretion	Main Actions
Amylase	Salivary glands, pancreas	Converts carbohydrates, starch, and glycogen to simple disaccharides
Cholecystokinin (CCK)	Duodenum, jejunum	Stimulates pancreatic enzyme secretion and gallbladder contraction
Chymotrypsinogen	Pancreas	Breaks down proteins into proteases and peptides
Enteroglucagon	Duodenum, small intestine	Inhibits pancreatic enzyme secretion and bowel motility
Gastric inhibitory peptide (GIP)	Small intestine	Decreases gastric motility and stimulates insulin secretion
Gastrin	Stomach, duodenum	Stimulates gastric acid secretion and mucosal growth
Glucagon	Pancreas	Stimulates hepatic glycogenolysis and inhibits motility
Lipase	Pancreas	Hydrolyzes short-chain and medium-chain triglycerides, involved in fat absorption
Pancreatic polypeptide	Pancreas	Inhibits gallbladder contraction and pancreatic and biliary secretion
Pepsinogen	Stomach	Converts large proteins into polypeptides
Secretin	Small intestine	Stimulates hepatic and pancreatic water and bicarbonate
Trypsinogen	Pancreas	Breaks down proteins into proteases and peptides
Vasoactive inhibitory peptide (VIP)	Small intestine, pancreas	Vasodilator; stimulates water and bicarbonate secretion, release of insulin and glucagon, and production of small intestinal juice

is a multistep process that includes the transfer of a nutrient across the intestinal cell membrane. The nutrient ultimately reaches the systemic circulation through the portal venous or splanchnic lymphatic systems, provided the GI or biliary tract does not excrete it. Ingested nutrients are primarily large polymers that cannot be absorbed by the intestinal cell membrane unless they are transformed into an absorbable molecular form. In addition, a coordinated interplay of GI motility and neurohormonal secretion is required to facilitate adequate digestion and absorption.

Nutrient digestion involves the complex coordination of multiple mechanical, enzymatic, and physicochemical processes.[1–3] Mechanical dissolution of food occurs by chewing, mixing, and grinding of the stomach contents. Food stimulates the secretion of numerous neurohormones and enzymes from the salivary glands, stomach, liver and biliary system, pancreas, and intestines (Table 138–1). As food passes along the gut lumen, these neurohormones modulate GI motility and the secretions from subsequent organs of the digestive system. Nutrient digestion occurs within the gut lumen and is a specific function of the intestinal cell membrane, which is comprised of finger-like pro-

jections called the villi. Each individual villus is made up of epithelial cells called enterocytes. The enterocyte surface contains special luminal projections called microvilli, which provide an increased surface area that is referred to as the brush border membrane.

Digestion and absorption of carbohydrate, fat, and protein within the small intestine is illustrated in Fig. 138–1. Carbohydrates are presented to the small intestine as either a digestible or nondigestible form. Polysaccharides (starches) and oligosaccharides (sucrose and lactose) undergo enzymatic digestion within the small intestine to produce simple sugars. The simple sugars are absorbed via active and passive transport mechanisms and are eventually released into the portal vein. Polysaccharides such as cellulose complexes and other fiber components pass undigested to the colon, where they are digested by bacteria and enzymes to short-chain fatty acids (SCFAs).[4] Absorption of SCFAs by the colon stimulates sodium and water reabsorption, serves as an energy source, and provides nourishment to the colonic mucosa cells.

Fat is presented to the small intestine as long-chain triglycerides (LCTs).[5] Its digestion requires pancreatic enzyme release and

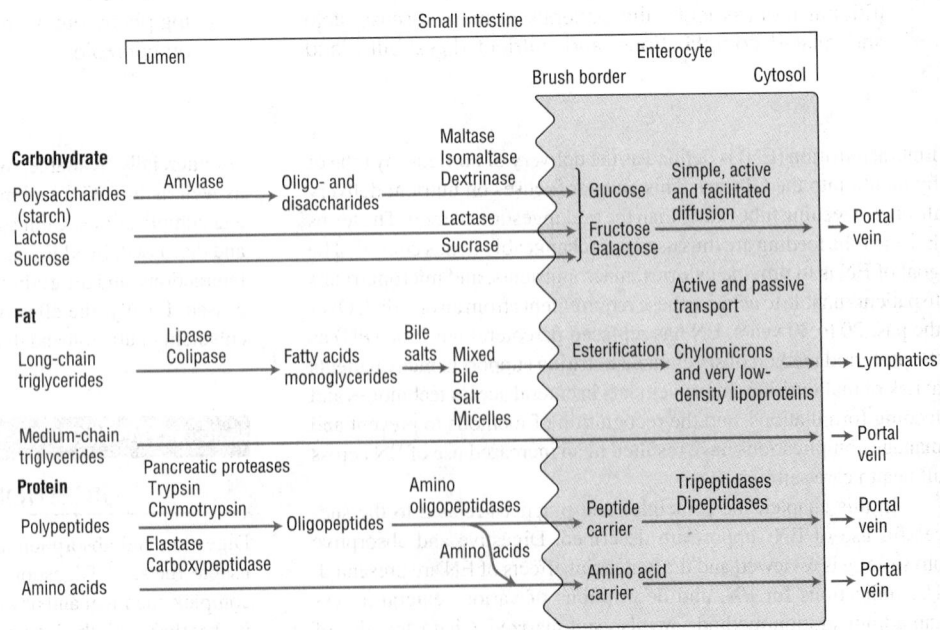

FIGURE 138–1. Schematic representation of carbohydrate, fat, and protein digestion.

TABLE 138–2. Factors Affecting Intestinal Nutrient Absorption

Method of ingestion
Digestibility
Gastric emptying
Intraluminal digestive capacity of the pancreas and the bile
Transit time
Contact surface
  Length
  Surface of villi
  Brush border enzyme content
  Carrier function
  Diffusion barrier thickness (unstirred layer)

formation of mixed bile salt micelles, which then facilitate absorption across the intestinal enterocyte. Within the enterocyte, triglycerides are re-esterified and packaged into chylomicrons for release into the lymphatic system. Medium-chain triglycerides (MCTs) can be absorbed intact by the mucosal membrane and are acted on by intracellular lipase within the enterocyte to release free fatty acids which pass directly into the portal vein.

Protein is presented to the small intestine primarily as large polypeptides and to a small extent as free amino acids due to the denaturation of protein within the stomach. Luminal polypeptide digestion generates oligopeptides, which are further hydrolyzed to dipeptides and tripeptides. Absorption of peptides occurs via a peptide transport system while free amino acids are carried via specific amino acid transport systems. The carriers for the peptides have proven to be very efficient, whereas absorption of free amino acids appears to be more limited and less efficient.[3] Understanding the mechanisms of digestive and absorptive physiology can greatly enhance the rational use of EN support during conditions of normal or altered GI anatomy and/or function. Several circumstances may alter the efficacy of nutrient digestion and absorption (Table 138–2). For example, the functional immaturity of the neonatal gut may lead to clinical problems associated with inadequate digestion and absorption of EN. These factors, as they relate to successful EN practice, are discussed in detail throughout this chapter.

GUT HOST DEFENSE MECHANISMS

Besides digesting and absorbing nutrients to maintain nutritional health, the GI tract is actively involved in defending the host from toxins and antigens by means of nonimmunologic and immunologic mechanisms (Table 138–3).[6] These gut host defense mechanisms are

TABLE 138–3. Gut Host Defense Mechanisms

Nonimmunologic	Immunologic
Mechanical	Gut-associated lymphoid tissue (GALT)
Epithelial cell	Secretory immunoglobulin A
Epithelial mucus gel layer	Hepatic Kupffer cells
Peristalsis	
Gastric acid	
Bile salts	
Salivary secretions	
Indigenous microflora	
Limits microbial	
proliferation	
Microbial antagonism	

also collectively referred to as the gut barrier function. The gut barrier acts to prevent the spread of intraluminal bacteria and endotoxin to systemic organs and tissues. Hydrochloric acid secreted by the stomach kills the majority of the bacteria ingested with food. Under normal circumstances, a mucus gel layer coats the intestinal epithelium and thereby alters the adherence of bacteria to the cells of the GI tract and provides a favorable environment for anaerobic bacteria. Anaerobic bacteria, which normally colonize the mucus layer, aid in preventing tissue colonization by potential pathogens. Small bowel peristalsis further prevents bacterial stasis and overgrowth. The gut barrier function is also maintained by the intestinal immune system, known as the gut-associated lymphoid tissue (GALT). This GALT regulates the local immune response to antigens within the GI tract. Specific immunoglobulins are secreted to kill remaining organisms and neutralize any toxins they produce. The hepatic Kupffer cells help to maintain gut barrier function by clearing the portal blood of gut-derived bacteria and endotoxins. The integrity of gut barrier function may be affected by numerous pathogenic insults such as physiologic stress and ischemia, and a variety of drugs, including chemotherapeutic agents. The nutritional aspects that influence the maintenance of the gut barrier will be addressed later in this chapter.

INDICATIONS FOR ENTERAL NUTRITION

The decision to initiate EN is based on a variety of factors as outlined in Fig. 136–1 in Chap. 136. Suitable candidates are those who cannot or will not eat a sufficient amount to meet nutritional requirements, those who exhibit a sufficient functioning GI tract to allow the absorption of nutrients, and those in whom a method of enteral access can be safely obtained.[7,8] Enteral nutrition may be indicated in a variety of conditions or disease states (Table 138–4). For example, patients who have certain neurologic disorders, such as following a cerebrovascular accident, and have difficulty swallowing

TABLE 138–4. Potential Indications for Enteral Nutrition

Neoplastic disease	**Gastrointestinal disease**
Chemotherapy	Inflammatory bowel disease
Radiation therapy	Short bowel syndrome
Upper gastrointestinal tumors	Esophageal motility disorder
Cancer cachexia	Pancreatitis
Organ failure	Fistulas
Hepatic	Gastroesophageal reflux disease
Renal	Esophageal atresia
Cardiac cachexia	**Neurologic impairment**
Pulmonary	Comatose state
Bronchopulmonary dysplasia	Cerebrovascular accident
Congenital heart disease	Demyelinating disease
Hypermetabolic states	Severe depression
Closed head injury	Failure to thrive
Burns	Cerebral palsy
Trauma	**Other indications**
Postoperative major surgery	Acquired immune deficiency
Sepsis	syndrome
	Anorexia nervosa
	Complications during pregnancy
	Geriatric patients with multiple
	chronic diseases
	Organ transplantation
	Inborn errors of metabolism
	Cystic fibrosis
	Extreme prematurity

often require EN. Patients unable to eat due to conditions such as facial or jaw injuries, lesions of the oral cavity or esophagus, esophageal stricture, or head and neck cancer may be candidates for EN delivered distal to the affected site. Extreme prematurity necessitates tube feeding because the suck-swallow mechanism has not yet developed sufficiently to allow safe oral intake.

Critically ill patients who are endotracheally intubated for mechanical ventilation represent a large percentage of patients requiring EN. Many of these patients may have reduced gastric motility and emptying caused by sepsis, postoperative anesthetic agents, opioid analgesics, and underlying pathology such as diabetic gastroparesis. However, successful EN can often be achieved by bypassing the stomach and placing the tip of the feeding tube beyond the pylorus into the duodenum, or preferably into the jejunum.

The use of EN during acute pancreatitis has increased. Concerns that feeding may exacerbate the disease process by stimulating exocrine pancreatic secretion historically led to the widespread use of PN and bowel rest in these patients. However, EN is well tolerated in patients with pancreatitis if the GI tract is otherwise functioning normally.[9] The degree of pancreatic stimulation depends on the location of the tip of the feeding tube and the composition of the feeding formulation. The more distally the feeding is delivered, the less pancreatic stimulation occurs. Jejunal feeding is associated with fewer complications than PN in patients with acute pancreatitis and has not been shown to exacerbate the disease. When patients with pancreatitis require specialized nutrition support, EN should be attempted prior to initiating PN.[7]

The only absolute contraindications for EN are mechanical obstruction[8] and necrotizing enterocolitis.[10] However, conditions such as severe diarrhea, protracted vomiting, enteric fistulae, severe GI hemorrhage, and intestinal dysmotility may result in significant challenges to the successful use of EN.

BENEFITS OF ENTERAL NUTRITION

The importance of maintaining nutrient delivery through the GI tract in patients without contraindication to its use is well supported. The possible reasons for the apparent beneficial effects of EN when compared to PN will be discussed. Another factor contributing to the beneficial effects of EN, specifically in the critically ill patient, is related to when it is initiated. Initiating EN within 24 to 48 hours of admission to an intensive care unit may be beneficial.

ENTERAL VERSUS PARENTERAL NUTRITION

A considerable body of laboratory and clinical evidence supports the importance and potential advantages of using EN when compared to PN. Clinical studies comparing EN to PN in the critically ill or injured patient often demonstrate improved outcomes from EN in terms of decreased infectious complications.[11–13] The precise mechanism that accounts for the apparent beneficial effects is not clear. One suggested explanation for the decrease in infectious complications is that EN prevents bacterial translocation.

Bacterial translocation is the migration of bacteria, fungi, or endotoxins from the GI tract through the mucosal barrier. Without intraluminal fuels, it has been proposed that the integrity and function of the GI tract may deteriorate, and under stress, allow for the translocation of microbes or endotoxins.[14] It is further proposed that endotoxin release can activate inflammatory pathways and thereby contribute to the development of multisystem organ failure. Provision of enteral nutrients appears to help maintain intestinal mucosal structure and

function.[15] It has been suggested that this will prevent translocation of gut bacteria to the portal or lymphatic circulation. However, this theory is primarily limited to data supporting the occurrence of bacterial translocation in the animal model and human studies are not available. There is no direct evidence to suggest that EN prevents or modifies bacterial translocation in humans; only indirect evidence exists.[14,16,17] Enteral nutrition appears to play some type of role in maintaining gut mucosal growth and development to preserve gut barrier function, but the mechanism remains unclear.

Critical reviews of available randomized controlled trials comparing EN to PN in the critically ill adult patient with an intact GI tract suggest a significant reduction in infectious complications associated with EN.[7,13] Decreased infectious complications have been documented in patients with abdominal trauma, burns, or severe head injury given EN compared to PN. The use of EN has been recommended over PN as the preferred route of feeding in the critically ill patient requiring specialized nutrition support.[7,13]

Enteral nutrition is more physiologic than PN in terms of nutrient utilization and is therefore generally associated with fewer metabolic complications. A metabolic advantage of enteral feeding compared with the parenteral route is improved glucose tolerance and lower insulin requirements to maintain normoglycemia.[18] It has been proposed that better blood glucose control occurs during enteral administration because the insulin released is absorbed with the glucose via the portal vein and is handled by the liver. The enteral route is also as effective as the parenteral route in maintaining or promoting repletion of nutritional indices among several patient populations.[19] An additional physiologic benefit of enteral feeding is that it stimulates bile flow through the biliary tract and hence reduces the development of gallbladder sludge and stone formation, which has been associated with long-term PN and bowel rest.[20] Also, EN avoids the potential infectious and technical complications associated with the placement and use of a central venous access device typically required for PN. Finally, EN is less costly than PN when all factors are considered.

EARLY VERSUS DELAYED INITIATION

The optimal timing of initiation of EN is a controversial issue. It has been suggested that initiating EN early in the course of illness may attenuate the stress response and improve feeding tolerance. Clinical studies demonstrating a decrease in infectious complications with the use of EN compared to PN in the critically ill patient initiated feeding within 24 to 48 hours of hospital admission.[21,22] It appears that the benefits of decreased infectious complications are not apparent when the initiation of EN is delayed. A review of available studies comparing early versus delayed EN in critically ill patients showed a trend toward a reduction in infectious complications with early EN.[13] In addition, a trend toward reduction in mortality associated with early EN was noted.

In critically ill patients who are hemodynamically unstable, early EN may result in gut ischemia due to poor gut blood flow and increased oxygen demand. It is therefore recommended to delay initiation of EN until the patient is fluid resuscitated and has an adequate perfusion pressure. Once this goal is obtained, often within 6 hours of hospitalization, the initiation of low rates of EN is considered appropriate as long as close clinical monitoring for GI intolerance is maintained.[23,24] Therefore, early EN (within 24 to 48 hours after hospital admission) has been recommended in critically ill patients.[13]

Early initiation of EN does not apply to the mild to moderately stressed patient who is otherwise well nourished. It is reasonable to delay the initiation of EN in these patients until oral intake is inadequate for 7 to 14 days or expected to be inadequate over a 7- to 14-day period.[7]

TABLE 138–5. Options and Considerations in the Selection of Enteral Access

Access	Indications	Tube Placement Options	Advantages	Disadvantages
Nasogastric or orogastric	Short-term Intact gag reflex Normal gastric emptying	Manually at bedside	Ease of placement Allows for all methods of administration Inexpensive Multiple commercially available tubes and sizes	Potential tube displacement Potential increased aspiration risk
Nasoduodenal or nasojejunal	Short-term Impaired gastric motility or emptying High risk of GER or aspiration	Manually at bedside Fluoroscopically Endoscopically	Potential reduced aspiration risk Allows for early postinjury or postoperative feeding Multiple commercially available tubes and sizes	Manual transpyloric passage requires greater skill Potential tube displacement or clogging Bolus or intermittent feeding not tolerated
Gastrostomy	Long-term Normal gastric emptying	Surgically Endoscopically Radiologically Laparoscopically	Allows for all methods of administration Large-bore tubes less likely to clog Multiple commercially available tubes and sizes Low-profile buttons available	Attendant risks associated with each type of procedure Potential increased aspiration risk Requires stoma site care
Jejunostomy	Long-term Impaired gastric motility or gastric emptying High risk of GER or aspiration	Surgically Endoscopically Radiologically Laparoscopically	Allows for early postinjury or postoperative feeding Potential reduced aspiration risk Multiple commercially available tubes and sizes	Attendant risks associated with each type of procedure Bolus or intermittent feeding not tolerated Requires stoma site care

GER, gastroesophageal reflux.

ENTERAL ACCESS

Recent advances in enteral access techniques have contributed to the expanded use of EN for conditions in which PN had previously been used. In particular, improved methods of achieving jejunal access for feeding have allowed for the use of EN during the early postoperative and postinjury period when gastric motility is typically delayed. As outlined in Table 138–5, various factors influence the selection of access site, including anticipated duration of use (short-term or long-term) and whether to feed into the stomach or small bowel. A review

of the various enteral access options is important because it influences the overall success of achieving nutrient goals by the enteral route. Illustrations of enteral access options are shown in Fig. 138–2.

SHORT-TERM ACCESS

Short-term enteral access is generally easier, less invasive, and less costly than long-term access.[25] The most frequently used routes for short-term enteral access are those accessed by inserting a tube through the nose and passing the tip into the stomach

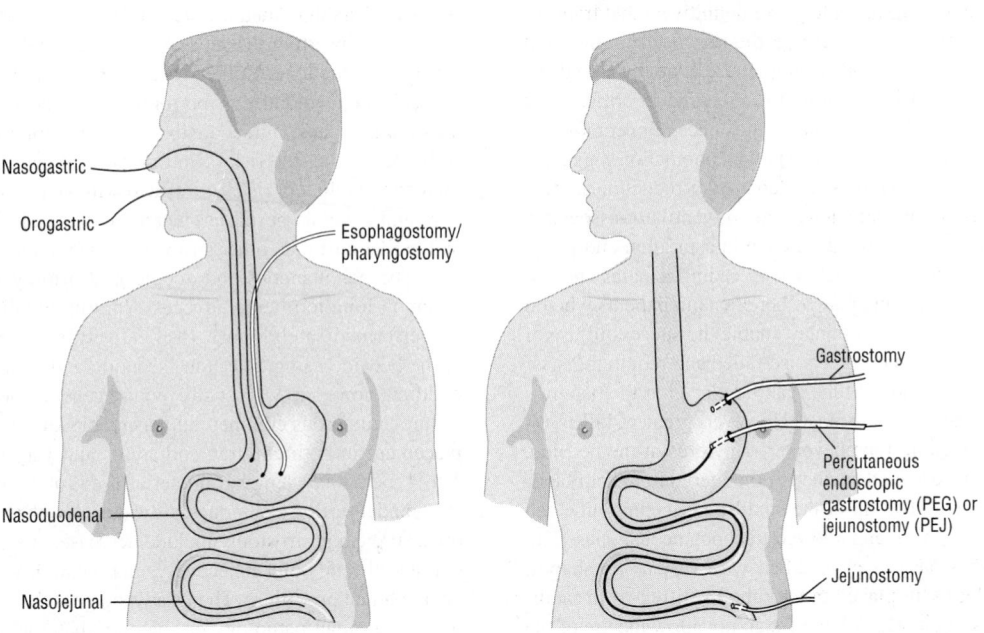

FIGURE 138–2. Access sites for tube feeding.

(nasogastric; NG), duodenum (nasoduodenal; ND), or jejunum (nasojejunal; NJ). In general, these tubes are used in the hospitalized patient when the anticipated tube feeding duration is less than 4 to 6 weeks. The orogastric (OG) route is generally reserved for patients in whom the nasopharyngeal area is inaccessible or in young infants who are obligate nasal breathers. These routes do not require surgical intervention and therefore are the least invasive. The feeding tube is frequently held in place only by a piece of tape on the nose or face, and therefore can be inadvertently pulled out relatively easily.

Nasogastric tubes vary in diameter size and stiffness. The large-bore ($\geq$14French [F]) rigid NG tubes are used primarily to decompress the stomach, but can also be used for feeding. There is a low incidence of clogging with these tubes, and they provide a reliable way to measure gastric residual volumes. The major disadvantage associated with the use of these tubes is patient discomfort. Small-bore nasal tubes designed solely for feeding are available in varying lengths (16 to 60 inches) and diameter sizes (5 to 12F) to accommodate both pediatric (including neonates) and adult patients. The tip of the tube can be placed into the stomach, duodenum, or jejunum. These tubes consist of a lightweight, pliable silicone or polyurethane material that is comfortable to the patient. A disadvantage of the small-bore tubes is that they may become occluded, often due to improper medication or tube flushing technique. Another disadvantage to the use of these tubes is that they do not allow a reliable way to monitor gastric residual volumes, as they will collapse when aspiration of gastric contents is attempted. Therefore when the monitoring of gastric residual volumes is important, such as in a critically ill patient, a large-bore NG tube is preferred.

◄ In general, the stomach is the least expensive and the least labor-intensive access site to use for enteral feeding; however, feeding into the stomach is not always tolerated. Patients with impaired gastric motility may be predisposed to aspiration and pneumonia when feedings are delivered into the stomach. Many critically ill, injured, and postoperative patients exhibit delayed gastric emptying, limiting their ability to tolerate gastric feeding. In addition, patients with diabetic gastroparesis or patients with severe gastroesophageal reflux disease or intractable vomiting are at a higher risk for aspiration of gastric contents resulting in pneumonia. In these patients, placing the tip of the tube into the duodenum or jejunum (also referred to as transpyloric placement) may be required to enable successful enteral feeding. However, studies have yet to prove definitively that transpyloric tube feedings actually do decrease the risk of aspiration and pneumonia, but are limited by small sample size. One meta-analysis of studies comparing gastric to transpyloric feeding in critically ill patients demonstrated no difference in the incidence of pneumonia,[26] while another critical review of the same patient population suggested that small bowel feedings were associated with a reduction in gastroesophageal regurgitation and a lower rate of ventilator-associated pneumonia.[27] Therefore, the true difference in aspiration and pneumonia risk between gastric and small bowel feeding remains unclear. However, the transpyloric route may be beneficial in patients who do not tolerate gastric feeding. Its use may enable the successful use of EN in patients who would have otherwise failed and required PN.

The NG, OG, ND, and NJ tubes can be placed at the patient's bedside by trained medical personnel. However, greater skill is required to place the feeding tube beyond the pylorus at the bedside. Several techniques have been described in the literature to help facilitate bedside placement. The tip of the small-bore feeding tube can be inserted into the stomach and allowed to spontaneously pass into the duodenum. Tubes have been modified with various tip shapes, weights, and a stylet (wire placed in the tube to stiffen it) to facilitate transpyloric insertion. Many facilities do not allow the use of the stylet at the bedside, however, due to the risk of inadvertent tube place-

ment into the lung. Prokinetic agents, such as metoclopramide and erythromycin, have been given prior to insertion to increase GI motility and facilitate spontaneous passage of the tube from the stomach into the small intestine.[28,29] Variable success rates have been reported with these techniques and is likely largely dependent on clinician experience. Alternatively, a variety of endoscopic and fluoroscopic techniques have been described to insert transpyloric tubes.[25] Radiographic confirmation of NG or transpyloric feeding tubes placed by bedside techniques should be obtained prior to use to verify appropriate tip placement.[7]

LONG-TERM ACCESS

Feeding tubes used for short-term enteral access are usually not optimal for long-term use due to patient discomfort, long-term complications, and mechanical failures that develop over time. Long-term access should generally be considered when EN is anticipated for longer than 4 to 6 weeks. Many techniques can be used to establish long-term enteral access, including laparotomy, laparoscopy, endoscopy, and fluoroscopy. The ability to perform the various techniques will be somewhat dependent on the expertise and facilities available within each institution. Long-term enteral access options include esophagostomy, pharyngostomy, gastrostomy, and jejunostomy.

Pharyngostomies and esophagostomies are invasive because the tube is located in the neck and passes through the skin into the esophagus or the pharynx. Historically, they have been used in patients with head and neck malignancies or patients with impaired swallowing due to neuromuscular disorders. However, better long-term enteral access techniques have replaced the need for the pharyngostomy and esophagotomy routes. They are rarely performed today due to the high complication rate and extreme difficulty associated with their care.[30]

A gastrostomy is the most common type of long-term enteral access. It eliminates the nasal irritation and discomfort associated with an NG, OG, ND, or NJ feeding tube and inadvertent removal is unlikely. In addition, since feeding gastrostomies utilize large-bore tubes, clogging is typically not a problem. Multiple techniques for insertion of a gastrostomy tube have been described, including surgical laparotomy, endoscopy, radiography, and laparoscopy. Surgical placement of a gastrostomy tube can be done at the time of a laparotomy for an unrelated problem, or it can be performed for the sole purpose of inserting the tube. Advantages of the open surgical gastrostomy compared to other gastrostomy techniques include a high success rate, avoidance of perforation and laceration of other intra-abdominal organs, and secure fixation of the stomach to the abdominal wall (decreasing the risk of intraperitoneal leakage). Disadvantages include the inherent risks associated with an invasive surgical procedure and general anesthesia, increased pain, a longer recovery time, and higher cost than other gastrostomy techniques.

The percutaneous endoscopic gastrostomy (PEG) is the most common long-term enteral access. It is minimally invasive and can be performed safely and cost-effectively in an endoscopy suite or at the bedside using conscious sedation and local anesthesia. Small children, however, will usually require general anesthesia for the procedure. Numerous commercially available kits are available for PEG placement in both children and adults and vary in size (12 to 28F; 1 to 4.5 cm shaft lengths), material used, internal and external bolsters, and insertion techniques. Advantages of the PEG compared with open surgical gastrostomy include decreased cost, avoidance of general anesthesia, quicker recovery, and the ability to be performed as an outpatient procedure. The disadvantage is the inability to visualize intra-abdominal pathology or anatomy that could lead to laceration or perforation of other organs. Also, early dislodgment of the PEG can lead to intra-abdominal leakage and peritonitis if the tract has not matured, because the only thing holding the stomach to the abdominal wall is the internal bolster. A review combining the results of 95 studies evaluating the use of the PEG procedure showed a 96.5% success rate and 0.7% procedure-related mortality rate.[30] However, the 30-day mortality rate was 10.5% and significantly higher than the open surgical gastrostomy, indicating that the procedure is being performed in patients who have existing severe comorbid conditions. The ethical implications regarding determination of appropriate candidates for PEG placement has been a topic of considerable interest in the literature.[30–32] The PEG tube is often placed inappropriately based on unrealistic and inaccurate expectations of what EN can accomplish in patients unable to eat. Patients with an unclear prognosis should be carefully selected and may benefit from a 60-day trial of small-bore NG feedings prior to PEG placement.[33]

Newer techniques for gastrostomy placement may be considered if the stomach cannot be accessed via endoscopy, including the percutaneous radiologic gastrostomy and laparoscopic gastrostomy.[30,34,35] The percutaneous radiologic gastrostomy (PRG) technique has been described using fluoroscopy, ultrasound, or computed tomography scan. These procedures are performed by interventional radiologists and involve distending the stomach and percutaneously cannulating the stomach with a needle to allow gastrostomy insertion. Placement requires a radiologist skilled in the procedure and use of local anesthesia with or without conscious sedation. The tubes used are usually smaller than a PEG (9 to 14F), so they may become more easily occluded. The laparoscopic gastrostomy is performed in the operating room, usually under general anesthesia. It provides another option to the open surgical gastrostomy if a PEG or PRG is not possible due to altered anatomy or other complications.

Once the gastrostomy tract has matured, a low-profile skin-level gastrostomy device may be placed for patient convenience and comfort. This device, a "gastric button," consists of a short silicone self-retaining conduit with either a mushroom tip or a balloon at the internal end and a one-way valve and small flange at the external end. It offers the convenience of avoiding having a tube end protruding when not in use, so it tends to be preferred in children or ambulatory adults who are receiving intermittent feedings. The exit site of all gastrostomies requires general stoma care to prevent inflammation and infection. When a gastrostomy tube is no longer needed, it can be easily removed. In adults, a common practice is to cut off the tube at skin level and allow retained components to pass through the GI tract. This technique has been associated with serious complications in children, including esophageal perforation and death, and therefore is not recommended in children.[36–38] Gastrostomy removal by traction or endoscopy (if there is an internal bolster) is associated with few complications. The gastrocutaneous fistula closes spontaneously in more than 70% of patients. If leaking continues, most cases will respond to use of histamine$_2$-antagonist therapy and silver nitrate cautery. Surgical closure is required in up to 23% of cases.[35] In general, the longer the tube is in place, the more likely it is that the fistulous tract will require surgical closure. Patients whose tubes are in place for less than 11 months are more likely to have spontaneous closure than those whose tubes are in for longer than 11 months.[36]

In patients at high risk of gastroesophageal reflux disease and aspiration who require long-term enteral access, a jejunostomy may be the most appropriate option.[39] Jejunostomies may also be indicated in patients unable to tolerate gastric feeding due to impaired gastric motility or delayed gastric emptying. These tubes can be inserted surgically, endoscopically, radiologically, or laparoscopically. The most appropriate technique depends on the skill, expertise, and facilities available. A surgical jejunostomy may be preferred if the patient requires a laparotomy or laparoscopy for other reasons. Endoscopic

placement of a jejunostomy can be done by various methods. Typically, a small-bore jejunal extension tube (6, 8, or 10F) is inserted through a PEG and advanced through the pylorus into the duodenum or jejunum. This procedure has been referred to as percutaneous endoscopic jejunostomy (PEJ), but this is misleading. The PEJ designation implies a direct opening from the skin into the jejunum. The more appropriate name is percutaneous endoscopic gastrojejunostomy or PEG with a jejunal extension tube. In addition, laparoscopically and radiologically placed jejunostomies are described in the literature.[39] Because jejunostomies are smaller-bore tubes, occlusion occurs more commonly than with gastrostomy tubes.

ADMINISTRATION METHODS

Enteral nutrition may be administered by continuous, cyclic, bolus, or intermittent methods and may be accomplished by bolus, gravity, or infusion pump–controlled techniques. The method of delivery depends on the location of the tip of the feeding tube, the clinical condition and intestinal function of the patient, the environment in which the patient resides, and the patient's tolerance to the tube feeding.

CONTINUOUS

Continuous tube feeding is characterized by the administration of an enteral feeding formulation via a delivery system generally 24 hours per day, allowing for occasional interruption of the feeding for medication administration, procedures, and other treatments. In the hospitalized patient, the continuous administration of tube feeding is the method most commonly used for initiation, and is generally the preferred method in critically ill patients.[40] When initiating feeding into the stomach, the continuous method of delivery is considered less likely to result in abdominal distention, vomiting, and diarrhea than the intermittent bolus method. Once tolerance is established, a conversion to intermittent bolus administration may be warranted. When feeding into the small intestine, the continuous method is recommended to enhance tolerance. The rapid delivery of feeding into the small intestine, especially hyperosmotic formulations, may contribute to abdominal distention, cramps, hyperperistalsis, and diarrhea. Therefore conversion to intermittent bolus administration is not recommended when feeding into the duodenum or jejunum. Continuous feeding may also be preferred in patients who have limited absorptive capacity due to rapid GI transit or severely impaired digestion. Slow continuous administration in such patients allows greater time for digestion and absorption of nutrients as they pass through the intestine.

The delivery system for a continuous infusion generally includes a feeding reservoir or bag attached to an extension set that is connected to an infusion pump. The delivery system is then attached to the patient's enteral access tube. Continuous infusion may increase nursing time because routine checks of the enteral infusion are needed, but this disadvantage may be negated by the potential for improved tolerance. For adults, infusion rates generally range from 50 to 125 mL/h, although higher infusion rates have been reported without complications. In children, initial infusion rates of 1 to 2 mL/kg per hour or 20 to 25 mL/kg per day with similar rate advancements every 4 to 8 hours or more depending on patient characteristics to the goal rate needed to meet caloric needs usually are tolerated well. The primary disadvantage to this method of administration is the cost and inconvenience associated with the pump and administration sets. In the home care setting, ambulatory enteral pumps are available to free the patient from the infusion pole and allow greater mobility.

CYCLIC

It may be warranted to infuse EN by way of a continuous infusion over a fixed time period rather than over the entire day. A patient who is not eating well during the day because of complaints of fullness and lack of appetite may benefit from a trial of stopping the enteral feeding during the day and infusing only at night. In addition, the infusion of EN only at night will free the patient from the pump during the day and allow for greater mobility. This may be particularly useful for the home patient or patient requiring rehabilitation. Since a pump controls the rate of infusion, this method of administration may be used in patients with either gastric or small bowel access.

BOLUS

The bolus administration of EN is most commonly used in the long-term setting in patients who have a gastrostomy. The administration technique involves the rapid delivery of the enteral feeding formulation, usually over 5 to 10 minutes. Essentially the only equipment needed is a syringe to instill the feeding solution into the tube. Depending on the patient's nutritional requirements, a volume of 240 to 500 mL is generally given per feeding and repeated 4 to 6 times/day. From a convenience standpoint, it is generally preferable to dose the bolus volume in increments of the feeding formulation can size (usually 240 mL). The volume in children is usually 20 to 25 mL/kg per feeding until adult volumes are reached. For convenience and by convention, feedings in children are often dosed based on increments of one-half to 1 ounce. Although many patients tolerate the rapid administration of the feeding into the stomach, the bolus technique may result in cramping, nausea, vomiting, aspiration, and diarrhea. Its use should be avoided in patients with delayed gastric emptying or patients at high risk of aspiration. Its use is also not recommended in patients with duodenal or jejunal access because the rapid delivery of a feeding formulation into the small intestine is generally not tolerated.

INTERMITTENT

The intermittent technique is similar to the bolus technique except that the prescribed volume of feeding is administered over a longer time period, generally 20 to 60 minutes. Like bolus feeding, its use should be limited to patients with gastric enteral access. The desired volume of feeding formulation is emptied into a reservoir bag or container and infused by an infusion pump or gravity drip using a roller clamp. Compared to the bolus technique, more equipment is required for intermittent administration. However, if a patient is experiencing intolerance to bolus administration, a switch to the slower infusion period may be warranted. Both bolus and intermittent administration are more consistent physiologically with normal eating patterns than the continuous method. One study in infants demonstrated that normal gallbladder emptying did not occur with continuous infusion feedings, but was normal in those infants receiving bolus feedings.[41] This has implications in patients receiving both EN and long-term PN, especially children, and the development of cholestatic liver disease.

ENTERAL FEEDING FORMULATION SELECTION

Historically, enteral formulas were created to provide essential nutrients. Over the years, enhancements have been made to meet specific patient needs and improve tolerance. For example, enteral formulas have been modified in nutrient composition by changing the content of the amino acids (such as glutamine and arginine), changing the omega-3 polyunsaturated fatty acid content, and adding ribonucleic acid to promote a favorable physiologic effect that improves disease outcome. These specific nutrients have been called nutraceuticals or pharmaconutrients due to the intent of their use to modify the disease process and improve clinical outcome. Currently, enteral feeding formulations are categorized by the Food and Drug Administration (FDA) as medical foods. They are considered components of supportive care and are simply regulated to ensure sanitary manufacture. Unfortunately, they are not subject to rules governing health claims, and the issue of using medical foods for therapeutic intent is an unrecognized area by the FDA.[42,43]

The macronutrient content of enteral formulas (namely, protein, carbohydrate, and fat) varies in nutrient complexity (Table 138–6). Nutrient complexity refers to the amount of hydrolysis and digestion

TABLE 138–6. Enteral Formula Nutrient Complexity

Nutrient	Polymeric or Intact	Partially Hydrolyzed or Elemental

Carbohydrate	Starches
	  Fruit, vegetable, cereal solids
	Glucose polymers
	  Corn syrup solids
	  Polysaccharides
		Oligosaccharides
		Maltodextrins
		Disaccharides
		  Maltose, sucrose, lactose
		Monosaccharides
		  Glucose
		  Galactose

Fat	Long-chain triglycerides
	Polyunsaturated fatty acids
	  Corn oil
	  Safflower oil
	  Soybean oil
	  Butterfat
	  Menhaden oil
	  Fish oils
		Medium-chain triglycerides
		  Coconut oil
		  Palm kernel oil
		Free fatty acids
		  Linoleic

Protein	Whole
	  Egg, milk, wheat, whey
	Isolates
	  Caseinate salts
	  Lactalbumin
		Oligopeptides
		Dipeptides
		Tripeptides
		L-Amino acids

a substrate source requires prior to intestinal absorption. Polymeric or intact substrates are of similar molecular form as the food we eat. Enteral formulas that contain partially hydrolyzed or elemental substrates are characterized as elemental, or defined-formula diets. The caloric contribution of each of the macronutrients is as follows: carbohydrates, 4 kcal/g; protein, 4 kcal/g; and fat, 9 kcal/g. Micronutrients, including electrolytes, vitamins, trace elements, and water, do not contribute to caloric content.

PROTEIN COMPOSITION

Important factors concerning the protein within enteral formulas are the quantity, quality, and molecular form of protein. The essential amino acid content of the protein source determines the quality of the protein, and most commercially available enteral feeding formulations contain proteins of high quality. The molecular form of the protein source in enteral formulas will determine the amount of digestion that is required for absorption within the small bowel. Polymeric or intact protein sources require digestion to smaller peptides and free amino acids before they are absorbed from the GI tract. Therefore enteral formulation protein sources such as meat, milk, eggs, and caseinates require digestion by hydrochloric acid, specific protein enzymes, and pancreatic enzymes. Enteral formulations may also contain protein sources that are partially hydrolyzed as peptides or L-amino acids. As the molecular form of protein is reduced in size, the osmotic load within the enteral formula is increased. Many commercially available enteral feeding formulations contain combinations of intact and partially hydrolyzed protein sources.

CONDITIONALLY ESSENTIAL AMINO ACIDS

Glutamine and arginine are normally considered nonessential amino acids. However, during periods of high physiologic stress, glutamine and arginine may become deficient and therefore have been characterized as conditionally essential. They are usually absent or present in only low amounts in enteral feeding formulations. Therefore certain enteral formulations targeted for the critically ill have been supplemented with glutamine and/or arginine.

Glutamine serves as a key fuel for rapidly dividing cells, including enterocytes, endothelial cells, lymphocytes, and fibroblasts. The primary site of glutamine production is skeletal muscle. During critical illness, the catabolism of skeletal muscle provides an increased supply of glutamine, but this may not be enough to meet the high rate of glutamine use by cells of the immune system and other cells involved in recovery and repair. Glutamine depletion may result, particularly during prolonged periods of metabolic stress. However, it is unclear whether the supplementation of glutamine to enteral formulations plays a role in preserving normal intestinal morphology and function or preserving immune function.[44,45] Questions still remain about whether glutamine may enhance the growth of some tumors in that it may act as a tumor stimulator. Further research and investigation are required to determine the potential benefits and harm associated with glutamine-enriched enteral feeding formulations.

Like glutamine, arginine is an amino acid that may not be synthesized in sufficient quantity during states of trauma or stress. Supplementing the diet with arginine in healthy volunteers results in stimulation of T-cell blastogenesis. In animals, supplemental arginine has been shown to decrease protein catabolism, enhance nitrogen retention following injury, and also accelerate wound healing. While arginine supplementation has been shown to improve survival in various animal models and improve a number of in vitro measures of immune function in humans, prospective trials evaluating the effect of arginine on clinical outcomes in humans are lacking.[46] Arginine is added to selected enteral formulations in the range of 4.5 to 14 g/L.

CARBOHYDRATE COMPOSITION

The carbohydrate component of enteral feeding formulations usually provides the major source of nonprotein calories. Polymeric or intact enteral formulations contain starches and numerous types of glucose polymers, which require digestion to the monosaccharide moieties prior to intestinal absorption (see Fig. 138–1). As the hydrolysis of carbohydrate increases within an enteral formulation, the osmolality of the formulation increases. Elemental carbohydrates such as glucose and galactose contribute significantly to the osmolality of enteral formulations, which may contribute to feeding intolerance. Therefore polymeric entities, rather than elemental sugars, are preferred in enteral formulas. Glucose polymers provide a useful carbohydrate source that is tolerated by most individuals (see Table 138–6). The polymers are large chains that provide minimal osmotic load, yet are absorbed easily in the intestine. The one shortcoming of glucose polymers and oligosaccharides is that they are not as sweet as simple glucose and thus may decrease the palatability of orally consumed products. Finally, almost all commercially available enteral feeding formulations used in adults are lactose-free because some ethnic populations are lactase deficient and disaccharidase production within the gut lumen is reduced during illness or bowel rest. Infant formulas are available with or without lactose.

FAT AND FATTY ACID COMPOSITION

Fat is an important constituent in the diet because it provides a concentrated calorie source and serves as a carrier for fat-soluble vitamins. Sufficient linoleic acid is required to prevent essential fatty acid deficiency and should approximate 1% to 3% of total daily calories. The most common sources of fat in enteral feeding formulations are vegetable oils (soy or corn) rich in polyunsaturated fatty acids. The concentration of fat varies between less than 2% to 45% of total calories. High fat content of the diet has been associated with delayed gastric emptying. Enteral feeding formulations can also contain fat in the form of medium-chain triglycerides (MCTs), derived from palm kernel or coconut oils. Because MCTs do not contain linoleic acid, most enteral formulations that contain MCTs will also contain a source of LCTs to provide essential fatty acids. Potential advantages of MCTs compared to LCTs are that they are more water soluble, they undergo rapid hydrolysis, they require little to no pancreatic lipase or bile salt for absorption, and they do not require carnitine for transport into the mitochondria where they are converted to energy. They also do not require chylomicron formation for small bowel enterocyte absorption.

The source of long-chain fat within some enteral formulations has been modified from omega-6 to omega-3 fatty acids in an effort to modulate the inflammatory response to metabolic stress.[46,47] The omega-6 fatty acids serve as precursors to certain cytokines that have been shown to be potent inflammatory mediators and also to decrease cell-mediated immune response. The omega-6 fatty acids are high in linoleic acid and are derived from vegetable oil, whereas the omega-3 fatty acids, derived from coldwater fish oils, are high in linolenic acid. It has been proposed that if the dietary proportion of omega-3 fatty acids is increased and omega-6 fatty acids is decreased, less inflammation and immunosuppression may occur during metabolic stress.

Docosahexaenoic acid (DHA) and arachidonic acid (ARA) are two fatty acids abundant in human milk, but until recently, were not contained in commercial infant formulas. While the role of ARA supplementation is unclear, DHA is known to be important in both brain and eye development. In some studies, DHA and ARA supplementation has been shown to provide benefits to a child's visual function and/or cognitive and behavioral development.[48–51] Other studies have shown no difference with DHA and ARA supplementation.[52] The FDA has classified the plant-based fatty acid blends of DHA and ARA (DHASCO, ARASCO; Martek Biosciences Corporation) as generally recognized as safe in infant formulas.

FIBER CONTENT

Fiber, in the form of soy polysaccharides, has been added to several enteral feeding formulations intended for use in both children and adults in amounts ranging from 5.9 g to 24 g of dietary fiber per liter. Infant formulas do not contain fiber, with the exception of one formula intended for use in infants with diarrhea (Similac Isomil DF, Ross Products Division, Abbott Laboratories). Fiber supplementation is common in clinical practice, primarily because fiber-free enteral formulations have been implicated as a contributing factor to both diarrhea and constipation. Ingested fiber undergoes bacterial degradation within the colon to produce short-chain fatty acids (SCFAs). Potential benefits of fiber are the trophic effects on the colonic mucosa as well as promotion of sodium and water absorption within the colon.[4] It may help regulate bowel function in both normal individuals and those with altered colonic motility conditions. In addition, the resulting SCFAs are an excellent energy source. Although beneficial effects of fiber supplementation have not been clearly proven in clinical studies, there is experimental evidence that fiber may play an integral role in normal human nutrition and risk is generally minimal.[53] Fiber supplementation may be beneficial when long-term EN is required or in patients who experience diarrhea or constipation while receiving a fiber-free enteral formulation. In intensive care units, however, drugs and metabolic stress seem to be more powerful determinants of bowel function than the presence or absence of fiber.

OSMOLALITY AND RENAL SOLUTE LOAD

The osmolality and the renal solute load can affect tolerance to enteral feeding formulations. The osmolality of a given enteral formulation is a function of the size and quantity of ionic and molecular particles, primarily related to the protein, carbohydrate, electrolyte, and mineral content within a given volume. The unit of measure of osmolality is milliosmoles per kilogram (mOsm/kg). Iso-osmolar is considered approximately 300 mOsm/kg. Enteral formulations with greater amounts of partially hydrolyzed or elemental substrates have a higher osmolality than formulations containing polymeric or intact substrate forms. Therefore formulations that contain sucrose or glucose, dipeptides and tripeptides, and amino acids are considered hyperosmolar. Increased caloric density also increases the osmolality of an enteral formulation. In general, the osmolality of commercially available enteral feeding formulations ranges from 300 to 900 mOsm/kg. The American Academy of Pediatrics recommends that enteral formulations for use in infants have an osmolality of approximately 450 mOsm/kg. An extensive review of the osmolality of formulas and medications commonly used in neonatal intensive care units has been published.[54]

Symptoms of gastric retention, diarrhea, abdominal distention, nausea, and vomiting have been attributed to enteral formulations having high osmolality. This is based on the assumption that a higher osmolality will draw water into the gut lumen. However, clinical evidence to support the relationship between osmolality and GI tolerance is lacking.[54] The practice of diluting hyperosmolar formulations has not been shown to enhance tolerance and should be discouraged unless dilution is done to increase fluid intake.[55] Factors such as concurrent antibiotic therapy, method of enteral feeding administration, and the formulation's composition are likely to play a greater role in GI tolerance.

The renal solute load is made up collectively of the protein, sodium, potassium, and chloride content of the enteral formulation. Formulations that contain a greater solute load increase the obligatory water loss via the kidney. It is estimated that 40 to 60 mL of water is the minimal amount necessary to excrete 1 g of nitrogen.[56] Those receiving high-protein enteral formulations unable to ingest more water, such as a geriatric patient or a patient with altered mental status, may be at risk for significant dehydration.

CLASSIFICATION OF ENTERAL FEEDING FORMULATIONS

⑤ Although the majority of a patient's needs can probably be met using three or four different formulations, certain disease states or clinical conditions may warrant the use of a specialty feeding formulation. Development of an effective formulary system should avoid the duplication of enteral feeding formulations and use only those specialty formulations with an established role. Categorizing enteral feeding formulations according to therapeutic class is necessary in developing a formulary system (Tables 138–7 and 138–8).

STANDARD POLYMERIC

A large number of commercially available enteral feeding formulations fall within the category of a standard polymeric formulation. These formulations are approximately isotonic (300 mOsm/L), provide about 1 kcal/mL, and are composed of intact nutrients in a well-proportioned mix of carbohydrate, fat, and protein. They are provided with or without dietary fiber. The nutrient requirements of the majority of adult patients and children older than 10 years of age receiving EN can generally be met using feeding formulations in this category. The nonprotein calorie:nitrogen ratio (NPC:N) of these products is approximately 125:1 to 150:1. This ratio is a useful parameter for assessing protein density in relation to calories provided. Certain feeding formulations in this category may be promoted as high nitrogen, but fall within standard protein amounts. To maintain their isotonicity, products within this category are not sweetened. Therefore they are not very palatable and generally only suited for tube feeding and not oral supplementation; however, flavored products are available.

HIGH PROTEIN

Enteral feeding formulations with an NPC:N ratio less than 125:1 can be categorized as high protein. The lower the ratio, the higher the protein density in relation to calories provided. In patients with high protein requirements, it is generally not acceptable to use a feeding formulation with standard protein amounts because the volume necessary to meet protein requirements will often result in excessive calorie intake. Patients who may be candidates for a high-protein feeding formulation are those with trauma, burns, pressure sores, surgical wounds, high fistula output, and other critically ill patients. In general, adult patients with estimated protein requirements exceeding 1.5 g/kg per day may benefit from a high-protein formulation.

TABLE 138–7. Adult Enteral Feeding Formulation Classification System

Category	Features	Product Examples

Standard polymeric	Isotonic
	1–1.2 kcal/mL
	NPC:N 125:1 to 150:1
	May contain fiber
		Osmolite 1 Cal, Isocal (MJ), Isocal HN (MJ)
		  Osmolite 1 Cal (R), Jevity 1 Cal (R), Ultracal
		  (MJ), Jevity 1.2 Cal (R),
		  Nutren 1.0 (N), Isosource (No),
		  Nutren w/Fiber (N), Fibersource (No)

High protein	NPC:N <125:1
	May contain fiber
		Promote (R), Replete (N),
		  Promote w/Fiber (R), Replete w/Fiber (N),
		  TraumaCal (MJ), Isosource VHN (No)

High caloric density	1.5–2 kcal/mL
	Lower electrolyte content per calorie
	Hypertonic
		Nutren 1.5 (N), Deliver 2.0 (MJ),
		  Two-Cal HN (R), Nutren 2.0 (N),
		  Novasource 2.0 (No)

Elemental	High proportion of free amino acids Low in fat	Tolerex (No), Criticare HN (MJ), Vital HN (R), Vivonex TEN (No)

Peptide-based	Contains dipeptides and tripeptides
	Contain MCTs
		Peptamen (N), Subdue (MJ),
		  Peptamen VHP (N), Subdue Plus (MJ),
		  Perative (R), Crucial (N), Peptinex DT (No)

Disease-specific		

Renal	Caloric dense
	Protein content varies
	Low electrolyte content
		Suplena (R), Magnacal Renal (MJ),
		  Nepro (R), Novasource Renal (No),
		  Renalcal (N), NutriRenal (N)

Hepatic	Increased branched-chain and decreased aromatic amino acids	Nutri-Hep (N)

Pulmonary	High fat, low carbohydrate	Pulmocare (R), Oxepa (R),
		  Respalor (MJ), Novasource Pulmonary (No),
		  NutriVent (N)

Diabetic	High fat, low carbohydrate	Glucerna (R), Resource Diabetic (No),
		  Choice DM (MJ), Glytrol (N),
		  Diabetisource AC (No)

Metabolic stress	Supplemented with glutamine, arginine,
	  nucleotides, and/or omega-3 fatty acids
		Impact varieties (No), Perative (R),
		  Crucial (N), AlitraQ (R)

Oral supplement	Sweetened for taste
	Hypertonic
		Ensure varieties (R), Boost (MJ),
		  Resource varieties (No), ProSure (R),
		  NuBasic varieties (N)

Manufacturers: MJ, Mead Johnson Nutritionals: R, Ross Products Division, Abbott Laboratories; N, Nestlé Clinical Nutrition; No, Novartis; MCT, medium-chain triglyceride; NPC:N, nonprotein calorie:nitrogen ratio.

HIGH CALORIC DENSITY

High caloric density formulations are concentrated to provide less fluid and electrolyte intake in comparison to a standard polymeric formulation. They provide approximately 2 kcal/mL and will achieve similar calorie and protein intake to a standard polymeric formulation, using half the volume. Although generally well tolerated as a tube feeding, the osmolality of caloric dense formulations is about double that of standard isotonic formulations. High caloric density formulations are indicated in patients requiring fluid and/or electrolyte restriction, such as those with renal insufficiency or congestive heart failure. Although specialty enteral formulations targeted for acute and chronic renal failure are also available, many patients with renal failure can be managed using a product in this category.

ELEMENTAL/PEPTIDE-BASED

Formulations in this category contain protein and/or fat components that are hydrolyzed into smaller, predigested forms. Traditionally, enteral formulations in this category were referred to as elemental and contained a high proportion of protein in the form of free amino acids and contained a low amount of fat. Although still commercially available, many of these formulations have been replaced in clinical practice with formulations containing a portion of the protein in the form of dipeptides and tripeptides and less free amino acids. The formula-

tions have been referred to as peptide-based. The alteration was made in an effort to optimize protein absorption in patients with impaired digestive or absorptive capacity. The results from human and animal intestinal perfusion studies indicate that the partially hydrolyzed sources of protein have an absorptive advantage over formulas that contain free amino acids.[57] Peptide-based formulations are generally higher in fat content than the older, elemental formulations, and use MCTs in varying proportions as the fat source.

Indications for use of peptide-based formulations are not clearly established. Unfortunately, there are few controlled data on the nutritional efficacy of the peptide-based or free amino acid formulations in humans. The routine use of peptide-based or free amino acid formulations is generally not recommended. Patients who do not tolerate standard, intact nutrient formulations due to malabsorption may be candidates for a trial of a peptide-based formulation. In addition, elemental or peptide-based products that have higher percentages of MCTs and small amounts of LCTs may be beneficial for patients with severe pancreatic insufficiency such as chronic pancreatitis and cystic fibrosis, severe abnormalities of the intestinal mucosa such as untreated celiac disease, or chylothorax.

DISEASE-SPECIFIC

Newer enteral feeding formulations have been designed to meet specific nutrient requirements and manage metabolic abnormalities

TABLE 138–8. Pediatric Enteral Feeding Formulation Classification System

Formula Type	Product Examples	Indications
Polymeric: Infants		
Cow's milk–based	Enfamil LIPIL,[a] Enfamil Lactofree LIPIL, Enfamil A.R. LIPIL (MJ); Similac Advance,[b] Similac Lactose Free Advance (R); Nestlé Good Start Supreme (N)	Normal, healthy infant
Soy protein–based	Enfamil ProSobee LIPIL (MJ); Similac Isomil Advance, Similac Isomil DF[c] (R); Nestlé Good Start Supreme Soy (N)	Lactase deficiency or intolerance, galactosemia
Prematurity	Enfamil Premature LIPIL (MJ); Similac Special Care Advance 20 Advance, Similac Special Care Advance 24 Advance (R)	Preterm infant less than 2–3 kg
Transition	Enfamil EnfaCare LIPIL (MJ); Similac NeoSure Advance (R)	Preterm infants less than 3 kg ready for discharge
Toddlers	Next Step, Next Step Soy (MJ); Similac 2, Isomil 2 (R); Nestlé Good Start 2 Essentials, Nestlé Good Start 2 Essentials Soy	Infants ready to transition to cow's milk
Special diets	Similac PM 60/40 (R)	Renal, cardiac, or endocrine disorders
Polymeric: Children 1–10 years		
	Enfamil Kindercal[d] (MJ); PediaSure, PediaSure with Fiber (R); Nutren Jr, Nutren Jr with Fiber (N), Resource Just for Kids (No)	Functioning GI tract requiring tube feedings
Monomeric: Infants		
	Enfamil Nutramigen LIPIL, Enfamil Pregestimil, Portagen (MJ); Similac Alimentum Advance (R); Neocate (SHS); EleCare (R)	Malabsorption, cow's milk protein allergy, chylothorax, cystic fibrosis, biliary atresia
Monomeric: Children 1–10 years		
	Vivonex Pediatric, Pediatric Peptinex DT, Pediatric Peptinex DT with Fiber (No); Peptamen Jr (N); Neocate Junior, Neocate One +, Pepdite One + (SHS); EleCare (R)	Same as above

Manufacturers: MJ, Mead Johnson Nutritionals: R, Ross Nutritional Products Division, Abbott Laboratories; N, Nestlé Clinical Nutrition; No, Novartis; SHS, SHS International Ltd.

[a]LIPIL signifies Mead Johnson products with docosahexaenoic acid and arachidonic acid supplementation.
[b]Advance signifies Ross products with docosahexaenoic acid and arachidonic acid supplementation.
[c]Diarrhea formula contains soy fiber 0.9 g per 100 kcal.
[d]Contains soy fiber 5.9 g per 1000 kcal.

associated with specific disease states. Conditions for which specialized enteral feeding formulations exist include renal failure, hepatic failure, pulmonary disease including acute respiratory distress syndrome (ARDS), diabetes mellitus, wound healing, and metabolic stress. Specific nutrient concerns during organ failure are discussed in Chap. 139. Unfortunately, scientific and clinical research supporting the efficacy of specialized enteral feeding formulations is minimal. A critical evaluation is necessary to determine when, or if, a role exists for their use.

Specialized enteral formulations designed to modulate the inflammatory response in patients with severe metabolic stress have been referred to as immune-enhancing formulations or immunonutrition. These specialized formulations are supplemented with nutrients such as glutamine, arginine, branched-chain amino acids, nucleotides, and omega-3 polyunsaturated fatty acids, due to their potential role in regulating immune function. Systematic literature reviews evaluating the clinical outcome of immune-enhancing formulations compared to standard formulations in critically ill patients have been published.[13,58–61] A meta-analysis of 12 clinical trials (cumulative n = 1482) demonstrated a significant reduction in infection rate and length of hospital stay for trauma, septic, or surgical patients re-

ceiving immunonutrition formulations.[58] Likewise, a meta-analysis of 10 clinical trials (cumulative n = 1009) demonstrated significant reductions in infectious complications and overall length of hospital stay for critically ill or cancer patients receiving immunonutrition formulations.[60] No effect on mortality with immunonutrition was demonstrated from either of the meta-analyses. However, one study documented increased mortality in patients receiving immune-enhancing formulations.[62] Unfortunately, available studies provide no insight as to which nutrient(s), if any, contributed to any potential improvement in clinical outcome.

CLINICAL CONTROVERSY

The role of immune-enhancing enteral formulations in critically ill patients is controversial. While some clinicians recommend their use based on studies suggesting improvement in measures of immune function, others await more evidence to support safety and improvement in clinical outcome measures. In addition, parameters for determining those critically ill patients most likely to benefit from the use of immune-enhancing enteral formulations are not clearly defined.

In patients with ARDS, improved outcomes have been documented using a low carbohydrate formulation supplemented with specific fatty acids (eicosapentaenoic acid and gamma-linolenic acid) and antioxidants.[63] When compared with a high fat formulation, the specialized diet was associated with fewer days of ventilatory support, fewer ICU days, and fewer new organ failures. Therefore it has been recommended that this specialized formulation be considered for patients with ARDS.[13,64]

There are no disease-specific enteral products currently marketed for use in infants or children from 1 to 10 years of age. The use of modular supplements is often necessary in children with special nutrition needs (see section on modular supplements, below).

ORAL SUPPLEMENTS

In general, oral supplements are not intended for tube feeding, but to enhance an oral diet. They are sweetened to improve taste and are therefore hypertonic (about 450 to 700 mOsm/kg). This is generally not a problem in the patient with a functioning GI tract. However, in the tube-fed patient, a sweetened product is not necessary and may contribute to GI intolerance, particularly diarrhea. Powder supplements that are mixed with milk should be avoided in lactose-intolerant patients. In addition to liquid supplements, puddings, gelatins, bars, and milkshake-like supplements are available.

MODULAR PRODUCTS

A module is a powder or liquid allowing addition of nutrients (i.e., protein, carbohydrate, or fat) to supplement a commercially available enteral formulation (Table 138–9). Addition of a modular product may be necessary, especially in children, to achieve a nutrient mix not supplied by a single commercially available product.[65] Alternatively, formulations available in powder or concentrate can be mixed with less water than needed for the standard dilution to deliver more nutrients in less volume. Infant formulas generally are concentrated beyond their standard concentration (standard varies depending on type) in this way. However, keep in mind the mixing process required for modular components increases the potential for introducing bacterial contamination. This problem has been particularly identified with the use of blenders and reconstitution of powders.[66,67] Human milk fortifiers are available for supplementation of human milk so that it meets the needs of a premature infant. Human milk fortifiers add additional calories, protein, and minerals and have been shown to improve nutritional outcomes in human milk–fed premature infants.[68–70]

TABLE 138–9. Modular Enteral Products

Primary Nutrient Supplied	Example Products (Mfg[a])
Carbohydrate	Moducal (MJ), Polycose (R)
Protein	ProMod (R), Casec (MJ)
Fat	MCT Oil (MJ), Microlipid (MJ)
Human milk fortifier	Enfamil Human Milk Fortifier (MJ), Similac Human Milk Fortifier (R)
Pectin/carbohydrate/potassium	Banana Flakes (K)
Carbohydrate and fat	Duocal (SHS)

[a]Manufacturers: R, Ross Products Division, Abbott Laboratories; MJ, Mead Johnson Nutritionals; K, Kanana; SHS, SHS International, Ltd.

REHYDRATION

Oral rehydration formulations are useful in maintaining hydration or treating dehydration in adult and pediatric patients with high GI output. Such formulations are available commercially in powder or liquid form or can be extemporaneously compounded. They can be administered orally or given via a feeding tube. The glucose content of oral rehydration solutions is important because it stimulates active transport systems, which in turn stimulate passive sodium and water uptake simultaneously with the glucose. Therefore oral or enteral administration of rehydration solutions may decrease fecal water loss and generate a positive electrolyte balance.

FORMULARY AND DELIVERY SYSTEM CONSIDERATIONS

In general, no more than one product is necessary per category of enteral feeding formulations and it may be possible to omit certain categories based on the specific population and physician prescribing practices within a given institution. The selection of product should be based on meeting patient nutritional requirements. Additional selection criteria include container size and type, liquid or powder form, shelf life, ease of use, and cost.

The majority of enteral products are available as ready-to-use, prepackaged liquids, whereas others are in a dehydrated, powdered state and require reconstitution prior to use. Advantages of ready-to-use liquid formulations are convenience and lower susceptibility to microbiologic contamination due to less required manipulation. One of the disadvantages is that more storage space is required. The ease or convenience of a ready-to-use liquid is especially important for self-care patients, the disabled, and those who have difficulty receiving or following printed instructions. Ready-to-use liquid enteral formulations are generally available in either cans or closed, ready-to-hang bags or rigid containers. Bolus administration of EN is usually achieved using formulas available in cans. However, when formula from a can is used for continuous or cyclic administration it must first be poured into a bag or bottle to allow for infusion via a pump. This "open system" differs from the closed, ready-to-hang containers from the standpoint of microbial contamination risk. The use of a powder formula is also considered an open system of delivery.

Contaminated enteral feeding formulations have been identified as a potential source of infectious complications.[66,67,71,72] The GI tract may serve as a portal of entry for bacteria into the systemic circulation, especially in patients who are receiving multiple antibiotics, have undergone a surgical procedure, or have GI tract stasis from a variety of causes. The contamination of enteral feeding formulations has been associated with a lack of attention to proper handling techniques, inability to disinfect preparation equipment, and nonsterile or contaminated tube feeding additives. Unlike liquid formulations, powdered products are not guaranteed to be sterile by the manufacturer. This is due to the inability to properly sterilize the powder without destruction of some of its components. Contamination of one infant formula with *Enterobacter sakazakii* at the manufacturing site was implicated in the death of an infant in a neonatal ICU that prompted FDA warnings regarding the use of powdered formulations in premature neonates and other immunocompromised infants. Because powder formulations require reconstitution, often in a blender that is difficult to sterilize, they are also more susceptible to contamination at the time of preparation. Stringent handling procedures are recommended during all aspects of enteral feeding preparation and delivery to minimize contamination risk. The closed-system containers supply a ready-to-hang, prefilled, sterile supply of formula in volumes of 1 to 1.5 L, and their use will decrease manipulation required for feeding administration. Numerous, but not all, enteral formulations intended for use in adults are available in the closed-administration system. The closed-administration system also offers the advantage of not requiring refrigeration and allowing hang times beyond 24 to 36 hours, whereas the conventional open delivery system necessitates hang times of generally 4 to 8 hours. If manipulation of a closed-system container is required for the addition of water, electrolytes, or medication, it should follow guidelines for an open system. In that case, use of cans is generally more cost-effective.

INITIATION AND ADVANCEMENT PROTOCOL

Guidelines for the initiation and advancement of enteral feeding formulations vary greatly and scientific support for any of the guidelines is weak or nonexistent. The typical recommendation for continuous administration of EN for adults is to start at 20 to 50 mL/h and advance by 10 to 25 mL/h every 4 to 8 hours until the desired goal is achieved. For intermittent administration, the typical recommendation is to start at 120 mL every 4 hours and advance by 30 to 60 mL every 8 to 12 hours.[55] In children, the recommendation for continuous administration is initiation of 1 to 2 mL/kg per hour or 20 to 25 mL/kg per bolus with advancement every 4 to 12 hours of similar volumes. In premature infants, feedings are initiated at lower rates or volumes, usually 10 to 20 mL/kg per day. Schedules for progression of tube feeding from initial to target rates are important and may influence tolerance. Conversely, if the protocol is too conservative, it may take an excessively long period of time to reach nutrient goals. The advancement of enteral feeding should be individualized for specific patient issues. As previously discussed, the practice of diluting enteral feeding formulations is not routinely recommended unless necessary to increase fluid intake.[55] The development of an EN protocol within an institution that outlines initiation and advancement criteria may be a useful strategy to optimize achievement of reaching nutrient goals.[13]

Such a protocol should incorporate assessment of GI tolerance and allow nursing to advance the rate based on pre-established, specific criteria.

COMPLICATIONS AND MONITORING

The majority of complications associated with EN can be categorized as metabolic, GI, and mechanical. The early detection and management of potential complications is necessary to allow for the successful use of EN. In addition, measures to avoid complications should be incorporated into the management of all patients receiving EN and require close monitoring (Table 138–10). The potential causes and guidelines for the prevention and treatment of complications will be discussed.

METABOLIC COMPLICATIONS

Metabolic complications associated with EN are similar to those associated with PN, but the occurrence tends to be lower. Complications related to hydration and electrolyte imbalance and altered glucose control are observed more frequently in patients with underlying organ dysfunction. The micronutrient and water content within enteral feeding formulations are in fixed amounts intended to meet recommended dietary allowances for the average patient. Therefore the frequency of clinical and laboratory assessment to monitor hydration, electrolyte, organ function, and glucose control adequately for a patient who is critically ill is greater than for a stable patient residing in a rehabilitation unit or at home. Patients receiving long-term EN at home may only require laboratory monitoring every 2 to 3 months depending on their clinical status. In addition to macronutrient content, it is important to evaluate the actual content of water and micronutrients provided by the enteral formulations, especially in critically ill patients at high risk for metabolic complications. Supplemental fluid and electrolytes may be required in some patients. Conversely, for patients who have fluid retention or increased serum electrolytes,

TABLE 138–10. Suggested Monitoring for EN Patients to Prevent the Development of Complications

Parameter	During Initiation of EN Therapy	During Stable EN Therapy
Vital signs	Every 4–6 h	As needed
Clinical assessment		
Weight	Daily	Weekly
Length/height (children)	Weekly–monthly	Monthly
Head circumference (<3 y of age)	Weekly–monthly	Monthly
Total intake/output	Daily	As needed
Tube feeding intake	Daily	Daily
Enterostomy tube site assessment	Daily	Daily
GI tolerance		
Stool frequency/volume	Daily	Daily
Abdomen assessment	Daily	Daily
Nausea or vomiting	Daily	Daily
Gastric residual volumes	Every 4–8 h (varies)	As needed
Tube placement	Prior to starting, then ongoing	Ongoing
Laboratory		
Electrolytes, BUN/S_{cr}, glucose	Daily	As needed
Calcium, magnesium, phosphorus	3–7 times/wk	As needed
Liver function tests	Weekly	As needed
Trace elements, vitamins	Patient-specific	Patient-specific

BUN, blood urea nitrogen; S_{cr}, serum creatinine.

the enteral formulation may need to be changed to one that is more concentrated or provides less of a particular nutrient.

GASTROINTESTINAL COMPLICATIONS

The GI complications associated with tube feeding include high gastric residuals, nausea, vomiting, abdominal distention, cramping, aspiration, diarrhea, and constipation. In general, these side effects can be attributed to drug-related, patient-related, or tube feeding–related factors.

A gastric residual volume refers to the volume of contents in the stomach and is measured by using a syringe and aspirating from a large-bore NG or gastrostomy tube. For patients receiving tube feeding into the stomach, gastric residual volumes are widely used as an indicator of tolerance. It is believed, although not well documented, that patients with high gastric residual volumes are at higher risk of vomiting and/or aspiration. It is generally suggested to measure residual volumes every 4 hours in hospitalized patients receiving continuous tube feeding into the stomach.[73,74]

CLINICAL CONTROVERSY

Clinicians argue about what constitutes an excessive gastric residual volume. In adults, the definition of a high residual volume ranges from greater than 200 mL to greater than 500 mL. In children, residual volumes greater than twice the bolus volume or twice the hourly infusion rate for continuous gastric feedings are considered excessive.

If high gastric residuals occur, the response is often to withhold tube feeding. However, frequent interruptions in the delivery of EN can adversely impact meeting nutrient goals. Because gastric residual volumes are unreliable, symptoms such as abdominal distention, fullness, bloating, and discomfort should also be assessed. A trend in elevated gastric residual volumes is generally more important than an isolated high measurement. If symptoms are present and residual volumes are elevated, a decrease in tube feeding rate may be warranted. It has been recommended that abruptly stopping tube feeding be reserved for patients with overt regurgitation or aspiration.[73] Gastric residual volumes should generally be returned to the patient unless they are excessive (greater than 500 mL in adults).[73] It may be beneficial to initiate a prokinetic agent such as metoclopramide to increase gastric emptying and enhance tolerance.[75,76] If high gastric residual volumes persist, a transpyloric feeding tube may be considered for feeding into the small bowel. Other interventions may include a trial of a proton pump inhibitor or histamine$_2$-receptor antagonist to decrease the volume of gastric secretions, and minimizing the use of narcotics, sedatives, or other agents that may delay gastric emptying.[55]

Aspiration pneumonia is considered the most serious complication associated with tube feeding and is potentially life-threatening. While aspiration is a fairly common event for critically ill patients on tube feeding, progression to aspiration pneumonia is difficult to predict. Risk factors for aspiration include a previous aspiration episode, decreased level of consciousness, neuromuscular disease, structural airway or GI tract abnormalities, endotracheal intubation, vomiting, persistently high gastric residual volumes, and prolonged supine position.[77] Identification of these risk factors along with close monitoring of gastric residual volumes is recommended for the management of critically ill patients receiving tube feeding. Traditionally, blue food coloring had been added to enteral formulations in an at-

tempt to detect aspiration. However, due to its low sensitivity for detection and association with several serious adverse events, including death, the addition of blue food dye to enteral formulations should no longer be used.[77,78] An alternative to blue dye is to test the tracheobronchial secretions for glucose (the glucose oxidase strip method). This method assumes that the glucose concentration of these secretions is normally less than 5 mg/dL and that higher concentrations are consistent with aspiration of a feeding formulation. Unfortunately, false-positives can occur using this technique due to blood in the specimen or when formulas containing low glucose concentrations (i.e., <200 mg/dL) are used.[78,79]

Strategies to decrease aspiration risk include those mentioned in the management of high gastric residual volumes. Keeping the patient's head of the bed elevated to a 30- to 45-degree angle during feeding and for 30 to 60 minutes after intermittent boluses is also recommended. This makes it more difficult for feeding to migrate up the esophagus against gravity. Changing from bolus or intermittent to continuous administration may also reduce the risk. Additionally, good oral care is strongly recommended. Aspiration may also occur with improper feeding tube placement or displacement. Therefore regular assessment of tube position is recommended.[77]

The reported incidence of diarrhea in patients receiving EN ranges from 20% to 70% and varies greatly due to the lack of a standard definition.[55,80] When monitoring for diarrhea, stool frequency, consistency, and volume should be evaluated and previous bowel habits should be considered. One definition of diarrhea is more than three to five liquid stools per day or more than 250 to 500 mL/day (10 mL/kg per day in children) stool output for at least two consecutive days.[80] A single loose stool does not constitute diarrhea or require intervention.

Diarrhea in patients receiving tube feeding may be caused by a number of factors, many of which are unrelated to the feeding. Management should be directed at identifying and correcting the most likely cause(s). Drug therapy is a common cause, particularly broad-spectrum antibiotics. Another drug-related cause is the sorbitol contained in many liquid medication formulations. Sorbitol is used as a sweetening agent to enhance palatability, but acts as an osmotic laxative at a certain dose. In addition, many drugs available in a liquid form are hyperosmolar, which may also contribute to diarrhea. Since many patients receiving tube feeding also receive medications in a liquid form, all medications should be evaluated for their potential contribution. Infectious causes of diarrhea, such as antibiotic-induced bacterial overgrowth by *Clostridium difficile* or other intestinal flora, need to be considered when diarrhea develops. Diarrhea also may occur as a result of malabsorption, owing to the underlying disease state or condition.

Tube feeding–related factors that may contribute to diarrhea include too rapid delivery or advancement of formula, intolerance to the formula composition, administering large volumes of feeding into the small bowel, and formula contamination. Measures to prevent or manage the development of diarrhea related directly to the tube feeding should address these potential causes.[81] If diarrhea occurs when using a fiber-free formulation, consider switching to a fiber-containing formulation. If using a high fat formulation, it may be beneficial to switch to a formulation lower in fat or having a proportion of the fat supplied as MCTs. If protein malabsorption is suspected, switching from an intact protein to a peptide-based source may be beneficial. Avoid lactose-containing enteral formulations, although the majority of products designed for tube feeding are lactose-free. Finally, assess the risk of bacterial contamination of the formula and take steps to minimize any potential risk factors. Once infectious etiologies have been excluded, pharmacologic intervention may be required to control severe diarrhea, including the use of opiates, diphenoxylate, and loperamide.

MECHANICAL COMPLICATIONS

Mechanical complications of EN are those associated with the feeding tube, including tube occlusion or malposition, and nasopulmonary intubation. Feeding tube occlusion is usually due to the improper administration of medications and/or flushing technique. Kinking of the tube may also cause occlusion. The tube should be flushed with at least 30 mL of water before and after administering any medication. The recommended volume used in children is generally less than 30 mL and depends on the size of the tube. The frequency of flushing should be at least every 8 hours during continuous feeding and before and after each intermittent feeding. If tube occlusion occurs, an attempt to irrigate the tube with warm water should be made. Other fluids such as colas and cranberry juice have been used to irrigate occluded tubes but have not been shown to be any better than warm water. Some success in re-establishing patency has also been shown with the use of pancreatic enzymes mixed in sodium bicarbonate.[82] In addition, declogging devices specifically designed to unclog feeding tubes are available. They have been designed to either mechanically break through or remove the occlusion or provide an applicator and syringe prefilled with pancreatic enzymes and various powders targeted to restore patency.

Inadvertent tube removal or displacement has been reported to occur in greater than 50% of patients receiving enteral tube feeding.[83] An agitated or confused patient may pull at the feeding tube and cause its removal or malposition. Measures to decrease agitation and confusion should be attempted. Various manipulations done to the patient throughout the day may also cause malposition. Securing the tube with tape may be helpful, as well as marking the tube with permanent ink at the exit site to assess for change in position.

When a feeding tube is inserted nasally or orally, there is a risk that the tube may inadvertently enter the tracheobronchial tree. The risk may be higher in patients who have an impaired cough or gag reflex and when a stylet is used for tube insertion. Proper positioning of the tube should always be confirmed by x-ray prior to feeding initiation to avoid inadvertent administration of enteral formula into the lung.

OTHER COMPLICATIONS

A unique complication of tube feedings in children, especially in the first year of life, is the development of feeding disorders due to oral hypersensitivity, poor oral/motor skills, and food aversion. In these children, transitioning from tube to oral nutrition is often difficult and protracted. The involvement of an occupational or speech therapist, behavioral psychologist, or other trained individual, as well as perseverance by the family often is necessary to improve oral intake. Avoidance of a strict nothing by mouth (NPO) status, if possible, and oral stimulation programs for those children who must remain NPO are recommended to avoid this complication.[84]

DRUG DELIVERY VIA FEEDING TUBE

Using enteral feeding tubes to deliver drugs is a common practice. It offers an alternative to parenteral administration in patients unable to take drugs by the oral route. However, in addition to complications of tube occlusion, effects on drug bioavailability and other potential interactions need to be considered when using this route. Medications have been given as a concomitant bolus administration via the feeding tube or admixed with the enteral feeding formulation.

CONCOMITANT DRUG ADMINISTRATION

Concomitant administration of medications with enteral feedings requires awareness of certain limitations. First, determination of tube tip placement should be considered. Medications delivered directly into the stomach allow for the normal capacity of drug dissolution. Medications delivered into the small bowel may result in alterations of drug dissolution because the stomach is bypassed. In addition, therapeutic effect designed to occur within the stomach, such as with antacids and sucralfate, may be influenced by feeding tube route. Because many drugs are best absorbed in the fasted state, they should be administered on an empty stomach as much as possible. Patients receiving bolus gastric feedings may receive medications appropriately spaced between the feedings, but patients receiving continuous feeding will require interruption for drug administration.

Selecting the proper medication dosage form for coadministration with the feeding is another important consideration. Medications in sublingual form, sustained-released capsules or tablets, and enteric-coated tablets should not be crushed and therefore should not be administered via enteral feeding tubes. An extensive list of oral dosage forms that should not be crushed is available in the literature.[85,86] Solid dosage forms that are appropriate to crush should be prepared as a very fine powder and mixed with 15 to 30 mL of water or other appropriate solvent before administering through the tube. In addition, the content of many capsules may be opened and administered in the same manner. Pellets contained inside microencapsulated dosage forms should generally not be crushed. It may be acceptable to administer intact pellets through the feeding tube, provided that the pellets are small enough and drug absorption is not compromised.[87,88] To avoid the need to crush a solid dosage form and mix with water, liquid dosage preparations have been used for administration through the feeding tube. However, the risk of GI intolerance should be considered due to hyperosmolality of the liquid formulation and possible sorbitol content.[87,88] Although the use of a liquid dosage preparation may be more convenient than a solid dosage form, it may not be the best choice if GI intolerance is an issue.

As previously mentioned, adherence to proper flushing technique is necessary to prevent occlusion when administering medication through a feeding tube. At least 30 mL of water in adults and usually 10 to 15 mL in children should be given before and after medication administration to clear the drug through the tube and help get the drug into the stomach. If more than one medication is scheduled for a given time, each should be administered separately and the tube should be flushed with at least 5 mL water between them.[86,87]

ADMIXTURE OF DRUGS WITH ENTERAL FEEDING

Mixing liquid medications with certain enteral feeding formulations has been associated with several types of physical incompatibilities including granulation, gel formation, separation, and precipitation.[86,87] Not only can these physical incompatibilities inhibit drug absorption, gel formation potentially may clog small-bore enteral feeding tubes. Physical incompatibility with medications is more common in formulations that contain intact protein than in those with hydrolyzed protein. Also, medication and enteral formula incompatibilities are more common with the use of acidic pharmaceutical syrups. The most prudent recommendation is to avoid the routine admixture whenever possible, especially for nonaqueous preparations and syrups. In the

TABLE 138–11. Medications with Special Considerations for Enteral Feeding Tube Administration

Drug	Interaction	Comments
Phenytoin	Reduced bioavailability in the presence of EN	A suggestion to minimize interaction is to hold tube feeding 1–2 h before and after phenytoin, but this has no proven benefit Adjust tube feeding rate to account for time held for phenytoin administration Monitor phenytoin serum concentrations and clinical response closely Consider switching to IV phenytoin route if unable to reach therapeutic level
Antibiotics (selected)	Potential for reduced bioavailability due to complexation of drug with divalent and trivalent cations found in enteral feeding	May influence quinolone antibiotics, penicillin, tetracycline, isoniazid, and rifampin Consider holding tube feeding before and after administration Avoid jejunal administration of ciprofloxacin Monitor clinical response
Warfarin	Decreased absorption of warfarin due to enteral feeding; therapeutic effect antagonized by vitamin K content of enteral formulations	Adjust warfarin dose based on INR Anticipate need to increase warfarin dose when enteral feedings are started and decrease dose when enteral feedings are stopped
Antacids	Altered pharmacologic effect of antacid if administered into the small bowel	Administer antacids only into a feeding tube with the tip placed in the stomach
Omeprazole	When omeprazole granules are crushed, the drug rapidly degrades in acid environment of stomach	Omeprazole granules become sticky when moistened with water, but can be mixed with acidic juices to avoid clumping; may be given via large-bore tube, but may occlude small-bore tubes An oral liquid suspension can be extemporaneously prepared for administration via a feeding tube[a]

[a]From Phillips et al,[92] and Quercia et al.[93]
EN, enteral nutrition; INR, International Normalized Ratio.

clinical setting exceptions do exist, such as adding electrolyte injections of potassium or sodium to enteral formulas to assist in maintaining or repleting the electrolyte requirements for a patient.

DRUG-NUTRIENT INTERACTIONS

9 The most significant drug and nutrient interactions that can occur during continuous enteral feeding are those in which the bioavailability of the drug is reduced and the desired pharmacologic effect is not achieved (Table 138–11). Unfortunately, limited clinical studies are available to document the extent of this problem with enteral feeding. Most of the observations are anecdotal case reports involving few patients. One of the most studied interactions has been the interaction between phenytoin and enteral feeding that results in decreased phenytoin bioavailability. The interaction was first reported in 1982, yet the precise mechanism for the interaction has not been identified.[89] Phenytoin serum concentrations may decrease by as much as 50% to 75% when phenytoin is given concomitantly with EN. Patients typically require higher than normal phenytoin doses while receiving EN.[87–90] The patient's clinical response and phenytoin serum concentrations should be monitored closely if phenytoin is given enterally during continuous enteral feeding and after its discontinuation.

CLINICAL CONTROVERSY

A number of methods to minimize the interaction between phenytoin and continuous enteral feeding have been suggested, but no consensus exists. Some clinicians choose holding the feeding for 1 to 2 hours before and after phenytoin administration to minimize the interaction. But since this has not been proven effective and may result in suboptimal nutrition, others choose not to interrupt the feeding.

Decreased bioavailability of certain antibiotics, particularly quinolones, has been documented when coadministered with enteral feeding.[87,88,91] Although the practice to hold tube feeding for 30 minutes before and 30 minutes after quinolone administration has been recommended, it has not been shown to ultimately improve drug absorption. There is evidence to suggest that ciprofloxacin absorption is significantly decreased when given via a jejunostomy tube, so this practice should be avoided.[91] Warfarin resistance has been documented during enteral feeding, possibly due to decreased absorption or the antagonist effects of vitamin K. Prior to 1980, it was thought that the content of vitamin K in dosages of up to 1330 mcg/1000 kcal of enteral feeding formula was contributing to the pharmacologic interaction with warfarin. Subsequently, the vitamin K content within formulas intended for use in adults has been reformulated to less than 200 mcg/1000 kcal. However, warfarin resistance has continued to be reported and a warfarin dosage increase may be required in patients receiving EN.[87,88] The patient's International Normalized Ratio should be closely monitored in patients receiving warfarin and enteral feedings. Conversely, when EN is discontinued, a reduction in warfarin dose may be required.

NUTRITION OUTCOME GOALS

Nutrition outcome goals of EN are to reverse protein-calorie malnutrition, maintain an adequate nutritional state, or promote growth and development of infants and children. Assessing the outcome of EN includes monitoring objective measures of body composition, protein and energy balance, and subjective outcome for physiologic muscle function and wound healing (Table 138–12). Besides an improvement in nutrition outcome, another goal of EN is to reduce disease-related morbidity and mortality. Measures of disease-related morbidity include length of hospital stay, infectious complications, and the

TABLE 138–12. Parameters Used to Monitor Enteral Nutrition Efficacy

Parameter	Comments
Anthropometrics	Weight (at least weekly; daily in neonates and infants)
	Serial measurement of triceps skinfold and midarm muscle circumference can be useful in patients on long-term enteral nutrition
Muscle function	Physical endurance
	Grip strength
Metabolic	Visceral proteins (albumin and transferrin) at least monthly
	24-hour urine urea nitrogen weekly to monthly
	Indirect calorimetry tailored to patient-specific situations
Nutrition intake	Calories, protein, fluid, electrolytes, trace elements, and vitamins
Skin integrity	Wound healing
	Pressure sores

patient's sense of well-being. Such clinical outcome goals are extremely difficult to document with the use of EN, in part because other factors such as age, underlying comorbidities, extent of injury, immunocompetence, and end-organ complications also affect disease outcome. However, no disease process improves significantly with prolonged starvation. Ultimately, the successful use of EN can avoid the need for PN in patients unable to meet nutrient requirements with an oral diet.

PHARMACOECONOMIC CONSIDERATIONS

Enteral nutrition has consistently been shown to be less expensive than PN. The pharmacoeconomic comparison between EN and PN should include an evaluation of therapeutic outcome relative to the cumulative cost associated with providing the therapy. Therapy costs should include costs related to placement and maintenance of enteral or parenteral access; costs of nutrients and related supplies; the time spent by professional staff in ordering, compounding, delivering, administering, and managing therapy; costs of laboratory monitoring; and costs of managing complications that result from therapy. However, it is very difficult to capture all of these costs and separate cost from charge-based estimates. None of the existing pharmacoeconomic analyses have incorporated all costs related to EN and PN therapy, but selected cost comparisons derived from clinical research trials in institutional settings have been published.[94–96] The cost of EN has been reported to be approximately one-fourth to one-half that of PN. Incorporating the cost of managing complications related to therapy greatly increases the overall cost of PN compared with EN.[96] In situations in which improved outcome has not been demonstrated with PN, EN appears preferable on a cost basis.[7]

ABBREVIATIONS

ARA: arachidonic acid
ARDS: acute respiratory distress syndrome
DHA: docosahexaenoic acid
EN: enteral nutrition
GALT: gut-associated lymphoid tissue
LCT: long-chain triglyceride

MCT: medium-chain triglyceride
ND: nasoduodenal
NG: nasogastric
NJ: nasojejunal
NPC:N: nonprotein calorie:nitrogen ratio
NPO: nothing by mouth
OG: orogastric
PEG: percutaneous endoscopic gastrostomy
PEJ: percutaneous endoscopic jejunostomy
PRG: percutaneous radiologic gastrostomy
PN: parenteral nutrition
SCFA: short-chain fatty acid

ACKNOWLEDGMENTS

We gratefully acknowledge Doug Janson, Pharm.D., BCNSP, for his contribution to the previous edition of this chapter.

Review Questions and other resources can be found at *www.pharmacotherapyonline.com.*

REFERENCES

1. Caspary WF. Physiology and pathophysiology of intestinal absorption. Am J Clin Nutr 1992;55:299S–308S.
2. DeLegge MH, Ridley C. Nutrient digestion, absorption, and excretion. In: Gottschlich MM, ed. The Science and Practice of Nutrition Support: A Case-Based Core Curriculum. Dubuque, IA, Kendall/Hunt, 2001:1–16.
3. Marsh MN, Riley SA. Digestion and absorption of nutrients and vitamins. In: Feldman M, Scharschmidt BF, Sleisenger MH, eds. Sleisenger & Fordtran's Gastrointestinal and Liver Disease: Pathophysiology/Diagnosis/Management, 6th ed. Philadelphia, WB Saunders, 1998:1471–1500.
4. Rombeau JL, Kripke SA. Metabolic and intestinal effects of short-chain fatty acids. JPEN J Parenter Enteral Nutr 1990;14(Suppl):181S–185S.
5. Frakenfield D. Energy and macrosubstrate requirements. In: Gottschlich MM, ed. The Science and Practice of Nutrition Support: A Case-Based Curriculum. Dubuque, IA, Kendall/Hunt, 2001:31–52.
6. Jabbar A, Chang WK, Dryden GW, McClave S. Gut immunology and the differential response to feeding and starvation. Nutr Clin Pract 2003;18:461–482.
7. A.S.P.E.N. Board of Directors and The Clinical Guidelines Task Force. Guidelines for the use of parenteral and enteral nutrition in adult and pediatric patients. JPEN J Parenter Enteral Nutr 2002;26(1 Suppl):1SA–138SA.
8. Kirby DF, DeLegge MH, Fleming CR. American Gastroenterological Association technical review on tube feeding for enteral nutrition. Gastroenterology 1995;108:1282–1301.
9. Abou-Assi S, O'Keefe SJ. Nutrition support during acute pancreatitis. Nutrition 2002;18:938–943.
10. Coit AK. Necrotizing enterocolitis. J Perinat Neonat Nurs 1999;12:53–66.
11. Barton RG. Nutrition support in critical illness. Nutr Clin Pract 1994;9:127–139.
12. Huckleberry Y. Nutrition support and the surgical patient. Am J Health-Syst Pharm 2004;61:671–684.
13. Heyland DK, Dhaliwal R, Drover JW, et al. Canadian clinical practice guidelines for nutrition support in mechanically ventilated, critically ill adult patients. JPEN J Parenter Enteral Nutr 2003;27:355–373.
14. Lipman TO. Bacterial translocation and enteral nutrition in humans: An outsider looks in. JPEN J Parenter Enteral Nutr 1995;19:156–165.
15. Hernandez G, Velasco N, Wainstein C, et al. Gut mucosal atrophy after a short enteral fasting period in critically ill patients. J Crit Care 1999;14:73–77.

16. Wernerman J, Hammarqvist F. Bacterial translocation: Effects of artificial feeding. Curr Opin Clin Nutr Metab Care 2002;5:163–166.

17. Alpers DH. Enteral feeding and gut atrophy. Curr Opin Clin Nutr Metab Care 2002;5:679–683.

18. van den Berghe G, Wouters PJ, Bouillon R, et al. Outcome benefit of intensive insulin therapy in the critically ill: Insulin dose versus glycemic control. Crit Care Med 2003;31:359–366.

19. Kudsk KA, Croce MA, Fabian TC, et al. Enteral versus parenteral feeding: Effects on septic morbidity after blunt and penetrating abdominal trauma. Ann Surg 1992;215:503–513.

20. Btaiche IF, Khalidi N. Parenteral nutrition-associated liver complications in children. Pharmacotherapy 2002;22:188–211.

21. Kudsk KA. Clinical applications of enteral nutrition. Nutr Clin Pract 1994;9:165–171.

22. Marik PE, Zaloga GP. Early enteral nutrition in acutely ill patients: A systemic review. Crit Care Med 2001;29:2264–2270.

23. McClave SA, Wei-Kuo Chang. Feeding the hypotensive patient: Does enteral feeding precipitate or protect against ischemic bowel? Nutr Clin Pract 2003;18:279–284.

24. Zaloga GP, Roberts PR, Marik P. Feeding the hemodynamically unstable patient: A critical evaluation of the evidence. Nutr Clin Pract 2003;18:285–293.

25. Vanek VW. Ins and outs of enteral access. Part 1: Short-term enteral access. Nutr Clin Pract 2002;17:275–283.

26. Marik PE, Zaloga GP. Gastric versus post-pyloric feeding: A systematic review. Crit Care 2003;7:46–51.

27. Heyland DK, Drover JW, Dkaliwal R, Greenwood J. Optimizing the benefits and minimizing the risks of enteral nutrition in the critically ill: Role of small bowel feeding. JPEN J Parenter Enteral Nutr 2002;26(6 Suppl):S51–S55.

28. Heiselman DE, Hofer, T, Vidovich RR. Enteral feeding tube placement success with intravenous metoclopramide administration in ICU patients. Chest 1995;107:1686–1688.

29. Kalliafas S, Choban PS, Ziegler D, et al. Erythromycin facilitates post-pyloric placement of nasoduodenal feeding tubes in intensive care unit patients: Randomized, double-blinded, placebo-controlled trial. JPEN J Parenter Enteral Nutr 1996;20:385–388.

30. Vanek VW. Ins and outs of enteral access. Part 2: Long-term access-esophagostomy and gastrostomy. Nutr Clin Pract 2003;18:50–74.

31. Angus F, Burakoff R. The percutaneous endoscopic gastrostomy tube. Medical and ethical issues in placement. Am J Gastroenterol 2003;98:272–277.

32. Gauderer MW. Percutaneous endoscopic gastrostomy and the evolution of contemporary long-term enteral access. Clin Nutr 2002;21:103–110.

33. Clarkston WK, Smith OJ, Walden JM. Percutaneous endoscopic gastrostomy and early mortality. South Med J 1990;83:1433–1436.

34. Ozmen MN, Akhan O. Percutaneous radiologic gastrostomy. Eur J Radiol 2002;43:186–195.

35. Dormann AJ, Huchzermeyer H. Endoscopic techniques for enteral nutrition: standards and innovations. Dig Dis 2002;20:145–153.

36. Kobak GE, McClenathan DT, Schurman SJ. Complications of removing percutaneous endoscopic gastrostomy tubes in children. J Pediatr Gastroenterol Nutr 2000;30:404–407.

37. Yaseen M, Steele MI, Grunow JE. Nonendoscopic removal of percutaneous endoscopic gastrostomy tubes: Morbidity and mortality in children. Gastrointest Endosc 1996;44:235–238.

38. Peitersen-Oberndorff KE, Vos GD, Baeten CG. Serous complications after incomplete removal of percutaneous endoscopic gastrostomy catheters. J Pediatr Gastroenterol Nutr 1999;2:230–232.

39. Vanek VW. Ins and outs of enteral access. Part 3: Long-term access-jejunostomy. Nutr Clin Pract 2003;18:201–220.

40. Clevenger FW, Rodriguez DJ. Decision-making for enteral feeding administration: The why behind where and how. Nutr Clin Pract 1995;10:104–113.

41. Jawaheer G, Shaw NJ, Pierro A. Continuous enteral feeding impairs gallbladder emptying in infants. J Pediatr 2001;138:822–825.

42. Mueller C, Nestle M. Regulation of medical foods: Toward a rational policy. Nutr Clin Pract 1995;10:8–15.

43. Heymsfield SB. Enteral solutions: Is there a solution? Nutr Clin Pract 1995;10:4–7.

44. Buchman AL. Glutamine: Commercially essential or conditionally essential? A critical appraisal of the human data. Am J Clin Nutr 2001;74:25–32.

45. Wilmore DW. The effect of glutamine supplementation in patients following elective surgery and accidental injury. J Nutr 2001;131:2543S–2549S.

46. Barton RG. Immune-enhancing enteral formulas: Are they beneficial in critically ill patients? Nutr Clin Pract 1997;12:51–62.

47. Matarese LE. Rationale and efficacy of specialized enteral nutrition. Nutr Clin Pract 1995;9:58–64.

48. O'Connor DL, Hall R, Adamkin D, et al. Growth and development in preterm infants fed long-chain polyunsaturated fatty acids: A prospective, randomized controlled trial. Pediatrics 2001;108:359–371.

49. Birch EE, Hoffman DR, Castañeda YS, et al. A randomized controlled trial of long-chain polyunsaturated fatty acid supplementation of formula in term infants after weaning at 6 weeks of age. Am J Clin Nutr 2002;75:570–580.

50. Lucas A, Stafford M, Morley R, et al. Efficacy and safety of long-chain polyunsaturated fatty acid supplementation of infant-formula milk: A randomised trial. Lancet 1999;354:1948–1954.

51. Innis SM, Adamkin DH, Hall RT, et al. Docosahexaenoic acid and arachidonic acid enhance growth with no adverse effects in preterm infants fed formula. J Pediatr 2002;140:547–554.

52. Heird WC. The role of polyunsaturated fatty acids in term and preterm infants and breastfeeding mothers. Pediatr Clin North Am 2001;48:173–188.

53. Scheppach WM, Bartram HP. Experimental evidence for and clinical implications of fiber and artificial enteral nutrition. Nutrition 1993;9:399–405.

54. Jew R, Owen D, Kaufman D, et al. Osmolality of commonly used medications and formulas in the neonatal intensive care unit. Nutr Clin Pract 1997;12:158–163.

55. Parrish CR. Enteral feeding: The art and the science. Nutr Clin Pract 2003;18:76–85.

56. MacBurney MM, Russell C, Young LS. Formulas. In: Rombeau JL, Caldwell MD, eds. Clinical Nutrition: Enteral and Tube Feeding, 2nd ed. Philadelphia, Saunders, 1990:149–173.

57. Silk DBA, Grimble GK. Relevance of physiology of nutrient absorption to formulation of enteral diets. Nutrition 1992;8:1–12.

58. Montejo JC, Zarazaga A, Lopez-Martinez J, et al. Immunonutrition in the intensive care unit. A systematic review and consensus statement. Clin Nutr 2003;22:221–233.

59. Beale RJ, Bryg DJ, Bihari DJ. Immunonutrition in the critically ill: A systematic review of clinical outcome. Crit Care Med 1999;27:2799–2805.

60. Heys SD, Walker LG, Smith I, Eremin O. Enteral nutritional supplementation with key nutrients in patients with critical illness and cancer: A meta-analysis of randomized controlled clinical trials. Ann Surg 1999;229:467–477.

61. Heyland DK, Novak F, Drover JW, et al. Should immunonutrition become routine in critically ill patients? A systematic review of the evidence. JAMA 2001;286:944–953.

62. Bower RH, Cerra FB, Bershadsky B, et al. Early enteral administration of a formula (Impact) supplemented with arginine, nucleotides, and fish oil in intensive care unit patients: Results of a multicenter, prospective, randomized, clinical trial. Crit Care Med 1995;23:436–449.

63. Gadek JE, DeMichele SJ, Karlstad MD, et al. Effect of enteral feeding with eicosapentaenoic acid, gamma-linolenic acid, and antioxidants in patients with acute respiratory distress syndrome. Crit Care Med 1999;27:1409–1420.

64. Russell MK, Charney P. Is there a role for specialized enteral nutrition in the intensive care unit? Nutr Clin Pract 2002;17:156–168.

65. Davis A, Baker S. The use of modular nutrients in pediatrics. JPEN J Parenter Enter Nutr 1996;20:228–236.

66. Navajas MF-C, Chacon DJ, Solvas JRG, et al. Bacterial contamination of enteral feeds as a possible risk of nosocomial infection. J Hosp Infect 1992;21:111–120.

67. Oliviera MH, Bonelli R, Aidoo KE, Batista CR. Microbiological quality of reconstituted enteral formulations used in hospitals. Nutrition 2000;16:729–733.

68. Atkinson SA. Human milk feeding of the micropremie. Clin Perinatol 2000;27:235–247.

69. Porcelli P, Schanler R, Greer F, et al. Growth in human milk-fed very low birth weight infants receiving a new human milk fortifier. Ann Nutr Metab 2000;44:2–10.

70. Sankaran K, Papageorgiou A, Ninan A, Sankaran R. A randomized, controlled evaluation of two commercially available human breast milk fortifiers in health preterm neonates. J Am Diet Assoc 1996;96:1145–1149.

71. Mehall JR, Kite CA, Saltzman DA, et al. Prospective study of the incidence and complications of bacterial contamination of enteral feeding in neonates. J Pediatr Surg 2002;37:1177–1182.

72. Thurn J, Crossley K, Gerdts A, et al. Enteral hyperalimentation as a source of nosocomial infection. J Hosp Infect 1990;15:203–217.

73. McClave SA, Snider HL. Clinical use of gastric residual volumes as a monitor for patients on enteral tube feeding. JPEN J Parenter Enteral Nutr 2002;26(6 Suppl):S43–S50.

74. Davis AM. Pediatrics. In: Matarese LE, Gottschlich MM, eds. Contemporary Nutrition Support Practice: A Clinical Guide. Philadelphia, Saunders, 1998:347–364.

75. MacLaren R. Intolerance to intragastric enteral nutrition in critically ill patients: Complications and management. Pharmacotherapy 2000;20:1486–1498.

76. Booth CM, Heyland DK, Paterson WG. Gastrointestinal promotility drugs in the critical care setting: A systematic review of the evidence. Crit Care Med 2002;30:1429–1435.

77. McClave SA, DeMeo MT, DeLegge MH, et al. North American Summit on Aspiration in the Critically Ill Patient: Consensus statement. JPEN J Parenter Enteral Nutr 2002;26(6 Suppl):S80–S85.

78. Maloney JP, Ryan TA, Brasel KJ, et al. Food dye use in enteral feedings: A review and a call for a moratorium. Nutr Clin Pract 2002;17:168–181.

79. Metheny NA, Clouse RE. Bedside methods for detecting aspiration in tube-fed patients. Chest 1997;111:724–731.

80. Bliss DZ, Guenter PA, Settle RG. Defining and reporting diarrhea in tube-fed patients—what a mess! Am J Clin Nutr 1992;55:753–759.

81. Eisenberg PG. Causes of diarrhea in tube-fed patients: A comprehensive approach to diagnosis and management. Nutr Clin Pract 1993;8:119–123.

82. Frankel EH, Enow NB, Jackson KC, et al. Methods of restoring patency to occluded feeding tubes. Nutr Clin Pract 1998;13:129–131.

83. Cabre E, Gassull MA. Complications of enteral feeding. Nutrition 1993;9:1–9.

84. Bayzyk S. Factors associated with transition to oral feedings in infants fed by nasogastric tubes. Am J Occup Ther 1990;44:1070–1078.

85. Mitchell JF. Oral dosage forms that should not be crushed: 2000 update. Hosp Pharm 2000;35:553–557.

86. Engle KK, Hannawa TE. Techniques for administering oral medications to critical care patients receiving continuous enteral nutrition. Am J Health-Syst Pharm 1999;56:1441–1444.

87. Beckwith MC, Feddema SS, Barton RG, Graves C. A guide to drug therapy in patients with enteral feeding tubes: Dosage form selection and administration methods. Hosp Pharm 2004;39:225–237.

88. Dickerson RN. Medication administration considerations for patients receiving enteral tube feedings. Hosp Pharm 2004;39:84–89, 96.

89. Bauer LA. Interference of oral phenytoin absorption by continuous nasogastric feedings. Neurology 1982;32:570–572.

90. Gilbert S, Hatton J, Magnuson B. How to minimize interaction between phenytoin and enteral feedings: Two approaches. Nutr Clin Pract 1996;11:28–31.

91. Nyffeler MS. Ciprofloxacin use in the enterally fed patient. Nutr Clin Pract 1999;14:73–77.

92. Phillips JO, Metzler MH, Palmieri MT, et al. A prospective study of simplified omeprazole suspension for the prophylaxis of stress-related mucosal damage. Crit Care Med 1996;24:1793–1800.

93. Quercia RA, Fan C, Liu X, et al. Stability of omeprazole in an extemporaneously prepared oral liquid. Am J Health-Syst Pharm 1997;54:1833–1836.

94. Senkel M, Mumme A, Eickhoff U, et al. Early postoperative enteral immunonutrition: Clinical outcome and cost-comparison analyses in surgical patients. Crit Care Med 1997;25:1489–1496.

95. McClave SA, Greene LM, Snider HL, et al. Comparison of the safety of early enteral vs parenteral nutrition in mild acute pancreatitis. JPEN J Parenter Enter Nutr 1996;21:14–20.

96. Trice S, Melnik G, Page CP. Complications and costs of early postoperative parenteral versus enteral nutrition in trauma patients. Nutr Clin Pract 1997;12:114–119.

139
NUTRITIONAL CONSIDERATIONS IN MAJOR ORGAN FAILURE

Renee M. DeHart and Sunshine J. Yocom

Learning Objectives and other resources can be found at *www.pharmacotherapyonline.com.*

KEY CONCEPTS

1 Lipid intolerance is common in acute renal failure, requiring careful monitoring of serum triglyceride concentrations before and during intravenous lipid administration.

2 Carbohydrate calories absorbed and protein lost via renal replacement therapy must be accounted for when designing a parenteral or enteral nutrition regimen for the patient with renal disease.

3 Standard mixed amino acids should be used rather than essential amino acid preparations in patients with acute renal failure.

4 Patients with renal failure will typically require lower amounts of potassium, magnesium, and phosphorus in the nutritional regimen unless refeeding syndrome is present or continuous renal replacement therapies are used.

5 Patients with alcoholic hepatitis or cirrhosis are frequently hypermetabolic when energy requirements are adjusted for lean body mass.

6 Hyperglycemia is common in cirrhosis. Patients with fulminant hepatitis are, however, prone instead to hypoglycemia.

7 Folic acid and thiamine supplementation is important in patients with liver disease for the prevention of anemia and Wernicke's encephalopathy, respectively.

8 In short bowel syndrome, parenteral nutrition should be used to meet nutritional needs in the immediate postoperative period after intestinal resection.

9 Increased fluid and electrolyte replacement may be necessary in short bowel syndrome patients to replace gastrointestinal losses. Patients may need increased calcium, magnesium, zinc, and other trace elements due to decreased absorption and/or excessive gastrointestinal losses.

10 Patients with ileal resection commonly develop vitamin B_{12} deficiency, necessitating therapy with parenteral cyanocobalamin.

11 As small bowel adaptation occurs, some short bowel syndrome patients receiving parenteral nutrition can be transitioned successfully to enteral nutrition. Early initiation of enteral intake affects adaptation because intraluminal nutrients are a stimulus for this process.

12 When a patient is fed with carbohydrates, the amount of carbon dioxide produced markedly exceeds the amount of oxygen consumed in comparison to proteins and fats, which can result in increased ventilatory demand in patients with pulmonary disease. Therefore higher-fat enteral formulas should be considered for use in these patients and overfeeding should be avoided.

13 Excessive fluid administration should be avoided in patients with pulmonary disease because it may exacerbate already compromised pulmonary function.

14 Phosphorus is essential in respiratory disease for its role in the synthesis of adenosine triphosphate, inadequate stores of which can lead to respiratory muscle weakness. Critically ill, malnourished patients are at risk for phosphorus depletion.

Because organ failure may alter absorption, use, and excretion of nutrients, administration of standard nutrients to patients with organ dysfunction may be inappropriate. Individualization of a nutritional regimen for these patients often requires a planned, disease-specific approach. Different laboratory tests or more frequent monitoring of traditional markers may be necessary to ensure that the desired therapeutic goals are achieved. For example, it is impossible to collect a 24-hour urine specimen to measure urea nitrogen and nitrogen balance in an anuric patient. In this situation, an alternative method of calculating urea nitrogen appearance is required.

Patients with acute organ failure requiring nutrition support often are hospitalized in intensive care units (ICUs). With advances in treating chronic organ failure, increasing numbers of older, chronically ill patients will require nutritional support on a long-term basis. It therefore will become increasingly common for nutrition support to be provided in community and ambulatory settings. Regardless of the setting, the clinician needs a firm pathophysiologic foundation on which to build a pharmaceutical care plan to ensure appropriate outcomes for patients requiring nutritional support.

This chapter discusses the nutritional needs of patients with renal, hepatic, gastrointestinal, and pulmonary failure. The predominant approaches to ensure delivery of safe and efficacious nutrients to patients with these disorders are critically reviewed.

RENAL FAILURE

Major differences exist between the metabolic, fluid, and electrolyte management of patients with acute versus chronic kidney disease (CKD). For example, positive nitrogen balance is more difficult to achieve in patients with acute renal failure (ARF) due to the increased rate of protein catabolism. Additionally, patients with acute renal failure are more likely to develop hyperglycemia during nutritional support and frequently are dialyzed by modalities that are not used commonly for the patient with end-stage kidney disease (ESKD). Because of these differences, the nutritional management of patients with ARF is discussed separately.

ACUTE RENAL FAILURE

EPIDEMIOLOGY

Acute renal failure occurs in approximately 5% of all hospitalized patients. The mortality rate of ARF patients who require renal replacement therapy ranges from 40% to as high as 80%.[1] Severe malnutrition has been found in 42% of patients with ARF and is an independent predictor of in-hospital mortality and increased morbidity from sepsis, shock, dysrhythmias, and acute respiratory failure.[2] Since malnutrition is an important contributor to mortality from ARF, nutrition support remains a cornerstone in the treatment of these patients.[3]

PATHOPHYSIOLOGY

Energy Requirements

Energy requirements in this patient population ideally should be measured by indirect calorimetry (see Chap. 135) because energy expenditures of patients with ARF are highly variable. Energy expenditure is close to normal in patients with uncomplicated ARF, but resting energy expenditure (REE) increases by 30% in the presence of sepsis and ARF.[3] Typically, ARF patients without underlying hypermetabolic conditions should receive 25 to 30 kcal/kg per day. Those with underlying hypermetabolic conditions can receive up to 35 kcal/kg per day, unless indirect calorimetry indicates otherwise.[4]

Carbohydrate

Hyperglycemia and peripheral insulin resistance are common in ARF. These patients usually have a superimposed illness that may cause glucose intolerance. The etiology of glucose intolerance in ARF is thought to be due to increased levels of glucagon, growth hormone, and catecholamines, all known antagonists of insulin. Other proposed mechanisms include an elevated glucagon:insulin ratio secondary to impaired degradation of these hormones and elevated secretion of inflammatory cytokines.

Fat

Intolerance to intravenous lipid emulsion (IVLE), evidenced by increased serum triglyceride concentrations, is common in ARF. Hypertriglyceridemia is thought to be caused by decreased catabolism of triglycerides and increased synthesis from free fatty acids (FFAs).[5] Hepatic triglyceride lipase and peripheral lipoprotein lipase activity may be reduced significantly in ARF patients.[3] Insulin resistance and metabolic acidosis may contribute to this process by inhibiting lipoprotein lipase.[6] Triglyceride concentrations therefore should be measured before administering IVLE to patients with ARF. FFA concentrations also are elevated in ARF.

Protein

Urea, the end product of nitrogen metabolism, accumulates rapidly in ARF. Most patients with ARF have a primary stressful illness that results in ureagenesis, and thus protein breakdown is markedly accelerated.[1] Protein catabolism in ARF may be stimulated as the result of insulin resistance, metabolic acidosis, circulating proteases and inflammatory mediators, and the effects of uremic toxins.[7] The mechanism may be direct, via modulation of protein synthesis, or indirect, by inhibiting the action of anabolic hormones.[8]

Significant amounts of protein and amino acids are also removed by dialysis. Amino acid losses of 5.2 g per conventional hemodialysis (HD), 7.3 g per high-flux HD, and up to 13 to 16 g/day during continuous renal replacement therapy (CRRT) have been reported.[9] In one study, CRRT removed urea nitrogen to the same degree as functionally normal kidneys.[10] The clearance of histidine and tryptophan are enhanced, whereas the clearance of phenylalanine and valine are reduced in nondialyzed patients with ARF.[11] In patients undergoing CRRT, glutamine represents roughly one-third of all amino acid dialysate losses. Serum glutamine concentrations decrease significantly early during CRRT but return to baseline subsequently, suggesting altered glutamine metabolism early in the course of CRRT.[12]

Fluid, Electrolyte, and Acid-Base Disorders

The volume status of patients with ARF depends primarily on residual urine output and the type of dialysis received, if any. The patient with oliguric ARF will have impaired excretion of sodium and water. In nonoliguric ARF, considerable sodium may be lost in the urine, necessitating replacement to maintain sodium balance. This also applies to the patient who is losing considerable gastric fluids. Patients on CRRT will lose sodium via hemofiltration or dialysis and should be given sodium as part of their CRRT replacement fluid regimen.

Hyperkalemia is observed frequently in ARF secondary to protein catabolism and intracellular potassium release. Hyperkalemia also results from the impaired secretion and excretion of potassium by the kidney and the endogenous release secondary to tissue breakdown. If this is severe, emergent dialysis may be indicated. Patients on CRRT, however, usually will require potassium replacement to avoid hypokalemia due to dialytic potassium losses.

Because phosphorus is excreted renally, hyperphosphatemia is common in ARF. Like potassium, large amounts of phosphorus are released into the circulation secondary to tissue breakdown during ARF. Control of hyperphosphatemia is important because as the calcium-phosphorus product (serum calcium in milligrams per deciliter multiplied by serum phosphorus in milligrams per deciliter) exceeds 55, the risk of developing metastatic calcification increases (see Chap. 44). Conversely, with initiation of dialysis, particularly CRRT, patients must be monitored for dialysis-induced hypophosphatemia.

The net removal of calcium during the continuous dialysis modalities depends on the calcium concentration of the dialysate fluid.[13] Severe hypocalcemia has been reported when regional citrate anticoagulation has been used for CRRT in ARF and hepatic failure patients.[14]

Hypermagnesemia is common in ARF secondary to impaired excretion and endogenous release from tissue breakdown. Both magnesium and calcium losses via CRRT have been quantified recently:

average losses were of 24 mmol and 70 mmol of magnesium and calcium, respectively.[10]

Patients with ARF usually have metabolic acidosis because of impaired excretion of organic acids. If potassium and sodium are needed in the PN regimen, they should be added as acetate salts, which will be converted to bicarbonate in the liver. This increase in bicarbonate will partially compensate their metabolic acidosis. Intermittent and continuous dialytic therapies also may help improve the metabolic acidosis accompanying ARF by increasing the removal of these endogenously generated acids, as well as by increasing serum bicarbonate levels as the result of diffusion from the dialysate into the blood. Correction of acidosis was greatest when lactate buffers (lactate > bicarbonate > acetate) were used in one study employing continuous veno-venous hemofiltration (CVVH).[15]

Trace Elements

The requirements for trace elements during nutritional support of ARF patients are not well established because trace element accumulation or losses during ARF have not been characterized. Additionally, many of the trace element alterations in ARF may in fact represent an "acute phase reaction."[4] Zinc and chromium are excreted by the kidney and theoretically can accumulate due to reduced excretion and increased intake secondary to impurities in dialysate or intravenous fluids.[16] In ARF patients undergoing CRRT, zinc intake via nutrition support has been shown to exceed patient losses.[10] Selenium concentrations are reduced in ARF patients and may result in a decrease in thyroxine concentrations.[17,18] Because manganese and copper are excreted in bile and zinc and copper are removed by peritoneal dialysis (PD) and HD, most ARF patients receiving parenteral nutrition (PN) should receive trace element supplementation.[19] At least one investigator has recommended giving this supplementation only twice weekly, but not all investigators have agreed on this point.[4]

Vitamins

Little information is available concerning alterations in vitamin requirements in ARF. Reduced plasma concentrations of vitamin A, ascorbate, vitamin D, and vitamin E have been reported in patients with ARF, whereas vitamin K concentrations are relatively increased.[20] Losses of vitamins via dialysis also must be considered. Traditional HD clears several water-soluble vitamins such as folic acid, vitamins C and B_{12}, and pyridoxine, but not the highly protein-bound vitamins A and D.[19] The clinical significance of these findings in ARF is unknown. Currently, it seems prudent to administer vitamins at least daily in doses recommended by the Nutrition Advisory Group of the American Medical Association for patients receiving PN (see Chap. 137).[4] Administration of ascorbic acid should be restricted to under 200 mg/day to avoid secondary oxalosis which may worsen renal function.[4] If the enteral route is used for nutritional support, vitamin administration should at least meet the recommended daily allowances (RDAs).

▶ TREATMENT: Acute Renal Failure

■ ADMINISTRATION ROUTES

Most patients with ARF have a superimposed illness that requires nutritional support by the parenteral route. Enteral nutrition (EN) should be considered when patients with ARF have functional gastrointestinal tracts. The products used frequently during EN in ARF are the calorically dense, electrolyte-free or electrolyte-reduced formulas (Table 139–1). These formulas are useful in patients with fluid overload, hyperkalemia, and hyperphosphatemia. Unfortunately, EN is impossible for many patients with ARF because they are critically ill and have an ileus.

■ SPECIALTY PRODUCTS

Based on the available data, it appears appropriate to use standard mixed amino acids rather than essential amino acid (EAA) solutions in ARF.[4] Improved survival and return of renal function were observed decades ago when EAAs plus glucose were compared with glucose alone in patients with ARF.[21] This led to the marketing of parenteral amino acids containing predominantly or solely EAAs. These products were formulated on the hypothesis that significant nitrogen reuse (urea recycling) occurs during ARF to synthesize nonessential amino acids. Subsequently, several prospective, double-blind studies

TABLE 139–1. Enteral Nutrition Products for Patients with Renal Failure

Product	Flavors	Caloric Density (kcal/mL)	Protein (g/L)	Potassium (mg/1000 kcal)	Phosphorus (mg/1000 kcal)
Deliver 2.0 (Mead Johnson)	V	2	75	845	505
Magnacal Renal (Mead Johnson)	V	2	70	635	400
Nepro (Ross)	V, C, BP	2	70	527	347
Nutren (Nestle)	V	2	80	960	670
NutriRenal (Nestlé)	V	2	70	628	350
Renalcal Diet (Nestlé)	V, Ch, O, Ca, I	2	34.4	N/A	N/A
Re/Neph (Ross)	V, S	2	67	63	N/A
Re/Neph Reduced Sugar (Ross)	V	2	76	84	N/A
Suplena (Ross)	V	2	30	510	365
TwoCal HN (Ross)	V, BP	2	83.5	1225	527

BP, butter pecan; Ca, cappuccino; C, cherry; Ch, chocolate; I, irish cream; O, orange; S, strawberry, V, vanilla.

TABLE 139–2. Empirie Parenteral Nutrition Formulas for Patients with Organ Failure

	Acute Renal Failure	Chronic Renal Failure	Hepatic Failure	Hepatic Transplant	Short Bowel	Pulmonary Failure
Dextrose (%)[a]	40	30	25	15	20	20
CAAs (%)[a]	Variable	4	5[b]	5	5	5
Lipids (%)[a]	1	2	2	2	2	3
NaCl (mEq/L)	0	0	0	0	80[c]	10
Na acetate (mEq/L)	0	30	0	0	0	0
Na phosphate (mEq/L)	0[d]	7.5	15	15	7.5	30
K acetate (mEq/L)	0[d]	0	50	0	60	20
K chloride (mEq/L)	0	10	0	40	0	20
Ca gluconate (mEq/L)	5[d]	5	5	10	10	5
Magnesium sulfate (mEq/L)	0[d]	6	16	20	10	5
Multivitamins (mL/day)	10	10	10	10	10	10
Zinc (mg/day)	3	3–6	8	3–6	10	3
Copper (mg/day)	1.2	1.2	<1.2	1.2	1.2	1.2
Manganese (mcg/day)	300	300	<300	300	≤300	300
Chromium (mcg/day)	12	12	<12	12	20	12
Selenium (mcg/day)	—	40	40	40	60	40

CAA, crystalline amino acid.

[a]Final concentrations after admixture.

[b]Hepatamine 4% when criteria for use are met.

[c]Does not include 0.45% sodium chloride injection or lipid.

[d]The continuous renal replacement therapies frequently require variable additions of electrolytes.

indicated no significant reduction in mortality when the EAA formulations were used.[21]

DESIGN AND INITIATION OF THE NUTRITIONAL REGIMEN

Patients with ARF typically require 25 to 35 kcal/kg per day, and a higher caloric intake may be necessary if hypermetabolism is present. In the absence of dialysis, the nutritional formula should be concentrated in a small volume and contain minimal sodium (Table 139–2). In the oliguric patient receiving PD or HD, these restrictions may be lessened, but the formula generally will need to be concentrated. When using these high-dextrose-concentration formulas, careful monitoring of glucose homeostasis (every 6 hours) is important because of the predisposition toward hyperglycemia in ARF and glucose intake should not exceed 5 g/kg per day.[4] Additionally, CRRT, which is increasingly popular in the treatment of ARF (see Chap. 42), contributes significant calories to a nutritional regimen. This is a direct result of the absorption of glucose from the dialysate or ultrafiltrate replacement fluids: Net uptakes of up to 355 g/day have been reported.[22]

Acute renal failure is not a contraindication to IVLE use, despite the changes in lipid metabolism seen in ARF. When the serum triglyceride concentration is less than 300 mg/dL, IVLE (3 to 7 kcal/kg per day) is recommended to prevent essential fatty acid deficiency and to provide a balanced caloric intake. Typically, doses of less than 1 g fat/kg per day will not significantly worsen triglyceride concentrations.[4]

Although individual patient assessment for presence of hypercatabolism and dialytic losses is necessary, it is not uncommon for patients to require 2.5 g/kg per day of protein or more to approach nitrogen balance.[23] Protein restriction to reduce the urea nitrogen appearance (UNA) rate from exogenous protein intake should not be used unless the ARF is thought to be very temporary and no hypercatabolism is present.[4] Once dialysis therapy is instituted, protein intake should be liberalized to 1 to 1.3 g/kg per day for noncatabolic patients and at least 1.2 to 1.5 g/kg per day for catabolic patients.[4] Patients undergoing CRRT may require up to 2.5 g/kg per day of

protein. Although this can be done safely while providing a greater percentage of patients with a positive nitrogen balance, a reduction in mortality has not been documented.[24]

Several electrolytes (i.e., phosphorus, magnesium, and potassium) warrant special attention when designing the initial nutritional regimen/formula for the ARF patient. During early ARF, PN solutions should not contain potassium unless the patient is hypokalemic or undergoing CRRT. After several days, the serum potassium concentrations tend to decrease, often necessitating cautious addition of potassium to the PN solution. If the enteral route is used, formulas with minimal potassium may be needed. Serum potassium concentrations may decrease more rapidly in patients receiving CRRT. Potassium losses during CRRT are proportional to the potassium gradient between blood and dialysate. Therefore cautious additions of potassium may be considered earlier in the course of ARF for those patients treated with CRRT. Serum magnesium concentrations do not decrease as quickly as potassium concentrations in patients receiving electrolyte-free nutrition regimens. As serum concentrations decrease toward normal and/or renal function returns, magnesium should be added to the PN solution in small amounts (4 to 6 mEq/L).

Phosphorus can be omitted from the nutritional formula of patients receiving PN until the phosphorus level approaches normal (<5 mg/dL). It is prudent to monitor phosphorus concentrations daily and to add phosphorus in small doses once the serum concentration is below 4 mg/dL. Failure to do so can lead to severe hypophosphatemia (see Chap. 49) despite continued renal failure, especially in the patient treated with CRRT. Patients with persistently high serum phosphorus concentrations who have a functional gastrointestinal tract (GIT) can be prescribed phosphate-binding therapy (see Chap. 44) and enteral feedings low in phosphorus to minimize the absorption of exogenous phosphorus.

EVALUATION OF THERAPEUTIC OUTCOMES

Despite recent advances in treatment, acute renal failure is still associated with significant mortality.[3]

To date, there is no clear consensus regarding a benefit of nutritional supplementation on the outcome parameters of renal recovery or mortality. While data suggest that malnourished ARF patients experience significantly higher mortality rates (odds ratio of in-hospital mortality of 7.21) than ARF patients without malnutrition,[2] not all studies have shown a survival benefit from aggressive nutritional support.[24] When nutrition support is used, the evaluation tools used in monitoring ARF patients are similar to those used for other patients receiving PN and EN (see Chaps. 137 and 138).

CHRONIC KIDNEY DISEASE

Chronic kidney disease (CKD), as evidenced by the inability of the kidneys to excrete nitrogenous and other waste products, usually develops over months to years (see Chap. 43). Malnutrition secondary to reduced oral nutrient intake frequently is evident when the glomerular filtration rate (GFR) drops below 20 to 25 mL/min. Patients with CKD are considered to have ESKD when the GFR falls below 15 mL/min (see Chap. 44). Malnutrition is also a common occurrence in ESKD, not only because of decreased oral intake, but also due to increased nutrient losses via the various renal replacement therapies. Because of its chronicity, malnutrition in these patients is treated most frequently in the ambulatory setting with EN.

EPIDEMIOLOGY

Protein-energy malnutrition is very common in the ESKD patient population. Significant malnutrition has been noted in 20% to 36% of ESKD patients undergoing HD and in up to 45% of patients commencing continuous ambulatory peritoneal dialysis (CAPD) or cycling peritoneal dialysis (CPD).[25,26] In one of the larger studies to date (n = 1397), mean dietary calorie and protein intake in those 50 years of age and older was 22 kcal/kg per day and 0.9 g/kg per day, respectively.[27] Both these values are lower than published recommendations for patients with CKD.[28] Protein-energy malnutrition is a significant predictor of morbidity and mortality in most studies of patients with ESKD. However, there appears to be a gender difference in nutritional status in ESKD patients: women tend to have a higher prevalence of malnutrition[26] and poorer nutritional outcomes, yet a lower mortality rate.[29]

PATHOPHYSIOLOGY

Carbohydrate

In general, ESKD patients are not as nutritionally stressed as patients with ARF; however, more than one-half of ESKD patients have insulin resistance and hyperglycemia. This has been attributed to the increased glucagon:insulin ratio, resulting in protein breakdown and gluconeogenesis. In patients with normal peritoneal transport on CAPD, roughly 60% of glucose in the dialysate is absorbed. One method of estimating the quantity of glucose absorbed is: glucose absorbed (g/day) = $0.89x$ (g/day) − 43, where x is the total amount of dialysate glucose instilled daily. This dialysate glucose absorption can worsen existing hyperglycemia and contribute significantly to the patient's energy intake. Therefore, kwashiorkor-type malnutrition is common. Although glucose control is not problematic unless the patient is diabetic, infected, or subjected to operative stress, insulin can be added to CAPD bags to control hyperglycemia (see Chap. 45).

Fat

Hypertriglyceridemia is common in ESKD patients.[30] This is mainly due to decreased catabolism of triglycerides secondary to decreased hepatic lipoprotein lipase activity.[5] Most ESKD patients receiving HD also receive heparin, which activates lipoprotein lipase and converts triglycerides to FFAs and glycerol. Carnitine, an amino acid necessary for the transport of long-chain fatty acids across mitochondria where oxidation results in energy production, is removed by HD and CAPD, and therefore serum carnitine concentrations typically are reduced in ESKD.[31]

Current guidelines do not advocate carnitine administration for the treatment of hypertriglyceridemia.[32] Studies of carnitine for this indication have varied widely in duration and have used both oral and intravenous administration in varying doses (1 mg/kg to 2 g/day intravenously, 10 mg/kg per day to 3 g/day orally). Patients receiving long-term dialysis treatment also have been shown to accumulate remnants of triglyceride-rich lipoproteins. This lipoprotein abnormality can result in type III hyperlipidemia with increased intermediate-density lipoprotein.

Leptin, which is produced and secreted by fat cells, appears to function as a lipostat mechanism via regulation of satiety (see Chap. 140). Leptin concentrations often are elevated in ESKD patients, particularly those undergoing CAPD.[33] Hyperleptinemia in ESKD patients may correlate positively with body fat mass[34] and negatively with lean body mass.[33] Further study is required to define the relationship between leptin concentrations and nutrition status in patients with CKD.[35]

Protein

Secondary analysis of the Modification of Diet in Renal Disease Study indicated that in nondiabetics, a reduction of dietary protein intake may slow the rate of renal disease progression and ultimately delay the onset of dialysis[36] (see Chap. 43). Meta-analyses of diabetic as well as nondiabetic patients suggest that dietary protein restriction to 0.5 to 0.85 g/kg per day is weakly associated with slowing of the progression of renal disease.[37] The recent National Kidney Foundation Kidney Disease Outcomes Quality Initiative guidelines for nutrition in patients with CKD recommend a diet providing 0.6 g/kg of protein per day for those with a GFR of less than 25 mL/min.[32] Although the safety of low-protein diets has been questioned, one analysis strongly suggests that for carefully selected and monitored patients, protein intakes of as low as 0.3 g/kg per day supplemented with EAAs can be used safely.[38] Although it has been suggested that vegetable-based low-protein diets may further slow progression of renal failure beyond that of animal-based low-protein diets, not all studies have found this to be true.[39]

ESKD patients receiving CAPD require special attention due to protein losses across the peritoneal membrane. Peritoneal protein losses typically range from 5 to 15 g/day in patients treated by CAPD.[32] PD protein losses, however, do not predict risk for malnutrition (as measured by serum albumin concentration) in all patients.[32] Nonetheless, these losses should be taken into consideration when designing the PN or EN formula for the CAPD patient. Recent guidelines suggest that dietary protein intake of at least 1.2 to 1.3 g/kg per day (at least 50% of high biologic value) is needed to consistently achieve neutral or positive nitrogen balance in nonacutely ill CAPD patients and clinically stable HD patients.[32] Dialysate protein losses also must be examined for the ESKD patient undergoing HD. The amount of protein lost via HD depends on the dialysis membrane used and whether the dialyzer is being reused. Typical losses are 10 to 12 g per dialysis session, but this may be increased by up to 50% with dialyzer reuse.[32] These losses must be considered when designing the protein regimen for the patient.

Fluid and Electrolytes

Hyponatremia, often due to overhydration, is common in CKD, but usually does not require additional administration of sodium. Regular dialysis is the principal means for control of body water and serum sodium concentration in the ESKD patient.

Patients with CKD or ESKD who develop hyperkalemia generally have ingested excessive potassium relative to the potassium-removing capacity of the failing kidney (and dialysis, in the case of ESKD). The undernourished CKD or ESKD patient receiving PN, however, may require considerable potassium as new body cell mass is synthesized. When inappropriately low amounts of potassium are given during refeeding, hypokalemia may develop.

Patients with CKD or ESKD often are treated for hyperphosphatemia with phosphorus-restricted diets and phosphate binding agents (see Chaps. 43 and 44). When these patients receive aggressive nutritional support, the combination of refeeding (cellular uptake of phosphorus for synthesis of body cell mass) and vigorous phosphate-binding therapy can result in hypophosphatemia.

Clinically significant hypermagnesemia is less common in patients with CKD and ESKD compared with ARF. It is usually added to the PN solution in reduced doses (4 mEq/L or less), and serum concentrations need to be monitored.

Metabolic acidosis, a common complication of ESKD, is associated with increased protein degradation and decreased synthesis of albumin.[32] Correction of acidosis in ESKD patients may be associated with increases in serum albumin, body weight, and midarm muscle circumference, and fewer hospitalizations.[40,41] Appropriate stabilization of serum bicarbonate concentrations (>22 mEq/L) via alteration of the dialysate bicarbonate concentration or administration of oral bicarbonate salts thus seems a prudent nutritional intervention in these patients (see Chap. 44 and 51).

Trace Elements

There are considerable data regarding trace element requirements in patients with ESKD.[19] Decreased zinc concentrations in dialysis patients have been linked to taste disturbances and sexual dysfunction.[16] Zinc supplementation, however, has not universally reversed these anomalies. Although serum concentrations of this trace element are decreased, total body stores of zinc in ESKD often are increased.[16] This suggests a redistribution of zinc or increased need to maintain normal enzymatic function in ESKD.

Serum chromium concentrations are elevated in chronic HD and CAPD patients,[16] perhaps due to the fact that needles used during HD and the peritoneal and hemodialysate fluids are sources of chromium. Both HD and CAPD patients have been found to have decreased selenium concentrations[42] that can be increased with oral selenium supplements of 135 to 140 mcg/day in HD patients.[43] It appears that for patients undergoing HD, significant selenium losses occur during dialysis.[44]

The trace element with the most established significance in ESKD is aluminum. Central nervous system toxicity is linked to the presence of aluminum in the dialysate or the excessive use of aluminum-containing medications. Consequently, the concentration of aluminum in dialysis solutions has been reduced and aluminum-containing antacids are no longer routinely used as phosphate binders. Aluminum toxicity can be treated with deferoxamine, as discussed in Chap. 44.

Vitamins

Vitamin status is better defined in CKD patients than those with ARF. CKD patients are prone to develop water-soluble vitamin deficiencies because of decreased dietary intake secondary to anorexia and restriction of certain foods because of their protein, potassium, or phosphorus content. Additionally, in the ESKD patient, HD losses of ascorbic acid, folic acid, and pyridoxine are common. Plasma ascorbic acid concentrations have been found to be normal in CAPD patients[45] but significantly reduced in HD patients.[46] The highly protein-bound vitamins (A, D, and B_{12}) are not removed significantly by HD.[19] Vitamin D deficiency is correlated with decreased serum albumin concentrations, and supplementation of vitamin D has increased serum albumin concentrations significantly in deficient patients.[47] Vitamin A concentrations often are elevated in CKD and ESKD and can lead to hypervitaminosis A and its cirrhosis-like syndrome. Conversely, vitamin E supplementation may have a distinct benefit to patients with ESKD. Increased oxidative stress in ESKD may contribute to the accelerated atherosclerosis in these patients. Vitamin E in doses of 800 international units per day has been shown to decrease low-density lipoprotein oxidation in patients with ESKD, especially in patients undergoing CAPD.[48] Thiamine concentrations decrease during dialysis; supplementation within the RDA recommendations is sufficient to keep concentrations in the normal range.[49] Elevated concentrations of homocysteine are associated with an increased risk of cardiovascular disease. Hyperhomocysteinemia is common in patients with ESKD. Folate doses from 2.5 mg three times weekly to 60 mg/day have lowered homocysteine concentrations in ESKD patients, but have not completely reduced concentrations to normal.[50,51]

▶ TREATMENT: Chronic Kidney Disease

▪ ADMINISTRATION ROUTES

CKD and ESKD patients who require nutritional support rarely need PN because their GIT usually is functional. The calorically dense low-electrolyte enteral formulas (see Table 139–1) are particularly useful. Even though ESKD patients receive regular dialysis, many are anuric between dialysis sessions, so excess fluid intake is a potential problem. Nepro, Magnacal Renal, NutriRenal, and Re/Neph are marketed specifically (due to their high caloric density and low electrolyte content) for the ESKD patient who receives regular dialysis. Suplena and Renalcal Diet, which are lower in protein, can be used in protein-restricted CKD patients not yet undergoing HD or CAPD. If there is superimposed illness that precludes EN, standard mixed amino acids should be used as the protein component of the PN solution.

The association of poor nutritional status and increased morbidity and mortality in ESKD has led to the development of alternative nutritional delivery systems for the ESKD patient. One such approach is intradialytic parenteral nutrition (IDPN), or the provision of glucose–amino acid–lipid admixture during HD. IDPN typically allows for the infusion of 650 to 1100 kcal per session (250 mL of 50% to 70% dextrose and 250 mL of 10% to 20% lipids) and 50 to 90 g of protein (500 mL of 10% to 15% amino acids).[52] An evidence-based evaluation of 24 studies employing IDPN found that the use of IDPN was associated with decreased mortality, but only 3 of the 24 studies were randomized.[53] Because of the weaknesses of the data, IDPN should be reserved for malnourished patients who have: serum albumin <3.4 g/dL, weight loss >10% of ideal body weight, dietary history of intake of <25 kcal/kg per day, and failed attempts at oral supplements and enteral tube feedings.[52]

Amino acid dialysate (AAD) is the IDPN counterpart for the CAPD patient. This technique entails using a 1.1% amino acid solution in place of one or two of the dextrose-containing PD exchanges per day. Improvements in serum transferrin and total protein concentrations have been observed in malnourished CAPD patients; however, no beneficial effect has been noted on patient mortality.[54] Adverse effects of this therapy have included exacerbations of uremic symptoms (due to increases in blood urea nitrogen) and metabolic acidosis. Not all studies have demonstrated benefits from this intervention.[55] In summary, AAD may be useful in the treatment of malnourished CAPD patients, but better designed studies are needed.

TABLE 139–3. Initial Enteral Nutrition Prescription for Patients with End-Stage Kidney Disease

Nutrient	Recommendation
Nonprotein calories	30–35 kcal/kg per day for HD
	25–35 kcal/kg per day CAPD (including calories from glucose absorption of dialysate)
Protein	1.1–1.4 g/kg IBW for HD
	1.2–1.5 g/kg IBW for CAPD
Sodium	2–3 g/day for HD[a]
	2–4 g/day for CAPD[a]
Potassium	40 mg/kg IBW[a]
Phosphorus	Less than 17 mg/kg IBW[a]
Calcium	1000–1500 mg/day[a]
Fluid	500–750 mL + daily urine output for HD
	To maintain appropriate fluid balance for CAPD

[a]Individualized based on patient's laboratory values.
CAPD, continuous ambulatory peritoneal dialysis; HD, hemodialysis; IBW, ideal body weight.
From Wiggins et al.[28]

Recombinant human growth hormone (rhGH) in doses of 0.2 international unit/kg per day subcutaneously has been used experimentally in adults with ESKD to enhance anabolism; weight gain equal to 1.2 kg and increased transferrin concentrations have been reported after 4 weeks.[56] In the future there may be a role for rhGH in the treatment of ESKD patients who have inadequate oral

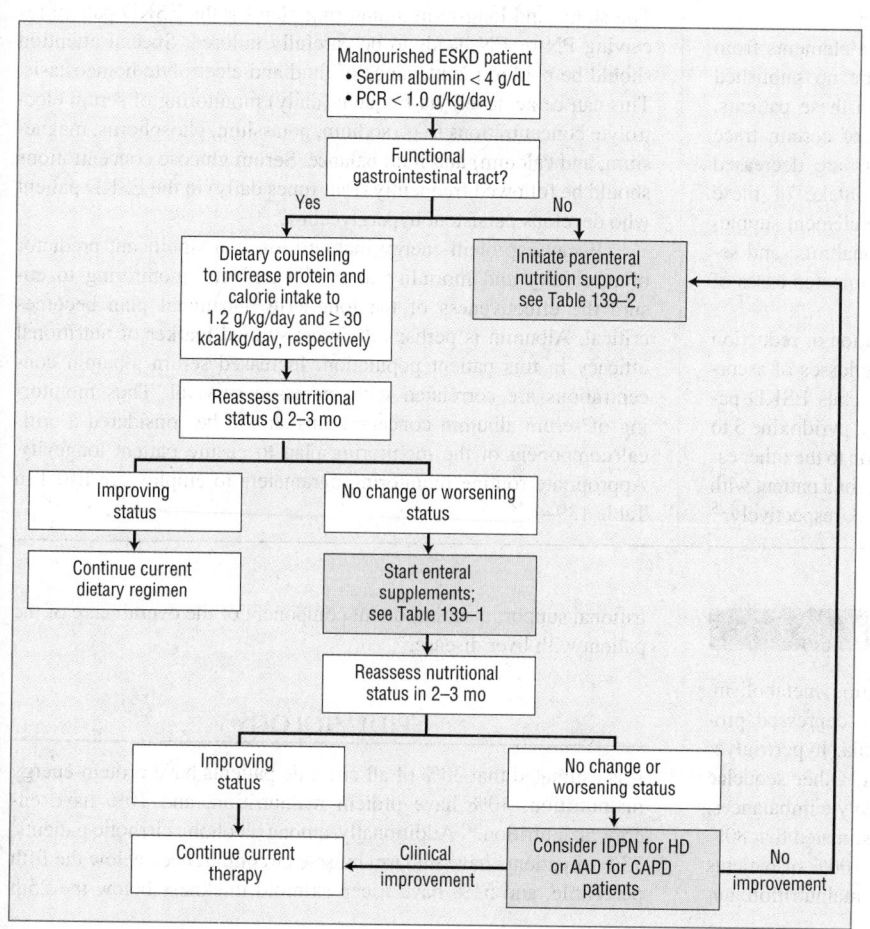

FIGURE 139–1. An algorithmic approach to nutritional support in the patient with end-stage renal disease.

intake despite appropriate dietary counseling and oral supplements.[57]

DESIGN AND INITIATION OF THE NUTRITIONAL REGIMEN

Current recommendations that factor in concurrent illnesses and the likelihood of preexisting malnutrition advocate 35 kcal/kg per day and 1.2 g/kg per day of protein for chronic HD patients and 1.2 to 1.3 g/kg per day of protein for CAPD patients.[32] This is higher than the spontaneous dietary intake in most dialysis patients, as previously discussed. Therefore dietary counseling is important to encourage compliance with these recommendations.

Several electrolytes warrant special attention when providing PN or EN to a patient with CKD or ESKD. Generally, sodium should be administered to CKD patients during nutritional support only to replace losses in order to avoid overhydration. Although these patients also are predisposed to hyperkalemia, once anabolism is attained in CKD patients, potassium requirements may be as high as 40 to 80 mEq/day. This dose needs to be given carefully and requires serum potassium concentration monitoring. Clinically significant hypermagnesemia is less common in patients with CKD compared with ARF. It is usually added to the PN solution in reduced doses (4 mEq/L).

◀ Patients with CKD or ESKD often are treated for hyperphosphatemia. With aggressive nutritional support, the combination of refeeding and phosphate-binding therapy can result in hypophosphatemia. Decreasing or temporarily discontinuing the phosphate-binding therapy is appropriate if this occurs. Thereafter conservative amounts of phosphorus may need to be administered.

Some practitioners advocate withholding trace elements from CKD and ESKD patients receiving PN. There are no published guidelines specific for the use of trace elements in these patients. Because serum concentrations in ESKD patients of certain trace elements are normal (e.g., manganese) and others are decreased (e.g., zinc and selenium), the standard dietary intake of these trace elements is recommended, and standard trace element supplements should be added to PN regimens.[19] Additional zinc and selenium supplementation may be considered in documented cases of deficiency.

During PN in CKD or ESKD patients, elimination or reduction of the dose of vitamin A is recommended. Dialytic losses of ascorbic acid, folic acid, and pyridoxine are common. Thus ESKD patients should receive ascorbic acid 50 to 100 mg/day, pyridoxine 5 to 10 mg/day, and at least 1 mg/day folic acid in addition to the other essential vitamins.[19] Typical PN and EN prescriptions for a patient with ESKD are presented in Table 139–2 and Table 139–3, respectively.[28]

TABLE 139–4. Routine Nutritional Monitoring in Patients with End-Stage Kidney Disease

Parameter	Frequency
Predialysis serum albumin	Monthly
Percentage of usual postdialysis or postdrain body weight	Monthly
Subjective global assessment	Every 6 months
Protein equivalent of total nitrogen appearance (PNA)[a]	Monthly for HD, every 3–4 months for CAPD
Dietary interview and/or diary	Every 6 months
Predialysis prealbumin	As needed
Anthropometry	As needed
Dual energy x-ray absorptiometry	As needed

BUN, blood urea nitrogen. CAPD, continuous ambulatory peritoneal dialysis; HD, hemodialysis.
[a]Beginning of week PNA = Co/[36.3 + (5.48) (spKt/V) + (53.5/spKt/V)] = 0.168, where Co is predialysis BUN and spKt/V, the single-pool index of hemodialysis adequacy = Ln(R − 0.08 × t) + [4 − (3.5 × R)] × UF/W (R is postdialysis: predialysis BUN ratio, t is dialysis session in hours, UF is ultrafiltration in liters, and W is postdialysis weight in kilograms) (see Chap. 45).
From National Kidney Foundation.[32]

An algorithmic approach to improve nutritional status and ensure optimal outcomes is presented in Fig. 139–1.[58]

EVALUATION OF THERAPEUTIC OUTCOMES

The short- and long-term monitoring plan for the ESKD patient receiving PN or EN needs to be carefully tailored. Special attention should be paid to maintenance of fluid and electrolyte homeostasis. This can be achieved via frequent (daily) monitoring of serum electrolyte concentrations (e.g., sodium, potassium, phosphorus, magnesium, and calcium) and fluid balance. Serum glucose concentrations should be followed frequently (four times daily) in the ESKD patient who develops persistent hyperglycemia.

Because protein-energy malnutrition is a significant predictor of morbidity and mortality in ESKD patients, monitoring to ensure the effectiveness of the long-term nutritional plan becomes critical. Albumin is perhaps the most studied marker of nutritional efficacy in this patient population. Increased serum albumin concentrations are correlated with increased survival. Thus monitoring of serum albumin concentrations should be considered a critical component of the monitoring plan to ensure patient longevity. Appropriate routine monitoring parameters to employ are listed in Table 139–4.[32]

HEPATIC FAILURE

The liver is the primary organ involved in the digestion, metabolism, and storage of nutrients. When functional capacity is depressed, profound nutrient intolerance (hyper- or hypoglycemia, hypertriglyceridemia, and hepatic encephalopathy) may result. Other sequelae that accompany the failing liver are fluid and electrolyte imbalances, vitamin deficiencies, and malnutrition. Since it is estimated that 80% of patients with alcoholic liver disease and almost 100% of patients awaiting liver transplantation have some degree of malnutrition, nutritional support is an important component of the overall care of the patient with liver disease.[59]

EPIDEMIOLOGY

It is estimated that 30% of all cirrhotic patients have protein-energy malnutrition, 40% have protein malnutrition, and 10% have energy malnutrition.[60] Additionally, among alcoholic cirrhotic patients, 73% of patients have midarm muscle circumferences below the fifth percentile, and 51% have tricep skinfold thickness below the 25th percentile, which is indicative of protein and energy malnutrition, respectively.[61] Aggressive support is thus imperative to optimize their outcomes and to increase the likelihood of liver transplantation success.

PATHOPHYSIOLOGY

ENERGY

5 Resting energy requirements in stable cirrhotics can appear to be normal, but most are hypermetabolic when the alterations in lean body mass are factored in.[59] The Harris-Benedict equation for estimating caloric needs usually underestimates their needs by 15% to 20%.[62] This underscores the need for patient-specific regimen design and monitoring. An initial energy provision of 25 to 35 kcal/kg per day for cirrhotic patients without underlying malnutrition and 35 to 40 kcal/kg per day for those with concurrent malnutrition is recommended.[59]

CARBOHYDRATE

In healthy adults, approximately 60% of absorbed glucose is taken up by the liver and used for glycogen synthesis, triglyceride synthesis, and glycolysis. In general, glycogen synthesis and glycolysis are enhanced by insulin, whereas gluconeogenesis and glycogen breakdown are controlled by glucagon.

6 Hyperglycemia is common in cirrhosis as a result of peripheral insulin resistance, which is mediated by a decreased binding to insulin receptors and defective postreceptor signal handling in peripheral tissues. Plasma concentrations of insulin are elevated with or without a glucose stimulus. This makes administration of large doses of glucose problematic because administration of insulin to control hyperglycemia may not improve use substantially.

Patients with fulminant hepatitis are prone to hypoglycemia because hepatic glucose production is depressed secondary to decreased glycogen stores and diminished gluconeogenesis. Also, impaired degradation of insulin by the damaged liver may contribute to this disorder. A continuous intravenous infusion of glucose usually prevents hypoglycemia in acute hepatitis, but concentrations greater than 10% glucose may be needed in more severe cases.

FAT

The liver is responsible for synthesis of cholesterol, high-density lipoproteins, and very-low-density lipoproteins. The enzymes lipoprotein lipase and lecithin-cholesterol acyltransferase also are synthesized in this organ. Increased serum triglyceride and FFA concentrations are encountered in patients with hepatic failure, primarily due to the increased lipolysis. The significant insulin resistance that can be seen in cirrhosis causes a shift to lipids as a fuel source.[59] Whereas only 35% of total calories are derived from fat in normal patients after an overnight fast, this can increase to 75% in patients with cirrhosis.[62] Incorporation of late evening snacks in patients with liver cirrhosis may correct abnormal substrate metabolism, increase carbohydrate, and decrease fat oxidation rates.[63,64]

Patients with severe liver failure may be at increased risk for essential fatty acid deficiency: the ratio of nonessential to essential fatty acids was found to be increased in patients with acute and chronic liver failure. Poor oral intake of fat and dietary fat malabsorption in patients with cirrhosis both contribute to essential fatty acid deficiency. These changes were due to decreased linoleic acid and increased serum

oleic acid concentrations.[65] The concentrations of linoleic acid can be increased with administration of an average of 33 g/day of IVLE supplementation.[66] Despite concerns of impaired clearance of long-chain triglycerides in IVLE due to impaired synthesis of apoprotein CII in cirrhotic patents, IVLE solutions have been given safely to patients with fulminant hepatic failure.[59]

Diarrhea and steatorrhea are common in patients with hepatic cholestasis because of intestinal malabsorption (due in part to mucosal edema from hypoalbuminemia), inadequate bile acid delivery to the duodenum, and pancreatic dysfunction with decreased secretion of lipase.[62] Micelle formation is impeded, and thus the long-chain fatty acids pass through the colon, resulting in a foul-smelling, soapy diarrhea.

PROTEIN

Nitrogen requirements for the patient with liver failure are not unlike those of normal subjects, but intolerance to protein is common, and protein restriction has been used successfully as part of the therapy. A dilemma arises when the diet becomes so restrictive that malnutrition results, and the patient becomes susceptible to infection and other complications. Overzealous use of protein to correct nutritional deficits invariably results in hepatic encephalopathy.

Because the liver metabolizes the aromatic amino acids (i.e., phenylalanine, tyrosine, and tryptophan), methionine, and glutamine, the plasma concentrations of these amino acids are elevated in cirrhotic patients. Plasma concentrations of the branched-chain amino acids (BCAAs) (i.e., valine, leucine, and isoleucine) often are depressed because these amino acids are metabolized by skeletal muscle. This altered plasma aminogram contributes to the development of hepatic encephalopathy.

FLUID AND ELECTROLYTES

Patients with severe cirrhosis often have ascites and peripheral edema. The excess of total body sodium in the presence of an even greater excess of total body water results in hyponatremia. Salt and fluid restrictions are required in order to avoid exacerbating this overhydrated state (see Chap. 49). Caution must be exercised, however, because severe sodium and fluid restriction may result in intravascular depletion, which may cause or exacerbate hepatic encephalopathy.

Hypokalemia is common in the patient with liver failure who has normal renal function. Poor nutritional intake and vomiting may initiate this disorder. Severe vomiting may lead to volume contraction metabolic alkalosis, with increased renal excretion of potassium. Secondary hyperaldosteronism, seen in the liver failure patient with intravascular depletion, also increases renal excretion of potassium. Loop diuretic therapy causes increased renal excretion of potassium, whereas diarrhea from lactulose therapy increases fecal excretion of potassium. All these conditions can lead to profound hypokalemia. Therefore, potassium requirements in the liver failure patient receiving specialized nutritional support often are increased substantially.

Poor nutritional intake secondary to alcohol abuse and increased excretion of magnesium secondary to diuretic therapy contribute to hypomagnesemia. Even in cirrhotic patients with normal serum magnesium concentrations, muscle magnesium has been found to be depleted and independently associated with hepatic encephalopathy.[67] During nutrition support, requirements for phosphorus are also substantially supranormal because synthesis of body cell mass occurs. Therefore this population is at risk for developing hypophosphatemia during refeeding.

TRACE ELEMENTS

Many patients with liver failure have a malabsorption syndrome and chronic diarrhea. Chronic diarrhea causes zinc deficiency because stool contains substantial quantities of zinc. Cytokines such as tumor necrosis factor, interleukin-1, and interleukin-6 may stimulate metallothionein, an intestinal zinc-binding protein, thereby inhibiting zinc absorption. Considering the importance of zinc in metalloenzyme reactions, wound healing, immunocompetence, and the senses of taste and smell, patients with chronic diarrhea or large ostomy losses should be suspected of having zinc deficiency; measurement of serum concentrations may be used to confirm such deficiencies. Patients receiving a protein-restricted diet may be at additional risk because substantial amounts of zinc are found in red meat.

Because copper and manganese are excreted in the bile, it has been recommended that these two trace elements not be administered or be administered in reduced doses to patients with serious cholestasis. Direct measurements of manganese in the globus pallidus of cirrhotic patients who died in hepatic coma were two- to sevenfold higher than expected.[68] These findings suggest that reduced quantities of manganese should be provided in the nutritional formulation to avoid exacerbating encephalopathy in the patient with chronic liver disease.

An association between alcoholism and low serum selenium concentrations has been reported.[69] Because selenium is important in maintaining the enzyme glutathione peroxidase, a deficiency of this trace element has been implicated as a cause of hepatic injury in the alcoholic patient. However, because human serum contains at least three fractions of selenium, the use of serum selenium concentrations as an accurate marker for selenium deficiency is controversial.

VITAMINS

Folic acid deficiency, the most common vitamin deficiency, may lead to megaloblastic anemia, whereas thiamine deficiency may result in Wernicke's encephalopathy after rehydration with intravenous glucose. Depletion of hepatic stores of vitamin A, pyridoxine, folic acid, riboflavin, pantothenic acid, vitamin B_{12}, and thiamine have been reported in patients with hepatic failure. Poor intake and malabsorption are the principal causes of vitamin deficiencies in patients with chronic liver disease.

Because vitamin D is metabolized to one of the active forms, 25-hydroxyvitamin D, in the liver, low concentrations of this vitamin are seen in patients with biliary cirrhosis. Impaired absorption of dietary vitamin D also may contribute to these low serum concentrations and the resulting osteoporosis. It is unclear whether vigorous supplementation of these fat-soluble vitamins should be provided during nutritional support, but clearly, therapeutic doses are indicated when a deficiency is documented.

▶ TREATMENT: Hepatic Failure

▦ ADMINISTRATION ROUTE

If the GIT is functional and accessible, EN should be attempted. The indications for PN in the patient with liver failure are similar to those for general hospitalized patients. In most cases, PN in the patient with liver failure can be accomplished via the administration of standard mixed amino acids (Fig. 139–2).

An enteral product is marketed as a supplement for patients with hepatic encephalopathy (NutriHep). It has increased amounts of BCAAs and reduced amounts of aromatic amino acids (AAAs) and methionine. NutriHep meets the U.S. RDA vitamin and mineral requirements, contains a high percentage of medium-chain triglycerides (MCTs), and is supplemented with carnitine. Clinical trials using BCAA products have yielded inconsistent outcomes with regard to both short-term improvement in encephalopathy as well as mortality benefit.[70] Studies investigating the longer-term effects of using BCAAs preferentially are lacking to date.

There has been considerable interest in the use of vegetable-protein diets in the chronic management of patients with cirrhosis and hepatic encephalopathy. Enthusiasm for this therapy is based on the reduced amounts of AAAs and methionine in vegetable protein. The

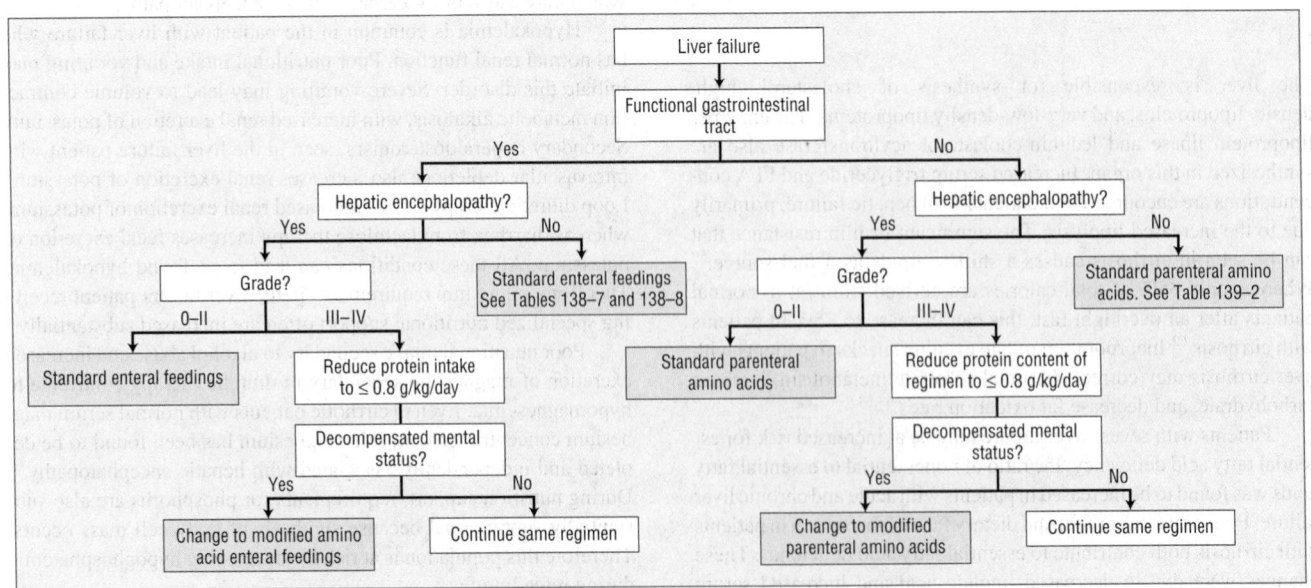

FIGURE 139–2. An algorithmic approach to nutritional support for the patient with hepatic failure.

beneficial effects of vegetable protein also may result from decreased nitrogen absorption in response to decreased gastrointestinal transit time or an increased fecal nitrogen excretion by colonic bacterial flora. However, compliance is more difficult to achieve with vegetable-based than animal-based protein diets in a large number of patients.

SPECIALTY PRODUCTS

The major controversy in nutritional support of the patient with liver failure has centered around the use of protein products. Modified amino acid solutions for PN (HepatAmine, others) are marketed for patients with liver failure and hepatic encephalopathy. They are enriched with BCAAs and have reduced amounts of AAAs and methionine. The products are formulated on the basis of the false neurotransmitter hypothesis, which concludes that hepatic encephalopathy may be due to increased AAA concentrations in the central nervous system.

BCAA products have not universally improved nitrogen balance. Standard amino acid mixtures can be used successfully without worsening encephalopathy. Studies examining improvement in encephalopathy or mortality rates with use of these modified amino acids have yielded conflicting results. This, coupled with the increased cost of these products, has led most clinicians to reserve these products for patients with severe encephalopathy who decompensate on standard amino acids despite continued lactulose-neomycin therapy.

CLINICAL CONTROVERSY

While specialty BCAA solutions have been shown to improve encephalopathy and reduce mortality in the short term, many clinicians reserve their use for patients who decompensate on standard amino acid solutions or fail temporary protein restriction attempts.

DESIGN AND INITIATION OF THE NUTRITIONAL REGIMEN

Patients with alcoholic hepatitis or cirrhosis are frequently hypermetabolic. Indirect calorimetry quantification may be preferred to empiric estimates of caloric requirements in this setting to avoid under- or overfeeding calories. Excessive calorie provision actually may promote liver dysfunction and increased production of carbon dioxide with an associated increased work of breathing. When dextrose-based PN is started in these patients, additional thiamine may be needed to prevent Wernicke's encephalopathy.

IVLE should be used in patients with liver failure only to prevent essential fatty acid deficiency when initial serum triglyceride concentrations exceed 300 mg/dL. If serum triglyceride concentrations are low or normal, IVLE should be used as a calorie source. Monitoring serum triglyceride concentration and FFA oxidation (not available in all facilities) to ensure that lipid is both cleared and oxidized appropriately has been suggested. Triglyceride concentrations are the only available marker in most clinical practices at this time. Oral MCTs have been used occasionally with success because they do not require pancreatic enzymes or micelle formation before absorption. However, these products do not provide essential fatty acids.

Most clinicians routinely use standard mixed amino acids and reserve BCAA products for patients with severe encephalopathy who decompensate on standard amino acids despite continued lactulose-neomycin therapy. Protein restriction temporarily to ≤0.8 g/kg per day is usually attempted before BCAA products in the patient with severe encephalopathy (see Fig. 139–2).

The electrolytes that warrant the most careful monitoring in liver disease include sodium, potassium, phosphorus, and magnesium. During fluid and salt restriction, patients (especially those receiving concurrent lactulose therapy) should be observed for symptoms of volume depletion (e.g., increased pulse rate, decreased blood pressure, or dry mucous membranes). The magnesium dose should be individualized to maintain concentrations in the normal range. This often requires magnesium concentrations as high as 24 mEq/L in the PN solution, which is two to three times the standard daily dose.

Trace elements that warrant individual attention include zinc, copper, and manganese. Oral supplementation of zinc sulfate (600 mg/day) capsules or intravenous zinc chloride may be needed to prevent deficiency or correct deficits. For patients receiving PN, withholding copper from the solution until a copper serum concentration in the normal range is documented or the cholestasis resolves is appropriate. Patients who have chronic cholestasis may require copper in reduced doses (e.g., 0.6 mg/day); however, they should have serum copper concentrations checked regularly (once per month in the acute care setting and every 6 months in the ambulatory setting). Manganese restriction also may be required in these patients. The nutritional requirements of patients with liver failure secondary to cirrhosis are

TABLE 139–5. Nutrition Recommendations for Patients with Liver Disease

Patient Type	Calorie Energy (kcal/kg per day)	Protein (g/kg per day)	Comments
Compensated cirrhosis	25–35	1–1.2	Use a bedtime snack and frequent small meals
Decompensated cirrhosis	25–35	0.5–1.5 for mild encephalopathy; 0.5 for severe encephalopathy	Use BCAAs for refractory cases of encephalopathy unresponsive to protein restriction
Decompenstated cirrhosis with malnutrition	35–40	1.5	May have to temporarily decrease protein for encephalopathy worsening

Decompensated cirrhosis: cirrhosis accompanied by significant ascites or encephalopathy.
BCAA, branched-chain amino acid.
From Matos et al[59] and Dudrick et al.[62]

listed in Table 139–5 and an empiric PN formula for the patient with hepatic failure is presented in Table 139–2.[59,62]

EVALUATION OF THERAPEUTIC OUTCOMES

Prealbumin and retinol-binding protein, traditionally sensitive markers of protein-energy malnutrition, may not be as reliable in patients with hepatic failure. Liver failure can cause decreased concentrations of both, independent of nutritional status.[71] Indeed, many of the commonly used markers of nutritional status correlate poorly with body cell mass in those with end-stage liver disease. Midarm muscle circumference and handgrip strength have been found to be the best

HEPATIC TRANSPLANTATION

Orthotopic liver transplantation (OLT) has become an important intervention for the patient with end-stage liver disease. Many patients receive nutrition support following this operation because of their poor preoperative nutritional status and the postoperative stress. Although hypermetabolism in the early postoperative period has been reported, a caloric intake of only 1.2 times basal energy expenditure (BEE) typically meets caloric needs in the short-term after transplantation.[72] Increased protein catabolism has been noted in response to the stress of liver transplantation and the administration of large doses of corticosteroids following surgical intervention.[73]

EPIDEMIOLOGY

The percentage of OLT patients requiring nutritional support has been well documented. In one report of 427 OLT patients, 32.7% received at least one form of nutritional support: 8.9% received tube feedings alone, 11.9% received PN alone, and a combination of tube feedings and PN was provided to 11.9%. In one group of patients undergoing elective OLT, 79% were at or below the 25th percentile of anthropometric measurements and 28% were below the fifth percentile.[74] This indicates a high prevalence of malnutrition in patients awaiting OLT. Severe malnutrition as assessed by subjective global assessment pre-OLT is associated with increased packed red blood cells, fresh frozen plasma, and cryoprecipitate transfusions, as well as longer postoperative hospital stays.[75] However, whether preoperative nutritional interventions improve outcomes post-OLT is still an area of controversy.

CLINICAL CONTROVERSY

Despite the high incidence of malnutrition pre-OLT, data supporting a mortality benefit from pre-OLT nutrition support are relatively lacking. Studies thus far have been limited by small sample size, so it is uncertain whether nutritional interventions in these patients truly convey a survival benefit long term. Larger controlled clinical trials are needed.

The majority of pre-OLT nutrition intervention studies demonstrate a morbidity benefit post-OLT (per anthropometric tests, hospital stay, and postoperative infections), but typically fail to demonstrate a mortality benefit that reaches statistical significance (although this may be due to small sample sizes).[72,73,76] Preoperative obesity is known to increase morbidity,[77] and in some studies, mortality perioperatively.[76] It is for these reasons that some centers consider

predictors of body cell mass.[71] The poor correlation of other markers suggests that they are of limited value for patients with changing hepatic function.

QUALITY-OF-LIFE ISSUES

Nutritional supplementation provided to patients with alcoholic cirrhosis has been demonstrated to reduce the frequency of hospitalizations. Therefore nutrition supplementation in liver failure should be viewed as a method of reducing nutrition-related complications, as well as improving quality of life and decreasing cost of care.

morbid obesity a relative contraindication to OLT and a reason for advocating weight loss pre-OLT in this patient group.

PATHOPHYSIOLOGY

CARBOHYDRATE, PROTEIN, AND FAT

Postoperative hyperglycemia is common after OLT. Corticosteroids administered to prevent organ rejection may contribute to the hyperglycemia observed during the postoperative period. Alterations in glucose uptake in peripheral tissue also may be present in these patients and thereby contribute to hyperglycemia after OLT.[78]

Most patients will tolerate standard amino acids following OLT because the new liver is functioning properly, and hepatic encephalopathy is not problematic. The excessive nitrogen losses associated with this procedure warrant the provision of 1.3 to 2 g/kg per day of protein immediately post-OLT.[72] Modified amino acids should be reserved for patients with marginal hepatic function associated with rejection or hepatic encephalopathy.

A combination of MCTs and long-chain triglycerides (LCTs) has been studied in post-OLT patients. No significant differences in carbohydrate or lipid oxidation rates were seen, thus suggesting that MCT-specific emulsion is not needed for the PN regimen of the OLT patient.[79] Large amounts of LCTs should be given cautiously, however, since it has been suggested that LCTs may impair reticuloendothelial function/recovery after OLT, which could contribute to increased postoperative infections.[80]

FLUID, ELECTROLYTE, AND ACID-BASE DISORDERS

Patients undergoing OLT receive a substantial amount of crystalloid and blood products during the operative procedure. This often results in an edematous state in the postoperative period, especially in patients who had ascites preoperatively. The large citrate load from administered blood products has been implicated in causing hypocalcemia (due to citrate binding of ionized calcium) and metabolic alkalosis (due to conversion of citrate to bicarbonate) in the postoperative period. Low serum concentrations of magnesium are common in the postoperative period.[72] Reduced intake from restricted diets and increased urinary excretion secondary to cyclosporine therapy contribute to hypomagnesemia.

TRACE ELEMENTS AND VITAMINS

Low serum concentrations of zinc are common in the postoperative period. Restricted diets before surgery and hyperzincuria secondary to liver disease both contribute to hypozincemia in this population. Serum zinc concentrations have been found to recover rapidly after transplantation, obviating the need for further supplementation.[81] On the other hand, patients who have severe cholestasis before and after OLT should have copper and manganese restricted because they are excreted in the bile and thus serum concentrations may be elevated.

Low serum vitamin A concentrations are present in many patients with chronic liver disease. Mean serum vitamin A concentrations measure less than one-half normal in pre-OLT patients, but normalize within 2 weeks after transplantation.[82]

Osteoporosis and fracture risk increase in patients after liver transplantation. Patients awaiting OLT have a 15% to 40% incidence of osteoporosis.[73] This incidence increases to as much as 46% post-OLT, with roughly 20% of patients experiencing a fracture within 1 year of transplant. Poor diets, lack of physical activity, reduced serum 25-hydroxyvitamin D and 1,25-dihydroxyvitamin D, and abnormal parathyroid hormone concentrations are all thought to contribute pretransplant.[73] Post-OLT corticosteroid therapy will also negatively impact bone metabolism, but may not be the sole reason for continued bone loss post-OLT. Mean bone mineral density (BMD) has taken a mean of 85 months to return to pre-OLT levels.[83] Single-dose bisphosphonate infusion did not alter bone formation or resorption in the early (30 days) post-OLT period.[84] It is likely that lowering steroid doses, BMD screening, preventive measures, and calcium and vitamin D supplementation will be the mainstay treatment options for this problem.[85]

▶ TREATMENT: Hepatic Transplantation

■ ADMINISTRATION ROUTES

The least invasive method of feeding should always be employed pre-OLT. If oral intake is inadequate, enteral feedings should be given via small-bore nasogastric or nasojejunal feeding tubes, unless the patient has active esophageal variceal bleeding. More permanently placed feeding tubes (gastrostomy, others) in patients with ascites should be avoided to minimize infection and fluid leakage risks.[72]

Post-OLT, if patients were not malnourished to start, oral diets with liquid supplements as needed can be attempted. In patients with pre-existing malnutrition, enteral nutrition via feeding tube is the therapy of choice; however, small bowel access is needed for this to occur, since postoperative gastric ileus is common. This would necessitate placement of a nasoduodenal or nasojejunal tube during or immediately after surgery. Calorie counts of oral intake can be used to determine when oral intake is sufficient to discontinue tube feedings. If no bowel function is present postoperatively, PN therapy is appropriate.

■ DESIGN AND INITIATION OF THE NUTRITIONAL REGIMEN

OLT patients should be given a nutritional formula that provides at least 1.2 times BEE per day postoperatively, with a mix of energy sources (typically 70% of calories given as carbohydrates once at goal rate). Because of the significant incidence of hyperglycemia immediately postoperatively, it is recommended to wait 24 hours if using PN, or to begin very slowly with a relatively low concentration of dextrose (e.g., 10% or 15% dextrose in water) and titrate as tolerated over a week.[72] These patients also should be provided with at least 1.3 g/kg per day dry weight of protein via standard amino acid solutions. Because OLT patients frequently are edematous postoperatively, the nutritional regimen may need to be volume-restricted. Citrate-containing blood products bind ionized calcium, mandating supplemental doses of calcium in PN. Supplemental doses of potassium and phosphorus may also be needed if refeeding occurs in the malnourished OLT patient. Additionally, OLT patients receiving cyclosporine therapy often will require magnesium in amounts that exceed standard doses during postoperative nutritional support. Lastly, routine multivitamin and trace element supplements should be given daily in the PN formula as outlined in Chap. 137. An example empiric PN for the OLT patient is presented in Table 139–2.

Given the increased rates of obesity seen post-OLT, dietary counseling on the long-term appropriateness of a low-fat, lean meat diet that is low in sodium and rich in calcium and vitamin D should be provided to these patients.[73] If intake of calcium and vitamin D is inadequate, supplements should be given to assure a total intake of 1,500 mg of elemental calcium and 400 to 800 international units of vitamin D.

■ EVALUATION OF THERAPEUTIC OUTCOMES

The monitoring plan of the OLT patient needs to be individualized. Patients receiving cyclosporine or corticosteroids should be monitored closely (at least every 6 hours) for hyperglycemia. Following successful OLT, hepatic encephalopathy is no longer problematic. Thus nitrogen balance should be evaluated to determine the optimal amount of protein to be provided. Fluid balance should be followed carefully to avoid volume overload, especially in patients who received large volumes of fluids intraoperatively. Serum magnesium levels should be monitored daily or more frequently if deficiency is documented, especially in patients receiving cyclosporine therapy. Serum potassium and phosphorus concentrations should also be followed carefully in the malnourished OLT patient because of the risk of the refeeding syndrome (see Chap. 137).

SHORT BOWEL SYNDROME

An intact functional GIT is essential for complete absorption and digestion of nutrients. Short bowel syndrome (SBS) is a disease state imposed by significant resection of the small bowel, which results in the malabsorption of nutrients and fluids. Morbidity and mortality due to gastrointestinal failure in SBS patients has been improved by interventional nutrition with PN and EN. The goal of nutritional support with parenteral and enteral nutrition is to maintain nutritional status and/or correct nutritional deficiencies.

EPIDEMIOLOGY

In the United States there are at least 10,000 patients who have SBS.[86] In adults, the most common etiologies of surgery leading to SBS are Crohn's disease, mesenteric vascular disease, and cancer. In infants, necrotizing enterocolitis, midgut volvulus, and intestinal atresia are the most common etiologies for resection leading to SBS.[87] This condition also may be functional as opposed to anatomic and occur in individuals who have not had resections, but who have a decreased small bowel absorptive capacity due to etiologies such as radiation enteritis or severe inflammatory bowel disease.[88] Symptoms of SBS may vary between patients, but generally include diarrhea, dehydration, electrolyte disturbances, and progressive malnutrition.[87,88]

PATHOPHYSIOLOGY

The average length of small intestine in adults is 600 cm. The majority of nutrients are absorbed in this part of the GIT, and the general consensus is that a diagnosis of SBS should occur when greater than 70% of the small intestine has been resected. Losing this absorptive capacity leads to deficiencies in multiple nutrients which requires the initiation of interventional nutrition.

8 PN must be used at least during the phase immediately following resection of the small intestine while the GIT is healing. EN may be used later during the transition to oral feedings since other areas of the intestinal tract are able to compensate with time.[86] The length and type of nutritional support a patient may require long term is based on such factors as the length of remaining small intestine and the presence or absence of a functional colon. Wilmore and colleagues estimate that for adult patients to transition off of PN, the residual jejunum-ileum length needs to be greater than 120 cm for individuals without a colon, or greater than 60 cm if a portion of the colon is in continuity with the remaining small intestine.[88] Factors that may predict a poor outcome include older age, disease in the residual bowel, and removal of the ileocecal valve, the physiologic sphincter that controls the rate of passage of intestinal contents from small to large bowel and prevents small bowel bacterial overgrowth.[87]

INTESTINAL ADAPTATION

The adaptation process of the residual small intestine to compensate for the resected area begins 12 to 24 hours after bowel resection.[88] The changes in the GIT to compensate for the lost absorptive area are gradual and may continue to occur for 1 to 2 years. Factors that act as stimuli for adaptation include luminal nutrients, pancreaticobiliary secretions, and intestinal hormones.[87,88] The ability of the remaining intestine to adjust after resection is also influenced by the area of bowel loss. The jejunum is the primary site for absorption of most nutrients, but if it is removed the ileum usually can accommodate and take on the structural characteristics and functional roles. Even with this compensation, patients with less than 50 to 60 cm of jejunum will typically need indefinite PN. With ileal resection, the jejunum has a decreased capacity to adapt and perform the functions of the ileum.[86,89]

ENERGY REQUIREMENTS

Caloric intake and energy needs of SBS patients are variable. Individuals who have lost more than 50% of their small intestine typically require an EN input of 30 to 40 kcal/kg of ideal body weight per day.[87] The average recommendation for patients with SBS who are receiving PN is 32 kcal/kg of ideal body weight per day.[86]

CARBOHYDRATE

Carbohydrate malabsorption plays a major role in diarrhea associated with SBS. Unabsorbed carbohydrates are broken down by intestinal bacteria to short-chain fatty acids (SCFAs), producing an osmotic load in the distal small intestine and colon that can lead to protracted diarrhea.[90] However, the colon is able to use these SCFAs as a source of energy, thus complex carbohydrates may provide a significant caloric source for patients with a massive resection and a preserved colon.[90,91]

FAT

Fat malabsorption is common in SBS as well. The pathophysiology of this problem is complex and related to alterations in pancreatic enzyme secretion and bile salt absorption. The ileum is the major site of the latter process, and with its removal bile salt malabsorption is common. Eventually, the total bile salt pool may be depleted, resulting in increased fat malabsorption and steatorrhea.[89] There has been much debate regarding the restriction of oral fats, which may decrease steatorrhea, number of stools, and stool weight in some patients. Fats have the highest number of kilocalories per gram, make the diet more palatable, and patients with SBS without a colon should not be restricted in the amount of fats they take in. Small bowel patients with continuity of healthy colon have shown that a diet higher in complex carbohydrates and lower in fat may have less stool volume and electrolyte loss, so this type diet may be more beneficial.[87] However, there is concern with patients on long-term PN with regard to the development of essential fatty acid deficiency. Biochemical evidence of this deficiency has been proven, even with appropriate intake of long-chain fatty acid lipid emulsions in grams per kilogram per day.[92]

PROTEIN

Protein typically is well tolerated as a caloric source in SBS patients. For those SBS patients on EN it is controversial what molecular form of the macronutrient maximizes protein absorption. In the past, EN often was initiated with elemental products that contained free amino acids as the protein source because the efficiency of protein uptake was perceived to be better. However, total protein absorption is faster and more complete with dipeptide and tripeptide formulations.[90] It appears that the absorption of free amino acids by the enteral route is a saturable process, whereas the absorption of small peptides is not. These more complex protein sources also may stimulate intestinal adaptation.[90]

FLUID, ELECTROLYTE, AND ACID-BASE DISORDERS

9 After substantial resections of the small bowel, the postoperative course is complicated by fluid and electrolyte imbalances that typically last 1 to 3 weeks.[87] Patients may have high-volume gastric fluid loss from nasogastric tubes and small intestine fluid loss from ostomies. Sodium content usually is elevated in these secretions, with concentrations of approximately 80 to 100 mEq/L.[90] Acute gastric hypersecretion may occur after massive resection and contribute significantly to these deficits.[87] Secretory diarrhea also results in fluid and electrolyte losses that may be difficult to quantify.

Patients with end jejunostomies or proximal ileostomies can have recurrent dehydration and electrolyte deficiencies. A high jejunostomy can have output of 3 L/day of fluid, with sodium loss of 90 mEq/L. To overcome the net secretion of sodium and water into the jejunum, the sodium content of fluids within the GI lumen must reach 90 mEq/L. In patients who have small intestine in continuity with the colon, the malabsorbed bile and fatty acids stimulate sodium and water excretion into the large bowel, but in general these patients are at less risk for sodium and water depletion.[91]

Patients with a jejunostomy are at risk of hypokalemia as well, so potassium levels must be monitored closely for supplementation. Other patients at risk for potassium depletion include individuals with long-term sodium depletion, magnesium deficiency, or excessive loss from diarrhea.[91] Metabolic alkalosis, which may occur when a patient becomes dehydrated, accelerates the renal excretion of potassium, as all hydrogen ions are conserved in an attempt to correct the acid-base disorder. As bicarbonate ions are excreted renally, potassium is taken with them to maintain osmotic balance.

The unusually large amount of unabsorbed fatty acids within the remaining intestine and colon of the patient with SBS will cause increased binding to calcium, resulting in a deficiency. This also may result in hyperoxaluria because dietary oxalate usually complexes with the intraluminal calcium and is excreted in the stool. As the result of decreased calcium available for binding, more oxalate is absorbed and available for renal excretion and formation of calcium oxalate renal stones.[88] Vitamin D deficiency results in insufficient calcium absorption; thus SBS patients requiring long-term PN are at risk for metabolic bone disease. Other potential causes of this disorder include aluminum toxicity, suppression of parathyroid hormone by parenteral vitamin D, disruption of parathyroid hormone regulation, and cytokine effects on bone resorption.[93]

Magnesium deficiency is common in SBS patients with large ostomy or diarrheal losses. This deficiency should be corrected aggressively because of the correlation between low magnesium and potassium concentrations, and magnesium supplementation decreases the formation of calcium oxalate kidney stones. Serum concentrations are most commonly monitored, but urinary magnesium concentrations may decrease earlier with deficiency, and may be a better estimate of total body stores than serum levels. Oral supplementation may be difficult because it can contribute to increased diarrhea or ostomy output. However, repletion is necessary to correct potassium deficits in addition to magnesium losses.[86]

SBS patients can lose substantial amounts of chloride (60 to 140 mEq/L) in addition to sodium from ostomy output. Dehydration occurs when there are stable losses from an ostomy that are not replaced, or when the patient is noncompliant with a restricted diet, resulting in loss of more fluid than is taken in. These individuals have a high risk of developing hypochloremic metabolic alkalosis.

Noncompliance with the infusion of appropriately prescribed fluids also can lead to dehydration. Patients who have SBS complicated by a pancreatic fistula and severe diarrhea lose considerable potassium and bicarbonate and may develop metabolic acidosis. Patients with severe diarrhea who have an intact colon will conserve sodium and chloride, resulting in considerable loss of potassium and bicarbonate and the development of metabolic acidosis. Quantifying fluid losses with particular attention to the sources of loss will aid in the acid-base management of these patients (see Chap. 51).

Lactic acidosis can occur in patients with SBS and may result in symptoms of ataxia and delirium.[94] D-Lactic acid is produced by the fermentation of malabsorbed carbohydrates by colonic bacteria, and increased concentrations are associated with small bowel bacterial overgrowth.[87,94] The diagnosis of D-lactic acidosis should be considered in patients with a functional colon who have an unexplained metabolic acidosis and an elevated anion gap.[87]

TRACE ELEMENTS

Patients with SBS are particularly prone to zinc deficiency as a result of excessive losses from stool, ostomy outputs, and fistula drainage. Signs of inadequate zinc include acrodermatitis and impaired wound healing. Although serum zinc concentrations are not always reflective of body zinc status, a low serum zinc concentration requires an adjustment in replacement amount.[91] Significant bowel resection, GI losses, and impaired intestinal absorption also contribute to imbalances of other trace elements, such as copper, selenium, and manganese. Trace element deficiencies and the need for supplementation of these micronutrients are essential for SBS patients, including those receiving PN, EN, or an adequate diet.[86]

VITAMINS

Patients with ileal resection commonly develop vitamin B_{12} deficiency, necessitating therapy with parenteral cyanocobalamin. Most other water-soluble vitamins are absorbed in the proximal jejunum, and deficits of these vitamins are found only in more severe SBS.[87] Small bowel bacterial overgrowth can contribute to diminished vitamin B_{12} because bacteria may metabolize the nutrient within the intestine, decreasing its availability for absorption.[88] SBS patients with fat malabsorption can acquire deficiencies in vitamins A, D, E, and K. These fat-soluble vitamins depend on bile salt micelles for effective absorption, and malabsorption with depletion of the bile salt pool can lead to their deficits.[89]

▶ TREATMENT: Short Bowel Syndrome

◼ ADMINISTRATION ROUTES

After intestinal resection, the clinical course and nutritional management of SBS patients may be described in three stages, or phases. The first stage, or acute phase, occurs during the initial postoperative period. This phase lasts at least 1 week, and may continue from 3 weeks to 3 months. It is complicated by major fluid and electrolyte losses (up to 5 L/day) and the parenteral route should be used to supply nutritional needs.

The second stage lasts from a few months to over a year, and institution of enteral or oral intake early during this stage is important because intraluminal nutrients are essential stimuli for intestinal adaptation. As the amount of enteral/oral nutrition is advanced as the patient tolerates, the duration of the daily infusion of PN may be decreased. In the third and final stage, adaptation is maximized and the patient is maintained with nutritional support tailored for long-term ambulatory management. If patients are unable to achieve full oral nutrition, home PN may be used. However, PN may not be required on a daily basis. If a PN regimen is to be reduced or discontinued, it should be done slowly; initially one to two nights of PN may be eliminated each week. Eventually, some patients may be able to tolerate administration on an every-other or every-third-night basis.[86,87,90] During the different phases of management PN is administered through a peripherally inserted central catheter or surgically placed indwelling central venous catheter[88] (see Chap. 137). Use of proper aseptic technique is vital in the care of these access sites because SBS patients have been shown to have significantly higher rates of catheter sepsis.[95]

DESIGN AND INITIATION OF NUTRITIONAL REGIMEN

The early phase of SBS is associated with large day-to-day variations in fluid and electrolyte losses. Strict output records should be assessed, as well as all intake including intravenous medications. Initially, it is recommended to start a standard PN solution that meets the patient's maintenance metabolic, fluid, and electrolyte needs, and a separate intravenous replacement solution is typically necessary to keep the patient euvolemic based on actual fluid losses.[95] Insensible losses should be estimated between 300 and 800 mL/day above measured output,[87,95] and daily urine output should be kept at least 1 L.[87] As fluid and electrolyte losses stabilize over time it becomes possible to incorporate these replacement requirements into the PN solution. The PN solution typically is composed of standard crystalline amino acids, glucose, and intravenous lipids. A generic caloric breakdown for SBS patients based on a need of 30 to 40 kcal/kg per day may be 1.5 g/kg of protein per day, approximately 20% to 30% of calories from intravenous lipids, and the remainder of calories from carbohydrates.[86] An example of a PN formula for the patient with SBS is given in Table 139–2.

The amounts of chloride versus acetate salt forms chosen for cation delivery should be based on assessment of the acid-base balance of the patient and sources of GI losses. More proximal GI losses generally are associated with increased chloride needs and more dis-

tal outputs with increased bicarbonate (i.e., acetate) requirements. Sodium losses may be extreme in SBS patients as already mentioned, requiring supplementation above what a typical PN patient requires. In addition, supplementation of potassium, calcium, magnesium, zinc, or other micronutrients over their maintenance amounts may be necessary to meet replacement needs.[86–88]

The transition from PN to enteral feedings is desirable because it is a stimulus for adaptation, and should be instituted as the patient progresses throughout the postoperative period. EN, given as a continuous infusion through a nasogastric or gastric feeding tube, may be advantageous over bolus feedings because it can maximize absorptive capacity, and may decrease recovery time and minimize diarrhea.[86,87] Formulas with protein hydrolysates and a combination of MCTs and LCTs, as well as elemental formulas have been suggested for these patients.[90,96] Because SBS may exacerbate lactose intolerance, lactose-free isotonic polymeric enteral formulas also have been recommended.[87]

Oral intake should be considered in small amounts, but must be regulated carefully at this point. Small volumes (600 to 1000 mL/day) of oral electrolyte solutions such as low-carbohydrate sports drinks and sugar- and caffeine-free beverages are optimal. Frequent, small amounts of solid food composed primarily of complex carbohydrates and proteins (600 to 1000 kcal/day) have been recommended, with avoidance of concentrated sweets and dairy products.[88,95] When a patient begins to consume greater than 1000 kcal/day orally without protracted diarrhea, PN may begin to be tapered, as well as EN (Fig. 139–3). Many factors must be considered once a patient begins to transition off interventional nutrition when determining the content of a long-term oral diet for an SBS patient. Factors such as the site and length of remaining intestine, tolerance, and patient acceptance must be considered. Fat generally is not restricted in patients without

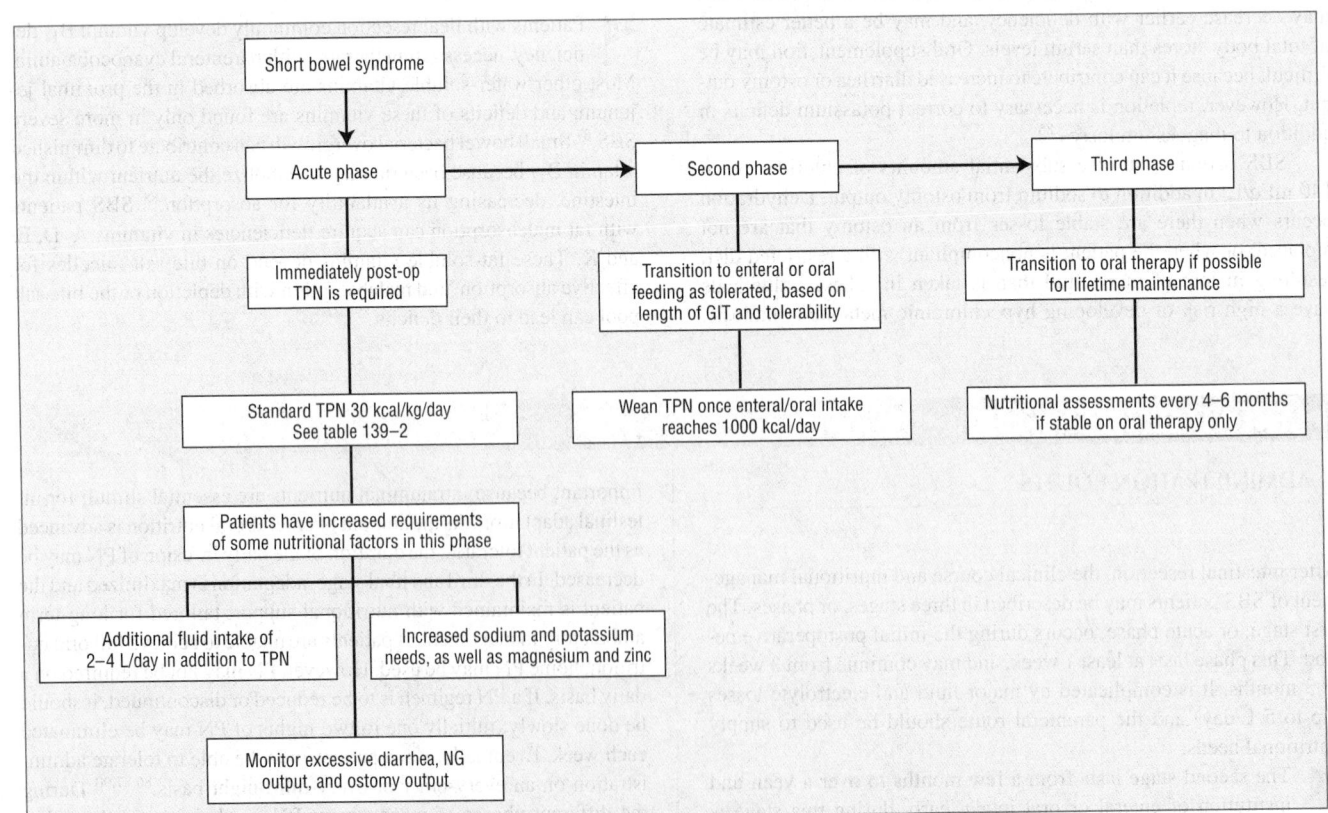

FIGURE 139–3. An algorithmic approach to nutritional support for the patient with short bowel syndrome.

a colon. However, patients with a colon may experience more diarrhea with a high-fat diet and may benefit from oral intake that has more calories from carbohydrates and less fat content.[87] The oral diet for patients with remaining functional colon also must account for oxalate content, and patients should avoid foods with high amounts of oxalate (e.g., spinach, parsley, rhubarb, cocoa, and tea) to decrease calcium oxalate renal stones.[91] Finally, oral diets in SBS patients often need to be supplemented to maintain electrolyte, mineral, vitamin, and trace element balance.

DRUG THERAPY

The delivery of medications to patients with SBS may present many challenges, not the least of which is the questionable absorption of oral therapies. It is important to avoid oral products that contain sorbitol or mannitol as inactive ingredients to avoid medication-related diarrhea. Loperamide and octreotide may be used to control diarrhea (see Chap. 36), and proton pump inhibitors and H_2-receptor antagonists are frequently required to reduce gastric hypersecretion (see Chap. 33).

The use of specialized nutrients and growth factors to enhance small bowel adaptation has been a focus of recent research. The amino acid glutamine is a fuel for intestinal cells, and may be necessary for maintaining intestinal structure in normal and stressed states.[88] Byrne and colleagues published an uncontrolled clinical study of patients who received glutamine in combination with recombinant human growth hormone (rhGH) and a high-carbohydrate/low-fat diet.[97] Recombinant growth hormone was added to the regimen because of its stimulant properties in bowel adaptation. Initial results showed that use resulted in significantly increased protein absorption in several patients and after a follow-up period of 1 year, 40% of patients were able to maintain nutrition status off PN with a continued high-carbohydrate and low-fat diet and glutamine supplementation.[97]

Other researchers have investigated the effects of glutamine and rhGH, with and without high-carbohydrate/low-fat diets, on body composition and intestinal absorption. In these randomized, double-blind, placebo-controlled crossover studies, which were done in small numbers of patients, the beneficial results of glutamine and rhGH were not duplicated.[98–100]

CLINICAL CONTROVERSY

Despite the lack of controlled clinical trials supporting its use, many clinicians supplement PN therapy with glutamine and recombinant growth hormone in an attempt to increase intestinal absorption and facilitate transition off PN. Recombinant growth hormone is a costly product with adverse effects, but PN is more costly and also has a serious adverse-effect profile. Larger controlled clinical trials are needed to determine the benefit of glutamine and rhGH in this patient population.

SURGICAL THERAPY AND INTESTINAL TRANSPLANTATION

The surgeon is one of the primary specialists caring for the SBS patient. Initially surgical management focuses on preventing GI resections and then preserving as much GIT as possible.[101] Intestinal transplantation is currently considered a high-risk proposition, and is reserved for those patients with life-threatening complications of their intestinal failure, including irreversible PN-related liver disease, or lack of venous access.[102] Over 500 patients have received an intestinal transplant, the majority being children. The overall survival rate is almost 60%, with 77% of the survivors achieving full nutritional autonomy. Partial gastrointestinal recoveries have been documented in approximately 15%, resulting in a rehabilitation rate greater than 90% in survivors. The majority of deaths were due to postoperative infections. In the absence of life-threatening complications, intestinal transplantation is difficult to justify at this time except for selected SBS patients.[103]

EVALUATION OF THERAPEUTIC OUTCOMES

Therapeutic monitoring of SBS patients for metabolic complications should follow the guidelines outlined in Chap. 137. This patient population differs in that serum electrolytes should be obtained daily until the patient has stabilized postoperatively. Special consideration should also be given to the fluid status of SBS patients, especially in the period immediately following surgery, when fluid losses are extreme. Monitoring of stool output is such a large factor it must be taken into consideration throughout the acute phase, as well as the entire life of all SBS patients. Because many patients with SBS remain on PN for extended periods of time, clinicians must be careful to monitor for elevations in liver enzymes, and cycling PN for 12 to 14 hours daily should be considered in those patients receiving IV nutrition to minimize these complications. Obtaining a serum fatty acid profile may be judicious in those patients on long-term PN without oral intake to ensure they do not have essential fatty acid deficiency.[95]

Long-term outcomes of adults with SBS on PN have been examined. Survival rates have been reported at 2 and 5 years to be 86% and 75%, respectively. In these same patients, the probability of requiring continued PN support was 49% at 2 years and 45% at 5 years.[104] Dependence on PN was related to residual intestinal length of less than 100 cm and absence of the terminal ileum and/or colon in continuity with the remaining small intestine.

The most comprehensive and thorough analysis of the clinical outcomes of patients receiving home PN or EN comes from Medicare and the North American Home Parenteral and Enteral Patient Registry.[105] It was estimated that 40,000 and 152,000 patients in the United States were receiving home PN and EN support, respectively. Patients with GI failure, which included those with Crohn's disease, ischemic bowel disease, motility disorders, and congenital bowel defects had relatively good outcomes, especially when compared with the groups with cancer or AIDS. The patients with GI failure had an 87% annual survival rate and a 50% to 75% likelihood of complete rehabilitation. Sepsis, metabolic disorders, and mechanical problems with catheters resulted in one to two hospitalizations per year for all patients.[105]

QUALITY-OF-LIFE ISSUES

Education of patients with SBS and their caregivers is essential, particularly in the setting of home PN and/or EN with its associated technology. In addition, quality-of-life (QOL) issues should be addressed with these individuals. Initially those patients on extended

PN therapy have a significant gain in QOL when transitioning from the hospital to their home setting. This is often followed by the reality of restrictions in daily living, dehydration and malnutrition despite PN, and complications such as sepsis and liver dysfunction. Patients with SBS on home PN have been shown to report that QOL is signif- icantly reduced in comparison to those with anatomic or functional SBS not on home PN.[106] Preparing patients and their caregivers for the possible stresses associated with this therapy (e.g., financial chal- lenges, fatigue, depression, complications, and social or emotional problems) may help to increase QOL.

PULMONARY FAILURE

The provision of nutritional support plays a direct role in the man- agement of patients with significant pulmonary disease. Patients with malnutrition are at increased risk of acute respiratory distress syn- drome (ARDS), and malnutrition in patients with chronic obstructive pulmonary disease (COPD) is well documented. There has also been a proven correlation between the outcomes of patients with alterations in nutritional status and pulmonary diseases.[107] Loss of lean muscle mass is detrimental because the depletion of diaphragm and inter- costal muscles make the effort of breathing harder, and progression of weight loss leads to muscle fatigue and respiratory failure. The ventilatory drive, as well as compensation to hypoxia, is depressed in COPD patients who are malnourished, and nutritional support plays a key role in optimizing respiratory muscle function in patients with pulmonary disease.[108]

EPIDEMIOLOGY

Greater than 10% of the U.S. population older than 45 years of age suffers from COPD, resulting in significant cost to the health care system.[108] Weight loss and protein-calorie malnutrition may occur in up to one-half of those patients suffering from COPD, and weight loss often progresses with disease progression.[108,109] In those patients suf- fering from acute respiratory failure, nutritional abnormalities have been reported in up to 70%.[110] Engelen and colleagues studied body composition in patients with COPD, specifically emphysema and chronic bronchitis. They found a higher incidence of lean mass de- pletion in those with emphysema compared to those with chronic bronchitis. Body weight and body mass index (BMI) were also lower in the group with emphysema.[111] In a further evaluation of these pa- tients, the same investigators reported that skeletal muscle weakness was associated with wasting of extremity fat free mass (FFM) that was independent of COPD subtype.[112] Regarding mortality, a rela- tionship has been shown between COPD patients with decreasing BMI, especially in more severe cases of COPD.[113]

PATHOPHYSIOLOGY

ENERGY

Several mechanisms have been proposed for the weight loss and mal- nutrition associated with COPD. First, several studies have shown that patients with COPD have an increased resting energy expenditure (REE). Those who are losing weight tend to have significantly higher REE adjusted for FFM compared with weight-stable patients.[114] Total daily energy expenditure (TDEE) also was found to be ele- vated in clinically stable COPD patients with both normal and in- creased REE. The cause of elevated TDEE despite a normal REE is still unknown, although factors that may contribute include oxy- gen cost of breathing, acute or chronic systemic inflammation, and medications.[115,116] Hypermetabolism through elevated REE and TDEE may be partially at fault for decreased body weight and FFM, although it has been shown that in this patient population intake may be suboptimal. During meals hypoxic patients tend to experi- ence decreases in oxygen saturation and increased dyspnea. Gastric filling may also be impaired due to diaphragmatic expansion and a false feeling of fullness.[110] These problems, combined with increased daily requirements, may result in the negative energy balance seen in many COPD patients. Several specialized equations have been devel- oped to estimate requirements in this patient population, and indirect calorimetry may be used, but clinical benefit is questionable. Patients with acute respiratory failure also may have alterations in energy ex- penditure, but the situation is similar in that predictive formulas for energy needs exist, and indirect calorimetry may be used, but there is no optimal approach to estimate energy needs in this patient popula- tion. Providing excess calories to the acutely ill patient in respiratory failure should be avoided because this may increase carbon dioxide production and associated work of breathing.[108]

CARBOHYDRATE

⓬ Malnutrition in patients with pulmonary disease and failure has been consistently identified in the literature, and nutrition sup- port should be considered as part of the overall treatment plan. How- ever, increasing nutritional intake can be complicated because it may elevate the respiratory quotient (RQ), which may lead to a correspond- ing increase in work of breathing and resulting hypercapnia. The RQ is the ratio of the amount of CO_2 produced divided by the amount of O_2 consumed. This is in response to the metabolism of macronutri- ents by the human body. Carbohydrates generate 1 mole of CO_2 for every mole of O_2 consumed (the RQ for carbohydrate is 1). Protein and fat metabolism produce RQs of 0.8 and 0.7, respectively. When a subject is overfed, the amount of CO_2 produced markedly exceeds the amount of O_2 consumed, which can result in increased ventilatory demand.[117] Ventilatory drive may be improved in some patients with pulmonary disease with moderate infusions of carbohydrates; how- ever, administration of glucose formulas >5 mg/kg per minute has been shown to increase production of CO_2, and has been associated with the inability to wean from mechanical ventilation.[108]

FAT

Fats have the lowest RQ, but administration of intravenous fat emul- sions to mechanically ventilated patients may have the potential to ad- versely affect pulmonary gas exchange in some clinical conditions.[116]

CLINICAL CONTROVERSY

There are conflicting data on the safety of administration of lipid emulsions to patients with ARDS. Discrepancies in trial data may be due to the use of differing lipid infusion rates and duration, as well as pre-existing lung status.

The administration of lipid emulsions to patients with ARDS either has no effect on oxygenation, or may possibly decrease oxygenation. A recent trial assessing both long-chain triglyceride and combination long-chain triglyceride/medium-chain triglyceride administration showed that there was no deleterious affect on oxygenation. Discrepancies in trial data may be due to differing lipid infusion rates and duration, and pre-existing lung status.[118] Rapid administration of intravenous lipids should be avoided; a rate of 3 mg/kg per minute has been shown to increase pulmonary vascular resistance in patients with ARDS.[107] In a review of nutritional intervention in ambulatory COPD patients, studies investigating the effects of dietary intake with varying percentages of fat content were evaluated. Diets high in fat were found to place a lower demand on the respiratory system in comparison to diets with a higher carbohydrate content, both immediately after a meal and when continued for a short duration (~2 weeks).[119] In addition to an improvement in forced expiratory volume, the number of breaths needed per minute has been shown to decrease within 3 weeks in COPD patients who switched to a high-fat/low-carbohydrate diet.[117]

PROTEIN

Undernourished patients have demonstrated a blunted response to hypercapnia that improves after as little as 1 week of adequate nutritional support. This response is thought to result from protein administration, as evidenced by decreased partial CO_2 pressure, increased minute ventilation, and improved breathing patterns after the start of PN. Protein administration also may influence ventilatory demand by increased ventilatory response to hypoxia and hypercapnia. This stimulation may be altered by the amino acid composition of the protein source, with increased amounts of BCAAs having a greater effect compared with standard amino acids.[116] Although this protein effect is potentially beneficial in some patients, excessive protein administration could theoretically lead to increased work of breathing and fatigue.[108]

FLUID, ELECTROLYTE, AND ACID-BASE DISORDERS

In patients with ARDS or pulmonary edema, excessive fluid intake should be avoided, and fluid accumulation is associated with a poor outcome. It may be beneficial to restrict fluid intake.[108] Patients in the ICU often receive substantial fluid loads from medica-tion administration, and when possible it is important to limit intake by concentrating these sources.

Alteration of micronutrient requirements in respiratory failure is commonly focused on phosphorus replacement. Phosphorus has an essential role in the synthesis of adenosine triphosphate (ATP) and 2,3-diphosphoglycerate (2,3-DPG). Inadequate stores of ATP can lead to respiratory muscle weakness, and normal contractility of the diaphragm muscles is dependent on phosphate.[108] Finally, a significant percentage of critically ill patients can experience hypophosphatemia from refeeding.[120] Most patients with moderate to severe hypophosphatemia and respiratory failure should be treated with intravenous sodium or potassium phosphate. Correction of hypophosphatemia in ICU patients receiving nutritional support with a graduated weight-based dosing scheme of phosphorus replacement has been reported (see Chap. 49). Clark and associates reported that use of this dosing regimen in ICU patients receiving nutritional support resulted in significant increases in serum phosphorus at all levels of deficiency.[121]

Ventilator-dependent patients and those with stable COPD often have respiratory acidosis. A balanced mixture of chloride and acetate salts often is appropriate in these patients. The acid-base status of the ICU patient with pulmonary compromise should be monitored daily, whereas every 2 to 3 days may be adequate for the stable COPD patient.

VITAMINS AND TRACE ELEMENTS

Patients with pulmonary disease usually do not have significant alterations in vitamin and trace element requirements, and they can receive standard doses of these micronutrients. There are some data that support the additional supplementation of antioxidants vitamin C, vitamin E, and β-carotene in pulmonary patients due to a correlation with moderately improved pulmonary function.[122] COPD patients may have an increased burden of oxidants from cigarette smoke or release of oxygen free radicals from inflammatory leukocytes in the lungs, and deficiencies of antioxidants may contribute to oxidant/antioxidant imbalances in these individuals.[123] The value of supplementation of these substances in COPD will require further clarification.

▶ TREATMENT: Pulmonary Failure

■ ADMINISTRATION ROUTES

When oral feedings are not adequate, the enteral route is preferred for nutritional support in pulmonary patients who have a functional gut and can meet their needs through this route. In acute respiratory failure PN is often recommended when the GI tract is not usable, or as a supplement to EN if sufficient energy intake is otherwise not possible.[108]

■ SPECIALTY PRODUCTS

Most general EN formulas contain an equal balance of nonprotein energy between carbohydrate and fat. Elemental or chemically defined products are the exception because they are intended to be high-carbohydrate, low-fat formulas to enhance absorption and digestion. In pulmonary patients administration of a high-carbohydrate formula may result in a significant increase in minute ventilation, heat production, and CO_2 production when compared with a high-fat formula. Because most general formulas contain balanced nonprotein calories, moderate doses of these products may be appropriate in most patients with pulmonary disease.

Enteral formulas (e.g., Pulmocare, NutriVent, and Respalor) marketed for use specifically by patients with pulmonary disease are also available. In comparison with standard formulas, these products contain a higher percentage of nonprotein calories as fat (>50%). Several studies have evaluated the use of these high-fat/low-carbohydrate products in patients with COPD and acute respiratory failure, and general results have been favorable.[117,124–126] These specialized pulmonary EN products are calorically dense (1.5 kcal/mL), which may be helpful in feeding patients with severe ARDS or pulmonary edema and in others who may require fluid restriction.

An additional concentrated formula (Oxepa) has been marketed specifically for critically ill patients on mechanical ventilation. The macronutrient composition of Oxepa is similar to that of the other specialized pulmonary enteral formulas, with 55% of caloric content from fat. However, the lipid blend in the formula has been altered to potentially decrease the production of proinflammatory cytokines by including eicosapentaenoic acid from fish oil and γ-linolenic acid from borage oil. Nutrients with antioxidant properties (i.e., vitamin C, vitamin E, and β-carotene) also have been supplemented in the product.[127]

DESIGN AND INITIATION OF THE NUTRITIONAL REGIMEN

In the patient with pulmonary failure, nutritional support should be given to meet energy and protein requirements and limit wasting of respiratory muscles. No major alterations in substrate disposition have been noted in patients with pulmonary failure; thus moderate doses of carbohydrate, fat, and protein are appropriate in most conditions. Total calorie provision 30% above BEE does not have any untoward effects on pulmonary status, although patients who are overfed two times BEE produce excessive CO_2, even in uncomplicated respiratory failure. In patients with borderline ventilatory status the nutritional regimen should be monitored closely to prevent excessive CO_2 production, and increasing the proportion of nonprotein calories as fat to the amount of carbohydrates may be beneficial in some patients to decrease CO_2 production.[108] In general, patients with ARDS who need PN may receive nonprotein calories administered within the following ranges: 55% to 80% carbohydrate and 20% to 45% lipid. A reasonable protein dose is 1 to 1.5 g/kg per day for the patient with stable COPD. Patients who are mechanically ventilated with superimposed illness may require higher doses of protein (1.5 to 2.5 g/kg per day). An approach to the patient with respiratory failure requiring PN or EN support is shown in Fig. 139–4. An empirical PN formula for the patient with respiratory failure is shown in Table 139–2.

DRUG THERAPY

Recombinant human growth hormone is known to induce general muscle growth, lipolysis, and protein anabolism. When used as adjunctive therapy to EN support, COPD patients have shown improvements in lean body mass, maximal inspiratory pressure, and exercise capacity.[128] The benefit of rhGH is debatable, with trials having differing results, but body mass and FFM typically will increase in patients after use of this product. The benefit in pulmonary patients as shown by improvements in respiratory muscle function and pulmonary function testing is questionable. The effects of anabolic steroids have also been evaluated for use in COPD as an adjunct to nutritional intervention. Patients on anabolic steroids tend to have larger increases in FFM and more favorable distributions in weight gain in comparison to interventional nutrition alone.[129] More studies are needed to characterize the benefits of rhGH, as well as anabolic steroids, and to determine the risk associated with the possible clinical benefits.

EVALUATION OF THERAPEUTIC OUTCOMES

Pulmonary patients are at extreme risk of malnutrition, therefore monitoring the progression of the patient on interventional nutrition is extremely important. Therapeutic monitoring of pulmonary patients on PN for metabolic complications should follow the guidelines presented in Chapter 137, and those patients on EN should be monitored as described in Chapter 138. Pulmonary status must be assessed for any changes, especially with the initiation of higher carbohydrate formulas of PN or EN. Weights should be charted frequently, and it

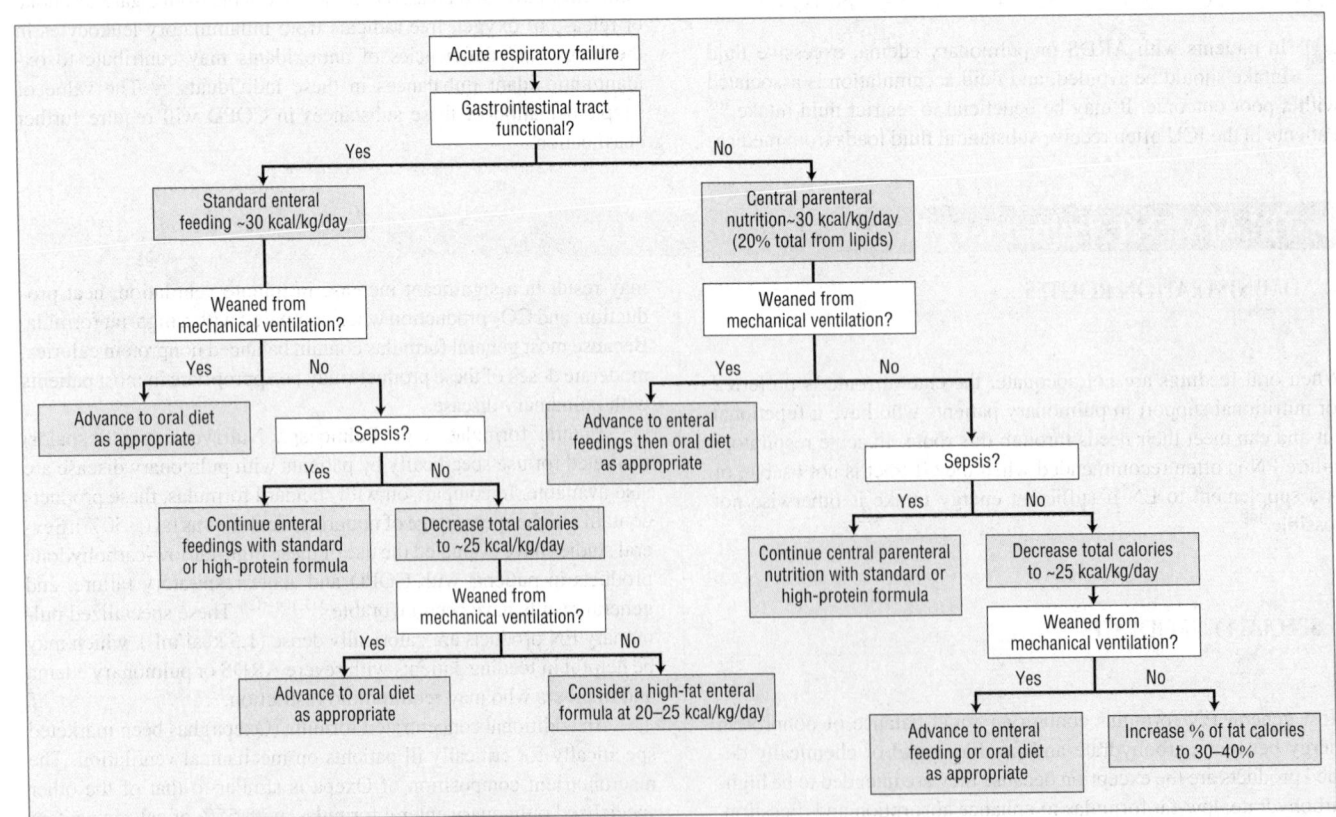

FIGURE 139–4. An algorithmic approach to nutritional support for the patient with acute respiratory failure.

is important that pre-albumin concentrations are assessed weekly for those patients in the hospital. It is important to remember that patients with ARDS in critical care units are prone to fluid overload due to medication administration, so careful monitoring of intake and output is necessary to avoid pulmonary edema. Nutritional status should be monitored every 4 to 6 months for those patients with stable pulmonary disease and COPD.

Long-term outcome assessments of pulmonary patients on PN are not available or applicable because PN is typically a short-term intervention in this patient population. There is an abundance of literature supporting interventional nutrition due to the improvement of FFM, body weight, and respiratory function in ambulatory pulmonary patients. In addition, a low BMI in this patient population has been shown to be associated with increased mortality rates in some patients, but with appropriate intervention the negative effects of low body weight may be reversed.[130]

QUALITY-OF-LIFE ISSUES

Patients with FFM depletion have shown through subjective testing that they have a decreased health-related QOL. Decreased activity and exercise capacity appeared to be associated with low FFM, which appears to be related to decreasing patient satisfaction.[110] Dyspnea has also been shown to be correlated strongly with health-related QOL in patients with decreased FFM, and may be the strongest predictor of patient satisfaction in correlation with malnutrition.[131]

ABBREVIATIONS

AAA: aromatic amino acid
AAD: amino acid dialysate
ARDS: acute respiratory distress syndrome
ARF: acute renal failure
ATP: adenosine triphosphate
BCAA: branched-chain amino acid
BEE: basal energy expenditure
BMD: bone mineral density
BMI: body mass index
CAPD: continuous ambulatory peritoneal dialysis
CKD: chronic kidney disease
COPD: chronic obstructive pulmonary disease
CPD: cycling peritoneal dialysis
CRRT: continuous renal replacement therapy
CVVH: continuous veno-venous hemofiltration
EAA: essential amino acid
EN: enteral nutrition
ESKD: end-stage kidney disease
FFA: free fatty acid
FFM: fat free mass
GFR: glomerular filtration rate
GIT: gastrointestinal tract
HD: hemodialysis
ICU: intensive care unit
IDPN: intradialytic parenteral nutrition
IVLE: intravenous lipid emulsion
LCT: long-chain triglyceride
MCT: medium-chain triglyceride
OLT: orthotopic liver transplantation
PD: peritoneal dialysis
PN: parenteral nutrition
QOL: quality-of-life
RDA: recommended daily allowance
REE: resting energy expenditure
rhGH: recombinant human growth hormone
RQ: respiratory quotient
SCFA: short-chain fatty acid
SBS: short bowel syndrome
TDEE: total daily energy expenditure
UNA: urea nitrogen appearance

Review Questions and other resources can be found at www.pharmacotherapyonline.com.

REFERENCES

1. Ikizler TA, Himmelfarb J. Nutrition in acute renal failure patients. Adv Ren Replace Ther 1997;4(2 Suppl 1):54–63.
2. Fiaccadori E, et al. Prevalence and clinical outcome associated with pre-existing malnutrition in acute renal failure: A prospective cohort study. J Am Soc Nephrol 1999;10:581–593.
3. Bozfakioglu S. Nutrition in patients with acute renal failure. Nephrol Dial Transplant 2001;16(Suppl 6):21–22.
4. Druml W. Nutritional management of acute renal failure. Am J Kidney Dis 2001;37(1 Suppl 2):S89–S94.
5. Keane WF. Lipids and the kidney. Kidney Int 1994;46:910–920.
6. Maheux P, et al. Relationship between insulin-mediated glucose disposal and regulation of plasma and adipose tissue lipoprotein lipase. Diabetologia 1997;40:850–858.
7. Druml W. Protein metabolism in acute renal failure. Miner Electrolyte Metab 1998;24:47–54.
8. Cooney RN, Kimball SR, Vary TC. Regulation of skeletal muscle protein turnover during sepsis: Mechanisms and mediators. Shock 1997;7:1–16.
9. Maxvold NJ, et al. Amino acid loss and nitrogen balance in critically ill children with acute renal failure: A prospective comparison between classic hemofiltration and hemofiltration with dialysis. Crit Care Med 2000;28:1161–1165.
10. Klein CJ, et al. Magnesium, calcium, zinc, and nitrogen loss in trauma patients during continuous renal replacement therapy. JPEN J Parenter Enteral Nutr 2002;26:77–92, discussion 92–93.
11. Druml W, et al. Elimination of amino acids in renal failure. Am J Clin Nutr 1994;60:418–423.
12. Novak I, et al. Glutamine and other amino acid losses during continuous venovenous hemodiafiltration. Artif Organs 1997;21:359–363.
13. Locatelli F, Pontoriero G, Di Filippo S. Electrolyte disorders and substitution fluid in continuous renal replacement therapy. Kidney Int Suppl 1998;66:S151–S155.
14. Meier-Kriesche HU, et al. Unexpected severe hypocalcemia during continuous venovenous hemodialysis with regional citrate anticoagulation. Am J Kidney Dis 1999;33:e8.
15. Heering P, et al. The use of different buffers during continuous hemofiltration in critically ill patients with acute renal failure. Intensive Care Med 1999;25:1244–1251.
16. Gallieni M, et al. Trace elements in renal failure: Are they clinically important? Nephrol Dial Transplant 1996;11:1232–1235.
17. Metnitz GH, et al. Impact of acute renal failure on antioxidant status in multiple organ failure. Acta Anaesthesiol Scand 2000;44:236–240.
18. Makropoulos W, Heintz B, Stefanidis I. Selenium deficiency and thyroid function in acute renal failure. Ren Fail 1997;19:129–136.
19. Wolk R. Micronutrition in dialysis. Nutr Clin Pract 1993;8:267–276.
20. Druml W, et al. Fat-soluble vitamins in patients with acute renal failure. Miner Electrolyte Metab 1998;24:220–226.
21. Seidner DL, Matarese LE, Steiger E. Nutritional care of the critically ill patient with renal failure. Semin Nephrol 1994;14:53–63.

22. Bellomo R, et al. Continuous arteriovenous haemodiafiltration in the critically ill: Influence on major nutrient balances. Intensive Care Med 1991;17:399–402.

23. Bellomo R, et al. High protein intake during continuous hemodiafiltration: Impact on amino acids and nitrogen balance. Int J Artif Organs 2002;25:261–268.

24. Bellomo R, et al. A prospective comparative study of moderate versus high protein intake for critically ill patients with acute renal failure. Ren Fail 1997;19:111–120.

25. Aparicio M, et al. Nutritional status of haemodialysis patients: A French national cooperative study. French Study Group for Nutrition in Dialysis. Nephrol Dial Transplant 1999;14:1679–1686.

26. Chung SH, Lindholm B, Lee HB. Influence of initial nutritional status on continuous ambulatory peritoneal dialysis patient survival. Perit Dial Int 2000;20:19–26.

27. Burrowes JD, et al. Cross-sectional relationship between dietary protein and energy intake, nutritional status, functional status, and comorbidity in older versus younger hemodialysis patients. J Ren Nutr 2002;12:87–95.

28. Wiggins KL, Harvey KS. A review of guidelines for nutrition care of renal patients. J Ren Nutr 2002;12:190–196.

29. Sehgal AR. Outcomes of renal replacement therapy among blacks and women. Am J Kidney Dis 2000;35(4 Suppl 1):S148–S152.

30. Gao H, Lew SQ, Bosch JP. Biochemical parameters, nutritional status and efficiency of dialysis in CAPD and CCPD patients. Am J Nephrol 1999;19:7–12.

31. Evans AM, et al. Pharmacokinetics of L-carnitine in patients with end-stage renal disease undergoing long-term hemodialysis. Clin Pharmacol Ther 2000;68:238–249.

32. National Kidney Foundation. Clinical practice guidelines for nutrition in chronic renal failure. K/DOQI, National Kidney Foundation. Am J Kidney Dis 2000;35(6 Suppl 2):S1–S140.

33. Stenvinkel P, et al. Increases in serum leptin levels during peritoneal dialysis are associated with inflammation and a decrease in lean body mass. J Am Soc Nephrol 2000;11:1303–1309.

34. Nishikawa M, et al. Measurement of serum leptin in patients with chronic renal failure on hemodialysis. Clin Nephrol 1999;51:296–303.

35. Norton PA. Affect of serum leptin on nutritional status in renal disease. J Am Diet Assoc 2002;102:1119–1125.

36. Levey AS, et al. Effects of dietary protein restriction on the progression of advanced renal disease in the Modification of Diet in Renal Disease Study. Am J Kidney Dis 1996;27:652–663.

37. Kasiske BL, et al. A meta-analysis of the effects of dietary protein restriction on the rate of decline in renal function. Am J Kidney Dis 1998; 31:954–961.

38. Aparicio M, Chauveau P, Combe C. Are supplemented low-protein diets nutritionally safe? Am J Kidney Dis 2001;37(1 Suppl 2):S71–S76.

39. Soroka N, et al. Comparison of a vegetable-based (soya) and an animal-based low-protein diet in predialysis chronic renal failure patients. Nephron 1998;79:173–180.

40. Lofberg E, et al. Correction of acidosis in dialysis patients increases branched-chain and total essential amino acid levels in muscle. Clin Nephrol 1997;48:230–237.

41. Stein A, et al. Role of an improvement in acid-base status and nutrition in CAPD patients. Kidney Int 1997;52:1089–1095.

42. Zima T, et al. Trace elements in hemodialysis and continuous ambulatory peritoneal dialysis patients. Blood Purif 1998;16:253–260.

43. Temple KA, Smith AM, Cockram DB. Selenate-supplemented nutritional formula increases plasma selenium in hemodialysis patients. J Ren Nutr 2000;10:16–23.

44. Bogye G, Tompos G, Alfthan G. Selenium depletion in hemodialysis patients treated with polysulfone membranes. Nephron 2000;84: 119–123.

45. Mydlik M, et al. Peritoneal clearance and peritoneal transfer of oxalic acid, vitamin C, and vitamin B_6 during continuous ambulatory peritoneal dialysis. Artif Organs 1998;22:784–788.

46. Wang S, et al. Plasma ascorbic acid in patients undergoing chronic haemodialysis. Eur J Clin Pharmacol 1999;55:527–532.

47. Yonemura K, et al. Vitamin D deficiency is implicated in reduced serum albumin concentrations in patients with end-stage renal disease. Am J Kidney Dis 2000;36:337–344.

48. Islam KN, et al. Alpha-tocopherol supplementation decreases the oxidative susceptibility of LDL in renal failure patients on dialysis therapy. Atherosclerosis 2000;150:217–224.

49. Frank T, et al. Assessment of thiamin status in chronic renal failure patients, transplant recipients and hemodialysis patients receiving a multivitamin supplementation. Int J Vitam Nutr Res 2000;70:159–166.

50. Dierkes J, et al. Response of hyperhomocysteinemia to folic acid supplementation in patients with end-stage renal disease. Clin Nephrol 1999; 51:108–115.

51. Sunder-Plassmann G, et al. Effect of high dose folic acid therapy on hyperhomocysteinemia in hemodialysis patients: Results of the Vienna multicenter study. J Am Soc Nephrol 2000;11:1106–1116.

52. Serna-Thome MG, Padilla-Rosciano AE, Suchil-Bernal L. Practical aspects of intradialytic nutritional support. Curr Opin Clin Nutr Metab Care 2002;5:293–296.

53. Foulks CJ. An evidence-based evaluation of intradialytic parenteral nutrition. Am J Kidney Dis 1999;33:186–192.

54. Jones M, et al. Treatment of malnutrition with 1.1% amino acid peritoneal dialysis solution: Results of a multicenter outpatient study. Am J Kidney Dis 1998;32:761–769.

55. Jones CH, et al. Fasting plasma amino acids are not normalized by 12-month amino acid-based dialysate in CAPD patients. Perit Dial Int 1999;19:174–177.

56. Iglesias P, et al. Recombinant human growth hormone therapy in malnourished dialysis patients: A randomized controlled study. Am J Kidney Dis 1998;32:454–463.

57. Caglar K, Hakim RM, Ikizler TA. Approaches to the reversal of malnutrition, inflammation, and atherosclerosis in end-stage renal disease. Nutr Rev 2002;60:378–387.

58. Ikizler TA, Hakim RM. Nutrition in end-stage renal disease. Kidney Int 1996;50:343–357.

59. Matos C, et al. Nutrition and chronic liver disease. J Clin Gastroenterol 2002;35:391–397.

60. Moriwaki H, et al. Nutritional pharmacotherapy of chronic liver disease: From support of liver failure to prevention of liver cancer. J Gastroenterol 2000;35(Suppl 12):13–17.

61. Campillo B, et al. Influence of liver failure, ascites, and energy expenditure on the response to oral nutrition in alcoholic liver cirrhosis. Nutrition 1997;13(7–8):613–621.

62. Dudrick SJ, Kavic SM. Hepatobiliary nutrition: History and future. J Hepatobiliary Pancreat Surg 2002;9:459–468.

63. Okamoto M, et al. Effect of a late evening snack on the blood glucose level and energy metabolism in patients with liver cirrhosis. Hepatol Res 2003;27:45–50.

64. Miwa Y, et al. Improvement of fuel metabolism by nocturnal energy supplementation in patients with liver cirrhosis. Hepatol Res 2000;18: 184–189.

65. Clemmesen JO, et al. Plasma phospholipid fatty acid pattern in severe liver disease. J Hepatol 2000;32:481–487.

66. Duerksen DR, et al. Essential fatty acid deficiencies in patients with chronic liver disease are not reversed by short-term intravenous lipid supplementation. Dig Dis Sci 1999;44:1342–1348.

67. Chacko RT, Chacko A. Serum and muscle magnesium in Indians with cirrhosis of liver. Indian J Med Res 1997;106:469–474.

68. Layrargues GP, et al. Role of manganese in the pathogenesis of portal-systemic encephalopathy. Metab Brain Dis 1998;13:311–317.

69. Sher L. Role of selenium depletion in the etiopathogenesis of depression in patients with alcoholism. Med Hypotheses 2002;59:330–333.

70. Nompleggi DJ, Bonkovsky HL. Nutritional supplementation in chronic liver disease: An analytical review. Hepatology 1994;19:518–533.

71. Calamita A, et al. Plasma levels of transthyretin and retinol-binding protein in Child-A cirrhotic patients in relation to protein-calorie status and plasma amino acids, zinc, vitamin A and plasma thyroid hormones. Arq Gastroenterol 1997;34:139–147.

72. Campos AC, Matias JE, Coelho JC. Nutritional aspects of liver transplantation. Curr Opin Clin Nutr Metab Care 2002;5:297–307.

73. Vintro AQ, Krasnoff JB, Painter P. Roles of nutrition and physical activity in musculoskeletal complications before and after liver transplantation. AACN Clin Issues 2002;13:333–347.

74. Harrison J, McKiernan J, Neuberger JM. A prospective study on the effect of recipient nutritional status on outcome in liver transplantation. Transpl Int 1997;10:369–374.

75. Stephenson GR, et al. Malnutrition in liver transplant patients: Preoperative subjective global assessment is predictive of outcome after liver transplantation. Transplantation 2001;72:666–670.

76. Cabre E, Gassull MA. Nutritional aspects of liver disease and transplantation. Curr Opin Clin Nutr Metab Care 2001;4:581–589.

77. Hade AM, et al. Both under-nutrition and obesity increase morbidity following liver transplantation. Ir Med J 2003;96:140–142.

78. Konrad T, et al. Evidence for impaired glucose effectiveness in cirrhotic patients after liver transplantation. Metabolism 2000;49:367–372.

79. Delafosse B, et al. Long- and medium-chain triglycerides during parenteral nutrition in critically ill patients. Am J Physiol 1997;272(4 Pt 1): E550–E555.

80. Kuse ER, et al. Hepatic reticuloendothelial function during parenteral nutrition including an MCT/LCT or LCT emulsion after liver transplantation—a double-blind study. Transpl Int 2002;15:272–277.

81. Pescovitz MD, et al. Zinc deficiency and its repletion following liver transplantation in humans. Clin Transplant 1996;10:256–260.

82. Janczewska I, Ericzon BG, Eriksson LS. Influence of orthotopic liver transplantation on serum vitamin A levels in patients with chronic liver disease. Scand J Gastroenterol 1995;30:68–71.

83. Feller RB, et al. Evidence of continuing bone recovery at a mean of 7 years after liver transplantation. Liver Transpl Surg 1999;5:407–413.

84. Bishop NJ, et al. Changes in calcium homoeostasis in patients undergoing liver transplantation: Effects of a single infusion of pamidronate administered pre-operatively. Clin Sci (Lond) 1999;97:157–163.

85. Ng TM, Bajjoka IE. Treatment options for osteoporosis in chronic liver disease patients requiring liver transplantation. Ann Pharmacother 1999;33:233–235.

86. Sundaram A, Koutkia P, Apovian CM. Nutritional management of short bowel syndrome in adults. J Clin Gastroenterol 2002;34:207–220.

87. Scolapio JS, Fleming CR. Short bowel syndrome. Gastroenterol Clin North Am 1998;27:467–479, viii.

88. Wilmore DW, Byrne TA, Persinger RL. Short bowel syndrome: New therapeutic approaches. Curr Probl Surg 1997;34:389–444.

89. Kvietys PR. Intestinal physiology relevant to short-bowel syndrome. Eur J Pediatr Surg 1999;9:196–199.

90. Vanderhoof JA, Langnas AN. Short-bowel syndrome in children and adults. Gastroenterology 1997;113:1767–1778.

91. Forbes A, Chadwick C. Short bowel syndrome. In: Souba WW, et al, eds. The A.S.P.E.N. Nutrition Support Practice Manual. Silver Springs, American Society for Parenteral and Enteral Nutrition, 1998:1–10.

92. Ling PR, et al. Disturbances in essential fatty acid metabolism in patients receiving long-term home parenteral nutrition. Dig Dis Sci 2002; 47:1679–1685.

93. Jeejeebhoy KN. Metabolic bone disease and total parenteral nutrition: A progress report. Am J Clin Nutr 1998;67:186–187.

94. Vanderhoof JA, et al. Treatment strategies for small bowel bacterial overgrowth in short bowel syndrome. J Pediatr Gastroenterol Nutr 1998; 27:155–160.

95. Lord LM, et al. Management of the patient with short bowel syndrome. AACN Clin Issues 2000;11:604–618.

96. Shanbhogue LK, Molenaar JC. Short bowel syndrome: Metabolic and surgical management. Br J Surg 1994;81:486–499.

97. Byrne TA, et al. A new treatment for patients with short-bowel syndrome. Growth hormone, glutamine, and a modified diet. Ann Surg 1995; 222:243–255.

98. Ellegard L, et al. Low-dose recombinant human growth hormone increases body weight and lean body mass in patients with short bowel syndrome. Ann Surg 1997;225:88–96.

99. Scolapio JS. Effect of growth hormone, glutamine, and diet on body composition in short bowel syndrome: A randomized, controlled study. JPEN J Parenter Enteral Nutr 1999;23:309–312, discussion 312–313.

100. Szkudlarek J, Jeppesen PB, Mortensen PB. Effect of high dose growth hormone with glutamine and no change in diet on intestinal absorption in short bowel patients: A randomised, double blind, crossover, placebo controlled study. Gut 2000;47:199–205.

101. Platell CF, et al. The management of patients with the short bowel syndrome. World J Gastroenterol 2002;8:13–20.

102. Grant D. Intestinal transplantation: 1997 report of the international registry. Intestinal Transplant Registry. Transplantation 1999;67: 1061–1064.

103. Goulet O, et al. Intestinal transplantation: Indications, results and strategy. Curr Opin Clin Nutr Metab Care 2000;3:329–338.

104. Messing B, et al. Long-term survival and parenteral nutrition dependence in adult patients with the short bowel syndrome. Gastroenterology 1999;117:1043–1050.

105. Howard L, et al. Current use and clinical outcome of home parenteral and enteral nutrition therapies in the United States. Gastroenterology 1995; 109:355–365.

106. Jeppesen PB, Langholz E, Mortensen PB. Quality of life in patients receiving home parenteral nutrition. Gut 1999;44:844–852.

107. Sher L. Effects of selenium status on mood and behaviour: Role of thyroid hormones. Aust N Z J Psychiatry 2002;36:559–560.

108. Berry JK, Baum CL. Malnutrition in chronic obstructive pulmonary disease: Adding insult to injury. AACN Clin Issues 2001;12:210–219.

109. Foley RJ, ZuWallack R. The impact of nutritional depletion in chronic obstructive pulmonary disease. J Cardiopulm Rehabil 2001;21: 288–295.

110. Schols AM, Wouters EF. Nutritional abnormalities and supplementation in chronic obstructive pulmonary disease. Clin Chest Med 2000;21: 753–762.

111. Engelen MP, et al. Different patterns of chronic tissue wasting among patients with chronic obstructive pulmonary disease. Clin Nutr 1999; 18:275–280.

112. Engelen MP, et al. Skeletal muscle weakness is associated with wasting of extremity fat-free mass but not with airflow obstruction in patients with chronic obstructive pulmonary disease. Am J Clin Nutr 2000;71: 733–738.

113. Landbo C, et al. Prognostic value of nutritional status in chronic obstructive pulmonary disease. Am J Respir Crit Care Med 1999;160: 1856–1861.

114. Creutzberg EC, et al. Prevalence of an elevated resting energy expenditure in patients with chronic obstructive pulmonary disease in relation to body composition and lung function. Eur J Clin Nutr 1998;52: 396–401.

115. Baarends EM, et al. Total daily energy expenditure relative to resting energy expenditure in clinically stable patients with COPD. Thorax 1997; 52:780–785.

116. Donahoe M. Nutritional support in advanced lung disease. The pulmonary cachexia syndrome. Clin Chest Med 1997;18:547–561.

117. Cai B, et al. Effect of supplementing a high-fat, low-carbohydrate enteral formula in COPD patients. Nutrition 2003;19:229–232.

118. Faucher M, et al. Cardiopulmonary effects of lipid emulsions in patients with ARDS. Chest 2003;124:285–291.

119. Ferreira I, et al. Nutritional intervention in COPD: A systematic overview. Chest 2001;119:353–363.

120. Crook MA, Hally V, Panteli JV. The importance of the refeeding syndrome. Nutrition 2001;17(7–8):632–637.

121. Clark CL, et al. Treatment of hypophosphatemia in patients receiving specialized nutrition support using a graduated dosing scheme: Results from a prospective clinical trial. Crit Care Med 1995;23:1504–1511.

122. Tabak C, et al. Dietary factors and pulmonary function: A cross sectional study in middle aged men from three European countries. Thorax 1999;54:1021–1026.

123. MacNee W. Oxidants/antioxidants and COPD. Chest 2000;117 (5 Suppl 1):303S–317S.

124. Efthimiou J, et al. Effect of carbohydrate rich versus fat rich loads on gas exchange and walking performance in patients with chronic obstructive lung disease. Thorax 1992;47:451–456.

125. Akrabawi SS, et al. Gastric emptying, pulmonary function, gas exchange, and respiratory quotient after feeding a moderate versus high fat enteral formula meal in chronic obstructive pulmonary disease patients. Nutrition 1996;12:260–265.

126. van den Berg B, Bogaard JM, Hop WC. High fat, low carbohydrate, enteral feeding in patients weaning from the ventilator. Intensive Care Med 1994;20:470–475.

127. Gadek JE, et al. Effect of enteral feeding with eicosapentaenoic acid, gamma-linolenic acid, and antioxidants in patients with acute respiratory distress syndrome. Enteral Nutrition in ARDS Study Group. Crit Care Med 1999;27:1409–1420.

128. Burdet L, et al. Administration of growth hormone to underweight patients with chronic obstructive pulmonary disease. A prospective, randomized, controlled study. Am J Respir Crit Care Med 1997;156:1800–1806.

129. Schols AM. Nutrition in chronic obstructive pulmonary disease. Curr Opin Pulm Med 2000;6:110–115.

130. Schols AM, et al. Weight loss is a reversible factor in the prognosis of chronic obstructive pulmonary disease. Am J Respir Crit Care Med, 1998;157(6 Pt 1):1791–1797.

131. Shoup R, et al. Body composition and health-related quality of life in patients with obstructive airways disease. Eur Respir J 1997;10:1576–1580.

140
OBESITY

John V. St. Peter and Mehmood A. Khan

Learning Objectives and other resources can be found at *www.pharmacotherapyonline.com.*

KEY CONCEPTS

1. Two clinical measures of excess body fat, regardless of sex, are the body mass index (BMI) and the waist circumference (WC). BMI and WC provide a better assessment of total body fat than weight alone and are independent predictors of obesity-related disease risk.

2. Excessive central adiposity increases risk for development of type 2 diabetes, hypertension, and dyslipidemia.

3. Weight loss of as little as 5% of total body weight can significantly improve blood pressure, lipid levels, and glucose tolerance in overweight and obese patients.

4. It is appropriate to consider medication therapy if 6 months of diet, exercise, and behavioral modification fail to stimulate weight loss.

5. A sufficient degree of obesity (BMI = 30 kg/m² and/or WC = 40 inches for males or 35 inches for females, or BMI of 27 to 30 kg/m² with concurrent risk factors) should be present before pharmacotherapy-facilitated weight loss is considered.

6. Some herbal and food supplement diet agents contain sources of pharmacologically active substances that should be used with caution or avoided in obese patients with conditions such as diabetes, hypertension, and significant cardiovascular disease.

7. The FDA does not regulate labeling of herbal and food supplement diet agents, and content is not guaranteed.

8. There is a high probability of weight regain when obesity pharmacotherapy is discontinued.

It is now estimated that over 95 million adults are overweight or obese in the United States.[1] Additionally, significant numbers of adolescents are developing overweight and obesity status.[1–4] Overweight and obesity significantly increase risk for development of many diseases, worsen outcomes in the presence of comorbid disease states, and most likely increase health care costs (Table 140–1).[5] Observational epidemiologic studies show that overall mortality parallels body weight increases above an optimal level.[6–8] This evidence is strongest for adults between the ages of 30 and 44 years. In older age groups, excess body weight increases the risk of death, but the degree of impact diminishes with age.[9] Annually, an estimated 15% to 35% of the American population resolve to lose weight, spending between $30 and $50 billion with little or no documented improvement.[10–12] The recent report of the Surgeon General and the inclusion of several aggressive Healthy People 2010 goals have helped to stimulate national initiatives aimed at reversing the rising rate of obesity through implementation of consensus guidelines and best practices.[13–16] This chapter reviews the epidemiology, pathophysiology, and therapeutic approaches for the management of obesity. Although nonpharmacologic treatment modalities are discussed, the pharmacotherapy of obesity is highlighted, and the role of pharmacotherapy relative to the other therapeutic options is discussed.[17]

EPIDEMIOLOGY

Obesity is increasing in prevalence in the United States. The National Health and Nutrition Examination Survey (NHANES) II data (1976–1980) estimated a prevalence of overweight persons in the United States at 25.4% of adults, representing 34 million individuals. During NHANES III (1988–1991), the prevalence had increased to 33.3%, representing 55 million American adults.[1] The prevention of obesity therefore is a public health priority.[14] This has been further emphasized by the continued pursuit of safe and effective long-term therapy for obesity. Individuals who were "fat" as children tend to remain overweight as adults.[4,18] Recent data from a large British study have provided further evidence for the relationship between an overweight childhood and subsequent excess weight as an adult.[19] In contrast to body weight, adult BMI was not well predicted from childhood weight. The fattest children had the highest risks of adult obesity. However, most obese adults had not been fat at earlier ages: Only 17% and 18% of obese 33-year-old men and women, respectively, had been fat at age 7 years. Thus most obese adults were not fat children. In contrast, early adulthood may be an important time for intervention to prevent future obesity. Of 4519 men and 4806 women in the study by Power and associates, obesity increased in prevalence from 2% to 11% in men and from 3% to 12% in women during the 10-year period between ages 23 and 33 years.[19] The prevalence of overweight varies between races within the United States.[20–22] Mexican-American women and black women had the highest prevalence, 48.1% and 49.1%, respectively. The prevalence of obesity also increases with age, reaching a maximum by the sixth decade in women and the seventh decade for men. Beyond this age, the prevalence progressively falls for both genders. Socioeconomic status also affects the prevalence of obesity in those between the ages of 25 and 54 years. The prevalence of overweight in nonpregnant women for

TABLE 140–1. Conditions More Prevalent in Obese Populations

Cardiovascular	**Musculoskeletal**
Hypertension	Degenerative joint disease
Left ventricular hypertrophy	**Skin**
Congestive heart failure	Acanthosis nigricans
Coronary artery disease	Stretch marks
Stroke	Hirsutism
Pulmonary	Skin tags
Obstructive airway disease	**Gastrointestinal**
Sleep apnea	Cholelithiasis
Pulmonary hypertension	Esophageal reflux
Metabolic	Hiatus hernia
Hypercholesterolemia	**Psychological**
Hypertriglyceridemia	Eating disorders
Low serum high-density lipoprotein	Depression
Diabetes mellitus and glucose	Affective disorders
intolerance	Social stigma
Hyperinsulinemia	**Neoplasm**
Polycystic ovary syndrome	Breast cancer
Increased serum urate	Colon cancer

each respective decade of life—25 to 34 years, 35 to 44 years, and 45 to 54 years—is 30.8%, 49.1%, and 54.1% of women with incomes below the poverty line versus 18.4%, 23.7%, and 30.3% of those above the poverty line.[19] Educational achievement, which is linked to socioeconomic status, is also correlated with the fraction of people who are overweight; prevalence of overweight is greatest in those with less than a high school education versus those with some college education.

ETIOLOGY

The etiology of obesity in the vast majority of individuals is unknown. However, studies in twins confirm the presence of genetic contributions.[23] It is likely multifactorial in origin, with genetic, environmental, and physiologic factors contributing to various degrees in different individuals. A definitive diagnosis of an underlying medical condition can be made in only a small minority of individuals. Even then, the diagnosed condition may or may not be treatable. One of the current controversies is the extent that genetic traits influence the risk of developing obesity, as well as how these genetic traits interact with environmental factors to cause obesity.[24]

GENETIC PREDISPOSITION

Family studies show a clear correlation of body weight between parents and children. The correlation between siblings is even higher. In monozygotic twins, BMI is almost always identical, and there is a strong correlation in the accumulation of visceral fat. These twin studies demonstrate the strong role of genetics in determining both obesity and distribution of body fat. The incidence of obesity in adopted individuals relative to their adopted parents provides insight into the role of genetics versus family environment. These studies show a clear correlation between the BMI of adult adoptees and their biologic parents. This relationship does not exist between an adoptee and his or her adoptive parent. These observations further support the notion that genes are primarily responsible for determining adult body weight. The relative impact of genetic versus environmental factors varies between persons. In some individuals, genetic factors are the primary determinants of obesity, whereas in others, the obesity may be caused primarily by environmental factors. The actual variance in body fat

between individuals determined by genes is not known. Estimates for this variance range from 20% to a high of almost 80%. Yet, clearly, without adequate caloric intake, obesity cannot occur. Thus the role of the environment is to facilitate expression of an underlying genetic trait for obesity. However, the specific gene or genes that code for obesity are unknown.[25] Most investigators would agree that more than one gene is involved in the development of human obesity.

ENVIRONMENTAL FACTORS

Economic development is associated with lifestyle changes.[3] Many of these societal changes may contribute to the observed rise in the prevalence of obesity throughout the world. Those which are most probably related to obesity include reduced physical activity or work (sedentary lifestyle), abundant and readily available food supply, increased fat intake, increased consumption of refined simple sugars, and decreased ingestion of vegetables, fruits, and complex carbohydrates. These changes in our environment likely contribute to a state of positive energy balance in many individuals (Fig. 140–1).[26] Observations from public health studies support this concept. For example, the prevalence of obesity in Copenhagen remained stable during the period between 1925 and 1942 at approximately 0.1%. However, since the end of World War II, there has been a steady increase in the prevalence of obesity.[26] These observational data suggest an environmental role for the development of obesity.

NUTRITION

Decades of research have led to several thousand publications regarding nutrition therapy for obesity. Yet the appropriate diet that leads to long-term weight loss in ambulatory self-sufficient individuals is not known. The consensus is that weight regain is almost always inevitable. It is clear that excess caloric intake is a prerequisite to weight gain and obesity, but not all individuals with high caloric intake gain weight. There is an ongoing debate whether the primary consideration is total calorie intake or macronutrient composition of the diet (i.e., percentage of calories as carbohydrates, protein, or fat). Of the three macronutrients, dietary fat has received the most attention. Both animals and humans prefer and often will seek out foods high in fat. High-fat foods have a desirable texture and sensory characteristics in the mouth. Although fat is itself tasteless, fats enhance the flavor of

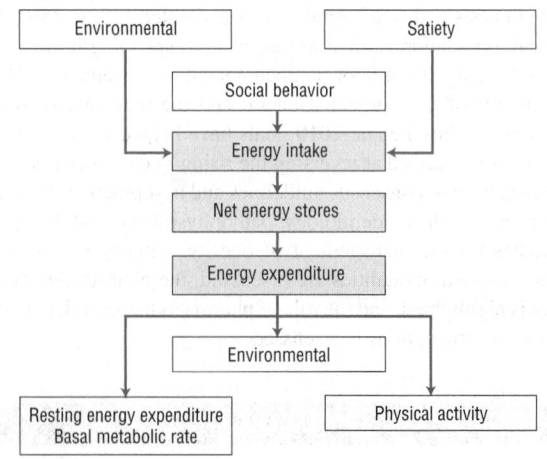

FIGURE 140–1. Net energy stores are determined by various inputs and outputs. Simply stated, obesity occurs when imbalance occurs between energy intake and expenditure.

other foods. Clearly, one way that fatty foods promote weight gain is by increased energy intake because fat is more energy dense than other macronutrients. Furthermore, fats are stored with greater efficiency than protein or carbohydrates. Nutritional management of obesity as discussed in this chapter is based on reducing calorie intake. Because the Western diet is high in fat, and because fat contains more than twice the calories per gram of carbohydrate and protein, in almost all diets the fat content is reduced by necessity.[27]

APPETITE

Central Receptor Systems

Multiple receptor systems, including those of the biogenic amines, are known to either stimulate or decrease food intake in both animals and humans. Serotonin, also known as 5-hydroxytryptamine (5-HT), and cells known to respond to 5-HT are found throughout the central nervous system and the periphery. At least seven distinct subfamilies of 5-HT receptors have been cloned to date, with each of these seven exhibiting one or more subtypes. Currently, two major noradrenergic receptor subtypes are recognized (α and β), each with multiple subtypes. Histamine and dopamine also demonstrate multiple receptor subtypes, but their role in regulation of human eating behaviors and food intake is less well documented. Direct stimulation of 5-HT$_{1A}$ and noradrenergic α_2-receptors will increase food intake, whereas the opposite occurs with 5-HT$_{2C}$ and noradrenergic α_1- or β_2-receptor activation. In animal models, stimulating histamine receptor subtypes 1 or 3 and dopamine receptor subtypes 1 or 2 results in lowering of food intake. Table 140–2 summarizes the major effects of direct receptor stimulation, inhibition, or changes in synaptic cleft amine concentrations on food intake.

Peptides

Since the 1950s, it has been conjectured that weight is controlled via a hormone interaction at the level of the hypothalamus.[28] The protein product of the mouse obese gene (ob) described in 1994 appears to be the signaling mechanism between peripheral energy storage and hypothalamic feeding centers.[28,29] This protein was called leptin (after leptos, the Greek word for "thin"). The ob/ob genetically obese

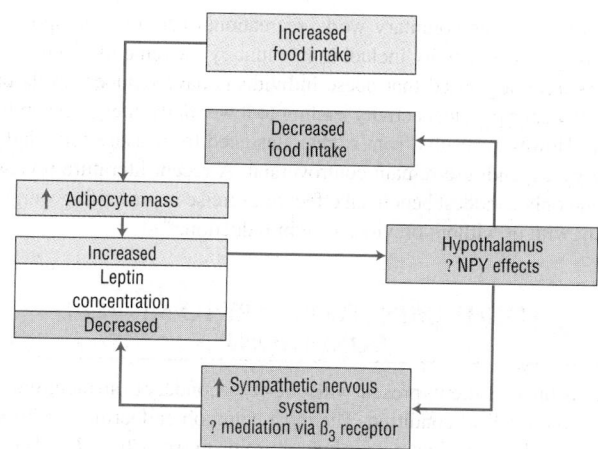

FIGURE 140–2. Effects of food intake on leptin concentrations and proposed feedback loops controlling food intake and leptin concentration. NPY, neuropeptide Y.

mouse does not produce leptin, and this animal's marked hyperphagia subsides with leptin supplementation. Adrenalectomy reverses the obese phenotype and restores the hypothalamic melanocortin tone in the ob/ob mouse, suggesting that glucocorticoids have a facilitative role in the development of obesity.[30] The human leptin homologue has been cloned, and various animal studies have demonstrated that leptin is produced in the periphery by white and possibly brown adipocytes. Additionally, it appears that the sympathetic nervous system (SNS), via β_3-adrenoceptors, inhibits leptin expression (Fig. 140–2). Unlike the leptin-deficient ob/ob mouse, obese human serum leptin levels increase as fat cell mass increases. There is a direct relationship between serum leptin concentrations and various markers of obesity such as percentage of body fat, BMI, and serum insulin concentrations. Thus humans appear to be resistant to the satiety effects of leptin, and recent studies of leptin supplementation in humans have not significantly decreased obesity.[31] Figure 140–2 shows the peripheral link that leptin appears to provide in signaling the central nervous system about the status of fat cell mass. However, there is increasing evidence of the complicated nature of leptin effects both within and outside the central nervous system.[32–34] A second peptide, neuropeptide Y (NPY), is being studied intensely for its effects on feeding.[35] NPY elicits many effects both peripherally and centrally, including appetite stimulation. Messenger RNA for two new appetite-stimulating proteins called orexins has been observed to be concentrated in the lateral hypothalamus.[36] An understanding of the relationships between the sympathetic nervous system, leptin, NPY, orexins, and other hormones such as insulin and glucocorticoids is still evolving.[37] Exogenous manipulation of these proteins may provide future pharmacotherapeutic approaches to obesity management.

ACTIVITY

It is generally accepted that increased physical activity is an important component in the management of obesity.[38] Similarly, a sedentary lifestyle predisposes to weight gain and obesity. Yet the question of whether obese individuals are less physically active compared with age-matched lean individuals remains unanswered. Some studies show no difference in physical activity between lean and obese individuals, whereas others suggest that obese persons are less active. Although some studies suggest that obese persons are less active, it is unclear whether less physical activity leads to obesity or physical inactivity is itself secondary to the physical effects of obesity. Physical

TABLE 140–2. Effects of Various Neurotransmitters, Receptors, and Peptides on Food Intake

Neurotransmitter/Receptor/Peptide	Action	Food Intake
Norepinephrine	Increase concentration	Decrease
α_1	Stimulate receptor	Decrease
α_2	Stimulate receptor	Increase
β_2	Stimulate receptor	Decrease
Serotonin	Increase concentration	Decrease
5-HT$_{1A}$	Stimulate receptor	Increase
5-HT$_{1B}$	Stimulate receptor	Decrease
5-HT$_{2C}$	Stimulate receptor	Decrease
Histamine		
H$_1$	Stimulate receptor	Decrease
H$_3$	Stimulate receptor	Decrease
Dopamine		
D$_1$	Stimulate receptor	Decrease
D$_2$	Stimulate receptor	Decrease
Leptin	Increase concentration	Decrease
Neuropeptide Y	Increase concentration	Increase
Galanin	Increase concentration	Increase

activity includes voluntary work, recreational activity, and spontaneous physical activity including involuntary movements. Some authors have suggested that obese individuals have reduced levels of spontaneous physical activity leading to lower daily energy expenditure. However, results from studies designed to measure total daily energy expenditure remain controversial. A recent literature review found only a modest beneficial effect of exercise in preventing weight gain, with or without previous weight reduction.[39]

WEIGHT GAIN SECONDARY TO MEDICAL CONDITIONS

Occasionally patients present with obesity secondary to an identifiable acquired medical condition. The most common endocrine condition associated with weight gain is hypothyroidism (see Chap. 73). These patients lose significant weight within weeks of thyroxin replacement therapy. However, many patients will not achieve a normal or ideal body weight despite adequate thyroid hormone replacement. Indeed, it is not uncommon for patients to request higher than physiologic replacement doses of thyroxin to artificially suppress their weight. It is important to remember that excess thyroid therapy can be associated with complications, including osteoporosis and cardiac disorders. Cushing's syndrome, another cause of obesity, is seen most commonly in patients receiving exogenous glucocorticoid therapy. These agents often are prescribed for a chronic condition such as chronic obstructive pulmonary disease (COPD), organ transplantation, or arthritis. Idiopathic Cushing's disease due to excess endogeneous steroid secretion is, in contrast, very rare. In both iatrogenic and idiopathic Cushing's disease, the weight gain is in part due to fluid retention as well as increased adiposity. The adiposity associated with glucocorticoid excess has a particular body distribution in that it is central with relative loss of body muscle mass and thinning of the skin, leading to the characteristic purple skin striae and a buffalo hump behind the neck.

Occasionally patients can present with lesions of the hypothalamus that lead to hyperphagia and obesity. This disorder is rare and should not be confused with behavioral disorders of eating that are associated with psychopathology. These include binge eating disorders, which may respond to psychotherapy and in some cases pharmacotherapy (see Chap. 62). Obesity is itself associated with a higher prevalence of affective disorders, which if untreated may impair the success of any weight loss program. The clinician managing obesity must be aware of the presence of psychosocial disorders both as a cause and effect of obesity. Counseling strategies need to be incorporated into the management of selected obese individuals.[40] Furthermore, medications used to manage affective disorders, such as the selective serotonin reuptake inhibitors, have not been studied extensively with regard to combination use with appetite suppressant agents.

GENETIC SYNDROMES

Syndromes in which obesity is a major component are extremely rare. Prader-Willi, Simpson-Goabi-Behmel, Cohen's, Bardet-Biedl, Carpenter's, Börjeson's, and Wilson-Turner syndromes have all been associated with obesity. Of these, Prader-Willi syndrome is the most common and has a frequency of 1 in 20,000 live births. Other phenotypic features include changes in stature, mental retardation, and developmental abnormalities (e.g., hypogonadism). Because the incidence of thes syndromes is rare, even collectively they contribute very little to the incidence of obesity. The clinician evaluating a patient for obesity needs to be aware of their existence, and the physical examination of obese patients always should include an assessment for secondary causes of obesity including genetic syndromes (Fig. 140–3).

PATHOPHYSIOLOGY

ENERGY BALANCE

The net balance of energy ingested relative to energy expended by an individual over time determines the degree of obesity. Figure 140–1 represents the interplay between energy intake and expenditure. Energy stores will increase if there is imbalance between intake and expenditure. An individual's metabolic rate is the single largest determinant of energy expenditure. It is important to determine metabolic rate under standardized conditions, giving rise to terms such as resting energy expenditure (REE) and basal metabolic rate (BMR). REE is defined as the energy expended by a person at rest under conditions of thermal neutrality. BMR is more precisely defined as the REE measured soon after awakening in the morning, at least 12 hours after the last meal. Metabolic rate increases after eating, based on the size and composition of the meal. It reaches a maximum approximately 1 hour after the meal is consumed and is essentially back to basal levels 4 hours after the meal. This increase in metabolic rate is known as the *thermogenic effect of food*. The REE may include the residual thermic effect of a previous meal and may be lower than BMR during quiet sleep. In practice, BMR and REE differ by less than 10%, and the terms frequently are used interchangeably.

PERIPHERAL STORAGE AND THERMOGENESIS

Adipose tissue generally is divided into two major types, white and brown. The primary function of white adipose tissue is lipid manufacture, storage, and release. Lipid storage occurs in response to insulin with lipid release occurring during periods of calorie restriction, when insulin levels are suppressed. Brown-type tissue is notable for its ability to dissipate energy via a process of uncoupled mitochondrial respiration.[41] Currently, the exact roles of each of these tissue subtypes are better defined in animal models than in humans. Adipose tissue is highly innervated by the sympathetic nervous system, and adrenergic stimulation is known to activate lipolysis in fat cells as well as increase energy expenditure in adipose tissue and skeletal muscle. These properties provide a potential pharmacologic avenue for altering energy balance and changing weight status. A major focus of research in obesity pharmacotherapy has centered on the activity of adrenergic receptors and their effect on adipose tissue with respect to energy storage and expenditure or thermogenesis.[42] All three subtypes of β-adrenergic receptors (β_1, β_2, and β_3) appear to be active in fat cell function. The β_3-receptor appears to be less responsive than β_1 and β_2 with respect to activation via norepinephrine. This has led to the development of specific β_3-adrenoceptor agonists. However, apparent differences in selectivity and responsiveness between animal and human β_3-receptors have complicated the drug development process. In vivo studies in humans suggest that the β_3-receptor may be largely responsible for adipose tissue adrenergic-mediated increases in thermogenesis.[43] Genetic polymorphisms have been identified in both the β_2- and β_3-receptor systems that are associated with obesity or excess weight gain.[44] Thus genetic susceptibility for excess weight status may in part be related to adrenergic dysfunction. The development of effective pharmacotherapies involving these receptor

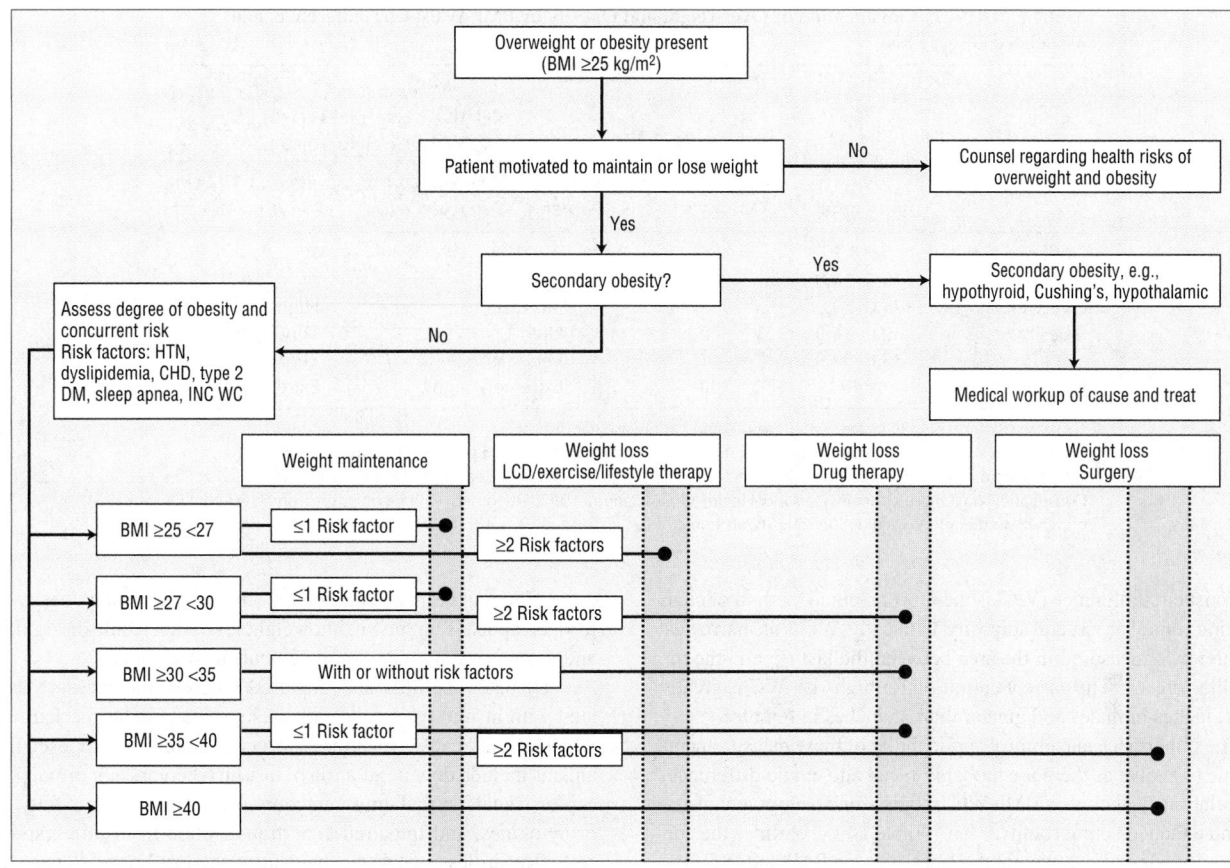

FIGURE 140–3. Pharmacotherapy treatment algorithm. A select population of individuals, based on BMI and WC together with concurrent risk factors, may benefit from medication therapy as an adjunct to a program of weight loss that includes diet, exercise, and behavioral modification. Abbreviations: WC, waist circumference; INC WC, >40 inches for males and >35 inches for females; BMI, body mass index; CHD, coronary heart disease; DM, diabetes mellitus; HTN, hypertension; LCD, low-calorie diet.

systems may be delayed pending definitive identification of receptor subtype contributions.

CLINICAL PRESENTATION

A consistent and reproducible description of weight status is essential in the diagnosis and management of obesity. For over two decades a clear distinction has been made between obesity and overweight by the National Center for Health Statistics (NCHS), yet clinicians and researchers often use the two terms interchangeably. *Overweight* refers to an excess body weight relative to a person's height. In contrast, *obesity* refers to a state of excess body fat as determined by measures of skinfold thickness, body density using underwater body weight, bioelectric impedance and conductivity, dual-energy x-ray absorptiometry (DEXA), computed tomography (CT), and magnetic resonance imaging (MRI). Many of these measurement techniques that determine body fat directly are too expensive and time-consuming to be used in population studies or for application in clinical medicine. Two measures which have been recognized as acceptable markers of excess body fat and have application regardless of sex are the body mass index (BMI) and the waist circumference (WC). While BMI and WC are related, each measure independently predicts disease risk. Both measurements should be taken at initial assessment and during routine follow-up of therapy for obesity.

Notably, epidemiologic studies demonstrate that WC adds little in terms of risk prediction once BMI reaches 35 kg/m². Thus, routine collection of WC should be implemented in those with BMI between 25 and 35 kg/m².

BMI is a measure of total body weight relative to height. Using metric units, it is defined as weight in kilograms divided by height in meters squared (kg/m²). Using pounds and inches, BMI (kg/m²) is estimated as: weight [pounds]/height [inches²] × 703. The BMI may overestimate the degree of excess body fat in various clinical situations (edematous states, extreme muscularity, muscle wasting, short-stature, etc), therefore clinical judgment is required.

Weight relative to height (BMI) is an acceptable measure of obesity; however, it does not always correspond to excess fat. Generally, central obesity reflects high levels of intra-abdominal or visceral fat. Intra-abdominal fat is best estimated by imaging techniques such as CT or MRI. More recent studies suggest that subcutaneous fat may be heterogeneous in its metabolic effects. In these studies, superficial subcutaneous fat had a weak association with metabolic markers of insulin production and release resistance, whereas deep subcutaneous fat had a strong relationship with insulin resistance.[45] This pattern of obesity is associated with an increased propensity for the development of hypertension, dyslipidemia, type 2 diabetes, and cardiovascular disease. Thus, in addition to the absolute excess fat mass, the distribution of this fat regionally in the body has an important effect on the mortality of obese individuals.

TABLE 140–3. Classification of Overweight and Obesity by BMI, Waist Circumference, and Associated Disease Risk

	BMI (kg/m^2)	Obesity Class	Disease Risk[a] (Relative to Normal Weight and Waist Circumference)	
			Men ≤40 in (≤102 cm) Women ≤35 in (≤88 cm)	>40 in (>102 cm) >35 in (>88 cm)
Underweight	<18.5		—	—
Normal[b]	18.5–24.9		—	—
Overweight	25.0–29.9		Increased	High
Obesity	30.0–34.9	I	High	Very high
	35.0–39.9	II	Very high	Very high
Extreme obesity	≥40	III	Extremely high	Extremely high

[a]Disease risk for type 2 diabetes, hypertension, and cardiovascular disease.
[b]Increased waist circumference can also be a marker for increased risk even in persons of normal weight.
Adapted from Preventing and Managing the Global Epidemic of Obesity. Report of the World Health Organization Consultation on Obesity. Geneva, World Health Organization, 1997. Reprinted with permission from NLH-NHLBI, http://www.nhlbi.nih.gov/guidelines/obesity/ob_home.htm

Waist circumference (WC) is the most practical method of characterizing central or visceral adiposity. Clinically, WC is the narrowest circumference measured in the area between the last rib and the top of the iliac crest.[27] The current definition for high-risk WC is greater than 40 inches in males and greater than 35 inches in females.[27]

The importance and clinical applicability of these measurements continue to evolve as there are probably racial and ethnic differences in the relationship between BMI, WC, and risk for development of disease and enhanced comorbidity.[20–22,46] Table 140–3 outlines the current classification of overweight and obesity using BMI and WC. The table identifies risk for development of type 2 diabetes, hypertension, or cardiovascular disease at various stages of BMI or WC. Note that increased WC confers increased risk even in normal-weight individuals.

COMORBIDITIES

Obesity is associated with serious health risks and increased mortality. Several disease states and/or conditions are more prevalent in obese patients (see Table 140–1). Increased body fat, increased total body weight, and a central distribution of body fat are all associated with an increased incidence of mortality, primarily due to cardiovascular disease. Hypertension, hyperlipidemia, insulin resistance, and glucose intolerance are all known cardiac risk factors that tend to cluster in obese individuals. Therefore, the obese individual is exposed to multiple risk factors. Some of the earliest studies from Framingham have confirmed the relationship between obesity and increased risk of stroke and coronary heart disease in both men and women.[47] This increased mortality is seen even with modest excess body weight. Blood pressure frequently is elevated in obese individuals and may in part explain the increased incidence of stroke and cardiovascular disease observed with obesity. Hypertension in lean individuals is associated with concentric hypertrophy due to an increased afterload, which increases the risk of cardiac ischemia. In contrast, with obesity eccentric dilatation is observed, leading to an increased volume load. This dilated cardiomyopathy is associated with a reduction in ventricular ejection fraction and a high-output cardiac state. The combination of obesity and hypertension is associated with thickening of the ventricular wall, ischemia, and increased heart volume. This leads more rapidly to heart failure and has been recognized for more than two decades.[48] Alterations in pulmonary function are common in patients with obesity. Most significant and costly in terms of morbidity and mortality is sleep apnea.[49] This disorder is more common in men. The exact mechanism by which obesity leads to sleep apnea is unknown, but weight loss often results in significant and sometimes dramatic improvements in sleep apnea.

Diabetes mellitus and impaired glucose tolerance are associated with insulin resistance and obesity. The cellular mechanism by which obesity causes insulin resistance is unknown. Proposed mechanisms include downregulation of insulin receptors, abnormal postreceptor signals, circulating antagonists to insulin such as fatty acids or cytokines, and impaired gene transcription in insulin-responsive cells. Regardless of the mechanism of the insulin resistance, as insulin response becomes impaired, the pancreatic β cells respond by increasing insulin production and release, resulting in a state of relative hyperinsulinemia. Although hyperinsulinemia is known to be associated with an increased risk of cardiovascular disease, it is not known whether the increased insulin levels contribute directly to cardiac disease or if they are just a marker for the underlying defect of insulin resistance and glucose intolerance. Insulin resistance in turn also frequently leads to impaired lipid metabolism (increased cholesterol, increased triglycerides, and low circulating high-density lipoprotein) and hypertension. As with cardiovascular disease, fat distribution is an important factor in determining the risk of developing type 2 diabetes. Central obesity has been shown to increase the risk of diabetes. Intentional weight loss has been shown to reduce mortality substantially in obese individuals with diabetes.[50]

Osteoarthritis in weight-bearing joints, such as the knees, may be related directly to the mechanical effects of excess body weight and the resulting forces exerted on these joint surfaces. The increase of osteoarthritis in non–weight-bearing joints, however, suggests that obesity may lead to altered cartilage, collagen, and even bone metabolism. Osteoarthritis and its symptoms, such as pain, are a significant barrier to physical activity and a key impediment to sustained weight loss.

Obesity affects the human reproductive system in a number of ways. Obesity is associated with earlier menarche in girls and hyperandrogenism, hirsutism, and anovulatory menstrual cycles in women. In some women this disorder manifests as overt polycystic ovary syndrome (PCOS).[51] Insulin resistance is common in these women. Weight loss, and more recently therapy with insulin-sensitizing drugs such as the thiazolidinediones and biguanides, can restore normal ovulation in some women.[51] These observations suggest that insulin resistance plays a part in the causation of PCOS-associated with obesity.

▶ TREATMENT: Obesity

▦ DESIRED OUTCOME

◀ Weight management is commonly considered successful when a predefined amount of weight has been lost such that a final goal is achieved. However, desired outcomes are fully dependent upon the clinical situation. Success may also include endpoints of decreasing the rate of weight gain or maintaining a weight-neutral status. A significant number of web-based resources for supporting both patient and practitioner weight management activities are available.[14,16,27,52–54]

▦ GENERAL APPROACH TO TREATMENT

The success of obesity therapy has been measured most often as weight loss over study periods of up to 12 months. Successful obesity treatment plans have incorporated diet, exercise, behavior modification (with or without pharmacologic therapy), and/or surgical intervention. Figure 140–4 shows the sites of action of these therapies within the energy intake, storage, and expenditure cycle.

Patients seeking help for obesity do so for many reasons, including improvement in their quality of life, a reduction in associated morbidity, and to prolong their life. Yet numerous individuals seek therapy for obesity primarily for cosmetic purposes and often have unreasonable goals and expectations. Aggressive marketing of weight loss programs, therapies, and diets—parallel to the fashion industry's standards of desirable body profiles—has led many individuals to set impossible goals and expectations. In some cases these persons will go to extreme measures to achieve weight loss, even at the risk of injury to themselves. Clinicians therefore must be careful not only to fully discuss risks of therapies, but also to clearly define achievable benefits and magnitude of weight loss. Criteria for weight loss vary from the most aggressive goal of trying to achieve an "ideal weight" to the more reasonable goals of modest (e.g., loss of 5% of body weight) but sustained weight loss. In practice, the goal has to be set based on many factors, including initial body weight, patient motivation and desire, presence of comorbid conditions, and age. For example, in patients with diabetes, even modest weight loss can improve glucose control and reduce mortality significantly,[50,51] yet in individuals with osteoarthritis, significantly more weight reduction may be required to improve symptoms. Indeed, dietary modification and exercise have been shown to ameliorate hyperglycemia, hyperlipidemia, and hypertension with weight loss of less than 5% of initial body weight. These data emphasize the importance of defining endpoints and measures of success in any weight loss plan.

Most weight loss interventions consist of a combination of lifestyle changes, diet, drug therapy if indicated, and in some cases surgery (see Fig. 140–3). Prior to recommending any therapy, the clinician must evaluate the patient for the presence of secondary causes of obesity. If a secondary cause is suspected, then a more complete diagnostic work-up and appropriate therapy are paramount. The next step in the patient evaluation is to determine the presence and severity of other medical conditions either directly associated with obesity

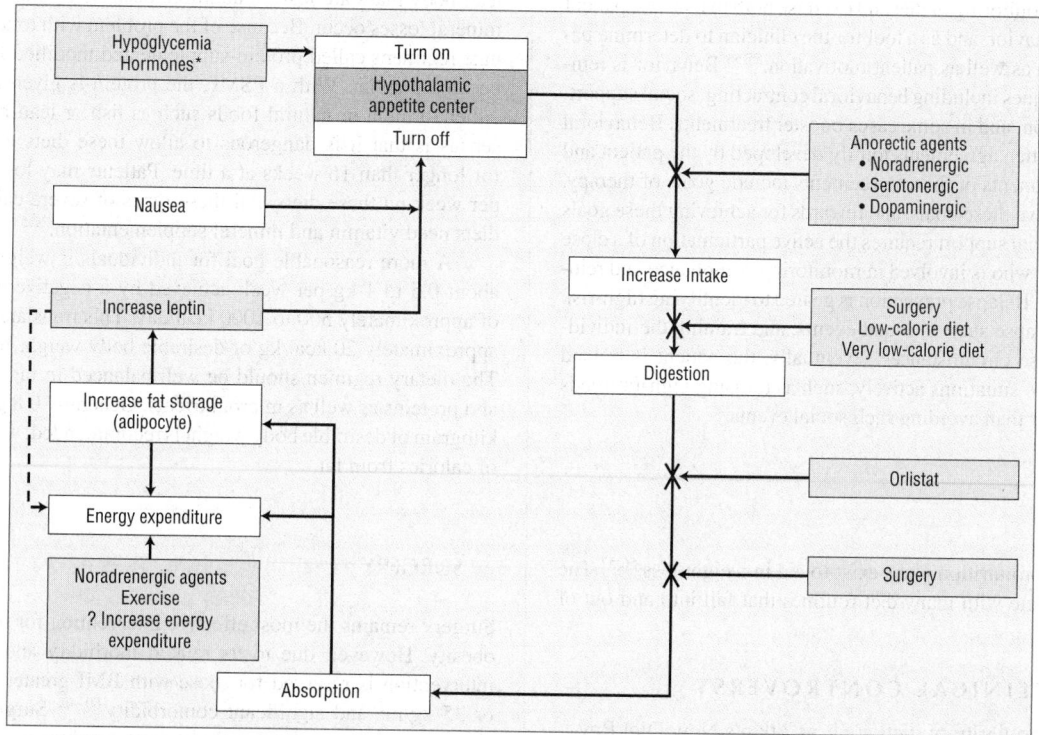

FIGURE 140–4. Hypothalamic appetite centers in the brain modulate both central and peripheral signals. This figure demonstrates the sites of action for various obesity treatment modalities within the cycle of energy intake and storage. Leptin, while signaling the central nervous system of the status of peripheral fat cell mass, may also have functions with regard to energy expenditure. Some appetite suppressant agents, alone or in combination, also modulate energy expenditure. *Including insulin, thyroxine, glucocorticoids, and progesterones.

(e.g., diabetes), or which have an impact on therapeutic decision making (e.g., history of liver disease or cardiac arrhythmia). Appropriate laboratory tests to exclude and/or quantify the degree of specific conditions such as diabetes, liver dysfunction, and nephropathy should be done as indicated by the history and physical examination. Based on the outcome of this medical evaluation, the patient then should be counseled on treatment options, benefits, and risks. The ultimate goals of treatment must be defined clearly. These goals may be absolute weight loss if obesity is present without other comorbid conditions. If improvement in blood glucose, blood cholesterol, and hypertension are primary goals, then these must be defined appropriately, such as target levels for low-density-lipoprotein cholesterol, glycosylated hemoglobin, or blood pressure. For these patients, weight loss goals may be as little as 5% of starting weight. In contrast, if obesity is causing physical problems such as impaired mobility, osteoarthritis, or sleep apnea, then 10% to 20% of starting weight may be more appropriate. All too often patients expect to lose weight overnight, only to be disappointed. Thus it is important to set a time course for the plan. A reasonable rate of weight loss is typically about 0.5 kg per week.

NONPHARMACOLOGIC THERAPY

BEHAVIORAL MODIFICATION

Behavior modification is common to almost all weight loss interventions. The primary aim is to help patients choose lifestyles that are conducive to safe and sustained weight loss. Behavioral therapy is based on principles of human learning and therefore attempts to substitute learned undesirable habits with desirable behaviors using a combination of stimulus control and reinforcement. Most such programs use self-monitoring of diet and exercise both to increase patient awareness of behavior, and as a tool for the clinician to determine patient compliance as well as patient motivation.[55,56] Behavior is reinforced by techniques including behavioral contracting, social support, relapse prevention, and in some cases booster treatments. Behavioral contracts are written agreements jointly developed by the patient and clinician. Components of these agreements include goals of therapy, methods to achieve these goals, and rewards for achieving these goals successfully. Social support requires the active participation of a close friend or relative who is involved in monitoring compliance and reinforcing behavior. Relapse prevention is geared to identifying high-risk situations for relapse such as social events, and training the individual to avoid these circumstances. Eventually, the patient is trained to deal with these situations actively, such as refusing high-fat foods assertively rather than avoiding such social events.

DIET

Numerous diet or nutrition plans exist to aid in weight loss.[56,57] The lay press is replete with many diet routines that fall into and out of favor.

CLINICAL CONTROVERSY

Due to the popularity of diets such as Atkin's New Diet Revolution (high fat, low carbohydrate, high protein) and The New Pritikin Program (low fat, high carbohydrate, medium protein), there is extensive discussion in the lay media and academic circles regarding the risks, benefits, and outcomes related to diets that preferentially employ macronutrient extremes (i.e., high protein vs. high carbohydrate vs. low fat). Ultimately, overall energy balance will determine the rate and extent of weight change.

Few, if any, of the popular "fad" diets have been objectively studied in a randomized, controlled fashion, with sufficient power to clearly determine their acute and chronic effects on human physiology. Additionally, the relative efficiency of these diets for weight loss and chronic weight maintenance remain ill-defined. However, recent efforts to better understand the acute and chronic effects of these extremes in macronutrient intake are being reported.[58,59] Whichever diet program is selected, it is clear that energy consumption must be less than energy expenditure to achieve weight loss (see Fig. 140–1). The challenge has been to develop a diet plan that leads to consistent adherence by the patient and therefore sustained weight loss and/or maintenance. Two broad categories of diet have been used in clinical practice: low calorie and very low calorie. The low-calorie diet (LCD) or Step 1 Diet, is recommended as part of the recent National Heart, Lung and Blood Institute (NHLBI) Obesity Education Initiative. This LCD recommends from 1000 to 1200 kcal/day for women and 1200 to 1600 kcal/day for men, based on estimated needs and weight maintenance or reduction goals. Very-low-calorie diets (VLCDs) generally contain less than 800 kcal/day. These highly restrictive diets often result in early weight loss, but have been disappointing in the long term in part because it is difficult for individuals to maintain compliance. Additionally, VLCDs require intensive medical monitoring, and are no more effective and possibly less effective for long-term weight reduction than LCDs. Other investigators have proposed total or modified fasts. The obvious problem with total fasts is that both fat and lean body mass are lost. In addition, because of diuresis, significant mineral losses occur. Because of the problem with total fasting, alternate regimens called protein-supplemented modified fasts (PSMFs), became popular. With a PSMF, the protein is given in the form of either formula or natural foods such as fish or lean meat. The consensus is that it is dangerous to allow these diets to be continued for longer than 16 weeks at a time. Patients may lose 1.5 to 2.3 kg per week on these diets. All these types of severe calorie-restricted diets need vitamin and mineral supplementation.[27,53]

A more reasonable goal for individuals is weight reduction of about 0.5 to 1 kg per week achieved by a negative calorie balance of approximately 500 to 1000 kcal/day. This translates into a diet of approximately 20 kcal/kg of desirable body weight for most adults. The dietary regimen should be well balanced in fat, carbohydrates, and proteins as well as micronutrients. Generally 0.8 g of protein per kilogram of desirable body weight is recommended, with at most 30% of calories from fat.

SURGERY

Surgery remains the most effective intervention for the treatment of obesity. However, due to its related morbidity and mortality, this intervention is reserved for those with BMI greater than 40 kg/m^2 or 35 kg/m^2 and significant comorbidity.[60–62] Surgical procedures either reduce the stomach volume and/or reduce the absorptive surface of the alimentary tract, resulting in some degree of malabsorption. Currently, the three major types of procedures are: stapled gastroplasty, adjustable gastric banding, and conventional Roux-en-Y gastric bypass.[63]

CLINICAL CONTROVERSY

The superiority of conventional Roux-en-Y bypass versus adjustable gastric banding in terms of efficacy, morbidity, and mortality is actively debated. However, given the nature of bariatric surgery and available alternatives, the probability that randomized controlled trials will be completed to answer these questions is low.

Gastroplasty and adjustable gastric banding are designed to reduce the volume of the stomach and thus restrict the rate of nutrient intake. Conventional bypass combines a restrictive approach with a degree of malabsorption induced by excluding 90% to 95% of the stomach, the entire duodenum, and a portion of the proximal jejunum. Conventional Roux-en-Y bypass yields greater and more long-lasting weight loss than the other two methods. Ultimately, reductions in total body weight of approximately 35% can be achieved. Less optimal weight loss, late weight gain, the need for surgical revision in 15% to 20% for outlet stenosis or severe reflux, and long-term failure rates of up to 80% have dampened interest in gastroplasty.[63] Similarly, gastric banding is plagued by frequent reoperation for stenosis and erosion or both of the band. Improvements in the peri- and postoperative care of gastric surgery patients has reduced morbidity and mortality with conventional bypass to approximately 10% and 1%, respectively.[63] Some of the most common early complications of conventional gastric bypass include: deep venous thrombosis, anastomotic leaks, and wound infections. Approximately one-third of patients develop significant vitamin B_{12} and iron deficiency with a large proportion demonstrating microcytic anemia. Dumping syndrome, characterized by colic, nausea, diarrhea, and bloating, does occur in a small number of patients and can complicate provision of drug therapy in some cases. Classically, Roux-en-Y gastric bypass was only performed as an open surgical procedure. However, recent developments in surgical technique have allowed this procedure to be performed via laparoscope.[62] Long-term results comparing the outcomes of open versus laparoscopic methods are not yet available. After experiencing weight loss, many gastric surgery patients are able to discontinue pharmacotherapy for glucose lowering, dyslipidemia, and hypertension. Frequently however, hypertension medications must be restarted at various time periods postsurgery, in spite of the fact that weight regain has not or has only minimally occurred. The reasons and mechanisms for this are unclear, but reiterate the need for intensive follow-up by all clinical specialties involved in the care of these patients.

Selection of the appropriate patients for surgery and subsequently identifying the most appropriate procedure for each patient is critical. The input of an experienced surgeon working with a multidisciplinary team is invaluable.

CLINICAL CONTROVERSY

The debate regarding the appropriateness of obesity pharmacotherapy remains heated, fueled by the recognized national need to treat a growing epidemic, the lack of long-term outcomes studies, and the medical and litigious fallout from the failed use of fen-phen (fenfluramine-phentermine) and dexfenfluramine (Redux).

PHARMACOLOGIC THERAPY

The debate regarding the appropriateness of obesity pharmacotherapy remains heated, fueled by the recognized national need to treat a growing epidemic and the medical and litigious fallout from the failed use of fen-phen (fenfluramine-phentermine) and dexfenfluramine (Redux).[64,65] Strategies for the pharmacologic management of obesity have been focused on modulating central and/or peripheral sites that regulate human energy balance. Figure 140–4 depicts sites of action and Table 140–4 lists the most common classes of agents currently in use. Since the 1970s, numerous studies of the effects of central appetite suppressant agents on weight status have been completed.[17] The National Task Force on the Prevention and Treatment of Obesity concluded that short-term anorexic agent use was difficult to justify because of the predictable weight regain that occurs on discontinuation of pharmacotherapy.[66] However, long-term pharmacotherapy may have a place in the treatment of obesity for

TABLE 140–4. Pharmacotherapeutic Agents for Weight Loss

Class	Availability	Status	Daily Dosages (mg)
Gastrointestinal lipase inhibitor			
Orlistat (Xenical)	Rx	Long-term use	360
Noradrenergic/serotonergic agent			
Sibutramine (Meridia)	Rx	Long-term use	5–15
Noradrenergic agents			
Phendimetrazine (Prelu-2, Bontril, Plegine, X-Trazine)	Rx	Short-term use	70–105
Phentermine (Fastin, Oby-trim, Adipex-P, Ionamin)	Rx	Short-term use	15–37.5
Diethylpropion (Tenuate, Tenuate Dospan)	Rx	Short-term use	75
Methamphetamine HCl (desoxyephedrine HCl)	Rx[a]	Not recommended	5–15
Amphetamine sulfate	Rx[a]	Not recommended	5–30
Dextroamphetamine sulfate (Dexedrine)	Rx[a]	Not recommended	5–30
Amphetamine/dextroamphetamine mixtures (Adderall)	Rx[a]	Not recommended	5–30
Benzphetamine (Didrex)	Rx[a]	Not recommended	25–150
Ephedrine (various)	OTC	Unlabeled use	20–60
Serotonergic agents			
Fluoxetine (Prozac)	Rx	Unlabeled use	60
Sertraline (Zoloft)	Rx	Unlabeled use	200

[a]High abuse potential.

patients who have no obvious contraindications to available drug therapy.[17,27,66] Additionally, the American Association of Clinical Endocrinologists (AACE) and the American College of Endocrinology (ACE) have developed a guideline for multidisciplinary obesity team approach to therapy.[67] Most recently, the U.S. Preventive Services Task Force has recently published an exhaustive summary of evidence related to screening and interventions for adult obesity that incorporates a graded assessment of obesity pharmacotherapy randomized controlled trials.[56] Routine implementation awaits the development of medications that are effective and safe with long-term exposure. The discovery of cardiac valve disease in relation to serotonergic appetite suppressant use and its resulting multibillion dollar class action litigation affirms the task force's warning for further study of available therapies prior to widespread implementation of routine obesity pharmacotherapy.[64,65] A recent five-state survey demonstrated the relatively common concurrent use of both prescription and nonprescription weight loss medications.[68] Therefore, clinicians should maintain a high degree of sensitivity towards the potential polypharmacy practices of patients with obesity. The next sections outline the recent and current status of pharmacologic agents for obesity therapy, focusing on proposed mechanisms, dosing recommendations, potential side effects, and monitoring parameters.

LIPASE INHIBITORS

Orlistat

The percentage of dietary intake as fat has been implicated as a contributing factor in the development of obesity. Fat represents an extremely dense energy source; 9 kcal/g as compared with approximately 4 kcal/g from protein or carbohydrate. In humans, most of accumulated body fat excess is derived from dietary sources because of a limited capacity to synthesize fat from carbohydrate. Gastrointestinal (gastric, pancreatic, and carboxylester) lipases are essential in the absorption of the long-chain triglycerides commonly found in Western diets. Additionally, lipase is known to play a role in facilitating gastric emptying and secretion of other pancreaticobiliary substances. Orlistat (Xenical, RO 18-0647) is a synthetic derivative of lipstatin, a natural lipase inhibitor produced by *Streptomyces toxytrincini*. Orlistat is minimally absorbed and selectively inhibits gastrointestinal lipases. Lipase inhibition results in decreased formation of free fatty acids from dietary triglyceride. Additionally, lower luminal free fatty acid concentrations result in malabsorption of cholesterol. Orlistat induces weight loss by a persistent lowering of dietary fat absorption. Clinical studies employing orlistat as an adjunct to diet therapy demonstrate dose-dependent reductions in fat absorption. Up to 30% reduction in fat absorption occurred with daily doses of 360 mg.[69] No additional decreases in fat absorption occur with doses above 400 mg/day. The drug must be taken with foods that contain fat in order to exert its effect.

At least one gastrointestinal complaint (soft stools, abdominal pain/colic, flatulence, fecal urgency, or incontinence) is reported initially in up to 80% of individuals using orlistat. These complaints are most common in the first 1 to 2 months of therapy, are mild to moderate in severity, and tend to improve with continued orlistat use. Appropriately limiting dietary fat prior to initiation of orlistat therapy may be beneficial in decreasing initial gastrointestinal complaints. Orlistat-induced malabsorption of fat-soluble vitamins has been documented.[69] Therefore, vitamin supplementation should be considered during therapy with this agent. Orlistat does not appear to change the pharmacokinetic or dynamic profiles of numerous other agents including oral contraceptives, digoxin, glyburide, phenytoin, paravastatin, warfarin, nifedipine, captopril, atenolol, furosemide, and ethanol. A notable exception is cyclosporine, wherein case reports suggest significant decreases in cyclosporine serum concentrations with concurrent orlistat use.[69]

Overall, results from clinical trials demonstrate that orlistat effectively increases the amount of weight lost and decreases the amount of weight regained during medically supervised weight loss programs.[70,71] Significant improvements in lipid profile, glucose control, and other markers of metabolism are seen in spite of the relatively small 2- to 4-kg differences in weight lost when using orlistat in addition to diet. In patients with impaired glucose tolerance, weight loss using orlistat significantly decreased the rate of conversion to type 2 diabetes.[72] Additionally, improved glycemic control can be attained in patients with type 2 diabetes by inducing or increasing weight loss with orlistat in addition to diet management. In some cases, dosages or the number of agents required for glucose lowering may be deceased.[73] Finally, orlistat is the first agent for the chronic treatment of obesity with an indication for use in adolescents aged 12 to 16 years.

NORADRENERGIC-SEROTONERGIC AGENTS

Sibutramine

An orally active racemic mixture, sibutramine, became available in the United States in early 1998.[74] The parent compound and two active metabolites appear to increase synaptic concentrations of serotonin, norepinephrine (NE), and dopamine via reuptake inhibition. The active metabolites (M_1 and M_2) are more potent than the parent sibutramine. Reuptake inhibition appears to be greatest for NE, followed by serotonin, with dopamine the least inhibited. Sibutramine, M_1, and M_2 do not directly stimulate serotonergic (5-HT$_1$ or 5-HT$_2$), noradrenergic (α_1, α_2, β_1, β_2, and β_3), or dopamine receptors. It is thought that sibutramine induces weight loss by both decreasing appetite and maintaining or increasing thermogenesis via the combined effects on 5-HT and NE reuptake inhibition. In humans, the degree to which these effects can be attributed to central versus peripheral activity is currently unknown. Sibutramine is subject to hepatic first-pass metabolism via cytochrome P450 3A4. Moderate changes in sibutramine and/or metabolite disposition have been seen with ketoconazole coadminstration. M_1 and M_2 area under the curve increased by 58% and 20%, respectively, with concurrent ketoconazole (200 mg twice daily for 7 days). Smaller changes have been noted with concurrent erythromycin and cimetidine. The active metabolites M_1 and M_2 exhibit elimination half-lives of 14 and 16 hours, respectively. Further metabolism of the active metabolites results in conjugates that are eliminated renally. The pharmacokinetics of sibutramine allow for once-daily oral dosing.

Sibutramine has been studied in clinical trials in doses from 1 to 30 mg daily and demonstrates a relatively clear dose-response relationship. Weight loss from daily doses of 1 mg is, on average, no different than from placebo. The recommended starting dose is 10 mg daily, with a recommended dose range of 5 to 15 mg daily. Dry mouth, anorexia, insomnia, constipation, appetite increase, dizziness, and nausea were noted two- to threefold more frequently in sibutramine-treated subjects than in placebo-treated subjects. Significant increases in both systolic and diastolic blood pressure and pulse rate have been noted with sibutramine use.[74] Baseline blood pressure should be established prior to beginning therapy, and close monitoring is required when using this agent. Sibutramine product labeling indicates that it should not be used in patients with a history of coronary artery disease, stroke, congestive heart failure, or arrhythmias. Like other centrally acting appetite suppressants, sibutramine should not be used in patients receiving MAO inhibitor therapies. Sibutramine is listed as a schedule IV prescription substance despite being noted as having no street value by recreational substance users. Primary pulmonary hypertension has not been reported with sibutramine use. Echocardiographic assessments of a small cohort of patients from clinical trials with approximately 6 months of exposure do not demonstrate the cardiac valve problems seen with the fenfluramine derivatives. Based on 12-month clinical trials, weight loss with sibutramine therapy appears to be most significant during the first 6 months of therapy. Twenty-nine percent of placebo-treated patients in these trials attained a 5% reduction in total body weight after 12 months. Using sibutramine at 10 and 15 mg/day resulted in 56% and 65% of patients, respectively, achieving at least a 5% reduction in total body weight. A 10% reduction in body weight was achieved by 8% of placebo-treated patients, whereas 30% and 39% of those taking sibutramine 10 and 15 mg/day, respectively, obtained this level of weight reduction. There is, on average, a tendency for weight regain after 6 months of treatment. As with other centrally active appetite suppressants, weight regain occurs with cessation of therapy. Safety and efficacy beyond 1 year of exposure to sibutramine are currently uncertain.

NORADRENERGIC AGENTS

Phentermine

Phentermine is structurally similar to amphetamine, but it has less severe CNS stimulation and a lower abuse potential. Its mechanism of action is related to enhanced norepinephrine and dopamine neurotransmission. Phentermine is available in both immediate-release and sustained-release formulations. However, the value of sustained-release formulations can be questioned based on the reported phentermine plasma half-life of 12 to 24 hours.[17] Phentermine is an effective adjunct to diet, exercise, and behavior modification for producing weight loss in excess of that seen with placebo.[17] Intermittent phentermine therapy appears to elicit comparable weight loss when compared with continuous use. However, most individuals experience weight regains during therapy and generally always after discontinuing use.[17] A single dose of 30 mg once daily in the morning provides effective appetite suppression throughout the day. Divided doses of 8 mg immediately prior to meals, however, are common. Doses above 30 mg daily do not improve effectiveness.[75] Evening or nighttime dosing should be avoided because of insomnia. Significant increases in blood pressure, palpitations, and arrhythmias can occur with phentermine administration. Use is not advisable in hypertensive patients and those with unstable cardiovascular function. The potential for hypertensive crisis with coadministration of phentermine and monoamine oxidase (MAO) inhibitors is noted in product labeling because of the documented cases of this syndrome seen with coadministration of amphetamine or noradrenergic derivatives and MAO inhibitors.[76] Similar warnings have been noted regarding concomitant use of tricyclic antidepressants, but this is less well documented. With MAO inhibitors, a minimum washout time of 14 days prior to use of any adrenergic agent is suggested to avoid excessive adrenergic stimulation syndromes. Phentermine use is contraindicated in patients who are abusers of substances such as cocaine, phencyclidine, and methamphetamine, again because of the potential for excessive adrenergic stimulation syndromes and abuse potential. Mydriasis from adrenergic stimulation can worsen glaucoma, and patients diagnosed with glaucoma should not receive phentermine. Diabetic patients may

experience altered insulin or oral hypoglycemic dosage requirements soon after beginning therapy and prior to any substantial weight loss.

Phentermine currently remains on the market as a short-term pharmacotherapy for obesity despite recognition of cardiac valvulopathy in a high percentage of patients who used phentermine in combination with fenfluramine derivatives. Phentermine remains one of the most widely prescribed weight management medications in spite of product labeling that indicates short-term, monotherapy use only.[77] This usage pattern persists in spite of the current federal recommendations that promote only long-term drug intervention when obesity pharmacotherapy is appropriate.[53]

Mazindol

Chemically distinct from amphetamines and phentermine, mazindol's tricyclic structure resulted in amphetamine-like appetite suppression.[17] Despite demonstrated efficacy as a short-term therapy for weight reduction, mazindol is no longer available in the United States.[78]

Diethylpropion

Diethylpropion stimulates norepinephrine release from presynaptic storage granules. Increased adrenergic neurotransmitter concentrations activate hypothalamic centers, which result in decreased appetite and food intake. This drug undergoes extensive first-pass hepatic metabolism. Active metabolites are eliminated renally and account for approximately 70% of the administered dose. The elimination half-life of these metabolites is approximately 8 hours.[75] Less than 10% of the parent compound is recovered in urine. No specific dosing recommendations exist for use in patients with renal or hepatic insufficiency. Diethylpropion can be taken in divided daily doses, generally 25 mg three times daily before meals. An extended-release formulation is also employed by some clinicians, usually as 75 mg taken once daily in the morning or midmorning. Both dosing regimens are effective in achieving short-term weight loss in excess of placebo.[17] Complaints of insomnia increase if late afternoon dosing is used. Diethylpropion causes less CNS stimulation than mazindol and generally causes less insomnia than phentermine. Patients with severe hypertension or significant cardiovascular disease should not receive diethylpropion. Diabetic patients may experience decreased insulin or oral hypoglycemic dosage requirements soon after beginning therapy and prior to any substantial weight loss. More frequent blood glucose self-monitoring and medical follow-up are warranted when treating diabetic patients with diethylpropion.

Amphetamines

Appetite suppressant effects of the amphetamines were well recognized in the 1930s. Amphetamines activate central noradrenergic receptor systems as well as dopaminergic pathways at higher doses, by stimulating neurotransmitter release. Increases in blood pressure and mild bronchodilation are attributed to peripheral α- and β-receptor activation. The central nervous system stimulant and addiction potential of amphetamine relative to other compounds has been described as amphetamine > methamphetamine > phentermine > mazindol > diethylpropion.[67] The powerful stimulant and addictive potential of the amphetamines relative to other available agents has resulted in their general avoidance for the treatment of obesity.[67]

Phenylpropanolamine

Although commonly classified as a noradrenergic anorexic, phenyl-propanolamine (PPA) is atypical with regard to its mechanism and site of action. PPA racemates, D- and L-norephedrine, have chemical structures quite similar to amphetamine.[17] PPA has been used for many years as a constituent of over-the-counter appetite suppressants and various cough and cold preparations. However, because of persistent case reports of hemorrhagic stroke related to PPA exposure, the U.S. Food and Drug Administration and pharmaceutical manufacturers partnered to complete a case-control study known as the Hemorrhagic Stroke Project (HSP) during the 1990s. In October 2000, the Nonprescription Drugs Advisory Committee discussed the HSP report and concluded that PPA was not safe for continued use. A peer-reviewed publication based on the HSP report suggests that PPA in appetite suppressants and possibly cough and cold preparations appears to increase the risk of hemorrhagic stroke in women.[79] No increased risk was noted in men. Based on the accepted background prevalence of stroke and the odds ratios defined by the HSP report, Kernan and colleagues estimate that 1 woman may experience PPA-related stroke for every 107,000 to 3,268,000 women exposed to PPA appetite suppressants.[79] Despite the very low risk of hemorrhagic stroke, the FDA believes that a favorable risk-benefit no longer exists for any PPA-containing products. As such, PPA-containing products have either been reformulated without PPA or removed from the market in the United States. However, due to the voluntary nature of the request for reformulation or removal from the market, the FDA recommends that all consumers review product labels to ensure the absence of PPA from weight loss and cough or cold preparations.[80]

Ephedrine

Chemically related to PPA (± norephedrine), ephedrine may be a viable obesity pharmacotherapy. It appears to suppress appetite and increase energy expenditure via release of presynaptic norepinephrine and direct stimulation of thermogenic β-adrenergic receptors.[81] The efficiency of ephedrine stimulation is somewhat blunted by physiologic feedback systems involving adenosine and various prostaglandins. This notion has stimulated research to characterize the effect of ephedrine in the presence of adenosine and prostaglandin antagonists such as caffeine and aspirin.[82] Ephedrine in combination with caffeine has enhanced appetite suppression and thermogenesis as compared with placebo and other anorectics over time periods of up to 6 months.[81,83] Oral doses of 20 mg ephedrine and 200 mg caffeine up to three times daily have been studied.[84] The spectrum of side effects with ephedrine and ephedrine-caffeine combinations is similar to that seen with other noradrenergic agents. Side effects are more notable at higher doses and most commonly include tremor, agitation, nervousness, increased sweating, and insomnia; palpitations and tachycardia have also been reported. Patients with diabetes, hypertension, or cardiovascular disease (including arrhythmic conditions) should not self-medicate with ephedrine-containing products without evaluation by a qualified physician. Ephedrine is available both with and without a prescription; neither form is labeled by the FDA for use as an obesity therapy.

SEROTONERGIC AGENTS

Serotonin is an important neurotransmitter involved in many human physiologic systems. Sleep-wake cycles, sensitivity to pain, blood pressure, mood, and eating behaviors have links to serotonin activity. Increasing central serotonin levels decreases the amount of food consumed and prolongs the time between food intake. Some serotonergic agents increase central serotonin concentrations via stimulating release of presynaptic stores and/or inhibition of reuptake into storage granules. Additionally, either the parent compound or metabolites of these agents also may stimulate postsynaptic 5-HT receptors directly. Peripheral serotonin effects that have an impact on appetite, such as slowing gastric motility, also have been described. A major distinction between serotonergic and noradrenergic anorexiants is that serotonergic agents lack the central stimulant effects and thus the abuse potential seen with the noradrenergic compounds.[17] Conversely, decreased wakefulness, altered sleep patterns, and changes in affect can be seen.

Antidepressants: Selective Serotonin Reuptake Inhibitors

It is interesting to note that some of the serotonergic appetite-suppressing agents were first studied as antidepressants and then noted subsequently to have effects on weight. As a class, the serotonin reuptake inhibitors generally are weight neutral as opposed to other commonly used compounds such as the tricyclic antidepressants (see Chap. 67). The National Task Force on the Prevention and Treatment of Obesity has reviewed multiple randomized, double-blinded, placebo-controlled weight loss clinical trials using fluoxetine and one with sertraline.[66,85] Patients receiving fluoxetine (60 mg/day) demonstrate initial weight loss of up to 2 to 4 kg on average, but weight regain occurs despite continued medication use such that no difference is noted between fluoxetine and placebo over periods of up to 1 year.[86] Similar findings are noted using sertraline (200 mg/day) as an adjunct to help maintain weight lost with a very-low-calorie diet.[85] A direct relationship exists between amount of weight lost and the sum of fluoxetine and norfluoxetine plasma concentrations. Higher plasma concentrations are associated with greater weight loss. The antidepressant serotonin reuptake inhibitors are not approved by the FDA as weight management agents and are not recommended currently for routine treatment of obesity. Some practitioners continue to prescribe these agents for the treatment of obesity "off label" either alone or in combination with phentermine.[87] The safety and efficacy of phentermine-serotonin reuptake inhibitor combinations is currently unclear. A case report of adverse experiences (e.g., impaired mentation, tremor, hyperreflexia, and gastrointestinal symptoms) with unintentional concurrent use of phentermine and fluoxetine reinforces the need for caution by prescribers of unlabeled combination therapy.[88] Serious adverse effects such as primary pulmonary hypertension and cardiac valve abnormalities in excess of background prevalence have not been reported in relation to selective serotonin reuptake inhibitor use for obesity therapy.

Fenfluramine and Dexfenfluramine

Fenfluramine is an orally active racemic mixture (D, L-fenfluramine) that was used extensively as monotherapy for appetite suppression for many years. Its D-isomer, dexfenfluramine, was used extensively in Europe prior to its release in the United States in 1996, and was the first agent in the United States to receive labeling for chronic use. Both agents increased synaptic serotonin concentration via reuptake inhibition and possibly by increasing serotonin release. In studies sponsored by the National Institutes of Health (NIH), it was demonstrated that the combination of fenfluramine with phentermine (fen-phen) resulted in significant weight loss with fewer side effects, using

TABLE 140–5. Herbal/Natural Products and Food Supplements Used for Weight Loss[a]

Herbal/Natural/Food Supplements	Active Moiety	Proposed Mechanism
Chromium picolinate	Chromium	Unclear
St. John's wort	Hypericin	Serotonergic/monoamine oxidase inhibition
Hoodia	P57	Unclear
White willow bark	Salicylate	Inhibit norepinephrine breakdown
Calcium pyruvate	Pyruvate	Unclear
Guarana extract	Caffeine	Noradrenergic
Various tea extracts	Caffeine	Noradrenergic
Garcinia gambogia extract (citrin)	Hydroxycitric acid	Unclear
Chitosan	Cationic polysaccharide	Block fat absorption

[a]Safety and efficacy not documented.

doses lower than commonly employed individually.[89] These placebo-controlled studies stimulated widespread use of fen-phen. Outside of product labeling, some clinicians also chose to use dexfenfluramine in combination with phentermine. Both fenfluramine derivatives were withdrawn from worldwide markets in 1997 due to a relationship with cardiac valvular insufficiency, valvular structural abnormalities, and pulmonary hypertension.[90,91]

PEPTIDES

Multiple different endogenous peptides, which play a role in the regulation of food intake, have been identified in animals and humans. Leptin originates in the adipocyte and is proposed to function as a peripheral feedback messenger with respect to fat storage (discussed earlier in the chapter). NPY and galanin are two CNS peptides that appear to similarly stimulate food consumption, but have differing effects on preference of carbohydrate or fat, as well as substrate metabolism.[37,92] Currently, NPY and galanin are thought to exert minimal effects on protein intake, but a third, less well-described CNS peptide, growth hormone-releasing factor, stimulates protein ingestion. Carbohydrate ingestion and use are related to NPY hypothalamic activity, specifically in the arcuate and medial paraventricular nucleus.[37,92] Galanin activity, centering in the lateral paraventricular nucleus and medial preoptic areas, increases both carbohydrate and fat intake with preferential effects on fat consumption and utilization.[37] NPY enhances fat synthesis via increased respiratory quotient and use of carbohydrate. Galanin appears to slow energy expenditure. NPY and galanin modulate the release of insulin, corticosterone, and vasopressin, further affecting nutrient intake behaviors and substrate metabolism. NPY is associated with increased levels of insulin, corticosterone, and vasopressin, whereas decreases are seen with galanin.[37] The macronutrient intake, energy use, and endocrine effects of NPY are most consistent with those seen in chronic obesity. Future pharmacotherapies may be developed based on knowledge of the effects of these endogenous peptides.

HERBAL, NATURAL, AND FOOD SUPPLEMENT WEIGHT LOSS THERAPIES

⬤ ⬤ Many individuals choose to undertake weight loss regimens that incorporate the ingestion of herbal, natural, or food supplement products without medical monitoring. It is important to remember that the FDA does not strictly regulate the manufacture and

labeling of these products. The problem with many marketed products is the lack of consistency in labeling versus actual product content. Table 140–5 lists some of the common constituents found in many of these products.

CHROMIUM

The inclusion of chromium as an effective agent for weight loss is unclear. The hexavalent form of this trace element is thought to be carcinogenic, whereas the trivalent form found in human food sources is essentially nontoxic.[93] Chromium is considered an essential nutrient and experimentally in animals is an insulin cofactor active in carbohydrate, protein, and lipid metabolism.[93] In humans, insulin resistance has been reported in a few cases of apparent severe chromium deficiency during long-term total parenteral nutrition (see Chap. 137). Currently, there is no reliable means of assessing total body chromium status, making diagnosis of deficiency difficult. The tryptophan metabolite, picolinic acid, forms a complex with trivalent chromium, which improves bioavailability. Food sources with highly available chromium include brewer's yeast, calf liver, American cheese, and wheat germ.[93] A double-blind, placebo-controlled study of chromium picolinate as a supplement to aerobic exercise in the treatment of obesity failed to demonstrate any effectiveness.[94]

EPHEDRA ALKALOIDS

Based on the known effects of ephedrine (see ephedrine, above), dietary supplements claiming weight management effects have employed plant sources of ephedra alkaloids. Various parts of the Ephedraceae, ma huang, *Sida cordifolia*, and *Pinellia ternata* plants are known to produce ephedra alkaloids, including L-ephedrine, D-pseudoephedrine, L-norephedrine, D-norpseudoephedrine, L-*N*-methylephedrine, and D-*N*-methylpseudoephedrine.[95] Common names routinely included in dietary supplement labeling for these alkaloid sources include joint fir, popotillo, country mallow, sea grape, and yellow horse. From 1994 through July 1997, the FDA received over 800 reports of serious adverse events, including seizures, stroke, and death, coincident with ephedrine alkaloid-containing dietary supplement use. An in-depth review of 140 reports of adverse events related to ephedrine alkaloid-containing dietary supplements demonstrated that approximately half the reports involved cardiovascular symptoms.[96] As of 2004, the FDA has determined that all sources of ephedra alkaloids must be excluded from dietary supplements because they present an unreasonabl high health risk.[97]

ST. JOHN'S WORT

A perennial flowering plant (*Hypericum perforatum*), St. John's wort has been employed as a medicinal herb for thousands of years. Its use in weight loss and herbal supplements probably is based on the proposed effects of its constituent naphthodianthrones (hypericin and pseudohypericin). These are thought to be inhibitors of MAO and would be expected to increase synaptic concentrations of monoamines such as serotonin and NE. Consistent with these assumptions, *Hypericum* extracts appear to be more effective than placebo in the treatment of depression.[98] However, in vitro studies have not been able to substantiate direct MAO inhibition at physiologic hypericin concentrations, and recognized antidepressant effects may be due to other constituents.[99] The risks of concurrent use of *Hypericum* derivatives and other adrenergic and serotonergic compounds have not been characterized. Currently, St. John's wort has not been studied with respect to its role in obesity management, and its safety and efficacy as a treatment modality in the self-management of obesity are unclear.

PYRUVATE

Pyruvate is a commonly listed ingredient in many herbal weight management preparations. Multiple salt forms are used, including sodium, magnesium, potassium, and calcium. Other names include α-ketopropionic acid, 2-oxypropanoic acid, and acetylformic acid. Pyruvate is a three-carbon intermediate formed during normal glucose metabolism and/or during glycolysis. It is advertised in the lay press for its ability to "increase metabolism" and thus promote weight loss. Objective data documenting these effects are lacking. While most pyruvate nutritional weight management supplements contain less than 2 g per dose, large exposures (more than 20 g) are known to cause noticeable gastrointestinal side effects including bloating and diarrhea.

HOODIA

Hoodia is a desert cactus of the Apocynaceae plant family. Natives indigenous to the Kalahari Desert are purported to consume the stems and roots of this plant for their appetite suppressant effects. Other names appearing on product labels include Kalahari cactus, Hoodia cactus or extract, Hoodia gordonii cactus, and Kalahari diet. Hoodia extract, sometimes also referred to as P57, is rumored to elicit weight loss; however, no peer-reviewed reports of effectiveness are currently available.

WHITE WILLOW BARK

White willow bark is a source of salicylate, a prostaglandin inhibitor. Prostaglandin inhibition may enhance adrenergic stimulation via inhibition of NE breakdown (see the earlier discussion of ephedrine).

GUARANA EXTRACT AND VARIOUS TEA EXTRACTS

Guarana and tea are sources of caffeine that have inherent adrenergic properties as well as increasing the effects of stimulant substances such as ephedrine or ephedra alkaloids (see the earlier discussion of ephedrine).

CHITOSAN

Chitosan is a cationic polysaccharide, specifically a partially *N*-deacetylated form of chitin. This nonhydrolyzable fiber exhibits properties similar to those of cellulose.[100] In vitro and preclinical data have indicated that chitosan may be effective in blocking absorption of fat from the gut. It has been suggested that orally administered chitosan may be an effective weight reduction agent by blocking calories ingested as fat. Chitosan is a major constituent in several heavily advertised weight management food supplements and over-the-counter preparations. However, a small number of properly randomized and blinded or open-label investigations currently demonstrate that orally administered chitosan is not an effective inhibitor of fat absorption in humans.[101,102] While further research may be warranted with respect to the appropriate dose in humans needed to impair fat absorption, current claims of chitosan effectiveness in humans are unsubstantiated.

PHARMACOECONOMIC CONSIDERATIONS

There are few data regarding economic consequences of treating obesity. One study evaluated the savings in prescription costs following a 12-week weight reduction program in 40 type 2 diabetic patients. Patients lost an average of 33.7 lb over the study period. A cost analysis was completed on 32 of 40 patients who were taking antihypertensive and/or antidiabetic medications using the out-of-pocket costs for these medications at the beginning of the study and after 1 year. The patients sustained a mean weight loss of 19.8 lb over the next year. The average cost of these prescriptions at the beginning as compared to the 1-year follow-up was $63.30 versus $32.50 per month. The estimated annual average saving in prescription costs per patient was $443. A more objective assessment of costs related to orlistat use has been published based on data obtained from three peer-reviewed publications. In this report from the United Kingdom, the cost utility of orlistat was estimated at £46,000 (approximately $75,000) per quality-adjusted life year gained. Sensitivity analysis from this report demonstrated variability in this estimate of £14,000 to £132,000 (approximately $23,000 to $215,200). The authors raised questions about the potential long-term value of pharmacotherapy for obesity.[103]

Finally, Martin and colleagues compared the costs associated with medical and surgical treatment of obesity.[104] Medical therapy groups received diet therapy only (no medications), and cost included weekly clinic visits for behavioral modification. A successful outcome was defined as loss of at least one-third of excess body weight above ideal body weight. They monitored all patients for 2 years and some for as long as 7 years so that long-term weight control could be addressed. As expected, the costs of surgery were much higher than medical therapy over the first 2 years ($24,000 vs. $3,000). However, when costs were extrapolated out to 6 years, the cost per pound lost for medical therapy exceeded surgical therapy (about $313 vs. $261 per pound lost). It is clear from the preceding data that weight loss can be expensive for the consumer. Prospectively designed cost-benefit or cost-effectiveness analyses are needed to determine if costs of weight loss therapy or surgery are balanced by lower costs of hospitalizations for other medical problems associated with obesity or the additional life years gained. Quality-of-life measures also need to be taken into consideration when evaluating these types of data.

Third-party payor and insurance reimbursement for provision of obesity treatment services continues to be inconsistent. However, these issues are under active discussion and specific information regarding reimbursement for obesity treatment from multiple different perspectives including the Centers for Medicaid and Medicare Services and the IRS are freely available via the Web.[105–107]

EVALUATION OF THERAPEUTIC OUTCOMES

MONITORING THE PHARMACEUTICAL CARE PLAN

Outcome Measures

Specific weight goals should be established that are consistent with medical needs and patient personal desire. For most obese patients, a weight loss goal of 5% to 10% to no more than 30% of initial weight is reasonable. An average rate of weight loss after the first month of therapy is around 1 lb per week. Patients should not be allowed to attain weight less than their estimated ideal weight. Assessment of patient progress should be documented in a health care setting once or twice monthly for 1 to 2 months and then monthly thereafter.[27,67] Each encounter should document weight, WC, BMI, blood pressure, medical history, and patient assessment of obesity medication tolerability.[27,67] Chronic use of obesity medications should be consistent with the approved product labeling. Medication therapy should be discontinued after 3 to 4 months if the patient has failed to demonstrate weight loss or maintenance of prior weight. A recent AACE/ACE statement on obesity provides a patient evaluation checklist, a validated survey of general well-being, and sample informed consent that could be used in screening and follow-up of patients receiving obesity pharmacotherapy as part of a weight loss program.[67] Additionally, numerous tools for both patient and practitioner are readily available through the Department of Human Services, NIH-NHLIB Obesity Education Initiative, and several other agencies.[16] The Short Form 36 (SF-36) also has been used as a quality-of-life evaluation tool for obese patients undergoing programmatic weight loss. Quarterly assessments of well-being and quality of life using validated assessment tools can be helpful in objectively quantifying the effectiveness of therapy as well as potential drug-induced side effects (e.g., depression).[67]

Diabetic patients receiving weight loss medication require more intense medical monitoring and self-monitoring of blood glucose. Some centrally acting weight loss agents, such as the serotonergic agents, have direct effects that immediately improve glucose tolerance, even prior to significant weight loss. Insulin therapy therefore may need to be adjusted with the start of obesity medication therapy. Peripherally active agents, such as orlistat, have also been shown to decrease oral hypoglycemic agent requirements in type 2 diabetic patients.[73] However, this effect was noted later in therapy and correlated more directly with weight loss. Some diabetic patients may require daily telephone contact with a health care provider to assist in adjusting their hypoglycemic therapy. Weekly patient visits to a health care setting may be necessary for 1 to 2 months until the effects of diet, exercise, and weight loss medication become more predictable. As frequent as quarterly assessment of hemoglobin A_{1c} may be appropriate in type 2 diabetics who lose weight to aid in adjustment of hypoglycemic therapy. Lipid profiles can normalize or improve with weight loss. Lipid status should be assessed semiannually or annually in patients with hyperlipidemia to determine need for continued hyperlipidemia therapies. Weight loss also can result in normalization of blood pressure in hypertensive obese patients. Assessment of appropriateness of antihypertensive therapy should occur with each follow-up visit.

An expert committee of the National Institutes of Health, Heart, Lung, and Blood Institute has completed an extensive summary of clinical guidelines for the assessment and treatment of obesity.[53] This report provides guidance with evidence-based, graded assessment and treatment recommendations from an extensive meta-analysis of the available obesity literature to date. The evaluation and management of a patient with obesity requires careful clinical, biochemical, and if necessary psychological evaluation. The evaluation must include an assessment of current medical conditions and medications the patient uses. Clearly, a multidisciplinary team including but not limited to a physician, nutritionist, psychologist, and pharmacist best achieves this. The algorithm in Figure 140–3 shows an approach to determining appropriate types of treatment for the overweight individual. The decision to treat any overweight/obese patient depends on the degree and distribution of obesity present, the motivation of the patient to lose weight, and the potential benefits and risks of weight loss. The initial step in this process should be to verify the presence of clinically significant excess body weight. In the clinical setting, this is done most often by measuring height, weight, and WC of the individual and calculating BMI. If the BMI is greater than 25 kg/m² and/or WC is greater than 40 inches for males or 35 inches for females, it is likely that the patient will benefit from weight maintenance or loss. The next step is to assess whether the patient actually is motivated to lose weight. No matter what the treatment options are, they all require significant effort on the part of the patient to change lifestyle and comply with the management plan. If it is clear that the patient is not yet ready to meet these expectations, then early counseling will reduce the chance of frustration for the patient, clinician, and in some cases other family members. This does not exclude the possibility of educating the patient about potential risks of obesity and the benefits of weight loss. This type of basic information in certain cases can lead to a significant change in motivation and desire to lose weight and improved compliance.

Pharmacotherapy may be appropriate for some overweight individuals (e.g., those with a BMI of 30 kg/m² or more without weight-related, immediate life-threatening medical conditions). It also should be considered for those with BMI of 27 kg/m² or more or an increased WC who have two or more risk factors. From the health care providers' perspective, drug therapy for obesity always should be considered as a supplement to an integrated program of diet, exercise, and behavior modification (including group support). A complete medical and medication history is essential in determining appropriate obesity drug therapy. Consideration must be given to alcohol, nicotine, caffeine, and herbal or food supplement use as well as prescription and nonprescription drugs.

CONCLUSIONS

The prevalence of obesity has increased dramatically in the latter part of this century. Obesity is determined by a combination of genetic and environmental factors. Epidemiologic studies provide evidence for a causative role of environmental factors in the development of obesity in those individuals who are genetically susceptible. Furthermore, there are clear differences in racial susceptibility to obesity and its complications such as diabetes. The precise role of genetic and environmental factors in the development is unknown. It is clear, though, that obesity is a lifelong condition. Currently, orlistat and sibutramine are available in the United States and are indicated for the long-term treatment of overweight and obesity. However, clinicians should keep in mind that long-term results over periods of 3 or more years regarding these therapies will require further research. Weight regain occurs in the majority of individuals regardless of the therapeutic modalities used. Nevertheless, in recent years, increasingly effective treatments have been developed. These agents have augmented the role of lifestyle changes and diet and therefore serve a useful role as adjunct therapies for obesity.

Every patient seeking help for the management of obesity should be evaluated for secondary causes of obesity. Although a secondary cause is rare, it is important to identify and manage. Treatment of obesity needs to be individualized. It is important to consider factors such as patient desires, age, degree and duration of obesity, and the presence or absence of medical conditions both directly related to obesity and those which may have an impact on the therapeutic decisions. Whatever combinations of therapeutic modalities are used, it is clear that management is a lifelong process requiring patient support and careful monitoring for safety and efficacy.

ABBREVIATIONS

AACE: American Association of Clinical Endocrinologists
ACE: American College of Endocrinology
5-HT: 5-hydroxytryptamine (serotonin)
BMI: body mass index
BMR: basal metabolic rate
COPD: chronic obstructive pulmonary disease
CT: computed tomography
DEXA: dual-energy x-ray absorptiometry
HSP: Hemorrhagic Stroke Project
LCD: low-calorie diet
MAO: monoamine oxidase
MRI: magnetic resonance imaging
NCHS: National Center for Health Statistics
NHANES: National Health and Nutrition Examination Survey
NHLBI: National Heart, Lung and Blood Institute
NIH: National Institutes of Health
NPY: neuropeptide Y
PCOS: polycystic ovary syndrome
PPA: phenylpropanolamine
PSMF: protein-supplemented modified fast
REE: resting energy expenditure
SF-36: Short Form 36
SNS: sympathetic nervous system
VLCD: very-low-calorie diet
WC: waist circumference

Review Questions and other resources can be found at *www.pharmacotherapyonline.com.*

REFERENCES

1. Kuczmarski RJ, Carroll MD, Flegal KM, Troiano RP. Varying body mass index cutoff points to describe overweight prevalence among U.S. adults: NHANES III (1988 to 1994). Obes Res 1997;5:542–548.
2. Folsom AR, Jacobs DRJ, Wagenknecht LE, et al. Increase in fasting insulin and glucose over seven years with increasing weight and inactivity of young adults. The CARDIA Study. Coronary Artery Risk Development in Young Adults. Am J Epidemiol 1996;144:235–246.
3. Crespo CJ, Smit E, Troiano RP, et al. Television watching, energy intake, and obesity in US children: Results from the third National Health and Nutrition Examination Survey, 1988–1994. Arch Pediatr Adolesc Med 2001;155:360–365.
4. Troiano RP, Flegal KM. Overweight children and adolescents: Description, epidemiology, and demographics. Pediatrics 1998;101:497–504.
5. Allison DB, Zannolli R, Narayan KM. The direct health care costs of obesity in the United States. Am J Pub Health 1999;89:1194–1199.
6. Kassirer JP, Angell M. Losing weight—an ill-fated New Year's resolution. N Engl J Med 1998;338:52–54.
7. Allison DB, Fontaine KR, Manson JE, et al. Annual deaths attributable to obesity in the United States. JAMA 1999;282:1530–1538.
8. Zhu S, Heo M, Plankey M, et al. Associations of body mass index and anthropometric indicators of fat mass and fat free mass with all-cause mortality among women in the first and second National Health and Nutrition Examination Surveys follow-up studies. Ann Epidemiol 2003;13:286–293.
9. Stevens J, Cai J, Pamuk ER, et al. The effect of age on the association between body-mass index and mortality. N Engl J Med 1998;338:1–7.
10. Williamson DF, Pamuk E, Thun M, et al. Prospective study of intentional weight loss and mortality in never-smoking overweight US white women aged 40–64 years [published erratum appears in Am J Epidemiol 1995;142:369]. Am J Epidemiol 1995;141:1128–1141.
11. Lissner L, Odell PM, D'Agostino RB, et al. Variability of body weight and health outcomes in the Framingham population. N Engl J Med 1991;324:1839–1844.
12. The painful Business of Losing Weight. Economist August 27, 1997;45–47.
13. Office of the Surgeon General. Overweight and obesity. http://www.surgeongeneral.gov/topics/obesity/2003.
14. U.S. Department of Health and Human Services. Healthy People 2010; Chapter 19, Nutrition and Overweight. http://www.healthypeople.gov/Document/HTML/Volume2/19Nutrition.htm#_edn16, 2003.
15. U.S. Preventive Services Task Force. Screening for obesity in adults: Recommendations and rationale. Ann Intern Med 2003;139:930–932.
16. U.S. Department of Health and Human Services, NIH-NHLBI. Obesity Education Initiative. http://www.nhlbi.nih.gov/about/oei/index.htm, 2003.
17. Bray GA, Greenway FL. Current and potential drugs for treatment of obesity. Endocrine Rev 1999;20:805–875.
18. Ogden CL, Troiano RP, Briefel RR, et al. Prevalence of overweight among preschool children in the United States, 1971 through 1994. Pediatrics 1997;99:E1.
19. Power C, Lake JK, Cole TJ. Body mass index and height from childhood to adulthood in the 1958 British born cohort. Am J Clin Nutr 1997;66:1094–1101.
20. Fernandez JR, Allison DB. Understanding racial differences in obesity and metabolic syndrome traits. Nutr Rev 2003;61:316–319.
21. Fernandez JR, Heo M, Heymsfield SB, et al. Is percentage body fat differentially related to body mass index in Hispanic Americans, African Americans, and European Americans? Am J Clin Nutr 2003;77:71–75.
22. Park YW, Allison DB, Heymsfield SB, Gallagher D. Larger amounts of visceral adipose tissue in Asian Americans. Obes Res 2001;9:381–387.
23. Hainer V, Stunkard A, Kunesova M, et al. A twin study of weight loss and metabolic efficiency. Int J Obes Relat Metab Disord 2001;25:533–537.
24. West DB. Genetics of obesity in humans and animal models. Endocrinol Metab Clin North Am 1996;25:801–813.
25. Comuzzie AG, Allison DB. The search for human obesity genes. Science 1998;280:1374–1377.
26. Hill JO, Peters JC. Environmental contributions to the obesity epidemic. Science 1998;280:1371–1374.
27. U.S. Department of Health and Human Services, NIH-NHLBI. Clinical Guidelines on the Identification, Evaluation, and Treatment of Overweight and Obesity in Adults; Practical Guide. http://www.nhlbi.nih.gov/guidelines/obesity/ob_home.htm, 2003.
28. Caro JF, Sinha MK, Kolaczynski JW, et al. Leptin: The tale of an obesity gene. Diabetes 1996;45:1455–1462.
29. Misra A, Garg A, Leptin, its receptor and obesity. J Investig Med 1996;44:540–548.

30. Makimura H, Mizuno TM, Roberts J, et al. Adrenalectomy reverses obese phenotype and restores hypothalamic melanocortin tone in leptin-deficient ob/ob mice. Diabetes 2000;49:1917–1923.

31. Proietto J, Thorburn AW. The therapeutic potential of leptin. Exp Opin Investig Drugs 2003;12:373–378.

32. Zabeau L, Lavens D, Peelman F, et al. The ins and outs of leptin receptor activation. FEBS Lett 2003;546:45–50.

33. Harvey J, Ashford ML. Leptin in the CNS: Much more than a satiety signal. Neuropharmacology 2003;44:845–854.

34. Juge-Aubry CE, Meier CA. Immunomodulatory actions of leptin. Molec Cell Endocrinol 2002;194:1–7.

35. Magni P. Hormonal control of the neuropeptide Y system. Curr Protein Peptide Sci 2003;4:45–57.

36. Barinaga M. New appetite-boosting peptides found. Science 1998;279:1134.

37. Woods SC, Seeley RJ, Porte DJ, Schwartz MW. Signals that regulate food intake and energy homeostasis. Science 1998;280:1378–1383.

38. Slentz CA, Duscha BD, Johnson JL, et al. Effects of the amount of exercise on body weight, body composition, and measures of central obesity: STRRIDE—a randomized controlled study. Arch Intern Med 2004;164:31–39.

39. Fogelholm M, Kukkonen-Harjula K. Does physical activity prevent weight gain; a systematic review. Obes Rev 2000;1:95–111.

40. Faith MS, Fontaine KR, Cheskin LJ, Allison DB. Behavioral approaches to the problems of obesity. Behav Modif 2000;24:459–493.

41. Chung WK, Luke A, Cooper RS, et al. The long isoform uncoupling protein-3 (UCP3L) in human energy homeostasis. Int J Obes Relat Metab Disord 1999;23(Suppl 6):S49–S50.

42. de Souza CJ, Burkey BF. Beta 3-adrenoceptor agonists as anti-diabetic and anti-obesity drugs in humans. Curr Pharm Des 2001;7:1433–1749.

43. Collins S, Surwit RS. The beta-adrenergic receptors and the control of adipose tissue metabolism and thermogenesis. Rec Prog Horm Res 2001;56:309–328.

44. Arner P, Hoffstedt J. Adrenoceptor genes in human obesity. J Intern Med 1999;245:667–672.

45. Kelley DE, Thaete FL, Troost F, et al. Subdivisions of subcutaneous abdominal adipose tissue and insulin resistance. Am J Physiol Endocrinol Metab 2000;278:E941–E948.

46. Fernandez JR, Shriver MD, Beasley TM, et al. Association of African genetic admixture with resting metabolic rate and obesity among women. Obes Res 2003;11:904–911.

47. Hubert HB, Feinleib M, McNamara PM, Castelli WP. Obesity as an independent risk factor for cardiovascular disease: A 26-year follow-up of participants in the Framingham Heart Study. Circulation 1983;67:968–977.

48. Messerli FH. Cardiovascular effects of obesity and hypertension. Lancet 1982;1:1165–1168.

49. Flier JS, Foster DW. Eating disorders: Obesity, anorexia nervosa, bulimia nervosa. In: Wilson JD, Foster DW, Kronenberg HM, Larsen PR, eds. Williams Textbook of Endocrinology. Philadelphia, WB Saunders, 1998:1061–1097.

50. Williamson DF, Thompson TJ, Thun M, et al. Intentional weight loss and mortality among overweight individuals with diabetes. Diabetes Care 2000;23:1499–1504.

51. Diamanti-Kandarakis E, Zapanti E. Insulin sensitizers and antiandrogens in the treatment of polycystic ovary syndrome. Ann N Y Acad Sci 2000;900:203–212.

52. U.S. Department of Health and Human Services, NIH-NHLBI. Aim for a healthy weight, Information for Patients and Health Professionals. http://www.nhlbi.nih.gov/health/public/heart/obesity/lose_wt/index.htm. Accessed May, 2004.

53. U.S. Department of Health and Human Services, NIH-NHLBI. Clinical Guidelines on the Identification, Evaluation, and Treatment of Overweight and Obesity in Adults, Full Report. http://www.nhlbi.nih.gov/guidelines/obesity/ob_home.htm, 2003.

54. American Heart Association. Physical activity and healthy eating program for women. http://www.s2mw.com/choosetomove/index.html, 2004.

55. Williamson DA, Perrin LA. Behavioral therapy for obesity. Endocrinol Metab Clin North Am 1996;25:943–954.

56. McTigue KM, Harris R, Hemphill B, et al. Screening and interventions for obesity in adults: Summary of the evidence for the U.S. Preventive Services Task Force. Ann Intern Med 2003;139:933–949.

57. National Institute of Diabetes and Digestive and Kidney Diseases (NIDDK) Health Information, Weight Loss and Control. http://www.niddk.nih.gov/health/nutrit/nutrit.htm, 2003.

58. Hays NP, Starling RD, Liu X, et al. Effects of an ad libitum low-fat, high-carbohydrate diet on body weight, body composition, and fat distribution in older men and women: A randomized controlled trial. Arch Intern Med 2004;164:210–217.

59. Foster GD, Wyatt HR, Hill JO, et al. A randomized trial of a low-carbohydrate diet for obesity. N Engl J Med 2003;348:2082–2090.

60. Waitman JA, Aronne LJ. Obesity surgery: Pros and cons. J Endocrinol Invest 2002;25:925–928.

61. O'Brien PE, Dixon JB. Laparoscopic adjustable gastric banding in the treatment of morbid obesity. Arch Surg 2003;138:376–382.

62. Cottam DR, Mattar SG, Schauer PR. Laparoscopic era of operations for morbid obesity. Arch Surg 2003;138:367–375.

63. Brolin RE. Bariatric surgery and long-term control of morbid obesity. JAMA 2002;288:2793–2796.

64. Khan MA, Herzog CA, St. Peter JV, et al. The prevalence of cardiac valvular insufficiency assessed by transthoracic echocardiography in obese patients treated with appetite-suppressant drugs. N Engl J Med 1998;339:713–718.

65. AHP Diet Drug Settlement. http://www.settlementdietdrugs.com/, 2003.

66. National Task Force on the Prevention and Treatment of Obesity. Long-term pharmacotherapy in the management of obesity. JAMA 1996;276:1907–1915.

67. Bray GA. AACE/ACE Obesity statement. Endocr Pract 1997;3:163–208.

68. Blanck HM, Khan LK, Serdula MK. Use of nonprescription weight loss products: results from a multistate survey. JAMA 2001;286:930–935.

69. Leung WY, Neil TG, Chan JC, Tomlinson B. Weight management and current options in pharmacotherapy: Orlistat and sibutramine. Clin Ther 2003;25:58–80.

70. Hauptman J, Lucas C, Boldrin MN, et al. Orlistat in the long-term treatment of obesity in primary care settings. Arch Fam Med 2000;9:160–167.

71. Rossner S, Sjostrom L, Noack R, et al. Weight loss, weight maintenance, and improved cardiovascular risk factors after 2 years treatment with orlistat for obesity. European Orlistat Obesity Study Group. Obes Res 2000;8:49–61.

72. Heymsfield SB, Segal KR, Hauptman J, et al. Effects of weight loss with orlistat on glucose tolerance and progression to type 2 diabetes in obese adults. Arch Intern Med 2000;160:1321–1326.

73. Hollander PA, Elbein SC, Hirsch IB, et al. Role of orlistat in the treatment of obese patients with type 2 diabetes. A 1-year randomized double-blind study. Diabetes Care 1998;21:1288–1294.

74. Arterburn DE, Crane PK, Veenstra DL. The efficacy and safety of sibutramine for weight loss: A systematic review. Arch Intern Med 2004;164:994–1003.

75. Silverstone T. Appetite suppressants. A review. Drugs 1992;43:820–836.

76. Dawson JK, Earnshaw SM, Graham CS. Dangerous monoamine oxidase inhibitor interactions are still occurring in the 1990s. J Accid Emerg Med 1995;12:49–51.

77. Stafford RS, Radley DC. National trends in antiobesity medication use. Arch Intern Med 2003;163:1046–1050.

78. U.S. FDA Center for Drug Evaluation and Research, Prescription and Over-the-Counter Drug Product List. http://www.fda.gov/cder/rxotcdpl/pdpl_200206.htm, 2003.

79. Kernan WN, Viscoli CM, Brass LM, et al. Phenylpropanolamine and the risk of hemorrhagic stroke. N Engl J Med 2000;343:1826–1832.

80. Food and Drug Administration. Phenylpropanolamine (PPA) information page. http://www.fda.gov/cder/drug/infopage/ppa/default.htm, 2003.

81. Astrup A, Breum L, Toubro S. Pharmacological and clinical studies of ephedrine and other thermogenic agonists. Obes Res 1995;3(Suppl 4):537S–40S.

82. Dulloo AG, Seydoux J, Girardier L. Potentiation of the thermogenic antiobesity effects of ephedrine by dietary methylxanthines: Adenosine antagonism or phosphodiesterase inhibition? Metabolism 1992;41:1233–1241.

83. Breum L, Pedersen JK, Ahlstrom F, Frimodt-Moller J. Comparison of an ephedrine/caffeine combination and dexfenfluramine in the treatment of obesity. A double-blind multi-centre trial in general practice. Int J Obes Relat Metab Disord 1994;18:99–103.

84. Astrup A, Breum L, Toubro S, et al. The effect and safety of an ephedrine/caffeine compound compared to ephedrine, caffeine and placebo in obese subjects on an energy restricted diet. A double blind trial. Int J Obes Relat Metab Disord 1992;16:269–277.

85. Wadden TA, Bartlett SJ, Foster GD, et al. Sertraline and relapse prevention training following treatment by very-low-calorie diet: A controlled clinical trial. Obes Res 1995;3:549–557.

86. Goldstein DJ, Rampey AHJ, Enas GG, et al. Fluoxetine: A randomized clinical trial in the treatment of obesity. Int J Obes Relat Metab Disord 1994;18:129–135.

87. Anchors M. Fluoxetine is a safer alternative to fenfluramine in the medical treatment of obesity. Arch Intern Med 1997;157:1270.

88. Bostwick JM, Brown TM. A toxic reaction from combining fluoxetine and phentermine. J Clin Psychopharmacol 1996;16:189–190.

89. Weintraub M. Long-term weight control study: Conclusions. Clin Pharmacol Ther 1992;51:642–646.

90. Food and Drug Administration. Fen-phen Safety Update Information; fenfluramine, phentermine, dexfenfluramine. http://www.fda.gov/cder/news/feninfo.htm, 2003.

91. Abenhaim L, Moride Y, Brenot F, et al. Appetite-suppressant drugs and the risk of primary pulmonary hypertension. International Primary Pulmonary Hypertension Study Group. N Engl J Med 1996;335:609–616.

92. Pedrazzini T, Pralong F, Grouzmann E. Neuropeptide Y: The universal soldier. Cell Molec Life Sci 2003;60:350–377.

93. National Research Council. Trace Elements. Recommended Dietary Allowances. Washington, National Academy Press, 1998:195–246.

94. Trent LK, Thieding-Cancel D. Effects of chromium picolinate on body composition. J Sports Med Phys Fitness 1995;35:273–280.

95. Betz JM, Gay ML, Mossoba MM, et al. Chiral gas chromatographic determination of ephedrine-type alkaloids in dietary supplements containing Ma Huang. J AOAC Int 1997;80:303–315.

96. Haller CA, Benowitz NL. Adverse cardiovascular and central nervous system events associated with dietary supplements containing ephedra alkaloids. N Engl J Med 2000;343:1833–1838.

97. Department of Health and Human Services, Food and Drug Administration. Final rule declaring dietary supplements containing ephedrine alkaloids as adulterated because they represent an unreasonable risk. Fed Regist 2004;69:6788–6854.

98. Linde K, Ramirez G, Mulrow CD, et al. St John's wort for depression—an overview and meta-analysis of randomised clinical trials. BMJ 1996;313:253–258.

99. Cott JM. In vitro receptor binding and enzyme inhibition by *Hypericum perforatum* extract. Pharmacopsychiatry 1997;30(Suppl 2):108–112.

100. Kanauchi O, Deuchi K, Imasato Y, et al. Mechanism for the inhibition of fat digestion by chitosan and for the synergistic effect of ascorbate. Biosci Biotech Biochem 1995;59:786–790.

101. Pittler MH, Abbot NC, Harkness EF, Ernst E. Randomized, double-blind trial of chitosan for body weight reduction. Eur J Clin Nutr 1999;53:379–381.

102. Stern JS, Gades MD, Halsted CH. Chitosan does not block fat absorption in men fed a high fat diet. Obes Res 2000;8:91S.

103. Foxcroft DR, Milne R. Orlistat for the treatment of obesity: Rapid review and cost-effectiveness model. Obes Rev 2000;1:121–126.

104. Martin LF, Tan TL, Horn JR, et al. Comparison of the costs associated with medical and surgical treatment of obesity. Surgery 1995;118:599–606.

105. Porter S. Dealing with obesity: Reimbursement remains an obstacle. FP Report: December 2000. FP Report 2004;6.

106. Centers for Medicare & Medicaid Services. Obesity as an Illness (#CAG-00108N). Medicare Coverage Policy, National Coverage Determinations: Tracking Sheet and Coverage Issues Manual, sections 35–26, 35–33. http://www.cms.hhs.gov/mcd/viewtrackingsheet.asp?id=57. Accessed May, 2004.

107. Internal Revenue Service. Publication 502: Medical and dental expenses for use in preparing 2003 returns. www.irs.gov, 2004.

GLOSSARY

2,3-bisphosphoglycerate—An intermediate in the Rapoport-Luebering shunt, formed between 1,3-bisphosphoglycerate and 3-phosphoglycerate; an important regulator of the affinity of hemoglobin for oxygen.

5α-reductase—Enzyme responsible for conversion of testosterone to its active metabolite dihydrotesterone. Two types of this enzyme exist. Type 2 is predominant in prostate cells.

α-hydroxy acids—Exfoliating products such as lactic, glycolic, malic, mandelic, and tartaric acid used in cosmetics.

β-hydroxy acid—Salicylic acid.

Abscess—A purulent collection of fluid separated from surrounding tissue by a wall comprised of inflammatory cells and adjacent organs. It usually contains necrotic debris, bacteria, and inflammatory cells.

Abstinence—Refraining from the indulgence in something, as sexual intercourse or substances, by one's own choice. The absence of genital contact that could permit a pregnancy (i.e., penile penetration into the vagina).

Acetabular—Relating to the acetabulum, the hollow, cuplike portion of the pelvis into which the head of the thigh bone (femur) fits.

Acne—Inflammatory eruption of the sebaceous gland.

Acnegenicity—Product effect that causes irritation of follicles resulting in papules and pustules.

Acquired resistance—See *Secondary resistance.*

Acromegaly—A pathologic condition characterized by excessive production of growth hormone.

Activities of daily living—Dressing, bathing, getting around inside the home, feeding, toileting, and grooming. See also *Instrumental activities of daily living.*

Acute coronary syndrome (ACS)—Ischemic chest discomfort at rest most often accompanied by ST-segment elevation, ST-segment depression or T-wave inversion on the 12-lead electrocardiogram and caused by plaque rupture and partial or complete occlusion of the coronary artery by thrombus. Acute coronary syndromes include infarction and unstable angina. Former terms used to describe types of ACS include *Q-wave myocardial infarction, non-Q-wave myocardial infarction* and *unstable angina.*

Acute pain—May be a useful physiologic process warning individuals of disease states and potentially harmful situations. Severe, unremitting, undertreated, acute pain, when it outlives its biologic usefulness, can produce many deleterious effects (e.g., psychological problems). It usually subsides when the healing process decreases the pain-producing stimuli.

Acute pancreatitis—Acute inflammation of the pancreas which may be mild with minimal or no organ dysfunction or severe with organ failure and local complications.

Acute stress disorder—The development of characteristic anxiety, dissociative, and other symptoms that occur within 1 month after exposure to an extreme traumatic stressor.

Acute tubular necrosis—Acute renal failure as the result of renal tubular epithelial cell damage, which may be caused by either direct toxic or ischemic effects of drugs.

Addiction—A primary, chronic, neurobiologic disease, with genetic, psychosocial, and environmental factors influencing its development and manifestations. It is characterized by behaviors that include one or more of the following: impaired control over drug use, compulsive use, continued use despite harm, and craving.

Adolescents—Pediatric patients who are 12 to 16 years of age.

Adoptive immunotherapy—Administration of immune cells for the purpose of cancer treatment.

Adrenergic—Neuronal or neurologic activity caused by neurotransmitters such as epinephrine, norepinephrine, and dopamine.

Adrenocorticotropic hormone (ACTH)—A polypeptide hormone secreted by the anterior pituitary that controls secretion of cortisol from the adrenal glands.

Adverse drug events—Injuries resulting from administration of a drug or other circumstances surrounding use of the drug, but not necessarily caused by the drug itself. See also *Adverse drug reaction.*

Adverse drug reaction—Any noxious, unintended, and undesired effect of a drug that occurs at doses used in humans for prophylaxis, diagnosis, or therapy.

Affect—Pattern of behaviors that a clinician can observe that expresses a person's current state of emotion.

Afterload—The pressure or the "load" the heart must generate to eject blood into the systemic circulation. Although approximated by the systemic vascular resistance, it is a complex measure that includes blood viscosity, aortic impedance, and ventricular wall thickness. Along with preload, it is an important determinant of cardiac output.

Aganglionosis—The state of being without ganglia.

Agnosia—Cardinal symptom of Alzheimer's disease; inability to recognize or identify a familiar object in the absence of impaired sensory function.

Agoraphobia—Anxiety about, or avoidance of, places or situations from which escape might be difficult (or embarrassing) or in which help may not be available in the event of having a panic attack or panic-like symptoms.

Akathisia—The sensation of inner restlessness resulting in the need to make movements such as pacing or moving the legs. Akathisia has subjective and objective components.

Albumin—The major protein in plasma, with a molecular weight of 65 kDa.

Albuminuria—A condition where a large amount of albumin (>300 mg/day) is present in the urine, often indicating glomerular damage in the kidney.

Alcoholism—A chronic, progressive, and potentially fatal biogenic and psychosocial disease characterized by tolerance and physical dependence and manifested by a total loss of control, as well as diverse personality changes and social consequences.

Allergic interstitial nephritis—Inflammation of the interstitial region of the kidney often associated with acute onset of renal insufficiency.

Allergic salute—Constant upward rubbing of the nose as a result of allergies.

Allergic shiners—Dark circles under the eyes as a result of nasal congestion leading to venous pooling.

Allodynia—Painful response to normally non-noxious stimuli.

Allogeneic transplantation—Transfer of cells between different individuals.

Allograft—An organ or tissue transplanted from one individual to another.

Alloimmunization—Rapid consumption of transfused platelets via an immune mediated reaction.

Amenorrhea—Absence of menstruation.

American Urological Association (AUA) symptom index—Validated questionnaire in which the patient assesses the level of annoyance of 7 obstructive and irritative voiding symptoms.

Amygdala—A small almond-shaped temporal lobe structure, which plays a role in emotions and fear control.

Anaphylactoid—Anaphylaxis-like reactions that do not involve IgE-medicated mechanisms.

Anaphylaxis—Acute, life-threatening allergic reaction involving multiple organ systems.

Anastomosis—The surgical connection of two tubular structures, such as blood vessels, in a transplanted organ.

Anemia of chronic disease—Mild to moderate anemia not associated with blood loss or hemolysis. Usually with normal cell size. May be seen with chronic inflammation (e.g., rheumatoid arthritis, chronic infection) or malignancy.

Anemia of chronic kidney disease—A decrease in red blood cell production caused by a deficiency in the hormone erythropoietin normally produced by progenitor cells of the kidney. As kidney function declines, less erythropoietin is available to stimulate red blood cell production (erythropoiesis) in the bone marrow. Contributing factors include iron deficiency and a shortened red blood cell lifespan.

Angioedema—An allergic reaction characterized by edema of a tissue such as the lips, eyes, mouth, joints or other structures due to leak of fluid from blood vessels.

Anhedonia—A lack of pleasure or interest in usual activities.

Anisocytosis—Considerable variation in the size of cells that are normally uniform, especially with reference to red blood cells.

Ankylosis—Bony fusion resulting from chronic joint inflammation.

Antibiogram—A summary of antimicrobial susceptibilities.

Anticipatory anxiety—The fear of having an anxiety attack, which is often a trigger by itself; "fear of fear."

Antimicrobial cycling—A predetermined change in an antimicrobial recommendation for empiric therapy of a specific infection at a predetermined time.

Antimycotic—Inhibiting fungal growth.

Antithrombotic—A pharmacologic agent that prevents thrombus/clot formation. This category includes both antiplatelet agents and anticoagulants.

Anuria—Production of less than 50 mL of urine/day.

Anxiety—A state of apprehension, uncertainty, and fear resulting from the anticipation of a realistic or fantasized threatening event or situation, often impairing physical and psychological functioning.

Aphasia—Cardinal symptom of Alzheimer's disease; inability to generate or comprehend spoken language.

Aphthous ulcers—Small ulcers (canker sores) that form on the inside of the mouth.

Apical pulse—Point at the apex (bottom portion) of the heart impacts the chest wall.

Appendageal—Referring to hair, sweat glands, and nails.

Apraxia—Cardinal symptom of Alzheimer's disease; inability to carry out a motor task in the absence of impaired motor function.

Arteriovenous malformations—A tangle of blood vessels, both arterial and venous, that can rupture and cause hemorrhage in the brain.

Arthrodesis—The surgical immobilization of a joint (i.e., joint fusion).

Ascites—Abnormal buildup of fluid in the abdomen.

Aspiration pneumonitis—The inflammation of lung tissue caused by the aspiration of fluids and gastric contents that often leads to dyspnea, pulmonary edema, secondary infections and adult respiratory distress syndrome. Hydrocarbon pneumonitis is caused by the pulmonary aspiration of hydrocarbons such as kerosene and gasoline.

Ataxia—An inability to coordinate muscle activity during voluntary movement; most often due to disorders of the cerebellum or the posterior columns of the spinal cord; may involve the limbs, head, or trunk.

Atelectasis—Pulmonary parenchymal collapse due to alveolar or bronchial obstruction.

Atopic dermatitis—Skin inflammation that causes itching, scales, and erythema.

Atopy—An allergic syndrome characterized by asthma, hay fever, and urticaria or eczema.

Atrial fibrillation—Rapid beating of the atria which results in variable ventricular rates.

Atropinism—Symptoms of poisoning by atropine or belladonna.

Aura—Sensory or somatosensory alteration without loss of consciousness.

Auscultation—Listening to the heart or other organs with a stethoscope.

Autologous transplantation—Readministration of the same person's cells which were previously collected.

Autosomal—Pertaining to a chromosome.

Azotemia—Term referring to elevated levels of urea in the serum or blood.

Azotorrhea—An excessive loss of protein in the feces.

Bacteremia—Presence of viable bacteria (fungi) in the bloodstream.

Bacterial prostatitis—An inflammation of the prostate gland and surrounding tissue as a result of infection.

Bacteriuria—The presence of bacteria in the urine.

Barrett esophagus—Inflammatory changes in the esophagus resulting in replacement of epithelial lining by columnar-type cells that can lead to stricture or adenocarcinoma.

Benign prostatic hyperplasia—Nonmalignant enlargement of the prostate gland in elderly men.

Biliverdin—A green bile pigment formed from the oxidation of heme.

Binge eating—Excessive intake of calorie laden food over a short period of time.

Biochemical markers—Intracellular macromolecules released into the peripheral circulation from necrotic myocytes as a result of myocardial cell death (infarction). These laboratory tests are used in the diagnosis of myocardial infarction. Examples include troponin I, troponin T, creatinine kinase MB and myoglobin.

Biofilm—A population or community of microorganisms adhering to a surface by a secreted coating. This coating also reduces microorganism vulnerability to antibiotics.

Biopsy—A procedure in which a tiny piece of a body part, such as the kidney or bladder, is removed for examination under a microscope.

Bipolar I—Characterized by one or more manic or mixed episodes, and is usually accompanied by major depressive episodes.

Bipolar II—Characterized by one or more major depressive episodes and accompanied by at least one hypomanic episode.

Blood-brain barrier (BBB)—The relative lack of permeability of large molecules (and those molecules lacking lipid solubility) into the central nervous system because of the nonfenestrated capillary beds of the cerebral vasculature.

Blood urea nitrogen (BUN)—A waste product in the blood that comes from the breakdown of food protein. The kidneys filter blood to remove urea and thus maintain homeostasis. As kidney function decreases, the BUN level increases.

Borborygmi—Rumbling or gurgling noises produced by movement of gas, fluid, or both in the alimentary canal, and audible at a distance.

Bradykinesia—Slowness of motor movements as seen in Parkinsonism.

Breakthrough bleeding—The unpredictable and irregular bleeding associated with hormone therapy.

Bronchiectasis—Dilation of a bronchus or bronchi, usually related to excessive secretions.

Bronchioles—A subdivision of bronchi; smaller in diameter and without cartilage.

Bronchiolitis—Inflammation of the bronchioles; the small elements of the tracheobronchial tree.

Bronchoalveolar lavage—Instilling and then removing a lavage fluid to reveal the secretory and/or cellular contents from deep in the lung.

Bronchorrhea—Excessive bronchial secretions that can impair pulmonary ventilation.

Bruit—An abnormal and often harsh sound heard over a blood vessel, usually an artery, on examination with a stethoscope caused by turbulent blood flow.

Bursitis—Inflammation of the bursa, a fluid-filled soft tissue structure which usually results in pain and swelling.

Caffeinism—A clinical syndrome produced by acute or chronic overuse of caffeine characterized by anxiety, psychomotor alterations, sleep disturbances, mood changes, and psychophysiologic complaints.

Calcimimetics—A class of agents that stimulate calcium-sensing receptors on the parathyhroid gland and "mimic" the effects of extracellular calcium. They suppress PTH release and increase the sensitivity of the receptor to extracellular calcium.

Calcium-sensing receptor—The calcium receptor on the chief cells of the parathyroid gland, activation of which leads to suppression of PTH release.

Candidiasis—Fungal infection involving *Candida*.

Cardiac index—Cardiac output standardized for body surface area. Mathematically, cardiac index = cardiac output/body surface area.

Cardiac output—The volume of blood pumped by the heart per unit of time. Cardiac output is the product of heart rate and stroke volume.

Cardioembolic stroke—An ischemic stroke thought to be caused by an embolism arising from the heart. Cardioembolic stroke can be assumed in patients with significant cardiovascular disease including atrial fibrillation, dilated cardiomyopathy, prosthetic valves, recent MI and patent foramen ovale.

Cardiopulmonary arrest—The abrupt cessation of spontaneous and effective ventilation and circulation following a cardiac or respiratory event.

Cardiopulmonary bypass—The use of extracorporeal devices to pump blood and oxygenate the blood while the heart or lungs are not functional. Extracorporeal membrane oxygenation (ECMO) is a form of long-term cardiopulmonary bypass that is typically used for days to weeks.

Carotid Doppler—A technique that provides information about the presence and severity of atherosclerosis of the carotid artery, using noninvasive sound wave technology.

Carotid endarterectomy—Removal of the atherosclerotic plaque from the inside of a stenotic carotid artery by a surgical technique. The vessel is surgically opened and sewn and/or patched after removal of the plaque.

Case-control study—An observational study of persons with the disease of interest (cases) and a suitable control group of persons without the disease to establish the extent of association between exposure(s) of interest and disease.

Cataplexy—Sudden loss of bilateral muscle tone resulting in an individual collapsing, and precipitated by situations resulting from high emotion (e.g., laughter, anger, excitement).

Cellulitis—An acute, infectious process that initially affects the epidermis and dermis and may subsequently spread within the superficial fascia.

Centrilobular—Affecting the central portion of the lobe.

Cerebral autoregulation—The process by which cerebral blood flow is maintained in a tight range over a wide range of peripheral blood pressures. It is accomplished by reactive dilation and constriction of cerebral arteries.

Cerebral blood flow (CBF)—The volume of blood perfusing a given brain mass as a function of time.

Cerebral blood volume (CBV)—The total volume of blood within the cerebral vasculature at a given point in time.

Cerebral metabolic rate of oxygen consumption (CMRO$_2$)—The cerebral metabolic rate for oxygen calculated as the mean hemispheric CBF and the arteriojugular venous O$_2$ difference (AVDO$_2$).

Cerebral microdialysis—A sampling method which allows continuous acquisition of small volume cerebral extracellular fluid specimens utilizing a microdialysis probe inserted into the brain.

Cerebral oxygen delivery (CDO$_2$)—The product of CBF and arterial oxygen content.

Cerebral perfusion pressure (CPP)—The difference between mean arterial pressure (MAP) and intracranial pressure (ICP).

Cerebrospinal fluid—The clear, colorless fluid that bathes and cushions the brain and spinal cord.

Cervical cap—A thimble-shaped latex rubber device which is held on the cervix by suction, thus acting as a barrier to reduce the risk of pregnancy.

Cervical effacement—During the first stage of labor, as the cervix is opening, it is also thinning. The thinning of the cervix is termed effacement.

Cervical ripening—Prior to inducing labor, the cervix must be favorable, approximately 2 cm dilated and 80% thinned out. If this is not the case, an agent must be used to induce histochemical changes to make the cervix more favorable.

Cervicitis—Inflammation of the cervix.

Chancre—A sore or ulcer, the dermal lesion of primary syphilis.

Chancroid—A venereal dermal lesion caused by agents other than syphilis.

Children—Pediatric patients who are 1 to 11 years of age.

Cholinesterase inhibitors—Class of medication that inhibits enzymatic activity of acetylcholinesterase, butyrylcholinesterase, or both in order to prevent the degradation of acetylcholine.

Chronic condition—An illness or impairment that cannot be cured.

Chronic kidney disease (CKD)—Slow and progressive loss of kidney function that takes several years, often resulting in permanent kidney failure requiring dialysis or transplantation.

Chronic pain/persistent pain—Pain persisting for months to years.

Chronic pancreatitis—Chronic inflammation of the pancreas caused by the many sequelae of long-standing pancreatic injury leading to irreversible pancreatic damage.

Chvostek's sign—A facial twitch produced by tapping on the cheek over the branches of the facial nerve.

Circumstantial speech—Speech pattern whereby the expressed ideas are characterized by unnecessary detail. The speaker ultimately makes his or her point, but in a very roundabout manner.

Clinical proteinuria—Total protein in the urine in amounts greater than 300 mg/day.

Clinical resistance—Refers to failure of an antifungal agent in the treatment of a fungal infection, that arises from factors other than microbial resistance, such as failure of the antifungal agent to reach the site of infection, or inability of a patient's immune system to eradicate a fungus whose growth is retarded by an antifungal agent.

Cognitive-behavioral therapy—A form of psychotherapy that is instructional in approach and is based on the theory that thoughts cause feelings and behaviors, not external influences such as people, situations, and events. Patients learn to identify the thinking that causes the negative feelings and behaviors and then learn how to replace the thinking with thoughts that lead to more desirable reactions.

Cohort study—Assembly of a group of persons without a disease(s) of interest at the onset of the study, determination of the exposure status of each person, and observation of the cohort over time to determine the development of disease in exposed and nonexposed persons.

Colectomy—Surgical removal of the colon.

Colonization resistance—Preservation of anaerobic flora by selective gut decontamination to prevent colonization by potentially pathogenic gram-negative organisms.

Colony-stimulating factors—Proteins that regulate the proliferation, maturation, and differentiation of stem cells to red blood cells, white blood cells, and platelets.

Coma—A state of unconsciousness whereby a patient is not opening his or her eyes, not obeying commands, and not uttering understandable words.

Comedo, comedones (pl.)—Plug of sebum and keratinous material in a hair follicle; blackhead.

Comedogenicity—Product effect that causes follicular plugging resulting in comedones.

Comedolytic—Prevents shed keratinocytes from aggregating in follicle and clogging pores.

Comorbidity—The presence of co-existing diseases.

Complex partial seizure—A seizure beginning in one hemisphere of the brain. It is manifested by automatisms, periods of memory loss, or aberrations of behavior.

Compulsion—Repetitive ritualistic behavior such as ordering or hand washing or a mental act such as repeating words silently with the intent of preventing or reducing distress or some dreaded event or situation. Actions performed in response to the obsessions or to control anxiety associated with the obsession.

Condom—A sheath, usually made of thin rubber, used to cover the penis during sexual intercourse to prevent conception or infection.

Confounding—A situation in which the effects of two processes are not separated. The distortion of the apparent effect of an exposure on risk brought about by the association of other factors that can influence the outcome.

Continuation therapy—The second phase in drug therapy during which the goal is to eliminate any remaining symptoms and prevent a relapse.

Continuous-combined estrogen-progestogen therapy—Daily administration of both estrogen and a progestogen.

Continuous-long cycle estrogen-progestogen therapy—Estrogen is given daily and a progestogen is given six times a year (every other month for 12 to 14 days).

Convulsion—Specific seizure type where the seizure is manifested by involuntary muscle contractions.

Corneocytes—Flattened, dead, keratin filled epidermal cells.

Coronary artery bypass graft surgery (CABGS)—Thoracic surgery where parts of a saphenous vein from a leg or internal mammary artery from the arm are placed as conduits to restore blood flow between the aorta and one or more coronary arteries to "bypass" the coronary artery stenosis (occlusion).

Cor pulmonale—Right-sided heart failure caused by lung disease.

Corpus cavernosum—Two chambers on the dorsal side of the penis. Chambers composed of sinusoidal tissue, which can fill with arterial blood to produce an erection.

Corpus spongiosum—One chamber on the ventral side of the penis. Chamber is composed of sinusoidal tissue, which can fill with arterial blood to produce an erection. The urethra passes through the corpus spongiosum.

Cortical necrosis—Acute renal failure secondary to ischemic necrosis of the renal cortex usually caused by significantly diminished renal arterial perfusion.

Corticotropin-releasing hormone (CRH)—A trophic hormone released by the hypothalmus that stimulates release of adrenocorticotropic hormone (ACTH).

Cost-effectiveness ratio—The outcome of cost-effective analysis. The numerator of the ratio summarizes the costs and financial savings associated with the therapy, including the costs of the therapy itself, side effects, medical costs and savings from avoided illness and disability. The denominator of the cost-effectiveness ratio reflects the health effect of the intervention. The year of life saved is probably the most commonly used measure of the health effect.

Craniectomy (for stroke)—Removal of part of the skull overlying an area of injury in order to relieve the pressure of cerebral edema.

C-reactive protein—An endogenous marker released by the body in response to inflammation.

Creatine kinase, creatine kinase MB—Creatine kinase (CK) enzymes are found in many isoforms, with varying concentrations depending on the type of tissue. Creatine kinase is a general term used to describe the non-specific total release of all types of CK, including that found in skeletal muscle (MM), brain (BB) and heart (MB). Creatine kinase MB is released into the blood from necrotic myocytes in response to infarction and is a useful laboratory test for diagnosing myocardial infarction. If the total CK is elevated, then the relative index (RI), or fraction of the total that is composed of CK MB, is calculated as follows:

$$RI = (CK\ MB\ /\ CK\ total) \times 100$$
A RI greater than 2 is typically diagnostic of infarction.

Creatinine—The breakdown of protein metabolic by-product obtained from the diet or generated from muscle of the body. Creatinine is removed from blood by the kidneys; as kidney disease progresses, the level of creatinine in the blood increases.

Creatinine clearance—A test that measures how efficiently the kidneys excrete creatinine. Low creatinine clearance usually indicates the presence of kidney damage.

Crepitus—A crinkly, crackling, or grating feeling or sound in the joints, skin, or lungs.

Crossmatch—A test to determine if a recipient has antibodies against donor antigens. A positive crossmatch indicates that the recipient has antibodies against the donor and the two are incompatible. A negative crossmatch means the recipient does not have antibodies against the donor and the two are considered compatible.

Crust—Dried exudate, secretion or hemorrhage; scab.

Culture negative endocarditis—Describes a patient in whom a clinical diagnosis of infective endocarditis is likely, but blood cultures do not yield a pathogen.

Cutaneous—Pertaining to the skin.

Cutis—Skin.

Cyanosis—Bluish tint to the skin or mucous membranes due to lack of oxygen.

Cyclic estrogen-progestogen therapy—Estrogen is taken continuously, with a progestogen added cyclically the last 10 to 14 days during each 28-day cycle.

Cyst—Sac or closed cavity containing fluid, semifluid, or solid material.

Cystitis—Inflammation of the bladder, usually caused by infection.

Cytokine—Any of numerous hormone-like, low-molecular-weight proteins secreted by various cell types (e.g., T-lymphocytes or monocytes) that regulate the intensity and duration of immune response and mediate cell-cell communication.

Dactylitis—Erythema and swollen hand, feet, fingers, and toes. Also known as *hand and foot syndrome*.

Defibrillation—The therapeutic use of electric current in an attempt to completely depolarize the myocardium and provide an opportunity for the natural pacemaker centers of the heart to resume normal activity.

Delayed cerebral ischemia—A worsening in neurologic function in a subarachnoid hemorrhage patient, occurring several days after the initial bleed, not due to another cause.

Delusion—Fixed, false beliefs that are not based in reality or consistent with the patient's religion or culture. Delusions can be classified as paranoid, somatic, or grandiose in nature. Delusions are often unshakable.

Dementia—A decrease in cognitive function, usually with memory and intellectual deficits and confusion.

Depersonalization—A change in an individual's self-awareness, during anxiety disorder, such that one feels detached from his or her own experiences, with the self, body, and mind seeming alien or distant. Persistent or recurrent experiences as if one is an outside observer of one's mental processes or body (e.g., feeling like one is in a dream).

Derealization—A feeling of estrangement or detachment from one's environment.

Dermatitis—Inflammation of the skin.

Dermatophyte—Fungal infection of the skin.

Dermis—The inner layer of skin between the epidermis and hypodermis.

Desensitization—Administration of increasing doses of drug to achieve patient tolerance and avoidance of hypersensitivity reactions.

Detoxification programs—A medically supervised treatment program for alcohol or drug addiction designed to purge the body of intoxicating or addictive substances. Such a program is used as a first step in overcoming physiological or psychological addiction.

Detumescence—Process by which an erect penis becomes flaccid.

Diaphragm—(1) A flexible ring covered with rubber or other plastic material, fitted over the cervix of the uterus to prevent pregnancy. (2) Muscular membrane separating the abdominal and thoracic cavities, used for respiration.

Diffusion-weighted imaging—A type of MRI that can sensitively detect changes in water movement in tissue. It is particularly sensitive to the early changes seen during brain ischemia.

Digital clubbing—Rounded and swollen tip of finger usually associated with long-term pulmonary disease.

Dihydrotestosterone—Metabolic conversion of testosterone by 5α reductase produces dihydrotestosterone. This is the primary androgen stimulant of prostate cell growth.

Disinhibition—A physiologic effect that occurs during psychoactive substance use characterized by a loss of normal, executive functioning and normal behavior. An increase in behaviors with the propensity to harm the individual is common.

Dissociative amnesia—Inability to remember some important aspect of an event.

Diverticulitis—Inflammation of a diverticulum, especially of the small pockets in the wall of the colon which fill with stagnant fecal material and become inflamed; rarely, they may cause obstruction, perforation, or bleeding.

Dopamine—A monoamine neurotransmitter formed in the brain by the decarboxylation of dopa and essential to the normal functioning of the central nervous system.

Drug addiction—A chronic disorder characterized by the compulsive use of a substance resulting in physical, psychological, or social harm to the user and continued use despite that harm.

Dysentery—Diarrhea characterized by blood, mucus, and leukocytes in the stool with tenesmus and fever.

Dyskinesia—Choreiform abnormal involuntary movements involving usually the face, neck, trunk, and extremities.

Dysmenorrhea—Difficult and painful menstruation with cramps and backache at the onset of menses.

Dyspepsia—Literally means "bad digestion," but refers to persistent or recurrent pain or discomfort centered in the upper abdomen. Symptoms may include epigastric pain, bloating, abdominal distention, postprandial fullness, early satiety, and nausea.

Dysphoria or dysphoric—A feeling of discomfort or an unpleasant mood, such as sadness, anxiety, or irritability.

Dystonia—Sustained muscular spasm or abnormal postures.

Early empirical therapy—The administration of systemic antifungal agents at the onset of fever and neutropenia.

Edema—Accumulation of fluid in tissues.

Effective renal plasma flow (ERPF)—The flow of plasma through the kidneys; often measured by para-amino hippurate (PAH) clearance and expressed in volume per unit of time (mL/min). The ERPF is less than the true renal plasma flow (RPF) because plasma flow through renal connective and adipose tissue is not measured and the extraction of PAH, although high (>0.9), is not complete.

Electroencephalogram (EEG)—Used to evaluate brain electrical activity.

Electroencephalography—A test that measures electrical brain wave activity through the use of multiple scalp electrodes.

Electromyography—Test of muscle function due to either primary muscle disease or secondary to nerve injury.

Elevated—An exaggerated feeling of well-being, euphoria, or elation.

Emergency contraception—Any method of contraception that acts after intercourse to prevent pregnancy.

Emesis—See *Vomiting.*

Empirical therapy—With systemic antifungal agents is administered to granulocytopenic patients with persistent or recurrent fever despite the administration of appropriate antimicrobial therapy.

Encephalitis—Inflammation of the brain tissue.

Endocarditis—An inflammation of the endocardium, the membrane lining the chambers of the heart and covering the cusps of the heart valves.

Enkephalins—Pentapeptide endorphins, found in many parts of the brain, that bind to specific receptor sites, some of which may be pain-related opiate receptors.

Enteric fever—Intestinal inflammation and ulceration with high fever and abdominal complaints caused by infection.

Enterocolitis—Inflammation of the small intestine and colon.

Enterotoxin—A cholera-like disease that produces secretory diarrhea.

Enuresis—Urinary incontinence, especially at night.

Enzymuria—Presence of enzymes in the urine.

Epidermis—The outer layer of skin.

Epilepsy—Two or more unprovoked seizures, symptoms of disturbed electrical activity in the brain.

Epilepsy syndrome—The combination of seizure type with other components of the patient history such as age of onset, intellectual development, findings on neurologic examination, and results of neuroimaging.

Epithelial cells—Cells that make up epithelium.

Epithelium—Layer of avascular cells covering body surfaces.

Erectile dysfunction—Failure to achieve a penile erection suitable for sexual intercourse. Also known as *impotence*.

Erysipelas—Infection of the more superficial layers of the skin and cutaneous lymphatics.

Erythema—Redness.

Erythema multiforme—Symmetrical patches of raised, red skin.

Erythema nodosum—Raised, red, tender nodules on the skin that vary in size from 1 cm to several centimeters.

Erythroderma—Generalized redness of the skin.

Erythropoiesis—The production of erythrocytes (red blood cells) within the bone marrow.

Erythropoietic agents—Agents developed with recombinant DNA technology that have the same biological activity as endogenous erythropoietin to stimulate red blood cell production. Available agents in the United States include epoetin alfa and darbepoetin alfa.

Erythropoietin—A hormone made by the kidneys that is required for red blood cell formation in the bone marrow. Lack of this hormone leads to anemia.

Esophageal—Involving the esophagus.

Esophagitis—Inflammation of the esophagus.

Estrogen therapy—Unopposed estrogen regimens administered to postmenopausal women following hysterectomy.

Euphoria—A mood state characterized by an exaggerated, superficial sense of well-being, characterized extreme happiness, sometimes more than is reasonable in a particular situation.

Euthymia or euthymic—A mood in a "normal" range without depression or mood elevation.

Evoked potentials—EEG-based technique involving measurement of brain wave activity in response to stimuli, usually visual or auditory.

Fasciculations—The localized contractions of muscle groups, often visible through the skin, due to excessive neuronal discharge.

Fear—A direct, focused response to a specific event or object of which an individual is consciously aware.

Felty's syndrome—Rheumatoid arthritis associated with splenomegaly and neutropenia.

Fibrosis—Formation of fibrous tissue as a reparative or reactive process.

Fistula—An abnormal connection between two internal organs or between an internal organ and the skin.

Flight of ideas—An accelerated flow of speech with thoughts that change rapidly from one topic to another. An almost continuous flow of pressured and rapid speech that abruptly changes from topic to topic. The associations between the topics are usually understandable.

Focal seizures—Partial seizures.

Follicle-stimulating hormone (FSH)—A polypeptide hormone secreted by the anterior pituitary gland that promotes ovarian follicle development and stimulates estradiol and progesterone.

Fungemia—The presence of fungi in the blood.

"Freezing"—Intermittent immobility lasting a few seconds, particularly in walking, seen in Parkinsonism.

Gamma-aminobutyric acid (GABA)—The major inhibitory neurotransmitter in the central nervous system.

Gastroesophageal reflux disease (GERD)—Symptomatic clinical condition or histologic alteration that results from episodes of gastroesophageal reflux.

Generalized anxiety disorder (GAO)—Excessive anxiety and worry occurring more days than not for a period of at least 6 months.

Generalized seizures—Seizures occurring in both hemispheres of the brain. They may be primary or secondarily generalized.

Genotypes—The structure of deoxyribonucleic acid (DNA) that determines the expression of a trait.

Genu valgum—A deformity marked by lateral angulation of the leg in relation to the thigh.

Genu varum—A deformity marked by medial angulation of the leg in relation to the thigh; an outward bowing of the legs.

Gigantism—Excess secretion of growth hormone prior to epiphyseal closure in children.

Glaucoma—Any of a group of ocular disorders that lead to an optic neuropathy characterized by changes in the optic nerve head (optic disk) that is associated with loss of visual sensitivity and field. Open angle and closed angle are the two major types of glaucoma.

Glomerular filtration rate (GFR)—The primary index of overall kidney function; the volume of plasma that is filtered by the glomerulus per unit of time; often reported in mL/min or mL/min/1.73 m^2.

Glomerulonephritis—Glomerular lesions characterized by inflammation of the capillary loops in the glomerulus caused by immunologic, vascular, and other idiopathic diseases (may be diffuse or membranoproliferative).

Glomerulosclerosis—Fibrosis of the glomeruli.

Glomerulus—A coiled capillary bed in the kidney that is responsible for filtering water and small molecular weight substances from the blood.

Gonadotropin-releasing hormone (GnRH)—A trophic hormone released by the hypothalamus that stimulates release of follicle-stimulating hormone (FSH) and luteinizing hormone (LH).

Gout—A disease spectrum that includes hyperuricemia, recurrent attacks of acute arthritis associated with monosodium urate crystals in leukocytes found in synovial fluid, deposits of monosodium urate crystals in tissues (tophi), interstitial renal disease, and uric acid nephrolithiasis.

gp120—The glycoprotein structure on the surface of HIV that binds to CD4 on human cells.

Grandiosity—An inflated self-appraisal of one's status, power, or identity.

Granuloma inguinale—Granuloma lesions affecting the genital area.

Growth hormone (GH)—A polypeptide hormone secreted by the anterior pituitary gland that stimulates IGF-I production and promotes growth of all body cells.

Growth hormone-releasing hormone (GH-RH)—A trophic hormone released by the hypothalmus that stimulates release of growth hormone.

Gumma—A granulomatous lesion found in organs or tissues as a result of syphilis.

Hallucinations—Abnormal sensory perceptions that occur while a person is awake and conscious and without external stimulation of the relevant sensory organ. Some common hallucinations are hearing voices when no one has spoken, seeing patterns, lights, beings or objects that aren't there, or feeling a crawling sensation on the skin. Many recreational drugs, including psychedelic drugs such as LSD and certain potent types of marijuana, can cause hallucinations.

Haptocorrin—A group of carrier proteins which bind with vitamin B_{12} in the blood and aid in its transport.

Haptoglobin—A group of α_2-globulins in human serum, so called because of their ability to combine with hemoglobin, preventing loss in the urine; levels are decreased in hemolytic disorders and increased in inflammatory conditions or with tissue damage.

Hay fever—See *Rhinitis*.

Heart failure—A clinical syndrome that can result from any disorder that impairs the ability of the heart to fill with or eject blood. Although heart failure may be caused by numerous cardiac disorders, the primary clinical signs and symptoms of dyspnea, fatigue, and volume overload are similar regardless of the initial cause.

Heinz bodies—Intracellular inclusions usually attached to the red cell membrane, composed of denatured hemoglobin.

Hematemesis—Vomiting up blood that may be bright red or similar to coffee grounds in appearance.

Hematochezia—The presence of blood in the stool.

Hematopoiesis—The formation and maturation of blood cells and their derivatives.

Hematopoietic growth factors—See *Colony-stimulating factors*.

Hematuria—Presence of red blood cells in the urine.

Homocysteine—A homolog of cysteine, produced by the demethylation of methionine, and an intermediate in the biosynthesis of l-cysteine from l-methionine via l-cystathionine. Elevated levels of homocysteine have been associated with certain forms of heart disease.

Hemolytic uremic syndrome—A condition characterized by the breakup of red blood cells (hemolysis) and kidney failure. Platelets clump together within the kidney's small blood vessels resulting in ischemia leading to kidney failure.

Hemosiderin—A golden yellow or yellow-brown insoluble protein produced by phagocytic digestion of hematin; found in most tissues, especially in the liver, spleen, and bone marrow, in the form of granules much larger than ferritin molecules (of which they are believed to be aggregates), but with a higher content, as much as 37%, of iron.

Hepatosplenic candidiasis—Clinical presentation often manifested only as fever while a patient remains neutropenic (<1000 WBC/mm^3). When the WBC count increases to >1000 cells/mm^3, imaging studies can detect the presence of abscess or microabscesses in the liver and spleen, often found with acute suppurative and granulomatous reactions. Infection may persist for months and ultimately cause the patient's death despite aggressive systemic therapy with antifungal agents. Also known as *chronic systemic candidiasis*.

Heterozygous—Presence of different (alleles) genes at one location.

Hippocampus—A sea horse–shaped structure located within the brain that is an important part of the limbic system. The hippocampus is involved in some aspects of memory, in the control of the autonomic functions, and in emotional expression.

Hollenhorst plaque—Cholesterol emboli that usually dislodges from the carotid arteries, or calcific fragments from a stenosed aortic valve that can be visualized on a retinal exam.

Homozygous—Presence of identical genes (alleles) at one location.

Hormone therapy—Either estrogen-only therapy or combined estrogen/progestogen therapy.

Hot flashes—A sensation of warmth, frequently accompanied by skin flushing and perspiration.

Human leukocyte antigens (HLA)—The "self antigens," the histocompatibility antigens found on human leukocytes and tissues that enable the body to differentiate "self" from "foreign" cells. The HLA antigens are used in histocompatibility testing to determine the suitability of an organ for transplant.

Hyperalgesia—Exaggerated painful response to normally noxious stimuli.

Hyperarousal—A state of elevated or increased alertness, awareness, or wakefulness.

Hypercapnia—Elevation of carbon dioxide gas in the blood.

Hyperkalemia—Serum potassium concentration above 5.5 mEq/L.

Hypermagnesemia—Serum magnesium concentration above 1.8 mEq/L or 2.3 mg/dL.

Hyperpigmentation—Excess pigment in skin causing an area of darker color than surrounding skin.

Hyperprolactinemia—A state of persistent serum prolactin elevation characterized by prolactin concentrations greater than 20 micrograms/liter observed on multiple occasions.

Hyperresponsiveness—In the airways, the characteristic of an exaggerated response to stimuli.

Hypervigilance—An enhanced state of sensory sensitivity accompanied by an exaggerated intensity of behaviors whose purpose it is to detect threats.

Hypnagogic hallucinations—Dreamlike experiences on the threshold of sleep that intrude into wakefulness.

Hypnopompic hallucinations—Dreamlike experiences on the threshold of awakening that intrude into wakefulness.

Hypochlorhydria—Presence of an abnormally small amount of hydrochloric acid in the stomach.

Hypokalemia—Serum potassium concentration below 3.5 mEq/L.

Hypomagnesemia—Serum magnesium concentration below 1.4 mEq/L or 1.7 mg/dL.

Hypomania—An abnormally and persistently elevated, expansive, or irritable mood that lasts at least 4 days, but does not cause marked impairment in functioning.

Hypomimia—Decreased facial expression often associated with decreased blink rate.

Hypophonia—Decreased volume of speech.

Hypothalamus—A small region at the base of the brain that controls the release of hormones from the anterior and posterior regions of the pituitary gland and regulates limbic functions, fluid balance, body temperature, cardiovascular function, respiratory function, and diurnal rhythms.

Iatrogenesis or iatrogenic disease—A disease produced as a consequence of medical or surgical treatment.

Ictal—The period during a seizure.

Icteric—Relating to or marked by jaundice.

Ileitis—Inflammation of the ileus.

Illusions—Visual perceptions that are misinterpreted but have a real sensory stimulus.

Immunocompromised host—A patient with defects in host defenses that predisposes him or her to infection (risk factors may include neutropenia, immune system defects from disease or immunosuppressive drug therapy, compromise of natural host defenses, environmental contamination, and changes in normal flora of the host).

Immunoglobulin—Structurally related glycoproteins that function as antibodies and are divided into classes on the basis of structure/biological activity.

Impaction—An immovable packing; a lodgment of something in a strait or passage of the body; as, impaction of the fetal head in the strait of the pelvis; impaction of food or feces in the intestines of man or beast.

Impetigo—A superficial skin infection that is seen most commonly in children.

Inanition—Severe weakness and wasting as occurs from lack of food, defect in assimilation, or neoplastic disease.

Induction—Administration of a highly intense level of immunosuppression in the perioperative period or use of antibody therapy to provide enough immunosuppression to delay administration of nephrotoxic calcineurin inhibitors.

Infant mortality—Deaths occurring before the age of one year per 1000 live births.

Infants—Pediatric patients who are 1 month to 1 year of age.

Infection—Inflammatory response to invasion of normally sterile host tissue by the microorganisms.

Information bias—A flaw in measuring exposure or outcome data that results in systematic differences in the quality of information gathered for study and comparison groups. See also *Selection bias.*

Instrumental activities of daily living—Housekeeping chores, shopping, going outside, medication management. See also *Activities of daily living.*

Insulin-like growth factor-I—An anabolic peptide that acts as a direct stimulator of cell proliferation and growth in all body cells.

Integumentary system—Skin, subcutaneous tissue, and skin appendages.

Interleukin—A type cytokine, usually influencing a white blood cell.

Intermittent-combined estrogen-progestogen therapy—A regimen that combines a daily estrogen with a progestogen administered intermittently in cycles of 3 days on and 3 days off (which is then repeated without interruption).

Interpersonal psychotherapy (IP)—IP is a psychological intervention that focuses on interpersonal relationships and psychosocial functioning.

Intertriginous areas—Body fold areas (e.g., between buttocks, beneath breasts, between toes, under arms).

Intoxication—The development of a substance-specific syndrome after recent ingestion and presence in the body of a substance, and it is associated with maladaptive behavior during the waking state caused by the effect of the substance on the central nervous system.

Intracavernosal injection—Injection into the corpus spongiosum.

Intracranial pressure—The pressure of the cerebral spinal fluid that is essentially the same as the pressure within the brain tissue (i.e., intraparenchymal pressure).

Intrauterine device—A device inserted in the uterus to prevent pregnancy, either through spermicidal action (copper device) or thickening cervical mucus to inhibit sperm penetration and migration (progesterone device).

Intrinsic resistance—See *Primary resistance.*

Intussusception—Invagination of one portion of the intestine into an adjacent part of the intestines.

Inulin—A fructose polysaccharide that is filtered by the glomerulus; its clearance is often used as an index of GFR.

Iothalamate—A nonradiolabeled or radiolabeled iodinated contrast agent that is filtered by the glomerulus; its clearance is often used as an index of GFR.

Irritable—Easily annoyed and provoked to anger.

Janeway lesion—These lesions appear as flat, painless, red to bluish-red spots on the palms and soles of patients with acute bacterial endocarditis.

Jarisch-Herxheimer reaction—An increase in symptoms of spirochetal disease caused by the initiation of treatment.

Jugular venous oxygen saturation (SjvO$_2$)—Oxygen hemoglobin saturation of blood in the jugular bulb which is a key element in estimating CMRO$_2$.

K complexes—Electronegative waves followed by electropositive waves seen on the EEG during sleep.

Keratinization—Keratin formation.

Keratinized—Skin that has developed thicker areas of keratin in the stratum corneum.

Keratinocyte—Cell of the epidermis that produces keratin.

Keratoconjunctivitis sicca—Dry itchy eyes resulting from atrophy of the lacrimal ducts, which may be seen in inflammatory arthritis.

Keratolytic—Agent that solubilizes intracellular cement of keratin cells in the stratum corneum.

Ketogenic diet—A special antiseizure diet that is high in fat and low in carbohydrates and protein.

Kleptomania—An impulse-control disorder whereby patients have an uncontrollable urge to steal, along with recurrent failure to resist these urges.

Lactation—The production of milk.

Lanugo—Fine body hair normally found on a fetus. The hair develops in patients with anorexia nervosa when they are very underweight and malnourished.

Laryngospasm—The spasmodic closure of the larynx due to a variety of causes such as allergic reactions, response to irritants, and pharmacologic actions.

Lavage—Washing out.

Left ventricular ejection fraction—Also known simply as the *ejection fraction*, it is the fraction or percentage of the end diastolic blood volume ejected by the left ventricle during systole. It is a measurement of cardiac systolic function with a normal ejection being >60%. It can be determined noninvasively by an echocardiogram.

Left ventricular hypertrophy—Enlargement of the left ventricle, which is seen in heart failure and may give rise to arrhythmias.

Leptospirosis—A bacterial disease that affects humans and animals caused by the genus *Leptospira*.

Lichenification—Thickening of epidermis due to irritation.

Lipid peroxidation—A pathophysiologic process involving the iron-catalyzed attack of lipid membranes by reactive oxygen species.

Liposomes—Spherical amphiphilic vesicles capable of sustained release of water-soluble substances.

Locus ceruleus—A small area in the brainstem containing norepinephrine neurons that is considered to be a key brain center for anxiety and fear.

Lower urinary tract symptoms—Term that collectively refers to obstructive and irritative urinary voiding symptoms of benign prostatic hypertrophy (BPH).

Lumbar puncture—The procedure used to withdraw cerebrospinal fluid via a needle inserted in the lumbar region of the spinal column.

Luteinizing hormone (LH)—A polypeptide hormone secreted by the anterior pituitary gland that stimulates ovulation and maintains the corpus luteum.

Lymphangitis—An inflammation involving the subcutaneous lymphatic channels.

Lymphocytosis—Increased blood concentration of lymphocytes ($> 4 \times 10^9$ cells/L) commonly observed in mononucleosis, pertussis, measles, chickenpox or lymphoid malignancies.

Lymphogranuloma venereum—Inflammation of the lymph nodes caused by *Chlamydia trachomatis* resulting in destruction and scarring of tissue.

Macule—Flat, nonpalpable, variable colored lesion.

Maculopapular—Skin eruption containing both macules and papules.

Magnetic resonance angiography (MRA)—A noninvasive method to evaluate the patency of blood vessels using magnetic resonance imaging.

Magnetic resonance imaging (MRI)—An imaging technique based upon the magnetic properties of the hydrogen atom. It provides an accurate, computer-processed image that can be more sensitive than computed tomography.

Major histocompatibility complex (MHC)—A set of genes responsible for most of the proteins on the surface of cells in the body that are responsible for recognition of "self."

Mania—An abnormally and persistently elevated, expansive, or irritable mood that lasts at least one week, and causes marked impairment in functioning.

Mass effect—An increase in intracranial pressure due to a space-occupying lesion in the brain, usually leading to a "shift" in brain contents, evident by imaging techniques.

Mastalgia or mastodynia—Pain in the breast.

Mean arterial pressure—The mean arterial pressure is the product of the cardiac output and systemic vascular resistance. Since the cardiac output is pulsatile, rather than continuous, and since 2/3 of the normal cardiac cycle is spent in diastole, the mean arterial pressure is not the arithmetic mean of the systolic and diastolic blood pressures. Mean arterial pressure = diastolic blood pressure + 1/3 (systolic blood pressure–diastolic blood pressure).

Meconium ileus—Intestinal obstruction due to meconium.

Megakaryocytes—Precursors of platelets.

Melanin—Dark pigment that is part of determining skin color.

Melena—Dark-colored stools resulting from upper gastrointestinal bleed.

Membrane stripping—When the cervix is dilated, a practitioner can use a hand to separate the amniotic membranes from the uterus. This technique has been shown to reduce the need for labor induction.

Menarche—The time of the first menstrual period or flow.

Meningitis—Inflammation, usually infectious, of the meninges, a covering of the brain.

Menopause—The permanent cessation of menses following the loss of ovarian follicular activity.

Menses—Periodic bloody discharge from the uterus.

Methionine—The l-isomer is a nutritionally essential amino acid and the most important natural source of "active methyl" groups in the body, hence usually involved in methylations in vivo.

Microalbuminuria—A condition in which a small amount of albumin (30 to 300 mg/day) is present in the urine; indicative of an early stage of chronic kidney disease (CKD).

Microcomedo—Microscopic lesion formed from the combination of sloughed, clumping keratinocytes reacting with sebum and fatty acids from the sebaceous gland.

Micrographia—Handwriting that is small, trails off in size, or very slow.

Midsystolic—Middle of systole.

Milia—Small, white, cysts containing keratin.

Mixed states—Rapidly alternating mood states (mania and major depressive episodes) that last at least one week, and cause marked impairment in functioning.

Molds—Fungal organisms that grow as multicellular branching, thread-like filaments (hyphae) that are either *septate* (divided by transverse walls) or *coenocytic* (multinucleate without cross walls). On agar media, molds grow outward from the point of inoculation by extension of the tips of filaments, and then branch repeatedly, interweaving to form fuzzy, matted growths called *mycelium*. Germ tubes are the beginning of *hyphae*, which arise as perpendicular extensions from the yeast cell, with no constriction at their point of origin.

Molybdenum (Mo)—A bioelement found in a number of proteins.

Mood—A more pervasive and sustained emotional state that colors a person's perception of the world.

Morbilliform—Maculopapular lesions that becomes confluent on the face and body.

Mucolytic—The ability to break down mucus.

Mucositis—Inflammation of the mucosa.

Multiple organ dysfunction syndrome (MODS)—Presence of altered organ function requiring intervention to maintain homeostasis.

Multiple sclerosis (MS)—A demyelinating disease, caused by inflammation, leading to neurologic deficits and often, disability.

Mutism—A state in which a person either had the inability or they refuse to speak or vocalize sounds.

Myoclonic seizures—Brief shock-like muscular contractions of the face, trunk, and extremities. They usually begin in adolescence and are referred to as *juvenile myoclonic epilepsy* (JME).

Myoclonus—A sudden twitching of muscles or parts of muscles, without any rhythm or pattern.

Mycotic—A fungal infection.

National Kidney Foundation (NKF)—A voluntary health organization that seeks to prevent kidney and urinary tract diseases, improve the health and well being of individuals and families affected by these diseases, and increase the availability of all organs for transplantation.

Nausea—An unpleasant sensation associated with an awareness of the urge to vomit.

Necrosis—Local death of cells or tissue.

Necrotizing fasciitis—A rare, but very severe infection of the subcutaneous tissue that may be caused by aerobic and/or anaerobic bacteria and results in progressive destruction of the superficial fascia and subcutaneous fat.

Neonates—Newborns who are 1 day to 1 month of age.

Nephritis—Inflammation of the kidney.

Nephrolithiasis—Presence of one or more stones in the renal pelvis, collecting system, or ureters.

Nephron—The working unit of the kidney that is comprised of a glomerulus and tubule. Each kidney is made up of about 1 million nephrons, which collectively remove drugs, toxins, and fluid from the blood.

Nephropathy—Refers to a pathologic alteration of the kidney.

Nephrotic range proteinuria—Proteinuria >3 grams/day associated with glomerular disease and nephrotic syndrome.

Nephrotoxicity—Toxic insult to the kidney.

Nerve conduction studies—Measurement of the speed of electrical conduction through a nerve.

Neuritic plaques—Hallmark pathological marker of Alzheimer's disease comprised of beta amyloid protein and masses of broken neurites.

Neurofibrillary tangles—Hallmark pathological marker of Alzheimer's disease derived from abnormal phosphorylation of tau protein filaments.

Neuropathic pain—Pain sustained by abnormal processing of sensory input by the peripheral or central nervous system.

Neutropenia—An abnormally reduced number of neutrophils circulating in peripheral blood; although exact definitions of neutropenia often vary, an absolute neutrophil count of <1000 cells/mm^3 indicates a reduction sufficient to predispose patients to infection.

N-methyl-D aspartate antagonists (NMDA)—Class of medications that decreases the activity of synaptic glutamate, thus decreasing the likelihood of cell death.

N-methyl-D-aspartate (NMDA) receptor—A cellular receptor complex involved in the intracellular passage of calcium into CNS cells upon stimulation by amines such as glutamate and aspartate.

Nocturia—Frequent nighttime urination (>2 micturitions per night).

Nodule—Elevated, palpable, solid, round or oval lesion more than 0.5 cm in diameter.

Nonoliguria—Production of >450 mL urine/day.

Nonulcer dyspepsia—Ulcer-like dyspepsia that has been investigated, but endoscopic findings yield no evidence of mucosal injury (ulcer).

Norepinephrine (NE)—A hormone secreted by the adrenal medulla and also released at synapses.

Nosocomial infection—An infection acquired in a health care facility.

NSAID—Nonsteroidal anti-inflammatory drug.

Oblique lie—The fetus is at an angle to the cervix. The head is not the presenting part, and often the patient will need to be delivered by cesarean section.

Obsession—Recurrent and persistent thoughts, images, or impulses experienced as intrusive and distressing. Unwanted thoughts or ideas that intrude into a person's thinking.

Obsessive-compulsive disorder (OCD)—An anxiety disorder characterized by obsessions and/or compulsions that are time-consuming and interfere significantly with normal routine, social, or occupational functioning or relationships.

Oliguria—Diminished volume of urine output (volume <400 to 500 mL/day).

Onychomycosis—Fungal infection of the nail apparatus.

Ophthalmia neonatorum—Inflammation of the conjunctiva resulting from acquisition of gonococcal infection at birth.

Opportunistic infection (OI)—Infection with microorganism that occurs due to altered physiologic state of the patient.

Organic erectile dysfunction—Term used to refer to erectile dysfunction that is due to vascular, neurologic, and/or hormonal causes.

Orthopnea—Difficulty breathing after lying down.

Orthostatic hypotension—A reduction of blood pressure when the patient changes position, usually from lying down to sitting up; often indicative of hypovolemia.

Osler's nodes—Osler's nodes are red, raised tender nodules usually 5 mm in diameter on the pulps of toes or fingers. Seen in patients with endocarditis, they are thought to be due to the deposition of immune complexes.

Osteomalacia—A disease characterized by abnormal bone mineralization (e.g., gradual softening and bending of the bones) with varying severity of pain. Referred to as *rickets* in children.

Osteopenia—Low bone density, DXA T score of -1 to -2.5

Osteophyte—A bony outgrowth or protuberance.

Osteoporosis—(1) Reduced bone mass associated with architectural deterioration of the skeleton and increased risk for fracture. (2) A chronic, progressive disease characterized by very low bone density (DXA T score <-2.5), microarchitectural deterioration and decreased bone strength, bone fragility, and a consequent increase in fracture risk.

Osteotomy—The surgical cutting of a bone.

Otitis media—Inflammation of the middle ear.

Oxytocin—A polypeptide hormone secreted by the posterior pituitary gland that stimulates uterine contraction.

Pain—An unpleasant sensory and emotional experience associated with actual or potential tissue damage or described in terms of such damage.

Palpation—Touching the skin to feel the outline of an organ.

Pan- or holo-systolic—Throughout the end time of systole.

Pancreatitis—An acute or chronic inflammation of the pancreas with variable involvement of local tissues and remote organs.

Panel of reactive antibodies (PRA)—The percentage of cells from a panel of donors with which a potential recipient's blood stream reacts. The more antibodies in the recipient's blood stream, the higher the PRA. The higher the PRA, the higher the risk for a positive crossmatch.

Panhypopituitarism—A condition of complete or partial loss of anterior and posterior pituitary function resulting in a complex disorder characterized by multiple pituitary-hormone deficiencies.

Panic attack—A discrete period in which there is the sudden onset of intense apprehension, fearfulness, or terror, often associated with feelings of impending doom.

Panic disorder—The presence of recurrent, unexpected panic attacks followed by at least 1 month of persistent concern about having another panic attack, worry about the possible implications or consequences of the panic attacks, or a significant behavioral change related to the attacks.

Panlobular—Affecting the entire lobe.

Papillary—Upper layer of the dermis.

Papule—Solid, elevated, lesion more than 0.5 cm in diameter.

Papulosquamous—Raised plaque or papule with scaling.

Para-aminohippurate (PAH)—A small molecule which is completely secreted from the tubules into urine, so that blood leaving the kidney is virtually free of PAH; a marker that is often used to measure renal plasma flow (RPF).

Parenchyma—Specific cells or tissue of an organ.

Paresthesia—An abnormal sensation, such as of burning, pricking, tickling, or tingling.

Parkinsonism—A constellation of symptoms with atypical features such that a diagnosis of idiopathic Parkinson's disease cannot be made.

Parous—Having borne one or more children.

Paroxysmal nocturnal dyspnea—Onset of difficulty breathing after lying down for several hours.

Partial seizure—A seizure that begins in one hemisphere of the brain. It may be simple, complex, or secondarily generalized.

Patch—Large macule (more than 2 cm in diameter).

Pelvic inflammatory disease (PID)—Infection of the lining of the uterus, the fallopian tubes, or the ovaries.

Penumbra (ischemic)—The area of brain tissue around the core of the infarct that has decreased function but remains viable. It is proposed that reperfusion of this tissue will allow survival of the affected neurons and other brain cells.

Peptic ulcer—Cellular distribution of the gastrointestinal mucosa, submucosa, and muscular layer. Chronic peptic ulcers usually occur as a "single hole" and are found most often in the stomach and duodenum.

Percussion—Tapping on a structure to elicit a sound.

Percussion and postural drainage—Tapping on the thorax to physically loosen pulmonary secretions and posturing the body to facilitate expectoration.

Percutaneous coronary intervention (PCI)—A minimally invasive procedure whereby access to the coronary arteries is obtained through the femoral artery up the aorta to the coronary os. Contrast media is used to visualize the coronary artery stenosis using a coronary angiogram. A guidewire is used to cross the stenosis and small balloon is inflated and/or stent is deployed to break up atherosclerotic plaque and restore coronary artery blood flow. The stent is left in place to prevent restenosis of the coronary artery.

Perimenopause—The period immediately prior to the menopause and the first year after menopause. Reflects the transition to menopause (with irregular menstrual cycles) and includes the 3 to 5 years before and 1 year after the cessation of menstrual flow.

Perioral dermatitis—Rash around the mouth. In patients with anorexia nervosa or bulimia nervosa, the rash is secondary to repeated vomiting that creates skin irritation from exposure to the gastric contents.

Peripheral arterial disease (PAD)—Atherosclerotic occlusive disease of the extremities, usually diagnosed by symptoms (claudication) or assessment of the blood flow to an extremity.

Peripheral blood progenitor cells—Immature blood cells, which are capable of producing white blood cells, platelets, and red blood cells.

Peritonitis—The acute, inflammatory response of the peritoneal lining to microorganisms, chemicals, irradiation, or foreign body injury.

Perseveration—Persistent repetition of the same verbal or motor response despite differing stimuli.

Petechiae—Pinpoint, flat, round, red spots under the skin caused by intradermal hemorrhage.

Pharmacoepidemiology—The study of the use of and the effects of drugs in large numbers of people with the purpose of supporting safe and effective drug therapies. This type of observational research is useful when more rigorous, experimental designs are not feasible.

Pharyngitis—An acute infection of the oropharynx or nasopharynx.

Pharmacovigilance—The science and activities relating to the detection, assessment, understanding and prevention of adverse effects or any other drug related problems.

Phenotypes—How a gene is expressed (e.g., eye color, height, drug metabolism capacity). The expression of genetic alleles (genotype) as an observable physical or biochemical trait.

Phobia—A persistent, abnormal, and irrational fear of a specific thing or situation that compels one to avoid it, despite the awareness and reassurance that it is not dangerous.

Photic stimulation—Stimulation of the visual cortex through visual stimulation with bright and alternating light.

Photoallergy—Photosensitivity disorder of skin (light and photoallergic agent).

Phototoxicity—Photosensitivity disorder of skin (light and phototoxic agent).

Physical dependence—(1) A state of adaptation that is manifested by a drug class specific withdrawal syndrome that can be produced by abrupt cessation, rapid dose reduction, decreasing blood level of the drug, and/or administration of an antagonist. (2) A pharmacologic effect of a drug defined by the occurrence of an abstinence syndrome following administration of an antagonist drug or abrupt dose reduction or discontinuation.

Pilonidal—Hair-containing cyst.

Pilosebaceous—Sebaceous gland and adjacent hair follicle.

Placenta previa—The placenta is located over the cervical opening. In this situation, the mother and baby can hemorrhage because the placenta will separate from the uterus before the baby is born. Women who have a placenta previa must be delivered by cesarean section.

Plaque—Raised, flat lesion (more than 2 cm in diameter).

Pneumonitis—Inflammation of lung tissue.

Poikilocytosis—The presence of irregularly shaped red blood cells in the peripheral blood.

Poikilothermia—Inability to maintain normal body temperature.

Polyarteritis nodosa—A systemic necrotizing vasculitis of small and medium-sized arteries.

Polycythemia—An increase in the number of red cells present in the blood.

Porphyria—A group of disorders involving heme biosynthesis, characterized by excessive excretion of porphyrins or their precursors; may be inherited or may be acquired, as from the effects of certain chemical agents.

Porphyrins—Pigments widely distributed throughout nature (e.g., heme, bile pigments, cytochromes) consisting of four pyrroles joined in a ring (porphin) structure.

Postrenal ARF—Acute renal failure with an anatomical cause that is in the urinary tract.

Postictal—The recovery period after a seizure, where a patient may be lethargic or confused. Duration can be variable.

Posttraumatic stress disorder—An anxiety disorder in which exposure to an exceptional mental or physical stressor is followed by persistent re-experiencing of the event, avoidance of reminders of the event, and arousal symptoms.

Postvoid residual urine volume—Urine left in the bladder after the patient has been asked to completely empty urine out of the bladder. Normally the postvoid residual urine volume should be zero. A high postvoid residual urine volume is associated with recurrent urinary tract infection.

Preload—Along with afterload, it is an important determinant of cardiac output. It is the degree of stretch of the myocardial fibers (sarcomeres) at the end of diastole. As the sarcomeres are stretched, the force of contraction increases. Preload is approximated by the left ventricular end diastolic volume or pressure.

Premature infants—Those born before 37 weeks' gestational age.

Premature ovarian failure—Amenorrhea, sex-steroid deficiency, and infertility in women younger than 40 years of age.

Premenstrual dysphoric disorder (PMDD)—A severe form of premenstrual syndrome and is listed in the appendix of the *Diagnostic and Statistical Manual of Mental Disorders*, Fourth Edition Revised. The diagnostic criteria require prospective documentation of symptoms, a specific constellation of symptoms, and functional impairment.

Premenstrual molimina—Includes premenstrual symptoms such as breast tenderness, pelvic heaviness or bloating, and food cravings that are not distressing and do not interfere with daily functioning.

Premenstrual syndrome (PMS)—Variably defined and usually requires a history of a single physical or mood symptom that occurs cyclically during the luteal phase of the menstrual cycle.

Prerenal ARF—Acute renal failure caused by a reduction of renal blood flow. Often associated with volume depletion or poor cardiac function.

Presbycusis—Progressive bilateral loss of hearing that occurs in the aged.

Pressured speech—More and faster speech that is difficult or impossible to interrupt.

Priapism—Painful prolonged erection.

Primary amenorrhea—Absence of menses in a girl who has reached the age of 16.

Primary hypogonadism—Failure of the testes to produce an adequate supply of testosterone to meet physiologic needs.

Primary lesion—Basic skin lesion that appears at the beginning of skin disorder.

Primary resistance—Refers to resistance recorded prior to drug exposure in vitro or in vivo, as determined by in vitro susceptibility testing using standardized methodology.

Progestogen—A term referring to progesterone and the synthetic progestational compounds (sometimes referred to as *progestins*).

Prolactin—A polypeptide hormone secreted by the anterior pituitary gland that stimulates lactation.

Proprioception—A sense or perception, usually at a subconscious level, of the movements and position of the body and especially its limbs, independent of vision; this sense is gained primarily from input from sensory nerve terminals in muscles and tendons and the fibrous capsule of joints combined with input from the vestibular apparatus.

Protease—An enzyme in HIV that cleaves large precursor polypeptides into functional proteins that are necessary to produce a complete virus.

Proteinuria—A condition in which the urine contains measurable amounts of protein (>150 mg/day); often a sign of glomerular or tubular damage in the kidney.

Proteolytic—The ability to break down protein.

Pruritus—Itching.

Pseudoaddiction—Behavior suggestive of addiction but caused by unrelieved pain.

Pseudoallergic—Adverse reactions that appear like allergic reactions but do not have an immunologic mechanism.

Pseudocyst—Collection of pancreatic juice and tissue debris enclosed by a wall of fibrous or granulation tissue.

Pseudomembranous colitis—Inflammation of the colon caused by the toxin of *Clostridium difficile* and resulting in bloody diarrhea.

Psychogenic erectile dysfunction—Erectile dysfunction due to failure of central nervous system to perceive or process sexually stimulating information.

Psychomotor retardation—A slowing or limitation of motor functioning or muscular movements.

Psychosocial stressor—Any significant life event or change that may be associated with the onset, occurrence, or exacerbation of a mental disorder.

Psychotherapy—A general term used to describe a form of treatment based on talking with a therapist. Psychotherapy aims to relieve distress by discussing and expressing feelings, to help the patient to change attitudes, behavior and habits and to develop better ways of coping.

Pulmonary artery occlusion pressure—It is usually determined by a balloon-tipped Swan-Ganz catheter that is advanced into a distal branch of the pulmonary artery. Inflation of the balloon at the catheter tip occludes the pulmonary artery and allows measurement of the left atrial pressure which reflects the left ventricular diastolic pressure. Therefore, it is a measure of the left ventricular preload.

Pulmonary aspiration—The inhalation of fluids and gastric contents into the lungs that may cause aspiration pneumonitis.

Pulseless electrical activity (PEA)—The absence of a detectable pulse and the presence of some type of electrical activity other than ventricular fibrillation (VF) or paroxysmal ventricular tachycardia (PVT).

Purgatives—An agent used for purging the bowels.

Purpura—Discoloration of skin due to hemorrhagic spot more than 0.5 cm in diameter.

Pustule—Small, raised lesion containing pus or exudates.

Pyelonephritis—An infection involving the kidneys and representing upper tract infection.

Pyoderma—Purulent skin disease.

Pyoderma gangrenosum—Skin ulceration with necrotic edges.

Pyuria—Presence of pus or white blood cells in the urine.

Quality-adjusted life year (QALY)—A humanistic assessment of quantity and quality of life. An adjusted life year is calculated by multiplying the number of years by the "utility" of the health state. For patients who have had a moderate stroke, the "utility" of their health state is usually less than 0.5. This means that it would take 2 years at their health state to equal one year at normal health (utility of 1.0).

Rational polytherapy—The concurrent use of two or more drugs for patients not responding to monotherapy. The combination of drugs is based on a consideration of mechanism of action, clinical pharmacokinetics, adverse reactions, and drug interactions.

Rebound vasodilation or congestion—See *Rhinitis medicamentosa*.

Rejection—The response of the immune system, usually involving T or B lymphocytes, to the recognition of foreign antigens in transplanted tissue, which destroys the cells in the transplanted organ and ultimately leads to organ failure, if not treated successfully.

Relative risk reduction—The amount of risk reduced when compared to a control. When one sees a 5% event rate in the control group and a 4% event rate in the treatment group, the relative risk reduction is 20%. The absolute risk reduction is 1%.

Renal—General term referring to the kidneys.

Renal osteodystrophy (ROD)—The condition resulting from sustained metabolic changes that occur with chronic kidney disease including secondary hyperparathyroidism, hyperphosphatemia, hypocalcemia, and vitamin D deficiency. The skeletal complications associated with ROD include osteitis fibrosa cystica (high bone turnover disease), osteomalacia (low bone turnover disease), adynamic bone disease, and mixed bone disorders.

Renal replacement therapy—Any form of dialysis or hemofiltration used to support patients without adequate kidney function. Goals of renal replacement therapy are to remove excess fluid; remove waste products and toxins; and control electrolyte concentrations.

Renovascular—Pertaining to blood vessels located within the kidney, such as the afferent and efferent arterioles, and renal arteries.

Retching—Contractions of the diaphragm, thoracic and abdominal muscles without expulsion of gastric contents.

Retinitis—Inflammation of the retina, often due to infection with cytomegalovirus.

Retrograde pyelography—A procedure where radiocontrast dye is injected into the ureter to produce detailed x-ray pictures of the ureter and kidneys.

Reverse transcriptase—The enzyme in HIV that synthesizes a complementary strand of DNA.

Rhabdomyolysis—The breakdown of muscle tissue and release of myoglobin and intracellular electrolytes into the circulation due to a variety of causes such as crush injuries, drug-induced immobilization, and status epilepticus. It often leads to acute renal failure.

Rheumatoid arthritis (RA)— A systemic, symmetric autoimmune disease with swelling, pain, and inflammation of joints as key findings.

Rhinitis—Inflammation of the nasal mucous membrane. Can be seasonal ("hay fever") or perennial (increasingly called *intermittent* or *persistent*).

Rhinitis medicamentosa—Nasal congestion associated with tolerance to and resulting overuse of topical decongestants. Also known as *rebound vasodilation* or *rebound congestion*.

Rickets—See *Osteomalacia*.

Rigidity—Increased muscular resistance to passive range of motion.

Roth's spot—A hemorrhage in the retina with a white center. Roth's spots are often associated with bacterial endocarditis.

Russell's sign—Callus on dorsum of the hand secondary to self-induced vomiting.

Salicylism—Poisoning by salicylic acid or any of its compounds.

Scale—Flake of stratum corneum.

Scar—Fibrous tissue formed during healing of injury to skin.

Scleritis—Inflammation of the white portion of the eyeball which may be superficial (episcleritis) or involve deeper layers of the eye.

Sebaceous gland—Gland that secretes sebum.

Sebosuppressive—Decreasing amount of sebum produced by the sebaceous gland.

Sebum—Oil produced by the sebaceous gland.

Secondary amenorrhea—Cessation of menses in a woman previously menstruating for 6 months or more.

Secondary hypogonadism—Failure of hypothalamus or pituitary gland to produce adequate amount of luteinizing hormone-releasing hormone (LHRH) or luteinizing hormone (LH). Thus, testicular production of testosterone is reduced.

Secondary prophylaxis (or suppressive therapy)—Refers to administration of systemic antifungal agents (generally prior to and throughout the period of granulocytopenia) to prevent relapse of a documented invasive fungal infection that was treated during a previous episode of granulocytopenia.

Secondary resistance—Develops upon exposure to an antifungal agent and can be either reversible, due to transient adaptation, or acquired as a result of one or more genetic alterations.

Seizure—Paroxysmal disorder of central nervous system, characterized by abnormal neuronal discharges with or without loss of consciousness. They vary in cause, presentation, consequences, duration, and management.

Selection bias—Systematic differences in characteristics between those selected for study and those who are not. See also *Information bias*.

Sepsis—The systemic inflammatory response syndrome (SIRS) secondary to infection. See also *Systemic inflammatory response syndrome*.

Septic shock—Sepsis with persistent hypotension despite fluid resuscitation, along with the presence of perfusion abnormalities. Patients who are on inotropic or vasopressor agents may not be hypotensive at the time perfusion abnormalities are measured.

Serotonin [5-hydroxytryptomine (5-HT)]—An inhibitory neurotransmitter originating in the raphe nucleus of the brainstem and projecting diffusely throughout the brain.

Serum urea nitrogen (SUN)—See *Blood urea nitrogen*.

Severe sepsis—Sepsis associated with organ dysfunction, hypoperfusion, or hypotension. Hypoperfusion and perfusion abnormalities may include, but are not limited to, lactic acidosis, oliguria, or acute alteration in mental status.

Short stature—A broad term describing a condition commonly defined by a physical height that is more than two standard deviations below the population mean and lower than the third percentile for height in a specific age group.

Sickle cell disease—A group of inherited RBC disorder in which HbS is present. Hemolytic anemia and painful vaso-occlusion are the main features.

Simple partial seizure—A seizure beginning in one hemisphere of the brain. It is manifested by alterations in motor functions, sensory or somatosensory symptoms without loss of consciousness. It may progress to a complex partial seizure or to a secondarily generalized seizure with loss of consciousness.

Single nephron GFR (SNGFR)—The rate of filtration through a single glomerulus of a nephron; often reported in nL/min.

Sinus ostia—The pathways that drain the sinuses.

Sinusitis—An inflammation and/or infection of the paranasal sinus mucosa.

Sjogren's syndrome—Rheumatoid arthritis with keratoconjunctivitis sicca.

Sleep spindles—Brief burst of electrical activity seen on the EEG, 12–14 Hz.

Slipped capital femoral epiphysis (SCFE)—Increased width of the femoral plate observed during GH treatment resulting in hip or knee pain.

Social anxiety disorder (SAD)—A disorder characterized by clinically significant anxiety provoked by exposure to certain types of social or performance situations, often leading to avoidance behavior.

Social phobia—See *Social anxiety disorder*.

Somatic pain—Pain arising from skin, bone, joint, muscle, or connective tissue.

Specific phobia—A phobia characterized by clinically significant anxiety provoked by exposure to a specific feared object or situation, often leading to avoidance behavior.

Spermicide—A substance (nonoxynol-9 in the United States) placed in the vagina to inhibit the activity of sperm, thus reducing the risk of pregnancy; available as vaginal creams, films, foams, gels, suppositories, sponges, and tablets.

Spirochete—The class of microorganism that is the agent of syphilis (*Treponema pallidum*).

Status epilepticus—30 minutes of continuous seizure activity or sequential seizures without full recovery between seizures.

Steatorrhea—Excessive loss of fat in stool.

Stevens-Johnson syndrome—A serious dermatologic reaction characterized by blistering of the mucous membranes (mouth, eyes, vagina) with patchy rashes that can cover most of the body. Patients may also experience fever, headache, and cough.

Stress-related mucosal damage—Superficial gastritis-like lesions associated with critical illness in hospitalized patients.

Striae—Linear, atrophic, pink, purple, or white lesions of skin secondary to changes in connective tissue.

Stroke—A sudden onset, focal neurologic deficit, of presumed vascular origin, lasting longer than 24 hours.

Stroke volume—The volume of blood ejected from the heart during systole.

Subarachnoid hemorrhage—Bleeding into the subarachnoid space, where cerebrospinal fluid resides. It is often due to an aneurysm rupture or trauma.

Substance abuse—A maladaptive pattern of substance use indicated by repeated adverse consequences related to the repeated use of the substance. Examples include failure to fulfill important obligations at work, school, or home; repeated use in situations in which it is physically dangerous, such as driving under the influence; legal problems; and social or interpersonal problems such as arguments and fights.

Substance dependence—The continued use of the substance despite adverse substance-related problems. The criteria for substance dependence are the same for each of the drugs or drug classes, varying only to fit the unique pharmacologic properties of each drug.

Suppressive therapy—See *Secondary prophylaxis*.

Swan-Ganz catheter—A catheter (tube) inserted into the heart to measure pressure and cardiac output.

Symptomatic intracerebral hemorrhage—Collection of blood in the brain, usually after an ischemic stroke, that is associated with neurologic worsening.

Syncope—Fainting.

Synechiae—A "creeping" angle closure that sometimes occurs in patients between attacks of closed-angle glaucoma.

Synergism—The combination of two drugs (such as antibiotics) that produces an effect greater than the sum of the two drugs if used alone.

Synesthesias—The overflow of one sensory modality to another. For example, colors are heard, sounds are seen.

Synovitis—Inflammation of the synovial lining of the joint. It is usually painful, particularly on motion, and is characterized by a fluctuating swelling due to effusion within a synovial sac.

Synovium—Synovial membrane, the inner of the two layers of the articular capsule of a synovial joint, composed of loose connective tissue and having a free smooth surface that lines the joint cavity. It secretes the synovial fluid.

Systemic inflammatory response syndrome (SIRS)—Systemic inflammatory response to a variety of clinical insults, which can be of infectious or noninfectious etiology.

Systemic vascular resistance (SVR)—The resistance to blood flow that is primarily determined by the vascular tone of the arteriolar blood vessels.

Tangential speech—Speech pattern whereby the connections between expressed ideas are unrelated or have little relationship to each other.

Taper—To gradually decrease the dosage of a drug over a period of time.

Tendonitis—Inflammation of tendons.

Tenesmus—A painful spasm of the urogenital diaphragm with an urgent desire to evacuate the bowel or bladder, involuntary straining, and the passage of little fecal matter or urine.

TEWL (transepidermal water loss)—The rate of water loss by evaporation from the skin.

Thalassemia—Any of a group of inherited disorders of hemoglobin metabolism in which there is impaired synthesis of one or more of the polypeptide chains of globin.

Third-spacing—The shift of fluid and protein into the peritoneal cavity and bowel wall lumen that occurs as a result of peritonitis.

Thought blocking—Interruption of a train of thought whereby the person stops speaking suddenly and without warning, even in the middle of a sentence. Person may report that the thoughts were taken out of his or her head.

Thought broadcasting—Belief that one's thoughts are audible to others.

Thrombopoiesis—The process of platelet production from immature cells.

Thrombotic thrombocytopenic purpura—A life-threatening disease involving embolism and thrombosis of the small blood vessels in the brain and kidney.

Thrush—Fungal infection of the oral mucosa.

Thyroid-stimulating hormone (TSH)—A polypeptide hormone secreted by the anterior pituitary gland that stimulates iodine uptake and thyroid hormone synthesis.

Thyrotropin-releasing hormone (TRH)—A trophic hormone released by the hypothalamus that stimulates release of thyroid-stimulating hormone (TSH).

Tibia vara—See *Genu valgum* and *Genu varum*.

Tinea barbae—Fungal infection of the hair follicles of the beard or mustache.

Tinea capitis—Fungal infection of the scalp, hair follicles, or adjacent skin.

Tinea corporis—Fungal infection of the glabrous skin of the trunk and extremities.

Tinea cruris—Fungal infection of the proximal thighs and buttocks.

Tinea manuum—Fungal infection of the palmar surface of the hands.

Tinea pedis—Fungal infection of the feet.

Tinnitus—A noise in the ears, as ringing, buzzing, roaring, clicking, etc. Such sounds may at times be heard by those other than the patient.

Tolerance—(1) A state of adaptation in which exposure to a drug induces changes that result in a diminution of one or more of the drug's effects over time. (2) The ability of the immune system to accept a transplanted allograft as part of "self."

Tonic-clonic seizure—Sharp tonic contraction of muscles followed by a period of rigidity and clonic movement.

Tophi—Urate deposits.

Toxic epidermal necrolysis—A syndrome similar to Stevens-Johnson syndrome characterized by blistering of skin and mucous membranes in response to administration of a drug. Large areas of skin may peel off.

Toxic megacolon—A segmental or total colonic distension of >6 cm with acute colitis and signs of systemic toxicity.

Toxic shock syndrome—Sudden onset of fever, muscle ache, vomiting and diarrhea, accompanied by a peeling rash and followed by low body temperature and shock; caused by staphylococcal endotoxin, especially from infection of the vagina associated with tampon use.

Toxoplasmosis—Clinical infection with *Toxoplasma gondii*.

Transverse lie—The fetus is perpendicular to the mother. Usually the shoulder is the presenting part. Fetuses in this position must be delivered by cesarean section.

Traveler's diarrhea—Diarrhea caused by contaminated food or water and usually attributed to enterotoxic *Escherichia coli* (ETEC), *Shigella*, *Campylobacter*, *Salmonella*, or viruses.

Troponin—A protein found predominately in cardiac, but not skeletal, muscle which regulates calcium-mediated interaction of actin and myosin. Troponin I and T are released into the blood from the myocytes at the time of myocardial cell necrosis secondary to infarction. These biochemical markers become elevated and are used in the diagnosis of myocardial infarction. Troponin I and T are more sensitive and specific for infarction that creatinine kinase which is found in both skeletal and myocardial cells. The exact value of troponin I or T which is diagnostic of infarction differs based upon assay.

Trousseau's sign—A hand spasm produced by placing a blood pressure cuff over the forearm and inflating the pressure above the systolic pressure for 3 minutes.

Tubule—Section of the nephron that is responsible for secretion and reabsorption of water, electrolytes, and drugs.

Tumor—Elevated, solid lesion.

Tumor necrosis factor alpha (TNF-α)—A proinflammatory cytokine.

Type I reaction—An immediate, IgE-mediated allergic reaction.

Ulcer—Loss of epidermis and dermis caused by sloughing of necrotic tissue.

Upper respiratory tract infection—Otitis media, sinusitis, pharyngitis, laryngitis (croup), rhinitis, or epiglottitis.

Uremia—An array of symptoms associated with accumulation of metabolic by-products and endogenous toxins in the blood due to impaired kidney function. Symptoms include nausea, vomiting, loss of appetite, weakness, and mental confusion.

Urethritis—Inflammation of the urethra.

Urinalysis—The diagnostic analysis of urine and its components; can be microscopic or macroscopic in nature.

Urinary incontinence—Involuntary leakage of urine. May result from urethral underactivity (stress urinary incontinence), urethral overactivity (overflow incontinence), or mixed pathophysiologic mechanisms.

Urine—Fluid waste resulting from filtration of blood by the kidneys; transferred to the bladder by ureters and expelled from the body through the urethra by the act of voiding or urinating.

Urticaria—A dermatologic reaction noted by elevated, erythematous patches that are pruritic.

Vacuum erection device—Medical device used to manually induce an erection.

Vagal nerve stimulator (VNS)—A medical device that is surgically implanted in patients with refractory epilepsy.

Vasculitis—A hypersensitivity process characterized by inflammation and necrosis of blood vessels.

Vasopressin—A posterior pituitary hormone that controls fluid balance by acting on the renal collecting ducts to prevent water loss.

Vegetation—Bacterial growth on heart valves.

Ventricular remodeling—Alterations in myocardial cells and the extracellular matrix that result in changes in the size, shape, structure, and function of the heart. The remodeling process leads to reductions in myocardial systolic and/or diastolic function that, in turn, leads to further myocardial injury, perpetuating the remodeling process and the decline in ventricular dysfunction and progression of heart failure.

Vesicle—Clear blister (<0.5 cm in diameter) filled with fluid.

Visceral pain—Pain arising from internal organs such as the large intestine or pancreas.

Vomiting—Contraction of the abdominal muscles, descent of the diaphragm, and opening of the gastric cardia resulting in expulsion of stomach contents from the mouth.

Vulgaris—Ordinary, common.

Withdrawal—The development of a substance-specific syndrome after cessation of or reduction in intake of a substance that was used regularly by the individual to induce a state of intoxication. Withdrawal causes significant distress to the individual and is associated with impairment in social, occupational, or other areas of functioning. Withdrawal is usually associated with substance dependence. Withdrawal generally is also associated with a craving to readminister the drug to relieve the symptoms.

Withdrawal bleeding—The predictable bleeding that results from cessation of a progestogen.

Withdrawal syndrome—The onset of a predictable constellation of signs and symptoms involving alerted activity of the central nervous system after the abrupt discontinuation of, or rapid decrease in, dosage of a drug.

Xerosis—Dry skin.

Xerostomia—Oral mucosal dryness.

Yeasts—Oval or spherically shaped unicellular forms that generally produce pasty or mucoid colonies on agar media, similar to those observed with bacterial cultures. Yeasts have rigid cell walls that reproduce by budding, a process in which daughter cells arise from pinching off a portion of the parent cell.

Zeitgebers—Environmental cues.

Zollinger-Ellison syndrome—Gastric acid hypersecretory disease caused by a gastrin-secreting tumor and leading to multiple, severe duodenal ulcers.

INDEX

Note: Page numbers followed by "f" refer to illustrations; page numbers followed by "t" refer to tables.